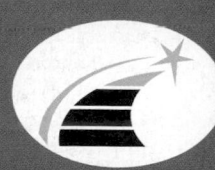

2022

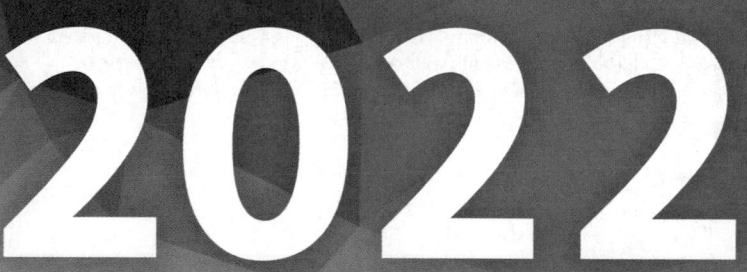

BUCK'S

ICD-10-CM
FOR HOSPITALS

Jackie L. Koesterman, CPC
Coding and Reimbursement Specialist
JDK Medical Coding EDU, LLC
Grand Forks, North Dakota

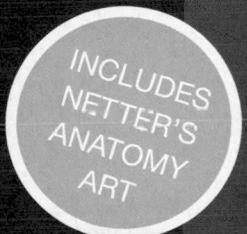

INCLUDES
NETTER'S
ANATOMY
ART

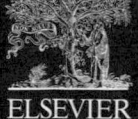

ELSEVIER

Elsevier
3251 Riverport Lane
St. Louis, Missouri 63043

BUCK'S 2022 ICD-10-CM FOR HOSPITALS   ISBN: 978-0-323-79034-5

Copyright © 2022, Elsevier Inc. All rights reserved.

Notice

Previous editions copyrighted 2021, 2020, 2019, 2018, 2017, 2016, 2015, 2014, 2013, 2010

International Standard Book Number: 978-0-323-79034-5

Senior Content Strategist: Brandi Graham
Senior Content Development Manager: Luke E. Held
Senior Content Development Specialist: Joshua S. Rapplean
Publishing Services Manager: Shereen Jameel
Senior Project Manager: Kamatchi Madhavan
Senior Book Designer: Maggie Reid

Printed in the United States of America

Last digit is the print number: 9 8 7 6 5 4 3 2 1

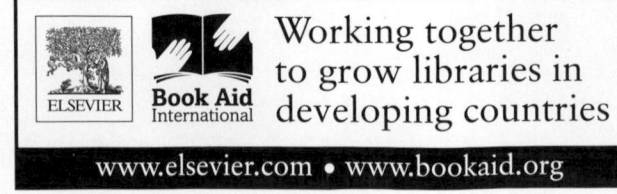

DEDICATION

To all the brave medical coders who transitioned the nation into a new coding system.
Decades of waiting finally concluded with the implementation of I-10,
and you have been the pioneers leading the way.

With greatest appreciations for your efforts!

Carol J. Buck, MS

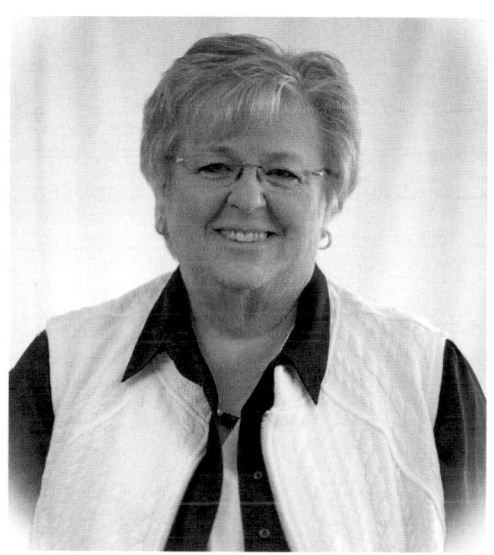

CONTENTS

ICD-10-CM

GUIDE TO USING THE 2022 ICD-10-CM FOR HOSPITALS

Medical coding has long been a part of the health care profession. Through the years medical coding systems have become more complex and extensive. Today, medical coding is an intricate and immense process that is present in every health care setting. The increased use of electronic submissions for health care services only increases the need for coders who understand the coding process.

2022 ICD-10-CM for Hospitals, Professional Edition was developed to help meet the needs of coding professionals at all levels by offering a comprehensive coding text at a reasonable price.

All material strictly adheres to the latest government versions available at the time of printing. Updates from the *Definitions of Medicare Code Edits* (MCE) will be posted to the companion website (www. codingupdates.com) when available.

Illustrations and Items

The ICD-10-CM Tabular List contains illustrations, pictures, and items to assist you in understanding difficult terminology, diseases/conditions, or coding in a specific category. Items are always printed in ▮▮▮▮▮▮ ink so that the added material is not mistaken for official notations or instructions. ▮▮▮▮▮▮ ink is used for other annotations in the text. Your ideas on what other descriptions or illustrations should be in future editions of this text are always appreciated.

Instructional Notations

Includes Notes

Includes
The word "Includes" appears immediately under certain categories to further define, or give examples of, the content of the category.

Excludes Notes

The ICD-10-CM has two types of excludes notes. Each note has a different definition for use, but they are both similar in that they indicate that codes excluded from each other are independent of each other.

Excludes1
A type 1 Excludes note is a pure excludes. It means "NOT CODED HERE!" An Excludes1 note indicates that the code excluded should never be used at the same time as the code above the Excludes1 note. An Excludes1 is for use when two conditions cannot occur together, such as a congenital form versus an acquired form of the same condition.

Excludes2
A type 2 Excludes note represents "NOT INCLUDED HERE." An Excludes2 note indicates that the condition excluded is not part of the condition it is excluded from, but a patient may have both conditions at the same time. When an Excludes2 note appears under a code, it is acceptable to use both the code and the excluded code together.

Code First/Use Additional Code notes (etiology/manifestation paired codes)

Certain conditions have both an underlying etiology and multiple body system manifestations due to the underlying etiology. For such conditions the ICD-10-CM has a coding convention that requires the underlying condition be sequenced first, followed by the manifestation. Wherever such a combination exists, there is a "use additional code" note at the etiology code, and a "code first" note at the manifestation code. These instructional notes indicate the proper sequencing order of the codes, etiology followed by manifestation.

In most cases the manifestation codes will have in the code title, "in diseases classified elsewhere." Codes with this title are a component of the etiology/manifestation convention. The code title indicates that it is a manifestation code. "In diseases classified elsewhere" codes are never permitted to be used as first-listed or principal diagnosis codes. They must be used in conjunction with an underlying condition code, and they must be listed following the underlying condition.

Use additional
The words indicate an instructional note that another code may be needed.

Code first
The words indicate an instructional note that directs the coder to sequence the underlying condition before the manifestation.

Code also
A "code also" note instructs that two codes may be required to fully describe a condition, but the sequencing of the two codes is discretionary, depending on the severity of the conditions and the reason for the encounter.

7th characters and placeholder X

For codes less than 6 characters that require a 7th character, a placeholder X should be assigned for all characters less than 6. The 7th character must always be the 7th character of a code.

Annotated

Throughout the manual, revisions, additions, and deleted codes or words are indicated by the following symbols:

➠ **Revised:** Revisions within the line or code from the previous edition are indicated by the arrow.

▶ **New:** Additions to the previous edition are indicated by the triangle.

~~deleted~~ **Deleted:** Deletions from the previous edition are struck through.

ICD-10-CM Tabular List Symbols

● **Use Additional Character(s):** The red stop sign cautions that the code requires additional character(s) to ensure the greatest specificity.

X For codes less than 6 characters that require a 7th character, a placeholder X should be assigned for all characters less than 6. The 7th character must always be the 7th character of a code.

● **Unacceptable Principal Diagnosis:** These codes have a blue dot before them and give additional information or describe the circumstances affecting the health care encounter but are unacceptable as principal diagnosis in the *Definitions of Medicare Code Edits* (MCE) for inpatient admission.

OGCR The *Official Guidelines for Coding and Reporting* symbol includes the placement of a portion of a guideline as that guideline pertains to the code by which it is located. The complete OGCR are located in Part I.

🄲🄼 Indicates **complications and comorbidities** and **major complications and comorbidities** according to the *Medicare Severity Diagnosis Related Groups (MS-DRGs), Definitions Manual.*

(Ex:) Indicates **exclusions** to complications and comorbidities (CC) and major complications and comorbidities (MCC) for both primary and secondary diagnoses, according to the *Medicare Severity Diagnosis Related Groups (MS-DRGs), Definitions Manual.* Each exclusion will indicate the corresponding PDX Collection, and the collections that list all of the excluded codes appear in Appendix A.

PDX as its own CC/MCC Indicates a combination code that when assigned as the Principal Diagnosis, it includes a condition that also qualifies as a CC/MCC according to the *Medicare Severity Diagnosis Related Groups (MS-DRGs), Definitions Manual.*

HAC is a **Hospital-Acquired Condition** that, when present as a secondary diagnosis in an inpatient setting, is a higher cost, higher volume, or both and results in a higher MS-DRG assignment according to the *Medicare Severity Diagnosis Related Groups (MS-DRGs), Definitions Manual.*

The **Hierarchical condition category (HCC)** was initiated in 2004 for the reimbursement for patients with Medicare Advantage plans (Medicare Part C). HCC is based on a list of chronic or severity of illness diagnosis codes that CMS uses to determine reimbursements to Medicare Advantage plans. The HCC risk adjustment factor data is calculated for an entire year for encounters of the patient's care.

Manifestation Code: Describes the manifestation of an underlying disease, not the disease itself, and therefore should not be assigned as a principal diagnosis, according to the *Definitions of Medicare Code Edits* (MCE).

Age conflict: The *Definitions of Medicare Code Edits* (MCE) detects inconsistencies between a patient's age and diagnosis. For example, a 5-year-old patient with benign prostatic hypertrophy or a 78-year-old pregnant female.

The diagnosis is clinically and virtually impossible in a patient of the stated age. Therefore, either the diagnosis or the age is presumed to be incorrect. There are four age categories for diagnoses in the *Definitions of Medicare Code Edits* (MCE):

N • Newborn. Age of 0 years; a subset of diagnoses intended only for newborns and neonates (e.g., fetal distress, perinatal jaundice).

P • Pediatric. Age range is 0-17 years inclusive (e.g., Reye's syndrome, routine child health exam).

M • Maternity. Age range is 9-64 years inclusive (e.g., diabetes in pregnancy, antepartum pulmonary complication).

A • Adult. Age range is 15-124 years inclusive (e.g., senile delirium, mature cataract).

♀♂ **Sex conflict:** *Definitions of Medicare Code Edits* (MCE) detects inconsistencies between a patient's sex and any diagnosis or procedure on the patient's record. For example, a male patient with cervical cancer (diagnosis) or a female patient with a prostatectomy (procedure). In both instances, the indicated diagnosis or the procedure conflicts with the stated sex of the patient. Therefore, either the patient's diagnosis, procedure, or sex is presumed to be incorrect.

Key words

Highlight identifies key words within similar code descriptions in a particular category.

Coding Clinic Identifies the year, quarter, and page number that presents information about an ICD-10-CM code in the American Hospital Association's *Coding Clinic*® for ICD-10-CM.

Visit codingupdates.com for the full list of 2022 Present on Admission codes.

SYMBOLS AND CONVENTIONS

ICD-10-CM Tabular

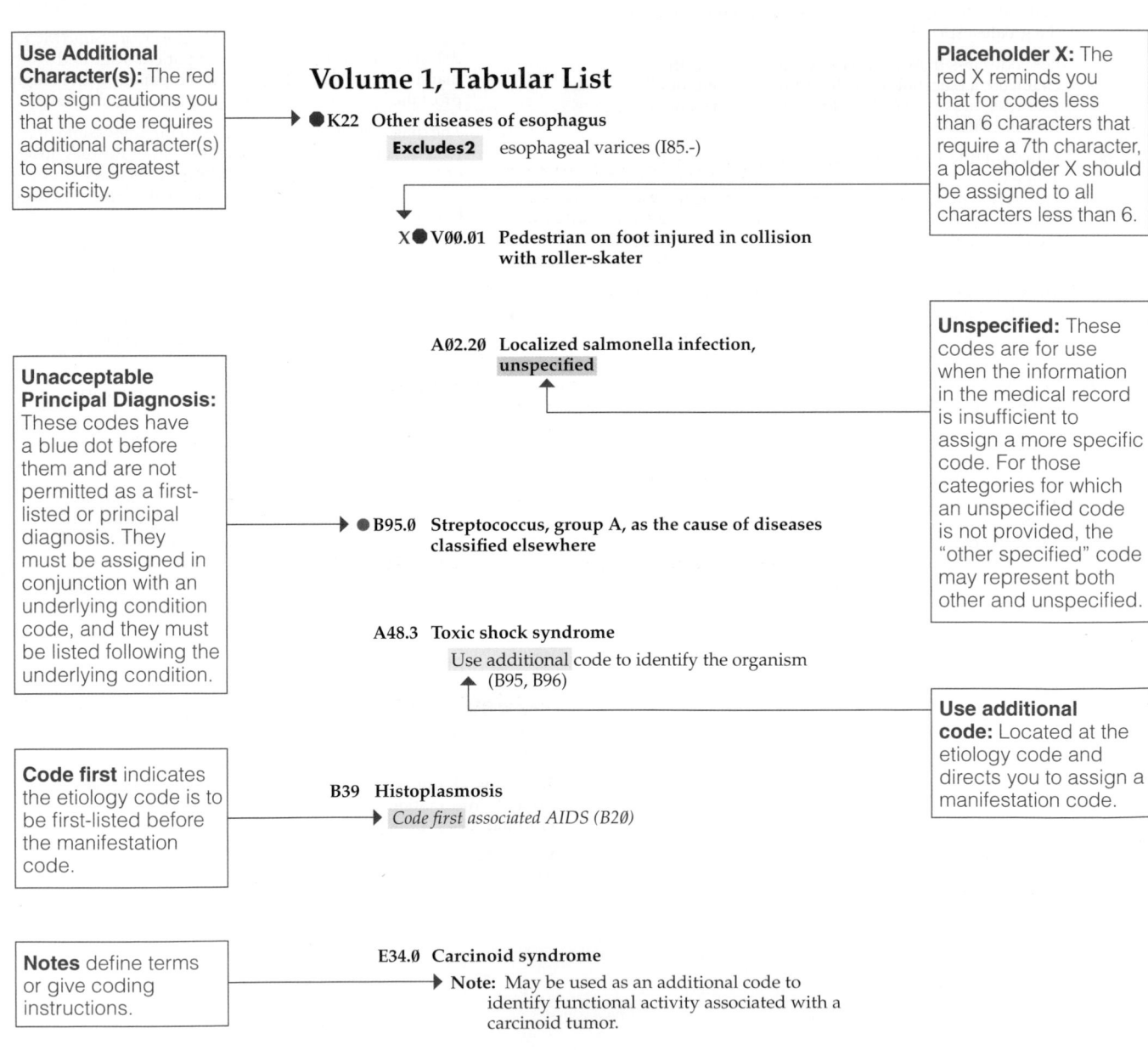

Use Additional Character(s): The red stop sign cautions you that the code requires additional character(s) to ensure greatest specificity.

Placeholder X: The red X reminds you that for codes less than 6 characters that require a 7th character, a placeholder X should be assigned to all characters less than 6.

Volume 1, Tabular List

● **K22   Other diseases of esophagus**

    Excludes2 esophageal varices (I85.-)

X● **V00.01   Pedestrian on foot injured in collision with roller-skater**

A02.20   Localized salmonella infection, unspecified

Unspecified: These codes are for use when the information in the medical record is insufficient to assign a more specific code. For those categories for which an unspecified code is not provided, the "other specified" code may represent both other and unspecified.

Unacceptable Principal Diagnosis: These codes have a blue dot before them and are not permitted as a first-listed or principal diagnosis. They must be assigned in conjunction with an underlying condition code, and they must be listed following the underlying condition.

● **B95.0   Streptococcus, group A, as the cause of diseases classified elsewhere**

A48.3   Toxic shock syndrome

    Use additional code to identify the organism (B95, B96)

Use additional code: Located at the etiology code and directs you to assign a manifestation code.

Code first indicates the etiology code is to be first-listed before the manifestation code.

B39   Histoplasmosis

    Code first associated AIDS (B20)

Notes define terms or give coding instructions.

E34.0   Carcinoid syndrome

    Note: May be used as an additional code to identify functional activity associated with a carcinoid tumor.

Codes or index entries are for purposes of illustration only and may not be current.

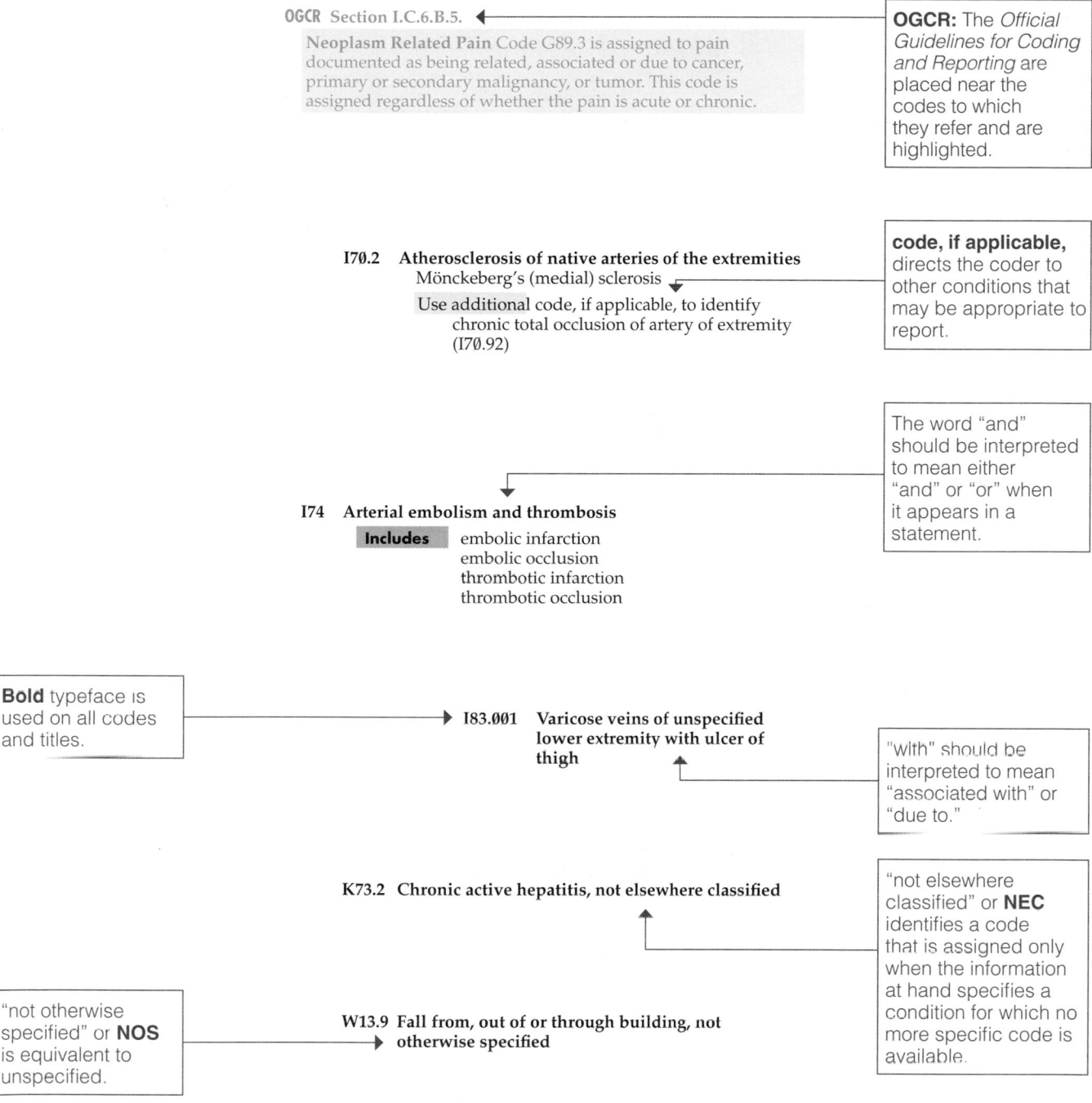

OGCR Section I.C.6.B.5.

Neoplasm Related Pain Code G89.3 is assigned to pain documented as being related, associated or due to cancer, primary or secondary malignancy, or tumor. This code is assigned regardless of whether the pain is acute or chronic.

OGCR: The *Official Guidelines for Coding and Reporting* are placed near the codes to which they refer and are highlighted.

I70.2   **Atherosclerosis of native arteries of the extremities**
Mönckeberg's (medial) sclerosis

Use additional code, if applicable, to identify chronic total occlusion of artery of extremity (I70.92)

code, if applicable, directs the coder to other conditions that may be appropriate to report.

The word "and" should be interpreted to mean either "and" or "or" when it appears in a statement.

I74   **Arterial embolism and thrombosis**
Includes   embolic infarction
embolic occlusion
thrombotic infarction
thrombotic occlusion

Bold typeface is used on all codes and titles.

I83.001   **Varicose veins of unspecified lower extremity with ulcer of thigh**

"with" should be interpreted to mean "associated with" or "due to."

K73.2   **Chronic active hepatitis, not elsewhere classified**

"not elsewhere classified" or **NEC** identifies a code that is assigned only when the information at hand specifies a condition for which no more specific code is available.

"not otherwise specified" or **NOS** is equivalent to unspecified.

W13.9   **Fall from, out of or through building, not otherwise specified**

Codes or index entries are for purposes of illustration only and may not be current.

Excludes1 means "NOT CODED HERE!" An Excludes1 note indicates that the code excluded should never be assigned at the same time as the code above the Excludes1 note.

M19 Other and unspecified osteoarthritis
> **Excludes1**   polyarthritis (M15.-)
> **Excludes2**   arthrosis of spine (M47.-)
>   hallux rigidus (M20.2)
>   osteoarthritis of spine (M47.-)

Excludes2 represents "NOT INCLUDED HERE." An Excludes2 note indicates that the condition excluded is not part of the condition represented by the code, but a patient may have both conditions at the same time and it is acceptable to use both the code and the excluded code together, when appropriate.

Includes: This note appears immediately under a three-character code title to further define, or give examples of, the content.

A06 Amebiasis
> **Includes**   infection due to Entamoeba histolytica

E26.01 Conn's syndrome
        Code also adrenal adenoma (D35.0)

Code also instructs that two codes may be required to fully describe a condition, but this note does not provide sequencing direction.

Codes titled "other" or "other specified" are for use when the information in the medical record provides detail for which a specific code does not exist.

E25.8 Other adrenogenital disorders

O00.2 Ovarian pregnancy   M

Maternity DX (Diagnosis) for ages 9-64 according to the *Definitions of Medicare Code Edits* (MCE).

P02.20 Newborn (suspected to be) affected
        by unspecified morphological and
        functional abnormalities of placenta   N

Newborn, Age 0, according to the *Definitions of Medicare Code Edits* (MCE).

L21.0 Seborrhea capitis   P
       Cradle cap

Pediatric Age, 0-17, according to the *Definitions of Medicare Code Edits* (MCE).

G30.1 Alzheimer's disease with late onset   A

Adult Age, 15-124, according to the *Definitions of Medicare Code Edits* (MCE).

Females Only according to the *Definitions of Medicare Code Edits* (MCE).

B37.3 Candidiasis of vulva and vagina ♀

C60.1 Malignant neoplasm of glans penis ♂

Males Only according to the *Definitions of Medicare Code Edits* (MCE).

Codes or index entries are for purposes of illustration only and may not be current.

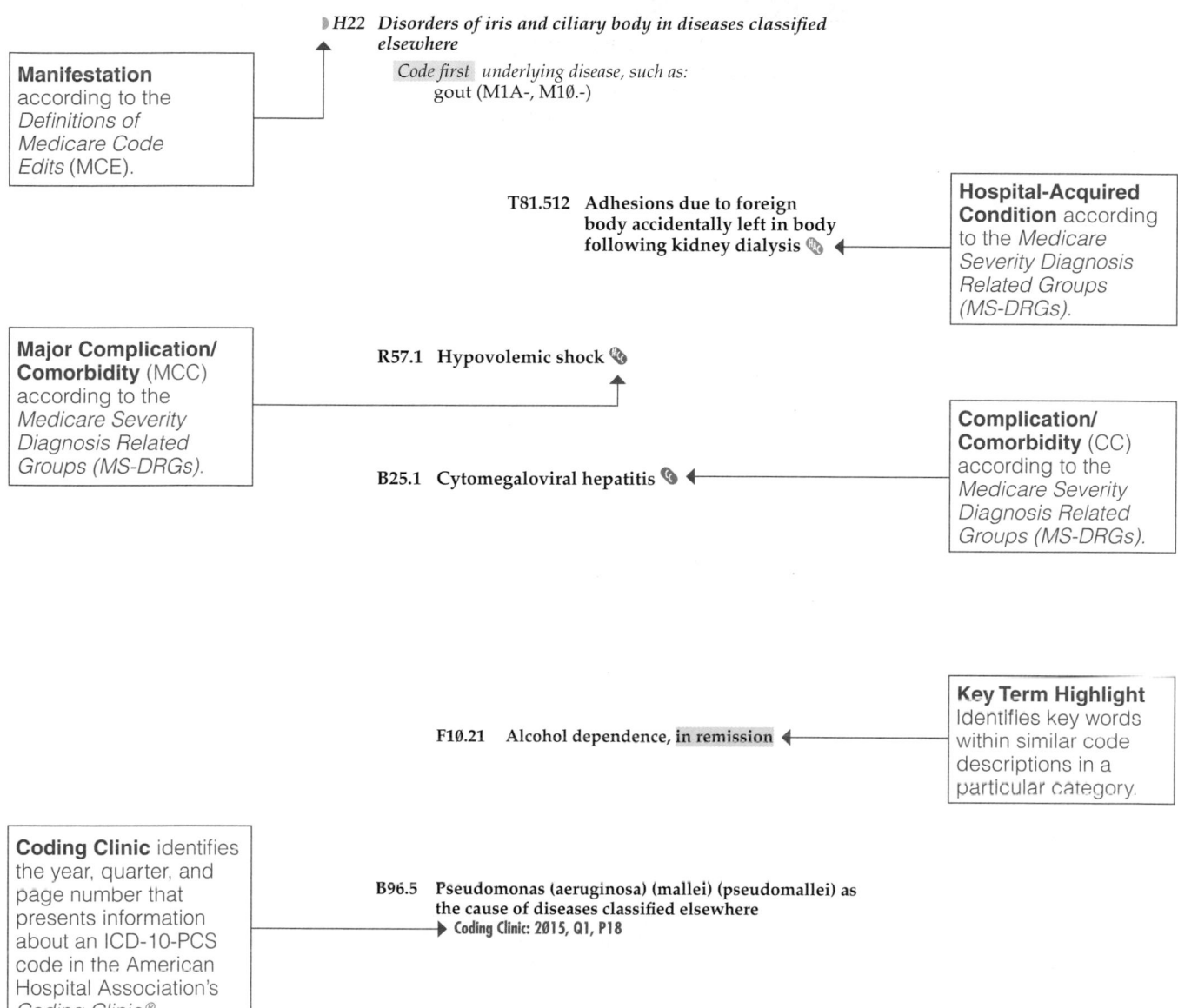

Manifestation according to the *Definitions of Medicare Code Edits* (MCE).

⟩H22 *Disorders of iris and ciliary body in diseases classified elsewhere*
    Code first underlying disease, such as:
        gout (M1A-, M1Ø.-)

T81.512 **Adhesions due to foreign body accidentally left in body following kidney dialysis**

Hospital-Acquired Condition according to the *Medicare Severity Diagnosis Related Groups (MS-DRGs)*.

Major Complication/ Comorbidity (MCC) according to the *Medicare Severity Diagnosis Related Groups (MS-DRGs)*.

R57.1 **Hypovolemic shock**

B25.1 **Cytomegaloviral hepatitis**

Complication/ Comorbidity (CC) according to the *Medicare Severity Diagnosis Related Groups (MS-DRGs)*.

F10.21 Alcohol dependence, **in remission**

Key Term Highlight Identifies key words within similar code descriptions in a particular category.

Coding Clinic identifies the year, quarter, and page number that presents information about an ICD-10-PCS code in the American Hospital Association's *Coding Clinic®*.

B96.5 **Pseudomonas (aeruginosa) (mallei) (pseudomallei) as the cause of diseases classified elsewhere**
    ⟩ **Coding Clinic: 2015, Q1, P18**

Codes or index entries are for purposes of illustration only and may not be current.

Alphabetic Index

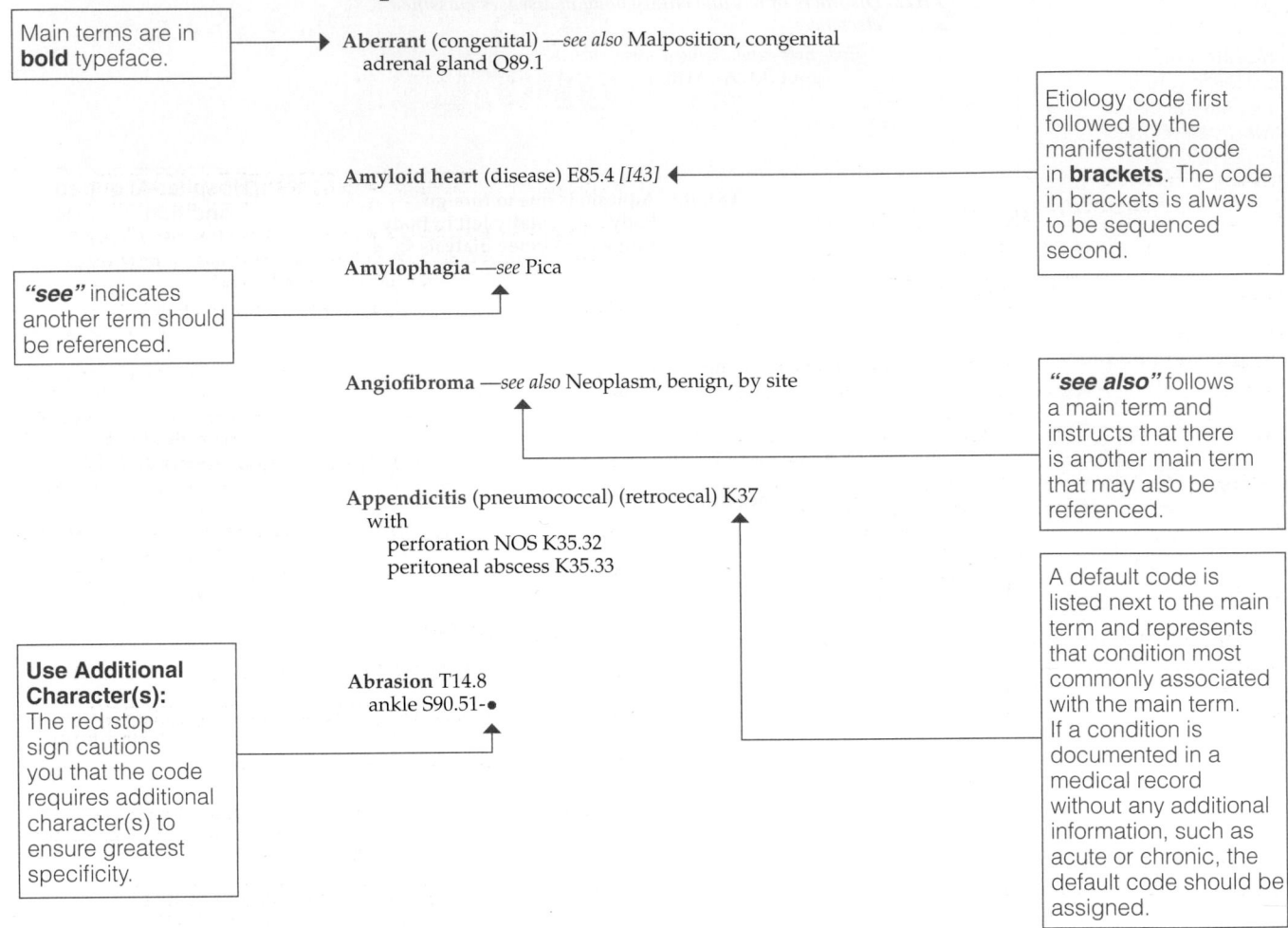

Main terms are in **bold** typeface.

Aberrant (congenital) —*see also* Malposition, congenital adrenal gland Q89.1

Etiology code first followed by the manifestation code in **brackets**. The code in brackets is always to be sequenced second.

Amyloid heart (disease) E85.4 *[I43]*

"see" indicates another term should be referenced.

Amylophagia —*see* Pica

Angiofibroma —*see also* Neoplasm, benign, by site

"see also" follows a main term and instructs that there is another main term that may also be referenced.

Appendicitis (pneumococcal) (retrocecal) K37
　with
　　perforation NOS K35.32
　　peritoneal abscess K35.33

A default code is listed next to the main term and represents that condition most commonly associated with the main term. If a condition is documented in a medical record without any additional information, such as acute or chronic, the default code should be assigned.

Use Additional Character(s):
The red stop sign cautions you that the code requires additional character(s) to ensure greatest specificity.

Abrasion T14.8
　ankle S90.51-●

Codes or index entries are for purposes of illustration only and may not be current.

No Change **CHAPTER 1**

No Change **CERTAIN INFECTIOUS AND PARASITIC DISEASES (A00-B99)**

No Change **OTHER BACTERIAL DISEASES (A30-A49)**

No Change **A37** Whooping cough

No Change **A37.0** Whooping cough due to Bordetella pertussis

No Change **A37.00** Whooping cough due to Bordetella pertussis without pneumonia

Add Paroxysmal cough due to Bordetella pertussis without pneumonia

No Change **A37.01** Whooping cough due to Bordetella pertussis with pneumonia

Add Paroxysmal cough due to Bordetella pertussis with pneumonia

No Change **RICKETTSIOSES (A75-A79)**

No Change **A77** Spotted fever [tick-borne rickettsioses]

No Change **A77.4** Ehrlichiosis

No Change **Excludes1**

Delete Rickettsiosis due to Ehrlichia sennetsu (A79.81)

Add anaplasmosis [A. phagocytophilum] (A79.82)

Add rickettsiosis due to Ehrlichia sennetsu (A79.81)

No Change **A79** Other rickettsioses

No Change **A79.8** Other specified rickettsioses

Add **A79.82** Anaplasmosis [A. phagocytophilum]

Add Transfusion transmitted A. phagocytophilum

No Change **VIRAL AND PRION INFECTIONS OF THE CENTRAL NERVOUS SYSTEM (A80-A89)**

No Change **A80** Acute poliomyelitis

Add **Excludes1** acute flaccid myelitis (G04.82)

No Change **HELMINTHIASES (B65-B83)**

No Change **B74** Filariasis

No Change **Excludes2**

Revise from tropical (pulmonary) eosinophilia NOS (J82)

Revise to tropical (pulmonary) eosinophilia NOS (J82.89)

No Change **SEQUELAE OF INFECTIOUS AND PARASITIC DISEASES (B90-B94)**

No Change **B94** Sequelae of other and unspecified infectious and parasitic diseases

No Change **B94.9** Sequelae of unspecified infectious and parasitic disease

Add **Excludes2** post COVID-19 condition (U09.9)

No Change **BACTERIAL AND VIRAL INFECTIOUS AGENTS (B95-B97)**

No Change **B97** Viral agents as the cause of diseases classified elsewhere

No Change **B97.4** Respiratory syncytial virus as the cause of diseases classified elsewhere

Delete **Excludes2** acute bronchiolitis due to respiratory syncytial virus (RSV) (J21.0)

Delete acute bronchitis due to respiratory syncytial virus (RSV) (J20.5)

Delete respiratory syncytial virus (RSV) pneumonia (J12.1)

Add **Excludes1** acute bronchiolitis due to respiratory syncytial virus (RSV) (J21.0)

Add acute bronchitis due to respiratory syncytial virus (RSV) (J20.5)

Add respiratory syncytial virus (RSV) pneumonia (J12.1)

No Change **CHAPTER 2**

No Change **NEOPLASMS (C00-D49)**

No Change **MALIGNANT NEOPLASMS OF DIGESTIVE ORGANS (C15-C26)**

No Change **C25** Malignant neoplasm of pancreas

No Change Code also

Revise from exocrine pancreatic insufficiency (K86.81)

Revise to if applicable exocrine pancreatic insufficiency (K86.81)

No Change **MALIGNANT NEOPLASMS OF RESPIRATORY AND INTRATHORACIC ORGANS (C30-C39)**

No Change **C30** Malignant neoplasm of nasal cavity and middle ear

No Change **C30.0** Malignant neoplasm of nasal cavity

No Change **Excludes1**

Revise from other and unspecified malignant neoplasm of skin of nose C44.301, C44.311, C44.321, C44.391)

Revise to other and unspecified malignant neoplasm of skin of nose (C44.301, C44.311, C44.321, C44.391)

No Change **MALIGNANT NEOPLASMS OF FEMALE GENITAL ORGANS (C51-C58)**

No Change **C56** Malignant neoplasm of ovary

Add **C56.3** Malignant neoplasm of bilateral ovaries

No Change **MALIGNANT NEOPLASMS OF ILL-DEFINED, OTHER SECONDARY AND UNSPECIFIED SITES (C76-C80)**

No Change **C79** Secondary malignant neoplasm of other and unspecified sites

No Change **C79.6** Secondary malignant neoplasm of ovary

Add **C79.63** Secondary malignant neoplasm of bilateral ovaries

No Change		**MALIGNANT NEOPLASMS OF LYMPHOID, HEMATOPOIETIC AND RELATED TISSUE (C81-C96)**
No Change	**C84**	Mature T/NK-cell lymphomas
No Change	C84.7	Anaplastic large cell lymphoma, ALK-negative
Add		**C84.7A Anaplastic large cell lymphoma, ALK-negative, breast**
Add		Breast implant associated anaplastic large cell lymphoma (BIA-ALCL)
Add		Use Additional code to identify:
Add		breast implant status (Z98.82)
Add		personal history of breast implant removal (Z98.86)

No Change		**IN SITU NEOPLASMS (D00-D09)**
No Change	**D02**	Carcinoma in situ of middle ear and respiratory system
No Change	D02.3	Carcinoma in situ of other parts of respiratory system
No Change		Excludes1
Revise from		carcinoma in situ of nose NOS D09.8
Revise to		carcinoma in situ of nose NOS (D09.8)

No Change		**NEOPLASMS OF UNCERTAIN BEHAVIOR, POLYCYTHEMIA VERA AND MYELODYSPLASTIC SYNDROMES (D37-D48)**
No Change	**D47**	Other neoplasms of uncertain behavior of lymphoid, hematopoietic and related tissue
No Change	D47.3	Essential (hemorrhagic) thrombocythemia
Add		Primary thrombocytosis
Add		Excludes2 reactive thrombocytosis (D75.838)
Add		secondary thrombocytosis (D75.838)
Add		thrombocythemia NOS (D75.839)
Add		thrombocytosis NOS (D75.839)
No Change	D47.Z	Other specified neoplasms of uncertain behavior of lymphoid, hematopoietic and related tissue
No Change		D47.Z2 Castleman disease
No Change		Code also
Revise from		if applicable human herpesvirus 8 infection (B10.89)
Revise to		, if applicable, human herpesvirus 8 infection (B10.89)

No Change	**CHAPTER 3**

No Change	**DISEASES OF THE BLOOD AND BLOOD-FORMING ORGANS AND CERTAIN DISORDERS INVOLVING THE IMMUNE MECHANISM (D50-D89)**

No Change		**HEMOLYTIC ANEMIAS (D55-D59)**
No Change	**D55**	Anemia due to enzyme disorders
No Change	D55.2	Anemia due to disorders of glycolytic enzymes
Delete		Hemolytic nonspherocytic (hereditary) anemia, type II
Delete		Hexokinase deficiency anemia
Delete		Pyruvate kinase [PK] deficiency anemia
Delete		Triose-phosphate isomerase deficiency anemia
Add		**D55.21 Anemia due to pyruvate kinase deficiency**
Add		PK deficiency anemia
Add		Pyruvate kinase deficiency anemia
Add		**D55.29 Anemia due to other disorders of glycolytic enzymes**
Add		Hexokinase deficiency anemia
Add		Triose-phosphate isomerase deficiency anemia

No Change	**D57**		Sickle-cell disorders
No Change		D57.4	Sickle-cell thalassemia
No Change			D57.41 Sickle-cell thalassemia, unspecified, with crisis
No Change			D57.419 Sickle-cell thalassemia, unspecified, with crisis
Revise from			Sickle-cell thalassemia with vasoocclusive pain
Revise to			Sickle-cell thalassemia with vasoocclusive pain NOS
No Change			D57.43 Sickle-cell thalassemia beta zero with crisis
No Change			D57.439 Sickle-cell thalassemia beta zero with crisis, unspecified
Revise from			Sickle-cell thalassemia beta zero with vasoocclusive pain
Revise to			Sickle-cell thalassemia beta zero with vasoocclusive pain NOS
No Change			D57.45 Sickle-cell thalassemia beta plus with crisis
No Change			D57.459 Sickle-cell thalassemia beta plus with crisis, unspecified
Revise from			Sickle-cell thalassemia beta plus with vasoocclusive pain
Revise to			Sickle-cell thalassemia beta plus with vasoocclusive pain NOS

No Change		**APLASTIC AND OTHER ANEMIAS AND OTHER BONE MARROW FAILURE SYNDROMES (D60-D64)**
No Change	**D64**	Other anemias
No Change	D64.8	Other specified anemias
No Change		D64.81 Anemia due to antineoplastic chemotherapy
Delete		Excludes1 aplastic anemia due to antineoplastic chemotherapy (D61.1)
Add		Excludes2 aplastic anemia due to antineoplastic chemotherapy (D61.1)

No Change		**COAGULATION DEFECTS, PURPURA AND OTHER HEMORRHAGIC CONDITIONS (D65-D69)**
No Change	**D68**	Other coagulation defects
No Change	D68.5	Primary thrombophilia
No Change		Excludes1
Revise from		thrombotic thrombocytopenic purpura (M31.1)
Revise to		thrombotic thrombocytopenic purpura (M31.19)
No Change	**D69**	Purpura and other hemorrhagic conditions
No Change		Excludes1
Revise from		thrombotic thrombocytopenic purpura (M31.1)
Revise to		thrombotic thrombocytopenic purpura (M31.19)

No Change		**OTHER DISORDERS OF BLOOD AND BLOOD-FORMING ORGANS (D70-D77)**
No Change	**D72**	Other disorders of white blood cells
No Change	D72.1	Eosinophilia
No Change		Excludes2
Revise from		Löffler's syndrome (J82)
Revise to		Löffler's syndrome (J82.89)
Revise from		pulmonary eosinophilia (J82)
Revise to		pulmonary eosinophilia (J82.-)

No Change	D75		Other and unspecified diseases of blood and blood-forming organs
No Change		D75.8	Other specified diseases of blood and blood-forming organs
Add			D75.83 Thrombocytosis
Add			Excludes2 essential thrombocythemia (D47.3)
Add			D75.838 Other thrombocytosis
Add			Reactive thrombocytosis
Add			Secondary thrombocytosis
Add			Code also underlying condition, if known and applicable
Add			D75.839 Thrombocytosis, unspecified
Add			Thrombocythemia NOS
Add			Thrombocytosis NOS

No Change **CERTAIN DISORDERS INVOLVING THE IMMUNE MECHANISM (D80-D89)**

No Change	D89		Other disorders involving the immune mechanism, not elsewhere classified
No Change		D89.4	Mast cell activation syndrome and related disorders
Add			D89.44 Hereditary alpha tryptasemia
Add			Use additional code if applicable, for:
Add			allergy status, other than to drugs and biological substances (Z91.0-)
Add			personal history of anaphylaxis (Z87.892)

No Change **CHAPTER 4**

No Change # ENDOCRINE, NUTRITIONAL AND METABOLIC DISEASES (E00-E89)

No Change **DISORDERS OF OTHER ENDOCRINE GLANDS (E20-E35)**

No Change	E21		Hyperparathyroidism and other disorders of parathyroid gland
Delete			Excludes1 familial hypocalciuric hypercalcemia (E83.52)
Add			Excludes2 familial hypocalciuric hypercalcemia (E83.52)

No Change **OTHER NUTRITIONAL DEFICIENCIES (E50-E64)**

No Change	E63		Other nutritional deficiencies
Delete			Excludes1 dehydration (E86.0)
Delete			failure to thrive, adult (R62.7)
Delete			failure to thrive, child (R62.51)
Delete			feeding problems in newborn (P92.-)
Delete			sequelae of malnutrition and other nutritional deficiencies (E64.-)
Add			Excludes2 dehydration (E86.0)
Add			failure to thrive, adult (R62.7)
Add			failure to thrive, child (R62.51)
Add			feeding problems in newborn (P92.-)
Add			sequelae of malnutrition and other nutritional deficiencies (E64.-)

No Change **METABOLIC DISORDERS (E70-E88)**

Delete			Excludes1 Ehlers-Danlos syndromes (Q79.6-)
Add			Excludes2 Ehlers-Danlos syndromes (Q79.6-)
No Change	E75		Disorders of sphingolipid metabolism and other lipid storage disorders
No Change		E75.2	Other sphingolipidosis
No Change			E75.24 Niemann-Pick disease
Add			Acid sphingomyelinase deficiency (ASMD)

No Change			E75.240 Niemann-Pick disease type A
Add			Acid sphingomyelinase deficiency type A (ASMD type A)
Add			Infantile neurovisceral acid sphingomyelinase deficiency
No Change			E75.241 Niemann-Pick disease type B
Add			Acid sphingomyelinase deficiency type B (ASMD type B)
Add			Chronic visceral acid sphingomyelinase deficiency
Add			E75.244 Niemann-Pick disease type A/B
Add			Acid sphingomyelinase deficiency type A/B (ASMD type A/B)
Add			Chronic neurovisceral acid sphingomyelinase deficiency
No Change			E75.249 Niemann-Pick disease, unspecified
Add			Acid sphingomyelinase deficiency (ASMD) NOS

No Change	E87		Other disorders of fluid, electrolyte and acid-base balance
No Change		E87.2	Acidosis
No Change			Excludes1
Revise from			diabetic acidosis - see categories E08-E10, E13 with ketoacidosis
Revise to			diabetic acidosis - see categories E08-E10, E11, E13 with ketoacidosis

No Change **CHAPTER 5**

No Change # MENTAL, BEHAVIORAL AND NEURODEVELOPMENTAL DISORDERS (F01-F99)

No Change **MOOD [AFFECTIVE] DISORDERS (F30-F39)**

Revise from	F32		Major depressive disorder, single episode
Revise to	F32		Depressive episode
No Change		F32.9	Major depressive disorder, single episode, unspecified
Delete			Depression NOS
Delete			Depressive disorder NOS
Add		F32.A	Depression, unspecified
Add			Depression NOS
Add			Depressive disorder NOS

No Change **BEHAVIORAL SYNDROMES ASSOCIATED WITH PHYSIOLOGICAL DISTURBANCES AND PHYSICAL FACTORS (F50-F59)**

No Change	F50		Eating disorders
Delete			Excludes1 feeding difficulties (R63.3)
Add			Excludes2 feeding difficulties (R63.3)

No Change **INTELLECTUAL DISABILITIES (F70-F79)**

No Change	F78		Other intellectual disabilities
Add		F78.A	Other genetic related intellectual disabilities
Add			F78.A1 SYNGAP1-related intellectual disability
Add			*Code also, if applicable, any associated:*
Add			autism spectrum disorder (F84.0)
Add			autistic disorder (F84.0)
Add			encephalopathy (G93.4-)
Add			epilepsy and recurrent seizures (G40.-)
Add			other pervasive developmental disorders (F84.8)
Add			pervasive developmental disorder, NOS (F84.9)

Add		F78.A9 Other genetic related intellectual disability
Add		*Code also, if applicable, any associated disorders*

No Change **PERVASIVE AND SPECIFIC DEVELOPMENTAL DISORDERS (F80-F89)**

No Change	F84	Pervasive developmental disorders
Delete		Use Additional code to identify any associated medical condition and intellectual disabilities.
Add		Code also any associated medical condition and intellectual disabilities

No Change **BEHAVIORAL AND EMOTIONAL DISORDERS WITH ONSET USUALLY OCCURRING IN CHILDHOOD AND ADOLESCENCE (F90-F98)**

No Change	F98	Other behavioral and emotional disorders with onset usually occurring in childhood and adolescence
No Change		F98.2 Other feeding disorders of infancy and childhood
Delete		Excludes1 feeding difficulties (R63.3)
Add		Excludes2 feeding difficulties (R63.3)

No Change **CHAPTER 6**

No Change **DISEASES OF THE NERVOUS SYSTEM (G00-G99)**

No Change **INFLAMMATORY DISEASES OF THE CENTRAL NERVOUS SYSTEM (G00-G09)**

No Change	G02	Meningitis in other infectious and parasitic diseases classified elsewhere
No Change		Excludes1
Revise from		infectious mononucleosis complicated by meningitis (B27.- with fourth character 2)
Revise to		infectious mononucleosis complicated by meningitis (B27.- with fifth character 2)
No Change	G04	Encephalitis, myelitis and encephalomyelitis
No Change		Excludes2
Revise from		toxic encephalitis (G92)
Revise to		toxic encephalitis (G92.8)
Revise from		toxic encephalopathy (G92)
Revise to		toxic encephalopathy (G92.8)
No Change		G04.8 Other encephalitis, myelitis and encephalomyelitis
Add		G04.82 Acute flaccid myelitis
Add		Excludes1 transverse myelitis (G37.3)
No Change	G05	Encephalitis, myelitis and encephalomyelitis in diseases classified elsewhere
Add		*Code first* congenital toxoplasmosis encephalitis, myelitis and encephalomyelitis (P37.1)
Add		cytomegaloviral encephalitis, myelitis and encephalomyelitis (B25.8)
Add		encephalitis, myelitis and encephalomyelitis (in) systemic lupus erythematosus (M32.19)
Add		eosinophilic meningoencephalitis (B83.2)
Delete		Excludes1 congenital toxoplasmosis encephalitis, myelitis and encephalomyelitis (P37.1)
Delete		cytomegaloviral encephalitis, myelitis and encephalomyelitis (B25.8)
Delete		encephalitis, myelitis and encephalomyelitis (in) systemic lupus erythematosus (M32.19)
Delete		eosinophilic meningoencephalitis (B83.2)

No Change **DEMYELINATING DISEASES OF THE CENTRAL NERVOUS SYSTEM (G35-G37)**

No Change	G37	Other demyelinating diseases of central nervous system
No Change		G37.3 Acute transverse myelitis in demyelinating disease of central nervous system
Add		Excludes1 acute flaccid myelitis (G04.82)

No Change **EPISODIC AND PAROXYSMAL DISORDERS (G40-G47)**

No Change	G44	Other headache syndromes
No Change		G44.8 Other specified headache syndromes
Add		G44.86 Cervicogenic headache
Add		Code also associated cervical spinal condition, if known

No Change **NERVE, NERVE ROOT AND PLEXUS DISORDERS (G50-G59)**

No Change	G55	Nerve root and plexus compressions in diseases classified elsewhere
No Change		Excludes1
Revise from		nerve root compression (due to) (in) spondylosis (M47.0-M47.2.-)
Revise to		nerve root compression (due to) (in) spondylosis (M47.0-, M47.2.-)

No Change **POLYNEUROPATHIES AND OTHER DISORDERS OF THE PERIPHERAL NERVOUS SYSTEM (G60-G65)**

No Change	G63	Polyneuropathy in diseases classified elsewhere
No Change		Excludes1
Revise from		infectious mononucleosis (B27.0-B27.9 with 1)
Revise to		infectious mononucleosis complicated by polyneuropathy (B27.0-B27.9 with fifth character 1)

No Change **DISEASES OF MYONEURAL JUNCTION AND MUSCLE (G70-G73)**

No Change	G71	Primary disorders of muscles
No Change		G71.2 Congenital myopathies
Revise from		G71.20 Congenital myopathy, unspecifed
Revise to		G71.20 Congenital myopathy, unspecified
No Change	G73	Disorders of myoneural junction and muscle in diseases classified elsewhere
No Change		G73.7 Myopathy in diseases classified elsewhere
No Change		Excludes1
Revise from		sicca syndrome [Sjögren] (M35.03)
Revise to		Sjögren syndrome (M35.03)

No Change **OTHER DISORDERS OF THE NERVOUS SYSTEM (G89-G99)**

No Change	G89	Pain, not elsewhere classified
No Change		Excludes2
Revise from		lumbar region pain (M54.5)
Revise to		lumbar region pain (M54.5-)
No Change	G92	Toxic encephalopathy
Delete		Toxic encephalitis
Delete		Toxic metabolic encephalopathy
Delete		*Code first* , if applicable, drug induced (T36-T50) or use (T51-T65) to identify toxic agent
Add		G92.0 Immune effector cell-associated neurotoxicity syndrome
Add		*Code first underlying cause such as:*
Add		complications of immune effector cellular therapy (T80.82)
Add		Code also associated signs and symptoms, such as seizures and cerebral edema
Add		Code also, if applicable:
Add		cerebral edema (G93.6)
Add		unspecified convulsions (R56.9)

Add		G92.00	**Immune effector cell-associated neurotoxicity syndrome, grade unspecified**
Add			ICANS, grade unspecified
Add		G92.01	**Immune effector cell-associated neurotoxicity syndrome, grade 1**
Add			ICANS, grade 1
Add		G92.02	**Immune effector cell-associated neurotoxicity syndrome, grade 2**
Add			ICANS, grade 2
Add		G92.03	**Immune effector cell-associated neurotoxicity syndrome, grade 3**
Add			ICANS, grade 3
Add		G92.04	**Immune effector cell-associated neurotoxicity syndrome, grade 4**
Add			ICANS, grade 4
Add		G92.05	**Immune effector cell-associated neurotoxicity syndrome, grade 5**
Add			ICANS, grade 5
Add	G92.8		**Other toxic encephalopathy**
Add			Toxic encephalitis
Add			Toxic metabolic encephalopathy
Add			*Code first poisoning due to drug or toxin, if applicable, (T36-T65 with fifth or sixth character 1-4 or 6)*
Add			Use Additional code for adverse effect, if applicable, to identify drug (T36-T50 with fifth or sixth character 5)
Add	G92.9		**Unspecified toxic encephalopathy**
Add			*Code first poisoning due to drug or toxin, if applicable, (T36-T65 with fifth or sixth character 1-4 or 6)*
Add			Use Additional code for adverse effect, if applicable, to identify drug (T36-T50 with fifth or sixth character 5)
No Change	G93		**Other disorders of brain**
No Change	G93.4		**Other and unspecified encephalopathy**
No Change			**Excludes2**
Revise from			toxic (metabolic) encephalopathy (G92)
Revise to			toxic (metabolic) encephalopathy (G92.8)
No Change	G93.5		**Compression of brain**
No Change			**Excludes1**
Delete			diffuse traumatic compression of brain (S06.2-)
Delete			focal traumatic compression of brain (S06.3-)
Add			traumatic compression of brain (S06.A-)

No Change **CHAPTER 7**

No Change **DISEASES OF THE EYE AND ADNEXA (H00-H59)**

No Change **DISORDERS OF CHOROID AND RETINA (H30-H36)**

No Change	H35		**Other retinal disorders**
No Change		H35.0	**Background retinopathy and retinal vascular changes**
No Change			Code also
Revise from			any associated hypertension (I10.-)
Revise to			any associated hypertension (I10)

No Change **CHAPTER 9**

No Change **DISEASES OF THE CIRCULATORY SYSTEM (I00-I99)**

This chapter contains the following blocks:

Revise from	I30-I52	Other forms of heart disease
Revise to	I30-I5A	Other forms of heart disease

No Change **ISCHEMIC HEART DISEASES (I20-I25)**

Delete			Use Additional code to identify presence of hypertension (I10-I16)
Add			Code also the presence of hypertension (I10-I16)
No Change	I24		**Other acute ischemic heart diseases**
Add			**Excludes2** non-ischemic myocardial injury (I5A)
No Change	I25		**Chronic ischemic heart disease**
Add			**Excludes2** non-ischemic myocardial injury (I5A)

Delete	**OTHER FORMS OF HEART DISEASE (I30-I52)**
Add	**OTHER FORMS OF HEART DISEASE (I30-I5A)**

No Change	I50		**Heart failure**
Delete			**Excludes1** neonatal cardiac failure (P29.0)
Add			**Excludes2** neonatal cardiac failure (P20.0)
Add		I5A	**Non-ischemic myocardial injury (non-traumatic)**
Add			Acute (non-ischemic) myocardial injury
Add			Chronic (non-ischemic) myocardial injury
Add			Unspecified (non-ischemic) myocardial injury
Add			*Code first the underlying cause, if known and applicable, such as:*
Add			acute kidney failure (N17.-)
Add			acute myocarditis (I40.-)
Add			cardiomyopathy (I42.-)
Add			chronic kidney disease (CKD) (N18.-)
Add			heart failure (I50.-)
Add			hypertensive urgency (I16.0)
Add			nonrheumatic aortic valve disorders (I35.-)
Add			paroxysmal tachycardia (I47.-)
Add			pulmonary embolism (I26.-)
Add			pulmonary hypertension (I27.0, I27.2-)
Add			sepsis (A41.-)
Add			takotsubo syndrome (I51.81)
Add			**Excludes1** acute myocardial infarction (I21.-)
Add			injury of heart (S26.-)
Add			**Excludes2** other acute ischemic heart diseases (I24.-)

No Change **DISEASES OF VEINS, LYMPHATIC VESSELS AND LYMPH NODES, NOT ELSEWHERE CLASSIFIED (I80-I89)**

No Change	I83		**Varicose veins of lower extremities**
Delete			**Excludes1** varicose veins complicating pregnancy (O22.0-)
Delete			varicose veins complicating the puerperium (O87.4)
Add			**Excludes2** varicose veins complicating pregnancy (O22.0-)
Add			varicose veins complicating the puerperium (O87.4)

No Change **CHAPTER 10**

No Change **DISEASES OF THE RESPIRATORY SYSTEM (J00-J99)**

No Change **ACUTE UPPER RESPIRATORY INFECTIONS (J00-J06)**

No Change	J05		**Acute obstructive laryngitis [croup] and epiglottitis**
No Change			Code also
Revise from			, if present, such as:
Revise to			, influenza, if present, such as:

No Change	**CHRONIC LOWER RESPIRATORY DISEASES (J40-J47)**	

No Change	J44	Other chronic obstructive pulmonary disease
No Change		**Includes:**
Revise from		chronic bronchitis with airways obstruction
Revise to		chronic bronchitis with airway obstruction

No Change	J47	Bronchiectasis
No Change	J47.0	Bronchiectasis with acute lower respiratory infection
Delete		Use Additional code to identify the infection
Add		Code also to identify infection, if applicable

No Change	**OTHER DISEASES OF THE RESPIRATORY SYSTEM (J96-J99)**

No Change	J99	Respiratory disorders in diseases classified elsewhere
No Change		**Excludes1**
Revise from		sicca syndrome (M35.02)
Revise to		Sjögren syndrome (M35.02)

No Change **CHAPTER 11**

No Change
DISEASES OF THE DIGESTIVE SYSTEM (K00-K95)

No Change	**DISEASES OF ORAL CAVITY AND SALIVARY GLANDS (K00-K14)**

No Change	K11	Diseases of salivary glands
No Change	K11.8	Other diseases of salivary glands
No Change		**Excludes1**
Revise from		sicca syndrome [Sjögren] (M35.0-)
Revise to		Sjögren syndrome (M35.0-)

No Change	**DISEASES OF ESOPHAGUS, STOMACH AND DUODENUM (K20-K31)**

No Change	K22	Other diseases of esophagus
No Change	K22.8	Other specified diseases of esophagus
Delete		Hemorrhage of esophagus NOS
Add	K22.81	Esophageal polyp
Add		**Excludes1** benign neoplasm of esophagus (D13.0)
Add	K22.82	Esophagogastric junction polyp
Add		**Excludes1** benign neoplasm of stomach (D13.1)
Add	K22.89	Other specified disease of esophagus
Add		Hemorrhage of esophagus NOS

No Change	K31	Other diseases of stomach and duodenum
Add	K31.A	Gastric intestinal metaplasia
Add	K31.A0	Gastric intestinal metaplasia, unspecified
Add		Gastric intestinal metaplasia indefinite for dysplasia
Add		Gastric intestinal metaplasia NOS
Add	K31.A1	Gastric intestinal metaplasia without dysplasia
Add	K31.A11	Gastric intestinal metaplasia without dysplasia, involving the antrum
Add	K31.A12	Gastric intestinal metaplasia without dysplasia, involving the body (corpus)
Add	K31.A13	Gastric intestinal metaplasia without dysplasia, involving the fundus
Add	K31.A14	Gastric intestinal metaplasia without dysplasia, involving the cardia
Add	K31.A15	Gastric intestinal metaplasia without dysplasia, involving multiple sites
Add	K31.A19	Gastric intestinal metaplasia without dysplasia, unspecified site

Add	K31.A2	Gastric intestinal metaplasia with dysplasia
Add	K31.A21	Gastric intestinal metaplasia with low grade dysplasia
Add	K31.A22	Gastric intestinal metaplasia with high grade dysplasia
Add	K31.A29	Gastric intestinal metaplasia with dysplasia, unspecified

No Change	**DISEASES OF APPENDIX (K35-K38)**

No Change	K37	Unspecified appendicitis
No Change		**Excludes1**
Revise from		-unspecified appendicitis with peritonitis (K35.2-, K35.3-)
Revise to		unspecified appendicitis with peritonitis (K35.2-, K35.3-)

No Change	**NONINFECTIVE ENTERITIS AND COLITIS (K50-K52)**

No Change	K52	Other and unspecified noninfective gastroenteritis and colitis
No Change	K52.2	Allergic and dietetic gastroenteritis and colitis
Delete		**Excludes2** food protein-induced proctocolitis (K52.82)
No Change	K52.29	Other allergic and dietetic gastroenteritis and colitis
Add		Allergic proctocolitis
Add		Food-induced eosinophilic proctocolitis
Add		Food protein-induced proctocolitis
Add		Milk protein-induced proctocolitis
No Change	K52.8	Other specified noninfective gastroenteritis and colitis
No Change	K52.82	Eosinophilic colitis
Delete		Allergic proctocolitis
Delete		Food-induced eosinophilic proctocolitis
Delete		Food protein-induced proctocolitis
Delete		Milk protein-induced proctocolitis
Add		**Excludes2** allergic proctocolitis (K52.29)
Add		food-induced eosinophilic proctocolitis (K52.29)
Add		food protein-induced enterocolitis syndrome (FPIES) (K52.21)
Add		food protein-induced proctocolitis (K52.29)
Add		milk protein-induced proctocolitis (K52.29)

No Change	**OTHER DISEASES OF INTESTINES (K55-K64)**

No Change	K59	Other functional intestinal disorders
No Change	K59.0	Constipation
No Change	K59.03	Drug induced constipation
No Change		Use Additional
Revise from		code for adverse effect, if applicable, to identify drug (T36-T50 with fifth or sixth character 5
Revise to		code for adverse effect, if applicable, to identify drug (T36-T50 with fifth or sixth character 5)

No Change	**DISEASES OF LIVER (K70-K77)**

No Change	K72	Hepatic failure, not elsewhere classified
No Change	K72.1	Chronic hepatic failure
Add		End stage liver disease
No Change	K77	Liver disorders in diseases classified elsewhere
Add		*Code first infectious mononucleosis with liver disease (B27.0-B27.9 with .9)*
Delete		**Excludes1** infectious mononucleosis with liver disease (B27.0-B27.9 with .9)

No Change **CHAPTER 12**

No Change
DISEASES OF THE SKIN AND SUBCUTANEOUS TISSUE (L00-L99)

No Change
DERMATITIS AND ECZEMA (L20-L30)

No Change **L24** Irritant contact dermatitis

No Change **L24.A** Irritant contact dermatitis due to friction or contact with body fluids

Add   Excludes1   virritant contact dermatitis related to stoma or fistula (L24.B-)

Add   Excludes2   erythema intertrigo (L30.4)

Add   **L24.A0** Irritant contact dermatitis due to friction or contact with body fluids, unspecified

Add   **L24.A1** Irritant contact dermatitis due to saliva

Add   **L24.A2** Irritant contact dermatitis due to fecal, urinary or dual incontinence

Add   Excludes1   diaper dermatitis (L22)

Add   **L24.A9** Irritant contact dermatitis due friction or contact with other specified body fluids

Add   Irritant contact dermatitis related to endotracheal tube

Add   Wound fluids, exudate

Add   **L24.B** Irritant contact dermatitis related to stoma or fistula

Add   Use Additional code to identify any artificial opening status (Z93.-), if applicable, for contact dermatitis related to stoma secretions

Add   **L24.B0** Irritant contact dermatitis related to unspecified stoma or fistula

Add   Irritant contact dermatitis related to fistula NOS

Add   Irritant contact dermatitis related to stoma NOS

Add   **L24.B1** Irritant contact dermatitis related to digestive stoma or fistula

Add   Irritant contact dermatitis related to gastrostomy

Add   Irritant contact dermatitis related to jejunostomy

Add   Irritant contact dermatitis related to saliva or spit fistula

Add   **L24.B2** Irritant contact dermatitis related to respiratory stoma or fistula

Add   Irritant contact dermatitis related to tracheostomy

Add   **L24.B3** Irritant contact dermatitis related to fecal or urinary stoma or fistula

Add   Irritant contact dermatitis related to colostomy

Add   Irritant contact dermatitis related to enterocutaneous fistula

Add   Irritant contact dermatitis related to ileostomy

No Change
OTHER DISORDERS OF THE SKIN AND SUBCUTANEOUS TISSUE (L80-L99)

No Change **L89** Pressure ulcer

No Change **L89.0** Pressure ulcer of elbow

No Change   **L89.01** Pressure ulcer of right elbow

No Change   **L89.019** Pressure ulcer of right elbow, unspecified stage

Revise from   Healing pressure right of elbow NOS

Revise to   Healing pressure ulcer of right elbow NOS

Delete   Healing pressure ulcer of right elbow, unspecified stage

No Change   **L89.02** Pressure ulcer of left elbow

No Change   **L89.029** Pressure ulcer of left elbow, unspecified stage

Revise from   Healing pressure ulcer of left of elbow NOS

Revise to   Healing pressure ulcer of left elbow NOS

Delete   Healing pressure ulcer of left elbow, unspecified stage

No Change **L99** Other disorders of skin and subcutaneous tissue in diseases classified elsewhere

No Change   Excludes1

Revise from   skin disorders in diabetes (E08-E13 with .62)

Revise to   skin disorders in diabetes (E08-E13 with .62-)

No Change **CHAPTER 13**

No Change
DISEASES OF THE MUSCULOSKELETAL SYSTEM AND CONNECTIVE TISSUE (M00-M99)

No Change
SYSTEMIC CONNECTIVE TISSUE DISORDERS (M30-M36)

No Change **M31** Other necrotizing vasculopathies

No Change **M31.1** Thrombotic microangiopathy

Delete   Thrombotic thrombocytopenic purpura

Add   **M31.10** Thrombotic microangiopathy, unspecified

Add   **M31.11** Hematopoietic stem cell transplantation-associated thrombotic microangiopathy [HSCT-TMA]

Add   Transplant-associated thrombotic microangiopathy [TA-TMA]

Add   Code first if applicable:

Add   complications of bone marrow transplant (T86.0-)

Add   complications of stem cell transplant (T86.5)

Add   Use Additional code to identify specific organ dysfunction, such as:

Add   acute kidney failure (N17.-)

Add   acute respiratory distress syndrome (J80)

Add   capillary leak syndrome (I78.8)

Add   diffuse alveolar hemorrhage (R04.89)

Add   encephalopathy (metabolic) (septic) (G93.41)

Add   fluid overload, unspecified (E87.70)

Add   graft versus host disease (D89.81-)

Add   hemolytic uremic syndrome (D59.3)

Add   hepatic failure (K72.-)

Add   hepatic veno-occlusive disease (K76.5)

Add   idiopathic interstitial pneumonia (J84.11-)

Add   sinusoidal obstruction syndrome (K76.5)

Add   **M31.19** Other thrombotic microangiopathy

Add   Thrombotic thrombocytopenic purpura

No Change **M34** Systemic sclerosis [scleroderma]

No Change **M34.8** Other forms of systemic sclerosis

No Change   **M34.81** Systemic sclerosis with lung involvement

Add   Code also if applicable:

Add   other interstitial pulmonary diseases (J84.89)

Add   secondary pulmonary arterial hypertension (I27.21)

No Change	M35	Other systemic involvement of connective tissue
Revise from	M35.0	Sicca syndrome [Sjögren]
Revise to	M35.0	Sjögren syndrome
Add		Sicca syndrome
Add		Use Additional code to identify associated manifestations
Add		**Excludes1** dry mouth, unspecified (R68.2)
Revise from	M35.00	Sicca syndrome, unspecified
Revise to	M35.00	Sjögren syndrome, unspecified
Revise from	M35.01	Sicca syndrome with keratoconjunctivitis
Revise to	M35.01	Sjögren syndrome with keratoconjunctivitis
Revise from	M35.02	Sicca syndrome with lung involvement
Revise to	M35.02	Sjögren syndrome with lung involvement
Revise from	M35.03	Sicca syndrome with myopathy
Revise to	M35.03	Sjögren syndrome with myopathy
Revise from	M35.04	Sicca syndrome with tubulo-interstitial nephropathy
Revise to	M35.04	Sjögren syndrome with tubulo-interstitial nephropathy
Add	M35.05	Sjögren syndrome with inflammatory arthritis
Add	M35.06	Sjögren syndrome with peripheral nervous system involvement
Add	M35.07	Sjögren syndrome with central nervous system involvement
Add	M35.08	Sjögren syndrome with gastrointestinal involvement
Add	M35.0A	Sjögren syndrome with glomerular disease
Add	M35.0B	Sjögren syndrome with vasculitis
Add	M35.0C	Sjögren syndrome with dental involvement
Revise from	M35.09	Sicca syndrome with other organ involvement
Revise to	M35.09	Sjögren syndrome with other organ involvement
No Change	M35.7	Hypermobility syndrome
Delete		**Excludes1** Ehlers-Danlos syndromes (Q79.6-)
Add		**Excludes2** Ehlers-Danlos syndromes (Q79.6-)
No Change	M35.8	Other specified systemic involvement of connective tissue
No Change	M35.81	Multisystem inflammatory syndrome
No Change		Use Additional
Delete		sequelae of COVID-19 (B94.8)
Add		post COVID-19 condition (U09.9)

DEFORMING DORSOPATHIES (M40-M43)   No Change

No Change	M40	Kyphosis and lordosis
Add		*Code first* underlying disease
No Change	M41	Scoliosis
Delete		**Excludes1** postprocedural scoliosis (M96.-)
Add		**Excludes2** postprocedural scoliosis (M96.-)
No Change	M41.5	Other secondary scoliosis
Add		*Code first* underlying disease

SPONDYLOPATHIES (M45-M49)   No Change

No Change	M45	Ankylosing spondylitis
Add	M45.A	Non-radiographic axial spondyloarthritis
Add	M45.A0	Non-radiographic axial spondyloarthritis of unspecified sites in spine
Add	M45.A1	Non-radiographic axial spondyloarthritis of occipito-atlanto-axial region
Add	M45.A2	Non-radiographic axial spondyloarthritis of cervical region
Add	M45.A3	Non-radiographic axial spondyloarthritis of cervicothoracic region
Add	M45.A4	Non-radiographic axial spondyloarthritis of thoracic region
Add	M45.A5	Non-radiographic axial spondyloarthritis of thoracolumbar region
Add	M45.A6	Non-radiographic axial spondyloarthritis of lumbar region
Add	M45.A7	Non-radiographic axial spondyloarthritis of lumbosacral region
Add	M45.A8	Non-radiographic axial spondyloarthritis of sacral and sacrococcygeal region
Add	M45.AB	Non-radiographic axial spondyloarthritis of multiple sites in spine

OTHER DORSOPATHIES (M50-M54)   No Change

No Change	M54	Dorsalgia
No Change	M54.5	Low back pain
Delete		Loin pain
Delete		Lumbago NOS
Add	M54.50	Low back pain, unspecified
Add		Loin pain
Add		Lumbago NOS
Add	M54.51	Vertebrogenic low back pain
Add		Low back vertebral endplate pain
Add	M54.59	Other low back pain
Add	M54.8	Other dorsalgia
No Change		**Excludes1**
Revise from		low back pain (M54.5)
Revise to		low back pain (M54.5-)

No Change **CHAPTER 14**

No Change **DISEASES OF THE GENITOURINARY SYSTEM (N00-N99)**

RENAL TUBULO-INTERSTITIAL DISEASES (N10-N16)   No Change

No Change	N16	Renal tubulo-interstitial disorders in diseases classified elsewhere
No Change		**Excludes1**
Revise from		pyelonephritis and tubulo-interstitial nephritis in sicca syndrome [Sjogren's] (M35.04)
Revise to		pyelonephritis and tubulo-interstitial nephritis in Sjogren syndrome (M35.04)

OTHER DISEASES OF THE URINARY SYSTEM (N30-N39)   No Change

Delete		**Excludes1** urinary infection (complicating):
Delete		abortion or ectopic or molar pregnancy (O00-O07, O08.8)
Delete		pregnancy, childbirth and the puerperium (O23.-, O75.3, O86.2-)
Add		**Excludes2** urinary infection (complicating):
Add		abortion or ectopic or molar pregnancy (O00-O07, O08.8)
Add		pregnancy, childbirth and the puerperium (O23.-, O75.3, O86.2-)
No Change	N39	Other disorders of urinary system
No Change	N39.4	Other specified urinary incontinence
No Change	N39.44	Nocturnal enuresis
Add		**Excludes2** nocturnal polyuria (R35.81)

NONINFLAMMATORY DISORDERS OF FEMALE GENITAL TRACT (N80-N98)   No Change

No Change	N97	Female infertility
Delete		**Excludes1** female infertility associated with:
Delete		hypopituitarism (E23.0)
Delete		Stein-Leventhal syndrome (E28.2)
Add		**Excludes2** female infertility associated with:
Add		hypopituitarism (E23.0)
Add		Stein-Leventhal syndrome (E28.2)

No Change **CHAPTER 15**

No Change
PREGNANCY, CHILDBIRTH AND THE PUERPERIUM (O00-O9A)

No Change
OTHER MATERNAL DISORDERS PREDOMINANTLY RELATED TO PREGNANCY (O20-O29)

No Change **O22** Venous complications and hemorrhoids in pregnancy

No Change   **O22.3** Deep phlebothrombosis in pregnancy

No Change   Use Additional

Revise from   code to identify the deep vein thrombosis (I82.4-, I82.5-, I82.62-. I82.72-)

Revise to   code to identify the deep vein thrombosis (I82.4-, I82.5-, I82.62-, I82.72-)

No Change
COMPLICATIONS PREDOMINANTLY RELATED TO THE PUERPERIUM (O85-O92)

No Change **O87** Venous complications and hemorrhoids in the puerperium

No Change   **O87.1** Deep phlebothrombosis in the puerperium

No Change   Use Additional

Revise from   code to identify the deep vein thrombosis (I82.4-, I82.5-, I82.62-. I82.72-)

Revise to   code to identify the deep vein thrombosis (I82.4-, I82.5-, I82.62-, I82.72-)

No Change **CHAPTER 16**

No Change
CERTAIN CONDITIONS ORIGINATING IN THE PERINATAL PERIOD (P00-P96)

No Change
NEWBORN AFFECTED BY MATERNAL FACTORS AND BY COMPLICATIONS OF PREGNANCY, LABOR, AND DELIVERY (P00–P04)

No Change **P00** Newborn affected by maternal conditions that may be unrelated to present pregnancy

No Change   **P00.2** Newborn affected by maternal infectious and parasitic diseases

Add   **Excludes2** newborn affected by (positive) maternal group B streptococcus (GBS) colonization (P00.82)

No Change   **P00.8** Newborn affected by other maternal conditions

Add   **P00.82** Newborn affected by (positive) maternal group B streptococcus (GBS) colonization

Add   Contact with positive maternal group B streptococcus

No Change   **P00.89** Newborn affected by other maternal conditions

Add   **Excludes2** newborn affected by positive maternal group B streptococcus (GBS) colonization (P00.82)

No Change **P04** Newborn affected by noxious substances transmitted via placenta or breast milk

Add   *Code first any current condition in newborn, if applicable*

No Change
DISORDERS OF NEWBORN RELATED TO LENGTH OF GESTATION AND FETAL GROWTH (P05-P08)

No Change **P08** Disorders of newborn related to long gestation and high birth weight

No Change   **P08.1** Other heavy for gestational age newborn

No Change   **Excludes1**

Revise from   syndrome of infant of mother with gestational diabetes (P70.0).

Revise to   syndrome of infant of mother with gestational diabetes (P70.0)

No Change
ABNORMAL FINDINGS ON NEONATAL SCREENING (P09)

No Change **P09** Abnormal findings on neonatal screening

Delete   Use Additional code to identify signs, symptoms and conditions associated with the screening

Add   **Includes:** Abnormal findings on state mandated newborn screens

Add   Failed newborn screening

Add   **P09.1** Abnormal findings on neonatal screening for inborn errors of metabolism

Add   **P09.2** Abnormal findings on neonatal screening for congenital endocrine disease

Add   Abnormal findings on neonatal screening for congenital adrenal hyperplasia

Add   Abnormal findings on neonatal screening for hypothyroidism screen

Add   **P09.3** Abnormal findings on neonatal screening for congenital hematologic disorders

Add   Abnormal findings for hemoglobinothies screen

Add   Abnormal findings on red cell membrane defects screen

Add   Abnormal findings on sickle cell screen

Add   **P09.4** Abnormal findings on neonatal screening for cystic fibrosis

Add   **P09.5** Abnormal findings on neonatal screening for critical congenital heart disease

Add   Neonatal congenital heart disease screening failure

Add   **P09.6** Abnormal findings on neonatal screening for neonatal hearing loss

Add   **Excludes2** encounter for hearing examination following failed hearing screening (Z01.110)

Add   **P09.8** Other abnormal findings on neonatal screening

Add   **P09.9** Abnormal findings on neonatal screening, unspecified

No Change
RESPIRATORY AND CARDIOVASCULAR DISORDERS SPECIFIC TO THE PERINATAL PERIOD (P19-P29)

No Change **P29** Cardiovascular disorders originating in the perinatal period

Delete   **Excludes1** congenital malformations of the circulatory system (Q20-Q28)

Add   **Excludes2** congenital malformations of the circulatory system (Q20-Q28)

No Change
OTHER DISORDERS ORIGINATING IN THE PERINATAL PERIOD (P90-P96)

No Change **P92** Feeding problems of newborn

Delete   **Excludes1** feeding problems in child over 28 days old (R63.3)

Add   **Excludes2** feeding problems in child over 28 days old (R63.3)

No Change **CHAPTER 17**

No Change
CONGENITAL MALFORMATIONS, DEFORMATIONS AND CHROMOSOMAL ABNORMALITIES (Q00-Q99)

No Change
CONGENITAL MALFORMATIONS OF THE CIRCULATORY SYSTEM (Q20-Q28)

No Change   Q21 Congenital malformations of cardiac septa

No Change   **Q21.8** Other congenital malformations of cardiac septa

No Change   Code also

Revise from   if applicable:

Revise to   , if applicable:

No Change	**CONGENITAL MALFORMATIONS OF THE URINARY SYSTEM (Q60-Q64)**		

No Change **Q61**	Cystic kidney disease		
No Change	Q61.5	Medullary cystic kidney	
Revise from		Nephronopthisis	
Revise to		Nephronophthisis	

No Change **CHAPTER 18**

No Change
SYMPTOMS, SIGNS AND ABNORMAL CLINICAL AND LABORATORY FINDINGS, NOT ELSEWHERE CLASSIFIED (R00-R99)

No Change	**SYMPTOMS AND SIGNS INVOLVING THE CIRCULATORY AND RESPIRATORY SYSTEMS (R00-R09)**		

No Change **R05**	Cough		
No Change	**Excludes1**		
Delete		cough with hemorrhage (R04.2)	
Add		paroxysmal cough due to Bordetella pertussis (A37.0-)	
Add	**Excludes2** cough with hemorrhage (R04.2)		
Add	R05.1	Acute cough	
Add	R05.2	Subacute cough	
Add	R05.3	Chronic cough	
Add		Persistent cough	
Add		Refractory cough	
Add		Unexplained cough	
Add	R05.4	Cough syncope	
Add		*Code first syncope and collapse (R55)*	
Add	R05.8	Other specified cough	
Add	R05.9	Cough, unspecified	

No Change	**SYMPTOMS AND SIGNS INVOLVING THE GENITOURINARY SYSTEM (R30-R39)**		

No Change **R35**	Polyuria		
No Change	R35.8	Other polyuria	
Delete		Polyuria NOS	
Add		R35.81	Nocturnal polyuria
Add			**Excludes2** nocturnal enuresis (N39.44)
Add		R35.89	Other polyuria
Add			Polyuria NOS

No Change	**SYMPTOMS AND SIGNS INVOLVING COGNITION, PERCEPTION, EMOTIONAL STATE AND BEHAVIOR (R40-R46)**		

No Change **R45**	Symptoms and signs involving emotional state		
No Change	R45.8	Other symptoms and signs involving emotional state	
Add		R45.88	Nonsuicidal self-harm
Add			Nonsuicidal self-injury
Add			Nonsuicidal self-mutilation
Add			Self-inflicted injury without suicidal intent
Add			Code also injury, if known

No Change	**GENERAL SYMPTOMS AND SIGNS (R50-R69)**		

No Change **R52**	Pain, unspecified		
No Change	**Excludes1**		
Revise from		lumbar region pain (M54.5)	
Revise to		lumbar region pain (M54.5-)	
No Change **R57**	Shock, not elsewhere classified		
No Change	**Excludes1**		
Delete		anesthetic shock (T88.3)	
Add		shock due to anesthesia (T88.2)	

No Change **R63**	Symptoms and signs concerning food and fluid intake		
No Change	R63.3	Feeding difficulties	
Delete		Feeding problem (elderly) (infant) NOS	
Delete		Picky eater	
Delete		**Excludes1** eating disorders (F50.-)	
Delete		feeding problems of newborn (P92.-)	
Delete		infant feeding disorder of nonorganic origin (F98.2-)	
Add		**Excludes2** eating disorders (F50.-)	
Add		feeding problems of newborn (P92.-)	
Add		infant feeding disorder of nonorganic origin (F98.2-)	
Add		R63.30	Feeding difficulties, unspecified
Add		R63.31	Pediatric feeding disorder, acute
Add			Pediatric feeding dysfunction, acute
Add			Code also, if applicable, associated conditions such as:
Add			aspiration pneumonia (J69.0)
Add			dysphagia (R13.1-)
Add			gastro-esophageal reflux disease (K21.-)
Add			malnutrition (E40-E46)
Add		R63.32	Pediatric feeding disorder, chronic
Add			Pediatric feeding dysfunction, chronic
Add			Code also, if applicable, associated conditions such as:
Add			aspiration pneumonia (J69.0)
Add			dysphagia (R13.1-)
Add			gastro-esophageal reflux disease (K21.-)
Add			malnutrition (E40-E46)
Add		R63.39	Other feeding difficulties
Add			Feeding problem (elderly) (infant) NOS
Add			Picky eater

No Change **R68**	Other general symptoms and signs		
No Change	R68.2	Dry mouth, unspecified	
No Change	**Excludes1**		
Revise from		dry mouth due to sicca syndrome [Sjögren] (M35.0-)	
Revise to		dry mouth due to Sjögren syndrome (M35.0-)	

No Change	**ABNORMAL FINDINGS ON EXAMINATION OF BLOOD, WITHOUT DIAGNOSIS (R70-R79)**		

No Change **R79**	Other abnormal findings of blood chemistry		
No Change	R79.8	Other specified abnormal findings of blood chemistry	
Add		R79.83	Abnormal findings of blood amino-acid level
Add			Homocysteinemia
Add			**Excludes1** disorders of amino-acid metabolism (E70-E72)

No Change **CHAPTER 19**

No Change
INJURY, POISONING AND CERTAIN OTHER CONSEQUENCES OF EXTERNAL CAUSES (S00-T88)

No Change	**INJURIES TO THE HEAD (S00-S09)**		

No Change **S00**	Superficial injury of head		
No Change	S00.1	Contusion of eyelid and periocular area	
No Change	**Excludes2**		
Revise from		contusion of eyeball and orbital tissues (S05.1)	
Revise to		contusion of eyeball and orbital tissues (S05.1-)	

No Change	**S01**	**Open wound of head**		
No Change		**S01.0**	**Open wound of scalp**	
No Change			Excludes1	
Revise from				avulsion of scalp (S08.0)
Revise to				avulsion of scalp (S08.0-)
No Change	**S06**	**Intracranial injury**		
No Change		**S06.2**	**Diffuse traumatic brain injury**	
Add			Use Additional code, if applicable, for traumatic brain compression or herniation (S06.A-)	
No Change		**S06.3**	**Focal traumatic brain injury**	
Add			Use Additional code, if applicable, for traumatic brain compression or herniation (S06.A-)	
No Change		**S06.5**	**Traumatic subdural hemorrhage**	
Add			Use Additional code, if applicable, for traumatic brain compression or herniation (S06.A-)	
No Change		**S06.6**	**Traumatic subarachnoid hemorrhage**	
Add			Use Additional code, if applicable, for traumatic brain compression or herniation (S06.A-)	
Add		**S06.A**	**Traumatic brain compression and herniation**	
Add			Traumatic cerebral compression	
Add			*Code first the underlying traumatic brain injury, such as:*	
Add			diffuse traumatic brain injury (S06.2-)	
Add			focal traumatic brain injury (S06.3-)	
Add			traumatic subdural hemorrhage (S06.5-)	
Add			traumatic subarachnoid hemorrhage (S06.6-)	
Add			**S06.A0**	**Traumatic brain compression without herniation**
Add				Traumatic brain compression NOS
Add				Traumatic cerebral compression NOS
Add			**S06.A1**	**Traumatic brain compression with herniation**
Add				Traumatic brain herniation
Add				Traumatic brainstem compression with herniation
Add				Traumatic cerebellar compression with herniation
Add				Traumatic cerebral compression with herniation

INJURIES TO THE THORAX (S20-S29)

No Change			
No Change	**S23**	**Dislocation and sprain of joints and ligaments of thorax**	
No Change		**S23.1**	**Subluxation and dislocation of thoracic vertebra**
No Change			Code also
Revise from			any associated
Revise to			any associated:

INJURIES TO THE KNEE AND LOWER LEG (S80-S89)

No Change	**S82**	**Fracture of lower leg, including ankle**	
No Change		Excludes2	
Revise from			periprosthetic fracture of prosthetic implant of knee (M97.0-)
Revise to			periprosthetic fracture around internal prosthetic implant of knee joint (M97.1-)

INJURIES TO THE ANKLE AND FOOT (S90-S99)

No Change			
No Change	**S92**	**Fracture of foot and toe, except ankle**	
Delete		Excludes1	traumatic amputation of ankle and foot (S98.-)
Add		Excludes2	traumatic amputation of ankle and foot (S98.-)

No Change		**POISONING BY, ADVERSE EFFECTS OF AND UNDERDOSING OF DRUGS, MEDICAMENTS AND BIOLOGICAL SUBSTANCES (T36-T50)**		
No Change	**T40**	**Poisoning by, adverse effect of and underdosing of narcotics and psychodysleptics [hallucinogens]**		
No Change		**T40.7**	**Poisoning by, adverse effect of and underdosing of cannabis (derivatives)**	
Add			**T40.71**	**Poisoning by, adverse effect of and underdosing of cannabis (derivatives)**
Add				**T40.711** Poisoning by cannabis, accidental (unintentional)
Add				**T40.712** Poisoning by cannabis, intentional self-harm
Add				**T40.713** Poisoning by cannabis, assault
Add				**T40.714** Poisoning by cannabis, undetermined
Add				**T40.715** Adverse effect of cannabis
Add				**T40.716** Underdosing of cannabis
Add			**T40.72**	**Poisoning by, adverse effect of and underdosing of synthetic cannabinoids**
Add				**T40.721** Poisoning by synthetic cannabinoids, accidental (unintentional)
Add				**T40.722** Poisoning by synthetic cannabinoids, intentional self-harm
Add				**T40.723** Poisoning by synthetic cannabinoids, assault
Add				**T40.724** Poisoning by synthetic cannabinoids, undetermined
Add				**T40.725** Adverse effect of synthetic cannabinoids
Add				**T40.726** Underdosing of synthetic cannabinoids
Delete			**T40.7X**	Poisoning by, adverse effect of and underdosing of cannabis (derivatives)
Delete				**T40.7X1** Poisoning by cannabis (derivatives), accidental (unintentional)
Delete				Poisoning by cannabis NOS
Delete				**T40.7X2** Poisoning by cannabis (derivatives), intentional self-harm
Delete				**T40.7X3** Poisoning by cannabis (derivatives), assault
Delete				**T40.7X4** Poisoning by cannabis (derivatives), undetermined
Delete				**T40.7X5** Adverse effect of cannabis (derivatives)
Delete				**T40.7X6** Underdosing of cannabis (derivatives)
No Change	**T44**	**Poisoning by, adverse effect of and underdosing of drugs primarily affecting the autonomic nervous system**		
No Change		**T44.8**	**Poisoning by, adverse effect of and underdosing of centrally-acting and adrenergic-neuron-blocking agents**	
Delete			Excludes1	poisoning by, adverse effect of and underdosing of clonidine (T46.5)
Delete				poisoning by, adverse effect of and underdosing of guanethidine (T46.5)
Add			Excludes2	poisoning by, adverse effect of and underdosing of clonidine (T46.5)
Add				poisoning by, adverse effect of and underdosing of guanethidine (T46.5)

No Change		**TOXIC EFFECTS OF SUBSTANCES CHIEFLY NONMEDICINAL AS TO SOURCE (T51-T65)**	
No Change **T63**	Toxic effect of contact with venomous animals and plants		
No Change	**T63.6**	Toxic effect of contact with other venomous marine animals	
Revise from		T63.61	Toxic effect of contact with Portugese Man-o-war
Revise to		T63.61	Toxic effect of contact with Portuguese Man-o-war
Revise from			T63.611 Toxic effect of contact with Portugese Man-o-war, accidental (unintentional)
Revise to			T63.611 Toxic effect of contact with Portuguese Man-o-war, accidental (unintentional)
Revise from			T63.612 Toxic effect of contact with Portugese Man-o-war, intentional self-harm
Revise to			T63.612 Toxic effect of contact with Portuguese Man-o-war, intentional self-harm
Revise from			T63.613 Toxic effect of contact with Portugese Man-o-war, assault
Revise to			T63.613 Toxic effect of contact with Portuguese Man-o-war, assault
Revise from			T63.614 Toxic effect of contact with Portugese Man-o-war, undetermined
Revise to			T63.614 Toxic effect of contact with Portuguese Man-o-war, undetermined

CERTAIN EARLY COMPLICATIONS OF TRAUMA (T79)

No Change **T79**	Certain early complications of trauma, not elsewhere classified	
No Change	**T79.4 Traumatic shock**	
No Change	**Excludes1**	
Delete		anesthetic shock (T88.2)
Add		shock due to anesthesia (T88.2)

COMPLICATIONS OF SURGICAL AND MEDICAL CARE, NOT ELSEWHERE CLASSIFIED (T80-T88)

No Change **T80**	Complications following infusion, transfusion and therapeutic injection		
No Change	**T80.8**	Other complications following infusion, transfusion and therapeutic injection	
Add		T80.82	Complication of immune effector cellular therapy
Add			Complication of chimeric antigen receptor (CAR-T) cell therapy
Add			Complication of IEC therapy
Add			**Excludes2** complication of bone marrow transplant (T86.0)
Add			complication of stem cell transplant (T86.5)
Add			Use Additional code to identify the
Add			specific complication, such as:
Add			cytokine release syndrome (D89.83-)
Add			immune effector cell-associated neurotoxicity syndrome (G92.0-)
No Change **T81**	Complications of procedures, not elsewhere classified		
No Change	**T81.1**	Postprocedural shock	
No Change		**Excludes1**	
Delete			anesthetic shock (T88.2)
Add			shock due to anesthesia (T88.2)

No Change	**T86 Complications of transplanted organs and tissue**		
No Change		**T86.2**	**Complications of heart transplant**
No Change		**Excludes1**	
Revise from			artificial heart device (T82.5)
Revise to			artificial heart device (T82.5-)
Revise from			heart-lung transplant (T86.3)
Revise to			heart-lung transplant (T86.3-)

No Change **CHAPTER 20**

No Change **EXTERNAL CAUSES OF MORBIDITY (V00-Y99)**

SLIPPING, TRIPPING, STUMBLING AND FALLS (W00-W19)

No Change **W13**	Fall from, out of or through building or structure		
No Change	**W13.4**	Fall from, out of or through window	
No Change		**Excludes2**	
Revise from			fall with subsequent striking against sharp glass (W01.110)
Revise to			fall with subsequent striking against sharp glass (W01.110-)

EXPOSURE TO INANIMATE MECHANICAL FORCES (W20-W49)

No Change **W25**	Contact with sharp glass	
No Change	**Excludes1**	
Revise from		fall on same level due to slipping, tripping and stumbling with subsequent striking against sharp glass (W01.110)
Revise to		fall on same level due to slipping, tripping and stumbling with subsequent striking against sharp glass (W01.110-)
Revise from		striking against sharp glass with subsequent fall (W18.02)
Revise to		striking against sharp glass with subsequent fall (W18.02-)
No Change	**Excludes2**	
Revise from		glass embedded in skin (W45)
Revise to		glass embedded in skin (W45.-)
No Change **W26**	Contact with other sharp objects	
No Change	**Excludes2**	
Revise from		sharp object(s) embedded in skin (W45)
Revise to		sharp object(s) embedded in skin (W45.-)

LEGAL INTERVENTION, OPERATIONS OF WAR, MILITARY OPERATIONS, AND TERRORISM (Y35-Y38)

No Change **Y35**	Legal intervention		
No Change	**Y35.8**	Legal intervention involving other specified means	
No Change		**Y35.89**	Legal intervention involving other specified means
Add			Y35.899 Legal intervention involving other specified means, unspecified person injured

No Change **CHAPTER 21**

No Change **FACTORS INFLUENCING HEALTH STATUS AND CONTACT WITH HEALTH SERVICES (Z00-Z99)**

PERSONS ENCOUNTERING HEALTH SERVICES FOR EXAMINATIONS (Z00-Z13)

No Change **Z01**	Encounter for other special examination without complaint, suspected or reported diagnosis	
No Change	**Z01.0**	Encounter for examination of eyes and vision

No Change	Z01.02	Encounter for examination of eyes and vision following failed vision screening
No Change		**Excludes1**
Revise from		examination for examination of eyes and vision with abnormal findings (Z01.01)
Revise to		encounter for examination of eyes and vision with abnormal findings (Z01.01)
Revise from		examination for examination of eyes and vision without abnormal findings (Z01.00)
Revise to		encounter for examination of eyes and vision without abnormal findings (Z01.00)

No Change Z09		Encounter for follow-up examination after completed treatment for conditions other than malignant neoplasm
No Change		Use Additional
Revise from		code to identify any applicable history of disease code (Z86.-. Z87.-)
Revise to		code to identify any applicable history of disease code (Z86.-, Z87.-)

No Change Z13		Encounter for screening for other diseases and disorders
No Change	Z13.2	Encounter for screening for nutritional, metabolic and other endocrine disorders
No Change	Z13.29	Encounter for screening for other suspected endocrine disorder
Delete		**Excludes1** encounter for screening for diabetes mellitus (Z13.1)
Add		**Excludes2** encounter for screening for diabetes mellitus (Z13.1)

PERSONS WITH POTENTIAL HEALTH HAZARDS RELATED TO COMMUNICABLE DISEASES (Z20-Z29)

No Change

No Change Z23		Encounter for immunization
Add		Code also, if applicable, encounter for immunization safety counseling (Z71.85)

No Change Z28		Immunization not carried out and underimmunization status
Add		Code also, if applicable, encounter for immunization safety counseling (Z71.85)

PERSONS ENCOUNTERING HEALTH SERVICES IN CIRCUMSTANCES RELATED TO REPRODUCTION (Z30-Z39)

No Change

No Change Z31		Encounter for procreative management
Delete		**Excludes1** complications associated with artificial fertilization (N98.-)
Delete		female infertility (N97.-)
Delete		male infertility (N46.-)
Add		**Excludes2** complications associated with artificial fertilization (N98.-)
Add		female infertility (N97.-)
Add		male infertility (N46.-)

No Change Z3A		Weeks of gestation
No Change		Code first
Delete		complications of pregnancy, childbirth and the puerperium (O09-O9A)
Add		obstetric condition or encounter for delivery (O09-O60, O80-O82)

ENCOUNTERS FOR OTHER SPECIFIC HEALTH CARE (Z40-Z53)

No Change

No Change Z45		Encounter for adjustment and management of implanted device
No Change	Z45.8	Encounter for adjustment and management of other implanted devices
No Change	Z45.81	Encounter for adjustment or removal of breast implant
Revise from		Encounter removal of tissue expander with or without synchronous insertion of permanent implant
Revise to		Encounter for removal of tissue expander with or without synchronous insertion of permanent implant

PERSONS WITH POTENTIAL HEALTH HAZARDS RELATED TO SOCIOECONOMIC AND PSYCHOSOCIAL CIRCUMSTANCES (Z55-Z65)

No Change

No Change Z55		Problems related to education and literacy
Add	Z55.5	Less than a high school diploma
		No general equivalence degree (GED)

Add Z58		Problems related to physical environment
Add		**Excludes2** occupational exposure (Z57.-)
Add	Z58.6	Inadequate drinking-water supply
Add		Lack of safe drinking water
Add		**Excludes2** deprivation of water (T73.1)

No Change Z59		Problems related to housing and economic circumstances
No Change	Z59.0	Homelessness
Add	Z59.00	Homelessness unspecified
Add	Z59.01	Sheltered homelessness
Add		Doubled up
Add		Living in a shelter such as: motel, scattered site housing, temporary or transitional living situation
Add	Z59.02	Unsheltered homelessness
Add		Residing in place not meant for human habitation such as: abandoned buildings, cars, parks, sidewalk
Add		Residing on the street
Revise from	Z59.4	Lack of adequate food and safe drinking water
Revise to	Z59.4	Lack of adequate food
Delete		Inadequate drinking water supply
Delete		**Excludes1** effects of hunger (T73.0)
Delete		inappropriate diet or eating habits (Z72.4)
Delete		malnutrition (E40-E46)
Add		**Excludes2** deprivation of food (T73.0)
Add		effects of hunger (T73.0)
Add		inappropriate diet or eating habits (Z72.4)
Add		malnutrition (E40-E46)
Add	Z59.41	Food insecurity
Add	Z59.48	Other specified lack of adequate food
Add		Inadequate food
Add		Lack of food
No Change	Z59.8	Other problems related to housing and economic circumstances
Delete		Foreclosure on loan
Delete		Isolated dwelling
Delete		Problems with creditors
Add	Z59.81	Housing instability, housed
Add		Foreclosure on home loan
Add		Past due on rent or mortgage
Add		Unwanted multiple moves in the last 12 months
Add	Z59.811	Housing instability, housed, with risk of homelessness
Add		Imminent risk of homelessness
Add	Z59.812	Housing instability, housed, homelessness in past 12 months
Add	Z59.819	Housing instability, housed unspecified

Add	Z59.89	**Other problems related to housing and economic circumstances**
Add		Foreclosure on loan
Add		Isolated dwelling
		Problems with creditors

No Change   **PERSONS ENCOUNTERING HEALTH SERVICES IN OTHER CIRCUMSTANCES (Z69-Z76)**

No Change **Z71**		**Persons encountering health services for other counseling and medical advice, not elsewhere classified**
No Change	**Z71.8**	**Other specified counseling**
Add		**Z71.85** **Encounter for immunization safety counseling**
Add		Encounter for vaccine product safety counseling
Add		Code also, if applicable, encounter for immunization (Z23)
Add		Code also, if applicable, immunization not carried out (Z28.-)
Add		**Excludes1** encounter for health counseling related to travel (Z71.84)

No Change **Z72**		**Problems related to lifestyle**
No Change	**Z72.4**	**Inappropriate diet and eating habits**
No Change		**Excludes1**
Revise from		lack of adequate food (Z59.4)
Revise to		lack of adequate food (Z59.48)

No Change **Z76**		**Persons encountering health services in other circumstances**
No Change	**Z76.4**	**Other boarder to healthcare facility**
No Change		**Excludes1**
Revise from		homelessness (Z59.0)
Revise to		homelessness (Z59.0-)

No Change   **PERSONS WITH POTENTIAL HEALTH HAZARDS RELATED TO FAMILY AND PERSONAL HISTORY AND CERTAIN CONDITIONS INFLUENCING HEALTH STATUS (Z77-Z99)**

No Change **Z79**		**Long term (current) drug therapy**
No Change	**Z79.4**	**Long term (current) use of insulin**
Delete		**Excludes1** long term (current) use of oral antidiabetic drugs (Z79.84)
Delete		long term (current) use of oral hypoglycemic drugs (Z79.84)
Add		**Excludes2** long term (current) use of oral hypoglycemic drugs (Z79.84)
Add		long term (current) use of oral antidiabetic drugs (Z79.84)

No Change **Z82**		**Family history of certain disabilities and chronic diseases (leading to disablement)**
No Change	**Z82.4**	**Family history of ischemic heart disease and other diseases of the circulatory system**
Revise from		Conditions classifiable to I00-I52, I65-I99
Revise to		Conditions classifiable to I00-I5A, I65-I99

No Change **Z86**		**Personal history of certain other diseases**
No Change	**Z86.1**	**Personal history of infectious and parasitic diseases**
No Change		**Z86.16** **Personal history of COVID-19**
Add		**Excludes1** post COVID-19 condition (U09.9)

No Change **Z87**		**Personal history of other diseases and conditions**
No Change	**Z87.8**	**Personal history of other specified conditions**
No Change		**Excludes2**
Revise from		personal history of self harm (Z91.5)
Revise to		personal history of self harm (Z91.5-)

No Change **Z91**		**Personal risk factors, not elsewhere classified**
No Change	**Z91.0**	**Allergy status, other than to drugs and biological substances**
No Change		**Z91.01** **Food allergy status**
Add		**Z91.014** **Allergy to mammalian meats**
Add		Allergy to beef
Add		Allergy to lamb
Add		Allergy to pork
Add		Allergy to red meats
No Change	**Z91.5**	**Personal history of self-harm**
Delete		Personal history of parasuicide
Delete		Personal history of self-poisoning
Delete		Personal history of suicide attempt
Add		Code also mental health disorder, if known
Add		**Z91.51** **Personal history of suicidal behavior**
Add		Personal history of parasuicide
Add		Personal history of self-poisoning
Add		Personal history of suicide attempt
Add		**Z91.52** **Personal history of nonsuicidal self-harm**
Add		Personal history of nonsuicidal self-injury
Add		Personal history of self-inflicted injury without suicidal intent
Add		Personal history of self-mutilation

No Change **Z92**		**Personal history of medical treatment**
No Change	**Z92.2**	**Personal history of drug therapy**
Revise from		**Z92.25** **Personal history of immunosupression therapy**
Revise to		**Z92.25** **Personal history of immunosuppression therapy**
No Change	**Z92.8**	**Personal history of other medical treatment**
Add		**Z92.85** **Personal history of cellular therapy**
Add		**Z92.850** **Personal history of Chimeric Antigen Receptor T-cell therapy**
Add		Personal history of CAR T-cell therapy
Add		**Z92.858** **Personal history of other cellular therapy**
Add		**Z92.859** **Personal history of cellular therapy, unspecified**
Add		**Z92.86** **Personal history of gene therapy**

No Change **Z99**		**Dependence on enabling machines and devices, not elsewhere classified**
Delete		**Excludes1** cardiac pacemaker status (Z95.0)

No Change # CHAPTER 22

No Change # CODES FOR SPECIAL PURPOSES (U00-U85)

No Change   **PROVISIONAL ASSIGNMENT OF NEW DISEASES OF UNCERTAIN ETIOLOGY OR EMERGENCY USE (U00-U49)**

Add	U09	**Post COVID-19 condition**
Add		**U09.9** **Post COVID-19 condition, unspecified**
Add		**Note:** This code enables establishment of a link with COVID-19.
Add		This code is not to be used in cases that are still presenting with active COVID-19.
Add		However, an exception is made in cases of re-infection with COVID-19, occurring with a condition related to prior COVID-19.
Add		Post-acute sequela of COVID-19
Add		*Code first the specific condition related to COVID-19 if known, such as:*
Add		chronic respiratory failure (J96.1-)
Add		loss of smell (R43.8)
Add		loss of taste (R43.8)
Add		multisystem inflammatory syndrome (M35.81)
Add		pulmonary embolism (I26.-)
Add		pulmonary fibrosis (J84.10)

PART I

Introduction

ICD-10-CM Official Guidelines for Coding and Reporting FY2022 (October 1, 2021 - September 30, 2022)

Narrative changes appear in **bold** text
Items <u>underlined</u> have been moved within the guidelines since the 2021 version
Italics are used to indicate revisions to heading changes

The Centers for Medicare and Medicaid Services (CMS) and the National Center for Health Statistics (NCHS), two departments within the U.S. Federal Government's Department of Health and Human Services (DHHS), provide the following guidelines for coding and reporting using the International Classification of Diseases, 10th Revision, Clinical Modification (ICD-10-CM). These guidelines should be used as a companion document to the official version of the ICD-10-CM as published on the NCHS website. The ICD-10-CM is a morbidity classification published by the United States for classifying diagnoses and reason for visits in all health care settings. The ICD-10-CM is based on the ICD-10, the statistical classification of disease published by the World Health Organization (WHO).

These guidelines have been approved by the four organizations that make up the Cooperating Parties for the ICD-10-CM: the American Hospital Association (AHA), the American Health Information Management Association (AHIMA), CMS, and NCHS.

These guidelines are a set of rules that have been developed to accompany and complement the official conventions and instructions provided within the ICD-10-CM itself. The instructions and conventions of the classification take precedence over guidelines. These guidelines are based on the coding and sequencing instructions in the Tabular List and Alphabetic Index of ICD-10-CM, but provide additional instruction. Adherence to these guidelines when assigning ICD-10-CM diagnosis codes is required under the Health Insurance Portability and Accountability Act (HIPAA). The diagnosis codes (Tabular List and Alphabetic Index) have been adopted under HIPAA for all health care settings. A joint effort between the health care provider and the coder is essential to achieve complete and accurate documentation, code assignment, and reporting of diagnoses and procedures. These guidelines have been developed to assist both the health care provider and the coder in identifying those diagnoses that are to be reported. The importance of consistent, complete documentation in the medical record cannot be overemphasized. Without such documentation accurate coding cannot be achieved. The entire record should be reviewed to determine the specific reason for the encounter and the conditions treated.

The term "encounter" is used for all settings, including hospital admissions. In the context of these guidelines, the term "provider" is used throughout the guidelines to mean physician or any qualified health care practitioner who is legally accountable for establishing the patient's diagnosis. Only this set of guidelines, approved by the Cooperating Parties, is official.

The guidelines are organized into sections. Section I includes the structure and conventions of the classification and general guidelines that apply to the entire classification, and chapter-specific guidelines that correspond to the chapters as they are arranged in the classification. Section II includes guidelines for selection of principal diagnosis for non-outpatient settings. Section III includes guidelines for reporting additional diagnoses in non-outpatient settings. Section IV is for outpatient coding and reporting. It is necessary to review all sections of the guidelines to fully understand all of the rules and instructions needed to code properly.

ICD-10-CM Official Guidelines for Coding and Reporting

Section I. Conventions, General Coding Guidelines and Chapter Specific Guidelines

A. Conventions for the ICD-10-CM
1. The Alphabetic Index and Tabular List
2. Format and Structure:
3. Use of codes for reporting purposes
4. Placeholder character
5. 7th Characters
6. Abbreviations
   a. Alphabetic Index abbreviations
   b. Tabular List abbreviations
7. Punctuation
8. Use of "and"
9. Other and Unspecified codes
   a. "Other" codes
   b. "Unspecified" codes
10. Includes Notes
11. Inclusion terms
12. Excludes Notes
    a. Excludes1
    b. Excludes2
13. Etiology/manifestation convention ("code first", "use additional code" and "in diseases classified elsewhere" notes)
14. "And"
15. "With"
16. "See" and "See Also"
17. "Code also note"
18. Default codes
19. Code assignment and Clinical Criteria

B. General Coding Guidelines
1. Locating a code in the ICD-10-CM
2. Level of Detail in Coding
3. Code or codes from A00.0 through T88.9, *Z00-Z99.8, U00-U85*
4. Signs and symptoms
5. Conditions that are an integral part of a disease process
6. Conditions that are not an integral part of a disease process
7. Multiple coding for a single condition
8. Acute and Chronic Conditions
9. Combination Code
10. Sequela (Late Effects)
11. Impending or Threatened Condition
12. Reporting Same Diagnosis Code More than Once
13. Laterality
14. Documentation *by Clinicians Other than the Patient's Provider*
15. Syndromes
16. Documentation of Complications of Care
17. Borderline Diagnosis
18. Use of Sign/Symptom/Unspecified Codes
19. Coding for Healthcare Encounters in Hurricane Aftermath
    a. Use of External Cause of Morbidity Codes
    b. Sequencing of External Causes of Morbidity Codes

   c. Other External Causes of Morbidity Code Issues
   d. Use of Z codes

C. Chapter-Specific Coding Guidelines
1. Chapter 1: Certain Infectious and Parasitic Diseases (A00-B99, U07.1, *U09.9*)
   a. Human Immunodeficiency Virus (HIV) Infections
   b. Infectious agents as the cause of diseases classified to other chapters
   c. Infections resistant to antibiotics
   d. Sepsis, Severe Sepsis, and Septic Shock *infection resistant to antibiotics*
   e. Methicillin Resistant *Staphylococcus aureus* (MRSA) Conditions
   f. Zika virus infection
   g. Coronavirus infections
2. Chapter 2: Neoplasms (C00-D49)
   a. Treatment directed at the malignancy
   b. Treatment of secondary site
   c. Coding and sequencing of complications
   d. Primary malignancy previously excised
   e. Admissions/Encounters involving chemotherapy, immunotherapy and radiation therapy
   f. Admission/encounter to determine extent of malignancy
   g. Symptoms, signs, and abnormal findings listed in Chapter 18 associated with neoplasms
   h. Admission/encounter for pain control/management
   i. Malignancy in two or more noncontiguous sites
   j. Disseminated malignant neoplasm, unspecified
   k. Malignant neoplasm without specification of site
   l. Sequencing of neoplasm codes
   m. Current malignancy versus personal history of malignancy
   n. Leukemia, Multiple Myeloma, and Malignant Plasma Cell Neoplasms in remission versus personal history
   o. Aftercare following surgery for neoplasm
   p. Follow-up care for completed treatment of a malignancy
   q. Prophylactic organ removal for prevention of malignancy
   r. Malignant neoplasm associated with transplanted organ
   s. Breast Implant Associated Anaplastic Large Cell Lymphoma
3. Chapter 3: Disease of the Blood and Blood-Forming Organs and Certain Disorders Involving the Immune Mechanism (D50-D89)
4. Chapter 4: Endocrine, Nutritional, and Metabolic Diseases (E00-E89)
   a. Diabetes mellitus
5. Chapter 5: Mental, Behavioral, and Neurodevelopmental disorders (F01 – F99)
   a. Pain disorders related to psychological factors
   b. Mental and behavioral disorders due to psychoactive substance use
   c. Factitious Disorder
6. Chapter 6: Diseases of the Nervous System (G00-G99)
   a. Dominant/nondominant side
   b. Pain - Category G89

GUIDELINES (ICD-10-CM)

Section II. Selection of Principal Diagnosis

Section III. Reporting Additional Diagnoses

Section IV. Diagnostic Coding and Reporting Guidelines for Outpatient Services

Appendix I: Present on Admission Reporting Guidelines

Section I. Conventions, General Coding Guidelines, and Chapter Specific Guidelines

The conventions, general guidelines, and chapter-specific guidelines are applicable to all health care settings unless otherwise indicated. The conventions and instructions of the classification take precedence over guidelines.

A. Conventions for the ICD-10-CM

The conventions for the ICD-10-CM are the general rules for use of the classification independent of the guidelines. These conventions are incorporated within the Alphabetic Index and Tabular List of the ICD-10-CM as instructional notes.

1. **The Alphabetic Index and Tabular List**

   The ICD-10-CM is divided into the Alphabetic Index, an alphabetical list of terms and their corresponding code, and the Tabular List, a structured list of codes divided into chapters based on body system or condition. The Alphabetic Index consists of the following parts: the Index of Diseases and Injury, the Index of External Causes of Injury, the Table of Neoplasms, and the Table of Drugs and Chemicals.

   See Section I.C2. General guidelines
   See Section I.C.19. Adverse effects, poisoning, underdosing and toxic effects

2. **Format and Structure:**

   The ICD-10-CM Tabular List contains categories, subcategories and codes. Characters for categories, subcategories and codes may be either a letter or a number. All categories are 3 characters. A 3-character category that has no further subdivision is equivalent to a code. Subcategories are either 4 or 5 characters. Codes may be 3, 4, 5, 6 or 7 characters. That is, each level of subdivision after a category is a subcategory. The final level of subdivision is a code. Codes that have applicable 7th characters are still referred to as codes, not subcategories. A code that has an applicable 7th character is considered invalid without the 7th character.

   The ICD-10-CM uses an indented format for ease in reference

3. **Use of codes for reporting purposes**

   For reporting purposes only codes are permissible, not categories or subcategories, and any applicable 7th character is required.

4. **Placeholder character**

   The ICD-10-CM utilizes a placeholder character "X". The "X" is used as a placeholder at certain codes to allow for future expansion. An example of this is at the poisoning, adverse effect and underdosing codes, categories T36-T50. Where a placeholder exists, the X must be used in order for the code to be considered a valid code.

5. **7th Characters**

   Certain ICD-10-CM categories have applicable 7th characters. The applicable 7th character is required for all codes within the category, or as the notes in the Tabular List instruct. The 7th character must always be the 7th character in the data field. If a

GUIDELINES (ICD-10-CM)

code that requires a 7th character is not 6 characters, a placeholder X must be used to fill in the empty characters.

6. **Abbreviations**

   a. **Alphabetic Index abbreviations**

      NEC "Not elsewhere classifiable"
      This abbreviation in the Alphabetic Index represents "other specified". When a specific code is not available for a condition the Alphabetic Index directs the coder to the "other specified" code in the Tabular List.

      NOS "Not otherwise specified"
      This abbreviation is the equivalent of unspecified.

   b. **Tabular List abbreviations**

      NEC "Not elsewhere classifiable"
      This abbreviation in the Tabular List represents "other specified". When a specific code is not available for a condition, the Tabular List includes an NEC entry under a code to identify the code as the "other specified" code.

      NOS "Not otherwise specified"
      This abbreviation is the equivalent of unspecified.

7. **Punctuation**

   [ ] Brackets are used in the Tabular List to enclose synonyms, alternative wording or explanatory phrases. Brackets are used in the Alphabetic Index to identify manifestation codes.

   ( ) Parentheses are used in both the Alphabetic Index and Tabular List to enclose supplementary words that may be present or absent in the statement of a disease or procedure without affecting the code number to which it is assigned. The terms within the parentheses are referred to as nonessential modifiers. The nonessential modifiers in the Alphabetic Index to Diseases apply to subterms following a main term except when a nonessential modifier and a subentry are mutually exclusive, the subentry takes precedence. For example, in the ICD-10-CM Alphabetic Index under the main term Enteritis, "acute" is a nonessential modifier and "chronic" is a subentry. In this case, the nonessential modifier "acute" does not apply to the subentry "chronic".

   : Colons are used in the Tabular List after an incomplete term which needs one or more of the modifiers following the colon to make it assignable to a given category.

8. **Use of "and".**
   See Section I.A.14. Use of the term "And"

9. **Other and Unspecified codes**

   a. **"Other" codes**
   Codes titled "other" or "other specified" are for use when the information in the medical record provides detail for which a specific code does not exist. Alphabetic Index entries with NEC in the line designate "other" codes in the Tabular List.

These Alphabetic Index entries represent specific disease entities for which no specific code exists so the term is included within an "other" code.

   b. **"Unspecified" codes**
   Codes titled "unspecified" are for use when the information in the medical record is insufficient to assign a more specific code. For those categories for which an unspecified code is not provided, the "other specified" code may represent both other and unspecified.
   See Section I.B.18 Use of signs/symptoms/unspecified codes

10. **Includes Notes**
    This note appears immediately under a 3-character code title to further define, or give examples of, the content of the category.

11. **Inclusion terms**
    List of terms is included under some codes. These terms are the conditions for which that code is to be used. The terms may be synonyms of the code title, or, in the case of "other specified" codes, the terms are a list of the various conditions assigned to that code. The inclusion terms are not necessarily exhaustive. Additional terms found only in the Alphabetic Index may also be assigned to a code.

12. **Excludes Notes**
    The ICD-10-CM has two types of excludes notes. Each type of note has a different definition for use, but they are all similar in that they indicate that codes excluded from each other are independent of each other.

    a. **Excludes1**
    A type 1 Excludes note is a pure excludes note. It means "NOT CODED HERE!" An Excludes1 note indicates that the code excluded should never be used at the same time as the code above the Excludes1 note. An Excludes1 is used when two conditions cannot occur together, such as a congenital form versus an acquired form of the same condition.

    An exception to the Excludes1 definition is the circumstance when the two conditions are unrelated to each other. If it is not clear whether the two conditions involving an Excludes1 note are related or not, query the provider. For example, code F45.8, Other somatoform disorders, has an Excludes1 note for "sleep related teeth grinding (G47.63)" because "teeth grinding" is an inclusion term under F45.8. Only one of these two codes should be assigned for teeth grinding. However, psychogenic dysmenorrhea is also an inclusion term under F45.8, and a patient could have both this condition and sleep-related teeth grinding. In this case, the two conditions are clearly unrelated to each other, and so it would be appropriate to report F45.8 and G47.63 together.

    b. **Excludes2**
    A Type 2 Excludes note represents "Not included here." An excludes2 note indicates that the condition excluded is not part of the condition represented by the code, but a patient may

have both conditions at the same time. When an Excludes2 note appears under a code, it is acceptable to use both the code and the excluded code together, when appropriate.

13. **Etiology/manifestation convention ("code first", "use additional code" and "in diseases classified elsewhere" notes)**

Certain conditions have both an underlying etiology and multiple body system manifestations due to the underlying etiology. For such conditions, the ICD-10-CM has a coding convention that requires the underlying condition be sequenced first, if applicable, followed by the manifestation. Wherever such a combination exists, there is a "use additional code" note at the etiology code, and a "code first" note at the manifestation code. These instructional notes indicate the proper sequencing order of the codes, etiology followed by manifestation.

In most cases the manifestation codes will have in the code title, "in diseases classified elsewhere." Codes with this title are a component of the etiology/manifestation convention. The code title indicates that it is a manifestation code. "In diseases classified elsewhere" codes are never permitted to be used as first-listed or principal diagnosis codes. They must be used in conjunction with an underlying condition code and they must be listed following the underlying condition. See category F02, Dementia in other diseases classified elsewhere, for an example of this convention.

There are manifestation codes that do not have "in diseases classified elsewhere" in the title. For such codes, there is a "use additional code" note at the etiology code and a "code first" note at the manifestation code and the rules for sequencing apply.

In addition to the notes in the Tabular List, these conditions also have a specific Alphabetic Index entry structure. In the Alphabetic Index both conditions are listed together with the etiology code first followed by the manifestation codes in brackets. The code in brackets is always to be sequenced second.

An example of the etiology/manifestation convention is dementia in Parkinson's disease. In the Alphabetic Index, code G20 is listed first, followed by code F02.80 or F02.81 in brackets. Code G20 represents the underlying etiology, Parkinson's disease, and must be sequenced first, whereas code F02.80 and F02.81 represent the manifestation of dementia in diseases classified elsewhere, with or without behavioral disturbance.

"Code first" and "Use additional code" notes are also used as sequencing rules in the classification for certain codes that are not part of an etiology/manifestation combination.

See Section I.B.7. Multiple coding for a single condition.

14. **"And"**

The word "and" should be interpreted to mean either "and" or "or" when it appears in a title.

For example, cases of "tuberculosis of bones", "tuberculosis of joints" and "tuberculosis of bones

and joints" are classified to subcategory A18.0, Tuberculosis of bones and joints.

15. **"With"**

The word "with" or "in" should be interpreted to mean "associated with" or "due to" when it appears in a code title, the Alphabetic Index, (either under a main term or subterm) or an instructional note in the Tabular List. The classification presumes a causal relationship between the two conditions linked by these terms in the Alphabetic Index or Tabular List. These conditions should be coded as related even in the absence of provider documentation explicitly linking them, unless the documentation clearly states the conditions are unrelated or when another guideline exists that specifically requires a documented linkage between two conditions (e.g., sepsis guideline for "acute organ dysfunction that is not clearly associated with the sepsis").

For conditions not specifically linked by these relational terms in the classification or when a guideline requires that a linkage between two conditions be explicitly documented provider documentation must link the conditions in order to code them as related.

The word "with" in the Alphabetic Index is sequenced immediately following the main term or subterm, not in alphabetical order.

16. **"See" and "See Also"**

The "see" instruction following a main term in the Alphabetic Index indicates that another term should be referenced. It is necessary to go to the main term referenced with the "see" note to locate the correct code.

A "see also" instruction following a main term in the Alphabetic Index instructs that there is another main term that may also be referenced that may provide additional Alphabetic Index entries that may be useful. It is not necessary to follow the "see also" note when the original main term provides the necessary code.

17. **"Code also" note**

A "code also" note instructs that two codes may be required to fully describe a condition, but this note does not provide sequencing direction. The sequencing depends on the circumstances of the encounter.

18. **Default codes**

A code listed next to a main term in the ICD-10-CM Alphabetic Index is referred to as a default code. The default code represents that condition that is most commonly associated with the main term, or is the unspecified code for the condition. If a condition is documented in a medical record (for example, appendicitis) without any additional information, such as acute or chronic, the default code should be assigned.

19. **Code assignment and Clinical Criteria**

The assignment of a diagnosis code is based on the provider's diagnostic statement that the condition exists. The provider's statement that the patient has a particular condition is sufficient. Code

assignment is not based on clinical criteria used by the provider to establish the diagnosis.

B. General Coding Guidelines

1. Locating a code in the ICD-10-CM

To select a code in the classification that corresponds to a diagnosis or reason for visit documented in a medical record, first locate the term in the Alphabetic Index, and then verify the code in the Tabular List. Read and be guided by instructional notations that appear in both the Alphabetic Index and the Tabular List.

It is essential to use both the Alphabetic Index and Tabular List when locating and assigning a code. The Alphabetic Index does not always provide the full code. Selection of the full code, including laterality and any applicable 7th character can only be done in the Tabular List. A dash (-) at the end of an Alphabetic Index entry indicates that additional characters are required. Even if a dash is not included at the Alphabetic Index entry, it is necessary to refer to the Tabular List to verify that no 7th character is required.

2. Level of Detail in Coding

Diagnosis codes are to be used and reported at their highest number of characters available **and to the highest level of specificity documented in the medical record.**

ICD-10-CM diagnosis codes are composed of codes with 3, 4, 5, 6, or 7 characters. Codes with three characters are included in ICD-10-CM as the heading of a category of codes that may be further subdivided by the use of 4th and/or 5th characters and/or 6th characters, which provide greater detail.

A 3-character code is to be used only if it is not further subdivided. A code is invalid if it has not been coded to the full number of characters required for that code, including the 7th character, if applicable.

3. Code or codes from A00.0 through T88.9, Z00-Z99.8, U00-U85

The appropriate code or codes from A00.0 through T88.9, Z00-Z99.8 **and U00-U85** must be used to identify diagnoses, symptoms, conditions, problems, complaints or other reason(s) for the encounter/visit.

4. Signs and symptoms

Codes that describe symptoms and signs, as opposed to diagnoses, are acceptable for reporting purposes when a related definitive diagnosis has not been established (confirmed) by the provider. Chapter 18 of ICD-10-CM, Symptoms, Signs, and Abnormal Clinical and Laboratory Findings, Not Elsewhere Classified (codes R00.0 - R99) contains many, but not all codes for symptoms.

See Section I.B.18 Use of signs/symptoms/unspecified codes

5. Conditions that are an integral part of a disease process

Signs and symptoms that are associated routinely with a disease process should not be assigned as additional codes, unless otherwise instructed by the classification.

6. Conditions that are not an integral part of a disease process

Additional signs and symptoms that may not be associated routinely with a disease process should be coded when present.

7. Multiple coding for a single condition

In addition to the etiology/manifestation convention that requires two codes to fully describe a single condition that affects multiple body systems, there are other single conditions that also require more than one code. "Use additional code" notes are found in the Tabular List at codes that are not part of an etiology/manifestation pair where a secondary code is useful to fully describe a condition. The sequencing rule is the same as the etiology/manifestation pair, "use additional code" indicates that a secondary code should be added, if known.

For example, for bacterial infections that are not included in Chapter 1, a secondary code from category B95, Streptococcus, Staphylococcus, and Enterococcus, as the cause of diseases classified elsewhere, or B96, Other bacterial agents as the cause of diseases classified elsewhere, may be required to identify the bacterial organism causing the infection. A "use additional code" note will normally be found at the infectious disease code, indicating a need for the organism code to be added as a secondary code.

"Code first" notes are also under certain codes that are not specifically manifestation codes but may be due to an underlying cause. When there is a "code first" note and an underlying condition is present, the underlying condition should be sequenced first, if known.

"Code, if applicable, any causal condition first," notes indicate that this code may be assigned as a principal diagnosis when the causal condition is unknown or not applicable. If a causal condition is known, then the code for that condition should be sequenced as the principal or first-listed diagnosis.

Multiple codes may be needed for sequela, complication codes and obstetric codes to more fully describe a condition. See the specific guidelines for these conditions for further instruction.

8. Acute and Chronic Conditions

If the same condition is described as both acute (subacute) and chronic, and separate subentries exist in the Alphabetic Index at the same indentation level, code both and sequence the acute (subacute) code first.

9. Combination Code

A combination code is a single code used to classify:
    Two diagnoses, or
    A diagnosis with an associated secondary process (manifestation)
    A diagnosis with an associated complication
    Combination codes are identified by referring to subterm entries in the Alphabetic Index and by reading the inclusion and exclusion notes in the Tabular List.

Assign only the combination code when that code fully identifies the diagnostic conditions involved or when the Alphabetic Index so directs. Multiple coding should not be used when the classification provides a combination code that clearly identifies all of the elements documented in the diagnosis. When the combination code lacks necessary specificity in describing the manifestation or complication, an additional code should be used as a secondary code.

10. **Sequela (Late Effects)**
    A sequela is the residual effect (condition produced) after the acute phase of an illness or injury has terminated. There is no time limit on when a sequela code can be used. The residual may be apparent early, such as in cerebral infarction, or it may occur months or years later, such as that due to a previous injury. Examples of sequela include: scar formation resulting from a burn, deviated septum due to a nasal fracture, and infertility due to tubal occlusion from old tuberculosis. Coding of sequela generally requires two codes sequenced in the following order: the condition or nature of the sequela is sequenced first. The sequela code is sequenced second.
    An exception to the above guidelines are those instances where the code for the sequela is followed by a manifestation code identified in the Tabular List and title, or the sequela code has been expanded (at the 4th, 5th, or 6th character levels) to include the manifestation(s). The code for the acute phase of an illness or injury that led to the sequela is never used with a code for the late effect.
    See Section I.C.9. Sequelae of cerebrovascular disease
    See Section I.C.15. Sequelae of complication of pregnancy, childbirth and the puerperium
    See Section I.C.19. Application of 7th characters for Chapter 19

11. **Impending or Threatened Condition**
    Code any condition described at the time of discharge as "impending" or "threatened" as follows:
    If it did occur, code as confirmed diagnosis.
    If it did not occur, reference the Alphabetic Index to determine if the condition has a subentry term for "impending" or "threatened" and also reference main term entries for "Impending" and for "Threatened."
    If the subterms are listed, assign the given code.
    If the subterms are not listed, code the existing underlying condition(s) and not the condition described as impending or threatened.

12. **Reporting Same Diagnosis Code More Than Once**
    Each unique ICD-10-CM diagnosis code may be reported only once for an encounter. This applies to bilateral conditions when there are no distinct codes identifying laterality or two different conditions classified to the same ICD-10-CM diagnosis code.

13. **Laterality**
    Some ICD-10-CM codes indicate laterality, specifying whether the condition occurs on the left, right or is bilateral. If no bilateral code is provided and the condition is bilateral, assign separate codes for both the left and right side. If the side is not identified in the medical record, assign the code for the unspecified side.
    When a patient has a bilateral condition and each side is treated during separate encounters, assign the "bilateral" code (as the condition still exists on both sides), including for the encounter to treat the first side. For the second encounter for treatment after one side has previously been treated and the condition no longer exists on that side, assign the appropriate unilateral code for the side where the condition still exists (e.g., cataract surgery performed on each eye in separate encounters). The bilateral code would not be assigned for the subsequent encounter, as the patient no longer has the condition in the previously-treated site. If the treatment on the first side did not completely resolve the condition, then the bilateral code would still be appropriate.
    When laterality is not documented by the patient's provider, code assignment for the affected side may be based on medical record documentation from other clinicians. If there is conflicting medical record documentation regarding the affected side, the patient's attending provider should be queried for clarification. Codes for "unspecified" side should rarely be used, such as when the documentation in the record is insufficient to determine the affected side and it is not possible to obtain clarification.

14. **Documentation by Clinicians Other than the Patient's Provider**
    Code assignment is based on the documentation by **the** patient's provider (i.e., physician or other qualified healthcare practitioner legally accountable for establishing the patient's diagnosis). There are a few exceptions **when** code assignment may be based on medical record documentation from clinicians who are not the patient's provider (i.e., physician or other qualified healthcare practitioner legally accountable for establishing the patient's diagnosis).
    In this context, "clinicians" other than the patient's provider refer to healthcare professionals permitted, based on regulatory or accreditation requirements or internal hospital policies, to document in a patient's official medical record.

    These exceptions include codes for:
    - **Body Mass Index (BMI)**
    - **Depth of non-pressure chronic ulcers**
    - **Pressure ulcer stage**
    - **Coma scale**
    - **NIH stroke scale (NIHSS)**
    - **Social determinants of health (SDOH)**
    - **Laterality**
    - **Blood alcohol level**

    This information is typically, **or may be,** documented by other clinicians involved in the care of the patient (e.g., a dietitian often documents

the BMI, a nurse often documents the pressure ulcer stages, and an emergency medical technician often documents the coma scale). However, the associated diagnosis (such as overweight, obesity, acute stroke, pressure ulcer, **or a condition classifiable to category F10, Alcohol related disorders**) must be documented by the patient's provider. If there is conflicting medical record documentation, either from the same clinician or different clinicians, the patient's attending provider should be queried for clarification.

The BMI, coma scale, and NIHSS **blood alcohol level** codes and **codes for social determinants of health** should only be reported as secondary diagnoses.

See Section I.C.21.c.17 for additional information regarding coding social determinants of health.

15. **Syndromes**

Follow the Alphabetic Index guidance when coding syndromes. In the absence of Alphabetic Index guidance, assign codes for the documented manifestations of the syndrome. Additional codes for manifestations that are not an integral part of the disease process may also be assigned when the condition does not have a unique code.

16. **Documentation of Complications of Care**

Code assignment is based on the provider's documentation of the relationship between the condition and the care or procedure, unless otherwise instructed by the classification. The guideline extends to any complications of care, regardless of the chapter the code is located in. It is important to note that not all conditions that occur during or following medical care or surgery are classified as complications. There must be a cause-and-effect relationship between the care provided and the condition, and an indication in the documentation that it is a complication. Query the provider for clarification, if the complication is not clearly documented.

17. **Borderline Diagnosis**

If the provider documents a "borderline" diagnosis at the time of discharge, the diagnosis is coded as confirmed, unless the classification provides a specific entry (e.g., borderline diabetes). If a borderline condition has a specific index entry in ICD-10-CM, it should be coded as such. Since borderline conditions are not uncertain diagnoses, no distinction is made between the care setting (inpatient versus outpatient). Whenever the documentation is unclear regarding a borderline condition, coders are encouraged to query for clarification.

18. **Use of Sign/Symptom/Unspecified Codes**

Sign/symptom and "unspecified" codes have acceptable, even necessary, uses. While specific diagnosis codes should be reported when they are supported by the available medical record documentation and clinical knowledge of the patient's health condition, there are instances when signs/symptoms or unspecified codes are the best

choices for accurately reflecting the healthcare encounter. Each healthcare encounter should be coded to the level of certainty known for that encounter.

As stated in the introductory section of these official coding guidelines, a joint effort between the healthcare provider and the coder is essential to achieve complete and accurate documentation, code assignment, and reporting of diagnoses and procedures. The importance of consistent, complete documentation in the medical record cannot be overemphasized. Without such documentation accurate coding cannot be achieved. The entire record should be reviewed to determine the specific reason for the encounter and the conditions treated.

If a definitive diagnosis has not been established by the end of the encounter, it is appropriate to report codes for sign(s) and/or symptom(s) in lieu of a definitive diagnosis. When sufficient clinical information isn't known or available about a particular health condition to assign a more specific code, it is acceptable to report the appropriate "unspecified" code (e.g., a diagnosis of pneumonia has been determined, but not the specific type). Unspecified codes should be reported when they are the codes that most accurately reflect what is known about the patient's condition at the time of that particular encounter. It would be inappropriate to select a specific code that is not supported by the medical record documentation or conduct medically unnecessary diagnostic testing in order to determine a more specific code.

19. **Coding for Healthcare Encounters in Hurricane Aftermath**

a. **Use of External Cause of Morbidity Codes**

An external cause of morbidity code should be assigned to identify the cause of the injury(ies) incurred as a result of the hurricane. The use of external cause of morbidity codes is supplemental to the application of ICD-10-CM codes. External cause of morbidity codes are never to be recorded as a principal diagnosis (first-listed in non-inpatient settings). The appropriate injury code should be sequenced before any external cause codes. The external cause of morbidity codes capture how the injury or health condition happened (cause), the intent (unintentional or accidental; or intentional, such as suicide or assault), the place where the event occurred, the activity of the patient at the time of the event, and the person's status (e.g., civilian, military). They should not be assigned for encounters to treat hurricane victims' medical conditions when no injury, adverse effect or poisoning is involved. External cause of morbidity codes should be assigned for each encounter for care and treatment of the injury. External cause of morbidity codes may be assigned in all health care settings. For the purpose of capturing complete and accurate ICD-10-CM data in the aftermath of the hurricane, a healthcare setting should be considered as

any location where medical care is provided by licensed healthcare professionals.

b. Sequencing of External Causes of Morbidity Codes

Codes for cataclysmic events, such as a hurricane, take priority over all other external cause codes except child and adult abuse and terrorism and should be sequenced before other external cause of injury codes. Assign as many external cause of morbidity codes as necessary to fully explain each cause. For example, if an injury occurs as a result of a building collapse during the hurricane, external cause codes for both the hurricane and the building collapse should be assigned, with the external causes code for hurricane being sequenced as the first external cause code. For injuries incurred as a direct result of the hurricane, assign the appropriate code(s) for the injuries, followed by the code X37.0-, Hurricane (with the appropriate 7th character), and any other applicable external cause of injury codes. Code X37.0- also should be assigned when an injury is incurred as a result of flooding caused by a levee breaking related to the hurricane. Code X38.-, Flood (with the appropriate 7th character), should be assigned when an injury is from flooding resulting directly from the storm. Code X36.0-, Collapse of dam or man-made structure, should not be assigned when the cause of the collapse is due to the hurricane. Use of code X36.0- is limited to collapses of man-made structures due to earth surface movements, not due to storm surges directly from a hurricane.

c. Other External Causes of Morbidity Code Issues

For injuries that are not a direct result of the hurricane, such as an evacuee that has incurred an injury as a result of a motor vehicle accident, assign the appropriate external cause of morbidity code(s) to describe the cause of the injury, but do not assign code X37.0-, Hurricane. If it is not clear whether the injury was a direct result of the hurricane, assume the injury is due to the hurricane and assign code X37.0-, Hurricane, as well as any other applicable external cause of morbidity codes. In addition to code X37.0-, Hurricane, other possible applicable external cause of morbidity codes include:

X30-	Exposure to excessive natural heat
X31-	Exposure to excessive natural cold
X38-	Flood

d. Use of Z codes

Z codes (other reasons for healthcare encounters) may be assigned as appropriate to further explain the reasons for presenting for healthcare services, including transfers between healthcare facilities **or provide additional information relevant to a patient encounter**. The ICD-10-CM Official Guidelines for Coding and Reporting identify which codes maybe assigned as principal or first-listed diagnosis only, secondary diagnosis only, or principal/first-listed or secondary (depending on the circumstances). Possible applicable Z codes include:

Z59.0-	Homelessness
Z59.1	Inadequate housing
Z59.5	Extreme poverty
Z75.1	Person awaiting admission to adequate facility elsewhere
Z75.3	Unavailability and inaccessibility of health-care facilities
Z75.4	Unavailability and inaccessibility of other helping agencies
Z76.2	Encounter for health supervision and care of other healthy infant and child
Z99.12	Encounter for respirator [ventilator] dependence during power failure

The external cause of morbidity codes and the Z codes listed above are not an all-inclusive list. Other codes may be applicable to the encounter based upon the documentation. Assign as many codes as necessary to fully explain each healthcare encounter. Since patient history information may be very limited, use any available documentation to assign the appropriate external cause of morbidity and Z codes.

C. Chapter-Specific Coding Guidelines

In addition to general coding guidelines, there are guidelines for specific diagnoses and/or conditions in the classification. Unless otherwise indicated, these guidelines apply to all health care settings. Please refer to Section II for guidelines on the selection of principal diagnosis.

1. Chapter 1: Certain Infectious and Parasitic Diseases (A00-B99, U07.1, *U09.9*)

a. Human Immunodeficiency Virus (HIV) Infections

1) Code only confirmed cases

Code only confirmed cases of HIV infection/illness. This is an exception to the hospital inpatient guideline Section II, H.

In this context, "confirmation" does not require documentation of positive serology or culture for HIV; the provider's diagnostic statement that the patient is HIV positive, or has an HIV-related illness is sufficient.

2) Selection and sequencing of HIV codes

(a) Patient admitted for HIV-related condition

If a patient is admitted for an HIV-related condition, the principal diagnosis should be B20, Human immunodeficiency virus [HIV] disease followed by additional diagnosis codes for all reported HIV-related conditions.

(b) Patient with HIV disease admitted for unrelated condition

If a patient with HIV disease is admitted for an unrelated condition (such as a traumatic injury), the code for the unrelated condition (e.g., the nature of injury code) should be the principal diagnosis. Other diagnoses would be B20 followed by additional diagnosis codes for all reported HIV-related conditions.

(c) Whether the patient is newly diagnosed

Whether the patient is newly diagnosed or has had previous admissions/encounters for HIV conditions is irrelevant to the sequencing decision.

(d) Asymptomatic human immunodeficiency virus

Z21, Asymptomatic human immunodeficiency virus [HIV] infection status, is to be applied when the patient without any documentation of symptoms is listed as being "HIV positive," "known HIV," "HIV test positive," or similar terminology. Do not use this code if the term "AIDS" **or "HIV disease"** is used or if the patient is treated for any HIV-related illness or is described as having any condition(s) resulting from his/her HIV positive status; use B20 in these cases.

(e) Patients with inconclusive HIV serology

Patients with inconclusive HIV serology, but no definitive diagnosis or manifestations of the illness, may be assigned code R75, Inconclusive laboratory evidence of human immunodeficiency virus [HIV].

(f) Previously diagnosed HIV-related illness

Patients with any known prior diagnosis of an HIV-related illness should be coded to B20. Once a patient has developed an HIV-related illness, the patient should always be assigned code B20 on every subsequent admission/encounter. Patients previously diagnosed with any HIV illness (B20) should never be assigned to R75 or Z21, Asymptomatic human immunodeficiency virus [HIV] infection status.

(g) HIV Infection in Pregnancy, Childbirth and the Puerperium

During pregnancy, childbirth or the puerperium, a patient admitted (or presenting for a health care encounter) because of an HIV-related illness should receive a principal diagnosis code of O98.7-, Human immunodeficiency [HIV] disease complicating pregnancy, childbirth and the puerperium, followed by B20 and the code(s) for the HIV-related illness(es). Codes from Chapter 15 always take sequencing priority.

Patients with asymptomatic HIV infection status admitted (or presenting for a health care encounter) during pregnancy, childbirth, or the puerperium should receive codes of O98.7- and Z21.

(h) Encounters for testing for HIV

If a patient is being seen to determine his/her HIV status, use code Z11.4, Encounter for screening for human immunodeficiency virus [HIV]. Use additional codes for any associated high-risk behavior, **if applicable.**

If a patient with signs or symptoms is being seen for HIV testing, code the signs and symptoms. An additional counseling code Z71.7, Human immunodeficiency virus [HIV] counseling, may be used if counseling is provided during the encounter for the test.

When a patient returns to be informed of his/her HIV test results and the test result is negative, use code Z71.7, Human immunodeficiency virus [HIV] counseling.

If the results are positive, see previous guidelines and assign codes as appropriate.

(i) History of HIV managed by medication

If a patient with documented history of HIV disease is currently managed on antiretroviral medications, assign code B20, Human immunodeficiency virus [HIV] disease. Code Z79.899, Other long term (current) drug therapy, may be assigned as an additional code to identify the long-term (current) use of antiretroviral medications.

b. Infectious agents as the cause of diseases classified to other chapters

Certain infections are classified in chapters other than Chapter 1 and no organism is identified as part of the infection code. In these instances, it is necessary to use an additional code from Chapter 1 to identify the organism. A code from category B95, Streptococcus, Staphylococcus, and Enterococcus as the cause of diseases classified to other chapters, B96, Other bacterial agents as the cause of diseases classified to other chapters, or B97, Viral agents as the cause of diseases classified to other chapters, is to be used as an additional code to identify the organism. An instructional note will be found at the infection code advising that an additional organism code is required.

c. Infections resistant to antibiotics

Many bacterial infections are resistant to current antibiotics. It is necessary to identify all infections documented as antibiotic resistant. Assign a code from category Z16, Resistance to antimicrobial drugs, following the infection code only if the infection code does not identify drug resistance.

d. Sepsis, Severe Sepsis, and Septic Shock

1) Coding of Sepsis and Severe Sepsis

(a) Sepsis

For a diagnosis of sepsis, assign the appropriate code for the underlying systemic infection. If the type of infection or causal organism is not further specified, assign code A41.9, Sepsis, unspecified organism.

A code from subcategory R65.2, Severe sepsis, should not be assigned unless severe sepsis or an associated acute organ dysfunction is documented.

(i) Negative or inconclusive blood cultures and sepsis
Negative or inconclusive blood cultures do not preclude a diagnosis of sepsis in patients with clinical evidence of the condition, however, the provider should be queried.

(ii) Urosepsis
The term urosepsis is a nonspecific term. It is not to be considered synonymous with sepsis. It has no default code in the Alphabetic Index. Should a provider use this

11

ICD-10-CM HOSPITAL EDITION

GUIDELINES (ICD-10-CM)

term, he/she must be queried for clarification.

(iii) **Sepsis with organ dysfunction**
If a patient has sepsis and associated acute organ dysfunction or multiple organ dysfunction (MOD), follow the instructions for coding severe sepsis.

(iv) **Acute organ dysfunction that is not clearly associated with the sepsis**
If a patient has sepsis and an acute organ dysfunction, but the medical record documentation indicates that the acute organ dysfunction is related to a medical condition other than the sepsis, do not assign a code from subcategory R65.2, Severe sepsis. An acute organ dysfunction must be associated with the sepsis in order to assign the severe sepsis code. If the documentation is not clear as to whether an acute organ dysfunction is related to the sepsis or another medical condition, query the provider.

(b) Severe sepsis
The coding of severe sepsis requires a minimum of 2 codes: first a code for the underlying systemic infection, followed by a code from subcategory R65.2, Severe sepsis. If the causal organism is not documented, assign code A41.9, Sepsis, unspecified organism, for the infection. Additional code(s) for the associated acute organ dysfunction are also required.

Due to the complex nature of severe sepsis, some cases may require querying the provider prior to assignment of the codes.

2) Septic shock

(a) Septic shock generally refers to circulatory failure associated with severe sepsis, and therefore, it represents a type of acute organ dysfunction.

For all cases of septic shock, the code for the systemic infection should be sequenced first, followed by code R65.21, Severe sepsis with septic shock or code T81.12, Postprocedural septic shock. Any additional codes for the other acute organ dysfunctions should also be assigned. As noted in the sequencing instructions in the Tabular List, the code for septic shock cannot be assigned as a principal diagnosis.

3) Sequencing of severe sepsis
If severe sepsis is present on admission, and meets the definition of principal diagnosis, the underlying systemic infection should be assigned as principal diagnosis followed by the appropriate code from subcategory R65.2 as required by the sequencing rules in the Tabular List. A code from subcategory R65.2 can never be assigned as a principal diagnosis.

When severe sepsis develops during an encounter (it was not present on admission) the underlying systemic infection and the appropriate code from subcategory R65.2 should be assigned as secondary diagnoses.

Severe sepsis may be present on admission but the diagnosis may not be confirmed until sometime after admission. If the documentation is not clear whether severe sepsis was present on admission, the provider should be queried.

4) Sepsis or severe sepsis with a localized infection
If the reason for admission is sepsis or severe sepsis and a localized infection, such as pneumonia or cellulitis, a code(s) for the underlying systemic infection should be assigned first and the code for the localized infection should be assigned as a secondary diagnosis. If the patient has severe sepsis, a code from subcategory R65.2 should also be assigned as a secondary diagnosis. If the patient is admitted with a localized infection, such as pneumonia, and sepsis/severe sepsis doesn't develop until after admission, the localized infection should be assigned first, followed by the appropriate sepsis/severe sepsis codes.

5) Sepsis due to a postprocedural infection

(a) Documentation of causal relationship
As with all postprocedural complications, code assignment is based on the provider's documentation of the relationship between the infection and the procedure.

(b) Sepsis due to a postprocedural infection
For infections following a procedure, a code from T81.40, to T81.43. Infection following a procedure, or a code from O86.00 to O86.03, Infection of obstetric surgical wound, that identifies the site of the infection should be coded first, if known. Assign an additional code for sepsis following a procedure (T81.44) or sepsis following an obstetrical procedure (O86.04). Use an additional code to identify the infectious agent. If the patient has severe sepsis the appropriate code from subcategory R65.2 should also be assigned with the additional code(s) for any acute organ dysfunction.

For infections following infusion, transfusion, therapeutic injection, or immunization, a code from subcategory T80.2, Infections following infusion, transfusion, and therapeutic injection, or code T88.0-, Infection following immunization, should be coded first, followed by the code for the specific infection. If the patient has severe sepsis, the appropriate code from subcategory R65.2 should also be assigned, with the additional codes(s) for any acute organ dysfunction.

(c) Postprocedural infection and postprocedural septic shock
If a postprocedural infection has resulted in postprocedural septic shock, assign the codes indicated above for sepsis due to a postprocedural infection, followed by code T81.12-, Postprocedural septic shock. Do not assign code R65.21, Severe sepsis with septic shock. Additional code(s) should

12

be assigned
for any acute organ dysfunction.

6) Sepsis and severe sepsis associated with a noninfectious process (condition)

In some cases a noninfectious process (condition), such as trauma, may lead to an infection which can result in sepsis or severe sepsis. If sepsis or severe sepsis is documented as associated with a noninfectious condition, such as a burn or serious injury, and this condition meets the definition for principal diagnosis, the code for the noninfectious condition should be sequenced first, followed by the code for the resulting infection. If severe sepsis is present, a code from subcategory R65.2 should also be assigned with any associated organ dysfunction(s) codes. It is not necessary to assign a code from subcategory R65.1, Systemic inflammatory response syndrome (SIRS) of non-infectious origin, for these cases.

If the infection meets the definition of principal diagnosis it should be sequenced before the non-infectious condition. When both the associated non-infectious condition and the infection meet the definition of principal diagnosis either may be assigned as principal diagnosis.

Only one code from category R65, Symptoms and signs specifically associated with systemic inflammation and infection, should be assigned. Therefore, when a non-infectious condition leads to an infection resulting in severe sepsis, assign the appropriate code from subcategory R65.2, Severe sepsis. Do not additionally assign a code from subcategory R65.1, Systemic inflammatory response syndrome (SIRS) of non-infectious origin.

See Section I.C.18. SIRS due to non-infectious process

7) Sepsis and septic shock complicating abortion, pregnancy, childbirth, and the puerperium

See Section I.C.15. Sepsis and septic shock complicating abortion, pregnancy, childbirth and the puerperium

8) Newborn sepsis

See Section I.C.16. f. Bacterial sepsis of Newborn

e. Methicillin Resistant Staphylococcus aureus (MRSA) Conditions

1) Selection and sequencing of MRSA codes

(a) Combination codes for MRSA infection

When a patient is diagnosed with an infection that is due to methicillin resistant *Staphylococcus aureus* (MRSA), and that infection has a combination code that includes the causal organism (e.g., sepsis, pneumonia) assign the appropriate combination code for the condition (e.g., code A41.02, Sepsis due to Methicillin resistant Staphylococcus aureus or code J15.212, Pneumonia due to Methicillin resistant Staphylococcus aureus). Do not assign code B95.62, Methicillin resistant Staphylococcus aureus infection as the cause of diseases classified elsewhere, as an additional code because the combination code includes the type of infection and the MRSA organism. Do not assign a code from subcategory Z16.11, Resistance to penicillins, as an additional diagnosis.

See Section C.1. for instructions on coding and sequencing of sepsis and severe sepsis.

(b) Other codes for MRSA infection

When there is documentation of a current infection (e.g., wound infection, stitch abscess, urinary tract infection) due to MRSA, and that infection does not have a combination code that includes the causal organism, assign the appropriate code to identify the condition along with code B95.62, Methicillin resistant Staphylococcus aureus infection as the cause of diseases classified elsewhere for the MRSA infection. Do not assign a code from subcategory Z16.11, Resistance to penicillins.

(c) Methicillin susceptible Staphylococcus aureus (MSSA) and MRSA colonization

The condition or state of being colonized or carrying MSSA or MRSA is called colonization or carriage, while an individual person is described as being colonized or being a carrier. Colonization means that MSSA or MSRA is present on or in the body without necessarily causing illness. A positive MRSA colonization test might be documented by the provider as "MRSA screen positive" or "MRSA nasal swab positive".

Assign code Z22.322, Carrier or suspected carrier of Methicillin resistant Staphylococcus aureus, for patients documented as having MRSA colonization. Assign code Z22.321, Carrier or suspected carrier of Methicillin susceptible Staphylococcus aureus, for patients documented as having MSSA colonization. Colonization is not necessarily indicative of a disease process or as the cause of a specific condition the patient may have unless documented as such by the provider.

(d) MRSA colonization and infection

If a patient is documented as having both MRSA colonization and infection during a hospital admission, code Z22.322, Carrier or suspected carrier of Methicillin resistant Staphylococcus aureus, and a code for the MRSA infection may both be assigned.

f. Zika virus infections

1) Code only confirmed cases

Code only a confirmed diagnosis of Zika virus (A92.5, Zika virus disease) as documented by the provider. This is an exception to the hospital inpatient guideline Section II, H.

In this context, "confirmation" does not require documentation of the type of test performed; the provider's diagnostic statement that the condition is confirmed is sufficient. This code should be assigned regardless of the stated mode of transmission.

If the provider documents "suspected", "possible" or "probable" Zika, do not assign code A92.5. Assign a code(s) explaining the reason for encounter (such as fever, rash, or joint pain) or Z20.821, Contact with and (suspected) exposure to Zika virus.

g. *Coronavirus infections*

1) COVID-19 infection (infection due to SARS-CoV-2)

(a) Code only confirmed cases

Code only a confirmed diagnosis of the 2019 novel coronavirus disease (COVID-19) as documented by the provider, or documentation of a positive COVID-19 test result. For a confirmed diagnosis, assign code U07.1, COVID-19. This is an exception to the hospital inpatient guideline Section II, H. In this context, "confirmation" does not require documentation of a positive test result for COVID-19; the provider's documentation that the individual has COVID-19 is sufficient.

If the provider documents "suspected," "possible," "probable," or "inconclusive" COVID-19, do not assign code U07.1. Instead, code the signs and symptoms reported. See guideline I.C.1.g.1.g.

(b) *Sequencing of codes*

When COVID-19 meets the definition of principal diagnosis, code U07.1, COVID-19, should be sequenced first, followed by the appropriate codes for associated manifestations, except when another guideline requires that certain codes be sequenced first, such as obstetrics, sepsis, or transplant complications.

For a COVID-19 infection that progresses to sepsis, see Section I.C.1.d. Sepsis, Severe Sepsis, and Septic Shock

See Section I.C.15.s. for COVID-19 infection in pregnancy, childbirth, and the puerperium

See Section I.C.16.h. for COVID-19 infection in newborn

For a COVID-19 infection in a lung transplant patient, see Section I.C.19.g.3.a. Transplant complications other than kidney.

(c) *Acute respiratory manifestations of COVID-19*

When the reason for the encounter/admission is a respiratory manifestation of COVID-19, assign code U07.1, COVID-19, as the principal/first-listed diagnosis and assign code(s) for the respiratory manifestation(s) as additional diagnoses.

The following conditions are examples of common respiratory manifestations of COVID-19.

(i) *Pneumonia*
For a patient with pneumonia confirmed as due to COVID-19, assign codes U07.1, COVID-19, and J12.89, Other viral pneumonia.

(ii) *Acute bronchitis*
For a patient with acute bronchitis confirmed as due to COVID-19, assign codes U07.1, and J20.8, Acute bronchitis due to other specified organisms.
Bronchitis not otherwise specified (NOS) due to COVID-19 should be coded using code U07.1 and J40, Bronchitis, not specified as acute or chronic.

(iii) *Lower respiratory infection*
If the COVID-19 is documented as being associated with a lower respiratory infection, not otherwise specified (NOS), or an acute respiratory infection, NOS, codes U07.1 and J22, Unspecified acute lower respiratory infection, should be assigned.
If the COVID-19 is documented as being associated with a respiratory infection, NOS, codes U07.1 and J98.8, Other specified respiratory disorders, should be assigned.

(iv) *Acute respiratory distress syndrome*
For acute respiratory distress syndrome (ARDS) due to COVID-19, assign codes U07.1, and J80, Acute respiratory distress syndrome.

(v) *Acute respiratory failure*
For acute respiratory failure due to COVID-19, assign code U07.1, and code J96.0-, Acute respiratory failure.

(d) *Non-respiratory manifestations of COVID-19*

When the reason for the encounter/admission is a non-respiratory manifestation (e.g., viral enteritis) of COVID-19, assign code U07.1, COVID-19, as the principal/first-listed diagnosis and assign code(s) for the manifestation(s) as additional diagnoses.

(e) *Exposure to COVID-19*

For asymptomatic individuals with actual or suspected exposure to COVID-19, assign code Z20.828, Contact with and (suspected) exposure to other viral communicable diseases.

For symptomatic individuals with actual or suspected exposure to COVID-19 and the infection has been ruled out, or test results are inconclusive or unknown, assign code Z20.828, Contact with and (suspected) exposure to other viral communicable diseases. See guideline I.C.21.c.1, Contact/Exposure, for additional guidance regarding the use of category Z20 codes.

If COVID-19 is confirmed, see guideline I.C.1.g.1.a.

(f) *Screening for COVID-19*

During the COVID-19 pandemic, a screening code is generally not appropriate. For encounters for COVID-19 testing, including preoperative testing, code as exposure to COVID-19 (guideline I.C.1.g.1.e).

Coding guidance will be updated as new information concerning any changes in the pandemic status becomes available.

(g) *Signs and symptoms without definitive diagnosis of COVID-19*

For patients presenting with any signs/symptoms associated with COVID-19 (such as fever, etc.) but a definitive diagnosis has not been established, assign the appropriate code(s) for each of the presenting signs and symptoms such as:
- **R05.1, Acute cough,** or **R05.9, Cough, unspecified**
- **R06.02 Shortness of breath**
- **R50.9 Fever, unspecified**

If a patient with signs/symptoms associated with COVID-19 also has an actual or suspected contact with or exposure to COVID-19, assign Z20.828, Contact with and (suspected) exposure to other viral communicable diseases, as an additional code.

(h) Asymptomatic individuals who test positive for COVID-19

For asymptomatic individuals who test positive for COVID-19, see guideline I.C.1.g.1.a. Although the individual is asymptomatic, the individual has tested positive and is considered to have the COVID-19 infection.

(i) Personal history of COVID-19

For patients with a history of COVID-19, assign code Z86.19, Personal history of other infectious and parasitic diseases.

(j) Follow-up visits after COVID-19 infection has resolved

For individuals who previously had COVID-19 without residual symptom(s) or condition(s), and are being seen for follow-up evaluation, and COVID-19 test results are negative, assign codes Z09, Encounter for follow-up examination after completed treatment for conditions other than malignant neoplasm, and Z86.19, Personal history of other infectious and parasitic diseases.

For follow-up visits for individuals with symptom(s) or condition(s) related to a previous COVID-19 infection, see guideline I.C.1.g.1.m.

See Section I.C.21.c.8, Factors influencing health states and contact with health services, Follow-up

(k) Encounter for antibody testing

For an encounter for antibody testing that is not being performed to confirm a current COVID-19 infection, nor is a follow-up test after resolution of COVID-19, assign Z01.84, Encounter for antibody response examination.

Follow the applicable guidelines above if the individual is being tested to confirm a current COVID-19 infection.

For follow-up testing after a COVID-19 infection, see guideline I.C.1.g.1.j.

(l) Multisystem Inflammatory Syndrome

For individuals with multisystem inflammatory syndrome (MIS) and COVID-19, assign code U07.1, COVID-19, as the principal/first-listed diagnosis and assign code M35.81, Multisystem inflammatory syndrome, as an additional diagnosis.

If an individual with a history of COVID-19 develops MIS, assign codes M35.81, Multisystem inflammatory syndrome, and U09.9, Post COVID-19 condition, unspecified.

If an individual with a known or suspected exposure to COVID-19, and no current COVID-19 infection or history of COVID-19, develops MIS, assign codes M35.81, Multisystem inflammatory syndrome, and Z20.822, Contact with and (suspected) exposure to COVID-19.

Additional codes should be assigned for any associated complications of MIS.

(m) Post COVID-19 Condition

For sequela of COVID-19, or associated symptoms or conditions that develop following a previous COVID-19 infection, assign a code(s) for the specific symptom(s) or condition(s) related to the previous COVID-19 infection, if known, and code U09.9, Post COVID-19 condition, unspecified.

Code U09.9 should not be assigned for manifestations of an active (current) COVID-19 infection.

If a patient has a condition(s) associated with a previous COVID-19 infection and develops a new active (current) COVID-19 infection, code U09.9 may be assigned in conjunction with code U07.1, COVID-19, to identify that the patient also has a condition(s) associated with a previous COVID-19 infection. Code(s) for the specific condition(s) associated with the previous COVID-19 infection and code(s) for manifestation(s) of the new active (current) COVID-19 infection should also be assigned.

2. **Chapter 2: Neoplasms (C00-D49)**
   General guidelines

Chapter 2 of the ICD-10-CM contains the codes for most benign and all malignant neoplasms. Certain benign neoplasms, such as prostatic adenomas, may be found in the specific body system chapters. To properly code a neoplasm it is necessary to determine from the record if the neoplasm is benign, in-situ, malignant, or of uncertain histologic behavior. If malignant, any secondary (metastatic) sites should also be determined.

Primary malignant neoplasms overlapping site boundaries

A primary malignant neoplasm that overlaps two or more contiguous (next to each other) sites should be classified to the subcategory/code .8 ("overlapping lesion"), unless the combination is specifically indexed elsewhere. For multiple neoplasms of the same site that are not contiguous such as tumors in different quadrants of the same breast, codes for each site should be assigned.

Malignant neoplasm of ectopic tissue

Malignant neoplasms of ectopic tissue are to be coded to the site of origin mentioned (e.g., ectopic pancreatic malignant neoplasms involving the stomach are coded to malignant neoplasm of pancreas, unspecified) (C25.9).

The neoplasm table in the Alphabetic Index should be referenced first. However, if the

histological term is documented, that term should be referenced first, rather than going immediately to the Neoplasm Table, in order to determine which column in the Neoplasm Table is appropriate. For example, if the documentation indicates "adenoma," refer to the term in the Alphabetic Index to review the entries under this term and the instructional note to "see also neoplasm, by site, benign." The table provides the proper code based on the type of neoplasm and the site. It is important to select the proper column in the table that corresponds to the type of neoplasm. The Tabular List should then be referenced to verify that the correct code has been selected from the table and that a more specific site code does not exist.

See Section I.C.21. Factors influencing health status and contact with health services, Status, for information regarding Z15.0, codes for genetic susceptibility to cancer.

a. Treatment directed at the malignancy

If the treatment is directed at the malignancy, designate the malignancy as the principal diagnosis.

The only exception to this guideline is if a patient admission/encounter is solely for the administration of chemotherapy, immunotherapy or external beam radiation therapy, assign the appropriate Z51.— code as the first-listed or principal diagnosis, and the diagnosis or problem for which the service is being performed as a secondary diagnosis.

b. Treatment of secondary site

When a patient is admitted because of a primary neoplasm with metastasis and treatment is directed toward the secondary site only, the secondary neoplasm is designated as the principal diagnosis even though the primary malignancy is still present.

c. Coding and sequencing of complications

Coding and sequencing of complications associated with the malignancies or with the therapy thereof are subject to the following guidelines:

1) Anemia associated with malignancy

When admission/encounter is for management of an anemia associated with the malignancy, and the treatment is only for anemia, the appropriate code for the malignancy is sequenced as the principal or first-listed diagnosis followed by the appropriate code for the anemia (such as code D63.0, Anemia in neoplastic disease).

2) Anemia associated with chemotherapy, immunotherapy and radiation therapy

When the admission/encounter is for management of an anemia associated with an adverse effect of the administration of chemotherapy or immunotherapy and the only treatment is for the anemia, the anemia code is sequenced first followed by the appropriate codes for the neoplasm and the adverse effect (T45.1X5, Adverse effect of antineoplastic and immunosuppressive drugs).

When the admission/encounter is for management of an anemia associated with an adverse effect of radiotherapy, the anemia code should be sequenced first, followed by the appropriate neoplasm code and code Y84.2, Radiological procedure and radiotherapy as the cause of abnormal reaction of the patient, or of later complication, without mention of misadventure at the time of the procedure.

3) Management of dehydration due to the malignancy

When the admission/encounter is for management of dehydration due to the malignancy and only the dehydration is being treated (intravenous rehydration), the dehydration is sequenced first, followed by the code(s) for the malignancy.

4) Treatment of a complication resulting from a surgical procedure

When the admission/encounter is for treatment of a complication resulting from a surgical procedure, designate the complication as the principal or first-listed diagnosis if treatment is directed at resolving the complication.

d. Primary malignancy previously excised

When a primary malignancy has been previously excised or eradicated from its site and there is no further treatment directed to that site and there is no evidence of any existing primary malignancy, at that site a code from category Z85, Personal history of malignant neoplasm, should be used to indicate the former site of the malignancy. Any mention of extension, invasion, or metastasis to another site is coded as a secondary malignant neoplasm to that site. The secondary site may be the principal or first-listed diagnosis with the Z85 code used as a secondary code.

e. Admissions/Encounters involving chemotherapy, immunotherapy and radiation therapy

1) Episode of care involves surgical removal of neoplasm

When an episode of care involves the surgical removal of a neoplasm, primary or secondary site, followed by adjunct chemotherapy or radiation treatment during the same episode of care, the code for the neoplasm should be assigned as principal or first-listed diagnosis.

2) Patient admission/encounter solely for administration of chemotherapy, immunotherapy and radiation therapy

If a patient admission/encounter is solely for the administration of chemotherapy, immunotherapy or external beam radiation therapy assign code Z51.0, Encounter for antineoplastic radiation therapy, or Z51.11, Encounter for antineoplastic chemotherapy, or Z51.12, Encounter for antineoplastic immunotherapy as the first-listed or principal diagnosis. If a patient receives more than one of these therapies during the same admission

more than one of these codes may be assigned, in any sequence.

The malignancy for which the therapy is being administered should be assigned as a secondary diagnosis.

If a patient admission/encounter is for the insertion or implantation of radioactive elements (e.g., brachytherapy) the appropriate code for the malignancy is sequenced as the principal or first-listed diagnosis. Code Z51.0 should not be assigned.

3) Patient admitted for radiation therapy, chemotherapy or immunotherapy and develops complications

When a patient is admitted for the purpose of external beam radiotherapy, immunotherapy or chemotherapy and develops complications such as uncontrolled nausea and vomiting or dehydration, the principal or first-listed diagnosis is Z51.0, Encounter for antineoplastic radiation therapy, or Z51.11, Encounter for antineoplastic chemotherapy, or Z51.12, Encounter for antineoplastic immunotherapy followed by any codes for the complications.

When a patient is admitted for the purpose of insertion or implantation of radioactive elements (e.g., brachytherapy) and develops complications such as uncontrolled nausea and vomiting or dehydration, the principal or first-listed diagnosis is the appropriate code for the malignancy followed by any codes for the complications.

f. Admission/encounter to determine extent of malignancy

When the reason for admission/encounter is to determine the extent of the malignancy, or for a procedure such as paracentesis or thoracentesis, the primary malignancy or appropriate metastatic site is designated as the principal or first-listed diagnosis, even though chemotherapy or radiotherapy is administered.

g. Symptoms, signs, and abnormal findings listed in Chapter 18 associated with neoplasms

Symptoms, signs, and ill-defined conditions listed in Chapter 18 characteristic of, or associated with, an existing primary or secondary site malignancy cannot be used to replace the malignancy as principal or first-listed diagnosis, regardless of the number of admissions or encounters for treatment and care of the neoplasm.

See Section I.C.21. Factors influencing health status and contact with health services, Encounter for prophylactic organ removal.

h. Admission/encounter for pain control/management

See Section I.C.6. for information on coding admission/encounter for pain control/management.

i. Malignancy in two or more noncontiguous sites

A patient may have more than one malignant tumor in the same organ. These tumors may represent different primaries or metastatic disease, depending on the site. Should the documentation be unclear, the provider should be queried as to the status of each tumor so that the correct codes can be assigned.

j. Disseminated malignant neoplasm, unspecified

Code C80.0, Disseminated malignant neoplasm, unspecified, is for use only in those cases where the patient has advanced metastatic disease and no known primary or secondary sites are specified. It should not be used in place of assigning codes for the primary site and all known secondary sites.

k. Malignant neoplasm without specification of site

Code C80.1, Malignant (primary) neoplasm, unspecified, equates to Cancer, unspecified. This code should only be used when no determination can be made as to the primary site of a malignancy. This code should rarely be used in the inpatient setting.

l. Sequencing of neoplasm codes

1) Encounter for treatment of primary malignancy

If the reason for the encounter is for treatment of a primary malignancy, assign the malignancy as the principal/first-listed diagnosis. The primary site is to be sequenced first, followed by any metastatic sites.

2) Encounter for treatment of secondary malignancy

When an encounter is for a primary malignancy with metastasis and treatment is directed toward the metastatic (secondary) site(s) only, the metastatic site(s) is designated as the principal/first-listed diagnosis. The primary malignancy is coded as an additional code.

3) Malignant neoplasm in a pregnant patient

When a pregnant **patient** has a malignant neoplasm, a code from subcategory O9A.1-, Malignant neoplasm complicating pregnancy, childbirth, and the puerperium, should be sequenced first, followed by the appropriate code from Chapter 2 to indicate the type of neoplasm.

4) Encounter for complication associated with a neoplasm

When an encounter is for management of a complication associated with a neoplasm, such as dehydration, and the treatment is only for the complication, the complication is coded first, followed by the appropriate code(s) for the neoplasm.

The exception to this guideline is anemia. When the admission/encounter is for management of an anemia associated with the malignancy, and the treatment is only for anemia, the appropriate code for the malignancy is sequenced as the principal or first-listed diagnosis followed by code D63.0, Anemia in neoplastic disease.

5) Complication from surgical procedure for treatment of a neoplasm

When an encounter is for treatment of a complication resulting from a surgical procedure performed for the treatment of the neoplasm, designate the complication as the principal/first-listed diagnosis. See the guideline regarding

the coding of a current malignancy versus personal history to determine if the code for the neoplasm should also be assigned.

6) Pathologic fracture due to a neoplasm
When an encounter is for a pathological fracture due to a neoplasm, and the focus of treatment is the fracture, a code from subcategory M84.5, Pathological fracture in neoplastic disease, should be sequenced first, followed by the code for the neoplasm.

If the focus of treatment is the neoplasm with an associated pathological fracture, the neoplasm code should be sequenced first, followed by a code from M84.5 for the pathological fracture.

m. Current malignancy versus personal history of malignancy
When a primary malignancy has been excised but further treatment, such as an additional surgery for the malignancy, radiation therapy or chemotherapy is directed to that site, the primary malignancy code should be used until treatment is completed.

When a primary malignancy has been previously excised or eradicated from its site, there is no further treatment (of the malignancy) directed to that site, and there is no evidence of any existing primary malignancy at that site, a code from category Z85, Personal history of malignant neoplasm, should be used to indicate the former site of the malignancy.

Codes from subcategories Z85.0 – Z85.85 should only be assigned for the former site of a primary malignancy, not the site of a secondary malignancy. Code Z85.89, may be assigned for the former site(s) of either a primary or secondary malignancy.

See Section I.C.21. Factors influencing health status and contact with health services, History (of)

n. Leukemia, Multiple Myeloma, and Malignant Plasma Cell Neoplasms in remission versus personal history
The categories for leukemia, and category C90, Multiple myeloma and malignant plasma cell neoplasms, have codes indicating whether or not the leukemia has achieved remission. There are also codes Z85.6, Personal history of leukemia, and Z85.79, Personal history of other malignant neoplasms of lymphoid, hematopoietic and related tissues. If the documentation is unclear, as to whether the leukemia has achieved remission, the provider should be queried.

See Section I.C.21. Factors influencing health status and contact with health services, History (of)

o. Aftercare following surgery for neoplasm
See Section I.C.21. Factors influencing health status and contact with health services, Aftercare

p. Follow-up care for completed treatment of a malignancy
See Section I.C.21. Factors influencing health status and contact with health services, Follow-up

q. Prophylactic organ removal for prevention of malignancy

See Section I.C. 21, Factors influencing health status and contact with health services, Prophylactic organ removal

r. Malignant neoplasm associated with transplanted organ
A malignant neoplasm of a transplanted organ should be coded as a transplant complication. Assign first the appropriate code from category T86.-, Complications of transplanted organs and tissue, followed by code C80.2, Malignant neoplasm associated with transplanted organ. Use an additional code for the specific malignancy.

s. Breast Implant Associated Anaplastic Large Cell Lymphoma
Breast implant associated anaplastic large cell lymphoma (BIA-ALCL) is a type of lymphoma that can develop around breast implants. Assign code C84.7A, Anaplastic large cell lymphoma, ALK-negative, breast, for BIA-ALCL. Do not assign a complication code from chapter 19.

3. Chapter 3: Disease of the blood and blood-forming organs and certain disorders involving the immune mechanism (D50-D89)
Reserved for future guideline expansion

4. Chapter 4: Endocrine, Nutritional, and Metabolic Diseases (E00-E89)
a. Diabetes mellitus
The diabetes mellitus codes are combination codes that include the type of diabetes mellitus, the body system affected, and the complications affecting that body system. As many codes within a particular category as are necessary to describe all of the complications of the disease may be used. They should be sequenced based on the reason for a particular encounter. Assign as many codes from categories E08 – E13 as needed to identify all of the associated conditions that the patient has.

1) Type of diabetes
The age of a patient is not the sole determining factor, though most type 1 diabetics develop the condition before reaching puberty. For this reason type 1 diabetes mellitus is also referred to as juvenile diabetes.

2) Type of diabetes mellitus not documented
If the type of diabetes mellitus is not documented in the medical record the default is E11.-, Type 2 diabetes mellitus.

3) Diabetes mellitus and the use of insulin, oral hypoglycemics, *and injectable non-insulin drugs*
If the documentation in a medical record does not indicate the type of diabetes but does indicate that the patient uses insulin, code E11, Type 2 diabetes mellitus, should be assigned. Additional code(s) should be assigned from category Z79 to identify the long-term (current) use of insulin or oral hypoglycemic drugs, **or injectable non-insulin antidiabetic, as follows:** If the patient is treated with both oral medications and insulin, **both code Z79.4, Long term (current) use of insulin, and code Z79.84, Long term (current) use of oral hypoglycemic drugs,** should be assigned. **If the patient is treated**

with both insulin and an injectable non-insulin antidiabetic drug, assign codes Z79.4, Long-term (current) use of insulin, and Z79.899, Other long term (current) drug therapy. If the patient is treated with both oral hypoglycemic drugs and an injectable non-insulin antidiabetic drug, assign codes Z79.84, Long-term (current) use of oral hypoglycemic drugs, and Z79.899, Other long-term (current) drug therapy. Code Z79.4 should not be assigned if insulin is given temporarily to bring a type 2 patient's blood sugar under control during an encounter.

4) Diabetes mellitus in pregnancy and gestational diabetes

See Section I.C.15. Diabetes mellitus in pregnancy.
See Section I.C.15. Gestational (pregnancy induced) diabetes

5) Complications due to insulin pump malfunction

(a) Underdose of insulin due to insulin pump failure

An underdose of insulin due to an insulin pump failure should be assigned to a code from subcategory T85.6, Mechanical complication of other specified internal and external prosthetic devices, implants and grafts, that specifies the type of pump malfunction, as the principal or first-listed code, followed by code T38.3X6-, Underdosing of insulin and oral hypoglycemic [antidiabetic] drugs. Additional codes for the type of diabetes mellitus and any associated complications due to the underdosing should also be assigned.

(b) Overdose of insulin due to insulin pump failure

The principal or first-listed code for an encounter due to an insulin pump malfunction resulting in an overdose of insulin, should also be T85.6-, Mechanical complication of other specified internal and external prosthetic devices, implants and grafts, followed by code T38.3X1-, Poisoning by insulin and oral hypoglycemic [antidiabetic] drugs, accidental (unintentional).

6) Secondary diabetes mellitus

Codes under categories E08, Diabetes mellitus due to underlying condition, E09, Drug or chemical induced diabetes mellitus and E13, Other specified diabetes mellitus, identify complications/manifestations associated with secondary diabetes mellitus. Secondary diabetes is always caused by another condition or event (e.g., cystic fibrosis, malignant neoplasm of pancreas, pancreatectomy, adverse effect of drug, or poisoning).

(a) Secondary diabetes mellitus and the use of insulin or hypoglycemic drugs

For patients with secondary diabetes mellitus who routinely use insulin or oral hypoglycemic drugs, **or injectable non-insulin drugs,** an additional code(s) from category Z79 should be assigned to identify the long-term (current) use of insulin or oral hypoglycemic drugs, **or non-injectable non-insulin drugs as follows:** If the patient is treated with both oral medications and insulin, **both code Z79.4, Long term (current) use of insulin, and code Z79.84, Long term (current) use of oral hypoglycemic drugs,** should be assigned. If the patient is treated with both insulin and an injectable non- insulin antidiabetic drug, assign codes Z79.4, Long- term (current) use of insulin, and Z79.899, Other long term (current) drug therapy. If the patient is treated with both oral hypoglycemic drugs and an injectable non-insulin antidiabetic drug, assign codes Z79.84, Long-term (current) use of oral hypoglycemic drugs, and Z79.899, Other long-term (current) drug therapy. Code Z79.4 should not be assigned if insulin is given temporarily to bring a type 2 patient's blood sugar under control during an encounter.

(b) Assigning and sequencing secondary diabetes codes and its causes

The sequencing of the secondary diabetes codes in relationship to codes for the cause of the diabetes is based on the Tabular List instructions for categories E08, E09 and E13.

(i) Secondary diabetes mellitus due to pancreatectomy For postpancreatectomy diabetes mellitus (lack of insulin due to the surgical removal of all or part of the pancreas), assign code E89.1, Postprocedural hypoinsulinemia. Assign a code from category E13 and a code from subcategory Z90.41-, Acquired absence of pancreas, as additional codes.

(ii) Secondary diabetes due to drugs Secondary diabetes may be caused by an adverse effect of correctly administered medications, poisoning or sequela of poisoning.

See Section I.C.19.e for coding of adverse effects and poisoning, and Section I.C.20 for external cause code reporting.

5. Chapter 5: Mental, Behavioral and Neurodevelopmental disorders (F01 – F99)

a. Pain disorders related to psychological factors

Assign code F45.41, for pain that is exclusively related to psychological disorders. As indicated by the Excludes1 note under category G89, a code from category G89 should not be assigned with code F45.41

Code F45.42, Pain disorders with related psychological factors, should be used with a code from category G89, Pain, not elsewhere classified, if there is documentation of a psychological component for a patient with acute or chronic pain.
See Section I.C.6. Pain

b. Mental and behavioral disorders due to psychoactive substance use

1) In Remission

Selection of codes for "in remission" for categories F10-F19, Mental and behavioral disorders due to psychoactive substance use (categories

F10-F19 with -11, -.21) requires the provider's clinical judgment. The appropriate codes for "in remission" are assigned only on the basis of provider documentation (as defined in the Official Guidelines for Coding and Reporting), unless otherwise instructed by the classification.

Mild substance use disorders in early or sustained remission are classified to the appropriate codes for substance abuse in remission, and moderate or severe substance use disorders in early or sustained remission are classified to the appropriate codes for substance dependence in remission.

2) Psychoactive Substance Use, Abuse and Dependence

When the provider documentation refers to use, abuse and dependence of the same substance (e.g., alcohol, opioid, cannabis, etc.), only one code should be assigned to identify the pattern of use based on the following hierarchy:
- If both use and abuse are documented, assign only the code for abuse
- If both abuse and dependence are documented, assign only the code for dependence
- If use, abuse and dependence are all documented, assign only the code for dependence
- If both use and dependence are documented, assign only the code for dependence.

3) Psychoactive Substance Use, Unspecified

As with all other unspecified diagnoses, the codes for unspecified psychoactive substance use disorders (F10.9-, F11.9-, F12.9-, F13.9-, F14.9-, F15.9-, F16.9-, F18.9-, F19.9-) should only be assigned based on provider documentation and when they meet the definition of a reportable diagnosis (see Section III, Reporting Additional Diagnoses). These codes are to be used only when the psychoactive substance use is associated 1with a **substance related disorder (chapter 5 such as sexual dysfunction and sleep disorder,** or a mental or behavioral disorder) **or medical condition**, and such a relationship is documented by the provider.

4) Medical Conditions Due to Psychoactive Substance Use, Abuse and Dependence

Medical conditions due to substance use, abuse, and dependence are not classified as substance-induced disorders. Assign the diagnosis code for the medical condition as directed by the Alphabetical Index along with the appropriate psychoactive substance use, abuse or dependence code. For example, for alcoholic pancreatitis due to alcohol dependence, assign the appropriate code from subcategory K85.2, Alcohol induced acute pancreatitis, and the appropriate code from subcategory F10.2, such as code F10.20, Alcohol dependence, uncomplicated. It would not be appropriate to assign code F10.288, Alcohol dependence with other alcohol-induced disorder.

5) Blood Alcohol Level

A code from category Y90, Evidence of alcohol involvement determined by blood alcohol level, may be assigned when this information is documented and the patient's provider has documented a condition classifiable to category F10, Alcohol related disorders. The blood alcohol level does not need to be documented by the patient's provider in order for it to be coded.

c. Factitious Disorder

Factitious disorder imposed on self or Munchausen's syndrome is a disorder in which a person falsely reports or causes his or her own physical or psychological signs or symptoms. For patients with documented factitious disorder on self or Munchausen's syndrome, assign the appropriate code from subcategory F68.1-, Factitious disorder imposed on self.

Munchausen's syndrome by proxy (MSBP) is a disorder in which a caregiver (perpetrator) falsely reports or causes an illness or injury in another person (victim) under his or her care, such as a child, an elderly adult, or a person who has a disability. The condition is also referred to as "factitious disorder imposed on another" or "factitious disorder by proxy." The perpetrator, not the victim, receives this diagnosis. Assign code F68.A, Factitious disorder imposed on another, to the perpetrator's record. For the victim of a patient suffering from MSBP, assign the appropriate code from categories T74, Adult and child abuse, neglect and other maltreatment, confirmed, or T76, Adult and child abuse, neglect and other maltreatment, suspected.

See Section I.C.19.f. Adult and child abuse, neglect and other maltreatment

6. Chapter 6: Diseases of the Nervous System (G00-G99)

a. Dominant/nondominant side

Codes from category G81, Hemiplegia and hemiparesis, and subcategories, G83.1, Monoplegia of lower limb, G83.2, Monoplegia of upper limb, and G83.3, Monoplegia, unspecified, identify whether the dominant or nondominant side is affected. Should the affected side be documented, but not specified as dominant or nondominant, and the classification system does not indicate a default, code selection is as follows:
- For ambidextrous patients, the default should be dominant.
- If the left side is affected, the default is non-dominant.
- If the right side is affected, the default is dominant.

b. Pain - Category G89

1) General coding information

Codes in category G89, Pain, not elsewhere classified, may be used in conjunction with codes from other categories and chapters to provide more detail about acute or chronic pain and neoplasm-related pain, unless otherwise indicated below.

If the pain is not specified as acute or chronic, post-thoracotomy, postprocedural, or neoplasm-related, do not assign codes from category G89.

A code from category G89 should not be assigned if the underlying (definitive) diagnosis is known, unless the reason for the encounter is pain control/management and not management of the underlying condition.

When an admission or encounter is for a procedure aimed at treating the underlying condition (e.g., spinal fusion, kyphoplasty), a code for the underlying condition (e.g., vertebral fracture, spinal stenosis) should be assigned as the principal diagnosis. No code from category G89 should be assigned.

(a) Category G89 Codes as Principal or First-Listed Diagnosis

Category G89 codes are acceptable as principal diagnosis or the first-listed code:

- When pain control or pain management is the reason for the admission/encounter (e.g., a patient with displaced intervertebral disc, nerve impingement and severe back pain presents for injection of steroid into the spinal canal). The underlying cause of the pain should be reported as an additional diagnosis, if known.
- When a patient is admitted for the insertion of a neurostimulator for pain control, assign the appropriate pain code as the principal or first-listed diagnosis. When an admission or encounter is for a procedure aimed at treating the underlying condition and a neurostimulator is inserted for pain control during the same admission/encounter, a code for the underlying condition should be assigned as the principal diagnosis and the appropriate pain code should be assigned as a secondary diagnosis.

(b) Use of Category G89 Codes in Conjunction with Site-Specific Pain Codes

(i) Assigning Category G89 and Site-Specific Pain Codes

Codes from category G89 may be used in conjunction with codes that identify the site of pain (including codes from Chapter 18) if the category G89 code provides additional information. For example, if the code describes the site of the pain, but does not fully describe whether the pain is acute or chronic, then both codes should be assigned.

(ii) Sequencing of Category G89 Codes with Site-Specific Pain Codes

The sequencing of category G89 codes with site-specific pain codes (including Chapter 18 codes), is dependent on the circumstances of the encounter/admission as follows:

- If the encounter is for pain control or pain management, assign the code from category G89 followed by the code identifying the

specific site of pain (e.g., encounter for pain management for acute neck pain from trauma is assigned code G89.11, Acute pain due to trauma, followed by code M54.2, Cervicalgia, to identify the site of pain).
- If the encounter is for any other reason except pain control or pain management, and a related definitive diagnosis has not been established (confirmed) by the provider, assign the code for the specific site of pain first, followed by the appropriate code from category G89.

2) Pain due to devices, implants and grafts

See Section I.C.19. Pain due to medical devices

3) Postoperative Pain

The provider's documentation should be used to guide the coding of postoperative pain, as well as *Section III. Reporting Additional Diagnoses* and *Section IV. Diagnostic Coding and Reporting in the Outpatient Setting.*

The default for post-thoracotomy and other postoperative pain not specified as acute or chronic is the code for the acute form.

Routine or expected postoperative pain immediately after surgery should not be coded.

(a) Postoperative pain not associated with specific postoperative complication

Postoperative pain not associated with a specific postoperative complication is assigned to the appropriate postoperative pain code in category G89.

(b) Postoperative pain associated with specific postoperative complication

Postoperative pain associated with a specific postoperative complication (such as painful wire sutures) is assigned to the appropriate code(s) found in Chapter 19, Injury, poisoning, and certain other consequences of external causes. If appropriate, use additional code(s) from category G89 to identify acute or chronic pain (G89.18 or G89.28).

4) Chronic pain

Chronic pain is classified to subcategory G89.2. There is no time frame defining when pain becomes chronic pain. The provider's documentation should be used to guide use of these codes.

5) Neoplasm Related Pain

Code G89.3 is assigned to pain documented as being related, associated or due to cancer, primary or secondary malignancy, or tumor. This code is assigned regardless of whether the pain is acute or chronic.

This code may be assigned as the principal or first-listed code when the stated reason for the admission/encounter is documented as pain control/pain management. The underlying neoplasm should be reported as an additional diagnosis.

When the reason for the admission/encounter is management of the neoplasm and the pain associated with the neoplasm is also documented, code G89.3 may be assigned as an additional

diagnosis. It is not necessary to assign an additional code for the site of the pain.

See Section I.C.2 for instructions on the sequencing of neoplasms for all other stated reasons for the admission/ encounter (except for pain control/pain management).

6) Chronic pain syndrome

Central pain syndrome (G89.Ø) and chronic pain syndrome (G89.4) are different than the term "chronic pain," and therefore codes should only be used when the provider has specifically documented this condition.

See Section I.C.5. Pain disorders related to psychological factors

7. Chapter 7: Diseases of the Eye and Adnexa (HØØ-H59)

a. Glaucoma

1) Assigning Glaucoma Codes

Assign as many codes from category H4Ø, Glaucoma, as needed to identify the type of glaucoma, the affected eye, and the glaucoma stage.

2) Bilateral glaucoma with same type and stage

When a patient has bilateral glaucoma and both eyes are documented as being the same type and stage, and there is a code for bilateral glaucoma, report only the code for the type of glaucoma, bilateral, with the seventh character for the stage.

When a patient has bilateral glaucoma and both eyes are documented as being the same type and stage, and the classification does not provide a code for bilateral glaucoma (i.e., subcategories H4Ø.1Ø, H4Ø.11 and H4Ø.2Ø) report only one code for the type of glaucoma with the appropriate seventh character for the stage.

3) Bilateral glaucoma stage with different types or stages

When a patient has bilateral glaucoma and each eye is documented as having a different type or stage, and the classification distinguishes laterality, assign the appropriate code for each eye rather than the code for bilateral glaucoma.

When a patient has bilateral glaucoma and each eye is documented as having a different type, and the classification does not distinguish laterality (i.e., subcategories H4Ø.1Ø, H4Ø.11 and H4Ø.2Ø), assign one code for each type of glaucoma with the appropriate 7th character for the stage.

When a patient has bilateral glaucoma and each eye is documented as having the same type, but different stage, and the classification does not distinguish laterality (i.e., subcategories H4Ø.1Ø, H4Ø.11 and H4Ø.2Ø), assign a code for the type of glaucoma for each eye with the 7th character for the specific glaucoma stage documented for each eye.

4) Patient admitted with glaucoma and stage evolves during the admission

If a patient is admitted with glaucoma and the stage progresses during the admission, assign the code for highest stage documented.

5) Indeterminate stage glaucoma

Assignment of the 7th character "4" for "indeterminate stage" should be based on the clinical documentation. The 7th character "4" is used for glaucomas whose stage cannot be clinically determined. This 7th character should not be confused with the 7th character "Ø", unspecified, which should be assigned when there is no documentation regarding the stage of the glaucoma.

b. Blindness

If "blindness" or "low vision" of both eyes is documented but the visual impairment category is not documented, assign code H54.3, Unqualified visual loss, both eyes. If "blindness" or "low vision" in one eye is documented but the visual impairment category is not documented, assign a code from H54.6-, Unqualified visual loss, one eye. If "blindness" or "visual loss" is documented without any information about whether one or both eyes are affected, assign code H54.7, Unspecified visual loss.

8. Chapter 8: Diseases of the Ear and Mastoid Process (H6Ø-H95)

Reserved for future guideline expansion

9. Chapter 9: Diseases of the Circulatory System (IØØ-I99)

a. Hypertension

The classification presumes a causal relationship between hypertension and heart involvement and between hypertension and kidney involvement, as the two conditions are linked by the term "with" in the Alphabetic Index. These conditions should be coded as related even in the absence of provider documentation explicitly linking them, unless the documentation clearly states the conditions are unrelated.

For hypertension and conditions not specifically linked by relational terms such as "with," "associated with" or "due to" in the classification, provider documentation must link the conditions in order to code them as related.

1) Hypertension with Heart Disease

Hypertension with heart conditions classified to I5Ø.- or I51.4-I51.7, I51.89, I51.9, are assigned to, a code from category I11, Hypertensive heart disease. Use additional code(s) from category I5Ø, Heart failure, to identify the type(s) of heart failure in those patients with heart failure.

The same heart conditions (I5Ø.-, I51.4-I51.7, I51.89, I51.9) with hypertension are coded separately if the provider has documented they are unrelated to the hypertension. Sequence according to the circumstances of the admission/encounter.

2) Hypertensive Chronic Kidney Disease

Assign codes from category I12, Hypertensive chronic kidney disease, when both hypertension and a condition classifiable to category N18, Chronic kidney disease (CKD), are present. CKD should not be coded as hypertensive if the provider indicates the CKD is not related to the hypertension.

The appropriate code from category N18 should be used as a secondary code with a code from

category I12 to identify the stage of chronic kidney disease.

See Section I.C.14. Chronic kidney disease.

If a patient has hypertensive chronic kidney disease and acute renal failure, the acute renal failure should also be coded. Sequence according to the circumstances of the admission/encounter.

3) Hypertensive Heart and Chronic Kidney Disease

Assign codes from combination category I13, Hypertensive heart and chronic kidney disease, when there is hypertension with both heart and kidney involvement. If heart failure is present, assign an additional code from category I50 to identify the type of heart failure.

The appropriate code from category N18, Chronic kidney disease, should be used as a secondary code with a code from category I13 to identify the stage of chronic kidney disease.

See Section I.C.14. Chronic kidney disease.

The codes in category I13, Hypertensive heart and chronic kidney disease, are combination codes that include hypertension, heart disease and chronic kidney disease. The Includes note at I13 specifies that the conditions included at I11 and I12 are included together in I13. If a patient has hypertension, heart disease and chronic kidney disease then a code from I13 should be used, not individual codes for hypertension, heart disease and chronic kidney disease, or codes from I11 or I12.

For patients with both acute renal failure and chronic kidney disease the acute renal failure should also be coded. Sequence according to the circumstances of the admission/encounter.

4) Hypertensive Cerebrovascular Disease

For hypertensive cerebrovascular disease, first assign the appropriate code from categories I60-I69, followed by the appropriate hypertension code.

5) Hypertensive Retinopathy

Subcategory H35.0, Background retinopathy and retinal vascular changes, should be used with a code from category I10 – I15, Hypertensive disease to include the systemic hypertension. The sequencing is based on the reason for the encounter.

6) Hypertension, Secondary

Secondary hypertension is due to an underlying condition. Two codes are required: one to identify the underlying etiology and one from category I15 to identify the hypertension. Sequencing of codes is determined by the reason for admission/encounter.

7) Hypertension, Transient

Assign code R03.0, Elevated blood pressure reading without diagnosis of hypertension, unless patient has an established diagnosis of hypertension. Assign code O13.-, Gestational [pregnancy-induced] hypertension without significant proteinuria, or O14.-, Pre-eclampsia, for transient hypertension of pregnancy.

8) Hypertension, Controlled

This diagnostic statement usually refers to an existing state of hypertension under control by therapy. Assign the appropriate code from categories I10-I15, Hypertensive diseases.

9) Hypertension, Uncontrolled

Uncontrolled hypertension may refer to untreated hypertension or hypertension not responding to current therapeutic regimen. In either case, assign the appropriate code from categories I10-I15, Hypertensive diseases.

10) Hypertensive Crisis

Assign a code from category I16, Hypertensive crisis, for documented hypertensive urgency, hypertensive emergency or unspecified hypertensive crisis. Code also any identified hypertensive disease (I10-I15). The sequencing is based on the reason for the encounter.

11) Pulmonary Hypertension

Pulmonary hypertension is classified to category I27, Other pulmonary heart diseases. For secondary pulmonary hypertension (I27.1, I27.2-), code also any associated conditions or adverse effects of drugs or toxins. The sequencing is based on the reason for the encounter, except for adverse effects of drugs.

See Section I.C.19.e

b. Atherosclerotic Coronary Artery Disease and Angina

ICD-10-CM has combination codes for atherosclerotic heart disease with angina pectoris. The subcategories for these codes are I25.11, Atherosclerotic heart disease of native coronary artery with angina pectoris and I25.7, Atherosclerosis of coronary artery bypass graft(s) and coronary artery of transplanted heart with angina pectoris.

When using one of these combination codes it is not necessary to use an additional code for angina pectoris. A causal relationship can be assumed in a patient with both atherosclerosis and angina pectoris, unless the documentation indicates the angina is due to something other than the atherosclerosis.

If a patient with coronary artery disease is admitted due to an acute myocardial infarction (AMI), the AMI should be sequenced before the coronary artery disease.

See Section I.C.9. Acute myocardial infarction (AMI)

c. Intraoperative and Postprocedural Cerebrovascular Accident

Medical record documentation should clearly specify the cause-and-effect relationship between the medical intervention and the cerebrovascular accident in order to assign a code for intraoperative or postprocedural cerebrovascular accident.

Proper code assignment depends on whether it was an infarction or hemorrhage and whether it occurred intraoperatively or postoperatively. If it was a cerebral hemorrhage, code assignment depends on the type of procedure performed.

d. Sequelae of Cerebrovascular Disease

1) Category I69, Sequelae of Cerebrovascular disease

Category I69 is used to indicate conditions classifiable to categories I60-I67 as the causes of sequela (neurologic deficits), themselves classified elsewhere. These "late effects" include neurologic deficits that persist after initial onset of conditions classifiable to categories I60-I67. The neurologic deficits caused by cerebrovascular disease may be present from the onset or may arise at any time after the onset of the condition classifiable to categories I60-I67.

Codes from category I69, Sequelae of cerebrovascular disease, that specify hemiplegia, hemiparesis and monoplegia identify whether the dominant or nondominant side is affected. Should the affected side be documented, but not specified as dominant or nondominant, and the classification system does not indicate a default, code selection is as follows:

- For ambidextrous patients, the default should be dominant.
- If the left side is affected, the default is non-dominant.
- If the right side is affected, the default is dominant.

2) Codes from category I69 with codes from I60-I67

Codes from category I69 may be assigned on a health care record with codes from I60-I67, if the patient has a current cerebrovascular disease and deficits from an old cerebrovascular disease.

3) Codes from category I69 and Personal history of transient ischemic attack (TIA) and cerebral infarction (Z86.73)

Codes from category I69 should not be assigned if the patient does not have neurologic deficits.

See Section I.C.21. 4. History (of) for use of personal history codes

e. Acute myocardial infarction (AMI)

1) Type 1 ST elevation myocardial infarction (STEMI) and non ST elevation myocardial infarction (NSTEMI)

The ICD-10-CM codes for type 1 acute myocardial infarction (AMI) identify the site, such as anterolateral wall or true posterior wall. Subcategories I21.0-I21.2 and code I21.3 are used for type 1 ST elevation myocardial infarction (STEMI). Code I21.4, Non-ST elevation (NSTEMI) myocardial infarction, is used for type 1 non ST elevation myocardial infarction (NSTEMI) and nontransmural MIs.

If a type 1 NSTEMI evolves to STEMI, assign the STEMI code. If a type 1 STEMI converts to NSTEMI due to thrombolytic therapy, it is still coded as STEMI.

For encounters occurring while the myocardial infarction is equal to, or less than, 4 weeks old, including transfers to another acute setting or a postacute setting, and the myocardial infarction meets the definition for "other diagnoses" (see Section III, Reporting Additional Diagnoses), codes

from category I21 may continue to be reported. For encounters after the 4 week time frame and the patient is still receiving care related to the myocardial infarction, the appropriate aftercare code should be assigned, rather than a code from category I21. For old or healed myocardial infarctions not requiring further care, code I25.2, Old myocardial infarction, may be assigned.

2) Acute myocardial infarction, unspecified

Code I21.9, Acute myocardial infarction, unspecified, is the default for unspecified acute myocardial infarction or unspecified type. If only type 1 STEMI or transmural MI without the site is documented, assign code I21.3, ST elevation (STEMI) myocardial infarction of unspecified site.

3) AMI documented as nontransmural or subendocardial but site provided

If an AMI is documented as nontransmural or subendocardial, but the site is provided, it is still coded as a subendocardial AMI.

See Section I.C.21.3 for information on coding status post administration of tPA in a different facility within the last 24 hours.

4) Subsequent acute myocardial infarction

A code from category I22, Subsequent ST elevation (STEMI) and non ST elevation (NSTEMI) myocardial infarction, is to be used when a patient who has suffered a type 1 or unspecified AMI has a new AMI within the 4 week time frame of the initial AMI. A code from category I22 must be used in conjunction with a code from category I21. The sequencing of the I22 and I21 codes depends on the circumstances of the encounter.

Do not assign code I22 for subsequent myocardial infarctions other than type 1 or unspecified. For subsequent type 2 AMI assign only code I21.A1. For subsequent type 4 or type 5 AMI, assign only code I21.A9.

If a subsequent myocardial infarction of one type occurs within 4 weeks of a myocardial infarction of a different type, assign the appropriate codes from category I21 to identify each type. Do not assign a code from I22. Codes from category I22 should only be assigned if both the initial and subsequent myocardial infarctions are type 1 or unspecified.

5) Other Types of Myocardial Infarction

The ICD-10-CM provides codes for different types of myocardial infarction. Type 1 myocardial infarctions are assigned to codes I21.0-I21.4.

Type 2 myocardial infarction (myocardial infarction due to demand ischemia or secondary to ischemic imbalance) is assigned to code I21.A1, Myocardial infarction type 2 with the underlying cause coded first. Do not assign code I24.8, Other forms of acute ischemic heart disease, for the demand ischemia. If a type 2 AMI is described as NSTEMI or STEMI, only assign code I21.A1. Codes I21.01-I21.4 should only be assigned for type 1 AMIs.

Acute myocardial infarctions type 3, 4a, 4b, 4c, and 5 are assigned to code I21.A9, Other myocardial infarction type.

The "Code also" and "Code first" notes should be followed related to complications, and for coding of postprocedural myocardial infarctions during or following cardiac surgery.

10. **Chapter 10: Diseases of the Respiratory System (J00-J99, _U07.1_)**

   a. **Chronic Obstructive Pulmonary Disease [COPD] and Asthma**

   1) **Acute exacerbation of chronic obstructive bronchitis and asthma**

The codes in categories J44 and J45 distinguish between uncomplicated cases and those in acute exacerbation. An acute exacerbation is a worsening or a decompensation of a chronic condition. An acute exacerbation is not equivalent to an infection superimposed on a chronic condition, though an exacerbation may be triggered by an infection.

   b. **Acute Respiratory Failure**

   1) **Acute respiratory failure as principal diagnosis**

A code from subcategory J96.0, Acute respiratory failure, or subcategory J96.2, Acute and chronic respiratory failure, may be assigned as a principal diagnosis when it is the condition established after study to be chiefly responsible for occasioning the admission to the hospital, and the selection is supported by the Alphabetic Index and Tabular List. However, chapter-specific coding guidelines (such as obstetrics, poisoning, HIV, newborn) that provide sequencing direction take precedence.

   2) **Acute respiratory failure as secondary diagnosis**

Respiratory failure may be listed as a secondary diagnosis if it occurs after admission, or if it is present on admission, but does not meet the definition of principal diagnosis.

   3) **Sequencing of acute respiratory failure and another acute condition**

When a patient is admitted with respiratory failure and another acute condition (e.g., myocardial infarction, cerebrovascular accident, aspiration pneumonia), the principal diagnosis will not be the same in every situation. This applies whether the other acute condition is a respiratory or nonrespiratory condition. Selection of the principal diagnosis will be dependent on the circumstances of admission. If both the respiratory failure and the other acute condition are equally responsible for occasioning the admission to the hospital, and there are no chapter-specific sequencing rules, the guideline regarding two or more diagnoses that equally meet the definition for principal diagnosis _(Section II, C.)_ may be applied in these situations.

If the documentation is not clear as to whether acute respiratory failure and another condition are equally responsible for occasioning the admission, query the provider for clarification.

   c. **Influenza due to certain identified influenza viruses**

Code only confirmed cases of influenza due to certain identified influenza viruses (category J09), and due to other identified influenza virus (category J10). This is an exception to the hospital inpatient guideline Section II, H. (Uncertain Diagnosis).

In this context, "confirmation" does not require documentation of positive laboratory testing specific for avian or other novel influenza A or other identified influenza virus. However, coding should be based on the provider's diagnostic statement that the patient has avian influenza, or other novel influenza A, for category J09, or has another particular identified strain of influenza, such as H1N1 or H3N2, but not identified as novel or variant, for category J10.

If the provider records "suspected" or "possible" or "probable" avian influenza, or novel influenza, or other identified influenza, then the appropriate influenza code from category J11, Influenza due to unidentified influenza virus, should be assigned. A code from category J09, Influenza due to certain identified influenza viruses, should not be assigned nor should a code from category J10, Influenza due to other identified influenza virus.

   d. **Ventilator associated Pneumonia**

   1) **Documentation of Ventilator associated Pneumonia**

As with all procedural or postprocedural complications, code assignment is based on the provider's documentation of the relationship between the condition and the procedure.

Code J95.851, Ventilator associated pneumonia, should be assigned only when the provider has documented ventilator associated pneumonia (VAP). An additional code to identify the organism (e.g., Pseudomonas aeruginosa, code B96.5) should also be assigned. Do not assign an additional code from categories J12-J18 to identify the type of pneumonia.

Code J95.851 should not be assigned for cases where the patient has pneumonia and is on a mechanical ventilator and the provider has not specifically stated that the pneumonia is ventilator-associated pneumonia. If the documentation is unclear as to whether the patient has a pneumonia that is a complication attributable to the mechanical ventilator, query the provider.

   2) **Ventilator associated Pneumonia Develops after Admission**

A patient may be admitted with one type of pneumonia (e.g., code J13, Pneumonia due to Streptococcus pneumonia) and subsequently develop VAP. In this instance, the principal diagnosis would be the appropriate code from categories J12-J18 for the pneumonia diagnosed at the time of admission. Code J95.851, Ventilator associated pneumonia, would be assigned as an additional

diagnosis when the provider has also documented the presence of ventilator associated pneumonia.

e. Vaping-related disorders

For patients presenting with condition(s) related to vaping, assign code U07.0, Vaping-related disorder, as the principal diagnosis. For lung injury due to vaping, assign only code U07.0. Assign additional codes for other manifestations, such as acute respiratory failure (subcategory J96.0-) or pneumonitis (code J68.0).

Associated respiratory signs and symptoms due to vaping, such as cough, shortness of breath, etc., are not coded separately, when a definitive diagnosis has been established. However, it would be appropriate to code separately any gastrointestinal symptoms, such as diarrhea and abdominal pain.

11. **Chapter 11: Diseases of the Digestive System (K00-K95)**
Reserved for future guideline expansion

12. **Chapter 12: Diseases of the Skin and Subcutaneous Tissue (L00-L99)**

a. **Pressure ulcer stage codes**

1) **Pressure ulcer stages**
Codes in category L89, Pressure ulcer, identify the site and stage of the pressure ulcer.

The ICD-10-CM classifies pressure ulcer stages based on severity, which is designated by stages 1-4, deep tissue pressure injury, unspecified stage, and unstageable.

Assign as many codes from category L89 as needed to identify all the pressure ulcers the patient has, if applicable.

See Section I.B.14 for pressure ulcer stage documentation by clinicians other than patient's provider

2) **Unstageable pressure ulcers**
Assignment of the code for unstageable pressure ulcer (L89.--0) should be based on the clinical documentation. These codes are used for pressure ulcers whose stage cannot be clinically determined (e.g., the ulcer is covered by eschar or has been treated with a skin or muscle graft). This code should not be confused with the codes for unspecified stage (L89.--9). When there is no documentation regarding the stage of the pressure ulcer, assign the appropriate code for unspecified stage (L89.9).

If during an encounter, the stage of an unstageable pressure ulcer is revealed after debridement, assign only the code for the stage revealed following debridement.

3) **Documented pressure ulcer stage**
Assignment of the pressure ulcer stage code should be guided by clinical documentation of the stage or documentation of the terms found in the Alphabetic Index. For clinical terms describing the stage that are not found in the Alphabetic Index, and there is no documentation of the stage, the provider should be queried.

4) **Patients admitted with pressure ulcers documented as healed**
No code is assigned if the documentation states that the pressure ulcer is completely healed at the time of admission.

5) **Pressure ulcers documented as healing**
Pressure ulcers described as healing should be assigned the appropriate pressure ulcer stage code based on the documentation in the medical record. If the documentation does not provide information about the stage of the healing pressure ulcer, assign the appropriate code for unspecified stage.

If the documentation is unclear as to whether the patient has a current (new) pressure ulcer or if the patient is being treated for a healing pressure ulcer, query the provider.

For ulcers that were present on admission but healed at the time of discharge, assign the code for the site and stage of the pressure ulcer at the time of admission.

6) **Patient admitted with pressure ulcer evolving into another stage during the admission**
If a patient is admitted to an inpatient hospital with a pressure ulcer at one stage and it progresses to a higher stage, two separate codes should be assigned: one code for the site and stage of the ulcer on admission and a second code for the same ulcer site and the highest stage reported during the stay.

7) **Pressure-induced deep tissue damage**
For pressure-induced deep tissue damage or deep tissue pressure injury, assign only the appropriate code for pressure-induced deep tissue damage (L89.--6).

b. **Non-Pressure Chronic Ulcers**

1) **Patients admitted with non-pressure ulcers documented as healed**
No code is assigned if the documentation states that the non-pressure ulcer is completely healed at the time of admission.

2) **Non-pressure ulcers documented as healing**
Non-pressure ulcers described as healing should be assigned the appropriate non-pressure ulcer code based on the documentation in the medical record. If the documentation does not provide information about the severity of the healing non-pressure ulcer, assign the appropriate code for unspecified severity.

If the documentation is unclear as to whether the patient has a current (new) non-pressure ulcer or if the patient is being treated for a healing non-pressure ulcer, query the provider.

For ulcers that were present on admission but healed at the time of discharge, assign the code for the site and severity of the non-pressure ulcer at the time of admission.

3) **Patient admitted with non-pressure ulcer that progresses to another severity level during the admission**

If a patient is admitted to an inpatient hospital with a non-pressure ulcer at one severity level and it progresses to a higher severity level, two separate codes should be assigned: one code for the site and severity level of the ulcer on admission and a second code for the same ulcer site and the highest severity level reported during the stay.

See Section I.B.14 for pressure ulcer stage documentation by clinicians other than patient's provider

13. **Chapter 13: Diseases of the Musculoskeletal System and Connective Tissue (M00-M99)**

    a. **Site and laterality**

    Most of the codes within Chapter 13 have site and laterality designations. The site represents the bone, joint or the muscle involved. For some conditions where more than one bone, joint or muscle is usually involved, such as osteoarthritis, there is a "multiple sites" code available. For categories where no multiple site code is provided and more than one bone, joint or muscle is involved, multiple codes should be used to indicate the different sites involved.

       1) **Bone versus joint**

       For certain conditions, the bone may be affected at the upper or lower end (e.g., avascular necrosis of bone, M87, Osteoporosis, M80, M81). Though the portion of the bone affected may be at the joint, the site designation will be the bone, not the joint.

    b. **Acute traumatic versus chronic or recurrent musculoskeletal conditions**

    Many musculoskeletal conditions are a result of previous injury or trauma to a site, or are recurrent conditions. Bone, joint or muscle conditions that are the result of a healed injury are usually found in Chapter 13. Recurrent bone, joint or muscle conditions are also usually found in Chapter 13. Any current, acute injury should be coded to the appropriate injury code from Chapter 19. Chronic or recurrent conditions should generally be coded with a code from Chapter 13. If it is difficult to determine from the documentation in the record which code is best to describe a condition, query the provider.

    c. **Coding of Pathologic Fractures**

    Seventh character A is for use as long as the patient is receiving active treatment for the fracture. While the patient may be seen by a new or different provider over the course of treatment for a pathological fracture, assignment of the 7th character is based on whether the patient is undergoing active treatment and not whether the provider is seeing the patient for the first time.

    Seventh character, D is to be used for encounters after the patient has completed active treatment for the fracture and is receiving routine care for the fracture during the healing or recovery phase. The other 7th characters, listed under each subcategory in the Tabular List, are to be used for subsequent encounters for treatment of problems associated with the healing, such as malunions, nonunions, and sequelae.

    Care for complications of surgical treatment for fracture repairs during the healing or recovery phase should be coded with the appropriate complication codes.

    See Section I.C.19. Coding of traumatic fractures

    d. **Osteoporosis**

    Osteoporosis is a systemic condition, meaning that all bones of the musculoskeletal system are affected. Therefore, site is not a component of the codes under category M81, Osteoporosis without current pathological fracture. The site codes under category M80, Osteoporosis with current pathological fracture, identify the site of the fracture, not the osteoporosis.

       1) **Osteoporosis without pathological fracture**

       Category M81, Osteoporosis without current pathological fracture, is for use for patients with osteoporosis who do not currently have a pathologic fracture due to the osteoporosis, even if they have had a fracture in the past. For patients with a history of osteoporosis fractures, status code Z87.310, Personal history of (healed) osteoporosis fracture, should follow the code from M81.

       2) **Osteoporosis with current pathological fracture**

       Category M80, Osteoporosis with current pathological fracture, is for patients who have a current pathologic fracture at the time of an encounter. The codes under M80 identify the site of the fracture. A code from category M80, not a traumatic fracture code, should be used for any patient with known osteoporosis who suffers a fracture, even if the patient had a minor fall or trauma, if that fall or trauma would not usually break a normal, healthy bone.

    e. **Multisystem Inflammatory Syndrome**

       See Section I.C.1.g.1.l for Multisystem Inflammatory Syndrome

14. **Chapter 14: Diseases of Genitourinary System (N00-N99)**

    a. **Chronic kidney disease**

       1) **Stages of chronic kidney disease (CKD)**

       The ICD-10-CM classifies CKD based on severity. The severity of CKD is designated by stages 1-5. Stage 2, code N18.2, equates to mild CKD; stage 3, codes N18.30-N18.32, equate to moderate CKD; and stage 4, code N18.4, equates to severe CKD. Code N18.6, End stage renal disease (ESRD), is assigned when the provider has documented end-stage-renal disease (ESRD).

       If both a stage of CKD and ESRD are documented, assign code N18.6 only.

       2) **Chronic kidney disease and kidney transplant status**

       Patients who have undergone kidney transplant may still have some form of chronic kidney disease (CKD) because the kidney transplant may not fully restore kidney function. Therefore, the presence

of CKD alone does not constitute a transplant complication. Assign the appropriate N18 code for the patient's stage of CKD and code Z94.0, Kidney transplant status. If a transplant complication such as failure or rejection or other transplant complication is documented, see Section I.C.19.g for information on coding complications of a kidney transplant. If the documentation is unclear as to whether the patient has a complication of the transplant, query the provider.

3) Chronic kidney disease with other conditions
Patients with CKD may also suffer from other serious conditions, most commonly diabetes mellitus and hypertension. The sequencing of the CKD code in relationship to codes for other contributing conditions is based on the conventions in the Tabular List.

See I.C.9. Hypertensive chronic kidney disease.
See I.C.19. Chronic kidney disease and kidney transplant complications.

15. Chapter 15: Pregnancy, Childbirth, and the Puerperium (O00-O9A)
a. General Rules for Obstetric Cases
1) Codes from Chapter 15 and sequencing priority
Obstetric cases require codes from Chapter 15, codes in the range O00-O9A, Pregnancy, Childbirth, and the Puerperium. Chapter 15 codes have sequencing priority over codes from other chapters. Additional codes from other chapters may be used in conjunction with Chapter 15 codes to further specify conditions. Should the provider document that the pregnancy is incidental to the encounter, then code Z33.1, Pregnant state, incidental, should be used in place of any Chapter 15 codes. It is the provider's responsibility to state that the condition being treated is not affecting the pregnancy.

2) Chapter 15 codes used only on the maternal record
Chapter 15 codes are to be used only on the maternal record, never on the record of the newborn.

3) Final character for trimester
The majority of codes in Chapter 15 have a final character indicating the trimester of pregnancy. The time frames for the trimesters are indicated at the beginning of the chapter. If trimester is not a component of a code it is because the condition always occurs in a specific trimester, or the concept of trimester of pregnancy is not applicable. Certain codes have characters for only certain trimesters because the condition does not occur in all trimesters, but it may occur in more than just one.

Assignment of the final character for trimester should be based on the provider's documentation of the trimester (or number of weeks) for the current admission/encounter. This applies to the assignment of trimester for pre-existing conditions as well as those that develop during or are due to the pregnancy. The provider's documentation of the number of weeks may be used to assign the appropriate code identifying the trimester.

Whenever delivery occurs during the current admission, and there is an "in childbirth" option for the obstetric complication being coded, the "in childbirth" code should be assigned.

When the classification does not provide an obstetric code with an "in childbirth" option, it is appropriate to assign a code describing the current trimester.

4) Selection of trimester for inpatient admissions that encompass more than one trimester
In instances when a patient is admitted to a hospital for complications of pregnancy during one trimester and remains in the hospital into a subsequent trimester, the trimester character for the antepartum complication code should be assigned on the basis of the trimester when the complication developed, not the trimester of the discharge. If the condition developed prior to the current admission/encounter or represents a pre-existing condition, the trimester character for the trimester at the time of the admission/encounter should be assigned.

5) Unspecified trimester
Each category that includes codes for trimester has a code for "unspecified trimester." The "unspecified trimester" code should rarely be used, such as when the documentation in the record is insufficient to determine the trimester and it is not possible to obtain clarification.

6) 7th character for Fetus Identification
Where applicable, a 7th character is to be assigned for certain categories (O31, O32, O33.3 - O33.6, O35, O36, O40, O41, O60.1, O60.2, O64, and O69) to identify the fetus for which the complication code applies.

Assign 7th character "0":
- For single gestations
- When the documentation in the record is insufficient to determine the fetus affected and it is not possible to obtain clarification.
- When it is not possible to clinically determine which fetus is affected.

b. Selection of OB Principal or First-listed Diagnosis
1) Routine outpatient prenatal visits
For routine outpatient prenatal visits when no complications are present, a code from category Z34, Encounter for supervision of normal pregnancy, should be used as the first-listed diagnosis. These codes should not be used in conjunction with Chapter 15 codes.

2) Supervision of High-Risk Pregnancy
Codes from category O09, Supervision of high-risk pregnancy, are intended for use only during the prenatal period. For complications during the labor or delivery episode as a result

of a high-risk pregnancy, assign the applicable complication codes from Chapter 15. If there are no complications during the labor or delivery episode, assign code O80, Encounter for full-term uncomplicated delivery.

For routine prenatal outpatient visits for patients with high-risk pregnancies, a code from category O09, Supervision of high-risk pregnancy, should be used as the first-listed diagnosis. Secondary Chapter 15 codes may be used in conjunction with these codes if appropriate.

3) Episodes when no delivery occurs
In episodes when no delivery occurs, the principal diagnosis should correspond to the principal complication of the pregnancy which necessitated the encounter. Should more than one complication exist, all of which are treated or monitored, any of the complication codes may be sequenced first.

4) When a delivery occurs
When an obstetric patient is admitted and delivers during that admission, the condition that prompted the admission should be sequenced as the principal diagnosis. If multiple conditions prompted the admission, sequence the one most related to the delivery as the principal diagnosis. A code for any complication of the delivery should be assigned as an additional diagnosis. In cases of cesarean delivery, if the patient was admitted with a condition that resulted in the performance of a cesarean procedure, that condition should be selected as the principal diagnosis. If the reason for the admission was unrelated to the condition resulting in the cesarean delivery, the condition related to the reason for the admission should be selected as the principal diagnosis.

5) Outcome of delivery
A code from category Z37, Outcome of delivery, should be included on every maternal record when a delivery has occurred. These codes are not to be used on subsequent records or on the newborn record.

c. Pre-existing conditions versus conditions due to the pregnancy
Certain categories in Chapter 15 distinguish between conditions of the mother that existed prior to pregnancy (pre-existing) and those that are a direct result of pregnancy. When assigning codes from Chapter 15, it is important to assess if a condition was pre-existing prior to pregnancy or developed during or due to the pregnancy in order to assign the correct code.

Categories that do not distinguish between pre-existing and pregnancy-related conditions may be used for either. It is acceptable to use codes specifically for the puerperium with codes complicating pregnancy and childbirth if a condition arises postpartum during the delivery encounter.

d. Pre-existing hypertension in pregnancy

Category O10, Pre-existing hypertension complicating pregnancy, childbirth and the puerperium, includes codes for hypertensive heart and hypertensive chronic kidney disease. When assigning one of the O10 codes that includes hypertensive heart disease or hypertensive chronic kidney disease, it is necessary to add a secondary code from the appropriate hypertension category to specify the type of heart failure or chronic kidney disease.

See Section I.C.9. Hypertension.

e. Fetal Conditions Affecting the Management of the Mother
1) Codes from categories O35 and O36
Codes from categories O35, Maternal care for known or suspected fetal abnormality and damage, and O36, Maternal care for other fetal problems, are assigned only when the fetal condition is actually responsible for modifying the management of the mother, i.e., by requiring diagnostic studies, additional observation, special care, or termination of pregnancy. The fact that the fetal condition exists does not justify assigning a code from this series to the mother's record.

2) In utero surgery
In cases when surgery is performed on the fetus, a diagnosis code from category O35, Maternal care for known or suspected fetal abnormality and damage, should be assigned identifying the fetal condition. Assign the appropriate procedure code for the procedure performed.

No code from Chapter 16, the perinatal codes, should be used on the mother's record to identify fetal conditions. Surgery performed in utero on a fetus is still to be coded as an obstetric encounter.

f. HIV Infection in Pregnancy, Childbirth and the Puerperium
During pregnancy, childbirth or the puerperium, a patient admitted because of an HIV-related illness should receive a principal diagnosis from subcategory O98.7-, Human immunodeficiency [HIV] disease complicating pregnancy, childbirth and the puerperium, followed by the code(s) for the HIV-related illness(es).

Patients with asymptomatic HIV infection status admitted during pregnancy, childbirth, or the puerperium should receive codes of O98.7- and Z21, Asymptomatic human immunodeficiency virus [HIV] infection status.

g. Diabetes mellitus in pregnancy
Diabetes mellitus is a significant complicating factor in pregnancy. Pregnant women who are diabetic should be assigned a code from category O24, Diabetes mellitus in pregnancy, childbirth, and the puerperium, first, followed by the appropriate diabetes code(s) (E08-E13) from Chapter 4.

h. Long-term use of insulin and oral hypoglycemics

See Section I.C.4.a.3 for information on the long term use of insulin and oral hypoglycemics.

i. Gestational (pregnancy induced) diabetes
Gestational (pregnancy induced) diabetes can occur during the second and third trimester of pregnancy in **patients** who were not diabetic prior to pregnancy. Gestational diabetes can cause complications in the pregnancy similar to those of pre-existing diabetes mellitus. It also puts the **patient** at greater risk of developing diabetes after the pregnancy. Codes for gestational diabetes are in subcategory O24.4, Gestational diabetes mellitus. No other code from category O24, Diabetes mellitus in pregnancy, childbirth, and the puerperium, should be used with a code from O24.4.

The codes under subcategory O24.4 include diet controlled, insulin controlled, and controlled by oral hypoglycemic drugs. If a patient with gestational diabetes is treated with both diet and insulin, only the code for insulin-controlled is required. If a patient with gestational diabetes is treated with both diet and oral hypoglycemic medications, only the code for "controlled by oral hypoglycemic drugs" is required. Code Z79.4, Long-term (current) use of insulin or code Z79.84, Long-term (current) use of oral hypoglycemic drugs, should not be assigned with codes from subcategory O24.4.

An abnormal glucose tolerance in pregnancy is assigned a code from subcategory O99.81, Abnormal glucose complicating pregnancy, childbirth, and the puerperium.

j. Sepsis and septic shock complicating abortion, pregnancy, childbirth and the puerperium
When assigning a Chapter 15 code for sepsis complicating abortion, pregnancy, childbirth, and the puerperium, a code for the specific type of infection should be assigned as an additional diagnosis. If severe sepsis is present, a code from subcategory R65.2, Severe sepsis, and code(s) for associated organ dysfunction(s) should also be assigned as additional diagnoses.

k. Puerperal sepsis
Code O85, Puerperal sepsis, should be assigned with a secondary code to identify the causal organism (e.g., for a bacterial infection, assign a code from category B95-B96, Bacterial infections in conditions classified elsewhere). A code from category A40, Streptococcal sepsis, or A41, Other sepsis, should not be used for puerperal sepsis. If applicable, use additional codes to identify severe sepsis (R65.2-) and any associated acute organ dysfunction.

Code O85 should not be assigned for sepsis following an obstetrical procedure (See Section I.C.1.d.5.b., Sepsis due to a postprocedural infection).

l. Alcohol, tobacco and drug use during pregnancy, childbirth and the puerperium

1) Alcohol use during pregnancy, childbirth and the puerperium

Codes under subcategory O99.31, Alcohol use complicating pregnancy, childbirth, and the puerperium, should be assigned for any pregnancy case when a mother uses alcohol during the pregnancy or postpartum. A secondary code from category F10, Alcohol related disorders, should also be assigned to identify manifestations of the alcohol use.

2) Tobacco use during pregnancy, childbirth and the puerperium
Codes under subcategory O99.33, Smoking (tobacco) complicating pregnancy, childbirth, and the puerperium, should be assigned for any pregnancy case when a mother uses any type of tobacco product during the pregnancy or postpartum. A secondary code from category F17, Nicotine dependence, should also be assigned to identify the type of nicotine dependence.

3) Drug use during pregnancy, childbirth and the puerperium
Codes under subcategory O99.32, Drug use complicating pregnancy, childbirth, and the puerperium, should be assigned for any pregnancy case when a mother uses drugs during the pregnancy or postpartum. This can involve illegal drugs, or inappropriate use or abuse of prescription drugs. Secondary code(s) from categories F11-F16 and F18-F19 should also be assigned to identify manifestations of the drug use.

m. Poisoning, toxic effects, adverse effects and underdosing in a pregnant patient
A code from subcategory O9A.2, Injury, poisoning and certain other consequences of external causes complicating pregnancy, childbirth, and the puerperium, should be sequenced first, followed by the appropriate injury, poisoning, toxic effect, adverse effect or underdosing code, and then the additional code(s) that specifies the condition caused by the poisoning, toxic effect, adverse effect or underdosing.

See Section I.C.19. Adverse effects, poisoning, underdosing and toxic effects.

n. Normal Delivery, Code O80

1) Encounter for full term uncomplicated delivery
Code O80 should be assigned when a woman is admitted for a full-term normal delivery and delivers a single, healthy infant without any complications antepartum, during the delivery, or postpartum during the delivery episode. Code O80 is always a principal diagnosis. It is not to be used if any other code from Chapter 15 is needed to describe a current complication of the antenatal, delivery, or postnatal period. Additional codes from other chapters may be used with code O80 if they are not related to or are in any way complicating the pregnancy.

2) Uncomplicated delivery with resolved antepartum complication
Code O80 may be used if the patient had a complication at some point during the pregnancy,

but the complication is not present at the time of the admission for delivery.

3) Outcome of delivery for O8Ø

Z37.Ø, Single live birth, is the only outcome of delivery code appropriate for use with O8Ø.

o. The Peripartum and Postpartum Periods

1) Peripartum and Postpartum periods

The postpartum period begins immediately after delivery and continues for 6 weeks following delivery. The peripartum period is defined as the last month of pregnancy to 5 months postpartum.

2) Peripartum and postpartum complication

A postpartum complication is any complication occurring within the 6-week period.

3) Pregnancy-related complications after 6-week period

Chapter 15 codes may also be used to describe pregnancy-related complications after the peripartum or postpartum period if the provider documents that a condition is pregnancy related.

4) Admission for routine postpartum care following delivery outside hospital

When the mother delivers outside the hospital prior to admission and is admitted for routine postpartum care and no complications are noted, code Z39.Ø, Encounter for care and examination of mother immediately after delivery, should be assigned as the principal diagnosis.

5) Pregnancy associated cardiomyopathy

Pregnancy associated cardiomyopathy, code O9Ø.3, is unique in that it may be diagnosed in the third trimester of pregnancy but may continue to progress months after delivery. For this reason, it is referred to as peripartum cardiomyopathy. Code O9Ø.3 is only for use when the cardiomyopathy develops as a result of pregnancy in a woman who did not have pre-existing heart disease.

p. Code O94, Sequelae of complication of pregnancy, childbirth, and the puerperium

1) Code O94

Code O94, Sequelae of complication of pregnancy, childbirth, and the puerperium, is for use in those cases when an initial complication of a pregnancy develops a **sequela** or sequelae requiring care or treatment at a future date.

2) After the initial postpartum period

This code may be used at any time after the initial postpartum period.

3) Sequencing of Code O94

This code, like all sequela codes, is to be sequenced following the code describing the sequelae of the complication.

q. Termination of Pregnancy and Spontaneous abortions

1) Abortion with Liveborn Fetus

When an attempted termination of pregnancy results in a liveborn fetus assign code Z33.2, Encounter for elective termination of pregnancy and a code from category Z37, Outcome of Delivery.

2) Retained Products of Conception following an abortion

Subsequent encounters for retained products of conception following a spontaneous abortion or elective termination of pregnancy, without complications are assigned O03.4, Incomplete spontaneous, abortion without complication or codes O07.4, Failed attempted termination of pregnancy without complication. This advice is appropriate even when the patient was discharged previously with a discharge diagnosis of complete abortion. If the patient has a specific complication associated with the spontaneous abortion or elective termination of pregnancy in addition to retained products of conception, assign the appropriate complication code (e.g., O03.-, O04.-, O07.-) instead of code O03.4 or O07.4

3) Complications leading to abortion

Codes from Chapter 15 may be used as additional codes to identify any documented complications of the pregnancy in conjunction with codes in categories in O04, O07 and O08.

r. Abuse in a pregnant patient

For suspected or confirmed cases of abuse of a pregnant patient, a code(s) from subcategories O9A.3, Physical abuse complicating pregnancy, childbirth, and the puerperium, O9A.4, Sexual abuse complicating pregnancy, childbirth, and the puerperium, and O9A.5, Psychological abuse complicating pregnancy, childbirth, and the puerperium, should be sequenced first, followed by the appropriate codes (if applicable) to identify any associated current injury due to physical abuse, sexual abuse, and the perpetrator of abuse.

See Section I.C.19. Adult and child abuse, neglect and other maltreatment.

s. *COVID-19 infection in pregnancy, childbirth, and the puerperium*

During pregnancy, childbirth or the puerperium, when COVID-19 is the reason for admission/ encounter, code O98.5-, Other viral diseases complicating pregnancy, childbirth and the puerperium, should be sequenced as the principal/ first-listed diagnosis, and code U07.1, COVID-19, and the appropriate codes for associated manifestation(s) should be assigned as additional diagnoses. Codes from Chapter 15 always take sequencing priority.

If the reason for admission/encounter is unrelated to COVID-19 but the patient tests positive for COVID-19 during the admission/ encounter, the appropriate code for the reason for admission/encounter should be sequenced as the principal/first-listed diagnosis, and codes O98.5- and U07.1, as well as the appropriate codes for associated COVID-19 manifestations, should be assigned as additional diagnoses.

16. Chapter 16: Certain Conditions Originating in the Perinatal Period (P00-P96)

For coding and reporting purposes the perinatal period is defined as before birth through the 28th day following birth. The following guidelines are provided for reporting purposes

a. General Perinatal Rules

1) Use of Chapter 16 Codes

Codes in this chapter are for use on the maternal record. Codes from Chapter 15, the obstetric chapter, are never permitted on the newborn record. Chapter 16 codes may be used throughout the life of the patient if the condition is still present.

2) Principal Diagnosis for Birth Record

When coding the birth episode in a newborn record, assign a code from category Z38, Liveborn infants according to place of birth and type of delivery, as the principal diagnosis. A code from category Z38 is assigned only once, to a newborn at the time of birth. If a newborn is transferred to another institution, a code from category Z38 should not be used at the receiving hospital.

A code from category Z38 is used only on the newborn record, not on the mother's record.

3) Use of Codes from other Chapters with Codes from Chapter 16

Codes from other chapters may be used with codes from Chapter 16 if the codes from the other chapters provide more specific detail. Codes for signs and symptoms may be assigned when a definitive diagnosis has not been established. If the reason for the encounter is a perinatal condition, the code from Chapter 16 should be sequenced first.

4) Use of Chapter 16 Codes after the Perinatal Period

Should a condition originate in the perinatal period, and continue throughout the life of the patient, the perinatal code should continue to be used regardless of the patient's age.

5) Birth process or community acquired conditions

If a newborn has a condition that may be either due to the birth process or community acquired and the documentation does not indicate which it is, the default is due to the birth process and the code from Chapter 16 should be used. If the condition is community-acquired, a code from Chapter 16 should not be assigned.

For COVID-19 infection in a newborn, see guideline I.C.16.h.

6) Code all clinically significant conditions

All clinically significant conditions noted on routine newborn examination should be coded. A condition is clinically significant if it requires:
- clinical evaluation; or
- therapeutic treatment; or
- diagnostic procedures; or
- extended length of hospital stay; or
- increased nursing care and/or monitoring; or
- has implications for future health care needs

Note: The perinatal guidelines listed above are the same as the general coding guidelines for "additional diagnoses", except for the final point regarding implications for future health care needs. Codes should be assigned for conditions that have been specified by the provider as having implications for future health care needs.

b. Observation and Evaluation of Newborns for Suspected Conditions not Found

1) Use of Z05 codes

Assign a code from category Z05, Observation and evaluation of newborns and infants for suspected conditions ruled out, to identify those instances when a healthy newborn is evaluated for a suspected condition that is determined after study not to be present. Do not use a code from category Z05 when the patient has identified signs or symptoms of a suspected problem; in such cases code the sign or symptom.

2) Z05 on other than the birth record

A code from category Z05 may also be assigned as a principal or first-listed code for readmissions or encounters when the code from category Z38 code no longer applies. Codes from category Z05 are for use only for healthy newborns and infants for which no condition after study is found to be present.

3) Z05 on a birth record

A code from category Z05 is to be used as a secondary code after the code from category Z38, Liveborn infants according to place of birth and type of delivery.

c. Coding Additional Perinatal Diagnoses

1) Assigning codes for conditions that require treatment

Assign codes for conditions that require treatment or further investigation, prolong the length of stay, or require resource utilization.

2) Codes for conditions specified as having implications for future health care needs

Assign codes for conditions that have been specified by the provider as having implications for future health care needs.

Note: This guideline should not be used for adult patients.

d. Prematurity and Fetal Growth Retardation

Providers utilize different criteria in determining prematurity. A code for prematurity should not be assigned unless it is documented. Assignment of codes in categories P05, Disorders of newborn related to slow fetal growth and fetal malnutrition, and P07, Disorders of newborn related to short gestation and low birth weight, not elsewhere classified, should be based on the recorded birth weight and estimated gestational age.

When both birth weight and gestational age are available, two codes from category P07 should be assigned, with the code for birth weight sequenced before the code for gestational age.

e. Low birth weight and immaturity status

Codes from category P07, Disorders of newborn related to short gestation and low birth weight, not elsewhere classified, are for use for a child or adult who was premature or had a low birth weight as a newborn and this is affecting the patient's current health status.

See Section I.C.21. Factors influencing health status and contact with health services, Status.

f. Bacterial Sepsis of Newborn
Category P36, Bacterial sepsis of newborn, includes congenital sepsis. If a perinate is documented as having sepsis without documentation of congenital or community acquired, the default is congenital and a code from category P36 should be assigned. If the P36 code includes the causal organism, an additional code from category B95, Streptococcus, Staphylococcus, and Enterococcus as the cause of diseases classified elsewhere, or B96, Other bacterial agents as the cause of diseases classified elsewhere, should not be assigned. If the P36 code does not include the causal organism, assign an additional code from category B96. If applicable, use additional codes to identify severe sepsis (R65.2-) and any associated acute organ dysfunction.

g. Stillbirth
Code P95, Stillbirth, is only for use in institutions that maintain separate records for stillbirths. No other code should be used with P95. Code P95 should not be used on the mother's record.

h. COVID-19 Infection in Newborn
For a newborn that tests positive for COVID-19, assign code U07.1, COVID-19, and the appropriate codes for associated manifestation(s) in neonates/newborns in the absence of documentation indicating a specific type of transmission. For a newborn that tests positive for COVID-19 and the provider documents the condition was contracted in utero or during the birth process, assign codes P35.8, Other congenital viral diseases, and U07.1, COVID-19. When coding the birth episode in a newborn record, the appropriate code from category Z38, Liveborn infants according to place of birth and type of delivery, should be assigned as the principal diagnosis.

17. Chapter 17: Congenital Malformations, Deformations, and Chromosomal Abnormalities (Q00-Q99)
Assign an appropriate code(s) from categories Q00-Q99, Congenital malformations, deformations, and chromosomal abnormalities when a malformation/deformation or chromosomal abnormality is documented. A malformation/deformation/or chromosomal abnormality may be the principal/first-listed diagnosis on a record or a secondary diagnosis.

When a malformation/deformation/or chromosomal abnormality does not have a unique code assignment, assign additional code(s) for any manifestations that may be present.

When the code assignment specifically identifies the malformation/deformation/or chromosomal abnormality, manifestations that are an inherent component of the anomaly should not be coded separately. Additional codes should be assigned for manifestations that are not an inherent component.

Codes from Chapter 17 may be used throughout the life of the patient. If a congenital malformation or deformity has been corrected, a personal history code should be used to identify the history of the malformation or deformity. Although present at birth, a malformation/deformation/or chromosomal abnormality may not be identified until later in life. Whenever the condition is diagnosed by the provider, it is appropriate to assign a code from codes Q00-Q99.

For the birth admission, the appropriate code from category Z38, Liveborn infants, according to place of birth and type of delivery, should be sequenced as the principal diagnosis, followed by any congenital anomaly codes, Q00-Q99.

18. Chapter 18: Symptoms, Signs, and Abnormal Clinical and Laboratory Findings, Not Elsewhere Classified (R00-R99)
Chapter 18 includes symptoms, signs, abnormal results of clinical or other investigative procedures, and ill-defined conditions regarding which no diagnosis classifiable elsewhere is recorded. Signs and symptoms that point to a specific diagnosis have been assigned to a category in other chapters of the classification.

a. Use of symptom codes
Codes that describe symptoms and signs are acceptable for reporting purposes when a related definitive diagnosis has not been established (confirmed) by the provider.

b. Use of a symptom code with a definitive diagnosis code
Codes for signs and symptoms may be reported in addition to a related definitive diagnosis when the sign or symptom is not routinely associated with that diagnosis, such as the various signs and symptoms associated with complex syndromes. The definitive diagnosis code should be sequenced before the symptom code.

Signs or symptoms that are associated routinely with a disease process should not be assigned as additional codes, unless otherwise instructed by the classification.

c. Combination codes that include symptoms
ICD-10-CM contains a number of combination codes that identify both the definitive diagnosis and common symptoms of that diagnosis. When using one of these combination codes, an additional code should not be assigned for the symptom.

d. Repeated falls
Code R29.6, Repeated falls, is for use for encounters when a patient has recently fallen and the reason for the fall is being investigated.

Code Z91.81, History of falling, is for use when a patient has fallen in the past and is at risk for future falls. When appropriate, both codes R29.6 and Z91.81 may be assigned together.

e. Coma

Code R40.20, Unspecified coma, may be assigned in conjunction with codes for any medical condition.

Do not report codes for **unspecified coma**, individual or total Glasgow coma scale scores for a patient with a medically induced coma or a sedated patient.

The coma scale codes (R40.21- to R40.24-) can be used in conjunction with traumatic brain injury codes. These codes are primarily for use by trauma registries, but they may be used in any setting where this information is collected. The coma scale codes should be sequenced after the diagnosis code(s).

These codes, one from each subcategory, are needed to complete the scale. The 7th character indicates when the scale was recorded. The 7th character should match for all three codes.

At a minimum, report the initial score documented on presentation at your facility. This may be a score from the emergency medicine technician (EMT) or in the emergency department. If desired, a facility may choose to capture multiple coma scale scores.

Assign code R40.24, Glasgow coma scale, total score, when only the total score is documented in the medical record and not the individual score(s).

If multiple coma scores are captured within the first 24 hours after hospital admission, assign only the code for the score at the time of admission. ICD-10-CM does not classify coma scores that are reported after admission but less than 24 hours later.

See Section I.B.14 for coma scale documentation by clinicians other than patient's provider

f. Functional quadriplegia
GUIDELINE HAS BEEN DELETED EFFECTIVE OCTOBER 1, 2017

g. SIRS due to Non-Infectious Process
The systemic inflammatory response syndrome (SIRS) can develop as a result of certain non-infectious disease processes, such as trauma, malignant neoplasm, or pancreatitis. When SIRS is documented with a noninfectious condition, and no subsequent infection is documented, the code for the underlying condition, such as an injury, should be assigned, followed by code R65.10, Systemic inflammatory response syndrome (SIRS) of non-infectious origin without acute organ dysfunction, or code R65.11, Systemic inflammatory response syndrome (SIRS) of non-infectious origin with acute organ dysfunction. If an associated acute organ dysfunction is documented, the appropriate code(s) for the specific type of organ dysfunction(s) should be assigned in addition to code R65.11. If acute organ dysfunction is documented, but it cannot be determined if the acute organ dysfunction is associated with SIRS or due to another condition (e.g., directly due to the trauma), the provider should be queried.

h. Death NOS

Code R99, Ill-defined and unknown cause of mortality, is only for use in the very limited circumstance when a patient who has already died is brought into an emergency department or other healthcare facility and is pronounced dead upon arrival. It does not represent the discharge disposition of death.

i. NIHSS Stroke Scale
The NIH stroke scale (NIHSS) codes (R29.7- -) can be used in conjunction with acute stroke codes (I63) to identify the patient's neurological status and the severity of the stroke. The stroke scale codes should be sequenced after the acute stroke diagnosis code(s).

At a minimum, report the initial score documented. If desired, a facility may choose to capture multiple stroke scale scores.

See Section I.B.14 for NIHSS stroke scale documentation by clinicians other than patient's provider

19. **Chapter 19: Injury, Poisoning, and Certain Other Consequences of External Causes (S00-T88)**

a. Application of 7th Characters in Chapter 19
Most categories in Chapter 19 have a 7th character requirement for each applicable code. Most categories in this chapter have three 7th character values (with the exception of fractures): A, initial encounter, D, subsequent encounter and S, sequela. Categories for traumatic fractures have additional 7th character values. While the patient may be seen by a new or different provider over the course of treatment for an injury, assignment of the 7th character is based on whether the patient is undergoing active treatment and not whether the provider is seeing the patient for the first time.

For complication codes, active treatment refers to treatment for the condition described by the code, even though it may be related to an earlier precipitating problem. For example, code T84.50XA, Infection and inflammatory reaction due to unspecified internal joint prosthesis, initial encounter, is used when active treatment is provided for the infection, even though the condition relates to the prosthetic device, implant or graft that was placed at a previous encounter.

7th character "A", initial encounter is used for each encounter where the patient is receiving active treatment for the condition.

7th character "D" subsequent encounter is used for encounters after the patient has completed active treatment of the condition and is receiving routine care for the condition during the healing or recovery phase.

The aftercare Z codes should not be used for aftercare for conditions such as injuries or poisonings, where 7th characters are provided to identify subsequent care. For example, for aftercare of an injury, assign the acute injury code with the 7th character "D" (subsequent encounter).

7th character "S", sequela, is for use for complications or conditions that arise as a direct result of a condition, such as scar formation after a burn. The scars are sequelae of the burn. When using 7th character "S", it is necessary to use both

the injury code that precipitated the sequela and the code for the sequela itself. The "S" is added only to the injury code, not the sequela code. The 7th character "S" identifies the injury responsible for the sequela. The specific type of sequela (e.g., scar) is sequenced first, followed by the injury code.

See Section I.B.10. Sequelae, (Late Effects)

b. Coding of Injuries

When coding injuries, assign separate codes for each injury unless a combination code is provided, in which case the combination code is assigned. Codes from category T07, Unspecified multiple injuries should not be assigned in the inpatient setting unless information for a more specific code is not available. Traumatic injury codes (S00-T14.9) are not to be used for normal, healing surgical wounds or to identify complications of surgical wounds.

The code for the most serious injury, as determined by the provider and the focus of treatment, is sequenced first.

1) Superficial injuries

Superficial injuries such as abrasions or contusions are not coded when associated with more severe injuries of the same site.

2) Primary injury with damage to nerves/ blood vessels

When a primary injury results in minor damage to peripheral nerves or blood vessels, the primary injury is sequenced first with additional code(s) for injuries to nerves and spinal cord (such as category S04), and/or injury to blood vessels (such as category S15). When the primary injury is to the blood vessels or nerves, that injury should be sequenced first.

3) Iatrogenic injuries

Injury codes from Chapter 19 should not be assigned for injuries that occur during, or as a result of, a medical intervention. Assign the appropriate complication code(s).

c. Coding of Traumatic Fractures

The principles of multiple coding of injuries should be followed in coding fractures. Fractures of specified sites are coded individually by site in accordance with both the provisions within categories S02, S12, S22, S32, S42, S49, S52, S59, S62, S72, S79, S82, S89, S92 and the level of detail furnished by medical record content.

A fracture not indicated as open or closed should be coded to closed. A fracture not indicated whether displaced or not displaced should be coded to displaced.

More specific guidelines are as follows:

1) Initial vs. subsequent encounter for fractures

Traumatic fractures are coded using the appropriate 7th character for initial encounter (A, B, C) for each encounter where the patient is receiving active treatment for the fracture. The appropriate 7th character for initial encounter should also be assigned for a patient who delayed seeking treatment for the fracture or nonunion.

Fractures are coded using the appropriate 7th character for subsequent care for encounters after the patient has completed active treatment of the fracture and is receiving routine care for the fracture during the healing or recovery phase.

Care for complications of surgical treatment for fracture repairs during the healing or recovery phase should be coded with the appropriate complication codes.

Care of complications of fractures, such as malunion and nonunion, should be reported with the appropriate 7th character for subsequent care with nonunion (K, M, N,) or subsequent care with malunion (P, Q, R).

Malunion/nonunion: The appropriate 7th character for initial encounter should also be assigned for a patient who delayed seeking treatment for the fracture or nonunion.

The open fracture designations in the assignment of the 7th character for fractures of the forearm, femur and lower leg, including ankle are based on the Gustilo open fracture classification. When the Gustilo classification type is not specified for an open fracture, the 7th character for open fracture type I or II should be assigned (B, E, H, M, Q).

A code from category M80, not a traumatic fracture code, should be used for any patient with known osteoporosis who suffers a fracture, even if the patient had a minor fall or trauma, if that fall or trauma would not usually break a normal, healthy bone.

See Section I.C.13. Osteoporosis.

The aftercare Z codes should not be used for aftercare for traumatic fractures. For aftercare of a traumatic fracture, assign the acute fracture code with the appropriate 7th character.

2) Multiple fractures sequencing

Multiple fractures are sequenced in accordance with the severity of the fracture.

3) Physeal fractures

For physeal fractures, assign only the code identifying the type of physeal fracture. Do not assign a separate code to identify the specific bone that is fractured.

d. Coding of Burns and Corrosions

The ICD-10-CM makes a distinction between burns and corrosions. The burn codes are for thermal burns, except sunburns, that come from a heat source, such as a fire or hot appliance. The burn codes are also for burns resulting from electricity and radiation. Corrosions are burns due to chemicals. The guidelines are the same for burns and corrosions.

Current burns (T20-T25) are classified by depth, extent and by agent (X code). Burns are classified by depth as first degree (erythema), second degree (blistering), and third degree (full-thickness involvement). Burns of the eye and internal organs (T26-T28) are classified by site, but not by degree.

1) Sequencing of burn and related condition codes

Sequence first the code that reflects the highest degree of burn when more than one burn is present.

    a. When the reason for the admission or encounter is for treatment of external multiple burns, sequence first the code

that reflects the burn of the highest degree.

b. When a patient has both internal and external burns, the circumstances of admission govern the selection of the principal diagnosis or first-listed diagnosis.

c. When a patient is admitted for burn injuries and other related conditions such as smoke inhalation and/or respiratory failure, the circumstances of admission govern the selection of the principal or first-listed diagnosis.

2) Burns of the same anatomic site

Classify burns of the same anatomic site and on the same side but of different degrees to the subcategory identifying the highest degree recorded in the diagnosis (e.g., for second and third degree burns of right thigh, assign only code T24.311-).

3) Non-healing burns

Non-healing burns are coded as acute burns.
Necrosis of burned skin should be coded as a non-healed burn.

4) Infected burn

For any documented infected burn site, use an additional code for the infection.

5) Assign separate codes for each burn site

When coding burns, assign separate codes for each burn site. Category T30, Burn and corrosion, body region unspecified is extremely vague and should rarely be used.

Codes for burns of "multiple sites" should only be assigned when the medical record documentation does not specify the individual sites.

6) Burns and corrosions classified according to extent of body surface involved

Assign codes from category T31, Burns classified according to extent of body surface involved, or T32, Corrosions classified according to extent of body surface involved, **for acute burns or corrosions** when the site of the burn **or corrosion** is not specified or when there is a need for additional data. It is advisable to use category T31 as additional coding when needed to provide data for evaluating burn mortality, such as that needed by burn units. It is also advisable to use category T31 as an additional code for reporting purposes when there is mention of a third-degree burn involving 20 percent or more of the body surface. **Codes from categories T31 and T32 should not be used for sequelae of burns or corrosions.**

Categories T31 and T32 are based on the classic "rule of nines" in estimating body surface involved: head and neck are assigned nine percent, each arm nine percent, each leg 18 percent, the anterior trunk 18 percent, posterior trunk 18 percent, and genitalia 1 percent. Providers may change these percentage assignments where necessary to accommodate infants and children who have proportionately larger heads than adults, and patients who have large buttocks, thighs, or abdomen that involve burns.

7) Encounters for treatment of sequela of burns

Encounters for the treatment of the late effects of burns or corrosions (i.e., scars or joint contractures) should be coded with a burn or corrosion code with the 7th character "S" for sequela.

8) Sequelae with a late effect code and current burn

When appropriate, both a code for a current burn or corrosion with 7th character "A" or "D" and a burn or corrosion code with 7th character "S" may be assigned on the same record (when both a current burn and sequelae of an old burn exist). Burns and corrosions do not heal at the same rate and a current healing wound may still exist with sequela of a healed burn or corrosion.

See Section I.B.10. Sequela, (Late Effects)

9) Use of an external cause code with burns and corrosions

An external cause code should be used with burns and corrosions to identify the source and intent of the burn, as well as the place where it occurred.

e. Adverse Effects, Poisoning, Underdosing and Toxic Effects

Codes in categories T36-T65 are combination codes that include the substance that was taken as well as the intent. No additional external cause code is required for poisonings, toxic effects, adverse effects and underdosing codes.

1) Do not code directly from the Table of Drugs

Do not code directly from the Table of Drugs and Chemicals. Always refer back to the Tabular List.

2) Use as many codes as necessary to describe

Use as many codes as necessary to describe completely all drugs, medicinal or biological substances.

3) If the same code would describe the causative agent

If the same code would describe the causative agent for more than one adverse reaction, poisoning, toxic effect or underdosing, assign the code only once.

4) If two or more drugs, medicinal or biological substances

If two or more drugs, medicinal or biological substances are taken, code each individually unless a combination code is listed in the Table of Drugs and Chemicals.

If multiple unspecified drugs, medicinal or biological substances were taken, assign the appropriate code from subcategory T50.91, Poisoning by, adverse effect of and underdosing of multiple unspecified drugs, medicaments and biological substances.

5) The occurrence of drug toxicity is classified in ICD-10-CM as follows:

(a) Adverse Effect

When coding an adverse effect of a drug that has been correctly prescribed and properly administered, assign the appropriate code for the nature of the adverse effect followed by the appropriate code for the adverse effect of the drug (T36-T50). The code for the drug should

have a 5th or 6th character "5" (for example T36.0X5-) Examples of the nature of an adverse effect are tachycardia, delirium, gastrointestinal hemorrhaging, vomiting, hypokalemia, hepatitis, renal failure, or respiratory failure.

(b) Poisoning

When coding a poisoning or reaction to the improper use of a medication (e.g., overdose, wrong substance given or taken in error, wrong route of administration), first assign the appropriate code from categories T36-T50. The poisoning codes have an associated intent as their 5th or 6th character (accidental, intentional self-harm, assault and undetermined). If the intent of the poisoning is unknown or unspecified, code the intent as accidental intent. The undetermined intent is only for use if the documentation in the record specifies that the intent cannot be determined. Use additional code(s) for all manifestations of poisonings.

If there is also a diagnosis of abuse or dependence of the substance, the abuse or dependence is assigned as an additional code.

Examples of poisoning include:

(i) Error was made in drug prescription Errors made in drug prescription or in the administration of the drug by provider, nurse, patient, or other person.

(ii) Overdose of a drug intentionally taken If an overdose of a drug was intentionally taken or administered and resulted in drug toxicity, it would be coded as a poisoning.

(iii) Nonprescribed drug taken with correctly prescribed and properly administered drug. If a nonprescribed drug or medicinal agent was taken in combination with a correctly prescribed and properly administered drug, any drug toxicity or other reaction resulting from the interaction of the two drugs would be classified as a poisoning.

(iv) Interaction of drug(s) and alcohol. When a reaction results from the interaction of a drug(s) and alcohol, this would be classified as poisoning.

See Section I.C.4. if poisoning is the result of insulin pump malfunctions.

(c) Underdosing

Underdosing refers to taking less of a medication than is prescribed by a provider or a manufacturer's instruction. Discontinuing the use of a prescribed medication on the patient's own initiative (not directed by the patient's provider) is also classified as an underdosing. For underdosing, assign the code from categories T36-T50 (5th or 6th character "6").

Codes for underdosing should never be assigned as principal or first-listed codes. If a patient has a relapse or exacerbation of the medical condition for which the drug is prescribed because of the reduction in dose, then the medical condition itself should be coded.

Noncompliance (Z91.12-, Z91.13- and Z91.14-) or complication of care (Y63.6-Y63.9) codes are to be used with an underdosing code to indicate intent, if known.

(d) Toxic Effects

When a harmful substance is ingested or comes in contact with a person, this is classified as a toxic effect. The toxic effect codes are in categories T51-T65.

Toxic effect codes have an associated intent: accidental, intentional self-harm, assault and undetermined.

f. Adult and child abuse, neglect and other maltreatment

Sequence first the appropriate code from categories T74 (Adult and child abuse, neglect and other maltreatment, confirmed) or T76 (Adult and child abuse, neglect and other maltreatment, suspected) for abuse, neglect and other maltreatment, followed by any accompanying mental health or injury code(s).

If the documentation in the medical record states abuse or neglect it is coded as confirmed (T74.-). It is coded as suspected if it is documented as suspected (T76.-).

For cases of confirmed abuse or neglect an external cause code from the assault section (X92-Y09) should be added to identify the cause of any physical injuries. A perpetrator code (Y07) should be added when the perpetrator of the abuse is known. For suspected cases of abuse or neglect, do not report external cause or perpetrator code.

If a suspected case of abuse, neglect or mistreatment is ruled out during an encounter code Z04.71, Encounter for examination and observation following alleged physical adult abuse, ruled out, or code Z04.72, Encounter for examination and observation following alleged child physical abuse, ruled out, should be used, not a code from T76.

If a suspected case of alleged rape or sexual abuse is ruled out during an encounter code Z04.41, Encounter for examination and observation following alleged adult rape or code Z04.42, Encounter for examination and observation following alleged child rape, should be used, not a code from T76.

If a suspected case of forced sexual exploitation or forced labor exploitation is ruled out during an encounter, code Z04.81, Encounter for examination and observation of victim following forced sexual exploitation, or code Z04.82, Encounter for examination and observation of victim following forced labor exploitation, should be used, not a code from T76.

See Section I.C.15. Abuse in a pregnant patient.

g. Complications of care

1) General guidelines for complications of care

(a) Documentation of complications of care

See Section I.B.16. for information on documentation of complications of care.

2) Pain due to medical devices

Pain associated with devices, implants or grafts left in a surgical site (for example painful hip prosthesis) is assigned to the appropriate code(s) found in Chapter 19, Injury, poisoning, and certain other consequences of external causes. Specific codes for pain due to medical devices are found in the T code section of the ICD-10-CM. Use additional code(s) from category G89 to identify acute or chronic pain due to presence of the device, implant or graft (G89.18 or G89.28).

3) Transplant complications

(a) Transplant complications other than kidney

Codes under category T86, Complications of transplanted organs and tissues, are for use for both complications and rejection of transplanted organs. A transplant complication code is only assigned if the complication affects the function of the transplanted organ. Two codes are required to fully describe a transplant complication: the appropriate code from category T86 and a secondary code that identifies the complication.

Pre-existing conditions or conditions that develop after the transplant are not coded as complications unless they affect the function of the transplanted organs.

See Section I.C.21. for transplant organ removal status
See Section I.C.2. for malignant neoplasm associated with transplanted organ.

(b) Kidney transplant complications

Patients who have undergone kidney transplant may still have some form of chronic kidney disease (CKD) because the kidney transplant may not fully restore kidney function. Code T86.1- should be assigned for documented complications of a kidney transplant, such as transplant failure or rejection or other transplant complication. Code T86.1- should not be assigned for post kidney transplant patients who have chronic kidney (CKD) unless a transplant complication such as transplant failure or rejection is documented. If the documentation is unclear as to whether the patient has a complication of the transplant, query the provider.

Conditions that affect the function of the transplanted kidney, other than CKD, should be assigned a code from subcategory T86.1, Complications of transplanted organ, Kidney, and a secondary code that identifies the complication.

For patients with CKD following a kidney transplant, but who do not have a complication such as failure or rejection, *see Section I.C.14. Chronic kidney disease and kidney transplant status.*

4) Complication codes that include the external cause

As with certain other T codes, some of the complications of care codes have the external cause included in the code. The code includes the nature of the complication as well as the type of procedure that caused the complication. No external cause code indicating the type of procedure is necessary for these codes.

5) Complications of care codes within the body system chapters

Intraoperative and postprocedural complication codes are found within the body system chapters with codes specific to the organs and structures of that body system. These codes should be sequenced first, followed by a code(s) for the specific complication, if applicable.

Complication codes from the body system chapters should be assigned for intraoperative and postprocedural complications (e.g., the appropriate complication code from Chapter 9 would be assigned for a vascular intraoperative or postprocedural complication) unless the complication is specifically indexed to a T code in Chapter 19.

20. **Chapter 20: External Causes of Morbidity (V00-Y99)**

The external causes of morbidity codes should never be sequenced as the first-listed or principal diagnosis.

External cause codes are intended to provide data for injury research and evaluation of injury prevention strategies. These codes capture how the injury or health condition happened (cause), the intent (unintentional or accidental; or intentional, such as suicide or assault), the place where the event occurred the activity of the patient at the time of the event, and the person's status (e.g., civilian, military).

There is no national requirement for mandatory ICD-10-CM external cause code reporting. Unless a provider is subject to a state-based external cause code reporting mandate or these codes are required by a particular payer, reporting of ICD-10-CM codes in Chapter 20, External Causes of Morbidity, is not required. In the absence of a mandatory reporting requirement, providers are encouraged to voluntarily report external cause codes, as they provide valuable data for injury research and evaluation of injury prevention strategies.

a. **General External Cause Coding Guidelines**

1) Used with any code in the range of A00.0-T88.9, Z00-Z99

An external cause code may be used with any code in the range of A00.0-T88.9, Z00-Z99, classification that represents a health condition due to an external cause. Though they are most applicable to injuries, they are also valid for use with such things as infections or diseases due to an external source, and other health conditions, such as a heart attack that occurs during strenuous physical activity.

2) External cause code used for length of treatment

Assign the external cause code, with the appropriate 7th character (initial encounter, subsequent

encounter or sequela) for each encounter for which the injury or condition is being treated.

Most categories in Chapter 20 have a 7th character requirement for each applicable code. Most categories in this chapter have three 7th character values: A, initial encounter, D, subsequent encounter and S, sequela. While the patient may be seen by a new or different provider over the course of treatment for an injury or condition, assignment of the 7th character for external cause should match the 7th character of the code assigned for the associated injury or condition for the encounter.

3) Use the full range of external cause codes
Use the full range of external cause codes to completely describe the cause, the intent, the place of occurrence and if applicable, the activity of the patient at the time of the event, and the patient's status, for all injuries, and other health conditions due to an external cause.

4) Assign as many external cause codes as necessary
Assign as many external cause codes as necessary to fully explain each cause. If only one external code can be recorded, assign the code most related to the principal diagnosis.

5) The selection of the appropriate external cause code
The selection of the appropriate external cause code is guided by the Alphabetic Index of External Causes and by Inclusion and Exclusion notes in the Tabular List.

6) External cause code can never be a principal diagnosis
An external cause code can never be a principal (first-listed) diagnosis.

7) Combination external cause codes
Certain of the external cause codes are combination codes that identify sequential events that result in an injury, such as a fall which results in striking against an object. The injury may be due to either event or both. The combination external cause code used should correspond to the sequence of events regardless of which caused the most serious injury.

8) No external cause code needed in certain circumstances
No external cause code from Chapter 20 is needed if the external cause and intent are included in a code from another chapter (e.g., T36.0X1- Poisoning by penicillins, accidental (unintentional)).

b. Place of Occurrence Guideline
Codes from category Y92, Place of occurrence of the external cause, are secondary codes for use after other external cause codes to identify the location of the patient at the time of injury or other condition.

Generally, a place of occurrence code is assigned only once, at the initial encounter for treatment. However, in the rare instance that a new injury occurs during hospitalization, an additional place of occurrence code may be assigned. No 7th characters are used for Y92. Only one code from Y92 should be recorded on a medical record.

Do not use place of occurrence code Y92.9 if the place is not stated or is not applicable.

c. Activity Code
Assign a code from category Y93, Activity code, to describe the activity of the patient at the time the injury or other health condition occurred.

An activity code is used only once, at the initial encounter for treatment. Only one code from Y93 should be recorded on a medical record.

The activity codes are not applicable to poisonings, adverse effects, misadventures or sequela.

Do not assign Y93.9, Unspecified activity, if the activity is not stated.

A code from category Y93 is appropriate for use with external cause and intent codes if identifying the activity provides additional information about the event.

d. Place of Occurrence, Activity, and Status Codes Used with other External Cause Code
When applicable, place of occurrence, activity, and external cause status codes are sequenced after the main external cause code(s). Regardless of the number of external cause codes assigned, there should be only one place of occurrence code, one activity code, and one external cause status code assigned to an encounter.

e. If the Reporting Format Limits the Number of External Cause Codes
If the reporting format limits the number of external cause codes that can be used in reporting clinical data, report the code for the cause/intent most related to the principal diagnosis. If the format permits capture of additional external cause codes, the cause/intent, including medical misadventures, of the additional events should be reported rather than the codes for place, activity, or external status.

f. Multiple External Cause Coding Guidelines
More than one external cause code is required to fully describe the external cause of an illness or injury. The assignment of external cause codes should be sequenced in the following priority:

If two or more events cause separate injuries, an external cause code should be assigned for each cause. The first-listed external cause code will be selected in the following order:

External codes for child and adult abuse take priority over all other external cause codes.
See Section I.C.19., Child and Adult abuse guidelines.
External codes for terrorism events take priority over all other external cause codes except child and adult abuse.
External cause codes for cataclysmic events take priority over all other external cause codes except child and adult abuse and terrorism.
External cause codes for transport accidents take priority over all other external cause codes except cataclysmic events, child and adult abuse and terrorism.
Activity and external cause status codes are assigned following all causal (intent) external cause codes.
The first-listed external cause code should correspond to the cause of the most serious

diagnosis due to an assault, accident, or self-harm, following the order of hierarchy listed above.

g. Child and Adult Abuse Guideline

Adult and child abuse, neglect and maltreatment are classified as assault. Any of the assault codes may be used to indicate the external cause of any injury resulting from the confirmed abuse.

For confirmed cases of abuse, neglect and maltreatment, when the perpetrator is known, a code from Y07, Perpetrator of maltreatment and neglect, should accompany any other assault codes.

See Section I.C.19. Adult and child abuse, neglect and other maltreatment

h. Unknown or Undetermined Intent Guideline

If the intent (accident, self-harm, assault) of the cause of an injury or other condition is unknown or unspecified, code the intent as accidental intent. All transport accident categories assume accidental intent.

1) Use of undetermined intent

External cause codes for events of undetermined intent are only for use if the documentation in the record specifies that the intent cannot be determined.

i. Sequelae (Late Effects) of External Cause Guidelines

1) Sequelae external cause codes

Sequela are reported using the external cause code with the 7th character "S" for sequela. These codes should be used with any report of a late effect or sequela resulting from a previous injury.

See Section I.B.10. Sequela (Late Effects)

2) Sequela external cause code with a related current injury

A sequela external cause code should never be used with a related current nature of injury code.

3) Use of sequela external cause codes for subsequent visits

Use a late effect external cause code for subsequent visits when a late effect of the initial injury is being treated. Do not use a late effect external cause code for subsequent visits for follow-up care (e.g., to assess healing, to receive rehabilitative therapy) of the injury when no late effect of the injury has been documented.

j. Terrorism Guidelines

1) Cause of injury identified by the Federal Government (FBI) as terrorism

When the cause of an injury is identified by the Federal Government (FBI) as terrorism, the first-listed external cause code should be a code from category Y38, Terrorism. The definition of terrorism employed by the FBI is found at the inclusion note at the beginning of category Y38. Use additional code for place of occurrence (Y92.-). More than one Y38 code may be assigned if the injury is the result of more than one mechanism of terrorism.

2) Cause of an injury is suspected to be the result of terrorism

When the cause of an injury is suspected to be the result of terrorism a code from category Y38 should not be assigned. Suspected cases should be classified as assault.

3) Code Y38.9, Terrorism, secondary effects

Assign code Y38.9, Terrorism, secondary effects, for conditions occurring subsequent to the terrorist event. This code should not be assigned for conditions that are due to the initial terrorist act.

It is acceptable to assign code Y38.9 with another code from Y38 if there is an injury due to the initial terrorist event and an injury that is a subsequent result of the terrorist event.

k. External Cause Status

A code from category Y99, External cause status, should be assigned whenever any other external cause code is assigned for an encounter, including an Activity code, except for the events noted below. Assign a code from category Y99, External cause status, to indicate the work status of the person at the time the event occurred. The status code indicates whether the event occurred during military activity, whether a non-military person was at work, whether an individual including a student or volunteer was involved in a non-work activity at the time of the causal event.

A code from Y99, External cause status, should be assigned, when applicable, with other external cause codes, such as transport accidents and falls. The external cause status codes are not applicable to poisonings, adverse effects, misadventures or late effects.

Do not assign a code from category Y99 if no other external cause codes (cause, activity) are applicable for the encounter.

An external cause status code is used only once, at the initial encounter for treatment. Only one code from Y99 should be recorded on a medical record.

Do not assign code Y99.9, Unspecified external cause status, if the status is not stated.

21. Chapter 21: Factors Influencing Health Status and Contact with Health Services (Z00-Z99)

Note: The chapter-specific guidelines provide additional information about the use of Z codes for specified encounters.

a. Use of Z Codes in Any Healthcare Setting

Z codes are for use in any healthcare setting. Z codes may be used as either a first-listed (principal diagnosis code in the inpatient setting) or secondary code, depending on the circumstances of the encounter. Certain Z codes may only be used as first-listed or principal diagnosis.

b. Z Codes Indicate a Reason for an Encounter

Z codes are not procedure codes. A corresponding procedure code must accompany a Z code to describe any procedure performed.

c. Categories of Z Codes

1) Contact/Exposure

Category Z20 indicates contact with, and suspected exposure to, communicable diseases. These codes are for patients who are suspected to have been exposed to a disease by close personal contact with an infected individual or are in an area where a disease is epidemic.

Category Z77, Other contact with and (suspected) exposures hazardous to health, indicates contact with and suspected exposures hazardous to health.

Contact/exposure codes may be used as a first-listed code to explain an encounter for testing, or, more commonly, as a secondary code to identify a potential risk.

2) Inoculations and vaccinations

Code Z23 is for encounters for inoculations and vaccinations. It indicates that a patient is being seen to receive a prophylactic inoculation against a disease. Procedure codes are required to identify the actual administration of the injection and the type(s) of immunizations given. Code Z23 may be used as a secondary code if the inoculation is given as a routine part of preventive health care, such as a well-baby visit.

3) Status

Status codes indicate that a patient is either a carrier of a disease or has the sequelae or residual of a past disease or condition. This includes such things as the presence of prosthetic or mechanical devices resulting from past treatment. A status code is informative, because the status may affect the course of treatment and its outcome. A status code is distinct from a history code. The history code indicates that the patient no longer has the condition.

A status code should not be used with a diagnosis code from one of the body system chapters, if the diagnosis code includes the information provided by the status code. For example, code Z94.1, Heart transplant status, should not be used with a code from subcategory T86.2, Complications of heart transplant. The status code does not provide additional information. The complication code indicates that the patient is a heart transplant patient.

For encounters for weaning from a mechanical ventilator, assign a code from subcategory J96.1, Chronic respiratory failure, followed by code Z99.11, Dependence on respirator [ventilator] status.

The status Z codes/categories are:
Z14 Genetic carrier
Genetic carrier status indicates that a person carries a gene, associated with a particular disease, which may be passed to offspring who may develop that disease. The person does not have the disease and is not at risk of developing the disease.
Z15 Genetic susceptibility to disease Genetic susceptibility indicates that a person has

a gene that increases the risk of that person developing the disease.

Codes from category Z15 should not be used as principal or first-listed codes. If the patient has the condition to which he/she is susceptible, and that condition is the reason for the encounter, the code for the current condition should be sequenced first. If the patient is being seen for follow-up after completed treatment for this condition, and the condition no longer exists, a follow-up code should be sequenced first, followed by the appropriate personal history and genetic susceptibility codes. If the purpose of the encounter is genetic counseling associated with procreative management, code Z31.5, Encounter for genetic counseling, should be assigned as the first-listed code, followed by a code from category Z15. Additional codes should be assigned for any applicable family or personal history.

Z16 Resistance to antimicrobial drugs
This code indicates that a patient has a condition that is resistant to antimicrobial drug treatment. Sequence the infection code first.
Z17 Estrogen receptor status
Z18 Retained foreign body fragments
Z19 Hormone sensitivity malignancy status
Z21 Asymptomatic HIV infection status This code indicates that a patient has tested positive for HIV but has manifested no signs or symptoms of the disease.
Z22 Carrier of infectious disease Carrier status indicates that a person harbors the specific organisms of a disease without manifest symptoms and is capable of transmitting the infection.
Z28.3 Underimmunization status
Z33.1 Pregnant state, incidental This code is a secondary code only for use when the pregnancy is in no way complicating the reason for visit. Otherwise, a code from the obstetric chapter is required.
Z66 Do not resuscitate
This code may be used when it is documented by the provider that a patient is on do not resuscitate status at any time during the stay.
Z67 Blood type
Z68 Body mass index (BMI)
BMI codes should only be assigned when there is an associated reportable diagnosis (such as obesity). Do not assign BMI codes during pregnancy.
See Section I.B.14 for BMI documentation by clinicians other than the patient's provider.
Z74.01 Bed confinement status
Z76.82 Awaiting organ transplant status
Z78 Other specified health status
Code Z78.1, Physical restraint status, may be used when it is documented by the provider that a patient has been put in restraints during the current encounter. Please note that this code should

not be reported when it is documented by the provider that a patient is temporarily restrained during a procedure.

Z79   Long-term (current) drug therapy

Codes from this category indicate a patient's continuous use of a prescribed drug (including such things as aspirin therapy) for the long-term treatment of a condition or for prophylactic use. It is not for use for patients who have addictions to drugs. This subcategory is not for use of medications for detoxification or maintenance programs to prevent withdrawal symptoms (e.g., methadone maintenance for opiate dependence). Assign the appropriate code for the drug use, abuse, or dependence instead.

Assign a code from Z79 if the patient is receiving a medication for an extended period as a prophylactic measure (such as for the prevention of deep vein thrombosis) or as treatment of a chronic condition (such as arthritis) or a disease requiring a lengthy course of treatment (such as cancer). Do not assign a code from category Z79 for medication being administered for a brief period of time to treat an acute illness or injury (such as a course of antibiotics to treat acute bronchitis).

Z88	Allergy status to drugs, medicaments and biological substances Except: Z88.9, Allergy status to unspecified drugs, medicaments and biological substances status
Z89	Acquired absence of limb
Z90	Acquired absence of organs, not elsewhere classified
Z91.0-	Allergy status, other than to drugs and biological substances
Z92.82	Status post administration of tPA (rtPA) in a different facility within the last 24 hours prior to admission to a current facility Assign code Z92.82, Status post administration of tPA (rtPA) in a different facility within the last 24 hours prior to admission to current facility, as a secondary diagnosis when a patient is received by transfer into a facility and documentation indicates they were administered tissue plasminogen activator (tPA) within the last 24 hours prior to admission to the current facility. This guideline applies even if the patient is still receiving the tPA at the time they are received into the current facility. The appropriate code for the condition for which the tPA was administered (such as cerebrovascular disease or myocardial infarction) should be assigned first. Code Z92.82 is only applicable to the receiving facility record and not to the transferring facility record.
Z93	Artificial opening status
Z94	Transplanted organ and tissue status
Z95	Presence of cardiac and vascular implants and grafts
Z96	Presence of other functional implants

Z97	Presence of other devices
Z98	Other postprocedural states

Assign code Z98.85, Transplanted organ removal status, to indicate that a transplanted organ has been previously removed. This code should not be assigned for the encounter in which the transplanted organ is removed. The complication necessitating removal of the transplant organ should be assigned for that encounter.

See Section I.C.19. for information on the coding of organ transplant complications.

Z99	Dependence on enabling machines and devices, not elsewhere classified

Note: Categories Z89-Z90 and Z93-Z99 are for use only if there are no complications or malfunctions of the organ or tissue replaced, the amputation site or the equipment on which the patient is dependent.

4) History (of)

There are two types of history Z codes, personal and family. Personal history codes explain a patient's past medical condition that no longer exists and is not receiving any treatment, but that has the potential for recurrence, and therefore may require continued monitoring.

Family history codes are for use when a patient has a family member(s) who has had a particular disease that causes the patient to be at higher risk of also contracting the disease.

Personal history codes may be used in conjunction with follow-up codes and family history codes may be used in conjunction with screening codes to explain the need for a test or procedure. History codes are also acceptable on any medical record regardless of the reason for visit. A history of an illness, even if no longer present, is important information that may alter the type of treatment ordered.

The reason for the encounter (for example, screening or counseling) should be sequenced first and the appropriate personal and/or family history code(s) should be assigned as additional diagnos(es).

The history Z code categories are:

Z80	Family history of primary malignant neoplasm
Z81	Family history of mental and behavioral disorders
Z82	Family history of certain disabilities and chronic diseases (leading to disablement)
Z83	Family history of other specific disorders
Z84	Family history of other conditions
Z85	Personal history of malignant neoplasm
Z86	Personal history of certain other diseases
Z87	Personal history of other diseases and conditions
Z91.4-	Personal history of psychological trauma, not elsewhere classified
Z91.5	Personal history of self-harm

Z91.81 History of falling
Z91.82 Personal history of military
        deployment
Z92   Personal history of medical treatment
        Except: Z92.0, Personal history of
        contraception Except: Z92.82, Status
        post administration of tPA (rtPA) in a
        different facility within the last 24 hours
        prior to admission to a current facility

5) Screening

Screening is the testing for disease or disease precursors in seemingly well individuals so that early detection and treatment can be provided for those who test positive for the disease (e.g., screening mammogram).

The testing of a person to rule out or confirm a suspected diagnosis because the patient has some sign or symptom is a diagnostic examination, not a screening. In these cases, the sign or symptom is used to explain the reason for the test.

A screening code may be a first-listed code if the reason for the visit is specifically the screening exam. It may also be used as an additional code if the screening is done during an office visit for other health problems. A screening code is not necessary if the screening is inherent to a routine examination, such as a pap smear done during a routine pelvic examination.

Should a condition be discovered during the screening then the code for the condition may be assigned as an additional diagnosis.

The Z code indicates that a screening exam is planned. A procedure code is required to confirm that the screening was performed.

The screening Z codes/categories:

Z11   Encounter for screening for infectious
        and parasitic diseases
Z12   Encounter for screening for malignant
        neoplasms
Z13   Encounter for screening for other
        diseases and disorders Except: Z13.9,
        Encounter for screening, unspecified
Z36   Encounter for antenatal screening for
        mother

6) Observation

There are three observation Z code categories. They are for use in very limited circumstances when a person is being observed for a suspected condition that is ruled out. The observation codes are not for use if an injury or illness or any signs or symptoms related to the suspected condition are present. In such cases the diagnosis/symptom code is used with the corresponding external cause code.

The observation codes are primarily to be used as a principal/first-listed diagnosis. An observation code may be assigned as a secondary diagnosis code when the patient is being observed for a condition that is ruled out and is unrelated to the principal/first-listed diagnosis (e.g., patient presents for treatment following injuries sustained in a motor vehicle accident and is also observed for suspected COVID-19 infection that is subsequently

ruled out). Also, when the principal diagnosis is required to be a code from category Z38, Liveborn infants according to place of birth and type of delivery, then a code from category Z05, Encounter for observation and evaluation of newborn for suspected diseases and conditions ruled out, is sequenced after the Z38 code. Additional codes may be used in addition to the observation code, but only if they are unrelated to the suspected condition being observed.

Codes from subcategory Z03.7 Encounter for suspected maternal and fetal conditions ruled out, may either be used as a first-listed or as an additional code assignment depending on the case. They are for use in very limited circumstances on a maternal record when an encounter is for a suspected maternal or fetal condition that is ruled out during that encounter (for example, a maternal or fetal condition may be suspected due to an abnormal test result). These codes should not be used when the condition is confirmed. In those cases, the confirmed condition should be coded. In addition, these codes are not for use if an illness or any signs or symptoms related to the suspected condition or problem are present. In such cases the diagnosis/symptom code is used.

Additional codes may be used in addition to the code from subcategory Z03.7, but only if they are unrelated to the suspected condition being evaluated.

Codes from subcategory Z03.7 may not be used for encounters for antenatal screening of mother. *See Section I.C.21. Screening.*

For encounters for suspected fetal condition that are inconclusive following testing and evaluation, assign the appropriate code from category O35, O36, O40 or O41.

The observation Z code categories:

Z03   Encounter for medical observation for
        suspected diseases and conditions ruled
        out
Z04   Encounter for examination and
        observation for other reasons Except:
        Z04.9, Encounter for examination and
        observation for unspecified reason
Z05   Encounter for observation and
        evaluation of newborn for suspected
        diseases and conditions ruled out

7) Aftercare

Aftercare visit codes cover situations when the initial treatment of a disease has been performed and the patient requires continued care during the healing or recovery phase, or for the long-term consequences of the disease. The aftercare Z code should not be used if treatment is directed at a current, acute disease. The diagnosis code is to be used in these cases.

Exceptions to this rule are codes Z51.0, Encounter for antineoplastic radiation therapy, and codes from subcategory Z51.1, Encounter for antineoplastic chemotherapy and immunotherapy. These codes are to be first-listed, followed by the

diagnosis code when a patient's encounter is solely to receive radiation therapy, chemotherapy, or immunotherapy for the treatment of a neoplasm. If the reason for the encounter is more than one type of antineoplastic therapy, code Z51.0 and a code from subcategory Z51.1 may be assigned together, in which case one of these codes would be reported as a secondary diagnosis.

The aftercare Z codes should also not be used for aftercare for injuries. For aftercare of an injury, assign the acute injury code with the appropriate 7th character (for subsequent encounter).

The aftercare codes are generally first-listed to explain the specific reason for the encounter. An aftercare code may be used as an additional code when some type of aftercare is provided in addition to the reason for admission and no diagnosis code is applicable. An example of this would be the closure of a colostomy during an encounter for treatment of another condition.

Aftercare codes should be used in conjunction with other aftercare codes or diagnosis codes to provide better detail on the specifics of an aftercare encounter visit, unless otherwise directed by the classification. The sequencing of multiple aftercare codes depends on the circumstances of the encounter.

Certain aftercare Z code categories need a secondary diagnosis code to describe the resolving condition or sequelae. For others, the condition is included in the code title.

Additional Z code aftercare category terms include fitting and adjustment, and attention to artificial openings.

Status Z codes may be used with aftercare Z codes to indicate the nature of the aftercare. For example code Z95.1, Presence of aortocoronary bypass graft, may be used with code Z48.812, Encounter for surgical aftercare following surgery on the circulatory system, to indicate the surgery for which the aftercare is being performed. A status code should not be used when the aftercare code indicates the type of status, such as using Z43.0, Encounter for attention to tracheostomy, with Z93.0, Tracheostomy status.

The aftercare Z category/codes:

Z42   Encounter for plastic and reconstructive surgery following medical procedure or healed injury
Z43   Encounter for attention to artificial openings
Z44   Encounter for fitting and adjustment of external prosthetic device
Z45   Encounter for adjustment and management of implanted device
Z46   Encounter for fitting and adjustment of other devices
Z47   Orthopedic aftercare
Z48   Encounter for other postprocedural aftercare
Z49   Encounter for care involving renal dialysis

Z51   Encounter for other aftercare and medical care

8) Follow-up
The follow-up codes are used to explain continuing surveillance following completed treatment of a disease, condition, or injury. They imply that the condition has been fully treated and no longer exists. They should not be confused with aftercare codes, or injury codes with a 7th character for subsequent encounter, that explain ongoing care of a healing condition or its sequelae. Follow-up codes may be used in conjunction with history codes to provide the full picture of the healed condition and its treatment. The follow-up code is sequenced first, followed by the history code.

A follow-up code may be used to explain multiple visits. Should a condition be found to have recurred on the follow-up visit, then the diagnosis code for the condition should be assigned in place of the follow-up code.

The follow-up Z code categories:

Z08   Encounter for follow-up examination after completed treatment for malignant neoplasm
Z09   Encounter for follow-up examination after completed treatment for conditions other than malignant neoplasm
Z39   Encounter for maternal postpartum care and examination

9) Donor
Codes in category Z52, Donors of organs and tissues, are used for living individuals who are donating blood or other body tissue. These codes are only for individuals donating for others, **as well as** not for self-donations. They are not used to identify cadaveric donations.

10) Counseling
Counseling Z codes are used when a patient or family member receives assistance in the aftermath of an illness or injury, or when support is required in coping with family or social problems.

The counseling Z codes/categories:

Z30.0-   Encounter for general counseling and advice on contraception
Z31.5   Encounter for procreative genetic counseling
Z31.6-   Encounter for general counseling and advice on procreation
Z32.2   Encounter for childbirth instruction
Z32.3   Encounter for childcare instruction
Z69   Encounter for mental health services for victim and perpetrator of abuse
Z70   Counseling related to sexual attitude, behavior and orientation
Z71   Persons encountering health services for other counseling and medical advice, not elsewhere classified
        Note: Code Z71.84, Encounter for health counseling related to travel, is to be used for health risk and safety counseling for future travel purposes.

Code Z71.85, Encounter for immunization safety counseling, is to be used for counseling of the patient or caregiver regarding the safety of a vaccine. This code should not be used for the provision of general information regarding risks and potential side effects during routine encounters for the administration of vaccines.

Z76.81 Expectant mother prebirth pediatrician visit

11) Encounters for Obstetrical and Reproductive Services

See Section I.C.15. Pregnancy, childbirth, and the puerperium, for further instruction on the use of these codes.

Z codes for pregnancy are for use in those circumstances when none of the problems or complications included in the codes from the Obstetrics chapter exist (a routine prenatal visit or postpartum care). Codes in category Z34, Encounter for supervision of normal pregnancy, are always first listed and are not to be used with any other code from the OB chapter.

Codes in category Z3A, Weeks of gestation, may be assigned to provide additional information about the pregnancy. Category Z3A codes should not be assigned for pregnancies with abortive outcomes (categories O00-O08), elective termination of pregnancy (code Z33.2), nor for postpartum conditions, as category Z3A is not applicable to these conditions. The date of the admission should be used to determine weeks of gestation for inpatient admissions that encompass more than one gestational week.

The outcome of delivery, category Z37, should be included on all maternal delivery records. It is always a secondary code. Codes in category Z37 should not be used on the newborn record.

Z codes for family planning (contraceptive) or procreative management and counseling should be included on an obstetric record either during the pregnancy or the postpartum stage, if applicable.

Z codes/categories for obstetrical and reproductive services:

Z30   Encounter for contraceptive management
Z31   Encounter for procreative management
Z32.2 Encounter for childbirth instruction
Z32.3 Encounter for childcare instruction
Z33   Pregnant state
Z34   Encounter for supervision of normal pregnancy
Z36   Encounter for antenatal screening of mother
Z3A   Weeks of gestation
Z37   Outcome of delivery
Z39   Encounter for maternal postpartum care and examination
Z76.81 Expectant mother prebirth pediatrician visit

12) Newborns and Infants

See Section I.C.16. Newborn (Perinatal) guidelines, for further instruction on the use of these codes.

Newborn Z codes/categories:

Z76.1 Encounter for health supervision and care of foundling
Z00.1- Encounter for routine child health examination
Z38   Liveborn infants according to place of birth and type of delivery

13) Routine and Administrative Examinations

The Z codes allow for the description of encounters for routine examinations, such as, a general check-up, or, examinations for administrative purposes, such as, a pre-employment physical. The codes are not to be used if the examination is for diagnosis of a suspected condition or for treatment purposes. In such cases the diagnosis code is used. During a routine exam, should a diagnosis or condition be discovered, it should be coded as an additional code. Pre-existing and chronic conditions and history codes may also be included as additional codes as long as the examination is for administrative purposes and not focused on any particular condition.

Some of the codes for routine health examinations distinguish between "with" and "without" abnormal findings. Code assignment depends on the information that is known at the time the encounter is being coded. For example, if no abnormal findings were found during the examination, but the encounter is being coded before test results are back, it is acceptable to assign the code for "without abnormal findings." When assigning a code for "with abnormal findings," additional code(s) should be assigned to identify the specific abnormal finding(s).

Pre-operative examination and pre-procedural laboratory examination Z codes are for use only in those situations when a patient is being cleared for a procedure or surgery and no treatment is given.

The Z codes/categories for routine and administrative examinations:

Z00   Encounter for general examination without complaint, suspected or reported diagnosis
Z01   Encounter for other special examination without complaint, suspected or reported diagnosis
Z02   Encounter for administrative examination
      Except: Z02.9, Encounter for administrative examinations, unspecified
Z32.0- Encounter for pregnancy test

14) Miscellaneous Z Codes

The miscellaneous Z codes capture a number of other health care encounters that do not fall into one of the other categories. Certain of these codes identify the reason for the encounter; others are for use as additional codes that provide useful information on circumstances that may affect a patient's care and treatment.

Prophylactic Organ Removal

For encounters specifically for prophylactic removal of an organ (such as prophylactic removal of breasts due to a genetic susceptibility to cancer or a family history of cancer), the principal or first-listed code should be a code from category Z40, Encounter for prophylactic surgery, followed by the appropriate codes to identify the associated risk factor (such as genetic susceptibility or family history).

If the patient has a malignancy of one site and is having prophylactic removal at another site to prevent either a new primary malignancy or metastatic disease, a code for the malignancy should also be assigned in addition to a code from subcategory Z40.0, Encounter for prophylactic surgery for risk factors related to malignant neoplasms. A Z40.0 code should not be assigned if the patient is having organ removal for treatment of a malignancy, such as the removal of the testes for the treatment of prostate cancer.

Miscellaneous Z codes/categories:

Z28	Immunization not carried out Except: Z28.3, Underimmunization status
Z29	Encounter for other prophylactic measures
Z40	Encounter for prophylactic surgery
Z41	Encounter for procedures for purposes other than remedying health state Except: Z41.9, Encounter for procedure for purposes other than remedying health state, unspecified
Z53	Persons encountering health services for specific procedures and treatment, not carried out
Z55	Problems related to education and literacy
Z56	Problems related to employment and unemployment
Z57	Occupational exposure to risk factors
Z58	Problems related to physical environment
Z59	Problems related to housing and economic circumstances
Z60	Problems related to social environment
Z62	Problems related to upbringing
Z63	Other problems related to primary support group, including family circumstances
Z64	Problems related to certain psychosocial circumstances
Z65	Problems related to other psychosocial circumstances
Z72	Problems related to lifestyle Note: These codes should be assigned only when the documentation specifies that the patient has an associated problem
Z73	Problems related to life management difficulty
Z74	Problems related to care provider dependency Except: Z74.01, Bed confinement status
Z75	Problems related to medical facilities and other health care
Z76.0	Encounter for issue of repeat prescription
Z76.3	Healthy person accompanying sick person
Z76.4	Other boarder to healthcare facility
Z76.5	Malingerer [conscious simulation]
Z91.1-	Patient's noncompliance with medical treatment and regimen
Z91.83	Wandering in diseases classified elsewhere
Z91.84-	Oral health risk factors
Z91.89	Other specified personal risk factors, not elsewhere classified

See Section I.B.14 for Z55-Z65 Persons with potential health hazards related to socioeconomic and psychosocial circumstances, documentation by clinicians other than the patient's provider

15) Nonspecific Z Codes

Certain Z codes are so non-specific, or potentially redundant with other codes in the classification, that there can be little justification for their use in the inpatient setting. Their use in the outpatient setting should be limited to those instances when there is no further documentation to permit more precise coding. Otherwise, any sign or symptom or any other reason for visit that is captured in another code should be used.

Nonspecific Z codes/categories:

Z02.9	Encounter for administrative examinations, unspecified
Z04.9	Encounter for examination and observation for unspecified reason
Z13.9	Encounter for screening, unspecified
Z41.9	Encounter for procedure for purposes other than remedying health state, unspecified
Z52.9	Donor of unspecified organ or tissue
Z86.59	Personal history of other mental and behavioral disorders
Z88.9	Allergy status to unspecified drugs, medicaments and biological substances status
Z92.0	Personal history of contraception

16) Z Codes That May Only be Principal/First-Listed Diagnosis

The following Z codes/categories may only be reported as the principal/first-listed diagnosis, except when there are multiple encounters on the same day and the medical records for the encounters are combined:

Z00	Encounter for general examination without complaint, suspected or reported diagnosis Except: Z00.6
Z01	Encounter for other special examination without complaint, suspected or reported diagnosis
Z02	Encounter for administrative examination
Z04	Encounter for examination and observation for other reasons
Z33.2	Encounter for elective termination of pregnancy

Z31.81 Encounter for male factor infertility in female patient

Z31.83 Encounter for assisted reproductive fertility procedure cycle

Z31.84 Encounter for fertility preservation procedure

Z34 Encounter for supervision of normal pregnancy

Z39 Encounter for maternal postpartum care and examination

Z38 Liveborn infants according to place of birth and type of delivery

Z40 Encounter for prophylactic surgery

Z42 Encounter for plastic and reconstructive surgery following medical procedure or healed injury

Z51.0 Encounter for antineoplastic radiation therapy

Z51.1- Encounter for antineoplastic chemotherapy and immunotherapy

Z52 Donors of organs and tissues Except: Z52.9, Donor of unspecified organ or tissue

Z76.1 Encounter for health supervision and care of foundling

Z76.2 Encounter for health supervision and care of other healthy infant and child

Z99.12 Encounter for respirator [ventilator] dependence during power failure

17) Social Determinants of Health
Codes describing social determinants of health (SDOH) should be assigned when this information is documented.

For social determinants of health, such as information found in categories Z55-Z65, Persons with potential health hazards related to socioeconomic and psychosocial circumstances, code assignment may be based on medical record documentation from clinicians involved in the care of the patient who are not the patient's provider since this information represents social information, rather than medical diagnoses.

For example, coding professionals may utilize documentation of social information from social workers, community health workers, case managers, or nurses, if their documentation is included in the official medical record.

Patient self-reported documentation may be used to assign codes for social determinants of health, as long as the patient self-reported information is signed-off by and incorporated into the medical record by either a clinician or provider.

Social determinants of health codes are located primarily in these Z code categories:

Z55 **Problems related to education and literacy**

Z56 **Problems related to employment and unemployment**

Z57 **Occupational exposure to risk factors**

Z58 **Problems related to physical environment**

Z59 **Problems related to housing and economic circumstances**

Z60 **Problems related to social environment**

Z62 **Problems related to upbringing**

Z63 **Other problems related to primary support group, including family circumstances**

Z64 **Problems related to certain psychosocial circumstances**

Z65 **Problems related to other psychosocial circumstances**

See Section I.B.14. Documentation by Clinicians Other than the Patient's Provider.

22. *Chapter 22: Codes for Special Purposes (U00-U85)*

U07.0 Vaping-related disorder (see Section I.C.10.e., Vaping-related disorders)

U07.1 COVID-19 (see Section I.C.1.g.1., COVID-19 infection)

U09.9 **Post COVID-19 condition, unspecified (see Section I.C.1.g.1.m)**

Section II. Selection of Principal Diagnosis

The circumstances of inpatient admission always govern the selection of principal diagnosis. The principal diagnosis is defined in the Uniform Hospital Discharge Data Set (UHDDS) as "that condition established after study to be chiefly responsible for occasioning the admission of the patient to the hospital for care."

The UHDDS definitions are used by hospitals to report inpatient data elements in a standardized manner. These data elements and their definitions can be found in the July 31, 1985, Federal Register (Vol. 50, No, 147), pp. 31038-40.

Since that time, the application of the UHDDS definitions has been expanded to include all nonoutpatient settings (acute care, short term, long term care and psychiatric hospitals; home health agencies; rehab facilities; nursing homes, etc...). The UHDDS definitions also apply to hospice services (all levels of care).

In determining principal diagnosis, coding conventions in the ICD-10-CM, the Tabular List and Alphabetic Index take precedence over these official coding guidelines. *(See Section I.A., Conventions for the ICD-10-CM)*

The importance of consistent, complete documentation in the medical record cannot be overemphasized. Without such documentation the application of all coding guidelines is a difficult, if not impossible, task.

A. **Codes for symptoms, signs, and ill-defined conditions**
   Codes for symptoms, signs, and ill-defined conditions from Chapter 18 are not to be used as principal diagnosis when a related definitive diagnosis has been established.

B. **Two or more interrelated conditions, each potentially meeting the definition for principal diagnosis.**
   When there are two or more interrelated conditions (such as diseases in the same ICD-10-CM chapter or manifestations characteristically associated with a certain disease) potentially meeting the definition of principal diagnosis, either condition may be sequenced first, unless the circumstances of the

admission, the therapy provided, the Tabular List, or the Alphabetic Index indicate otherwise.

C. Two or more diagnoses that equally meet the definition for principal diagnosis

In the unusual instance when two or more diagnoses equally meet the criteria for principal diagnosis as determined by the circumstances of admission, diagnostic workup and/or therapy provided, and the Alphabetic Index, Tabular List, or another coding guidelines does not provide sequencing direction, any one of the diagnoses may be sequenced first.

D. Two or more comparative or contrasting conditions.

In those rare instances when two or more contrasting or comparative diagnoses are documented as "either/or" (or similar terminology), they are coded as if the diagnoses were confirmed and the diagnoses are sequenced according to the circumstances of the admission. If no further determination can be made as to which diagnosis should be principal, either diagnosis may be sequenced first.

E. A symptom(s) followed by contrasting/ comparative diagnoses

GUIDELINE HAS BEEN DELETED EFFECTIVE OCTOBER 1, 2014

F. Original treatment plan not carried out

Sequence as the principal diagnosis the condition, which after study occasioned the admission to the hospital, even though treatment may not have been carried out due to unforeseen circumstances.

G. Complications of surgery and other medical care

When the admission is for treatment of a complication resulting from surgery or other medical care, the complication code is sequenced as the principal diagnosis. If the complication is classified to the T80-T88 series and the code lacks the necessary specificity in describing the complication, an additional code for the specific complication should be assigned.

H. Uncertain Diagnosis

If the diagnosis documented at the time of discharge is qualified as "probable," "suspected," "likely," "questionable," "possible," or "still to be ruled out," "compatible with," "consistent with," or other similar terms indicating uncertainty, code the condition as if it existed or was established. The bases for these guidelines are the diagnostic workup, arrangements for further workup or observation, and initial therapeutic approach that correspond most closely with the established diagnosis.

Note: This guideline is applicable only to inpatient admissions to short-term, acute, long-term care and psychiatric hospitals.

I. Admission from Observation Unit

1. Admission Following Medical Observation

When a patient is admitted to an observation unit for a medical condition, which either worsens or does not improve, and is subsequently admitted as an inpatient of the same hospital for this same medical condition, the principal diagnosis would be the medical condition which led to the hospital admission.

2. Admission Following Post-Operative Observation

When a patient is admitted to an observation unit to monitor a condition (or complication) that develops following outpatient surgery, and then is subsequently admitted as an inpatient of the same hospital, hospitals should apply the Uniform Hospital Discharge Data Set (UHDDS) definition of principal diagnosis as "that condition established after study to be chiefly responsible for occasioning the admission of the patient to the hospital for care."

J. Admission from Outpatient Surgery

When a patient receives surgery in the hospital's outpatient surgery department and is subsequently admitted for continuing inpatient care at the same hospital, the following guidelines should be followed in selecting the principal diagnosis for the inpatient admission:

- If the reason for the inpatient admission is a complication, assign the complication as the principal diagnosis.
- If no complication, or other condition, is documented as the reason for the inpatient admission, assign the reason for the outpatient surgery as the principal diagnosis.
- If the reason for the inpatient admission is another condition unrelated to the surgery, assign the unrelated condition as the principal diagnosis.

K. Admissions/Encounters for Rehabilitation

When the purpose for the admission/encounter is rehabilitation, sequence first the code for the condition for which the service is being performed. For example, for an admission/encounter for rehabilitation for right-sided dominant hemiplegia following a cerebrovascular infarction, report code I69.351, Hemiplegia and hemiparesis following cerebral infarction affecting right dominant side, as the first-listed or principal diagnosis.

If the condition for which the rehabilitation service is no longer present, report the appropriate aftercare code as the first-listed or principal diagnosis, unless the rehabilitation service is being provided following an injury. For rehabilitation services following active treatment of an injury, assign the injury code with the appropriate seventh character for subsequent encounter as the first-listed or principal diagnosis. For example, if a patient with severe degenerative osteoarthritis of the hip, underwent hip replacement and the current encounter/admission is for rehabilitation, report code Z47.1, Aftercare following joint replacement surgery, as the first-listed or principal diagnosis. If the patient requires rehabilitation post hip replacement for right intertrochanteric femur fracture, report code S72.141D, Displaced intertrochanteric fracture of right femur, subsequent encounter for closed fracture with routine healing, as the first-listed or principal diagnosis.

See Section I.C.21.c.7, Factors influencing health states and contact with health services, Aftercare.
See Section I.C.19.a, for additional information about the use of 7th characters for injury codes.

Section III. Reporting Additional Diagnoses

GENERAL RULES FOR OTHER (ADDITIONAL) DIAGNOSES

For reporting purposes the definition for "other diagnoses" is interpreted as additional conditions that affect patient care in terms of requiring:

clinical evaluation; or
therapeutic treatment; or
diagnostic procedures; or
extended length of hospital stay; or
increased nursing care and/or monitoring.

The UHDDS item #11-b defines Other Diagnoses as "all conditions that coexist at the time of admission, that develop subsequently, or that affect the treatment received and/or the length of stay. Diagnoses that relate to an earlier episode which have no bearing on the current hospital stay are to be excluded." UHDDS definitions apply to inpatients in acute care, short-term, long term care and psychiatric hospital setting. The UHDDS definitions are used by acute care short-term hospitals to report inpatient data elements in a standardized manner. These data elements and their definitions can be found in the July 31, 1985, Federal Register (Vol. 50, No, 147), pp. 31038-40.

Since that time, the application of the UHDDS definitions has been expanded to include all nonoutpatient settings (acute care, short term, long term care and psychiatric hospitals; home health agencies; rehab facilities; nursing homes, etc. . .). The UHDDS definitions also apply to hospice services (all levels of care).

The following guidelines are to be applied in designating "other diagnoses" when neither the Alphabetic Index nor the Tabular List in ICD-10-CM provide direction. The listing of the diagnoses in the patient record is the responsibility of the attending provider.

A. Previous conditions

If the provider has included a diagnosis in the final diagnostic statement, such as the discharge summary or the face sheet, it should ordinarily be coded. Some providers include in the diagnostic statement resolved conditions or diagnoses and status-post procedures from previous admissions that have no bearing on the current stay. Such conditions are not to be reported and are coded only if required by hospital policy.

However, history codes (categories Z80-Z87) may be used as secondary codes if the historical condition or family history has an impact on current care or influences treatment.

B. Abnormal findings

Abnormal findings (laboratory, x-ray, pathologic, and other diagnostic results) are not coded and reported unless the provider indicates their clinical significance. If the findings are outside the normal range and the attending provider has ordered other tests to evaluate the condition or prescribed treatment, it is appropriate to ask the provider whether the abnormal finding should be added.

Please note: This differs from the coding practices in the outpatient setting for coding encounters for diagnostic tests that have been interpreted by a provider.

C. Uncertain Diagnosis

If the diagnosis documented at the time of discharge is qualified as "probable," "suspected," "likely," "questionable," "possible," or "still to be ruled out," "compatible with," "consistent with," or other similar terms indicating uncertainty, code the condition as if it existed or was established. The bases for these guidelines are the diagnostic workup, arrangements for further workup or observation, and initial therapeutic approach that correspond most closely with the established diagnosis.

Note: This guideline is applicable only to inpatient admissions to short-term, acute, long-term care and psychiatric hospitals.

Section IV. Diagnostic Coding and Reporting Guidelines for Outpatient Services

These coding guidelines for outpatient diagnoses have been approved for use by hospitals/ providers in coding and reporting hospital-based outpatient services and provider-based office visits. Guidelines in Section I, Conventions, general coding guidelines and chapter-specific guidelines, should also be applied for outpatient services and office visits.

Information about the use of certain abbreviations, punctuation, symbols, and other conventions used in the ICD-10-CM Tabular List (code numbers and titles), can be found in Section IA of these guidelines, under "Conventions Used in the Tabular List." Section I.B. contains general guidelines that apply to the entire classification. Section I.C. contains chapter-specific guidelines that correspond to the chapters as they are arranged in the classification. Information about the correct sequence to use in finding a code is also described in Section I.

The terms encounter and visit are often used interchangeably in describing outpatient service contacts and, therefore, appear together in these guidelines without distinguishing one from the other.

Though the conventions and general guidelines apply to all settings, coding guidelines for outpatient and provider reporting of diagnoses will vary in a number of instances from those for inpatient diagnoses, recognizing that:

The Uniform Hospital Discharge Data Set (UHDDS) definition of principal diagnosis does not apply to hospital-based outpatient services and provider-based office visits.

Coding guidelines for inconclusive diagnoses (probable, suspected, rule out, etc.) were developed for inpatient reporting and do not apply to outpatients.

A. Selection of first-listed condition

In the outpatient setting, the term first-listed diagnosis is used in lieu of principal diagnosis.

In determining the first-listed diagnosis the coding conventions of ICD-10-CM, as well as the

general and disease specific guidelines take precedence over the outpatient guidelines.

Diagnoses often are not established at the time of the initial encounter/visit. It may take two or more visits before the diagnosis is confirmed.

The most critical rule involves beginning the search for the correct code assignment through the Alphabetic Index. Never begin searching initially in the Tabular List as this will lead to coding errors.

1. Outpatient Surgery

When a patient presents for outpatient surgery (same day surgery), code the reason for the surgery as the first-listed diagnosis (reason for the encounter), even if the surgery is not performed due to a contraindication.

2. Observation Stay

When a patient is admitted for observation for a medical condition, assign a code for the medical condition as the first-listed diagnosis.

When a patient presents for outpatient surgery and develops complications requiring admission to observation, code the reason for the surgery as the first reported diagnosis (reason for the encounter), followed by codes for the complications as secondary diagnoses.

B. Codes from A00.0 through T88.9, Z00-Z99, U00-U85

The appropriate code(s) from A00.0 through T88.9, Z00-Z99, **and U00-U85** must be used to identify diagnoses, symptoms, conditions, problems, complaints, or other reason(s) for the encounter/visit.

C. Accurate reporting of ICD-10-CM diagnosis codes

For accurate reporting of ICD-10-CM diagnosis codes, the documentation should describe the patient's condition, using terminology which includes specific diagnoses as well as symptoms, problems, or reasons for the encounter. There are ICD-10-CM codes to describe all of these.

D. Codes that describe symptoms and signs

Codes that describe symptoms and signs, as opposed to diagnoses, are acceptable for reporting purposes when a diagnosis has not been established (confirmed) by the provider. Chapter 18 of ICD-10-CM, Symptoms, Signs, and Abnormal Clinical and Laboratory Findings Not Elsewhere Classified (codes R00-R99) contains many, but not all codes for symptoms.

E. Encounters for circumstances other than a disease or injury

ICD-10-CM provides codes to deal with encounters for circumstances other than a disease or injury. The Factors Influencing Health Status and Contact with Health Services codes (Z00-Z99) are provided to deal with occasions when circumstances other than a disease or injury are recorded as diagnosis or problems.

See Section I.C.21., Factors influencing health status and contact with health services.

F. Level of Detail in Coding

1. ICD-10-CM codes with 3, 4, 5, 6 or 7 characters

ICD-10-CM is composed of codes with 3, 4, 5, 6 or 7 characters. Codes with three characters are included in ICD-10-CM as the heading of a category of codes that may be further subdivided by the use of 4th, 5th, 6th or 7th characters to provide greater specificity.

2. Use of full number of characters required for a code

A 3-character code is to be used only if it is not further subdivided. A code is invalid if it has not been coded to the full number of characters required for that code, including the 7th character, if applicable.

3. Highest level of specificity

Code to the highest level of specificity when supported by the medical record documentation.

G. ICD-10-CM code for the diagnosis, condition, problem, or other reason for encounter/visit

List first the ICD-10-CM code for the diagnosis, condition, problem, or other reason for encounter/visit shown in the medical record to be chiefly responsible for the services provided. List additional codes that describe any coexisting conditions. In some cases the first-listed diagnosis may be a symptom when a diagnosis has not been established (confirmed) by the provider.

H. Uncertain diagnosis

Do not code diagnoses documented as "probable," "suspected," "questionable," "ruled out," "compatible with," "consistent with," or "working diagnosis" or other similar terms indicating uncertainty. Rather, code the condition(s) to the highest degree of certainty for that encounter/visit, such as symptoms, signs, abnormal test results, or other reason for the visit.

Please note: This differs from the coding practices used by short-term, acute care, long-term care and psychiatric hospitals.

I. Chronic diseases

Chronic diseases treated on an ongoing basis may be coded and reported as many times as the patient receives treatment and care for the condition(s)

J. Code all documented conditions that coexist

Code all documented conditions that coexist at the time of the encounter/visit, and require or affect patient care treatment or management. Do not code conditions that were previously treated and no longer exist. However, history codes (categories Z80-Z87) may be used as secondary codes if the historical condition or family history has an impact on current care or influences treatment.

K. Patients receiving diagnostic services only

For patients receiving diagnostic services only during an encounter/visit, sequence first the diagnosis, condition, problem, or other reason for encounter/visit shown in the medical record to be chiefly responsible for the outpatient services provided during the encounter/visit. Codes for other diagnoses (e.g., chronic conditions) may be sequenced as additional diagnoses.

For encounters for routine laboratory/radiology testing in the absence of any signs, symptoms, or associated diagnosis, assign Z01.89, Encounter for other specified special examinations. If routine testing is performed during the same encounter as a test to evaluate a sign, symptom, or diagnosis, it is appropriate to assign both the Z code and the code describing the reason for the non-routine test.

For outpatient encounters for diagnostic tests that have been interpreted by a physician, and the final report is available at the time of coding, code any confirmed or definitive diagnosis(es) documented in the interpretation. Do not code related signs and symptoms as additional diagnoses.

Please note: This differs from the coding practice in the hospital inpatient setting regarding abnormal findings on test results.

L. Patients receiving therapeutic services only

For patients receiving therapeutic services only during an encounter/visit, sequence first the diagnosis, condition, problem, or other reason for encounter/visit shown in the medical record to be chiefly responsible for the outpatient services provided during the encounter/visit. Codes for other diagnoses (e.g., chronic conditions) may be sequenced as additional diagnoses.

The only exception to this rule is that when the primary reason for the admission/encounter is chemotherapy or radiation therapy, the appropriate Z code for the service is listed first, and the diagnosis or problem for which the service is being performed listed second.

M. Patients receiving preoperative evaluations only

For patients receiving preoperative evaluations only, sequence first a code from subcategory Z01.81, Encounter for pre-procedural examinations, to describe the pre-op consultations. Assign a code for the condition to describe the reason for the surgery as an additional diagnosis. Code also any findings related to the pre-op evaluation.

N. Ambulatory surgery

For ambulatory surgery, code the diagnosis for which the surgery was performed. If the postoperative diagnosis is known to be different from the preoperative diagnosis at the time the diagnosis is confirmed, select the postoperative diagnosis for coding, since it is the most definitive.

O. Routine outpatient prenatal visits

See Section I.C.15., Routine outpatient prenatal visits.

P. Encounters for general medical examinations with abnormal findings

The subcategories for encounters for general medical examinations, Z00.0- and encounter for routine child health examination, Z00.12-, provide codes for with and without abnormal findings. Should a general medical examination result in an abnormal finding, the code for general medical examination with abnormal finding should be assigned as the first-listed diagnosis. An examination with abnormal findings refers to a condition/diagnosis that is newly identified or a change in severity of a chronic condition (such as uncontrolled hypertension, or an acute exacerbation of chronic obstructive pulmonary disease) during a routine physical examination. A secondary code for the abnormal finding should also be coded.

Q. Encounters for routine health screenings

See Section I.C.21., Factors influencing health status and contact with health services, Screening

Appendix I
Present on Admission Reporting Guidelines

Introduction

These guidelines are to be used as a supplement to the *ICD-10-CM Official Guidelines for Coding and Reporting* to facilitate the assignment of the Present on Admission (POA) indicator for each diagnosis and external cause of injury code reported on claim forms (UB-04 and 837 Institutional).

These guidelines are not intended to replace any guidelines in the main body of the *ICD-10-CM Official Guidelines for Coding and Reporting*. The POA guidelines are not intended to provide guidance on when a condition should be coded, but rather, how to apply the POA indicator to the final set of diagnosis codes that have been assigned in accordance with Sections I, II, and III of the official coding guidelines. Subsequent to the assignment of the ICD-10-CM codes, the POA indicator should then be assigned to those conditions that have been coded.

As stated in the Introduction to the ICD-10-CM Official Guidelines for Coding and Reporting, a joint effort between the healthcare provider and the coder is essential to achieve complete and accurate documentation, code assignment, and reporting of diagnoses and procedures. The importance of consistent, complete documentation in the medical record cannot be overemphasized. Medical record documentation from any provider involved in the care and treatment of the patient may be used to support the determination of whether a condition was present on admission or not. In the context of the official coding guidelines, the term "provider" means a physician or any qualified healthcare practitioner who is legally accountable for establishing the patient's diagnosis.

These guidelines are not a substitute for the provider's clinical judgment as to the determination of whether a condition was/was not present on admission. The provider should be queried regarding issues related to the linking of signs/symptoms, timing of test results, and the timing of findings.

Please see the CDC website for the detailed list of ICD-10-CM codes that do not require the use of a POA indicator (https://www.cdc.gov/nchs/icd/icd10cm.htm) (https://www.cms.gov/Medicare/Coding/ICD10/2018-ICD-10-CM-and-GEMs.html). The codes and categories on this exempt list are for circumstances regarding the healthcare encounter or factors influencing health status that do not represent a current disease or injury or that describe conditions that are always present on admission.

General Reporting Requirements

All claims involving inpatient admissions to general acute care hospitals or other facilities that are subject to a law or regulation mandating collection of present on admission information.

Present on admission is defined as present at the time the order for inpatient admission occurs—conditions that develop during an outpatient encounter, including emergency department, observation, or outpatient surgery, are considered as present on admission.

POA indicator is assigned to principal and secondary diagnoses (as defined in Section II of the Official Guidelines for Coding and Reporting) and the external cause of injury codes.

Issues related to inconsistent, missing, conflicting or unclear documentation must still be resolved by the provider.

If a condition would not be coded and reported based on UHDDS definitions and current official coding guidelines, then the POA indicator would not be reported.

Reporting Options

Y - Yes

N - No

U - Unknown

W - Clinically undetermined

Unreported/Not used - (Exempt from POA reporting)

Reporting Definitions

Y = present at the time of inpatient admission

N = not present at the time of inpatient admission

U = documentation is insufficient to determine if condition is present on admission

W = provider is unable to clinically determine whether condition was present on admission or not

Timeframe for POA Identification and Documentation

There is no required timeframe as to when a provider (per the definition of "provider" used in these guidelines) must identify or document a condition to be present on admission. In some clinical situations, it may not be possible for a provider to make a definitive diagnosis (or a condition may not be recognized or reported by the patient) for a period of time after admission. In some cases it may be several days before the provider arrives at a definitive diagnosis. This does not mean that the condition was not present on admission. Determination of whether the condition was present on admission or not will be based on the applicable POA guideline as identified in this document, or on the provider's best clinical judgment.

If at the time of code assignment the documentation is unclear as to whether a condition was present on admission or not, it is appropriate to query the provider for clarification.

Assigning the POA Indicator

Condition is on the "Exempt from Reporting" list

Leave the "present on admission" field blank if the condition is on the list of ICD-10-CM codes for which this field is not applicable. This is the only circumstance in which the field may be left blank.

POA Explicitly Documented

Assign "Y" for any condition the provider explicitly documents as being present on admission.

Assign "N" for any condition the provider explicitly documents as not present at the time of admission.

Conditions diagnosed prior to inpatient admission

Assign "Y" for conditions that were diagnosed prior to admission (example: hypertension, diabetes mellitus, asthma)

Conditions diagnosed during the admission but clearly present before admission

Assign "Y" for conditions diagnosed during the admission that were clearly present but not diagnosed until after admission occurred.

Diagnoses subsequently confirmed after admission are considered present on admission if at the time of admission they are documented as suspected, possible, rule out, differential diagnosis, or constitute an underlying cause of a symptom that is present at the time of admission.

Condition develops during outpatient encounter prior to inpatient admission

Assign "Y" for any condition that develops during an outpatient encounter prior to a written order for inpatient admission.

Documentation does not indicate whether condition was present on admission

Assign "U" when the medical record documentation is unclear as to whether the condition was present on admission. "U" should not be routinely assigned and used only in very limited circumstances. Coders are encouraged to query the providers when the documentation is unclear.

Documentation states that it cannot be determined whether the condition was or was not present on admission

Assign "W" when the medical record documentation indicates that it cannot be clinically determined whether or not the condition was present on admission.

Chronic condition with acute exacerbation during the admission

If a single code identifies both the chronic condition and the acute exacerbation, see POA guidelines pertaining to codes that contain multiple clinical concepts.

If a single code only identifies the chronic condition and not the acute exacerbation (e.g., acute exacerbation of chronic leukemia), assign "Y."

Conditions documented as possible, probable, suspected, or rule out at the time of discharge

If the final diagnosis contains a possible, probable, suspected, or rule out diagnosis, and this diagnosis was based on signs, symptoms or clinical findings suspected at the time of inpatient admission, assign "Y."

If the final diagnosis contains a possible, probable, suspected, or rule out diagnosis, and this diagnosis was based on signs, symptoms or clinical findings that were not present on admission, assign "N".

Conditions documented as impending or threatened at the time of discharge

If the final diagnosis contains an impending or threatened diagnosis, and this diagnosis is based on symptoms or clinical findings that were present on admission, assign "Y".

If the final diagnosis contains an impending or threatened diagnosis, and this diagnosis is based on symptoms or clinical findings that were not present on admission, assign "N".

Acute and Chronic Conditions

Assign "Y" for acute conditions that are present at time of admission and "N" for acute conditions that are not present at time of admission.

Assign "Y" for chronic conditions, even though the condition may not be diagnosed until after admission.

If a single code identifies both an acute and chronic condition, see the POA guidelines for codes that contain multiple clinical concepts.

Codes That Contain Multiple Clinical Concepts

Assign "N" if at least one of the clinical concepts included in the code was not present on admission (e.g., COPD with acute exacerbation and the exacerbation was not present on admission; gastric ulcer that does not start bleeding until after admission; asthma patient develops status asthmaticus after admission).

Assign "Y" if all of the clinical concepts included in the code were present on admission (e.g., duodenal ulcer that perforates prior to admission).

For infection codes that include the causal organism, assign "Y" if the infection (or signs of the infection) were present on admission, even though the culture results may not be known until after admission (e.g., patient is admitted with pneumonia and the provider documents Pseudomonas as the causal organism a few days later).

Same Diagnosis Code for Two or More Conditions

When the same ICD-10-CM diagnosis code applies to two or more conditions during the same encounter (e.g., two separate conditions classified to the same ICD-10-CM diagnosis code):

Assign "Y" if all conditions represented by the single ICD-10-CM code were present on admission (e.g., bilateral unspecified age-related cataracts).

Assign "N" if any of the conditions represented by the single ICD-10-CM code was not present on admission (e.g., traumatic secondary and recurrent hemorrhage and seroma is assigned to a single code T79.2, but only one of the conditions was present on admission).

Obstetrical conditions

Whether or not the patient delivers during the current hospitalization does not affect assignment of the POA indicator. The determining factor for POA assignment is whether the pregnancy complication or obstetrical condition described by the code was present at the time of admission or not.

If the pregnancy complication or obstetrical condition was present on admission (e.g., patient admitted in preterm labor), assign "Y".

If the pregnancy complication or obstetrical condition was not present on admission (e.g., 2nd degree laceration during delivery, postpartum hemorrhage that occurred during current hospitalization, fetal distress develops after admission), assign "N".

If the obstetrical code includes more than one diagnosis and any of the diagnoses identified by the code were not present on admission assign "N".

(e.g., Category O11, Pre-existing hypertension with pre-eclampsia)

Perinatal conditions

Newborns are not considered to be admitted until after birth. Therefore, any condition present at birth or that developed in utero is considered present at admission and should be assigned "Y". This includes conditions that occur during delivery (e.g., injury during delivery, meconium aspiration, exposure to streptococcus B in the vaginal canal).

Congenital conditions and anomalies

Assign "Y" for congenital conditions and anomalies except for categories Q00-Q99, Congenital anomalies, which are on the exempt list. Congenital conditions are always considered present on admission.

External cause of injury codes

Assign "Y" for any external cause code representing an external cause of morbidity that occurred prior to inpatient admission (e.g., patient fell out of bed at home, patient fell out of bed in emergency room prior to admission).

Assign "N" for any external cause code representing an external cause of morbidity that occurred during inpatient hospitalization (e.g., patient fell out of hospital bed during hospital stay, patient experienced an adverse reaction to a medication administered after inpatient admission).

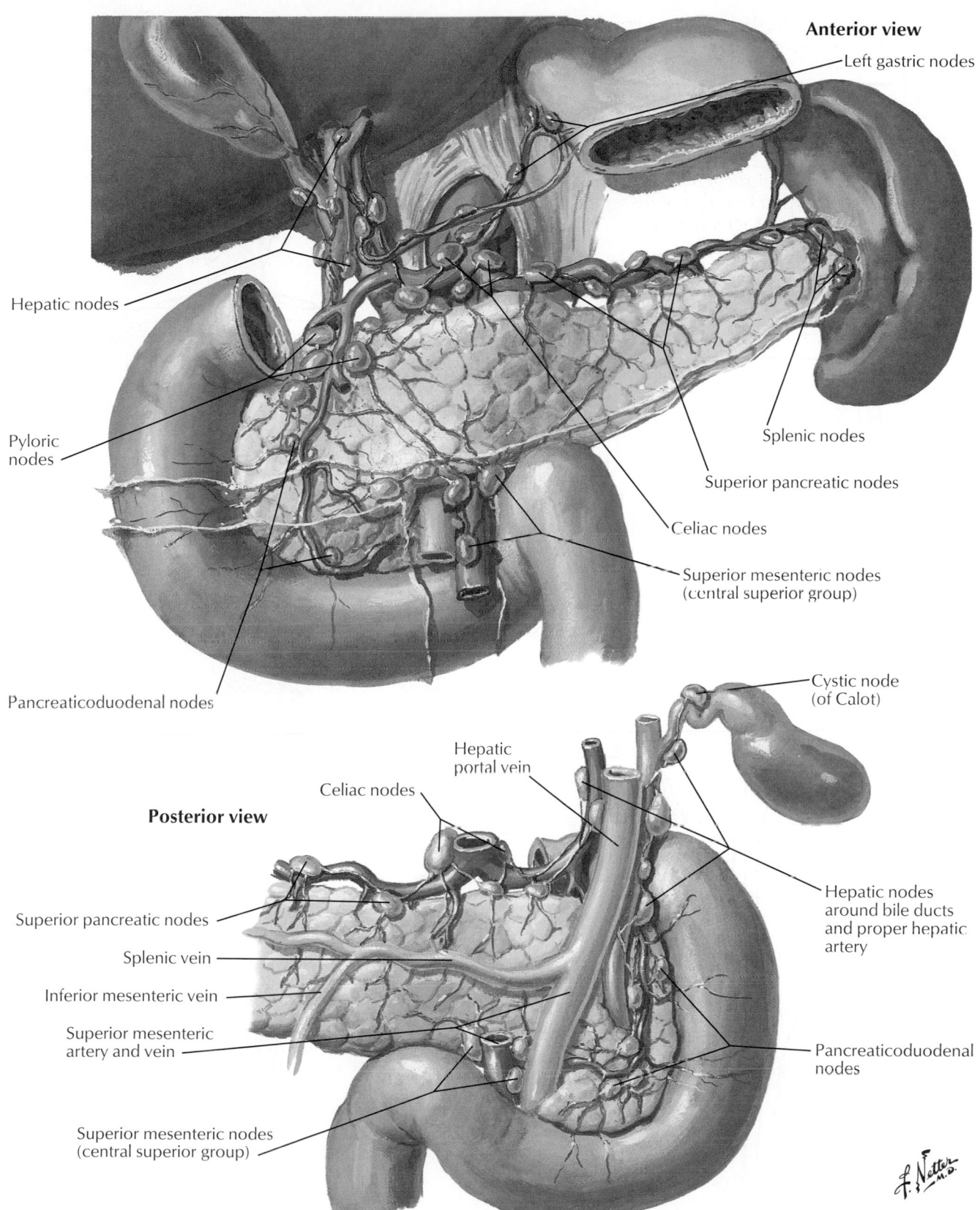

Anterior view

Left gastric nodes

Hepatic nodes

Pyloric nodes

Pancreaticoduodenal nodes

Splenic nodes

Superior pancreatic nodes

Celiac nodes

Superior mesenteric nodes (central superior group)

Cystic node (of Calot)

Hepatic portal vein

Celiac nodes

Posterior view

Superior pancreatic nodes

Splenic vein

Inferior mesenteric vein

Superior mesenteric artery and vein

Superior mesenteric nodes (central superior group)

Hepatic nodes around bile ducts and proper hepatic artery

Pancreaticoduodenal nodes

Plate 1   Lymph Vessels and Nodes of Pancreas. (Netter: Atlas of Human Anatomy, 4 ed, 2006, Saunders. Plate 315)

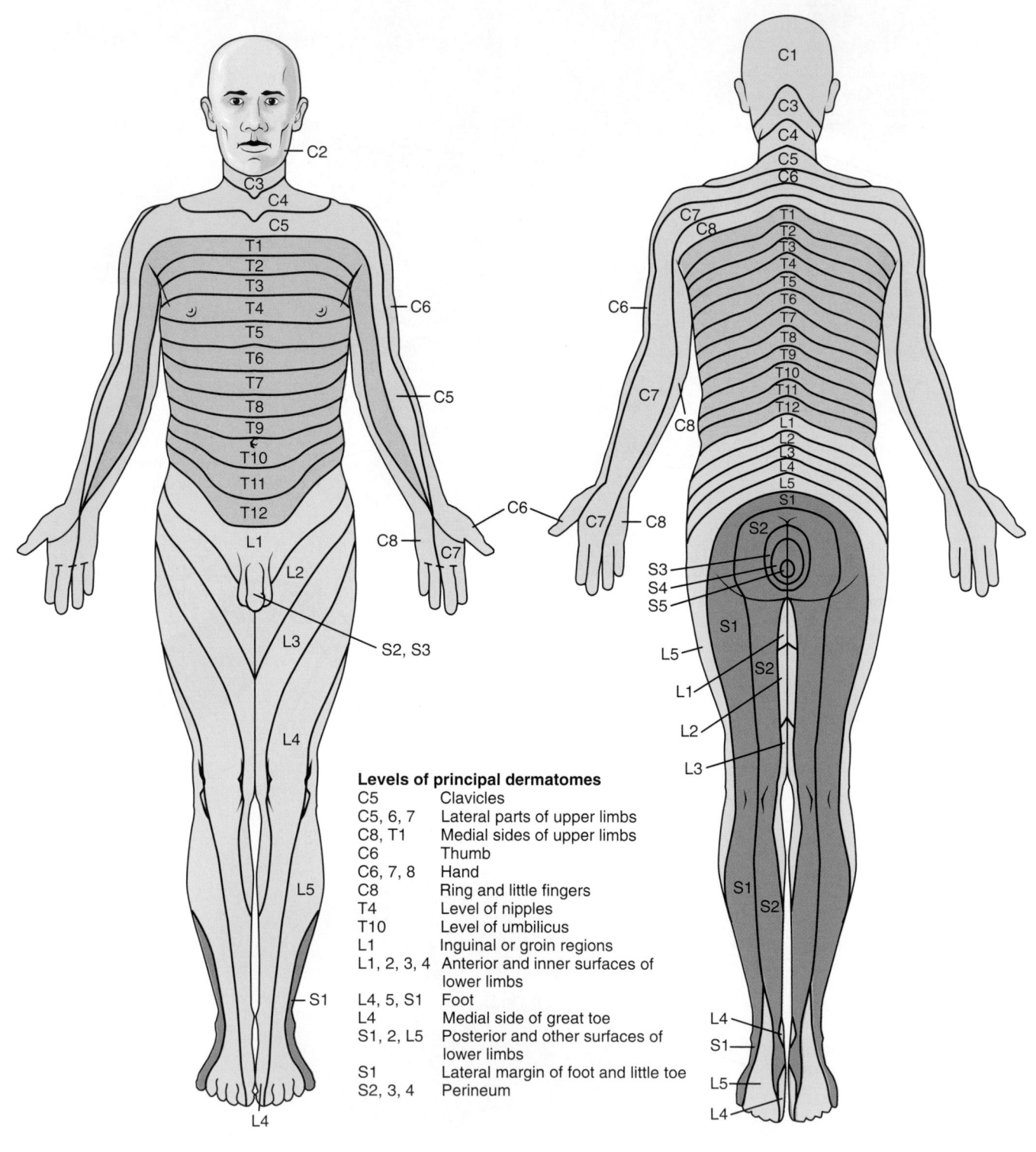

Levels of principal dermatomes

C5	Clavicles
C5, 6, 7	Lateral parts of upper limbs
C8, T1	Medial sides of upper limbs
C6	Thumb
C6, 7, 8	Hand
C8	Ring and little fingers
T4	Level of nipples
T10	Level of umbilicus
L1	Inguinal or groin regions
L1, 2, 3, 4	Anterior and inner surfaces of lower limbs
L4, 5, S1	Foot
L4	Medial side of great toe
S1, 2, L5	Posterior and other surfaces of lower limbs
S1	Lateral margin of foot and little toe
S2, 3, 4	Perineum

Plate 2 Schematic demarcation of Dermatomes. (Miller MD, Hart JA, MacKnight JM: Essential Orthopaedics, ed 2, Philadelphia, 2020, Elsevier.)

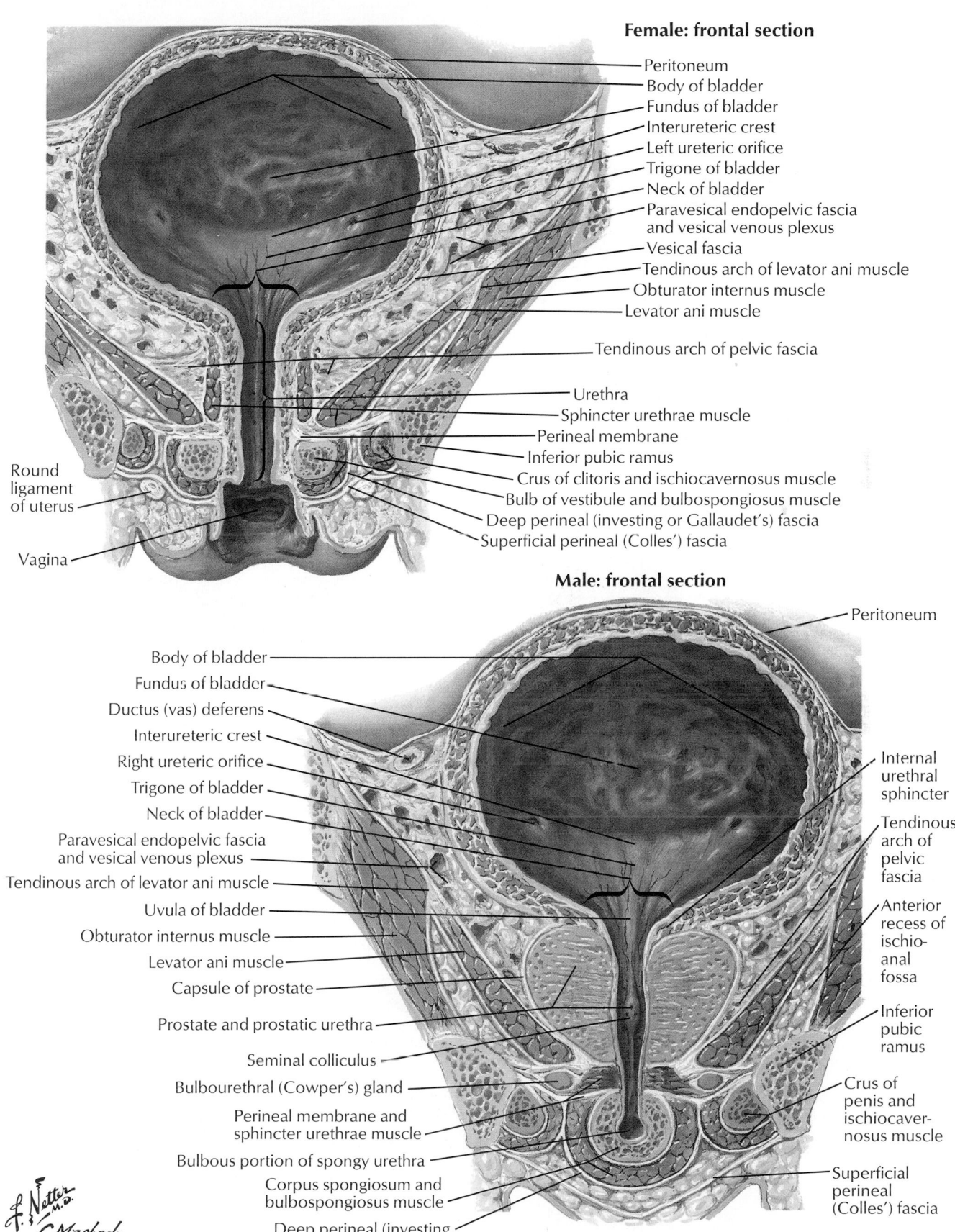

Female: frontal section

- Peritoneum
- Body of bladder
- Fundus of bladder
- Interureteric crest
- Left ureteric orifice
- Trigone of bladder
- Neck of bladder
- Paravesical endopelvic fascia and vesical venous plexus
- Vesical fascia
- Tendinous arch of levator ani muscle
- Obturator internus muscle
- Levator ani muscle
- Tendinous arch of pelvic fascia
- Urethra
- Sphincter urethrae muscle
- Perineal membrane
- Inferior pubic ramus
- Crus of clitoris and ischiocavernosus muscle
- Bulb of vestibule and bulbospongiosus muscle
- Deep perineal (investing or Gallaudet's) fascia
- Superficial perineal (Colles') fascia

- Round ligament of uterus
- Vagina

Male: frontal section

- Peritoneum

- Body of bladder
- Fundus of bladder
- Ductus (vas) deferens
- Interureteric crest
- Right ureteric orifice
- Trigone of bladder
- Neck of bladder
- Paravesical endopelvic fascia and vesical venous plexus
- Tendinous arch of levator ani muscle
- Uvula of bladder
- Obturator internus muscle
- Levator ani muscle
- Capsule of prostate
- Prostate and prostatic urethra
- Seminal colliculus
- Bulbourethral (Cowper's) gland
- Perineal membrane and sphincter urethrae muscle
- Bulbous portion of spongy urethra
- Corpus spongiosum and bulbospongiosus muscle
- Deep perineal (investing or Gallaudet's) fascia

- Internal urethral sphincter
- Tendinous arch of pelvic fascia
- Anterior recess of ischio-anal fossa
- Inferior pubic ramus
- Crus of penis and ischiocavernosus muscle
- Superficial perineal (Colles') fascia

Plate 3 Urinary Bladder: Female and Male. (Netter: Atlas of Human Anatomy, 4 ed, 2006, Saunders. Plate 366.)

ANATOMY ILLUSTRATIONS

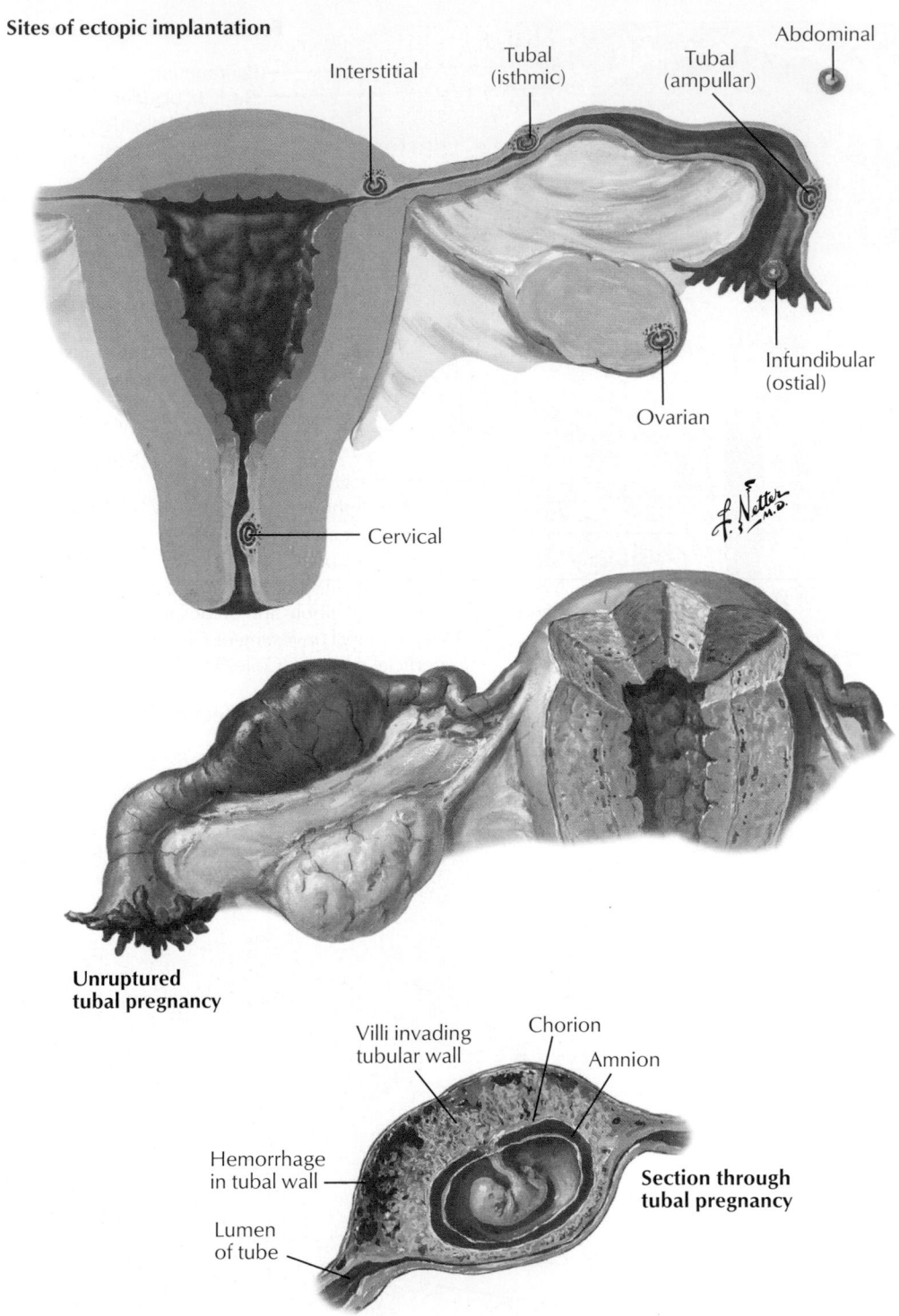

Sites of ectopic implantation

Interstitial

Tubal
(isthmic)

Tubal
(ampullar)

Abdominal

Infundibular
(ostial)

Ovarian

Cervical

**Unruptured
tubal pregnancy**

Villi invading
tubular wall

Chorion

Amnion

Hemorrhage
in tubal wall

Lumen
of tube

**Section through
tubal pregnancy**

Plate 4   Ectopic Pregnancy. (Netter: Atlas of Human Anatomy, 4 ed, 2006, Saunders. Plate 375)

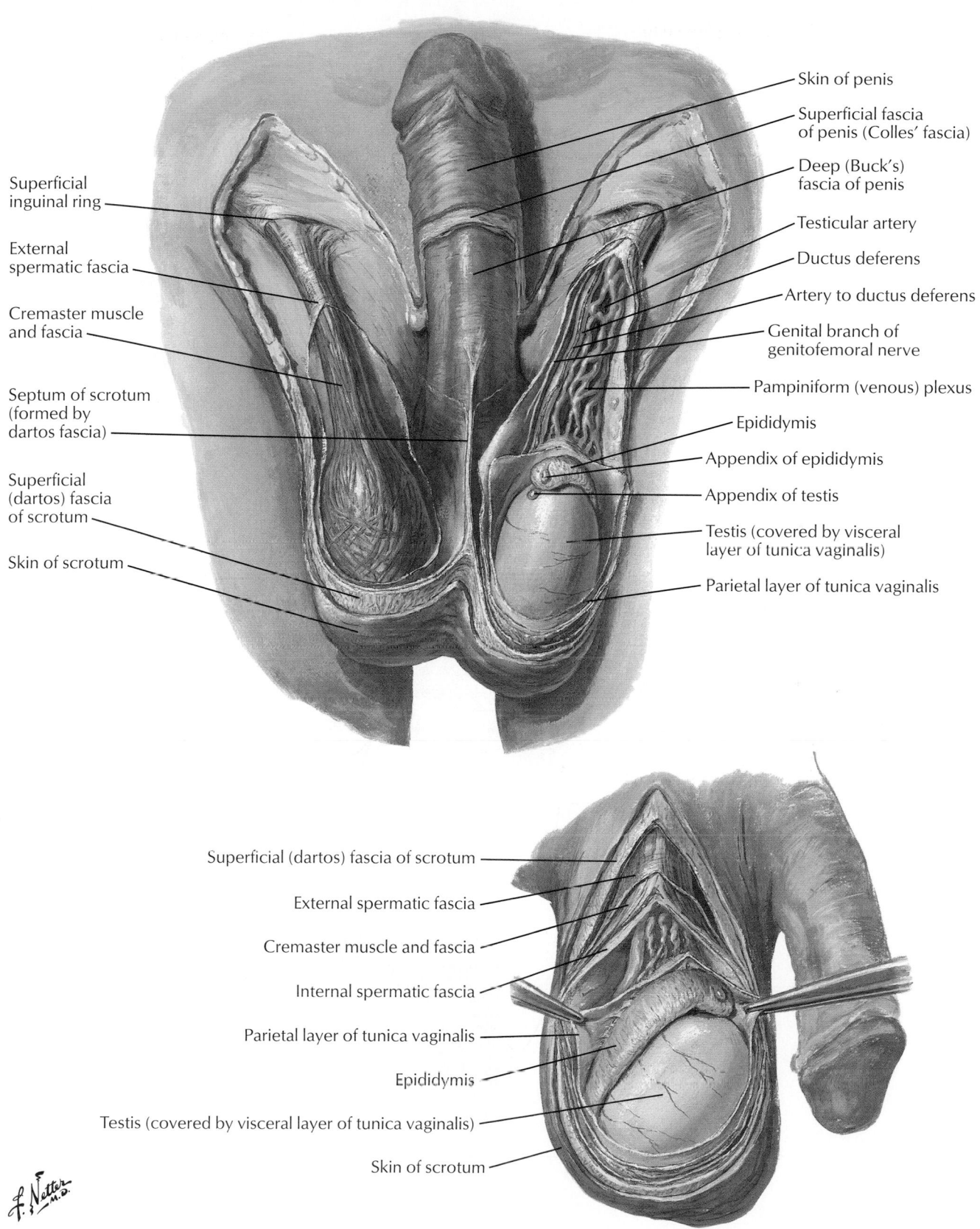

Superficial
inguinal ring

External
spermatic fascia

Cremaster muscle
and fascia

Septum of scrotum
(formed by
dartos fascia)

Superficial
(dartos) fascia
of scrotum

Skin of scrotum

Skin of penis

Superficial fascia
of penis (Colles' fascia)

Deep (Buck's)
fascia of penis

Testicular artery

Ductus deferens

Artery to ductus deferens

Genital branch of
genitofemoral nerve

Pampiniform (venous) plexus

Epididymis

Appendix of epididymis

Appendix of testis

Testis (covered by visceral
layer of tunica vaginalis)

Parietal layer of tunica vaginalis

Superficial (dartos) fascia of scrotum

External spermatic fascia

Cremaster muscle and fascia

Internal spermatic fascia

Parietal layer of tunica vaginalis

Epididymis

Testis (covered by visceral layer of tunica vaginalis)

Skin of scrotum

Plate 5 Scrotum and Contents. (Netter: Atlas of Human Anatomy, 4 ed, 2006, Saunders. Plate 387)

ANATOMY ILLUSTRATIONS

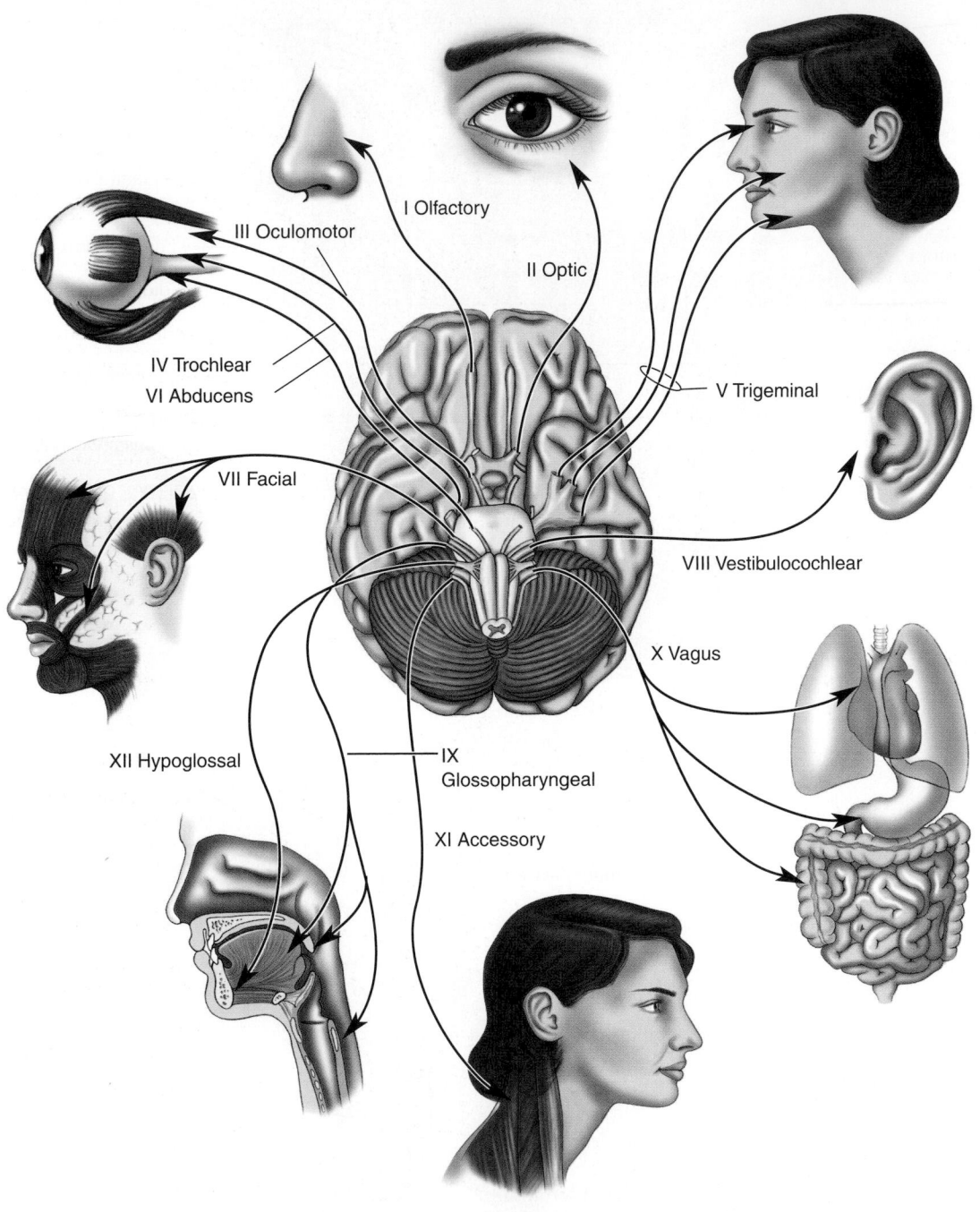

I Olfactory

III Oculomotor

II Optic

IV Trochlear
VI Abducens

V Trigeminal

VII Facial

VIII Vestibulocochlear

X Vagus

XII Hypoglossal

IX
Glossopharyngeal

XI Accessory

Plate 6 Cranial Nerves (12 pairs) are known by their numbers (Roman numerals) and names. (Herlihy BL: The Human Body in Health and Illness, ed 6, St. Louis, 2018, Elsevier.)

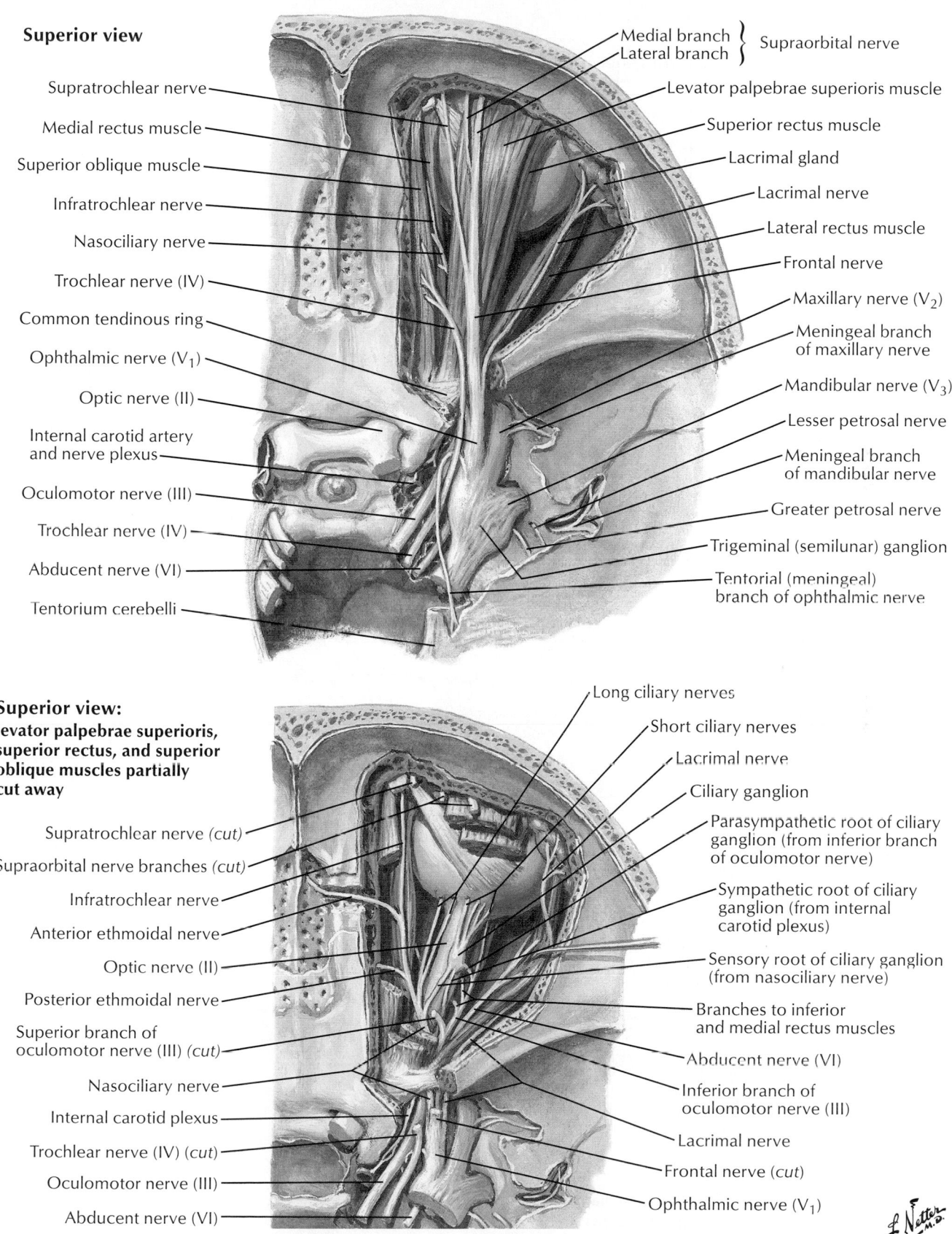

Superior view

Supratrochlear nerve

Medial rectus muscle

Superior oblique muscle

Infratrochlear nerve

Nasociliary nerve

Trochlear nerve (IV)

Common tendinous ring

Ophthalmic nerve (V₁)

Optic nerve (II)

Internal carotid artery and nerve plexus

Oculomotor nerve (III)

Trochlear nerve (IV)

Abducent nerve (VI)

Tentorium cerebelli

Medial branch } Supraorbital nerve
Lateral branch

Levator palpebrae superioris muscle

Superior rectus muscle

Lacrimal gland

Lacrimal nerve

Lateral rectus muscle

Frontal nerve

Maxillary nerve (V₂)

Meningeal branch of maxillary nerve

Mandibular nerve (V₃)

Lesser petrosal nerve

Meningeal branch of mandibular nerve

Greater petrosal nerve

Trigeminal (semilunar) ganglion

Tentorial (meningeal) branch of ophthalmic nerve

Superior view:
levator palpebrae superioris, superior rectus, and superior oblique muscles partially cut away

Supratrochlear nerve (cut)

Supraorbital nerve branches (cut)

Infratrochlear nerve

Anterior ethmoidal nerve

Optic nerve (II)

Posterior ethmoidal nerve

Superior branch of oculomotor nerve (III) (cut)

Nasociliary nerve

Internal carotid plexus

Trochlear nerve (IV) (cut)

Oculomotor nerve (III)

Abducent nerve (VI)

Long ciliary nerves

Short ciliary nerves

Lacrimal nerve

Ciliary ganglion

Parasympathetic root of ciliary ganglion (from inferior branch of oculomotor nerve)

Sympathetic root of ciliary ganglion (from internal carotid plexus)

Sensory root of ciliary ganglion (from nasociliary nerve)

Branches to inferior and medial rectus muscles

Abducent nerve (VI)

Inferior branch of oculomotor nerve (III)

Lacrimal nerve

Frontal nerve (cut)

Ophthalmic nerve (V₁)

ANATOMY ILLUSTRATIONS

Plate 7 Nerves of Orbit. (Netter: Atlas of Human Anatomy, 4 ed, 2006, Saunders. Plate 86)

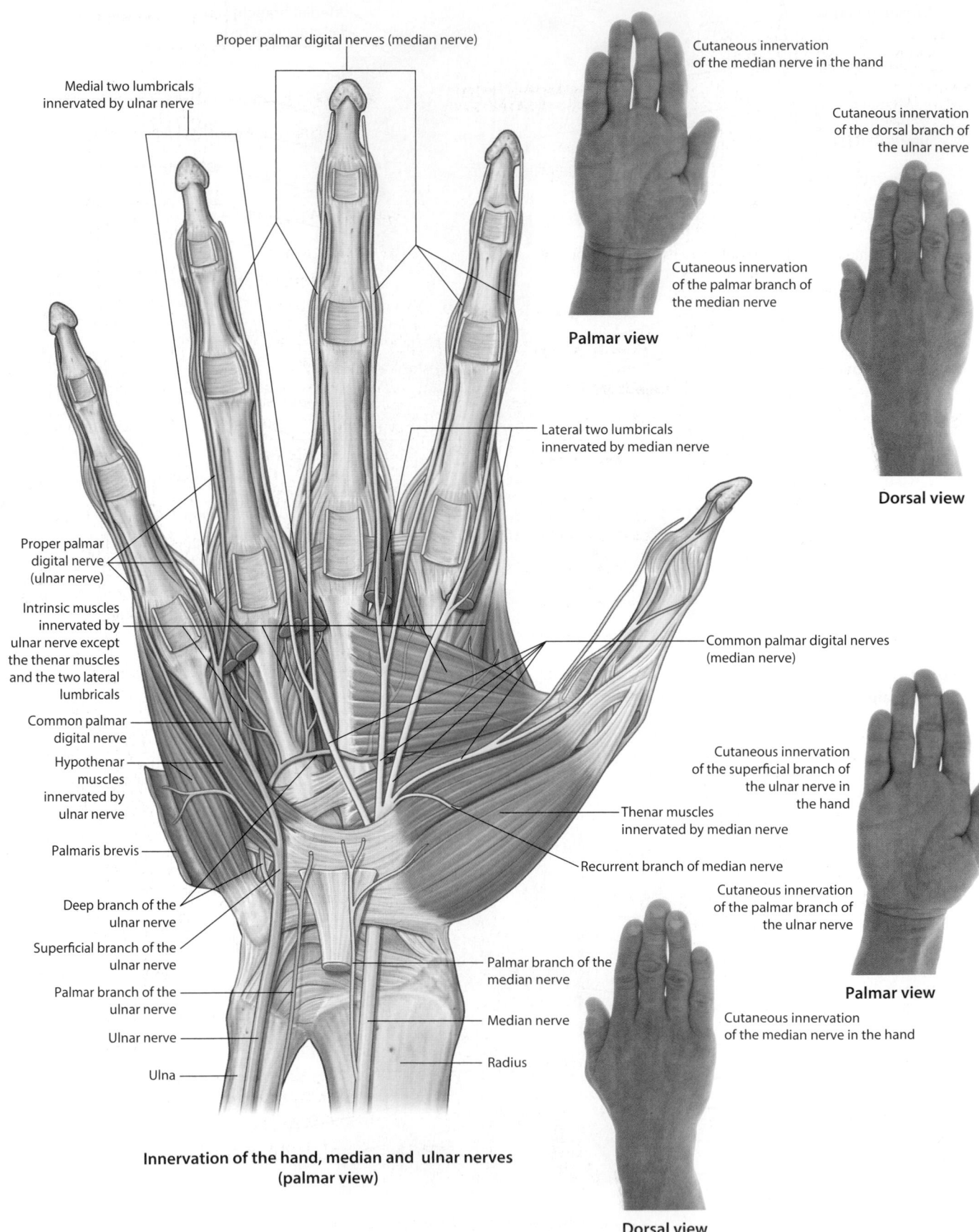

Proper palmar digital nerves (median nerve)

Medial two lumbricals innervated by ulnar nerve

Cutaneous innervation of the median nerve in the hand

Cutaneous innervation of the dorsal branch of the ulnar nerve

Cutaneous innervation of the palmar branch of the median nerve

Palmar view

Dorsal view

Lateral two lumbricals innervated by median nerve

Proper palmar digital nerve (ulnar nerve)

Intrinsic muscles innervated by ulnar nerve except the thenar muscles and the two lateral lumbricals

Common palmar digital nerves (median nerve)

Common palmar digital nerve

Hypothenar muscles innervated by ulnar nerve

Palmaris brevis

Cutaneous innervation of the superficial branch of the ulnar nerve in the hand

Thenar muscles innervated by median nerve

Recurrent branch of median nerve

Deep branch of the ulnar nerve

Superficial branch of the ulnar nerve

Palmar branch of the ulnar nerve

Ulnar nerve

Ulna

Palmar branch of the median nerve

Median nerve

Radius

Cutaneous innervation of the palmar branch of the ulnar nerve

Palmar view

Cutaneous innervation of the median nerve in the hand

Innervation of the hand, median and ulnar nerves (palmar view)

Dorsal view

Plate 8   Innervation of the Hand: Median and Ulnar Nerves (From Drake RL, Vogl AW, Mitchell AWM, Tibbitts RM, Richardson PE: Gray's Atlas of Anatomy, ed 2, Philadelphia, 2015, Churchill Livingstone.)

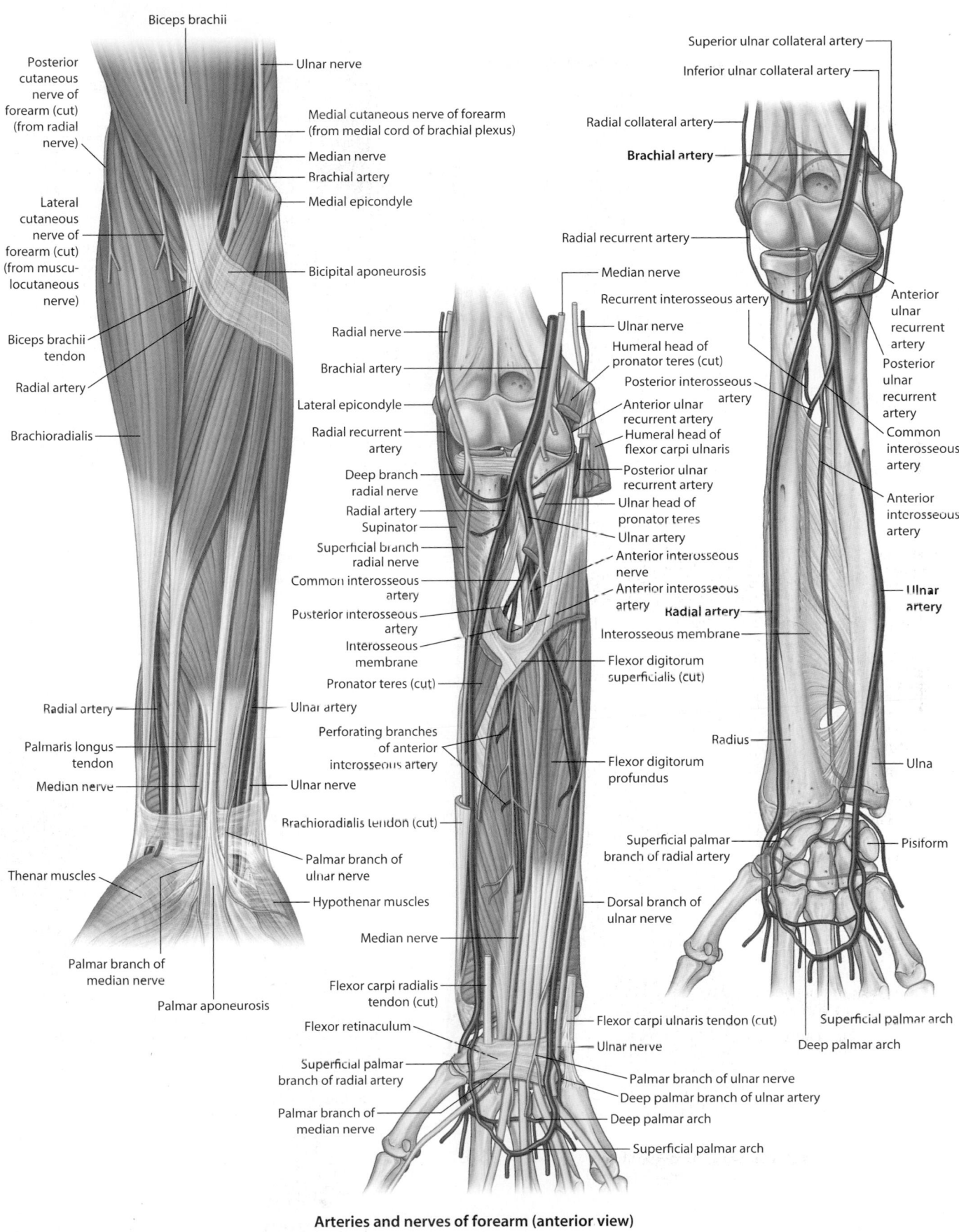

Biceps brachii

Posterior cutaneous nerve of forearm (cut) (from radial nerve)

Ulnar nerve

Medial cutaneous nerve of forearm (from medial cord of brachial plexus)

Median nerve

Brachial artery

Medial epicondyle

Lateral cutaneous nerve of forearm (cut) (from musculocutaneous nerve)

Bicipital aponeurosis

Biceps brachii tendon

Radial artery

Brachioradialis

Radial artery

Palmaris longus tendon

Median nerve

Thenar muscles

Palmar branch of median nerve

Palmar aponeurosis

Radial nerve

Brachial artery

Lateral epicondyle

Radial recurrent artery

Deep branch radial nerve

Radial artery

Supinator

Superficial branch radial nerve

Common interosseous artery

Posterior interosseous artery

Interosseous membrane

Pronator teres (cut)

Ulnar artery

Perforating branches of anterior interosseous artery

Brachioradialis tendon (cut)

Palmar branch of ulnar nerve

Hypothenar muscles

Median nerve

Flexor carpi radialis tendon (cut)

Flexor retinaculum

Superficial palmar branch of radial artery

Palmar branch of median nerve

Median nerve

Recurrent interosseous artery

Ulnar nerve

Humeral head of pronator teres (cut)

Posterior interosseous artery

Anterior ulnar recurrent artery

Humeral head of flexor carpi ulnaris

Posterior ulnar recurrent artery

Ulnar head of pronator teres

Ulnar artery

Anterior interosseous nerve

Anterior interosseous artery

Radial artery

Interosseous membrane

Flexor digitorum superficialis (cut)

Flexor digitorum profundus

Dorsal branch of ulnar nerve

Flexor carpi ulnaris tendon (cut)

Ulnar nerve

Palmar branch of ulnar nerve

Deep palmar branch of ulnar artery

Deep palmar arch

Superficial palmar arch

Superior ulnar collateral artery

Inferior ulnar collateral artery

Radial collateral artery

Brachial artery

Radial recurrent artery

Anterior ulnar recurrent artery

Posterior ulnar recurrent artery

Common interosseous artery

Anterior interosseous artery

Ulnar artery

Radial artery

Radius

Ulna

Superficial palmar branch of radial artery

Pisiform

Superficial palmar arch

Deep palmar arch

Arteries and nerves of forearm (anterior view)

ANATOMY ILLUSTRATIONS

Plate 9   Arteries and Nerves of the Forearm (Anterior View) (From Drake RL, Vogl AW, Mitchell AWM, Tibbitts RM, Richardson PE: Gray's Atlas of Anatomy, ed 2, Philadelphia, 2015, Churchill Livingstone.)

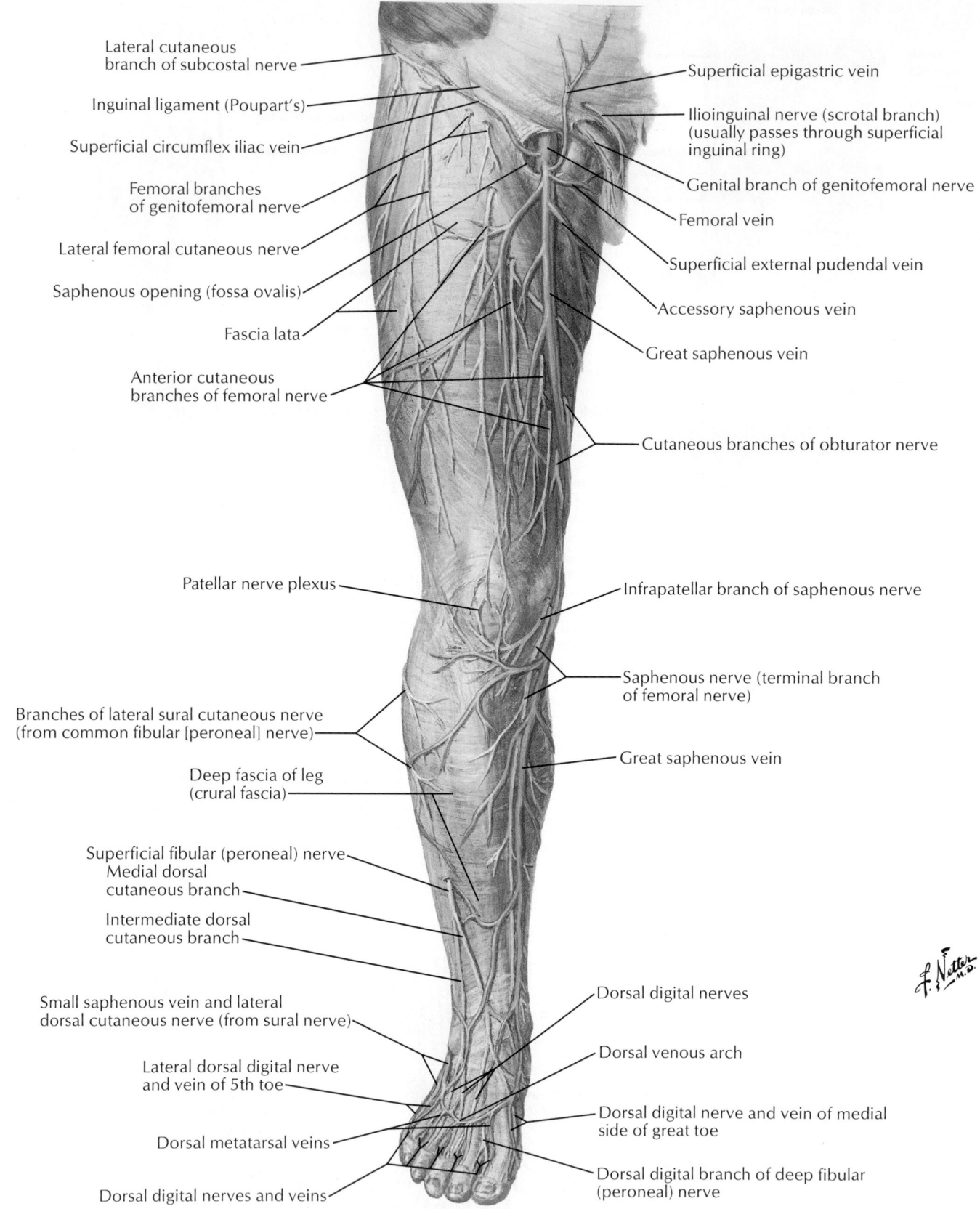

Lateral cutaneous branch of subcostal nerve

Inguinal ligament (Poupart's)

Superficial circumflex iliac vein

Femoral branches of genitofemoral nerve

Lateral femoral cutaneous nerve

Saphenous opening (fossa ovalis)

Fascia lata

Anterior cutaneous branches of femoral nerve

Patellar nerve plexus

Branches of lateral sural cutaneous nerve (from common fibular [peroneal] nerve)

Deep fascia of leg (crural fascia)

Superficial fibular (peroneal) nerve
Medial dorsal cutaneous branch

Intermediate dorsal cutaneous branch

Small saphenous vein and lateral dorsal cutaneous nerve (from sural nerve)

Lateral dorsal digital nerve and vein of 5th toe

Dorsal metatarsal veins

Dorsal digital nerves and veins

Superficial epigastric vein

Ilioinguinal nerve (scrotal branch) (usually passes through superficial inguinal ring)

Genital branch of genitofemoral nerve

Femoral vein

Superficial external pudendal vein

Accessory saphenous vein

Great saphenous vein

Cutaneous branches of obturator nerve

Infrapatellar branch of saphenous nerve

Saphenous nerve (terminal branch of femoral nerve)

Great saphenous vein

Dorsal digital nerves

Dorsal venous arch

Dorsal digital nerve and vein of medial side of great toe

Dorsal digital branch of deep fibular (peroneal) nerve

Plate 10 Superficial Nerves and Veins of Lower Limb: Anterior View. (Netter: Atlas of Human Anatomy, 4 ed, 2006, Saunders. Plate 544)

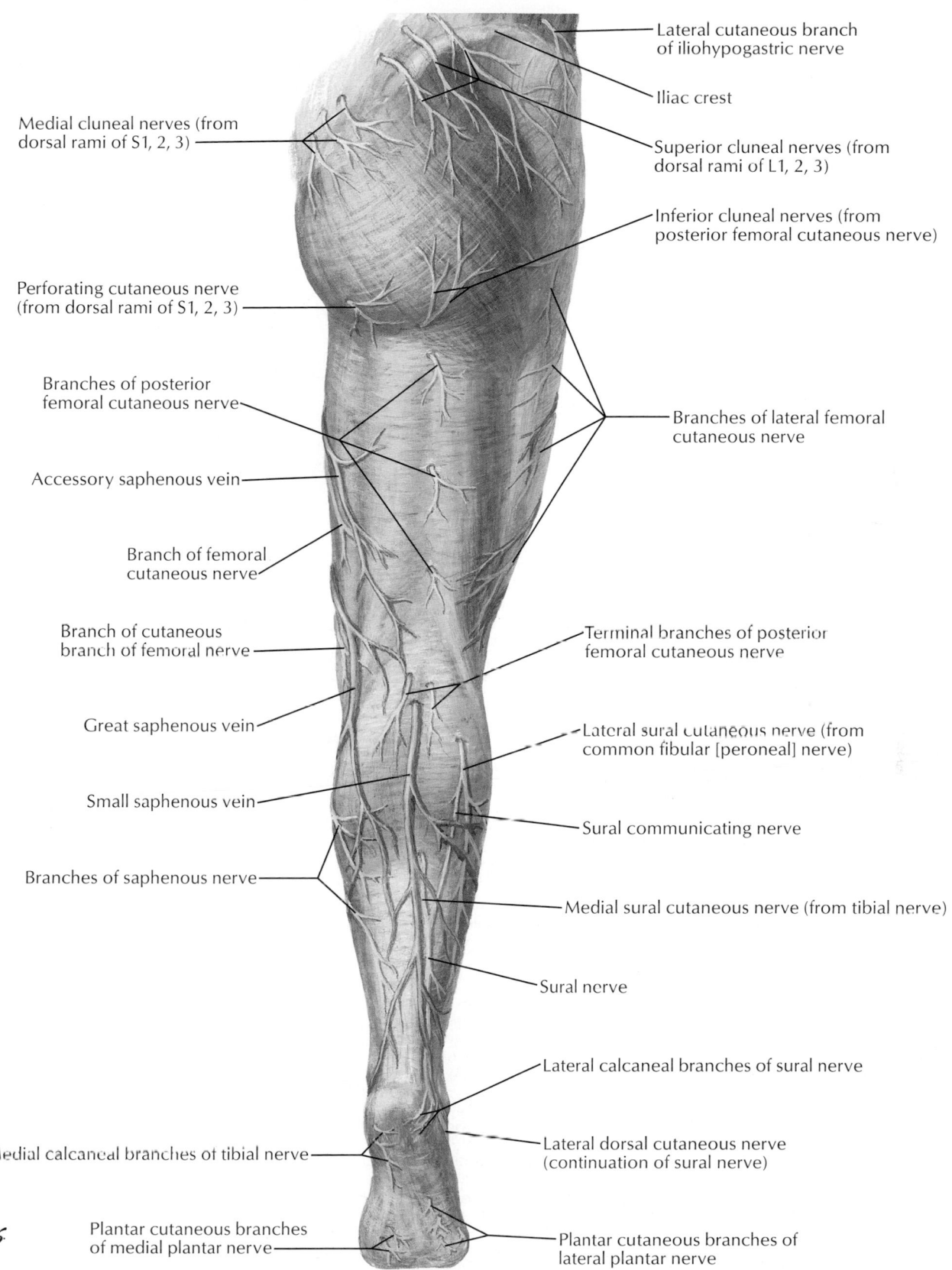

Lateral cutaneous branch
of iliohypogastric nerve

Iliac crest

Medial cluneal nerves (from
dorsal rami of S1, 2, 3)

Superior cluneal nerves (from
dorsal rami of L1, 2, 3)

Inferior cluneal nerves (from
posterior femoral cutaneous nerve)

Perforating cutaneous nerve
(from dorsal rami of S1, 2, 3)

Branches of posterior
femoral cutaneous nerve

Accessory saphenous vein

Branches of lateral femoral
cutaneous nerve

Branch of femoral
cutaneous nerve

Branch of cutaneous
branch of femoral nerve

Terminal branches of posterior
femoral cutaneous nerve

Great saphenous vein

Lateral sural cutaneous nerve (from
common fibular [peroneal] nerve)

Sural communicating nerve

Small saphenous vein

Branches of saphenous nerve

Medial sural cutaneous nerve (from tibial nerve)

Sural nerve

Lateral calcaneal branches of sural nerve

Medial calcaneal branches of tibial nerve

Lateral dorsal cutaneous nerve
(continuation of sural nerve)

Plantar cutaneous branches
of medial plantar nerve

Plantar cutaneous branches of
lateral plantar nerve

Plate 11 Superficial Nerves and Veins of Lower Limb: Posterior View. (Netter: Atlas of Human Anatomy, 4 ed, 2006, Saunders. Plate 545)

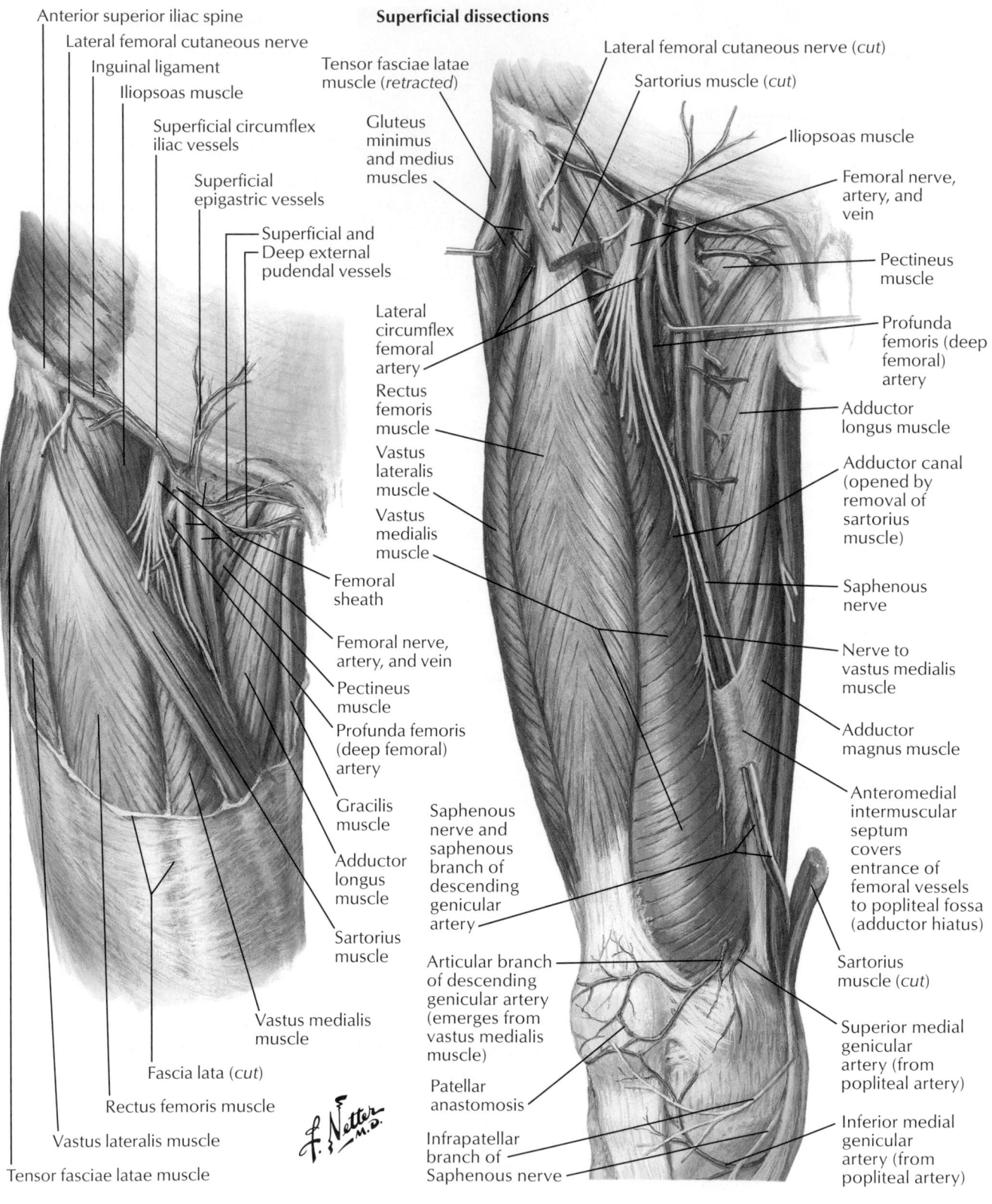

Anterior superior iliac spine
Lateral femoral cutaneous nerve
Inguinal ligament
Iliopsoas muscle
Superficial circumflex iliac vessels
Superficial epigastric vessels
Superficial and Deep external pudendal vessels

Superficial dissections

Tensor fasciae latae muscle (*retracted*)
Gluteus minimus and medius muscles

Lateral femoral cutaneous nerve (*cut*)
Sartorius muscle (*cut*)
Iliopsoas muscle
Femoral nerve, artery, and vein
Pectineus muscle

Lateral circumflex femoral artery
Rectus femoris muscle
Vastus lateralis muscle
Vastus medialis muscle
Femoral sheath
Femoral nerve, artery, and vein
Pectineus muscle
Profunda femoris (deep femoral) artery
Gracilis muscle
Adductor longus muscle
Sartorius muscle
Vastus medialis muscle
Fascia lata (*cut*)
Rectus femoris muscle
Vastus lateralis muscle
Tensor fasciae latae muscle

Saphenous nerve and saphenous branch of descending genicular artery
Articular branch of descending genicular artery (emerges from vastus medialis muscle)
Patellar anastomosis
Infrapatellar branch of Saphenous nerve

Profunda femoris (deep femoral) artery
Adductor longus muscle
Adductor canal (opened by removal of sartorius muscle)
Saphenous nerve
Nerve to vastus medialis muscle
Adductor magnus muscle
Anteromedial intermuscular septum covers entrance of femoral vessels to popliteal fossa (adductor hiatus)
Sartorius muscle (*cut*)
Superior medial genicular artery (from popliteal artery)
Inferior medial genicular artery (from popliteal artery)

Plate 12   Arteries and Nerves of Thigh: Anterior Views. (Netter: Atlas of Human Anatomy, 4 ed, 2006, Saunders. Plate 500)

Deep dissection

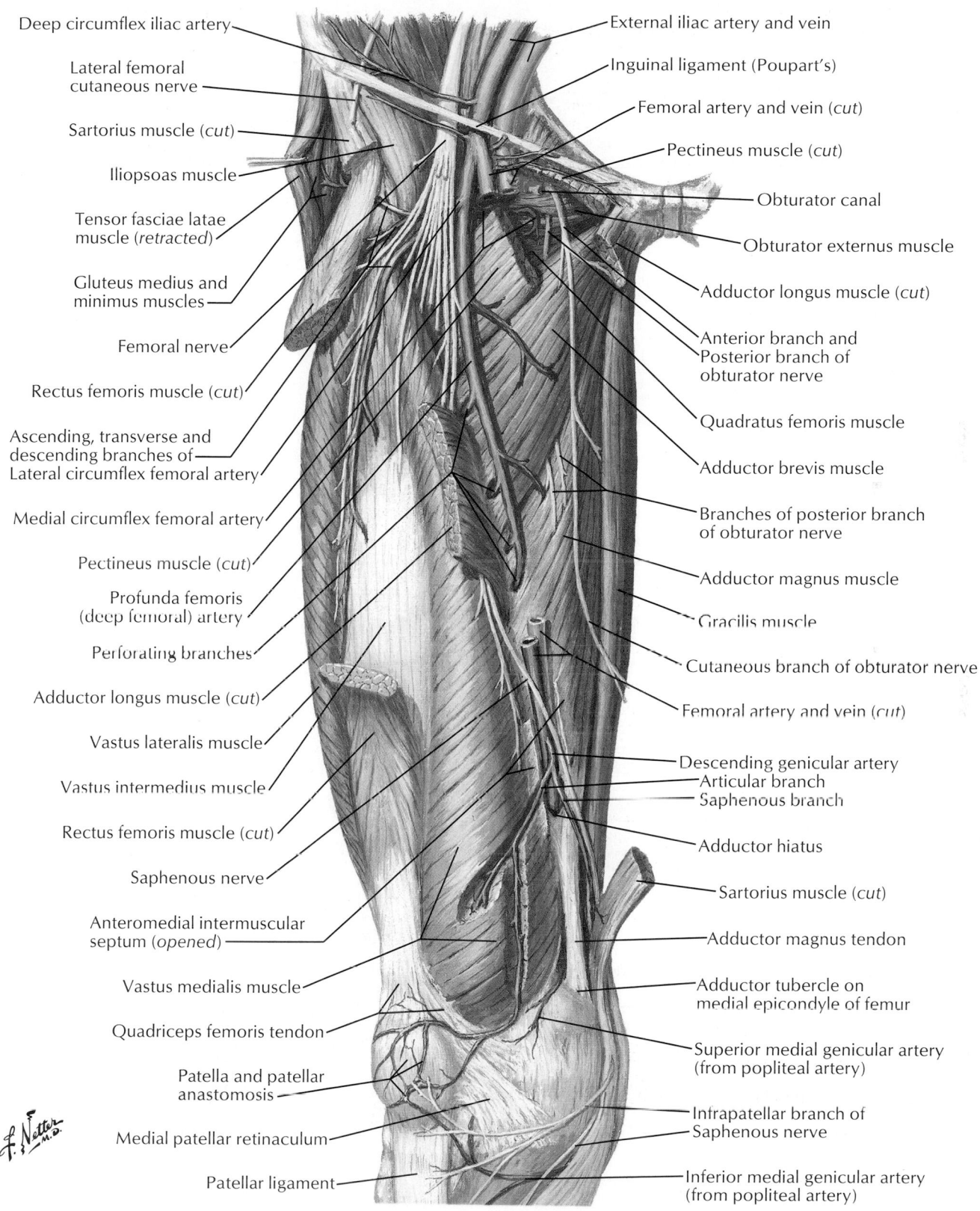

Deep circumflex iliac artery

Lateral femoral
cutaneous nerve

Sartorius muscle (*cut*)

Iliopsoas muscle

Tensor fasciae latae
muscle (*retracted*)

Gluteus medius and
minimus muscles

Femoral nerve

Rectus femoris muscle (*cut*)

Ascending, transverse and
descending branches of
Lateral circumflex femoral artery

Medial circumflex femoral artery

Pectineus muscle (*cut*)

Profunda femoris
(deep femoral) artery

Perforating branches

Adductor longus muscle (*cut*)

Vastus lateralis muscle

Vastus intermedius muscle

Rectus femoris muscle (*cut*)

Saphenous nerve

Anteromedial intermuscular
septum (*opened*)

Vastus medialis muscle

Quadriceps femoris tendon

Patella and patellar
anastomosis

Medial patellar retinaculum

Patellar ligament

External iliac artery and vein

Inguinal ligament (Poupart's)

Femoral artery and vein (*cut*)

Pectineus muscle (*cut*)

Obturator canal

Obturator externus muscle

Adductor longus muscle (*cut*)

Anterior branch and
Posterior branch of
obturator nerve

Quadratus femoris muscle

Adductor brevis muscle

Branches of posterior branch
of obturator nerve

Adductor magnus muscle

Gracilis muscle

Cutaneous branch of obturator nerve

Femoral artery and vein (*cut*)

Descending genicular artery
Articular branch
Saphenous branch

Adductor hiatus

Sartorius muscle (*cut*)

Adductor magnus tendon

Adductor tubercle on
medial epicondyle of femur

Superior medial genicular artery
(from popliteal artery)

Intrapatellar branch of
Saphenous nerve

Inferior medial genicular artery
(from popliteal artery)

f. Netter
M.D.

ANATOMY ILLUSTRATIONS

Plate 13 Arteries and Nerves of Thigh: Posterior View. (Netter: Atlas of Human Anatomy, 4 ed, 2006, Saunders. Plate 501)

Deep dissection

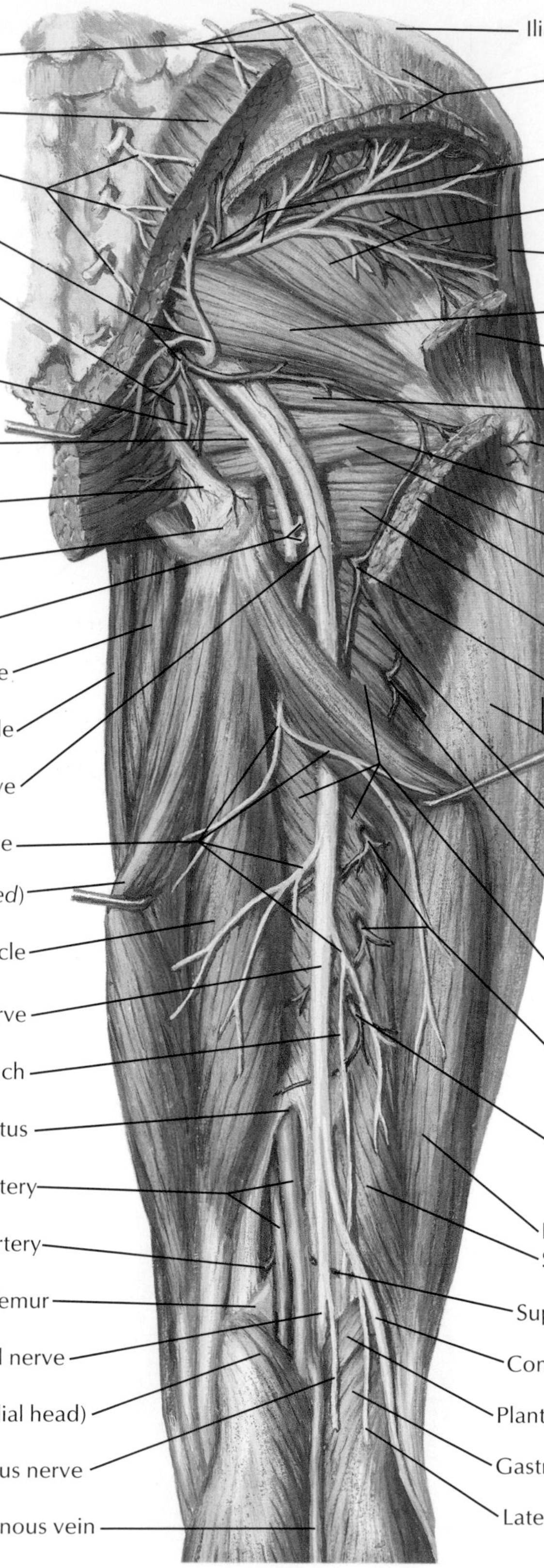

Superior cluneal nerves

Gluteus maximus muscle (cut)

Medial cluneal nerves

Inferior gluteal artery and nerve

Pudendal nerve

Nerve to obturator internus (and superior gemellus)

Posterior femoral cutaneous nerve

Sacrotuberous ligament

Ischial tuberosity

Inferior cluneal nerves (cut)

Adductor magnus muscle

Gracilis muscle

Sciatic nerve

Muscular branches of sciatic nerve

Semitendinosus muscle (retracted)

Semimembranosus muscle

Sciatic nerve

Articular branch

Adductor hiatus

Popliteal vein and artery

Superior medial genicular artery

Medial epicondyle of femur

Tibial nerve

Gastrocnemius muscle (medial head)

Medial sural cutaneous nerve

Small saphenous vein

Iliac crest

Gluteal aponeurosis and gluteus medius muscle (cut)

Superior gluteal artery and nerve

Gluteus minimus muscle

Tensor fasciae latae muscle

Piriformis muscle

Gluteus medius muscle (cut)

Superior gemellus muscle

Greater trochanter of femur

Obturator internus muscle

Inferior gemellus muscle

Gluteus maximus muscle (cut)

Quadratus femoris muscle

Medial circumflex femoral artery

Vastus lateralis muscle and iliotibial tract

Adductor minimus part of adductor magnus muscle

1st perforating artery (from profunda femoris artery)

Adductor magnus muscle

2nd and 3rd perforating arteries (from profunda femoris artery)

4th perforating artery (from profunda femoris artery)

Long head (retracted)
Short head
} Biceps femoris muscle

Superior lateral genicular artery

Common fibular (peroneal) nerve

Plantaris muscle

Gastrocnemius muscle (lateral head)

Lateral sural cutaneous nerve

Plate 14 Arteries and Nerves of Thigh: Posterior View. (Netter: Atlas of Human Anatomy, 4 ed, 2006, Saunders. Plate 502)

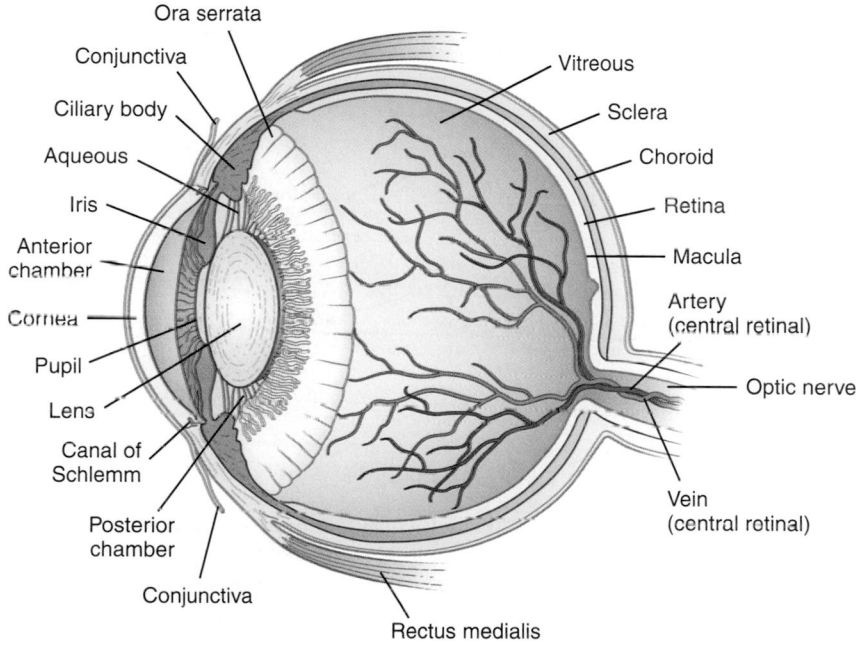

Ora serrata

Conjunctiva

Ciliary body

Aqueous

Iris

Anterior chamber

Cornea

Pupil

Lens

Canal of Schlemm

Posterior chamber

Conjunctiva

Rectus medialis

Vitreous

Sclera

Choroid

Retina

Macula

Artery (central retinal)

Optic nerve

Vein (central retinal)

Plate 15 Anatomy of the eye. (Dehn RW, Asprey DP: Essential Clinical Procedures, ed 3, Philadelphia, 2013, Saunders.)

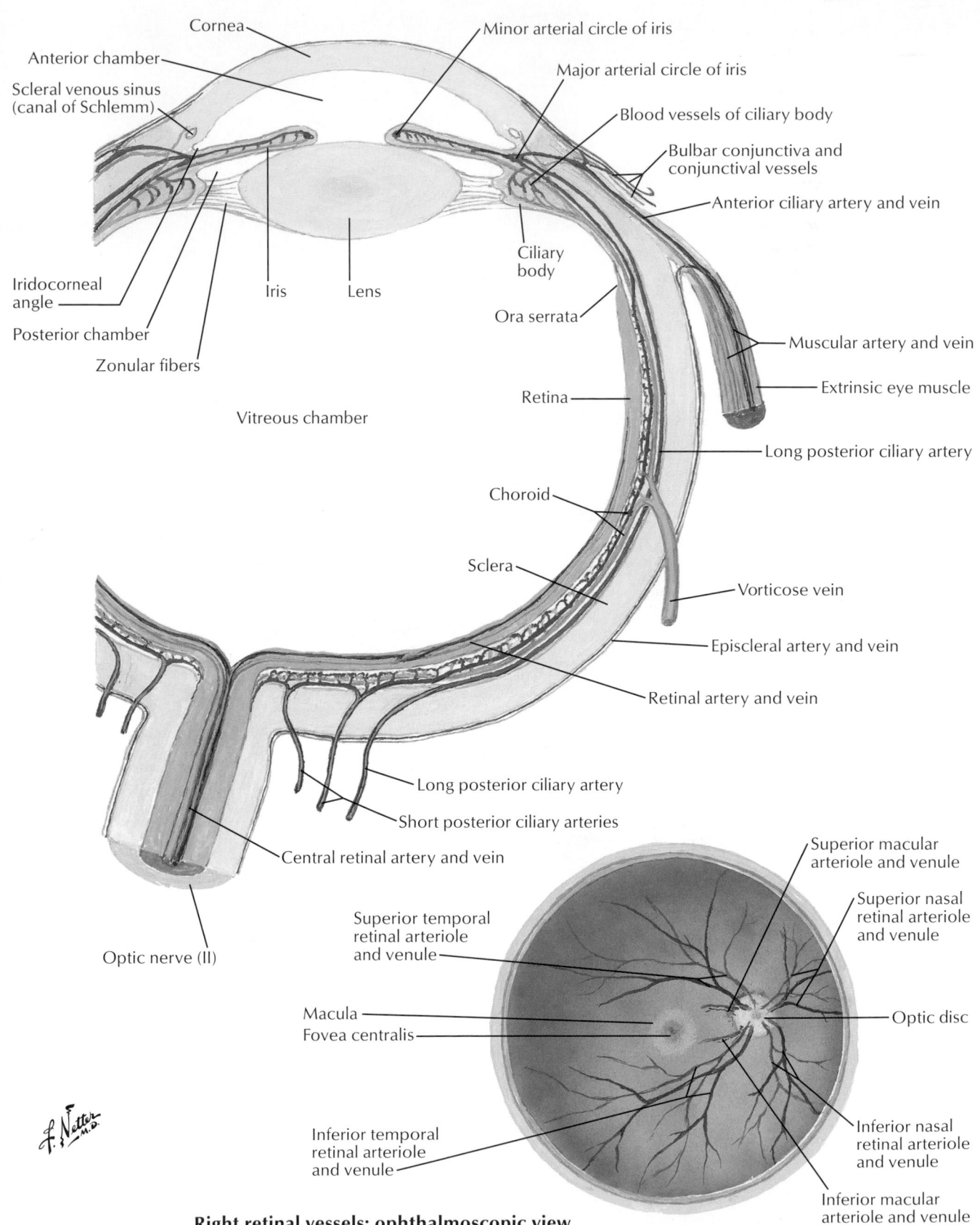

Cornea

Minor arterial circle of iris

Anterior chamber

Major arterial circle of iris

Scleral venous sinus
(canal of Schlemm)

Blood vessels of ciliary body

Bulbar conjunctiva and
conjunctival vessels

Anterior ciliary artery and vein

Iridocorneal
angle

Iris

Lens

Ciliary
body

Posterior chamber

Ora serrata

Muscular artery and vein

Zonular fibers

Extrinsic eye muscle

Vitreous chamber

Retina

Long posterior ciliary artery

Choroid

Sclera

Vorticose vein

Episcleral artery and vein

Retinal artery and vein

Long posterior ciliary artery

Short posterior ciliary arteries

Central retinal artery and vein

Optic nerve (II)

Superior macular
arteriole and venule

Superior nasal
retinal arteriole
and venule

Superior temporal
retinal arteriole
and venule

Macula

Optic disc

Fovea centralis

Inferior nasal
retinal arteriole
and venule

Inferior temporal
retinal arteriole
and venule

Inferior macular
arteriole and venule

Right retinal vessels: ophthalmoscopic view

Plate 16 Intrinsic Arteries and Veins of Eye. (Netter: Atlas of Human Anatomy, 4 ed, 2006, Saunders. Plate 90)

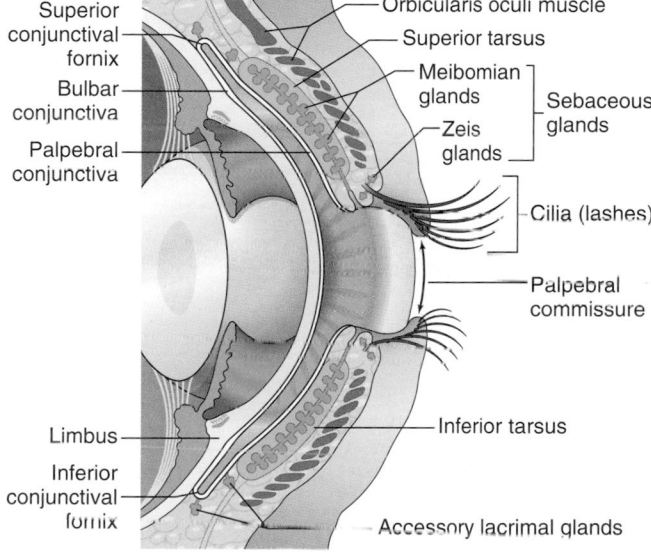

Plate 17 Anatomy of the conjunctiva and eyelids. (Kumar V, Abbas AK, Aster JC: Robbins and Cotran Pathologic Basis of Disease, ed 9, Philadelphia, 2015, Saunders.)

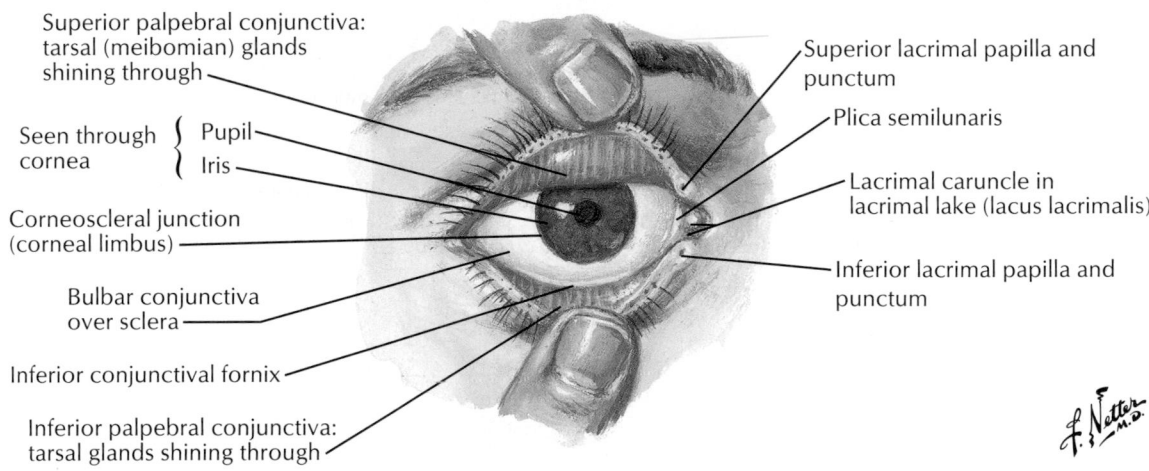

Superior palpebral conjunctiva: tarsal (meibomian) glands shining through

Seen through cornea { Pupil / Iris

Corneoscleral junction (corneal limbus)

Bulbar conjunctiva over sclera

Inferior conjunctival fornix

Inferior palpebral conjunctiva: tarsal glands shining through

Superior lacrimal papilla and punctum

Plica semilunaris

Lacrimal caruncle in lacrimal lake (lacus lacrimalis)

Inferior lacrimal papilla and punctum

Plate 18   Eyelid. (Netter: Atlas of Human Anatomy, 4 ed, 2006, Saunders. Plate 81, Upper)

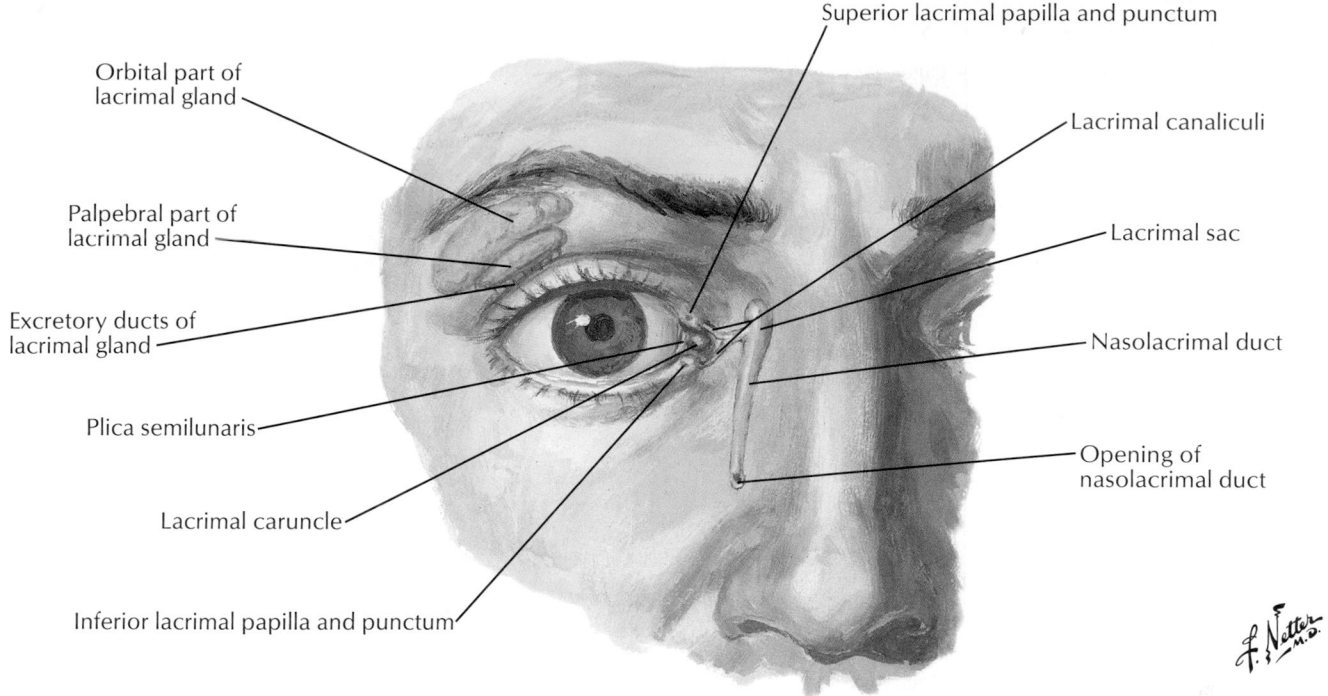

Orbital part of lacrimal gland

Palpebral part of lacrimal gland

Excretory ducts of lacrimal gland

Plica semilunaris

Lacrimal caruncle

Inferior lacrimal papilla and punctum

Superior lacrimal papilla and punctum

Lacrimal canaliculi

Lacrimal sac

Nasolacrimal duct

Opening of nasolacrimal duct

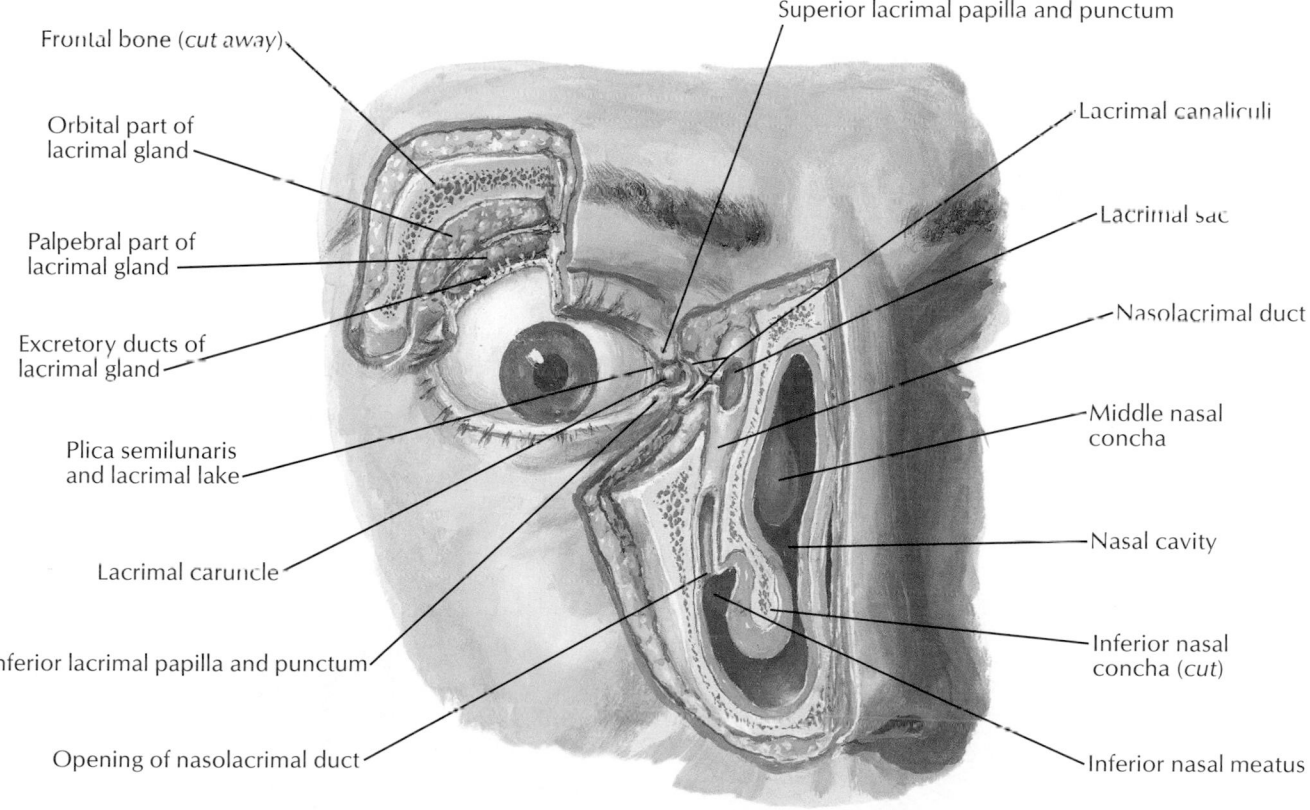

Frontal bone (*cut away*)

Orbital part of lacrimal gland

Palpebral part of lacrimal gland

Excretory ducts of lacrimal gland

Plica semilunaris and lacrimal lake

Lacrimal caruncle

Inferior lacrimal papilla and punctum

Opening of nasolacrimal duct

Superior lacrimal papilla and punctum

Lacrimal canaliculi

Lacrimal sac

Nasolacrimal duct

Middle nasal concha

Nasal cavity

Inferior nasal concha (*cut*)

Inferior nasal meatus

Plate 19 Lacrimal Apparatus. (Netter: Atlas of Human Anatomy, 4 ed, 2006, Saunders. Plate 82)

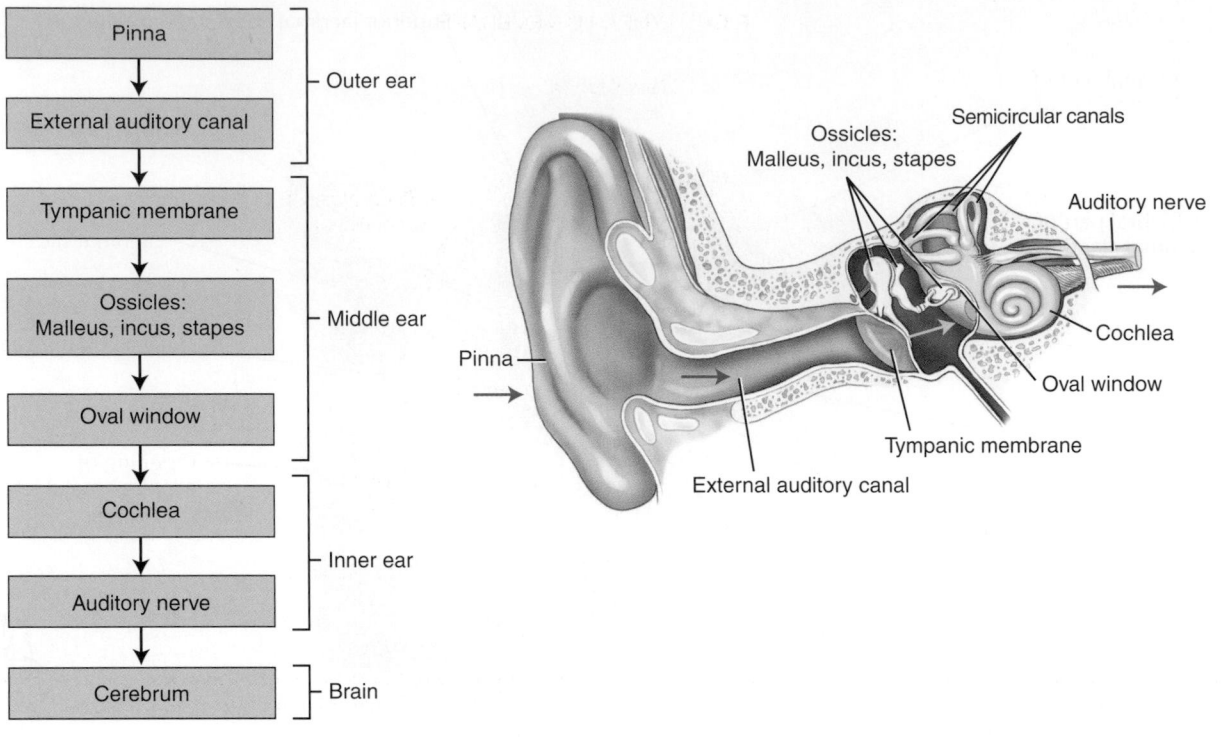

Pinna → External auditory canal — Outer ear

Tympanic membrane → Ossices: Malleus, incus, stapes → Oval window — Middle ear

Cochlea → Auditory nerve — Inner ear

Cerebrum — Brain

Plate 20 Pathway of Sound. (LaFleur Brooks D, LaFleur Brooks M: Basic Medical Language, ed 4, St. Louis, 2013, Mosby.)

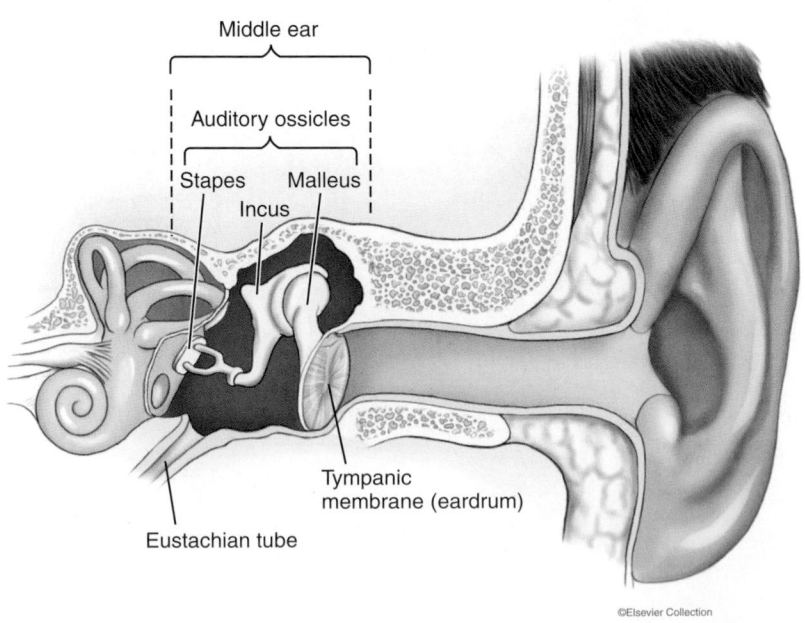

©Elsevier Collection

Plate 21 Middle ear structures. (©Elsevier Collection.)

RIGHT TYMPANIC MEMBRANE

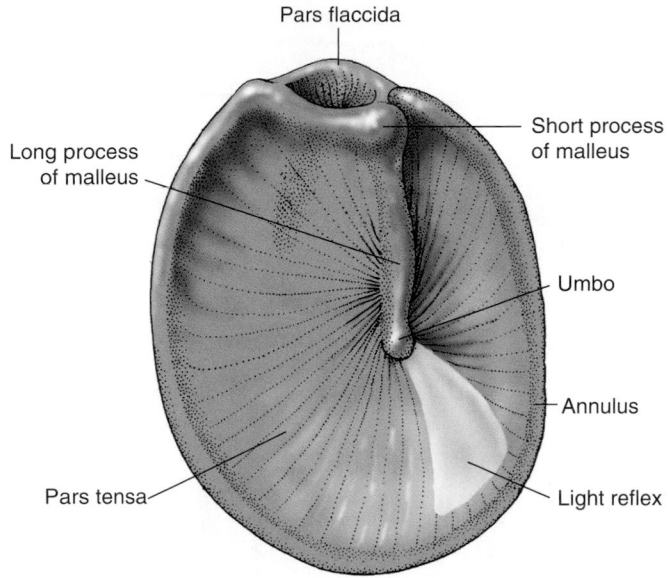

Pars flaccida

Short process
of malleus

Long process
of malleus

Umbo

Annulus

Pars tensa

Light reflex

Plate 22   Structural landmarks of tympanic membrane. (Ignatavicius DD, Workman ML: Medical-Surgical Nursing: Patient-Centered Collaborative Care, ed 7, St. Louis, 2013, Saunders.)

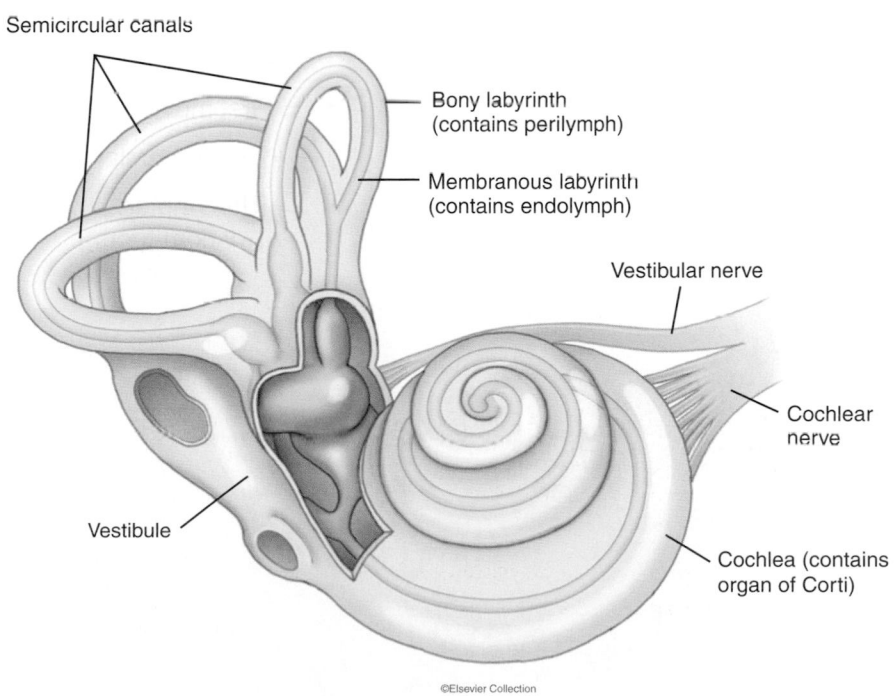

Semicircular canals

Bony labyrinth
(contains perilymph)

Membranous labyrinth
(contains endolymph)

Vestibular nerve

Cochlear
nerve

Vestibule

Cochlea (contains
organ of Corti)

©Elsevier Collection

Plate 23   Inner ear structures. (©Elsevier Collection.)

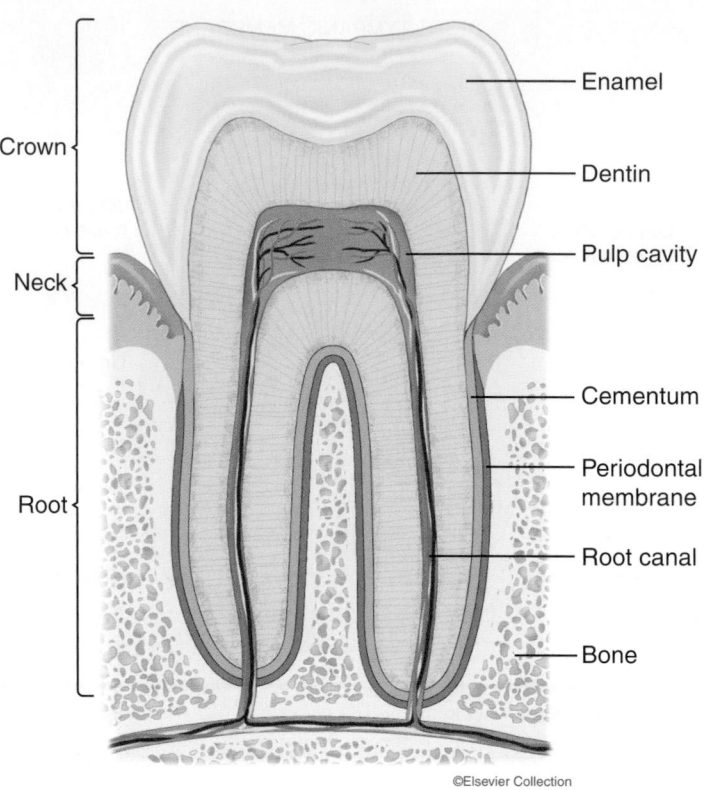

Crown

Neck

Root

Enamel

Dentin

Pulp cavity

Cementum

Periodontal membrane

Root canal

Bone

©Elsevier Collection

Plate 24 The Tooth. (©Elsevier Collection).

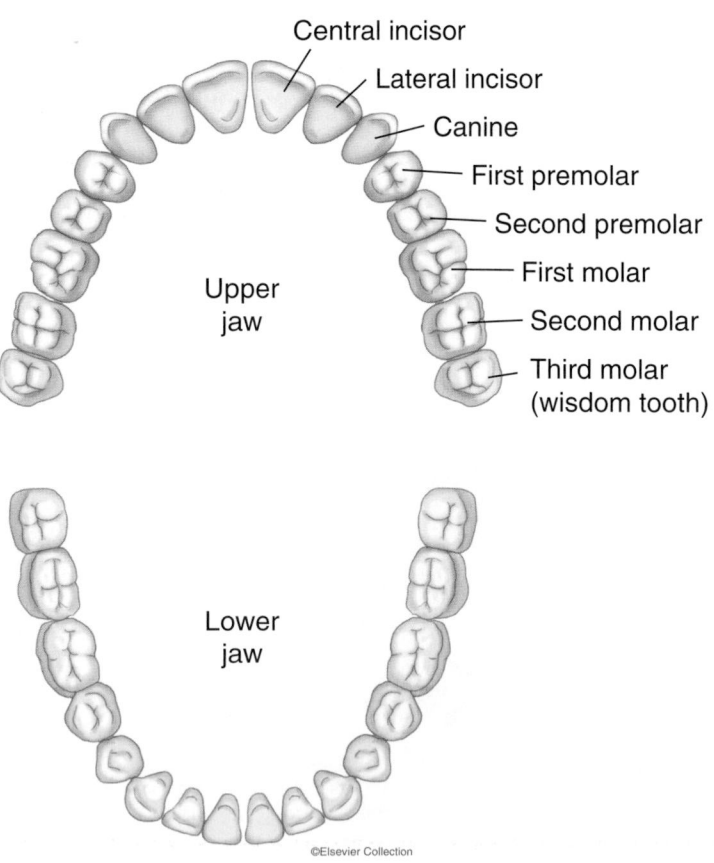

Central incisor

Lateral incisor

Canine

First premolar

Second premolar

First molar

Second molar

Third molar (wisdom tooth)

Upper jaw

Lower jaw

©Elsevier Collection

Plate 25 Adult Teeth. (©Elsevier Collection).

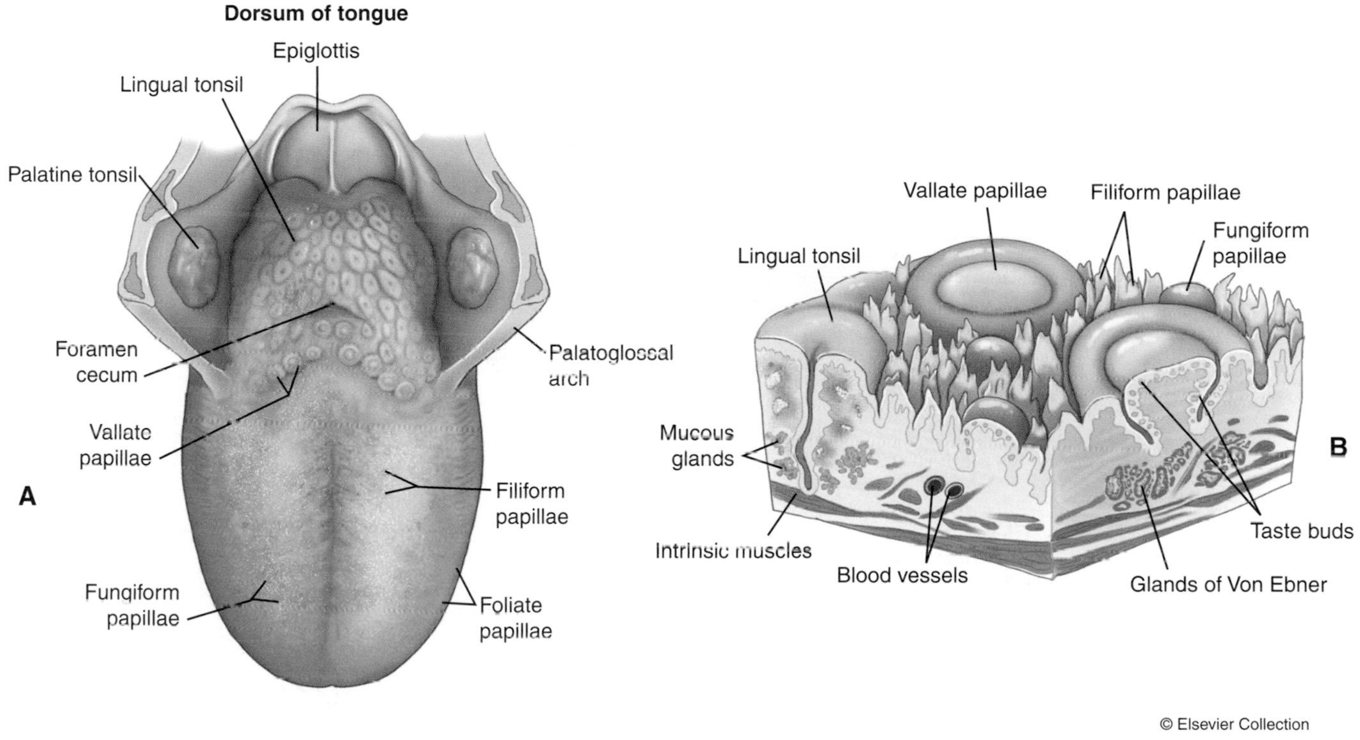

Dorsum of tongue

Epiglottis

Lingual tonsil

Palatine tonsil

Foramen cecum

Vallate papillae

A

Fungiform papillae

Filiform papillae

Foliate papillae

Palatoglossal arch

Vallate papillae

Filiform papillae

Fungiform papillae

Lingual tonsil

Mucous glands

Intrinsic muscles

Blood vessels

Taste buds

Glands of Von Ebner

B

© Elsevier Collection

Plate 26 A, Dorsal view of tongue showing the roughened large lingual tonsils on the posterior of the tongue and the foliate papillae on the side. B, Section of dorsal of the tongue showing a cutaway through lingual papillae and showing von Ebner's glands at the base of the vallate papilla. (Brand RW, Isselhard DE: Anatomy of Orofacial Structures: A Comprehensive Approach, ed 8, St. Louis, 2019, Elsevier.)

ANATOMY ILLUSTRATIONS

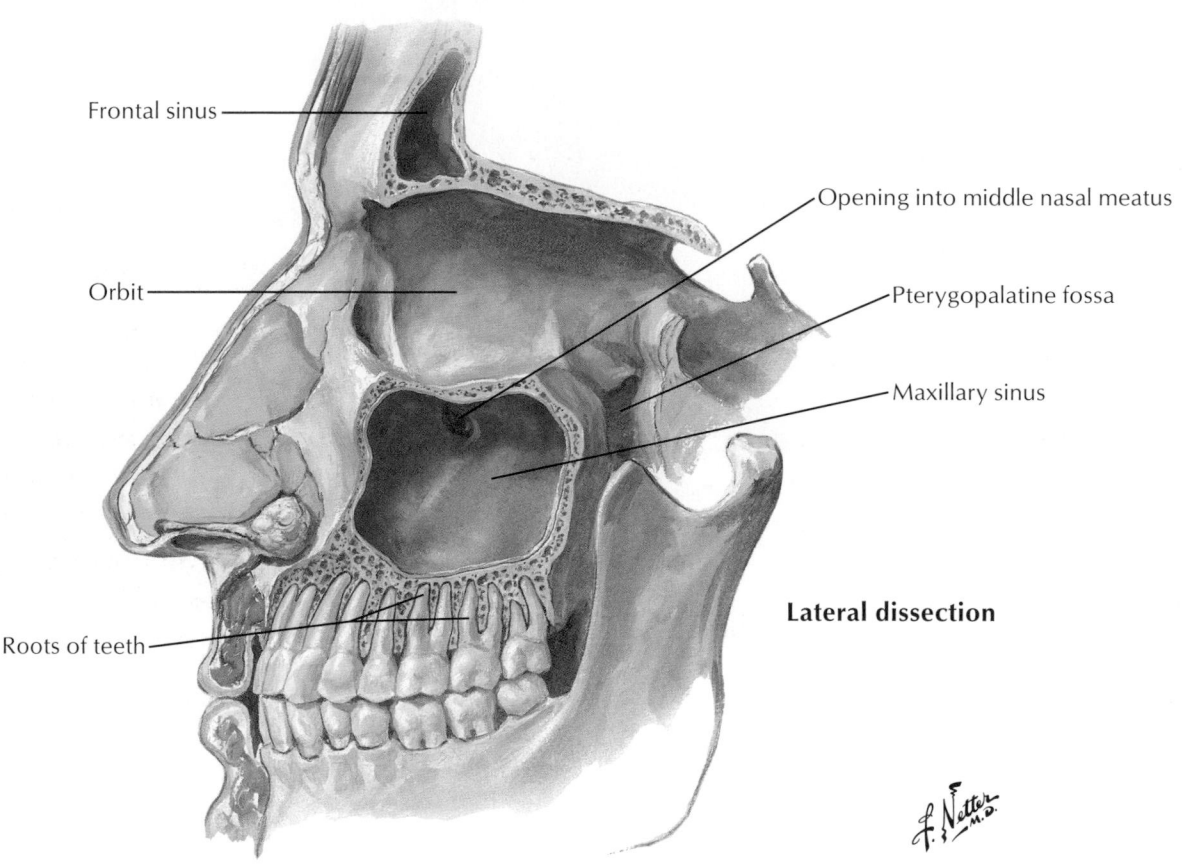

Frontal sinus

Orbit

Opening into middle nasal meatus

Pterygopalatine fossa

Maxillary sinus

Lateral dissection

Roots of teeth

Plate 27 Paranasal Sinuses. (Netter: Atlas of Human Anatomy, 4 ed, 2006, Saunders. Plate 49)

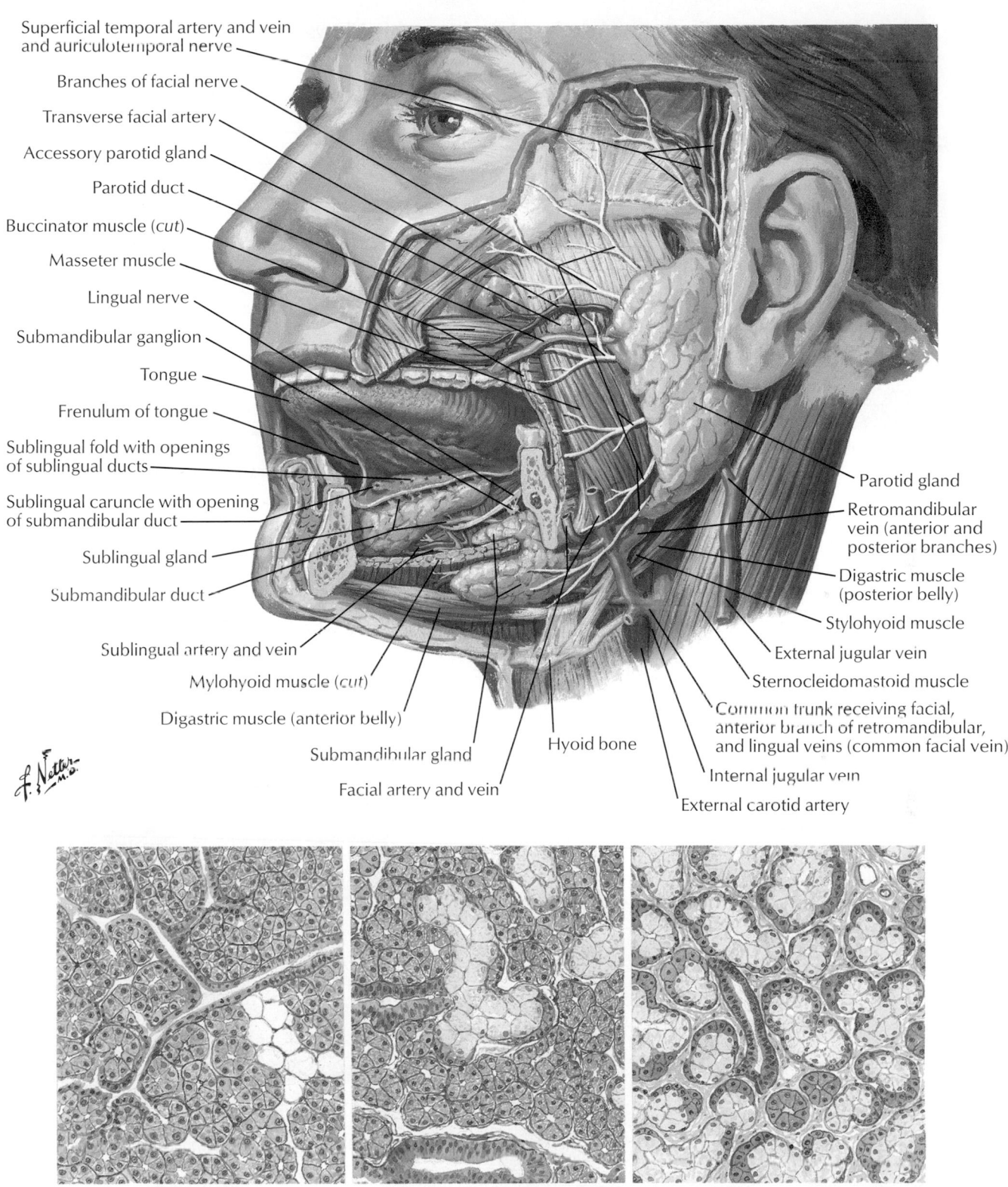

Superficial temporal artery and vein and auriculotemporal nerve

Branches of facial nerve

Transverse facial artery

Accessory parotid gland

Parotid duct

Buccinator muscle (*cut*)

Masseter muscle

Lingual nerve

Submandibular ganglion

Tongue

Frenulum of tongue

Sublingual fold with openings of sublingual ducts

Sublingual caruncle with opening of submandibular duct

Sublingual gland

Submandibular duct

Sublingual artery and vein

Mylohyoid muscle (*cut*)

Digastric muscle (anterior belly)

Submandibular gland

Facial artery and vein

Hyoid bone

Parotid gland

Retromandibular vein (anterior and posterior branches)

Digastric muscle (posterior belly)

Stylohyoid muscle

External jugular vein

Sternocleidomastoid muscle

Common trunk receiving facial, anterior branch of retromandibular, and lingual veins (common facial vein)

Internal jugular vein

External carotid artery

Parotid gland:
totally serous

Submandibular gland:
mostly serous, partially mucous

Sublingual gland:
almost completely mucous

Plate 28   Salivary Glands. (Netter: Atlas of Human Anatomy, 4 ed, 2006, Saunders. Plate 61)

Coronary Arteries: Arteriographic Views

Right coronary artery: left anterior oblique view

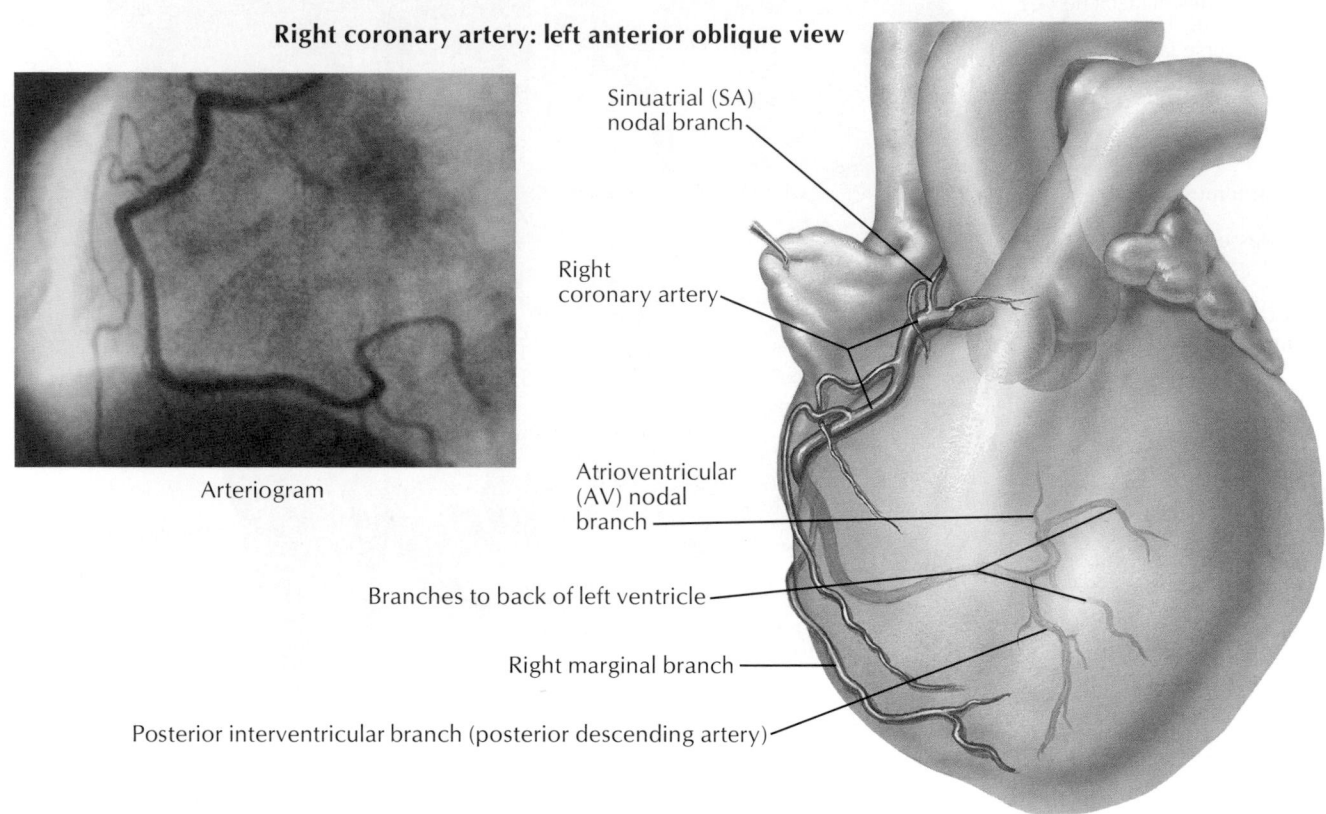

Sinuatrial (SA) nodal branch

Right coronary artery

Atrioventricular (AV) nodal branch

Branches to back of left ventricle

Right marginal branch

Posterior interventricular branch (posterior descending artery)

Arteriogram

Right coronary artery: right anterior oblique view

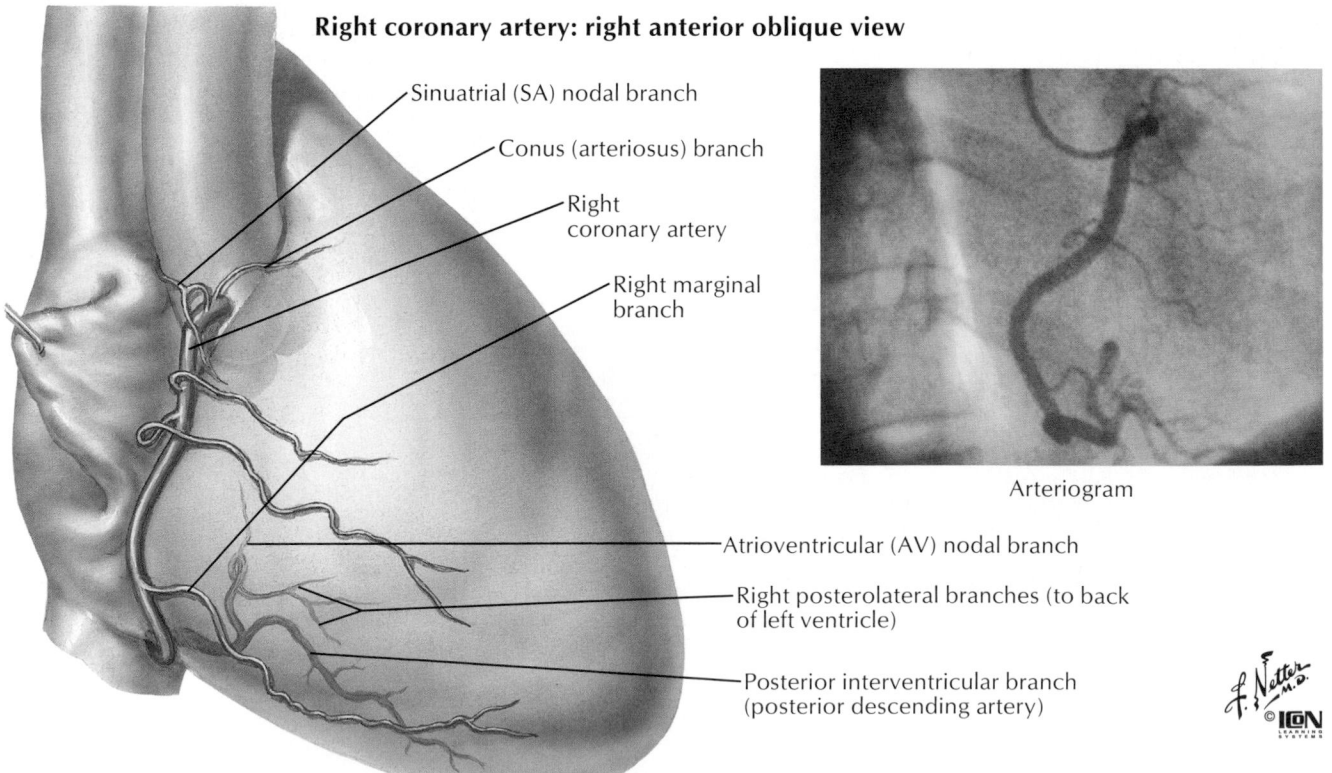

Sinuatrial (SA) nodal branch

Conus (arteriosus) branch

Right coronary artery

Right marginal branch

Atrioventricular (AV) nodal branch

Right posterolateral branches (to back of left ventricle)

Posterior interventricular branch (posterior descending artery)

Arteriogram

Plate 29 Coronary Arteries: Arteriographic Views. (Netter: Atlas of Human Anatomy, 4 ed, 2006, Saunders. Plate 218)

80

ANATOMY ILLUSTRATIONS

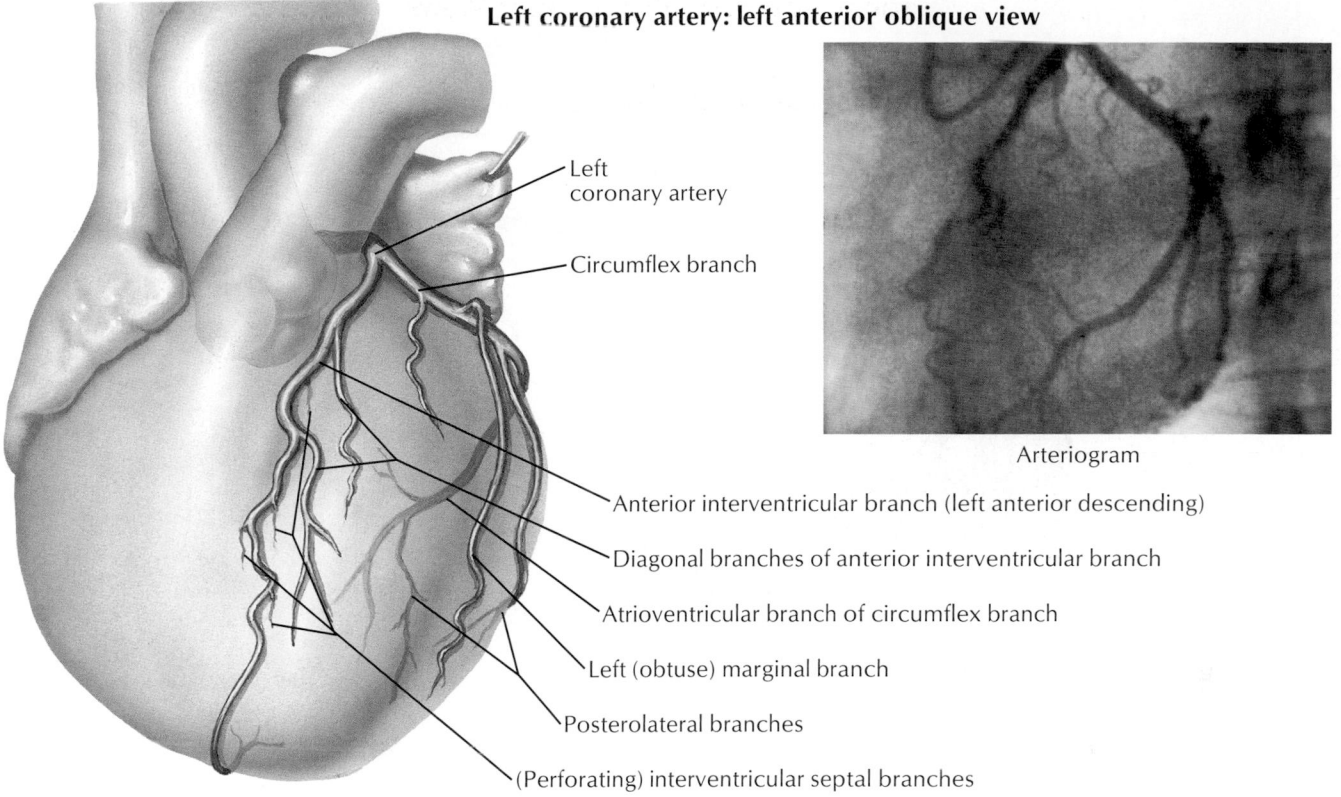

Left coronary artery: left anterior oblique view

Left coronary artery

Circumflex branch

Arteriogram

Anterior interventricular branch (left anterior descending)

Diagonal branches of anterior interventricular branch

Atrioventricular branch of circumflex branch

Left (obtuse) marginal branch

Posterolateral branches

(Perforating) interventricular septal branches

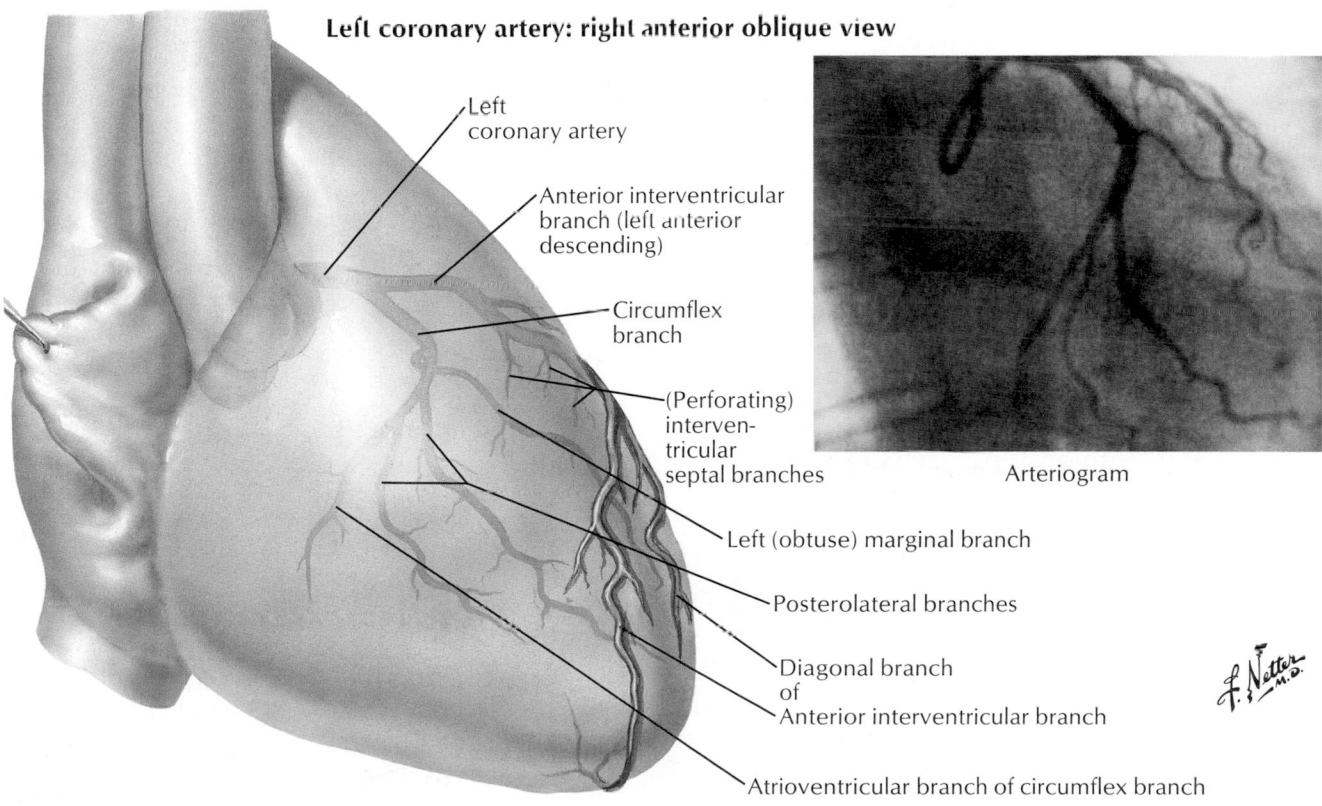

Left coronary artery: right anterior oblique view

Left coronary artery

Anterior interventricular branch (left anterior descending)

Circumflex branch

(Perforating) interventricular septal branches

Left (obtuse) marginal branch

Posterolateral branches

Diagonal branch of Anterior interventricular branch

Atrioventricular branch of circumflex branch

Arteriogram

Plate 30   Coronary Arteries: Arteriographic Views. (Netter: Atlas of Human Anatomy, 4 ed, 2006, Saunders. Plate 219)

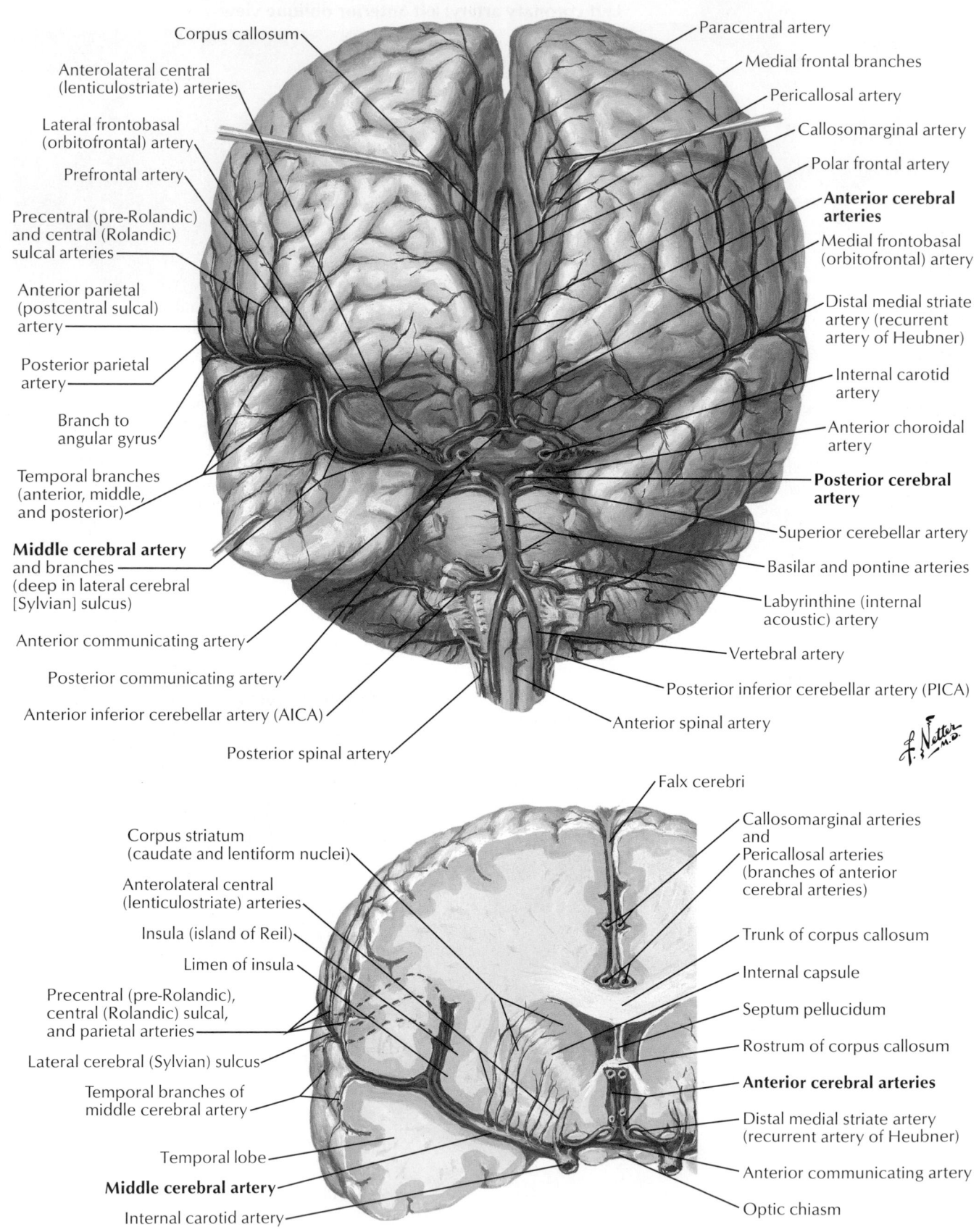

Corpus callosum

Anterolateral central
(lenticulostriate) arteries

Lateral frontobasal
(orbitofrontal) artery

Prefrontal artery

Precentral (pre-Rolandic)
and central (Rolandic)
sulcal arteries

Anterior parietal
(postcentral sulcal)
artery

Posterior parietal
artery

Branch to
angular gyrus

Temporal branches
(anterior, middle,
and posterior)

Middle cerebral artery
and branches
(deep in lateral cerebral
[Sylvian] sulcus)

Anterior communicating artery

Posterior communicating artery

Anterior inferior cerebellar artery (AICA)

Posterior spinal artery

Paracentral artery

Medial frontal branches

Pericallosal artery

Callosomarginal artery

Polar frontal artery

**Anterior cerebral
arteries**

Medial frontobasal
(orbitofrontal) artery

Distal medial striate
artery (recurrent
artery of Heubner)

Internal carotid
artery

Anterior choroidal
artery

**Posterior cerebral
artery**

Superior cerebellar artery

Basilar and pontine arteries

Labyrinthine (internal
acoustic) artery

Vertebral artery

Posterior inferior cerebellar artery (PICA)

Anterior spinal artery

Corpus striatum
(caudate and lentiform nuclei)

Anterolateral central
(lenticulostriate) arteries

Insula (island of Reil)

Limen of insula

Precentral (pre-Rolandic),
central (Rolandic) sulcal,
and parietal arteries

Lateral cerebral (Sylvian) sulcus

Temporal branches of
middle cerebral artery

Temporal lobe

Middle cerebral artery

Internal carotid artery

Falx cerebri

Callosomarginal arteries
and
Pericallosal arteries
(branches of anterior
cerebral arteries)

Trunk of corpus callosum

Internal capsule

Septum pellucidum

Rostrum of corpus callosum

Anterior cerebral arteries

Distal medial striate artery
(recurrent artery of Heubner)

Anterior communicating artery

Optic chiasm

Plate 31   Arteries of Brain: Frontal View and Section. (Netter: Atlas of Human Anatomy, 4 ed, 2006, Saunders. Plate 141)

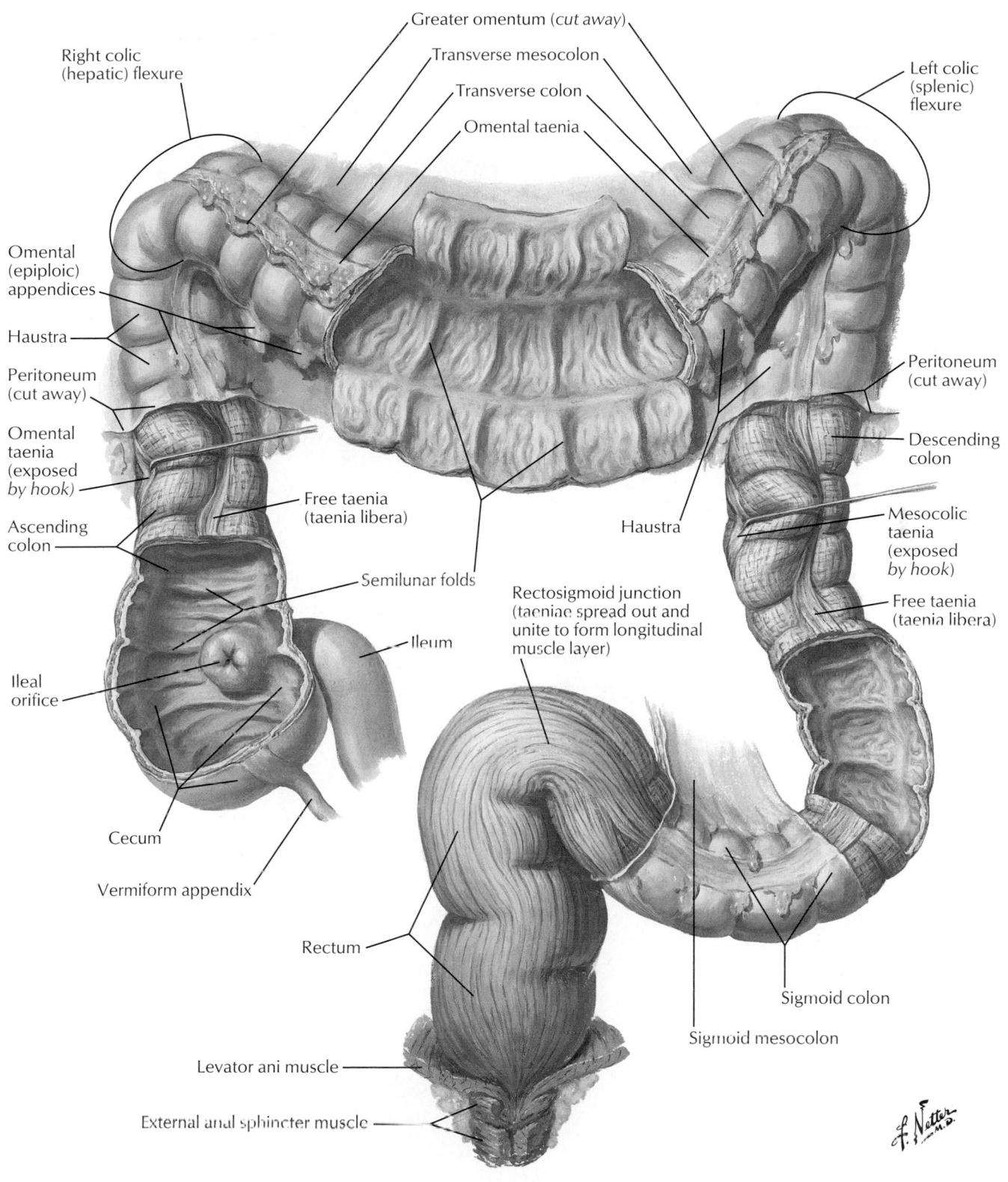

Right colic (hepatic) flexure

Greater omentum (cut away)

Transverse mesocolon

Transverse colon

Omental taenia

Left colic (splenic) flexure

Omental (epiploic) appendices

Haustra

Peritoneum (cut away)

Omental taenia (exposed by hook)

Ascending colon

Free taenia (taenia libera)

Semilunar folds

Ileal orifice

Cecum

Vermiform appendix

Ileum

Haustra

Peritoneum (cut away)

Descending colon

Mesocolic taenia (exposed by hook)

Free taenia (taenia libera)

Rectosigmoid junction (taeniae spread out and unite to form longitudinal muscle layer)

Rectum

Levator ani muscle

External anal sphincter muscle

Sigmoid colon

Sigmoid mesocolon

f. Netter M.D.

Plate 32 Mucosa and Musculature of Large Intestine. (Netter: Atlas of Human Anatomy, 4 ed, 2006, Saunders. Plate 284)

Transverse Section: T3–4 Intervertebral Disc, Manubrium

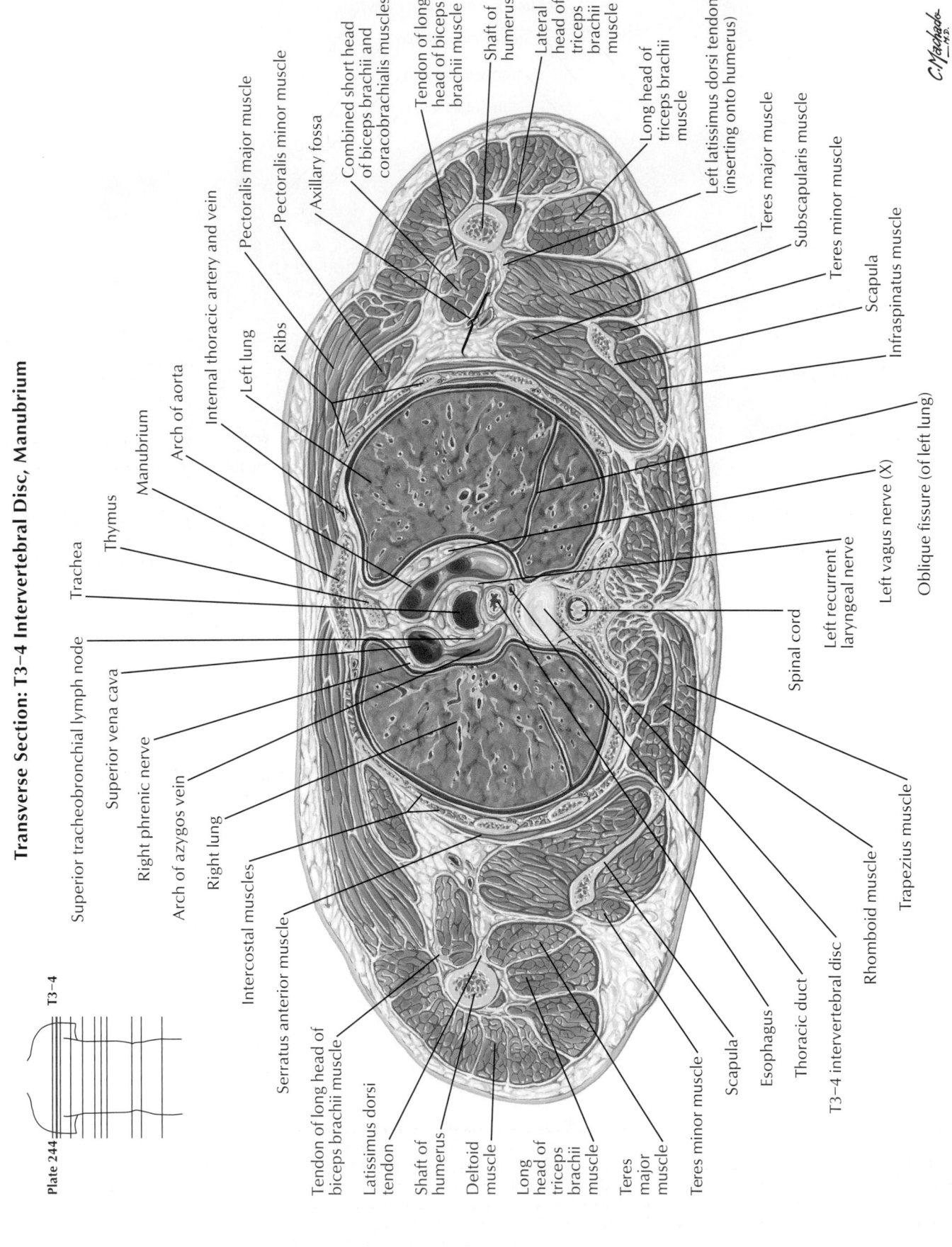

Plate 244

T3-4

Superior tracheobronchial lymph node

Superior vena cava

Right phrenic nerve

Arch of azygos vein

Right lung

Trachea

Thymus

Manubrium

Arch of aorta

Internal thoracic artery and vein

Left lung

Ribs

Pectoralis major muscle

Pectoralis minor muscle

Axillary fossa

Combined short head of biceps brachii and coracobrachialis muscles

Tendon of long head of biceps brachii muscle

Shaft of humerus

Lateral head of triceps brachii muscle

Long head of triceps brachii muscle

Left latissimus dorsi tendon (inserting onto humerus)

Teres major muscle

Subscapularis muscle

Teres minor muscle

Scapula

Infraspinatus muscle

Oblique fissure (of left lung)

Left vagus nerve (X)

Left recurrent laryngeal nerve

Spinal cord

Trapezius muscle

Rhomboid muscle

T3–4 intervertebral disc

Thoracic duct

Esophagus

Scapula

Teres minor muscle

Teres major muscle

Long head of triceps brachii muscle

Deltoid muscle

Shaft of humerus

Latissimus dorsi tendon

Tendon of long head of biceps brachii muscle

Serratus anterior muscle

Intercostal muscles

C. Machado _M.D.

Plate 33 Cross Section of Thorax at T3-4 Disc Level. (Netter: Atlas of Human Anatomy, 4 ed, 2006, Saunders. Plate 244)

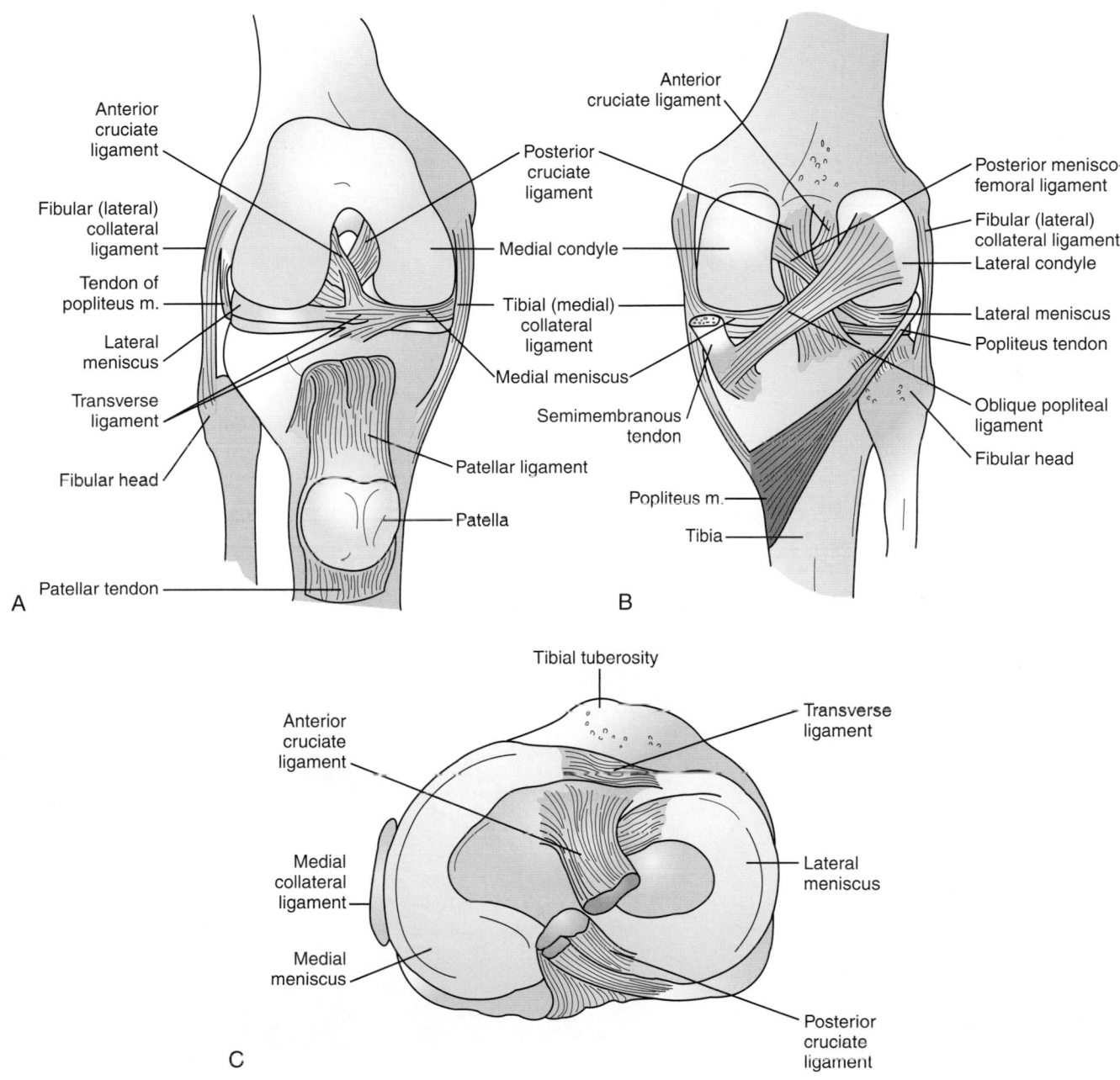

Anterior cruciate ligament

Fibular (lateral) collateral ligament

Tendon of popliteus m.

Lateral meniscus

Transverse ligament

Fibular head

Patellar tendon

A

Posterior cruciate ligament

Medial condyle

Tibial (medial) collateral ligament

Medial meniscus

Patellar ligament

Patella

Anterior cruciate ligament

Posterior meniscofemoral ligament

Fibular (lateral) collateral ligament

Lateral condyle

Lateral meniscus

Popliteus tendon

Oblique popliteal ligament

Fibular head

Semimembranous tendon

Popliteus m.

Tibia

B

Tibial tuberosity

Anterior cruciate ligament

Medial collateral ligament

Medial meniscus

Transverse ligament

Lateral meniscus

Posterior cruciate ligament

C

Plate 34 Knee joint opened; anterior, posterior, and proximal views. A, Anterior view of the knee joint, opened by folding the patella and patellar ligament inferiorly. On the lateral side is the fibular collateral ligament, separated by the popliteal tendon from the lateral meniscus. On the medial side, the tibial collateral ligament is attached to the medial meniscus. The anterior and posterior cruciate ligaments are seen between the femoral condyles. B, Posterior view of the opened knee joint with a more complete view of the posterior cruciate ligament. C, The femur is removed, showing the proximal (articular) end of the right tibia. On the medial side is the gently curved medial meniscus; on the lateral side is the more tightly curved lateral meniscus. The anterior end of the medial meniscus is anchored to the surface of the tibia by the transverse ligament. The cut ends of the anterior and posterior cruciate ligaments are shown, as well as the meniscofemoral ligament. (Fritz S: Mosby's Essential Sciences for Therapeutic Massage: Anatomy, Physiology, Biomechanics, and Pathology, ed 5, St. Louis, 2017, Elsevier.)

Paramedian (sagittal) dissection

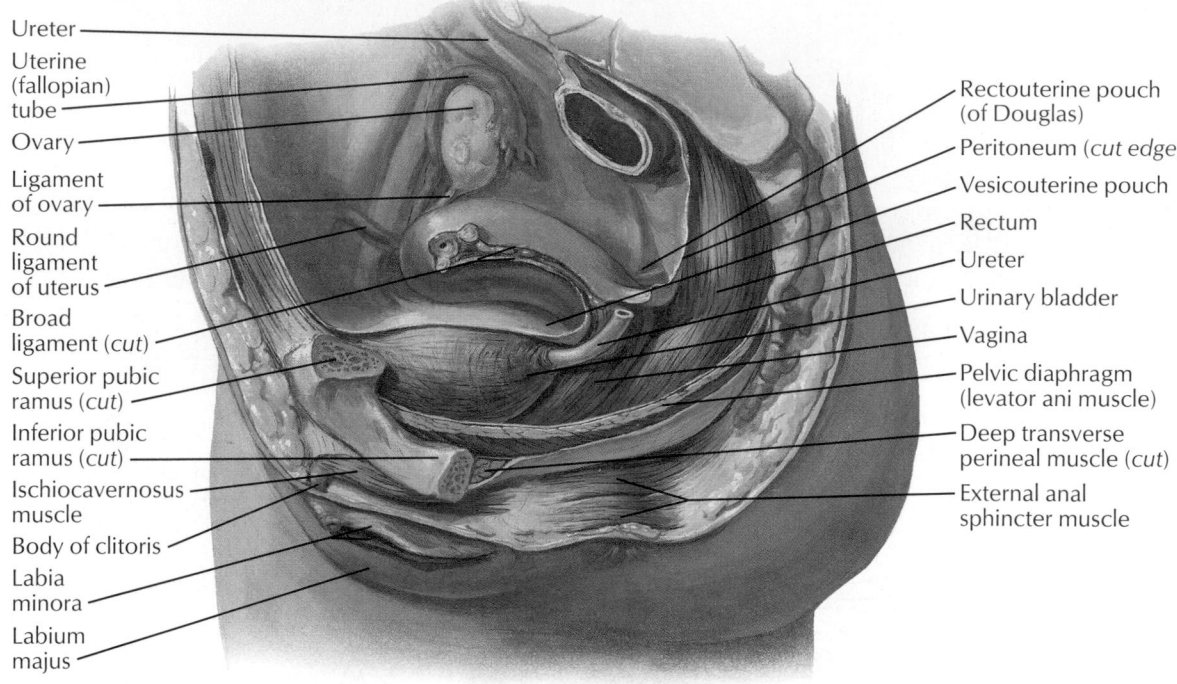

Ureter

Uterine (fallopian) tube

Ovary

Ligament of ovary

Round ligament of uterus

Broad ligament (*cut*)

Superior pubic ramus (*cut*)

Inferior pubic ramus (*cut*)

Ischiocavernosus muscle

Body of clitoris

Labia minora

Labium majus

Rectouterine pouch (of Douglas)

Peritoneum (*cut edge*)

Vesicouterine pouch

Rectum

Ureter

Urinary bladder

Vagina

Pelvic diaphragm (levator ani muscle)

Deep transverse perineal muscle (*cut*)

External anal sphincter muscle

Median (sagittal) section

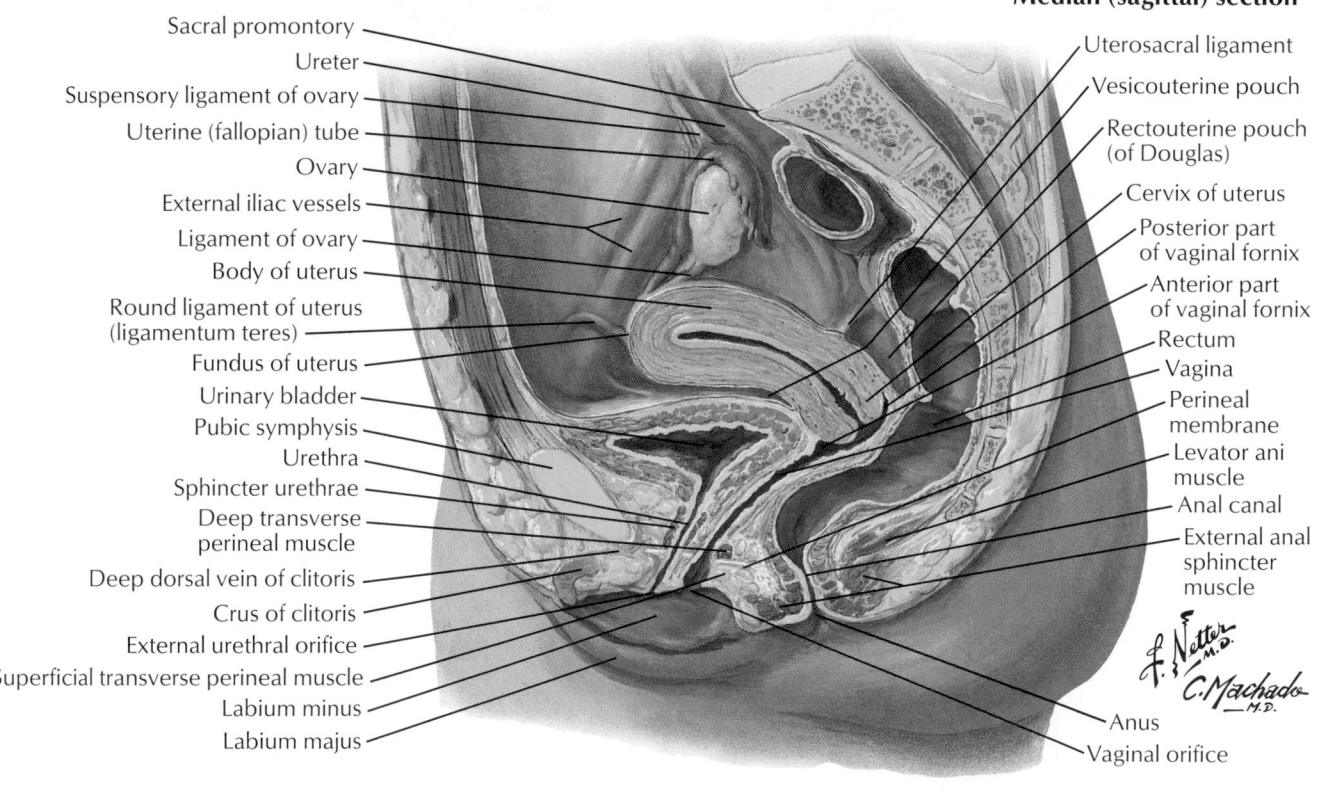

Sacral promontory

Ureter

Suspensory ligament of ovary

Uterine (fallopian) tube

Ovary

External iliac vessels

Ligament of ovary

Body of uterus

Round ligament of uterus (ligamentum teres)

Fundus of uterus

Urinary bladder

Pubic symphysis

Urethra

Sphincter urethrae

Deep transverse perineal muscle

Deep dorsal vein of clitoris

Crus of clitoris

External urethral orifice

Superficial transverse perineal muscle

Labium minus

Labium majus

Uterosacral ligament

Vesicouterine pouch

Rectouterine pouch (of Douglas)

Cervix of uterus

Posterior part of vaginal fornix

Anterior part of vaginal fornix

Rectum

Vagina

Perineal membrane

Levator ani muscle

Anal canal

External anal sphincter muscle

Anus

Vaginal orifice

Plate 35   Pelvic Viscera and Perineum: Female. (Netter: Atlas of Human Anatomy, 4 ed, 2006, Saunders. Plate 360)

PART II

Alphabetic Index

A

Aarskog's syndrome Q87.19
Abandonment —*see* Maltreatment
Abasia (-astasia) (hysterical) F44.4
Abderhalden-Kaufmann-Lignac syndrome
　(cystinosis) E72.04
Abdomen, abdominal —*see also* condition
　acute R10.0
　angina K55.1
　muscle deficiency syndrome Q79.4
Abdominalgia —*see* Pain, abdominal
Abduction contracture, hip or other joint —*see*
　Contraction, joint
Aberrant (congenital) —*see also* Malposition,
　congenital
　adrenal gland Q89.1
　artery (peripheral) Q27.8
　　basilar NEC Q28.1
　　cerebral Q28.3
　　coronary Q24.5
　　digestive system Q27.8
　　eye Q15.8
　　lower limb Q27.8
　　precerebral Q28.1
　　pulmonary Q25.79
　　renal Q27.2
　　retina Q14.1
　　specified site NEC Q27.8
　　subclavian Q27.8
　　upper limb Q27.8
　　vertebral Q28.1
　breast Q83.8
　endocrine gland NEC Q89.2
　hepatic duct Q44.5
　pancreas Q45.3
　parathyroid gland Q89.2
　pituitary gland Q89.2
　sebaceous glands, mucous membrane,
　　mouth, congenital Q38.6
　spleen Q89.09
　subclavian artery Q27.8
　thymus (gland) Q89.2
　thyroid gland Q89.2
　vein (peripheral) NEC Q27.8
　　cerebral Q28.3
　　digestive system Q27.8
　　lower limb Q27.8
　　precerebral Q28.1
　　specified site NEC Q27.8
　　upper limb Q27.8
Aberration
　distantal —*see* Disturbance, visual
　mental F99
Abetalipoproteinemia E78.6
Abiotrophy R68.89
Ablatio, ablation
　retinae —*see* Detachment, retina
Ablepharia, ablepharon Q10.3
Abnormal, abnormality, abnormalities —*see*
　　also Anomaly
　acid-base balance (mixed) E87.4
　albumin R77.0
　alphafetoprotein R77.2
　alveolar ridge K08.9
　anatomical relationship Q89.9
　apertures, congenital, diaphragm Q79.1
　auditory perception H93.29-●
　　diplacusis —*see* Diplacusis
　　hyperacusis —*see* Hyperacusis
　　recruitment —*see* Recruitment, auditory
　　threshold shift —*see* Shift, auditory
　　　threshold
　autosomes Q99.9
　　fragile site Q95.5
　basal metabolic rate R94.8
　biosynthesis, testicular androgen
　　E29.1
　bleeding time R79.1
▶blood amino-acid level R79.83

Abnormal, abnormality, abnormalities —
　(Continued)
　blood level (of)
　　cobalt R79.0
　　copper R79.0
　　iron R79.0
　　lithium R78.89
　　magnesium R79.0
　　mineral NEC R79.0
　　zinc R79.0
　blood pressure
　　elevated R03.0
　　low reading (nonspecific) R03.1
　blood sugar R73.09
　blood-gas level R79.81
　bowel sounds R19.15
　　absent R19.11
　　hyperactive R19.12
　brain scan R94.02
　breathing R06.9
　caloric test R94.138
　cerebrospinal fluid R83.9
　　cytology R83.6
　　drug level R83.2
　　enzyme level R83.0
　　hormones R83.1
　　immunology R83.4
　　microbiology R83.5
　　nonmedicinal level R83.3
　　specified type NEC R83.8
　chemistry, blood R79.9
　　C-reactive protein R79.82
　　drugs —*see* Findings, abnormal, in blood
　　gas level R79.81
　　minerals R79.0
　　pancytopenia D61.818
　　PTT R79.1
　　specified NEC R79.89
　　toxins —*see* Findings, abnormal, in
　　　blood
　chest sounds (friction) (rales) R09.89
　chromosome, chromosomal Q99.9
　　with more than three X chromosomes,
　　　female Q97.1
　　analysis result R89.8
　　　bronchial washings R84.8
　　　cerebrospinal fluid R83.8
　　　cervix uteri NEC R87.89
　　　nasal secretions R84.8
　　　nipple discharge R89.8
　　　peritoneal fluid R85.89
　　　pleural fluid R84.8
　　　prostatic secretions R86.8
　　　saliva R85.89
　　　seminal fluid R86.8
　　　sputum R84.8
　　　synovial fluid R89.8
　　　throat scrapings R84.8
　　　vagina R87.89
　　　vulva R87.89
　　　wound secretions R89.8
　　dicentric replacement Q93.2
　　ring replacement Q93.2
　　sex Q98.8
　　　female phenotype Q97.9
　　　　specified NEC Q97.8
　　　male phenotype Q98.9
　　　　specified NEC Q98.8
　　　structural male Q98.6
　　specified NEC Q99.8
　clinical findings NEC R68.89
　coagulation D68.9
　　newborn, transient P61.6
　　profile R79.1
　　time R79.1
　communication —*see* Fistula
　conjunctiva, vascular H11.41-●
　coronary artery Q24.5
　cortisol-binding globulin E27.8
　course, eustachian tube Q17.8

Abnormal, abnormality, abnormalities —
　(Continued)
　creatinine clearance R94.4
　cytology
　　anus R85.619
　　　atypical squamous cells cannot
　　　　exclude high grade squamous
　　　　intraepithelial lesion (ASC-H)
　　　　R85.611
　　　atypical squamous cells of undetermined
　　　　significance (ASC-US) R85.610
　　　cytologic evidence of malignancy
　　　　R85.614
　　　high grade squamous intraepithelial
　　　　lesion (HGSIL) R85.613
　　　human papillomavirus (HPV) DNA test
　　　　high risk positive R85.81
　　　　low risk postive R85.82
　　　inadequate smear R85.615
　　　low grade squamous intraepithelial
　　　　lesion (LGSIL) R85.612
　　　satisfactory anal smear but lacking
　　　　transformation zone R85.616
　　　specified NEC R85.618
　　　unsatisfactory smear R85.615
　　female genital organs —*see* Abnormal,
　　　Papanicolaou (smear)
　dark adaptation curve H53.61
　dentofacial NEC —*see* Anomaly, dentofacial
　development, developmental Q89.9
　　central nervous system Q07.9
　diagnostic imaging
　　abdomen, abdominal region NEC R93.5
　　biliary tract R93.2
　　bladder R93.41
　　breast R92.8
　　central nervous system NEC R90.89
　　cerebrovascular NEC R90.89
　　coronary circulation R93.1
　　digestive tract NEC R93.3
　　gastrointestinal (tract) R93.3
　　genitourinary organs R93.89
　　head R93.0
　　heart R93.1
　　intrathoracic organ NEC R93.89
　　kidney R93.42-●
　　limbs R93.6
　　liver R93.2
　　lung (field) R91.8
　　musculoskeletal system NEC R93.7
　　renal pelvis R93.41
　　retroperitoneum R93.5
　　site specified NEC R93.89
　　skin and subcutaneous tissue R93.89
　　skull R93.0
　　testis R93.81-●
　　urinary organs specified NEC R93.49
　　ureter R93.41
　direction, teeth, fully erupted M26.30
　ear ossicles, acquired NEC H74.39-●
　　ankylosis —*see* Ankylosis, ear ossicles
　　discontinuity —*see* Discontinuity, ossicles,
　　　ear
　　partial loss —*see* Loss, ossicles, ear (partial)
　Ebstein Q22.5
　echocardiogram R93.1
　echoencephalogram R90.81
　echogram —*see* Abnormal, diagnostic
　　imaging
　electrocardiogram [ECG] [EKG] R94.31
　electroencephalogram [EEG] R94.01
　electrolyte —*see* Imbalance, electrolyte
　electromyogram [EMG] R94.131
　electro-oculogram [EOG] R94.110
　electrophysiological intracardiac studies
　　R94.39
　electroretinogram [ERG] R94.111
　erythrocytes
　　congenital, with perinatal jaundice D58.9
　feces (color) (contents) (mucus) R19.5

Abnormal, abnormality, abnormalities —
(Continued)
  finding —see Findings, abnormal, without
    diagnosis
  fluid
    amniotic —see Abnormal, specimen,
      specified
    cerebrospinal —see Abnormal,
      cerebrospinal fluid
    peritoneal —see Abnormal, specimen,
      digestive organs
    pleural —see Abnormal, specimen,
      respiratory organs
    synovial —see Abnormal, specimen,
      specified
    thorax (bronchial washings) (pleural
      fluid) —see Abnormal, specimen,
      respiratory organs
    vaginal —see Abnormal, specimen, female
      genital organs
  form
    teeth K00.2
    uterus —see Anomaly, uterus
  function studies
    auditory R94.120
    bladder R94.8
    brain R94.09
    cardiovascular R94.30
    ear R94.128
    endocrine NEC R94.7
    eye NEC R94.118
    kidney R94.4
    liver R94.5
    nervous system
      central NEC R94.09
      peripheral NEC R94.138
    pancreas R94.8
    placenta R94.8
    pulmonary R94.2
    special senses NEC R94.128
    spleen R94.8
    thyroid R94.6
    vestibular R94.121
  gait —see Gait
    hysterical F44.4
  gastrin secretion E16.4
  globulin R77.1
    cortisol-binding E27.8
    thyroid-binding E07.89
  glomerular, minor —see also N00-N07 with
    fourth character .0 N05.0
  glucagon secretion E16.3
  glucose tolerance (test) (non-fasting)
    R73.09
  gravitational (G) forces or states (effect of)
    T75.81
  hair (color) (shaft) L67.9
    specified NEC L67.8
  hard tissue formation in pulp (dental)
    K04.3
  head movement R25.0
  heart
    rate R00.9
      specified NEC R00.8
    shadow R93.1
    sounds NEC R01.2
  hemoglobin (disease) —see also Disease,
    hemoglobin D58.2
    trait —see Trait, hemoglobin, abnormal
  histology NEC R89.7
  immunological findings R89.4
    in serum R76.9
      specified NEC R76.8
  increase in appetite R63.2
  involuntary movement —see Abnormal,
    movement, involuntary
  jaw closure M26.51
  karyotype R89.8
  kidney function test R94.4
  knee jerk R29.2
  leukocyte (cell) (differential) NEC D72.9

Abnormal, abnormality, abnormalities —
(Continued)
  liver function test (see also Elevated, liver
    function, test) R79.89
  loss of
    height R29.890
    weight R63.4
  mammogram NEC R92.8
    calcification (calculus) R92.1
    microcalcification R92.0
  Mantoux test R76.11
  movement (disorder) —see also Disorder,
    movement
    head R25.0
    involuntary R25.9
      fasciculation R25.3
      of head R25.0
      spasm R25.2
      specified type NEC R25.8
      tremor R25.1
  myoglobin (Aberdeen) (Annapolis) R89.7
  neonatal screening P09.9
    for
      congenital adrenal hyperplasia P09.2
      congenital endocrine disease P09.2
      congenital hematologic disorders P09.3
      critical congenital heart disease P09.5
      cystic fibrosis P09.4
      hemoglobinothies P09.3
      hypothyroidism P09.2
      inborn errors of metabolism P09.1
      neonatal hearing loss P09.6
      red cell membrane defects P09.3
      sickle cell P09.3
      specified NEC P09.8
  oculomotor study R94.113
  palmar creases Q82.8
  Papanicolaou (smear)
    anus R85.619
      atypical squamous cells cannot
        exclude high grade squamous
        intraepithelial lesion (ASC-H)
        R85.611
      atypical squamous cells of undetermined
        significance (ASC-US) R85.610
      cytologic evidence of malignancy
        R85.614
      high grade squamous intraepithelial
        lesion (HGSIL) R85.613
      human papillomavirus (HPV) DNA test
        high risk positive R85.81
        low risk postive R85.82
      inadequate smear R85.615
      low grade squamous intraepithelial
        lesion (LGSIL) R85.612
      satisfactory anal smear but lacking
        transformation zone R85.616
      specified NEC R85.618
      unsatisfactory smear R85.615
    bronchial washings R84.6
    cerebrospinal fluid R83.6
    cervix R87.619
      atypical squamous cells cannot
        exclude high grade squamous
        intraepithelial lesion (ASC-H)
        R87.611
      atypical squamous cells of undetermined
        significance (ASC-US) R87.610
      cytologic evidence of malignancy
        R87.614
      high grade squamous intraepithelial
        lesion (HGSIL) R87.613
      inadequate smear R87.615
      low grade squamous intraepithelial
        lesion (LGSIL) R87.612
      non-atypical endometrial cells R87.618
      satisfactory cervical smear but lacking
        transformation zone R87.616
      specified NEC R87.618
      thin preparaton R87.619
      unsatisfactory smear R87.615

Abnormal, abnormality, abnormalities —
(Continued)
  Papanicolaou (smear) (Continued)
    nasal secretions R84.6
    nipple discharge R89.6
    peritoneal fluid R85.69
    pleural fluid R84.6
    prostatic secretions R86.6
    saliva R85.69
    seminal fluid R86.6
    sites NEC R89.6
    sputum R84.6
    synovial fluid R89.6
    throat scrapings R84.6
    vagina R87.629
      atypical squamous cells cannot
        exclude high grade squamous
        intraepithelial lesion (ASC-H)
        R87.621
      atypical squamous cells of undetermined
        significance (ASC-US) R87.620
      cytologic evidence of malignancy
        R87.624
      high grade squamous intraepithelial
        lesion (HGSIL) R87.623
      inadequate smear R87.625
      low grade squamous intraepithelial
        lesion (LGSIL) R87.622
      specified NEC R87.628
      thin preparation R87.629
      unsatisfactory smear R87.625
    vulva R87.69
    wound secretions R89.6
  partial thromboplastin time (PTT) R79.1
  pelvis (bony) —see Deformity, pelvis
  percussion, chest (tympany) R09.89
  periods (grossly) —see Menstruation
  phonocardiogram R94.39
  plantar reflex R29.2
  plasma
    protein R77.9
      specified NEC R77.8
    viscosity R70.1
  pleural (folds) Q34.0
  posture R29.3
  product of conception O02.9
    specified type NEC O02.89
  prothrombin time (PT) R79.1
  pulmonary
    artery, congenital Q25.79
    function, newborn P28.89
    test results R94.2
  pulsations in neck R00.2
  pupillary H21.56-●
    function (reaction) (reflex) —see Anomaly,
      pupil, function
  radiological examination —see Abnormal,
    diagnostic imaging
  red blood cell(s) (morphology) (volume)
    R71.8
  reflex —see Reflex
  renal function test R94.4
  response to nerve stimulation R94.130
  retinal correspondence H53.31
  retinal function study R94.111
  rhythm, heart —see also Arrhythmia
  saliva —see Abnormal, specimen, digestive
    organs
  scan
    kidney R94.4
    liver R93.2
    thyroid R94.6
  secretion
    gastrin E16.4
    glucagon E16.3
  semen, seminal fluid —see Abnormal,
    specimen, male genital organs
  serum level (of)
    acid phosphatase R74.8
    alkaline phosphatase R74.8
    amylase R74.8

Abnormal, abnormality, abnormalities — *(Continued)*
  serum level (of) *(Continued)*
    enzymes R74.9
      specified NEC R74.8
    lipase R74.8
    triacylglycerol lipase R74.8
  shape
    gravid uterus —*see* Anomaly, uterus
  sinus venosus Q21.1
  size, tooth, teeth K00.2
  spacing, tooth, teeth, fully erupted M26.30
  specimen
    digestive organs (peritoneal fluid) (saliva) R85.9
      cytology R85.69
      drug level R85.2
      enzyme level R85.0
      histology R85.7
      hormones R85.1
      immunology R85.4
      microbiology R85.5
      nonmedicinal level R85.3
      specified type NEC R85.89
    female genital organs (secretions) (smears) R87.9
      cytology R87.69
        cervix R87.619
          human papillomavirus (HPV) DNA test
            high risk positive R87.810
            low risk positive R87.820
          inadequate (unsatisfactory) smear R87.615
          non-atypical endometrial cells R87.618
          specified NEC R87.618
        vagina R87.629
          human papillomavirus (HPV) DNA test
            high risk positive R87.811
            low risk positive R87.821
          inadequate (unsatisfactory) smear R87.625
        vulva R87.69
      drug level R87.2
      enzyme level R87.0
      histological R87.7
      hormones R87.1
      immunology R87.4
      microbiology R87.5
      nonmedicinal level R87.3
      specified type NEC R87.89
    male genital organs (prostatic secretions) (semen) R86.9
      cytology R86.6
      drug level R86.2
      enzyme level R86.0
      histological R86.7
      hormones R86.1
      immunology R86.4
      microbiology R86.5
      nonmedicinal level R86.3
      specified type NEC R86.8
    nipple discharge —*see* Abnormal, specimen, specified
    respiratory organs (bronchial washings) (nasal secretions) (pleural fluid) (sputum) R84.9
      cytology R84.6
      drug level R84.2
      enzyme level R84.0
      histology R84.7
      hormones R84.1
      immunology R84.4
      microbiology R84.5
      nonmedicinal level R84.3
      specified type NEC R84.8
    specified organ, system and tissue NOS R89.9
      cytology R89.6

Abnormal, abnormality, abnormalities — *(Continued)*
  specimen *(Continued)*
    specified organ, system and tissue NOS *(Continued)*
      drug level R89.2
      enzyme level R89.0
      histology R89.7
      hormones R89.1
      immunology R89.4
      microbiology R89.5
      nonmedicinal level R89.3
      specified type NEC R89.8
    synovial fluid —*see* Abnormal, specimen, specified
    thorax (bronchial washings) (pleural fluids) —*see* Abnormal, specimen, respiratory organs
    vagina (secretion) (smear) R87.629
    vulva (secretion) (smear) R87.69
    wound secretion —*see* Abnormal, specimen, specified
  spermatozoa —*see* Abnormal, specimen, male genital organs
  sputum (amount) (color) (odor) R09.3
  stool (color) (contents) (mucus) R19.5
    bloody K92.1
    guaiac positive R19.5
  synchondrosis Q78.8
  thermography —*see also* Abnormal, diagnostic imaging R93.89
  thyroid-binding globulin E07.89
  tooth, teeth (form) (size) K00.2
  toxicology (findings) R78.9
  transport protein E88.09
  tumor marker NEC R97.8
  ultrasound results —*see* Abnormal, diagnostic imaging
  umbilical cord complicating delivery O69.9
  urination NEC R39.198
  urine (constituents) R82.90
    bile R82.2
    cytological examination R82.89
    drugs R82.5
    fat R82.0
    glucose R81
    heavy metals R82.6
    hemoglobin R82.3
    histological examination R82.89
    ketones R82.4
    microbiological examination (culture) R82.79
    myoglobin R82.1
    positive culture R82.79
    protein —*see* Proteinuria
    specified substance NEC R82.998
      chromoabnormality NEC R82.91
    substances nonmedical R82.6
  uterine hemorrhage —*see* Hemorrhage, uterus
  vectorcardiogram R94.39
  visually evoked potential (VEP) R94.112
  white blood cells D72.9
    specified NEC D72.89
  X-ray examination —*see* Abnormal, diagnostic imaging
Abnormity (any organ or part) —*see* Anomaly
Abocclusion M26.29
  hemolytic disease (newborn) P55.1
  incompatibility reaction ABO —*see* Complication(s), transfusion, incompatibility reaction, ABO
Abolition, language R48.8
Aborter, habitual or recurrent —*see* Loss (of), pregnancy, recurrent
Abortion (complete) (spontaneous) O03.9
  with
    retained products of conception —*see* Abortion, incomplete
  attempted (elective) (failed) O07.4
    complicated by O07.30
      afibrinogenemia O07.1
      cardiac arrest O07.36

Abortion *(Continued)*
  attempted *(Continued)*
    complicated by *(Continued)*
      chemical damage of pelvic organ(s) O07.34
      circulatory collapse O07.31
      cystitis O07.38
      defibrination syndrome O07.1
      electrolyte imbalance O07.33
      embolism (air) (amniotic fluid) (blood clot) (fat) (pulmonary) (septic) (soap) O07.2
      endometritis O07.0
      genital tract and pelvic infection O07.0
      hemolysis O07.1
      hemorrhage (delayed) (excessive) O07.1
      infection
        genital tract or pelvic O07.0
        urinary tract tract O07.38
      intravascular coagulation O07.1
      laceration of pelvic organ(s) O07.34
      metabolic disorder O07.33
      oliguria O07.32
      oophoritis O07.0
      parametritis O07.0
      pelvic peritonitis O07.0
      perforation of pelvic organ(s) O07.34
      renal failure or shutdown O07.32
      salpingitis or salpingo-oophoritis O07.0
      sepsis O07.37
      shock O07.31
      specified condition NEC O07.39
      tubular necrosis (renal) O07.32
      uremia O07.32
      urinary tract infection O07.38
      venous complication NEC O07.35
        embolism (air) (amniotic fluid) (blood clot) (fat) (pulmonary) (septic) (soap) O07.2
  complicated (by) (following) O03.80
    afibrinogenemia O03.6
    cardiac arrest O03.86
    chemical damage of pelvic organ(s) O03.84
    circulatory collapse O03.81
    cystitis O03.88
    defibrination syndrome O03.6
    electrolyte imbalance O03.83
    embolism (air) (amniotic fluid) (blood clot) (fat) (pulmonary) (septic) (soap) O03.7
    endometritis O03.5
    genital tract and pelvic infection O03.5
    hemolysis O03.6
    hemorrhage (delayed) (excessive) O03.6
    infection
      genital tract or pelvic O03.5
      urinary tract O03.88
    intravascular coagulation O03.6
    laceration of pelvic organ(s) O03.84
    metabolic disorder O03.83
    oliguria O03.82
    oophoritis O03.5
    parametritis O03.5
    pelvic peritonitis O03.5
    perforation of pelvic organ(s) O03.84
    renal failure or shutdown O03.82
    salpingitis or salpingo-oophoritis O03.5
    sepsis O03.87
    shock O03.81
    specified condition NEC O03.89
    tubular necrosis (renal) O03.82
    uremia O03.82
    urinary tract infection O03.88
    venous complication NEC O03.85
      embolism (air) (amniotic fluid) (blood clot) (fat) (pulmonary) (septic) (soap) O03.7
  failed —*see* Abortion, attempted
  habitual or recurrent N96
    with current abortion —*see* categories O03-O04
    without current pregnancy N96
    care in current pregnancy O26.2-●

▶ New   ➠ Revised   ~~deleted~~ Deleted   ● Use Additional Character(s)

Abortion *(Continued)*
incomplete (spontaneous) O03.4
  complicated (by) (following) O03.30
    afibrinogenemia O03.1
    cardiac arrest O03.36
    chemical damage of pelvic organ(s) O03.34
    circulatory collapse O03.31
    cystitis O03.38
    defibrination syndrome O03.1
    electrolyte imbalance O03.33
    embolism (air) (amniotic fluid) (blood clot) (fat) (pulmonary) (septic) (soap) O03.2
    endometritis O03.0
    genital tract and pelvic infection O03.0
    hemolysis O03.1
    hemorrhage (delayed) (excessive) O03.1
    infection
      genital tract or pelvic O03.0
      urinary tract O03.38
    intravascular coagulation O03.1
    laceration of pelvic organ(s) O03.34
    metabolic disorder O03.33
    oliguria O03.32
    oophoritis O03.0
    parametritis O03.0
    pelvic peritonitis O03.0
    perforation of pelvic organ(s) O03.34
    renal failure or shutdown O03.32
    salpingitis or salpingo-oophoritis O03.0
    sepsis O03.37
    shock O03.31
    specified condition NEC O03.39
    tubular necrosis (renal) O03.32
    uremia O03.32
    urinary infection O03.38
    venous complication NEC O03.35
      embolism (air) (amniotic fluid) (blood clot) (fat) (pulmonary) (septic) (soap) O03.2
induced (encounter for) Z33.2
  complicated by O04.80
    afibrinogenemia O04.6
    cardiac arrest O04.86
    chemical damage of pelvic organ(s) O04.84
    circulatory collapse O04.81
    cystitis O04.88
    defibrination syndrome O04.6
    electrolyte imbalance O04.83
    embolism (air) (amniotic fluid) (blood clot) (fat) (pulmonary) (septic) (soap) O04.7
    endometritis O04.5
    genital tract and pelvic infection O04.5
    hemolysis O04.6
    hemorrhage (delayed) (excessive) O04.6
    infection
      genital tract or pelvic O04.5
      urinary tract O04.88
    intravascular coagulation O04.6
    laceration of pelvic organ(s) O04.84
    metabolic disorder O04.83
    oliguria O04.82
    oophoritis O04.5
    parametritis O04.5
    pelvic peritonitis O04.5
    perforation of pelvic organ(s) O04.84
    renal failure or shutdown O04.82
    salpingitis or salpingo-oophoritis O04.5
    sepsis O04.87
    shock O04.81
    specified condition NEC O04.89
    tubular necrosis (renal) O04.82
    uremia O04.82
    urinary tract infection O04.88
    venous complication NEC O04.85
      embolism (air) (amniotic fluid) (blood clot) (fat) (pulmonary) (septic) (soap) O04.7
inevitable O03.4
missed O02.1

Abortion *(Continued)*
spontaneous —*see* Abortion (complete) (spontaneous)
  threatened O20.0
threatened (spontaneous) O20.0
tubal O00.10-●
  with intrauterine pregnancy O00.11-
Abortus fever A23.1
Aboulomania F60.7
Abrami's disease D59.8
Abramov-Fiedler myocarditis (acute isolated myocarditis) I40.1
Abrasion T14.8
abdomen, abdominal (wall) S30.811
alveolar process S00.512
ankle S90.51-●
antecubital space —*see* Abrasion, elbow
anus S30.817
arm (upper) S40.81-●
auditory canal —*see* Abrasion, ear
auricle —*see* Abrasion, ear
axilla —*see* Abrasion, arm
back, lower S30.810
breast S20.11-●
brow S00.81
buttock S30.810
calf —*see* Abrasion, leg
canthus —*see* Abrasion, eyelid
cheek S00.81
  internal S00.512
chest wall —*see* Abrasion, thorax
chin S00.81
clitoris S30.814
cornea S05.0-●
costal region —*see* Abrasion, thorax
dental K03.1
digit(s)
  foot —*see* Abrasion, toe
  hand —*see* Abrasion, finger
ear S00.41-●
elbow S50.31-●
epididymis S30.813
epigastric region S30.811
epiglottis S10.11
esophagus (thoracic) S27.818
  cervical S10.11
eyebrow —*see* Abrasion, eyelid
eyelid S00.21-●
face S00.81
finger(s) S60.41-●
  index S60.41-●
  little S60.41-●
  middle S60.41-●
  ring S60.41-●
flank S30.811
foot (except toe(s) alone) S90.81-●
  toe —*see* Abrasion, toe
forearm S50.81-●
  elbow only —*see* Abrasion, elbow
forehead S00.81
genital organs, external
  female S30.816
  male S30.815
groin S30.811
gum S00.512
hand S60.51-●
head S00.91
  ear —*see* Abrasion, ear
  eyelid —*see* Abrasion, eyelid
  lip S00.511
  nose S00.31
  oral cavity S00.512
  scalp S00.01
  specified site NEC S00.81
heel —*see* Abrasion, foot
hip S70.21-●
inguinal region S30.811
interscapular region S20.419
jaw S00.81
knee S80.21-●
labium (majus) (minus) S30.814

Abrasion *(Continued)*
larynx S10.11
leg (lower) S80.81-●
  knee —*see* Abrasion, knee
  upper —*see* Abrasion, thigh
lip S00.511
lower back S30.810
lumbar region S30.810
malar region S00.81
mammary —*see* Abrasion, breast
mastoid region S00.81
mouth S00.512
nail
  finger —*see* Abrasion, finger
  toe —*see* Abrasion, toe
nape S10.81
nasal S00.31
neck S10.91
  specified site NEC S10.81
  throat S10.11
nose S00.31
occipital region S00.01
oral cavity S00.512
orbital region —*see* Abrasion, eyelid
palate S00.512
palm —*see* Abrasion, hand
parietal region S00.01
pelvis S30.810
penis S30.812
perineum
  female S30.814
  male S30.810
periocular area —*see* Abrasion, eyelid
phalanges
  finger —*see* Abrasion, finger
  toe —*see* Abrasion, toe
pharynx S10.11
pinna —*see* Abrasion, ear
popliteal space —*see* Abrasion, knee
prepuce S30.812
pubic region S30.810
pudendum
  female S30.816
  male S30.815
sacral region S30.810
scalp S00.01
scapular region —*see* Abrasion, shoulder
scrotum S30.813
shin —*see* Abrasion, leg
shoulder S40.21-●
skin NEC T14.8
sternal region S20.319
submaxillary region S00.81
submental region S00.81
subungual
  finger(s) —*see* Abrasion, finger
  toe(s) —*see* Abrasion, toe
supraclavicular fossa S10.81
supraorbital S00.81
temple S00.81
temporal region S00.81
testis S30.813
thigh S70.31-●
thorax, thoracic (wall) S20.91
  back S20.41-●
  front S20.31-●
throat S10.11
thumb S60.31-●
toe(s) (lesser) S90.416
  great S90.41-●
tongue S00.512
tooth, teeth (dentifrice) (habitual) (hard tissues) (occupational) (ritual) (traditional) K03.1
trachea S10.11
tunica vaginalis S30.813
tympanum, tympanic membrane —*see* Abrasion, ear
uvula S00.512
vagina S30.814
vocal cords S10.11

Abrasion (Continued)
  vulva S30.814
  wrist S60.81-•
Abrism —see Poisoning, food, noxious, plant
Abruptio placentae O45.9-•
  with
    afibrinogenemia O45.01-•
    coagulation defect O45.00-•
      specified NEC O45.09-•
    disseminated intravascular coagulation
      O45.02-•
    hypofibrinogenemia O45.01-•
  specified NEC O45.8-•
Abruption, placenta —see Abruptio placentae
Abscess (connective tissue) (embolic) (fistulous)
    (infective) (metastatic) (multiple)
    (pernicious) (pyogenic) (septic) L02.91
  with
    diverticular disease (intestine) K57.80
      with bleeding K57.81
      large intestine K57.20
        with
          bleeding K57.21
          small intestine K57.40
            with bleeding K57.41
      small intestine K57.00
        with
          bleeding K57.01
          large intestine K57.40
            with bleeding K57.41
    lymphangitis - code by site under Abscess
  abdomen, abdominal
    cavity K65.1
    wall L02.211
  abdominopelvic K65.1
  accessory sinus —see Sinusitis
  adrenal (capsule) (gland) E27.8
  alveolar K04.7
    with sinus K04.6
  amebic A06.4
    brain (and liver or lung abscess) A06.6
    genitourinary tract A06.82
    liver (without mention of brain or lung
      abscess) A06.4
    lung (and liver) (without mention of brain
      abscess) A06.5
    specified site NEC A06.89
    spleen A06.89
  anerobic A48.0
  ankle —see Abscess, lower limb
  anorectal K61.2
  antecubital space —see Abscess, upper limb
  antrum (chronic) (Highmore) —see Sinusitis,
    maxillary
  anus K61.0
  apical (tooth) K04.7
    with sinus (alveolar) K04.6
  appendix K35.33
  areola (acute) (chronic) (nonpuerperal)
    N61.1
    puerperal, postpartum or gestational —see
      Infection, nipple
  arm (any part) —see Abscess, upper limb
  artery (wall) I77.89
  atheromatous I77.2
  auricle, ear —see Abscess, ear, external
  axilla (region) L02.41-•
    lymph gland or node L04.2
  back (any part, except buttock) L02.212
  Bartholin's gland N75.1
    with
      abortion —see Abortion, by type
        complicated by, sepsis
      ectopic or molar pregnancy O08.0
      following ectopic or molar pregnancy O08.0
  Bezold's —see Mastoiditis, acute
  bilharziasis B65.1
  bladder (wall) —see Cystitis, specified type
    NEC
  bone (subperiosteal) —see also Osteomyelitis,
    specified type NEC

Abscess (Continued)
  bone (Continued)
    accessory sinus (chronic) —see Sinusitis
    chronic or old —see Osteomyelitis, chronic
    jaw (lower) (upper) M27.2
    mastoid —see Mastoiditis, acute,
      subperiosteal
    petrous —see Petrositis
    spinal (tuberculous) A18.01
      nontuberculous —see Osteomyelitis,
        vertebra
  bowel K63.0
  brain (any part) (cystic) (otogenic) G06.0
    amebic (with abscess of any other site) A06.6
    gonococcal A54.82
    pheomycotic (chromomycotic) B43.1
    tuberculous A17.81
  breast (acute) (chronic) (nonpuerperal)
    N61.1
    newborn P39.0
    puerperal, postpartum, gestational —see
      Mastitis, obstetric, purulent
  broad ligament N73.2
    acute N73.0
    chronic N73.1
  Brodie's (localized) (chronic) M86.8X-•
  bronchi J98.09
  buccal cavity K12.2
  bulbourethral gland N34.0
  bursa M71.00
    ankle M71.07-•
    elbow M71.02-•
    foot M71.07-•
    hand M71.04-•
    hip M71.05-•
    knee M71.06-•
    multiple sites M71.09
    pharyngeal J39.1
    shoulder M71.01-•
    specified site NEC M71.08
    wrist M71.03-•
  buttock L02.31
  canthus —see Blepharoconjunctivitis
  cartilage —see Disorder, cartilage, specified
    type NEC
  cecum K35.33
  cerebellum, cerebellar G06.0
    sequelae G09
  cerebral (embolic) G06.0
    sequelae G09
  cervical (meaning neck) L02.11
    lymph gland or node L04.0
  cervix (stump) (uteri) —see Cervicitis
  cheek (external) L02.01
    inner K12.2
  chest J86.9
    with fistula J86.0
    wall L02.213
  chin L02.01
  choroid —see Inflammation, chorioretinal
  circumtonsillar J36
  cold (lung) (tuberculous) —see also
    Tuberculosis, abscess, lung
    articular —see Tuberculosis, joint
  colon (wall) K63.0
  colostomy K94.02
  conjunctiva —see Conjunctivitis, acute
  cornea H16.31-•
  corpus
    cavernosum N48.21
    luteum —see Oophoritis
  Cowper's gland N34.0
  cranium G06.0
  cul-de-sac (Douglas') (posterior) —see
    Peritonitis, pelvic, female
  cutaneous —see Abscess, by site
  dental K04.7
    with sinus (alveolar) K04.6
  dentoalveolar K04.7
    with sinus K04.6
  diaphragm, diaphragmatic K65.1

Abscess (Continued)
  Douglas' cul-de-sac or pouch —see
    Peritonitis, pelvic, female
  Dubois A50.59
  ear (middle) —see also Otitis, media,
    suppurative
    acute —see Otitis, media, suppurative,
      acute
    external H60.0-•
  entamebic —see Abscess, amebic
  enterostomy K94.12
  epididymis N45.4
  epidural G06.2
    brain G06.0
    spinal cord G06.1
  epiglottis J38.7
  epiploon, epiploic K65.1
  erysipelatous —see Erysipelas
  esophagus K20.80
  ethmoid (bone) (chronic) (sinus) J32.2
  external auditory canal —see Abscess, ear,
    external
  extradural G06.2
    brain G06.0
      sequelae G09
    spinal cord G06.1
  extraperitoneal K68.19
  eye —see Endophthalmitis, purulent
  eyelid H00.03-•
  face (any part, except ear, eye and nose) L02.01
  fallopian tube —see Salpingitis
  fascia M72.8
  fauces J39.1
  fecal K63.0
  femoral (region) —see Abscess, lower limb
  filaria, filarial —see Infestation, filarial
  finger (any) —see also Abscess, hand
    nail —see Cellulitis, finger
  foot L02.61-•
  forehead L02.01
  frontal sinus (chronic) J32.1
  gallbladder K81.0
  genital organ or tract
    female (external) N76.4
    male N49.9
      multiple sites N49.8
      specified NEC N49.8
  gestational mammary O91.11-•
  gestational subareolar O91.11-•
  gingival —see Periodontitis, localized
  gland, glandular (lymph) (acute) —see
    Lymphadenitis, acute
  gluteal (region) L02.31
  gonorrheal —see Gonococcus
  groin L02.214
  gum —see Periodontitis, localized
  hand L02.51-•
  head NEC L02.811
    face (any part, except ear, eye and nose)
      L02.01
  heart —see Carditis
  heel —see Abscess, foot
  helminthic —see Infestation, helminth
  hepatic (cholangitic) (hematogenic)
    (lymphogenic) (pylephlebitic) K75.0
    amebic A06.4
  hip (region) —see Abscess, lower limb
  horseshoe K61.31
  ileocecal K35.33
  ileostomy (bud) K94.12
  iliac (region) L02.214
    fossa K35.33
  infraclavicular (fossa) —see Abscess, upper
    limb
  inguinal (region) L02.214
    lymph gland or node L04.1
  intersphincteric K61.4
  intestine, intestinal NEC K63.0
    rectal K61.1
  intra-abdominal —see also Abscess,
    peritoneum K65.1

▶ New   ➡ Revised   ~~deleted~~ Deleted   • Use Additional Character(s)

Abscess *(Continued)*
   intra-abdominal *(Continued)*
     following procedure T81.43
      obstetrical O86.03
     postprocedural T81.43
     retroperitoneal K68.11
   intracranial G06.0
   intramammary —*see* Abscess, breast
   intramuscular, following procedure
     T81.44
     obstetrical O86.02
   intraorbital —*see* Abscess, orbit
   intraperitoneal K65.1
   intrasphincteric (anus) K61.4
   intraspinal G06.1
   intratonsillar J36
   ischiorectal (fossa) (specified NEC) K61.39
   jaw (bone) (lower) (upper) M27.2
   joint —*see* Arthritis, pyogenic or pyemic
     spine (tuberculous) A18.01
      nontuberculous —*see* Spondylopathy,
       infective
   kidney N15.1
     with calculus N20.0
      with hydronephrosis N13.6
     puerperal (postpartum) O86.21
   knee —*see also* Abscess, lower limb
     joint M00.9
   labium (majus) (minus) N76.4
   lacrimal
     caruncle —*see* Inflammation, lacrimal,
      passages, acute
     gland —*see* Dacryoadenitis
     passages (duct) (sac) —*see* Inflammation,
      lacrimal, passages, acute
   lacunar N34.0
   larynx J38.7
   lateral (alveolar) K04.7
     with sinus K04.6
   leg (any part) —*see* Abscess, lower limb
   lens H27.8
   lingual K14.0
     tonsil J36
   lip K13.0
   Littre's gland N34.0
   liver (cholangitic) (hematogenic) (lymphogenic)
     (pylephlebitic) (pyogenic) K75.0
     amebic (due to Entamoeba histolytica)
      (dysenteric) (tropical) A06.4
      with
       brain abscess (and liver or lung
        abscess) A06.6
       lung abscess A06.5
   loin (region) L02.211
   lower limb L02.41-●
   lumbar (tuberculous) A18.01
     nontuberculous L02.212
   lung (miliary) (putrid) J85.2
     with pneumonia J85.1
      due to specified organism (*see*
       Pneumonia, in (due to))
     amebic (with liver abscess) A06.5
      with
       brain abscess A06.6
       pneumonia A06.5
   lymph, lymphatic, gland or node (acute) —*see
     also* Lymphadenitis, acute
     mesentery I88.0
   malar M27.2
   mammary gland —*see* Abscess, breast
   marginal, anus K61.0
   mastoid —*see* Mastoiditis, acute
   maxilla, maxillary M27.2
     molar (tooth) K04.7
      with sinus K04.6
     premolar K04.7
     sinus (chronic) J32.0
   mediastinum J85.3
   meibomian gland —*see* Hordeolum
   meninges G06.2
   mesentery, mesenteric K65.1
   mesosalpinx —*see* Salpingitis

Abscess *(Continued)*
   mons pubis L02.215
   mouth (floor) K12.2
   muscle —*see* Myositis, infective
   myocardium I40.0
   nabothian (follicle) —*see* Cervicitis
   nasal J32.9
   nasopharyngeal J39.1
   navel L02.216
     newborn P38.9
      with mild hemorrhage P38.1
      without hemorrhage P38.9
   neck (region) L02.11
     lymph gland or node L04.0
   nephritic —*see* Abscess, kidney
   nipple N61.1
     associated with
      lactation —*see* Pregnancy, complicated by
      pregnancy —*see* Pregnancy, complicated
       by
   nose (external) (fossa) (septum) J34.0
     sinus (chronic) —*see* Sinusitis
   omentum K65.1
   operative wound T81.49
   orbit, orbital —*see* Cellulitis, orbit
   otogenic G06.0
   ovary, ovarian (corpus luteum) —*see* Oophoritis
   oviduct —*see* Oophoritis
   palate (soft) K12.2
     hard M27.2
   palmar (space) —*see* Abscess, hand
   pancreas (duct) —*see* Pancreatitis, acute
   parafrenal N48.21
   parametric, parametrium N73.2
     acute N73.0
     chronic N73.1
   paranephric N15.1
   parapancreatic —*see* Pancreatitis, acute
   parapharyngeal J39.0
   pararectal K61.1
   parasinus —*see* Sinusitis
   parauterine (*see also* Disease, pelvis,
     inflammatory) N73.2
   paravaginal —*see* Vaginitis
   parietal region (scalp) L02.811
   parodontal —*see* Periodontitis, aggressive,
     localized
   parotid (duct) (gland) K11.3
     region K12.2
   pectoral (region) L02.213
   pelvis, pelvic
     female —*see* Disease, pelvis, inflammatory
     male, peritoneal K65.1
   penis N48.21
     gonococcal (accessory gland) (periurethral)
      A54.1
   perianal K61.0
   periapical K04.7
     with sinus (alveolar) K04.6
   periappendicular K35.33
   pericardial I30.1
   pericecal K35.33
   pericemental —*see* Periodontitis, aggressive,
     localized
   pericholecystic —*see* Cholecystitis, acute
   pericoronal —*see* Periodontitis, aggressive,
     localized
   peridental —*see* Periodontitis, aggressive,
     localized
   perimetric —*see also* Disease, pelvis,
     inflammatory N73.2
   perinephric, perinephritic —*see* Abscess,
     kidney
   perineum, perineal (superficial) L02.215
     urethra N34.0
   periodontal (parietal) —*see* Periodontitis,
     aggressive, localized
     apical K04.7
   periosteum, periosteal —*see also*
     Osteomyelitis, specified type NEC
     with osteomyelitis —*see also* Osteomyelitis,
      specified type NEC

Abscess *(Continued)*
   periosteum, periosteal *(Continued)*
     acute —*see* Osteomyelitis, acute
     chronic —*see* Osteomyelitis, chronic
   peripharyngeal J39.0
   peripleuritic J86.9
     with fistula J86.0
   periprostatic N41.2
   perirectal K61.1
   perirenal (tissue) —*see* Abscess, kidney
   perisinuous (nose) —*see* Sinusitis
   peritoneum, peritoneal (perforated)
     (ruptured) K65.1
     with appendicitis (*see also* Appendicitis)
      K35.33
     pelvic
      female —*see* Peritonitis, pelvic, female
      male K65.1
     postoperative T81.49
     puerperal, postpartum, childbirth O85
     tuberculous A18.31
   peritonsillar J36
   perityphlic K35.33
   periureteral N28.89
   periurethral N34.0
     gonococcal (accessory gland) (periurethral)
      A54.1
   periuterine —*see also* Disease, pelvis,
     inflammatory N73.2
   perivesical —*see* Cystitis, specified type NEC
   petrous bone —*see* Petrositis
   phagedenic NOS L02.91
     chancroid A57
   pharynx, pharyngeal (lateral) J39.1
   pilonidal L05.01
   pituitary (gland) E23.6
   pleura J86.9
     with fistula J86.0
   popliteal —*see* Abscess, lower limb
   postcecal K35.33
   postlaryngeal J38.7
   postnasal J34.0
   postoperative (any site) (*see also* Infection,
     postoperative wound) T81.49
     retroperitoneal K68.11
   postpharyngeal J39.0
   posttonsillar J36
   post-typhoid A01.09
   pouch of Douglas —*see* Peritonitis, pelvic,
     female
   premammary —*see* Abscess, breast
   prepatellar —*see* Abscess, lower limb
▶   presacral K68.19
   prostate N41.2
     gonococcal (acute) (chronic) A54.22
   psoas muscle K68.12
   puerperal - code by site under Puerperal,
     abscess
   pulmonary —*see* Abscess, lung
   pulp, pulpal (dental) K04.01
     irreversible K04.02
     reversible K04.01
   rectovaginal septum K63.0
   rectovesical —*see* Cystitis, specified
     type NEC
   rectum K61.1
   renal —*see* Abscess, kidney
   retina —*see* Inflammation, chorioretinal
   retrobulbar —*see* Abscess, orbit
   retrocecal K65.1
   retrolaryngeal J38.7
   retromammary —*see* Abscess, breast
   retroperitoneal NEC K68.19
     postprocedural K68.11
   retropharyngeal J39.0
   retrouterine —*see* Peritonitis, pelvic, female
   retrovesical —*see* Cystitis, specified type NEC
   root, tooth K04.7
     with sinus (alveolar) K04.6
   round ligament —*see also* Disease, pelvis,
     inflammatory N73.2
   rupture (spontaneous) NOS L02.91

Abscess *(Continued)*
　sacrum (tuberculous)
　　nontuberculous M46.28
　salivary (duct) (gland) K11.3
　scalp (any part) L02.811
　scapular —*see* Osteomyelitis, specified type
　　NEC
　sclera —*see* Scleritis
　scrofulous (tuberculous) A18.2
　scrotum N49.2
　seminal vesicle N49.0
　septal, dental K04.7
　　with sinus (alveolar) K04.6
　serous —*see* Periostitis
　shoulder (region) —*see* Abscess, upper limb
　sigmoid K63.0
　sinus (accessory) (chronic) (nasal) —*see also*
　　Sinusitis
　　intracranial venous (any) G06.0
　Skene's duct or gland N34.0
　skin —*see* Abscess, by site
　specified site NEC L02.818
　spermatic cord N49.1
　sphenoidal (sinus) (chronic) J32.3
　spinal cord (any part) (staphylococcal) G06.1
　　tuberculous A17.81
　spine (column) (tuberculous) A18.01
　　epidural G06.1
　　nontuberculous —*see* Osteomyelitis, vertebra
　spleen D73.3
　　amebic A06.89
　stitch T81.41
　　following an obstetrical procedure O86.01
　subarachnoid G06.2
　　brain G06.0
　　spinal cord G06.1
　subareolar —*see* Abscess, breast
　subcecal K35.33
　subcutaneous —*see also* Abscess, by site
　　following procedure T81.41
　　　obstetrical O86.01
　　pheomycotic (chromomycotic) B43.2
　subdiaphragmatic K65.1
　subdural G06.2
　　brain G06.0
　　　sequelae G09
　　spinal cord G06.1
　sub-fascial, following an obstetrical
　　procedure O86.02
　subgaleal L02.811
　subhepatic K65.1
　sublingual K12.2
　　gland K11.3
　submammary —*see* Abscess, breast
　submandibular (region) (space) (triangle) K12.2
　　gland K11.3
　submaxillary (region) L02.01
　　gland K11.3
　submental L02.01
　　gland K11.3
　subperiosteal —*see* Osteomyelitis, specified
　　type NEC
　subphrenic K65.1
　　following an obstetrical procedure O86.03
　　postoperative T81.43
　suburethral N34.0
　sudoriparous L75.8
　supraclavicular (fossa) —*see* Abscess, upper
　　limb
　supralevator K61.5
　suprapelvic, acute N73.0
　suprarenal (capsule) (gland) E27.8
　sweat gland L74.8
　tear duct —*see* Inflammation, lacrimal,
　　passages, acute
　temple L02.01
　temporal region L02.01
　temporosphenoidal G06.0
　tendon (sheath) M65.00
　　ankle M65.07-•
　　foot M65.07-•
　　forearm M65.03-•
　　hand M65.04-•

Abscess *(Continued)*
　tendon (sheath) *(Continued)*
　　lower leg M65.06-•
　　pelvic region M65.05-•
　　shoulder region M65.01-•
　　specified site NEC M65.08
　　thigh M65.05-•
　　upper arm M65.02-•
　testis N45.4
　thigh —*see* Abscess, lower limb
　thorax J86.9
　　with fistula J86.0
　throat J39.1
　thumb —*see also* Abscess, hand
　　nail —*see* Cellulitis, finger
　thymus (gland) E32.1
　thyroid (gland) E06.0
　toe (any) —*see also* Abscess, foot
　　nail —*see* Cellulitis, toe
　tongue (staphylococcal) K14.0
　tonsil(s) (lingual) J36
　tonsillopharyngeal J36
　tooth, teeth (root) K04.7
　　with sinus (alveolar) K04.6
　　supporting structures NEC —*see*
　　　Periodontitis, aggressive, localized
　trachea J39.8
　trunk L02.219
　　abdominal wall L02.211
　　back L02.212
　　chest wall L02.213
　　groin L02.214
　　perineum L02.215
　　umbilicus L02.216
　tubal —*see* Salpingitis
　tuberculous —*see* Tuberculosis, abscess
　tubo-ovarian —*see* Salpingo-oophoritis
　tunica vaginalis N49.1
　umbilicus L02.216
　upper
　　limb L02.41-•
　　respiratory J39.8
　urethral (gland) N34.0
　urinary N34.0
　uterus, uterine (wall) —*see also* Endometritis
　　ligament —*see also* Disease, pelvis,
　　　inflammatory N73.2
　　neck —*see* Cervicitis
　uvula K12.2
　vagina (wall) —*see* Vaginitis
　vaginorectal —*see* Vaginitis
　vas deferens N49.1
　vermiform appendix K35.33
　vertebra (column) (tuberculous) A18.01
　　nontuberculous —*see* Osteomyelitis,
　　　vertebra
　vesical —*see* Cystitis, specified type NEC
　vesico-uterine pouch —*see* Peritonitis, pelvic,
　　female
　vitreous (humor) —*see* Endophthalmitis,
　　purulent
　vocal cord J38.3
　von Bezold's —*see* Mastoiditis, acute
　vulva N76.4
　vulvovaginal gland N75.1
　web space —*see* Abscess, hand
　wound T81.49
　wrist —*see* Abscess, upper limb
Absence (of) (organ or part) (complete or
　partial)
　adrenal (gland) (congenital) Q89.1
　　acquired E89.6
　albumin in blood E88.09
　alimentary tract (congenital) Q45.8
　　upper Q40.8
　alveolar process (acquired) —*see* Anomaly,
　　alveolar
　ankle (acquired) Z89.44-•
　anus (congenital) Q42.3
　　with fistula Q42.2
　aorta (congenital) Q25.41
　appendix, congenital Q42.8

Absence *(Continued)*
　arm (acquired) Z89.20-•
　　above elbow Z89.22-•
　　　congenital (with hand present) —*see*
　　　　Agenesis, arm, with hand present
　　　　and hand —*see* Agenesis, forearm,
　　　　and hand
　　below elbow Z89.21-•
　　　congenital (with hand present) —*see*
　　　　Agenesis, arm, with hand present
　　　　and hand —*see* Agenesis, forearm,
　　　　and hand
　　congenital —*see* Defect, reduction, upper
　　　limb
　　shoulder (following explantation of
　　　shoulder joint prosthesis) (joint) (with
　　　or without presence of antibiotic-
　　　impregnated cement spacer) Z89.23-•
　　congenital (with hand present) —*see*
　　　Agenesis, arm, with hand present
　artery (congenital) (peripheral) Q27.8
　　brain Q28.3
　　coronary Q24.5
　　pulmonary Q25.79
　　specified NEC Q27.8
　　umbilical Q27.0
　atrial septum (congenital) Q21.1
　auditory canal (congenital) (external) Q16.1
　auricle (ear), congenital Q16.0
　bile, biliary duct, congenital Q44.5
　bladder (acquired) Z90.6
　　congenital Q64.5
　bowel sounds R19.11
　brain Q00.0
　　part of Q04.3
　breast(s) (and nipple(s)) (acquired) Z90.1-•
　　congenital Q83.8
　broad ligament Q50.6
　bronchus (congenital) Q32.4
　canaliculus lacrimalis, congenital Q10.4
　cerebellum (vermis) Q04.3
　cervix (acquired) (with uterus) Z90.710
　　with remaining uterus Z90.712
　　congenital Q51.5
　chin, congenital Q18.8
　cilia (congenital) Q10.3
　　acquired —*see* Madarosis
　clitoris (congenital) Q52.6
　coccyx, congenital Q76.49
　cold sense R20.8
　congenital
　　lumen —*see* Atresia
　　organ or site NEC —*see* Agenesis
　　septum —*see* Imperfect, closure
　corpus callosum Q04.0
　cricoid cartilage, congenital Q31.8
　diaphragm (with hernia), congenital Q79.1
　digestive organ(s) or tract, congenital Q45.8
　　acquired NEC Z90.49
　　upper Q40.8
　ductus arteriosus Q28.8
　duodenum (acquired) Z90.49
　　congenital Q41.0
　ear, congenital Q16.9
　　acquired H93.8-•
　　auricle Q16.0
　　external Q16.0
　　inner Q16.5
　　lobe, lobule Q17.8
　　middle, except ossicles Q16.4
　　　ossicles Q16.3
　　ossicles Q16.3
　ejaculatory duct (congenital) Q55.4
　endocrine gland (congenital) NEC Q89.2
　　acquired E89.89
　epididymis (congenital) Q55.4
　　acquired Z90.79
　epiglottis, congenital Q31.8
　esophagus (congenital) Q39.8
　　acquired (partial) Z90.49
　eustachian tube (congenital) Q16.2
　extremity (acquired) Z89.9
　　congenital Q73.0

▶ New　⇒ Revised　~~deleted~~ Deleted　• Use Additional Character(s)

Absence *(Continued)*
extremity (acquired) *(Continued)*
knee (following explantation of knee joint prosthesis) (joint) (with or without presence of antibiotic-impregnated cement spacer) Z89.52-•
lower (above knee) Z89.619
below knee Z89.51-•
upper —*see* Absence, arm
eye (acquired) Z90.01
congenital Q11.1
muscle (congenital) Q10.3
eyeball (acquired) Z90.01
eyelid (fold) (congenital) Q10.3
acquired Z90.01
face, specified part NEC Q18.8
fallopian tube(s) (acquired) Z90.79
congenital Q50.6
family member (causing problem in home) NEC —*see also* Disruption, family Z63.32
femur, congenital —*see* Defect, reduction, lower limb, longitudinal, femur
fibrinogen (congenital) D68.2
acquired D65
finger(s) (acquired) Z89.02-•
congenital —*see* Agenesis, hand
foot (acquired) Z89.43-•
congenital —*see* Agenesis, foot
forearm (acquired) —*see* Absence, arm, below elbow
gallbladder (acquired) Z90.49
congenital Q44.0
gamma globulin in blood D80.1
hereditary D80.0
genital organs
acquired (female) (male) Z90.79
female, congenital Q52.8
external Q52.71
internal NEC Q52.8
male, congenital Q55.8
genitourinary organs, congenital NEC
female Q52.8
male Q55.8
globe (acquired) Z90.01
congenital Q11.1
glottis, congenital Q31.8
hand and wrist (acquired) Z89.11-•
congenital —*see* Agenesis, hand
head, part (acquired) NEC Z90.09
heat sense R20.8
hip (following explantation of hip joint prosthesis) (joint) (with or without presence of antibiotic-impregnated cement spacer) Z89.62-•
hymen (congenital) Q52.4
ileum (acquired) Z90.49
congenital Q41.2
immunoglobulin, isolated NEC D80.3
IgA D80.2
IgG D80.3
IgM D80.4
incus (acquired) —*see* Loss, ossicles, ear
congenital Q16.3
inner ear, congenital Q16.5
intestine (acquired) (small) Z90.49
congenital Q41.9
specified NEC Q41.8
large Z90.49
congenital Q42.9
specified NEC Q42.8
iris, congenital Q13.1
jejunum (acquired) Z90.49
congenital Q41.1
joint
acquired
hip (following explantation of hip joint prosthesis) (with or without presence of antibiotic-impregnated cement spacer) Z89.62-•
knee (following explantation of knee joint prosthesis) (with or without presence of antibiotic-impregnated cement spacer) Z89.52-•

Absence *(Continued)*
joint *(Continued)*
acquired *(Continued)*
shoulder (following explantation of shoulder joint prosthesis) (with or without presence of antibiotic-impregnated cement spacer) Z89.23-•
congenital NEC Q74.8
kidney(s) (acquired) Z90.5
congenital Q60.2
bilateral Q60.1
unilateral Q60.0
knee (following explantation of knee joint prosthesis) (joint) (with or without presence of antibiotic-impregnated cement spacer) Z89.52-•
labyrinth, membranous Q16.5
larynx (congenital) Q31.8
acquired Z90.02
leg (above knee) Z89.61-•
below knee (acquired) Z89.51-•
congenital —*see* Defect, reduction, lower limb
lens (acquired) —*see also* Aphakia
congenital Q12.3
post cataract extraction Z98.4-•
limb (acquired) —*see* Absence, extremity
lip Q38.6
liver (congenital) Q44.7
lung (fissure) (lobe) (bilateral) (unilateral) (congenital) Q33.3
acquired (any part) Z90.2
menstruation —*see* Amenorrhea
muscle (congenital) (pectoral) Q79.8
ocular Q10.3
neck, part Q18.8
neutrophil —*see* Agranulocytosis
nipple(s) (with breast(s)) (acquired) Z90.1-•
congenital Q83.2
nose (congenital) Q30.1
acquired Z90.09
organ
of Corti, congenital Q16.5
or site, congenital NEC Q89.8
acquired NEC Z90.89
osseous meatus (ear) Q16.4
ovary (acquired)
bilateral Z90.722
congenital
bilateral Q50.02
unilateral Q50.01
unilateral Z90.721
oviduct (acquired)
bilateral Z90.722
congenital Q50.6
unilateral Z90.721
pancreas (congenital) Q45.0
acquired Z90.410
complete Z90.410
partial Z90.411
total Z90.410
parathyroid gland (acquired) E89.2
congenital Q89.2
patella, congenital Q74.1
penis (congenital) Q55.5
acquired Z90.79
pericardium (congenital) Q24.8
pituitary gland (congenital) Q89.2
acquired E89.3
prostate (acquired) Z90.79
congenital Q55.4
pulmonary valve Q22.0
punctum lacrimale (congenital) Q10.4
radius, congenital —*see* Defect, reduction, upper limb, longitudinal, radius
rectum (congenital) Q42.1
with fistula Q42.0
acquired Z90.49
respiratory organ NOS Q34.9
rib (acquired) Z90.89
congenital Q76.6
sacrum, congenital Q76.49

Absence *(Continued)*
salivary gland(s), congenital Q38.4
scrotum, congenital Q55.29
seminal vesicles (congenital) Q55.4
acquired Z90.79
septum
atrial (congenital) Q21.1
between aorta and pulmonary artery Q21.4
ventricular (congenital) Q20.4
sex chromosome
female phenotype Q97.8
male phenotype Q98.8
skull bone (congenital) Q75.8
with
anencephaly Q00.0
encephalocele —*see* Encephalocele
hydrocephalus Q03.9
with spina bifida —*see* Spina bifida, by site, with hydrocephalus
microcephaly Q02
spermatic cord, congenital Q55.4
spine, congenital Q76.49
spleen (congenital) Q89.01
acquired Z90.81
sternum, congenital Q76.7
stomach (acquired) (partial) Z90.3
congenital Q40.2
superior vena cava, congenital Q26.8
teeth, tooth (congenital) K00.0
acquired (complete) K08.109
class I K08.101
class II K08.102
class III K08.103
class IV K08.104
due to
caries K08.139
class I K08.131
class II K08.132
class III K08.133
class IV K08.134
periodontal disease K08.129
class I K08.121
class II K08.122
class III K08.123
class IV K08.124
specified NEC K08.199
class I K08.191
class II K08.192
class III K08.193
class IV K08.194
trauma K08.119
class I K08.111
class II K08.112
class III K08.113
class IV K08.114
partial K08.409
class I K08.401
class II K08.402
class III K08.403
class IV K08.404
due to
caries K08.439
class I K08.431
class II K08.432
class III K08.433
class IV K08.434
periodontal disease K08.429
class I K08.421
class II K08.422
class III K08.423
class IV K08.424
specified NEC K08.499
class I K08.491
class II K08.492
class III K08.493
class IV K08.494
trauma K08.419
class I K08.411
class II K08.412
class III K08.413
class IV K08.414
tendon (congenital) Q79.8

▶ New   ⇒ Revised   ~~deleted~~ Deleted   • Use Additional Character(s)

Absence *(Continued)*
testis (congenital) Q55.0
  acquired Z90.79
thumb (acquired) Z89.01-•
  congenital —*see* Agenesis, hand
thymus gland Q89.2
thyroid (gland) (acquired) E89.0
  cartilage, congenital Q31.8
  congenital E03.1
toe(s) (acquired) Z89.42-•
  with foot —*see* Absence, foot and ankle
  congenital —*see* Agenesis, foot
  great Z89.41-•
tongue, congenital Q38.3
trachea (cartilage), congenital Q32.1
transverse aortic arch, congenital Q25.49
tricuspid valve Q22.4
umbilical artery, congenital Q27.0
upper arm and forearm with hand present,
  congenital —*see* Agenesis, arm, with
  hand present
ureter (congenital) Q62.4
  acquired Z90.6
urethra, congenital Q64.5
uterus (acquired) Z90.710
  with cervix Z90.710
  with remaining cervical stump Z90.711
  congenital Q51.0
uvula, congenital Q38.5
vagina, congenital Q52.0
vas deferens (congenital) Q55.4
  acquired Z90.79
vein (peripheral) congenital NEC Q27.8
  cerebral Q28.3
  digestive system Q27.8
  great Q26.8
  lower limb Q27.8
  portal Q26.5
  precerebral Q28.1
  specified site NEC Q27.8
  upper limb Q27.8
vena cava (inferior) (superior), congenital
  Q26.8
ventricular septum Q20.4
vertebra, congenital Q76.49
vulva, congenital Q52.71
wrist (acquired) Z89.12-•
Absorbent system disease I87.8
Absorption
carbohydrate, disturbance K90.49
chemical —*see* Table of Drugs and Chemicals
  through placenta (newborn) P04.9
    environmental substance P04.6
    nutritional substance P04.5
    obstetric anesthetic or analgesic drug P04.0
drug NEC —*see* Table of Drugs and Chemicals
  addictive
    through placenta (newborn) *(see also*
      Newborn, affected by, maternal,
      use of) P04.40
      cocaine P04.41
      hallucinogens P04.42
      specified drug NEC P04.49
  medicinal
    through placenta (newborn) P04.19
  through placenta (newborn) P04.19
    obstetric anesthetic or analgesic drug P04.0
fat, disturbance K90.49
  pancreatic K90.3
noxious substance —*see* Table of Drugs and
  Chemicals
protein, disturbance K90.49
starch, disturbance K90.49
toxic substance —*see* Table of Drugs and
  Chemicals
uremic —*see* Uremia
Abstinence symptoms, syndrome
alcohol F10.239
  with delirium F10.231
cocaine F14.23
neonatal P96.1
nicotine —*see* Dependence, drug, nicotine,
  with, withdrawal

Abstinence symptoms, syndrome *(Continued)*
opioid F11.93
  with dependence F11.23
psychoactive NEC F19.939
  with
    delirium F19.931
    dependence F19.239
      with
        delirium F19.231
        perceptual disturbance F19.232
      uncomplicated F19.230
    perceptual disturbance F19.932
  uncomplicated F19.930
sedative F13.939
  with
    delirium F13.931
    dependence F13.239
      with
        delirium F13.231
        perceptual disturbance F13.232
      uncomplicated F13.230
    perceptual disturbance F13.932
  uncomplicated F13.930
stimulant NEC F15.93
  with dependence F15.23
Abulia R68.89
Abulomania F60.7
Abuse
adult —*see* Maltreatment, adult
  as reason for
    couple seeking advice (including
      offender) Z63.0
alcohol (non-dependent) F10.10
  with
    anxiety disorder F10.180
    intoxication F10.129
      with delirium F10.121
      uncomplicated F10.120
    mood disorder F10.14
    other specified disorder F10.188
    psychosis F10.159
      delusions F10.150
      hallucinations F10.151
    sexual dysfunction F10.181
    sleep disorder F10.182
    unspecified disorder F10.19
    withdrawal F10.139
      with
        perceptual disturbance F10.132
      delirium F10.131
      uncomplicated F10.130
  counseling and surveillance Z71.41
  in remission (early) (sustained) F10.11
amphetamine (or related substance) —*see also*
  Abuse, drug, stimulant NEC
  stimulant NEC F15.10
    with
      anxiety disorder F15.180
      intoxication F15.129
        with
          delirium F15.121
          perceptual disturbance F15.122
      withdrawal F15.13
analgesics (non-prescribed) (over the counter)
  F55.8
antacids F55.0
antidepressants —*see* Abuse, drug,
  psychoactive NEC
anxiolytic —*see* Abuse, drug, sedative
barbiturates —*see* Abuse, drug, sedative
caffeine —*see* Abuse, drug, stimulant NEC
cannabis, cannabinoids —*see* Abuse, drug,
  cannabis
child —*see* Maltreatment, child
cocaine —*see* Abuse, drug, cocaine
drug NEC (non-dependent) F19.10
  with sleep disorder F19.182
  amphetamine type —*see* Abuse, drug,
    stimulant NEC
  analgesics (non-prescribed) (over the
    counter) F55.8
  antacids F55.0
  antidepressants —*see* Abuse, drug,
    psychoactive NEC

Abuse *(Continued)*
drug NEC *(Continued)*
  anxiolytics —*see* Abuse, drug, sedative
  barbiturates —*see* Abuse, drug, sedative
  caffeine —*see* Abuse, drug, stimulant NEC
  cannabis F12.10
    with
      anxiety disorder F12.180
      intoxication F12.129
        with
          delirium F12.121
          perceptual disturbance F12.122
        uncomplicated F12.120
      other specified disorder F12.188
      psychosis F12.159
        delusions F12.150
        hallucinations F12.151
      unspecified disorder F12.19
      withdrawal F12.13
    in remission (early) (sustained) F12.11
  cocaine F14.10
    with
      anxiety disorder F14.180
      intoxication F14.129
        with
          delirium F14.121
          perceptual disturbance F14.122
        uncomplicated F14.120
      mood disorder F14.14
      other specified disorder F14.188
      psychosis F14.159
        delusions F14.150
        hallucinations F14.151
      sexual dysfunction F14.181
      sleep disorder F14.182
      unspecified disorder F14.19
      withdrawal F14.13
    in remission (early) (sustained) F14.11
  counseling and surveillance Z71.51
  hallucinogen F16.10
    with
      anxiety disorder F16.180
      flashbacks F16.183
      intoxication F16.129
        with
          delirium F16.121
          perceptual disturbance F16.122
        uncomplicated F16.120
      mood disorder F16.14
      other specified disorder F16.188
      perception disorder, persisting F16.183
      psychosis F16.159
        delusions F16.150
        hallucinations F16.151
      unspecified disorder F16.19
    in remission (early) (sustained) F16.11
  hashish —*see* Abuse, drug, cannabis
  herbal or folk remedies F55.1
  hormones F55.3
  hypnotics —*see* Abuse, drug, sedative
  inhalant F18.10
    with
      anxiety disorder F18.180
      dementia, persisting F18.17
      intoxication F18.129
        with delirium F18.121
        uncomplicated F18.120
      mood disorder F18.14
      other specified disorder F18.188
      psychosis F18.159
        delusions F18.150
        hallucinations F18.151
      unspecified disorder F18.19
    in remission (early) (sustained) F18.11
  in remission (early) (sustained) F19.11
  laxatives F55.2
  LSD —*see* Abuse, drug, hallucinogen
  marihuana —*see* Abuse, drug, cannabis
  morphine type (opioids) —*see* Abuse, drug,
    opioid

▶ New   ⇒ Revised   ~~deleted~~ Deleted   • Use Additional Character(s)

Abuse *(Continued)*
  drug NEC *(Continued)*
    opioid F11.10
      with
        intoxication F11.129
          with
            delirium F11.121
            perceptual disturbance F11.122
          uncomplicated F11.120
        mood disorder F11.14
        other specified disorder F11.188
        psychosis F11.159
          delusions F11.150
          hallucinations F11.151
        sexual dysfunction F11.181
        sleep disorder F11.182
        unspecified disorder F11.19
        withdrawal F11.13
      in remission (early) (sustained) F11.11
    PCP (phencyclidine) (or related substance) —
        see Abuse, drug, hallucinogen
    psychoactive NEC F19.10
      with
        amnestic disorder F19.16
        anxiety disorder F19.180
        dementia F19.17
        intoxication F19.129
          with
            delirium F19.121
            perceptual disturbance F19.122
          uncomplicated F19.120
        mood disorder F19.14
        other specified disorder F19.188
        psychosis F19.159
          delusions F19.150
          hallucinations F19.151
        sexual dysfunction F19.181
        sleep disorder F19.182
        unspecified disorder F19.19
        withdrawal F19.139
          with
            perceptual disturbance F19.132
          delirium F19.131
          uncomplicated F19.130
    sedative, hypnotic or anxiolytic F13.10
      with
        anxiety disorder F13.180
        intoxication F13.129
          with delirium F13.121
          uncomplicated F13.120
        mood disorder F13.14
        other specified disorder F13.188
        psychosis F13.159
          delusions F13.150
          hallucinations F13.151
        sexual dysfunction F13.181
        sleep disorder F13.182
        unspecified disorder F13.19
        withdrawal F13.139
          with
            perceptual disturbance F13.132
          delirium F13.131
          uncomplicated F13.130
      in remission (early) (sustained) F13.11
    solvent — see Abuse, drug, inhalant
    steroids F55.3
    stimulant NEC F15.10
      with
        anxiety disorder F15.180
        intoxication F15.129
          with
            delirium F15.121
            perceptual disturbance F15.122
          uncomplicated F15.120
        mood disorder F15.14
        other specified disorder F15.188
        psychosis F15.159
          delusions F15.150
          hallucinations F15.151
        sexual dysfunction F15.181
        sleep disorder F15.182
        unspecified disorder F15.19
        withdrawal F15.13
      in remission (early) (sustained) F15.11

Abuse *(Continued)*
  drug NEC *(Continued)*
    tranquilizers —see Abuse, drug, sedative
    vitamins F55.4
  hallucinogens —see Abuse, drug, hallucinogen
  hashish —see Abuse, drug, cannabis
  herbal or folk remedies F55.1
  hormones F55.3
  hypnotic —see Abuse, drug, sedative
  inhalant —see Abuse, drug, inhalant
  laxatives F55.2
  LSD —see Abuse, drug, hallucinogen
  marihuana —see Abuse, drug, cannabis
  morphine type (opioids) —see Abuse, drug,
      opioid
  non-psychoactive substance NEC F55.8
    antacids F55.0
    folk remedies F55.1
    herbal remedies F55.1
    hormones F55.3
    laxatives F55.2
    steroids F55.3
    vitamins F55.4
  opioids —see Abuse, drug, opioid
  PCP (phencyclidine) (or related substance) —
      see Abuse, drug, hallucinogen
  physical (adult) (child) —see Maltreatment
  psychoactive substance —see Abuse, drug,
      psychoactive NEC
  psychological (adult) (child) —see Maltreatment
  sedative —see Abuse, drug, sedative
  sexual —see Maltreatment
  solvent —see Abuse, drug, inhalant
  steroids F55.3
  vitamins F55.4
Acalculia R48.8
  developmental F81.2
Acanthamebiasis (with) B60.10
  conjunctiva B60.12
  keratoconjunctivitis B60.13
  meningoencephalitis B60.11
  other specified B60.19
Acanthocephaliasis B83.8
Acanthocheilonemiasis B74.4
Acanthocytosis E78.6
Acantholysis L11.9
Acanthosis (acquired) (nigricans) L83
  benign Q82.8
  congenital Q82.8
  seborrheic L82.1
    inflamed L82.0
  tongue K14.3
Acapnia E87.3
Acarbia E87.2
Acardia, acardius Q89.8
Acardiacus amorphus Q89.8
Acardiotrophia I51.4
Acariasis B88.0
  scabies B86
Acarodermatitis (urticarioides) B88.0
Acarophobia F40.218
Acatalasemia, acatalasia E80.3
Acathisia (drug induced) G25.71
Accelerated atrioventricular conduction I45.6
Accentuation of personality traits (type A) Z73.1
Accessory (congenital)
  adrenal gland Q89.1
  anus Q43.4
  appendix Q43.4
  atrioventricular conduction I45.6
  auditory ossicles Q16.3
  auricle (ear) Q17.0
  biliary duct or passage Q44.5
  bladder Q64.79
  blood vessels NEC Q27.9
    coronary Q24.5
  bone NEC Q79.8
  breast tissue, axilla Q83.1
  carpal bones Q74.0
  cecum Q43.4
  chromosome(s) NEC (nonsex) Q92.9

Accessory *(Continued)*
  chromosome(s) NEC (nonsex) *(Continued)*
    with complex rearrangements NEC Q92.5
      seen only at prometaphase Q92.8
    13 —see Trisomy, 13
    18 —see Trisomy, 18
    21 —see Trisomy, 21
    partial Q92.9
    sex
      female phenotype Q97.8
  coronary artery Q24.5
  cusp(s), heart valve NEC Q24.8
    pulmonary Q22.3
  cystic duct Q44.5
  digit(s) Q69.9
  ear (auricle) (lobe) Q17.0
  endocrine gland NEC Q89.2
  eye muscle Q10.3
  eyelid Q10.3
  face bone(s) Q75.8
  fallopian tube (fimbria) (ostium) Q50.6
  finger(s) Q69.0
  foreskin N47.8
  frontonasal process Q75.8
  gallbladder Q44.1
  genital organ(s)
    female Q52.8
      external Q52.79
      internal NEC Q52.8
    male Q55.8
  genitourinary organs NEC Q89.8
    female Q52.8
    male Q55.8
  hallux Q69.2
  heart Q24.8
    valve NEC Q24.8
      pulmonary Q22.3
  hepatic ducts Q44.5
  hymen Q52.4
  intestine (large) (small) Q43.4
  kidney Q63.0
  lacrimal canal Q10.6
  leaflet, heart valve NEC Q24.8
  ligament, broad Q50.6
  liver Q44.7
    duct Q44.5
  lobule (ear) Q17.0
  lung (lobe) Q33.1
  muscle Q79.8
  navicular of carpus Q74.0
  nervous system, part NEC Q07.8
  nipple Q83.3
  nose Q30.8
  organ or site not listed —see Anomaly, by site
  ovary Q50.31
  oviduct Q50.6
  pancreas Q45.3
  parathyroid gland Q89.2
  parotid gland (and duct) Q38.4
  pituitary gland Q89.2
  preauricular appendage Q17.0
  prepuce N47.8
  renal arteries (multiple) Q27.2
  rib Q76.6
    cervical Q76.5
  roots (teeth) K00.2
  salivary gland Q38.4
  sesamoid bones Q74.8
    foot Q74.2
    hand Q74.0
  skin tags Q82.8
  spleen Q89.09
  sternum Q76.7
  submaxillary gland Q38.4
  tarsal bones Q74.2
  teeth, tooth K00.1
  tendon Q79.8
  thumb Q69.1
  thymus gland Q89.2
  thyroid gland Q89.2
  toes Q69.2

▶ New ⇒ Revised ~~deleted~~ Deleted ● Use Additional Character(s) 97

Accessory *(Continued)*
  tongue Q38.3
  tooth, teeth K00.1
  tragus Q17.0
  ureter Q62.5
  urethra Q64.79
  urinary organ or tract NEC Q64.8
  uterus Q51.28
  vagina Q52.10
  valve, heart NEC Q24.8
    pulmonary Q22.3
  vertebra Q76.49
  vocal cords Q31.8
  vulva Q52.79
Accident
  birth —*see* Birth, injury
  cardiac —*see* Infarct, myocardium
  cerebral I63.9
  cerebrovascular (embolic) (ischemic)
      (thrombotic) I63.9
    aborted I63.9
    hemorrhagic —*see* Hemorrhage,
        intracranial, intracerebral
    old (without sequelae) Z86.73
      with sequelae (of) —*see* Sequelae,
          infarction, cerebral
  coronary —*see* Infarct, myocardium
  craniovascular I63.9
  vascular, brain I63.9
Accidental —*see* condition
Accommodation (disorder) —*see also* condition
  hysterical paralysis of F44.89
  insufficiency of H52.4
  paresis —*see* Paresis, of accommodation
  spasm —*see* Spasm, of accommodation
Accouchement —*see* Delivery
Accreta placenta O43.21-●
Accretio cordis (nonrheumatic) I31.0
Accretions, tooth, teeth K03.6
Acculturation difficulty Z60.3
Accumulation secretion, prostate N42.89
Acephalia, acephalism, acephalus, acephaly
    Q00.0
Acephalobrachia monster Q89.8
Acephalochirus monster Q89.8
Acephalogaster Q89.8
Acephalostomus monster Q89.8
Acephalothorax Q89.8
Acerophobia F40.298
Acetonemia R79.89
  in Type 1 diabetes E10.10
    with coma E10.11
Acetonuria R82.4
Achalasia (cardia) (esophagus) K22.0
  congenital Q39.5
  pylorus Q40.0
  sphincteral NEC K59.89
Ache(s) —*see* Pain
Acheilia Q38.6
Achillobursitis —*see* Tendinitis, Achilles
Achillodynia —*see* Tendinitis, Achilles
Achlorhydria, achlorhydric (neurogenic) K31.83
  anemia D50.8
  diarrhea K31.83
  psychogenic F45.8
  secondary to vagotomy K91.1
Achluophobia F40.228
Acholia K82.8
Acholuric jaundice (familial)
      (splenomegalic) —*see also* Spherocytosis
    acquired D59.8
Achondrogenesis Q77.0
Achondroplasia (osteosclerosis congenita)
    Q77.4
Achroma, cutis L80
Achromat (ism), achromatopsia (acquired)
      (congenital) H53.51
Achromia, congenital —*see* Albinism
Achromia parasitica B36.0
Achylia gastrica K31.89
  psychogenic F45.8

Acid
  burn —*see* Corrosion
  deficiency
    amide nicotinic E52
    ascorbic E54
    folic E53.8
    nicotinic E52
    pantothenic E53.8
  intoxication E87.2
  peptic disease K30
  phosphatase deficiency E83.39
  stomach K30
    psychogenic F45.8
Acidemia E87.2
  argininosuccinic E72.22
  isovaleric E71.110
  metabolic (newborn) P19.9
    first noted before onset of labor P19.0
    first noted during labor P19.1
    noted at birth P19.2
  methylmalonic E71.120
  pipecolic E72.3
  propionic E71.121
Acidity, gastric (high) K30
  psychogenic F45.8
Acidocytopenia —*see* Agranulocytosis
Acidocytosis D72.10
Acidopenia —*see* Agranulocytosis
Acidosis (lactic) (respiratory) E87.2
  in Type 1 diabetes E10.10
    with coma E10.11
  kidney, tubular N25.89
  lactic E87.2
  metabolic NEC E87.2
    hyperchloremic, of newborn P74.421
    with respiratory acidosis E87.4
    late, of newborn P74.0
  mixed metabolic and respiratory, newborn P84
  newborn P84
  renal (hyperchloremic) (tubular) N25.89
  respiratory E87.2
    complicated by
      metabolic
        acidosis E87.4
        alkalosis E87.4
Aciduria
  4-hydroxybutyric E72.81
  argininosuccinic E72.22
  gamma-hydroxybutyric E72.81
  glutaric (type I) E72.3
    type II E71.313
    type III E71.5-●
  orotic (congenital) (hereditary) (pyrimidine
      deficiency) E79.8
    anemia D53.0
Acladiosis (skin) B36.0
Aclasis, diaphyseal Q78.6
Acleistocardia Q21.1
Aclusion —*see* Anomaly, dentofacial,
    malocclusion
Acne L70.9
  artificialis L70.8
  atrophica L70.2
  cachecticorum (Hebra) L70.8
  conglobata L70.1
  cystic L70.0
  decalvans L66.2
  excoriée (des jeunes filles) L70.5
  frontalis L70.2
  indurata L70.0
  infantile L70.4
  keloid L73.0
  lupoid L70.2
  necrotic, necrotica (miliaris) L70.2
  neonatal L70.4
  nodular L70.0
  occupational L70.8
  picker's L70.5
  pustular L70.0
  rodens L70.2
  rosacea L71.9

Acne *(Continued)*
  specified NEC L70.8
  tropica L70.3
  varioliformis L70.2
  vulgaris L70.0
Acnitis (primary) A18.4
Acosta's disease T70.29
Acoustic —*see* condition
Acousticophobia F40.298
ACPO (acute colonic pseudo-obstruction) K59.81
Acquired —*see also* condition
  immunodeficiency syndrome (AIDS) B20
Acrania Q00.0
Acroangiodermatitis I78.9
Acroasphyxia, chronic I73.89
Acrobystitis N47.7
Acrocephalopolysyndactyly Q87.0
Acrocephalosyndactyly Q87.0
Acrocephaly Q75.0
Acrochondrohyperplasia —*see* Syndrome,
    Marfan's
Acrocyanosis I73.89
  newborn P28.2
    meaning transient blue hands and feet -
        omit code
Acrodermatitis L30.8
  atrophicans (chronica) L90.4
  continua (Hallopeau) L40.2
  enteropathica (hereditary) E83.2
  Hallopeau's L40.2
  infantile papular L44.4
  perstans L40.2
  pustulosa continua L40.2
  recalcitrant pustular L40.2
Acrodynia —*see* Poisoning, mercury
Acromegaly, acromegalia E22.0
Acromelalgia I73.81
Acromicria, acromikria Q79.8
Acronyx L60.0
Acropachy, thyroid —*see* Thyrotoxicosis
Acroparesthesia (simple) (vasomotor) I73.89
Acropathy, thyroid —*see* Thyrotoxicosis
Acrophobia F40.241
Acroposthitis N47.7
Acroscleriasis, acroscleroderma,
    acrosclerosis —*see* Sclerosis, systemic
Acrosphacelus I96
Acrospiroma, eccrine —*see* Neoplasm, skin,
    benign
Acrostealgia —*see* Osteochondropathy
Acrotrophodynia —*see* Immersion
ACTH ectopic syndrome E24.3
Actinic —*see* condition
Actinobacillosis, actinobacillus A28.8
  mallei A24.0
  muris A25.1
Actinomyces israelii (infection) —*see*
    Actinomycosis
Actinomycetoma (foot) B47.1
Actinomycosis, actinomycotic A42.9
  with pneumonia A42.0
  abdominal A42.1
  cervicofacial A42.2
  cutaneous A42.89
  gastrointestinal A42.1
  pulmonary A42.0
  sepsis A42.7
  specified site NEC A42.89
Actinoneuritis G62.82
Action, heart
  disorder I49.9
  irregular I49.9
    psychogenic F45.8
Activated protein C resistance D68.51
Activation
  mast cell (disorder) (syndrome) D89.40
    idiopathic D89.42
    monoclonal D89.41
    secondary D89.43
    specified type NEC D89.49
Active —*see* condition

Acute —*see also* condition
  abdomen R10.0
  gallbladder —*see* Cholecystitis, acute
Acyanotic heart disease (congenital) Q24.9
Acystia Q64.5
Adair-Dighton syndrome (brittle bones and
  blue sclera, deafness) Q78.0
Adamantinoblastoma —*see* Ameloblastoma
Adamantinoma —*see also* Cyst, calcifying
  odontogenic
  long bones C40.90
    lower limb C40.2-●
    upper limb C40.0-●
  malignant C41.1
    jaw (bone) (lower) C41.1
      upper C41.0
  tibial C40.2-●
Adamantoblastoma —*see* Ameloblastoma
Adams-Stokes (-Morgagni) disease or
  syndrome I45.9
Adaption reaction —*see* Disorder, adjustment
Addiction —*see also* Dependence F19.20
  alcohol, alcoholic (ethyl) (methyl) (wood)
    (without remission) F10.20
    with remission F10.21
  drug —*see* Dependence, drug
  ethyl alcohol (without remission) F10.20
    with remission F10.21
  heroin —*see* Dependence, drug, opioid
  methyl alcohol (without remission) F10.20
    with remission F10.21
  methylated spirit (without remission) F10.20
    with remission F10.21
  morphine(-like substances) —*see*
    Dependence, drug, opioid
  nicotine —*see* Dependence, drug, nicotine
  opium and opioids —*see* Dependence, drug,
    opioid
  tobacco —*see* Dependence, drug, nicotine
Addisonian crisis E27.2
Addison's
  anemia (pernicious) D51.0
  disease (bronze) or syndrome E27.1
    tuberculous A18.7
  keloid L94.0
Addison-Biermer anemia (pernicious) D51.0
Addison-Schilder complex E71.528
Additional —*see also* Accessory
  chromosome(s) Q99.8
    21 —*see* Trisomy, 21
    sex —*see* Abnormal, chromosome, sex
Adduction contracture, hip or other joint —*see*
  Contraction, joint
Adenitis —*see also* Lymphadenitis
  acute, unspecified site L04.9
  axillary I88.9
    acute L04.2
    chronic or subacute I88.1
  Bartholin's gland N75.8
  bulbourethral gland —*see* Urethritis
  cervical I88.9
    acute L04.0
    chronic or subacute I88.1
  chancroid (Hemophilus ducreyi) A57
  chronic, unspecified site I88.1
  Cowper's gland —*see* Urethritis
  due to Pasteurella multocida (P. septica) A28.0
  epidemic, acute B27.09
  gangrenous L04.9
  gonorrheal NEC A54.89
  groin I88.9
    acute L04.1
    chronic or subacute I88.1
  infectious (acute) (epidemic) B27.09
  inguinal I88.9
    acute L04.1
    chronic or subacute I88.1
  lymph gland or node, except mesenteric I88.9
    acute —*see* Lymphadenitis, acute
    chronic or subacute I88.1
  mesenteric (acute) (chronic) (nonspecific)
    (subacute) I88.0

Adenitis (Continued)
  parotid gland (suppurative) —*see*
    Sialoadenitis
  salivary gland (any) (suppurative) —*see*
    Sialoadenitis
  scrofulous (tuberculous) A18.2
  Skene's duct or gland —*see* Urethritis
  strumous, tuberculous A18.2
  subacute, unspecified site I88.1
  sublingual gland (suppurative) —*see*
    Sialoadenitis
  submandibular gland (suppurative) —*see*
    Sialoadenitis
  submaxillary gland (suppurative) —*see*
    Sialoadenitis
  tuberculous —*see* Tuberculosis, lymph gland
  urethral gland —*see* Urethritis
  Wharton's duct (suppurative) —*see*
    Sialoadenitis
Adenoacanthoma —*see* Neoplasm, malignant,
  by site
Adenoameloblastoma —*see* Cyst, calcifying
  odontogenic
Adenocarcinoid (tumor) —*see* Neoplasm,
  malignant, by site
Adenocarcinoma —*see also* Neoplasm,
  malignant, by site
  acidophil
    specified site —*see* Neoplasm, malignant,
      by site
    unspecified site C75.1
  adrenal cortical C74.0-●
  alveolar —*see* Neoplasm, lung, malignant
  apocrine
    breast —*see* Neoplasm, breast, malignant
    in situ
      breast D05.8-●
      specified site NEC —*see* Neoplasm, skin,
        in situ
      unspecified site D04.9
    specified site NEC —*see* Neoplasm, skin,
      malignant
    unspecified site C44.99
  basal cell
    specified site —*see* Neoplasm, skin,
      malignant
    unspecified site C08.9
  basophil
    specified site —*see* Neoplasm, malignant,
      by site
    unspecified site C75.1
  bile duct type C22.1
    liver C22.1
    specified site NEC —*see* Neoplasm,
      malignant, by site
    unspecified site C22.1
  bronchiolar —*see* Neoplasm, lung,
    malignant
  bronchioloalveolar —*see* Neoplasm, lung,
    malignant
  ceruminous C44.29-●
  cervix, in situ (*see also* Carcinoma, cervix
    uteri, in situ) D06.9
  chromophobe
    specified site —*see* Neoplasm, malignant,
      by site
    unspecified site C75.1
  diffuse type
    specified site —*see* Neoplasm, malignant,
      by site
    unspecified site C16.9
  duct
    infiltrating
      with Paget's disease —*see* Neoplasm,
        breast, malignant
      specified site —*see* Neoplasm,
        malignant, by site
      unspecified site (female) C50.91-●
        male C50.92-●
    specified site —*see* Neoplasm, malignant,
      by site

Adenocarcinoma (Continued)
  duct (Continued)
    unspecified site
      female C56.9
      male C61
  eosinophil
    specified site —*see* Neoplasm, malignant,
      by site
    unspecified site C75.1
  follicular
    with papillary C73
    moderately differentiated C73
    specified site —*see* Neoplasm, malignant,
      by site
    trabecular C73
    unspecified site C73
    well differentiated C73
  Hurthle cell C73
  in
    adenomatous
      polyposis coli C18.9
  infiltrating duct
    with Paget's disease —*see* Neoplasm,
      breast, malignant
    specified site —*see* Neoplasm,
      malignant, by site
    unspecified site (female)
      C50.91-●
    male C50.92-●
  inflammatory
    specified site —*see* Neoplasm,
      malignant, by site
    unspecified site (female)
      C50.91-●
    male C50.92-●
  intestinal type
    specified site —*see* Neoplasm,
      malignant, by site
    unspecified site C16.9
  intracystic papillary
  intraductal
    breast D05.1-●
    noninfiltrating
      breast D05.1-●
      papillary
        with invasion
          specified site —*see* Neoplasm,
            malignant, by site
          unspecified site (female)
            C50.91-●
          male C50.92-●
        breast D05.1-●
        specified site NEC —*see* Neoplasm, in
          situ, by site
        unspecified site D05.1-●
      specified site NEC —*see* Neoplasm, in
        situ, by site
      unspecified site D05.1-●
    papillary
      with invasion
        specified site —*see* Neoplasm,
          malignant, by site
        unspecified site (female)
          C50.91-●
        male C50.92-●
      breast D05.1-●
      specified site —*see* Neoplasm, in situ,
        by site
      Hurthle cell C73
      unspecified site D05.1-●
    specified site NEC —*see* Neoplasm, in situ,
      by site
    unspecified site D05.1-●
  islet cell
    with exocrine, mixed
      specified site —*see* Neoplasm,
        malignant, by site
      unspecified site C25.9
    pancreas C25.4
    specified site NEC —*see* Neoplasm,
      malignant, by site
    unspecified site C25.4

Adenocarcinoma (Continued)
  lobular
    in situ
      breast D05.0-●
      specified site NEC —see Neoplasm, in
        situ, by site
      unspecified site D05.0-●
    specified site —see Neoplasm, malignant,
      by site
    unspecified site (female) C50.91-●
      male C50.92-●
  mucoid —see also Neoplasm, malignant,
    by site
    cell
      specified site —see Neoplasm,
        malignant, by site
      unspecified site C75.1
  nonencapsulated sclerosing C73
  papillary
    with follicular C73
    follicular variant C73
    intraductal (noninfiltrating)
      with invasion
        specified site —see Neoplasm,
          malignant, by site
        unspecified site (female) C50.91-●
          male C50.92-●
      breast D05.1-●
      specified site NEC —see Neoplasm, in
        situ, by site
      unspecified site D05.1-●
    serous
      specified site —see Neoplasm,
        malignant, by site
      unspecified site C56.9
  papillocystic
    specified site —see Neoplasm, malignant,
      by site
    unspecified site C56.9
  pseudomucinous
    specified site —see Neoplasm, malignant,
      by site
    unspecified site C56.9
  renal cell C64-●
  sebaceous —see Neoplasm, skin, malignant,
    by site
  serous —see also Neoplasm, malignant, by site
    papillary
      specified site —see Neoplasm,
        malignant, by site
      unspecified site C56.9
  sweat gland —see Neoplasm, skin, malignant
  water-clear cell C75.0
Adenocarcinoma-in-situ —see also Neoplasm,
  in situ, by site
  breast D05.9-●
Adenofibroma
  clear cell —see Neoplasm, benign, by site
  endometrioid D27.9
    borderline malignancy D39.10
    malignant C56-●
  mucinous
    specified site —see Neoplasm, benign, by
      site
    unspecified site D27.9
  papillary
    specified site —see Neoplasm, benign, by
      site
    unspecified site D27.9
  prostate —see Enlargement, enlarged,
    prostate
  serous
    specified site —see Neoplasm, benign, by
      site
    unspecified site D27.9
  specified site —see Neoplasm, benign,
    by site
  unspecified site D27.9
Adenofibrosis
  breast —see Fibroadenosis, breast
  endometrioid N80.0

Adenoiditis (chronic) J35.02
  with tonsillitis J35.03
  acute J03.90
    recurrent J03.91
    specified organism NEC J03.80
      recurrent J03.81
    staphylococcal J03.80
      recurrent J03.81
    streptococcal J03.00
      recurrent J03.01
Adenoids —see condition
Adenolipoma —see Neoplasm, benign,
  by site
Adenolipomatosis, Launois-Bensaude E88.89
Adenolymphoma
  specified site —see Neoplasm, benign, by site
  unspecified site D11.9
Adenoma —see also Neoplasm, benign, by site
  acidophil
    specified site —see Neoplasm, benign, by
      site
    unspecified site D35.2
  acidophil-basophil, mixed
    specified site —see Neoplasm, benign, by
      site
    unspecified site D35.2
  adrenal (cortical) D35.00
    clear cell D35.00
    compact cell D35.00
    glomerulosa cell D35.00
    heavily pigmented variant D35.00
    mixed cell D35.00
  alpha-cell
    pancreas D13.7
    specified site NEC —see Neoplasm, benign,
      by site
    unspecified site D13.7
  alveolar D14.30
  apocrine
    breast D24-●
    specified site NEC —see Neoplasm, skin,
      benign, by site
    unspecified site D23.9
  basal cell D11.9
  basophil
    specified site —see Neoplasm, benign,
      by site
    unspecified site D35.2
  basophil-acidophil, mixed
    specified site —see Neoplasm, benign, by
      site
    unspecified site D35.2
  beta-cell
    pancreas D13.7
    specified site NEC —see Neoplasm, benign,
      by site
    unspecified site D13.7
  bile duct D13.4
    common D13.5
    extrahepatic D13.5
    intrahepatic D13.4
    specified site NEC —see Neoplasm, benign,
      by site
    unspecified site D13.4
  black D35.00
  bronchial D38.1
    cylindroid type —see Neoplasm, lung,
      malignant
  ceruminous D23.2-●
  chief cell D35.1
  chromophobe
    specified site —see Neoplasm, benign, by
      site
    unspecified site D35.2
  colloid
    specified site —see Neoplasm, benign, by
      site
    unspecified site D34
  ~~duct~~
  eccrine, papillary —see Neoplasm, skin,
    benign

Adenoma (Continued)
  endocrine, multiple
    single specified site —see Neoplasm,
      uncertain behavior, by site
    two or more specified sites D44-●
    unspecified site D44.9
  endometrioid —see also Neoplasm, benign
    borderline malignancy —see Neoplasm,
      uncertain behavior, by site
  eosinophil
    specified site —see Neoplasm, malignant,
      by site
    unspecified site D35.2
  fetal
    specified site —see Neoplasm, benign, by
      site
    unspecified site D34
  follicular
    specified site —see Neoplasm, benign, by
      site
    unspecified site D34
  hepatocellular D13.4
  Hurthle cell D34
  islet cell
    pancreas D13.7
    specified site NEC —see Neoplasm, benign,
      by site
    unspecified site D13.7
  liver cell D13.4
  macrofollicular
    specified site —see Neoplasm, benign, by site
    unspecified site D34
  malignant, malignum —see Neoplasm,
    malignant, by site
  microcystic
    pancreas D13.6
    specified site NEC —see Neoplasm, benign,
      by site
    unspecified site D13.6
  microfollicular
    specified site —see Neoplasm, benign, by
      site
    unspecified site D34
  mucoid cell
    specified site —see Neoplasm, benign, by
      site
    unspecified site D35.2
  multiple endocrine
    single specified site —see Neoplasm,
      uncertain behavior, by site
    two or more specified sites D44-●
    unspecified site D44.9
  nipple D24-●
  papillary —see also Neoplasm, benign, by site
    eccrine —see Neoplasm, skin, benign, by
      site
  Pick's tubular
    specified site —see Neoplasm, benign, by
      site
    unspecified site
      female D27.9
      male D29.20
  pleomorphic
    carcinoma in —see Neoplasm, salivary
      gland, malignant
      specified site —see Neoplasm,
        malignant, by site
      unspecified site C08.9
  polypoid —see also Neoplasm, benign
    adenocarcinoma in —see Neoplasm,
      malignant, by site
    adenocarcinoma in situ —see Neoplasm, in
      situ, by site
  prostate —see Neoplasm, benign, prostate
  rete cell D29.20
  sebaceous —see Neoplasm, skin, benign
  Sertoli cell
    specified site —see Neoplasm, benign, by site
    unspecified site
      female D27.9
      male D29.20

  ▶ New   ➡ Revised   ~~deleted~~ Deleted   ● Use Additional Character(s)

Adenoma *(Continued)*
skin appendage —*see* Neoplasm, skin, benign
sudoriferous gland —*see* Neoplasm, skin, benign
sweat gland —*see* Neoplasm, skin, benign
testicular
  specified site —*see* Neoplasm, benign, by site
  unspecified site
    female D27.9
    male D29.20
tubular —*see also* Neoplasm, benign, by site
  adenocarcinoma in —*see* Neoplasm, malignant, by site
  adenocarcinoma in situ —*see* Neoplasm, in situ, by site
  Pick's
    specified site —*see* Neoplasm, benign
    unspecified site
      female D27.9
      male D29.20
tubulovillous —*see also* Neoplasm, benign, by site
  adenocarcinoma in —*see* Neoplasm, malignant, by site
  adenocarcinoma in situ —*see* Neoplasm, in situ, by site
villous —*see* Neoplasm, uncertain behavior, by site
  adenocarcinoma in —*see* Neoplasm, malignant, by site
  adenocarcinoma in situ —*see* Neoplasm, in situ, by site
water-clear cell D35.1
Adenomatosis
endocrine (multiple) E31.20
  single specified site —*see* Neoplasm, uncertain behavior, by site
erosive of nipple D24-●
pluriendocrine —*see* Adenomatosis, endocrine
pulmonary D38.1
  malignant —*see* Neoplasm, lung, malignant
specified site —*see* Neoplasm, benign, by site
unspecified site D12.6
Adenomatous
goiter (nontoxic) E04.9
  with hyperthyroidism —*see* Hyperthyroidism, with, goiter, nodular
  toxic —*see* Hyperthyroidism, with, goiter, nodular
Adenomyoma —*see also* Neoplasm, benign, by site
prostate —*see* Enlarged, prostate
Adenomyometritis N80.0
Adenomyosis N80.0
Adenopathy (lymph gland) R59.9
generalized R59.1
inguinal R59.0
localized R59.0
mediastinal R59.0
mesentery R59.0
syphilitic (secondary) A51.49
tracheobronchial R59.0
  tuberculous A15.4
    primary (progressive) A15.7
tuberculous —*see also* Tuberculosis, lymph gland
  tracheobronchial A15.4
    primary (progressive) A15.7
Adenosalpingitis —*see* Salpingitis
Adenosarcoma —*see* Neoplasm, malignant, by site
Adenosclerosis I88.8
Adenosis (sclerosing) **breast** —*see* Fibroadenosis, breast
Adenovirus, as cause of disease classified elsewhere B97.0
Adentia (complete) (partial) —*see* Absence, teeth

Adherent —*see also* Adhesions
labia (minora) N90.89
pericardium (nonrheumatic) I31.0
  rheumatic I09.2
placenta (with hemorrhage) O72.0
  without hemorrhage O73.0
prepuce, newborn N47.0
scar (skin) L90.5
tendon in scar L90.5
Adhesions, adhesive (postinfective) K66.0
with intestinal obstruction K56.50
  complete K56.52
  incomplete K56.51
  partial K56.51
abdominal (wall) —*see* Adhesions, peritoneum
appendix K38.8
bile duct (common) (hepatic) K83.8
bladder (sphincter) N32.89
bowel —*see* Adhesions, peritoneum
cardiac I31.0
  rheumatic I09.2
cecum —*see* Adhesions, peritoneum
cervicovaginal N88.1
  congenital Q52.8
  postpartal O90.89
    old N88.1
cervix N88.1
ciliary body NEC —*see* Adhesions, iris
clitoris N90.89
colon —*see* Adhesions, peritoneum
common duct K83.8
congenital —*see also* Anomaly, by site
  fingers —*see* Syndactylism, complex, fingers
  omental, anomalous Q43.3
  peritoneal Q43.3
  tongue (to gum or roof of mouth) Q38.3
conjunctiva (acquired) H11.21-●
  congenital Q15.8
cystic duct K82.8
diaphragm —*see* Adhesions, peritoneum
due to foreign body —*see* Foreign body
duodenum —*see* Adhesions, peritoneum
ear
  middle H74.1-●
epididymis N50.89
epidural —*see* Adhesions, meninges
epiglottis J38.7
eyelid H02.59
female pelvis N73.6
gallbladder K82.8
globe H44.89
heart I31.0
  rheumatic I09.2
ileocecal (coil) —*see* Adhesions, peritoneum
ileum —*see* Adhesions, peritoneum
intestine —*see also* Adhesions, peritoneum
  with obstruction K56.50
    complete K56.52
    incomplete K56.51
    partial K56.51
intra-abdominal —*see* Adhesions, peritoneum
iris H21.50-●
  anterior H21.51-●
  goniosynechiae H21.52-●
  posterior H21.54-●
  to corneal graft T85.898
joint —*see* Ankylosis
  knee M23.8X
  temporomandibular M26.61-●
labium (majus) (minus), congenital Q52.5
liver —*see* Adhesions, peritoneum
lung J98.4
mediastinum J98.59
meninges (cerebral) (spinal) G96.12
  congenital Q07.8
  tuberculous (cerebral) (spinal) A17.0
mesenteric —*see* Adhesions, peritoneum
nasal (septum) (to turbinates) J34.89
ocular muscle —*see* Strabismus, mechanical
omentum —*see* Adhesions, peritoneum

Adhesions, adhesive *(Continued)*
ovary N73.6
  congenital (to cecum, kidney or omentum) Q50.39
paraovarian N73.6
pelvic (peritoneal)
  female N73.6
    postprocedural N99.4
  male —*see* Adhesions, peritoneum
  postpartal (old) N73.6
  tuberculous A18.17
penis to scrotum (congenital) Q55.8
periappendiceal —*see also* Adhesions, peritoneum
pericardium (nonrheumatic) I31.0
  focal I31.8
  rheumatic I09.2
  tuberculous A18.84
pericholecystic K82.8
perigastric —*see* Adhesions, peritoneum
periovarian N73.6
periprostatic N42.89
perirectal —*see* Adhesions, peritoneum
perirenal N28.89
peritoneum, peritoneal (postinfective) K66.0
  with obstruction (intestinal) K56.50
    complete K56.52
    incomplete K56.51
    partial K56.51
  congenital Q43.3
  pelvic, female N73.6
    postprocedural N99.4
  postpartal, pelvic N73.6
  postprocedural K66.0
  to uterus N73.6
peritubal N73.6
periureteral N28.89
periuterine N73.6
perivesical N32.89
perivesicular (seminal vesicle) N50.89
pleura, pleuritic J94.8
  tuberculous NEC A15.6
pleuropericardial J94.8
postoperative (gastrointestinal tract) K66.0
  with obstruction —*see also* Obstruction, intestine, postoperative K91.30
  due to foreign body accidentally left in wound —*see* Foreign body, accidentally left during a procedure
  pelvic peritoneal N99.4
  urethra —*see* Stricture, urethra, postprocedural
  vagina N99.2
postpartal, old (vulva or perineum) N90.89
preputial, prepuce N47.5
pulmonary J98.4
pylorus —*see* Adhesions, peritoneum
sciatic nerve —*see* Lesion, nerve, sciatic
seminal vesicle N50.89
shoulder (joint) —*see* Capsulitis, adhesive
sigmoid flexure —*see* Adhesions, peritoneum
spermatic cord (acquired) N50.89
  congenital Q55.4
spinal canal G96.12
stomach —*see* Adhesions, peritoneum
subscapular —*see* Capsulitis, adhesive
temporomandibular M26.61-●
tendinitis —*see also* Tenosynovitis, specified type NEC
  shoulder —*see* Capsulitis, adhesive
testis N44.8
tongue, congenital (to gum or roof of mouth) Q38.3
  acquired K14.8
trachea J39.8
tubo-ovarian N73.6
tunica vaginalis N44.8
uterus N73.6
  internal N85.6
  to abdominal wall N73.6

Adhesions, adhesive (Continued)
vagina (chronic) N89.5
postoperative N99.2
vitreomacular H43.82-●
vitreous H43.89
vulva N90.89
Adiaspiromycosis B48.8
Adie (-Holmes) pupil or syndrome —see
Anomaly, pupil, function, tonic pupil
Adiponecrosis neonatorum P83.88
Adiposis —see also Obesity
cerebralis E23.6
dolorosa E88.2
Adiposity —see also Obesity
heart —see Degeneration, myocardial
localized E65
Adiposogenital dystrophy E23.6
Adjustment
disorder —see Disorder, adjustment
implanted device —see Encounter (for),
adjustment (of)
prosthesis, external —see Fitting
reaction —see Disorder, adjustment
Administration of tPA (rtPA) in a different
facility within the last 24 hours prior to
admission to current facility Z92.82
Admission (for) —see also Encounter (for)
adjustment (of)
artificial
arm Z44.00-●
complete Z44.01-●
partial Z44.02-●
eye Z44.2
leg Z44.10-●
complete Z44.11-●
partial Z44.12-●
brain neuropacemaker Z46.2
implanted Z45.42
breast
implant Z45.81
prosthesis (external) Z44.3
colostomy belt Z46.89
contact lenses Z46.0
cystostomy device Z46.6
dental prosthesis Z46.3
device NEC
abdominal Z46.89
implanted Z45.89
cardiac Z45.09
defibrillator (with synchronous
cardiac pacemaker) Z45.02
pacemaker (cardiac
resynchronization therapy
(CRT-P)) Z45.018
pulse generator Z45.010
resynchronization therapy
defibrillator (CRT-D) Z45.02
hearing device Z45.328
bone conduction Z45.320
cochlear Z45.321
infusion pump Z45.1
nervous system Z45.49
CSF drainage Z45.41
hearing device —see Admission,
adjustment, device, implanted,
hearing device
neuropacemaker Z45.42
visual substitution Z45.31
specified NEC Z45.89
vascular access Z45.2
visual substitution Z45.31
nervous system Z46.2
implanted —see Admission,
adjustment, device, implanted,
nervous system
orthodontic Z46.4
prosthetic Z44.9
arm —see Admission, adjustment,
artificial, arm
breast Z44.3
dental Z46.3

Admission (Continued)
adjustment (Continued)
device NEC (Continued)
prosthetic (Continued)
eye Z44.2
leg —see Admission, adjustment,
artificial, leg
specified type NEC Z44.8
substitution
auditory Z46.2
implanted —see Admission,
adjustment, device, implanted,
hearing device
nervous system Z46.2
implanted —see Admission,
adjustment, device, implanted,
nervous system
visual Z46.2
implanted Z45.31
urinary Z46.6
hearing aid Z46.1
implanted —see Admission, adjustment,
device, implanted, hearing device
ileostomy device Z46.89
intestinal appliance or device NEC Z46.89
neuropacemaker (brain) (peripheral nerve)
(spinal cord) Z46.2
implanted Z45.42
orthodontic device Z46.4
orthopedic (brace) (cast) (device) (shoes)
Z46.89
pacemaker (cardiac resynchronization
therapy (CRT-P))
cardiac Z45.018
pulse generator Z45.010
nervous system Z46.2
implanted Z45.42
portacath (port-a-cath) Z45.2
prosthesis Z44.9
arm —see Admission, adjustment,
artificial, arm
breast Z44.3
dental Z46.3
eye Z44.2
leg —see Admission, adjustment,
artificial, leg
specified NEC Z44.8
spectacles Z46.0
aftercare (see also Aftercare) Z51.89
postpartum
immediately after delivery Z39.0
routine follow-up Z39.2
radiation therapy (antineoplastic) Z51.0
attention to artificial opening (of) Z43.9
artificial vagina Z43.7
colostomy Z43.3
cystostomy Z43.5
enterostomy Z43.4
gastrostomy Z43.1
ileostomy Z43.2
jejunostomy Z43.4
nephrostomy Z43.6
specified site NEC Z43.8
intestinal tract Z43.4
urinary tract Z43.6
tracheostomy Z43.0
ureterostomy Z43.6
urethrostomy Z43.6
breast augmentation or reduction Z41.1
breast reconstruction following mastectomy
Z42.1
change of
dressing (nonsurgical) Z48.00
neuropacemaker device (brain) (peripheral
nerve) (spinal cord) Z46.2
implanted Z45.42
surgical dressing Z48.01
circumcision, ritual or routine (in absence of
diagnosis) Z41.2
clinical research investigation (control)
(normal comparison) (participant) Z00.6

Admission (Continued)
contraceptive management Z30.9
cosmetic surgery NEC Z41.1
counseling (see also Counseling)
dietary Z71.3
gestational carrier Z31.7
HIV Z71.7
human immunodeficiency virus Z71.7
nonattending third party Z71.0
procreative management NEC Z31.69
delivery, full-term, uncomplicated O80
cesarean, without indication O82
desensitization to allergens Z51.6
dietary surveillance and counseling Z71.3
ear piercing Z41.3
examination at health care facility (adult) —
see also Examination Z00.00
with abnormal findings Z00.01
clinical research investigation (control)
(normal comparison) (participant)
Z00.6
dental Z01.20
with abnormal findings Z01.21
donor (potential) Z00.5
ear Z01.10
with abnormal findings NEC Z01.118
following failed vision screening
Z01.020
with abnormal findings Z01.021
eye Z01.00
with abnormal findings Z01.01
general, specified reason NEC Z00.8
hearing Z01.10
with abnormal findings NEC Z01.118
infant or child (over 28 days old) Z00.129
with abnormal findings Z00.121
postpartum checkup Z39.2
psychiatric (general) Z00.8
requested by authority Z04.6
vision Z01.00
with abnormal findings Z01.01
following failed vision screening
Z01.020
with abnormal findings Z01.021
infant or child (over 28 days old) Z00.129
with abnormal findings Z00.121
fitting (of)
artificial
arm —see Admission, adjustment,
artificial, arm
eye Z44.2
leg —see Admission, adjustment,
artificial, leg
brain neuropacemaker Z46.2
implanted Z45.42
breast prosthesis (external) Z44.3
colostomy belt Z46.89
contact lenses Z46.0
cystostomy device Z46.6
dental prosthesis Z46.3
dentures Z46.3
device NEC
abdominal Z46.89
nervous system Z46.2
implanted —see Admission,
adjustment, device, implanted,
nervous system
orthodontic Z46.4
prosthetic Z44.9
breast Z44.3
dental Z46.3
eye Z44.2
substitution
auditory Z46.2
implanted —see Admission,
adjustment, device, implanted,
hearing device
nervous system Z46.2
implanted —see Admission,
adjustment, device, implanted,
nervous system

Admission *(Continued)*
  fitting (of) *(Continued)*
    device NEC *(Continued)*
      substitution *(Continued)*
        visual Z46.2
          implanted Z45.31
      hearing aid Z46.1
      ileostomy device Z46.89
      intestinal appliance or device NEC Z46.89
      neuropacemaker (brain) (peripheral nerve) (spinal cord) Z46.2
        implanted Z45.42
      orthodontic device Z46.4
      orthopedic device (brace) (cast) (shoes) Z46.89
      prosthesis Z44.9
        arm —*see* Admission, adjustment, artificial, arm
        breast Z44.3
        dental Z46.3
        eye Z44.2
        leg —*see* Admission, adjustment, artificial, leg
        specified type NEC Z44.8
      spectacles Z46.0
  follow-up examination Z09
  intrauterine device management Z30.431
    initial prescription Z30.014
  mental health evaluation Z00.8
    requested by authority Z04.6
  observation —*see* Observation
  Papanicolaou smear, cervix Z12.4
    for suspected malignant neoplasm Z12.4
  plastic and reconstructive surgery following medical procedure or healed injury NEC Z42.8
  plastic surgery, cosmetic NEC Z41.1
  postpartum observation
    immediately after delivery Z39.0
    routine follow-up Z39.2
  poststerilization (for restoration) Z31.0
    aftercare Z31.42
  procreative management Z31.9
  prophylactic (measure) —*see also* Encounter, prophylactic measures
    organ removal Z40.00
      breast Z40.01
      fallopian tube(s) Z40.03
        with ovary(s) Z40.02
      ovary(s) Z40.02
      specified organ NEC Z40.09
      testes Z40.09
    vaccination Z23
  psychiatric examination (general) Z00.8
    requested by authority Z04.6
  radiation therapy (antineoplastic) Z51.0
  reconstructive surgery following medical procedure or healed injury NEC Z42.8
  removal of
    cystostomy catheter Z43.5
    drains Z48.03
    dressing (nonsurgical) Z48.00
    implantable subdermal contraceptive Z30.46
    intrauterine contraceptive device Z30.432
    neuropacemaker (brain) (peripheral nerve) (spinal cord) Z46.2
      implanted Z45.42
    staples Z48.02
    surgical dressing Z48.01
    sutures Z48.02
    ureteral stent Z46.6
  respirator [ventilator] use during power failure Z99.12
  restoration of organ continuity (poststerilization) Z31.0
    aftercare Z31.42
  sensitivity test —*see also* Test, skin
    allergy NEC Z01.82
    Mantoux Z11.1

Admission *(Continued)*
  tuboplasty following previous sterilization Z31.0
    aftercare Z31.42
  vasoplasty following previous sterilization Z31.0
    aftercare Z31.42
  vision examination Z01.00
    with abnormal findings Z01.01
      following failed vision screening Z01.020
        with abnormal findings Z01.021
    infant or child (over 28 days old) Z00.129
      with abnormal findings Z00.121
  waiting period for admission to other facility Z75.1
Adnexitis (suppurative) —*see* Salpingo-oophoritis
Adolescent X-linked adrenoleukodystrophy E71.521
Adrenal (gland) —*see* condition
Adrenalism, tuberculous A18.7
Adrenalitis, adrenitis E27.8
  autoimmune E27.1
  meningococcal, hemorrhagic A39.1
Adrenarche, premature E27.0
Adrenocortical syndrome —*see* Cushing's, syndrome
Adrenogenital syndrome E25.9
  acquired E25.8
  congenital E25.0
  salt loss E25.0
Adrenogenitalism, congenital E25.0
Adrenoleukodystrophy E71.529
  neonatal E71.511
  X-linked E71.529
    Addison only phenotype E71.528
    Addison-Schilder E71.528
    adolescent E71.521
    adrenomyeloneuropathy E71.522
    childhood cerebral E71.520
    other specified E71.528
Adrenomyeloneuropathy E71.522
Adventitious bursa —*see* Bursopathy, specified type NEC
Adverse effect —*see* Table of Drugs and Chemicals, categories T36-T50, with 6th character 5
Advice —*see* Counseling
Adynamia (episodica) (hereditary) (periodic) G72.3
Aeration lung imperfect, newborn —*see* Atelectasis
Aerobullosis T70.3
Aerocele —*see* Embolism, air
Aerodermectasia
  subcutaneous (traumatic) T79.7
Aerodontalgia T70.29
Aeroembolism T70.3
Aerogenes capsulatus infection A48.0
Aero-otitis media T70.0
Aerophagy, aerophagia (psychogenic) F45.8
Aerophobia F40.228
Aerosinusitis T70.1
Aerotitis T70.0
Affection —*see* Disease
Afibrinogenemia —*see also* Defect, coagulation D68.8
  acquired D65
  congenital D68.2
  following ectopic or molar pregnancy O08.1
  in abortion —*see* Abortion, by type, complicated by, afibrinogenemia
  puerperal O72.3
African
  sleeping sickness B56.9
  tick fever A68.1
  trypanosomiasis B56.9
    gambian B56.0
    rhodesian B56.1

Aftercare —*see also* Care Z51.89
  following surgery (for) (on)
    amputation Z47.81
    attention to
      drains Z48.03
      dressings (nonsurgical) Z48.00
        surgical Z48.01
      sutures Z48.02
    circulatory system Z48.812
    delayed (planned) wound closure Z48.1
    digestive system Z48.815
    explantation of joint prosthesis (staged procedure)
      hip Z47.32
      knee Z47.33
      shoulder Z47.31
    genitourinary system Z48.816
    joint replacement Z47.1
    neoplasm Z48.3
    nervous system Z48.811
    oral cavity Z48.814
    organ transplant
      bone marrow Z48.290
      heart Z48.21
      heart-lung Z48.280
      kidney Z48.22
      liver Z48.23
      lung Z48.24
      multiple organs NEC Z48.288
      specified NEC Z48.298
    orthopedic NEC Z47.89
    planned wound closure Z48.1
    removal of internal fixation device Z47.2
    respiratory system Z48.813
    scoliosis Z47.82
    sense organs Z48.810
    skin and subcutaneous tissue Z48.817
    specified body system
      circulatory Z48.812
      digestive Z48.815
      genitourinary Z48.816
      nervous Z48.811
      oral cavity Z48.814
      respiratory Z48.813
      sense organs Z48.810
      skin and subcutaneous tissue Z48.817
      teeth Z48.814
    specified NEC Z48.89
    spinal Z47.89
    teeth Z48.814
  fracture — code to fracture with seventh character D
  involving
    removal of
      drains Z48.03
      dressings (nonsurgical) Z48.00
      staples Z48.02
      surgical dressings Z48.01
      sutures Z48.02
  neuropacemaker (brain) (peripheral nerve) (spinal cord) Z46.2
    implanted Z45.42
  orthopedic NEC Z47.89
  postprocedural —*see* Aftercare, following surgery
After-cataract —*see* Cataract, secondary
Agalactia (primary) O92.3
  elective, secondary or therapeutic O92.5
Agammaglobulinemia (acquired (secondary)) (nonfamilial) D80.1
  with
    immunoglobulin-bearing B-lymphocytes D80.1
    lymphopenia D81.9
  autosomal recessive (Swiss type) D80.0
  Bruton's X-linked D80.0
  common variable (CVAgamma) D80.1
  congenital sex-linked D80.0
  hereditary D80.0
  lymphopenic D81.9
  Swiss type (autosomal recessive) D80.0

Agammaglobulinemia (Continued)
  X-linked (with growth hormone deficiency) (Bruton) D80.0
Aganglionosis (bowel) (colon) Q43.1
Age (old) —*see* Senility
Agenesis
  adrenal (gland) Q89.1
  alimentary tract (complete) (partial) NEC Q45.8
    upper Q40.8
  anus, anal (canal) Q42.3
    with fistula Q42.2
  aorta Q25.41
  appendix Q42.8
  arm (complete) Q71.0-●
    with hand present Q71.1-●
  artery (peripheral) Q27.9
    brain Q28.3
    coronary Q24.5
    pulmonary Q25.79
    specified NEC Q27.8
    umbilical Q27.0
  auditory (canal) (external) Q16.1
  auricle (ear) Q16.0
  bile duct or passage Q44.5
  bladder Q64.5
  bone Q79.9
  brain Q00.0
    part of Q04.3
  breast (with nipple present) Q83.8
    with absent nipple Q83.0
  bronchus Q32.4
  canaliculus lacrimalis Q10.4
  carpus —*see* Agenesis, hand
  cartilage Q79.9
  cecum Q42.8
  cerebellum Q04.3
  cervix Q51.5
  chin Q18.8
  cilia Q10.3
  circulatory system, part NOS Q28.9
  clavicle Q74.0
  clitoris Q52.6
  coccyx Q76.49
  colon Q42.9
    specified NEC Q42.8
  corpus callosum Q04.0
  cricoid cartilage Q31.8
  diaphragm (with hernia) Q79.1
  digestive organ(s) or tract (complete) (partial) NEC Q45.8
    upper Q40.8
  ductus arteriosus Q28.8
  duodenum Q41.0
  ear Q16.9
    auricle Q16.0
    lobe Q17.8
  ejaculatory duct Q55.4
  endocrine (gland) NEC Q89.2
  epiglottis Q31.8
  esophagus Q39.8
  eustachian tube Q16.2
  eye Q11.1
    adnexa Q15.8
  eyelid (fold) Q10.3
  face
    bones NEC Q75.8
    specified part NEC Q18.8
  fallopian tube Q50.6
  femur —*see* Defect, reduction, lower limb, longitudinal, femur
  fibula —*see* Defect, reduction, lower limb, longitudinal, fibula
  finger (complete) (partial) —*see* Agenesis, hand
  foot (and toes) (complete) (partial) Q72.3-●
  forearm (with hand present) —*see* Agenesis, arm, with hand present
    and hand Q71.2-●
  gallbladder Q44.0
  gastric Q40.2

Agenesis (Continued)
  genitalia, genital (organ(s))
    female Q52.8
      external Q52.71
      internal NEC Q52.8
    male Q55.8
  glottis Q31.8
  hair Q84.0
  hand (and fingers) (complete) (partial) Q71.3-●
  heart Q24.8
    valve NEC Q24.8
      pulmonary Q22.0
  hepatic Q44.7
  humerus —*see* Defect, reduction, upper limb
  hymen Q52.4
  ileum Q41.2
  incus Q16.3
  intestine (small) Q41.9
    large Q42.9
      specified NEC Q42.8
  iris (dilator fibers) Q13.1
  jaw M26.09
  jejunum Q41.1
  kidney(s) (partial) Q60.2
    bilateral Q60.1
    unilateral Q60.0
  labium (majus) (minus) Q52.71
  labyrinth, membranous Q16.5
  lacrimal apparatus Q10.4
  larynx Q31.8
  leg (complete) Q72.0-●
    with foot present Q72.1-●
    lower leg (with foot present) —*see* Agenesis, leg, with foot present
      and foot Q72.2-●
  lens Q12.3
  limb (complete) Q73.0
    lower —*see* Agenesis, leg
    upper —*see* Agenesis, arm
  lip Q38.0
  liver Q44.7
  lung (fissure) (lobe) (bilateral) (unilateral) Q33.3
  mandible, maxilla M26.09
  metacarpus —*see* Agenesis, hand
  metatarsus —*see* Agenesis, foot
  muscle Q79.8
    eyelid Q10.3
    ocular Q15.8
  musculoskeletal system NEC Q79.8
  nail(s) Q84.3
  neck, part Q18.8
  nerve Q07.8
  nervous system, part NEC Q07.8
  nipple Q83.2
  nose Q30.1
  nuclear Q07.8
  organ
    of Corti Q16.5
    or site not listed —*see* Anomaly, by site
  osseous meatus (ear) Q16.1
  ovary
    bilateral Q50.02
    unilateral Q50.01
  oviduct Q50.6
  pancreas Q45.0
  parathyroid (gland) Q89.2
  parotid gland(s) Q38.4
  patella Q74.1
  pelvic girdle (complete) (partial) Q74.2
  penis Q55.5
  pericardium Q24.8
  pituitary (gland) Q89.2
  prostate Q55.4
  punctum lacrimale Q10.4
  radioulnar —*see* Defect, reduction, upper limb
  radius —*see* Defect, reduction, upper limb, longitudinal, radius
  rectum Q42.1
    with fistula Q42.0

Agenesis (Continued)
  renal Q60.2
    bilateral Q60.1
    unilateral Q60.0
  respiratory organ NEC Q34.8
  rib Q76.6
  roof of orbit Q75.8
  round ligament Q52.8
  sacrum Q76.49
  salivary gland Q38.4
  scapula Q74.0
  scrotum Q55.29
  seminal vesicles Q55.4
  septum
    atrial Q21.1
    between aorta and pulmonary artery Q21.4
    ventricular Q20.4
  shoulder girdle (complete) (partial) Q74.0
  skull (bone) Q75.8
    with
      anencephaly Q00.0
      encephalocele —*see* Encephalocele
      hydrocephalus Q03.9
        with spina bifida —*see* Spina bifida, by site, with hydrocephalus
      microcephaly Q02
  spermatic cord Q55.4
  spinal cord Q06.0
  spine Q76.49
  spleen Q89.01
  sternum Q76.7
  stomach Q40.2
  submaxillary gland(s) (congenital) Q38.4
  tarsus —*see* Agenesis, foot
  tendon Q79.8
  testicle Q55.0
  thymus (gland) Q89.2
  thyroid (gland) E03.1
    cartilage Q31.8
  tibia —*see* Defect, reduction, lower limb, longitudinal, tibia
  tibiofibular —*see* Defect, reduction, lower limb, specified type NEC
  toe (and foot) (complete) (partial) —*see* Agenesis, foot
  tongue Q38.3
  trachea (cartilage) Q32.1
  ulna —*see* Defect, reduction, upper limb, longitudinal, ulna
  upper limb —*see* Agenesis, arm
  ureter Q62.4
  urethra Q64.5
  urinary tract NEC Q64.8
  uterus Q51.0
  uvula Q38.5
  vagina Q52.0
  vas deferens Q55.4
  vein(s) (peripheral) Q27.9
    brain Q28.3
    great NEC Q26.8
    portal Q26.5
  vena cava (inferior) (superior) Q26.8
  vermis of cerebellum Q04.3
  vertebra Q76.49
  vulva Q52.71
Ageusia R43.2
Agitated —*see* condition
Agitation R45.1
Aglossia (congenital) Q38.3
Aglossia-adactylia syndrome Q87.0
Aglycogenosis E74.00
Agnosia (body image) (other senses) (tactile) R48.1
  developmental F88
  verbal R48.1
    auditory R48.1
      developmental F80.2
    developmental F80.2
  visual (object) R48.3

A

▶ New   ⇒ Revised   ~~deleted~~ Deleted   ● Use Additional Character(s)

Agoraphobia F40.00
　with panic disorder F40.01
　without panic disorder F40.02
Agrammatism R48.8
Agranulocytopenia —see Agranulocytosis
Agranulocytosis (chronic) (cyclical) (genetic)
　　(infantile) (periodic) (pernicious) (see also
　　Neutropenia) D70.9
　congenital D70.0
　cytoreductive cancer chemotherapy sequela
　　D70.1
　drug-induced D70.2
　　due to cytoreductive cancer chemotherapy
　　　D70.1
　due to infection D70.3
　secondary D70.4
　　drug-induced D70.2
　　　due to cytoreductive cancer
　　　　chemotherapy D70.1
Agraphia (absolute) R48.8
　with alexia R48.0
　developmental F81.81
Ague (dumb) —see Malaria
Agyria Q04.3
Ahumada-del Castillo syndrome E23.0
Aichomophobia F40.298
AIDS (related complex) B20
Ailment heart —see Disease, heart
Ailurophobia F40.218
Ainhum (disease) L94.6
AIN —see Neoplasia, intraepithelial, anal
AIPHI (acute idiopathic pulmonary hemorrhage
　　in infants (over 28 days old)) R04.81
Air
　anterior mediastinum J98.2
　compressed, disease T70.3
　conditioner lung or pneumonitis J67.7
　embolism (artery) (cerebral) (any site)
　　　T79.0
　　with ectopic or molar pregnancy O08.2
　　due to implanted device NEC —see
　　　Complications, by site and type,
　　　specified NEC
　　following
　　　abortion —see Abortion by type,
　　　　complicated by, embolism
　　　ectopic or molar pregnancy O08.2
　　　infusion, therapeutic injection or
　　　　transfusion T80.0
　　in pregnancy, childbirth or puerperium —
　　　see Embolism, obstetric
　　traumatic T79.0
　hunger, psychogenic F45.8
　rarefied, effects of —see Effect, adverse, high
　　altitude
　sickness T75.3
Airplane sickness T75.3
Akathisia (drug-induced) (treatment- induced)
　　G25.71
　neuroleptic induced (acute) G25.71
　tardive G25.71
Akinesia R29.898
Akinetic mutism R41.89
Akureyri's disease G93.3
Alactasia, congenital E73.0
Alagille's syndrome Q44.7
Alastrim B03
Albers-Schönberg syndrome Q78.2
Albert's syndrome —see Tendinitis,
　　Achilles
Albinism, albino E70.30
　with hematologic abnormality E70.339
　　Chédiak-Higashi syndrome E70.330
　　Hermansky-Pudlak syndrome E70.331
　　other specified E70.338
　　I E70.320
　　II E70.321
　ocular E70.319
　　autosomal recessive E70.311
　　other specified E70.318
　　X-linked E70.310

Albinism, albino (Continued)
　oculocutaneous E70.329
　　other specified E70.328
　　tyrosinase (ty) negative E70.320
　　tyrosinase (ty) positive E70.321
　other specified E70.39
Albinismus E70.30
Albright (-McCune)(-Sternberg) syndrome
　　Q78.1
Albuminous —see condition
Albuminuria, albuminuric (acute) (chronic)
　　(subacute) —see also Proteinuria R80.9
　complicating pregnancy —see Proteinuria,
　　gestational
　with
　　gestational hypertension —see
　　　Pre-eclampsia
　　pre-existing hypertension —see
　　　Hypertension, complicating
　　　pregnancy, pre-existing, with,
　　　pre-eclampsia
　gestational —see Proteinuria, gestational
　with
　　gestational hypertension —see
　　　Pre-eclampsia
　　pre-existing hypertension —see
　　　Hypertension, complicating
　　　pregnancy, pre-existing, with,
　　　pre-eclampsia
　orthostatic R80.2
　postural R80.2
　pre-eclamptic —see Pre-eclampsia
　scarlatinal A38.8
Albuminurophobia F40.298
Alcaptonuria E70.29
Alcohol, alcoholic, alcohol-induced
　addiction (without remission) F10.20
　　with remission F10.21
　amnestic disorder, persisting F10.96
　　with dependence F10.26
　anxiety disorder F10.980
　bipolar and related disorder F10.94
　brain syndrome, chronic F10.97
　　with dependence F10.27
　cardiopathy I42.6
　counseling and surveillance
　　　Z71.41
　　family member Z71.42
　delirium (acute) (tremens) (withdrawal)
　　　F10.231
　　with intoxication F10.921
　　in
　　　abuse F10.121
　　　dependence F10.221
　dementia F10.97
　　with dependence F10.27
　depressive disorder F10.94
　deterioration F10.97
　　with dependence F10.27
　hallucinosis (acute) F10.951
　　in
　　　abuse F10.151
　　　dependence F10.251
　insanity F10.959
　intoxication (acute) (without dependence)
　　　F10.129
　　with
　　　delirium F10.121
　　　dependence F10.229
　　　　with delirium F10.221
　　　　uncomplicated F10.220
　　uncomplicated F10.120
　jealousy F10.988
　Korsakoff's, Korsakov's, Korsakow's F10.26
　liver K70.9
　　acute —see Disease, liver, alcoholic,
　　　hepatitis
　major neurocognitive disorder, amnestic-
　　confabulatory type F10.96
　major neurocognitive disorder, nonamnestic-
　　confabulatory type F10.97

Alcohol, alcoholic, alcohol-induced (Continued)
　mania (acute) (chronic) F10.959
　mild neurocognitive disorder F10.988
　paranoia, paranoid (type) psychosis F10.950
　pellagra E52
　poisoning, accidental (acute) NEC —see
　　　Table of Drugs and Chemicals, alcohol,
　　　poisoning
　psychosis —see Psychosis, alcoholic
　psychotic disorder F10.959
　sexual dysfunction F10.981
　sleep disorder F10.982
　withdrawal (without convulsions) F10.239
　　with delirium F10.231
Alcoholism (chronic) (without remission) F10.20
　with
　　psychosis —see Psychosis, alcoholic
　　remission F10.21
　Korsakov's F10.96
　　with dependence F10.26
Alder (-Reilly) anomaly or syndrome
　　(leukocyte granulation) D72.0
Aldosteronism E26.9
　familial (type I) E26.02
　glucocorticoid-remediable E26.02
　primary (due to (bilateral) adrenal
　　hyperplasia) E26.09
　primary NEC E26.09
　secondary E26.1
　specified NEC E26.89
Aldosteronoma D44.10
Aldrich(-Wiskott) syndrome (eczema-
　　thrombocytopenia) D82.0
Alektorophobia F40.218
Aleppo boil B55.1
Aleukemic —see condition Aleukia
　congenital D70.0
　hemorrhagica D61.9
　　congenital D61.09
　splenica D73.1
Alexia R48.0
　developmental F81.0
　secondary to organic lesion R48.0
Algoneurodystrophy M89.00
　ankle M89.07-●
　foot M89.07-●
　forearm M89.03-●
　hand M89.04-●
　lower leg M89.06-●
　multiple sites M89.0-●
　shoulder M89.01-●
　specified site NEC M89.08
　thigh M89.05-●
　upper arm M89.02-●
Algophobia F40.298
Alienation, mental —see Psychosis
Alkalemia E87.3
Alkalosis E87.3
　metabolic E87.3
　　with respiratory acidosis E87.4
　of newborn P74.41
　respiratory E87.3
Alkaptonuria E70.29
Allen-Masters syndrome N83.8
Allergy, allergic (reaction) (to) T78.40
　air-borne substance NEC (rhinitis) J30.89
　alveolitis (extrinsic) J67.9
　　due to
　　　Aspergillus clavatus J67.4
　　　Cryptostroma corticale J67.6
　　　organisms (fungal, thermophilic
　　　　actinomycete) growing in
　　　　ventilation (air conditioning)
　　　　systems J67.7
　　specified type NEC J67.8
　anaphylactic reaction or shock T78.2
　angioneurotic edema T78.3
　animal (dander) (epidermal) (hair) (rhinitis)
　　　J30.81
　bee sting (anaphylactic shock) —see Toxicity,
　　venom, arthropod, bee

Allergy, allergic *(Continued)*
  biological —*see* Allergy, drug
  colitis —*see also* Colitis, allergic K52.29
  dander (animal) (rhinitis) J30.81
  dandruff (rhinitis) J30.81
  dental restorative material (existing) K08.55
  dermatitis —*see* Dermatitis, contact, allergic
  diathesis —*see* History, allergy
  drug, medicament & biological (any)
    (external) (internal) T78.40
    correct substance properly administered —
      see Table of Drugs and Chemicals, by
      drug, adverse effect
    wrong substance given or taken NEC (by
      accident) —*see* Table of Drugs and
      Chemicals, by drug, poisoning
  due to pollen J30.1
  dust (house) (stock) (rhinitis) J30.89
    with asthma —*see* Asthma, allergic extrinsic
  eczema —*see* Dermatitis, contact, allergic
  epidermal (animal) (rhinitis) J30.81
  feathers (rhinitis) J30.89
  food (any) (ingested) NEC T78.1
    anaphylactic shock —*see* Shock,
      anaphylactic, due to food
    dermatitis —*see* Dermatitis, due to, food
    dietary counseling and surveillance Z71.3
    in contact with skin L23.6
    rhinitis J30.5
    status (without reaction) Z91.018
    ▶beef Z91.014
      eggs Z91.012
    ▶lamb Z91.014
    ▶mammalian meats Z91.014
      milk products Z91.011
      peanuts Z91.010
    ▶pork Z91.014
    ▶red meats Z91.014
      seafood Z91.013
      specified NEC Z91.018
  gastrointestinal —*see also* specific type of
    allergic reaction
    meaning colitis —*see also* Colitis, allergic)
      K52.29
    meaning gastroenteritis —*see also*
      Gastroenteritis, allergic) K52.29
    meaning other adverse food reaction not
      elsewhere classified T78.1
  grain J30.1
  grass (hay fever) (pollen) J30.1
    asthma —*see* Asthma, allergic extrinsic
  hair (animal) (rhinitis) J30.81
  history (of) —*see* History, allergy
  horse serum —*see* Allergy, serum
  inhalant (rhinitis) J30.89
    pollen J30.1
  kapok (rhinitis) J30.89
  medicine —*see* Allergy, drug
  milk protein —*see also* Allergy, food Z91.011
    anaphylactic reaction T78.07
    dermatitis L27.2
    enterocolitis syndrome K52.21
    enteropathy K52.22
    gastroenteritis K52.29
    gastroesophageal reflux —*see also* Reaction,
      adverse, food) K21.9
      with esophagitis without bleeding K21.00
        with bleeding K21.01
    ➡proctocolitis K52.29
  nasal, seasonal due to pollen J30.1
  pneumonia J82.89
  pollen (any) (hay fever) J30.1
    asthma —*see* Asthma, allergic extrinsic
  primrose J30.1
  primula J30.1
  ➡proctocolitis K52.29
  purpura D69.0
  ragweed (hay fever) (pollen) J30.1
    asthma —*see* Asthma, allergic extrinsic
  rose (pollen) J30.1
  seasonal NEC J30.2

Allergy, allergic *(Continued)*
  Senecio jacobae (pollen) J30.1
  serum —*see also* Reaction, serum T80.69
    anaphylactic shock T80.59
  shock (anaphylactic) T78.2
    due to
      administration of blood and blood
        products T80.51
      adverse effect of correct medicinal
        substance properly administered
        T88.6
      immunization T80.52
      serum NEC T80.59
      vaccination T80.52
    specific NEC T78.49
  tree (any) (hay fever) (pollen) J30.1
    asthma —*see* Asthma, allergic extrinsic
  upper respiratory J30.9
  urticaria L50.0
  vaccine —*see* Allergy, serum
  wheat —*see* Allergy, food
Allescheriasis B48.2
Alligator skin disease Q80.9
Allocheiria, allochiria R20.8
Almeida's disease —*see*
  Paracoccidioidomycosis
Alopecia (hereditaria) (seborrheica) L65.9
  androgenic L64.9
    drug-induced L64.0
    specified NEC L64.8
  areata L63.9
    ophiasis L63.2
    specified NEC L63.8
    totalis L63.0
    universalis L63.1
  cicatricial L66.9
    specified NEC L66.8
  circumscripta L63.9
  congenital, congenitalis Q84.0
  due to cytotoxic drugs NEC L65.8
  mucinosa L65.2
  postinfective NEC L65.8
  postpartum L65.0
  premature L64.8
  specific (syphilitic) A51.32
  specified NEC L65.8
  syphilitic (secondary) A51.32
  totalis (capitis) L63.0
  universalis (entire body) L63.1
  X-ray L58.1
Alpers' disease G31.81
Alpine sickness T70.29
Alport syndrome Q87.81
ALTE (apparent life threatening event) in
  newborn and infant R68.13
Alteration (of), **Altered**
  awareness
    transient R40.4
    unintended under general anesthesia,
      during procedure T88.53
  mental status R41.82
  pattern of family relationships affecting child
    Z62.898
  sensation
    following
      cerebrovascular disease I69.998
        cerebral infarction I69.398
        intracerebral hemorrhage I69.198
        nontraumatic intracranial hemorrhage
          NEC I69.298
        specified disease NEC I69.898
        subarachnoid hemorrhage I69.098
Alternating —*see* condition
Altitude, high (effects) —*see* Effect, adverse,
  high altitude
Aluminosis (of lung) J63.0
Alveolitis
  allergic (extrinsic) —*see* Pneumonitis,
    hypersensitivity
  due to
    Aspergillus clavatus J67.4
    Cryptostroma corticale J67.6

Alveolitis *(Continued)*
  fibrosing (cryptogenic) (idiopathic) J84.112
  jaw M27.3
  sicca dolorosa M27.3
Alveolus, alveolar —*see* condition
Alymphocytosis D72.810
  thymic (with immunodeficiency) D82.1
Alymphoplasia, thymic D82.1
Alzheimer's disease or sclerosis —*see* Disease,
  Alzheimer's
Amastia (with nipple present) Q83.8
  with absent nipple Q83.0
Amathophobia F40.228
Amaurosis (acquired) (congenital) —*see also*
  Blindness
  fugax G45.3
  hysterical F44.6
  Leber's congenital H35.50
  uremic —*see* Uremia
Amaurotic idiocy (infantile) (juvenile) (late)
  E75.4
Amaxophobia F40.248
Ambiguous genitalia Q56.4
Amblyopia (congenital) (ex anopsia) (partial)
  (suppression) H53.00-●
  anisometropic —*see* Amblyopia, refractive
  deprivation H53.01-●
  hysterical F44.6
  nocturnal —*see also* Blindness, night
    vitamin A deficiency E50.5
  refractive H53.02-●
  strabismic H53.03-●
  suspect H53.04-●
  tobacco H53.8
  toxic NEC H53.8
  uremic —*see* Uremia
Ameba, amebic (histolytica) —*see also* Amebiasis
  abscess (liver) A06.4
Amebiasis A06.9
  with abscess —*see* Abscess, amebic
  acute A06.0
  chronic (intestine) A06.1
    with abscess —*see* Abscess, amebic
  cutaneous A06.7
  cutis A06.7
  cystitis A06.81
  genitourinary tract NEC A06.82
  hepatic —*see* Abscess, liver, amebic
  intestine A06.0
  nondysenteric colitis A06.2
  skin A06.7
  specified site NEC A06.89
Ameboma (of intestine) A06.3
Amelia Q73.0
  lower limb —*see* Agenesis, leg
  upper limb —*see* Agenesis, arm
Ameloblastoma —*see also* Cyst, calcifying
  odontogenic
  long bones C40.9-●
    lower limb C40.2-●
    upper limb C40.0-●
  malignant C41.1
    jaw (bone) (lower) C41.1
      upper C41.0
  tibial C40.2-●
Amelogenesis imperfecta K00.5
  nonhereditaria (segmentalis) K00.4
Amenorrhea N91.2
  hyperhormonal E28.8
  primary N91.0
  secondary N91.1
Amentia —*see* Disability, intellectual
  Meynert's (nonalcoholic) F04
American
  leishmaniasis B55.2
  mountain tick fever A93.2
Ametropia —*see* Disorder, refraction
AMH (asymptomatic microscopic hematuria)
  R31.21
Amianthosis J61
Amimia R48.8

    ▶ New   ⇒ Revised   ~~deleted~~ Deleted   ● Use Additional Character(s)

Amino-acid disorder E72.9
  anemia D53.0
Aminoacidopathy E72.9
Aminoaciduria E72.9
Amnes (t)ic syndrome (post-traumatic) F04
  induced by
    alcohol F10.96
      with dependence F10.26
    psychoactive NEC F19.96
      with
        abuse F19.16
        dependence F19.26
    sedative F13.96
      with dependence F13.26
Amnesia R41.3
  anterograde R41.1
  auditory R48.8
  dissociative F44.0
    with dissociative fugue F44.1
  hysterical F44.0
  postictal in epilepsy —see Epilepsy
  psychogenic F44.0
  retrograde R41.2
  transient global G45.4
Amnion, amniotic —see condition
Amnionitis —see Pregnancy, complicated by
Amok F68.8
Amoral traits F60.89
Amphetamine (or other stimulant) —
    induced
  anxiety disorder F15.980
  bipolar and related disorder F15.94
  delirium F15.921
  depressive disorder F15.94
  obsessive-compulsive and related disorder
    F15.988
  psychotic disorder F15.959
  sexual dysfunction F15.981
  sleep disorder F15.982
  stimulant withdrawal F15.23
Ampulla
  lower esophagus K22.89
  phrenic K22.89
Amputation —see also Absence, by site,
    acquired
  neuroma (postoperative) (traumatic) —see
      Complications, amputation stump,
      neuroma
  stump (surgical)
    abnormal, painful, or with complication
        (late) —see Complications, amputation
        stump
    healed or old NOS Z89.9
  traumatic (complete) (partial)
    arm (upper) (complete) S48.91-●
      at
        elbow S58.01-●
          partial S58.02-●
        shoulder joint (complete) S48.01-●
          partial S48.02-●
      between
        elbow and wrist (complete) S58.11-●
          partial S58.12-●
        shoulder and elbow (complete)
            S48.11-●
          partial S48.12-●
      partial S48.92-●
    breast (complete) S28.21-●
      partial S28.22-●
    clitoris (complete) S38.211
      partial S38.212
    ear (complete) S08.11-●
      partial S08.12-●
    finger (complete) (metacarpophalangeal)
        S68.11-●
      index S68.11-●
      little S68.11-●
      middle S68.11-●
      partial S68.12-●
        index S68.12-●
        little S68.12-●

Amputation (Continued)
  traumatic (Continued)
    finger (Continued)
      partial (Continued)
        middle S68.12-●
        ring S68.12-●
      ring S68.11-●
      thumb —see Amputation, traumatic,
          thumb
      transphalangeal (complete) S68.61-●
        index S68.61-●
        little S68.61-●
        middle S68.61-●
        partial S68.62-●
          index S68.62-●
          little S68.62-●
          middle S68.62-●
          ring S68.62-●
        ring S68.61-●
    foot (complete) S98.91-●
      at ankle level S98.01-●
        partial S98.02-●
      midfoot S98.31-●
        partial S98.32-●
      partial S98.92-●
    forearm (complete) S58.91-●
      at elbow level (complete) S58.01-●
        partial S58.02-●
      between elbow and wrist (complete)
          S58.11-●
        partial S58.12-●
      partial S58.92-●
    genital organ(s) (external)
      female (complete) S38.211
        partial S38.212
      male
        penis (complete) S38.221
          partial S38.222
        scrotum (complete) S38.231
          partial S38.232
        testes (complete) S38.231
          partial S38.232
    hand (complete) (wrist level) S68.41-●
      finger(s) alone —see Amputation,
          traumatic, finger
      partial S68.42-●
      thumb alone —see Amputation,
          traumatic, thumb
    transmetacarpal (complete) S68.71-●
      partial S68.72-●
    head
      ear —see Amputation, traumatic, ear
      nose (partial) S08.812
        complete S08.811
      part S08.89
        scalp S08.0
    hip (and thigh) (complete) S78.91-●
      at hip joint (complete) S78.01-●
        partial S78.02-●
      between hip and knee (complete)
          S78.11-●
        partial S78.12-●
      partial S78.92-●
    labium (majus) (minus) (complete)
        S38.21-●
      partial S38.21-●
    leg (lower) S88.91-●
      at knee level S88.01-●
        partial S88.02-●
      between knee and ankle S88.11-●
        partial S88.12-●
      partial S88.92-●
    nose (partial) S08.812
      complete S08.811
    penis (complete) S38.221
      partial S38.222
    scrotum (complete) S38.231
      partial S38.232
    shoulder —see Amputation, traumatic, arm
      at shoulder joint —see Amputation,
          traumatic, arm, at shoulder joint

Amputation (Continued)
  traumatic (Continued)
    testes (complete) S38.231
      partial S38.232
    thigh —see Amputation, traumatic, hip
    thorax, part of S28.1
      breast —see Amputation, traumatic, breast
    thumb (complete) (metacarpophalangeal)
        S68.01-●
      partial S68.02-●
      transphalangeal (complete) S68.51-●
        partial S68.52-●
    toe (lesser) S98.13-●
      great S98.11-●
        partial S98.12-●
      more than one S98.21-●
        partial S98.22-●
      partial S98.14-●
    vulva (complete) S38.211
      partial S38.212
Amputee (bilateral) (old) Z89.9
Amsterdam dwarfism Q87.19
Amusia R48.8
  developmental F80.89
Amyelencephalus, amyelencephaly Q00.0
Amyelia Q06.0
Amygdalitis —see Tonsillitis
Amygdalolith J35.8
Amyloid heart (disease) E85.4 [I43]
Amyloidosis (generalized) (primary) E85.9
  with lung involvement E85.4 [J99]
  familial E85.2
  genetic E85.2
  heart E85.4 [I43]
  hemodialysis-associated E85.3
  light chain (AL) E85.81
  liver E85.4 [K77]
  localized E85.4
  neuropathic heredofamilial E85.1
  non-neuropathic heredofamilial E85.0
  organ limited E85.4
  Portuguese E85.1
  pulmonary E85.4 [J99]
  secondary systemic E85.3
  senile systemic (SSA) E85.82
  skin (lichen) (macular) E85.4 [L99]
  specified NEC E85.89
  subglottic E85.4 [J99]
  wild-type transthyretin-related (ATTR) E85.82
Amylopectinosis (brancher enzyme deficiency)
    E74.03
Amylophagia —see Pica
Amyoplasia congenita Q79.8
Amyotonia M62.89
  congenita G70.2
Amyotrophia, amyotrophy, amyotrophic G71.8
  congenita Q79.8
  diabetic —see Diabetes, amyotrophy
  lateral sclerosis G12.21
  neuralgic G54.5
  spinal progressive G12.25
Anacidity, gastric K31.83
  psychogenic F45.8
Anaerosis of newborn P28.89
Analbuminemia E88.09
Analgesia —see Anesthesia
Analphalipoproteinemia E78.6
Anaphylactic
  purpura D69.0
  shock or reaction —see Shock, anaphylactic
Anaphylactoid shock or reaction —see Shock,
    anaphylactic
Anaphylactoid syndrome of pregnancy
    O88.01-●
Anaphylaxis —see Shock, anaphylactic
Anaplasia cervix —see also Dysplasia, cervix
    N87.9
Anaplasmosis, human A77.49
Anaplasmosis [A. phagocytophilum]
    (transfusion transmitted) A79.82
  human A77.49

Anarthria R47.1
Anasarca R60.1
  cardiac —*see* Failure, heart, congestive
  lung J18.2
  newborn P83.2
  nutritional E43
  pulmonary J18.2
  renal N04.9
Anastomosis
  aneurysmal —*see* Aneurysm
  arteriovenous ruptured brain I60.8
  intestinal K63.89
    complicated NEC K91.89
      involving urinary tract N99.89
  intracerebral I61.8
  intraparenchymal I61.8
  intraventricular I61.5
  retinal and choroidal vessels (congenital) Q14.8
  subarachnoid I60.8
Anatomical narrow angle H40.03-●
Ancylostoma, ancylostomiasis (braziliense)
    (caninum) (ceylanicum) (duodenale) B76.0
  Necator americanus B76.1
Andersen's disease (glycogen storage) E74.09
Anderson-Fabry disease E75.21
Andes disease T70.29
Andrews' disease (bacterid) L08.89
Androblastoma
  benign
    specified site —*see* Neoplasm, benign, by
      site
    unspecified site
      female D27.9
      male D29.20
  malignant
    specified site —*see* Neoplasm, malignant,
      by site
    unspecified site
      female C56.9
      male C62.90
  specified site —*see* Neoplasm, uncertain
      behavior, by site
  tubular
    with lipid storage
      specified site —*see* Neoplasm, benign,
        by site
      unspecified site
        female D27.9
        male D29.20
    specified site —*see* Neoplasm, benign, by site
    unspecified site
      female D27.9
      male D29.20
  unspecified site
    female D39.10
    male D40.10
Androgen insensitivity syndrome —*see also*
    Syndrome, androgen insensitivity E34.50
Androgen resistance syndrome —*see also*
    Syndrome, androgen insensitivity E34.50
Android pelvis Q74.2
  with disproportion (fetopelvic) O33.3
    causing obstructed labor O65.3
Androphobia F40.290
Anectasis, pulmonary (newborn) —*see* Atelectasis
Anemia (essential) (general) (hemoglobin
    deficiency) (infantile) (primary) (profound)
    D64.9
  with (due to) (in)
    disorder of
      ⇒ anaerobic glycolysis D55.29
      pentose phosphate pathway D55.1
    koilonychia D50.9
  achlorhydric D50.8
  achrestic D53.1
  Addison (-Biermer) (pernicious) D51.0
  agranulocytic —*see* Agranulocytosis
  amino-acid-deficiency D53.0
  aplastic D61.9
    congenital D61.09
    drug-induced D61.1

Anemia *(Continued)*
  aplastic *(Continued)*
    due to
      drugs D61.1
      external agents NEC D61.2
      infection D61.2
      radiation D61.2
    idiopathic D61.3
    red cell (pure) D60.9
      chronic D60.0
      congenital D61.01
      specified type NEC D60.8
      transient D60.1
    specified type NEC D61.89
    toxic D61.2
  aregenerative
    congenital D61.09
  asiderotic D50.9
  atypical (primary) D64.9
  Baghdad spring D55.29
  Balantidium coli A07.0
  Biermer's (pernicious) D51.0
  blood loss (chronic) D50.0
    acute D62
  bothriocephalus B70.0 *[D63.8]*
  brickmaker's B76.9 *[D63.8]*
  cerebral I67.89
  childhood D58.9
  chlorotic D50.8
  chronic
    blood loss D50.0
    hemolytic D58.9
      idiopathic D59.9
    simple D53.9
  chronica congenita aregenerativa D61.09
  combined system disease NEC D51.0 *[G32.0]*
    due to dietary vitamin B12 deficiency
      D51.3 *[G32.0]*
  complicating pregnancy, childbirth
      or puerperium —*see* Pregnancy,
      complicated by (management affected
      by), anemia
  congenital P61.4
    aplastic D61.09
    due to isoimmunization NOS P55.9
    dyserythropoietic, dyshematopoietic D64.4
    following fetal blood loss P61.3
    Heinz body D58.2
    hereditary hemolytic NOS D58.9
    pernicious D51.0
    spherocytic D58.0
  Cooley's (erythroblastic) D56.1
  cytogenic D51.0
  deficiency D53.9
    ⇒ 2, 3 diphosphoglycurate mutase D55.29
    ⇒ 2, 3 PG D55.29
    6 phosphogluconate dehydrogenase D55.1
    6-PGD D55.1
    amino-acid D53.0
    combined B12 and folate D53.1
    enzyme D55.9
      drug-induced (hemolytic) D59.2
      glucose-6-phosphate dehydrogenase
        (G6PD) D55.0
      ⇒ glycolytic D55.29
      nucleotide metabolism D55.3
      related to hexose monophosphate
        (HMP) shunt pathway NEC D55.1
      specified type NEC D55.8
    erythrocytic glutathione D55.1
    folate D52.9
      dietary D52.0
      drug-induced D52.1
    folic acid D52.9
      dietary D52.0
      drug-induced D52.1
    G SH D55.1
    G6PD D55.0
    GGS-R D55.1
    glucose-6-phosphate dehydrogenase D55.0
    glutathione reductase D55.1

Anemia *(Continued)*
  deficiency *(Continued)*
    ⇒ glyceraldehyde phosphate dehydrogenase
        D55.29
    ⇒ hexokinase D55.29
    iron D50.9
      secondary to blood loss (chronic) D50.0
    nutritional D53.9
      with
        poor iron absorption D50.8
        specified deficiency NEC D53.8
    ⇒ phosphofructo-aldolase D55.29
    ⇒ phosphoglycerate kinase D55.29
    ⇒ PK D55.21
    protein D53.0
    ⇒ pyruvate kinase D55.21
    transcobalamin II D55.22
    ⇒ triose-phosphate isomerase D55.29
    vitamin B12 NOS D51.9
      dietary D51.3
      due to
        intrinsic factor deficiency D51.0
        selective vitamin B12 malabsorption
          with proteinuria D51.1
      pernicious D51.0
      specified type NEC D51.8
  Diamond-Blackfan (congenital hypoplastic)
      D61.01
  dibothriocephalus B70.0 *[D63.8]*
  dimorphic D53.1
  diphasic D53.1
  Diphyllobothrium (Dibothriocephalus) B70.0
      [D63.8]
  due to (in) (with)
    antineoplastic chemotherapy D64.81
    blood loss (chronic) D50.0
      acute D62
    chemotherapy, antineoplastic D64.81
    chronic disease classified elsewhere NEC
        D63.8
    chronic kidney disease D63.1
    deficiency
      amino-acid D53.0
      copper D53.8
      folate (folic acid) D52.9
        dietary D52.0
        drug-induced D52.1
      molybdenum D53.8
      protein D53.0
      zinc D53.8
    dietary vitamin B12 deficiency D51.3
    disorder of
      glutathione metabolism D55.1
      nucleotide metabolism D55.3
    drug —*see* Anemia, by type —*see also* Table
        of Drugs and Chemicals
    end stage renal disease D63.1
    enzyme disorder D55.9
    fetal blood loss P61.3
    fish tapeworm (D latum) infestation B70.0
        [D63.8]
    hemorrhage (chronic) D50.0
      acute D62
    impaired absorption D50.9
    loss of blood (chronic) D50.0
      acute D62
    myxedema E03.9 *[D63.8]*
    Necator americanus B76.1 *[D63.8]*
    prematurity P61.2
    selective vitamin B12 malabsorption with
        proteinuria D51.1
    transcobalamin II deficiency D51.2
  Dyke-Young type (secondary) (symptomatic)
      D59.19
  dyserythropoietic (congenital) D64.4
  dyshematopoietic (congenital) D64.4
  Egyptian B76.9 *[D63.8]*
  elliptocytosis —*see* Elliptocytosis
  enzyme-deficiency, drug-induced D59.2
  epidemic —*see also* Ancylostomiasis B76.9
      [D63.8]

Anemia *(Continued)*
erythroblastic
familial D56.1
newborn —*see also* Disease, hemolytic
P55.9
of childhood D56.1
erythrocytic glutathione deficiency D55.1
erythropoietin-resistant anemia (EPO
resistant anemia) D63.1
Faber's (achlorhydric anemia) D50.9
factitious (self-induced blood letting) D50.0
familial erythroblastic D56.1
Fanconi's (congenital pancytopenia) D61.09
favism D55.0
fish tapeworm (D. latum) infestation B70.0
[D63.8]
folate (folic acid) deficiency D52.9
glucose-6-phosphate dehydrogenase (G6PD)
deficiency D55.0
glutathione-reductase deficiency D55.1
goat's milk D52.0
granulocytic —*see* Agranulocytosis
Heinz body, congenital D58.2
hemolytic D58.9
acquired D59.9
with hemoglobinuria NEC D59.6
autoimmune NEC D59.19
infectious D59.4
specified type NEC D59.8
toxic D59.4
acute D59.9
due to enzyme deficiency specified type
NEC D55.8
Lederer's D59.19
autoimmune D59.10
cold D59.12
drug-induced D59.0
mixed D59.13
warm D59.11
chronic D58.9
idiopathic D59.9
cold type (secondary) (symptomatic)
D59.12
congenital (spherocytic) —*see*
Spherocytosis
due to
cardiac conditions D59.4
drugs (nonautoimmune) D59.2
autoimmune D59.0
enzyme disorder D55.9
drug-induced D59.2
presence of shunt or other internal
prosthetic device D59.4
familial D58.9
hereditary D58.9
due to enzyme disorder D55.9
specified type NEC D55.8
specified type NEC D58.8
idiopathic (chronic) D59.9
mechanical D59.4
microangiopathic D59.4
mixed type (primary) (secondary)
(symptomatic) D59.13
nonautoimmune D59.4
drug-induced D59.2
nonspherocytic
congenital or hereditary NEC D55.8
glucose-6-phosphate dehydrogenase
deficiency D55.0
pyruvate kinase deficiency D55.21
type
I D55.1
II D55.29
type
I D55.1
II D55.29
primary
autoimmune
cold type D59.12
mixed type D59.13
warm type D59.11

hemolytic *(Continued)*
secondary D59.4
autoimmune
cold type D59.12
mixed type D59.13
warm type D59.11
specified (hereditary) type NEC D58.8
Stransky-Regala type —*see also*
Hemoglobinopathy D58.8
symptomatic D59.4
autoimmune
cold type D59.12
mixed type D59.13
warm type D59.11
toxic D59.4
warm type (primary) (secondary)
(symptomatic) D59.11
hemorrhagic (chronic) D50.0
acute D62
Herrick's D57.1
hexokinase deficiency D55.29
hookworm B76.9 [D63.8]
hypochromic (idiopathic) (microcytic)
(normoblastic) D50.9
due to blood loss (chronic) D50.0
acute D62
familial sex-linked D64.0
pyridoxine-responsive D64.3
sideroblastic, sex-linked D64.0
hypoplasia, red blood cells D61.9
congenital or familial D61.01
hypoplastic (idiopathic) D61.9
congenital or familial (of childhood)
D61.01
hypoproliferative (refractive) D61.9
idiopathic D64.9
aplastic D61.3
hemolytic, chronic D59.9
in (due to) (with)
chronic kidney disease D63.1
end stage renal disease D63.1
failure, kidney (renal) D63.1
neoplastic disease —*see also* Neoplasm
D63.0
intertropical —*see also* Ancylostomiasis
D63.8
iron deficiency D50.9
secondary to blood loss (chronic) D50.0
acute D62
specified type NEC D50.8
Joseph-Diamond-Blackfan (congenital
hypoplastic) D61.01
Lederer's (hemolytic) D59.19
leukoerythroblastic D61.82
macrocytic D53.9
nutritional D52.0
tropical D52.8
malarial (*see also* Malaria) B54 [D63.8]
malignant (progressive) D51.0
malnutrition D53.9
marsh (*see also* Malaria) B54 [D63.8]
Mediterranean (with other
hemoglobinopathy) D56.9
megaloblastic D53.9
combined B12 and folate deficiency
D53.1
hereditary D51.1
nutritional D52.0
orotic aciduria D53.0
refractory D53.1
specified type NEC D53.1
megalocytic D53.1
microcytic (hypochromic) D50.9
due to blood loss (chronic) D50.0
acute D62
familial D56.8
microdrepanocytosis D57.40
microelliptopoikilocytic (Rietti-Greppi-
Micheli) D56.9
miner's B76.9 [D63.8]

myelodysplastic D46.9
myelofibrosis D75.81
myelogenous D64.89
myelopathic D64.89
myelophthisic D61.82
myeloproliferative D47.Z9
newborn P61.4
due to
ABO (antibodies, isoimmunization,
maternal/fetal incompatibility)
P55.1
Rh (antibodies, isoimmunization,
maternal/fetal incompatibility)
P55.0
following fetal blood loss P61.3
posthemorrhagic (fetal) P61.3
nonspherocytic hemolytic —*see* Anemia,
hemolytic, nonspherocytic
normocytic (infectional) D64.9
due to blood loss (chronic) D50.0
acute D62
myelophthisic D61.82
nutritional (deficiency) D53.9
with
poor iron absorption D50.8
specified deficiency NEC D53.8
megaloblastic D52.0
of prematurity P61.2
orotaciduric (congenital) (hereditary)
D53.0
osteosclerotic D64.89
ovalocytosis (hereditary) —*see* Elliptocytosis
paludal —*see also* Malaria B54 [D63.8]
pernicious (congenital) (malignant)
(progressive) D51.0
pleochromic D64.89
of sprue D52.8
posthemorrhagic (chronic) D50.0
acute D62
newborn P61.3
postoperative (postprocedural)
due to (acute) blood loss D62
chronic blood loss D50.0
specified NEC D64.89
postpartum O90.81
pressure D64.89
progressive D64.9
malignant D51.0
pernicious D51.0
protein-deficiency D53.0
pseudoleukemica infantum D64.89
pure red cell D60.9
congenital D61.01
pyridoxine-responsive D64.3
pyruvate kinase deficiency D55.21
refractory D46.4
with
excess of blasts D46.20
1 (RAEB 1) D46.21
2 (RAEB 2) D46.22
in transformation (RAEB T) —*see*
Leukemia, acute myeloblastic
hemochromatosis D46.1
sideroblasts (ring) (RARS) D46.1
without ring sideroblasts, so stated
D46.0
without sideroblasts without excess of
blasts D46.0
megaloblastic D53.1
sideroblastic D46.1
sideropenic D50.9
Rietti-Greppi-Micheli D56.9
scorbutic D53.2
secondary to
blood loss (chronic) D50.0
acute D62
hemorrhage (chronic) D50.0
acute D62
semiplastic D61.89
sickle-cell —*see* Disease, sickle-cell

Anemia *(Continued)*
   sideroblastic D64.3
      hereditary D64.0
      hypochromic, sex-linked D64.0
      pyridoxine-responsive NEC D64.3
      refractory D46.1
      secondary (due to)
         disease D64.1
         drugs and toxins D64.2
      specified type NEC D64.3
   sideropenic (refractory) D50.9
      due to blood loss (chronic) D50.0
         acute D62
   simple chronic D53.9
   specified type NEC D64.89
   spherocytic (hereditary) —*see* Spherocytosis
   splenic D64.89
   splenomegalic D64.89
   stomatocytosis D58.8
   syphilitic (acquired) (late) A52.79 *[D63.8]*
   target cell D64.89
   thalassemia D56.9
   thrombocytopenic —*see* Thrombocytopenia
   toxic D61.2
   tropical B76.9 *[D63.8]*
      macrocytic D52.8
   tuberculous A18.89 *[D63.8]*
   vegan D51.3
   vitamin
      B6-responsive D64.3
      B12 deficiency (dietary) pernicious
         D51.0
   von Jaksch's D64.89
   Witts' (achlorhydric anemia) D50.8
Anemophobia F40.228
Anencephalus, anencephaly Q00.0
Anergasia —*see* Psychosis, organic
Anesthesia, anesthetic R20.0
   complication or reaction NEC —*see also*
      Complications, anesthesia T88.59
      due to
         correct substance properly
            administered —*see* Table of Drugs
            and Chemicals, by drug, adverse
            effect
         overdose or wrong substance given —*see*
            Table of Drugs and Chemicals, by
            drug, poisoning
         unintended awareness under general
            anesthesia during procedure
            T88.53
            personal history of Z92.84
   cornea H18.81-●
   dissociative F44.6
   functional (hysterical) F44.6
   hyperesthetic, thalamic G89.0
   hysterical F44.6
   local skin lesion R20.0
   sexual (psychogenic) F52.1
   shock (due to) T88.2
   skin R20.0
   testicular N50.9
Anetoderma (maculosum) (of) L90.8
   Jadassohn-Pellizzari L90.2
   Schweniger-Buzzi L90.1
Aneurin deficiency E51.9
Aneurysm (anastomotic) (artery) (cirsoid)
      (diffuse) (false) (fusiform) (multiple)
      (saccular) I72.9
   abdominal (aorta) I71.4
      ruptured I71.3
      syphilitic A52.01
   aorta, aortic (nonsyphilitic) I71.9
      abdominal I71.4
         ruptured I71.3
      arch I71.2
         ruptured I71.1
      arteriosclerotic I71.9
         ruptured I71.8
      ascending I71.2
         ruptured I71.1

Aneurysm *(Continued)*
   aorta, aortic (nonsyphilitic) *(Continued)*
      congenital Q25.43
      descending I71.9
         abdominal I71.4
            ruptured I71.3
         ruptured I71.8
         thoracic I71.2
            ruptured I71.1
      root Q25.43
      ruptured I71.8
      sinus, congenital Q25.43
      syphilitic A52.01
      thoracic I71.2
         ruptured I71.1
      thoracoabdominal I71.6
         ruptured I71.5
      thorax, thoracic (arch) I71.2
         ruptured I71.1
      transverse I71.2
         ruptured I71.1
      valve (heart) —*see also* Endocarditis, aortic
         I35.8
   arteriosclerotic I72.9
      cerebral I67.1
         ruptured —*see* Hemorrhage, intracranial,
            subarachnoid
   arteriovenous (congenital) —*see also*
      Malformation, arteriovenous
      acquired I77.0
         brain I67.1
            ruptured —*see* Aneurysm,
               arteriovenous, brain, ruptured
         coronary I25.41
         pulmonary I28.0
      brain Q28.2
         ruptured I60.8
            intracerebral I61.8
            intraparenchymal I61.8
            intraventricular I61.5
            subarachnoid I60.8
      peripheral —*see* Malformation,
         arteriovenous, peripheral
      precerebral vessels Q28.0
      specified site NEC —*see also* Malformation,
         arteriovenous
         acquired I77.0
   basal —*see* Aneurysm, brain
   basilar (trunk) I72.5
   berry (congenital) (nonruptured) I67.1
      ruptured I60.7
   brain I67.1
      arteriosclerotic I67.1
         ruptured —*see* Hemorrhage, intracranial,
            subarachnoid
      arteriovenous (congenital) (nonruptured)
         Q28.2
         acquired I67.1
            ruptured —*see* Aneurysm,
               arteriorvenous, brain, ruptured
               I60.8-
         ruptured —*see* Aneurysm,
            arteriorvenous, brain, ruptured
            I60.8-
      berry (congenital) (nonruptured) I67.1
         ruptured —*see also* Hemorrhage,
            intracranial, subarachnoid I60.7
      congenital Q28.3
         aorta (root) (sinus) Q25.43
         ruptured I60.7
      meninges I67.1
         ruptured I60.8
      miliary (congenital) (nonruptured) I67.1
         ruptured —*see also* Hemorrhage,
            intracranial, subarachnoid I60.7
      mycotic I33.0
      ruptured —*see* Hemorrhage, intracranial,
         subarachnoid
      syphilitic (hemorrhage) A52.05
   cardiac (false) —*see also* Aneurysm, heart
      I25.3

Aneurysm *(Continued)*
   carotid artery (common) (external) I72.0
      internal (intracranial) I67.1
         extracranial portion I72.0
      ruptured into brain I60.0-●
      syphilitic A52.09
         intracranial A52.05
   cavernous sinus I67.1
      arteriovenous (congenital) (nonruptured)
         Q28.3
         ruptured I60.8
   celiac I72.8
   central nervous system, syphilitic A52.05
   cerebral —*see* Aneurysm, brain
   chest —*see* Aneurysm, thorax
   circle of Willis I67.1
      congenital Q28.3
         ruptured I60.6
      ruptured I60.6
   common iliac artery I72.3
   congenital (peripheral) Q27.8
      aorta (root) (sinus) Q25.43
      brain Q28.3
         ruptured I60.7
      coronary Q24.5
      digestive system Q27.8
      lower limb Q27.8
      pulmonary Q25.79
      retina Q14.1
      specified site NEC Q27.8
      upper limb Q27.8
   conjunctiva —*see* Abnormality, conjunctiva,
      vascular
   conus arteriosus —*see* Aneurysm, heart
   coronary (arteriosclerotic) (artery) I25.41
      arteriovenous, congenital Q24.5
      congenital Q24.5
      ruptured —*see* Infarct, myocardium
      syphilitic A52.06
      vein I25.89
   cylindroid (aorta) I71.9
      ruptured I71.8
      syphilitic A52.01
   ductus arteriosus Q25.0
   endocardial, infective (any valve) I33.0
   femoral (artery) (ruptured) I72.4
   gastroduodenal I72.8
   gastroepiploic I72.8
   heart (wall) (chronic or with a stated duration
      of over 4 weeks) I25.3
      valve —*see* Endocarditis
   hepatic I72.8
   iliac (common) (artery) (ruptured) I72.3
   infective I72.9
      endocardial (any valve) I33.0
   innominate (nonsyphilitic) I72.8
      syphilitic A52.09
   interauricular septum —*see* Aneurysm,
      heart
   interventricular septum —*see* Aneurysm,
      heart
   intrathoracic (nonsyphilitic) I71.2
      ruptured I71.1
      syphilitic A52.01
   lower limb I72.4
   lung (pulmonary artery) I28.1
   mediastinal (nonsyphilitic) I72.8
      syphilitic A52.09
   miliary (congenital) I67.1
      ruptured —*see* Hemorrhage, intracerebral,
         subarachnoid, intracranial
   mitral (heart) (valve) I34.8
   mural —*see* Aneurysm, heart
   mycotic I72.9
      endocardial (any valve) I33.0
      ruptured, brain —*see* Hemorrhage,
         intracerebral, subarachnoid
   myocardium —*see* Aneurysm, heart
   neck I72.0
   pancreaticoduodenal I72.8
   patent ductus arteriosus Q25.0

▶ New   ⇒ Revised   ~~deleted~~ Deleted   ● Use Additional Character(s)

Aneurysm *(Continued)*
  peripheral NEC I72.8
    congenital Q27.8
      digestive system Q27.8
      lower limb Q27.8
      specified site NEC Q27.8
      upper limb Q27.8
  popliteal (artery) (ruptured) I72.4
  precerebral
    congrenital (nonruptured) Q28.1
    specified site, NEC I72.5
  pulmonary I28.1
    arteriovenous Q25.72
      acquired I28.0
    syphilitic A52.09
    valve (heart) —*see* Endocarditis, pulmonary
  racemose (peripheral) I72.9
    congenital —*see* Aneurysm, congenital
  radial I72.1
  Rasmussen NEC A15.0
  renal (artery) I72.2
  retina —*see also* Disorder, retina,
      microaneurysms
    congenital Q14.1
    diabetic —*see* E08-E13 with .3-•
  sinus of Valsalva Q25.49
  specified NEC I72.8
  spinal (cord) I72.8
    syphilitic (hemorrhage) A52.09
  splenic I72.8
  subclavian (artery) (ruptured) I72.8
    syphilitic A52.09
  superior mesenteric I72.8
  syphilitic (aorta) A52.01
    central nervous system A52.05
    congenital (late) A50.54 [I79.0]
    spine, spinal A52.09
  thoracoabdominal (aorta) I71.6
    ruptured I71.5
    syphilitic A52.01
  thorax, thoracic (aorta) (arch) (nonsyphilitic)
      I71.2
    ruptured I71.1
    syphilitic A52.01
  traumatic (complication) (early), specified
      site —*see* Injury, blood vessel
  tricuspid (heart) (valve) I07.8
  ulnar I72.1
  upper limb (ruptured) I72.1
  valve, valvular —*see* Endocarditis
  visceral NEC I72.8
  venous —*see also* Varix I86.8
    congenital Q27.8
      digestive system Q27.8
      lower limb Q27.8
      specified site NEC Q27.8
      upper limb Q27.8
  ventricle —*see* Aneurysm, heart
  vertebral artery I72.6
  visceral NEC I72.8
Angelman syndrome Q93.51
Anger R45.4
Angiectasis, angiectopia I99.8
Angiitis I77.6
  allergic granulomatous M30.1
  hypersensitivity M31.0
  necrotizing M31.9
    specified NEC M31.8
  nervous system, granulomatous I67.7
Angina (attack) (cardiac) (chest) (heart)
    (pectoris) (syndrome) (vasomotor) I20.9
  with
    atherosclerotic heart disease —*see*
      Arteriosclerosis, coronary (artery)
    documented spasm I20.1
  abdominal K55.1
  accelerated —*see* Angina, unstable
  agranulocytic —*see* Agranulocytosis
  angiospastic —*see* Angina, with documented
      spasm
  aphthous B08.5

Angina *(Continued)*
  crescendo —*see* Angina, unstable
  croupous J05.0
  cruris I73.9
  de novo effort —*see* Angina, unstable
  diphtheritic, membranous A36.0
  equivalent I20.8
  exudative, chronic J37.0
  following acute myocardial infarction I23.7
  gangrenous diphtheritic A36.0
  intestinal K55.1
  Ludovici K12.2
  Ludwig's K12.2
  malignant diphtheritic A36.0
  membranous J05.0
    diphtheritic A36.0
    Vincent's A69.1
  mesenteric K55.1
  monocytic —*see* Mononucleosis, infectious
  of effort —*see* Angina, specified NEC
  phlegmonous J36
    diphtheritic A36.0
  post-infarctional I23.7
  pre-infarctional —*see* Angina, unstable
  Prinzmetal —*see* Angina, with documented
      spasm
  progressive —*see* Angina, unstable
  pseudomembranous A69.1
  pultaceous, diphtheritic A36.0
  spasm-induced —*see* Angina, with
      documented spasm
  specified NEC I20.8
  stable I20.8
  stenocardia —*see* Angina, specified NEC
  stridulous, diphtheritic A36.2
  tonsil J36
  trachealis J05.0
  unstable I20.0
  variant —*see* Angina, with documented spasm
  Vincent's A69.1
  worsening effort —*see* Angina, unstable
Angioblastoma —*see* Neoplasm, connective
    tissue, uncertain behavior
Angiocholecystitis —*see* Cholecystitis, acute
Angiocholitis —*see also* Cholecystitis, acute
    K83.09
Angiodysgenesis spinalis G95.19
Angiodysplasia (cecum) (colon) K55.20
  with bleeding K55.21
  duodenum (and stomach) K31.819
    with bleeding K31.811
  stomach (and duodenum) K31.819
    with bleeding K31.811
Angioedema (allergic) (any site) (with urticaria)
    T78.3
  episodic, with eosinophilia D72.118
  hereditary D84.1
Angioendothelioma —*see* Neoplasm, uncertain
    behavior, by site
  benign D18.00
    intra-abdominal D18.03
    intracranial D18.02
    skin D18.01
    specified site NEC D18.09
  bone —*see* Neoplasm, bone, malignant
  Ewing's —*see* Neoplasm, bone, malignant
Angioendotheliomatosis C85.8-•
Angiofibroma —*see also* Neoplasm, benign, by
    site
  juvenile
    specified site —*see* Neoplasm, benign, by
      site
    unspecified site D10.6
Angiohemophilia (A) (B) D68.0
Angioid streaks (choroid) (macula) (retina)
    H35.33
Angiokeratoma —*see* Neoplasm, skin, benign
  corporis diffusum E75.21
Angioleiomyoma —*see* Neoplasm, connective
    tissue, benign
Angiolipoma —*see also* Lipoma
  infiltrating —*see* Lipoma

Angioma —*see also* Hemangioma, by site
  capillary I78.1
  hcmorrhagicum hereditaria I78.0
  intra-abdominal D18.03
  intracranial D18.02
  malignant —*see* Neoplasm, connective tissue,
      malignant
  plexiform D18.00
    intra-abdominal D18.03
    intracranial D18.02
    skin D18.01
    specified site NEC D18.09
  senile I78.1
  serpiginosum L81.7
  skin D18.01
  specified site NEC D18.09
  spider I78.1
  stellate I78.1
  venous Q28.3
Angiomatosis Q82.8
  bacillary A79.89
  encephalotrigeminal Q85.8
  hemorrhagic familial I78.0
  hereditary familial I78.0
  liver K76.4
Angiomyolipoma —*see* Lipoma
Angiomyoliposarcoma —*see* Neoplasm,
    connective tissue, malignant
Angiomyoma —*see* Neoplasm, connective
    tissue, benign
Angiomyosarcoma —*see* Neoplasm, connective
    tissue, malignant
Angiomyxoma —*see* Neoplasm, connective
    tissue, uncertain behavior
Angioneurosis F45.8
Angioneurotic edema (allergic) (any site) (with
    urticaria) T78.3
  hereditary D84.1
Angiopathia, angiopathy I99.9
  cerebral I67.9
    amyloid E85.4 [I68.0]
  diabetic (peripheral) —*see* Diabetes,
      angiopathy
  peripheral I73.9
    diabetic —*see* Diabetes, angiopathy
    specified type NEC I73.89
  retinae syphilitica A52.05
  retinalis (juvenilis)
    diabetic —*see* Diabetes, retinopathy
    proliferative —*see* Retinopathy, proliferative
Angiosarcoma —*see also* Neoplasm, connective
    tissue, malignant
  liver C22.3
Angiosclerosis —*see* Arteriosclerosis
Angiospasm (peripheral) (traumatic) (vessel)
    I73.9
  brachial plexus G54.0
  cerebral G45.9
  cervical plexus G54.2
  nerve
    arm —*see* Mononeuropathy, upper limb
      axillary G54.0
      median —*see* Lesion, nerve, median
      ulnar —*see* Lesion, nerve, ulnar
    axillary G54.0
    leg —*see* Mononeuropathy, lower limb
    median —*see* Lesion, nerve, median
    plantar —*see* Lesion, nerve, plantar
    ulnar —*see* Lesion, nerve, ulnar
Angiospastic disease or edema I73.9
Angiostrongyliasis
  due to
    Parastrongylus
      cantonensis B83.2
      costaricensis B81.3
  intestinal B81.3
Anguillulosis —*see* Strongyloidiasis
Angulation
  cecum —*see* Obstruction, intestine
  coccyx (acquired) —*see also* subcategory M43.8
    congenital NEC Q76.49

Angulation (*Continued*)
  femur (acquired) —*see also* Deformity, limb, specified type NEC, thigh
    congenital Q74.2
  intestine (large) (small) —*see* Obstruction, intestine
  sacrum (acquired) —*see also* subcategory M43.8
    congenital NEC Q76.49
  sigmoid (flexure) —*see* Obstruction, intestine
  spine —*see* Dorsopathy, deforming, specified NEC
  tibia (acquired) —*see also* Deformity, limb, specified type NEC, lower leg
    congenital Q74.2
  ureter N13.5
    with infection N13.6
  wrist (acquired) —*see also* Deformity, limb, specified type NEC, forearm
    congenital Q74.0
Angulus infectiosus (lips) K13.0
Anhedonia R45.84
  sexual F52.0
Anhidrosis L74.4
Anhydration E86.0
Anhydremia E86.0
Anidrosis L74.4
Aniridia (congenital) Q13.1
Anisakiasis (infection) (infestation) B81.0
Anisakis larvae infestation B81.0
Aniseikonia H52.32
Anisocoria (pupil) H57.02
  congenital Q13.2
Anisocytosis R71.8
Anisometropia (congenital) H52.31
Ankle —*see* condition
Ankyloblepharon (eyelid) (acquired) —*see also* Blepharophimosis
  filiforme (adnatum) (congenital) Q10.3
  total Q10.3
Ankyloglossia Q38.1
Ankylosis (fibrous) (osseous) (joint) M24.60
  ankle M24.67-●
  arthrodesis status Z98.1
  cricoarytenoid (cartilage) (joint) (larynx) J38.7
  dental K03.5
  ear ossicles H74.31-●
  elbow M24.62-●
  foot M24.67-●
  hand M24.64-●
  hip M24.65-●
  incostapedial joint (infectional) —*see* Ankylosis, ear ossicles
  jaw (temporomandibular) M26.61-●
  knee M24.66-●
  lumbosacral (joint) M43.27
  postoperative (status) Z98.1
  produced by surgical fusion, status Z98.1
  sacro-iliac (joint) M43.28
  shoulder M24.61-●
  specified site NEC M24.69
  spine (joint) —*see also* Fusion, spine
    spondylitic —*see* Spondylitis, ankylosing
  surgical Z98.1
  temporomandibular M26.61-●
  tooth, teeth (hard tissues) K03.5
  wrist M24.63-●
Ankylostoma —*see* Ancylostoma
Ankylostomiasis —*see* Ancylostomiasis
Ankylurethria —*see* Stricture, urethra
Annular —*see also* condition
  detachment, cervix N88.8
  organ or site, congenital NEC —*see* Distortion
  pancreas (congenital) Q45.1
Anodontia (complete) (partial) (vera) K00.0
  acquired K08.10
Anomaly, anomalous (congenital) (unspecified type) Q89.9
  abdominal wall NEC Q79.59
  acoustic nerve Q07.8
  adrenal (gland) Q89.1
  Alder (-Reilly) (leukocyte granulation) D72.0

Anomaly, anomalous (*Continued*)
  alimentary tract Q45.9
    upper Q40.9
  alveolar M26.70
    hyperplasia M26.79
      mandibular M26.72
      maxillary M26.71
    hypoplasia M26.79
      mandibular M26.74
      maxillary M26.73
    ridge (process) M26.79
    specified NEC M26.79
  ankle (joint) Q74.2
  anus Q43.9
  aorta (arch) NEC Q25.40
    coarctation (preductal) (postductal) Q25.1
  aortic cusp or valve Q23.9
  appendix Q43.8
  apple peel syndrome Q41.1
  aqueduct of Sylvius Q03.0
    with spina bifida —*see* Spina bifida, with hydrocephalus
  arm Q74.0
  arteriovenous NEC
    coronary Q24.5
    gastrointestinal Q27.33
      acquired —*see* Angiodysplasia
  artery (peripheral) Q27.9
    basilar NEC Q28.1
    cerebral Q28.3
    coronary Q24.5
    digestive system Q27.8
    eye Q15.8
    great Q25.9
      specified NEC Q25.8
    lower limb Q27.8
    peripheral Q27.9
      specified NEC Q27.8
    pulmonary NEC Q25.79
    renal Q27.2
    retina Q14.1
    specified site NEC Q27.8
    subclavian Q27.8
      origin Q25.48
    umbilical Q27.0
    upper limb Q27.8
    vertebral NEC Q28.1
  aryteno-epiglottic folds Q31.8
  atrial
    bands or folds Q20.8
    septa Q21.1
  atrioventricular
    excitation I45.6
    septum Q21.0
  auditory canal Q17.8
  auricle
    ear Q17.8
      causing impairment of hearing Q16.9
    heart Q20.8
  Axenfeld's Q15.0
  back Q89.9
  band
    atrial Q20.8
    heart Q24.8
    ventricular Q24.8
  Bartholin's duct Q38.4
  biliary duct or passage Q44.5
  bladder Q64.70
    absence Q64.5
    diverticulum Q64.6
    exstrophy Q64.10
      cloacal Q64.12
      extroversion Q64.19
      specified type NEC Q64.19
      supravesical fissure Q64.11
    neck obstruction Q64.31
    specified type NEC Q64.79
  bone Q79.9
    arm Q74.0
    face Q75.9
    leg Q74.2

Anomaly, anomalous (*Continued*)
  bone (*Continued*)
    pelvic girdle Q74.2
    shoulder girdle Q74.0
    skull Q75.9
      with
        anencephaly Q00.0
        encephalocele —*see* Encephalocele
        hydrocephalus Q03.9
          with spina bifida —*see* Spina bifida, by site, with hydrocephalus
        microcephaly Q02
  brain (multiple) Q04.9
    vessel Q28.3
  breast Q83.9
  broad ligament Q50.6
  bronchus Q32.4
  bulbus cordis Q21.9
  bursa Q79.9
  canal of Nuck Q52.4
  canthus Q10.3
  capillary Q27.9
  cardiac Q24.9
    chambers Q20.9
      specified NEC Q20.8
    septal closure Q21.9
      specified NEC Q21.8
    valve NEC Q24.8
      pulmonary Q22.3
  cardiovascular system Q28.8
  carpus Q74.0
  caruncle, lacrimal Q10.6
  cascade stomach Q40.2
  cauda equina Q06.3
  cecum Q43.9
  cerebral Q04.9
    vessels Q28.3
  cervix Q51.9
  Chédiak-Higashi(-Steinbrinck) (congenital gigantism of peroxidase granules) E70.330
  cheek Q18.9
  chest wall Q67.8
    bones Q76.9
  chin Q18.9
  chordae tendineae Q24.8
  choroid Q14.3
    plexus Q07.8
  chromosomes, chromosomal Q99.9
    D (1) —*see* condition, chromosome 13
    E (3) —*see* condition, chromosome 18
    G —*see* condition, chromosome 21
    sex
      female phenotype Q97.8
      gonadal dysgenesis (pure) Q99.1
      Klinefelter's Q98.4
      male phenotype Q98.9
      Turner's Q96.9
    specified NEC Q99.8
  cilia Q10.3
  circulatory system Q28.9
  clavicle Q74.0
  clitoris Q52.6
  coccyx Q76.49
  colon Q43.9
  common duct Q44.5
  communication
    coronary artery Q24.5
    left ventricle with right atrium Q21.0
  concha (ear) Q17.3
  connection
    portal vein Q26.5
    pulmonary venous Q26.4
      partial Q26.3
      total Q26.2
    renal artery with kidney Q27.2
  cornea (shape) Q13.4
  coronary artery or vein Q24.5
  cranium —*see* Anomaly, skull
  cricoid cartilage Q31.8
  cystic duct Q44.5

▶ New   ➡ Revised   ~~deleted~~ Deleted   ● Use Additional Character(s)

Anomaly, anomalous (Continued)
  dental
    alveolar —see Anomaly, alveolar
    arch relationship M26.20
      specified NEC M26.29
  dentofacial M26.9
    alveolar —see Anomaly, alveolar
    dental arch relationship M26.20
      specified NEC M26.29
    functional M26.50
      specified NEC M26.59
    jaw-cranial base relationship M26.10
      asymmetry M26.12
        maxillary M26.11
      specified type NEC M26.19
    jaw size M26.00
      macrogenia M26.05
      mandibular
        hyperplasia M26.03
        hypoplasia M26.04
      maxillary
        hyperplasia M26.01
        hypoplasia M26.02
      microgenia M26.06
      specified type NEC M26.09
    malocclusion M26.4
      dental arch relationship NEC M26.29
      jaw-cranial base relationship —see
          Anomaly, dentofacial, jaw-cranial
          base relationship
      jaw size —see Anomaly, dentofacial, jaw
          size
    specified type NEC M26.89
    temporomandibular joint M26.60-●
      adhesions M26.61-●
      ankylosis M26.61-●
      arthralgia M26.62-●
      articular disc M26.63-●
      specified type NEC M26.69
    tooth position, fully erupted M26.30
      specified NEC M26.39
  dermatoglyphic Q82.8
  diaphragm (apertures) NEC Q79.1
  digestive organ(s) or tract Q45.9
    lower Q43.9
    upper Q40.9
  distance, interarch (excessive) (inadequate)
      M26.25
  distribution, coronary artery Q24.5
  ductus
    arteriosus Q25.0
    botalli Q25.0
  duodenum Q43.9
  dura (brain) Q04.9
    spinal cord Q06.9
  ear (external) Q17.9
    causing impairment of hearing Q16.9
    inner Q16.5
    middle (causing impairment of hearing)
        Q16.4
      ossicles Q16.3
  Ebstein's (heart) (tricuspid valve) Q22.5
  ectodermal Q82.9
  Eisenmenger's (ventricular septal defect)
      Q21.8
  ejaculatory duct Q55.4
  elbow Q74.0
  endocrine gland NEC Q89.2
  epididymis Q55.4
  epiglottis Q31.8
  esophagus Q39.9
  eustachian tube Q17.8
  eye Q15.9
    anterior segment Q13.9
      specified NEC Q13.89
    posterior segment Q14.9
      specified NEC Q14.8
    ptosis (eyelid) Q10.0
    specified NEC Q15.8
  eyebrow Q18.8
  eyelid Q10.3
    ptosis Q10.0

Anomaly, anomalous (Continued)
  face Q18.9
    bone(s) Q75.9
  fallopian tube Q50.6
  fascia Q79.9
  femur NEC Q74.2
  fibula NEC Q74.2
  finger Q74.0
  fixation, intestine Q43.3
  flexion (joint) NOS Q74.9
    hip or thigh Q65.89
  foot NEC Q74.2
    varus (congenital) Q66.3-●
  foramen
    Botalli Q21.1
    ovale Q21.1
  forearm Q74.0
  forehead Q75.8
  form, teeth K00.2
  fovea centralis Q14.1
  frontal bone —see Anomaly, skull
  gallbladder (position) (shape) (size)
      Q44.1
  Gartner's duct Q52.4
  gastrointestinal tract Q45.9
  genitalia, genital organ(s) or system
    female Q52.9
      external Q52.70
      internal NOS Q52.9
    male Q55.9
      hydrocele P83.5
      specified NEC Q55.8
  genitourinary NEC
    female Q52.9
    male Q55.9
  Gerbode Q21.0
  glottis Q31.8
  granulation or granulocyte, genetic
      (constitutional) (leukocyte) D72.0
  gum Q38.6
  gyri Q07.9
  hair Q84.2
  hand Q74.0
  hard tissue formation in pulp K04.3
  head —see Anomaly, skull
  heart Q24.9
    auricle Q20.8
    bands or folds Q24.8
    fibroelastosis cordis I42.4
    obstructive NEC Q22.6
    patent ductus arteriosus (Botalli) Q25.0
    septum Q21.9
      auricular Q21.1
      interatrial Q21.1
      interventricular Q21.0
        with pulmonary stenosis or atresia,
            dextraposition of aorta and
            hypertrophy of right ventricle
            Q21.3
      specified NEC Q21.8
      ventricular Q21.0
        with pulmonary stenosis or atresia,
            dextraposition of aorta and
            hypertrophy of right ventricle
            Q21.3
    tetralogy of Fallot Q21.3
    valve NEC Q24.8
      aortic
        bicuspid valve Q23.1
        insufficiency Q23.1
        stenosis Q23.0
          subaortic Q24.4
      mitral
        insufficiency Q23.3
        stenosis Q23.2
      pulmonary Q22.3
        atresia Q22.0
        insufficiency Q22.2
        stenosis Q22.1
          infundibular Q24.3
          subvalvular Q24.3

Anomaly, anomalous (Continued)
  heart (Continued)
    valve NEC (Continued)
      tricuspid
        atresia Q22.4
        stenosis Q22.4
      ventricle Q20.8
  heel NEC Q74.2
  Hegglin's D72.0
  hemianencephaly Q00.0
  hemicephaly Q00.0
  hemicrania Q00.0
  hepatic duct Q44.5
  hip NEC Q74.2
  hourglass stomach Q40.2
  humerus Q74.0
  hydatid of Morgagni
    female Q50.5
    male (epididymal) Q55.4
      testicular Q55.29
  hymen Q52.4
  hypersegmentation of neutrophils, hereditary
      D72.0
  hypophyseal Q89.2
  ileocecal (coil) (valve) Q43.9
  ileum Q43.9
  ilium NEC Q74.2
  integument Q84.9
    specified NEC Q84.8
  interarch distance (excessive) (inadequate)
      M26.25
  intervertebral cartilage or disc Q76.49
  intestine (large) (small) Q43.9
    with anomalous adhesions, fixation or
        malrotation Q43.3
  iris Q13.2
  ischium NEC Q74.2
  jaw —see Anomaly, dentofacial
    alveolar —see Anomaly, alveolar
    jaw-cranial base relationship —see Anomaly,
        dentofacial, jaw-cranial base relationship
  jejunum Q43.8
  joint Q74.9
    specified NEC Q74.8
  Jordan's D72.0
  kidney(s) (calyx) (pelvis) Q63.9
    artery Q27.2
    specified NEC Q63.8
  Klippel-Feil (brevicollis) Q76.1
  knee Q74.1
  labium (majus) (minus) Q52.70
  labyrinth, membranous Q16.5
  lacrimal apparatus or duct Q10.6
  larynx, laryngeal (muscle) Q31.9
    web (bed) Q31.0
  lens Q12.9
  leukocytes, genetic D72.0
    granulation (constitutional) D72.0
  lid (fold) Q10.3
  ligament Q79.9
    broad Q50.6
    round Q52.8
  limb Q74.9
    lower NEC Q74.2
      reduction deformity —see Defect,
          reduction, lower limb
    upper Q74.0
  lip Q38.0
  liver Q44.7
    duct Q44.5
  lower limb NEC Q74.2
  lumbosacral (joint) (region) Q76.49
    kyphosis —see Kyphosis, congenital
    lordosis —see Lordosis, congenital
  lung (fissure) (lobe) Q33.9
  mandible —see Anomaly, dentofacial
  maxilla —see Anomaly, dentofacial
  May (-Hegglin) D72.0
  meatus urinarius NEC Q64.79
  meningeal bands or folds Q07.9
    constriction of Q07.8
    spinal Q06.9

Anomaly, anomalous (Continued)
  meninges Q07.9
    cerebral Q04.8
    spinal Q06.9
  meningocele Q05.9
  mesentery Q45.9
  metacarpus Q74.0
  metatarsus NEC Q74.2
  middle ear Q16.4
    ossicles Q16.3
  mitral (leaflets) (valve) Q23.9
    insufficiency Q23.3
    specified NEC Q23.8
    stenosis Q23.2
  mouth Q38.6
  Müllerian —see also Anomaly, by site
    uterus NEC Q51.818
  multiple NEC Q89.7
  muscle Q79.9
    eyelid Q10.3
  musculoskeletal system, except limbs Q79.9
  myocardium Q24.8
  nail Q84.6
  narrowness, eyelid Q10.3
  nasal sinus (wall) Q30.8
  neck (any part) Q18.9
  nerve Q07.9
    acoustic Q07.8
    optic Q07.8
  nervous system (central) Q07.9
  nipple Q83.9
  nose, nasal (bones) (cartilage) (septum)
      (sinus) Q30.9
    specified NEC Q30.8
  ocular muscle Q15.8
  omphalomesenteric duct Q43.0
  opening, pulmonary veins Q26.4
  optic
    disc Q14.2
    nerve Q07.8
  opticociliary vessels Q13.2
  orbit (eye) Q10.7
  organ Q89.9
    of Corti Q16.5
  origin
    artery
      innominate Q25.8
      pulmonary Q25.79
      renal Q27.2
      subclavian Q25.48
  osseous meatus (ear) Q16.1
  ovary Q50.39
  oviduct Q50.6
  palate (hard) (soft) NEC Q38.5
  pancreas or pancreatic duct Q45.3
  papillary muscles Q24.8
  parathyroid gland Q89.2
  paraurethral ducts Q64.79
  parotid (gland) Q38.4
  patella Q74.1
  Pelger-Huët (hereditary hyposegmentation)
      D72.0
  pelvic girdle NEC Q74.2
  pelvis (bony) NEC Q74.2
    rachitic E64.3
  penis (glans) Q55.69
  pericardium Q24.8
  peripheral vascular system Q27.9
  Peter's Q13.4
  pharynx Q38.8
  pigmentation L81.9
    congenital Q82.8
  pituitary (gland) Q89.2
  pleural (folds) Q34.0
  portal vein Q26.5
    connection Q26.5
  position, tooth, teeth, fully erupted M26.30
    specified NEC M26.39
  precerebral vessel Q28.1
  prepuce Q55.69
  prostate Q55.4

Anomaly, anomalous (Continued)
  pulmonary Q33.9
    artery NEC Q25.79
    valve Q22.3
      atresia Q22.0
      insufficiency Q22.2
      specified type NEC Q22.3
      stenosis Q22.1
        infundibular Q24.3
        subvalvular Q24.3
    venous connection Q26.4
      partial Q26.3
      total Q26.2
  pupil Q13.2
    function H57.00
      anisocoria H57.02
      Argyll Robertson pupil H57.01
      miosis H57.03
      mydriasis H57.04
      specified type NEC H57.09
      tonic pupil H57.05-●
  pylorus Q40.3
  radius Q74.0
  rectum Q43.9
  reduction (extremity) (limb)
    femur (longitudinal) —see Defect,
        reduction, lower limb, longitudinal,
        femur
    fibula (longitudinal) —see Defect,
        reduction, lower limb, longitudinal,
        fibula
    lower limb —see Defect, reduction, lower
        limb
    radius (longitudinal) —see Defect,
        reduction, upper limb, longitudinal,
        radius
    tibia (longitudinal) —see Defect, reduction,
        lower limb, longitudinal, tibia
    ulna (longitudinal) —see Defect, reduction,
        upper limb, longitudinal, ulna
    upper limb —see Defect, reduction, upper
        limb
  refraction —see Disorder, refraction
  renal Q63.9
    artery Q27.2
    pelvis Q63.9
      specified NEC Q63.8
  respiratory system Q34.9
    specified NEC Q34.8
  retina Q14.1
  rib Q76.6
    cervical Q76.5
  Rieger's Q13.81
  rotation —see Malrotation
    hip or thigh Q65.89
  round ligament Q52.8
  sacroiliac (joint) NEC Q74.2
  sacrum NEC Q76.49
    kyphosis —see Kyphosis, congenital
    lordosis —see Lordosis, congenital
  saddle nose, syphilitic A50.57
  salivary duct or gland Q38.4
  scapula Q74.0
  scrotum —see Malformation, testis and
      scrotum
  sebaceous gland Q82.9
  seminal vesicles Q55.4
  sense organs NEC Q07.8
  sex chromosomes NEC —see also Anomaly,
      chromosomes
    female phenotype Q97.8
    male phenotype Q98.9
  shoulder (girdle) (joint) Q74.0
  sigmoid (flexure) Q43.9
  simian crease Q82.8
  sinus of Valsalva Q25.49
  skeleton generalized Q78.9
  skin (appendage) Q82.9
  skull Q75.9
    with
      anencephaly Q00.0
      encephalocele —see Encephalocele

Anomaly, anomalous (Continued)
  skull (Continued)
    with (Continued)
      hydrocephalus Q03.9
        with spina bifida —see Spina bifida, by
            site, with hydrocephalus
      microcephaly Q02
  specified organ or site NEC Q89.8
  spermatic cord Q55.4
  spine, spinal NEC Q76.49
    column NEC Q76.49
      kyphosis —see Kyphosis, congenital
      lordosis —see Lordosis, congenital
    cord Q06.9
    nerve root Q07.8
  spleen Q89.09
    agenesis Q89.01
  stenonian duct Q38.4
  sternum NEC Q76.7
  stomach Q40.3
  submaxillary gland Q38.4
  tarsus NEC Q74.2
  tendon Q79.9
  testis —see Malformation, testis and scrotum
  thigh NEC Q74.2
  thorax (wall) Q67.8
    bony Q76.9
  throat Q38.8
  thumb Q74.0
  thymus gland Q89.2
  thyroid (gland) Q89.2
    cartilage Q31.8
  tibia NEC Q74.2
    saber A50.56
  toe Q74.2
  tongue Q38.3
  tooth, teeth K00.9
    eruption K00.6
    position, fully erupted M26.30
    spacing, fully erupted M26.30
  trachea (cartilage) Q32.1
  tragus Q17.9
  tricuspid (leaflet) (valve) Q22.9
    atresia or stenosis Q22.4
    Ebstein's Q22.5
  Uhl's (hypoplasia of myocardium, right
      ventricle) Q24.8
  ulna Q74.0
  umbilical artery Q27.0
  union
    cricoid cartilage and thyroid cartilage
        Q31.8
    thyroid cartilage and hyoid bone Q31.8
    trachea with larynx Q31.8
  upper limb Q74.0
  urachus Q64.4
  ureter Q62.8
    obstructive NEC Q62.39
      cecoureterocele Q62.32
      orthotopic ureterocele Q62.31
  urethra Q64.70
    absence Q64.5
    double Q64.74
    fistula to rectum Q64.73
    obstructive Q64.39
      stricture Q64.32
    prolapse Q64.71
    specified type NEC Q64.79
  urinary tract Q64.9
  uterus Q51.9
    with only one functioning horn Q51.4
  uvula Q38.5
  vagina Q52.4
  valleculae Q31.8
  valve (heart) NEC Q24.8
    coronary sinus Q24.5
    inferior vena cava Q24.8
    pulmonary Q22.3
    sinus coronarius Q24.5
    venae cavae inferioris Q24.8
  vas deferens Q55.4

▶ New   ⇒ Revised   ~~deleted~~ Deleted   ● Use Additional Character(s)

Anomaly, anomalous *(Continued)*
  vascular Q27.9
    brain Q28.3
    ring Q25.45
  vein(s) (peripheral) Q27.9
    brain Q28.3
    cerebral Q28.3
    coronary Q24.5
    developmental Q28.3
    great Q26.9
      specified NEC Q26.8
  vena cava (inferior) (superior) Q26.9
  venous —*see* Anomaly, vein(s)
  venous return Q26.8
  ventricular
    bands or folds Q24.8
    septa Q21.1
  vertebra Q76.49
    kyphosis —*see* Kyphosis, congenital
    lordosis —*see* Lordosis, congenital
  vesicourethral orifice Q64.79
  vessel(s) Q27.9
    optic papilla Q14.2
    precerebral Q28.1
  vitelline duct Q43.0
  vitreous body or humor Q14.0
  vulva Q52.70
  wrist (joint) Q74.0
Anomia R48.8
Anonychia (congenital) Q84.3
  acquired L60.8
Anophthalmos, anophthalmus (congenital)
  (globe) Q11.1
  acquired Z90.01
Anopia, anopsia H53.46-●
  quadrant H53.46-●
Anorchia, anorchism, anorchidism Q55.0
Anorexia R63.0
  hysterical F44.89
  nervosa F50.00
    atypical F50.9
    binge eating type F50.2
      with purging F50.02
    restricting type F50.01
Anorgasmy, psychogenic (female)
  F52.31
  male F52.32
Anosmia R43.0
  hysterical F44.6
  postinfectional J39.8
Anosognosia R41.89
Anosteoplasia Q78.9
Anovulatory cycle N97.0
Anoxemia R09.02
  newborn P84
Anoxia (pathological) R09.02
  altitude T70.29
  cerebral G93.1
    complicating
      anesthesia (general) (local) or other
        sedation T88.59
        in labor and delivery O74.3
        in pregnancy O29.21-●
        postpartum, puerperal O89.2
      delivery (cesarean) (instrumental)
        O75.4
    during a procedure G97.81
    newborn P84
    resulting from a procedure G97.82
  due to
    drowning T75.1
    high altitude T70.29
  heart —*see* Insufficiency, coronary
  intrauterine P84
  myocardial —*see* Insufficiency, coronary
  newborn P84
  spinal cord G95.11
  systemic (by suffocation) (low content in
    atmosphere) —*see* Asphyxia,
    traumatic
Anteflexion —*see* Anteversion

Antenatal
  care (normal pregnancy) Z34.90
  screening (encounter for) of mother —*see also*
    Encounter, antenatal screening Z36.9
Antepartum —*see* condition
Anterior —*see* condition
Antero-occlusion M26.220
Anteversion
  cervix —*see* Anteversion, uterus
  femur (neck), congenital Q65.89
  uterus, uterine (cervix) (postinfectional)
    (postpartal, old) N85.4
    congenital Q51.818
    in pregnancy or childbirth —*see* Pregnancy,
      complicated by
Anthophobia F40.228
Anthracosilicosis J60
Anthracosis (lung) (occupational) J60
  lingua K14.3
Anthrax A22.9
  with pneumonia A22.1
  cerebral A22.8
  colitis A22.2
  cutaneous A22.0
  gastrointestinal A22.2
  inhalation A22.1
  intestinal A22.2
  meningitis A22.8
  pulmonary A22.1
  respiratory A22.1
  sepsis A22.7
  specified manifestation NEC A22.8
Anthropoid pelvis Q74.2
  with disproportion (fetopelvic) O33.0
Anthropophobia F40.10
  generalized F40.11
Antibodies, maternal (blood group) —*see*
  Isoimmunization, affecting management of
  pregnancy
anti-D —*see* Isoimmunization, affecting
  management of pregnancy, Rh
  newborn P55.0
Antibody
  anticardiolipin R76.0
    with
      hemorrhagic disorder D68.312
      hypercoagulable state D68.61
  antiphosphatidylglycerol R76.0
    with
      hemorrhagic disorder D68.312
      hypercoagulable state D68.61
  antiphosphatidylinositol R76.0
    with
      hemorrhagic disorder D68.312
      hypercoagulable state D68.61
  antiphosphatidylserine R76.0
    with
      hemorrhagic disorder D68.312
      hypercoagulable state D68.61
  antiphospholipid R76.0
    with
      hemorrhagic disorder D68.312
      hypercoagulable state D68.61
Anticardiolipin syndrome D68.61
Anticoagulant, circulating (intrinsic) —*see also* -
  Disorder, hemorrhagic D68.318
  drug-induced (extrinsic) —*see also* - Disorder,
    hemorrhagic D68.32
  iatrogenic D68.32
Antidiuretic hormone syndrome E22.2
Antimonial cholera —*see* Poisoning,
  antimony
Antiphospholipid
  antibody
    with hemorrhagic disorder D68.312
    syndrome D68.61
Antisocial personality F60.2
Antithrombinemia —*see* Circulating
  anticoagulants
Antithromboplastinemia D68.318
Antithromboplastinogenemia D68.318

Antitoxin complication or reaction —*see*
  Complications, vaccination
Antlophobia F40.228
Antritis J32.0
  maxilla J32.0
    acute J01.00
      recurrent J01.01
  stomach K29.60
    with bleeding K29.61
Antrum, antral —*see* condition
Anuria R34
  calculus (impacted) (recurrent) —*see also*
    Calculus, urinary N20.9
  following
    abortion —*see* Abortion by type
      complicated by, renal failure
    ectopic or molar pregnancy O08.4
  newborn P96.0
  postprocedural N99.0
  postrenal N13.8
  traumatic (following crushing) T79.5
Anus, anal —*see* condition
Anusitis K62.89
Anxiety F41.9
  depression F41.8
  episodic paroxysmal F41.0
  generalized F41.1
  hysteria F41.8
  neurosis F41.1
  panic type F41.0
  reaction F41.1
  separation, abnormal (of childhood) F93.0
  specified NEC F41.8
  state F41.1
Aorta, aortic —*see* condition
Aortectasia —*see* Ectasia, aorta
  with aneurysm —*see* Aneurysm, aorta
Aortitis (nonsyphilitic) (calcific) I77.6
  arteriosclerotic I70.0
  Doehle-Heller A52.02
  luetic A52.02
  rheumatic —*see* Endocarditis, acute,
    rheumatic
  specific (syphilitic) A52.02
  syphilitic A52.02
    congenital A50.54 *[I79.1]*
Apathetic thyroid storm —*see* Thyrotoxicosis
Apathy R45.3
Apeirophobia F40.228
Apepsia K30
  psychogenic F45.8
Aperistalsis, esophagus K22.0
Apertognathia M26.29
Apert's syndrome Q87.0
Aphagia R13.0
  psychogenic F50.9
Aphakia (acquired) (postoperative) H27.0-●
  congenital Q12.3
Aphasia (amnestic) (global) (nominal)
  (semantic) (syntactic) R47.01
  acquired, with epilepsy (Landau-Kleffner
    syndrome) —*see* Epilepsy, specified
    NEC
  auditory (developmental) F80.2
  developmental (receptive type) F80.2
    expressive type F80.1
    Wernicke's F80.2
  following
    cerebrovascular disease I69.920
      cerebral infarction I69.320
      intracerebral hemorrhage I69.120
      nontraumatic intracranial hemorrhage
        NEC I69.220
      specified disease NEC I69.820
      subarachnoid hemorrhage I69.020
  primary progressive G31.01 *[F02.80]*
    with behavioral disturbance G31.01
      [F02.81]
  progressive isolated G31.01 *[F02.80]*
    with behavioral disturbance G31.01
      [F02.81]

Aphasia *(Continued)*
  sensory F80.2
  syphilis, tertiary A52.19
  Wernicke's (developmental) F80.2
Aphonia (organic) R49.1
  hysterical F44.4
  psychogenic F44.4
Aphthae, aphthous —*see also* condition
  Bednar's K12.0
  cachectic K14.0
  epizootic B08.8
  fever B08.8
  oral (recurrent) K12.0
  stomatitis (major) (minor) K12.0
  thrush B37.0
  ulcer (oral) (recurrent) K12.0
    genital organ(s) NEC
      female N76.6
      male N50.89
    larynx J38.7
Apical —*see* condition
Apiphobia F40.218
Aplasia —*see also* Agenesis
  abdominal muscle syndrome Q79.4
  alveolar process (acquired) —*see* Anomaly,
      alveolar
    congenital Q38.6
  aorta (congenital) Q25.41
  axialis extracorticalis (congenita) E75.29
  bone marrow (myeloid) D61.9
    congenital D61.01
  brain Q00.0
    part of Q04.3
  bronchus Q32.4
  cementum K00.4
  cerebellum Q04.3
  cervix (congenital) Q51.5
  congenital pure red cell D61.01
  corpus callosum Q04.0
  cutis congenita Q84.8
  erythrocyte congenital D61.01
  extracortical axial E75.29
  eye Q11.1
  fovea centralis (congenital) Q14.1
  gallbladder, congenital Q44.0
  iris Q13.1
  labyrinth, membranous Q16.5
  limb (congenital) Q73.8
    lower —*see* Defect, reduction, lower limb
    upper —*see* Agenesis, arm
  lung, congenital (bilateral) (unilateral)
      Q33.3
  pancreas Q45.0
  parathyroid-thymic D82.1
  Pelizaeus-Merzbacher E75.29
  penis Q55.5
  prostate Q55.4
  red cell (with thymoma) D60.9
    acquired D60.9
      due to drugs D60.9
    adult D60.9
    chronic D60.0
    congenital D61.01
    constitutional D61.01
    due to drugs D60.9
    hereditary D61.01
    of infants D61.01
    primary D61.01
    pure D61.01
      due to drugs D60.9
    specified type NEC D60.8
    transient D60.1
  round ligament Q52.8
  skin Q84.8
  spermatic cord Q55.4
  spleen Q89.01
  testicle Q55.0
  thymic, with immunodeficiency D82.1
  thyroid (congenital) (with myxedema) E03.1
  uterus Q51.0
  ventral horn cell Q06.1

Apnea, apneic (of) (spells) R06.81
  newborn NEC P28.4
    obstructive P28.4
    sleep (central) (obstructive) (primary) P28.3
  prematurity P28.4
  sleep G47.30
    central (primary) G47.31
      idiopathic G47.31
      in conditions classified elsewhere G47.37
    obstructive (adult) (pediatric) G47.33
      hypopnea G47.33
    primary central G47.31
    specified NEC G47.39
Apneumatosis, newborn P28.0
Apocrine metaplasia (breast) —*see* Dysplasia,
    mammary, specified type NEC
Apophysitis (bone) —*see also*
    Osteochondropathy
  calcaneus M92.8
  juvenile M92.9
Apoplectiform convulsions (cerebral ischemia)
    I67.82
Apoplexia, apoplexy, apoplectic
  adrenal A39.1
  heart (auricle) (ventricle) —*see* Infarct,
      myocardium
  heat T67.01
  hemorrhagic (stroke) —*see* Hemorrhage,
      intracranial
  meninges, hemorrhagic —*see* Hemorrhage,
      intracranial, subarachnoid
  uremic N18.9 [I68.8]
Appearance
  bizarre R46.1
  specified NEC R46.89
  very low level of personal hygiene R46.0
Appendage
  epididymal (organ of Morgagni) Q55.4
  intestine (epiploic) Q43.8
  preauricular Q17.0
  testicular (organ of Morgagni) Q55.29
Appendicitis (pneumococcal) (retrocecal) K37
  with
    gangrene K35.891
    perforation NOS K35.32
    peritoneal abscess K35.33
    peritonitis NEC K35.33
      generalized (with perforation or
          rupture) K35.20
        with abscess K35.21
      localized K35.30
        with
          gangrene K35.32
          perforation K35.32
            and abscess K35.33
      ruptured NOS (with localized
          peritonitis) K35.32
  acute (catarrhal) (fulminating) (gangrenous)
      (obstructive) (retrocecal) (suppurative)
      K35.80
    with
      gangrene K35.891
      peritoneal abscess K35.33
      peritonitis NEC K35.33
        generalized (with perforation or
            rupture) K35.20
          with abscess K35.21
        localized K35.30
          with
            gangrene K35.32
            perforation K35.32
              and abscess K35.33
      specified NEC K35.890
        with gangrene K35.891
  amebic A06.89
  chronic (recurrent) K36
  exacerbation —*see* Appendicitis, acute
  gangrenous —*see* Appendicitis, acute
  healed (obliterative) K36
  interval K36
  neurogenic K36

Appendicitis *(Continued)*
  obstructive K36
  recurrent K36
  relapsing K36
    ruptured NOS (with localized peritonitis)
        K35.32
  subacute (adhesive) K36
  subsiding K36
  suppurative —*see* Appendicitis, acute
  tuberculous A18.32
Appendicopathia oxyurica B80
Appendix, appendicular —*see also* condition
  epididymis Q55.4
  Morgagni
    female Q50.5
    male (epididymal) Q55.4
      testicular Q55.29
  testis Q55.29
Appetite
  depraved —*see* Pica
  excessive R63.2
  lack or loss —*see also* Anorexia R63.0
    nonorganic origin F50.89
    psychogenic F50.89
  perverted (hysterical) —*see* Pica
Apple peel syndrome Q41.1
Apprehension state F41.1
Apprehensiveness, abnormal F41.9
Approximal wear K03.0
Apraxia (classic) (ideational) (ideokinetic)
    (ideomotor) (motor) (verbal) R48.2
  following
    cerebrovascular disease I69.990
      cerebral infarction I69.390
      intracerebral hemorrhage I69.190
      nontraumatic intracranial hemorrhage
          NEC I69.290
      specified disease NEC I69.890
      subarachnoid hemorrhage I69.090
  oculomotor, congenital H51.8
Aptyalism K11.7
Apudoma —*see* Neoplasm, uncertain behavior,
    by site
Aqueous misdirection H40.83-●
Arabicum elephantiasis —*see* Infestation, filarial
Arachnitis —*see* Meningitis
Arachnodactyly —*see* Syndrome, Marfan's
Arachnoiditis (acute) (adhesive) (basal) (brain)
    (cerebrospinal) —*see* Meningitis
Arachnophobia F40.210
Arboencephalitis, Australian A83.4
Arborization block (heart) I45.5
ARC (AIDS-related complex) B20
Arch
  aortic Q25.49
  bovine Q25.49
Arches —*see* condition
Arcuate uterus Q51.810
Arcuatus uterus Q51.810
Arcus (cornea) senilis —*see* Degeneration,
    cornea, senile
Arc-welder's lung J63.4
Areflexia R29.2
Areola —*see* condition
Argentaffinoma —*see also* Neoplasm, uncertain
    behavior, by site
  malignant —*see* Neoplasm, malignant, by site
  syndrome E34.0
Argininemia E72.21
Arginosuccinic aciduria E72.22
Argyll Robertson phenomenon, pupil or
    syndrome (syphilitic) A52.19
  atypical H57.09
  nonsyphilitic H57.09
Argyria, argyriasis
  conjunctival H11.13-●
  from drug or medicament —*see* Table of
      Drugs and Chemicals, by substance
Argyrosis, conjunctival H11.13-●
Arhinencephaly Q04.1
Ariboflavinosis E53.0

▶ New   ⇒ Revised   ~~deleted~~ Deleted   ● Use Additional Character(s)

Arm —*see* condition
Arnold-Chiari disease, obstruction or
    syndrome (type II) Q07.00
  with
    hydrocephalus Q07.02
      with spina bifida Q07.03
    spina bifida Q07.01
      with hydrocephalus Q07.03
  type III —*see* Encephalocele
  type IV Q04.8
Aromatic amino-acid metabolism disorder E70.9
  specified NEC E70.89
Arousals, confusional G47.51
Arrest, arrested
  cardiac I46.9
    complicating
      abortion —*see* Abortion, by type,
        complicated by, cardiac arrest
      anesthesia (general) (local) or other
        sedation —*see* Table of Drugs and
        Chemicals, by drug
      in labor and delivery O74.2
      in pregnancy O29.11-●
      postpartum, puerperal O89.1
      delivery (cesarean) (instrumental) O75.4
    due to
      cardiac condition I46.2
      specified condition NEC I46.8
    intraoperative I97.71-●
    newborn P29.81
    personal history, successfully resuscitated
      Z86.74
    postprocedural I97.12-●
      obstetric procedure O75.4
  cardiorespiratory —*see* Arrest, cardiac
  circulatory —*see* Arrest, cardiac
  deep transverse O64.0
  development or growth
    bone —*see* Disorder, bone, development or
      growth
    child R62.50
    tracheal rings Q32.1
  epiphyseal
    complete
      femur M89.15-●
      humerus M89.12-●
      tibia M89.16-●
      ulna M89.13-●
      forearm M89.13-●
      specified NEC M89.13-●
      ulna —*see* Arrest, epiphyseal, by type,
        ulna
      lower leg M89.16-●
      specified NEC M89.168
      tibia —*see* Arrest, epiphyseal, by type,
        tibia
    partial
      femur M89.15-●
      humerus M89.12-●
      tibia M89.16-●
      ulna M89.13-●
    specified NEC M89.18
  granulopoiesis —*see* Agranulocytosis
  growth plate —*see* Arrest, epiphyseal
  heart —*see* Arrest, cardiac
  legal, anxiety concerning Z65.3
  physeal —*see* Arrest, epiphyseal
  respiratory R09.2
    newborn P28.81
  sinus I45.5
  spermatogenesis (complete) —*see*
    Azoospermia
    incomplete —*see* Oligospermia
  transverse (deep) O64.0
Arrhenoblastoma
  benign
    specified site —*see* Neoplasm, benign, by
      site
    unspecified site
      female D27.9
      male D29.20

Arrhenoblastoma (*Continued*)
  malignant
    specified site —*see* Neoplasm, malignant,
      by site
    unspecified site
      female C56.9
      male C62.90
  specified site —*see* Neoplasm, uncertain
    behavior, by site
  unspecified site
    female D39.10
    male D40.10
Arrhythmia (auricle)(cardiac) (juvenile)(nodal)
  (reflex)(supraventricular)(transitory)
  (ventricle) I49.9
  block I45.9
  extrasystolic I49.49
  newborn
    bradycardia P29.12
    occurring before birth P03.819
      before onset of labor P03.810
      during labor P03.811
    tachycardia P29.11
  psychogenic F45.8
  sinus I49.8
  specified NEC I49.8
  vagal R55
  ventricular re-entry I47.0
Arrillaga-Ayerza syndrome (pulmonary
  sclerosis with pulmonary hypertension)
  I27.0
Arsenical pigmentation L81.8
  from drug or medicament —*see* Table of
    Drugs and Chemicals
Arsenism —*see* Poisoning, arsenic
Arterial —*see* condition
Arteriofibrosis —*see* Arteriosclerosis
Arteriolar sclerosis —*see* Arteriosclerosis
Arteriolith —*see* Arteriosclerosis
Arteriolitis I77.6
  necrotizing, kidney I77.5
  renal —*see* Hypertension, kidney
Arteriolosclerosis —*see* Arteriosclerosis
Arterionephrosclerosis —*see* Hypertension,
  kidney
Arteriopathy I77.9
  cerebral autosomal dominant,
    with subcortical infarcts and
    leukoencephalopathy
    (CADASIL) I67.850
Arteriosclerosis, arteriosclerotic (diffuse)
  (obliterans) (of) (senile) (with calcification)
  I70.90
  with
    chronic limb-threatening ischemia —*see*
      Arteriosclerosis, with critical limb
      ischemia
    critical limb ischemia
      bypass graft I70.329
        autologous vein graft I70.429
          leg I70.429
            with
              gangrene (and intermittent
                claudication, rest pain,
                and ulcer) I70.469
              rest pain (and intermittent
                claudication) I70.429
          bilateral I70.423
            with
              gangrene (and intermittent
                claudication, rest pain,
                and ulcer) I70.463
              rest pain (and intermittent
                claudication) I70.423
          left I70.422
            with
              gangrene (and intermittent
                claudication, rest pain,
                and ulcer) I70.462
              rest pain (and intermittent
                claudication) I70.422

Arteriosclerosis, arteriosclerotic (*Continued*)
  chronic limb-threatening ischemia
    (*Continued*)
    critical limb ischemia (*Continued*)
      bypass graft (*Continued*)
        autologous vein graft (*Continued*)
          leg (*Continued*)
            left (*Continued*)
              with (*Continued*)
                ulceration (and intermittent
                  claudication and rest
                  pain) I70.449
                ankle I70.443
                calf I70.442
                foot site NEC I70.445
                heel I70.444
                lower leg NEC I70.448
                mid foot I70.444
                thigh I70.441
            right I70.421
              with
                gangrene (and intermittent
                  claudication, rest pain,
                  and ulcer) I70.461
                rest pain (and intermittent
                  claudication) I70.421
                ulceration (and intermittent
                  claudication and rest
                  pain) I70.439
                ankle I70.433
                calf I70.432
                foot site NEC I70.435
                heel I70.434
                lower leg NEC I70.438
                midfoot I70.434
                thigh I70.431
        leg I70.329
          with
            gangrene (and intermittent
               claudication, rest pain, and
               ulcer) I70.369
            rest pain (and intermittent
               claudication) I70.329
        bilateral I70.323
          with
            gangrene (and intermittent
               claudication, rest pain,
               and ulcer) I70.363
            rest pain (and intermittent
               claudication) I70.323
        left I70.322
          with
            rest pain (and intermittent
               claudication) I70.322
            ulceration (and intermittent
               claudication and rest
              pain) I70.349
            ankle I70.343
            calf I70.342
            foot site NEC I70.345
            heel I70.344
            lower leg NEC I70.348
            midfoot I70.344
            thigh I70.341
        right I70.321
          with
            gangrene (and intermittent
               claudication, rest pain,
               and ulcer) I70.361
            rest pain (and intermittent
               claudication) I70.321
            ulceration (and intermittent
               claudication and rest
              pain) I70.339
            ankle I70.333
            calf I70.332
            foot site NEC I70.335
            heel I70.334
            lower leg NEC I70.338
            midfoot I70.334
            thigh I70.331

Arteriosclerosis, arteriosclerotic *(Continued)*
  chronic limb-threatening ischemia
    (Continued)
    critical limb ischemia *(Continued)*
      bypass graft *(Continued)*
        nonautologous biological graft I70.529
          leg I70.529
            with
              gangrene (and intermittent
                claudication, rest pain,
                and ulcer) I70.569
              rest pain (and intermittent
                claudication) I70.529
          bilateral I70.523
            with
              gangrene (and intermittent
                claudication, rest pain,
                and ulcer) I70.563
              rest pain (and intermittent
                 claudication) I70.523
          left I70.522
            with
              gangrene (and intermittent
                 claudication, rest pain,
                 and ulcer) I70.562
              rest pain (and intermittent
                 claudication) I70.522
              ulceration (and intermittent
                claudication and rest
                pain) I70.549
                ankle I70.543
                calf I70.542
                foot site NEC I70.545
                heel I70.544
                lower leg NEC I70.548
                midfoot I70.544
                thigh I70.541
          right I70.521
            with
              gangrene (and intermittent
                claudication, rest pain,
                and ulcer) I70.561
              rest pain (and intermittent
                 claudication) I70.521
              ulceration (and intermittent
                claudication and rest
                pain) I70.539
                ankle I70.533
                calf I70.532
                foot site NEC I70.535
                heel I70.534
                lower leg NEC I70.538
                midfoot I70.534
                thigh I70.531
        nonbiological graft I70.629
          leg I70.629
            with
              gangrene (and intermittent
                claudication, rest pain,
                and ulcer) I70.669
              rest pain (and intermittent
                 claudication) I70.629
          bilateral I70.623
            with
              gangrene (and intermittent
                claudication, rest pain,
                and ulcer) I70.663
              rest pain (and intermittent
                 claudication) I70.623
          left I70.622
            with
              gangrene (and intermittent
                claudication, rest pain,
                and ulcer) I70.662
              rest pain (and intermittent
                 claudication) I70.622
              ulceration (and intermittent
                claudication and rest
                pain) I70.649
                ankle I70.643
                calf I70.642

Arteriosclerosis, arteriosclerotic *(Continued)*
  chronic limb-threatening ischemia
    (Continued)
    critical limb ischemia *(Continued)*
      bypass graft *(Continued)*
        nonbiological graft *(Continued)*
          leg *(Continued)*
            left *(Continued)*
              with *(Continued)*
                ulceration *(Continued)*
                  foot site NEC I70.645
                  heel I70.644
                  lower leg NEC I70.648
                  midfoot I70.644
                  thigh I70.641
          right I70.621
            with
              gangrene (and intermittent
                claudication, rest pain,
                and ulcer) I70.661
              rest pain (and intermittent
                 claudication) I70.621
              ulceration (and intermittent
                claudication and rest
                pain) I70.639
                ankle I70.633
                calf I70.632
                foot site NEC I70.635
                heel I70.634
                lower leg NEC I70.638
                midfoot I70.634
                thigh I70.631
        specified graft NEC I70.729
          leg I70.729
            with
              gangrene (and intermittent
                claudication, rest pain,
                and ulcer) I70.769
              rest pain (and intermittent
                 claudication) I70.729
          bilateral I70.723
            with
              gangrene (and intermittent
                claudication, rest pain,
                and ulcer) I70.763
              rest pain (and intermittent
                 claudication) I70.723
          left I70.722
            with
              gangrene (and intermittent
                claudication, rest pain,
                and ulcer) I70.762
              rest pain (and intermittent
                 claudication) I70.722
              ulceration (and intermittent
                claudication and rest
                pain) I70.749
                ankle I70.743
                calf I70.742
                foot site NEC I70.745
                heel I70.744
                lower leg NEC I70.748
                midfoot I70.744
                thigh I70.741
          right I70.721
            with
              gangrene (and intermittent
                claudication, rest pain,
                and ulcer) I70.761
              rest pain (and intermittent
                 claudication) I70.721
              ulceration (and intermittent
                claudication and rest
                pain) I70.739
                ankle I70.733
                calf I70.732
                foot site NEC I70.735
                heel I70.734
                lower leg NEC I70.738
                midfoot I70.734
                thigh I70.731

Arteriosclerosis, arteriosclerotic *(Continued)*
  chronic limb-threatening ischemia
    (Continued)
    critical limb ischemia *(Continued)*
      leg I70.229
        with
          gangrene (and intermittent
            claudication, rest pain, and
            ulcer) I70.269
          rest pain (and intermittent
            claudication) I70.229
      bilateral I70.223
        with
          gangrene (and intermittent
            claudication, rest pain, and
            ulcer) I70.263
          rest pain (and intermittent
            claudication) I70.223
      left I70.222
        with
          gangrene (and intermittent
            claudication, rest pain, and
            ulcer) I70.262
          rest pain (and intermittent
            claudication) I70.222
          ulceration (and intermittent
            claudication and rest pain)
            I70.249
          ankle I70.243
          calf I70.242
          foot site NEC I70.245
          heel I70.244
          lower leg NEC I70.248
          midfoot I70.244
          thigh I70.241
      right I70.221
        with
          gangrene (and intermittent
            claudication, rest pain, and
            ulcer) I70.261
          rest pain (and intermittent
            claudication) I70.221
          ulceration (and intermittent
            claudication and rest pain)
            I70.239
          ankle I70.233
          calf I70.232
          foot site NEC I70.235
          heel I70.234
          lower leg NEC I70.238
          midfoot I70.234
          thigh I70.231
  aorta I70.0
  arteries of extremities —*see* Arteriosclerosis,
    extremities
    with
      chronic limb-threatening ischemia —*see*
        Arteriosclerosis, with critical limb
        ischemia
      critical limb ischemia —*see*
        Arteriosclerosis, with critical limb
        ischemia
  brain I67.2
  bypass graft
    with
      chronic limb-threatening ischemia —*see*
        Arteriosclerosis, with critical limb
        ischemia
      critical limb ischemia —*see*
        Arteriosclerosis, with critical limb
        ischemia
    coronary —*see* Arteriosclerosis, coronary,
      bypass graft
    extremities —*see* Arteriosclerosis,
      extremities, bypass graft
  cardiac —*see* Disease, heart, ischemic,
    atherosclerotic
  cardiopathy —*see* Disease, heart, ischemic,
    atherosclerotic
  cardiorenal —*see* Hypertension,
    cardiorenal

▶ New   ⇒ Revised   ~~deleted~~ Deleted   ● Use Additional Character(s)

Arteriosclerosis, arteriosclerotic *(Continued)*
cardiovascular —*see* Disease, heart, ischemic,
atherosclerotic
carotid —*see also* Occlusion, artery, carotid
I65.2-●
central nervous system I67.2
cerebral I67.2
cerebrovascular I67.2
coronary (artery) I25.10
bypass graft I25.810
with
angina pectoris I25.709
with documented spasm I25.701
specified type NEC I25.708
unstable I25.700
ischemic chest pain I25.709
autologous artery I25.810
with
angina pectoris I25.729
with documented spasm
I25.721
specified type I25.728
unstable I25.720
ischemic chest pain I25.729
autologous vein I25.810
with
angina pectoris I25.719
with documented spasm
I25.711
specified type I25.718
unstable I25.710
ischemic chest pain I25.719
nonautologous biological I25.810
with
angina pectoris I25.739
with documented spasm
I25.731
specified type I25.738
unstable I25.730
ischemic chest pain I25.739
specified type NEC I25.810
with
angina pectoris I25.799
with documented spasm I25.791
specified type I25.798
unstable I25.790
ischemic chest pain I25.799
due to
calcified coronary lesion (severely)
I25.84
lipid rich plaque I25.83
native vessel
with
angina pectoris I25.119
with documented spasm I25.111
specified type NEC I25.118
unstable I25.110
ischemic chest pain I25.119
transplanted heart I25.811
bypass graft I25.812
with
angina pectoris I25.769
with documented spasm I25.761
specified type I25.768
unstable I25.760
ischemic chest pain I25.769
native coronary artery I25.811
with
angina pectoris I25.759
with documented spasm I25.751
specified type I25.758
unstable I25.750
ischemic chest pain I25.759
extremities (native arteries) I70.209
with
chronic limb-threatening ischemia —*see*
Arteriosclerosis, with critical limb
ischemia
critical limb ischemia —*see*
Arteriosclerosis, with critical limb
ischemia

Arteriosclerosis, arteriosclerotic *(Continued)*
extremities *(Continued)*
bypass graft I70.309
with
chronic limb-threatening ischemia —
see Arteriosclerosis, with critical
limb ischemia
critical limb ischemia —*see*
Arteriosclerosis, with critical limb
ischemia
autologous vein graft I70.409
leg I70.409
with
gangrene (and intermittent
claudication, rest pain and
ulcer) I70.469
intermittent claudication I70.419
rest pain (and intermittent
claudication) I70.429
bilateral I70.403
with
gangrene (and intermittent
claudication, rest pain and
ulcer) I70.463
intermittent claudication
I70.413
rest pain (and intermittent
claudication) I70.423
specified type NEC I70.493
left I70.402
with
gangrene (and intermittent
claudication, rest pain and
ulcer) I70.462
intermittent claudication I70.412
rest pain (and intermittent
claudication) I70.422
ulceration (and intermittent
claudication and rest
pain) I70.449
ankle I70.443
calf I70.442
foot site NEC I70.445
heel I70.444
lower leg NEC I70.448
midfoot I70.444
thigh I70.441
specified type NEC I70.492
right I70.401
with
gangrene (and intermittent
claudication, rest pain and
ulcer) I70.461
intermittent claudication
I70.411
rest pain (and intermittent
claudication) I70.421
ulceration (and intermittent
claudication and rest
pain) I70.439
ankle I70.433
calf I70.432
foot site NEC I70.435
heel I70.434
lower leg NEC I70.438
midfoot I70.434
thigh I70.431
specified type NEC I70.491
specified type NEC I70.499
specified NEC I70.408
with
gangrene (and intermittent
claudication, rest pain and
ulcer) I70.468
intermittent claudication I70.418
rest pain (and intermittent
claudication) I70.428
ulceration (and intermittent
claudication and rest pain)
I70.45
specified type NEC I70.498

Arteriosclerosis, arteriosclerotic *(Continued)*
extremities *(Continued)*
bypass graft *(Continued)*
leg I70.309
with
gangrene (and intermittent
claudication, rest pain and
ulcer) I70.369
intermittent claudication I70.319
rest pain (and intermittent
claudication) I70.329
bilateral I70.303
with
gangrene (and intermittent
claudication, rest pain and
ulcer) I70.363
intermittent claudication I70.313
rest pain (and intermittent
claudication) I70.323
specified type NEC I70.393
left I70.302
with
gangrene (and intermittent
claudication, rest pain and
ulcer) I70.362
intermittent claudication I70.312
rest pain (and intermittent
claudication) I70.322
ulceration (and intermittent
claudication and rest pain)
I70.349
ankle I70.343
calf I70.342
foot site NEC I70.345
heel I70.344
lower leg NEC I70.348
midfoot I70.344
thigh I70.341
specified type NEC I70.392
right I70.301
with
gangrene (and intermittent
claudication, rest pain and
ulcer) I70.361
intermittent claudication
I70.311
rest pain (and intermittent
claudication) I70.321
ulceration (and intermittent
claudication and rest pain)
I70.339
ankle I70.333
calf I70.332
foot site NEC I70.335
heel I70.334
lower leg NEC I70.338
midfoot I70.334
thigh I70.331
specified type NEC I70.391
specified type NEC I70.399
nonautologous biological graft
I70.509
leg I70.509
with
gangrene (and intermittent
claudication, rest pain and
ulcer) I70.569
intermittent claudication
I70.519
rest pain (and intermittent
claudication) I70.529
bilateral I70.503
with
gangrene (and intermittent
claudication, rest pain and
ulcer) I70.563
intermittent claudication
I70.513
rest pain (and intermittent
claudication) I70.523
specified type NEC I70.593

Arteriosclerosis, arteriosclerotic (Continued)
  extremities (Continued)
    bypass graft (Continued)
      nonautologous biological graft
        (Continued)
        leg (Continued)
          left I70.502
            with
              gangrene (and intermittent
                claudication, rest pain and
                ulcer) I70.562
              intermittent claudication
                I70.512
              rest pain (and intermittent
                claudication) I70.522
              ulceration (and intermittent
                claudication and rest
                pain) I70.549
              ankle I70.543
              calf I70.542
              foot site NEC I70.545
              heel I70.544
              lower leg NEC I70.548
              midfoot I70.544
              thigh I70.541
            specified type NEC
              I70.592
          right I70.501
            with
              gangrene (and intermittent
                claudication, rest pain and
                ulcer) I70.561
              intermittent claudication
                I70.511
              rest pain (and intermittent
                claudication) I70.521
              ulceration (and intermittent
                claudication and rest
                pain) I70.539
              ankle I70.533
              calf I70.532
              foot site NEC I70.535
              heel I70.534
              lower leg NEC I70.538
              midfoot I70.534
              thigh I70.531
            specified type NEC I70.591
          specified type NEC I70.599
        specified NEC I70.508
          with
            gangrene (and intermittent
              claudication, rest pain and
              ulcer) I70.568
            intermittent claudication
              I70.518
            rest pain (and intermittent
              claudication) I70.528
            ulceration (and intermittent
              claudication and rest pain)
              I70.55
          specified type NEC I70.598
      nonbiological graft I70.609
        leg I70.609
          with
            gangrene (and intermittent
              claudication, rest pain and
              ulcer) I70.669
            intermittent claudication
              I70.619
            rest pain (and intermittent
              claudication) I70.629
          bilateral I70.603
            with
              gangrene (and intermittent
               claudication, rest pain and
               ulcer) I70.663
             intermittent claudication
              I70.613
             rest pain (and intermittent
               claudication) I70.623
           specified type NEC I70.693

Arteriosclerosis, arteriosclerotic (Continued)
  extremities (Continued)
    bypass graft (Continued)
      nonbiological graft (Continued)
        leg (Continued)
          left I70.602
            with
              gangrene (and intermittent
                claudication, rest pain and
                ulcer) I70.662
              intermittent claudication
                I70.612
              rest pain (and intermittent
                claudication) I70.622
              ulceration (and intermittent
                claudication and rest
                pain) I70.649
              ankle I70.643
              calf I70.642
              foot site NEC I70.645
              heel I70.644
              lower leg NEC I70.648
              midfoot I70.644
              thigh I70.641
            specified type NEC I70.692
          right I70.601
            with
              gangrene (and intermittent
                claudication, rest pain and
                ulcer) I70.661
              intermittent claudication
                I70.611
              rest pain (and intermittent
                claudication) I70.621
              ulceration (and intermittent
                claudication and rest
                pain) I70.639
              ankle I70.633
              calf I70.632
              foot site NEC I70.635
              heel I70.634
              lower leg NEC I70.638
              midfoot I70.634
              thigh I70.631
            specified type NEC I70.691
          specified type NEC I70.699
        specified NEC I70.608
          with
            gangrene (and intermittent
              claudication, rest pain and
              ulcer) I70.668
            intermittent claudication I70.618
            rest pain (and intermittent
              claudication) I70.628
            ulceration (and intermittent
              claudication and rest pain)
              I70.65
          specified type NEC I70.698
      specified graft NEC I70.709
        leg I70.709
          with
            gangrene (and intermittent
              claudication, rest pain and
              ulcer) I70.769
            intermittent claudication I70.719
            rest pain (and intermittent
              claudication) I70.729
          bilateral I70.703
            with
              gangrene (and intermittent
               claudication, rest pain and
               ulcer) I70.763
             intermittent claudication I70.713
             rest pain (and intermittent
               claudication) I70.723
            specified type NEC I70.793
          left I70.702
            with
              gangrene (and intermittent
                claudication, rest pain and
                ulcer) I70.762

Arteriosclerosis, arteriosclerotic (Continued)
  extremities (Continued)
    bypass graft (Continued)
      specified graft NEC (Continued)
        leg (Continued)
          left (Continued)
            with (Continued)
              intermittent claudication I70.712
              rest pain (and intermittent
                claudication) I70.722
              ulceration (and intermittent
                claudication and rest
                pain) I70.749
              ankle I70.743
              calf I70.742
              foot site NEC I70.745
              heel I70.744
              lower leg NEC I70.748
              midfoot I70.744
              thigh I70.741
            specified type NEC I70.792
          right I70.701
            with
              gangrene (and intermittent
                claudication, rest pain and
                ulcer) I70.761
              intermittent claudication I70.711
              rest pain (and intermittent
                claudication) I70.721
              ulceration (and intermittent
                claudication and rest
                pain) I70.739
              ankle I70.733
              calf I70.732
              foot site NEC I70.735
              heel I70.734
              lower leg NEC I70.738
              midfoot I70.734
              thigh I70.731
            specified type NEC I70.791
          specified type NEC I70.799
        specified NEC I70.708
          with
            gangrene (and intermittent
              claudication, rest pain and
              ulcer) I70.768
            intermittent claudication I70.718
            rest pain (and intermittent
              claudication) I70.728
            ulceration (and intermittent
              claudication and rest pain)
              I70.75
          specified type NEC I70.798
      specified NEC I70.308
        with
          gangrene (and intermittent
            claudication, rest pain and
            ulcer) I70.368
         intermittent claudication I70.318
         rest pain (and intermittent
          claudication) I70.328
         ulceration (and intermittent
          claudication and rest pain)
          I70.35
        specified type NEC I70.398
    leg I70.209
      with
        gangrene (and intermittent
          claudication, rest pain and ulcer)
          I70.269
        intermittent claudication I70.219
        rest pain (and intermittent
          claudication) I70.229
      bilateral I70.203
        with
          gangrene (and intermittent
           claudication, rest pain and
           ulcer) I70.263
        intermittent claudication I70.213
        rest pain (and intermittent
          claudication) I70.223
        specified type NEC I70.293

▶ New   ⇒ Revised   ~~deleted~~ Deleted   ● Use Additional Character(s)

Arteriosclerosis, arteriosclerotic *(Continued)*
  extremities *(Continued)*
    leg *(Continued)*
      left I70.202
        with
          gangrene (and intermittent
            claudication, rest pain and
            ulcer) I70.262
          intermittent claudication I70.212
          rest pain (and intermittent
            claudication) I70.222
          ulceration (and intermittent
            claudication and rest pain)
            I70.249
            ankle I70.243
            calf I70.242
            foot site NEC I70.245
            heel I70.244
            lower leg NEC I70.248
            midfoot I70.244
            thigh I70.241
        specified type NEC I70.292
      right I70.201
        with
          gangrene (and intermittent
            claudication, rest pain and
            ulcer) I70.261
          intermittent claudication I70.211
          rest pain (and intermittent
            claudication) I70.221
          ulceration (and intermittent
            claudication and rest pain)
            I70.239
            ankle I70.233
            calf I70.232
            foot site NEC I70.235
            heel I70.234
            lower leg NEC I70.238
            midfoot I70.234
            thigh I70.231
        specified type NEC I70.291
      specified type NEC I70.299
    specified site NEC I70.208
      with
        gangrene (and intermittent claudication,
          rest pain and ulcer) I70.268
        intermittent claudication I70.218
        rest pain (and intermittent
          claudication) I70.228
        ulceration (and intermittent
          claudication and rest pain) I70.25
        specified type NEC I70.298
  generalized I70.91
  heart (disease) —*see* Arteriosclerosis,
    coronary (artery)
  kidney —*see* Hypertension, kidney
  medial —*see* Arteriosclerosis, extremities
  mesenteric (artery) K55.1
  Mönckeberg's —*see* Arteriosclerosis,
    extremities
  myocarditis I51.4
  peripheral (of extremities) —*see*
    Arteriosclerosis, extremities
  pulmonary (idiopathic) I27.0
  renal (arterioles) —*see also* Hypertension,
    kidney
    artery I70.1
  retina (vascular) I70.8 [H35.0-•]
  specified artery NEC I70.8
  spinal (cord) G95.19
  vertebral (artery) I67.2
Arteriospasm I73.9
Arteriovenous —*see* condition
Arteritis I77.6
  allergic M31.0
  aorta (nonsyphilitic) I77.6
    syphilitic A52.02
  aortic arch M31.4
  brachiocephalic M31.4
  brain I67.7
    syphilitic A52.04

Arteritis *(Continued)*
  cerebral I67.7
    in
      diseases classified elsewhere I68.2
      systemic lupus erythematosus M32.19
    listerial A32.89
    syphilitic A52.04
    tuberculous A18.89
  coronary (artery) I25.89
    rheumatic I01.8
      chronic I09.89
    syphilitic A52.06
  cranial (left) (right), giant cell M31.6
  deformans —*see* Arteriosclerosis
  giant cell NEC M31.6
    with polymyalgia rheumatica M31.5
  necrosing or necrotizing M31.9
    specified NEC M31.8
  nodosa M30.0
  obliterans —*see* Arteriosclerosis
  pulmonary I28.8
  rheumatic —*see* Fever, rheumatic
  senile —*see* Arteriosclerosis
  suppurative I77.2
  syphilitic (general) A52.09
    brain A52.04
    coronary A52.06
    spinal A52.09
  temporal, giant cell M31.6
  young female aortic arch syndrome M31.4
Artery, arterial —*see also* condition
  abscess I77.89
  single umbilical Q27.0
Arthralgia (allergic) —*see also* Pain, joint
  in caisson disease T70.3
  temporomandibular M26.62
Arthritis, arthritic (acute) (chronic)
  (nonpyogenic) (subacute) M19.90
  allergic —*see* Arthritis, specified form NEC
  ankylosing (crippling) (spine) —*see also*
    Spondylitis, ankylosing
    sites other than spine —*see* Arthritis,
      specified form NEC
  atrophic —*see* Osteoarthritis
    spine —*see* Spondylitis, ankylosing
  back —*see* Spondylopathy, inflammatory
  blennorrhagic (gonococcal) A54.42
  Charcot's —*see* Arthropathy, neuropathic
    diabetic —*see* Diabetes, arthropathy,
      neuropathic
    syringomyelic G95.0
  chylous (filarial) —*see also* category M01 B74.9
  climacteric (any site) NEC —*see* Arthritis,
    specified form NEC
  crystal (-induced) —*see* Arthritis, in, crystals
  deformans —*see* Osteoarthritis
  degenerative —*see* Osteoarthritis
  due to or associated with
    acromegaly E22.0
    brucellosis —*see* Brucellosis
    caisson disease T70.3
    diabetes —*see* Diabetes, arthropathy
    dracontiasis —*see also* category M01 B72
    enteritis NEC
      regional —*see* Enteritis, regional
    erysipelas —*see also* category M01 A46
    erythema
      epidemic A25.1
      nodosum L52
    filariasis NOS B74.9
    glanders A24.0
    helminthiasis —*see also* category M01 B83.9
    hemophilia D66 [M36.2]
    Henoch-(Schönlein) purpura D69.0 [M36.4]
    human parvovirus —*see also* category M01
      B97.6
    infectious disease NEC —*see* category M01
    leprosy (*see also* category M01) —*see also*
      Leprosy A30.9
    Lyme disease A69.23
    mycobacteria —*see also* category M01 A31.8

Arthritis, arthritic *(Continued)*
  due to or associated with *(Continued)*
    parasitic disease NEC —*see also* category
      M01 B89
    paratyphoid fever (*see also* category M01)
      —*see also* Fever, paratyphoid A01.4
    rat bite fever —*see also* category M01 A25.1
    regional enteritis —*see* Enteritis, regional
    respiratory disorder NOS J98.9
    serum sickness —*see also* Reaction, serum
      T80.69
    syringomyelia G95.0
    typhoid fever A01.04
  epidemic erythema A25.1
  ▶ facet joint (*see also* Spondylosis) M47.819
  febrile —*see* Fever, rheumatic
  gonococcal A54.42
  gouty (acute) —*see* Gout
  in (due to)
    acromegaly —*see also* subcategory
      M14.8-• E22.0
    amyloidosis —*see also* subcategory
      M14.8-• E85.4
    bacterial disease —*see also* subcategory
      M01 A49.9
    Behçet's syndrome M35.2
    caisson disease —*see also* subcategory
      M14.8-• T70.3
    coliform bacilli (Escherichia coli) —*see*
      Arthritis, in, pyogenic organism NEC
    crystals M11.9
      dicalcium phosphate —*see* Arthritis, in,
        crystals, specified type NEC
      hydroxyapatite M11.0-•
      pyrophosphate —*see* Arthritis, in,
        crystals, specified type NEC
      specified type NEC M11.80
        ankle M11.87-•
        elbow M11.82-•
        foot joint M11.87-•
        hand joint M11.84-•
        hip M11.85-•
        knee M11.86-•
        multiple sites M11.8-•
        shoulder M11.81-•
        vertebrae M11.88
        wrist M11.83-•
    dermatoarthritis, lipoid E78.81
    dracontiasis (dracunculiasis) —*see also*
      category M01 B72
    endocrine disorder NEC —*see also*
      subcategory M14.8-• E34.9
    enteritis, infectious NEC —*see also* category
      M01 A09
      specified organism NEC —*see also*
        category M01 A08.8
    erythema
      multiforme —*see also* subcategory
        M14.8-• L51.9
      nodosum —*see also* subcategory M14.8-•
        L52
    gout —*see* Gout
    helminthiasis NEC —*see also* category M01
      B83.9
    hemochromatosis —*see also* subcategory
      M14.8-• E83.118
    hemoglobinopathy NEC D58.2 [M36.3]
    hemophilia NEC D66 [M36.2]
    Hemophilus influenzae M00.8-• [B96.3]
    Henoch(-Schönlein) purpura D69.0 [M36.4]
    hyperparathyroidism NEC —*see also*
      subcategory M14.8-• E21.3
    hypersensitivity reaction NEC T78.49
      [M36.4]
    hypogammaglobulinemia —*see also*
      subcategory M14.8-• D80.1
    hypothyroidism NEC —*see also*
      subcategory M14.8-• E03.9
    infection —*see* Arthritis, pyogenic or
      pyemic
      spine —*see* Spondylopathy, infective
    infectious disease NEC —*see* category M01

Arthritis, arthritic *(Continued)*
  in *(Continued)*
    leprosy —*see also* category M01 A30.9
    leukemia NEC C95.9-● *[M36.1]*
    lipoid dermatoarthritis E78.81
    Lyme disease A69.23
    Mediterranean fever, familial —*see also*
      subcategory M14.8-● M04.1
    Meningococcus A39.83
    metabolic disorder NEC —*see also*
      subcategory M14.8-● E88.9
    multiple myelomatosis C90.0-● *[M36.1]*
    mumps B26.85
    mycosis NEC —*see also* category M01 B49
    myelomatosis (multiple) C90.0-● *[M36.1]*
    neurological disorder NEC G98.0
    ochronosis —*see also* subcategory M14.8-●
      E70.29
    O'nyong-nyong —*see also* category M01
      A92.1
    parasitic disease NEC —*see also* category
      M01 B89
    paratyphoid fever —*see also* category M01
      A01.4
    Pseudomonas —*see* Arthritis, pyogenic,
      bacterial NEC
    psoriasis L40.50
    pyogenic organism NEC —*see* Arthritis,
      pyogenic, bacterial NEC
    Reiter's disease —*see* Reiter's disease
    respiratory disorder NEC —*see also*
      subcategory M14.8-● J98.9
    reticulosis, malignant —*see also*
      subcategory M14.8-● C86.0
    rubella B06.82
    Salmonella (arizonae) (cholerae-suis)
      (enteritidis) (typhimurium)
      A02.23
    sarcoidosis D86.86
    specified bacteria NEC —*see* Arthritis,
      pyogenic, bacterial NEC
    sporotrichosis B42.82
    syringomyelia G95.0
    thalassemia NEC D56.9 *[M36.3]*
    tuberculosis —*see* Tuberculosis, arthritis
    typhoid fever A01.04
    urethritis, Reiter's —*see* Reiter's disease
    viral disease NEC —*see also* category M01
      B34.9
  infectious or infective —*see also* Arthritis,
    pyogenic or pyemic
    spine —*see* Spondylopathy, infective
  juvenile M08.90
    with systemic onset —*see* Still's disease
    ankle M08.97-●
    elbow M08.92-●
    foot joint M08.97-●
    hand joint M08.94-●
    hip M08.95-●
    knee M08.96-●
    multiple site M08.99
    pauciarticular M08.40
      ankle M08.47-●
      elbow M08.42-●
      foot joint M08.47-●
      hand joint M08.44-●
      hip M08.45-●
      knee M08.46-●
      shoulder M08.41-●
      specified site NEC M08.4A
      vertebrae M08.48
      wrist M08.43-●
    psoriatic L40.54
    rheumatoid —*see* Arthritis, rheumatoid,
      juvenile
    shoulder M08.91-●
    specified site NEC M08.9A
    specified type NEC M08.80
      ankle M08.87-●
      elbow M08.82-●
      foot joint M08.87-●

Arthritis, arthritic *(Continued)*
  juvenile *(Continued)*
    specified type NEC *(Continued)*
      hand joint M08.84-●
      hip M08.85-●
      knee M08.86-●
      multiple site M08.89
      shoulder M08.81-●
      specified joint NEC M08.88
      vertebrae M08.88
      wrist M08.83-●
    vertebra M08.98
    wrist M08.93-●
  meaning osteoarthritis —*see* Osteoarthritis
  meningococcal A39.83
  menopausal (any site) NEC —*see* Arthritis,
    specified form NEC
  mutilans (psoriatic) L40.52
  mycotic NEC —*see also* category M01 B49
  neuropathic (Charcot) —*see* Arthropathy,
    neuropathic
    diabetic —*see* Diabetes, arthropathy,
      neuropathic
    nonsyphilitic NEC G98.0
    syringomyelic G95.0
  ochronotic —*see also* subcategory M14.8-●
    E70.29
  palindromic (any site) —*see* Rheumatism,
    palindromic
  pneumococcal M00.10
    ankle M00.17-●
    elbow M00.12-●
    foot joint —*see* Arthritis, pneumococcal,
      ankle
    hand joint M00.14-●
    hip M00.15-●
    knee M00.16-●
    multiple site M00.19
    shoulder M00.11-●
    vertebra M00.18
    wrist M00.13-●
  postdysenteric —*see* Arthropathy,
    postdysenteric
  postmeningococcal A39.84
  postrheumatic, chronic —*see* Arthropathy,
    postrheumatic, chronic
  primary progressive —*see also* Arthritis,
    specified form NEC
    spine —*see* Spondylitis, ankylosing
  psoriatic L40.50
  purulent (any site except spine) —*see*
    Arthritis, pyogenic or pyemic
    spine —*see* Spondylopathy, infective
  pyogenic or pyemic (any site except spine)
    M00.9
    bacterial NEC M00.80
      ankle M00.87-●
      elbow M00.82-●
      foot joint —*see* Arthritis, pyogenic,
        bacterial NEC, ankle
      hand joint M00.84-●
      hip M00.85-●
      knee M00.86-●
      multiple site M00.89
      shoulder M00.81-●
      vertebra M00.88
      wrist M00.83-●
    pneumococcal —*see* Arthritis,
      pneumococcal
    spine —*see* Spondylopathy, infective
    staphylococcal —*see* Arthritis,
      staphylococcal
    streptococcal —*see* Arthritis, streptococcal
      NEC
      pneumococcal —*see* Arthritis,
        pneumococcal
  reactive —*see* Reiter's disease
  rheumatic —*see also* Arthritis,
    rheumatoid
    acute or subacute —*see* Fever,
      rheumatic

Arthritis, arthritic *(Continued)*
  rheumatoid M06.9
    with
      carditis —*see* Rheumatoid, carditis
      endocarditis —*see* Rheumatoid, carditis
      heart involvement NEC —*see*
        Rheumatoid, carditis
      lung involvement —*see* Rheumatoid, lung
      myocarditis —*see* Rheumatoid, carditis
      myopathy —*see* Rheumatoid, myopathy
      pericarditis —*see* Rheumatoid, carditis
      polyneuropathy —*see* Rheumatoid,
        polyneuropathy
      rheumatoid factor —*see* Arthritis,
        rheumatoid, seropositive
      splenoadenomegaly and leukopenia —
        see Felty's syndrome
      vasculitis —*see* Rheumatoid, vasculitis
      visceral involvement NEC —*see*
        Rheumatoid, arthritis, with
        involvement of organs NEC
    juvenile (with or without rheumatoid
      factor) M08.00
      with systemic onset —*see* Still's disease
      ankle M08.07-●
      elbow M08.02-●
      foot joint M08.07-●
      hand joint M08.04-●
      hip M08.05-●
      knee M08.06-●
      multiple site M08.09
      shoulder M08.01-●
      specified site NEC M08.0A
      vertebra M08.08
      wrist M08.03-●
    seronegative M06.00
      ankle M06.07-●
      elbow M06.02-●
      foot joint M06.07-●
      hand joint M06.04-●
      hip M06.05-●
      knee M06.06-●
      multiple sites M06.09
      shoulder M06.01-●
      specified site NEC M06.0A
      vertebra M06.08
      wrist M06.03-●
    seropositive M05.9
      without organ involvement M05.70
        ankle M05.77-●
        elbow M05.72-●
        foot joint M05.77-●
        hand joint M05.74-●
        hip M05.75-●
        knee M05.76-●
        multiple sites M05.79
        shoulder M05.71-●
        specified site NEC M05.7A
        vertebra —*see* Spondylitis, ankylosing
        wrist M05.73-●
      specified NEC M05.80
        ankle M05.87-●
        elbow M05.82-●
        foot joint M05.87-●
        hand joint M05.84-●
        hip M05.85-●
        knee M05.86-●
        multiple sites M05.89
        specified site NEC M05.8A
        shoulder M05.81-●
        vertebra —*see* Spondylitis, ankylosing
        wrist M05.83-●
      specified type NEC M06.80
        ankle M06.87-●
        elbow M06.82-●
        foot joint M06.87-●
        hand joint M06.84-●
        hip M06.85-●
        knee M06.86-●
        multiple site M06.89
        shoulder M06.81-●

▶ New   ⇒ Revised   ~~deleted~~ Deleted   ● Use Additional Character(s)

Arthritis, arthritic *(Continued)*
  rheumatoid *(Continued)*
    specified type NEC *(Continued)*
      specified site NEC M06.8A
      vertebra M06.88
      wrist M06.83-●
    spine —*see* Spondylitis, ankylosing
  rubella B06.82
  scorbutic —*see also* subcategory M14.8-● E54
  senile or senescent —*see* Osteoarthritis
  septic (any site except spine) —*see* Arthritis,
    pyogenic or pyemic
    spine —*see* Spondylopathy, infective
  serum (nontherapeutic) (therapeutic) —*see*
    Arthropathy, postimmunization
  specified form NEC M13.80
    ankle M13.87-●
    elbow M13.82-●
    foot joint M13.87-●
    hand joint M13.84-●
    hip M13.85-●
    knee M13.86-●
    multiple site M13.89
    shoulder M13.81-●
    specified joint NEC M13.88
    wrist M13.83-●
  spine —*see also* Spondylosis
    infectious or infective NEC —*see*
      Spondylopathy, infective
    Marie-Strümpell —*see* Spondylitis,
      ankylosing
    pyogenic —*see* Spondylopathy, infective
    rheumatoid —*see* Spondylitis, ankylosing
    traumatic (old) —*see* Spondylopathy,
      traumatic
    tuberculous A18.01
  staphylococcal M00.00
    ankle M00.07-●
    elbow M00.02 ●
    foot joint —*see* Arthritis, staphylococcal,
      ankle
    hand joint M00.04-●
    hip M00.05-●
    knee M00.06-●
    multiple site M00.09
    shoulder M00.01-●
    vertebra M00.08
    wrist M00.03-●
  streptococcal NEC M00.20
    ankle M00.27-●
    elbow M00.22-●
    foot joint —*see* Arthritis, streptococcal, ankle
    hand joint M00.24-●
    hip M00.25-●
    knee M00.26-●
    multiple site M00.29
    shoulder M00.21-●
    vertebra M00.28
    wrist M00.23-●
  suppurative —*see* Arthritis, pyogenic or
    pyemic
  syphilitic (late) A52.16
    congenital A50.55 *[M12.80]*
  syphilitica deformans (Charcot) A52.16
  temporomandibular joint M26.65-●
  toxic of menopause (any site) —*see* Arthritis,
    specified form NEC
  transient —*see* Arthropathy, specified form
    NEC
  traumatic (chronic) —*see* Arthropathy,
    traumatic
  tuberculous A18.02
    spine A18.01
  uratic —*see* Gout
  urethritica (Reiter's) —*see* Reiter's disease
  vertebral —*see* Spondylopathy, inflammatory
  villous (any site) —*see* Arthropathy, specified
    form NEC
Arthrocele —*see* Effusion, joint
Arthrodesis status Z98.1
Arthrodynia —*see also* Pain, joint

Arthrodysplasia Q74.9
Arthrofibrosis, joint —*see* Ankylosis
Arthrogryposis (congenital) Q68.8
  multiplex congenita Q74.3
Arthrokatadysis M24.7
Arthropathy (*see also* Arthritis) M12.9
  Charcot's —*see* Arthropathy, neuropathic
    diabetic —*see* Diabetes, arthropathy,
      neuropathic
    syringomyelic G95.0
  cricoarytenoid J38.7
  crystal(-induced) —*see* Arthritis, in, crystals
  diabetic NEC —*see* Diabetes, arthropathy
  distal interphalangeal, psoriatic L40.51
  enteropathic M07.60
    ankle M07.67-●
    elbow M07.62-●
    foot joint M07.67-●
    hand joint M07.64-●
    hip M07.65-●
    knee M07.66-●
    multiple site M07.69
    shoulder M07.61-●
    vertebra M07.68
    wrist M07.63-●
  ▶ facet joint (*see also* Spondylosis) M47.819
  following intestinal bypass M02.00
    ankle M02.07-●
    elbow M02.02-●
    foot joint M02.07-●
    hand joint M02.04-●
    hip M02.05-●
    knee M02.06-●
    multiple site M02.09
    shoulder M02.01-●
    vertebra M02.08
    wrist M02.03-●
  gouty —*see also* Gout
    in (due to)
      Lesch-Nyhan syndrome E79.1 *[M14.8-●]*
      sickle-cell disorders D57-● *[M14.8-●]*
  hemophilic NEC D66 *[M36.2]*
    in (due to)
      hyperparathyroidism NEC E21.3
        [M14.8-●]
      metabolic disease NOS E88.9 *[M14.8-●]*
  in (due to)
    acromegaly E22.0 *[M14.8-●]*
    amyloidosis E85.4 *[M14.8-●]*
    blood disorder NOS D75.9 *[M36.3]*
    diabetes —*see* Diabetes, arthropathy
    endocrine disease NOS E34.9 *[M14.8 ●]*
    erythema
      multiforme L51.9 *[M14.8-●]*
      nodosum L52 *[M14.8-●]*
  hemochromatosis E83.118 *[M14.8-●]*
    hemoglobinopathy NEC D58.2 *[M36.3]*
    hemophilia NEC D66 *[M36.2]*
    Henoch-Schönlein purpura D69.0 *[M36.4]*
    hyperthyroidism E05.90 *[M14.8-●]*
    hypothyroidism E03.9 *[M14.8-●]*
    infective endocarditis I33.0 *[M12.80]*
    leukemia NEC C95.9-● *[M36.1]*
    malignant histiocytosis C96.A *[M36.1]*
    metabolic disease NOS E88.9 *[M14.8-●]*
    multiple myeloma C90.0-● *[M36.1]*
    neoplastic disease NOS (*see also* Neoplasm)
      D49.9 *[M36.1]*
    nutritional deficiency —*see also*
      subcategory M14.8-● E63.9
    psoriasis NOS L40.50
    sarcoidosis D86.86
    syphilis (late) A52.77
      congenital A50.55 *[M12.80]*
    thyrotoxicosis —*see also* subcategory
      M14.8-● E05.90
    ulcerative colitis K51.90 *[M07.60]*
    viral hepatitis (postinfectious) NEC B19.9
      [M12.80]
    Whipple's disease —*see also* subcategory
      M14.8-● K90.81

Arthropathy *(Continued)*
  Jaccoud —*see* Arthropathy, postrheumatic,
    chronic
  juvenile —*see* Arthritis, juvenile
    psoriatic L40.54
  mutilans (psoriatic) L40.52
  neuropathic (Charcot) M14.60
    ankle M14.67-●
    diabetic —*see* Diabetes, arthropathy,
      neuropathic
    elbow M14.62-●
    foot joint M14.67-●
    hand joint M14.64-●
    hip M14.65-●
    knee M14.66-●
    multiple site M14.69
    nonsyphilitic NEC G98.0
    shoulder M14.61-●
    syringomyelic G95.0
    vertebra M14.68
    wrist M14.63-●
  osteopulmonary —*see* Osteoarthropathy,
    hypertrophic, specified NEC
  postdysenteric M02.10
    ankle M02.17-●
    elbow M02.12-●
    foot joint M02.17-●
    hand joint M02.14-●
    hip M02.15-●
    knee M02.16-●
    multiple site M02.19
    shoulder M02.11-●
    vertebra M02.18
    wrist M02.13-●
  postimmunization M02.20
    ankle M02.27-●
    elbow M02.22-●
    foot joint M02.27-●
    hand joint M02.24-●
    hip M02.25-●
    knee M02.26-●
    multiple site M02.29
    shoulder M02.21-●
    vertebra M02.28
    wrist M02.23-●
  postinfectious NEC B99 *[M12.80]*
    in (due to)
      enteritis due to Yersinia enterocolitica
        A04.6 *[M12.80]*
      syphilis A52.77
      viral hepatitis NEC B19.9 *[M12.80]*
  postrheumatic, chronic (Jaccoud)
    M12.00
    ankle M12.07-●
    elbow M12.02-●
    foot joint M12.07-●
    hand joint M12.04-●
    hip M12.05-●
    knee M12.06-●
    multiple site M12.09
    shoulder M12.01-●
    specified joint NEC M12.08
    vertebrae M12.08
    wrist M12.03-●
  psoriatic NEC L40.59
    interphalangeal, distal L40.51
  reactive M02.9
    in (due to)
      infective endocarditis I33.0
        [M02.9]
    specified type NEC M02.80
      ankle M02.87-●
      elbow M02.82-●
      foot joint M02.87-●
      hand joint M02.84-●
      hip M02.85-●
      knee M02.86-●
      multiple site M02.89
      shoulder M02.81-●
      vertebra M02.88
      wrist M02.83-●

Arthropathy (Continued)
  specified form NEC M12.80
    ankle M12.87-●
    elbow M12.82-●
    foot joint M12.87-●
    hand joint M12.84-●
    hip M12.85-●
    knee M12.86-●
    multiple site M12.89
    shoulder M12.81-●
    specified joint NEC M12.88
    vertebrae M12.88
    wrist M12.83-●
  syringomyelic G95.0
  tabes dorsalis A52.16
  tabetic A52.16
  temporomandibular joint M26.65-●
  transient —see Arthropathy, specified form
      NEC
  traumatic M12.50
    ankle M12.57-●
    elbow M12.52-●
    foot joint M12.57-●
    hand joint M12.54-●
    hip M12.55-●
    knee M12.56-●
    multiple site M12.59
    shoulder M12.51-●
    specified joint NEC M12.58
    vertebrae M12.58
    wrist M12.53-●
Arthropyosis —see Arthritis, pyogenic or
    pyemic
Arthrosis (deformans) (degenerative)
    (localized) —see also Osteoarthritis
    M19.90
  spine —see Spondylosis
Arthus' phenomenon or reaction T78.41
  due to
    drug —see Table of Drugs and Chemicals,
        by drug
Articular —see condition
Articulation, reverse (teeth) M26.24
Artificial
  insemination complication —see
      Complications, artificial, fertilization
  opening status (functioning) (without
      complication) Z93.9
    anus (colostomy) Z93.3
    colostomy Z93.3
    cystostomy Z93.50
      appendico-vesicostomy Z93.52
      cutaneous Z93.51
      specified NEC Z93.59
    enterostomy Z93.4
    gastrostomy Z93.1
    ileostomy Z93.2
    intestinal tract NEC Z93.4
    jejunostomy Z93.4
    nephrostomy Z93.6
    specified site NEC Z93.8
    tracheostomy Z93.0
    ureterostomy Z93.6
    urethrostomy Z93.6
    urinary tract NEC Z93.6
    vagina Z93.8
  vagina status Z93.8
Arytenoid —see condition
Asbestosis (occupational) J61
ASC-H (atypical squamous cells cannot exclude
    high grade squamous intraepithelial lesion
    on cytologic smear)
  anus R85.611
  cervix R87.611
  vagina R87.621
ASC-US (atypical squamous cells of
    undetermined significance on cytologic
    smear)
  anus R85.610
  cervix R87.610
  vagina R87.620

Ascariasis B77.9
  with
    complications NEC B77.89
    intestinal complications B77.0
    pneumonia, pneumonitis B77.81
Ascaridosis, ascaridiasis —see Ascariasis
Ascaris (infection) (infestation)
    (lumbricoides) —see Ascariasis
Ascending —see condition
Aschoff's bodies —see Myocarditis, rheumatic
Ascites (abdominal) R18.8
  cardiac —see also Failure, heart, right I50.810
  chylous (nonfilarial) I89.8
    filarial —see Infestation, filarial
  due to
    cirrhosis, alcoholic K70.31
    hepatitis
      alcoholic K70.11
      chronic active K71.51
    S. japonicum B65.2
  heart —see also Failure, heart, right I50.810
  malignant R18.0
  pseudochylous R18.8
  syphilitic A52.74
  tuberculous A18.31
Aseptic —see condition
Asherman's syndrome N85.6
Asialia K11.7
Asiatic cholera —see Cholera
Asimultagnosia (simultanagnosia) R48.3
Askin's tumor —see Neoplasm, connective
    tissue, malignant
Asocial personality F60.2
Asomatognosia R41.4
Aspartylglucosaminuria E77.1
Asperger's disease or syndrome F84.5
Aspergilloma —see Aspergillosis
Aspergillosis (with pneumonia) B44.9
  bronchopulmonary, allergic B44.81
  disseminated B44.7
  generalized B44.7
  pulmonary NEC B44.1
    allergic B44.81
    invasive B44.0
  specified NEC B44.89
  tonsillar B44.2
Aspergillus (flavus) (fumigatus) (infection)
    (terreus) —see Aspergillosis
Aspermatogenesis —see Azoospermia
Aspermia (testis) —see Azoospermia
Asphyxia, asphyxiation (by) R09.01
  antenatal P84
  birth P84
  bunny bag —see Asphyxia, due to,
      mechanical threat to breathing, trapped
      in bed clothes
  crushing S28.0
  drowning T75.1
  gas, fumes, or vapor —see Table of Drugs and
      Chemicals
  inhalation —see Inhalation
  intrauterine P84
  local I73.00
    with gangrene I73.01
  mucus —see also Foreign body, respiratory
      tract, causing asphyxia
  newborn P84
  pathological R09.01
  postnatal P84
    mechanical —see Asphyxia, due to,
        mechanical threat to breathing
  prenatal P84
  reticularis R23.1
  strangulation —see Asphyxia, due to,
      mechanical threat to breathing
  submersion T75.1
  traumatic T71.9
    due to
      crushed chest S28.0
      foreign body (in) —see Foreign body,
          respiratory tract, causing asphyxia

Asphyxia, asphyxiation (Continued)
  traumatic (Continued)
    due to (Continued)
      low oxygen content of ambient air
          T71.20
        due to
          being trapped in
            low oxygen environment
                T71.29
            in car trunk T71.221
              circumstances undetermined
                  T71.224
              done with intent to harm by
                  another person T71.223
                self T71.222
            in refrigerator T71.231
              circumstances undetermined
                  T71.234
              done with intent to
                  harm by
                another person T71.233
                self T71.232
          cave-in T71.21
      mechanical threat to breathing
          (accidental) T71.191
        circumstances undetermined T71.194
        done with intent to harm by
            another person T71.193
          self T71.192
        hanging T71.161
          circumstances undetermined
              T71.164
          done with intent to harm by
              another person T71.163
            self T71.162
        plastic bag T71.121
          circumstances undetermined T71.124
          done with intent to harm by
              another person T71.123
            self T71.122
        smothering
          in furniture T71.151
            circumstances undetermined
                T71.154
            done with intent to harm by
                another person T71.153
              self T71.152
          under
            another person's body T71.141
              circumstances undetermined
                  T71.144
              done with intent to harm
                  T71.143
            pillow T71.111
              circumstances undetermined
                  T71.114
              done with intent to harm by
                  another person T71.113
                self T71.112
        trapped in bed clothes T71.131
          circumstances undetermined
              T71.134
          done with intent to harm by
              another person T71.133
            self T71.132
  vomiting, vomitus —see Foreign body,
      respiratory tract, causing asphyxia
Aspiration
  amniotic (clear) fluid (newborn) P24.10
    with
      pneumonia (pneumonitis) P24.11
      respiratory symptoms P24.11
  blood
    newborn (without respiratory symptoms)
        P24.20
      with
        pneumonia (pneumonitis) P24.21
        respiratory symptoms P24.21
    specified age NEC —see Foreign body,
        respiratory tract
  bronchitis J69.0

▶ New   ⇒ Revised   ~~deleted~~ Deleted   ● Use Additional Character(s)

Aspiration *(Continued)*
⟹food or foreign body —*see* Foreign body,
   by site
  liquor (amnii) (newborn) P24.10
    with
      pneumonia (pneumonitis) P24.11
      respiratory symptoms P24.11
  meconium (newborn) (without respiratory
    symptoms) P24.00
    with
      pneumonitis (pneumonitis) P24.01
      respiratory symptoms P24.01
  milk (newborn) (without respiratory
    symptoms) P24.30
    with
      pneumonia (pneumonitis) P24.31
      respiratory symptoms P24.31
    specified age NEC —*see* Foreign body,
      respiratory tract
  mucus —*see also* Foreign body, by site,
    causing asphyxia
    newborn P24.10
      with
        pneumonia (pneumonitis) P24.11
        respiratory symptoms P24.11
  neonatal P24.9
    specific NEC (without respiratory
      symptoms) P24.80
    with
      pneumonia (pneumonitis) P24.81
      respiratory symptoms P24.81
  newborn P24.9
    specific NEC (without respiratory
      symptoms) P24.80
    with
      pneumonia (pneumonitis) P24.81
      respiratory symptoms P24.81
  pneumonia J69.0
  pneumonitis J69.0
  syndrome of newborn —*see* Aspiration, by
    substance, with pneumonia
  vernix caseosa (newborn) P24.80
    with
      pneumonia (pneumonitis) P24.81
      respiratory symptoms P24.81
  vomitus —*see also* Foreign body, respiratory
    tract
    newborn (without respiratory symptoms)
      P24.30
    with
      pneumonia (pneumonitis) P24.31
      respiratory symptoms P24.31
Asplenia (congenital) Q89.01
  postsurgical Z90.81
Assam fever B55.0
Assault, sexual —*see* Maltreatment
Assmann's focus NEC A15.0
Astasia (-abasia) (hysterical) F44.4
Asteatosis cutis L85.3
Astereognosia, astereognosis R48.1
Asterixis R27.8
  in liver disease K71.3
Asteroid hyalitis —*see* Deposit, crystalline
Asthenia, asthenic R53.1
  cardiac —*see also* Failure, heart I50.9
    psychogenic F45.8
  cardiovascular —*see also* Failure, heart I50.9
    psychogenic F45.8
  heart —*see also* Failure, heart I50.9
    psychogenic F45.8
  hysterical F44.4
  myocardial —*see also* Failure, heart I50.9
    psychogenic F45.8
  nervous F48.8
  neurocirculatory F45.8
  neurotic F48.8
  psychogenic F48.8
  psychoneurotic F48.8
  psychophysiologic F48.8
  reaction (psychophysiologic) F48.8
  senile R54

Asthenopia —*see also* Discomfort, visual
  hysterical F44.6
  psychogenic F44.6
Asthenospermia —*see* Abnormal, specimen,
  male genital organs
Asthma, asthmatic (bronchial) (catarrh)
  (spasmodic) J45.909
  with
    chronic obstructive bronchitis J44.9
      with
        acute lower respiratory infection
          J44.0
        exacerbation (acute) J44.1
    chronic obstructive pulmonary disease
      J44.9
      with
        acute lower respiratory infection
          J44.0
        exacerbation (acute) J44.1
    exacerbation (acute) J45.901
  hay fever —*see* Asthma, allergic extrinsic
  rhinitis, allergic —*see* Asthma, allergic
    extrinsic
    status asthmaticus J45.902
  allergic extrinsic J45.909
    with
      exacerbation (acute) J45.901
      status asthmaticus J45.902
  atopic —*see* Asthma, allergic extrinsic
  cardiac —*see* Failure, ventricular, left
  cardiobronchial I50.1
  childhood J45.909
    with
      exacerbation (acute) J45.901
      status asthmaticus J45.902
  chronic obstructive J44.9
    with
      acute lower respiratory infection J44.0
      exacerbation (acute) J44.1
  collier's J60
  cough variant J45.991
  detergent J69.8
  due to
    detergent J69.8
    inhalation of fumes J68.3
  eosinophilic J82.83
  extrinsic, allergic —*see* Asthma, allergic
    extrinsic
  grinder's J62.8
  hay —*see* Asthma, allergic extrinsic
  heart I50.1
  idiosyncratic —*see* Asthma, nonallergic
  intermittent (mild) J45.20
    with
      exacerbation (acute) J45.21
      status asthmaticus J45.22
  intrinsic, nonallergic —*see* Asthma,
    nonallergic
  Kopp's E32.8
  late-onset J45.909
    with
      exacerbation (acute) J45.901
      status asthmaticus J45.902
  mild intermittent J45.20
    with
      exacerbation (acute) J45.21
      status asthmaticus J45.22
  mild persistent J45.30
    with
      exacerbation (acute) J45.31
      status asthmaticus J45.32
  Millar's (laryngismus stridulus) J38.5
  miner's J60
  mixed J45.909
    with
      exacerbation (acute) J45.901
      status asthmaticus J45.902
  moderate persistent J45.40
    with
      exacerbation (acute) J45.41
      status asthmaticus J45.42

Asthma, asthmatic *(Continued)*
  nervous —*see* Asthma, nonallergic
  nonallergic (intrinsic) J45.909
    with
      exacerbation (acute) J45.901
      status asthmaticus J45.902
    persistent
      mild J45.30
        with
          exacerbation (acute) J45.31
          status asthmaticus J45.32
      moderate J45.40
        with
          exacerbation (acute) J45.41
          status asthmaticus J45.42
      severe J45.50
        with
          exacerbation (acute) J45.51
          status asthmaticus J45.52
  platinum J45.998
  pneumoconiotic NEC J64
  potter's J62.8
  predominantly allergic J45.909
  psychogenic F54
  pulmonary eosinophilic J82.83
  red cedar J67.8
  Rostan's I50.1
  sandblaster's J62.8
  sequoiosis J67.8
  severe persistent J45.50
    with
      exacerbation (acute) J45.51
      status asthmaticus J45.52
  specified NEC J45.998
  stonemason's J62.8
  thymic E32.8
  tuberculous —*see* Tuberculosis, pulmonary
  Wichmann's (laryngismus stridulus) J38.5
  wood J67.8
Astigmatism (compound) (congenital)
  H52.20-●
  irregular H52.21-●
  regular H52.22-●
Astraphobia F40.220
Astroblastoma
  specified site —*see* Neoplasm, malignant, by
    site
  unspecified site C71.9
Astrocytoma (cystic)
  anaplastic
    specified site —*see* Neoplasm, malignant,
      by site
    unspecified site C71.9
  fibrillary
    specified site —*see* Neoplasm, malignant,
      by site
    unspecified site C71.9
  fibrous
    specified site —*see* Neoplasm, malignant,
      by site
    unspecified site C71.9
  gemistocytic
    specified site —*see* Neoplasm, malignant,
      by site
    unspecified site C71.9
  juvenile
    specified site —*see* Neoplasm, malignant,
      by site
    unspecified site C71.9
  pilocytic
    specified site —*see* Neoplasm, malignant,
      by site
    unspecified site C71.9
  piloid
    specified site —*see* Neoplasm, malignant,
      by site
    unspecified site C71.9
  protoplasmic
    specified site —*see* Neoplasm, malignant,
      by site
    unspecified site C71.9

Astrocytoma (Continued)
  specified site NEC —see Neoplasm,
      malignant, by site
  subependymal D43.2
    giant cell
      specified site —see Neoplasm, uncertain
          behavior, by site
      unspecified site D43.2
    specified site —see Neoplasm, uncertain
        behavior, by site
    unspecified site D43.2
  unspecified site C71.9
Astroglioma
  specified site —see Neoplasm, malignant, by
      site
  unspecified site C71.9
Asymbolia R48.8
Asymmetry —see also Distortion
  between native and reconstructed breast N65.1
  face Q67.0
  jaw (lower) —see Anomaly, dentofacial, jaw-
      cranial base relationship, asymmetry
Asynergia, asynergy R27.8
  ventricular I51.89
Asystole (heart) —see Arrest, cardiac
At risk
  for
    dental caries Z91.849
      high Z91.843
      low Z91.841
      moderate Z91.842
    falling Z91.81
Ataxia, ataxy, ataxic R27.0
  acute R27.8
  autosomal recessive Friedreich G11.11
  brain (hereditary) G11.9
  cerebellar (hereditary) G11.9
    with defective DNA repair G11.3
      alcoholic G31.2
      early-onset G11.10
        with
          essential tremor G11.19
          myoclonus [Hunt's ataxia] G11.19
          retained tendon reflexes G11.19
        in
          alcoholism G31.2
          myxedema E03.9 [G13.2]
          neoplastic disease —see also Neoplasm
              D49.9 [G32.81]
          specified disease NEC G32.81
      late-onset (Marie's) G11.2
  cerebral (hereditary) G11.9
  congenital nonprogressive G11.0
  family, familial —see Ataxia, hereditary
  following
    cerebrovascular disease I69.993
      cerebral infarction I69.393
      intracerebral hemorrhage I69.193
      nontraumatic intracranial hemorrhage
          NEC I69.293
      specified disease NEC I69.893
      subarachnoid hemorrhage I69.093
  Friedreich's (heredofamilial) (cerebellar)
      (spinal) G11.11
  gait R26.0
    hysterical F44.4
  general R27.8
  gluten M35.9 [G32.81]
    with celiac disease K90.0 [G32.81]
  hereditary G11.9
    with neuropathy G60.2
    cerebellar —see Ataxia, cerebellar
    spastic G11.4
    specified NEC G11.8
    spinal (Friedreich's) G11.11
  heredofamilial —see Ataxia, hereditary
  Hunt's G11.19
  hysterical F44.4
  locomotor (progressive) (syphilitic) (partial)
      (spastic) A52.11
    diabetic —see Diabetes, ataxia

Ataxia, ataxy, ataxic (Continued)
  Marie's (cerebellar) (heredofamilial)
      (late- onset) G11.2
  nonorganic origin F44.4
  nonprogressive, congenital G11.0
  psychogenic F44.4
  Roussy-Lévy G60.0
  Sanger-Brown's (hereditary) G11.2
  spastic hereditary G11.4
  spinal
    hereditary (Friedreich's) G11.11
    progressive (syphilitic) A52.11
  spinocerebellar, X-linked recessive
      G11.19
  telangiectasia (Louis-Bar) G11.3
Ataxia-telangiectasia (Louis-Bar) G11.3
Atelectasis (massive) (partial) (pressure)
    (pulmonary) J98.11
  newborn P28.10
    due to resorption P28.11
    partial P28.19
    primary P28.0
    secondary P28.19
  primary (newborn) P28.0
  tuberculous —see Tuberculosis, pulmonary
Atelocardia Q24.9
Atelomyelia Q06.1
Atheroembolism
  of
    extremities
      lower I75.02-●
      upper I75.01-●
    kidney I75.81
    specified NEC I75.89
Atheroma, atheromatous —see also
    Arteriosclerosis I70.90
  aorta, aortic I70.0
    valve —see also Endocarditis,
        aortic I35.8
  aorto-iliac I70.0
  artery —see Arteriosclerosis
  basilar (artery) I67.2
  carotid (artery) (common) (internal)
      I67.2
  cerebral (arteries) I67.2
  coronary (artery) I25.10
    with angina pectoris —see Arteriosclerosis,
        coronary (artery)
  degeneration —see Arteriosclerosis
  heart, cardiac —see Disease, heart, ischemic,
      atherosclerotic
  mitral (valve) I34.8
  myocardium, myocardial —see Disease, heart,
      ischemic, atherosclerotic
  pulmonary valve (heart) —see also
      Endocarditis, pulmonary I37.8
  tricuspid (heart) (valve) I36.8
  valve, valvular —see Endocarditis
  vertebral (artery) I67.2
Atheromatosis —see Arteriosclerosis
Atherosclerosis —see also Arteriosclerosis
  coronary
    artery I25.10
      with angina pectoris —see
          Arteriosclerosis, coronary (artery),
      due to
        calcified coronary lesion (severely)
            I25.84
        lipid rich plaque I25.83
    transplanted heart I25.811
      bypass graft I25.812
        with angina pectoris —see
            Arteriosclerosis, coronary (artery)
      native coronary artery I25.811
        with angina pectoris —see
            Arteriosclerosis, coronary (artery)
Athetosis (acquired) R25.8
  bilateral (congenital) G80.3
  congenital (bilateral) (double) G80.3
  double (congenital) G80.3
  unilateral R25.8

Athlete's
  foot B35.3
  heart I51.7
Athrepsia E41
Athyrea (acquired) —see also Hypothyroidism
  congenital E03.1
Atonia, atony, atonic
  bladder (sphincter) (neurogenic) N31.2
  capillary I78.8
  cecum K59.89
    psychogenic F45.8
  colon —see Atony, intestine
  congenital P94.2
➡ esophagus K22.89
  intestine K59.89
    psychogenic F45.8
  stomach K31.89
    neurotic or psychogenic F45.8
  uterus (during labor) O62.2
    with hemorrhage (postpartum) O72.1
    postpartum (with hemorrhage) O72.1
      without hemorrhage O75.89
Atopy —see History, allergy
Atransferrinemia, congenital E88.09
Atresia, atretic
  alimentary organ or tract NEC Q45.8
    upper Q40.8
  ani, anus, anal (canal) Q42.3
    with fistula Q42.2
  aorta (ring) Q25.29
  aortic (orifice) (valve) Q23.0
    arch Q25.21
    congenital with hypoplasia of ascending
        aorta and defective development of
        left ventricle (with mitral stenosis)
        Q23.4
    in hypoplastic left heart syndrome Q23.4
  aqueduct of Sylvius Q03.0
    with spina bifida —see Spina bifida, with
        hydrocephalus
  artery NEC Q27.8
    cerebral Q28.3
    coronary Q24.5
    digestive system Q27.8
    eye Q15.8
    lower limb Q27.8
    pulmonary Q25.5
    specified site NEC Q27.8
    umbilical Q27.0
    upper limb Q27.8
  auditory canal (external) Q16.1
  bile duct (common) (congenital) (hepatic)
      Q44.2
    acquired —see Obstruction, bile duct
  bladder (neck) Q64.39
    obstruction Q64.31
  bronchus Q32.4
  cecum Q42.8
  cervix (acquired) N88.2
    congenital Q51.828
    in pregnancy or childbirth —see Anomaly,
        cervix, in pregnancy or childbirth
        causing obstructed labor O65.5
  choana Q30.0
  colon Q42.9
    specified NEC Q42.8
  common duct Q44.2
  cricoid cartilage Q31.8
  cystic duct Q44.2
    acquired K82.8
      with obstruction K82.0
  digestive organs NEC Q45.8
  duodenum Q41.0
  ear canal Q16.1
  ejaculatory duct Q55.4
  epiglottis Q31.8
  esophagus Q39.0
    with tracheoesophageal fistula Q39.1
  eustachian tube Q17.8
  fallopian tube (congenital) Q50.6
    acquired N97.1

▶ New   ⇒ Revised   ~~deleted~~ Deleted   ● Use Additional Character(s)

Atresia, atretic *(Continued)*
  follicular cyst N83.0-●
  foramen of
    Luschka Q03.1
      with spina bifida —*see* Spina bifida, with
        hydrocephalus
    Magendie Q03.1
      with spina bifida —*see* Spina bifida, with
        hydrocephalus
  gallbladder Q44.1
  genital organ
    external
      female Q52.79
      male Q55.8
    internal
      female Q52.8
      male Q55.8
  glottis Q31.8
  gullet Q39.0
    with tracheoesophageal fistula Q39.1
  heart valve NEC Q24.8
    pulmonary Q22.0
    tricuspid Q22.4
  hymen Q52.3
    acquired (postinfective) N89.6
  ileum Q41.2
  intestine (small) Q41.9
    large Q42.9
      specified NEC Q42.8
  iris, filtration angle Q15.0
  jejunum Q41.1
  lacrimal apparatus Q10.4
  larynx Q31.8
  meatus urinarius Q64.33
  mitral valve Q23.2
    in hypoplastic left heart syndrome Q23.4
  nares (anterior) (posterior) Q30.0
  nasopharynx Q34.8
  nose, nostril Q30.0
    acquired J34.89
  organ or site NEC Q89.8
  osseous meatus (ear) Q16.1
  oviduct (congenital) Q50.6
    acquired N97.1
  parotid duct Q38.4
    acquired K11.8
  pulmonary (artery) Q25.5
    valve Q22.0
  pulmonic Q22.0
  pupil Q13.2
  rectum Q42.1
    with fistula Q42.0
  salivary duct Q38.4
    acquired K11.8
  sublingual duct Q38.4
    acquired K11.8
  submandibular duct Q38.4
    acquired K11.8
  submaxillary duct Q38.4
    acquired K11.8
  thyroid cartilage Q31.8
  trachea Q32.1
  tricuspid valve Q22.4
  ureter Q62.10
    pelvic junction Q62.11
    vesical orifice Q62.12
  ureteropelvic junction Q62.11
  ureterovesical orifice Q62.12
  urethra (valvular) Q64.39
    stricture Q64.32
  urinary tract NEC Q64.8
  uterus Q51.818
    acquired N85.8
  vagina (congenital) Q52.4
    acquired (postinfectional) (senile) N89.5
  vas deferens Q55.3
  vascular NEC Q27.8
    cerebral Q28.3
    digestive system Q27.8
    lower limb Q27.8
    specified site NEC Q27.8
    upper limb Q27.8

Atresia, atretic *(Continued)*
  vein NEC Q27.8
    digestive system Q27.8
    great Q26.8
    lower limb Q27.8
    portal Q26.5
    pulmonary Q26.4
      partial Q26.3
      total Q26.2
    specified site NEC Q27.8
    upper limb Q27.8
  vena cava (inferior) (superior) Q26.8
  vesicourethral orifice Q64.31
  vulva Q52.79
    acquired N90.5
Atrichia, atrichosis —*see* Alopecia
Atrophia —*see also* Atrophy
  cutis senilis L90.8
    due to radiation L57.8
  gyrata of choroid and retina H31.23
  senilis R54
    dermatological L90.8
      due to radiation (nonionizing) (solar)
        L57.8
  unguium L60.3
    congenita Q84.6
Atrophie blanche (en plaque) (de Milian) L95.0
Atrophoderma, atrophodermia (of) L90.9
  diffusum (idiopathic) L90.4
  maculatum L90.8
    et striatum L90.8
      due to syphilis A52.79
    syphilitic A51.39
  neuriticum L90.8
  Pasini and Pierini L90.3
  pigmentosum Q82.1
  reticulatum symmetricum faciei L66.4
  senile L90.8
    due to radiation (nonionizing) (solar) L57.8
  vermiculata (cheeks) L66.4
Atrophy, atrophic (of)
  adrenal (capsule) (gland) E27.49
    primary (autoimmune) E27.1
  alveolar process or ridge (edentulous) K08.20
  anal sphincter (disuse) N81.84
  appendix K38.8
  arteriosclerotic —*see* Arteriosclerosis
  bile duct (common) (hepatic) K83.8
  bladder N32.89
    neurogenic N31.8
  blanche (en plaque) (of Milian) L95.0
  bone (senile) NEC —*see also* Disorder, bone,
    specified type NEC
    due to
      tabes dorsalis (neurogenic) A52.11
  brain (cortex) (progressive) G31.9
    frontotemporal circumscribed G31.01
      [F02.80]
      with behavioral disturbance G31.01
        [F02.81]
    senile NEC G31.1
  breast N64.2
    obstetric —*see* Disorder, breast, specified
      type NEC
  buccal cavity K13.79
  cardiac —*see* Degeneration, myocardial
  cartilage (infectional) (joint) —*see* Disorder,
    cartilage, specified NEC
  cerebellar —*see* Atrophy, brain
  cerebral —*see* Atrophy, brain
  cervix (mucosa) (senile) (uteri) N88.8
    menopausal N95.8
  Charcot-Marie-Tooth G60.0
  choroid (central) (macular) (myopic) (retina)
    H31.10-●
    diffuse secondary H31.12-●
    gyrate H31.23
    senile H31.11-●
  ciliary body —*see* Atrophy, iris
  conjunctiva (senile) H11.89
  corpus cavernosum N48.89

Atrophy, atrophic *(Continued)*
  cortical —*see* Atrophy, brain
  cystic duct K82.8
  Déjérine-Thomas G23.8
  disuse NEC —*see* Atrophy, muscle
  Duchenne-Aran G12.21
  ear H93.8-●
  edentulous alveolar ridge K08.20
  endometrium (senile) N85.8
    cervix N88.8
  enteric K63.89
  epididymis N50.89
  eyeball —*see* Disorder, globe, degenerated
    condition, atrophy
  eyelid (senile) —*see* Disorder, eyelid,
    degenerative
  facial (skin) L90.9
  fallopian tube (senile) N83.32-●
    with ovary N83.33-●
  fascioscapulohumeral (Landouzy-Déjérine)
    G71.02
  fatty, thymus (gland) E32.8
  gallbladder K82.8
  gastric K29.40
    with bleeding K29.41
  gastrointestinal K63.89
  glandular I89.8
  globe H44.52-●
  gum —*see* Recession, gingival
  hair L67.8
  heart (brown) —*see* Degeneration, myocardial
  hemifacial Q67.4
    Romberg G51.8
  infantile E41
    paralysis, acute —*see* Poliomyelitis,
      paralytic
  intestine K63.89
  iris (essential) (progressive) H21.26-●
    specified NEC H21.29
  kidney (senile) (terminal) —*see also* Sclerosis,
    renal N26.1
    congenital or infantile Q60.5
      bilateral Q60.4
      unilateral Q60.3
    hydronephrotic —*see* Hydronephrosis
  lacrimal gland (primary) H04.14-●
    secondary H04.15-●
  Landouzy-Déjérine G71.02
  laryngitis, infective J37.0
  larynx J38.7
  Leber's optic (hereditary) H47.22
  lip K13.0
  liver (yellow) K72.90
    with coma K72.91
    acute, subacute K72.00
      with coma K72.01
    chronic K72.10
      with coma K72.11
  lung (senile) J98.4
  macular (dermatological) L90.8
    syphilitic, skin A51.39
      striated A52.79
  mandible (edentulous) K08.20
    minimal K08.21
    moderate K08.22
    severe K08.23
  maxilla K08.20
    minimal K08.24
    moderate K08.25
    severe K08.26
  muscle, muscular (diffuse) (general)
    (idiopathic) (primary) M62.50
    ankle M62.57-●
    Duchenne-Aran G12.21
    foot M62.57-●
    forearm M62.53-●
    hand M62.54-●
    infantile spinal G12.0
    lower leg M62.56-●
    multiple sites M62.59
    myelopathic —*see* Atrophy, muscle, spinal

Atrophy, atrophic (Continued)
   muscle, muscular (Continued)
      myotonic G71.11
      neuritic G58.9
      neuropathic (peroneal) (progressive) G60.0
      pelvic (disuse) N81.84
      peroneal G60.0
      progressive (bulbar) G12.21
         adult G12.1
         infantile (spinal) G12.0
         spinal G12.25
            adult G12.1
            infantile G12.0
      pseudohypertrophic G71.02
      shoulder region M62.51-●
      specified site NEC M62.58
      spinal G12.9
         adult form G12.1
         Aran-Duchenne G12.21
         childhood form, type II G12.1
         distal G12.1
         hereditary NEC G12.1
         infantile, type I (Werdnig-Hoffmann)
            G12.0
         juvenile form, type III (Kugelberg-
            Welander) G12.1
         progressive G12.25
         scapuloperoneal form G12.1
         specified NEC G12.8
      syphilitic A52.78
      thigh M62.55-●
      upper arm M62.52-●
   myocardium —see Degeneration, myocardial
   myometrium (senile) N85.8
      cervix N88.8
   myopathic NEC —see Atrophy, muscle
   myotonia G71.11
   nail L60.3
   nasopharynx J31.1
   nerve —see also Disorder, nerve
      abducens —see Strabismus, paralytic, sixth
         nerve
      accessory G52.8
      acoustic or auditory —see subcategory
         H93.3
      cranial G52.9
         eighth (auditory) —see subcategory
            H93.3
         eleventh (accessory) G52.8
         fifth (trigeminal) G50.8
         first (olfactory) G52.0
         fourth (trochlear) —see Strabismus,
            paralytic, fourth nerve
         second (optic) H47.20
         sixth (abducens) —see Strabismus,
            paralytic, sixth nerve
         tenth (pneumogastric) (vagus) G52.2
         third (oculomotor) —see Strabismus,
            paralytic, third nerve
         twelfth (hypoglossal) G52.3
      hypoglossal G52.3
      oculomotor —see Strabismus, paralytic,
         third nerve
      olfactory G52.0
      optic (papillomacular bundle)
         syphilitic (late) A52.15
           congenital A50.44
      pneumogastric G52.2
      trigeminal G50.8
      trochlear —see Strabismus, paralytic,
         fourth nerve
      vagus (pneumogastric) G52.2
   neurogenic, bone, tabetic A52.11
   ⇒ nutritional E43
     ▶ with marasmus E41
   old age R54
   olivopontocerebellar G23.8
   optic (nerve) H47.20
      glaucomatous H47.23-●
      hereditary H47.22
      primary H47.21-●

Atrophy, atrophic (Continued)
   optic (Continued)
      specified type NEC H47.29-●
      syphilitic (late) A52.15
         congenital A50.44
   orbit H05.31-●
   ovary (senile) N83.31-●
      with fallopian tube N83.33-●
   oviduct (senile) —see Atrophy, fallopian tube
   palsy, diffuse (progressive) G12.22
   pancreas (duct) (senile) K86.89
   parotid gland K11.0
   pelvic muscle N81.84
   penis N48.89
   pharynx J39.2
   pluriglandular E31.8
      autoimmune E31.0
   polyarthritis M15.9
   prostate N42.89
   pseudohypertrophic (muscle) G71.02
   renal —see also Sclerosis, renal N26.1
   retina, retinal (postinfectional) H35.89
   rhinitis J31.0
   salivary gland K11.0
   scar L90.5
   sclerosis, lobar (of brain) G31.09 [F02.80]
      with behavioral disturbance G31.09 [F02.81]
   scrotum N50.89
   seminal vesicle N50.89
   senile R54
      due to radiation (nonionizing) (solar) L57.8
   skin (patches) (spots) L90.9
      degenerative (senile) L90.8
      due to radiation (nonionizing) (solar) L57.8
      senile L90.8
   spermatic cord N50.89
   spinal (acute) (cord) G95.89
      muscular —see Atrophy, muscle, spinal
      paralysis G12.20
         acute —see Poliomyelitis, paralytic
         meaning progressive muscular atrophy
            G12.25
   spine (column) —see Spondylopathy,
      specified NEC
   spleen (senile) D73.0
   stomach K29.40
      with bleeding K29.41
   striate (skin) L90.6
      syphilitic A52.79
   subcutaneous L90.9
   sublingual gland K11.0
   submandibular gland K11.0
   submaxillary gland K11.0
   Sudeck's —see Algoneurodystrophy
   suprarenal (capsule) (gland) E27.49
      primary E27.1
   systemic affecting central nervous system
      in
         myxedema E03.9 [G13.2]
         neoplastic disease —see also Neoplasm
            D49.9 [G13.1]
         specified disease NEC G13.8
   tarso-orbital fascia, congenital Q10.3
   testis N50.0
   thenar, partial —see Syndrome, carpal tunnel
   thymus (fatty) E32.8
   thyroid (gland) (acquired) E03.4
      with cretinism E03.1
      congenital (with myxedema) E03.1
   tongue (senile) K14.8
      papillae K14.4
   trachea J39.8
   tunica vaginalis N50.89
   turbinate J34.89
   tympanic membrane (nonflaccid) H73.82-●
      flaccid H73.81-●
   upper respiratory tract J39.8
   uterus, uterine (senile) N85.8
      cervix N88.8
      due to radiation (intended effect) N85.8
         adverse effect or misadventure N99.89

Atrophy, atrophic (Continued)
   vagina (senile) N95.2
   vas deferens N50.89
   vascular I99.8
   vertebra (senile) —see Spondylopathy,
      specified NEC
   vulva (senile) N90.5
   Werdnig-Hoffmann G12.0
   yellow —see Failure, hepatic
Attack, attacks
   with alteration of consciousness (with
      automatisms) —see Epilepsy,
      localization-related, symptomatic, with
      complex partial seizures
   without alteration of consciousness —
      see Epilepsy, localization-related,
      symptomatic, with simple partial
      seizures
   Adams-Stokes I45.9
   akinetic —see Epilepsy, generalized, specified
      NEC
   angina —see Angina
   atonic —see Epilepsy, generalized, specified
      NEC
   benign shuddering G25.83
   cataleptic —see Catalepsy
   coronary —see Infarct, myocardium
   cyanotic, newborn P28.2
   drop NEC R55
   epileptic —see Epilepsy
   heart —see infarct, myocardium
   hysterical F44.9
   jacksonian —see Epilepsy, localization-
      related, symptomatic, with simple
      partial seizures
   myocardium, myocardial —see Infarct,
      myocardium
   myoclonic —see Epilepsy, generalized,
      specified NEC
   panic F41.0
   psychomotor —see Epilepsy, localization-
      related, symptomatic, with complex
      partial seizures
   salaam —see Epilepsy, spasms
   schizophreniform, brief F23
   shuddering, benign G25.83
   Stokes-Adams I45.9
   syncope R55
   transient ischemic (TIA) G45.9
      specified NEC G45.8
   unconsciousness R55
      hysterical F44.89
   vasomotor R55
   vasovagal (paroxysmal) (idiopathic) R55
Attention (to)
   artificial
      opening (of) Z43.9
         digestive tract NEC Z43.4
            colon Z43.3
            ilium Z43.2
            stomach Z43.1
         specified NEC Z43.8
         trachea Z43.0
         urinary tract NEC Z43.6
            cystostomy Z43.5
            nephrostomy Z43.6
            ureterostomy Z43.6
            urethrostomy Z43.6
         vagina Z43.7
   colostomy Z43.3
   cystostomy Z43.5
   deficit disorder or syndrome F98.8
      with hyperactivity —see Disorder,
         attention-deficit hyperactivity
   gastrostomy Z43.1
   ileostomy Z43.2
   jejunostomy Z43.4
   nephrostomy Z43.6
   surgical dressings Z48.01
   sutures Z48.02
   tracheostomy Z43.0

Attention (Continued)
  ureterostomy Z43.6
  urethrostomy Z43.6
Attrition
  gum —see Recession, gingival
  tooth, teeth (excessive) (hard tissues) K03.0
Atypical, atypism —see also condition
  cells (on cytolgocial smear) (endocervical)
      (endometrial) (glandular)
    cervix R87.619
    vagina R87.629
  cervical N87.9
  endometrium N85.9
    hyperplasia N85.00
  parenting situation Z62.9
Auditory —see condition
Aujeszky's disease B33.8
Aurantiasis, cutis E67.1
Auricle, auricular —see also condition
  cervical Q18.2
Auriculotemporal syndrome G50.8
Austin Flint murmur (aortic insufficiency)
    I35.1
Australian
  Q fever A78
  X disease A83.4
Autism, autistic (childhood) (infantile) F84.0
  atypical F84.9
  spectrum disorder F84.0
Autodigestion R68.89
Autoerythrocyte sensitization (syndrome)
    D69.2
Autographism L50.3
Autoimmune
  disease (systemic) M35.9
  inhibitors to clotting factors D68.311
  lymphoproliferative syndrome [ALPS]
      D89.82
  thyroiditis E06.3
Autointoxication R68.89
Automatism G93.89
  with temporal sclerosis G93.81
  epileptic —see Epilepsy, localization- related,
      symptomatic, with complex partial
      seizures
  paroxysmal, idiopathic —see Epilepsy,
      localization-related, symptomatic, with
      complex partial seizures

Autonomic, autonomous
  bladder (neurogenic) N31.2
  hysteria seizure F44.5
Autosensitivity, erythrocyte D69.2
Autosensitization, cutaneous L30.2
Autosome —see condition by chromosome
    involved
Autotopagnosia R48.1
Autotoxemia R68.89
Autumn —see condition
Avellis' syndrome G46.8
Aversion
⇒ oral R63.39
    newborn P92.-●
    nonorganic origin F98.2
  sexual F52.1
Aviator's
  disease or sickness —see Effect, adverse, high
      altitude
  ear T70.0
Avitaminosis (multiple) —see also Deficiency,
    vitamin E56.9
  B E53.9
    with
      beriberi E51.11
      pellagra E52
  B2 E53.0
  B6 E53.1
  B12 E53.8
  D E55.9
    with rickets E55.0
  G E53.0
  K E56.1
  nicotinic acid E52
AVNRT (atrioventricular nodal re-entrant
    tachycardia) I47.1
AVRT (atrioventricular nodal re-entrant
    tachycardia) I47.1
Avulsion (traumatic)
  blood vessel —see Injury, blood vessel
  bone —see Fracture, by site
  cartilage —see also Dislocation, by site
    symphyseal (inner), complicating delivery
        O71.6
  external site other than limb —see Wound,
      open, by site
  eye S05.7-●

Avulsion (Continued)
  head (intracranial)
    external site NEC S08.89
    scalp S08.0
  internal organ or site —see Injury, by site
  joint —see also Dislocation, by site
    capsule —see Sprain, by site
  kidney S37.06-●
  ligament —see Sprain, by site
  limb —see also Amputation, traumatic,
      by site
    skin and subcutaneous tissue —see Wound,
        open, by site
  muscle —see Injury, muscle
  nerve (root) —see Injury, nerve
  scalp S08.0
  skin and subcutaneous tissue —see Wound,
      open, by site
  spleen S36.032
  symphyseal cartilage (inner), complicating
      delivery O71.6
  tendon —see Injury, muscle
  tooth S03.2
Awareness of heart beat R00.2
Axenfeld's
  anomaly or syndrome Q15.0
  degeneration (calcareous) Q13.4
Axilla, axillary —see also condition
  breast Q83.1
Axonotmesis —see Injury, nerve
Ayerza's disease or syndrome (pulmonary
      artery sclerosis with pulmonary
      hypertension) I27.0
Azoospermia (organic) N46.01
  due to
    drug therapy N46.021
    efferent duct obstruction N46.023
    infection N46.022
    radiation N46.024
    specified cause NEC N46.029
    systemic disease N46.025
Azotemia R79.89
  meaning uremia N19
Aztec ear Q17.3
Azygos
  continuation inferior vena cava Q26.8
  lobe (lung) Q33.1

B

Baastrup's disease —*see* Kissing spine
Babesiosis B60.00
  due to
    Babesia
      divergens B60.03
      duncani B60.02
      KO-1 B60.09
      microti B60.01
      MO-1 B60.03
      species
        unspecified B60.00
      venatorum B60.09
    specified NEC B60.09
Babington's disease (familial hemorrhagic
  telangiectasia) I78.0
Babinski's syndrome A52.79
Baby
  crying constantly R68.11
  floppy (syndrome) P94.2
Bacillary —*see* condition
Bacilluria R82.71
Bacillus —*see also* Infection, bacillus
  abortus infection A23.1
  anthracis infection A22.9
  coli infection —*see also* Escherichia coli B96.20
  Flexner's A03.1
  mallei infection A24.0
  Shiga's A03.0
  suipestifer infection —*see* Infection, salmonella
Back —*see* condition
Backache (postural) M54.9
  sacroiliac M53.3
  specified NEC M54.89
Backflow —*see* Reflux
Backward reading (dyslexia) F81.0
Bacteremia R78.81
  with sepsis —*see* Sepsis
Bactericholia —*see* Cholecystitis, acute
Bacterid, bacteride (pustular) L40.3
Bacterium, bacteria, bacterial
  agent NEC, as cause of disease classified
    elsewhere B96.89
  in blood —*see* Bacteremia
  in urine —*see* Bacteriuria
Bacteriuria, bacteruria R82.71
  asymptomatic R82.71
Bacteroides
  fragilis, as cause of disease classified
    elsewhere B96.6
Bad
  heart —*see* Disease, heart
  trip
    due to drug abuse —*see* Abuse, drug,
      hallucinogen
    due to drug dependence —*see* Dependence,
      drug, hallucinogen
Baelz's disease (cheilitis glandularis
  apostematosa) K13.0
Baerensprung's disease (eczema marginatum)
  B35.6
Bagasse disease or pneumonitis J67.1
Bagassosis J67.1
Baker's cyst —*see* Cyst, Baker's
Bakwin-Krida syndrome (metaphyseal
  dysplasia) Q78.5
Balancing side interference M26.56
Balanitis (circinata) (erosiva) (gangrenosa)
  (phagedenic) (vulgaris) N48.1
  amebic A06.82
  candidal B37.42
  due to Haemophilus ducreyi A57
  gonococcal (acute) (chronic) A54.23
  xerotica obliterans N48.0
Balanoposthitis N47.6
  gonococcal (acute) (chronic) A54.23
  ulcerative (specific) A63.8
Balanorrhagia —*see* Balanitis
Balantidiasis, balantidiosis A07.0
Bald tongue K14.4

Baldness —*see also* Alopecia
  male-pattern —*see* Alopecia, androgenic
Balkan grippe A78
Balloon disease —*see* Effect, adverse, high
  altitude
Balo's disease (concentric sclerosis) G37.5
Bamberger-Marie disease —*see* Osteoarthropathy,
  hypertrophic, specified type NEC
Bancroft's filariasis B74.0
Band(s)
  adhesive —*see* Adhesions, peritoneum
  anomalous or congenital —*see also* Anomaly,
    by site
    heart (atrial) (ventricular) Q24.8
    intestine Q43.3
    omentum Q43.3
  cervix N88.1
  constricting, congenital Q79.8
  gallbladder (congenital) Q44.1
  intestinal (adhesive) —*see* Adhesions,
    peritoneum
  obstructive
    intestine K56.50
      complete K56.52
      incomplete K56.51
      partial K56.51
    peritoneum K56.50
      complete K56.52
      incomplete K56.51
      partial K56.51
  periappendiceal, congenital Q43.3
  peritoneal (adhesive) —*see* Adhesions,
    peritoneum
  uterus N73.6
    internal N85.6
  vagina N89.5
Bandemia D72.825
Bandl's ring (contraction), **complicating
  delivery** O62.4
Bangkok hemorrhagic fever A91
Bang's disease (brucella abortus) A23.1
Bankruptcy, anxiety concerning Z59.89
Bannister's disease T78.3
  hereditary D84.1
Banti's disease or syndrome (with cirrhosis)
  (with portal hypertension) K76.6
Bar, median, prostate —*see* Enlargement,
  enlarged, prostate
Barcoo disease or rot —*see* Ulcer, skin
Barlow's disease E54
Barodontalgia T70.29
Baron Münchausen syndrome —*see* Disorder,
  factitious
Barosinusitis T70.1
Barotitis T70.0
Barotrauma T70.29
  odontalgia T70.29
  otitic T70.0
  sinus T70.1
Barraquer (-Simons) disease or syndrome
  (progressive lipodystrophy) E88.1
Barré-Guillain disease or syndrome G61.0
Barré-Liéou syndrome (posterior cervical
  sympathetic) M53.0
Barrel chest M95.4
Barrett's
  disease —*see* Barrett's, esophagus
  esophagus K22.70
    with dysplasia K22.719
      high grade K22.711
      low grade K22.710
    without dysplasia K22.70
  syndrome —*see* Barrett's, esophagus
  ulcer K22.10
    with bleeding K22.11
    without bleeding K22.10
Barth syndrome E78.71
Bársony (-Polgár) (-Teschendorf) **syndrome**
  (corkscrew esophagus) K22.4
Bartholinitis (suppurating) N75.8
  gonococcal (acute) (chronic) (with abscess)
    A54.1

Bartonellosis A44.9
  cutaneous A44.1
  mucocutaneous A44.1
  specified NEC A44.8
  systemic A44.0
Barton's fracture S52.56-●
Bartter's syndrome E26.81
Basal —*see* condition
Basan's (hidrotic) **ectodermal dysplasia** Q82.4
Baseball finger —*see* Dislocation, finger
Basedow's disease (exophthalmic goiter) —*see*
  Hyperthyroidism, with, goiter
Basic —*see* condition
Basilar —*see* condition
Bason's (hidrotic) **ectodermal dysplasia** Q82.4
Basopenia —*see* Agranulocytosis
Basophilia D72.824
Basophilism (cortico-adrenal) (Cushing's)
  (pituitary) E24.0
Bassen-Kornzweig disease or syndrome E78.6
Bat ear Q17.5
Bateman's
  disease B08.1
  purpura (senile) D69.2
Bathing cramp T75.1
Bathophobia F40.248
Batten (-Mayou) disease E75.4
  retina E75.4 *[H36]*
Batten-Steinert syndrome G71.11
Battered —*see* Maltreatment
Battey Mycobacterium infection A31.0
Battle exhaustion F43.0
Battledore placenta O43.19-●
Baumgarten-Cruveilhier cirrhosis, disease or
  syndrome K74.69
Bauxite fibrosis (of lung) J63.1
Bayle's disease (general paresis) A52.17
Bazin's disease (primary) (tuberculous) A18.4
Beach ear —*see* Swimmer's, ear
Beaded hair (congenital) Q84.1
Béal conjunctivitis or syndrome B30.2
Beard's disease (neurasthenia) F48.8
Beat(s)
  atrial, premature I49.1
  ectopic I49.49
  elbow —*see* Bursitis, elbow
  escaped, heart I49.49
  hand —*see* Bursitis, hand
  knee —*see* Bursitis, knee
  premature I49.40
    atrial I49.1
    auricular I49.1
    supraventricular I49.1
Beau's
  disease or syndrome —*see* Degeneration,
    myocardial
  lines (transverse furrows on fingernails) L60.4
Bechterev's syndrome —*see* Spondylitis,
  ankylosing
Beck's syndrome (anterior spinal artery
  occlusion) I65.8
Becker's
  cardiomyopathy I42.8
  disease
    idiopathic mural endomyocardial disease
      I42.3
    myotonia congenita, recessive form G71.12
  dystrophy G71.01
  pigmented hairy nevus D22.5
Beckwith-Wiedemann syndrome Q87.3
Bed confinement status Z74.01
Bed sore —*see* Ulcer, pressure, by site
Bedbug bite(s) —*see* Bite(s), by site, superficial,
  insect
Bedclothes, asphyxiation or suffocation
  by —*see* Asphyxia, traumatic, due to,
    mechanical, trapped
Bednar's
  aphthae K12.0
  tumor —*see* Neoplasm, malignant, by site
Bedridden Z74.01

▶ New ⇒ Revised ~~deleted~~ Deleted ● Use Additional Character(s)

Bedsore —*see* Ulcer, pressure, by site
Bedwetting —*see* Enuresis
Bee sting (with allergic or anaphylactic shock) —*see* Toxicity, venom, arthropod, bee
Beer drinker's heart (disease) I42.6
Begbie's disease (exophthalmic goiter) —*see* Hyperthyroidism, with, goiter
Behavior
  antisocial
    adult Z72.811
    child or adolescent Z72.810
  disorder, disturbance —*see* Disorder, conduct
  disruptive —*see* Disorder, conduct
  drug seeking Z76.5
  inexplicable R46.2
  marked evasiveness R46.5
  obsessive-compulsive R46.81
  overactivity R46.3
  poor responsiveness R46.4
  self-damaging (life-style) Z72.89
  sleep-incompatible Z72.821
  slowness R46.4
  specified NEC R46.89
  strange (and inexplicable) R46.2
  suspiciousness R46.5
  type A pattern Z73.1
  undue concern or preoccupation with stressful events R46.6
  verbosity and circumstantial detail obscuring reason for contact R46.7
Behcet's disease or syndrome M35.2
Behr's disease —*see* Degeneration, macula
Beigel's disease or morbus (white piedra) B36.2
Bejel A65
Bekhterev's syndrome —*see* Spondylitis, ankylosing
Belching —*see* Eructation
Bell's
  mania F30.8
  palsy, paralysis G51.0
    infant or newborn P11.3
  spasm G51.3-•
Bence Jones albuminuria or proteinuria NEC R80.3
Bends T70.3
Benedikt's paralysis or syndrome G46.3
Benign (*see also* condition)
  prostatic hyperplasia —*see* Hyperplasia, prostate
Bennett's fracture (displaced) S62.21-•
Benson's disease —*see* Deposit, crystalline
Bent
  back (hysterical) F44.4
  nose M95.0
    congenital Q67.4
Bereavement (uncomplicated) Z63.4
Bergeron's disease (hysterical chorea) F44.4
Berger's disease —*see* Nephropathy, IgA
Beriberi (dry) E51.11
  heart (disease) E51.12
  polyneuropathy E51.11
  wet E51.12
    involving circulatory system E51.11
Berlin's disease or edema (traumatic) S05.8X-•
Berlock (berloque) dermatitis L56.2
Bernard-Horner syndrome G90.2
Bernard-Soulier disease or thrombopathia D69.1
Bernhardt (-Roth) disease —*see* Mononeuropathy, lower limb, meralgia paresthetica
Bernheim's syndrome —*see* Failure, heart, right
Bertielliasis B71.8
Berylliosis (lung) J63.2
Besnier-Boeck (-Schaumann) disease —*see* Sarcoidosis
Besnier's
  lupus pernio D86.3
  prurigo L20.0
Bestiality F65.89
Best's disease H35.50

Beta-mercaptolactate-cysteine disulfiduria E72.09
Betalipoproteinemia, broad or floating E78.2
Betting and gambling Z72.6
  pathological (compulsive) F63.0
Bezoar T18.9
  intestine T18.3
  stomach T18.2
Bezold's abscess —*see* Mastoiditis, acute
Bianchi's syndrome R48.8
Bicornate or bicornis uterus Q51.3
  in pregnancy or childbirth O34.00
    causing obstructed labor O65.5
Bicuspid aortic valve Q23.1
Biedl-Bardet syndrome Q87.89
Bielschowsky (-Jansky) disease E75.4
Biermer's (pernicious) anemia or disease D51.0
Biett's disease L93.0
Bifid (congenital)
  apex, heart Q24.8
  clitoris Q52.6
  kidney Q63.8
  nose Q30.2
  patella Q74.1
  scrotum Q55.29
  toe NEC Q74.2
  tongue Q38.3
  ureter Q62.8
  uterus Q51.3
  uvula Q35.7
Biforis uterus (suprasimplex) Q51.3
Bifurcation (congenital)
  gallbladder Q44.1
  kidney pelvis Q63.8
  renal pelvis Q63.8
  rib Q76.6
  tongue, congenital Q38.3
  trachea Q32.1
  ureter Q62.8
  urethra Q64.74
  vertebra Q76.49
Big spleen syndrome D73.1
Bigeminal pulse R00.8
Bilateral —*see* condition
Bile
  duct —*see* condition
  pigments in urine R82.2
Bilharziasis —*see also* Schistosomiasis
  chyluria B65.0
  cutaneous B65.3
  galacturia B65.0
  hematochyluria B65.0
  intestinal B65.1
  lipemia B65.9
  lipuria B65.0
  oriental B65.2
  piarhemia B65.9
  pulmonary NOS B65.9 *[J99]*
    pneumonia B65.9 *[J17]*
  tropical hematuria B65.0
  vesical B65.0
Biliary —*see* condition
Bilirubin metabolism disorder E80.7
  specified NEC E80.6
Bilirubinemia, familial nonhemolytic E80.4
Bilirubinuria R82.2
Biliuria R82.2
Bilocular stomach K31.2
Binswanger's disease I67.3
Biparta, bipartite
  carpal scaphoid Q74.0
  patella Q74.1
  vagina Q52.10
Bird
  face Q75.8
  fancier's disease or lung J67.2
Birt-Hogg-Dube syndrome Q87.89
Birth
  complications in mother —*see* Delivery, complicated
  compression during NOS P15.9

Birth (*Continued*)
  defect —*see* Anomaly
  immature (less than 37 completed weeks) —*see* Preterm, newborn
    extremely (less than 28 completed weeks) —*see* Immaturity, extreme
  inattention, at or after —*see* Maltreatment, child, neglect
  injury NOS P15.9
    basal ganglia P11.1
    brachial plexus NEC P14.3
    brain (compression) (pressure) P11.2
    central nervous system NOS P11.9
    cerebellum P11.1
    cerebral hemorrhage P10.1
    external genitalia P15.5
    eye P15.3
    face P15.4
    fracture
      bone P13.9
        specified NEC P13.8
      clavicle P13.4
      femur P13.2
      humerus P13.3
      long bone, except femur P13.3
      radius and ulna P13.3
      skull P13.0
      spine P11.5
      tibia and fibula P13.3
    intracranial P11.2
      laceration or hemorrhage P10.9
        specified NEC P10.8
    intraventricular hemorrhage P10.2
    laceration
      brain P10.1
      by scalpel P15.8
      peripheral nerve P14.9
    liver P15.0
    meninges
      brain P11.1
      spinal cord P11.5
    nerve
      brachial plexus P14.3
      cranial NEC (except facial) P11.4
      facial P11.3
      peripheral P14.9
      phrenic (paralysis) P14.2
    paralysis
      facial nerve P11.3
      spinal P11.5
    penis P15.5
    rupture
      spinal cord P11.5
    scalp P12.9
    scalpel wound P15.8
    scrotum P15.5
    skull NEC P13.1
      fracture P13.0
    specified type NEC P15.8
    spinal cord P11.5
    spine P11.5
    spleen P15.1
    sternomastoid (hematoma) P15.2
    subarachnoid hemorrhage P10.3
    subcutaneous fat necrosis P15.6
    subdural hemorrhage P10.0
    tentorial tear P10.4
    testes P15.5
    vulva P15.5
  lack of care, at or after —*see* Maltreatment, child, neglect
  neglect, at or after —*see* Maltreatment, child, neglect
  palsy or paralysis, newborn, NOS (birth injury) P14.9
  premature (infant) —*see* Preterm, newborn
  shock, newborn P96.89
  trauma —*see* Birth, injury
  weight
    4000 grams to 4499 grams P08.1
    4500 grams or more P08.0

Birth (Continued)
  weight (Continued)
    low (2499 grams or less) —see Low,
        birthweight
      extremely (999 grams or less) —see Low,
          birthweight, extreme
Birthmark Q82.5
Bisalbuminemia E88.09
Biskra's button B55.1
Bite(s) (animal) (human)
  abdomen, abdominal
    wall S31.159
      with penetration into peritoneal cavity
          S31.659
      epigastric region S31.152
        with penetration into peritoneal cavity
            S31.652
      left
        lower quadrant S31.154
          with penetration into peritoneal
              cavity S31.654
        upper quadrant S31.151
          with penetration into peritoneal
              cavity S31.651
      periumbilic region S31.155
        with penetration into peritoneal cavity
            S31.655
      right
        lower quadrant S31.153
          with penetration into peritoneal
              cavity S31.653
        upper quadrant S31.150
          with penetration into peritoneal
              cavity S31.650
      superficial NEC S30.871
        insect S30.861
  alveolar (process) —see Bite, oral cavity
  amphibian (venomous) —see Venom, bite,
      amphibian
  animal —see also Bite, by site
    venomous —see Venom
  ankle S91.05-●
    superficial NEC S90.57-●
      insect S90.56-●
  antecubital space —see Bite, elbow
  anus S31.835
    superficial NEC S30.877
      insect S30.867
  arm (upper) S41.15-●
    lower —see Bite, forearm
    superficial NEC S40.87-●
      insect S40.86-●
  arthropod NEC —see Venom, bite, arthropod
  auditory canal (external) (meatus) —
      see Bite, ear
  auricle, ear —see Bite, ear
  axilla —see Bite, arm
  back —see also Bite, thorax, back
    lower S31.050
      with penetration into retroperitoneal
          space S31.051
      superficial NEC S30.870
        insect S30.860
  bedbug —see Bite(s), by site, superficial,
      insect
  breast S21.05-●
    superficial NEC S20.17-●
      insect S20.16-●
  brow —see Bite, head, specified site NEC
  buttock S31.805
    left S31.825
    right S31.815
    superficial NEC S30.870
      insect S30.860
  calf —see Bite, leg
  canaliculus lacrimalis —see Bite, eyelid
  canthus, eye —see Bite, eyelid
  centipede —see Toxicity, venom, arthropod,
      centipede
  cheek (external) S01.45-●
    internal —see Bite, oral cavity
    superficial NEC S00.87
      insect S00.86

Bite (Continued)
  chest wall —see Bite, thorax
  chigger B88.0
  chin —see Bite, head, specified site NEC
  clitoris —see Bite, vulva
  costal region —see Bite, thorax
  digit(s)
    hand —see Bite, finger
    toe —see Bite, toe
  ear (canal) (external) S01.35-●
    superficial NEC S00.47-●
      insect S00.46-●
  elbow S51.05-●
    superficial NEC S50.37-●
      insect S50.36-●
  epididymis —see Bite, testis
  epigastric region —see Bite, abdomen
  epiglottis —see Bite, neck, specified site NEC
  esophagus, cervical S11.25
    superficial NEC S10.17
      insect S10.16
  eyebrow —see Bite, eyelid
  eyelid S01.15-●
    superficial NEC S00.27-●
      insect S00.26-●
  face NEC —see Bite, head, specified site NEC
  finger(s) S61.259
    with
      damage to nail S61.359
    index S61.258
      with
        damage to nail S61.358
      left S61.251
        with
          damage to nail S61.351
      right S61.250
        with
          damage to nail S61.350
      superficial NEC S60.478
        insect S60.46-●
    little S61.25-●
      with
        damage to nail S61.35-●
      superficial NEC S60.47-●
        insect S60.46-●
    middle S61.25-●
      with
        damage to nail S61.35-●
      superficial NEC S60.47-●
        insect S60.46-●
    ring S61.25-●
      with
        damage to nail S61.35-●
      superficial NEC S60.47-●
        insect S60.46-●
    superficial NEC S60.479
      insect S60.469
    thumb —see Bite, thumb
  flank —see Bite, abdomen, wall
  flea —see Bite, by site, superficial,
      insect
  foot (except toe(s) alone) S91.35-●
    superficial NEC S90.87-●
      insect S90.86-●
    toe —see Bite, toe
  forearm S51.85-●
    elbow only —see Bite, elbow
    superficial NEC S50.87-●
      insect S50.86-●
  forehead —see Bite, head, specified site
      NEC
  genital organs, external
    female S31.552
      superficial NEC S30.876
        insect S30.866
      vagina and vulva —see Bite, vulva
    male S31.551
      penis —see Bite, penis
      scrotum —see Bite, scrotum
      superficial NEC S30.875
        insect S30.865
      testes —see Bite, testis
  groin —see Bite, abdomen, wall

Bite (Continued)
  gum —see Bite, oral cavity
  hand S61.45-●
    finger —see Bite, finger
    superficial NEC S60.57-●
      insect S60.56-●
    thumb —see Bite, thumb
  head S01.95
    cheek —see Bite, cheek
    ear —see Bite, ear
    eyelid —see Bite, eyelid
    lip —see Bite, lip
    nose —see Bite, nose
    oral cavity —see Bite, oral cavity
    scalp —see Bite, scalp
    specified site NEC S01.85
      superficial NEC S00.87
        insect S00.86
    superficial NEC S00.97
      insect S00.96
    temporomandibular area —see Bite, cheek
  heel —see Bite, foot
  hip S71.05-●
    superficial NEC S70.27-●
      insect S70.26-●
  hymen S31.45
  hypochondrium —see Bite, abdomen, wall
  hypogastric region —see Bite, abdomen, wall
  inguinal region —see Bite, abdomen, wall
  insect —see Bite, by site, superficial, insect
  instep —see Bite, foot
  interscapular region —see Bite, thorax, back
  jaw —see Bite, head, specified site NEC
  knee S81.05-●
    superficial NEC S80.27-●
      insect S80.26-●
  labium (majus) (minus) —see Bite, vulva
  lacrimal duct —see Bite, eyelid
  larynx S11.015
    superficial NEC S10.17
      insect S10.16
  leg (lower) S81.85-●
    ankle —see Bite, ankle
    foot —see Bite, foot
    knee —see Bite, knee
    superficial NEC S80.87-●
      insect S80.86-●
    toe —see Bite, toe
    upper —see Bite, thigh
  lip S01.551
    superficial NEC S00.571
      insect S00.561
  lizard (venomous) —see Venom, bite, reptile
  loin —see Bite, abdomen, wall
  lower back —see Bite, back, lower
  lumbar region —see Bite, back, lower
  malar region —see Bite, head, specified site
      NEC
  mammary —see Bite, breast
  marine animals (venomous) —see Toxicity,
      venom, marine animal
  mastoid region —see Bite, head, specified site
      NEC
  mouth —see Bite, oral cavity
  nail
    finger —see Bite, finger
    toe —see Bite, toe
  nape —see Bite, neck, specified site NEC
  nasal (septum) (sinus) —see Bite, nose
  nasopharynx —see Bite, head, specified site
      NEC
  neck S11.95
    involving
      cervical esophagus —see Bite,
          esophagus, cervical
      larynx —see Bite, larynx
      pharynx —see Bite, pharynx
      thyroid gland S11.15
      trachea —see Bite, trachea
    specified site NEC S11.85
      superficial NEC S10.87
        insect S10.86

▶ New   ⇒ Revised   ~~deleted~~ Deleted   ● Use Additional Character(s)

Bite *(Continued)*
 neck *(Continued)*
  superficial NEC S10.97
   insect S10.96
  throat S11.85
   superficial NEC S10.17
    insect S10.16
 nose (septum) (sinus) S01.25
  superficial NEC S00.37
   insect S00.36
 occipital region —*see* Bite, scalp
 oral cavity S01.552
  superficial NEC S00.572
   insect S00.562
 orbital region —*see* Bite, eyelid
 palate —*see* Bite, oral cavity
 palm —*see* Bite, hand
 parietal region —*see* Bite, scalp
 pelvis S31.050
  with penetration into retroperitoneal space S31.051
  superficial NEC S30.870
   insect S30.860
 penis S31.25
  superficial NEC S30.872
   insect S30.862
 perineum
  female —*see* Bite, vulva
  male —*see* Bite, pelvis
 periocular area (with or without lacrimal passages) —*see* Bite, eyelid
 phalanges
  finger —*see* Bite, finger
  toe —*see* Bite, toe
 pharynx S11.25
  superficial NEC S10.17
   insect S10.16
 pinna —*see* Bite, ear
 poisonous —*see* Venom
 popliteal space —*see* Bite, knee
 prepuce —*see* Bite, penis
 pubic region —*see* Bite, abdomen, wall
 rectovaginal septum —*see* Bite, vulva
 red bug B88.0
 reptile NEC —*see also* Venom, bite, reptile
  nonvenomous —*see* Bite, by site
  snake —*see* Venom, bite, snake
 sacral region —*see* Bite, back, lower
 sacroiliac region —*see* Bite, back, lower
 salivary gland —*see* Bite, oral cavity
 scalp S01.05
  superficial NEC S00.07
   insect S00.06
 scapular region —*see* Bite, shoulder
 scrotum S31.35
  superficial NEC S30.873
   insect S30.863
 sea-snake (venomous) —*see* Toxicity, venom, snake, sea snake
 shin —*see* Bite, leg
 shoulder S41.05-●
  superficial NEC S40.27-●
   insect S40.26-●
 snake —*see also* Venom, bite, snake
  nonvenomous —*see* Bite, by site
 spermatic cord —*see* Bite, testis
 spider (venomous) —*see* Toxicity, venom, spider
  nonvenomous —*see* Bite, by site, superficial, insect
 sternal region —*see* Bite, thorax, front
 submaxillary region —*see* Bite, head, specified site NEC
 submental region —*see* Bite, head, specified site NEC
 subungual
  finger(s) —*see* Bite, finger
  toe —*see* Bite, toe
 superficial —*see* Bite, by site, superficial
 supraclavicular fossa S11.85

Bite *(Continued)*
 supraorbital —*see* Bite, head, specified site NEC
 temple, temporal region —*see* Bite, head, specified site NEC
 temporomandibular area —*see* Bite, cheek
 testis S31.35
  superficial NEC S30.873
   insect S30.863
 thigh S71.15-●
  superficial NEC S70.37-●
   insect S70.36-●
 thorax, thoracic (wall) S21.95
  back S21.25-●
   with penetration into thoracic cavity S21.45-●
  breast —*see* Bite, breast
  front S21.15-●
   with penetration into thoracic cavity S21.35-●
  superficial NEC S20.97
   back S20.47-●
   front S20.37-●
   insect S20.96
    back S20.46-●
    front S20.36-●
 throat —*see* Bite, neck, throat
 thumb S61.05-●
  with
   damage to nail S61.15-●
  superficial NEC S60.37-●
   insect S60.36-●
 thyroid S11.15
  superficial NEC S10.87
   insect S10.86
 toe(s) S91.15-●
  with
   damage to nail S91.25-●
  great S91.15-●
   with
    damage to nail S91.25-●
  lesser S91.15-●
   with
    damage to nail S91.25-●
  superficial NEC S90.47-●
   great S90.47-●
   insect S90.46-●
    great S90.46-●
 tongue S01.552
 trachea S11.025
  superficial NEC S10.17
   insect S10.16
 tunica vaginalis —*see* Bite, testis
 tympanum, tympanic membrane —*see* Bite, ear
 umbilical region S31.155
 uvula —*see* Bite, oral cavity
 vagina —*see* Bite, vulva
 venomous —*see* Venom
 vocal cords S11.035
  superficial NEC S10.17
   insect S10.16
 vulva S31.45
  superficial NEC S30.874
   insect S30.864
 wrist S61.55-●
  superficial NEC S60.87-●
   insect S60.86-●
Biting, cheek or lip K13.1
Biventricular failure (heart) I50.82
Björck (-Thorson) syndrome (malignant carcinoid) E34.0
Black
 death A20.9
 eye S00.1-●
 hairy tongue K14.3
 heel (foot) S90.3-●
 lung (disease) J60
 palm (hand) S60.22-●
Blackfan-Diamond anemia or syndrome (congenital hypoplastic anemia) D61.01

Blackhead L70.0
Blackout R55
Bladder —*see* condition
Blast (air) (hydraulic) (immersion) (underwater)
 blindness S05.8X-●
 injury
  abdomen or thorax —*see* Injury, by site
  ear (acoustic nerve trauma) —*see* Injury, nerve, acoustic, specified type NEC
  syndrome NEC T70.8
Blastoma —*see* Neoplasm, malignant, by site
 pulmonary —*see* Neoplasm, lung, malignant
Blastomycosis, blastomycotic B40.9
 Brazilian —*see* Paracoccidioidomycosis
 cutaneous B40.3
 disseminated B40.7
 European —*see* Cryptococcosis
 generalized B40.7
 keloidal B48.0
 North American B40.9
 primary pulmonary B40.0
 pulmonary B40.2
  acute B40.0
  chronic B40.1
 skin B40.3
 South American —*see* Paracoccidioidomycosis
 specified NEC B40.89
Bleb(s) R23.8
 emphysematous (lung) (solitary) J43.9
 endophthalmitis H59.43
 filtering (vitreous), after glaucoma surgery Z98.83
 inflammed (infected), postprocedural H59.40
  stage 1 H59.41
  stage 2 H59.42
  stage 3 H59.43
 lung (ruptured) J43.9
  congenital —*see* Atelectasis
  newborn P25.8
 subpleural (emphysematous) J43.9
Blebitis, postprocedural H59.40
 stage 1 H59.41
 stage 2 H59.42
 stage 3 H59.43
Bleeder (familial) (hereditary) —*see* Hemophilia
Bleeding —*see also* Hemorrhage
 anal K62.5
 anovulatory N97.0
 atonic, following delivery O72.1
 capillary I78.8
  puerperal O72.2
 contact (postcoital) N93.0
 due to uterine subinvolution N85.3
 ear —*see* Otorrhagia
 excessive, associated with menopausal onset N92.4
 familial —*see* Defect, coagulation
 following intercourse N93.0
 gastrointestinal K92.2
 hemorrhoids —*see* Hemorrhoids
 intermenstrual (regular) N92.3
  irregular N92.1
 intraoperative —*see* Complication, intraoperative, hemorrhage
 irregular N92.6
 menopausal N92.4
 newborn, intraventricular —*see* Newborn, affected by, hemorrhage, intraventricular
 nipple N64.59
 nose R04.0
 ovulation N92.3
 perimenopausal N92.4
 postclimacteric N95.0
 postcoital N93.0
 postmenopausal N95.0
 postoperative —*see* Complication, postprocedural, hemorrhage
 preclimacteric N92.4
 pre-pubertal vaginal N93.1
 puberty (excessive, with onset of menstrual periods) N92.2

Bleeding *(Continued)*
rectum, rectal K62.5
newborn P54.2
tendencies —*see* Defect, coagulation
throat R04.1
tooth socket (post-extraction) K91.840
umbilical stump P51.9
uterus, uterine NEC N93.9
climacteric N92.4
dysfunctional or functional N93.8
menopausal N92.4
preclimacteric or premenopausal N92.4
unrelated to menstrual cycle N93.9
vagina, vaginal (abnormal) N93.9
dysfunctional or functional N93.8
newborn P54.6
pre-pubertal N93.1
vicarious N94.89
Blennorrhagia, blennorrhagic —*see* Gonorrhea
Blennorrhea (acute) (chronic) —*see also*
Gonorrhea
inclusion (neonatal) (newborn) P39.1
lower genitourinary tract (gonococcal) A54.00
neonatorum (gonococcal ophthalmia) A54.31
Blepharelosis —*see* Entropion
Blepharitis (angularis) (ciliaris) (eyelid)
(marginal) (nonulcerative) H01.009
herpes zoster B02.39
left H01.006
lower H01.005
upper H01.004
upper and lower H01.00B
right H01.003
lower H01.002
upper H01.001
upper and lower H01.00A
squamous H01.029
left H01.026
lower H01.025
upper H01.024
upper and lower H01.02B
right H01.023
lower H01.022
upper H01.021
upper and lower H01.02A
ulcerative H01.019
left H01.016
lower H01.015
upper H01.014
upper and lower H01.01B
right H01.013
lower H01.012
upper H01.011
upper and lower H01.01B
Blepharochalasis H02.30
congenital Q10.0
left H02.36
lower H02.35
upper H02.34
right H02.33
lower H02.32
upper H02.31
Blepharoclonus H02.59
Blepharoconjunctivitis H10.50-●
angular H10.52-●
contact H10.53-●
ligneous H10.51-●
Blepharophimosis (eyelid) H02.529
congenital Q10.3
left H02.526
lower H02.525
upper H02.524
right H02.523
lower H02.522
upper H02.521
Blepharoptosis H02.40-●
congenital Q10.0
mechanical H02.41-●
myogenic H02.42-●
neurogenic H02.43-●
paralytic H02.43-●
Blepharopyorrhea, gonococcal A54.39

Blepharospasm G24.5
drug induced G24.01
Blighted ovum O02.0
Blind —*see also* Blindness
bronchus (congenital) Q32.4
loop syndrome K90.2
congenital Q43.8
sac, fallopian tube (congenital) Q50.6
spot, enlarged —*see* Defect, visual field,
localized, scotoma, blind spot area
tract or tube, congenital NEC —*see* Atresia,
by site
Blindness (acquired) (congenital) (both eyes)
H54.0X-●
blast S05.8X-●
color —*see* Deficiency, color vision
concussion S05.8X-●
cortical H47.619
left brain H47.612
right brain H47.611
day H53.11
due to injury (current episode) S05.9-●
sequelae — code to injury with seventh
character S
eclipse (total) —*see* Retinopathy, solar
emotional (hysterical) F44.6
face H53.16
hysterical F44.6
legal (both eyes) (USA definition) H54.8
mind R48.8
night H53.60
abnormal dark adaptation curve H53.61
acquired H53.62
congenital H53.63
specified type NEC H53.69
vitamin A deficiency E50.5
one eye (other eye normal) H54.40
left (normal vision on right) H54.42-●
low vision on right H54.12-●
low vision, other eye H54.10
right (normal vision on left) H54.41-●
low vision on left H54.11-●
psychic R48.8
river B73.01
snow —*see* Photokeratitis
sun, solar —*see* Retinopathy, solar
transient —*see* Disturbance, vision, subjective,
loss, transient
traumatic (current episode) S05.9-●
word (developmental) F81.0
acquired R48.0
secondary to organic lesion R48.0
Blister (nonthermal)
abdominal wall S30.821
alveolar process S00.522
ankle S90.52-●
antecubital space —*see* Blister, elbow
anus S30.827
arm (upper) S40.82-●
auditory canal —*see* Blister, ear
auricle —*see* Blister, ear
axilla —*see* Blister, arm
back, lower S30.820
beetle dermatitis L24.89
breast S20.12-●
brow S00.82
calf —*see* Blister, leg
canthus —*see* Blister, eyelid
cheek S00.82
internal S00.522
chest wall —*see* Blister, thorax
chin S00.82
costal region —*see* Blister, thorax
digit(s)
foot —*see* Blister, toe
hand —*see* Blister, finger
due to burn —*see* Burn, by site, second degree
ear S00.42-●
elbow S50.32-●
epiglottis S10.12
esophagus, cervical S10.12
eyebrow —*see* Blister, eyelid

Blister *(Continued)*
eyelid S00.22-●
face S00.82
fever B00.1
finger(s) S60.429
index S60.42-●
little S60.42-●
middle S60.42-●
ring S60.42-●
foot (except toe(s) alone) S90.82-●
toe —*see* Blister, toe
forearm S50.82-●
elbow only —*see* Blister, elbow
forehead S00.82
fracture - omit code
genital organ
female S30.826
male S30.825
gum S00.522
hand S60.52-●
head S00.92
ear —*see* Blister, ear
eyelid —*see* Blister, eyelid
lip S00.521
nose S00.32
oral cavity S00.522
scalp S00.02
specified site NEC S00.82
heel —*see* Blister, foot
hip S70.22-●
interscapular region S20.429
jaw S00.82
knee S80.22-●
larynx S10.12
leg (lower) S80.82-●
knee —*see* Blister, knee
upper —*see* Blister, thigh
lip S00.521
malar region S00.82
mammary —*see* Blister, breast
mastoid region S00.82
mouth S00.522
multiple, skin, nontraumatic R23.8
nail
finger —*see* Blister, finger
toe —*see* Blister, toe
nasal S00.32
neck S10.92
specified site NEC S10.82
throat S10.12
nose S00.32
occipital region S00.02
oral cavity S00.522
orbital region —*see* Blister, eyelid
palate S00.522
palm —*see* Blister, hand
parietal region S00.02
pelvis S30.820
penis S30.822
periocular area —*see* Blister, eyelid
phalanges
finger —*see* Blister, finger
toe —*see* Blister, toe
pharynx S10.12
pinna —*see* Blister, ear
popliteal space —*see* Blister, knee
scalp S00.02
scapular region —*see* Blister, shoulder
scrotum S30.823
shin —*see* Blister, leg
shoulder S40.22-●
sternal region S20.329
submaxillary region S00.82
submental region S00.82
subungual
finger(s) —*see* Blister, finger
toe(s) —*see* Blister, toe
supraclavicular fossa S10.82
supraorbital S00.82
temple S00.82
temporal region S00.82
testis S30.823

▶ New   ⇒ Revised   ~~deleted~~ Deleted   ● Use Additional Character(s)

Blister *(Continued)*
thermal —*see* Burn, second degree, by site
thigh S70.32-●
thorax, thoracic (wall) S20.92
back S20.42-●
front S20.32-●
throat S10.12
thumb S60.32-●
toe(s) S90.42-●
great S90.42-●
tongue S00.522
trachea S10.12
tympanum, tympanic membrane —*see* Blister, ear
upper arm —*see* Blister, arm (upper)
uvula S00.522
vagina S30.824
vocal cords S10.12
vulva S30.824
wrist S60.82-●
Bloating R14.0
Bloch-Sulzberger disease or syndrome Q82.3
Block, blocked
alveolocapillary J84.10
arborization (heart) I45.5
arrhythmic I45.9
atrioventricular (incomplete) (partial) I44.30
with atrioventricular dissociation I44.2
complete I44.2
congenital Q24.6
congenital Q24.6
first degree I44.0
second degree (types I and II) I44.1
specified NEC I44.39
third degree I44.2
types I and II I44.1
auriculoventricular —*see* Block, atrioventricular
bifascicular (cardiac) I45.2
bundle-branch (complete) (false) (incomplete) I45.4
bilateral I45.2
left I44.7
with right bundle branch block I45.2
hemiblock I44.60
anterior I44.4
posterior I44.5
incomplete I44.7
with right bundle branch block I45.2
right I45.10
with
left bundle branch block I45.2
left fascicular block I45.2
specified NEC I45.19
Wilson's type I45.19
cardiac I45.9
conduction I45.9
complete I44.2
fascicular (left) I44.60
anterior I44.4
posterior I44.5
right I45.0
specified NEC I44.69
foramen Magendie (acquired) G91.1
congenital Q03.1
with spina bifida —*see* Spina bifida, by site, with hydrocephalus
heart I45.9
bundle branch I45.4
bilateral I45.2
complete (atrioventricular) I44.2
congenital Q24.6
first degree (atrioventricular) I44.0
second degree (atrioventricular) I44.1
specified type NEC I45.5
third degree (atrioventricular) I44.2
hepatic vein I82.0
intraventricular (nonspecific) I45.4
bundle branch
bilateral I45.2
kidney N28.9
postcystoscopic or postprocedural N99.0

Block, blocked *(Continued)*
Mobitz (types I and II) I44.1
myocardial —*see* Block, heart
nodal I45.5
organ or site, congenital NEC —*see* Atresia, by site
portal (vein) I81
second degree (types I and II) I44.1
sinoatrial I45.5
sinoauricular I45.5
third degree I44.2
trifascicular I45.3
tubal N97.1
vein NOS I82.90
Wenckebach (types I and II) I44.1
Blockage —*see* Obstruction
Blocq's disease F44.4
Blood
constituents, abnormal R78.9
disease D75.9
donor —*see* Donor, blood
dyscrasia D75.9
with
abortion —*see* Abortion, by type, complicated by, hemorrhage
ectopic pregnancy O08.1
molar pregnancy O08.1
following ectopic or molar pregnancy O08.1
newborn P61.9
puerperal, postpartum O72.3
flukes NEC —*see* Schistosomiasis
in
feces K92.1
occult R19.5
urine —*see* Hematuria
mole O02.0
occult in feces R19.5
pressure
decreased, due to shock following injury T79.4
examination only Z01.30
fluctuating I99.8
high —*see* Hypertension
borderline R03.0
incidental reading, without diagnosis of hypertension R03.0
low —*see also* Hypotension
incidental reading, without diagnosis of hypotension R03.1
spitting —*see* Hemoptysis
staining cornea —*see* Pigmentation, cornea, stromal
transfusion
reaction or complication —*see* Complications, transfusion
type
A (Rh positive) Z67.10
Rh negative Z67.11
AB (Rh positive) Z67.30
Rh negative Z67.31
B (Rh positive) Z67.20
Rh negative Z67.21
O (Rh positive) Z67.40
Rh negative Z67.41
Rh (positive) Z67.90
negative Z67.91
vessel rupture —*see* Hemorrhage
vomiting —*see* Hematemesis
Blood-forming organs, disease D75.9
Bloodgood's disease —*see* Mastopathy, cystic
Bloom (-Machacek)(-Torre) **syndrome** Q82.8
Blount disease or osteochondrosis M92.51-●
Blue
baby Q24.9
diaper syndrome E72.09
dome cyst (breast) —*see* Cyst, breast
dot cataract Q12.0
nevus D22.9

Blue *(Continued)*
sclera Q13.5
with fragility of bone and deafness Q78.0
toe syndrome I75.02-●
Blueness —*see* Cyanosis
Blues, postpartal O90.6
baby O90.6
Blurring, visual H53.8
Blushing (abnormal) (excessive) R23.2
BMI —*see* Body, mass index
Boarder, hospital NEC Z76.4
accompanying sick person Z76.3
healthy infant or child Z76.2
foundling Z76.1
Bockhart's impetigo L01.02
Bodechtel-Guttman disease (subacute sclerosing panencephalitis) A81.1
Boder-Sedgwick syndrome (ataxia-telangiectasia) G11.3
Body, bodies
Aschoff's —*see* Myocarditis, rheumatic
asteroid, vitreous —*see* Deposit, crystalline
cytoid (retina) —*see* Occlusion, artery, retina
drusen (degenerative) (macula) (retinal) —*see also* Degeneration, macula, drusen
optic disc —*see* Drusen, optic disc
foreign —*see* Foreign body
loose
joint, except knee —*see* Loose, body, joint
knee M23.4-●
sheath, tendon —*see* Disorder, tendon, specified type NEC
mass index (BMI)
adult
19.9 or less Z68.1
20.0-20.9 Z68.20
21.0-21.9 Z68.21
22.0-22.9 Z68.22
23.0-23.9 Z68.23
24.0-24.9 Z68.24
25.0-25.9 Z68.25
26.0-26.9 Z68.26
27.0-27.9 Z68.27
28.0-28.9 Z68.28
29.0-29.9 Z68.29
30.0-30.9 Z68.30
31.0-31.9 Z68.31
32.0-32.9 Z68.32
33.0-33.9 Z68.33
34.0-34.9 Z68.34
35.0-35.9 Z68.35
36.0-36.9 Z68.36
37.0-37.9 Z68.37
38.0-38.9 Z68.38
39.0-39.9 Z68.39
40.0-44.9 Z68.41
45.0-49.9 Z68.42
50.0-59.9 Z68.43
60.0-69.9 Z68.44
70 and over Z68.45
pediatric
5th percentile to less than 85th percentile for age Z68.52
85th percentile to less than 95th percentile for age Z68.53
greater than or equal to ninety-fifth percentile for age Z68.54
less than fifth percentile for age Z68.51
Mooser's A75.2
rice —*see also* Loose, body, joint
knee M23.4-●
rocking F98.4
Boeck's
disease or sarcoid —*see* Sarcoidosis
lupoid (miliary) D86.3
Boerhaave's syndrome (spontaneous esophageal rupture) K22.3
Boggy
cervix N88.8
uterus N85.8

Boil —see also Furuncle, by site
　Aleppo B55.1
　Baghdad B55.1
　Delhi B55.1
　lacrimal
　　gland —see Dacryoadenitis
　　passages (duct) (sac) —see Inflammation,
　　　lacrimal, passages, acute
　Natal B55.1
　orbit, orbital —see Abscess, orbit
　tropical B55.1
Bold hives —see Urticaria
Bombé, iris —see Membrane, pupillary
Bone —see condition
Bonnevie-Ullrich syndrome —see also Turner's
　syndrome Q87.19
Bonnier's syndrome —see subcategory H81.8
Bonvale dam fever T73.3
Bony block of joint —see Ankylosis
BOOP (bronchiolitis obliterans organized
　pneumonia) J84.89
Borderline
　diabetes mellitus R73.03
　hypertension R03.0
　osteopenia M85.8-●
　pelvis, with obstruction during labor O65.1
　personality F60.3
Borna disease A83.9
Bornholm disease B33.0
Boston exanthem A88.0
Botalli, ductus (patent) (persistent) Q25.0
Bothriocephalus latus infestation B70.0
Botulism (foodborne intoxication) A05.1
　infant A48.51
　non-foodborne A48.52
　wound A48.52
Bouba —see Yaws
Bouchard's nodes (with arthropathy) M15.2
Bouffée délirante F23
Bouillaud's disease or syndrome (rheumatic
　heart disease) I01.9
Bourneville's disease Q85.1
Boutonniere deformity (finger) —see
　Deformity, finger, boutonniere
Bouveret (-Hoffmann) syndrome (paroxysmal
　tachycardia) I47.9
Bovine heart —see Hypertrophy, cardiac
Bowel —see condition
Bowen's
　dermatosis (precancerous) —see Neoplasm,
　　skin, in situ
　disease —see Neoplasm, skin, in situ
　epithelioma —see Neoplasm, skin, in situ
　type
　　epidermoid carcinoma-in-situ —see
　　　Neoplasm, skin, in situ
　　intraepidermal squamous cell carcinoma —
　　　see Neoplasm, skin, in situ
Bowing
　femur —see also Deformity, limb, specified
　　type NEC, thigh
　　congenital Q68.3
　fibula —see also Deformity, limb, specified
　　type NEC, lower leg
　　congenital Q68.4
　forearm —see Deformity, limb, specified type
　　NEC, forearm
　leg(s), long bones, congenital Q68.5
　radius —see Deformity, limb, specified type
　　NEC, forearm
　tibia —see also Deformity, limb, specified type
　　NEC, lower leg
　　congenital Q68.4
Bowleg(s) (acquired) M21.16-●
　congenital Q68.5
　rachitic E64.3
Boyd's dysentery A03.2
Brachial —see condition
Brachycardia R00.1
Brachycephaly Q75.0
Bradley's disease A08.19

Bradyarrhythmia, cardiac I49.8
Bradycardia (sinoatrial) (sinus) (vagal) R00.1
　neonatal P29.12
　reflex G90.09
　tachycardia syndrome I49.5
Bradykinesia R25.8
Bradypnea R06.89
Bradytachycardia I49.5
Brailsford's disease or osteochondrosis —see
　Osteochondrosis, juvenile, radius
Brain —see also condition
　death G93.82
　syndrome —see Syndrome, brain
Branched-chain amino-acid disorder E71.2
Branchial —see condition
　cartilage, congenital Q18.2
Branchiogenic remnant (in neck) Q18.0
Brandt's syndrome (acrodermatitis
　enteropathica) E83.2
Brash (water) R12
Bravais-Jacksonian epilepsy —see Epilepsy,
　localization-related, symptomatic, with
　simple partial seizures
Braxton Hicks contractions —see False, labor
Brazilian leishmaniasis B55.2
BRBPR K62.5
Break, retina (without detachment) H33.30-●
　with retinal detachment —see Detachment,
　　retina
　horseshoe tear H33.31-●
　multiple H33.33-●
　round hole H33.32-●
Breakdown
　device, graft or implant —see also
　　Complications, by site and type,
　　mechanical T85.618
　arterial graft NEC —see Complication,
　　cardiovascular device, mechanical,
　　vascular
　breast (implant) T85.41
　catheter NEC T85.618
　　cystostomy T83.010
　　dialysis (renal) T82.41
　　　intraperitoneal T85.611
　　Hopkins T83.018
　　ileostomy T83.018
　　infusion NEC T82.514
　　　cranial T85.610
　　　epidural T85.610
　　　intrathecal T85.610
　　　spinal T85.610
　　　subarachnoid T85.610
　　　subdural T85.610
　　nephrostomy T83.012
　　urethral indwelling T83.011
　　urinary NEC T83.018
　　urostomy T83.018
　electronic (electrode) (pulse generator)
　　(stimulator)
　　bone T84.310
　　cardiac T82.119
　　　electrode T82.110
　　　pulse generator T82.111
　　　specified type NEC T82.118
　　nervous system —see Complication,
　　　prosthetic device, mechanical,
　　　electronic nervous system stimulator
　　urinary —see Complication,
　　　genitourinary, device, urinary,
　　　mechanical
　fixation, internal (orthopedic) NEC —
　　see Complication, fixation device,
　　mechanical
　gastrointestinal —see Complications,
　　prosthetic device, mechanical,
　　gastrointestinal device
　genital NEC T83.418
　　intrauterine contraceptive device T83.31
　　penile prosthesis (cylinder) (implanted)
　　　(pump) (resevoir) T83.410
　　testicular prosthesis T83.411

Breakdown (Continued)
　device, graft or implant (Continued)
　　heart NEC —see Complication,
　　　cardiovascular device, mechanical
　　intrathecal infusion pump T85.615
　　joint prosthesis —see Complications..., joint
　　　prosthesis, internal, mechanical, by site
　　nervous system, specified device NEC
　　　T85.615
　　ocular NEC —see Complications, prosthetic
　　　device, mechanical, ocular device
　　orthopedic NEC —see Complication,
　　　orthopedic, device, mechanical
　　specified NEC T85.618
　　subcutaneous device pocket
　　　nervous system prosthetic device,
　　　　implant, or graft T85.890
　　　other internal prosthetic device, implant,
　　　　or graft T85.898
　　sutures, permanent T85.612
　　　used in bone repair —see Complications,
　　　　fixation device, internal
　　　　(orthopedic), mechanical
　　urinary NEC T83.118
　　　graft T83.21
　　　sphincter, implanted T83.111
　　　stent (ileal conduit) (nephroureteral)
　　　　T83.113
　　　ureteral indwelling T83.112
　　vascular NEC —see Complication,
　　　cardiovascular device, mechanical
　　ventricular intracranial shunt T85.01
　nervous F48.8
　perineum O90.1
　respirator J95.850
　　specified NEC J95.859
　ventilator J95.850
　　specified NEC J95.859
Breast —see also condition
　buds E30.1
　　in newborn P96.89
　dense R92.2
　nodule —see also Lump, breast N63.0
Breath
　foul R19.6
　holder, child R06.89
　holding spell R06.89
　shortness R06.02
Breathing
　labored —see Hyperventilation
　mouth R06.5
　　causing malocclusion M26.5
　periodic R06.3
　　high altitude G47.32
Breathlessness R06.81
Breda's disease —see Yaws
Breech presentation (mother) O32.1
　causing obstructed labor O64.1
　footling O32.8
　　causing obstructed labor O64.8
　incomplete O32.8
　　causing obstructed labor O64.8
Breisky's disease N90.4
Brennemann's syndrome I88.0
Brenner
　tumor (benign) D27.9
　　borderline malignancy D39.1-●
　　malignant C56
　　proliferating D39.1
Bretonneau's disease or angina A36.0
Breus' mole O02.0
Brevicollis Q76.49
Brickmakers' anemia B76.9 [D63.8]
Bridge, myocardial Q24.5
Bright red blood per rectum (BRBPR)
　K62.5
Bright's disease —see also Nephritis
　arteriosclerotic —see Hypertension, kidney
Brill (-Zinsser) disease (recrudescent typhus)
　A75.1
Brill-Symmers' disease C82.90

Brion-Kayser disease —*see* Fever, parathyroid
Briquet's disorder or syndrome F45.0
Brissaud's
  infantilism or dwarfism E23.0
  motor-verbal tic F95.2
Brittle
  bones disease Q78.0
  nails L60.3
    congenital Q84.6
Broad —*see also* condition
  beta disease E78.2
  ligament laceration syndrome N83.8
Broad- or floating-betalipoproteinemia E78.2
Brock's syndrome (atelectasis due to enlarged
    lymph nodes) J98.19
Brocq-Duhring disease (dermatitis
    herpetiformis) L13.0
Brodie's abscess or disease M86.8X-●
Broken
  arches —*see also* Deformity, limb, flat foot
  arm (meaning upper limb) —*see* Fracture, arm
  back —*see* Fracture, vertebra
  bone —*see* Fracture
  implant or internal device —*see*
    Complications, by site and type,
    mechanical
  leg (meaning lower limb) —*see* Fracture, leg
  nose S02.2
  tooth, teeth —*see* Fracture, tooth
Bromhidrosis, bromidrosis L75.0
➡ Bromidism, bromism G92.8
  chronic (dependence) F13.20
  due to
    correct substance properly administered —
      see Table of Drugs and Chemicals, by
      drug, adverse effect
    overdose or wrong substance given
      or taken —*see* Table of Drugs and
      Chemicals, by drug, poisoning
Bromidrosiphobia F40.298
Bronchi, bronchial —*see* condition
Bronchiectasis (cylindrical) (diffuse) (fusiform)
    (localized) (saccular) J47.9
  with
    acute
      bronchitis J47.0
      lower respiratory infection J47.0
    exacerbation (acute) J47.1
  congenital Q33.4
  tuberculous NEC —*see* Tuberculosis,
    pulmonary
Bronchiolectasis —*see* Bronchiectasis
Bronchiolitis (acute) (infective) (subacute) J21.9
  with
    bronchospasm or obstruction J21.9
    influenza, flu or grippe —*see* Influenza,
      with, respiratory manifestations NEC
    chemical (chronic) J68.4
      acute J68.0
    chronic (fibrosing) (obliterative) J44.9
    due to
      external agent —*see* Bronchitis, acute,
        due to
      human metapneumovirus J21.1
      respiratory syncytial virus (RSV) J21.0
      specified organism NEC J21.8
    fibrosa obliterans J44.9
    influenzal —*see* Influenza, with, respiratory
      manifestations NEC
    obliterans J42
      with organizing pneumonia (BOOP) J84.89
    obliterative (chronic) (subacute) J44.9
      due to chemicals, gases, fumes or vapors
        (inhalation) J68.4
      due to fumes or vapors J68.4
    respiratory, interstitial lung disease J84.115
Bronchitis (diffuse) (fibrinous) (hypostatic)
    (infective) (membranous) J40
  with
    influenza, flu or grippe —*see* Influenza,
      with, respiratory manifestations NEC

Bronchitis (*Continued*)
  with (*Continued*)
    obstruction (airway) (lung) J44.9
    tracheitis (15 years of age and above) J40
      acute or subacute J20.9
      chronic J42
      under 15 years of age J20.9
  acute or subacute (with bronchospasm or
      obstruction) J20.9
    with
      bronchiectasis J47.0
      chronic obstructive pulmonary disease
        J44.0
      chemical (due to gases, fumes or vapors)
        J68.0
    due to
      fumes or vapors J68.0
      Haemophilus influenzae J20.1
      Mycoplasma pneumoniae J20.0
      radiation J70.0
      specified organism NEC J20.8
      Streptococcus J20.2
      virus
        coxsackie J20.3
        echovirus J20.7
        parainfluenzae J20.4
        respiratory syncytial (RSV) J20.5
        rhinovirus J20.6
    viral NEC J20.8
  allergic (acute) J45.909
    with
      exacerbation (acute) J45.901
      status asthmaticus J45.902
  arachidic T17.528
  aspiration (due to food and vomit) J69.0
  asthmatic J45.9
    chronic J44.9
      with
        acute lower respiratory infection J44.0
        exacerbation (acute) J44.1
  capillary —*see* Pneumonia, broncho
  caseous (tuberculous) A15.5
  Castellani's A69.8
  catarrhal (15 years of age and above) J40
    acute —*see* Bronchitis, acute
    chronic J41.0
    under 15 years of age J20.9
  chemical (acute) (subacute) J68.0
    chronic J68.4
    due to fumes or vapors J68.0
      chronic J68.4
  chronic J42
    with
      airways obstruction J44.9
      tracheitis (chronic) J42
    asthmatic (obstructive) J44.9
    catarrhal J41.0
    chemical (due to fumes or vapors) J68.4
    due to
      chemicals, gases, fumes or vapors
        (inhalation) J68.4
      radiation J70.1
      tobacco smoking J41.0
    emphysematous J44.9
    mucopurulent J41.1
    non-obstructive J41.0
    obliterans J44.9
    obstructive J44.9
    purulent J41.1
    simple J41.0
  croupous —*see* Bronchitis, acute
  due to gases, fumes or vapors (chemical)
    J68.0
  emphysematous (obstructive) J44.9
  exudative —*see* Bronchitis, acute
  fetid J41.1
  grippal —*see* Influenza, with, respiratory
    manifestations NEC
  in those under 15 years age —*see* Bronchitis,
    acute
    chronic —*see* Bronchitis, chronic

Bronchitis (*Continued*)
  influenzal —*see* Influenza, with, respiratory
    manifestations NEC
  mixed simple and mucopurulent J41.8
  moulder's J62.8
  mucopurulent (chronic) (recurrent) J41.1
    acute or subacute J20.9
    simple (mixed) J41.8
  obliterans (chronic) J44.9
  obstructive (chronic) (diffuse) J44.9
  pituitous J41.1
  pneumococcal, acute or subacute J20.2
  pseudomembranous, acute or subacute —*see*
    Bronchitis, acute
  purulent (chronic) (recurrent) J41.1
    acute or subacute —*see* Bronchitis, acute
  putrid J41.1
  senile (chronic) J42
  simple and mucopurulent (mixed) J41.8
  smokers' J41.0
  spirochetal NEC A69.8
  subacute —*see* Bronchitis, acute
  suppurative (chronic) J41.1
    acute or subacute —*see* Bronchitis, acute
  tuberculous A15.5
  under 15 years of age —*see* Bronchitis, acute
    chronic —*see* Bronchitis, chronic
  viral NEC, acute or subacute —*see also*
    Bronchitis, acute J20.8
Bronchoalveolitis J18.0
Bronchoaspergillosis B44.1
Bronchocele meaning goiter E04.0
Broncholithiasis J98.09
  tuberculous NEC A15.5
Bronchomalacia J98.09
  congenital Q32.2
Bronchomycosis NOS B49 [*J99*]
  candidal B37.1
Bronchopleuropneumonia —*see* Pneumonia,
  broncho
Bronchopneumonia —*see* Pneumonia, broncho
Bronchopneumonitis —*see* Pneumonia,
  broncho
Bronchopulmonary —*see* condition
Bronchopulmonitis —*see* Pneumonia, broncho
Bronchorrhagia (*see* Hemoptysis)
Bronchorrhea J98.09
  acute J20.9
  chronic (infective) (purulent) J12
Bronchospasm (acute) J98.01
  with
    bronchiolitis, acute J21.9
    bronchitis, acute (conditions in J20) —*see*
      Bronchitis, acute
  due to external agent —*see* condition,
    respiratory, acute, due to
  exercise induced J45.990
Bronchospirochetosis A69.8
  Castellani A69.8
Bronchostenosis J98.09
Bronchus —*see* condition
Brontophobia F40.220
Bronze baby syndrome P83.88
Brooke's tumor —*see* Neoplasm, skin, benign
Brown enamel of teeth (hereditary) K00.5
Brown's sheath syndrome H50.61-●
Brown-Séquard disease, paralysis or
    syndrome G83.81
Bruce sepsis A23.0
Brucellosis (infection) A23.9
  abortus A23.1
  canis A23.3
  dermatitis A23.9
  melitensis A23.0
  mixed A23.8
  sepsis A23.9
    melitensis A23.0
    specified NEC A23.8
  suis A23.2
Bruck-de Lange disease Q87.19
Bruck's disease —*see* Deformity, limb

BRUE (brief resolved unexplained event) R68.13
Brugsch's syndrome Q82.8
Bruise (skin surface intact) —see also Contusion
with
  open wound —see Wound, open
  internal organ —see Injury, by site
  newborn P54.5
  scalp, due to birth injury, newborn P12.3
  umbilical cord O69.5
Bruit (arterial) R09.89
  cardiac R01.1
Brush burn —see Abrasion, by site
Bruton's X-linked agammaglobulinemia D80.0
Bruxism
  psychogenic F45.8
  sleep related G47.63
Bubbly lung syndrome P27.0
Bubo I88.8
  blennorrhagic (gonococcal) A54.89
  chancroidal A57
  climatic A55
  due to Haemophilus ducreyi A57
  gonococcal A54.89
  indolent (nonspecific) I88.8
  inguinal (nonspecific) I88.8
    chancroidal A57
    climatic A55
    due to H. ducreyi A57
    infective I88.8
  scrofulous (tuberculous) A18.2
  soft chancre A57
  suppurating —see Lymphadenitis, acute
  syphilitic (primary) A51.0
    congenital A50.07
  tropical A55
  virulent (chancroidal) A57
Bubonic plague A20.0
Bubonocele —see Hernia, inguinal
Buccal —see condition
Buchanan's disease or osteochondrosis M91.0
Buchem's syndrome (hyperostosis corticalis)
  M85.2
Bucket-handle fracture or tear (semilunar
  cartilage) —see Tear, meniscus
Budd-Chiari syndrome (hepatic vein
  thrombosis) I82.0
Budgerigar fancier's disease or lung
  J67.2
Buds
  breast E30.1
    in newborn P96.89
Buerger's disease (thromboangiitis obliterans)
  I73.1
Bulbar —see condition
Bulbus cordis (left ventricle) (persistent) Q21.8
Bulimia (nervosa) F50.2
  atypical F50.9
  normal weight F50.9
Bulky
  stools R19.5
  uterus N85.2
Bulla (e) R23.8
  lung (emphysematous) (solitary) J43.9
    newborn P25.8
Bullet wound —see also Wound, open
  fracture - code as Fracture, by site
  internal organ —see Injury, by site
Bundle
  branch block (complete) (false)
    (incomplete) —see Block, bundle-branch
  of His —see condition
Bunion M21.61-●
  tailor's M21.62-●
Bunionette M21.62-●
Buphthalmia, buphthalmos (congenital) Q15.0
Burdwan fever B55.0
Bürger-Grütz disease or syndrome E78.3
Buried
  penis (congenital) Q55.64
    acquired N48.83
  roots K08.3

Burke's syndrome K86.89
Burkitt
  cell leukemia C91.0-●
  lymphoma (malignant) C83.7-●
    small noncleaved, diffuse C83.7-●
    spleen C83.77
    undifferentiated C83.7-●
  tumor C83.7-●
  type
    acute lymphoblastic leukemia C91.0-●
    undifferentiated C83.7-●
Burn (electricity) (flame) (hot gas, liquid or hot
  object) (radiation) (steam) (thermal) T30.0
  abdomen, abdominal (muscle) (wall)
    T21.02
    first degree T21.12
    second degree T21.22
    third degree T21.32
  above elbow T22.039
    first degree T22.139
    left T22.032
      first degree T22.132
      second degree T22.232
      third degree T22.332
    right T22.031
      first degree T22.131
      second degree T22.231
      third degree T22.331
    second degree T22.239
    third degree T22.339
  acid (caustic) (external) (internal) —see
    Corrosion, by site
  alimentary tract NEC T28.2
    esophagus T28.1
    mouth T28.0
    pharynx T28.0
  alkaline (caustic) (external) (internal) —see
    Corrosion, by site
  ankle T25.019
    first degree T25.119
    left T25.012
      first degree T25.112
      second degree T25.212
      third degree T25.312
    multiple with foot —see Burn, lower, limb,
      multiple, ankle and foot
    right T25.011
      first degree T25.111
      second degree T25.211
      third degree T25.311
    second degree T25.219
    third degree T25.319
  anus —see Burn, buttock
  arm (lower) (upper) —see Burn, upper,
    limb
  axilla T22.049
    first degree T22.149
    left T22.042
      first degree T22.142
      second degree T22.242
      third degree T22.342
    right T22.041
      first degree T22.141
      second degree T22.241
      third degree T22.341
    second degree T22.249
    third degree T22.349
  back (lower) T21.04
    first degree T21.14
    second degree T21.24
    third degree T21.34
    upper T21.03
      first degree T21.13
      second degree T21.23
      third degree T21.33
  blisters - code as Burn, second degree, by site
  breast(s) —see Burn, chest wall
  buttock(s) T21.05
    first degree T21.15
    second degree T21.25
    third degree T21.35

Burn (Continued)
  calf T24.039
    first degree T24.139
    left T24.032
      first degree T24.132
      second degree T24.232
      third degree T24.332
    right T24.031
      first degree T24.131
      second degree T24.231
      third degree T24.331
    second degree T24.239
    third degree T24.339
  canthus (eye) —see Burn, eyelid
  caustic acid or alkaline —see Corrosion, by
    site
  cervix T28.3
  cheek T20.06
    first degree T20.16
    second degree T20.26
    third degree T20.36
  chemical (acids) (alkalines) (caustics) (external)
    (internal) —see Corrosion, by site
  chest wall T21.01
    first degree T21.11
    second degree T21.21
    third degree T21.31
  chin T20.03
    first degree T20.13
    second degree T20.23
    third degree T20.33
  colon T28.2
  conjunctiva (and cornea) —see Burn, cornea
  cornea (and conjunctiva) T26.1-●
    chemical —see Corrosion, cornea
  corrosion (external) (internal) —see
    Corrosion, by site
  deep necrosis of underlying tissue - code as
    Burn, third degree, by site
  dorsum of hand T23.069
    first degree T23.169
    left T23.062
      first degree T23.162
      second degree T23.262
      third degree T23.362
    right T23.061
      first degree T23.161
      second degree T23.261
      third degree T23.361
    second degree T23.269
    third degree T23.369
  due to ingested chemical agent —see
    Corrosion, by site
  ear (auricle) (external) (canal) T20.01
    first degree T20.11
    second degree T20.21
    third degree T20.31
  elbow T22.029
    first degree T22.129
    left T22.022
      first degree T22.122
      second degree T22.222
      third degree T22.322
    right T22.021
      first degree T22.121
      second degree T22.221
      third degree T22.321
    second degree T22.229
    third degree T22.329
  epidermal loss - code as Burn, second degree,
    by site
  erythema, erythematous - code as Burn, first
    degree, by site
  esophagus T28.1
  extent (percentage of body surface)
    less than 10 percent T31.0
    10-19 percent T31.10
      with 0-9 percent third degree burns
        T31.10
      with 10-19 percent third degree burns
        T31.11

▶ New   ⇒ Revised   ~~deleted~~ Deleted   ● Use Additional Character(s)

Burn *(Continued)*
  extent *(Continued)*
    20-29 percent T31.20
      with 0-9 percent third degree burns
        T31.20
      with 10-19 percent third degree burns
        T31.21
      with 20-29 percent third degree burns
        T31.22
    30-39 percent T31.30
      with 0-9 percent third degree burns
        T31.30
      with 10-19 percent third degree burns
        T31.31
      with 20-29 percent third degree burns
        T31.32
      with 30-39 percent third degree burns
        T31.33
    40-49 percent T31.40
      with 0-9 percent third degree burns
        T31.40
      with 10-19 percent third degree burns
        T31.41
      with 20-29 percent third degree burns
        T31.42
      with 30-39 percent third degree burns
        T31.43
      with 40-49 percent third degree burns
        T31.44
    50-59 percent T31.50
      with 0-9 percent third degree burns T31.50
      with 10-19 percent third degree burns
        T31.51
      with 20-29 percent third degree burns
        T31.52
      with 30-39 percent third degree burns
        T31.53
      with 40-49 percent third degree burns
        T31.54
      with 50-59 percent third degree burns
        T31.55
    60-69 percent T31.60
      with 0-9 percent third degree burns T31.60
      with 10-19 percent third degree burns
        T31.61
      with 20-29 percent third degree burns
        T31.62
      with 30-39 percent third degree burns
        T31.63
      with 40-49 percent third degree burns
        T31.64
      with 50-59 percent third degree burns
        T31.65
      with 60-69 percent third degree burns
        T31.66
    70-79 percent T31.70
      with 0-9 percent third degree burns T31.70
      with 10-19 percent third degree burns
        T31.71
      with 20-29 percent third degree burns
        T31.72
      with 30-39 percent third degree burns
        T31.73
      with 40-49 percent third degree burns
        T31.74
      with 50-59 percent third degree burns
        T31.75
      with 60-69 percent third degree burns
        T31.76
      with 70-79 percent third degree burns
        T31.77
    80-89 percent T31.80
      with 0-9 percent third degree burns T31.80
      with 10-19 percent third degree burns
        T31.81
      with 20-29 percent third degree burns
        T31.82
      with 30-39 percent third degree burns
        T31.83
      with 40-49 percent third degree burns
        T31.84

Burn *(Continued)*
  extent *(Continued)*
    80-89 percent T31.80 *(Continued)*
      with 50-59 percent third degree burns
        T31.85
      with 60-69 percent third degree burns
        T31.86
      with 70-79 percent third degree burns
        T31.87
      with 80-89 percent third degree burns
        T31.88
    90 percent or more T31.90
      with 0-9 percent third degree burns T31.90
      with 10-19 percent third degree burns
        T31.91
      with 20-29 percent third degree burns
        T31.92
      with 30-39 percent third degree burns
        T31.93
      with 40-49 percent third degree burns
        T31.94
      with 50-59 percent third degree burns
        T31.95
      with 60-69 percent third degree burns
        T31.96
      with 70-79 percent third degree burns
        T31.97
      with 80-89 percent third degree burns
        T31.98
      with 90 percent or more third degree
        burns T31.99
  extremity —*see* Burn, limb
  eye(s) and adnexa T26.4-●
    with resulting rupture and destruction of
      eyeball T26.2-●
    conjunctival sac —*see* Burn, cornea
    cornea —*see* Burn, cornea
    lid —*see* Burn, eyelid
    periocular area —*see* Burn, eyelid
    specified site NEC T26.3-●
  eyeball —*see* Burn, eye
  eyelid(s) T26.0-●
    chemical —*see* Corrosion, eyelid
  face —*see* Burn, head
  finger T23.029
    first degree T23.129
    left T23.022
      first degree T23.122
      second degree T23.222
      third degree T23.322
    multiple sites (without thumb) T23.039
      with thumb T23.049
        first degree T23.149
        left T23.042
          first degree T23.142
          second degree T23.242
          third degree T23.342
        right T23.041
          first degree T23.141
          second degree T23.241
          third degree T23.341
        second degree T23.249
        third degree T23.349
      first degree T23.139
      left T23.032
        first degree T23.132
        second degree T23.232
        third degree T23.332
      right T23.031
        first degree T23.131
        second degree T23.231
        third degree T23.331
      second degree T23.239
      third degree T23.339
    right T23.021
      first degree T23.121
      second degree T23.221
      third degree T23.321
    second degree T23.229
    third degree T23.329
  flank —*see* Burn, abdominal wall

Burn *(Continued)*
  foot T25.029
    first degree T25.129
    left T25.022
      first degree T25.122
      second degree T25.222
      third degree T25.322
    multiple with ankle —*see* Burn, lower,
      limb, multiple, ankle and foot
    right T25.021
      first degree T25.121
      second degree T25.221
      third degree T25.321
    second degree T25.229
    third degree T25.329
  forearm T22.019
    first degree T22.119
    left T22.012
      first degree T22.112
      second degree T22.212
      third degree T22.312
    right T22.011
      first degree T22.111
      second degree T22.211
      third degree T22.311
    second degree T22.219
    third degree T22.319
  forehead T20.06
    first degree T20.16
    second degree T20.26
    third degree T20.36
  fourth degree - code as Burn, third degree,
    by site
  friction —*see* Burn, by site
  from swallowing caustic or corrosive
    substance NEC —*see* Corrosion,
    by site
  full thickness skin loss - code as Burn, third
    degree, by site
  gastrointestinal tract NEC T28.2
    from swallowing caustic or corrosive
      substance T28.7
  genital organs
    external
      female T21.07
        first degree T21.17
        second degree T21.27
        third degree T21.37
      male T21.06
        first degree T21.16
        second degree T21.26
        third degree T21.36
    internal T28.3
      from caustic or corrosive substance
        T28.8
  groin —*see* Burn, abdominal wall
  hand(s) T23.009
    back —*see* Burn, dorsum of hand
    finger —*see* Burn, finger
    first degree T23.109
    left T23.002
      first degree T23.102
      second degree T23.202
      third degree T23.302
    multiple sites with wrist T23.099
      first degree T23.199
      left T23.092
        first degree T23.192
        second degree T23.292
        third degree T23.392
      right T23.091
        first degree T23.191
        second degree T23.291
        third degree T23.391
      second degree T23.299
      third degree T23.399
    palm —*see* Burn, palm
    right T23.001
      first degree T23.101
      second degree T23.201
      third degree T23.301

Burn *(Continued)*
  hand *(Continued)*
    second degree T23.209
    third degree T23.309
    thumb —*see* Burn, thumb
  head (and face) (and neck) T20.00
    cheek —*see* Burn, cheek
    chin —*see* Burn, chin
    ear —*see* Burn, ear
    eye(s) only —*see* Burn, eye
    first degree T20.10
    forehead —*see* Burn, forehead
    lip —*see* Burn, lip
    multiple sites T20.09
      first degree T20.19
      second degree T20.29
      third degree T20.39
    neck —*see* Burn, neck
    nose —*see* Burn, nose
    scalp —*see* Burn, scalp
    second degree T20.20
    third degree T20.30
  hip(s) —*see* Burn, thigh
  inhalation —*see* Burn, respiratory tract
    caustic or corrosive substance (fumes) —*see*
      Corrosion, respiratory tract
  internal organ(s) T28.40
    alimentary tract T28.2
      esophagus T28.1
    eardrum T28.41
    esophagus T28.1
    from caustic or corrosive substance
      (swallowing) NEC —*see* Corrosion,
      by site
    genitourinary T28.3
    mouth T28.0
    pharynx T28.0
    respiratory tract —*see* Burn, respiratory
      tract
    specified organ NEC T28.49
  interscapular region —*see* Burn, back,
    upper
  intestine (large) (small) T28.2
  knee T24.029
    first degree T24.129
    left T24.022
      first degree T24.122
      second degree T24.222
      third degree T24.322
    right T24.021
      first degree T24.121
      second degree T24.221
      third degree T24.321
    second degree T24.229
    third degree T24.329
  labium (majus) (minus) —*see* Burn, genital
    organs, external, female
  lacrimal apparatus, duct, gland or sac —*see*
    Burn, eye, specified site NEC
  larynx T27.0
    with lung T27.1
  leg(s) (lower) (upper) —*see* Burn, lower,
    limb
  lightning —*see* Burn, by site
  limb(s)
    lower (except ankle or foot alone) —*see*
      Burn, lower, limb
    upper —*see* Burn, upper limb
  lip(s) T20.02
    first degree T20.12
    second degree T20.22
    third degree T20.32
  lower
    back —*see* Burn, back
    limb T24.009
      ankle —*see* Burn, ankle
      calf —*see* Burn, calf
      first degree T24.109
      foot —*see* Burn, foot
      hip —*see* Burn, thigh
      knee —*see* Burn, knee

Burn *(Continued)*
  lower *(Continued)*
    limb *(Continued)*
      left T24.002
        first degree T24.102
        second degree T24.202
        third degree T24.302
      multiple sites, except ankle and foot
        T24.099
        ankle and foot T25.099
          first degree T25.199
          left T25.092
            first degree T25.192
            second degree T25.292
            third degree T25.392
          right T25.091
            first degree T25.191
            second degree T25.291
            third degree T25.391
          second degree T25.299
          third degree T25.399
        first degree T24.199
        left T24.092
          first degree T24.192
          second degree T24.292
          third degree T24.392
        right T24.091
          first degree T24.191
          second degree T24.291
          third degree T24.391
        second degree T24.299
        third degree T24.399
      right T24.001
        first degree T24.101
        second degree T24.201
        third degree T24.301
      second degree T24.209
      thigh —*see* Burn, thigh
      third degree T24.309
      toe —*see* Burn, toe
  lung (with larynx and trachea) T27.1
  mouth T28.0
  neck T20.07
    first degree T20.17
    second degree T20.27
    third degree T20.37
  nose (septum) T20.04
    first degree T20.14
    second degree T20.24
    third degree T20.34
  ocular adnexa —*see* Burn, eye
  orbit region —*see* Burn, eyelid
  palm T23.059
    first degree T23.159
    left T23.052
      first degree T23.152
      second degree T23.252
      third degree T23.352
    right T23.051
      first degree T23.151
      second degree T23.251
      third degree T23.351
    second degree T23.259
    third degree T23.359
  ~~partial thickness - code as Burn, degree, by site~~
  ▶partial thickness - code as Burn, by site,
    second degree
  pelvis —*see* Burn, trunk
  penis —*see* Burn, genital organs, external,
    male
  perineum
    female —*see* Burn, genital organs, external,
      female
    male —*see* Burn, genital organs, external,
      male
  periocular area —*see* Burn, eyelid
  pharynx T28.0
  rectum T28.2
  respiratory tract T27.3
    larynx —*see* Burn, larynx
    specified part NEC T27.2
    trachea —*see* Burn, trachea

Burn *(Continued)*
  sac, lacrimal —*see* Burn, eye, specified site
    NEC
  scalp T20.05
    first degree T20.15
    second degree T20.25
    third degree T20.35
  scapular region T22.069
    first degree T22.169
    left T22.062
      first degree T22.162
      second degree T22.262
      third degree T22.362
    right T22.061
      first degree T22.161
      second degree T22.261
      third degree T22.361
    second degree T22.269
    third degree T22.369
  sclera —*see* Burn, eye, specified site NEC
  scrotum —*see* Burn, genital organs, external,
    male
  shoulder T22.059
    first degree T22.159
    left T22.052
      first degree T22.152
      second degree T22.252
      third degree T22.352
    right T22.051
      first degree T22.151
      second degree T22.251
      third degree T22.351
    second degree T22.259
    third degree T22.359
  stomach T28.2
  temple —*see* Burn, head
  testis —*see* Burn, genital organs, external, male
  thigh T24.019
    first degree T24.119
    left T24.012
      first degree T24.112
      second degree T24.212
      third degree T24.312
    right T24.011
      first degree T24.111
      second degree T24.211
      third degree T24.311
    second degree T24.219
    third degree T24.319
  thorax (external) —*see* Burn, trunk
  throat (meaning pharynx) T28.0
  thumb(s) T23.019
    first degree T23.119
    left T23.012
      first degree T23.112
      second degree T23.212
      third degree T23.312
    multiple sites with fingers T23.049
      first degree T23.149
      left T23.042
        first degree T23.142
        second degree T23.242
        third degree T23.342
      right T23.041
        first degree T23.141
        second degree T23.241
        third degree T23.341
      second degree T23.249
      third degree T23.349
    right T23.011
      first degree T23.111
      second degree T23.211
      third degree T23.311
    second degree T23.219
    third degree T23.319
  toe T25.039
    first degree T25.139
    left T25.032
      first degree T25.132
      second degree T25.232
      third degree T25.332

▶ New   ⇒ Revised   ~~deleted~~ Deleted   ● Use Additional Character(s)

Burn (*Continued*)
  toe (*Continued*)
    right T25.031
      first degree T25.131
      second degree T25.231
      third degree T25.331
    second degree T25.239
    third degree T25.339
  tongue T28.0
  tonsil(s) T28.0
  trachea T27.0
    with lung T27.1
  trunk T21.00
    abdominal wall —*see* Burn, abdominal wall
    anus —*see* Burn, buttock
    axilla —*see* Burn, upper limb
    back —*see* Burn, back
    breast —*see* Burn, chest wall
    buttock —*see* Burn, buttock
    chest wall —*see* Burn, chest wall
    first degree T21.10
    flank —*see* Burn, abdominal wall
    genital
      female —*see* Burn, genital organs, external, female
      male —*see* Burn, genital organs, external, male
    groin —*see* Burn, abdominal wall
    interscapular region —*see* Burn, back, upper
    labia —*see* Burn, genital organs, external, female
    lower back —*see* Burn, back
    penis —*see* Burn, genital organs, external, male
    perineum
      female —*see* Burn, genital organs, external, female
      male —*see* Burn, genital organs, external, male
    scapula region —*see* Burn, scapular region
    scrotum —*see* Burn, genital organs, external, male
    second degree T21.20
    specified site NEC T21.09
      first degree T21.19
      second degree T21.29
      third degree T21.39
    testes —*see* Burn, genital organs, external, male
    third degree T21.30
    upper back —*see* Burn, back, upper
    vulva —*see* Burn, genital organs, external, female
  unspecified site with extent of body surface involved specified
    less than 10 percent T31.0
    10-19 percent (0-9 percent third degree) T31.10
      with 10-19 percent third degree T31.11
    20-29 percent (0-9 percent third degree) T31.20
      with
        10-19 percent third degree T31.21
        20-29 percent third degree T31.22
    30-39 percent (0-9 percent third degree) T31.30
      with
        10-19 percent third degree T31.31
        20-29 percent third degree T31.32
        30-39 percent third degree T31.33
    40-49 percent (0-9 percent third degree) T31.40
      with
        10-19 percent third degree T31.41
        20-29 percent third degree T31.42
        30-39 percent third degree T31.43
        40-49 percent third degree T31.44

Burn (*Continued*)
  unspecified site with extent of body surface involved specified (*Continued*)
    50-59 percent (0-9 percent third degree) T31.50
      with
        10-19 percent third degree T31.51
        20-29 percent third degree T31.52
        30-39 percent third degree T31.53
        40-49 percent third degree T31.54
        50-59 percent third degree T31.55
    60-69 percent (0-9 percent third degree) T31.60
      with
        10-19 percent third degree T31.61
        20-29 percent third degree T31.62
        30-39 percent third degree T31.63
        40-49 percent third degree T31.64
        50-59 percent third degree T31.65
        60-69 percent third degree T31.66
    70-79 percent (0-9 percent third degree) T31.70
      with
        10-19 percent third degree T31.71
        20-29 percent third degree T31.72
        30-39 percent third degree T31.73
        40-49 percent third degree T31.74
        50-59 percent third degree T31.75
        60-69 percent third degree T31.76
        70-79 percent third degree T31.77
    80-89 percent (0-9 percent third degree) T31.80
      with
        10-19 percent third degree T31.81
        20-29 percent third degree T31.82
        30-39 percent third degree T31.83
        40-49 percent third degree T31.84
        50-59 percent third degree T31.85
        60-69 percent third degree T31.86
        70-79 percent third degree T31.87
        80-89 percent third degree T31.88
    90 percent or more (0-9 percent third degree) T31.90
      with
        10-19 percent third degree T31.91
        20-29 percent third degree T31.92
        30-39 percent third degree T31.93
        40-49 percent third degree T31.94
        50-59 percent third degree T31.95
        60-69 percent third degree T31.96
        70-79 percent third degree T31.97
        80-89 percent third degree T31.98
        90-99 percent third degree T31.99
  upper limb T22.00
    above elbow —*see* Burn, above elbow
    axilla —*see* Burn, axilla
    elbow —*see* Burn, elbow
    first degree T22.10
    forearm —*see* Burn, forearm
    hand —*see* Burn, hand
    interscapular region —*see* Burn, back, upper
    multiple sites T22.099
      first degree T22.199
      left T22.092
        first degree T22.192
        second degree T22.292
        third degree T22.392
      right T22.091
        first degree T22.191
        second degree T22.291
        third degree T22.391
      second degree T22.299
      third degree T22.399
    scapular region —*see* Burn, scapular region
    second degree T22.20
    shoulder —*see* Burn, shoulder
    third degree T22.30
    wrist —*see* Burn, wrist
  uterus T28.3
  vagina T28.3

Burn (*Continued*)
  vulva —*see* Burn, genital organs, external, female
  wrist T23.079
    first degree T23.179
    left T23.072
      first degree T23.172
      second degree T23.272
      third degree T23.372
    multiple sites with hand T23.099
      first degree T23.199
      left T23.092
        first degree T23.192
        second degree T23.292
        third degree T23.392
      right T23.091
        first degree T23.191
        second degree T23.291
        third degree T23.391
      second degree T23.299
      third degree T23.399
    right T23.071
      first degree T23.171
      second degree T23.271
      third degree T23.371
    second degree T23.279
    third degree T23.379
Burnett's syndrome E83.52
Burning
  feet syndrome E53.9
  sensation R20.8
  tongue K14.6
Burn-out (state) Z73.0
Burns' disease or osteochondrosis —*see* Osteochondrosis, juvenile, ulna
Bursa —*see* condition
Bursitis M71.9
  Achilles —*see* Tendinitis, Achilles
  adhesive —*see* Bursitis, specified NEC
  ankle —*see* Enthesopathy, lower limb, ankle, specified type NEC
  calcaneal —*see* Enthesopathy, foot, specified type NEC
  collateral ligament, tibial —*see* Bursitis, tibial collateral
  due to use, overuse, pressure —*see also* Disorder, soft tissue, due to use, specified type NEC
    specified NEC —*see* Disorder, soft tissue, due to use, specified NEC
  Duplay's M75.0
  elbow NEC M70.3-●
    olecranon M70.2-●
  finger —*see* Disorder, soft tissue, due to use, specified type NEC, hand
  foot —*see* Enthesopathy, foot, specified type NEC
  gonococcal A54.49
  gouty —*see* Gout
  hand M70.1-●
  hip NEC M70.7-●
    trochanteric M70.6-●
  infective NEC M71.10
    abscess —*see* Abscess, bursa
    ankle M71.17-●
    elbow M71.12-●
    foot M71.17-●
    hand M71.14-●
    hip M71.15-●
    knee M71.16-●
    multiple sites M71.19
    shoulder M71.11-●
    specified site NEC M71.18
    wrist M71.13-●
  ischial —*see* Bursitis, hip
  knee NEC M70.5-●
    prepatellar M70.4-●
  occupational NEC —*see also* Disorder, soft tissue, due to, use
  olecranon —*see* Bursitis, elbow, olecranon
  pharyngeal J39.1

Bursitis *(Continued)*
  popliteal —*see* Bursitis, knee
  prepatellar M70.4-●
➧radiohumeral M70.3-●
  rheumatoid M06.20
    ankle M06.27-●
    elbow M06.22-●
    foot joint M06.27-●
    hand joint M06.24-●
    hip M06.25-●
    knee M06.26-●
    multiple site M06.29
    shoulder M06.21-●
    vertebra M06.28
    wrist M06.23-●
  scapulohumeral —*see* Bursitis, shoulder
  semimembranous muscle (knee) —*see*
      Bursitis, knee
  shoulder M75.5-●
    adhesive —*see* Capsulitis, adhesive
  specified NEC M71.50
    ankle M71.57-●
    due to use, overuse or pressure —*see*
        Disorder, soft tissue, due to, use
    elbow M71.52-●
    foot M71.57-●
    hand M71.54-●

Bursitis *(Continued)*
  specified NEC *(Continued)*
    hip M71.55-●
    knee M71.56-●
    shoulder —*see* Bursitis, shoulder
    specified site NEC M71.58
    tibial collateral M76.4-●
    wrist M71.53-●
  subacromial —*see* Bursitis, shoulder
  subcoracoid —*see* Bursitis, shoulder
  subdeltoid —*see* Bursitis, shoulder
  syphilitic A52.78
  Thornwaldt, Tornwaldt J39.2
  tibial collateral M76.4-●
  toe —*see* Enthesopathy, foot, specified type
      NEC
  trochanteric (area) —*see* Bursitis, hip,
      trochanteric
  wrist —*see* Bursitis, hand
Bursopathy M71.9
  specified type NEC M71.80
    ankle M71.87-●
    elbow M71.82-●
    foot M71.87-●
    hand M71.84-●
    hip M71.85-●
    knee M71.86-●

Bursopathy *(Continued)*
  specified type NEC *(Continued)*
    multiple sites M71.89
    shoulder M71.81-●
    specified site NEC M71.88
    wrist M71.83-●
Burst stitches or sutures (complication of
    surgery) T81.31
  external operation wound T81.31
  internal operation wound T81.32
Buruli ulcer A31.1
Bury's disease L95.1
Buschke's
  disease —*see* Cryptococcosis by site
  scleredema —*see* Sclerosis, systemic
Busse-Buschke disease —*see* Cryptococcosis
    by site
Buttock —*see* condition
Button
  Biskra B55.1
  Delhi B55.1
  oriental B55.1
Buttonhole deformity (finger) —*see* Deformity,
    finger, boutonniere
Bwamba fever A92.8
Byssinosis J66.0
Bywaters' syndrome T79.5

C

Cachexia R64
  cancerous R64
  cardiac —see Disease, heart
  dehydration E86.0
  due to malnutrition R64
  exophthalmic —see Hyperthyroidism
  heart —see Disease, heart
  hypophyseal E23.0
  hypopituitary E23.0
  lead —see Poisoning, lead
  malignant R64
  marsh —see Malaria
  nervous F48.8
  old age R54
  paludal —see Malaria
  pituitary E23.0
▶ pulmonary R64
  renal N28.9
  saturnine —see Poisoning, lead
  senile R54
  Simmonds' E23.0
  splenica D73.0
  strumipriva E03.4
  tuberculous NEC —see Tuberculosis
CADASIL (cerebral autosomal dominant
    arteriopathy with subcortical infarcts
    and leukoencephalopathy) I67.850
Café au lait spots L81.3
Caffeine-induced
  anxiety disorder F15.980
  sleep disorder F15.982
Caffey's syndrome Q78.8
Caisson disease T70.3
Cake kidney Q63.1
Caked breast (puerperal, postpartum) O92.79
Calabar swelling B74.3
Calcaneal spur —see Spur, bone, calcaneal
Calcaneo-apophysitis M92.8
Calcareous —see condition
Calcicosis J62.8
Calciferol (vitamin D) deficiency E55.9
  with rickets E55.0
Calcification
  adrenal (capsule) (gland) E27.49
    tuberculous E35 [B90.8]
  aorta I70.0
  artery (annular) —see Arteriosclerosis
  auricle (ear) —see Disorder, pinna, specified
    type NEC
  basal ganglia G23.8
  bladder N32.89
    due to Schistosoma hematobium B65.0
  brain (cortex) —see Calcification, cerebral
  bronchus J98.09
  bursa M71.40
    ankle M71.47-●
    elbow M71.42-●
    foot M71.47-●
    hand M71.44-●
    hip M71.45-●
    knee M71.46-●
    multiple sites M71.49
    shoulder M75.3-●
    specified site NEC M71.48
    wrist M71.43-●
  cardiac —see Degeneration, myocardial
  cerebral (cortex) G93.89
    artery I67.2
  cervix (uteri) N88.8
  choroid plexus G93.89
  conjunctiva —see Concretion, conjunctiva
  corpora cavernosa (penis) N48.89
  cortex (brain) —see Calcification, cerebral
  dental pulp (nodular) K04.2
  dentinal papilla K00.4
  fallopian tube N83.8
  falx cerebri G96.198
  gallbladder K82.8
  general E83.59
  heart —see also Degeneration, myocardial
    valve —see Endocarditis

Calcification (Continued)
  idiopathic infantile arterial (IIAC) Q28.8
  intervertebral cartilage or disc
      (postinfective) —see Disorder, disc,
      specified NEC
  intracranial —see Calcification, cerebral
  joint —see Disorder, joint, specified type
      NEC
  kidney N28.89
    tuberculous N29 [B90.1]
  larynx (senile) J38.7
  lens —see Cataract, specified NEC
  lung (active) (postinfectional) J98.4
    tuberculous B90.9
  lymph gland or node (postinfectional) I89.8
    tuberculous —see also Tuberculosis, lymph
        gland B90.8
  mammographic R92.1
  massive (paraplegic) —see Myositis,
      ossificans, in, quadriplegia
  medial —see Arteriosclerosis, extremities
  meninges (cerebral) (spinal) G96.198
  metastatic E83.59
  Mönckeberg's —see Arteriosclerosis,
      extremities
  muscle M61.9
    due to burns —see Myositis, ossificans, in,
        burns
    paralytic —see Myositis, ossificans, in,
        quadriplegia
    specified type NEC M61.40
      ankle M61.47-●
      foot M61.47-●
      forearm M61.43-●
      hand M61.44-●
      lower leg M61.46-●
      multiple sites M61.49
      pelvic region M61.45-●
      shoulder region M61.41-●
      specified site NEC M61.48
      thigh M61.45-●
      upper arm M61.42-●
  myocardium, myocardial —see Degeneration,
      myocardial
  ovary N83.8
  pancreas K86.89
  penis N48.89
  periarticular —see Disorder, joint, specified
      type NEC
  pericardium —see also Pericarditis I31.1
  pineal gland E34.8
  pleura J94.8
    postinfective J94.8
    tuberculous NEC B90.9
  pulpal (dental) (nodular) K04.2
  sclera H15.89
  spleen D73.89
  subcutaneous L94.2
  suprarenal (capsule) (gland) E27.49
  tendon (sheath) —see also Tenosynovitis,
      specified type NEC
    with bursitis, synovitis or tenosynovitis —
        see Tendinitis, calcific
  trachea J39.8
  ureter N28.89
  vitreous —see Deposit, crystalline
Calcified —see Calcification
Calcinosis (interstitial) (tumoral) (universalis)
    E83.59
  with Raynaud's phenomenon, esophageal
      dysfunction, sclerodactyly, telangiectasia
      (CREST syndrome) M34.1
  circumscripta (skin) L94.2
  cutis L94.2
Calciphylaxis —see also Calcification, by site
    E83.59
Calcium
  deposits —see Calcification, by site
  metabolism disorder E83.50
  salts or soaps in vitreous —see Deposit,
      crystalline

Calciuria R82.994
Calculi —see Calculus
Calculosis, intrahepatic —see Calculus, bile
    duct
Calculus, calculi, calculous
  ampulla of Vater —see Calculus, bile duct
  anuria (impacted) (recurrent) —see also
      Calculus, urinary N20.9
  appendix K38.1
  bile duct (common) (hepatic) K80.50
    with
      calculus of gallbladder —see Calculus,
          gallbladder and bile duct
      cholangitis K80.30
        with
          cholecystitis —see Calculus, bile
              duct, with cholecystitis
          obstruction K80.31
          acute K80.32
            with
              chronic cholangitis K80.36
                with obstruction K80.37
              obstruction K80.33
          chronic K80.34
            with
              acute cholangitis K80.36
                with obstruction K80.37
              obstruction K80.35
      cholecystitis (with cholangitis) K80.40
        with obstruction K80.41
        acute K80.42
          with
            chronic cholecystitis K80.46
              with obstruction K80.47
            obstruction K80.43
        chronic K80.44
          with
            acute cholecystitis K80.46
              with obstruction K80.47
            obstruction K80.45
      obstruction K80.51
  biliary —see also Calculus, gallbladder
    specified NEC K80.80
      with obstruction K80.81
  bilirubin, multiple —see Calculus,
      gallbladder
  bladder (encysted) (impacted) (urinary)
      (diverticulum) N21.0
  bronchus J98.09
  calyx (kidney) (renal) —see Calculus, kidney
  cholesterol (pure) (solitary) —see Calculus,
      gallbladder
  common duct (bile) —see Calculus, bile duct
  conjunctiva —see Concretion, conjunctiva
  cystic N21.0
    duct —see Calculus, gallbladder
  dental (subgingival) (supragingival)
      K03.6
  diverticulum
    bladder N21.0
    kidney N20.0
  epididymis N50.89
  gallbladder K80.20
    with
      bile duct calculus —see Calculus,
          gallbladder and bile duct
      cholecystitis K80.10
        with obstruction K80.11
        acute K80.00
          with
            chronic cholecystitis K80.12
              with obstruction K80.13
            obstruction K80.01
        chronic K80.10
          with
            acute cholecystitis K80.12
              with obstruction K80.13
            obstruction K80.11
        specified NEC K80.18
          with obstruction K80.19
      obstruction K80.21

Calculus, calculi, calculous *(Continued)*
- gallbladder and bile duct K80.70
  - with
    - cholecystitis K80.60
      - with obstruction K80.61
      - acute K80.62
        - with
          - chronic cholecystitis K80.66
            - with obstruction K80.67
          - obstruction K80.63
        - chronic K80.64
          - with
            - acute cholecystitis K80.66
              - with obstruction K80.67
            - obstruction K80.65
      - obstruction K80.71
- hepatic (duct) —*see* Calculus, bile duct
- hepatobiliary K80.80
  - with obstruction K80.81
- ileal conduit N21.8
- intestinal (impaction) (obstruction) K56.49
- kidney (impacted) (multiple) (pelvis) (recurrent) (staghorn) N20.0
  - with calculus, ureter N20.2
  - congenital Q63.8
- lacrimal passages —*see* Dacryolith
- liver (impacted) —*see* Calculus, bile duct
- lung J98.4
- mammographic R92.1
- nephritic (impacted) (recurrent) —*see* Calculus, kidney
- nose J34.89
- pancreas (duct) K86.89
- parotid duct or gland K11.5
- pelvis, encysted —*see* Calculus, kidney
- prostate N42.0
- pulmonary J98.4
- pyelitis (impacted) (recurrent) N20.0
  - with hydronephrosis N13.6
- pyelonephritis (impacted) (recurrent) —*see* category N20
  - with hydronephrosis N13.6
- renal (impacted) (recurrent) —*see* Calculus, kidney
- salivary (duct) (gland) K11.5
- seminal vesicle N50.89
- staghorn —*see* Calculus, kidney
- Stensen's duct K11.5
- stomach K31.89
- sublingual duct or gland K11.5
  - congenital Q38.4
- submandibular duct, gland or region K11.5
- submaxillary duct, gland or region K11.5
- suburethral N21.8
- tonsil J35.8
- tooth, teeth (subgingival) (supragingival) K03.6
- tunica vaginalis N50.89
- ureter (impacted) (recurrent) N20.1
  - with calculus, kidney N20.2
    - with hydronephrosis N13.2
      - with infection N13.6
- ureteropelvic junction N20.1
- urethra (impacted) N21.1
- urinary (duct) (impacted) (passage) (tract) N20.9
  - with hydronephrosis N13.2
    - with infection N13.6
  - in (due to)
  - lower N21.9
    - specified NEC N21.8
- vagina N89.8
- vesical (impacted) N21.0
- Wharton's duct K11.5
- xanthine E79.8 *[N22]*

Calicectasis N28.89
Caliectasis N28.89
California
- disease B38.9
- encephalitis A83.5
Caligo cornea —*see* Opacity, cornea, central
Callositas, callosity (infected) L84

Callus (infected) L84
- bone —*see* Osteophyte
  - excessive, following fracture - code as Sequelae of fracture
CALME (childhood asymmetric labium majus enlargement) N90.61
Calorie deficiency or malnutrition —*see also* Malnutrition E46
Calvé-Perthes disease —*see* Legg-Calve-Perthes disease
Calvé's disease —*see* Osteochondrosis, juvenile, spine
Calvities —*see* Alopecia, androgenic
Cameroon fever —*see* Malaria
Camptocormia (hysterical) F44.4
Camurati-Engelmann syndrome Q78.3
Canal —*see also* condition
- atrioventricular common Q21.2
Canaliculitis (lacrimal) (acute) (subacute) H04.33-●
- Actinomyces A42.89
- chronic H04.42-●
Canavan's disease E75.29
Canceled procedure (surgical) Z53.9
- because of
  - contraindication Z53.09
    - smoking Z53.01
  - left against medical advice (AMA) Z53.29
  - patient's decision Z53.20
    - for reasons of belief or group pressure Z53.1
    - specified reason NEC Z53.29
  - specified reason NEC Z53.8
Cancer —*see also* Neoplasm, by site, malignant
- bile duct type, liver C22.1
- blood —*see* Leukemia
- breast —*see also* Neoplasm, breast, malignant C50.91-●
- hepatocellular C22.0
- lung —*see also* Neoplasm, lung, malignant C34.90-●
- ovarian —*see also* Neoplasm, ovary, malignant C56.9-●
- unspecified site (primary) C80.1
Cancer (o)phobia F45.29
Cancerous —*see* Neoplasm, malignant, by site
Cancrum oris A69.0
Candidiasis, candidal B37.9
- balanitis B37.42
- bronchitis B37.1
- cheilitis B37.83
- congenital P37.5
- cystitis B37.41
- disseminated B37.7
- endocarditis B37.6
- enteritis B37.82
- esophagitis B37.81
- intertrigo B37.2
- lung B37.1
- meningitis B37.5
- mouth B37.0
- nails B37.2
- neonatal P37.5
- onychia B37.2
- oral B37.0
- osteomyelitis B37.89
- otitis externa B37.84
- paronychia B37.2
- perionyxis B37.2
- pneumonia B37.1
- proctitis B37.82
- pulmonary B37.1
- pyelonephritis B37.49
- sepsis B37.7
- skin B37.2
- specified site NEC B37.89
- stomatitis B37.0
- systemic B37.7
- urethritis B37.41
- urogenital site NEC B37.49
- vagina B37.3
- vulva B37.3
- vulvovaginitis B37.3

Candidid L30.2
Candidosis —*see* Candidiasis
Candiru infection or infestation B88.8
Canities (premature) L67.1
- congenital Q84.2
Canker (mouth) (sore) K12.0
- rash A38.9
Cannabinosis J66.2
Cannabis induced
- anxiety disorder F12.980
- psychotic disorder F12.959
- sleep disorder F12.988
Canton fever A75.9
Cantrell's syndrome Q87.89
Capillariasis (intestinal) B81.1
- hepatic B83.8
Capillary —*see* condition
Caplan's syndrome —*see* Rheumatoid, lung
Capsule —*see* condition
Capsulitis (joint) —*see also* Enthesopathy
- adhesive (shoulder) M75.0-●
- hepatic K65.8
- labyrinthine —*see* Otosclerosis, specified NEC
- thyroid E06.9
Caput
- crepitus Q75.8
- medusae I86.8
- succedaneum P12.81
Car sickness T75.3
Carapata (disease) A68.0
Carate —*see* Pinta
Carbon lung J60
Carbuncle L02.93
- abdominal wall L02.231
- anus K61.0
- auditory canal, external —*see* Abscess, ear, external
- auricle ear —*see* Abscess, ear, external
- axilla L02.43-●
- back (any part) L02.232
- breast N61.1
- buttock L02.33
- cheek (external) L02.03
- chest wall L02.233
- chin L02.03
- corpus cavernosum N48.21
- ear (any part) (external) (middle) —*see* Abscess, ear, external
- external auditory canal —*see* Abscess, ear, external
- eyelid —*see* Abscess, eyelid
- face NEC L02.03
- femoral (region) —*see* Carbuncle, lower limb
- finger —*see* Carbuncle, hand
- flank L02.231
- foot L02.63-●
- forehead L02.03
- genital —*see* Abscess, genital
- gluteal (region) L02.33
- groin L02.234
- hand L02.53-●
- head NEC L02.831
- heel —*see* Carbuncle, foot
- hip —*see* Carbuncle, lower limb
- kidney —*see* Abscess, kidney
- knee —*see* Carbuncle, lower limb
- labium (majus) (minus) N76.4
- lacrimal
  - gland —*see* Dacryoadenitis
  - passages (duct) (sac) —*see* Inflammation, lacrimal, passages, acute
- leg —*see* Carbuncle, lower limb
- lower limb L02.43-●
- malignant A22.0
- navel L02.236
- neck L02.13
- nose (external) (septum) J34.0
- orbit, orbital —*see* Abscess, orbit
- palmar (space) —*see* Carbuncle, hand
- partes posteriores L02.33
- pectoral region L02.233
- penis N48.21

▶ New   ⇒ Revised   ~~deleted~~ Deleted   ● Use Additional Character(s)

Carbuncle *(Continued)*
  perineum L02.235
  pinna —*see* Abscess, ear, external
  popliteal —*see* Carbuncle, lower limb
  scalp L02.831
  seminal vesicle N49.0
  shoulder —*see* Carbuncle, upper limb
  specified site NEC L02.838
  temple (region) L02.03
  thumb —*see* Carbuncle, hand
  toe —*see* Carbuncle, foot
  trunk L02.239
    abdominal wall L02.231
    back L02.232
    chest wall L02.233
    groin L02.234
    perineum L02.235
    umbilicus L02.236
  umbilicus L02.236
  upper limb L02.43-●
  urethra N34.0
  vulva N76.4
Carbunculus —*see* Carbuncle
Carcinoid (tumor) —*see* Tumor, carcinoid
Carcinoidosis E34.0
Carcinoma (malignant) —*see also* Neoplasm,
  by site, malignant
  acidophil
    specified site —*see* Neoplasm, malignant,
      by site
    unspecified site C75.1
  acidophil-basophil, mixed
    specified site —*see* Neoplasm, malignant,
      by site
    unspecified site C75.1
  adnexal (skin) —*see* Neoplasm, skin, malignant
  adrenal cortical C74.0-●
  alveolar —*see* Neoplasm, lung, malignant
    cell —*see* Neoplasm, lung, malignant
  ameloblastic C41.1
    upper jaw (bone) C41.0
  apocrine
    breast —*see* Neoplasm, breast, malignant
    specified site NEC —*see* Neoplasm, skin,
      malignant
    unspecified site C44.99
  basal cell (pigmented) (*see also* Neoplasm,
    skin, malignant) C44.91
    fibro-epithelial —*see* Neoplasm, skin,
      malignant
    morphea —*see* Neoplasm, skin, malignant
    multicentric —*see* Neoplasm, skin,
      malignant
  basaloid
  basal-squamous cell, mixed —*see* Neoplasm,
    skin, malignant
  basophil
    specified site —*see* Neoplasm, malignant,
      by site
    unspecified site C75.1
  basophil-acidophil, mixed
    specified site —*see* Neoplasm, malignant,
      by site
    unspecified site C75.1
  basosquamous —*see* Neoplasm, skin, malignant
  bile duct
    with hepatocellular, mixed C22.0
    liver C22.1
    specified site NEC —*see* Neoplasm,
      malignant, by site
    unspecified site C22.1
  branchial or branchiogenic C10.4
  bronchial or bronchogenic —*see* Neoplasm,
    lung, malignant
  bronchiolar —*see* Neoplasm, lung, malignant
  bronchioloalveolar —*see* Neoplasm, lung,
    malignant
  C cell
    specified site —*see* Neoplasm, malignant,
      by site
    unspecified site C73
  ceruminous C44.29-●

Carcinoma *(Continued)*
  cervix uteri
    in situ D06.9
      endocervix D06.0
      exocervix D06.1
      specified site NEC D06.7
  chorionic
    specified site —*see* Neoplasm, malignant,
      by site
    unspecified site
      female C58
      male C62.90
  chromophobe
    specified site —*see* Neoplasm, malignant,
      by site
    unspecified site C75.1
  cloacogenic
    specified site —*see* Neoplasm, malignant,
      by site
    unspecified site C21.2
  diffuse type
    specified site —*see* Neoplasm, malignant,
      by site
    unspecified site C16.9
  duct (cell)
    with Paget's disease —*see* Neoplasm,
      breast, malignant
    infiltrating
      with lobular carcinoma (in situ)
        specified site —*see* Neoplasm,
          malignant, by site
        unspecified site (female) C50.91-●
          male C50.92-●
      specified site —*see* Neoplasm,
        malignant, by site
      unspecified site (female) C50.91-●
        male C50.92-●
  ductal
    with lobular
      specified site —*see* Neoplasm,
        malignant, by site
      unspecified site (female) C50.91-●
        male C50.92-●
  ductular, infiltrating
    specified site —*see* Neoplasm, malignant,
      by site
    unspecified site (female) C50.91-●
      male C50.92-●
  embryonal
    liver C22.7
  endometrioid
    specified site —*see* Neoplasm, malignant,
      by site
    unspecified site
      female C56.9
      male C61
  eosinophil
    specified site —*see* Neoplasm, malignant,
      by site
    unspecified site C75.1
  epidermoid —*see also* Neoplasm, skin
    malignant
    in situ, Bowen's type —*see* Neoplasm, skin,
      in situ
  fibroepithelial, basal cell —*see* Neoplasm,
    skin, malignant
  follicular
    with papillary (mixed) C73
    moderately differentiated C73
    pure follicle C73
    specified site —*see* Neoplasm, malignant,
      by site
    trabecular C73
    unspecified site C73
    well differentiated C73
  generalized, with unspecified primary site
    C80.0
  glycogen-rich —*see* Neoplasm, breast,
    malignant
  granulosa cell C56-●
  hepatic cell C22.0

Carcinoma *(Continued)*
  hepatocellular C22.0
    with bile duct, mixed C22.0
    fibrolamellar C22.0
  hepatocholangiolitic C22.0
  Hurthle cell C73
  in
    adenomatous
      polyposis coli C18.9
    pleomorphic adenoma —*see* Neoplasm,
      salivary glands, malignant
    situ —*see* Carcinoma-in-situ
  infiltrating
    duct
      with lobular
        specified site —*see* Neoplasm,
          malignant, by site
        unspecified site (female) C50.91-●
          male C50.92-●
      with Paget's disease —*see* Neoplasm,
        breast, malignant
      specified site —*see* Neoplasm,
        malignant
      unspecified site (female) C50.91-●
        male C50.92-●
    ductular
      specified site —*see* Neoplasm,
        malignant
      unspecified site (female) C50.91-●
        male C50.92-●
    lobular
      specified site —*see* Neoplasm,
        malignant
      unspecified site (female) C50.91-●
        male C50.92-●
  inflammatory
    specified site —*see* Neoplasm, malignant
    unspecified site (female) C50.91 ●
      male C50.92-●
  intestinal type
    specified site —*see* Neoplasm, malignant,
      by site
    unspecified site C16.9
  intracystic
    noninfiltrating —*see* Neoplasm, in situ,
      by site
  intraductal (noninfiltrating)
    with Paget's disease —*see* Neoplasm,
      breast, malignant
    breast D05.1-●
    papillary
      with invasion
        specified site —*see* Neoplasm,
          malignant, by site
        unspecified site (female) C50.91 ●
          male C50.92-●
      breast D05.1-●
      specified site NEC —*see* Neoplasm,
        in situ, by site
      unspecified site (female) D05.1-●
    specified site NEC —*see* Neoplasm,
      in situ, by site
    unspecified site (female) D05.1-●
  intraepidermal —*see* Neoplasm, in situ
    squamous cell, Bowen's type —*see*
      Neoplasm, skin, in situ
  intraepithelial —*see* Neoplasm, in situ,
    by site
    squamous cell —*see* Neoplasm, in situ,
      by site
  intraosseous C41.1
    upper jaw (bone) C41.0
  islet cell
    with exocrine, mixed
      specified site —*see* Neoplasm,
        malignant, by site
      unspecified site C25.9
    pancreas C25.4
    specified site NEC —*see* Neoplasm,
      malignant, by site
    unspecified site C25.4

Carcinoma *(Continued)*
  juvenile, breast —*see* Neoplasm, breast,
    malignant
  large cell
    small cell
      specified site —*see* Neoplasm,
        malignant, by site
      unspecified site C34.90
  Leydig cell (testis)
    specified site —*see* Neoplasm, malignant,
      by site
    unspecified site
      female C56.9
      male C62.90
  lipid-rich (female) C50.91-•
    male C50.92-•
  liver cell C22.0
  liver NEC C22.7
  lobular (infiltrating)
    with intraductal
      specified site —*see* Neoplasm,
        malignant, by site
      unspecified site (female) C50.91-•
        male C50.92-•
    noninfiltrating
      breast D05.0-•
      specified site NEC —*see* Neoplasm, in
        situ, by site
      unspecified site D05.0-•
    specified site —*see* Neoplasm, malignant,
      by site
    unspecified site (female) C50.91-•
      male C50.92-•
  medullary
    with
      amyloid stroma
        specified site —*see* Neoplasm,
          malignant, by site
        unspecified site C73
      lymphoid stroma
        specified site —*see* Neoplasm,
          malignant, by site
        unspecified site (female) C50.91-•
          male C50.92-•
  Merkel cell C4A.9
    anal margin C4A.51
    anal skin C4A.51
    canthus C4A.1-•
    ear and external auricular canal C4A.2-•
    external auricular canal C4A.2-•
    eyelid, including canthus C4A.1-•
    face C4A.30
      specified NEC C4A.39
    hip C4A.7-•
    lip C4A.0
    lower limb, including hip C4A.7-•
    neck C4A.4
    nodal presentation C7B.1
    nose C4A.31
    overlapping sites C4A.8
    perianal skin C4A.51
    scalp C4A.4
    secondary C7B.1
    shoulder C4A.6-•
    skin of breast C4A.52
    trunk NEC C4A.59
    upper limb, including shoulder C4A.6-•
    visceral metastatic C7B.1
  metastatic —*see* Neoplasm, secondary
  metatypical —*see* Neoplasm, skin, malignant
  morphea, basal cell —*see* Neoplasm, skin,
    malignant
  mucoid
    cell
      specified site —*see* Neoplasm,
        malignant, by site
      unspecified site C75.1
  neuroendocrine —*see also* Tumor,
    neuroendocrine
    high grade, any site C7A.1
    poorly differentiated, any site C7A.1

Carcinoma *(Continued)*
  nonencapsulated sclerosing C73
  noninfiltrating
    intracystic —*see* Neoplasm, in situ, by site
    intraductal
      breast D05.1-•
      papillary
        breast D05.1-•
        specified site NEC —*see* Neoplasm, in
          situ, by site
        unspecified site D05.1-•
      specified site —*see* Neoplasm, in situ,
        by site
      unspecified site D05.1-•
    lobular
      breast D05.0-•
      specified site NEC —*see* Neoplasm, in
        situ, by site
      unspecified site (female) D05.0-•
  oat cell
    specified site —*see* Neoplasm, malignant,
      by site
    unspecified site C34.90
  odontogenic C41.1
    upper jaw (bone) C41.0
  papillary
    with follicular (mixed) C73
    follicular variant C73
    intraductal (noninfiltrating)
      with invasion
        specified site —*see* Neoplasm,
          malignant, by site
        unspecified site (female) C50.91-•
          male C50.92-•
      breast D05.1-•
      specified site NEC —*see* Neoplasm, in
        situ, by site
      unspecified site D05.1-•
    serous
      specified site —*see* Neoplasm,
        malignant, by site
      surface
        specified site —*see* Neoplasm,
          malignant, by site
        unspecified site C56.9
      unspecified site C56.9
  papillocystic
    specified site —*see* Neoplasm, malignant,
      by site
    unspecified site C56.9
  parafollicular cell
    specified site —*see* Neoplasm, malignant,
      by site
    unspecified site C73
  pilomatrix —*see* Neoplasm, skin, malignant
  pseudomucinous
    specified site —*see* Neoplasm, malignant,
      by site
    unspecified site C56.9
  renal cell C64-•
  Schmincke —*see* Neoplasm, nasopharynx,
    malignant
  Schneiderian
    specified site —*see* Neoplasm, malignant,
      by site
    unspecified site C30.0
  sebaceous —*see* Neoplasm, skin, malignant
  secondary —*see also* Neoplasm, secondary,
    by site
    Merkel cell C7B.1
  secretory, breast —*see* Neoplasm, breast,
    malignant
  serous
    papillary
      specified site —*see* Neoplasm,
        malignant, by site
      unspecified site C56.9
    surface, papillary
      specified site —*see* Neoplasm,
        malignant, by site
      unspecified site C56.9

Carcinoma *(Continued)*
  Sertoli cell
    specified site —*see* Neoplasm, malignant,
      by site
    unspecified site C62.90
      female C56.9
      male C62.90
  skin appendage —*see* Neoplasm, skin,
    malignant
  small cell
    fusiform cell
      specified site —*see* Neoplasm,
        malignant, by site
      unspecified site C34.90
    intermediate cell
      specified site —*see* Neoplasm,
        malignant, by site
      unspecified site C34.90
    large cell
      specified site —*see* Neoplasm,
        malignant, by site
      unspecified site C34.90
  solid
    with amyloid stroma
      specified site —*see* Neoplasm,
        malignant, by site
      unspecified site C73
    microinvasive
      specified site —*see* Neoplasm,
        malignant, by site
      unspecified site C53.9
  sweat gland —*see* Neoplasm, skin,
    malignant
  theca cell C56.-•
  thymic C37
  unspecified site (primary) C80.1
  water-clear cell C75.0
Carcinoma-in-situ —*see also* Neoplasm, in situ,
  by site
  breast NOS D05.9-•
    specified type NEC D05.8-•
  epidermoid —*see also* Neoplasm, in situ, by
    site
    with questionable stromal invasion
      cervix D06.9
      specified site NEC —*see* Neoplasm, in
        situ, by site
      unspecified site D06.9
    Bowen's type —*see* Neoplasm, skin,
      in situ
  intraductal
    breast D05.1-•
    specified site NEC —*see* Neoplasm, in situ,
      by site
    unspecified site D05.1-•
  lobular
    with
      infiltrating duct
        breast (female) C50.91-•
          male C50.92-•
        specified site NEC —*see* Neoplasm,
          malignant
        unspecified site (female) C50.91-•
          male C50.92-•
      intraductal
        breast D05.8-•
        specified site NEC —*see* Neoplasm, in
          situ, by site
        unspecified site (female) D05.8-•
    breast D05.0-•
    specified site NEC —*see* Neoplasm, in situ,
      by site
    unspecified site D05.0-•
  squamous cell —*see also* Neoplasm, in situ,
    by site
    with questionable stromal invasion
      cervix D06.9
      specified site NEC —*see* Neoplasm, in
        situ, by site
      unspecified site D06.9
Carcinomaphobia F45.29

▶ New   ⇒ Revised   ~~deleted~~ Deleted   • Use Additional Character(s)

Carcinomatosis C80.0
  peritonei C78.6
  unspecified site (primary) (secondary) C80.0
Carcinosarcoma —see Neoplasm, malignant,
    by site
  embryonal —see Neoplasm, malignant, by site
Cardia, cardial —see condition
Cardiac —see also condition
  death, sudden —see Arrest, cardiac
  pacemaker
    in situ Z95.0
      management or adjustment Z45.018
  tamponade I31.4
Cardialgia —see Pain, precordial
Cardiectasis —see Hypertrophy, cardiac
Cardiochalasia K21.9
Cardiomalacia I51.5
Cardiomegalia glycogenica diffusa E74.02 [143]
Cardiomegaly —see also Hypertrophy, cardiac
  congenital Q24.8
  glycogen E74.02 [143]
  idiopathic I51.7
Cardiomyoliposis I51.5
Cardiomyopathy (familial) (idiopathic) I42.9
  alcoholic I42.6
  amyloid E85.4 [143]
    transthyretin-related (ATTR) familial E85.4
      [143]
  arteriosclerotic —see Disease, heart, ischemic,
    atherosclerotic
  beriberi E51.12
  cobalt-beer I42.6
  congenital I42.4
  congestive I42.0
  constrictive NOS I42.5
  dilated I42.0
  due to
    alcohol I42.6
    beriberi E51.12
    cardiac glycogenosis E74.02 [143]
    drugs I42.7
    external agents NEC I42.7
    Friedreich's ataxia G11.11
    myotonia atrophica G71.11 [143]
    progressive muscular dystrophy G71.09
      [143]
  glycogen storage E74.02 [143]
  hypertensive —see Hypertension, heart
  hypertrophic (nonobstructive) I42.2
    obstructive I42.1
      congenital Q24.8
  in
    Chagas' disease (chronic) B57.2
      acute B57.0
    sarcoidosis D86.85
  ischemic I25.5
  metabolic E88.9 [143]
    thyrotoxic E05.90 [143]
      with thyroid storm E05.91 [143]
  newborn I42.8
    congenital I42.4
  non-ischemic (see also by cause) I42.8
  nutritional E63.9 [143]
    beriberi E51.12
  obscure of Africa I42.8
  peripartum O90.3
  postpartum O90.3
  restrictive NEC I42.5
  rheumatic I09.0
  secondary I42.9
  specified NEC I42.8
  stress induced I51.81
  takotsubo I51.81
  thyrotoxic E05.90 [143]
    with thyroid storm E05.91 [143]
  toxic NEC I42.7
  transthyretin-related (ATTR) familial amyloid
    E85.4
  tuberculous A18.84
  viral B33.24
Cardionephritis —see Hypertension,
    cardiorenal

Cardionephropathy —see Hypertension,
    cardiorenal
Cardionephrosis —see Hypertension, cardiorenal
Cardiopathia nigra I27.0
Cardiopathy —see also Disease, heart I51.9
  idiopathic I42.9
  mucopolysaccharidosis E76.3 [152]
Cardiopericarditis —see Pericarditis
Cardiophobia F45.29
Cardiorenal —see condition
Cardiorrhexis —see Infarct, myocardium
Cardiosclerosis —see Disease, heart, ischemic,
    atherosclerotic
Cardiosis —see Disease, heart
Cardiospasm (esophagus) (reflex) (stomach)
    K22.0
  congenital Q39.5
    with megaesophagus Q39.5
Cardiostenosis —see Disease, heart
Cardiosymphysis I31.0
Cardiovascular —see condition
Carditis (acute) (bacterial) (chronic) (subacute)
    I51.89
  meningococcal A39.50
  rheumatic —see Disease, heart, rheumatic
  rheumatoid —see Rheumatoid, carditis
  viral B33.20
Care (of) (for) (following)
  child (routine) Z76.2
  family member (handicapped) (sick)
    creating problem for family Z63.6
    provided away from home for holiday
      relief Z75.5
    unavailable, due to
      absence (person rendering care)
        (sufferer) Z74.2
      inability (any reason) of person
        rendering care Z74.2
  foundling Z76.1
  holiday relief Z75.5
  improper —see Maltreatment
  lack of (at or after birth) (infant) —see
    Maltreatment, child, neglect
  lactating mother Z39.1
  palliative Z51.5
  postpartum
    immediately after delivery Z39.0
    routine follow-up Z39.2
  respite Z75.5
  unavailable, due to
    absence of person rendering care Z74.2
    inability (any reason) of person rendering
      care Z74.2
  well-baby Z76.2
Caries
  bone NEC A18.03
  dental (dentino enamel junction) (early
    childhood) (of dentine) (pre-eruptive)
    (recurrent) (to the pulp) K02.9
    arrested (coronal) (root) K02.3
    chewing surface
      limited to enamel K02.51
      penetrating into dentin K02.52
      penetrating into pulp K02.53
    coronal surface
      chewing surface
        limited to enamel K02.51
        penetrating into dentin K02.52
        penetrating into pulp K02.53
      pit and fissure surface
        limited to enamel K02.51
        penetrating into dentin K02.52
        penetrating into pulp K02.53
      smooth surface
        limited to enamel K02.61
        penetrating into dentin K02.62
        penetrating into pulp K02.63
    pit and fissure surface
      limited to enamel K02.51
      penetrating into dentin K02.52
      penetrating into pulp K02.53

Caries (Continued)
  dental (Continued)
    primary, cervical origin K02.52
    root K02.7
    smooth surface
      limited to enamel K02.61
      penetrating into dentin K02.62
      penetrating into pulp K02.63
  external meatus —see Disorder, ear, external,
    specified type NEC
  hip (tuberculous) A18.02
  initial (tooth)
    chewing surface K02.51
    pit and fissure surface K02.51
    smooth surface K02.61
  knee (tuberculous) A18.02
  labyrinth —see subcategory H83.8
  limb NEC (tuberculous) A18.03
  mastoid process (chronic) —see Mastoiditis,
    chronic
    tuberculous A18.03
  middle ear —see subcategory H74.8
  nose (tuberculous) A18.03
  orbit (tuberculous) A18.03
  ossicles, ear —see Abnormal, ear ossicles
  petrous bone —see Petrositis
  root (dental) (tooth) K02.7
  sacrum (tuberculous) A18.01
  spine, spinal (column) (tuberculous) A18.01
  syphilitic A52.77
    congenital (early) A50.02 [M90.80]
  tooth, teeth —see Caries, dental
  tuberculous A18.03
  vertebra (column) (tuberculous) A18.01
Carious teeth —see Caries, dental
Carneous mole O02.0
Carnitine insufficiency E71.40
Carotenemia (dietary) E67.1
Carotenosis (cutis) (skin) E67.1
Carotid body or sinus syndrome G90.01
Carotidynia G90.01
Carpal tunnel syndrome —see Syndrome,
    carpal tunnel
Carpenter's syndrome Q87.0
Carpopedal spasm —see Tetany
Carr-Barr-Plunkett syndrome Q97.1
Carrier (suspected) of
  amebiasis Z22.1
  bacterial disease NEC Z22.39
    diphtheria Z22.2
    intestinal infectious NEC Z22.1
      typhoid Z22.0
    meningococcal Z22.31
    sexually transmitted Z22.4
    specified NEC Z22.39
    staphylococcal (Methicillin susceptible)
      Z22.321
      Methicillin resistant Z22.322
    streptococcal Z22.338
      group B Z22.330
        complicating pregnancy or delivery
          O99.82-●
    typhoid Z22.0
  cholera Z22.1
  diphtheria Z22.2
  gastrointestinal pathogens NEC Z22.1
  genetic Z14.8
    cystic fibrosis Z14.1
    hemophilia A (asymptomatic) Z14.01
      symptomatic Z14.02
  gestational, pregnant Z33.1
  gonorrhea Z22.4
  HAA (hepatitis Australian-antigen) B18.8
  HB (c)(s)-AG B18.1
  hepatitis (viral) B18.9
    Australia-antigen (HAA) B18.8
    B surface antigen (HBsAg) B18.1
      with acute delta- (super)infection B17.0
    C B18.2
    specified NEC B18.8
  human T-cell lymphotropic virus type-1
    (HTLV-1) infection Z22.6

Carrier of (Continued)
  infectious organism Z22.9
    specified NEC Z22.8
  meningococci Z22.31
  Salmonella typhosa Z22.0
  serum hepatitis —see Carrier, hepatitis
  staphylococci (Methicillin susceptible) Z22.321
    Methicillin resistant Z22.322
  streptococci Z22.338
    group B Z22.330
      complicating pregnancy or delivery
        O99.82-●
  syphilis Z22.4
  typhoid Z22.0
  venereal disease NEC Z22.4
Carrion's disease A44.0
Carter's relapsing fever (Asiatic) A68.1
Cartilage —see condition
Caruncle (inflamed)
  conjunctiva (acute) —see Conjunctivitis, acute
  labium (majus) (minus) N90.89
  lacrimal —see Inflammation, lacrimal,
      passages
  myrtiform N89.8
  urethral (benign) N36.2
Cascade stomach K31.2
Caseation lymphatic gland (tuberculous) A18.2
Cassidy (-Scholte) **syndrome** (malignant
    carcinoid) E34.0
Castellani's disease A69.8
Castration, traumatic, male S38.231
Casts in urine R82.998
Cat
  cry syndrome Q93.4
  ear Q17.3
  eye syndrome Q92.8
Catabolism, senile R54
Catalepsy (hysterical) F44.2
  schizophrenic F20.2
Cataplexy (idiopathic) —see Narcolepsy
Cataract (cortical) (immature) (incipient) H26.9
  with
    neovascularization —see Cataract,
        complicated
  age-related —see Cataract, senile
  anterior
    and posterior axial embryonal Q12.0
    pyramidal Q12.0
  associated with
    galactosemia E74.21 [H28]
    myotonic disorders G71.19 [H28]
  blue Q12.0
  central Q12.0
  cerulean Q12.0
  complicated H26.20
    with
      neovascularization H26.21-●
      ocular disorder H26.22-●
      glaucomatous flecks H26.23-●
  congenital Q12.0
  coraliform Q12.0
  coronary Q12.0
  crystalline Q12.0
  diabetic —see Diabetes, cataract
  drug-induced H26.3-●
  due to
    ocular disorder —see Cataract, complicated
    radiation H26.8
  electric H26.8
  extraction status Z98.4-●
  glass-blower's H26.8
  heat ray H26.8
  heterochromic —see Cataract, complicated
  hypermature —see Cataract, senile,
      morgagnian type
  in (due to)
    chronic iridocyclitis —see Cataract,
        complicated
    diabetes —see Diabetes, cataract
    endocrine disease E34.9 [H28]
    eye disease —see Cataract, complicated

Cataract (Continued)
  in (due to) (Continued)
    hypoparathyroidism E20.9 [H28]
    malnutrition-dehydration E46 [H28]
    metabolic disease E88.9 [H28]
    myotonic disorders G71.19 [H28]
    nutritional disease E63.9 [H28]
  infantile —see Cataract, presenile
  irradiational —see Cataract, specified NEC
  juvenile —see Cataract, presenile
  malnutrition-dehydration E46 [H28]
  morgagnian —see Cataract, senile,
      morgagnian type
  myotonic G71.19 [H28]
  myxedema E03.9 [H28]
  nuclear
    embryonal Q12.0
    sclerosis —see Cataract, senile, nuclear
  presenile H26.00-●
    combined forms H26.06-●
    cortical H26.01-●
    lamellar —see Cataract, presenile, cortical
    nuclear H26.03-●
    specified NEC H26.09
    subcapsular polar (anterior) H26.04-●
      posterior H26.05-●
    zonular —see Cataract, presenile, cortical
  secondary H26.40
    Soemmering's ring H26.41-●
    specified NEC H26.49-●
    to eye disease —see Cataract, complicated
  senile H25.9
    brunescens —see Cataract, senile, nuclear
    combined forms H25.81-●
    coronary —see Cataract, senile, incipient
    cortical H25.01-●
    hypermature —see Cataract, senile,
        morgagnian type
    incipient (mature) (total) H25.09-●
      cortical —see Cataract, senile, cortical
      subcapsular —see Cataract, senile,
          subcapsular
    morgagnian type (hypermature) H25.2-●
    nuclear (sclerosis) H25.1-●
    polar subcapsular (anterior) (posterior) —
        see Cataract, senile, incipient
    punctate —see Cataract, senile, incipient
    specified NEC H25.89
    subcapsular polar (anterior) H25.03-●
      posterior H25.04-●
  snowflake —see Diabetes, cataract
  specified NEC H26.8
  toxic —see Cataract, drug-induced
  traumatic H26.10-●
    localized H26.11-●
    partially resolved H26.12-●
    total H26.13-●
  zonular (perinuclear) Q12.0
Cataracta —see also Cataract
  brunescens —see Cataract, senile, nuclear
  centralis pulverulenta Q12.0
  cerulea Q12.0
  complicata —see Cataract, complicated
  congenita Q12.0
  coralliformis Q12.0
  coronaria Q12.0
  diabetic —see Diabetes, cataract
  membranacea
    accreta —see Cataract, secondary
    congenita Q12.0
  nigra —see Cataract, senile, nuclear
  sunflower —see Cataract, complicated
Catarrh, catarrhal (acute) (febrile) (infectious)
    (inflammation) (see also condition) J00
  bronchial —see Bronchitis
  chest —see Bronchitis
  chronic J31.0
  due to congenital syphilis A50.03
  enteric —see Enteritis
  eustachian H68.009
  fauces —see Pharyngitis

Catarrh, catarrhal (Continued)
  gastrointestinal —see Enteritis
  gingivitis K05.00
    nonplaque induced K05.01
    plaque induced K05.00
  hay —see Fever, hay
  intestinal —see Enteritis
  larynx, chronic J37.0
  liver B15.9
    with hepatic coma B15.0
  lung —see Bronchitis
  middle ear, chronic —see Otitis, media,
      nonsuppurative, chronic, serous
  mouth K12.1
  nasal (chronic) —see Rhinitis
  nasobronchial J31.1
  nasopharyngeal (chronic) J31.1
    acute J00
  pulmonary —see Bronchitis
  spring (eye) (vernal) —see Conjunctivitis,
      acute, atopic
  summer (hay) —see Fever, hay
  throat J31.2
  tubotympanal —see also Otitis, media,
      nonsuppurative
    chronic —see Otitis, media,
        nonsuppurative, chronic, serous
Catatonia (schizophrenic) F20.2
Catatonic
  disorder due to known physiologic condition
    F06.1
  schizophrenia F20.2
  stupor R40.1
Cat-scratch —see also Abrasion
  disease or fever A28.1
Cauda equina —see condition
Cauliflower ear M95.1-●
Causalgia (upper limb) G56.4-●
  lower limb G57.7-●
Cause
  external, general effects T75.89
Caustic burn —see Corrosion, by site
Cavare's disease (familial periodic paralysis)
    G72.3
Cave-in, injury
  crushing (severe) —see Crush
  suffocation —see Asphyxia, traumatic, due to
      low oxygen, due to cave-in
Cavernitis (penis) N48.29
Cavernositis N48.29
Cavernous —see condition
Cavitation of lung —see also Tuberculosis,
    pulmonary
  nontuberculous J98.4
Cavities, dental —see Caries, dental
Cavity
  lung —see Cavitation of lung
  optic papilla Q14.2
  pulmonary —see Cavitation of lung
Cavovarus foot, congenital Q66.1-●
Cavus foot (congenital) Q66.7-●
  acquired —see Deformity, limb, foot, specified
      NEC
Cazenave's disease L10.2
**CDKL5 (Cyclin-Dependent Kinase-Like 5
    Deficiency Disorder)** G40.42
Cecitis K52.9
  with perforation, peritonitis, or rupture K65.8
Cecoureterocele Q62.32
Cecum —see condition
Celiac
  artery compression syndrome I77.4
  disease (with steatorrhea) K90.0
  infantilism K90.0
Cell(s), cellular —see also condition
  in urine R82.998
Cellulitis (diffuse) (phlegmonous) (septic)
    (suppurative) L03.90
  abdominal wall L03.311
  anaerobic A48.0
  ankle —see Cellulitis, lower limb
  anus K61.0

C

▶ New   ⟹ Revised   ~~deleted~~ Deleted   ● Use Additional Character(s)

Cellulitis *(Continued)*
  arm —*see* Cellulitis, upper limb
  auricle (ear) —*see* Cellulitis, ear
  axilla L03.11-●
  back (any part) L03.312
  breast (acute) (nonpuerperal) (subacute)
      N61.0
    nipple N61.0
  broad ligament
    acute N73.0
  buttock L03.317
  cervical (meaning neck) L03.221
  cervix (uteri) —*see* Cervicitis
  cheek (external) L03.211
    internal K12.2
  chest wall L03.313
  chronic L03.90
  clostridial A48.0
  corpus cavernosum N48.22
  digit
    finger —*see* Cellulitis, finger
    toe —*see* Cellulitis, toe
  Douglas' cul-de-sac or pouch
    acute N73.0
  drainage site (following operation) T81.49
  ear (external) H60.1-●
  eosinophilic (granulomatous) L98.3
  erysipelatous —*see* Erysipelas
  external auditory canal —*see* Cellulitis, ear
  eyelid —*see* Abscess, eyelid
  face NEC L03.211
  finger (intrathecal) (periosteal)
      (subcutaneous) (subcuticular) L03.01-●
  foot —*see* Cellulitis, lower limb
  gangrenous —*see* Gangrene
  genital organ NEC
    female (external) N76.4
    male N49.9
      multiple sites N49.8
      specified NEC N49.8
  gluteal (region) L03.317
  gonococcal A54.89
  groin L03.314
  hand —*see* Cellulitis, upper limb
  head NEC L03.811
    face (any part, except ear, eye and nose)
        L03.211
  heel —*see* Cellulitis, lower limb
  hip —*see* Cellulitis, lower limb
  jaw (region) L03.211
  knee —*see* Cellulitis, lower limb
  labium (majus) (minus) —*see* Vulvitis
  lacrimal passages —*see* Inflammation,
      lacrimal, passages
  larynx J38.7
  leg —*see* Cellulitis, lower limb
  lip K13.0
  lower limb L03.11-●
    toe —*see* Cellulitis, toe
  mouth (floor) K12.2
  multiple sites, so stated L03.90
  nasopharynx J39.1
  navel L03.316
    newborn P38.9
      with mild hemorrhage P38.1
      without hemorrhage P38.9
  neck (region) L03.221
  nipple (acute) (nonpuerperal) (subacute) N61.0
  nose (septum) (external) J34.0
  orbit, orbital H05.01-●
  palate (soft) K12.2
  pectoral (region) L03.313
  pelvis, pelvic (chronic)
    female —*see also* Disease, pelvis,
        inflammatory N73.2
      acute N73.0
    following ectopic or molar pregnancy O08.0
    male K65.0
  penis N48.22
  perineal, perineum L03.315
  periorbital L03.213

Cellulitis *(Continued)*
  perirectal K61.1
  peritonsillar J36
  periurethral N34.0
  periuterine —*see also* Disease, pelvis,
      inflammatory N73.2
    acute N73.0
  pharynx J39.1
  preseptal L03.213
  rectum K61.1
  retroperitoneal K68.9
  round ligament
    acute N73.0
  scalp (any part) L03.811
  scrotum N49.2
  seminal vesicle N49.0
  shoulder —*see* Cellulitis, upper limb
  specified site NEC L03.818
  submandibular (region) (space) (triangle)
      K12.2
    gland K11.3
  submaxillary (region) K12.2
    gland K11.3
  thigh —*see* Cellulitis, lower limb
  thumb (intrathecal) (periosteal)
      (subcutaneous) (subcuticular) —*see*
      Cellulitis, finger
  toe (intrathecal) (periosteal) (subcutaneous)
      (subcuticular) L03.03-●
  tonsil J36
  trunk L03.319
    abdominal wall L03.311
    back (any part) L03.312
    buttock L03.317
    chest wall L03.313
    groin L03.314
    perineal, perineum L03.315
    umbilicus L03.316
  tuberculous (primary) A18.4
  umbilicus L03.316
  upper limb L03.11-●
    axilla —*see* Cellulitis, axilla
    finger —*see* Cellulitis, finger
    thumb —*see* Cellulitis, finger
  vaccinal T88.0
  vocal cord J38.3
  vulva —*see* Vulvitis
  wrist —*see* Cellulitis, upper limb
Cementoblastoma, benign —*see* Cyst,
    calcifying odontogenic
Cementoma —*see* Cyst, calcifying odontogenic
Cementoperiostitis —*see* Periodontitis
Cementosis K03.4
Central auditory processing disorder H93.25
Central pain syndrome G89.0
Cephalematocele, cephal (o)hematocele
  newborn P52.8
    birth injury P10.8
  traumatic —*see* Hematoma, brain
Cephalematoma, cephalhematoma (calcified)
  newborn (birth injury) P12.0
  traumatic —*see* Hematoma, brain
Cephalgia, cephalalgia —*see also* Headache
  histamine G44.009
    intractable G44.001
    not intractable G44.009
  trigeminal autonomic (TAC) NEC G44.099
    intractable G44.091
    not intractable G44.099
Cephalic —*see* condition
Cephalitis —*see* Encephalitis
Cephalocele —*see* Encephalocele
Cephalomenia N94.89
Cephalopelvic —*see* condition
Cerclage (with cervical incompetence) in
    pregnancy —*see* Incompetence, cervix, in
    pregnancy
Cerebellitis —*see* Encephalitis
Cerebellum, cerebellar —*see* condition
Cerebral —*see* condition
Cerebritis —*see* Encephalitis

Cerebro-hepato-renal syndrome Q87.89
Cerebromalacia —*see* Softening, brain
    sequelae of cerebrovascular disease I69.398
Cerebroside lipidosis E75.22
Cerebrospasticity (congenital) G80.1
Cerebrospinal —*see* condition
Cerebrum —*see* condition
Ceroid-lipofuscinosis, neuronal E75.4
Cerumen (accumulation) (impacted) H61.2-●
Cervical —*see also* condition
  auricle Q18.2
  dysplasia in pregnancy —*see* Abnormal,
      cervix, in pregnancy or childbirth
  erosion in pregnancy —*see* Abnormal, cervix,
      in pregnancy or childbirth
  fibrosis in pregnancy —*see* Abnormal, cervix,
      in pregnancy or childbirth
  fusion syndrome Q76.1
  rib Q76.5
  shortening (complicating pregnancy) O26.87-●
Cervicalgia M54.2
Cervicitis (acute) (chronic) (nonvenereal)
    (senile (atrophic)) (subacute) (with
    ulceration) N72
  with
    abortion —*see* Abortion, by type complicated
        by genital tract and pelvic infection
    ectopic pregnancy O08.0
    molar pregnancy O08.0
  chlamydial A56.09
  gonococcal A54.03
  herpesviral A60.03
  puerperal (postpartum) O86.11
  syphilitic A52.76
  trichomonal A59.09
  tuberculous A18.16
Cervicocolpitis (emphysematosa) (*see also*
    Cervicitis) N72
Cervix —*see* condition
Cesarean delivery, previous, affecting
    management of pregnancy O34.219
  classical (vertical) scar O34.212
  isthmocele O34.22
  low transverse scar O34.211
  mid-transverse T incision O34.218
  scar
    defect (isthmocele) O34.22
    specified type NEC O34.218
Céstan (-Chenais) paralysis or syndrome G46.3
Céstan-Raymond syndrome I65.8
Cestode infestation B71.9
  specified type NEC B71.8
Cestodiasis B71.9
Chabert's disease A22.9
Chacaleh E53.8
Chafing L30.4
Chagas' (-Mazza) disease (chronic) B57.2
  with
    cardiovascular involvement NEC B57.2
    digestive system involvement B57.30
      megacolon B57.32
      megaesophagus B57.31
      other specified B57.39
    megacolon B57.32
    megaesophagus B57.31
    myocarditis B57.2
    nervous system involvement B57.40
      meningitis B57.41
      meningoencephalitis B57.42
      other specified B57.49
    specified organ involvement NEC B57.5
  acute (with) B57.1
    cardiovascular NEC B57.0
    myocarditis B57.0
Chagres fever B50.9
Chairridden Z74.09
Chalasia (cardiac sphincter) K21.9
Chalazion H00.19
  left H00.16
    lower H00.15
    upper H00.14

Chalazion (Continued)
  right H00.13
    lower H00.12
    upper H00.11
Chalcosis —see also Disorder, globe,
    degenerative, chalcosis
  cornea —see Deposit, cornea
  crystalline lens —see Cataract, complicated
  retina H35.89
Chalicosis (pulmonum) J62.8
Chancre (any genital site) (hard) (hunterian)
    (mixed) (primary) (seronegative)
    (seropositive) (syphilitic) A51.0
  congenital A50.07
  conjunctiva NEC A51.2
  Ducrey's A57
  extragenital A51.2
  eyelid A51.2
  lip A51.2
  nipple A51.2
  Nisbet's A57
  of
    carate A67.0
    pinta A67.0
    yaws A66.0
  palate, soft A51.2
  phagedenic A57
  simple A57
  soft A57
    bubo A57
    palate A51.2
  urethra A51.0
  yaws A66.0
Chancroid (anus) (genital) (penis) (perineum)
    (rectum) (urethra) (vulva) A57
Chandler's disease (osteochondritis dissecans,
    hip) —see Osteochondritis, dissecans, hip
Change(s) (in) (of) —see also Removal
  arteriosclerotic —see Arteriosclerosis
  bone —see also Disorder, bone
    diabetic —see Diabetes, bone change
  bowel habit R19.4
  cardiorenal (vascular) —see Hypertension,
    cardiorenal
  cardiovascular —see Disease, cardiovascular
  circulatory I99.9
  cognitive (mild) (organic) R41.89
  color, tooth, teeth
    during formation K00.8
    posteruptive K03.7
  contraceptive device Z30.433
  corneal membrane H18.30
    Bowman's membrane fold or rupture
      H18.31-●
    Descemet's membrane
      fold H18.32-●
      rupture H18.33-●
  coronary —see Disease, heart, ischemic
  degenerative, spine or vertebra —see
    Spondylosis
  dental pulp, regressive K04.2
  dressing (nonsurgical) Z48.00
    surgical Z48.01
  heart —see Disease, heart
  hip joint —see Derangement, joint, hip
  hyperplastic larynx J38.7
  hypertrophic
    nasal sinus J34.89
    turbinate, nasal J34.3
    upper respiratory tract J39.8
  indwelling catheter Z46.6
  inflammatory —see also Inflammation
    sacroiliac M46.1
  job, anxiety concerning Z56.1
  joint —see Derangement, joint
  life —see Menopause
  mental status R41.82
  minimal (glomerular) —see also N00-N07
    with fourth character .0 N05.0
  myocardium, myocardial —see Degeneration,
    myocardial - of life —see Menopause
  pacemaker Z45.018
    pulse generator Z45.010

Change (Continued)
  personality (enduring) F68.8
    due to (secondary to)
      general medical condition F07.0
    secondary (nonspecific) F60.89
  regressive, dental pulp K04.2
  renal —see Disease, renal
  retina H35.9
    myopic —see also Myopia, degenerative
      H44.2-●
  sacroiliac joint M53.3
  senile —see also condition R54
  sensory R20.8
  skin R23.9
    acute, due to ultraviolet radiation L56.9
      specified NEC L56.8
    chronic, due to nonionizing radiation L57.9
      specified NEC L57.8
    cyanosis R23.0
    flushing R23.2
    pallor R23.1
    petechiae R23.3
    specified change NEC R23.8
    swelling —see Mass, localized
    texture R23.4
  trophic
    arm —see Mononeuropathy, upper limb
    leg —see Mononeuropathy, lower limb
  vascular I99.9
  vasomotor I73.9
  voice R49.9
    psychogenic F44.4
    specified NEC R49.8
Changing sleep-work schedule, affecting sleep
    G47.26
Changuinola fever A93.1
Chapping skin T69.8
Charcot-Marie-Tooth disease, paralysis or
    syndrome G60.0
Charcot's
  arthropathy —see Arthropathy, neuropathic
  cirrhosis K74.3
  disease (tabetic arthropathy) A52.16
  joint (disease) (tabetic) A52.16
    diabetic —see Diabetes, with, arthropathy
    syringomyelic G95.0
  syndrome (intermittent claudication) I73.9
CHARGE association Q89.8
Charley-horse (quadriceps) M62.831
    traumatic (quadriceps) S76.11-●
Charlouis' disease —see Yaws
Cheadle's disease E54
Checking (of)
  cardiac pacemaker (battery) (electrode(s))
    Z45.018
    pulse generator Z45.010
  implantable subdermal contraceptive Z30.46
  intrauterine contraceptive device Z30.431
  wound Z48.0-●
    due to injury - code to Injury, by site, using
      appropriate seventh character for
      subsequent encounter
Check-up —see Examination
Chédiak-Higashi (-Steinbrinck) **syndrome**
    (congenital gigantism of peroxidase
    granules) E70.330
Cheek —see condition
Cheese itch B88.0
Cheese-washer's lung J67.8
Cheese-worker's lung J67.8
Cheilitis (acute) (angular) (catarrhal) (chronic)
    (exfoliative) (gangrenous) (glandular)
    (infectional) (suppurative) (ulcerative)
    (vesicular) K13.0
  actinic (due to sun) L56.8
    other than from sun L59.8
  candidal B37.83
Cheilodynia K13.0
Cheiloschisis —see Cleft, lip
Cheilosis (angular) K13.0
  with pellagra E52
  due to
    vitamin B2 (riboflavin) deficiency E53.0

Cheiromegaly M79.89
Cheiropompholyx L30.1
Cheloid —see Keloid
Chemical burn —see Corrosion, by site
Chemodectoma —see Paraganglioma,
    nonchromaffin
Chemosis, conjunctiva —see Edema,
    conjunctiva
Chemotherapy (session) (for)
  cancer Z51.11
  neoplasm Z51.11
Cherubism M27.8
Chest —see condition
Cheyne-Stokes breathing (respiration) R06.3
Chiari's
  disease or syndrome (hepatic vein
    thrombosis) I82.0
  malformation
    type I G93.5
    type II —see Spina bifida
  net Q24.8
Chicago disease B40.9
Chickenpox —see Varicella
Chiclero ulcer or sore B55.1
Chigger (infestation) B88.0
Chignon (disease) B36.8
  newborn (from vacuum extraction) (birth
    injury) P12.1
Chilaiditi's syndrome (subphrenic
    displacement, colon) Q43.3
Chilblain(s) (lupus) T69.1
Child
  custody dispute Z65.3
Childbirth —see Delivery
Childhood
  cerebral X-linked adrenoleukodystrophy
    E71.520
  period of rapid growth Z00.2
Chill(s) R68.83
  with fever R50.9
  without fever R68.83
  congestive in malarial regions B54
Chilomastigiasis A07.8
Chimera 46,XX/46,XY Q99.0
Chin —see condition
Chinese dysentery A03.9
Chionophobia F40.228
Chitral fever A93.1
Chlamydia, chlamydial A74.9
  cervicitis A56.09
  conjunctivitis A74.0
  cystitis A56.01
  endometritis A56.11
  epididymitis A56.19
  female
    pelvic inflammatory disease A56.11
    pelviperitonitis A56.11
  orchitis A56.19
  peritonitis A74.81
  pharyngitis A56.4
  proctitis A56.3
  psittaci (infection) A70
  salpingitis A56.11
  sexually-transmitted infection NEC A56.8
  specified NEC A74.89
  urethritis A56.01
  vulvovaginitis A56.02
Chlamydiosis —see Chlamydia
Chloasma (skin) (idiopathic) (symptomatic)
    L81.1
  eyelid H02.719
    hyperthyroid E05.90 [H02.719]
      with thyroid storm E05.91 [H02.719]
    left H02.716
      lower H02.715
      upper H02.714
    right H02.713
      lower H02.712
      upper H02.711
Chloroma C92.3-●
Chlorosis D50.9
  Egyptian B76.9 [D63.8]
  miner's B76.9 [D63.8]

▶ New   ⇒ Revised   ~~deleted~~ Deleted   ● Use Additional Character(s)

Chlorotic anemia D50.8
Chocolate cyst (ovary) N80.1
Choked
  disc or disk —see Papilledema
  on food, phlegm, or vomitus NOS —see
    Foreign body, by site
  while vomiting NOS —see Foreign body, by
    site
Chokes (resulting from bends) T70.3
Choking sensation R09.89
Cholangiectasis K83.8
Cholangiocarcinoma
  with hepatocellular carcinoma, combined
    C22.0
  liver C22.1
  specified site NEC —see Neoplasm,
    malignant, by site
  unspecified site C22.1
Cholangiohepatitis K83.8
  due to fluke infestation B66.1
Cholangiohepatoma C22.0
Cholangiolitis (acute) (chronic) (extrahepatic)
    (gangrenous) (intrahepatic) K83.09
  paratyphoidal —see Fever, paratyphoid
  typhoidal A01.09
Cholangioma D13.4
  malignant —see Cholangiocarcinoma
Cholangitis (ascending) (primary) (recurrent)
    (sclerosing) (secondary) (stenosing)
    (suppurative) K83.09
  with calculus, bile duct —see Calculus, bile
    duct, with cholangitis
  chronic nonsuppurative destructive K74.3
  primary K83.09
    sclerosing K83.01
  sclerosing K83.09
Cholecystectasia K82.8
Cholecystitis K81.9
  with
    calculus, stones in
      bile duct (common) (hepatic) —
        see Calculus, bile duct, with
        cholecystitis
      cystic duct —see Calculus, gallbladder,
        with cholecystitis
      gallbladder —see Calculus, gallbladder,
        with cholecystitis
      choledocholithiasis —see Calculus, bile
        duct, with cholecystitis
      cholelithiasis —see Calculus, gallbladder,
        with cholecystitis
    gangrene of gallbladder K82.A1
    perforation of gallbladder K82.A2
  acute (emphysematous) (gangrenous)
    (suppurative) K81.0
  with
    calculus, stones in
      cystic duct —see Calculus, gallbladder,
        with cholecystitis, acute
      gallbladder —see Calculus, gallbladder,
        with cholecystitis, acute
      choledocholithiasis —see Calculus, bile
        duct, with cholecystitis, acute
      cholelithiasis —see Calculus, gallbladder,
        with cholecystitis, acute
    chronic cholecystitis K81.2
      with gallbladder calculus K80.12
        with obstruction K80.13
  chronic K81.1
    with acute cholecystitis K81.2
      with gallbladder calculus K80.12
        with obstruction K80.13
  emphysematous (acute) —see Cholecystitis,
    acute
  gangrenous —see Cholecystitis, acute
  paratyphoidal, current A01.4
  suppurative —see Cholecystitis, acute
  typhoidal A01.09
Cholecystolithiasis —see Calculus, gallbladder
Choledochitis (suppurative) K83.09
Choledocholith —see Calculus, bile duct

Choledocholithiasis (common duct) (hepatic
    duct) —see Calculus, bile duct
  cystic —see Calculus, gallbladder
  typhoidal A01.09
Cholelithiasis (cystic duct) (gallbladder)
    (impacted) (multiple) —see Calculus,
    gallbladder
  bile duct (common) (hepatic) —see Calculus,
    bile duct
  hepatic duct —see Calculus, bile duct
  specified NEC K80.80
    with obstruction K80.81
Cholemia —see also Jaundice
  familial (simple) (congenital) E80.4
  Gilbert's E80.4
Choleperitoneum, choleperitonitis K65.3
Cholera (Asiatic) (epidemic) (malignant) A00.9
  antimonial —see Poisoning, antimony
  classical A00.0
  due to Vibrio cholerae 01 A00.9
    biovar cholerae A00.0
    biovar eltor A00.1
    el tor A00.1
  el tor A00.1
Cholerine —see Cholera
Cholestasis NEC K83.1
  with hepatocyte injury K71.0
  due to total parenteral nutrition (TPN) K76.89
  pure K71.0
Cholesteatoma (ear) (middle) (with reaction)
    H71.9-●
  attic H71.0-●
  external ear (canal) H60.4-●
  mastoid H71.2-●
  postmastoidectomy cavity (recurrent) —see
    Complications, postmastoidectomy,
    recurrent cholesteatoma
  recurrent (postmastoidectomy) —see
    Complications, postmastoidectomy,
    recurrent cholesteatoma
  tympanum H71.1-●
Cholesteatosis, diffuse H71.3-●
Cholesteremia E78.00
Cholesterin in vitreous —see Deposit, crystalline
Cholesterol
  deposit
    retina H35.89
    vitreous —see Deposit, crystalline
  elevated (high) E78.00
    with elevated (high) triglycerides E78.2
    screening for Z13.220
  imbibition of gallbladder K82.4
Cholesterolemia (essential) (pure) E78.00
  familial E78.01
  hereditary E78.01
Cholesterolosis, cholesterosis (gallbladder)
    K82.4
  cerebrotendinous E75.5
Cholocolic fistula K82.3
Choluria R82.2
Chondritis M94.8X9
  aurical H61.03-●
  costal (Tietze's) M94.0
  external ear H61.03-●
  patella, posttraumatic —see Chondromalacia,
    patella
  pinna H61.03-●
  purulent M94.8X-●
  tuberculous NEC A18.02
    intervertebral A18.01
Chondroblastoma —see also Neoplasm, bone,
    benign
  malignant —see Neoplasm, bone, malignant
Chondrocalcinosis M11.20
  ankle M11.27-●
  elbow M11.22-●
  familial M11.10
    ankle M11.17-●
    elbow M11.12-●
    foot joint M11.17-●
    hand joint M11.14-●

Chondrocalcinosis (Continued)
  familial (Continued)
    hip M11.15-●
    knee M11.16-●
    multiple site M11.19
    shoulder M11.11-●
    vertebrae M11.18
    wrist M11.13-●
  foot joint M11.27-●
  hand joint M11.24-●
  hip M11.25-●
  knee M11.26-●
  multiple site M11.29
  shoulder M11.21-●
  specified type NEC M11.20
    ankle M11.27-●
    elbow M11.22-●
    foot joint M11.27-●
    hand joint M11.24-●
    hip M11.25-●
    knee M11.26-●
    multiple site M11.29
    shoulder M11.21-●
    vertebrae M11.28
    wrist M11.23-●
  vertebrae M11.28
  wrist M11.23-●
Chondrodermatitis nodularis helicis or
    anthelicis —see Perichondritis, ear
Chondrodysplasia Q78.9
  with hemangioma Q78.4
  calcificans congenita Q77.3
  fetalis Q77.4
  metaphyseal (Jansen's) (McKusick's)
    (Schmid's) Q78.8
  punctata Q77.3
Chondrodystrophy, chondrodystrophia
    (familial) (fetalis) (hypoplastic) Q78.9
  calcificans congenita Q77.3
  myotonic (congenital) G71.13
  punctata Q77.3
Chondroectodermal dysplasia Q77.6
Chondrogenesis imperfecta Q77.4
Chondrolysis M94.35-●
Chondroma —see also Neoplasm, cartilage,
    benign
  juxtacortical —see Neoplasm, bone, benign
  periosteal —see Neoplasm, bone, benign
Chondromalacia (systemic) M94.20
  acromioclavicular joint M94.21-●
  ankle M94.27-●
  elbow M94.22-●
  foot joint M94.27-●
  glenohumeral joint M94.21-●
  hand joint M94.24-●
  hip M94.25-●
  knee M94.26-●
    patella M22.4-●
  multiple sites M94.29
  patella M22.4-●
  rib M94.28
  sacroiliac joint M94.259
  shoulder M94.21-●
  sternoclavicular joint M94.21-●
  vertebral joint M94.28
  wrist M94.23-●
Chondromatosis —see also Neoplasm, cartilage,
    uncertain behavior
  internal Q78.4
Chondromyxosarcoma —see Neoplasm,
    cartilage, malignant
Chondro-osteodysplasia (Morquio-Brailsford
    type) E76.219
Chondro-osteodystrophy E76.29
Chondro-osteoma —see Neoplasm, bone, benign
Chondropathia tuberosa M94.0
Chondrosarcoma —see Neoplasm, cartilage,
    malignant
  juxtacortical —see Neoplasm, bone, malignant
  mesenchymal —see Neoplasm, connective
    tissue, malignant
  myxoid —see Neoplasm, cartilage, malignant

Chordee (nonvenereal) N48.89
  congenital Q54.4
  gonococcal A54.09
Chorditis (fibrinous) (nodosa) (tuberosa) J38.2
Chordoma —see Neoplasm, vertebral (column), malignant
Chorea (chronic) (gravis) (posthemiplegic) (senile) (spasmodic) G25.5
  with
    heart involvement I02.0
      active or acute (conditions in I01- ●) I02.0
      rheumatic I02.9
        with valvular disorder I02.0
      rheumatic heart disease (chronic) (inactive) (quiescent) — code to rheumatic heart condition involved
  drug-induced G25.4
  habit F95.8
  hereditary G10
  Huntington's G10
  hysterical F44.4
  minor I02.9
    with heart involvement I02.0
  progressive G25.5
    hereditary G10
  rheumatic (chronic) I02.9
    with heart involvement I02.0
  Sydenham's I02.9
    with heart involvement —see Chorea, with rheumatic heart disease
    nonrheumatic G25.5
Choreoathetosis (paroxysmal) G25.5
Chorioadenoma (destruens) D39.2
Chorioamnionitis O41.12- ●
Chorioangioma D26.7
Choriocarcinoma —see Neoplasm, malignant, by site
  combined with
    embryonal carcinoma —see Neoplasm, malignant, by site
    other germ cell elements —see Neoplasm, malignant, by site
    teratoma —see Neoplasm, malignant, by site
  specified site —see Neoplasm, malignant, by site
  unspecified site
    female C58
    male C62.90
Chorioencephalitis (acute) (lymphocytic) (serous) A87.2
Chorioepithelioma —see Choriocarcinoma
Choriomeningitis (acute) (lymphocytic) (serous) A87.2
Chorionepithelioma —see Choriocarcinoma
Chorioretinitis —see also Inflammation, chorioretinal
  disseminated —see also Inflammation, chorioretinal, disseminated
    in neurosyphilis A52.19
  Egyptian B76.9 [D63.8]
  focal —see also Inflammation, chorioretinal, focal
  histoplasmic B39.9 [H32]
  in (due to)
    histoplasmosis B39.9 [H32]
    syphilis (secondary) A51.43
      late A52.71
    toxoplasmosis (acquired) B58.01
      congenital (active) P37.1 [H32]
    tuberculosis A18.53
  juxtapapillary, juxtapapillaris —see Inflammation, chorioretinal, focal, juxtapapillary
  leprous A30.9 [H32]
  miner's B76.9 [D63.8]
  progressive myopia (degeneration) —see also Myopia, degenerative H44.2- ●
  syphilitic (secondary) A51.43
    congenital (early) A50.01 [H32]
      late A50.32
    late A52.71
  tuberculous A18.53

Chorioretinopathy, central serous H35.71- ●
Choroid —see condition
Choroideremia H31.21
Choroiditis —see Chorioretinitis
Choroidopathy —see Disorder, choroid
Choroidoretinitis —see Chorioretinitis
Choroidoretinopathy, central serous —see Chorioretinopathy, central serous
Christian-Weber disease M35.6
Christmas disease D67
Chromaffinoma —see also Neoplasm, benign, by site
  malignant —see Neoplasm, malignant, by site
Chromatopsia —see Deficiency, color vision
Chromhidrosis, chromidrosis L75.1
Chromoblastomycosis —see Chromomycosis
Chromoconversion R82.91
Chromomycosis B43.9
  brain abscess B43.1
  cerebral B43.1
  cutaneous B43.0
  skin B43.0
  specified NEC B43.8
  subcutaneous abscess or cyst B43.2
Chromophytosis B36.0
Chromosome —see condition by chromosome involved
  D (1) —see condition, chromosome 13
  E (3) —see condition, chromosome 18
  G —see condition, chromosome 21
Chromotrichomycosis B36.8
Chronic —see condition
  fracture —see Fracture, pathological
Churg-Strauss syndrome M30.1
Chyle cyst, mesentery I89.8
Chylocele (nonfilarial) I89.8
  filarial —see also Infestation, filarial B74.9 [N51]
  tunica vaginalis N50.89
    filarial —see also Infestation, filarial B74.9 [N51]
Chylomicronemia (fasting) (with hyperprebetalipoproteinemia) E78.3
Chylopericardium I31.3
  acute I30.9
➡ Chylothorax (nonfilarial) J94.0
  filarial —see also Infestation, filarial B74.9 [J91.8]
Chylous —see condition
Chyluria (nonfilarial) R82.0
  due to
    bilharziasis B65.0
    Brugia (malayi) B74.1
      timori B74.2
    schistosomiasis (bilharziasis) B65.0
    Wuchereria (bancrofti) B74.0
  filarial —see Infestation, filarial
Cicatricial (deformity) —see Cicatrix
Cicatrix (adherent) (contracted) (painful) (vicious) —see also Scar L90.5
  adenoid (and tonsil) J35.8
  alveolar process M26.79
  anus K62.89
  auricle —see Disorder, pinna, specified type NEC
  bile duct (common) (hepatic) K83.8
  bladder N32.89
  bone —see Disorder, bone, specified type NEC
  brain G93.89
  cervix (postoperative) (postpartal) N88.1
  common duct K83.8
  cornea H17.9
    tuberculous A18.59
  duodenum (bulb), obstructive K31.5
  esophagus K22.2
  eyelid —see Disorder, eyelid function
  hypopharynx J39.2
  lacrimal passages —see Obstruction, lacrimal
  larynx J38.7
  lung J98.4
  middle ear —see subcategory H74.8
  mouth K13.79

Cicatrix (Continued)
  muscle M62.89
    with contracture —see Contraction, muscle NEC
  nasopharynx J39.2
  palate (soft) K13.79
  penis N48.89
  pharynx J39.2
  prostate N42.89
  rectum K62.89
  retina —see Scar, chorioretinal
  semilunar cartilage —see Derangement, meniscus
  seminal vesicle N50.89
  skin L90.5
    infected L08.89
    postinfective L90.5
    tuberculous B90.8
  specified site NEC L90.5
  throat J39.2
  tongue K14.8
  tonsil (and adenoid) J35.8
  trachea J39.8
  tuberculous NEC B90.9
  urethra N36.8
  uterus N85.8
  vagina N89.8
    postoperative N99.2
  vocal cord J38.3
  wrist, constricting (annular) L90.5
CIDP (chronic inflammatory demyelinating polyneuropathy) G61.81
CIN —see Neoplasia, intraepithelial, cervix
CINCA (chronic infantile neurological, cutaneous and articular syndrome) M04.2
Cinchonism —see Deafness, ototoxic
  correct substance properly administered —see Table of Drugs and Chemicals, by drug, adverse effect
  overdose or wrong substance given or taken —see Table of Drugs and Chemicals, by drug, poisoning
Circle of Willis —see condition
Circular —see condition
Circulating anticoagulants —see also - Disorder, hemorrhagic D68.318
  due to drugs —see also - Disorder, hemorrhagic D68.32
  following childbirth O72.3
Circulation
  collateral, any site I99.8
  defective (lower extremity) I99.9
    congenital Q28.9
  embryonic Q28.9
  failure (peripheral) R57.9
    newborn P29.89
  fetal, persistent P29.38
  heart, incomplete Q28.9
Circulatory system —see condition
Circulus senilis (cornea) —see Degeneration, cornea, senile
Circumcision (in absence of medical indication) (ritual) (routine) Z41.2
Circumscribed —see condition
Circumvallate placenta O43.11- ●
Cirrhosis, cirrhotic (hepatic) (liver) K74.60
  alcoholic K70.30
    with ascites K70.31
  atrophic —see Cirrhosis, liver
  Baumgarten-Cruveilhier K74.69
  biliary (cholangiolitic) (cholangitic) (hypertrophic) (obstructive) (pericholangiolitic) K74.5
    due to
      Clonorchiasis B66.1
      flukes B66.3
    primary K74.3
    secondary K74.4
  cardiac (of liver) K76.1
  Charcot's K74.3

▶ New   ➡ Revised   ~~deleted~~ Deleted   ● Use Additional Character(s)

Cirrhosis, cirrhotic *(Continued)*
  cholangiolitic, cholangitic, cholostatic
    (primary) K74.3
  congestive K76.1
  Cruveilhier-Baumgarten K74.69
  cryptogenic (liver) K74.69
  due to
    hepatolenticular degeneration E83.01
    Wilson's disease E83.01
    xanthomatosis E78.2
  fatty K76.0
    alcoholic K70.0
  Hanot's (hypertrophic) K74.3
  hepatic —*see* Cirrhosis, liver
  hypertrophic K74.3
  Indian childhood K74.69
  kidney —*see* Sclerosis, renal
  Laennec's K70.30
    with ascites K70.31
    alcoholic K70.30
      with ascites K70.31
    nonalcoholic K74.69
  liver K74.60
    alcoholic K70.30
      with ascites K70.31
      fatty K70.0
    congenital P78.81
    syphilitic A52.74
  lung (chronic) J84.10
  macronodular K74.69
    alcoholic K70.30
      with ascites K70.31
  micronodular K74.69
    alcoholic K70.30
      with ascites K70.31
  mixed type K74.69
  monolobular K74.3
  nephritis —*see* Sclerosis, renal
  nutritional K74.69
    alcoholic K70.30
      with ascites K70.31
  obstructive —*see* Cirrhosis, biliary
  ovarian N83.8
  pancreas (duct) K86.89
  pigmentary E83.110
  portal K74.69
    alcoholic K70.30
      with ascites K70.31
  postnecrotic K74.69
    alcoholic K70.30
      with ascites K70.31
  pulmonary J84.10
  renal —*see* Sclerosis, renal
  spleen D73.2
  stasis K76.1
  Todd's K74.3
  unilobar K74.3
  xanthomatous (biliary) K74.5
    due to xanthomatosis (familial) (metabolic)
      (primary) E78.2
Cistern, subarachnoid R93.0
Citrullinemia E72.23
Citrullinuria E72.23
Civatte's disease or poikiloderma L57.3
Clam digger's itch B65.3
Clammy skin R23.1
Clap —*see* Gonorrhea
Clarke-Hadfield syndrome (pancreatic
  infantilism) K86.89
Clark's paralysis G80.9
Clastothrix L67.8
Claude Bernard-Horner syndrome G90.2
  traumatic —*see* Injury, nerve, cervical
    sympathetic
Claude's disease or syndrome G46.3
Claudicatio venosa intermittens I87.8
Claudication (intermittent) I73.9
  cerebral (artery) G45.9
  spinal cord (arteriosclerotic) G95.19
    syphilitic A52.09
  venous (axillary) I87.8

Claustrophobia F40.240
Clavus (infected) L84
Clawfoot (congenital) Q66.89
  acquired —*see* Deformity, limb, clawfoot
Clawhand (acquired) —*see also* Deformity, limb,
  clawhand
  congenital Q68.1
Clawtoe (congenital) Q66.89
  acquired —*see* Deformity, toe, specified NEC
Clay eating —*see* Pica
Cleansing of artificial opening —*see* Attention
  to, artificial, opening
Cleft (congenital) —*see also* Imperfect, closure
  alveolar process M26.79
  branchial (persistent) Q18.2
  cyst Q18.0
    fistula Q18.0
    sinus Q18.0
  cricoid cartilage, posterior Q31.8
  foot Q72.7
  hand Q71.6
  lip (unilateral) Q36.9
    with cleft palate Q37.9
      hard Q37.1
        with soft Q37.5
      soft Q37.3
        with hard Q37.5
    bilateral Q36.0
      with cleft palate Q37.8
        hard Q37.0
          with soft Q37.4
        soft Q37.2
          with hard Q37.4
    median Q36.1
  nose Q30.2
  palate Q35.9
    with cleft lip (unilateral) Q37.9
      bilateral Q37.8
    hard Q35.1
      with
        cleft lip (unilateral) Q37.1
          bilateral Q37.0
        soft Q35.5
          with cleft lip (unilateral) Q37.5
            bilateral Q37.4
    medial Q35.5
    soft Q35.3
      with
        cleft lip (unilateral) Q37.3
          bilateral Q37.2
        hard Q35.5
          with cleft lip (unilateral) Q37.5
            bilateral Q37.4
  penis Q55.69
  scrotum Q55.29
  thyroid cartilage Q31.8
  uvula Q35.7
Cleidocranial dysostosis Q74.0
Cleptomania F63.2
Clicking hip (newborn) R29.4
Climacteric (female) —*see also* Menopause
  arthritis (any site) NEC —*see* Arthritis,
    specified form NEC
  depression (single episode) F32.89
    recurrent episode F33.8
  male (symptoms) (syndrome) NEC N50.89
  melancholia (single episode) F32.89
    recurrent episode F33.8
  paranoid state F22
  polyarthritis NEC —*see* Arthritis, specified
    form NEC
  symptoms (female) N95.1
Clinical research investigation (clinical trial)
  (control subject) (normal comparison)
  (participant) Z00.6
Clitoris —*see* condition Cloaca (persistent)
  Q43.7
Clonorchiasis, clonorchis infection (liver)
  B66.1
Clonus R25.8
Closed bite M26.29

Clostridium (C.) perfringens, as cause of
  disease classified elsewhere B96.7
Closure
  congenital, nose Q30.0
  cranial sutures, premature Q75.0
  defective or imperfect NEC —*see* Imperfect,
    closure
  fistula, delayed —*see* Fistula
  foramen ovale, imperfect Q21.1
  hymen N89.6
  interauricular septum, defective Q21.1
  interventricular septum, defective Q21.0
  lacrimal duct —*see also* Stenosis, lacrimal,
    duct
    congenital Q10.5
  nose (congenital) Q30.0
    acquired M95.0
  of artificial opening —*see* Attention to,
    artificial, opening
  primary angle, without glaucoma damage
    H40.06-●
  vagina N89.5
  valve —*see* Endocarditis
  vulva N90.5
Clot (blood) —*see also* Embolism
  artery (obstruction) (occlusion) —*see*
    Embolism
  bladder N32.89
  brain (intradural or extradural) —*see*
    Occlusion, artery, cerebral
  circulation I74.9
  heart —*see also* Infarct, myocardium
    not resulting in infarction I51.3
  vein —*see* Thrombosis
Clouded state R40.1
  epileptic —*see* Epilepsy, specified NEC
  paroxysmal —*see* Epilepsy, specified NEC
Cloudy antrum, antra J32.0
Clouston's (hidrotic) ectodermal dysplasia
  Q82.4
Clubbed nail pachydermoperiostosis M89.40
  [L62]
Clubbing of finger(s) (nails) R68.3
Clubfinger R68.3
  congenital Q68.1
Clubfoot (congenital) Q66.89
  acquired —*see* Deformity, limb, clubfoot
  equinovarus Q66.0-●
  paralytic —*see* Deformity, limb, clubfoot
Clubhand (congenital) (radial) Q71.4-●
  acquired —*see* Deformity, limb, clubhand
Clubnail R68.3
  congenital Q84.6
Clump, kidney Q63.1
Clumsiness, clumsy child syndrome F82
Cluttering F98.81
Clutton's joints A50.51 [M12.80]
Coagulation, intravascular (diffuse)
  (disseminated) —*see also* Defibrination
    syndrome
  complicating abortion —*see* Abortion, by
    type, complicated by, intravascular
    coagulation
  following ectopic or molar pregnancy
    O08.1
Coagulopathy —*see also* Defect, coagulation
  consumption D65
  intravascular D65
  newborn P60
Coalition
  calcaneo-scaphoid Q66.89
  tarsal Q66.89
Coalminer's
  elbow —*see* Bursitis, elbow, olecranon
  lung or pneumoconiosis J60
Coalworker's lung or pneumoconiosis
  J60
Coarctation
  aorta (preductal) (postductal) Q25.1
  pulmonary artery Q25.71
Coated tongue K14.3

Coats' disease (exudative retinopathy) —see
  Retinopathy, exudative
Cocaine-induced
  anxiety disorder F14.980
  bipolar and related disorder F14.94
  depressive disorder F14.94
  obsessive-compulsive and related disorder
    F14.988
  psychotic disorder F14.959
  sleep disorder F14.982
  sexual dysfunction F14.981
Cocainism —see Disorder, cocaine use
Coccidioidomycosis B38.9
  cutaneous B38.3
  disseminated B38.7
  generalized B38.7
  meninges B38.4
  prostate B38.81
  pulmonary B38.2
    acute B38.0
    chronic B38.1
  skin B38.3
  specified NEC B38.89
Coccidioidosis —see Coccidioidomycosis
Coccidiosis (intestinal) A07.3
Coccydynia, coccygodynia M53.3
Coccyx —see condition
Cochin-China diarrhea K90.1
Cockayne's syndrome Q87.19
Cocked up toe —see Deformity, toe, specified
  NEC
Cock's peculiar tumor L72.3
Codman's tumor —see Neoplasm, bone, benign
Coenurosis B71.8
Coffee-worker's lung J67.8
Cogan's syndrome H16.32-●
  oculomotor apraxia H51.8
Coitus, painful (female) N94.10
  male N53.12
  psychogenic F52.6
Cold J00
  with influenza, flu, or grippe —see Influenza,
    with, respiratory manifestations NEC
  agglutinin disease or hemoglobinuria
    (chronic) D59.12
  bronchial —see Bronchitis
  chest —see Bronchitis
  common (head) J00
  effects of T69.9
    specified effect NEC T69.8
  excessive, effects of T69.9
    specified effect NEC T69.8
  exhaustion from T69.8
  exposure to T69.9
    specified effect NEC T69.8
  head J00
  injury syndrome (newborn) P80.0
  on lung —see Bronchitis
  rose J30.1
  sensitivity, auto-immune D59.12
  symptoms J00
  virus J00
Coldsore B00.1
Colibacillosis A49.8
  as the cause of other disease (see also
    Escherichia coli) B96.20
  generalized A41.50
Colic (bilious) (infantile) (intestinal) (recurrent)
  (spasmodic) R10.83
  abdomen R10.83
    psychogenic F45.8
  appendix, appendicular K38.8
  bile duct —see Calculus, bile duct
  biliary —see Calculus, bile duct
  common duct —see Calculus, bile duct
  cystic duct —see Calculus, gallbladder
  Devonshire NEC —see Poisoning, lead
  gallbladder —see Calculus, gallbladder
  gallstone —see Calculus, gallbladder
    gallbladder or cystic duct —see Calculus,
      gallbladder

Colic (Continued)
  hepatic (duct) —see Calculus, bile duct
  hysterical F45.8
  kidney N23
  lead NEC —see Poisoning, lead
  mucous K58.9
    with diarrhea K58.0
    psychogenic F54
  nephritic N23
  painter's NEC —see Poisoning, lead
  pancreas K86.89
  psychogenic F45.8
  renal N23
  saturnine NEC —see Poisoning, lead
  ureter N23
  urethral N36.8
    due to calculus N21.1
  uterus NEC N94.89
    menstrual —see Dysmenorrhea
  worm NOS B83.9
Colicystitis —see Cystitis
Colitis (acute) (catarrhal) (chronic)
  (noninfective) (hemorrhagic) (see also
  Enteritis) K52.9
  allergic K52.29
    with
      food protein-induced enterocolitis
        syndrome K52.21
      ➡proctocolitis K52.29
  amebic (acute) —see also Amebiasis A06.0
    nondysenteric A06.2
  anthrax A22.2
  bacillary —see Infection, Shigella
  balantidial A07.0
  Clostridium difficile
    not specified as recurrent A04.72
    recurrent A04.71
  coccidial A07.3
  collagenous K52.831
  cystica superficialis K52.89
  dietary counseling and surveillance (for) Z71.3
  dietetic —see also Colitis, allergic K52.29
  drug-induced K52.1
  due to radiation K52.0
  eosinophilic K52.82
  food hypersensitivity —see also Colitis,
    allergic K52.29
  giardial A07.1
  granulomatous —see Enteritis, regional, large
    intestine
  infectious —see Enteritis, infectious
  indeterminate, so stated K52.3
  ischemic K55.9
    acute (subacute) —see also Ischemia,
      intestine, acute K55.039
    chronic K55.1
    due to mesenteric artery insufficiency K55.1
    fulminant (acute) —see also Ischemia,
      intestine, acute K55.039
  left sided K51.50
    with
      abscess K51.514
      complication K51.519
        specified NEC K51.518
      fistula K51.513
      obstruction K51.512
      rectal bleeding K51.511
  lymphocytic K52.832
  membranous
    psychogenic F54
  microscopic K52.839
    specified NEC K52.838
  mucous —see Syndrome, irritable, bowel
    psychogenic F54
  noninfective K52.9
    specified NEC K52.89
  polyposa —see Polyp, colon, inflammatory
  protozoal A07.9
  pseudomembranous
    not specified as recurrent A04.72
    recurrent A04.71

Colitis (Continued)
  pseudomucinous —see Syndrome, irritable,
    bowel
  regional —see Enteritis, regional, large intestine
    infectious A09
  segmental —see Enteritis, regional, large
    intestine
  septic —see Enteritis, infectious
  spastic K58.9
    with diarrhea K58.0
    psychogenic F54
  staphylococcal A04.8
    foodborne A05.0
  subacute ischemic —see also Ischemia,
    intestine, acute K55.039
  thromboulcerative —see also Ischemia,
    intestine, acute K55.039
  toxic NEC K52.1
    due to Clostridium difficile
      not specified as recurrent A04.72
      recurrent A04.71
  transmural —see Enteritis, regional, large
    intestine
  trichomonal A07.8
  tuberculous (ulcerative) A18.32
  ulcerative (chronic) K51.90
    with
      complication K51.919
        abscess K51.914
        fistula K51.913
        obstruction K51.912
        rectal bleeding K51.911
        specified complication NEC K51.918
    enterocolitis —see Enterocolitis, ulcerative
    ileocolitis —see Ileocolitis, ulcerative
    mucosal proctocolitis —see Proctocolitis,
      mucosal
    proctitis —see Proctitis, ulcerative
    pseudopolyposis —see Polyp, colon,
      inflammatory
    psychogenic F54
    rectosigmoiditis —see Rectosigmoiditis,
      ulcerative
    specified type NEC K51.80
      with
        complication K51.819
          abscess K51.814
          fistula K51.813
          obstruction K51.812
          rectal bleeding K51.811
          specified complication NEC K51.818
Collagenosis, collagen disease (nonvascular)
  (vascular) M35.9
  cardiovascular I42.8
  reactive perforating L87.1
  specified NEC M35.89
Collapse R55
  adrenal E27.2
  cardiorespiratory R57.0
  cardiovascular R57.0
    newborn P29.89
  circulatory (peripheral) R57.9
    during or after labor and delivery O75.1
    following ectopic or molar pregnancy O08.3
    newborn P29.89
  during or
    after labor and delivery O75.1
    resulting from a procedure, not elsewhere
      classified T81.10
  external ear canal —see Stenosis, external ear
    canal
  general R55
  heart —see Disease, heart
  heat T67.1
  hysterical F44.89
  labyrinth, membranous (congenital) Q16.5
  lung (massive) —see also Atelectasis J98.19
    pressure due to anesthesia (general) (local)
      or other sedation T88.2
      during labor and delivery O74.1
      in pregnancy O29.02-●
      postpartum, puerperal O89.09

▶ New   ➡ Revised   ~~deleted~~ Deleted   ● Use Additional Character(s)

Collapse *(Continued)*
  myocardial —*see* Disease, heart
  nervous F48.8
  neurocirculatory F45.8
  nose M95.0
  postoperative T81.10
  pulmonary —*see also* Atelectasis J98.19
    newborn —*see* Atelectasis
  trachea J39.8
  tracheobronchial J98.09
  valvular —*see* Endocarditis
  vascular (peripheral) R57.9
    during or after labor and delivery O75.1
    following ectopic or molar pregnancy O08.3
    newborn P29.89
  vertebra M48.50-●
    cervical region M48.52-●
    cervicothoracic region M48.53-●
    in (due to)
      metastasis —*see* Collapse, vertebra, in, specified disease NEC
      osteoporosis —*see also* Osteoporosis M80.88
        cervical region M80.88
        cervicothoracic region M80.88
        lumbar region M80.88
        lumbosacral region M80.88
        multiple sites M80.88
        occipito-atlanto-axial region M80.88
        sacrococcygeal region M80.88
        thoracic region M80.88
        thoracolumbar region M80.88
      specified disease NEC M48.50-●
        cervical region M48.52-●
        cervicothoracic region M48.53-●
        lumbar region M48.56-●
        lumbosacral region M48.57-●
        occipito-atlanto-axial region M48.51-●
        sacrococcygeal region M48.58-●
        thoracic region M48.54-●
        thoracolumbar region M48.55-●
    lumbar region M48.56-●
    lumbosacral region M48.57-●
    occipito-atlanto-axial region M48.51-●
    sacrococcygeal region M48.58-●
    thoracic region M48.54-●
    thoracolumbar region M48.55-●
Collateral —*see also* condition
  circulation (venous) I87.8
  dilation, veins I87.8
Colles' fracture S52.53-●
Collet (-Sicard) **syndrome** G52.7
Collier's asthma or lung J60
Collodion baby Q80.2
Colloid nodule (of thyroid) (cystic) E04.1
Coloboma (iris) Q13.0
  eyelid Q10.3
  fundus Q14.8
  lens Q12.2
  optic disc (congenital) Q14.2
    acquired H47.31-●
Coloenteritis —*see* Enteritis
Colon —*see* condition
Colonization
  MRSA (Methicillin resistant Staphylococcus aureus) Z22.322
  MSSA (Methicillin susceptible Staphylococcus aureus) Z22.321
  status —*see* Carrier (suspected) of
Coloptosis K63.4
Color blindness —*see* Deficiency, color vision
Colostomy
  attention to Z43.3
  fitting or adjustment Z46.89
  malfunctioning K94.03
  status Z93.3
Colpitis (acute) —*see* Vaginitis
Colpocele N81.5
Colpocystitis —*see* Vaginitis
Colpospasm N94.2
Column, spinal, vertebral —*see* condition

Coma R40.20
  with
    motor response (none) R40.231
      abnormal R40.233
      abnormal extensor posturing to pain or noxious stimuli (<2 years of age) R40.232
      abnormal flexure posturing to pain or noxious stimuli (0-5 years of age) R40.233
      extension R40.232
      extensor posturing to pain or noxious stimuli (2-5 years of age) R40.232
      flexion/decorticate posturing (<2 years of age) R40.233
      flexion withdrawal R40.234
      localizes pain (2-5 years of age) R40.235
      normal or spontaneous movement (<2 years of age) R40.236
      obeys commands (2-5 years of age) R40.236
      score of
        1 R40.231
        2 R40.232
        3 R40.233
        4 R40.234
        5 R40.235
        6 R40.236
      withdraws from pain or noxious stimuli (0-5 years of age) R40.234
      withdraws to touch (<2 years of age) R40.235
    opening of eyes (never) R40.211
      in response to
        pain R40.212
        sound R40.213
      score of
        1 R40.211
        2 R40.212
        3 R40.213
        4 R40.214
      spontaneous R40.214
    verbal response (none) R40.221
      confused conversation R40.224
      cooing or babbling or crying appropriately (<2 years of age) R40.225
      inappropriate crying or screaming (<2 years of age) R40.223
      inappropriate words R40.223
      inappropriate words (2-5 years of age) R40.224
      incomprehensible sounds (2-5 years of age) R40.222
      incomprehensible words R40.222
      irritable cries (<2 years of age) R40.224
      moans/grunts to pain; restless (<2 years old) R40.222
      oriented R40.225
      score of
        1 R40.221
        2 R40.222
        3 R40.223
        4 R40.224
        5 R40.225
      screaming (2-5 years of age) R40.223
      uses appropriate words (2-5 years of age) R40.225
  eclamptic —*see* Eclampsia
  epileptic —*see* Epilepsy
  Glasgow, scale score —*see* Glasgow coma scale
  hepatic —*see* Failure, hepatic, by type, with coma
  hyperglycemic (diabetic) —*see* Diabetes, by type, with hyperosmolarity, with coma
  hyperosmolar (diabetic) —*see* Diabetes, by type, with hyperosmolarity, with coma
  hypoglycemic (diabetic) —*see* Diabetes, by type, with hypoglycemia, with coma
  nondiabetic E15

Coma *(Continued)*
  in diabetes —*see* Diabetes, coma
  insulin-induced —*see* Coma, hypoglycemic
  ketoacidotic (diabetic) —*see* Diabetes, by type, with ketoacidosis, with coma
  myxedematous E03.5
  newborn P91.5
  persistent vegetative state R40.3
  specified NEC, without documented Glasgow coma scale score, or with partial Glasgow coma scale score reported R40.244
Comatose —*see* Coma
Combat fatigue F43.0
Combined —*see* condition
Comedo, comedones (giant) L70.0
Comedocarcinoma —*see also* Neoplasm, breast, malignant
  noninfiltrating
    breast D05.8-●
    specified site —*see* Neoplasm, in situ, by site
    unspecified site D05.8-●
Comedomastitis —*see* Ectasia, mammary duct
Comminuted fracture - code as Fracture, closed
Common
  arterial trunk Q20.0
  atrioventricular canal Q21.2
  atrium Q21.1
  cold (head) J00
  truncus (arteriosus) Q20.0
  variable immunodeficiency —*see* Immunodeficiency, common variable
  ventricle Q20.4
Commotio, commotion (current)
  brain —*see* Injury, intracranial, concussion
  cerebri —*see* Injury, intracranial, concussion
  retinae S05.8X-●
  spinal cord —*see* Injury, spinal cord, by region
  spinalis —*see* Injury, spinal cord, by region
Communication
  between
    base of aorta and pulmonary artery Q21.4
    left ventricle and right atrium Q20.5
    pericardial sac and pleural sac Q34.8
    pulmonary artery and pulmonary vein, congenital Q25.72
  congenital between uterus and digestive or urinary tract Q51.7
Compartment syndrome (deep) (posterior) (traumatic) T79.A0
  abdomen T79.A3
  lower extremity (hip, buttock, thigh, leg, foot, toes) T79.A2
  nontraumatic
    abdomen M79.A3
    lower extremity (hip, buttock, thigh, leg, foot, toes) M79.A2-●
    specified site NEC M79.A9
    upper extremity (shoulder, arm, forearm, wrist, hand, fingers) M79.A1-●
  specified site NEC T79.A9
  upper extremity (shoulder, arm, forearm, wrist, hand, fingers) T79.A1
Compensation
  failure —*see* Disease, heart
  neurosis, psychoneurosis —*see* Disorder, factitious
Complaint —*see also* Disease
  bowel, functional K59.9
    psychogenic F45.8
  intestine, functional K59.9
    psychogenic F45.8
  kidney —*see* Disease, renal
  miners' J60
Complete —*see* condition
Complex
  Addison-Schilder E71.528
  cardiorenal —*see* Hypertension, cardiorenal
  Costen's M26.69
  disseminated mycobacterium avium-intracellulare (DMAC) A31.2

Complex *(Continued)*
  Eisenmenger's (ventricular septal defect) I27.83
  hypersexual F52.8
  jumped process, spine —*see* Dislocation, vertebra
  primary, tuberculous A15.7
  Schilder-Addison E71.528
  subluxation (vertebral) M99.19
    abdomen M99.19
    acromioclavicular M99.17
    cervical region M99.11
    cervicothoracic M99.11
    costochondral M99.18
    costovertebral M99.18
    head region M99.10
    hip M99.15
    lower extremity M99.16
    lumbar region M99.13
    lumbosacral M99.13
    occipitocervical M99.10
    pelvic region M99.15
    pubic M99.15
    rib cage M99.18
    sacral region M99.14
    sacrococcygeal M99.14
    sacroiliac M99.14
    specified NEC M99.19
    sternochondral M99.18
    sternoclavicular M99.17
    thoracic region M99.12
    thoracolumbar M99.12
    upper extremity M99.17
  Taussig-Bing (transposition, aorta and overriding pulmonary artery) Q20.1
Complication(s) (from) (of)
  accidental puncture or laceration during a procedure (of) —*see* Complications, intraoperative (intraprocedural), puncture or laceration
  amputation stump (surgical) (late) NEC T87.9
    dehiscence T87.81
    infection or inflammation T87.40
      lower limb T87.4-●
      upper limb T87.4-●
    necrosis T87.50
      lower limb T87.5-●
      upper limb T87.5-●
    neuroma T87.30
      lower limb T87.3-●
      upper limb T87.3-●
    specified type NEC T87.89
  anastomosis (and bypass) —*see also* Complications, prosthetic device or implant
    intestinal (internal) NEC K91.89
      involving urinary tract N99.89
    urinary tract (involving intestinal tract) N99.89
    vascular —*see* Complications, cardiovascular device or implant
  anesthesia, anesthetic —*see also* Anesthesia, complication T88.59
    brain, postpartum, puerperal O89.2
    cardiac
      in
        labor and delivery O74.2
        pregnancy O29.19-●
      postpartum, puerperal O89.1
    central nervous system
      in
        labor and delivery O74.3
        pregnancy O29.29-●
      postpartum, puerperal O89.2
    difficult or failed intubation T88.4
      in pregnancy O29.6-●
    failed sedation (conscious) (moderate) during procedure T88.52
    general, unintended awareness during procedure T88.53
    hyperthermia, malignant T88.3
    hypothermia T88.51
    intubation failure T88.4

Complication *(Continued)*
  anesthesia, anesthetic *(Continued)*
    malignant hyperthermia T88.3
    pulmonary
      in
        labor and delivery O74.1
        pregnancy NEC O29.09-●
      postpartum, puerperal O89.09
    shock T88.2
    spinal and epidural
      in
        labor and delivery NEC O74.6
          headache O74.5
        pregnancy NEC O29.5X-●
      postpartum, puerperal NEC O89.5
        headache O89.4
    unintended awareness under general anesthesia during procedure T88.53
  anti-reflux device —*see* Complications, esophageal anti-reflux device
  aortic (bifurcation) graft —*see* Complications, graft, vascular
  aortocoronary (bypass) graft —*see* Complications, coronary artery (bypass) graft
  aortofemoral (bypass) graft —*see* Complications, extremity artery (bypass) graft
  arteriovenous
    fistula, surgically created T82.9
      embolism T82.818
      fibrosis T82.828
      hemorrhage T82.838
      infection or inflammation T82.7
      mechanical
        breakdown T82.510
        displacement T82.520
        leakage T82.530
        malposition T82.520
        obstruction T82.590
        perforation T82.590
        protrusion T82.590
      pain T82.848
      specified type NEC T82.898
      stenosis T82.858
      thrombosis T82.868
    shunt, surgically created T82.9
      embolism T82.818
      fibrosis T82.828
      hemorrhage T82.838
      infection or inflammation T82.7
      mechanical
        breakdown T82.511
        displacement T82.521
        leakage T82.531
        malposition T82.521
        obstruction T82.591
        perforation T82.591
        protrusion T82.591
      pain T82.848
      specified type NEC T82.898
      stenosis T82.858
      thrombosis T82.868
  arthroplasty —*see* Complications, joint prosthesis
  artificial
    fertilization or insemination N98.9
      attempted introduction (of)
        embryo in embryo transfer N98.3
        ovum following in vitro fertilization N98.2
      hyperstimulation of ovaries N98.1
      infection N98.0
      specified NEC N98.8
    heart T82.9
      embolism T82.817
      fibrosis T82.827
      hemorrhage T82.837
      infection or inflammation T82.7
      mechanical
        breakdown T82.512
        displacement T82.522
        leakage T82.532

Complication *(Continued)*
  artificial *(Continued)*
    heart *(Continued)*
      mechanical *(Continued)*
        malposition T82.522
        obstruction T82.592
        perforation T82.592
        protrusion T82.592
      pain T82.847
      specified type NEC T82.897
      stenosis T82.857
      thrombosis T82.867
    opening
      cecostomy —*see* Complications, colostomy
      colostomy —*see* Complications, colostomy
      cystostomy —*see* Complications, cystostomy
      enterostomy —*see* Complications, enterostomy
      gastrostomy —*see* Complications, gastrostomy
      ileostomy —*see* Complications, enterostomy
      jejunostomy —*see* Complications, enterostomy
      nephrostomy —*see* Complications, stoma, urinary tract
      tracheostomy —*see* Complications, tracheostomy
      ureterostomy —*see* Complications, stoma, urinary tract
      urethrostomy —*see* Complications, stoma, urinary tract
  balloon implant or device
    gastrointestinal T85.9
      embolism T85.818
      fibrosis T85.828
      hemorrhage T85.838
      infection and inflammation T85.79
      pain T85.848
      specified type NEC T85.898
      stenosis T85.858
      thrombosis T85.868
    vascular (counterpulsation) T82.9
      embolism T82.818
      fibrosis T82.828
      hemorrhage T82.838
      infection or inflammation T82.7
      mechanical
        breakdown T82.513
        displacement T82.523
        leakage T82.533
        malposition T82.523
        obstruction T82.593
        perforation T82.593
        protrusion T82.593
      pain T82.848
      specified type NEC T82.898
      stenosis T82.858
      thrombosis T82.868
  bariatric procedure
    gastric band procedure K95.09
      infection K95.01
    specified procedure NEC K95.89
      infection K95.81
  bile duct implant (prosthetic) T85.9
    embolism T85.818
    fibrosis T85.828
    hemorrhage T85.838
    infection and inflammation T85.79
    mechanical
      breakdown T85.510
      displacement T85.520
      malfunction T85.510
      malposition T85.520
      obstruction T85.590
      perforation T85.590
      protrusion T85.590
      specified NEC T85.590
    pain T85.848
    specified type NEC T85.898

▶ New   ⮕ Revised   ~~deleted~~ Deleted   ● Use Additional Character(s)

Complication *(Continued)*
bile duct implant *(Continued)*
  stenosis T85.858
  thrombosis T85.868
bladder device (auxiliary) —*see*
  Complications, genitourinary, device or
  implant, urinary system
bleeding (postoperative) —*see* Complication,
  postoperative, hemorrhage
  intraoperative —*see* Complication,
   intraoperative, hemorrhage
blood vessel graft —*see* Complications, graft,
  vascular
bone
  device NEC T84.9
   embolism T84.81
   fibrosis T84.82
   hemorrhage T84.83
   infection or inflammation T84.7
   mechanical
    breakdown T84.318
    displacement T84.328
    malposition T84.328
    obstruction T84.398
    perforation T84.398
    protrusion T84.398
   pain T84.84
   specified type NEC T84.89
   stenosis T84.85
   thrombosis T84.86
  graft —*see* Complications, graft, bone
  growth stimulator (electrode) —*see*
   Complications, electronic stimulator
   device, bone
  marrow transplant —*see* Complications,
   transplant, bone, marrow
brain neurostimulator (electrode) —*see*
  Complications, electronic stimulator
  device, brain
breast implant (prosthetic) T85.9
  capsular contracture T85.44
  embolism T85.818
  fibrosis T85.828
  hemorrhage T85.838
  infection and inflammation T85.79
  mechanical
   breakdown T85.41
   displacement T85.42
   leakage T85.43
   malposition T85.42
   obstruction T85.49
   perforation T85.49
   protrusion T85.49
   specified NEC T85.49
  pain T85.848
  specified type NEC T85.898
  stenosis T85.858
  thrombosis T85.868
bypass —*see also* Complications, prosthetic
  device or implant
  aortocoronary —*see* Complications,
   coronary artery (bypass) graft
  arterial —*see also* Complications, graft,
   vascular
   extremity —*see* Complications, extremity
    artery (bypass) graft
cardiac —*see also* Disease, heart
  device, implant or graft T82.9
   embolism T82.817
   fibrosis T82.827
   hemorrhage T82.837
   infection or inflammation T82.7
    valve prosthesis T82.6
   mechanical
    breakdown T82.519
     specified device NEC T82.518
    displacement T82.529
     specified device NEC T82.528
    leakage T82.539
     specified device NEC T82.538
    malposition T82.529
     specified device NEC T82.528

Complication *(Continued)*
cardiac *(Continued)*
  device, implant or graft *(Continued)*
   mechanical *(Continued)*
    obstruction T82.599
     specified device NEC T82.598
    perforation T82.599
     specified device NEC T82.598
    protrusion T82.599
     specified device NEC T82.598
   pain T82.847
   specified type NEC T82.897
   stenosis T82.857
   thrombosis T82.867
cardiovascular device, graft or implant T82.9
  aortic graft —*see* Complications, graft,
   vascular
  arteriovenous
   fistula, artificial —*see* Complication,
    arteriovenous, fistula, surgically
    created
   shunt —*see* Complication, arteriovenous,
    shunt, surgically created
  artificial heart —*see* Complication,
   artificial, heart
  balloon (counterpulsation) device —*see*
   Complication, balloon implant,
   vascular
  carotid artery graft —*see* Complications,
   graft, vascular
  coronary bypass graft —*see* Complication,
   coronary artery (bypass) graft
  dialysis catheter (vascular) —*see*
   Complication, catheter, dialysis
  electronic T82.9
   electrode T82.9
    embolism T82.817
    fibrosis T82.827
    hemorrhage T82.837
    infection T82.7
    mechanical
     breakdown T82.110
     displacement T82.120
     leakage T82.190
     obstruction T82.190
     perforation T82.190
     protrusion T82.190
     specified type NEC T82.190
    pain T82.847
    specified NEC T82.897
    stenosis T82.857
    thrombosis T82.867
   embolism T82.817
   fibrosis T82.827
   hemorrhage T82.837
   infection T82.7
   mechanical
    breakdown T82.119
    displacement T82.129
    leakage T82.199
    obstruction T82.199
    perforation T82.199
    protrusion T82.199
    specified type NEC T82.199
   pain T82.847
   pulse generator T82.9
    embolism T82.817
    fibrosis T82.827
    hemorrhage T82.837
    infection T82.7
    mechanical
     breakdown T82.111
     displacement T82.121
     leakage T82.191
     obstruction T82.191
     perforation T82.191
     protrusion T82.191
     specified type NEC T82.191
    pain T82.847
    specified NEC T82.897
    stenosis T82.857
    thrombosis T82.867

Complication *(Continued)*
cardiovascular device, graft or implant
  (Continued)
  electronic *(Continued)*
   specified condition NEC T82.897
   specified device NEC T82.9
    embolism T82.817
    fibrosis T82.827
    hemorrhage T82.837
    infection T82.7
    mechanical
     breakdown T82.118
     displacement T82.128
     leakage T82.198
     obstruction T82.198
     perforation T82.198
     protrusion T82.198
     specified type NEC T82.198
    pain T82.847
    specified NEC T82.897
    stenosis T82.857
    thrombosis T82.867
   stenosis T82.857
   thrombosis T82.867
  extremity artery graft —*see* Complication,
   extremity artery (bypass) graft
  femoral artery graft —*see* Complication,
   extremity artery (bypass) graft
  heart
   transplant —*see* Complication,
    transplant, heart
   valve —*see* Complication, prosthetic
    device, heart valve
    graft —*see* Complication, heart, valve,
     graft
  heart-lung transplant —*see* Complication,
   transplant, heart, with lung
  infection or inflammation T82.7
  umbrella device —*see* Complication,
   umbrella device, vascular
  vascular graft (or anastomosis) —*see*
   Complication, graft, vascular
carotid artery (bypass) graft —*see*
  Complications, graft, vascular
catheter (device) NEC —*see also*
  Complications, prosthetic device or
  implant
  cranial infusion
   infection and inflammation T85.735
   mechanical
    breakdown T85.610
    displacement T85.620
    leakage T85.630
    malfunction T85.690
    malposition T85.620
    obstruction T85.690
    perforation T85.690
    protrusion T85.690
    specified NEC T85.690
  cystostomy T83.9
   embolism T83.81
   fibrosis T83.82
   hemorrhage T83.83
   infection and inflammation T83.510
   mechanical
    breakdown T83.010
    displacement T83.020
    leakage T83.030
    malposition T83.020
    obstruction T83.090
    perforation T83.090
    protrusion T83.090
    specified NEC T83.090
   pain T83.84
   specified type NEC T83.89
   stenosis T83.85
   thrombosis T83.86
  dialysis (vascular) T82.9
   embolism T82.818
   fibrosis T82.828
   hemorrhage T82.838

Complication (*Continued*)
  catheter NEC (*Continued*)
    dialysis (*Continued*)
      infection and inflammation T82.7
      intraperitoneal —*see* Complications,
          catheter, intraperitoneal
      mechanical
        breakdown T82.41
        displacement T82.42
        leakage T82.43
        malposition T82.42
        obstruction T82.49
        perforation T82.49
        protrusion T82.49
      pain T82.848
      specified type NEC T82.898
      stenosis T82.858
      thrombosis T82.868
    epidural infusion T85.9
      embolism T85.810
      fibrosis T85.820
      hemorrhage T85.830
      infection and inflammation T85.735
      mechanical
        breakdown T85.610
        displacement T85.620
        leakage T85.630
        malfunction T85.610
        malposition T85.620
        obstruction T85.690
        perforation T85.690
        protrusion T85.690
        specified NEC T85.690
      pain T85.840
      specified type NEC T85.890
      stenosis T85.850
      thrombosis T85.860
    intraperitoneal dialysis T85.9
      embolism T85.818
      fibrosis T85.828
      hemorrhage T85.838
      infection and inflammation T85.71
      mechanical
        breakdown T85.611
        displacement T85.621
        leakage T85.631
        malfunction T85.611
        malposition T85.621
        obstruction T85.691
        perforation T85.691
        protrusion T85.691
        specified NEC T85.691
      pain T85.848
      specified type NEC T85.898
      stenosis T85.858
      thrombosis T85.868
    intrathecal infusion
      infection and inflammation T85.735
      mechanical
        breakdown T85.610
        displacement T85.620
        leakage T85.630
        malfunction T85.690
        malposition T85.620
        obstruction T85.690
        perforation T85.690
        protrusion T85.690
        specified NEC T85.690
    intravenous infusion T82.9
      embolism T82.818
      fibrosis T82.828
      hemorrhage T82.838
      infection or inflammation T82.7
      mechanical
        breakdown T82.514
        displacement T82.524
        leakage T82.534
        malposition T82.524
        obstruction T82.594
        perforation T82.594
        protrusion T82.594
      pain T82.848

Complication (*Continued*)
  catheter NEC (*Continued*)
    intravenous infusion (*Continued*)
      specified type NEC T82.898
      stenosis T82.858
      thrombosis T82.868
    spinal infusion
      infection and inflammation T85.735
      mechanical
        breakdown T85.610
        displacement T85.620
        leakage T85.630
        malfunction T85.690
        malposition T85.620
        obstruction T85.690
        perforation T85.690
        protrusion T85.690
        specified NEC T85.690
    subarachnoid infusion
      infection and inflammation
          T85.735
      mechanical
        breakdown T85.610
        displacement T85.620
        leakage T85.630
        malfunction T85.690
        malposition T85.620
        obstruction T85.690
        perforation T85.690
        protrusion T85.690
        specified NEC T85.690
    subdural infusion T85.9
      embolism T85.810
      fibrosis T85.820
      hemorrhage T85.830
      infection and inflammation T85.735
      mechanical
        breakdown T85.610
        displacement T85.620
        leakage T85.630
        malfunction T85.610
        malposition T85.620
        obstruction T85.690
        perforation T85.690
        protrusion T85.690
        specified NEC T85.690
      pain T85.840
      specified type NEC T85.890
      stenosis T85.850
      thrombosis T85.860
    urethral T83.9
      displacement T83.028
      embolism T83.81
      fibrosis T83.82
      hemorrhage T83.83
      indwelling
        breakdown T83.011
        displacement T83.021
        infection and inflammation T83.511
        leakage T83.031
        specified complication NEC T83.091
      infection and inflammation T83.511
      leakage T83.038
      malposition T83.028
      mechanical
        breakdown T83.011
      obstruction (mechanical) T83.091
      pain T83.84
      perforation T83.091
      protrusion T83.091
      specified type NEC T83.091
      stenosis T83.85
      thrombosis T83.86
    urinary NEC
      breakdown T83.018
      displacement T83.028
      infection and inflammation T83.518
      leakage T83.038
      specified complication NEC T83.098
    cecostomy (stoma) —*see* Complications,
        colostomy

Complication (*Continued*)
  cesarean delivery wound NEC O90.89
    disruption O90.0
    hematoma O90.2
    infection (following delivery) O86.00
  chemotherapy (antineoplastic) NEC T88.7
  ▶chimeric antigen receptor (CAR-T) cell
      therapy T80.82
  chin implant (prosthetic) —*see* Complication,
      prosthetic device or implant, specified
      NEC
  circulatory system I99.8
    intraoperative I97.88
    postprocedural I97.89
      following cardiac surgery —*see also*
          Infarct, myocardium, associated with
          revascularization procedure I97.19-●
        postcardiotomy syndrome I97.0
      hypertension I97.3
      lymphedema after mastectomy I97.2
      postcardiotomy syndrome I97.0
      specified NEC I97.89
  colostomy (stoma) K94.00
    hemorrhage K94.01
    infection K94.02
    malfunction K94.03
    mechanical K94.03
    specified complication NEC K94.09
  contraceptive device, intrauterine —
      see Complications, intrauterine,
      contraceptive device
  cord (umbilical) —*see* Complications,
      umbilical cord
  corneal graft —*see* Complications, graft, cornea
  coronary artery (bypass) graft T82.9
    atherosclerosis —*see* Arteriosclerosis,
        coronary (artery)
    embolism T82.818
    fibrosis T82.828
    hemorrhage T82.838
    infection and inflammation T82.7
    mechanical
      breakdown T82.211
      displacement T82.212
      leakage T82.213
      malposition T82.212
      obstruction T82.218
      perforation T82.218
      protrusion T82.218
      specified NEC T82.218
    pain T82.848
    specified type NEC T82.898
    stenosis T82.858
    thrombosis T82.868
  counterpulsation device (balloon), intra-
      aortic —*see* Complications, balloon
      implant, vascular
  cystostomy (stoma) N99.518
    catheter —*see* Complications, catheter,
        cystostomy
    hemorrhage N99.510
    infection N99.511
    malfunction N99.512
    specified type NEC N99.518
  delivery —*see also* Complications, obstetric
      O75.9
    procedure (instrumental) (manual)
        (surgical) O75.4
    specified NEC O75.89
  dialysis (peritoneal) (renal) —*see also*
      Complications, infusion
    catheter (vascular) —*see* Complication,
        catheter, dialysis
      peritoneal, intraperitoneal —*see*
          Complications, catheter,
          intraperitoneal
  dorsal column (spinal) neurostimulator —*see*
      Complications, electronic stimulator
      device, spinal cord
  drug NEC T88.7
  ear procedure —*see also* Disorder, ear
    intraoperative H95.88-●

▶ New   ⇒ Revised   ~~deleted~~ Deleted   ● Use Additional Character(s)

Complication *(Continued)*
  ear procedure *(Continued)*
    intraoperative *(Continued)*
      hematoma —*see* Complications,
        intraoperative, hematoma (of), ear
      hemorrhage —*see* Complications,
        intraoperative, hemorrhage (of), ear
      laceration —*see* Complications,
        intraoperative, puncture or
        laceration..., ear
      seroma —*see* Complications,
        postprocedural, seroma (of),
        mastoid process
      specified NEC H95.88-●
    postoperative H95.89-●
      external ear canal stenosis H95.81-●
      hematoma —*see* Complications,
        postprocedural, hemorrhage
        (hematoma) (of), ear
      hemorrhage —*see* Complications,
        postprocedural, hemorrhage
        (hematoma) (of), ear
      postmastoidectomy —*see* Complications,
        postmastoidectomy
      specified NEC H95.89-●
  ectopic pregnancy O08.9
    damage to pelvic organs O08.6
    embolism O08.2
    genital infection O08.0
    hemorrhage (delayed) (excessive) O08.1
    metabolic disorder O08.5
    renal failure O08.4
    shock O08.3
    specified type NEC O08.0
    venous complication NEC O08.7
  electronic stimulator device
    bladder (urinary) —*see* Complications,
      electronic stimulator device, urinary
    bone T84.9
      breakdown T84.310
      displacement T84.320
      embolism T84.81
      fibrosis T84.82
      hemorrhage T84.83
      infection or inflammation T84.7
      malfunction T84.310
      malposition T84.320
      mechanical NEC T84.390
      obstruction T84.390
      pain T84.84
      perforation T84.390
      protrusion T84.390
      specified type NEC T84.89
      stenosis T84.85
      thrombosis T84.86
    brain T85.9
      embolism T85.810
      fibrosis T85.820
      hemorrhage T85.830
      infection and inflammation T85.731
      mechanical
        breakdown T85.110
        displacement T85.120
        leakage T85.190
        malposition T85.120
        obstruction T85.190
        perforation T85.190
        protrusion T85.190
        specified NEC T85.190
      pain T85.840
      specified type NEC T85.890
      stenosis T85.850
      thrombosis T85.860
    cardiac (defibrillator) (pacemaker) —*see*
      Complications, cardiovascular device
      or implant, electronic
    generator (brain) (gastric) (peripheral)
      (sacral) (spinal)
      breakdown T85.113
      displacement T85.123
      leakage T85.193

Complication *(Continued)*
  electronic stimulator device *(Continued)*
    generator *(Continued)*
      malposition T85.123
      obstruction T85.193
      perforation T85.193
      protrusion T85.193
      specified type NEC T85.193
    muscle T84.9
      breakdown T84.418
      displacement T84.428
      embolism T84.81
      fibrosis T84.82
      hemorrhage T84.83
      infection or inflammation T84.7
      mechanical NEC T84.498
      pain T84.84
      specified type NEC T84.89
      stenosis T84.85
      thrombosis T84.86
    nervous system T85.9
      brain —*see* Complications, electronic
        stimulator device, brain
      cranial nerve —*see* Complications,
        electronic stimulator device,
        peripheral nerve
      embolism T85.810
      fibrosis T85.820
      gastric nerve —*see* Complications,
        electronic stimulator device,
        peripheral nerve
      hemorrhage T85.830
      infection and inflammation T85.738
      mechanical
        breakdown T85.118
        displacement T85.128
        leakage T85.199
        malposition T85.128
        obstruction T85.199
        perforation T85.199
        protrusion T85.199
        specified NEC T85.199
      pain T85.840
      peripheral nerve —*see* Complications,
        electronic stimulator device,
        peripheral nerve
      sacral nerve —*see* Complications, electronic
        stimulator device, peripheral nerve
      specified type NEC T85.890
      spinal cord —*see* Complications, electronic
        stimulator device, spinal cord
      stenosis T85.850
      thrombosis T85.860
      vagal nerve —*see* Complications, electronic
        stimulator device, peripheral nerve
    peripheral nerve T85.9
      embolism T85.810
      fibrosis T85.820
      hemorrhage T85.830
      infection and inflammation T85.732
      mechanical
        breakdown T85.111
        displacement T85.121
        leakage T85.191
        malposition T85.121
        obstruction T85.191
        perforation T85.191
        protrusion T85.191
        specified NEC T85.191
      pain T85.840
      specified type NEC T85.890
      stenosis T85.850
      thrombosis T85.860
    spinal cord T85.9
      embolism T85.810
      fibrosis T85.820
      hemorrhage T85.830
      infection and inflammation T85.733
      mechanical
        breakdown T85.112
        displacement T85.122

Complication *(Continued)*
  electronic stimulator device *(Continued)*
    spinal cord *(Continued)*
      mechanical *(Continued)*
        leakage T85.192
        malposition T85.122
        obstruction T85.192
        perforation T85.192
        protrusion T85.192
        specified NEC T85.192
      pain T85.840
      specified type NEC T85.890
      stenosis T85.850
      thrombosis T85.860
    urinary T83.9
      embolism T83.81
      fibrosis T83.82
      hemorrhage T83.83
      infection and inflammation T83.598
      mechanical
        breakdown T83.110
        displacement T83.120
        malposition T83.120
        perforation T83.190
        protrusion T83.190
        specified NEC T83.190
      pain T83.84
      specified type NEC T83.89
      stenosis T83.85
      thrombosis T83.86
  electroshock therapy T88.9
    specified NEC T88.8
  endocrine E34.9
    postprocedural
      adrenal hypofunction E89.6
      hypoinsulinemia E89.1
      hypoparathyroidism E89.2
      hypopituitarism E89.3
      hypothyroidism E89.0
      ovarian failure E89.40
        asymptomatic E89.40
        symptomatic E89.41
      specified NEC E89.89
      testicular hypofunction E89.5
  endodontic treatment NEC M27.59
  enterostomy (stoma) K94.10
    hemorrhage K94.11
    infection K94.12
    malfunction K94.13
    mechanical K94.13
    specified complication NEC K94.19
  episiotomy, disruption O90.1
  esophageal anti-reflux device T85.9
    embolism T85.818
    fibrosis T85.828
    hemorrhage T85.838
    infection and inflammation T85.79
    mechanical
      breakdown T85.511
      displacement T85.521
      malfunction T85.511
      malposition T85.521
      obstruction T85.591
      perforation T85.591
      protrusion T85.591
      specified NEC T85.591
    pain T85.848
    specified type NEC T85.898
    stenosis T85.858
    thrombosis T85.868
  esophagostomy K94.30
    hemorrhage K94.31
    infection K94.32
    malfunction K94.33
    mechanical K94.33
    specified complication NEC K94.39
  extracorporeal circulation T80.90
  extremity artery (bypass) graft T82.9
    arteriosclerosis —*see* Arteriosclerosis,
      extremities, bypass graft
    embolism T82.818
    fibrosis T82.828

Complication *(Continued)*
  extremity artery (bypass) graft *(Continued)*
    hemorrhage T82.838
    infection and inflammation T82.7
    mechanical
      breakdown T82.318
        femoral artery T82.312
      displacement T82.328
        femoral artery T82.322
      leakage T82.338
        femoral artery T82.332
      malposition T82.328
        femoral artery T82.322
      obstruction T82.398
        femoral artery T82.392
      perforation T82.398
        femoral artery T82.392
      protrusion T82.398
        femoral artery T82.392
    pain T82.848
    specified type NEC T82.898
    stenosis T82.858
    thrombosis T82.868
  eye H57.9
    corneal graft —*see* Complications, graft, cornea
    implant (prosthetic) T85.9
      embolism T85.818
      fibrosis T85.828
      hemorrhage T85.838
      infection and inflammation T85.79
      mechanical
        breakdown T85.318
        displacement T85.328
        leakage T85.398
        malposition T85.328
        obstruction T85.398
        perforation T85.398
        protrusion T85.398
        specified NEC T85.398
      pain T85.848
      specified type NEC T85.898
      stenosis T85.858
      thrombosis T85.868
    intraocular lens —*see* Complications, intraocular lens
    orbital prosthesis —*see* Complications, orbital prosthesis
  female genital N94.9
    device, implant or graft NEC —*see* Complications, genitourinary, device or implant, genital tract
  femoral artery (bypass) graft —*see* Complication, extremity artery (bypass) graft
  fixation device, internal (orthopedic) T84.9
    infection and inflammation T84.60
      arm T84.61-●
        humerus T84.61-●
        radius T84.61-●
        ulna T84.61-●
      leg T84.629
        femur T84.62-●
        fibula T84.62-●
        tibia T84.62-●
      specified site NEC T84.69
      spine T84.63
    mechanical
      breakdown
        limb T84.119
          carpal T84.210
          femur T84.11-●
          fibula T84.11-●
          humerus T84.11-●
          metacarpal T84.210
          metatarsal T84.213
          phalanx
            foot T84.213
            hand T84.210
          radius T84.11-●
          tarsal T84.213

Complication *(Continued)*
  fixation device, internal *(Continued)*
    mechanical *(Continued)*
      breakdown *(Continued)*
        limb *(Continued)*
          tibia T84.11-●
          ulna T84.11-●
        specified bone NEC T84.218
        spine T84.216
      displacement
        limb T84.129
          carpal T84.220
          femur T84.12-●
          fibula T84.12-●
          humerus T84.12-●
          metacarpal T84.220
          metatarsal T84.223
          phalanx
            foot T84.223
            hand T84.220
          radius T84.12-●
          tarsal T84.223
          tibia T84.12-●
          ulna T84.12-●
        specified bone NEC T84.228
        spine T84.226
      malposition —*see* Complications, fixation device, internal, mechanical, displacement
      obstruction —*see* Complications, fixation device, internal, mechanical, specified type NEC
      perforation —*see* Complications, fixation device, internal, mechanical, specified type NEC
      protrusion —*see* Complications, fixation device, internal, mechanical, specified type NEC
      specified type NEC
        limb T84.199
          carpal T84.290
          femur T84.19-●
          fibula T84.19-●
          humerus T84.19-●
          metacarpal T84.290
          metatarsal T84.293
          phalanx
            foot T84.293
            hand T84.290
          radius T84.19-●
          tarsal T84.293
          tibia T84.19-●
          ulna T84.19-●
        specified bone NEC T84.298
        vertebra T84.296
    specified type NEC T84.89
      embolism T84.81
      fibrosis T84.82
      hemorrhage T84.83
      pain T84.84
      specified complication NEC T84.89
      stenosis T84.85
      thrombosis T84.86
  following
    acute myocardial infarction NEC I23.8
      aneurysm (false) (of cardiac wall) (of heart wall) (ruptured) I23.3
      angina I23.7
      atrial
        septal defect I23.1
        thrombosis I23.6
      cardiac wall rupture I23.3
      chordae tendinae rupture I23.4
      defect
        septal
          atrial (heart) I23.1
          ventricular (heart) I23.2
      hemopericardium I23.0
      papillary muscle rupture I23.5
      rupture
        cardiac wall I23.3
          with hemopericardium I23.0

Complication *(Continued)*
  following *(Continued)*
    acute myocardial infarction NEC *(Continued)*
      rupture *(Continued)*
        chordae tendineae I23.4
        papillary muscle I23.5
      specified NEC I23.8
      thrombosis
        atrium I23.6
        auricular appendage I23.6
        ventricle (heart) I23.6
      ventricular
        septal defect I23.2
        thrombosis I23.6
    ectopic or molar pregnancy O08.9
      cardiac arrest O08.81
      sepsis O08.82
      specified type NEC O08.89
      urinary tract infection O08.83
    termination of pregnancy —*see* Abortion
  gastrointestinal K92.9
    bile duct prosthesis —*see* Complications, bile duct implant
    esophageal anti-reflux device —*see* Complications, esophageal anti-reflux device
    postoperative
      colostomy —*see* Complications, colostomy
      dumping syndrome K91.1
      enterostomy —*see* Complications, enterostomy
      gastrostomy —*see* Complications, gastrostomy
      malabsorption NEC K91.2
      obstruction —*see also* Obstruction, intestine, postoperative K91.30
      postcholecystectomy syndrome K91.5
      specified NEC K91.89
      vomiting after GI surgery K91.0
    prosthetic device or implant
      bile duct prosthesis —*see* Complications, bile duct implant
      esophageal anti-reflux device —*see* Complications, esophageal anti-reflux device
      specified type NEC
        embolism T85.818
        fibrosis T85.828
        hemorrhage T85.838
        mechanical
          breakdown T85.518
          displacement T85.528
          malfunction T85.518
          malposition T85.528
          obstruction T85.598
          perforation T85.598
          protrusion T85.598
          specified NEC T85.598
        pain T85.848
        specified complication NEC T85.898
        stenosis T85.858
        thrombosis T85.868
  gastrostomy (stoma) K94.20
    hemorrhage K94.21
    infection K94.22
    malfunction K94.23
    mechanical K94.23
    specified complication NEC K94.29
  genitourinary
    device or implant T83.9
      genital tract T83.9
        infection or inflammation T83.69
        intrauterine contraceptive device —*see* Complications, intrauterine, contraceptive device
        mechanical —*see* Complications, by device, mechanical
        mesh —*see* Complications, prosthetic device or implant, mesh
        penile prosthesis —*see* Complications, prosthetic device, penile

▶ New   ⇒ Revised   ~~deleted~~ Deleted   ● Use Additional Character(s)

Complication *(Continued)*
  genitourinary *(Continued)*
    device or implant *(Continued)*
      genital tract *(Continued)*
        specified type NEC T83.89
          embolism T83.81
          fibrosis T83.82
          hemorrhage T83.83
          pain T83.84
          specified complication NEC T83.89
          stenosis T83.85
          thrombosis T83.86
      vaginal mesh —*see* Complications,
        prosthetic device or implant, mesh
    urinary system T83.9
      cystostomy catheter —*see*
        Complication, catheter,
        cystostomy
      electronic stimulator —*see*
        Complications, electronic
        stimulator device, urinary
      indwelling urethral catheter —*see*
        Complications, catheter, urethral,
        indwelling
      infection or inflammation T83.598
        indwelling urethral catheter T83.511
      kidney transplant —*see* Complication,
        transplant, kidney
      organ graft —*see* Complication, graft,
        urinary organ
      specified type NEC T83.89
        embolism T83.81
        fibrosis T83.82
        hemorrhage T83.83
        mechanical T83.198
          breakdown T83.118
          displacement T83.128
          malfunction T83.118
          malposition T83.128
          obstruction T83.198
          perforation T83.198
          protrusion T83.198
          specified NEC T83.198
      sphincter, implanted T83.191
      stent (ileal conduit) (nephroureteral)
        T83.193
        ureteral indwelling T83.192
      pain T83.84
      specified complication NEC T83.89
      stenosis T83.85
      thrombosis T83.86
      sphincter implant —*see* Complications,
        implant, urinary sphincter
  postprocedural
    pelvic peritoneal adhesions N99.4
    renal failure N99.0
    specified NEC N99.89
    stoma —*see* Complications, stoma,
      urinary tract
    urethral stricture —*see* Stricture, urethra,
      postprocedural
    vaginal
      adhesions N99.2
      vault prolapse N99.3
  graft (bypass) (patch) —*see also*
    Complications, prosthetic device or
    implant
    aorta —*see* Complications, graft, vascular
    arterial —*see* Complication, graft, vascular
    bone T86.839
      failure T86.831
      infection T86.832
      mechanical T84.318
        breakdown T84.318
        displacement T84.328
        protrusion T84.398
        specified type NEC T84.398
      rejection T86.830
      specified type NEC T86.838
    carotid artery —*see* Complications, graft,
      vascular

Complication *(Continued)*
  graft *(Continued)*
    cornea T86.849-
      failure T86.841-
      infection T86.842-
      mechanical T85.398
        breakdown T85.318
        displacement T85.328
        protrusion T85.398
        specified type NEC T85.398
      rejection T86.840-
      retroprosthetic membrane T85.398
      specified type NEC T86.848-
    femoral artery (bypass) —*see* Complication,
      extremity artery (bypass) graft
    genital organ or tract —*see* Complications,
      genitourinary, device or implant,
      genital tract
    muscle T84.9
      breakdown T84.410
      displacement T84.420
      embolism T84.81
      fibrosis T84.82
      hemorrhage T84.83
      infection and inflammation T84.7
      mechanical NEC T84.490
      pain T84.84
      specified type NEC T84.89
      stenosis T84.85
      thrombosis T84.86
    nerve —*see* Complication, prosthetic device
      or implant, specified NEC
    skin —*see* Complications, prosthetic device
      or implant, skin graft
    tendon T84.9
      breakdown T84.410
      displacement T84.420
      embolism T84.81
      fibrosis T84.82
      hemorrhage T84.83
      infection and inflammation T84.7
      mechanical NEC T84.490
      pain T84.84
      specified type NEC T84.89
      stenosis T84.85
      thrombosis T84.86
    urinary organ T83.9
      embolism T83.81
      fibrosis T83.82
      hemorrhage T83.83
      infection and inflammation T83.598
        indwelling urethral catheter T83.511
      mechanical
        breakdown T83.21
        displacement T83.22
        erosion T83.24
        exposure T83.25
        leakage T83.23
        malposition T83.22
        obstruction T83.29
        perforation T83.29
        protrusion T83.29
        specified NEC T83.29
      pain T83.84
      specified type NEC T83.89
      stenosis T83.85
      thrombosis T83.86
    vascular T82.9
      embolism T82.818
      femoral artery —*see* Complication,
        extremity artery (bypass) graft
      fibrosis T82.828
      hemorrhage T82.838
      mechanical
        breakdown T82.319
          aorta (bifurcation) T82.310
          carotid artery T82.311
          specified vessel NEC T82.318
        displacement T82.329
          aorta (bifurcation) T82.320
          carotid artery T82.321
          specified vessel NEC T82.328

Complication *(Continued)*
  graft *(Continued)*
    vascular *(Continued)*
      mechanical *(Continued)*
        leakage T82.339
          aorta (bifurcation) T82.330
          carotid artery T82.331
          specified vessel NEC T82.338
        malposition T82.329
          aorta (bifurcation) T82.320
          carotid artery T82.321
          specified vessel NEC T82.328
        obstruction T82.399
          aorta (bifurcation) T82.390
          carotid artery T82.391
          specified vessel NEC T82.398
        perforation T82.399
          aorta (bifurcation) T82.390
          carotid artery T82.391
          specified vessel NEC T82.398
        protrusion T82.399
          aorta (bifurcation) T82.390
          carotid artery T82.391
          specified vessel NEC T82.398
      pain T82.848
      specified complication NEC T82.898
      stenosis T82.858
      thrombosis T82.868
  heart I51.9
    assist device
      infection and inflammation T82.7
    following acute myocardial infarction —
      see Complications, following, acute
      myocardial infarction
    postoperative —*see* Complications,
      circulatory system
    transplant —*see* Complication, transplant,
      heart
      and lung(s) —*see* Complications,
        transplant, heart, with lung
    valve
      graft (biological) T82.9
        embolism T82.817
        fibrosis T82.827
        hemorrhage T82.837
        infection and inflammation T82.7
        mechanical T82.228
          breakdown T82.221
          displacement T82.222
          leakage T82.223
          malposition T82.222
          obstruction T82.228
          perforation T82.228
          protrusion T82.228
        pain T82.847
        specified type NEC T82.897
        stenosis T82.857
        thrombosis T82.867
      prosthesis T82.9
        embolism T82.817
        fibrosis T82.827
        hemorrhage T82.837
        infection or inflammation T82.6
        mechanical T82.09
          breakdown T82.01
          displacement T82.02
          leakage T82.03
          malposition T82.02
          obstruction T82.09
          perforation T82.09
          protrusion T82.09
        pain T82.847
        specified type NEC T82.897
          mechanical T82.09
        stenosis T82.857
        thrombosis T82.867
  hematoma
    intraoperative —*see* Complication,
      intraoperative, hemorrhage
    postprocedural —*see* Complication,
      postprocedural, hematoma
  hemodialysis —*see* Complications, dialysis

Complication *(Continued)*
hemorrhage
intraoperative *—see* Complication, intraoperative, hemorrhage
postprocedural *—see* Complication, postprocedural, hemorrhage
▶IEC (immune effector cellular) therapy T8Ø.82
ileostomy (stoma) *—see* Complications, enterostomy
▶immune effector cellular (IEC) therapy T8Ø.82
immunization (procedure) *—see* Complications, vaccination
implant *—see also* Complications, by site and type
urinary sphincter T83.9
embolism T83.81
fibrosis T83.82
hemorrhage T83.83
infection and inflammation T83.591
mechanical
breakdown T83.111
displacement T83.121
leakage T83.191
malposition T83.121
obstruction T83.191
perforation T83.191
protrusion T83.191
specified NEC T83.191
pain T83.84
specified type NEC T83.89
stenosis T83.85
thrombosis T83.86
infusion (procedure) T8Ø.9Ø
air embolism T8Ø.Ø
blood *—see* Complications, transfusion
catheter *—see* Complications, catheter
infection T8Ø.29
pump *—see* Complications, cardiovascular, device or implant
sepsis T8Ø.29
serum reaction *—see also* Reaction, serum T8Ø.69
anaphylactic shock *—see also* Shock, anaphylactic T8Ø.59
specified type NEC T8Ø.89
inhalation therapy NEC T81.81
injection (procedure) T8Ø.9Ø
drug reaction *—see* Reaction, drug
infection T8Ø.29
sepsis T8Ø.29
serum (prophylactic) (therapeutic) *—see* Complications, vaccination
specified type NEC T8Ø.89
vaccine (any) *—see* Complications, vaccination
inoculation (any) *—see* Complications, vaccination
insulin pump
infection and inflammation T85.72
mechanical
breakdown T85.614
displacement T85.624
leakage T85.633
malposition T85.624
obstruction T85.694
perforation T85.694
protrusion T85.694
specified NEC T85.694
intestinal pouch NEC K91.858
intraocular lens (prosthetic) T85.9
embolism T85.818
fibrosis T85.828
hemorrhage T85.838
infection and inflammation T85.79
mechanical
breakdown T85.21
displacement T85.22
malposition T85.22
obstruction T85.29
perforation T85.29
protrusion T85.29
specified NEC T85.29

Complication *(Continued)*
intraocular lens *(Continued)*
pain T85.848
specified type NEC T85.898
stenosis T85.858
thrombosis T85.868
intraoperative (intraprocedural)
cardiac arrest *—see also* Infarct, myocardium, associated with revascularization procedure
during cardiac surgery I97.71Ø
during other surgery I97.711
cardiac functional disturbance NEC *—see also* Infarct, myocardium, associated with revascularization procedure
during cardiac surgery I97.79Ø
during other surgery I97.791
hemorrhage (hematoma) (of)
circulatory system organ or structure
during cardiac bypass I97.411
during cardiac catheterization I97.41Ø
during other circulatory system procedure I97.418
during other procedure I97.42
digestive system organ
during procedure on digestive system K91.61
during procedure on other organ K91.62
ear
during procedure on ear and mastoid process H95.21
during procedure on other organ H95.22
endocrine system organ or structure
during procedure on endocrine system organ or structure E36.Ø1
during procedure on other organ E36.Ø2
eye and adnexa
during ophthalmic procedure H59.11-●
during other procedure H59.12-●
genitourinary organ or structure
during procedure on genitourinary organ or structure N99.61
during procedure on other organ N99.62
mastoid process
during procedure on ear and mastoid process H95.21
during procedure on other organ H95.22
musculoskeletal structure
during musculoskeletal surgery M96.81Ø
during non-orthopedic surgery M96.811
during orthopedic surgery M96.81Ø
nervous system
during a nervous system procedure G97.31
during other procedure G97.32
respiratory system
during other procedure J95.62
during procedure on respiratory system organ or structure J95.61
skin and subcutaneous tissue
during a dermatologic procedure L76.Ø1
during a procedure on other organ L76.Ø2
spleen
during a procedure on other organ D78.Ø2
during a procedure on the spleen D78.Ø1
puncture or laceration (accidental) (unintentional) (of)
brain
during a nervous system procedure G97.48
during other procedure G97.49

Complication *(Continued)*
intraoperative *(Continued)*
puncture or laceration *(Continued)*
circulatory system organ or structure
during circulatory system procedure I97.51
during other procedure I97.52
digestive system
during procedure on digestive system K91.71
during procedure on other organ K91.72
ear
during procedure on ear and mastoid process H95.31
during procedure on other organ H95.32
endocrine system organ or structure
during procedure on endocrine system organ or structure E36.11
during procedure on other organ E36.12
eye and adnexa
during ophthalmic procedure H59.21-●
during other procedure H59.22-●
genitourinary organ or structure
during procedure on genitourinary organ or structure N99.71
during procedure on other organ N99.72
mastoid process
during procedure on ear and mastoid process H95.31
during procedure on other organ H95.32
musculoskeletal structure
during musculoskeletal surgery M96.82Ø
during non-orthopedic surgery M96.821
during orthopedic surgery M96.82Ø
nervous system
during a nervous system procedure G97.48
during other procedure G97.49
respiratory system
during other procedure J95.72
during procedure on respiratory system organ or structure J95.71
skin and subcutaneous tissue
during a dermatologic procedure L76.11
during a procedure on other organ L76.12
spleen
during a procedure on other organ D78.12
during a procedure on the spleen D78.11
specified NEC
circulatory system I97.88
digestive system K91.81
ear H95.88
endocrine system E36.8
eye and adnexa H59.88
genitourinary system N99.81
mastoid process H95.88
musculoskeletal structure M96.89
nervous system G97.81
respiratory system J95.88
skin and subcutaneous tissue L76.81
spleen D78.81
intraperitoneal catheter (dialysis) ➡(infusion) *—see* Complication(s), catheter, intraperitoneal dialysis
intrathecal infusion pump
infection and inflammation T85.738
mechanical
breakdown T85.615
displacement T85.625
leakage T85.635
malfunction T85.695
malposition T85.625
obstruction T85.695

▶ New ➡ Revised ~~deleted~~ Deleted ● Use Additional Character(s)

Complication *(Continued)*
  intrathecal infusion pump *(Continued)*
    mechanical *(Continued)*
      perforation T85.695
      protrusion T85.695
      specified NEC T85.695
  intrauterine
    contraceptive device
      embolism T83.81
      fibrosis T83.82
      hemorrhage T83.83
      infection and inflammation T83.69
      mechanical
        breakdown T83.31
        displacement T83.32
        malposition T83.32
        obstruction T83.39
        perforation T83.39
        protrusion T83.39
        specified NEC T83.39
      pain T83.84
      specified type NEC T83.89
      stenosis T83.85
      thrombosis T83.86
    procedure (fetal), to newborn P96.5
  jejunostomy (stoma) —*see* Complications,
    enterostomy
  joint prosthesis, internal T84.9
    breakage (fracture) T84.01-●
    dislocation T84.02-●
    fracture T84.01-●
    infection or inflammation T84.50
      hip T84.5-●
      knee T84.5-●
      specified joint NEC T84.59
    instability T84.02-●
    malposition —*see* Complications, joint
      prosthesis, mechanical, displacement
    mechanical
      breakage, broken T84.01-●
      dislocation T84.02-●
      fracture T84.01-●
      instability T84.02-●
      leakage —*see* Complications, joint
        prosthesis, mechanical, specified NEC
      loosening T84.039
        hip T84.03-●
        knee T84.03-●
        specified joint NEC T84.038
      obstruction —*see* Complications, joint
        prosthesis, mechanical, specified
        NEC
      perforation —*see* Complications, joint
        prosthesis, mechanical, specified
        NEC
      osteolysis T84.059
        hip T84.05-●
        knee T84.05-●
        other specified joint T84.058
      ~~periprosthetic T84.059~~
    ▶ periprosthetic osteolysis T84.059
      protrusion —*see* Complications, joint
        prosthesis, mechanical, specified
        NEC
      specified complication NEC T84.099
        hip T84.09-●
        knee T84.09-●
        other specified joint T84.098
      subluxation T84.02-●
      wear of articular bearing surface T84.069
        hip T84.06-●
        knee T84.06-●
        other specified joint T84.068
    specified joint NEC T84.89
      embolism T84.81
      fibrosis T84.82
      hemorrhage T84.83
      pain T84.84
      specified complication NEC T84.89
      stenosis T84.85
      thrombosis T84.86
    subluxation T84.02-●

Complication *(Continued)*
  kidney transplant —*see* Complications,
    transplant, kidney
  labor O75.9
    specified NEC O75.89
  liver transplant (immune or nonimmune) —
    see Complications, transplant,
    liver
  lumbar puncture G97.1
    cerebrospinal fluid leak G97.0
    headache or reaction G97.1
  lung transplant —*see* Complications,
    transplant, lung
    and heart —*see* Complications, transplant,
      lung, with heart
  male genital N50.9
    device, implant or graft —*see*
      Complications, genitourinary,
      device or implant, genital tract
    postprocedural or postoperative —*see*
      Complications, genitourinary,
      postprocedural
      specified NEC N99.89
  mastoid (process) procedure
    intraoperative H95.88-●
      hematoma —*see* Complications,
        intraoperative, hemorrhage
        (hematoma) (of), mastoid process
      hemorrhage —*see* Complications,
        intraoperative, hemorrhage
        (hematoma) (of), mastoid process
      laceration —*see* Complications,
        intraoperative, puncture or
        laceration..., mastoid process
      specified NEC H95.88-●
    postmastoidectomy —*see* Complications,
      postmastoidectomy
    postoperative H95.89-●
      external ear canal stenosis H95.81-●
      hematoma —*see* Complications...,
        postprocedural, hematoma (of),
        mastoid process
      hemorrhage —*see* Complications...,
        postprocedural, hemorrhage (of),
        mastoid process
      postmastoidectomy —*see* Complications,
        postmastoidectomy
      seroma —*see* Complications,
        postprocedural, seroma (of),
        mastoid process
      specified NEC H95.89-●
  mastoidectomy cavity —*see* Complications,
    postmastoidectomy
  mechanical —*see* Complications, by site and
    type, mechanical
  medical procedures (*see also* Complication(s),
    intraoperative) T88.9
  metabolic E88.9
    postoperative E89.89
      specified NEC E89.89
  molar pregnancy NOS O08.9
    damage to pelvic organs O08.6
    embolism O08.2
    genital infection O08.0
    hemorrhage (delayed) (excessive) O08.1
    metabolic disorder O08.5
    renal failure O08.4
    shock O08.3
    specified type NEC O08.0
    venous complication NEC O08.7
  musculoskeletal system —*see also*
    Complication, intraoperative
    (intraprocedural), by site
    device, implant or graft NEC —*see*
      Complications, orthopedic, device or
      implant
    internal fixation (nail) (plate) (rod) —*see*
      Complications, fixation device,
      internal
    joint prosthesis —*see* Complications, joint
      prosthesis

Complication *(Continued)*
  musculoskeletal system *(Continued)*
    postoperative (postprocedural) M96.89
      with osteoporosis —*see* Osteoporosis
      fracture following insertion of device —
        see Fracture, following insertion of
        orthopedic implant, joint prosthesis
        or bone plate
      joint instability after prosthesis removal
        M96.89
      lordosis M96.4
      postlaminectomy syndrome NEC M96.1
        kyphosis M96.2
      pseudarthrosis M96.0
      specified complication NEC M96.89
    post radiation M96.89
      kyphosis M96.3
      scoliosis M96.5
      specified complication NEC M96.89
  nephrostomy (stoma) —*see* Complications,
    stoma, urinary tract, external NEC
  nervous system G98.8
    central G96.9
    device, implant or graft —*see also*
      Complication, prosthetic device or
      implant, specified NEC
      electronic stimulator (electrode(s)) —*see*
        Complications, electronic stimulator
        device
      specified NEC
        infection and inflammation T85.738
        mechanical T85.695
          breakdown T85.615
          displacement T85.625
          leakage T85.635
          malfunction T85.695
          malposition T85.625
          obstruction T85.695
          perforation T85.695
          protrusion T85.695
          specified NEC T85.695
      ventricular shunt —*see* Complications,
        ventricular shunt
    electronic stimulator (electrode(s)) —*see*
      Complications, electronic stimulator
      device
    postprocedural G97.82
      intracranial hypotension G97.2
      specified NEC G97.82
      spinal fluid leak G97.0
  newborn, due to intrauterine (fetal)
    procedure P96.5
  nonabsorbable (permanent) sutures —*see*
    Complication, sutures, permanent
  obstetric O75.9
    procedure (instrumental) (manual)
      (surgical) specified NEC O75.4
    specified NEC O75.89
    surgical wound NEC O90.89
      hematoma O90.2
      infection O86.00
  ocular lens implant —*see* Complications,
    intraocular lens
  ophthalmologic
    postprocedural bleb —*see* Blebitis
  orbital prosthesis T85.9
    embolism T85.818
    fibrosis T85.828
    hemorrhage T85.838
    infection and inflammation T85.79
    mechanical
      breakdown T85.31-●
      displacement T85.32-●
      malposition T85.32-●
      obstruction T85.39-●
      perforation T85.39-●
      protrusion T85.39-●
      specified NEC T85.39-●
    pain T85.848
    specified type NEC T85.898
    stenosis T85.858
    thrombosis T85.868

Complication *(Continued)*
  organ or tissue transplant (partial) (total) —
    see Complications, transplant
  orthopedic —*see also* Disorder, soft tissue
    device or implant T84.9
      bone
        device or implant —*see* Complication,
          bone, device NEC
        graft —*see* Complication, graft, bone
      breakdown T84.418
      displacement T84.428
      electronic bone stimulator —*see*
        Complications, electronic stimulator
        device, bone
      embolism T84.81
      fibrosis T84.82
      fixation device —*see* Complication,
        fixation device, internal
      hemorrhage T84.83
      infection or inflammation T84.7
      joint prosthesis —*see* Complication, joint
        prosthesis, internal
      malfunction T84.418
      malposition T84.428
      mechanical NEC T84.498
      muscle graft —*see* Complications, graft,
        muscle
      obstruction T84.498
      pain T84.84
      perforation T84.498
      protrusion T84.498
      specified complication NEC T84.89
      stenosis T84.85
      tendon graft —*see* Complications, graft,
        tendon
      thrombosis T84.86
    fracture (following insertion of device) —
      see Fracture, following insertion of
      orthopedic implant, joint prosthesis or
      bone plate
    postprocedural M96.89
      fracture —*see* Fracture, following
        insertion of orthopedic implant,
        joint prosthesis or bone plate
      postlaminectomy syndrome NEC M96.1
        kyphosis M96.3
        lordosis M96.4
      postradiation
        kyphosis M96.2
        scoliosis M96.5
      pseudarthrosis post-fusion M96.0
      specified type NEC M96.89
  pacemaker (cardiac) —*see* Complications,
    cardiovascular device or implant,
    electronic
  pancreas transplant —*see* Complications,
    transplant, pancreas
  penile prosthesis (implant) —*see*
    Complications, prosthetic device, penile
  perfusion NEC T80.90
  perineal repair (obstetrical) NEC O90.89
    disruption O90.1
    hematoma O90.2
    infection (following delivery) O86.09
  phototherapy T88.9
    specified NEC T88.8
  postmastoidectomy NEC H95.19-●
    cyst, mucosal H95.13-●
    granulation H95.12-●
    inflammation, chronic H95.11-●
    recurrent cholesteatoma H95.0-●
  postoperative —*see* Complications,
    postprocedural
    circulatory —*see* Complications, circulatory
      system
    ear —*see* Complications, ear
    endocrine —*see* Complications,
      endocrine
    eye —*see* Complications, eye
    lumbar puncture G97.1
      cerebrospinal fluid leak G97.0

Complication *(Continued)*
  postoperative *(Continued)*
    nervous system (central) (peripheral) —*see*
      Complications, nervous system
    respiratory system —*see* Complications,
      respiratory system
  postprocedural —*see also* Complications,
    surgical procedure
    cardiac arrest —*see also* Infarct,
      myocardium, associated with
      revascularization procedure
      following cardiac surgery I97.120
      following other surgery I97.121
    cardiac functional disturbance NEC —*see*
      also Infarct, myocardium, associated
      with revascularization procedure
      following cardiac surgery I97.190
      following other surgery I97.191
    cardiac insufficiency
      following cardiac surgery I97.110
      following other surgery I97.111
    chorioretinal scars following retinal
      surgery H59.81-●
    following cataract surgery
      cataract (lens) fragments H59.02-●
      cystoid macular edema H59.03-●
      specified NEC H59.09-●
      vitreous (touch) syndrome H59.01-●
    heart failure
      following cardiac surgery I97.130
      following other surgery I97.131
    hematoma (of)
      circulatory system organ or structure
        following cardiac bypass I97.631
        following cardiac catheterization
          I97.630
        following other circulatory system
          procedure I97.638
        following other procedure I97.621
      digestive system
        following procedure on digestive
          system K91.870
        following procedure on other organ
          K91.871
      ear
        following other procedure H95.52
        following procedure on ear and
          mastoid process H95.51
      endocrine system
        following endocrine system procedure
          E89.820
        following other procedure E89.821
      eye and adnexa
        following ophthalmic procedure
          H59.33-●
        following other procedure H59.34-●
      genitourinary organ or structure
        following procedure on genitourinary
          organ or structure N99.840
        following procedure on other organ
          N99.841
      mastoid process
        following other procedure H95.52
        following procedure on ear and
          mastoid process H95.51
      musculoskeletal structure
        following musculoskeletal surgery
          M96.840
        following non-orthopedic surgery
          M96.841
        following orthopedic surgery M96.840
      nervous system
        following nervous system procedure
          G97.61
        following other procedure G97.62
      respiratory system
        following other procedure J95.861
        following procedure on respiratory
          system organ or structure J95.860
      skin and subcutaneous tissue
        following dermatologic procedure
          L76.31

Complication *(Continued)*
  postprocedural *(Continued)*
    hematoma *(Continued)*
      skin and subcutaneous tissue *(Continued)*
        following procedure on other organ
          L76.32
      spleen
        following procedure on other organ
          D78.32
        following procedure on the spleen
          D78.31
    hemorrhage (of)
      circulatory system organ or structure
        following cardiac bypass I97.611
        following cardiac catheterization
          I97.610
        following other circulatory system
          procedure I97.618
        following other procedure I97.620
      digestive system
        following procedure on digestive
          system K91.840
        following procedure on other organ
          K91.841
      ear
        following other procedure H95.42
        following procedure on ear and
          mastoid process H95.41
      endocrine system
        following endocrine system procedure
          E89.810
        following other procedure E89.811
      eye and adnexa
        following ophthalmic procedure
          H59.31-●
        following other procedure H59.32-●
      genitourinary organ or structure
        following procedure on genitourinary
          organ or structure N99.820
        following procedure on other organ
          N99.821
      mastoid process
        following other procedure H95.42
        following procedure on ear and
          mastoid process H95.41
      musculoskeletal structure
        following musculoskeletal surgery
          M96.830
        following non-orthopedic surgery
          M96.831
        following orthopedic surgery M96.830
      nervous system
        following nervous system procedure
          G97.51
        following other procedure G97.52
      respiratory system
        following other procedure J95.831
        following procedure on respiratory
          system organ or structure J95.830
      skin and subcutaneous tissue
        following dermatologic procedure
          L76.21
        following a procedure on other organ
          L76.22
      spleen
        following procedure on other organ
          D78.22
        following procedure on the spleen
          D78.21
    seroma (of)
      circulatory system organ or structure
        following cardiac bypass I97.641
        following cardiac catheterization
          I97.640
        following other circulatory system
          procedure I97.648
        following other procedure I97.622
      digestive system
        following procedure on digestive
          system K91.872
        following procedure on other organ
          K91.873

▶ New   ⇒ Revised   ~~deleted~~ Deleted   ● Use Additional Character(s)

Complication *(Continued)*
  postprocedural *(Continued)*
    seroma *(Continued)*
      ear
        following other procedure H95.54
        following procedure on ear and
          mastoid process H95.53
      endocrine system
        following endocrine system procedure
          E89.822
        following other procedure E89.823
      eye and adnexa
        following ophthalmic procedure
          H59.35-•
        following other procedure H59.36-•
      genitourinary organ or structure
        following procedure on genitourinary
          organ or structure N99.842
        following procedure on other organ
          N99.843
      mastoid process
        following other procedure H95.54
        following procedure on ear and
          mastoid process H95.53
      musculoskeletal structure
        following musculoskeletal surgery
          M96.842
        following non-orthopedic surgery
          M96.843
        following orthopedic surgery M96.842
      nervous system
        following nervous system procedure
          G97.63
        following other procedure G97.64
      respiratory system
        following other procedure J95.863
        following procedure on respiratory
          system organ or structure J95.862
      skin and subcutaneous tissue
        following dermatologic procedure
          L76.33
        following procedure on other organ
          L76.34
      spleen
        following procedure on other organ
          D78.34
        following procedure on the spleen
          D78.33
    specified NEC
      circulatory system I97.89
      digestive K91.89
      ear H95.89
      endocrine E89.89
      eye and adnexa H59.89
      genitourinary N99.89
      mastoid process H95.89
      metabolic E89.89
      musculoskeletal structure M96.89
      nervous system G97.82
      respiratory system J95.89
      skin and subcutaneous tissue L76.82
      spleen D78.89
  pregnancy NEC —*see* Pregnancy,
    complicated by
  prosthetic device or implant T85.9
    bile duct —*see* Complications, bile duct
      implant
    breast —*see* Complications, breast
      implant
    bulking agent
      ureteral
        erosion T83.714
        exposure T83.724
      urethral
        erosion T83.713
        exposure T83.723
    cardiac and vascular NEC —*see*
      Complications, cardiovascular device
      or implant
    corneal transplant —*see* Complications,
      graft, cornea

Complication *(Continued)*
  prosthetic device or implant *(Continued)*
    electronic nervous system stimulator —*see*
      Complications, electronic stimulator
      device
    epidural infusion catheter —*see*
      Complications, catheter, epidural
    esophageal anti-reflux device —*see*
      Complications, esophageal anti-reflux
      device
    genital organ or tract —*see* Complications,
      genitourinary, device or implant,
      genital tract
      specified NEC T83.79
    heart valve —*see* Complications, heart,
      valve, prosthesis
    infection or inflammation T85.79
      intestine transplant T86.892
      liver transplant T86.43
      lung transplant T86.812
      pancreas transplant T86.892
      skin graft T86.822
    intraocular lens —*see* Complications,
      intraocular lens
    ⟹ intraperitoneal (dialysis) catheter —*see*
      Complication(s), catheter,
      intraperitoneal dialysis
    joint —*see* Complications, joint prosthesis,
      internal
    mechanical NEC T85.698
      dialysis catheter (vascular) —*see also*
        Complication, catheter, dialysis,
        mechanical
        ⟹ peritoneal —*see* Complication(s),
          catheter, intraperitoneal dialysis
      gastrointestinal device T85.598
      ocular device T85.398
      subdural (infusion) catheter T85.690
      suture, permanent T85.692
        that for bone repair —*see*
          Complications, fixation device,
          internal (orthopedic), mechanical
      ventricular shunt
        breakdown T85.01
        displacement T85.02
        leakage T85.03
        malposition T85.02
        obstruction T85.09
        perforation T85.09
        protrusion T85.09
        specified NEC T85.09
    mesh
      erosion (to surrounding organ or tissue)
        T83.718
        urethral (into pelvic floor muscles)
          T83.712
        vaginal (into pelvic floor muscles)
          T83.711
      exposure (into surrounding organ or
        tissue) T83.728
        urethral (through urethral wall)
          T83.722
        vaginal (into vagina) (through vaginal
          wall) T83.721
    orbital —*see* Complications, orbital
      prosthesis
    penile T83.9
      embolism T83.81
      fibrosis T83.82
      hemorrhage T83.83
      infection and inflammation T83.61
      mechanical
        breakdown T83.410
        displacement T83.420
        leakage T83.490
        malposition T83.420
        obstruction T83.490
        perforation T83.490
        protrusion T83.490
        specified NEC T83.490
      pain T83.84

Complication *(Continued)*
  prosthetic device or implant *(Continued)*
    penile *(Continued)*
      specified type NEC T83.89
      stenosis T83.85
      thrombosis T83.86
    prosthetic materials NEC
      erosion (to surrounding organ or tissue)
        T83.718
      exposure (into surrounding organ or
        tissue) T83.728
    skin graft T86.829
      artificial skin or decellularized
        allodermis
        embolism T85.818
        fibrosis T85.828
        hemorrhage T85.838
        infection and inflammation T85.79
        mechanical
          breakdown T85.613
          displacement T85.623
          malfunction T85.613
          malposition T85.623
          obstruction T85.693
          perforation T85.693
          protrusion T85.693
          specified NEC T85.693
        pain T85.848
        specified type NEC T85.898
        stenosis T85.858
        thrombosis T85.868
      failure T86.821
      infection T86.822
      rejection T86.820
      specified NEC T86.828
    sling
      urethral (female) (male)
        erosion T83.712
        exposure T83.722
    specified NEC T85.9
      embolism T85.818
      fibrosis T85.828
      hemorrhage T85.838
      infection and inflammation T85.79
      mechanical
        breakdown T85.618
        displacement T85.628
        leakage T85.638
        malfunction T85.618
        malposition T85.628
        obstruction T85.698
        perforation T85.698
        protrusion T85.698
        specified NEC T85.698
      pain T85.848
      specified type NEC T85.898
      stenosis T85.858
      thrombosis T85.868
    subdural infusion catheter —*see*
      Complications, catheter, subdural
    sutures —*see* Complications, sutures
    urinary organ or tract NEC —*see*
      Complications, genitourinary, device
      or implant, urinary system
    vascular —*see* Complications,
      cardiovascular device or implant
    ventricular shunt —*see* Complications,
      ventricular shunt (device)
  puerperium —*see* Puerperal
  puncture, spinal G97.1
    cerebrospinal fluid leak G97.0
    headache or reaction G97.1
  pyelogram N99.89
  radiation
    kyphosis M96.2
    scoliosis M96.5
  reattached
    extremity (infection) (rejection)
      lower T87.1X-•
      upper T87.0X-•
    specified body part NEC T87.2

Complication *(Continued)*
  reconstructed breast
    asymmetry between native and
        reconstructed breast N65.1
    deformity N65.0
    disproportion between native and
        reconstructed breast N65.1
    excess tissue N65.0
    misshappen N65.0
  reimplant NEC —*see also* Complications,
      prosthetic device or implant
    limb (infection) (rejection) —*see*
        Complications, reattached,
        extremity
    organ (partial) (total) —*see* Complications,
        transplant
    prosthetic device NEC —*see* Complications,
        prosthetic device
  renal N28.9
    allograft —*see* Complications, transplant,
        kidney
    dialysis —*see* Complications, dialysis
  respirator
    mechanical J95.850
      specified NEC J95.859
  respiratory system J98.9
    device, implant or graft —*see*
        Complication, prosthetic device or
        implant, specified NEC
    lung transplant —*see* Complications,
        prosthetic device or implant, lung
        transplant
    postoperative J95.89
      air leak J95.812
      Mendelson's syndrome (chemical
          pneumonitis) J95.4
      pneumothorax J95.811
      pulmonary insufficiency (acute) (after
          nonthoracic surgery) J95.2
        chronic J95.3
        following thoracic surgery J95.1
      respiratory failure (acute) J95.821
        acute and chronic J95.822
      specified NEC J95.89
      subglottic stenosis J95.5
      tracheostomy complication —*see*
          Complications, tracheostomy
    therapy T81.89
  sedation during labor and delivery O74.9
    cardiac O74.2
    central nervous system O74.3
    pulmonary NEC O74.1
  shunt —*see also* Complications, prosthetic
      device or implant
    arteriovenous —*see* Complications,
        arteriovenous, shunt
    ventricular (communicating) —*see*
        Complications, ventricular shunt
  skin
    graft T86.829
      failure T86.821
      infection T86.822
      rejection T86.820
      specified type NEC T86.828
  spinal
    anesthesia —*see* Complications, anesthesia,
        spinal
    catheter (epidural) (subdural) —*see*
        Complications, catheter
    puncture or tap G97.1
      cerebrospinal fluid leak G97.0
      headache or reaction G97.1
  stent
    bile duct —*see* Complications, bile duct
        prosthesis
    ureteral indwelling
      breakdown T83.112
      displacement T83.122
      leakage T83.192
      malposition T83.122

Complication *(Continued)*
  stent *(Continued)*
    ureteral indwelling *(Continued)*
      obstruction T83.192
      perforation T83.192
      protrusion T83.192
      specified NEC T83.192
    urinary (ileal conduit) (nephroureteral)
        T83.193
      embolism T83.81
      fibrosis T83.82
      hemorrhage T83.83
      infection and inflammation T83.593
      mechanical
        breakdown T83.113
        displacement T83.123
        leakage T83.193
        malposition T83.123
        obstruction T83.193
        perforation T83.193
        protrusion T83.193
        specified NEC T83.193
      pain T83.84
      specified type NEC T83.89
      stenosis T83.85
      thrombosis T83.86
    vascular
      end stent stenosis —*see* Restenosis,
          stent
      in stent stenosis —*see* Restenosis, stent
  stoma
    digestive tract
      colostomy —*see* Complications,
          colostomy
      enterostomy —*see* Complications,
          enterostomy
      esophagostomy —*see* Complications,
          esophagostomy
      gastrostomy —*see* Complications,
          gastrostomy
    urinary tract N99.528
      continent N99.538
        hemorrhage N99.530
        herniation N99.533
        infection N99.531
        malfunction N99.532
        specified type NEC N99.538
        stenosis N99.534
      cystostomy —*see* Complications,
          cystostomy
      external NOS N99.528
      hemorrhage N99.520
      herniation N99.523
      incontinent N99.528
        hemorrhage N99.520
        herniation N99.523
        infection N99.521
        malfunction N99.522
        specified type NEC N99.528
        stenosis N99.524
      infection N99.521
      malfunction N99.522
      specified type NEC N99.528
      stenosis N99.524
    stomach banding —*see* Complication(s),
        bariatric procedure
    stomach stapling —*see* Complication(s),
        bariatric procedure
  surgical material, nonabsorbable —*see*
      Complication, suture, permanent
  surgical procedure (on) T81.9
    amputation stump (late) —*see*
        Complications, amputation stump
    cardiac —*see* Complications, circulatory
        system
    cholesteatoma, recurrent —*see*
        Complications, postmastoidectomy,
        recurrent cholesteatoma
    circulatory (early) —*see* Complications,
        circulatory system

Complication *(Continued)*
  surgical procedure *(Continued)*
    digestive system —*see* Complications,
        gastrointestinal
    dumping syndrome (postgastrectomy)
        K91.1
    ear —*see* Complications, ear
    elephantiasis or lymphedema I97.89
        postmastectomy I97.2
    emphysema (surgical) T81.82
    endocrine —*see* Complications, endocrine
    eye —*see* Complications, eye
    fistula (persistent postoperative) T81.83
    foreign body inadvertently left in wound
        (sponge) (suture) (swab) —*see* Foreign
        body, accidentally left during a
        procedure
    gastrointestinal —*see* Complications,
        gastrointestinal
    genitourinary NEC N99.89
    hematoma
      intraoperative —*see* Complication,
          intraoperative, hemorrhage
      postprocedural —*see* Complication,
          postprocedural, hematoma
    hemorrhage
      intraoperative —*see* Complication,
          intraoperative, hemorrhage
      postprocedural —*see* Complication,
          postprocedural, hemorrhage
    hepatic failure K91.82
    hyperglycemia (postpancreatectomy) E89.1
    hypoinsulinemia (postpancreatectomy)
        E89.1
    hypoparathyroidism
        (postparathyroidectomy) E89.2
    hypopituitarism (posthypophysectomy)
        E89.3
    hypothyroidism (post-thyroidectomy)
        E89.0
    intestinal obstruction —*see also*
        Obstruction, intestine, postoperative
        K91.30
    intracranial hypotension following
        ventricular shunting
        (ventriculostomy) G97.2
    lymphedema I97.89
        postmastectomy I97.2
    malabsorption (postsurgical) NEC K91.2
      osteoporosis —*see* Osteoporosis,
          postsurgical malabsorption
    mastoidectomy cavity NEC —*see*
        Complications, postmastoidectomy
    metabolic E89.89
      specified NEC E89.89
    musculoskeletal —*see* Complications,
        musculoskeletal system
    nervous system (central) (peripheral) —*see*
        Complications, nervous system
    ovarian failure E89.40
      asymptomatic E89.40
      symptomatic E89.41
    peripheral vascular —*see* Complications,
        surgical procedure, vascular
    postcardiotomy syndrome I97.0
    postcholecystectomy syndrome K91.5
    postcommissurotomy syndrome I97.0
    postgastrectomy dumping syndrome K91.1
    postlaminectomy syndrome NEC M96.1
      kyphosis M96.3
    postmastectomy lymphedema syndrome
        I97.2
    postmastoidectomy cholesteatoma —*see*
        Complications, postmastoidectomy,
        recurrent cholesteatoma
    postvagotomy syndrome K91.1
    postvalvulotomy syndrome I97.0
    pulmonary insufficiency (acute) J95.2
      chronic J95.3
      following thoracic surgery J95.1

▶ New   ⇒ Revised   ~~deleted~~ Deleted   ● Use Additional Character(s)

Complication *(Continued)*
 surgical procedure *(Continued)*
  reattached body part —*see* Complications,
    reattached
  respiratory —*see* Complications,
    respiratory system
  shock (hypovolemic) T81.19
  spleen (postoperative) D78.89
   intraoperative D78.81
  stitch abscess T81.41
  subglottic stenosis (postsurgical) J95.5
  testicular hypofunction E89.5
  transplant —*see* Complications, organ or
    tissue transplant
  urinary NEC N99.89
  vaginal vault prolapse (posthysterectomy)
    N99.3
  vascular (peripheral)
   artery T81.719
    mesenteric T81.710
    renal T81.711
    specified NEC T81.718
   vein T81.72
  wound infection T81.49
 suture, permanent (wire) NEC T85.9
  with repair of bone —*see* Complications,
    fixation device, internal
  embolism T85.818
  fibrosis T85.828
  hemorrhage T85.838
  infection and inflammation T85.79
  mechanical
   breakdown T85.612
   displacement T85.622
   malfunction T85.612
   malposition T85.622
   obstruction T85.692
   perforation T85.692
   protrusion T85.692
   specified NEC T85.692
  pain T85.848
  specified type NEC T85.898
  stenosis T85.858
  thrombosis T85.868
 tracheostomy J95.00
  granuloma J95.09
  hemorrhage J95.01
  infection J95.02
  malfunction J95.03
  mechanical J95.03
  obstruction J95.03
  specified type NEC J95.09
  tracheo-esophageal fistula J95.04
 transfusion (blood) (lymphocytes) (plasma)
   T80.92
  air embolism T80.0
  circulatory overload E87.71
  febrile nonhemolytic transfusion reaction
    R50.84
  hemochromatosis E83.111
  hemolysis T80.89
  hemolytic reaction (antigen unspecified)
    T80.919
  incompatibility reaction (antigen
    unspecified) T80.919
   ABO T80.30
    delayed serologic (DSTR) T80.39
    hemolytic transfusion reaction
      (HTR) (unspecified time after
      transfusion) T80.319
     acute (AHTR) (less than 24 hours
       after transfusion) T80.310
     delayed (DHTR) (24 hours or
       more after transfusion)
       T80.311
    specified NEC T80.39
   acute (antigen unspecified) T80.910
   delayed (antigen unspecified)
     T80.911
   delayed serologic (DSTR) T80.89

Complication *(Continued)*
 transfusion *(Continued)*
  incompatibility reaction *(Continued)*
   Non-ABO (minor antigens (Duffy)
     (K) (Kell) (Kidd) (Lewis) (M) (N)
     (P) (S)) T80.A0
    delayed serologic (DSTR) T80.A9
    hemolytic transfusion reaction
      (HTR) (unspecified time after
      transfusion) T80.A19
     acute (AHTR) (less than 24 hours
       after transfusion) T80.A10
     delayed (DHTR) (24 hours or more
       after transfusion) T80.A11
    specified NEC T80.A9
   Rh (antigens (C) (c) (D) (E) (e)) (factor)
     T80.40
    delayed serologic (DSTR) T80.49
    hemolytic transfusion reaction
      (HTR) (unspecified time after
      transfusion) T80.419
     acute (AHTR) (less than 24 hours
       after transfusion) T80.410
     delayed (DHTR) (24 hours or more
       after transfusion) T80.411
    specified NEC T80.49
  infection T80.29
   acute T80.22
  reaction NEC T80.89
  sepsis T80.29
  shock T80.89
 transplant T86.90
  bone T86.839
   failure T86.831
   infection T86.832
   rejection T86.830
   specified type NEC T86.838
  bone marrow T86.00
   failure T86.02
   infection T86.03
   rejection T86.01
   specified type NEC T86.09
  cornea T86.849-
   failure T86.841
   infection T86.842-
   rejection T86.840-
   specified type NEC T86.848-
  failure T86.92
  heart T86.20
   with lung T86.30
   cardiac allograft vasculopathy T86.290
    failure T86.32
    infection T86.33
    rejection T86.31
    specified type NEC T86.39
   failure T86.22
   infection T86.23
   rejection T86.21
   specified type NEC T86.298
  infection T86.93
  intestine T86.859
   failure T86.851
   infection T86.852
   rejection T86.850
   specified type NEC T86.858
  kidney T86.10
   failure T86.12
   infection T86.13
   rejection T86.11
   specified type NEC T86.19
  liver T86.40
   failure T86.42
   infection T86.43
   rejection T86.41
   specified type NEC T86.49
  lung T86.819
   with heart T86.30
    failure T86.32
    infection T86.33
    rejection T86.31
    specified type NEC T86.39

Complication *(Continued)*
 transplant *(Continued)*
  lung *(Continued)*
   failure T86.811
   infection T86.812
   rejection T86.810
   specified type NEC T86.818
  malignant neoplasm C80.2
  pancreas T86.899
   failure T86.891
   infection T86.892
   rejection T86.890
   specified type NEC T86.898
  peripheral blood stem cells T86.5
  post-transplant lymphoproliferative
    disorder (PTLD) D47.Z1
  rejection T86.91
  skin T86.829
   failure T86.821
   infection T86.822
   rejection T86.820
   specified type NEC T86.828
  specified
   tissue T86.899
    failure T86.891
    infection T86.892
    rejection T86.890
    specified type NEC T86.898
   type NEC T86.99
  stem cell (from peripheral blood) (from
    umbilical cord) T86.5
  umbilical cord stem cells T86.5
 trauma (early) T79.9
  specified NEC T79.8
 ultrasound therapy NEC T88.9
 umbilical cord NEC
  complicating delivery O69.9
   specified NEC O69.89
 umbrella device, vascular T82.9
  embolism T82.818
  fibrosis T82.828
  hemorrhage T82.838
  infection or inflammation T82.7
  mechanical
   breakdown T82.515
   displacement T82.525
   leakage T82.535
   malposition T82.525
   obstruction T82.595
   perforation T82.595
   protrusion T82.595
  pain T82.848
  specified type NEC T82.898
  stenosis T82.858
  thrombosis T82.868
 urethral catheter —*see* Complications,
   catheter, urethral, indwelling
 vaccination T88.1
  anaphylaxis NEC T80.52
  arthropathy —*see* Arthropathy,
    postimmunization
  cellulitis T88.0
  encephalitis or encephalomyelitis
    G04.02
  infection (general) (local) NEC T88.0
  meningitis G03.8
  myelitis G04.02
  protein sickness T80.62
  rash T88.1
  reaction (allergic) T88.1
   serum T80.62
  sepsis T88.0
  serum intoxication, sickness, rash, or other
    serum reaction NEC T80.62
   anaphylactic shock T80.52
  shock (allergic) (anaphylactic) T80.52
  vaccinia (generalized) (localized) T88.1
 vas deferens device or implant —*see*
   Complications, genitourinary, device or
   implant, genital tract

Complication (Continued)
vascular I99.9
  device or implant T82.9
    embolism T82.818
    fibrosis T82.828
    hemorrhage T82.838
    infection or inflammation T82.7
    mechanical
      breakdown T82.519
        specified device NEC T82.518
      displacement T82.529
        specified device NEC T82.528
      leakage T82.539
        specified device NEC T82.538
      malposition T82.529
        specified device NEC T82.528
      obstruction T82.599
        specified device NEC T82.598
      perforation T82.599
        specified device NEC T82.598
      protrusion T82.599
        specified device NEC T82.598
    pain T82.848
    specified type NEC T82.898
    stenosis T82.858
    thrombosis T82.868
  dialysis catheter —*see* Complication,
      catheter, dialysis
  following infusion, therapeutic injection or
      transfusion T80.1
  graft T82.9
    embolism T82.818
    fibrosis T82.828
    hemorrhage T82.838
    mechanical
      breakdown T82.319
        aorta (bifurcation) T82.310
        carotid artery T82.311
        specified vessel NEC T82.318
      displacement T82.329
        aorta (bifurcation) T82.320
        carotid artery T82.321
        specified vessel NEC T82.328
      leakage T82.339
        aorta (bifurcation) T82.330
        carotid artery T82.331
        specified vessel NEC T82.338
      malposition T82.329
        aorta (bifurcation) T82.320
        carotid artery T82.321
        specified vessel NEC T82.328
      obstruction T82.399
        aorta (bifurcation) T82.390
        carotid artery T82.391
        specified vessel NEC T82.398
      perforation T82.399
        aorta (bifurcation) T82.390
        carotid artery T82.391
        specified vessel NEC T82.398
      protrusion T82.399
        aorta (bifurcation) T82.390
        carotid artery T82.391
        specified vessel NEC T82.398
    pain T82.848
    specified complication NEC T82.898
    stenosis T82.858
    thrombosis T82.868
  postoperative —*see* Complications,
      postoperative, circulatory
  vena cava device (filter) (sieve) (umbrella) —
      see Complications, umbrella device,
      vascular
  ventilation therapy NEC T81.81
  ventilator
    mechanical J95.850
      specified NEC J95.859
  ventricular (communicating) shunt (device)
      T85.9
    embolism T85.810
    fibrosis T85.820
    hemorrhage T85.830
    infection and inflammation T85.730

Complication (Continued)
ventricular shunt (Continued)
  mechanical
    breakdown T85.01
    displacement T85.02
    leakage T85.03
    malposition T85.02
    obstruction T85.09
    perforation T85.09
    protrusion T85.09
    specified NEC T85.09
  pain T85.840
  specified type NEC T85.890
  stenosis T85.850
  thrombosis T85.860
wire suture, permanent (implanted) —*see*
    Complications, suture, permanent
Compressed air disease T70.3
Compression
with injury - code by Nature of injury
artery I77.1
  celiac, syndrome I77.4
brachial plexus G54.0
brain (stem) G93.5
  due to
    ➠contusion (diffuse) (*see also* Injury,
        intracranial, diffuse) S06.A0
      ▶with herniation S06.A1
    ➠focal (*see also* Injury, intracranial, focal)
        S06.A0
      ▶ with herniation S06.A1
    ➠injury NEC (*see also* Injury, intracranial,
        diffuse) S06.A0
  ▶nontraumatic G93.5
  ➠traumatic (*see also* Injury, intracranial,
      diffuse) S06.A0
    ▶with herniation S06.A1
bronchus J98.09
cauda equina G83.4
celiac (artery) (axis) I77.4
cerebral —*see* Compression, brain
cervical plexus G54.2
cord
  spinal —*see* Compression, spinal
  umbilical —*see* Compression, umbilical cord
cranial nerve G52.9
  eighth —*see* subcategory H93.3
  eleventh G52.8
  fifth G50.8
  first G52.0
  fourth —*see* Strabismus, paralytic, fourth
      nerve
  ninth G52.1
  second —*see* Disorder, nerve, optic
  seventh G51.8
  sixth —*see* Strabismus, paralytic, sixth nerve
  tenth G52.2
  third —*see* Strabismus, paralytic, third nerve
  twelfth G52.3
diver's squeeze T70.3
during birth (newborn) P15.9
esophagus K22.2
eustachian tube —*see* Obstruction, eustachian
    tube, cartilaginous
facies Q67.1
fracture
  nontraumatic NOS —*see* Collapse, vertebra
  pathological —*see* Fracture, pathological
  traumatic —*see* Fracture, traumatic
heart —*see* Disease, heart
intestine —*see* Obstruction, intestine
laryngeal nerve, recurrent G52.2
  with paralysis of vocal cords and larynx
      J38.00
    bilateral J38.02
    unilateral J38.01
lumbosacral plexus G54.1
lung J98.4
lymphatic vessel I89.0
medulla —*see* Compression, brain
nerve —*see also* Disorder, nerve G58.9
  arm NEC —*see* Mononeuropathy, upper limb

Compression (Continued)
nerve (Continued)
  axillary G54.0
  cranial —*see* Compression, cranial nerve
  leg NEC —*see* Mononeuropathy, lower
      limb
  median (in carpal tunnel) —*see* Syndrome,
      carpal tunnel
  optic —*see* Disorder, nerve, optic
  plantar —*see* Lesion, nerve, plantar
  posterior tibial (in tarsal tunnel) —*see*
      Syndrome, tarsal tunnel
  root or plexus NOS (in) G54.9
    intervertebral disc disorder NEC —
        see Disorder, disc, with,
        radiculopathy
      with myelopathy —*see* Disorder, disc,
          with, myelopathy
    neoplastic disease —*see also* Neoplasm
        D49.9 *[G55]*
    spondylosis —*see* Spondylosis, with
        radiculopathy
  sciatic (acute) —*see* Lesion, nerve, sciatic
  sympathetic G90.8
  traumatic —*see* Injury, nerve
  ulnar —*see* Lesion, nerve, ulnar
  upper extremity NEC —*see*
      Mononeuropathy, upper limb
spinal (cord) G95.20
  by displacement of intervertebral disc
      NEC —*see also* Disorder, disc, with,
      myelopathy
  nerve root NOS G54.9
    due to displacement of intervertebral
        disc NEC —*see* Disorder, disc, with,
        radiculopathy
      with myelopathy —*see* Disorder, disc,
          with, myelopathy
  specified NEC G95.29
  spondylogenic (cervical) (lumbar,
      lumbosacral) (thoracic) —*see*
      Spondylosis, with myelopathy NEC
  anterior —*see* Syndrome, anterior, spinal
      artery, compression
  traumatic —*see* Injury, spinal cord, by
      region
subcostal nerve (syndrome) —*see*
    Mononeuropathy, upper limb, specified
    NEC
sympathetic nerve NEC G90.8
syndrome T79.5
trachea J39.8
ulnar nerve (by scar tissue) —*see* Lesion,
    nerve, ulnar
umbilical cord
  complicating delivery O69.2
    cord around neck O69.1
      prolapse O69.0
    specified NEC O69.2
ureter N13.5
vein I87.1
vena cava (inferior) (superior) I87.1
Compulsion, compulsive
gambling F63.0
neurosis F42.8
personality F60.5
states F42.8
swearing F42.8
  in Gilles de la Tourette's syndrome F95.2
tics and spasms F95.9
Concato's disease (pericardial polyserositis)
    A19.9
nontubercular I31.1
pleural —*see* Pleurisy, with effusion
Concavity chest wall M95.4
Concealed penis Q55.64
Concern (normal) **about sick person in family**
    Z63.6
Concrescence (teeth) K00.2
Concretio cordis I31.1
rheumatic I09.2

▶ New   ➠ Revised   ~~deleted~~ Deleted   ● Use Additional Character(s)

Concretion —see also Calculus
  appendicular K38.1
  canaliculus —see Dacryolith
  clitoris N90.89
  conjunctiva H11.12-●
  eyelid —see Disorder, eyelid, specified type NEC
  lacrimal passages —see Dacryolith
  prepuce (male) N47.8
  salivary gland (any) K11.5
  seminal vesicle N50.89
  tonsil J35.8
Concussion (brain) (cerebral) (current)
    S06.0X9
  with
    loss of consciousness of 30 minutes or less
        S06.0X1
    loss of consciousness of unspecified
        duration S06.0X9
  blast (air) (hydraulic) (immersion)
      (underwater)
    abdomen or thorax —see Injury, blast, by
        site
    ear with acoustic nerve injury —see Injury,
        nerve, acoustic, specified type NEC
  cauda equina S34.3
  conus medullaris S34.02
  ocular S05.8X-●
  spinal (cord)
    cervical S14.0
    lumbar S34.01
    sacral S34.02
    thoracic S24.0
  syndrome F07.81
  without loss of consciousness S06.0X0
Condition —see also Disease
  post COVID-19 U09.9
Conditions arising in the perinatal period —
    see Newborn, affected by
Conduct disorder —see Disorder, conduct
Condyloma A63.0
  acuminatum A63.0
  gonorrheal A54.09
  latum A51.31
  syphilitic A51.31
    congenital A50.07
  venereal, syphilitic A51.31
Conflagration —see also Burn
  asphyxia (by inhalation of gases, fumes or
      vapors) —see also Table of Drugs and
      Chemicals T59.9-●
Conflict (with) —see also Discord
  family Z73.9
  marital Z63.0
    involving divorce or estrangement Z63.5
  parent-child Z62.820
    parent-adopted child Z62.821
    parent-biological child Z62.820
    parent-foster child Z62.822
  social role NEC Z73.5
Confluent —see condition
Confusion, confused R41.0
  epileptic F05
  mental state (psychogenic) F44.89
  psychogenic F44.89
  reactive (from emotional stress, psychological
      trauma) F44.89
Confusional arousals G47.51
Congelation T69.9
Congenital —see also condition
  aortic septum Q25.49
  intrinsic factor deficiency D51.0
  malformation —see Anomaly
Congestion, congestive
  bladder N32.89
  bowel K63.89
  brain G93.89
  breast N64.59
  bronchial J98.09
  catarrhal J31.0
  chest R09.89
  chill, malarial —see Malaria

Congestion, congestive (Continued)
  circulatory NEC I99.8
  duodenum K31.89
  eye —see Hyperemia, conjunctiva
  facial, due to birth injury P15.4
  general R68.89
  glottis J37.0
  heart —see Failure, heart, congestive
  hepatic K76.1
  hypostatic (lung) —see Edema, lung
  intestine K63.89
  kidney N28.89
  labyrinth —see subcategory H83.8
  larynx J37.0
  liver K76.1
  lung R09.89
    active or acute —see Pneumonia
  malaria, malarial —see Malaria
  nasal R09.81
  nose R09.81
  orbit, orbital —see also Exophthalmos
    inflammatory (chronic) —see Inflammation,
        orbit
  ovary N83.8
  pancreas K86.89
  pelvic, female N94.89
  pleural J94.8
  prostate (active) N42.1
  pulmonary —see Congestion, lung
  renal N28.89
  retina H35.81
  seminal vesicle N50.1
  spinal cord G95.19
  spleen (chronic) D73.2
  stomach K31.89
  trachea —see Tracheitis
  urethra N36.8
  uterus N85.8
    with subinvolution N85.3
  venous (passive) I87.8
  viscera R68.89
Congestive —see Congestion
Conical
  cervix (hypertrophic elongation) N88.4
  cornea —see Keratoconus
  teeth K00.2
Conjoined twins Q89.4
Conjugal maladjustment Z63.0
  involving divorce or estrangement Z63.5
Conjunctiva —see condition
Conjunctivitis (staphylococcal) (streptococcal)
    NOS H10.9
  Acanthamoeba B60.12
  acute H10.3-●
    atopic H10.1-●
    chemical —see also Corrosion, cornea
        H10.21-●
    mucopurulent H10.02-●
      follicular H10.01-●
    pseudomembranous H10.22-●
    serous except viral H10.23-●
      viral —see Conjunctivitis, viral
    toxic H10.21-●
  adenoviral (acute) (follicular) B30.1
  allergic (acute) —see Conjunctivitis, acute,
      atopic
    chronic H10.45
      vernal H10.44
  anaphylactic —see Conjunctivitis, acute,
      atopic
  Apollo B30.3
  atopic (acute) —see Conjunctivitis, acute,
      atopic
  Béal's B30.2
  blennorrhagic (gonococcal) (neonatorum)
      A54.31
  chemical (acute) —see also Corrosion, cornea
      H10.21-●
  chlamydial A74.0
    due to trachoma A71.1
    neonatal P39.1

Conjunctivitis (Continued)
  chronic (nodosa) (petrificans) (phlyctenular)
      H10.40-●
    allergic H10.45
      vernal H10.44
    follicular H10.43-●
    giant papillary H10.41-●
    simple H10.42-●
    vernal H10.44
  coxsackievirus 24 B30.3
  diphtheritic A36.86
  due to
    dust —see Conjunctivitis, acute, atopic
    filariasis B74.9
    mucocutaneous leishmaniasis B55.2
  enterovirus type 70 (hemorrhagic) B30.3
  epidemic (viral) B30.9
    hemorrhagic B30.3
  gonococcal (neonatorum) A54.31
  granular (trachomatous) A71.1
    sequelae (late effect) B94.0
  hemorrhagic (acute) (epidemic) B30.3
  herpes zoster B02.31
  in (due to)
    Acanthamoeba B60.12
    adenovirus (acute) (follicular) B30.1
    Chlamydia A74.0
    coxsackievirus 24 B30.3
    diphtheria A36.86
    enterovirus type 70 (hemorrhagic) B30.3
    filariasis B74.9
    gonococci A54.31
    herpes (simplex) virus B00.53
      zoster B02.31
    infectious disease NEC B99
    meningococci A39.89
    mucocutaneous leishmaniasis B55.2
    rosacea H10.82-●
    syphilis (late) A52.71
    zoster B02.31
  inclusion A74.0
  infantile P39.1
    gonococcal A54.31
  Koch-Weeks' —see Conjunctivitis, acute,
      mucopurulent
  light —see Conjunctivitis, acute, atopic
  ligneous —see Blepharoconjunctivitis,
      ligneous
  meningococcal A39.89
  mucopurulent —see Conjunctivitis, acute,
      mucopurulent
  neonatal P39.1
    gonococcal A54.31
  Newcastle B30.8
  of Béal B30.2
  parasitic
    filariasis B74.9
    mucocutaneous leishmaniasis B55.2
  Parinaud's H10.89
  petrificans H10.89
  rosacea H10.82-●
  specified NEC H10.89
  swimming-pool B30.1
  trachomatous A71.1
    acute A71.0
    sequelae (late effect) B94.0
  traumatic NEC H10.89
  tuberculous A18.59
  tularemic A21.1
  tularensis A21.1
  viral B30.9
    due to
      adenovirus B30.1
      enterovirus B30.3
    specified NEC B30.8
Conjunctivochalasis H11.82-●
Connective tissue —see condition
Conn's syndrome E26.01
Conradi (-Hunermann) **disease** Q77.3
Consanguinity Z84.3
  counseling Z71.89

Conscious simulation (of illness) Z76.5
Consecutive —*see* condition
Consolidation lung (base) —*see* Pneumonia, lobar
Constipation (atonic) (neurogenic) (simple) (spastic) K59.00
  chronic K59.09
    idiopathic K59.04
  drug-induced K59.03
  functional K59.04
  outlet dysfunction K59.02
  psychogenic F45.8
  slow transit K59.01
  specified NEC K59.09
Constitutional —*see also* condition
  substandard F60.7
Constitutionally substandard F60.7
Constriction —*see also* Stricture
  auditory canal —*see* Stenosis, external ear canal
  bronchial J98.09
  duodenum K31.5
  esophagus K22.2
  external
    abdomen, abdominal (wall) S30.841
    alveolar process S00.542
    ankle S90.54-●
    antecubital space —*see* Constriction, external, forearm
    arm (upper) S40.84-●
    auricle —*see* Constriction, external, ear
    axilla —*see* Constriction, external, arm
    back, lower S30.840
    breast S20.14-●
    brow S00.84
    buttock S30.840
    calf —*see* Constriction, external, leg
    canthus —*see* Constriction, external, eyelid
    cheek S00.84
      internal S00.542
    chest wall —*see* Constriction, external, thorax
    chin S00.84
    clitoris S30.844
    costal region —*see* Constriction, external, thorax
    digit(s)
      foot —*see* Constriction, external, toe
      hand —*see* Constriction, external, finger
    ear S00.44-●
    elbow S50.34-●
    epididymis S30.843
    epigastric region S30.841
    esophagus, cervical S10.14
    eyebrow —*see* Constriction, external, eyelid
    eyelid S00.24-●
    face S00.84
    finger(s) S60.44-●
      index S60.44-●
      little S60.44-●
      middle S60.44-●
      ring S60.44-●
    flank S30.841
    foot (except toe(s) alone) S90.84-●
      toe —*see* Constriction, external, toe
    forearm S50.84-●
      elbow only —*see* Constriction, external, elbow
    forehead S00.84
    genital organs, external
      female S30.846
      male S30.845
    groin S30.841
    gum S00.542
    hand S60.54-●
    head S00.94
      ear —*see* Constriction, external, ear
      eyelid —*see* Constriction, external, eyelid
      lip S00.541
      nose S00.34
      oral cavity S00.542

Constriction *(Continued)*
  external *(Continued)*
    head *(Continued)*
      scalp S00.04
      specified site NEC S00.84
    heel —*see* Constriction, external, foot
    hip S70.24-●
    inguinal region S30.841
    interscapular region S20.449
    jaw S00.84
    knee S80.24-●
    labium (majus) (minus) S30.844
    larynx S10.14
    leg (lower) S80.84-●
      knee —*see* Constriction, external, knee
      upper —*see* Constriction, external, thigh
    lip S00.541
    lower back S30.840
    lumbar region S30.840
    malar region S00.84
    mammary —*see* Constriction, external, breast
    mastoid region S00.84
    mouth S00.542
    nail
      finger —*see* Constriction, external, finger
      toe —*see* Constriction, external, toe
    nasal S00.34
    neck S10.94
      specified site NEC S10.84
      throat S10.14
    nose S00.34
    occipital region S00.04
    oral cavity S00.542
    orbital region —*see* Constriction, external, eyelid
    palate S00.542
    palm —*see* Constriction, external, hand
    parietal region S00.04
    pelvis S30.840
    penis S30.842
    perineum
      female S30.844
      male S30.840
    periocular area —*see* Constriction, external, eyelid
    phalanges
      finger —*see* Constriction, external, finger
      toe —*see* Constriction, external, toe
    pharynx S10.14
    pinna —*see* Constriction, external, ear
    popliteal space —*see* Constriction, external, knee
    prepuce S30.842
    pubic region S30.840
    pudendum
      female S30.846
      male S30.845
    sacral region S30.840
    scalp S00.04
    scapular region —*see* Constriction, external, shoulder
    scrotum S30.843
    shin —*see* Constriction, external, leg
    shoulder S40.24-●
    sternal region S20.349
    submaxillary region S00.84
    submental region S00.84
    subungual
      finger(s) —*see* Constriction, external, finger
      toe(s) —*see* Constriction, external, toe
    supraclavicular fossa S10.84
    supraorbital S00.84
    temple S00.84
    temporal region S00.84
    testis S30.843
    thigh S70.34-●
    thorax, thoracic (wall) S20.94
      back S20.44-●
      front S20.34-●
    throat S10.14

Constriction *(Continued)*
  external *(Continued)*
    thumb S60.34-●
    toe(s) (lesser) S90.44-●
      great S90.44-●
    tongue S00.542
    trachea S10.14
    tunica vaginalis S30.843
    uvula S00.542
    vagina S30.844
    vulva S30.844
    wrist S60.84-●
  gallbladder —*see* Obstruction, gallbladder
  intestine —*see* Obstruction, intestine
  larynx J38.6
    congenital Q31.8
      specified NEC Q31.8
      subglottic Q31.1
  organ or site, congenital NEC —*see* Atresia, by site
  prepuce (acquired) (congenital) N47.1
  pylorus (adult hypertrophic) K31.1
    congenital or infantile Q40.0
    newborn Q40.0
  ring dystocia (uterus) O62.4
  spastic —*see also* Spasm
    ureter N13.5
  ureter N13.5
    with infection N13.6
  urethra —*see* Stricture, urethra
  visual field (peripheral) (functional) —*see* Defect, visual field
Constrictive —*see* condition
Consultation
  without complaint or sickness Z71.9
    feared complaint unfounded Z71.1
    specified reason NEC Z71.89
  medical —*see* Counseling, medical
  religious Z71.81
  specified reason NEC Z71.89
  spiritual Z71.81
Consumption —*see* Tuberculosis
Contact (with) —*see also* Exposure (to)
  acariasis Z20.7
  AIDS virus Z20.6
  air pollution Z77.110
  algae and algae toxins Z77.121
  algae bloom Z77.121
  anthrax Z20.810
  aromatic (hazardous) compounds NEC Z77.028
  aromatic amines Z77.020
  aromatic dyes NOS Z77.028
  arsenic Z77.010
  asbestos Z77.090
  bacterial disease NEC Z20.818
  benzene Z77.021
  blue-green algae bloom Z77.121
  body fluids (potentially hazardous) Z77.21
  brown tide Z77.121
  chemicals (chiefly nonmedicinal) (hazardous) NEC Z77.098
  cholera Z20.09
  chromium compounds Z77.018
  communicable disease Z20.9
    bacterial NEC Z20.818
    specified NEC Z20.89
    viral NEC Z20.828
    Zika virus Z20.821
  coronavirus (disease) (novel) 2019 Z20.822
  COVID-19 Z20.822
  cyanobacteria bloom Z77.121
  dyes Z77.098
  Escherichia coli (E. coli) Z20.01
  fiberglass —*see* Table of Drugs and Chemicals, fiberglass
  German measles Z20.4
  gonorrhea Z20.2
  hazardous metals NEC Z77.018
  hazardous substances NEC Z77.29
  hazards in the physical environment NEC Z77.128
  hazards to health NEC Z77.9

Contact *(Continued)*
HIV Z20.6
HTLV-III/LAV Z20.6
human immunodeficiency virus (HIV) Z20.6
infection Z20.9
  specified NEC Z20.89
infestation (parasitic) NEC Z20.7
intestinal infectious disease NEC Z20.09
  Escherichia coli (E. coli) Z20.01
lead Z77.011
meningococcus Z20.811
mold (toxic) Z77.120
nickel dust Z77.018
noise Z77.122
parasitic disease Z20.7
pediculosis Z20.7
pfiesteria piscicida Z77.121
poliomyelitis Z20.89
pollution
  air Z77.110
  environmental NEC Z77.118
  soil Z77.112
  water Z77.111
polycyclic aromatic hydrocarbons Z77.028
▶ positive maternal group B streptococcus P00.82
rabies Z20.3
radiation, naturally occurring NEC Z77.123
radon Z77.123
red tide (Florida) Z77.121
rubella Z20.4
SARS-CoV-2 Z20.822
sexually-transmitted disease Z20.2
smallpox (laboratory) Z20.89
syphilis Z20.2
tuberculosis Z20.1
uranium Z77.012
varicella Z20.820
venereal disease Z20.2
viral disease NEC Z20.828
viral hepatitis Z20.5
water pollution Z77.111
Zika virus Z20.821
Contamination, food —*see* Intoxication, foodborne
Contraception, contraceptive
advice Z30.09
counseling Z30.09
device (intrauterine) (in situ) Z97.5
  causing menorrhagia T83.83
  checking Z30.431
  complications —*see* Complications,
    intrauterine, contraceptive device
  in place Z97.5
  initial prescription Z30.014
  reinsertion Z30.433
  removal Z30.432
  replacement Z30.433
emergency (postcoital) Z30.012
initial prescription Z30.019
  barrier Z30.018
  diaphragm Z30.018
  injectable Z30.013
  intrauterine device Z30.014
  pills Z30.011
  postcoital (emergency) Z30.012
  specified type NEC Z30.018
  subdermal implantable Z30.017
  transdermal patch hormonal Z30.016
  vaginal ring hormonal Z30.015
maintenance Z30.40
  barrier Z30.49
  diaphragm Z30.49
  examination Z30.8
  injectable Z30.42
  intrauterine device Z30.431
  pills Z30.41
  specified type NEC Z30.49
  subdermal implantable Z30.46
  transdermal patch hormonal Z30.45
  vaginal ring hormonal Z30.44
management Z30.9
  specified NEC Z30.8
postcoital (emergency) Z30.012

Contraception, contraceptive *(Continued)*
prescription Z30.019
  repeat Z30.40
sterilization Z30.2
surveillance (drug) —*see* Contraception,
  maintenance
Contraction(s), contracture, contracted
Achilles tendon —*see also* Short, tendon,
  Achilles
  congenital Q66.89
amputation stump (surgical) (flexion) (late)
  next proximal joint T87.89
anus K59.89
bile duct (common) (hepatic) K83.8
bladder N32.89
  neck or sphincter N32.0
bowel, cecum, colon or intestine, any part —
  see Obstruction, intestine
Braxton Hicks —*see* False, labor
breast implant, capsular T85.44
bronchial J98.09
burn (old) —*see* Cicatrix
cervix —*see* Stricture, cervix
cicatricial —*see* Cicatrix
conjunctiva, trachomatous, active A71.1
  sequelae (late effect) B94.0
Dupuytren's M72.0
eyelid —*see* Disorder, eyelid function
fascia (lata) (postural) M72.8
  Dupuytren's M72.0
  palmar M72.0
  plantar M72.2
finger NEC —*see also* Deformity, finger
  congenital Q68.1
  joint —*see* Contraction, joint, hand
flaccid —*see* Contraction, paralytic
gallbladder K82.0
heart valve —*see* Endocarditis
hip —*see* Contraction, joint, hip
hourglass
  bladder N32.89
    congenital Q64.79
  gallbladder K82.0
    congenital Q44.1
  stomach K31.89
    congenital Q40.2
    psychogenic F45.8
  uterus (complicating delivery) O62.4
hysterical F44.4
internal os —*see* Stricture, cervix
joint (abduction) (acquired) (adduction)
  (flexion) (rotation) M24.50
  ankle M24.57-●
  congenital NEC Q68.8
    hip Q65.89
  elbow M24.52-●
  foot joint M24.57-●
  hand joint M24.54-●
  hip M24.55-●
    congenital Q65.89
  hysterical F44.4
  knee M24.56-●
  shoulder M24.51-●
  specified site NEC M24.59
  wrist M24.53-●
kidney (granular) (secondary) N26.9
  congenital Q63.8
  hydronephritic —*see* Hydronephrosis
  Page N26.2
  pyelonephritic —*see* Pyelitis, chronic
  tuberculous A18.11
ligament —*see also* Disorder, ligament
  congenital Q79.8
muscle (postinfective) (postural) NEC M62.40
  with contracture of joint —*see* Contraction,
    joint
  ankle M62.47-●
  congenital Q79.8
    sternocleidomastoid Q68.0
  extraocular —*see* Strabismus
  eye (extrinsic) —*see* Strabismus
  foot M62.47-●

Contraction, contracture, contracted
(Continued)
  muscle *(Continued)* forearm M62.43-●
    hand M62.44-●
    hysterical F44.4
    ischemic (Volkmann's) T79.6
    lower leg M62.46-●
    multiple sites M62.49
    pelvic region M62.45-●
    posttraumatic —*see* Strabismus, paralytic
    psychogenic F45.8
      conversion reaction F44.4
    shoulder region M62.41-●
    specified site NEC M62.48
    thigh M62.45-●
    upper arm M62.42-●
neck —*see* Torticollis
ocular muscle —*see* Strabismus
organ or site, congenital NEC —*see* Atresia,
  by site
outlet (pelvis) —*see* Contraction, pelvis
palmar fascia M72.0
paralytic
  joint —*see* Contraction, joint
  muscle —*see also* Contraction, muscle NEC
    ocular —*see* Strabismus, paralytic
pelvis (acquired) (general) M95.5
  with disproportion (fetopelvic) O33.1
    causing obstructed labor O65.1
  inlet O33.2
  mid-cavity O33.3
  outlet O33.3
plantar fascia M72.2
premature
  atrium I49.1
  auriculoventricular I49.49
  heart I49.49
  junctional I49.2
  supraventricular I49.1
  ventricular I49.3
prostate N42.89
pylorus NEC —*see also* Pylorospasm
  psychogenic F45.8
rectum, rectal (sphincter) K59.89
ring (Bandl's) (complicating delivery) O62.4
scar —*see* Cicatrix
spine —*see* Dorsopathy, deforming
sternocleidomastoid (muscle), congenital
  Q68.0
stomach K31.89
  hourglass K31.89
    congenital Q40.2
    psychogenic F45.8
  psychogenic F45.8
tendon (sheath) M62.40
  with contracture of joint —*see* Contraction,
    joint
  Achilles —*see* Short, tendon, Achilles
  ankle M62.47-●
    Achilles —*see* Short, tendon, Achilles
  foot M62.47-●
  forearm M62.43-●
  hand M62.44-●
  lower leg M62.46-●
  multiple sites M62.49
  neck M62.48
  pelvic region M62.45-●
  shoulder region M62.41-●
  specified site NEC M62.48
  thigh M62.45-●
  thorax M62.48
  trunk M62.48
  upper arm M62.42-●
toe —*see* Deformity, toe, specified NEC
ureterovesical orifice (postinfectional) N13.5
  with infection N13.6
urethra —*see also* Stricture, urethra
  orifice N32.0
uterus N85.8
  abnormal NEC O62.9
  clonic (complicating delivery) O62.4
  dyscoordinate (complicating delivery) O62.4

Contraction, contracture, contracted
  (Continued)
  uterus *(Continued)*
    hourglass (complicating delivery) O62.4
    hypertonic O62.4
    hypotonic NEC O62.2
    inadequate
      primary O62.0
      secondary O62.1
    incoordinate (complicating delivery) O62.4
    poor O62.2
    tetanic (complicating delivery) O62.4
  vagina (outlet) N89.5
  vesical N32.89
    neck or urethral orifice N32.0
  visual field —*see* Defect, visual field,
    generalized
  Volkmann's (ischemic) T79.6
Contusion (skin surface intact) T14.8
  abdomen, abdominal (muscle) (wall) S30.1
  adnexa, eye NEC S05.8X-●
  adrenal gland S37.812
  alveolar process S00.532
  ankle S90.0-●
  antecubital space —*see* Contusion, forearm
  anus S30.3
  arm (upper) S40.02-●
    lower (with elbow) —*see* Contusion,
      forearm
  auditory canal —*see* Contusion, ear
  auricle —*see* Contusion, ear
  axilla —*see* Contusion, arm, upper
  back —*see also* Contusion, thorax, back
    lower S30.0
  bile duct S36.13
  bladder S37.22
  bone NEC T14.8
  brain (diffuse) —*see* Injury, intracranial, diffuse
    focal —*see* Injury, intracranial, focal
  brainstem S06.38-●
  breast S20.0-●
  broad ligament S37.892
  brow S00.83
  buttock S30.0
  canthus, eye S00.1-●
  cauda equina S34.3
  cerebellar, traumatic S06.37-●
  cerebral S06.33-●
    left side S06.32-●
    right side S06.31-●
  cheek S00.83
    internal S00.532
  chest (wall) —*see* Contusion, thorax
  chin S00.83
  clitoris S30.23
  colon —*see* Injury, intestine, large, contusion
  common bile duct S36.13
  conjunctiva S05.1-●
    with foreign body (in conjunctival sac) —
      see Foreign body, conjunctival sac
  conus medullaris (spine) S34.139
  cornea —*see* Contusion, eyeball
    with foreign body —*see* Foreign body,
      cornea
  corpus cavernosum S30.21
  cortex (brain) (cerebral) —*see* Injury,
    intracranial, diffuse
    focal —*see* Injury, intracranial, focal
  costal region —*see* Contusion, thorax
  cystic duct S36.13
  diaphragm S27.802
  duodenum S36.420
  ear S00.43-●
  elbow S50.0-●
    with forearm —*see* Contusion, forearm
  epididymis S30.22
  epigastric region S30.1
  epiglottis S10.0
  esophagus (thoracic) S27.812
    cervical S10.0
  eyeball S05.1-●

Contusion *(Continued)*
  eyebrow S00.1-●
  eyelid (and periocular area) S00.1-●
  face NEC S00.83
  fallopian tube S37.529
    bilateral S37.522
    unilateral S37.521
  femoral triangle S30.1
  finger(s) S60.00
    with damage to nail (matrix) S60.10
    index S60.02-●
      with damage to nail S60.12-●
    little S60.05-●
      with damage to nail S60.15-●
    middle S60.03-●
      with damage to nail S60.13-●
    ring S60.04-●
      with damage to nail S60.14-●
    thumb —*see* Contusion, thumb
  flank S30.1
  foot (except toe(s) alone) S90.3-●
    toe —*see* Contusion, toe
  forearm S50.1-●
    elbow only —*see* Contusion, elbow
  forehead S00.83
  gallbladder S36.122
  genital organs, external
    female S30.202
    male S30.201
  globe (eye) —*see* Contusion, eyeball
  groin S30.1
  gum S00.532
  hand S60.22-●
    finger(s) —*see* Contusion, finger
    wrist —*see* Contusion, wrist
  head S00.93
    ear —*see* Contusion, ear
    eyelid —*see* Contusion, eyelid
    lip S00.531
    nose S00.33
    oral cavity S00.532
    scalp S00.03
    specified part NEC S00.83
  heart —*see also* Injury, heart S26.91
  heel —*see* Contusion, foot
  hepatic duct S36.13
  hip S70.0-●
  ileum S36.428
  iliac region S30.1
  inguinal region S30.1
  interscapular region S20.229
  intra-abdominal organ S36.92
    colon —*see* Injury, intestine, large, contusion
    liver S36.112
    pancreas —*see* Contusion, pancreas
    rectum S36.62
    small intestine —*see* Injury, intestine, small,
      contusion
    specified organ NEC S36.892
    spleen —*see* Contusion, spleen
    stomach S36.32
  iris (eye) —*see* Contusion, eyeball
  jaw S00.83
  jejunum S36.428
  kidney S37.01-●
    major (greater than 2 cm) S37.02-●
    minor (less than 2 cm) S37.01-●
  knee S80.0-●
  labium (majus) (minus) S30.23
  lacrimal apparatus, gland or sac S05.8X-●
  larynx S10.0
  leg (lower) S80.1-●
    knee —*see* Contusion, knee
  lens —*see* Contusion, eyeball
  lip S00.531
  liver S36.112
  lower back S30.0
  lumbar region S30.0
  lung S27.329
    bilateral S27.322
    unilateral S27.321

Contusion *(Continued)*
  malar region S00.83
  mastoid region S00.83
  membrane, brain —*see* Injury, intracranial,
    diffuse
    focal —*see* Injury, intracranial, focal
  mesentery S36.892
  mesosalpinx S37.892
  mouth S00.532
  muscle —*see* Contusion, by site
  nail
    finger —*see* Contusion, finger, with
      damage to nail
    toe —*see* Contusion, toe, with damage to
      nail
  nasal S00.33
  neck S10.93
    specified site NEC S10.83
    throat S10.0
  nerve —*see* Injury, nerve
  newborn P54.5
  nose S00.33
  occipital
    lobe (brain) —*see* Injury, intracranial,
      diffuse
      focal —*see* Injury, intracranial,
        focal
    region (scalp) S00.03
  orbit (region) (tissues) S05.1-●
  ovary S37.429
    bilateral S37.422
    unilateral S37.421
  palate S00.532
  pancreas S36.229
    body S36.221
    head S36.220
    tail S36.222
  parietal
    lobe (brain) —*see* Injury, intracranial,
      diffuse
      focal —*see* Injury, intracranial, focal
    region (scalp) S00.03
  pelvic organ S37.92
    adrenal gland S37.812
    bladder S37.22
    fallopian tube —*see* Contusion, fallopian
      tube
    kidney —*see* Contusion, kidney
    ovary —*see* Contusion, ovary
    prostate S37.822
    specified organ NEC S37.892
    ureter S37.12
    urethra S37.32
    uterus S37.62
  pelvis S30.0
  penis S30.21
  perineum
    female S30.23
    male S30.0
  periocular area S00.1-●
  peritoneum S36.81
  periurethral tissue —*see* Contusion,
    urethra
  pharynx S10.0
  pinna —*see* Contusion, ear
  popliteal space —*see* Contusion, knee
  prepuce S30.21
  prostate S37.822
  pubic region S30.1
  pudendum
    female S30.202
    male S30.201
  quadriceps femoris —*see* Contusion, thigh
  rectum S36.62
  retroperitoneum S36.892
  round ligament S37.892
  sacral region S30.0
  scalp S00.03
    due to birth injury P12.3
  scapular region —*see* Contusion, shoulder
  sclera —*see* Contusion, eyeball

▶ New   ⇒ Revised   ~~deleted~~ Deleted   ● Use Additional Character(s)

Contusion *(Continued)*
  scrotum S30.22
  seminal vesicle S37.892
  shoulder S40.01-•
  skin NEC T14.8
  small intestine —*see* Injury, intestine, small,
    contusion
  spermatic cord S30.22
  spinal cord —*see* Injury, spinal cord,
    by region
    cauda equina S34.3
    conus medullaris S34.139
  spleen S36.029
    major S36.021
    minor S36.020
  sternal region S20.219
  stomach S36.32
  subconjunctival S05.1-•
  subcutaneous NEC T14.8
  submaxillary region S00.83
  submental region S00.83
  subperiosteal NEC T14.8
  subungual
    finger —*see* Contusion, finger, with
      damage to nail
    toe —*see* Contusion, toe, with damage to
      nail
  supraclavicular fossa S10.83
  supraorbital S00.83
  suprarenal gland S37.812
  temple (region) S00.83
  temporal
    lobe (brain) —*see* Injury, intracranial,
      diffuse
      focal —*see* Injury, intracranial, focal
    region S00.83
  testis S30.22
  thigh S70.1-•
  thorax (wall) S20.20
    back S20.22-•
    front S20.21-•
  throat S10.0
  thumb S60.01-•
    with damage to nail S60.11-•
  toe(s) (lesser) S90.12-•
    with damage to nail S90.22-•
    great S90.11-•
      with damage to nail S90.21-•
  tongue S00.532
  trachea (cervical) S10.0
    thoracic S27.52
  tunica vaginalis S30.22
  tympanum, tympanic membrane —*see*
    Contusion, ear
  ureter S37.12
  urethra S37.32
  urinary organ NEC S37.892
  uterus S37.62
  uvula S00.532
  vagina S30.23
  vas deferens S37.892
  vesical S37.22
  vocal cord(s) S10.0
  vulva S30.23
  wrist S60.21-•
Conus (congenital) (any type) Q14.8
  cornea —*see* Keratoconus
  medullaris syndrome G95.81
Conversion hysteria, neurosis or reaction
  F44.9
Converter, tuberculosis (test reaction) R76.11
Conviction (legal), anxiety concerning
  Z65.0
  with imprisonment Z65.1
Convulsions (idiopathic) —*see also* Seizure(s)
  R56.9
  apoplectiform (cerebral ischemia) I67.82
  dissociative F44.5
  epileptic —*see* Epilepsy
  epileptiform, epileptoid —*see* Seizure,
    epileptiform

Convulsions *(Continued)*
  ether (anesthetic) —*see* Table of Drugs and
    Chemicals, by drug
  febrile R56.00
    with status epilepticus G40.901
    complex R56.01
      with status epilepticus G40.901
    simple R56.00
  hysterical F44.5
  infantile P90
    epilepsy —*see* Epilepsy
  jacksonian —*see* Epilepsy, localization-
    related, symptomatic, with simple
    partial seizures
  myoclonic G25.3
  newborn P90
  obstetrical (nephritic) (uremic) —*see*
    Eclampsia
  paretic A52.17
  post traumatic R56.1
  psychomotor —*see* Epilepsy, localization-
    related, symptomatic, with complex
    partial seizures
  recurrent R56.9
  reflex R25.8
  scarlatinal A38.8
  tetanus, tetanic —*see* Tetanus
  thymic E32.8
Convulsive —*see also* Convulsions
Cooley's anemia D56.1
Coolie itch B76.9
Cooper's
  disease —*see* Mastopathy, cystic
  hernia —*see* Hernia, abdomen, specified site
    NEC
Cupra itch B88.0
Coprophagy F50.89
Coprophobia F40.298
Coproporphyria, hereditary E80.29
Cor
  biloculare Q20.8
  bovis, bovinum —*see* Hypertrophy, cardiac
  pulmonale (chronic) I27.81
    acute I26.09
  triatriatum, triatrium Q24.2
  triloculare Q20.8
    biatrium Q20.4
    biventriculare Q21.1
Corbus' disease (gangrenous balanitis) N48.1
Cord —*see also* condition
  around neck
    complicating delivery O69.81
      with compression O69.1
  bladder G95.89
    tabetic A52.19
Cordis ectopia Q24.8
Corditis (spermatic) N49.1
Corectopia Q13.2
Cori's disease (glycogen storage) E74.03
Corkhandler's disease or lung J67.3
Corkscrew esophagus K22.4
Corkworker's disease or lung J67.3
Corn (infected) L84
Cornea —*see also* condition
  donor Z52.5
  plana Q13.4
Cornelia de Lange syndrome Q87.19
Cornu cutaneum L85.8
Cornual gestation or pregnancy O00.80
  with intrauterine pregnancy O00.81
Coronary (artery) —*see* condition
Coronavirus (infection)
  as cause of disease classified elsewhere
    B97.29
  coronavirus-19 U07.1
  COVID-19 U07.1
  SARS-associated B97.21
Corpora —*see also* condition
  amylacea, prostate N42.89
  cavernosa —*see* condition
Corpulence —*see* Obesity

Corpus —*see* condition
Corrected transposition Q20.5
Corrosion (injury) (acid) (caustic) (chemical)
  (lime) (external) (internal) T30.4
  abdomen, abdominal (muscle) (wall)
    T21.42
    first degree T21.52
    second degree T21.62
    third degree T21.72
  above elbow T22.439
    first degree T22.539
    left T22.432
      first degree T22.532
      second degree T22.632
      third degree T22.732
    right T22.431
      first degree T22.531
      second degree T22.631
      third degree T22.731
    second degree T22.639
    third degree T22.739
  alimentary tract NEC T28.7
  ankle T25.419
    first degree T25.519
    left T25.412
      first degree T25.512
      second degree T25.612
      third degree T25.712
    multiple with foot —*see* Corrosion, lower,
      limb, multiple, ankle and foot
    right T25.411
      first degree T25.511
      second degree T25.611
      third degree T25.711
    second degree T25.619
    third degree T25.719
  anus —*see* Corrosion, buttock
  arm(s) (meaning upper limb(s)) —*see*
    Corrosion, upper limb
  axilla T22.449
    first degree T22.549
    left T22.442
      first degree T22.542
      second degree T22.642
      third degree T22.742
    right T22.441
      first degree T22.541
      second degree T22.641
      third degree T22.741
    second degree T22.649
    third degree T22.749
  back (lower) T21.44
    first degree T21.54
    second degree T21.64
    third degree T21.74
    upper T21.43
      first degree T21.53
      second degree T21.63
      third degree T21.73
  blisters - code as Corrosion, second degree,
    by site
  breast(s) —*see* Corrosion, chest wall
  buttock(s) T21.45
    first degree T21.55
    second degree T21.65
    third degree T21.75
  calf T24.439
    first degree T24.539
    left T24.432
      first degree T24.532
      second degree T24.632
      third degree T24.732
    right T24.431
      first degree T24.531
      second degree T24.631
      third degree T24.731
    second degree T24.639
    third degree T24.739
  canthus (eye) —*see* Corrosion, eyelid
  cervix T28.8

Corrosion (*Continued*)
  cheek T20.46
    first degree T20.56
    second degree T20.66
    third degree T20.76
  chest wall T21.41
    first degree T21.51
    second degree T21.61
    third degree T21.71
  chin T20.43
    first degree T20.53
    second degree T20.63
    third degree T20.73
  colon T28.7
  conjunctiva (and cornea) —*see* Corrosion,
      cornea
  cornea (and conjunctiva) T26.6-●
  deep necrosis of underlying tissue -
      code as Corrosion, third degree,
      by site
  dorsum of hand T23.469
    first degree T23.569
    left T23.462
      first degree T23.562
      second degree T23.662
      third degree T23.762
    right T23.461
      first degree T23.561
      second degree T23.661
      third degree T23.761
    second degree T23.669
    third degree T23.769
  ear (auricle) (external) (canal) T20.41
    drum T28.91
    first degree T20.51
    second degree T20.61
    third degree T20.71
  elbow T22.429
    first degree T22.529
    left T22.422
      first degree T22.522
      second degree T22.622
      third degree T22.722
    right T22.421
      first degree T22.521
      second degree T22.621
      third degree T22.721
    second degree T22.629
    third degree T22.729
  entire body —*see* Corrosion, multiple body
      regions
  epidermal loss - code as Corrosion, second
      degree, by site
  epiglottis T27.4
  erythema, erythematous - code as Corrosion,
      first degree, by site
  esophagus T28.6
  extent (percentage of body surface)
    less than 10 percent T32.0
    10-19 percent (0-9 percent third degree)
        T32.10
      with 10-19 percent third degree
          T32.11
    20-29 percent (0-9 percent third degree)
        T32.20
      with
        10-19 percent third degree T32.21
        20-29 percent third degree T32.22
    30-39 percent (0-9 percent third degree)
        T32.30
      with
        10-19 percent third degree T32.31
        20-29 percent third degree T32.32
        30-39 percent third degree T32.33
    40-49 percent (0-9 percent third degree)
        T32.40
      with
        10-19 percent third degree T32.41
        20-29 percent third degree T32.42
        30-39 percent third degree T32.43
        40-49 percent third degree T32.44

Corrosion (*Continued*)
  extent (*Continued*)
    50-59 percent (0-9 percent third degree)
        T32.50
      with
        10-19 percent third degree T32.51
        20-29 percent third degree T32.52
    50-59 percent (*Continued*)
      with (*Continued*)
        30-39 percent third degree T32.53
        40-49 percent third degree T32.54
        50-59 percent third degree T32.55
    60-69 percent (0-9 percent third degree)
        T32.60
      with
        10-19 percent third degree T32.61
        20-29 percent third degree T32.62
        30-39 percent third degree T32.63
        40-49 percent third degree T32.64
        50-59 percent third degree T32.65
        60-69 percent third degree T32.66
    70-79 percent (0-9 percent third degree)
        T32.70
      with
        10-19 percent third degree T32.71
        20-29 percent third degree T32.72
        30-39 percent third degree T32.73
        40-49 percent third degree T32.74
        50-59 percent third degree T32.75
        60-69 percent third degree T32.76
        70-79 percent third degree T32.77
    80-89 percent (0-9 percent third degree)
        T32.80
      with
        10-19 percent third degree T32.81
        20-29 percent third degree T32.82
        30-39 percent third degree T32.83
        40-49 percent third degree T32.84
        50-59 percent third degree T32.85
        60-69 percent third degree T32.86
        70-79 percent third degree T32.87
        80-89 percent third degree T32.88
    90 percent or more (0-9 percent third
        degree) T32.90
      with
        10-19 percent third degree T32.91
        20-29 percent third degree T32.92
        30-39 percent third degree T32.93
        40-49 percent third degree T32.94
        50-59 percent third degree T32.95
        60-69 percent third degree T32.96
        70-79 percent third degree T32.97
        80-89 percent third degree T32.98
        90-99 percent third degree T32.99
  extremity —*see* Corrosion, limb
  eye(s) and adnexa T26.9-●
    with resulting rupture and destruction of
        eyeball T26.7-●
    conjunctival sac —*see* Corrosion,
        cornea
    cornea —*see* Corrosion, cornea
    lid —*see* Corrosion, eyelid
    periocular area —*see* Corrosion eyelid
    specified site NEC T26.8-●
  eyeball —*see* Corrosion, eye
  eyelid(s) T26.5-●
  face —*see* Corrosion, head
  finger T23.429
    first degree T23.529
    left T23.422
      first degree T23.522
      second degree T23.622
      third degree T23.722
    multiple sites (without thumb)
        T23.439
      with thumb T23.449
        first degree T23.549
        left T23.442
          first degree T23.542
          second degree T23.642
          third degree T23.742

Corrosion (*Continued*)
  finger (*Continued*)
    multiple sites (*Continued*)
      with thumb (*Continued*)
        right T23.441
          first degree T23.541
          second degree T23.641
          third degree T23.741
        second degree T23.649
        third degree T23.749
      first degree T23.539
      left T23.432
        first degree T23.532
        second degree T23.632
        third degree T23.732
      right T23.431
        first degree T23.531
        second degree T23.631
        third degree T23.731
      second degree T23.639
      third degree T23.739
    right T23.421
      first degree T23.521
      second degree T23.621
      third degree T23.721
    second degree T23.629
    third degree T23.729
  flank —*see* Corrosion, abdomen
  foot T25.429
    first degree T25.529
    left T25.422
      first degree T25.522
      second degree T25.622
      third degree T25.722
    multiple with ankle —*see* Corrosion, lower,
        limb, multiple, ankle and foot
    right T25.421
      first degree T25.521
      second degree T25.621
      third degree T25.721
    second degree T25.629
    third degree T25.729
  forearm T22.419
    first degree T22.519
    left T22.412
      first degree T22.512
      second degree T22.612
      third degree T22.712
    right T22.411
      first degree T22.511
      second degree T22.611
      third degree T22.711
    second degree T22.619
    third degree T22.719
  forehead T20.46
    first degree T20.56
    second degree T20.66
    third degree T20.76
  fourth degree - code as Corrosion, third
      degree, by site
  full thickness skin loss - code as Corrosion,
      third degree, by site
  gastrointestinal tract NEC T28.7
  genital organs
    external
      female T21.47
        first degree T21.57
        second degree T21.67
        third degree T21.77
      male T21.46
        first degree T21.56
        second degree T21.66
        third degree T21.76
    internal T28.8
  groin —*see* Corrosion, abdominal wall
  hand(s) T23.409
    back —*see* Corrosion, dorsum of hand
    finger —*see* Corrosion, finger
    first degree T23.509
    left T23.402
      first degree T23.502
      second degree T23.602
      third degree T23.702

▶ New   ⇒ Revised   ~~deleted~~ Deleted   ● Use Additional Character(s)

Corrosion (Continued)
  hand(s) (Continued)
    multiple sites with wrist T23.499
      first degree T23.599
      left T23.492
        first degree T23.592
        second degree T23.692
        third degree T23.792
      right T23.491
        first degree T23.591
        second degree T23.691
        third degree T23.791
      second degree T23.699
      third degree T23.799
    palm —see Corrosion, palm
    right T23.401
      first degree T23.501
      second degree T23.601
      third degree T23.701
    second degree T23.609
    third degree T23.709
    thumb —see Corrosion, thumb
  head (and face) (and neck) T20.40
    cheek —see Corrosion, cheek
    chin —see Corrosion, chin
    ear —see Corrosion, ear
    eye(s) only —see Corrosion, eye
    first degree T20.50
    forehead —see Corrosion, forehead
    lip —see Corrosion, lip
    multiple sites T20.49
      first degree T20.59
      second degree T20.69
      third degree T20.79
    neck —see Corrosion, neck
    nose —see Corrosion, nose
    scalp —see Corrosion, scalp
    second degree T20.60
    third degree T20.70
  hip(s) —see Corrosion, lower, limb
  inhalation —see Corrosion, respiratory
      tract
  internal organ(s) (see also Corrosion, by site)
      T28.90
    alimentary tract T28.7
      esophagus T28.6
    esophagus T28.6
    genitourinary T28.8
    mouth T28.5
    pharynx T28.5
    specified organ NEC T28.99
  interscapular region —see Corrosion, back,
      upper
  intestine (large) (small) T28.7
  knee T24.429
    first degree T24.529
    left T24.422
      first degree T24.522
      second degree T24.622
      third degree T24.722
    right T24.421
      first degree T24.521
      second degree T24.621
      third degree T24.721
    second degree T24.629
    third degree T24.729
  labium (majus) (minus) —see Corrosion,
      genital organs, external, female
  lacrimal apparatus, duct, gland or sac —see
      Corrosion, eye, specified site NEC
  larynx T27.4
    with lung T27.5
  leg(s) (meaning lower limb(s)) —see
      Corrosion, lower limb
  limb(s)
    lower —see Corrosion, lower, limb
    upper —see Corrosion, upper limb
  lip(s) T20.42
    first degree T20.52
    second degree T20.62
    third degree T20.72

Corrosion (Continued)
  lower
    back —see Corrosion, back
    limb T24.409
      ankle —see Corrosion, ankle
      calf —see Corrosion, calf
      first degree T24.509
      foot —see Corrosion, foot
      hip —see Corrosion, thigh
      knee —see Corrosion, knee
      left T24.402
        first degree T24.502
        second degree T24.602
        third degree T24.702
      multiple sites, except ankle and foot
          T24.499
        ankle and foot T25.499
          first degree T25.599
          left T25.492
            first degree T25.592
            second degree T25.692
            third degree T25.792
          right T25.491
            first degree T25.591
            second degree T25.691
            third degree T25.791
          second degree T25.699
          third degree T25.799
        first degree T24.599
        left T24.492
          first degree T24.592
          second degree T24.692
          third degree T24.792
        right T24.491
          first degree T24.591
          second degree T24.691
          third degree T24.791
        second degree T24.699
        third degree T24.799
      right T24.401
        first degree T24.501
        second degree T24.601
        third degree T24.701
      second degree T24.609
      thigh —see Corrosion, thigh
      third degree T24.709
  lung (with larynx and trachea) T27.5
  mouth T28.5
  neck T20.47
    first degree T20.57
    second degree T20.67
    third degree T20.77
  nose (septum) T20.44
    first degree T20.54
    second degree T20.64
    third degree T20.74
  ocular adnexa —see Corrosion, eye
  orbit region —see Corrosion, eyelid
  palm T23.459
    first degree T23.559
    left T23.452
      first degree T23.552
      second degree T23.652
      third degree T23.752
    right T23.451
      first degree T23.551
      second degree T23.651
      third degree T23.751
    second degree T23.659
    third degree T23.759
  partial thickness - code as Corrosion,
      unspecified degree, by site
  pelvis —see Corrosion, trunk
  penis —see Corrosion, genital organs,
      external, male
  perineum
    female —see Corrosion, genital organs,
        external, female
    male —see Corrosion, genital organs,
        external, male
  periocular area —see Corrosion, eyelid

Corrosion (Continued)
  pharynx T28.5
  rectum T28.7
  respiratory tract T27.7
    larynx —see Corrosion, larynx
    specified part NEC T27.6
    trachea —see Corrosion, larynx
  sac, lacrimal —see Corrosion, eye,
      specified site NEC
  scalp T20.45
    first degree T20.55
    second degree T20.65
    third degree T20.75
  scapular region T22.469
    first degree T22.569
    left T22.462
      first degree T22.562
      second degree T22.662
      third degree T22.762
    right T22.461
      first degree T22.561
      second degree T22.661
      third degree T22.761
    second degree T22.669
    third degree T22.769
  sclera —see Corrosion, eye, specified site NEC
  scrotum —see Corrosion, genital organs,
      external, male
  shoulder T22.459
    first degree T22.559
    left T22.452
      first degree T22.552
      second degree T22.652
      third degree T22.752
    right T22.451
      first degree T22.551
      second degree T22.651
      third degree T22.751
    second degree T22.659
    third degree T22.759
  stomach T28.7
  temple —see Corrosion, head
  testis —see Corrosion, genital organs,
      external, male
  thigh T24.419
    first degree T24.519
    left T24.412
      first degree T24.512
      second degree T24.612
      third degree T24.712
    right T24.411
      first degree T24.511
      second degree T24.611
      third degree T24.711
    second degree T24.619
    third degree T24.719
  thorax (external) —see Corrosion, trunk
  throat (meaning pharynx) T28.5
  thumb(s) T23.419
    first degree T23.519
    left T23.412
      first degree T23.512
      second degree T23.612
      third degree T23.712
    multiple sites with fingers T23.449
      first degree T23.549
      left T23.442
        first degree T23.542
        second degree T23.642
        third degree T23.742
      right T23.441
        first degree T23.541
        second degree T23.641
        third degree T23.741
      second degree T23.649
      third degree T23.749
    right T23.411
      first degree T23.511
      second degree T23.611
      third degree T23.711
    second degree T23.619
    third degree T23.719

Corrosion (Continued)
toe T25.439
first degree T25.539
left T25.432
first degree T25.532
second degree T25.632
third degree T25.732
right T25.431
first degree T25.531
second degree T25.631
third degree T25.731
second degree T25.639
third degree T25.739
tongue T28.5
tonsil(s) T28.5
total body —see Corrosion, multiple body regions
trachea T27.4
with lung T27.5
trunk T21.40
abdominal wall —see Corrosion, abdominal wall
anus —see Corrosion, buttock
axilla —see Corrosion, upper limb
back —see Corrosion, back
breast —see Corrosion, chest wall
buttock —see Corrosion, buttock
chest wall —see Corrosion, chest wall
first degree T21.50
flank —see Corrosion, abdominal wall
genital
female —see Corrosion, genital organs, external, female
male —see Corrosion, genital organs, external, male
groin —see Corrosion, abdominal wall
interscapular region —see Corrosion, back, upper
labia —see Corrosion, genital organs, external, female
lower back —see Corrosion, back
penis —see Corrosion, genital organs, external, male
perineum
female —see Corrosion, genital organs, external, female
male —see Corrosion, genital organs, external, male
scapular region —see Corrosion, upper limb
scrotum —see Corrosion, genital organs, external, male
second degree T21.60
shoulder —see Corrosion, upper limb
specified site NEC T21.49
first degree T21.59
second degree T21.69
third degree T21.79
testes —see Corrosion, genital organs, external, male
third degree T21.70
upper back —see Corrosion, back, upper
vagina T28.8
vulva —see Corrosion, genital organs, external, female
unspecified site with extent of body surface involved specified
less than 10 percent T32.0
10-19 percent (0-9 percent third degree) T32.10
with 10-19 percent third degree T32.11
20-29 percent (0-9 percent third degree) T32.20
with
10-19 percent third degree T32.21
20-29 percent third degree T32.22
30-39 percent (0-9 percent third degree) T32.30
with
10-19 percent third degree T32.31
20-29 percent third degree T32.32
30-39 percent third degree T32.33

Corrosion (Continued)
unspecified site with extent of body surface involved specified (Continued)
40-49 percent (0-9 percent third degree) T32.40
with
10-19 percent third degree T32.41
20-29 percent third degree T32.42
30-39 percent third degree T32.43
40-49 percent third degree T32.44
50-59 percent (0-9 percent third degree) T32.50
with
10-19 percent third degree T32.51
20-29 percent third degree T32.52
30-39 percent third degree T32.53
40-49 percent third degree T32.54
50-59 percent third degree T32.55
60-69 percent (0-9 percent third degree) T32.60
with
10-19 percent third degree T32.61
20-29 percent third degree T32.62
30-39 percent third degree T32.63
40-49 percent third degree T32.64
50-59 percent third degree T32.65
60-69 percent third degree T32.66
70-79 percent (0-9 percent third degree) T32.70
with
10-19 percent third degree T32.71
20-29 percent third degree T32.72
30-39 percent third degree T32.73
40-49 percent third degree T32.74
50-59 percent third degree T32.75
60-69 percent third degree T32.76
70-79 percent third degree T32.77
80-89 percent (0-9 percent third degree) T32.80
with
10-19 percent third degree T32.81
20-29 percent third degree T32.82
30-39 percent third degree T32.83
40-49 percent third degree T32.84
50-59 percent third degree T32.85
60-69 percent third degree T32.86
70-79 percent third degree T32.87
80-89 percent third degree T32.88
90 percent or more (0-9 percent third degree) T32.90
with
10-19 percent third degree T32.91
20-29 percent third degree T32.92
30-39 percent third degree T32.93
40-49 percent third degree T32.94
50-59 percent third degree T32.95
60-69 percent third degree T32.96
70-79 percent third degree T32.97
80-89 percent third degree T32.98
90-99 percent third degree T32.99
upper limb (axilla) (scapular region) T22.40
above elbow —see Corrosion, above elbow
axilla —see Corrosion, axilla
elbow —see Corrosion, elbow
first degree T22.50
forearm —see Corrosion, forearm
hand —see Corrosion, hand
interscapular region —see Corrosion, back, upper
multiple sites T22.499
first degree T22.599
left T22.492
first degree T22.592
second degree T22.692
third degree T22.792
right T22.491
first degree T22.591
second degree T22.691
third degree T22.791
second degree T22.699
third degree T22.799
scapular region —see Corrosion, scapular region

Corrosion (Continued)
upper limb (axilla) (scapular region) (Continued)
second degree T22.60
shoulder —see Corrosion, shoulder
third degree T22.70
wrist —see Corrosion, hand
uterus T28.8
vagina T28.8
vulva —see Corrosion, genital organs, external, female
wrist T23.479
first degree T23.579
left T23.472
first degree T23.572
second degree T23.672
third degree T23.772
multiple sites with hand T23.499
first degree T23.599
left T23.492
first degree T23.592
second degree T23.692
third degree T23.792
right T23.491
first degree T23.591
second degree T23.691
third degree T23.791
second degree T23.699
third degree T23.799
right T23.471
first degree T23.571
second degree T23.671
third degree T23.771
second degree T23.679
third degree T23.779
Corrosive burn —see Corrosion
Corsican fever —see Malaria
Cortical —see condition
Cortico-adrenal —see condition
Coryza (acute) J00
with grippe or influenza —see Influenza, with, respiratory manifestations NEC
syphilitic
congenital (chronic) A50.05
Costen's syndrome or complex M26.69
Costiveness —see Constipation
Costochondritis M94.0
Cot death R99
Cotard's syndrome F22
Cotia virus B08.8
Cotton wool spots (retinal) H35.81
Cotungo's disease —see Sciatica
Cough (affected) (epidemic) (nervous) R05.9
with hemorrhage —see Hemoptysis
acute R05.1
bronchial R05.8
with grippe or influenza —see Influenza, with, respiratory manifestations NEC
chronic R05.3
functional F45.8
hysterical F45.8
laryngeal, spasmodic R05.8
paroxysmal, due to Bordetella pertussis (without pneumonia) A37.00
with pneumonia A37.01
persistent R05.3
refractory R05.3
psychogenic F45.8
smokers' J41.0
specified NEC R05.8
subacute R05.2
syncope R05.4
tea taster's B49
unexplained R05.3
Counseling (for) Z71.9
abuse NEC
perpetrator Z69.82
victim Z69.81
alcohol abuser Z71.41
family Z71.42
child abuse
nonparental
perpetrator Z69.021
victim Z69.020

▶ New   ⇒ Revised   ~~deleted~~ Deleted   ● Use Additional Character(s)

Counseling *(Continued)*
  parental
    perpetrator Z69.011
    victim Z69.010
  consanguinity Z71.89
  contraceptive Z30.09
  dietary Z71.3
  drug abuser Z71.51
    family member Z71.52
  exercise Z71.82
  family Z71.89
  fertility preservation (prior to cancer therapy)
    (prior to removal of gonads) Z31.62
  for non-attending third party Z71.0
    related to sexual behavior or orientation Z70.2
  genetic
    nonprocreative Z71.83
    procreative NEC Z31.5
  gestational carrier Z31.7
  health (advice) (education) (instruction) —*see*
    Counseling, medical
    risk for travel (international) Z71.84
  human immunodeficiency virus (HIV) Z71.7
▶ immunization safety Z71.85
  impotence Z70.1
  insulin pump use Z46.81
  medical (for) Z71.9
    boarding school resident Z59.3
    consanguinity Z71.89
    feared complaint and no disease found Z71.1
    human immunodeficiency virus (HIV) Z71.7
    institutional resident Z59.3
    on behalf of another Z71.0
      related to sexual behavior or orientation
        Z70.2
    person living alone Z60.2
    specified reason NEC Z71.89
  natural family planning
    procreative Z31.61
    to avoid pregnancy Z30.02
  perpetrator (of)
    abuse NEC Z69.82
    child abuse
      non-parental Z69.021
      parental Z69.011
    rape NEC Z69.82
    spousal abuse Z69.12
  procreative NEC Z31.69
    fertility preservation (prior to cancer therapy)
      (prior to removal of gonads) Z31.62
    using natural family planning Z31.61
  promiscuity Z70.1
  rape victim Z69.81
  religious Z71.81
  safety for travel (international) Z71.84
  sex, sexual (related to) Z70.9
    attitude(s) Z70.0
    behavior or orientation Z70.1
    combined concerns Z70.3
    non-responsiveness Z70.1
    on behalf of third party Z70.2
    specified reason NEC Z70.8
  specified reason NEC Z71.89
  spiritual Z71.81
  spousal abuse (perpetrator) Z69.12
    victim Z69.11
  substance abuse Z71.89
    alcohol Z71.41
    drug Z71.51
    tobacco Z71.6
  travel (international) Z71.84
  tobacco use Z71.6
  use (of)
    insulin pump Z46.81
▶ vaccine product safety Z71.85
  victim (of)
    abuse Z69.81
    child abuse
      by parent Z69.010
      non-parental Z69.020
    rape NEC Z69.81
Coupled rhythm R00.8

Couvelaire syndrome or uterus (complicating
  delivery) O45.8X-●
COVID-19 U07.1
▶ condition post U09.9
  contact (with) Z20.822
  exposure (to) Z20.822
  history of (personal) Z86.16
▶ long (haul) U09.9
  pneumonia J12.82
  screening Z11.52
▶ sequelae (post acute) U09.9
Cowperitis —*see* Urethritis
Cowper's gland —*see* condition
Cowpox B08.010
  due to vaccination T88.1
Coxa
  magna M91.4-●
  plana M91.2-●
  valga (acquired) —*see also* Deformity, limb,
    specified type NEC, thigh
    congenital Q65.81
    sequelae (late effect) of rickets E64.3
  vara (acquired) —*see also* Deformity, limb,
    specified type NEC, thigh
    congenital Q65.82
    sequelae (late effect) of rickets E64.3
Coxalgia, coxalgic (nontuberculous) —*see also*
  Pain, joint, hip
  tuberculous A18.02
Coxitis —*see* Monoarthritis, hip
Coxsackie (virus) (infection) B34.1
  as cause of disease classified elsewhere B97.11
  carditis B33.20
  central nervous system NEC A88.8
  endocarditis B33.21
  enteritis A08.39
  meningitis (aseptic) A87.0
  myocarditis B33.22
  pericarditis B33.23
  pharyngitis B08.5
  pleurodynia B33.0
  specific disease NEC B33.8
Crabs, meaning pubic lice B85.3
Crack baby P04.41
Cracked nipple N64.0
  associated with
    lactation O92.13
    pregnancy O92.11-●
    puerperium O92.12
Cracked tooth K03.81
Cradle cap L21.0
Craft neurosis F48.8
Cramp(s) R25.2
  abdominal —*see* Pain, abdominal
  bathing T75.1
  colic R10.83
    psychogenic F45.8
  due to immersion T75.1
  fireman T67.2
  heat T67.2
  immersion T75.1
  intestinal —*see* Pain, abdominal
    psychogenic F45.8
  leg, sleep related G47.62
  limb (lower) (upper) NEC R25.2
    sleep related G47.62
  linotypist's F48.8
    organic G25.89
  muscle (limb) (general) R25.2
    due to immersion T75.1
    psychogenic F45.8
  occupational (hand) F48.8
    organic G25.89
  salt-depletion E87.1
  sleep related, leg G47.62
  stoker's T67.2
  swimmer's T75.1
  telegrapher's F48.8
    organic G25.89
  typist's F48.8
    organic G25.89
  uterus N94.89
    menstrual —*see* Dysmenorrhea

Cramp(s) *(Continued)*
  writer's F48.8
    organic G25.89
Cranial —*see* condition
Craniocleidodysostosis Q74.0
Craniofenestria (skull) Q75.8
Craniolacunia (skull) Q75.8
Craniopagus Q89.4
Craniopathy, metabolic M85.2
Craniopharyngeal —*see* condition
Craniopharyngioma D44.4
Craniorachischisis (totalis) Q00.1
Cranioschisis Q75.8
Craniostenosis Q75.0
Craniosynostosis Q75.0
Craniotabes (cause unknown) M83.8
  neonatal P96.3
  rachitic E64.3
  syphilitic A50.56
Cranium —*see* condition
Craw-craw —*see* Onchocerciasis
Creaking joint —*see* Derangement, joint,
  specified type NEC
Creeping
  eruption B76.9
  palsy or paralysis G12.22
Crenated tongue K14.8
Creotoxism A05.9
Crepitus
  caput Q75.8
  joint —*see* Derangement, joint, specified type
    NEC
Crescent or conus choroid, congenital Q14.3
CREST syndrome M34.1
Cretin, cretinism (congenital) (endemic)
  (nongoitrous) (sporadic) E00.9
  pelvis
    with disproportion (fetopelvic) O33.0
      causing obstructed labor O65.0
  type
    hypothyroid E00.1
    mixed E00.2
    myxedematous E00.1
    neurological E00.0
Creutzfeldt-Jakob disease or syndrome (with
  dementia) A81.00
  familial A81.09
  iatrogenic A81.09
  specified NEC A81.09
  sporadic A81.09
  variant (vCJD) A81.01
Crib death R99
Cribriform hymen Q52.3
Cri-du-chat syndrome Q93.4
Crigler-Najjar disease or syndrome E80.5
Crime, victim of Z65.4
Crimean hemorrhagic fever A98.0
Criminalism F60.2
Crisis
  abdomen R10.0
  acute reaction F43.0
  addisonian E27.2
  adrenal (cortical) E27.2
  celiac K90.0
  Dietl's N13.8
  emotional —*see also* Disorder, adjustment
    acute reaction to stress F43.0
    specific to childhood and adolescence F93.8
  glaucomatocyclitic —*see* Glaucoma,
    secondary, inflammation
  heart —*see* Failure, heart
  nitritoid I95.2
    correct substance properly administered —
      see Table of Drugs and Chemicals, by
      drug, adverse effect
    overdose or wrong substance given
      or taken —*see* Table of Drugs and
      Chemicals, by drug, poisoning
  oculogyric H51.8
    psychogenic F45.8
  Pel's (tabetic) A52.11
  psychosexual identity F64.2
  renal N28.0

Crisis *(Continued)*
  sickle-cell D57.00
    with
      acute chest syndrome D57.01
      cerebral vascular involvement D57.03
      crisis (painful) D57.00
        with complication specified NEC D57.09
      splenic sequestration D57.02
      vasoocclusive pain D57.00
  state (acute reaction) F43.0
  tabetic A52.11
  thyroid —*see* Thyrotoxicosis with thyroid
      storm
  thyrotoxic —*see* Thyrotoxicosis with thyroid
      storm
Crocq's disease (acrocyanosis) I73.89
Crohn's disease —*see* Enteritis, regional
Crooked septum, nasal J34.2
Cross syndrome E70.328
Crossbite (anterior) (posterior) M26.24
Cross-eye —*see* Strabismus, convergent
    concomitant
Croup, croupous (catarrhal) (infectious)
    (inflammatory) (nondiphtheritic) J05.0
  bronchial J20.9
  diphtheritic A36.2
  false J38.5
  spasmodic J38.5
    diphtheritic A36.2
  stridulous J38.5
    diphtheritic A36.2
Crouzon's disease Q75.1
Crowding, tooth, teeth, fully erupted M26.31
CRST syndrome M34.1
Cruchet's disease A85.8
Cruelty in children —*see also* Disorder, conduct
Crural ulcer —*see* Ulcer, lower limb
Crush, crushed, crushing T14.8
  abdomen S38.1
  ankle S97.0-●
  arm (upper) (and shoulder) S47.-●
  axilla —*see* Crush, arm
  back, lower S38.1
  buttock S38.1
  cheek S07.0
  chest S28.0
  cranium S07.1
  ear S07.0
  elbow S57.0-●
  extremity
    lower
      ankle —*see* Crush, ankle
      below knee —*see* Crush, leg
      foot —*see* Crush, foot
      hip —*see* Crush, hip
      knee —*see* Crush, knee
      thigh —*see* Crush, thigh
      toe —*see* Crush, toe
    upper
      below elbow S67.9-●
      elbow —*see* Crush, elbow
      finger —*see* Crush, finger
      forearm —*see* Crush, forearm
      hand —*see* Crush, hand
      thumb —*see* Crush, thumb
      upper arm —*see* Crush, arm
      wrist —*see* Crush, wrist
  face S07.0
  finger(s) S67.1-●
    with hand (and wrist) —*see* Crush, hand,
        specified site NEC
    index S67.19-●
    little S67.19-●
    middle S67.19-●
    ring S67.19-●
    thumb —*see* Crush, thumb
  foot S97.8-●
    toe —*see* Crush, toe
  forearm S57.8-●
  genitalia, external
    female S38.002
      vagina S38.03
      vulva S38.03

Crush, crushed, crushing *(Continued)*
  genitalia, external *(Continued)*
    male S38.001
      penis S38.01
      scrotum S38.02
      testis S38.02
  hand (except fingers alone) S67.2-●
    with wrist S67.4-●
  head S07.9
    specified NEC S07.8
  heel —*see* Crush, foot
  hip S77.0-●
    with thigh S77.2-●
  internal organ (abdomen, chest, or pelvis)
      NEC T14.8
  knee S87.0-●
  labium (majus) (minus) S38.03
  larynx S17.0
  leg (lower) S87.8-●
    knee —*see* Crush, knee
  lip S07.0
  lower
    back S38.1
    leg —*see* Crush, leg
  neck S17.9
  nerve —*see* Injury, nerve
  nose S07.0
  pelvis S38.1
  penis S38.01
  scalp S07.8
  scapular region —*see* Crush, arm
  scrotum S38.02
  severe, unspecified site T14.8
  shoulder (and upper arm) —*see* Crush, arm
  skull S07.1
  syndrome (complication of trauma) T79.5
  testis S38.02
  thigh S77.1-●
    with hip S77.2-●
  throat S17.8
  thumb S67.0-●
    with hand (and wrist) —*see* Crush, hand,
        specified site NEC
  toe(s) S97.10-●
    great S97.11-●
    lesser S97.12-●
  trachea S17.0
  vagina S38.03
  vulva S38.03
  wrist S67.3-●
    with hand S67.4-●
Crusta lactea L21.0
Crusts R23.4
Crutch paralysis —*see* Injury, brachial plexus
Cruveilhier-Baumgarten cirrhosis, disease or
    syndrome K74.69
Cruveilhier's atrophy or disease G12.8
Crying (constant) (continuous) (excessive)
  child, adolescent, or adult R45.83
  infant (baby) (newborn) R68.11
Cryofibrinogenemia D89.2
Cryoglobulinemia (essential) (idiopathic)
    (mixed) (primary) (purpura) (secondary)
    (vasculitis) D89.1
  with lung involvement D89.1 *[J99]*
Cryptitis (anal) (rectal) K62.89
Cryptococcosis, cryptococcus (infection)
    (neoformans) B45.9
  bone B45.3
  cerebral B45.1
  cutaneous B45.2
  disseminated B45.7
  generalized B45.7
  meningitis B45.1
  meningocerebralis B45.1
  osseous B45.3
  pulmonary B45.0
  skin B45.2
  specified NEC B45.8
Cryptopapillitis (anus) K62.89
Cryptophthalmos Q11.2
  syndrome Q87.0

Cryptorchid, cryptorchism, cryptorchidism Q53.9
  bilateral Q53.20
    abdominal Q53.211
    perineal Q53.22
  unilateral Q53.10
    abdominal Q53.111
    perineal Q53.12
Cryptosporidiosis A07.2
  hepatobiliary B88.8
  respiratory B88.8
Cryptostromosis J67.6
Crystalluria R82.998
Cubitus
  congenital Q68.8
  valgus (acquired) M21.0-●
    congenital Q68.8
    sequelae (late effect) of rickets E64.3
  varus (acquired) M21.1-●
    congenital Q68.8
    sequelae (late effect) of rickets E64.3
Cultural deprivation or shock Z60.3
Curling esophagus K22.4
Curling's ulcer —*see* Ulcer, peptic, acute
Curschmann (-Batten) (-Steinert) **disease or**
    syndrome G71.11
Curse, Ondine's —*see* Apnea, sleep
Curvature
  organ or site, congenital NEC —*see* Distortion
  penis (lateral) Q55.61
  Pott's (spinal) A18.01
  radius, idiopathic, progressive (congenital)
      Q74.0
  spine (acquired) (angular) (idiopathic)
      (incorrect) (postural) —*see* Dorsopathy,
      deforming
    congenital Q67.5
    due to or associated with
      Charcot-Marie-Tooth disease —*see also*
          subcategory M49.8 G60.0
      osteitis
        deformans M88.88
        fibrosa cystica —*see also* subcategory
            M49.8 E21.0
      tuberculosis (Pott's curvature) A18.01
    sequelae (late effect) of rickets E64.3
    tuberculous A18.01
Cushingoid due to steroid therapy E24.2
  correct substance properly administered —*see*
      Table of Drugs and Chemicals, by drug,
      adverse effect
  overdose or wrong substance given
      or taken —*see* Table of Drugs and
      Chemicals, by drug, poisoning
Cushing's
  syndrome or disease E24.9
    drug-induced E24.2
    iatrogenic E24.2
    pituitary-dependent E24.0
    specified NEC E24.8
  ulcer —*see* Ulcer, peptic, acute
Cusp, Carabelli - omit code
Cut (external) —*see also* Laceration
  muscle —*see* Injury, muscle
Cutaneous —*see also* condition
  hemorrhage R23.3
  larva migrans B76.9
Cutis —*see also* condition
  hyperelastica Q82.8
    acquired L57.4
  laxa (hyperelastica) —*see* Dermatolysis
  marmorata R23.8
  osteosis L94.2
  pendula —*see* Dermatolysis
  rhomboidalis nuchae L57.2
  verticis gyrata Q82.8
    acquired L91.8
Cyanosis R23.0
  due to
    patent foramen botalli Q21.1
    persistent foramen ovale Q21.1
  enterogenous D74.8
  paroxysmal digital —*see* Raynaud's disease
    with gangrene I73.01
  retina, retinal H35.89

Cyanotic heart disease I24.9
  congenital Q24.9
Cycle
  anovulatory N97.0
  menstrual, irregular N92.6
Cyclencephaly Q04.9
Cyclical vomiting, in migraine (see also
    Vomiting, cyclical) G43.A0
  psychogenic F50.89
Cyclitis —see also Iridocyclitis H20.9
  chronic —see Iridocyclitis, chronic
  Fuchs' heterochromic H20.81-●
  granulomatous —see Iridocyclitis, chronic
  lens-induced —see Iridocyclitis,
      lens-induced
  posterior H30.2-●
Cycloid personality F34.0
Cyclophoria H50.54
Cyclopia, cyclops Q87.0
Cyclopism Q87.0
Cyclosporiasis A07.4
Cyclothymia F34.0
Cyclothymic personality F34.0
Cyclotropia H50.41-●
Cylindroma —see also Neoplasm, malignant,
    by site
  eccrine dermal —see Neoplasm, skin, benign
  skin —see Neoplasm, skin, benign
Cylindruria R82.998
Cynanche
  diphtheritic A36.2
  tonsillaris J36
Cynophobia F40.218
Cynorexia R63.2
Cyphosis —see Kyphosis
Cyprus fever —see Brucellosis
Cyst (colloid) (mucous) (simple) (retention)
  adenoid (infected) J35.8
  adrenal gland E27.8
    congenital Q89.1
  air, lung J98.4
  allantoic Q64.4
  alveolar process (jaw bone) M27.40
  amnion, amniotic O41.8X-●
  aneurysmal M27.49
  anterior
    chamber (eye) —see Cyst, iris
    nasopalatine K09.1
  antrum J34.1
  anus K62.89
  apical (tooth) (periodontal) K04.8
  appendix K38.8
  arachnoid, brain (acquired) G93.0
    congenital Q04.6
  arytenoid J38.7
  Baker's M71.2-●
    ruptured M66.0
    tuberculous A18.02
  Bartholin's gland N75.0
  bile duct (common) (hepatic) K83.5
  bladder (multiple) (trigone) N32.89
  blue dome (breast) —see Cyst, breast
  bone (local) NEC M85.60
    aneurysmal M85.50
      ankle M85.57-●
      foot M85.57-●
      forearm M85.53-●
      hand M85.54-●
      jaw M27.49
      lower leg M85.56-●
      multiple site M85.59
      neck M85.58
      rib M85.58
      shoulder M85.51-●
      skull M85.58
      specified site NEC M85.58
      thigh M85.55-●
      toe M85.57-●
      upper arm M85.52-●
      vertebra M85.58
    solitary M85.40
      ankle M85.47-●
      fibula M85.46-●

Cyst (Continued)
  bone NEC (Continued)
    solitary (Continued)
      foot M85.47-●
      hand M85.44-●
      humerus M85.42-●
      jaw M27.49
      neck M85.48
      pelvis M85.45-●
      radius M85.43-●
      rib M85.48
      shoulder M85.41-●
      skull M85.48
      specified site NEC M85.48
      tibia M85.46-●
      toe M85.47-●
      ulna M85.43-●
      vertebra M85.48
    specified type NEC M85.60
      ankle M85.67-●
      foot M85.67-●
      forearm M85.63-●
      hand M85.64-●
      jaw M27.40
        developmental (nonodontogenic) K09.1
        odontogenic K09.0
        latent M27.0
      lower leg M85.66-●
      multiple site M85.69
      neck M85.68
      rib M85.68
      shoulder M85.61-●
      skull M85.68
      specified site NEC M85.68
      thigh M85.65-●
      toe M85.67-●
      upper arm M85.62-●
      vertebra M85.68
  brain (acquired) G93.0
    congenital Q04.6
    hydatid B67.99 [G94]
    third ventricle (colloid), congenital
        Q04.6
  branchial (cleft) Q18.0
  branchiogenic Q18.0
  breast (benign) (blue dome) (pedunculated)
      (solitary) N60.0-●
    involution —see Dysplasia, mammary,
        specified type NEC
    sebaceous —see Dysplasia, mammary,
        specified type NEC
  broad ligament (benign) N83.8
  bronchogenic (mediastinal) (sequestration)
      J98.4
    congenital Q33.0
  buccal K09.8
  bulbourethral gland N36.8
  bursa, bursal NEC M71.30
    with rupture —see Rupture, synovium
    ankle M71.37-●
    elbow M71.32-●
    foot M71.37-●
    hand M71.34-●
    hip M71.35-●
    multiple sites M71.39
    pharyngeal J39.2
    popliteal space —see Cyst, Baker's
    shoulder M71.31-●
    specified site NEC M71.38
    wrist M71.33-●
  calcifying odontogenic D16.5
    upper jaw (bone) (maxilla) D16.4
  canal of Nuck (female) N94.89
    congenital Q52.4
  canthus —see Cyst, conjunctiva
  carcinomatous —see Neoplasm, malignant,
      by site
  cauda equina G95.89
  cavum septi pellucidi —see Cyst, brain
  celomic (pericardium) Q24.8
  cerebellopontine (angle) —see Cyst, brain
  cerebellum —see Cyst, brain
  cerebral —see Cyst, brain

Cyst (Continued)
  cervical lateral Q18.0
  cervix NEC N88.8
    embryonic Q51.6
    nabothian N88.8
  chiasmal optic NEC —see Disorder, optic,
      chiasm
  chocolate (ovary) N80.1
  choledochus, congenital Q44.4
  chorion O41.8X-●
  choroid plexus G93.0
    congenital Q04.6
  ciliary body —see Cyst, iris
  clitoris N90.7
  colon K63.89
  common (bile) duct K83.5
  congenital NEC Q89.8
    adrenal gland Q89.1
    epiglottis Q31.8
    esophagus Q39.8
    fallopian tube Q50.4
    kidney Q61.00
      more than one (multiple) Q61.02
        specified as polycystic Q61.3
          adult type Q61.2
          infantile type NEC Q61.19
            collecting duct dilation Q61.11
      solitary Q61.01
    larynx Q31.8
    liver Q44.6
    lung Q33.0
    mediastinum Q34.1
    ovary Q50.1
    oviduct Q50.4
    periurethral (tissue) Q64.79
    prepuce Q55.69
    salivary gland (any) Q38.4
    sublingual Q38.6
    submaxillary gland Q38.6
    thymus (gland) Q89.2
    tongue Q38.3
    ureterovesical orifice Q62.8
    vulva Q52.79
  conjunctiva H11.44-●
  cornea H18.89-●
  corpora quadrigemina G93.0
  corpus
    albicans N83.29-●
    luteum (hemorrhagic) (ruptured) N83.1-●
  Cowper's gland (benign) (infected) N36.8
  cranial meninges G93.0
  craniobuccal pouch E23.6
  craniopharyngeal pouch E23.6
  cystic duct K82.8
  Cysticercus —see Cysticercosis
  Dandy-Walker Q03.1
    with spina bifida —see Spina bifida
  dental (root) K04.8
    developmental K09.0
    eruption K09.0
    primordial K09.0
  dentigerous (mandible) (maxilla) K09.0
  dermoid —see Neoplasm, benign, by site
    with malignant transformation C56.-●
    implantation
      external area or site (skin) NEC L72.0
      iris —see Cyst, iris, implantation
      vagina N89.8
      vulva N90.7
    mouth K09.8
    oral soft tissue K09.8
    sacrococcygeal —see Cyst, pilonidal
  developmental K09.1
    odontogenic K09.0
    oral region (nonodontogenic) K09.1
    ovary, ovarian Q50.1
  dura (cerebral) G93.0
    spinal G96.198
  ear (external) Q18.1
  echinococcal —see Echinococcus
  embryonic
    cervix uteri Q51.6
    fallopian tube Q50.4

Cyst *(Continued)*
  embryonic *(Continued)*
    vagina Q52.4
  endometrium, endometrial (uterus) N85.8
    ectopic —*see* Endometriosis
  enterogenous Q43.8
  epidermal, epidermoid (inclusion) *(see also*
    Cyst, skin)* L72.0
    mouth K09.8
    oral soft tissue K09.8
  epididymis N50.3
  epiglottis J38.7
  epiphysis cerebri E34.8
  epithelial (inclusion) L72.0
  epoophoron Q50.5
  eruption K09.0
➧ esophagus K22.89
  ethmoid sinus J34.1
  external female genital organs NEC N90.7
  eye NEC H57.89
    congenital Q15.8
  eyelid (sebaceous) H02.829
    infected —*see* Hordeolum
    left H02.826
      lower H02.825
      upper H02.824
    right H02.823
      lower H02.822
      upper H02.821
  fallopian tube N83.8
    congenital Q50.4
  fimbrial (twisted) Q50.4
  fissural (oral region) K09.1
  follicle (graafian) (hemorrhagic) N83.0-●
    nabothian N88.8
  follicular (atretic) (hemorrhagic) (ovarian)
    N83.0-●
    dentigerous K09.0
    odontogenic K09.0
    skin L72.9
      specified NEC L72.8
  frontal sinus J34.1
  gallbladder K82.8
  ganglion —*see* Ganglion
  Gartner's duct Q52.4
  gingiva K09.0
  gland of Moll —*see* Cyst, eyelid
  globulomaxillary K09.1
  graafian follicle (hemorrhagic) N83.0-●
  granulosal lutein (hemorrhagic) N83.1-●
  hemangiomatous D18.00
    intra-abdominal D18.03
    intracranial D18.02
    skin D18.01
    specified site NEC D18.09
  hemorrhagic M27.49
  hydatid —*see also* Echinococcus B67.90
    brain B67.99 *[G94]*
    liver —*see also* Cyst, liver, hydatid B67.8
    lung NEC B67.99 *[J99]*
    Morgagni
      female Q50.5
      male (epididymal) Q55.4
        testicular Q55.29
    specified site NEC B67.99
  hymen N89.8
    embryonic Q52.4
  hypopharynx J39.2
  hypophysis, hypophyseal (duct) (recurrent)
    E23.6
    cerebri E23.6
  implantation (dermoid)
    external area or site (skin) NEC L72.0
    iris —*see* Cyst, iris, implantation
    vagina N89.8
    vulva N90.7
  incisive canal K09.1
  inclusion (epidermal) (epithelial)
    (epidermoid) (squamous) L72.0
    not of skin - code under Cyst, by site
  intestine (large) (small) K63.89
  intracranial —*see* Cyst, brain

Cyst *(Continued)*
  intraligamentous —*see also* Disorder, ligament
    knee —*see* Derangement, knee
  intrasellar E23.6
  iris H21.309
    exudative H21.31-●
    idiopathic H21.30-●
    implantation H21.32-●
    parasitic H21.33-●
    pars plana (primary) H21.34-●
      exudative H21.35-●
  jaw (bone) M27.40
    aneurysmal M27.49
    developmental (odontogenic) K09.0
    fissural K09.1
    hemorrhagic M27.49
    traumatic M27.49
  joint NEC —*see* Disorder, joint, specified type
    NEC
  kidney (acquired) N28.1
    calyceal —*see* Hydronephrosis
    congenital Q61.00
    more than one (multiple) Q61.02
      specified as polycystic Q61.3
        adult type (autosomal dominant)
          Q61.2
        infantile type (autosomal recessive)
          NEC Q61.19
            collecting duct dilation Q61.11
    pyelogenic —*see* Hydronephrosis
    simple N28.1
    solitary (single) Q61.01
      acquired N28.1
  labium (majus) (minus) N90.7
    sebaceous N90.7
  lacrimal —*see also* Disorder, lacrimal system,
    specified NEC
    gland H04.13-●
    passages or sac —*see* Disorder, lacrimal
      system, specified NEC
  larynx J38.7
  lateral periodontal K09.0
  lens H27.8
    congenital Q12.8
  lip (gland) K13.0
  liver (idiopathic) (simple) K76.89
    congenital Q44.6
    hydatid B67.8
      granulosus B67.0
      multilocularis B67.5
  lung J98.4
    congenital Q33.0
    giant bullous J43.9
  lutein N83.1-●
  lymphangiomatous D18.1
  lymphoepithelial, oral soft tissue K09.8
  macula —*see* Degeneration, macula, hole
  malignant —*see* Neoplasm, malignant, by site
  mammary gland —*see* Cyst, breast
  mandible M27.40
    dentigerous K09.0
    radicular K04.8
  maxilla M27.40
    dentigerous K09.0
    radicular K04.8
  medial, face and neck Q18.8
  median
    anterior maxillary K09.1
    palatal K09.1
  mediastinum, congenital Q34.1
  meibomian (gland) —*see* Chalazion
    infected —*see* Hordeolum
  membrane, brain G93.0
  meninges (cerebral) G93.0
    spinal G96.198
  meniscus, knee —*see* Derangement, knee,
    meniscus, cystic
  mesentery, mesenteric K66.8
    chyle I89.8
  mesonephric duct
    female Q50.5
    male Q55.4
  milk N64.89

Cyst *(Continued)*
  Morgagni (hydatid)
    female Q50.5
    male (epididymal) Q55.4
      testicular Q55.29
  mouth K09.8
  Müllerian duct Q50.4
    appendix testis Q55.29
    cervix Q51.6
    fallopian tube Q50.4
    female Q50.4
    male Q55.29
    prostatic utricle Q55.4
    vagina (embryonal) Q52.4
  multilocular (ovary) D39.10
    benign —*see* Neoplasm, benign, by site
  myometrium N85.8
  nabothian (follicle) (ruptured) N88.8
  nasoalveolar K09.1
  nasolabial K09.1
  nasopalatine (anterior) (duct) K09.1
  nasopharynx J39.2
  neoplastic —*see* Neoplasm, uncertain
    behavior, by site
    benign —*see* Neoplasm, benign, by site
  nerve root
    cervical G96.191
    lumbar G96.191
    sacral G96.191
    thoracic G96.191
  nervous system NEC G96.89
  neuroenteric (congenital) Q06.8
  nipple —*see* Cyst, breast
  nose (turbinates) J34.1
    sinus J34.1
  odontogenic, developmental K09.0
  omentum (lesser) K66.8
    congenital Q45.8
  ora serrata —*see* Cyst, retina, ora serrata
  oral
    region K09.9
      developmental (nonodontogenic) K09.1
      specified NEC K09.8
    soft tissue K09.9
      specified NEC K09.8
  orbit H05.81-●
  ovary, ovarian (twisted) N83.20-●
    adherent N83.20-●
    chocolate N80.1
    corpus
      albicans N83.29-●
      luteum (hemorrhagic) N83.1-●
    dermoid D27.9
    developmental Q50.1
    due to failure of involution NEC N83.20-●
    endometrial N80.1
    follicular (graafian) (hemorrhagic) N83.0-●
    hemorrhagic N83.20-●
    in pregnancy or childbirth O34.8-●
      with obstructed labor O65.5
    multilocular D39.10
    pseudomucinous D27.9
    retention N83.29-●
    serous N83.20-●
    specified NEC N83.29-●
    theca lutein (hemorrhagic) N83.1-●
    tuberculous A18.18
  oviduct N83.8
  palate (median) (fissural) K09.1
  palatine papilla (jaw) K09.1
  pancreas, pancreatic (hemorrhagic) (true) K86.2
    congenital Q45.2
    false K86.3
  paralabral
    hip M24.85-●
    shoulder S43.43-●
  paramesonephric duct Q50.4
    female Q50.4
    male Q55.29
  paranephric N28.1
  paraphysis, cerebri, congenital Q04.6
  parasitic B89
  parathyroid (gland) E21.4

Cyst *(Continued)*
paratubal N83.8
paraurethral duct N36.8
paroophoron Q50.5
parotid gland K11.6
parovarian Q50.5
pelvis, female N94.89
in pregnancy or childbirth O34.8-●
causing obstructed labor O65.5
penis (sebaceous) N48.89
periapical K04.8
pericardial (congenital) Q24.8
acquired (secondary) I31.8
pericoronal K09.0
perineural G96.191
periodontal K04.8
lateral K09.0
peripelvic (lymphatic) N28.1
peritoneum K66.8
chylous I89.8
periventricular, acquired, newborn P91.1
pharynx (wall) J39.2
pilar L72.11
pilonidal (infected) (rectum) L05.91
with abscess L05.01
malignant C44.59-●
pituitary (duct) (gland) E23.6
placenta O43.19-●
pleura J94.8
popliteal —*see* Cyst, Baker's
porencephalic Q04.6
acquired G93.0
postanal (infected) —*see* Cyst, pilonidal
postmastoidectomy cavity (mucosal) —*see*
Complications, postmastoidectomy, cyst
preauricular Q18.1
prepuce N47.4
congenital Q55.69
primordial (jaw) K09.0
prostate N42.83
pseudomucinous (ovary) D27.9
pupillary, miotic H21.27-●
radicular (residual) K04.8
radiculodental K04.8
ranular K11.8
Rathke's pouch E23.6
rectum (epithelium) (mucous) K62.89
renal —*see* Cyst, kidney
residual (radicular) K04.8
retention (ovary) N83.29-●
salivary gland K11.6
retina H33.19-●
ora serrata H33.11-●
parasitic H33.12-●
retroperitoneal K68.9
sacrococcygeal (dermoid) —*see* Cyst,
pilonidal
salivary gland or duct (mucous extravasation
or retention) K11.6
Sampson's N80.1
sclera H15.89
scrotum L72.9
sebaceous L72.3
sebaceous (duct) (gland) L72.3
breast —*see* Dysplasia, mammary, specified
type NEC
eyelid —*see* Cyst, eyelid
genital organ NEC
female N94.89
male N50.89
scrotum L72.3
semilunar cartilage (knee) (multiple) —*see*
Derangement, knee, meniscus, cystic
seminal vesicle N50.89
serous (ovary) N83.20-●
sinus (accessory) (nasal) J34.1
Skene's gland N36.8
skin L72.9
breast —*see* Dysplasia, mammary, specified
type NEC
epidermal, epidermoid L72.0
epithelial L72.0
eyelid —*see* Cyst, eyelid

Cyst *(Continued)*
skin *(Continued)*
genital organ NEC
female N90.7
male N50.89
inclusion L72.0
scrotum L72.9
sebaceous L72.3
sweat gland or duct L74.8
solitary
bone —*see* Cyst, bone, solitary
jaw M27.40
kidney N28.1
spermatic cord N50.89
sphenoid sinus J34.1
spinal meninges G96.198
spleen NEC D73.4
congenital Q89.09
hydatid —*see also* Echinococcus B67.99 *[D77]*
Stafne's M27.0
subarachnoid intrasellar R93.0
subcutaneous, pheomycotic (chromomycotic)
B43.2
subdural (cerebral) G93.0
spinal cord G96.198
sublingual gland K11.6
submandibular gland K11.6
submaxillary gland K11.6
suburethral N36.8
suprarenal gland E27.8
suprasellar —*see* Cyst, brain
sweat gland or duct L74.8
synovial —*see also* Cyst, bursa
ruptured —*see* Rupture, synovium
Tarlov G96.191
tarsal —*see* Chalazion
tendon (sheath) —*see* Disorder, tendon,
specified type NEC
testis N44.2
tunica albuginea N44.1
theca lutein (ovary) N83.1-●
Thornwaldt's J39.2
thymus (gland) E32.8
thyroglossal duct (infected) (persistent) Q89.2
thyroid (gland) E04.1
thyrolingual duct (infected) (persistent) Q89.2
tongue K14.8
tonsil J35.8
tooth —*see* Cyst, dental
Tornwaldt's J39.2
trichilemmal (proliferating) L72.12
trichodermal L72.12
tubal (fallopian) N83.8
inflammatory —*see* Salpingitis, chronic
tubo-ovarian N83.8
inflammatory N70.13
tunica
albuginea testis N44.1
vaginalis N50.89
turbinate (nose) J34.1
Tyson's gland N48.89
urachus, congenital Q64.4
ureter N28.89
ureterovesical orifice N28.89
urethra, urethral (gland) N36.8
uterine ligament N83.8
uterus (body) (corpus) (recurrent)
N85.8
embryonic Q51.818
cervix Q51.6
vagina, vaginal (implantation) (inclusion)
(squamous cell) (wall) N89.8
embryonic Q52.4
vallecula, vallecular (epiglottis) J38.7
vesical (orifice) N32.89
vitreous body H43.89
vulva (implantation) (inclusion) N90.7
congenital Q52.79
sebaceous gland N90.7
vulvovaginal gland N90.7
wolffian
female Q50.5
male Q55.4

Cystadenocarcinoma —*see* Neoplasm,
malignant, by site
bile duct C22.1
endometrioid —*see* Neoplasm, malignant,
by site
specified site —*see* Neoplasm, malignant,
by site
unspecified site
female C56.9
male C61
mucinous
papillary
specified site —*see* Neoplasm,
malignant, by site
unspecified site C56.9
specified site —*see* Neoplasm, malignant,
by site
unspecified site C56.9
papillary
mucinous
specified site —*see* Neoplasm,
malignant, by site
unspecified site C56.9
pseudomucinous
specified site —*see* Neoplasm,
malignant, by site
unspecified site C56.9
serous
specified site —*see* Neoplasm,
malignant, by site
unspecified site C56.9
specified site —*see* Neoplasm, malignant,
by site
unspecified site C56.9
pseudomucinous
papillary
specified site —*see* Neoplasm,
malignant, by site
unspecified site C56.9
specified site —*see* Neoplasm, malignant,
by site
unspecified site C56.9
serous
papillary
specified site —*see* Neoplasm,
malignant, by site
unspecified site C56.9
specified site —*see* Neoplasm, malignant,
by site
unspecified site C56.9
Cystadenofibroma
clear cell —*see* Neoplasm, benign, by site
endometrioid D27.9
borderline malignancy D39.1-●
malignant C56.-●
mucinous
specified site —*see* Neoplasm, benign, by site
unspecified site D27.9
serous
specified site —*see* Neoplasm, benign, by site
unspecified site D27.9
specified site —*see* Neoplasm, benign, by site
unspecified site D27.9
Cystadenoma —*see also* Neoplasm, benign, by
site
bile duct D13.4
endometrioid —*see* Neoplasm, benign, by site
borderline malignancy —*see* Neoplasm,
uncertain behavior, by site
malignant —*see* Neoplasm, malignant, by site
mucinous
borderline malignancy
ovary C56.-●
specified site NEC —*see* Neoplasm,
uncertain behavior, by site
unspecified site C56.9
papillary
borderline malignancy
ovary C56.-●
specified site NEC —*see* Neoplasm,
uncertain behavior, by site
unspecified site C56.9

Cystadenoma (Continued)
  mucinous (Continued)
    papillary (Continued)
      specified site —see Neoplasm, benign,
        by site
      unspecified site D27.9
    specified site —see Neoplasm, benign, by site
    unspecified site D27.9
  papillary
    borderline malignancy
      ovary C56-•
      specified site NEC —see Neoplasm,
        uncertain behavior, by site
      unspecified site C56.9
    lymphomatosum
      specified site —see Neoplasm, benign,
        by site
      unspecified site D11.9
    mucinous
      borderline malignancy
        ovary C56.-•
        specified site NEC —see Neoplasm,
          uncertain behavior, by site
        unspecified site C56.9
      specified site —see Neoplasm, benign,
        by site
      unspecified site D27.9
    pseudomucinous
      borderline malignancy
        ovary C56.-•
        specified site NEC —see Neoplasm,
          uncertain behavior, by site
        unspecified site C56.9
      specified site —see Neoplasm, benign,
        by site
      unspecified site D27.9
    serous
      borderline malignancy
        ovary C56.-•
        specified site NEC —see Neoplasm,
          uncertain behavior, by site
        unspecified site C56.9
      specified site —see Neoplasm, benign,
        by site
      unspecified site D27.9
    specified site —see Neoplasm, benign, by site
    unspecified site D27.9
  pseudomucinous
    borderline malignancy
      ovary C56.-•
      specified site NEC —see Neoplasm,
        uncertain behavior, by site
      unspecified site C56.9
    papillary
      borderline malignancy
        ovary C56.-•
        specified site NEC —see Neoplasm,
          uncertain behavior, by site
        unspecified site C56.9
      specified site —see Neoplasm, benign,
        by site
      unspecified site D27.9
    specified site —see Neoplasm, benign, by site
    unspecified site D27.9
  serous
    borderline malignancy
      ovary C56.-•
      specified site NEC —see Neoplasm,
        uncertain behavior, by site
      unspecified site C56.9
    papillary
      borderline malignancy
        ovary C56.-•
        specified site NEC —see Neoplasm,
          uncertain behavior, by site
        unspecified site C56.9
      specified site —see Neoplasm, benign,
        by site
      unspecified site D27.9
    specified site —see Neoplasm, benign, by site
    unspecified site D27.9

Cystathionine synthase deficiency E72.11
Cystathioninemia E72.19
Cystathioninuria E72.19
Cystic —see also condition
  breast (chronic) —see Mastopathy, cystic
  corpora lutea (hemorrhagic) N83.1-•
  duct —see condition
  eyeball (congenital) Q11.0
  fibrosis —see Fibrosis, cystic
  kidney (congenital) Q61.9
    adult type Q61.2
    infantile type NEC Q61.19
      collecting duct dilatation Q61.11
    medullary Q61.5
  liver, congenital Q44.6
  lung disease J98.4
    congenital Q33.0
  mastitis, chronic —see Mastopathy, cystic
  medullary, kidney Q61.5
  meniscus —see Derangement, knee,
    meniscus, cystic
  ovary N83.20-•
Cysticercosis, cysticerciasis B69.9
  with
    epileptiform fits B69.0
    myositis B69.81
  brain B69.0
  central nervous system B69.0
  cerebral B69.0
  ocular B69.1
  specified NEC B69.89
Cysticercus cellulose infestation —see
    Cysticercosis
Cystinosis (malignant) E72.04
Cystinuria E72.01
Cystitis (exudative) (hemorrhagic) (septic)
    (suppurative) N30.90
  with
    fibrosis —see Cystitis, chronic, interstitial
    hematuria N30.91
    leukoplakia —see Cystitis, chronic,
      interstitial
    malakoplakia —see Cystitis, chronic,
      interstitial
    metaplasia —see Cystitis, chronic, interstitial
    prostatitis N41.3
  acute N30.00
    with hematuria N30.01
    of trigone N30.30
      with hematuria N30.31
  allergic —see Cystitis, specified type NEC
  amebic A06.81
  bilharzial B65.9 [N33]
  blennorrhagic (gonococcal) A54.01
  bullous —see Cystitis, specified type NEC
  calculous N21.0
  chlamydial A56.01
  chronic N30.20
    with hematuria N30.21
    interstitial N30.10
      with hematuria N30.11
    of trigone N30.30
      with hematuria N30.31
    specified NEC N30.20
      with hematuria N30.21
  cystic (a) —see Cystitis, specified type NEC
  diphtheritic A36.85
  echinococcal
    granulosus B67.39
    multilocularis B67.69
  emphysematous —see Cystitis, specified type
    NEC
  encysted —see Cystitis, specified type NEC
  eosinophilic —see Cystitis, specified type
    NEC
  follicular —see Cystitis, of trigone
  gangrenous —see Cystitis, specified type
    NEC
  glandularis —see Cystitis, specified type
    NEC

Cystitis (Continued)
  gonococcal A54.01
  incrusted —see Cystitis, specified type
    NEC
  interstitial (chronic) —see Cystitis, chronic,
    interstitial
  irradiation N30.40
    with hematuria N30.41
  irritation —see Cystitis, specified type
    NEC
  malignant —see Cystitis, specified type
    NEC
  of trigone N30.30
    with hematuria N30.31
  panmural —see Cystitis, chronic, interstitial
  polyposa —see Cystitis, specified type NEC
  prostatic N41.3
  puerperal (postpartum) O86.22
  radiation —see Cystitis, irradiation
  specified type NEC N30.80
    with hematuria N30.81
  subacute —see Cystitis, chronic
  submucous —see Cystitis, chronic, interstitial
  syphilitic (late) A52.76
  trichomonal A59.03
  tuberculous A18.12
  ulcerative —see Cystitis, chronic, interstitial
Cystocele (-urethrocele)
  female N81.10
    with prolapse of uterus —see Prolapse,
      uterus
    lateral N81.12
    midline N81.11
    paravaginal N81.12
  in pregnancy or childbirth O34.8-•
    causing obstructed labor O65.5
  male N32.89
Cystolithiasis N21.0
Cystoma —see also Neoplasm, benign, by site
  endometrial, ovary N80.1
  mucinous
    specified site —see Neoplasm, benign, by site
    unspecified site D27.9
  serous
    specified site —see Neoplasm, benign, by site
    unspecified site D27.9
  simple (ovary) N83.29-•
Cystoplegia N31.2
Cystoptosis N32.89
Cystopyelitis —see Pyelonephritis
Cystorrhagia N32.89
Cystosarcoma phyllodes D48.6-•
  benign D24-•
  malignant —see Neoplasm, breast, malignant
Cystostomy
  attention to Z43.5
  complication —see Complications, cystostomy
  status Z93.50
    appendico-vesicostomy Z93.52
    cutaneous Z93.51
    specified NEC Z93.59
Cystourethritis —see Urethritis
Cystourethrocele —see also Cystocele
  female N81.10
    with uterine prolapse —see Prolapse,
      uterus
    lateral N81.12
    midline N81.11
    paravaginal N81.12
  male N32.89
Cytomegalic inclusion disease
  congenital P35.1
Cytomegalovirus infection B25.9
Cytomycosis (reticuloendothelial) B39.4
Cytopenia D75.9
  refractory
    with multilineage dysplasia D46.A
      and ring sideroblasts (RCMD RS) D46.B
Czerny's disease (periodic hydrarthrosis of the
  knee) —see Effusion, joint, knee

▶ New   ⇒ Revised   ~~deleted~~ Deleted   • Use Additional Character(s)

D

Daae (-Finsen) disease (epidemic pleurodynia) B33.0
Dabney's grip B33.0
Da Costa's syndrome F45.8
Dacryoadenitis, dacryadenitis H04.00-●
  acute H04.01-●
  chronic H04.02-●
Dacryocystitis H04.30-●
  acute H04.32-●
  chronic H04.41-●
  neonatal P39.1
  phlegmonous H04.31-●
  syphilitic A52.71
    congenital (early) A50.01
  trachomatous, active A71.1
    sequelae (late effect) B94.0
Dacryocystoblenorrhea —see Inflammation, lacrimal, passages, chronic
Dacryocystocele —see Disorder, lacrimal system, changes
Dacryolith, dacryolithiasis H04.51-●
Dacryoma —see Disorder, lacrimal system, changes
Dacryopericystitis —see Dacryocystitis
Dacryops H04.11-●
Dacryostenosis —see also Stenosis, lacrimal
  congenital Q10.5
Dactylitis
  bone —see Osteomyelitis
  sickle-cell D57.00
    Hb C D57.219
    Hb SS D57.00
    specified NEC D57.819
  skin L08.9
  syphilitic A52.77
  tuberculous A18.03
Dactylolysis spontanea (ainhum) L94.6
Dactylosymphysis Q70.9
  fingers —see Syndactylism, complex, fingers
  toes —see Syndactylism, complex, toes
Damage
  arteriosclerotic —see Arteriosclerosis
  brain (nontraumatic) G93.9
    anoxic, hypoxic G93.1
      resulting from a procedure G97.82
    child NEC G80.9
    due to birth injury P11.2
  cardiorenal (vascular) —see Hypertension, cardiorenal
  cerebral NEC —see Damage, brain
  coccyx, complicating delivery O71.6
  coronary —see Disease, heart, ischemic
  deep tissue, pressure-induced —see also L89
    with final character .6
  eye, birth injury P15.3
  liver (nontraumatic) K76.9
    alcoholic K70.9
    due to drugs —see Disease, liver, toxic
    toxic —see Disease, liver, toxic
  lung
    dabbing (related) U07.0
    electronic cigarette (related) U07.0
    vaping (associated) (device) (product) (use) U07.0
  medication T88.7
  organ
    dabbing (related) U07.0
    electronic cigarette (related) U07.0
    vaping (associated) (device) (product) (use) U07.0
  pelvic
    joint or ligament, during delivery O71.6
    organ NEC
      during delivery O71.5
      following ectopic or molar pregnancy O08.6
  renal —see Disease, renal
  subendocardium, subendocardial —see Degeneration, myocardial
  vascular I99.9

Dana-Putnam syndrome (subacute combined sclerosis with pernicious anemia) —see Degeneration, combined
Danbolt (-Cross) syndrome (acrodermatitis enteropathica) E83.2
Dandruff L21.0
Dandy-Walker syndrome Q03.1
  with spina bifida —see Spina bifida
Danlos' syndrome (see also Syndrome, Ehler-Danlos) Q79.60
Darier (-White) disease (congenital) Q82.8
  meaning erythema annulare centrifugum L53.1
Darier-Roussy sarcoid D86.3
Darling's disease or histoplasmosis B39.4
Darwin's tubercle Q17.8
Dawson's (inclusion body) encephalitis A81.1
De Beurmann (-Gougerot) disease B42.1
De la Tourette's syndrome F95.2
De Lange's syndrome Q87.19
De Morgan's spots (senile angiomas) I78.1
De Quervain's
  disease (tendon sheath) M65.4
  syndrome E34.51
  thyroiditis (subacute granulomatous thyroiditis) E06.1
De Toni-Fanconi (-Debré) syndrome E72.09
  with cystinosis E72.04
Dead
  fetus, retained (mother) O36.4
    early pregnancy O02.1
  labyrinth —see subcategory H83.2
  ovum, retained O02.0
Deaf nonspeaking NEC H91.3
Deafmutism (acquired) (congenital) NEC H91.3
  hysterical F44.6
  syphilitic, congenital —see also subcategory H94.8 A50.09
Deafness (acquired) (complete) (hereditary) (partial) H91.9-●
  with blue sclera and fragility of bone Q78.0
  auditory fatigue —see Deafness, specified type NEC
  aviation T70.0
    nerve injury —see Injury, nerve, acoustic, specified type NEC
  boilermaker's —see subcategory H83.3
  central —see Deafness, sensorineural
  conductive H90.2
    and sensorineural
      mixed H90.8
        bilateral H90.6
      bilateral H90.0
      unilateral H90.1-●
        with restricted hearing on the contralateral side H90.A-●
  congenital H90.5
    with blue sclera and fragility of bone Q78.0
  due to toxic agents —see Deafness, ototoxic
  emotional (hysterical) F44.6
  functional (hysterical) F44.6
  high frequency H91.9-●
  hysterical F44.6
  low frequency H91.9-●
  mental R48.8
  mixed conductive and sensorineural H90.8
    bilateral H90.6
    unilateral H90.7-●
  nerve —see Deafness, sensorineural
  neural —see Deafness, sensorineural
  noise-induced —see also subcategory H83.3
    nerve injury —see Injury, nerve, acoustic, specified type NEC
  nonspeaking H91.3
  ototoxic —see subcategory H91.0
  perceptive —see Deafness, sensorineural
  psychogenic (hysterical) F44.6
  sensorineural H90.5
    and conductive
      mixed H90.8
        bilateral H90.6
      bilateral H90.3

Deafness (Continued)
  sensorineural (Continued)
    unilateral H90.4-●
      with restricted hearing on the contralateral side H90.A-●
    sensory —see Deafness, sensorineural
    specified type NEC —see subcategory H91.8
    sudden (idiopathic) H91.2-●
    syphilitic A52.15
    transient ischemic H93.01-●
    traumatic —see Injury, nerve, acoustic, specified type NEC
    word (developmental) H93.25
Death (cause unknown) (of) (unexplained) (unspecified cause) R99
  brain G93.82
  cardiac (sudden) (with successful resuscitation) — code to underlying disease
    family history of Z82.41
    personal history of Z86.74
  family member (assumed) Z63.4
Debility (chronic) (general) (nervous) R53.81
  congenital or neonatal NOS P96.9
  nervous R53.81
  old age R54
  senile R54
Débove's disease (splenomegaly) R16.1
Decalcification
  bone —see Osteoporosis
  teeth K03.89
Decapsulation, kidney N28.89
Decay
  dental —see Caries, dental
  senile R54
  tooth, teeth —see Caries, dental
Deciduitis (acute)
  following ectopic or molar pregnancy O08.0
Decline (general) —see Debility
  cognitive, age-associated R41.81
Decompensation
  cardiac (acute) (chronic) —see Disease, heart
  cardiovascular —see Disease, cardiovascular
  heart —see Disease, heart
  hepatic —see Failure, hepatic
  myocardial (acute) (chronic) —see Disease, heart
  respiratory J98.8
Decompression sickness T70.3
Decrease (d)
  absolute neutrophile count —see Neutropenia
  blood
    platelets —see Thrombocytopenia
    pressure R03.1
      due to shock following
        injury T79.4
        operation T81.19
  estrogen E28.39
    postablative E89.40
      asymptomatic E89.40
      symptomatic E89.41
  fragility of erythrocytes D58.8
  function
    lipase (pancreatic) K90.3
    ovary in hypopituitarism E23.0
    parenchyma of pancreas K86.89
    pituitary (gland) (anterior) (lobe) E23.0
      posterior (lobe) E23.0
  functional activity R68.89
  glucose R73.09
  hematocrit R71.0
  hemoglobin R71.0
  leukocytes D72.819
    specified NEC D72.818
  libido R68.82
  lymphocytes D72.810
  platelets D69.6
  respiration, due to shock following injury T79.4
  sexual desire R68.82
  tear secretion NEC —see Syndrome, dry eye

Decrease *(Continued)*
  tolerance
    fat K90.49
    glucose R73.09
    pancreatic K90.3
    salt and water E87.8
  vision NEC H54.7
  white blood cell count D72.819
    specified NEC D72.818
Decubitus (ulcer) —*see* Ulcer, pressure, by site
  cervix N86
Deepening acetabulum —*see* Derangement,
  joint, specified type NEC, hip
Defect, defective Q89.9
  3-beta-hydroxysteroid dehydrogenase E25.0
  11-hydroxylase E25.0
  21-hydroxylase E25.0
  abdominal wall, congenital Q79.59
  antibody immunodeficiency D80.9
  aorticopulmonary septum Q21.4
  atrial septal (ostium secundum type) Q21.1
    following acute myocardial infarction
      (current complication) I23.1
    ostium primum type Q21.2
  atrioventricular
    canal Q21.2
    septum Q21.2
  auricular septal Q21.1
  bilirubin excretion NEC E80.6
  biosynthesis, androgen (testicular) E29.1
  bulbar septum Q21.0
  catalase E80.3
  cell membrane receptor complex (CR3) D71
  circulation I99.9
    congenital Q28.9
    newborn Q28.9
  coagulation (factor) —*see also* Deficiency,
    factor D68.9
    with
      ectopic pregnancy O08.1
      molar pregnancy O08.1
    acquired D68.4
    antepartum with hemorrhage —*see*
      Hemorrhage, antepartum, with
      coagulation defect
    due to
      liver disease D68.4
      vitamin K deficiency D68.4
    hereditary NEC D68.2
    intrapartum O67.0
    newborn, transient P61.6
    postpartum O99.13
      with hemorrhage O72.3
    specified type NEC D68.8
  complement system D84.1
  conduction (heart) I45.9
    bone —*see* Deafness, conductive
  congenital, organ or site not listed —*see*
    Anomaly, by site
  coronary sinus Q21.1
  cushion, endocardial Q21.2
  degradation, glycoprotein E77.1
  dental bridge, crown, fillings —*see* Defect,
    dental restoration
  dental restoration K08.50
    specified NEC K08.59
  dentin (hereditary) K00.5
  Descemet's membrane, congenital Q13.89
  developmental —*see also* Anomaly
    cauda equina Q06.3
  diaphragm
    with elevation, eventration or hernia —*see*
      Hernia, diaphragm
    congenital Q79.1
      with hernia Q79.0
      gross (with hernia) Q79.0
  ectodermal, congenital Q82.9
  Eisenmenger's Q21.8
  enzyme
    catalase E80.3
    peroxidase E80.3

Defect, defective *(Continued)*
  esophagus, congenital Q39.9
  extensor retinaculum M62.89
  fibrin polymerization D68.2
  filling
    bladder R93.41
    kidney R93.42-●
    renal pelvis R93.41
    stomach R93.3
    ureter R93.41
    urinary organs, specified NEC R93.49
  GABA (gamma aminobutyric acid) metabolic
    E72.81
  Gerbode Q21.0
  glucose transport, blood-brain barrier E74.810
  glycoprotein degradation E77.1
  Hageman (factor) D68.2
  hearing —*see* Deafness
  high grade F70
  interatrial septal Q21.1
  interauricular septal Q21.1
  interventricular septal Q21.0
    with dextroposition of aorta, pulmonary
      stenosis and hypertrophy of right
      ventricle Q21.3
    in tetralogy of Fallot Q21.3
  learning (specific) —*see* Disorder, learning
  lymphocyte function antigen-1 (LFA-1) D84.0
  lysosomal enzyme, post-translational
    modification E77.0
  major osseous M89.70
    ankle M89.77-●
    carpus M89.74-●
    clavicle M89.71-●
    femur M89.75-●
    fibula M89.76-●
    fingers M89.74-●
    foot M89.77-●
    forearm M89.73-●
    hand M89.74-●
    humerus M89.72-●
    lower leg M89.76-●
    metacarpus M89.74-●
    metatarsus M89.77-●
    multiple sites M89.79
    pelvic region M89.75-●
    pelvis M89.75-●
    radius M89.73-●
    scapula M89.71-●
    shoulder region M89.71-●
    specified NEC M89.78
    tarsus M89.77-●
    thigh M89.75-●
    tibia M89.76-●
    toes M89.77-●
    ulna M89.73-●
  mental —*see* Disability, intellectual
  modification, lysosomal enzymes, post-
    translational E77.0
  obstructive, congenital
    renal pelvis Q62.39
    ureter Q62.39
      atresia —*see* Atresia, ureter
      cecoureterocele Q62.32
      megaureter Q62.2
      orthotopic ureterocele Q62.31
  osseous, major M89.70
    ankle M89.77-●
    carpus M89.74-●
    clavicle M89.71-●
    femur M89.75-●
    fibula M89.76-●
    fingers M89.74-●
    foot M89.77-●
    forearm M89.73-●
    hand M89.74-●
    humerus M89.72-●
    lower leg M89.76-●
    metacarpus M89.74-●
    metatarsus M89.77-●
    multiple sites M89.9

Defect, defective *(Continued)*
  osseous, major *(Continued)*
    pelvic region M89.75-●
    pelvis M89.75-●
    radius M89.73-●
    scapula M89.71-●
    shoulder region M89.71-●
    specified NEC M89.78
    tarsus M89.77-●
    thigh M89.75-●
    tibia M89.76-●
    toes M89.77-●
    ulna M89.73-●
  osteochondral NEC —*see also* Deformity
    M95.8-●
  ostium
    primum Q21.2
    secundum Q21.1
  peroxidase E80.3
  placental blood supply —*see* Insufficiency,
    placental
  platelets, qualitative D69.1
    constitutional D68.0
  postural NEC, spine —*see* Dorsopathy,
    deforming
  reduction
    limb Q73.8
      lower Q72.9-●
        absence —*see* Agenesis, leg
        foot —*see* Agenesis, foot
        longitudinal
          femur Q72.4-●
          fibula Q72.6-●
          tibia Q72.5-●
        specified type NEC Q72.89-●
        split foot Q72.7-●
      specified type NEC Q73.8
      upper Q71.9-●
        absence —*see* Agenesis, arm
        forearm —*see* Agenesis, forearm
        hand —*see* Agenesis, hand
        lobster-claw hand Q71.6-●
        longitudinal
          radius Q71.4-●
          ulna Q71.5-●
        specified type NEC Q71.89-●
  renal pelvis Q63.8
    obstructive Q62.39
  respiratory system, congenital Q34.9
  restoration, dental K08.50
    specified NEC K08.59
  retinal nerve bundle fibers H35.89
  septal (heart) NOS Q21.9
    acquired (atrial) (auricular) (ventricular)
      (old) I51.0
    atrial Q21.1
      concurrent with acute myocardial
        infarction —*see* Infarct,
        myocardium
      following acute myocardial infarction
        (current complication) I23.1
      ventricular —*see also* Defect, ventricular
        septal Q21.0
    sinus venosus Q21.1
  speech —*see* Disorder, speech
    developmental F80.9
    specified NEC R47.89
  Taussig-Bing (aortic transposition and
    overriding pulmonary artery)
    Q20.1
  teeth, wedge K03.1
  vascular (local) I99.9
    congenital Q27.9
  ventricular septal Q21.0
    concurrent with acute myocardial
      infarction —*see* Infarct,
      myocardium
    following acute myocardial infarction
      (current complication) I23.2
    in tetralogy of Fallot Q21.3
  vision NEC H54.7

▶ New   ⇒ Revised   ~~deleted~~ Deleted   ● Use Additional Character(s)

Defect, defective (Continued)
visual field H53.40
  bilateral
    heteronymous H53.47
    homonymous H53.46-●
    generalized contraction H53.48-●
    localized
      arcuate H53.43-●
      scotoma (central area) H53.41-●
        blind spot area H53.42-●
      sector H53.43-●
      specified type NEC H53.45-●
voice R49.9
  specified NEC R49.8
wedge, tooth, teeth (abrasion) K03.1
Deferentitis N49.1
gonorrheal (acute) (chronic) A54.23
Defibrination (syndrome) D65
antepartum —see Hemorrhage, antepartum,
  with coagulation defect, disseminated
  intravascular coagulation
following ectopic or molar pregnancy O08.1
intrapartum O67.0
newborn P60
postpartum O72.3
Deficiency, deficient
3-beta hydroxysteroid dehydrogenase E25.0
11-hydroxylase E25.0
21-hydroxylase E25.0
5-alpha reductase (with male
  pseudohermaphroditism) E29.1
AADC (aromatic L-amino acid
  decarboxylase) E70.81
abdominal muscle syndrome Q79.4
AC globulin (congenital) (hereditary) D68.2
  acquired D68.4
accelerator globulin (Ac G) (blood) D68.2
acid phosphatase E83.39
▶ acid sphingomyelinase (ASMD) E75.249
  ▶ type
    ▶ A E75.240
    ▶ A/B E75.244
    ▶ B E75.241
activating factor (blood) D68.2
ADA2 (adenosine deaminase 2) D81.32
adenosine deaminase (ADA) D81.30
  with severe combined immunodeficiency
    (SCID) D81.31
  partial (type 1) D81.39
  specified NEC D81.39
  type 1 (without SCID) (without severe
    combined immunodeficiency) D81.39
  type 2 D81.32
aldolase (hereditary) E74.19
alpha-1-antitrypsin E88.01
amino-acids E72.9
anemia —see Anemia
aneurin E51.9
antibody with
  hyperimmunoglobulinemia D80.6
  near-normal immunoglobins D80.6
antidiuretic hormone E23.2
anti-hemophilic
  factor (A) D66
    B D67
    C D68.1
  globulin (AHG) NEC D66
antithrombin (antithrombin III) D68.59
aromatic L-amino acid decarboxylase
  (AADC) E70.81
ascorbic acid E54
attention (disorder) (syndrome) F98.8
  with hyperactivity —see Disorder,
    attention-deficit hyperactivity
autoprothrombin
  I D68.2
  II D67
  C D68.2
beta-glucuronidase E76.29
biotin E53.8
biotin-dependent carboxylase D81.819
biotinidase D81.810

Deficiency, deficient (Continued)
brancher enzyme (amylopectinosis) E74.03
C1 esterase inhibitor (C1-INH) D84.1
calciferol E55.9
  with
    adult osteomalacia M83.8
    rickets —see Rickets
calcium (dietary) E58
calorie, severe E43
  with marasmus E41
    and kwashiorkor E42
cardiac —see Insufficiency, myocardial
carnitine E71.40
  due to
    hemodialysis E71.43
    inborn errors of metabolism E71.42
    Valproic acid therapy E71.43
  iatrogenic E71.43
  muscle palmityltransferase E71.314
  primary E71.41
  secondary E71.448
carotene E50.9
central nervous system G96.89
ceruloplasmin (Wilson) E83.01
choline E53.8
Christmas factor D67
chromium E61.4
▶ chronic neurovisceral acid sphingomyelinase
  E75.244
▶ chronic visceral acid sphingomyelinase
  E75.241
clotting (blood) —see also Deficiency,
  coagulation factor D68.9
clotting factor NEC (hereditary) —see also
  Deficiency, factor D68.2
coagulation NOS D68.9
  with
    ectopic pregnancy O08.1
    molar pregnancy O08.1
  acquired (any) D68.4
  antepartum hemorrhage —see Hemorrhage,
    antepartum, with coagulation defect
  clotting factor NEC —see also Deficiency,
    factor D68.2
  due to
    hyperprothrombinemia D68.4
    liver disease D68.4
    vitamin K deficiency D68.4
  newborn, transient P61.6
  postpartum O72.3
  specified NEC D68.8
cognitive F09
color vision H53.50
  achromatopsia H53.51
  acquired H53.52
  deuteranomaly H53.53
  protanomaly H53.54
  specified type NEC H53.59
  tritanomaly H53.55
combined glucocorticoid and
  mineralocorticoid E27.49
contact factor D68.2
copper (nutritional) E61.0
corticoadrenal E27.40
  primary E27.1
craniofacial axis Q75.0
cyanocobalamin E53.8
debrancher enzyme (limit dextrinosis) E74.03
dehydrogenase
  long chain/very long chain acyl CoA
    E71.310
  medium chain acyl CoA E71.311
  short chain acyl CoA E71.312
diet E63.9
dihydropyrimidine dehydrogenase (DPD)
  E88.89
disaccharidase E73.9
edema —see Malnutrition, severe
endocrine E34.9
energy-supply —see Malnutrition
enzymes, circulating NEC E88.09

Deficiency, deficient (Continued)
ergosterol E55.9
  with
    adult osteomalacia M83.8
    rickets —see Rickets
essential fatty acid (EFA) E63.0
eye movements
  saccadic H55.81
  smooth pursuit H55.82
factor —see also Deficiency, coagulation
  Hageman D68.2
  I (congenital) (hereditary) D68.2
  II (congenital) (hereditary) D68.2
  IX (congenital) (functional) (hereditary)
    (with functional defect) D67
  multiple (congenital) D68.8
    acquired D68.4
  V (congenital) (hereditary) D68.2
  VII (congenital) (hereditary) D68.2
  VIII (congenital) (functional) (hereditary)
    (with functional defect) D66
    with vascular defect D68.0
  X (congenital) (hereditary) D68.2
  XI (congenital) (hereditary) D68.1
  XII (congenital) (hereditary) D68.2
  XIII (congenital) (hereditary) D68.2
femoral, proximal focal (congenital) —
  see Defect, reduction, lower limb,
  longitudinal, femur
fibrin-stabilizing factor (congenital)
  (hereditary) D68.2
  acquired D68.4
fibrinase D68.2
fibrinogen (congenital) (hereditary) D68.2
  acquired D65
folate E53.8
folic acid E53.8
foreskin N47.3
fructokinase E74.11
fructose 1,6 diphosphatase E74.19
fructose-1-phosphate aldolase E74.19
GABA (gamma aminobutyric acid)
  transaminase E72.81
GABA-T (gamma aminobutyric acid
  transaminase) E72.81
galactokinase E74.29
galactose-1-phosphate uridyl transferase
  E74.29
gammaglobulin in blood D80.1
  hereditary D80.0
glass factor D68.2
glucocorticoid E27.49
  mineralocorticoid E27.49
glucose-6-phosphatase E74.01
glucose-6-phosphate dehydrogenase anemia
  anemia D55.0
  without anemia D75.A
glucose transporter protein type 1 E74.810
glucuronyl transferase E80.5
Glut1 E74.810
glycogen synthetase E74.09
gonadotropin (isolated) E23.0
growth hormone (idiopathic) (isolated) E23.0
Hageman factor D68.2
hemoglobin D64.9
hepatophosphorylase E74.09
homogentisate 1,2-dioxygenase E70.29
hormone
  anterior pituitary (partial) NEC E23.0
    growth E23.0
  growth (isolated) E23.0
  pituitary E23.0
  testicular E29.1
hypoxanthine-(guanine)-
  phosphoribosyltransferase (HG-PRT)
  (total HG-PRT) E79.1
immunity D84.9
  cell-mediated D84.89
    with thrombocytopenia and eczema
      D82.0
  combined D81.9

Deficiency, deficient (Continued)
immunity (Continued)
  humoral D80.9
  IgA (secretory) D80.2
  IgG D80.3
  IgM D80.4
immuno —see Immunodeficiency
immunoglobulin, selective
  A (IgA) D80.2
  G (IgG) (subclasses) D80.3
  M (IgM) D80.4
▶infantile neurovisceral acid sphingomyelinase
  E75.240
inositol (B complex) E53.8
intrinsic
  factor (congenital) D51.0
  sphincter N36.42
    with urethral hypermobility N36.43
iodine E61.8
  congenital syndrome —see Syndrome,
    iodine-deficiency, congenital
iron E61.1
  anemia D50.9
kalium E87.6
kappa-light chain D80.8
labile factor (congenital) (hereditary) D68.2
  acquired D68.4
lacrimal fluid (acquired) —see also Syndrome,
  dry eye
  congenital Q10.6
lactase
  congenital E73.0
  secondary E73.1
Laki-Lorand factor D68.2
lecithin cholesterol acyltransferase E78.6
lipocaic K86.89
lipoprotein (familial) (high density) E78.6
liver phosphorylase E74.09
lysosomal alpha-1, 4 glucosidase E74.02
magnesium E61.2
major histocompatibility complex
  class I D81.6
  class II D81.7
manganese E61.3
menadione (vitamin K) E56.1
  newborn P53
mental (familial) (hereditary) —see Disability,
  intellectual
methylenetetrahydrofolate reductase
  (MTHFR) E72.12
mevalonate kinase M04.1
mineral NEC E61.8
mineralocorticoid E27.49
  with glucocorticoid E27.49
molybdenum (nutritional) E61.5
moral F60.2
multiple nutrient elements E61.7
multiple sulfatase (MSD) E75.26
muscle
  carnitine (palmityltransferase) E71.314
  phosphofructokinase E74.09
myoadenylate deaminase E79.2
myocardial —see Insufficiency, myocardial
myophosphorylase E74.04
NADH diaphorase or reductase (congenital)
  D74.0
NADH-methemoglobin reductase
  (congenital) D74.0
natrium E87.1
niacin (amide) (-tryptophan) E52
nicotinamide E52
nicotinic acid E52
number of teeth —see Anodontia
nutrient element E61.9
  multiple E61.7
  specified NEC E61.8
nutrition, nutritional E63.9
  sequelae —see Sequelae, nutritional
    deficiency
  specified NEC E63.8
of interleukin 1 receptor antagonist [DIRA]
  M04.8

Deficiency, deficient (Continued)
ornithine transcarbamylase E72.4
ovarian E28.39
oxygen —see Anoxia
pantothenic acid E53.8
parathyroid (gland) E20.9
perineum (female) N81.89
phenylalanine hydroxylase E70.1
phosphoenolpyruvate carboxykinase E74.4
phosphofructokinase E74.19
phosphomannomutase E74.818
phosphomannose isomerase E74.818
phosphomannosyl mutase E74.818
phosphorylase kinase, liver E74.09
pituitary hormone (isolated) E23.0
plasma thromboplastin
  antecedent (PTA) D68.1
  component (PTC) D67
plasminogen (type 1) (type 2) E88.02
platelet NEC D69.1
  constitutional D68.0
polyglandular E31.8
  autoimmune E31.0
potassium (K) E87.6
prepuce N47.3
proaccelerin (congenital) (hereditary) D68.2
  acquired D68.4
proconvertin factor (congenital) (hereditary)
  D68.2
  acquired D68.4
protein —see also Malnutrition E46
  anemia D53.0
  C D68.59
  S D68.59
prothrombin (congenital) (heredItary) D68.2
  acquired D68.4
Prower factor D68.2
pseudocholinesterase E88.09
PTA (plasma thromboplastin antecedent) D68.1
PTC (plasma thromboplastin component) D67
purine nucleoside phosphorylase (PNP) D81.5
pyracin (alpha) (beta) E53.1
pyridoxal E53.1
pyridoxamine E53.1
pyridoxine (derivatives) E53.1
pyruvate
  carboxylase E74.4
  dehydrogenase E74.4
riboflavin (vitamin B2) E53.0
salt E87.1
secretion
  ovary E28.39
  salivary gland (any) K11.7
  urine R34
selenium (dietary) E59
serum antitrypsin, familial E88.01
short stature homeobox gene (SHOX)
  with
    dyschondrosteosis Q78.8
    short stature (idiopathic) E34.3
    Turner's syndrome Q96.9
sodium (Na) E87.1
SPCA (factor VII) D68.2
sphincter, intrinsic N36.42
  with urethral hypermobility N36.43
stable factor (congenital) (hereditary) D68.2
  acquired D68.4
Stuart-Prower (factor X) D68.2
succinic semialdehyde dehydrogenase
  E72.81
sucrase E74.39
sulfatase E75.26
sulfite oxidase E72.19
thiamin, thiaminic (chloride) E51.9
  beriberi (dry) E51.11
    wet E51.12
thrombokinase D68.2
  newborn P53
thyroid (gland) —see Hypothyroidism
tocopherol E56.0
tooth bud K00.0
transcobalamine II (anemia) D51.2

Deficiency, deficient (Continued)
vanadium E61.6
vascular I99.9
vasopressin E23.2
vertical ridge K06.8
viosterol —see Deficiency, calciferol
vitamin (multiple) NOS E56.9
  A E50.9
    with
      Bitot's spot (corneal) E50.1
      follicular keratosis E50.8
      keratomalacia E50.4
      manifestations NEC E50.8
      night blindness E50.5
      scar of cornea, xerophthalmic E50.6
      xeroderma E50.8
      xerophthalmia E50.7
      xerosis
        conjunctival E50.0
          and Bitot's spot E50.1
        cornea E50.2
          and ulceration E50.3
    sequelae E64.1
  B (complex) NOS E53.9
    with
      beriberi (dry) E51.11
        wet E51.12
      pellagra E52
  B1 NOS E51.9
    beriberi (dry) E51.11
      with circulatory system
        manifestations E51.11
      wet E51.12
  B12 E53.8
  B2 (riboflavin) E53.0
  B6 E53.1
  C E54
    sequelae E64.2
  D E55.9
    with
      adult osteomalacia M83.8
      rickets —see Rickets
    25-hydroxylase E83.32
  E E56.0
  folic acid E53.8
  G E53.0
  group B E53.9
    specified NEC E53.8
  H (biotin) E53.8
  K E56.1
    of newborn P53
  nicotinic E52
  P E56.8
  PP (pellagra-preventing) E52
  specified NEC E56.8
  thiamin E51.9
    beriberi —see Beriberi
zinc, dietary E60
Deficit —see also Deficiency
attention and concentration R41.840
  following
    cerebral infarction I69.310
    cerebrovascular disease I69.910
      specified disease NEC I69.810
    nontraumatic
      intracerebral hemorrhage I69.110
      specified intracranial hemorrhage
        NEC I69.210
      subarachnoid hemorrhage I69.010
  disorder —see Attention, deficit
cognitive
  communication R41.841
  emotional
    following
      cerebral infarction I69.315
      cerebrovascular disease I69.915
        specified disease NEC I69.815
      nontraumatic
        intracerebral hemorrhage I69.115
        specified intracranial hemorrhage
          NEC I69.215
        subarachnoid hemorrhage I69.015

Deficit *(Continued)*
  cognitive *(Continued)*
    following
      cerebral infarction I69.319
      cerebrovascular disease I69.919
        specified disease NEC I69.819
      nontraumatic
        intracerebral hemorrhage I69.119
        specified intracranial hemorrhage
          NEC I69.219
        subarachnoid hemorrhage I69.019
    social
      following
        cerebral infarction I69.315
        cerebrovascular disease I69.915
          specified disease NEC I69.815
        nontraumatic
          intracerebral hemorrhage I69.115
          specified intracranial hemorrhage
            NEC I69.215
          subarachnoid hemorrhage I69.015
  cognitive NEC R41.89
    following
      cerebral infarction I69.318
      cerebrovascular disease I69.918
        specified disease NEC I69.818
      nontraumatic
        intracerebral hemorrhage I69.118
        specified intracranial hemorrhage
          NEC I69.218
        subarachnoid hemorrhage I69.018
  concentration R41.840
  executive function R41.844
    following
      cerebral infarction I69.314
      cerebrovascular disease I69.914
        specified disease NEC I69.814
      nontraumatic
        intracerebral hemorrhage I69.114
        specified intracranial hemorrhage
          NEC I69.214
        subarachnoid hemorrhage I69.014
  frontal lobe R41.844
    following
      cerebral infarction I69.314
      cerebrovascular disease I69.914
        specified disease NEC I69.814
      nontraumatic
        intracerebral hemorrhage I69.114
        specified intracranial hemorrhage
          NEC I69.214
        subarachnoid hemorrhage I69.014
  memory
    following
      cerebral infarction I69.311
      cerebrovascular disease I69.911
        specified disease NEC I69.811
      nontraumatic
        intracerebral hemorrhage
          I69.111
        specified intracranial hemorrhage
          NEC I69.211
        subarachnoid hemorrhage I69.011
  neurologic NEC R29.818
    ischemic
      reversible (RIND) I63.9
        prolonged (PRIND) I63.9
  oxygen R09.02
  prolonged reversible ischemic neurologic
    (PRIND) I63.9
  psychomotor R41.843
    following
      cerebral infarction I69.313
      cerebrovascular disease I69.913
        specified disease NEC I69.813
      nontraumatic
        intracerebral hemorrhage I69.113
        specified intracranial hemorrhage
          NEC I69.213
        subarachnoid hemorrhage
          I69.013

Deficit *(Continued)*
  visuospatial R41.842
    following
      cerebral infarction I69.312
      cerebrovascular disease I69.912
        specified disease NEC I69.812
      nontraumatic
        intracerebral hemorrhage I69.112
        specified intracranial hemorrhage
          NEC I69.212
        subarachnoid hemorrhage
          I69.012
Deflection
  radius —*see* Deformity, limb, specified type
    NEC, forearm
  septum (acquired) (nasal) (nose) J34.2
  spine —*see* Curvature, spine
  turbinate (nose) J34.2
Defluvium
  capillorum —*see* Alopecia
  ciliorum —*see* Madarosis
  unguium L60.8
Deformity Q89.9
  abdomen, congenital Q89.9
  abdominal wall
    acquired M95.8
    congenital Q79.59
  acquired (unspecified site) M95.9
  adrenal gland Q89.1
  alimentary tract, congenital Q45.9
    upper Q40.9
  ankle (joint) (acquired) —*see also* Deformity,
    limb, lower leg
    abduction —*see* Contraction, joint, ankle
    congenital Q68.8
    contraction —*see* Contraction, joint, ankle
    specified type NEC —*see* Deformity, limb,
      foot, specified NEC
  anus (acquired) K62.89
    congenital Q43.9
  aorta (arch) (congenital) Q25.40
    acquired I77.89
  aortic
    arch, acquired I77.89
    cusp or valve (congenital) Q23.8
      acquired —*see also* Endocarditis, aortic
        I35.8
  arm (acquired) (upper) —*see also* Deformity,
    limb, upper arm
    congenital Q68.8
    forearm —*see* Deformity, limb, forearm
  artery (congenital) (peripheral) NOS Q27.9
    acquired I77.89
    coronary (acquired) I25.9
      congenital Q24.5
    umbilical Q27.0
  atrial septal Q21.1
  auditory canal (external) (congenital) —*see*
    also Malformation, ear, external
    acquired —*see* Disorder, ear, external,
      specified type NEC
  auricle
    ear (congenital) —*see also* Malformation,
      ear, external
      acquired —*see* Disorder, pinna,
        deformity
  back —*see* Dorsopathy, deforming
  bile duct (common) (congenital) (hepatic)
    Q44.5
    acquired K83.8
  biliary duct or passage (congenital) Q44.5
    acquired K83.8
  bladder (neck) (trigone) (sphincter)
    (acquired) N32.89
    congenital Q64.79
  bone (acquired) NOS M95.9
    congenital Q79.9
    turbinate M95.0
  brain (congenital) Q04.9
    acquired G93.89
    reduction Q04.3

Deformity *(Continued)*
  breast (acquired) N64.89
    congenital Q83.9
    reconstructed N65.0
  bronchus (congenital) Q32.4
    acquired NEC J98.09
  bursa, congenital Q79.9
  canaliculi (lacrimalis) (acquired) —*see also*
    Disorder, lacrimal system, changes
    congenital Q10.6
  canthus, acquired —*see* Disorder, eyelid,
    specified type NEC
  capillary (acquired) I78.8
  cardiovascular system, congenital Q28.9
  caruncle, lacrimal (acquired) —*see also*
    Disorder, lacrimal system, changes
    congenital Q10.6
  cascade, stomach K31.2
  cecum (congenital) Q43.9
    acquired K63.89
  cerebral, acquired G93.89
    congenital Q04.9
  cervix (uterus) (acquired) NEC N88.8
    congenital Q51.9
  cheek (acquired) M95.2
    congenital Q18.9
  chest (acquired) (wall) M95.4
    congenital Q67.8
    sequelae (late effect) of rickets E64.3
  chin (acquired) M95.2
    congenital Q18.9
  choroid (congenital) Q14.3
    acquired H31.8
    plexus Q07.8
      acquired G96.198
  cicatricial —*see* Cicatrix
  cilia, acquired —*see* Disorder, eyelid,
    specified type NEC
  clavicle (acquired) M95.8
    congenital Q68.8
  clitoris (congenital) Q52.6
    acquired N90.89
  clubfoot —*see* Clubfoot
  coccyx (acquired) —*see* subcategory
    M43.8
  colon (congenital) Q43.9
    acquired K63.89
  concha (ear), congenital —*see also*
    Malformation, ear, external
    acquired —*see* Disorder, pinna, deformity
  cornea (acquired) H18.70
    congenital Q13.4
    descemetocele —*see* Descemetocele
    ectasia —*see* Ectasia, cornea
    specified NEC H18.79-●
    staphyloma —*see* Staphyloma, cornea
  coronary artery (acquired) I25.9
    congenital Q24.5
  cranium (acquired) —*see* Deformity, skull
  cricoid cartilage (congenital) Q31.8
    acquired J38.7
  cystic duct (congenital) Q44.5
    acquired K82.8
  Dandy-Walker Q03.1
    with spina bifida —*see* Spina bifida
  diaphragm (congenital) Q79.1
    acquired J98.6
  digestive organ NOS Q45.9
  ductus arteriosus Q25.0
  duodenal bulb K31.89
  duodenum (congenital) Q43.9
    acquired K31.89
  dura —*see* Deformity, meninges
  ear (acquired) —*see also* Disorder, pinna,
    deformity
    congenital (external) Q17.9
      internal Q16.5
      middle Q16.4
        ossicles Q16.3
      ossicles Q16.3
  ectodermal (congenital) NEC Q84.9

Deformity *(Continued)*

ejaculatory duct (congenital) Q55.4
    acquired N50.89
elbow (joint) (acquired) —*see also* Deformity,
    limb, upper arm
    congenital Q68.8
    contraction —*see* Contraction, joint, elbow
endocrine gland NEC Q89.2
epididymis (congenital) Q55.4
    acquired N50.89
epiglottis (congenital) Q31.8
    acquired J38.7
esophagus (congenital) Q39.9
  ➜acquired K22.89
eustachian tube (congenital) NEC Q17.8
eye, congenital Q15.9
eyebrow (congenital) Q18.8
eyelid (acquired) —*see also* Disorder, eyelid,
    specified type NEC
    congenital Q10.3
face (acquired) M95.2
    congenital Q18.9
fallopian tube, acquired N83.8
femur (acquired) —*see* Deformity, limb,
    specified type NEC, thigh
fetal
    with fetopelvic disproportion O33.7
    causing obstructed labor O66.3
finger (acquired) M20.00-●
    boutonniere M20.02-●
    congenital Q68.1
    flexion contracture —*see* Contraction, joint,
      hand
    mallet finger M20.01-●
    specified NEC M20.09-●
    swan-neck M20.03-●
flexion (joint) (acquired) —*see also* Deformity,
    limb, flexion M21.20
    congenital NOS Q74.9
    hip Q65.89
foot (acquired) —*see also* Deformity, limb,
    lower leg
    cavovarus (congenital) Q66.1-●
    congenital NOS Q66.9-●
      specified type NEC Q66.89
    specified type NEC —*see* Deformity, limb,
      foot, specified NEC
    valgus (congenital) Q66.6
      acquired —*see* Deformity, valgus, ankle
    varus (congenital) NEC Q66.3-●
      acquired —*see* Deformity, varus, ankle
forearm (acquired) —*see also* Deformity, limb,
    forearm
    congenital Q68.8
forehead (acquired) M95.2
    congenital Q75.8
frontal bone (acquired) M95.2
    congenital Q75.8
gallbladder (congenital) Q44.1
    acquired K82.8
gastrointestinal tract (congenital) NOS Q45.9
    acquired K63.89
genitalia, genital organ(s) or system NEC
    female (congenital) Q52.9
      acquired N94.89
      external Q52.70
    male (congenital) Q55.9
      acquired N50.89
globe (eye) (congenital) Q15.8
    acquired H44.89
gum, acquired NEC K06.8
hand (acquired) —*see* Deformity, limb, hand
    congenital Q68.1
head (acquired) M95.2
    congenital Q75.8
heart (congenital) Q24.9
    septum Q21.9
      auricular Q21.1
      ventricular Q21.0
    valve (congenital) NEC Q24.8
      acquired —*see* Endocarditis

Deformity *(Continued)*

heel (acquired) —*see* Deformity, foot
hepatic duct (congenital) Q44.5
    acquired K83.8
hip (joint) (acquired) —*see also* Deformity,
    limb, thigh
    congenital Q65.9
    due to (previous) juvenile
      osteochondrosis —*see* Coxa, plana
    flexion —*see* Contraction, joint, hip
hourglass —*see* Contraction, hourglass
humerus (acquired) M21.82-●
    congenital Q74.0
hypophyseal (congenital) Q89.2
ileocecal (coil) (valve) (acquired) K63.89
    congenital Q43.9
ileum (congenital) Q43.9
    acquired K63.89
ilium (acquired) M95.5
    congenital Q74.2
integument (congenital) Q84.9
intervertebral cartilage or disc (acquired) —
    see Disorder, disc, specified NEC
intestine (large) (small) (congenital) NOS
    Q43.9
    acquired K63.89
intrinsic minus or plus (hand) —*see*
    Deformity, limb, specified type NEC,
    forearm
iris (acquired) H21.89
    congenital Q13.2
ischium (acquired) M95.5
    congenital Q74.2
jaw (acquired) (congenital) M26.9
joint (acquired) NEC M21.90
    congenital Q68.8
    elbow M21.92-●
    hand M21.94-●
    hip M21.95-●
    knee M21.96-●
    shoulder M21.92-●
    wrist M21.93-●
kidney(s) (calyx) (pelvis) (congenital) Q63.9
    acquired N28.89
    artery (congenital) Q27.2
      acquired I77.89
Klippel-Feil (brevicollis) Q76.1
knee (acquired) NEC —*see also* Deformity,
    limb, lower leg
    congenital Q68.2
labium (majus) (minus) (congenital) Q52.79
    acquired N90.89
lacrimal passages or duct (congenital) NEC
    Q10.6
    acquired —*see* Disorder, lacrimal system,
      changes
larynx (muscle) (congenital) Q31.8
    acquired J38.7
    web (glottic) Q31.0
leg (upper) (acquired) NEC —*see also*
    Deformity, limb, thigh
    congenital Q68.8
    lower leg —*see* Deformity, limb, lower leg
lens (acquired) H27.8
    congenital Q12.9
lid (fold) (acquired) —*see also* Disorder,
    eyelid, specified type NEC
    congenital Q10.3
ligament (acquired) —*see* Disorder, ligament
    congenital Q79.9
limb (acquired) M21.90
    clawfoot M21.53-●
    clawhand M21.51-●
    clubfoot M21.54-●
    clubhand M21.52-●
    congenital, except reduction deformity
      Q74.9
    flat foot M21.4-●
    flexion M21.20
      ankle M21.27-●
      elbow M21.22-●

Deformity *(Continued)*

limb *(Continued)*
    flexion *(Continued)*
      finger M21.24-●
      hip M21.25-●
      knee M21.26-●
      shoulder M21.21-●
      toe M21.27-●
      wrist M21.23-●
    foot
      claw —*see* Deformity, limb, clawfoot
      club —*see* Deformity, limb, clubfoot
      drop M21.37-●
      flat —*see* Deformity, limb, flat foot
      specified NEC M21.6X-●
    forearm M21.93-●
    hand M21.94-●
    lower leg M21.96-●
    specified type NEC M21.80
      forearm M21.83-●
      lower leg M21.86-●
      thigh M21.85-●
      upper arm M21.82-●
    thigh M21.95-●
    unequal length M21.70
      short site is
        femur M21.75-●
        fibula M21.76-●
        humerus M21.72-●
        radius M21.73-●
        tibia M21.76-●
        ulna M21.73-●
    upper arm M21.92-●
    valgus —*see* Deformity, valgus
    varus —*see* Deformity, varus
    wrist drop M21.33-●
lip (acquired) NEC K13.0
    congenital Q38.0
liver (congenital) Q44.7
    acquired K76.89
lumbosacral (congenital) (joint) (region)
    Q76.49
    acquired —*see* subcategory M43.8
    kyphosis —*see* Kyphosis, congenital
    lordosis —*see* Lordosis, congenital
lung (congenital) Q33.9
    acquired J98.4
lymphatic system, congenital Q89.9
Madelung's (radius) Q74.0
mandible (acquired) (congenital) M26.9
maxilla (acquired) (congenital) M26.9
meninges or membrane (congenital) Q07.9
    cerebral Q04.8
      acquired G96.198
  ➜spinal cord (congenital) Q06.-●
      acquired G96.198
metacarpus (acquired) —*see* Deformity, limb,
    forearm
    congenital Q74.0
metatarsus (acquired) —*see* Deformity, foot
    congenital Q66.9-●
middle ear (congenital) Q16.4
    ossicles Q16.3
mitral (leaflets) (valve) I05.8
    parachute Q23.2
    stenosis, congenital Q23.2
mouth (acquired) K13.79
    congenital Q38.6
multiple, congenital NEC Q89.7
muscle (acquired) M62.89
    congenital Q79.9
      sternocleidomastoid Q68.0
musculoskeletal system (acquired) M95.9
    congenital Q79.9
    specified NEC M95.8
nail (acquired) L60.8
    congenital Q84.6
nasal —*see* Deformity, nose
neck (acquired) M95.3
    congenital Q18.9
      sternocleidomastoid Q68.0

▶ New   ➜ Revised   ~~deleted~~ Deleted   ● Use Additional Character(s)

Deformity *(Continued)*
  nervous system (congenital) Q07.9
  nipple (congenital) Q83.9
    acquired N64.89
  nose (acquired) (cartilage) M95.0
    bone (turbinate) M95.0
    congenital Q30.9
      bent or squashed Q67.4
    saddle M95.0
      syphilitic A50.57
    septum (acquired) J34.2
      congenital Q30.8
    sinus (wall) (congenital) Q30.8
      acquired M95.0
    syphilitic (congenital) A50.57
      late A52.73
  ocular muscle (congenital) Q10.3
    acquired —*see* Strabismus, mechanical
  opticociliary vessels (congenital) Q13.2
  orbit (eye) (acquired) H05.30
    atrophy —*see* Atrophy, orbit
    congenital Q10.7
    due to
      bone disease NEC H05.32-•
      trauma or surgery H05.33-•
    enlargement —*see* Enlargement, orbit
    exostosis —*see* Exostosis, orbit
  organ of Corti (congenital) Q16.5
  ovary (congenital) Q50.39
    acquired N83.8
  oviduct, acquired N83.8
  palate (congenital) Q38.5
    acquired M27.8
    cleft (congenital) —*see* Cleft, palate
  pancreas (congenital) Q45.3
    acquired K86.89
  parathyroid (gland) Q89.2
  parotid (gland) (congenital) Q38.4
    acquired K11.8
  patella (acquired) —*see* Disorder, patella,
      specified NEC
  pelvis, pelvic (acquired) (bony) M95.5
    with disproportion (fetopelvic) O33.0
      causing obstructed labor O65.0
    congenital Q74.2
    rachitic sequelae (late effect) E64.3
  penis (glans) (congenital) Q55.69
    acquired N48.89
  pericardium (congenital) Q24.8
    acquired —*see* Pericarditis
  pharynx (congenital) Q38.8
    acquired J39.2
  pinna, acquired —*see also* Disorder, pinna,
      deformity
    congenital Q17.9
  pituitary (congenital) Q89.2
  posture —*see* Dorsopathy, deforming
  prepuce (congenital) Q55.69
    acquired N47.8
  prostate (congenital) Q55.4
    acquired N42.89
  pupil (congenital) Q13.2
    acquired —*see* Abnormality, pupillary
  pylorus (congenital) Q40.3
    acquired K31.89
  rachitic (acquired), old or healed E64.3
  radius (acquired) —*see also* Deformity, limb,
      forearm
    congenital Q68.8
  rectum (congenital) Q43.9
    acquired K62.89
  reduction (extremity) (limb), congenital (*see
      also* condition and site) Q73.8
    brain Q04.3
    lower —*see* Defect, reduction, lower limb
    upper —*see* Defect, reduction, upper limb
  renal —*see* Deformity, kidney
  respiratory system (congenital) Q34.9
  rib (acquired) M95.4
    congenital Q76.6
      cervical Q76.5

Deformity *(Continued)*
  rotation (joint) (acquired) —*see* Deformity,
      limb, specified site NEC
    congenital Q74.9
    hip —*see* Deformity, limb, specified type
      NEC, thigh
      congenital Q65.89
  sacroiliac joint (congenital) Q74.2
    acquired —*see* subcategory M43.8
  sacrum (acquired) —*see* subcategory M43.8
  saddle
    back —*see* Lordosis
    nose M95.0
      syphilitic A50.57
  salivary gland or duct (congenital) Q38.4
    acquired K11.8
  scapula (acquired) M95.8
    congenital Q68.8
  scrotum (congenital) —*see also* Malformation,
      testis and scrotum
    acquired N50.89
  seminal vesicles (congenital) Q55.4
    acquired N50.89
  septum, nasal (acquired) J34.2
  shoulder (joint) (acquired) —*see* Deformity,
      limb, upper arm
    congenital Q74.0
    contraction —*see* Contraction, joint,
      shoulder
  sigmoid (flexure) (congenital) Q43.9
    acquired K63.89
  skin (congenital) Q82.9
  skull (acquired) M95.2
    congenital Q75.8
      with
        anencephaly Q00.0
        encephalocele —*see* Encephalocele
        hydrocephalus Q03.9
          with spina bifida —*see* Spina bifida,
            by site, with hydrocephalus
        microcephaly Q02
  soft parts, organs or tissues (of pelvis)
    in pregnancy or childbirth NEC O34.8-•
      causing obstructed labor O65.5
  spermatic cord (congenital) Q55.4
    acquired N50.89
    torsion —*see* Torsion, spermatic cord
  spinal —*see* Dorsopathy, deforming
    column (acquired) —*see* Dorsopathy,
      deforming
    congenital Q67.5
    cord (congenital) Q06.9
      acquired G95.89
    nerve root (congenital) Q07.9
  spine (acquired) —*see also* Dorsopathy,
      deforming
    congenital Q67.5
    rachitic E64.3
    specified NEC —*see* Dorsopathy,
      deforming, specified NEC
  spleen
    acquired D73.89
    congenital Q89.09
  Sprengel's (congenital) Q74.0
  sternocleidomastoid (muscle), congenital
      Q68.0
  sternum (acquired) M95.4
    congenital NEC Q76.7
  stomach (congenital) Q40.3
    acquired K31.89
  submandibular gland (congenital) Q38.4
  submaxillary gland (congenital) Q38.4
    acquired K11.8
  talipes —*see* Talipes
  testis (congenital) —*see also* Malformation,
      testis and scrotum
    acquired N44.8
    torsion —*see* Torsion, testis
  thigh (acquired) —*see also* Deformity, limb,
      thigh
    congenital NEC Q68.8

Deformity *(Continued)*
  thorax (acquired) (wall) M95.4
    congenital Q67.8
    sequelae of rickets E64.3
  thumb (acquired) —*see also* Deformity, finger
    congenital NEC Q68.1
  thymus (tissue) (congenital) Q89.2
  thyroid (gland) (congenital) Q89.2
    cartilage Q31.8
      acquired J38.7
  tibia (acquired) —*see also* Deformity, limb,
      specified type NEC, lower leg
    congenital NEC Q68.8
    saber (syphilitic) A50.56
  toe (acquired) M20.6-•
    congenital Q66.9-•
    hallux rigidus M20.2-•
    hallux valgus M20.1-•
    hallux varus M20.3-•
    hammer toe M20.4-•
    specified NEC M20.5X-•
  tongue (congenital) Q38.3
    acquired K14.8
  tooth, teeth K00.2
  trachea (rings) (congenital) Q32.1
    acquired J39.8
  transverse aortic arch (congenital)
      Q25.49
  tricuspid (leaflets) (valve) I07.8
    atresia or stenosis Q22.4
    Ebstein's Q22.5
  trunk (acquired) M95.8
    congenital Q89.9
  ulna (acquired) —*see also* Deformity, limb,
      forearm
    congenital NEC Q68.8
  urachus, congenital Q64.4
  ureter (opening) (congenital) Q62.8
    acquired N28.89
  urethra (congenital) Q64.79
    acquired N36.8
  urinary tract (congenital) Q64.9
    urachus Q64.4
  uterus (congenital) Q51.9
    acquired N85.8
  uvula (congenital) Q38.5
  vagina (acquired) N89.8
    congenital Q52.4
  valgus NEC M21.00
    ankle M21.07-•
    elbow M21.02-•
    hip M21.05-•
    knee M21.06-•
  valve, valvular (congenital) (heart) Q24.8
    acquired —*see* Endocarditis
  varus NEC M21.10
    ankle M21.17-•
    elbow M21.12-•
    hip M21.15
    knee M21.16-•
    tibia —*see* Osteochondrosis, juvenile, tibia
  vas deferens (congenital) Q55.4
    acquired N50.89
  vein (congenital) Q27.9
    great Q26.9
  vertebra —*see* Dorsopathy, deforming
  vertical talus (congenital) Q66.80
    left foot Q66.82
    right foot Q66.81
  vesicourethral orifice (acquired) N32.89
    congenital NEC Q64.79
  vessels of optic papilla (congenital) Q14.2
  visual field (contraction) —*see* Defect, visual
      field
  vitreous body, acquired H43.89
  vulva (congenital) Q52.79
    acquired N90.89
  wrist (joint) (acquired) —*see also* Deformity,
      limb, forearm
    congenital Q68.8
    contraction —*see* Contraction, joint, wrist

Degeneration, degenerative
- adrenal (capsule) (fatty) (gland) (hyaline) (infectional) E27.8
- amyloid —*see also* Amyloidosis E85.9
- anterior cornua, spinal cord G12.29
- anterior labral S43.49-•
- aorta, aortic I70.0
  - fatty I77.89
- aortic valve (heart) —*see* Endocarditis, aortic
- arteriovascular —*see* Arteriosclerosis
- artery, arterial (atheromatous) (calcareous) — *see also* Arteriosclerosis
  - cerebral, amyloid E85.4 [I68.0]
  - medial —*see* Arteriosclerosis, extremities
- articular cartilage NEC —*see* Derangement, joint, articular cartilage, by site
- atheromatous —*see* Arteriosclerosis
- basal nuclei or ganglia G23.9
  - specified NEC G23.8
- bone NEC —*see* Disorder, bone, specified type NEC
- brachial plexus G54.0
- brain (cortical) (progressive) G31.9
  - alcoholic G31.2
  - arteriosclerotic I67.2
  - childhood G31.9
    - specified NEC G31.89
  - cystic G31.89
    - congenital Q04.6
  - in
    - alcoholism G31.2
    - beriberi E51.2
    - cerebrovascular disease I67.9
    - congenital hydrocephalus Q03.9
      - with spina bifida —*see also* Spina bifida
    - Fabry-Anderson disease E75.21
    - Gaucher's disease E75.22
    - Hunter's syndrome E76.1
    - lipidosis
      - cerebral E75.4
      - generalized E75.6
    - mucopolysaccharidosis —*see* Mucopolysaccharidosis
    - myxedema E03.9 [G32.89]
    - neoplastic disease —*see also* Neoplasm D49.6 [G32.89]
    - Niemann-Pick disease E75.249 [G32.89]
    - sphingolipidosis E75.3 [G32.89]
    - vitamin B12 deficiency E53.8 [G32.89]
  - senile NEC G31.1
- breast N64.89
- Bruch's membrane —*see* Degeneration, choroid
- capillaries (fatty) I78.8
  - amyloid E85.89 [I79.8]
- cardiac —*see also* Degeneration, myocardial
  - valve, valvular —*see* Endocarditis
- cardiorenal —*see* Hypertension, cardiorenal
- cardiovascular —*see also* Disease, cardiovascular
  - renal —*see* Hypertension, cardiorenal
- cerebellar NOS G31.9
  - alcoholic G31.2
  - primary (hereditary) (sporadic) G11.9
- cerebral —*see* Degeneration, brain
- cerebrovascular I67.9
  - due to hypertension I67.4
- cervical plexus G54.2
- cervix N88.8
  - due to radiation (intended effect) N88.8
    - adverse effect or misadventure N99.89
- chamber angle H21.21-•
- changes, spine or vertebra —*see* Spondylosis
- chorioretinal —*see also* Degeneration, choroid hereditary H31.20
- choroid (colloid) (drusen) H31.10-•
  - atrophy —*see* Atrophy, choroidal
  - hereditary —*see* Dystrophy, choroidal, hereditary

Degeneration, degenerative (*Continued*)
- ciliary body H21.22-•
- cochlear —*see* subcategory H83.8
- combined (spinal cord) (subacute) E53.8 [G32.0]
  - with anemia (pernicious) D51.0 [G32.0]
    - due to dietary vitamin B12 deficiency D51.3 [G32.0]
  - in (due to)
    - vitamin B12 deficiency E53.8 [G32.0]
    - anemia D51.9 [G32.0]
- conjunctiva H11.10
  - concretions —*see* Concretion, conjunctiva
  - deposits —*see* Deposit, conjunctiva
  - pigmentations —*see* Pigmentation, conjunctiva
  - pinguecula —*see* Pinguecula
  - xerosis —*see* Xerosis, conjunctiva
- cornea H18.40
  - calcerous H18.43
    - band keratopathy H18.42-•
  - familial, hereditary —*see* Dystrophy, cornea
  - hyaline (of old scars) H18.49
  - keratomalacia —*see* Keratomalacia
  - nodular H18.45-•
  - peripheral H18.46-•
  - senile H18.41-•
  - specified type NEC H18.49
- cortical (cerebellar) (parenchymatous) G31.89
  - alcoholic G31.2
  - diffuse, due to arteriopathy I67.2
- corticobasal G31.85
- cutis L98.8
  - amyloid E85.4 [L99]
- dental pulp K04.2
- disc disease —*see* Degeneration, intervertebral disc NEC
- dorsolateral (spinal cord) —*see* Degeneration, combined
- extrapyramidal G25.9
- eye, macular —*see also* Degeneration, macula congenital or hereditary —*see* Dystrophy, retina
- facet joints —*see* Spondylosis
- fatty
  - liver NEC K76.0
    - alcoholic K70.0
- grey matter (brain) (Alpers') G31.81
- heart —*see also* Degeneration, myocardial
  - amyloid E85.4 [I43]
  - atheromatous —*see* Disease, heart, ischemic, atherosclerotic
  - ischemic —*see* Disease, heart, ischemic
- hepatolenticular (Wilson's) E83.01
- hepatorenal K76.7
- hyaline (diffuse) (generalized)
  - localized —*see* Degeneration, by site
- infrapatellar fat pad M79.4
- intervertebral disc NOS
  - with
    - myelopathy —*see* Disorder, disc, with, myelopathy
    - radiculitis or radiculopathy —*see* Disorder, disc, with, radiculopathy
  - cervical, cervicothoracic —*see* Disorder, disc, cervical, degeneration
    - with
      - myelopathy —*see* Disorder, disc, cervical, with myelopathy
      - neuritis, radiculitis or radiculopathy —*see* Disorder, disc, cervical, with neuritis
  - lumbar region M51.36
    - with
      - myelopathy M51.06
      - neuritis, radiculitis, radiculopathy or sciatica M51.16
  - lumbosacral region M51.37
    - with
      - neuritis, radiculitis, radiculopathy or sciatica M51.17

Degeneration, degenerative (*Continued*)
- intervertebral disc (*Continued*)
  - sacrococcygeal region M53.3
  - thoracic region M51.34
    - with
      - myelopathy M51.04
      - neuritis, radiculitis, radiculopathy M51.14
  - thoracolumbar region M51.35
    - with
      - myelopathy M51.05
      - neuritis, radiculitis, radiculopathy M51.15
- intestine, amyloid E85.4
- iris (pigmentary) H21.23-•
- ischemic —*see* Ischemia
- joint disease —*see* Osteoarthritis
- kidney N28.89
  - amyloid E85.4 [N29]
  - cystic, congenital Q61.9
  - fatty N28.89
  - polycystic Q61.3
    - adult type (autosomal dominant) Q61.2
    - infantile type (autosomal recessive) NEC Q61.19
    - collecting duct dilatation Q61.11
- Kuhnt-Junius —*see also* Degeneration, macula H35.32-•
- lens —*see* Cataract
- lenticular (familial) (progressive) (Wilson's) (with cirrhosis of liver) E83.01
- liver (diffuse) NEC K76.89
  - amyloid E85.4 [K77]
  - cystic K76.89
    - congenital Q44.6
  - fatty NEC K76.0
    - alcoholic K70.0
  - hypertrophic K76.89
  - parenchymatous, acute or subacute K72.00
    - with coma K72.01
  - pigmentary K76.89
  - toxic (acute) K71.9
- lung J98.4
- lymph gland I89.8
  - hyaline I89.8
- macula, macular (acquired) (age-related) (senile) H35.30
  - angioid streaks H35.33
  - atrophic age-related H35.31-•
  - congenital or hereditary —*see* Dystrophy, retina
  - cystoid H35.35-•
  - drusen H35.36-•
  - dry age-related H35.31-•
  - exudative H35.32-•
  - hole H35.34-•
  - nonexudative H35.31-•
  - puckering H35.37-•
  - toxic H35.38-•
  - wet age-related H35.32-•
- membranous labyrinth, congenital (causing impairment of hearing) Q16.5
- meniscus —*see* Derangement, meniscus
- mitral —*see* Insufficiency, mitral
- Mönckeberg's —*see* Arteriosclerosis, extremities
- motor centers, senile G31.1
- multi-system G90.3
- mural —*see* Degeneration, myocardial
- muscle (fatty) (fibrous) (hyaline) (progressive) M62.89
  - heart —*see* Degeneration, myocardial
- myelin, central nervous system G37.9
- myocardial, myocardium (fatty) (hyaline) (senile) I51.5
  - with rheumatic fever (conditions in I00) I09.0
    - active, acute or subacute I01.2
      - with chorea I02.0
    - inactive or quiescent (with chorea) I09.0

▶ New   ⇒ Revised   ~~deleted~~ Deleted   • Use Additional Character(s)

Degeneration, degenerative *(Continued)*
  myocardial, myocardium *(Continued)*
    hypertensive —*see* Hypertension, heart
    rheumatic —*see* Degeneration, myocardial,
      with rheumatic fever
    syphilitic A52.06
  nasal sinus (mucosa) J32.9
    frontal J32.1
    maxillary J32.0
  nerve —*see* Disorder, nerve
  nervous system G31.9
    alcoholic G31.2
    amyloid E85.4 *[G99.8]*
    autonomic G90.9
    fatty G31.89
    specified NEC G31.89
  nipple N64.89
  olivopontocerebellar (hereditary) (familial)
    G23.8
  osseous labyrinth —*see* subcategory H83.8
  ovary N83.8
    cystic N83.20-●
    microcystic N83.20-●
  pallidal pigmentary (progressive) G23.0
  pancreas K86.89
    tuberculous A18.83
  penis N48.89
  pigmentary (diffuse) (general)
    localized —*see* Degeneration, by site
    pallidal (progressive) G23.0
  pineal gland E34.8
  pituitary (gland) E23.6
  popliteal fat pad M79.4
  posterolateral (spinal cord) —*see*
    Degeneration, combined
  pulmonary valve (heart) I37.8
  pulp (tooth) K04.2
  pupillary margin H21.24-●
  renal —*see* Degeneration, kidney
  retina H35.9
    hereditary (cerebroretinal) (congenital)
      (juvenile) (macula) (peripheral)
      (pigmentary) —*see* Dystrophy, retina
    Kuhnt-Junius —*see also* Degeneration,
      macula H35.32-●
    macula (cystic) (exudative) (hole)
      (nonexudative) (pseudohole) (senile)
      (toxic) —*see* Degeneration, macula
    peripheral H35.40
      lattice H35.41-●
      microcystoid H35.42-●
      paving stone H35.43-●
      secondary
        pigmentary H35.45-●
        vitreoretinal H35.46-●
      senile reticular H35.44-●
    pigmentary (primary) —*see also* Dystrophy,
      retina
    secondary —*see* Degeneration, retina,
      peripheral, secondary
    posterior pole —*see* Degeneration, macula
  saccule, congenital (causing impairment of
    hearing) Q16.5
  senile R54
    brain G31.1
    cardiac, heart or myocardium —*see*
      Degeneration, myocardial
    motor centers G31.1
    vascular —*see* Arteriosclerosis
  sinus (cystic) —*see also* Sinusitis
    polypoid J33.1
  skin L98.8
    amyloid E85.4 *[L99]*
    colloid L98.8
  spinal (cord) G31.89
    amyloid E85.4 *[G32.89]*
    combined (subacute) —*see* Degeneration,
      combined
    dorsolateral —*see* Degeneration, combined
    familial NEC G31.89
    fatty G31.89

Degeneration, degenerative *(Continued)*
  spinal *(Continued)*
    funicular —*see* Degeneration, combined
    posterolateral —*see* Degeneration,
      combined
    subacute combined —*see* Degeneration,
      combined
    tuberculous A17.81
  spleen D73.0
    amyloid E85.4 *[D77]*
  stomach K31.89
  striatonigral G23.2
  suprarenal (capsule) (gland) E27.8
  synovial membrane (pulpy) —*see* Disorder,
    synovium, specified type NEC
  tapetoretinal —*see* Dystrophy, retina
  thymus (gland) E32.8
    fatty E32.8
  thyroid (gland) E07.89
  tricuspid (heart) (valve) I07.9
  tuberculous NEC —*see* Tuberculosis
  turbinate J34.89
  uterus (cystic) N85.8
  vascular (senile) —*see* Arteriosclerosis
    hypertensive —*see* Hypertension
  vitreoretinal, secondary —*see* Degeneration,
    retina, peripheral, secondary, vitreoretinal
  vitreous (body) H43.81-●
  Wallerian —*see* Disorder, nerve
  Wilson's hepatolenticular E83.01
Deglutition
  paralysis R13.0
    hysterical F44.4
  pneumonia J69.0
Degos' disease I77.89
Dehiscence (of)
  amputation stump T87.81
  cesarean wound O90.0
  closure of
    cornea T81.31
    craniotomy T81.32
    fascia (muscular) (superficial) T81.32
    internal organ or tissue T81.32
    laceration (external) (internal) T81.33
    ligament T81.32
    mucosa T81.31
    muscle or muscle flap T81.32
    ribs or rib cage T81.32
    skin and subcutaneous tissue (full-
      thickness) (superficial) T81.31
    skull T81.32
    sternum (sternotomy) T81.32
    tendon T81.32
    traumatic laceration (external) (internal)
      T81.33
  episiotomy O90.1
  operation wound NEC T81.31
    external operation wound (superficial)
      T81.31
    internal operation wound (deep)
      T81.32
  perineal wound (postpartum) O90.1
  traumatic injury wound repair T81.33
  wound T81.30
    traumatic repair T81.33
Dehydration E86.0
  newborn P74.1
Déjérine-Roussy syndrome G93.89
Déjérine-Sottas disease or neuropathy
  (hypertrophic) G60.0
Déjérine-Thomas atrophy G23.8
Delay, delayed
  any plane in pelvis
    complicating delivery O66.9
  birth or delivery NOS O63.9
  closure, ductus arteriosus (Botalli) P29.38
  coagulation —*see* Defect, coagulation
  conduction (cardiac) (ventricular)
    I45.9
  delivery, second twin, triplet, etc
    O63.2

Delay, delayed *(Continued)*
  development R62.50
    global F88
    intellectual (specific) F81.9
    language F80.9
      due to hearing loss F80.4
    learning F81.9
    pervasive F84.9
    physiological R62.50
      specified stage NEC R62.0
    reading F81.0
    sexual E30.0
    speech F80.9
      due to hearing loss F80.4
    spelling F81.81
  ejaculation F52.32
  gastric emptying K30
  menarche E30.0
  menstruation (cause unknown) N91.0
  milestone R62.0
  passage of meconium (newborn)
    P76.0
  primary respiration P28.9
  puberty (constitutional) E30.0
  separation of umbilical cord P96.82
  sexual maturation, female E30.0
  sleep phase syndrome G47.21
  union, fracture —*see* Fracture, by site
  vaccination Z28.9
Deletion(s)
  autosome Q93.9
    identified by fluorescence in situ
      hybridization (FISH) Q93.89
    identified by in situ hybridization (ISH)
      Q93.89
  chromosome
    with complex rearrangements NEC
      Q93.7
    part of NEC Q93.59
    seen only at prometaphase Q93.89
    short arm
      4 Q93.3
      5p Q93.4
      22q11.2 Q93.81
    specified NEC Q93.89
  long arm chromosome 18 or 21 Q93.89
    with complex rearrangements NEC Q93.7
  microdeletions NEC Q93.88
Delhi boil or button B55.1
Delinquency (juvenile) (neurotic) F91.8
  group Z72.810
Delinquent immunization status Z28.3
Delirious (acute or subacute) (not alcohol or
  drug-induced) (with dementia) R41.0
  alcoholic (acute) (tremens) (withdrawal)
    F10.921
    with intoxication F10.921
      in
        abuse F10.121
        dependence F10.221
  due to (secondary to)
    alcohol
      intoxication F10.921
        in
          abuse F10.121
          dependence F10.221
      withdrawal F10.231
    amphetamine intoxication F15.921
      in
        abuse F15.121
        dependence F15.221
    anxiolytic
      intoxication F13.921
        in
          abuse F13.121
          dependence F13.221
      withdrawal F13.231
    cannabis intoxication (acute) F12.921
      in
        abuse F12.121
        dependence F12.221

Delirious *(Continued)*
  due to *(Continued)*
    cocaine intoxication (acute) F14.921
      in
        abuse F14.121
        dependence F14.221
    general medical condition F05
    hallucinogen intoxication F16.921
      in
        abuse F16.121
        dependence F16.221
    hypnotic
      intoxication F13.921
        in
          abuse F13.121
          dependence F13.221
      withdrawal F13.231
    inhalant intoxication (acute) F18.921
      in
        abuse F18.121
        dependence F18.221
    multiple etiologies F05
    opioid intoxication (acute) F11.921
      in
        abuse F11.121
        dependence F11.221
    other (or unknown) substance
      F19.921
    phencyclidine intoxication (acute)
      F16.921
      in
        abuse F16.121
        dependence F16.221
    psychoactive substance NEC intoxication
      (acute) F19.921
      in
        abuse F19.121
        dependence F19.221
    sedative
      intoxication F13.921
        in
          abuse F13.121
          dependence F13.221
      withdrawal F13.231
    unknown etiology R41.0
  exhaustion F43.0
  hysterical F44.89
  postprocedural (postoperative) F05
  puerperal F05
  thyroid —*see* Thyrotoxicosis with thyroid
    storm
  traumatic —*see* Injury, intracranial
  tremens (alcohol-induced) F10.231
    sedative-induced F13.231
Delivery (childbirth) (labor)
  arrested active phase O62.1
  cesarean (for)
    without indication O82
    abnormal
      pelvis (bony) (deformity) (major) NEC
        with disproportion (fetopelvic)
          O33.0
        with obstructed labor O65.0
        presentation or position O32.9
    abruptio placentae —*see also* Abruptio
      placentae 045.9-●
    acromion presentation O32.2
    atony, uterus O62.2
    breech presentation O32.1
      incomplete O32.8
    brow presentation O32.3
    cephalopelvic disproportion O33.9
    cerclage O34.3-●
    chin presentation O32.3
    cicatrix of cervix O34.4-●
    contracted pelvis (general)
      inlet O33.2
      outlet O33.3
    cord presentation or prolapse
      O69.0
    cystocele O34.8-●

Delivery *(Continued)*
  cesarean *(Continued)*
    deformity (acquired) (congenital)
      pelvic organs or tissues NEC O34.8-●
      pelvis (bony) NEC O33.0
    disproportion NOS O33.9
    eclampsia —*see* Eclampsia
    face presentation O32.3
    failed
      forceps O66.5
      induction of labor O61.9
        instrumental O61.1
        mechanical O61.1
        medical O61.0
        specified NEC O61.8
        surgical O61.1
      trial of labor NOS O66.40
        following previous cesarean delivery
          O66.41
      vacuum extraction O66.5
      ventouse O66.5
    fetal-maternal hemorrhage O43.01-●
    hemorrhage (intrapartum) O67.9
      with coagulation defect O67.0
      specified cause NEC O67.8
    high head at term O32.4
    hydrocephalic fetus O33.6
    incarceration of uterus O34.51-●
    incoordinate uterine action O62.4
    increased size, fetus O33.5
    inertia, uterus O62.2
      primary O62.0
      secondary O62.1
    isthmocele O34.22
    lateroversion, uterus O34.59-●
    mal lie O32.9
    malposition
      fetus O32.9
      pelvic organs or tissues NEC O34.8-●
      uterus NEC O34.59-●
    malpresentation NOS O32.9
    oblique presentation O32.2
    occurring after 37 completed weeks of
      gestation but before 39 completed
      weeks gestation due to (spontaneous)
      onset of labor O75.82
    oversize fetus O33.5
    pelvic tumor NEC O34.8-●
    placenta previa O44.0-●
      complete O44.0-●
      with hemorrhage O44.1-●
    placental insufficiency O36.51-●
    planned, occurring after 37 completed
      weeks of gestation but before 39
      completed weeks gestation due to
      (spontaneous) onset of labor O75.82
    polyp, cervix O34.4-●
      causing obstructed labor O65.5
    poor dilatation, cervix O62.0
    pre-eclampsia O14.94
      mild O14.04
      moderate O14.04
      severe O14.14
        with hemolysis, elevated liver
          enzymes and low platelet count
          (HELLP) O14.24
    previous
      cesarean delivery O34.219
        classical (vertical) scar O34.212
        isthmocele O34.22
        low transverse scar O34.211
        mid-transverse T incision O34.218
        scar
          defect (isthmocele) O34.22
          specified type NEC O34.218
      surgery (to)
        cervix O34.4-●
        gynecological NEC O34.8-●
        rectum O34.7-●
        uterus O34.29
        vagina O34.6-●

Delivery *(Continued)*
  cesarean *(Continued)*
    prolapse
      arm or hand O32.2
      uterus O34.52-●
    prolonged labor NOS O63.9
    rectocele O34.8-●
    retroversion
      uterus O34.53-●
    rigid
      cervix O34.4-●
      pelvic floor O34.8-●
      perineum O34.7-●
      vagina O34.6-●
      vulva O34.7-●
    sacculation, pregnant uterus O34.59-●
    scar(s)
      cervix O34.4-●
      cesarean delivery O34.219
        classical (vertical) O34.212
        isthmocele O34.22
        low transverse O34.211
        mid-transverse T incision O34.218
        scar
          defect (isthmocele) O34.22
          specified type NEC O34.218
      defect (isthmocele) O34.22
      transmural uterine O34.29
      uterus O34.29
    Shirodkar suture in situ O34.3-●
    shoulder presentation O32.2
    stenosis or stricture, cervix O34.4-●
    streptococcus group B (GBS) carrier state
      O99.824
    transmural uterine scar O34.29
    transverse presentation or lie O32.2
    tumor, pelvic organs or tissues NEC O34.8-●
      cervix O34.4-●
    umbilical cord presentation or prolapse
      O69.0
  completely normal case O80
  complicated O75.9
    by
      abnormal, abnormality (of)
        forces of labor O62.9
          specified type NEC O62.8
        glucose O99.814
        uterine contractions NOS O62.9
      abruptio placentae —*see also* Abruptio
        placentae O45.9-●
      abuse
        physical O9A.32
        psychological O9A.52
        sexual O9A.42
      adherent placenta O72.0
        without hemorrhage O73.0
      alcohol use O99.314
      anemia (pre-existing) O99.02
      anesthetic death O74.8
      annular detachment of cervix O71.3
      atony, uterus O62.2
      attempted vacuum extraction and
        forceps O66.5
      Bandl's ring O62.4
      bariatric surgery status O99.844
      biliary tract disorder O26.62
      bleeding —*see* Delivery, complicated by,
        hemorrhage
      blood disorder NEC O99.12
      cervical dystocia (hypotonic) O62.2
        primary O62.0
        secondary O62.1
      circulatory system disorder O99.42
      compression of cord (umbilical) NEC
        O69.2
      condition NEC O99.892
      contraction, contracted ring O62.4
      cord (umbilical)
        around neck
          with compression O69.1
          without compression O69.81

  ▶ New   ⇒ Revised   ~~deleted~~ Deleted   ● Use Additional Character(s)

Delivery *(Continued)*
  complicated *(Continued)*
    by *(Continued)*
      cord *(Continued)*
        bruising O69.5
        complication O69.9
          specified NEC O69.89
        compression NEC O69.2
        entanglement O69.2
          without compression O69.82
        hematoma O69.5
        presentation O69.0
        prolapse O69.0
        short O69.3
        thrombosis (vessels) O69.5
        vascular lesion O69.5
      Couvelaire uterus O45.8X-●
      damage to (injury to) NEC
        perineum O71.82
        periurethral tissue O71.82
        vulva O71.82
      delay following rupture of membranes
        (spontaneous) —*see* Pregnancy,
        complicated by, premature rupture
        of membranes
      depressed fetal heart tones O76
      diabetes O24.92
        gestational O24.429
          diet controlled O24.420
          insulin controlled O24.424
          oral drug controlled (antidiabetic)
            (hypoglycemic) O24.425
        pre-existing O24.32
          specified NEC O24.82
          type 1 O24.02
          type 2 O24.12
      diastasis recti (abdominis) O71.89
      dilatation
        bladder O66.8
        cervix incomplete, poor or slow O62.0
      disease NEC O99.892
      disruptio uteri —*see* Delivery,
        complicated by, rupture, uterus
      drug use O99.324
      dysfunction, uterus NOS O62.9
        hypertonic O62.4
        hypotonic O62.2
          primary O62.0
          secondary O62.1
        incoordinate O62.4
      eclampsia O15.1
      embolism (pulmonary) —*see* Embolism,
        obstetric
      endocrine, nutritional or metabolic
        disease NEC O99.284
      failed
        attempted vaginal birth after previous
          cesarean delivery O66.41
        induction of labor O61.9
          instrumental O61.1
          mechanical O61.1
          medical O61.0
          specified NEC O61.8
          surgical O61.1
        trial of labor O66.40
      female genital mutilation O65.5
      fetal
        abnormal acid-base balance O68
        acidemia O68
        acidosis O68
        alkalosis O68
        death, early O02.1
        deformity O66.3
        heart rate or rhythm (abnormal) (non-
          reassuring) O76
        hypoxia O77.8
        stress O77.9
          due to drug administration O77.1
          electrocardiographic evidence of
            O77.8
          specified NEC O77.8
          ultrasound evidence of O77.8

Delivery *(Continued)*
  complicated *(Continued)*
    by *(Continued)*
      fever during labor O75.2
      gastric banding status O99.844
      gastric bypass status O99.844
      gastrointestinal disease NEC O99.62
      gestational
        diabetes O24.429
          diet controlled O24.420
          insulin (and diet) controlled
            O24.424
          oral drug controlled (antidiabetic)
            (hypoglycemic) O24.425
        edema O12.04
          with proteinuria O12.24
        proteinuria O12.14
      gonorrhea O98.22
      hematoma O71.7
        ischial spine O71.7
        pelvic O71.7
        vagina O71.7
        vulva or perineum O71.7
      hemorrhage (uterine) O67.9
        associated with
          afibrinogenemia O67.0
          coagulation defect O67.0
          hyperfibrinolysis O67.0
          hypofibrinogenemia O67.0
        due to
          low implantation of placenta
            O44.5-●
          low-lying placenta O44.5-●
          placenta previa O44.1-●
            marginal O44.3-●
            partial O44.3-●
          premature separation of placenta
            (normally implanted) (*see also*
            Abruptio placentae) O45.9-●
          retained placenta O72.0
          uterine leiomyoma O67.8
        placenta NEC O67.8
        postpartum NEC (atonic) (immediate)
          O72.1
          with retained or trapped placenta
            O72.0
          delayed O72.2
          secondary O72.2
          third stage O72.0
      hourglass contraction, uterus O62.4
      hypertension, hypertensive (pre-
        existing) —*see* Hypertension,
        complicated by, childbirth (labor)
      hypotension O26.5-●
      incomplete dilatation (cervix)
        O62.0
      incoordinate uterus contractions
        O62.4
      inertia, uterus O62.2
        during latent phase of labor O62.0
        primary O62.0
        secondary O62.1
      infection (maternal) O98.92
        carrier state NEC O99.834
        gonorrhea O98.22
        human immunodeficiency virus (HIV)
          O98.72
        sexually transmitted NEC O98.32
        specified NEC O98.82
        syphilis O98.12
        tuberculosis O98.02
        viral hepatitis O98.42
        viral NEC O98.52
      injury (to mother) (*see also* Delivery,
        complicated, by, damage to)
        O71.9
        nonobstetric O9A.22
          caused by abuse —*see* Delivery,
            complicated by, abuse
      intrauterine fetal death, early O02.1
      inversion, uterus O71.2

Delivery *(Continued)*
  complicated *(Continued)*
    by *(Continued)*
      laceration (perineal) O70.9
        anus (sphincter) O70.4
          with third degree laceration —*see*
            also Delivery, complicated, by,
            laceration, perineum, third
            degree O70.20
          with mucosa O70.3
          without third degree laceration
            O70.4
        bladder (urinary) O71.5
        bowel O71.5
        cervix (uteri) O71.3
        fourchette O70.0
        hymen O70.0
        labia O70.0
        pelvic
          floor O70.1
          organ NEC O71.5
        perineum, perineal O70.9
          first degree O70.0
          fourth degree O70.3
          muscles O70.1
          second degree O70.1
          skin O70.0
          slight O70.0
          third degree O70.20
           with
            both external anal sphincter
             (EAS) and internal anal
             sphincter (IAS) torn (IIIc)
             O70.23
            less than 50% of external anal
             sphincter (EAS) thickness
             torn (IIIa) O70.21
            more than 50% external anal
             sphincter (EAS) thickness
             torn (IIIb) O70.22
           IIIa O70.21
           IIIb O70.22
           IIIc O70.23
        peritoneum (pelvic) O71.5
        rectovaginal (septum) (without
          perineal laceration) O71.4
          with perineum —*see also* Delivery,
            complicated, by, laceration,
            perineum, third degree
            O70.20
            with anal or rectal mucosa
             O70.3
        specified NEC O71.89
        sphincter ani —*see* Delivery,
          complicated, by, laceration, anus
          (sphincter)
        urethra O71.5
        uterus O71.81
          before labor O71.81
        vagina, vaginal (deep) (high)
          (without perineal laceration)
          O71.4
          with perineum O70.0
          muscles, with perineum O70.1
        vulva O70.0
      liver disorder O26.62
      malignancy O9A.12
      malnutrition O25.2
      malposition, malpresentation
        without obstruction O32.9 —*see*
          also Delivery, complicated by,
          obstruction
        breech O32.1
        compound O32.6
        face (brow) (chin) O32.3
        footling O38.8
        high head O32.4
        oblique O32.2
        specified NEC O32.8
        transverse O32.2
        unstable lie O32.0

Delivery *(Continued)*
  complicated *(Continued)*
    by *(Continued)*
      malposition, malpresentation
          (Continued)
        placenta O44.0-●
          with hemorrhage O44.1-●
        uterus or cervix O65.5
      meconium in amniotic fluid O77.0
      mental disorder NEC O99.344
      metrorrhexis —*see* Delivery, complicated
          by, rupture, uterus
      nervous system disorder O99.354
      obesity (pre-existing) O99.214
      obesity surgery status O99.844
      obstetric trauma O71.9
        specified NEC O71.89
      obstructed labor
        due to
          breech (complete) (frank)
              presentation O64.1
            incomplete O64.8
          brow presentation O64.3
          buttock presentation O64.1
          chin presentation O64.2
          compound presentation O64.5
          contracted pelvis O65.1
          deep transverse arrest O64.0
          deformed pelvis O65.0
          dystocia (fetal) O66.9
            due to
              conjoined twins O66.3
              fetal
                abnormality NEC O66.3
                ascites O66.3
                hydrops O66.3
                meningomyelocele O66.3
                sacral teratoma O66.3
                tumor O66.3
              hydrocephalic fetus O66.3
          shoulder O66.0
          face presentation O64.2
          fetopelvic disproportion O65.4
          footling presentation O64.8
          impacted shoulders O66.0
          incomplete rotation of fetal head
              O64.0
          large fetus O66.2
          locked twins O66.1
          malposition O64.9
            specified NEC O64.8
          malpresentation O64.9
            specified NEC O64.8
          multiple fetuses NEC O66.6
          pelvic
            abnormality (maternal) O65.9
              organ O65.5
              specified NEC O65.8
            contraction
              inlet O65.2
              mid-cavity O65.3
              outlet O65.3
          persistent (position)
            occipitoiliac O64.0
            occipitoposterior O64.0
            occipitosacral O64.0
            occipitotransverse O64.0
          prolapsed arm O64.4
          shoulder presentation O64.4
          specified NEC O66.8
      pathological retraction ring, uterus
          O62.4
      penetration, pregnant uterus by
          instrument O71.1
      perforation —*see* Delivery, complicated
          by, laceration
      placenta, placental
        ablatio —*see also* Abruptio placentae
            O45.9-●
        abnormality O43.9-●
          specified NEC O43.89-●

Delivery *(Continued)*
  complicated *(Continued)*
    by *(Continued)*
      placenta, placental *(Continued)*
        abruptio —*see also* Abruptio placentae
            O45.9-●
        accreta O43.21-●
        adherent (with hemorrhage) O72.0
          without hemorrhage O73.0
        detachment (premature) —*see also*
            Abruptio placentae O45.9-●
        disorder O43.9-●
          specified NEC O43.89-●
        hemorrhage NEC O67.8
        increta O43.22-●
        low (implantation) (lying) O44.4-●
          with hemorrhage O44.5-●
        malformation O43.10-●
        malposition O44.0-●
          without hemorrhage O44.1-●
        percreta O43.23-●
        previa (central) (complete) (lateral)
            (total) O44.0-●
          with hemorrhage O44.1-●
            marginal O44.2-●
              with hemorrhage O44.3-●
            partial O44.2-●
              with hemorrhage O44.3-●
        retained (with hemorrhage)
            O72.0
          without hemorrhage O73.0
        separation (premature) O45.9-●
          specified NEC O45.8X-●
        vicious insertion O44.1-●
      precipitate labor O62.3
      premature rupture, membranes (see
          also Pregnancy, complicated by,
          premature rupture of membranes)
          O42.90
      prolapse
        arm or hand O32.2
        cord (umbilical) O69.0
        foot or leg O32.8
        uterus O34.52-●
      prolonged labor O63.9
        first stage O63.0
        second stage O63.1
      protozoal disease (maternal) O98.62
      respiratory disease NEC O99.52
      retained membranes or portions of
          placenta O72.2
        without hemorrhage O73.1
      retarded birth O63.9
      retention of secundines (with
          hemorrhage) O72.0
        without hemorrhage O73.0
        partial O72.2
          without hemorrhage O73.1
      rupture
        bladder (urinary) O71.5
        cervix O71.3
        pelvic organ NEC O71.5
        urethra O71.5
        uterus (during or after labor)
            O71.1
          before labor O71.0-●
      separation, pubic bone (symphysis
          pubis) O71.6
      shock O75.1
      shoulder presentation O64.4
      skin disorder NEC O99.72
      spasm, cervix O62.4
      stenosis or stricture, cervix O65.5
      streptococcus group B (GBS) carrier state
          O99.824
      subluxation of symphysis (pubis)
          O26.72
      syphilis (maternal) O98.12
      tear —*see* Delivery, complicated by,
          laceration
      tetanic uterus O62.4

Delivery *(Continued)*
  complicated *(Continued)*
    by *(Continued)*
      trauma (obstetrical) —*see also* Delivery,
          complicated, by, damage to O71.9
        non-obstetric O9A.22
        periurethral O71.82
        specified NEC O71.89
      tuberculosis (maternal) O98.02
      tumor, pelvic organs or tissues NEC
          O65.5
      umbilical cord around neck
        with compression O69.1
        without compression O69.81
      uterine inertia O62.2
        during latent phase of labor O62.0
        primary O62.0
        secondary O62.1
      vasa previa O69.4
      velamentous insertion of cord O43.12-●
    specified complication NEC O75.89
  delayed NOS O63.9
    following rupture of membranes
        artificial O75.5
    second twin, triplet, etc. O63.2
  forceps, low following failed vacuum
      extraction O66.5
  missed (at or near term) O36.4
  normal O80
  obstructed —*see* Delivery, complicated by,
      obstructed labor
  precipitate O62.3
  preterm —*see also* Pregnancy, complicated by,
      preterm labor O60.10
  spontaneous O80
  term pregnancy NOS O80
  uncomplicated O80
  vaginal, following previous cesarean delivery
      O34.219
    classical (vertical) scar O34.212
    low transverse scar O34.211
    mid-transverse T incision O34.218
    scar
      defect (isthmocele) O34.22
      specified type NEC O34.218]
Delusions (paranoid) —*see* Disorder, delusional
Dementia (degenerative (primary)) (old age)
    (persisting) F03.90
  with
    aggressive behavior F03.91
    behavioral disturbance F03.91
    combative behavior F03.91
    Lewy bodies G31.83 *[F02.80]*
      with behavioral disturbance G31.83
          [F02.81]
    Parkinson's disease G20 *[F02.80]*
      with behavioral disturbance G20
          [F02.81]
    Parkinsonism G31.83 *[F02.80]*
      with behavioral disturbance G31.83
          [F02.81]
    violent behavior F03.91
  alcoholic F10.97
    with dependence F10.27
  Alzheimer's type —*see* Disease, Alzheimer's
  arteriosclerotic —*see* Dementia, vascular
  atypical, Alzheimer's type —*see* Disease,
      Alzheimer's, specified NEC
  congenital —*see* Disability, intellectual
  frontal (lobe) G31.09 *[F02.80]*
    with behavioral disturbance G31.09
        [F02.81]
  frontotemporal G31.09 *[F02.80]*
    with behavioral disturbance G31.09
        [F02.81]
    specified NEC G31.09 *[F02.80]*
      with behavioral disturbance G31.09
          [F02.81]
  in (due to)
    alcohol F10.97
      with dependence F10.27

Dementia *(Continued)*
in *(Continued)*
Alzheimer's disease —*see* Disease,
Alzheimer's
arteriosclerotic brain disease —*see*
Dementia, vascular
cerebral lipidoses E75.-● *[F02.80]*
with behavioral disturbance
E75.-● *[F02.81]*
Creutzfeldt-Jakob disease —*see also*
Creutzfeldt-Jakob disease or
syndrome (with dementia) A81.00
epilepsy G40.-● *[F02.80]*
with behavioral disturbance
G40.-● *[F02.81]*
hepatolenticular degeneration E83.01
[F02.80]
with behavioral disturbance E83.01
[F02.81]
human immunodeficiency virus (HIV)
disease B20 *[F02.80]*
with behavioral disturbance B20 *[F02.81]*
Huntington's disease or chorea G10 *[F02.80]*
with behavioral disturbance G10 *[F02.81]*
hypercalcemia E83.52 *[F02.80]*
with behavioral disturbance E83.52
[F02.81]
hypothyroidism, acquired E03.9 *[F02.80]*
with behavioral disturbance E03.9
[F02.81]
due to iodine deficiency E01.8 *[F02.80]*
with behavioral disturbance E01.8
[F02.81]
inhalants F18.97
with dependence F18.27
multiple
etiologies F03
sclerosis G35 *[F02.80]*
with behavioral disturbance G35
[F02.81]
neurosyphilis A52.17 *[F02.80]*
with behavioral disturbance A52.17
[F02.81]
juvenile A50.49 *[F02.80]*
with behavioral disturbance A50.49
[F02.81]
niacin deficiency E52 *[F02.80]*
with behavioral disturbance E52 *[F02.81]*
paralysis agitans G20 *[F02.80]*
with behavioral disturbance G20 *[F02.81]*
Parkinson's disease G20 *[F02.80]*
pellagra E52 *[F02.80]*
with behavioral disturbance E52 *[F02.81]*
Pick's G31.01 *[F02.80]*
with behavioral disturbance G31.01
[F02.81]
polyarteritis nodosa M30.0 *[F02.80]*
with behavioral disturbance M30.0
[F02.81]
psychoactive drug F19.97
with dependence F19.27
inhalants F18.97
with dependence F18.27
sedatives, hypnotics or anxiolytics
F13.97
with dependence F13.27
sedatives, hypnotics or anxiolytics
F13.97
with dependence F13.27
systemic lupus erythematosus
M32.-● *[F02.80]*
with behavioral disturbance
M32.-● *[F02.81]*
trypanosomiasis
African B56.9 *[F02.80]*
with behavioral disturbance B56.9
[F02.81]
unknown etiology F03
vitamin B12 deficiency E53.8 *[F02.80]*
with behavioral disturbance E53.8
[F02.81]

Dementia *(Continued)*
vitamin B12 deficiency *(Continued)*
volatile solvents F18.97
with dependence F18.27
infantile, infantilis F84.3
Lewy body G31.83 *[F02.80]*
with behavioral disturbance G31.83
[F02.81]
multi-infarct —*see* Dementia, vascular
paralytica, paralytic (syphilitic) A52.17
[F02.80]
with behavioral disturbance A52.17
[F02.81]
juvenilis A50.45
paretic A52.17
praecox —*see* Schizophrenia
presenile F03
Alzheimer's type —*see* Disease,
Alzheimer's, early onset
primary degenerative F03
progressive, syphilitic A52.17
senile F03
with acute confusional state F05
Alzheimer's type —*see* Disease,
Alzheimer's, late onset
depressed or paranoid type F03
vascular (acute onset) (mixed) (multi-infarct)
(subcortical) F01.50
with behavioral disturbance F01.51
Demineralization, bone —*see* Osteoporosis
Demodex folliculorum (infestation) B88.0
Demophobia F40.248
Demoralization R45.3
Demyelination, demyelinization
central nervous system G37.9
specified NEC G37.8
corpus callosum (central) G37.1
disseminated, acute G36.9
specified NEC G36.8
global G35
in optic neuritis G36.0
Dengue (classical) (fever) A90
hemorrhagic A91
sandfly A93.1
Dennie-Marfan syphilitic syndrome
A50.45
Dens evaginatus, in dente or invaginatus
K00.2
Dense breasts R92.2
Density
increased, bone (disseminated) (generalized)
(spotted) —*see* Disorder, bone, density
and structure, specified type NEC
lung (nodular) J98.4
Dental —*see also* condition
examination Z01.20
with abnormal findings Z01.21
restoration
aesthetically inadequate or displeasing
K08.56
defective K08.50
specified NEC K08.59
failure of marginal integrity K08.51
failure of periodontal anatomical integrity
K08.54
Dentia praecox K00.6
Denticles (pulp) K04.2
Dentigerous cyst K09.0
Dentin
irregular (in pulp) K04.3
opalescent K00.5
secondary (in pulp) K04.3
sensitive K03.89
Dentinogenesis imperfecta K00.5
Dentinoma —*see* Cyst, calcifying odontogenic
Dentition (syndrome) K00.7
delayed K00.6
difficult K00.7
precocious K00.6
premature K00.6
retarded K00.6

Dependence (on) (syndrome) F19.20
with remission F19.21
alcohol (ethyl) (methyl) (without remission)
F10.20
with
amnestic disorder, persisting F10.26
anxiety disorder F10.280
dementia, persisting F10.27
intoxication F10.229
with delirium F10.221
uncomplicated F10.220
mood disorder F10.24
psychotic disorder F10.259
with
delusions F10.250
hallucinations F10.251
remission F10.21
sexual dysfunction F10.281
sleep disorder F10.282
specified disorder NEC F10.288
withdrawal F10.239
with
delirium F10.231
perceptual disturbance F10.232
uncomplicated F10.230
counseling and surveillance Z71.41
▶in remission F10.21
amobarbital —*see* Dependence, drug,
sedative
amphetamine(s) (type) —*see* Dependence,
drug, stimulant NEC
amytal (sodium) —*see* Dependence, drug,
sedative
analgesic NEC F55.8
anesthetic (agent) (gas) (general) (local)
NEC —*see* Dependence, drug,
psychoactive NEC
anxiolytic NEC —*see* Dependence, drug,
sedative
barbital(s) —*see* Dependence, drug, sedative
barbiturate(s) (compounds) (drugs
classifiable to T42) —*see* Dependence,
drug, sedative
benzedrine —*see* Dependence, drug,
stimulant NEC
bhang —*see* Dependence, drug, cannabis
bromide(s) NEC —*see* Dependence, drug,
sedative
caffeine —*see* Dependence, drug, stimulant
NEC
cannabis (sativa) (indica) (resin) (derivatives)
(type) —*see* Dependence, drug, cannabis
chloral (betaine) (hydrate) —*see* Dependence,
drug, sedative
chlordiazepoxide —*see* Dependence, drug,
sedative
coca (leaf) (derivatives) —*see* Dependence,
drug, cocaine
cocaine —*see* Dependence, drug, cocaine
codeine —*see* Dependence, drug, opioid
combinations of drugs F19.20
dagga —*see* Dependence, drug, cannabis
demerol —*see* Dependence, drug, opioid
dexamphetamine —*see* Dependence, drug,
stimulant NEC
dexedrine —*see* Dependence, drug, stimulant
NEC
dextromethorphan —*see* Dependence, drug,
opioid
dextromoramide —*see* Dependence, drug,
opioid
dextro-nor-pseudo-ephedrine —*see*
Dependence, drug, stimulant NEC
dextrorphan —*see* Dependence, drug,
opioid
diazepam —*see* Dependence, drug,
sedative
dilaudid —*see* Dependence, drug,
opioid
D-lysergic acid diethylamide —*see*
Dependence, drug, hallucinogen

Dependence *(Continued)*
  drug NEC F19.20
    with sleep disorder F19.282
    cannabis F12.20
      with
        anxiety disorder F12.280
        intoxication F12.229
          with
            delirium F12.221
            perceptual disturbance F12.222
          uncomplicated F12.220
        other specified disorder F12.288
        psychosis F12.259
          delusions F12.250
          hallucinations F12.251
        unspecified disorder F12.29
        withdrawal F12.23
      in remission F12.21
    cocaine F14.20
      with
        anxiety disorder F14.280
        intoxication F14.229
          with
            delirium F14.221
            perceptual disturbance F14.222
          uncomplicated F14.220
        mood disorder F14.24
        other specified disorder F14.288
        psychosis F14.259
          delusions F14.250
          hallucinations F14.251
        sexual dysfunction F14.281
        sleep disorder F14.282
        unspecified disorder F14.29
        withdrawal F14.23
      in remission F14.21
      withdrawal symptoms in newborn P96.1
    counseling and surveillance Z71.51
    hallucinogen F16.20
      with
        anxiety disorder F16.280
        flashbacks F16.283
        intoxication F16.229
          with delirium F16.221
          uncomplicated F16.220
        mood disorder F16.24
        other specified disorder F16.288
        perception disorder, persisting F16.283
        psychosis F16.259
          delusions F16.250
          hallucinations F16.251
        unspecified disorder F16.29
      in remission F16.21
    in remission F19.21
    inhalant F18.20
      with
        anxiety disorder F18.280
        dementia, persisting F18.27
        intoxication F18.229
          with delirium F18.221
          uncomplicated F18.220
        mood disorder F18.24
        other specified disorder
          F18.288
        psychosis F18.259
          delusions F18.250
          hallucinations F18.251
        unspecified disorder F18.29
      in remission F18.21
    nicotine F17.200
      with disorder F17.209
        in remission F17.201
        specified disorder NEC
          F17.208
        withdrawal F17.203
      chewing tobacco F17.220
        with disorder F17.229
          in remission F17.221
          specified disorder NEC
            F17.228
          withdrawal F17.223

Dependence *(Continued)*
  drug NEC *(Continued)*
    nicotine *(Continued)*
      cigarettes F17.210
        with disorder F17.219
          in remission F17.211
          specified disorder NEC F17.218
          withdrawal F17.213
      specified product NEC F17.290
        with disorder F17.299
          remission F17.291
          specified disorder NEC F17.298
          withdrawal F17.293
    opioid F11.20
      with
        intoxication F11.229
          with
            delirium F11.221
            perceptual disturbance F11.222
          uncomplicated F11.220
        mood disorder F11.24
        other specified disorder F11.288
        psychosis F11.259
          delusions F11.250
          hallucinations F11.251
        sexual dysfunction F11.281
        sleep disorder F11.282
        unspecified disorder F11.29
        withdrawal F11.23
      in remission F11.21
    psychoactive NEC F19.20
      with
        amnestic disorder F19.26
        anxiety disorder F19.280
        dementia F19.27
        intoxication F19.229
          with
            delirium F19.221
            perceptual disturbance F19.222
          uncomplicated F19.220
        mood disorder F19.24
        other specified disorder F19.288
        psychosis F19.259
          delusions F19.250
          hallucinations F19.251
        sexual dysfunction F19.281
        sleep disorder F19.282
        unspecified disorder F19.29
        withdrawal F19.239
          with
            delirium F19.231
            perceptual disturbance F19.232
          uncomplicated F19.230
      in remission F13.21
    sedative, hypnotic or anxiolytic F13.20
      with
        amnestic disorder F13.26
        anxiety disorder F13.280
        dementia, persisting F13.27
        intoxication F13.229
          with delirium F13.221
          uncomplicated F13.220
        mood disorder F13.24
        other specified disorder F13.288
        psychosis F13.259
          delusions F13.250
          hallucinations F13.251
        sexual dysfunction F13.281
        sleep disorder F13.282
        unspecified disorder F13.29
        withdrawal F13.239
          with
            delirium F13.231
            perceptual disturbance F13.232
          uncomplicated F13.230
      in remission F13.21
    stimulant NEC F15.20
      with
        anxiety disorder F15.280
        intoxication F15.229
          with
            delirium F15.221
            perceptual disturbance F15.222
          uncomplicated F15.220

Dependence *(Continued)*
  methyl *(Continued)*
    stimulant NEC *(Continued)*
      with *(Continued)*
        mood disorder F15.24
        other specified disorder F15.288
        psychosis F15.259
          delusions F15.250
          hallucinations F15.251
        sexual dysfunction F15.281
        sleep disorder F15.282
        unspecified disorder F15.29
        withdrawal F15.23
      in remission F15.21
  ethyl
    alcohol (without remission) F10.20
      with remission F10.21
    bromide —*see* Dependence, drug,
      sedative
    carbamate F19.20
    chloride F19.20
    morphine —*see* Dependence, drug, opioid
  ganja —*see* Dependence, drug, cannabis
  glue (airplane) (sniffing) —*see* Dependence,
    drug, inhalant
  glutethimide —*see* Dependence, drug,
    sedative
  hallucinogenics —*see* Dependence, drug,
    hallucinogen
  hashish —*see* Dependence, drug, cannabis
  hemp —*see* Dependence, drug, cannabis
  heroin (salt) (any) —*see* Dependence, drug,
    opioid
  hypnotic NEC —*see* Dependence, drug,
    sedative
  Indian hemp —*see* Dependence, drug,
    cannabis
  inhalants —*see* Dependence, drug, inhalant
  khat —*see* Dependence, drug, stimulant NEC
  laudanum —*see* Dependence, drug, opioid
  LSD (-25) (derivatives) —*see* Dependence,
    drug, hallucinogen
  luminal —*see* Dependence, drug, sedative
  lysergic acid —*see* Dependence, drug,
    hallucinogen
  maconha —*see* Dependence, drug, cannabis
  marihuana —*see* Dependence, drug, cannabis
  meprobamate —*see* Dependence, drug,
    sedative
  mescaline —*see* Dependence, drug,
    hallucinogen
  methadone —*see* Dependence, drug, opioid
  methamphetamine(s) —*see* Dependence,
    drug, stimulant NEC
  methaqualone —*see* Dependence, drug,
    sedative
  methyl
    alcohol (without remission) F10.20
      with remission F10.21
    bromide —*see* Dependence, drug, sedative
    morphine —*see* Dependence, drug, opioid
    phenidate —*see* Dependence, drug,
      stimulant NEC
    sulfonal —*see* Dependence, drug, sedative
  morphine (sulfate) (sulfite) (type) —*see*
    Dependence, drug, opioid
  narcotic (drug) NEC —*see* Dependence, drug,
    opioid
  nembutal —*see* Dependence, drug, sedative
  neraval —*see* Dependence, drug, sedative
  neravan —*see* Dependence, drug, sedative
  neurobarb —*see* Dependence, drug, sedative
  nicotine —*see* Dependence, drug, nicotine
  nitrous oxide F19.20
  nonbarbiturate sedatives and tranquilizers
    with similar effect —*see* Dependence,
    drug, sedative
  on
    artificial heart (fully implantable)
      (mechanical) Z95.812
    aspirator Z99.0

▶ New   ⇒ Revised   ~~deleted~~ Deleted   ● Use Additional Character(s)

Dependence *(Continued)*
on *(Continued)*
care provider (because of) Z74.9
impaired mobility Z74.09
need for
assistance with personal care Z74.1
continuous supervision Z74.3
no other household member able to
render care Z74.2
specified reason NEC Z74.8
machine Z99.89
enabling NEC Z99.89
specified type NEC Z99.89
renal dialysis (hemodialysis) (peritoneal)
Z99.2
respirator Z99.11
ventilator Z99.11
wheelchair Z99.3
opiate —*see* Dependence, drug, opioid
opioids —*see* Dependence, drug, opioid
opium (alkaloids) (derivatives) (tincture) —
see Dependence, drug, opioid
oxygen (long-term) (supplemental) Z99.81
paraldehyde —*see* Dependence, drug,
sedative
paregoric —*see* Dependence, drug, opioid
PCP (phencyclidine) (or related substance) —
see Dependence, drug, hallucinogen
pentobarbital —*see* Dependence, drug,
sedative
pentobarbitone (sodium) —*see* Dependence,
drug, sedative
pentothal —*see* Dependence, drug, sedative
peyote —*see* Dependence, drug, hallucinogen
phencyclidine (PCP) (or related substance) —
see Dependence, drug, hallucinogen
phenmetrazine —*see* Dependence, drug,
stimulant NEC
phenobarbital —*see* Dependence, drug,
sedative
polysubstance F19.20
psilocibin, psilocin, psilocyn, psilocyline —*see*
Dependence, drug, hallucinogen
psychostimulant NEC —*see* Dependence,
drug, stimulant NEC
secobarbital —*see* Dependence, drug, sedative
seconal —*see* Dependence, drug, sedative
sedative NEC —*see* Dependence, drug,
sedative
specified drug NEC —*see* Dependence, drug
stimulant NEC —*see* Dependence, drug,
stimulant NEC
substance NEC —*see* Dependence, drug
supplemental oxygen Z99.81
tobacco —*see* Dependence, drug, nicotine
counseling and surveillance Z71.6
tranquilizer NEC —*see* Dependence, drug,
sedative
vitamin B6 E53.1
volatile solvents —*see* Dependence, drug,
inhalant
Dependency
care-provider Z74.9
passive F60.7
reactions (persistent) F60.7
Depersonalization (in neurotic state) (neurotic)
(syndrome) F48.1
Depletion
extracellular fluid E86.9
plasma E86.1
potassium E87.6
nephropathy N25.89
salt or sodium E87.1
causing heat exhaustion or prostration
T67.4
nephropathy N28.9
volume NOS E86.9
Deployment (current) (military) status Z56.82
in theater or in support of military war,
peacekeeping and humanitarian
operations Z56.82

Deployment *(Continued)*
personal history of Z91.82
military war, peacekeeping and
humanitarian deployment (current or
past conflict) Z91.82
returned from Z91.82
Depolarization, premature I49.40
atrial I49.1
junctional I49.2
specified NEC I49.49
ventricular I49.3
Deposit
bone in Boeck's sarcoid D86.89
calcareous, calcium —*see* Calcification
cholesterol
retina H35.89
vitreous (body) (humor) —*see* Deposit,
crystalline
conjunctiva H11.11-●
cornea H18.00-●
argentous H18.02-●
due to metabolic disorder H18.03-●
Kayser-Fleischer ring H18.04-●
pigmentation —*see* Pigmentation, cornea
crystalline, vitreous (body) (humor) H43.2-●
hemosiderin in old scars of cornea —*see*
Pigmentation, cornea, stromal
metallic in lens —*see* Cataract, specified NEC
skin R23.8
tooth, teeth (betel) (black) (green) (materia
alba) (orange) (tobacco) K03.6
urate, kidney —*see* Calculus, kidney
Depraved appetite —*see* Pica
Depressed
HDL cholesterol E78.6
➡ **Depression** (acute) (mental) F32.A
agitated (single episode) F32.2
anaclitic —*see* Disorder, adjustment
anxiety F41.8
persistent F34.1
arches —*see also* Deformity, limb, flat foot
atypical (single episode) F32.89
recurrent episode F33.8
basal metabolic rate R94.8
bone marrow D75.89
central nervous system R09.2
cerebral R29.818
newborn P91.4
cerebrovascular I67.9
chest wall M95.4
climacteric (single episode) F32.89
recurrent episode F33.8
endogenous (without psychotic symptoms)
F33.2
with psychotic symptoms F33.3
functional activity R68.89
hysterical F44.89
involutional (single episode) F32.89
recurrent episode F33.8
major F32.9
with psychotic symptoms F32.3
recurrent —*see* Disorder, depressive,
recurrent
manic-depressive —*see* Disorder, depressive,
recurrent
masked (single episode) F32.89
medullary G93.89
menopausal (single episode) F32.89
recurrent episode F33.8
metatarsus —*see* Depression, arches
monopolar F33.9
nervous F34.1
neurotic F34.1
nose M95.0
postnatal (NOS) F53.0
postpartum (NOS) F53.0
post-psychotic of schizophrenia F32.89
post-schizophrenic F32.89
psychogenic (reactive) (single episode)
F32.9
psychoneurotic F34.1

Depression *(Continued)*
psychotic (single episode) F32.3
recurrent F33.3
reactive (psychogenic) (single episode) F32.9
psychotic (single episode) F32.3
recurrent —*see* Disorder, depressive, recurrent
respiratory center G93.89
seasonal —*see* Disorder, depressive, recurrent
senile F03
severe, single episode F32.2
situational F43.21
skull Q67.4
specified NEC (single episode) F32.89
sternum M95.4
visual field —*see* Defect, visual field
vital (recurrent) (without psychotic
symptoms) F33.2
with psychotic symptoms F33.3
single episode F32.2
Deprivation
cultural Z60.3
effects NOS T73.9
specified NEC T73.8
emotional NEC Z65.8
affecting infant or child —*see*
Maltreatment, child, psychological
food T73.0
protein —*see* Malnutrition
sleep Z72.820
social Z60.4
affecting infant or child —*see*
Maltreatment, child, psychological
specified NEC T73.8
vitamins —*see* Deficiency, vitamin
water T73.1
Derangement
ankle (internal) —*see* Derangement, joint,
ankle
cartilage (articular) NEC —*see* Derangement,
joint, articular cartilage, by site
recurrent —*see* Dislocation, recurrent
cruciate ligament, anterior, current injury —
see Sprain, knee, cruciate, anterior
elbow (internal) —*see* Derangement, joint,
elbow
hip (joint) (internal) (old) —*see* Derangement,
joint, hip
joint (internal) M24.9
ankylosis —*see* Ankylosis
articular cartilage M24.10
ankle M24.17-●
elbow M24.12-●
foot M24.17-●
hand M24.14-●
hip M24.15-●
knee NEC M23.9-●
loose body —*see* Loose, body
shoulder M24.11-●
specified site NEC M24.19
wrist M24.13-●
contracture —*see* Contraction, joint
current injury —*see also* Dislocation
knee, meniscus or cartilage —*see* Tear,
meniscus
dislocation
pathological —*see* Dislocation,
pathological
recurrent —*see* Dislocation, recurrent
knee —*see* Derangement, knee
ligament —*see* Disorder, ligament
loose body —*see* Loose, body
recurrent —*see* Dislocation, recurrent
specified type NEC M24.80
ankle M24.87-●
elbow M24.82-●
foot joint M24.87-●
hand joint M24.84-●
hip M24.85-●
shoulder M24.81-●
specified site NEC M24.89
wrist M24.83-●
temporomandibular M26.69

Derangement (Continued)
  knee (recurrent) M23.9-●
    ligament disruption, spontaneous M23.60-●
      anterior cruciate M23.61-●
      capsular M23.67-●
      instability, chronic M23.5-●
      lateral collateral M23.64-●
      medial collateral M23.63-●
      posterior cruciate M23.62-●
    loose body M23.4-●
    meniscus M23.30-●
      cystic M23.00-●
        lateral M23.002
          anterior horn M23.04-●
          posterior horn M23.05-●
          specified NEC M23.06-●
        medial M23.005
          anterior horn M23.01-●
          posterior horn M23.02-●
          specified NEC M23.03-●
      degenerate —see Derangement, knee, meniscus, specified NEC
      detached —see Derangement, knee, meniscus, specified NEC
      due to old tear or injury M23.20-●
        lateral M23.20-●
          anterior horn M23.24-●
          posterior horn M23.25-●
          specified NEC M23.26-●
        medial M23.20-●
          anterior horn M23.21-●
          posterior horn M23.22-●
          specified NEC M23.23-●
      retained —see Derangement, knee, meniscus, specified NEC
      specified NEC M23.30-●
        lateral M23.30-●
          anterior horn M23.34-●
          posterior horn M23.35-●
          specified NEC M23.36-●
        medial M23.30-●
          anterior horn M23.31-●
          posterior horn M23.32-●
          specified NEC M23.33-●
    old M23.8X-●
    specified NEC —see subcategory M23.8
  low back NEC —see Dorsopathy, specified NEC
  meniscus —see Derangement, knee, meniscus
  mental —see Psychosis
  patella, specified NEC —see Disorder, patella, derangement NEC
  semilunar cartilage (knee) —see Derangement, knee, meniscus, specified NEC
  shoulder (internal) —see Derangement, joint, shoulder
Dercum's disease E88.2
Derealization (neurotic) F48.1
Dermal —see condition
Dermaphytid —see Dermatophytosis
Dermatitis (eczematous) L30.9
  ab igne L59.0
  acarine B88.0
  actinic (due to sun) L57.8
    other than from sun L59.8
  allergic —see Dermatitis, contact, allergic
  ambustionis, due to burn or scald —see Burn
  amebic A06.7
  ammonia L22
  arsenical (ingested) L27.8
  artefacta L98.1
    psychogenic F54
  atopic L20.9
    psychogenic F54
    specified NEC L20.89
  autoimmune progesterone L30.8
  berlock, berloque L56.2
  blastomycotic B40.3
  blister beetle L24.89
  bullous, bullosa L13.9
    mucosynechial, atrophic L12.1
    seasonal L30.8
    specified NEC L13.8

Dermatitis (Continued)
  calorica L59.0
    due to burn or scald —see Burn
  caterpillar L24.89
  cercarial B65.3
  combustionis L59.0
    due to burn or scald —see Burn
  congelationis T69.1
  contact (occupational) L25.9
    allergic L23.9
      due to
        adhesives L23.1
        cement L23.5
        chemical products NEC L23.5
        chromium L23.0
        cosmetics L23.2
        dander (cat) (dog) L23.81
        drugs in contact with skin L23.3
        dyes L23.4
        food in contact with skin L23.6
        hair (cat) (dog) L23.81
        insecticide L23.5
        metals L23.0
        nickel L23.0
        plants, non-food L23.7
        plastic L23.5
        rubber L23.5
        specified agent NEC L23.89
    due to
      cement L25.3
      chemical products NEC L25.3
      cosmetics L25.0
      dander (cat) (dog) L23.81
      drugs in contact with skin L25.1
      dyes L25.2
      food in contact with skin L25.4
      hair (cat) (dog) L23.81
      plants, non-food L25.5
      specified agent NEC L25.8
    irritant L24.9
      due to
        ▶body fluids L24.A0
          ▶incontinence (dual) (fecal) (urinary) L24.A2
          ▶saliva L24.A1
          ▶specified NEC L24.A9
        cement L24.5
        chemical products NEC L24.5
        cosmetics L24.3
        detergents L24.0
        drugs in contact with skin L24.4
        food in contact with skin L24.6
        oils and greases L24.1
        plants, non-food L24.7
        ▶related to
          ▶colostomy L24.B3
          ▶endotracheal tube L24.A9
          ▶enterocutaneous
          ▶fistula L24.B3
          ▶gastrostomy L24.B1
          ▶ileostomy L24.B3
          ▶jejunostomy L24.B1
          ▶saliva or spit fistula L24.B1
          ▶stoma or fistula L24.B0
            ▶digestive L24.B1
            ▶fecal or urinary L24.B3
            ▶respiratory L24.B2
          ▶tracheostomy L24.B2
         solvents L24.2
        specified agent NEC L24.89
  contusiformis L52
  desquamative L30.8
  diabetic —see E08-E13 with .620
  diaper L22
  diphtheritica A36.3
  dry skin L85.3
  due to
    acetone (contact) (irritant) L24.2
    acids (contact) (irritant) L24.5
    adhesive(s) (allergic) (contact) (plaster) L23.1
      irritant L24.5

Dermatitis (Continued)
  due to (Continued)
    alcohol (irritant) (skin contact) (substances in category T51) L24.2
      taken internally L27.8
    alkalis (contact) (irritant) L24.5
    arsenic (ingested) L27.8
    carbon disulfide (contact) (irritant) L24.2
    caustics (contact) (irritant) L24.5
    cement (contact) L25.3
    cereal (ingested) L27.2
    chemical(s) NEC L25.3
      taken internally L27.8
    chlorocompounds L24.2
    chromium (contact) (irritant) L24.81
    coffee (ingested) L27.2
    cold weather L30.8
    cosmetics (contact) L25.0
      allergic L23.2
      irritant L24.3
    cyclohexanes L24.2
    dander (cat) (dog) L23.81
    Demodex species B88.0
    Dermanyssus gallinae B88.0
    detergents (contact) (irritant) L24.0
    dichromate L24.81
    drugs and medicaments (generalized) (internal use) L27.0
      external —see Dermatitis, due to, drugs, in contact with skin
      in contact with skin L25.1
        allergic L23.3
        irritant L24.4
      localized skin eruption L27.1
      specified substance —see Table of Drugs and Chemicals
    dyes (contact) L25.2
      allergic L23.4
      irritant L24.89
    epidermophytosis —see Dermatophytosis
    esters L24.2
    external irritant NEC L24.9
    fish (ingested) L27.2
    flour (ingested) L27.2
    food (ingested) L27.2
      in contact with skin L25.4
    fruit (ingested) L27.2
    furs (allergic) (contact) L23.81
    glues —see Dermatitis, due to, adhesives
    glycols L24.2
    greases NEC (contact) (irritant) L24.1
    hair (cat) (dog) L23.81
    hot
      objects and materials —see Burn
      weather or places L59.0
    hydrocarbons L24.2
    infrared rays L59.8
    ingestion, ingested substance L27.9
      chemical NEC L27.8
      drugs and medicaments —see Dermatitis, due to, drugs
      food L27.2
      specified NEC L27.8
    insecticide in contact with skin L24.5
    internal agent L27.9
      drugs and medicaments (generalized) —see Dermatitis, due to, drugs
      food L27.2
    irradiation —see Dermatitis, due to, radioactive substance
    ketones L24.2
    lacquer tree (allergic) (contact) L23.7
    light (sun) NEC L57.8
      acute L56.8
      other L59.8
    Liponyssoides sanguineus B88.0
    low temperature L30.8
    meat (ingested) L27.2
    metals, metal salts (contact) (irritant) L24.81
    milk (ingested) L27.2

  ▶ New   ⇛ Revised   ~~deleted~~ Deleted   ● Use Additional Character(s)

Dermatitis *(Continued)*
  due to *(Continued)*
    nickel (contact) (irritant) L24.81
    nylon (contact) (irritant) L24.5
    oils NEC (contact) (irritant) L24.1
    paint solvent (contact) (irritant) L24.2
    petroleum products (contact) (irritant) (substances in T52) L24.2
    plants NEC (contact) L25.5
      allergic L23.7
      irritant L24.7
    plasters (adhesive) (any) (allergic) (contact) L23.1
      irritant L24.5
    plastic (contact) L25.3
    preservatives (contact) —*see* Dermatitis, due to, chemical, in contact with skin
    primrose (allergic) (contact) L23.7
    primula (allergic) (contact) L23.7
    radiation L59.8
      nonionizing (chronic exposure) L57.8
      sun NEC L57.8
        acute L56.8
    radioactive substance L58.9
      acute L58.0
      chronic L58.1
    radium L58.9
      acute L58.0
      chronic L58.1
    ragweed (allergic) (contact) L23.7
    Rhus (allergic) (contact) (diversiloba) (radicans) (toxicodendron) (venenata) (verniciflua) L23.7
    rubber (contact) L24.5
    Senecio jacobaea (allergic) (contact) L23.7
    solvents (contact) (irritant) (substances in categories T52) L24.2
    specified agent NEC (contact) L25.8
      allergic L23.89
      irritant L24.89
    sunshine NEC L57.8
      acute L56.8
    tetrachlorethylene (contact) (irritant) L24.2
    toluene (contact) (irritant) L24.2
    turpentine (contact) L24.2
    ultraviolet rays (sun NEC) (chronic exposure) L57.8
      acute L56.8
    vaccine or vaccination L27.0
      specified substance —*see* Table of Drugs and Chemicals
    varicose veins —*see* Varix, leg, with, inflammation
    X-rays L58.9
      acute L58.0
      chronic L58.1
  dyshydrotic L30.1
  dysmenorrheica N94.6
  escharotica —*see* Burn
  exfoliative, exfoliativa (generalized) L26
    neonatorum L00
  eyelid —(*see also* Dermatosis, eyelid) H01.9
    allergic H01.119
      left H01.116
        lower H01.115
        upper H01.114
      right H01.113
        lower H01.112
        upper H01.111
    contact —*see* Dermatitis, eyelid, allergic
    due to
      Demodex species B88.0
      herpes (zoster) B02.39
        simplex B00.59
    eczematous H01.139
      left H01.136
        lower H01.135
        upper H01.134
      right H01.133
        lower H01.132
        upper H01.131
    specified NEC H01.8

Dermatitis *(Continued)*
  facta, factitia, factitial L98.1
    psychogenic F54
  flexural NEC L20.82
  friction L30.4
  fungus B36.9
    specified type NEC B36.8
  gangrenosa, gangrenous infantum L08.0
  harvest mite B88.0
  heat L59.0
  herpesviral, vesicular (ear) (lip) B00.1
  herpetiformis (bullous) (erythematous) (pustular) (vesicular) L13.0
    juvenile L12.2
    senile L12.0
  hiemalis L30.8
  hypostatic, hypostatica —*see* Varix, leg, with, inflammation
  infectious eczematoid L30.3
  infective L30.3
  irritant —*see* Dermatitis, contact, irritant
  Jacquet's (diaper dermatitis) L22
  Leptus B88.0
  lichenified NEC L28.0
  medicamentosa (generalized) (internal use) —*see* Dermatitis, due to drugs
  mite B88.0
  multiformis L13.0
    juvenile L12.2
  napkin L22
  neurotica L13.0
  nummular L30.0
  papillaris capillitii L73.0
  pellagrous E52
  perioral L71.0
  photocontact L56.2
  polymorpha dolorosa L13.0
  pruriginosa L13.0
  pruritic NEC L30.8
  psychogenic F54
  purulent L08.0
  pustular
    contagious B08.02
    subcorneal L13.1
  pyococcal L08.0
  pyogenica L08.0
  repens L40.2
  Ritter's (exfoliativa) L00
  Schamberg's L81.7
  schistosome B65.3
  seasonal bullous L30.8
  seborrheic L21.9
    infantile L21.1
    specified NEC L21.8
  sensitization NOS L23.9
  septic L08.0
  solare L57.8
  specified NEC L30.8
  stasis I87.2
    with
      varicose ulcer —*see* Varix, leg, with ulcer, with inflammation
      varicose veins —*see* Varix, leg, with, inflammation
    due to postthrombotic syndrome —*see* Syndrome, postthrombotic
  suppurative L08.0
  traumatic NEC L30.4
  trophoneurotica L13.0
  ultraviolet (sun) (chronic exposure) L57.8
    acute L56.8
  varicose —*see* Varix, leg, with, inflammation
  vegetans L10.1
  verrucosa B43.0
  vesicular, herpesviral B00.1
Dermatoarthritis, lipoid E78.81
Dermatochalasis, eyelid H02.839
  left H02.836
    lower H02.835
    upper H02.834
  right H02.833
    lower H02.832
    upper H02.831

Dermatofibroma (lenticulare) —*see* Neoplasm, skin, benign
  protuberans —*see* Neoplasm, skin, uncertain behavior
Dermatofibrosarcoma (pigmented) (protuberans) —*see* Neoplasm, skin, malignant
Dermatographia L50.3
Dermatolysis (exfoliativa) (congenital) Q82.8
  acquired L57.4
  eyelids —*see* Blepharochalasis
  palpebrarum —*see* Blepharochalasis
  senile L57.4
Dermatomegaly NEC Q82.8
Dermatomucosomyositis M33.10
  with
    myopathy M33.12
    respiratory involvement M33.11
    specified organ involvement NEC M33.19
Dermatomycosis B36.9
  furfuracea B36.0
  specified type NEC B36.8
Dermatomyositis (acute) (chronic) —*see also* Dermatopolymyositis
  adult —*see also* Dermatomyositis, specified NEC M33.10
  in (due to) neoplastic disease —*see also* Neoplasm D49.9 *[M36.0]*
  juvenile M33.00
    with
      myopathy M33.02
      respiratory involvement M33.01
      specified organ involvement NEC M33.09
    without myopathy M33.03
  specified NEC M33.10
    with
      myopathy M33.12
      respiratory involvement M33.11
      specified organ involvement NEC M33.19
    without myopathy M33.13
Dermatoneuritis of children —*see* Poisoning, mercury
Dermatophilosis A48.8
Dermatophytid L30.2
Dermatophytide —*see* Dermatophytosis
Dermatophytosis (epidermophyton) (infection) (Microsporum) (tinea) (Trichophyton) B35.9
  beard B35.0
  body B35.4
  capitis B35.0
  corporis B35.4
  deep-seated B35.8
  disseminated B35.8
  foot B35.3
  granulomatous B35.8
  groin B35.6
  hand B35.2
  nail B35.1
  perianal (area) B35.6
  scalp B35.0
  specified NEC B35.8
Dermatopolymyositis M33.90
  with
    myopathy M33.92
    respiratory involvement M33.91
    specified organ involvement NEC M33.99
  in neoplastic disease —*see also* Neoplasm D49.9 *[M36.0]*
  juvenile M33.00
    with
      myopathy M33.02
      respiratory involvement M33.01
      specified organ involvement NEC M33.09
  specified NEC M33.10
    myopathy M33.12
    respiratory involvement M33.11
    specified organ involvement NEC M33.19
  without myopathy M33.93
Dermatopolyneuritis —*see* Poisoning, mercury
Dermatorrhexis (*see also* Syndrome, Ehlers-Danlos) Q79.60
  acquired L57.4

Dermatosclerosis —*see also* Scleroderma
  localized L94.0
Dermatosis L98.9
  Andrews' L08.89
  Bowen's —*see* Neoplasm, skin, in situ
  bullous L13.9
    specified NEC L13.8
  exfoliativa L26
➡ eyelid (noninfectious) (*see also* Dermatitis,
      eyelid) H01.9
    ~~dermatitis —see Dermatitis, eyelid~~
    discoid lupus erythematosus —*see* Lupus,
        erythematosus, eyelid
    xeroderma —*see* Xeroderma, acquired,
        eyelid
  factitial L98.1
  febrile neutrophilic L98.2
  gonococcal A54.89
  herpetiformis L13.0
    juvenile L12.2
  linear IgA L13.8
  menstrual NEC L98.8
  neutrophilic, febrile L98.2
  occupational —*see* Dermatitis, contact
  papulosa nigra L82.1
  pigmentary L81.9
    progressive L81.7
    Schamberg's L81.7
  psychogenic F54
  purpuric, pigmented L81.7
  pustular, subcorneal L13.1
  transient acantholytic L11.1
Dermographia, dermographism L50.3
Dermoid (cyst) —*see also* Neoplasm, benign,
      by site
    with malignant transformation C56-●
    due to radiation (nonionizing) L57.8
Dermopathy
  infiltrative with thyrotoxicosis —*see*
      Thyrotoxicosis
  nephrogenic fibrosing L90.8
Dermophytosis —*see* Dermatophytosis
Descemetocele H18.73-●
Descemet's membrane —*see* condition
Descending —*see* condition
Descensus uteri —*see* Prolapse, uterus
Desert
  rheumatism B38.0
  sore —*see* Ulcer, skin
Desertion (newborn) —*see* Maltreatment
Desmoid (extra-abdominal) (tumor) —*see*
      Neoplasm, connective tissue, uncertain
      behavior
    abdominal D48.1
➡ **Despondency** F32.A
Desquamation, skin R23.4
Destruction, destructive —*see also* Damage
  articular facet —*see also* Derangement, joint,
      specified type NEC
    knee M23.8X-●
    vertebra —*see* Spondylosis
  bone —*see also* Disorder, bone, specified type
      NEC
    syphilitic A52.77
  joint —*see also* Derangement, joint, specified
      type NEC
    sacroiliac M53.3
  rectal sphincter K62.89
  septum (nasal) J34.89
  tuberculous NEC —*see* Tuberculosis
  tympanum, tympanic membrane
      (nontraumatic) —*see* Disorder, tympanic
      membrane, specified NEC
  vertebral disc —*see* Degeneration,
      intervertebral disc
Destructiveness —*see also* Disorder, conduct
  adjustment reaction —*see* Disorder, adjustment
Desultory labor O62.2
Detachment
  cartilage —*see* Sprain
  cervix, annular N88.8
    complicating delivery O71.3

Detachment (*Continued*)
  choroid (old) (postinfectional) (simple)
      (spontaneous) H31.40-●
    hemorrhagic H31.41-●
    serous H31.42-●
  ligament —*see* Sprain
  meniscus (knee) —*see also* Derangement,
      knee, meniscus, specified NEC
    current injury —*see* Tear, meniscus
    due to old tear or injury —*see*
        Derangement, knee, meniscus, due to
        old tear
  retina (without retinal break) (serous)
      H33.2-●
    with retinal:
      break H33.00-●
        giant H33.03-●
        multiple H33.02-●
        single H33.01-●
      dialysis H33.04-●
    pigment epithelium —*see* Degeneration,
        retina, separation of layers, pigment
        epithelium detachment
    rhegmatogenous —*see* Detachment, retina,
        with retinal, break
    specified NEC H33.8
    total H33.05-●
    traction H33.4-●
  vitreous (body) H43.81
Detergent asthma J69.8
Deterioration
  epileptic F06.8
  general physical R53.81
  heart, cardiac —*see* Degeneration,
      myocardial
  mental —*see* Psychosis
  myocardial, myocardium —*see* Degeneration,
      myocardial
  senile (simple) R54
Deuteranomaly (anomalous trichromat) H53.53
Deuteranopia (complete) (incomplete) H53.53
Development
  abnormal, bone Q79.9
  arrested R62.50
    bone —*see* Arrest, development or growth,
        bone
    child R62.50
    due to malnutrition E45
  defective, congenital —*see also* Anomaly, by
      site
    cauda equina Q06.3
    left ventricle Q24.8
      in hypoplastic left heart syndrome Q23.4
    valve Q24.8
      pulmonary Q22.3
  delayed (*see also* Delay, development) R62.50
    arithmetical skills F81.2
    language (skills) (expressive) F80.1
    learning skill F81.9
    mixed skills F88
    motor coordination F82
    reading F81.0
    specified learning skill NEC F81.89
    speech F80.9
    spelling F81.81
    written expression F81.81
  imperfect, congenital —*see also* Anomaly, by
      site
    heart Q24.9
    lungs Q33.6
  incomplete
    bronchial tree Q32.4
    organ or site not listed —*see* Hypoplasia,
        by site
    respiratory system Q34.9
  sexual, precocious NEC E30.1
  tardy, mental (*see also* Disability, intellectual)
      F79
Developmental —*see* condition
  testing, infant or child —*see* Examination,
      child

Devergie's disease (pityriasis rubra pilaris) L44.0
Deviation (in)
  conjugate palsy (eye) (spastic) H51.0
➡ esophagus (acquired) K22.89
  eye, skew H51.8
  midline (jaw) (teeth) (dental arch) M26.29
    specified site NEC —*see* Malposition
  nasal septum J34.2
    congenital Q67.4
  opening and closing of the mandible M26.53
  organ or site, congenital NEC —*see*
      Malposition, congenital
  septum (nasal) (acquired) J34.2
    congenital Q67.4
  sexual F65.9
    bestiality F65.89
    erotomania F52.8
    exhibitionism F65.2
    fetishism, fetishistic F65.0
      transvestism F65.1
    frotteurism F65.81
    masochism F65.51
    multiple F65.89
    necrophilia F65.89
    nymphomania F52.8
    pederosis F65.4
    pedophilia F65.4
    sadism, sadomasochism F65.52
    satyriasis F52.8
    specified type NEC F65.89
    transvestism F64.1
    voyeurism F65.3
  teeth, midline M26.29
  trachea J39.8
  ureter, congenital Q62.61
Device
  cerebral ventricle (communicating) in situ Z98.2
  contraceptive —*see* Contraceptive, device
  drainage, cerebrospinal fluid, in situ Z98.2
Devic's disease G36.0
Devil's
  grip B33.0
  pinches (purpura simplex) D69.2
Devitalized tooth K04.90
Devonshire colic —*see* Poisoning, lead
Dextraposition, aorta Q20.3
  in tetralogy of Fallot Q21.3
Dextrinosis, limit (debrancher enzyme
      deficiency) E74.03
Dextrocardia (true) Q24.0
  with
    complete transposition of viscera Q89.3
    situs inversus Q89.3
Dextrotransposition, aorta Q20.3
d-glycericacidemia E72.59
Dhat syndrome F48.8
Dhobi itch B35.6
Di George's syndrome D82.1
Di Guglielmo's disease C94.0-●
Diabetes, diabetic (mellitus) (sugar) E11.9
  with
    amyotrophy E11.44
    arthropathy NEC E11.618
    autonomic (poly)neuropathy E11.43
    cataract E11.36
    Charcot's joints E11.610
    chronic kidney disease E11.22
    circulatory complication NEC E11.59
  ▶ coma due to
      ▶ hyperosmolarity E11.01
      ▶ hypoglycemia E11.641
      ▶ ketoacidosis E11.11
    complication E11.8
      specified NEC E11.69
    dermatitis E11.620
    foot ulcer E11.621
    gangrene E11.52
    gastroparalysis E11.43
    gastroparesis E11.43
    glomerulonephrosis, intracapillary E11.21
    glomerulosclerosis, intercapillary E11.21
    hyperglycemia E11.65

▶ New   ➡ Revised   ~~deleted~~ Deleted   ● Use Additional Character(s)

Diabetes, diabetic *(Continued)*
 insulin dependent — code to type of diabetes
 juvenile-onset —*see* Diabetes, type 1
 ketosis-prone —*see* Diabetes, type 1
 latent R73.03
 neonatal (transient) P70.2
 non-insulin dependent — code to type of
  diabetes
 out of control — code to Diabetes, by type,
  with hyperglycemia
 phosphate E83.39
 poorly controlled — code to Diabetes, by
  type, with hyperglycemia
 postpancreatectomy —*see* Diabetes, specified
  type NEC
 postprocedural —*see* Diabetes, specified type
  NEC
 secondary diabetes mellitus NEC —*see*
  Diabetes, specified type NEC
 specified type NEC E13.9
  with
   amyotrophy E13.44
   arthropathy NEC E13.618
   autonomic (poly)neuropathy E13.43
   cataract E13.36
   Charcot's joints E13.610
   chronic kidney disease E13.22
   circulatory complication NEC E13.59
   complication E13.8
    specified NEC E13.69
   dermatitis E13.620
   foot ulcer E13.621
   gangrene E13.52
   gastroparalysis E13.43
   gastroparesis E13.43
   glomerulonephrosis, intracapillary
    E13.21
   glomerulosclerosis, intercapillary E13.21
   hyperglycemia E13.65
   hyperosmolarity E13.00
    with coma E13.01
   hypoglycemia E13.649
    with coma E13.641
   ketoacidosis E13.10
    with coma E13.11
   kidney complications NEC E13.29
   Kimmelsteil-Wilson disease E13.21
   mononeuropathy E13.41
   myasthenia E13.44
   necrobiosis lipoidica E13.620
   nephropathy E13.21
   neuralgia E13.42
   neurologic complication NEC E13.49
   neuropathic arthropathy E13.610
   neuropathy E13.40
   ophthalmic complication NEC E13.39
   oral complication NEC E13.638
   periodontal disease E13.630
   peripheral angiopathy E13.51
    with gangrene E13.52
   polyneuropathy E13.42
   renal complication NEC E13.29
   renal tubular degeneration E13.29
   retinopathy E13.319
    with macular edema E13.311
     resolved following treatment
      E13.37
    nonproliferative E13.329
     with macular edema E13.321
     mild E13.329
      with macular edema E13.321
     moderate E13.339
      with macular edema E13.331
     severe E13.349
      with macular edema E13.341
    proliferative E13.359
     with
      combined traction retinal
       detachment and
       rhegmatogenous retinal
       detachment E13.354

Diabetes, diabetic *(Continued)*
 specified type NEC *(Continued)*
  with *(Continued)*
   retinopathy *(Continued)*
    proliferative *(Continued)*
     with *(Continued)*
      macular edema E13.351
      stable proliferative diabetic
       retinopathy E13.355
      traction retinal detachment
       involving the macula
       E13.352
      traction retinal detachment not
       involving the macula
       E13.353
   skin complication NEC E13.628
   skin ulcer E13.622
 steroid-induced —*see* Diabetes, due to, drug
  or chemical
 type 1 E10.9
  with
   amyotrophy E10.44
   arthropathy NEC E10.618
   autonomic (poly)neuropathy E10.43
   cataract E10.36
   Charcot's joints E10.610
   chronic kidney disease E10.22
   circulatory complication NEC E10.59
  ▶coma due to
   ▶hypoglycemia E11.641
   ▶ketoacidosis E11.11
   complication E10.8
    specified NEC E10.69
   dermatitis E10.620
   foot ulcer E10.621
   gangrene E10.52
   gastroparalysis E10.43
   gastroparesis E10.43
   glomerulonephrosis, intracapillary E10.21
   glomerulosclerosis, intercapillary E10.21
   hyperglycemia E10.65
   hypoglycemia E10.649
    with coma E10.641
   ketoacidosis E10.10
    with coma E10.11
   kidney complications NEC E10.29
   Kimmelsteil-Wilson disease E10.21
   mononeuropathy E10.41
   myasthenia E10.44
   necrobiosis lipoidica E10.620
   nephropathy E10.21
   neuralgia E10.42
   neurologic complication NEC E10.49
   neuropathic arthropathy E10.610
   neuropathy E10.40
   ophthalmic complication NEC E10.39
   oral complication NEC E10.638
   osteomyelitis E10.69
   periodontal disease E10.630
   peripheral angiopathy E10.51
    with gangrene E10.52
   polyneuropathy E10.42
   renal complication NEC E10.29
   renal tubular degeneration E10.29
   retinopathy E10.319
    with macular edema E10.311
     resolved following treatment E10.37
    nonproliferative E10.329
     with macular edema E10.321
     mild E10.329
      with macular edema E10.321
     moderate E10.339
      with macular edema E10.331
     severe E10.349
      with macular edema E10.341
    proliferative E10.359
     with
      combined traction retinal
       detachment and
       rhegmatogenous retinal
       detachment E13.354

Diabetes, diabetic *(Continued)*
 type 1 *(Continued)*
  with *(Continued)*
   retinopathy *(Continued)*
    proliferative *(Continued)*
     with *(Continued)*
      macular edema E13.351
      stable proliferative diabetic
       retinopathy E13.355
      traction retinal detachment
       involving the macula E13.352
      traction retinal detachment not
       involving the macula E13.353
   skin complication NEC E10.628
   skin ulcer NEC E10.622
 type 2 E11.9
  with
   amyotrophy E11.44
   arthropathy NEC E11.618
   autonomic (poly)neuropathy E11.43
   cataract E11.36
   Charcot's joints E11.610
   chronic kidney disease E11.22
   circulatory complication NEC E11.59
  ▶coma due to
   ▶hyperosmolarity E11.01
   ▶hypoglycemia E11.641
   ▶ketoacidosis E11.11
   complication E11.8
    specified NEC E11.69
   dermatitis E11.620
   foot ulcer E11.621
   gangrene E11.52
   gastroparalysis E11.43
   gastroparesis E11.43
   glomerulonephrosis, intracapillary E11.21
   glomerulosclerosis, intercapillary E11.21
   hyperglycemia E11.65
   hyperosmolarity E11.00
    with coma E11.01
   hypoglycemia E11.649
    with coma E11.641
   ketoacidosis E11.10
    with coma E11.11
   kidney complications NEC E11.29
   Kimmelsteil-Wilson disease E11.21
   mononeuropathy E11.41
   myasthenia E11.44
   necrobiosis lipoidica E11.620
   nephropathy E11.21
   neuralgia E11.42
   neurologic complication NEC E11.49
   neuropathic arthropathy E11.610
   neuropathy E11.40
   ophthalmic complication NEC E11.39
   oral complication NEC E11.638
   osteomyelitis E11.69
   periodontal disease E11.630
   peripheral angiopathy E11.51
    with gangrene E11.52
   polyneuropathy E11.42
   renal complication NEC E11.29
   renal tubular degeneration E11.29
   retinopathy E11.319
    with macular edema E11.311
     resolved following treatment E11.37
    nonproliferative E11.329
     with macular edema E11.321
     mild E11.329
      with macular edema E11.321
     moderate E11.339
      with macular edema E11.331
     severe E11.349
      with macular edema E11.341
    proliferative E11.359
     with
      combined traction retinal
       detachment and
       rhegmatogenous retinal
       detachment E11.354
      macular edema E11.351

Diabetes, diabetic *(Continued)*
　type 2 *(Continued)*
　　with *(Continued)*
　　　retinopathy *(Continued)*
　　　　proliferative *(Continued)*
　　　　　with *(Continued)*
　　　　　　stable proliferative diabetic
　　　　　　　retinopathy E11.355
　　　　　　traction retinal detachment
　　　　　　　involving the macula E11.352
　　　　　　traction retinal detachment not
　　　　　　　involving the macula E11.353
　　　　skin complication NEC E11.628
　　　　skin ulcer NEC E11.622
　　uncontrolled
　　　meaning
　　　　hyperglycemia —*see* Diabetes, by type,
　　　　　with, hyperglycemia
　　　　hypoglycemia —*see* Diabetes, by type,
　　　　　with, hypoglycemia
Diacyclothrombopathia D69.1
Diagnosis deferred R69
Dialysis (intermittent) (treatment)
　noncompliance (with) Z91.15
　renal (hemodialysis) (peritoneal), status Z99.2
　retina, retinal —*see* Detachment, retina, with
　　retinal, dialysis
Diamond-Blackfan anemia (congenital
　　hypoplastic) D61.01
Diamond-Gardener syndrome
　　(autoerythrocyte sensitization) D69.2
Diaper rash L22
Diaphoresis (excessive) R61
Diaphragm —*see* condition
Diaphragmalgia R07.1
Diaphragmatitis, diaphragmitis J98.6
Diaphysial aclasis Q78.6
Diaphysitis —*see* Osteomyelitis, specified type
　　NEC
Diarrhea, diarrheal (disease) (infantile)
　　(inflammatory) R19.7
　achlorhydric K31.83
　allergic K52.29
　　due to
　　　colitis —*see* Colitis, allergic
　　　enteritis —*see* Enteritis, allergic
　amebic —*see also* Amebiasis A06.0
　　with abscess —*see* Abscess, amebic
　　acute A06.0
　　chronic A06.1
　　nondysenteric A06.2
　bacillary —*see* Dysentery, bacillary
　balantidial A07.0
　cachectic NEC K52.89
　Chilomastix A07.8
　choleriformis A00.1
　chronic (noninfectious) K52.9
　coccidial A07.3
　Cochin-China K90.1
　　strongyloidiasis B78.0
　Dientamoeba A07.8
　dietetic —*see also* Diarrhea, allergic K52.29
　drug-induced K52.1
　due to
　　bacteria A04.9
　　　specified NEC A04.8
　　Campylobacter A04.5
　　Capillaria philippinensis B81.1
　　Clostridium difficile
　　　not specified as recurrent A04.72
　　　recurrent A04.71
　　Clostridium perfringens (C) (F) A04.8
　　Cryptosporidium A07.2
　　drugs K52.1
　　Escherichia coli A04.4
　　　enteroaggregative A04.4
　　　enterohemorrhagic A04.3
　　　enteroinvasive A04.2
　　　enteropathogenic A04.0
　　　enterotoxigenic A04.1
　　　specified NEC A04.4

Diarrhea, diarrheal *(Continued)*
　due to *(Continued)*
　　food hypersensitivity —*see also* Diarrhea,
　　　allergic K52.29
　　Necator americanus B76.1
　　S. japonicum B65.2
　　specified organism NEC A08.8
　　　bacterial A04.8
　　　viral A08.39
　　Staphylococcus A04.8
　　Trichuris trichiuria B79
　　virus —*see* Enteritis, viral
　　Yersinia enterocolitica A04.6
　dysenteric A09
　endemic A09
　epidemic A09
　flagellate A07.9
　Flexner's (ulcerative) A03.1
　functional K59.1
　　following gastrointestinal surgery K91.89
　　psychogenic F45.8
　Giardia lamblia A07.1
　giardial A07.1
　hill K90.1
　infectious A09
　malarial —*see* Malaria
　mite B88.0
　mycotic NEC B49
　neonatal (noninfectious) P78.3
　nervous F45.8
　neurogenic K59.1
　noninfectious K52.9
　postgastrectomy K91.1
　postvagotomy K91.1
　protozoal A07.9
　　specified NEC A07.8
　psychogenic F45.8
　specified
　　bacterium NEC A04.8
　　virus NEC A08.39
　strongyloidiasis B78.0
　toxic K52.1
　trichomonal A07.8
　tropical K90.1
　tuberculous A18.32
　viral —*see* Enteritis, viral
Diastasis
　cranial bones M84.88
　　congenital NEC Q75.8
　joint (traumatic) —*see* Dislocation
　muscle M62.00
　　ankle M62.07-●
　　congenital Q79.8
　　foot M62.07-●
　　forearm M62.03-●
　　hand M62.04-●
　　lower leg M62.06-●
　　pelvic region M62.05-●
　　shoulder region M62.01-●
　　specified site NEC M62.08
　　thigh M62.05-●
　　upper arm M62.02-●
　recti (abdomen)
　　complicating delivery O71.89
　　congenital Q79.59
Diastema, tooth, teeth, fully erupted M26.32
Diastematomyelia Q06.2
Diataxia, cerebral G80.4
Diathesis
　allergic —*see* History, allergy
　bleeding (familial) D69.9
　cystine (familial) E72.00
　gouty —*see* Gout
　hemorrhagic (familial) D69.9
　　newborn NEC P53
　spasmophilic R29.0
Diaz's disease or osteochondrosis (juvenile)
　　(talus) —*see* Osteochondrosis, juvenile,
　　tarsus
Dibothriocephalus, dibothriocephaliasis
　　(latus) (infection) (infestation) B70.0
　larval B70.1

Dicephalus, dicephaly Q89.4
Dichotomy, teeth K00.2
Dichromat, dichromatopsia (congenital) —*see*
　　Deficiency, color vision
Dichuchwa A65
Dicroceliasis B66.2
Didelphia, didelphys —*see* Double uterus
Didymytis N45.1
　with orchitis N45.3
Dietary
　inadequacy or deficiency E63.9
　surveillance and counseling Z71.3
Dietl's crisis N13.8
Dieulafoy lesion (hemorrhagic)
　duodenum K31.82
⮞esophagus K22.89
　intestine (colon) K63.81
　stomach K31.82
Difficult, difficulty (in)
　acculturation Z60.3
⮞feeding R63.30
　　newborn P92.9
　　　breast P92.5
　　　specified NEC P92.8
　　nonorganic (infant or child) F98.29
　　▶specified NEC R63.39
　intubation, in anesthesia T88.4
　mechanical, gastroduodenal stoma K91.89
　　causing obstruction —*see also* Obstruction,
　　　intestine, postoperative K91.30
　micturition
　　need to immediately re-void R39.191
　　position dependent R39.192
　　specified NEC R39.198
　reading (developmental) F81.0
　　secondary to emotional disorders F93.9
　spelling (specific) F81.81
　　with reading disorder F81.89
　　due to inadequate teaching Z55.8
　swallowing —*see* Dysphagia
　walking R26.2
　work
　　conditions NEC Z56.5
　　schedule Z56.3
Diffuse —*see* condition
DiGeorge's syndrome (thymic hypoplasia) D82.1
Digestive —*see* condition
Dihydropyrimidine dehydrogenase disease
　　(DPD) E88.89
Diktyoma —*see* Neoplasm, malignant, by site
Dilaceration, tooth K00.4
Dilatation
　anus K59.89
　　venule —*see* Hemorrhoids
　aorta (focal) (general) —*see* Ectasia, aorta
　　with aneurysm —*see* Aneurysm, aorta
　　congenital Q25.44
　artery —*see* Aneurysm
　bladder (sphincter) N32.89
　　congenital Q64.79
　blood vessel I99.8
　bronchial J47.9
　　with
　　　exacerbation (acute) J47.1
　　　lower respiratory infection J47.0
⮞calyx N28.89
　　▶due to obstruction —*see* Hydronephosis
　capillaries I78.8
　cardiac (acute) (chronic) —*see also*
　　Hypertrophy, cardiac
　　congenital Q24.8
　　　valve NEC Q24.8
　　　　pulmonary Q22.3
　　valve —*see* Endocarditis
　cavum septi pellucidi Q06.8
　cervix (uteri) —*see also* Incompetency, cervix
　　incomplete, poor, slow complicating
　　　delivery O62.0
　colon K59.39
　　congenital Q43.1
　　psychogenic F45.8
　　toxic K59.31

Dilatation (*Continued*)
  common duct (acquired) K83.8
    congenital Q44.5
  cystic duct (acquired) K82.8
    congenital Q44.5
  duct, mammary —*see* Ectasia, mammary duct
  duodenum K59.89
  esophagus K22.89
    congenital Q39.5
    due to achalasia K22.0
  eustachian tube, congenital Q17.8
  gallbladder K82.8
  gastric —*see* Dilatation, stomach
  heart (acute) (chronic) —*see also* Hypertrophy,
      cardiac
    congenital Q24.8
    valve —*see* Endocarditis
  ileum K59.89
    psychogenic F45.8
  jejunum K59.89
    psychogenic F45.8
  kidney (calyx) (collecting structures) (cystic)
      (parenchyma) (pelvis) (idiopathic) N28.89
    ▶due to obstruction —*see* Hydronephrosis
  lacrimal passages or duct —*see* Disorder,
      lacrimal system, changes
  lymphatic vessel I89.0
  mammary duct —*see* Ectasia, mammary duct
  Meckel's diverticulum (congenital) Q43.0
    malignant —*see* Table of Neoplasms, small
        intestine, malignant
  myocardium (acute) (chronic) —*see*
      Hypertrophy, cardiac organ or site,
      congenital NEC —*see* Distortion
  pancreatic duct K86.89
  pericardium —*see* Pericarditis
  pharynx J39.2
  prostate N42.89
  pulmonary
    artery (idiopathic) I28.8
    valve, congenital Q22.3
  pupil H57.04
  rectum K59.39
  saccule, congenital Q16.5
  salivary gland (duct) K11.8
  sphincter ani K62.89
  stomach K31.89
    acute K31.0
    psychogenic F45.8
  submaxillary duct K11.8
  trachea, congenital Q32.1
  ureter (idiopathic) N28.82
    congenital Q62.2
    due to obstruction N13.4
  urethra (acquired) N36.8
  vasomotor I73.9
  vein I86.8
  ventricular, ventricle (acute) (chronic) —*see
      also* Hypertrophy, cardiac
    cerebral, congenital Q04.8
  venule NEC I86.8
  vesical orifice N32.89
Dilated, dilation —*see* Dilatation
Diminished, diminution
  hearing (acuity) —*see* Deafness
  sense or sensation (cold) (heat) (tactile)
      (vibratory) R20.8
  vision NEC H54.7
  vital capacity R94.2
Diminuta taenia B71.0
Dimitri-Sturge-Weber disease Q85.8
Dimple
  congenital sacral Q82.6
  parasacral Q82.6
  pilonidal or postanal —*see* Cyst, pilonidal
Dioctophyme renalis (infection) (infestation)
    B83.8
Dipetalonemiasis B74.4
Diphallus Q55.69
Diphtheria, diphtheritic (gangrenous)
    (hemorrhagic) A36.9

Diphtheria, diphtheritic (*Continued*)
  carrier (suspected) Z22.2
  cutaneous A36.3
  faucial A36.0
  infection of wound A36.3
  laryngeal A36.2
  myocarditis A36.81
  nasal, anterior A36.89
  nasopharyngeal A36.1
  neurological complication A36.89
  pharyngeal A36.0
  specified site NEC A36.89
  tonsillar A36.0
Diphyllobothriasis (intestine) B70.0
  larval B70.1
Diplacusis H93.22-●
Diplegia (upper limbs) G83.0
  congenital (cerebral) G80.8
  facial G51.0
  lower limbs G82.20
  spastic G80.1
Diplococcus, diplococcal —*see* condition
Diplopia H53.2
Dipsomania F10.20
  with
    psychosis —*see* Psychosis, alcoholic
    remission F10.21
Dipylidiasis B71.1
DIRA (deficiency of interleukin 1 receptor
    antagonist) M04.8
Direction, teeth, abnormal, fully erupted M26.30
Dirofilariasis B74.8
Dirt-eating child F98.3
Disability, disabilities
  heart —*see* Disease, heart
  intellectual F79
    with
      autistic features F84.9
        ▶pathogenic CHAMP1 (genetic)
            (variant) F78.A9
        ▶pathogenic HNRNPH2 (genetic)
            (variant) F78.A9
        ▶pathogenic SATB2 (genetic) (variant)
            F78.A9
        ▶pathogenic SETBP1 (genetic) (variant)
            F78.A9
        ▶pathogenic STXBP1 (genetic) (variant)
            F78.A9
        ▶pathogenic SYNGAP1 (genetic)
            (variant) F78.A1
    ▶autosomal dominant F78.A9
    ▶autosomal recessive F78.A9
    ▶genetic related F78.A9
      ▶with
        ▶pathogenic CHAMP1 (variant) F78.
            A9
        ▶pathogenic HNRNPH2 (variant)
            F78.A9
        ▶pathogenic SATB2 (variant) F78.A9
        ▶pathogenic SETBP1 (variant) F78.A9
        ▶pathogenic STXBP1 (variant) F78.A9
        ▶pathogenic SYNGAP1 (variant) F78.
            A1
      ▶specified NEC F78.A9
      ▶SYNGAP1-related F78.A1
    ▶in
      ▶autosomal dominant mental
          retardation F78.A9
      ▶autosomal recessive mental
          retardation F78.A9
      ▶SATB2-associated syndrome F78.A9
      ▶SETBP1 disorder F78.A9
      ▶STXBP1 encephalopathy with epilepsy
          (see also Encephalopathy; and
          see also Epilepsy) F78.A9
      ▶X-linked mental retardation
          (syndromic) (Bain type) F78.A9
    mild (I.Q. 50-69) F70
    moderate (I.Q. 35-49) F71
    profound (I.Q. under 20) F73
    severe (I.Q. 20-34) F72

Disability, disabilities (*Continued*)
  intellectual (*Continued*)
    ▶specified level NEC F78.A9
    ▶SYNGAP1-related F78.A1
    ▶X-linked (syndromic) (Bain type) F78.A9
  knowledge acquisition F81.9
  learning F81.9
  limiting activities Z73.6
  spelling, specific F81.81
Disappearance of family member Z63.4
Disarticulation —*see* Amputation
  meaning traumatic amputation —*see*
      Amputation, traumatic
Discharge (from)
  abnormal finding in —*see* Abnormal, specimen
  breast (female) (male) N64.52
  diencephalic autonomic idiopathic —*see*
      Epilepsy, specified NEC
  ear —*see also* Otorrhea
    blood —*see* Otorrhagia
  excessive urine R35.89
  nipple N64.52
  penile R36.9
  postnasal R09.82
  prison, anxiety concerning Z65.2
  urethral R36.9
    without blood R36.0
    hematospermia R36.1
  vaginal N89.8
Discitis, diskitis M46.40
  cervical region M46.42
  cervicothoracic region M46.43
  lumbar region M46.46
  lumbosacral region M46.47
  multiple sites M46.49
  occipito-atlanto-axial region M46.41
  pyogenic —*see* Infection, intervertebral
      disc, pyogenic
  sacrococcygeal region M46.48
  thoracic region M46.44
  thoracolumbar region M46.45
Discoid
  meniscus (congenital) Q68.6
  semilunar cartilage (congenital) —*see*
      Derangement, knee, meniscus,
      specified NEC
Discoloration
  nails L60.8
  teeth (posteruptive) K03.7
    during formation K00.8
Discomfort
  chest R07.89
  visual H53.14-●
Discontinuity, ossicles, ear H74.2-●
Discord (with)
  boss Z56.4
  classmates Z55.4
  counselor Z64.4
  employer Z56.4
  family Z63.8
  fellow employees Z56.4
  in-laws Z63.1
  landlord Z59.2
  lodgers Z59.2
  neighbors Z59.2
  probation officer Z64.4
  social worker Z64.4
  teachers Z55.4
  workmates Z56.4
Discordant connection
  atrioventricular (congenital) Q20.5
  ventriculoarterial Q20.3
Discrepancy
  centric occlusion maximum intercuspation
      M26.55
  leg length (acquired) —*see* Deformity, limb,
      unequal length
    congenital —*see* Defect, reduction, lower
        limb
  uterine size date O26.84-●
Discrimination
  ethnic Z60.5
  political Z60.5

▶ New ⇰ Revised ~~deleted~~ Deleted ● Use Additional Character(s)

Discrimination *(Continued)*
  racial Z60.5
  religious Z60.5
  sex Z60.5
Disease, diseased —*see also* Syndrome
  absorbent system I87.8
  acid-peptic K30
  Acosta's T70.29
  Adams-Stokes (-Morgagni) (syncope with
    heart block) I45.9
  Addison's anemia (pernicious) D51.0
  adenoids (and tonsils) J35.9
  adrenal (capsule) (cortex) (gland) (medullary)
    E27.9
    hyperfunction E27.0
    specified NEC E27.8
  ainhum L94.6
  airway
    obstructive, chronic J44.9
      due to
        cotton dust J66.0
        specific organic dusts NEC J66.8
    reactive —*see* Asthma
  akamushi (scrub typhus) A75.3
  Albers-Schönberg (marble bones) Q78.2
  Albert's —*see* Tendinitis, Achilles
  alimentary canal K63.9
  alligator-skin Q80.9
    acquired L85.0
  alpha heavy chain C88.3
  alpine T70.29
  altitude T70.20
  alveolar ridge
    edentulous K06.9
      specified NEC K06.8
  alveoli, teeth K08.9
  Alzheimer's G30.9 *[F02.80]*
    with behavioral disturbance G30.9 *[F02.81]*
    early onset G30.0 *[F02.80]*
      with behavioral disturbance G30.0 *[F02.81]*
    late onset G30.1 *[F02.80]*
      with behavioral disturbance G30.1 *[F02.81]*
    specified NEC G30.8 *[F02.80]*
      with behavioral disturbance G30.8 *[F02.81]*
  amyloid —*see* Amyloidosis
  Andersen's (glycogenosis IV) E74.09
  Andes T70.29
  Andrews' (bacterid) L08.89
  angiospastic I73.9
    cerebral G45.9
    vein I87.8
  anterior
    chamber H21.9
    horn cell G12.29
  antiglomerular basement membrane
    (anti-GBM) antibody M31.0
    tubulo-interstitial nephritis N12
  antral —*see* Sinusitis, maxillary
  anus K62.9
    specified NEC K62.89
  aorta (nonsyphilitic) I77.9
    syphilitic NEC A52.02
  aortic (heart) (valve) I35.9
    rheumatic I06.9
  Apollo B30.3
  aponeuroses —*see* Enthesopathy
  appendix K38.9
    specified NEC K38.8
  aqueous (chamber) H21.9
  Arnold-Chiari —*see* Arnold-Chiari disease
  arterial I77.9
    occlusive —*see* Occlusion, by site
      due to stricture or stenosis I77.1
    peripheral I73.9
  arteriocardiorenal —*see* Hypertension,
    cardiorenal
  arteriolar (generalized) (obliterative) I77.9
  arteriorenal —*see* Hypertension, kidney
  arteriosclerotic —*see also* Arteriosclerosis
    cardiovascular —*see* Disease, heart,
      ischemic, atherosclerotic
    coronary (artery) —*see* Disease, heart,
      ischemic, atherosclerotic

Disease, diseased *(Continued)*
  arteriosclerotic *(Continued)*
    heart —*see* Disease, heart, ischemic,
      atherosclerotic
  artery I77.9
    cerebral I67.9
    coronary I25.10
      with angina pectoris —*see*
        Arteriosclerosis, coronary (artery)
    peripheral I73.9
  arthropod-borne NOS (viral) A94
    specified type NEC A93.8
  atticoantral, chronic H66.20
    left H66.22
      with right H66.23
    right H66.21
      with left H66.23
  auditory canal —*see* Disorder, ear, external
  auricle, ear NEC —*see* Disorder, pinna
  Australian X A83.4
  autoimmune (systemic) NOS M35.9
    hemolytic D59.10
      cold type (primary) (secondary)
        (symptomatic) D59.12
      drug-induced D59.0
      mixed type (primary) (secondary)
        (symptomatic) D59.13
      warm type (primary) (secondary)
        (symptomatic) D59.11
    thyroid E06.3
  autoinflammatory M04.9
    NOD2-associated M04.8
    specified type NEC M04.8
  aviator's —*see* Effect, adverse, high altitude
  Ayerza's (pulmonary artery sclerosis with
    pulmonary hypertension) I27.0
  Babington's (familial hemorrhagic
    telangiectasia) I78.0
  bacterial A49.9
    specified NEC A48.8
    zoonotic A28.9
      specified type NEC A28.8
  Baelz's (cheilitis glandularis apostematosa)
    K13.0
  bagasse J67.1
  balloon —*see* Effect, adverse, high altitude
  Bang's (brucella abortus) A23.1
  Bannister's T78.3
  barometer makers' —*see* Poisoning, mercury
  Barraquer (-Simons') (progressive
    lipodystrophy) E88.1
  Barrett's —*see* Barrett's, esophagus
  Bartholin's gland N75.9
  basal ganglia G25.9
    degenerative G23.9
      specified NEC G23.8
    specified NEC G25.89
  Basedow's (exophthalmic goiter) —*see*
    Hyperthyroidism, with, goiter (diffuse)
  Bateman's B08.1
  Batten-Steinert G71.11
  Battey A31.0
  Beard's (neurasthenia) F48.8
  Becker
    idiopathic mural endomyocardial I42.3
    myotonia congenita G71.12
  Begbie's (exophthalmic goiter) —*see*
    Hyperthyroidism, with, goiter (diffuse)
  behavioral, organic F07.9
  Beigel's (white piedra) B36.2
  Benson's —*see* Deposit, crystalline
  Bernard-Soulier (thrombopathy) D69.1
  Bernhardt (-Roth) —*see* Mononeuropathy,
    lower limb, meralgia paresthetica
  Biermer's (pernicious anemia) D51.0
  bile duct (common) (hepatic) K83.9
    with calculus, stones —*see* Calculus, bile duct
    specified NEC K83.8
  biliary (tract) K83.9
    specified NEC K83.8
  Billroth's —*see* Spina bifida
  bird fancier's J67.2
  black lung J60

Disease, diseased *(Continued)*
  bladder N32.9
    in (due to)
      schistosomiasis (bilharziasis) B65.0 *[N33]*
    specified NEC N32.89
  bleeder's D66
  blood D75.9
    forming organs D75.9
    vessel I99.9
  Bloodgood's —*see* Mastopathy, cystic
  Blount M92.51-●
  Bodechtel-Guttmann (subacute sclerosing
    panencephalitis) A81.1
  bone —*see also* Disorder, bone
    aluminum M83.4
    fibrocystic NEC
      jaw M27.49
  bone-marrow D75.9
  Borna A83.9
  Bornholm (epidemic pleurodynia) B33.0
  Bouchard's (myopathic dilatation of the
    stomach) K31.0
  Bouillaud's (rheumatic heart disease) I01.9
  Bourneville (-Brissaud) (tuberous sclerosis)
    Q85.1
  Bouveret (-Hoffmann) (paroxysmal
    tachycardia) I47.9
  bowel K63.9
    functional K59.9
      psychogenic F45.8
  brain G93.9
    arterial, artery I67.9
    arteriosclerotic I67.2
    congenital Q04.9
    degenerative —*see* Degeneration, brain
    inflammatory —*see* Encephalitis
    organic G93.9
      arteriosclerotic I67.2
    parasitic NEC B71.9 *[G94]*
    senile NEC G31.1
    specified NEC G93.89
  breast *(see also* Disorder, breast) N64.9
    cystic (chronic) —*see* Mastopathy, cystic
    fibrocystic —*see* Mastopathy, cystic
    Paget's
      female, unspecified side C50.91-●
      male, unspecified side C50.92-●
    specified NEC N64.89
  Breda's —*see* Yaws
  Bretonneau's (diphtheritic malignant angina)
    A36.0
  Bright's —*see* Nephritis
    arteriosclerotic —*see* Hypertension, kidney
  Brill's (recrudescent typhus) A75.1
  Brill-Zinsser (recrudescent typhus) A75.1
  Brion-Kayser —*see* Fever, paratyphoid
  broad
    beta E78.2
    ligament (noninflammatory) N83.9
      inflammatory —*see* Disease, pelvis,
        inflammatory
      specified NEC N83.8
  Brocq-Duhring (dermatitis herpetiformis) L13.0
  Brocq's
    meaning
      dermatitis herpetiformis L13.0
      prurigo L28.2
  bronchopulmonary J98.4
  bronchus NEC J98.09
  bronze Addison's E27.1
    tuberculous A18.7
  budgerigar fancier's J67.2
  Buerger's (thromboangiitis obliterans) I73.1
  bullous L13.9
    chronic of childhood L12.2
    specified NEC L13.8
  Bürger-Grütz (essential familial
    hyperlipemia) E78.3
  bursa —*see* Bursopathy
  caisson T70.3
  California —*see* Coccidioidomycosis
  capillaries I78.9
    specified NEC I78.8

Disease, diseased (*Continued*)
  Carapata A68.0
  cardiac —*see* Disease, heart
  cardiopulmonary, chronic I27.9
  cardiorenal (hepatic) (hypertensive)
      (vascular) —*see* Hypertension,
      cardiorenal
  cardiovascular (atherosclerotic) I25.10
      with angina pectoris —*see* Arteriosclerosis,
          coronary (artery),
      congenital Q28.9
      hypertensive —*see* Hypertension, heart
      newborn P29.9
          specified NEC P29.89
      renal (hypertensive) —*see* Hypertension,
          cardiorenal
      syphilitic (asymptomatic) A52.00
  cartilage —*see* Disorder, cartilage
  Castellani's A69.8
  Castleman (unicentric) (multicentric)
      D47.Z2
      HHV-8-associated —*see also* Herpesvirus,
          human, 8 D47.Z2
  cat-scratch A28.1
  Cavare's (familial periodic paralysis) G72.3
  cecum K63.9
  celiac (adult) (infantile) (with steatorrhea)
      K90.0
  cellular tissue L98.9
  central core G71.29
  cerebellar, cerebellum —*see* Disease, brain
  cerebral —*see also* Disease, brain
      degenerative —*see* Degeneration, brain
  cerebrospinal G96.9
  cerebrovascular I67.9
      acute I67.89
          embolic I63.4-●
          thrombotic I63.3-●
      arteriosclerotic I67.2
      hereditary NEC I67.858
      specified NEC I67.89
  cervix (uteri) (noninflammatory) N88.9
      inflammatory —*see* Cervicitis
      specified NEC N88.8
  Chabert's A22.9
  Chandler's (osteochondritis dissecans, hip) —
      see Osteochondritis, dissecans, hip
  Charlouis —*see* Yaws
  Chédiak-Steinbrinck (-Higashi) (congenital
      gigantism of peroxidase granules) E70.330
  chest J98.9
  Chiari's (hepatic vein thrombosis) I82.0
  Chicago B40.9
  Chignon B36.8
  chigo, chigoe B88.1
  childhood granulomatous D71
  Chinese liver fluke B66.1
  chlamydial A74.9
      specified NEC A74.89
  cholecystic K82.9
  choroid H31.9
      specified NEC H31.8
  Christmas D67
  chronic bullous of childhood L12.2
  chylomicron retention E78.3
  ciliary body H21.9
      specified NEC H21.89
  circulatory (system) NEC I99.8
      newborn P29.9
      syphilitic A52.00
          congenital A50.54
  coagulation factor deficiency (congenital) —
      see Defect, coagulation
  coccidioidal —*see* Coccidioidomycosis
  cold
      agglutinin or hemoglobinuria D59.12
          paroxysmal D59.6
      hemagglutinin (chronic) D59.12
  collagen NOS (nonvascular) (vascular) M35.9
      specified NEC M35.89
  colon K63.9
      functional K59.9
          congenital Q43.2

Disease, diseased (*Continued*)
  colon K63.9(*Continued*)
      ischemic —*see also* Ischemia, intestine,
          acute K55.039
  colonic inflammatory bowel, unclassified
      (IBDU) K52.3
  combined system —*see* Degeneration,
      combined
  compressed air T70.3
  Concato's (pericardial polyserositis) A19.9
      nontubercular I31.1
      pleural —*see* Pleurisy, with effusion
  conjunctiva H11.9
      chlamydial A74.0
      specified NEC H11.89
      viral B30.9
          specified NEC B30.8
  connective tissue, systemic (diffuse) M35.9
      in (due to)
          hypogammaglobulinemia D80.1 [*M36.8*]
          ochronosis E70.29 [*M36.8*]
      specified NEC M35.89
  Conor and Bruch's (boutonneuse fever) A77.1
  Cooper's —*see* Mastopathy, cystic
  Cori's (glycogenosis III) E74.03
  corkhandler's or corkworker's J67.3
  cornea H18.9
      specified NEC H18.89-●
  coronary (artery) —*see* Disease, heart,
      ischemic, atherosclerotic
      congenital Q24.5
      ostial, syphilitic (aortic) (mitral)
          (pulmonary) A52.03
  corpus cavernosum N48.9
      specified NEC N48.89
  Cotugno's —*see* Sciatica
  COVID-19 U07.1
  coxsackie (virus) NEC B34.1
  cranial nerve NOS G52.9
  Creutzfeldt-Jakob —*see* Creutzfeldt-Jakob
      disease or syndrome
  Crocq's (acrocyanosis) I73.89
  Crohn's —*see* Enteritis, regional
  Curschmann G71.11
  cystic
      breast (chronic) —*see* Mastopathy, cystic
      kidney, congenital Q61.9
      liver, congenital Q44.6
      lung J98.4
          congenital Q33.0
  cytomegalic inclusion (generalized) B25.9
      with pneumonia B25.0
      congenital P35.1
  cytomegaloviral B25.9
      specified NEC B25.8
  Czerny's (periodic hydrarthrosis of the
      knee) —*see* Effusion, joint, knee
  Daae (-Finsen) (epidemic pleurodynia) B33.0
  Darling's —*see* Histoplasmosis capsulati
  Débove's (splenomegaly) R16.1
  deer fly —*see* Tularemia
  Degos' I77.8
  demyelinating, demyelinizating (nervous
      system) G37.9
      multiple sclerosis G35
      specified NEC G37.8
  dense deposit —*see also* N00-N07 with fourth
      character .6 N05.6
  deposition, hydroxyapatite —*see* Disease,
      hydroxyapatite deposition
  de Quervain's (tendon sheath) M65.4
      thyroid (subacute granulomatous
          thyroiditis) E06.1
  Devergie's (pityriasis rubra pilaris) L44.0
  Devic's G36.0
  diaphorase deficiency D74.0
  diaphragm J98.6
  diarrheal, infectious NEC A09
  digestive system K92.9
      specified NEC K92.89
  disc, degenerative —*see* Degeneration,
      intervertebral disc

Disease, diseased (*Continued*)
  discogenic —*see also* Displacement,
      intervertebral disc NEC
      with myelopathy —*see* Disorder, disc, with,
          myelopathy
  diverticular —*see* Diverticula
  Dubois (thymus) A50.59 [*E35*]
  Duchenne-Griesinger G71.01
  Duchenne's
      muscular dystrophy G71.01
      pseudohypertrophy, muscles G71.01
  ductless glands E34.9
  Duhring's (dermatitis herpetiformis) L13.0
  duodenum K31.9
      specified NEC K31.89
  Dupré's (meningism) R29.1
  Dupuytren's (muscle contracture) M72.0
  Durand-Nicholas-Favre (climatic bubo) A55
  Duroziez's (congenital mitral stenosis) Q23.2
  ear —*see* Disorder, ear
  Eberth's —*see* Fever, typhoid
  Ebola (virus) A98.4
  Ebstein's heart Q22.5
  Echinococcus —*see* Echinococcus
  echovirus NEC B34.1
  Eddowes' (brittle bones and blue sclera) Q78.0
  edentulous (alveolar) ridge K06.9
      specified NEC K06.8
  Edsall's T67.2
  Eichstedt's (pityriasis versicolor) B36.0
  Eisenmenger's (irreversible) I27.83
  Ellis-van Creveld (chondroectodermal
      dysplasia) Q77.6
  end stage renal (ESRD) N18.6
      due to hypertension I12.0
  endocrine glands or system NEC E34.9
  endomyocardial (eosinophilic) I42.3
  English (rickets) E55.0
  enteroviral, enterovirus NEC B34.1
      central nervous system NEC A88.8
  epidemic B99.9
      specified NEC B99.8
  epididymis N50.9
  Erb (-Landouzy) G71.02
  Erdheim-Chester (ECD) E88.89
  esophagus K22.9
      functional K22.4
      psychogenic F45.8
      ⮕specified NEC K22.89
  Eulenburg's (congenital paramyotonia) G71.19
  eustachian tube —*see* Disorder, eustachian tube
  external
      auditory canal —*see* Disorder, ear, external
      ear —*see* Disorder, ear, external
  extrapyramidal G25.9
      specified NEC G25.89
  eye H57.9
      anterior chamber H21.9
      inflammatory NEC H57.89
      muscle (external) —*see* Strabismus
      specified NEC H57.89
      syphilitic —*see* Oculopathy, syphilitic
  eyeball H44.9
      specified NEC H44.89
  eyelid —*see* Disorder, eyelid
      specified NEC —*see* Disorder, eyelid,
          specified type NEC
  eyeworm of Africa B74.3
  facial nerve (seventh) G51.9
      newborn (birth injury) P11.3
  Fahr (of brain) G23.8
  Fahr Volhard (of kidney) I12.-●
  fallopian tube (noninflammatory) N83.9
      inflammatory —*see* Salpingo-oophoritis
      specified NEC N83.8
  familial periodic paralysis G72.3
  Fanconi's (congenital pancytopenia) D61.09
  fascia NEC —*see also* Disorder, muscle
      inflammatory —*see* Myositis
      specified NEC M62.89
  Fauchard's (periodontitis) —*see* Periodontitis
  Favre-Durand-Nicolas (climatic bubo) A55
  Fede's K14.0

▶ New   ⮕ Revised   ~~deleted~~ Deleted   ● Use Additional Character(s)

Disease, diseased *(Continued)*
    Feer's —*see* Poisoning, mercury
    female pelvic inflammatory —*see also* Disease,
        pelvis, inflammatory N73.9
        syphilitic (secondary) A51.42
        tuberculous A18.17
    Fernels' (aortic aneurysm) I71.9
    fibrocaseous of lung —*see* Tuberculosis,
        pulmonary
    fibrocystic —*see* Fibrocystic disease
    Fiedler's (leptospiral jaundice) A27.0
    fifth B08.3
    file-cutter's —*see* Poisoning, lead
    fish-skin Q80.9
        acquired L85.0
    Flajani (-Basedow) (exophthalmic goiter) —
        see Hyperthyroidism, with, goiter (diffuse)
    flax-dresser's J66.1
    fluke —*see* Infestation, fluke
    foot and mouth B08.8
    foot process N04.9
    Forbes' (glycogenosis III) E74.03
    Fordyce-Fox (apocrine miliaria) L75.2
    Fordyce's (ectopic sebaceous glands) (mouth)
        Q38.6
    Forestier's (rhizomelic pseudopolyarthritis)
        M35.3
        meaning ankylosing hyperostosis —*see*
            Hyperostosis, ankylosing
    Fothergill's
        neuralgia —*see* Neuralgia, trigeminal
        scarlatina anginosa A38.9
    Fournier (gangrene) N49.3
        female N76.89
    fourth B08.8
    Fox (-Fordyce) (apocrine miliaria) L75.2
    Francis' —*see* Tularemia
    Franklin C88.2
    Frei's (climatic bubo) A55
    Friedreich's
        combined systemic or ataxia G11.11
        myoclonia G25.3
    frontal sinus —*see* Sinusitis, frontal
    fungus NEC B49
    Gaisböck's (polycythemia hypertonica) D75.1
    gallbladder K82.9
        calculus —*see* Calculus, gallbladder
        cholecystitis —*see* Cholecystitis
        cholesterolosis K82.4
        fistula —*see* Fistula, gallbladder
        hydrops K82.1
        obstruction —*see* Obstruction, gallbladder
        perforation K82.2
        specified NEC K82.8
    gamma heavy chain C88.2
    Gamna's (siderotic splenomegaly) D73.2
    Gamstorp's (adynamia episodica hereditaria)
        G72.3
    Gandy-Nanta (siderotic splenomegaly) D73.2
    ganister J62.8
    gastric —*see* Disease, stomach
    gastroesophageal reflux (GERD) K21.9
        with esophagitis (without bleeding) K21.00
        with bleeding K21.01
    gastrointestinal (tract) K92.9
        amyloid E85.4
        functional K59.9
            psychogenic F45.8
        specified NEC K92.89
    Gee (-Herter) (-Heubner) (-Thaysen)
        (nontropical sprue) K90.0
    genital organs
        female N94.9
        male N50.9
    Gerhardt's (erythromelalgia) I73.81
    Gibert's (pityriasis rosea) L42
    Gierke's (glycogenosis I) E74.01
    Gilles de la Tourette's (motor-verbal tic) F95.2
    gingiva K06.9
        plaque induced K05.00
        specified NEC K06.8
    gland (lymph) I89.9

Disease, diseased *(Continued)*
    Glanzmann's (hereditary hemorrhagic
        thrombasthenia) D69.1
    glass-blower's (cataract) —*see* Cataract,
        specified NEC
        salivary gland hypertrophy K11.1
    Glisson's —*see* Rickets
    globe H44.9
        specified NEC H44.89
    glomerular —*see also* Glomerulonephritis
        with edema —*see* Nephrosis
        acute —*see* Nephritis, acute
        chronic —*see* Nephritis, chronic
        minimal change N05.0
        rapidly progressive N01.9
    glycogen storage E74.00
        Andersen's E74.09
        Cori's E74.03
        Forbes' E74.03
        generalized E74.00
        glucose-6-phosphatase deficiency E74.01
        heart E74.02 *[I43]*
        hepatorenal E74.09
        Hers' E74.09
        liver and kidney E74.09
        McArdle's E74.04
        muscle phosphofructokinase E74.09
        myocardium E74.02 *[I43]*
        Pompe's E74.02
        Tauri's E74.09
        type 0 E74.09
        type I E74.01
        type II E74.02
        type III E74.03
        type IV E74.09
        type V E74.04
        type VI XI E74.09
        Von Gierke's E74.01
    Goldstein's (familial hemorrhagic
        telangiectasia) I78.0
    gonococcal NOS A54.9
    graft-versus-host (GVH) D89.813
        acute D89.810
        acute on chronic D89.812
        chronic D89.811
    grainhandler's J67.8
    granulomatous (childhood) (chronic) D71
    Graves' (exophthalmic goiter) —*see*
        Hyperthyroidism, with, goiter (diffuse)
    Griesinger's —*see* Ancylostomiasis
    Grisel's M43.6
    Gruby's (tinea tonsurans) B35.0
    Guillain-Barré G61.0
    Guinon's (motor-verbal tic) F95.2
    gum K06.9
    gynecological N94.9
    H (Hartnup's) E72.02
    Haff —*see* Poisoning, mercury
    Hageman (congenital factor XII deficiency)
        D68.2
    hair (color) (shaft) L67.9
        follicles L73.9
            specified NEC L73.8
    Hamman's (spontaneous mediastinal
        emphysema) J98.2
    hand, foot and mouth B08.4
    Hansen's —*see* Leprosy
    Hantavirus, with pulmonary manifestations
        B33.4
        with renal manifestations A98.5
    Harada's H30.81- •
    Hartnup (pellagra-cerebellar ataxia-renal
        aminoaciduria) E72.02
    Hart's (pellagra-cerebellar ataxia-renal
        aminoaciduria) E72.02
    Hashimoto's (struma lymphomatosa) E06.3
    Hb —*see* Disease, hemoglobin
    heart (organic) I51.9
        with
            pulmonary edema (acute) —*see also*
                Failure, ventricular, left I50.1

Disease, diseased *(Continued)*
    heart *(Continued)*
        rheumatic fever (conditions in I00)
            active I01.9
                with chorea I02.0
                specified NEC I01.8
            inactive or quiescent (with chorea) I09.9
                specified NEC I09.89
        amyloid E85.4 *[I43]*
        aortic (valve) I35.9
        arteriosclerotic or sclerotic (senile) —*see*
            Disease, heart, ischemic, atherosclerotic
        artery, arterial —*see* Disease, heart,
            ischemic, atherosclerotic
        beer drinkers' I42.6
        beriberi (wet) E51.12
        black I27.0
        congenital Q24.9
            cyanotic Q24.9
            specified NEC Q24.8
        coronary —*see* Disease, heart, ischemic
        cryptogenic I51.9
        fibroid —*see* Myocarditis
        functional I51.89
            psychogenic F45.8
        glycogen storage E74.02 *[I43]*
        gonococcal A54.83
        hypertensive —*see* Hypertension, heart
        hyperthyroid —*see also* Hyperthyroidism
            E05.90 *[I43]*
            with thyroid storm E05.91 *[I43]*
        ischemic (chronic or with a stated duration
            of over 4 weeks) I25.9
            atherosclerotic (of) I25.10
                with angina pectoris —*see*
                    Arteriosclerosis, coronary (artery)
                coronary artery bypass graft —*see*
                    Arteriosclerosis, coronary (artery),
            cardiomyopathy I25.5
            diagnosed on ECG or other special
                investigation, but currently
                presenting no symptoms I25.6
            silent I25.6
            specified form NEC I25.89
        kyphoscoliotic I27.1
        meningococcal A39.50
            endocarditis A39.51
            myocarditis A39.52
            pericarditis A39.53
        mitral I05.9
            specified NEC I05.8
        muscular —*see* Degeneration, myocardial
        psychogenic (functional) F45.8
        pulmonary (chronic) I27.9
            in schistosomiasis B65.9 *[I52]*
            specified NEC I27.89
        rheumatic (chronic) (inactive) (old)
            (quiescent) (with chorea) I09.9
            active or acute I01.9
                with chorea (acute) (rheumatic)
                    (Sydenham's) I02.0
            specified NEC I09.89
        senile —*see* Myocarditis
        syphilitic A52.06
            aortic A52.03
                aneurysm A52.01
            congenital A50.54 *[I52]*
        thyrotoxic —*see also* Thyrotoxicosis E05.90
            [I43]
            with thyroid storm E05.91 *[I43]*
        valve, valvular (obstructive)
            (regurgitant) —*see also* Endocarditis
            congenital NEC Q24.8
                pulmonary Q22.3
        vascular —*see* Disease, cardiovascular
    heavy chain NEC C88.2
        alpha C88.3
        gamma C88.2
        mu C88.2
    Hebra's
        pityriasis
            maculata et circinata L42
            rubra pilaris L44.0

Disease, diseased *(Continued)*
  Hebra's *(Continued)*
    prurigo L28.2
  hematopoietic organs D75.9
  hemoglobin or Hb
    abnormal (mixed) NEC D58.2
      with thalassemia D56.9
    AS genotype D57.3
    Bart's D56.0
    C (Hb-C) D58.2
      with other abnormal hemoglobin NEC
        D58.2
      elliptocytosis D58.1
      Hb-S D57.2-●
      sickle-cell D57.2-●
      thalassemia D56.8
    Constant Spring D58.2
    D (Hb-D) D58.2
    E (Hb-E) D58.2
    E-beta thalassemia D56.5
    elliptocytosis D58.1
    H (Hb-H) (thalassemia) D56.0
      with other abnormal hemoglobin NEC
        D56.9
      Constant Spring D56.0
    I thalassemia D56.9
    M D74.0
    S or SS D57.1
      with
        acute chest syndrome D57.01
        cerebral vascular involvement D57.03
        crisis (painful) D57.00
          with complication specified NEC
            D57.09
        splenic sequestration D57.02
        vasoocclusive pain D57.00
      beta plus D57.44
        with
          acute chest syndrome D57.451
          cerebral vascular involvement
            D57.453
          crisis D57.459
            with specified complication NEC
              D57.458
          splenic sequestration D57.452
          vasoocclusive pain D57.459
        without crisis D57.44
      beta zero D57.42
        with
          acute chest syndrome D57.431
          cerebral vascular involvement
            D57.433
          crisis D57.439
            with specified complication NEC
              D57.438
          splenic sequestration D57.432
          vasoocclusive pain D57.439
        without crisis D57.42
    SC D57.2-●
    SD D57.8-●
    SE D57.8-●
    spherocytosis D58.0
    unstable, hemolytic D58.2
  hemolytic (newborn) P55.9
    autoimmune D59.10
      cold type (primary) (secondary)
        (symptomatic) D59.12
      mixed type (primary) (secondary)
        (symptomatic) D59.13
      warm type (primary) (secondary)
        (symptomatic) D59.11
    drug-induced D59.0
    due to or with
      incompatibility
        ABO (blood group) P55.1
        blood (group) (Duffy) (K) (Kell)
          (Kidd) (Lewis) (M) (S) NEC P55.8
        Rh (blood group) (factor) P55.0
        Rh negative mother P55.0
    specified type NEC P55.8
    unstable hemoglobin D58.2
  hemorrhagic D69.9
    newborn P53

Disease, diseased *(Continued)*
  Henoch (-Schönlein) (purpura nervosa)
    D69.0
  hepatic —*see* Disease, liver
  hepatobiliary K83.9
    toxic K71.9
  hepatolenticular E83.01
  heredodegenerative NEC
    spinal cord G95.89
  herpesviral, disseminated B00.7
  Hers' (glycogenosis VI) E74.09
  Herter (-Gee) (-Heubner) (nontropical sprue)
    K90.0
  Heubner-Herter (nontropical sprue) K90.0
  high fetal gene or hemoglobin thalassemia
    D56.9
  Hildenbrand's —*see* Typhus
  hip (joint) M25.9
    congenital Q65.89
    suppurative M00.9
    tuberculous A18.02
  His (-Werner) (trench fever) A79.0
  Hodgson's I71.2
    ruptured I71.1
  Holla —*see* Spherocytosis
  hookworm B76.9
    specified NEC B76.8
  host-versus-graft D89.813
    acute D89.810
    acute on chronic D89.812
    chronic D89.811
  human immunodeficiency virus (HIV) B20
  Huntington's G10
    with dementia G10 [F02.80]
  Hutchinson's (cheiropompholyx) —*see*
    Hutchinson's disease
  hyaline (diffuse) (generalized)
    membrane (lung) (newborn) P22.0
    adult J80
  hydatid —*see* Echinococcus
  hydroxyapatite deposition M11.00
    ankle M11.07-●
    elbow M11.02-●
    foot joint M11.07-●
    hand joint M11.04-●
    hip M11.05-●
    knee M11.06-●
    multiple site M11.09
    shoulder M11.01-●
    vertebra M11.08
    wrist M11.03-●
  hyperkinetic —*see* Hyperkinesia
  hypertensive —*see* Hypertension
  hypophysis E23.7
  Iceland G93.3
  I-cell E77.0
  immune D89.9
  immunoproliferative (malignant) C88.9
    small intestinal C88.3
    specified NEC C88.8
  inclusion B25.9
    salivary gland B25.9
  infectious, infective B99.9
    congenital P37.9
      specified NEC P37.8
      viral P35.9
        specified type NEC P35.8
    specified NEC B99.8
  inflammatory
    penis N48.29
      abscess N48.21
      cellulitis N48.22
    prepuce N47.7
      balanoposthitis N47.6
    tubo-ovarian —*see* Salpingo-oophoritis
  intervertebral disc —*see also* Disorder, disc
    with myelopathy —*see* Disorder, disc, with,
      myelopathy
    cervical, cervicothoracic —*see* Disorder,
      disc, cervical
      with
        myelopathy —*see* Disorder, disc,
          cervical, with myelopathy

Disease, diseased *(Continued)*
  cervical, cervicothoracic *(Continued)*
        neuritis, radiculitis or
          radiculopathy —*see* Disorder,
          disc, cervical, with neuritis
        specified NEC —*see* Disorder, disc,
          cervical, specified type NEC
    lumbar (with)
      myelopathy M51.06
      neuritis, radiculitis, radiculopathy or
        sciatica M51.16
      specified NEC M51.86
    lumbosacral (with)
      neuritis, radiculitis, radiculopathy or
        sciatica M51.17
      specified NEC M51.87
  intervertebral disc *(Continued)*
    specified NEC —*see* Disorder, disc,
      specified NEC
    thoracic (with)
      myelopathy M51.04
      neuritis, radiculitis or radiculopathy
        M51.14
      specified NEC M51.84
    thoracolumbar (with)
      myelopathy M51.05
      neuritis, radiculitis or radiculopathy
        M51.15
      specified NEC M51.85
  intestine K63.9
    functional K59.9
      psychogenic F45.8
      specified NEC K59.89
    organic K63.9
    protozoal A07.9
    specified NEC K63.89
  iris H21.9
    specified NEC H21.89
  iron metabolism or storage E83.10
  island (scrub typhus) A75.3
  itai-itai —*see* Poisoning, cadmium
  Jakob-Creutzfeldt —*see* Creutzfeldt-Jakob
    disease or syndrome
  jaw M27.9
    fibrocystic M27.49
    specified NEC M27.8
  jigger B88.1
  joint —*see also* Disorder, joint
    Charcot's —*see* Arthropathy, neuropathic
      (Charcot)
    degenerative —*see* Osteoarthritis
      multiple M15.9
      spine —*see* Spondylosis
    ▶facet joint (*see also* Spondylosis) M47.819
    hypertrophic —*see* Osteoarthritis
    sacroiliac M53.3
    specified NEC —*see* Disorder, joint,
      specified type NEC
    spine NEC —*see* Dorsopathy
    suppurative —*see* Arthritis, pyogenic or
      pyemic
  Jourdain's (acute gingivitis) K05.00
    nonplaque induced K05.01
    plaque induced K05.00
  Kaschin-Beck (endemic polyarthritis) M12.10
    ankle M12.17-●
    elbow M12.12-●
    foot joint M12.17-●
    hand joint M12.14-●
    hip M12.15-●
    knee M12.16-●
    multiple site M12.19
    shoulder M12.11-●
    vertebra M12.18
    wrist M12.13-●
  Katayama B65.2
  Kedani (scrub typhus) A75.3
  Keshan E59
  kidney (functional) (pelvis) N28.9
    chronic N18.9
      hypertensive —*see* Hypertension, kidney
      stage 1 N18.1
      stage 2 (mild) N18.2

▶ New　　⇒ Revised　　~~deleted~~ Deleted　　● Use Additional Character(s)

Disease, diseased *(Continued)*
  kidney *(Continued)*
    stage 3 (moderate) N18.30
      stage 3a N18.31
      stage 3b N18.32
    stage 4 (severe) N18.4
    stage 5 N18.5
    complicating pregnancy —*see* Pregnancy,
      complicated by, renal disease
    cystic (congenital) Q61.9
    diabetic —*see* E08-E13 with .22
    fibrocystic (congenital) Q61.8
    hypertensive —*see* Hypertension, kidney
    in (due to)
      schistosomiasis (bilharziasis) B65.9 *[N29]*
    multicystic Q61.4
    polycystic Q61.3
      adult type Q61.2
      childhood type NEC Q61.19
        collecting duct dilatation Q61.11
    Kimmelstiel (-Wilson) (intercapillary
      polycystic (congenital)
      glomerulosclerosis) —*see* E08-E13 with .21
    Kimura D21.9
      specified site (see Neoplasm, connective
        tissue benign)
    Kinnier Wilson's (hepatolenticular
      degeneration) E83.01
    kissing —*see* Mononucleosis, infectious
    Klebs' —*see also* Glomerulonephritis N05.- ●
    Klippel-Feil (brevicollis) Q76.1
    Köhler-Pellegrini-Stieda (calcification, knee
      joint) —*see* Bursitis, tibial collateral
    Kok Q89.8
    König's (osteochondritis dissecans) —*see*
      Osteochondritis, dissecans
    Korsakoff's (nonalcoholic) F04
      alcoholic F10.96
      with dependence F10.26
    Kostmann's (infantile genetic
      agranulocytosis) D70.0
    kuru A81.81
    Kyasanur Forest A98.2
    labyrinth, ear —*see* Disorder, ear, inner
    lacrimal system —*see* Disorder, lacrimal
      system
    Lafora's —*see* Epilepsy, generalized,
      idiopathic
    Lancereaux-Mathieu (leptospiral jaundice)
      A27.0
    Landry's G61.0
    Larrey-Weil (leptospiral jaundice) A27.0
    larynx J38.7
    legionnaires' A48.1
      nonpneumonic A48.2
    Lenegre's I44.2
    lens H27.9
      specified NEC H27.8
    Lev's (acquired complete heart block) I44.2
    Lewy body (dementia) G31.83 *[F02.80]*
      with behavioral disturbance G31.83
        [F02.81]
    Lichtheim's (subacute combined sclerosis
      with pernicious anemia) D51.0
    Lightwood's (renal tubular acidosis)
      N25.89
    Lignac's (cystinosis) E72.04
    lip K13.0
    lipid-storage E75.6
      specified NEC E75.5
    Lipschütz's N76.6
    liver (chronic) (organic) K76.9
      alcoholic (chronic) K70.9
        acute —*see* Disease, liver, alcoholic,
          hepatitis
        cirrhosis K70.30
          with ascites K70.31
        failure K70.40
          with coma K70.41
        fatty liver K70.0
        fibrosis K70.2
        hepatitis K70.10
          with ascites K70.11

Disease, diseased *(Continued)*
  liver *(Continued)*
    sclerosis K70.2
    cystic, congenital Q44.6
    drug-induced (idiosyncratic) (toxic)
      (predictable) (unpredictable) —*see*
      Disease, liver, toxic
    ➡ end stage K72.10
      due to hepatitis —*see* Hepatitis
      ▶ with coma K72.11
    fatty, nonalcoholic (NAFLD) K76.0
      alcoholic K70.0
    fibrocystic (congenital) Q44.6
    fluke
      Chinese B66.1
      oriental B66.1
      sheep B66.3
    gestational alloimmune (GALD) P78.84
    glycogen storage E74.09 *[K77]*
    in (due to)
      schistosomiasis (bilharziasis) B65.9 *[K77]*
    inflammatory K75.9
      alcoholic K70.1
      specified NEC K75.89
    polycystic (congenital) Q44.6
    toxic K71.9
      with
        cholestasis K71.0
        cirrhosis (liver) K71.7
        fibrosis (liver) K71.7
        focal nodular hyperplasia K71.8
        hepatic granuloma K71.8
        hepatic necrosis K71.10
          with coma K71.11
        hepatitis NEC K71.6
          acute K71.2
          chronic
            active K71.50
              with ascites K71.51
            lobular K71.4
            persistent K71.3
          lupoid K71.50
            with ascites K71.51
        peliosis hepatis K71.8
        veno-occlusive disease (VOD) of liver
          K71.8
    veno-occlusive K76.5
  Lobo's (keloid blastomycosis) B48.0
  Lobstein's (brittle bones and blue sclera)
    Q78.0
  Ludwig's (submaxillary cellulitis) K12.2
  lumbosacral region M53.87
  lung J98.4
    black J60
    congenital Q33.9
    cystic J98.4
      congenital Q33.0
    dabbing (related) U07.0
    electronic cigarette (related) U07.0
    fibroid (chronic) —*see* Fibrosis, lung
    fluke B66.4
      oriental B66.4
    in
      amyloidosis E85.4 *[J99]*
      sarcoidosis D86.0
      Sjögren's syndrome M35.02
      systemic
        lupus erythematosus M32.13
        sclerosis M34.81
    interstitial J84.9
      of childhood, specified NEC J84.848
      respiratory bronchiolitis J84.115
      specified NEC J84.89
      with progressive fibrotic phenotype, in
        diseases classified elsewhere J84.170
    obstructive (chronic) J44.9
      with
        acute
          bronchitis J44.0
          exacerbation NEC J44.1
          lower respiratory infection J44.0
        alveolitis, allergic J67.9
        asthma J44.9

Disease, diseased *(Continued)*
  lung *(Continued)*
    obstructive (chronic) *(Continued)*
      bronchiectasis J47.9
        with
          exacerbation (acute) J47.1
          lower respiratory infection J47.0
        bronchitis J44.9
        with
          exacerbation (acute) J44.1
          lower respiratory infection J44.0
        emphysema J43.9
        hypersensitivity pneumonitis J67.9
      decompensated J44.1
        with
          exacerbation (acute) J44.1
    polycystic J98.4
      congenital Q33.0
    rheumatoid (diffuse) (interstitial) —*see*
      Rheumatoid, lung
    vaping (associated) (device) (product) (use)
      U07.0
  Lutembacher's (atrial septal defect with
    mitral stenosis) Q21.1
  Lyme A69.20
  lymphatic (gland) (system) (channel) (vessel)
    I89.9
  lymphoproliferative D47.9
    specified NEC D47.Z9
    T-gamma D47.Z9
    X-linked D82.3
  Magitot's M27.2
  malarial —*see* Malaria
  malignant —*see also* Neoplasm, malignant,
    by site
  Manson's B65.1
  maple bark J67.6
  maple-syrup-urine E71.0
  Marburg (virus) A98.3
  Marion's (bladder neck obstruction) N32.0
  Marsh's (exophthalmic goiter) —*see*
    Hyperthyroidism, with, goiter (diffuse)
  mastoid (process) —*see* Disorder, ear, middle
  Mathieu's (leptospiral jaundice) A27.0
  Maxcy's A75.2
  McArdle (-Schmid-Pearson) (glycogenosis
    V) E74.04
  mediastinum J98.59
  medullary center (idiopathic) (respiratory)
    G93.89
  Meige's (chronic hereditary edema) Q82.0
  meningococcal —*see* Infection, meningococcal
  mental F99
    organic F09
  mesenchymal M35.9
  mesenteric embolic —*see also* Ischemia,
    intestine, acute K55.039
  metabolic, metabolism E88.9
    bilirubin E80.7
  metal-polisher's J62.8
  metastatic —*see also* Neoplasm, secondary, by
    site C79.9
  microvascular — code to condition
  microvillus
    atrophy Q43.8
    inclusion (MVD) Q43.8
  middle ear —*see* Disorder, ear, middle
  Mikulicz' (dryness of mouth, absent or
    decreased lacrimation) K11.8
  Milroy's (chronic hereditary edema) Q82.0
  Minamata —*see* Poisoning, mercury
  minicore G71.29
  Minor's G95.19
  Minot's (hemorrhagic disease, newborn)
    P53
  Minot-von Willebrand-Jürgens
    (angiohemophilia) D68.0
  Mitchell's (erythromelalgia) I73.81
  mitral (valve) I05.9
    nonrheumatic I34.9
  mixed connective tissue M35.1

Disease, diseased *(Continued)*
  moldy hay J67.0
  Monge's T70.29
  Morgagni-Adams-Stokes (syncope with heart block) I45.9
  Morgagni's (syndrome) (hyperostosis frontalis interna) M85.2
  Morton's (with metatarsalgia) —*see* Lesion, nerve, plantar
  Morvan's G60.8
  motor neuron (bulbar) (mixed type) (spinal) G12.20
    amyotrophic lateral sclerosis G12.21
    familial G12.24
    progressive bulbar palsy G12.22
    specified NEC G12.29
  moyamoya I67.5
  mu heavy chain disease C88.2
  multicore G71.29
  multiminicore G71.29
  muscle —*see also* Disorder, muscle
    inflammatory —*see* Myositis
    ocular (external) —*see* Strabismus
  musculoskeletal system, soft tissue —*see also* Disorder, soft tissue
    specified NEC —*see* Disorder, soft tissue, specified type NEC
  mushroom workers' J67.5
  mycotic B49
  ⮩myelodysplastic, not classified *(see also* Syndrome, myelodysplasia) C94.6
  myeloproliferative, not classified C94.6
    chronic D47.1
  myocardium, myocardial —*see also* Degeneration, myocardial I51.5
    primary (idiopathic) I42.9
  myoneural G70.9
  Naegeli's D69.1
  nails L60.9
    specified NEC L60.8
  Nairobi (sheep virus) A93.8
  nasal J34.9
  nemaline body G71.21
  nerve —*see* Disorder, nerve
  nervous system G98.8
    autonomic G90.9
    central G96.9
      specified NEC G96.89
    congenital Q07.9
    parasympathetic G90.9
    specified NEC G98.8
    sympathetic G90.9
    vegetative G90.9
  neuromuscular system G70.9
  Newcastle B30.8
  Nicolas (-Durand)-Favre (climatic bubo) A55
  nipple N64.9
    Paget's C50.01-●
      female C50.01-●
      male C50.02-●
  Nishimoto (-Takeuchi) I67.5
  nonarthropod-borne NOS (viral) B34.9
    enterovirus NEC B34.1
  nonautoimmune hemolytic D59.4
    drug-induced D59.2
  Nonne-Milroy-Meige (chronic hereditary edema) Q82.0
  nose J34.9
  nucleus pulposus —*see* Disorder, disc
  nutritional E63.9
  oast-house-urine E72.19
    ocular
      herpesviral B00.50
      zoster B02.30
  obliterative vascular I77.1
  Ohara's —*see* Tularemia
  Opitz's (congestive splenomegaly) D73.2
  Oppenheim-Urbach (necrobiosis lipoidica diabeticorum) —*see* E08-E13 with .620
  optic nerve NEC —*see* Disorder, nerve, optic
    orbit —*see* Disorder, orbit

Disease, diseased *(Continued)*
  organ
    dabbing (related) U07.0
    electronic cigarette (related) U07.0
    vaping (associated) (device) (product) (use) U07.0
  Oriental liver fluke B66.1
  Oriental lung fluke B66.4
  Ormond's N13.5
  Oropouche virus A93.0
  Osler-Rendu (familial hemorrhagic telangiectasia) I78.0
  osteofibrocystic E21.0
  Otto's M24.7
  outer ear —*see* Disorder, ear, external
  ovary (noninflammatory) N83.9
    cystic N83.20-●
    inflammatory —*see* Salpingo-oophoritis
    polycystic E28.2
    specified NEC N83.8
  Owren's (congenital) —*see* Defect, coagulation
  pancreas K86.9
    cystic K86.2
    fibrocystic E84.9
    specified NEC K86.89
  panvalvular I08.9
    specified NEC I08.8
  parametrium (noninflammatory) N83.9
  parasitic B89
    cerebral NEC B71.9 *[G94]*
    intestinal NOS B82.9
    mouth B37.0
    skin NOS B88.9
    specified type —*see* Infestation
    tongue B37.0
  parathyroid (gland) E21.5
    specified NEC E21.4
  Parkinson's G20
  parodontal K05.6
  Parrot's (syphilitic osteochondritis) A50.02
  Parry's (exophthalmic goiter) —*see* Hyperthyroidism, with, goiter (diffuse)
  Parson's (exophthalmic goiter) —*see* Hyperthyroidism, with, goiter (diffuse)
  Paxton's (white piedra) B36.2
  pearl-worker's —*see* Osteomyelitis, specified type NEC
  Pellegrini-Stieda (calcification, knee joint) — *see* Bursitis, tibial collateral
  pelvis, pelvic
    female NOS N94.9
      specified NEC N94.89
    gonococcal (acute) (chronic) A54.24
    inflammatory (female) N73.9
      acute N73.0
      chlamydial A56.11
      chronic N73.1
      specified NEC N73.8
      syphilitic (secondary) A51.42
        late A52.76
      tuberculous A18.17
    organ, female N94.9
    peritoneum, female NEC N94.89
  penis N48.9
    inflammatory N48.29
      abscess N48.21
      cellulitis N48.22
    specified NEC N48.89
  periapical tissues NOS K04.90
  periodontal K05.6
    specified NEC K05.5
  periosteum —*see* Disorder, bone, specified type NEC
  peripheral
    arterial I73.9
    autonomic nervous system G90.9
    nerves —*see* Polyneuropathy
    vascular NOS I73.9

Disease, diseased *(Continued)*
  peritoneum K66.9
    pelvic, female NEC N94.89
    specified NEC K66.8
  persistent mucosal (middle ear) H66.20
    left H66.22
      with right H66.23
    right H66.21
      with left H66.23
  Petit's —*see* Hernia, abdomen, specified site NEC
  pharynx J39.2
    specified NEC J39.2
  Phocas' —*see* Mastopathy, cystic
  photochromogenic (acid-fast bacilli) (pulmonary) A31.0
    nonpulmonary A31.9
  Pick's G31.01 *[F02.80]*
    with behavioral disturbance G31.01 *[F02.81]*
    brain G31.01 *[F02.80]*
      with behavioral disturbance G31.01 *[F02.81]*
    of pericardium (pericardial pseudocirrhosis of liver) I31.1
  pigeon fancier's J67.2
  pineal gland E34.8
  pink —*see* Poisoning, mercury
  Pinkus' (lichen nitidus) L44.1
  pinworm B80
  Piry virus A93.8
  pituitary (gland) E23.7
  pituitary-snuff-taker's J67.8
  pleura (cavity) J94.9
    specified NEC J94.8
  pneumatic drill (hammer) T75.21
  Pollitzer's (hidradenitis suppurativa) L73.2
  polycystic
    kidney or renal Q61.3
      adult type Q61.2
      childhood type NEC Q61.19
        collecting duct dilatation Q61.11
    liver or hepatic Q44.6
    lung or pulmonary J98.4
      congenital Q33.0
    ovary, ovaries E28.2
    spleen Q89.09
  polyethylene T84.05-●
  Pompe's (glycogenosis II) E74.02
  Posadas-Wernicke B38.9
  Potain's (pulmonary edema) —*see* Edema, lung
  prepuce N47.8
    inflammatory N47.7
      balanoposthitis N47.6
  Pringle's (tuberous sclerosis) Q85.1
  prion, central nervous system A81.9
    specified NEC A81.89
  prostate N42.9
    specified NEC N42.89
  protozoal B64
    acanthamebiasis —*see* Acanthamebiasis
    African trypanosomiasis —*see* African trypanosomiasis
    babesiosis —*(see also* Babesiosis) B60.00
    Chagas disease —*see* Chagas disease
    intestine, intestinal A07.9
    leishmaniasis —*see* Leishmaniasis
    malaria —*see* Malaria
    naegleriasis B60.2
    pneumocystosis B59
    specified organism NEC B60.8
    toxoplasmosis —*see* Toxoplasmosis
  pseudo-Hurler's E77.0
  psychiatric F99
  psychotic —*see* Psychosis
  Puente's (simple glandular cheilitis) K13.0
  puerperal —*see also* Puerperal O90.89

Disease, diseased *(Continued)*
  pulmonary —*see also* Disease, lung
    artery I28.9
    chronic obstructive J44.9
      with
        acute bronchitis J44.0
        exacerbation (acute) J44.1
        lower respiratory infection (acute)
          J44.0
      decompensated J44.1
        with
          exacerbation (acute) J44.1
    heart I27.9
      specified NEC I27.89
    hypertensive (vascular) —*see also*
      Hypertension, pulmonary I27.20
      primary (idiopathic) I27.0
    valve I37.9
      rheumatic I09.89
  pulp (dental) NOS K04.90
  pulseless M31.4
  Putnam's (subacute combined sclerosis with
    pernicious anemia) D51.0
  Pyle (-Cohn) (metaphyseal dysplasia) Q78.5
  ragpicker's or ragsorter's A22.1
  Raynaud's —*see* Raynaud's disease
  reactive airway —*see* Asthma
  Reclus' (cystic) —*see* Mastopathy, cystic
  rectum K62.9
    specified NEC K62.89
  Refsum's (heredopathia atactica
    polyneuritiformis) G60.1
  renal (functional) (pelvis) —*see also* Disease,
    kidney N28.9
    with
      edema —*see* Nephrosis
      glomerular lesion —*see*
        Glomerulonephritis
        with edema —*see* Nephrosis
      interstitial nephritis N12
    acute N28.9
    chronic —*see also* Disease, kidney, chronic
      N18.9
    cystic, congenital Q61.9
    diabetic —*see* E08-E13 with .22
    end-stage (failure) N18.6
      due to hypertension I12.0
    fibrocystic (congenital) Q61.8
    hypertensive —*see* Hypertension, kidney
    lupus M32.14
    phosphate-losing (tubular) N25.0
    polycystic (congenital) Q61.3
      adult type Q61.2
      childhood type NEC Q61.19
        collecting duct dilatation Q61.11
    rapidly progressive N01.9
    subacute N01.9
  Rendu-Osler-Weber (familial hemorrhagic
    telangiectasia) I78.0
  renovascular (arteriosclerotic) —*see*
    Hypertension, kidney
  respiratory (tract) J98.9
    acute or subacute NOS J06.9
      due to
        chemicals, gases, fumes or vapors
          (inhalation) J68.3
        external agent J70.9
          specified NEC J70.8
        radiation J70.0
        smoke inhalation J70.5
      noninfectious J39.8
    chronic NOS J98.9
      due to
        chemicals, gases, fumes or vapors
          J68.4
        external agent J70.9
          specified NEC J70.8
        radiation J70.1
    newborn P27.9
      specified NEC P27.8

Disease, diseased *(Continued)*
  respiratory (tract) *(Continued)*
    due to
      chemicals, gases, fumes or vapors J68.9
        acute or subacute NEC J68.3
        chronic J68.4
      external agent J70.9
        specified NEC J70.8
    newborn P28.9
      specified type NEC P28.89
    upper J39.9
      acute or subacute J06.9
      noninfectious NEC J39.8
      specified NEC J39.8
      streptococcal J06.9
  retina, retinal H35.9
    Batten's or Batten-Mayou E75.4 *[H36]*
    specified NEC H35.89
  rheumatoid —*see* Arthritis, rheumatoid
  rickettsial NOS A79.9
    specified type NEC A79.89
  Riga (-Fede) (cachectic aphthae) K14.0
  Riggs' (compound periodontitis) —*see*
    Periodontitis
  Ritter's L00
  Rivalta's (cervicofacial actinomycosis) A42.2
  rod body G71.21
  Robles' (onchocerciasis) B73.01
  Roger's (congenital interventricular septal
    defect) Q21.0
  Rosenthal's (factor XI deficiency) D68.1
  Ross River B33.1
  Rossbach's (hyperchlorhydria) K31.89
    psychogenic F45.8
  Rotes Quérol —*see* Hyperostosis, ankylosing
  Roth (-Bernhardt) —*see* Mononeuropathy,
    lower limb, meralgia paresthetica
  Runeberg's (progressive pernicious anemia)
    D51.0
  sacroiliac NEC M53.3
  salivary gland or duct K11.9
    inclusion B25.9
    specified NEC K11.8
    virus B25.9
  sandworm B76.9
  Schimmelbusch's —*see* Mastopathy, cystic
  Schmorl's —*see* Schmorl's disease or nodes
  Schönlein (-Henoch) (purpura rheumatica)
    D69.0
  Schottmüller's —*see* Fever, paratyphoid
  Schultz's (agranulocytosis) —*see*
    Agranulocytosis
  Schwalbe-Ziehen-Oppenheim G24.1
  Schwartz-Jampel G71.13
  sclera H15.9
    specified NEC H15.89
  scrofulous (tuberculous) A18.2
  scrotum N50.9
  sebaceous glands L73.9
  semilunar cartilage, cystic —*see also*
    Derangement, knee, meniscus, cystic
  seminal vesicle N50.9
  serum NEC —*see also* Reaction, serum T80.69
  sexually transmitted A64
    anogenital
      herpesviral infection —*see* Herpes,
        anogenital
      warts A63.0
    chancroid A57
    chlamydial infection —*see* Chlamydia
    gonorrhea —*see* Gonorrhea
    granuloma inguinale A58
    specified organism NEC A63.8
    syphilis —*see* Syphilis
    trichomoniasis —*see* Trichomoniasis
  Sézary C84.1-•
  shimamushi (scrub typhus) A75.3
  shipyard B30.0
  sickle-cell D57.1
    with
      acute chest syndrome D57.01

Disease, diseased *(Continued)*
  sickle-cell *(Continued)*
      cerebral vascular involvement D57.03
      crisis (painful) D57.00
        with complication specified NEC
          D57.09
      splenic sequestration D57.02
      vasoocclusive pain D57.00
    elliptocytosis D57.8-•
    Hb-C D57.20
      with
        acute chest syndrome D57.211
        cerebral vascular involvement D57.213
        crisis (painful) D57.219
          with specified complication NEC
            D57.218
        splenic sequestration D57.212
        vasoocclusive pain D57.219
      without crisis D57.20
    Hb-SD D57.80
      with
        acute chest syndrome D57.811
        cerebral vascular involvement D57.813
        crisis (painful) D57.819
          with complication specified NEC
            D57.818
        splenic sequestration D57.812
        vasoocclusive pain D57.819
      without crisis D57.80
    Hb-SE D57.80
      with
        acute chest syndrome D57.811
        cerebral vascular involvement D57.813
        crisis (painful) D57.819
          with complication specified NEC
            D57.818
        splenic sequestration D57.812
        vasoocclusive pain D57.819
      without crisis D57.80
    specified NEC D57.80
      with
        acute chest syndrome D57.811
        cerebral vascular involvement
          D57.813
        crisis (painful) D57.819
          with complication specified NEC
            D57.818
        splenic sequestration D57.812
        vasoocclusive pain D57.819
      without crisis D57.80
    spherocytosis D57.80
      with
        acute chest syndrome D57.811
        cerebral vascular involvement D57.813
        crisis (painful) D57.819
          with complication specified NEC
            D57.818
        splenic sequestration D57.812
        vasoocclusive pain D57.819
      without crisis D57.80
    thalassemia D57.40
      with
        acute chest syndrome D57.411
        cerebral vascular involvement D57.413
        crisis (painful) D57.419
          with specified complication NEC
            D57.418
        splenic sequestration D57.412
        vasoocclusive pain D57.419
    beta plus D57.44
      with
        acute chest syndrome D57.451
        cerebral vascular involvement
          D57.453
        crisis D57.459
          with specified complication NEC
            D57.458
        splenic sequestration D57.452
        vasoocclusive pain D57.459
      without crisis D57.44

Disease, diseased *(Continued)*
  sickle-cell *(Continued)*
    thalassemia *(Continued)*
      beta zero D57.42
        with
          acute chest syndrome D57.431
          cerebral vascular involvement
            D57.433
          crisis D57.439
            with specified complication NEC
              D57.438
          splenic sequestration D57.432
          vasoocclusive pain D57.439
        without crisis D57.42
  silo-filler's J68.8
    bronchitis J68.0
    pneumonitis J68.0
    pulmonary edema J68.1
  simian B B00.4
  Simons' (progressive lipodystrophy) E88.1
  sin nombre virus B33.4
  sinus —*see* Sinusitis
  Sirkari's B55.0
  sixth B08.20
    due to human herpesvirus 6 B08.21
    due to human herpesvirus 7 B08.22
  skin L98.9
    due to metabolic disorder NEC
      E88.9 *[L99]*
    specified NEC L98.8
  slim (HIV) B20
  small vessel I73.9
  Sneddon-Wilkinson (subcorneal pustular
    dermatosis) L13.1
  South African creeping B88.0
  spinal (cord) G95.9
    congenital Q06.9
    specified NEC G95.89
  spine —*see also* Spondylopathy
    joint —*see* Dorsopathy
    tuberculous A18.01
  spinocerebellar (hereditary) G11.9
    specified NEC G11.8
  spleen D73.9
    amyloid E85.4 *[D77]*
    organic D73.9
    polycystic Q89.09
    postinfectional D73.89
  sponge-diver's —*see* Toxicity, venom, marine
    animal, sea anemone
  Startle Q89.8
  Steinert's G71.11
  Sticker's (erythema infectiosum) B08.3
  Stieda's (calcification, knee joint) —*see*
    Bursitis, tibial collateral
  Stokes' (exophthalmic goiter) —*see*
    Hyperthyroidism, with, goiter
    (diffuse)
  Stokes-Adams (syncope with heart block)
    I45.9
  stomach K31.9
    functional, psychogenic F45.8
    specified NEC K31.89
  stonemason's J62.8
  storage
    glycogen —*see* Disease, glycogen storage
    mucopolysaccharide —*see*
      Mucopolysaccharidosis
  striatopallidal system NEC G25.89
  Stuart-Prower (congenital factor X deficiency)
    D68.2
  Stuart's (congenital factor X deficiency)
    D68.2
  subcutaneous tissue —*see* Disease, skin
  supporting structures of teeth K08.9
    specified NEC K08.89
  suprarenal (capsule) (gland) E27.9
    hyperfunction E27.0
    specified NEC E27.8
  sweat glands L74.9
    specified NEC L74.8

Disease, diseased *(Continued)*
  Sweeley-Klionsky E75.21
  Swift (-Feer) —*see* Poisoning, mercury
  swimming-pool granuloma A31.1
  Sylvest's (epidemic pleurodynia) B33.0
  sympathetic nervous system G90.9
  synovium —*see* Disorder, synovium
  syphilitic —*see* Syphilis
  systemic tissue mast cell D47.02
  tanapox (virus) B08.71
  Tangier E78.6
  Tarral-Besnier (pityriasis rubra pilaris) L44.0
  Tauri's E74.09
  tear duct —*see* Disorder, lacrimal system
  tendon, tendinous —*see also* Disorder, tendon
    nodular —*see* Trigger finger
  terminal vessel I73.9
  testis N50.9
  thalassemia Hb-S —*see* Disease, sickle-cell,
    thalassemia
  Thaysen-Gee (nontropical sprue) K90.0
  Thomsen G71.12
  throat J39.2
    septic J02.0
  thromboembolic —*see* Embolism
  thymus (gland) E32.9
    specified NEC E32.8
  thyroid (gland) E07.9
    heart —*see also* Hyperthyroidism
      E05.90 *[I43]*
      with thyroid storm E05.91 *[I43]*
    specified NEC E07.8
  Tietze's M94.0
  tongue K14.9
    specified NEC K14.89
  tonsils, tonsillar (and adenoids) J35.9
  tooth, teeth K08.9
    hard tissues K03.9
      specified NEC K03.89
    pulp NEC K04.99
    specified NEC K08.89
  Tourette's F95.2
  trachea NEC J39.8
  tricuspid I07.9
    nonrheumatic I36.9
  triglyceride-storage E75.5
  trophoblastic —*see* Mole, hydatidiform
  tsutsugamushi A75.3
  tube (fallopian) (noninflammatory) N83.9
    inflammatory —*see* Salpingitis
    specified NEC N83.8
  tuberculous NEC —*see* Tuberculosis
  tubo-ovarian (noninflammatory) N83.9
    inflammatory —*see* Salpingo-oophoritis
    specified NEC N83.8
  tubotympanic, chronic —*see* Otitis, media,
    suppurative, chronic, tubotympanic
  tubulo-interstitial N15.9
    specified NEC N15.8
  tympanum —*see* Disorder, tympanic
    membrane
  Uhl's Q24.8
  Underwood's (sclerema neonatorum) P83.0
  Unverricht (-Lundborg) —*see* Epilepsy,
    generalized, idiopathic
  Urbach-Oppenheim (necrobiosis lipoidica
    diabeticorum) —*see* E08-E13 with .620
  ureter N28.9
    in (due to)
      schistosomiasis (bilharziasis)
        B65.0 *[N29]*
  urethra N36.9
    specified NEC N36.8
  urinary (tract) N39.9
    bladder N32.9
      specified NEC N32.89
    specified NEC N39.8
  uterus (noninflammatory) N85.9
    infective —*see* Endometritis
    inflammatory —*see* Endometritis
    specified NEC N85.8

Disease, diseased *(Continued)*
  uveal tract (anterior) H21.9
    posterior H31.9
  vagabond's B85.1
  vagina, vaginal (noninflammatory) N89.9
    inflammatory NEC N76.89
    specified NEC N89.8
  valve, valvular I38
    multiple I08.9
      specified NEC I08.8
  van Creveld-von Gierke (glycogenosis I)
    E74.01
  vas deferens N50.9
  vascular I99.9
    arteriosclerotic —*see* Arteriosclerosis
    ciliary body NEC —*see* Disorder, iris,
      vascular
    hypertensive —*see* Hypertension
    iris NEC —*see* Disorder, iris, vascular
    obliterative I77.1
      peripheral I73.9
    occlusive I99.8
    peripheral (occlusive) I73.9
      in diabetes mellitus —*see* E08-E13 with .51
  vasomotor I73.9
  vasospastic I73.9
  vein I87.9
  venereal —*see also* Disease, sexually
    transmitted A64
    chlamydial NEC A56.8
      anus A56.3
      genitourinary NOS A56.2
      pharynx A56.4
      rectum A56.3
    fifth A55
    sixth A55
    specified nature or type NEC A63.8
  vertebra, vertebral —*see also* Spondylopathy
    disc —*see* Disorder, disc
  vibration —*see* Vibration, adverse effects
  viral, virus —*see also* Disease, by type of virus
    B34.9
    arbovirus NOS A94
    arthropod-borne NOS A94
    congenital P35.9
      specified NEC P35.8
    Hanta (with renal manifestations)
      (Dobrava) (Puumala) (Seoul) A98.5
      with pulmonary manifestations (Andes)
        (Bayou) (Bermejo) (Black Creek
        Canal) (Choclo) (Juquitiba) (Laguna
        negra) (Lechiguanas) (New York)
        (Oran) (Sin nombre) B33.4
    Hantaan (Korean hemorrhagic fever) A98.5
    human immunodeficiency (HIV) B20
    Kunjin A83.4
    nonarthropod-borne NOS B34.9
    Powassan A84.81
    Rocio (encephalitis) A83.6
    Sin nombre (Hantavirus) (cardio)-
      pulmonary syndrome B33.4
    Tahyna B33.8
    vesicular stomatitis A93.8
  vitreous H43.9
    specified NEC H43.89
  vocal cord J38.3
  Volkmann's, acquired T79.6
  von Eulenburg's (congenital paramyotonia)
    G71.19
  von Gierke's (glycogenosis I) E74.01
  von Graefe's —*see* Strabismus, paralytic,
    ophthalmoplegia, progressive
  von Willebrand (-Jürgens) (angiohemophilia)
    D68.0
  Vrolik's (osteogenesis imperfecta) Q78.0
  vulva (noninflammatory) N90.9
    inflammatory NEC N76.89
    specified NEC N90.89
  Wallgren's (obstruction of splenic vein with
    collateral circulation) I87.8
  Wassilieff's (leptospiral jaundice) A27.0

Disease, diseased (Continued)
  wasting NEC R64
    due to malnutrition E43
      with marasmus E41
  Waterhouse-Friderichsen A39.1
  Wegner's (syphilitic osteochondritis) A50.02
  Weil's (leptospiral jaundice of lung) A27.0
  Weir Mitchell's (erythromelalgia) I73.81
  Werdnig-Hoffmann G12.0
  Wermer's E31.21
  Werner-His (trench fever) A79.0
  Werner-Schultz (neutropenic splenomegaly)
    D73.81
  Wernicke-Posadas B38.9
  whipworm B79
  white blood cells D72.9
    specified NEC D72.89
  white matter R90.82
  white-spot, meaning lichen sclerosus et
    atrophicus L90.0
    penis N48.0
    vulva N90.4
  Wilkie's K55.1
  Wilkinson-Sneddon (subcorneal pustular
    dermatosis) L13.1
  Willis' —see Diabetes
  Wilson's (hepatolenticular degeneration) E83.01
  woolsorter's A22.1
  yaba monkey tumor B08.72
  yaba pox (virus) B08.72
  Zika virus A92.5
  zoonotic, bacterial A28.9
    congenital P35.4
    specified type NEC A28.8
Disfigurement (due to scar) L90.5
Disgerminoma —see Dysgerminoma
DISII (diffuse idiopathic skeletal
  hyperostosis) —see Hyperostosis, ankylosing
Disinsertion, retina —see Detachment, retina
Dislocatable hip, congenital Q65.6
Dislocation (articular)
  with fracture —see Fracture
  acromioclavicular (joint) S43.10 ●
    with displacement
      100%-200% S43.12-●
      more than 200% S43.13-●
    inferior S43.14-●
    posterior S43.15-●
  ankle S93.0-●
  astragalus —see Dislocation, ankle
  atlantoaxial S13.121
  atlantooccipital S13.111
  atloidooccipital S13.111
  breast bone S23.29
  capsule, joint code by site under Dislocation
  carpal (bone) —see Dislocation, wrist
  carpometacarpal (joint) NEC S63.05-●
    thumb S63.04-●
  cartilage (joint) - code by site under
    Dislocation
  cervical spine (vertebra) —see Dislocation,
    vertebra, cervical
  chronic —see Dislocation, recurrent
  clavicle —see Dislocation, acromioclavicular
    joint
  coccyx S33.2
  congenital NEC Q68.8
  coracoid —see Dislocation, shoulder
  costal cartilage S23.29
  costochondral S23.29
  cricoarytenoid articulation S13.29
  cricothyroid articulation S13.29
  dorsal vertebra —see Dislocation, vertebra,
    thoracic
  ear ossicle —see Discontinuity, ossicles, ear
  elbow S53.10-●
    congenital Q68.8
    pathological —see Dislocation, pathological
      NEC, elbow
    radial head alone —see Dislocation, radial
      head

Dislocation (Continued)
  elbow (Continued)
    recurrent —see Dislocation, recurrent,
      elbow
    traumatic S53.10-●
      anterior S53.11-●
      lateral S53.14-●
      medial S53.13-●
      posterior S53.12-●
      specified type NEC S53.19-●
  eye, nontraumatic —see Luxation, globe
  eyeball, nontraumatic —see Luxation, globe
  femur
    distal end —see Dislocation, knee
    proximal end —see Dislocation, hip
  fibula
    distal end —see Dislocation, ankle
    proximal end —see Dislocation, knee
  finger S63.25-●
    index S63.25-●
    interphalangeal S63.27-●
      distal S63.29-●
        index S63.29-●
        little S63.29-●
        middle S63.29-●
        ring S63.29-●
      index S63.27-●
      little S63.27-●
      middle S63.27-●
      proximal S63.28-●
        index S63.28-●
        little S63.28-●
        middle S63.28-●
        ring S63.28-●
      ring S63.27-●
    little S63.25-●
    metacarpophalangeal S63.26-●
      index S63.26-●
      little S63.26-●
      middle S63.26-●
      ring S63.26-●
    middle S63.25-●
    recurrent —see Dislocation, recurrent,
      finger
    ring S63.25-●
    thumb —see Dislocation, thumb
  foot S93.30-●
    recurrent —see Dislocation, recurrent,
      foot
    specified site NEC S93.33-●
    tarsal joint S93.31-●
    tarsometatarsal joint S93.32-●
    toe —see Dislocation, toe
  fracture —see Fracture
  glenohumeral (joint) —see Dislocation,
    shoulder
  glenoid —see Dislocation, shoulder
  habitual —see Dislocation, recurrent
  hip S73.00-●
    anterior S73.03-●
      obturator S73.02-●
    central S73.04-●
    congenital (total) Q65.2
      bilateral Q65.1
      partial Q65.5
        bilateral Q65.4
        unilateral Q65.3-●
      unilateral Q65.0-●
    developmental M24.85-●
    pathological —see Dislocation, pathological
      NEC, hip
    posterior S73.01-●
    recurrent —see Dislocation, recurrent,
      hip
  humerus, proximal end —see Dislocation,
    shoulder
  incomplete —see Subluxation, by site
  incus —see Discontinuity, ossicles,
    ear
  infracoracoid —see Dislocation,
    shoulder

Dislocation (Continued)
  innominate (pubic junction) (sacral
    junction) S33.39
    acetabulum —see Dislocation, hip
  interphalangeal (joint(s))
    finger S63.279
      distal S63.29-●
        index S63.29-●
        little S63.29-●
        middle S63.29-●
        ring S63.29-●
      index S63.27-●
      little S63.27-●
      middle S63.27-●
      proximal S63.28-●
        index S63.28-●
        little S63.28-●
        middle S63.28-●
        ring S63.28-●
      ring S63.27-●
    foot or toe —see Dislocation, toe
    thumb S63.12-●
  jaw (cartilage) (meniscus) S03.0-●
  joint prosthesis —see Complications, joint
    prosthesis, mechanical, displacement,
    by site
  knee S83.106
    cap —see Dislocation, patella
    congenital Q68.2
    old M23.8X-●
    patella —see Dislocation, patella
    pathological —see Dislocation, pathological
      NEC, knee
    proximal tibia
      anteriorly S83.11-●
      laterally S83.14-●
      medially S83.13-●
      posteriorly S83.12-●
    recurrent —see also Derangement, knee,
      specified NEC
    specified type NEC S83.19-●
  lacrimal gland H04.16-●
  lens (complete) H27.10-●
    anterior H27.12-●
    congenital Q12.1
    ocular implant —see Complications,
      intraocular lens
    partial H27.11-●
    posterior H27.13-●
    traumatic S05.8X-●
  ligament code by site under Dislocation
  lumbar (vertebra) —see Dislocation, vertebra,
    lumbar
  lumbosacral (vertebra) —see also Dislocation,
    vertebra, lumbar
    congenital Q76.49
  mandible S03.0-●
  meniscus (knee) —see Tear, meniscus
    other sites code by site under
      Dislocation
  metacarpal (bone)
    distal end —see Dislocation, finger
    proximal end S63.06-●
  metacarpophalangeal (joint)
    finger S63.26-●
      index S63.26-●
      little S63.26-●
      middle S63.26-●
      ring S63.26-●
    thumb S63.11-●
  metatarsal (bone) —see Dislocation, foot
  metatarsophalangeal (joint(s)) —see
    Dislocation, toe
  midcarpal (joint) S63.03-●
  midtarsal (joint) —see Dislocation, foot
  neck S13.20
    specified site NEC S13.29
    vertebra —see Dislocation, vertebra,
      cervical
  nose (septal cartilage) S03.1
  occipitoatloid S13.111

Dislocation (*Continued*)
old —*see* Derangement, joint, specified type
NEC
ossicles, ear —*see* Discontinuity, ossicles, ear
partial —*see* Subluxation, by site
patella S83.006
congenital Q74.1
lateral S83.01-●
recurrent (nontraumatic) M22.0-●
incomplete M22.1-●
specified type NEC S83.09-●
pathological NEC M24.30
ankle M24.37-●
elbow M24.32-●
foot joint M24.37-●
hand joint M24.34-●
hip M24.35-●
knee M24.36-●
lumbosacral joint —*see* subcategory M53.2
pelvic region —*see* Dislocation,
pathological, hip
sacroiliac —*see* subcategory M53.2
shoulder M24.31-●
specified site NEC M24.39
wrist M24.33-●
pelvis NEC S33.30
specified NEC S33.39
phalanx
finger or hand —*see* Dislocation, finger
foot or toe —*see* Dislocation, toe
prosthesis, internal —*see* Complications,
prosthetic device, by site, mechanical
radial head S53.006
anterior S53.01-●
posterior S53.02-●
specified type NEC S53.09-●
radiocarpal (joint) S63.02-●
radiohumeral (joint) —*see* Dislocation, radial
head
radioulnar (joint)
distal S63.01-●
proximal —*see* Dislocation, elbow
radius
distal end —*see* Dislocation, wrist
proximal end —*see* Dislocation, radial head
recurrent M24.40
ankle M24.47-●
elbow M24.42-●
finger M24.44-●
foot joint M24.47-●
hand joint M24.44-●
hip M24.45-●
knee M24.46-●
patella —*see* Dislocation, patella,
recurrent
patella —*see* Dislocation, patella,
recurrent
sacroiliac —*see* subcategory M53.2
shoulder M24.41-●
specified site NEC M24.49
toe M24.47-●
vertebra —*see also* subcategory M43.5
atlantoaxial M43.4
with myelopathy M43.3
wrist M24.43-●
rib (cartilage) S23.29
sacrococcygeal S33.2
sacroiliac (joint) (ligament) S33.2
congenital Q74.2
recurrent —*see* subcategory M53.2
sacrum S33.2
scaphoid (bone) (hand) (wrist) —*see*
Dislocation, wrist
foot —*see* Dislocation, foot
scapula —*see* Dislocation, shoulder, girdle,
scapula
semilunar cartilage, knee —*see* Tear,
meniscus
septal cartilage (nose) S03.1
septum (nasal) (old) J34.2
sesamoid bone code by site under Dislocation

Dislocation (*Continued*)
shoulder (blade) (ligament) (joint) (traumatic)
S43.006
acromioclavicular —*see* Dislocation,
acromioclavicular
chronic —*see* Dislocation, recurrent,
shoulder
congenital Q68.8
girdle S43.30-●
scapula S43.31-●
specified site NEC S43.39-●
humerus S43.00-●
anterior S43.01-●
inferior S43.03-●
posterior S43.02-●
pathological —*see* Dislocation, pathological
NEC, shoulder
recurrent —*see* Dislocation, recurrent,
shoulder
specified type NEC S43.08-●
spine
cervical —*see* Dislocation, vertebra, cervical
congenital Q76.49
due to birth trauma P11.5
lumbar —*see* Dislocation, vertebra, lumbar
thoracic —*see* Dislocation, vertebra,
thoracic
spontaneous —*see* Dislocation, pathological
sternoclavicular (joint) S43.206
anterior S43.21-●
posterior S43.22-●
sternum S23.29
subglenoid —*see* Dislocation, shoulder
symphysis pubis S33.4
talus —*see* Dislocation, ankle
tarsal (bone(s)) (joint(s)) —*see* Dislocation,
foot
tarsometatarsal (joint(s)) —*see* Dislocation,
foot
temporomandibular (joint) S03.0-●
thigh, proximal end —*see* Dislocation, hip
thorax S23.20
specified site NEC S23.29
vertebra —*see* Dislocation, vertebra
thumb S63.10-●
interphalangeal joint —*see* Dislocation,
interphalangeal (joint), thumb
metacarpophalangeal joint —*see*
Dislocation, metacarpophalangeal
(joint), thumb
thyroid cartilage S13.29
tibia
distal end —*see* Dislocation, ankle
proximal end —*see* Dislocation, knee
tibiofibular (joint)
distal —*see* Dislocation, ankle
superior —*see* Dislocation, knee
toe(s) S93.106
great S93.10-●
interphalangeal joint S93.11-●
metatarsophalangeal joint S93.12-●
interphalangeal joint S93.119
lesser S93.106
interphalangeal joint S93.11-●
metatarsophalangeal joint S93.12-●
metatarsophalangeal joint S93.12-●
tooth S03.2
trachea S23.29
ulna
distal end S63.07-●
proximal end —*see* Dislocation, elbow
ulnohumeral (joint) —*see* Dislocation, elbow
vertebra (articular process) (body)
(traumatic)
cervical S13.101
atlantoaxial joint S13.121
atlantooccipital joint S13.111
atloidooccipital joint S13.111
joint between
C0 and C1 S13.111
C1 and C2 S13.121

Dislocation (*Continued*)
vertebra (*Continued*)
cervical (*Continued*)
joint between (*Continued*)
C2 and C3 S13.131
C3 and C4 S13.141
C4 and C5 S13.151
C5 and C6 S13.161
C6 and C7 S13.171
C7 and T1 S13.181
occipitoatloid joint S13.111
congenital Q76.49
lumbar S33.101
joint between
L1 and L2 S33.111
L2 and L3 S33.121
L3 and L4 S33.131
L4 and L5 S33.141
nontraumatic —*see* Displacement,
intervertebral disc
partial —*see* Subluxation, by site
recurrent NEC —*see* subcategory
M43.5
thoracic S23.101
joint between
T1 and T2 S23.111
T2 and T3 S23.121
T3 and T4 S23.123
T4 and T5 S23.131
T5 and T6 S23.133
T6 and T7 S23.141
T7 and T8 S23.143
T8 and T9 S23.151
T9 and T10 S23.153
T10 and T11 S23.161
T11 and T12 S23.163
T12 and L1 S23.171
wrist (carpal bone) S63.006
carpometacarpal joint —*see* Dislocation,
carpometacarpal (joint)
distal radioulnar joint —*see* Dislocation,
radioulnar (joint), distal
metacarpal bone, proximal —*see*
Dislocation, metacarpal (bone),
proximal end
midcarpal —*see* Dislocation, midcarpal
(joint)
radiocarpal joint —*see* Dislocation,
radiocarpal (joint)
recurrent —*see* Dislocation, recurrent,
wrist
specified site NEC S63.09-●
ulna —*see* Dislocation, ulna, distal end
xiphoid cartilage S23.29
Disorder (of) —*see also* Disease
acantholytic L11.9
specified NEC L11.8
acute
psychotic —*see* Psychosis, acute
stress F43.0
adjustment (grief) F43.20
with
anxiety F43.22
with depressed mood F43.23
conduct disturbance F43.24
with emotional disturbance
F43.25
depressed mood F43.21
with anxiety F43.23
other specified symptom F43.29
adrenal (capsule) (gland) (medullary)
E27.9
specified NEC E27.8
adrenogenital E25.9
drug-induced E25.8
iatrogenic E25.8
idiopathic E25.8
adult personality (and behavior) F69
specified NEC F68.8
affective (mood) —*see* Disorder, mood
aggressive, unsocialized F91.1

▶ New ➠ Revised ~~deleted~~ Deleted ● Use Additional Character(s)

Disorder *(Continued)*
  cholesterol and bile acid metabolism E78.70
    Barth syndrome E78.71
    other specified E78.79
    Smith-Lemli-Opitz syndrome E78.72
  choroid H31.9
    atrophy —*see* Atrophy, choroid
    degeneration —*see* Degeneration, choroid
    detachment —*see* Detachment, choroid
    dystrophy —*see* Dystrophy, choroid
    hemorrhage —*see* Hemorrhage, choroid
    rupture —*see* Rupture, choroid
    scar —*see* Scar, chorioretinal
    solar retinopathy —*see* Retinopathy, solar
    specified type NEC H31.8
  ciliary body —*see* Disorder, iris
    degeneration —*see* Degeneration, ciliary
      body
  coagulation (factor) (*see also* Defect,
      coagulation) D68.9
    newborn, transient P61.6
  cocaine use
    mild F14.10
      with
        amphetamine, cocaine, or other
          stimulant intoxication
          with perceptual disturbances
            F14.122
          without perceptual disturbances
            F14.129
        cocaine-induced
          anxiety disorder F14.180
          bipolar and related disorder
            F14.14
          depressive disorder F14.14
          obsessive-compulsive and related
            disorder F14.188
          psychotic disorder F14.159
          sexual dysfunction F14.181
          sleep disorder F14.182
        cocaine intoxication delirium F14.121
      in remission (early) (sustained) F14.11
    moderate or severe F14.20
      with
        amphetamine, cocaine, or other
          stimulant intoxication
          with perceptual disturbances
            F14.222
          without perceptual disturbances
            F14.229
        cocaine-induced
          anxiety disorder F14.280
          bipolar and related disorder
            F14.24
          depressive disorder F14.24
          obsessive-compulsive and related
            disorder F14.288
          psychotic disorder F14.259
          sexual dysfunction F14.281
          sleep disorder F14.282
        cocaine intoxication delirium F14.221
      in remission (early) (sustained) F14.21
  coccyx NEC M53.3
  cognitive F09
    due to (secondary to) general medical
        condition F09
    persisting R41.89
      due to
        alcohol F10.97
          with dependence F10.27
        anxiolytics F13.97
          with dependence F13.27
        hypnotics F13.97
          with dependence F13.27
        sedatives F13.97
          with dependence F13.27
        specified substance NEC
          F19.97
          with
            abuse F19.17
            dependence F19.27

Disorder *(Continued)*
  communication F80.9
    social pragmatic F80.82
  conduct (childhood) F91.9
    adjustment reaction —*see* Disorder,
      adjustment
    adolescent onset type F91.2
    childhood onset type F91.1
    compulsive F63.9
    confined to family context F91.0
    depressive F91.8
    group type F91.2
    hyperkinetic —*see* Disorder, attention-
      deficit hyperactivity
    oppositional defiance F91.3
    socialized F91.2
    solitary aggressive type F91.1
    specified NEC F91.8
    unsocialized (aggressive) F91.1
  conduction, heart I45.9
  congenital glycosylation (CDG) E74.89
  conjunctiva H11.9
    infection —*see* Conjunctivitis
  connective tissue, localized L94.9
    specified NEC L94.8
  conversion (functional neurological symptom
      disorder)
    with
      abnormal movement F44.4
      anesthesia or sensory loss F44.6
      attacks or seizures F44.5
      mixed symptoms F44.7
      special sensory symptoms F44.6
      speech symptoms F44.4
      swallowing symptoms F44.4
      weakness or paralysis F44.4
  convulsive (secondary) —*see* Convulsions
  cornea H18.9
    deformity —*see* Deformity, cornea
    degeneration —*see* Degeneration, cornea
    deposits —*see* Deposit, cornea
    due to contact lens H18.82-●
      specified as edema —*see* Edema, cornea
    edema —*see* Edema, cornea
    keratitis —*see* Keratitis
    keratoconjunctivitis —*see*
      Keratoconjunctivitis
    membrane change —*see* Change, corneal
      membrane
    neovascularization —*see*
      Neovascularization, cornea
    scar —*see* Opacity, cornea
    specified type NEC H18.89-●
    ulcer —*see* Ulcer, cornea
  corpus cavernosum N48.9
  cranial nerve —*see* Disorder, nerve, cranial
  Cyclin-Dependent Kinase-Like 5 Deficiency
    (CDKL5) G40.42
  cyclothymic F34.0
  defiant oppositional F91.3
  delusional (persistent) (systematized) F22
    induced F24
  depersonalization F48.1
➡ depressive F32.A
    due to known physiological condition
      with
        depressive features F06.31
        major depressive-like episode F06.32
        mixed features F06.34
    major F32.9
      with psychotic symptoms F32.3
      in remission (full) F32.5
        partial F32.4
      recurrent F33.9
        with psychotic features F33.3
      single episode F32.9
        mild F32.0
        moderate F32.1
        severe (without psychotic symptoms)
          F32.2
        with psychotic symptoms F32.3

Disorder *(Continued)*
  depressive *(Continued)*
    organic F06.31
    persistent F34.1
    recurrent F33.9
      current episode
        mild F33.0
        moderate F33.1
        severe (without psychotic symptoms)
          F33.2
        with psychotic symptoms F33.3
      in remission F33.40
        full F33.42
        partial F33.41
      specified NEC F33.8
    single episode —*see* Episode, depressive
    specified NEC F32.89
  developmental F89
    arithmetical skills F81.2
    coordination (motor) F82
    expressive writing F81.81
    language F80.9
      expressive F80.1
      mixed receptive and expressive
        F80.2
      receptive type F80.2
      specified NEC F80.89
    learning F81.9
      arithmetical F81.2
      reading F81.0
    mixed F88
    motor coordination or function F82
    pervasive F84.9
      specified NEC F84.8
    phonological F80.0
    reading F81.0
    scholastic skills —*see also* Disorder,
      learning
      mixed F81.89
    specified NEC F88
    speech F80.9
      articulation F80.0
      specified NEC F80.89
    written expression F81.81
  diaphragm J98.6
  digestive (system) K92.9
    newborn P78.9
      specified NEC P78.89
    postprocedural —*see* Complication,
      gastrointestinal
  psychogenic F45.8
  disc (intervertebral) M51.9
    with
      myelopathy
        cervical region M50.00
        cervicothoracic region M50.03
        high cervical region M50.01
        lumbar region M51.06
        mid-cervical region M50.020
        sacrococcygeal region M53.3
        thoracic region M51.04
        thoracolumbar region M51.05
      radiculopathy
        cervical region M50.10
        cervicothoracic region M50.13
        high cervical region M50.11
        lumbar region M51.16
        lumbosacral region M51.17
        mid-cervical region M50.120
        sacrococcygeal region M53.3
        thoracic region M51.14
        thoracolumbar region M51.15
    cervical M50.90
      with
        myelopathy M50.00
          C2-C3 M50.01
          C3-C4 M50.01
          C4-C5 M50.021
          C5-C6 M50.022
          C6-C7 M50.023
          C7-T1 M50.03

Disorder *(Continued)*
 disc *(Continued)*
  cervical *(Continued)*
   with *(Continued)*
    myelopathy *(Continued)*
     cervicothoracic region M50.03
     high cervical region M50.01
     mid-cervical region M50.020
    neuritis, radiculitis or radiculopathy
      M50.10
     C2-C3 M50.11
     C3-C4 M50.11
     C4-C5 M50.121
     C5-C6 M50.122
     C6-C7 M50.123
     C7-T1 M50.13
     cervicothoracic region M50.13
     high cervical region M50.11
     mid-cervical region M50.120
   C2-C3 M50.91
   C3-C4 M50.91
   C4-C5 M50.921
   C5-C6 M50.922
   C6-C7 M50.923
   C7-T1 M50.93
   cervicothoracic region M50.93
   degeneration M50.30
    C2-C3 M50.31
    C3-C4 M50.31
    C4-C5 M50.321
    C5-C6 M50.322
    C6-C7 M50.323
    C7-T1 M50.33
    cervicothoracic region M50.33
    high cervical region M50.31
    mid-cervical region M50.320
   displacement M50.20
    C2-C3 M50.21
    C3-C4 M50.21
    C4-C5 M50.221
    C5-C6 M50.222
    C6-C7 M50.223
    C7-T1 M50.23
    cervicothoracic region M50.23
    high cervical region M50.21
    mid-cervical region M50.220
   high cervical region M50.91
   mid-cervical region M50.920
   specified type NEC M50.80
    C2-C3 M50.81
    C3-C4 M50.81
    C4-C5 M50.821
    C5-C6 M50.822
    C6-C7 M50.823
    C7-T1 M50.83
    cervicothoracic region M50.83
    high cervical region M50.81
    mid-cervical region M50.820
  specified NEC
   lumbar region M51.86
   lumbosacral region M51.87
   sacrococcygeal region M53.3
   thoracic region M51.84
   thoracolumbar region M51.85
 disinhibited attachment (childhood) F94.2
 disintegrative, childhood NEC F84.3
 disruptive F91.9
  mood dysregulation F34.81
  specified NEC F91.8
 disruptive behavior —*see* Disorder, conduct
 dissocial personality F60.2
 dissociative F44.9
  affecting
   motor function F44.4
    and sensation F44.7
   sensation F44.6
    and motor function F44.7
  brief reactive F43.0
  due to (secondary to) general medical
    condition F06.8
  mixed F44.7

Disorder *(Continued)*
 dissociative *(Continued)*
  organic F06.8
  other specified NEC F44.89
 double heterozygous sickling —*see* Disease,
    sickle-cell
 dream anxiety F51.5
 drug induced hemorrhagic D68.32
 drug related F19.99
  abuse —*see* Abuse, drug
  dependence —*see* Dependence, drug
 dysmorphic body F45.22
 dysthymic F34.1
 ear H93.9-●
  bleeding —*see* Otorrhagia
  deafness —*see* Deafness
  degenerative H93.09-●
  discharge —*see* Otorrhea
  external H61.9-●
   auditory canal stenosis —*see* Stenosis,
     external ear canal
   exostosis —*see* Exostosis, external ear
     canal
   impacted cerumen —*see* Impaction,
     cerumen
   otitis —*see* Otitis, externa
   perichondritis —*see* Perichondritis, ear
   pinna —*see* Disorder, pinna
   specified type NEC H61.89-●
    in diseases classified elsewhere
      H62.8X-●
  inner H83.9-●
   vestibular dysfunction —*see* Disorder,
     vestibular function
  middle H74.9-●
   adhesive H74.1-●
   ossicle —*see* Abnormal, ear ossicles
   polyp —*see* Polyp, ear (middle)
   specified NEC, in diseases classified
     elsewhere H75.8-●
  postprocedural —*see* Complications, ear,
    procedure
  specified NEC, in diseases classified
    elsewhere H94.8-●
 eating (adult) (psychogenic) F50.9
  anorexia —*see* Anorexia
  binge F50.81
  bulimia F50.2
  child F98.29
   pica F98.3
   rumination disorder F98.21
  pica F50.89
   childhood F98.3
 electrolyte (balance) NEC E87.8
  with
   abortion —*see* Abortion by type
     complicated by specified condition
     NEC
   ectopic pregnancy O08.5
   molar pregnancy O08.5
  acidosis (metabolic) (respiratory) E87.2
  alkalosis (metabolic) (respiratory) E87.3
 elimination, transepidermal L87.9
  specified NEC L87.8
 emotional (persistent) F34.9
  of childhood F93.9
   specified NEC F93.8
 endocrine E34.9
  postprocedural E89.89
  specified NEC E89.89
 erectile (male) (organic) —*see also*
    Dysfunction, sexual, male, erectile N52.9
  nonorganic F52.21
 erythematous —*see* Erythema
 esophagus K22.9
  functional K22.4
  psychogenic F45.8
 eustachian tube H69.9-●
  infection —*see* Salpingitis, eustachian
  obstruction —*see* Obstruction, eustachian
    tube

Disorder *(Continued)*
 eustachian tube *(Continued)*
  patulous —*see* Patulous, eustachian tube
  specified NEC H69.8-●
 exhibitionistic F65.2
 extrapyramidal G25.9
  in diseases classified elsewhere —*see*
    category G26
  specified type NEC G25.89
 eye H57.9
  postprocedural —*see* Complication,
    postprocedural, eye
 eyelid H02.9
  cyst —*see* Cyst, eyelid
  degenerative H02.70
   chloasma —*see* Chloasma, eyelid
   madarosis —*see* Madarosis
   specified type NEC H02.79
   vitiligo —*see* Vitiligo, eyelid
   xanthelasma —*see* Xanthelasma
  dermatochalasis —*see* Dermato-chalasis
  edema —*see* Edema, eyelid
  elephantiasis —*see* Elephantiasis, eyelid
  foreign body, retained —*see* Foreign body,
    retained, eyelid
  function H02.59
   abnormal innervation syndrome —
     see Syndrome, abnormal
     innervation
   blepharochalasis —*see* Blepharochalasis
   blepharoclonus —*see* Blepharoclonus
   blepharophimosis —*see*
     Blepharophimosis
   blepharoptosis —*see* Blepharoptosis
   lagophthalmos —*see* Lagophthalmos
   lid retraction —*see* Retraction, lid
  hypertrichosis —*see* Hypertrichosis,
    eyelid
  specified type NEC H02.89
  vascular H02.879
   left H02.876
    lower H02.875
    upper H02.874
   right H02.873
    lower H02.872
    upper H02.871
 factitious
  by proxy F68.A
  imposed on another F68.A
  imposed on self F68.10
   with predominantly
    psychological symptoms F68.11
     with physical symptoms F68.13
    physical symptoms F68.12
     with psychological symptoms F68.13
 factor, coagulation —*see* Defect,
    coagulation
 fatty acid
  metabolism E71.30
   specified NEC E71.39
  oxidation
   LCAD E71.310
   MCAD E71.311
   SCAD E71.312
   specified deficiency NEC E71.318
 feeding (infant or child) —*see also* Disorder,
  ▦ eating R63.30
  or eating disorder F50.9
  ▶ pediatric
   ▶ acute R63.31
   ▶ chronic R63.32
  specified NEC F50.9
 feigned (with obvious motivation)
    Z76.5
  without obvious motivation —
    see Disorder, factitious
 female
  hypoactive sexual desire F52.0
  orgasmic F52.31
  sexual interest/arousal F52.22
 fetishistic F65.0
 fibroblastic M72.9
  specified NEC M72.8

▶ New   ⇒ Revised   ~~deleted~~ Deleted   ● Use Additional Character(s)

Disorder *(Continued)*
  fluency
    adult onset F98.5
    childhood onset F80.81
    following
      cerebral infarction I69.323
      cerebrovascular disease I69.923
        specified disease NEC I69.823
      intracerebral hemorrhage I69.123
      nontraumatic intracranial hemorrhage
        NEC I69.223
      subarachnoid hemorrhage I69.023
    in conditions classified elsewhere
      R47.82
  fluid balance E87.8
  follicular (skin) L73.9
    specified NEC L73.8
  frotteuristic F65.81
  fructose metabolism E74.10
    essential fructosuria E74.11
    fructokinase deficiency E74.11
    fructose-1, 6-diphosphatase deficiency
      E74.19
    hereditary fructose intolerance E74.12
    other specified E74.19
  functional polymorphonuclear neutrophils
    D71
  gallbladder, biliary tract and pancreas in
    diseases classified elsewhere K87
  gambling F63.0
  gamma aminobutyric acid (GABA)
    metabolism E72.89
  gamma-glutamyl cycle E72.89
  gastric (functional) K31.9
    motility K30
    psychogenic F45.8
    secretion K30
  gastrointestinal (functional) NOS K92.9
    newborn P78.9
    psychogenic F45.8
  gender-identity or -role F64.9
    childhood F64.2
    effect on relationship F66
    of adolescence or adulthood F64.0
      nontranssexual F64.8
    specified NEC F64.8
    uncertainty F66
  genito-pelvic pain penetration F52.6
  genitourinary system
    female N94.9
    male N50.9
    psychogenic F45.8
  globe H44.9
    degenerated condition H44.50
      absolute glaucoma H44.51-●
      atrophy H44.52-●
      leucocoria H44.53-●
    degenerative H44.30
      chalcosis H44.31-●
      myopia —*see also* Myopia, degenerative
        H44.2-●
      siderosis H44.32-●
      specified type NEC H44.39-●
    endophthalmitis —*see* Endophthalmitis
    foreign body, retained —*see* Foreign body,
      intraocular, old, retained
    hemophthalmos —*see* Hemophthalmos
    hypotony H44.40
      due to
        ocular fistula H44.42-●
        specified disorder NEC H44.43-●
      flat anterior chamber H44.41-●
      primary H44.44-●
    luxation —*see* Luxation, globe
    specified type NEC H44.89
  glomerular (in) N05.9
    amyloidosis E85.4 *[N08]*
    cryoglobulinemia D89.1 *[N08]*
    disseminated intravascular coagulation
      D65 *[N08]*
    Fabry's disease E75.21 *[N08]*

Disorder *(Continued)*
  glomerular *(Continued)*
    familial lecithin cholesterol acyltransferase
      deficiency E78.6 *[N08]*
    Goodpasture's syndrome M31.0
    hemolytic-uremic syndrome D59.3
    Henoch (-Schönlein) purpura D69.0
      [N08]
    malariae malaria B52.0
    microscopic polyangiitis M31.7 *[N08]*
    multiple myeloma C90.0-● *[N08]*
    mumps B26.83
    schistosomiasis B65.9 *[N08]*
    sepsis NEC A41.-● *[N08]*
      streptococcal A40.-● *[N08]*
    sickle-cell disorders D57.-● *[N08]*
    strongyloidiasis B78.9 *[N08]*
    subacute bacterial endocarditis I33.0
      [N08]
    syphilis A52.75
    systemic lupus erythematosus M32.14
  ➡thrombotic thrombocytopenic purpura
      M31.19 *[N08]*
    Waldenström macroglobulinemia C88.0
      [N08]
    Wegener's granulomatosis M31.31
  gluconeogenesis E74.4
  glucosaminoglycan metabolism —
    see Disorder, metabolism,
    glucosaminoglycan
  glucose transport E74.819
    specified NEC E74.818
  glycine metabolism E72.50
    d-glycericacidemia E72.59
    hyperhydroxyprolinemia E72.59
    hyperoxaluria R82.992
      primary E72.53
    hyperprolinemia E72.59
    non ketotic hyperglycinemia E72.51
    oxalosis E72.53
    oxaluria E72.53
    sarcosinemia E72.59
    trimethylaminuria E72.52
  glycoprotein metabolism E77.9
    specified NEC E77.8
  habit (and impulse) F63.9
    involving sexual behavior NEC F65.9
    specified NEC F63.89
  hallucinogen use
    mild F16.10
      with
        hallucinogen-induced
          anxiety disorder F16.180
          bipolar and related disorder
            F16.14
          depressive disorder F16.14
          psychotic disorder F16.159
        hallucinogen intoxication delirium
          F16.121
        other hallucinogen intoxication
          F16.129
      in remission (early) (sustained) F16.11
    moderate or severe F16.20
      with
        hallucinogen-induced
          anxiety disorder F16.280
          bipolar and related disorder
            F16.24
          depressive disorder F16.24
          psychotic disorder F16.259
        hallucinogen intoxication delirium
          F16.221
        other hallucinogen intoxication
          F16.229
      in remission (early) (sustained)
        F16.21
  heart action I49.9
  hematological D75.9
    newborn (transient) P61.9
    specified NEC P61.8
  hematopoietic organs D75.9

Disorder *(Continued)*
  hemorrhagic NEC D69.9
    drug-induced D68.32
    due to
      extrinsic circulating anticoagulants
        D68.32
      increase in
        anti-IIa D68.32
        anti-Xa D68.32
      intrinsic
        circulating anticoagulants D68.318
        increase in
          antithrombin D68.318
          anti-VIIIa D68.318
          anti-IXa D68.318
          anti-XIa D68.318
    following childbirth O72.3
  hemostasis —*see* Defect, coagulation
  histidine metabolism E70.40
    histidinemia E70.41
    other specified E70.49
  hoarding F42.3
  hyperkinetic —*see* Disorder, attention-deficit
    hyperactivity
  hyperleucine-isoleucinemia E71.19
  hypervalinemia E71.19
  hypoactive sexual desire F52.0
  hypochondriacal F45.20
    body dysmorphic F45.22
    neurosis F45.21
    other specified F45.29
  identity
    dissociative F44.81
    illness anxiety F45.21
    of childhood F93.8
  immune mechanism (immunity) D89.9
    specified type NEC D89.89
  impaired renal tubular function N25.9
    specified NEC N25.89
  impulse (control) F63.9
  inflammatory
    pelvic, in diseases classified elsewhere —
      see category N74
    penis N48.29
      abscess N48.21
      cellulitis N48.22
  inhalant use
    mild F18.10
      with
        inhalant-induced
          anxiety disorder F18.180
          depressive disorder F18.14
          major neurocognitive disorder
            F18.17
          mild neurocognitive disorder
            F18.188
          psychotic disorder F18.159
        inhalant intoxication F18.129
        inhalant intoxication delirium F18.121
      in remission (early) (sustained) F18.11
    moderate or severe F18.20
      with
        inhalant-induced
          anxiety disorder F18.280
          depressive disorder F18.24
          major neurocognitive disorder
            F18.27
          mild neurocognitive disorder
            F18.288
          psychotic disorder F18.259
        inhalant intoxication F18.229
        inhalant intoxication delirium F18.221
      in remission (early) (sustained) F18.21
  integument, newborn P83.9
    specified NEC P83.88
  intermittent explosive F63.81
  internal secretion pancreas —*see* Increased,
    secretion, pancreas, endocrine
  intestine, intestinal
    carbohydrate absorption NEC E74.39
      postoperative K91.2

Disorder *(Continued)*
   intestine, intestinal *(Continued)*
      functional NEC K59.9
         postoperative K91.89
      psychogenic F45.8
      vascular K55.9
         chronic K55.1
         specified NEC K55.8
   intraoperative (intraprocedural) —*see*
      Complications, intraoperative
   involuntary emotional expression (IEED) F48.2
   iris H21.9
      adhesions —*see* Adhesions, iris
      atrophy —*see* Atrophy, iris
      chamber angle recession —*see* Recession,
         chamber angle
      cyst —*see* Cyst, iris
      degeneration —*see* Degeneration, iris
      in diseases classified elsewhere H22
      iridodialysis —*see* Iridodialysis
      iridoschisis —*see* Iridoschisis
      miotic pupillary cyst —*see* Cyst, pupillary
      pupillary
         abnormality —*see* Abnormality, pupillary
         membrane —*see* Membrane, pupillary
      specified type NEC H21.89
      vascular NEC H21.1X-●
   iron metabolism E83.10
      specified NEC E83.19
   isovaleric acidemia E71.110
   jaw, developmental M27.0
      temporomandibular —*see also* Anomaly,
         dentofacial, temporomandibular joint
         M26.60-●
   joint M25.9
      derangement —*see* Derangement, joint
      effusion —*see* Effusion, joint
      fistula —*see* Fistula, joint
      hemarthrosis —*see* Hemarthrosis
      instability —*see* Instability, joint
      osteophyte —*see* Osteophyte
      pain —*see* Pain, joint
      psychogenic F45.8
      specified type NEC M25.80
         ankle M25.87-●
         elbow M25.82-●
         foot joint M25.87-●
         hand joint M25.84-●
         hip M25.85-●
         knee M25.86-●
         shoulder M25.81-●
         wrist M25.83-●
      stiffness —*see* Stiffness, joint
   ketone metabolism E71.32
   kidney N28.9
      functional (tubular) N25.9
      in
         schistosomiasis B65.9 [N29]
      tubular function N25.9
         specified NEC N25.89
   lacrimal system H04.9
      changes H04.69
         fistula —*see* Fistula, lacrimal
      gland H04.19
         atrophy —*see* Atrophy, lacrimal gland
         cyst —*see* Cyst, lacrimal, gland
         dacryops —*see* Dacryops
         dislocation —*see* Dislocation, lacrimal
            gland
         dry eye syndrome —*see* Syndrome, dry
            eye
         infection —*see* Dacryoadenitis
         granuloma —*see* Granuloma, lacrimal
         inflammation —*see* Inflammation, lacrimal
         obstruction —*see* Obstruction, lacrimal
      specified NEC H04.89
   lactation NEC O92.79
   language (developmental) F80.9
      expressive F80.1
      mixed receptive and expressive F80.2
      receptive F80.2

Disorder *(Continued)*
   late luteal phase dysphoric N94.89
   learning (specific) F81.9
      acalculia R48.8
      alexia R48.0
      mathematics F81.2
      reading F81.0
      specified
         with impairment in
            mathematics F81.2
            reading F81.0
            written expression F81.81
      specified NEC F81.89
      spelling F81.81
      written expression F81.81
   lens H27.9
      aphakia —*see* Aphakia
      cataract —*see* Cataract
      dislocation —*see* Dislocation, lens
      specified type NEC H27.8
   ligament M24.20
      ankle M24.27-●
      attachment, spine —*see* Enthesopathy,
         spinal
      elbow M24.22-●
      foot joint M24.27-●
      hand joint M24.24-●
      hip M24.25-●
      knee —*see* Derangement, knee, specified
         NEC
      shoulder M24.21-●
      specified site NEC M24.29
      vertebra M24.28
      wrist M24.23-●
   ligamentous attachments —*see also*
      Enthesopathy
      spine —*see* Enthesopathy, spinal
   lipid
      metabolism, congenital E78.9
      storage E75.6
         specified NEC E75.5
   lipoprotein
      deficiency (familial) E78.6
      metabolism E78.9
         specified NEC E78.89
   liver K76.9
      malarial B54 [K77]
   low back —*see also* Dorsopathy, specified NEC
   lumbosacral
      plexus G54.1
      root (nerve) NEC G54.4
   lung, interstitial, drug-induced J70.4
      acute J70.2
      chronic J70.3
      dabbing (related) U07.0
      e-cigarette (related) U07.0
      electronic cigarette (related) U07.0
      vaping (associated) (device) (product)
         (related) (use) U07.0
   lymphoproliferative, post-transplant (PTLD)
      D47.Z1
   lysine and hydroxylysine metabolism E72.3
   major neurocognitive —*see* Dementia, in
      (due to)
   male
      erectile (organic) —*see also* Dysfunction,
         sexual, male, erectile N52.9
         nonorganic F52.21
      hypoactive sexual desire F52.0
      orgasmic F52.32
   manic F30.9
      organic F06.33
   mast cell activation —*see* Activation, mast cell
   mastoid —*see also* Disorder, ear, middle
      postprocedural —*see* Complications, ear,
         procedure
   meninges, specified type NEC G96.198
   meniscus —*see* Derangement, knee,
      meniscus
   menopausal N95.9
      specified NEC N95.8

Disorder *(Continued)*
   menstrual N92.6
      psychogenic F45.8
      specified NEC N92.5
   mental (or behavioral) (nonpsychotic) F99
      due to (secondary to)
         amphetamine
            due to drug abuse —*see* Abuse, drug,
               stimulant
            due to drug dependence —*see*
               Dependence, drug, stimulant
         brain disease, damage and dysfunction
            F09
         caffeine use
            due to drug abuse —*see* Abuse, drug,
               stimulant
            due to drug dependence —*see*
               Dependence, drug, stimulant
         cannabis use
            due to drug abuse —*see* Abuse, drug,
               cannabis
            due to drug dependence —*see*
               Dependence, drug, cannabis
         general medical condition F09
         sedative or hypnotic use
            due to drug abuse —*see* Abuse, drug,
               sedative
            due to drug dependence —*see*
               Dependence, drug, sedative
         tobacco (nicotine) use —*see* Dependence,
            drug, nicotine
      following organic brain damage F07.9
         frontal lobe syndrome F07.0
         personality change F07.0
         postconcussional syndrome F07.81
         specified NEC F07.89
      infancy, childhood or adolescence F98.9
      neurotic —*see* Neurosis
      organic or symptomatic F09
      presenile, psychotic F03
      problem NEC
      psychoneurotic —*see* Neurosis
      psychotic —*see* Psychosis
      puerperal F53.0
      senile, psychotic NEC F03
   metabolic, amino acid, transitory, newborn
      P74.8
   metabolism NOS E88.9
      amino-acid E72.9
         aromatic E70.9
            albinism —*see* Albinism
            histidine E70.40
               histidinemia E70.41
               other specified E70.49
            hyperphenylalaninemia E70.1
               classical phenylketonuria E70.0
            other specified E70.89
            tryptophan E70.5
            tyrosine E70.20
             hypertyrosinemia E70.21
             other specified E70.29
         branched chain E71.2
            3-methylglutaconic aciduria E71.111
            hyperleucine-isoleucinemia E71.19
            hypervalinemia E71.19
            isovaleric acidemia E71.110
            maple syrup urine disease E71.0
            methylmalonic acidemia E71.120
            organic aciduria NEC E71.118
            other specified E71.19
            proprionate NEC E71.128
            proprionic acidemia E71.121
         glycine E72.50
            d-glycericacidemia E72.59
            hyperhydroxyprolinemia E72.59
            hyperoxaluria R82.992
             primary E72.53
            hyperprolinemia E72.59
            non-ketotic hyperglycinemia
             E72.51
            other specified E72.59

▶ New   ⇒ Revised   ~~deleted~~ Deleted   ● Use Additional Character(s)

Disorder *(Continued)*
  metabolism *(Continued)*
    amino-acid *(Continued)*
      glycine *(Continued)*
        sarcosinemia E72.59
        trimethylaminuria E72.52
      hydroxylysine E72.3
      lysine E72.3
      ornithine E72.4
      other specified E72.89
        beta-amino acid E72.89
        gamma-glutamyl cycle E72.89
      straight-chain E72.89
      sulfur-bearing E72.10
        homocystinuria E72.11
        methylenetetrahydrofolate reductase deficiency E72.12
      other specified E72.19
    bile acid and cholesterol metabolism E78.70
    bilirubin E80.7
      specified NEC E80.6
    calcium E83.50
      hypercalcemia E83.52
      hypocalcemia E83.51
      other specified E83.59
    carbohydrate E74.9
      specified NEC E74.89
    cholesterol and bile acid metabolism E78.70
    congenital E88.9
    copper E83.00
      specified type NEC E83.09
      Wilson's disease E83.01
    cystinuria E72.01
    fructose E74.10
    galactose E74.20
    glucosaminoglycan E76.9
      mucopolysaccharidosis —*see* Mucopolysaccharidosis
      specified NEC E76.8
    glutamine E72.89
    glycine E72.50
    glycogen storage (hepatorenal) E74.09
    glycoprotein E77.9
      specified NEC E77.8
    glycosaminoglycan E76.9
      specified NEC E76.8
    in labor and delivery O75.89
    iron E83.10
    isoleucine E71.19
    leucine E71.19
    lipoid E78.9
    lipoprotein E78.9
      specified NEC E78.89
    magnesium E83.40
      hypermagnesemia E83.41
      hypomagnesemia E83.42
      other specified E83.49
    mineral E83.9
      specified NEC E83.89
    mitochondrial E88.40
      MELAS syndrome E88.41
      MERRF syndrome (myoclonic epilepsy associated with ragged-red fibers) E88.42
      other specified E88.49
    ornithine E72.4
    phosphatases E83.30
    phosphorus E83.30
      acid phosphatase deficiency E83.39
      hypophosphatasia E83.39
      hypophosphatemia E83.39
        familial E83.31
      other specified E83.39
      pseudovitamin D deficiency E83.32
    plasma protein NEC E88.09
    porphyrin —*see* Porphyria
    postprocedural E89.89
      specified NEC E89.89
    purine E79.9
      specified NEC E79.8

Disorder *(Continued)*
  metabolism *(Continued)*
    pyrimidine E79.9
      specified NEC E79.8
    pyruvate E74.4
    serine E72.89
    sodium E87.8
    specified NEC E88.89
    threonine E72.89
    valine E71.19
    zinc E83.2
    methylmalonic acidemia E71.120
    micturition NEC —*see also* Difficulty, micturition R39.198
      feeling of incomplete emptying R39.14
      hesitancy R39.11
      poor stream R39.12
      psychogenic F45.8
      split stream R39.13
      straining R39.16
      urgency R39.15
    mild neurocognitive G31.84
    mitochondrial metabolism E88.40
    mitral (valve) —*see* Endocarditis, mitral
    mixed
      anxiety and depressive F41.8
      of scholastic skills (developmental) F81.89
      receptive expressive language F80.2
    mood F39
      bipolar —*see* Disorder, bipolar
      depressive —*see* Disorder, depressive
      due to (secondary to)
        alcohol F10.94
        amphetamine F15.94
          in
            abuse F15.14
            dependence F15.24
        anxiolytic F13.94
          in
            abuse F13.14
            dependence F13.24
        cocaine F14.94
          in
            abuse F14.14
            dependence F14.24
        general medical condition F06.30
        hallucinogen F16.94
          in
            abuse F16.14
            dependence F16.24
        hypnotic F13.94
          in
            abuse F13.14
            dependence F13.24
        inhalant F18.94
          in
            abuse F18.14
            dependence F18.24
        opioid F11.94
          in
            abuse F11.14
            dependence F11.24
        phencyclidine (PCP) F16.94
          in
            abuse F16.14
            dependence F16.24
        physiological condition F06.30
          with
            depressive features F06.31
            major depressive-like episode F06.32
            manic features F06.33
            mixed features F06.34
        psychoactive substance NEC F19.94
          in
            abuse F19.14
            dependence F19.24
        sedative F13.94
          in
            abuse F13.14
            dependence F13.24

Disorder *(Continued)*
  mood *(Continued)*
    due to *(Continued)*
      volatile solvents F18.94
        in
          abuse F18.14
          dependence F18.24
    manic episode F30.9
      with psychotic symptoms F30.2
      without psychotic symptoms F30.10
        mild F30.11
        moderate F30.12
        severe F30.13
      in remission (full) F30.4
        partial F30.3
      specified type NEC F30.8
    organic F06.30
      right hemisphere F07.89
    persistent F34.9
      cyclothymia F34.0
      dysthymia F34.1
      specified type NEC F34.89
    recurrent F39
    right hemisphere organic F07.89
  movement G25.9
    drug-induced G25.70
      akathisia G25.71
      specified NEC G25.79
    hysterical F44.4
    in diseases classified elsewhere —*see* category G26
    periodic limb G47.61
      sleep related G47.61
    sleep related NEC G47.69
    specified NEC G25.89
    stereotyped F98.4
    treatment-induced G25.9
  multiple personality F44.81
  muscle M62.9
    attachment, spine —*see* Enthesopathy, spinal
    in trichinellosis —*see* Trichinellosis, with muscle disorder
    psychogenic F45.8
    specified type NEC M62.89
    tone, newborn P94.9
      specified NEC P94.8
  muscular
    attachments —*see also* Enthesopathy
      spine —*see* Enthesopathy, spinal
    urethra N36.44
  musculoskeletal system, soft tissue —*see* Disorder, soft tissue
    postprocedural M96.89
    psychogenic F45.8
  myoneural G70.9
    due to lead G70.1
    specified NEC G70.89
    toxic G70.1
  myotonic NEC G71.19
  nail, in diseases classified elsewhere L62
  neck region NEC —*see* Dorsopathy, specified NEC
  neonatal onset multisystemic inflammatory (NOMID) M04.2
  nerve G58.9
    abducent NEC —*see* Strabismus, paralytic, sixth nerve
    accessory G52.8
    acoustic —*see* subcategory H93.3
    auditory —*see* subcategory H93.3
    auriculotemporal G50.8
    axillary G54.0
    cerebral —*see* Disorder, nerve, cranial
    cranial G52.9
      eighth —*see* subcategory H93.3
      eleventh G52.8
      fifth G50.9
      first G52.0
      fourth NEC —*see* Strabismus, paralytic, fourth nerve

Disorder *(Continued)*
  nerve *(Continued)*
    cranial *(Continued)*
      multiple G52.7
      ninth G52.1
      second NEC —*see* Disorder, nerve,
        optic
      seventh NEC G51.8
      sixth NEC —*see* Strabismus, paralytic,
        sixth nerve
      specified NEC G52.8
      tenth G52.2
      third NEC —*see* Strabismus, paralytic,
        third nerve
      twelfth G52.3
    entrapment —*see* Neuropathy,
      entrapment
    facial G51.9
      specified NEC G51.8
    femoral —*see* Lesion, nerve, femoral
    glossopharyngeal NEC G52.1
    hypoglossal G52.3
    intercostal G58.0
    lateral
      cutaneous of thigh —*see*
        Mononeuropathy, lower limb,
        meralgia paresthetica
      popliteal —*see* Lesion, nerve, popliteal
    lower limb —*see* Mononeuropathy, lower
      limb
    medial popliteal —*see* Lesion, nerve,
      popliteal, medial
    median NEC —*see* Lesion, nerve,
      median
    multiple G58.7
    oculomotor NEC —*see* Strabismus,
      paralytic, third nerve
    olfactory G52.0
    optic NEC H47.09-●
      hemorrhage into sheath —*see*
        Hemorrhage, optic nerve
      ischemic H47.01-●
    peroneal —*see* Lesion, nerve, popliteal
    phrenic G58.8
    plantar —*see* Lesion, nerve, plantar
    pneumogastric G52.2
    posterior tibial —*see* Syndrome, tarsal
      tunnel
    radial —*see* Lesion, nerve, radial
    recurrent laryngeal G52.2
    root G54.9
      cervical G54.2
      lumbosacral G54.1
      specified NEC G54.8
      thoracic G54.3
    sciatic NEC —*see* Lesion, nerve, sciatic
    specified NEC G58.8
      lower limb —*see* Mononeuropathy,
        lower limb, specified NEC
      upper limb —*see* Mononeuropathy,
        upper limb, specified NEC
    sympathetic G90.9
    tibial —*see* Lesion, nerve, popliteal,
      medial
    trigeminal G50.9
      specified NEC G50.8
    trochlear NEC —*see* Strabismus, paralytic,
      fourth nerve
    ulnar —*see* Lesion, nerve, ulnar
    upper limb —*see* Mononeuropathy, upper
      limb
    vagus G52.2
  nervous system G98.8
    autonomic (peripheral) G90.9
      specified NEC G90.8
    central G96.9
      specified NEC G96.89
    parasympathetic G90.9
    specified NEC G98.8
    sympathetic G90.9
    vegetative G90.9

  neurocognitive R41.9
    major
      with
        aggressive behavior F01.51
        combative behavior F01.51
        violent behavior F01.51
      due to vascular disease, with behavioral
        disturbance F01.51
      in (due to) (other diseases classified
        elsewhere) —*see also* Dementia, in
        (due to) F02.80
        with
          aggressive behavior F02.81
          combative behavior F02.81
          violent behavior F02.81
        without behavioral disturbance F01.50
    mild G31.84
  neurodevelopmental F89
    specified NEC F88
  neurohypophysis NEC E23.3
  neurological NEC R29.818
  neuromuscular G70.9
    hereditary NEC G71.9
    specified NEC G70.89
    toxic G70.1
  neurotic F48.9
    specified NEC F48.8
  neutrophil, polymorphonuclear D71
  nicotine use —*see* Dependence, drug, nicotine
  nightmare F51.5
  non-rapid eye movement sleep arousal
    sleep terror type F51.4
    sleepwalking type F51.3
  nose J34.9
    specified NEC J34.89
  obsessive-compulsive F42.9
    and related disorder due to a known
      physiological condition F06.8
  odontogenesis NOS K00.9
  opioid use
    with
      opioid-induced psychotic disorder
        F11.959
        with
          delusions F11.950
          hallucinations F11.951
    due to drug abuse —*see* Abuse, drug,
      opioid
    due to drug dependence —*see* Dependence,
      drug, opioid
    mild F11.10
      with
        opioid-induced
          anxiety disorder F11.188
          depressive disorder F11.14
          sexual dysfunction F11.181
        opioid intoxication
          with perceptual disturbances
            F11.122
          delirium F11.121
          without perceptual disturbances
            F11.129
      in remission (early) (sustained) F11.11
    moderate or severe F11.20
      with
        opioid-induced
          anxiety disorder F11.288
          anxiety disorder F11.988
          depressive disorder F11.24
          depressive disorder F11.94
          sexual dysfunction F11.281
          sexual dysfunction F11.981
        opioid intoxication
          with perceptual disturbances
            F11.222
          delirium F11.221
          without perceptual disturbances
            F11.229
      in remission (early) (sustained) F11.21
  oppositional defiant F91.3

  optic
    chiasm H47.49
      due to
        inflammatory disorder H47.41
        neoplasm H47.42
        vascular disorder H47.43
    disc H47.39-●
      coloboma —*see* Coloboma, optic disc
      drusen —*see* Drusen, optic disc
      pseudopapilledema —*see*
        Pseudopapilledema
      radiations —*see* Disorder, visual, pathway
      tracts —*see* Disorder, visual, pathway
  orbit H05.9
    cyst —*see* Cyst, orbit
    deformity —*see* Deformity, orbit
    edema —*see* Edema, orbit
    enophthalmos —*see* Enophthalmos
    exophthalmos —*see* Exophthalmos
    hemorrhage —*see* Hemorrhage, orbit
    inflammation —*see* Inflammation, orbit
    myopathy —*see* Myopathy, extraocular
      muscles
    retained foreign body —*see* Foreign body,
      orbit, old
    specified type NEC H05.89
  organic
    anxiety F06.4
    catatonic F06.1
    delusional F06.2
    dissociative F06.8
    emotionally labile (asthenic) F06.8
    mood (affective) F06.30
    schizophrenia-like F06.2
  orgasmic (female) F52.31
    male F52.32
  ornithine metabolism E72.4
  overanxious F41.1
    of childhood F93.8
  pain
    with related psychological factors F45.42
    exclusively related to psychological factors
      F45.41
    genito-pelvic penetration disorder F52.6
  pancreatic internal secretion E16.9
    specified NEC E16.8
  panic F41.0
    with agoraphobia F40.01
  papulosquamous L44.9
    in diseases classified elsewhere L45
    specified NEC L44.8
  paranoid F22
    induced F24
    shared F24
  paraphilic F65.9
    specified NEC F65.89
  parathyroid (gland) E21.5
    specified NEC E21.4
  parietoalveolar NEC J84.09
  paroxysmal, mixed R56.9
  patella M22.9-●
    chondromalacia —*see* Chondromalacia,
      patella
    derangement NEC M22.3X-●
    recurrent
      dislocation —*see* Dislocation, patella,
        recurrent
      subluxation —*see* Dislocation, patella,
        recurrent, incomplete
    specified NEC M22.8X-●
  patellofemoral M22.2X-●
  pedophilic F65.4
  pentose phosphate pathway with anemia
    D55.1
  perception, due to hallucinogens
    F16.983
    in
      abuse F16.183
      dependence F16.283
  peripheral nervous system NEC G64

▶ New   ⇒ Revised   ~~deleted~~ Deleted   ● Use Additional Character(s)

Disorder *(Continued)*
  peroxisomal E71.50
    biogenesis
      neonatal adrenoleukodystrophy
        E71.511
      specified disorder NEC E71.518
      Zellweger syndrome E71.510
    rhizomelic chondrodysplasia punctata
      E71.540
    specified form NEC E71.548
      group 1 E71.518
      group 2 E71.53
      group 3 E71.542
    X-linked adrenoleukodystrophy E71.529
      adolescent E71.521
      adrenomyeloneuropathy E71.522
      childhood E71.520
      specified form NEC E71.528
    Zellweger-like syndrome E71.541
  persistent
    (somatoform) pain F45.41
    affective (mood) F34.9
  personality —*see also* Personality F60.9
    affective F34.0
    aggressive F60.3
    amoral F60.2
    anankastic F60.5
    antisocial F60.2
    anxious F60.6
    asocial F60.2
    asthenic F60.7
    avoidant F60.6
    borderline F60.3
    change (secondary) due to general medical
      condition F07.0
    compulsive F60.5
    cyclothymic F34.0
    dependent (passive) F60.7
    depressive F34.1
    dissocial F60.2
    emotional instability F60.3
    expansive paranoid F60.0
    explosive F60.3
    following organic brain damage F07.9
    histrionic F60.4
    hyperthymic F34.0
    hypothymic F34.1
    hysterical F60.4
    immature F60.89
    inadequate F60.7
    labile F60.3
    mixed (nonspecific) F60.89
    moral deficiency F60.2
    narcissistic F60.81
    negativistic F60.89
    obsessional F60.5
    obsessive (-compulsive) F60.5
    organic F07.9
    overconscientious F60.5
    paranoid F60.0
    passive (-dependent) F60.7
    passive-aggressive F60.89
    pathological NEC F60.9
    pseudosocial F60.2
    psychopathic F60.2
    schizoid F60.1
    schizotypal F21
    self-defeating F60.7
    specified NEC F60.89
    type A F60.5
    unstable (emotional) F60.3
  pervasive, developmental F84.9
  phencyclidine use
    mild F16.10
      with
        phencyclidine-induced
          anxiety disorder F16.180
          bipolar and related disorder
            F16.14
          depressive disorder F16.14
          psychotic disorder F16.159

Disorder *(Continued)*
  phencyclidine use *(Continued)*
    mild *(Continued)*
      with *(Continued)*
        phencyclidine intoxication F16.129
        phencyclidine intoxication delirium
          F16.121
      in remission (early) (sustained) F16.11
    moderate or severe F16.20
      with
        phencyclidine-induced
          anxiety disorder F16.280
          bipolar and related disorder F16.24
          depressive disorder F16.24
          psychotic disorder F16.259
        phencyclidine intoxication F16.229
        phencyclidine intoxication delirium
          F16.221
      in remission (early) (sustained) F16.21
  phobic anxiety, childhood F40.8
  phosphate-losing tubular N25.0
  pigmentation L81.9
    choroid, congenital Q14.3
    diminished melanin formation L81.6
    iron L81.8
    specified NEC L81.8
  pinna (noninfective) H61.10-●
    deformity, acquired H61.11-●
    hematoma H61.12-●
    perichondritis —*see* Perichondritis, ear
    specified type NEC H61.19-●
  pituitary gland E23.7
    iatrogenic (postprocedural) E89.3
    specified NEC E23.6
  platelets D69.1
  plexus G54.9
    specified NEC G54.8
  polymorphonuclear neutrophils D71
  porphyrin metabolism —*see* Porphyria
  postconcussional F07.81
  posthallucinogen perception F16.983
    in
      abuse F16.183
      dependence F16.283
  postmenopausal N95.9
    specified NEC N95.8
  postprocedural (postoperative) —*see*
    Complications, postprocedural
  post-transplant lymphoproliferative D47.z1
  post-traumatic stress (PTSD) F43.10
    acute F43.11
    chronic F43.12
  premenstrual dysphoric (PMDD) F32.81
  prepuce N47.8
  propionic acidemia E71.121
  prostate N42.9
    specified NEC N42.89
  psychogenic NOS —*see also* condition F45.9
    anxiety F41.8
    appetite F50.9
    asthenic F48.8
    cardiovascular (system) F45.8
    compulsive F42.8
    cutaneous F54
    depressive F32.9
    digestive (system) F45.8
    dysmenorrheic F45.8
    dyspneic F45.8
    endocrine (system) F54
    eye NEC F45.8
    feeding —*see* Disorder, eating
    functional NEC F45.8
    gastric F45.8
    gastrointestinal (system) F45.8
    genitourinary (system) F45.8
    heart (function) (rhythm) F45.8
    hyperventilatory F45.8
    hypochondriacal —*see* Disorder,
      hypochondriacal
    intestinal F45.8
    joint F45.8

Disorder *(Continued)*
  psychogenic NOS *(Continued)*
    learning F81.9
    limb F45.8
    lymphatic (system) F45.8
    menstrual F45.8
    micturition F45.8
    monoplegic NEC F44.4
    motor F44.4
    muscle F45.8
    musculoskeletal F45.8
    neurocirculatory F45.8
    obsessive F42.8
    occupational F48.8
    organ or part of body NEC F45.8
    paralytic NEC F44.4
    phobic F40.9
    physical NEC F45.8
    rectal F45.8
    respiratory (system) F45.8
    rheumatic F45.8
    sexual (function) F52.9
    skin (allergic) (eczematous) F54
    sleep F51.9
    specified part of body NEC F45.8
    stomach F45.8
  psychological F99
    associated with
      disease classified elsewhere F54
      sexual
        development F66
        relationship F66
      uncertainty about gender identity F64.9
  psychomotor NEC F44.4
    hysterical F44.4
  psychoneurotic —*see also* Neurosis
    mixed NEC F48.8
  psychophysiologic —*see* Disorder,
    somatoform
  psychosexual F65.9
    development F66
    identity of childhood F64.2
  psychosomatic NOS —*see* Disorder,
    somatoform
    multiple F45.0
    undifferentiated F45.1
  psychotic —*see* Psychosis
    transient (acute) F23
  puberty E30.9
    specified NEC E30.8
  pulmonary (valve) —*see* Endocarditis,
    pulmonary
  purine metabolism E79.9
  pyrimidine metabolism E79.9
  pyruvate metabolism E74.4
  reactive attachment (childhood) F94.1
  reading R48.0
    developmental (specific) F81.0
  receptive language F80.2
  receptor, hormonal, peripheral —*see also*
    Syndrome, androgen insensitivity E34.50
  recurrent brief depressive F33.8
  reflex R29.2
  refraction H52.7
    aniseikonia H52.32
    anisometropia H52.31
    astigmatism —*see* Astigmatism
    hypermetropia —*see* Hypermetropia
    myopia —*see* Myopia
    presbyopia H52.4
    specified NEC H52.6
  relationship F68.8
    due to sexual orientation F66
  REM sleep behavior G47.52
  renal function, impaired (tubular) N25.9
  resonance R49.9
    specified NEC R49.8
  respiratory function, impaired —*see also*
    Failure, respiration
    postprocedural —*see* Complication,
      postoperative, respiratory system
    psychogenic F45.8

Disorder (Continued)

retina H35.9

  angioid streaks H35.33

  changes in vascular appearance H35.01-●

  degeneration —see Degeneration, retina

  dystrophy (hereditary) —see Dystrophy, retina

  edema H35.81

  hemorrhage —see Hemorrhage, retina

  ischemia H35.82

  macular degeneration —see Degeneration, macula

  microaneurysms H35.04-●

  microvascular abnormality NEC H35.09

  neovascularization —see Neovascularization, retina

  retinopathy —see Retinopathy

  separation of layers H35.70

    central serous chorioretinopathy H35.71-●

    pigment epithelium detachment (serous) H35.72-●

      hemorrhagic H35.73-●

    specified type NEC H35.89

  telangiectasis —see Telangiectasis, retina

  vasculitis —see Vasculitis, retina

retroperitoneal K68.9

right hemisphere organic affective F07.89

rumination (infant or child) F98.21

sacrum, sacrococcygeal NEC M53.3

schizoaffective F25.9

  bipolar type F25.0

  depressive type F25.1

  manic type F25.0

  mixed type F25.0

  specified NEC F25.8

schizoid of childhood F84.5

schizophrenia spectrum and other psychotic disorder F29

  specified NEC F28

schizophreniform F20.81

  brief F23

schizotypal (personality) F21

secretion, thyrocalcitonin E07.0

sedative, hypnotic, or anxiolytic use

  mild F13.10

    with

      sedative, hypnotic, or anxiolytic-induced

        anxiety disorder F13.180

        bipolar and related disorder F13.14

        depressive disorder F13.14

        psychotic disorder F13.159

        sexual dysfunction F13.181

      sedative, hypnotic, or anxiolytic intoxication F13.129

      sedative, hypnotic, or anxiolytic intoxication delirium F13.121

    in remission (early) (sustained) F13.11

  moderate or severe F13.20

    with

      sedative, hypnotic, or anxiolytic-induced

        anxiety disorder F13.280

        bipolar and related disorder F13.24

        depressive disorder F13.24

        major neurocognitive disorder F13.27

        mild neurocognitive disorder F13.288

        psychotic disorder F13.259

        sexual dysfunction F13.281

      sedative, hypnotic, or anxiolytic intoxication F13.229

      sedative, hypnotic, or anxiolytic intoxication delirium F13.221

    in remission (early) (sustained) F13.21

seizure —see also Epilepsy G40.909

  intractable G40.919

    with status epilepticus G40.911

semantic pragmatic F80.89

  with autism F84.0

sense of smell R43.1

  psychogenic F45.8

separation anxiety, of childhood F93.0

sexual

  arousal, female F52.22

  aversion F52.1

  function, psychogenic F52.9

  interest/arousal, female F52.22

  masochism F65.51

  maturation F66

  nonorganic F52.9

  preference —see also Deviation, sexual F65.9

    fetishistic transvestism F65.1

  relationship F66

  sadism F65.52

shyness, of childhood and adolescence F40.10

sibling rivalry F93.8

sickle-cell (sickling) (homozygous) —see Disease, sickle-cell

  heterozygous D57.3

  specified type NEC D57.8-●

  trait D57.3

sinus (nasal) J34.9

  specified NEC J34.89

skin L98.9

  atrophic L90.9

    specified NEC L90.8

  granulomatous L92.9

    specified NEC L92.8

  hypertrophic L91.9

    specified NEC L91.8

  infiltrative NEC L98.6

  newborn P83.9

    specified NEC P83.88

  picking F42.4

  psychogenic (allergic) (eczematous) F54

sleep G47.9

  breathing-related —see Apnea, sleep

  circadian rhythm G47.20

    advance sleep phase type G47.22

    delayed sleep phase type G47.21

    due to

      alcohol

        abuse F10.182

        dependence F10.282

        use F10.982

      amphetamines

        abuse F15.182

        dependence F15.282

        use F15.982

      caffeine

        abuse F15.182

        dependence F15.282

        use F15.982

      cocaine

        abuse F14.182

        dependence F14.282

        use F14.982

      drug NEC

        abuse F19.182

        dependence F19.282

        use F19.982

      opioid

        abuse F11.182

        dependence F11.282

        use F11.982

      psychoactive substance NEC

        abuse F19.182

        dependence F19.282

        use F19.982

      sedative, hypnotic, or anxiolytic

        abuse F13.182

        dependence F13.282

        use F13.982

      stimulant NEC

        abuse F15.182

        dependence F15.282

        use F15.982

    free running type G47.24

sleep (Continued)

  circadian rhythm (Continued)

    in conditions classified elsewhere G47.27

    irregular sleep wake type G47.23

    jet lag type G47.25

    non-24-hour sleep-wake type G47.24

    shift work type G47.26

    specified NEC G47.29

  due to

    alcohol

      abuse F10.182

      dependence F10.282

      use F10.982

    amphetamine

      abuse F15.182

      dependence F15.282

      use F15.982

    anxiolytic

      abuse F13.182

      dependence F13.282

      use F13.982

    caffeine

      abuse F15.182

      dependence F15.282

      use F15.982

    cocaine

      abuse F14.182

      dependence F14.282

      use F14.982

    drug NEC

      abuse F19.182

      dependence F19.282

      use F19.982

    hypnotic

      abuse F13.182

      dependence F13.282

      use F13.982

    opioid

      abuse F11.182

      dependence F11.282

      use F11.982

    psychoactive substance NEC

      abuse F19.182

      dependence F19.282

      use F19.982

    sedative

      abuse F13.182

      dependence F13.282

      use F13.982

    stimulant NEC

      abuse F15.182

      dependence F15.282

      use F15.982

  emotional F51.9

  excessive somnolence —see Hypersomnia

  hypersomnia type —see Hypersomnia

  initiating or maintaining —see Insomnia

  nightmares F51.5

  nonorganic F51.9

    specified NEC F51.8

  parasomnia type G47.50

  specified NEC G47.8

  terrors F51.4

  walking F51.3

sleep-wake pattern or schedule —see also Disorder, sleep, circadian rhythm G47.9

  specified NEC G47.8

social

  anxiety (of childhood) F40.10

    generalized F40.11

  functioning in childhood F94.9

    specified NEC F94.8

  pragmatic F80.82

soft tissue M79.9

  ankle M79.9

  due to use, overuse and pressure M70.90

    ankle M70.97-●

    bursitis —see Bursitis

    foot M70.97-●

▶ New   ⇒ Revised   ~~deleted~~ Deleted   ● Use Additional Character(s)

Disorder *(Continued)*
  soft tissue *(Continued)*
    due to use, overuse and pressure *(Continued)*
      forearm M70.93-●
      hand M70.94-●
      lower leg M70.96-●
      multiple sites M70.99
      pelvic region M70.95-●
      shoulder region M70.91-●
      specified site NEC M70.98
      specified type NEC M70.80
        ankle M70.87-●
        foot M70.87-●
        forearm M70.83-●
        hand M70.84-●
        lower leg M70.86-●
        multiple sites M70.89
        pelvic region M70.85-●
        shoulder region M70.81-●
        specified site NEC M70.88
        thigh M70.85-●
        upper arm M70.82-●
      thigh M70.95-●
      upper arm M70.92-●
    foot M79.9
    forearm M79.9
    hand M79.9
    lower leg M79.9
    multiple sites M79.9
    occupational —*see* Disorder, soft tissue, due to use, overuse and pressure
    pelvic region M79.9
    shoulder region M79.9
    specified type NEC M79.89
    thigh M79.9
    upper arm M79.9
  somatic symptom F45.1
  somatization F45.0
  somatoform F45.9
    pain (persistent) F45.41
    somatization (multiple) (long-lasting) F45.0
    specified NEC F45.8
    undifferentiated F45.1
  somnolence, excessive —*see* Hypersomnia
  specific
    arithmetical F81.2
    developmental, of motor F82
    reading F81.0
    speech and language F80.9
    spelling F81.81
    written expression F81.81
  speech R47.9
    articulation (functional) (specific) F80.0
    developmental F80.9
    specified NEC R47.89
  speech-sound F80.0
  spelling (specific) F81.81
  spine —*see also* Dorsopathy
    ligamentous or muscular attachments, peripheral —*see* Enthesopathy, spinal
    specified NEC —*see* Dorsopathy, specified NEC
  stereotyped, habit or movement F98.4
  stimulant use (other) (unspecified)
    mild F15.10
      in remission (early) (sustained) F15.11
    moderate or severe F15.20
      in remission (early) (sustained) F15.21
  stomach (functional) —*see* Disorder, gastric
  stress F43.9
    acute F43.0
    post-traumatic F43.10
      acute F43.11
      chronic F43.12
  substance use (other) (unknown)
    mild F19.10
      with substance-induced
        anxiety disorder F19.180
        bipolar and related disorder F19.14

Disorder *(Continued)*
  substance use (other) (unknown) *(Continued)*
    mild *(Continued)*
      with substance-induced *(Continued)*
        depressive disorder F19.14
        major neurocognitive disorder F19.17
        mild neurocognitive disorder F19.188
        obsessive-compulsive and related disorder F19.188
        sexual dysfunction F19.181
      substance intoxication F19.129
      substance intoxication delirium F19.121
    moderate or severe F19.20
      with substance-induced
        anxiety disorder F19.280
        bipolar and related disorder F19.24
        depressive disorder F19.24
        major neurocognitive disorder F19.27
        mild neurocognitive disorder F19.288
        obsessive-compulsive and related disorder F19.288
        sexual dysfunction F19.281
      in remission (early) (sustained) F19.21
      substance intoxication F19.229
      substance intoxication delirium F19.221
  sulfur-bearing amino-acid metabolism E72.10
  sweat gland (eccrine) L74.9
    apocrine L75.9
      specified NEC L75.8
    specified NEC L74.8
  synovium M67.90
    acromioclavicular M67.91-●
    ankle M67.97-●
    elbow M67.92-●
    foot M67.97-●
    forearm M67.93-●
    hand M67.94-●
    hip M67.95-●
    knee M67.96-●
    multiple sites M67.99
    rupture —*see* Rupture, synovium
    shoulder M67.91-●
    specified type NEC M67.80
      acromioclavicular M67.81-●
      ankle M67.87-●
      elbow M67.82-●
      foot M67.87-●
      hand M67.84-●
      hip M67.85-●
      knee M67.86-●
      multiple sites M67.89
      wrist M67.83-●
    synovitis —*see* Synovitis
    upper arm M67.92-●
    wrist M67.93-●
  temperature regulation, newborn P81.9
    specified NEC P81.8
  temporomandibular joint M26.60-●
  tendon M67.90
    acromioclavicular M67.91-●
    ankle M67.97-●
    contracture —*see* Contracture, tendon
    elbow M67.92-●
    foot M67.97-●
    forearm M67.93-●
    hand M67.94-●
    hip M67.95-●
    knee M67.96-●
    multiple sites M67.99
    rupture —*see* Rupture, tendon
    shoulder M67.91-●
    specified type NEC M67.80
      acromioclavicular M67.81-●
      ankle M67.87-●
      elbow M67.82-●
      foot M67.87-●
      hand M67.84-●
      hip M67.85-●
      knee M67.86-●
      multiple sites M67.89

Disorder *(Continued)*
  tendon *(Continued)*
    specified type NEC *(Continued)*
      trunk M67.88
      wrist M67.83-●
    synovitis —*see* Synovitis
    tendinitis —*see* Tendinitis
    tenosynovitis —*see* Tenosynovitis
    trunk M67.98
    upper arm M67.92-●
    wrist M67.93-●
  thoracic root (nerve) NEC G54.3
  thyrocalcitonin hypersecretion E07.0
  thyroid (gland) E07.9
    function NEC, neonatal, transitory P72.2
    iodine-deficiency related E01.8
    specified NEC E07.89
  tic —*see* Tic
  tobacco use
    chewing tobacco (mild) (moderate) (severe) F17.220
      in remission (early) (sustained) F17.221
    cigarettes (mild) (moderate) (severe)
      in remission (early) (sustained) F17.211
    mild F17.200
      in remission (early) (sustained) F17.201
    moderate F17.200
      in remission (early) (sustained) F17.201
    severe F17.200
      in remission (early) (sustained) F17.201
    specified product NEC (mild) (moderate) (severe)
      in remission (early) (sustained) F17.291
  tooth K08.9
    development K00.9
      specified NEC K00.8
    eruption K00.6
  Tourette's F95.2
  trance and possession F44.89
  transvestic F65.1
  trauma and stressor-related F43.9
    other specified F43.8
  tricuspid (valve) —*see* Endocarditis, tricuspid
  tryptophan metabolism E70.5
  tubular, phosphate-losing N25.0
  tubulo-interstitial (in)
    brucellosis A23.9 *[N16]*
    cystinosis E72.04
    diphtheria A36.84
    glycogen storage disease E74.00 *[N16]*
    leukemia NEC C95.9-● *[N16]*
    lymphoma NEC C85.9-● *[N16]*
    mixed cryoglobulinemia D89.1 *[N16]*
    multiple myeloma C90.0-● *[N16]*
    Salmonella infection A02.25
    sarcoidosis D86.84
    sepsis A41.9 *[N16]*
      streptococcal A40.9 *[N16]*
    systemic lupus erythematosus M32.15
    toxoplasmosis B58.83
    transplant rejection T86.91 *[N16]*
    Wilson's disease E83.01 *[N16]*
  tubulo-renal function, impaired N25.9
    specified NEC N25.89
  tympanic membrane H73.9-●
    atrophy —*see* Atrophy, tympanic membrane
    infection —*see* Myringitis
    perforation —*see* Perforation, tympanum
    specified NEC H73.89-●
  unsocialized aggressive F91.1
  urea cycle metabolism E72.20
    argininemia E72.21
    arginosuccinic aciduria E72.22
    citrullinemia E72.23
    ornithine transcarbamylase deficiency E72.4
    other specified E72.29
  ureter (in) N28.9
    schistosomiasis B65.0 *[N29]*
    tuberculosis A18.11
  urethra N36.9
    specified NEC N36.8

Disorder *(Continued)*
  urinary system N39.9
    specified NEC N39.8
  valve, heart
    aortic —*see* Endocarditis, aortic
    mitral —*see* Endocarditis, mitral
    pulmonary —*see* Endocarditis, pulmonary
    rheumatic
      aortic —*see* Endocarditis, aortic,
        rheumatic
      mitral —*see* Endocarditis, mitral
      pulmonary —*see* Endocarditis,
        pulmonary, rheumatic
      tricuspid —*see* Endocarditis, tricuspid
    tricuspid —*see* Endocarditis, tricuspid
  vestibular function H81.9-•
    specified NEC —*see* subcategory H81.8
      in diseases classified elsewhere H82.-•
    vertigo —*see* Vertigo
  vision, binocular H53.30
    abnormal retinal correspondence H53.31
    diplopia H53.2
    fusion with defective stereopsis H53.32
    simultaneous perception H53.33
    suppression H53.34
  visual
    cortex
      blindness H47.619
        left brain H47.612
        right brain H47.611
      due to
        inflammatory disorder H47.629
          left brain H47.622
          right brain H47.621
        neoplasm H47.639
          left brain H47.632
          right brain H47.631
        vascular disorder H47.649
          left brain H47.642
          right brain H47.641
    pathway H47.9
      due to
        inflammatory disorder H47.51-•
        neoplasm H47.52-•
        vascular disorder H47.53-•
    optic chiasm —*see* Disorder, optic,
      chiasm
  vitreous body H43.9
    crystalline deposits —*see* Deposit,
      crystalline
    degeneration —*see* Degeneration, vitreous
    hemorrhage —*see* Hemorrhage, vitreous
    opacities —*see* Opacity, vitreous
    prolapse —*see* Prolapse, vitreous
    specified type NEC H43.89
  voice R49.9
    specified type NEC R49.8
  volatile solvent use
    due to drug abuse —*see* Abuse, drug,
      inhalant
    due to drug dependence —*see* Dependence,
      drug, inhalant
  voyeuristic F65.3
  white blood cells D72.9
    specified NEC D72.89
  withdrawing, child or adolescent
    F40.10
Disorientation R41.0
Displacement, displaced
  acquired traumatic of bone, cartilage, joint,
    tendon NEC —*see* Dislocation
  adrenal gland (congenital) Q89.1
  appendix, retrocecal (congenital) Q43.8
  auricle (congenital) Q17.4
  bladder (acquired) N32.89
    congenital Q64.19
  brachial plexus (congenital) Q07.8
  brain stem, caudal (congenital) Q04.8
  canaliculus (lacrimalis), congenital Q10.6
  cardia through esophageal hiatus (congenital)
    Q40.1

Displacement, displaced *(Continued)*
  cerebellum, caudal (congenital) Q04.8
  cervix —*see* Malposition, uterus
  colon (congenital) Q43.3
  device, implant or graft —*see also*
    Complications, by site and type,
    mechanical T85.628
    arterial graft NEC —*see* Complication,
      cardiovascular device, mechanical,
      vascular
    breast (implant) T85.42
    catheter NEC T85.628
      dialysis (renal) T82.42
        intraperitoneal T85.621
      infusion NEC T82.524
        spinal (epidural) (subdural) T85.620
      urinary
        cystostomy T83.020
        Hopkins T83.028
        ileostomy T83.028
        indwelling T83.021
        nephrostomy T83.022
        specified NEC T83.028
        urostomy T83.028
    electronic (electrode) (pulse generator)
      (stimulator) —*see* Complication,
      electronic stimulator
    fixation, internal (orthopedic) NEC —
      see Complication, fixation device,
      mechanical
    gastrointestinal —*see* Complications,
      prosthetic device, mechanical,
      gastrointestinal device
    genital NEC T83.428
      intrauterine contraceptive device (string)
        T83.32
      penile prosthesis (cylinder) (implanted)
        (pump) (resevoir) T83.420
      testicular prosthesis T83.421
    heart NEC —*see* Complication,
      cardiovascular device, mechanical
    joint prosthesis —*see* Complications, joint
      prosthesis, mechanical
    ocular —*see* Complications, prosthetic
      device, mechanical, ocular device
    orthopedic NEC —*see* Complication,
      orthopedic, device or graft,
      mechanical
    specified NEC T85.628
    urinary NEC T83.128
      graft T83.22
      sphincter, implanted T83.121
      stent (ileal conduit) (nephroureteral)
        T83.123
      ureteral indwelling T83.122
    vascular NEC —*see* Complication,
      cardiovascular device, mechanical
    ventricular intracranial shunt T85.02
  electronic stimulator
    bone T84.320
    cardiac —*see* Complications, cardiac
      device, electronic
    nervous system —*see* Complication,
      prosthetic device, mechanical,
      electronic nervous system
      stimulator
    urinary —*see* Complications, electronic
      stimulator, urinary
  esophageal mucosa into cardia of stomach,
    congenital Q39.8
  esophagus (acquired) K22.89
    congenital Q39.8
  eyeball (acquired) (lateral) (old) —*see*
    Displacement, globe
    congenital Q15.8
    current —*see* Avulsion, eye
  fallopian tube (acquired) N83.4-•
    congenital Q50.6
    opening (congenital) Q50.6
  gallbladder (congenital) Q44.1
  gastric mucosa (congenital) Q40.2

Displacement, displaced *(Continued)*
  globe (acquired) (old) (lateral) H05.21-•
    current —*see* Avulsion, eye
  heart (congenital) Q24.8
    acquired I51.89
  hymen (upward) (congenital) Q52.4
  intervertebral disc NEC
    with myelopathy —*see* Disorder, disc, with,
      myelopathy
    cervical, cervicothoracic (with)
      M50.20
      myelopathy —*see* Disorder, disc,
        cervical, with myelopathy
      neuritis, radiculitis or radiculopathy —
        see Disorder, disc, cervical, with
        neuritis
    due to trauma —*see* Dislocation, vertebra
    lumbar region M51.26
      with
        neuritis, radiculitis, radiculopathy or
          sciatica M51.16
    lumbosacral region M51.27
      with
        myelopathy M51.07
        neuritis, radiculitis, radiculopathy or
          sciatica M51.17
    sacrococcygeal region M53.3
    thoracic region M51.24
      with
        myelopathy M51.04
        neuritis, radiculitis, radiculopathy
          M51.14
    thoracolumbar region M51.25
      with
        myelopathy M51.05
        neuritis, radiculitis, radiculopathy
          M51.15
  intrauterine device (string) T83.32
  kidney (acquired) N28.83
    congenital Q63.2
  lachrymal, lacrimal apparatus or duct
    (congenital) Q10.6
  lens, congenital Q12.1
  macula (congenital) Q14.1
  Meckel's diverticulum Q43.0
    malignant —*see* Table of Neoplasms, small
      intestine, malignant
  nail (congenital) Q84.6
    acquired L60.8
  opening of Wharton's duct in mouth Q38.4
  organ or site, congenital NEC —*see*
    Malposition, congenital
  ovary (acquired) N83.4-•
    congenital Q50.39
    free in peritoneal cavity (congenital)
      Q50.39
    into hernial sac N83.4-•
  oviduct (acquired) N83.4-•
    congenital Q50.6
  parathyroid (gland) E21.4
  parotid gland (congenital) Q38.4
  punctum lacrimale (congenital) Q10.6
  sacro-iliac (joint) (congenital) Q74.2
    current injury S33.2
    old —*see* subcategory M53.2
  salivary gland (any) (congenital) Q38.4
  spleen (congenital) Q89.09
  stomach, congenital Q40.2
  sublingual duct Q38.4
  tongue (downward) (congenital) Q38.3
  tooth, teeth, fully erupted M26.30
    horizontal M26.33
    vertical M26.34
  trachea (congenital) Q32.1
  ureter or ureteric opening or orifice
    (congenital) Q62.62
  uterine opening of oviducts or fallopian tubes
    Q50.6
  uterus, uterine —*see* Malposition, uterus
  ventricular septum Q21.0
    with rudimentary ventricle Q20.4

▶ New　⇒ Revised　~~deleted~~ Deleted　• Use Additional Character(s)

Disproportion
  between native and reconstructed breast
      N65.1
  fiber-type G71.20
      congenital G71.29
Disruptio uteri —*see* Rupture, uterus
Disruption (of)
  ciliary body NEC H21.89
  closure of
      cornea T81.31
      craniotomy T81.32
      fascia (muscular) (superficial) T81.32
      internal organ or tissue T81.32
      laceration (external) (internal) T81.33
      ligament T81.32
      mucosa T81.31
      muscle or muscle flap T81.32
      ribs or rib cage T81.32
      skin and subcutaneous tissue (full-
          thickness) (superficial) T81.31
      skull T81.32
      sternum (sternotomy) T81.32
      tendon T81.32
      traumatic laceration (external) (internal)
          T81.33
  family Z63.8
      due to
          absence of family member due to
              military deployment Z63.31
          absence of family member NEC
              Z63.32
          alcoholism and drug addiction in
              family Z63.72
          bereavement Z63.4
          death (assumed) or disappearance of
              family member Z63.4
          divorce or separation Z63.5
          drug addiction in family Z63.72
          return of family member from military
              deployment (current or past
              conflict) Z63.71
          stressful life events NEC Z63.79
  iris NEC H21.89
  ligament(s) —*see also* Sprain
      knee
          current injury —*see* Dislocation, knee
          old (chronic) —*see* Derangement, knee,
              ligament, instability, chronic
          spontaneous NEC —*see* Derangement,
              knee, disruption ligament
  ossicular chain —*see* Discontinuity, ossicles,
      ear
  pelvic ring (stable) S32.810
      unstable S32.811
  traumatic injury wound repair T81.33
  wound T81.30
      episiotomy O90.1
      operation T81.31
          cesarean O90.0
          external operation wound (superficial)
              T81.31
          internal operation wound (deep)
              T81.32
      perineal (obstetric) O90.1
  traumatic injury repair T81.33
Dissatisfaction with
  employment Z56.9
  school environment Z55.4
Dissecting —*see* condition
Dissection
  aorta I71.00
      abdominal I71.02
      thoracic I71.01
      thoracoabdominal I71.03
  artery I77.70
      basilar (trunk) I77.75
      carotid I77.71
      cerebral (nonruptured) I67.0
          ruptured —*see* Hemorrhage, intracranial,
              subarachnoid
      coronary I25.42

Dissection (*Continued*)
  artery (*Continued*)
      extremity
          lower I77.77
          upper I77.76
      iliac I77.72
      precerebral
          congenital (nonruptured) Q28.1
          specified site NEC I77.75
      renal I77.73
      specified NEC I77.79
      vertebral I77.74
  precerebral artery, congenital (nonruptured)
      Q28.1
      Heartland A93.8
  traumatic —*see* Wound, open, by site
  vascular I99.8
  wound —*see* Wound, open
Disseminated —*see* condition
Dissociation
  auriculoventricular or atrioventricular (AV)
      (any degree) (isorhythmic) I45.89
      with heart block I44.2
  interference I45.89
Dissociative reaction, state F44.9
Dissolution, vertebra —*see* Osteoporosis
Distension, distention
  abdomen R14.0
  bladder N32.89
  cecum K63.89
  colon K63.89
  gallbladder K82.8
  intestine K63.89
  kidney N28.89
  liver K76.89
  seminal vesicle N50.89
  stomach K31.89
      acute K31.0
      psychogenic F45.8
  ureter —*see* Dilatation, ureter
  uterus N85.8
Distoma hepaticum infestation B66.3
Distomiasis B66.9
  bile passages B66.3
  hemic B65.9
  hepatic B66.3
      due to Clonorchis sinensis B66.1
  intestinal B66.5
  liver B66.3
      due to Clonorchis sinensis B66.1
  lung B66.4
  pulmonary B66.4
Distomolar (fourth molar) K00.1
Disto-occlusion (Division I) (Division II)
      M26.212
Distortion(s) (congenital)
  adrenal (gland) Q89.1
  arm NEC Q68.8
  bile duct or passage Q44.5
  bladder Q64.79
  brain Q04.9
  cervix (uteri) Q51.9
  chest (wall) Q67.8
      bones Q76.8
  clavicle Q74.0
  clitoris Q52.6
  coccyx Q76.49
  common duct Q44.5
  coronary Q24.5
  cystic duct Q44.5
  ear (auricle) (external) Q17.3
      inner Q16.5
      middle Q16.4
          ossicles Q16.3
  endocrine NEC Q89.2
  eustachian tube Q17.8
  eye (adnexa) Q15.8
  face bone(s) NEC Q75.8
  fallopian tube Q50.6
  femur NEC Q68.8
  fibula NEC Q68.8

Distortion (*Continued*)
  finger(s) Q68.1
  foot Q66.9-●
  genitalia, genital organ(s)
      female Q52.8
          external Q52.79
          internal NEC Q52.8
  gyri Q04.8
  hand bone(s) Q68.1
  heart (auricle) (ventricle) Q24.8
      valve (cusp) Q24.8
  hepatic duct Q44.5
  humerus NEC Q68.8
  hymen Q52.4
  intrafamilial communications Z63.8
  jaw NEC M26.89
  labium (majus) (minus) Q52.79
  leg NEC Q68.8
  lens Q12.8
  liver Q44.7
  lumbar spine Q76.49
      with disproportion O33.8
          causing obstructed labor O65.0
  lumbosacral (joint) (region) Q76.49
      kyphosis —*see* Kyphosis, congenital
      lordosis —*see* Lordosis, congenital
  nerve Q07.8
  nose Q30.8
  organ
      of Corti Q16.5
      or site not listed —*see* Anomaly, by site
          ossicles, ear Q16.3
  oviduct Q50.6
  pancreas Q45.3
  parathyroid (gland) Q89.2
  pituitary (gland) Q89.2
  radius NEC Q68.8
  sacroiliac joint Q74.2
  sacrum Q76.49
  scapula Q74.0
  shoulder girdle Q74.0
  skull bone(s) NEC Q75.8
      with
          anencephalus Q00.0
          encephalocele —*see* Encephalocele
          hydrocephalus Q03.9
              with spina bifida —*see* Spina bifida,
                  with hydrocephalus
          microcephaly Q02
  spinal cord Q06.8
  spine Q76.49
      kyphosis —*see* Kyphosis, congenital
      lordosis —*see* Lordosis, congenital
  spleen Q89.09
  sternum NEC Q76.7
  thorax (wall) Q67.8
      bony Q76.8
  thymus (gland) Q89.2
  thyroid (gland) Q89.2
  tibia NEC Q68.8
  toe(s) Q66.9-●
  tongue Q38.3
  trachea (cartilage) Q32.1
  ulna NEC Q68.8
  ureter Q62.8
  urethra Q64.79
      causing obstruction Q64.39
  uterus Q51.9
  vagina Q52.4
  vertebra Q76.49
      kyphosis —*see* Kyphosis, congenital
      lordosis —*see* Lordosis, congenital
  visual —*see also* Disturbance, vision
      shape and size H53.15
  vulva Q52.79
  wrist (bones) (joint) Q68.8
Distress
  abdomen —*see* Pain, abdominal
  acute respiratory R06.03
      syndrome (adult) (child) J80
  epigastric R10.13

Distress (*Continued*)
fetal P84
  complicating pregnancy —*see* Stress, fetal
gastrointestinal (functional) K30
  psychogenic F45.8
intestinal (functional) NOS K59.9
  psychogenic F45.8
maternal, during labor and delivery O75.0
relationship, with spouse or intimate partner Z63.0
respiratory (adult) (child) R06.03
  newborn P22.9
    specified NEC P22.8
  orthopnea R06.01
  psychogenic F45.8
  shortness of breath R06.02
  specified type NEC R06.09
Distribution vessel, atypical Q27.9
coronary artery Q24.5
precerebral Q28.1
Distichiasis L68.8
Disturbance(s) —*see also* Disease
absorption K90.9
  calcium E58
  carbohydrate K90.49
  fat K90.49
    pancreatic K90.3
  protein K90.49
  starch K90.49
  vitamin —*see* Deficiency, vitamin
acid-base equilibrium E87.8
  mixed E87.4
activity and attention (with hyperkinesis) —*see* Disorder, attention-deficit hyperactivity
amino acid transport E72.00
assimilation, food K90.9
auditory nerve, except deafness —*see* subcategory H93.3
behavior —*see* Disorder, conduct
blood clotting (mechanism) —*see also* Defect, coagulation D68.9
cerebral
  nerve —*see* Disorder, nerve, cranial
  status, newborn P91.9
    specified NEC P91.88
circulatory I99.9
conduct —*see also* Disorder, conduct F91.9
  adjustment reaction —*see* Disorder, adjustment
  compulsive F63.9
  disruptive F91.9
  hyperkinetic —*see* Disorder, attention-deficit hyperactivity
  socialized F91.2
  specified NEC F91.8
  unsocialized F91.1
coordination R27.8
cranial nerve —*see* Disorder, nerve, cranial
deep sensibility —*see* Disturbance, sensation
digestive K30
  psychogenic F45.8
electrolyte —*see also* Imbalance, electrolyte
  newborn, transitory P74.49
    hyperammonemia P74.6
    hyperchloremia P74.421
    hyperchloremic metabolic acidosis P74.421
    hypochloremia P74.422
    potassium balance
      hyperkalemia P74.31
      hypokalemia P74.32
    sodium balance
      hypernatremia P74.21
      hyponatremia P74.22
    specified type NEC P74.49
emotions specific to childhood and adolescence F93.9
  with
    anxiety and fearfulness NEC F93.8
    elective mutism F94.0

Disturbance (*Continued*)
emotions specific to childhood and adolescence (*Continued*)
  with (*Continued*)
    oppositional disorder F91.3
    sensitivity (withdrawal) F40.10
    shyness F40.10
    social withdrawal F40.10
  involving relationship problems F93.8
  mixed F93.8
  specified NEC F93.8
endocrine (gland) E34.9
  neonatal, transitory P72.9
    specified NEC P72.8
equilibrium R42
fructose metabolism E74.10
gait —*see* Gait
  hysterical F44.4
  psychogenic F44.4
gastrointestinal (functional) K30
  psychogenic F45.8
habit, child F98.9
hearing, except deafness and tinnitus —*see* Abnormal, auditory perception
heart, functional (conditions in I44-I50)
  due to presence of (cardiac) prosthesis I97.19-●
  postoperative I97.89
    cardiac surgery —*see also* Infarct, myocardium, associated with revascularization procedure I97.19-●
hormones E34.9
innervation uterus (parasympathetic) (sympathetic) N85.8
keratinization NEC
  gingiva K05.10
    nonplaque induced K05.11
    plaque induced K05.10
  lip K13.0
  oral (mucosa) (soft tissue) K13.29
  tongue K13.29
learning (specific) —*see* Disorder, learning
memory —*see* Amnesia
  mild, following organic brain damage F06.8
mental F99
  associated with diseases classified elsewhere F54
metabolism E88.9
  with
    abortion —*see* Abortion, by type with other specified complication
    ectopic pregnancy O08.5
    molar pregnancy O08.5
  amino-acid E72.9
    aromatic E70.9
    branched-chain E71.2
    straight-chain E72.89
    sulfur-bearing E72.10
  ammonia E72.20
  arginine E72.21
  argininosuccinic acid E72.22
  carbohydrate E74.9
  cholesterol E78.9
  citrulline E72.23
  cystathionine E72.19
  general E88.9
  glutamine E72.89
  histidine E70.40
  homocystine E72.19
  hydroxylysine E72.3
  in labor or delivery O75.89
  iron E83.10
  lipoid E78.9
  lysine E72.3
  methionine E72.19
  neonatal, transitory P74.9
    calcium and magnesium P71.9
      specified type NEC P71.8
    carbohydrate metabolism P70.9
      specified type NEC P70.8
    specified NEC P74.8

Disturbance (*Continued*)
metabolism (*Continued*)
  ornithine E72.4
  phosphate E83.39
  sodium NEC E87.8
  threonine E72.89
  tryptophan E70.5
  tyrosine E70.20
  urea cycle E72.20
motor R29.2
nervous, functional R45.0
neuromuscular mechanism (eye), due to syphilis A52.15
nutritional E63.9
  nail L60.3
ocular motion H51.9
  psychogenic F45.8
oculogyric H51.8
  psychogenic F45.8
oculomotor H51.9
  psychogenic F45.8
olfactory nerve R43.1
optic nerve NEC —*see* Disorder, nerve, optic
oral epithelium, including tongue NEC K13.29
perceptual due to
  alcohol withdrawal F10.232
  amphetamine intoxication F15.922
    in
      abuse F15.122
      dependence F15.222
  anxiolytic withdrawal F13.232
  cannabis intoxication (acute) F12.922
    in
      abuse F12.122
      dependence F12.222
  cocaine intoxication (acute) F14.922
    in
      abuse F14.122
      dependence F14.222
  hypnotic withdrawal F13.232
  opioid intoxication (acute) F11.922
    in
      abuse F11.122
      dependence F11.222
  phencyclidine intoxication (acute) F16.122
  sedative withdrawal F13.232
personality (pattern) (trait) —*see also* Disorder, personality F60.9
  following organic brain damage F07.9
polyglandular E31.9
  specified NEC E31.8
potassium balance, newborn
  hyperkalemia P74.31
  hypokalemia P74.32
psychogenic F45.9
psychomotor F44.4
psychophysical visual H53.16
pupillary —*see* Anomaly, pupil, function
reflex R29.2
rhythm, heart I49.9
salivary secretion K11.7
sensation (cold) (heat) (localization) (tactile discrimination) (texture) (vibratory) NEC R20.9
  hysterical F44.6
  skin R20.9
    anesthesia R20.0
    hyperesthesia R20.3
    hypoesthesia R20.1
    paresthesia R20.2
    specified type NEC R20.8
  smell R43.9
    and taste (mixed) R43.8
    anosmia R43.0
    parosmia R43.1
    specified NEC R43.8
  taste R43.9
    and smell (mixed) R43.8
    parageusia R43.2
    specified NEC R43.8

▶ New   ⇒ Revised   ~~deleted~~ Deleted   ● Use Additional Character(s)

Disturbance *(Continued)*
  sensory —*see* Disturbance, sensation
  situational (transient) —*see also* Disorder,
    adjustment
    acute F43.0
  sleep G47.9
    nonorganic origin F51.9
  smell —*see* Disturbance, sensation, smell
  sociopathic F60.2
  sodium balance, newborn
    hypernatremia P74.21
    hyponatremia P74.22
  speech R47.9
    developmental F80.9
    specified NEC R47.89
  stomach (functional) K31.9
  sympathetic (nerve) G90.9
  taste —*see* Disturbance, sensation, taste
  temperature
    regulation, newborn P81.9
      specified NEC P81.8
    sense R20.8
      hysterical F44.6
  tooth
    eruption K00.6
    formation K00.4
    structure, hereditary NEC K00.5
  touch —*see* Disturbance, sensation
  vascular I99.9
    arteriosclerotic —*see* Arteriosclerosis
  vasomotor I73.9
  vasospastic I73.9
  vision, visual H53.9
    following
      cerebral infarction I69.398
      cerebrovascular disease I69.998
        specified NEC I69.898
      intracerebral hemorrhage I69.198
      nontraumatic intracranial hemorrhage
        NEC I69.298
      specified disease NEC I69.898
      subarachnoid hemorrhage I69.098
    psychophysical H53.16
    specified NEC H53.8
    subjective H53.10
      day blindness H53.11
      discomfort H53.14-●
      distortions of shape and size H53.15
      loss
        sudden H53.13-●
        transient H53.12-●
      specified type NEC H53.19
  voice R49.9
    psychogenic F44.4
    specified NEC R49.8
Diuresis R35.89
Diver's palsy, paralysis or squeeze T70.3
Diverticulitis (acute) K57.92
  bladder —*see* Cystitis
  ileum —*see* Diverticulitis, intestine, small
  intestine K57.92
    with
      abscess, perforation K57.80
        with bleeding K57.81
      bleeding K57.93
      congenital Q43.8
      large K57.32
        with
          abscess, perforation K57.20
            with bleeding K57.21
          bleeding K57.33
          small intestine K57.52
            with
              abscess, perforation K57.40
                with bleeding K57.41
              bleeding K57.53
      small K57.12
        with
          abscess, perforation K57.00
            with bleeding K57.01
          bleeding K57.13

Diverticulitis *(Continued)*
  intestine *(Continued)*
    small *(Continued)*
      with *(Continued)*
        large intestine K57.52
          with
            abscess, perforation K57.40
              with bleeding K57.41
            bleeding K57.53
Diverticulosis K57.90
  with bleeding K57.91
  large intestine K57.30
    with
      bleeding K57.31
      small intestine K57.50
        with bleeding K57.51
  small intestine K57.10
    with
      bleeding K57.11
      large intestine K57.50
        with bleeding K57.51
Diverticulum, diverticula (multiple) K57.90
  appendix (noninflammatory) K38.2
  bladder (sphincter) N32.3
    congenital Q64.6
  bronchus (congenital) Q32.4
    acquired J98.09
  calyx, calyceal (kidney) N28.89
  cardia (stomach) K31.4
  cecum —*see* Diverticulosis, intestine, large
    congenital Q43.8
  colon —*see* Diverticulosis, intestine, large
    congenital Q43.8
  duodenum —*see* Diverticulosis, intestine,
    small
    congenital Q43.8
  epiphrenic (esophagus) K22.5
  esophagus (congenital) Q39.6
    acquired (epiphrenic) (pulsion) (traction)
      K22.5
  eustachian tube —*see* Disorder, eustachian
    tube, specified NEC
  fallopian tube N83.8
  gastric K31.4
  heart (congenital) Q24.8
  ileum —*see* Diverticulosis, intestine, small
  jejunum —*see* Diverticulosis, intestine, small
  kidney (pelvis) (calyces) N28.89
    with calculus —*see* Calculus, kidney
  Meckel's (displaced) (hypertrophic) Q43.0
    malignant —*see* Table of Neoplasms, small
      intestine, malignant
  midthoracic K22.5
  organ or site, congenital NEC —*see* Distortion
  pericardium (congenital) (cyst) Q24.8
    acquired I31.8
  pharyngoesophageal (congenital) Q39.6
    acquired K22.5
  pharynx (congenital) Q38.7
  rectosigmoid —*see* Diverticulosis, intestine,
    large
    congenital Q43.8
  rectum —*see* Diverticulosis, intestine,
    large
  Rokitansky's K22.5
  seminal vesicle N50.89
  sigmoid —*see* Diverticulosis, intestine,
    large
    congenital Q43.8
  stomach (acquired) K31.4
    congenital Q40.2
  trachea (acquired) J39.8
  ureter (acquired) N28.89
    congenital Q62.8
  ureterovesical orifice N28.89
  urethra (acquired) N36.1
    congenital Q64.79
  ventricle, left (congenital) Q24.8
  vesical N32.3
    congenital Q64.6
  Zenker's (esophagus) K22.5

Division
  cervix uteri (acquired) N88.8
  glans penis Q55.69
  labia minora (congenital) Q52.79
  ligament (partial or complete) (current) —*see
    also* Sprain
    with open wound —*see* Wound, open
  muscle (partial or complete) (current) —*see
    also* Injury, muscle
    with open wound —*see* Wound, open
  nerve (traumatic) —*see* Injury, nerve
  spinal cord —*see* Injury, spinal cord,
    by region
  vein I87.8
Divorce, causing family disruption Z63.5
Dix-Hallpike neurolabyrinthitis —*see*
  Neuronitis, vestibular
Dizziness R42
  hysterical F44.89
  psychogenic F45.8
DMAC (disseminated mycobacterium avium-
  intracellulare complex) A31.2
DNR (do not resuscitate) Z66
Doan-Wiseman syndrome (primary splenic
  neutropenia) —*see* Agranulocytosis
Doehle-Heller aortitis A52.02
Dog bite —*see* Bite
Dohle body panmyelopathic syndrome D72.0
Dolichocephaly Q67.2
Dolichocolon Q43.8
Dolichostenomelia —*see* Syndrome, Marfan's
Donohue's syndrome E34.8
Donor (organ or tissue) Z52.9
  blood (whole) Z52.000
    autologous Z52.010
    specified component (lymphocytes)
      (platelets) NEC Z52.008
      autologous Z52.018
      specified donor NEC Z52.098
    specified donor NEC Z52.090
    stem cells Z52.001
      autologous Z52.011
      specified donor NEC Z52.091
  bone Z52.20
    autologous Z52.21
    marrow Z52.3
    specified type NEC Z52.29
  cornea Z52.5
  egg (Oocyte) Z52.819
    age 35 and over Z52.812
      anonymous recipient Z52.812
      designated recipient Z52.813
    under age 35 Z52.810
      anonymous recipient Z52.810
      designated recipient Z52.811
  kidney Z52.4
  liver Z52.6
  lung Z52.89
  lymphocyte —*see* Donor, blood, specified
    components NEC
  Oocyte —*see* Donor, egg
  platelets Z52.008
  potential, examination of Z00.5
  semen Z52.89
  skin Z52.10
    autologous Z52.11
    specified type NEC Z52.19
  specified organ or tissue NEC Z52.89
  sperm Z52.89
Donovanosis A58
Dorsalgia M54.9
  psychogenic F45.41
  specified NEC M54.89
Dorsopathy M53.9
  deforming M43.9
    specified NEC —*see* subcategory M43.8
  specified NEC M53.80
    cervical region M53.82
    cervicothoracic region M53.83
    lumbar region M53.86
    lumbosacral region M53.87

▶ New   ⇒ Revised   ~~deleted~~ Deleted   ● Use Additional Character(s)

Dorsopathy *(Continued)*
  specified NEC *(Continued)*
    occipito-atlanto-axial region M53.81
    sacrococcygeal region M53.88
    thoracic region M53.84
    thoracolumbar region M53.85
Double
  albumin E88.09
  aortic arch Q25.45
  auditory canal Q17.8
  auricle (heart) Q20.8
  bladder Q64.79
  cervix Q51.820
    with doubling of uterus (and vagina)
      Q51.10
      with obstruction Q51.11
  inlet ventricle Q20.4
  kidney with double pelvis (renal) Q63.0
  meatus urinarius Q64.75
  monster Q89.4
  outlet
    left ventricle Q20.2
    right ventricle Q20.1
  pelvis (renal) with double ureter Q62.5
  tongue Q38.3
  ureter (one or both sides) Q62.5
    with double pelvis (renal) Q62.5
  urethra Q64.74
  urinary meatus Q64.75
  uterus Q51.28
    with
      doubling of cervix (and vagina) Q51.10
        with obstruction Q51.11
      complete Q51.21
      in pregnancy or childbirth O34.0-●
        causing obstructed labor O65.5
      partial Q51.22
      specified NEC Q51.28
  vagina Q52.10
    with doubling of uterus (and cervix)
      Q51.10
      with obstruction Q51.11
  vision H53.2
  vulva Q52.79
▶ **Doubled up** Z59.01
Douglas' pouch, cul-de-sac —*see* condition
Down syndrome Q90.9
  meiotic nondisjunction Q90.0
  mitotic nondisjunction Q90.1
  mosaicism Q90.1
  translocation Q90.2
DPD (dihydropyrimidine dehydrogenase
    deficiency) E88.89
Dracontiasis B72
Dracunculiasis, dracunculosis B72
Dream state, hysterical F44.89
Drepanocytic anemia —*see* Disease,
    sickle-cell
Dresbach's syndrome (elliptocytosis)
    D58.1
Dreschlera (hawaiiensis) (infection)
    B43.8
Dressler's syndrome I24.1
Drift, ulnar —*see* Deformity, limb, specified
    type NEC, forearm
Drinking (alcohol)
  excessive, to excess NEC (without
    dependence) F10.10
    habitual (continual) (without remission)
      F10.20
      with remission F10.21
Drip, postnasal (chronic) R09.82
  due to
    allergic rhinitis —*see* Rhinitis, allergic
    common cold J00
    gastroesophageal reflux —*see* Reflux,
      gastroesophageal
    nasopharyngitis —*see* Nasopharyngitis
    other known condition — code to
      condition
    sinusitis —*see* Sinusitis

Droop
  facial R29.810
    cerebrovascular disease I69.992
      cerebral infarction I69.392
      intracerebral hemorrhage I69.192
      nontraumatic intracranial hemorrhage
        NEC I69.292
      specified disease NEC I69.892
      subarachnoid hemorrhage I69.092
Drop (in)
  attack NEC R55
  finger —*see* Deformity, finger
  foot —*see* Deformity, limb, foot, drop
  hematocrit (precipitous) R71.0
  hemoglobin R71.0
  toe —*see* Deformity, toe, specified NEC
  wrist —*see* Deformity, limb, wrist drop
Dropped heart beats I45.9
Dropsy, dropsical —*see also* Hydrops
  abdomen R18.8
  brain —*see* Hydrocephalus
  cardiac, heart —*see* Failure, heart, congestive
  gangrenous —*see* Gangrene
  heart —*see* Failure, heart, congestive
  kidney —*see* Nephrosis
  lung —*see* Edema, lung
  newborn due to isoimmunization P56.0
  pericardium —*see* Pericarditis
Drowned, drowning (near) T75.1
Drowsiness R40.0
Drug
  abuse counseling and surveillance Z71.51
  addiction —*see* Dependence
  dependence —*see* Dependence
  habit —*see* Dependence
  harmful use —*see* Abuse, drug
  induced fever R50.2
  overdose —*see* Table of Drugs and Chemicals,
    by drug, poisoning
  poisoning —*see* Table of Drugs and
    Chemicals, by drug, poisoning
  resistant organism infection —*see also*
    Resistant, organism, to, drug Z16.30
  therapy
    long term (current) (prophylactic) —*see*
      Therapy, drug long-term (current)
      (prophylactic)
    short term - omit code
  wrong substance given or taken in error —*see*
    Table of Drugs and Chemicals, by drug,
    poisoning
Drunkenness (without dependence) F10.129
  acute in alcoholism F10.229
  chronic (without remission) F10.20
    with remission F10.21
  pathological (without dependence) F10.129
    with dependence F10.229
  sleep F51.9
Drusen
  macula (degenerative) (retina) —*see*
    Degeneration, macula, drusen
  optic disc H47.32-●
Dry, dryness —*see also* condition
  larynx J38.7
  mouth R68.2
    due to dehydration E86.0
  nose J34.89
  socket (teeth) M27.3
  throat J39.2
DSAP L56.5
Duane's syndrome H50.81-●
Dubin-Johnson disease or syndrome E80.6
Dubois' disease (thymus gland) A50.59 *[E35]*
Dubowitz' syndrome Q87.19
Duchenne-Aran muscular atrophy G12.21
Duchenne-Griesinger disease G71.01
Duchenne's
  disease or syndrome
    motor neuron disease G12.22
    muscular dystrophy G71.01
  locomotor ataxia (syphilitic) A52.11

Duchenne's *(Continued)*
  paralysis
    birth injury P14.0
    due to or associated with
      motor neuron disease G12.22
      muscular dystrophy G71.01
Ducrey's chancre A57
Duct, ductus —*see* condition
Duhring's disease (dermatitis herpetiformis)
    L13.0
Dullness, cardiac (decreased) (increased) R01.2
Dumb ague —*see* Malaria
Dumbness —*see* Aphasia
Dumdum fever B55.0
Dumping syndrome (postgastrectomy) K91.1
Duodenitis (nonspecific) (peptic) K29.80
  with bleeding K29.81
Duodenocholangitis —*see* Cholangitis
Duodenum, duodenal —*see* condition
➠ **Duplay's bursitis or periarthritis** M75.0
Duplication, duplex —*see also* Accessory
  alimentary tract Q45.8
  anus Q43.4
  appendix (and cecum) Q43.4
  biliary duct (any) Q44.5
  bladder Q64.79
  cecum (and appendix) Q43.4
  cervix Q51.820
  chromosome NEC
    with complex rearrangements NEC Q92.5
    seen only at prometaphase Q92.8
  cystic duct Q44.5
  digestive organs Q45.8
  esophagus Q39.8
  frontonasal process Q75.8
  intestine (large) (small) Q43.4
  kidney Q63.0
  liver Q44.7
  pancreas Q45.3
  penis Q55.69
  respiratory organs NEC Q34.8
  salivary duct Q38.4
  spinal cord (incomplete) Q06.2
  stomach Q40.2
Dupré's disease (meningism) R29.1
Dupuytren's contraction or disease M72.0
Durand-Nicolas-Favre disease A55
Durotomy (inadvertent) (incidental) G97.41
Duroziez's disease (congenital mitral stenosis)
    Q23.2
Dutton's relapsing fever (West African)
    A68.1
Dwarfism E34.3
  achondroplastic Q77.4
  congenital E34.3
  constitutional E34.3
  hypochondroplastic Q77.4
  hypophyseal E23.0
  infantile E34.3
  Laron-type E34.3
  Lorain (-Levi) type E23.0
  metatropic Q77.8
  nephrotic-glycosuric (with
    hypophosphatemic rickets) E72.09
  nutritional E45
  pancreatic K86.89
  pituitary E23.0
  renal N25.0
  thanatophoric Q77.1
Dyke-Young anemia (secondary)
    (symptomatic) D59.19
Dysacusis —*see* Abnormal, auditory
    perception
Dysadrenocortism E27.9
  hyperfunction E27.0
Dysarthria R47.1
  following
    cerebral infarction I69.322
    cerebrovascular disease I69.922
      specified disease NEC I69.822
    intracerebral hemorrhage I69.122

▶ New   ➠ Revised   ~~deleted~~ Deleted   ● Use Additional Character(s)

Dysarthria *(Continued)*
  following *(Continued)*
    nontraumatic intracranial hemorrhage
      NEC I69.222
    subarachnoid hemorrhage I69.022
Dysautonomia (familial) G90.1
Dysbarism T70.3
Dysbasia R26.2
  angiosclerotica intermittens I73.9
  hysterical F44.4
  lordotica (progressiva) G24.1
  nonorganic origin F44.4
  psychogenic F44.4
Dysbetalipoproteinemia (familial) E78.2
Dyscalculia R48.8
  developmental F81.2
Dyschezia K59.00
Dyschondroplasia (with hemangiomata) Q78.4
Dyschromia (skin) L81.9
Dyscollagenosis M35.9
Dyscranio-pygo-phalangy Q87.0
Dyscrasia
  blood (with) D75.9
    antepartum hemorrhage —*see* Hemorrhage,
      antepartum, with coagulation defect
    intrapartum hemorrhage O67.0
    newborn P61.9
      specified type NEC P61.8
    puerperal, postpartum O72.3
  polyglandular, pluriglandular E31.9
Dysendocrinism E34.9
Dysentery, dysenteric (catarrhal) (diarrhea)
      (epidemic) (hemorrhagic) (infectious)
      (sporadic) (tropical) A09
  abscess, liver A06.4
  amebic —*see also* Amebiasis A06.0
    with abscess —*see* Abscess, amebic
    acute A06.0
    chronic A06.1
  arthritis —*see also* category M01 A09
    bacillary —*see also* category M01 A03.9
  bacillary A03.9
    arthritis —*see also* category M01 A03.9
    Boyd A03.2
    Flexner A03.1
    Schmitz (-Stutzer) A03.0
    Shiga (-Kruse) A03.0
    Shigella A03.9
      boydii A03.2
      dysenteriae A03.0
      flexneri A03.1
      group A A03.0
      group B A03.1
      group C A03.2
      group D A03.3
      sonnei A03.3
      specified type NEC A03.8
    Sonne A03.3
    specified type NEC A03.8
  balantidial A07.0
  Balantidium coli A07.0
  Boyd's A03.2
  candidal B37.82
  Chilomastix A07.8
  Chinese A03.9
  coccidial A07.3
  Dientamoeba (fragilis) A07.8
  Embadomonas A07.8
  Entamoeba, entamebic —*see* Dysentery,
    amebic
  Flexner-Boyd A03.2
  Flexner's A03.1
  Giardia lamblia A07.1
  Hiss-Russell A03.1
  Lamblia A07.1
  leishmanial B55.0
  malarial —*see* Malaria
  metazoal B82.0
  monilial B37.82
  protozoal A07.9
  Salmonella A02.0

Dysentery, dysenteric *(Continued)*
  schistosomal B65.1
  Schmitz (-Stutzer) A03.0
  Shiga (-Kruse) A03.0
  Shigella NOS —*see* Dysentery, bacillary
  Sonne A03.3
  strongyloidiasis B78.0
  trichomonal A07.8
  viral —*see also* Enteritis, viral A08.4
Dysequilibrium R42
Dysesthesia R20.8
  hysterical F44.6
Dysfibrinogenemia (congenital) D68.2
Dysfunction
  adrenal E27.9
    hyperfunction E27.0
  autonomic
    due to alcohol G31.2
    somatoform F45.8
  bladder N31.9
    neurogenic NOS —*see* Dysfunction,
      bladder, neuromuscular
    neuromuscular NOS N31.9
      atonic (motor) (sensory) N31.2
      autonomous N31.2
      flaccid N31.2
      nonreflex N31.2
      reflex N31.1
      specified NEC N31.8
      uninhibited N31.0
  bleeding, uterus N93.8
  cerebral G93.89
  colon K59.9
    psychogenic F45.8
  colostomy K94.03
  cystic duct K82.8
  cystostomy (stoma) —*see* Complications,
    cystostomy
  ejaculatory N53.19
    anejaculatory orgasm N53.13
    painful N53.12
    premature F52.4
    retarded N53.11
  endocrine NOS E34.9
  endometrium N85.8
  enterostomy K94.13
  erectile —*see* Dysfunction, sexual, male, erectile
▶feeding, pediatric
  ▶acute R63.31
  ▶chronic R63.32
  gallbladder K82.8
  gastrostomy (stoma) K94.23
  gland, glandular NOS E34.9
    meibomian, of eyelid -see Dysfunction,
      meibomian gland
  heart I51.89
  hemoglobin D75.89
  hepatic K76.89
  hypophysis E23.7
  hypothalamic NEC E23.3
  ileostomy (stoma) K94.13
  jejunostomy (stoma) K94.13
  kidney —*see* Disease, renal
  labyrinthine —*see* subcategory H83.2
  left ventricular, following sudden emotional
    stress I51.81
  liver K76.89
  male —*see* Dysfunction, sexual, male
  meibomian gland, of eyelid H02.889
    left H02.886
      lower H02.885
      upper H02.884
      upper and lower eyelids H02.88B
    right H02.883
      lower H02.882
      upper H02.881
      upper and lower eyelids H02.88A
  orgasmic (female) F52.31
    male F52.32
  ovary E28.9
    specified NEC E28.8
  papillary muscle I51.89
  parathyroid E21.4

Dysfunction *(Continued)*
  physiological NEC R68.89
    psychogenic F59
  pineal gland E34.8
  pituitary (gland) E23.3
  platelets D69.1
  polyglandular E31.9
    specified NEC E31.8
  psychophysiologic F59
  psychosexual F52.9
    with
      dyspareunia F52.6
      premature ejaculation F52.4
      vaginismus F52.5
  pylorus K31.9
  rectum K59.9
    psychogenic F45.8
  reflex (sympathetic) —*see* Syndrome, pain,
    complex regional I
  segmental —*see* Dysfunction, somatic
  senile R54
  sexual (due to) R37
    alcohol F10.981
    amphetamine F15.981
      in
        abuse F15.181
        dependence F15.281
    anxiolytic F13.981
      in
        abuse F13.181
        dependence F13.281
    cocaine F14.981
      in
        abuse F14.181
        dependence F14.281
    excessive sexual drive F52.8
    failure of genital response (male) F52.21
      female F52.22
    female N94.9
      aversion F52.1
      dyspareunia N94.10
        psychogenic F52.6
      frigidity F52.22
      nymphomania F52.8
      orgasmic F52.31
      psychogenic F52.9
        aversion F52.1
        dyspareunia F52.6
        frigidity F52.22
        nymphomania F52.8
        orgasmic F52.31
        vaginismus F52.5
      vaginismus N94.2
        psychogenic F52.5
    hypnotic F13.981
      in
        abuse F13.181
        dependence F13.281
    inhibited orgasm (female) F52.31
      male F52.32
    lack
      of sexual enjoyment F52.1
      or loss of sexual desire F52.0
    male N53.9
      anejaculatory orgasm N53.13
      ejaculatory N53.19
        painful N53.12
        premature F52.4
        retarded N53.11
      erectile N52.9
        drug induced N52.2
        due to
          disease classified elsewhere N52.1
          drug N52.2
        postoperative (postprocedural) N52.39
          following
            cryotherapy N52.37
            interstitial seed therapy N52.36
            prostate ablative therapy N52.37
            prostatectomy N52.34
              radical N52.31

Dysfunction *(Continued)*
  sexual *(Continued)*
    male *(Continued)*
      erectile *(Continued)*
        postoperative *(Continued)*
          following *(Continued)*
            radiation therapy N52.35
            radical cystectomy N52.32
            ultrasound ablative therapy N52.37
            urethral surgery N52.33
        psychogenic F52.21
        specified cause NEC N52.8
        vasculogenic
          arterial insufficiency N52.01
            with corporo-venous occlusive N52.03
          corporo-venous occlusive N52.02
            with arterial insufficiency N52.03
      impotence —*see* Dysfunction, sexual, male, erectile
      psychogenic F52.9
        aversion F52.1
        erectile F52.21
        orgasmic F52.32
        premature ejaculation F52.4
        satyriasis F52.8
        specified type NEC F52.8
      specified type NEC N53.8
    nonorganic F52.9
      specified NEC F52.8
    opioid F11.981
      in
        abuse F11.181
        dependence F11.281
    orgasmic dysfunction (female) F52.31
      male F52.32
    premature ejaculation F52.4
    psychoactive substances NEC F19.981
      in
        abuse F19.181
        dependence F19.281
    psychogenic F52.9
    sedative F13.981
      in
        abuse F13.181
        dependence F13.281
    sexual aversion F52.1
    vaginismus (nonorganic) (psychogenic) F52.5
  sinoatrial node I49.5
  somatic M99.09
    abdomen M99.09
    acromioclavicular M99.07
    cervical region M99.01
    cervicothoracic M99.01
    costochondral M99.08
    costovertebral M99.08
    head region M99.00
    hip M99.05
    lower extremity M99.06
    lumbar region M99.03
    lumbosacral M99.03
    occipitocervical M99.00
    pelvic region M99.05
    pubic M99.05
    rib cage M99.08
    sacral region M99.04
    sacrococcygeal M99.04
    sacroiliac M99.04
    specified NEC M99.09
    sternochondral M99.08
    sternoclavicular M99.07
    thoracic region M99.02
    thoracolumbar M99.02
    upper extremity M99.07
  somatoform autonomic F45.8
  stomach K31.89
    psychogenic F45.8
  suprarenal E27.9
    hyperfunction E27.0

Dysfunction *(Continued)*
  symbolic R48.9
    specified type NEC R48.8
  temporomandibular (joint) M26.69
    joint-pain syndrome M26.62-●
  testicular (endocrine) E29.9
    specified NEC E29.8
  thymus E32.9
  thyroid E07.9
  ureterostomy (stoma) —*see* Complications, stoma, urinary tract
  urethrostomy (stoma) —*see* Complications, stoma, urinary tract
  uterus, complicating delivery O62.9
    hypertonic O62.4
    hypotonic O62.2
      primary O62.0
      secondary O62.1
  ventricular I51.9
    with congestive heart failure —*see also* Failure, heart I50.9
    left, reversible, following sudden emotional stress I51.81
Dysgenesis
  gonadal (due to chromosomal anomaly) Q96.9
    pure Q99.1
  renal Q60.5
    bilateral Q60.4
    unilateral Q60.3
  reticular D72.0
  tidal platelet D69.3
Dysgerminoma
  specified site —*see* Neoplasm, malignant, by site
  unspecified site
    female C56.9
    male C62.90
Dysgeusia R43.2
Dysgraphia R27.8
Dyshidrosis, dysidrosis L30.1
Dyskaryotic cervical smear R87.619
Dyskeratosis L85.8
  cervix —*see* Dysplasia, cervix
  congenital Q82.8
  uterus NEC N85.8
Dyskinesia G24.9
  biliary (cystic duct or gallbladder) K82.8
  drug induced
    orofacial G24.01
  esophagus K22.4
  hysterical F44.4
  intestinal K59.89
  nonorganic origin F44.4
  orofacial (idiopathic) G24.4
    drug induced G24.01
  psychogenic F44.4
  subacute, drug induced G24.01
  tardive G24.01
    neuroleptic induced G24.01
  trachea J39.8
  tracheobronchial J98.09
Dyslalia (developmental) F80.0
Dyslexia R48.0
  developmental F81.0
Dyslipidemia E78.5
  depressed HDL cholesterol E78.6
  elevated fasting triglycerides E78.1
Dysmaturity —*see also* Light for dates
  pulmonary (newborn) (Wilson-Mikity) P27.0
Dysmenorrhea (essential) (exfoliative) N94.6
  congestive (syndrome) N94.6
  primary N94.4
  psychogenic F45.8
  secondary N94.5
Dysmetabolic syndrome X E88.81
Dysmetria R27.8
Dysmorphism (due to)
  alcohol Q86.0
  exogenous cause NEC Q86.8
  hydantoin Q86.1
  warfarin Q86.2

Dysmorphophobia (nondelusional) F45.22
  delusional F22
Dysnomia R47.01
Dysorexia R63.0
  psychogenic F50.89
Dysostosis
  cleidocranial, cleidocranialis Q74.0
  craniofacial Q75.1
  Fairbank's (idiopathic familial generalized osteophytosis) Q78.9
  mandibulofacial (incomplete) Q75.4
  multiplex E76.01
  oculomandibular Q75.5
Dyspareunia (female) N94.10
  deep N94.12
  male N53.12
  nonorganic F52.6
  psychogenic F52.6
  secondary N94.19
  specified NEC N94.19
  superficial (introital) N94.11
Dyspepsia R10.13
  atonic K30
  functional (allergic) (congenital) (gastrointestinal) (occupational) (reflex) K30
  intestinal K59.89
  nervous F45.8
  neurotic F45.8
  psychogenic F45.8
Dysphagia R13.10
  cervical R13.19
  following
    cerebral infarction I69.391
    cerebrovascular disease I69.991
      specified NEC I69.891
    intracerebral hemorrhage I69.191
    nontraumatic intracranial hemorrhage NEC I69.291
    specified disease NEC I69.891
    subarachnoid hemorrhage I69.091
  functional (hysterical) F45.8
  hysterical F45.8
  nervous (hysterical) F45.8
  neurogenic R13.19
  oral phase R13.11
  oropharyngeal phase R13.12
  pharyngeal phase R13.13
  pharyngoesophageal phase R13.14
  psychogenic F45.8
  sideropenic D50.1
  spastica K22.4
  specified NEC R13.19
Dysphagocytosis, congenital D71
Dysphasia R47.02
  developmental
    expressive type F80.1
    receptive type F80.2
  following
    cerebrovascular disease I69.921
      cerebral infarction I69.321
      intracerebral hemorrhage I69.121
    nontraumatic intracranial hemorrhage NEC I69.221
      specified disease NEC I69.821
      subarachnoid hemorrhage I69.021
Dysphonia R49.0
  functional F44.4
  hysterical F44.4
  psychogenic F44.4
  spastica J38.3
Dysphoria
  gender F64.9
    in
      adolescence and adulthood F64.0
      children F64.2
    specified NEC F64.8
    postpartal O90.6
Dyspituitarism E23.3

Dysplasia —see also Anomaly
  acetabular, congenital Q65.89
  alveolar capillary, with vein misalignment
      J84.843
  anus (histologically confirmed) (mild)
      (moderate) K62.82
    severe D01.3
  arrhythmogenic right ventricular I42.8
  arterial, fibromuscular I77.3
  asphyxiating thoracic (congenital) Q77.2
  brain Q07.9
  bronchopulmonary, perinatal P27.1
  cervix (uteri) N87.9
    mild N87.0
    moderate N87.1
    severe D06.9
  chondroectodermal Q77.6
  colon D12.6
  craniometaphyseal Q78.58
  dentinal K00.5
  diaphyseal, progressive Q78.3
  dystrophic Q77.5
  ectodermal (anhidrotic) (congenital)
      (hereditary) Q82.4
    hydrotic Q82.8
  epithelial, uterine cervix —see Dysplasia,
      cervix
  eye (congenital) Q11.2
  fibrous
    bone NEC (monostotic) M85.00
      ankle M85.07-●
      foot M85.07-●
      forearm M85.03-●
      hand M85.04-●
      lower leg M85.06-●
      multiple site M85.09
      neck M85.08
      rib M85.08
      shoulder M85.01-●
      skull M85.08
      specified site NEC M85.08
      thigh M85.05-●
      toe M85.07-●
      upper arm M85.02-●
      vertebra M85.08
    diaphyseal, progressive Q78.3
    jaw M27.8
    polyostotic Q78.1
  florid osseous —see also Cyst, calcifying
      odontogenic
  high grade, focal D12.6
  hip, congenital Q65.89
  joint, congenital Q74.8
  kidney Q61.4
    multicystic Q61.4
  leg Q74.2
  lung, congenital (not associated with short
      gestation) Q33.6
  mammary (gland) (benign) N60.9-●
    cyst (solitary) —see Cyst, breast
    cystic —see Mastopathy, cystic
    duct ectasia —see Ectasia, mammary duct
    fibroadenosis —see Fibroadenosis, breast
    fibrosclerosis —see Fibrosclerosis, breast
    specified type NEC N60.8-●
  metaphyseal Q78.5
  muscle Q79.8
  oculodentodigital Q87.0
  periapical (cemental) (cemento-osseous) —see
      Cyst, calcifying odontogenic
  periosteum —see Disorder, bone, specified
      type NEC
  polyostotic fibrous Q78.1
  prostate —see also Neoplasia, intraepithelial,
      prostate N42.30
    severe D07.5
    specified type NEC N42.39
  renal Q61.4
    multicystic Q61.4
  retinal, congenital Q14.1
  right ventricular, arrhythmogenic I42.8

Dysplasia (Continued)
  septo-optic Q04.4
  skin L98.8
  spinal cord Q06.1
  spondyloepiphyseal Q77.7
  thymic, with immunodeficiency D82.1
  vagina N89.3
    mild N89.0
    moderate N89.1
    severe NEC D07.2
  vulva N90.3
    mild N90.0
    moderate N90.1
    severe NEC D07.1
Dysplasminogenemia E88.02
Dyspnea (nocturnal) (paroxysmal) R06.00
  asthmatic (bronchial) J45.909
    with
      bronchitis J45.909
        with
          exacerbation (acute) J45.901
          status asthmaticus J45.902
        chronic J44.9
      exacerbation (acute) J45.901
      status asthmaticus J45.902
  cardiac —see Failure, ventricular, left
  cardiac —see Failure, ventricular, left
  functional F45.8
  hyperventilation R06.4
  hysterical F45.8
  newborn P28.89
  psychogenic F45.8
  shortness of breath R06.02
  specified type NEC R06.09
Dyspraxia R27.8
  developmental (syndrome) F82
Dysproteinemia E88.09
Dysreflexia, autonomic G90.4
Dysrhythmia
  cardiac I49.9
    newborn
      bradycardia P29.12
        occurring before birth P03.819
          before onset of labor P03.810
          during labor P03.811
      tachycardia P29.11
    postoperative I97.89
  cerebral or cortical —see Epilepsy
Dyssomnia —see Disorder, sleep
Dyssynergia
  biliary K83.8
  bladder sphincter N36.44
  cerebellaris myoclonica (Hunt's ataxia) G11.19
Dysthymia F34.1
Dysthyroidism E07.9
Dystocia O66.9
  affecting newborn P03.1
  cervical (hypotonic) O62.2
    affecting newborn P03.6
    primary O62.0
    secondary O62.1
  contraction ring O62.4
  fetal O66.9
    abnormality NEC O66.3
    conjoined twins O66.3
    oversize O66.2
  maternal O66.9
  positional O64.9
  shoulder (girdle) O66.0
    causing obstructed labor O66.0
  uterine NEC O62.4
Dystonia G24.9
  cervical G24.3
  deformans progressiva G24.1
  drug induced NEC G24.09
    acute G24.02
    specified NEC G24.09
  familial G24.1
  idiopathic G24.1
    familial G24.1
    nonfamilial G24.2
    orofacial G24.4

Dystonia (Continued)
  lenticularis G24.8
  musculorum deformans G24.1
  neuroleptic induced (acute) G24.02
  orofacial (idiopathic) G24.4
  oromandibular G24.4
    due to drug G24.01
  specified NEC G24.8
  torsion (familial) (idiopathic) G24.1
    acquired G24.8
    genetic G24.1
    symptomatic (nonfamilial) G24.2
Dystonic movements R25.8
Dystrophy, dystrophia
  adiposogenital E23.6
  autosomal recessive, childhood type,
      muscular dystrophy resembling
      Duchenne or Becker G71.01
  Becker's type G71.01
  cervical sympathetic G90.2
  choroid (hereditary) H31.20
    central areolar H31.22
    choroideremia H31.21
    gyrate atrophy H31.23
    specified type NEC H31.29
  cornea (hereditary) H18.50-●
    endothelial H18.51-●
    epithelial H18.52-●
    granular H18.53-●
    lattice H18.54-●
    macular H18.55-●
    specified type NEC H18.59-●
  Duchenne's type G71.01
  due to malnutrition E45
  Erb's G71.02
  Fuchs' H18.51-●
  Gower's muscular G71.01
  hair L67.8
  infantile neuraxonal G31.89
  Landouzy-Déjérine G71.02
  Leyden-Möbius G71.09
  muscular G71.00
    autosomal recessive, childhood type,
        muscular dystrophy resembling
        Duchenne or Becker G71.01
    benign (Becker type) G71.01
      scapuloperoneal with early contractures
          [Emery-Dreifuss] G71.09
    congenital (hereditary) (progressive) (with
        specific morphological abnormalities
        of the muscle fiber) G71.09
      myotonic G71.11
    distal G71.09
    Duchenne type G71.01
    Emery-Dreifuss G71.09
    Erb type G71.02
    facioscapulohumeral G71.02
    Gower's G71.01
    hereditary (progressive) G71.09
    Landouzy-Déjérine type G71.02
    limb-girdle G71.09
    myotonic G71.11
    progressive (hereditary) G71.09
      Charcot-Marie (-Tooth) type G60.0
    pseudohypertrophic (infantile) G71.01
    scapulohumeral G71.02
    scapuloperoneal G71.09
    severe (Duchenne type) G71.01
    specified type NEC G71.09
  myocardium, myocardial —see
      Degeneration, myocardial
  nail L60.3
    congenital Q84.6
  nutritional E45
  ocular G71.09
  oculocerebrorenal E72.03
  oculopharyngeal G71.09
  ovarian N83.8
  polyglandular E31.8
  reflex (neuromuscular) (sympathetic) —
      see Syndrome, pain, complex regional I

Dystrophy, dystrophia *(Continued)*
  retinal (hereditary) H35.50
    in
      lipid storage disorders E75.6 *[H36]*
      systemic lipidoses E75.6 *[H36]*
    involving
      pigment epithelium H35.54
      sensory area H35.53
    pigmentary H35.52
    vitreoretinal H35.51

Dystrophy, dystrophia *(Continued)*
  Salzmann's nodular —*see* Degeneration,
    cornea, nodular
  scapuloperoneal G71.09
  skin NEC L98.8
  sympathetic (reflex) —*see* Syndrome, pain,
    complex regional I
    cervical G90.2
  tapetoretinal H35.54

Dystrophy, dystrophia *(Continued)*
  thoracic, asphyxiating Q77.2
  unguium L60.3
    congenital Q84.6
  vitreoretinal H35.51
  vulva N90.4
  yellow (liver) —*see* Failure, hepatic
Dysuria R30.0
  psychogenic F45.8

▶ New   ⇒ Revised   ~~deleted~~ Deleted   ● Use Additional Character(s)

E

Eales' disease H35.06-•
Ear —*see also* condition
  piercing Z41.3
  tropical NEC B36.9 *[H62.40]*
  in
    aspergillosis B44.89
    candidiasis B37.84
    moniliasis B37.84
  wax (impacted) H61.20
    left H61.22
      with right H61.23
    right H61.21
      with left H61.23
Earache —*see* subcategory H92.0
Early satiety R68.81
Eaton-Lambert syndrome—*see* Syndrome,
  Lambert-Eaton
Eberth's disease (typhoid fever) A01.00
Ebola virus disease A98.4
Ebstein's anomaly or syndrome (heart) Q22.5
Eccentro-osteochondrodysplasia E76.29
Ecchondroma —*see* Neoplasm, bone, benign
Ecchondrosis D48.0
Ecchymosis R58
  conjunctiva —*see* Hemorrhage, conjunctiva
  eye (traumatic) —*see* Contusion, eyeball
  eyelid (traumatic) —*see* Contusion, eyelid
  newborn P54.5
  spontaneous R23.3
  traumatic —*see* Contusion
Echinococciasis —*see* Echinococcus
Echinococcosis —*see* Echinococcus
Echinococcus (infection) B67.90
  granulosus B67.4
    bone B67.2
    liver B67.0
    lung B67.1
    multiple sites B67.32
    specified site NEC B67.39
    thyroid B67.31
  liver NOS B67.8
    granulosus B67.0
    multilocularis B67.5
  lung NEC B67.99
    granulosus B67.1
    multilocularis B67.69
  multilocularis B67.7
    liver B67.5
    multiple sites B67.61
    specified site NEC B67.69
  specified site NEC B67.99
    granulosus B67.39
    multilocularis B67.69
  thyroid NEC B67.99
    granulosus B67.31
    multilocularis B67.69 *[E35]*
Echinorhynchiasis B83.8
Echinostomiasis B66.8
Echolalia R48.8
Echovirus, as cause of disease classified
  elsewhere B97.12
Eclampsia, eclamptic (coma) (convulsions)
  (delirium) (with hypertension) NEC O15.9
  complicating
    labor and delivery O15.1
    postpartum O15.2
    pregnancy O15.0-•
    puerperium O15.2
Economic circumstances affecting care Z59.9
Economo's disease A85.8
Ectasia, ectasis
  annuloaortic I35.8
  aorta I77.819
    with aneurysm —*see* Aneurysm, aorta
    abdominal I77.811
    thoracic I77.810
    thoracoabdominal I77.812
  breast —*see* Ectasia, mammary duct
  capillary I78.8
  cornea H18.71-•

Ectasia, ectasis *(Continued)*
  gastric antral vascular (GAVE) K31.819
    with hemorrhage K31.811
    without hemorrhage K31.819
  mammary duct N60.4-•
  salivary gland (duct) K11.8
  sclera —*see* Sclerectasia
Ecthyma L08.0
  contagiosum B08.02
  gangrenosum L08.0
  infectiosum B08.02
Ectocardia Q24.8
Ectodermal dysplasia (anhidrotic) Q82.4
Ectodermosis erosiva pluriorificialis
  L51.1
Ectopic, ectopia (congenital)
  abdominal viscera Q45.8
    due to defect in anterior abdominal wall
      Q79.59
  ACTH syndrome E24.3
  adrenal gland Q89.1
  anus Q43.5
  atrial beats I49.1
  beats I49.49
    atrial I49.1
    ventricular I49.3
  bladder Q64.10
  bone and cartilage in lung Q33.5
  brain Q04.8
  breast tissue Q83.8
  cardiac Q24.8
  cerebral Q04.8
  cordis Q24.8
  endometrium —*see* Endometriosis
  gastric mucosa Q40.2
  gestation —*see* Pregnancy, by site
  heart Q24.8
  hormone secretion NEC E34.2
  kidney (crossed) (pelvis) Q63.2
  lens, lentis Q12.1
  mole —*see* Pregnancy, by site
  organ or site NEC —*see* Malposition,
    congenital
  pancreas Q45.3
  pregnancy —*see* Pregnancy, ectopic
  pupil —*see* Abnormality, pupillary
  renal Q63.2
  sebaceous glands of mouth Q38.6
  spleen Q89.09
  testis Q53.00
    bilateral Q53.02
    unilateral Q53.01
  thyroid Q89.2
  tissue in lung Q33.5
  ureter Q62.63
  ventricular beats I49.3
  vesicae Q64.10
Ectromelia Q73.8
  lower limb —*see* Defect, reduction, limb,
    lower, specified type NEC
  upper limb —*see* Defect, reduction, limb,
    upper, specified type NEC
Ectropion H02.109
  cervix N86
    with cervicitis N72
  congenital Q10.1
  eyelid H02.109
    cicatricial H02.119
      left H02.116
        lower H02.115
        upper H02.114
      right H02.113
        lower H02.112
        upper H02.111
    congenital Q10.1
    left H02.106
      lower H02.105
      upper H02.104
    mechanical H02.129
      left H02.126
        lower H02.125
        upper H02.124

Ectropion *(Continued)*
  eyelid *(Continued)*
    mechanical *(Continued)*
      right H02.123
        lower H02.122
        upper H02.121
    paralytic H02.159
      left H02.156
        lower H02.155
        upper H02.154
      right H02.153
        lower H02.152
        upper H02.151
    right H02.103
      lower H02.102
      upper H02.101
    senile H02.139
      left H02.136
        lower H02.135
        upper H02.134
      right H02.133
        lower H02.132
        upper H02.131
    spastic H02.149
      left H02.146
        lower H02.145
        upper H02.144
      right H02.143
        lower H02.142
        upper H02.141
  iris H21.89
  lip (acquired) K13.0
    congenital Q38.0
  urethra N36.8
  uvea H21.89
Eczema (acute) (chronic) (erythematous)
  (fissum) (rubrum) (squamous) (*see also*
  Dermatitis) L30.9
  contact —*see* Dermatitis, contact
  dyshydrotic L30.1
  external ear —*see* Otitis, externa, acute,
    eczematoid
  flexural L20.82
  herpeticum B00.0
  hypertrophicum L28.0
  hypostatic —*see* Varix, leg, with,
    inflammation
  impetiginous L01.1
  infantile (due to any substance) L20.83
    intertriginous L21.1
    seborrheic L21.1
  intertriginous NEC L30.4
    infantile L21.1
  intrinsic (allergic) L20.84
  lichenified NEC L28.0
  marginatum (hebrae) B35.6
  pustular L30.3
  stasis I87.2
    with varicose veins —*see* Varix, leg, with,
      inflammation
  vaccination, vaccinatum T88.1
  varicose —*see* Varix, leg, with, inflammation
Eczematid L30.2
Eddowes (-Spurway) **syndrome** Q78.0
Edema, edematous (infectious) (pitting)
  (toxic) R60.9
  with nephritis —*see* Nephrosis
  allergic T78.3
  amputation stump (surgical) (sequelae
    (late effect)) T87.89
  angioneurotic (allergic) (any site) (with
    urticaria) T78.3
    hereditary D84.1
  angiospastic I73.9
  Berlin's (traumatic) S05.8X-•
  brain (cytotoxic) (vasogenic) G93.6
    due to birth injury P11.0
    newborn (anoxia or hypoxia) P52.4
      birth injury P11.0
    traumatic —*see* Injury, intracranial,
      cerebral edema
  cardiac —*see* Failure, heart, congestive

Edema, edematous (Continued)
cardiovascular —see Failure, heart, congestive
cerebral —see Edema, brain
cerebrospinal —see Edema, brain
cervix (uteri) (acute) N88.8
  puerperal, postpartum O90.89
chronic hereditary Q82.0
circumscribed, acute T78.3
  hereditary D84.1
conjunctiva H11.42-●
cornea H18.2-●
  idiopathic H18.22-●
  secondary H18.23-●
    due to contact lens H18.21-●
due to
  lymphatic obstruction I89.0
  salt retention E87.0
epiglottis —see Edema, glottis
essential, acute T78.3
  hereditary D84.1
extremities, lower —see Edema, legs
eyelid NEC H02.849
  left H02.846
    lower H02.845
    upper H02.844
  right H02.843
    lower H02.842
    upper H02.841
familial, hereditary Q82.0
famine —see Malnutrition, severe
generalized R60.1
glottis, glottic, glottidis (obstructive) (passive)
    J38.4
  allergic T78.3
    hereditary D84.1
heart —see Failure, heart, congestive
heat T67.7
hereditary Q82.0
inanition —see Malnutrition, severe
intracranial G93.6
iris H21.89
joint —see Effusion, joint
larynx —see Edema, glottis
legs R60.0
  due to venous obstruction I87.1
  hereditary Q82.0
localized R60.0
  due to venous obstruction I87.1
lower limbs —see Edema, legs
lung J81.1
  with heart condition or failure —see
    Failure, ventricular, left
  acute J81.0
  chemical (acute) J68.1
    chronic J68.1
  chronic J81.1
    due to
      chemicals, gases, fumes or vapors
        (inhalation) J68.1
      external agent J70.9
        specified NEC J70.8
      radiation J70.1
  due to
    chemicals, fumes or vapors (inhalation)
      J68.1
    external agent J70.9
      specified NEC J70.8
    high altitude T70.29
    near drowning T75.1
    radiation J70.0
  meaning failure, left ventricle I50.1
lymphatic I89.0
  due to mastectomy I97.2
macula H35.81
  cystoid, following cataract surgery —see
    Complications, postprocedural,
    following cataract surgery
  diabetic —see Diabetes, by type, with,
    retinopathy, with macular edema
malignant —see Gangrene, gas
Milroy's Q82.0

Edema, edematous (Continued)
nasopharynx J39.2
newborn P83.30
  hydrops fetalis —see Hydrops, fetalis
  specified NEC P83.39
nutritional —see also Malnutrition, severe
  with dyspigmentation, skin and hair E40
optic disc or nerve —see Papilledema
orbit H05.22-●
pancreas K86.89
papilla, optic —see Papilledema
penis N48.89
periodic T78.3
  hereditary D84.1
pharynx J39.2
pulmonary —see Edema, lung
Quincke's T78.3
  hereditary D84.1
renal —see Nephrosis
retina H35.81
  diabetic —see Diabetes, by type, with,
    retinopathy, with macular edema
salt E87.0
scrotum N50.89
seminal vesicle N50.89
spermatic cord N50.89
spinal (cord) (vascular) (nontraumatic) G95.19
starvation —see Malnutrition, severe
stasis —see Hypertension, venous, (chronic)
subglottic —see Edema, glottis
supraglottic —see Edema, glottis
testis N44.8
tunica vaginalis N50.89
vas deferens N50.89
vulva (acute) N90.89
Edentulism —see Absence, teeth, acquired
Edsall's disease T67.2
Educational handicap Z55.9
▶less than a high school diploma Z55.5
▶no general equivalence degree (GED) Z55.5
  specified NEC Z55.8
Edward's syndrome —see Trisomy, 18
Effect, adverse
abnormal gravitational (G) forces or states
    T75.81
abuse —see Maltreatment
air pressure T70.9
  specified NEC T70.8
altitude (high) —see Effect, adverse, high
    altitude
anesthesia —see also Anesthesia T88.59
  in labor and delivery O74.9
  local, toxic
    in labor and delivery O74.4-●
    in pregnancy NEC O29.3-●
    postpartum, puerperal O89.3
  postpartum, puerperal O89.9
  specified NEC T88.59
    in labor and delivery O74.8
    postpartum, puerperal O89.8
  spinal and epidural T88.59
    headache T88.59
      in labor and delivery O74.5
      postpartum, puerperal O89.4
    specified NEC
      in labor and delivery O74.6
      postpartum, puerperal O89.5
antitoxin —see Complications, vaccination
atmospheric pressure T70.9
  due to explosion T70.8
  high T70.3
  low —see Effect, adverse, high altitude
  specified effect NEC T70.8
biological, correct substance properly
    administered —see Effect, adverse, drug
blood (derivatives) (serum) (transfusion) —
    see Complications, transfusion
chemical substance —see Table of Drugs and
    Chemicals
cold (temperature) (weather) T69.9
  chilblains T69.1
  frostbite —see Frostbite
  specified effect NEC T69.8

Effect, adverse (Continued)
drugs and medicaments T88.7
  specified drug —see Table of Drugs and
    Chemicals, by drug, adverse effect
  specified effect — code to condition
electric current, electricity (shock) T75.4
  burn —see Burn
exertion (excessive) T73.3
exposure —see Exposure
external cause NEC T75.89
foodstuffs T78.1
  allergic reaction —see Allergy, food
    causing anaphylaxis —see Shock,
      anaphylactic, due to food
  noxious —see Poisoning, food, noxious
gases, fumes, or vapors T59.9-●
  specified agent —see Table of Drugs and
    Chemicals
glue (airplane) sniffing
  due to drug abuse —see Abuse, drug,
    inhalant
  due to drug dependence —see Dependence,
    drug, inhalant
heat —see Heat
high altitude NEC T70.29
  anoxia T70.29
  on
    ears T70.0
    sinuses T70.1
  polycythemia D75.1
high pressure fluids T70.4
hot weather —see Heat
hunger T73.0
immersion, foot —see Immersion
immunization —see Complications,
    vaccination
immunological agents —see Complications,
    vaccination
infrared (radiation) (rays) NOS T66
  dermatitis or eczema L59.8
infusion —see Complications, infusion
lack of care of infants —see Maltreatment,
    child
lightning —see Lightning
medical care T88.9
  specified NEC T88.8
medicinal substance, correct, properly
    administered —see Effect, adverse, drug
motion T75.3
noise, on inner ear —see subcategory H83.3
overheated places —see Heat
psychosocial, of work environment Z56.5
radiation (diagnostic) (infrared) (natural
    source) (therapeutic) (ultraviolet) (X-ray)
    NOS T66
  dermatitis or eczema —see Dermatitis, due
    to, radiation
  fibrosis of lung J70.1
  pneumonitis J70.0
  pulmonary manifestations
    acute J70.0
    chronic J70.1
  skin L59.9
radioactive substance NOS
  dermatitis or eczema —see Radiodermatitis
reduced temperature T69.9
  immersion foot or hand —see Immersion
  specified effect NEC T69.8
serum NEC (see also Reaction, serum) T80.69
specified NEC T78.8
  external cause NEC T75.89
strangulation —see Asphyxia, traumatic
submersion T75.1
thirst T73.1
toxic —see Toxicity
transfusion —see Complications, transfusion
ultraviolet (radiation) (rays) NOS T66
  burn —see Burn
  dermatitis or eczema —see Dermatitis, due
    to, ultraviolet rays
    acute L56.8

▶ New   ⇒ Revised   ~~deleted~~ Deleted   ● Use Additional Character(s)

Effect, adverse (Continued)
vaccine (any) —see Complications, vaccination
vibration —see Vibration, adverse effects
water pressure NEC T70.9
specified NEC T70.8
weightlessness T75.82
whole blood —see Complications, transfusion
work environment Z56.5
Effect(s) (of) (from) —see Effect, adverse NEC
Effects, late —see Sequelae
Effluvium
anagen L65.1
telogen L65.0
Effort syndrome (psychogenic) F45.8
Effusion
➡ amniotic fluid —see Pregnancy, complicated
by, premature rupture of membranes
brain (serous) G93.6
bronchial —see Bronchitis
cerebral G93.6
cerebrospinal —see also Meningitis
vessel G93.6
chest —see Effusion, pleura
chylous, chyliform (pleura) J94.0
intracranial G93.6
joint M25.40
ankle M25.47-●
elbow M25.42-●
foot joint M25.47-●
hand joint M25.44-●
hip M25.45-●
knee M25.46-●
shoulder M25.41-●
specified joint NEC M25.48
wrist M25.43-●
malignant pleural J91.0
meninges —see Meningitis
pericardium, pericardial (noninflammatory)
I31.3
acute —see Pericarditis, acute
peritoneal (chronic) R18.8
pleura, pleurisy, pleuritic, pleuropericardial
J90
chylous, chyliform J94.0
due to systemic lupus erythematosis
M32.13
in conditions classified elsewhere J91.8
influenzal —see Influenza, with, respiratory
manifestations NEC
malignant J91.0
newborn P28.89
tuberculous NEC A15.6
primary (progressive) A15.7
spinal —see Meningitis
thorax, thoracic —see Effusion, pleura
Egg shell nails L60.3
congenital Q84.6
EGPA (eosinophilic granulomatosis with
polyangiitis) M30.1
Egyptian splenomegaly B65.1
Ehlers-Danlos syndrome (see also Syndrome,
Ehlers-Danlos) Q79.60
Ehrlichiosis A77.40
due to
E. chafeensis A77.41
E. ewingii A77.49
E. muris euclairensis A77.49
E. sennetsu A79.81
specified organism NEC A77.49
Eichstedt's disease B36.0
Eisenmenger's
complex or syndrome I27.83
defect Q21.8
Ejaculation
delayed F52.32
painful N53.12
premature F52.4
retarded N53.11
retrograde N53.14
semen, painful N53.12
psychogenic F52.6

Ekbom's syndrome (restless legs) G25.81
Ekman's syndrome (brittle bones and blue
sclera) Q78.0
Elastic skin Q82.8
acquired L57.4
Elastofibroma —see Neoplasm, connective
tissue, benign
Elastoma (juvenile) Q82.8
Miescher's L87.2
Elastomyofibrosis I42.4
Elastosis
actinic, solar L57.8
atrophicans (senile) L57.4
perforans serpiginosa L87.2
senilis L57.4
Elbow —see condition
Electric current, electricity, effects (concussion)
(fatal) (nonfatal) (shock) T75.4
burn —see Burn
Electric feet syndrome E53.8
Electrocution T75.4
from electroshock gun (taser) T75.4
Electrolyte imbalance E87.8
with
abortion —see Abortion by type,
complicated by, electrolyte imbalance
ectopic pregnancy O08.5
molar pregnancy O08.5
Elephantiasis (nonfilarial) I89.0
arabicum —see Infestation, filarial
bancroftian B74.0
congenital (any site) (hereditary) Q82.0
due to
Brugia (malayi) B74.1
timori B74.2
mastectomy I97.2
Wuchereria (bancrofti) B74.0
eyelid H02.859
left H02.856
lower H02.855
upper H02.854
right H02.853
lower H02.852
upper H02.851
filarial, filariensis —see Infestation, filarial
glandular I89.0
graecorum A30.9
lymphangiectatic I89.0
lymphatic vessel I89.0
due to mastectomy I97.2
scrotum (nonfilarial) I89.0
streptococcal I89.0
surgical I97.89
postmastectomy I97.2
telangiectodes I89.0
vulva (nonfilarial) N90.89
Elevated, elevation
alanine transaminase (ALT) R74.01
ALT (alanine transaminase) R74.01
antibody titer R76.0
aspartate transaminase (AST) R74.01
AST (aspartate transaminase) R74.01
basal metabolic rate R94.8
blood pressure —see also Hypertension
reading (incidental) (isolated) (nonspecific),
no diagnosis of hypertension R03.0
blood sugar R73.9
body temperature (of unknown origin) R50.9
C-reactive protein (CRP) R79.82
cancer antigen 125 [CA 125] R97.1
carcinoembryonic antigen [CEA] R97.0
cholesterol E78.00
with high triglycerides E78.2
conjugate, eye H51.0
diaphragm, congenital Q79.1
erythrocyte sedimentation rate R70.0
fasting glucose R73.01
fasting triglycerides E78.1
finding on laboratory examination —see
Findings, abnormal, inconclusive,
without diagnosis, by type of exam

Elevated, elevation (Continued)
GFR (glomerular filtration rate) —see
Findings, abnormal, inconclusive,
without diagnosis, by type of exam
glucose tolerance (oral) R73.02
immunoglobulin level R76.8
indoleacetic acid R82.5
lactic acid dehydrogenase (LDH) level R74.02
leukocytes D72.829
lipoprotein a (Lp(a)) level E78.41
liver function
study R94.5
test R79.89
alkaline phosphatase R74.8
aminotransferase R74.01
bilirubin R17
hepatic enzyme R74.8
lactate dehydrogenase R74.02
(Lp(a)) (lipoprotein(a)) E78.41
lymphocytes D72.820
prostate specific antigen [PSA] R97.20
Rh titer —see Complication(s), transfusion,
incompatibility reaction, Rh (factor)
scapula, congenital Q74.0
sedimentation rate R70.0
SGOT R74.01
SGPT R74.01
transaminase level R74.01
triglycerides E78.1
with high cholesterol E78.2
troponin R77.8
tumor associated antigens [TAA] NEC R97.8
tumor specific antigens [TSA] NEC R97.8
urine level of
17-ketosteroids R82.5
catecholamine R82.5
indoleacetic acid R82.5
steroids R82.5
vanillylmandelic acid (VMA) R82.5
venous pressure I87.8
white blood cell count D72.829
specified NEC D72.828
Elliptocytosis (congenital) (hereditary) D58.1
Hb C (disease) D58.1
hemoglobin disease D58.1
sickle-cell (disease) D57.8-●
trait D57.3
Ellison-Zollinger syndrome E16.4
Ellis-van Creveld syndrome
(chondroectodermal dysplasia) Q77.6
Elongated, elongation (congenital) —see also
Distortion
bone Q79.9
cervix (uteri) Q51.828
acquired N88.4
hypertrophic N88.4
colon Q43.8
common bile duct Q44.5
cystic duct Q44.5
frenulum, penis Q55.69
labia minora (acquired) N90.69
ligamentum patellae Q74.1
petiolus (epiglottidis) Q31.8
tooth, teeth K00.2
uvula Q38.6
Eltor cholera A00.1
➡ **Emaciation** R64
▶ due to malnutrition E43
Embadomoniasis A07.8
Embedded tooth, teeth K01.0
root only K08.3
Embolic —see condition
Embolism (multiple) (paradoxical) I74.9
air (any site) (traumatic) T79.0
following
abortion —see Abortion by type
complicated by embolism
ectopic pregnancy O08.2
infusion, therapeutic injection or
transfusion T80.0
molar pregnancy O08.2

Embolism *(Continued)*
  air *(Continued)*
    following *(Continued)*
      procedure NEC
        artery T81.719
          mesenteric T81.710
          renal T81.711
          specified NEC T81.718
        vein T81.72
    in pregnancy, childbirth or puerperium —*see* Embolism, obstetric
  amniotic fluid (pulmonary) —*see also* Embolism, obstetric
    following
      abortion —*see* Abortion by type complicated by embolism
      ectopic pregnancy O08.2
      molar pregnancy O08.2
  aorta, aortic I74.10
    abdominal I74.09
      saddle I74.01
    bifurcation I74.09
    saddle I74.01
    thoracic I74.11
  artery I74.9
    auditory, internal I65.8
    basilar —*see* Occlusion, artery, basilar
    carotid (common) (internal) —*see* Occlusion, artery, carotid
    cerebellar (anterior inferior) (posterior inferior) (superior) I66.3
    cerebral —*see* Occlusion, artery, cerebral
    choroidal (anterior) I65.8
    communicating posterior I65.8
    coronary —*see also* Infarct, myocardium
      not resulting in infarction I24.0
    extremity I74.4
      lower I74.3
      upper I74.2
    hypophyseal I65.8
    iliac I74.5
    limb I74.4
      lower I74.3
      upper I74.2
    mesenteric (with gangrene) —*see also* Ischemia, intestine, acute K55.09
    ophthalmic —*see* Occlusion, artery, retina
    peripheral I74.4
    pontine I65.8
    precerebral —*see* Occlusion, artery, precerebral
    pulmonary —*see* Embolism, pulmonary
    renal N28.0
    retinal —*see* Occlusion, artery, retina
    septic I76
    specified NEC I74.8
    vertebral —*see* Occlusion, artery, vertebral
  basilar (artery) I65.1
  blood clot
    following
      abortion —*see* Abortion by type complicated by embolism
      ectopic or molar pregnancy O08.2
    in pregnancy, childbirth or puerperium —*see* Embolism, obstetric
  brain —*see also* Occlusion, artery, cerebral
    following
      abortion —*see* Abortion by type complicated by embolism
      ectopic or molar pregnancy O08.2
    puerperal, postpartum, childbirth —*see* Embolism, obstetric
  capillary I78.8
  cardiac —*see also* Infarct, myocardium
    not resulting in infarction I51.3
  carotid (artery) (common) (internal) —*see* Occlusion, artery, carotid
  cavernous sinus (venous) —*see* Embolism, intracranial venous sinus
  cerebral —*see* Occlusion, artery, cerebral
  cholesterol —*see* Atheroembolism

Embolism *(Continued)*
  coronary (artery or vein) (systemic) —*see* Occlusion, coronary
  due to device, implant or graft —*see also* Complications, by site and type, specified NEC
    arterial graft NEC T82.818
    breast (implant) T85.818
    catheter NEC T85.818
      dialysis (renal) T82.818
        intraperitoneal T85.818
      infusion NEC T82.818
        spinal (epidural) (subdural) T85.810
      urinary (indwelling) T83.81
    electronic (electrode) (pulse generator) (stimulator)
      bone T84.81
      cardiac T82.817
      nervous system (brain) (peripheral nerve) (spinal) T85.810
      urinary T83.81
    fixation, internal (orthopedic) NEC T84.81
    gastrointestinal (bile duct) (esophagus) T85.818
    genital NEC T83.81
    heart (graft) (valve) T82.817
    joint prosthesis T84.81
    ocular (corneal graft) (orbital implant) T85.818
    orthopedic (bone graft) NEC T86.838
    specified NEC T85.818
    urinary (graft) NEC T83.81
    vascular NEC T82.818
    ventricular intracranial shunt T85.810
  extremities
    lower —*see* Embolism, vein, lower extremity
      arterial I74.3
    upper I74.2
  eye H34.9
  fat (cerebral) (pulmonary) (systemic) T79.1
    complicating delivery —*see* Embolism, obstetric
    following
      abortion —*see* Abortion by type complicated by embolism
      ectopic or molar pregnancy O08.2
  following
    abortion —*see* Abortion by type complicated by embolism
    ectopic or molar pregnancy O08.2
    infusion, therapeutic injection or transfusion air T80.0
  heart (fatty) —*see also* Infarct, myocardium
    not resulting in infarction I51.3
  hepatic (vein) I82.0
  in pregnancy, childbirth or puerperium —*see* Embolism, obstetric
  intestine (artery) (vein) (with gangrene) —*see also* Ischemia, intestine, acute K55.039
  intracranial —*see also* Occlusion, artery, cerebral
    venous sinus (any) G08
      nonpyogenic I67.6
  intraspinal venous sinuses or veins G08
    nonpyogenic G95.19
  kidney (artery) N28.0
  lateral sinus (venous) —*see* Embolism, intracranial, venous sinus
  leg —*see* Embolism, vein, lower extremity
    arterial I74.3
  longitudinal sinus (venous) —*see* Embolism, intracranial, venous sinus
  lung (massive) —*see* Embolism, pulmonary
  meninges I66.8
  mesenteric (artery) (vein) (with gangrene) —*see also* Ischemia, intestine, acute K55.059
  obstetric (in) (pulmonary)
    childbirth O88.22
      air O88.02
      amniotic fluid O88.12

Embolism *(Continued)*
  obstetric *(Continued)*
    childbirth *(Continued)*
      blood clot O88.22
      fat O88.82
      pyemic O88.32
      septic O88.32
      specified type NEC O88.82
    pregnancy O88.21-●
      air O88.01-●
      amniotic fluid O88.11-●
      blood clot O88.21-●
      fat O88.81-●
      pyemic O88.31-●
      septic O88.31-●
      specified type NEC O88.81-●
    puerperal O88.23
      air O88.03
      amniotic fluid O88.13
      blood clot O88.23
      fat O88.83
      pyemic O88.33
      septic O88.33
      specified type NEC O88.83
  ophthalmic —*see* Occlusion, artery, retina
  penis N48.81
  peripheral artery NOS I74.4
  pituitary E23.6
  popliteal (artery) I74.3
  portal (vein) I81
  postoperative, postprocedural
    artery T81.719
      mesenteric T81.710
      renal T81.711
      specified NEC T81.718
    vein T81.72
  precerebral artery —*see* Occlusion, artery, precerebral
  puerperal —*see* Embolism, obstetric
  pulmonary (acute) (artery) (vein) I26.99
    with acute cor pulmonale I26.09
    chronic I27.82
    following
      abortion —*see* Abortion by type complicated by embolism
      ectopic or molar pregnancy O08.2
    healed or old Z86.711
    in pregnancy, childbirth or puerperium —*see* Embolism, obstetric
    multiple subsegmental without acute cor pulmonale I26.94
    personal history of Z86.711
    saddle I26.92
      with acute cor pulmonale I26.02
    septic I26.90
      with acute cor pulmonale I26.01
    single subsegmental without acute cor pulmonale I26.93
    subsegmental NOS I26.93
  pyemic (multiple) I76
    following
      abortion —*see* Abortion by type complicated by embolism
      ectopic or molar pregnancy O08.2
    Hemophilus influenzae A41.3
    pneumococcal A40.3
      with pneumonia J13
    puerperal, postpartum, childbirth (any organism) —*see* Embolism, obstetric
    specified organism NEC A41.89
    staphylococcal A41.2
    streptococcal A40.9
  renal (artery) N28.0
    vein I82.3
  retina, retinal —*see* Occlusion, artery, retina
  saddle
    abdominal aorta I74.01
    pulmonary artery I26.92
      with acute cor pulmonale I26.02

▶ New   ➡ Revised   ~~deleted~~ Deleted   ● Use Additional Character(s)

Embolism *(Continued)*
 septic (arterial) I76
  complicating abortion —*see* Abortion, by
   type, complicated by, embolism
 sinus —*see* Embolism, intracranial, venous
  sinus
 soap complicating abortion —*see* Abortion,
  by type, complicated by, embolism
 spinal cord G95.19
  pyogenic origin G06.1
 spleen, splenic (artery) I74.8
 upper extremity I74.2
 vein (acute) I82.90
  antecubital I82.61-●
   chronic I82.71-●
  axillary I82.A1-●
   chronic I82.A2-●
  basilic I82.61-●
   chronic I82.71-●
  brachial I82.62-●
   chronic I82.72-●
  brachiocephalic (innominate) I82.290
   chronic I82.291
  cephalic I82.61-●
   chronic I82.71-●
  chronic I82.91
  deep (DVT) I82.40-●
   calf I82.4Z-●
    chronic I82.5Z-●
   lower leg I82.4Z-●
    chronic I82.5Z-●
   thigh I82.4Y-●
    chronic I82.5Y-●
   upper leg I82.4Y
    chronic I82.5y--●
  femoral I82.41-●
   chronic I82.51 ●
  iliac (iliofemoral) I82.42-●
   chronic I82.52-●
  innominate I82.290
   chronic I82.291
  internal jugular I82.C1-●
   chronic I82.C2-●
  lower extremity
   deep I82.40-●
    chronic I82.50-●
    specified NEC I82.49-●
     chronic NEC I82.59-●
   distal
    deep I82.4Z-●
   proximal
    deep I82.4Y-●
     chronic I82.5Y-●
   superficial I82.81-●
  popliteal I82.43-●
   chronic I82.53-●
  radial I82.62-●
   chronic I82.72-●
  renal I82.3
  saphenous (greater) (lesser) I82.81-●
  specified NEC I82.890
   chronic NEC I82.891
  subclavian I82.B1-●
   chronic I82.B2-●
  thoracic NEC I82.290
   chronic I82.291
  tibial I82.44-●
   chronic I82.54-●
  ulnar I82.62-●
   chronic I82.72-●
  upper extremity I82.60-●
   chronic I82.70-●
   deep I82.62-●
    chronic I82.72-●
   superficial I82.61-●
    chronic I82.71-●
 vena cava
  inferior (acute) I82.220
   chronic I82.221
  superior (acute) I82.210
   chronic I82.211

Embolism *(Continued)*
 venous sinus G08
 vessels of brain —*see* Occlusion, artery,
  cerebral
Embolus —*see* Embolism
Embryoma —*see also* Neoplasm, uncertain
  behavior, by site
 benign —*see* Neoplasm, benign, by site
 kidney C64.-●
 liver C22.0
 malignant —*see also* Neoplasm, malignant,
  by site
  kidney C64.-●
  liver C22.0
  testis C62.9-●
   descended (scrotal) C62.1-●
   undescended C62.0-●
 testis C62.9-●
  descended (scrotal) C62.1-●
  undescended C62.0-●
Embryonic
 circulation Q28.9
 heart Q28.9
 vas deferens Q55.4
Embryopathia NOS Q89.9
Embryotoxon Q13.4
Emesis —*see* Vomiting
Emotional lability R45.86
Emotionality, pathological F60.3
Emotogenic disease —*see* Disorder,
  psychogenic
Emphysema (atrophic) (bullous) (chronic)
  (interlobular) (lung) (obstructive)
  (pulmonary) (senile) (vesicular) J43.9
 cellular tissue (traumatic) T79.7
  surgical T81.82
 centrilobular J43.2
 compensatory J98.3
 congenital (interstitial) P25.0
 conjunctiva H11.89
 connective tissue (traumatic) T79.7
  surgical T81.82
 due to chemicals, gases, fumes or vapors J68.4
 eyelid(s) —*see* Disorder, eyelid, specified type
   NEC
  surgical T81.82
  traumatic T79.7
 interstitial J98.2
  congenital P25.0
  perinatal period P25.0
 laminated tissue T79.7
  surgical T81.82
 mediastinal J98.2
  newborn P25.2
 orbit, orbital —*see* Disorder, orbit, specified
   type NEC
 panacinar J43.1
 panlobular J43.1
 specified NEC J43.8
 subcutaneous (traumatic) T79.7
  nontraumatic J98.2
  postprocedural T81.82
  surgical T81.82
 surgical T81.82
 thymus (gland) (congenital) E32.8
 traumatic (subcutaneous) T79.7
 unilateral J43.0
Empty nest syndrome Z60.0
Empyema (acute) (chest) (double) (pleura)
  (supradiaphragmatic) (thorax) J86.9
 with fistula J86.0
 accessory sinus (chronic) —*see* Sinusitis
 antrum (chronic) —*see* Sinusitis, maxillary
 brain (any part) —*see* Abscess, brain
 ethmoidal (chronic) (sinus) —*see* Sinusitis,
   ethmoidal
 extradural —*see* Abscess, extradural
 frontal (chronic) (sinus) —*see* Sinusitis, frontal
 gallbladder K81.0
 mastoid (process) (acute) —*see* Mastoiditis,
   acute
 maxilla, maxillary M27.2

Empyema *(Continued)*
 sinus (chronic) —*see* Sinusitis, maxillary
 nasal sinus (chronic) —*see* Sinusitis
 sinus (accessory) (chronic) (nasal) —*see*
   Sinusitis
 sphenoidal (sinus) (chronic) —*see* Sinusitis,
   sphenoidal
 subarachnoid —*see* Abscess, extradural
 subdural —*see* Abscess, subdural
 tuberculous A15.6
 ureter —*see* Ureteritis
 ventricular —*see* Abscess, brain
En coup de sabre lesion L94.1
Enamel pearls K00.2
Enameloma K00.2
Enanthema, viral B09
Encephalitis (chronic) (hemorrhagic)
  (idiopathic) (nonepidemic) (spurious)
  (subacute) G04.90
 acute —*see also* Encephalitis, viral A86
  disseminated G04.00
   infectious G04.01
   noninfectious G04.81
   postimmunization (postvaccination)
     G04.02
   postinfectious G04.01
  inclusion body A85.8
  necrotizing hemorrhagic G04.30
   postimmunization G04.32
   postinfectious G04.31
   specified NEC G04.39
 arboviral, arbovirus NEC A85.2
 arthropod-borne NEC (viral) A85.2
 Australian A83.4
 California (virus) A83.5
 Central European (tick-borne) A84.1
 Czechoslovakian A84.1
 Dawson's (inclusion body) A81.1
 diffuse sclerosing A81.1
 disseminated, acute G04.00
 due to
  cat scratch disease A28.1
  human immunodeficiency virus (HIV)
    disease B20 *[G05.3]*
  malaria —*see* Malaria
  rickettsiosis —*see* Rickettsiosis
  smallpox inoculation G04.02
  typhus —*see* Typhus
 Eastern equine A83.2
 endemic (viral) A86
 epidemic NEC (viral) A86
 equine (acute) (infectious) (viral) A83.9
  Eastern A83.2
  Venezuelan A92.2
  Western A83.1
 Far Eastern (tick-borne) A84.0
 following vaccination or other immunization
    procedure G04.02
 herpes zoster B02.0
 herpesviral B00.4
  due to herpesvirus 6 B10.01
  due to herpesvirus 7 B10.09
  specified NEC B10.09
 Ilheus (virus) A83.8
 in (due to)
  actinomycosis A42.82
  adenovirus A85.1
  African trypanosomiasis B56.9 *[G05.3]*
  Chagas' disease (chronic) B57.42
  cytomegalovirus B25.8
  enterovirus A85.0
  herpes (simplex) virus B00.4
   due to herpesvirus 6 B10.01
   due to herpesvirus 7 B10.09
   specified NEC B10.09
  infectious disease NEC B99 *[G05.3]*
  influenza —*see* Influenza, with,
    encephalopathy
  listeriosis A32.12
  measles B05.0
  mumps B26.2
  naegleriasis B60.2

Encephalitis *(Continued)*
  in *(Continued)*
    parasitic disease NEC B89 *[G05.3]*
    poliovirus A80.9 *[G05.3]*
    rubella B06.01
    syphilis
      congenital A50.42
      late A52.14
    systemic lupus erythematosus M32.19
    toxoplasmosis (acquired) B58.2
      congenital P37.1
    tuberculosis A17.82
    zoster B02.0
  inclusion body A81.1
  infectious (acute) (virus) NEC A86
  Japanese (B type) A83.0
  La Crosse A83.5
  lead —*see* Poisoning, lead
  lethargica (acute) (infectious) A85.8
  louping ill A84.89
  lupus erythematosus, systemic M32.19
  lymphatica A87.2
  Mengo A85.8
  meningococcal A39.81
  Murray Valley A83.4
  otitic NEC H66.40 *[G05.3]*
  parasitic NOS B71.9
  periaxial G37.0
  periaxialis (concentrica) (diffuse) G37.5
  postchickenpox B01.11
  postexanthematous NEC B09
  postimmunization G04.02
  postinfectious NEC G04.01
  postmeasles B05.0
  postvaccinal G04.02
  postvaricella B01.11
  postviral NEC A86
  Powassan A84.81
  Rasmussen G04.81
  Rio Bravo A85.8
  Russian
    autumnal A83.0
    spring-summer (taiga) A84.0
  saturnine —*see* Poisoning, lead
  specified NEC G04.81
  St. Louis A83.3
  subacute sclerosing A81.1
  summer A83.0
  suppurative G04.81
  tick-borne A84.9
  Torula, torular (cryptococcal) B45.1
  ➡toxic NEC G92.8
  trichinosis B75 *[G05.3]*
  type
    B A83.0
    C A83.3
  van Bogaert's A81.1
  Venezuelan equine A92.2
  Vienna A85.8
  viral, virus A86
    arthropod-borne NEC A85.2
      mosquito-borne A83.9
        Australian X disease A83.4
        California virus A83.5
        Eastern equine A83.2
        Japanese (B type) A83.0
        Murray Valley A83.4
        specified NEC A83.8
        St. Louis A83.3
        type B A83.0
        type C A83.3
        Western equine A83.1
      tick-borne A84.9
        biundulant A84.1
        central European A84.1
        Czechoslovakian A84.1
        diphasic meningoencephalitis A84.1
        Far Eastern A84.0
        Russian spring-summer (taiga) A84.0
        specified NEC A84.89
      specified type NEC A85.8
      tick-borne, specified NEC A84.89
  Western equine A83.1

Encephalocele Q01.9
  frontal Q01.0
  nasofrontal Q01.1
  occipital Q01.2
  specified NEC Q01.8
Encephalocystocele —*see* Encephalocele
Encephaloduroarteriomyosynangiosis
  (EDAMS) I67.5
Encephalomalacia (brain) (cerebellar)
  (cerebral) —*see* Softening, brain
Encephalomeningitis —*see*
  Meningoencephalitis
Encephalomeningocele —*see* Encephalocele
Encephalomeningomyelitis —*see*
  Meningoencephalitis
Encephalomyelitis —*see also* Encephalitis G04.90
  acute disseminated G04.00
    infectious G04.01
    noninfectious G04.81
    postimmunization G04.02
    postinfectious G04.01
  acute necrotizing hemorrhagic G04.30
    postimmunization G04.32
    postinfectious G04.31
    specified NEC G04.39
  benign myalgic G93.3
  equine A83.9
    Eastern A83.2
    Venezuelan A92.2
    Western A83.1
  in diseases classified elsewhere G05.3
  myalgic, benign G93.3
  postchickenpox B01.11
  postinfectious NEC G04.01
  postmeasles B05.0
  postvaccinal G04.02
  postvaricella B01.11
  rubella B06.01
  specified NEC G04.81
  Venezuelan equine A92.2
Encephalomyelocele —*see* Encephalocele
Encephalomyelomeningitis —*see*
  Meningoencephalitis
Encephalomyelopathy G96.9
Encephalomyeloradiculitis (acute) G61.0
Encephalomyeloradiculoneuritis (acute)
  (Guillain-Barré) G61.0
Encephalomyeloradiculopathy G96.9
Encephalopathia hyperbilirubinemica,
  newborn P57.9
  due to isoimmunization (conditions in P55)
    P57.0
Encephalopathy (acute) G93.40
  acute necrotizing hemorrhagic G04.30
    postimmunization G04.32
    postinfectious G04.31
    specified NEC G04.39
  alcoholic G31.2
  anoxic —*see* Damage, brain, anoxic
  arteriosclerotic I67.2
  centrolobar progressive (Schilder) G37.0
  congenital Q07.9
  degenerative, in specified disease NEC G32.89
  due to
    ➡drugs (*see also* Table of Drugs and
      Chemicals) G92.8
  demyelinating callosal G37.1
  hepatic —*see* Failure, hepatic
  hyperbilirubinemic, newborn P57.9
    due to isoimmunization (conditions in P55)
      P57.0
  hypertensive I67.4
  hypoglycemic E16.2
  hypoxic —*see* Damage, brain, anoxic
  hypoxic ischemic P91.60
    mild P91.61
    moderate P91.62
    severe P91.63
  in (due to) (with)
    birth injury P11.1
    hyperinsulinism E16.1 *[G94]*

Encephalopathy *(Continued)*
  in *(Continued)*
    influenza —*see* Influenza, with,
      encephalopathy
    lack of vitamin (*see also* Deficiency, vitamin)
      E56.9 *[G32.89]*
    neoplastic disease (*see also* Neoplasm)
      D49.9 *[G13.1]*
    serum (*see also* Reaction, serum) T80.69
    syphilis A52.17
    trauma (postconcussional) F07.81
      current injury —*see* Injury, intracranial
    vaccination G04.02
  lead —*see* Poisoning, lead
  metabolic G93.41
  ➡drug induced G92.8
  ➡toxic G92.8
  myoclonic, early, symptomatic —*see* Epilepsy,
    generalized, specified NEC
  necrotizing, subacute (Leigh) G31.82
  neonatal P91.819
    in diseases classified elsewhere P91.811
  pellagrous E52 *[G32.89]*
  portosystemic —*see* Failure, hepatic
  postcontusional F07.81
    current injury —*see* Injury, intracranial,
      diffuse
  posthypoglycemic (coma) E16.1 *[G94]*
  postradiation G93.89
  saturnine —*see* Poisoning, lead
  septic G93.41
  specified NEC G93.49
  spongiform, subacute (viral) A81.09
  ➡toxic G92.8
  ➡metabolic G92.8
  traumatic (postconcussional) F07.81
    current injury —*see* Injury, intracranial
  vitamin B deficiency NEC E53.9 *[G32.89]*
    vitamin B1 E51.2
  Wernicke's E51.2
Encephalorrhagia —*see* Hemorrhage,
  intracranial, intracerebral
Encephalosis, posttraumatic F07.81
Enchondroma —*see also* Neoplasm, bone,
  benign
Enchondromatosis (cartilaginous) (multiple)
  Q78.4
Encopresis R15.9
  functional F98.1
  nonorganic origin F98.1
  psychogenic F98.1
Encounter (with health service) (for) Z76.89
  adjustment and management (of)
    breast implant Z45.81
    implanted device NEC Z45.89
    myringotomy device (stent) (tube)
      Z45.82
    neurostimulator (brain) (gastric)
      (peripheral nerve) (sacral nerve)
      (spinal cord) (vagus nerve) Z45.42
  administrative purpose only Z02.9
    examination for
      adoption Z02.82
      armed forces Z02.3
      disability determination Z02.71
      driving license Z02.4
      employment Z02.1
      insurance Z02.6
      medical certificate NEC Z02.79
      paternity testing Z02.81
      residential institution admission Z02.2
      school admission Z02.0
      sports Z02.5
      specified reason NEC Z02.89
  aftercare —*see* Aftercare
  antenatal screening Z36.9
    cervical length Z36.86
    chromosomal anomalies Z36.0
    congenital cardiac abnormalities Z36.83
    elevated maternal serum alphafetoprotein
      level Z36.1

▶ New   ⇒ Revised   ~~deleted~~ Deleted   ● Use Additional Character(s)

Encounter *(Continued)*
  antenatal screening *(Continued)*
    fetal growth retardation Z36.4
    fetal lung maturity Z36.84
    fetal macrosomia Z36.88
    hydrops fetalis Z36.81
    intrauterine growth restriction (IUGR)/
      small-for-dates Z36.4
    isoimmunization Z36.5
    large-for-dates Z36.88
    malformations Z36.3
    non-visualized anatomy on a previous scan
      Z36.2
    nuchal translucency Z36.82
    raised alphafetoprotein level Z36.1
    risk of pre-term labor Z36.86
    specified type NEC Z36.89
    specified follow-up NEC Z36.2
    specified genetic defects NEC Z36.8A
    Streptococcus B Z36.85
    suspected anomaly Z36.3
    uncertain dates Z36.87
  assisted reproductive fertility procedure cycle
    Z31.83
  blood typing Z01.83
    Rh typing Z01.83
  breast augmentation or reduction Z41.1
  breast implant exchange (different material)
    (different size) Z45.81
  breast reconstruction following mastectomy
    Z42.1
  check-up —*see* Examination
  chemotherapy for neoplasm Z51.11
  colonoscopy, screening Z12.11
  counseling —*see* Counseling
  delivery, full-term, uncomplicated O80
    cesarean, without indication O82
  desensitization to allergens Z51.6
  ear piercing Z41.3
  examination —*see* Examination
  expectant parent(s) (adoptive) pre-birth
    pediatrician visit Z76.81
  fertility preservation procedure (prior to
    cancer therapy) (prior to removal of
    gonads) Z31.84
  fitting (of) —*see* Fitting (and adjustment) (of)
  genetic
    counseling
      nonprocreative Z71.83
      procreative Z31.5
    testing —*see* Test, genetic
  hearing conservation and treatment Z01.12
  immunotherapy for neoplasm Z51.12
  in vitro fertilization cycle Z31.83
  instruction (in)
    child care (postpartal) (prenatal) Z32.3
    childbirth Z32.2
    natural family planning
      procreative Z31.61
      to avoid pregnancy Z30.02
  insulin pump titration Z46.81
  joint prosthesis insertion following prior
    explantation of joint prosthesis (staged
    procedure)
    hip Z47.32
    knee Z47.33
    shoulder Z47.31
  laboratory (as part of a general medical
    examination) Z00.00
    with abnormal findings Z00.01
  mental health services (for)
    abuse NEC
      perpetrator Z69.82
      victim Z69.81
    child abuse
      nonparental
        perpetrator Z69.021
        victim Z69.020
      parental
        perpetrator Z69.011
        victim Z69.010

Encounter *(Continued)*
  mental health services *(Continued)*
    child neglect
      nonparental
        perpetrator Z69.021
        victim Z69.020
      parental
        perpetrator Z69.011
        victim Z69.010
    child psychological abuse
      nonparental
        perpetrator Z69.021
        victim Z69.020
      parental
        perpetrator Z69.011
        victim Z69.010
    child sexual abuse
      nonparental
        perpetrator Z69.021
        victim Z69.020
      parental
        perpetrator Z69.011
        victim Z69.010
    non-spousal adult abuse
      perpetrator Z69.82
      victim Z69.81
    spousal or partner
      abuse
        perpetrator Z69.12
        victim Z69.11
      neglect
        perpetrator Z69.12
        victim Z69.11
      psychological abuse
        perpetrator Z69.12
        victim Z69.11
      violence
        perpetrator (physical) (sexual)
          Z69.12
        victim (physical) Z69.11
          sexual Z69.81
  observation (for) (ruled out)
    exposure to (suspected)
      anthrax Z03.810
      biological agent NEC Z03.818
  pediatrician visit, by expectant parent(s)
    (adoptive) Z76.81
  placental sample (taken vaginally) —*see also*
    Encounter, antenatal screening Z36.9
  plastic and reconstructive surgery following
    medical procedure or healed injury NEC
    Z42.8
  pregnancy
    supervision of —*see* Pregnancy,
      supervision of
    test Z32.00
      result negative Z32.02
      result positive Z32.01
  procreative management and counseling for
    gestational carrier Z31.7
  prophylactic measures Z29.9
    antivenin Z29.12
    fluoride administration Z29.3
    immunotherapy for respiratory syncytial
      virus (RSV) Z29.11
    rabies immune globin Z29.14
    Rho (D) immune globulin Z29.13
    specified NEC Z29.8
  radiation therapy (antineoplastic) Z51.0
  radiological (as part of a general medical
    examination) Z00.00
    with abnormal findings Z00.01
  reconstructive surgery following medical
    procedure or healed injury NEC
    Z42.8
  removal (of) —*see also* Removal
    artificial
      arm Z44.00-•
        complete Z44.01-•
        partial Z44.02-•
      eye Z44.2-•

Encounter *(Continued)*
  removal *(Continued)*
    artificial *(Continued)*
      leg Z44.10-•
        complete Z44.11-•
        partial Z44.12-•
    breast implant Z45.81
      tissue expander (with or without
        synchronous insertion of permanent
        implant) Z45.81
    device Z46.9
      specified NEC Z46.89
    external
      fixation device — code to fracture with
        seventh character D
      prosthesis, prosthetic device Z44.9
        breast Z44.3-•
        specified NEC Z44.8
    implanted device NEC Z45.89
    insulin pump Z46.81
    internal fixation device Z47.2
    myringotomy device (stent) (tube) Z45.82
    nervous system device NEC Z46.2
      brain neuropacemaker Z46.2
      visual substitution device Z46.2
        implanted Z45.31
    non-vascular catheter Z46.82
    orthodontic device Z46.4
    stent
      ureteral Z46.6
    urinary device Z46.6
  repeat cervical smear to confirm findings of
    recent normal smear following initial
    abnormal smear Z01.42
  respirator [ventilator] use during power
    failure (Z99.12)
  Rh typing Z01.83
  screening —*see* Screening
  specified NEC Z76.89
  sterilization Z30.2
  suspected condition, ruled out
    amniotic cavity and membrane Z03.71
    cervical shortening Z03.75
    fetal anomaly Z03.73
    fetal growth Z03.74
    maternal and fetal conditions NEC
      Z03.79
    oligohydramnios Z03.71
    placental problem Z03.72
    polyhydramnios Z03.71
  suspected exposure (to), ruled out
    anthrax Z03.810
    biological agents NEC Z03.818
  termination of pregnancy, elective Z33.2
  testing —*see* Test
  therapeutic drug level monitoring Z51.81
  titration, insulin pump Z46.81
  to determine fetal viability of pregnancy
    O36.80
  training
    insulin pump Z46.81
  X-ray of chest (as part of a general medical
    examination Z00.00)
    with abnormal findings Z00.01
Encystment —*see* Cyst
Endarteritis (bacterial, subacute) (infective)
  I77.6
  brain I67.7
  cerebral or cerebrospinal I67.7
  deformans —*see* Arteriosclerosis
  embolic —*see* Embolism
  obliterans —*see also* Arteriosclerosis
    pulmonary I28.8
  pulmonary I28.8
  retina —*see* Vasculitis, retina
  senile —*see* Arteriosclerosis
  syphilitic A52.09
    brain or cerebral A52.04
    congenital A50.54 *[I79.8]*
  tuberculous A18.89
Endemic —*see* condition

Endocarditis (chronic) (marantic) (nonbacterial)
(thrombotic) (valvular) I38
  with rheumatic fever (conditions in I00)
    active —*see* Endocarditis, acute,
      rheumatic
    inactive or quiescent (with chorea) I09.1
  acute or subacute I33.9
    infective I33.0
    rheumatic (aortic) (mitral) (pulmonary)
      (tricuspid) I01.1
      with chorea (acute) (rheumatic)
        (Sydenham's) I02.0
  aortic (heart) (nonrheumatic) (valve) I35.8
    with
      mitral disease I08.0
        with tricuspid (valve) disease I08.3
        active or acute I01.1
          with chorea (acute) (rheumatic)
            (Sydenham's) I02.0
        rheumatic fever (conditions in I00)
          active —*see* Endocarditis, acute,
            rheumatic
          inactive or quiescent (with chorea)
            I06.9
      tricuspid (valve) disease I08.2
        with mitral (valve) disease I08.3
    acute or subacute I33.9
    arteriosclerotic I35.8
    rheumatic I06.9
      with mitral disease I08.0
        with tricuspid (valve) disease I08.3
        active or acute I01.1
          with chorea (acute) (rheumatic)
            (Sydenham's) I02.0
      active or acute I01.1
        with chorea (acute) (rheumatic)
          (Sydenham's) I02.0
      specified NEC I06.8
    specified cause NEC I35.8
    syphilitic A52.03
  arteriosclerotic I38
  atypical verrucous (Libman-Sacks) M32.11
  bacterial (acute) (any valve) (subacute) I33.0
  candidal B37.6
  congenital Q24.8
  constrictive I33.0
  Coxiella burnetii A78 [*I39*]
  Coxsackie B33.21
  due to
    prosthetic cardiac valve T82.6
    Q fever A78 [*I39*]
    Serratia marcescens I33.0
    typhoid (fever) A01.02
  gonococcal A54.83
  infectious or infective (acute) (any valve)
    (subacute) I33.0
  lenta (acute) (any valve) (subacute) I33.0
  Libman-Sacks M32.11
  listerial A32.82
  Löffler's I42.3
  malignant (acute) (any valve) (subacute) I33.0
  meningococcal A39.51
  mitral (chronic) (double) (fibroid) (heart)
    (inactive) (valve) (with chorea) I05.9
    with
      aortic (valve) disease I08.0
        with tricuspid (valve) disease I08.3
        active or acute I01.1
          with chorea (acute) (rheumatic)
            (Sydenham's) I02.0
      rheumatic fever (conditions in I00)
        active —*see* Endocarditis, acute,
          rheumatic
        inactive or quiescent (with chorea)
          I05.9
      tricuspid (valve) disease I08.1
        with aortic (valve) disease I08.3
    active or acute I01.1
      with chorea (acute) (rheumatic)
        (Sydenham's) I02.0
    bacterial I33.0

Endocarditis (*Continued*)
  mitral (*Continued*)
    arteriosclerotic I34.8
    nonrheumatic I34.8
      acute or subacute I33.9
    specified NEC I05.8
  monilial B37.6
  multiple valves I08.9
    specified disorders I08.8
  mycotic (acute) (any valve) (subacute) I33.0
  pneumococcal (acute) (any valve) (subacute)
    I33.0
  pulmonary (chronic) (heart) (valve) I37.8
    with rheumatic fever (conditions in I00)
      active —*see* Endocarditis, acute,
        rheumatic
      inactive or quiescent (with chorea) I09.89
        with aortic, mitral or tricuspid disease
          I08.8
    acute or subacute I33.9
      rheumatic I01.1
        with chorea (acute) (rheumatic)
          (Sydenham's) I02.0
    arteriosclerotic I37.8
    congenital Q22.2
    rheumatic (chronic) (inactive) (with chorea)
      I09.89
      active or acute I01.1
        with chorea (acute) (rheumatic)
          (Sydenham's) I02.0
    syphilitic A52.03
  purulent (acute) (any valve) (subacute) I33.0
  Q fever A78 [*I39*]
  rheumatic (chronic) (inactive) (with chorea)
    I09.1
    active or acute (aortic) (mitral)
      (pulmonary) (tricuspid) I01.1
      with chorea (acute) (rheumatic)
        (Sydenham's) I02.0
  rheumatoid —*see* Rheumatoid, carditis
  septic (acute) (any valve) (subacute) I33.0
  streptococcal (acute) (any valve) (subacute)
    I33.0
  subacute —*see* Endocarditis, acute
  suppurative (acute) (any valve) (subacute)
    I33.0
  syphilitic A52.03
  toxic I33.9
  tricuspid (chronic) (heart) (inactive)
    (rheumatic) (valve) (with chorea) I07.9
    with
      aortic (valve) disease I08.2
        mitral (valve) disease I08.3
      mitral (valve) disease I08.1
        aortic (valve) disease I08.3
      rheumatic fever (conditions in I00)
        active —*see* Endocarditis, acute,
          rheumatic
        inactive or quiescent (with chorea)
          I07.8
    active or acute I01.1
      with chorea (acute) (rheumatic)
        (Sydenham's) I02.0
    arteriosclerotic I36.8
    nonrheumatic I36.8
      acute or subacute I33.9
    specified cause, except rheumatic I36.8
  tuberculous —*see* Tuberculosis, endocarditis
  typhoid A01.02
  ulcerative (acute) (any valve) (subacute) I33.0
  vegetative (acute) (any valve) (subacute) I33.0
  verrucous (atypical) (nonbacterial)
    (nonrheumatic) M32.11
Endocardium, endocardial —*see also* condition
  cushion defect Q21.2
Endocervicitis —*see also* Cervicitis
  due to intrauterine (contraceptive) device
    T83.69
  hyperplastic N72
Endocrine —*see* condition
Endocrinopathy, pluriglandular E31.9

Endodontic
  overfill M27.52
  underfill M27.53
Endodontitis K04.01
  irreversible K04.02
  reversible K04.01
Endomastoiditis —*see* Mastoiditis
Endometrioma N80.9
Endometriosis N80.9
  appendix N80.5
  bladder N80.8
  bowel N80.5
  broad ligament N80.3
  cervix N80.0
  colon N80.5
  cul-de-sac (Douglas') N80.3
  exocervix N80.0
  fallopian tube N80.2
  female genital organ NEC N80.8
  gallbladder N80.8
  in scar of skin N80.6
  internal N80.0
  intestine N80.5
  lung N80.8
  myometrium N80.0
  ovary N80.1
  parametrium N80.3
  pelvic peritoneum N80.3
  peritoneal (pelvic) N80.3
  rectovaginal septum N80.4
  rectum N80.5
  round ligament N80.3
  skin (scar) N80.6
  specified site NEC N80.8
  stromal D39.0
  thorax N80.8
  umbilicus N80.8
  uterus (internal) N80.0
  vagina N80.4
  vulva N80.8
Endometritis (decidual) (nonspecific) (purulent)
  (senile (atrophic) (suppurative) N71.9
  with ectopic pregnancy O08.0
  acute N71.0
  blenorrhagic (gonococcal) (acute) (chronic)
    A54.24
  cervix, cervical (with erosion or ectropion) —
    see also Cervicitis
    hyperplastic N72
  chlamydial A56.11
  chronic N71.1
  following
    abortion —*see* Abortion by type
      complicated by genital infection
    ectopic or molar pregnancy O08.0
  gonococcal, gonorrheal (acute) (chronic) A54.24
  hyperplastic —*see also* Hyperplasia,
    endometrial N85.00-●
    cervix N72
  puerperal, postpartum, childbirth O86.12
  subacute N71.0
  tuberculous A18.17
Endometrium —*see* condition
Endomyocardiopathy, South African I42.3
Endomyocarditis —*see* Endocarditis
Endomyofibrosis I42.3
Endomyometritis —*see* Endometritis
Endopericarditis —*see* Endocarditis
Endoperineuritis —*see* Disorder, nerve
Endophlebitis —*see* Phlebitis
Endophthalmia —*see* Endophthalmitis,
  purulent
Endophthalmitis (acute) (infective) (metastatic)
  (subacute) H44.009
  bleb associated H59.4 —*see also* Bleb,
    inflamed (infected), postprocedural
  gonorrheal A54.39
  in (due to)
    cysticercosis B69.1
    onchocerciasis B73.01
    toxocariasis B83.0

▶ New   ⇒ Revised   ~~deleted~~ Deleted   ● Use Additional Character(s)

Endophthalmitis *(Continued)*
  panuveitis —*see* Panuveitis
  parasitic H44.12-●
  purulent H44.00-●
    panophthalmitis —*see* Panophthalmitis
    vitreous abscess H44.02-●
  specified NEC H44.19
  sympathetic —*see* Uveitis, sympathetic
Endosalpingioma D28.2
Endosalpingiosis N94.89
Endosteitis —*see* Osteomyelitis
Endothelioma, bone —*see* Neoplasm, bone, malignant
Endotheliosis (hemorrhagic infectional) D69.8
Endotoxemia — code to condition
Endotrachelitis —*see* Cervicitis
Engelmann (-Camurati) **syndrome** Q78.3
English disease —*see* Rickets
Engman's disease L30.3
Engorgement
  breast N64.59
    newborn P83.4
    puerperal, postpartum O92.79
  lung (passive) —*see* Edema, lung
  pulmonary (passive) —*see* Edema, lung
  stomach K31.89
  venous, retina —*see* Occlusion, retina, vein, engorgement
Enlargement, enlarged —*see also* Hypertrophy
  adenoids J35.2
    with tonsils J35.3
  alveolar ridge K08.89
    congenital —*see* Anomaly, alveolar
  apertures of diaphragm (congenital) Q79.1
  gingival K06.1
  heart, cardiac —*see* Hypertrophy, cardiac
  labium majus, childhood asymmetric (CALME) N90.61
  lacrimal gland, chronic H04.03-●
  liver —*see* Hypertrophy, liver
  lymph gland or node R59.9
    generalized R59.1
    localized R59.0
  orbit H05.34-●
  organ or site, congenital NEC —*see* Anomaly, by site
  parathyroid (gland) E21.0
  pituitary fossa R93.0
  prostate N40.0
    with lower urinary tract symptoms (LUTS) N40.1
    without lower urinary tract symptoms (LUTS) N40.0
  sella turcica R93.0
  spleen —*see* Splenomegaly
  thymus (gland) (congenital) E32.0
  thyroid (gland) —*see* Goiter
  tongue K14.8
  tonsils J35.1
    with adenoids J35.3
  uterus N85.2
  vestibular aqueduct Q16.5
Enophthalmos H05.40-●
  due to
    orbital tissue atrophy H05.41-●
    trauma or surgery H05.42-●
Enostosis M27.8
Entamebic, entamebiasis —*see* Amebiasis
Entanglement
  umbilical cord(s) O69.82
    with compression O69.2
    around neck (with compression) O69.81
      with compression O69.1
      without compression O69.81
    of twins in monoamniotic sac O69.2
    without compression O69.82
Enteralgia —*see* Pain, abdominal
Enteric —*see* condition

Enteritis (acute) (diarrheal) (hemorrhagic) (noninfective) K52.9
  adenovirus A08.2
  aertrycke infection A02.0
  allergic K52.29
    with
      eosinophilic gastritis or gastroenteritis K52.81
      food protein-induced enterocolitis syndrome K52.21
      food protein-induced enteropathy K52.22
      FPIES K52.21
  amebic (acute) A06.0
    with abscess —*see* Abscess, amebic
    chronic A06.1
      with abscess —*see* Abscess, amebic
      nondysenteric A06.2
    nondysenteric A06.2
  astrovirus A08.32
  bacillary NOS A03.9
  bacterial A04.9
    specified NEC A04.8
  calicivirus A08.31
  candidal B37.82
  Chilomastix A07.8
  choleriformis A00.1
  chronic (noninfectious) K52.9
    ulcerative —*see* Colitis, ulcerative
  cicatrizing (chronic) —*see* Enteritis, regional, small intestine
  Clostridium
    botulinum (food poisoning) A05.1
    difficile
      not specified as recurrent A04.72
      recurrent A04.71
  coccidial A07.3
  coxsackie virus A08.39
  dietetic —*see also* Enteritis, allergic K52.29
  drug-induced K52.1
  due to
    astrovirus A08.32
    calicivirus A08.31
    coxsackie virus A08.39
    drugs K52.1
    echovirus A08.39
    enterovirus NEC A08.39
    food hypersensitivity —*see also* Enteritis, allergic K52.29
    infectious organism (bacterial) (viral) —*see* Enteritis, infectious
    torovirus A08.39
    Yersinia enterocolitica A04.6
  echovirus A08.39
  eltor A00.1
  enterovirus NEC A08.39
  eosinophilic K52.81
  epidemic (infectious) A09
  fulminant —*see also* Ischemia, intestine, acute K55.019
  gangrenous —*see* Enteritis, infectious
  giardial A07.1
  infectious NOS A09
    due to
      adenovirus A08.2
      Aerobacter aerogenes A04.8
      Arizona (bacillus) A02.0
      bacteria NOS A04.9
        specified NEC A04.8
      Campylobacter A04.5
      Clostridium difficile
        not specified as recurrent A04.72
        recurrent A04.71
      Clostridium perfringens A04.8
      Enterobacter aerogenes A04.8
      enterovirus A08.39
      Escherichia coli A04.4
        enteroaggregative A04.4
        enterohemorrhagic A04.3
        enteroinvasive A04.2
        enteropathogenic A04.0
        enterotoxigenic A04.1
        specified NEC A04.4

Enteritis *(Continued)*
  infectious NOS *(Continued)*
    due to *(Continued)*
      specified
        bacteria NEC A04.8
        virus NEC A08.39
      Staphylococcus A04.8
      virus NEC A08.4
        specified type NEC A08.39
      Yersinia enterocolitica A04.6
    specified organism NEC A08.8
  influenzal —*see* Influenza, with, digestive manifestations
  ischemic K55.9
    acute —*see also* Ischemia, intestine, acute K55.019
    chronic K55.1
  microsporidial A07.8
  mucomembranous, myxomembranous —*see* Syndrome, irritable bowel
  mucous —*see* Syndrome, irritable bowel
  necroticans A05.2
  necrotizing of newborn —*see* Enterocolitis, necrotizing, in newborn
  neurogenic —*see* Syndrome, irritable bowel
  newborn necrotizing —*see* Enterocolitis, necrotizing, in newborn
  noninfectious K52.9
  norovirus A08.11
  parasitic NEC B82.9
  paratyphoid (fever) —*see* Fever, paratyphoid
  protozoal A07.9
    specified NEC A07.8
  radiation K52.0
  regional (of) K50.90
    with
      complication K50.919
        abscess K50.914
        fistula K50.913
        intestinal obstruction K50.912
        rectal bleeding K50.911
        specified complication NEC K50.918
    colon —*see* Enteritis, regional, large intestine
    duodenum —*see* Enteritis, regional, small intestine
    ileum —*see* Enteritis, regional, small intestine
    jejunum —*see* Enteritis, regional, small intestine
    large bowel —*see* Enteritis, regional, large intestine
    large intestine (colon) (rectum) K50.10
      with
        complication K50.119
          abscess K50.114
          fistula K50.113
          intestinal obstruction K50.112
          rectal bleeding K50.111
          small intestine (duodenum) (ileum) (jejunum) involvement K50.80
          with
            complication K50.819
              abscess K50.814
              fistula K50.813
              intestinal obstruction K50.812
              rectal bleeding K50.811
              specified complication NEC K50.818
          specified complication NEC K50.118
    rectum —*see* Enteritis, regional, large intestine
    small intestine (duodenum) (ileum) (jejunum) K50.00
      with
        complication K50.019
          abscess K50.014
          fistula K50.013
          intestinal obstruction K50.012

Enteritis (Continued)
  regional (Continued)
    small intestine (Continued)
      with (Continued)
        complication (Continued)
          large intestine (colon) (rectum)
            involvement K50.80
            with
              complication K50.819
                abscess K50.814
                fistula K50.813
                intestinal obstruction
                  K50.812
                rectal bleeding K50.811
                specified complication NEC
                  K50.818
            rectal bleeding K50.011
            specified complication NEC
              K50.018
  rotaviral A08.0
  Salmonella, salmonellosis (arizonae)
    (cholerae-suis) (enteritidis)
    (typhimurium) A02.0
  segmental —see Enteritis, regional
  septic A09
  Shigella —see Infection, Shigella
  small round structured NEC A08.19
  spasmodic, spastic —see Syndrome, irritable
    bowel
  staphylococcal A04.8
    due to food A05.0
  torovirus A08.39
  toxic NEC K52.1
    due to Clostridium difficile
      not specified as recurrent A04.72
      recurrent A04.71
  trichomonal A07.8
  tuberculous A18.32
  typhosa A01.00
  ulcerative (chronic) —see Colitis, ulcerative
  viral A08.4
    adenovirus A08.2
    enterovirus A08.39
    Rotavirus A08.0
    small round structured NEC A08.19
    specified NEC A08.39
    virus specified NEC A08.39
Enterobiasis B80
Enterobius vermicularis (infection) (infestation)
  B80
Enterocele —see also Hernia, abdomen
  pelvic, pelvis (acquired) (congenital) N81.5
  vagina, vaginal (acquired) (congenital)
    NEC N81.5
Enterocolitis —see also Enteritis K52.9
  due to Clostridium difficile
    not specified as recurrent A04.72
    recurrent A04.71
  fulminant ischemic —see also Ischemia,
    intestine, acute K55.059
  granulomatous —see Enteritis, regional
  hemorrhagic (acute) —see also Ischemia,
    intestine, acute K55.059
    chronic K55.1
  infectious NEC A09
  ischemic K55.9
  necrotizing K55.30
    with
      perforation K55.33
      pneumatosis K55.32
      and perforation K55.33
    due to Clostridium difficile
      not specified as recurrent A04.72
      recurrent A04.71
    in non-newborn K55.30
      stage 1 (without pneumatosis, without
        perforation) K55.31
      stage 2 (with pneumatosis, without
        perforation) K55.32
      stage 3 (with pneumatosis, with
        perforation) K55.33

Enterocolitis (Continued)
  necrotizing (Continued)
    in newborn P77.9
      stage 1 (without pneumatosis, without
        perforation) P77.1
      stage 2 (with pneumatosis, without
        perforation) P77.2
      stage 3 (with pneumatosis, with
        perforation) P77.3
    without pneumatosis or perforation K55.31
  noninfectious K52.9
    newborn —see Enterocolitis, necrotizing, in
      newborn
  pseudomembranous (newborn)
    not specified as recurrent A04.72
    recurrent A04.71
  radiation K52.0
    newborn —see Enterocolitis, necrotizing, in
      newborn
  ulcerative (chronic) —see Pancolitis,
    ulcerative (chronic)
Enterogastritis —see Enteritis
Enteropathy K63.9
  celiac-gluten-sensitive K90.0
    non-celiac K90.41
  food protein-induced K52.22
  hemorrhagic, terminal —see also Ischemia,
    intestine, acute K55.059
  protein-losing K90.49
Enteroperitonitis —see Peritonitis
Enteroptosis K63.4
Enterorrhagia K92.2
Enterospasm —see also Syndrome, irritable,
  bowel
  psychogenic F45.8
Enterostenosis —see also Obstruction, intestine,
  specified NEC K56.699
Enterostomy
  complication —see Complication,
    enterostomy
  status Z93.4
Enterovirus, as cause of disease classified
  elsewhere B97.10
  coxsackievirus B97.11
  echovirus B97.12
  other specified B97.19
Enthesopathy (peripheral) M77.5-•
  Achilles tendinitis —see Tendinitis, Achilles
  ankle and tarsus M77.9
    specified type NEC —see Enthesopathy,
      foot, specified type NEC
  anterior tibial syndrome M76.81-•
  calcaneal spur —see Spur, bone, calcaneal
  elbow region M77.8
    lateral epicondylitis —see Epicondylitis,
      lateral
    medial epicondylitis —see Epicondylitis,
      medial
  foot NEC M77.8
    metatarsalgia —see Metatarsalgia
    specified type NEC M77.5-•
  forearm M77.8
  gluteal tendinitis —see Tendinitis, gluteal
  hand M77.8
  hip —see Enthesopathy, lower limb, specified
    type NEC
  iliac crest spur —see Spur, bone, iliac crest
  iliotibial band syndrome —see Syndrome,
    iliotibial band
  knee —see Enthesopathy, lower limb, lower
    leg, specified type NEC
  lateral epicondylitis —see Epicondylitis,
    lateral
  lower limb (excluding foot) M76.9
    Achilles tendinitis —see Tendinitis, Achilles
    ankle and tarsus M77.5-
      specified type NEC - see Enthesopathy,
        foot, specified type NEC
    anterior tibial syndrome M76.81-•
    gluteal tendinitis —see Tendinitis, gluteal
    iliac crest spur —see Spur, bone, iliac crest

Enthesopathy (Continued)
  lower limb (Continued)
    iliotibial band syndrome —see Syndrome,
      iliotibial band
    patellar tendinitis —see Tendinitis, patellar
    pelvic region —see Enthesopathy, lower
      limb, specified type NEC
    peroneal tendinitis —see Tendinitis,
      peroneal
    posterior tibial syndrome M76.82-•
    psoas tendinitis —see Tendinitis, psoas
    specified type NEC M76.89-•
    tibial collateral bursitis —see Bursitis, tibial
      collateral
  medial epicondylitis —see Epicondylitis,
    medial
  multiple sites M77.8
  patellar tendinitis —see Tendinitis, patellar
  pelvis M77.8
  periarthritis of wrist —see Periarthritis, wrist
  peroneal tendinitis —see Tendinitis, peroneal
  posterior tibial syndrome M76.82-•
  psoas tendinitis —see Tendinitis, psoas
  shoulder M77.8
  shoulder region —see Lesion, shoulder
  specified type NEC M77.8
  spinal M46.00
    cervical region M46.02
    cervicothoracic region M46.03
    lumbar region M46.06
    lumbosacral region M46.07
    multiple sites M46.09
    occipito-atlanto-axial region M46.01
    sacrococcygeal region M46.08
    thoracic region M46.04
    thoracolumbar region M46.05
  tibial collateral bursitis —see Bursitis, tibial
    collateral
  upper arm M77.8
  wrist and carpus NEC M77.8
    calcaneal spur —see Spur, bone, calcaneal
    periarthritis of wrist —see Periarthritis,
      wrist
Entomophobia F40.218
Entomophthoromycosis B46.8
Entrance, air into vein —see Embolism, air
Entrapment, nerve —see Neuropathy,
  entrapment
Entropion (eyelid) (paralytic) H02.009
  cicatricial H02.019
    left H02.016
      lower H02.015
      upper H02.014
    right H02.013
      lower H02.012
      upper H02.011
  congenital Q10.2
  left H02.006
    lower H02.005
    upper H02.004
  mechanical H02.029
    left H02.026
      lower H02.025
      upper H02.024
    right H02.023
      lower H02.022
      upper H02.021
  right H02.003
    lower H02.002
    upper H02.001
  senile H02.039
    left H02.036
      lower H02.035
      upper H02.034
    right H02.033
      lower H02.032
      upper H02.031
  spastic H02.049
    left H02.046
      lower H02.045
      upper H02.044

▶ New   ⇒ Revised   ~~deleted~~ Deleted   • Use Additional Character(s)

Entropion *(Continued)*
  spastic *(Continued)*
    right H02.043
      lower H02.042
      upper H02.041
Enucleated eye (traumatic, current) S05.7-•
Enuresis R32
  functional F98.0
  habit disturbance F98.0
  nocturnal N39.44
    psychogenic F98.0
  nonorganic origin F98.0
  psychogenic F98.0
Eosinopenia *—see* Agranulocytosis
Eosinophilia (allergic) (idiopathic) (secondary)
    D72.10
  with
    angiolymphoid hyperplasia (ALHE)
      D18.01
  familial D72.19
  hereditary D72.19
  in disease classified elsewhere D72.18
  infiltrative *—see* Eosinophilia, pulmonary
    Löffler's J82.89
  peritoneal *—see* Peritonitis, eosinophilic
  pulmonary NEC J82.89
    acute J82.82
    asthmatic J82.83
    chronic J82.81
    specified NEC D72.19
  tropical (pulmonary) J82.89
Eosinophilia-myalgia syndrome M35.89
Ependymitis (acute) (cerebral) (chronic)
    (granular) *—see* Encephalomyelitis
Ependymoblastoma
  specified site *—see* Neoplasm, malignant, by
    site
  unspecified site C71.9
Ependymoma (epithelial) (malignant)
  anaplastic
    specified site *—see* Neoplasm, malignant,
      by site
    unspecified site C71.9
  benign
    specified site *—see* Neoplasm, benign, by
      site
    unspecified site D33.2
  myxopapillary D43.2
    specified site *—see* Neoplasm, uncertain
      behavior, by site
    unspecified site D43.2
  papillary D43.2
    specified site *—see* Neoplasm, uncertain
      behavior, by site
    unspecified site D43.2
  specified site *—see* Neoplasm, malignant, by
    site
  unspecified site C71.9
Ependymopathy G93.89
Ephelis, ephelides L81.2
Epiblepharon (congenital) Q10.3
Epicanthus, epicanthic fold (eyelid)
    (congenital) Q10.3
Epicondylitis (elbow)
  lateral M77.1-•
  medial M77.0-•
Epicystitis *—see* Cystitis
Epidemic *—see* condition
Epidermidalization, cervix *—see* Dysplasia,
    cervix
Epidermis, epidermal *—see* condition
Epidermodysplasia verruciformis B07.8
Epidermolysis
  bullosa (congenital) Q81.9
    acquired L12.30
      drug-induced L12.31
      specified cause NEC L12.35
    dystrophica Q81.2
    letalis Q81.1
    simplex Q81.0
    specified NEC Q81.8

Epidermolysis *(Continued)*
  necroticans combustiformis L51.2
    due to drug *—see* Table of Drugs and
      Chemicals, by drug
Epidermophytid *—see* Dermatophytosis
Epidermophytosis (infected) *—see*
    Dermatophytosis
Epididymis *—see* condition
Epididymitis (acute) (nonvenereal) (recurrent)
    (residual) N45.1
  with orchitis N45.3
  blennorrhagic (gonococcal) A54.23
  caseous (tuberculous) A18.15
  chlamydial A56.19
  filarial *—see also* Infestation, filarial B74.9
    [N51]
  gonococcal A54.23
  syphilitic A52.76
  tuberculous A18.15
Epididymo-orchitis *—see also* Epididymitis
    N45.3
Epidural *—see* condition
Epigastrium, epigastric *—see* condition
Epigastrocele *—see* Hernia, ventral
Epiglottis *—see* condition
Epiglottitis, epiglottiditis (acute) J05.10
  with obstruction J05.11
  chronic J37.0
Epignathus Q89.4
Epilepsia partialis continua *—see also*
    Kozhevnikof's epilepsy G40.1-•
Epilepsy, epileptic, epilepsia (attack) (cerebral)
    (convulsion) (fit) (seizure) G40.909

> Note: the following terms are to be
> considered equivalent to intractable:
> pharmacoresistant (pharmacologically
> resistant), treatment resistant, refractory
> (medically) and poorly controlled

  with
    complex partial seizures *—see* Epilepsy,
      localization-related, symptomatic,
      with complex partial seizures
    grand mal seizures on awakening —
      see Epilepsy, generalized, specified
      NEC
    myoclonic absences *—see* Epilepsy,
      generalized, specified NEC
    myoclonic-astatic seizures *—see* Epilepsy,
      generalized, specified NEC
    simple partial seizures *—see* Epilepsy,
      localization-related, symptomatic,
      with simple partial seizures
  akinetic *—see* Epilepsy, generalized, specified
    NEC
  benign childhood with centrotemporal EEG
    spikes *—see* Epilepsy, localization-
    related, idiopathic
  benign myoclonic in infancy G40.80-•
  Bravais-jacksonian *—see* Epilepsy,
    localization-related, symptomatic,
    with simple partial seizures
  childhood
    with occipital EEG paroxysms *—see*
      Epilepsy, localization-related,
      idiopathic
    absence G40.A09
      intractable G40.A19
        with status epilepticus G40.A11
        without status epilepticus G40.A19
      not intractable G40.A09
        with status epilepticus G40.A01
        without status epilepticus G40.A09
  climacteric *—see* Epilepsy, specified NEC
  cysticercosis B69.0
  deterioration (mental) F06.8
  due to syphilis A52.19
  focal *—see* Epilepsy, localization-related,
    symptomatic, with simple partial
    seizures

Epilepsy, epileptic, epilepsia *(Continued)*
  generalized
    idiopathic G40.309
      intractable G40.319
        with status epilepticus G40.311
        without status epilepticus G40.319
      not intractable G40.309
        with status epilepticus G40.301
        without status epilepticus G40.309
    specified NEC G40.409
      intractable G40.419
        with status epilepticus G40.411
        without status epilepticus G40.419
      not intractable G40.409
        with status epilepticus G40.401
        without status epilepticus G40.409
  impulsive petit mal *—see* Epilepsy, juvenile
    myoclonic
  intractable G40.919
    with status epilepticus G40.911
    without status epilepticus G40.919
  juvenile absence G40.A09
    intractable G40.A19
      with status epilepticus G40.A11
      without status epilepticus G40.A19
    not intractable G40.A09
      with status epilepticus G40.A01
      without status epilepticus G40.A09
  juvenile myoclonic G40.B11
    intractable G40.B19
      with status epilepticus G40.B11
      without status epilepticus G40.B19
    not intractable G40.B09
      with status epilepticus G40.B01
      without status epilepticus G40.B09
  localization-related (focal) (partial)
    idiopathic G40.009
      with seizures of localized onset G40.009
        intractable G40.019
          with status epilepticus G40.011
          without status epilepticus G40.019
        not intractable G40.009
          with status epilepticus G40.001
          without status epilepticus G40.009
    symptomatic
      with complex partial seizures G40.209
        intractable G40.219
          with status epilepticus G40.211
          without status epilepticus G40.219
        not intractable G40.209
          with status epilepticus G40.201
          without status epilepticus
            G40.209
      with simple partial seizures G40.109
        intractable G40.119
          with status epilepticus G40.111
          without status epilepticus
            G40.119
        not intractable G40.109
          with status epilepticus G40.101
          without status epilepticus G40.109
  myoclonus, myoclonic *—see also* Epilepsy,
    generalized, specified NEC
    progressive *—see* Epilepsy, generalized,
      idiopathic
    severe, in infancy (SMEI) G40.83-•
  not intractable G40.909
    with status epilepticus G40.901
    without status epilepticus G40.909
  on awakening *—see* Epilepsy, generalized,
    specified NEC
  parasitic NOS B71.9 *[G94]*
  partialis continua *—see also* Kozhevnikof's
    epilepsy G40.1-•
  peripheral *—see* Epilepsy, specified NEC
  polymorphic, in infancy (PMEI) G40.83-•
  procursiva *—see* Epilepsy, localization-
    related, symptomatic, with simple
    partial seizures
  progressive (familial) myoclonic *—see*
    Epilepsy, generalized, idiopathic

Epilepsy, epileptic, epilepsia (Continued)
reflex —see Epilepsy, specified NEC
related to
alcohol G40.509
not intractable G40.509
with status epilepticus G40.501
without status epliepticus G40.509
drugs G40.509
not intractable G40.509
with status epilepticus G40.501
without status epliepticus G40.509
external causes G40.509
not intractable G40.509
with status epilepticus G40.501
without status epliepticus G40.509
hormonal changes G40.509
not intractable G40.509
with status epilepticus G40.501
without status epilepticus G40.509
sleep deprivation G40.509
not intractable G40.509
with status epilepticus G40.501
without status epliepticus G40.509
stress G40.509
not intractable G40.509
with status epilepticus G40.501
without status epliepticus G40.509
somatomotor —see Epilepsy, localization-
related, symptomatic, with simple
partial seizures
somatosensory —see Epilepsy, localization-
related, symptomatic, with simple
partial seizures
spasms G40.822
intractable G40.824
with status epilepticus G40.823
without status epilepticus G40.824
not intractable G40.822
with status epilepticus G40.821
without status epilepticus G40.822
specified NEC G40.802
intractable G40.804
with status epilepticus G40.803
without status epilepticus G40.804
not intractable G40.802
with status epilepticus G40.801
without status epilepticus G40.802
syndromes
generalized
idiopathic G40.309
intractable G40.319
with status epilepticus G40.311
without status epilepticus G40.319
not intractable G40.309
with status epilepticus G40.301
without status epilepticus G40.309
specified NEC G40.409
intractable G40.419
with status epilepticus G40.411
without status epilepticus G40.419
not intractable G40.409
with status epilepticus G40.401
without status epilepticus G40.409
localization-related (focal) (partial)
idiopathic G40.009
with seizures of localized onset
G40.009
intractable G40.019
with status epilepticus G40.011
without status epilepticus
G40.019
not intractable G40.009
with status epilepticus G40.001
without status epilepticus
G40.009
symptomatic
with complex partial seizures
G40.209
intractable G40.219
with status epilepticus G40.211
without status epilepticus G40.219

Epilepsy, epileptic, epilepsia (Continued)
syndromes (Continued)
localization-related (Continued)
symptomatic (Continued)
with complex partial seizures
(Continued)
not intractable G40.209
with status epilepticus G40.201
without status epilepticus
G40.209
with simple partial seizures G40.109
intractable G40.119
with status epilepticus G40.111
without status epilepticus
G40.119
not intractable G40.109
with status epilepticus G40.101
without status epilepticus
G40.109
specified NEC G40.802
intractable G40.804
with status epilepticus G40.803
without status epilepticus G40.804
not intractable G40.802
with status epilepticus G40.801
without status epilepticus G40.802
tonic (-clonic) —see Epilepsy, generalized,
specified NEC
twilight F05
uncinate (gyrus) —see Epilepsy, localization-
related, symptomatic, with complex
partial seizures
Unverricht (-Lundborg) (familial myoclonic) —
see Epilepsy, generalized, idiopathic
visceral —see Epilepsy, specified NEC
visual —see Epilepsy, specified NEC
Epiloia Q85.1
Epimenorrhea N92.0
Epipharyngitis —see Nasopharyngitis
Epiphora H04.20-●
due to
excess lacrimation H04.21-●
insufficient drainage H04.22-●
Epiphyseal arrest —see Arrest, epiphyseal
Epiphyseolysis, epiphysiolysis —see
Osteochondropathy
Epiphysitis —see also Osteochondropathy
juvenile M92.9
syphilitic (congenital) A50.02
Epiplocele —see Hernia, abdomen
Epiploitis —see Peritonitis
Epiplosarcomphalocele —see Hernia,
umbilicus
Episcleritis (suppurative) H15.10-●
in (due to)
syphilis A52.71
tuberculosis A18.51
nodular H15.12-●
periodica fugax H15.11-●
angioneurotic —see Edema, angioneurotic
syphilitic (late) A52.71
tuberculous A18.51
Episode
affective, mixed F39
depersonalization (in neurotic state) F48.1
⮞ depressive F32.A
major F32.9
mild F32.0
moderate F32.1
severe (without psychotic symptoms)
F32.2
with psychotic symptoms F32.3
recurrent F33.9
brief F33.8
specified NEC F32.89
hypomanic F30.8
manic F30.9
with
psychotic symptoms F30.2
remission (full) F30.4
partial F30.3

Episode (Continued)
manic (Continued)
without psychotic symptoms F30.10
mild F30.11
moderate F30.12
severe (without psychotic symptoms)
F30.13
with psychotic symptoms F30.2
other specified F30.8
recurrent F31.89
psychotic F23
organic F06.8
schizophrenic (acute) NEC, brief F23
Epispadias (female) (male) Q64.0
Episplenitis D73.89
Epistaxis (multiple) R04.0
hereditary I78.0
vicarious menstruation N94.89
Epithelioma (malignant) —see also Neoplasm,
malignant, by site
adenoides cysticum —see Neoplasm, skin,
benign
basal cell —see Neoplasm, skin, malignant
benign —see Neoplasm, benign, by site
Bowen's —see Neoplasm, skin, in situ
calcifying, of Malherbe —see Neoplasm, skin,
benign
external site —see Neoplasm, skin, malignant
intraepidermal, Jadassohn —see Neoplasm,
skin, benign
squamous cell —see Neoplasm, malignant,
by site
Epitheliomatosis pigmented Q82.1
Epitheliopathy, multifocal placoid pigment
H30.14-●
Epithelium, epithelial —see condition
Epituberculosis (with atelectasis) (allergic)
A15.7
Eponychia Q84.6
Epstein's
nephrosis or syndrome —see Nephrosis
pearl K09.8
Epulis (gingiva) (fibrous) (giant cell) K06.8
Equinia A24.0
Equinovarus (congenital) (talipes) Q66.0-●
acquired —see Deformity, limb, clubfoot
Equivalent
convulsive (abdominal) —see Epilepsy,
specified NEC
epileptic (psychic) —see Epilepsy,
localization-related, symptomatic, with
complex partial seizures
Erb (-Duchenne) **paralysis** (birth injury)
(newborn) P14.0
Erb's
disease G71.02
palsy, paralysis (brachial) (birth) (newborn)
P14.0
spinal (spastic) syphilitic A52.17
pseudohypertrophic muscular dystrophy
G71.02
Erb-Goldflam disease or syndrome G70.00
with exacerbation (acute) G70.01
in crisis G70.01
Erdheim's syndrome (acromegalic
macrospondylitis) E22.0
Erection, painful (persistent) —see Priapism
Ergosterol deficiency (vitamin D) E55.9
with
adult osteomalacia M83.8
rickets —see Rickets
Ergotism —see also Poisoning, food, noxious,
plant
from ergot used as drug (migraine therapy) —
see Table of Drugs and Chemicals
Erosio interdigitalis blastomycetica B37.2
Erosion
artery I77.2
without rupture I77.89
bone —see Disorder, bone, density and
structure, specified NEC

▶ New ⮞ Revised ~~deleted~~ Deleted ● Use Additional Character(s)

Erosion (Continued)
  bronchus J98.09
  cartilage (joint) —see Disorder, cartilage,
      specified type NEC
  cervix (uteri) (acquired) (chronic) (congenital)
      N86
    with cervicitis N72
  cornea (nontraumatic) —see Ulcer, cornea
    recurrent H18.83-●
    traumatic —see Abrasion, cornea
  dental (idiopathic) (occupational) (due to
      diet, drugs or vomiting) K03.2
  duodenum, postpyloric —see Ulcer,
      duodenum
  esophagus K22.10
    with bleeding K22.11
  gastric —see Ulcer, stomach
  gastrojejunal —see Ulcer, gastrojejunal
  ⇒ implanted mesh —see Complications,
      prosthetic device or implant, mesh
  intestine K63.3
  lymphatic vessel I89.8
  pylorus, pyloric (ulcer) —see Ulcer, stomach
  spine, aneurysmal A52.09
  stomach —see Ulcer, stomach
  subcutaneous device pocket
    nervous system prosthetic device, implant,
        or graft T85.890
    other internal prosthetic device, implant, or
        graft T85.898
  teeth (idiopathic) (occupational) (due to diet,
      drugs or vomiting) K03.2
  urethra N36.8
  uterus N85.8
Erotomania F52.8
Error
  metabolism, inborn —see Disorder, metabolism
  refractive —see Disorder, refraction
Eructation R14.2
  nervous or psychogenic F45.8
Eruption
  creeping B76.9
  drug (generalized) (taken internally) L27.0
    fixed L27.1
    in contact with skin —see Dermatitis, due
        to drugs
    localized L27.1
  Hutchinson, summer L56.4
  Kaposi's varicelliform B00.0
  napkin L22
  polymorphous light (sun) L56.4
  recalcitrant pustular L13.8
  ringed R23.8
  skin (nonspecific) R21
    creeping (meaning hookworm) B76.9
    due to inoculation/vaccination
        (generalized) —see also Dermatitis,
        due to, vaccine L27.0
      localized L27.1
    erysipeloid A26.0
    feigned L98.1
    Kaposi's varicelliform B00.0
    lichenoid L28.0
    meaning dermatitis —see Dermatitis
    toxic NEC L53.0
  tooth, teeth, abnormal (incomplete) (late)
      (premature) (sequence) K00.6
  vesicular R23.8
Erysipelas (gangrenous) (infantile) (newborn)
    (phlegmonous) (suppurative) A46
  external ear A46 [H62.40]
  puerperal, postpartum O86.89
Erysipeloid A26.9
  cutaneous (Rosenbach's) A26.0
  disseminated A26.8
  sepsis A26.7
  specified NEC A26.8
Erythema, erythematous (infectional)
    (inflammation) L53.9
  ab igne L59.0

Erythema, erythematous (Continued)
  annulare (centrifugum) (rheumaticum) L53.1
  arthriticum epidemicum A25.1
  brucellum —see Brucellosis
  chronic figurate NEC L53.3
  chronicum migrans (Borrelia burgdorferi)
      A69.20
  diaper L22
  due to
    chemical NEC L53.0
      in contact with skin L24.5
    drug (internal use) —see Dermatitis, due
        to, drugs
  elevatum diutinum L95.1
  endemic E52
  epidemic, arthritic A25.1
  figuratum perstans L53.3
  gluteal L22
  heat - code by site under Burn, first degree
  ichthyosiforme congenitum bullous
      Q80.3
  in diseases classified elsewhere L54
  induratum (nontuberculous) L52
    tuberculous A18.4
  infectiosum B08.3
  intertrigo L30.4
  iris L51.9
  marginatum L53.2
    in (due to) acute rheumatic fever I00
  medicamentosum —see Dermatitis, due to,
      drugs
  migrans A26.0
    chronicum A69.20
    tongue K14.1
  multiforme (major) (minor) L51.9
    bullous, bullosum L51.1
    conjunctiva L51.1
    nonbullous L51.0
    pemphigoides L12.0
    specified NEC L51.8
  napkin L22
  neonatorum P83.88
    toxic P83.1
  nodosum L52
    tuberculous A18.4
  palmar L53.8
  pernio T69.1
  rash, newborn P83.88
  scarlatiniform (recurrent) (exfoliative)
      L53.8
  solare L55.0
  specified NEC L53.8
  toxic, toxicum NEC L53.0
    newborn P83.1
  tuberculous (primary) A18.4
Erythematous, erythematosus —see condition
Erythermalgia (primary) I73.81
Erythralgia I73.81
Erythrasma L08.1
Erythredema (polyneuropathy) —see Poisoning,
    mercury
Erythremia (acute) C94.0-●
  chronic D45
  secondary D75.1
Erythroblastopenia —see also Aplasia, red cell
    D60.9
  congenital D61.01
Erythroblastophthisis D61.09
Erythroblastosis (fetalis) (newborn) P55.9
  due to
    ABO (antibodies) (incompatibility)
        (isoimmunization) P55.1
    Rh (antibodies) (incompatibility)
        (isoimmunization) P55.0
Erythrocyanosis (crurum) I73.89
Erythrocythemia —see Erythremia
Erythrocytosis (megalosplenic) (secondary)
    D75.1
  familial D75.0
  oval, hereditary —see Elliptocytosis

Erythrocytosis (Continued)
  secondary D75.1
  stress D75.1
Erythroderma (secondary) —see also Erythema
    L53.9
  bullous ichthyosiform, congenital Q80.3
  desquamativum L21.1
  ichthyosiform, congenital (bullous) Q80.3
  neonatorum P83.88
  psoriaticum L40.8
Erythrodysesthesia, palmar plantar (PPE)
    L27.1
Erythrogenesis imperfecta D61.09
Erythroleukemia C94.0-●
Erythromelalgia I73.81
Erythrophagocytosis D75.89
Erythrophobia F40.298
Erythroplakia, oral epithelium, and tongue
    K13.29
Erythroplasia (Queyrat) D07.4
  specified site —see Neoplasm, skin, in situ
  unspecified site D07.4
Escherichia coli (E. coli), as cause of disease
    classified elsewhere B96.20
  non-O157 Shiga toxin-producing (with
      known O group) B96.22
  non-Shiga toxin-producing B96.29
  O157 with confirmation of Shiga toxin when
      H antigen is unknown, or is not H7
      B96.21
  O157:H- (nonmotile) with confirmation of
      Shiga toxin B96.21
  Shiga toxin-producing (with unspecified O
      group) (STEC) B96.23
  O157 B96.21
  O157:H7 with or without confirmation of
      Shiga toxin-production B96.21
  specified NEC B96.29
Esophagismus K22.4
Esophagitis (acute) (alkaline) (chemical)
    (chronic) (infectional) (necrotic) (peptic)
    (postoperative) (without bleeding)
    K20.90
  with bleeding K20.91
  candidal B37.81
  due to gastrointestinal reflux disease (without
      bleeding) K21.00
    with bleeding K21.01
  eosinophilic K20.0
  reflux K21.00
  specified NEC (without bleeding) K20.80
    with bleeding K21.81
  tuberculous A18.83
  ulcerative K22.10
    with bleeding K22.11
Esophagocele K22.5
⇒ **Esophagomalacia** K22.89
Esophagospasm K22.4
Esophagostenosis K22.2
Esophagostomiasis B81.8
Esophagotracheal —see condition
Esophagus —see condition
Esophoria H50.51
  convergence, excess H51.12
  divergence, insufficiency H51.8
Esotropia —see Strabismus, convergent
    concomitant
Espundia B55.2
Essential —see condition
Esthesioneuroblastoma C30.0
Esthesioneurocytoma C30.0
Esthesioneuroepithelioma C30.0
Esthiomene A55
Estivo-autumnal malaria (fever) B50.9
Estrangement (marital) Z63.5
  parent-child NEC Z62.890
Estriasis —see Myiasis
Ethanolism —see Alcoholism
Etherism —see Dependence, drug, inhalant
Ethmoid, ethmoidal —see condition

Ethmoiditis (chronic) (nonpurulent)
  (purulent) —*see also* Sinusitis, ethmoidal
  influenzal —*see* Influenza, with, respiratory
    manifestations NEC
  Woakes' J33.1
Ethylism —*see* Alcoholism
Eulenburg's disease (congenital paramyotonia)
  G71.19
Eumycetoma B47.0
Eunuchoidism E29.1
  hypogonadotropic E23.0
European blastomycosis —*see* Cryptococcosis
Eustachian —*see* condition
Evaluation (for) (of)
  development state
    adolescent Z00.3
    period of
      delayed growth in childhood Z00.70
        with abnormal findings Z00.71
      rapid growth in childhood Z00.2
    puberty Z00.3
  growth and developmental state (period of
      rapid growth) Z00.2
    delayed growth Z00.70
      with abnormal findings Z00.71
  mental health (status) Z00.8
    requested by authority Z04.6
  period of
    delayed growth in childhood Z00.70
      with abnormal findings Z00.71
    rapid growth in childhood Z00.2
  suspected condition —*see* Observation
Evans syndrome D69.41
Event
  apparent life threatening in newborn and
      infant (ALTE) R68.13
  brief resolved unexplained event (BRUE)
      R68.13
Eventration —*see also* Hernia, ventral
  colon into chest —*see* Hernia, diaphragm
  diaphragm (congenital) Q79.1
Eversion
  bladder N32.89
  cervix (uteri) N86
    with cervicitis N72
  foot NEC —*see also* Deformity, valgus, ankle
    congenital Q66.6
  punctum lacrimale (postinfectional) (senile)
      H04.52-•
  ureter (meatus) N28.89
  urethra (meatus) N36.8
  uterus N81.4
Evidence
  cytologic
    of malignancy on anal smear R85.614
    of malignancy on cervical smear R87.614
    of malignancy on vaginal smear R87.624
Evisceration
  birth injury P15.8
  traumatic NEC
    eye —*see* Enucleated eye
Evulsion —*see* Avulsion
Ewing's sarcoma or tumor —*see* Neoplasm,
  bone, malignant
Examination (for) (following) (general) (of)
  (routine) Z00.00
  with abnormal findings Z00.01
  abuse, physical (alleged), ruled out
    adult Z04.71
    child Z04.72
  adolescent (development state) Z00.3
  alleged rape or sexual assault (victim), ruled
    out
    adult Z04.41
    child Z04.42
  allergy Z01.82
  annual (adult) (periodic) (physical) Z00.00
    with abnormal findings Z00.01
    gynecological Z01.419
      with abnormal findings Z01.411
  antibody response Z01.84

Examination (*Continued*)
  blood —*see* Examination, laboratory
  blood pressure Z01.30
    with abnormal findings Z01.31
  cancer staging —*see* Neoplasm, malignant,
      by site
  cervical Papanicolaou smear Z12.4
    as part of routine gynecological
        examination Z01.419
      with abnormal findings Z01.411
  child (over 28 days old) Z00.129
    with abnormal findings Z00.121
    under 28 days old —*see* Newborn,
        examination
  clinical research control or normal
      comparison (control) (participant)
      Z00.6
  contraceptive (drug) maintenance (routine)
      Z30.8
    device (intrauterine) Z30.431
  dental Z01.20
    with abnormal findings Z01.21
  developmental —*see* Examination, child
  donor (potential) Z00.5
  ear Z01.10
    with abnormal findings NEC Z01.118
  eye Z01.00
    with abnormal findings Z01.01
    following failed vision screening Z01.020
      with abnormal findings Z01.021
  following
    accident NEC Z04.3
      transport Z04.1
      work Z04.2
    assault, alleged, ruled out
      adult Z04.71
      child Z04.72
    motor vehicle accident Z04.1
    treatment (for) Z09
      combined NEC Z09
        fracture Z09
        malignant neoplasm Z08
      malignant neoplasm Z08
      mental disorder Z09
      specified condition NEC Z09
  follow-up (routine) (following) Z09
    chemotherapy NEC Z09
      malignant neoplasm Z08
    fracture Z09
    malignant neoplasm Z08
    postpartum Z39.2
    psychotherapy Z09
    radiotherapy NEC Z09
      malignant neoplasm Z08
    surgery NEC Z09
      malignant neoplasm Z08
  forced sexual exploitation Z04.81
  forced labor exploitation Z04.82
  gynecological Z01.419
    with abnormal findings Z01.411
    for contraceptive maintenance Z30.8
  health —*see* Examination, medical
  hearing Z01.10
    with abnormal findings NEC Z01.118
    infant or child (over 28 days old) Z00.129
      with abnormal findings Z00.121
    following failed hearing screening
        Z01.110
  immunity status testing Z01.84
  laboratory (as part of a general medical
      examination) Z00.00
    with abnormal findings Z00.01
    preprocedural Z01.812
  lactating mother Z39.1
  medical (adult) (for) (of) Z00.00
    with abnormal findings Z00.01
    administrative purpose only Z02.9
      specified NEC Z02.89
    admission to
      armed forces Z02.3
      old age home Z02.2

Examination (*Continued*)
  medical (*Continued*)
    admission to (*Continued*)
      prison Z02.89
      residential institution Z02.2
      school Z02.0
        following illness or medical treatment
            Z02.0
      summer camp Z02.89
    adoption Z02.82
    blood alcohol or drug level Z02.83
    camp (summer) Z02.89
    clinical research, normal subject (control)
        (participant) Z00.6
    control subject in clinical research (normal
        comparison) (participant) Z00.6
    donor (potential) Z00.5
    driving license Z02.4
    general (adult) Z00.00
      with abnormal findings Z00.01
    immigration Z02.89
    insurance purposes Z02.6
    marriage Z02.89
    medicolegal reasons NEC Z04.89
    naturalization Z02.89
    participation in sport Z02.5
    paternity testing Z02.81
    population survey Z00.8
    pre-employment Z02.1
    pre-operative —*see* Examination,
        pre-procedural
    pre-procedural
      cardiovascular Z01.810
      respiratory Z01.811
      specified NEC Z01.818
    preschool children
      for admission to school Z02.0
    prisoners
      for entrance into prison Z02.89
    recruitment for armed forces Z02.3
    specified NEC Z00.8
    sport competition Z02.5
  medicolegal reason NEC Z04.89
    forced sexual exploitation Z04.81
    forced labor exploitation Z04.82
  newborn —*see* Newborn, examination
  pelvic (annual) (periodic) Z01.419
    with abnormal findings Z01.411
  period of rapid growth in childhood Z00.2
  periodic (adult) (annual) (routine) Z00.00
    with abnormal findings Z00.01
  physical (adult) —*see also* Examination,
      medical Z00.00
    sports Z02.5
  postpartum
    immediately after delivery Z39.0
    routine follow-up Z39.2
  pre-chemotherapy (antineoplastic) Z01.818
  prenatal (normal pregnancy) —*see also*
      Pregnancy, normal Z34.9-•
  pre-procedural (pre-operative)
    cardiovascular Z01.810
    laboratory Z01.812
    respiratory Z01.811
    specified NEC Z01.818
  prior to chemotherapy (antineoplastic) Z01.818
  psychiatric NEC Z00.8
    follow-up not needing further care Z09
    requested by authority Z04.6
  radiological (as part of a general medical
      examination) Z00.00
    with abnormal findings Z00.01
  repeat cervical smear to confirm findings of
      recent normal smear following initial
      abnormal smear Z01.42
  skin (hypersensitivity) Z01.82
  special —*see also* Examination, by type Z01.89
    specified type NEC Z01.89
  specified type or reason NEC Z04.89
  teeth Z01.20
    with abnormal findings Z01.21

▶ New ⇒ Revised ~~deleted~~ Deleted • Use Additional Character(s)

Examination *(Continued)*
   urine —*see* Examination, laboratory
   vision Z01.00
      with abnormal findings Z01.01
         following failed vision screening Z01.020
            with abnormal findings Z01.021
         infant or child (over 28 days old) Z00.129
            with abnormal findings Z00.121
Exanthem, exanthema —*see also* Rash
   with enteroviral vesicular stomatitis B08.4
   Boston A88.0
   epidemic with meningitis A88.0 [G02]
   subitum B08.20
      due to human herpesvirus 6 B08.21
      due to human herpesvirus 7 B08.22
   viral, virus B09
      specified type NEC B08.8
Excess, excessive, excessively
   alcohol level in blood R78.0
   androgen (ovarian) E28.1
   attrition, tooth, teeth K03.0
   carotene, carotin (dietary) E67.1
   cold, effects of T69.9
      specified effect NEC T69.8
   convergence H51.12
   crying
      in child, adolescent, or adult R45.83
      in infant R68.11
   development, breast N62
   divergence H51.8
   drinking (alcohol) NEC (without
         dependence) F10.10
      habitual (continual) (without remission)
         F10.20
   eating R63.2
   estrogen E28.0
   fat —*see also* Obesity
      in heart —*see* Degeneration, myocardial
      localized E65
   foreskin N47.8
   gas R14.0
   glucagon E16.3
   heat —*see* Heat
   intermaxillary vertical dimension of fully
         erupted teeth M26.37
   interocclusal distance of fully erupted teeth
         M26.37
   kalium E87.5
   large
      colon K59.39
         congenital Q43.8
      infant P08.0
      organ or site, congenital NEC —*see*
         Anomaly, by site
   long
      organ or site, congenital NEC —*see*
         Anomaly, by site
   menstruation (with regular cycle) N92.0
      with irregular cycle N92.1
   napping Z72.821
   natrium E87.0
   number of teeth K00.1
   nutrient (dietary) NEC R63.2
   potassium (K) E87.5
   salivation K11.7
   secretion —*see also* Hypersecretion
      milk O92.6
      sputum R09.3
      sweat R61
   sexual drive F52.8
   short
      organ or site, congenital NEC —*see*
         Anomaly, by site
      umbilical cord in labor or delivery O69.3
   skin L98.7
      and subcutaneous tissue L98.7
      eyelid (acquired) —*see* Blepharochalasis
         congenital Q10.3
   sodium (Na) E87.0
   spacing of fully erupted teeth M26.32
   sputum R09.3

Excess, excessive, excessively *(Continued)*
   sweating R61
   thirst R63.1
      due to deprivation of water T73.1
   tuberosity of jaw M26.07
   vitamin
      A (dietary) E67.0
         administered as drug (prolonged
            intake) —*see* Table of Drugs and
            Chemicals, vitamins, adverse
            effect
         overdose or wrong substance given
            or taken —*see* Table of Drugs and
            Chemicals, vitamins, poisoning
      D (dietary) E67.3
         administered as drug (prolonged
            intake) —*see* Table of Drugs and
            Chemicals, vitamins, adverse
            effect
         overdose or wrong substance given
            or taken —*see* Table of Drugs and
            Chemicals, vitamins, poisoning
   weight
      gain R63.5
      loss R63.4
Excitability, abnormal, under minor stress
      (personality disorder) F60.3
Excitation
   anomalous atrioventricular I45.6
   psychogenic F30.8
   reactive (from emotional stress, psychological
         trauma) F30.8
Excitement
   hypomanic F30.8
   manic F30.9
   mental, reactive (from emotional stress,
         psychological trauma) F30.8
   state, reactive (from emotional stress,
         psychological trauma) F30.8
Excoriation (traumatic) —*see also* Abrasion
   neurotic L98.1
   skin picking disorder F42.4
Exfoliation
   due to erythematous conditions according to
         extent of body surface involved L49.0
      10-19 percent of body surface L49.1
      20-29 percent of body surface L49.2
      30-39 percent of body surface L49.3
      40-49 percent of body surface L49.4
      50-59 percent of body surface L49.5
      60-69 percent of body surface L49.6
      70-79 percent of body surface L49.7
      80-89 percent of body surface L49.8
      90-99 percent of body surface L49.9
      less than 10 percent of body surface L49.0
   teeth, due to systemic causes K08.0
Exfoliative —*see* condition
Exhaustion, exhaustive (physical NEC) R53.83
   battle F43.0
   cardiac —*see* Failure, heart
   delirium F43.0
   due to
      cold T69.8
      excessive exertion T73.3
      exposure T73.2
      neurasthenia F48.8
   heart —*see* Failure, heart
   heat —*see also* Heat, exhaustion T67.5
      due to
         salt depletion T67.4
         water depletion T67.3
   maternal, complicating delivery O75.81
   mental F48.8
   myocardium, myocardial —*see* Failure, heart
   nervous F48.8
   old age R54
   psychogenic F48.8
   psychosis F43.0
   senile R54
   vital NEC Z73.0
Exhibitionism F65.2

Exocervicitis —*see* Cervicitis
Exomphalos Q79.2
   meaning hernia —*see* Hernia, umbilicus
Exophoria H50.52
   convergence, insufficiency H51.11
   divergence, excess H51.8
Exophthalmos H05.2-●
   congenital Q15.8
   constant NEC H05.24-●
   displacement, globe —*see* Displacement,
      globe
   due to thyrotoxicosis (hyperthyroidism) —*see*
      Hyperthyroidism, with, goiter (diffuse)
   dysthyroid —*see* Hyperthyroidism, with,
      goiter (diffuse)
   goiter —*see* Hyperthyroidism, with, goiter
      (diffuse)
   intermittent NEC H05.25-●
   malignant —*see* Hyperthyroidism, with,
      goiter (diffuse)
   orbital
      edema —*see* Edema, orbit
      hemorrhage —*see* Hemorrhage, orbit
   pulsating NEC H05.26-●
   thyrotoxic, thyrotropic —*see*
      Hyperthyroidism, with, goiter (diffuse)
Exostosis —*see also* Disorder, bone
   cartilaginous —*see* Neoplasm, bone, benign
   congenital (multiple) Q78.6
   external ear canal H61.81-●
   gonococcal A54.49
   jaw (bone) M27.8
   multiple, congenital Q78.6
   orbit H05.35-●
   osteocartilaginous —*see* Neoplasm, bone,
      benign
   syphilitic A52.77
Exotropia —*see* Strabismus, divergent
   concomitant
Explanation of
   investigation finding Z71.2
   medication Z71.89
▶**Exploitation**
   ▶labor
      ▶confirmed
         ▶adult forced T74.61
         ▶child forced T74.62
      ▶suspected
         ▶adult forced T76.61
         ▶child forced T76.62
   ▶sexual
      ▶confirmed
         ▶adult forced T74.51
         ▶child T74.52
      ▶suspected
         ▶adult forced T76.51
         ▶child T76.52
Exposure (to) —*see also* Contact, with
      T75.89
   acariasis Z20.7
   AIDS virus Z20.6
   air pollution Z77.110
   algae and algae toxins Z77.121
   algae bloom Z77.121
   anthrax Z20.810
   aromatic amines Z77.020
   aromatic (hazardous) compounds NEC
      Z77.028
   aromatic dyes NOS Z77.028
   arsenic Z77.010
   asbestos Z77.090
   bacterial disease NEC Z20.818
   benzene Z77.021
   blue-green algae bloom Z77.121
   body fluids (potentially hazardous)
      Z77.21
   brown tide Z77.121
   chemicals (chiefly nonmedicinal) (hazardous)
      NEC Z77.098
   cholera Z20.09
   chromium compounds Z77.018

Exposure *(Continued)*
  cold, effects of T69.9
    specified effect NEC T69.8
  communicable disease Z20.9
    bacterial NEC Z20.818
    specified NEC Z20.89
    viral NEC Z20.828
    Zika virus Z20.821
    ▶coronavirus (disease) (novel) 2019 Z20.822
  cyanobacteria bloom Z77.121
  disaster Z65.5
  discrimination Z60.5
  dyes Z77.098
  effects of T73.9
  environmental tobacco smoke (acute)
      (chronic) Z77.22
  Escherichia coli (E. coli) Z20.01
  exhaustion due to T73.2
  fiberglass —*see* Table of Drugs and
      Chemicals, fiberglass
  German measles Z20.4
  gonorrhea Z20.2
  hazardous metals NEC Z77.018
  hazardous substances NEC Z77.29
  hazards in the physical environment NEC
      Z77.128
  hazards to health NEC Z77.9
  human immunodeficiency virus (HIV)
      Z20.6
  human T-lymphotropic virus type-1 (HTLV-1)
      Z20.89
  implanted
    mesh —*see* Complications, prosthetic
        device or implant, mesh
    prosthetic materials NEC —*see*
        Complications, prosthetic materials
        NEC
  infestation (parasitic) NEC Z20.7
  intestinal infectious disease NEC Z20.09
    Escherichia coli (E. coli) Z20.01
  lead Z77.011
  meningococcus Z20.811
  mold (toxic) Z77.120
  nickel dust Z77.018
  noise Z77.122
  occupational
    air contaminants NEC Z57.39
    dust Z57.2
    environmental tobacco smoke Z57.31
    extreme temperature Z57.6
    noise Z57.0

Exposure *(Continued)*
  radiation Z57.1
  risk factors Z57.9
    specified NEC Z57.8
  toxic agents (gases) (liquids) (solids)
      (vapors) in agriculture Z57.4
  toxic agents (gases) (liquids) (solids)
      (vapors) in industry NEC Z57.5
  vibration Z57.7
  parasitic disease NEC Z20.7
  pediculosis Z20.7
  persecution Z60.5
  pfiesteria piscicida Z77.121
  poliomyelitis Z20.89
  pollution
    air Z77.110
    environmental NEC Z77.118
    soil Z77.112
    water Z77.111
  polycyclic aromatic hydrocarbons Z77.028
  prenatal (drugs) (toxic chemicals) —*see*
      Newborn, affected by, noxious substances
      transmitted via placenta or breast milk
  rabies Z20.3
  radiation, naturally occurring NEC Z77.123
  radon Z77.123
  red tide (Florida) Z77.121
  rubella Z20.4
  second hand tobacco smoke (acute) (chronic)
      Z77.22
    in the perinatal period P96.81
  sexually-transmitted disease Z20.2
  smallpox (laboratory) Z20.89
  syphilis Z20.2
  terrorism Z65.4
  torture Z65.4
  tuberculosis Z20.1
  uranium Z77.012
  varicella Z20.820
  venereal disease Z20.2
  viral disease NEC Z20.828
  war Z65.5
  water pollution Z77.111
    Zika virus Z20.821
Exsanguination —*see* Hemorrhage
Exstrophy
  abdominal contents Q45.8
  bladder Q64.10
    cloacal Q64.12
    specified type NEC Q64.19
    supravesical fissure Q64.11

Extensive —*see* condition
Extra —*see also* Accessory
  marker chromosomes (normal individual)
      Q92.61
    in abnormal individual Q92.62
  rib Q76.6
    cervical Q76.5
Extrasystoles (supraventricular) I49.49
  atrial I49.1
  auricular I49.1
  junctional I49.2
  ventricular I49.3
Extrauterine gestation or pregnancy —*see*
    Pregnancy, by site
Extravasation
  blood R58
  chyle into mesentery I89.8
  pelvicalyceal N13.8
  pyelosinus N13.8
  urine (from ureter) R39.0
  vesicant agent
    antineoplastic chemotherapy T80.810
    other agent NEC T80.818
Extremity —*see* condition, limb
Extrophy —*see* Exstrophy
Extroversion
  bladder Q64.19
  uterus N81.4
    complicating delivery O71.2
    postpartal (old) N81.4
Extruded tooth (teeth) M26.34
Extrusion
  breast implant (prosthetic) T85.42
  eye implant (globe) (ball) T85.328
  intervertebral disc —*see* Displacement,
      intervertebral disc
  ocular lens implant (prosthetic) —*see*
      Complications, intraocular lens
  vitreous —*see* Prolapse, vitreous
Exudate
  pleural —*see* Effusion, pleura
  retina H35.89
  ▶wound fluids L24.A9
Exudative —*see* condition
Eye, eyeball, eyelid —*see* condition
Eyestrain —*see* Disturbance, vision, subjective
Eyeworm disease of Africa B74.3

▶ New   ⇒ Revised   ~~deleted~~ Deleted   • Use Additional Character(s)

F

Faber's syndrome (achlorhydric anemia) D50.9
Fabry (-Anderson) disease E75.21
Facet syndrome M47.89-●
Faciocephalalgia, autonomic —see also
    Neuropathy, peripheral, autonomic G90.09
Factor(s)
  psychic, associated with diseases classified
    elsewhere F54
  psychological
    affecting physical conditions F54
    or behavioral
      affecting general medical condition F54
      associated with disorders or diseases
        classified elsewhere F54
Fahr disease (of brain) G23.8
Fahr Volhard disease (of kidney) I12.-●
Failure, failed
  abortion —see Abortion, attempted
  aortic (valve) I35.8
    rheumatic I06.8
  attempted abortion —see Abortion, attempted
  biventricular I50.82
    due to left heart failure I50.814
  bone marrow —see Anemia, aplastic
  cardiac —see Failure, heart
  cardiorenal (chronic) —see also Failure, renal,
    and Failure, heart I50.9
    hypertensive I13.2
  cardiorespiratory (see also Failure, heart) R09.2
  cardiovascular (chronic) —see Failure, heart
  cerebrovascular I67.9
  cervical dilatation in labor O62.0
  circulation, circulatory (peripheral) R57.9
    newborn P29.89
  compensation —see Disease, heart
  compliance with medical treatment or
    regimen —see Noncompliance
  congestive —see Failure, heart, congestive
  dental implant (endosseous) M27.69
    due to
      failure of dental prosthesis M27.63
      lack of attached gingiva M27.62
      occlusal trauma (poor prosthetic design)
        M27.62
      parafunctional habits M27.62
      periodontal infection (peri-implantitis)
        M27.62
      poor oral hygiene M27.62
    osseointegration M27.61
      due to
        complications of systemic disease
          M27.61
        poor bone quality M27.61
      iatrogenic M27.61
      post-osseointegration
        biological M27.62
        due to complications of systemic disease
          M27.62
        iatrogenic M27.62
        mechanical M27.63
      pre-integration M27.61
      pre-osseointegration M27.61
    specified NEC M27.69
  descent of head (at term) of pregnancy
    (mother) O32.4
  endosseous dental implant —see Failure,
    dental implant
  engagement of head (term of pregnancy)
    (mother) O32.4
  erection (penile) —see also Dysfunction,
    sexual, male, erectile N52.9
    nonorganic F52.21
  examination(s), anxiety concerning Z55.2
  expansion terminal respiratory units
    (newborn) (primary) P28.0
  forceps NOS (with subsequent cesarean
    delivery) O66.5
  gain weight (child over 28 days old) R62.51
    adult R62.7
    newborn P92.6

Failure, failed (Continued)
  genital response (male) F52.21
    female F52.22
  heart (acute) (senile) (sudden) I50.9
    with
      acute pulmonary edema —see Failure,
        ventricular, left
      decompensation I50.9
        with
          normal ejection fraction I50.33
          preserved ejection fraction I50.33
          reduced ejection fraction I50.23
            with diastolic dysfunction I50.43
        combined systolic and diastolic
          I50.43
        diastolic I50.33
        right I50.813
        systolic I50.23
    dilatation —see Disease, heart
    hypertension —see Hypertension, heart
    normal ejection fraction —see Failure,
      heart, diastolic
    preserved ejection fraction —see Failure,
      heart, diastolic
    reduced ejection fraction —see Failure,
      heart, systolic
    arteriosclerotic I70.90
    biventricular I50.82
      due to left heart failure I50.814
    combined left-right sided I50.82
      due to left heart failure I50.814
    compensated —see also Failure, heart, by
      type as diastolic or systolic, chronic
      I50.9
    complicating
      anesthesia (general) (local) or other
        sedation
        in labor and delivery O74.2
        in pregnancy O29.12-●
        postpartum, puerperal O89.1
      delivery (cesarean) (instrumental) O75.4
    congestive I50.9
      with rheumatic fever (conditions in I00)
        active I01.8
        inactive or quiescent (with chorea)
          I09.81
      newborn P29.0
      rheumatic (chronic) (inactive) (with
        chorea) I09.81
        active or acute I01.8
        with chorea I02.0
    decompensated —see also Failure, heart, by
      type as diastolic or systolic, acute and
      chronic I50.9
    degenerative —see Degeneration, myocardial
    diastolic (congestive) (left ventricular) I50.30
      acute (congestive) I50.31
        and (on) chronic (congestive) I50.33
      chronic (congestive) I50.32
        and (on) acute (congestive) I50.33
      combined with systolic (congestive)
        I50.40
      acute (congestive) I50.41
        and (on) chronic (congestive) I50.43
      chronic (congestive) I50.42
        and (on) acute (congestive) I50.43
    due to presence of cardiac prosthesis I97.13-●
    end stage —see also Failure, heart, by type
      as diastolic or systolic, chronic I50.84
    following cardiac surgery I97.13-●
    high output NOS I50.83
    hypertensive —see Hypertension, heart
    left (ventricular) —see also Failure,
      ventricular, left
      combined diastolic and systolic —see
        Failure, heart, diastolic, combined
        with systolic
      diastolic —see Failure, heart, diastolic
      systolic —see Failure, heart, systolic
    low output (syndrome) NOS I50.9
    newborn P29.0
    organic —see Disease, heart
    peripartum O90.3

Failure, failed (Continued)
  heart (Continued)
    postprocedural I97.13-●
    rheumatic (chronic) (inactive) I09.9
    right (isolated) (ventricular) I50.810
      acute I50.811
        and (on) chronic I50.813
      chronic I50.812
        and acute I50.813
      secondary to left heart failure I50.814
    specified NEC I50.89

> Note: heart failure stages A, B, C, and
> D are based on the American College of
> Cardiology and American Heart Association
> stages of heart failure, which complement
> and should not be confused with the New
> York Heart Association Classification of
> Heart Failure, into Class I, Class II, Class III,
> and Class IV

    stage A Z91.89
    stage B (see also Failure, heart, by type as
      diastolic or systolic) I50.9
    stage C (see also Failure, heart, by type as
      diastolic or systolic) I50.9
    stage D (see also Failure, heart, by type
      as diastolic or systolic, chronic)
      I50.84
    systolic (congestive) (left ventricular)
      I50.20
      acute (congestive) I50.21
        and (on) chronic (congestive) I50.23
      chronic (congestive) I50.22
        and (on) acute (congestive) I50.23
      combined with diastolic (congestive)
        I50.40
      acute (congestive) I50.41
        and (on) chronic (congestive)
          I50.43
      chronic (congestive) I50.42
        and (on) acute (congestive) I50.43
    thyrotoxic (see also Thyrotoxicosis) E05.90
      [I43]
      with
        high output (see also Thyrotoxicosis)
          I50.83
        thyroid storm E05.91 [I43]
          high output (see also
            Thyrotoxicosis) I50.83
    valvular —see Endocarditis
  hepatic K72.90
    with coma K72.91
    acute or subacute K72.00
      with coma K72.01
      due to drugs K71.10
        with coma K71.11
    alcoholic (acute) (chronic) (subacute)
      K70.40
      with coma K70.41
    chronic K72.10
      with coma K72.11
      due to drugs (acute) (subacute) (chronic)
        K71.10
        with coma K71.11
    due to drugs (acute) (subacute) (chronic)
      K71.10
      with coma K71.11
    postprocedural K91.82
  hepatorenal K76.7
  induction (of labor) O61.9
    abortion —see Abortion, attempted
    by
      oxytocic drugs O61.0
      prostaglandins O61.0
    instrumental O61.1
    mechanical O61.1
    medical O61.0
    specified NEC O61.8
    surgical O61.1

Failure, failed *(Continued)*
  intubation during anesthesia T88.4
    in pregnancy O29.6-●
    labor and delivery O74.7
    postpartum, puerperal O89.6
  involution, thymus (gland) E32.0
  kidney —*see also* Disease, kidney, chronic N19
    acute —*see also* Failure, renal, acute N17.9-●
    diabetic —*see* E08-E13 with .22
  lactation (complete) O92.3
    partial O92.4
  Leydig's cell, adult E29.1
  liver —*see* Failure, hepatic
  menstruation at puberty N91.0
  mitral I05.8
  myocardial, myocardium —*see also* Failure, heart I50.9
    chronic —*see also* Failure, heart, congestive I50.9
    congestive —*see also* Failure, heart, congestive I50.9
▶newborn screening —*see* Abnormal, neonatal screening
▶neonatal congenital heart disease P09.5
  orgasm (female) (psychogenic) F52.31
    male F52.32
  ovarian (primary) E28.39
    iatrogenic E89.40
      asymptomatic E89.40
      symptomatic E89.41
    postprocedural (postablative) (postirradiation) (postsurgical) E89.40
      asymptomatic E89.40
      symptomatic E89.41
  ovulation causing infertility N97.0
  polyglandular, autoimmune E31.0
  prosthetic joint implant —*see* Complications, joint prosthesis, mechanical, breakdown, by site
  renal N19
    with
      tubular necrosis (acute) N17.0
    acute N17.9
      with
        cortical necrosis N17.1
        medullary necrosis N17.2
        tubular necrosis N17.0
      specified NEC N17.8
    chronic N18.9
      hypertensive —*see* Hypertension, kidney
    congenital P96.0
    end stage (chronic) N18.6
      due to hypertension I12.0
    following
      abortion —*see* Abortion by type
        complicated by specified condition NEC
      crushing T79.5
      ectopic or molar pregnancy O08.4
      labor and delivery (acute) O90.4
    hypertensive —*see* Hypertension, kidney
    postprocedural N99.0
  respiration, respiratory J96.90
    with
      hypercapnia J96.92
      hypercarbia J96.02
      hypoxia J96.91
    acute J96.00
      with
        hypercapnia J96.02
        hypercarbia J96.92
        hypoxia J96.01
    acute and (on) chronic J96.20
      with
        hypercapnia J96.22
        hypercarbia J96.22
        hypoxia J96.21
    center G93.89
    chronic J96.10
      with
        hypercapnia J96.12
        hypercarbia J96.12
        hypoxia J96.11

Failure, failed *(Continued)*
  respiration, respiratory *(Continued)*
    newborn P28.5
    postprocedural (acute) J95.821
      acute and chronic J95.822
  rotation
    cecum Q43.3
    colon Q43.3
    intestine Q43.3
    kidney Q63.2
  sedation (conscious) (moderate) during procedure T88.52
    history of Z92.83
  segmentation —*see also* Fusion
    fingers —*see* Syndactylism, complex, fingers
    vertebra Q76.49
      with scoliosis Q76.3
  seminiferous tubule, adult E29.1
  senile (general) R54
  sexual arousal (male) F52.21
    female F52.22
  testicular endocrine function E29.1
  to thrive (child over 28 days old) R62.51
    adult R62.7
    newborn P92.6
  transplant T86.92
    bone T86.831
      marrow T86.02
    cornea T86.841-●
    heart T86.22
      with lung(s) T86.32
    intestine T86.851
    kidney T86.12
    liver T86.42
    lung(s) T86.811
      with heart T86.32
    pancreas T86.891
    skin (allograft) (autograft) T86.821
    specified organ or tissue NEC T86.891
    stem cell (peripheral blood) (umbilical cord) T86.5
  trial of labor (with subsequent cesarean delivery) O66.40
    following previous cesarean delivery O66.41
  tubal ligation N99.89
  urinary —*see* Disease, kidney, chronic
  vacuum extraction NOS (with subsequent cesarean delivery) O66.5
  vasectomy N99.89
  ventouse NOS (with subsequent cesarean delivery) O66.5
  ventricular —*see also* Failure, heart I50.9
    left —*see also* Failure, heart, left I50.1
      with rheumatic fever (conditions in I00)
        active I01.8
          with chorea I02.0
        inactive or quiescent (with chorea) I09.81
      rheumatic (chronic) (inactive) (with chorea) I09.81
        active or acute I01.8
          with chorea I02.0
    right —*see* Failure, heart, right
  vital centers, newborn P91.88
Fainting (fit) R55
Fallen arches —*see* Deformity, limb, flat foot
Falling, falls (repeated) R29.6
  any organ or part —*see* Prolapse
Fallopian
  insufflation Z31.41
  tube —*see* condition
Fallot's
  pentalogy Q21.8
  tetrad or tetralogy Q21.3
  triad or trilogy Q22.3
False —*see also* condition
  croup J38.5
  joint —*see* Nonunion, fracture

False *(Continued)*
  labor (pains) O47.9
    at or after 37 completed weeks of gestation O47.1
    before 37 completed weeks of gestation O47.0-●
  passage, urethra (prostatic) N36.5
  pregnancy F45.8
Family, familial —*see also* condition
  disruption Z63.8
    involving divorce or separation Z63.5
  Li-Fraumeni (syndrome) Z15.01
  planning advice Z30.09
  problem Z63.9
    specified NEC Z63.8
  retinoblastoma C69.2-●
Famine (effects of) T73.0
  edema —*see* Malnutrition, severe
Fanconi (-de Toni)(-Debré) **syndrome** E72.09
  with cystinosis E72.04
Fanconi's anemia (congenital pancytopenia) D61.09
Farber's disease or syndrome E75.29
Farcy A24.0
Farmer's
  lung J67.0
  skin L57.8
Farsightedness —*see* Hypermetropia
Fascia —*see* condition
Fasciculation R25.3
Fasciitis M72.9
  diffuse (eosinophilic) M35.4
  infective M72.8
    necrotizing M72.6
  necrotizing M72.6
  nodular M72.4
  perirenal (with ureteral obstruction) N13.5
    with infection N13.6
  plantar M72.2
  specified NEC M72.8
  traumatic (old) M72.8
    current - code by site under Sprain
Fascioliasis B66.3
Fasciolopsis, fasciolopsiasis (intestinal) B66.5
Fascioscapulohumeral myopathy G71.02
Fast pulse R00.0
Fat
  embolism —*see* Embolism, fat
  excessive —*see also* Obesity
    in heart —*see* Degeneration, myocardial
  in stool R19.5
  localized (pad) E65
    heart —*see* Degeneration, myocardial
    knee M79.4
    retropatellar M79.4
  necrosis
    breast N64.1
    mesentery K65.4
    omentum K65.4
  pad E65
    knee M79.4
Fatigue R53.83
  auditory deafness —*see* Deafness
  chronic R53.82
  combat F43.0
  general R53.83
    psychogenic F48.8
  heat (transient) T67.6
  muscle M62.89
  myocardium —*see* Failure, heart
  neoplasm-related R53.0
  nervous, neurosis F48.8
  operational F48.8
  psychogenic (general) F48.8
  senile R54
  voice R49.8
Fatness —*see* Obesity

Fatty —see also condition
  apron E65
  degeneration —see Degeneration, fatty
  heart (enlarged) —see Degeneration,
    myocardial
  liver NEC K76.0
    alcoholic K70.0
    nonalcoholic K76.0
    necrosis —see Degeneration, fatty
Fauces —see condition
Fauchard's disease (periodontitis) —see
    Periodontitis
Faucitis J02.9
Favism (anemia) D55.0
Favus —see Dermatophytosis
Fazio-Londe disease or syndrome
    G12.1
Fear complex or reaction F40.9
Fear of —see Phobia
Feared complaint unfounded Z71.1
Febris, febrile —see also Fever
  flava —see also Fever, yellow A95.9
  melitensis A23.0
  pestis —see Plague
  recurrens —see Fever, relapsing
  rubra A38.9
Fecal
  incontinence R15.9
  smearing R15.1
  soiling R15.1
  urgency R15.2
Fecalith (impaction) K56.41
  appendix K38.1
  congenital P76.8
Fede's disease K14.0
Feeble rapid pulse due to shock following
    injury T79.4
Feeble-minded F70
Feeding
  difficulties R63.30
  problem (elderly) (infant) R63.39
    newborn P92.9
      specified NEC P92.8
    nonorganic (adult) —see Disorder,
      eating
Feeling (of)
  foreign body in throat R09.89
Feer's disease —see Poisoning, mercury
Feet —see condition
Feigned illness Z76.5
Feil-Klippel syndrome (brevicollis) Q76.1
Feinmesser's (hidrotic) ectodermal dysplasia
    Q82.4
Felinophobia F40.218
Felon —see also Cellulitis, digit
  with lymphangitis —see Lymphangitis,
    acute, digit
Felty's syndrome M05.00
  ankle M05.07-●
  elbow M05.02-●
  foot joint M05.07-●
  hand joint M05.04-●
  hip M05.05-●
  knee M05.06-●
  multiple site M05.09
  shoulder M05.01-●
  vertebra —see Spondylitis, ankylosing
  wrist M05.03-●
Female genital cutting status —see Female
    genital mutilation status (FGM)
Female genital mutilation status (FGM)
    N90.810
  specified NEC N90.818
  type I (clitorectomy status) N90.811
  type II (clitorectomy with excision
    of labia minora status)
    N90.812
  type III (infibulation status)
    N90.813
  type IV N90.818
Femur, femoral —see condition

Fenestration, fenestrated —see also Imperfect,
    closure
  aortico-pulmonary Q21.4
  cusps, heart valve NEC Q24.8
    pulmonary Q22.3
  pulmonic cusps Q22.3
Fernell's disease (aortic aneurysm) I71.9
Fertile eunuch syndrome E23.0
Fetid
  breath R19.6
  sweat L75.0
Fetishism F65.0
  transvestic F65.1
Fetus, fetal —see also condition
  alcohol syndrome (dysmorphic) Q86.0
  compressus O31.0-●
  hydantoin syndrome Q86.1
  lung tissue P28.0
  papyraceous O31.0-●
Fever (inanition) (of unknown origin)
    (persistent) (with chills) (with rigor) R50.9
  abortus A23.1
  Aden (dengue) A90
  African tick bite A77.8
  African tick-borne A68.1
  American
    mountain (tick) A93.2
    spotted A77.0
  aphthous B08.8
  arbovirus, arboviral A94
    hemorrhagic A94
    specified NEC A93.8
  Argentinian hemorrhagic A96.0
  Assam B55.0
  Australian Q A78
  Bangkok hemorrhagic A91
  Barmah forest A92.8
  Bartonella A44.0
  bilious, hemoglobinuric B50.8
  blackwater B50.8
  blister B00.1
  Bolivian hemorrhagic A96.1
  Bonvale dam T73.3
  boutonneuse A77.1
  brain — see Encephalitis
  Brazilian purpuric A48.4
  breakbone A90
  Bullis A77.0
  Bunyamwera A92.8
  Burdwan B55.0
  Bwamba A92.8
  Cameroon —see Malaria
  Canton A75.9
  catarrhal (acute) J00
    chronic J31.0
  cat-scratch A28.1
  Central Asian hemorrhagic A98.0
  cerebral —see Encephalitis
  cerebrospinal meningococcal A39.0
  Chagres B50.9
  Chandipura A92.8
  Changuinola A93.1
  Charcot's (biliary) (hepatic) (intermittent) —
    see Calculus, bile duct
  Chikungunya (viral) (hemorrhagic) A92.0
  Chitral A93.1
  Colombo —see Fever, paratyphoid
  Colorado tick (virus) A93.2
  congestive (remittent) —see Malaria
  Congo virus A98.0
  continued malarial B50.9
  Corsican —see Malaria
  Crimean-Congo hemorrhagic A98.0
  Cyprus —see Brucellosis
  dandy A90
  deer fly —see Tularemia
  dengue (virus) A90
    hemorrhagic A91
    sandfly A93.1
  desert B38.0
  drug induced R50.2

Fever (Continued)
  due to
    conditions classified elsewhere R50.81
    heat T67.01
  enteric A01.00
  enteroviral exanthematous (Boston
    exanthem) A88.0
  ephemeral (of unknown origin) R50.9
  epidemic hemorrhagic A98.5
  erysipelatous —see Erysipelas
  estivo-autumnal (malarial) B50.9
  famine A75.0
  five day A79.0
  following delivery O86.4
  Fort Bragg A27.89
  gastroenteric A01.00
  gastromalarial —see Malaria
  Gibraltar —see Brucellosis
  glandular —see Mononucleosis, infectious
  Guama (viral) A92.8
  Haverhill A25.1
  hay (allergic) J30.1
    with asthma (bronchial) J45.909
      with
        exacerbation (acute) J45.901
        status asthmaticus J45.902
      due to
        allergen other than pollen J30.89
        pollen, any plant or tree J30.1
  heat (effects) T67.01
  hematuric, bilious B50.8
  hemoglobinuric (malarial) (bilious) B50.8
  hemorrhagic (arthropod-borne) NOS A94
    with renal syndrome A98.5
    arenaviral A96.9
      specified NEC A96.8
    Argentinian A96.0
    Bangkok A91
    Bolivian A96.1
    Central Asian A98.0
    Chikungunya A92.0
    Crimean-Congo A98.0
    dengue (virus) A91
    epidemic A98.5
    Junin (virus) A96.0
    Korean A98.5
    Kyasanur forest A98.2
    Machupo (virus) A96.1
    mite-borne A93.8
    mosquito-borne A92.8
    Omsk A98.1
    Philippine A91
    Russian A98.5
    Singapore A91
    Southeast Asia A91
    Thailand A91
    tick-borne NEC A93.8
    viral A99
      specified NEC A98.8
  hepatic —see Cholecystitis
  herpetic —see Herpes
  icterohemorrhagic A27.0
  Indiana A93.8
  infective B99.9
    specified NEC B99.8
  intermittent (bilious) —see also Malaria
    of unknown origin R50.9
    pernicious B50.9
  iodide R50.2
  Japanese river A75.3
  jungle —see also Malaria
    yellow A95.0
  Junin (virus) hemorrhagic A96.0
  Katayama B65.2
  kedani A75.3
  Kenya (tick) A77.1
  Kew Garden A79.1
  Korean hemorrhagic A98.5
  Lassa A96.2
  Lone Star A77.0
  Machupo (virus) hemorrhagic A96.1

Fever (Continued)
  malaria, malarial —see Malaria
  Malta A23.9
  Marseilles A77.1
  marsh —see Malaria
  Mayaro (viral) A92.8
  Mediterranean —see also Brucellosis A23.9
    familial M04.1
    tick A77.1
  meningeal —see Meningitis
  Meuse A79.0
  Mexican A75.2
  mianeh A68.1
  miasmatic —see Malaria
  mosquito-borne (viral) A92.9
    hemorrhagic A92.8
  mountain —see also Brucellosis
    meaning Rocky Mountain spotted fever A77.0
    tick (American) (Colorado) (viral) A93.2
  Mucambo (viral) A92.8
  mud A27.9
  Neapolitan —see Brucellosis
  neutropenic D70.9
  newborn P81.9
    environmental P81.0
  Nine-Mile A78
  non-exanthematous tick A93.2
  North Asian tick-borne A77.2
  Omsk hemorrhagic A98.1
  O'nyong-nyong (viral) A92.1
  Oropouche (viral) A93.0
  Oroya A44.0
  pacific coast tick A77.8
  paludal —see Malaria
  Panama (malarial) B50.9
  Pappataci A93.1
  paratyphoid A01.4
    A A01.1
    B A01.2
    C A01.3
  parrot A70
  periodic (Mediterranean) M04.1
  persistent (of unknown origin) R50.9
  petechial A39.0
  pharyngoconjunctival B30.2
  Philippine hemorrhagic A91
  phlebotomus A93.1
  Piry (virus) A93.8
  Pixuna (viral) A92.8
  Plasmodium ovale B53.0
  polioviral (nonparalytic) A80.4
  Pontiac A48.2
  postimmunization R50.83
  postoperative R50.82
    due to infection T81.40
  posttransfusion R50.84
  postvaccination R50.83
  presenting with conditions classified elsewhere R50.81
  pretibial A27.89
  puerperal O86.4
  Q A78
  quadrilateral A78
  quartan (malaria) B52.9
  Queensland (coastal) (tick) A77.3
  quintan A79.0
  rabbit —see Tularemia
  rat-bite A25.9
    due to
      Spirillum A25.0
      Streptobacillus moniliformis A25.1
  recurrent —see Fever, relapsing
  relapsing (Borrelia) A68.9
    Carter's (Asiatic) A68.1
    Dutton's (West African) A68.1
    Koch's A68.9
    louse-borne A68.0
    Novy's
      louse-borne A68.0
      tick-borne A68.1

Fever (Continued)
  relapsing (Borrelia) (Continued)
    Obermeyer's (European) A68.0
    tick-borne A68.1
  remittent (bilious) (congestive) (gastric) —see Malaria
  rheumatic (active) (acute) (chronic) (subacute) I00
    with central nervous system involvement I02.9
    active with heart involvement —see category I01
    inactive or quiescent with
      cardiac hypertrophy I09.89
      carditis I09.9
      endocarditis I09.1
        aortic (valve) I06.9
          with mitral (valve) disease I08.0
        mitral (valve) I05.9
          with aortic (valve) disease I08.0
        pulmonary (valve) I09.89
        tricuspid (valve) I07.8
      heart disease NEC I09.89
      heart failure (congestive) (conditions in category I50.) I09.81
      left ventricular failure (conditions in I50.1-I50.4-) I09.81
      myocarditis, myocardial degeneration (conditions in I51.4) I09.0
      pancarditis I09.9
      pericarditis I09.2
  Rift Valley (viral) A92.4
  Rocky Mountain spotted A77.0
  rose J30.1
  Ross River B33.1
  Russian hemorrhagic A98.5
  San Joaquin (Valley) B38.0
  sandfly A93.1
  Sao Paulo A77.0
  scarlet A38.9
  seven day (leptospirosis) (autumnal) (Japanese) A27.89
    dengue A90
  shin-bone A79.0
  Singapore hemorrhagic A91
  solar A90
  Songo A98.5
  sore B00.1
  South African tick-bite A68.1
  Southeast Asia hemorrhagic A91
  spinal —see Meningitis
  spirillary A25.0
  splenic —see Anthrax
  spotted A77.9
    American A77.0
    Brazilian A77.0
    cerebrospinal meningitis A39.0
    Colombian A77.0
    due to Rickettsia
      africae (African tick bite fever) A77.8
      australis A77.3
      conorii A77.1
      parkeri A77.8
      rickettsii A77.0
      sibirica A77.2
      specified type NEC A77.8
    Ehrlichiosis A77.40
      due to
        E. chafeensis A77.41
        specified organism NEC A77.49
    Rocky Mountain A77.0
  steroid R50.2
  streptobacillary A25.1
  subtertian B50.9
  Sumatran mite A75.3
  sun A90
  swamp A27.9
  swine A02.8
  sylvatic, yellow A95.0
  Tahyna B33.8
  tertian —see Malaria, tertian

Fever (Continued)
  Thailand hemorrhagic A91
  thermic T67.01
  three-day A93.1
  tick
    American mountain A93.2
    Colorado A93.2
    Kemerovo A93.8
    Mediterranean A77.1
    mountain A93.2
    nonexanthematous A93.2
    Quaranfil A93.8
  tick-bite NEC A93.8
  tick-borne (hemorrhagic) NEC A93.8
  trench A79.0
  tsutsugamushi A75.3
  typhogastric A01.00
  typhoid (abortive) (hemorrhagic) (intermittent) (malignant) A01.00
    complicated by
      arthritis A01.04
      heart involvement A01.02
      meningitis A01.01
      osteomyelitis A01.05
      pneumonia A01.03
      specified NEC A01.09
  typhomalarial —see Malaria
  typhus —see Typhus (fever)
  undulant —see Brucellosis
  unknown origin R50.9
  uveoparotid D86.89
  valley B38.0
  Venezuelan equine A92.2
  vesicular stomatitis A93.8
  viral hemorrhagic —see Fever, hemorrhagic, by type of virus
  Volhynian A79.0
  Wesselsbron (viral) A92.8
  West
    African B50.8
    Nile (viral) A92.30
      with
        complications NEC A92.39
        cranial nerve disorders A92.32
        encephalitis A92.31
        encephalomyelitis A92.31
        neurologic manifestation NEC A92.32
        optic neuritis A92.32
        polyradiculitis A92.32
  Whitmore's —see Melioidosis
  Wolhynian A79.0
  worm B83.9
  yellow A95.9
    jungle A95.0
    sylvatic A95.0
    urban A95.1
  Zika virus A92.5
Fibrillation
  atrial or auricular (established) I48.91
    chronic I48.20
      persistent I48.19
    paroxysmal I48.0
    permanent I48.21
    persistent (chronic) (NOS) (other) I48.19
      longstanding I48.11
  cardiac I49.8
  heart I49.8
  muscular M62.89
  ventricular I49.01
Fibrin
  ball or bodies, pleural (sac) J94.1
  chamber, anterior (eye) (gelatinous exudate) —see Iridocyclitis, acute
Fibrinogenolysis —see Fibrinolysis
Fibrinogenopenia D68.8
  acquired D65
  congenital D68.2
Fibrinolysis (hemorrhagic) (acquired) D65
  antepartum hemorrhage —see Hemorrhage, antepartum, with coagulation defect

▶ New   ⟹ Revised   ~~deleted~~ Deleted   ● Use Additional Character(s)

Fibrinolysis *(Continued)*
  following
    abortion —*see* Abortion by type
      complicated by hemorrhage
    ectopic or molar pregnancy O08.1
  intrapartum O67.0
  newborn, transient P60
  postpartum O72.3
Fibrinopenia (hereditary) D68.2
  acquired D68.4
Fibrinopurulent —*see* condition
Fibrinous —*see* condition
Fibroadenoma
  cellular intracanalicular D24-●
  giant D24-●
  intracanalicular
    cellular D24-●
    giant D24-●
    specified site —*see* Neoplasm, benign, by
      site
    unspecified site D24-●
  juvenile D24-●
  pericanalicular
    specified site —*see* Neoplasm, benign, by
      site
    unspecified site D24-●
  phyllodes D24-●
  prostate D29.1
  specified site NEC —*see* Neoplasm, benign,
    by site
  unspecified site D24-●
Fibroadenosis, breast (chronic) (cystic) (diffuse)
  (periodic) (segmental) N60.2-●
Fibroangioma —*see also* Neoplasm, benign, by
  site
  juvenile
    specified site —*see* Neoplasm, benign, by
      site
    unspecified site D10.6
Fibrochondrosarcoma —*see* Neoplasm,
  cartilage, malignant
Fibrocystic
  disease —*see also* Fibrosis, cystic
    breast —*see* Mastopathy, cystic
    jaw M27.49
    kidney (congenital) Q61.8
    liver Q44.6
    pancreas E84.9
  kidney (congenital) Q61.8
Fibrodysplasia ossificans progressiva —*see*
  Myositis, ossificans, progressiva
Fibroelastosis (cordis) (endocardial)
  (endomyocardial) I42.4
Fibroid (tumor) —*see also* Neoplasm, connective
  tissue, benign
  disease, lung (chronic) —*see* Fibrosis, lung
  heart (disease) —*see* Myocarditis
  in pregnancy or childbirth O34.1-●
    causing obstructed labor O65.5
  induration, lung (chronic) —*see* Fibrosis, lung
  lung —*see* Fibrosis, lung
  pneumonia (chronic) —*see* Fibrosis, lung
  uterus —*see also* Leiomyoma, uterus D25.9
Fibrolipoma —*see* Lipoma
Fibroliposarcoma —*see* Neoplasm, connective
  tissue, malignant
Fibroma —*see also* Neoplasm, connective tissue,
  benign
  ameloblastic —*see* Cyst, calcifying odontogenic
  bone (nonossifying) —*see* Disorder, bone,
    specified type NEC
    ossifying —*see* Neoplasm, bone, benign
  cementifying —*see* Neoplasm, bone, benign
  chondromyxoid —*see* Neoplasm, bone,
    benign
  desmoplastic —*see* Neoplasm, connective
    tissue, uncertain behavior
  durum —*see* Neoplasm, connective tissue,
    benign
  fascial —*see* Neoplasm, connective tissue,
    benign

Fibroma *(Continued)*
  invasive —*see* Neoplasm, connective tissue,
    uncertain behavior
  molle —*see* Lipoma
  myxoid —*see* Neoplasm, connective tissue,
    benign
  nasopharynx, nasopharyngeal (juvenile)
    D10.6
  nonosteogenic (nonossifying) —*see* Dysplasia,
    fibrous
  odontogenic (central) —*see* Cyst, calcifying
    odontogenic
  ossifying —*see* Neoplasm, bone, benign
  periosteal —*see* Neoplasm, bone, benign
  soft —*see* Lipoma
Fibromatosis M72.9
  abdominal —*see* Neoplasm, connective tissue,
    uncertain behavior
  aggressive —*see* Neoplasm, connective tissue,
    uncertain behavior
  congenital generalized —*see* Neoplasm,
    connective tissue, uncertain behavior
  Dupuytren's M72.0
  gingival K06.1
  palmar (fascial) M72.0
  plantar (fascial) M72.2
  pseudosarcomatous (proliferative)
    (subcutaneous) M72.4
  retroperitoneal D48.3
  specified NEC M72.8
Fibromyalgia M79.7
Fibromyoma —*see also* Neoplasm, connective
  tissue, benign
  uterus (corpus) —*see also* Leiomyoma, uterus
    in pregnancy or childbirth —*see* Fibroid, in
      pregnancy or childbirth
    causing obstructed labor O65.5
Fibromyositis M79.7
Fibromyxolipoma D17.9
Fibromyxoma —*see* Neoplasm, connective
  tissue, benign
Fibromyxosarcoma —*see* Neoplasm, connective
  tissue, malignant
Fibro-odontoma, ameloblastic —*see* Cyst,
  calcifying odontogenic
Fibro-osteoma —*see* Neoplasm, bone, benign
Fibroplasia, retrolental H35.17
Fibropurulent —*see* condition
Fibrosarcoma —*see also* Neoplasm, connective
  tissue, malignant
  ameloblastic C41.1
    upper jaw (bone) C41.0
  congenital —*see* Neoplasm, connective tissue,
    malignant
  fascial —*see* Neoplasm, connective tissue,
    malignant
  infantile —*see* Neoplasm, connective tissue,
    malignant
  odontogenic C41.1
    upper jaw (bone) C41.0
  periosteal —*see* Neoplasm, bone, malignant
Fibrosclerosis
  breast N60.3-●
  multifocal M35.5
  penis (corpora cavernosa) N48.6
Fibrosis, fibrotic
  adrenal (gland) E27.8
  amnion O41.8X-●
  anal papillae K62.89
  arteriocapillary —*see* Arteriosclerosis
  bladder N32.89
    interstitial —*see* Cystitis, chronic,
      interstitial
    localized submucosal —*see* Cystitis,
      chronic, interstitial
    panmural —*see* Cystitis, chronic, interstitial
  breast —*see* Fibrosclerosis, breast
  capillary —*see also* Arteriosclerosis I70.90
    lung (chronic) —*see* Fibrosis, lung
  cardiac —*see* Myocarditis
  cervix N88.8

Fibrosis, fibrotic *(Continued)*
  chorion O41.8X-●
  corpus cavernosum (sclerosing) N48.6
  cystic (of pancreas) E84.9
    with
      distal intestinal obstruction syndrome
        E84.19
      fecal impaction E84.19
      intestinal manifestations NEC E84.19
      pulmonary manifestations E84.0
      specified manifestations NEC E84.8
  due to device, implant or graft —*see also*
    Complications, by site and type,
    specified NEC T85.828
    arterial graft NEC T82.828
    breast (implant) T85.828
    catheter NEC T85.828
      dialysis (renal) T82.828
        intraperitoneal T85.828
      infusion NEC T82.828
        spinal (epidural) (subdural)
          T85.820
      urinary (indwelling) T83.82
    electronic (electrode) (pulse generator)
      (stimulator)
      bone T84.82
      cardiac T82.827
      nervous system (brain) (peripheral
        nerve) (spinal) T85.820
      urinary T83.82
    fixation, internal (orthopedic) NEC T84.82
    gastrointestinal (bile duct) (esophagus)
      T85.828
    genital NEC T83.82
    heart NEC T82.827
    joint prosthesis T84.82
    ocular (corneal graft) (orbital implant)
      NEC T85.828
    orthopedic NEC T84.82
    specified NEC T85.828
    urinary NEC T83.82
    vascular NEC T82.828
    ventricular intracranial shunt T85.820
  ejaculatory duct N50.89
  endocardium —*see* Endocarditis
  endomyocardial (tropical) I42.3
  epididymis N50.89
  eye muscle —*see* Strabismus, mechanical
  heart —*see* Myocarditis
  hepatic —*see* Fibrosis, liver
  hepatolienal (portal hypertension) K76.6
  hepatosplenic (portal hypertension) K76.6
  infrapatellar fat pad M79.4
  intrascrotal N50.89
  kidney N26.9
  liver K74.00
    with sclerosis K74.2
    advanced K74.02
    alcoholic K70.2
    early K74.01
    stage
      F1 or F2 K74.01
      F3 K74.02
  lung (atrophic) (chronic) (confluent)
    (massive) (perialveolar) (peribronchial)
    J84.10
    with
      anthracosilicosis J60
      anthracosis J60
      asbestosis J61
      bagassosis J67.1
      bauxite J63.1
      berylliosis J63.2
      byssinosis J66.0
      calcicosis J62.8
      chalicosis J62.8
      dust reticulation J64
      farmer's lung J67.0
      ganister disease J62.8
      graphite J63.3
      pneumoconiosis NOS J64

Fibrosis, fibrotic *(Continued)*
  lung *(Continued)*
    with *(Continued)*
      siderosis J63.4
      silicosis J62.8
    capillary J84.10
    congenital P27.8
    diffuse (idiopathic) J84.10
      chemicals, gases, fumes or vapors
        (inhalation) J68.4
      interstitial J84.10
        acute J84.114
      talc J62.0
    following radiation J70.1
    idiopathic J84.112
    postinflammatory J84.10
    silicotic J62.8
    tuberculous —*see* Tuberculosis, pulmonary
  lymphatic gland I89.8
  median bar —*see* Hyperplasia, prostate
  mediastinum (idiopathic) J98.59
  meninges G96.198
  myocardium, myocardial —*see* Myocarditis
  ovary N83.8
  oviduct N83.8
  pancreas K86.89
  penis NEC N48.6
  pericardium I31.0
  perineum, in pregnancy or childbirth O34.7-●
    causing obstructed labor O65.5
  pleura J94.1
  popliteal fat pad M79.4
  prostate (chronic) —*see* Hyperplasia, prostate
  pulmonary —*see also* Fibrosis, lung J84.10
    congenital P27.8
    idiopathic J84.112
  rectal sphincter K62.89
  retroperitoneal, idiopathic (with ureteral
    obstruction) N13.5
    with infection N13.6
  sclerosing mesenteric (idiopathic) K65.4
  scrotum N50.89
  seminal vesicle N50.89
  senile R54
  skin L90.5
  spermatic cord N50.89
  spleen D73.89
    in schistosomiasis (bilharziasis) B65.9 [D77]
  subepidermal nodular —*see* Neoplasm, skin,
    benign
  submucous (oral) (tongue) K13.5
  testis N44.8
    chronic, due to syphilis A52.76
  thymus (gland) E32.8
  tongue, submucous K13.5
  tunica vaginalis N50.89
  uterus (non-neoplastic) N85.8
  vagina N89.8
  valve, heart —*see* Endocarditis
  vas deferens N50.89
  vein I87.8
Fibrositis (periarticular) M79.7
  nodular, chronic (Jaccoud's) (rheumatoid) —
    see Arthropathy, postrheumatic, chronic
Fibrothorax J94.1
Fibrotic —*see* Fibrosis
Fibrous —*see* condition
Fibroxanthoma —*see also* Neoplasm, connective
  tissue, benign
  atypical —*see* Neoplasm, connective tissue,
    uncertain behavior
  malignant —*see* Neoplasm, connective tissue,
    malignant
Fibroxanthosarcoma —*see* Neoplasm,
  connective tissue, malignant
Fiedler's
  disease (icterohemorrhagic leptospirosis) A27.0
  myocarditis (acute) I40.1
Fifth disease B08.3
  venereal A55
Filaria, filarial, filariasis —*see* Infestation, filarial

Filatov's disease —*see* Mononucleosis, infectious
File-cutter's disease —*see* Poisoning, lead
Filling defect
  biliary tract R93.2
  bladder R93.41
  duodenum R93.3
  gallbladder R93.2
  gastrointestinal tract R93.3
  intestine R93.3
  kidney R93.42-●
  stomach R93.3
  ureter R93.41
  urinary organs, specified NEC R93.49
Fimbrial cyst Q50.4
Financial problem affecting care NOS Z59.9
  ⮕bankruptcy Z59.89
  ⮕foreclosure on loan Z59.89
  ▶home loan Z59.81-●
Findings, abnormal, inconclusive, without
  diagnosis —*see also* Abnormal
  17-ketosteroids, elevated R82.5
  acetonuria R82.4
  alcohol in blood R78.0
  anisocytosis R71.8
  antenatal screening of mother O28.9
    biochemical O28.1
    chromosomal O28.5
    cytological O28.2
    genetic O28.5
    hematological O28.0
    radiological O28.4
    specified NEC O28.8
    ultrasonic O28.3
  antibody titer, elevated R76.0
  anticardiolipin antibody R76.0
  antiphosphatidylglycerol antibody R76.0
  antiphosphatidylinositol antibody R76.0
  antiphosphatidylserine antibody R76.0
  antiphospholipid antibody R76.0
  bacteriuria R82.71
  bicarbonate E87.8
  bile in urine R82.2
  blood sugar R73.09
    high R73.9
    low (transient) E16.2
  body fluid or substance, specified NEC
    R88.8
  casts, urine R82.998
  catecholamines R82.5
  cells, urine R82.998
  chloride E87.8
  cholesterol E78.9
    high E78.00
      with high triglycerides E78.2
  chyluria R82.0
  cloudy
    dialysis effluent R88.0
    urine R82.90
  creatinine clearance R94.4
  crystals, urine R82.998
  culture
    blood R78.81
    positive —*see* Positive, culture
  echocardiogram R93.1
  electrolyte level, urinary R82.998
  function study NEC R94.8
    bladder R94.8
    endocrine NEC R94.7
      thyroid R94.6
    kidney R94.4
    liver R94.5
    pancreas R94.8
    placenta R94.8
    pulmonary R94.2
    spleen R94.8
  gallbladder, nonvisualization R93.2
  glucose (tolerance test) (non-fasting) R73.09
  glycosuria R81
  heart
    shadow R93.1
    sounds R01.2
  hematinuria R82.3

Findings, abnormal, inconclusive, without
  diagnosis *(Continued)*
  hematocrit drop (precipitous) R71.0
  hemoglobinuria R82.3
  human papillomavirus (HPV) DNA test
    positive
    cervix
      high risk R87.810
      low risk R87.820
    vagina
      high risk R87.811
      low risk R87.821
  in blood (of substance not normally found in
    blood) R78.9
    addictive drug NEC R78.4
    alcohol (excessive level) R78.0
    cocaine R78.2
    hallucinogen R78.3
    heavy metals (abnormal level) R78.79
    lead R78.71
    lithium (abnormal level) R78.89
    opiate drug R78.1
    psychotropic drug R78.5
    specified substance NEC R78.89
    steroid agent R78.6
  indoleacetic acid, elevated R82.5
  ketonuria R82.4
  lactic acid dehydrogenase (LDH) R74.02
  ⮕liver function test (*see also* Elevated, liver
    function, test) R79.89
  mammogram NEC R92.8
    calcification (calculus) R92.1
    inconclusive result (due to dense breasts)
      R92.2
    microcalcification R92.0
  mediastinal shift R93.89
  melanin, urine R82.998
  myoglobinuria R82.1
  ⮕neonatal screening —*see* Abnormal, neonatal
    screening
  ▶newborn screens, state mandated —*see*
    Abnormal, neonatal screening
  nonvisualization of gallbladder R93.2
  odor of urine NOS R82.90
  Papanicolaou cervix R87.619
    non-atypical endometrial cells R87.618
  pneumoencephalogram R93.0
  poikilocytosis R71.8
  potassium (deficiency) E87.6
    excess E87.5
  PPD R76.11
  radiologic (X-ray) R93.89
    abdomen R93.5
    biliary tract R93.2
    breast R92.8
    gastrointestinal tract R93.3
    genitourinary organs R93.89
    head R93.0
    inconclusive due to excess body fat of
      patient R93.9
    intrathoracic organs NEC R93.1
    musculoskeletal
      limbs R93.6
      other than limb R93.7
    placenta R93.89
    retroperitoneum R93.5
    skin R93.89
    skull R93.0
    subcutaneous tissue R93.89
    testis R93.81-●
  red blood cell (count) (morphology) (sickling)
    (volume) R71.8
  scan NEC R94.8
    bladder R94.8
    bone R94.8
    kidney R94.4
    liver R93.2
    lung R94.2
    pancreas R94.8
    placental R94.8
    spleen R94.8
    thyroid R94.6
  sedimentation rate, elevated R70.0

▶ New   ⮕ Revised   ~~deleted~~ Deleted   ● Use Additional Character(s)

Findings, abnormal, inconclusive, without
      diagnosis (Continued)
SGOT R74.Ø1
SGPT R74.Ø1
sodium (deficiency) E87.1
      excess E87.Ø
specified body fluid NEC R88.8
stress test R94.39
thyroid (function) (metabolic rate) (scan)
      (uptake) R94.6
transaminase (level) R74.Ø1
triglycerides E78.9
      high E78.1
            with high cholesterol E78.2
tuberculin skin test (without active
      tuberculosis) R76.11
urine R82.9Ø
      acetone R82.4
      bacteria R82.71
      bile R82.2
      casts or cells R82.998
      chyle R82.Ø
      culture positive R82.79
      glucose R81
      hemoglobin R82.3
      ketone R82.4
      sugar R81
vanillylmandelic acid (VMA), elevated
      R82.5
vectorcardiogram (VCG) R94.39
ventriculogram R93.Ø
white blood cell (count) (differential)
      (morphology) D72.9
xerography R92.8
Finger —see condition
Fire, Saint Anthony's —see Erysipelas
Fire-setting
      pathological (compulsive) F63.1
Fish hook stomach K31.89
Fishmeal-worker's lung J67.8
Fissure, fissured
      anus, anal K6Ø.2
            acute K6Ø.Ø
            chronic K6Ø.1
            congenital Q43.8
      ear, lobule, congenital Q17.8
      epiglottis (congenital) Q31.8
      larynx J38.7
            congenital Q31.8
      lip K13.Ø
            congenital —see Cleft, lip
      nipple N64.Ø
            associated with
                  lactation O92.13
                  pregnancy O92.11-•
                  puerperium O92.12
      nose Q3Ø.2
      palate (congenital) —see Cleft, palate
      skin R23.4
      spine (congenital) —see also Spina bifida
            with hydrocephalus —see Spina bifida, by
                  site, with hydrocephalus
      tongue (acquired) K14.5
            congenital Q38.3
Fistula (cutaneous) L98.8
      abdomen (wall) K63.2
            bladder N32.2
            intestine NEC K63.2
            ureter N28.89
            uterus N82.5
      abdominorectal K63.2
      abdominosigmoidal K63.2
      abdominothoracic J86.Ø
      abdominouterine N82.5
            congenital Q51.7
      abdominovesical N32.2
      accessory sinuses —see Sinusitis
      actinomycotic —see Actinomycosis
      alveolar antrum —see Sinusitis, maxillary
      alveolar process KØ4.6
      anorectal K6Ø.5
      antrobuccal —see Sinusitis, maxillary
      antrum —see Sinusitis, maxillary

Fistula (Continued)
      anus, anal (recurrent) (infectional) K6Ø.3
            congenital Q43.6
                  with absence, atresia and stenosis Q42.2
            tuberculous A18.32
      aorta-duodenal I77.2
      appendix, appendicular K38.3
      arteriovenous (acquired) (nonruptured) I77.Ø
            brain I67.1
                  congenital Q28.2
                        ruptured —see Fistula, arteriovenous,
                              brain, ruptured
                  ruptured I6Ø.8
                        intracerebral I61.8
                        intraparenchymal I61.8
                        intraventricular I61.5
                        subarachnoid I6Ø.8
            cerebral —see Fistula, arteriovenous, brain
            congenital (peripheral) —see also
                  Malformation, arteriovenous
                  brain Q28.2
                        ruptured —see Fistula, arteriovenous,
                              brain, ruptured
                  coronary Q24.5
                  pulmonary Q25.72
            coronary I25.41
                  congenital Q24.5
            pulmonary I28.Ø
                  congenital Q25.72
            surgically created (for dialysis) Z99.2
                  complication —see Complication,
                        arteriovenous, fistula, surgically
                        created
            traumatic —see Injury, blood vessel
      artery I77.2
      aural (mastoid) —see Mastoiditis, chronic
      auricle —see also Disorder, pinna, specified
            type NEC
            congenital Q18.1
      Bartholin's gland N82.8
      bile duct (common) (hepatic) K83.3
            with calculus, stones —see also Calculus,
                  bile duct K83.3
      biliary (tract) —see Fistula, bile duct
      bladder (sphincter) NEC —see also Fistula,
            vesico- N32.2
            into seminal vesicle N32.2
      bone —see also Disorder, bone, specified type
            NEC
            with osteomyelitis, chronic —see
                  Osteomyelitis, chronic, with draining
                  sinus
      brain G93.89
            arteriovenous (acquired) (see Fistula,
                  arteriovenous, brain) I67.1
            congenital Q28.2
      branchial (cleft) Q18.Ø
      branchiogenous Q18.Ø
      breast N61.Ø
            puerperal, postpartum or gestational, due
                  to mastitis (purulent) —see Mastitis,
                  obstetric, purulent
      bronchial J86.Ø
      bronchocutaneous, bronchomediastinal,
            bronchopleural, bronchopleuromediastinal
            (infective) J86.Ø
            tuberculous NEC A15.5
      bronchoesophageal J86.Ø
            congenital Q39.2
                  with atresia of esophagus Q39.1
      bronchovisceral J86.Ø
      buccal cavity (infective) K12.2
      cecosigmoidal K63.2
      cecum K63.2
      cerebrospinal (fluid) G96.Ø8
      cervical, lateral Q18.1
      cervicoaural Q18.1
      cervicosigmoidal N82.4
      cervicovesical N82.1
      cervix N82.8
      chest (wall) J86.Ø

Fistula (Continued)
      cholecystenteric —see Fistula, gallbladder
      cholecystocolic —see Fistula, gallbladder
      cholecystocolonic —see Fistula, gallbladder
      cholecystoduodenal —see Fistula, gallbladder
      cholecystogastric —see Fistula, gallbladder
      cholecystointestinal —see Fistula, gallbladder
      choledochoduodenal —see Fistula, bile duct
      cholocolic K82.3
      coccyx —see Sinus, pilonidal
      colon K63.2
      colostomy K94.Ø9
      colovesical N32.1
      common duct —see Fistula, bile duct
      congenital, site not listed —see Anomaly, by
            site
      coronary, arteriovenous I25.41
            congenital Q24.5
      costal region J86.Ø
      cul-de-sac, Douglas' N82.8
      cystic duct —see also Fistula, gallbladder
            congenital Q44.5
      dental KØ4.6
      diaphragm J86.Ø
      duodenum K31.6
      ear (external) (canal) —see Disorder, ear,
            external, specified type NEC
      enterocolic K63.2
      enterocutaneous K63.2
      enterouterine N82.4
            congenital Q51.7
      enterovaginal N82.4
            congenital Q52.2
            large intestine N82.3
            small intestine N82.2
      enterovesical N32.1
      epididymis N5Ø.89
            tuberculous A18.15
      esophagobronchial J86.Ø
            congenital Q39.2
                  with atresia of esophagus Q39.1
⮕esophagocutaneous K22.89
      esophagopleural-cutaneous J86.Ø
      esophagotracheal J86.Ø
            congenital Q39.2
                  with atresia of esophagus Q39.1
⮕esophagus K22.89
            congenital Q39.2
                  with atresia of esophagus Q39.1
      ethmoid —see Sinusitis, ethmoidal
      eyeball (cornea) (sclera) —see Disorder, globe,
            hypotony
      eyelid HØ1.8
      fallopian tube, external N82.5
      fecal K63.2
            congenital Q43.6
      from periapical abscess KØ4.6
      frontal sinus —see Sinusitis, frontal
      gallbladder K82.3
            with calculus, cholelithiasis, stones —see
                  Calculus, gallbladder
      gastric K31.6
      gastrocolic K31.6
            congenital Q4Ø.2
            tuberculous A18.32
      gastroenterocolic K31.6
      gastroesophageal K31.6
      gastrojejunal K31.6
      gastrojejunocolic K31.6
      genital tract (female) N82.9
            specified NEC N82.8
            to intestine NEC N82.4
            to skin N82.5
      hepatic artery-portal vein, congenital Q26.6
      hepatopleural J86.Ø
      hepatopulmonary J86.Ø
      ileorectal or ileosigmoidal K63.2
      ileovaginal N82.2
      ileovesical N32.1
      ileum K63.2
      in ano K6Ø.3
            tuberculous A18.32

Fistula *(Continued)*
   inner ear (labyrinth) —*see* subcategory H83.1
   intestine NEC K63.2
   intestinocolonic (abdominal) K63.2
   intestinoureteral N28.89
   intestinouterine N82.4
   intestinovaginal N82.4
     large intestine N82.3
     small intestine N82.2
   intestinovesical N32.1
   ischiorectal (fossa) K61.39
   jejunum K63.2
   joint M25.10
     ankle M25.17-●
     elbow M25.12-●
     foot joint M25.17-●
     hand joint M25.14-●
     hip M25.15-●
     knee M25.16-●
     shoulder M25.11-●
     specified joint NEC M25.18
     tuberculous —*see* Tuberculosis, joint
     vertebrae M25.18
     wrist M25.13-●
   kidney N28.89
   labium (majus) (minus) N82.8
   labyrinth —*see* subcategory H83.1
   lacrimal (gland) (sac) H04.61-●
   lacrimonasal duct —*see* Fistula, lacrimal
   laryngotracheal, congenital Q34.8
   larynx J38.7
   lip K13.0
     congenital Q38.0
   lumbar, tuberculous A18.01
   lung J86.0
   lymphatic I89.8
   mammary (gland) N61.0
   mastoid (process) (region) —*see* Mastoiditis,
     chronic
   maxillary J32.0
   medial, face and neck Q18.8
   mediastinal J86.0
   mediastinobronchial J86.0
   mediastinocutaneous J86.0
   middle ear —*see* subcategory H74.8
   mouth K12.2
   nasal J34.89
     sinus —*see* Sinusitis
   nasopharynx J39.2
   nipple N64.0
   nose J34.89
   oral (cutaneous) K12.2
     maxillary J32.0
     nasal (with cleft palate) —*see* Cleft, palate
   orbit, orbital —*see* Disorder, orbit, specified
     type NEC
   oroantral J32.0
   oviduct, external N82.5
   palate (hard) M27.8
   pancreatic K86.89
   pancreaticoduodenal K86.89
   parotid (gland) K11.4
     region K12.2
   penis N48.89
   perianal K60.3
   pericardium (pleura) (sac) —*see* Pericarditis
   pericecal K63.2
   perineorectal K60.4 perineosigmoidal K63.2
   perineosigmoidal K63.2
   perineum, perineal (with urethral
     involvement) NEC N36.0
     tuberculous A18.13
     ureter N28.89
   perirectal K60.4
     tuberculous A18.32
   peritoneum K65.9
   pharyngoesophageal J39.2
   pharynx J39.2
     branchial cleft (congenital) Q18.0
   pilonidal (infected) (rectum) —*see* Sinus,
     pilonidal

Fistula *(Continued)*
   pleura, pleural, pleurocutaneous,
     pleuroperitoneal J86.0
     tuberculous NEC A15.6
   pleuropericardial I31.8
   portal vein-hepatic artery, congenital Q26.6
   postauricular H70.81-●
   postoperative, persistent T81.83
     specified site —*see* Fistula, by site
   preauricular (congenital) Q18.1
   prostate N42.89
   pulmonary J86.0
     arteriovenous I28.0
       congenital Q25.72
     tuberculous —*see* Tuberculosis, pulmonary
   pulmonoperitoneal J86.0
   rectolabial N82.4
   rectosigmoid (intercommunicating) K63.2
   rectoureteral N28.89
   rectourethral N36.0
     congenital Q64.73
   rectouterine N82.4
     congenital Q51.7
   rectovaginal N82.3
     congenital Q52.2
     tuberculous A18.18
   rectovesical N32.1
     congenital Q64.79
   rectovesicovaginal N82.3
   rectovulval N82.4
     congenital Q52.79
   rectum (to skin) K60.4
     congenital Q43.6
       with absence, atresia and stenosis Q42.0
     tuberculous A18.32
   renal N28.89
   retroauricular —*see* Fistula, postauricular
   salivary duct or gland (any) K11.4
     congenital Q38.4
   scrotum (urinary) N50.89
     tuberculous A18.15
   semicircular canals —*see* subcategory H83.1
   sigmoid K63.2
     to bladder N32.1
   sinus —*see* Sinusitis
   skin L98.8
     to genital tract (female) N82.5
   splenocolic D73.89
   stercoral K63.2
   stomach K31.6
   sublingual gland K11.4
   submandibular gland K11.4
   submaxillary (gland) K11.4
     region K12.2
   thoracic J86.0
     duct I89.8
   thoracoabdominal J86.0
   thoracogastric J86.0
   thoracointestinal J86.0
   thorax J86.0
   thyroglossal duct Q89.2
   thyroid E07.89
   trachea, congenital (external) (internal) Q32.1
   tracheoesophageal J86.0
     congenital Q39.2
       with atresia of esophagus Q39.1
     following tracheostomy J95.04
   traumatic arteriovenous —*see* Injury, blood
     vessel, by site
   tuberculous - code by site under Tuberculosis
   typhoid A01.09
   umbilicourinary Q64.8
   urachus, congenital Q64.4
   ureter (persistent) N28.89
   ureteroabdominal N28.89
   ureterorectal N28.89
   ureterosigmoido-abdominal N28.89
   ureterovaginal N82.1
   ureterovesical N32.2
   urethra N36.0
     congenital Q64.79
     tuberculous A18.13

Fistula *(Continued)*
   urethroperineal N36.0
   urethroperineovesical N32.2
   urethrorectal N36.0
     congenital Q64.73
   urethroscrotal N50.89
   urethrovaginal N82.1
   urethrovesical N32.2
   urinary (tract) (persistent) (recurrent)
     N36.0
   uteroabdominal N82.5
     congenital Q51.7
   uteroenteric, uterointestinal N82.4
     congenital Q51.7
   uterorectal N82.4
     congenital Q51.7
   uteroureteric N82.1
   uterourethral Q51.7
   uterovaginal N82.8
   uterovesical N82.1
     congenital Q51.7
   uterus N82.8
   vagina (postpartal) (wall) N82.8
   vaginocutaneous (postpartal) N82.5
   vaginointestinal NEC N82.4
     large intestine N82.3
     small intestine N82.2
   vaginoperineal N82.5
   vasocutaneous, congenital Q55.7
   vesical NEC N32.2
   vesicoabdominal N32.2
   vesicocervicovaginal N82.1
   vesicocolic N32.1
   vesicocutaneous N32.2
   vesicoenteric N32.1
   vesicointestinal N32.1
   vesicometrorectal N82.4
   vesicoperineal N32.2
   vesicorectal N32.1
     congenital Q64.79
   vesicosigmoidal N32.1
   vesicosigmoidovaginal N82.3
   vesicoureteral N32.2
   vesicoureterovaginal N82.1
   vesicourethral N32.2
   vesicourethrorectal N32.1
   vesicouterine N82.1
     congenital Q51.7
   vesicovaginal N82.0
   vulvorectal N82.4
     congenital Q52.79
Fit R56.9
   epileptic —*see* Epilepsy
   fainting R55
   hysterical F44.5
   newborn P90
Fitting (and adjustment) (of)
   artificial
     arm —*see* Admission, adjustment, artificial,
       arm
     breast Z44.3
     eye Z44.2
     leg —*see* Admission, adjustment, artificial,
       leg
   automatic implantable cardiac defibrillator
     (with synchronous cardiac pacemaker)
     Z45.02
   brain neuropacemaker Z46.2
     implanted Z45.42
   cardiac defibrillator —*see* Fitting (and
     adjustment) (of), automatic implantable
     cardiac defibrillator
   catheter, non-vascular Z46.82
   colostomy belt Z46.89
   contact lenses Z46.0
   CRT-D (resynchronization therapy
     defibrillator) Z45.02
   CRT-P (cardiac resynchronization therapy
     pacemaker) Z45.018
     pulse generator Z45.010
   cystostomy device Z46.6

    ▶ New   ⇒ Revised   ~~deleted~~ Deleted   ● Use Additional Character(s)

Fitting *(Continued)*
  defibrillator, cardiac —*see* Fitting (and
     adjustment) (of), automatic implantable
     cardiac defibrillator
  dentures Z46.3
  device NOS Z46.9
    abdominal Z46.89
    gastrointestinal NEC Z46.59
    implanted NEC Z45.89
    nervous system Z46.2
      implanted —*see* Admission, adjustment,
       device, implanted, nervous system
    orthodontic Z46.4
    orthoptic Z46.0
    orthotic Z46.89
    prosthetic (external) Z44.9
      breast Z44.3
      dental Z46.3
      eye Z44.2
      specified NEC Z44.8
    specified NEC Z46.89
    substitution
      auditory Z46.2
        implanted —*see* Admission,
         adjustment, device, implanted,
         hearing device
      nervous system Z46.2
        implanted —*see* Admission,
         adjustment, device, implanted,
         nervous system
      visual Z46.2
        implanted Z45.31
    urinary Z46.6
  gastric lap band Z46.51
  gastrointestinal appliance NEC Z46.59
  glasses (reading) Z46.0
  hearing aid Z46.1
  ileostomy device Z46.89
  insulin pump Z46.81
  intestinal appliance NEC Z46.89
  myringotomy device (stent) (tube) Z45.82
  neuropacemaker Z46.2
    implanted Z45.42
  non-vascular catheter Z46.82
  orthodontic device Z46.4
  orthopedic device (brace) (cast) (corset)
    (shoes) Z46.89
  pacemaker (cardiac) (cardiac
    resynchronization therapy (CRT-P))
    Z45.018
    nervous system (brain) (peripheral nerve)
      (spinal cord) Z46.2
      implanted Z45.42
    pulse generator Z45.010
  portacath (port-a-cath) Z45.2
  prosthesis (external) Z44.9
    arm —*see* Admission, adjustment, artificial,
      arm
    breast Z44.3
    dental Z46.3
    eye Z44.2
    leg —*see* Admission, adjustment, artificial,
      leg
    specified NEC Z44.8
  spectacles Z46.0
  wheelchair Z46.89
Fitzhugh-Curtis syndrome
  due to
    Chlamydia trachomatis A74.81
    Neisseria gonorrhorea (gonococcal
      peritonitis) A54.85
Fitz's syndrome (acute hemorrhagic
  pancreatitis) —*see also* Pancreatitis,
  acute K85.80
Fixation
  joint —*see* Ankylosis
  larynx J38.7
  stapes —*see* Ankylosis, ear ossicles
    deafness —*see* Deafness, conductive
  uterus (acquired) —*see* Malposition, uterus
  vocal cord J38.3

Flabby ridge K06.8
Flaccid —*see also* condition
  palate, congenital Q38.5
Flail
  chest S22.5-●
    newborn (birth injury) P13.8
  joint (paralytic) M25.20
    ankle M25.27-●
    elbow M25.22-●
    foot joint M25.27-●
    hand joint M25.24-●
    hip M25.25-●
    knee M25.26-●
    shoulder M25.21-●
    specified joint NEC M25.28
    wrist M25.23-●
Flajani's disease —*see* Hyperthyroidism, with,
  goiter (diffuse)
Flap, liver K71.3
Flashbacks (residual to hallucinogen use)
  F16.283
Flat
  chamber (eye) —*see* Disorder, globe,
    hypotony, flat anterior chamber
  chest, congenital Q67.8
  foot (acquired) (fixed type) (painful)
    (postural) —*see also* Deformity, limb,
    flat foot
    congenital (rigid) (spastic (everted))
      Q66.5-●
    rachitic sequelae (late effect) E64.3
  organ or site, congenital NEC —*see* Anomaly,
    by site
  pelvis M95.5
    with disproportion (fetopelvic) O33.0
      causing obstructed labor O65.0
    congenital Q74.2
Flatau-Schilder disease G37.0
Flatback syndrome M40.30
  lumbar region M40.36
  lumbosacral region M40.37
  thoracolumbar region M40.35
Flattening
  head, femur M89.8X5
  hip —*see* Coxa, plana
  lip (congenital) Q18.8
  nose (congenital) Q67.4
    acquired M95.0
Flatulence R14.3
  psychogenic F45.8
Flatus R14.3
  vaginalis N89.8
Flax-dresser's disease J66.1
Flea bite —*see* Injury, bite, by site, superficial,
  insect
Flecks, glaucomatous (subcapsular) —*see*
  Cataract, complicated
Fleischer (-Kayser) **ring** (cornea) H18.04-●
Fleshy mole O02.0
Flexibilitas cerea —*see* Catalepsy
Flexion
  amputation stump (surgical) T87.89
  cervix —*see* Malposition, uterus
  contracture, joint —*see* Contraction, joint
  deformity, joint —*see also* Deformity, limb,
    flexion M21.20
    hip, congenital Q65.89
  uterus —*see also* Malposition, uterus
    lateral —*see* Lateroversion, uterus
Flexner-Boyd dysentery A03.2
Flexner's dysentery A03.1
Flexure —*see* Flexion
Flint murmur (aortic insufficiency) I35.1
Floater, vitreous —*see* Opacity, vitreous
Floating
  cartilage (joint) —*see also* Loose, body, joint
    knee —*see* Derangement, knee, loose body
  gallbladder, congenital Q44.1
  kidney N28.89
    congenital Q63.8
  spleen D73.89

Flooding N92.0
Floor —*see* condition
Floppy
  baby syndrome (nonspecific) P94.2
  iris syndrome (intraoperative) (IFIS) H21.81
  nonrheumatic mitral valve syndrome I34.1
Flu —*see also* Influenza
  avian —*see also* Influenza, due to, identified
    novel influenza A virus J09.X2
  bird —*see also* Influenza, due to, identified
    novel influenza A virus J09.X2
  intestinal NEC A08.4
  swine (viruses that normally cause infections
    in pigs) —*see also* Influenza, due to,
    identified novel influenza A virus J09.X2
Fluctuating blood pressure I99.8
Fluid
  abdomen R18.8
  chest J94.8
  heart —*see* Failure, heart, congestive
  joint —*see* Effusion, joint
  loss (acute) E86.9
  lung —*see* Edema, lung
  overload E87.70
    specified NEC E87.79
  peritoneal cavity R18.8
  pleural cavity J94.8
  retention R60.9
Flukes NEC —*see also* Infestation, fluke
  blood NEC —*see* Schistosomiasis
  liver B66.3
Fluor (vaginalis) N89.8
  trichomonal or due to Trichomonas
    (vaginalis) A59.00
Fluorosis
  dental K00.3
  skeletal M85.10
    ankle M85.17-●
    foot M85.17-●
    forearm M85.13-●
    hand M85.14-●
    lower leg M85.16-●
    multiple site M85.19
    neck M85.18
    rib M85.18
    shoulder M85.11-●
    skull M85.18
    specified site NEC M85.18
    thigh M85.15-●
    toe M85.17-●
    upper arm M85.12-●
    vertebra M85.18
Flush syndrome E34.0
Flushing R23.2
  menopausal N95.1
Flutter
  atrial or auricular I48.92
    atypical I48.4
    type I I48.3
    type II I48.4
    typical I48.3
  heart I49.8
    atrial or auricular I48.92
      atypical I48.4
      type I I48.3
      type II I48.4
      typical I48.3
    ventricular I49.02
  ventricular I49.02
FNHTR (febrile nonhemolytic transfusion
  reaction) R50.84
Fochier's abscess - code by site under Abscess
Focus, Assmann's —*see* Tuberculosis,
  pulmonary
Fogo selvagem L10.3
Foix-Alajouanine syndrome G95.19
Fold, folds (anomalous) —*see also* Anomaly,
  by site
  Descemet's membrane —*see* Change, corneal
    membrane, Descemet's, fold
  epicanthic Q10.3
  heart Q24.8

Folie à deux F24
Follicle
  cervix (nabothian) (ruptured) N88.8
  graafian, ruptured, with hemorrhage N83.0-●
  nabothian N88.8
Follicular —*see* condition
Folliculitis (superficial) L73.9
  abscedens et suffodiens L66.3
  cyst N83.0-●
  decalvans L66.2
  deep —*see* Furuncle, by site
  gonococcal (acute) (chronic) A54.01
  keloid, keloidalis L73.0
  pustular L01.02
  ulerythematosa reticulata L66.4
Folliculome lipidique
  specified site —*see* Neoplasm, benign, by site
  unspecified site
    female D27.9
    male D29.20
Folling's disease E70.0
Follow-up —*see* Examination, follow-up
Fong's syndrome (hereditary osteo-
    onychodysplasia) Q87.2
Food
  allergy L27.2
  asphyxia (from aspiration or inhalation) —*see*
      Foreign body, by site
  choked on —*see* Foreign body, by site
  deprivation T73.0
    specified kind of food NEC E63.8
▶ insecurity Z59.41
  intoxication —*see* Poisoning, food
  lack of T73.0
  poisoning —*see* Poisoning, food
  rejection NEC —*see* Disorder, eating
  strangulation or suffocation —*see* Foreign
      body, by site
  toxemia —*see* Poisoning, food
Foot —*see* condition
Foramen ovale (nonclosure) (patent)
    (persistent) Q21.1
Forbes' glycogen storage disease E74.03
Fordyce-Fox disease L75.2
Fordyce's disease (mouth) Q38.6
Forearm —*see* condition
▶ **Foreclosure on loan** Z59.89
Foreign body
  with
    laceration —*see* Laceration, by site, with
        foreign body
    puncture wound —*see* Puncture, by site,
        with foreign body
  accidentally left following a procedure
      T81.509
    aspiration T81.506
      resulting in
        adhesions T81.516
        obstruction T81.526
        perforation T81.536
        specified complication NEC
            T81.596
    cardiac catheterization T81.505
      resulting in
        acute reaction T81.60
          aseptic peritonitis T81.61
          specified NEC T81.69
        adhesions T81.515
        obstruction T81.525
        perforation T81.535
        specified complication NEC
            T81.595
    causing
      acute reaction T81.60
        aseptic peritonitis T81.61
        specified complication NEC T81.69
      adhesions T81.519
      aseptic peritonitis T81.61
      obstruction T81.529
      perforation T81.539
      specified complication NEC T81.599

Foreign body *(Continued)*
  accidentally left following a procedure
      (Continued)
    endoscopy T81.504
      resulting in
        adhesions T81.514
        obstruction T81.524
        perforation T81.534
        specified complication NEC T81.594
    immunization T81.503
      resulting in
        adhesions T81.513
        obstruction T81.523
        perforation T81.533
        specified complication NEC T81.593
    infusion T81.501
      resulting in
        adhesions T81.511
        obstruction T81.521
        perforation T81.531
        specified complication NEC T81.591
    injection T81.503
      resulting in
        adhesions T81.513
        obstruction T81.523
        perforation T81.533
        specified complication NEC T81.593
    kidney dialysis T81.502
      resulting in
        adhesions T81.512
        obstruction T81.522
        perforation T81.532
        specified complication NEC T81.592
    packing removal T81.507
      resulting in
        acute reaction T81.60
          aseptic peritonitis T81.61
          specified NEC T81.69
        adhesions T81.517
        obstruction T81.527
        perforation T81.537
        specified complication NEC T81.597
    puncture T81.506
      resulting in
        adhesions T81.516
        obstruction T81.526
        perforation T81.536
        specified complication NEC T81.596
    specified procedure NEC T81.508
      resulting in
        acute reaction T81.60
          aseptic peritonitis T81.61
          specified NEC T81.69
        adhesions T81.518
        obstruction T81.528
        perforation T81.538
        specified complication NEC T81.598
    surgical operation T81.500
      resulting in
        acute reaction T81.60
          aseptic peritonitis T81.61
          specified NEC T81.69
        adhesions T81.510
        obstruction T81.520
        perforation T81.530
        specified complication NEC T81.590
    transfusion T81.501
      resulting in
        adhesions T81.511
        obstruction T81.521
        perforation T81.531
        specified complication NEC T81.591
  alimentary tract T18.9
    anus T18.5
    colon T18.4
    esophagus —*see* Foreign body, esophagus
    mouth T18.0
    multiple sites T18.8
    rectosigmoid (junction) T18.5
    rectum T18.5
    small intestine T18.3

Foreign body *(Continued)*
  alimentary tract *(Continued)*
    specified site NEC T18.8
    stomach T18.2
  anterior chamber (eye) S05.5-●
  auditory canal —*see* Foreign body, entering
      through orifice, ear
  bronchus T17.508
    causing
      asphyxiation T17.500
        food (bone) (seed) T17.520
        gastric contents (vomitus) T17.510
        specified type NEC T17.590
      injury NEC T17.508
        food (bone) (seed) T17.528
        gastric contents (vomitus) T17.518
        specified type NEC T17.598
  canthus —*see* Foreign body, conjunctival sac
  ciliary body (eye) S05.5-●
  conjunctival sac T15.1-●
  cornea T15.0-●
  entering through orifice
    accessory sinus T17.0
    alimentary canal T18.9
      multiple parts T18.8
      specified part NEC T18.8
    alveolar process T18.0
    antrum (Highmore's) T17.0
    anus T18.5
    appendix T18.4
    auditory canal —*see* Foreign body, entering
        through orifice, ear
    auricle —*see* Foreign body, entering
        through orifice, ear
    bladder T19.1
    bronchioles —*see* Foreign body, respiratory
        tract, specified site NEC
    bronchus (main) —*see* Foreign body,
        bronchus
    buccal cavity T18.0
    canthus (inner) —*see* Foreign body,
        conjunctival sac
    cecum T18.4
    cervix (canal) (uteri) T19.3
    colon T18.4
    conjunctival sac —*see* Foreign body,
        conjunctival sac
    cornea —*see* Foreign body, cornea
    digestive organ or tract NOS T18.9
      multiple parts T18.8
      specified part NEC T18.8
    duodenum T18.3
    ear (external) T16.-●
    esophagus —*see* Foreign body, esophagus
    eye (external) NOS T15.9-●
      conjunctival sac —*see* Foreign body,
          conjunctival sac
      cornea —*see* Foreign body, cornea
      specified part NEC T15.8-●
    eyeball —*see also* Foreign body, entering
        through orifice, eye, specified part
        NEC
      with penetrating wound —*see* Puncture,
          eyeball
    eyelid —*see also* Foreign body, conjunctival
        sac
      with
        laceration —*see* Laceration, eyelid,
            with foreign body
        puncture —*see* Puncture, eyelid, with
            foreign body
        superficial injury —*see* Foreign body,
            superficial, eyelid
    gastrointestinal tract T18.9
      multiple parts T18.8
      specified part NEC T18.8
    genitourinary tract T19.9
      multiple parts T19.8
      specified part NEC T19.8
    globe —*see* Foreign body, entering through
        orifice, eyeball

Foreign body *(Continued)*
    entering through orifice *(Continued)*
        gum T18.0
        Highmore's antrum T17.0
        hypopharynx —*see* Foreign body, pharynx
        ileum T18.3
        intestine (small) T18.3
            large T18.4
        lacrimal apparatus (punctum) —*see*
            Foreign body, entering through orifice,
            eye, specified part NEC
        large intestine T18.4
        larynx —*see* Foreign body, larynx
        lung —*see* Foreign body, respiratory tract,
            specified site NEC
        maxillary sinus T17.0
        mouth T18.0
        nasal sinus T17.0
        nasopharynx —*see* Foreign body, pharynx
        nose (passage) T17.1
        nostril T17.1
        oral cavity T18.0
        palate T18.0
        penis T19.4
        pharynx —*see* Foreign body, pharynx
        piriform sinus —*see* Foreign body, pharynx
        rectosigmoid (junction) T18.5
        rectum T18.5
        respiratory tract —*see* Foreign body,
            respiratory tract
        sinus (accessory) (frontal) (maxillary)
            (nasal) T17.0
            piriform —*see* Foreign body, pharynx
        small intestine T18.3
        stomach T18.2
        suffocation by —*see* Foreign body, by site
        tear ducts or glands —*see* Foreign body,
            entering through orifice, eye, specified
            part NEC
        throat —*see* Foreign body, pharynx
        tongue T18.0
        tonsil, tonsillar (fossa) —*see* Foreign body,
            pharynx
        trachea —*see* Foreign body, trachea
        ureter T19.8
        urethra T19.0
        uterus (any part) T19.3
        vagina T19.2
        vulva T19.2
    esophagus T18.108
        causing
            injury NEC T18.108
                food (bone) (seed) T18.128
                gastric contents (vomitus) T18.118
                specified type NEC T18.198
            tracheal compression T18.100
                food (bone) (seed) T18.120
                gastric contents (vomitus) T18.110
                specified type NEC T18.190
    feeling of, in throat R09.89
    fragment —*see* Retained, foreign body
        fragments (type of)
    genitourinary tract T19.9
        bladder T19.1
        multiple parts T19.8
        penis T19.4
        specified site NEC T19.8
        urethra T19.0
        uterus T19.3
            IUD Z97.5
        vagina T19.2
            contraceptive device Z97.5
        vulva T19.2
    granuloma (old) (soft tissue) —*see also*
        Granuloma, foreign body
        skin L92.3
    in
        laceration —*see* Laceration, by site, with
            foreign body
        puncture wound —*see* Puncture, by site,
            with foreign body
        soft tissue (residual) M79.5

Foreign body *(Continued)*
    inadvertently left in operation wound —*see*
        Foreign body, accidentally left during a
        procedure
    ingestion, ingested NOS T18.9
    inhalation or inspiration —*see* Foreign body,
        by site
    internal organ, not entering through a natural
        orifice - code as specific injury with
        foreign body
    intraocular S05.5-●
        old, retained (nonmagnetic) H44.70-●
            anterior chamber H44.71-●
            ciliary body H44.72-●
            iris H44.72-●
            lens H44.73-●
            magnetic H44.60-●
                anterior chamber H44.61-●
                ciliary body H44.62-●
                iris H44.62-●
                lens H44.63-●
                posterior wall H44.64-●
                specified site NEC H44.69-●
                vitreous body H44.65-●
            posterior wall H44.74-●
            specified site NEC H44.79-●
            vitreous body H44.75-●
    iris —*see* Foreign body, intraocular
    lacrimal punctum —*see* Foreign body,
        entering through orifice, eye, specified
        part NEC
    larynx T17.308
        causing
            asphyxiation T17.300
                food (bone) (seed) T17.320
                gastric contents (vomitus) T17.310
                specified type NEC T17.390
            injury NEC T17.308
                food (bone) (seed) T17.328
                gastric contents (vomitus) T17.318
                specified type NEC T17.398
    lens —*see* Foreign body, intraocular
    ocular muscle S05.4-●
        old, retained —*see* Foreign body, orbit, old
    old or residual
        soft tissue (residual) M79.5
    operation wound, left accidentally —*see*
        Foreign body, accidentally left during a
        procedure
    orbit S05.4-●
        old, retained H05.5-●
    pharynx T17.208
        causing
            asphyxiation T17.200
                food (bone) (seed) T17.220
                gastric contents (vomitus)
                    T17.210
                specified type NEC T17.290
            injury NEC T17.208
                food (bone) (seed) T17.228
                gastric contents (vomitus)
                    T17.218
                specified type NEC T17.298
        larynx —*see* Foreign body, larynx
        lung —*see* Foreign body, respiratory tract,
            specified site NEC
        multiple parts —*see* Foreign body,
            respiratory tract, specified site NEC

Foreign body *(Continued)*
    respiratory tract *(Continued)*
        nasal sinus T17.0
        nasopharynx —*see* Foreign body,
            pharynx
        nose T17.1
        nostril T17.1
        pharynx —*see* Foreign body, pharynx
        specified site NEC T17.808
            causing
                asphyxiation T17.800
                    food (bone) (seed) T17.820
                    gastric contents (vomitus) T17.810
                    specified type NEC T17.890
                injury NEC T17.808
                    food (bone) (seed) T17.828
                    gastric contents (vomitus) T17.818
                    specified type NEC T17.898
        throat —*see* Foreign body, pharynx
        trachea —*see* Foreign body, trachea
    retained (old) (nonmagnetic) (in)
        anterior chamber (eye) —*see* Foreign body,
            intraocular, old, retained, anterior
            chamber
            magnetic —*see* Foreign body, intraocular,
                old, retained, magnetic, anterior
                chamber
        ciliary body —*see* Foreign body,
            intraocular, old, retained, ciliary body
            magnetic —*see* Foreign body, intraocular,
                old, retained, magnetic, ciliary body
        eyelid H02.819
            left H02.816
                lower H02.815
                upper H02.814
            right H02.813
                lower H02.812
                upper H02.811
        fragments —*see* Retained, foreign body
            fragments (type of)
        globe —*see* Foreign body, intraocular, old,
            retained
            magnetic —*see* Foreign body, intraocular,
                old, retained, magnetic
        intraocular —*see* Foreign body, intraocular,
            old, retained
            magnetic —*see* Foreign body, intraocular,
                old, retained, magnetic
        iris —*see* Foreign body, intraocular, old,
            retained, iris
            magnetic —*see* Foreign body, intraocular,
                old, retained, magnetic, iris
        lens —*see* Foreign body, intraocular, old,
            retained, lens
            magnetic —*see* Foreign body, intraocular,
                old, retained, magnetic, lens
        muscle —*see* Foreign body, retained, soft
            tissue
        orbit —*see* Foreign body, orbit, old
        posterior wall of globe —*see* Foreign body,
            intraocular, old, retained, posterior
            wall
            magnetic —*see* Foreign body, intraocular,
                old, retained, magnetic, posterior
                wall
        retrobulbar —*see* Foreign body, orbit, old,
            retrobulbar
        soft tissue M79.5
        vitreous —*see* Foreign body, intraocular,
            old, retained, vitreous body
            magnetic —*see* Foreign body, intraocular,
                old, retained, magnetic, vitreous
                body
    retina S05.5-●
    superficial, without open wound
        abdomen, abdominal (wall) S30.851
        alveolar process S00.552
        ankle S90.55-●
        antecubital space —*see* Foreign body,
            superficial, forearm
        anus S30.857

Foreign body *(Continued)*
superficial, without open wound *(Continued)*
arm (upper) S40.85-●
auditory canal —*see* Foreign body, superficial, ear
auricle —*see* Foreign body, superficial, ear
axilla —*see* Foreign body, superficial, arm
back, lower S30.850
breast S20.15-●
brow S00.85
buttock S30.850
calf —*see* Foreign body, superficial, leg
canthus —*see* Foreign body, superficial, eyelid
cheek S00.85
internal S00.552
chest wall —*see* Foreign body, superficial, thorax
chin S00.85
clitoris S30.854
costal region —*see* Foreign body, superficial, thorax
digit(s)
foot —*see* Foreign body, superficial, toe
hand —*see* Foreign body, superficial, finger
ear S00.45-●
elbow S50.35-●
epididymis S30.853
epigastric region S30.851
epiglottis S10.15
esophagus, cervical S10.15
eyebrow —*see* Foreign body, superficial, eyelid
eyelid S00.25-●
face S00.85
finger(s) S60.459
index S60.45-●
little S60.45-●
middle S60.45-●
ring S60.45-●
flank S30.851
foot (except toe(s) alone) S90.85-●
toe —*see* Foreign body, superficial, toe
forearm S50.85-●
elbow only —*see* Foreign body, superficial, elbow
forehead S00.85
genital organs, external
female S30.856
male S30.855
groin S30.851
gum S00.552
hand S60.55-●
head S00.95
ear —*see* Foreign body, superficial, ear
eyelid —*see* Foreign body, superficial, eyelid
lip S00.551
nose S00.35
oral cavity S00.552
scalp S00.05
specified site NEC S00.85
heel —*see* Foreign body, superficial, foot
hip S70.25-●
inguinal region S30.851
interscapular region S20.459
jaw S00.85
knee S80.25-●
labium (majus) (minus) S30.854
larynx S10.15
leg (lower) S80.85-●
knee —*see* Foreign body, superficial, knee
upper —*see* Foreign body, superficial, thigh
lip S00.551
lower back S30.850
lumbar region S30.850
malar region S00.85
mammary —*see* Foreign body, superficial, breast

Foreign body *(Continued)*
superficial, without open wound *(Continued)*
mastoid region S00.85
mouth S00.552
nail
finger —*see* Foreign body, superficial, finger
toe —*see* Foreign body, superficial, toe
nape S00.85
nasal S00.35
neck S10.95
specified site NEC S10.85
throat S10.15
nose S00.35
occipital region S00.05
oral cavity S00.552
orbital region —*see* Foreign body, superficial, eyelid
palate S00.552
palm —*see* Foreign body, superficial, hand
parietal region S00.05
pelvis S30.850
penis S30.852
perineum
female S30.854
male S30.850
periocular area —*see* Foreign body, superficial, eyelid
phalanges
finger —*see* Foreign body, superficial, finger
toe —*see* Foreign body, superficial, toe
pharynx S10.15
pinna —*see* Foreign body, superficial, ear
popliteal space —*see* Foreign body, superficial, knee
prepuce S30.852
pubic region S30.850
pudendum
female S30.856
male S30.855
sacral region S30.850
scalp S00.05
scapular region —*see* Foreign body, superficial, shoulder
scrotum S30.853
shin —*see* Foreign body, superficial, leg
shoulder S40.25-●
sternal region S20.359
submaxillary region S00.85
submental region S00.85
subungual
finger(s) —*see* Foreign body, superficial, finger
toe(s) —*see* Foreign body, superficial, toe
supraclavicular fossa S10.85
supraorbital S00.85
temple S00.85
temporal region S00.85
testis S30.853
thigh S70.35-●
thorax, thoracic (wall) S20.95
back S20.45-●
front S20.35-●
throat S10.15
thumb S60.35-●
toe(s) (lesser) S90.456
great S90.45-●
tongue S00.552
trachea S10.15
tunica vaginalis S30.853
tympanum, tympanic membrane —*see* Foreign body, superficial, ear
uvula S00.552
vagina S30.854
vocal cords S10.15
vulva S30.854
wrist S60.85-●
swallowed T18.9

Foreign body *(Continued)*
trachea T17.408
causing
asphyxiation T17.400
food (bone) (seed) T17.420
gastric contents (vomitus) T17.410
specified type NEC T17.490
injury NEC T17.408
food (bone) (seed) T17.428
gastric contents (vomitus) T17.418
specified type NEC T17.498
type of fragment —*see* Retained, foreign body fragments (type of)
vitreous (humor) S05.5-●
Forestier's disease (rhizomelic pseudopolyarthritis) M35.3-●
meaning ankylosing hyperostosis —*see* Hyperostosis, ankylosing
Formation
hyalin in cornea —*see* Degeneration, cornea
sequestrum in bone (due to infection) —*see* Osteomyelitis, chronic
valve
colon, congenital Q43.8
ureter (congenital) Q62.39
Formication R20.2
Fort Bragg fever A27.89
Fossa —*see also* condition
pyriform —*see* condition
Foster-Kennedy syndrome H47.14-●
Fothergill's
disease (trigeminal neuralgia) —*see also* Neuralgia, trigeminal
scarlatina anginosa A38.9
Foul breath R19.6
Foundling Z76.1
Fournier disease or gangrene N49.3
female N76.89
Fourth
cranial nerve —*see* condition
molar K00.1
Foville's (peduncular) **disease or syndrome** G46.3
Fox (-Fordyce) **disease** (apocrine miliaria) L75.2
FPIES (food protein-induced enterocolitis syndrome) K52.21
Fracture, burst —*see* Fracture, traumatic, by site
Fracture, chronic —*see* Fracture, pathological, by site
Fracture, insufficiency —*see* Fracture, pathological, by site
Fracture, nontraumatic, NEC
atypical
femur M84.750-●
complete
oblique M84.759
left side M84.758
right side M84.757
transverse M84.756
left side M84.755
right side M84.754
incomplete M84.753
left side M84.752
right side M84.751
Fracture, pathological (pathologic) —*see also* Fracture, traumatic M84.40
ankle M84.47-●
carpus M84.44-●
clavicle M84.41-●
compression (not due to trauma) —*see also* Collapse, vertebra M48.50-●
dental implant M27.63
dental restorative material K08.539
with loss of material K08.531
without loss of material K08.530
due to
neoplastic disease NEC —*see also* Neoplasm M84.50
ankle M84.57-●
carpus M84.54-●
clavicle M84.51-●
femur M84.55-●

▶ New　⇒ Revised　~~deleted~~ Deleted　● Use Additional Character(s)

Fracture, pathological *(Continued)*
  due to *(Continued)*
    neoplastic disease NEC *(Continued)*
      fibula M84.56-●
      finger M84.54-●
      hip M84.559
      humerus M84.52-●
      ilium M84.550
      ischium M84.550
      metacarpus M84.54-●
      metatarsus M84.57-●
      neck M84.58
      pelvis M84.550
      radius M84.53-●
      rib M84.58
      scapula M84.51-●
      skull M84.58
      specified site NEC M84.58
      tarsus M84.57-●
      tibia M84.56-●
      toe M84.57-●
      ulna M84.53-●
      vertebra M84.58
    osteoporosis M80.00
      disuse —*see* Osteoporosis, specified type NEC, with pathological fracture
      drug-induced —*see* Osteoporosis, drug induced, with pathological fracture
      idiopathic —*see* Osteoporosis, specified type NEC, with pathological fracture
      postmenopausal —*see* Osteoporosis, postmenopausal, with pathological fracture
      postoophorectomy —*see* Osteoporosis, postoophorectomy, with pathological fracture
      postsurgical malabsorption —*see* Osteoporosis, specified type NEC, with pathological fracture
      specified cause NEC —*see* Osteoporosis, specified type NEC, with pathological fracture
    specified disease NEC M84.60
      ankle M84.67-●
      carpus M84.64-●
      clavicle M84.61-●
      femur M84.65-●
      fibula M84.66-●
      finger M84.64-●
      hip M84.65-●
      humerus M84.62-●
      ilium M84.650
      ischium M84.650
      metacarpus M84.64-●
      metatarsus M84.67-●
      neck M84.68
      radius M84.63-●
      rib M84.68
      scapula M84.61-●
      skull M84.68
      tarsus M84.67-●
      tibia M84.66-●
      toe M84.67-●
      ulna M84.63-●
      vertebra M84.68
  femur M84.45-●
  fibula M84.46-●
  finger M84.44-●
  hip M84.459
  humerus M84.42-●
  ilium M84.454
  ischium M84.454
  joint prosthesis —*see* Complications, joint prosthesis, mechanical, breakdown, by site
  periprosthetic —*see* Fracture, pathological, periprosthetic
  metacarpus M84.44-●
  metatarsus M84.47-●
  neck M84.48

Fracture, pathological *(Continued)*
  pelvis M84.454
  periprosthetic M97.9
    ankle M97.2-●
    elbow M97.4-●
    finger M97.8
    hip M97.0-●
    knee M97.1-●
    other specified joint M97.8
    shoulder M97.3-●
    spinal joint M97.8
    toe joint M97.8
    wrist joint M97.8
  radius M84.43-●
  restorative material (dental) K08.539
    with loss of material K08.531
    without loss of material K08.530
  rib M84.48
  scapula M84.41-●
  skull M84.48
  tarsus M84.47-●
  tibia M84.46-●
  toe M84.47-●
  ulna M84.43-●
  vertebra M84.48
Fracture, traumatic (abduction) (adduction) (separation) —*see also* Fracture, pathological T14.8
  acetabulum S32.40-●
    column
      anterior (displaced) (iliopubic) S32.43-●
        nondisplaced S32.436
      posterior (displaced) (ilioischial) S32.443
        nondisplaced S32.44-●
    dome (displaced) S32.48-●
      nondisplaced S32.48
    specified NEC S32.49-●
    transverse (displaced) S32.45-●
      with associated posterior wall fracture (displaced) S32.46-●
        nondisplaced S32.46-●
      nondisplaced S32.45-●
    wall
      anterior (displaced) S32.41-●
        nondisplaced S32.41-●
      medial (displaced) S32.47-●
        nondisplaced S32.47-●
      posterior (displaced) S32.42-●
        with associated transverse fracture (displaced) S32.46-●
        nondisplaced S32.46-●
        nondisplaced S32.42-●
  acromion —*see* Fracture, scapula, acromial process
  ankle S82.899
    bimalleolar (displaced) S82.84-●
      nondisplaced S82.84-●
    lateral malleolus only (displaced) S82.6-●
      nondisplaced S82.6-●
    medial malleolus (displaced) S82.5-●
      associated with Maisonneuve's fracture —*see* Fracture, Maisonneuve's
      nondisplaced S82.5-●
    talus —*see* Fracture, tarsal, talus
    trimalleolar (displaced) S82.85-●
      nondisplaced S82.85-●
  arm (upper) —*see also* Fracture, humerus, shaft
    humerus —*see* Fracture, humerus
    radius —*see* Fracture, radius
    ulna —*see* Fracture, ulna
  astragalus —*see* Fracture, tarsal, talus
  atlas —*see* Fracture, neck, cervical vertebra, first
  axis —*see* Fracture, neck, cervical vertebra, second
  back —*see* Fracture, vertebra
  Barton's —*see* Barton's fracture
  base of skull —*see* Fracture, skull, base

Fracture, traumatic *(Continued)*
  basicervical (basal) (femoral) S72.0
  Bennett's —*see* Bennett's fracture
  bimalleolar —*see* Fracture, ankle, bimalleolar
  blow-out S02.3-●
  bone NEC T14.8
    birth injury P13.9
    following insertion of orthopedic implant, joint prosthesis or bone plate —*see* Fracture, following insertion of orthopedic implant, joint prosthesis or bone plate
    in (due to) neoplastic disease NEC — *see* Fracture, pathological, due to, neoplastic disease
    pathological (cause unknown) —*see* Fracture, pathological
  breast bone —*see* Fracture, sternum
  buckle —*see* Fracture, by site, torus
  bucket handle (semilunar cartilage) —*see* Tear, meniscus
  burst —*see* Fracture, traumatic, by site
  calcaneus —*see* Fracture, tarsal, calcaneus
  carpal bone(s) S62.10-●
    capitate (displaced) S62.13-●
      nondisplaced S62.13-●
    cuneiform —*see* Fracture, carpal bone, triquetrum
    hamate (body) (displaced) S62.143
      hook process (displaced) S62.15-●
        nondisplaced S62.15-●
      nondisplaced S62.14-●
    larger multangular —*see* Fracture, carpal bones, trapezium
    lunate (displaced) S62.12-●
      nondisplaced S62.12-●
    navicular S62.00-●
      distal pole (displaced) S62.01-●
        nondisplaced S62.01-●
      middle third (displaced) S62.02-●
        nondisplaced S62.02-●
      proximal third (displaced) S62.03-●
        nondisplaced S62.03-●
      volar tuberosity —*see* Fracture, carpal bones, navicular, distal pole
    os magnum —*see* Fracture, carpal bones, capitate
    pisiform (displaced) S62.16-●
      nondisplaced S62.16-●
    semilunar —*see* Fracture, carpal bones, lunate
    smaller multangular —*see* Fracture, carpal bones, trapezoid
    trapezium (displaced) S62.17-●
      nondisplaced S62.17-●
    trapezoid (displaced) S62.18-●
      nondisplaced S62.18-●
    triquetrum (displaced) S62.11-●
      nondisplaced S62.11-●
    unciform —*see* Fracture, carpal bones, hamate
  cervical —*see* Fracture, vertebra, cervical
  clavicle S42.00-●
    acromial end (displaced) S42.03-●
      nondisplaced S42.03-●
    birth injury P13.4
    lateral end —*see* Fracture, clavicle, acromial end
    shaft (displaced) S42.02-●
      nondisplaced S42.02-●
    sternal end (anterior) (displaced) S42.01-●
      nondisplaced S42.01-●
      posterior S42.01-●
  coccyx S32.2
  collapsed —*see* Collapse, vertebra
  collar bone —*see* Fracture, clavicle
  Colles' —*see* Colles' fracture
  coronoid process —*see* Fracture, ulna, upper end, coronoid process
  corpus cavernosum penis S39.840

► New   ⇒ Revised   ~~deleted~~ Deleted   ● Use Additional Character(s)

Fracture, traumatic *(Continued)*
  foot *(Continued)*
    sesamoid S92.81-●
    specified NEC S92.81-●
    talus —*see* Fracture, tarsal, talus
    tarsal —*see* Fracture, tarsal
    toe —*see* Fracture, toe
  forearm S52.9-●
    radius —*see* Fracture, radius
    ulna —*see* Fracture, ulna
  fossa (anterior) (middle) (posterior) S02.19
  fragility —*see* Fracture, pathological, due to
      osteoporosis
  frontal (bone) (skull) S02.0
    sinus S02.19
  glenoid (cavity) (scapula) —*see* Fracture,
      scapula, glenoid cavity
  greenstick —*see* Fracture, by site
  hallux —*see* Fracture, toe, great
  hand S62.9-●
    carpal —*see* Fracture, carpal bone
    finger (except thumb) —*see* Fracture,
        finger
    metacarpal —*see* Fracture, metacarpal
    navicular (scaphoid) (hand) —*see* Fracture,
        carpal bone, navicular
    thumb —*see* Fracture, thumb
  healed or old
    with complications - code by Nature of the
        complication
  heel bone —*see* Fracture, tarsal, calcaneus
  Hill-Sachs S42.29-●
  hip —*see* Fracture, femur, neck
  humerus S42.30-●
    anatomical neck —*see* Fracture, humerus,
        upper end
    articular process —*see* Fracture, humerus,
        lower end
    capitellum —*see* Fracture, humerus, lower
        end, condyle, lateral
    distal end —*see* Fracture, humerus, lower
        end
    epiphysis
      lower —*see* Fracture, humerus, lower
          end, physeal
      upper —*see* Fracture, humerus, upper
          end, physeal
    external condyle —*see* Fracture, humerus,
        lower end, condyle, lateral
    following insertion of implant, prosthesis
        or plate M96.62-●
    great tuberosity —*see* Fracture, humerus,
        upper end, greater tuberosity
    intercondylar —*see* Fracture, humerus,
        lower end
    internal epicondyle —*see* Fracture, humerus,
        lower end, epicondyle, medial
    lesser tuberosity —*see* Fracture, humerus,
        upper end, lesser tuberosity
    lower end S42.40-●
      condyle
        lateral (displaced) S42.45-●
          nondisplaced S42.45-●
        medial (displaced) S42.46-●
          nondisplaced S42.46-●
      epicondyle
        lateral (displaced) S42.43-●
          nondisplaced S42.43-●
        medial (displaced) S42.44-●
          incarcerated S42.44-●
          nondisplaced S42.44-●
      physeal S49.10-●
        Salter-Harris
          Type I S49.11-●
          Type II S49.12-●
          Type III S49.13-●
          Type IV S49.14-●
          specified NEC S49.19-●
      specified NEC (displaced)
          S42.49-●
        nondisplaced S42.49-●

Fracture, traumatic *(Continued)*
  humerus *(Continued)*
    lower end *(Continued)*
      supracondylar (simple) (displaced)
          S42.41-●
        with intercondylar fracture —*see*
            Fracture, humerus, lower end
        comminuted (displaced) S42.42-●
          nondisplaced S42.42-●
        nondisplaced S42.41-●
      torus S42.48-●
      transcondylar (displaced) S42.47-●
        nondisplaced S42.47-●
    proximal end —*see* Fracture, humerus,
        upper end
    shaft S42.30-●
      comminuted (displaced) S42.35-●
        nondisplaced S42.35-●
      greenstick S42.31-●
      oblique (displaced) S42.33-●
        nondisplaced S42.33-●
      segmental (displaced) S42.36-●
        nondisplaced S42.36-●
      specified NEC S42.39-●
      spiral (displaced) S42.34-●
        nondisplaced S42.34-●
      transverse (displaced) S42.32-●
        nondisplaced S42.32-●
    supracondylar —*see* Fracture, humerus,
        lower end
    surgical neck —*see* Fracture, humerus,
        upper end, surgical neck
    trochlea —*see* Fracture, humerus, lower
        end, condyle, medial
    tuberosity —*see* Fracture, humerus, upper
        end
    upper end S42.20-●
      anatomical neck —*see* Fracture,
          humerus, upper end, specified NEC
      articular head —*see* Fracture, humerus,
          upper end, specified NEC
      epiphysis —*see* Fracture, humerus,
          upper end, physeal
      greater tuberosity (displaced) S42.25-●
        nondisplaced S42.25-●
      lesser tuberosity (displaced) S42.26-●
        nondisplaced S42.26-●
      physeal S49.00-●
        Salter-Harris
          Type I S49.01-●
          Type II S49.02-●
          Type III S49.03-●
          Type IV S49.04-●
          specified NEC S49.09-●
      specified NEC (displaced) S42.29-●
        nondisplaced S42.29-●
      surgical neck (displaced) S42.21-●
        four-part S42.24-●
        nondisplaced S42.21-●
        three-part S42.23-●
        two-part (displaced) S42.22-●
          nondisplaced S42.22-●
      torus S42.27-●
      transepiphyseal —*see* Fracture, humerus,
          upper end, physeal
  hyoid bone S12.8
  ilium S32.30-●
    with disruption of pelvic ring —*see*
        Disruption, pelvic ring
    avulsion (displaced) S32.31-●
      nondisplaced S32.31-●
    specified NEC S32.39-●
  impaction, impacted - code as Fracture, by
      site
  innominate bone —*see* Fracture, ilium
  instep —*see* Fracture, foot
  ischium S32.60-●
    with disruption of pelvic ring —*see*
        Disruption, pelvic ring
    avulsion (displaced) S32.61-●
      nondisplaced S32.61-●
    specified NEC S32.69-●

Fracture, traumatic *(Continued)*
  jaw (bone) (lower) —*see* Fracture, mandible
    upper —*see* Fracture, maxilla
  joint prosthesis —*see* Complications, joint
        prosthesis, mechanical, breakdown,
        by site
    periprosthetic —*see* Fracture, traumatic,
        periprosthetic
  knee cap —*see* Fracture, patella
  larynx S12.8
  late effects —*see* Sequelae, fracture
  leg (lower) S82.9-●
    ankle —*see* Fracture, ankle
    femur —*see* Fracture, femur
    fibula —*see* Fracture, fibula
    malleolus —*see* Fracture, ankle
    patella —*see* Fracture, patella
    specified site NEC S82.89-●
    tibia —*see* Fracture, tibia
  lumbar spine —*see* Fracture, vertebra, lumbar
  lumbosacral spine S32.9
  Maisonneuve's (displaced) S82.86-●
    nondisplaced S82.86-●
  malar bone —*see also* Fracture, maxilla
        S02.400
    left side S02.40B
    right side S02.40A
  malleolus —*see* Fracture, ankle
  malunion —*see* Fracture, by site
  mandible (lower jawbone) S02.609
    alveolus S02.67-●
    angle (of jaw) S02.65-●
    body, unspecified S02.600-●
      left side S02.602
      right side S02.601
    condylar process S02.61-●
    coronoid process S02.63-●
    ramus, unspecified S02.64-●
    specified site NEC S02.69
    subcondylar process S02.62-●
    symphysis S02.66
  manubrium (sterni) S22.21
    dissociation from sternum S22.23
  march —*see* Fracture, traumatic, stress, by site
  maxilla, maxillary (bone) (sinus) (superior)
        (upper jaw) S02.401
    alveolus S02.42
    inferior —*see* Fracture, mandible
    LeFort I S02.411
    LeFort II S02.412
    LeFort III S02.413
    left side S02.40D
    right side S02.40C
  metacarpal S62.309
    base (displaced) S62.319
      nondisplaced S62.349
    fifth S62.30-●
      base (displaced) S62.31-●
        nondisplaced S62.34-●
      neck (displaced) S62.33-●
        nondisplaced S62.36-●
      shaft (displaced) S62.32-●
        nondisplaced S62.35-●
      specified NEC S62.398
    first S62.20-●
      base NEC (displaced) S62.23-●
        nondisplaced S62.23-●
      Bennett's —*see* Bennett's fracture
      neck (displaced) S62.25-●
        nondisplaced S62.25-●
      shaft (displaced) S62.24-●
        nondisplaced S62.24-●
      specified NEC S62.29-●
    fourth S62.30-●
      base (displaced) S62.31-●
        nondisplaced S62.34-●
      neck (displaced) S62.33-●
        nondisplaced S62.36-●
      shaft (displaced) S62.32-●
        nondisplaced S62.35-●
      specified NEC S62.39-●

Fracture, traumatic *(Continued)*
  metacarpal *(Continued)*
    neck (displaced) S62.33-●
      nondisplaced S62.36-●
    Rolando's —*see* Rolando's fracture
    second S62.30-●
      base (displaced) S62.31-●
        nondisplaced S62.34-●
      neck (displaced) S62.33-●
        nondisplaced S62.36-●
      shaft (displaced) S62.32-●
        nondisplaced S62.35-●
      specified NEC S62.39-●
    shaft (displaced) S62.32-●
      nondisplaced S62.35-●
    specified NEC S62.399
    third S62.30-●
      base (displaced) S62.31-●
        nondisplaced S62.34-●
      neck (displaced) S62.33-●
        nondisplaced S62.36-●
      shaft (displaced) S62.32-●
        nondisplaced S62.35-●
      specified NEC S62.39-●
  metaphyseal —*see* Fracture, traumatic, by
    site, shaft
  metastatic —*see* Fracture, pathological,
    due to, neoplastic disease —*see also*
    Neoplasm
  metatarsal bone S92.30-●
    fifth (displaced) S92.35-●
      nondisplaced S92.35-●
    first (displaced) S92.31-●
      nondisplaced S92.31-●
    fourth (displaced) S92.34-●
      nondisplaced S92.34-●
    physeal S99.10-●
      Salter-Harris
        Type I S99.11-●
        Type II S99.12-●
        Type III S99.13-●
        Type IV S99.14-●
      specified NEC S99.19-●
    second (displaced) S92.32-●
      nondisplaced S92.32-●
    third (displaced) S92.33-●
      nondisplaced S92.33-●
  Monteggia's —*see* Monteggia's fracture
  multiple
    hand (and wrist) NEC —*see* Fracture,
      by site
    ribs —*see* Fracture, rib, multiple
  nasal (bone(s)) S02.2
  navicular (scaphoid) (foot) —*see also* Fracture,
    tarsal, navicular
    hand —*see* Fracture, carpal, navicular
  neck S12.9
    cervical vertebra S12.9
      fifth (displaced) S12.400
        nondisplaced S12.401
        specified type NEC (displaced)
          S12.490
          nondisplaced S12.491
      first (displaced) S12.000
        burst (stable) S12.01
          unstable S12.02
        lateral mass (displaced)
          S12.040
          nondisplaced S12.041
        nondisplaced S12.001
        posterior arch (displaced)
          S12.030
          nondisplaced S12.031
        specified type NEC (displaced)
          S12.090
          nondisplaced S12.091
      fourth (displaced) S12.300
        nondisplaced S12.301
        specified type NEC (displaced)
          S12.390
          nondisplaced S12.391

Fracture, traumatic *(Continued)*
  neck *(Continued)*
    cervical vertebra *(Continued)*
      second (displaced) S12.100
        dens (anterior) (displaced) (type II)
          S12.110
          nondisplaced S12.112
          posterior S12.111
          specified type NEC (displaced)
            S12.120
            nondisplaced S12.121
        nondisplaced S12.101
        specified type NEC (displaced)
          S12.190
          nondisplaced S12.191
      seventh (displaced) S12.600
        nondisplaced S12.601
        specified type NEC (displaced)
          S12.690
          nondisplaced S12.691
      sixth (displaced) S12.500
        nondisplaced S12.501
        specified type NEC (displaced)
          S12.590
          nondisplaced S12.591
      third (displaced) S12.200
        nondisplaced S12.201
        specified type NEC (displaced)
          S12.290
          nondisplaced S12.291
    hyoid bone S12.8
    larynx S12.8
    specified site NEC S12.8
    thyroid cartilage S12.8
    trachea S12.8
  neoplastic NEC —*see* Fracture, pathological,
    due to, neoplastic disease
  neural arch —*see* Fracture, vertebra
  newborn —*see* Birth, injury, fracture
  nontraumatic —*see* Fracture, pathological
  nonunion —*see* Nonunion, fracture
  nose, nasal (bone) (septum) S02.2
  occiput —*see* Fracture, skull, base,
    occiput
  odontoid process —*see* Fracture, neck,
    cervical vertebra, second
  olecranon (process) (ulna) —*see* Fracture,
    ulna, upper end, olecranon process
  orbit, orbital (bone) (region) S02.85
    floor (blow-out) S02.3-●
    roof S02.12-●
    wall S02.85
      lateral S02.84-●
      medial S02.83-●
  os
    calcis —*see* Fracture, tarsal,
      calcaneus
    magnum —*see* Fracture, carpal,
      capitate
    pubis —*see* Fracture, pubis
  palate S02.8-●
  parietal bone (skull) S02.0
  patella S82.00-●
    comminuted (displaced) S82.04-●
      nondisplaced S82.04-●
    longitudinal (displaced) S82.02-●
      nondisplaced S82.02-●
    osteochondral (displaced) S82.01-●
      nondisplaced S82.01-●
    specified NEC S82.09-●
    transverse (displaced) S82.03-●
      nondisplaced S82.03-●
  pedicle (of vertebral arch) —*see* Fracture,
    vertebra
  pelvis, pelvic (bone) S32.9
    acetabulum —*see* Fracture, acetabulum
    circle —*see* Disruption, pelvic ring
    following insertion of implant, prosthesis
      or plate M96.65
    ilium —*see* Fracture, ilium
    ischium —*see* Fracture, ischium

Fracture, traumatic *(Continued)*
  pelvis, pelvic *(Continued)*
    multiple
      with disruption of pelvic ring (circle) —
        see Disruption, pelvic ring
      without disruption of pelvic ring (circle)
        S32.82
    pubis —*see* Fracture, pubis
    sacrum —*see* Fracture, sacrum
    specified site NEC S32.89
  periprosthetic, around internal prosthetic
    joint M97.9
    ankle M97.2-●
    elbow M97.4-●
    finger M97.8
    hip M97.0-●
    knee M97.1-●
    shoulder M97.3-●
    specified joint NEC M97.8
    spine M97.8
    toe M97.8
    wrist M97.8
  phalanx
    foot —*see* Fracture, toe
    hand —*see* Fracture, finger
  pisiform —*see* Fracture, carpal, pisiform
  pond —*see* Fracture, skull
  prosthetic device, internal —*see*
    Complications, prosthetic device, by site,
    mechanical
  pubis S32.50-●
    with disruption of pelvic ring —*see*
      Disruption, pelvic ring
    specified site NEC S32.59-●
    superior rim S32.59-●
  radius S52.9-●
    distal end —*see* Fracture, radius, lower end
    following insertion of implant, prosthesis
      or plate M96.63-●
    head —*see* Fracture, radius, upper end,
      head
    lower end S52.50-●
      Barton's —*see* Barton's fracture
      Colles' —*see* Colles' fracture
      extraarticular NEC S52.55-●
      intraarticular NEC S52.57-●
      physeal S59.20-●
        Salter-Harris
          Type I S59.21-●
          Type II S59.22-●
          Type III S59.23-●
          Type IV S59.24-●
        specified NEC S59.29-●
      Smith's —*see* Smith's fracture
      specified NEC S52.59-●
      styloid process (displaced) S52.51-●
        nondisplaced S52.51-●
      torus S52.52-●
    neck —*see* Fracture, radius, upper end
    proximal end —*see* Fracture, radius, upper
      end
    shaft S52.30-●
      bent bone S52.38-●
      comminuted (displaced) S52.35-●
        nondisplaced S52.35-●
      Galeazzi's —*see* Galeazzi's fracture
      greenstick S52.31-●
      oblique (displaced) S52.33-●
        nondisplaced S52.33-●
      segmental (displaced) S52.36-●
        nondisplaced S52.36-●
      specified NEC S52.39-●
      spiral (displaced) S52.34-●
        nondisplaced S52.34-●
      transverse (displaced) S52.32-●
        nondisplaced S52.32-●
    upper end S52.10-●
      head (displaced) S52.12-●
        nondisplaced S52.12-●
      neck (displaced) S52.13-●
        nondisplaced S52.13-●

▶ New   ⇒ Revised   ~~deleted~~ Deleted   ● Use Additional Character(s)

Fracture, traumatic *(Continued)*
  radius *(Continued)*
    upper end *(Continued)*
      physeal S59.10-●
        Salter-Harris
          Type I S59.11-●
          Type II S59.12-●
          Type III S59.13-●
          Type IV S59.14-●
        specified NEC S59.19-●
      specified NEC S52.18-●
      torus S52.11-●
  ramus
    inferior or superior, pubis —*see* Fracture, pubis
    mandible —*see* Fracture, mandible
  restorative material (dental) K08.539
    with loss of material K08.531
    without loss of material K08.530
  rib S22.3-●
    with flail chest —*see* Flail, chest
    multiple S22.4-●
      with flail chest —*see* Flail, chest
  root, tooth —*see* Fracture, tooth
  sacrum S32.10
    specified NEC S32.19
    Type
      1 S32.14
      2 S32.15
      3 S32.16
      4 S32.17
    Zone
      I S32.119
        displaced (minimally) S32.111
          severely S32.112
        nondisplaced S32.110
      II S32.129
        displaced (minimally) S32.121
          severely S32.122
        nondisplaced S32.120
      III S32.139
        displaced (minimally) S32.131
          severely S32.132
        nondisplaced S32.130
  scaphoid (hand) —*see also* Fracture, carpal, navicular
    foot —*see* Fracture, tarsal, navicular
  scapula S42.10-●
    acromial process (displaced) S42.12-●
      nondisplaced S42.12-●
    body (displaced) S42.11-●
      nondisplaced S42.11-●
    coracoid process (displaced) S42.13 ●
      nondisplaced S42.13-●
    glenoid cavity (displaced) S42.14-●
      nondisplaced S42.14-●
    neck (displaced) S42.15-●
      nondisplaced S42.15-●
    specified NEC S42.19-●
  semilunar bone, wrist —*see* Fracture, carpal, lunate
  sequelae —*see* Sequelae, fracture
  sesamoid bone
    foot S92.81-●
    hand —*see* Fracture, carpal
    other —*see* Fracture, traumatic, by site
  shepherd's —*see* Fracture, tarsal, talus
  shoulder (girdle) S42.9-●
    blade —*see* Fracture, scapula
  sinus (ethmoid) (frontal) S02.19
  skull S02.91
    base S02.10-●
      occiput S02.119
        condyle S02.113
          type I S02.110
            left side S02.11B
            right side S02.11A
          type II S02.111
            left side S02.11D
            right side S02.11C

Fracture, traumatic *(Continued)*
  skull *(Continued)*
    base *(Continued)*
      occiput *(Continued)*
        condyle *(Continued)*
          type III S02.112
            left side S02.11F
            right side S02.11E
          specified NEC S02.118
            left side S02.11H
            right side S02.11G
        specified NEC S02.19-●
    birth injury P13.0
    frontal bone S02.0
    parietal bone S02.0
    specified site NEC S02.8
    temporal bone S02.19
    vault S02.0
  Smith's —*see* Smith's fracture
  sphenoid (bone) (sinus) S02.19
  spine —*see* Fracture, vertebra
  spinous process —*see* Fracture, vertebra
  spontaneous (cause unknown) —*see* Fracture, pathological
  stave (of thumb) —*see* Fracture, metacarpal, first
  sternum S22.20
    with flail chest —*see* Flail, chest
    body S22.22
    manubrium S22.21
    xiphoid (process) S22.24
  stress M84.30
    ankle M84.37-●
    carpus M84.34 ●
    clavicle M84.31-●
    femoral neck M84.359
    femur M84.35-●
    fibula M84.36-●
    finger M84.34-●
    hip M84.359
    humerus M84.32-●
    ilium M84.350
    ischium M84.350
    metacarpus M84.34-●
    metatarsus M84.37-●
    neck —*see* Fracture, fatigue, vertebra
    pelvis M84.350
    radius M84.33-●
    rib M84.38
    scapula M84.31-●
    skull M84.38
    tarsus M84.37-●
    tibia M84.36-●
    toe M84.37-●
    ulna M84.33-●
    vertebra —*see* Fracture, fatigue, vertebra
  supracondylar, elbow —*see* Fracture, humerus, lower end, supracondylar
  symphysis pubis —*see* Fracture, pubis
  talus (ankle bone) —*see* Fracture, tarsal, talus
  tarsal bone(s) S92.20-●
    astragalus —*see* Fracture, tarsal, talus
    calcaneus S92.00-●
      anterior process (displaced) S92.02-●
        nondisplaced S92.02-●
      body (displaced) S92.01-●
        nondisplaced S92.01-●
      extraarticular NEC (displaced) S92.05-●
        nondisplaced S92.05-●
      intraarticular (displaced) S92.06-●
        nondisplaced S92.06-●
      physeal S99.00-●
        Salter-Harris
          Type I S99.01-●
          Type II S99.02-●
          Type III S99.03-●
          Type IV S99.04-●
        specified NEC S99.09-●

Fracture, traumatic *(Continued)*
  tarsal bone(s) *(Continued)*
    calcaneus *(Continued)*
      tuberosity (displaced) S92.04-●
        avulsion (displaced) S92.03-●
          nondisplaced S92.03-●
        nondisplaced S92.04-●
    cuboid (displaced) S92.21-●
      nondisplaced S92.21-●
    cuneiform
      intermediate (displaced) S92.23-●
        nondisplaced S92.23-●
      lateral (displaced) S92.22-●
        nondisplaced S92.22-●
      medial (displaced) S92.24-●
        nondisplaced S92.24-●
    navicular (displaced) S92.25-●
      nondisplaced S92.25-●
    scaphoid —*see* Fracture, tarsal, navicular
    talus S92.10-●
      avulsion (displaced) S92.15-●
        nondisplaced S92.15-●
      body (displaced) S92.12-●
        nondisplaced S92.12-●
      dome (displaced) S92.14-●
        nondisplaced S92.14-●
      head (displaced) S92.12-●
        nondisplaced S92.12-●
      lateral process (displaced) S92.14-●
        nondisplaced S92.14-●
      neck (displaced) S92.11-●
        nondisplaced S92.11-●
      posterior process (displaced) S92.13-●
        nondisplaced S92.13-●
      specified NEC S92.19-●
  temporal bone (styloid) S02.19
  thorax (bony) S22.9
    with flail chest —*see* Flail, chest
    rib S22.3-●
      multiple S22.4-●
        with flail chest —*see* Flail, chest
    sternum S22.20
      body S22.22
      manubrium S22.21
      xiphoid process S22.24
    vertebra (displaced) S22.009
      burst (stable) S22.001
        unstable S22.002
      eighth S22.069
        burst (stable) S22.061
          unstable S22.062
        specified type NEC S22.068
        wedge compression S22.060
      eleventh S22.089
        burst (stable) S22.081
          unstable S22.082
        specified type NEC S22.088
        wedge compression S22.080
      fifth S22.059
        burst (stable) S22.051
          unstable S22.052
        specified type NEC S22.058
        wedge compression S22.050
      first S22.019
        burst (stable) S22.011
          unstable S22.012
        specified type NEC S22.018
        wedge compression S22.010
      fourth S22.049
        burst (stable) S22.041
          unstable S22.042
        specified type NEC S22.048
        wedge compression S22.040
      ninth S22.079
        burst (stable) S22.071
          unstable S22.072
        specified type NEC S22.078
        wedge compression S22.070
      nondisplaced S22.001

▶ New   ⇨ Revised   ~~deleted~~ Deleted   ● Use Additional Character(s)

F

Fracture, traumatic *(Continued)*
  vertebra, vertebral *(Continued)*
    metastatic —*see* Collapse, vertebra, in,
      specified disease NEC —*see also*
      Neoplasm
    newborn (birth injury) P11.5
    sacrum S32.10
      specified NEC S32.19
      Type
        1 S32.14
        2 S32.15
        3 S32.16
        4 S32.17
      Zone
        I S32.119
          displaced (minimally) S32.111
            severely S32.112
          nondisplaced S32.110
        II S32.129
          displaced (minimally) S32.121
            severely S32.122
          nondisplaced S32.120
        III S32.139
          displaced (minimally) S32.131
            severely S32.132
          nondisplaced S32.130
    thoracic —*see* Fracture, thorax, vertebra
  vertex S02.0
  vomer (bone) S02.2
  wrist S62.10-●
    carpal —*see* Fracture, carpal bone
    navicular (scaphoid) (hand) —*see* Fracture,
      carpal, navicular
  xiphisternum, xiphoid (process) S22.24
  zygoma S02.442
    left side S02.40F
    right side S02.40E
Fragile, fragility
  autosomal site Q95.5
  bone, congenital (with blue sclera) Q78.0
  capillary (hereditary) D69.8
  hair L67.8
  nails L60.3
  non-sex chromosome site Q95.5
  X chromosome Q99.2
Fragilitas
  crinium L67.8
  ossium (with blue sclerae) (hereditary) Q78.0
  unguium L60.3
    congenital Q84.6
Fragments, cataract (lens), following cataract
  surgery H59.02-●
  retained foreign body —*see* Retained, foreign
    body fragments (type of)
Frailty (frail) R54
  mental R41.81
Frambesia, frambesial (tropica) —*see also* Yaws
  initial lesion or ulcer A66.0
  primary A66.0
Frambeside
  gummatous A66.4
  of early yaws A66.2
Frambesioma A66.1
Franceschetti-Klein (-Wildervanck) disease or
  syndrome Q75.4
Francis' disease —*see* Tularemia
Franklin disease C88.2
Frank's essential thrombocytopenia D69.3
Fraser's syndrome Q87.0
Freckle(s) L81.2
  malignant melanoma in —*see* Melanoma
  melanotic (Hutchinson's) —*see* Melanoma,
    in situ
  retinal D49.81
Frederickson's hyperlipoproteinemia, type
  I and V E78.3
  IIA E78.00
  IIB and III E78.2
  IV E78.1
Freeman Sheldon syndrome Q87.0
Freezing —*see also* Effect, adverse, cold T69.9

Freiberg's disease (infraction of metatarsal head
  or osteochondrosis) —*see* Osteochondrosis,
  juvenile, metatarsus
Frei's disease A55
Fremitus, friction, cardiac R01.2
Frenum, frenulum
  external os Q51.828
  tongue (shortening) (congenital) Q38.1
Frequency micturition (nocturnal) R35.0
  psychogenic F45.8
Frey's syndrome
  auriculotemporal G50.8
  hyperhidrosis L74.52
Friction
  burn —*see* Burn, by site
  fremitus, cardiac R01.2
  precordial R01.2
  sounds, chest R09.89
Friderichsen-Waterhouse syndrome or disease
  A39.1
Friedländer's B (bacillus) NEC —*see also*
  condition A49.8
Friedreich's
  ataxia G11.11
  combined systemic disease G11.11
  facial hemihypertrophy Q67.4
  sclerosis (cerebellum) (spinal cord)
    G11.11
Frigidity F52.22
Fröhlich's syndrome E23.6
Frontal —*see also* condition
  lobe syndrome F07.0
Frostbite (superficial) T33.90
  with
    partial thickness skin loss —*see* Frostbite
      (superficial), by site
    tissue necrosis T34.90
  abdominal wall T33.3
    with tissue necrosis T34.3
  ankle T33.81-●
    with tissue necrosis T34.81-●
  arm T33.4-●
  with tissue necrosis T34.4-●
    finger(s) —*see* Frostbite, finger
    hand —*see* Frostbite, hand
    wrist —*see* Frostbite, wrist
  ear T33.01-●
    with tissue necrosis T34.01-●
  face T33.09
    with tissue necrosis T34.09
  finger T33.53-●
    with tissue necrosis T34.53-●
  foot T33.82-●
    with tissue necrosis T34.82-●
  hand T33.52-●
    with tissue necrosis T34.52-●
  head T33.09
    with tissue necrosis T34.09
    ear —*see* Frostbite, ear
    nose —*see* Frostbite, nose
  hip (and thigh) T33.6-●
    with tissue necrosis T34.6-●
  knee T33.7-●
    with tissue necrosis T34.7-●
  leg T33.9-●
    with tissue necrosis T34.9-●
    ankle —*see* Frostbite, ankle
    foot —*see* Frostbite, foot
    knee —*see* Frostbite, knee
    lower T33.7-●
      with tissue necrosis T34.7-●
    thigh —*see* Frostbite, hip
    toe —*see* Frostbite, toe
  limb
    lower T33.99
      with tissue necrosis T34.99
    upper —*see* Frostbite, arm
  neck T33.1
    with tissue necrosis T34.1
  nose T33.02
    with tissue necrosis T34.02

Frostbite *(Continued)*
  pelvis T33.3
    with tissue necrosis T34.3
  specified site NEC T33.99
    with tissue necrosis T34.99
  thigh —*see* Frostbite, hip
  thorax T33.2
    with tissue necrosis T34.2
  toes T33.83-●
    with tissue necrosis T34.83-●
  trunk T33.99
    with tissue necrosis T34.99
  wrist T33.51-●
    with tissue necrosis T34.51-●
Frotteurism F65.81
Frozen —*see also* Effect, adverse, cold T69.9
  pelvis (female) N94.89
    male K66.8
  shoulder —*see* Capsulitis, adhesive
Fructokinase deficiency E74.11
Fructose 1,6 diphosphatase deficiency E74.19
Fructosemia (benign) (essential) E74.12
Fructosuria (benign) (essential) E74.11
Fuchs'
  black spot (myopic) —*see also* Myopia,
    degenerative H44.2-●
  dystrophy (corneal endothelium) H18.51-●
  heterochromic cyclitis —*see* Cyclitis, Fuchs'
    heterochromic
Fucosidosis E77.1
Fugue R68.89
  dissociative F44.1
  hysterical (dissociative) F44.1
  postictal in epilepsy —*see* Epilepsy
  reaction to exceptional stress (transient)
    F43.0
Fulminant, fulminating —*see* condition
Functional —*see also* condition
  bleeding (uterus) N93.8
Functioning, intellectual, borderline R41.83
Fundus —*see* condition
Fungemia NOS B49
Fungus, fungous
  cerebral G93.89
  disease NOS B49
  infection —*see* Infection, fungus
Funiculitis (acute) (chronic) (endemic)
  N49.1
  gonococcal (acute) (chronic) A54.23
  tuberculous A18.15
Funnel
  breast (acquired) M95.4
    congenital Q67.6
    sequelae (late effect) of rickets E64.3
  chest (acquired) M95.4
    congenital Q67.6
    sequelae (late effect) of rickets E64.3
  pelvis (acquired) M95.5
    with disproportion (fetopelvic) O33.3
      causing obstructed labor O65.3
    congenital Q74.2
FUO (fever of unknown origin) R50.9
Furfur L21.0
  microsporon B36.0
Furrier's lung J67.8
Furrowed K14.5
  nail(s) (transverse) L60.4
    congenital Q84.6
  tongue K14.5
    congenital Q38.3
Furuncle L02.92
  abdominal wall L02.221
  ankle —*see* Furuncle, lower limb
  antecubital space —*see* Furuncle, upper
    limb
  anus K61.0
  arm —*see* Furuncle, upper limb
  auditory canal, external —*see* Abscess, ear,
    external
  auricle (ear) —*see* Abscess, ear, external
  axilla (region) L02.42-●

Furuncle (Continued)
  back (any part) L02.222
  breast N61.1
  buttock L02.32
  cheek (external) L02.02
  chest wall L02.223
  chin L02.02
  corpus cavernosum N48.21
  ear, external —see Abscess, ear, external
  external auditory canal —see Abscess, ear,
      external
  eyelid —see Abscess, eyelid
  face L02.02
  femoral (region) —see Furuncle, lower
      limb
  finger —see Furuncle, hand
  flank L02.221
  foot L02.62-●
  forehead L02.02
  gluteal (region) L02.32
  groin L02.224
  hand L02.52-●
  head L02.821
      face L02.02
  hip —see Furuncle, lower limb
  kidney —see Abscess, kidney
  knee —see Furuncle, lower limb
  labium (majus) (minus) N76.4
  lacrimal
      gland —see Dacryoadenitis
      passages (duct) (sac) —see Inflammation,
          lacrimal, passages, acute
  leg (any part) —see Furuncle, lower limb
  lower limb L02.42-●
  malignant A22.0
  mouth K12.2
  navel L02.226
  neck L02.12
  nose J34.0
  orbit, orbital —see Abscess, orbit
  palmar (space) —see Furuncle, hand
  partes posteriores L02.32
  pectoral region L02.223
  penis N48.21
  perineum L02.225

Furuncle (Continued)
  pinna —see Abscess, ear, external
  popliteal —see Furuncle, lower limb
  prepatellar —see Furuncle, lower limb
  scalp L02.821
  seminal vesicle N49.0
  shoulder —see Furuncle, upper limb
  specified site NEC L02.828
  submandibular K12.2
  temple (region) L02.02
  thumb —see Furuncle, hand
  toe —see Furuncle, foot
  trunk L02.229
      abdominal wall L02.221
      back L02.222
      chest wall L02.223
      groin L02.224
      perineum L02.225
      umbilicus L02.226
  umbilicus L02.226
  upper limb L02.42-●
  vulva N76.4
Furunculosis —see Furuncle
Fused —see Fusion, fused
Fusion, fused (congenital)
  astragaloscaphoid Q74.2
  atria Q21.1
  auditory canal Q16.1
  auricles, heart Q21.1
  binocular with defective stereopsis H53.32
  bone Q79.8
  cervical spine M43.22
  choanal Q30.0
  commissure, mitral valve Q23.2
  cusps, heart valve NEC Q24.8
      mitral Q23.2
      pulmonary Q22.1
      tricuspid Q22.4
  ear ossicles Q16.3
  fingers Q70.0-●
  hymen Q52.3
  joint (acquired) —see also Ankylosis
      congenital Q74.8
  kidneys (incomplete) Q63.1
  labium (majus) (minus) Q52.5

Fusion, fused (Continued)
  larynx and trachea Q34.8
  limb, congenital Q74.8
      lower Q74.2
      upper Q74.0
  lobes, lung Q33.8
  lumbosacral (acquired) M43.27
      arthrodesis status Z98.1
      congenital Q76.49
      postprocedural status Z98.1
  nares, nose, nasal, nostril(s) Q30.0
  organ or site not listed —see Anomaly, by site
  ossicles Q79.9
      auditory Q16.3
  pulmonic cusps Q22.1
  ribs Q76.6
  sacroiliac (joint) (acquired) M43.28
      arthrodesis status Z98.1
      congenital Q74.2
      postprocedural status Z98.1
  spine (acquired) NEC M43.20
      arthrodesis status Z98.1
      cervical region M43.22
      cervicothoracic region M43.23
      congenital Q76.49
      lumbar M43.26
      lumbosacral region M43.27
      occipito-atlanto-axial region M43.21
      postoperative status Z98.1
      sacrococcygeal region M43.28
      thoracic region M43.24
      thoracolumbar region M43.25
  sublingual duct with submaxillary duct at
      opening in mouth Q38.4
  testes Q55.1
  toes Q70.2
  tooth, teeth K00.2
  trachea and esophagus Q39.8
  twins Q89.4
  vagina Q52.4
  ventricles, heart Q21.0
  vertebra (arch) —see Fusion, spine
  vulva Q52.5
Fusospirillosis (mouth) (tongue) (tonsil) A69.1
Fussy baby R68.12

▶ New   ⇒ Revised   ~~deleted~~ Deleted   ● Use Additional Character(s)

G

Gain in weight (abnormal) (excessive) —*see also* Weight, gain
Gaisböck's disease (polycythemia hypertonica) D75.1
Gait abnormality R26.9
  ataxic R26.0
  falling R29.6
  hysterical (ataxic) (staggering) F44.4
  paralytic R26.1
  spastic R26.1
  specified type NEC R26.89
  staggering R26.0
  unsteadiness R26.81
  walking difficulty NEC R26.2
Galactocele (breast) N64.89
  puerperal, postpartum O92.79
Galactokinase deficiency E74.29
Galactophoritis N61.0
  gestational, puerperal, postpartum O91.2-•
Galactorrhea O92.6
  not associated with childbirth N64.3
Galactosemia (classic) (congenital) E74.21
Galactosuria E74.29
Galacturia R82.0
  schistosomiasis (bilharziasis) B65.0
GALD (gestational alloimmune liver disease) P78.84
Galeazzi's fracture S52.37-•
Galen's vein —*see* condition
Galeophobia F40.218
Gall duct —*see* condition
Gallbladder —*see also* condition
  acute K81.0
Gallop rhythm R00.8
Gallstone (colic) (cystic duct) (gallbladder) (impacted) (multiple) —*see also* Calculus, gallbladder
  with
    cholecystitis —*see* Calculus, gallbladder, with cholecystitis
  bile duct (common) (hepatic) —*see* Calculus, bile duct
  causing intestinal obstruction K56.3
  specified NEC K80.80
    with obstruction K80.81
Gambling Z72.6
  pathological (compulsive) F63.0
Gammopathy (of undetermined significance [MGUS]) D47.2
  associated with lymphoplasmacytic dyscrasia D47.2
  monoclonal D47.2
  polyclonal D89.0
Gamna's disease (siderotic splenomegaly) D73.1
Gamophobia F40.298
Gampsodactylia (congenital) Q66.7-•
Gamstorp's disease (adynamia episodica hereditaria) G72.3
Gandy-Nanta disease (siderotic splenomegaly) D73.1
Gang
  membership offenses Z72.810
Gangliocytoma D36.10
Ganglioglioma —*see* Neoplasm, uncertain behavior, by site
Ganglion (compound) (diffuse) (joint) (tendon) (sheath) M67.40
  ankle M67.47-•
  foot M67.47-•
  forearm M67.43-•
  hand M67.44-•
  lower leg M67.46-•
  multiple sites M67.49
  of yaws (early) (late) A66.6
  pelvic region M67.45-•
  periosteal —*see* Periostitis
  shoulder region M67.41-•
  specified site NEC M67.48

Ganglion (*Continued*)
  thigh region M67.45-•
  tuberculous A18.09
  upper arm M67.42-•
  wrist M67.43-•
Ganglioneuroblastoma —*see* Neoplasm, nerve, malignant
Ganglioneuroma D36.10
  malignant —*see* Neoplasm, nerve, malignant
Ganglioneuromatosis D36.10
Ganglionitis
  fifth nerve —*see* Neuralgia, trigeminal
  gasserian (postherpetic) (postzoster) B02.21
  geniculate G51.1
    newborn (birth injury) P11.3
    postherpetic, postzoster B02.21
  herpes zoster B02.21
  postherpetic geniculate B02.21
Gangliosidosis E75.10
  GM1 E75.19
  GM2 E75.00
    other specified E75.09
    Sandhoff disease E75.01
    Tay-Sachs disease E75.02
  GM3 E75.19
  mucolipidosis IV E75.11
Gangosa A66.5
Gangrene, gangrenous (connective tissue) (dropsical) (dry) (moist) (skin) (ulcer) —*see also* Necrosis I96
➠with diabetes (mellitus) —*see* Diabetes, with gangrene
  abdomen (wall) I96
  alveolar M27.3
  appendix K35.80
    with
      peritonitis, localized (*see also* Appendicitis) K35.31
  arteriosclerotic (general) (senile) —*see* Arteriosclerosis, extremities, with, gangrene
  auricle I96
  Bacillus welchii A48.0
  bladder (infectious) —*see* Cystitis, specified type NEC
  bowel, cecum, or colon —*see* Gangrene, intestine
  Clostridium perfringens or welchii A48.0
  cornea H18.89-•
  corpora cavernosa N48.29
    noninfective N48.89
  cutaneous, spreading I96
  decubital —*see* Ulcer, pressure, by site
➠diabetic (any site) —*see* Diabetes, with gangrene
  emphysematous —*see* Gangrene, gas
  epidemic —*see* Poisoning, food, noxious, plant
  epididymis (infectional) N45.1
  erysipelas —*see* Erysipelas
  extremity (lower) (upper) I96
  Fournier N49.3
    female N76.89
  fusospirochetal A69.0
  gallbladder —*see* Cholecystitis, acute
  gas (bacillus) A48.0
    following
      abortion —*see* Abortion by type complicated by infection
      ectopic or molar pregnancy O08.0
  glossitis K14.0
  hernia —*see* Hernia, by site, with gangrene
  intestine, intestinal (hemorrhagic) (massive) —*see also* Infarct, intestine K55.069
    with
      mesenteric embolism —*see also* Infarct, intestine K55.069
      obstruction —*see* Obstruction, intestine
  laryngitis J04.0
  limb (lower) (upper) I96

Gangrene, gangrenous (*Continued*)
  lung J85.0
    spirochetal A69.8
  lymphangitis I89.1
  Meleney's (synergistic) —*see* Ulcer, skin
  mesentery —*see also* Infarct, intestine K55.069
    with
      embolism —*see also* Infarct, intestine K55.069
      intestinal obstruction —*see* Obstruction, intestine
  mouth A69.0
  ovary —*see* Oophoritis
  pancreas —*see* Pancreatitis, acute
  penis N48.29
    noninfective N48.89
  perineum I96
  pharynx —*see also* Pharyngitis
    Vincent's A69.1
  presenile I73.1
  progressive synergistic —*see* Ulcer, skin
  pulmonary J85.0
  pulpal (dental) K04.1
  quinsy J36
  Raynaud's (symmetric gangrene) I73.01
  retropharyngeal J39.2
  scrotum N49.3
    noninfective N50.89
  senile (atherosclerotic) —*see* Arteriosclerosis, extremities, with, gangrene
  spermatic cord N49.1
    noninfective N50.89
  spine I96
  spirochetal NEC A69.8
  spreading cutaneous I96
  stomatitis A69.0
  symmetrical I73.01
  testis (infectional) N45.2
    noninfective N44.8
  throat —*see also* Pharyngitis
    diphtheritic A36.0
    Vincent's A69.1
  thyroid (gland) E07.89
  tooth (pulp) K04.1
  tuberculous NEC —*see* Tuberculosis
  tunica vaginalis N49.1
    noninfective N50.89
  umbilicus I96
  uterus —*see* Endometritis
  uvulitis K12.2
  vas deferens N49.1
    noninfective N50.89
  vulva N76.89
Ganister disease J62.8
Ganser's syndrome (hysterical) F44.89
Gardner-Diamond syndrome (autoerythrocyte sensitization) D69.2
Gargoylism E76.01
Garré's disease, osteitis (sclerosing), **osteomyelitis** —*see* Osteomyelitis, specified type NEC
Garrod's pad, knuckle M72.1
Gartner's duct
  cyst Q52.4
  persistent Q50.6
Gas R14.3
  asphyxiation, inhalation, poisoning, suffocation NEC —*see* Table of Drugs and Chemicals
  excessive R14.0
  gangrene A48.0
    following
      abortion —*see* Abortion by type complicated by infection
      ectopic or molar pregnancy O08.0
  on stomach R14.0
  pains R14.1
Gastralgia —*see also* Pain, abdominal
Gastrectasis K31.0
  psychogenic F45.8

Gastric —*see* condition
Gastrinoma
  malignant
    pancreas C25.4
    specified site NEC —*see* Neoplasm,
      malignant, by site
    unspecified site C25.4
  specified site —*see* Neoplasm, uncertain
    behavior
  unspecified site D37.9
Gastritis (simple) K29.70
  with bleeding K29.71
  acute (erosive) K29.00
    with bleeding K29.01
  alcoholic K29.20
    with bleeding K29.21
  allergic K29.60
    with bleeding K29.61
  atrophic (chronic) K29.40
    with bleeding K29.41
  chronic (antral) (fundal) K29.50
    with bleeding K29.51
    atrophic K29.40
      with bleeding K29.41
    superficial K29.30
      with bleeding K29.31
  dietary counseling and surveillance Z71.3
  due to diet deficiency E63.9
  eosinophilic K52.81
  giant hypertrophic K29.60
    with bleeding K29.61
  granulomatous K29.60
    with bleeding K29.61
  hypertrophic (mucosa) K29.60
    with bleeding K29.61
  nervous F54
  spastic K29.60
    with bleeding K29.61
  specified NEC K29.60
    with bleeding K29.61
  superficial chronic K29.30
    with bleeding K29.31
  tuberculous A18.83
  viral NEC A08.4
Gastrocarcinoma —*see* Neoplasm, malignant,
  stomach
Gastrocolic —*see* condition
Gastrodisciasis, gastrodiscoidiasis B66.8
Gastroduodenitis K29.90
  with bleeding K29.91
  virus, viral A08.4
    specified type NEC A08.39
Gastrodynia —*see* Pain, abdominal
Gastroenteritis (acute) (chronic) (noninfectious)
  (*see also* Enteritis) K52.9
  allergic K52.29
  with
    eosinophilic gastritis or gastroenteritis
      K52.81
    food protein-induced enterocolitis
      syndrome K52.21
    food protein-induced enteropathy K52.22
  dietetic —*see also* Gastroenteritis, allergic
    K52.29
  drug-induced K52.1
  due to
    Cryptosporidium A07.2
    drugs K52.1
    food poisoning —*see* Intoxication,
      foodborne
    radiation K52.0
  eosinophilic K52.81
  epidemic (infectious) A09
  food hypersensitivity —*see also*
    Gastroenteritis, allergic K52.29
  infectious —*see* Enteritis, infectious
  influenzal —*see* Influenza, with
    gastroenteritis
  noninfectious K52.9
    specified NEC K52.89
  rotaviral A08.0

Gastroenteritis (*Continued*)
  Salmonella A02.0
  toxic K52.1
  viral NEC A08.4
    acute infectious A08.39
      type Norwalk A08.11
    infantile (acute) A08.39
    Norwalk agent A08.11
    rotaviral A08.0
    severe of infants A08.39
    specified type NEC A08.39
Gastroenteropathy —*see also* Gastroenteritis K52.9
  acute, due to Norovirus A08.11
  acute, due to Norwalk agent A08.11
  infectious A09
Gastroenteroptosis K63.4
Gastroesophageal laceration-hemorrhage
  syndrome K22.6
Gastrointestinal —*see* condition
Gastrojejunal —*see* condition
Gastrojejunitis —*see also* Enteritis K52.9
Gastrojejunocolic —*see* condition
Gastroliths K31.89
Gastromalacia K31.89
Gastroparalysis K31.84
  diabetic —*see* Diabetes, gastroparalysis
Gastroparesis K31.84
  diabetic —*see* Diabetes, by type, with
    gastroparesis
Gastropathy K31.9
  ➡congestive portal (*see also*, Hypertension,
    portal) K31.89
  erythematous K29.70
  exudative K90.89
  ➡portal hypertensive (*see also*, Hypertension,
    portal) K31.89
Gastroptosis K31.89
Gastrorrhagia K92.2
  psychogenic F45.8
Gastroschisis (congenital) Q79.3
Gastrospasm (neurogenic) (reflex) K31.89
  neurotic F45.8
  psychogenic F45.8
Gastrostaxis —*see* Gastritis, with bleeding
Gastrostenosis K31.89
Gastrostomy
  attention to Z43.1
  status Z93.1
Gastrosuccorrhea (continuous) (intermittent)
  K31.89
  neurotic F45.8
  psychogenic F45.8
Gatophobia F40.218
Gaucher's disease or splenomegaly (adult)
  (infantile) E75.22
Gee (-Herter)(-Thaysen) **disease** (nontropical
  sprue) K90.0
Gélineau's syndrome G47.419
  with cataplexy G47.411
Gemination, tooth, teeth K00.2
Gemistocytoma
  specified site —*see* Neoplasm, malignant, by
    site
  unspecified site C71.9
General, generalized —*see* condition
Genetic
  carrier (status)
    cystic fibrosis Z14.1
    hemophilia A (asymptomatic) Z14.01
      symptomatic Z14.02
    specified NEC Z14.8
  susceptibility to disease NEC Z15.89
    malignant neoplasm Z15.09
      breast Z15.01
      endometrium Z15.04
      ovary Z15.02
      prostate Z15.03
      specified NEC Z15.09
    multiple endocrine neoplasia Z15.81
Genital —*see* condition
Genito-anorectal syndrome A55

Genitourinary system —*see* condition
Genu
  congenital Q74.1
  extrorsum (acquired) —*see also* Deformity,
    varus, knee
    congenital Q74.1
    sequelae (late effect) of rickets E64.3
  introrsum (acquired) —*see also* Deformity,
    valgus, knee
    congenital Q74.1
    sequelae (late effect) of rickets E64.3
  rachitic (old) E64.3
  recurvatum (acquired) —*see also* Deformity,
    limb, specified type NEC, lower leg
    congenital Q68.2
    sequelae (late effect) of rickets E64.3
  valgum (acquired) (knock-knee) M21.06-●
    congenital Q74.1
    sequelae (late effect) of rickets E64.3
  varum (acquired) (bowleg) M21.16-●
    congenital Q74.1
    sequelae (late effect) of rickets E64.3
Geographic tongue K14.1
Geophagia —*see* Pica
Geotrichosis B48.3
  stomatitis B48.3
Gephyrophobia F40.242
Gerbode defect Q21.0
GERD (gastroesophageal reflux disease) K21.9
Gerhardt's
  disease (erythromelalgia) I73.81
  syndrome (vocal cord paralysis) J38.00
    bilateral J38.02
    unilateral J38.01
German measles —*see also* Rubella
  exposure to Z20.4
Germinoblastoma (diffuse) C85.9-●
  follicular C82.9-●
Germinoma —*see* Neoplasm, malignant, by site
Gerontoxon —*see* Degeneration, cornea, senile
Gerstmann-Sträussler-Scheinker syndrome
  (GSS) A81.82
Gerstmann's syndrome R48.8
  developmental F81.2
Gestation (period) —*see also* Pregnancy
  ectopic —*see* Pregnancy, by site
  multiple O30.9-●
    greater than quadruplets —*see* Pregnancy,
      multiple (gestation), specified NEC
    specified NEC —*see* Pregnancy, multiple
      (gestation), specified NEC
Gestational
  mammary abscess O91.11-●
  purulent mastitis O91.11-●
  subareolar abscess O91.11-●
Ghon tubercle, primary infection A15.7
Ghost
  teeth K00.4
  vessels (cornea) H16.41-●
Ghoul hand A66.3
Gianotti-Crosti disease L44.4
Giant
  cell
    epulis K06.8
    peripheral granuloma K06.8
  esophagus, congenital Q39.5
  kidney, congenital Q63.3
  urticaria T78.3
    hereditary D84.1
Giardiasis A07.1
Gibert's disease or pityriasis L42
Giddiness R42
  hysterical F44.89
  psychogenic F45.8
Gierke's disease (glycogenosis I) E74.01
Gigantism (cerebral) (hypophyseal) (pituitary)
  E22.0
  constitutional E34.4
Gilbert's disease or syndrome E80.4
Gilchrist's disease B40.9
Gilford-Hutchinson disease E34.8

▶ New   ⮕ Revised   ~~deleted~~ Deleted   ● Use Additional Character(s)

Gilles de la Tourette's disease or syndrome (motor-verbal tic) F95.2
Gingivitis K05.10
  acute (catarrhal) K05.00
    necrotizing A69.1
    nonplaque induced K05.01
    plaque induced K05.00
  chronic (desquamative) (hyperplastic) (simple marginal) (pregnancy associated) (ulcerative) K05.10
    nonplaque induced K05.11
    plaque induced K05.10
  expulsiva —see Periodontitis
  necrotizing ulcerative (acute) A69.1
  pellagrous E52
    acute necrotizing A69.1
  Vincent's A69.1
Gingivoglossitis K14.0
Gingivopericementitis —see Periodontitis
Gingivosis —see Gingivitis, chronic
Gingivostomatitis K05.10
  herpesviral B00.2
  necrotizing ulcerative (acute) A69.1
Gland, glandular —see condition
Glanders A24.0
Glanzmann (-Naegeli) disease or thrombasthenia D69.1
Glasgow coma scale
  total score
    3-8 R40.243
    9-12 R40.242
    13-15 R40.241
Glass-blower's disease (cataract) —see Cataract, specified NEC
Glaucoma H40.9
  with
    increased episcleral venous pressure H40.81-●
    pseudoexfoliation of lens —see Glaucoma, open angle, primary, capsular
  absolute H44.51-●
  angle-closure (primary) H40.20-●
    acute (attack) (crisis) H40.21-●
    chronic H40.22-●
    intermittent H40.23-●
    residual stage H40.24-●
  borderline H40.00-●
  capsular (with pseudoexfoliation of lens) —see Glaucoma, open angle, primary, capsular
  childhood Q15.0
  closed angle —see Glaucoma, angle-closure
  congenital Q15.0
  corticosteroid-induced —see Glaucoma, secondary, drugs
  hypersecretion H40.82-●
  in (due to)
    amyloidosis E85.4 [H42]
    aniridia Q13.1 [H42]
    concussion of globe —see Glaucoma, secondary, trauma
    dislocation of lens —see Glaucoma, secondary
    disorder of lens NEC —see Glaucoma, secondary
    drugs —see Glaucoma, secondary, drugs
    endocrine disease NOS E34.9 [H42]
    eye
      inflammation —see Glaucoma, secondary, inflammation
      trauma —see Glaucoma, secondary, trauma
    hypermature cataract —see Glaucoma, secondary
    iridocyclitis —see Glaucoma, secondary, inflammation
    lens disorder —see Glaucoma, secondary, Lowe's syndrome E72.03 [H42]
    metabolic disease NOS E88.9 [H42]
    ocular disorders NEC —see Glaucoma, secondary

Glaucoma (Continued)
  in (due to) (Continued)
    onchocerciasis B73.02
    pupillary block —see Glaucoma, secondary
    retinal vein occlusion —see Glaucoma, secondary
    Rieger's anomaly Q13.81 [H42]
    rubeosis of iris —see Glaucoma, secondary
    tumor of globe —see Glaucoma, secondary
  infantile Q15.0
  low tension —see Glaucoma, open angle, primary, low-tension
  malignant H40.83-●
  narrow angle —see Glaucoma, angle-closure
  newborn Q15.0
  noncongestive (chronic) —see Glaucoma, open angle
  nonobstructive —see Glaucoma, open angle
  obstructive —see also Glaucoma, angle-closure
    due to lens changes —see Glaucoma, secondary
  open angle H40.10-●
    primary H40.11-●
      capsular (with pseudoexfoliation of lens) H40.14-●
      low-tension H40.12-●
      pigmentary H40.13-●
      residual stage H40.15-●
  phacolytic —see Glaucoma, secondary
  pigmentary —see Glaucoma, open angle, primary, pigmentary
  postinfectious —see Glaucoma, secondary, inflammation
  secondary (to) H40.5-●
    drugs H40.6-●
    inflammation H40.4-●
    trauma H40.3-●
  simple (chronic) H40.11-●
  simplex H40.11-●
  specified type NEC H40.89
  suspect H40.00-●
  syphilitic A52.71
  traumatic —see also Glaucoma, secondary, trauma
    newborn (birth injury) P15.3
  tuberculous A18.59
Glaucomatous flecks (subcapsular) —see Cataract, complicated
Glazed tongue K14.4
Gleet (gonococcal) A54.01
Glénard's disease K63.4
Glioblastoma (multiforme)
  with sarcomatous component
    specified site —see Neoplasm, malignant, by site
    unspecified site C71.9
  giant cell
    specified site —see Neoplasm, malignant, by site
    unspecified site C71.9
  specified site —see Neoplasm, malignant, by site
  unspecified site C71.9
Glioma (malignant)
  astrocytic
    specified site —see Neoplasm, malignant, by site
    unspecified site C71.9
  mixed
    specified site —see Neoplasm, malignant, by site
    unspecified site C71.9
  nose Q30.8
  specified site NEC —see Neoplasm, malignant, by site
  subependymal D43.2
    specified site —see Neoplasm, uncertain behavior, by site
    unspecified site D43.2
  unspecified site C71.9
Gliomatosis cerebri C71.0

Glioneuroma —see Neoplasm, uncertain behavior, by site
Gliosarcoma
  specified site —see Neoplasm, malignant, by site
  unspecified site C71.9
Gliosis (cerebral) G93.89
  spinal G95.89
Glisson's disease —see Rickets
Globinuria R82.3
Globus (hystericus) F45.8
Glomangioma D18.00
  intra-abdominal D18.03
  intracranial D18.02
  skin D18.01
  specified site NEC D18.09
Glomangiomyoma D18.00
  intra-abdominal D18.03
  intracranial D18.02
  skin D18.01
  specified site NEC D18.09
Glomangiosarcoma —see Neoplasm, connective tissue, malignant
Glomerular
  disease in syphilis A52.75
  nephritis —see Glomerulonephritis
Glomerulitis —see Glomerulonephritis
Glomerulonephritis —see also Nephritis N05.9
  with
    C3
      glomerulonephritis N05.A
      glomerulopathy N05.A
        with dense deposit disease N05.6
    edema —see Nephrosis
    minimal change N05.0
    minor glomerular abnormality N05.0
  acute N00.9
  chronic N03.9
  crescentic (diffuse) NEC —see also N00-N07 with fourth character .7 N05.7
  dense deposit —see also N00-N07 with fourth character .6 N05.6
  diffuse
    crescentic —see also N00-N07 with fourth character .7 N05.7
    endocapillary proliferative —see also N00N07 with fourth character .4 N05.4
    membranous —see also N00-N07 with fourth character .2 N05.2
    mesangial proliferative —see also N00-N07 with fourth character .3 N05.3
    mesangiocapillary —see also N00-N07 with fourth character .5 N05.5
    sclerosing N18.9
  endocapillary proliferative (diffuse) NEC —see also N00-N07 with fourth character .4 N05.4
  extracapillary NEC —see also N00-N07 with fourth character .7 N05.7
  focal (and segmental) —see also N00-N07 with fourth character .1 N05.1
  hypocomplementemic —see Glomerulonephritis, membranoproliferative
  IgA —see Nephropathy, IgA
  immune complex (circulating) NEC N05.8
  in (due to)
    amyloidosis E85.4 [N08]
    bilharziasis B65.9 [N08]
    cryoglobulinemia D89.1 [N08]
    defibrination syndrome D65 [N08]
    diabetes mellitus —see Diabetes, glomerulosclerosis
    disseminated intravascular coagulation D65 [N08]
    Fabry (-Anderson) disease E75.21 [N08]
    Goodpasture's syndrome M31.0
    hemolytic-uremic syndrome D59.3
    Henoch (-Schönlein) purpura D69.0 [N08]
    lecithin cholesterol acyltransferase deficiency E78.6 [N08]

Glomerulonephritis (Continued)
  in (Continued)
    microscopic polyangiitis M31.7 [N08]
    multiple myeloma C90.0-● [N08]
    Plasmodium malariae B52.0
    schistosomiasis B65.9 [N08]
    sepsis A41.9-● [N08]
      streptococcal A40-● [N08]
    sickle-cell disorders D57.-● [N08]
    strongyloidiasis B78.9 [N08]
    subacute bacterial endocarditis I33.0
      [N08]
    syphilis (late) congenital A50.59 [N08]
    systemic lupus erythematosus M32.14
  ➡thrombotic thrombocytopenic purpura
    M31.19 [N08]
    typhoid fever A01.09
    Waldenström macroglobulinemia C88.0
      [N08]
    Wegener's granulomatosis M31.31
  latent or quiescent N03.9
  lobular, lobulonodular —
    see Glomerulonephritis,
    membranoproliferative
  membranoproliferative (diffuse) (type 1
    or 3) —see also N00-N07 with fourth
    character .5 N05.5
    dense deposit (type 2) NEC —see also
      N00-N07 with fourth character .6
      N05.6
  membranous (diffuse) NEC —see also
    N00-N07 with fourth character .2 N05.2
  mesangial
    IgA/IgG —see Nephropathy, IgA
    proliferative (diffuse) NEC —see also
      N00-N07 with fourth character .3
      N05.3
  mesangiocapillary (diffuse) NEC —see also
    N00-N07 with fourth character .5 N05.5
  necrotic, necrotizing NEC —see also N00-N07
    with fourth character .8 N05.8
  nodular —see Glomerulonephritis,
    membranoproliferative
  poststreptococcal NEC N05.9
    acute N00.9
    chronic N03.9
    rapidly progressive N01.9
  proliferative NEC —see also N00-N07 with
    fourth character .8 N05.8
    diffuse (lupus) M32.14
  rapidly progressive N01.9
  sclerosing, diffuse N18.9
  specified pathology NEC —see also N00-N07
    with fourth character .8 N05.8
  subacute N01.9
Glomerulopathy —see Glomerulonephritis
Glomerulosclerosis —see also Sclerosis, renal
  intercapillary (nodular) (with diabetes) —see
    Diabetes, glomerulosclerosis
  intracapillary —see Diabetes, glomerulosclerosis
Glossagra K14.6
Glossalgia K14.6
Glossitis (chronic superficial) (gangrenous)
  (Moeller's) K14.0
  areata exfoliativa K14.1
  atrophic K14.4
  benign migratory K14.1
  cortical superficial, sclerotic K14.0
  Hunter's D51.0
  interstitial, sclerous K14.0
  median rhomboid K14.2
  pellagrous E52
  superficial, chronic K14.0
Glossocele K14.8
Glossodynia K14.6
  exfoliativa K14.4
Glossoncus K14.8
Glossopathy K14.9
Glossophytia K14.3
Glossoplegia K14.8
Glossoptosis K14.8

Glossopyrosis K14.6
Glossotrichia K14.3
Glossy skin L90.8
Glottis —see condition
Glottitis —see also Laryngitis J04.0
Glucagonoma
  pancreas
    benign D13.7
    malignant C25.4
    uncertain behavior D37.8
  specified site NEC
    benign —see Neoplasm, benign, by site
    malignant —see Neoplasm, malignant, by
      site
    uncertain behavior —see Neoplasm,
      uncertain behavior, by site
  unspecified site
    benign D13.7
    malignant C25.4
    uncertain behavior D37.8
Glucoglycinuria E72.51
Glucose-galactose malabsorption E74.39
Glue
  ear —see Otitis, media, nonsuppurative,
    chronic, mucoid
  sniffing (airplane) —see Abuse, drug, inhalant
    dependence —see Dependence, drug,
      inhalant
GLUT1 deficiency syndrome 1, infantile onset
  E74.810
GLUT1 deficiency syndrome 2, childhood
  onset E74.810
Glutaric aciduria E72.3
Glycinemia E72.51
Glycinuria (renal) (with ketosis) E72.09
Glycogen
  infiltration —see Disease, glycogen storage
  storage disease —see Disease, glycogen storage
Glycogenosis (diffuse) (generalized) —see also
  Disease, glycogen storage
  cardiac E74.02 [I43]
  diabetic, secondary —see Diabetes,
    glycogenosis, secondary
  pulmonary interstitial J84.842
Glycopenia E16.2
Glycosuria R81
  renal (familial) E74.818
Gnathostoma spinigerum (infection)
  (infestation), **gnathostomiasis** (wandering
  swelling) B83.1
Goiter (plunging) (substernal) E04.9
  with
    hyperthyroidism (recurrent) —see
      Hyperthyroidism, with, goiter
    thyrotoxicosis —see Hyperthyroidism,
      with, goiter
  adenomatous —see Goiter, nodular
  cancerous C73
  congenital (nontoxic) E03.0
    diffuse E03.0
    parenchymatous E03.0
    transitory, with normal functioning P72.0
  cystic E04.2
    due to iodine-deficiency E01.1
  due to
    enzyme defect in synthesis of thyroid
      hormone E07.1
    iodine-deficiency (endemic) E01.2
  dyshormonogenetic (familial) E07.1
  endemic (iodine-deficiency) E01.2
    diffuse E01.0
    multinodular E01.1
  exophthalmic —see Hyperthyroidism, with,
    goiter
  iodine-deficiency (endemic) E01.2
    diffuse E01.0
    multinodular E01.1
    nodular E01.1
  lingual Q89.2
  lymphadenoid E06.3
  malignant C73

Goiter (Continued)
  multinodular (cystic) (nontoxic) E04.2
    toxic or with hyperthyroidism E05.20
      with thyroid storm E05.21
  neonatal NEC P72.0
  nodular (nontoxic) (due to) E04.9
    with
      hyperthyroidism E05.20
        with thyroid storm E05.21
      thyrotoxicosis E05.20
        with thyroid storm E05.21
    endemic E01.1
    iodine-deficiency E01.1
    sporadic E04.9
    toxic E05.20
      with thyroid storm E05.21
  nontoxic E04.9
    diffuse (colloid) E04.0
    multinodular E04.2
    simple E04.0
    specified NEC E04.8
    uninodular E04.1
  simple E04.0
  toxic —see Hyperthyroidism, with, goiter
  uninodular (nontoxic) E04.1
    toxic or with hyperthyroidism E05.10
      with thyroid storm E05.11
Goiter-deafness syndrome E07.1
Goldberg syndrome Q89.8
Goldberg-Maxwell syndrome E34.51
Goldblatt's hypertension or kidney I70.1
Goldenhar (-Gorlin) **syndrome** Q87.0
Goldflam-Erb disease or syndrome G70.00
  with exacerbation (acute) G70.01
  in crisis G70.01
Goldscheider's disease Q81.8
Goldstein's disease (familial hemorrhagic
  telangiectasia) I78.0
Golfer's elbow —see Epicondylitis, medial
Gonadoblastoma
  specified site —see Neoplasm, uncertain
    behavior, by site
  unspecified site
    female D39.10
    male D40.10
Gonecystitis —see Vesiculitis
Gongylonemiasis B83.8
Goniosynechiae —see Adhesions, iris,
  goniosynechiae
Gonococcemia A54.86
Gonococcus, gonococcal (disease) (infection)
  —see also condition A54.9
  anus A54.6
  bursa, bursitis A54.49
  conjunctiva, conjunctivitis (neonatorum)
    A54.31
  endocardium A54.83
  eye A54.30
    conjunctivitis A54.31
    iridocyclitis A54.32
    keratitis A54.33
    newborn A54.31
    other specified A54.39
  fallopian tubes (acute) (chronic) A54.24
  genitourinary (organ) (system) (tract) (acute)
    lower A54.00
      with abscess (accessory gland)
        (periurethral) A54.1
    upper —see also condition A54.29
  heart A54.83
  iridocyclitis A54.32
  joint A54.42
  lymphatic (gland) (node) A54.89
  meninges, meningitis A54.81
  musculoskeletal A54.40
    arthritis A54.42
    osteomyelitis A54.43
    other specified A54.49
    spondylopathy A54.41
  pelviperitonitis A54.24
  pelvis (acute) (chronic) A54.24

▶ New   ➡ Revised   ~~deleted~~ Deleted   ● Use Additional Character(s)

Gonococcus, gonococcal *(Continued)*
  pharynx A54.5
  proctitis A54.6
  pyosalpinx (acute) (chronic) A54.24
  rectum A54.6
  skin A54.89
  specified site NEC A54.89
  tendon sheath A54.49
  throat A54.5
  urethra (acute) (chronic) A54.01
    with abscess (accessory gland)
        (periurethral) A54.1
  vulva (acute) (chronic) A54.02
Gonocytoma
  specified site —*see* Neoplasm, uncertain
      behavior, by site
  unspecified site
    female D39.10
    male D40.10
Gonorrhea (acute) (chronic) A54.9
  Bartholin's gland (acute) (chronic) (purulent)
      A54.02
    with abscess (accessory gland)
        (periurethral) A54.1
  bladder A54.01
  cervix A54.03
  conjunctiva, conjunctivitis (neonatorum)
      A54.31
  contact Z20.2
  Cowper's gland (with abscess) A54.1
  exposure to Z20.2
  fallopian tube (acute) (chronic) A54.24
  kidney (acute) (chronic) A54.21
  lower genitourinary tract A54.00
    with abscess (accessory gland)
        (periurethral) A54.1
  ovary (acute) (chronic) A54.24
  pelvis (acute) (chronic) A54.24
    female pelvic inflammatory disease A54.24
  penis A54.09
  prostate (acute) (chronic) A54.22
  seminal vesicle (acute) (chronic) A54.23
  specified site not listed —*see also* Gonococcus
      A54.89
  spermatic cord (acute) (chronic) A54.23
  urethra A54.01
    with abscess (accessory gland)
        (periurethral) A54.1
  vagina A54.02
  vas deferens (acute) (chronic) A54.23
  vulva A54.02
Goodall's disease A08.19
Goodpasture's syndrome M31.0
Gopalan's syndrome (burning feet) E53.0
Gorlin-Chaudry-Moss syndrome Q87.0
Gottron's papules L94.4
Gougerot's syndrome (trisymptomatic) L81.7
Gougerot-Blum syndrome (pigmented
    purpuric lichenoid dermatitis) L81.7
Gougerot-Carteaud disease or syndrome
    (confluent reticulate papillomatosis) L83
Gouley's syndrome (constrictive pericarditis)
    I31.1
Goundou A66.6
Gout, chronic (*see also* Gout, gouty) M1A.9-●
  drug-induced M1A.20
    ankle M1A.27-●
    elbow M1A.22-●
    foot joint M1A.27-●
    hand joint M1A.24-●
    hip M1A.25-●
    knee M1A.26-●
    multiple site M1A.29
    shoulder M1A.21-●
    vertebrae M1A.28
    wrist M1A.23-●
  idiopathic M1A.00
    ankle M1A.07-●
    elbow M1A.02-●
    foot joint M1A.07-●
    hand joint M1A.04-●

Gout, chronic *(Continued)*
  idiopathic *(Continued)*
    hip M1A.05-●
    knee M1A.06-●
    multiple site M1A.09
    shoulder M1A.01-●
    vertebrae M1A.08
    wrist M1A.03-●
  in (due to) renal impairment M1A.30
    ankle M1A.37-●
    elbow M1A.32-●
    foot joint M1A.37-●
    hand joint M1A.34-●
    hip M1A.35-●
    knee M1A.36-●
    multiple site M1A.39
    shoulder M1A.31-●
    vertebrae M1A.38
    wrist M1A.33-●
  lead-induced M1A.10
    ankle M1A.17-●
    elbow M1A.12-●
    foot joint M1A.17-●
    hand joint M1A.14-●
    hip M1A.15-●
    knee M1A.16-●
    multiple site M1A.19
    shoulder M1A.11-●
    vertebrae M1A.18
    wrist M1A.13-●
  primary —*see* Gout, chronic, idiopathic
  saturnine —*see* Gout, chronic, lead-induced
  secondary NEC M1A.40
    ankle M1A.47-●
    elbow M1A.42-●
    foot joint M1A.47-●
    hand joint M1A.44-●
    hip M1A.45-●
    knee M1A.46-●
    multiple site M1A.49
    shoulder M1A.41-●
    vertebrae M1A.48
    wrist M1A.43-●
  syphilitic —*see also* subcategory M14.8-●
      A52.77
  tophi M1A.9
Gout, gouty (acute) (attack) (flare) —*see also*
    Gout, chronic M10.9-●
  drug-induced M10.20
    ankle M10.27-●
    elbow M10.22-●
    foot joint M10.27-●
    hand joint M10.24-●
    hip M10.25-●
    knee M10.26-●
    multiple site M10.29
    shoulder M10.21-●
    vertebrae M10.28
    wrist M10.23-●
  idiopathic M10.00
    ankle M10.07-●
    elbow M10.02-●
    foot joint M10.07-●
    hand joint M10.04-●
    hip M10.05-●
    knee M10.06-●
    multiple site M10.09
    shoulder M10.01-●
    vertebrae M10.08
    wrist M10.03-●
  in (due to) renal impairment M10.30
    ankle M10.37-●
    elbow M10.32-●
    foot joint M10.37-●
    hand joint M10.34-●
    hip M10.35-●
    knee M10.36-●
    multiple site M10.39
    shoulder M10.31-●
    vertebrae M10.38
    wrist M10.33-●

Gout, gouty *(Continued)*
  lead-induced M10.10
    ankle M10.17-●
    elbow M10.12-●
    foot joint M10.17-●
    hand joint M10.14-●
    hip M10.15-●
    knee M10.16-●
    multiple site M10.19
    shoulder M10.11-●
    vertebrae M10.18
    wrist M10.13-●
  primary —*see* Gout, idiopathic
  saturnine —*see* Gout, lead-induced
  secondary NEC M10.40
    ankle M10.47-●
    elbow M10.42-●
    foot joint M10.47-●
    hand joint M10.44-●
    hip M10.45-●
    knee M10.46-●
    multiple site M10.49
    shoulder M10.41-●
    vertebrae M10.48
    wrist M10.43-●
  syphilitic —*see also* subcategory M14.8-●
      A52.77
  tophi NEC —*see* Gout, chronic
Gower's
  muscular dystrophy G71.01
  syndrome (vasovagal attack) R55
Gradenigo's syndrome —*see* Otitis, media,
    suppurative, acute
Graefe's disease —*see* Strabismus, paralytic,
    ophthalmoplegia, progressive
Graft-versus-host disease D89.813
  acute D89.810
  acute on chronic D89.812
  chronic D89.811
Grain mite (itch) B88.0
Grainhandler's disease or lung J67.8
Grand mal —*see* Epilepsy, generalized,
    specified NEC
Grand multipara status only (not pregnant)
    Z64.1
  pregnant —*see* Pregnancy, complicated by,
    grand multiparity
Granite worker's lung J62.8
Granular —*see also* condition
  inflammation, pharynx J31.2
  kidney (contracting) —*see* Sclerosis, renal
  liver K74.69
Granulation tissue (abnormal) (excessive) L92.9
  postmastoidectomy cavity —*see*
      Complications, postmastoidectomy,
      granulation
Granulocytopenia (primary) (malignant) —*see*
    Agranulocytosis
Granuloma L92.9
  abdomen K66.8
    from residual foreign body L92.3
    pyogenicum L98.0
  actinic L57.5
  annulare (perforating) L92.0
  apical K04.5
  aural —*see* Otitis, externa, specified NEC
  beryllium (skin) L92.3
  bone
    eosinophilic C96.6
    from residual foreign body —*see*
        Osteomyelitis, specified type NEC
    lung C96.6
  brain (any site) G06.0
    schistosomiasis B65.9 *[G07]*
  canaliculus lacrimalis —*see* Granuloma,
      lacrimal
  candidal (cutaneous) B37.2
  cerebral (any site) G06.0
  coccidioidal (primary) (progressive) B38.7
    lung B38.1
    meninges B38.4

Granuloma (*Continued*)
    colon K63.89
    conjunctiva H11.22-●
    dental K04.5
    ear, middle —*see* Cholesteatoma
    eosinophilic C96.6
        bone C96.6
        lung C96.6
        oral mucosa K13.4
        skin L92.2
    eyelid H01.8
    facial (e) L92.2
    foreign body (in soft tissue) NEC M60.20
        ankle M60.27-●
        foot M60.27-●
        forearm M60.23-●
        hand M60.24-●
        in operation wound —*see* Foreign body,
            accidentally left during a procedure
        lower leg M60.26-●
        pelvic region M60.25-●
        shoulder region M60.21-●
        skin L92.3
        specified site NEC M60.28
        subcutaneous tissue L92.3
        thigh M60.25-●
        upper arm M60.22-●
    gangraenescens M31.2
    genito-inguinale A58
    giant cell (central) (reparative) (jaw) M27.1
        gingiva (peripheral) K06.8
    gland (lymph) I88.8
    hepatic NEC K75.3
        in (due to)
            berylliosis J63.2 [*K77*]
            sarcoidosis D86.89
    Hodgkin C81.9
    ileum K63.89
    infectious B99.9
        specified NEC B99.8
    inguinale (Donovan) (venereal) A58
    intestine NEC K63.89
    intracranial (any site) G06.0
    intraspinal (any part) G06.1
    iridocyclitis —*see* Iridocyclitis, chronic
    jaw (bone) (central) M27.1
        reparative giant cell M27.1
    kidney —*see also* Infection, kidney N15.8
    lacrimal H04.81-●
    larynx J38.7
    lethal midline (faciale (e)) M31.2
    liver NEC —*see* Granuloma, hepatic
    lung (infectious) —*see also* Fibrosis, lung
        coccidioidal B38.1
        eosinophilic C96.6
    Majocchi's B35.8
    malignant (facial (e)) M31.2
    mandible (central) M27.1
    midline (lethal) M31.2
    monilial (cutaneous) B37.2
    nasal sinus —*see* Sinusitis
    operation wound T81.89
        foreign body —*see* Foreign body,
            accidentally left during a procedure
        stitch T81.89
        talc —*see* Foreign body, accidentally left
            during a procedure
    oral mucosa K13.4
    orbit, orbital H05.11-●
    paracoccidioidal B41.8
    penis, venereal A58
    periapical K04.5
    peritoneum K66.8
        due to ova of helminths NOS —*see also*
            Helminthiasis B83.9 [*K67*]
    postmastoidectomy cavity —*see*
        Complications, postmastoidectomy,
        recurrent cholesteatoma
    prostate N42.89
    pudendi (ulcerating) A58
    pulp, internal (tooth) K03.3

Granuloma (*Continued*)
    pyogenic, pyogenicum (of) (skin) L98.0
        gingiva K06.8
        maxillary alveolar ridge K04.5
        oral mucosa K13.4
    rectum K62.89
    reticulohistiocytic D76.3
    rubrum nasi L74.8
    Schistosoma —*see* Schistosomiasis
    septic (skin) L98.0
    silica (skin) L92.3
    sinus (accessory) (infective) (nasal) —*see*
        Sinusitis
    skin L92.9
        from residual foreign body L92.3
        pyogenicum L98.0
    spine
        syphilitic (epidural) A52.19
        tuberculous A18.01
    stitch (postoperative) T81.89
    suppurative (skin) L98.0
    swimming pool A31.1
    talc —*see also* Granuloma, foreign body
        in operation wound —*see* Foreign body,
            accidentally left during a procedure
    telangiectaticum (skin) L98.0
    tracheostomy J95.09
    trichophyticum B35.8
    tropicum A66.4
    umbilical P83.81
    umbilicus P83.81
    urethra N36.8
    uveitis —*see* Iridocyclitis, chronic
    vagina A58
    venereum A58
    vocal cord J38.3
Granulomatosis L92.9
    with polyangiitis M31.3
    eosinophilic, with polyangiitis [EGPA] M30.1
    lymphoid C83.8-●
    miliary (listerial) A32.89
    necrotizing, respiratory M31.30
    progressive septic D71
    specified NEC L92.8
    Wegener's M31.30
        with renal involvement M31.31
Granulomatous tissue (abnormal) (excessive)
    L92.9
Granulosis rubra nasi L74.8
Graphite fibrosis (of lung) J63.3
Graphospasm F48.8
    organic G25.89
Grating scapula M89.8X1
Gravel (urinary) —*see* Calculus, urinary
Graves' disease —*see* Hyperthyroidism, with,
    goiter
Gravis —*see* condition
Grawitz tumor C64.-●
Gray syndrome (newborn) P93.0
Grayness, hair (premature) L67.1
    congenital Q84.2
Green sickness D50.8
Greenfield's disease
    meaning
        concentric sclerosis (encephalitis periaxialis
            concentrica) G37.5
        metachromatic leukodystrophy E75.25
Greenstick fracture - code as Fracture, by site
Grey syndrome (newborn) P93.0
Grief F43.21
    prolonged F43.29
    reaction —*see also* Disorder, adjustment F43.20
Griesinger's disease B76.0
Grinder's lung or pneumoconiosis J62.8
Grinding, teeth
    psychogenic F45.8
    sleep related G47.63
Grip
    Dabney's B33.0
    devil's B33.0
Grippe, grippal —*see also* Influenza
    Balkan A78
    summer, of Italy A93.1

Grisel's disease M43.6
Groin —*see* condition
Grooved tongue K14.5
Ground itch B76.9
Grover's disease or syndrome L11.1
Growing pains, children R29.898
Growth (fungoid) (neoplastic) (new) —*see also*
    Neoplasm
    adenoid (vegetative) J35.8
    benign —*see* Neoplasm, benign, by site
    malignant —*see* Neoplasm, malignant, by site
    rapid, childhood Z00.2
    secondary —*see* Neoplasm, secondary, by site
Gruby's disease B35.0
Gubler-Millard paralysis or syndrome G46.3
Guerin-Stern syndrome Q74.3
Guidance, insufficient anterior (occlusal) M26.54
Guillain-Barré disease or syndrome G61.0
    sequelae G65.0
Guinea worms (infection) (infestation) B72
Guinon's disease (motor-verbal tic) F95.2
Gull's disease E03.4
Gum —*see* condition
Gumboil K04.7
    with sinus K04.6
Gumma (syphilitic) A52.79
    artery A52.09
        cerebral A52.04
    bone A52.77
        of yaws (late) A66.6
    brain A52.19
    cauda equina A52.19
    central nervous system A52.3
    ciliary body A52.71
    congenital A50.59
    eyelid A52.71
    heart A52.06
    intracranial A52.19
    iris A52.71
    kidney A52.75
    larynx A52.73
    leptomeninges A52.19
    liver A52.74
    meninges A52.19
    myocardium A52.06
    nasopharynx A52.73
    neurosyphilitic A52.3
    nose A52.73
    orbit A52.71
    palate (soft) A52.79
    penis A52.76
    pericardium A52.06
    pharynx A52.73
    pituitary A52.79
    scrofulous (tuberculous) A18.4
    skin A52.79
    specified site NEC A52.79
    spinal cord A52.19
    tongue A52.79
    tonsil A52.73
    trachea A52.73
    tuberculous A18.4
    ulcerative due to yaws A66.4
    ureter A52.75
    yaws A66.4
        bone A66.6
Gunn's syndrome Q07.8
Gunshot wound —*see also* Puncture, open
    fracture - code as Fracture, by site
    internal organs —*see* Injury, by site
Gynandrism Q56.0
Gynandroblastoma
    specified site —*see* Neoplasm, uncertain
        behavior, by site
    unspecified site
        female D39.10
        male D40.10
Gynecological examination (periodic) (routine)
    Z01.419
    with abnormal findings Z01.411
Gynecomastia N62
Gynephobia F40.291
Gyrate scalp Q82.8

H

H (Hartnup's) disease E72.02
Haas' disease or osteochondrosis (juvenile) (head of humerus) —see Osteochondrosis, juvenile, humerus
Habit, habituation
  bad sleep Z72.821
  chorea F95.8
  disturbance, child F98.9
  drug —see Dependence, drug
  irregular sleep Z72.821
  laxative F55.2
  spasm —see Tic
  tic —see Tic
Haemophilus (H.) influenzae, as cause of disease classified elsewhere B96.3
Haff disease —see Poisoning, mercury
Hageman's factor defect, deficiency or disease D68.2
Haglund's disease or osteochondrosis (juvenile) (os tibiale externum) —see Osteochondrosis, juvenile, tarsus
Hailey-Hailey disease Q82.8
Hair —see also condition
  plucking F63.3
    in stereotyped movement disorder F98.4
  tourniquet syndrome —see also Constriction, external, by site
    finger S60.44-●
    penis S30.842
    thumb S60.34-●
    toe S90.44-●
Hairball in stomach T18.2
Hair-pulling, pathological (compulsive) F63.3
Hairy black tongue K14.3
Half vertebra Q76.49
Halitosis R19.6
Hallerman-Streiff syndrome Q87.0
Hallervorden-Spatz disease G23.0
Hallopeau's acrodermatitis or disease L40.2
Hallucination R44.3
  auditory R44.0
  gustatory R44.2
  olfactory R44.2
  specified NEC R44.2
  tactile R44.2
  visual R44.1
Hallucinosis (chronic) F28
  alcoholic (acute) F10.951
    in
      abuse F10.151
      dependence F10.251
  drug-induced F19.951
    cannabis F12.951
    cocaine F14.951
    hallucinogen F16.151
      in
        abuse F19.151
          cannabis F12.151
          cocaine F14.151
          hallucinogen F16.151
          inhalant F18.151
          opioid F11.151
          sedative, anxiolytic or hypnotic F13.151
          stimulant NEC F15.151
        dependence F19.251
          cannabis F12.251
          cocaine F14.251
          hallucinogen F16.251
          inhalant F18.251
          opioid F11.251
          sedative, anxiolytic or hypnotic F13.251
          stimulant NEC F15.251
    inhalant F18.951
    opioid F11.951
    sedative, anxiolytic or hypnotic F13.951
    stimulant NEC F15.951
  organic F06.0

Hallux
  deformity (acquired) NEC M20.5X-●
  limitus M20.5X-●
  malleus (acquired) NEC M20.3-●
  rigidus (acquired) M20.2-●
    congenital Q74.2
    sequelae (late effect) of rickets E64.3
  valgus (acquired) M20.1-●
    congenital Q66.6
  varus (acquired) M20.3-●
    congenital Q66.3-●
Halo, visual H53.19
Hamartoma, hamartoblastoma Q85.9
  epithelial (gingival), odontogenic, central or peripheral —see Cyst, calcifying odontogenic
Hamartosis Q85.9
Hamman-Rich syndrome J84.114
Hammer toe (acquired) NEC —see also Deformity, toe, hammer toe
  congenital Q66.89
  sequelae (late effect) of rickets E64.3
Hand —see condition
Hand-foot syndrome L27.1
Handicap, handicapped
  educational Z55.9
  specified NEC Z55.8
Hand-Schüller-Christian disease or syndrome C96.5
Hanging (asphyxia) (strangulation) (suffocation) —see Asphyxia, traumatic, due to mechanical threat
Hangnail —see also Cellulitis, digit
  with lymphangitis —see Lymphangitis, acute, digit
Hangover (alcohol) F10.129
Hanhart's syndrome Q87.0
Hanot-Chauffard (-Troisier) syndrome E83.19
Hanot's cirrhosis or disease K74.3
Hansen's disease —see Leprosy
Hantaan virus disease (Korean hemorrhagic fever) A98.5
Hantavirus disease (with renal manifestations) (Dobrava) (Puumala) (Seoul) A98.5
  with pulmonary manifestations (Andes) (Bayou) (Bermejo) (Black Creek Canal) (Choclo) (Juquitiba) (Laguna negra) (Lechiguanas) (New York) (Oran) (Sin nombre) B33.4
Happy puppet syndrome Q93.59
Harada's disease or syndrome H30.81-●
Hardening
  artery —see Arteriosclerosis
  brain G93.89
Harelip (complete) (incomplete) —see Cleft, lip
Harlequin (newborn) Q80.4
Harley's disease D59.6
Harmful use (of)
  alcohol F10.10
  anxiolytics —see Abuse, drug, sedative
  cannabinoids —see Abuse, drug, cannabis
  cocaine —see Abuse, drug, cocaine
  drug —see Abuse, drug
  hallucinogens —see Abuse, drug, hallucinogen
  hypnotics —see Abuse, drug, sedative -
  opioids —see Abuse, drug, opioid
  PCP (phencyclidine) —see Abuse, drug, hallucinogen
  sedatives —see Abuse, drug, sedative
  stimulants NEC —see Abuse, drug, stimulant
Harris' lines —see Arrest, epiphyseal
Hartnup's disease E72.02
Harvester's lung J67.0
Harvesting ovum for in vitro fertilization Z31.83
Hashimoto's disease or thyroiditis E06.3
Hashitoxicosis (transient) E06.3
Hassal-Henle bodies or warts (cornea) H18.49
Haut mal —see Epilepsy, generalized, specified NEC
Haverhill fever A25.1

Hay fever —see also Fever, hay J30.1
Hayem-Widal syndrome D59.8
Haygarth's nodes M15.8
Haymaker's lung J67.0
Hb (abnormal)
  Bart's disease D56.0
  disease —see Disease, hemoglobin
  trait —see Trait
Head —see condition
Headache R51.9
  with
    orthostatic component NEC R51.0
    positional component NEC R51.0
  allergic NEC G44.89
  associated with sexual activity G44.82
▶ cervicogenic G44.86
  chronic daily R51.9
  cluster G44.009
    chronic G44.029
      intractable G44.021
      not intractable G44.029
    episodic G44.019
      intractable G44.011
      not intractable G44.019
    intractable G44.001
    not intractable G44.009
  cough (primary) G44.83
  daily chronic R51.9
  drug-induced NEC G44.40
    intractable G44.41
    not intractable G44.40
  exertional (primary) G44.84
  histamine G44.009
    intractable G44.001
    not intractable G44.009
  hypnic G44.81
  lumbar puncture G97.1
  medication overuse G44.40
    intractable G44.41
    not intractable G44.40
  menstrual —see Migraine, menstrual
  migraine (type) —see also Migraine G43.909
  nasal septum R51.9
  neuralgiform, short lasting unilateral, with conjunctival injection and tearing (SUNCT) G44.059
    intractable G44.051
    not intractable G44.059
  new daily persistent (NDPH) G44.52
  orgasmic G44.82
  periodic syndromes in adults and children G43.C0
    with refractory migraine G43.C1
      intractable G43.C1
      not intractable G43.C0
    without refractory migraine G43.C0
  postspinal puncture G97.1
  post-traumatic G44.309
    acute G44.319
      intractable G44.311
      not intractable G44.319
    chronic G44.329
      intractable G44.321
      not intractable G44.329
    intractable G44.301
    not intractable G44.309
  pre-menstrual —see Migraine, menstrual
  preorgasmic G44.82
  primary
    cough G44.83
    exertional G44.84
    stabbing G44.85
    thunderclap G44.53
  rebound G44.40
    intractable G44.41
    not intractable G44.40
  short lasting unilateral neuralgiform, with conjunctival injection and tearing (SUNCT) G44.059
    intractable G44.051
    not intractable G44.059
  specified syndrome NEC G44.89

Headache (Continued)
  spinal and epidural anesthesia - induced T88.59
    in labor and delivery O74.5
    in pregnancy O29.4-●
    postpartum, puerperal O89.4
  spinal fluid loss (from puncture) G97.1
  stabbing (primary) G44.85
  tension (-type) G44.209
    chronic G44.229
      intractable G44.221
      not intractable G44.229
    episodic G44.219
      intractable G44.211
      not intractable G44.219
    intractable G44.201
    not intractable G44.209
  thunderclap (primary) G44.53
  vascular NEC G44.1
Healthy
  infant
    accompanying sick mother Z76.3
    receiving care Z76.2
  person accompanying sick person Z76.3
Hearing examination Z01.10
  with abnormal findings NEC Z01.118
  infant or child (over 28 days old) Z00.129
    with abnormal findings Z00.121
  following failed hearing screening Z01.110
  for hearing conservation and treatment Z01.12
Heart —see condition
Heart beat
  abnormality R00.9
    specified NEC R00.8
  awareness R00.2
  rapid R00.0
  slow R00.1
Heartburn R12
  psychogenic F45.8
Heartland virus disease A93.8
Heat (effects) T67.9
  apoplexy T67.01
  burn —see also Burn L55.9
  collapse T67.1
  cramps T67.2
  dermatitis or eczema L59.0
  edema T67.7
  erythema - code by site under Burn, first degree
  excessive T67.9
    specified effect NEC T67.8
  exhaustion T67.5
    anhydrotic T67.3
    due to
      salt (and water) depletion T67.4
      water depletion T67.3
        with salt depletion T67.4
  fatigue (transient) T67.6
  fever T67.01
  hyperpyrexia T67.01
  prickly L74.0
  prostration —see Heat, exhaustion
  pyrexia T67.01
  rash L74.0
  specified effect NEC T67.8
  stroke T67.01
    exertional T67.02
    specified NEC T67.09
  sunburn —see Sunburn
  syncope T67.1
Heavy-for-dates NEC (infant) (4000g to 4499g) P08.1
  exceptionally (4500g or more) P08.0
Hebephrenia, hebephrenic (schizophrenia) F20.1
Heberden's disease or nodes (with arthropathy) M15.1
Hebra's
  pityriasis L26
  prurigo L28.2
Heel —see condition
Heerfordt's disease D86.89
Hegglin's anomaly or syndrome D72.0
Heilmeyer-Schoner disease D45

Heine-Medin disease A80.9
Heinz body anemia, congenital D58.2
Heliophobia F40.228
Heller's disease or syndrome F84.3
HELLP syndrome (hemolysis, elevated liver enzymes and low platelet count) O14.2-●
  complicating
    childbirth O14.24
    puerperium O14.25
Helminthiasis —see also Infestation, helminth
  Ancylostoma B76.0
  intestinal B82.0
    mixed types (types classifiable to more than one of the titles B65.0-B81.3 and B81.8) B81.4
    specified type NEC B81.8
  mixed types (intestinal) (types classifiable to more than one of the titles B65.0-B81.3 and B81.8) B81.4
  Necator (americanus) B76.1
  specified type NEC B83.8
Heloma L84
Hemangioblastoma —see Neoplasm, connective tissue, uncertain behavior
  malignant —see Neoplasm, connective tissue, malignant
Hemangioendothelioma —see also Neoplasm, uncertain behavior, by site
  benign D18.00
    intra-abdominal D18.03
    intracranial D18.02
    skin D18.01
    specified site NEC D18.09
  bone (diffuse) —see Neoplasm, bone, malignant
  epithelioid —see also Neoplasm, uncertain behavior, by site
    malignant —see Neoplasm, malignant, by site
  malignant —see Neoplasm, connective tissue, malignant
Hemangiofibroma —see Neoplasm, benign, by site
Hemangiolipoma —see Lipoma
Hemangioma D18.00
  arteriovenous D18.00
    intra-abdominal D18.03
    intracranial D18.02
    skin D18.01
    specified site NEC D18.09
  capillary I78.1
    intra-abdominal D18.03
    intracranial D18.02
    skin D18.01
    specified site NEC D18.09
  cavernous D18.00
    intra-abdominal D18.03
    intracranial D18.02
    skin D18.01
    specified site NEC D18.09
  epithelioid D18.00
    intra-abdominal D18.03
    intracranial D18.02
    skin D18.01
    specified site NEC D18.09
  histiocytoid D18.00
    intra-abdominal D18.03
    intracranial D18.02
    skin D18.01
    specified site NEC D18.09
  infantile D18.00
    intra-abdominal D18.03
    intracranial D18.02
    skin D18.01
    specified site NEC D18.09
  intra-abdominal D18.03
  intracranial D18.02
  intramuscular D18.00
    intra-abdominal D18.03
    intracranial D18.02
    skin D18.01
    specified site NEC D18.09

Hemangioma (Continued)
  intrathoracic structures D18.09
  juvenile D18.00
  malignant —see Neoplasm, connective tissue, malignant
  plexiform D18.00
    intra-abdominal D18.03
    intracranial D18.02
    skin D18.01
    specified site NEC D18.09
  racemose D18.00
    intra-abdominal D18.03
    intracranial D18.02
    skin D18.01
    specified site NEC D18.09
  sclerosing —see Neoplasm, skin, benign
  simplex D18.00
    intra-abdominal D18.03
    intracranial D18.02
    skin D18.01
    specified site NEC D18.09
  skin D18.01
  specified site NEC D18.09
  venous D18.00
    intra-abdominal D18.03
    intracranial D18.02
    skin D18.01
    specified site NEC D18.09
  verrucous keratotic D18.00
    intra-abdominal D18.03
    intracranial D18.02
    skin D18.01
    specified site NEC D18.09
Hemangiomatosis (systemic) I78.8
  involving single site —see Hemangioma
Hemangiopericytoma —see also Neoplasm, connective tissue, uncertain behavior
  benign —see Neoplasm, connective tissue, benign
  malignant —see Neoplasm, connective tissue, malignant
Hemangiosarcoma —see Neoplasm, connective tissue, malignant
Hemarthrosis (nontraumatic) M25.00
  ankle M25.07-●
  elbow M25.02-●
  foot joint M25.07-●
  hand joint M25.04-●
  hip M25.05-●
  in hemophilic arthropathy —see Arthropathy, hemophilic
  knee M25.06-●
  shoulder M25.01-●
  specified joint NEC M25.08
  traumatic —see Sprain, by site
  vertebrae M25.08
  wrist M25.03-●
Hematemesis K92.0
  with ulcer - code by site under Ulcer, with hemorrhage K27.4
  newborn, neonatal P54.0
    due to swallowed maternal blood P78.2
Hematidrosis L74.8
Hematinuria —see also Hemoglobinuria
  malarial B50.8
Hematobilia K83.8
Hematocele
  female NEC N94.89
    with ectopic pregnancy O00.90
      with intrauterine pregnancy O00.91
  ovary N83.8
  male N50.1
Hematochezia —see also Melena K92.1
Hematochyluria —see also Infestation, filarial
  schistosomiasis (bilharziasis) B65.0
Hematocolpos (with hematometra or hematosalpinx) N89.7
Hematocornea —see Pigmentation, cornea, stromal
Hematogenous —see condition

▶ New   ⇒ Revised   ~~deleted~~ Deleted   ● Use Additional Character(s)

Hematoma (traumatic) (skin surface intact) —
see also Contusion
  with
    injury of internal organs —see Injury, by site
    open wound —see Wound, open
  amputation stump (surgical) (late) T87.89
  aorta, dissecting I71.00
    abdominal I71.02
    thoracic I71.01
    thoracoabdominal I71.03
  aortic intramural —see Dissection, aorta
  arterial (complicating trauma) —see Injury,
    blood vessel, by site
  auricle —see Contusion, ear
    nontraumatic —see Disorder, pinna,
      hematoma
  birth injury NEC P15.8
  brain (traumatic)
    with
      cerebral laceration or contusion
        (diffuse) —see Injury, intracranial,
        diffuse
      focal —see Injury, intracranial, focal
    cerebellar, traumatic S06.37-●
    intracerebral, traumatic —see Injury,
      intracranial, intracerebral hemorrhage
    newborn NEC P52.4
      birth injury P10.1
    nontraumatic —see Hemorrhage,
      intracranial
    subarachnoid, arachnoid, traumatic —see
      Injury, intracranial, subarachnoid
      hemorrhage
    subdural, traumatic —see Injury,
      intracranial, subdural hemorrhage
  breast (nontraumatic) N64.89
  broad ligament (nontraumatic) N83.7
    traumatic S37.892
  cerebellar, traumatic S06.37-●
  cerebral —see Hematoma, brain
  cerebrum S06.36-●
    left S06.35-●
    right S06.34-●
  cesarean delivery wound O90.2
  complicating delivery (perineal) (pelvic)
    (vagina) (vulva) O71.7
  corpus cavernosum (nontraumatic) N48.89
  epididymis (nontraumatic) N50.1
  epidural (traumatic) —see Injury, intracranial,
    epidural hemorrhage
    spinal —see Injury, spinal cord, by region
  episiotomy O90.2
  face, birth injury P15.4
  genital organ NEC (nontraumatic)
    female (nonobstetric) N94.89
      traumatic S30.202
    male N50.1
      traumatic S30.201
  internal organs —see Injury, by site
  intracerebral, traumatic —see Injury,
    intracranial, intracerebral hemorrhage
  intraoperative —see Complications,
    intraoperative, hemorrhage
  labia (nontraumatic) (nonobstetric) N90.8
  liver (subcapsular) (nontraumatic) K76.89
    birth injury P15.0
  mediastinum —see Injury, intrathoracic
  mesosalpinx (nontraumatic) N83.7
    traumatic S37.898
  muscle - code by site under Contusion
  nontraumatic
    muscle M79.81
    soft tissue M79.81
  obstetrical surgical wound O90.2
  orbit, orbital (nontraumatic) —see also
    Hemorrhage, orbit
    traumatic —see Contusion, orbit
  pelvis (female) (nontraumatic) (nonobstetric)
    N94.89
    obstetric O71.7
    traumatic —see Injury, by site

Hematoma (Continued)
  penis (nontraumatic) N48.89
    birth injury P15.5
  perianal (nontraumatic) K64.5
  perineal S30.23
    complicating delivery O71.7
  perirenal —see Injury, kidney
  pinna —see Contusion, ear
    nontraumatic —see Disorder, pinna,
      hematoma
  placenta O43.89-●
  postoperative (postprocedural) —see
    Complication, postprocedural,
    hematoma
  retroperitoneal (nontraumatic) K66.1
    traumatic S36.892
  scrotum, superficial S30.22
    birth injury P15.5
  seminal vesicle (nontraumatic) N50.1
    traumatic S37.892
  spermatic cord (traumatic) S37.892
    nontraumatic N50.1
  spinal (cord) (meninges) —see also Injury,
    spinal cord, by region
    newborn (birth injury) P11.5
  spleen D73.5
    intraoperative —see Complications,
      intraoperative, hemorrhage, spleen
    postprocedural (postoperative) —see
      Complications, postprocedural,
      hemorrhage, spleen
  sternocleidomastoid, birth injury P15.2
  sternomastoid, birth injury P15.2
  subarachnoid (traumatic) —see Injury,
    intracranial, subarachnoid hemorrhage
    newborn (nontraumatic) P52.5
      due to birth injury P10.3
    nontraumatic —see Hemorrhage,
      intracranial, subarachnoid
  subdural (traumatic) —see Injury, intracranial,
    subdural hemorrhage
    newborn (localized) P52.8
      birth injury P10.0
    nontraumatic —see Hemorrhage,
      intracranial, subdural
  superficial, newborn P54.5
  testis (nontraumatic) N50.1
    birth injury P15.5
  tunica vaginalis (nontraumatic) N50.1
  umbilical cord, complicating delivery O69.5
  uterine ligament (broad) (nontraumatic) N83.7
    traumatic S37.892
  vagina (ruptured) (nontraumatic) N89.8
    complicating delivery O71.7
  vas deferens (nontraumatic) N50.1
    traumatic S37.892
  vitreous —see Hemorrhage, vitreous
  vulva (nontraumatic) (nonobstetric) N90.89
    complicating delivery O71.7
    newborn (birth injury) P15.5
Hematometra N85.7
  with hematocolpos N89.7
Hematomyelia (central) G95.19
  newborn (birth injury) P11.5
  traumatic T14.8
Hematomyelitis G04.90
Hematoperitoneum —see Hemoperitoneum
Hematophobia F40.230
Hematopneumothorax (see Hemothorax)
Hematopoiesis, cyclic D70.4
Hematoporphyria —see Porphyria
Hematorachis, hematorrhachis G95.19
  newborn (birth injury) P11.5
Hematosalpinx N83.6
  with
    hematocolpos N89.7
    hematometra N85.7
      with hematocolpos N89.7
  infectional —see Salpingitis
Hematospermia R36.1
Hematothorax (see Hemothorax)

Hematuria R31.9
  benign (familial) (of childhood) —see also
    Hematuria, idiopathic
    essential microscopic R31.1
  due to sulphonamide, sulfonamide —see Table
    of Drugs and Chemicals, by drug
  endemic —see also Schistosomiasis B65.0
  gross R31.0
  idiopathic N02.9
    with glomerular lesion
      C3
        glomerulonephritis N02.A
        glomerulopathy N02.A
          with dense deposit disease N02.6
      crescentic (diffuse) glomerulonephritis
        N02.7
      dense deposit disease N02.6
      endocapillary proliferative
        glomerulonephritis N02.4
      focal and segmental hyalinosis or
        sclerosis N02.1
      membranoproliferative (diffuse) N02.5
      membranous (diffuse) N02.2
      mesangial proliferative (diffuse) N02.3
      mesangiocapillary (diffuse) N02.5
      minor abnormality N02.0
      proliferative NEC N02.8
      specified pathology NEC N02.8
  intermittent —see Hematuria, idiopathic
  malarial B50.8
  microscopic NEC (with symptoms) R31.29
    asymptomatic R31.21
    benign essential R31.1
  paroxysmal —see also Hematuria, idiopathic
    nocturnal D59.5
  persistent —see Hematuria, idiopathic
  recurrent —see Hematuria, idiopathic
  tropical —see also Schistosomiasis B65.0
  tuberculous A18.13
Hemeralopia (day blindness) H53.11
  vitamin A deficiency E50.5
Hemi-akinesia R41.4
Hemianalgesia R20.0
Hemianencephaly Q00.0
Hemianesthesia R20.0
Hemianopia, hemianopsia (heteronymous)
  H53.47
  homonymous H53.46-●
  syphilitic A52.71
Hemiathetosis R25.8
Hemiatrophy R68.89
  cerebellar G31.9
  face, facial, progressive (Romberg) G51.8
  tongue K14.8
Hemiballism (us) G25.5
Hemicardia Q24.8
Hemicephalus, hemicephaly Q00.0
Hemichorea G25.5
Hemicolitis, left —see Colitis, left sided
Hemicrania
  congenital malformation Q00.0
  continua G44.51
  meaning migraine —see also Migraine G43.909
  paroxysmal G44.039
    chronic G44.049
      intractable G44.041
      not intractable G44.049
    episodic G44.039
      intractable G44.031
      not intractable G44.039
    intractable G44.031
    not intractable G44.039
Hemidystrophy —see Hemiatrophy
Hemiectromelia Q73.8
Hemihypalgesia R20.8
Hemihypesthesia R20.1
Hemi-inattention R41.4
Hemimelia Q73.8
  lower limb —see Defect, reduction, lower
    limb, specified type NEC
  upper limb —see Defect, reduction, upper
    limb, specified type NEC

▶ New   ⇒ Revised   ~~deleted~~ Deleted   ● Use Additional Character(s)

Hemorrhage, hemorrhagic *(Continued)*
cranial —*see* Hemorrhage, intracranial
cutaneous R23.3
  due to autosensitivity, erythrocyte D69.2
  newborn P54.5
delayed
  following ectopic or molar pregnancy
    O08.1
  postpartum O72.2
diathesis (familial) D69.9
disease D69.9
  newborn P53
  specified type NEC D69.8
due to or associated with
  afibrinogenemia or other coagulation defect
    (conditions in categories D65-D69)
    antepartum —*see* Hemorrhage,
      antepartum, with coagulation
      defect
    intrapartum O67.0
  dental implant M27.61
  device, implant or graft —*see also*
    Complications, by site and type,
    specified NEC T85.838
    arterial graft NEC T82.838
    breast T85.838
    catheter NEC T85.838
      dialysis (renal) T82.838
        intraperitoneal T85.838
      infusion NEC T82.838
        spinal (epidural) (subdural)
          T85.830
      urinary (indwelling) T83.83
    electronic (electrode) (pulse generator)
      (stimulator)
      bone T84.83
      cardiac T82.837
      nervous system (brain) (peripheral
        nerve) (spinal) T85.830
      urinary T83.83
    fixation, internal (orthopedic) NEC
      T84.83
    gastrointestinal (bile duct) (esophagus)
      T85.838
    genital NEC T83.83
    heart NEC T82.837
    joint prosthesis T84.83
    ocular (corneal graft) (orbital implant)
      NEC T85.838
    orthopedic NEC T84.83
      bone graft T86.838
    specified NEC T85.838
    urinary NEC T83.83
    vascular NEC T82.838
    ventricular intracranial shunt T85.838
duodenum, duodenal K92.2
  ulcer —*see* Ulcer, duodenum, with
    hemorrhage
dura mater —*see* Hemorrhage, intracranial,
  subdural
endotracheal —*see* Hemorrhage, lung
epicranial subaponeurotic (massive), birth
  injury P12.2
epidural (traumatic) —*see also* Injury,
  intracranial, epidural hemorrhage
  nontraumatic I62.1
⇒esophagus K22.89
  varix I85.01
    secondary I85.11
excessive, following ectopic gestation
  (subsequent episode) O08.1
extradural (traumatic) —*see* Injury,
  intracranial, epidural hemorrhage
  birth injury P10.8
  newborn (anoxic) (nontraumatic) P52.8
  nontraumatic I62.1
eye NEC H57.89
  fundus —*see* Hemorrhage, retina
  lid —*see* Disorder, eyelid, specified type
    NEC
fallopian tube N83.6

Hemorrhage, hemorrhagic *(Continued)*
fibrinogenolysis —*see* Fibrinolysis
fibrinolytic (acquired) —*see* Fibrinolysis
from
  ear (nontraumatic) —*see* Otorrhagia
  tracheostomy stoma J95.01
fundus, eye —*see* Hemorrhage, retina
funis —*see* Hemorrhage, umbilicus, cord
gastric —*see* Hemorrhage, stomach
gastroenteric K92.2
  newborn P54.3
gastrointestinal (tract) K92.2
  newborn P54.3
genital organ, male N50.1
genitourinary (tract) NOS R31.9
gingiva K06.8
globe (eye) —*see* Hemophthalmos
graafian follicle cyst (ruptured) N83.0-●
gum K06.8
heart I51.89
hypopharyngeal (throat) R04.1
intermenstrual (regular) N92.3
  irregular N92.1
internal (organs) NEC R58
  capsule I61.0
  ear —*see* subcategory H83.8
  newborn P54.8
intestine K92.2
  newborn P54.3
intra-abdominal R58
intra-alveolar (lung), newborn P26.8
intracerebral (nontraumatic) —*see*
  Hemorrhage, intracranial,
  intracerebral
intracranial (nontraumatic) I62.9
  birth injury P10.9
  epidural, nontraumatic I62.1
  extradural, nontraumatic I62.1
  intracerebral (nontraumatic) (in) I61.9
    brain stem I61.3
    cerebellum I61.4
    hemisphere I61.2
      cortical (superficial) I61.1
      subcortical (deep) I61.0
    intraoperative
      during a nervous system procedure
        G97.31
      during other procedure G97.32
    intraventricular I61.5
    multiple localized I61.6
    newborn P52.4
      birth injury P10.1
    postprocedural
      following a nervous system procedure
        G97.51
      following other procedure
        G97.52
    specified NEC I61.8
    superficial I61.1
    traumatic (diffuse) —*see* Injury,
      intracranial, diffuse
    focal —*see* Injury, intracranial, focal
  newborn P52.9
    specified NEC P52.8
  subarachnoid (nontraumatic) (from) I60.9
    intracranial (cerebral) artery I60.7
      anterior communicating I60.2
      basilar I60.4
      carotid siphon and bifurcation
        I60.0-●
      communicating I60.7
        anterior I60.2
        posterior I60.3-●
      middle cerebral I60.1-●
      posterior communicating I60.3-●
      specified artery NEC I60.6
      vertebral I60.5-●
    newborn P52.5
      birth injury P10.3
    specified NEC I60.8
    traumatic S06.6X-●

Hemorrhage, hemorrhagic *(Continued)*
intracranial *(Continued)*
  subdural (nontraumatic) I62.00
    acute I62.01
    birth injury P10.0
    chronic I62.03
    newborn (anoxic) (hypoxic) P52.8
      birth injury P10.0
    spinal G95.19
    subacute I62.02
    traumatic —*see* Injury, intracranial,
      subdural hemorrhage
  traumatic —*see* Injury, intracranial, focal
    brain injury
intramedullary NEC G95.19
intraocular —*see* Hemophthalmos
intraoperative, intraprocedural —*see*
  Complication, hemorrhage (hematoma),
  intraoperative (intraprocedural), by site
intrapartum —*see* Hemorrhage, complicating,
  delivery
intrapelvic
  female N94.89
  male K66.1
intraperitoneal K66.1
intrapontine I61.3
intraprocedural —*see* Complication,
  hemorrhage (hematoma), intraoperative
  (intraprocedural), by site
intrauterine N85.7
  complicating delivery —*see also* Hemorrhage,
    complicating, delivery O67.9
  postpartum —*see* Hemorrhage, postpartum
intraventricular I61.5
  newborn (nontraumatic) —*see also* Newborn,
    affected by, hemorrhage P52.3
    due to birth injury P10.2
    grade
      1 P52.0
      2 P52.1
      3 P52.21
      4 P52.22
intravesical N32.89
iris (postinfectional) (postinflammatory)
  (toxic) —*see* Hyphema
joint (nontraumatic) —*see* Hemarthrosis
kidney N28.89
knee (joint) (nontraumatic) —*see*
  Hemarthrosis, knee
labyrinth —*see* subcategory H83.8
lenticular striate artery I61.0
ligature, vessel —*see* Hemorrhage,
  postoperative
liver K76.89
lung R04.89
  newborn P26.9
    massive P26.1
    specified NEC P26.8
  tuberculous —*see* Tuberculosis, pulmonary
massive umbilical, newborn P51.0
mediastinum —*see* Hemorrhage, lung
medulla I61.3
membrane (brain) I60.8
  spinal cord —*see* Hemorrhage, spinal cord
meninges, meningeal (brain) (middle) I60.8
  spinal cord —*see* Hemorrhage, spinal cord
mesentery K66.1
metritis —*see* Endometritis
mouth K13.79
mucous membrane NEC R58
  newborn P54.8
muscle M62.89
nail (subungual) L60.8
nasal turbinate R04.0
  newborn P54.8
navel, newborn P51.9
newborn P54.9
  specified NEC P54.8
nipple N64.59
nose R04.0
  newborn P54.8

Hemorrhage, hemorrhagic (Continued)
  omentum K66.1
  optic nerve (sheath) H47.02-•
  orbit, orbital H05.23-•
  ovary NEC N83.8
  oviduct N83.6
  pancreas K86.89
  parathyroid (gland) (spontaneous) E21.4
  parturition —see Hemorrhage, complicating,
      delivery
  penis N48.89
  pericardium, pericarditis I31.2
  peritoneum, peritoneal K66.1
  peritonsillar tissue J35.8
    due to infection J36
  petechial R23.3
    due to autosensitivity, erythrocyte D69.2
  pituitary (gland) E23.6
  pleura —see Hemorrhage, lung
  polioencephalitis, superior E51.2
  polymyositis —see Polymyositis
  pons, pontine I61.3
  posterior fossa (nontraumatic) I61.8
    newborn P52.6
  postmenopausal N95.0
  postnasal R04.0
  postoperative —see Complications,
      postprocedural, hemorrhage, by site
  postpartum NEC (following delivery of
      placenta) O72.1
    delayed or secondary O72.2
    retained placenta O72.0
    third stage O72.0
  pregnancy —see Hemorrhage, antepartum
  preretinal —see Hemorrhage, retina
  prostate N42.1
  puerperal —see Hemorrhage, postpartum
    delayed or secondary O72.2
  pulmonary R04.89
    newborn P26.9
      massive P26.1
      specified NEC P26.8
    tuberculous —see Tuberculosis, pulmonary
  purpura (primary) D69.3
  rectum (sphincter) K62.5
    newborn P54.2
  recurring, following initial hemorrhage at
      time of injury T79.2
  renal N28.89
  respiratory passage or tract R04.9
    specified NEC R04.89
  retina, retinal (vessels) H35.6-•
    diabetic —see Diabetes, retinal, hemorrhage
  retroperitoneal R58
  scalp R58
  scrotum N50.1
  secondary (nontraumatic) R58
    following initial hemorrhage at time of
        injury T79.2
  seminal vesicle N50.1
  skin R23.3
    newborn P54.5
  slipped umbilical ligature P51.8
  spermatic cord N50.1
  spinal (cord) G95.19
    newborn (birth injury) P11.5
  spleen D73.5
    intraoperative —see Complications,
        intraoperative, hemorrhage, spleen
    postprocedural —see Complications,
        postprocedural, hemorrhage, spleen
  stomach K92.2
    newborn P54.3
    ulcer —see Ulcer, stomach, with
        hemorrhage
  subarachnoid (nontraumatic) —see
      Hemorrhage, intracranial, subarachnoid
  subconjunctival —see also Hemorrhage,
      conjunctiva
    birth injury P15.3
  subcortical (brain) I61.0

Hemorrhage, hemorrhagic (Continued)
  subcutaneous R23.3
  subdiaphragmatic R58
  subdural (acute) (nontraumatic) —see
      Hemorrhage, intracranial, subdural
  subependymal
    newborn P52.0
      with intraventricular extension P52.1
          and intracerebral extension P52.22
  subgaleal P12.2
  subhyaloid —see Hemorrhage, retina
  subperiosteal —see Disorder, bone, specified
      type NEC
  subretinal —see Hemorrhage, retina
  subtentorial —see Hemorrhage, intracranial,
      subdural
  subungual L60.8
  suprarenal (capsule) (gland) E27.49
    newborn P54.4
  tentorium (traumatic) NEC —see
      Hemorrhage, brain
    newborn (birth injury) P10.4
  testis N50.1
  third stage (postpartum) O72.0
  thorax —see Hemorrhage, lung
  throat R04.1
  thymus (gland) E32.8
  thyroid (cyst) (gland) E07.89
  tongue K14.8
  tonsil J35.8
  trachea —see Hemorrhage, lung
  tracheobronchial R04.89
    newborn P26.0
  traumatic — code to specific injury
    cerebellar —see Hemorrhage, brain
    intracranial —see Hemorrhage, brain
    recurring or secondary (following initial
        hemorrhage at time of injury) T79.2
  tuberculous NEC —see also Tuberculosis,
      pulmonary A15.0
  tunica vaginalis N50.1
  ulcer - code by site under Ulcer, with
      hemorrhage K27.4
  umbilicus, umbilical
    cord
      after birth, newborn P51.9
      complicating delivery O69.5
    newborn P51.9
      massive P51.0
      slipped ligature P51.8
    stump P51.9
  urethra (idiopathic) N36.8
  uterus, uterine (abnormal) N93.9
    climacteric N92.4
    complicating delivery —see Hemorrhage,
        complicating, delivery
    dysfunctional or functional N93.8
    intermenstrual (regular) N92.3
      irregular N92.1
    postmenopausal N95.0
    postpartum —see Hemorrhage, postpartum
    preclimacteric or premenopausal N92.4
    prepubertal N93.8
    pubertal N92.2
  vagina (abnormal) N93.9
    newborn P54.6
  vas deferens N50.1
  vasa previa O69.4
  ventricular I61.5
  vesical N32.89
  viscera NEC R58
    newborn P54.8
  vitreous (humor) (intraocular) H43.1-•
  vulva N90.89
Hemorrhoids (bleeding) (without mention of
    degree) K64.9
  1st degree (grade/stage I) (without prolapse
      outside of anal canal) K64.0
  2nd degree (grade/stage II) (that prolapse
      with straining but retract spontaneously)
      K64.1

Hemorrhoids (Continued)
  3rd degree (grade/stage III) (that prolapse
      with straining and require manual
      replacement back inside anal canal)
      K64.2
  4th degree (grade/stage IV) (with prolapsed
      tissue that cannot be manually replaced)
      K64.3
  complicating
    pregnancy O22.4
    puerperium O87.2
  external K64.4
    with
      thrombosis K64.5
  internal (without mention of degree) K64.8
  prolapsed K64.8
  skin tags
    anus K64.4
    residual K64.4
  specified NEC K64.8
  strangulated —see also Hemorrhoids, by
      degree K64.8
  thrombosed —see also Hemorrhoids, by
      degree K64.5
  ulcerated —see also Hemorrhoids, by degree
      K64.8
Hemosalpinx N83.6
  with
    hematocolpos N89.7
    hematometra N85.7
      with hematocolpos N89.7
Hemosiderosis (dietary) E83.19
  pulmonary, idiopathic E83.1 [J84.03]
  transfusion T80.89
Hemothorax (bacterial) (nontuberculous)
    J94.2
  newborn P54.8
  traumatic S27.1
    with pneumothorax S27.2
  tuberculous NEC A15.6
Henoch (-Schönlein) disease or syndrome
    (purpura) D69.0
Henpue, henpuye A66.6
Hepar lobatum (syphilitic) A52.74
Hepatalgia K76.89
Hepatitis K75.9
  acute B17.9
    with coma K72.01
    with hepatic failure —see Failure, hepatic
    alcoholic —see Hepatitis, alcoholic
    infectious B15.9
    non-viral K72.0
    viral B17.9
  alcoholic (acute) (chronic) K70.10
    with ascites K70.11
  amebic —see Abscess, liver, amebic
  anicteric (viral) —see Hepatitis, viral
  antigen-associated (HAA) —see Hepatitis, B
  Australia-antigen (positive) —see Hepatitis, B
  autoimmune K75.4
  B B19.10
    with hepatic coma B19.11
    acute B16.9
      with
        delta-agent (coinfection) (without
            hepatic coma) B16.1
          with hepatic coma B16.0
        hepatic coma (without delta-agent
            coinfection) B16.2
    chronic B18.1
      with delta-agent B18.0
  bacterial NEC K75.89
  C (viral) B19.20
    with hepatic coma B19.21
    acute B17.10
      with hepatic coma B17.11
    chronic B18.2
  catarrhal (acute) B15.9
    with hepatic coma B15.0
  cholangiolitic K75.89
  cholestatic K75.89

▶ New   ⇒ Revised   ~~deleted~~ Deleted   • Use Additional Character(s)

Hepatitis (Continued)
chronic K73.9
active NEC K73.2
lobular NEC K73.1
persistent NEC K73.0
specified NEC K73.8
cytomegaloviral B25.1
due to ethanol (acute) (chronic) —see
Hepatitis, alcoholic
epidemic B15.9
with hepatic coma B15.0
fulminant NEC (viral) —see Hepatitis, viral
granulomatous NEC K75.3
herpesviral B00.81
history of
B Z86.19
C Z86.19
homologous serum —see Hepatitis, viral,
type B
in (due to)
mumps B26.81
toxoplasmosis (acquired) B58.1
congenital (active) P37.1 [K77]
infectious, infective B15.9
acute (subacute) B17.9
chronic B18.9
inoculation —see Hepatitis, viral, type B
interstitial (chronic) K74.69
▶ischemia, ischemic K72.00
lupoid NEC K75.2
malignant NEC (with hepatic failure)
K72.90
with coma K72.91
neonatal giant cell P59.29
neonatal (idiopathic) (toxic) P59.29
newborn P59.29
postimmunization —see Hepatitis, viral,
type B
post-transfusion —see Hepatitis, viral, type B
reactive, nonspecific K75.2
serum —see Hepatitis, viral, type B
▶shock K72.00
specified type NEC
with hepatic failure —see Failure, hepatic
syphilitic (late) A52.74
congenital (early) A50.08 [K77]
late A50.59 [K77]
secondary A51.45
toxic —see also Disease, liver, toxic K71.6
tuberculous A18.83
viral, virus B19.9
with hepatic coma B19.0
acute B17.9
chronic B18.9
specified NEC B18.8
type
B B18.1
with delta-agent B18.0
C B18.2
congenital P35.3
coxsackie B33.8 [K77]
cytomegalic inclusion B25.1
in remission, any type — code to Hepatitis,
chronic, by type
non-A, non-B B17.8
specified type NEC (with or without coma)
B17.8
type
A B15.9
with hepatic coma B15.0
B B19.10
with hepatic coma B19.11
acute B16.9
with
delta-agent (coinfection) (without
hepatic coma) B16.1
with hepatic coma B16.0
hepatic coma (without delta-
agent coinfection) B16.2
chronic B18.1
with delta-agent B18.0

Hepatitis (Continued)
viral, virus (Continued)
type (Continued)
C B19.20
with hepatic coma B19.21
acute B17.10
with hepatic coma B17.11
chronic B18.2
E B17.2
non-A, non-B B17.8
Hepatization lung (acute) —see Pneumonia, lobar
Hepatoblastoma C22.2
Hepatocarcinoma C22.0
Hepatocholangiocarcinoma C22.0
Hepatocholangioma, benign D13.4
Hepatocholangitis K75.89
Hepatolenticular degeneration E83.01
Hepatoma (malignant) C22.0
benign D13.4
embryonal C22.0
Hepatomegaly —see also Hypertrophy, liver
with splenomegaly R16.2
congenital Q44.7
in mononucleosis
gammaherpesviral B27.09
infectious specified NEC B27.89
Hepatoptosis K76.89
**Hepatorenal syndrome following labor and
delivery** O90.4
Hepatosis K76.89
Hepatosplenomegaly R16.2
hyperlipemic (Bürger-Grütz type) E78.3 [K77]
Hereditary —see condition
▶**Hereditary alpha tryptasemia (syndrome)** D89.44
Heredodegeneration, macular —see Dystrophy,
retina
Heredopathia atactica polyneuritiformis G60.1
Heredosyphilis —see Syphilis, congenital
Herlitz' syndrome Q81.1
Hermansky-Pudlak syndrome E70.331
Hermaphrodite, hermaphroditism (true) Q56.0
46,XX with streak gonads Q99.1
46,XX/46,XY Q99.0
46,XY with streak gonads Q99.1
chimera 46,XX/46,XY Q99.0
Hernia, hernial (acquired) (recurrent) K46.9
with
gangrene —see Hernia, by site, with,
gangrene
incarceration —see Hernia, by site, with,
obstruction
irreducible —see Hernia, by site, with,
obstruction
obstruction —see Hernia, by site, with,
obstruction
strangulation —see Hernia, by site, with,
obstruction
abdomen, abdominal K46.9
with
gangrene (and obstruction) K46.1
obstruction K46.0
femoral —see Hernia, femoral
incisional —see Hernia, incisional
inguinal —see Hernia, inguinal
specified site NEC K45.8
with
gangrene (and obstruction) K45.1
obstruction K45.0
umbilical —see Hernia, umbilical
wall —see Hernia, ventral
appendix —see Hernia, abdomen
bladder (mucosa) (sphincter)
congenital (female) (male) Q79.51
female —see Cystocele
male N32.89
brain, congenital —see Encephalocele
cartilage, vertebra —see Displacement,
intervertebral disc
cerebral, congenital —see also Encephalocele
endaural Q01.8
ciliary body (traumatic) S05.2-●

Hernia, hernial (Continued)
colon —see Hernia, abdomen
Cooper's —see Hernia, abdomen, specified
site NEC
crural —see Hernia, femoral
diaphragm, diaphragmatic K44.9
with
gangrene (and obstruction) K44.1
obstruction K44.0
congenital Q79.0
direct (inguinal) —see Hernia, inguinal
diverticulum, intestine —see Hernia,
abdomen
double (inguinal) —see Hernia, inguinal,
bilateral
due to adhesions (with obstruction) K56.50
epigastric —see also Hernia, ventral K43.9
esophageal hiatus —see Hernia, hiatal
external (inguinal) —see Hernia, inguinal
fallopian tube N83.4-●
fascia M62.89
femoral K41.90
with
gangrene (and obstruction) K41.40
not specified as recurrent K41.40
recurrent K41.41
obstruction K41.30
not specified as recurrent K41.30
recurrent K41.31
bilateral K41.20
with
gangrene (and obstruction) K41.10
not specified as recurrent K41.10
recurrent K41.11
obstruction K41.00
not specified as recurrent K41.00
recurrent K41.01
not specified as recurrent K41.20
recurrent K41.21
not specified as recurrent K41.90
recurrent K41.91
unilateral K41.90
with
gangrene (and obstruction) K41.40
not specified as recurrent K41.40
recurrent K41.41
obstruction K41.30
not specified as recurrent K41.30
recurrent K41.31
not specified as recurrent K41.90
recurrent K41.91
foramen magnum G93.5
congenital Q01.8
funicular (umbilical) —see also Hernia,
umbilicus
spermatic (cord) —see Hernia, inguinal
gastrointestinal tract —see Hernia, abdomen
Hesselbach's —see Hernia, femoral, specified
site NEC
hiatal (esophageal) (sliding) K44.9
with
gangrene (and obstruction) K44.1
obstruction K44.0
congenital Q40.1
hypogastric —see Hernia, ventral
incarcerated —see also Hernia, by site, with
obstruction
with gangrene —see Hernia, by site, with
gangrene
incisional K43.92
with
gangrene (and obstruction) K43.1
obstruction K43.0
indirect (inguinal) —see Hernia, inguinal
inguinal (direct) (external) (funicular)
(indirect) (internal) (oblique) (scrotal)
(sliding) K40.90
with
gangrene (and obstruction) K40.40
not specified as recurrent K40.40
recurrent K40.41

Hernia, hernial *(Continued)*
  inguinal *(Continued)*
    with *(Continued)*
      obstruction K40.30
        not specified as recurrent K40.30
        recurrent K40.31
      bilateral K40.20
        with
          gangrene (and obstruction) K40.10
            not specified as recurrent K40.10
            recurrent K40.11
          obstruction K40.00
            not specified as recurrent K40.00
            recurrent K40.01
        not specified as recurrent K40.20
        recurrent K40.21
      not specified as recurrent K40.90
      recurrent K40.91
      unilateral K40.90
        with
          gangrene (and obstruction) K40.40
            not specified as recurrent K40.40
            recurrent K40.41
          obstruction K40.30
            not specified as recurrent K40.30
            recurrent K40.31
        not specified as recurrent K40.90
        recurrent K40.91
  internal —*see also* Hernia, abdomen
    inguinal —*see* Hernia, inguinal
  interstitial —*see* Hernia, abdomen
  intervertebral cartilage or disc —*see*
    Displacement, intervertebral disc
  intestine, intestinal —*see* Hernia, by site
  intra-abdominal —*see* Hernia, abdomen
  iris (traumatic) S05.2-●
  irreducible —*see also* Hernia, by site, with
    obstruction
    with gangrene —*see* Hernia, by site, with
      gangrene
  ischiatic —*see* Hernia, abdomen, specified
    site NEC
  ischiorectal —*see* Hernia, abdomen, specified
    site NEC
  lens (traumatic) S05.2-●
  linea (alba) (semilunaris) —*see* Hernia,
    ventral
  Littre's —*see* Hernia, abdomen
  lumbar —*see* Hernia, abdomen, specified site
    NEC
  lung (subcutaneous) J98.4
  mediastinum J98.59
  mesenteric (internal) —*see* Hernia, abdomen
  midline —*see* Hernia, ventral
  muscle (sheath) M62.89
  nucleus pulposus —*see* Displacement,
    intervertebral disc
  oblique (inguinal) —*see* Hernia, inguinal
  obstructive —*see also* Hernia, by site, with
    obstruction
    with gangrene —*see* Hernia, by site, with
      gangrene
  obturator —*see* Hernia, abdomen, specified
    site NEC
  omental —*see* Hernia, abdomen
  ovary N83.4-●
  oviduct N83.4-●
  paraesophageal —*see also* Hernia, diaphragm
    congenital Q40.1
  parastomal K43.5
    with
      gangrene (and obstruction) K43.4
      obstruction K43.3
  paraumbilical —*see* Hernia, umbilicus
  perineal —*see* Hernia, abdomen, specified
    site NEC
  Petit's —*see* Hernia, abdomen, specified site
    NEC
  postoperative —*see* Hernia, incisional
  pregnant uterus —*see* Abnormal, uterus in
    pregnancy or childbirth
  prevesical N32.89

Hernia, hernial *(Continued)*
  properitoneal —*see* Hernia, abdomen,
    specified site NEC
  pudendal —*see* Hernia, abdomen, specified
    site NEC
  rectovaginal N81.6
  retroperitoneal —*see* Hernia, abdomen,
    specified site NEC
  Richter's —*see* Hernia, abdomen, with
    obstruction
  Rieux's, Riex's —*see* Hernia, abdomen,
    specified site NEC
  sac condition (adhesion) (dropsy)
    (inflammation) (laceration)
    (suppuration) - code by site under
    Hernia
  sciatic —*see* Hernia, abdomen, specified site
    NEC
  scrotum, scrotal —*see* Hernia, inguinal
  sliding (inguinal) —*see also* Hernia, inguinal
    hiatus —*see* Hernia, hiatal
  spigelian —*see* Hernia, ventral
  spinal —*see* Spina bifida
  strangulated —*see also* Hernia, by site, with
    obstruction
    with gangrene —*see* Hernia, by site, with
      gangrene
  subxiphoid —*see* Hernia, ventral
  supra-umbilicus —*see* Hernia, ventral
  tendon —*see* Disorder, tendon, specified type
    NEC
  Treitz's (fossa) —*see* Hernia, abdomen,
    specified site NEC
  tunica vaginalis Q55.29
  umbilicus, umbilical K42.9
    with
      gangrene (and obstruction) K42.1
      obstruction K42.0
  ureter N28.89
  urethra, congenital Q64.79
  urinary meatus, congenital Q64.79
  uterus N81.4
    pregnant —*see* Abnormal, uterus in
      pregnancy or childbirth
  vaginal (anterior) (wall) —*see* Cystocele
  Velpeau's —*see* Hernia, femoral
  ventral K43.9
    with
      gangrene (and obstruction) K43.7
      obstruction K43.6
    incisional K43.2
      with
        gangrene (and obstruction) K43.1
        obstruction K43.0
      recurrent —*see* Hernia, incisional
    specified NEC K43.9
      with
        gangrene (and obstruction) K43.7
        obstruction K43.6
  vesical
    congenital (female) (male) Q79.51
    female —*see* Cystocele
    male N32.89
  vitreous (into wound) S05.2-●
    into anterior chamber —*see* Prolapse,
      vitreous
Herniation —*see also* Hernia
  brain (stem) G93.5
  ▶nontraumatic G93.5
  ▶traumatic S06.A1
    ▶cerebellar S06.A1
    ▶subfalcine (cingulate) S06.A1
    ▶tonsillar S06.A1
    ▶transtentorial (central) (upward
      cerebellar) S06.A1
    ▶uncal S06.A1
  cerebral G93.5
  ▶nontraumatic G93.5
  ▶traumatic S06.A1
  mediastinum J98.59
  nucleus pulposus —*see* Displacement,
    intervertebral disc
Herpangina B08.5

Herpes, herpesvirus, herpetic B00.9
  anogenital A60.9
    perianal skin A60.1
    rectum A60.1
    urogenital tract A60.00
      cervix A60.03
      male genital organ NEC A60.02
      penis A60.01
      specified site NEC A60.09
      vagina A60.04
      vulva A60.04
  blepharitis (zoster) B02.39
    simplex B00.59
  circinatus B35.4
    bullosus L12.0
  conjunctivitis (simplex) B00.53
    zoster B02.31
  cornea B02.33
  encephalitis B00.4
    due to herpesvirus 6 B10.01
    due to herpesvirus 7 B10.09
    specified NEC B10.09
  eye (zoster) B02.30
    simplex B00.50
  eyelid (zoster) B02.39
    simplex B00.59
  facialis B00.1
  febrilis B00.1
  geniculate ganglionitis B02.21
  genital, genitalis A60.00
    female A60.09
    male A60.02
  gestational, gestationis O26.4-●
  gingivostomatitis B00.2
  human B00.9
    1 —*see* Herpes, simplex
    2 —*see* Herpes, simplex
    3 —*see* Varicella
    4 —*see* Mononucleosis, Epstein-Barr (virus)
    5 —*see* Disease, cytomegalic inclusion
      (generalized)
    6
      encephalitis B10.01
      specified NEC B10.81
    7
      encephalitis B10.09
      specified NEC B10.82
    8 B10.89
  infection NEC B10.89
    Kaposi's sarcoma associated B10.89
  iridocyclitis (simplex) B00.51
    zoster B02.32
  iris (vesicular erythema multiforme) L51.9
  iritis (simplex) B00.51
  Kaposi's sarcoma associated B10.89
  keratitis (simplex) (dendritic) (disciform)
    (interstitial) B00.52
    zoster (interstitial) B02.33
  keratoconjunctivitis (simplex) B00.52
    zoster B02.33
  labialis B00.1
  lip B00.1
  meningitis (simplex) B00.3
    zoster B02.1
  ophthalmicus (zoster) NEC B02.30
    simplex B00.50
  penis A60.01
  perianal skin A60.1
  pharyngitis, pharyngotonsillitis B00.2
  rectum A60.1
  scrotum A60.02
  sepsis B00.7
  simplex B00.9
    complicated NEC B00.89
    congenital P35.2
    conjunctivitis B00.53
    external ear B00.1
    eyelid B00.59
    hepatitis B00.81
    keratitis (interstitial) B00.52
    myelitis B00.82
    specified complication NEC B00.89
    visceral B00.89

▶ New   ⇒ Revised   ~~deleted~~ Deleted   ● Use Additional Character(s)

Herpes, herpesvirus, herpetic (Continued)
stomatitis B00.2
tonsurans B35.0
visceral B00.89
vulva A60.04
whitlow B00.89
zoster —see also condition B02.9
auricularis B02.21
complicated NEC B02.8
conjunctivitis B02.31
disseminated B02.7
encephalitis B02.0
eye(lid) B02.39
geniculate ganglionitis B02.21
keratitis (interstitial) B02.33
meningitis B02.1
myelitis B02.24
neuritis, neuralgia B02.29
ophthalmicus NEC B02.30
oticus B02.21
polyneuropathy B02.23
specified complication NEC B02.8
trigeminal neuralgia B02.22
Herpesvirus (human) —see Herpes
Herpetophobia F40.218
Herrick's anemia —see Disease, sickle-cell
Hers' disease E74.09
Herter-Gee syndrome K90.0
Herxheimer's reaction R68.89
Hesitancy
of micturition R39.11
urinary R39.11
Hesselbach's hernia —see Hernia, femoral, specified site NEC
Heterochromia (congenital) Q13.2
cataract —see Cataract, complicated
cyclitis (Fuchs) —see Cyclitis, Fuchs' heterochromic
hair L67.1
iritis —see Cyclitis, Fuchs' heterochromic
retained metallic foreign body
(nonmagnetic) —see Foreign body, intraocular, old, retained
magnetic —see Foreign body, intraocular, old, retained, magnetic
uveitis —see Cyclitis, Fuchs' heterochromic
Heterophoria —see Strabismus, heterophoria
Heterophyes, heterophyiasis (small intestine) B66.8
Heterotopia, heterotopic —see also Malposition, congenital
cerebralis Q04.8
Heterotropia —see Strabismus
Heubner-Herter disease K90.0
Hexadactylism Q69.9
HGSIL (cytology finding) (high grade squamous intraepithelial lesion on cytologic smear) (Pap smear finding)
anus R85.613
cervix R87.613
biopsy (histology) finding — see Neoplasia, intraepithelial, cervix, grade II or grade III
vagina R87.623
biopsy (histology) finding — see Neoplasia, intraepithelial, vagina, grade II or grade III
Hibernoma —see Lipoma
Hiccup, hiccough R06.6
epidemic B33.0
psychogenic F45.8
Hidden penis (congenital) Q55.64
acquired N48.83
Hidradenitis (axillaris) (suppurative) L73.2
Hidradenoma (nodular) —see also Neoplasm, skin, benign
clear cell —see Neoplasm, skin, benign
papillary —see Neoplasm, skin, benign
Hidrocystoma —see Neoplasm, skin, benign

High
altitude effects T70.20
anoxia T70.29
on
ears T70.0
sinuses T70.1
polycythemia D75.1
arch
foot Q66.7-●
palate, congenital Q38.5
arterial tension —see Hypertension
basal metabolic rate R94.8
blood pressure —see also Hypertension
borderline R03.0
reading (incidental) (isolated)
(nonspecific), without diagnosis of hypertension R03.0
cholesterol E78.00
with high triglycerides E78.2
diaphragm (congenital) Q79.1
expressed emotional level within family Z63.8
head at term O32.4
palate, congenital Q38.5
risk
infant NEC Z76.2
sexual behavior (heterosexual) Z72.51
bisexual Z72.53
homosexual Z72.52
scrotal testis, testes
bilateral Q53.23
unilateral Q53.13
temperature (of unknown origin) R50.9
thoracic rib Q76.6
triglycerides E78.1
with high cholesterol E78.2
Hildenbrand's disease A75.0
Ilium —see condition
Hip —see condition
Hippel's disease Q85.8
Hippophobia F40.218
Hippus H57.09
Hirschsprung's disease or megacolon Q43.1
Hirsutism, hirsuties L68.0
Hirudiniasis
external B88.3
internal B83.4
Hiss-Russell dysentery A03.1
Histidinemia, histidinuria E70.41
Histiocytoma —see also Neoplasm, skin, benign
fibrous —see also Neoplasm, skin, benign
atypical —see Neoplasm, connective tissue, uncertain behavior
malignant —see Neoplasm, connective tissue, malignant
Histiocytosis D76.3
acute differentiated progressive C96.0
Langerhans' cell NEC C96.6
multifocal X
multisystemic (disseminated) C96.0
unisystemic C96.5
pulmonary, adult (adult PLCH) J84.82
unifocal (X) C96.6
lipid, lipoid D76.3
essential E75.29
malignant C96.A
mononuclear phagocytes NEC D76.1
Langerhans' cells C96.6
non-Langerhans cell D76.3
polyostotic sclerosing D76.3
sinus, with massive lymphadenopathy D76.3
syndrome NEC D76.3
X NEC C96.6
acute (progressive) C96.0
chronic C96.6
multifocal C96.5
multisystemic C96.0
unifocal C96.6
Histoplasmosis B39.9
with pneumonia NEC B39.2
African B39.5
American —see Histoplasmosis, capsulati

Histoplasmosis (Continued)
capsulati B39.4
disseminated B39.3
generalized B39.3
pulmonary B39.2
acute B39.0
chronic B39.1
Darling's B39.4
duboisii B39.5
lung NEC B39.2
History
family (of) —see also History, personal (of)
alcohol abuse Z81.1
allergy NEC Z84.89
anemia Z83.2
arthritis Z82.61
asthma Z82.5
blindness Z82.1
cardiac death (sudden) Z82.41
carrier of genetic disease Z84.81
chromosomal anomaly Z82.79
chronic
disabling disease NEC Z82.8
lower respiratory disease Z82.5
colonic polyps Z83.71
congenital malformations and deformations Z82.79
polycystic kidney Z82.71
consanguinity Z84.3
deafness Z82.2
diabetes mellitus Z83.3
disability NEC Z82.8
disease or disorder (of)
allergic NEC Z84.89
behavioral NEC Z81.8
blood and blood-forming organs Z83.2
cardiovascular NEC Z82.49
chronic disabling NEC Z82.8
digestive Z83.79
ear NEC Z83.52
elevated lipoprotein (a) (Lp(a)) Z83.430
endocrine NEC Z83.49
eye NEC Z83.518
glaucoma Z83.511
familial hypercholesterolemia Z83.42
genitourinary NEC Z84.2
glaucoma Z83.511
hematological Z83.2
immune mechanism Z83.2
infectious NEC Z83.1
ischemic heart Z82.49
kidney Z84.1
lipoprotein metabolism Z83.438
mental NEC Z81.8
metabolic Z83.49
musculoskeletal NEC Z82.69
neurological NEC Z82.0
nutritional Z83.49
parasitic NEC Z83.1
psychiatric NEC Z81.8
respiratory NEC Z83.6
skin and subcutaneous tissue NEC Z84.0
specified NEC Z84.89
drug abuse NEC Z81.3
elevated lipoprotein(a) (Lp (a)) Z83.430
epilepsy Z82.0
familial hypercholesterolemia Z83.42
genetic disease carrier Z84.81
glaucoma Z83.511
hearing loss Z82.2
human immunodeficiency virus (HIV) infection Z83.0
Huntington's chorea Z82.0
hyperlipidemia, familial combined Z83.438
intellectual disability Z81.0
leukemia Z80.6
lipidemia NEC Z83.438
malignant neoplasm (of) NOS Z80.9
bladder Z80.52
breast Z80.3
bronchus Z80.1

History (Continued)
   family (Continued)
      malignant neoplasm (Continued)
         digestive organ Z80.0
         gastrointestinal tract Z80.0
         genital organ Z80.49
            ovary Z80.41
            prostate Z80.42
            specified organ NEC Z80.49
            testis Z80.43
         hematopoietic NEC Z80.7
         intrathoracic organ NEC Z80.2
         kidney Z80.51
         lung Z80.1
         lymphatic NEC Z80.7
         ovary Z80.41
         prostate Z80.42
         respiratory organ NEC Z80.2
         specified site NEC Z80.8
         testis Z80.43
         trachea Z80.1
         urinary organ or tract Z80.59
            bladder Z80.52
            kidney Z80.51
      mental
         disorder NEC Z81.8
      multiple endocrine neoplasia (MEN)
         syndrome Z83.41
      osteoporosis Z82.62
      polycystic kidney Z82.71
      polyps (colon) Z83.71
      psychiatric disorder Z81.8
      psychoactive substance abuse NEC Z81.3
      respiratory condition NEC Z83.6
         asthma and other lower respiratory
            conditions Z82.5
      self-harmful behavior Z81.8
      SIDS (sudden infant death syndrome) Z84.82
      skin condition Z84.0
      specified condition NEC Z84.89
      stroke (cerebrovascular) Z82.3
      substance abuse NEC Z81.4
         alcohol Z81.1
         drug NEC Z81.3
         psychoactive NEC Z81.3
         tobacco Z81.2
      sudden
         cardiac death Z82.41
         infant death syndrome (SIDS) Z84.82
      tobacco abuse Z81.2
      violence, violent behavior Z81.8
      visual loss Z82.1
   personal (of) —see also History, family (of)
      abuse
         adult Z91.419
            forced labor or sexual exploitation
               Z91.42
            physical and sexual Z91.410
            psychological Z91.411
         childhood Z62.819
            forced labor or sexual exploitation in
               childhood Z62.813
            physical Z62.810
            psychological Z62.811
            sexual Z62.810
      alcohol dependence F10.21
      allergy (to) Z88.9
         analgesic agent NEC Z88.6
         anesthetic Z88.4
         antibiotic agent NEC Z88.1
         anti-infective agent NEC Z88.3
         contrast media Z91.041
         drugs, medicaments and biological
            substances Z88.9
            specified NEC Z88.8
         food Z91.018
            additives Z91.02
           ▶beef Z91.014
            eggs Z91.012
           ▶lamb Z91.014
           ▶mammalian meats Z91.014
            milk products Z91.011
            peanuts Z91.010

History (Continued)
   personal (Continued)
      allergy (Continued)
         food (Continued)
           ▶pork Z91.014
           ▶red meats Z91.014
            seafood Z91.013
            specified food NEC Z91.018
         insect Z91.038
            bee Z91.030
         latex Z91.040
         medicinal agents Z88.9
            specified NEC Z88.8
         narcotic agent NEC Z88.5
         nonmedicinal agents Z91.048
         penicillin Z88.0
         serum Z88.7
         specified NEC Z91.09
         sulfonamides Z88.2
         vaccine Z88.7
      anaphylactic shock Z87.892
      anaphylaxis Z87.892
      behavioral disorders Z86.59
      benign carcinoid tumor Z86.012
      benign neoplasm Z86.018
         brain Z86.011
         carcinoid Z86.012
         colonic polyps Z86.010
      brain injury (traumatic) Z87.820
      breast implant removal Z98.86
      calculi, renal Z87.442
      cancer —see History, personal (of),
         malignant neoplasm (of)
      cardiac arrest (death), successfully
         resuscitated Z86.74
      ▶CAR-T (Chimeric Antigen Receptor T-cell)
         therapy Z92.850
      ▶cellular therapy Z92.859
         ▶specified NEC Z92.858
      cerebral infarction without residual deficit
         Z86.73
      cervical dysplasia Z87.410
      chemotherapy for neoplastic condition
         Z92.21
      childhood abuse —see History, personal
         (of), abuse
      ▶Chimeric Antigen Receptor T-cell (CAR-T)
         therapy Z92.850
      cleft lip (corrected) Z87.730
      cleft palate (corrected) Z87.730
      collapsed vertebra (healed) Z87.311
         due to osteoporosis Z87.310
      combat and operational stress reaction
         Z86.51
      congenital malformation (corrected) Z87.798
         circulatory system (corrected) Z87.74
         digestive system (corrected) NEC
            Z87.738
         ear (corrected) Z87.721
         eye (corrected) Z87.720
         face and neck (corrected) Z87.790
         genitourinary system (corrected) NEC
            Z87.718
         heart (corrected) Z87.74
         integument (corrected) Z87.76
         limb(s) (corrected) Z87.76
         musculoskeletal system (corrected) Z87.76
         neck (corrected) Z87.790
         nervous system (corrected) NEC Z87.728
         respiratory system (corrected) Z87.75
         sense organs (corrected) NEC Z87.728
         specified NEC Z87.798
      contraception Z92.0
      coronavirus (disease) (novel) 2019 Z86.16
      COVID-19 Z86.16
      deployment (military) Z91.82
      diabetic foot ulcer Z86.31
      disease or disorder (of) Z87.898
         blood and blood-forming organs Z86.2
         circulatory system Z86.79
            specified condition NEC Z86.79
         connective tissue NEC Z87.39

History (Continued)
   personal (Continued)
      disease or disorder (of) (Continued)
         digestive system Z87.19
            colonic polyp Z86.010
            peptic ulcer disease Z87.11
            specified condition NEC Z87.19
         ear Z86.69
         endocrine Z86.39
            diabetic foot ulcer Z86.31
            gestational diabetes Z86.32
            specified type NEC Z86.39
         eye Z86.69
         genital (track) system NEC
            female Z87.42
            male Z87.438
         hematological Z86.2
         Hodgkin Z85.71
         immune mechanism Z86.2
         infectious Z86.19
            coronavirus (disease) (novel) 2019
               Z86.16
            COVID-19 Z86.16
            malaria Z86.13
            Methicillin resistant Staphylococcus
               aureus (MRSA) Z86.14
            poliomyelitis Z86.12
            SARS-CoV-2 Z86.16
            specified NEC Z86.19
            tuberculosis Z86.11
         mental NEC Z86.59
         metabolic Z86.39
            diabetic foot ulcer Z86.31
            gestational diabetes Z86.32
            specified type NEC Z86.39
         musculoskeletal NEC Z87.39
         nervous system Z86.69
         nutritional Z86.39
         parasitic Z86.19
         respiratory system NEC Z87.09
         sense organs Z86.69
         skin Z87.2
         specified site or type NEC Z87.898
         subcutaneous tissue Z87.2
         trophoblastic Z87.59
         urinary system NEC Z87.448
      drug dependence —see Dependence, drug,
         by type, in remission
      drug therapy
         antineoplastic chemotherapy Z92.21
         estrogen Z92.23
        ➥immunosuppression Z92.25
         inhaled steroids Z92.240
         monoclonal drug Z92.22
         specified NEC Z92.29
         steroid Z92.241
         systemic steroids Z92.241
      dysplasia
         cervical (mild) (moderate) Z87.410
            severe (grade III) Z86.001
         prostatic Z87.430
         vaginal (mild) (moderate) Z87.411
            severe (grade III) Z86.002
         vulvar (mild) (moderate) Z87.412
            severe (grade III) Z86.002
      embolism (venous) Z86.718
         pulmonary Z86.711
      encephalitis Z86.61
      estrogen therapy Z92.23
      extracorporeal membrane oxygenation
         (ECMO) Z92.81
      failed conscious sedation Z92.83
      failed moderate sedation Z92.83
      fall, falling Z91.81
      forced labor or sexual exploitation Z91.42
         in childhood Z62.813
      fracture (healed)
         fatigue Z87.312
         fragility Z87.310
         osteoporosis Z87.310
         pathological NEC Z87.311
         stress Z87.312
         traumatic Z87.81

▶ New   ⇨ Revised   ~~deleted~~ Deleted   ● Use Additional Character(s)

History *(Continued)*
  personal *(Continued)*
▶ gene therapy Z92.86
  gestational diabetes Z86.32
  hepatitis
    B Z86.19
    C Z86.19
  Hodgkin disease Z85.71
  hyperthermia, malignant Z88.4
  hypospadias (corrected) Z87.710
  hysterectomy Z90.710
⇒ immunosuppression therapy Z92.25
  in situ neoplasm
    breast Z86.000
    cervix uteri Z86.001
    digestive organs, specified NEC Z86.004
    esophagus Z86.003
    genital organs, specified NEC Z86.002
    melanoma Z86.006
    middle ear Z86.005
    oral cavity Z86.003
    respiratory system Z86.005
    skin Z86.007
    specified NEC Z86.008
    stomach Z86.003
  infection NEC Z86.19
    central nervous system Z86.61
    coronavirus (disease) (novel) 2019 Z86.16
    COVID-19 Z86.16
    latent tuberculosis Z86.15
    Methicillin resistant Staphylococcus aureus (MRSA) Z86.14
    SARS-CoV-2 Z86.16
    urinary (recurrent) (tract) Z87.41
  injury NEC Z87.828
  in utero procedure during pregnancy Z98.870
  in utero procedure while a fetus Z98.871
  irradiation Z92.3
  kidney stones Z87.442
  latent tuberculosis Z86.15
  leukemia Z85.6
  lymphoma (non-Hodgkin) Z85.72
  malignant melanoma (skin) Z85.820
  malignant neoplasm (of) Z85.9
    accessory sinuses Z85.22
    anus NEC Z85.048
      carcinoid Z85.040
    bladder Z85.51
    bone Z85.830
    brain Z85.841
    breast Z85.3
    bronchus NEC Z85.118
      carcinoid Z85.110
    carcinoid —*see* History, personal (of), malignant neoplasm, by site, carcinioid
    cervix Z85.41
    colon NEC Z85.038
      carcinoid Z85.030
    digestive organ Z85.00
      specified NEC Z85.09
    endocrine gland NEC Z85.858
    epididymis Z85.48
    esophagus Z85.01
    eye Z85.840
    gastrointestinal tract —*see* History, malignant neoplasm, digestive organ
    genital organ
      female Z85.40
        specified NEC Z85.44
      male Z85.45
        specified NEC Z85.49
    hematopoietic NEC Z85.79
    intrathoracic organ Z85.20-●
    kidney NEC Z85.528
      carcinoid Z85.520
    large intestine NEC Z85.038
      carcinoid Z85.030
    larynx Z85.21
    liver Z85.05
    lung NEC Z85.118
      carcinoid Z85.110

History *(Continued)*
  personal *(Continued)*
    malignant neoplasm (of) *(Continued)*
      mediastinum Z85.29
      Merkel cell Z85.821
      middle ear Z85.22
      nasal cavities Z85.22
      nervous system NEC Z85.848
        oral cavity Z85.819
        specified site NEC Z85.818
      ovary Z85.43
      pancreas Z85.07
      pelvis Z85.53
      pharynx Z85.819
        specified site NEC Z85.818
      pleura Z85.29
      prostate Z85.46
      rectosigmoid junction NEC Z85.048
        carcinoid Z85.040
      rectum NEC Z85.048
        carcinoid Z85.040
      respiratory organ Z85.20
      sinuses, accessory Z85.22
      skin NEC Z85.828
        melanoma Z85.820
        Merkel cell Z85.821
      small intestine NEC Z85.068
        carcinoid Z85.060
      soft tissue Z85.831
      specified site NEC Z85.89
      stomach NEC Z85.028
        carcinoid Z85.020
      testis Z85.47
      thymus NEC Z85.238
        carcinoid Z85.230
      thyroid Z85.850
      tongue Z85.810
      trachea Z85.12
      ureter Z85.54
      urinary organ or tract Z85.50
        specified NEC Z85.59
      uterus Z85.42
    maltreatment Z91.89
    medical treatment NEC Z92.89
    melanoma Z85.820
      in situ Z86.06
      malignant (skin) Z85.820
    meningitis Z86.61
    mental disorder Z86.59
    Merkel cell carcinoma (skin) Z85.821
    Methicillin resistant Staphylococcus aureus (MRSA) Z86.14
    military deployment Z91.82
    military war, peacekeeping and humanitarian deployment (current or past conflict) Z91.82
    myocardial infarction (old) I25.2
    neglect (in)
      adult Z91.412
      childhood Z62.812
    neoplasia
      anal intraepithelial, III [AIN III] Z86.004
      high-grade prostatic intraepithelial, III [HGPIN III] Z86.002
      vaginal intraepithelial, III [VAIN III] Z86.002
      vulvar intraepithelial, III [VIN III] Z86.002
    neoplasm
      benign Z86.018
        brain Z86.011
        colon polyp Z86.010
      in situ
        breast Z86.000
        cervix uteri Z86.001
        digestive organs, specified NEC Z86.004
        esophagus Z86.003
        genital organs, specified NEC Z86.002
        melanoma Z86.006
        middle ear Z86.005
        oral cavity Z86.003
        respiratory system Z86.005
        skin Z86.007
        specified NEC Z86.008

History *(Continued)*
  personal *(Continued)*
    neoplasm *(Continued)*
      in situ *(Continued)*
        stomach Z86.003
      malignant —*see* History of, malignant neoplasm
      uncertain behavior Z86.03
    nephrotic syndrome Z87.441
    nicotine dependence Z87.891
    noncompliance with medical treatment or regimen —*see* Noncompliance
    nutritional deficiency Z86.39
    obstetric complications Z87.59
      childbirth Z87.59
      pregnancy Z87.59
      pre-term labor Z87.51
      puerperium Z87.59
    osteoporosis fractures Z87.31
⇒ parasuicide (attempt) Z91.51
    physical trauma NEC Z87.828
    ⇒ self-harm or suicide attempt Z91.51
    pneumonia (recurrent) Z87.01
    poisoning NEC Z91.89
    ⇒ self-harm or suicide attempt Z91.51
    poor personal hygiene Z91.89
    preterm labor Z87.51
    procedure during pregnancy Z98.870
    procedure while a fetus Z98.871
    prolonged reversible ischemic neurologic deficit (PRIND) Z86.73
    prostatic dysplasia Z87.430
    psychiatric disorder NEC Z87.89
    psychological
      abuse
        adult Z91.411
        child Z62.811
      trauma, specified NEC Z91.49
    radiation therapy Z92.3
    removal
      implant
        breast Z98.86
    renal calculi Z87.442
    respiratory condition NEC Z87.09
    retained foreign body fully removed Z87.821
    risk factors NEC Z91.89
    SARS-CoV-2 infection Z86.16
⇒ self-harm
    ▶ nonsuicidal Z91.52
    ▶ suicidal Z91.51
▶ self-inflicted injury without suicidal intent Z91.52
▶ self-injury
    ▶ nonsuicidal Z91.52
▶ self-mutilation Z91.52
⇒ self-poisoning attempt Z91.51
    ▶ suicidal behavior Z91.51
    sex reassignment Z87.890
    sleep-wake cycle problem Z72.821
    specified NEC Z87.898
    steroid therapy (systemic) Z92.241
      inhaled Z92.240
    stroke without residual deficits Z86.73
    substance abuse NEC F10-F19
    sudden cardiac arrest Z86.74
    sudden cardiac death successfully resuscitated Z86.74
⇒ suicide attempt Z91.51
    surgery NEC Z98.890
      with uterine scar Z98.891
      sex reassignment Z87.890
      transplant —*see* Transplant
    thrombophlebitis Z86.72
    thrombosis (venous) Z86.718
      pulmonary Z86.711
    tobacco dependence Z87.891
    transient ischemic attack (TIA) without residual deficits Z86.73
    trauma (physical) NEC Z87.828
      psychological NEC Z91.49
    ⇒ self-harm Z91.51
    traumatic brain injury Z87.820

History *(Continued)*
  personal *(Continued)*
    tuberculosis, latent infection Z86.15
    unhealthy sleep-wake cycle Z72.821
    unintended awareness under general
      anesthesia Z92.84
    urinary (recurrent) (tract) infection(s) Z87.440
    urinary calculi Z87.42
    uterine scar from previous surgery Z98.891
    vaginal dysplasia Z87.411
    venous thrombosis or embolism Z86.718
      pulmonary Z86.711
    vulvar dysplasia Z87.412
His-Werner disease A79.0
HIV —*see also* Human, immunodeficiency virus
  B20
  laboratory evidence (nonconclusive) R75
  nonconclusive test (in infants) R75
  positive, seropositive Z21
Hives (bold) —*see* Urticaria
Hoarseness R49.0
⇒**Hobo** Z59.00
Hodgkin disease —*see* Lymphoma, Hodgkin
Hodgson's disease I71.2
  ruptured I71.1
Hoffa-Kastert disease E88.89
Hoffa's disease E88.89
Hoffmann-Bouveret syndrome I47.9
Hoffmann's syndrome E03.9 *[G73.7]*
Hole (round)
  macula H35.34-●
  retina (without detachment) —*see* Break,
    retina, round hole
    with detachment —*see* Detachment, retina,
      with retinal, break
Holiday relief care Z75.5
Hollenhorst's plaque —*see* Occlusion, artery,
  retina
Hollow foot (congenital) Q66.7-●
  acquired —*see* Deformity, limb, foot, specified
    NEC
Holoprosencephaly Q04.2
Holt-Oram syndrome Q87.2
⇒**Homelessness** Z59.00
  ▶sheltered Z59.01
  ▶unsheltered Z59.02
Homesickness —*see* Disorder, adjustment
▶**Homocysteinemia** R79.83
Homocystinemia, homocystinuria E72.11
Homogentisate 1,2-dioxygenase deficiency
  E70.29
Homologous serum hepatitis (prophylactic)
  (therapeutic) —*see* Hepatitis, viral, type B
Honeycomb lung J98.4
  congenital Q33.0
Hooded
  clitoris Q52.6
  penis Q55.69
Hookworm (disease) (infection) (infestation) B76.9
  with anemia B76.9 *[D63.8]*
  specified NEC B76.8
Hordeolum (eyelid) (externum) (recurrent)
  H00.019
  internum H00.029
    left H00.026
      lower H00.025
      upper H00.024
    right H00.023
      lower H00.022
      upper H00.021
  left H00.016
    lower H00.015
    upper H00.014
  right H00.013
    lower H00.012
    upper H00.011
Horn
  cutaneous L85.8
  nail L60.2
    congenital Q84.6
Horner (-Claude Bernard) **syndrome** G90.2
  traumatic —*see* Injury, nerve, cervical
    sympathetic

Horseshoe kidney (congenital) Q63.1
Horton's headache or neuralgia G44.099
  intractable G44.091
  not intractable G44.099
Hospital hopper syndrome —*see* Disorder,
  factitious
Hospitalism in children —*see* Disorder,
  adjustment
Hostility R45.5
  towards child Z62.3
Hot flashes
  menopausal N95.1
Hourglass (contracture) —*see also* Contraction,
  hourglass
  stomach K31.89
    congenital Q40.2
    stricture K31.2
Household, housing circumstance affecting
  care Z59.9
⇒specified NEC Z59.89
Housemaid's knee —*see* Bursitis, prepatellar
▶**HSCT-TMA (hematopoietic stem cell**
  transplantation-associated thrombotic
  microangiopathy) M31.11
Hudson (-Stähli) **line** (cornea) —*see*
  Pigmentation, cornea, anterior
Human
  bite (open wound) —*see also* Bite
    intact skin surface —*see* Bite, superficial
  herpesvirus —*see* Herpes
  immunodeficiency virus (HIV) disease
    (infection) B20
    asymptomatic status Z21
    contact Z20.6
    counseling Z71.7
    dementia B20 *[F02.80]*
      with behavioral disturbance B20 *[F02.81]*
    exposure to Z20.6
    laboratory evidence R75
    type-2 (HIV 2) as cause of disease classified
      elsewhere B97.35
  papillomavirus (HPV)
    DNA test positive
      high risk
        cervix R87.810
        vagina R87.811
      low risk
        cervix R87.820
        vagina R87.821
    screening for Z11.51
  T-cell lymphotropic virus
    type-1 (HTLV-I) infection B33.3
      as cause of disease classified elsewhere
        B97.33
      carrier Z22.6
    type-2 (HTLV-II) as cause of disease
      classified elsewhere B97.34
Humidifier lung or pneumonitis J67.7
Humiliation (experience) **in childhood** Z62.898
Humpback (acquired) —*see* Kyphosis
Hunchback (acquired) —*see* Kyphosis
Hunger T73.0
  air, psychogenic F45.8
Hungry bone syndrome E83.81
Hunner's ulcer —*see* Cystitis, chronic, interstitial
Hunter's
  glossitis D51.0
  syndrome E76.1
Huntington's disease or chorea G10
  with dementia G10 *[F02.80]*
    with behavioral disturbance G10 *[F02.81]*
Hunt's
  disease or syndrome (herpetic geniculate
    ganglionitis) B02.21
    dyssynergia cerebellaris myoclonica G11.19
  neuralgia B02.21
Hurler (-Scheie) **disease or syndrome** E76.02
Hurst's disease G36.1
Hurthle cell
  adenocarcinoma C73
  adenoma D34
  carcinoma C73
  tumor D34

Hutchinson-Boeck disease or syndrome —*see*
  Sarcoidosis
Hutchinson-Gilford disease or syndrome E34.8
Hutchinson's
  disease, meaning
    angioma serpiginosum L81.7
    pompholyx (cheiropompholyx) L30.1
    prurigo estivalis L56.4
    summer eruption or summer prurigo L56.4
  melanotic freckle —*see* Melanoma, in situ
    malignant melanoma in —*see* Melanoma
  teeth or incisors (congenital syphilis) A50.52
  triad (congenital syphilis) A50.53
Hyalin plaque, sclera, senile H15.89
Hyaline membrane (disease) (lung)
  (pulmonary) (newborn) P22.0
Hyalinosis
  cutis (et mucosae) E78.89
  focal and segmental (glomerular) —*see also*
    N00-N07 with fourth character .1 N05.1
Hyalitis, hyalosis, asteroid —*see also* Deposit,
  crystalline
  syphilitic (late) A52.71
Hydatid
  cyst or tumor —*see* Echinococcus
  mole —*see* Hydatidiform mole
  Morgagni
    female Q50.5
    male (epididymal) Q55.4
      testicular Q55.29
Hydatidiform mole (benign) (complicating
  pregnancy) (delivered) (undelivered) O01.9
  classical O01.0
  complete O01.0
  incomplete O01.1
  invasive D39.2
  malignant D39.2
  partial O01.1
Hydatidosis —*see* Echinococcus
Hydradenitis (axillaris) (suppurative) L73.2
Hydradenoma —*see* Hidradenoma
Hydramnios O40.-●
Hydrancephaly, hydranencephaly Q04.3
  with spina bifida —*see* Spina bifida, with
    hydrocephalus
Hydrargyrism NEC —*see* Poisoning, mercury
Hydrarthrosis —*see also* Effusion, joint
  gonococcal A54.42
  intermittent M12.40
    ankle M12.47-●
    elbow M12.42-●
    foot joint M12.47-●
    hand joint M12.44-●
    hip M12.45-●
    knee M12.46-●
    multiple site M12.49
    shoulder M12.41-●
    specified joint NEC M12.48
    wrist M12.43-●
  of yaws (early) (late) —*see also* subcategory
    M14.8-● A66.6
  syphilitic (late) A52.77
    congenital A50.55 *[M12.80]*
Hydremia D64.89
Hydrencephalocele (congenital) —*see*
  Encephalocele
Hydrencephalomeningocele (congenital) —*see*
  Encephalocele
Hydroa R23.8
  aestivale L56.4
  vacciniforme L56.4
Hydroadenitis (axillaris) (suppurative) L73.2
Hydrocalycosis —*see* Hydronephrosis
Hydrocele (spermatic cord) (testis) (tunica
  vaginalis) N43.3
  canal of Nuck N94.89
  communicating N43.2
    congenital P83.5
  congenital P83.5
  encysted N43.0
  female NEC N94.89
  infected N43.1
  newborn P83.5

Hydrocele *(Continued)*
round ligament N94.89
specified NEC N43.2
spinalis —*see* Spina bifida
vulva N90.89
Hydrocephalus (acquired) (external) (internal)
(malignant) (recurrent) G91.9
aqueduct Sylvius stricture Q03.0
causing disproportion O33.6
with obstructed labor O66.3
communicating G91.0
congenital (external) (internal) Q03.9
with spina bifida Q05.4
cervical Q05.0
dorsal Q05.1
lumbar Q05.2
lumbosacral Q05.2
sacral Q05.3
thoracic Q05.1
thoracolumbar Q05.1
specified NEC Q03.8
due to toxoplasmosis (congenital) P37.1
foramen Magendie block (acquired) G91.1
congenital —*see also* Hydrocephalus,
congenital Q03.1
in (due to)
infectious disease NEC B89 [*G91.4*]
neoplastic disease NEC (*see also* Neoplasm)
G91.4
parasitic disease B89 [*G91.4*]
newborn Q03.9
with spina bifida —*see* Spina bifida, with
hydrocephalus
noncommunicating G91.1
normal pressure G91.2
secondary G91.0
obstructive G91.1
otitic G93.2
post-traumatic NEC G91.3
secondary G91.4
post-traumatic G91.3
specified NEC G91.8
syphilitic, congenital A50.49
Hydrocolpos (congenital) N89.8
Hydrocystoma —*see* Neoplasm, skin, benign
Hydroencephalocele (congenital) —*see*
Encephalocele
Hydroencephalomeningocele (congenital) —
see Encephalocele
Hydrohematopneumothorax —*see* Hemothorax
Hydromeningitis —*see* Meningitis
Hydromeningocele (spinal) —*see also* Spina bifida
cranial —*see* Encephalocele
Hydrometra N85.8
Hydrometrocolpos N89.8
Hydromicrocephaly Q02
Hydromphalos (since birth) Q45.8
Hydromyelia Q06.4
Hydromyelocele —*see* Spina bifida
Hydronephrosis (atrophic) (early)
(functionless) (intermittent) (primary)
(secondary) **NEC** N13.30
with
infection N13.6
obstruction (by) (of)
renal calculus N13.2
with infection N13.6
ureteral NEC N13.1
with infection N13.6
calculus N13.2
with infection N13.6
ureteropelvic junction (congenital) Q62.11
acquired N13.0
with infection N13.6
ureteral stricture NEC N13.1
with infection N13.6
congenital Q62.0
due to acquired occlusion of ureteropelvic
junction N13.0
specified type NEC N13.39
tuberculous A18.11
Hydropericarditis —*see* Pericarditis
Hydropericardium —*see* Pericarditis

Hydroperitoneum R18.8
Hydrophobia —*see* Rabies
Hydrophthalmos Q15.0
Hydropneumohemothorax —*see* Hemothorax
Hydropneumopericarditis —*see* Pericarditis
Hydropneumopericardium —*see* Pericarditis
Hydropneumothorax J94.8
traumatic —*see* Injury, intrathoracic, lung
tuberculous NEC A15.6
Hydrops R60.9
abdominis R18.8
articulorum intermittens —*see* Hydrarthrosis,
intermittent
cardiac —*see* Failure, heart, congestive
causing obstructed labor (mother) O66.3
endolymphatic H81.0-●
fetal —*see* Pregnancy, complicated by,
hydrops, fetalis
Hydrops *(Continued)*
fetalis P83.2
due to
ABO isoimmunization P56.0
alpha thalassemia D56.0
hemolytic disease P56.90
specified NEC P56.99
isoimmunization (ABO) (Rh) P56.0
other specified nonhemolytic disease
NEC P83.2
Rh incompatibility P56.0
during pregnancy —*see* Pregnancy,
complicated by, hydrops, fetalis
gallbladder K82.1
joint —*see* Effusion, joint
labyrinth H81.0
newborn (idiopathic) P83.2
due to
ABO isoimmunization P56.0
alpha thalassemia D56.0
hemolytic disease P56.90
specified NEC P56.99
isoimmunization (ABO) (Rh) P56.0
Rh incompatibility P56.0
nutritional —*see* Malnutrition, severe
pericardium —*see* Pericarditis
pleura —*see* Hydrothorax
spermatic cord —*see* Hydrocele
Hydropyonephrosis N13.6
Hydrorachis Q06.4
Hydrorrhea (nasal) J34.89
pregnancy —*see* Rupture, membranes,
premature
Hydrosadenitis (axillaris) (suppurative) L73.2
Hydrosalpinx (fallopian tube) (follicularis) N70.11
Hydrothorax (double) (pleura) J94.8
chylous (nonfilarial) I89.8
filarial —*see also* Infestation, filarial B74.9
[*J91.8*]
traumatic —*see* Injury, intrathoracic
tuberculous NEC (non primary) A15.6
Hydroureter —*see also* Hydronephrosis N13.4
with infection N13.6
congenital Q62.39
Hydroureteronephrosis —*see* Hydronephrosis
Hydrourethra N36.8
Hydroxykynureninuria E70.89
Hydroxylysinemia E72.3
Hydroxyprolinemia E72.59
Hygiene, sleep
abuse Z72.821
inadequate Z72.821
poor Z72.821
Hygroma (congenital) (cystic) D18.1
praepatellar, prepatellar —*see* Bursitis,
prepatellar
Hymen —*see* condition
Hymenolepis, hymenolepiasis (diminuta)
(infection) (infestation) (nana) B71.0
Hypalgesia R20.8
Hyperacidity (gastric) K31.89
psychogenic F45.8
Hyperactive, hyperactivity F90.9
basal cell, uterine cervix —*see* Dysplasia, cervix
bowel sounds R19.12

Hyperactive, hyperactivity*(Continued)*
cervix epithelial (basal) —*see* Dysplasia, cervix
child F90.9
attention deficit —*see* Disorder, attention-
deficit hyperactivity
detrusor muscle N32.81
gastrointestinal K31.89
psychogenic F45.8
nasal mucous membrane J34.3
stomach K31.89
thyroid (gland) —*see* Hyperthyroidism
Hyperacusis H93.23-●
Hyperadrenalism E27.5
Hyperadrenocorticism E24.9
congenital E25.0
iatrogenic E24.2
correct substance properly administered —
see Table of Drugs and Chemicals, by
drug, adverse effect
overdose or wrong substance given
or taken —*see* Table of Drugs and
Chemicals, by drug, poisoning
not associated with Cushing's syndrome E27.0
pituitary-dependent E24.0
Hyperaldosteronism E26.9
familial (type I) E26.02
glucocorticoid-remediable E26.02
primary (due to (bilateral) adrenal
hyperplasia) E26.09
primary NEC E26.09
secondary E26.1
specified NEC E26.89
Hyperalgesia R20.8
Hyperalimentation R63.2
carotene, carotin E67.1
specified NEC E67.8
vitamin
A E67.0
D E67.3
Hyperaminoaciduria
arginine E72.21
cystine E72.01
lysine E72.3
ornithine E72.4
Hyperammonemia (congenital) E72.20
Hyperazotemia —*see* Uremia
Hyperbetalipoproteinemia (familial) E78.00
with prebetalipoproteinemia E78.2
Hyperbilirubinemia
constitutional E80.6
familial conjugated E80.6
neonatal (transient) —*see* Jaundice, newborn
Hypercalcemia, hypocalciuric, familial E83.52
Hypercalciuria, idiopathic R82.994
Hypercapnia R06.89
newborn P84
Hypercarotenemia (dietary) E67.1
Hypercementosis K03.4
Hyperchloremia E87.8
Hyperchlorhydria K31.89
neurotic F45.8
psychogenic F45.8
Hypercholesterinemia —*see*
Hypercholesterolemia
Hypercholesterolemia (essential) (primary)
(pure) E78.00
with hyperglyceridemia, endogenous E78.2
dietary counseling and surveillance Z71.3
familial E78.01
hereditary E78.01
Hyperchylia gastrica, psychogenic F45.8
Hyperchylomicronemia (familial) (primary) E78.3
with hyperbetalipoproteinemia E78.3
Hypercoagulable (state) D68.59
activated protein C resistance D68.51
antithrombin (III) deficiency D68.59
factor V Leiden mutation D68.51
primary NEC D68.59
protein C deficiency D68.59
protein S deficiency D68.59
prothrombin gene mutation D68.52
secondary D68.69
specified NEC D68.69

Hypercoagulation (state) D68.59
Hypercorticalism, pituitary-dependent E24.0
Hypercorticosolism —*see* Cushing's, syndrome
Hypercorticosteronism E24.2
  correct substance properly administered —*see* Table of Drugs and Chemicals, by drug, adverse effect
  overdose or wrong substance given or taken —*see* Table of Drugs and Chemicals, by drug, poisoning
Hypercortisonism E24.2
  correct substance properly administered —*see* Table of Drugs and Chemicals, by drug, adverse effect
  overdose or wrong substance given or taken —*see* Table of Drugs and Chemicals, by drug, poisoning
Hyperekplexia Q89.8
Hyperelectrolytemia E87.8
Hyperemesis R11.10
  with nausea R11.2
  gravidarum (mild) O21.0
    with
      carbohydrate depletion O21.1
      dehydration O21.1
      electrolyte imbalance O21.1
      metabolic disturbance O21.1
    severe (with metabolic disturbance) O21.1
  projectile R11.12
  psychogenic F45.8
Hyperemia (acute) (passive) R68.89
  anal mucosa K62.89
  bladder N32.89
  cerebral I67.89
  conjunctiva H11.43-•
  ear internal, acute —*see* subcategory H83.0
  enteric K59.89
  eye —*see* Hyperemia, conjunctiva
  eyelid (active) (passive) —*see* Disorder, eyelid, specified type NEC
  intestine K59.89
  iris —*see* Disorder, iris, vascular
  kidney N28.89
  labyrinth —*see* subcategory H83.0
  liver (active) K76.89
  lung (passive) —*see* Edema, lung
  pulmonary (passive) —*see* Edema, lung
  renal N28.89
  retina H35.89
  stomach K31.89
Hyperesthesia (body surface) R20.3
  larynx (reflex) J38.7
    hysterical F44.89
  pharynx (reflex) J39.2
    hysterical F44.89
Hyperestrogenism (drug-induced) (iatrogenic) E28.0
Hyperexplexia Q89.8
Hyperfibrinolysis —*see* Fibrinolysis
Hyperfructosemia E74.19
Hyperfunction
  adrenal cortex, not associated with Cushing's syndrome E27.0
  medulla E27.5
    adrenomedullary E27.5
  virilism E25.9
    congenital E25.0
  ovarian E28.8
  pancreas K86.89
  parathyroid (gland) E21.3
  pituitary (gland) (anterior) E22.9
    specified NEC E22.8
  polyglandular E31.1
  testicular E29.0
Hypergammaglobulinemia D89.2
  polyclonal D89.0
  Waldenström D89.0
Hypergastrinemia E16.4
Hyperglobulinemia R77.1
Hyperglycemia, hyperglycemic (transient) R73.9
  coma —*see* Diabetes, by type, with coma
  postpancreatectomy E89.1

Hyperglyceridemia (endogenous) (essential) (familial) (hereditary) (pure) E78.1
  mixed E78.3
Hyperglycinemia (non-ketotic) E72.51
Hypergonadism
  ovarian E28.8
  testicular (primary) (infantile) E29.0
Hyperheparinemia D68.32
Hyperhidrosis, hyperidrosis R61
  focal
    primary L74.519
      axilla L74.510
      face L74.511
      palms L74.512
      soles L74.513
    secondary L74.52
  generalized R61
  localized
    primary L74.519
      axilla L74.510
      face L74.511
      palms L74.512
      soles L74.513
    secondary L74.52
  psychogenic F45.8
  secondary R61
    focal L74.52
Hyperhistidinemia E70.41
Hyperhomocysteinemia E72.11
Hyperhydroxyprolinemia E72.59
Hyperinsulinism (functional) E16.1
  with
    coma (hypoglycemic) E15
    encephalopathy E16.1 [G94]
  ectopic E16.1
  therapeutic misadventure (from administration of insulin) —*see* subcategory T38.3
Hyperkalemia E87.5
Hyperkeratosis —*see also* Keratosis L85.9
  cervix N88.0
  due to yaws (early) (late) (palmar or plantar) A66.3
  follicularis Q82.8
    penetrans (in cutem) L87.0
  palmoplantaris climacterica L85.1
  pinta A67.1
  senile (with pruritus) L57.0
  universalis congenita Q80.8
  vocal cord J38.3
  vulva N90.4
Hyperkinesia, hyperkinetic (disease) (reaction) (syndrome) (childhood) (adolescence) —*see also* Disorder, attention-deficit hyperactivity
  heart I51.89
Hyperleucine-isoleucinemia E71.19
Hyperlipemia, hyperlipidemia E78.5
  combined E78.2
    familial E78.49
  group
    A E78.00
    B E78.1
    C E78.2
    D E78.3
  mixed E78.2
  specified NEC E78.49
Hyperlipidosis E75.6
  hereditary NEC E75.5
Hyperlipoproteinemia E78.5
  Fredrickson's type
    I E78.3
    IIa E78.00
    IIb E78.2
    III E78.2
    IV E78.1
    V E78.3
  low-density-lipoprotein-type (LDL) E78.00
  very-low-density-lipoprotein-type (VLDL) E78.1
Hyperlucent lung, unilateral J43.0
Hyperlysinemia E72.3
Hypermagnesemia E83.41
  neonatal P71.8

Hypermenorrhea N92.0
Hypermethioninemia E72.19
Hypermetropia (congenital) H52.0-•
Hypermobility, hypermotility
  cecum —*see* Syndrome, irritable bowel
  coccyx —*see* subcategory M53.2
  colon —*see* Syndrome, irritable bowel
    psychogenic F45.8
  ileum K58.9
  intestine —*see also* Syndrome, irritable bowel K58.9
    psychogenic F45.8
  meniscus (knee) —*see* Derangement, knee, meniscus
  scapula —*see* Instability, joint, shoulder
  stomach K31.89
    psychogenic F45.8
  syndrome M35.7
  urethra N36.41
    with intrinsic sphincter deficiency N36.43
Hypernasality R49.21
Hypernatremia E87.0
Hypernephroma C64.-•
Hyperopia —*see* Hypermetropia
Hyperorexia nervosa F50.2
Hyperornithinemia E72.4
Hyperosmia R43.1
Hyperosmolality E87.0
Hyperostosis (monomelic) —*see also* Disorder, bone, density and structure, specified NEC
  ankylosing (spine) M48.10
    cervical region M48.12
    cervicothoracic region M48.13
    lumbar region M48.16
    lumbosacral region M48.17
    multiple sites M48.19
    occipito-atlanto-axial region M48.11
    sacrococcygeal region M48.18
    thoracic region M48.14
    thoracolumbar region M48.15
  cortical (skull) M85.2
    infantile M89.8X-•
  frontal, internal of skull M85.2
  interna frontalis M85.2
  skeletal, diffuse idiopathic —*see* Hyperostosis, ankylosing
  skull M85.2
    congenital Q75.8
  vertebral, ankylosing —*see* Hyperostosis, ankylosing
Hyperovarism E28.8
Hyperoxaluria (primary) R82.992
Hyperparathyroidism E21.3
  primary E21.0
  secondary (renal) N25.81
    non-renal E21.1
  specified NEC E21.2
  tertiary E21.2
Hyperpathia R20.8
Hyperperistalsis R19.2
  psychogenic F45.8
Hyperpermeability, capillary I78.8
Hyperphagia R63.2
Hyperphenylalaninemia NEC E70.1
Hyperphoria (alternating) H50.53
Hyperphosphatemia E83.39
Hyperpiesis, hyperpiesia —*see* Hypertension
Hyperpigmentation —*see also* Pigmentation
  melanin NEC L81.4
  postinflammatory L81.0
Hyperpinealism E34.8
Hyperpituitarism E22.9
Hyperplasia, hyperplastic
  adenoids J35.2
  adrenal (capsule) (cortex) (gland) E27.8
    with
      sexual precocity (male) E25.9
        congenital E25.0
      virilism, adrenal E25.9
        congenital E25.0
      virilization (female) E25.9
        congenital E25.0

▶ New   ⇒ Revised   ~~deleted~~ Deleted   • Use Additional Character(s)

▶ New   ⇒ Revised   ~~deleted~~ Deleted   ● Use Additional Character(s)

Hypertension, hypertensive *(Continued)*
  benign, intracranial G93.2
  borderline R03.0
  cardiorenal (disease) I13.10
    with heart failure I13.0
      with stage 1 through stage 4 chronic
        kidney disease I13.0
      with stage 5 or end stage renal disease
        I13.2
    without heart failure I13.10
      with stage 1 through stage 4 chronic
        kidney disease I13.10
      with stage 5 or end stage renal disease
        I13.11
  cardiovascular
    disease (arteriosclerotic) (sclerotic) —*see*
      Hypertension, heart
    renal (disease) —*see* Hypertension,
      cardiorenal
  chronic venous —*see* Hypertension, venous
    (chronic)
  complicating
    childbirth (labor) O16.4
      pre-existing O10.92
        with
          heart disease O10.12
            with renal disease O10.32
          pre-eclampsia O11.4
          renal disease O10.22
            with heart disease O10.32
        essential O10.02
        secondary O10.42
    pregnancy O16.-●
      with edema —*see also* Pre-eclampsia
        O14.9-●
      gestational (pregnancy induced)
        (without proteinuria) O13.-●
        with proteinuria O14.9-●
          mild pre-eclampsia O14.0-●
          moderate pre-eclampsia O14.0-●
          severe pre-eclampsia O14.1-●
            with hemolysis, elevated liver
              enzymes and low platelet
              count (HELLP) O14.2-●
      pre-existing O10.91-●
        with
          heart disease O10.11-●
            with renal disease O10.31-●
          pre-eclampsia —*see* category O11
          renal disease O10.21-●
            with heart disease O10.31-●
          essential O10.01-●
          secondary O10.41-●
      transient O13.-●
    puerperium pre-existing O16.5
      pre-existing
        with
          heart disease O10.13
            with renal disease O10.33
          pre-eclampsia O11.5
          renal disease O10.23
            with heart disease O10.33
          essential O10.03
      pregnancy-induced O13.9
      secondary O10.43
  crisis I16.9
  due to
    endocrine disorders I15.2
    pheochromocytoma I15.2
    renal disorders NEC I15.1
      arterial I15.0
    renovascular disorders I15.0
    specified disease NEC I15.8
  emergency I16.1
  encephalopathy I67.4
  gestational (without significant proteinuria)
    (pregnancy-induced) (transient) O13.-●
    with significant proteinuria —*see*
      Pre-eclampsia
    complicating
      delivery O13.4
      puerperium O13.5

Hypertension, hypertensive *(Continued)*
  Goldblatt's I70.1
  heart (disease) (conditions in I51.4-I51.9 due
    to hypertension) I11.9
    with
      heart failure (congestive) I11.0
      kidney disease (chronic) —*see*
        Hypertension, cardiorenal
  intracranial, benign G93.2
  kidney I12.9
    with
      heart disease —*see* Hypertension,
        cardiorenal
      stage 1 through stage 4 chronic kidney
        disease I12.9
      stage 5 chronic kidney disease (CKD) or
        end stage renal disease (ESRD) I12.0
  lesser circulation I27.0
  maternal O16.-●
  newborn P29.2
    pulmonary (persistent) P29.30
  ocular H40.05-●
  pancreatic duct — code to underlying
    condition
    with chronic pancreatitis K86.1
  portal (due to chronic liver disease)
    (idiopathic) K76.6
    gastropathy K31.89
    in (due to) schistosomiasis (bilharziasis)
      B65.9 *[K77]*
  postoperative I97.3
  psychogenic F45.8
  pulmonary NEC I27.20
    with
      cor pulmonale (chronic) I27.29
        acute I26.09
      right heart ventricular strain/failure
        I27.29
        acute I26.09
      right to left shunt related to congenital
        heart disease I27.83
      unclear multifactorial mechanisms
        I27.29
    arterial (associated) (drug-induced) (toxin-
      induced) I27.21
    chronic thromboembolic I27.24
    due to
      hematologic disorders I27.29
▶   kyphoscoliotic heart disease I27.1
      left heart disease I27.22
      lung diseases and hypoxia I27.23
      metabolic disorders I27.29
      specified systemic disorders NEC I27.29
    group 1 (associated) (drug-induced) (toxin-
      induced) I27.21
    group 2 I27.22
    group 3 I27.23
    group 4 I27.24
    group 5 I27.29
    of newborn (persistent) P29.30
      secondary
        arterial I27.21
        specified NEC I27.29
    primary (idiopathic) I27.0
  renal —*see* Hypertension, kidney
  renovascular I15.0
  secondary NEC I15.9
    due to
      endocrine disorders I15.2
      pheochromocytoma I15.2
      renal disorders NEC I15.1
        arterial I15.0
      renovascular disorders I15.0
    specified NEC I15.8
  transient R03.0
    of pregnancy O13.●
  urgency I16.0
  venous (chronic)
    due to
      deep vein thrombosis —*see* Syndrome,
        postthrombotic

Hypertension, hypertensive *(Continued)*
  venous *(Continued)*
    idiopathic I87.309
      with
        inflammation I87.32-●
          with ulcer I87.33-●
        specified complication NEC I87.39-●
        ulcer I87.31-●
          with inflammation I87.33-●
      asymptomatic I87.30-●
Hypertensive urgency —*see* Hypertension
Hyperthecosis ovary E28.8
Hyperthermia (of unknown origin) —*see also*
  Hyperpyrexia
  malignant, due to anesthesia T88.3
  newborn P81.9
    environmental P81.0
Hyperthyroid (recurrent) —*see* Hyperthyroidism
Hyperthyroidism (latent) (pre-adult) (recurrent)
  E05.90
  with
    goiter (diffuse) E05.00
      with thyroid storm E05.01
      nodular (multinodular) E05.20
        with thyroid storm E05.21
        uninodular E05.10
          with thyroid storm E05.11
    storm E05.91
  due to ectopic thyroid tissue E05.30
    with thyroid storm E05.31
  neonatal, transitory P72.1
  specified NEC E05.80
    with thyroid storm E05.81
Hypertony, hypertonia, hypertonicity
  bladder N31.8
  congenital P94.1
  stomach K31.89
    psychogenic F45.8
  uterus, uterine (contractions) (complicating
    delivery) O62.4
Hypertrichosis L68.9
  congenital Q84.2
  eyelid H02.869
    left H02.866
      lower H02.865
      upper H02.864
    right H02.863
      lower H02.862
      upper H02.861
  lanuginosa Q84.2
    acquired L68.1
  localized L68.2
  specified NEC L68.8
Hypertriglyceridemia, essential E78.1
Hypertrophy, hypertrophic
  adenofibromatous, prostate —*see*
    Enlargement, enlarged, prostate
  adenoids (infective) J35.2
    with tonsils J35.3
  adrenal cortex E27.8
  alveolar process or ridge —*see* Anomaly,
    alveolar
  anal papillae K62.89
  artery I77.89
    congenital NEC Q27.8
      digestive system Q27.8
      lower limb Q27.8
      specified site NEC Q27.8
      upper limb Q27.8
  auricular —*see* Hypertrophy, cardiac
  Bartholin's gland N75.8
  bile duct (common) (hepatic) K83.8
  bladder (sphincter) (trigone) N32.89
  bone M89.30
    carpus M89.34-●
    clavicle M89.31-●
    femur M89.35-●
    fibula M89.36-●
    finger M89.34-●
    humerus M89.32-●
    ilium M89.359

Hypertrophy, hypertrophic (Continued)
  bone (Continued)
    ischium M89.359
    metacarpus M89.34-●
    metatarsus M89.37-●
    multiple sites M89.39
    neck M89.38
    radius M89.33-●
    rib M89.38
    scapula M89.31-●
    skull M89.38
    tarsus M89.37-●
    tibia M89.36-●
    toe M89.37-●
    ulna M89.33-●
    vertebra M89.38
  brain G93.89
  breast N62
    cystic —see Mastopathy, cystic
    newborn P83.4
    pubertal, massive N62
    puerperal, postpartum —see Disorder,
      breast, specified type NEC
    senile (parenchymatous) N62
  cardiac (chronic) (idiopathic) I51.7
    with rheumatic fever (conditions in I00)
      active I01.8
      inactive or quiescent (with chorea) I09.89
    congenital NEC Q24.8
    fatty —see Degeneration, myocardial
    hypertensive —see Hypertension, heart
    rheumatic (with chorea) I09.89
      active or acute I01.8
        with chorea I02.0
    valve —see Endocarditis
  cartilage —see Disorder, cartilage, specified
    type NEC
  cecum —see Megacolon
  cervix (uteri) N88.8
    congenital Q51.828
    elongation N88.4
  clitoris (cirrhotic) N90.89
    congenital Q52.6
  colon —see also Megacolon
    congenital Q43.2
  conjunctiva, lymphoid H11.89
  corpora cavernosa N48.89
  cystic duct K82.8
  duodenum K31.89
  endometrium (glandular) —see also
    Hyperplasia, endometrial N85.00-●
    cervix N88.8
  epididymis N50.89
  esophageal hiatus (congenital) Q79.1
    with hernia —see Hernia, hiatal
  eyelid —see Disorder, eyelid, specified type
    NEC
▶ facet joint (see also Spondylosis) M47.819
  fat pad E65
    knee (infrapatellar) (popliteal) (prepatellar)
      (retropatellar) M79.4
  foot (congenital) Q74.2
  frenulum, frenum (tongue) K14.8
    lip K13.0
  gallbladder K82.8
  gastric mucosa K29.60
    with bleeding K29.61
  gland, glandular R59.9
    generalized R59.1
    localized R59.0
  gum (mucous membrane) K06.1
  heart (idiopathic) —see also Hypertrophy,
    cardiac
    valve —see also Endocarditis I38
  hemifacial Q67.4
  hepatic —see Hypertrophy, liver
  hiatus (esophageal) Q79.1
  hilus gland R59.0
  hymen, congenital Q52.4
  ileum K63.89
  intestine NEC K63.89
  jejunum K63.89

Hypertrophy, hypertrophic (Continued)
  kidney (compensatory) N28.81
    congenital Q63.3
  labium (majus) (minus) N90.60
  ligament —see Disorder, ligament
  lingual tonsil (infective) J35.1
    with adenoids J35.3
  lip K13.0
    congenital Q18.6
  liver R16.0
    acute K76.89
    cirrhotic —see Cirrhosis, liver
    congenital Q44.7
    fatty —see Fatty, liver
  lymph, lymphatic gland R59.9
    generalized R59.1
    localized R59.0
    tuberculous —see Tuberculosis, lymph
      gland
  mammary gland —see Hypertrophy, breast
  Meckel's diverticulum (congenital) Q43.0
    malignant —see Table of Neoplasms, small
      intestine, malignant
  median bar —see Hyperplasia, prostate
  meibomian gland —see Chalazion
  meniscus, knee, congenital Q74.1
  metatarsal head —see Hypertrophy, bone,
    metatarsus
  metatarsus —see Hypertrophy, bone,
    metatarsus
  mucous membrane
    alveolar ridge K06.2
    gum K06.1
    nose (turbinate) J34.3
  muscle M62.89
  muscular coat, artery I77.89
  myocardium —see also Hypertrophy, cardiac
    idiopathic I42.2
  myometrium N85.2
  nail L60.2
    congenital Q84.5
  nasal J34.89
    alae J34.89
    bone J34.89
    cartilage J34.89
    mucous membrane (septum) J34.3
    sinus J34.89
    turbinate J34.3
  nasopharynx, lymphoid (infectional) (tissue)
    (wall) J35.2
  nipple N62
  organ or site, congenital NEC —see Anomaly,
    by site - ovary N83.8
  palate (hard) M27.8
    soft K13.79
  pancreas, congenital Q45.3
  parathyroid (gland) E21.0
  parotid gland K11.1
  penis N48.89
  pharyngeal tonsil J35.2
  pharynx J39.2
    lymphoid (infectional) (tissue) (wall)
      J35.2
  pituitary (anterior) (fossa) (gland) E23.6
  prepuce (congenital) N47.8
    female N90.89
  prostate —see Enlargement, enlarged,
    prostate
    congenital Q55.4
  pseudomuscular G71.09
  pylorus (adult) (muscle) (sphincter) K31.1
    congenital or infantile Q40.0
  rectal, rectum (sphincter) K62.89
  rhinitis (turbinate) J31.0
  salivary gland (any) K11.1
    congenital Q38.4
  scaphoid (tarsal) —see Hypertrophy, bone,
    tarsus
  scar L91.0
  scrotum N50.89
  seminal vesicle N50.89

Hypertrophy, hypertrophic (Continued)
  sigmoid —see Megacolon
  skin L91.9
    specified NEC L91.8
  spermatic cord N50.89
  spleen —see Splenomegaly
  spondylitis —see Spondylosis
  stomach K31.89
  sublingual gland K11.1
  submandibular gland K11.1
  suprarenal cortex (gland) E27.8
  synovial NEC M67.20
    acromioclavicular M67.21-●
    ankle M67.27-●
    elbow M67.22-●
    foot M67.27-●
    hand M67.24-●
    hip M67.25-●
    knee M67.26-●
    multiple sites M67.29
    specified site NEC M67.28
    wrist M67.23-●
  tendon —see Disorder, tendon, specified type
    NEC
  testis N44.8
    congenital Q55.29
  thymic, thymus (gland) (congenital)
    E32.0
  thyroid (gland) —see Goiter
  toe (congenital) Q74.2
    acquired —see also Deformity, toe, specified
      NEC
  tongue K14.8
    congenital Q38.2
    papillae (foliate) K14.3
  tonsils (faucial) (infective) (lingual)
    (lymphoid) J35.1
    with adenoids J35.3
  tunica vaginalis N50.89
  ureter N28.89
  urethra N36.8
  uterus N85.2
    neck (with elongation) N88.4
    puerperal O90.89
  uvula K13.79
  vagina N89.8
  vas deferens N50.89
  vein I87.8
  ventricle, ventricular (heart) —see also
    Hypertrophy, cardiac
    congenital Q24.8
    in tetralogy of Fallot Q21.3
  verumontanum N36.8
  vocal cord J38.3
  vulva N90.60
    stasis (nonfilarial) N90.69
Hypertropia H50.2-●
Hypertyrosinemia E70.21
Hyperuricemia (asymptomatic) E79.0
Hyperuricosuria R82.993
Hypervalinemia E71.19
Hyperventilation (tetany) R06.4
  hysterical F45.8
  psychogenic F45.8
  syndrome F45.8
Hypervitaminosis (dietary) NEC E67.8
  A E67.0
    administered as drug (prolonged intake) —
      see Table of Drugs and Chemicals,
      vitamins, adverse effect
    overdose or wrong substance given
      or taken —see Table of Drugs and
      Chemicals, vitamins, poisoning
  B6 E67.2
  D E67.3
    administered as drug (prolonged intake) —
      see Table of Drugs and Chemicals,
      vitamins, adverse effect
    overdose or wrong substance given
      or taken —see Table of Drugs and
      Chemicals, vitamins, poisoning

Hypervitaminosis NEC *(Continued)*
  K E67.8
    administered as drug (prolonged intake) —
      see Table of Drugs and Chemicals,
      vitamins, adverse effect
    overdose or wrong substance given
      or taken —*see* Table of Drugs and
      Chemicals, vitamins, poisoning
Hypervolemia E87.70
  specified NEC E87.79
Hypesthesia R20.1
  cornea —*see* Anesthesia, cornea
Hyphema H21.0-●
  traumatic S05.1-●
Hypoacidity, gastric K31.89
  psychogenic F45.8
Hypoadrenalism, hypoadrenia E27.40
  primary E27.1
  tuberculous A18.7
Hypoadrenocorticism E27.40
  pituitary E23.0
  primary E27.1
Hypoalbuminemia E88.09
Hypoaldosteronism E27.40
Hypoalphalipoproteinemia E78.6
Hypobarism T70.29
Hypobaropathy T70.29
Hypobetalipoproteinemia (familial) E78.6
Hypocalcemia E83.51
  dietary E58
  neonatal P71.1
    due to cow's milk P71.0
  phosphate-loading (newborn) P71.1
Hypochloremia E87.8
Hypochlorhydria K31.89
  neurotic F45.8
  psychogenic F45.8
Hypochondria, hypochondriac,
    hypochondriasis (reaction) F45.21
  sleep F51.03
Hypochondrogenesis Q77.0
Hypochondroplasia Q77.4
Hypochromasia, blood cells D50.8
Hypodontia —*see* Anodontia
Hypocitraturia R82.991
Hypoeosinophilia D72.89
Hypoesthesia R20.1
Hypofibrinogenemia D68.8
  acquired D65
  congenital (hereditary) D68.2
Hypofunction
  adrenocortical E27.40
    drug-induced E27.3
    postprocedural E89.6
    primary E27.1
  adrenomedullary, postprocedural E89.6
  cerebral R29.818
  corticoadrenal NEC E27.40
  intestinal K59.89
  labyrinth —*see* subcategory H83.2
  ovary E28.39
  pituitary (gland) (anterior) E23.0
  testicular E29.1
    postprocedural (postsurgical)
      (postirradiation) (iatrogenic) E89.5
Hypogalactia O92.4
Hypogammaglobulinemia —*see also*
    Agammaglobulinemia D80.1
  hereditary D80.0
  nonfamilial D80.1
  transient, of infancy D80.7
Hypogenitalism (congenital) —*see*
    Hypogonadism
Hypoglossia Q38.3
Hypoglycemia (spontaneous) E16.2
  coma E15
    diabetic —*see* Diabetes, by type, with
      hypoglycemia, with coma
  diabetic —*see* Diabetes, hypoglycemia
  dietary counseling and surveillance
    Z71.3

Hypoglycemia *(Continued)*
  drug-induced E16.0
    with coma (nondiabetic) E15
  due to insulin E16.0
    with coma (nondiabetic) E15
    therapeutic misadventure —*see*
      subcategory T38.3
  functional, nonhyperinsulinemic E16.1
  iatrogenic E16.0
    with coma (nondiabetic) E15
  in infant of diabetic mother P70.1
    gestational diabetes P70.0
  infantile E16.1
  leucine-induced E71.19
  neonatal (transitory) P70.4
    iatrogenic P70.3
  reactive (not drug-induced) E16.1
  transitory neonatal P70.4
Hypogonadism
  female E28.39
  hypogonadotropic E23.0
  male E29.1
  ovarian (primary) E28.39
  pituitary E23.0
  testicular (primary) E29.1
Hypohidrosis, hypoidrosis L74.4
Hypoinsulinemia, postprocedural E89.1
Hypokalemia E87.6
Hypoleukocytosis —*see* Agranulocytosis
Hypolipoproteinemia (alpha) (beta) E78.6
Hypomagnesemia E83.42
  neonatal P71.2
Hypomania, hypomanic reaction F30.8
Hypomenorrhea —*see* Oligomenorrhea
Hypometabolism R63.8
Hypomotility
  gastrointestinal (tract) K31.89
    psychogenic F45.8
  intestine K59.89
    psychogenic F45.8
  stomach K31.89
    psychogenic F45.8
Hyponasality R49.22
Hyponatremia E87.1
Hypo-osmolality E87.1
Hypo-ovarianism, hypo-ovarism
    E28.39
Hypoparathyroidism E20.9
  familial E20.8
  idiopathic E20.0
  neonatal, transitory P71.4
  postprocedural E89.2
  specified NEC E20.8
Hypoperfusion (in)
  newborn P96.89
Hypopharyngitis —*see* Laryngopharyngitis
Hypophoria H50.53
Hypophosphatemia, hypophosphatasia
    (acquired) (congenital) (renal) E83.39
  familial E83.31
Hypophyseal, hypophysis —*see also*
    condition
  dwarfism E23.0
  gigantism E22.0
Hypopiesis —*see* Hypotension
Hypopinealism E34.8
Hypopituitarism (juvenile) E23.0
  drug-induced E23.1
  due to
    hypophysectomy E89.3
    radiotherapy E89.3
  iatrogenic NEC E23.1
  postirradiation E89.3
  postpartum O99.285
  postprocedural E89.3
Hypoplasia, hypoplastic
  adrenal (gland), congenital Q89.1
  alimentary tract, congenital Q45.8
    upper Q40.8
  anus, anal (canal) Q42.3
    with fistula Q42.2

Hypoplasia, hypoplastic *(Continued)*
  aorta, aortic Q25.42
    ascending, in hypoplastic left heart
      syndrome Q23.4
    valve Q23.1
      in hypoplastic left heart syndrome
        Q23.4
  areola, congenital Q83.8
  arm (congenital) —*see* Defect, reduction,
    upper limb
  artery (peripheral) Q27.8
    brain (congenital) Q28.3
    coronary Q24.5
    digestive system Q27.8
    lower limb Q27.8
    pulmonary Q25.79
      functional, unilateral J43.0
    retinal (congenital) Q14.1
    specified site NEC Q27.8
    umbilical Q27.0
    upper limb Q27.8
  auditory canal Q17.8
    causing impairment of hearing Q16.9
  biliary duct or passage Q44.5
  bone NOS Q79.9
    face Q75.8
    marrow D61.9
      megakaryocytic D69.49
    skull —*see* Hypoplasia, skull
  brain Q02
    gyri Q04.3
    part of Q04.3
  breast (areola) N64.82
  bronchus Q32.4
  cardiac Q24.8
  carpus —*see* Defect, reduction, upper limb,
    specified type NEC
  cartilage hair Q78.8
  cecum Q42.8
  cementum K00.4
  cephalic Q02
  cerebellum Q04.3
  cervix (uteri), congenital Q51.821
  clavicle (congenital) Q74.0
  coccyx Q76.49
  colon Q42.9
    specified NEC Q42.8
  corpus callosum Q04.0
  cricoid cartilage Q31.2
  digestive organ(s) or tract NEC Q45.8
    upper (congenital) Q40.8
  ear (auricle) (lobe) Q17.2
    middle Q16.4
  enamel of teeth (neonatal) (postnatal)
    (prenatal) K00.4
  endocrine (gland) NEC Q89.2
  endometrium N85.8
  epididymis (congenital) Q55.4
  epiglottis Q31.2
  erythroid, congenital D61.01
  esophagus (congenital) Q39.8
  eustachian tube Q17.8
  eye Q11.2
  eyelid (congenital) Q10.3
  face Q18.8
    bone(s) Q75.8
  femur (congenital) —*see* Defect, reduction,
    lower limb, specified type NEC
  fibula (congenital) —*see* Defect, reduction,
    lower limb, specified type NEC
  finger (congenital) —*see* Defect, reduction,
    upper limb, specified type NEC
  focal dermal Q82.8
  foot —*see* Defect, reduction, lower limb,
    specified type NEC
  gallbladder Q44.0
  genitalia, genital organ(s)
    female, congenital Q52.8
      external Q52.79
      internal NEC Q52.8
    in adiposogenital dystrophy E23.6

▶ New   ⇒ Revised   ~~deleted~~ Deleted   ● Use Additional Character(s)

Hypotropia H50.2-●
Hypoventilation R06.89
  congenital central alveolar G47.35
  sleep related
    idiopathic nonobstructive alveolar
      G47.34
    in conditions classified elsewhere G47.36
Hypovitaminosis —*see* Deficiency, vitamin
Hypovolemia E86.1
  surgical shock T81.19
  traumatic (shock) T79.4

Hypoxemia R09.02
  newborn P84
  sleep related, in conditions classified
    elsewhere G47.36
Hypoxia —*see also* Anoxia R09.02
  cerebral, during a procedure NEC G97.81
    postprocedural NEC G97.82
  intrauterine P84
  myocardial —*see* Insufficiency, coronary
  newborn P84
  sleep-related G47.34

Hypsarhythmia —*see* Epilepsy, generalized,
  specified NEC
Hysteralgia, pregnant uterus O26.89-●
Hysteria, hysterical (conversion) (dissociative
  state) F44.9
  anxiety F41.8
  convulsions F44.5
  psychosis, acute F44.9
Hysteroepilepsy F44.5

I

IBDU (colonic inflammatory bowel disease unclassified) K52.3
▶ICANS (immune effector cell-associated neurotoxicity syndrome) —see Syndrome, immune effector cell-associated neurotoxicity
Ichthyoparasitism due to Vandellia cirrhosa B88.8
Ichthyosis (congenital) Q80.9
    acquired L85.0
    fetalis Q80.4
    hystrix Q80.8
    lamellar Q80.2
    lingual K13.29
    palmaris and plantaris Q82.8
    simplex Q80.0
    vera Q80.8
    vulgaris Q80.0
    X-linked Q80.1
Ichthyotoxism —see Poisoning, fish
    bacterial —see Intoxication, foodborne
Icteroanemia, hemolytic (acquired) D59.9
    congenital —see Spherocytosis
Icterus —see also Jaundice
    conjunctiva R17
    gravis, newborn P55.0
    hematogenous (acquired) D59.9
    hemolytic (acquired) D59.9
        congenital —see Spherocytosis
    hemorrhagic (acute) (leptospiral) (spirochetal) A27.0
        newborn P53
    infectious B15.9
        with hepatic coma B15.0
        leptospiral A27.0
        spirochetal A27.0
    neonatorum —see Jaundice, newborn
    newborn P59.9
    spirochetal A27.0
Ictus solaris, solis T67.01
Ideation
    homicidal R45.850
    suicidal R45.851
Identity disorder (child) F64.9
    gender role F64.2
    psychosexual F64.2
Idioglossia F80.0
Idiopathic —see condition
Idiot, idiocy (congenital) F73
    amaurotic (Bielschowsky(-Jansky)) (family) (infantile (late)) (juvenile (late)) (Vogt-Spielmeyer) E75.4
    microcephalic Q02
Id reaction (due to bacteria) L30.2
IgE asthma J45.909
IIAC (idiopathic infantile arterial calcification) Q28.8
Ileitis (chronic) (noninfectious) —see also Enteritis K52.9
    backwash —see Pancolitis, ulcerative (chronic)
    infectious A09
    regional (ulcerative) —see Enteritis, regional, small intestine
    segmental —see Enteritis, regional
    terminal (ulcerative) —see Enteritis, regional, small intestine
Ileocolitis —see also Enteritis K52.9
    infectious A09
    regional —see Enteritis, regional
    ulcerative K51.0-●
Ileostomy
    attention to Z43.2
    malfunctioning K94.13
    status Z93.2
        with complication —see Complications, enterostomy
Ileotyphus —see Typhoid
Ileum —see condition
Ileus (bowel) (colon) (inhibitory) (intestine) K56.7
    adynamic K56.0

Ileus (Continued)
    due to gallstone (in intestine) K56.3
    duodenal (chronic) K31.5
    gallstone K56.3
    mechanical NEC —see also Obstruction, intestine, specified K56.699
    meconium P76.0
        in cystic fibrosis E84.11
        meaning meconium plug (without cystic fibrosis) P76.0
    myxedema K59.89
    neurogenic K56.0
        Hirschsprung's disease or megacolon Q43.1
    newborn
        due to meconium P76.0
            in cystic fibrosis E84.11
            meaning meconium plug (without cystic fibrosis) P76.0
        transitory P76.1
    obstructive —see also Obstruction, intestine, specified K56.699
    paralytic K56.0
    postoperative K91.89
Iliac —see condition
Iliotibial band syndrome M76.3-●
Illiteracy Z55.0
Illness —see also Disease R69
    manic-depressive —see Disorder, bipolar
Imbalance R26.89
    autonomic G90.8
    constituents of food intake E63.1
    electrolyte E87.8
        with
            abortion —see Abortion by type, complicated by, electrolyte imbalance
            molar pregnancy O08.5
        due to hyperemesis gravidarum O21.1
        following ectopic or molar pregnancy O08.5
        neonatal, transitory NEC P74.49
            potassium
                hyperkalemia P74.31
                hypokalemia P74.32
            sodium
                hypernatremia P74.21
                hyponatremia P74.22
    endocrine E34.9
    eye muscle NOS H50.9
    hormone E34.9
    hysterical F44.4
    labyrinth —see subcategory H83.2
    posture R29.3
    protein-energy —see Malnutrition
    sympathetic G90.8
Imbecile, imbecility (I.Q. 35-49) F71
Imbedding, intrauterine device T83.39
Imbibition, cholesterol (gallbladder) K82.4
Imbrication, teeth, fully erupted M26.30
Imerslund (-Gräsbeck) syndrome D51.1
Immature —see also Immaturity
    birth (less than 37 completed weeks) —see Preterm, newborn
    extremely (less than 28 completed weeks) —see Immaturity, extreme
    personality F60.89
Immaturity (less than 37 completed weeks) —see also Preterm, newborn
    extreme of newborn (less than 28 completed weeks of gestation) (less than 196 completed days of gestation) (unspecified weeks of gestation) P07.20
        gestational age
            23 completed weeks (23 weeks, 0 days through 23 weeks, 6 days) P07.22
            24 completed weeks (24 weeks, 0 days through 24 weeks, 6 days) P07.23
            25 completed weeks (25 weeks, 0 days through 25 weeks, 6 days) P07.24
            26 completed weeks (26 weeks, 0 days through 26 weeks, 6 days) P07.25
            27 completed weeks (27 weeks, 0 days through 27 weeks, 6 days) P07.26
            less than 23 completed weeks P07.21

Immaturity (Continued)
    fetus or infant light-for-dates —see Light-for-dates
    lung, newborn P28.0
    organ or site NEC —see Hypoplasia
    pulmonary, newborn P28.0
    reaction F60.89
    sexual (female) (male), after puberty E30.0
Immersion T75.1
    foot T69.02-●
    hand T69.01-●
Immobile, immobility
    complete, due to severe physical disability or frailty R53.2
    intestine K59.89
    syndrome (paraplegic) M62.3
Immune reconstitution (inflammatory) syndrome [IRIS] D89.3
Immunization —see also Vaccination
    ABO —see Incompatibility, ABO
        in newborn P55.1
    appropriate for age
        child (over 28 days old) Z00.129
            with abnormal findings Z00.121
    complication —see Complications, vaccination
    encounter for Z23
    not done (not carried out) Z28.9
        because (of)
            acute illness of patient Z28.01
            allergy to vaccine (or component) Z28.04
            caregiver refusal Z28.82
            chronic illness of patient Z28.02
            contraindication NEC Z28.09
            delay in delivery of vaccine Z28.83
            group pressure Z28.1
            guardian refusal Z28.82
            immune compromised state of patient Z28.03
            lack of availability of vaccine Z28.83
            manufacturer delay of vaccine Z28.83
            parent refusal Z28.82
            patient's belief Z28.1
            patient had disease being vaccinated against Z28.81
            patient refusal Z28.21
            religious beliefs of patient Z28.1
            specified reason NEC Z28.89
                of patient Z28.29
            unavailability of vaccine Z28.83
            unspecified patient reason Z28.20
    Rh factor
        affecting management of pregnancy NEC O36.09-●
            anti-D antibody O36.01-●
        from transfusion —see Complication(s), transfusion, incompatibility reaction, Rh (factor)
Immunocompromised NOS D84.9
Immunocytoma C83.0-●
Immunodeficiency D84.9
    with
        adenosine-deaminase deficiency (see also Deficiency, adenosine deaminase) D81.30
        antibody defects D80.9
            specified type NEC D80.8
        hyperimmunoglobulinemia D80.6
        increased immunoglobulin M (IgM) D80.5
        major defect D82.9
            specified type NEC D82.8
        partial albinism D82.8
        short-limbed stature D82.2
        thrombocytopenia and eczema D82.0
    antibody with
        hyperimmunoglobulinemia D80.6
        near-normal immunoglobulins D80.6
    autosomal recessive, Swiss type D80.0

Immunodeficiency (Continued)
  combined D81.9
    biotin-dependent carboxylase D81.819
      biotinidase D81.810
      holocarboxylase synthetase D81.818
      specified type NEC D81.818
    severe (SCID) D81.9
      with
        low or normal B-cell numbers D81.2
        low T- and B-cell numbers D81.1
        reticular dysgenesis D81.0
    specified type NEC D81.89
  common variable D83.9
    with
      abnormalities of B-cell numbers and
        function D83.0
      autoantibodies to B- or T-cells D83.2
      immunoregulatory T-cell disorders
        D83.1
    specified type NEC D83.8
  due to
    conditions classified elsewhere D84.81
    drugs D84.821
    external causes D84.822
    medication (current or past) D84.821
  following hereditary defective response to
    Epstein-Barr virus (EBV) D82.3
  selective, immunoglobulin
    A (IgA) D80.2
    G (IgG) (subclasses) D80.3
    M (IgM) D80.4
  severe combined (SCID) D81.9
    due to adenosine deaminase deficiency
      D81.31
  specified type NEC D84.89
  X-linked, with increased IgM D80.5
Immunodeficient NOS D84.9
Immunosuppressed NOS D84.9
Immunotherapy (encounter for)
  antineoplastic Z51.12
Impaction, impacted
  bowel, colon, rectum —see also Impaction,
    fecal K56.49
    by gallstone K56.3
  calculus —see Calculus
  cerumen (ear) (external) H61.2-●
  cuspid —see Impaction, tooth
  dental (same or adjacent tooth) K01.1
  fecal, feces K56.41
  fracture —see Fracture, by site
  gallbladder —see Calculus, gallbladder
  gallstone(s) —see Calculus, gallbladder
    bile duct (common) (hepatic) —see
      Calculus, bile duct
    cystic duct —see Calculus, gallbladder
    in intestine, with obstruction (any part)
      K56.3
  intestine (calculous) NEC —see also
    Impaction, fecal K56.49
    gallstone, with ileus K56.3
  intrauterine device (IUD) T83.39
  molar —see Impaction, tooth
  shoulder, causing obstructed labor O66.0
  tooth, teeth K01.1
  turbinate J34.89
Impaired, impairment (function)
  auditory discrimination —see Abnormal,
    auditory perception
  cognitive, mild, so stated G31.84
  dual sensory Z73.82
  fasting glucose R73.01
  glucose tolerance (oral) R73.02
  hearing —see Deafness
  heart —see Disease, heart
  kidney N28.9
    disorder resulting from N25.9
      specified NEC N25.89
  liver K72.90
    with coma K72.91
  mastication K08.89
  mild cognitive, so stated G31.84

Impaired, impairment (Continued)
  mobility
    ear ossicles —see Ankylosis, ear ossicles
    requiring care provider Z74.09
  myocardium, myocardial —see Insufficiency,
    myocardial
  rectal sphincter R19.8
  renal (acute) (chronic) N28.9
    disorder resulting from N25.9
      specified NEC N25.89
  vision NEC H54.7
    both eyes H54.3
Impediment, speech (see also Disorder, speech)
    R47.9
  psychogenic (childhood) F98.8
  slurring R47.81
  specified NEC R47.89
Impending
  coronary syndrome I20.0
  delirium tremens F10.239
  myocardial infarction I20.0
Imperception auditory (acquired) —see also
    Deafness
  congenital H93.25
Imperfect
  aeration, lung (newborn) NEC —see
    Atelectasis
  closure (congenital)
    alimentary tract NEC Q45.8
      lower Q43.8
      upper Q40.8
    atrioventricular ostium Q21.2
    atrium (secundum) Q21.1
    branchial cleft NOS Q18.2
      cyst Q18.0
      fistula Q18.0
      sinus Q18.0
    choroid Q14.3
    cricoid cartilage Q31.8
    cusps, heart valve NEC Q24.8
      pulmonary Q22.3
    ductus
      arteriosus Q25.0
      Botalli Q25.0
    ear drum (causing impairment of hearing)
      Q16.4
    esophagus with communication to
      bronchus or trachea Q39.1
    eyelid Q10.3
    foramen
      botalli Q21.1
      ovale Q21.1
    genitalia, genital organ(s) or system
      female Q52.8
        external Q52.79
        internal NEC Q52.8
      male Q55.8
    glottis Q31.8
    interatrial ostium or septum Q21.1
    interauricular ostium or septum Q21.1
    interventricular ostium or septum Q21.0
    larynx Q31.8
    lip —see Cleft, lip
    nasal septum Q30.3
    nose Q30.2
    omphalomesenteric duct Q43.0
    optic nerve entry Q14.2
    organ or site not listed —see Anomaly,
      by site
    ostium
      interatrial Q21.1
      interauricular Q21.1
      interventricular Q21.0
    palate —see Cleft, palate
    preauricular sinus Q18.1
    retina Q14.1
    roof of orbit Q75.8
    sclera Q13.5
    septum
      aorticopulmonary Q21.4
      atrial (secundum) Q21.1

Imperfect (Continued)
  closure (Continued)
    septum (Continued)
      between aorta and pulmonary artery
        Q21.4
      heart Q21.9
      interatrial (secundum) Q21.1
      interauricular (secundum) Q21.1
      interventricular Q21.0
        in tetralogy of Fallot Q21.3
      nasal Q30.3
      ventricular Q21.0
        with pulmonary stenosis or atresia,
          dextraposition of aorta, and
          hypertrophy of right ventricle
          Q21.3
        in tetralogy of Fallot Q21.3
    skull Q75.0
      with
        anencephaly Q00.0
        encephalocele —see Encephalocele
        hydrocephalus Q03.9
          with spina bifida —see Spina bifida,
            by site, with hydrocephalus
        microcephaly Q02
    spine (with meningocele) —see Spina
      bifida
    trachea Q32.1
    tympanic membrane (causing impairment
      of hearing) Q16.4
    uterus Q51.818
    vitelline duct Q43.0
  erection —see Dysfunction, sexual, male,
    erectile
  fusion —see Imperfect, closure
  inflation, lung (newborn) —see Atelectasis
  posture R29.3
  rotation, intestine Q43.3
  septum, ventricular Q21.0
Imperfectly descended testis —see
    Cryptorchid
Imperforate (congenital) —see also Atresia
  anus Q42.3
    with fistula Q42.2
  cervix (uteri) Q51.828
  esophagus Q39.0
    with tracheoesophageal fistula Q39.1
  hymen Q52.3
  jejunum Q41.1
  pharynx Q38.8
  rectum Q42.1
    with fistula Q42.0
  urethra Q64.39
  vagina Q52.4
Impervious (congenital) —see also Atresia
  anus Q42.3
    with fistula Q42.2
  bile duct Q44.2
  esophagus Q39.0
    with tracheoesophageal fistula Q39.1
  intestine (small) Q41.9
    large Q42.9
      specified NEC Q42.8
  rectum Q42.1
    with fistula Q42.0
  ureter —see Atresia, ureter
  urethra Q64.39
Impetiginization of dermatoses L01.1
Impetigo (any organism) (any site) (circinate)
    (contagiosa) (simplex) (vulgaris) L01.00
  Bockhart's L01.02
  bullous, bullosa L01.03
  external ear L01.00 [H62.40]
  follicularis L01.02
  furfuracea L30.5
  herpetiformis L40.1
    nonobstetrical L40.1
  neonatorum L01.03
  nonbullous L01.01
  specified type NEC L01.09
  ulcerative L01.09

▶ New   ⇒ Revised   ~~deleted~~ Deleted   ● Use Additional Character(s)

Impingement (on teeth)
joint —*see* Disorder, joint, specified type NEC
soft tissue
anterior M26.81
posterior M26.82
Implant, endometrial N80.9
Implantation
anomalous —*see* Anomaly, by site
ureter Q62.63
cyst
external area or site (skin) NEC L72.0
iris —*see* Cyst, iris, implantation
vagina N89.8
vulva N90.7
dermoid (cyst) —*see* Implantation, cyst
Impotence (sexual) N52.9
counseling Z70.1
organic origin —*see also* Dysfunction, sexual,
male, erectile N52.9
psychogenic F52.21
Impression, basilar Q75.8
Imprisonment, anxiety concerning Z65.1
Improper care (child) (newborn) —*see*
Maltreatment
Improperly tied umbilical cord (causing
hemorrhage) P51.8
Impulsiveness (impulsive) R45.87
Inability to swallow —*see* Aphagia
Inaccessible, inaccessibility
health care NEC Z75.3
due to
waiting period Z75.2
for admission to facility elsewhere Z75.1
other helping agencies Z75.4
Inactive —*see* condition
Inadequate, inadequacy
aesthetics of dental restoration K08.56
biologic, constitutional, functional, or social
F60.7
development
child R62.50
genitalia
after puberty NEC E30.0
congenital
female Q52.8
external Q52.79
internal Q52.8
male Q55.8
lungs Q33.6
associated with short gestation P28.0
organ or site not listed —*see* Anomaly, by
site
diet (causing nutritional deficiency)
E63.9
▶ drinking-water supply Z58.6
eating habits Z72.4
environment, household Z59.1
family support Z63.8
⇒ food (supply) NEC Z59.48
hunger effects T73.0
functional F60.7
household care, due to
family member
handicapped or ill Z74.2
on vacation Z75.5
temporarily away from home Z74.2
technical defects in home Z59.1
temporary absence from home of person
rendering care Z74.2
housing (heating) (space) Z59.1
income (financial) Z59.6
intrafamilial communication Z63.8
material resources Z59.9
mental —*see* Disability, intellectual
parental supervision or control of child
Z62.0
personality F60.7
pulmonary
function R06.89
newborn P28.5
ventilation, newborn P28.5

Inadequate, inadequacy (*Continued*)
sample of cytologic smear
anus R85.615
cervix R87.615
vagina R87.625
social F60.7
insurance Z59.7
skills NEC Z73.4
supervision of child by parent Z62.0
teaching affecting education Z55.8
welfare support Z59.7
Inanition R64
with edema —*see* Malnutrition, severe
due to
deprivation of food T73.0
malnutrition —*see* Malnutrition
fever R50.9
Inappropriate
change in quantitative human chorionic
gonadotropin (hCG) in early pregnancy
O02.81
diet or eating habits Z72.4
level of quantitative human chorionic
gonadotropin (hCG) for gestational age
in early pregnancy O02.81
secretion
antidiuretic hormone (ADH) (excessive)
E22.2
deficiency E23.2
pituitary (posterior) E22.2
Inattention at or after birth —*see* Neglect
Incarceration, incarcerated
enterocele K46.0
gangrenous K46.1
epiplocele K46.0
gangrenous K46.1
exomphalos K42.0
gangrenous K42.1
hernia —*see also* Hernia, by site, with
obstruction
with gangrene —*see* Hernia, by site, with
gangrene
iris, in wound —*see* Injury, eye, laceration,
with prolapse
lens, in wound —*see* Injury, eye, laceration,
with prolapse
omphalocele K42.0
prison, anxiety concerning Z65.1
rupture —*see* Hernia, by site
sarcoepiplocele K46.0
gangrenous K46.1
sarcoepiplomphalocele K42.0
with gangrene K42.1
uterus N85.8
gravid O34.51-●
causing obstructed labor O65.5
Incised wound
external —*see* Laceration
internal organs —*see* Injury, by site
Incision, incisional
hernia K43.2
with
gangrene (and obstruction) K43.1
obstruction K43.0
surgical, complication —*see* Complications,
surgical procedure
traumatic
external —*see* Laceration
internal organs —*see* Injury, by site
Inclusion
azurophilic leukocytic D72.0
blennorrhea (neonatal) (newborn)
P39.1
gallbladder in liver (congenital) Q44.1
Incompatibility
ABO
affecting management of pregnancy
O36.11-●
anti-A sensitization O36.11-●
anti-B sensitization O36.19-●
specified NEC O36.19-●

Incompatibility (*Continued*)
ABO (*Continued*)
infusion or transfusion reaction —*see*
Complication(s), transfusion,
incompatibility reaction, ABO
newborn P55.1
blood (group) (Duffy) (K) (Kell) (Kidd)
(Lewis) (M) (S) NEC
affecting management of pregnancy
O36.11-●
anti-A sensitization O36.11-●
anti-B sensitization O36.19-●
infusion or transfusion reaction
T80.89
newborn P55.8
divorce or estrangement Z63.5
Rh (blood group) (factor) Z31.82
affecting management of pregnancy NEC
O36.09-●
anti-D antibody O36.01-●
infusion or transfusion reaction —*see*
Complication(s), transfusion,
incompatibility reaction, Rh (factor)
newborn P55.0
rhesus —*see* Incompatibility, Rh
Incompetency, incompetent, incompetence
annular
aortic (valve) —*see* Insufficiency, aortic
mitral (valve) I34.0
pulmonary valve (heart) I37.1
aortic (valve) —*see* Insufficiency, aortic
cardiac valve —*see* Endocarditis
cervix, cervical (os) N88.3
in pregnancy O34.3-●
chronotropic I45.89
with
autonomic dysfunction G90.8
ischemic heart disease I25.89
left ventricular dysfunction I51.89
sinus node dysfunction I49.8
esophagogastric (junction) (sphincter) K22.0
mitral (valve) —*see* Insufficiency, mitral
pelvic fundus N81.89
pubocervical tissue N81.82
pulmonary valve (heart) I37.1
congenital Q22.3
rectovaginal tissue N81.83
tricuspid (annular) (valve) —*see* Insufficiency,
tricuspid
valvular —*see* Endocarditis
congenital Q24.8
vein, venous (saphenous) (varicose) —*see*
Varix, leg
Incomplete —*see also* condition
bladder, emptying R33.9
defecation R15.0
expansion lungs (newborn) NEC —*see*
Atelectasis
rotation, intestine Q43.3
Inconclusive
diagnostic imaging due to excess body fat of
patient R93.9
findings on diagnostic imaging of breast NEC
R92.8
mammogram (due to dense breasts) R92.2
Incontinence R32
anal sphincter R15.9
coital N39.491
feces R15.9
nonorganic origin F98.1
insensible (urinary) N39.42
overflow N39.490
postural (urinary) N39.492
psychogenic F45.8
rectal R15.9
reflex N39.498
stress (female) (male) N39.3
and urge N39.46
urethral sphincter R32
urge N39.41
and stress (female) (male) N39.46

Incontinence (Continued)
  urine (urinary) R32
    continuous N39.45
    due to cognitive impairment, or severe
      physical disability or immobility
      R39.81
    functional R39.81
    insensible N39.42
    mixed (stress and urge) N39.46
    nocturnal N39.44
    nonorganic origin F98.0
    overflow N39.490
    post dribbling N39.43
    postural N39.492
    reflex N39.498
    specified NEC N39.498
    stress (female) (male) N39.3
      and urge N39.46
    total N39.498
    unaware N39.42
    urge N39.41
      and stress (female) (male) N39.46
Incontinentia pigmenti Q82.3
Incoordinate, incoordination
  esophageal-pharyngeal (newborn) —see
    Dysphagia
  muscular R27.8
  uterus (action) (contractions) (complicating
    delivery) O62.4
Increase, increased
  abnormal, in development R63.8
  androgens (ovarian) E28.1
  anticoagulants (antithrombin) (anti-VIIIa)
    (anti-IXa) (anti-Xa) (anti-XIa) —see
    Circulating anticoagulants
  cold sense R20.8
  estrogen E28.0
  function
    adrenal
      cortex —see Cushing's, syndrome
      medulla E27.5
    pituitary (gland) (anterior) (lobe) E22.9
      posterior E22.2
  heat sense R20.8
  intracranial pressure (benign) G93.2
  permeability, capillaries I78.8
  pressure, intracranial G93.2
  secretion
    gastrin E16.4
    glucagon E16.3
    pancreas, endocrine E16.9
      growth hormone-releasing hormone
        E16.8
      pancreatic polypeptide E16.8
      somatostatin E16.8
      vasoactive-intestinal polypeptide
        E16.8
  sphericity, lens Q12.4
  splenic activity D73.1
  venous pressure I87.8
    portal K76.6
Increta placenta O43.22-●
Incrustation, cornea, foreign body (lead)
  (zinc) —see Foreign body, cornea
Incyclophoria H50.54
Incyclotropia —see Cyclotropia
Indeterminate sex Q56.4
India rubber skin Q82.8
Indigestion (acid) (bilious) (functional)
  K30
  catarrhal K31.89
  due to decomposed food NOS A05.9
  nervous F45.8
  psychogenic F45.8
Indirect —see condition
Induratio penis plastica N48.6
Induration, indurated
  brain G93.89
  breast (fibrous) N64.51
    puerperal, postpartum O92.29
  broad ligament N83.8

Induration, indurated (Continued)
  chancre
    anus A51.1
      congenital A50.07
      extragenital NEC A51.2
  corpora cavernosa (penis) (plastic) N48.6
  liver (chronic) K76.89
  lung (black) (chronic) (fibroid) —see also
    Fibrosis, lung J84.10
    essential brown J84.03
  penile (plastic) N48.6
  phlebitic —see Phlebitis
  skin R23.4
Inebriety (without dependence) —see Alcohol,
  intoxication
Inefficiency, kidney N28.9
Inelasticity, skin R23.4
Inequality, leg (length) (acquired) —see also
  Deformity, limb, unequal length
  congenital —see Defect, reduction, lower limb
  lower leg —see Deformity, limb, unequal
    length
Inertia
  bladder (neurogenic) N31.2
  stomach K31.89
    psychogenic F45.8
  uterus, uterine during labor O62.2
    during latent phase of labor O62.0
    primary O62.0
    secondary O62.1
  vesical (neurogenic) N31.2
Infancy, infantile, infantilism —see also
  condition
  celiac K90.0
  genitalia, genitals (after puberty) E30.0
  Herter's (nontropical sprue) K90.0
  intestinal NEC K90.0
  Lorain E23.0
  pancreatic K86.89
  pelvis M95.5
    with disproportion (fetopelvic) O33.1
      causing obstructed labor O65.1
  pituitary E23.0
  renal N25.0
  uterus —see Infantile, genitalia
Infant(s) —see also Infancy
  excessive crying R68.11
  irritable child R68.12
  lack of care —see Neglect
  liveborn (singleton) Z38.2
    born in hospital Z38.00
      by cesarean Z38.01
    born outside hospital Z38.1
    multiple NEC Z38.8
      born in hospital Z38.68
        by cesarean Z38.69
      born outside hospital Z38.7
    quadruplet Z38.8
      born in hospital Z38.63
        by cesarean Z38.64
      born outside hospital Z38.7
    quintuplet Z38.8
      born in hospital Z38.65
        by cesarean Z38.66
      born outside hospital Z38.7
    triplet Z38.8
      born in hospital Z38.61
        by cesarean Z38.62
      born outside hospital Z38.7
    twin Z38.5
      born in hospital Z38.30
        by cesarean Z38.31
      born outside hospital Z38.4
  of diabetic mother (syndrome of) P70.1
    gestational diabetes P70.0
Infantile —see also condition
  genitalia, genitals E30.0
  os, uterine E30.0
  penis E30.0
  testis E29.1
  uterus E30.0

Infantilism —see Infancy
Infarct, infarction
  adrenal (capsule) (gland) E27.49
  appendices epiploicae —see also Infarct,
    intestine K55.069
  bowel —see also Infarct, intestine K55.069
  brain (stem) —see Infarct, cerebral
  breast N64.89
  brewer's (kidney) N28.0
  cardiac —see Infarct, myocardium
  cerebellar —see Infarct, cerebral
  cerebral (acute) (chronic) (see also Occlusion,
    artery cerebral or precerebral, with
    infarction) I63.9-●
    aborted I63.9
    cortical I63.9
    due to
      cerebral venous thrombosis,
        nonpyogenic I63.6
      embolism
        cerebral arteries I63.4-●
        precerebral arteries I63.1-●
      occlusion NEC
        cerebral arteries I63.5-●
        precerebral arteries I63.2-●
        small artery I63.81
      stenosis NEC
        cerebral arteries I63.5-●
        precerebral arteries I63.2-●
        small artery I63.81
      thrombosis
        cerebral artery I63.3-●
        precerebral artery I63.0-●
    intraoperative
      during cardiac surgery I97.810
      during other surgery I97.811
    neonatal P91.82-●
    perinatal (arterial ischemic) P91.82-●
    postprocedural
      following cardiac surgery I97.820
      following other surgery I97.821
    specified NEC I63.89
  colon (acute) (agnogenic) (embolic)
    (hemorrhagic) (nonocclusive)
    (nonthrombotic) (occlusive) (segmental)
    (thrombotic) (with gangrene) —see also
    Infarct, intestine K55.049
  coronary artery —see Infarct, myocardium
  embolic —see Embolism
  fallopian tube N83.8
  gallbladder K82.8
  heart —see Infarct, myocardium
  hepatic K76.3
  hypophysis (anterior lobe) E23.6
  impending (myocardium) I20.0
  intestine (acute) (agnogenic) (embolic)
    (hemorrhagic) (nonocclusive)
    (nonthrombotic) (occlusive) (thrombotic)
    (with gangrene) K55.069
    diffuse K55.062
    focal K55.061
    large K55.049
      diffuse K55.042
      focal K55.041
    small K55.029
      diffuse K55.022
      focal K55.021
  kidney N28.0
  lacunar I63.81
  liver K76.3
  lung (embolic) (thrombotic) —see Embolism,
    pulmonary
  lymph node I89.8
  mesentery, mesenteric (embolic) (thrombotic)
    (with gangrene) —see also Infarct,
    intestine K55.069
  muscle (ischemic) M62.20
    ankle M62.27-●
    foot M62.27-●
    forearm M62.23-●
    hand M62.24-●

▶ New   ⇒ Revised   ~~deleted~~ Deleted   ● Use Additional Character(s)

Infarct, infarction (Continued)
  muscle (Continued)
    lower leg M62.26-●
    pelvic region M62.25-●
    shoulder region M62.21-●
    specified site NEC M62.28
    thigh M62.25-●
    upper arm M62.22-●
  myocardium, myocardial (acute) (with stated
      duration of 4 weeks or less) I21.9
    associated with revascularization
        procedure I21.A9
    diagnosed on ECG, but presenting no
        symptoms I25.2
    due to
      demand ischemia I21.A1
      ischemic imbalance I21.A1
    healed or old I25.2
    intraoperative —see also Infarct,
        myocardium, associated with
        revascularization procedure
      during cardiac surgery I97.790
      during other surgery I97.791
    non-Q wave I21.4
    non-ST elevation (NSTEMI) I21.4
      subsequent I22.2
    nontransmural I21.4
    past (diagnosed on ECG or other
        investigation, but currently presenting
        no symptoms) I25.2
    postprocedural —see also Infarct,
        myocardium, associated with
        revascularization procedure
      following cardiac surgery —see also Infarct,
          myocardium, type 4 or type 5 I97.190
      following other surgery I97.191
    Q wave —see also Infarct, myocardium, by
        site I21.3
    secondary to
      demand ischemia I21.A1
      ischemic imbalance I21.A1
    ST elevation (STEMI) I21.3
      anterior (anteroapical) (anterolateral)
          (anteroseptal) (Q wave) (wall) I21.09
        subsequent I22.0
      inferior (diaphragmatic) (inferolateral)
          (inferoposterior) (wall) NEC I21.19
        subsequent I22.1
      inferoposterior transmural (Q wave) I21.11
      involving
        coronary artery of anterior wall NEC
            I21.09
        coronary artery of inferior wall NEC
            I21.19
        diagonal coronary artery I21.02
        left anterior descending coronary
            artery I21.02
        left circumflex coronary artery I21.21
        left main coronary artery I21.01
        oblique marginal coronary artery I21.21
        right coronary artery I21.11
      lateral (apical-lateral) (basal-lateral)
          (high) I21.29
        subsequent I22.8
      posterior (posterobasal) (posterolateral)
          (posteroseptal) (true) I21.29
        subsequent I22.8
      septal I21.29
        subsequent I22.8
      specified NEC I21.29
        subsequent I22.8
      subsequent I22.9
    subsequent (recurrent) (reinfarction) I22.9
      anterior (anteroapical) (anterolateral)
          (anteroseptal) (wall) I22.0
      diaphragmatic (wall) I22.1
      inferior (diaphragmatic) (inferolateral)
          (inferoposterior) (wall) I22.1
      lateral (apical-lateral) (basal-lateral)
          (high) I22.8
      non-ST elevation (NSTEMI) I22.2

Infarct, infarction (Continued)
  myocardium, myocardial (Continued)
    subsequent (Continued)
      posterior (posterobasal) (posterolateral)
          (posteroseptal) (true) I22.8
      septal I22.8
      specified NEC I22.8
      ST elevation I22.9
        anterior (anteroapical) (anterolateral)
            (anteroseptal) (wall) I22.0
        inferior (diaphragmatic) (inferolateral)
            (inferoposterior) (wall) I22.1
        specified NEC I22.8
      subendocardial I22.2
      transmural I21.3
        anterior (anteroapical) (anterolateral)
            (anteroseptal) (wall) I22.0
        diaphragmatic (wall) I22.1
        inferior (diaphragmatic) (inferolateral)
            (inferoposterior) (wall) I22.1
        lateral (apical-lateral) (basal-lateral)
            (high) I22.8
        posterior (posterobasal) (posterolateral)
            (posteroseptal) (true) I22.8
        specified NEC I22.8
      type 1 —see also Infarction, myocardial,
          subsequent, by site, or by ST
          elevation or non-ST elevation I22.9
      type 2 I21.A1
      type 3 I21.A9
      type 4 I21.A9
      type 5 I21.A9
    syphilitic A52.06
    transmural I21.9
      anterior (anteroapical) (anterolateral)
          (anteroseptal) (Q wave) (wall) NEC
          I21.09
      inferior (diaphragmatic) (inferolateral)
          (inferoposterior) (Q wave) (wall)
          NEC I21.19
      inferoposterior (Q wave) I21.11
      lateral (apical-lateral) (basal-lateral)
          (high) NEC I21.29
      posterior (posterobasal) (posterolateral)
          (posteroseptal) (true) NEC I21.29
      septal NEC I21.29
      specified NEC I21.29
      type 1 —see also Infarction, myocardial,
          by site, or by ST elevation or non-ST
          elevation I21.9
      type 2 I21.A1
      type 3 I21.A9
      type 4 (a) (b) (c) I21.A9
      type 5 I21.A9
    nontransmural I21.4
    omentum —see also Infarct, intestine
        K55.069
    ovary N83.8
    pancreas K86.89
    papillary muscle —see Infarct, myocardium
    parathyroid gland E21.4
    pituitary (gland) E23.6
    placenta O43.81-●
    prostate N42.89
    pulmonary (artery) (vein) (hemorrhagic) —
        see Embolism, pulmonary
    renal (embolic) (thrombotic) N28.0
    retina, retinal (artery) —see Occlusion, artery,
        retina
    spinal (cord) (acute) (embolic) (nonembolic)
        G95.11
    spleen D73.5
      embolic or thrombotic I74.8
    subendocardial (acute) (nontransmural) I21.4
    suprarenal (capsule) (gland) E27.49
    testis N50.1
    thrombotic —see also Thrombosis
      artery, arterial —see Embolism
    thyroid (gland) E07.89
    ventricle (heart) —see Infarct, myocardium
Infecting —see condition

Infection, infected, infective (opportunistic)
    B99.9
  with
    drug resistant organism —see Resistance
        (to), drug —see also specific organism
    lymphangitis —see Lymphangitis
    organ dysfunction (acute) R65.20
      with septic shock R65.21
  abscess (skin) - code by site under Abscess
  Absidia —see Mucormycosis
  Acanthamoeba —see Acanthamebiasis
  Acanthocheilonema (perstans) (streptocerca)
      B74.4
  accessory sinus (chronic) —see Sinusitis
  achorion —see Dermatophytosis
  Acremonium falciforme B47.0
  acromioclavicular M00.9
  Actinobacillus (actinomycetem-comitans)
      A28.8
    mallei A24.0
    muris A25.1
  Actinomadura B47.1
  Actinomyces (israelii) —see also
      Actinomycosis A42.9
  Actinomycetales —see Actinomycosis
  actinomycotic NOS —see Actinomycosis
  adenoid (and tonsil) J03.90
    chronic J35.02
  adenovirus NEC
    as cause of disease classified elsewhere
        B97.0
    unspecified nature or site B34.0
  aerogenes capsulatus A48.0
  aertrycke —see Infection, salmonella
  alimentary canal NOS —see Enteritis,
      infectious
  Allescheria boydii B48.2
  Alternaria B48.8
  alveolus, alveolar (process) K04.7
  Ameba, amebic (histolytica) —see Amebiasis
  amniotic fluid, sac or cavity O41.10-●
    chorioamnionitis O41.12-●
    placentitis O41.14-●
  amputation stump (surgical) —see
      Complication, amputation stump,
      infection
  Ancylostoma (duodenalis) B76.0
  Anisakiasis, Anisakis larvae B81.0
  anthrax —see Anthrax
  antrum (chronic) —see Sinusitis, maxillary
  anus, anal (papillae) (sphincter) K62.89
  arbovirus (arbor virus) A94
    specified type NEC A93.8
  artificial insemination N98.0
  Ascaris lumbricoides —see Ascariasis
  Ascomycetes B47.0
  Aspergillus (flavus) (fumigatus) (terreus) —
      see Aspergillosis
  atypical
    acid-fast (bacilli) —see Mycobacterium,
        atypical
    mycobacteria —see Mycobacterium, atypical
    virus A81.9
      specified type NEC A81.89
  auditory meatus (external) —see Otitis,
      externa, infective
  auricle (ear) —see Otitis, externa, infective
  axillary gland (lymph) L04.2
  Bacillus A49.9
    abortus A23.1
    anthracis —see Anthrax
    Ducrey's (any location) A57
    Flexner's A03.1
    Friedländer's NEC A49.8
    gas (gangrene) A48.0
    mallei A24.0
    melitensis A23.0
    paratyphoid, paratyphosus A01.4
      A A01.1
      B A01.2
      C A01.3

Infection, infected, infective *(Continued)*
  Bacillus *(Continued)*
    Shiga (-Kruse) A03.0
    suipestifer —*see* Infection, salmonella
    swimming pool A31.1
    typhosa A01.00
    welchii —*see* Gangrene, gas
  bacterial NOS A49.9
    as cause of disease classified elsewhere B96.89
      Bacteroides fragilis [B. fragilis] B96.6
      Clostridium perfringens [C. perfringens] B96.7
      Enterobacter sakazakii B96.89
      Enterococcus B95.2
      Escherichia coli [E. coli] (*see also* Escherichia coli) B96.20
      Helicobacter pylori [H.pylori] B96.81
      Hemophilus influenzae [H. influenzae] B96.3
      Klebsiella pneumoniae [K. pneumoniae] B96.1
      Mycoplasma pneumoniae [M. pneumoniae] B96.0
      Proteus (mirabilis) (morganii) B96.4
      Pseudomonas (aeruginosa) (mallei) (pseudomallei) B96.5
      Staphylococcus B95.8
        aureus (methicillin susceptible) (MSSA) B95.61
          methicillin resistant (MRSA) B95.62
        specified NEC B95.7
      Streptococcus B95.5
        group A B95.0
        group B B95.1
        pneumoniae B95.3
        specified NEC B95.4
        Vibrio vulnificus B96.82
    specified NEC A48.8
  Bacterium
    paratyphosum A01.4
      A A01.1
      B A01.2
      C A01.3
    typhosum A01.00
  Bacteroides NEC A49.8
    fragilis, as cause of disease classified elsewhere B96.6
  Balantidium coli A07.0
  Bartholin's gland N75.8
  Basidiobolus B46.8
  bile duct (common) (hepatic) —*see* Cholangitis
  bladder —*see* Cystitis
  Blastomyces, blastomycotic —*see also* Blastomycosis
    brasiliensis —*see* Paracoccidioidomycosis
    dermatitidis —*see* Blastomycosis
    European —*see* Cryptococcosis
    Loboi B48.0
    North American B40.9
    South American —*see* Paracoccidioidomycosis
  bleb, postprocedure —*see* Blebitis
  bone —*see* Osteomyelitis
  Bordetella —*see* Whooping cough
  Borrelia bergdorfi A69.20
  brain —*see also* Encephalitis G04.90
    membranes —*see* Meningitis
    septic G06.0
      meninges —*see* Meningitis, bacterial
  branchial cyst Q18.0
  breast —*see* Mastitis
  bronchus —*see* Bronchitis
  Brucella A23.9
    abortus A23.1
    canis A23.3
    melitensis A23.0
    mixed A23.8
    specified NEC A23.8
    suis A23.2

Infection, infected, infective *(Continued)*
  Brugia (malayi) B74.1
    timori B74.2
  bursa —*see* Bursitis, infective
  buttocks (skin) L08.9
  Campylobacter, intestinal A04.5
    as cause of disease classified elsewhere B96.81
  Candida (albicans) (tropicalis) —*see* Candidiasis
  candiru B88.8
  Capillaria (intestinal) B81.1
    hepatica B83.8
    philippinensis B81.1
  cartilage —*see* Disorder, cartilage, specified type NEC
  catheter-related bloodstream (CRBSI) T80.211
  cat liver fluke B66.0
  cellulitis - code by site under Cellulitis
  central line-associated T80.219
    bloodstream (CLABSI) T80.211
    specified NEC T80.218
  Cephalosporium falciforme B47.0
  cerebrospinal —*see* Meningitis
  cervical gland (lymph) L04.0
  cervix —*see* Cervicitis
  cesarean delivery wound (puerperal) O86.00
  cestodes —*see* Infestation, cestodes
  chest J22
  Chilomastix (intestinal) A07.8
  Chlamydia, chlamydial A74.9
    anus A56.3
    genitourinary tract A56.2
      lower A56.00
      specified NEC A56.19
    lymphogranuloma A55
    pharynx A56.4
    psittaci A70
    rectum A56.3
    sexually transmitted NEC A56.8
  cholera —*see* Cholera
  Cladosporium
    bantianum (brain abscess) B43.1
    carrionii B43.0
    castellanii B36.1
    trichoides (brain abscess) B43.1
    werneckii B36.1
  Clonorchis (sinensis) (liver) B66.1
  Clostridium NEC
    bifermentans A48.0
    botulinum (food poisoning) A05.1
      infant A48.51
      wound A48.52
    difficile
      as cause of disease classified elsewhere B96.89
      foodborne (disease)
        not specified as recurrent A04.72
        recurrent A04.71
      gas gangrene A48.0
      necrotizing enterocolitis
        not specified as recurrent A04.72
        recurrent A04.71
      sepsis A41.4
    gas-forming NEC A48.0
    histolyticum A48.0
    novyi, causing gas gangrene A48.0
    oedematiens A48.0
    perfringens
      as cause of disease classified elsewhere B96.7
      due to food A05.2
      foodborne (disease) A05.2
      gas gangrene A48.0
      sepsis A41.4
    septicum, causing gas gangrene A48.0
    sordellii, causing gas gangrene A48.0

Infection, infected, infective *(Continued)*
  Clostridium NEC *(Continued)*
    welchii
      as cause of disease classified elsewhere B96.7
      foodborne (disease) A05.2
      gas gangrene A48.0
      necrotizing enteritis A05.2
      sepsis A41.4
  Coccidioides (immitis) —*see* Coccidioidomycosis
  colon —*see* Enteritis, infectious
  colostomy K94.02
  common duct —*see* Cholangitis
  congenital P39.9
    Candida (albicans) P37.5
    cytomegalovirus P35.1
    hepatitis, viral P35.3
    herpes simplex P35.2
    infectious or parasitic disease P37.9
      specified NEC P37.8
    listeriosis (disseminated) P37.2
    malaria NEC P37.4
      falciparum P37.3
    Plasmodium falciparum P37.3
    poliomyelitis P35.8
    rubella P35.0
    skin P39.4
    toxoplasmosis (acute) (subacute) (chronic) P37.1
    tuberculosis P37.0
    urinary (tract) P39.3
    vaccinia P35.8
    virus P35.9
      specified type NEC P35.8
  Conidiobolus B46.8
  coronavirus-2019 U07.1
  coronavirus NEC B34.2
    as cause of disease classified elsewhere B97.29
    severe acute respiratory syndrome (SARS associated) B97.21
  corpus luteum —*see* Salpingo-oophoritis
  Corynebacterium diphtheriae —*see* Diphtheria
  cotia virus B08.8
  COVID-19 U07.1
  Coxiella burnetii A78
  coxsackie —*see* Coxsackie
  Cryptococcus neoformans —*see* Cryptococcosis
  Cryptosporidium A07.2
  Cunninghamella —*see* Mucormycosis
  cyst —*see* Cyst
  cystic duct —*see also* Cholecystitis K81.9
  Cysticercus cellulosae —*see* Cysticercosis
  cytomegalovirus, cytomegaloviral B25.9
    congenital P35.1
    maternal, maternal care for (suspected) damage to fetus O35.3
    mononucleosis B27.10
      with
        complication NEC B27.19
        meningitis B27.12
        polyneuropathy B27.11
  delta-agent (acute), in hepatitis B carrier B17.0
  dental (pulpal origin) K04.7
  Deuteromycetes B47.0
  Dicrocoelium dendriticum B66.2
  Dipetalonema (perstans) (streptocerca) B74.4
  diphtherial —*see* Diphtheria
  Diphyllobothrium (adult) (latum) (pacificum) B70.0
    larval B70.1
  Diplogonoporus (grandis) B71.8
  Dipylidium caninum B67.4
  Dirofilaria B74.8
  Dracunculus medinensis B72
  Drechslera (hawaiiensis) B43.8
  Ducrey Haemophilus (any location) A57

Infection, infected, infective *(Continued)*
  due to or resulting from
    artificial insemination N98.0
    Babesia
      divergens (-like) strain B60.03
      duncani (-type) species B60.02
      microti B60.01
      species
        specified NEC B60.09
    central venous catheter T80.219
      bloodstream T80.211
      exit or insertion site T80.212
      localized T80.212
      port or reservoir T80.212
      specified NEC T80.218
      tunnel T80.212
    device, implant or graft —*see also*
      Complications, by site and type,
      infection or inflammation T85.79
      arterial graft NEC T82.7
      breast (implant) T85.79
      catheter NEC T85.79
        dialysis (renal) T82.7
          central line T80.211
          intraperitoneal T85.71
        infusion NEC T82.7
          cranial T85.735
          intrathecal T85.735
          spinal (epidural) (subdural) T85.735
          subarachnoid T85.735
        urinary T83.518
          cystostomy T83.510
          Hopkins T83.518
          ileostomy T83.518
          nephrostomy T83.512
          specified NEC T83.518
          urethral indwelling T83.511
          urostomy T83.518
      electronic (electrode) (pulse generator)
        (stimulator)
        bone T84.7
        cardiac T82.7
        nervous system T85.738
          brain T85.731
          cranial nerve T85.732
          gastric nerve T85.732
          generator pocket T85.734
          neurostimulator generator
            T85.734
          peripheral nerve T85.732
          sacral nerve T85.732
          spinal cord T85.733
          vagal nerve T85.732
        urinary T83.590
      fixation, internal (orthopedic) NEC —
        see Complication, fixation device,
        infection
      gastrointestinal (bile duct) (esophagus)
        T85.79
        neurostimulator electrode (lead)
          T85.732
      genital NEC T83.69
      heart NEC T82.7
        valve (prosthesis) T82.6
          graft T82.7
      joint prosthesis —*see* Complication, joint
        prosthesis, infection
      ocular (corneal graft) (orbital implant)
        NEC T85.79
      orthopedic NEC T84.7
      penile (cylinder) (pump) (resevoir)
        T83.61
      specified NEC T85.79
      testicular T83.62
      urinary NEC T83.598
        ileal conduit stent T83.593
        implanted neurostimulation T83.590
        implanted sphincter T83.591
        indwelling ureteral stent T83.592
        nephroureteral stent T83.593
        specified stent NEC T83.593

Infection, infected, infective *(Continued)*
  due to or resulting from *(Continued)*
    device, implant or graft *(Continued)*
      vascular NEC T82.7
      ventricular intracranial (communicating)
        shunt T85.730
    Hickman catheter T80.219
      bloodstream T80.211
      localized T80.212
      specified NEC T80.218
    immunization or vaccination
      T88.0
    infusion, injection or transfusion
      NEC T80.29
      acute T80.22
    injury NEC - code by site under Wound,
      open
    peripherally inserted central catheter
      (PICC) T80.219
      bloodstream T80.211
      localized T80.212
      specified NEC T80.218
    portacath (port-a-cath) T80.219
      bloodstream T80.211
      localized T80.212
      specified NEC T80.218
    protozoa of the order Piroplasmida NEC
      B60.09
    pulmonary artery catheter —*see* Infection,
      due to or resulting from, central
      venous catheter
    surgery T81.40
    Swan Ganz catheter —*see* Infection, due
      to or resulting from, central venous
      catheter
    triple lumen catheter T80.219
      bloodstream T80.211
      localized T80.212
      specified NEC T80.218
    umbilical venous catheter T80.219
      bloodstream T80.211
      localized T80.212
      specified NEC T80.218
  during labor NEC O75.3
  ear (middle) —*see also* Otitis media
    external —*see* Otitis, externa, infective
    inner —*see* subcategory H83.0
  Eberthella typhosa A01.00
  Echinococcus —*see* Echinococcus
  echovirus
    as cause of disease classified elsewhere
      B97.12
    unspecified nature or site B34.1
  endocardium I33.0
  endocervix —*see* Cervicitis
  Entamoeba —*see* Amebiasis
  enteric —*see* Enteritis, infectious
  Enterobacter sakazakii B96.89
  Enterobius vermicularis B80
  enterostomy K94.12
  enterovirus B34.1
    as cause of disease classified elsewhere
      B97.10
      coxsackievirus B97.11
      echovirus B97.12
      specified NEC B97.19
  Entomophthora B46.8
  Epidermophyton —*see* Dermatophytosis
  epididymis —*see* Epididymitis
  episiotomy (puerperal) O86.09
  Erysipelothrix (insidiosa) (rhusiopathiae) —
    see Erysipeloid
  erythema infectiosum B08.3
  Escherichia (E.) coli NEC A49.8
    as cause of disease classified elsewhere —
      see also Escherichia coli B96.20
    congenital P39.8
      sepsis P36.4
    generalized A41.51
    intestinal —*see* Enteritis, infectious, due to,
      Escherichia coli

Infection, infected, infective *(Continued)*
  ethmoidal (chronic) (sinus) —*see* Sinusitis,
    ethmoidal
  eustachian tube (ear) —*see* Salpingitis,
    eustachian
  external auditory canal (meatus) NEC —*see*
    Otitis, externa, infective
  eye (purulent) —*see* Endophthalmitis, purulent
  eyelid —*see* Inflammation, eyelid
  fallopian tube —*see* Salpingo-oophoritis
  Fasciola (gigantica) (hepatica) (indica) B66.3
  Fasciolopsis (buski) B66.5
  filarial —*see* Infestation, filarial
  finger (skin) L08.9
    nail L03.01-●
      fungus B35.1
  fish tapeworm B70.0
    larval B70.1
  flagellate, intestinal A07.9
  fluke —*see* Infestation, fluke
  focal
    teeth (pulpal origin) K04.7
    tonsils J35.01
  Fonsecaea (compactum) (pedrosoi) B43.0
  food —*see* Intoxication, foodborne
  foot (skin) L08.9
    dermatophytic fungus B35.3
  Francisella tularensis —*see* Tularemia
  frontal (sinus) (chronic) —*see* Sinusitis, frontal
  fungus NOS B49
    beard B35.0
    dermatophytic —*see* Dermatophytosis
    foot B35.3
    groin B35.6
    hand B35.2
    nail B35.1
    pathogenic to compromised host only B48.8
    perianal (area) B35.6
    scalp B35.0
    skin B36.9
      foot B35.3
      hand B35.2
      toenails B35.1
  Fusarium B48.8
  gallbladder —*see* Cholecystitis
  gas bacillus —*see* Gangrene, gas
  gastrointestinal —*see* Enteritis, infectious
  generalized NEC —*see* Sepsis
  generator pocket, implanted electronic
    neurostimulator T85.734
  genital organ or tract
    female —*see* Disease, pelvis, inflammatory
    male N49.9
      multiple sites N49.8
      specified NEC N49.8
  Ghon tubercle, primary A15.7
  Giardia lamblia A07.1
  gingiva (chronic) K05.10
    acute K05.00
      nonplaque induced K05.01
      plaque induced K05.00
    nonplaque induced K05.11
    plaque induced K05.10
  glanders A24.0
  glenosporopsis B48.0
  Gnathostoma (spinigerum) B83.1
  Gongylonema B83.8
  gonococcal —*see* Gonococcus
  gram-negative bacilli NOS A49.9
  guinea worm B72
  gum (chronic) K05.10
    acute K05.00
      nonplaque induced K05.01
      plaque induced K05.00
    nonplaque induced K05.11
    plaque induced K05.10
  Haemophilus —*see* Infection, Hemophilus
  heart —*see* Carditis
  Helicobacter pylori A04.8
    as cause of disease classified elsewhere
      B96.81

Infection, infected, infective (Continued)
  helminths B83.9
    intestinal B82.0
      mixed (types classifiable to more than
        one of the titles B65.0-B81.3 and
        B81.8) B81.4
      specified type NEC B81.8
    specified type NEC B83.8
  Hemophilus
    aegyptius, systemic A48.4
    ducrey (any location) A57
    generalized A41.3
    influenzae NEC A49.2
      as cause of disease classified elsewhere
        B96.3
  herpes (simplex) —see also Herpes
    congenital P35.2
    disseminated B00.7
    zoster B02.9
  herpesvirus, herpesviral —see Herpes
  Heterophyes (heterophyes) B66.8
  hip (joint) NEC M00.9
    due to internal joint prosthesis
      left T84.52
      right T84.51
    skin NEC L08.9
  Histoplasma —see Histoplasmosis
    American B39.4
    capsulatum B39.4
  hookworm B76.9
  human
    papilloma virus A63.0
    T-cell lymphotropic virus type-1 (HTLV-1)
      B33.3
  hydrocele N43.0
  Hymenolepis B71.0
  hypopharynx —see Pharyngitis
  inguinal (lymph) glands L04.1
    due to soft chancre A57
  intervertebral disc, pyogenic M46.30
    cervical region M46.32
    cervicothoracic region M46.33
    lumbar region M46.36
    lumbosacral region M46.37
    multiple sites M46.39
    occipito-atlanto-axial region M46.31
    sacrococcygeal region M46.38
    thoracic region M46.34
    thoracolumbar region M46.35
  intestine, intestinal —see Enteritis, infectious
    specified NEC A08.8
  intra-amniotic affecting newborn NEC P39.2
  intrauterine inflammation O41.12-•
  Isospora belli or hominis A07.3
  Japanese B encephalitis A83.0
  jaw (bone) (lower) (upper) M27.2
  joint NEC M00.9
    due to internal joint prosthesis T84.50
  kidney (cortex) (hematogenous) N15.9
    with calculus N20.0
      with hydronephrosis N13.6
    following ectopic gestation O08.83
    pelvis and ureter (cystic) N28.85
    puerperal (postpartum) O86.21
    specified NEC N15.8
  Klebsiella (K.) pneumoniae NEC A49.8
    as cause of disease classified elsewhere
      B96.1
  knee (joint) NEC M00.9
    due to internal joint prosthesis
      left T84.54
      right T84.53
    joint M00.9
    skin L08.9
  Koch's —see Tuberculosis
  labia (majora) (minora) (acute) —see Vulvitis
  lacrimal
    gland —see Dacryoadenitis
    passages (duct) (sac) —see Inflammation,
      lacrimal, passages
  lancet fluke B66.2

Infection, infected, infective (Continued)
  larynx NEC J38.7
  leg (skin) NOS L08.9
  Legionella pneumophila A48.1
    nonpneumonic A48.2
  Leishmania —see also Leishmaniasis
    aethiopica B55.1
    braziliensis B55.2
    chagasi B55.0
    donovani B55.0
    infantum B55.0
    major B55.1
    mexicana B55.1
    tropica B55.1
  lentivirus, as cause of disease classified
    elsewhere B97.31
  Leptosphaeria senegalensis B47.0
  Leptospira interrogans A27.9
    autumnalis A27.89
    canicola A27.89
    hebdomadis A27.89
    icterohaemorrhagiae A27.0
    pomona A27.89
    specified type NEC A27.89
  leptospirochetal NEC —see Leptospirosis
  Listeria monocytogenes —see also Listeriosis
    congenital P37.2
  Loa loa B74.3
    with conjunctival infestation B74.3
    eyelid B74.3
  Loboa loboi B48.0
  local, skin (staphylococcal) (streptococcal)
    L08.9
    abscess - code by site under Abscess
    cellulitis - code by site under Cellulitis
    specified NEC L08.89
    ulcer —see Ulcer, skin
  Loefflerella mallei A24.0
  lung —see also Pneumonia J18.9
    atypical Mycobacterium A31.0
    spirochetal A69.8
    tuberculous —see Tuberculosis, pulmonary
    virus —see Pneumonia, viral
  lymph gland —see also Lymphadenitis, acute
    mesenteric I88.0
  lymphoid tissue, base of tongue or posterior
    pharynx, NEC (chronic) J35.03
  Madurella (grisea) (mycetomii) B47.0
  major
    following ectopic or molar pregnancy
      O08.0
    puerperal, postpartum, childbirth O85
  Malassezia furfur B36.0
  Malleomyces
    mallei A24.0
    pseudomallei (whitmori) —see Melioidosis
  mammary gland N61.0
  Mansonella (ozzardi) (perstans) (streptocerca)
    B74.4
  mastoid —see Mastoiditis
  maxilla, maxillary M27.2
    sinus (chronic) —see Sinusitis, maxillary
  mediastinum J98.51
  Medina (worm) B72
  meibomian cyst or gland —see Hordeolum
  meninges —see Meningitis, bacterial
  meningococcal —see also condition A39.9
    adrenals A39.1
    brain A39.81
    cerebrospinal A39.0
    conjunctiva A39.89
    endocardium A39.51
    heart A39.50
      endocardium A39.51
      myocardium A39.52
      pericardium A39.53
    joint A39.83
    meninges A39.0
    meningococcemia A39.4
      acute A39.2
      chronic A39.3

Infection, infected, infective (Continued)
  meningococcal (Continued)
    myocardium A39.52
    pericardium A39.53
    retrobulbar neuritis A39.82
    specified site NEC A39.89
  mesenteric lymph nodes or glands NEC
    I88.0
  Metagonimus B66.8
  metatarsophalangeal M00.9
  methicillin
    resistant Staphylococcus aureus (MRSA)
      A49.02
    susceptible Staphylococcus aureus (MSSA)
      A49.01
  Microsporum, microsporic —see
    Dermatophytosis
  mixed flora (bacterial) NEC A49.8
  Monilia —see Candidiasis
  Monosporium apiospermum B48.2
  mouth, parasitic B37.0
  Mucor —see Mucormycosis
  muscle NEC —see Myositis, infective
  mycelium NOS B49
  mycetoma B47.9
    actinomycotic NEC B47.1
    mycotic NEC B47.0
  Mycobacterium, mycobacterial —see
    Mycobacterium
  Mycoplasma NEC A49.3
    pneumoniae, as cause of disease classified
      elsewhere B96.0
  mycotic NOS B49
    pathogenic to compromised host only
      B48.8
    skin NOS B36.9
  myocardium NEC I40.0
  nail (chronic)
    with lymphangitis —see Lymphangitis,
      acute, digit
    finger L03.01-•
      fungus B35.1
    ingrowing L60.0
    toe L03.03-•
      fungus B35.1
  nasal sinus (chronic) —see Sinusitis
  nasopharynx —see Nasopharyngitis
  navel L08.82
  Necator americanus B76.1
  Neisseria —see Gonococcus
  Neotestudina rosatii B47.0
  newborn P39.9
    intra-amniotic NEC P39.2
    skin P39.4
    specified type NEC P39.8
  nipple N61.0
    associated with
      lactation O91.03
      pregnancy O91.01-•
      puerperium O91.02
  Nocardia —see Nocardiosis
  obstetrical surgical wound (puerperal)
    O86.00
    incisional site
      deep O86.02
      superficial O86.01
    organ and space site O86.03
    surgical site specified NEC O86.09
  Oesophagostomum (apiostomum)
    B81.8
  Oestrus ovis —see Myiasis
  Oidium albicans B37.9
  Onchocerca (volvulus) —see Onchocerciasis -
    oncovirus, as cause of disease classified
      elsewhere B97.32
  operation wound T81.49
  Opisthorchis (felineus) (viverrini) B66.0
  orbit, orbital —see Inflammation, orbit
  orthopoxvirus NEC B08.09
  ovary —see Salpingo-oophoritis
  Oxyuris vermicularis B80

▶ New   ⇒ Revised   ~~deleted~~ Deleted   • Use Additional Character(s)

Infection, infected, infective *(Continued)*
  pancreas (acute) —*see* Pancreatitis, acute
    abscess —*see* Pancreatitis, acute
    specified NEC —*see also* Pancreatitis, acute
      K85.80
  papillomavirus, as cause of disease classified
    elsewhere B97.7
  papovavirus NEC B34.4
  Paracoccidioides brasiliensis —*see*
    Paracoccidioidomycosis
  Paragonimus (westermani) B66.4
  parainfluenza virus B34.8
  parameningococcus NOS A39.9
  parapoxvirus B08.60
    specified NEC B08.69
  parasitic B89
  Parastrongylus
    cantonensis B83.2
    costaricensis B81.3
    paratyphoid A01.4
      Type A A01.1
      Type B A01.2
      Type C A01.3
  paraurethral ducts N34.2
  parotid gland —*see* Sialoadenitis
  parvovirus NEC B34.3
    as cause of disease classified elsewhere
      B97.6
  Pasteurella NEC A28.0
    multocida A28.0
    pestis —*see* Plague
    pseudotuberculosis A28.0
    septica (cat bite) (dog bite) A28.0
    tularensis —*see* Tularemia
  pelvic, female —*see* Disease, pelvis,
    inflammatory
  Penicillium (marneffei) B48.4
  penis (glans) (retention) NEC N48.29
  periapical K04.5
  peridental, periodontal K05.20
    generalized —*see* Periodontitis, aggressive,
      generalized
    localized —*see* Periodontitis, aggressive,
      localized
  perinatal period P39.9
    specified type NEC P39.8
  perineal repair (puerperal) O86.09
  periorbital —*see* Inflammation, orbit
  perirectal K62.89
  perirenal —*see* Infection, kidney
  peritoneal —*see* Peritonitis
  periureteral N28.89
  Petriellidium boydii B48.2
  pharynx —*see also* Pharyngitis
    coxsackievirus B08.5
    posterior, lymphoid (chronic) J35.03
  Phialophora
    gougerotii (subcutaneous abscess or cyst)
      B43.2
    jeanselmei (subcutaneous abscess or cyst)
      B43.2
    verrucosa (skin) B43.0
  Piedraia hortae B36.3
  pinta A67.9
    intermediate A67.1
    late A67.2
    mixed A67.3
    primary A67.0
  pinworm B80
  pityrosporum furfur B36.0
  pleuro-pneumonia-like organism (PPLO)
    NEC A49.3
    as cause of disease classified elsewhere
      B96.0
  pneumococcus, pneumococcal NEC A49.1
    as cause of disease classified elsewhere
      B95.3
    generalized (purulent) A40.3
      with pneumonia J13
  Pneumocystis carinii (pneumonia) B59
  Pneumocystis jiroveci (pneumonia) B59

Infection, infected, infective *(Continued)*
  port or reservoir T80.212
  postoperative T81.40
  postoperative wound T81.49
  postprocedural T81.40
    surgical site
      deep incisional T81.42
      organ and space T81.43
      specified NEC T81.49
      superficial incisional T81.41
  postvaccinal T88.0
  prepuce NEC N47.7
    with penile inflammation N47.6
  prion —*see* Disease, prion, central nervous
    system
  prostate (capsule) —*see* Prostatitis
  Proteus (mirabilis) (morganii) (vulgaris) NEC
    A49.8
    as cause of disease classified elsewhere
      B96.4
  protozoal NEC B64
    intestinal A07.9
      specified NEC A07.8
    specified NEC B60.8
  Pseudoallescheria boydii B48.2
  Pseudomonas NEC A49.8
    as cause of disease classified elsewhere
      B96.5
    mallei A24.0
    pneumonia J15.1
    pseudomallei —*see* Melioidosis
  puerperal O86.4
    genitourinary tract NEC O86.89
    major or generalized O85
    minor O86.4
    specified NEC O86.89
  pulmonary —*see* Infection, lung
  purulent —*see* Abscess
  Pyrenochaeta romeroi B47.0
  Q fever A78
  rectum (sphincter) K62.89
  renal —*see also* Infection, kidney
    pelvis and ureter (cystic) N28.85
  reovirus, as cause of disease classified
    elsewhere B97.5
  respiratory (tract) NEC J98.8
    acute J22
    chronic J98.8
    influenzal (upper) (acute) —*see* Influenza,
      with, respiratory manifestations
      NEC
    lower (acute) J22
      chronic —*see* Bronchitis, chronic
    rhinovirus J00
    syncytial virus (RSV) —*see* Infection, virus,
      respiratory syncytial (RSV)
    upper (acute) NOS J06.9
      chronic J39.8
      streptococcal J06.9
      viral NOS J06.9
        due to respiratory syncytial virus
          (RSV) J06.9 *[B97.1]*
  resulting from
    presence of internal prosthesis, implant,
      graft —*see* Complications, by site and
      type, infection
  retortamoniasis A07.8
  retroperitoneal NEC K68.9
  retrovirus B33.3
    as cause of disease classified elsewhere
      B97.30
    human
      immunodeficiency, type 2 (HIV 2)
        B97.35
      T-cell lymphotropic
        type I (HTLV-I) B97.33
        type II (HTLV-II) B97.34
    lentivirus B97.31
    oncovirus B97.32
    specified NEC B97.39
  Rhinosporidium (seeberi) B48.1

Infection, infected, infective *(Continued)*
  rhinovirus
    as cause of disease classified elsewhere
      B97.89
    unspecified nature or site B34.8
  Rhizopus —*see* Mucormycosis
  rickettsial NOS A79.9
  roundworm (large) NEC B82.0
    Ascariasis —*see also* Ascariasis B77.9
  rubella —*see* Rubella
  Saccharomyces —*see* Candidiasis
  salivary duct or gland (any) —*see*
    Sialoadenitis
  Salmonella (aertrycke) (arizonae)
    (callinarum) (cholerae-suis) (enteritidis)
    (suipestifer) (typhimurium) A02.9
    with
      (gastro) enteritis A02.0
      sepsis A02.1
      specified manifestation NEC
        A02.8
    due to food (poisoning) A02.9
    hirschfeldii A01.3
    localized A02.20
      arthritis A02.23
      meningitis A02.21
      osteomyelitis A02.24
      pneumonia A02.22
      pyelonephritis A02.25
      specified NEC A02.29
    paratyphi A01.4
      A A01.1
      B A01.2
      C A01.3
    schottmuelleri A01.2
    typhi, typhosa —*see* Typhoid
  Sarcocystis A07.8
  scabies B86
  Schistosoma —*see* Infestation, Schistosoma
  scrotum (acute) NEC N49.2
  seminal vesicle —*see* Vesiculitis
  septic
    localized, skin —*see* Abscess
  sheep liver fluke B66.3
  Shigella A03.9
    boydii A03.2
    dysenteriae A03.0
    flexneri A03.1
    group
      A A03.0
      B A03.1
      C A03.2
      D A03.3
    Schmitz (-Stutzer) A03.0
    schmitzii A03.0
    shigae A03.0
    sonnei A03.3
    specified NEC A03.8
  shoulder (joint) NEC M00.9
    due to internal joint prosthesis
      T84.59
    skin NEC L08.9
  sinus (accessory) (chronic) (nasal) —*see also*
    Sinusitis
    pilonidal —*see* Sinus, pilonidal
    skin NEC L08.89
  Skene's duct or gland —*see* Urethritis
  skin (local) (staphylococcal) (streptococcal)
    L08.9
    abscess - code by site under Abscess
    cellulitis - code by site under Cellulitis
    due to fungus B36.9
      specified type NEC B36.8
    mycotic B36.9
      specified type NEC B36.8
    newborn P39.4
    ulcer —*see* Ulcer, skin
  slow virus A81.9
    specified NEC A81.89
  Sparganum (mansoni) (proliferum) (baxteri)
    B70.1

Infection, infected, infective (Continued)

specific —see also Syphilis
  to perinatal period —see Infection,
    congenital
specified NEC B99.8
spermatic cord NEC N49.1
sphenoidal (sinus) —see Sinusitis,
  sphenoidal
spinal cord NOS —see also Myelitis G04.91
  abscess G06.1
  meninges —see Meningitis
  streptococcal G04.89
Spirillum A25.0
spirochetal NOS A69.9
  lung A69.8
  specified NEC A69.8
Spirometra larvae B70.1
spleen D73.89
Sporotrichum, Sporothrix (schenckii) —see
  Sporotrichosis
staphylococcal, unspecified site
  aureus (methicillin susceptible) (MSSA)
    A49.01
    methicillin resistant (MRSA) A49.02
  as cause of disease classified elsewhere
    B95.8
    aureus (methicillin susceptible) (MSSA)
      B95.61
      methicillin resistant (MRSA)
        B95.62
    specified NEC B95.7
  food poisoning A05.0
  generalized (purulent) A41.2
  pneumonia —see Pneumonia,
    staphylococcal
Stellantchasmus falcatus B66.8
streptobacillus moniliformis A25.1
streptococcal NEC A49.1
  as cause of disease classified elsewhere
    B95.5
  B genitourinary complicating
    childbirth O98.82
    pregnancy O98.81-●
    puerperium O98.83
  congenital
    sepsis P36.10
      group B P36.0
      specified NEC P36.19
  generalized (purulent) A40.9
Streptomyces B47.1
Strongyloides (stercoralis) —see
  Strongyloidiasis
stump (amputation) (surgical) —see
  Complication, amputation stump,
  infection
subcutaneous tissue, local L08.9
suipestifer —see Infection, salmonella
swimming pool bacillus A31.1
Taenia —see Infestation, Taenia
Taeniarhynchus saginatus B68.1
tapeworm —see Infestation,
  tapeworm
tendon (sheath) —see Tenosynovitis, infective
  NEC
Ternidens diminutus B81.8
testis —see Orchitis
threadworm B80
throat —see Pharyngitis
thyroglossal duct K14.8
toe (skin) L08.9
  cellulitis L03.03-●
    fungus B35.1
  nail L03.03-●
    fungus B35.1
tongue NEC K14.0
  parasitic B37.0
tonsil (and adenoid) (faucial) (lingual)
  (pharyngeal) —see Tonsillitis
tooth, teeth K04.7
  irreversible K04.02
  periapical K04.7

Infection, infected, infective (Continued)

tooth, teeth (Continued)
  peridental, periodontal K05.20
    generalized —see Periodontitis,
      aggressive, generalized
    localized —see Periodontitis, aggressive,
      localized
  pulp K04.01
    irreversible K04.02
    reversible K04.01
TORCH —see Infection, congenital
  without active infection P00.2
Torula histolytica —see Cryptococcosis
Toxocara (canis) (cati) (felis) B83.0
Toxoplasma gondii —see Toxoplasma
trachea, chronic J42
trematode NEC —see Infestation, fluke
trench fever A79.0
Treponema pallidum —see Syphilis
Trichinella (spiralis) B75
Trichomonas A59.9
  cervix A59.09
  intestine A07.8
  prostate A59.02
  specified site NEC A59.8
  urethra A59.03
  urogenitalis A59.00
  vagina A59.01
  vulva A59.01
Trichophyton, trichophytic —see
  Dermatophytosis
Trichosporon (beigelii) cutaneum B36.2
Trichostrongylus B81.2
Trichuris (trichiura) B79
Trombicula (irritans) B88.0
Trypanosoma
  brucei
    gambiense B56.0
    rhodesiense B56.1
  cruzi —see Chagas' disease
tubal —see Salpingo-oophoritis
tuberculous
  latent (LTBI) Z22.7
  NEC —see Tuberculosis
tubo-ovarian —see Salpingo-oophoritis
tunica vaginalis N49.1
tunnel T80.212
tympanic membrane NEC —see Myringitis
typhoid (abortive) (ambulant) (bacillus) —see
  Typhoid
typhus A75.9
  flea-borne A75.2
  mite-borne A75.3
  recrudescent A75.1
  tick-borne A77.9
    African A77.1
    North Asian A77.2
umbilicus L08.82
ureter —see Ureteritis
urethra —see Urethritis
urinary (tract) N39.0
  bladder —see Cystitis
  complicating
    pregnancy O23.4-●
      specified type NEC O23.3-●
  kidney —see Infection, kidney
  newborn P39.3
  puerperal (postpartum) O86.20
  tuberculous A18.13
  urethra —see Urethritis
uterus, uterine —see Endometritis
vaccination T88.0
vaccinia not from vaccination B08.011
vagina (acute) —see Vaginitis
varicella B01.9
varicose veins —see Varix
vas deferens NEC N49.1
vesical —see Cystitis
Vibrio
  cholerae A00.0
    El Tor A00.1

Infection, infected, infective (Continued)

Vibrio (Continued)
  parahaemolyticus (food poisoning)
    A05.3
  vulnificus
    as cause of disease classified elsewhere
      B96.82
    foodborne intoxication A05.5
Vincent's (gum) (mouth) (tonsil) A69.1
virus, viral NOS B34.9
  adenovirus
    as cause of disease classified elsewhere
      B97.0
    unspecified nature or site B34.0
  arborvirus, arbovirus arthropod-borne
    A94
  as cause of disease classified elsewhere
    B97.89
    adenovirus B97.0
    coronavirus B97.29
      SARS-associated B97.21
    coxsackievirus B97.11
    echovirus B97.12
    enterovirus B97.10
      coxsackievirus B97.11
      echovirus B97.12
      specified NEC B97.19
    human
      immunodeficiency, type 2 (HIV 2)
        B97.35
      metapneumovirus B97.81
      T-cell lymphotropic,
        type I (HTLV-I) B97.33
        type II (HTLV-II) B97.34
    papillomavirus B97.7
    parvovirus B97.6
    reovirus B97.5
    respiratory syncytial (RSV) —see
      Infection virus, respiratory
      syncytial (RSV)
    retrovirus B97.30
      human
        immunodeficiency, type 2 (HIV 2)
          B97.35
        T-cell lymphotropic,
          type I (HTLV-I) B97.33
          type II (HTLV-II) B97.34
      lentivirus B97.31
      oncovirus B97.32
      specified NEC B97.39
    specified NEC B97.89
  central nervous system A89
    atypical A81.9
      specified NEC A81.89
    enterovirus NEC A88.8
      meningitis A87.0
    slow virus A81.9
      specified NEC A81.89
    specified NEC A88.8
  chest J98.8
  cotia B08.8
  COVID-19 U07.1
  coxsackie —see also Infection, coxsackie
    B34.1
    as cause of disease classified elsewhere
      B97.11
  ECHO
    as cause of disease classified elsewhere
      B97.12
    unspecified nature or site B34.1
  encephalitis, tick-borne A84.9
  enterovirus, as cause of disease classified
    elsewhere B97.10
    coxsackievirus B97.11
    echovirus B97.12
    specified NEC B97.19
  exanthem NOS B09
  human metapneumovirus as cause of
    disease classified elsewhere B97.81
  human papilloma as cause of disease
    classified elsewhere B97.7

▶ New   ⇒ Revised   ~~deleted~~ Deleted   ● Use Additional Character(s)

Infection, infected, infective *(Continued)*
  virus, viral NOS *(Continued)*
    intestine —*see* Enteritis, viral
    respiratory syncytial (RSV) —*see* Infection
        virus, respiratory syncytial (RSV)
      bronchiolitis J21.0
      bronchitis J20.5
      bronchopneumonia J12.1
      otitis media H65.-• *[B97.4]*
      pneumonia J12.1
      upper respiratory infection J06.9
          [B97.4]
    rhinovirus
      as cause of disease classified elsewhere
          B97.89
      unspecified nature or site B34.8
    slow A81.9
      specified NEC A81.89
    specified type NEC B33.8
      as cause of disease classified elsewhere
          B97.89
      unspecified nature or site B34.8
    unspecified nature or site B34.9
    West Nile —*see* Virus, West Nile
  vulva (acute) —*see* Vulvitis
  West Nile —*see* Virus, West Nile
  whipworm B79
  worms B83.9
    specified type NEC B83.8
  Wuchereria (bancrofti) B74.0
    malayi B74.1
  yatapoxvirus B08.70
    specified NEC B08.79
  yeast *(see also* Candidiasis) B37.9
  yellow fever —*see* Fever, yellow
  Yersinia
    enterocolitica (intestinal) A04.6
    pestis —*see* Plague
    pseudotuberculosis A28.2
  Zeis' gland —*see* Hordeolum
  Zika virus A92.5
    congenital P35.4
  zoonotic bacterial NOS A28.9
  Zopfia senegalensis B47.0
Infective, infectious —*see* condition
Infertility
  female N97.9
    age-related N97.8
    associated with
      anovulation N97.0
      cervical (mucus) disease or anomaly
          N88.3
      congenital anomaly
        cervix N88.3
        fallopian tube N97.1
        uterus N97.2
        vagina N97.8
      dysmucorrhea N88.3
      fallopian tube disease or anomaly
          N97.1
      pituitary-hypothalamic origin
          E23.0
      specified origin NEC N97.8
      Stein-Leventhal syndrome E28.2
      uterine disease or anomaly N97.2
      vaginal disease or anomaly N97.8
    due to
      cervical anomaly N88.3
      fallopian tube anomaly N97.1
      ovarian failure E28.39
      Stein-Leventhal syndrome
          E28.2
      uterine anomaly N97.2
      vaginal anomaly N97.8
    nonimplantation N97.2
    origin
      cervical N88.3
      tubal (block) (occlusion) (stenosis)
          N97.1
      uterine N97.2
      vaginal N97.8

Infertility *(Continued)*
  male N46.9
    azoospermia N46.01
      extratesticular cause N46.029
        drug therapy N46.021
        efferent duct obstruction N46.023
        infection N46.022
        radiation N46.024
        specified cause NEC N46.029
        systemic disease N46.025
    oligospermia N46.11
      extratesticular cause N46.129
        drug therapy N46.121
        efferent duct obstruction N46.123
        infection N46.122
        radiation N46.124
        specified cause NEC N46.129
        systemic disease N46.125
    specified type NEC N46.8
Infestation B88.9
  Acanthocheilonema (perstans) (streptocerca)
      B74.4
  Acariasis B88.0
    demodex folliculorum B88.0
    sarcoptes scabiei B86
    trombiculae B88.0
  Agamofilaria streptocerca B74.4
  Ancylostoma, ankylostoma (braziliense)
      (caninum) (ceylanicum) (duodenale)
      B76.0
    americanum B76.1
    new world B76.1
  Anisakis larvae, anisakiasis B81.0
  arthropod NEC B88.2
  Ascaris lumbricoides —*see* Ascariasis
  Balantidium coli A07.0
  beef tapeworm B68.1
  Bothriocephalus (latus) B70.0
    larval B70.1
  broad tapeworm B70.0
    larval B70.1
  Brugia (malayi) B74.1
    timori B74.2
  candiru B88.8
  Capillaria
    hepatica B83.8
    philippinensis B81.1
  cat liver fluke B66.0
  cestodes B71.9
    diphyllobothrium —*see* Infestation,
        diphyllobothrium
    dipylidiasis B71.1
    hymenolepiasis B71.0
    specified type NEC B71.8
  chigger B88.0
  chigo, chigoe B88.1
  Clonorchis (sinensis) (liver) B66.1
  coccidial A07.3
  crab-lice B85.3
  Cysticercus cellulosae —*see* Cysticercosis
  Demodex (folliculorum) B88.0
  Dermanyssus gallinae B88.0
  Dermatobia (hominis) —*see* Myiasis
  Dibothriocephalus (latus) B70.0
    larval B70.1
  Dicrocoelium dendriticum B66.2
  Diphyllobothrium (adult) (latum) (intestinal)
      (pacificum) B70.0
    larval B70.1
  Diplogonoporus (grandis) B71.8
  Dipylidium caninum B67.4
  Distoma hepaticum B66.3
  dog tapeworm B67.4
  Dracunculus medinensis B72
  dragon worm B72
  dwarf tapeworm B71.0
  Echinococcus —*see* Echinococcus
  Echinostomum ilocanum B66.8
  Entamoeba (histolytica) —*see* Infection,
      Ameba
  Enterobius vermicularis B80

Infestation *(Continued)*
  eyelid
    in (due to)
      leishmaniasis B55.1
      loiasis B74.3
      onchocerciasis B73.09
      phthiriasis B85.3
    parasitic NOS B89
  eyeworm B74.3
  Fasciola (gigantica) (hepatica) (indica) B66.3
  Fasciolopsis (buski) (intestine) B66.5
  filarial B74.9
    bancroftian B74.0
    conjunctiva B74.9
    due to
      Acanthocheilonema (perstans)
          (streptocerca) B74.4
      Brugia (malayi) B74.1
        timori B74.2
      Dracunculus medinensis B72
      guinea worm B72
      loa loa B74.3
      Mansonella (ozzardi) (perstans)
          (streptocerca) B74.4
      Onchocerca volvulus B73.00
        eye B73.00
        eyelid B73.09
      Wuchereria (bancrofti) B74.0
    Malayan B74.1
    ozzardi B74.4
    specified type NEC B74.8
  fish tapeworm B70.0
    larval B70.1
  fluke B66.9
    blood NOS —*see* Schistosomiasis
    cat liver B66.0
    intestinal B66.5
    lancet B66.2
    liver (sheep) B66.3
      cat B66.0
      Chinese B66.1
      due to clonorchiasis B66.1
      oriental B66.1
    lung (oriental) B66.4
    sheep liver B66.3
    specified type NEC B66.8
  fly larvae —*see* Myiasis
  Gasterophilus (intestinalis) —*see* Myiasis
  Gastrodiscoides hominis B66.8
  Giardia lamblia A07.1
  Gnathostoma (spinigerum) B83.1
  Gongylonema B83.8
  guinea worm B72
  helminth B83.9
    angiostrongyliasis B83.2
      intestinal B81.3
    gnathostomiasis B83.1
    hirudiniasis, internal B83.4
    intestinal B82.0
      angiostrongyliasis B81.3
      anisakiasis B81.0
      ascariasis —*see* Ascariasis
      capillariasis B81.1
      cysticercosis —*see* Cysticercosis
      diphyllobothriasis —*see* Infestation,
          diphyllobothriasis
      dracunculiasis B72
      echinococcus —*see* Echinococcosis
      enterobiasis B80
      filariasis —*see* Infestation, filarial
      fluke —*see* Infestation, fluke
      hookworm —*see* Infestation, hookworm
      mixed (types classifiable to more than
          one of the titles B65.0-B81.3 and
          B81.8) B81.4
      onchocerciasis —*see* Onchocerciasis
      schistosomiasis —*see* Infestation,
          schistosoma
      specified
        cestode NEC —*see* Infestation, cestode
        type NEC B81.8

Infestation (*Continued*)
  helminth (*Continued*)
    intestinal (*Continued*)
      strongyloidiasis —*see* Strongyloidiasis
      taenia —*see* Infestation, taenia
      trichinellosis B75
      trichostrongyliasis B81.2
      trichuriasis B79
     specified type NEC B83.8
     syngamiasis B83.3
     visceral larva migrans B83.0
   Heterophyes (heterophyes) B66.8
   hookworm B76.9
    ancylostomiasis B76.0
    necatoriasis B76.1
    specified type NEC B76.8
   Hymenolepis (diminuta) (nana) B71.0
   intestinal NEC B82.9
   leeches (aquatic) (land) —*see* Hirudiniasis
   Leishmania —*see* Leishmaniasis
   lice, louse —*see* Infestation, Pediculus
   Linguatula B88.8
   Liponyssoides sanguineus B88.0
   Loa loa B74.3
    conjunctival B74.3
    eyelid B74.3
   louse —*see* Infestation, Pediculus
   maggots —*see* Myiasis
   Mansonella (ozzardi) (perstans) (streptocerca) B74.4
   Medina (worm) B72
   Metagonimus (yokogawai) B66.8
   microfilaria streptocerca —*see* Onchocerciasis
    eye B73.00
    eyelid B73.09
   mites B88.9
    scabic B86
   Monilia (albicans) —*see* Candidiasis
   mouth B37.0
   Necator americanus B76.1
   nematode NEC (intestinal) B82.0
    Ancylostoma B76.0
    conjunctiva NEC B83.9
    Enterobius vermicularis B80
    Gnathostoma spinigerum B83.1
    physaloptera B80
    specified NEC B81.8
    trichostrongylus B81.2
    trichuris (trichuria) B79
   Oesophagostomum (apiostomum) B81.8
   Oestrus ovis —*see also* Myiasis B87.9
   Onchocerca (volvulus) —*see* Onchocerciasis
   Opisthorchis (felineus) (viverrini) B66.0
   orbit, parasitic NOS B89
   Oxyuris vermicularis B80
   Paragonimus (westermani) B66.4
   parasite, parasitic B89
    eyelid B89
    intestinal NOS B82.9
    mouth B37.0
    skin B88.9
    tongue B37.0
   Parastrongylus
    cantonensis B83.2
    costaricensis B81.3
   Pediculus B85.2
    body B85.1
    capitis (humanus) (any site) B85.0
    corporis (humanus) (any site) B85.1
    head B85.0
    mixed (classifiable to more than one of the titles B85.0-B85.3) B85.4
    pubis (any site) B85.3
   Pentastoma B88.8
   Phthirus (pubis) (any site) B85.3
    with any infestation classifiable to B85.0-B85.2 B85.4
   pinworm B80
   pork tapeworm (adult) B68.0

Infestation (*Continued*)
  protozoal NEC B64
   intestinal A07.9
    specified NEC A07.8
   specified NEC B60.8
  pubic, louse B85.3
  rat tapeworm B71.0
  red bug B88.0
  roundworm (large) NEC B82.0
   Ascariasis —*see also* Ascariasis B77.9
  sandflea B88.1
  Sarcoptes scabiei B86
  scabies B86
  Schistosoma B65.9
   bovis B65.8
   cercariae B65.3
   haematobium B65.0
   intercalatum B65.8
   japonicum B65.2
   mansoni B65.1
   mattheei B65.8
   mekongi B65.8
   specified type NEC B65.8
   spindale B65.8
  screw worms —*see* Myiasis
  skin NOS B88.9
  Sparganum (mansoni) (proliferum) (baxteri) B70.1
   larval B70.1
  specified type NEC B88.8
  Spirometra larvae B70.1
  Stellantchasmus falcatus B66.8
  Strongyloides stercoralis —*see* Strongyloidiasis
  Taenia B68.9
   diminuta B71.0
   echinococcus —*see* Echinococcus
   mediocanellata B68.1
   nana B71.0
   saginata B68.1
   solium (intestinal form) B68.0
    larval form —*see* Cysticercosis
  Taeniarhynchus saginatus B68.1
  tapeworm B71.9
   beef B68.1
   broad B70.0
    larval B70.1
   dog B67.4
   dwarf B71.0
   fish B70.0
    larval B70.1
   pork B68.0
   rat B71.0
  Ternidens diminutus B81.8
  Tetranychus molestissimus B88.0
  threadworm B80
  tongue B37.0
  Toxocara (canis) (cati) (felis) B83.0
  trematode(s) NEC —*see* Infestation, fluke
  Trichinella (spiralis) B75
  Trichocephalus B79
  Trichomonas —*see* Trichomoniasis
  Trichostrongylus B81.2
  Trichuris (trichiura) B79
  Trombicula (irritans) B88.0
  Tunga penetrans B88.1
  Uncinaria americana B76.1
  Vandellia cirrhosa B88.8
  whipworm B79
  worms B83.9
   intestinal B82.0
  Wuchereria (bancrofti) B74.0
Infiltrate, infiltration
  amyloid (generalized) (localized) —*see* Amyloidosis
  calcareous NEC R89.7
   localized —*see* Degeneration, by site
  calcium salt R89.7
  cardiac
   fatty —*see* Degeneration, myocardial
   glycogenic E74.02 [143]

Infiltrate, infiltration (*Continued*)
  corneal —*see* Edema, cornea
  eyelid —*see* Inflammation, eyelid
  glycogen, glycogenic —*see* Disease, glycogen storage
  heart, cardiac
   fatty —*see* Degeneration, myocardial
   glycogenic E74.02 [143]
  inflammatory in vitreous H43.89
  kidney N28.89
  leukemic —*see* Leukemia
  liver K76.89
   fatty —*see* Fatty, liver NEC
   glycogen —*see also* Disease, glycogen storage E74.03 [K77]
  lung R91.8
   eosinophilic —*see* Eosinophilia, pulmonary
  lymphatic —*see also* Leukemia, lymphatic C91.9-•
   gland I88.9
  muscle, fatty M62.89
  myocardium, myocardial
   fatty —*see* Degeneration, myocardial
   glycogenic E74.02 [143]
  on chest x-ray R91.8
  pulmonary R91.8
   with eosinophilia —*see* Eosinophilia, pulmonary
  skin (lymphocytic) L98.6
  thymus (gland) (fatty) E32.8
  urine R39.0
  vesicant agent
   antineoplastic chemotherapy T80.810
   other agent NEC T80.818
  vitreous body H43.89
Infirmity R68.89
  senile R54
Inflammation, inflamed, inflammatory (with exudation)
  abducent (nerve) —*see* Strabismus, paralytic, sixth nerve
  accessory sinus (chronic) —*see* Sinusitis
  adrenal (gland) E27.8
  alveoli, teeth M27.3
   scorbutic E54
  anal canal, anus K62.89
  antrum (chronic) —*see* Sinusitis, maxillary
  appendix —*see* Appendicitis
  arachnoid —*see* Meningitis
  areola N61.0
   puerperal, postpartum or gestational —*see* Infection, nipple
  areolar tissue NOS L08.9
  artery —*see* Arteritis
  auditory meatus (external) —*see* Otitis, externa
  Bartholin's gland N75.8
  bile duct (common) (hepatic) or passage —*see* Cholangitis
  bladder —*see* Cystitis
  bone —*see* Osteomyelitis
  brain —*see also* Encephalitis
   membrane —*see* Meningitis
  breast N61.0
   puerperal, postpartum, gestational —*see* Mastitis, obstetric
  broad ligament —*see* Disease, pelvis, inflammatory
  bronchi —*see* Bronchitis
  catarrhal J00
  cecum —*see* Appendicitis
  cerebral —*see also* Encephalitis
   membrane —*see* Meningitis
  cerebrospinal
   meningococcal A39.0
  cervix (uteri) —*see* Cervicitis
  chest J98.8
  chorioretinal H30.9-•
   cyclitis —*see* Cyclitis
   disseminated H30.10-•
    generalized H30.13-•
    peripheral H30.12-•
    posterior pole H30.11-•

Inflammation, inflamed, inflammatory
(Continued)
  chorioretinal *(Continued)*
    epitheliopathy —*see* Epitheliopathy
    focal H30.00-●
      juxtapapillary H30.01-●
      macular H30.04-●
      paramacular —*see* Inflammation,
        chorioretinal, focal, macular
      peripheral H30.03-●
      posterior pole H30.02-●
      specified type NEC H30.89-●
  choroid —*see* Inflammation, chorioretinal
  chronic, postmastoidectomy cavity —*see*
    Complications, postmastoidectomy,
    inflammation
  colon —*see* Enteritis
  connective tissue (diffuse) NEC —*see*
    Disorder, soft tissue, specified type NEC
  cornea —*see* Keratitis
  corpora cavernosa N48.29
  cranial nerve —*see* Disorder, nerve, cranial
  Douglas' cul-de-sac or pouch (chronic) N73.0
  due to device, implant or graft —*see also*
    Complications, by site and type,
    infection or inflammation
    arterial graft T82.7
    breast (implant) T85.79
    catheter T85.79
      dialysis (renal) T82.7
        intraperitoneal T85.71
      infusion T82.7
        cranial T85.735
        intrathecal T85.735
        spinal (epidural) (subdural) T85.735
        subarachnoid T85.735
      urinary T83.518
        cystostomy T83.510
        Hopkins T83.518
        ileostomy T83.518
        nephrostomy T83.512
        specified NEC T83.518
        urethral indwelling T83.511
        urostomy T83.518
    electronic (electrode) (pulse generator)
      (stimulator)
      bone T84.7
      cardiac T82.7
      nervous system T85.738
        brain T85.731
        cranial nerve T85.732
        gastric nerve T85.732
        neurostimulator generator T85.734
        peripheral nerve T85.732
        sacral nerve T85.732
        spinal cord T85.733
        vagal nerve T85.732
      urinary T83.590
    fixation, internal (orthopedic) NEC —
      see Complication, fixation device,
      infection
    gastrointestinal (bile duct) (esophagus)
      T85.79
    neurostimulator electrode (lead) T85.732
    genital NEC T83.69
    heart NEC T82.7
      valve (prosthesis) T82.6
        graft T82.7
    joint prosthesis —*see* Complication, joint
      prosthesis, infection
    ocular (corneal graft) (orbital implant)
      NEC T85.79
    orthopedic NEC T84.7
    penile (cylinder) (pump) (resevoir) T83.61
    specified NEC T85.79
    testicular T83.62
    urinary NEC T83.598
      ileal conduit stent T83.593
      implanted neurostimulation T83.590
      implanted sphincter T83.591
      indwelling ureteral stent T83.592

Inflammation, inflamed, inflammatory
(Continued)
  due to device, implant or graft *(Continued)*
  (Continued)
    urinary NEC *(Continued)*
      nephroureteral stent T83.593
      specified stent NEC T83.593
    vascular NEC T82.7
    ventricular intracranial (communicating)
      shunt T85.730
  duodenum K29.80
    with bleeding K29.81
  dura mater —*see* Meningitis
  ear (middle) —*see also* Otitis, media
    external —*see* Otitis, externa
    inner —*see* subcategory H83.0
  epididymis —*see* Epididymitis
  esophagus —*see* Esophagitis
  ethmoidal (sinus) (chronic) —*see* Sinusitis,
    ethmoidal
  eustachian tube (catarrhal) —*see* Salpingitis,
    eustachian
  eyelid H01.9
    abscess —*see* Abscess, eyelid
    blepharitis —*see* Blepharitis
    chalazion —*see* Chalazion
    dermatosis (noninfectious) —*see*
      Dermatosis, eyelid
    hordeolum —*see* Hordeolum
    specified NEC H01.8
  fallopian tube —*see* Salpingo-oophoritis
  fascia —*see* Myositis
  follicular, pharynx J31.2
  frontal (sinus) (chronic) —*see* Sinusitis, frontal
  gallbladder —*see* Cholecystitis
  gastric —*see* Gastritis
  gastrointestinal — *see* Enteritis
  genital organ (internal) (diffuse)
    female —*see* Disease, pelvis, inflammatory
    male N49.9
      multiple sites N49.8
      specified NEC N49.8
  gland (lymph) —*see* Lymphadenitis
  glottis —*see* Laryngitis
  granular, pharynx J31.2
  gum K05.10
    nonplaque induced K05.11
    plaque induced K05.10
  heart —*see* Carditis
  hepatic duct —*see* Cholangitis
  ileoanal (internal) pouch K91.850
  ileum —*see also* Enteritis
    regional or terminal —*see* Enteritis, regional
  intestinal pouch K91.850
  intestine (any part) —*see* Enteritis
  jaw (acute) (bone) (chronic) (lower)
    (suppurative) (upper) M27.2
  joint NEC —*see* Arthritis
    sacroiliac M46.1
  kidney —*see* Nephritis
  knee (joint) M13.169
    tuberculous A18.02
  labium (majus) (minus) —*see* Vulvitis
  lacrimal
    gland —*see* Dacryoadenitis
    passages (duct) (sac) —*see also* Dacryocystitis
      canaliculitis —*see* Canaliculitis, lacrimal
  larynx —*see* Laryngitis
  leg NOS L08.9
  lip K13.0
  liver (capsule) —*see also* Hepatitis
    chronic K73.9
    suppurative K75.0
  lung (acute) —*see also* Pneumonia
    chronic J98.4
  lymphatic vessel —*see* Lymphangitis
  lymph gland or node —*see* Lymphadenitis
  maxilla, maxillary M27.2
    sinus (chronic) —*see* Sinusitis, maxillary
  membranes of brain or spinal cord —*see*
    Meningitis

Inflammation, inflamed, inflammatory
(Continued)
  meninges —*see* Meningitis
  mouth K12.1
  muscle —*see* Myositis
  myocardium —*see* Myocarditis
  nasal sinus (chronic) —*see* Sinusitis
  nasopharynx —*see* Nasopharyngitis
  navel L08.82
  ➠nerve NEC —*see* Neuritis
  nipple N61.0
    puerperal, postpartum or gestational —*see*
      Infection, nipple
  nose —*see* Rhinitis
  oculomotor (nerve) —*see* Strabismus,
    paralytic, third nerve
  optic nerve —*see* Neuritis, optic
  orbit (chronic) H05.10
    acute H05.00
      abscess —*see* Abscess, orbit
      cellulitis —*see* Cellulitis, orbit
      osteomyelitis —*see* Osteomyelitis, orbit
      periostitis —*see* Periostitis, orbital
      tenonitis —*see* Tenonitis, eye
    granuloma —*see* Granuloma, orbit
    myositis —*see* Myositis, orbital
  ovary —*see* Salpingo-oophoritis
  oviduct —*see* Salpingo-oophoritis
  pancreas (acute) —*see* Pancreatitis
  parametrium N73.0
  parotid region L08.9
  pelvis, female —*see* Disease, pelvis,
    inflammatory
  penis (corpora cavernosa) N48.29
  perianal K62.89
  pericardium —*see* Pericarditis
  perineum (female) (male) L08.9
  perirectal K62.89
  peritoneum —*see* Peritonitis
  periuterine —*see* Disease, pelvis, inflammatory
  perivesical — *see* Cystitis
  petrous bone (acute) (chronic) —*see* Petrositis
  pharynx (acute) —*see* Pharyngitis
  pia mater —*see* Meningitis
  pleura —*see* Pleurisy
  polyp, colon —*see also* Polyp, colon,
    inflammatory K51.40
  prostate — *see also* Prostatitis
    specified type NEC N41.8
  rectosigmoid —*see* Rectosigmoiditis
  rectum —*see also* Proctitis K62.89
  respiratory, upper —*see also* Infection,
    respiratory, upper J06.9
    acute, due to radiation J70.0
    chronic, due to external agent —*see*
      condition, respiratory, chronic, due to
    due to
      chemicals, gases, fumes or vapors
        (inhalation) J68.2
      radiation J70.1
  retina —*see* Chorioretinitis
  retrocecal —*see* Appendicitis
  retroperitoneal —*see* Peritonitis
  salivary duct or gland (any) (suppurative) —
    see Sialoadenitis
  scorbutic, alveoli, teeth E54
  scrotum N49.2
  seminal vesicle —*see* Vesiculitis
  sigmoid —*see* Enteritis
  sinus —*see* Sinusitis
  Skene's duct or gland —*see* Urethritis
  skin L08.9
  spermatic cord N49.1
  sphenoidal (sinus) —*see* Sinusitis, sphenoidal
  spinal
    cord —*see* Encephalitis
    membrane —*see* Meningitis
    nerve —*see* Disorder, nerve
  spine —*see* Spondylopathy, inflammatory
  spleen (capsule) D73.89
  stomach —*see* Gastritis

Inflammation, inflamed, inflammatory
  (Continued)
  subcutaneous tissue L08.9
  suprarenal (gland) E27.8
  synovial —*see* Tenosynovitis
  tendon (sheath) NEC —*see* Tenosynovitis
  testis —*see* Orchitis
  throat (acute) —*see* Pharyngitis
  thymus (gland) E32.8
  thyroid (gland) —*see* Thyroiditis
  tongue K14.0
  tonsil —*see* Tonsillitis
  trachea —*see* Tracheitis
  trochlear (nerve) —*see* Strabismus, paralytic,
    fourth nerve
  tubal —*see* Salpingo-oophoritis
  tuberculous NEC —*see* Tuberculosis
  tubo-ovarian —*see* Salpingo-oophoritis
  tunica vaginalis N49.1
  tympanic membrane —*see* Tympanitis
  umbilicus, umbilical L08.82
  uterine ligament —*see* Disease, pelvis,
    inflammatory
  uterus (catarrhal) —*see* Endometritis
  uveal tract (anterior) NOS —*see also*
    Iridocyclitis
    posterior —*see* Chorioretinitis
  vagina —*see* Vaginitis
  vas deferens N49.1
  vein —*see also* Phlebitis
    intracranial or intraspinal (septic) G08
    thrombotic I80.9
      leg —*see* Phlebitis, leg
      lower extremity —*see* Phlebitis, leg
  vocal cord J38.3
  vulva —*see* Vulvitis
  Wharton's duct (suppurative) —*see*
    Sialoadenitis
Inflation, lung, imperfect (newborn) —*see*
  Atelectasis
Influenza (bronchial) (epidemic) (respiratory
  (upper)) (unidentified influenza virus) J11.1
  with
    digestive manifestations J11.2
    encephalopathy J11.81
    enteritis J11.2
    gastroenteritis J11.2
    gastrointestinal manifestations J11.2
    laryngitis J11.1
    myocarditis J11.82
    otitis media J11.83
    pharyngitis J11.1
    pneumonia J11.00
      specified type J11.08
    respiratory manifestations NEC J11.1
    specified manifestation NEC J11.89
  A (non-novel) J10-●
  A/H5N1 —*see also* Influenza, due to,
    identified novel influenza A virus J09.X2
  avian —*see also* Influenza, due to, identified
    novel influenza A virus J09.X2
  B J10-●
  bird —*see also* Influenza, due to, identified
    novel influenza A virus J09.X2
  C J10-●
  novel (2009) H1N1 influenza —*see also*
    Influenza, due to, identified influenza
    virus NEC J10.1
  novel influenza A/H1N1 —*see also* Influenza,
    due to, identified influenza virus NEC
    J10.1
  due to
    avian (*see also* Influenza, due to, identified
      novel influenza A virus) J09.X2
    identified influenza virus NEC J10.1
      with
        digestive manifestations J10.2
        encephalopathy J10.81
        enteritis J10.2
        gastroenteritis J10.2
        gastrointestinal manifestations J10.2

Influenza *(Continued)*
  due to *(Continued)*
    identified influenza virus NEC *(Continued)*
      with *(Continued)*
        laryngitis J10.1
        myocarditis J10.82
        otitis media J10.83
        pharyngitis J10.1
        pneumonia (unspecified type) J10.00
          with same identified influenza virus
            J10.01
          specified type NEC J10.08
        respiratory manifestations NEC J10.1
        specified manifestation NEC J10.89
    identified novel influenza A virus J09.X2
      with
        digestive manifestations J09.X3
        encephalopathy J09.X9
        enteritis J09.X3
        gastroenteritis J09.X3
        gastrointestinal manifestations J09.X3
        laryngitis J09.X2
        myocarditis J09.X9
        otitis media J09.X9
        pharyngitis J09.X2
        pneumonia J09.X1
        respiratory manifestations NEC
          J09.X2
        specified manifestation NEC J09.X9
        upper respiratory symptoms J09.X2
    of other animal origin, not bird or swine (*see*
      also Influenza, due to, identified novel
      influenza A virus) J09.X2
    swine (viruses that normally cause infections
      in pigs) —*see also* Influenza, due to,
      identified novel influenza A virus
      J09.X2
Influenza-like disease —*see* Influenza
Influenzal —*see* Influenza
Infraction, Freiberg's (metatarsal head) —*see*
  Osteochondrosis, juvenile, metatarsus
Infraeruption of tooth (teeth) M26.34
Infusion complication, misadventure, or
  reaction —*see* Complications, infusion
Ingestion
  chemical —*see* Table of Drugs and Chemicals,
    by substance, poisoning
  drug or medicament
    correct substance properly administered —
      see Table of Drugs and Chemicals, by
      drug, adverse effect
    overdose or wrong substance given
      or taken —*see* Table of Drugs and
      Chemicals, by drug, poisoning
  foreign body —*see* Foreign body, alimentary
    tract
  multiple drug —*see* Table of Drugs and
    Chemicals, multiple
  tularemia A21.3
Ingrowing
  hair (beard) L73.1
  nail (finger) (toe) L60.0
Inguinal —*see also* condition
  testicle Q53.9
    bilateral Q53.212
    unilateral Q53.112
Inhalant-induced
  anxiety disorder F18.980
  depressive disorder F18.94
  major neurocognitive disorder F18.97
  mild neurocognitive disorder F18.988
  psychotic disorder F18.959
Inhalation
  anthrax A22.1
  flame T27.3
  food or foreign body —*see* Foreign body, by
    site
  gases, fumes, or vapors T59.9-●
    specified agent NEC —*see* Table of Drugs
      and Chemicals, by substance
      T59.89-●

Inhalation *(Continued)*
  liquid or vomitus —*see* Asphyxia
  meconium (newborn) P24.00
    with
      with respiratory symptoms P24.01
      pneumonia (pneumonitis) P24.01
  mucus —*see* Asphyxia, mucus
  oil or gasoline (causing suffocation) —*see*
    Foreign body, by site
  smoke T59.81-●
    with respiratory conditions J70.5
      due to chemicals, gases, fumes and
        vapors J68.9
  ➠ steam (*see also* Burn, respiratory tract) T59.9-●
  stomach contents or secretions —*see* Foreign
    body, by site
    due to anesthesia (general) (local) or other
      sedation T88.59
      in labor and delivery O74.0
      in pregnancy O29.01-●
      postpartum, puerperal O89.01
Inhibition, orgasm
  female F52.31
  male F52.32
Inhibitor, systemic lupus erythematosus
  (presence of) D68.62
Iniencephalus, iniencephaly Q00.2
Injection, traumatic jet (air) (industrial) (water)
  (paint or dye) T70.4
Injury —*see also* specified injury type T14.90
  abdomen, abdominal S39.91
    blood vessel —*see* Injury, blood vessel,
      abdomen
    cavity —*see* Injury, intra-abdominal
    contusion S30.1
    internal —*see* Injury, intra-abdominal
    intra-abdominal organ —*see* Injury,
      intra-abdominal
    nerve —*see* Injury, nerve, abdomen
    open —*see* Wound, open, abdomen
    specified NEC S39.81
    superficial —*see* Injury, superficial,
      abdomen
  Achilles tendon S86.00-●
    laceration S86.02-●
    specified type NEC S86.09-●
    strain S86.01-●
  acoustic, resulting in deafness —*see* Injury,
    nerve, acoustic
  adrenal (gland) S37.819
    contusion S37.812
    laceration S37.813
    specified type NEC S37.818
  alveolar (process) S09.93
  ankle S99.91-●
    contusion —*see* Contusion, ankle
    dislocation —*see* Dislocation, ankle
    fracture —*see* Fracture, ankle
    nerve —*see* Injury, nerve, ankle
    open —*see* Wound, open, ankle
    specified type NEC S99.81-●
    sprain —*see* Sprain, ankle
    superficial —*see* Injury, superficial, ankle
  anterior chamber, eye —*see* Injury, eye,
    specified site NEC
  anus —*see* Injury, abdomen
  aorta (thoracic) S25.00
    abdominal S35.00
      laceration (minor) (superficial) S35.01
        major S35.02
      specified type NEC S35.09
    laceration (minor) (superficial) S25.01
      major S25.02
    specified type NEC S25.09
  arm (upper) S49.9-●
    blood vessel —*see* Injury, blood vessel,
      arm
    contusion —*see* Contusion, arm, upper
    fracture —*see* Fracture, humerus
    lower —*see* Injury, forearm
    muscle —*see* Injury, muscle, shoulder

  ▶ New   ➠ Revised   ~~deleted~~ Deleted   ● Use Additional Character(s)

Injury *(Continued)*
  arm *(Continued)*
    nerve —*see* Injury, nerve, arm
    open —*see* Wound, open, arm
    specified type NEC S49.8-●
    superficial —*see* Injury, superficial, arm
  artery (complicating trauma) —*see also* Injury, blood vessel, by site
    cerebral or meningeal —*see* Injury, intracranial
  auditory canal (external) (meatus) S09.91
  auricle, auris, ear S09.91
  axilla —*see* Injury, shoulder
  back —*see* Injury, back, lower
  bile duct S36.13
  birth —*see also* Birth, injury P15.9
  bladder (sphincter) S37.20
    at delivery O71.5
    contusion S37.22
    laceration S37.23
    obstetrical trauma O71.5
    specified type NEC S37.29
  blast (air) (hydraulic) (immersion) (underwater) NEC T14.8
    acoustic nerve trauma —*see* Injury, nerve, acoustic
    bladder —*see* Injury, bladder
    brain —*see* Concussion
    colon —*see* Injury, intestine, large, blast injury
    ear (primary) S09.31-●
      secondary S09.39-●
    generalized T70.8
    lung —*see* Injury, intrathoracic, lung, blast injury
    multiple body organs T70.8
    peritoneum S36.81
    rectum S36.61
    retroperitoneum S36.898
    small intestine S36.419
      duodenum S36.410
      specified site NEC S36.418
    specified
      intra-abdominal organ NEC S36.898
      pelvic organ NEC S37.899
  blood vessel NEC T14.8
    abdomen S35.9-●
      aorta —*see* Injury, aorta, abdominal
      celiac artery —*see* Injury, blood vessel, celiac artery
      iliac vessel —*see* Injury, blood vessel, iliac
      laceration S35.91
      mesenteric vessel —*see* Injury, mesenteric
      portal vein —*see* Injury, blood vessel, portal vein
      renal vessel —*see* Injury, blood vessel, renal
      specified vessel NEC S35.8X-●
      splenic vessel —*see* Injury, blood vessel, splenic
      vena cava —*see* Injury, vena cava, inferior
    ankle —*see* Injury, blood vessel, foot
    aorta (abdominal) (thoracic) —*see* Injury, aorta
    arm (upper) NEC S45.90-●
      forearm —*see* Injury, blood vessel, forearm
      laceration S45.91-●
      specified
        site NEC S45.80-●
          laceration S45.81-●
          specified type NEC S45.89-●
        type NEC S45.99-●
      superficial vein S45.30-●
        laceration S45.31-●
        specified type NEC S45.39-●
    axillary
      artery S45.00-●
        laceration S45.01-●
        specified type NEC S45.09-●

Injury *(Continued)*
  blood vessel NEC *(Continued)*
    axillary *(Continued)*
      vein S45.20-●
        laceration S45.21-●
        specified type NEC S45.29-●
    azygos vein —*see* Injury, blood vessel, thoracic, specified site NEC
    brachial
      artery S45.10-●
        laceration S45.11-●
        specified type NEC S45.19-●
      vein S45.20-●
        laceration S45.219
        specified type NEC S45.29-●
    carotid artery (common) (external) (internal, extracranial) S15.00-●
      internal, intracranial S06.8-●
      laceration (minor) (superficial) S15.01-●
        major S15.02-●
      specified type NEC S15.09-●
    celiac artery S35.219
      branch S35.299
        laceration (minor) (superficial) S35.291
          major S35.292
        specified NEC S35.298
      laceration (minor) (superficial) S35.211
        major S35.212
      specified type NEC S35.218
    cerebral —*see* Injury, intracranial
    deep plantar —*see* Injury, blood vessel, plantar artery
    digital (hand) —*see* Injury, blood vessel, finger
    dorsal
      artery (foot) S95.00 ●
        laceration S95.01-●
        specified type NEC S95.09-●
      vein (foot) S95.20 ●
        laceration S95.21-●
        specified type NEC S95.29-●
    due to accidental laceration during procedure —*see* Laceration, accidental complicating surgery
    extremity —*see* Injury, blood vessel, limb
    femoral
      artery (common) (superficial) S75.00-●
        laceration (minor) (superficial) S75.01-●
          major S75.02-●
        specified type NEC S75.09-●
      vein (hip level) (thigh level) S75.10-●
        laceration (minor) (superficial) S75.11-●
          major S75.12-●
        specified type NEC S75.19-●
    finger S65.50-●
      index S65.50-●
        laceration S65.51-●
        specified type NEC S65.59-●
      laceration S65.51-●
      little S65.50-●
        laceration S65.51-●
        specified type NEC S65.59-●
      middle S65.50-●
        laceration S65.51-●
        specified type NEC S65.59-●
      specified type NEC S65.59-●
      thumb —*see* Injury, blood vessel, thumb
    foot S95.90-●
      dorsal
        artery —*see* Injury, blood vessel, dorsal, artery
        vein —*see* Injury, blood vessel, dorsal, vein
      laceration S95.91-●
      plantar artery —*see* Injury, blood vessel, plantar artery
      specified
        site NEC S95.80-●
          laceration S95.81-●
          specified type NEC S95.89-●
        specified type NEC S95.99-●

Injury *(Continued)*
  blood vessel NEC *(Continued)*
    forearm S55.90-●
      laceration S55.91-●
      radial artery —*see* Injury, blood vessel, radial artery
      specified
        site NEC S55.80-●
          laceration S55.81-●
          specified type NEC S55.89-●
        type NEC S55.99-●
      ulnar artery —*see* Injury, blood vessel, ulnar artery
      vein S55.20-●
        laceration S55.21-●
        specified type NEC S55.29-●
    gastric
      artery —*see* Injury, mesenteric, artery, branch
      vein —*see* Injury, blood vessel, abdomen
    gastroduodenal artery —*see* Injury, mesenteric, artery, branch
    greater saphenous vein (lower leg level) S85.30-●
      hip (and thigh) level S75.20-●
        laceration (minor) (superficial) S75.21-●
          major S75.22-●
        specified type NEC S75.29-●
      laceration S85.31-●
      specified type NEC S85.39-●
    hand (level) S65.90-●
      finger —*see* Injury, blood vessel, finger
      laceration S65.91-●
      palmar arch —*see* Injury, blood vessel, palmar arch
      radial artery —*see* Injury, blood vessel, radial artery, hand
      specified
        site NEC S65.80-●
          laceration S65.81-●
          specified type NEC S65.89 ●
        type NEC S65.99-●
      thumb —*see* Injury, blood vessel, thumb
      ulnar artery —*see* Injury, blood vessel, ulnar artery, hand
    head S09.0
      intracranial —*see* Injury, intracranial
      multiple S09.0
    hepatic
      artery —*see* Injury, mesenteric, artery
      vein —*see* Injury, vena cava, inferior
    hip S75.90-●
      femoral artery —*see* Injury, blood vessel, femoral, artery
      femoral vein —*see* Injury, blood vessel, femoral, vein
      greater saphenous vein —*see* Injury, blood vessel, greater saphenous, hip level
      laceration S75.91-●
      specified
        site NEC S75.80-●
          laceration S75.81-●
          specified type NEC S75.89-●
        type NEC S75.99-●
    hypogastric (artery) (vein) —*see* Injury, blood vessel, iliac
    iliac S35.5-●
      artery S35.51-●
      specified vessel NEC S35.5-●
      uterine vessel —*see* Injury, blood vessel, uterine
      vein S35.51-●
    innominate —*see* Injury, blood vessel, thoracic, innominate
    intercostal (artery) (vein) —*see* Injury, blood vessel, thoracic, intercostal
    jugular vein (external) S15.20-●
      internal S15.30-●
        laceration (minor) (superficial) S15.31-●
          major S15.32-●
        specified type NEC S15.39-●

Injury *(Continued)*
  blood vessel NEC *(Continued)*
    jugular vein *(Continued)*
      laceration (minor) (superficial) S15.21-●
        major S15.22-●
      specified type NEC S15.29-●
    leg (level) (lower) S85.90-●
      greater saphenous —*see* Injury, blood
        vessel, greater saphenous
      laceration S85.91-●
      lesser saphenous —*see* Injury, blood
        vessel, lesser saphenous
      peroneal artery —*see* Injury, blood
        vessel, peroneal artery
      popliteal
        artery —*see* Injury, blood vessel,
          popliteal, artery
        vein —*see* Injury, blood vessel,
          popliteal, vein
      specified
        site NEC S85.80-●
          laceration S85.81-●
          specified type NEC S85.89-●
        type NEC S85.99-●
      thigh —*see* Injury, blood vessel, hip
      tibial artery —*see* Injury, blood vessel,
        tibial artery
    lesser saphenous vein (lower leg level)
      S85.40-●
      laceration S85.41-●
      specified type NEC S85.49-●
    limb
      lower —*see* Injury, blood vessel, leg
      upper —*see* Injury, blood vessel, arm
    lower back —*see* Injury, blood vessel,
      abdomen
      specified NEC —*see* Injury, blood vessel,
        abdomen, specified, site NEC
    mammary (artery) (vein) —*see* Injury, blood
      vessel, thoracic, specified site NEC
    mesenteric (inferior) (superior)
      artery —*see* Injury, mesenteric, artery
      vein —*see* Injury, mesenteric, vein
    neck S15.9
      specified site NEC S15.8
    ovarian (artery) (vein) —*see* subcategory
      S35.8
    palmar arch (superficial) S65.20-●
      deep S65.30-●
        laceration S65.31-●
        specified type NEC S65.39-●
      laceration S65.21-●
      specified type NEC S65.29-●
    pelvis —*see* Injury, blood vessel, abdomen
      specified NEC —*see* Injury, blood vessel,
        abdomen, specified, site NEC
    peroneal artery S85.20-●
      laceration S85.21-●
      specified type NEC S85.29-●
    plantar artery (deep) (foot) S95.10-●
      laceration S95.11-●
      specified type NEC S95.19-●
    popliteal
      artery S85.00-●
        laceration S85.01-●
        specified type NEC S85.09-●
      vein S85.50-●
        laceration S85.51-●
        specified type NEC S85.59-●
    portal vein S35.319
      laceration S35.311
      specified type NEC S35.318
    precerebral —*see* Injury, blood vessel, neck
    pulmonary (artery) (vein) —*see* Injury,
      blood vessel, thoracic, pulmonary
    radial artery (forearm level) S55.10-●
      hand and wrist (level) S65.10-●
        laceration S65.11-●
        specified type NEC S65.19-●
      laceration S55.11-●
      specified type NEC S55.19-●

Injury *(Continued)*
  blood vessel NEC *(Continued)*
    renal
      artery S35.40-●
        laceration S35.41-●
        specified NEC S35.49-●
      vein S35.40-●
        laceration S35.41-●
        specified NEC S35.49-●
    saphenous vein (greater) (lower leg
      level) —*see* Injury, blood vessel,
      greater saphenous
      hip and thigh level —*see* Injury, blood
        vessel, greater saphenous, hip level
      lesser —*see* Injury, blood vessel, lesser
        saphenous
    shoulder
      specified NEC —*see* Injury, blood vessel,
        arm, specified site NEC
      superficial vein —*see* Injury, blood
        vessel, arm, superficial vein
    specified NEC T14.8
    splenic
      artery —*see* Injury, blood vessel, celiac
        artery, branch
      vein S35.329
        laceration S35.321
        specified NEC S35.328
    subclavian —*see* Injury, blood vessel,
      thoracic, innominate
    thigh —*see* Injury, blood vessel, hip
    thoracic S25.90
      aorta S25.00
        laceration (minor) (superficial)
          S25.01
          major S25.02
        specified type NEC S25.09
      azygos vein —*see* Injury, blood vessel,
        thoracic, specified, site NEC
      innominate
        artery S25.10-●
          laceration (minor) (superficial)
            S25.11-●
            major S25.12-●
          specified type NEC S25.19-●
        vein S25.30-●
          laceration (minor) (superficial)
            S25.31-●
            major S25.32-●
          specified type NEC S25.39-●
      intercostal S25.50-●
        laceration S25.51-●
        specified type NEC S25.59-●
      laceration S25.91
      mammary vessel —*see* Injury, blood
        vessel, thoracic, specified, site NEC
      pulmonary S25.40-●
        laceration (minor) (superficial)
          S25.41-●
          major S25.42-●
        specified type NEC S25.49-●
      specified
        site NEC S25.80-●
          laceration S25.81-●
          specified type NEC S25.89-●
        type NEC S25.99
      subclavian —*see* Injury, blood vessel,
        thoracic, innominate
      vena cava (superior) S25.20
        laceration (minor) (superficial)
          S25.21
          major S25.22
        specified type NEC S25.29
    thumb S65.40-●
      laceration S65.41-●
      specified type NEC S65.49-●
    tibial artery S85.10-●
      anterior S85.13-●
        laceration S85.14-●
        specified injury NEC S85.15-●
      laceration S85.11-●

Injury *(Continued)*
  blood vessel NEC *(Continued)*
    tibial artery *(Continued)*
      posterior S85.16-●
        laceration S85.17-●
        specified injury NEC S85.18-●
      specified injury NEC S85.12-●
    ulnar artery (forearm level) S55.00-●
      hand and wrist (level) S65.00-●
        laceration S65.01-●
        specified type NEC S65.09-●
      laceration S55.01-●
      specified type NEC S55.09-●
    upper arm (level) —*see* Injury, blood vessel,
      arm
    superficial vein —*see* Injury, blood
      vessel, arm, superficial vein
    uterine S35.5-●
      artery S35.53-●
      vein S35.53-●
    vena cava —*see* Injury, vena cava
    vertebral artery S15.10-●
      laceration (minor) (superficial)
        S15.11-●
        major S15.12-●
      specified type NEC S15.19-●
    wrist (level) —*see* Injury, blood vessel,
      hand
  brachial plexus S14.3
    newborn P14.3
  brain (traumatic) S06.9-●
    diffuse (axonal) S06.2X-●
    focal S06.30-●
  brainstem S06.38-●
  breast NOS S29.9
  broad ligament —*see* Injury, pelvic organ,
    specified site NEC
  bronchus, bronchi —*see* Injury, intrathoracic,
    bronchus
  brow S09.90
  buttock S39.92
  canthus, eye S05.90
  cardiac plexus —*see* Injury, nerve, thorax,
    sympathetic
  cauda equina S34.3
  cavernous sinus —*see* Injury, intracranial
  cecum —*see* Injury, colon
  celiac ganglion or plexus —*see* Injury, nerve,
    lumbosacral, sympathetic
  cerebellum —*see* Injury, intracranial
  cerebral —*see* Injury, intracranial
  cervix (uteri) —*see* Injury, uterus
  cheek (wall) S09.93
  chest —*see* Injury, thorax
  childbirth (newborn) —*see also* Birth, injury
    maternal NEC O71.9
  chin S09.93
  choroid (eye) —*see* Injury, eye, specified site
    NEC
  clitoris S39.94
  coccyx —*see also* Injury, back, lower
    complicating delivery O71.6
  colon —*see* Injury, intestine, large
  common bile duct —*see* Injury, liver
  conjunctiva (superficial) —*see* Injury, eye,
    conjunctiva
  conus medullaris —*see* Injury, spinal, sacral
  cord
    spermatic (pelvic region) S37.898
      scrotal region S39.848
    spinal —*see* Injury, spinal cord, by region
  cornea —*see* Injury, eye, specified site NEC
    abrasion —*see* Injury, eye, cornea,
      abrasion
  cortex (cerebral) —*see also* Injury, intracranial
    visual —*see* Injury, nerve, optic
  costal region NEC S29.9
  costochondral NEC S29.9
  cranial
    cavity —*see* Injury, intracranial
    nerve —*see* Injury, nerve, cranial

    ▶ New   ⇒ Revised   ~~deleted~~ Deleted   ● Use Additional Character(s)

Injury *(Continued)*
    crushing —*see* Crush
    cutaneous sensory nerve
    cystic duct —*see* Injury, liver
    deep tissue —*see* Contusion, by site
        meaning pressure ulcer —*see* Ulcer,
            pressure L89 with final character .6
    delivery (newborn) P15.9
        maternal NEC O71.9
    Descemet's membrane —*see* Injury, eyeball,
        penetrating
    diaphragm —*see* Injury, intrathoracic,
        diaphragm
    duodenum —*see* Injury, intestine, small,
        duodenum
    ear (auricle) (external) (canal) S09.91
        abrasion —*see* Abrasion, ear
        bite —*see* Bite, ear
        blister —*see* Blister, ear
        bruise —*see* Contusion, ear
        contusion —*see* Contusion, ear
        external constriction —*see* Constriction,
            external, ear
        hematoma —*see* Hematoma, ear
        inner —*see* Injury, ear, middle
        laceration —*see* Laceration, ear
        middle S09.30-●
            blast —*see* Injury, blast, ear
            specified NEC S09.39-●
        puncture —*see* Puncture, ear
        superficial —*see* Injury, superficial, ear
    eighth cranial nerve (acoustic or auditory) —
        see Injury, nerve, acoustic
    elbow S59.90-●
        contusion —*see* Contusion, elbow
        dislocation —*see* Dislocation, elbow
        fracture —*see* Fracture, ulna, upper
            end
        open —*see* Wound, open, elbow
        specified NEC S59.80-●
        sprain —*see* Sprain, elbow
        superficial —*see* Injury, superficial,
            elbow
    eleventh cranial nerve (accessory) —*see*
        Injury, nerve, accessory
    epididymis S39.94
    epigastric region S39.91
    epiglottis NEC S19.89
    esophageal plexus —*see* Injury, nerve, thorax,
        sympathetic
    esophagus (thoracic part) —*see also* Injury,
        intrathoracic, esophagus
        cervical NEC S19.85
    eustachian tube S09.30-●
    eye S05.9-●
        avulsion S05.7-●
        ball —*see* Injury, eyeball
        conjunctiva S05.0-●
        cornea
            abrasion S05.0-●
        laceration S05.3-●
            with prolapse S05.2-●
        lacrimal apparatus S05.8X-●
        orbit penetration S05.4-●
        specified site NEC S05.8X-●
    eyeball S05.8X-●
        contusion S05.1-●
        penetrating S05.6-●
            with
                foreign body S05.5-●
                prolapse or loss of intraocular tissue
                    S05.2-●
                without prolapse or loss of intraocular
                    tissue S05.3-●
        specified type NEC S05.8-●
    eyebrow S09.93
    eyelid S09.93
        abrasion —*see* Abrasion, eyelid
        contusion —*see* Contusion, eyelid
        open —*see* Wound, open, eyelid
    face S09.93

Injury *(Continued)*
    fallopian tube S37.509
        bilateral S37.502
            blast injury S37.512
            contusion S37.522
            laceration S37.532
            specified type NEC S37.592
        blast injury (primary) S37.519
            bilateral S37.512
            secondary —*see* Injury, fallopian tube,
                specified type NEC
            unilateral S37.511
        contusion S37.529
            bilateral S37.522
            unilateral S37.521
        laceration S37.539
            bilateral S37.532
            unilateral S37.531
        specified type NEC S37.599
            bilateral S37.592
            unilateral S37.591
        unilateral S37.501
            blast injury S37.511
            contusion S37.521
            laceration S37.531
            specified type NEC S37.591
    fascia —*see* Injury, muscle
    fifth cranial nerve (trigeminal) —*see* Injury,
        nerve, trigeminal
    finger (nail) S69.9-●
        blood vessel —*see* Injury, blood vessel,
            finger
        contusion —*see* Contusion, finger
        dislocation —*see* Dislocation, finger
        fracture —*see* Fracture, finger
        muscle —*see* Injury, muscle, finger
        nerve —*see* Injury, nerve, digital, finger
        open —*see* Wound, open, finger
        specified NEC S69.8-●
        sprain —*see* Sprain, finger
        superficial —*see* Injury, superficial, finger
    first cranial nerve (olfactory) —*see* Injury,
        nerve, olfactory
    flank —*see* Injury, abdomen
    foot S99.92-●
        blood vessel —*see* Injury, blood vessel,
            foot
        contusion —*see* Contusion, foot
        dislocation —*see* Dislocation, foot
        fracture —*see* Fracture, foot
        muscle —*see* Injury, muscle, foot
        open —*see* Wound, open, foot
        specified type NEC S99.82-●
        sprain —*see* Sprain, foot
        superficial —*see* Injury, superficial, foot
    forceps NOS P15.9
    forearm S59.91-●
        blood vessel —*see* Injury, blood vessel,
            forearm
        contusion —*see* Contusion, forearm
        fracture —*see* Fracture, forearm
        muscle —*see* Injury, muscle, forearm
        nerve —*see* Injury, nerve, forearm
        open —*see* Wound, open, forearm
        specified NEC S59.81-●
        superficial —*see* Injury, superficial, forearm
    forehead S09.90
    fourth cranial nerve (trochlear) —*see* Injury,
        nerve, trochlear
    gallbladder S36.129
        contusion S36.122
        laceration S36.123
        specified NEC S36.128
    ganglion
        celiac, coeliac —*see* Injury, nerve,
            lumbosacral, sympathetic
        gasserian —*see* Injury, nerve, trigeminal
        stellate —*see* Injury, nerve, thorax,
            sympathetic
        thoracic sympathetic —*see* Injury, nerve,
            thorax, sympathetic

Injury *(Continued)*
    gasserian ganglion —*see* Injury, nerve,
        trigeminal
    gastric artery —*see* Injury, blood vessel, celiac
        artery, branch
    gastroduodenal artery —*see* Injury, blood
        vessel, celiac artery, branch
    gastrointestinal tract —*see* Injury,
        intra-abdominal
        with open wound into abdominal cavity —
            see Wound, open, with penetration
            into peritoneal cavity
        colon —*see* Injury, intestine, large
        rectum —*see* Injury, intestine, large, rectum
            with open wound into abdominal cavity
                S36.61
        small intestine —*see* Injury, intestine, small
        specified site NEC —*see* Injury, intra-
            abdominal, specified, site NEC
        stomach —*see* Injury, stomach
    genital organ(s)
        external S39.94
            specified NEC S39.848
        internal S37.90
            fallopian tube —*see* Injury, fallopian tube
            ovary —*see* Injury, ovary
            prostate —*see* Injury, prostate
            seminal vesicle —*see* Injury, pelvis,
                organ, specified site NEC
            uterus —*see* Injury, uterus
            vas deferens —*see* Injury, pelvis, organ,
                specified site NEC
    obstetrical trauma O71.9
    gland
        lacrimal laceration —*see* Injury, eye,
            specified site NEC
        salivary S09.93
        thyroid NEC S19.84
    globe (eye) S05.90
        specified NEC S05.8X-●
    groin —*see* Injury, abdomen
    gum S09.90
    hand S69.9-●
        blood vessel —*see* Injury, blood vessel,
            hand
        contusion —*see* Contusion, hand
        fracture —*see* Fracture, hand
        muscle —*see* Injury, muscle, hand
        nerve —*see* Injury, nerve, hand
        open —*see* Wound, open, hand
        specified NEC S69.8-●
        sprain —*see* Sprain, hand
        superficial —*see* Injury, superficial, hand
    head S09.90
        with loss of consciousness S06.9-●
        specified NEC S09.8-●
    heart (traumatic) S26.90
        with hemopericardium S26.00
            contusion S26.01
            laceration (mild) S26.020
                major S26.022
                moderate S26.021
            specified type NEC S26.09
        without hemopericardium S26.10
            contusion S26.11
            laceration S26.12
            specified type NEC S26.19
        contusion S26.91
        laceration S26.92
        non-traumatic (acute) (chronic) (non-
            ischemic) I5A
        specified type NEC S26.99
    heel —*see* Injury, foot
    hepatic
        artery —*see* Injury, blood vessel, celiac
            artery, branch
        duct —*see* Injury, liver
        vein —*see* Injury, vena cava, inferior
    hip S79.91-●
        blood vessel —*see* Injury, blood vessel, hip
        contusion —*see* Contusion, hip
        dislocation —*see* Dislocation, hip

Injury (Continued)
  hip (Continued)
    fracture —see Fracture, femur, neck
    muscle —see Injury, muscle, hip
    nerve —see Injury, nerve, hip
    open —see Wound, open, hip
    specified NEC S79.81-●
    sprain —see Sprain, hip
    superficial —see Injury, superficial, hip
  hymen S39.94
  hypogastric
    blood vessel —see Injury, blood vessel, iliac
    plexus —see Injury, nerve, lumbosacral,
      sympathetic
  ileum —see Injury, intestine, small
  iliac region S39.91
  instrumental (during surgery) —see
    Laceration, accidental complicating
    surgery
    birth injury —see Birth, injury
    nonsurgical —see Injury, by site
    obstetrical O71.9
      bladder O71.5
      cervix O71.3
      high vaginal O71.4
      perineal NOS O70.9
      urethra O71.5
      uterus O71.5
        with rupture or perforation O71.1
  internal T14.8
    aorta —see Injury, aorta
    bladder (sphincter) —see Injury, bladder
      with
        ectopic or molar pregnancy O08.6
        following ectopic or molar pregnancy
          O08.6
        obstetrical trauma O71.5
    bronchus, bronchi —see Injury,
      intrathoracic, bronchus
    cecum —see Injury, intestine, large
    cervix (uteri) —see also Injury, uterus
      with ectopic or molar pregnancy O08.6
      following ectopic or molar pregnancy
        O08.6
      obstetrical trauma O71.3
    chest —see Injury, intrathoracic
    gastrointestinal tract —see Injury,
      intra-abdominal
    heart —see Injury, heart
    intestine NEC —see Injury, intestine
    intrauterine —see Injury, uterus
    mesentery —see Injury, intra-abdominal,
      specified, site NEC
    pelvis, pelvic (organ) S37.90
      following ectopic or molar pregnancy
        (subsequent episode) O08.6
      obstetrical trauma NEC O71.5
        rupture or perforation O71.1
      specified NEC S39.83
    rectum —see Injury, intestine, large, rectum
    stomach —see Injury, stomach
    ureter —see Injury, ureter
    urethra (sphincter) following ectopic or
      molar pregnancy O08.6
    uterus —see Injury, uterus
  interscapular area —see Injury, thorax
  intestine
    large S36.509
      ascending (right) S36.500
        blast injury (primary) S36.510
          secondary S36.590
        contusion S36.520
        laceration S36.530
        specified type NEC S36.590
      blast injury (primary) S36.519
        ascending (right) S36.510
        descending (left) S36.512
        rectum S36.61
        sigmoid S36.513
        specified site NEC S36.518
        transverse S36.511

Injury (Continued)
  intestine (Continued)
    large (Continued)
      contusion S36.529
        ascending (right) S36.520
        descending (left) S36.522
        rectum S36.62
        sigmoid S36.523
        specified site NEC S36.528
        transverse S36.521
      descending (left) S36.502
        blast injury (primary) S36.512
          secondary S36.592
        contusion S36.522
        laceration S36.532
        specified type NEC S36.592
      laceration S36.539
        ascending (right) S36.530
        descending (left) S36.532
        rectum S36.63
        sigmoid S36.533
        specified site NEC S36.538
        transverse S36.531
      rectum S36.60
        blast injury (primary) S36.61
          secondary S36.69
        contusion S36.62
        laceration S36.63
        specified type NEC S36.69
      sigmoid S36.503
        blast injury (primary) S36.513
          secondary S36.593
        contusion S36.523
        laceration S36.533
        specified type NEC S36.593
      specified
        site NEC S36.508
          blast injury (primary)
            S36.518
            secondary S36.598
          contusion S36.528
          laceration S36.538
          specified type NEC S36.598
        type NEC S36.599
          ascending (right) S36.590
          descending (left) S36.592
          rectum S36.69
          sigmoid S36.593
          specified site NEC S36.598
          transverse S36.591
      transverse S36.501
        blast injury (primary) S36.511
          secondary S36.591
        contusion S36.521
        laceration S36.531
        specified type NEC S36.591
    small S36.409
      blast injury (primary) S36.419
        duodenum S36.410
        secondary S36.499
          duodenum S36.490
          specified site NEC S36.498
        specified site NEC S36.418
      contusion S36.429
        duodenum S36.420
        specified site NEC S36.428
      duodenum S36.400
        blast injury (primary) S36.410
          secondary S36.490
        contusion S36.420
        laceration S36.430
        specified NEC S36.490
      laceration S36.439
        duodenum S36.430
        specified site NEC S36.438
      specified
        site NEC S36.408
        type NEC S36.499
          duodenum S36.490
          specified site NEC
            S36.498

Injury (Continued)
  intra-abdominal S36.90
    adrenal gland —see Injury, adrenal gland
    bladder —see Injury, bladder
    colon —see Injury, intestine, large
    contusion S36.92
    fallopian tube —see Injury, fallopian tube
    gallbladder —see Injury, gallbladder
    intestine —see Injury, intestine
    kidney —see Injury, kidney
    laceration S36.93
    liver —see Injury, liver
    ovary —see Injury, ovary
    pancreas —see Injury, pancreas
    pelvic NOS S37.90
    peritoneum —see Injury, intra-abdominal,
      specified, site NEC
    prostate —see Injury, prostate
    rectum —see Injury, intestine, large, rectum
    retroperitoneum —see Injury, intra-
      abdominal, specified, site NEC
    seminal vesicle —see Injury, pelvis, organ,
      specified site NEC
    small intestine —see Injury, intestine, small
    specified
      pelvic S37.90
        specified
          site NEC S37.899
            specified type NEC S37.898
            type NEC S37.99
      site NEC S36.899
        contusion S36.892
        laceration S36.893
        specified type NEC S36.898
      type NEC S36.99
    spleen —see Injury, spleen
    stomach —see Injury, stomach
    ureter —see Injury, ureter
    urethra —see Injury, urethra
    uterus —see Injury, uterus
    vas deferens —see Injury, pelvis, organ,
      specified site NEC
  ⇒ intracranial (traumatic) (see also, if applicable,
    Compression, brain, traumatic) S06.9-●
    cerebellar hemorrhage, traumatic —see
      Injury, intracranial, focal
    cerebral edema, traumatic S06.1X-●
      diffuse S06.1X-●
      focal S06.1X-●
    diffuse (axonal) S06.2X-●
    epidural hemorrhage (traumatic) S06.4X-●
    focal brain injury S06.30-●
      contusion —see Contusion, cerebral
      laceration —see Laceration, cerebral
    intracerebral hemorrhage, traumatic
      S06.36-●
      left side S06.35-●
      right side S06.34-●
    subarachnoid hemorrhage, traumatic
      S06.6X-●
    subdural hemorrhage, traumatic
      S06.5X-●
  intraocular —see Injury, eyeball, penetrating
  intrathoracic S27.9
    bronchus S27.409
      bilateral S27.402
      blast injury (primary) S27.419
        bilateral S27.412
        secondary —see Injury, intrathoracic,
          bronchus, specified type NEC
        unilateral S27.411
      contusion S27.429
        bilateral S27.422
        unilateral S27.421
      laceration S27.439
        bilateral S27.432
        unilateral S27.431
      specified type NEC S27.499
        bilateral S27.492
        unilateral S27.491
      unilateral S27.401

  ▶ New   ⇒ Revised   ~~deleted~~ Deleted   ● Use Additional Character(s)

Injury (Continued)
  intrathoracic (Continued)
    diaphragm S27.809
      contusion S27.802
      laceration S27.803
      specified type NEC S27.808
    esophagus (thoracic) S27.819
      contusion S27.812
      laceration S27.813
      specified type NEC S27.818
    heart —see Injury, heart
    hemopneumothorax S27.2
    hemothorax S27.1
    lung S27.309
      aspiration J69.0
      bilateral S27.302
      blast injury (primary) S27.319
        bilateral S27.312
        secondary —see Injury, intrathoracic,
          lung, specified type NEC
        unilateral S27.311
      contusion S27.329
        bilateral S27.322
        unilateral S27.321
      laceration S27.339
        bilateral S27.332
        unilateral S27.331
      specified type NEC S27.399
        bilateral S27.392
        unilateral S27.391
      unilateral S27.301
    pleura S27.60
      laceration S27.63
      specified type NEC S27.69
    pneumothorax S27.0
    specified organ NEC S27.899
      contusion S27.892
      laceration S27.893
      specified type NEC S27.898
    thoracic duct —see Injury, intrathoracic,
      specified organ NEC
    thymus gland —see Injury, intrathoracic,
      specified organ NEC
    trachea, thoracic S27.50
      blast (primary) S27.51
      contusion S27.52
      laceration S27.53
      specified type NEC S27.59
  iris —see Injury, eye, specified site NEC
    penetrating —see Injury, eyeball,
      penetrating
  jaw S09.93
  jejunum —see Injury, intestine, small
  joint NOS T14.8
    old or residual —see Disorder, joint,
      specified type NEC
  kidney S37.00-●
    acute (nontraumatic) N17.9
    contusion —see Contusion, kidney
    laceration —see Laceration, kidney
    specified NEC S37.09-●
  knee S89.9-●
    contusion —see Contusion, knee
    dislocation —see Dislocation, knee
    meniscus (lateral) (medial) —see Sprain,
      knee, specified site NEC
      old injury or tear —see Derangement,
        knee, meniscus, due to old injury
    open —see Wound, open, knee
    specified NEC S89.8-●
    sprain —see Sprain, knee
    superficial —see Injury, superficial, knee
  labium (majus) (minus) S39.94
  labyrinth, ear S09.30-●
  lacrimal apparatus, duct, gland, or sac —see
    Injury, eye, specified site NEC
  larynx NEC S19.81
  leg (lower) S89.9-●
    blood vessel —see Injury, blood vessel, leg
    contusion —see Contusion, leg
    fracture —see Fracture, leg

Injury (Continued)
  leg (Continued)
    muscle —see Injury, muscle, leg
    nerve —see Injury, nerve, leg
    open —see Wound, open, leg
    specified NEC S89.8-●
    superficial —see Injury, superficial, leg
  lens, eye —see Injury, eye, specified site
    NEC
    penetrating —see Injury, eyeball,
      penetrating
  limb NEC T14.8
  lip S09.93
  liver S36.119
    contusion S36.112
    laceration S36.113
      major (stellate) S36.116
      minor S36.114
      moderate S36.115
    specified NEC S36.118
  lower back S39.92
    specified NEC S39.82
  lumbar, lumbosacral (region) S39.92
    plexus —see Injury, lumbosacral plexus
  lumbosacral plexus S34.4
  lung —see also Injury, intrathoracic, lung
    aspiration J69.0
    dabbing (related) U07.0
    electronic cigarette (related) U07.0
    EVALI - [e-cigarette, or vaping, product
      use associated] U07.0
    transfusion-related (TRALI) J95.84
    vaping (associated) (device) (product) (use)
      U07.0
  lymphatic thoracic duct —see Injury,
    intrathoracic, specified organ NEC
  malar region S09.93
  mastoid region S09.90
  maxilla S09.93
  mediastinum —see Injury, intrathoracic,
    specified organ NEC
  membrane, brain —see Injury, intracranial
  meningeal artery —see Injury, intracranial,
    subdural hemorrhage
  meninges (cerebral) —see Injury, intracranial
  mesenteric
    artery
      branch S35.299
        laceration (minor) (superficial) S35.291
        major S35.292
        specified NEC S35.298
      inferior S35.239
        laceration (minor) (superficial) S35.231
        major S35.232
        specified NEC S35.238
      superior S35.229
        laceration (minor) (superficial) S35.221
        major S35.222
        specified NEC S35.228
    plexus (inferior) (superior) —see Injury,
      nerve, lumbosacral, sympathetic
    vein
      inferior S35.349
        laceration S35.341
        specified NEC S35.348
      superior S35.339
        laceration S35.331
        specified NEC S35.338
  mesentery —see Injury, intra-abdominal,
    specified site NEC
  mesosalpinx —see Injury, pelvic organ,
    specified site NEC
  middle ear S09.30-●
  midthoracic region NOS S29.9
  mouth S09.93
  multiple NOS T07
  muscle (and fascia) (and tendon)
    abdomen S39.001
      laceration S39.021
      specified type NEC S39.091
      strain S39.011

Injury (Continued)
  muscle (Continued)
    abductor
      thumb, forearm level —see Injury,
        muscle, thumb, abductor
    adductor
      thigh S76.20-●
        laceration S76.22-●
        specified type NEC S76.29-●
        strain S76.21-●
    ankle —see Injury, muscle, foot
    anterior muscle group, at leg level (lower)
      S86.20-●
      laceration S86.22-●
      specified type NEC S86.29-●
      strain S86.21-●
    arm (upper) —see Injury, muscle,
      shoulder
    biceps (parts NEC) S46.20-●
      laceration S46.22-●
      long head S46.10-●
        laceration S46.12-●
        specified type NEC S46.19-●
        strain S46.11-●
      specified type NEC S46.29-●
      strain S46.21-●
    extensor
      finger(s) (other than thumb) —see Injury,
        muscle, finger by site, extensor
      forearm level, specified NEC —see
        Injury, muscle, forearm, extensor
      thumb —see Injury, muscle, thumb,
        extensor
      toe (large) (ankle level) (foot level) —see
        Injury, muscle, toe, extensor
    finger
      extensor (forearm level) S56.40-●
        hand level S66.309
          laceration S66.329
          specified type NEC S66.399
          strain S66.319
        laceration S56.429
        specified type NEC S56.499
        strain S56.419
      flexor (forearm level) S56.10-●
        hand level S66.109
          laceration S66.129
          specified type NEC S66.199
          strain S66.119
        laceration S56.129
        specified type NEC S56.199
        strain S56.119
      index
        extensor (forearm level)
          hand level S66.308
            laceration S66.32-●
            specified type NEC S66.39-●
            strain S66.31-●
          specified type NEC S56.492-●
        flexor (forearm level)
          hand level S66.108
            laceration S66.12-●
            specified type NEC
              S66.19-●
            strain S66.11-●
          specified type NEC S56.19-●
          strain S56.11-●
        intrinsic S66.50-●
          laceration S66.52-●
          specified type NEC S66.59-●
          strain S66.51-●
      intrinsic S66.509
        laceration S66.529
        specified type NEC S66.599
        strain S66.519
      little
        extensor (forearm level)
          hand level S66.30-●
            laceration S66.32-●
            specified type NEC S66.39-●
            strain S66.31-●

Injury *(Continued)*
  muscle *(Continued)*
    finger *(Continued)*
      little *(Continued)*
        extensor *(Continued)*
          laceration S56.42-•
          specified type NEC S56.49-•
          strain S56.41-•
        flexor (forearm level)
          hand level S66.10-•
            laceration S66.12-•
            specified type NEC S66.19-•
            strain S66.11-•
          laceration S56.12-•
          specified type NEC S56.19-•
          strain S56.11-•
        intrinsic S66.50-•
          laceration S66.52-•
          specified type NEC S66.59-•
          strain S66.51-•
      middle
        extensor (forearm level)
          hand level S66.30-•
            laceration S66.32-•
            specified type NEC
              S66.39-•
            strain S66.31-•
          laceration S56.42-•
          specified type NEC
            S56.49-•
          strain S56.41-•
        flexor (forearm level)
          hand level S66.10-•
            laceration S66.12-•
            specified type NEC
              S66.19-•
            strain S66.11-•
          laceration S56.12-•
          specified type NEC S56.19-•
          strain S56.11-•
        intrinsic S66.50-•
          laceration S66.52-•
          specified type NEC S66.59-•
          strain S66.51-•
      ring
        extensor (forearm level)
          hand level S66.30-•
            laceration S66.32-•
            specified type NEC S66.39-•
            strain S66.31-•
          laceration S56.42-•
          specified type NEC S56.49-•
          strain S56.41-•
        flexor (forearm level)
          hand level S66.10-•
            laceration S66.12-•
            specified type NEC S66.19-•
            strain S66.11-•
          laceration S56.12-•
          specified type NEC S56.19-•
          strain S56.11-•
        intrinsic S66.50-•
          laceration S66.52-•
          specified type NEC S66.59-•
          strain S66.51-•
    flexor
      finger(s) (other than thumb) — *see* Injury, muscle, finger
      forearm level, specified NEC — *see* Injury, muscle, forearm, flexor
      thumb —*see* Injury, muscle, thumb, flexor
      toe (long) (ankle level) (foot level) —*see* Injury, muscle, toe, flexor
    foot S96.90-•
      intrinsic S96.20-•
        laceration S96.22-•
        specified type NEC S96.29-•
        strain S96.21-•
      laceration S96.92-•

Injury *(Continued)*
  muscle *(Continued)*
    foot *(Continued)*
      long extensor, toe —*see* Injury, muscle, toe, extensor
      long flexor, toe —*see* Injury, muscle, toe, flexor
      specified
        site NEC S96.80-•
          laceration S96.82-•
          specified type NEC S96.89-•
          strain S96.81-•
        type NEC S96.99-•
      strain S96.91-•
    forearm (level) S56.90-•
      extensor S56.90-•
        laceration S56.52-•
        specified type NEC S56.59-•
        strain S56.51-•
      flexor S56.20-•
        laceration S56.22-•
        specified type NEC S56.29-•
        strain S56.21-•
      laceration S56.92-•
      specified S56.99-•
        site NEC S56.80-•
          laceration S56.82-•
          strain S56.81-•
        type NEC S56.89-•
      strain S56.91-•
    hand (level) S66.90-•
      laceration S66.92-•
      specified
        site NEC S66.80-•
          laceration S66.82-•
          specified type NEC S66.89-•
          strain S66.81-•
        type NEC S66.99-•
      strain S66.91-•
    head S09.10
      laceration S09.12
      specified type NEC S09.19
      strain S09.11
    hip NEC S76.00-•
      laceration S76.02-•
      specified type NEC S76.09-•
      strain S76.01-•
    intrinsic
      ankle and foot level —*see* Injury, muscle, foot, intrinsic
      finger (other than thumb) —*see* Injury, muscle, finger by site, intrinsic
      foot (level) —*see* Injury, muscle, foot, intrinsic
      thumb —*see* Injury, muscle, thumb, intrinsic
    leg (level) (lower) S86.90-•
      Achilles tendon —*see* Injury, Achilles tendon
      anterior muscle group —*see* Injury, muscle, anterior muscle group
      laceration S86.92-•
      peroneal muscle group —*see* Injury, muscle, peroneal muscle group
      posterior muscle group —*see* Injury, muscle, posterior muscle group, leg level
      specified
        site NEC S86.80-•
          laceration S86.82-•
          specified type NEC S86.89-•
          strain S86.81-•
        type NEC S86.99-•
      strain S86.91-•
    long
      extensor toe, at ankle and foot level —*see* Injury, muscle, toe, extensor
      flexor, toe, at ankle and foot level —*see* Injury, muscle, toe, flexor
      head, biceps —*see* Injury, muscle, biceps, long head

Injury *(Continued)*
  muscle *(Continued)*
    lower back S39.002
      laceration S39.022
      specified type NEC S39.092
      strain S39.012
    neck (level) S16.9
      laceration S16.2
      specified type NEC S16.8
      strain S16.1
    pelvis S39.003
      laceration S39.023
      specified type NEC S39.093
      strain S39.013
    peroneal muscle group, at leg level (lower) S86.30-•
      laceration S86.32-•
      specified type NEC S86.39-•
      strain S86.31-•
    posterior muscle (group)
      leg level (lower) S86.10-•
        laceration S86.12-•
        specified type NEC S86.19-•
        strain S86.11-•
      thigh level S76.30-•
        laceration S76.32-•
        specified type NEC S76.39-•
        strain S76.31-•
    quadriceps (thigh) S76.10-•
      laceration S76.12-•
      specified type NEC S76.19-•
      strain S76.11-•
    shoulder S46.90-•
      laceration S46.92-•
      rotator cuff —*see* Injury, rotator cuff
      specified site NEC S46.80-•
        laceration S46.82-•
        specified type NEC S46.89-•
        strain S46.81-•
      specified type NEC S46.99-•
      strain S46.91-•
    thigh NEC (level) S76.90-•
      adductor —*see* Injury, muscle, adductor, thigh
      laceration S76.92-•
      posterior muscle (group) —*see* Injury, muscle, posterior muscle, thigh level
      quadriceps —*see* Injury, muscle, quadriceps
      specified
        site NEC S76.80-•
          laceration S76.82-•
          specified type NEC S76.89-•
          strain S76.81-•
        type NEC S76.99-•
      strain S76.91-•
    thorax (level) S29.009
      back wall S29.002
      front wall S29.001
      laceration S29.029
        back wall S29.022
        front wall S29.021
      specified type NEC S29.099
        back wall S29.092
        front wall S29.091
      strain S29.019
        back wall S29.012
        front wall S29.011
    thumb
      abductor (forearm level) S56.30-•
        laceration S56.32-•
        specified type NEC S56.39-•
        strain S56.31-•
      extensor (forearm level) S56.30-•
        hand level S66.20-•
          laceration S66.22-•
          specified type NEC S66.29-•
          strain S66.21-•
        laceration S56.32-•
        specified type NEC S56.39-•
        strain S56.31-•

▶ New   ⟹ Revised   ~~deleted~~ Deleted   • Use Additional Character(s)

Injury (Continued)
  muscle (Continued)
    thumb (Continued)
      flexor (forearm level) S56.00-●
        hand level S66.00-●
          laceration S66.02-●
          specified type NEC S66.09-●
          strain S66.01-●
        laceration S56.02-●
        specified type NEC S56.09-●
        strain S56.01-●
        wrist level —see Injury, muscle, thumb, flexor, hand level
      intrinsic S66.40-●
        laceration S66.42-●
        specified type NEC S66.49-●
        strain S66.41-●
    toe —see also Injury, muscle, foot
      extensor, long S96.10-●
        laceration S96.12-●
        specified type NEC S96.19-●
        strain S96.11-●
      flexor, long S96.00-●
        laceration S96.02-●
        specified type NEC S96.09-●
        strain S96.01-●
    triceps S46.30-●
      laceration S46.32-●
      specified type NEC S46.39-●
      strain S46.31-●
    wrist (and hand) level —see Injury, muscle, hand
  musculocutaneous nerve —see Injury, nerve, musculocutaneous
▶myocardial (acute) (chronic) (non-ischemic) (non-traumatic) I5A
  ▶traumatic —see Injury, heart
⇒myocardium —see also Injury, heart
  ▶non-traumatic —see Injury, myocardial
nape —see Injury, neck
nasal (septum) (sinus) S09.92
nasopharynx S09.92
neck S19.9
  specified NEC S19.80
    specified site NEC S19.89
nerve NEC T14.8
  abdomen S34.9
    peripheral S34.6
    specified site NEC S34.8
  abducens S04.4-●
    contusion S04.4 ●
    laceration S04.4-●
    specified type NEC S04.4-●
  abducent —see Injury, nerve, abducens
  accessory S04.7-●
    contusion S04.7-●
    laceration S04.7-●
    specified type NEC S04.7-●
  acoustic S04.6-●
    contusion S04.6 ●
    laceration S04.6-●
    specified type NEC S04.6-●
  ankle S94.9-●
    cutaneous sensory S94.3-●
    specified site NEC —see subcategory S94.8
  anterior crural, femoral —see Injury, nerve, femoral
  arm (upper) S44.9-●
    axillary —see Injury, nerve, axillary
    cutaneous —see Injury, nerve, cutaneous, arm
    median —see Injury, nerve, median, upper arm
    musculocutaneous —see Injury, nerve, musculocutaneous
    radial —see Injury, nerve, radial, upper arm
    specified site NEC —see subcategory S44.8
    ulnar —see Injury, nerve, ulnar, arm
  auditory —see Injury, nerve, acoustic

Injury (Continued)
  nerve NEC (Continued)
    axillary S44.3-●
    brachial plexus —see Injury, brachial plexus
    cervical sympathetic S14.5
    cranial S04.9
      contusion S04.9
      eighth (acoustic or auditory) —see Injury, nerve, acoustic
      eleventh (accessory) —see Injury, nerve, accessory
      fifth (trigeminal) —see Injury, nerve, trigeminal
      first (olfactory) —see Injury, nerve, olfactory
      fourth (trochlear) —see Injury, nerve, trochlear
      laceration S04.9
      ninth (glossopharyngeal) —see Injury, nerve, glossopharyngeal
      second (optic) —see Injury, nerve, optic
      seventh (facial) —see Injury, nerve, facial
      sixth (abducent) —see Injury, nerve, abducens
      specified
        nerve NEC S04.89-●
          contusion S04.89-●
          laceration S04.89-●
          specified type NEC S04.89-●
        type NEC S04.9
      tenth (pneumogastric or vagus) —see Injury, nerve, vagus
      third (oculomotor) —see Injury, nerve, oculomotor
      twelfth (hypoglossal) —see Injury, nerve, hypoglossal
    cutaneous sensory
      ankle (level) S94.3-●
      arm (upper) (level) S44.5-●
      foot (level) —see Injury, nerve, cutaneous sensory, ankle
      forearm (level) S54.3-●
      hip (level) S74.2 ●
      leg (lower level) S84.2-●
      shoulder (level) —see Injury, nerve, cutaneous sensory, arm
      thigh (level) —see Injury, nerve, cutaneous sensory, hip
    deep peroneal —see Injury, nerve, peroneal, foot
    digital
      finger S64.4-●
        index S64.49-●
        little S64.49-●
        middle S64.49-●
        ring S64.49-●
      thumb S64.3-●
      toe —see Injury, nerve, ankle, specified site NEC
    eighth cranial (acoustic or auditory) —see Injury, nerve, acoustic
    eleventh cranial (accessory) —see Injury, nerve, accessory
    facial S04.5-●
      contusion S04.5-●
      laceration S04.5-●
      newborn P11.3
      specified type NEC S04.5-●
    femoral (hip level) (thigh level) S74.1-●
    fifth cranial (trigeminal) —see Injury, nerve, trigeminal
    finger (digital) —see Injury, nerve, digital, finger
    first cranial (olfactory) —see Injury, nerve, olfactory
    foot S94.9-●
      cutaneous sensory S94.3-●
      deep peroneal S94.2-●
      lateral plantar S94.0-●

Injury (Continued)
  nerve NEC (Continued)
    foot (Continued)
      medial plantar S94.1-●
      specified site NEC —see subcategory S94.8
    forearm (level) S54.9-●
      cutaneous sensory —see Injury, nerve, cutaneous sensory, forearm
      median —see Injury, nerve, median
      radial —see Injury, nerve, radial
      specified site NEC —see subcategory S54.8
      ulnar —see Injury, nerve, ulnar
    fourth cranial (trochlear) —see Injury, nerve, trochlear
    glossopharyngeal S04.89-●
      specified type NEC S04.89-●
    hand S64.9-●
      median —see Injury, nerve, median, hand
      radial —see Injury, nerve, radial, hand
      specified NEC —see subcategory S64.8
      ulnar —see Injury, nerve, ulnar, hand
    hip (level) S74.9-●
      cutaneous sensory —see Injury, nerve, cutaneous sensory, hip
      femoral —see Injury, nerve, femoral
      sciatic —see Injury, nerve, sciatic
      specified site NEC —see subcategory S74.8
    hypoglossal S04.89-●
      specified type NEC S04.89-●
    lateral plantar S94.0-●
    leg (lower) S84.9-●
      cutaneous sensory —see Injury, nerve, cutaneous sensory, leg
      peroneal —see Injury, nerve, peroneal
      specified site NEC —see subcategory S84.8
      tibial —see Injury, nerve, tibial
      upper —see Injury, nerve, thigh
    lower
      back —see Injury, nerve, abdomen, specified site NEC
      peripheral —see Injury, nerve, abdomen, peripheral
      limb —see Injury, nerve, leg
    lumbar plexus —see Injury, nerve, lumbosacral, sympathetic
⇒   lumbar spinal
▶   peripheral S34.6
  ▶ root S34.21
  ▶ sympathetic S34.5
    lumbosacral
      plexus —see Injury, nerve, lumbosacral, sympathetic
      sympathetic S34.5
    medial plantar S94.1-●
    median (forearm level) S54.1-●
      hand (level) S64.1-●
      upper arm (level) S44.1-●
      wrist (level) —see Injury, nerve, median, hand
    musculocutaneous S44.4-●
    musculospiral (upper arm level) —see Injury, nerve, radial, upper arm
    neck S14.9
      peripheral S14.4
      specified site NEC S14.8
      sympathetic S14.5
    ninth cranial (glossopharyngeal) —see Injury, nerve, glossopharyngeal
    oculomotor S04.1-●
      contusion S04.1-●
      laceration S04.1-●
      specified type NEC S04.1-●
    olfactory S04.81-●
      specified type NEC S04.81-●
    optic S04.01-●
      contusion S04.01-●
      laceration S04.01-●
      specified type NEC S04.01-●

Injury (Continued)
  nerve NEC (Continued)
    pelvic girdle —see Injury, nerve, hip
    pelvis —see Injury, nerve, abdomen,
      specified site NEC
      peripheral —see Injury, nerve, abdomen,
        peripheral
    peripheral NEC T14.8
      abdomen —see Injury, nerve, abdomen,
        peripheral
      lower back —see Injury, nerve, abdomen,
        peripheral
      neck —see Injury, nerve, neck, peripheral
      pelvis —see Injury, nerve, abdomen,
        peripheral
      specified NEC T14.8
    peroneal (lower leg level) S84.1-●
      foot S94.2-●
    plexus
      brachial —see Injury, brachial plexus
      celiac, coeliac —see Injury, nerve,
        lumbosacral, sympathetic
      mesenteric, inferior —see Injury, nerve,
        lumbosacral, sympathetic
      sacral —see Injury, lumbosacral plexus
      spinal
        brachial —see Injury, brachial plexus
        lumbosacral —see Injury, lumbosacral
          plexus
    pneumogastric —see Injury, nerve, vagus
    radial (forearm level) S54.2-●
      hand (level) S64.2-●
      upper arm (level) S44.2-●
      wrist (level) —see Injury, nerve, radial,
        hand
    root —see Injury, nerve, spinal, root
    sacral plexus —see Injury, lumbosacral
      plexus
    sacral spinal
    peripheral S34.6
      root S34.22
      sympathetic S34.5
    sciatic (hip level) (thigh level) S74.0-●
    second cranial (optic) —see Injury, nerve,
      optic
    self-inflicted, without suicidal intent
      R45.88
    seventh cranial (facial) —see Injury, nerve,
      facial
    shoulder —see Injury, nerve, arm
    sixth cranial (abducent) —see Injury, nerve,
      abducens
    spinal
      plexus —see Injury, nerve, plexus, spinal
      root
        cervical S14.2
        dorsal S24.2
        lumbar S34.21
        sacral S34.22
        thoracic —see Injury, nerve, spinal,
          root, dorsal
    splanchnic —see Injury, nerve, lumbosacral,
      sympathetic
    sympathetic NEC —see Injury, nerve,
      lumbosacral, sympathetic
      cervical —see Injury, nerve, cervical
        sympathetic
    tenth cranial (pneumogastric or vagus) —
      see Injury, nerve, vagus
    thigh (level) —see Injury, nerve, hip
      cutaneous sensory —see Injury, nerve,
        cutaneous sensory, hip
      femoral —see Injury, nerve, femoral
      sciatic —see Injury, nerve, sciatic
      specified NEC —see Injury, nerve, hip
    third cranial (oculomotor) —see Injury,
      nerve, oculomotor
    thorax S24.9
      peripheral S24.3
      specified site NEC S24.8
      sympathetic S24.4

Injury (Continued)
  nerve NEC (Continued)
    thumb, digital —see Injury, nerve, digital,
      thumb
    tibial (lower leg level) (posterior) S84.0-●
    toe —see Injury, nerve, ankle
    trigeminal S04.3-●
      contusion S04.3-●
      laceration S04.3-●
      specified type NEC S04.3-●
    trochlear S04.2-●
      contusion S04.2-●
      laceration S04.2-●
      specified type NEC S04.2-●
    twelfth cranial (hypoglossal) —see Injury,
      nerve, hypoglossal
    ulnar (forearm level) S54.0-●
      arm (upper) (level) S44.0-●
      hand (level) S64.0-●
      wrist (level) —see Injury, nerve, ulnar,
        hand
    vagus S04.89-●
      specified type NEC S04.89-●
    wrist (level) —see Injury, nerve, hand
  ninth cranial nerve (glossopharyngeal) —see
    Injury, nerve, glossopharyngeal
  nose (septum) S09.92
  obstetrical O71.9
    specified NEC O71.89
  occipital (region) (scalp) S09.90
    lobe —see Injury, intracranial
  optic chiasm S04.02
  optic radiation S04.03-●
  optic tract and pathways S04.03-●
  orbit, orbital (region) —see Injury, eye
    penetrating (with foreign body) —see
      Injury, eye, orbit, penetrating
    specified NEC —see Injury, eye, specified
      site NEC
  ovary, ovarian S37.409
    bilateral S37.402
      contusion S37.422
      laceration S37.432
      specified type NEC S37.492
    blood vessel —see Injury, blood vessel,
      ovarian
    contusion S37.429
      bilateral S37.422
      unilateral S37.421
    laceration S37.439
      bilateral S37.432
      unilateral S37.431
    specified type NEC S37.499
      bilateral S37.492
      unilateral S37.491
    unilateral S37.401
      contusion S37.421
      laceration S37.431
      specified type NEC S37.491
  palate (hard) (soft) S09.93
  pancreas S36.209
    body S36.201
      contusion S36.221
      laceration S36.231
        major S36.261
        minor S36.241
        moderate S36.251
      specified type NEC S36.291
    contusion S36.229
    head S36.200
      contusion S36.220
      laceration S36.230
        major S36.260
        minor S36.240
        moderate S36.250
      specified type NEC S36.290
    laceration S36.239
      major S36.269
      minor S36.249
      moderate S36.259
    specified type NEC S36.299
    tail S36.202
      contusion S36.222

Injury (Continued)
  pancreas (Continued)
    tail (Continued)
      laceration S36.232
        major S36.262
        minor S36.242
        moderate S36.252
      specified type NEC S36.292
  parietal (region) (scalp) S09.90
    lobe —see Injury, intracranial
  patellar ligament (tendon) S76.10-●
    laceration S76.12-●
    specified NEC S76.19-●
    strain S76.11-●
  pelvis, pelvic (floor) S39.93
    complicating delivery O70.1
    joint or ligament, complicating delivery
      O71.6
    organ S37.90
      with ectopic or molar pregnancy
        O08.6
      complication of abortion —see Abortion
      contusion S37.92
      following ectopic or molar pregnancy
        O08.6
      laceration S37.93
      obstetrical trauma NEC O71.5
      specified
        site NEC S37.899
          contusion S37.892
          laceration S37.893
          specified type NEC S37.898
        type NEC S37.99
    specified NEC S39.83
  penis S39.94
  perineum S39.94
  peritoneum S36.81
    laceration S36.893
  periurethral tissue —see Injury, urethra
    complicating delivery O71.82
  phalanges
    foot —see Injury, foot
    hand —see Injury, hand
  pharynx NEC S19.85
  pleura —see Injury, intrathoracic, pleura
  plexus
    brachial —see Injury, brachial plexus
    cardiac —see Injury, nerve, thorax,
      sympathetic
    celiac, coeliac —see Injury, nerve,
      lumbosacral, sympathetic
    esophageal —see Injury, nerve, thorax,
      sympathetic
    hypogastric —see Injury, nerve,
      lumbosacral, sympathetic
    lumbar, lumbosacral —see Injury,
      lumbosacral plexus
    mesenteric —see Injury, nerve, lumbosacral,
      sympathetic
    pulmonary —see Injury, nerve, thorax,
      sympathetic
  postcardiac surgery (syndrome) I97.0
  prepuce S39.94
  pressure
    injury —see Ulcer, pressure, by site
  prostate S37.829
    contusion S37.822
    laceration S37.823
    specified type NEC S37.828
  pubic region S39.94
  pudendum S39.94
  pulmonary plexus —see Injury, nerve, thorax,
    sympathetic
  rectovaginal septum NEC S39.83
  rectum —see Injury, intestine, large, rectum
  retina —see Injury, eye, specified site
    NEC
    penetrating —see Injury, eyeball,
      penetrating
  retroperitoneal —see Injury, intra-abdominal,
    specified site NEC

▶ New   ⇒ Revised   ~~deleted~~ Deleted   ● Use Additional Character(s)

Injury (Continued)

rotator cuff (muscle(s)) (tendon(s)) S46.00-●
   laceration S46.02-●
   specified type NEC S46.09-●
   strain S46.01-●
round ligament —see Injury, pelvic organ,
   specified site NEC
sacral plexus —see Injury, lumbosacral
   plexus
salivary duct or gland S09.93
scalp S09.90
   newborn (birth injury) P12.9
      due to monitoring (electrode) (sampling
         incision) P12.4
      specified NEC P12.89
         caput succedaneum P12.81
scapular region —see Injury, shoulder
sclera —see Injury, eye, specified site NEC
   penetrating —see Injury, eyeball,
      penetrating
scrotum S39.94
second cranial nerve (optic) —see Injury,
   nerve, optic
seminal vesicle —see Injury, pelvic organ,
   specified site NEC
seventh cranial nerve (facial) —see Injury,
   nerve, facial
shoulder S49.9-●
   blood vessel —see Injury, blood vessel,
      arm
   contusion —see Contusion, shoulder
   dislocation —see Dislocation, shoulder
   fracture —see Fracture, shoulder
   muscle —see Injury, muscle, shoulder
   nerve —see Injury, nerve, shoulder
   open —see Wound, open, shoulder
   specified type NEC S19.8-●
   sprain —see Sprain, shoulder girdle
   superficial —see Injury, superficial,
      shoulder
sinus
   cavernous —see Injury, intracranial
   nasal S09.92
sixth cranial nerve (abducent) —see Injury,
   nerve, abducens
skeleton, birth injury P13.9
   specified part NEC P13.8
skin NEC T14.8
   surface intact —see Injury, superficial
skull NEC S09.90
specified NEC T14.8
spermatic cord (pelvic region) S37.898
   scrotal region S39.848
spinal (cord)
   cervical (neck) S14.109
      anterior cord syndrome S14.139
         C1 level S14.131
         C2 level S14.132
         C3 level S14.133
         C4 level S14.134
         C5 level S14.135
         C6 level S14.136
         C7 level S14.137
         C8 level S14.138
      Brown-Séquard syndrome S14.149
         C1 level S14.141
         C2 level S14.142
         C3 level S14.143
         C4 level S14.144
         C5 level S14.145
         C6 level S14.146
         C7 level S14.147
         C8 level S14.148
      C1 level S14.101
      C2 level S14.102
      C3 level S14.103
      C4 level S14.104
      C5 level S14.105
      C6 level S14.106
      C7 level S14.107
      C8 level S14.108

Injury (Continued)

spinal (Continued)
   cervical (Continued)
      central cord syndrome
         S14.129
         C1 level S14.121
         C2 level S14.122
         C3 level S14.123
         C4 level S14.124
         C5 level S14.125
         C6 level S14.126
         C7 level S14.127
         C8 level S14.128
      complete lesion S14.119
         C1 level S14.111
         C2 level S14.112
         C3 level S14.113
         C4 level S14.114
         C5 level S14.115
         C6 level S14.116
         C7 level S14.117
         C8 level S14.118
      concussion S14.0
      edema S14.0
      incomplete lesion specified NEC
         S14.159
         C1 level S14.151
         C2 level S14.152
         C3 level S14.153
         C4 level S14.154
         C5 level S14.155
         C6 level S14.156
         C7 level S14.157
         C8 level S14.158
      posterior cord syndrome S14.159
         C1 level S14.151
         C2 level S14.152
         C3 level S14.153
         C4 level S14.154
         C5 level S14.155
         C6 level S14.156
         C7 level S14.157
         C8 level S14.158
   dorsal —see Injury, spinal, thoracic
   lumbar S34.109
      complete lesion S34.119
         L1 level S34.111
         L2 level S34.112
         L3 level S34.113
         L4 level S34.114
         L5 level S34.115
      concussion S34.01
      edema S34.01
      incomplete lesion S34.129
         L1 level S34.121
         L2 level S34.122
         L3 level S34.123
         L4 level S34.124
         L5 level S34.125
      L1 level S34.101
      L2 level S34.102
      L3 level S34.103
      L4 level S34.104
      L5 level S34.105
   nerve root NEC
      cervical —see Injury, nerve, spinal, root,
         cervical
      dorsal —see Injury, nerve, spinal, root,
         dorsal
      lumbar S34.21
      sacral S34.22
      thoracic —see Injury, nerve, spinal, root,
         dorsal
   plexus
      brachial —see Injury, brachial
         plexus
      lumbosacral —see Injury, lumbosacral
         plexus
   sacral S34.139
      complete lesion S34.131
      incomplete lesion S34.132

Injury (Continued)

spinal (Continued)
   thoracic S24.109
      anterior cord syndrome S24.139
         T1 level S24.131
         T2-T6 level S24.132
         T7-T10 level S24.133
         T11-T12 level S24.134
      Brown-Séquard syndrome
         S24.149
         T1 level S24.141
         T2-T6 level S24.142
         T7-T10 level S24.143
         T11-T12 level S24.144
      complete lesion S24.119
         T1 level S24.111
         T2-T6 level S24.112
         T7-T10 level S24.113
         T11-T12 level S24.114
      concussion S24.0
      edema S24.0
      incomplete lesion specified NEC
         S24.159
         T1 level S24.151
         T2-T6 level S24.152
         T7-T10 level S24.153
         T11-T12 level S24.154
      posterior cord syndrome S24.159
         T1 level S24.151
         T2-T6 level S24.152
         T7-T10 level S24.153
         T11-T12 level S24.154
      T1 level S24.101
      T2-T6 level S24.102
      T7-T10 level S24.103
      T11-T12 level S24.104
   splanchnic nerve —see Injury, nerve,
      lumbosacral, sympathetic
   spleen S36.00
      contusion S36.029
         major S36.021
         minor S36.020
      laceration S36.039
         major (massive) (stellate) S36.032
         moderate S36.031
         superficial (capsular) (minor) S36.030
      specified type NEC S36.09
   splenic artery —see Injury, blood vessel, celiac
      artery, branch
   stellate ganglion —see Injury, nerve, thorax,
      sympathetic
   sternal region S29.9
   stomach S36.30
      contusion S36.32
      laceration S36.33
      specified type NEC S36.39
   subconjunctival —see Injury, eye, conjunctiva
   subcutaneous NEC T14.8
   submaxillary region S09.93
   submental region S09.93
   subungual
      fingers —see Injury, hand
      toes —see Injury, foot
   superficial NEC T14.8
      abdomen, abdominal (wall) S30.92
         abrasion S30.811
         bite S30.871
            insect S30.861
         contusion S30.1
         external constriction S30.841
         foreign body S30.851
      abrasion —see Abrasion, by site
      adnexa, eye NEC —see Injury, eye,
         specified site NEC
      alveolar process —see Injury, superficial,
         oral cavity
      ankle S90.91-●
         abrasion —see Abrasion, ankle
         bite —see Bite, ankle
         blister —see Blister, ankle
         contusion —see Contusion, ankle

Injury (Continued)
　superficial NEC (Continued)
　　ankle (Continued)
　　　external constriction —see Constriction,
　　　　external, ankle
　　　foreign body —see Foreign body,
　　　　superficial, ankle
　　anus S30.98
　　arm (upper) S40.92-●
　　　abrasion —see Abrasion, arm
　　　bite —see Bite, superficial, arm
　　　blister —see Blister, arm (upper)
　　　contusion —see Contusion, arm
　　　external constriction —see Constriction,
　　　　external, arm
　　　foreign body —see Foreign body,
　　　　superficial, arm
　　auditory canal (external) (meatus) —see
　　　Injury, superficial, ear
　　auricle —see Injury, superficial, ear
　　axilla —see Injury, superficial, arm
　　back —see also Injury, superficial, thorax,
　　　back
　　　lower S30.91
　　　　abrasion S30.810
　　　　contusion S30.0
　　　　external constriction S30.840
　　　　superficial
　　　　　bite NEC S30.870
　　　　　　insect S30.860
　　　　　foreign body S30.850
　　bite NEC —see Bite, superficial NEC, by
　　　site
　　blister —see Blister, by site
　　breast S20.10-●
　　　abrasion —see Abrasion, breast
　　　bite —see Bite, superficial, breast
　　　contusion —see Contusion, breast
　　　external constriction —see Constriction,
　　　　external, breast
　　　foreign body —see Foreign body,
　　　　superficial, breast
　　brow —see Injury, superficial, head,
　　　specified NEC
　　buttock S30.91
　　calf —see Injury, superficial, leg
　　canthus, eye —see Injury, superficial,
　　　periocular area
　　cheek (external) —see Injury, superficial,
　　　head, specified NEC
　　　internal —see Injury, superficial, oral
　　　　cavity
　　chest wall —see Injury, superficial, thorax
　　chin —see Injury, superficial, head NEC
　　clitoris S30.95
　　conjunctiva —see Injury, eye, conjunctiva
　　　with foreign body (in conjunctival
　　　　sac) —see Foreign body,
　　　　conjunctival sac
　　contusion —see Contusion, by site
　　costal region —see Injury, superficial,
　　　thorax
　　digit(s)
　　　hand —see Injury, superficial, finger
　　ear (auricle) (canal) (external) S00.40-●
　　　abrasion —see Abrasion, ear
　　　bite —see Bite, superficial, ear
　　　contusion —see Contusion, ear
　　　external constriction —see Constriction,
　　　　external, ear
　　　foreign body —see Foreign body,
　　　　superficial, ear
　　elbow S50.90-●
　　　abrasion —see Abrasion, elbow
　　　bite —see Bite, superficial, elbow
　　　blister —see Blister, elbow
　　　contusion —see Contusion, elbow
　　　external constriction —see Constriction,
　　　　external, elbow
　　　foreign body —see Foreign body,
　　　　superficial, elbow

Injury (Continued)
　superficial NEC (Continued)
　　epididymis S30.94
　　epigastric region S30.92
　　epiglottis —see Injury, superficial, throat
　　esophagus
　　　cervical —see Injury, superficial,
　　　　throat
　　external constriction —see Constriction,
　　　external, by site
　　extremity NEC T14.8
　　eyeball NEC —see Injury, eye, specified
　　　site NEC
　　eyebrow —see Injury, superficial,
　　　periocular area
　　eyelid S00.20-●
　　　abrasion —see Abrasion, eyelid
　　　bite —see Bite, superficial, eyelid
　　　contusion —see Contusion, eyelid
　　　external constriction —see Constriction,
　　　　external, eyelid
　　　foreign body —see Foreign body,
　　　　superficial, eyelid
　　face NEC —see Injury, superficial, head,
　　　specified NEC
　　finger(s) S60.949
　　　abrasion —see Abrasion, finger
　　　bite —see Bite, superficial, finger
　　　blister —see Blister, finger
　　　contusion —see Contusion, finger
　　　external constriction —see Constriction,
　　　　external, finger
　　　foreign body —see Foreign body,
　　　　superficial, finger
　　　index S60.94-●
　　　insect bite —see Bite, by site, superficial,
　　　　insect
　　　little S60.94-●
　　　middle S60.94-●
　　　ring S60.94-●
　　flank S30.92
　　foot S90.92-●
　　　abrasion —see Abrasion, foot
　　　bite —see Bite, foot
　　　blister —see Blister, foot
　　　contusion —see Contusion, foot
　　　external constriction —see Constriction,
　　　　external, foot
　　　foreign body —see Foreign body,
　　　　superficial, foot
　　forearm S50.91-●
　　　abrasion —see Abrasion, forearm
　　　bite —see Bite, forearm, superficial
　　　blister —see Blister, forearm
　　　contusion —see Contusion, forearm
　　　elbow only —see Injury, superficial,
　　　　elbow
　　　external constriction —see Constriction,
　　　　external, forearm
　　　foreign body —see Foreign body,
　　　　superficial, forearm
　　forehead —see Injury, superficial, head
　　　NEC
　　foreign body —see Foreign body,
　　　superficial
　　genital organs, external
　　　female S30.97
　　　male S30.96
　　globe (eye) —see Injury, eye, specified site
　　　NEC
　　groin S30.92
　　gum —see Injury, superficial, oral
　　　cavity
　　hand S60.92-●
　　　abrasion —see Abrasion, hand
　　　bite —see Bite, superficial, hand
　　　contusion —see Contusion, hand
　　　external constriction —see Constriction,
　　　　external, hand
　　　foreign body —see Foreign body,
　　　　superficial, hand

Injury (Continued)
　superficial NEC (Continued)
　　head S00.90
　　　ear —see Injury, superficial, ear
　　　eyelid —see Injury, superficial, eyelid
　　　nose S00.30
　　　oral cavity S00.502
　　　scalp S00.00
　　　specified site NEC S00.80
　　heel —see Injury, superficial, foot
　　hip S70.91-●
　　　abrasion —see Abrasion, hip
　　　bite —see Bite, superficial, hip
　　　blister —see Blister, hip
　　　contusion —see Contusion, hip
　　　external constriction —see Constriction,
　　　　external, hip
　　　foreign body —see Foreign body,
　　　　superficial, hip
　　iliac region —see Injury, superficial,
　　　abdomen
　　inguinal region —see Injury, superficial,
　　　abdomen
　　insect bite —see Bite, by site, superficial,
　　　insect
　　interscapular region —see Injury,
　　　superficial, thorax, back
　　jaw —see Injury, superficial, head, specified
　　　NEC
　　knee S80.91-●
　　　abrasion —see Abrasion, knee
　　　bite —see Bite, superficial, knee
　　　blister —see Blister, knee
　　　contusion —see Contusion, knee
　　　external constriction —see Constriction,
　　　　external, knee
　　　foreign body —see Foreign body,
　　　　superficial, knee
　　labium (majus) (minus) S30.95
　　lacrimal (apparatus) (gland) (sac) —see
　　　Injury, eye, specified site NEC
　　larynx —see Injury, superficial, throat
　　leg (lower) S80.92-●
　　　abrasion —see Abrasion, leg
　　　bite —see Bite, superficial, leg
　　　contusion —see Contusion, leg
　　　external constriction —see Constriction,
　　　　external, leg
　　　foreign body —see Foreign body,
　　　　superficial, leg
　　　knee —see Injury, superficial, knee
　　limb NEC T14.8
　　lip S00.501
　　lower back S30.91
　　lumbar region S30.91
　　malar region —see Injury, superficial, head,
　　　specified NEC
　　mammary —see Injury, superficial, breast
　　mastoid region —see Injury, superficial,
　　　head, specified NEC
　　mouth —see Injury, superficial, oral cavity
　　muscle NEC T14.8
　　nail NEC T14.8
　　　finger —see Injury, superficial, finger
　　　toe —see Injury, superficial, toe
　　nasal (septum) —see Injury, superficial, nose
　　neck S10.90
　　　specified site NEC S10.80
　　nose (septum) S00.30
　　occipital region —see Injury, superficial,
　　　scalp
　　oral cavity S00.502
　　orbital region —see Injury, superficial,
　　　periocular area
　　palate —see Injury, superficial, oral
　　　cavity
　　palm —see Injury, superficial, hand
　　parietal region —see Injury, superficial,
　　　scalp
　　pelvis S30.91
　　　girdle —see Injury, superficial, hip

　　▶ New　⇒ Revised　~~deleted~~ Deleted　● Use Additional Character(s)

Injury *(Continued)*
  superficial NEC *(Continued)*
    penis S30.93
    perineum
      female S30.95
      male S30.91
    periocular area S00.20-●
      abrasion —*see* Abrasion, eyelid
      bite —*see* Bite, superficial, eyelid
      contusion —*see* Contusion, eyelid
      external constriction —*see* Constriction,
        external, eyelid
      foreign body —*see* Foreign body,
        superficial, eyelid
    phalanges
      finger —*see* Injury, superficial, finger
      toe —*see* Injury, superficial, toe
    pharynx —*see* Injury, superficial, throat
    pinna —*see* Injury, superficial, ear
    popliteal space —*see* Injury, superficial,
      knee
    prepuce S30.93
    pubic region S30.91
    pudendum
      female S30.97
      male S30.96
    sacral region S30.91
    scalp S00.00
    scapular region —*see* Injury, superficial,
      shoulder
    sclera —*see* Injury, eye, specified site NEC
    scrotum S30.94
    shin —*see* Injury, superficial, leg
    shoulder S40.91-●
      abrasion —*see* Abrasion, shoulder
      bite —*see* Bite, superficial, shoulder
      blister —*see* Blister, shoulder
      contusion —*see* Contusion, shoulder
      external constriction —*see* Constriction,
        external, shoulder
      foreign body —*see* Foreign body,
        superficial, shoulder
    skin NEC T14.8
    sternal region —*see* Injury, superficial,
      thorax, front
    subconjunctival —*see* Injury, eye, specified
      site NEC
    subcutaneous NEC T14.8
    submaxillary region —*see* Injury,
      superficial, head, specified NEC
    submental region —*see* Injury, superficial,
      head, specified NEC
    subungual
      finger(s) —*see* Injury, superficial, finger
      toe(s) —*see* Injury, superficial, toe
    supraclavicular fossa —*see* Injury,
      superficial, neck
    supraorbital —*see* Injury, superficial, head,
      specified NEC
    temple —*see* Injury, superficial, head,
      specified NEC
    temporal region —*see* Injury, superficial,
      head, specified NEC
    testis S30.94
    thigh S70.92-●
      abrasion —*see* Abrasion, thigh
      bite —*see* Bite, superficial, thigh
      blister —*see* Blister, thigh
      contusion —*see* Contusion, thigh
      external constriction —*see* Constriction,
        external, thigh
      foreign body —*see* Foreign body,
        superficial, thigh
    thorax, thoracic (wall) S20.90
      abrasion —*see* Abrasion, thorax
      back S20.40-●
      bite —*see* Bite, thorax, superficial
      blister —*see* Blister, thorax
      contusion —*see* Contusion, thorax
      external constriction —*see* Constriction,
        external, thorax

Injury *(Continued)*
  superficial NEC *(Continued)*
    thorax, thoracic *(Continued)*
      foreign body —*see* Foreign body,
        superficial, thorax
      front S20.30-●
    throat S10.10
      abrasion S10.11
      bite S10.17
        insect S10.16
      blister S10.12
      contusion S10.0
      external constriction S10.14
      foreign body S10.15
    thumb S60.93-●
      abrasion —*see* Abrasion, thumb
      bite —*see* Bite, superficial, thumb
      blister —*see* Blister, thumb
      contusion —*see* Contusion, thumb
      external constriction —*see* Constriction,
        external, thumb
      foreign body —*see* Foreign body,
        superficial, thumb
      insect bite —*see* Bite, by site, superficial,
        insect
      specified type NEC S60.39-●
    toe(s) S90.93-●
      abrasion —*see* Abrasion, toe
      bite —*see* Bite, toe
      blister —*see* Blister, toe
      contusion —*see* Contusion, toe
      external constriction —*see* Constriction,
        external, toe
      foreign body —*see* Foreign body,
        superficial, toe
      great S90.93-●
    tongue —*see* Injury, superficial, oral cavity
    tooth, teeth —*see* Injury, superficial, oral
      cavity
    trachea S10.10
    tunica vaginalis S30.94
    tympanum, tympanic membrane —*see*
      Injury, superficial, ear
    uvula —*see* Injury, superficial, oral cavity
    vagina S30.95
    vocal cords —*see* Injury, superficial, throat
    vulva S30.95
    wrist S60.91-●
  supraclavicular region —*see* Injury, neck
  supraorbital S09.93
  suprarenal gland (multiple) —*see* Injury,
    adrenal
  surgical complication (external or internal
    site) —*see* Laceration, accidental
    complicating surgery
  temple S09.90
  temporal region S09.90
  tendon —*see also* Injury, muscle, by site
    abdomen —*see* Injury, muscle, abdomen
    Achilles —*see* Injury, Achilles tendon
    lower back —*see* Injury, muscle, lower
      back
    pelvic organs —*see* Injury, muscle, pelvis
  tenth cranial nerve (pneumogastric or
    vagus) —*see* Injury, nerve, vagus
  testis S39.94
  thigh S79.92-●
    blood vessel —*see* Injury, blood vessel, hip
    contusion —*see* Contusion, thigh
    fracture —*see* Fracture, femur
    muscle —*see* Injury, muscle, thigh
    nerve —*see* Injury, nerve, thigh
    open —*see* Wound, open, thigh
    specified NEC S79.82-●
    superficial —*see* Injury, superficial, thigh
  third cranial nerve (oculomotor) —*see* Injury,
    nerve, oculomotor
  thorax, thoracic S29.9
    blood vessel —*see* Injury, blood vessel,
      thorax
    cavity —*see* Injury, intrathoracic

Injury *(Continued)*
  thorax, thoracic *(Continued)*
    dislocation —*see* Dislocation, thorax
    external (wall) S29.9
      contusion —*see* Contusion, thorax
      nerve —*see* Injury, nerve, thorax
      open —*see* Wound, open, thorax
      specified NEC S29.8
      sprain —*see* Sprain, thorax
      superficial —*see* Injury, superficial,
        thorax
    fracture —*see* Fracture, thorax
    internal —*see* Injury, intrathoracic
    intrathoracic organ —*see* Injury,
      intrathoracic
    sympathetic ganglion —*see* Injury, nerve,
      thorax, sympathetic
  throat —*see also* Injury, neck S19.9
  thumb S69.9-●
    blood vessel —*see* Injury, blood vessel,
      thumb
    contusion —*see* Contusion, thumb
    dislocation —*see* Dislocation, thumb
    fracture —*see* Fracture, thumb
    muscle —*see* Injury, muscle, thumb
    nerve —*see* Injury, nerve, digital, thumb
    open —*see* Wound, open, thumb
    specified NEC S69.8-●
    sprain —*see* Sprain, thumb
    superficial —*see* Injury, superficial, thumb
  thymus (gland) —*see* Injury, intrathoracic,
    specified organ NEC
  thyroid (gland) NEC S19.84
  toe S99.92-●
    contusion —*see* Contusion, toe
    dislocation —*see* Dislocation, toe
    fracture —*see* Fracture, toe
    muscle —*see* Injury, muscle, toe
    open —*see* Wound, open, toe
    specified type NEC S99.82-●
    sprain —*see* Sprain, toe
    superficial —*see* Injury, superficial, toe
  tongue S09.93
  tonsil S09.93
  tooth S09.93
  trachea (cervical) NEC S19.82
    thoracic —*see* Injury, intrathoracic, trachea,
      thoracic
  transfusion-related acute lung (TRALI)
    J95.84
  tunica vaginalis S39.94
  twelfth cranial nerve (hypoglossal) —*see*
    Injury, nerve, hypoglossal
  ureter S37.10
    contusion S37.12
    laceration S37.13
    specified type NEC S37.19
  urethra (sphincter) S37.30
    at delivery O71.5
    contusion S37.32
    laceration S37.33
    specified type NEC S37.38
  urinary organ S37.899
    contusion S37.92
    laceration S37.93
    specified
      site NEC S37.899
        contusion S37.892
        laceration S37.893
        specified type NEC S37.898
      type NEC S37.99
  uterus, uterine S37.60
    with ectopic or molar pregnancy O08.6
    blood vessel —*see* Injury, blood vessel, iliac
    contusion S37.62
    laceration S37.63
      cervix at delivery O71.3
    rupture associated with obstetrics —*see*
      Rupture, uterus
    specified type NEC S37.69
  uvula S09.93

Injury *(Continued)*
  vagina S39.93
    abrasion S30.814
    bite S31.45
      insect S30.864
      superficial NEC S30.874
    contusion S30.23
    crush S38.03
    during delivery —*see* Laceration, vagina,
      during delivery
    external constriction S30.844
    insect bite S30.864
    laceration S31.41
      with foreign body S31.42
    open wound S31.40
    puncture S31.43
      with foreign body S31.44
    superficial S30.95
      foreign body S30.854
  vas deferens —*see* Injury, pelvic organ,
    specified site NEC
  vascular NEC T14.8
  vein —*see* Injury, blood vessel
  vena cava (superior) S25.20
    inferior S35.10
      laceration (minor) (superficial) S35.11
        major S35.12
      specified type NEC S35.19
    laceration (minor) (superficial) S25.21
      major S25.22
    specified type NEC S25.29
  vesical (sphincter) —*see* Injury, bladder
  visual cortex S04.04-●
  vitreous (humor) S05.90
    specified NEC S05.8X-●
  vocal cord NEC S19.83
  vulva S39.94
    abrasion S30.814
    bite S31.45
      insect S30.864
      superficial NEC S30.874
    contusion S30.23
    crush S38.03
    during delivery —*see* Laceration,
      perineum, female, during delivery
    external constriction S30.844
    insect bite S30.864
    laceration S31.41
      with foreign body S31.42
    open wound S31.40
    puncture S31.43
      with foreign body S31.44
    superficial S30.95
      foreign body S30.854
  whiplash (cervical spine) S13.4
  wrist S69.9-●
    blood vessel —*see* Injury, blood vessel,
      hand
    contusion —*see* Contusion, wrist
    dislocation —*see* Dislocation, wrist
    fracture —*see* Fracture, wrist
    muscle —*see* Injury, muscle, hand
    nerve —*see* Injury, nerve, hand
    open —*see* Wound, open, wrist
    specified NEC S69.8-●
    sprain —*see* Sprain, wrist
    superficial —*see* Injury, superficial, wrist
Inoculation —*see also* Vaccination
  complication or reaction —*see* Complications,
    vaccination
Insanity, insane —*see also* Psychosis
  adolescent —*see* Schizophrenia
  confusional F28
    acute or subacute F05
  delusional F22
  senile F03
Insect
  bite —*see* Bite, by site, superficial, insect
  venomous, poisoning NEC (by) —*see* Venom,
    arthropod
► **Insecurity, food** Z59.41

Insensitivity
  adrenocorticotropin hormone (ACTH)
    E27.49
  androgen E34.50
    complete E34.51
    partial E34.52
Insertion
  cord (umbilical) lateral or velamentous
    O43.12-●
  intrauterine contraceptive device (encounter
    for) —*see* Intrauterine contraceptive
    device
Insolation (sunstroke) T67.01
Insomnia (organic) G47.00
  without objective findings F51.02
  adjustment F51.02
  adjustment disorder F51.02
  behavioral, of childhood Z73.819
    combined type Z73.812
    limit setting type Z73.811
    sleep-onset association type Z73.810
  childhood Z73.819
  chronic F51.04
    somatized tension F51.04
  conditioned F51.04
  due to
    alcohol
      abuse F10.182
      dependence F10.282
      use F10.982
    amphetamines
      abuse F15.182
      dependence F15.282
      use F15.982
    anxiety disorder F51.05
    caffeine
      abuse F15.182
      dependence F15.282
      use F15.982
    cocaine
      abuse F14.182
      dependence F14.282
      use F14.982
    depression F51.05
    drug NEC
      abuse F19.182
      dependence F19.282
      use F19.982
    medical condition G47.01
    mental disorder NEC F51.05
    opioid
      abuse F11.182
      dependence F11.282
      use F11.982
    psychoactive substance NEC
      abuse F19.182
      dependence F19.282
      use F19.982
    sedative, hypnotic, or anxiolytic
      abuse F13.182
      dependence F13.282
      use F13.982
    stimulant NEC
      abuse F15.182
      dependence F15.282
      use F15.982
  fatal familial (FFI) A81.83
  idiopathic F51.01
  learned F51.3
  nonorganic origin F51.01
  not due to a substance or known
    physiological condition F51.01
    specified NEC F51.09
  paradoxical F51.03
  primary F51.01
  psychiatric F51.05
  psychophysiologic F51.04
  related to psychopathology F51.05
  short-term F51.02
  specified NEC G47.09
  stress-related F51.02
  transient F51.02

Inspiration
  food or foreign body —*see* Foreign body, by site
  mucus —*see* Asphyxia, mucus
Inspissated bile syndrome (newborn) P59.1
Instability
  emotional (excessive) F60.3
► housing
  ► housed Z59.819
    ► with risk of homelessness Z59.811
    ► homelessness in past 12 months Z59.812
  joint (post-traumatic) M25.30
    ankle M25.37-●
    due to old ligament injury —*see* Disorder,
      ligament
    elbow M25.32-●
    flail —*see* Flail, joint
    foot M25.37-●
    hand M25.34-●
    hip M25.35-●
    knee M25.36-●
    lumbosacral —*see* subcategory M53.2
    prosthesis —*see* Complications, joint
      prosthesis, mechanical, displacement,
      by site
    sacroiliac —*see* subcategory M53.2
    secondary to
      old ligament injury —*see* Disorder,
        ligament
      removal of joint prosthesis M96.89
    shoulder (region) M25.31-●
    specified site NEC M25.39
    spine —*see* subcategory M53.2
    wrist M25.33-●
  knee (chronic) M23.5-●
  lumbosacral —*see* subcategory M53.2
  nervous F48.8
  personality (emotional) F60.3
  spine —*see* Instability, joint, spine
  vasomotor R55
Institutional syndrome (childhood) F94.2
Institutionalization, affecting child Z62.22
  disinhibited attachment F94.2
Insufficiency, insufficient
  accommodation, old age H52.4
  adrenal (gland) E27.40
    primary E27.1
  adrenocortical E27.40
    drug-induced E27.3
    iatrogenic E27.3
    primary E27.1
  anatomic crown height K08.89
  anterior (occlusal) guidance M26.54
  anus K62.89
  aortic (valve) I35.1
    with
      mitral (valve) disease I08.0
        with tricuspid (valve) disease I08.3
      stenosis I35.2
      tricuspid (valve) disease I08.2
        with mitral (valve) disease I08.3
    congenital Q23.1
    rheumatic I06.1
      with
        mitral (valve) disease I08.0
          with tricuspid (valve) disease I08.3
        stenosis I06.2
          with mitral (valve) disease I08.0
            with tricuspid (valve) disease
              I08.3
        tricuspid (valve) disease I08.2
          with mitral (valve) disease I08.3
    specified cause NEC I35.1
    syphilitic A52.03
  arterial I77.1
    basilar G45.0
    carotid (hemispheric) G45.1
    cerebral I67.81
    coronary (acute or subacute) I24.8
    mesenteric K55.1
    peripheral I73.9
    precerebral (multiple) (bilateral) G45.2
    vertebral G45.0

Insufficiency, insufficient *(Continued)*
  arteriovenous I99.8
  biliary K83.8
  cardiac —*see also* Insufficiency, myocardial
    due to presence of (cardiac) prosthesis
      I97.11-●
    postprocedural I97.11-●
  cardiorenal, hypertensive I13.2
  cardiovascular —*see* Disease, cardiovascular
  cerebrovascular (acute) I67.81
    with transient focal neurological signs and
      symptoms G45.8
  circulatory NEC I99.8
    newborn P29.89
  clinical crown length K08.89
  convergence H51.11
  coronary (acute or subacute) I24.8
    chronic or with a stated duration of over 4
      weeks I25.89
  corticoadrenal E27.40
    primary E27.1
  dietary E63.9
  divergence H51.8
  food T73.0
➠ gastroesophageal K22.89
  gonadal
    ovary E28.39
    testis E29.1
  heart —*see also* Insufficiency, myocardial
    newborn P29.0
    valve —*see* Endocarditis
  hepatic —*see* Failure, hepatic
  idiopathic autonomic G90.09
  interocclusal distance of fully erupted teeth
    (ridge) M26.36
  kidney N28.9
    acute N28.9
    chronic N18.9
  lacrimal (secretion) H04.12 ●
    passages —*see* Stenosis, lacrimal
  liver —*see* Failure, hepatic
  lung —*see* Insufficiency, pulmonary
  mental (congenital) *see* Disability,
    intellectual
  mesenteric K55.1
  mitral (valve) I34.0
    with
      aortic valve disease I08.0
        with tricuspid (valve) disease I08.3
      obstruction or stenosis I05.2
        with aortic valve disease I08.0
      tricuspid (valve) disease I08.1
        with aortic (valve) disease I08.3
    congenital Q23.3
    rheumatic I05.1
      with
        aortic valve disease I08.0
          with tricuspid (valve) disease I08.3
        obstruction or stenosis I05.2
          with aortic valve disease I08.0
            with tricuspid (valve) disease
              I08.3
        tricuspid (valve) disease I08.1
          with aortic (valve) disease I08.3
      active or acute I01.1
        with chorea, rheumatic (Sydenham's)
          I02.0
    specified cause, except rheumatic I34.0
  muscle —*see also* Disease, muscle
    heart —*see* Insufficiency, myocardial
    ocular NEC H50.9
  myocardial, myocardium (with
    arteriosclerosis) —*see also* Failure,
    heart I50.9
    with
      rheumatic fever (conditions in I00) I09.0
        active, acute or subacute I01.2
          with chorea I02.0
        inactive or quiescent (with chorea)
          I09.0
    congenital Q24.8

Insufficiency, insufficient *(Continued)*
  myocardial, myocardium *(Continued)*
    hypertensive —*see* Hypertension, heart
    newborn P29.0
    rheumatic I09.0
      active, acute, or subacute I01.2
    syphilitic A52.06
  nourishment T73.0
  pancreatic K86.89
    exocrine K86.81
  parathyroid (gland) E20.9
  peripheral vascular (arterial) I73.9
  pituitary E23.0
  placental (mother) O36.51-●
  platelets D69.6
  prenatal care affecting management of
    pregnancy O09.3-●
  progressive pluriglandular E31.0
  pulmonary J98.4
    acute, following surgery (nonthoracic)
      J95.2
      thoracic J95.1
    chronic, following surgery J95.3
    following
      shock J98.4
      trauma J98.4
    newborn P28.89
    valve I37.1
      with stenosis I37.2
      congenital Q22.2
      rheumatic I09.89
        with aortic, mitral or tricuspid (valve)
          disease I08.8
  pyloric K31.89
  renal (acute) N28.9
    chronic N18.9
  respiratory R06.89
    newborn P28.5
  rotation —*see* Malrotation
  sleep syndrome F51.12
  social insurance Z59.7
  suprarenal E27.40
    primary E27.1
  tarso-orbital fascia, congenital Q10.3
  testis E29.1
  thyroid (gland) (acquired) E03.9
    congenital E03.1
  tricuspid (valve) (rheumatic) I07.1
    with
      aortic (valve) disease I08.2
        with mitral (valve) disease I08.3
      mitral (valve) disease I08.1
        with aortic (valve) disease I08.3
      obstruction or stenosis I07.2
        with aortic (valve) disease I08.2
          with mitral (valve) disease I08.3
    congenital Q22.8
    nonrheumatic I36.1
      with stenosis I36.2
  urethral sphincter R32
  valve, valvular (heart) I38
    aortic —*see* Insufficiency, aortic (valve)
    mitral —*see* Insufficiency, mitral (valve)
    pulmonary —*see* Insufficiency, pulmonary,
      valve
    tricuspid —*see* Insufficiency, tricuspid
      (valve)
    congenital Q24.8
  vascular I99.8
    intestine K55.9
      acute —*see also* Ischemia, intestine, acute
        K55.059
    mesenteric K55.1
    peripheral I73.9
    renal —*see* Hypertension, kidney
  velopharyngeal
    acquired K13.79
    congenital Q38.8
  venous (chronic) (peripheral) I87.2
  ventricular —*see* Insufficiency, myocardial
  welfare support Z59.7

Insufflation, fallopian Z31.41
Insular —*see* condition
Insulinoma
  pancreas
    benign D13.7
    malignant C25.4
    uncertain behavior D37.8
  specified site
    benign —*see* Neoplasm, by site, benign
    malignant —*see* Neoplasm, by site,
      malignant
    uncertain behavior —*see* Neoplasm, by site,
      uncertain behavior
  unspecified site
    benign D13.7
    malignant C25.4
    uncertain behavior D37.8
Insuloma —*see* Insulinoma
Interference
  balancing side M26.56
  non-working side M26.56
Intermenstrual —*see* condition
Intermittent —*see* condition
Internal —*see* condition
Interrogation
  cardiac defibrillator (automatic) (implantable)
    Z45.02
  cardiac pacemaker Z45.018
  cardiac (event) (loop) recorder Z45.09
  infusion pump (implanted) (intrathecal) Z45.1
  neurostimulator Z46.2
Interruption
  aortic arch Q25.21
  phase-shift, sleep cycle —*see* Disorder, sleep,
    circadian rhythm
  sleep phase-shift, or 24 hour sleep-wake
    cycle —*see* Disorder, sleep, circadian
    rhythm
Interstitial —*see* condition
Intertrigo L30.4
  labialis K13.0
Intervertebral disc —*see* condition
Intestine, intestinal —*see* condition
Intolerance
  carbohydrate K90.49
  disaccharide, hereditary E73.0
  fat NEC K90.49
    pancreatic K90.3
  food K90.49
    dietary counseling and surveillance Z71.3
  fructose E74.10
    hereditary E74.12
  glucose(-galactose) E74.39
  gluten K90.01
  lactose E73.9
    specified NEC E73.8
  lysine E72.3
  milk NEC K90.49
    lactose E73.9
  protein K90.49
  starch NEC K90.49
  sucrose (-isomaltose) E74.31
Intoxicated NEC (without dependence) —*see*
  Alcohol, intoxication
Intoxication
  acid E87.2
  alcoholic (acute) (without dependence) —*see*
    Alcohol, intoxication
  alimentary canal K52.1
  amphetamine (without dependence) —*see*
    also Abuse, drug, stimulant, with
    intoxication
    stimulant NEC F15.10
      with
        anxiety disorder F15.180
        intoxication F15.129
          with
            delirium F15.121
            perceptual disturbance F15.122
      with dependence —*see* Dependence, drug,
        stimulant, with intoxication

Intoxication (Continued)
  anxiolytic (acute) (without dependence) —see
      Abuse, drug, sedative, with intoxication
    with dependence —see Dependence, drug,
        sedative, with intoxication
  caffeine F15.929
    with dependence —see Dependence, drug,
        stimulant, with intoxication
  cannabinoids (acute) (without
      dependence) —see Use, cannabis, with
      intoxication
    with
      abuse —see Abuse, drug, cannabis, with
          intoxication
      dependence —see Dependence, drug,
          cannabis, with intoxication
  chemical —see Table of Drugs and
      Chemicals
    via placenta or breast milk —see
        Absorption, chemical, through
        placenta
  cocaine (acute) (without dependence) —see
      Abuse, drug, cocaine, with intoxication
    with dependence —see Dependence, drug,
        cocaine, with intoxication
  drug
    acute (without dependence) —see Abuse,
        drug, by type with intoxication
      with dependence —see Dependence,
          drug, by type with intoxication
    addictive
      via placenta or breast milk —see
          Absorption, drug, addictive,
          through placenta
    newborn P93.8
      gray baby syndrome P93.0
    overdose or wrong substance given
        or taken —see Table of Drugs and
        Chemicals, by drug, poisoning
  enteric K52.1
  foodborne A05.9
    bacterial A05.9
    classical (Clostridium botulinum)
        A05.1
    due to
      Bacillus cereus A05.4
      bacterium A05.9
        specified NEC A05.8
      Clostridium
        botulinum A05.1
        perfringens A05.2
        welchii A05.2
      Salmonella A02.9
        with
          (gastro) enteritis A02.0
          localized infection(s) A02.20
            arthritis A02.23
            meningitis A02.21
            osteomyelitis A02.24
            pneumonia A02.22
            pyelonephritis A02.25
            specified NEC A02.29
          sepsis A02.1
          specified manifestation NEC
              A02.8
      Staphylococcus A05.0
      Vibrio
        parahaemolyticus A05.3
        vulnificus A05.5
    enterotoxin, staphylococcal A05.0
    noxious —see Poisoning, food, noxious
  gastrointestinal K52.1
  hallucinogenic (without dependence) —
      see Abuse, drug, hallucinogen, with
      intoxication
    with dependence —see Dependence, drug,
        hallucinogen, with intoxication
  hypnotic (acute) (without dependence) —see
      Abuse, drug, sedative, with intoxication
    with dependence —see Dependence, drug,
        sedative, with intoxication

Intoxication (Continued)
  inhalant (acute) (without dependence) —see
      Abuse, drug, inhalant, with intoxication
    with dependence —see Dependence, drug,
        inhalant, with intoxication
  meaning
    inebriation —see category F10
    poisoning —see Table of Drugs and
        Chemicals
  methyl alcohol (acute) (without
      dependence) —see Alcohol, intoxication
  opioid (acute) (without dependence) —see
      Abuse, drug, opioid, with intoxication
    with dependence —see Dependence, drug,
        opioid, with intoxication
  pathologic NEC (without dependence) —see
      Alcohol, intoxication
  phencyclidine (without dependence) —see
      Abuse, drug, hallucinogen, with
      intoxication
    with dependence —see Dependence, drug,
        hallucinogen, with intoxication
  potassium (K) E87.5
  psychoactive substance NEC (without
      dependence) —see Abuse, drug,
      psychoactive NEC, with intoxication
    with dependence —see Dependence, drug,
        psychoactive NEC, with intoxication
  sedative (acute) (without dependence) —see
      Abuse, drug, sedative, with intoxication
    with dependence —see Dependence, drug,
        sedative, with intoxication
  serum —see also Reaction, serum T80.69
  uremic —see Uremia
  volatile solvents (acute) (without
      dependence) —see Abuse, drug,
      inhalant, with intoxication
    with dependence —see Dependence, drug,
        inhalant, with intoxication
  water E87.79
Intraabdominal testis, testes
  bilateral Q53.211
  unilateral Q53.111
Intracranial —see condition
Intrahepatic gallbladder Q44.1
Intraligamentous —see condition
Intrathoracic —see also condition
  kidney Q63.2
Intrauterine contraceptive device
  checking Z30.431
  in situ Z97.5
  insertion Z30.430
    immediately following removal
        Z30.433
  management Z30.431
  reinsertion Z30.433
  removal Z30.432
  replacement Z30.433
  retention in pregnancy O26.3-●
Intraventricular —see condition
Intrinsic deformity —see Deformity
Intubation, difficult or failed T88.4
Intumescence, lens (eye) (cataract) —see
    Cataract
Intussusception (bowel) (colon) (enteric)
    (ileocecal) (ileocolic) (intestine) (rectum)
    K56.1
  appendix K38.8
  congenital Q43.8
  ureter (with obstruction) N13.5
Invagination (bowel, colon, intestine or rectum)
    K56.1
Inversion
  albumin-globulin (A-G) ratio E88.09
  bladder N32.89
  cecum —see Intussusception
  cervix N88.8
  chromosome in normal individual
      Q95.1
  circadian rhythm —see Disorder, sleep,
      circadian rhythm

Inversion (Continued)
  nipple N64.59
    congenital Q83.8
    gestational —see Retraction, nipple
    puerperal, postpartum —see Retraction,
        nipple
  nyctohemeral rhythm —see Disorder, sleep,
      circadian rhythm
  optic papilla Q14.2
  organ or site, congenital NEC —see Anomaly,
      by site
  sleep rhythm —see Disorder, sleep, circadian
      rhythm
  testis (congenital) Q55.29
  uterus (chronic) (postinfectional) (postpartal,
      old) N85.5
    postpartum O71.2
  vagina (posthysterectomy) N99.3
  ventricular Q20.5
Investigation —see also Examination Z04.9
  clinical research subject (control) (normal
      comparison) (participant) Z00.6
Involuntary movement, abnormal R25.9
Involution, involutional —see also condition
  breast, cystic —see Dysplasia, mammary,
      specified type NEC
  depression (single episode) F32.89
    recurrent episode F33.9
  melancholia (single episode) F32.89
    recurrent episode F33.8
  ovary, senile —see Atrophy, ovary
  thymus failure E32.8
I.Q.
  under 20 F73
  20-34 F72
  35-49 F71
  50-69 F70
IRDS (type I) P22.0
  type II P22.1
Irideremia Q13.1
Iridis rubeosis —see Disorder, iris, vascular
Iridochoroiditis (panuveitis) —see Panuveitis
Iridocyclitis H20.9-●
  acute H20.0-●
    hypopyon H20.05-●
    primary H20.01-●
    recurrent H20.02-●
    secondary (noninfectious) H20.04-●
      infectious H20.03-●
  chronic H20.1-●
  due to allergy —see Iridocyclitis, acute,
      secondary
  endogenous —see Iridocyclitis, acute,
      primary
  Fuchs' —see Cyclitis, Fuchs' heterochromic
  gonococcal A54.32
  granulomatous —see Iridocyclitis, chronic
  herpes, herpetic (simplex) B00.51
    zoster B02.32
  hypopyon —see Iridocyclitis, acute,
      hypopyon
  in (due to)
    ankylosing spondylitis M45.9
    gonococcal infection A54.32
    herpes (simplex) virus B00.51
      zoster B02.32
    infectious disease NOS B99
    parasitic disease NOS B89 [H22]
    sarcoidosis D86.83
    syphilis A51.43
    tuberculosis A18.54
    zoster B02.32
  lens-induced H20.2-●
  nongranulomatous —see Iridocyclitis, acute
  recurrent —see Iridocyclitis, acute, recurrent
  rheumatic —see Iridocyclitis, chronic
  subacute —see Iridocyclitis, acute
  sympathetic —see Uveitis, sympathetic
  syphilitic (secondary) A51.43
  tuberculous (chronic) A18.54
  Vogt-Koyanagi H20.82-●

▶ New   ⇒ Revised   ~~deleted~~ Deleted   ● Use Additional Character(s)

Iridocyclochoroiditis (panuveitis) —*see*
    Panuveitis
Iridodialysis H21.53-●
Iridodonesis H21.89
Iridoplegia (complete) (partial) (reflex) H57.09
Iridoschisis H21.25-●
Iris —*see also* condition
    bombé —*see* Membrane, pupillary
Iritis —*see also* Iridocyclitis
    chronic —*see* Iridocyclitis, chronic
    diabetic —*see* E08-E13 with .39
    due to
        herpes simplex B00.51
        leprosy A30.9 [H22]
    gonococcal A54.32
    gouty —*see also* Gout, by type M10.9 [H22]
    granulomatous —*see* Iridocyclitis, chronic
    lens induced —*see* Iridocyclitis, lens-induced
    papulosa (syphilitic) A52.71
    rheumatic —*see* Iridocyclitis, chronic
    syphilitic (secondary) A51.43
        congenital (early) A50.01
        late A52.71
    tuberculous A18.54
Iron —*see* condition
Iron-miner's lung J63.4
Irradiated enamel (tooth, teeth) K03.89
Irradiation effects, adverse T66
Irreducible, irreducibility —*see* condition
Irregular, irregularity
    action, heart I49.9
    alveolar process K08.89
    bleeding N92.6
    breathing R06.89
    contour of cornea (acquired) —*see* Deformity,
        cornea
        congenital Q13.4
    contour, reconstructed breast N65.0
    dentin (in pulp) K04.3
    eye movements H55.89
        deficient
            saccadic H55.81
            smooth H55.82
        nystagmus —*see* Nystagmus
    labor O62.2
    menstruation (cause unknown) N92.6
    periods N92.6
    prostate N42.9
    pupil —*see* Abnormality, pupillary
    reconstructed breast N65.0
    respiratory R06.89
    septum (nasal) J34.2
    shape, organ or site, congenital NEC —*see*
        Distortion
    sleep-wake pattern (rhythm) G47.23
Irritable, irritability R45.4
    bladder N32.89
    bowel (syndrome) K58.9
        with
            constipation K58.1
            diarrhea K58.0
        mixed K58.2
        psychogenic F45.8
        specified NEC K58.8
    bronchial —*see* Bronchitis
    cerebral, in newborn P91.3
    colon —*see also* Irritable, bowel K58.9
        with diarrhea K58.0
        psychogenic F45.8
    duodenum K59.89
    heart (psychogenic) F45.8
    hip —*see* Derangement, joint, specified type
        NEC, hip
    ileum K59.89
    infant R68.12
    jejunum K59.89
    rectum K59.89
    stomach K31.89
        psychogenic F45.8
    sympathetic G90.8
    urethra N36.8

Irritation
    anus K62.89
    axillary nerve G54.0
    bladder N32.89
    brachial plexus G54.0
    bronchial —*see* Bronchitis
    cervical plexus G54.2
    cervix —*see* Cervicitis
    choroid, sympathetic —*see* Endophthalmitis
    cranial nerve —*see* Disorder, nerve, cranial
    gastric K31.89
        psychogenic F45.8
    globe, sympathetic —*see* Uveitis, sympathetic
    labyrinth —*see* subcategory H83.2
    lumbosacral plexus G54.1
    meninges (traumatic) —*see* Injury, intracranial
        nontraumatic —*see* Meningismus
    nerve —*see* Disorder, nerve
    nervous R45.0
    penis N48.89
    perineum NEC L29.3
    peripheral autonomic nervous system G90.8
    peritoneum —*see* Peritonitis
    pharynx J39.2
    plantar nerve —*see* Lesion, nerve, plantar
    spinal (cord) (traumatic) —*see also* Injury,
        spinal cord, by region
        nerve G58.9
            root NEC —*see* Radiculopathy
        nontraumatic —*see* Myelopathy
    stomach K31.89
        psychogenic F45.8
    sympathetic nerve NEC G90.8
    ulnar nerve —*see* Lesion, nerve, ulnar
    vagina N89.8
Ischemia, ischemic I99.8
    bowel (transient)
        acute   *see also* Ischemia, intestine, acute
            K55.059
        chronic K55.1
        due to mesenteric artery insufficiency
            K55.1
    brain —*see* Ischemia, cerebral
    cardiac (*see* Disease, heart, ischemic)
    cardiomyopathy I25.5
    cerebral (chronic) (generalized) I67.82
        arteriosclerotic I67.2
        intermittent G45.9
        newborn P91.0
        recurrent focal G45.8
        transient G45.9
    colon chronic (due to mesenteric artery
        insufficiency) K55.1
    coronary —*see* Disease, heart, ischemic
    demand (coronary) —*see also* Angina
        I24.8
        with myocardial infarction I21.A1
        resulting in myocardial infarction
            I21.A1
    heart (chronic or with a stated duration of
        over 4 weeks) I25.9
        acute or with a stated duration of 4 weeks
            or less I24.9
        subacute I24.9
    infarction, muscle —*see* Infarct, muscle
    intestine (large) (small) (transient) K55.9
        acute K55.059
            diffuse K55.052
            focal K55.051
            large K55.039
                diffuse K55.032
                focal K55.031
            small K55.019
                diffuse K55.012
                focal K55.011
        chronic K55.1
        due to mesenteric artery insufficiency
            K55.1
    kidney N28.0
    limb, critical —*see* Arteriosclerosis, with
        critical limb ischemia

Ischemia, ischemic (*Continued*)
    limb-threatening, chronic —*see*
        Arteriosclerosis, with critical limb
        ischemia
    mesenteric, acute —*see also* Ischemia,
        intestine, acute K55.059
    muscle, traumatic T79.6
    myocardium, myocardial (chronic or with
        a stated duration of over 4 weeks)
        I25.9
        acute, without myocardial infarction
            I51.3
        silent (asymptomatic) I25.6
        transient of newborn P29.4
    renal N28.0
    retina, retinal —*see* Occlusion, artery, retina
    small bowel
        acute K55.019
            diffuse K55.012
            focal K55.011
        chronic K55.1
        due to mesenteric artery insufficiency
            K55.1
    spinal cord G95.11
    subendocardial —*see* Insufficiency,
        coronary
    supply (coronary) —*see also* Angina
        I25.9
        due to vasospasm I20.1
Ischial spine —*see* condition
Ischialgia —*see* Sciatica
Ischiopagus Q89.4
Ischium, ischial —*see* condition
Ischuria R34
Iselin's disease or osteochondrosis —*see*
    Osteochondrosis, juvenile, metatarsus
Islands of
    parotid tissue in
        lymph nodes Q38.6
        neck structures Q38.6
    submaxillary glands in
        fascia Q38.6
        lymph nodes Q38.6
        neck muscles Q38.6
Islet cell tumor, pancreas D13.7
Isoimmunization NEC —*see also*
    Incompatibility
    affecting management of pregnancy (ABO)
        (with hydrops fetalis) O36.11-●
        anti-A sensitization O36.11-●
        anti-B sensitization O36.19-●
        anti-c sensitization O36.09-●
        anti-C sensitization O36.09-●
        anti-e sensitization O36.09-●
        anti-E sensitization O36.09-●
        Rh NEC O36.09-●
            anti-D antibody O36.01-●
        specified NEC O36.19-●
    newborn P55.9
        with
            hydrops fetalis P56.0
            kernicterus P57.0
        ABO (blood groups) P55.1
        Rhesus (Rh) factor P55.0
        specified type NEC P55.8
Isolation, isolated
⇒ dwelling Z59.89
    family Z63.79
    social Z60.4
Isoleucinosis E71.19
Isomerism atrial appendages (with asplenia or
    polysplenia) Q20.6
Isosporiasis, isosporosis A07.3
Isovaleric acidemia E71.110
Issue of
    medical certificate Z02.79
        for disability determination Z02.71
    repeat prescription (appliance) (glasses)
        (medicinal substance, medicament,
        medicine) Z76.0
        contraception —*see* Contraception

Itch, itching —*see also* Pruritus
  baker's L23.6
  barber's B35.0
  bricklayer's L24.5
  cheese B88.0
  clam digger's B65.3
  coolie B76.9
  copra B88.0
  dew B76.9
  dhobi B35.6
  filarial —*see* Infestation, filarial
  grain B88.0
  grocer's B88.0

Itch, itching (*Continued*)
  ground B76.9
  harvest B88.0
  jock B35.6
  Malabar B35.5
    beard B35.0
    foot B35.3
    scalp B35.0
  meaning scabies B86
  Norwegian B86
  perianal L29.0
  poultrymen's B88.0

Itch, itching (*Continued*)
  sarcoptic B86
  scabies B86
  scrub B88.0
  straw B88.0
  swimmer's B65.3
  water B76.9
  winter L29.8
Ivemark's syndrome (asplenia with congenital
  heart disease) Q89.01
Ivory bones Q78.2
Ixodiasis NEC B88.8

▶ New   ⇒ Revised   ~~deleted~~ Deleted   ● Use Additional Character(s)

J

Jaccoud's syndrome —see Arthropathy, postrheumatic, chronic
Jackson's
  membrane Q43.3
  paralysis or syndrome G83.89
  veil Q43.3
Jacquet's dermatitis (diaper dermatitis) L22
Jadassohn-Pellizari's disease or anetoderma
  L90.2
Jadassohn's
  blue nevus —see Nevus
  intraepidermal epithelioma —see Neoplasm, skin, benign
Jaffe-Lichtenstein (-Uehlinger) syndrome —see Dysplasia, fibrous, bone NEC
Jakob-Creutzfeldt disease or syndrome —see Creutzfeldt-Jakob disease or syndrome
Jaksch-Luzet disease D64.89
Jamaican
⇒neuropathy G92.8
⇒paraplegic tropical ataxic-spastic syndrome G92.8
Janet's disease F48.8
Janiceps Q89.4
Jansky-Bielschowsky amaurotic idiocy E75.4
Japanese
  B-type encephalitis A83.0
  river fever A75.3
Jaundice (yellow) R17
  acholuric (familial) (splenomegalic) —see also Spherocytosis
    acquired D59.8
  breast-milk (inhibitor) P59.3
  catarrhal (acute) B15.9
    with hepatic coma B15.0
  cholestatic (benign) R17
  due to or associated with
    delayed conjugation P59.8
      associated with (due to) preterm delivery P59.0
    preterm delivery P59.0
  epidemic (catarrhal) B15.9
    with hepatic coma B15.0
    leptospiral A27.0
    spirochetal A27.0
  familial nonhemolytic (congenital) (Gilbert) E80.4
    Crigler-Najjar E80.5
  febrile (acute) B15.9
    with hepatic coma B15.0
    leptospiral A27.0
    spirochetal A27.0
  hematogenous D59.9
  hemolytic (acquired) D59.9
    congenital —see Spherocytosis

Jaundice (Continued)
  hemorrhagic (acute) (leptospiral) (spirochetal) A27.0
  infectious (acute) (subacute) B15.9
    with hepatic coma B15.0
    leptospiral A27.0
    spirochetal A27.0
  leptospiral (hemorrhagic) A27.0
  malignant (without coma) K72.90
    with coma K72.91
  neonatal —see Jaundice, newborn
  newborn P59.9
    due to or associated with
      ABO
        antibodies P55.1
        incompatibility, maternal/fetal P55.1
        isoimmunization P55.1
      absence or deficiency of enzyme system for bilirubin conjugation (congenital) P59.8
      bleeding P58.1
      breast milk inhibitors to conjugation P59.3
        associated with preterm delivery P59.0
      bruising P58.0
      Crigler-Najjar syndrome E80.5
      delayed conjugation P59.8
        associated with preterm delivery P59.0
      drugs or toxins
        given to newborn P58.42
        transmitted from mother P58.41
      excessive hemolysis P58.9
        due to
          bleeding P58.1
          bruising P58.0
          drugs or toxins
            given to newborn P58.42
            transmitted from mother P58.41
          infection P58.2
          polycythemia P58.3
          swallowed maternal blood P58.5
        specified type NEC P58.8
      galactosemia E74.21
      Gilbert syndrome E80.4
      hemolytic disease P55.9
        ABO isoimmunization P55.1
        Rh isoimmunization P55.0
        specified NEC P55.8
      hepatocellular damage P59.20
        specified NEC P59.29
      hereditary hemolytic anemia P58.8
      hypothyroidism, congenital E03.1
      incompatibility, maternal/fetal NOS P55.9
      infection P58.2

Jaundice (Continued)
  newborn (Continued)
    due to or associated with (Continued)
      inspissated bile syndrome P59.1
      isoimmunization NOS P55.9
      mucoviscidosis E84.9
      polycythemia P58.3
      preterm delivery P59.0
      Rh
        antibodies P55.0
        incompatibility, maternal/fetal P55.0
        isoimmunization P55.0
      specified cause NEC P59.8
      swallowed maternal blood P58.5
      spherocytosis (congenital) D58.0
    nonhemolytic congenital familial (Gilbert) E80.4
    nuclear, newborn —see also Kernicterus of newborn P57.9
    obstructive —see also Obstruction, bile duct K83.1
    post-immunization —see Hepatitis, viral, type, B
    post-transfusion —see Hepatitis, viral, type, B
    regurgitation —see also Obstruction, bile duct K83.1
    serum (homologous) (prophylactic) (therapeutic) —see Hepatitis, viral, type, B
    spirochetal (hemorrhagic) A27.0
    symptomatic R17
      newborn P59.9
Jaw —see condition
Jaw-winking phenomenon or syndrome Q07.8
Jealousy
  alcoholic F10.988
  childhood F93.8
  sibling F93.8
Jejunitis —see Enteritis
Jejunostomy status Z93.4
Jejunum, jejunal —see condition
Jensen's disease —see Inflammation, chorioretinal, focal, juxtapapillary
Jerks, myoclonic G25.3
Jervell-Lange-Nielsen syndrome I45.81
Jeune's disease Q77.2
Jigger disease B88.1
Job's syndrome (chronic granulomatous disease) D71
Joint —see also condition
  mice —see Loose, body, joint
    knee M23.4-●
Jordan's anomaly or syndrome D72.0
Joseph-Diamond-Blackfan anemia (congenital hypoplastic) D61.01
Jungle yellow fever A95.0
Jüngling's disease —see Sarcoidosis
Juvenile —see condition

K

Kahler's disease C90.0-●
Kakke E51.11
Kala-azar B55.0
Kallmann's syndrome E23.0
Kanner's syndrome (autism) —see Psychosis, childhood
Kaposi's
 dermatosis (xeroderma pigmentosum) Q82.1
 lichen ruber L44.0
  acuminatus L44.0
 sarcoma
  colon C46.4
  connective tissue C46.1
  gastrointestinal organ C46.4
  lung C46.5-●
  lymph node (multiple) C46.3
  palate (hard) (soft) C46.2
  rectum C46.4
  skin (multiple sites) C46.0
  specified site NEC C46.7
  stomach C46.4
  unspecified site C46.9
 varicelliform eruption B00.0
  vaccinia T88.1
Kartagener's syndrome or triad (sinusitis, bronchiectasis, situs inversus) Q89.3
Karyotype
 with abnormality except iso (Xq) Q96.2
 45,X Q96.0
 46,X
  iso (Xq) Q96.1
 46,XX Q98.3
  with streak gonads Q50.32
  hermaphrodite (true) Q99.1
  male Q98.3
 46,XY
  with streak gonads Q56.1
  female Q97.3
  hermaphrodite (true) Q99.1
 47,XXX Q97.0
 47,XXY Q98.0
 47,XYY Q98.5
Kaschin-Beck disease —see Disease, Kaschin-Beck
Katayama's disease or fever B65.2
Kawasaki's syndrome M30.3
Kayser-Fleischer ring (cornea) (pseudosclerosis) H18.04-●
Kaznelson's syndrome (congenital hypoplastic anemia) D61.01
Kearns-Sayre syndrome H49.81-●
Kedani fever A75.3
Kelis L91.0
Kelly (-Patterson) syndrome (sideropenic dysphagia) D50.1
Keloid, cheloid L91.0
 acne L73.0
 Addison's L94.0
 cornea —see Opacity, cornea
 Hawkin's L91.0
 scar L91.0
Keloma L91.0
Kenya fever A77.1
Keratectasia —see also Ectasia, cornea
 congenital Q13.4
Keratinization of alveolar ridge mucosa
 excessive K13.23
 minimal K13.22
Keratinized residual ridge mucosa
 excessive K13.23
 minimal K13.22
Keratitis (nodular) (nonulcerative) (simple) (zonular) H16.9
 with ulceration (central) (marginal) (perforated) (ring) —see Ulcer, cornea
 actinic —see Photokeratitis
 arborescens (herpes simplex) B00.52
 areolar H16.11-●
 bullosa H16.8

Keratitis (Continued)
 deep H16.309
  specified type NEC H16.399
 dendritic (a) (herpes simplex) B00.52
 disciform (is) (herpes simplex) B00.52
  varicella B01.81
 filamentary H16.12-●
 gonococcal (congenital or prenatal) A54.33
 herpes, herpetic (simplex) B00.52
  zoster B02.33
 in (due to)
  acanthamebiasis B60.13
  adenovirus B30.0
  exanthema —see also Exanthem B09
  herpes (simplex) virus B00.52
  measles B05.81
  syphilis A50.31
  tuberculosis A18.52
  zoster B02.33
 interstitial (nonsyphilitic) H16.30-●
  diffuse H16.32-●
  herpes, herpetic (simplex) B00.52
   zoster B02.33
  sclerosing H16.33-●
  specified type NEC H16.39-●
  syphilitic (congenital) (late) A50.31
  tuberculous A18.52
 macular H16.11-●
 nummular H16.11-●
 oyster shuckers' H16.8
 parenchymatous —see Keratitis, interstitial
 petrificans H16.8
 postmeasles B05.81
 punctata
  leprosa A30.9 [H16.14-●]
  syphilitic (profunda) A50.31
 punctate H16.14-●
 purulent H16.8
 rosacea L71.8
 sclerosing H16.33-●
 specified type NEC H16.8
 stellate H16.11-●
 striate H16.11-●
 superficial H16.10-●
  with conjunctivitis —see Keratoconjunctivitis
  due to light —see Photokeratitis
 suppurative H16.8
 syphilitic (congenital) (prenatal) A50.31
 trachomatous A71.1
  sequelae B94.0
 tuberculous A18.52
 vesicular H16.8
 xerotic —see also Keratomalacia H16.8
  vitamin A deficiency E50.4
Keratoacanthoma L85.8
Keratocele —see Descemetocele
Keratoconjunctivitis H16.20-●
 Acanthamoeba B60.13
 adenoviral B30.0
 epidemic B30.0
 exposure H16.21-●
 herpes, herpetic (simplex) B00.52
  zoster B02.33
 in exanthema —see also Exanthem B09
 infectious B30.0
 lagophthalmic —see Keratoconjunctivitis, specified type NEC
 neurotrophic H16.23-●
 phlyctenular H16.25-●
 postmeasles B05.81
 shipyard B30.0
 sicca (Sjogren's) M35.0-●
  not Sjogren's H16.22-●
 specified type NEC H16.29-●
 tuberculous (phlyctenular) A18.52
 vernal H16.26-●
Keratoconus H18.60-●
 congenital Q13.4
 stable H18.61-●
 unstable H18.62-●

Keratocyst (dental) (odontogenic) —see Cyst, calcifying odontogenic
Keratoderma, keratodermia (congenital) (palmaris et plantaris) (symmetrical) Q82.8
 acquired L85.1
  in diseases classified elsewhere L86
 climactericum L85.1
 gonococcal A54.89
 gonorrheal A54.89
 punctata L85.2
 Reiter's —see Reiter's disease
Keratodermatocele —see Descemetocele
Keratoglobus H18.79
 congenital Q15.8
  with glaucoma Q15.0
Keratohemia —see Pigmentation, cornea, stromal
Keratoiritis —see also Iridocyclitis
 syphilitic A50.39
 tuberculous A18.54
Keratoma L57.0
 palmaris and plantaris hereditarium Q82.8
 senile L57.0
Keratomalacia H18.44-●
 vitamin A deficiency E50.4
Keratomegaly Q13.4
Keratomycosis B49
 nigrans, nigricans (palmaris) B36.1
Keratopathy H18.9
 band H18.42-●
 bullous H18.1-●
 bullous (aphakic), following cataract surgery H59.01-●
Keratoscleritis, tuberculous A18.52
Keratosis L57.0
 actinic L57.0
 arsenical L85.8
 congenital, specified NEC Q80.8
 female genital NEC N94.89
 follicularis Q82.8
  acquired L11.0
  congenita Q82.8
  et parafollicularis in cutem penetrans L87.0
  spinulosa (decalvans) Q82.8
  vitamin A deficiency E50.8
 gonococcal A54.89
 male genital (external) N50.89
 nigricans L83
 obturans, external ear (canal) —see Cholesteatoma, external ear
 palmaris et plantaris (inherited) (symmetrical) Q82.8
  acquired L85.1
 penile N48.89
 pharynx J39.2
 pilaris, acquired L85.8
 punctata (palmaris et plantaris) L85.2
 scrotal N50.89
 seborrheic L82.1
  inflamed L82.0
 senile L57.0
 solar L57.0
 tonsillaris J35.8
 vagina N89.4
 vegetans Q82.8
 vitamin A deficiency E50.8
 vocal cord J38.3
Kerato-uveitis —see Iridocyclitis
Kerion (celsi) B35.0
Kernicterus of newborn (not due to isoimmunization) P57.9
 due to isoimmunization (conditions in P55.0-P55.9) P57.0
 specified type NEC P57.8
Kerunoparalysis T75.09
Keshan disease E59
Ketoacidosis E87.2
 diabetic —see Diabetes, by type, with ketoacidosis
Ketonuria R82.4

Ketosis NEC E88.89
  diabetic —*see* Diabetes, by type, with
    ketoacidosis
Kew Garden fever A79.1
Kidney —*see* condition
Kienböck's disease —*see also* Osteochondrosis,
    juvenile, hand, carpal lunate
  adult M93.1
Kimmelstiel (-Wilson) disease —*see* Diabetes,
    Kimmelstiel (-Wilson) disease
Kimura disease D21.9
  specified site (*see* Neoplasm, connective
    tissue benign)
Kink, kinking
  artery I77.1
  hair (acquired) L67.8
  ileum or intestine —*see* Obstruction,
    intestine
  Lane's —*see* Obstruction, intestine
  organ or site, congenital NEC —*see* Anomaly,
    by site
  ureter (pelvic junction) N13.5
    with
      hydronephrosis N13.1
        with infection N13.6
      pyelonephritis (chronic) N11.1
    congenital Q62.39
  vein(s) I87.8
    caval I87.1
    peripheral I87.1
Kinnier Wilson's disease (hepatolenticular
    degeneration) E83.01
Kissing spine M48.20
  cervical region M48.22
  cervicothoracic region M48.23
  lumbar region M48.26
  lumbosacral region M48.27
  occipito-atlanto-axial region M48.21
  thoracic region M48.24
  thoracolumbar region M48.25
Klatskin's tumor C24.0
Klauder's disease A26.8
Klebs' disease —*see also* Glomerulonephritis
    N05.-•
Klebsiella (K.) pneumoniae, as cause of
    disease classified elsewhere B96.1
Klein (e)-Levin syndrome G47.13
Kleptomania F63.2
Klinefelter's syndrome Q98.4
  karyotype 47,XXY Q98.0
  male with more than two X chromosomes
    Q98.1
Klippel-Feil deficiency, disease, or syndrome
    (brevicollis) Q76.1
Klippel's disease I67.2
Klippel-Trenaunay (-Weber) syndrome
    Q87.2
Klumpke (-Déjerine) palsy, paralysis (birth)
    (newborn) P14.1
Knee —*see* condition
Knock knee (acquired) M21.06-•
  congenital Q74.1

Knot(s)
  intestinal, syndrome (volvulus) K56.2
  surfer S89.8-•
  umbilical cord (true) O69.2
Knotting (of)
  hair L67.8
  intestine K56.2
Knuckle pad (Garrod's) M72.1
Koch's
  infection —*see* Tuberculosis
  relapsing fever A68.9
Koch-Weeks' conjunctivitis —*see*
    Conjunctivitis, acute, mucopurulent
Köebner's syndrome Q81.8
Köenig's disease (osteochondritis dissecans) —
    see Osteochondritis, dissecans
Köhler-Pellegrini-Steida disease or syndrome
    (calcification, knee joint) —*see* Bursitis,
    tibial collateral
Köhler's disease
  patellar —*see* Osteochondrosis, juvenile,
    patella
  tarsal navicular —*see* Osteochondrosis,
    juvenile, tarsus
Koilonychia L60.3
  congenital Q84.6
Kojevnikov's, epilepsy —*see* Kozhevnikof's
    epilepsy
Koplik's spots B05.9
Kopp's asthma E32.8
Korsakoff's (Wernicke) disease, psychosis or
    syndrome (alcoholic) F10.96
  with dependence F10.26
  drug-induced
    due to drug abuse —*see* Abuse, drug, by
      type, with amnestic disorder
    due to drug dependence —*see* Dependence,
      drug, by type, with amnestic disorder
  nonalcoholic F04
Korsakov's disease, psychosis or syndrome —
    see Korsakoff's disease
Korsakow's disease, psychosis or syndrome —
    see Korsakoff's disease
Kostmann's disease or syndrome (infantile
    genetic agranulocytosis) —*see*
    Agranulocytosis
Kozhevnikof's epilepsy G40.109
  intractable G40.119
    with status epilepticus G40.111
    without status epilepticus G40.119
  not intractable G40.109
    with status epilepticus G40.101
    without status epilepticus G40.109
Krabbe's
  disease E75.23
  syndrome, congenital muscle hypoplasia
    Q79.8
Kraepelin-Morel disease —*see* Schizophrenia
Kraft-Weber-Dimitri disease Q85.8
Kraurosis
  ani K62.89
  penis N48.0

Kraurosis (*Continued*)
  vagina N89.8
  vulva N90.4
Kreotoxism A05.9
Krukenberg's
  spindle —*see* Pigmentation, cornea, posterior
  tumor C79.6-•
Kufs' disease E75.4
Kugelberg-Welander disease G12.1
Kuhnt-Junius degeneration —*see also*
    Degeneration, macula H35.32-•
Kümmell's disease or spondylitis —*see*
    Spondylopathy, traumatic
Kupffer cell sarcoma C22.3
Kuru A81.81
Kussmaul's
  disease M30.0
  respiration E87.2
    in diabetic acidosis —*see* Diabetes, by type,
      with ketoacidosis
Kwashiorkor E40
  marasmic, marasmus type E42
Kyasanur Forest disease A98.2
Kyphoscoliosis, kyphoscoliotic (acquired) —
    see also Scoliosis M41.9
  congenital Q67.5
  heart (disease) I27.1
  sequelae of rickets E64.3
  tuberculous A18.01
Kyphosis, kyphotic (acquired) M40.209
  cervical region M40.202
  cervicothoracic region M40.203
  congenital Q76.419
    cervical region Q76.412
    cervicothoracic region Q76.413
    occipito-atlanto-axial region Q76.411
    thoracic region Q76.414
    thoracolumbar region Q76.415
  Morquio-Brailsford type (spinal) —*see also*
    subcategory M49.8 E76.219
  postlaminectomy M96.3
  postradiation therapy M96.2
  postural (adolescent) M40.00
    cervicothoracic region M40.03
    thoracic region M40.04
    thoracolumbar region M40.05
  secondary NEC M40.10
    cervical region M40.12
    cervicothoracic region M40.13
    thoracic region M40.14
    thoracolumbar region M40.15
  sequelae of rickets E64.3
  specified type NEC M40.299
    cervical region M40.292
    cervicothoracic region M40.293
    thoracic region M40.294
    thoracolumbar region M40.295
  syphilitic, congenital A50.56
  thoracic region M40.204
  thoracolumbar region M40.205
  tuberculous A18.01
Kyrle disease L87.0

L

Labia, labium —*see* condition
Labile
blood pressure R09.89
vasomotor system I73.9
Labioglossal paralysis G12.29
Labium leporinum —*see* Cleft, lip
Labor —*see* Delivery
Labored breathing —*see* Hyperventilation
Labyrinthitis (circumscribed) (destructive)
(diffuse) (inner ear) (latent) (purulent)
(suppurative) (*see also* subcategory)
H83.0
syphilitic A52.79
Laceration
with abortion —*see* Abortion, by type,
complicated by laceration of pelvic
organs
abdomen, abdominal
wall S31.119
with
foreign body S31.129
penetration into peritoneal cavity
S31.619
with foreign body S31.629
epigastric region S31.112
with
foreign body S31.122
penetration into peritoneal cavity
S31.612
with foreign body S31.622
left
lower quadrant S31.114
with
foreign body S31.124
penetration into peritoneal cavity
S31.614
with foreign body S31.624
upper quadrant S31.111
with
foreign body S31.121
penetration into peritoneal cavity
S31.611
with foreign body S31.621
periumbilic region S31.115
with
foreign body S31.125
penetration into peritoneal cavity
S31.615
with foreign body S31.625
right
lower quadrant S31.113
with
foreign body S31.123
penetration into peritoneal cavity
S31.613
with foreign body S31.623
upper quadrant S31.110
with
foreign body S31.120
penetration into peritoneal cavity
S31.610
with foreign body S31.620
accidental, complicating surgery —*see*
Complications, surgical, accidental
puncture or laceration
Achilles tendon S86.02-●
adrenal gland S37.813
alveolar (process) —*see* Laceration, oral cavity
ankle S91.01-●
with
foreign body S91.02-●
antecubital space —*see* Laceration, elbow
anus (sphincter) S31.831
with
ectopic or molar pregnancy O08.6
foreign body S31.832
complicating delivery —*see* Delivery,
complicated, by, laceration, anus
(sphincter)

Laceration (*Continued*)
anus (*Continued*)
following ectopic or molar pregnancy
O08.6
nontraumatic, nonpuerperal —*see* Fissure,
anus
arm (upper) S41.11-●
with foreign body S41.12-●
lower —*see* Laceration, forearm
auditory canal (external) (meatus) —*see*
Laceration, ear
auricle, ear —*see* Laceration, ear
axilla —*see* Laceration, arm
back —*see also* Laceration, thorax, back
lower S31.010
with
foreign body S31.020
with penetration into
retroperitoneal space S31.021
penetration into retroperitoneal space
S31.011
bile duct S36.13
bladder S37.23
with ectopic or molar pregnancy O08.6
following ectopic or molar pregnancy
O08.6
obstetrical trauma O71.5
blood vessel —*see* Injury, blood vessel
bowel —*see also* Laceration, intestine
with ectopic or molar pregnancy O08.6
complicating abortion —*see* Abortion,
by type, complicated by, specified
condition NEC
following ectopic or molar pregnancy
O08.6
obstetrical trauma O71.5
brain (any part) (cortex) (diffuse)
(membrane) —*see also* Injury,
intracranial, diffuse
during birth P10.8
with hemorrhage P10.1
focal —*see* Injury, intracranial, focal brain
injury
brainstem S06.38-●
breast S21.01-●
with foreign body S21.02-●
broad ligament S37.893
with ectopic or molar pregnancy O08.6
following ectopic or molar pregnancy
O08.6
laceration syndrome N83.8
obstetrical trauma O71.6
syndrome (laceration) N83.8
buttock S31.801
with foreign body S31.802
left S31.821
with foreign body S31.822
right S31.811
with foreign body S31.812
calf —*see* Laceration, leg
canaliculus lacrimalis —*see* Laceration,
eyelid
canthus, eye —*see* Laceration, eyelid
capsule, joint —*see* Sprain
causing eversion of cervix uteri (old) N86
central (perineal), complicating delivery
O70.9
cerebellum, traumatic S06.37-●
cerebral S06.33-●
during birth P10.8
with hemorrhage P10.1
left side S06.32-●
right side S06.31-●
cervix (uteri)
with ectopic or molar pregnancy O08.6
following ectopic or molar pregnancy
O08.6
nonpuerperal, nontraumatic N88.1
obstetrical trauma (current) O71.3
old (postpartal) N88.1
traumatic S37.63

Laceration (*Continued*)
cheek (external) S01.41-●
with foreign body S01.42-●
internal —*see* Laceration, oral cavity
chest wall —*see* Laceration, thorax
chin —*see* Laceration, head, specified site
NEC
chordae tendinae NEC I51.1
concurrent with acute myocardial
infarction —*see* Infarct, myocardium
following acute myocardial infarction
(current complication) I23.4
clitoris —*see* Laceration, vulva
colon —*see* Laceration, intestine, large,
colon
common bile duct S36.13
cortex (cerebral) —*see* Injury, intracranial,
diffuse
costal region —*see* Laceration, thorax
cystic duct S36.13
diaphragm S27.803
digit(s)
foot —*see* Laceration, toe
hand —*see* Laceration, finger
duodenum S36.430
ear (canal) (external) S01.31-●
with foreign body S01.32-●
drum S09.2-●
elbow S51.01-●
with
foreign body S51.02-●
epididymis —*see* Laceration, testis
epigastric region —*see* Laceration, abdomen,
wall, epigastric region
esophagus K22.89
traumatic
cervical S11.21
with foreign body S11.22
thoracic S27.813
eye (ball) S05.3-●
with prolapse or loss of intraocular tissue
S05.2-●
penetrating S05.6-●
eyebrow —*see* Laceration, eyelid
eyelid S01.11-●
with foreign body S01.12-●
face NEC —*see* Laceration, head, specified
site NEC
fallopian tube S37.539
bilateral S37.532
unilateral S37.531
finger(s) S61.219
with
damage to nail S61.319
with
foreign body S61.329
foreign body S61.229
index S61.218
with
damage to nail S61.318
with
foreign body S61.328
foreign body S61.228
left S61.211
with
damage to nail S61.311
with
foreign body S61.321
foreign body S61.221
right S61.210
with
damage to nail S61.310
with
foreign body S61.320
foreign body S61.220
little S61.218
with
damage to nail S61.318
with
foreign body S61.328
foreign body S61.228

▶ New　　⇒ Revised　　~~deleted~~ Deleted　　● Use Additional Character(s)

Laceration *(Continued)*
finger *(Continued)*
little *(Continued)*
left S61.217
with
damage to nail S61.317
with
foreign body S61.327
foreign body S61.227
right S61.216
with
damage to nail S61.316
with
foreign body S61.326
foreign body S61.226
middle S61.218
with
damage to nail S61.318
with
foreign body S61.328
foreign body S61.228
left S61.213
with
damage to nail S61.313
with
foreign body S61.323
foreign body S61.223
right S61.212
with
damage to nail S61.312
with
foreign body S61.322
foreign body S61.222
ring S61.218
with
damage to nail S61.318
with
foreign body S61.328
foreign body S61.228
left S61.215
with
damage to nail S61.315
with
foreign body S61.325
foreign body S61.225
right S61.214
with
damage to nail S61.314
with
foreign body S61.324
foreign body S61.224
flank S31.119
with foreign body S31.129
foot (except toe(s) alone) S91.319
with foreign body S91.329
left S91.312
with foreign body S91.322
right S91.311
with foreign body S91.321
toe —*see* Laceration, toe
forearm S51.819
with
foreign body S51.829
elbow only —*see* Laceration,
elbow
left S51.812
with
foreign body S51.822
right S51.811
with
foreign body S51.821
forehead S01.81
with foreign body S01.82
fourchette O70.0
with ectopic or molar pregnancy
O08.6
complicating delivery O70.0
following ectopic or molar pregnancy
O08.6
gallbladder S36.123

Laceration *(Continued)*
genital organs, external
female S31.512
with foreign body S31.522
vagina —*see* Laceration, vagina
vulva —*see* Laceration, vulva
male S31.511
with foreign body S31.521
penis —*see* Laceration, penis
scrotum —*see* Laceration, scrotum
testis —*see* Laceration, testis
groin —*see* Laceration, abdomen, wall
gum —*see* Laceration, oral cavity
hand S61.419
with
foreign body S61.429
finger —*see* Laceration, finger
left S61.412
with
foreign body S61.422
right S61.411
with
foreign body S61.421
thumb —*see* Laceration, thumb
head S01.91
with foreign body S01.92
cheek —*see* Laceration, cheek
ear —*see* Laceration, ear
eyelid —*see* Laceration, eyelid
lip —*see* Laceration, lip
nose —*see* Laceration, nose
oral cavity —*see* Laceration, oral
cavity
scalp S01.01
with foreign body S01.02
specified site NEC S01.81
with foreign body S01.82
temporomandibular area —*see* Laceration,
cheek
heart —*see* Injury, heart, laceration
heel —*see* Laceration, foot
hepatic duct S36.13
lip S71.019
with foreign body S71.029
left S71.012
with foreign body S71.022
right S71.011
with foreign body S71.021
hymen —*see* Laceration, vagina
hypochondrium —*see* Laceration, abdomen,
wall
hypogastric region —*see* Laceration,
abdomen, wall
ileum S36.438
inguinal region —*see* Laceration, abdomen,
wall
instep —*see* Laceration, foot
internal organ —*see* Injury, by site
interscapular region —*see* Laceration, thorax,
back
intestine
large
colon S36.539
ascending S36.530
descending S36.532
sigmoid S36.533
specified site NEC S36.538
rectum S36.63
transverse S36.531
small S36.439
duodenum S36.430
specified site NEC S36.438
intra-abdominal organ S36.93
intestine —*see* Laceration, intestine
liver —*see* Laceration, liver
pancreas —*see* Laceration, pancreas
peritoneum S36.81
specified site NEC S36.893
spleen —*see* Laceration, spleen
stomach —*see* Laceration, stomach

Laceration *(Continued)*
intracranial NEC —*see also* Injury,
intracranial, diffuse
birth injury P10.9
jaw —*see* Laceration, head, specified site NEC
jejunum S36.438
joint capsule —*see* Sprain, by site
kidney S37.03-●
major (greater than 3 cm) (massive)
(stellate) S37.06-●
minor (less than 1 cm) S37.04-●
moderate (1 to 3 cm) S37.05-●
multiple S37.06-●
knee S81.01-●
with foreign body S81.02-●
labium (majus) (minus) —*see* Laceration,
vulva
lacrimal duct —*see* Laceration, eyelid
large intestine —*see* Laceration, intestine,
large
larynx S11.011
with foreign body S11.012
leg (lower) S81.819
with foreign body S81.829
foot —*see* Laceration, foot
knee —*see* Laceration, knee
left S81.812
with foreign body S81.822
right S81.811
with foreign body S81.821
upper —*see* Laceration, thigh
ligament —*see* Sprain
lip S01.511
with foreign body S01.521
liver S36.113
major (stellate) S36.116
minor S36.114
moderate S36.115
loin —*see* Laceration, abdomen, wall
lower back —*see* Laceration, back, lower
lumbar region —*see* Laceration, back, lower
lung S27.339
bilateral S27.332
unilateral S27.331
malar region —*see* Laceration, head, specified
site NEC
mammary —*see* Laceration, breast
mastoid region —*see* Laceration, head,
specified site NEC
meninges —*see* Injury, intracranial, diffuse
meniscus —*see* Tear, meniscus
mesentery S36.893
mesosalpinx S37.893
mouth —*see* Laceration, oral cavity
muscle —*see* Injury, muscle, by site,
laceration
nail
finger —*see* Laceration, finger, with
damage to nail
toe —*see* Laceration, toe, with damage to nail
nasal (septum) (sinus) —*see* Laceration, nose
nasopharynx —*see* Laceration, head, specified
site NEC
neck S11.91
with foreign body S11.92
involving
cervical esophagus S11.21
with foreign body S11.22
larynx —*see* Laceration, larynx
pharynx —*see* Laceration, pharynx
thyroid gland —*see* Laceration, thyroid
gland
trachea —*see* Laceration, trachea
specified site NEC S11.81
with foreign body S11.82
nerve —*see* Injury, nerve
nose (septum) (sinus) S01.21
with foreign body S01.22
ocular NOS S05.3-●
adnexa NOS S01.11-●

▶ New   ⇒ Revised   ~~deleted~~ Deleted   ● Use Additional Character(s)

Laceration (Continued)
  trachea S11.021
    with foreign body S11.022
  tunica vaginalis —*see* Laceration, testis
  tympanum, tympanic membrane —*see*
    Laceration, ear, drum
  umbilical region S31.115
    with foreign body S31.125
  ureter S37.13
  urethra S37.33
    with or following ectopic or molar
      pregnancy O08.6
    obstetrical trauma O71.5
  urinary organ NEC S37.893
  uterus S37.63
    with ectopic or molar pregnancy O08.6
    following ectopic or molar pregnancy O08.6
    nonpuerperal, nontraumatic N85.8
    obstetrical trauma NEC O71.81
    old (postpartal) N85.8
  uvula —*see* Laceration, oral cavity
  vagina S31.41
    with
      ectopic or molar pregnancy O08.6
      foreign body S31.42
    during delivery O71.4
      with perineal laceration —*see* Laceration,
        perineum, female, during delivery
    following ectopic or molar pregnancy
      O08.6
    nonpuerperal, nontraumatic N89.8
    old (postpartal) N89.8
  vas deferens S37.893
  vesical —*see* Laceration, bladder
  vocal cords S11.031
    with foreign body S11.032
  vulva S31.41
    with
      ectopic or molar pregnancy O08.6
      foreign body S31.42
    complicating delivery O70.0
    following ectopic or molar pregnancy
      O08.6
    nonpuerperal, nontraumatic N90.89
    old (postpartal) N90.89
  wrist S61.519
    with
      foreign body S61.529
    left S61.512
      with
        foreign body S61.522
    right S61.511
      with
        foreign body S61.521
Lack of
  achievement in school Z55.3
  adequate
    ➠food Z59.48
    intermaxillary vertical dimension of fully
      erupted teeth M26.36
    sleep Z72.820
  appetite (*see* Anorexia) R63.0
  awareness R41.9
  care
    in home Z74.2
    of infant (at or after birth) T76.02
      confirmed T74.02
  cognitive functions R41.9
  coordination R27.9
    ataxia R27.0
    specified type NEC R27.8
  development (physiological) R62.50
    failure to thrive (child over 28 days old)
      R62.51
    adult R62.7
    newborn P92.6
    short stature R62.52
    specified type NEC R62.59
  energy R53.83
  financial resources Z59.6

Lack of (Continued)
  ➠food Z59.48
  growth R62.52
  heating Z59.1
  ➠housing (permanent) (temporary) Z59.00
    adequate Z59.1
  learning experiences in childhood Z62.898
  leisure time (affecting life-style) Z73.2
  material resources Z59.9
  memory —*see also* Amnesia
    mild, following organic brain damage
      F06.8
  ovulation N97.0
  parental supervision or control of child Z62.0
  person able to render necessary care Z74.2
  physical exercise Z72.3
  play experience in childhood Z62.898
  posterior occlusal support M26.57
  relaxation (affecting life-style) Z73.2
  ▶safe drinking water Z58.6
  sexual
    desire F52.0
    enjoyment F52.1
  ➠shelter Z59.02
  sleep (adequate) Z72.820
  supervision of child by parent Z62.0
  support, posterior occlusal M26.57
  water T73.1
    ▶safe drinking Z58.6
Lacrimal —*see* condition
Lacrimation, abnormal —*see* Epiphora
Lacrimonasal duct —*see* condition
Lactation, lactating (breast) (puerperal,
  postpartum)
  associated
    cracked nipple O92.13
    retracted nipple O92.03
  defective O92.4
  disorder NEC O92.79
  excessive O92.6
  failed (complete) O92.3
    partial O92.4
  mastitis NEC *see* Mastitis, obstetric
  mother (care and/or examination) Z39.1
  nonpuerperal N64.3
Lacticemia, excessive E87.2
Lacunar skull Q75.8
Laennec's cirrhosis K70.30
  with ascites K70.31
  nonalcoholic K74.69
Lafora's disease —*see* Epilepsy, generalized,
  idiopathic
Lag, lid (nervous) —*see* Retraction, lid
Lagophthalmos (eyelid) (nervous) H02.209
  bilateral, upper and lower eyelids H02.20C
  cicatricial H02.219
    bilateral, upper and lower eyelids H02.21C
    left H02.216
      lower H02.215
      upper H02.214
      upper and lower eyelids H02.21B
    right H02.213
      lower H02.212
      upper H02.211
      upper and lower eyelids H02.21A
  keratoconjunctivitis —*see* Keratoconjunctivitis
  left H02.206
    lower H02.205
    upper H02.204
    upper and lower eyelids H02.20B
  mechanical H02.229
    bilateral, upper and lower eyelids H02.22C
    left H02.226
      lower H02.225
      upper H02.224
      upper and lower eyelids H02.22B
    right H02.223
      lower H02.222
      upper H02.221
      upper and lower eyelids H02.22A

Lagophthalmos (Continued)
  paralytic H02.239
    bilateral, upper and lower eyelids H02.23C
    left H02.236
      lower H02.235
      upper H02.234
      upper and lower eyelids H02.23B
    right H02.233
      lower H02.232
      upper H02.231
      upper and lower eyelids H02.23A
    right H02.203
      lower H02.202
      upper H02.201
      upper and lower eyelids H02.20A
Laki-Lorand factor deficiency —*see* Defect,
  coagulation, specified type NEC
Lalling F80.0
Lambert-Eaton syndrome —*see* Syndrome,
  Lambert-Eaton
Lambliasis, lambliosis A07.1
Landau-Kleffner syndrome —*see* Epilepsy,
  specified NEC
**Landouzy-Déjérine dystrophy or
  facioscapulohumeral atrophy** G71.02
Landouzy's disease (icterohemorrhagic
  leptospirosis) A27.0
Landry-Guillain-Barré, syndrome or paralysis
  G61.0
Landry's disease or paralysis G61.0
Lane's
  band Q43.3
  kink —*see* Obstruction, intestine
  syndrome K90.2
Langdon Down's syndrome —*see* Trisomy, 21
Lapsed immunization schedule status Z28.3
Large
  baby (regardless of gestational age) (4000g to
    4499g) P08.1
  ear, congenital Q17.1
  physiological cup Q14.2
  stature R68.89
Large-for-dates NEC (infant) (4000g to 4499g)
  P08.1
  affecting management of pregnancy O36.6-●
  exceptionally (4500g or more) P08.0
Larsen-Johansson disease
  orosteochondrosis —*see* Osteochondrosis,
    juvenile, patella
Larsen's syndrome (flattened facies and
  multiple congenital dislocations) Q74.8
Larva migrans
  cutaneous B76.9
    Ancylostoma B76.0
  visceral B83.0
Laryngeal —*see* condition
Laryngismus (stridulus) J38.5
  congenital P28.89
  diphtheritic A36.2
Laryngitis (acute) (edematous) (fibrinous)
  (infective) (infiltrative) (malignant)
  (membranous) (phlegmonous)
  (pneumococcal) (pseudomembranous)
  (septic) (subglottic) (suppurative)
  (ulcerative) J04.0
  with
    influenza, flu, or grippe —*see* Influenza,
      with, laryngitis
    tracheitis (acute) —*see* Laryngotracheitis
  atrophic J37.0
  catarrhal J37.0
  chronic J37.0
    with tracheitis (chronic) J37.1
  diphtheritic A36.2
  due to external agent —*see* Inflammation,
    respiratory, upper, due to
  Hemophilus influenzae J04.0
  H. influenzae J04.0
  hypertrophic J37.0
  influenzal —*see* Influenza, with, respiratory
    manifestations NEC

Laryngitis *(Continued)*
  obstructive J05.0
  sicca J37.0
  spasmodic J05.0
    acute J04.0
  streptococcal J04.0
  stridulous J05.0
  syphilitic (late) A52.73
    congenital A50.59 *[J99]*
      early A50.03 *[J99]*
  tuberculous A15.5
  Vincent's A69.1
Laryngocele (congenital) (ventricular) Q31.3
Laryngofissure J38.7
  congenital Q31.8
Laryngomalacia (congenital) Q31.5
Laryngopharyngitis (acute) J06.0
  chronic J37.0
  due to external agent —*see* Inflammation,
    respiratory, upper, due to
Laryngoplegia J38.00
  bilateral J38.02
  unilateral J38.01
Laryngoptosis J38.7
Laryngospasm J38.5
Laryngostenosis J38.6
Laryngotracheitis (acute) (Infectional)
  (infective) (viral) J04.2
  atrophic J37.1
  catarrhal J37.1
  chronic J37.1
  diphtheritic A36.2
  due to external agent —*see* Inflammation,
    respiratory, upper, due to
  Hemophilus influenzae J04.2
  hypertrophic J37.1
  influenzal —*see* Influenza, with, respiratory
    manifestations NEC
  pachydermic J38.7
  sicca J37.1
  spasmodic J38.5
    acute J05.0
  streptococcal J04.2
  stridulous J38.5
  syphilitic (late) A52.73
    congenital A50.59 *[J99]*
      early A50.03 *[J99]*
  tuberculous A15.5
  Vincent's A69.1
Laryngotracheobronchitis —*see* Bronchitis
Larynx, laryngeal —*see* condition
Lassa fever A96.2
Lassitude —*see* Weakness
Late
  talker R62.0
  walker R62.0
Late effect(s) —*see* Sequelae
Latent —*see* condition
Laterocession —*see* Lateroversion
Lateroflexion —*see* Lateroversion
Lateroversion
  cervix —*see* Lateroversion, uterus
  uterus, uterine (cervix) (postinfectional)
    (postpartal, old) N85.4
    congenital Q51.818
    in pregnancy or childbirth O34.59-●
Lathyrism —*see* Poisoning, food, noxious,
  plant
Launois' syndrome (pituitary gigantism) E22.0
Launois-Bensaude adenolipomatosis E88.89
Laurence-Moon (-Bardet)-Biedl syndrome
  Q87.89
Lax, laxity —*see also* Relaxation
  ligament (ous) —*see also* Disorder, ligament
    familial M35.7
    knee —*see* Derangement, knee
  skin (acquired) L57.4
    congenital Q82.8
Laxative habit F55.2
Lazy leukocyte syndrome D70.8
Lead miner's lung J63.6

Leak, leakage
  air NEC J93.82
    postprocedural J95.812
  amniotic fluid —*see* Rupture, membranes,
    premature
  blood (microscopic), fetal, into maternal
    circulation affecting management
    of pregnancy —*see* Pregnancy,
    complicated by
  cerebrospinal fluid G96.00
    cranial
      postoperative G96.08
      specified NEC G96.08
      spontaneous G96.01
      traumatic G96.08
    from spinal (lumbar) puncture G97.0
    spinal
      postoperative G96.09
      post-traumatic G96.09
      specified NEC G96.09
      spontaneous G96.02
    spontaneous
      from
        skull base G96.01
      spine G96.02
  CSF —*see* Leak, cerebrospinal fluid
  device, implant or graft —*see also*
    Complications, by site and type,
    mechanical
    arterial graft NEC —*see* Complication,
      cardiovascular device, mechanical,
      vascular
    breast (implant) T85.43
    catheter NEC T85.638
      dialysis (renal) T82.43
        intraperitoneal T85.631
      infusion NEC T82.534
        spinal (epidural) (subdural)
          T85.630
      urinary T83.038
        cystostomy T83.030
        Hopkins T83.038
        ileostomy T83.038
        indwelling T83.031
        nephrostomy T83.032
        specified NEC T83.038
        urostomy T83.038
    gastrointestinal —*see* Complications,
      prosthetic device, mechanical,
      gastrointestinal device
    genital NEC T83.498
      penile prosthesis (cylinder) (implanted)
        (pump) (resevoir) T83.490
      testicular prosthesis T83.491
    heart NEC —*see* Complication,
      cardiovascular device, mechanical
    joint prosthesis —*see* Complications, joint
      prosthesis, mechanical, specified NEC,
      by site
    ocular NEC —*see* Complications, prosthetic
      device, mechanical, ocular device
    orthopedic NEC —*see* Complication,
      orthopedic, device, mechanical
    persistent air J93.82
    specified NEC T85.638
    urinary NEC —*see also* Complication,
      genitourinary, device, urinary,
      mechanical
      graft T83.23
    vascular NEC —*see* Complication,
      cardiovascular device, mechanical
    ventricular intracranial shunt T85.03
  urine —*see* Incontinence
Leaky heart —*see* Endocarditis
Learning defect (specific) F81.9
Leather bottle stomach C16.9
Leber's
  congenital amaurosis H35.50
  optic atrophy (hereditary) H47.22
Lederer's anemia D59.19
Leeches (external) —*see* Hirudiniasis

Leg —*see* condition
Legg (-Calvé)-**Perthes disease, syndrome or**
  osteochondrosis M91.1-●
Legionellosis A48.1
  nonpneumonic A48.2
Legionnaires'
  disease A48.1
    nonpneumonic A48.2
    pneumonia A48.1
Leigh's disease G31.82
Leiner's disease L21.1
Leiofibromyoma —*see* Leiomyoma
Leiomyoblastoma —*see* Neoplasm, connective
  tissue, benign
Leiomyofibroma —*see also* Neoplasm,
  connective tissue, benign
  uterus (cervix) (corpus) D25.9
Leiomyoma —*see also* Neoplasm, connective
  tissue, benign
  bizarre —*see* Neoplasm, connective tissue,
    benign
  cellular —*see* Neoplasm, connective tissue,
    benign
  epithelioid —*see* Neoplasm, connective
    tissue, benign
  uterus (cervix) (corpus) D25.9
    intramural D25.1
    submucous D25.0
    subserosal D25.2
  vascular —*see* Neoplasm, connective tissue,
    benign
Leiomyoma, leiomyomatosis (intravascular) —
  see Neoplasm, connective tissue, uncertain
  behavior
Leiomyosarcoma —*see also* Neoplasm,
  connective tissue, malignant
  epithelioid —*see* Neoplasm, connective
    tissue, malignant
  myxoid —*see* Neoplasm, connective tissue,
    malignant
Leishmaniasis B55.9
  American (mucocutaneous) B55.2
    cutaneous B55.1
  Asian Desert B55.1
  Brazilian B55.2
  cutaneous (any type) B55.1
  dermal —*see also* Leishmaniasis, cutaneous
    post-kala-azar B55.0
  eyelid B55.1
  infantile B55.0
  Mediterranean B55.0
  mucocutaneous (American) (New World)
    B55.2
  naso-oral B55.2
  nasopharyngeal B55.2
  old world B55.1
  tegumentaria diffusa B55.1
  visceral B55.0
Leishmanoid, dermal —*see also* Leishmaniasis,
  cutaneous
  post-kala-azar B55.0
Lenegre's disease I44.2
Lengthening, leg —*see* Deformity, limb,
  unequal length
Lennert's lymphoma —*see* Lymphoma,
  Lennert's
Lennox-Gastaut syndrome G40.812
  intractable G40.814
    with status epilepticus G40.813
    without status epilepticus G40.814
  not intractable G40.812
    with status epilepticus G40.811
    without status epilepticus G40.812
Lens —*see* condition
Lenticonus (anterior) (posterior) (congenital)
  Q12.8
Lenticular degeneration, progressive E83.01
Lentiglobus (posterior) (congenital) Q12.8
Lentigo (congenital) L81.4
  maligna —*see also* Melanoma, in situ
    melanoma —*see* Melanoma

▶ New   ⇒ Revised   ~~deleted~~ Deleted   ● Use Additional Character(s)

Lentivirus, as cause of disease classified
    elsewhere B97.31
Leontiasis
  ossium M85.2
  syphilitic (late) A52.78
    congenital A50.59
Lepothrix A48.8
Lepra —*see* Leprosy
Leprechaunism E34.8
Leprosy A30.-●
  with muscle disorder A30.9 [M63.80]
    ankle A30.9 [M63.87-●]
    foot A30.9 [M63.87-●]
    forearm A30.9 [M63.83-●]
    hand A30.9 [M63.84-●]
    lower leg A30.9 [M63.86-●]
    multiple sites A30.9 [M63.89]
    pelvic region A30.9 [M63.85-●]
    shoulder region A30.9 [M63.81-●]
    specified site NEC A30.9 [M63.88]
    thigh A30.9 [M63.85-●]
    upper arm A30.9 [M63.82-●]
  anesthetic A30.9
  BB A30.3
  BL A30.4
  borderline (infiltrated) (neuritic) A30.3
    lepromatous A30.4
    tuberculoid A30.2
  BT A30.2
  dimorphous (infiltrated) (neuritic) A30.3
  I A30.0
  indeterminate (macular) (neuritic) A30.0
  lepromatous (diffuse) (infiltrated) (macular)
    (neuritic) (nodular) A30.5
  LL A30.5
  macular (early) (neuritic) (simple) A30.9
  maculoanesthetic A30.9
  mixed A30.3
  neural A30.9
  nodular A30.5
  primary neuritic A30.3
  specified type NEC A30.8
  TT A30.1
  tuberculoid (major) (minor) A30.1
Leptocytosis, hereditary D56.9
Leptomeningitis (chronic) (circumscribed)
  (hemorrhagic) (nonsuppurative) —*see*
  Meningitis
Leptomeningopathy G96.198
Leptospiral —*see* condition
Leptospirochetal —*see* condition
Leptospirosis A27.9
  canicola A27.89
  due to Leptospira interrogans serovar
    icterohaemorrhagiae A27.0
  icterohemorrhagica A27.0
  pomona A27.89
  Weil's disease A27.0
Leptus dermatitis B88.0
Leriche's syndrome (aortic bifurcation
  occlusion) I74.09
Leri's pleonosteosis Q78.8
Leri-Weill syndrome Q77.8
Lermoyez' syndrome —*see* Vertigo, peripheral
  NEC
Lesch-Nyhan syndrome E79.1
Leser-Trélat disease L82.1
  inflamed L82.0
Lesion(s) (nontraumatic)
  abducens nerve —*see* Strabismus, paralytic,
    sixth nerve
  alveolar process K08.9
  angiocentric immunoproliferative
    D47.Z9
  anorectal K62.9
  aortic (valve) I35.9
  auditory nerve —*see* subcategory
    H93.3
  basal ganglion G25.9
  bile duct —*see* Disease, bile duct
  biomechanical M99.9

Lesion (*Continued*)
  biomechanical (*Continued*)
    specified type NEC M99.89
      abdomen M99.89
      acromioclavicular M99.87
      cervical region M99.81
      cervicothoracic M99.81
      costochondral M99.88
      costovertebral M99.88
      head region M99.80
      hip M99.85
      lower extremity M99.86
      lumbar region M99.83
      lumbosacral M99.83
      occipitocervical M99.80
      pelvic region M99.85
      pubic M99.85
      rib cage M99.88
      sacral region M99.84
      sacrococcygeal M99.84
      sacroiliac M99.84
      specified NEC M99.89
      sternochondral M99.88
      sternoclavicular M99.87
      thoracic region M99.82
      thoracolumbar M99.82
      upper extremity M99.87
  bladder N32.9
  bone —*see* Disorder, bone
  brachial plexus G54.0
  brain G93.9
    congenital Q04.9
    vascular I67.9
      degenerative I67.9
      hypertensive I67.4
  buccal cavity K13.79
  calcified —*see* Calcification
  canthus —*see* Disorder, eyelid
  carate —*see* Pinta, lesions
  cardia K31.9
  cardiac —*see also* Disease, heart I51.9
    congenital Q24.9
    valvular —*see* Endocarditis
  cauda equina G83.4
  cecum K63.9
  cerebral —*see* Lesion, brain
  cerebrovascular I67.9
    degenerative I67.9
    hypertensive I67.4
  cervical (nerve) root NEC G54.2
  chiasmal —*see* Disorder, optic, chiasm
  chorda tympani G51.8
  coin, lung R91.1
  colon K63.9
  combined periodontic - endodontic K05.5
  congenital —*see* Anomaly, by site
  conjunctiva H11.9
  conus medullaris —*see* Injury, conus
    medullaris
  coronary artery —*see* Ischemia, heart
  cranial nerve G52.9
    eighth —*see* Disorder, ear
    eleventh G52.9
    fifth G50.9
    first G52.0
    fourth —*see* Strabismus, paralytic, fourth
      nerve
    seventh G51.9
    sixth —*see* Strabismus, paralytic, sixth nerve
    tenth G52.2
    twelfth G52.3
  cystic —*see* Cyst
  degenerative —*see* Degeneration
  duodenum K31.9
  edentulous (alveolar) ridge, associated with
    trauma, due to traumatic occlusion K06.2
  en coup de sabre L94.1
  eyelid —*see* Disorder, eyelid
  gasserian ganglion G50.8
  gastric K31.9
  gastroduodenal K31.9

Lesion (*Continued*)
  gastrointestinal K63.9
  gingiva, associated with trauma K06.2
  glomerular
    focal and segmental —*see also* N00-N07
      with fourth character .1 N05.1
    minimal change —*see also* N00-N07 with
      fourth character .0 N05.0
  heart (organic) —*see* Disease, heart
  hyperchromic, due to pinta (carate) A67.1
  hyperkeratotic —*see* Hyperkeratosis
  hypothalamic E23.7
  ileocecal K63.9
  ileum K63.9
  iliohypogastric nerve G57.8-●
  inflammatory —*see* Inflammation
  intestine K63.9
  intracerebral —*see* Lesion, brain
  intrachiasmal (optic) —*see* Disorder, optic,
    chiasm
  intracranial, space-occupying R90.0
  joint —*see* Disorder, joint
    sacroiliac (old) M53.3
  keratotic —*see* Keratosis
  kidney —*see* Disease, renal
  laryngeal nerve (recurrent) G52.2
  lip K13.0
  liver K76.9
  lumbosacral
    plexus G54.1
    root (nerve) NEC G54.4
  lung (coin) R91.1
  maxillary sinus J32.0
  mitral I05.9
  Morel-Lavallée —*see* Hematoma,
    by site
  motor cortex NEC G93.89
  mouth K13.79
  nerve G58.9
    femoral G57.2-●
    median G56.1-●
      carpal tunnel syndrome —*see* Syndrome,
        carpal tunnel
    plantar G57.6-●
    popliteal (lateral) G57.3-●
      medial G57.4-●
    radial G56.3-●
    sciatic G57.0-●
    spinal —*see* Injury, nerve, spinal
    ulnar G56.2-●
  nervous system, congenital Q07.9
  nonallopathic —*see* Lesion, biomechanical
  nose (internal) J34.89
  obstructive —*see* Obstruction
  obturator nerve G57.8-●
  oral mucosa K13.70
  organ or site NEC —*see* Disease, by site
  osteolytic —*see* Osteolysis
  peptic K27.9
  periodontal, due to traumatic occlusion K05.5
  pharynx J39.2
  pigment, pigmented (skin) L81.9
  pinta —*see* Pinta, lesions
  polypoid —*see* Polyp
  prechiasmal (optic) —*see* Disorder, optic,
    chiasm
  primary —*see also* Syphilis, primary A51.0
    carate A67.0
    pinta A67.0
    yaws A66.0
  pulmonary J98.4
    valve I37.9
  pylorus K31.9
  rectosigmoid K63.9
  retina, retinal H35.9
  sacroiliac (joint) (old) M53.3
  salivary gland K11.9
    benign lymphoepithelial K11.8
  saphenous nerve G57.8-●
  sciatic nerve G57.0-●
  secondary —*see* Syphilis, secondary

Lesion (*Continued*)
   shoulder (region) M75.9-●
      specified NEC M75.8-●
   sigmoid K63.9
   sinus (accessory) (nasal) J34.89
   skin L98.9
      suppurative LØ8.Ø
   SLAP S43.43-●
   spinal cord G95.9
      congenital QØ6.9
   spleen D73.89
   stomach K31.9
   superior glenoid labrum S43.43-●
   syphilitic —*see* Syphilis
   tertiary —*see* Syphilis, tertiary
   thoracic root (nerve) NEC G54.3
   tonsillar fossa J35.9
   tooth, teeth KØ8.9
      white spot
         chewing surface KØ2.51
         pit and fissure surface KØ2.51
         smooth surface KØ2.61
   traumatic —*see* specific type of injury by site
   tricuspid (valve) IØ7.9
      nonrheumatic I36.9
   trigeminal nerve G5Ø.9
   ulcerated or ulcerative —*see* Ulcer, skin
   uterus N85.9
   vagina N89.8
   vulva N9Ø.89
   vagus nerve G52.2
   valvular —*see* Endocarditis
   vascular I99.9
      affecting central nervous system I67.9
      following trauma NEC T14.8
      umbilical cord, complicating delivery O69.5
   warty —*see* Verruca
   white spot (tooth)
      chewing surface KØ2.51
      pit and fissure surface KØ2.51
      smooth surface KØ2.61
▶**Less than a high school diploma** Z55.5
Lethargic —*see* condition
Lethargy R53.83
Letterer-Siwe's disease C96.Ø
Leukemia, leukemic C95.9-●
   acute basophilic C94.8-●
   acute bilineal C95.Ø-●
   acute erythroid C94.Ø-●
   acute lymphoblastic C91.Ø-●
   acute megakaryoblastic C94.2-●
   acute megakaryocytic C94.2-●
   acute mixed lineage C95.Ø-●
   acute monoblastic (monoblastic/monocytic)
      C93.Ø-●
   acute monocytic (monoblastic/monocytic)
      C93.Ø-●
   acute myeloblastic (minimal differentiation)
      (with maturation) C92.Ø-●
   acute myeloid, NOS C92.Ø-●
      with
         11q23-abnormality C92.6-●
         dysplasia of remaining hematopoesis
            and/or myelodysplastic disease in
            its history C92.A-●
         multilineage dysplasia C92.A-●
         variation of MLL-gene C92.6-●
      M6 (a)(b) C94.Ø-●
      M7 C94.2-●
   acute myelomonocytic C92.5-●
   acute promyelocytic C92.4-●
   adult T-cell (HTLV-1-associated) (acute
      variant) (chronic variant)
      (lymphomatoid variant) (smouldering
      variant) C91.5-●
   aggressive NK-cell C94.8-●
   AML (1/ETO) (MØ) (M1) (M2) (without a
      FAB classification) C92.Ø-●
   AML M3 C92.4-●
   AML M4 (Eo with inv(16) or t(16;16)) C92.5-●
   AML M5 C93.Ø-●

Leukemia, leukemic (*Continued*)
   AML M5a C93.Ø-●
   AML M5b C93.Ø-●
   AML Me with t (15;17) and variants C92.4-●
   atypical chronic myeloid, BCR/ABL-negative
      C92.2-●
   biphenotypic acute C95.Ø-●
   blast cell C95.Ø-●
   Burkitt-type, mature B-cell C91.A-●
   chronic eosinophilic (*see also* Syndrome,
      hypereosinophilic, myeloid) C94.8-●
   chronic lymphocytic, of B-cell type C91.1-●
   chronic monocytic C93.1-●
   chronic myelogenous (Philadelphia
      chromosome (Ph1) positive) (t(9;22))
      (q34;q11) (with crisis of blast cells)
      C92.1-●
   chronic myeloid, BCR/ABL-positive C92.1-●
      atypical, BCR/ABL-negative C92.2-●
   chronic myelomonocytic C93.1-●
   chronic neutrophilic D47.1
   CMML (-1) (-2) (with eosinophilia) C93.1-●
   granulocytic —*see also* Category C92 C92.9-●
   hairy-cell C91.4-●
   juvenile myelomonocytic C93.3-●
   lymphoid C91.9-●
      specified NEC C91.Z-●
   mast cell C94.3-●
   mature B-cell, Burkitt-type C91.A-●
   monocytic (subacute) C93.9-●
      specified NEC C93.Z-●
   myelogenous —*see also* Category
      C92 C92.9-●
   myeloid C92.9-●
      specified NEC C92.Z-●
   plasma cell C9Ø.1-●
   plasmacytic C9Ø.1-●
   prolymphocytic
      of B-cell type C91.3-●
      of T-cell type C91.6-●
   specified NEC C94.8-●
   stem cell, of unclear lineage C95.Ø-●
   subacute lymphocytic C91.9-●
   T-cell large granular lymphocytic C91.Z-●
   unspecified cell type C95.9-●
      acute C95.Ø-●
      chronic C95.1-●
Leukemoid reaction —*see also* Reaction,
   leukemoid D72.823-●
Leukoaraiosis (hypertensive) I67.81
Leukoariosis —*see* Leukoaraiosis
Leukocoria —*see* Disorder, globe, degenerated
   condition, leucocoria
Leukocytopenia D72.819
Leukocytosis D72.829
   eosinophilic D72.19
Leukoderma, leukodermia NEC L81.5
   syphilitic A51.39
      late A52.79
Leukodystrophy E75.29
Leukoedema, oral epithelium K13.29
Leukoencephalitis GØ4.81
   acute (subacute) hemorrhagic G36.1
      postimmunization or postvaccinal
         GØ4.Ø2
   postinfectious GØ4.Ø1
   subacute sclerosing A81.1
   van Bogaert's (sclerosing) A81.1
Leukoencephalopathy —*see also*
   Encephalopathy G93.49
   Binswanger's I67.3
⇒heroin vapor G92.8
   metachromatic E75.25
   multifocal (progressive) A81.2
   postimmunization and postvaccinal
      GØ4.Ø2
   progressive multifocal A81.2
   reversible, posterior G93.6
   van Bogaert's (sclerosing) A81.1
   vascular, progressive I67.3
Leukoerythroblastosis D75.9

Leukokeratosis —*see also* Leukoplakia
   mouth K13.21
   nicotina palati K13.24
   oral mucosa K13.21
   tongue K13.21
   vocal cord J38.3
Leukokraurosis vulva (e) N9Ø.4
Leukoma (cornea) —*see also* Opacity, cornea
   adherent H17.Ø-●
   interfering with central vision —*see* Opacity,
      cornea, central
Leukomalacia, cerebral, newborn P91.2
   periventricular P91.2
Leukomelanopathy, hereditary D72.Ø
Leukonychia (punctata) (striata) L6Ø.8
   congenital Q84.4
Leukopathia unguium L6Ø.8
   congenital Q84.4
Leukopenia D72.819
   basophilic D72.818
   chemotherapy (cancer) induced D7Ø.1
   congenital D7Ø.Ø
   cyclic D7Ø.Ø
   drug induced NEC D7Ø.2
      due to cytoreductive cancer chemotherapy
         D7Ø.1
   eosinophilic D72.818
   familial D7Ø.Ø
   infantile genetic D7Ø.Ø
   malignant D7Ø.9
   periodic D7Ø.Ø
   transitory neonatal P61.5
Leukopenic —*see* condition
Leukoplakia
   anus K62.89
   bladder (postinfectional) N32.89
   buccal K13.21
   cervix (uteri) N88.Ø
⇒esophagus K22.89
   gingiva K13.21
   hairy (oral mucosa) (tongue) K13.3
   kidney (pelvis) N28.89
   larynx J38.7
   lip K13.21
   mouth K13.21
   oral epithelium, including tongue (mucosa)
      K13.21
   palate K13.21
   pelvis (kidney) N28.89
   penis (infectional) N48.Ø
   rectum K62.89
   syphilitic (late) A52.79
   tongue K13.21
   ureter (postinfectional) N28.89
   urethra (postinfectional) N36.8
   uterus N85.8
   vagina N89.4
   vocal cord J38.3
   vulva N9Ø.4
Leukorrhea N89.8
   due to Trichomonas (vaginalis)
      A59.ØØ
   trichomonal A59.ØØ
Leukosarcoma C85.9
Levocardia (isolated) Q24.1
   with situs inversus Q89.3
Levotransposition Q2Ø.5
Lev's disease or syndrome (acquired complete
   heart block) I44.2
Levulosuria —*see* Fructosuria
Levurid L3Ø.2
Lewy body (ies) (dementia) (disease)
   G31.83
Leyden-Moebius dystrophy G71.Ø9
Leydig cell
   carcinoma
      specified site —*see* Neoplasm, malignant,
         by site
      unspecified site
         female C56.9-●
         male C62.9-●

▶ New   ⇒ Revised   ~~deleted~~ Deleted   ● Use Additional Character(s)

Leydig cell (Continued)
  tumor
    benign
      specified site —see Neoplasm, benign,
        by site
      unspecified site
        female D27.-●
        male D29.2-●
    malignant
      specified site —see Neoplasm,
        malignant, by site
      unspecified site
        female C56.-●
        male C62.9-●
    specified site —see Neoplasm, uncertain
        behavior, by site
    unspecified site
      female D39.1-●
      male D40.1-●
Leydig-Sertoli cell tumor
  specified site —see Neoplasm, benign,
      by site
  unspecified site
    female D27.-●
    male D29.2-●
LGSIL (Low grade squamous intraepithelial
    lesion on cytologic smear of)
  anus R85.612
  cervix R87.612
  vagina R87.622
Liar, pathologic F60.2
Libido
  decreased R68.82
Libman-Sacks disease M32.11
Lice (infestation) B85.2
  body (Pediculus corporis) B85.1
  crab B85.3
  head (Pediculus capitis) B85.0
  mixed (classifiable to more than one of the
      titles B85.0-B85.3) B85.4
  pubic (Phthirus pubis) B85.3
Lichen L28.0
  albus L90.0
    penis N48.0
    vulva N90.4
  amyloidosis E85.4 [L99]
  atrophicus L90.0
    penis N48.0
    vulva N90.4
  congenital Q82.8
  myxedematosus L98.5
  nitidus L44.1
  pilaris Q82.8
    acquired L85.8
  planopilaris L66.1
  planus (chronicus) L43.9
    annularis L43.8
    bullous L43.1
    follicular L66.1
    hypertrophic L43.0
    moniliformis L44.3
    of Wilson L43.9
    specified NEC L43.8
    subacute (active) L43.3
    tropicus L43.3
  ruber
    acuminatus L44.0
    moniliformis L44.3
    planus L43.9
  sclerosus (et atrophicus) L90.0
    penis N48.0
    vulva N90.4
  scrofulosus (primary) (tuberculous) A18.4
  simplex (chronicus) (circumscriptus)
      L28.0
  striatus L44.2
  urticatus L28.2
Lichenification L28.0
Lichenoides tuberculosis (primary) A18.4
Lichtheim's disease or syndrome D51.0
Lien migrans D73.89

Ligament —see condition
Light
  for gestational age —see Light for dates
  headedness R42
Light-for-dates (infant) P05.00
  with weight of
    499 grams or less P05.01
    500-749 grams P05.02
    750-999 grams P05.03
    1000-1249 grams P05.04
    1250-1499 grams P05.05
    1500-1749 grams P05.06
    1750-1999 grams P05.07
    2000-2499 grams P05.08
    2500 grams and over P05.09
  affecting management of pregnancy O36.59-●
  and small-for-dates —see Small for dates
  specified NEC P05.09
Lightning (effects) (stroke) (struck by) T75.00
  burn —see Burn
  foot E53.8
  shock T75.01
  specified effect NEC T75.09
Lightwood-Albright syndrome N25.89
Lightwood's disease or syndrome (renal
    tubular acidosis) N25.89
Lignac (-de Toni) (-Fanconi) (-Debré) disease or
    syndrome E72.09
  with cystinosis E72.04
Ligneous thyroiditis E06.5
Likoff's syndrome I20.8
Limb —see condition
Limbic epilepsy personality syndrome F07.0
Limitation, limited
  activities due to disability Z73.6
  cardiac reserve —see Disease, heart
  eye muscle duction, traumatic —see
      Strabismus, mechanical
  mandibular range of motion M26.52
Lindau (-von Hippel) disease Q85.8
Line(s)
  Beau's L60.4
  Harris' —see Arrest, epiphyseal
  Hudson's (cornea) —see Pigmentation,
      cornea, anterior
  Stähli's (cornea) —see Pigmentation, cornea,
      anterior
Linea corneae senilis —see Change, cornea,
    senile
Lingua
  geographica K14.1
  nigra (villosa) K14.3
  plicata K14.5
  tylosica K13.29
Lingual —see condition
Linguatulosis B88.8
Linitis (gastric) plastica C16.9
Lip —see condition
Lipedema —see Edema
Lipemia —see also Hyperlipidemia
  retina, retinalis E78.3
Lipidosis E75.6
  cerebral (infantile) (juvenile) (late) E75.4
  cerebroretinal E75.4
  cerebroside E75.22
  cholesterol (cerebral) E75.5
  glycolipid E75.21
  hepatosplenomegalic E78.3
  sphingomyelin —see Niemann-Pick disease
      or syndrome
  sulfatide E75.29
Lipoadenoma —see Neoplasm, benign, by site
Lipoblastoma —see Lipoma
Lipoblastomatosis —see Lipoma
Lipochondrodystrophy E76.01
Lipochrome histiocytosis (familial) D71
Lipodermatosclerosis —see Varix, leg, with,
    inflammation
  ulcerated —see Varix, leg, with, ulcer, with
    inflammation by site
Lipodystrophia progressiva E88.1

Lipodystrophy (progressive) E88.1
  insulin E88.1
  intestinal K90.81
  mesenteric K65.4
Lipofibroma —see Lipoma
Lipofuscinosis, neuronal (with ceroidosis)
    E75.4
Lipogranuloma, sclerosing L92.8
Lipogranulomatosis E78.89
Lipoid —see also condition
  histiocytosis D76.3
    essential E75.29
  nephrosis N04.9
  proteinosis of Urbach E78.89
Lipoidemia —see Hyperlipidemia
Lipoidosis —see Lipidosis
Lipoma D17.9
  fetal D17.9
    fat cell D17.9
  infiltrating D17.9
  intramuscular D17.9
  pleomorphic D17.9
  site classification
    arms (skin) (subcutaneous) D17.2-●
    connective tissue D17.30
      intra-abdominal D17.5
      intrathoracic D17.4
      peritoneum D17.79
      retroperitoneum D17.79
      specified site NEC D17.39
      spermatic cord D17.6
    face (skin) (subcutaneous) D17.0
    genitourinary organ NEC D17.72
    head (skin) (subcutaneous) D17.0
    intra-abdominal D17.5
    intrathoracic D17.4
    kidney D17.71
    legs (skin) (subcutaneous) D17.2-●
    neck (skin) (subcutaneous) D17.0
    peritoneum D17.79
    retroperitoneum D17.79
    skin D17.30
      specified site NEC D17.39
    specified site NEC D17.79
    spermatic cord D17.6
    subcutaneous D17.30
      specified site NEC D17.39
    trunk (skin) (subcutaneous) D17.1
    unspecified D17.9
  spindle cell D17.9
Lipomatosis E88.2
  dolorosa (Dercum) E88.2
  fetal —see Lipoma
  Launois-Bensaude E88.89
Lipomyoma —see Lipoma
Lipomyxoma —see Lipoma
Lipomyxosarcoma —see Neoplasm, connective
    tissue, malignant
Lipoprotein metabolism disorder E78.9
Lipoproteinemia E78.5
  broad-beta E78.2
  floating-beta E78.2
  hyper-pre-beta E78.1
Liposarcoma —see also Neoplasm, connective
    tissue, malignant
  dedifferentiated —see Neoplasm, connective
    tissue, malignant
  differentiated type —see Neoplasm,
    connective tissue, malignant
  embryonal —see Neoplasm, connective tissue,
    malignant
  mixed type —see Neoplasm, connective
    tissue, malignant
  myxoid —see Neoplasm, connective tissue,
    malignant
  pleomorphic —see Neoplasm, connective
    tissue, malignant
  round cell —see Neoplasm, connective tissue,
    malignant
  well differentiated type —see Neoplasm,
    connective tissue, malignant

Liposynovitis prepatellaris E88.89
Lipping, cervix N86
Lipschütz disease or ulcer N76.6
Lipuria R82.0
   schistosomiasis (bilharziasis) B65.0
Lisping F80.0
Lissauer's paralysis A52.17
Lissencephalia, lissencephaly Q04.3
Listeriosis, listerellosis A32.9
   congenital (disseminated) P37.2
   cutaneous A32.0
   neonatal, newborn (disseminated) P37.2
   oculoglandular A32.81
   specified NEC A32.89
Lithemia E79.0
Lithiasis —see Calculus
Lithosis J62.8
Lithuria R82.998
Litigation, anxiety concerning Z65.3
Little leaguer's elbow —see Epicondylitis, medial
Little's disease G80.9
Littre's
   gland —see condition
   hernia —see Hernia, abdomen
Littritis —see Urethritis
Livedo (annularis) (racemosa) (reticularis) R23.1
Liver —see condition
Living alone (problems with) Z60.2
   with handicapped person Z74.2
▶Living in a shelter (motel) (scattered site
     housing) (temporary or transitional living
     situation) Z59.01
Lloyd's syndrome —see Adenomatosis, endocrine
Loa loa, loaiasis, loasis B74.3
Lobar —see condition
Lobomycosis B48.0
Lobo's disease B48.0
Lobotomy syndrome F07.0
Lobstein (-Ekman) disease or syndrome Q78.0
Lobster-claw hand Q71.6-●
Lobulation (congenital) —see also Anomaly,
     by site
   kidney, Q63.1
   liver, abnormal Q44.7
   spleen Q89.09
Lobule, lobular —see condition
Local, localized —see condition
Locked twins causing obstructed labor O66.1
Locked-in state G83.5
Locking
   joint —see Derangement, joint, specified type
     NEC
   knee —see Derangement, knee
Lockjaw —see Tetanus
Löffler's
   endocarditis I42.3
   eosinophilia J82.89
   pneumonia J82.89
   syndrome (eosinophilic pneumonitis) J82.89
Loiasis (with conjunctival infestation) (eyelid)
     B74.3
Lone Star fever A77.0
Long
  ▶COVID (-19) (see also COVID-19) U09.9
   labor O63.9
     first stage O63.0
     second stage O63.1
   QT syndrome I45.81
Long-term (current) (prophylactic) drug
     therapy (use of)
   agents affecting estrogen receptors and
     estrogen levels NEC Z79.818
   anastrozole (Arimidex) Z79.811
   antibiotics Z79.2
     short-term use - omit code
   anticoagulants Z79.01
   anti-inflammatory, non-steroidal (NSAID)
     Z79.1
   antiplatelet Z79.02
   antithrombotics Z79.02
   aromatase inhibitors Z79.811
   aspirin Z79.82
   birth control pill or patch Z79.3

Long-term (Continued)
   bisphosphonates Z79.83
   contraceptive, oral Z79.3
   drug, specified NEC Z79.899
   estrogen receptor downregulators Z79.818
   Evista Z79.810
   exemestane (Aromasin) Z79.811
   Fareston Z79.810
   fulvestrant (Faslodex) Z79.818
   gonadotropin-releasing hormone (GnRH)
     agonist Z79.818
   goserelin acetate (Zoladex) Z79.818
   hormone replacement Z79.890
   insulin Z79.4
   letrozole (Femara) Z79.811
   leuprolide acetate (leuprorelin) (Lupron)
     Z79.818
   megestrol acetate (Megace) Z79.818
   methadone for pain management Z79.891
   Nolvadex Z79.810
  ▶non-insulin antidiabetic drug, injectable
     Z79.899
   non-steroidal anti-inflammatories (NSAID)
     Z79.1
   opiate analgesic Z79.891
   oral
     antidiabetic Z79.84
     contraceptive Z79.3
     hypoglycemic Z79.84
   raloxifene (Evista) Z79.810
   selective estrogen receptor modulators
     (SERMs) Z79.810
   steroids
     inhaled Z79.51
     systemic Z79.52
   tamoxifen (Nolvadex) Z79.810
   toremifene (Fareston) Z79.810
Longitudinal stripes or grooves, nails L60.8
   congenital Q84.6
Loop
   intestine —see Volvulus
   vascular on papilla (optic) Q14.2
Loose —see also condition
   body
     joint M24.00
       ankle M24.07-●
       elbow M24.02-●
       hand M24.04-●
       hip M24.05-●
       knee M23.4-●
       shoulder (region) M24.01-●
       specified site NEC M24.08
       toe M24.07-●
       vertebra M24.08
       wrist M24.03-●
     knee M23.4-●
     sheath, tendon —see Disorder, tendon,
       specified type NEC
   cartilage —see Loose, body, joint
   skin and subcutaneous tissue (following
     bariatric surgery weight loss) (following
     dietary weight loss) L98.7
   tooth, teeth K08.89
Loosening
   aseptic
     joint prosthesis —see Complications, joint
       prosthesis, mechanical, loosening,
       by site
   epiphysis —see Osteochondropathy
   mechanical
     joint prosthesis —see Complications, joint
       prosthesis, mechanical, loosening,
       by site
Looser-Milkman (-Debray) syndrome M83.8
Lop ear (deformity) Q17.3
Lorain (-Levi) short stature syndrome E23.0
Lordosis M40.50
   acquired —see Lordosis, specified type NEC
   congenital Q76.429
     lumbar region Q76.426
     lumbosacral region Q76.427
     sacral region Q76.428
     sacrococcygeal region Q76.428

Lordosis (Continued)
   congenital(Continued)
     thoracolumbar region Q76.425
   lumbar region M40.56
   lumbosacral region M40.57
   postsurgical M96.4
   postural —see Lordosis, specified type NEC
   rachitic (late effect) (sequelae) E64.3
   sequelae of rickets E64.3
   specified type NEC M40.40
     lumbar region M40.46
     lumbosacral region M40.47
     thoracolumbar region M40.45
   thoracolumbar region M40.55
   tuberculous A18.01
Loss (of)
   appetite (see Anorexia) R63.0
     hysterical F50.89
     nonorganic origin F50.89
     psychogenic F50.89
   blood —see Hemorrhage
   bone —see Loss, substance of, bone
   consciousness, transient R55
     traumatic —see Injury, intracranial
   control, sphincter, rectum R15.9
     nonorganic origin F98.1
   elasticity, skin R23.4
   family (member) in childhood Z62.898
   fluid (acute) E86.9
   function of labyrinth —see subcategory H83.2
   hair, nonscarring —see Alopecia
   hearing —see also Deafness
     central NOS H90.5
     conductive H90.2
       bilateral H90.0
       unilateral
         with
           restricted hearing on the
             contralateral side H90.A1-●
           unrestricted hearing on the
             contralateral side H90.1-●
     mixed conductive and sensorineural
       hearing loss H90.8
       bilateral H90.6
       unilateral
         with
           restricted hearing on the
             contralateral side H90.A3-●
           unrestricted hearing on the
             contralateral side H90.7-●
     neural NOS H90.5
     perceptive NOS H90.5
     sensorineural NOS H90.5
       bilateral H90.3
       unilateral
         with
           restricted hearing on the
             contralateral side H90.A2-●
           unrestricted hearing on the
             contralateral side H90.4-●
     sensory NOS H90.5
   height R29.890
   limb or member, traumatic, current —see
     Amputation, traumatic
   love relationship in childhood Z62.898
   memory —see also Amnesia
     mild, following organic brain damage F06.8
   mind —see Psychosis
   occlusal vertical dimension of fully erupted
     teeth M26.37
   organ or part —see Absence, by site, acquired
   ossicles, ear (partial) H74.32-●
   parent in childhood Z63.4
   pregnancy, recurrent N96
     without current pregnancy N96
     care in current pregnancy O26.2-●
   recurrent pregnancy —see Loss, pregnancy,
     recurrent
   self-esteem, in childhood Z62.898
   sense of
     smell —see Disturbance, sensation, smell
     taste —see Disturbance, sensation, taste
     touch R20.8

▶ New   ⇒ Revised   ~~deleted~~ Deleted   ● Use Additional Character(s)

Loss *(Continued)*
sensory R44.9
  dissociative F44.6
sexual desire F52.0
sight (acquired) (complete) (congenital) —*see* Blindness
substance of
  bone —*see* Disorder, bone, density and structure, specified NEC
    horizontal alveolar K06.3
  cartilage —*see* Disorder, cartilage, specified type NEC
    auricle (ear) —*see* Disorder, pinna, specified type NEC
    vitreous (humor) H15.89
tooth, teeth —*see* Absence, teeth, acquired
vision, visual H54.7
  both eyes H54.3
  one eye H54.60
    left (normal vision on right) H54.62
    right (normal vision on left) H54.61
  specified as blindness —*see* Blindness
  subjective
    sudden H53.13-●
    transient H53.12-●
vitreous —*see* Prolapse, vitreous
voice —*see* Aphonia
weight (abnormal) (cause unknown) R63.4
Louis-Bar syndrome (ataxia-telangiectasia) G11.3
Louping ill (encephalitis) A84.89
Louse, lousiness —*see* Lice
Low
achiever, school Z55.3
back syndrome M54.50
basal metabolic rate R94.8
birthweight (2499 grams or less) P07.10
  with weight of
    1000-1249 grams P07.14
    1250-1499 grams P07.15
    1500-1749 grams P07.16
    1750-1999 grams P07.17
    2000-2499 grams P07.18
  extreme (999 grams or less) P07.00
    with weight of
      499 grams or less P07.01
      500-749 grams P07.02
      750-999 grams P07.03
  for gestational age —*see* Light for dates
blood pressure —*see also* Hypotension
  reading (incidental) (isolated) (nonspecific) R03.1
cardiac reserve —*see* Disease, heart
function —*see also* Hypofunction
  kidney N28.9
hematocrit D64.9
hemoglobin D64.9
income Z59.6
level of literacy Z55.0
lying
  kidney N28.89
  organ or site, congenital —*see* Malposition, congenital
output syndrome (cardiac) —*see* Failure, heart
platelets (blood) —*see* Thrombocytopenia
reserve, kidney N28.89
salt syndrome E87.1
self esteem R45.81
set ears Q17.4
vision H54.2X-
  one eye (other eye normal) H54.50
    left (normal vision on right) H54.52A-
  other eye blind —*see* Blindness
    right (normal vision on left) H54.511-
Low-density-lipoprotein-type (LDL) **hyperlipoproteinemia** E78.00
Lowe's syndrome E72.03
Lown-Ganong-Levine syndrome I45.6

LSD reaction (acute) (without dependence) F16.90
  with dependence F16.20
L-shaped kidney Q63.8
LTBI (lantent tuberculosis infection) Z22.7
Ludwig's angina or disease K12.2
Lues (venerea), **luetic** —*see* Syphilis
Luetscher's syndrome (dehydration) E86.0
Lumbago, lumbalgia M54.50
  with sciatica M54.4-●
  due to intervertebral disc disorder M51.17
  due to displacement, intervertebral disc M51.27
    with sciatica M51.17
Lumbar —*see* condition
Lumbarization, vertebra, congenital Q76.49
Lumbermen's itch B88.0
Lump —*see also* Mass
breast N63.0
  axillary tail
    left N63.32
    right N63.31
  left
    lower inner quadrant N63.24
    lower outer quadrant N63.23
    overlapping quadrants N63.25
    unspecified quadrant N63.20
    upper inner quadrant N63.22
    upper outer quadrant N63.21
  right
    lower inner quadrant N63.14
    lower outer quadrant N63.13
    overlapping quadrants N63.15
    unspecified quadrant N63.10
    upper inner quadrant N63.12
    upper outer quadrant N63.11
  subareolar
    left N63.42
    right N63.41
Lunacy —*see* Psychosis
Lung —*see* condition
Lupoid (miliary) of Boeck D86.3
Lupus
anticoagulant D68.62
  with
    hemorrhagic disorder D68.312
    hypercoagulable state D68.62
  finding without diagnosis R76.0
discoid (local) L93.0
erythematosus (discoid) (local) L93.0
  disseminated —*see* Lupus, erythematosus, systemic
  eyelid H01.129
    left H01.126
      lower H01.125
      upper H01.124
    right H01.123
      lower H01.122
      upper H01.121
  profundus L93.2
  specified NEC L93.2
  subacute cutaneous L93.1
  systemic M32.9
    with organ or system involvement M32.10
      endocarditis M32.11
      lung M32.13
      pericarditis M32.12
      renal (glomerular) M32.14
        tubulo-interstitial M32.15
      specified organ or system NEC M32.19
    drug-induced M32.0
    inhibitor (presence of) D68.62
      with
        hemorrhagic disorder D68.312
        hypercoagulable state D68.62
      finding without diagnosis R76.0
    specified NEC M32.8
  exedens A18.4

Lupus *(Continued)*
hydralazine M32.0
  correct substance properly administered — *see* Table of Drugs and Chemicals, by drug, adverse effect
  overdose or wrong substance given or taken —*see* Table of Drugs and Chemicals, by drug, poisoning
nephritis (chronic) M32.14
nontuberculous, not disseminated L93.0
panniculitis L93.2
pernio (Besnier) D86.3
systemic —*see* Lupus, erythematosus, systemic
tuberculous A18.4
  eyelid A18.4
vulgaris A18.4
  eyelid A18.4
Luteinoma D27.-●
Lutembacher's disease or syndrome (atrial septal defect with mitral stenosis) Q21.1
Luteoma D27.-●
Lutz (-Splendore-de Almeida) **disease** —*see* Paracoccidioidomycosis
Luxation —*see also* Dislocation
eyeball (nontraumatic) —*see* Luxation, globe
  birth injury P15.3
globe, nontraumatic H44.82-●
lacrimal gland —*see* Dislocation, lacrimal gland
lens (old) (partial) (spontaneous)
  congenital Q12.1
  syphilitic A50.39
Lycanthropy F22
Lyell's syndrome L51.2
  due to drug L51.2
    correct substance properly administered — *see* Table of Drugs and Chemicals, by drug, adverse effect
    overdose or wrong substance given or taken —*see* Table of Drugs and Chemicals, by drug, poisoning
Lyme disease A69.20
Lymph
gland or node —*see* condition
scrotum —*see* Infestation, filarial
Lymphadenitis I88.9
with ectopic or molar pregnancy O08.0
acute L04.9
  axilla L04.2
  face L04.0
  head L04.0
  hip L04.3
  limb
    lower L04.3
    upper L04.2
  neck L04.0
  shoulder L04.2
  specified site NEC L04.8
  trunk L04.1
anthracosis (occupational) J60
any site, except mesenteric I88.9
  chronic I88.1
  subacute I88.1
breast
  gestational —*see* Mastitis, obstetric
  puerperal, postpartum (nonpurulent) O91.22
chancroidal (congenital) A57
chronic I88.1
  mesenteric I88.0
due to
  Brugia (malayi) B74.1
    timori B74.2
  chlamydial lymphogranuloma A55
  diphtheria (toxin) A36.89
  lymphogranuloma venereum A55
  Wuchereria bancrofti B74.0
following ectopic or molar pregnancy O08.0
gonorrheal A54.89
infective —*see* Lymphadenitis, acute

Lymphadenitis *(Continued)*
  mesenteric (acute) (chronic) (nonspecific) (subacute) I88.0
    due to Salmonella typhi A01.09
    tuberculous A18.39
  mycobacterial A31.8
  purulent —*see* Lymphadenitis, acute
  pyogenic —*see* Lymphadenitis, acute
  regional, nonbacterial I88.8
  septic —*see* Lymphadenitis, acute
  subacute, unspecified site I88.1
  suppurative —*see* Lymphadenitis, acute
  syphilitic (early) (secondary) A51.49
    late A52.79
  tuberculous —*see* Tuberculosis, lymph gland
  venereal (chlamydial) A55
Lymphadenoid goiter E06.3
Lymphadenopathy (generalized) R59.1
  angioimmunoblastic, with dysproteinemia (AILD) C86.5
  due to toxoplasmosis (acquired) B58.89
    congenital (acute) (subacute) (chronic) P37.1
  localized R59.0
  syphilitic (early) (secondary) A51.49
Lymphadenosis R59.1
Lymphangiectasis I89.0
  conjunctiva H11.89
  postinfectional I89.0
  scrotum I89.0
Lymphangiectatic elephantiasis, nonfilarial I89.0
Lymphangioendothelioma D18.1
  malignant —*see* Neoplasm, connective tissue, malignant
Lymphangioleiomyomatosis J84.81
Lymphangioma D18.1
  capillary D18.1
  cavernous D18.1
  cystic D18.1
  malignant —*see* Neoplasm, connective tissue, malignant
Lymphangiomyoma D18.1
Lymphangiomyomatosis J84.81
Lymphangiosarcoma —*see* Neoplasm, connective tissue, malignant
Lymphangitis I89.1
  with
    abscess - code by site under Abscess
    cellulitis - code by site under Cellulitis
    ectopic or molar pregnancy O08.0
  acute L03.91
    abdominal wall L03.321
    ankle —*see* Lymphangitis, acute, lower limb
    arm —*see* Lymphangitis, acute, upper limb
    auricle (ear) —*see* Lymphangitis, acute, ear
    axilla L03.12-●
    back (any part) L03.322
    buttock L03.327
    cervical (meaning neck) L03.222
    cheek (external) L03.212
    chest wall L03.323
    digit
      finger —*see* Lymphangitis, acute, finger
      toe —*see* Lymphangitis, acute, toe
    ear (external) H60.1-●
    external auditory canal —*see* Lymphangitis, acute, ear
    eyelid —*see* Abscess, eyelid
    face NEC L03.212
    finger (intrathecal) (periosteal) (subcutaneous) (subcuticular) L03.02-●
    foot —*see* Lymphangitis, acute, lower limb
    gluteal (region) L03.327
    groin L03.324
    hand —*see* Lymphangitis, acute, upper limb
    head NEC L03.891
      face (any part, except ear, eye and nose) L03.212

Lymphangitis *(Continued)*
  acute *(Continued)*
    heel —*see* Lymphangitis, acute, lower limb
    hip —*see* Lymphangitis, acute, lower limb
    jaw (region) L03.212
    knee —*see* Lymphangitis, acute, lower limb
    leg —*see* Lymphangitis, acute, lower limb
    lower limb L03.12-●
      toe —*see* Lymphangitis, acute, toe
    navel L03.326
    neck (region) L03.222
    orbit, orbital —*see* Cellulitis, orbit
    pectoral (region) L03.323
    perineal, perineum L03.325
    scalp (any part) L03.891
    shoulder —*see* Lymphangitis, acute, upper limb
    specified site NEC L03.898
    thigh —*see* Lymphangitis, acute, lower limb
    thumb (intrathecal) (periosteal) (subcutaneous) (subcuticular) —*see* Lymphangitis, acute, finger
    toe (intrathecal) (periosteal) (subcutaneous) (subcuticular) L03.04-●
    trunk L03.329
      abdominal wall L03.321
      back (any part) L03.322
      buttock L03.327
      chest wall L03.323
      groin L03.324
      perineal, perineum L03.325
      umbilicus L03.326
    umbilicus L03.326
    upper limb L03.12-●
      axilla —*see* Lymphangitis, acute, axilla
      finger —*see* Lymphangitis, acute, finger
      thumb —*see* Lymphangitis, acute, finger
    wrist —*see* Lymphangitis, acute, upper limb
  breast
    gestational —*see* Mastitis, obstetric
  chancroidal A57
  chronic (any site) I89.1
  due to
    Brugia (malayi) B74.1
      timori B74.2
    Wuchereria bancrofti B74.0
  following ectopic or molar pregnancy O08.89
  penis
    acute N48.29
    gonococcal (acute) (chronic) A54.09
  puerperal, postpartum, childbirth O86.89
  strumous, tuberculous A18.2
  subacute (any site) I89.1
  tuberculous —*see* Tuberculosis, lymph gland
Lymphatic (vessel) —*see* condition
Lymphatism E32.8
Lymphectasia I89.0
Lymphedema (acquired) —*see also* Elephantiasis
  congenital Q82.0
  hereditary (chronic) (idiopathic) Q82.0
  postmastectomy I97.2
  praecox I89.0
  secondary I89.0
  surgical NEC I97.89
    postmastectomy (syndrome) I97.2
Lymphoblastic —*see* condition
Lymphoblastoma (diffuse) —*see* Lymphoma, lymphoblastic (diffuse)
  giant follicular —*see* Lymphoma, lymphoblastic (diffuse)
  macrofollicular —*see* Lymphoma, lymphoblastic (diffuse)
Lymphocele I89.8
Lymphocytic
  chorioencephalitis (acute) (serous) A87.2
  choriomeningitis (acute) (serous) A87.2
  meningoencephalitis A87.2
Lymphocytoma, benign cutis L98.8

Lymphocytopenia D72.810
Lymphocytosis (symptomatic) D72.820
  infectious (acute) B33.8
Lymphoepithelioma —*see* Neoplasm, malignant, by site
Lymphogranuloma (malignant) —*see also* Lymphoma, Hodgkin
  chlamydial A55
  inguinale A55
  venereum (any site) (chlamydial) (with stricture of rectum) A55
Lymphogranulomatosis (malignant) —*see also* Lymphoma, Hodgkin
  benign (Boeck's sarcoid) (Schaumann's) D86.1
Lymphohistiocytosis, hemophagocytic (familial) D76.1
Lymphoid —*see* condition
Lymphoma (of) (malignant) C85.90
  adult T-cell (HTLV-1-associated) (acute variant) (chronic variant) (lymphomatoid variant) (smouldering variant) C91.5-●
  anaplastic large cell
    ALK-negative C84.7-●
    ALK-positive C84.6-●
    ▶breast implant associated (BIA-ALCL) C84.7A
    CD30-positive C84.6-●
    primary cutaneous C86.6
  angioimmunoblastic T-cell C86.5
  BALT C88.4
  B-cell C85.1-●
  B-precursor C83.5-●
  blastic NK-cell C86.4
  blastic plasmacytoid dendritic cell neoplasm (BPDCN) C86.4
  bronchial-associated lymphoid tissue [BALT-lymphoma] C88.4
  Burkitt (atypical) C83.7-●
  Burkitt-like C83.7-●
  centrocytic C83.1-●
  cutaneous follicle center C82.6-●
  cutaneous T-cell C84.A-●
  diffuse follicle center C82.5-●
  diffuse large cell C83.3-●
    anaplastic C83.3-●
    B-cell C83.3-●
    CD30-positive C83.3-●
    centroblastic C83.3-●
    immunoblastic C83.3-●
    plasmablastic C83.3-●
    subtype not specified C83.3-●
    T-cell rich C83.3-●
  enteropathy-type (associated) (intestinal) T-cell C86.2
  extranodal marginal zone B-cell lymphoma of mucosa-associated lymphoid tissue [MALT-lymphoma] C88.4
  extranodal NK/T-cell, nasal type C86.0
  follicular C82.9-●
    grade
      I C82.0-●
      II C82.1-●
      III C82.2-●
      IIIa C82.3-●
      IIIb C82.4-●
    specified NEC C82.8-●
  hepatosplenic T-cell (alpha-beta) (gamma-delta) C86.1
  histiocytic C85.9-●
    true C96.A
  Hodgkin C81.9
    lymphocyte-rich (classical) C81.4-●
    lymphocyte depleted (classical) C81.3-●
    mixed cellularity (classical) C81.2-●
    nodular sclerosis (classical) C81.1-●
    specified NEC (classical) C81.7-●
    lymphocyte-rich classical C81.4-●
    lymphocyte depleted classical C81.3-●
    mixed cellularity classical C81.2-●

▶ New   ⇒ Revised   ~~deleted~~ Deleted   ● Use Additional Character(s)

Lymphoma *(Continued)*
   Hodgkin *(Continued)*
      nodular
         lymphocyte predominant C81.0-●
         sclerosis (classical) C81.1-●
   intravascular large B-cell C83.8-●
   Lennert's C84.4-●
   lymphoblastic (diffuse) C83.5-●
   lymphoblastic B-cell C83.5-●
   lymphoblastic T-cell C83.5-●
   lymphoepithelioid C84.4-●
   lymphoplasmacytic C83.0-●
      with IgM-production C88.0
   MALT C88.4
   mantle cell C83.1-●
   mature T-cell NEC C84.4-●
   mature T/NK-cell C84.9-●
      specified NEC C84.Z-●
   mediastinal (thymic) large B-cell
      C85.2-●
   Mediterranean C88.3

Lymphoma *(Continued)*
   mucosa-associated lymphoid tissue
      [MALT-lymphoma] C88.4
   NK/T cell C84.9-●
   nodal marginal zone C83.0-●
   non-follicular (diffuse) C83.9-●
      specified NEC C83.8-●
   non-Hodgkin —*see also* Lymphoma, by type
      C85.9-●
      specified NEC C85.8-●
   non-leukemic variant of B-CLL C83.0-●
   peripheral T-cell, not classified C84.4-●
   primary cutaneous
      anaplastic large cell C86.6
      CD30-positive large T-cell C86.6
   primary effusion B-cell C83.8-●
   SALT C88.4
   skin-associated lymphoid tissue
      [SALT-lymphoma] C88.4
   small cell B-cell C83.0-●
   splenic marginal zone C83.0-●

Lymphoma *(Continued)*
   subcutaneous panniculitis-like T-cell
      C86.3
   T-precursor C83.5-●
   true histiocytic C96.A
Lymphomatosis —*see* Lymphoma
Lymphopathia venereum, veneris A55
Lymphopenia D72.810
Lymphoplasmacytic leukemia —*see* Leukemia,
   chronic lymphocytic, B-cell type
Lymphoproliferation, X-linked disease D82.3
Lymphoreticulosis, benign (of inoculation)
   A28.1
Lymphorrhea I89.8
Lymphosarcoma (diffuse) —*see also* Lymphoma
   C85.9-●
Lymphostasis I89.8
Lypemania —*see* Melancholia
Lysine and hydroxylysine metabolism
   disorder E72.3
Lyssa —*see* Rabies

M

Macacus ear Q17.3
Maceration, wet feet, tropical (syndrome) T69.02-●
MacLeod's syndrome J43.0
Macrocephalia, macrocephaly Q75.3
Macrocheilia, macrochilia (congenital)Q18.6
Macrocolon —see also Megacolon Q43.1
Macrocornea Q15.8
  with glaucoma Q15.0
Macrocytic —see condition
Macrocytosis D75.89
Macrodactylia, macrodactylism (fingers) (thumbs) Q74.0
  toes Q74.2
Macrodontia K00.2
Macrogenia M26.05
Macrogenitosomia (adrenal) (male) (praecox) E25.9
  congenital E25.0
Macroglobulinemia (idiopathic) (primary) C88.0
  monoclonal (essential) D47.2
  Waldenström C88.0
Macroglossia (congenital) Q38.2
  acquired K14.8
Macrognathia, macrognathism (congenital) (mandibular) (maxillary) M26.09
Macrogyria (congenital) Q04.8
Macrohydrocephalus —see Hydrocephalus
Macromastia —see Hypertrophy, breast
Macrophthalmos Q11.3
  in congenital glaucoma Q15.0
Macropsia H53.15
Macrosigmoid K59.39
  congenital Q43.2
Macrospondylitis, acromegalic E22.0
Macrostomia (congenital) Q18.4
Macrotia (external ear) (congenital) Q17.1
Macula
  cornea, corneal —see Opacity, cornea
  degeneration (atrophic) (exudative) (senile) —see also Degeneration, macula
  hereditary —see Dystrophy, retina
Maculae ceruleae — B85.1
Maculopathy, toxic —see Degeneration, macula, toxic
Madarosis (eyelid) H02.729
  left H02.726
    lower H02.725
    upper H02.724
  right H02.723
    lower H02.722
    upper H02.721
Madelung's
  deformity (radius) Q74.0
  disease
    radial deformity Q74.0
    symmetrical lipomas, neck E88.89
Madness —see Psychosis
Madura
  foot B47.9
    actinomycotic B47.1
    mycotic B47.0
Maduromycosis B47.0
Maffucci's syndrome Q78.4
Magnesium metabolism disorder —see Disorder, metabolism, magnesium
Main en griffe (acquired) —see also Deformity, limb, clawhand
  congenital Q74.0
Maintenance (encounter for)
  antineoplastic chemotherapy Z51.11
  antineoplastic radiation therapy Z51.0
  methadone F11.20
Majocchi's
  disease L81.7
  granuloma B35.8
Major —see condition
Malabar itch (any site) B35.5

Malabsorption K90.9
  calcium K90.89
  carbohydrate K90.49
  disaccharide K73.9
  fat K90.49
  galactose E74.20
  glucose(-galactose) E74.39
  intestinal K90.9
    specified NEC K90.89
  isomaltose E74.31
  lactose E73.9
  methionine E72.19
  monosaccharide E74.39
  postgastrectomy K91.2
  postsurgical K91.2
  protein K90.49
  starch K90.49
  sucrose E74.39
  syndrome K90.9
    postsurgical K91.2
Malacia, bone (adult) M83.9
  juvenile —see Rickets
Malacoplakia
  bladder N32.89
  pelvis (kidney) N28.89
  ureter N28.89
  urethra N36.8
Malacosteon, juvenile —see Rickets
Maladaptation —see Maladjustment
Maladie de Roger Q21.0
Maladjustment
  conjugal Z63.0
    involving divorce or estrangement Z63.5
  educational Z55.4
  family Z63.9
  marital Z63.0
    involving divorce or estrangement Z63.5
  occupational NEC Z56.89
  simple, adult —see Disorder, adjustment
  situational —see Disorder, adjustment
  social Z60.9
    due to
      acculturation difficulty Z60.3
      discrimination and persecution (perceived) Z60.5
      exclusion and isolation Z60.4
      life-cycle (phase of life) transition Z60.0
      rejection Z60.4
      specified reason NEC Z60.8
Malaise R53.81
Malakoplakia —see Malacoplakia
Malaria, malarial (fever) B54
  with
    blackwater fever B50.8
      hemoglobinuric (bilious) B50.8
    hemoglobinuria B50.8
  accidentally induced (therapeutically) - code by type under Malaria
  algid B50.9
  cerebral B50.0 [G94]
  clinically diagnosed (without parasitological confirmation) B54
  congenital NEC P37.4
    falciparum P37.3
  congestion, congestive B54
  continued (fever) B50.9
  estivo-autumnal B50.9
  falciparum B50.9
    with complications NEC B50.8
      cerebral B50.0 [G94]
    severe B50.8
  hemorrhagic B54
  malariae B52.9
    with
      complications NEC B52.8
      glomerular disorder B52.0
  malignant (tertian) —see Malaria, falciparum
  mixed infections — code to first listed type in B50-B53
  ovale B53.0
  parasitologically confirmed NEC B53.8

Malaria, malarial (Continued)
  pernicious, acute —see Malaria, falciparum
  Plasmodium (P.)
    falciparum NEC —see Malaria, falciparum
    malariae NEC B52.9
      with Plasmodium
        falciparum (and or vivax) —see Malaria, falciparum
        vivax —see also Malaria, vivax and falciparum —see Malaria, falciparum
    ovale B53.0
      with Plasmodium malariae —see also Malaria, malariae
      and vivax —see also Malaria, vivax and falciparum —see Malaria, falciparum
    simian B53.1
      with Plasmodium malariae —see also Malaria, malariae
      and vivax —see also Malaria, vivax and falciparum —see Malaria, falciparum
    vivax NEC B51.9
      with Plasmodium falciparum —see Malaria, falciparum
  quartan —see Malaria, malariae
  quotidian —see Malaria, falciparum
  recurrent B54
  remittent B54
  specified type NEC (parasitologically confirmed) B53.8
  spleen B54
  subtertian (fever) —see Malaria, falciparum
  tertian (benign) —see also Malaria, vivax
    malignant B50.9
  tropical B50.9
  typhoid B54
  vivax B51.9
    with
      complications NEC B51.8
      ruptured spleen B51.0
Malassez's disease (cystic) N50.89
Malassimilation K90.9
Mal de los pintos —see Pinta
Mal de mer T75.3
Maldescent, testis Q53.9
  bilateral Q53.20
    abdominal Q53.211
    perineal Q53.22
  unilateral Q53.10
    abdominal Q53.111
    perineal Q53.12
Maldevelopment —see also Anomaly
  brain Q07.9
  colon Q43.9
  hip Q74.2
    congenital dislocation Q65.2
      bilateral Q65.1
      unilateral Q65.0-●
  mastoid process Q75.8
  middle ear Q16.4
    except ossicles Q16.4
    ossicles Q16.3
  ossicles Q16.3
  spine Q76.49
  toe Q74.2
Male type pelvis Q74.2
  with disproportion (fetopelvic) O33.3
    causing obstructed labor O65.3
Malformation (congenital) —see also Anomaly
  adrenal gland Q89.1
  affecting multiple systems with skeletal changes NEC Q87.5
  alimentary tract Q45.9
    specified type NEC Q45.8
    upper Q40.9
      specified type NEC Q40.8
  aorta Q25.40
    absence Q25.41
    aneurysm, congenital Q25.43

▶ New   ➠ Revised   ~~deleted~~ Deleted   ● Use Additional Character(s)

Malformation *(Continued)*
 aorta *(Continued)*
  aplasia Q25.41
  atresia Q25.29
   aortic arch Q25.21
  coarctation (preductal) (postductal) Q25.1
  dilatation, congenital Q25.44
  hypoplasia Q25.42
  patent ductus arteriosus Q25.0
  specified type NEC Q25.49
  stenosis Q25.1
   supravalvular Q25.3
 aortic valve Q23.9
  specified NEC Q23.8
 arteriovenous, aneurysmatic (congenital)
   Q27.30
  brain Q28.2
   ruptured I60.8
    intracerebral I61.8
    intraparenchymal I61.8
    intraventricular I61.5
    subarachnoid I60.8
  cerebral (*see* Malformation, arteriovenous,
    brain) Q28.2
  peripheral Q27.30
   congenital Q27.33
   digestive system —*see* Angiodysplasia
   lower limb Q27.32
   other specified site Q27.39
   renal vessel Q27.34
   upper limb Q27.31
  precerebral vessels (nonruptured) Q28.0
 auricle
  ear (congenital) Q17.3
   acquired H61.119
    left H61.112
     with right H61.113
    right H61.111
     with left H61.113
 bile duct Q44.5
 bladder Q64.79
  aplasia Q64.5
  diverticulum Q64.6
  exstrophy —*see* Exstrophy, bladder
  neck obstruction Q64.31
 bone Q79.9
  face Q75.9
   specified type NEC Q75.8
  skull Q75.9
   specified type NEC Q75.8
 brain (multiple) Q04.9
  arteriovenous Q28.2
  specified type NEC Q04.8
 branchial cleft Q18.2
 breast Q83.9
  specified type NEC Q83.8
 broad ligament Q50.6
 bronchus Q32.4
 bursa Q79.9
 cardiac
  chambers Q20.9
   specified type NEC Q20.8
  septum Q21.9
   specified type NEC Q21.8
 cerebral Q04.9
  vessels Q28.3
 cervix uteri Q51.9
  specified type NEC Q51.828
 Chiari
  Type I G93.5
  Type II Q07.01
 choroid (congenital) Q14.3
  plexus Q07.8
 circulatory system Q28.9
 cochlea Q16.5
 cornea Q13.4
 coronary vessels Q24.5
 corpus callosum (congenital) Q04.0
 diaphragm Q79.1
 digestive system NEC, specified type NEC
   Q45.8

Malformation *(Continued)*
 dura Q07.9
  brain Q04.9
  spinal Q06.9
 ear Q17.9
  causing impairment of hearing Q16.9
  external Q17.9
   accessory auricle Q17.0
   causing impairment of hearing Q16.9
    absence of
     auditory canal Q16.1
     auricle Q16.0
   macrotia Q17.1
   microtia Q17.2
   misplacement Q17.4
   misshapen NEC Q17.3
   prominence Q17.5
   specified type NEC Q17.8
  inner Q16.5
  middle Q16.4
   absence of eustachian tube Q16.2
   ossicles (fusion) Q16.3
  ossicles Q16.3
  specified type NEC Q17.8
 epididymis Q55.4
 esophagus Q39.9
  specified type NEC Q39.8
 eye Q15.9
  lid Q10.3
  specified NEC Q15.8
 fallopian tube Q50.6
 genital organ —*see* Anomaly, genitalia
 great
  artery Q25.9
   aorta —*see* Malformation, aorta
   pulmonary artery —*see* Malformation,
     pulmonary, artery
   specified type NEC Q25.8
  vein Q26.9
   anomalous
    portal venous connection Q26.5
    pulmonary venous connection Q26.4
     partial Q26.3
     total Q26.2
   persistent left superior vena cava Q26.1
   portal vein-hepatic artery fistula Q26.6
   specified type NEC Q26.8
   vena cava stenosis, congenital Q26.0
 gum Q38.6
 hair Q84.2
 heart Q24.9
  specified type NEC Q24.8
 integument Q84.9
  specified type NEC Q84.8
 internal ear Q16.5
 intestine Q43.9
  specified type NEC Q43.8
 iris Q13.2
 joint Q74.9
  ankle Q74.2
  lumbosacral Q76.49
  sacroiliac Q74.2
  specified type NEC Q74.8
 kidney Q63.9
  accessory Q63.0
  giant Q63.3
  horseshoe Q63.1
  hydronephrosis Q62.0
  malposition Q63.2
  specified type NEC Q63.8
 lacrimal apparatus Q10.6
 lingual Q38.3
 lip Q38.0
 liver Q44.7
 lung Q33.9
 meninges or membrane (congenital) Q07.9
  cerebral Q04.8
  spinal (cord) Q06.9
 middle ear Q16.4
  ossicles Q16.3
 mitral valve Q23.9
  specified NEC Q23.8

Malformation *(Continued)*
 Mondini's (congenital) (malformation,
   cochlea) Q16.5
 mouth (congenital) Q38.6
 multiple types NEC Q89.7
 musculoskeletal system Q79.9
 myocardium Q24.8
 nail Q84.6
 nervous system (central) Q07.9
 nose Q30.9
  specified type NEC Q30.8
 optic disc Q14.2
 orbit Q10.7
 ovary Q50.39
 palate Q38.5
 parathyroid gland Q89.2
 pelvic organs or tissues NEC
  in pregnancy or childbirth O34.8-●
   causing obstructed labor O65.5
 penis Q55.69
  aplasia Q55.5
  curvature (lateral) Q55.61
  hypoplasia Q55.62
 pericardium Q24.8
 peripheral vascular system Q27.9
  specified type NEC Q27.8
 pharynx Q38.8
 precerebral vessels Q28.1
 prostate Q55.4
 pulmonary
  arteriovenous Q25.72
  artery Q25.9
   atresia Q25.5
   specified type NEC Q25.79
   stenosis Q25.6
  valve Q22.3
 renal artery Q27.2
 respiratory system Q34.9
 retina Q14.1
 scrotum —*see* Malformation, testis and scrotum
 seminal vesicles Q55.4
 sense organs NEC Q07.9
 skin Q82.9
 specified NEC Q89.8
 spinal
  cord Q06.9
  nerve root Q07.8
 spine Q76.49
  kyphosis —*see* Kyphosis, congenital
  lordosis —*see* Lordosis, congenital
 spleen Q89.09
 stomach Q40.3
  specified type NEC Q40.2
 teeth, tooth K00.9
 tendon Q79.9
 testis and scrotum Q55.20
  aplasia Q55.0
  hypoplasia Q55.1
  polyorchism Q55.21
  retractile testis Q55.22
  scrotal transposition Q55.23
  specified NEC Q55.29
 thorax, bony Q76.9
 throat Q38.8
 thyroid gland Q89.2
 tongue (congenital) Q38.3
  hypertrophy Q38.2
  tie Q38.1
 trachea Q32.1
 tricuspid valve Q22.9
  specified type NEC Q22.8
 umbilical cord NEC (complicating delivery)
   O69.89
 umbilicus Q89.9
 ureter Q62.8
  agenesis Q62.4
  duplication Q62.5
  malposition —*see* Malposition, congenital,
    ureter
  obstructive defect —*see* Defect, obstructive,
    ureter
  vesico-uretero-renal reflux Q62.7

Malformation (*Continued*)
  urethra Q64.79
    aplasia Q64.5
    duplication Q64.74
    posterior valves Q64.2
    prolapse Q64.71
    stricture Q64.32
  urinary system Q64.9
  uterus Q51.9
    specified type NEC Q51.818
  vagina Q52.4
  vascular system, peripheral Q27.9
  vas deferens Q55.4
    atresia Q55.3
  venous —*see* Anomaly, vein(s)
  vulva Q52.70
Malfunction —*see also* Dysfunction
  cardiac electronic device T82.119
    electrode T82.110
    pulse generator T82.111
    specified type NEC T82.118
  catheter device NEC T85.618
    cystostomy T83.010
    dialysis (renal) (vascular) T82.41
      intraperitoneal T85.611
    infusion NEC T82.514
      cranial T85.610
      epidural T85.610
      intrathecal T85.610
      spinal T85.610
      subarachnoid T85.610
      subdural T85.610
    urinary —*see also* Breakdown, device,
      catheter T83.018
  colostomy K94.03
    valve K94.03
  cystostomy (stoma) N99.512
    catheter T83.010
  enteric stoma K94.13
  enterostomy K94.13
  esophagostomy K94.33
  gastroenteric K31.89
  gastrostomy K94.23
  ileostomy K94.13
    valve K94.13
  intrathecal infusion pump T85.615
  jejunostomy K94.13
  nervous system device, implant or graft,
    specified NEC T85.615
  pacemaker —*see* Malfunction, cardiac
    electronic device
  prosthetic device, internal —*see*
    Complications, prosthetic device, by site,
    mechanical
  tracheostomy J95.03
  urinary device NEC —*see* Complication,
    genitourinary, device, urinary,
    mechanical
  valve
    colostomy K94.03
    heart T82.09
    ileostomy K94.13
  vascular graft or shunt NEC —*see*
    Complication, cardiovascular device,
    mechanical, vascular
  ventricular (communicating shunt) T85.01
Malherbe's tumor —*see* Neoplasm, skin,
  benign
Malibu disease L98.8-●
Malignancy —*see also* Neoplasm, malignant,
  by site
  unspecified site (primary) C80.1
Malignant —*see* condition
Malingerer, malingering Z76.5
Mallet finger (acquired) —*see* Deformity, finger,
  mallet finger
  congenital Q74.0
  sequelae of rickets E64.3
Malleus A24.0
Mallory's bodies R89.7
Mallory-Weiss syndrome K22.6

Malnutrition E46
  degree
    first E44.1
    mild (protein) E44.1
    moderate (protein) E44.0
    second E44.0
    severe (protein-energy) E43
      intermediate form E42
        with
          kwashiorkor (and marasmus) E42
          marasmus E41
    third E43
  following gastrointestinal surgery K91.2
  intrauterine
    light-for-dates —*see* Light for dates
    small-for-dates —*see* Small for dates
  lack of care, or neglect (child) (infant) T76.02
    confirmed T74.02
  malignant E40
  protein E46
    calorie E46
      mild E44.1
      moderate E44.0
      severe E43
        intermediate form E42
          with
            kwashiorkor (and marasmus)
              E42
            marasmus E41
    energy E46
      mild E44.1
      moderate E44.0
      severe E43
        intermediate form E42
          with
            kwashiorkor (and marasmus)
              E42
            marasmus E41
  severe (protein-energy) E43
    with
      kwashiorkor (and marasmus) E42
      marasmus E41
Malocclusion (teeth) M26.4
  Angle's M26.219
    class I M26.211
    class II M26.212
    class III M26.213
  due to
    abnormal swallowing M26.59
    mouth breathing M26.59
    tongue, lip or finger habits M26.59
  temporomandibular (joint) M26.69
Malposition
  cervix —*see* Malposition, uterus
  congenital
    adrenal (gland) Q89.1
    alimentary tract Q45.8
      lower Q43.8
      upper Q40.8
    aorta Q25.49
    appendix Q43.8
    arterial trunk Q20.0
    artery (peripheral) Q27.8
      coronary Q24.5
      digestive system Q27.8
      lower limb Q27.8
      pulmonary Q25.79
      specified site NEC Q27.8
      upper limb Q27.8
    auditory canal Q17.8
      causing impairment of hearing Q16.9
    auricle (ear) Q17.4
      causing impairment of hearing Q16.9
    cervical Q18.2
    biliary duct or passage Q44.5
    bladder (mucosa) —*see* Exstrophy,
      bladder
    brachial plexus Q07.8
    brain tissue Q04.8
    breast Q83.8
    bronchus Q32.4

Malposition (*Continued*)
  congenital (*Continued*)
    cecum Q43.8
    clavicle Q74.0
    colon Q43.8
    digestive organ or tract NEC Q45.8
      lower Q43.8
      upper Q40.8
    ear (auricle) (external) Q17.4
      ossicles Q16.3
    endocrine (gland) NEC Q89.2
    epiglottis Q31.8
    eustachian tube Q17.8
    eye Q15.8
    facial features Q18.8
    fallopian tube Q50.6
    finger(s) Q68.1
      supernumerary Q69.0
    foot Q66.9-●
    gallbladder Q44.1
    gastrointestinal tract Q45.8
    genitalia, genital organ(s) or tract
      female Q52.8
        external Q52.79
        internal NEC Q52.8
      male Q55.8
    glottis Q31.8
    hand Q68.1
    heart Q24.8
      dextrocardia Q24.0
        with complete transposition of viscera
          Q89.3
    hepatic duct Q44.5
    hip (joint) Q65.89
    intestine (large) (small) Q43.8
      with anomalous adhesions, fixation or
        malrotation Q43.3
    joint NEC Q68.8
    kidney Q63.2
    larynx Q31.8
    limb Q68.8
      lower Q68.8
      upper Q68.8
    liver Q44.7
    lung (lobe) Q33.8
    nail(s) Q84.6
    nerve Q07.8
    nervous system NEC Q07.8
    nose, nasal (septum) Q30.8
    organ or site not listed —*see* Anomaly,
      by site
    ovary Q50.39
    pancreas Q45.3
    parathyroid (gland) Q89.2
    patella Q74.1
    peripheral vascular system Q27.8
    pituitary (gland) Q89.2
    respiratory organ or system NEC
      Q34.8
    rib (cage) Q76.6
      supernumerary in cervical region
        Q76.5
    scapula Q74.0
    shoulder Q74.0
    spinal cord Q06.8
    spleen Q89.09
    sternum NEC Q76.7
    stomach Q40.2
    symphysis pubis Q74.2
    thymus (gland) Q89.2
    thyroid (gland) (tissue) Q89.2
      cartilage Q31.8
    toe(s) Q66.9-●
      supernumerary Q69.2
    tongue Q38.3
    trachea Q32.1
    ureter Q62.60
      deviation Q62.61
      displacement Q62.62
      ectopia Q62.63
      specified type NEC Q62.69

▶ New   ⇒ Revised   deleted Deleted   ● Use Additional Character(s)

Malposition (*Continued*)
  congenital (*Continued*)
    uterus Q51.818
    vein(s) (peripheral) Q27.8
      great Q26.8
    vena cava (inferior) (superior) Q26.8
  device, implant or graft —*see also*
      Complications, by site and type,
      mechanical T85.628
    arterial graft NEC —*see* Complication,
        cardiovascular device, mechanical,
        vascular
    breast (implant) T85.42
    catheter NEC T85.628
      cystostomy T83.020
      dialysis (renal) T82.42
        intraperitoneal T85.621
      infusion NEC T82.524
        spinal (epidural) (subdural) T85.620
      urinary —*see also* Displacement, device,
          catheter, urinary T83.028
    electronic (electrode) (pulse generator)
        (stimulator)
      bone T84.320
      cardiac T82.129
        electrode T82.120
        pulse generator T82.121
        specified type NEC T82.128
      nervous system —*see* Complication,
          prosthetic device, mechanical,
          electronic nervous system
          stimulator
      urinary —*see* Complication,
          genitourinary, device, urinary,
          mechanical
    fixation, internal (orthopedic) NEC —
        see Complication, fixation device,
        mechanical
    gastrointestinal —*see* Complications,
        prosthetic device, mechanical,
        gastrointestinal device
    genital NEC T83.428
      intrauterine contraceptive device (string)
          T83.32
      penile prosthesis (cylinder) (implanted)
          (pump) (resevoir) T83.420
      testicular prosthesis T83.421
    heart NEC —*see* Complication,
        cardiovascular device, mechanical
    joint prosthesis —*see* Complication, joint
        prosthesis, mechanical
    ocular NEC —*see* Complications,
        prosthetic device, mechanical,
        ocular device
    orthopedic NEC —*see* Complication,
        orthopedic, device, mechanical
    specified NEC T85.628
    urinary NEC —*see also* Complication,
        genitourinary, device, urinary,
        mechanical
      graft T83.22
    vascular NEC —*see* Complication,
        cardiovascular device, mechanical
    ventricular intracranial shunt T85.02
  fetus —*see* Pregnancy, complicated by
      (management affected by), presentation,
      fetal
  gallbladder K82.8
  gastrointestinal tract, congenital Q45.8
  heart, congenital NEC Q24.8
  joint prosthesis —*see* Complications, joint
      prosthesis, mechanical, displacement,
      by site
  stomach K31.89
    congenital Q40.2
  tooth, teeth, fully erupted M26.30
  uterus (acute) (acquired) (adherent)
      (asymptomatic) (postinfectional)
      (postpartal, old) N85.4
    anteflexion or anteversion N85.4
      congenital Q51.818

Malposition (*Continued*)
  uterus (*Continued*)
    flexion N85.4
      lateral —*see* Lateroversion, uterus
    inversion N85.5
    lateral (flexion) (version) —*see*
        Lateroversion, uterus
      in pregnancy or childbirth —*see*
          subcategory O34.5
    retroflexion or retroversion —*see*
        Retroversion, uterus
Malposture R29.3
Malrotation
  cecum Q43.3
  colon Q43.3
  intestine Q43.3
  kidney Q63.2
Malta fever —*see* Brucellosis
Maltreatment
  adult
    abandonment
      confirmed T74.01
      suspected T76.01
    bullying
      confirmed T74.31
      suspected T76.31
    confirmed T74.91
    history of Z91.419
    intimidation (through social media)
      confirmed T74.31
      suspected T76.31
    neglect
      confirmed T74.01
      suspected T76.01
    physical abuse
      confirmed T74.11
      suspected T76.11
    psychological abuse
      confirmed T74.31
      history of Z91.411
      suspected T76.31
    sexual abuse
      confirmed T74.21
      suspected T76.21
    suspected T76.91
  child
    abandonment
      confirmed T74.02
      suspected T76.02
    bullying
      confirmed T74.32
      suspected T76.32
    confirmed T74.92
    history of —*see* History, personal (of),
        abuse
    intimidation (through social media)
      confirmed T74.32
      suspected T76.32
    neglect
      confirmed T74.02
      history of —*see* History, personal (of),
          abuse
      suspected T76.02
    physical abuse
      confirmed T74.12
      history of —*see* History, personal (of),
          abuse
      suspected T76.12
    psychological abuse
      confirmed T74.32
      history of —*see* History, personal (of),
          abuse
      suspected T76.32
    sexual abuse
      confirmed T74.22
      history of —*see* History, personal (of),
          abuse
      suspected T76.22
    suspected T76.92
  personal history of Z91.89
Maltworker's lung J67.4

Malunion, fracture —*see* Fracture, by site
Mammillitis N61.0
  puerperal, postpartum O91.02
Mammitis —*see* Mastitis
Mammogram (examination) Z12.39
  routine Z12.31
Mammoplasia N62
Management (of)
  bone conduction hearing device (implanted)
      Z45.320
  cardiac pacemaker NEC Z45.018
  cerebrospinal fluid drainage device Z45.41
  cochlear device (implanted) Z45.321
  contraceptive Z30.9
    specified NEC Z30.8
  implanted device Z45.9
    specified NEC Z45.89
  infusion pump Z45.1
  procreative Z31.9
    male factor infertility in female Z31.81
    specified NEC Z31.89
  prosthesis (external) —*see also* Fitting
      Z44.9
    implanted Z45.9
      specified NEC Z45.89
  renal dialysis catheter Z49.01
  vascular access device Z45.2
Mangled —*see* specified injury by site
Mania (monopolar) —*see also* Disorder, mood,
    manic episode
  with psychotic symptoms F30.2
  without psychotic symptoms F30.10
    mild F30.11
    moderate F30.12
    severe F30.13
  Bell's F30.8
  chronic (recurrent) F31.89
  hysterical F44.89
  puerperal F30.8
  recurrent F31.89
Manic depression F31.9
**Manic-depressive insanity, psychosis, or
    syndrome** —*see* Disorder, bipolar
Mannosidosis E77.1
Mansonelliasis, mansonellosis B74.4
Manson's
  disease B65.1
  schistosomiasis B65.1
Manual —*see* condition
Maple-bark-stripper's lung (disease) J67.6
Maple-syrup-urine disease E71.0
Marable's syndrome (celiac artery
    compression) I77.4
Marasmus E41
  due to malnutrition E41
  intestinal E41
  nutritional E41
  senile R54
  tuberculous NEC —*see* Tuberculosis
Marble
  bones Q78.2
  skin R23.8
Marburg virus disease A98.3
March
  fracture —*see* Fracture, traumatic, stress, by
      site
  hemoglobinuria D59.6
Marchesani (-Weill) **syndrome** Q87.0
Marchiafava (-Bignami) **syndrome or disease**
    G37.1
Marchiafava-Micheli syndrome D59.5
Marcus Gunn's syndrome Q07.8
Marfan's syndrome —*see* Syndrome, Marfan's
Marie-Bamberger disease —*see*
    Osteoarthropathy, hypertrophic, specified
    NEC
**Marie-Charcot-Tooth neuropathic muscular
    atrophy** G60.0
Marie's
  cerebellar ataxia (late-onset) G11.2
  disease or syndrome (acromegaly) E22.0

M

Marie-Strümpell arthritis, disease or
  spondylitis —see Spondylitis, ankylosing
Marion's disease (bladder neck obstruction)
  N32.0
Marital conflict Z63.0
Mark
  port wine Q82.5
  raspberry Q82.5
  strawberry Q82.5
  stretch L90.6
  tattoo L81.8
Marker heterochromatin —see Extra, marker
  chromosomes
Maroteaux-Lamy syndrome (mild) (severe)
  E76.29
Marrow (bone)
  arrest D61.9
  poor function D75.89
Marseilles fever A77.1
Marsh fever —see Malaria
Marshall's (hidrotic) **ectodermal dysplasia**
  Q82.4
Marsh's disease (exophthalmic goiter)
  E05.00
  with storm E05.01
Masculinization (female) **with adrenal**
  hyperplasia E25.9
  congenital E25.0
Masculinovoblastoma D27.-●
Masochism (sexual) F65.51
Mason's lung J62.8
Mass
  abdominal R19.00
    epigastric R19.06
    generalized R19.07
    left lower quadrant R19.04
    left upper quadrant R19.02
    periumbilic R19.05
    right lower quadrant R19.03
    right upper quadrant R19.01
    specified site NEC R19.09
  breast —see also Lump, breast N63.0
  chest R22.2
  cystic —see Cyst
  ear H93.8-●
  head R22.0
  intra-abdominal (diffuse) (generalized) —see
    Mass, abdominal
  kidney N28.89
  liver R16.0
  localized (skin) R22.9
    chest R22.2
    head R22.0
    limb
      lower R22.4-●
      upper R22.3-●
    neck R22.1
    trunk R22.2
  lung R91.8
  malignant —see Neoplasm, malignant,
    by site
  neck R22.1
  pelvic (diffuse) (generalized) —see Mass,
    abdominal
  specified organ NEC —see Disease, by site
  splenic R16.1
  substernal thyroid —see Goiter
  superficial (localized) R22.9
  umbilical (diffuse) (generalized) R19.09
Massive —see condition
Mast cell
  disease, systemic tissue D47.02
  leukemia C94.3-●
  neoplasm
    malignant C96.20
      specified type NEC C96.29
    of uncertain behavior NEC D47.09
  sarcoma C96.22
  tumor D47.09
Mastalgia N64.4
Masters-Allen syndrome N83.8

Mastitis (acute) (diffuse) (nonpuerperal)
  (subacute) N61.0
  with abscess N61.1
  chronic (cystic) —see Mastopathy, cystic
  cystic (Schimmelbusch's type) —see
    Mastopathy, cystic
  fibrocystic —see Mastopathy, cystic
  granulomatous N61.2-●
  infective N61.0
    newborn P39.0
  interstitial, gestational or puerperal —see
    Mastitis, obstetric
  neonatal (noninfective) P83.4
    infective P39.0
  obstetric (interstitial) (nonpurulent)
    associated with
      lactation O91.23
      pregnancy O91.21-●
      puerperium O91.22
    purulent
      associated with
        lactation O91.13
        pregnancy O91.11-●
        puerperium O91.12
  periductal —see Ectasia, mammary duct
  phlegmonous —see Mastopathy, cystic
  plasma cell —see Ectasia, mammary duct
  without abscess N61.0
Mastocytoma (extracutaneous) D47.09
  malignant C96.29
  solitary D47.01
Mastocytosis D47.09
  aggressive systemic C96.21
  cutaneous (diffuse) (maculopapular) D47.01
    congenital Q82.2
    of neonatal onset Q82.2
    of newborn onset Q82.2
  indolent systemic D47.02
  isolated bone marrow D47.02
  malignant C96.29
  systemic (indolent) (smoldering)
    with an associated hematological
      non-mast cell lineage disease (SM-
      AHNMD) D47.02
Mastodynia N64.4
Mastoid —see condition
Mastoidalgia —see subcategory H92.0
Mastoiditis (coalescent) (hemorrhagic)
  (suppurative) H70.9-●
  acute, subacute H70.00-●
    complicated NEC H70.09-●
    subperiosteal H70.01-●
  chronic (necrotic) (recurrent) H70.1-●
  in (due to)
    infectious disease NEC B99 [H75.0-●]
    parasitic disease NEC B89 [H75.0-●]
    tuberculosis A18.03
  petrositis —see Petrositis
  postauricular fistula —see Fistula,
    postauricular
  specified NEC H70.89-●
  tuberculous A18.03
Mastopathy, mastopathia N64.9
  chronica cystica —see Mastopathy, cystic
  cystic (chronic) (diffuse) N60.1
    with epithelial proliferation N60.3-●
  diffuse cystic —see Mastopathy, cystic
  estrogenic, oestrogenica N64.89
  ovarian origin N64.89
Mastoplasia, mastoplastia N62
Masturbation (excessive) F98.8
Maternal care (for) —see Pregnancy
  (complicated by) (management affected by)
Matheiu's disease (leptospiral jaundice) A27.0
Mauclaire's disease or osteochondrosis —see
  Osteochondrosis, juvenile, hand, metacarpal
Maxcy's disease A75.2
Maxilla, maxillary —see condition
May (-Hegglin) **anomaly or syndrome** D72.0
McArdle (-Schmid)(-Pearson) **disease**
  (glycogen storage) E74.04

McCune-Albright syndrome Q78.1
McQuarrie's syndrome (idiopathic familial
  hypoglycemia) E16.2
Meadow's syndrome Q86.1
Measles (black) (hemorrhagic) (suppressed)
  B05.9
  with
    complications NEC B05.89
    encephalitis B05.0
    intestinal complications B05.4
    keratitis (keratoconjunctivitis) B05.81
    meningitis B05.1
    otitis media B05.3
    pneumonia B05.2
  French —see Rubella
  German —see Rubella
  Liberty —see Rubella
Meatitis, urethral —see Urethritis
Meatus, meatal —see condition
Meat-wrappers' asthma J68.9
Meckel-Gruber syndrome Q61.9
Meckel's diverticulitis, diverticulum
  (displaced) (hypertrophic) Q43.0
Meconium
  ileus, newborn P76.0
    in cystic fibrosis E84.11
    meaning meconium plug (without cystic
      fibrosis) P76.0
  obstruction, newborn P76.0
    due to fecaliths P76.0
    in mucoviscidosis E84.11
  peritonitis P78.0
  plug syndrome (newborn) NEC P76.0
Median —see also condition
  arcuate ligament syndrome I77.4
  bar (prostate) (vesical orifice) —see
    Hyperplasia, prostate
  rhomboid glossitis K14.2
Mediastinal shift R93.89
Mediastinitis (acute) (chronic) J98.51
  syphilitic A52.73
  tuberculous A15.8
Mediastinopericarditis —see also Pericarditis
  acute I30.9
  adhesive I31.0
  chronic I31.8
  rheumatic I09.2
Mediastinum, mediastinal —see condition
Medicine poisoning —see Table of Drugs and
  Chemicals, by drug, poisoning
Mediterranean
  fever —see Brucellosis
    familial M04.1
    tick A77.1
  kala-azar B55.0
  leishmaniasis B55.0
  tick fever A77.1
Medulla —see condition
Medullary cystic kidney Q61.5
Medullated fibers
  optic (nerve) Q14.8
  retina Q14.1
Medulloblastoma
  desmoplastic C71.6
  specified site —see Neoplasm, malignant, by
    site
  unspecified site C71.6
Medulloepithelioma —see also Neoplasm,
  malignant, by site
  teratoid —see Neoplasm, malignant, by site
Medullomyoblastoma
  specified site —see Neoplasm, malignant, by
    site
  unspecified site C71.6
Meekeren-Ehlers-Danlos syndrome —see also
  Syndrome, Ehlers-Danlos Q79.6
Megacolon (acquired) (functional) (not
  Hirschsprung's disease) (in) K59.39
  Chagas' disease B57.32
  congenital, congenitum (aganglionic) Q43.1
  Hirschsprung's (disease) Q43.1

▶ New   ⇒ Revised   ~~deleted~~ Deleted   ● Use Additional Character(s)

Megacolon (*Continued*)
toxic NEC K59.31
due to Clostridium difficile
not specified as recurrent A04.72
recurrent A04.71
Megaesophagus (functional) K22.0
congenital Q39.5
in (due to) Chagas' disease B57.31
Megalencephaly Q04.5
Megalerythema (epidemic) B08.3
Megaloappendix Q43.8
Megalocephalus, megalocephaly NEC Q75.3
Megalocornea Q15.8
with glaucoma Q15.0
Megalocytic anemia D53.1
Megalodactylia (fingers) (thumbs) (congenital)
Q74.0
toes Q74.2
Megaloduodenum Q43.8
Megaloesophagus (functional) K22.0
congenital Q39.5
Megalogastria (acquired) K31.89
congenital Q40.2
Megalophthalmos Q11.3
Megalopsia H53.15
Megalosplenia —*see* Splenomegaly
Megaloureter N28.82
congenital Q62.2
Megarectum K62.89
Megasigmoid K59.39
congenital Q43.2
Megaureter N28.82
congenital Q62.2
Megavitamin-B6 syndrome E67.2
Megrim —*see* Migraine
Meibomian
cyst, infected —*see* Hordeolum
gland —*see* condition
sty, stye —*see* Hordeolum
Meibomitis —*see* Hordeolum
Melge Milroy disease (chronic hereditary
edema) Q82.0
Meige's syndrome Q82.0
Melalgia, nutritional E53.8
Melancholia F32.A
climacteric (single episode) F32.89
recurrent episode F33.8
hypochondriac F45.29
intermittent (single episode) F32.89
recurrent episode F33.8
involutional (single episode) F32.89
recurrent episode F33.8
menopausal (single episode) F32.89
recurrent episode F33.8
puerperal F32.89
reactive (emotional stress or trauma) F32.3
recurrent F33.9
senile F03
stuporous (single episode) F32.89
recurrent episode F33.8
Melanemia R79.89
Melanoameloblastoma —*see* Neoplasm, bone,
benign
Melanoblastoma —*see* Melanoma
Melanocarcinoma —*see* Melanoma
Melanocytoma, eyeball D31.9-●
Melanocytosis, neurocutaneous Q82.8
Melanoderma, melanodermia L81.4
Melanodontia, infantile K03.89
Melanodontoclasia K03.89
Melanoepithelioma —*see* Melanoma
Melanoma (malignant) C43.9
acral lentiginous, malignant —*see* Melanoma,
skin, by site
amelanotic —*see* Melanoma, skin, by site
balloon cell —*see* Melanoma, skin, by site
benign —*see* Nevus
desmoplastic, malignant —*see* Melanoma,
skin, by site
epithelioid cell —*see* Melanoma, skin, by site
with spindle cell, mixed —*see* Melanoma,
skin, by site

Melanoma (*Continued*)
in
giant pigmented nevus —*see* Melanoma,
skin, by site
Hutchinson's melanotic freckle —*see*
Melanoma, skin, by site
junctional nevus —*see* Melanoma, skin,
by site
precancerous melanosis —*see* Melanoma,
skin, by site
in situ D03.9
abdominal wall D03.59
ala nasi D03.39
ankle D03.7-●
anus, anal (margin) (skin) D03.51
arm D03.6-●
auditory canal D03.2-●
auricle (ear) D03.2-●
auricular canal (external) D03.2-●
axilla, axillary fold D03.59
back D03.59
breast D03.52
brow D03.39
buttock D03.59
canthus (eye) D03.1-●
cheek (external) D03.39
chest wall D03.59
chin D03.39
choroid D03.8
conjunctiva D03.8
ear (external) D03.2-●
external meatus (ear) D03.2-●
eye D03.8
eyebrow D03.39
eyelid (lower) (upper) D03.1-●
face D03.30
specified NEC D03.39
female genital organ (external) NEC D03.8
finger D03.6-●
flank D03.59
foot D03.7-●
forearm D03.6-●
forehead D03.39
foreskin D03.8
gluteal region D03.59
groin D03.59
hand D03.6-●
heel D03.7-●
helix D03.2-●
hip D03.7-●
interscapular region D03.59
iris D03.8
jaw D03.39
knee D03.7-●
labium (majus) (minus) D03.8
lacrimal gland D03.8
leg D03.7-●
lip (lower) (upper) D03.0
lower limb NEC D03.7-●
male genital organ (external) NEC D03.8
nail D03.9
finger D03.6-●
toe D03.7-●
neck D03.4
nose (external) D03.39
orbit D03.8
penis D03.8
perianal skin D03.51
perineum D03.51
pinna D03.2-●
popliteal fossa or space D03.7-●
prepuce D03.8
pudendum D03.8
retina D03.8
retrobulbar D03.8
scalp D03.4
scrotum D03.8
shoulder D03.6-●
specified site NEC D03.8
submammary fold D03.52
temple D03.39

Melanoma (*Continued*)
in situ (*Continued*)
thigh D03.7-●
toe D03.7-●
trunk NEC D03.59
umbilicus D03.59
upper limb NEC D03.6-●
vulva D03.8
juvenile —*see* Nevus
malignant, of soft parts except skin —*see*
Neoplasm, connective tissue, malignant
metastatic
breast C79.81
genital organ C79.82
specified site NEC C79.89
neurotropic, malignant —*see* Melanoma, skin,
by site
nodular —*see* Melanoma, skin, by site
regressing, malignant —*see* Melanoma, skin,
by site
skin C43.9
abdominal wall C43.59
ala nasi C43.31
ankle C43.7-●
anus, anal (skin) C43.51
arm C43.6-●
auditory canal (external) C43.2-●
auricle (ear) C43.2-●
auricular canal (external) C43.2-●
axilla, axillary fold C43.59
back C43.59
breast (female) (male) C43.52
brow C43.39
buttock C43.59
canthus (eye) C43.1-●
cheek (external) C43.39
chest wall C43.59
chin C43.39
ear (external) C43.2-●
elbow C43.6-●
external meatus (ear) C43.2-●
eyebrow C43.39
eyelid (lower) (upper) C43.1-●
face C43.30
specified NEC C43.39
female genital organ (external) NEC C51.9
finger C43.6-●
flank C43.59
foot C43.7-●
forearm C43.6-●
forehead C43.39
foreskin C60.0
glabella C43.39
gluteal region C43.59
groin C43.59
hand C43.6-●
heel C43.7-●
helix C43.2-●
hip C43.7-●
interscapular region C43.59
jaw (external) C43.39
knee C43.7-●
labium C51.9
majus C51.0
minus C51.1
leg C43.7-●
lip (lower) (upper) C43.0
lower limb NEC C43.7-●
male genital organ (external) NEC C63.9
nail
finger C43.6-●
toe C43.7-●
nasolabial groove C43.39
nates C43.59
neck C43.4
nose (external) C43.31
overlapping site C43.8
palpebra C43.1-●
penis C60.9
perianal skin C43.51
perineum C43.51

Melanoma *(Continued)*
  skin *(Continued)*
    pinna C43.2-●
    popliteal fossa or space C43.7-●
    prepuce C60.0
    pudendum C51.9
    scalp C43.4
    scrotum C63.2
    shoulder C43.6-●
    skin NEC C43.9
    submammary fold C43.52
    temple C43.39
    thigh C43.7-●
    toe C43.7-●
    trunk NEC C43.59
    umbilicus C43.59
    upper limb NEC C43.6-●
    vulva C51.9
      overlapping sites C51.8
    spindle cell
      with epithelioid, mixed —*see* Melanoma, skin, by site
      type A C69.4-●
      type B C69.4-●
    superficial spreading —*see* Melanoma, skin, by site
Melanosarcoma —*see also* Melanoma
  epithelioid cell —*see* Melanoma
Melanosis L81.4
  addisonian E27.1
    tuberculous A18.7
  adrenal E27.1
  colon K63.89
  conjunctiva —*see* Pigmentation, conjunctiva
    congenital Q13.89
  cornea (presenile) (senile) —*see also* Pigmentation, cornea
    congenital Q13.4
  eye NEC H57.89
    congenital Q15.8
  lenticularis progressiva Q82.1
  liver K76.89
  precancerous —*see also* Melanoma, in situ
    malignant melanoma in —*see* Melanoma
  Riehl's L81.4
  sclera H15.89
    congenital Q13.89
  suprarenal E27.1
  tar L81.4
  toxic L81.4
Melanuria R82.998
MELAS syndrome E88.41
Melasma L81.1
  adrenal (gland) E27.1
  suprarenal (gland) E27.1
Melena K92.1
  with ulcer - code by site under Ulcer, with hemorrhage K27.4
  due to swallowed maternal blood P78.2
  newborn, neonatal P54.1
    due to swallowed maternal blood P78.2
Meleney's
  gangrene (cutaneous) —*see* Ulcer, skin
  ulcer (chronic undermining) —*see* Ulcer, skin
Melioidosis A24.9
  acute A24.1
  chronic A24.2
  fulminating A24.1
  pneumonia A24.1
  pulmonary (chronic) A24.2
    acute A24.1
    subacute A24.2
  sepsis A24.1
  specified NEC A24.3
  subacute A24.2
Melitensis, febris A23.0
Melkersson (-Rosenthal) syndrome G51.2
Mellitus, diabetes —*see* Diabetes
Melorheostosis (bone) —*see* Disorder, bone, density and structure, specified NEC
Meloschisis Q18.4

Melotia Q17.4
Membrana
  capsularis lentis posterior Q13.89
  epipapillaris Q14.2
Membranacea placenta O43.19-●
Membranaceous uterus N85.8
Membrane(s), membranous —*see also* condition
  cyclitic —*see* Membrane, pupillary
  folds, congenital —*see* Web
  Jackson's Q43.3
  over face of newborn P28.9
  premature rupture —*see* Rupture, membranes, premature
  pupillary H21.4-●
    persistent Q13.89
  retained (with hemorrhage) (complicating delivery) O72.2
    without hemorrhage O73.1
  secondary cataract —*see* Cataract, secondary
  unruptured (causing asphyxia) —*see* Asphyxia, newborn
  vitreous —*see* Opacity, vitreous, membranes and strands
Membranitis —*see* Chorioamnionitis
Memory disturbance, lack or loss —*see also* Amnesia
  mild, following organic brain damage F06.8
Menadione deficiency E56.1
Menarche
  delayed E30.0
  precocious E30.1
Mendacity, pathologic F60.2
Mendelson's syndrome (due to anesthesia) J95.4
  in labor and delivery O74.0
  in pregnancy O29.01-●
  obstetric O74.0
  postpartum, puerperal O89.01
Ménétrier's disease or syndrome K29.60
  with bleeding K29.61
Ménière's disease, syndrome or vertigo H81.0-●
Meninges, meningeal —*see* condition
Meningioma —*see also* Neoplasm, meninges, benign
  angioblastic —*see* Neoplasm, meninges, benign
  angiomatous —*see* Neoplasm, meninges, benign
  atypical —*see* Neoplasm, meninges, uncertain behavior
  endotheliomatous —*see* Neoplasm, meninges, benign
  fibroblastic —*see* Neoplasm, meninges, benign
  fibrous —*see* Neoplasm, meninges, benign
  hemangioblastic —*see* Neoplasm, meninges, benign
  hemangiopericytic —*see* Neoplasm, meninges, benign
  malignant —*see* Neoplasm, meninges, malignant
  meningiothelial —*see* Neoplasm, meninges, benign
  meningotheliomatous —*see* Neoplasm, meninges, benign
  mixed —*see* Neoplasm, meninges, benign
  multiple —*see* Neoplasm, meninges, uncertain behavior
  papillary —*see* Neoplasm, meninges, uncertain behavior
  psammomatous —*see* Neoplasm, meninges, benign
  syncytial —*see* Neoplasm, meninges, benign
  transitional —*see* Neoplasm, meninges, benign
Meningiomatosis (diffuse) —*see* Neoplasm, meninges, uncertain behavior
Meningism —*see* Meningismus
Meningismus (infectional) (pneumococcal) R29.1
  due to serum or vaccine R29.1
  influenzal —*see* Influenza, with, manifestations NEC

Meningitis (basal) (basic) (brain) (cerebral) (cervical) (congestive) (diffuse) (hemorrhagic) infantile) (membranous) (metastatic) (nonspecific) (pontine) (progressive) (simple) (spinal) (subacute) (sympathetic) (toxic) G03.9
  abacterial G03.0
  actinomycotic A42.81
  adenoviral A87.1
  arbovirus A87.8
  aseptic (acute) G03.0
  bacterial G00.9
    Escherichia coli (E. coli) G00.8
    Friedländer (bacillus) G00.8
    gram-negative G00.9
    H. influenzae G00.0
    Klebsiella G00.8
    pneumococcal G00.1
    specified organism NEC G00.8
    staphylococcal G00.3
    streptococcal (acute) G00.2
  benign recurrent (Mollaret) G03.2
  candidal B37.5
  caseous (tuberculous) A17.0
  cerebrospinal A39.0
  chronic NEC G03.1
  clear cerebrospinal fluid NEC G03.0
  coxsackievirus A87.0
  cryptococcal B45.1
  diplococcal (gram positive) A39.0
  echovirus A87.0
  enteroviral A87.0
  eosinophilic B83.2
  epidemic NEC A39.0
  Escherichia coli (E. coli) G00.8
  fibrinopurulent G00.9
    specified organism NEC G00.8
  Friedländer (bacillus) G00.8
  gonococcal A54.81
  gram-negative cocci G00.9
  gram-positive cocci G00.9
  Haemophilus (influenzae) G00.0
  H. influenzae G00.0
  in (due to)
    adenovirus A87.1
    African trypanosomiasis B56.9 *[G02]*
    anthrax A22.8
    bacterial disease NEC A48.8 *[G01]*
    Chagas' disease (chronic) B57.41
    chickenpox B01.0
    coccidioidomycosis B38.4
    Diplococcus pneumoniae G00.1
    enterovirus A87.0
    herpes (simplex) virus B00.3
      zoster B02.1
    infectious mononucleosis B27.92
    leptospirosis A27.81
    Listeria monocytogenes A32.11
    Lyme disease A69.21
    measles B05.1
    mumps (virus) B26.1
    neurosyphilis (late) A52.13
    parasitic disease NEC B89 *[G02]*
    poliovirus A80.9 *[G02]*
    preventive immunization, inoculation or vaccination G03.8
    rubella B06.02
    Salmonella infection A02.21
    specified cause NEC G03.8
    Streptococcal pneumoniae G00.1
    typhoid fever A01.01
    varicella B01.0
    viral disease NEC A87.8
    whooping cough A37.90
    zoster B02.1
  infectious G00.9
  influenzal (H. influenzae) G00.0
  Klebsiella G00.8
  leptospiral (aseptic) A27.81
  lymphocytic (acute) (benign) (serous) A87.2
  meningococcal A39.0

► New   ⇒ Revised   ~~deleted~~ Deleted   ● Use Additional Character(s)

Meningitis (Continued)
  Mima polymorpha G00.8
  Mollaret (benign recurrent) G03.2
  monilial B37.5
  mycotic NEC B49 *[G02]*
  Neisseria A39.0
  nonbacterial G03.0
  nonpyogenic NEC G03.0
  ossificans G96.198
  pneumococcal streptococcus pneumoniae
    G00.1
  poliovirus A80.9 *[G02]*
  postmeasles B05.1
  purulent G00.9
    specified organism NEC G00.8
  pyogenic G00.9
    specified organism NEC G00.8
  Salmonella (arizonae) (Cholerae-Suis)
    (enteritidis) (typhimurium) A02.21
  septic G00.9
    specified organism NEC G00.8
  serosa circumscripta NEC G03.0
  serous NEC G93.2
  specified organism NEC G00.8
  sporotrichosis B42.81
  staphylococcal G00.3
  sterile G03.0
  Streptococcal (acute) G00.2
    pneumoniae G00.1
  suppurative G00.9
    specified organism NEC G00.8
  syphilitic (late) (tertiary) A52.13
    acute A51.41
    congenital A50.41
    secondary A51.41
  Torula histolytica (cryptococcal) B45.1
  traumatic (complication of injury) T79.8
  tuberculous A17.0
  typhoid A01.01
  viral NEC A87.9
  Yersinia pestis A20.3
Meningocele (spinal) —*see also* Spina bifida
  with hydrocephalus —*see* Spina bifida, by
    site, with hydrocephalus
  acquired (traumatic) G96.198
  cerebral —*see* Encephalocele
Meningocerebritis —*see* Meningoencephalitis
Meningococcemia A39.4
  acute A39.2
  chronic A39.3
Meningococcus, meningococcal —*see also*
    condition A39.9
  adrenalitis, hemorrhagic A39.1
  carrier (suspected) of Z22.31
  meningitis (cerebrospinal) A39.0
Meningoencephalitis —*see also* Encephalitis
    G04.90
  acute NEC —*see also* Encephalitis, viral A86
  bacterial NEC G04.2
  California A83.5
  diphasic A84.1
  eosinophilic B83.2
  epidemic A39.81
  herpesviral, herpetic B00.4
    due to herpesvirus 6 B10.01
    due to herpesvirus 7 B10.09
    specified NEC B10.09
  in (due to)
    blastomycosis NEC B40.81
    diseases classified elsewhere G05.3
    free-living amebae B60.2
    Hemophilus influenzae (H. influenzae)
      G00.0
    herpes B00.4
      due to herpesvirus 6 B10.01
      due to herpesvirus 7 B10.09
      specified NEC B10.09
    H. influenzae G00.0
    Lyme disease A69.22
    mercury —*see* subcategory T56.1
    mumps B26.2

Meningoencephalitis (Continued)
  in (due to) (Continued)
    Naegleria (amebae) (organisms) (fowleri)
      B60.2
    Parastrongylus cantonensis B83.2
    toxoplasmosis (acquired) B58.2
      congenital P37.1
  infectious (acute) (viral) A86
  influenzal (H. influenzae) G00.0
  Listeria monocytogenes A32.12
  lymphocytic (serous) A87.2
  mumps B26.2
  parasitic NEC B89 *[G05.3]*
  pneumococcal G04.2
  primary amebic B60.2
  specific (syphilitic) A52.14
  specified organism NEC G04.81
  staphylococcal G04.2
  streptococcal G04.2
  syphilitic A52.14
⇨ toxic NEC G92.8
    due to mercury —*see* subcategory T56.1
  tuberculous A17.82
  virus NEC A86
Meningoencephalocele —*see also*
    Encephalocele
  syphilitic A52.19
    congenital A50.49
Meningoencephalomyelitis —*see also*
    Meningoencephalitis
  acute NEC (viral) A86
    disseminated G04.00
      postimmunization or postvaccination
        G04.02
      postinfectious G04.01
  due to
    actinomycosis A42.82
    Torula B45.1
    Toxoplasma or toxoplasmosis (acquired)
      B58.2
      congenital P37.1
  postimmunization or postvaccination
    G04.02
Meningoencephalomyelopathy G96.9
Meningoencephalopathy G96.9
Meningomyelitis —*see also*
    Meningoencephalitis
  bacterial NEC G04.2
  blastomycotic NEC B40.81
  cryptococcal B45.1
  in diseases classified elsewhere G05.4
  meningococcal A39.81
  syphilitic A52.14
  tuberculous A17.82
Meningomyelocele —*see also* Spina bifida
  syphilitic A52.19
Meningomyeloneuritis —*see*
    Meningoencephalitis
Meningoradiculitis —*see* Meningitis
Meningovascular —*see* condition
Menkes' disease or syndrome E83.09
  meaning maple-syrup-urine disease E71.0
Menometrorrhagia N92.1
Menopause, menopausal (asymptomatic)
    (state) Z78.0
  arthritis (any site) NEC —*see* Arthritis,
    specified form NEC
  bleeding N92.4
  depression (single episode) F32.89
    agitated (single episode) F32.2
      recurrent episode F33.9
    psychotic (single episode) F32.89
      zrecurrent episode F33.8
    recurrent episode F33.9
    melancholia (single episode) F32.89
      recurrent episode F33.8
  paranoid state F22
  premature E28.319
    asymptomatic E28.319
      postirradiation E89.40
      postsurgical E89.40

Menopause, menopausal (Continued)
  premature (Continued)
    symptomatic E28.310
      postirradiation E89.41
      postsurgical E89.41
  psychosis NEC F28
  symptomatic N95.1
  toxic polyarthritis NEC —*see* Arthritis,
    specified form NEC
Menorrhagia (primary) N92.0
  climacteric N92.4
    menopausal N92.4
  menopausal N92.4
  perimenopausal N92.4
  postclimacteric N95.0
  postmenopausal N95.0
  preclimacteric or premenopausal N92.4
  pubertal (menses retained) N92.2
Menostaxis N92.0
Menses, retention N94.89
Menstrual —*see* Menstruation
Menstruation
  absent —*see* Amenorrhea
  anovulatory N97.0
  cycle, irregular N92.6
  delayed N91.0
  disorder N93.9
    psychogenic F45.8
  during pregnancy O20.8
  excessive (with regular cycle) N92.0
    with irregular cycle N92.1
    at puberty N92.2
  frequent N92.0
  infrequent —*see* Oligomenorrhea
  irregular N92.6
    specified NEC N92.5
  latent N92.5
  membranous N92.5
  painful —*see also* Dysmenorrhea N94.6
    primary N94.4
    psychogenic F45.8
    secondary N94.5
  passage of clots N92.0
  precocious E30.1
  protracted N92.5
  rare —*see* Oligomenorrhea
  retained N94.89
  retrograde N92.5
  scanty —*see* Oligomenorrhea
  suppression N94.89
  vicarious (nasal) N94.89
Mental —*see also* condition
  deficiency —*see* Disability, intellectual
  deterioration —*see* Psychosis
  disorder —*see* Disorder, mental
  exhaustion F48.8
  insufficiency (congenital) —*see* Disability,
    intellectual
  observation without need for further medical
    care Z03.89
  retardation —*see* Disability, intellectual
  subnormality —*see* Disability, intellectual
  upset —*see* Disorder, mental
Meralgia paresthetica G57.1-●
Mercurial —*see* condition
Mercurialism —*see* subcategory T56.1
MERRF syndrome (myoclonic epilepsy
    associated with ragged-red fiber) E88.42
Merkel cell tumor —*see* Carcinoma, Merkel cell
Merocele —*see* Hernia, femoral
Meromelia
  lower limb —*see* Defect, reduction, lower
    limb
    intercalary
      femur —*see* Defect, reduction, lower
        limb, specified type NEC
        tibiofibular (complete) (incomplete) —
          see Defect, reduction, lower limb
  upper limb —*see* Defect, reduction, upper
    limb
    intercalary, humeral, radioulnar —*see*
      Agenesis, arm, with hand present

M

Merzbacher-Pelizaeus disease E75.29
Mesaortitis —see Aortitis
Mesarteritis —see Arteritis
Mesencephalitis —see Encephalitis
Mesenchymoma —see also Neoplasm,
    connective tissue, uncertain behavior
  benign —see Neoplasm, connective tissue,
    benign
  malignant —see Neoplasm, connective tissue,
    malignant
Mesenteritis
  retractile K65.4
  sclerosing K65.4
Mesentery, mesenteric —see condition
Mesiodens, mesiodentes K00.1
Mesio-occlusion M26.213
Mesocolon —see condition
Mesonephroma (malignant) —see Neoplasm,
    malignant, by site
  benign —see Neoplasm, benign, by site
Mesophlebitis —see Phlebitis
Mesostromal dysgenesia Q13.89
Mesothelioma (malignant) C45.9
  benign
    mesentery D19.1
    mesocolon D19.1
    omentum D19.1
    peritoneum D19.1
    pleura D19.0
    specified site NEC D19.7
    unspecified site D19.9
  biphasic C45.9
    benign
      mesentery D19.1
      mesocolon D19.1
      omentum D19.1
      peritoneum D19.1
      pleura D19.0
      specified site NEC D19.7
      unspecified site D19.9
  cystic D48.4
  epithelioid C45.9
    benign
      mesentery D19.1
      mesocolon D19.1
      omentum D19.1
      peritoneum D19.1
      pleura D19.0
      specified site NEC D19.7
      unspecified site D19.9
  fibrous C45.9
    benign
      mesentery D19.1
      mesocolon D19.1
      omentum D19.1
      peritoneum D19.1
      pleura D19.0
      specified site NEC D19.7
      unspecified site D19.9
  site classification
    liver C45.7
    lung C45.7
    mediastinum C45.7
    mesentery C45.1
    mesocolon C45.1
    omentum C45.1
    pericardium C45.2
    peritoneum C45.1
    pleura C45.0
      parietal C45.0
    retroperitoneum C45.7
    specified site NEC C45.7
    unspecified C45.9
Metabolic syndrome E88.81
Metagonimiasis B66.8
Metagonimus infestation (intestine)
    B66.8
Metal
  pigmentation L81.8
  polisher's disease J62.8
Metamorphopsia H53.15

Metaplasia
  apocrine (breast) —see Dysplasia, mammary,
    specified type NEC
  cervix (squamous) —see Dysplasia, cervix
  endometrium (squamous) (uterus) N85.8
  esophagus K22.7-●
▶ gastric intestinal K31.A0
  ▶ with dysplasia K31.A29
    ▶ high grade K31.A22
    ▶ low grade K31.A21
  ▶ indefinite for dysplasia K31.A0
  ▶ without dysplasia K31.A19
    ▶ involving
      ▶ antrum K31.A11
      ▶ body (corpus) K31.A12
      ▶ cardia K31.A14
      ▶ fundus K31.A13
      ▶ multiple sites K31.A15
  kidney (pelvis) (squamous) N28.89
  myelogenous D73.1
  myeloid (agnogenic) (megakaryocytic) D73.1
  spleen D73.1
  squamous cell, bladder N32.89
Metastasis, metastatic
  abscess —see Abscess
  calcification E83.59
  cancer
    from specified site —see Neoplasm,
      malignant, by site
    to specified site —see Neoplasm, secondary,
      by site
  deposits (in) —see Neoplasm, secondary, by site
  disease (see also Neoplasm, secondary, by site)
    C79.9
  spread (to) —see Neoplasm, secondary, by site
Metastrongyliasis B83.8
Metatarsalgia M77.4-●
  anterior G57.6-●
  Morton's G57.6-●
Metatarsus, metatarsal —see also condition
  adductus, congenital Q66.22-●
  valgus (abductus), congenital Q66.6
  varus (congenital) Q66.22-●
    primus Q66.21-●
Methadone use —see Use, opioid
Methemoglobinemia D74.9
  acquired (with sulfhemoglobinemia) D74.8
  congenital D74.0
  enzymatic (congenital) D74.0
  Hb M disease D74.0
  hereditary D74.0
  toxic D74.8
Methemoglobinuria —see Hemoglobinuria
Methioninemia E72.19
Methylmalonic acidemia E71.120
Metritis (catarrhal) (hemorrhagic) (septic)
    (suppurative) —see also Endometritis
  cervical —see Cervicitis
Metropathia hemorrhagica N93.8
Metroperitonitis —see Peritonitis, pelvic, female
Metrorrhagia N92.1
  climacteric N92.4
  menopausal N92.4
  perimenopausal N92.4
  postpartum NEC (atonic) (following delivery
    of placenta) O72.1
    delayed or secondary O72.2
  preclimacteric or premenopausal N92.4
  psychogenic F45.8
Metrorrhexis —see Rupture, uterus
Metrosalpingitis N70.91
Metrostaxis N93.8
Metrovaginitis —see Endometritis
Meyer-Schwickerath and Weyers syndrome
    Q87.0
Meynert's amentia (nonalcoholic) F04
  alcoholic F10.96
    with dependence F10.26
Mibelli's disease (porokeratosis) Q82.8
Mice, joint —see Loose, body, joint
  knee M23.4
Micrencephalon, micrencephaly Q02

Microalbuminuria R80.9
Microaneurysm, retinal —see also Disorder,
    retina, microaneurysms
  diabetic —see E08-E13 with .31
Microangiopathy (peripheral) I73.9
▶ thrombotic M31.10
    ▶ hematopoietic stem cell transplantation-
      associated [HSCT-TMA] M31.10
Microcalcifications, breast R92.0
Microcephalus, microcephalic, microcephaly
    Q02
  due to toxoplasmosis (congenital) P37.1
Microcheilia Q18.7
Microcolon (congenital) Q43.8
Microcornea (congenital) Q13.4
Microcytic —see condition D57.40
Microdeletions NEC Q93.88
Microdontia K00.2
Microdrepanocytosis D57.40
  with
    acute chest syndrome D57.411
    cerebral vascular involvement D57.413
    crisis (painful) D57.419
      with specified complication NEC D57.418
    splenic sequestration D57.412
    vasoocclusive pain D57.419
Microembolism
  atherothrombotic —see Atheroembolism
  retinal —see Occlusion, artery, retina
Microencephalon Q02
Microfilaria streptocerca infestation —see
    Onchocerciasis
Microgastria (congenital) Q40.2
Microgenia M26.06
Microgenitalia, congenital
  female Q52.8
  male Q55.8
Microglioma —see Lymphoma, non-Hodgkin,
    specified NEC
Microglossia (congenital) Q38.3
Micrognathia, micrognathism (congenital)
    (mandibular) (maxillary) M26.09
Microgyria (congenital) Q04.3
Microinfarct of heart —see Insufficiency, coronary
Microlentia (congenital) Q12.8
Microlithiasis, alveolar, pulmonary J84.02
Micromastia N64.82
Micromyelia (congenital) Q06.8
Micropenis Q55.62
Microphakia (congenital) Q12.8
Microphthalmos, microphthalmia (congenital)
    Q11.2
  due to toxoplasmosis P37.1
Micropsia H53.15
Microscopic polyangiitis (polyarteritis) M31.7
Microsporidiosis B60.8
  intestinal A07.8
Microsporon furfur infestation B36.0
Microsporosis —see also Dermatophytosis
  nigra B36.1
Microstomia (congenital) Q18.5
Microtia (congenital) (external ear) Q17.2
Microtropia H50.40
Microvillus inclusion disease (MVD) (MVID)
    Q43.8
Micturition
  disorder NEC —see also Difficulty, micturition
    R39.198
    psychogenic F45.8
  frequency R35.0
    psychogenic F45.8
  hesitancy R39.11
  incomplete emptying R39.14
  nocturnal R35.1
  painful R30.9
    dysuria R30.0
    psychogenic F45.8
    tenesmus R30.1
  poor stream R39.12
  position dependent R39.192
  split stream R39.13
  straining R39.16
  urgency R39.15

▶ New   ⇒ Revised   ~~deleted~~ Deleted   ● Use Additional Character(s)

Mid plane —see condition
Middle
 ear —see condition
 lobe (right) syndrome J98.19
Miescher's elastoma L87.2
Mietens' syndrome Q87.2
Migraine (idiopathic) G43.909
 with refractory migraine G43.919
  with status migrainosus G43.911
  without status migrainosus G43.919
 with aura (acute-onset) (prolonged) (typical)
   (without headache) G43.109
  with refractory migraine G43.119
   with status migrainosus G43.111
   without status migrainosus G43.119
  intractable G43.119
   with status migrainosus G43.111
   without status migrainosus G43.119
  not intractable G43.109
   with status migrainosus G43.101
   without status migrainosus G43.109
  persistent G43.509
   with cerebral infarction G43.609
    with refractory migraine G43.619
     with status migrainosus G43.611
     without status migrainosus G43.619
    intractable G43.619
     with status migrainosus G43.611
     without status migrainosus G43.619
    not intractable G43.609
     with status migrainosus G43.601
     without status migrainosus G43.609
    without refractory migraine G43.609
     with status migrainosus G43.601
     without status migrainosus G43.609
   without cerebral infarction G43.509
    with refractory migraine G43.519
     with status migrainosus G43.511
     without status migrainosus G43.519
    intractable G43.519
     with status migrainosus G43.511
     without status migrainosus G43.519
    not intractable G43.509
     with status migrainosus G43.501
     without status migrainosus G43.509
    without refractory migraine G43.509
     with status migrainosus G43.501
     without status migrainosus G43.509
  without mention of refractory migraine
    G43.109
   with status migrainosus G43.101
   without status migrainosus G43.109
 abdominal G43.D0
  with refractory migraine G43.D1
  intractable G43.D1
  not intractable G43.D0
  without refractory migraine G43.D0
 basilar —see Migraine, with aura
 classical —see Migraine, with aura
 common —see Migraine, without aura
 complicated G43.109
 equivalents —see Migraine, with aura
 familiar —see Migraine, hemiplegic
 hemiplegic G43.409
  with refractory migraine G43.419
   with status migrainosus G43.411
   without status migrainosus G43.419
  intractable G43.419
   with status migrainosus G43.411
   without status migrainosus G43.419
  not intractable G43.409
   with status migrainosus G43.401
   without status migrainosus G43.409
  without refractory migraine G43.409
   with status migrainosus G43.401
   without status migrainosus G43.409
 intractable G43.919
  with status migrainosus G43.911
  without status migrainosus G43.919
 menstrual G43.829
  with refractory migraine G43.839
   with status migrainosus G43.831
   without status migrainosus G43.839

Migraine (Continued)
 menstrual (Continued)
  intractable G43.839
   with status migrainosus G43.831
   without status migrainosus G43.839
  not intractable G43.829
   with status migrainosus G43.821
   without status migrainosus G43.829
  without refractory migraine G43.829
   with status migrainosus G43.821
   without status migrainosus G43.829
 menstrually related —see Migraine, menstrual
 not intractable G43.909
  with status migrainosus G43.901
  without status migrainosus G43.919
 ophthalmoplegic G43.B0
  with refractory migraine G43.B1
  intractable G43.B1
  not intractable G43.B0
   without refractory migraine G43.B0
 persistent aura (with, without) cerebral
   infarction —see Migraine, with aura,
   persistent
 preceded or accompanied by transient focal
   neurological phenomena —see Migraine,
   with aura
 pre-menstrual —see Migraine, menstrual
 pure menstrual —see Migraine, menstrual
 retinal —see Migraine, with aura
 specified NEC G43.809
  intractable G43.819
   with status migrainosus G43.811
   without status migrainosus G43.819
  not intractable G43.809
   with status migrainosus G43.801
   without status migrainosus G43.809
 sporadic —see Migraine, hemiplegic
 transformed —see Migraine, without aura,
   chronic
 triggered seizures —see Migraine, with aura
 without aura G43.009
  with refractory migraine G43.019
   with status migrainosus G43.011
   without status migrainosus G43.019
  chronic G43.709
   with refractory migraine G43.719
    with status migrainosus G43.711
    without status migrainosus G43.719
   intractable
    with status migrainosus G43.711
    without status migrainosus G43.719
   not intractable
    with status migrainosus G43.701
    without status migrainosus G43.709
   without refractory migraine G43.709
    with status migrainosus G43.701
    without status migrainosus G43.709
  intractable
   with status migrainosus G43.011
   without status migrainosus G43.019
  not intractable
   with status migrainosus G43.001
   without status migrainosus G43.009
  without mention of refractory migraine
    G43.009
   with status migrainosus G43.001
   without status migrainosus G43.009
  without refractory migraine G43.909
   with status migrainosus G43.901
   without status migrainosus G43.919
➥**Migrant, social** Z59.00
Migration, anxiety concerning Z60.3
Migratory, migrating —see also condition
➥person Z59.00
 testis Q55.29
Mikity-Wilson disease or syndrome P27.0
Mikulicz' disease or syndrome K11.8
Miliaria L74.3
 alba L74.1
 apocrine L75.2
 crystallina L74.1
 profunda L74.2
 rubra L74.0

Miliaria (Continued)
 tropicalis L74.2
Miliary —see condition
Milium L72.0
 colloid L57.8
Milk
 crust L21.0
 excessive secretion O92.6
 poisoning —see Poisoning, food, noxious
 retention O92.79
 sickness —see Poisoning, food, noxious
 spots I31.0
Milk-alkali disease or syndrome E83.52
Milk-leg (deep vessels) (nonpuerperal) —see
   Embolism, vein, lower extremity
 complicating pregnancy O22.3-●
 puerperal, postpartum, childbirth O87.1
Milkman's disease or syndrome M83.8
Milky urine —see Chyluria
Millard-Gubler (-Foville) **paralysis or**
   syndrome G46.3
Millar's asthma J38.5
Miller-Fisher syndrome G61.0
Mills' disease —see Hemiplegia
Millstone maker's pneumoconiosis J62.8
Milroy's disease (chronic hereditary edema)
   Q82.0
Minamata disease T56.1-●
Miners' asthma or lung J60
Minkowski-Chauffard syndrome —see
   Spherocytosis
Minor —see condition
Minor's disease (hematomyelia) G95.19
Minot's disease (hemorrhagic disease),
   newborn P53
Minot-von Willebrand-Jurgens disease or
   syndrome (angiohemophilia) D68.0
Minus (and plus) **hand** (intrinsic) —see Deformity,
   limb, specified type NEC, forearm
Miosis (pupil) H57.03
Mirizzi's syndrome (hepatic duct stenosis)
   K83.1
Mirror writing F81.0
MIS-A M35.81
MIS-C M35.81
Misadventure (of) (prophylactic) (therapeutic) —
   see also Complications T88.9
 administration of insulin (by accident) — see
   subcategory T38.3
 infusion —see Complications, infusion
 local applications (of fomentations, plasters,
   etc.) T88.9
  burn or scald —see Burn
  specified NEC T88.8
 medical care (early) (late) T88.9
  adverse effect of drugs or chemicals —see
   Table of Drugs and Chemicals
 medical care (early) (late)
  burn or scald —see Burn
  specified NEC T88.8
 specified NEC T88.8
 surgical procedure (early) (late) —see
   Complications, surgical procedure
 transfusion —see Complications, transfusion
 vaccination or other immunological
   procedure —see Complications,
   vaccination
Miscarriage O03.9
Misdirection, aqueous H40.83-●
Misperception, sleep state F51.02
Misplaced, misplacement
 ear Q17.4
 kidney (acquired) N28.89
  congenital Q63.2
 organ or site, congenital NEC —see
   Malposition, congenital
Missed
 abortion O02.1
 delivery O36.4
Missing —see also Absence
 string of intrauterine contraceptive device
   T83.32

Misuse of drugs F19.99
Mitchell's disease (erythromelalgia) I73.81
Mite(s) (infestation) B88.9
  diarrhea B88.0
  grain (itch) B88.0
  hair follicle (itch) B88.0
  in sputum B88.0
Mitral —*see* condition
Mittelschmerz N94.0
Mixed —*see* condition
MMN (multifocal motor neuropathy) G61.82
MNGIE (Mitochondrial Neurogastrointestinal
    Encephalopathy) syndrome E88.49
Mobile, mobility
  cecum Q43.3
  excessive —*see* Hypermobility
  gallbladder, congenital Q44.1
  kidney N28.89
  organ or site, congenital NEC —*see*
      Malposition, congenital
Mobitz heart block (atrioventricular) I44.1
Moebius, Möbius
  disease (ophthalmoplegic migraine) —*see*
      Migraine, ophthalmoplegic
  syndrome Q87.0
      congenital oculofacial paralysis (with other
          anomalies) Q87.0
      ophthalmoplegic migraine —*see* Migraine,
          ophthalmoplegic
Moeller's glossitis K14.0
Mohr's syndrome (Types I and II) Q87.0
Mola destruens D39.2
Molar pregnancy O02.0
Molarization of premolars K00.2
Molding, head (during birth) - omit code
Mole (pigmented) —*see also* Nevus
  blood O02.0
  Breus' O02.0
  cancerous —*see* Melanoma
  carneous O02.0
  destructive D39.2
  fleshy O02.0
  hydatid, hydatidiform (benign) (complicating
      pregnancy) (delivered) (undelivered)
      O01.9
    classical O01.0
    complete O01.0
    incomplete O01.1
    invasive D39.2
    malignant D39.2
    partial O01.1
  intrauterine O02.0
  invasive (hydatidiform) D39.2
  malignant
    meaning
        malignant hydatidiform mole D39.2
        melanoma —*see* Melanoma
  nonhydatidiform O02.0
  nonpigmented —*see* Nevus
  pregnancy NEC O02.0
  skin —*see* Nevus
  tubal O00.10-
    with intrauterine pregnancy O00.11-
  vesicular —*see* Mole, hydatidiform
Molimen, molimina (menstrual) N94.3
Molluscum contagiosum (epitheliale) B08.1
**Mönckeberg's arteriosclerosis, disease, or
    sclerosis** —*see* Arteriosclerosis, extremities
Mondini's malformation (cochlea) Q16.5
Mondor's disease I80.8
Monge's disease T70.29
Monilethrix (congenital) Q84.1
Moniliasis —*see also* Candidiasis B37.9
  neonatal P37.5
Monitoring (encounter for)
  therapeutic drug level Z51.81
Monkey malaria B53.1
Monkeypox B04
Monoarthritis M13.10
  ankle M13.17-●
  elbow M13.12-●

Monoarthritis (Continued)
  foot joint M13.17-●
  hand joint M13.14-●
  hip M13.15-●
  knee M13.16-●
  shoulder M13.11-●
  wrist M13.13-●
Monoblastic —*see* condition
Monochromat (ism), monochromatopsia
  (acquired) (congenital) H53.51
Monocytic —*see* condition
Monocytopenia D72.818
Monocytosis (symptomatic) D72.821
Monomania —*see* Psychosis
Mononeuritis G58.9
  cranial nerve —*see* Disorder, nerve,
      cranial
  femoral nerve G57.2-●
  lateral
    cutaneous nerve of thigh G57.1-●
    popliteal nerve G57.3-●
  lower limb G57.9-●
    specified nerve NEC G57.8-●
  medial popliteal nerve G57.4-●
  median nerve G56.1-●
  multiplex G58.7
  plantar nerve G57.6-●
  posterior tibial nerve G57.5-●
  radial nerve G56.3-●
  sciatic nerve G57.0-●
  specified NEC G58.8
  tibial nerve G57.4-●
  ulnar nerve G56.2-●
  upper limb G56.9-●
    specified nerve NEC G56.8-●
  vestibular —*see* subcategory H93.3
Mononeuropathy G58.9
  carpal tunnel syndrome —*see* Syndrome,
      carpal tunnel
  diabetic NEC —*see* E08-E13 with .41
  femoral nerve —*see* Lesion, nerve, femoral
  ilioinguinal nerve G57.8-●
  in diseases classified elsewhere —*see* category
      G59
  intercostal G58.0
  lower limb G57.9-●
    causalgia —*see* Causalgia, lower limb
    femoral nerve —*see* Lesion, nerve,
        femoral
    meralgia paresthetica G57.1-●
    plantar nerve —*see* Lesion, nerve, plantar
    popliteal nerve —*see* Lesion, nerve,
        popliteal
    sciatic nerve —*see* Lesion, nerve, sciatic
    specified NEC G57.8-●
    tarsal tunnel syndrome —*see* Syndrome,
        tarsal tunnel
  median nerve —*see* Lesion, nerve, median
  multiplex G58.7
  obturator nerve G57.8-●
  popliteal nerve —*see* Lesion, nerve, popliteal
  radial nerve —*see* Lesion, nerve, radial
  saphenous nerve G57.8-●
  specified NEC G58.8
  tarsal tunnel syndrome —*see* Syndrome,
      tarsal tunnel
  tuberculous A17.83
  ulnar nerve —*see* Lesion, nerve, ulnar
  upper limb G56.9-●
    carpal tunnel syndrome —*see* Syndrome,
        carpal tunnel
    causalgia —*see* Causalgia
    median nerve —*see* Lesion, nerve, median
    radial nerve —*see* Lesion, nerve, radial
    specified site NEC G56.8-●
    ulnar nerve —*see* Lesion, nerve, ulnar
Mononucleosis, infectious B27.90
  with
    complication NEC B27.99
    meningitis B27.92
    polyneuropathy B27.91

Mononucleosis, infectious (Continued)
  cytomegaloviral B27.10
    with
        complication NEC B27.19
        meningitis B27.12
        polyneuropathy B27.11
  Epstein-Barr (virus) B27.00
    with
        complication NEC B27.09
        meningitis B27.02
        polyneuropathy B27.01
  gammaherpesviral B27.00
    with
        complication NEC B27.09
        meningitis B27.02
        polyneuropathy B27.01
  specified NEC B27.80
    with
        complication NEC B27.89
        meningitis B27.82
        polyneuropathy B27.81
Monoplegia G83.3-●
  congenital (cerebral) G80.8
    spastic G80.1
  embolic (current episode) I63.4-●
  following
    cerebrovascular disease
      cerebral infarction
          lower limb I69.34-●
          upper limb I69.33-●
      intracerebral hemorrhage
          lower limb I69.14-●
          upper limb I69.13-●
      lower limb I69.94-●
      nontraumatic intracranial hemorrhage
          NEC
          lower limb I69.24-●
          upper limb I69.23-●
      specified disease NEC
          lower limb I69.84-●
          upper limb I69.83-●
      stroke NOS
          lower limb I69.34-●
          upper limb I69.33-●
      subarachnoid hemorrhage
          lower limb I69.04-●
          upper limb I69.03-●
      upper limb I69.93-●
  hysterical (transient) F44.4
  lower limb G83.1-●
  psychogenic (conversion reaction) F44.4
  thrombotic (current episode) I63.3-●
  transient R29.818
  upper limb G83.2-●
Monorchism, monorchidism Q55.0
Monosomy —*see also* Deletion, chromosome
    Q93.9
  specified NEC Q93.89
  whole chromosome
    meiotic nondisjunction Q93.0
    mitotic nondisjunction Q93.1
    mosaicism Q93.1
  X Q96.9
Monster, monstrosity (single) Q89.7
  acephalic Q00.0
  twin Q89.4
Monteggia's fracture (-dislocation) S52.27-●
Mooren's ulcer (cornea) —*see* Ulcer, cornea,
    Mooren's
Moore's syndrome —*see* Epilepsy, specified
    NEC
Mooser-Neill reaction A75.2
Mooser's bodies A75.2
Morbidity not stated or unknown R69
Morbilli —*see* Measles
Morbus —*see also* Disease
  angelicus, anglorum E55.0
  Beigel B36.2
  caducus —*see* Epilepsy
  celiacus K90.0
  comitialis —*see* Epilepsy

Morbus *(Continued)*
  cordis —*see also* Disease, heart I51.9
    valvulorum —*see* Endocarditis
  coxae senilis M16.9
    tuberculous A18.02
  hemorrhagicus neonatorum P53
  maculosus neonatorum P54.5
Morel (-Stewart)(-Morgagni) **syndrome**
  M85.2
Morel-Kraepelin disease —*see* Schizophrenia
Morel-Moore syndrome M85.2
Morgagni's
  cyst, organ, hydatid, or appendage
    female Q50.5
    male (epididymal) Q55.4
      testicular Q55.29
  syndrome M85.2
Morgagni-Stewart-Morel syndrome M85.2
Morgagni-Stokes-Adams syndrome I45.9
Morgagni-Turner (-Albright) **syndrome**
  Q96.9
Moria F07.0
Moron (I.Q. 50-69) F70
Morphea L94.0
Morphinism (without remission) F11.20
  with remission F11.21
Morphinomania (without remission) F11.20
  with remission F11.21
Morquio (-Ullrich)(-Brailsford) **disease or**
  syndrome —*see* Mucopolysaccharidosis
Mortification (dry) (moist) —*see* Gangrene
Morton's metatarsalgia (neuralgia)(neuroma)
  (syndrome) G57.6
Morvan's disease or syndrome G60.8
Mosaicism, mosaic (autosomal) (chromosomal)
  45,X/46,XX Q96.3
  45,X/other cell lines NEC with abnormal sex
    chromosome Q96.4
  sex chromosome
    female Q97.8
    lines with various numbers of
      X chromosomes Q97.2
    male Q98.7
  XY Q96.3
Moschowitz' disease M31.19
Mother yaw A66.0
Motion sickness (from travel, any vehicle)
  (from roundabouts or swings) T75.3
Mottled, mottling, teeth (enamel) (endemic)
  (nonendemic) K00.3
Mounier-Kuhn syndrome Q32.4
  with bronchiectasis J47.9
    exacerbation (acute) J47.1
    lower respiratory infection J47.0
  acquired J98.09
    with bronchiectasis J47.9
      with
        exacerbation (acute) J47.1
        lower respiratory infection J47.0
Mountain
  sickness T70.29
    with polycythemia , acquired (acute)
      D75.1
  tick fever A93.2
Mouse, joint —*see* Loose, body, joint
  knee M23.4-●
Mouth —*see* condition
Movable
  coccyx —*see* subcategory M53.2
  kidney N28.89
    congenital Q63.8
  spleen D73.89
Movements, dystonic R25.8
Moyamoya disease I67.5
MRSA (Methicillin resistant Staphylococcus
  aureus)
  infection A49.02
    as the cause of diseases classified
      elsewhere B95.62
  sepsis A41.02
MSD (multiple sulfatase deficiency) E75.26

MSSA (Methicillin susceptible Staphylococcus
  aureus)
  infection A49.01
    as the cause of diseases classified
      elsewhere B95.61
  sepsis A41.01
Mucha-Habermann disease L41.0
Mucinosis (cutaneous) (focal) (papular)
  (reticular erythematous) (skin) L98.5
  oral K13.79
Mucocele
  appendix K38.8
  buccal cavity K13.79
  gallbladder K82.1
  lacrimal sac, chronic H04.43-●
  nasal sinus J34.1
  nose J34.1
  salivary gland (any) K11.6
  sinus (accessory) (nasal) J34.1
  turbinate (bone) (middle) (nasal) J34.1
  uterus N85.8
Mucolipidosis
  I E77.1
  II, III E77.0
  IV E75.11
Mucopolysaccharidosis E76.3
  beta-gluduronidase deficiency E76.29
  cardiopathy E76.3 *[I52]*
  Hunter's syndrome E76.1
  Hurler's syndrome E76.01
  Hurler-Scheie syndrome E76.02
  Maroteaux-Lamy syndrome E76.29
  Morquio syndrome E76.219
    A E76.210
    B E76.211
    classic E76.210
  Sanfilippo syndrome E76.22
  Scheie's syndrome E76.03
  specified NEC E76.29
  type
    I
      Hurler's syndrome E76.01
      Hurler-Scheie syndrome E76.02
      Scheie's syndrome E76.03
    II E76.1
    III E76.22
    IV E76.219
    IVA E76.210
    IVB E76.211
    VI E76.29
    VII E76.29
Mucormycosis B46.5
  cutaneous B46.3
  disseminated B46.4
  gastrointestinal B46.2
  generalized B46.4
  pulmonary B46.0
  rhinocerebral B46.1
  skin B46.3
  subcutaneous B46.3
Mucositis (ulcerative) K12.30
  due to drugs NEC K12.32
  gastrointestinal K92.81
  mouth (oral) (oropharyngeal) K12.30
    due to antineoplastic therapy
      K12.31
    due to drugs NEC K12.32
    due to radiation K12.33
    specified NEC K12.39
    viral K12.39
  nasal J34.81
  oral cavity —*see* Mucositis, mouth
  oral soft tissues —*see* Mucositis, mouth
  vagina and vulva N76.81
Mucositis necroticans agranulocytica —*see*
  Agranulocytosis
Mucous —*see also* condition
  patches (syphilitic) A51.39
    congenital A50.07
Mucoviscidosis E84.9
  with meconium obstruction E84.11

Mucus
  asphyxia or suffocation —*see* Asphyxia, mucus
    in stool R19.5
  plug —*see* Asphyxia, mucus
Muguet B37.0
Mulberry molars (congenital syphilis) A50.52
Müllerian mixed tumor
  specified site —*see* Neoplasm, malignant, by
    site
  unspecified site C54.9
Multicystic kidney (development) Q61.4
Multiparity (grand) Z64.1
  affecting management of pregnancy, labor
    and delivery (supervision only)
    O09.4-●
  requiring contraceptive management —*see*
    Contraception
Multipartita placenta O43.19-●
Multiple, multiplex —*see also* condition
  digits (congenital) Q69.9
  endocrine neoplasia —*see* Neoplasia,
    endocrine, multiple [MEN]
  personality F44.81
Multisystem inflammatory syndrome (in
  adults) (in children) M35.81
Mumps B26.9
  arthritis B26.85
  complication NEC B26.89
  encephalitis B26.2
  hepatitis B26.81
  meningitis (aseptic) B26.1
  meningoencephalitis B26.2
  myocarditis B26.82
  oophoritis B26.89
  orchitis B26.0
  pancreatitis B26.3
  polyneuropathy B26.84
Mumu —*see also* Infestation, filarial B74.9 *[N51]*
Münchhausen's syndrome —*see* Disorder,
  factitious
Münchmeyer's syndrome —*see* Myositis,
  ossificans, progressiva
Mural —*see* condition
Murmur (cardiac) (heart) (organic) R01.1
  abdominal R19.15
  aortic (valve) —*see* Endocarditis, aortic
  benign R01.0
  diastolic —*see* Endocarditis
  Flint I35.1
  functional R01.0
  Graham Steell I37.1
  innocent R01.0
  mitral (valve) —*see* Insufficiency, mitral
  nonorganic R01.0
  presystolic, mitral —*see* Insufficiency, mitral
  pulmonic (valve) I37.8
  systolic R01.1
  tricuspid (valve) I07.9
  valvular —*see* Endocarditis
Murri's disease (intermittent hemoglobinuria)
  D59.6
Muscle, muscular —*see also* condition
  carnitine (palmityltransferase) deficiency
    E71.314
Musculoneuralgia —*see* Neuralgia
Mushroom-workers' (pickers') **disease or lung**
  J67.5
Mushrooming hip —*see* Derangement, joint,
  specified NEC, hip
Mutation(s)
  factor V Leiden D68.51
  surfactant, of lung J84.83
  prothrombin gene D68.52
Mutism —*see also* Aphasia
  deaf (acquired) (congenital) NEC H91.3
  elective (adjustment reaction) (childhood)
    F94.0
  hysterical F44.4
  selective (childhood) F94.0
MVD (microvillus inclusion disease) Q43.8
MVID (microvillus inclusion disease) Q43.8

M

Myalgia M79.10
  auxiliary muscles, head and neck M79.12
  epidemic (cervical) B33.0
  mastication muscle M79.11
  site specified NEC M79.18
  traumatic NEC T14.8
Myasthenia G70.9
  congenital G70.2
  cordis —see Failure, heart
  developmental G70.2
  gravis G70.00
    with exacerbation (acute) G70.01
    in crisis G70.01
    neonatal, transient P94.0
    pseudoparalytica G70.00
      with exacerbation (acute) G70.01
      in crisis G70.01
  stomach, psychogenic F45.8
  syndrome
    in
      diabetes mellitus —see E08-E13 with .44
      neoplastic disease —see also Neoplasm
          D49.9 [G73.3]
      pernicious anemia D51.0 [G73.3]
      thyrotoxicosis E05.90 [G73.3]
        with thyroid storm E05.91 [G73.3]
Myasthenic M62.81
Mycelium infection B49
Mycetismus —see Poisoning, food, noxious,
    mushroom
Mycetoma B47.9
  actinomycotic B47.1
  bone (mycotic) B47.9 [M90.80]
  eumycotic B47.0
  foot B47.9
    actinomycotic B47.1
    mycotic B47.0
  madurae NEC B47.9
    mycotic B47.0
  maduromycotic B47.0
  mycotic B47.0
  nocardial B47.1
Mycobacteriosis —see Mycobacterium
Mycobacterium, mycobacterial (infection)
    A31.9
  anonymous A31.9
  atypical A31.9
    cutaneous A31.1
    pulmonary A31.0
      tuberculous —see Tuberculosis,
          pulmonary
    specified site NEC A31.8
  avium (intracellulare complex) A31.0
  balnei A31.1
  Battey A31.0
  chelonei A31.8
  cutaneous A31.1
  extrapulmonary systemic A31.8
  fortuitum A31.8
  intracellulare (Battey bacillus) A31.0
  kakaferifu A31.8
  kansasii (yellow bacillus) A31.0
  kasongo A31.8
  leprae —see also Leprosy A30.9
  luciflavum A31.1
  marinum (M. balnei) A31.1
  nonspecific —see Mycobacterium, atypical
  pulmonary (atypical) A31.0
    tuberculous —see Tuberculosis, pulmonary
  scrofulaceum A31.8
  simiae A31.8
  systemic, extrapulmonary A31.8
  szulgai A31.8
  terrae A31.8
  triviale A31.8
  tuberculosis (human, bovine) —see
      Tuberculosis
  ulcerans A31.1
  xenopi A31.8
Mycoplasma (M.) **pneumoniae, as cause of**
    disease classified elsewhere B96.0

Mycosis, mycotic B49
  cutaneous NEC B36.9
  ear B36.9
    in
      aspergillosis B44.89
      candidiasis B37.84
      moniliasis B37.84
  fungoides (extranodal) (solid organ) C84.0-●
  mouth B37.0
  nails B35.1
  opportunistic B48.8
  skin NEC B36.9
  specified NEC B48.8
  stomatitis B37.0
  vagina, vaginitis (candidal) B37.3
Mydriasis (pupil) H57.04
Myelatelia Q06.1
Myelinolysis, pontine, central G37.2
Myelitis (acute) (ascending) (childhood)
    (chronic) (descending) (diffuse)
    (disseminated) (idiopathic) (pressure)
    (progressive) (spinal cord) (subacute) —see
    also Encephalitis G04.91
➠flaccid G04.82
  herpes simplex B00.82
  herpes zoster B02.24
  in diseases classified elsewhere G05.4
  necrotizing, subacute G37.4
  optic neuritis in G36.0
  postchickenpox B01.12
  postherpetic B02.24
  postimmunization G04.02
  postinfectious NEC G04.89
  postvaccinal G04.02
  specified NEC G04.89
  syphilitic (transverse) A52.14
➠toxic G92.9
  transverse (in demyelinating diseases of
      central nervous system) G37.3
  tuberculous A17.82
  varicella B01.12
Myeloblastic —see condition
Myeloblastoma
  granular cell —see also Neoplasm, connective
      tissue
    malignant —see Neoplasm, connective
        tissue, malignant
    tongue D10.1
Myelocele —see Spina bifida
Myelocystocele —see Spina bifida
Myelocytic —see condition
Myelodysplasia D46.9
  specified NEC D46.Z
  spinal cord (congenital) Q06.1
Myelodysplastic syndrome (see also Syndrome,
    myelodysplastic) D46.9
  with
    5q deletion D46.C
    isolated del (5q) chromosomal abnormality
        C46.C
  specified NEC D46.Z
Myeloencephalitis —see Encephalitis
Myelofibrosis D75.81
  with myeloid metaplasia D47.4
  acute C94.4-●
  idiopathic (chronic) D47.4
  primary D47.1
  secondary D75.81
    in myeloproliferative disease
        D47.4
Myelogenous —see condition
Myeloid —see condition
Myelokathexis D70.9
Myeloleukodystrophy E75.29
Myelolipoma —see Lipoma
Myeloma (multiple) C90.0-●
  monostotic C90.3
    plasma cell C90.0-●
  plasma cell C90.0-●
  solitary —see also Plasmacytoma, solitary
      C90.3-●

Myelomalacia G95.89
Myelomatosis C90.0-●
Myelomeningitis —see Meningoencephalitis
Myelomeningocele (spinal cord) —see Spina
    bifida
Myelo-osteo-musculodysplasia hereditaria
    Q79.8
Myelopathic
  anemia D64.89
  muscle atrophy —see Atrophy, muscle,
      spinal
  pain syndrome G89.0
Myelopathy (spinal cord) G95.9
  drug-induced G95.89
  in (due to)
    degeneration or displacement,
        intervertebral disc NEC —see
        Disorder, disc, with, myelopathy
    infection —see Encephalitis
    intervertebral disc disorder —see also
        Disorder, disc, with, myelopathy
    mercury —see subcategory T56.1
    neoplastic disease —see also Neoplasm
        D49.9 [G99.2]
    pernicious anemia D51.0 [G99.2]
    spondylosis —see Spondylosis, with,
        myelopathy NEC
  necrotic (subacute) (vascular) G95.19
  radiation-induced G95.89
  spondylogenic NEC —see Spondylosis, with
      myelopathy NEC
  toxic G95.89
  transverse, acute G37.3
  vascular G95.19
  vitamin B12 E53.8 [G32.0]
Myelophthisis D61.82
Myeloradiculitis G04.91
Myeloradiculodysplasia (spinal)
    Q06.1
Myelosarcoma C92.3-●
Myelosclerosis D75.89
  with myeloid metaplasia D47.4
  disseminated, of nervous system
      G35
  megakaryocytic D47.4
    with myeloid metaplasia
        D47.4
Myelosis
  acute C92.0-●
  aleukemic C92.9-●
  chronic D47.1
  erythremic (acute) C94.0-●
  megakaryocytic C94.2-●
  nonleukemic D72.828
  subacute C92.9-●
Myiasis (cavernous) B87.9
  aural B87.4
  creeping B87.0
  cutaneous B87.0
  dermal B87.0
  ear (external) (middle) B87.4
  eye B87.2
  genitourinary B87.81
  intestinal B87.82
  laryngeal B87.3
  nasopharyngeal B87.3
  ocular B87.2
  orbit B87.2
  skin B87.0
  specified site NEC B87.89
  traumatic B87.1
  wound B87.1
Myoadenoma, prostate —see Hyperplasia,
    prostate
Myoblastoma
  granular cell —see also Neoplasm, connective
      tissue, benign
    malignant —see Neoplasm, connective
        tissue, malignant
  tongue D10.1
Myocardial —see condition

▶ New   ➠ Revised   ~~deleted~~ Deleted   ● Use Additional Character(s)

Myocardiopathy (congestive) (constrictive) (familial) (hypertrophic nonobstructive) (idiopathic) (infiltrative) (obstructive) (primary) (restrictive) (sporadic) —*see also* Cardiomyopathy I42.9
  alcoholic I42.6
  cobalt-beer I42.6
  glycogen storage E74.02 [I43]
  hypertrophic obstructive I42.1
  in (due to)
    beriberi E51.12
    cardiac glycogenosis E74.02 [I43]
    Friedreich's ataxia G11.11 [I43]
    myotonia atrophica G71.11 [I43]
    progressive muscular dystrophy G71.03 [I43]
  obscure (African) I42.8
  secondary I42.9
  thyrotoxic E05.90 [I43]
    with storm E05.91 [I43]
  toxic NEC I42.7
Myocarditis (with arteriosclerosis) (chronic) (fibroid) (interstitial) (old) (progressive) (senile) I51.4
  with
    rheumatic fever (conditions in I00) I09.0
      active —*see* Myocarditis, acute, rheumatic
      inactive or quiescent (with chorea) I09.0
  active I40.9
    rheumatic I01.2
      with chorea (acute) (rheumatic) (Sydenham's) I02.0
  acute or subacute (interstitial) I40.9
    due to
      streptococcus (beta-hemolytic) I01.2
    idiopathic I40.1
    rheumatic I01.2
      with chorea (acute) (rheumatic) (Sydenham's) I02.0
    specified NEC I40.8
  aseptic of newborn B33.22
  bacterial (acute) I40.0
  Coxsackie (virus) B33.22
  diphtheritic A36.81
  eosinophilic I40.1
  epidemic of newborn (Coxsackie) B33.22
  Fiedler's (acute) (isolated) I40.1
  giant cell (acute) (subacute) I40.1
  gonococcal A54.83
  granulomatous (idiopathic) (isolated) (nonspecific) I40.1
  hypertensive —*see* Hypertension, heart
  idiopathic (granulomatous) I40.1
  in (due to)
    diphtheria A36.81
    epidemic louse-borne typhus A75.0 [I41]
    Lyme disease A69.29
    sarcoidosis D86.85
    scarlet fever A38.1
    toxoplasmosis (acquired) B58.81
    typhoid A01.02
    typhus NEC A75.9 [I41]
  infective I40.0
  influenzal —*see* Influenza, with, myocarditis
  isolated (acute) I40.1
  meningococcal A39.52
  mumps B26.82
  nonrheumatic, active I40.9
  parenchymatous I40.9
  pneumococcal I40.0
  rheumatic (chronic) (inactive) (with chorea) I09.0
    active or acute I01.2
      with chorea (acute) (rheumatic) (Sydenham's) I02.0
  rheumatoid —*see* Rheumatoid, carditis
  septic I40.0
  staphylococcal I40.0
  suppurative I40.0
  syphilitic (chronic) A52.06

Myocarditis (*Continued*)
  toxic I40.8
    rheumatic —*see* Myocarditis, acute, rheumatic
  tuberculous A18.84
  typhoid A01.02
  valvular —*see* Endocarditis
  virus, viral I40.0
    of newborn (Coxsackie) B33.22
Myocardium, myocardial —*see* condition
Myocardosis —*see* Cardiomyopathy
Myoclonus, myoclonic, myoclonia (familial) (essential) (multifocal) (simplex) G25.3
  drug-induced G25.3
  epilepsy —*see also* Epilepsy, generalized, specified NEC G40.4-●
    familial (progressive) G25.3
  epileptica G40.409
    with status epilepticus G40.401
  facial G51.3-●
  familial progressive G25.3
  Friedreich's G25.3
  jerks G25.3
  massive G25.3
  palatal G25.3
  pharyngeal G25.3
Myocytolysis I51.5
Myodiastasis —*see* Diastasis, muscle
Myoendocarditis —*see* Endocarditis
Myoepithelioma —*see* Neoplasm, benign, by site
Myofasciitis (acute) —*see* Myositis
Myofibroma —*see also* Neoplasm, connective tissue, benign
  uterus (cervix) (corpus) —*see* Leiomyoma
Myofibromatosis D48.1
  infantile Q89.8
Myofibrosis M62.89
  heart —*see* Myocarditis
  scapulohumeral —*see* Lesion, shoulder, specified NEC
Myofibrositis M79.7
  scapulohumeral —*see* Lesion, shoulder, specified NEC
Myoglobulinuria, myoglobinuria (primary) R82.1
Myokymia, facial G51.4
Myolipoma —*see* Lipoma
Myoma —*see also* Neoplasm, connective tissue, benign
  malignant —*see* Neoplasm, connective tissue, malignant
  prostate D29.1
  uterus (cervix) (corpus) —*see* Leiomyoma
Myomalacia M62.89
Myometritis —*see* Endometritis
Myometrium —*see* condition
Myonecrosis, clostridial A48.0
Myopathy G72.9
  acute
    necrotizing G72.81
    quadriplegic G72.81
  alcoholic G72.1
  benign congenital G71.20
  central core G71.29
  centronuclear G71.228
    autosomal (dominant) (recessive) G71.228
    other specified NEC G71.228
  congenital (benign) G71.20
  critical illness G72.81
  distal G71.09
  drug-induced G72.0
  endocrine NEC E34.9 [G73.7]
  extraocular muscles H05.82-●
  facioscapulohumeral G71.02
  hereditary G71.9
    specified NEC G71.8
  hyaline body G71.29
  myosin storage G71.29
  immune NEC G72.49

Myopathy (*Continued*)
  in (due to)
    Addison's disease E27.1 [G73.7]
    alcohol G72.1
    amyloidosis E85.0 [G73.7]
    cretinism E00.9 [G73.7]
    Cushing's syndrome E24.9 [G73.7]
    drugs G72.0
    endocrine disease NEC E34.9 [G73.7]
    giant cell arteritis M31.6 [G73.7]
    glycogen storage disease E74.00 [G73.7]
    hyperadrenocorticism E24.9 [G73.7]
    hyperparathyroidism NEC E21.3 [G73.7]
    hypoparathyroidism E20.9 [G73.7]
    hypopituitarism E23.0 [G73.7]
    hypothyroidism E03.9 [G73.7]
    infectious disease NEC B99 [G73.7]
    lipid storage disease E75.6 [G73.7]
    metabolic disease NEC E88.9 [G73.7]
    myxedema E03.9 [G73.7]
    parasitic disease NEC B89 [G73.7]
    polyarteritis nodosa M30.0 [G73.7]
    rheumatoid arthritis —*see* Rheumatoid, myopathy
    sarcoidosis D86.87
    scleroderma M34.82
    sicca syndrome M35.03
    Sjögren's syndrome M35.03
    systemic lupus erythematosus M32.19
    thyrotoxicosis (hyperthyroidism) E05.90 [G73.7]
      with thyroid storm E05.91 [G73.7]
    toxic agent NEC G72.2
  inflammatory NEC G72.49
  intensive care (ICU) G72.81
  limb-girdle G71.09
  mitochondrial NEC G71.3
  myosin storage G71.29
  myotonic, proximal (PROMM) G71.11
  myotubular (centronuclear) G71.220
    X-linked G71.220
  nemaline G71.21
  ocular G71.09
  oculopharyngeal G71.09
  of critical illness G72.81
  primary G71.9
    specified NEC G71.8
  progressive NEC G72.89
  proximal myotonic (PROMM) G71.11
  rod (body) G71.21
  scapulohumeral G71.02
  specified NEC G72.89
  toxic G72.2
Myopericarditis —*see also* Pericarditis
  chronic rheumatic I09.2
Myopia (axial) (congenital) H52.1-●
  degenerative (malignant) H44.20
    with
      choroidal neovascularization H44.2A-●
      foveoschisis H44.2D-●
      macular hole H44.2B-●
      retinal detachment H44.2C-●
      specified maculopathy NEC H44.2E-●
    bilateral H44.23
    left eye H44.22
    right eye H44.21
  malignant —*see also* Myopia, degenerative H44.2-●
  pernicious —*see also* Myopia, degenerative H44.2-●
  progressive high (degenerative) —*see also* Myopia, degenerative H44.2-●
Myosarcoma —*see* Neoplasm, connective tissue, malignant
Myosis (pupil) H57.03
  stromal (endolymphatic) D39.0
Myositis M60.9
  clostridial A48.0
  due to posture —*see* Myositis, specified type NEC

Myositis (*Continued*)
  epidemic B33.0
  fibrosa or fibrous (chronic), Volkmann's T79.6
  foreign body granuloma —*see* Granuloma,
    foreign body
  in (due to)
    bilharziasis B65.9 [*M63.8-•*]
    cysticercosis B69.81
    leprosy A30.9 [*M63.8-•*]
    mycosis B49 [*M63.8-•*]
    sarcoidosis D86.87
    schistosomiasis B65.9 [*M63.8-•*]
    syphilis
      late A52.78
      secondary A51.49
    toxoplasmosis (acquired) B58.82
    trichinellosis B75 [*M63.8-•*]
    tuberculosis A18.09
  inclusion body [IBM] G72.41
  infective M60.009
    arm M60.002
      left M60.001
      right M60.000
    leg M60.005
      left M60.004
      right M60.003
    lower limb M60.005
      ankle M60.07-•
      foot M60.07-•
      lower leg M60.06-•
      thigh M60.05-•
      toe M60.07-•
    multiple sites M60.09
    specified site NEC M60.08
    upper limb M60.002
      finger M60.04-•
      forearm M60.03-•
      hand M60.04-•
      shoulder region M60.01-•
      upper arm M60.02-•
  interstitial M60.10
    ankle M60.17-•
    foot M60.17-•
    forearm M60.13-•
    hand M60.14-•
    lower leg M60.16-•
    multiple sites M60.19
    shoulder region M60.11-•
    specified site NEC M60.18
    thigh M60.15-•
    upper arm M60.12-•
  mycotic B49 [*M63.8-•*]
  ossificans or ossifying (circumscripta) —*see*
    also Ossification, muscle, specified NEC
    in (due to)
      burns M61.30
        ankle M61.37-•
        foot M61.37-•
        forearm M61.33-•
        hand M61.34-•
        lower leg M61.36-•

Myositis (*Continued*)
  ossificans or ossifying (*Continued*)
    in (due to) (*Continued*)
      burns (*Continued*)
        multiple sites M61.39
        pelvic region M61.35-•
        shoulder region M61.31-•
        specified site NEC M61.38
        thigh M61.35-•
        upper arm M61.32-•
      quadriplegia or paraplegia M61.20
        ankle M61.27-•
        foot M61.27-•
        forearm M61.23-•
        hand M61.24-•
        lower leg M61.26-•
        multiple sites M61.29
        pelvic region M61.25-•
        shoulder region M61.21-•
        specified site NEC M61.28
        thigh M61.25-•
        upper arm M61.22-•
    progressiva M61.10
      ankle M61.17-•
      finger M61.14-•
      foot M61.17-•
      forearm M61.13-•
      hand M61.14-•
      lower leg M61.16-•
      multiple sites M61.19
      pelvic region M61.15-•
      shoulder region M61.11-•
      specified site NEC M61.18
      thigh M61.15-•
      toe M61.17-•
      upper arm M61.12-•
    traumatica M61.00
      ankle M61.07-•
      foot M61.07-•
      forearm M61.03-•
      hand M61.04-•
      lower leg M61.06-•
      multiple sites M61.09
      pelvic region M61.05-•
      shoulder region M61.01-•
      specified site NEC M61.08
      thigh M61.05-•
      upper arm M61.02-•
  purulent —*see* Myositis, infective
  specified type NEC M60.80
    ankle M60.87-•
    foot M60.87-•
    forearm M60.83-•
    hand M60.84-•
    lower leg M60.86-•
    multiple sites M60.89
    pelvic region M60.85-•
    shoulder region M60.81-•
    specified site NEC M60.88
    thigh M60.85-•
    upper arm M60.82-•

Myositis (*Continued*)
  suppurative —*see* Myositis, infective
  traumatic (old) —*see* Myositis, specified type
    NEC
Myospasia impulsiva F95.2
Myotonia (acquisita) (intermittens) M62.89
  atrophica G71.11
  chondrodystrophic G71.13
  congenita (acetazolamide responsive)
    (dominant) (recessive) G71.12
  drug-induced G71.14
  dystrophica G71.11
  fluctuans G71.19
  levior G71.12
  permanens G71.19
  symptomatic G71.19
Myotonic pupil —*see* Anomaly, pupil, function,
  tonic pupil
Myriapodiasis B88.2
Myringitis H73.2-•
  with otitis media —*see* Otitis, media
  acute H73.00-•
    bullous H73.01-•
    specified NEC H73.09-•
  bullous —*see* Myringitis, acute, bullous
  chronic H73.1-•
Mysophobia F40.228
Mytilotoxism —*see* Poisoning, fish
Myxadenitis labialis K13.0
Myxedema (adult) (idiocy) (infantile)
    (juvenile) —*see also* Hypothyroidism
    E03.9
  circumscribed E05.90
    with storm E05.91
  coma E03.5
  congenital E00.1
  cutis L98.5
  localized (pretibial) E05.90
    with storm E05.91
  papular L98.5
Myxochondrosarcoma —*see* Neoplasm,
  cartilage, malignant
Myxofibroma —*see* Neoplasm, connective
  tissue, benign
  odontogenic —*see* Cyst, calcifying
    odontogenic
Myxofibrosarcoma —*see* Neoplasm, connective
  tissue, malignant
Myxolipoma D17.9
Myxoliposarcoma —*see* Neoplasm, connective
  tissue, malignant
Myxoma —*see also* Neoplasm, connective tissue,
  benign
  nerve sheath —*see* Neoplasm, nerve,
    benign
  odontogenic —*see* Cyst, calcifying
    odontogenic
Myxosarcoma —*see* Neoplasm, connective
  tissue, malignant

▶ New   ⇒ Revised   ~~deleted~~ Deleted   • Use Additional Character(s)

N

Naegeli's
  disease Q82.8
  leukemia, monocytic C93.1-●
Naegleriasis (with meningoencephalitis)
    B60.2
Naffziger's syndrome G54.0
Naga sore —see Ulcer, skin
Nägele's pelvis M95.5
  with disproportion (fetopelvic) O33.0
    causing obstructed labor O65.0
Nail —see also condition
  biting F98.8
  patella syndrome Q87.2
Nanism, nanosomia —see Dwarfism
Nanophyetiasis B66.8
Nanukayami A27.89
Napkin rash L22
Narcolepsy G47.419
  with cataplexy G47.411
  in conditions classified elsewhere G47.429
    with cataplexy G47.421
Narcosis R06.89
Narcotism —see Dependence
NARP (Neuropathy, Ataxia and Retinitis
    pigmentosa) syndrome E88.49
Narrow
  anterior chamber angle H40.03-●
  gingival width (of periodontal soft tissue)
    K05.5
  pelvis —see Contraction, pelvis
Narrowing —see also Stenosis
  artery I77.1
    auditory, internal I65.8
    basilar —see Occlusion, artery, basilar
    carotid —see Occlusion, artery, carotid
    cerebellar —see Occlusion, artery, cerebellar
    cerebral —see Occlusion artery, cerebral
    choroidal —see Occlusion, artery,
        precerebral, specified NEC
    communicating posterior —see
        Occlusion, artery, precerebral,
        specified NEC
    coronary —see also Disease, heart, ischemic,
        atherosclerotic
      congenital Q24.5
        syphilitic A50.54 [I52]
      due to syphilis NEC A52.06
    hypophyseal —see Occlusion, artery,
        precerebral, specified NEC
    pontine —see Occlusion, artery, precerebral,
        specified NEC
    precerebral —see Occlusion, artery,
        precerebral
    vertebral —see Occlusion, artery, vertebral
  auditory canal (external) —see Stenosis,
      external ear canal
  eustachian tube —see Obstruction, eustachian
      tube
  eyelid —see Disorder, eyelid function
  larynx J38.6
  mesenteric artery —see also Ischemia,
      intestine, acute K55.059
  palate M26.89
  palpebral fissure —see Disorder, eyelid
      function
  ureter N13.5
    with infection N13.6
  urethra —see Stricture, urethra
Narrowness, abnormal, eyelid Q10.3
Nasal —see condition
Nasolachrymal, nasolacrimal —see condition
Nasopharyngeal —see also condition
  pituitary gland Q89.2
  torticollis M43.6
Nasopharyngitis (acute) (infective)
    (streptococcal) (subacute) J00
  chronic (suppurative) (ulcerative) J31.1
Nasopharynx, nasopharyngeal —see condition
Natal tooth, teeth K00.6

Nausea (without vomiting) R11.0
  with vomiting R11.2
  gravidarum —see Hyperemesis, gravidarum
  marina T75.3
  navalis T75.3
Navel —see condition
Neapolitan fever —see Brucellosis
Near drowning T75.1
Nearsightedness —see Myopia
Near-syncope R55
Nebula, cornea —see Opacity, cornea
Necator americanus infestation B76.1
Necatoriasis B76.1
Neck —see condition
Necrobiosis R68.89
  lipoidica NEC L92.1
    with diabetes —see E08-E13 with .620
Necrolysis, toxic epidermal L51.2
  due to drug
    correct substance properly administered —
        see Table of Drugs and Chemicals, by
        drug, adverse effect
    overdose or wrong substance given
        or taken —see Table of Drugs and
        Chemicals, by drug, poisoning
Necrophilia F65.89
Necrosis, necrotic (ischemic) —see also
    Gangrene
  adrenal (capsule) (gland) E27.49
  amputation stump (surgical) (late) T87.50
    arm T87.5-●
    leg T87.5-●
  antrum J32.0
  aorta (hyaline) —see also Aneurysm, aorta
    cystic medial —see Dissection, aorta
  artery I77.5
  bladder (aseptic) (sphincter) N32.89
  bone —see also Osteonecrosis M87.9
    aseptic or avascular —see Osteonecrosis
        idiopathic M87.00
    ethmoid J32.2
    jaw M27.2
    tuberculous —see Tuberculosis, bone
  brain I67.89
  breast (aseptic) (fat) (segmental) N64.1
  bronchus J98.09
  central nervous system NEC I67.89
  cerebellar I67.89
  cerebral I67.89
  colon —see also Infarct, intestine K55.049
  cornea H18.89-●
  cortical (acute) (renal) N17.1
  cystic medial (aorta) —see Dissection, aorta
  dental pulp K04.1
  esophagus K22.89
  ethmoid (bone) J32.2
  eyelid —see Disorder, eyelid, degenerative
  fat, fatty (generalized) —see also Disorder, soft
      tissue, specified type NEC
    abdominal wall K65.4
    breast (aseptic) (segmental) N64.1
    localized —see Degeneration, by site, fatty
    mesentery K65.4
    omentum K65.4
    pancreas K86.89
    peritoneum K65.4
    skin (subcutaneous), newborn P83.0
    subcutaneous, due to birth injury P15.6
  gallbladder —see Cholecystitis, acute
  heart —see Infarct, myocardium
  hip, aseptic or avascular —see Osteonecrosis,
      by type, femur
  intestine (acute) (hemorrhagic) (massive) —
      see also Infarct, intestine K55.069
  jaw M27.2
  kidney (bilateral) N28.0
    acute N17.9
    cortical (acute) (bilateral) N17.1
      with ectopic or molar pregnancy O08.4
    medullary (bilateral) (in acute renal failure)
        (papillary) N17.2

Necrosis, necrotic (Continued)
  kidney (Continued)
    papillary (bilateral) (in acute renal
        failure) N17.2
    tubular N17.0
      with ectopic or molar pregnancy
          O08.4
      complicating
        abortion —see Abortion, by type,
            complicated by, tubular necrosis
        ectopic or molar pregnancy O08.4
        pregnancy —see Pregnancy,
            complicated by, diseases of,
            specified type or system NEC
      following ectopic or molar pregnancy
          O08.4
    traumatic T79.5
  larynx J38.7
  liver (with hepatic failure) (cell) —see Failure,
      hepatic
  hemorrhagic, central K76.2
  lung J85.0
  lymphatic gland —see Lymphadenitis, acute
  mammary gland (fat) (segmental) N64.1
  mastoid (chronic) —see Mastoiditis, chronic
  medullary (acute) (renal) N17.2
  mesentery —see also Infarct, intestine
      K55.069
    fat K65.4
  mitral valve —see Insufficiency, mitral
  myocardium, myocardial —see Infarct,
      myocardium
  nose J34.0
  omentum (with mesenteric infarction) —see
      also Infarct, intestine K55.069
    fat K65.4
  orbit, orbital —see Osteomyelitis, orbit
  ossicles, ear —see Abnormal, ear ossicles
  ovary N70.92
  pancreas (aseptic) (duct) (fat) K86.89
    acute (infective) —see Pancreatitis, acute
    infective —see Pancreatitis, acute
  papillary (acute) (renal) N17.2
  perineum N90.89
  peritoneum (with mesenteric infarction) —see
      also Infarct, intestine K55.069
    fat K65.4
  pharynx J02.9
    in granulocytopenia —see Neutropenia
    Vincent's A69.1
  phosphorus —see subcategory T54.2
  pituitary (gland) E23.0
    postpartum O99.285
    Sheehan O99.285
  pressure —see Ulcer, pressure, by site
  pulmonary J85.0
  pulp (dental) K04.1
  radiation —see Necrosis, by site
  radium —see Necrosis, by site
  renal —see Necrosis, kidney
  sclera H15.89
  scrotum N50.89
  skin or subcutaneous tissue NEC I96
  spine, spinal (column) —see also
      Osteonecrosis, by type, vertebra
    cord G95.19
  spleen D73.5
  stomach K31.89
  stomatitis (ulcerative) A69.0
  subcutaneous fat, newborn P83.88
  subendocardial (acute) I21.4
    chronic I25.89
  suprarenal (capsule) (gland) E27.49
  testis N50.89
  thymus (gland) E32.8
  tonsil J35.8
  trachea J39.8
  tuberculous NEC —see Tuberculosis
  tubular (acute) (anoxic) (renal) (toxic)
      N17.0
    postprocedural N99.0

Necrosis, necrotic (Continued)
  vagina N89.8
  vertebra —see also Osteonecrosis, by type,
    vertebra
    tuberculous A18.01
  vulva N90.89
  X-ray —see Necrosis, by site
Necrospermia —see Infertility, male
Need (for)
  care provider because (of)
    assistance with personal care Z74.1
    continuous supervision required Z74.3
    impaired mobility Z74.09
    no other household member able to render
      care Z74.2
    specified reason NEC Z74.8
  immunization —see Vaccination
  vaccination —see Vaccination
Neglect
  adult
    confirmed T74.01
    history of Z91.412
    suspected T76.01
  child (childhood)
    confirmed T74.02
    history of Z62.812
    suspected T76.02
  emotional, in childhood Z62.898
  hemispatial R41.4
  left-sided R41.4
  sensory R41.4
  visuospatial R41.4
Neisserian infection NEC —see Gonococcus
Nelaton's syndrome G60.8
Nelson's syndrome E24.1
Nematodiasis (intestinal) B82.0
  Ancylostoma B76.0
Neonatal —see also Newborn
  acne L70.4
  bradycardia P29.12
  ➡ screening, abnormal findings on —see
    Abnormal, neonatal screening ~~P09~~
  tachycardia P29.11
  tooth, teeth K00.6
Neonatorum —see condition
Neoplasia
  endocrine, multiple (MEN) E31.20
    type I E31.21
    type IIA E31.22
    type IIB E31.23
  intraepithelial (histologically confirmed)
    anal (AIN) (histologically confirmed)
      K62.82
      grade I K62.82
      grade II K62.82
      severe D01.3
    cervical glandular (histologically
      confirmed) D06.9
    cervix (uteri) (CIN) (histologically
      confirmed) N87.9
      glandular D06.9
      grade I N87.0
      grade II N87.1
      grade III (severe dysplasia) —see also
        Carcinoma, cervix uteri, in situ
        D06.9
    prostate (histologically confirmed) (PIN)
      N42.31
      grade I N42.31
      grade II N42.31
      grade III (severe dysplasia) D07.5
    vagina (histologically confirmed) (VAIN)
      N89.3
      grade I N89.0
      grade II N89.1
      grade III (severe dysplasia) D07.2
    vulva (histologically confirmed) (VIN)
      N90.3
      grade I N90.0
      grade II N90.1
      grade III (severe dysplasia) D07.1

Neoplasm, neoplastic —see also Table of
  Neoplasms
  lipomatous, benign —see Lipoma
  malignant mast cell C96.20
    specified type NEC C96.29
  mast cell, of uncertain behavior NEC D47.09
Neovascularization
  ciliary body —see Disorder, iris, vascular
  cornea H16.40-●
    deep H16.44-●
    ghost vessels —see Ghost, vessels
    localized H16.43-●
    pannus —see Pannus
  iris —see Disorder, iris, vascular
  retina H35.05-●
Nephralgia N23
Nephritis, nephritic (albuminuric) (azotemic)
  (congenital) (disseminated) (epithelial)
  (familial) (focal) (granulomatous)
  (hemorrhagic) (infantile) (nonsuppurative,
  excretory) (uremic) N05.9
  with
    C3
      glomerulonephritis N05.A
      glomerulopathy N05.A
        with dense deposit disease N05.6
      dense deposit disease N05.6
      diffuse
        crescentic glomerulonephritis N05.7
        endocapillary proliferative
          glomerulonephritis N05.4
        membranous glomerulonephritis N05.2
        mesangial proliferative
          glomerulonephritis N05.3
        mesangiocapillary glomerulonephritis
          N05.5
      edema —see Nephrosis
      focal and segmental glomerular lesions
        N05.1
      foot process disease N04.9
      glomerular lesion
        diffuse sclerosing N05.8
        hypocomplementemic —see Nephritis,
          membranoproliferative
        IgA —see Nephropathy, IgA
        lobular, lobulonodular —see Nephritis,
          membranoproliferative
        nodular —see Nephritis,
          membranoproliferative
      lesion of
        glomerulonephritis, proliferative N05.8
        renal necrosis N05.9
      minor glomerular abnormality N05.0
      specified morphological changes NEC
        N05.8
  acute N00.9
    with
      C3
        glomerulonephritis N00.A
        glomerulopathy N00.A
          with dense deposit disease N00.6
        dense deposit disease N00.6
        diffuse
          crescentic glomerulonephritis N00.7
          endocapillary proliferative
            glomerulonephritis N00.4
          membranous glomerulonephritis
            N00.2
          mesangial proliferative
            glomerulonephritis N00.3
          mesangiocapillary glomerulonephritis
            N00.5
        focal and segmental glomerular lesions
          N00.1
        minor glomerular abnormality N00.0
        specified morphological changes NEC
          N00.8
  amyloid E85.4 [N08]
  antiglomerular basement membrane (anti-
    GBM) antibody NEC
    in Goodpasture's syndrome M31.0

Nephritis, nephritic (Continued)
  antitubular basement membrane (tubulo-
    interstitial) NEC N12
    toxic —see Nephropathy, toxic
  arteriolar —see Hypertension, kidney
  arteriosclerotic —see Hypertension, kidney
  ascending —see Nephritis, tubulo-interstitial
  atrophic N03.9
  Balkan (endemic) N15.0
  calculous, calculus —see Calculus,
    kidney
  cardiac —see Hypertension, kidney
  cardiovascular —see Hypertension,
    kidney
  chronic N03.9
    with
      C3
        glomerulonephritis N03.A
        glomerulopathy N03.A
          with dense deposit disease N03.6
        dense deposit disease N03.6
        diffuse
          crescentic glomerulonephritis
            N03.7
          endocapillary proliferative
            glomerulonephritis N03.4
          membranous glomerulonephritis
            N03.2
          mesangial proliferative
            glomerulonephritis N03.3
          mesangiocapillary glomerulonephritis
            N03.5
        focal and segmental glomerular lesions
          N03.1
        minor glomerular abnormality
          N03.0
        specified morphological changes
          NEC N03.8
    arteriosclerotic —see Hypertension,
      kidney
  cirrhotic N26.9
  complicating pregnancy O26.83-●
  croupous N00.9
  degenerative —see Nephrosis
  diffuse sclerosing N05.8
  due to
    diabetes mellitus —see E08-E13 with .21
    subacute bacterial endocarditis I33.0
    systemic lupus erythematosus (chronic)
      M32.14
    typhoid fever A01.09
  gonococcal (acute) (chronic) A54.21
  hypocomplementemic —see Nephritis,
    membranoproliferative
  IgA —see Nephropathy, IgA
  immune complex (circulating) NEC N05.8
  infective —see Nephritis, tubulo-interstitial
  interstitial —see Nephritis, tubulo-interstitial
  lead N14.3
  membranoproliferative (diffuse) (type 1
    or 3) —see also N00-N07 with fourth
    character .5 N05.5
    type 2 —see also N00-N07 with fourth
      character .6 N05.6
  minimal change N05.0
  necrotic, necrotizing NEC —see also N00-N07
    with fourth character .8 N05.8
  nephrotic —see Nephrosis
  nodular —see Nephritis,
    membranoproliferative
  polycystic Q61.3
    adult type Q61.2
    autosomal
      dominant Q61.2
      recessive NEC Q61.19
    childhood type NEC Q61.19
    infantile type NEC Q61.19
  poststreptococcal N05.9
    acute N00.9
    chronic N03.9
    rapidly progressive N01.9

▶ New   ➡ Revised   ~~deleted~~ Deleted   ● Use Additional Character(s)

Nephritis, nephritic (Continued)
  proliferative NEC —see also N00-N07 with
    fourth character .8 N05.8
  purulent —see Nephritis, tubulo-interstitial
  rapidly progressive N01.9
    with
      C3
        glomerulonephritis N01.A
        glomerulopathy N01.A
          with dense deposit disease N01.6
      dense deposit disease N01.6
      diffuse
        crescentic glomerulonephritis N01.7
        endocapillary proliferative
          glomerulonephritis N01.4
        membranous glomerulonephritis
          N01.2
        mesangial proliferative
          glomerulonephritis N01.3
        mesangiocapillary glomerulonephritis
          N01.5
      focal and segmental glomerular lesions
        N01.1
      minor glomerular abnormality N01.0
      specified morphological changes NEC
        N01.8
  salt losing or wasting NEC N28.89
  saturnine N14.3
  sclerosing, diffuse N05.8
  septic —see Nephritis, tubulo-interstitial
  specified pathology NEC —see also N00-N07
    with fourth character .8 N05.8
  subacute N01.9
  suppurative —see Nephritis,
    tubulo-interstitial
  syphilitic (late) A52.75
    congenital A50.59 [N08]
    early (secondary) A51.44
  toxic —see Nephropathy, toxic
  tubal, tubular —see Nephritis,
    tubulo-interstitial
  tuberculous A18.11
  tubulo-interstitial (in) N12
    acute (infectious) N10
    chronic (infectious) N11.9
      nonobstructive N11.8
        reflux-associated N11.0
      obstructive N11.1
      specified NEC N11.8
    due to
      brucellosis A23.9 [N16]
      cryoglobulinemia D89.1 [N16]
      glycogen storage disease E74.00 [N16]
      Sjögren's syndrome M35.04
  vascular —see Hypertension, kidney
  war N00.9
Nephroblastoma (epithelial) (mesenchymal)
  C64-●
Nephrocalcinosis E83.59 [N29]
Nephrocystitis, pustular —see Nephritis,
  tubulo-interstitial
Nephrolithiasis (congenital) (pelvis)
  (recurrent) —see also Calculus, kidney
Nephroma C64-●
  mesoblastic D41.0-●
Nephronephritis —see Nephrosis
Nephronophthisis Q61.5
Nephropathia epidemica A98.5
Nephropathy —see also Nephritis N28.9
  with
    edema —see Nephrosis
    glomerular lesion —see
      Glomerulonephritis
  amyloid, hereditary E85.0
  analgesic N14.0
    with medullary necrosis, acute N17.2
  Balkan (endemic) N15.0
  chemical —see Nephropathy, toxic
  diabetic —see E08-E13 with .21
  drug-induced N14.2
    specified NEC N14.1

Nephropathy (Continued)
  focal and segmental hyalinosis or sclerosis
    N02.1
  heavy metal-induced N14.3
  hereditary NEC N07.9
    with
      C3
        glomerulonephritis N07.A
        glomerulopathy N07.A
          with dense deposit disease N07.6
      dense deposit disease N07.6
      diffuse
        crescentic glomerulonephritis N07.7
        endocapillary proliferative
          glomerulonephritis N07.4
        membranous glomerulonephritis
          N07.2
        mesangial proliferative
          glomerulonephritis N07.3
        mesangiocapillary glomerulonephritis
          N07.5
      focal and segmental glomerular lesions
        N07.1
      minor glomerular abnormality N07.0
      specified morphological changes NEC
        N07.8
  hypercalcemic N25.89
  hypertensive —see Hypertension, kidney
  hypokalemic (vacuolar) N25.89
  IgA N02.8
    with glomerular lesion N02.9
      focal and segmental hyalinosis or
        sclerosis N02.1
      membranoproliferative (diffuse) N02.5
      membranous (diffuse) N02.2
      mesangial proliferative (diffuse) N02.3
      mesangiocapillary (diffuse) N02.5
      proliferative NEC N02.8
      specified pathology NEC N02.8
  lead N14.3
  membranoproliferative (diffuse) N02.5
  membranous (diffuse) N02.2
  mesangial (IgA/IgG) —see Nephropathy, IgA
    proliferative (diffuse) N02.3
  mesangiocapillary (diffuse) N02.5
  obstructive N13.8
  phenacetin N17.2
  phosphate-losing N25.0
  potassium depletion N25.89
  pregnancy-related O26.83-●
  proliferative NEC (see also N00-N07 with
    fourth character .8) N05.8
  protein-losing N25.89
  saturnine N14.3
  sickle-cell D57.-● [N08]
  toxic NEC N14.4
    due to
      drugs N14.2
        analgesic N14.0
        specified NEC N14.1
      heavy metals N14.3
  vasomotor N17.0
  water-losing N25.89
Nephroptosis N28.83
Nephropyosis —see Abscess, kidney
Nephrorrhagia N28.89
Nephrosclerosis (arteriolar) (arteriosclerotic)
  (chronic) (hyaline) —see also Hypertension,
    kidney
  hyperplastic —see Hypertension, kidney
  senile N26.9
Nephrosis, nephrotic (Epstein's) (syndrome)
  (congenital) N04.9
  with
    foot process disease N04.9
    glomerular lesion N04.1
    hypocomplementemic N04.5
  acute N04.9
  anoxic —see Nephrosis, tubular
  chemical —see Nephrosis, tubular
  cholemic K76.7

Nephrosis, nephrotic (Continued)
  diabetic —see E08-E13 with .21
  Finnish type (congenital) Q89.8
  hemoglobin N10
  hemoglobinuric —see Nephrosis, tubular
  in
    amyloidosis E85.4 [N08]
    diabetes mellitus —see E08-E13 with .21
    epidemic hemorrhagic fever A98.5
    malaria (malariae) B52.0
  ischemic —see Nephrosis, tubular
  lipoid N04.9
  lower nephron —see Nephrosis, tubular
  malarial (malariae) B52.0
  minimal change N04.0
  myoglobin N10
  necrotizing —see Nephrosis, tubular
  osmotic (sucrose) N25.89
  radiation N04.9
  syphilitic (late) A52.75
  toxic —see Nephrosis, tubular
  tubular (acute) N17.0
    postprocedural N99.0
    radiation N04.9
Nephrosonephritis, hemorrhagic (endemic)
  A98.5
Nephrostomy
  attention to Z43.6
  status Z93.6
Nerve —see also condition
  injury —see Injury, nerve, by body site
Nerves R45.0
Nervous —see also condition R45.0
  heart F45.8
  stomach F45.8
  tension R45.0
Nervousness R45.0
Nesidioblastoma
  pancreas D13.7
  specified site NEC —see Neoplasm, benign,
    by site
  unspecified site D13.7
Nettleship's syndrome —see Urticaria
  pigmentosa
Neumann's disease or syndrome L10.1
Neuralgia, neuralgic (acute) M79.2
  accessory (nerve) G52.8
  acoustic (nerve) —see subcategory H93.3
  auditory (nerve) —see subcategory H93.3
  ciliary G44.009
    intractable G44.001
    not intractable G44.009
  cranial
    nerve —see also Disorder, nerve, cranial
      fifth or trigeminal —see Neuralgia,
        trigeminal
    postherpetic, postzoster B02.29
  ear —see subcategory H92.0
  facialis vera G51.1
  Fothergill's —see Neuralgia, trigeminal
  glossopharyngeal (nerve) G52.1
  Horton's G44.099
    intractable G44.091
    not intractable G44.099
  Hunt's B02.21
  hypoglossal (nerve) G52.3
  infraorbital —see Neuralgia, trigeminal
  malarial —see Malaria
  migrainous G44.009
    intractable G44.001
    not intractable G44.009
  Morton's G57.6-●
  nerve, cranial —see Disorder, nerve, cranial
  nose G52.0
  occipital M54.81
  olfactory G52.0
  penis N48.9
  perineum R10.2
  postherpetic NEC B02.29
    trigeminal B02.22
  pubic region R10.2

Neuralgia, neuralgic *(Continued)*
scrotum R10.2
Sluder's G44.89
specified nerve NEC G58.8
spermatic cord R10.2
sphenopalatine (ganglion) G90.09
trifacial —*see* Neuralgia, trigeminal
trigeminal G50.0
postherpetic, postzoster B02.22
vagus (nerve) G52.2
writer's F48.8
organic G25.89
Neurapraxia —*see* Injury, nerve
Neurasthenia F48.8
cardiac F45.8
gastric F45.8
heart F45.8
Neurilemmoma —*see also* Neoplasm, nerve,
benign
acoustic (nerve) D33.3
malignant —*see also* Neoplasm, nerve,
malignant
acoustic (nerve) C72.4
Neurilemmosarcoma —*see* Neoplasm, nerve,
malignant
Neurinoma —*see* Neoplasm, nerve, benign
Neurinomatosis —*see* Neoplasm, nerve,
uncertain behavior
Neuritis (rheumatoid) M79.2
abducens (nerve) —*see* Strabismus, paralytic,
sixth nerve
accessory (nerve) G52.8
acoustic (nerve) —*see also* subcategory H93.3
in (due to)
infectious disease NEC B99 *[H94.0-●]*
parasitic disease NEC B89 *[H94.0-●]*
syphilitic A52.15
alcoholic G62.1
with psychosis —*see* Psychosis, alcoholic
amyloid, any site E85.4 *[G63]*
auditory (nerve) —*see* subcategory H93.3
brachial —*see* Radiculopathy
due to displacement, intervertebral disc —
see Disorder, disc, cervical, with neuritis
cranial nerve
due to Lyme disease A69.22
eighth or acoustic or auditory —*see*
subcategory H93.3
eleventh or accessory G52.8
fifth or trigeminal G51.0
first or olfactory G52.0
fourth or trochlear —*see* Strabismus,
paralytic, fourth nerve
second or optic —*see* Neuritis, optic
seventh or facial G51.8
newborn (birth injury) P11.3
sixth or abducent —*see* Strabismus,
paralytic, sixth nerve
tenth or vagus G52.2
third or oculomotor —*see* Strabismus,
paralytic, third nerve
twelfth or hypoglossal G52.3
Déjérine-Sottas G60.0
diabetic (mononeuropathy) —*see* E08-E13
with .41
polyneuropathy —*see* E08-E13 with .42
due to
beriberi E51.11
displacement, prolapse or rupture,
intervertebral disc —*see* Disorder, disc,
with, radiculopathy
herniation, nucleus pulposus M51.9 *[G55]*
endemic E51.11
facial G51.8
newborn (birth injury) P11.3
general —*see* Polyneuropathy
geniculate ganglion G51.1
due to herpes (zoster) B02.21
gouty —*see also* Gout, by type M10.9 *[G63]*
hypoglossal (nerve) G52.3
ilioinguinal (nerve) G57.9-●
infectious (multiple) NEC G61.0

Neuritis *(Continued)*
interstitial hypertrophic progressive G60.0
lumbar M54.16
lumbosacral M54.17
multiple —*see also* Polyneuropathy
endemic E51.11
infective, acute G61.0
multiplex endemica E51.11
nerve root —*see* Radiculopathy
oculomotor (nerve) —*see* Strabismus,
paralytic, third nerve
olfactory nerve G52.0
optic (nerve) (hereditary) (sympathetic) H46.9
with demyelination G36.0
in myelitis G36.0
nutritional H46.2
papillitis —*see* Papillitis, optic
retrobulbar H46.1-●
specified type NEC H46.8
toxic H46.3
peripheral (nerve) G62.9
multiple —*see* Polyneuropathy
single —*see* Mononeuritis
pneumogastric (nerve) G52.2
postherpetic, postzoster B02.29
progressive hypertrophic interstitial G60.0
retrobulbar —*see also* Neuritis, optic,
retrobulbar
in (due to)
late syphilis A52.15
meningococcal infection A39.82
meningococcal A39.82
syphilitic A52.15
sciatic (nerve) —*see also* Sciatica
due to displacement of intervertebral
disc —*see* Disorder, disc, with,
radiculopathy
serum —*see also* Reaction, serum T80.69
shoulder-girdle G54.5
specified nerve NEC G58.8
spinal (nerve) root —*see* Radiculopathy
syphilitic A52.15
thenar (median) G56.1-●
thoracic M54.14
toxic NEC G62.2
trochlear (nerve) —*see* Strabismus, paralytic,
fourth nerve
vagus (nerve) G52.2
Neuroastrocytoma —*see* Neoplasm, uncertain
behavior, by site
Neuroavitaminosis E56.9 *[G99.8]*
Neuroblastoma
olfactory C30.0
specified site —*see* Neoplasm, malignant, by
site
unspecified site C74.90
Neurochorioretinitis —*see* Chorioretinitis
Neurocirculatory asthenia F45.8
Neurocysticercosis B69.0
Neurocytoma —*see* Neoplasm, benign, by site
Neurodermatitis (circumscribed)
(circumscripta) (local) L28.0
atopic L20.81
diffuse (Brocq) L20.81
disseminated L20.81
Neuroencephalomyelopathy, optic G36.0
Neuroepithelioma —*see also* Neoplasm,
malignant, by site
olfactory C30.0
Neurofibroma —*see also* Neoplasm, nerve,
benign
melanotic —*see* Neoplasm, nerve, benign
multiple —*see* Neurofibromatosis
plexiform —*see* Neoplasm, nerve, benign
Neurofibromatosis (multiple) (nonmalignant)
Q85.00
acoustic Q85.02
malignant —*see* Neoplasm, nerve, malignant
specified NEC Q85.09
type 1 (von Recklinghausen) Q85.01
type 2 Q85.02

Neurofibrosarcoma —*see* Neoplasm, nerve,
malignant
Neurogenic —*see also* condition
bladder —*see also* Dysfunction, bladder,
neuromuscular N31.9
cauda equina syndrome G83.4
bowel NEC K59.2
heart F45.8
Neuroglioma —*see* Neoplasm, uncertain
behavior, by site
Neurolabyrinthitis (of Dix and Hallpike) —*see*
Neuronitis, vestibular
Neurolathyrism —*see* Poisoning, food, noxious,
plant
Neuroleprosy A30.9
Neuroma —*see also* Neoplasm, nerve, benign
acoustic (nerve) D33.3
amputation (stump) (traumatic) (surgical
complication) (late) T87.3-●
arm T87.3-●
leg T87.3-●
digital (toe) G57.6-●
interdigital G58.8
lower limb toe G57.8-●
upper limb G56.8-●
intermetatarsal G57.8-●
Morton's G57.6-●
nonneoplastic
arm G56.9-●
leg G57.9-●
lower extremity G57.9-●
upper extremity G56.9-●
optic (nerve) D33.3
plantar G57.6-●
plexiform —*see* Neoplasm, nerve,
benign
surgical (nonneoplastic)
arm G56.9-●
leg G57.9-●
lower extremity G57.9-●
upper extremity G56.9-●
Neuromyalgia —*see* Neuralgia
Neuromyasthenia (epidemic) (postinfectious)
G93.3
Neuromyelitis G36.9
ascending G61.0
optica G36.0
Neuromyopathy G70.9
paraneoplastic D49.9 *[G13.0]*
Neuromyotonia (Isaacs) G71.19
Neuronevus —*see* Nevus
Neuronitis G58.9
ascending (acute) G57.2-●
vestibular H81.2-●
Neuroparalytic —*see* condition
Neuropathy, neuropathic G62.9
acute motor G62.81
alcoholic G62.1
with psychosis —*see* Psychosis,
alcoholic
arm G56.9-●
autonomic, peripheral —*see* Neuropathy,
peripheral, autonomic
axillary G56.9-●
bladder N31.9
atonic (motor) (sensory) N31.2
autonomous N31.2
flaccid N31.2
nonreflex N31.2
reflex N31.1
uninhibited N31.0
brachial plexus G54.0
cervical plexus G54.2
chronic
progressive segmentally demyelinating
G62.89
relapsing demyelinating G62.89
Déjérine-Sottas G60.0
diabetic —*see* E08-E13 with .40
mononeuropathy —*see* E08-E13 with .41
polyneuropathy —*see* E08-E13 with .42

Neuropathy, neuropathic *(Continued)*
  entrapment G58.9
    iliohypogastric nerve G57.8-●
    ilioinguinal nerve G57.8-●
    lateral cutaneous nerve of thigh
      G57.1-●
    median nerve G56.0-●
    obturator nerve G57.8-●
    peroneal nerve G57.3-●
    posterior tibial nerve G57.5-●
    saphenous nerve G57.8-●
    ulnar nerve G56.2-●
  facial nerve G51.9
  hereditary G60.9
    motor and sensory (types I-IV) G60.0
    sensory G60.8
    specified NEC G60.8
  hypertrophic G60.0
    Charcot-Marie-Tooth G60.0
    Déjérine-Sottas G60.0
    interstitial progressive G60.0
    of infancy G60.0
    Refsum G60.1
  idiopathic G60.9
    progressive G60.3
    specified NEC G60.8
  in association with hereditary ataxia
    G60.2
  intercostal G58.0
  ischemic —*see* Disorder, nerve
  Jamaica (ginger) G62.2
  leg NEC G57.9-●
  lower extremity G57.9-●
  lumbar plexus G54.1
  median nerve G56.1-●
  motor and sensory —*see also* Polyneuropathy
    hereditary (types I-IV) G60.0
  multifocal motor (MMN) G61.82
  multiple (acute) (chronic) —*see*
    Polyneuropathy
  optic (nerve) —*see also* Neuritis, optic
    ischemic H47.01-●
  paraneoplastic (sensorial) (Denny Brown)
    D49.9 *[G13.0]*
  peripheral (nerve) —*see also* Polyneuropathy
    G62.9
    autonomic G90.9
      idiopathic G90.09
      in (due to)
        amyloidosis E85.4 *[G99.0]*
        diabetes mellitus —*see* E08-E13 with
          .43
        endocrine disease NEC E34.9 *[G99.0]*
        gout M10.00 *[G99.0]*
        hyperthyroidism E05.90 *[G99.0]*
          with thyroid storm E05.91 *[G99.0]*
        metabolic disease NEC E88.9 *[G99.0]*
    idiopathic G60.9
      progressive G60.3
    in (due to)
      antitetanus serum G62.0
      arsenic G62.2
      drugs NEC G62.0
      lead G62.2
      organophosphate compounds G62.2
      toxic agent NEC G62.2
  plantar nerves G57.6-●
  progressive
    hypertrophic interstitial G60.0
    inflammatory G62.81
  radicular NEC —*see* Radiculopathy
  sacral plexus G54.1
  sciatic G57.0-●
  serum G61.1
  toxic NEC G62.2
  trigeminal sensory G50.8
  ulnar nerve G56.2-●
  uremic N18.9 *[G63]*
  vitamin B12 E53.8 *[G63]*
    with anemia (pernicious) D51.0 *[G63]*
      due to dietary deficiency D51.3 *[G63]*

Neurophthisis —*see also* Disorder, nerve
  peripheral, diabetic —*see* E08-E13 with .42
Neuroretinitis —*see* Chorioretinitis
Neuroretinopathy, hereditary optic H47.22
Neurosarcoma —*see* Neoplasm, nerve, malignant
Neurosclerosis —*see* Disorder, nerve
Neurosis, neurotic F48.9
  anankastic F42.8
  anxiety (state) F41.1
    panic type F41.0
  asthenic F48.8
  bladder F45.8
  cardiac (reflex) F45.8
  cardiovascular F45.8
  character F60.9
  colon F45.8
  compensation F68.10
  compulsive, compulsion F42.8
  conversion F44.9
  craft F48.8
  cutaneous F45.8
  depersonalization F48.1
  depressive (reaction) (type) F34.1
  environmental F48.8
  excoriation L98.1
  fatigue F48.8
  functional —*see* Disorder, somatoform
  gastric F45.8
  gastrointestinal F45.8
  heart F45.8
  hypochondriacal F45.21
  hysterical F44.9
  incoordination F45.8
    larynx F45.8
    vocal cord F45.8
  intestine F45.8
  larynx (sensory) F45.8
    hysterical F44.4
  mixed NEC F48.8
  musculoskeletal F45.8
  obsessional F42.8
  obsessive-compulsive F42.8
  occupational F48.8
  ocular NEC F45.8
  organ —*see* Disorder, somatoform
  pharynx F45.8
  phobic F40.9
  posttraumatic (situational) F43.10
    acute F43.11
    chronic F43.12
  psychasthenic (type) F48.8
  railroad F48.8
  rectum F45.8
  respiratory F45.8
  rumination F45.8
  sexual F65.9
  situational F48.8
  social F40.10
    generalized F40.11
  specified type NEC F48.8
  state F48.9
    with depersonalization episode F48.1
  stomach F45.8
  traumatic F43.10
    acute F43.11
    chronic F43.12
  vasomotor F45.8
  visceral F45.8
  war F48.8
Neurospongioblastosis diffusa Q85.1
Neurosyphilis (arrested) (early) (gumma) (late)
  (latent) (recurrent) (relapse) A52.3
  with ataxia (cerebellar) (locomotor) (spastic)
    (spinal) A52.19
  aneurysm (cerebral) A52.05
  arachnoid (adhesive) A52.13
  arteritis (any artery) (cerebral) A52.04
  asymptomatic A52.2
  congenital A50.40
  dura (mater) A52.13
  general paresis A52.17

Neurosyphilis *(Continued)*
  hemorrhagic A52.05
  juvenile (asymptomatic) (meningeal)
    A50.40
  leptomeninges (aseptic) A52.13
  meningeal, meninges (adhesive) A52.13
  meningitis A52.13
  meningovascular (diffuse) A52.13
  optic atrophy A52.15
  parenchymatous (degenerative) A52.19
  paresis, paretic A52.17
    juvenile A50.45
  remission in (sustained) A52.3
  serological (without symptoms) A52.2
  specified nature or site NEC A52.19
  tabes, tabetic (dorsalis) A52.11
    juvenile A50.45
  taboparesis A52.17
    juvenile A50.45
  thrombosis (cerebral) A52.05
  vascular (cerebral) NEC A52.05
Neurothekeoma —*see* Neoplasm, nerve, benign
Neurotic —*see* Neurosis
Neurotoxemia —*see* Toxemia
Neutroclusion M26.211
Neutropenia, neutropenic (chronic) (genetic)
  (idiopathic) (immune) (infantile)
  (malignant) (pernicious) (splenic) D70.9
  congenital (primary) D70.0
  cyclic D70.4
  cytoreductive cancer chemotherapy sequela
    D70.1
  drug-induced D70.2
    due to cytoreductive cancer chemotherapy
      D70.1
  due to infection D70.3
  fever D70.9
  neonatal, transitory (isoimmune) (maternal
    transfer) P61.5
  periodic D70.4
  secondary (cyclic) (periodic) (splenic) D70.4
    drug-induced D70.2
    due to cytoreductive cancer
      chemotherapy D70.1
  toxic D70.8
Neutrophilia, hereditary giant D72.0
Nevocarcinoma —*see* Melanoma
Nevus D22.9
  achromic —*see* Neoplasm, skin, benign
  amelanotic —*see* Neoplasm, skin, benign
  angiomatous D18.00
    intra-abdominal D18.03
    intracranial D18.02
    skin D18.01
    specified site NEC D18.09
  araneus I78.1
  balloon cell —*see* Neoplasm, skin, benign
  bathing trunk D48.5
  blue —*see* Neoplasm, skin, benign
    cellular —*see* Neoplasm, skin, benign
    giant —*see* Neoplasm, skin, benign
    Jadassohn's —*see* Neoplasm, skin, benign
    malignant —*see* Melanoma
  capillary D18.00
    intra-abdominal D18.03
    intracranial D18.02
    skin D18.01
    specified site NEC D18.09
  cavernous D18.00
    intra-abdominal D18.03
    intracranial D18.02
    skin D18.01
    specified site NEC D18.09
  cellular —*see* Neoplasm, skin, benign
    blue —*see* Neoplasm, skin, benign
  choroid D31.3-●
  comedonicus Q82.5
  conjunctiva D31.0-●
  dermal —*see* Neoplasm, skin, benign
    with epidermal nevus —*see* Neoplasm,
      skin, benign

Nevus (Continued)
dysplastic —see Neoplasm, skin, benign
eye D31.9-●
flammeus Q82.5
hemangiomatous D18.00
  intra-abdominal D18.03
  intracranial D18.02
  skin D18.01
  specified site NEC D18.09
iris D31.4-●
lacrimal gland D31.5-●
lymphatic D18.1
magnocellular
  specified site —see Neoplasm, benign, by
    site
  unspecified site D31.40
malignant —see Melanoma
meaning hemangioma D18.00
  intra-abdominal D18.03
  intracranial D18.02
  skin D18.01
  specified site NEC D18.09
mouth (mucosa) D10.30
  specified site NEC D10.39
  white sponge Q38.6
multiplex Q85.1
non-neoplastic I78.1
oral mucosa D10.30
  specified site NEC D10.39
  white sponge Q38.6
orbit D31.6-●
pigmented
  giant —see also Neoplasm, skin, uncertain
    behavior D48.5
    malignant melanoma in —see Melanoma
portwine Q82.5
retina D31.2-●
retrobulbar D31.6-●
sanguineous Q82.5
senile I78.1
skin D22.9
  abdominal wall D22.5
  ala nasi D22.39
  ankle D22.7-●
  anus, anal D22.5
  arm D22.6-●
  auditory canal (external) D22.2-●
  auricle (ear) D22.2-●
  auricular canal (external) D22.2-●
  axilla, axillary fold D22.5
  back D22.5
  breast D22.5
  brow D22.39
  buttock D22.5
  canthus (eye) D22.1-●
  cheek (external) D22.39
  chest wall D22.5
  chin D22.39
  ear (external) D22.2-●
  external meatus (ear) D22.2-●
  eyebrow D22.39
  eyelid (lower) (upper) D22.1-●
  face D22.30
    specified NEC D22.39
  female genital organ (external) NEC D28.0
  finger D22.6-●
  flank D22.5
  foot D22.7-●
  forearm D22.6-●
  forehead D22.39
  foreskin D29.0
  genital organ (external) NEC
    female D28.0
    male D29.9
  gluteal region D22.5
  groin D22.5
  hand D22.6-●
  heel D22.7-●
  helix D22.2-●
  hip D22.7-●
  interscapular region D22.5

Nevus (Continued)
skin (Continued)
  jaw D22.39
  knee D22.7-●
  labium (majus) (minus) D28.0
  leg D22.7-●
  lip (lower) (upper) D22.0
  lower limb D22.7-●
  male genital organ (external) D29.9
  nail D22.9
    finger D22.6-●
    toe D22.7-●
  nasolabial groove D22.39
  nates D22.5
  neck D22.4
  nose (external) D22.39
  palpebra D22.1-●
  penis D29.0
  perianal skin D22.5
  perineum D22.5
  pinna D22.2-●
  popliteal fossa or space D22.7-●
  prepuce D29.0
  pudendum D28.0
  scalp D22.4
  scrotum D29.4
  shoulder D22.6-●
  submammary fold D22.5
  temple D22.39
  thigh D22.7-●
  toe D22.7-●
  trunk NEC D22.5
  umbilicus D22.5
  upper limb D22.6-●
  vulva D28.0
  specified site NEC —see Neoplasm, benign,
    by site
spider I78.1
stellar I78.1
strawberry Q82.5
Sutton's benign D22.9
unius lateris Q82.5
Unna's Q82.5
vascular Q82.5
verrucous Q82.5
Newborn (infant) (liveborn) (singleton)
  Z38.2
abstinence syndrome P96.1
acne L70.4
affected by
  abnormalities of membranes P02.9
    specified NEC P02.8
  abruptio placenta P02.1
  amino-acid metabolic disorder, transitory
    P74.8
  amniocentesis (while in utero) P00.6
  amnionitis P02.78
  apparent life threatening event (ALTE)
    R68.13
  bleeding (into)
    cerebral cortex P52.22
    germinal matrix P52.0
    ventricles P52.1
  breech delivery P03.0
  cardiac arrest P29.81
  cardiomyopathy I42.8
    congenital I42.4
  cerebral ischemia P91.0
  Cesarean delivery P03.4
  chemotherapy agents P04.11
  chorioamnionitis P02.78
  cocaine (crack) P04.41
  complications of labor and delivery P03.9
    specified NEC P03.89
  compression of umbilical cord NEC P02.5
  contracted pelvis P03.1
  cyanosis P28.2
  delivery P03.9
    Cesarean P03.4
    forceps P03.2
    vacuum extractor P03.3

Newborn (Continued)
affected by (Continued)
  drugs of addiction P04.40
    cocaine P04.41
    hallucinogens P04.42
    specified drug NEC P04.49
  entanglement (knot) in umbilical cord P02.5
  environmental chemicals P04.6
  fetal (intrauterine)
    growth retardation P05.9
    inflammatory response syndrome (FIRS)
      P02.70
    malnutrition not light or small for
      gestational age P05.2
  FIRS (fetal inflammatory response
    syndrome) P02.70
  forceps delivery P03.2
  heart rate abnormalities
    bradycardia P29.12
    intrauterine P03.819
      before onset of labor P03.810
      during labor P03.811
    tachycardia P29.11
  hemorrhage (antepartum) P02.1
    cerebellar (nontraumatic) P52.6
    intracerebral (nontraumatic) P52.4
    intracranial (nontraumatic) P52.9
      specified NEC P52.8
    intraventricular (nontraumatic) P52.3
      grade 1 P52.0
      grade 2 P52.1
      grade 3 P52.21
      grade 4 P52.22
    posterior fossa (nontraumatic) P52.6
    subarachnoid (nontraumatic) P52.5
    subependymal P52.0
      with intracerebral extension P52.22
      with intraventricular extension P52.1
        with enlargment of ventricles P52.21
      without intraventricular extension
        P52.0
  hypoxic ischemic encephalopathy [HIE]
    P91.60
    mild P91.61
    moderate P91.62
    severe P91.63
  induction of labor P03.89
  intestinal perforation P78.0
  intrauterine (fetal) blood loss P50.9
    due to (from)
      cut end of co-twin cord P50.5
      hemorrhage into
        co-twin P50.3
        maternal circulation P50.4
      placenta P50.2
      ruptured cord blood P50.1
      vasa previa P50.0
      specified NEC P50.8
  intrauterine (fetal) hemorrhage P50.9
  intrauterine (in utero) procedure P96.5
  malpresentation (malposition) NEC P03.1
  maternal (complication of) (use of)
    alcohol P04.3
    amphetamines P04.16
    analgesia (maternal) P04.0
    anesthesia (maternal) P04.0
    anticonvulsants P04.13
    antidepressants P04.15
    antineoplastic chemotherapy P04.11
    anxiolytics P04.1A
    blood loss P02.1
    cannabis P04.81
    circulatory disease P00.3
    condition P00.9
      specified NEC P00.89
    cytotoxic drugs P04.12
    delivery P03.9
      Cesarean P03.4
      forceps P03.2
      vacuum extractor P03.3
    diabetes mellitus (pre-existing) P70.1

▶ New   ⇒ Revised   ~~deleted~~ Deleted   ● Use Additional Character(s)

Newborn *(Continued)*
  affected by *(Continued)*
    maternal *(Continued)*
      disorder P00.9
        specified NEC P00.89
      drugs (addictive) (illegal) NEC P04.49
      ectopic pregnancy P01.4
      gestational diabetes P70.0
     ▶group B streptococcus (GBS)
        colonization (positive) P00.82
      hemorrhage P02.1
      hypertensive disorder P00.0
      incompetent cervix P01.0
      infectious disease P00.2
      injury P00.5
      labor and delivery P03.9
      malpresentation before labor P01.7
      maternal death P01.6
      medical procedure P00.7
      medication P04.19
        specified type NEC P04.18
      multiple pregnancy P01.5
      nutritional disorder P00.4
      oligohydramnios P01.2
      opiates P04.14
        administered for procedures during
          pregnancy or labor and delivery
          P04.0
      parasitic disease P00.2
      periodontal disease P00.81
      placenta previa P02.0
      polyhydramnios P01.3
      precipitate delivery P03.5
      pregnancy P01.9
        specified P01.8
      premature rupture of membranes P01.1
      renal disease P00.1
      respiratory disease P00.3
      sedative-hypnotics P04.17
      surgical procedure P00.6
      tranquilizers administered for
        procedures during pregnancy or
        labor and delivery P04.0
      urinary tract disease P00.1
      uterine contraction (abnormal) P03.6
    meconium peritonitis P78.0
    medication (legal) (maternal use)
      (prescribed) P04.19
    membrane abnormalities P02.9
      specified NEC P02.8
    membranitis P02.78
    methamphetamine(s) P04.49
    mixed metabolic and respiratory acidosis P84
    neonatal abstinence syndrome P96.1
    noxious substances transmitted via
      placenta or breast milk P04.9
      cannabis P04.81
      specified NEC P04.89
    nutritional supplements P04.5
    placenta previa P02.0
    placental
      abnormality (functional)
        (morphological) P02.20
        specified NEC P02.29
      dysfunction P02.29
      infarction P02.29
      insufficiency P02.29
      separation NEC P02.1
      transfusion syndromes P02.3
    placentitis P02.78
    precipitate delivery P03.5
    prolapsed cord P02.4
    respiratory arrest P28.81
    slow intrauterine growth P05.9
    tobacco P04.2
    twin to twin transplacental transfusion P02.3
    umbilical cord (tightly) around neck P02.5
    umbilical cord condition P02.60
      short cord P02.69
      specified NEC P02.69
    uterine contractions (abnormal) P03.6
    vasa previa P02.69
      from intrauterine blood loss P50.0

Newborn *(Continued)*
  apnea P28.4
    obstructive P28.4
    primary P28.3
    sleep (central) (obstructive) (primary) P28.3
  born in hospital Z38.00
    by cesarean Z38.01
  born outside hospital Z38.1
  breast buds P96.89
  breast engorgement P83.4
  check-up —*see* Newborn, examination
  convulsion P90
  dehydration P74.1
  examination
    8 to 28 days old Z00.111
    under 8 days old Z00.110
  fever P81.9
    environmentally-induced P81.0
  hyperbilirubinemia P59.9
    of prematurity P59.0
  hypernatremia P74.21
  hyponatremia P74.22
  infection P39.9
    candidal P37.5
    specified NEC P39.8
    urinary tract P39.3
  jaundice P59.9
    due to
      breast milk inhibitor P59.3
      hepatocellular damage P59.20
        specified NEC P59.29
      preterm delivery P59.0
    of prematurity P59.0
    specified NEC P59.8
  late metabolic acidosis P74.0
  mastitis P39.0
    infective P39.0
    noninfective P83.4
  multiple born NEC Z38.8
    born in hospital Z38.68
      by cesarean Z38.69
    born outside hospital Z38.7
  omphalitis P38.9
    with mild hemorrhage P38.1
    without hemorrhage P38.9
  post-term P08.21
  prolonged gestation (over 42 completed
    weeks) P08.22
  quadruplet Z38.8
    born in hospital Z38.63
      by cesarean Z38.64
    born outside hospital Z38.7
  quintuplet Z38.8
    born in hospital Z38.65
      by cesarean Z38.66
    born outside hospital Z38.7
  seizure P90
  sepsis (congenital) P36.9
    due to
      anaerobes NEC P36.5
      Escherichia coli P36.4
      Staphylococcus P36.30
        aureus P36.2
        specified NEC P36.39
      Streptococcus P36.10
        group B P36.0
        specified NEC P36.19
      specified NEC P36.8
  triplet Z38.8
    born in hospital Z38.61
      by cesarean Z38.62
    born outside hospital Z38.7
  twin Z38.5
    born in hospital Z38.30
      by cesarean Z38.31
    born outside hospital Z38.4
  vomiting P92.09
    bilious P92.01
  weight check Z00.111
Newcastle conjunctivitis or disease B30.8
Nezelof's syndrome (pure alymphocytosis) D81.4

Niacin (amide) **deficiency** E52
Nicolas (-Durand)-**Favre disease** A55
Nicotine —*see* Tobacco
Nicotinic acid deficiency E52
Niemann-Pick disease or syndrome E75.249
  specified NEC E75.248
  type
    A E75.240
   ▶A/B E75.244
    B E75.241
    C E75.242
    D E75.243
Night
  blindness —*see* Blindness, night
  sweats R61
  terrors (child) F51.4
Nightmares (REM sleep type) F51.5
NIHSS (National Institutes of Health Stroke
  Scale) **score** R29.7-●
Nipple —*see* condition
Nisbet's chancre A57
Nishimoto (-Takeuchi) **disease** I67.5
Nitritoid crisis or reaction —*see* Crisis,
  nitritoid
Nitrosohemoglobinemia D74.8
Njovera A65
▶**No general equivalence degree (GED)** Z55.5
Nocardiosis, nocardiasis A43.9
  cutaneous A43.1
  lung A43.0
  pneumonia A43.0
  pulmonary A43.0
  specified site NEC A43.8
Nocturia R35.1
  psychogenic F45.8
Nocturnal —*see* condition
Nodal rhythm I49.8
Node(s) —*see also* Nodule
  Bouchard's (with arthropathy) M15.2
  Haygarth's M15.8
  Heberden's (with arthropathy) M15.1
  larynx J38.7
  lymph —*see* condition
  milker's B08.03
  Osler's I33.0
  Schmorl's —*see* Schmorl's disease
  singer's J38.2
  teacher's J38.2
  tuberculous —*see* Tuberculosis, lymph
    gland
  vocal cord J38.2
Nodule(s), nodular
  actinomycotic —*see* Actinomycosis
  breast NEC —*see also* Lump, breast
    N63.0
  colloid (cystic), thyroid E04.1
  cutaneous —*see* Swelling, localized
  endometrial (stromal) D26.1
  Haygarth's M15.8
  inflammatory —*see* Inflammation
  juxta-articular
    syphilitic A52.77
    yaws A66.7
  larynx J38.7
  lung, solitary (subsegmental branch of the
    bronchial tree) R91.1
    multiple R91.8
  milker's B08.03
  prostate N40.2
    with lower urinary tract symptoms (LUTS)
      N40.3
    without lower urinary tract symptoms
      (LUTS) N40.2
  pulmonary, solitary (subsegmental branch of
    the bronchial tree) R91.1
  retrocardiac R09.89
  rheumatoid M06.30
    ankle M06.37-●
    elbow M06.32-●
    foot joint M06.37-●
    hand joint M06.34-●

Nodule(s), nodular *(Continued)*
  rheumatoid *(Continued)*
    hip M06.35-●
    knee M06.36-●
    multiple site M06.39
    shoulder M06.31-●
    vertebra M06.38
    wrist M06.33-●
  scrotum (inflammatory) N49.2
  singer's J38.2
  solitary, lung (subsegmental branch of the
    bronchial tree) R91.1
    multiple R91.8
  subcutaneous —*see* Swelling, localized
  teacher's J38.2
  thyroid (cold) (gland) (nontoxic) E04.1
    with thyrotoxicosis E05.20
      with thyroid storm E05.21
    toxic or with hyperthyroidism E05.20
      with thyroid storm E05.21
  vocal cord J38.2
Noma (gangrenous) (hospital) (infective)
  A69.0
  auricle I96
  mouth A69.0
  pudendi N76.89
  vulvae N76.89
➡ **Nomad, nomadism** Z59.00
NOMID (neonatal onset multisystemic
  inflammatory disorder) M04.2
Nonadherence to medical treatment Z91.19
Nonautoimmune hemolytic anemia D59.4
  drug-induced D59.2
Nonclosure —*see also* Imperfect, closure
  ductus arteriosus (Botallo's) Q25.0
  foramen
    botalli Q21.1
    ovale Q21.1
Noncompliance Z91.19
  with
    dialysis Z91.15
    dietary regimen Z91.11
    medical treatment Z91.19
    medication regimen NEC Z91.14
      underdosing —*see also* Table of Drugs
        and Chemicals, categories T36-T50,
        with final character 6 Z91.14
        intentional NEC Z91.128
          due to financial hardship of patient
            Z91.120
        unintentional NEC Z91.138
          due to patient's age related debility
            Z91.130
    renal dialysis Z91.15
Nondescent (congenital) —*see also* Malposition,
  congenital
  cecum Q43.3
  colon Q43.3

Nondescent *(Continued)*
  testicle Q53.9
    bilateral Q53.20
      abdominal Q53.211
      perineal Q53.22
    unilateral Q53.10
      abdominal Q53.111
      perineal Q53.12
Nondevelopment
  brain Q02
    part of Q04.3
  heart Q24.8
  organ or site, congenital NEC —*see*
    Hypoplasia
Nonengagement
  head NEC O32.4
    in labor, causing obstructed labor
      O64.8
Nonexanthematous tick fever A93.2
Nonexpansion, lung (newborn) P28.0
Nonfunctioning
  cystic duct —*see also* Disease, gallbladder
    K82.8
  gallbladder —*see also* Disease, gallbladder
    K82.8
  kidney N28.9
  labyrinth —*see* subcategory H83.2
Non-Hodgkin lymphoma NEC —*see*
  Lymphoma, non-Hodgkin
Nonimplantation, ovum N97.2
Noninsufflation, fallopian tube N97.1
Non-ketotic hyperglycinemia E72.51
Nonne-Milroy syndrome Q82.0
Nonovulation N97.0
Non-palpable testicle(s)
  bilateral R39.84
  unilateral R39.83
Nonpatent fallopian tube N97.1
Nonpneumatization, lung NEC P28.0
Nonrotation —*see* Malrotation
Nonsecretion, urine —*see* Anuria
Nonunion
  fracture —*see* Fracture, by site
  joint, following fusion or arthrodesis
    M96.0
  organ or site, congenital NEC —*see*
    Imperfect, closure
  symphysis pubis, congenital Q74.2
Nonvisualization, gallbladder R93.2
Nonvital, nonvitalized tooth K04.99
Non-working side interference
  M26.56
Noonan's syndrome Q87.19
Normocytic anemia (infectional) due to
  blood loss (chronic) D50.0
  acute D62
Norrie's disease (congenital) Q15.8
North American blastomycosis B40.9

Norwegian itch B86
Nose, nasal —*see* condition
Nosebleed R04.0
Nose-picking F98.8
Nosomania F45.21
Nosophobia F45.22
Nostalgia F43.20
Notch of iris Q13.2
Notching nose, congenital (tip)
  Q30.2
Nothnagel's
  syndrome —*see* Strabismus, paralytic, third
    nerve
  vasomotor acroparesthesia I73.89
Novy's relapsing fever A68.9
  louse-borne A68.0
  tick-borne A68.1
Noxious
  foodstuffs, poisoning by —*see* Poisoning,
    food, noxious, plant
  substances transmitted through placenta or
    breast milk P04.9
Nucleus pulposus —*see* condition
Numbness R20.0
Nuns' knee —*see* Bursitis, prepatellar
Nursemaid's elbow S53.03-●
Nutcracker esophagus K22.4
Nutmeg liver K76.1
Nutrient element deficiency E61.9
  specified NEC E61.8
Nutrition deficient or insufficient —*see also*
  Malnutrition E46
  due to
    insufficient food T73.0
    lack of
      care (child) T76.02
        adult T76.01
      food T73.0
Nutritional stunting E45
Nyctalopia (night blindness) —*see* Blindness,
  night
Nycturia R35.1
  psychogenic F45.8
Nymphomania F52.8
Nystagmus H55.00
  benign paroxysmal —*see* Vertigo, benign
    paroxysmal
  central positional H81.4
  congenital H55.01
  dissociated H55.04
  latent H55.02
  miners' H55.09
  positional
    benign paroxysmal H81.4
    central H81.4
  specified form NEC H55.09
  visual deprivation H55.03

▶ New   ➡ Revised   ~~deleted~~ Deleted   ● Use Additional Character(s)

O

Obermeyer's relapsing fever (European)
    A68.0
Obesity E66.9
  with alveolar hypoventilation E66.2
  adrenal E27.8
  complicating
    childbirth O99.214
    pregnancy O99.21-●
    puerperium O99.215
  constitutional E66.8
  dietary counseling and surveillance Z71.3
  drug-induced E66.1
  due to
    drug E66.1
    excess calories E66.09
      morbid E66.01
      severe E66.01
  endocrine E66.8
  endogenous E66.8
  exogenous E66.09
  familial E66.8
  glandular E66.8
  hypothyroid —see Hypothyroidism
  hypoventilation syndrome (OHS)
    E66.2
  morbid E66.01
    with
      alveolar hypoventilation E66.2
      obesity hypoventilation syndrome
        (OHS) E66.2
    due to excess calories E66.01
  nutritional E66.09
  pituitary E23.6
  severe E66.01
  specified type NEC E66.8
Oblique —see condition
Obliteration
  appendix (lumen) K38.8
  artery I77.1
  bile duct (noncalculous) K83.1
  common duct (noncalculous) K83.1
  cystic duct —see Obstruction, gallbladder
  disease, arteriolar I77.1
  endometrium N85.8
  eye, anterior chamber —see Disorder, globe,
    hypotony
  fallopian tube N97.1
  lymphatic vessel I89.0
    due to mastectomy I97.2
  organ or site, congenital NEC —see Atresia,
    by site
  ureter N13.5
    with infection N13.6
  urethra —see Stricture, urethra
  vein I87.8
  vestibule (oral) K08.89
Observation (following) (for) (without need for
    further medical care) Z04.9
  accident NEC Z04.3
    at work Z04.2
    transport Z04.1
  adverse effect of drug Z03.6
  alleged rape or sexual assault (victim),
    ruled out
    adult Z04.41
    child Z04.42
  criminal assault Z04.89
  development state
    adolescent Z00.3
    period of rapid growth in childhood Z00.2
    puberty Z00.3
  disease, specified NEC Z03.89
  following work accident Z04.2
  forced sexual exploitation Z04.81
  forced labor exploitation Z04.82
  growth and development state —see
    Observation, development state
  injuries (accidental) NEC —see also
    Observation, accident

Observation (Continued)
  newborn (for)
    suspected condition, related to exposure
      from the mother or birth process —
      see Newborn, affected by, maternal
    ruled out Z05.9
      cardiac Z05.0
      connective tissue Z05.73
      gastrointestinal Z05.5
      genetic Z05.41
      genitourinary Z05.6
      immunologic Z05.43
      infectious Z05.1
      metabolic Z05.42
      musculoskeletal Z05.72
      neurological Z05.2
      respiratory Z05.3
      skin and subcutaneous tissue Z05.71
      specified condition NEC Z05.8
  postpartum
    immediately after delivery Z39.0
    routine follow-up Z39.2
  pregnancy (normal) (without complication)
    Z34.9-●
    high risk O09.9-●
  suicide attempt, alleged NEC Z03.89
    self-poisoning Z03.6
  suspected, ruled out —see also Suspected
    condition, ruled out
    abuse, physical
      adult Z04.71
      child Z04.72
    accident at work Z04.2
    adult battering victim Z04.71
    child battering victim Z04.72
    condition NEC Z03.89
      newborn —see also Observation,
        newborn (for), suspected condition,
        ruled out Z05.9
    drug poisoning or adverse effect Z03.6
    exposure (to)
      anthrax Z03.810
      biological agent NEC Z03.818
    foreign body
      aspirated (inhaled) Z03.822
      ingested Z03.821
      inserted (injected), in (eye) (orifice)
        (skin) Z03.823
    inflicted injury NEC Z04.89
    suicide attempt, alleged Z03.89
      self-poisoning Z03.6
    toxic effects from ingested substance (drug)
      (poison) Z03.6
  toxic effects from ingested substance (drug)
    (poison) Z03.6
Obsession, obsessional state F42.8
  mixed thoughts and acts F42.2
Obsessive-compulsive neurosis or reaction
  F42.8
Obstetric embolism, septic —see Embolism,
  obstetric, septic
Obstetrical trauma (complicating delivery)
  O71.9
  with or following ectopic or molar pregnancy
    O08.6
  specified type NEC O71.89
Obstipation —see Constipation
Obstruction, obstructed, obstructive
  airway J98.8
    with
      allergic alveolitis J67.9
      asthma J45.909
        with
          exacerbation (acute) J45.901
          status asthmaticus J45.902
      bronchiectasis J47.9
        with
          exacerbation (acute) J47.1
          lower respiratory infection J47.0
      bronchitis (chronic) J44.9
      emphysema J43.9

Obstruction, obstructed, obstructive
  (Continued)
  airway (Continued)
    chronic J44.9
      with
        allergic alveolitis —see Pneumonitis,
          hypersensitivity
        bronchiectasis J47.9
          with
            exacerbation (acute) J47.1
            lower respiratory infection J47.0
      due to
        foreign body —see Foreign body, by site,
          causing asphyxia
        inhalation of fumes or vapors J68.9
        laryngospasm J38.5
  ampulla of Vater K83.1
  aortic (heart) (valve) —see Stenosis, aortic
  aortoiliac I74.09
  aqueduct of Sylvius G91.1
    congenital Q03.0
      with spina bifida —see Spina bifida, by
        site, with hydrocephalus
  Arnold-Chiari —see Arnold-Chiari disease
  artery (see also Atherosclerosis, artery) I70.9
    basilar (complete) (partial) —see Occlusion,
      artery, basilar
    carotid (complete) (partial) —see Occlusion,
      artery, carotid
    cerebellar —see Occlusion, artery, cerebellar
    cerebral (anterior) (middle) (posterior) —
      see Occlusion, artery, cerebral
    precerebral —see Occlusion, artery,
      precerebral
    renal N28.0
    retinal NEC —see Occlusion, artery, retina
    stent —see Restenosis, stent
    vertebral (complete) (partial) —see
      Occlusion, artery, vertebral
  band (intestinal) —see also Obstruction,
    intestine, specified NEC K56.699
  bile duct or passage (common) (hepatic)
    (noncalculous) K83.1
    with calculus K80.51
    congenital (causing jaundice) Q44.3
  biliary (duct) (tract) K83.1
    gallbladder K82.0
  bladder-neck (acquired) N32.0
    congenital Q64.31
    due to hyperplasia (hypertrophy) of
      prostate —see Hyperplasia, prostate
  bowel —see Obstruction, intestine
  bronchus J98.09
  canal, ear —see Stenosis, external ear canal
  cardia K22.2
  caval veins (inferior) (superior) I87.1
  cecum —see Obstruction, intestine
  circulatory I99.8
  colon —see Obstruction, intestine
  common duct (noncalculous) K83.1
  coronary (artery) —see Occlusion, coronary
  cystic duct —see also Obstruction, gallbladder
    with calculus K80.21
  device, implant or graft —see also
    Complications, by site and type,
    mechanical T85.698
    arterial graft NEC —see Complication,
      cardiovascular device, mechanical,
      vascular
    catheter NEC T85.628
      cystostomy T83.090
      dialysis (renal) T82.49
        intraperitoneal T85.691
      Hopkins T83.098
      ileostomy T83.098
      infusion NEC T82.594
        spinal (epidural) (subdural) T85.690
      nephrostomy T83.092
      urethral indwelling T83.091
      urinary T83.098
      urostomy T83.098

Obstruction, obstructed, obstructive
(Continued)
device, implant or graft (Continued)
due to infection T85.79
gastrointestinal —see Complications,
prosthetic device, mechanical,
gastrointestinal device
genital NEC T83.498
intrauterine contraceptive device T83.39
penile prosthesis (cylinder) (implanted)
(pump) (resevoir) T83.490
testicular prosthesis T83.491
heart NEC —see Complication,
cardiovascular device, mechanical
joint prosthesis —see Complications, joint
prosthesis, mechanical, specified NEC,
by site
orthopedic NEC —see Complication,
orthopedic, device, mechanical
specified NEC T85.628
urinary NEC —see also Complication,
genitourinary, device, urinary,
mechanical
graft T83.29
vascular NEC —see Complication,
cardiovascular device, mechanical
ventricular intracranial shunt T85.09
due to foreign body accidentally left in
operative wound T81.529
duodenum K31.5
ejaculatory duct N50.89
esophagus K22.2
eustachian tube (complete) (partial) H68.10-●
cartilagenous (extrinsic) H68.13-●
intrinsic H68.12-●
osseous H68.11-●
fallopian tube (bilateral) N97.1
fecal K56.41
with hernia —see Hernia, by site, with
obstruction
foramen of Monro (congenital) Q03.8
with spina bifida —see Spina bifida,
by site, with hydrocephalus
foreign body —see Foreign body
gallbladder K82.0
with calculus, stones K80.21
congenital Q44.1
gastric outlet K31.1
gastrointestinal —see Obstruction, intestine
hepatic K76.89
duct (noncalculous) K83.1
hepatobiliary K83.1
ileum —see Obstruction, intestine
iliofemoral (artery) I74.5
intestine K56.609
complete K56.601
incomplete K56.600
partial K56.600
with
adhesions (intestinal) (peritoneal) K56.50
complete K56.52
incomplete K56.51
partial K56.51
adynamic K56.0
by gallstone K56.3
congenital (small) Q41.9
large Q42.9
specified part NEC Q42.8
neurogenic K56.0
Hirschsprung's disease or megacolon
Q43.1
newborn P76.9
due to
fecaliths P76.8
inspissated milk P76.2
meconium (plug) P76.0
in mucoviscidosis E84.11
specified NEC P76.8
postoperative K91.30
complete K91.32
incomplete K91.31
partial K91.31

Obstruction, obstructed, obstructive
(Continued)
intestine (Continued)
reflex K56.0
specified NEC K56.699
complete K56.691
incomplete K56.690
partial K56.690
volvulus K56.2
intracardiac ball valve prosthesis T82.09
jejunum —see Obstruction, intestine
joint prosthesis —see Complications, joint
prosthesis, mechanical, specified NEC,
by site
⇒ kidney (calices) (see also Hydronephrosis)
N28.89
labor —see Delivery
lacrimal (passages) (duct)
by
dacryolith —see Dacryolith
stenosis —see Stenosis, lacrimal
congenital Q10.5
neonatal H04.53-●
lacrimonasal duct —see Obstruction, lacrimal
lacteal, with steatorrhea K90.2
laryngitis —see Laryngitis
larynx NEC J38.6
congenital Q31.8
lung J98.4
disease, chronic J44.9
lymphatic I89.0
meconium (plug)
newborn P76.0
due to fecaliths P76.0
in mucoviscidosis E84.11
mitral —see Stenosis, mitral
nasal J34.89
nasolacrimal duct —see also Obstruction,
lacrimal
congenital Q10.5
nasopharynx J39.2
nose J34.89
organ or site, congenital NEC —see Atresia,
by site
pancreatic duct K86.89
parotid duct or gland K11.8
pelviureteral junction N13.5
with hydronephrosis N13.0
congenital Q62.39
pharynx J39.2
portal (circulation) (vein) I81
prostate —see also Hyperplasia, prostate
valve (urinary) N32.0
pulmonary valve (heart) I37.0
pyelonephritis (chronic) N11.1
pylorus
adult K31.1
congenital or infantile Q40.0
rectosigmoid —see Obstruction, intestine
rectum K62.4
⇒ renal (see also Hydronephrosis) N28.89
outflow N13.8
pelvis, congenital Q62.39
respiratory J98.8
chronic J44.9
retinal (vessels) H34.9
salivary duct (any) K11.8
with calculus K11.5
sigmoid —see Obstruction, intestine
sinus (accessory) (nasal) J34.89
Stensen's duct K11.8
stomach NEC K31.89
acute K31.0
congenital Q40.2
due to pylorospasm K31.3
submandibular duct K11.8
submaxillary gland K11.8
with calculus K11.5
thoracic duct I89.0
thrombotic —see Thrombosis
trachea J39.8

Obstruction, obstructed, obstructive
(Continued)
tracheostomy airway J95.03
tricuspid (valve) —see Stenosis, tricuspid
upper respiratory, congenital Q34.8
ureter (functional) (pelvic junction) NEC N13.5
with
hydronephrosis N13.1
with infection N13.6
▶ congenital Q62.39
pyelonephritis (chronic) N11.1
congenital Q62.39
due to calculus —see Calculus, ureter
urethra NEC N36.8
congenital Q64.39
urinary (moderate) N13.9
due to hyperplasia (hypertrophy) of
prostate —see Hyperplasia, prostate
organ or tract (lower) N13.9
prostatic valve N32.0
specified NEC N13.8
uropathy N13.9
uterus N85.8
vagina N89.5
valvular —see Endocarditis
vein, venous I87.1
caval (inferior) (superior) I87.1
thrombotic —see Thrombosis
vena cava (inferior) (superior) I87.1
vesical NEC N32.0
vesicourethral orifice N32.0
congenital Q64.31
vessel NEC I99.8
stent —see Restenosis, stent
Obturator —see condition
Occlusal wear, teeth K03.0
Occlusio pupillae —see Membrane, pupillary
Occlusion, occluded
anus K62.4
congenital Q42.3
with fistula Q42.2
aortoiliac (chronic) I74.09
aqueduct of Sylvius G91.1
congenital Q03.0
with spina bifida —see Spina bifida, by
site, with hydrocephalus
artery —see also Atherosclerosis, artery I70.9
auditory, internal I65.8
basilar I65.1
with
infarction I63.22
due to
embolism I63.12
thrombosis I63.02
brain or cerebral I66.9
with infarction (due to) I63.5-●
embolism I63.4-●
thrombosis I63.3-●
carotid I65.2-●
with
infarction I63.23-●
due to
embolism I63.13-●
thrombosis I63.03-●
cerebellar (anterior inferior) (posterior
inferior) (superior) I66.3
with infarction I63.54-●
due to
embolism I63.44-●
thrombosis I63.34-●
cerebral I66.9
with infarction I63.50
due to
embolism I63.40
specified NEC I63.49
thrombosis I63.30
specified NEC I63.39
anterior I66.1-●
with infarction I63.52-●
due to
embolism I63.42-●
thrombosis I63.32-●

Occlusion, occluded *(Continued)*
  artery *(Continued)*
    cerebral *(Continued)*
      middle I66.0-●
        with infarction I63.51-●
          due to
            embolism I63.41-●
            thrombosis I63.31-●
      posterior I66.2-●
        with infarction I63.53-●
          due to
            embolism I63.43-●
            thrombosis I63.33-●
      specified NEC I66.8
        with infarction I63.59
          due to
            embolism I63.4-●
            thrombosis I63.3-●
    choroidal (anterior) —*see* Occlusion,
      artery, cerebral, specified NEC
    communicating posterior —*see* Occlusion,
      artery, precerebral, specified NEC
    complete
      coronary I25.82
      extremities I70.92
    coronary (acute) (thrombotic) (without
      myocardial infarction) I24.0
      with myocardial infarction —*see*
        Infarction, myocardium
      chronic total I25.82
      complete I25.82
      healed or old I25.2
      total (chronic) I25.82
    hypophyseal —*see* Occlusion, artery,
      precerebral, specified NEC
    iliac I74.5
    lower extremities due to stenosis or
      stricture I77.1
    mesenteric (embolic) (thrombotic) —*see also*
      Infarct, intestine K55.069
    perforating —*see* Occlusion, artery,
      cerebral, specified NEC
    peripheral I77.9
      thrombotic or embolic I74.4
    pontine —*see* Occlusion, artery, precerebral,
      specified NEC
    precerebral I65.9
      with infarction I63.20
        due to
          embolism I63.10
            specified NEC I63.19
          thrombosis I63.00
            specified NEC I63.09
          specified NEC I63.29
      basilar —*see* Occlusion, artery, basilar
      carotid —*see* Occlusion, artery, carotid
      puerperal O88.23
      specified NEC I65.8
        with infarction I63.29
          due to
            embolism I63.19
            thrombosis I63.09
      vertebral —*see* Occlusion, artery,
        vertebral
    renal N28.0
    retinal
      branch H34.23-●
      central H34.1-●
      partial H34.21-●
      transient H34.0-●
    spinal —*see* Occlusion, artery, precerebral,
      vertebral
    total (chronic)
      coronary I25.82
      extremities I70.92
    vertebral I65.0-●
      with
        infarction I63.21-●
          due to
            embolism I63.11-●
            thrombosis I63.01-●

Occlusion, occluded *(Continued)*
    basilar artery —*see* Occlusion, artery, basilar
    bile duct (common) (hepatic) (noncalculous)
      K83.1
    bowel —*see* Obstruction, intestine
    carotid (artery) (common) (internal) —*see*
      Occlusion, artery, carotid
    centric (of teeth) M26.59
      maximum intercuspation discrepancy
        M26.55
    cerebellar (artery) —*see* Occlusion, artery,
      cerebellar
    cerebral (artery) —*see* Occlusion, artery,
      cerebral
    cerebrovascular —*see also* Occlusion, artery,
      cerebral
      with infarction I63.5-●
    cervical canal —*see* Stricture, cervix
    cervix (uteri) —*see* Stricture, cervix
    choanal Q30.0
    choroidal (artery) —*see* Occlusion, artery,
      precerebral, specified NEC
    colon —*see* Obstruction, intestine
    communicating posterior artery —*see*
      Occlusion, artery, precerebral, specified
      NEC
    coronary (artery) (vein) (thrombotic) —*see*
      also Infarct, myocardium
      chronic total I25.82
      healed or old I25.2
      not resulting in infarction I24.0
      total (chronic) I25.82
    cystic duct —*see* Obstruction, gallbladder
    embolic —*see* Embolism
    fallopian tube N97.1
      congenital Q50.6
    gallbladder —*see also* Obstruction,
      gallbladder
      congenital (causing jaundice) Q44.1
    gingiva, traumatic K06.2
    hymen N89.6
      congenital Q52.3
    hypophyseal (artery) —*see* Occlusion, artery,
      precerebral, specified NEC
    iliac artery I74.5
    intestine —*see* Obstruction, intestine
    lacrimal passages —*see* Obstruction, lacrimal
    lung J98.4
    lymph or lymphatic channel I89.0
    mammary duct N64.89
    mesenteric artery (embolic) (thrombotic) —
      see also Infarct, intestine K55.069
    nose J34.89
      congenital Q30.0
    organ or site, congenital NEC —*see* Atresia,
      by site
    oviduct N97.1
      congenital Q50.6
    peripheral arteries
      due to stricture or stenosis I77.1
      upper extremity I74.2
    pontine (artery) —*see* Occlusion, artery,
      precerebral, specified NEC
    posterior lingual, of mandibular teeth M26.29
    precerebral artery —*see* Occlusion, artery,
      precerebral
    punctum lacrimale —*see* Obstruction,
      lacrimal
    pupil —*see* Membrane, pupillary
    pylorus, adult —*see also* Stricture, pylorus
      K31.1
    renal artery N28.0
    retina, retinal
      artery —*see* Occlusion, artery, retinal
      vein (central) H34.81-●
        engorgement H34.82-●
        tributary H34.83-●
        vessels H34.9
    spinal artery —*see* Occlusion, artery,
      precerebral, vertebral
    teeth (mandibular) (posterior lingual) M26.29

Occlusion, occluded *(Continued)*
    thoracic duct I89.0
    thrombotic —*see* Thrombosis, artery
    traumatic
      edentulous (alveolar) ridge K06.2
      gingiva K06.2
      periodontal K05.5
    tubal N97.1
    ureter (complete) (partial) N13.5
      congenital Q62.10
    ureteropelvic junction N13.5
      congenital Q62.11
    ureterovesical orifice N13.5
      congenital Q62.12
    urethra —*see* Stricture, urethra
    uterus N85.8
    vagina N89.5
    vascular NEC I99.8
    vein —*see* Thrombosis
      retinal —*see* Occlusion, retinal, vein
    vena cava (inferior) (superior) —*see*
      Embolism, vena cava
    ventricle (brain) NEC G91.1
    vertebral (artery) —*see* Occlusion, artery,
      vertebral
    vessel (blood) I99.8
    vulva N90.5
Occult
  blood in feces (stools) R19.5
Occupational
  problems NEC Z56.89
Ochlophobia —*see* Agoraphobia
Ochronosis (endogenous) E70.29
Ocular muscle —*see* condition
Oculogyric crisis or disturbance H51.8
  psychogenic F45.8
Oculomotor syndrome H51.9
Oculopathy
  syphilitic NEC A52.71
    congenital
      early A50.01
      late A50.30
    early (secondary) A51.43
    late A52.71
Oddi's sphincter spasm K83.4
Odontalgia K08.89
Odontoameloblastoma —*see* Cyst, calcifying
  odontogenic
Odontoclasia K03.89
Odontodysplasia, regional K00.4
Odontogenesis imperfecta K00.5
Odontoma (ameloblastic) (complex)
  (compound) (fibroameloblastic) —*see* Cyst,
  calcifying odontogenic
Odontomyelitis (closed) (open) K04.01
  irreversible K04.02
  reversible K04.01
Odontorrhagia K08.89
Odontosarcoma, ameloblastic C41.1
  upper jaw (bone) C41.0
Oestriasis —*see* Myiasis
Oguchi's disease H53.63
Ohara's disease —*see* Tularemia
OHS (obesity hypoventilation syndrome) E66.2

Oidiomycosis —*see* Candidiasis
Oidium albicans infection —*see* Candidiasis
Old (previous) myocardial infarction
  I25.2
Old age (without mention of debility) R54-●
  dementia F03
Olfactory —*see* condition
Oligemia —*see* Anemia
Oligoastrocytoma
  specified site —*see* Neoplasm, malignant,
    by site
  unspecified site C71.9
Oligocythemia D64.9
Oligodendroblastoma
  specified site —*see* Neoplasm, malignant
  unspecified site C71.9

Oligodendroglioma
  anaplastic type
    specified site —*see* Neoplasm, malignant,
      by site
    unspecified site C71.9
  specified site —*see* Neoplasm, malignant,
    by site
  unspecified site C71.9
Oligodontia —*see* Anodontia
Oligoencephalon Q02
Oligohidrosis L74.4
Oligohydramnios O41.0-●
Oligohydrosis L74.4
Oligomenorrhea N91.5
  primary N91.3
  secondary N91.4
Oligophrenia —*see also* Disability, intellectual
  phenylpyruvic E70.0
Oligospermia N46.11
  due to
    drug therapy N46.121
    efferent duct obstruction N46.123
    infection N46.122
    radiation N46.124
    specified cause NEC N46.129
    systemic disease N46.125
Oligotrichia —*see* Alopecia
Oliguria R34
  with, complicating or following ectopic or
    molar pregnancy O08.4
  postprocedural N99.0
Ollier's disease Q78.4
Omenotocele —*see* Hernia, abdomen, specified
    site NEC
Omentitis —*see* Peritonitis
Omentum, omental —*see* condition
Omphalitis (congenital) (newborn) P38.9
  with mild hemorrhage P38.1
  without hemorrhage P38.9
  not of newborn L08.82
  tetanus A33
Omphalocele Q79.2
Omphalomesenteric duct, persistent Q43.0
Omphalorrhagia, newborn P51.9
Omsk hemorrhagic fever A98.1
Onanism (excessive) F98.8
Onchocerciasis, onchocercosis B73.1
  with
    eye disease B73.00
      endophthalmitis B73.01
      eyelid B73.09
      glaucoma B73.02
      specified NEC B73.09
    eye NEC B73.00
    eyelid B73.09
Oncocytoma —*see* Neoplasm, benign, by site
Oncovirus, as cause of disease classified
    elsewhere B97.32
Ondine's curse —*see* Apnea, sleep
Oneirophrenia F23
Onychauxis L60.2
  congenital Q84.5
Onychia —*see also* Cellulitis, digit
  with lymphangitis —*see* Lymphangitis, acute,
    digit
  candidal B37.2
  dermatophytic B35.1
Onychitis —*see also* Cellulitis, digit
  with lymphangitis —*see* Lymphangitis, acute,
    digit
Onychocryptosis L60.0
Onychodystrophy L60.3
  congenital Q84.6
Onychogryphosis, onychogryposis L60.2
Onycholysis L60.1
Onychomadesis L60.8
Onychomalacia L60.3
Onychomycosis (finger) (toe) B35.1
Onycho-osteodysplasia Q87.2
Onychophagia F98.8
Onychophosis L60.8

Onychoptosis L60.8
Onychorrhexis L60.3
  congenital Q84.6
Onychoschizia L60.3
Onyxis (finger) (toe) L60.0
Onyxitis —*see also* Cellulitis, digit
  with lymphangitis —*see* Lymphangitis, acute,
    digit
Oophoritis (cystic) (infectional) (interstitial)
    N70.92
  with salpingitis N70.93
  acute N70.02
    with salpingitis N70.03
  chronic N70.12
    with salpingitis N70.13
  complicating abortion —*see* Abortion, by
    type, complicated by, oophoritis
Oophorocele N83.4-●
Opacity, opacities
  cornea H17.-●
    central H17.1-●
    congenital Q13.3
    degenerative —*see* Degeneration, cornea
    hereditary —*see* Dystrophy, cornea
    inflammatory —*see* Keratitis
    minor H17.81-●
    peripheral H17.82-●
    sequelae of trachoma (healed) B94.0
    specified NEC H17.89
  enamel (teeth) (fluoride) (nonfluoride) K00.3
  lens —*see* Cataract
  snowball —*see* Deposit, crystalline
  vitreous (humor) NEC H43.39-●
    congenital Q14.0
    membranes and strands H43.31-●
Opalescent dentin (hereditary) K00.5
Open, opening
  abnormal, organ or site, congenital —*see*
    Imperfect, closure
  angle with
    borderline
      findings
        high risk H40.02-●
        low risk H40.01-●
      intraocular pressure H40.00-●
    cupping of discs H40.01-●
    glaucoma (primary) —*see* Glaucoma, open
      angle
  bite
    anterior M26.220
    posterior M26.221
  false —*see* Imperfect, closure
  margin on tooth restoration K08.51
  restoration margins of tooth K08.51
  wound —*see* Wound, open
Operational fatigue F48.8
Operative —*see* condition
Operculitis —*see* Periodontitis
Operculum —*see* Break, retina
Ophiasis L63.2
Ophthalmia —*see also* Conjunctivitis H10.9
  actinic rays —*see* Photokeratitis
  allergic (acute) —*see* Conjunctivitis, acute,
    atopic
  blennorrhagic (gonococcal) (neonatorum)
    A54.31
  diphtheritic A36.86
  Egyptian A71.1
  electrica —*see* Photokeratitis
  gonococcal (neonatorum) A54.31
  metastatic —*see* Endophthalmitis, purulent
  migraine —*see* Migraine, ophthalmoplegic
  neonatorum, newborn P39.1
    gonococcal A54.31
  nodosa H16.24-●
  purulent —*see* Conjunctivitis, acute,
    mucopurulent
  spring —*see* Conjunctivitis, acute, atopic
  sympathetic —*see* Uveitis, sympathetic
Ophthalmitis —*see* Ophthalmia
Ophthalmocele (congenital) Q15.8

Ophthalmoneuromyelitis G36.0
Ophthalmoplegia —*see also* Strabismus, paralytic
  anterior internuclear —*see* Ophthalmoplegia,
    internuclear
  ataxia-areflexia G61.0
  diabetic —*see* E08-E13 with .39
  exophthalmic E05.00
    with thyroid storm E05.01
  external H49.88-●
    progressive H49.4-●
      with pigmentary retinopathy —*see*
        Kearns-Sayre syndrome
    total H49.3-●
  internal (complete) (total) H52.51-●
  internuclear H51.2-●
  migraine —*see* Migraine, ophthalmoplegic
  Parinaud's H49.88-●
  progressive external —*see* Ophthalmoplegia,
    external, progressive
  supranuclear, progressive G23.1
  total (external) —*see* Ophthalmoplegia,
    external, total
Opioid(s)
  abuse —*see* Abuse, drug, opioids
  dependence —*see* Dependence, drug, opioids
  induced, without use disorder
    anxiety disorder F11.988
    delirium F11.921
    depressive disorder F11.94
    sexual dysfunction F11.981
    sleep disorder F11.982
Opisthognathism M26.09
Opisthorchiasis (felineus) (viverrini) B66.0
Opitz' disease D73.2
Opiumism —*see* Dependence, drug, opioid
Oppenheim's disease G70.2
Oppenheim-Urbach disease (necrobiosis
    lipoidica diabeticorum) —*see* E08-E13 with
    .620
Optic nerve —*see* condition
Orbit —*see* condition
Orchioblastoma C62.9-●
Orchitis (gangrenous) (nonspecific) (septic)
    (suppurative) N45.2
  blennorrhagic (gonococcal) (acute) (chronic)
    A54.23
  chlamydial A56.19
  filarial —*see also* Infestation, filarial B74.9
    [N51]
  gonococcal (acute) (chronic) A54.23
  mumps B26.0
  syphilitic A52.76
  tuberculous A18.15
Orf (virus disease) B08.02
Organic —*see also* condition
  brain syndrome F09
  heart —*see* Disease, heart
  mental disorder F09
  psychosis F09
Orgasm
  anejaculatory N53.13
Oriental
  bilharziasis B65.2
  schistosomiasis B65.2
Orifice —*see* condition
Origin of both great vessels from right
    ventricle Q20.1
Ormond's disease (with ureteral obstruction)
    N13.5
  with infection N13.6
Ornithine metabolism disorder E72.4
Ornithinemia (Type I) (Type II) E72.4
Ornithosis A70
Orotaciduria, oroticaciduria (congenital)
    (hereditary) (pyrimidine deficiency) E79.8
  anemia D53.0
Orthodontics
  adjustment Z46.4
  fitting Z46.4
Orthopnea R06.01
Orthopoxvirus B08.09

Os, uterus —*see* condition
Osgood-Schlatter disease or osteochondrosis M92.52-●
Osler (-Weber)-Rendu disease I78.0
Osler's nodes I33.0
Osmidrosis L75.0
Osseous —*see* condition
Ossification
  artery —*see* Arteriosclerosis
  auricle (ear) —*see* Disorder, pinna, specified type NEC
  bronchial J98.09
  cardiac —*see* Degeneration, myocardial
  cartilage (senile) —*see* Disorder, cartilage, specified type NEC
  coronary (artery) —*see* Disease, heart, ischemic, atherosclerotic
  diaphragm J98.6
  ear, middle —*see* Otosclerosis
  falx cerebri G96.198
  fontanel, premature Q75.0
  heart —*see also* Degeneration, myocardial
    valve —*see* Endocarditis
  larynx J38.7
  ligament —*see* Disorder, tendon, specified type NEC
    posterior longitudinal —*see* Spondylopathy, specified NEC
  meninges (cerebral) (spinal) G96.198
  multiple, eccentric centers —*see* Disorder, bone, development or growth
  muscle —*see also* Calcification, muscle
    due to burns —*see* Myositis, ossificans, in, burns
    paralytic —*see* Myositis, ossificans, in, quadriplegia
    progressive —*see* Myositis, ossificans, progressiva
    specified NEC M61.50
      ankle M61.57-●
      foot M61.57-●
      forearm M61.53-●
      hand M61.54-●
      lower leg M61.56-●
      multiple sites M61.59
      pelvic region M61.55-●
      shoulder region M61.51-●
      specified site NEC M61.58
      thigh M61.55-●
      upper arm M61.52-●
    traumatic —*see* Myositis, ossificans, traumatica
  myocardium, myocardial —*see* Degeneration, myocardial
  penis N48.89
  periarticular —*see* Disorder, joint, specified type NEC
  pinna —*see* Disorder, pinna, specified type NEC
  rider's bone —*see* Ossification, muscle, specified NEC
  sclera H15.89
  subperiosteal, post-traumatic M89.8X-●
  tendon —*see* Disorder, tendon, specified type NEC
  trachea J39.8
  tympanic membrane —*see* Disorder, tympanic membrane, specified NEC
  vitreous (humor) —*see* Deposit, crystalline
Osteitis —*see also* Osteomyelitis
  alveolar M27.3
  condensans M85.30
    ankle M85.37-●
    foot M85.37-●
    forearm M85.33-●
    hand M85.34-●
    lower leg M85.36-●
    multiple site M85.39
    neck M85.38
    rib M85.38
    shoulder M85.31-●

Osteitis (Continued)
  condensans (Continued)
    skull M85.38
    specified site NEC M85.38
    thigh M85.35-●
    toe M85.37-●
    upper arm M85.32-●
    vertebra M85.38
  deformans M88.9
    in (due to)
      malignant neoplasm of bone C41.9 [M90.60]
      neoplastic disease —*see also* Neoplasm D49.9 [M90.60]
        carpus D49.9 [M90.64-●]
        clavicle D49.9 [M90.61-●]
        femur D49.9 [M90.65-●]
        fibula D49.9 [M90.66-●]
        finger D49.9 [M90.64-●]
        humerus D49.9 [M90.62-●]
        ilium D49.9 [M90.65-●]
        ischium D49.9 [M90.65-●]
        metacarpus D49.9 [M90.64-●]
        metatarsus D49.9 [M90.67-●]
        multiple sites D49.9 [M90.69]
        neck D49.9 [M90.68]
        radius D49.9 [M90.63-●]
        rib D49.9 [M90.68]
        scapula D49.9 [M90.61-●]
        skull D49.9 [M90.68]
        tarsus D49.9 [M90.67-●]
        tibia D49.9 [M90.66-●]
        toe D49.9 [M90.67-●]
        ulna D49.9 [M90.63-●]
        vertebra D49.9 [M90.68]
    skull M88.0
    specified NEC —*see* Paget's disease, bone, by site
    vertebra M88.1
  due to yaws A66.6
  fibrosa NEC —*see* Cyst, bone, by site
    circumscripta —*see* Dysplasia, fibrous, bone NEC
    cystica (generalisata) E21.0
    disseminata Q78.1
    osteoplastica E21.0
  fragilitans Q78.0
  Garr's (sclerosing) —*see* Osteomyelitis, specified type NEC
  jaw (acute) (chronic) (lower) (suppurative) (upper) M27.2
  parathyroid E21.0
  petrous bone (acute) (chronic) —*see* Petrositis
  sclerotic, nonsuppurative —*see* Osteomyelitis, specified type NEC
  tuberculosa A18.09
    cystica D86.89
    multiplex cystoides D86.89
Osteoarthritis M19.90
  ankle M19.07-●
  elbow M19.02-●
  foot joint M19.07-●
➡ generalized (multiple joints) M15.9
    erosive M15.4
    primary M15.0
    specified NEC M15.8
  hand joint M19.04-●
    first carpometacarpal joint M18.9-●
  hip M16.1-●
    bilateral M16.0
    due to hip dysplasia (unilateral) M16.3-●
      bilateral M16.2
  interphalangeal
    distal (Heberden) M15.1
    proximal (Bouchard) M15.2
  knee M17.1-●
    bilateral M17.0
  post-traumatic NEC M19.92
    ankle M19.17-●
    elbow M19.12-●
    foot joint M19.17-●

Osteoarthritis (Continued)
  post-traumatic NEC (Continued)
    hand joint M19.14-●
      first carpometacarpal joint M18.3-●
        bilateral M18.2
    hip M16.5-●
      bilateral M16.4
    knee M17.3-●
      bilateral M17.2
    shoulder M19.11-●
    specified site NEC M19.19
    wrist M19.13-●
  primary M19.91
    ankle M19.07-●
    elbow M19.02-●
    foot joint M19.07-●
    hand joint M19.04-●
      first carpometacarpal joint M18.1-●
        bilateral M18.0
    hip M16.1-●
      bilateral M16.0
    knee M17.1-●
      bilateral M17.0
➡   multiple sites M15.9
    shoulder M19.01-●
    spine —*see* Spondylosis
    wrist M19.03-●
  secondary M19.93
    ankle M19.27-●
    elbow M19.22-●
    foot joint M19.27-●
    hand joint M19.24-●
      first carpometacarpal joint M18.5-●
        bilateral M18.4
    hip M16.7
      bilateral M16.6
    knee M17.5
      bilateral M17.4
    multiple M15.3
    shoulder M19.21-●
    specified site NEC M19.29
    spine —*see* Spondylosis
    wrist M19.23-●
  shoulder M19.01-●
  specified site NEC M19.09
  spine —*see* Spondylosis
  wrist M19.03-●
Osteoarthropathy (hypertrophic) M19.90
  ankle —*see* Osteoarthritis, primary, ankle
  elbow —*see* Osteoarthritis, primary, elbow
  foot joint —*see* Osteoarthritis, primary, foot
  hand joint —*see* Osteoarthritis, primary, hand joint
  knee joint —*see* Osteoarthritis, primary, knee
  multiple site —*see* Osteoarthritis, primary, multiple joint
  pulmonary —*see also* Osteoarthropathy, specified type NEC
    hypertrophic —*see* Osteoarthropathy, hypertrophic, specified type NEC
  secondary —*see* Osteoarthropathy, specified type NEC
  secondary hypertrophic —*see* Osteoarthropathy, specified type NEC
  shoulder —*see* Osteoarthritis, primary, shoulder
  specified joint NEC —*see* Osteoarthritis, primary, specified joint NEC
  specified type NEC M89.40
    carpus M89.44-●
    clavicle M89.41-●
    femur M89.45-●
    fibula M89.46-●
    finger M89.44-●
    humerus M89.42-●
    ilium M89.459
    ischium M89.459
    metacarpus M89.44-●
    metatarsus M89.47-●
    multiple sites M89.49
    neck M89.48
    radius M89.43-●

Osteoarthropathy (Continued)
  specified type NEC (Continued)
    rib M89.48
    scapula M89.41-●
    skull M89.48
    tarsus M89.47-●
    tibia M89.46-●
    toe M89.47-●
    ulna M89.43-●
    vertebra M89.48
  spine —see Spondylosis
  wrist —see Osteoarthritis, primary, wrist
Osteoarthrosis (degenerative) (hypertrophic)
    (joint) —see also Osteoarthritis
  deformans alkaptonurica E70.29 [M36.8]
  erosive M15.4
  generalized M15.9
    primary M15.0
  polyarticular M15.9
  spine —see Spondylosis
Osteoblastoma —see Neoplasm, bone, benign
  aggressive —see Neoplasm, bone, uncertain
    behavior
Osteochondroarthrosis deformans
    endemica —see Disease, Kaschin-Beck
Osteochondritis —see also Osteochondropathy,
    by site
  Brailsford's —see Osteochondrosis, juvenile,
    radius
  dissecans M93.20
    ankle M93.27-●
    elbow M93.22-●
    foot M93.27-●
    hand M93.24-●
    hip M93.25-●
    knee M93.26-●
    multiple sites M93.29
    shoulder joint M93.21-●
    specified site NEC M93.28
    wrist M93.23-●
  juvenile M92.9
    patellar —see Osteochondrosis, juvenile,
      patella
  syphilitic (congenital) (early) A50.02
    [M90.80]
    ankle A50.02 [M90.87-●]
    elbow A50.02 [M90.82-●]
    foot A50.02 [M90.87-●]
    forearm A50.02 [M90.83-●]
    hand A50.02 [M90.84-●]
    hip A50.02 [M90.85-●]
    knee A50.02 [M90.86●-●]
    multiple sites A50.02 [M90.89]
    shoulder joint A50.02 [M90.81-●]
    specified site NEC A50.02 [M90.88]
Osteochondrodysplasia Q78.9
  with defects of growth of tubular bones and
    spine Q77.9
  specified NEC Q77.8
  specified NEC Q78.8
Osteochondrodystrophy E78.9
Osteochondrolysis —see Osteochondritis,
    dissecans
Osteochondroma —see Neoplasm, bone, benign
Osteochondromatosis D48.0
  syndrome Q78.4
Osteochondromyxosarcoma —see Neoplasm,
    bone, malignant
Osteochondropathy M93.90
  ankle M93.97-●
  elbow M93.92-●
  foot M93.97-●
  hand M93.94-●
  hip M93.95-●
  Kienböck's disease of adults M93.1
  knee M93.96-●
  multiple joints M93.99
  osteochondritis dissecans —see
    Osteochondritis, dissecans
  osteochondrosis —see Osteochondrosis
  shoulder region M93.91-●

Osteochondropathy (Continued)
  slipped upper femoral epiphysis —see
    Slipped, epiphysis, upper femoral
  specified joint NEC M93.98
  specified type NEC M93.80
    ankle M93.87-●
    elbow M93.82-●
    foot M93.87-●
    hand M93.84-●
    hip M93.85-●
    knee M93.86-●
    multiple joints M93.89
    shoulder region M93.81-●
    specified joint NEC M93.88
    wrist M93.83-●
  syphilitic, congenital
    early A50.02 [M90.80]
    late A50.56 [M90.80]
  wrist M93.93-●
Osteochondrosarcoma —see Neoplasm, bone,
    malignant
Osteochondrosis —see also Osteochondropathy,
    by site
  acetabulum (juvenile) M91.0
  adult —see Osteochondropathy, specified
    type NEC, by site
  astragalus (juvenile) —see Osteochondrosis,
    juvenile, tarsus
  ~~Blount's —see Osteochondrosis, juvenile, tibia~~
  Blount M92.51-●
  Buchanan's M91.0
  Burns' —see Osteochondrosis, juvenile, ulna
  calcaneus (juvenile) —see Osteochondrosis,
    juvenile, tarsus
  capitular epiphysis (femur) (juvenile) —see
    Legg-Calvé-Perthes disease
  carpal (juvenile) (lunate) (scaphoid) —see
    Osteochondrosis, juvenile, hand, carpal
    lunate
    adult M93.1
  coxae juvenilis —see Legg-Calvé-Perthes
    disease
  deformans juvenilis, coxae —see Legg-Calvé-
    Perthes disease
  Diaz's —see Osteochondrosis, juvenile, tarsus
  dissecans (knee) (shoulder) —see
    Osteochondritis, dissecans
  femoral capital epiphysis (juvenile) —see
    Legg-Calvé-Perthes disease
  femur (head), juvenile —see Legg-Calvé-
    Perthes disease
  fibula (juvenile) —see Osteochondrosis,
    juvenile, fibula
  foot NEC (juvenile) M92.8
  Freiberg's —see Osteochondrosis, juvenile,
    metatarsus
  Haas' (juvenile) —see Osteochondrosis,
    juvenile, humerus
  Haglund's —see Osteochondrosis, juvenile,
    tarsus
  hip (juvenile) —see Legg-Calvé-Perthes disease
  humerus (capitulum) (head) (juvenile) —see
    Osteochondrosis, juvenile, humerus
  ilium, iliac crest (juvenile) M91.0
  ischiopubic synchondrosis M91.0
  Iselin's —see Osteochondrosis, juvenile,
    metatarsus
  juvenile, juvenilis M92.9
    after congenital dislocation of hip
      reduction —see Osteochondrosis,
      juvenile, hip, specified NEC
    arm —see Osteochondrosis, juvenile, upper
      limb NEC
    capitular epiphysis (femur) —see Legg-
      Calvé-Perthes disease
    clavicle, sternal epiphysis —see
      Osteochondrosis, juvenile, upper limb
      NEC
    coxae —see Legg-Calvé-Perthes disease
    deformans M92.9
    fibula M92.50-●

Osteochondrosis (Continued)
  juvenile, juvenilis (Continued)
    foot NEC M92.8
    hand M92.20-●
      carpal lunate M92.21-●
      metacarpal head M92.22-●
      specified site NEC M92.29-●
    head of femur —see Legg-Calvé-Perthes
      disease
    hip and pelvis M91.9-●
      coxa plana —see Coxa, plana
      femoral head —see Legg-Calvé-Perthes
        disease
      pelvis M91.0
      pseudocoxalgia —see Pseudocoxalgia
      specified NEC M91.8-●
    humerus M92.0-●
    limb
      lower NEC M92.8
      upper NEC —see Osteochondrosis,
        juvenile, upper limb NEC
    medial cuneiform bone —see
      Osteochondrosis, juvenile, tarsus
    metatarsus M92.7-●
    patella M92.4-●
    radius M92.1-●
    specified
      site NEC M92.8
      type NEC M92.8
        tibia and fibula M92.59-●
    ~~specified site NEC M92.8~~
    spine M42.00
      cervical region M42.02
      cervicothoracic region M42.03
      lumbar region M42.06
      lumbosacral region M42.07
      multiple sites M42.09
      occipito-atlanto-axial region
        M42.01
      sacrococcygeal region M42.08
      thoracic region M42.04
      thoracolumbar region M42.05
    tarsus M92.6-●
    tibia M92.50-●
      proximal M92.51-●
      tubercle M92.52-●
    ulna M92.1-●
    upper limb NEC M92.3-●
    vertebra (body) (epiphyseal plates)
      (Calvé's) (Scheuermann's) —see
      Osteochondrosis, juvenile, spine
  Kienböck's —see Osteochondrosis, juvenile,
    hand, carpal lunate
    adult M93.1
  Köhler's
    patellar —see Osteochondrosis, juvenile,
      patella
    tarsal navicular —see Osteochondrosis,
      juvenile, tarsus
  Legg-Perthes (-Calvé's) (-Waldenström) —see
    Legg-Calvé-Perthes disease
  limb
    lower NEC (juvenile) M92.8
      tibia and fibula M92.59-●
    upper NEC (juvenile) —see
      Osteochondrosis, juvenile, upper limb
      NEC
  lunate bone (carpal) (juvenile) —see also
    Osteochondrosis, juvenile, hand, carpal
    lunate
    adult M93.1
  Mauclaire's —see Osteochondrosis, juvenile,
    hand, metacarpal
  metacarpal (head) (juvenile) —see
    Osteochondrosis, juvenile, hand,
    metacarpal
  metatarsus (fifth) (head) (juvenile)
    (second) —see Osteochondrosis, juvenile,
    metatarsus
  navicular (juvenile) —see Osteochondrosis,
    juvenile, tarsus

Osteochondrosis *(Continued)*
  os
    calcis (juvenile) —*see* Osteochondrosis,
      juvenile, tarsus
    tibiale externum (juvenile) —*see*
      Osteochondrosis, juvenile, tarsus
  Osgood-Schlatter M92.52-●
  Panner's —*see* Osteochondrosis, juvenile,
    humerus
  patellar center (juvenile) (primary)
    (secondary) —*see* Osteochondrosis,
    juvenile, patella
  pelvis (juvenile) M91.0
  Pierson's M91.0
  radius (head) (juvenile) —*see*
    Osteochondrosis, juvenile, radius
  Scheuermann's —*see* Osteochondrosis,
    juvenile, spine
  Sever's —*see* Osteochondrosis, juvenile, tarsus
  Sinding-Larsen —*see* Osteochondrosis,
    juvenile, patella
  spine M42.9
    adult M42.10
      cervical region M42.12
      cervicothoracic region M42.13
      lumbar region M42.16
      lumbosacral region M42.17
      multiple sites M42.19
      occipito-atlanto-axial region M42.11
      sacrococcygeal region M42.18
      thoracic region M42.14
      thoracolumbar region M42.15
    juvenile —*see* Osteochondrosis, juvenile,
      spine
  symphysis pubis (juvenile) M91.0
  syphilitic (congenital) A50.02
  talus (juvenile) —*see* Osteochondrosis,
    juvenile, tarsus
  tarsus (navicular) (juvenile) —*see*
    Osteochondrosis, juvenile, tarsus
  tibia (proximal) (tubercle) (juvenile) —*see*
    Osteochondrosis, juvenile, tibia
  tuberculous —*see* Tuberculosis, bone
  ulna (lower) (juvenile) —*see* Osteochondrosis,
    juvenile, ulna
  van Neck's M91.0
  vertebral —*see* Osteochondrosis, spine
Osteoclastoma D48.0
  malignant —*see* Neoplasm, bone, malignant
Osteodynia —*see* Disorder, bone, specified type
  NEC
Osteodystrophy Q78.9
  azotemic N25.0
  congenital Q78.9
  parathyroid, secondary E21.1
  renal N25.0
Osteofibroma —*see* Neoplasm, bone, benign
Osteofibrosarcoma —*see* Neoplasm, bone,
  malignant
Osteogenesis imperfecta Q78.0
Osteogenic —*see* condition
Osteolysis M89.50
  carpus M89.54-●
  clavicle M89.51-●
  femur M89.55-●
  fibula M89.56-●
  finger M89.54-●
  humerus M89.52-●
  ilium M89.559
  ischium M89.559
  joint prosthesis (periprosthetic) —*see*
    Complications, joint prosthesis,
    mechanical, periprosthetic, osteolysis,
    by site
  metacarpus M89.54-●
  metatarsus M89.57-●
  multiple sites M89.59
  neck M89.58
  periprosthetic —*see* Complications, joint
    prosthesis, mechanical, periprosthetic,
    osteolysis, by site

Osteolysis *(Continued)*
  radius M89.53-●
  rib M89.58
  scapula M89.51-●
  skull M89.58
  tarsus M89.57-●
  tibia M89.56-●
  toe M89.57-●
  ulna M89.53-●
  vertebra M89.58
Osteoma —*see also* Neoplasm, bone, benign
  osteoid —*see also* Neoplasm, bone, benign
    giant —*see* Neoplasm, bone, benign
Osteomalacia M83.9
  adult M83.9
    drug-induced NEC M83.5
    due to
      malabsorption (postsurgical) M83.2
      malnutrition M83.3
    specified NEC M83.8
  aluminium-induced M83.4
  infantile —*see* Rickets
  juvenile —*see* Rickets
  oncogenic E83.89
  pelvis M83.8
  puerperal M83.0
  senile M83.1
  vitamin-D-resistant in adults E83.31 *[M90.8-●]*
    carpus E83.31 *[M90.84-●]*
    clavicle E83.31 *[M90.81-●]*
    femur E83.31 *[M90.85-●]*
    fibula E83.31 *[M90.86-●]*
    finger E83.31 *[M90.84-●]*
    humerus E83.31 *[M90.82-●]*
    ilium E83.31 *[M90.859]*
    ischium E83.31 *[M90.859]*
    metacarpus E83.31 *[M90.84-●]*
    metatarsus E83.31 *[M90.87-●]*
    multiple sites E83.31 *[M90.89]*
    neck E83.31 *[M90.88]*
    radius E83.31 *[M90.83-●]*
    rib E83.31 *[M90.88]*
    scapula E83.31 *[M90.819]*
    skull E83.31 *[M90.88]*
    tarsus E83.31 *[M90.879]*
    tibia E83.31 *[M90.869]*
    toe E83.31 *[M90.879]*
    ulna E83.31 *[M90.839]*
    vertebra E83.31 *[M90.88]*
Osteomyelitis (general) (infective)
  (localized) (neonatal) (purulent)
  (septic) (staphylococcal) (streptococcal)
  (suppurative) (with periostitis) M86.9
  acute M86.10
    carpus M86.14-●
    clavicle M86.11-●
    femur M86.15-●
    fibula M86.16-●
    finger M86.14-●
    hematogenous M86.00
      carpus M86.04-●
      clavicle M86.01-●
      femur M86.05-●
      fibula M86.06-●
      finger M86.04-●
      humerus M86.02-●
➡   ilium M86.08
➡   ischium M86.08
      mandible M27.2
      metacarpus M86.04-●
      metatarsus M86.07-●
      multiple sites M86.09
      neck M86.08
      orbit H05.02-●
      petrous bone —*see* Petrositis
      radius M86.03-●
      rib M86.08
      scapula M86.01-●
      skull M86.08
      tarsus M86.07-●
      tibia M86.06-●

Osteomyelitis *(Continued)*
  acute *(Continued)*
    hematogenous *(Continued)*
      toe M86.07-●
      ulna M86.03-●
      vertebra —*see* Osteomyelitis, vertebra
    humerus M86.12-●
    ilium M86.18
    ischium M86.18
    mandible M27.2
    metacarpus M86.14-●
    metatarsus M86.17-●
    multiple sites M86.19
    neck M86.18
    orbit H05.02-●
    petrous bone —*see* Petrositis
    radius M86.13-●
    rib M86.18
    scapula M86.11-●
    skull M86.18
    tarsus M86.17-●
    tibia M86.16-●
    toe M86.17-●
    ulna M86.13-●
    vertebra —*see* Osteomyelitis, vertebra
  chronic (or old) M86.60
    with draining sinus M86.40
      carpus M86.44-●
      clavicle M86.41-●
      femur M86.45-●
      fibula M86.46-●
      finger M86.44-●
      humerus M86.42-●
      ilium M86.459
      ischium M86.459
      mandible M27.2
      metacarpus M86.44-●
      metatarsus M86.47-●
      multiple sites M86.49
      neck M86.48
      orbit H05.02-●
      petrous bone —*see* Petrositis
      radius M86.43-●
      rib M86.48
      scapula M86.41-●
      skull M86.48
      tarsus M86.47-●
      tibia M86.46-●
      toe M86.47-●
      ulna M86.43-●
      vertebra —*see* Osteomyelitis, vertebra
    carpus M86.64-●
    clavicle M86.61-●
    femur M86.65-●
    fibula M86.66-●
    finger M86.64-●
    hematogenous NEC M86.50
      carpus M86.54-●
      clavicle M86.51-●
      femur M86.55-●
      fibula M86.56-●
      finger M86.54-●
      humerus M86.52-●
      ilium M86.559
      ischium M86.559
      mandible M27.2
      metacarpus M86.54-●
      metatarsus M86.57-●
      multifocal M86.30
        carpus M86.34-●
        clavicle M86.31-●
        femur M86.35-●
        fibula M86.36-●
        finger M86.34-●
        humerus M86.32-●
        ilium M86.359
        ischium M86.359
        metacarpus M86.34-●
        metatarsus M86.37-●
        multiple sites M86.39
        neck M86.38

Osteomyelitis *(Continued)*
  chronic *(Continued)*
    hematogenous NEC *(Continued)*
      multifocal *(Continued)*
        radius M86.33-●
        rib M86.38
        scapula M86.31-●
        skull M86.38
        tarsus M86.37-●
        tibia M86.36-●
        toe M86.37-●
        ulna M86.33-●
        vertebra —*see* Osteomyelitis, vertebra
      multiple sites M86.59
      neck M86.58
      orbit H05.02-●
      petrous bone —*see* Petrositis
      radius M86.53-●
      rib M86.58
      scapula M86.51-●
      skull M86.58
      tarsus M86.57-●
      tibia M86.56-●
      toe M86.57-●
      ulna M86.53-●
      vertebra —*see* Osteomyelitis, vertebra
    humerus M86.62-●
    ilium M86.659
    ischium M86.659
    mandible M27.2
    metacarpus M86.64-●
    metatarsus M86.67-●
    multifocal —*see* Osteomyelitis, chronic, hematogenous, multifocal
    multiple sites M86.69
    neck M86.68
    orbit H05.02-●
    petrous bone —*see* Petrositis
    radius M86.63-●
    rib M86.68
    scapula M86.61-●
    skull M86.68
    tarsus M86.67-●
    tibia M86.66-●
    toe M86.67-●
    ulna M86.63-●
    vertebra —*see* Osteomyelitis, vertebra
  echinococcal B67.2
  Garr's —*see* Osteomyelitis, specified type NEC
  in diabetes mellitus —*see* E08-E13 with .69
  jaw (acute) (chronic) (lower) (neonatal) (suppurating) (upper) M27.2
  nonsuppurating —*see* Osteomyelitis, specified type NEC
  orbit H05.02-●
  petrous bone —*see* Petrositis
  Salmonella (arizonae) (cholerae-suis) (enteritidis) (typhimurium) A02.24
  sclerosing, nonsuppurative —*see* Osteomyelitis, specified type NEC
  specified type NEC —*see also* subcategory M86.8X-●
    mandible M27.2
    orbit H05.02-●
    petrous bone —*see* Petrositis
    vertebra —*see* Osteomyelitis, vertebra
  subacute M86.20
    carpus M86.24-●
    clavicle M86.21-●
    femur M86.25-●
    fibula M86.26-●
    finger M86.24-●
    humerus M86.22-●
    mandible M27.2
    metacarpus M86.24-●
    metatarsus M86.27-●
    multiple sites M86.29
    neck M86.28
    orbit H05.02-●
    petrous bone —*see* Petrositis
    radius M86.23-●

Osteomyelitis *(Continued)*
  subacute *(Continued)*
    rib M86.28
    scapula M86.21-●
    skull M86.28
    tarsus M86.27-●
    tibia M86.26-●
    toe M86.27-●
    ulna M86.23-●
    vertebra —*see* Osteomyelitis, vertebra
  syphilitic A52.77
    congenital (early) A50.02 [M90.80]
  tuberculous —*see* Tuberculosis, bone
  typhoid A01.05
  vertebra M46.20
    cervical region M46.22
    cervicothoracic region M46.23
    lumbar region M46.26
    lumbosacral region M46.27
    occipito-atlanto-axial region M46.21
    sacrococcygeal region M46.28
    thoracic region M46.24
    thoracolumbar region M46.25
Osteomyelofibrosis D47.4
Osteomyelosclerosis D75.89
Osteonecrosis M87.9
  due to
    drugs —*see* Osteonecrosis, secondary, due to, drugs
    trauma —*see* Osteonecrosis, secondary, due to, trauma
  idiopathic aseptic M87.00
    ankle M87.07-●
    carpus M87.03-●
    clavicle M87.01-●
    femur M87.05-●
    fibula M87.06-●
    finger M87.04-●
    humerus M87.02-●
    ilium M87.050
    ischium M87.050
    metacarpus M87.04-●
    metatarsus M87.07-●
    multiple sites M87.09
    neck M87.08
    pelvis M87.050
    radius M87.03-●
    rib M87.08
    scapula M87.01-●
    skull M87.08
    tarsus M87.07-●
    tibia M87.06-●
    toe M87.07-●
    ulna M87.03-●
    vertebra M87.08
  secondary NEC M87.30
    carpus M87.33-●
    clavicle M87.31-●
    due to
      drugs M87.10
        carpus M87.13-●
        clavicle M87.11-●
        femur M87.15-●
        fibula M87.16-●
        finger M87.14-●
        humerus M87.12-●
        ilium M87.159
        ischium M87.159
        jaw M87.180
        metacarpus M87.14-●
        metatarsus M87.17-●
        multiple sites M87.19
        neck M87.18
        radius M87.13-●
        rib M87.18
        scapula M87.11-●
        skull M87.18
        tarsus M87.17-●
        tibia M87.16-●
        toe M87.17-●
        ulna M87.13-●
        vertebra M87.18

Osteonecrosis *(Continued)*
  secondary NEC *(Continued)*
    due to *(Continued)*
      hemoglobinopathy NEC D58.2 [M90.50]
        carpus D58.2 [M90.54-●]
        clavicle D58.2 [M90.51-●]
        femur D58.2 [M90.55-●]
        fibula D58.2 [M90.56-●]
        finger D58.2 [M90.54-●]
        humerus D58.2 [M90.52-●]
        ilium D58.2 [M90.55-●]
        ischium D58.2 [M90.55-●]
        metacarpus D58.2 [M90.54-●]
        metatarsus D58.2 [M90.57-●]
        multiple sites D58.2 [M90.58]
        neck D58.2 [M90.58]
        radius D58.2 [M90.53-●]
        rib D58.2 [M90.58]
        scapula D58.2 [M90.51-●]
        skull D58.2 [M90.58]
        tarsus D58.2 [M90.57-●]
        tibia D58.2 [M90.56-●]
        toe D58.2 [M90.57-●]
        ulna D58.2 [M90.53-●]
        vertebra D58.2 [M90.58]
      trauma (previous) M87.20
        carpus M87.23-●
        clavicle M87.21-●
        femur M87.25-●
        fibula M87.26-●
        finger M87.24-●
        humerus M87.22-●
        ilium M87.25-●
        ischium M87.25-●
        metacarpus M87.24-●
        metatarsus M87.27-●
        multiple sites M87.29
        neck M87.28
        radius M87.23-●
        rib M87.28
        scapula M87.21-●
        skull M87.28
        tarsus M87.27-●
        tibia M87.26-●
        toe M87.27-●
        ulna M87.23-●
        vertebra M87.28
    femur M87.35-●
    fibula M87.36-●
    finger M87.34-●
    humerus M87.32
    ilium M87.350
    in
      caisson disease T70.3 [M90.50]
        carpus T70.3 [M90.54-●]
        clavicle T70.3 [M90.51-●]
        femur T70.3 [M90.55-●]
        fibula T70.3 [M90.56-●]
        finger T70.3 [M90.54-●]
        humerus T70.3 [M90.52-●]
        ilium T70.3 [M90.55-●]
        ischium T70.3 [M90.55-●]
        metacarpus T70.3 [M90.54-●]
        metatarsus T70.3 [M90.57-●]
        multiple sites T70.3 [M90.59]
        neck T70.3 [M90.58]
        radius T70.3 [M90.53-●]
        rib T70.3 [M90.58]
        scapula T70.3 [M90.51-●]
        skull T70.3 [M90.58]
        tarsus T70.3 [M90.57-●]
        tibia T70.3 [M90.56-●]
        toe T70.3 [M90.57-●]
        ulna T70.3 [M90.53-●]
        vertebra T70.3 [M90.58]
    ischium M87.350
    metacarpus M87.34-●
    metatarsus M87.37-●
    multiple site M87.39
    neck M87.38

▶ New   ⇒ Revised   ~~deleted~~ Deleted   ● Use Additional Character(s)

Osteonecrosis *(Continued)*
  secondary NEC *(Continued)*
    radius M87.33-●
    rib M87.38
    scapula M87.319
    skull M87.38
    tarsus M87.379
    tibia M87.366
    toe M87.379
    ulna M87.33-●
    vertebra M87.38
  specified type NEC M87.80
    carpus M87.83-●
    clavicle M87.81-●
    femur M87.85-●
    fibula M87.86-●
    finger M87.84-●
    humerus M87.82-●
    ilium M87.85-●
    ischium M87.85-●
    metacarpus M87.84-●
    metatarsus M87.87-●
    multiple sites M87.89
    neck M87.88
    radius M87.83-●
    rib M87.88-●
    scapula M87.81-●
    skull M87.88
    tarsus M87.87-●
    tibia M87.86-●
    toe M87.87-●
    ulna M87.83-●
    vertebra M87.88
Osteo-onycho-arthro-dysplasia Q87.2
Osteo-onychodysplasia, hereditary Q87.2
Osteopathia condensans disseminata Q78.8
Osteopathy —*see also* Osteomyelitis,
    Osteonecrosis, Osteoporosis
  after poliomyelitis M89.60
    carpus M89.64-●
    clavicle M89.61-●
    femur M89.65-●
    fibula M89.66-●
    finger M89.64-●
    humerus M89.62-●
    ilium M89.659
    ischium M89.659
    metacarpus M89.64-●
    metatarsus M89.67-●
    multiple sites M89.69
    neck M89.68
    radius M89.63-●
    rib M89.68
    scapula M89.61-●
    skull M89.68
    tarsus M89.67-●
    tibia M89.66-●
    toe M89.67-●
    ulna M89.63-●
    vertebra M89.68
  in (due to)
    renal osteodystrophy N25.0
    specified diseases classified elsewhere —
        see subcategory M90.8
Osteopenia M85.8-●
  borderline M85.8-●
Osteoperiostitis —*see* Osteomyelitis, specified
    type NEC
Osteopetrosis (familial) Q78.2
Osteophyte M25.70
  ankle M25.77-●
  elbow M25.72-●
  foot joint M25.77-●
  hand joint M25.74-●
  hip M25.75-●
  knee M25.76-●
  shoulder M25.71-●
  spine M25.78
  vertebrae M25.78
  wrist M25.73-●
Osteopoikilosis Q78.8

Osteoporosis (female) (male) M81.0
  with current pathological fracture M80.00
  age-related M81.0
    with current pathologic fracture M80.00
      carpus M80.04-●
      clavicle M80.01-●
      fibula M80.06-●
      finger M80.04-●
      humerus M80.02-●
      ilium M80.05-●
      ischium M80.05 ●
      metacarpus M80.04-●
      metatarsus M80.07-●
      pelvis M80.05-●
      radius M80.03-●
      scapula M80.01-●
      site specified NEC M80.0A
      tarsus M80.07-●
      tibia M80.06-●
      toe M80.07-●
      ulna M80.03-●
      vertebra M80.08
  disuse M81.8
    with current pathological fracture M80.80
      carpus M80.84-●
      clavicle M80.81-●
      fibula M80.86-●
      finger M80.84-●
      humerus M80.82-●
      ilium M80.85-●
      ischium M80.85-●
      metacarpus M80.84-●
      metatarsus M80.87-●
      pelvis M80 85-●
      radius M80.83-●
      scapula M80.81-●
      site specified NEC M80.8A
      tarsus M80.87-●
      tibia M80.86-●
      toe M80.87-●
      ulna M80.83-●
      vertebra M80.88
  drug induced —*see* Osteoporosis, specified
      type NEC
  idiopathic —*see* Osteoporosis, specified type
      NEC
  involutional —*see* Osteoporosis, age-related
  Lequesne M81.6
  localized M81.6
  postmenopausal M81.0
    with pathological fracture M80.00
      carpus M80.04-●
      clavicle M80.01-●
      fibula M80.06-●
      finger M80.04-●
      humerus M80.02-●
      ilium M80.05-●
      ischium M80.05-●
      metacarpus M80.04-●
      metatarsus M80.07-●
      pelvis M80.05-●
      radius M80.03-●
      scapula M80.01-●
      site specified NEC M80.0A
      tarsus M80.07-●
      tibia M80.06-●
      toe M80.07-●
      ulna M80.03-●
      vertebra M80.08
  postoophorectomy —*see* Osteoporosis,
      specified type NEC
  postsurgical malabsorption —*see*
      Osteoporosis, specified type NEC
  post-traumatic —*see* Osteoporosis, specified
      type NEC
  senile —*see* Osteoporosis, age-related
  specified type NEC M81.8
    with pathological fracture M80.80
      carpus M80.84-●
      clavicle M80.81-●
      fibula M80.86-●

Osteoporosis *(Continued)*
  specified type NEC *(Continued)*
    with pathological fracture *(Continued)*
      finger M80.84-●
      humerus M80.82-●
      ilium M80.85-●
      ischium M80.85-●
      metacarpus M80.84-●
      metatarsus M80.87-●
      pelvis M80.85-●
      radius M80.83-●
      scapula M80.81-●
      site specified NEC M80.8A
      tarsus M80.87-●
      tibia M80.86-●
      toe M80.87-●
      ulna M80.83-●
      vertebra M80.88
Osteopsathyrosis (idiopathica) Q78.0
Osteoradionecrosis, jaw (acute) (chronic)
    (lower) (suppurative) (upper) M27.2
Osteosarcoma (any form) —*see* Neoplasm,
    bone, malignant
Osteosclerosis Q78.2
  acquired M85.8-●
  congenita Q77.4
  fragilitas (generalisata) Q78.2
  myelofibrosis D75.81
Osteosclerotic anemia D64.89
Osteosis
  cutis L94.2
  renal fibrocystic N25.0
Österreicher-Turner syndrome Q87.2
Ostium
  atrioventriculare commune Q21.2
  primum (arteriosum) (defect) (persistent) Q21.2
  secundum (arteriosum) (defect) (patent)
    (persistent) Q21.1
Ostrum-Furst syndrome Q75.8
Otalgia —*see* subcategory H92.0
Otitis (acute) H66.90
  with effusion —*see also* Otitis, media,
      nonsuppurative
    purulent —*see* Otitis, media, suppurative
  adhesive —*see* subcategory H74.1
  chronic —*see also* Otitis, media, chronic
    with effusion —*see also* Otitis, media,
        nonsuppurative, chronic
  externa H60.9-●
    abscess —*see* Abscess, ear, external
    acute (noninfective) H60.50-●
      actinic H60.51-●
      chemical H60.52-●
      contact H60.53-●
      eczematoid H60.54-●
      infective —*see* Otitis, externa, infective
      reactive H60.55-●
      specified NEC H60.59-●
    cellulitis —*see* Cellulitis, ear
    chronic H60.6-●
    diffuse —*see* Otitis, externa, infective, diffuse
    hemorrhagic —*see* Otitis, externa, infective,
        hemorrhagic
    in (due to)
      aspergillosis B44.89
      candidiasis B37.84
      erysipelas A46 [*H62.40*]
      herpes (simplex) virus infection B00.1
          zoster B02.8
      impetigo L01.00 [*H62.40*]
      infectious disease NEC B99 [*H62.4-●*]
      mycosis NEC B36.9 [*H62.40*]
      parasitic disease NEC B89 [*H62.40*]
      viral disease NEC B34.9 [*H62.40*]
      zoster B02.8
    infective NEC H60.39-●
      abscess —*see* Abscess, ear, external
      cellulitis —*see* Cellulitis, ear
      diffuse H60.31-●
      hemorrhagic H60.32-●
      swimmer's ear —*see* Swimmer's, ear

Otitis (Continued)
  externa (Continued)
    malignant H60.2-●
    mycotic NEC B36.9 [H62.40]
      in
        aspergillosis B44.89
        candidiasis B37.84
        moniliasis B37.84
    necrotizing —see Otitis, externa,
      malignant
    Pseudomonas aeruginosa —see Otitis,
      externa, malignant
    reactive —see Otitis, externa, acute,
      reactive
    specified NEC —see subcategory
      H60.8
    tropical NEC B36.9 [H62.40]
      in
        aspergillosis B44.89
        candidiasis B37.84
        moniliasis B37.84
  insidiosa —see Otosclerosis
  interna —see subcategory H83.0
  media (hemorrhagic) (staphylococcal)
    (streptococcal) H66.9-●
    with effusion (nonpurulent) —see Otitis,
      media, nonsuppurative
    acute, subacute H66.90
      allergic —see Otitis, media,
        nonsuppurative, acute, allergic
      exudative —see Otitis, media,
        suppurative, acute
      mucoid —see Otitis, media,
        nonsuppurative, acute
      necrotizing —see also Otitis, media,
        suppurative, acute
        in
          measles B05.3
          scarlet fever A38.0
      nonsuppurative NEC —see Otitis, media,
        nonsuppurative, acute
      purulent —see Otitis, media,
        suppurative, acute
      sanguinous —see Otitis, media,
        nonsuppurative, acute
      secretory —see Otitis, media,
        nonsuppurative, acute, serous
      seromucinous —see Otitis, media,
        nonsuppurative, acute
      serous —see Otitis, media,
        nonsuppurative, acute, serous
      suppurative —see Otitis, media,
        suppurative, acute
    allergic —see Otitis, media, nonsuppurative
    catarrhal —see Otitis, media,
      nonsuppurative
    chronic H66.90
      with effusion (nonpurulent) —see Otitis,
        media, nonsuppurative, chronic
      allergic —see Otitis, media,
        nonsuppurative, chronic, allergic
      benign suppurative —see Otitis, media,
        suppurative, chronic, tubotympanic
      catarrhal —see Otitis, media,
        nonsuppurative, chronic, serous
      exudative —see Otitis, media,
        suppurative, chronic
      mucinous —see Otitis, media,
        nonsuppurative, chronic, mucoid
      mucoid —see Otitis, media,
        nonsuppurative, chronic, mucoid
      nonsuppurative NEC —see Otitis, media,
        nonsuppurative, chronic
      purulent —see Otitis, media,
        suppurative, chronic
      secretory —see Otitis, media,
        nonsuppurative, chronic, mucoid
      seromucinous —see Otitis, media,
        nonsuppurative, chronic
      serous —see Otitis, media,
        nonsuppurative, chronic, serous

Otitis (Continued)
  media (Continued)
    chronic (Continued)
      suppurative —see Otitis, media,
        suppurative, chronic
      transudative —see Otitis, media,
        nonsuppurative, chronic, mucoid
    exudative —see Otitis, media,
      nonsuppurative
    in (due to) (with)
      influenza —see Influenza, with, otitis
        media
      measles B05.3
      scarlet fever A38.0
      tuberculosis A18.6
      viral disease NEC B34.-● [H67.-●]
    mucoid —see Otitis, media,
      nonsuppurative
    nonsuppurative H65.9-●
      acute or subacute NEC H65.19-●
        allergic H65.11-●
          recurrent H65.11-●
        recurrent H65.19-●
        secretory —see Otitis, media,
          nonsuppurative, serous
        serous H65.0-●
          recurrent H65.0-●
      chronic H65.49-●
        allergic H65.41-●
        mucoid H65.3-●
        serous H65.2-●
    postmeasles B05.3
    purulent —see Otitis, media, suppurative
    secretory —see Otitis, media,
      nonsuppurative
    seromucinous —see Otitis, media,
      nonsuppurative
    serous —see Otitis, media, nonsuppurative
    suppurative H66.4-●
      acute H66.00-●
        with rupture of ear drum H66.01-●
        recurrent H66.00-●
          with rupture of ear drum H66.01-●
      chronic —see also subcategory H66.3
        atticoantral H66.2-●
        benign —see Otitis, media,
          suppurative, chronic,
          tubotympanic
        tubotympanic H66.1-●
    transudative —see Otitis, media,
      nonsuppurative
    tuberculous A18.6
Otocephaly Q18.2
Otolith syndrome —see subcategory H81.8
Otomycosis (diffuse) NEC B36.9 [H62.40]
  in
    aspergillosis B44.89
    candidiasis B37.84
    moniliasis B37.84
Otoporosis —see Otosclerosis
Otorrhagia (nontraumatic) H92.2-●
  traumatic - code by Type of injury
Otorrhea H92.1-●
  cerebrospinal (fluid) G96.01
    postoperative G96.08
    specified NEC G96.08
    spontaneous G96.01
    traumatic G96.08
Otosclerosis (general) H80.9-●
  cochlear (endosteal) H80.2-●
  involving
    otic capsule —see Otosclerosis, cochlear
    oval window
      nonobliterative H80.0-●
      obliterative H80.1-●
    round window —see Otosclerosis, cochlear
  nonobliterative —see Otosclerosis, involving,
    oval window, nonobliterative
  obliterative —see Otosclerosis, involving, oval
    window, obliterative
  specified NEC H80.8-●

Otospongiosis —see Otosclerosis
Otto's disease or pelvis M24.7
Outcome of delivery Z37.9
  multiple births Z37.9
    all liveborn Z37.50
      quadruplets Z37.52
      quintuplets Z37.53
      sextuplets Z37.54
      specified number NEC Z37.59
      triplets Z37.51
    all stillborn Z37.7
    some liveborn Z37.60
      quadruplets Z37.62
      quintuplets Z37.63
      sextuplets Z37.64
      specified number NEC Z37.69
      triplets Z37.61
  single NEC Z37.9
    liveborn Z37.0
    stillborn Z37.1
  twins NEC Z37.9
    both liveborn Z37.2
    both stillborn Z37.4
    one liveborn, one stillborn Z37.3
Outlet —see condition
Ovalocytosis (congenital) (hereditary) —see
  Elliptocytosis
Ovarian —see Condition
Ovariocele N83.4-●
Ovaritis (cystic) —see Oophoritis
Ovary, ovarian —see also condition
  resistant syndrome E28.39
  vein syndrome N13.8
Overactive —see also Hyperfunction
  adrenal cortex NEC E27.0
  bladder N32.81
  hypothalamus E23.3
  thyroid —see Hyperthyroidism
Overactivity R46.3
  child —see Disorder, attention-deficit
    hyperactivity
Overbite (deep) (excessive) (horizontal)
  (vertical) M26.29
Overbreathing —see Hyperventilation
Overconscientious personality F60.5
Overdevelopment —see Hypertrophy
Overdistension —see Distension
Overdose, overdosage (drug) —see Table of
  Drugs and Chemicals, by drug, poisoning
Overeating R63.2
  nonorganic origin F50.89
  psychogenic F50.89
Overexertion (effects) (exhaustion) T73.3
Overexposure (effects) T73.9
  exhaustion T73.2
Overfeeding —see Overeating
  newborn P92.4
Overfill, endodontic M27.52
Overgrowth, bone —see Hypertrophy, bone
Overhanging of dental restorative material
  (unrepairable) K08.52
Overheated (places) (effects) —see Heat
Overjet (excessive horizontal) M26.23
Overlaid, overlying (suffocation) —see Asphyxia,
  traumatic, due to mechanical threat
Overlap, excessive horizontal (teeth) M26.23
Overl apping toe (acquired) —see also
  Deformity, toe, specified NEC
  congenital (fifth toe) Q66.89
Overload
  circulatory, due to transfusion (blood) (blood
    components) (TACO) E87.71
  fluid E87.70
    due to transfusion (blood) (blood
      components) E87.71
    specified NEC E87.79
  iron, due to repeated red blood cell
    transfusions E83.111
  potassium (K) E87.5
  sodium (Na) E87.0
Overnutrition —see Hyperalimentation

Overproduction —*see also* Hypersecretion
  ACTH E27.0
  catecholamine E27.5
  growth hormone E22.0
Overprotection, child by parent Z62.1
Overriding
  aorta Q25.49
  finger (acquired) —*see* Deformity, finger
    congenital Q68.1
  toe (acquired) —*see also* Deformity, toe,
    specified NEC
      congenital Q66.89

Overstrained R53.83
  heart —*see* Hypertrophy, cardiac
Overuse, muscle NEC
  M70.8-●
Overweight E66.3
Overworked R53.83
Oviduct —*see* condition
Ovotestis Q56.0
Ovulation (cycle)
  failure or lack of N97.0
  pain N94.0

Ovum —*see* condition
Owren's disease or syndrome (parahemophilia)
  D68.2
Ox heart —*see* Hypertrophy, cardiac
Oxalosis E72.53
Oxaluria E72.53
Oxycephaly, oxycephalic Q75.0
  syphilitic, congenital A50.02
Oxyuriasis B80
Oxyuris vermicularis (infestation) B80
Ozena J31.0

P

Pachyderma, pachydermia L85.9
  larynx (verrucosa) J38.7
Pachydermatocele (congenital) Q82.8
Pachydermoperiostosis —*see also*
    Osteoarthropathy, hypertrophic, specified
    type NEC
  clubbed nail M89.40 [L62]
Pachygyria Q04.3
Pachymeningitis (adhesive) (basal) (brain)
    (cervical) (chronic) (circumscribed)
    (external) (fibrous) (hemorrhagic)
    (hypertrophic) (internal) (purulent) (spinal)
    (suppurative) —*see* Meningitis
Pachyonychia (congenital) Q84.5
Pacinian tumor —*see* Neoplasm, skin, benign
Pad, knuckle or Garrod's M72.1
Paget-Schroetter syndrome I82.890
Paget's disease
  with infiltrating duct carcinoma —*see*
      Neoplasm, breast, malignant
  bone M88.9
    carpus M88.84-•
    clavicle M88.81-•
    femur M88.85-•
    fibula M88.86-•
    finger M88.84-•
    humerus M88.82-•
    ilium M88.85-•
    in neoplastic disease —*see* Osteitis,
        deformans, in neoplastic disease
    ischium M88.85-•
    metacarpus M88.84-•
    metatarsus M88.87-•
    multiple sites M88.89
    neck M88.88
    radius M88.83-•
    rib M88.88
    scapula M88.81-•
    skull M88.0
    specified NEC M88.88
    tarsus M88.87-•
    tibia M88.86-•
    toe M88.87-•
    ulna M88.83-•
    vertebra M88.1
  breast (female) C50.01-•
    male C50.02-•
  extramammary —*see also* Neoplasm, skin,
      malignant
    anus C21.0
      margin C44.590
      skin C44.590
  intraductal carcinoma —*see* Neoplasm,
      breast, malignant
  malignant —*see* Neoplasm, skin, malignant
    breast (female) C50.01-•
      male C50.02-•
    unspecified site (female) C50.01-•
      male C50.02-•
  mammary —*see* Paget's disease, breast
  nipple —*see* Paget's disease, breast
  osteitis deformans —*see* Paget's disease, bone
Pain(s) —*see also* Painful R52
  abdominal R10.9
    colic R10.83
    generalized R10.84
      with acute abdomen R10.0
    lower R10.30
      left quadrant R10.32
      pelvic or perineal R10.2
      periumbilical R10.33
      right quadrant R10.31
    rebound —*see* Tenderness, abdominal,
        rebound
    severe with abdominal rigidity R10.0
    tenderness —*see* Tenderness, abdominal
    upper R10.10
      epigastric R10.13
      left quadrant R10.12
      right quadrant R10.11

Pain (*Continued*)
  acute R52
    due to trauma G89.11
    neoplasm related G89.3
    postprocedural NEC G89.18
    post-thoracotomy G89.12
    specified by site — code to Pain, by site
  adnexa (uteri) R10.2
  anginoid —*see* Pain, precordial
  anus K62.89
  arm —*see* Pain, limb, upper
  axillary (axilla) M79.62-•
  back (postural) M54.9
  bladder R39.89
    associated with micturition —*see*
        Micturition, painful
    chronic R39.82
  bone —*see* Disorder, bone, specified type NEC
  breast N64.4
  broad ligament R10.2
  cancer associated (acute) (chronic) G89.3
  cecum —*see* Pain, abdominal
  cervicobrachial M53.1
  chest (central) R07.9
    anterior wall R07.89
    atypical R07.89
    ischemic I20.9
    musculoskeletal R07.89
    non-cardiac R07.89
    on breathing R07.1
    pleurodynia R07.81
    precordial R07.2
    wall (anterior) R07.89
  chronic G89.29
    associated with significant psychosocial
        dysfunction G89.4
    due to trauma G89.21
    neoplasm related G89.3
    postoperative NEC G89.28
    postprocedural NEC G89.28
    post-thoracotomy G89.22
    specified NEC G89.29
  coccyx M53.3
  colon —*see* Pain, abdominal
  coronary —*see* Angina
  costochondral R07.1
  diaphragm R07.1
  due to cancer G89.3
  due to device, implant or graft —*see also*
      Complications, by site and type,
      specified NEC T85.848
    arterial graft NEC T82.848
    breast (implant) T85.848
    catheter NEC T85.848
      dialysis (renal) T82.848
        intraperitoneal T85.848
      infusion NEC T82.848
        spinal (epidural) (subdural) T85.840
      urinary (indwelling) T83.84
    electronic (electrode) (pulse generator)
        (stimulator)
      bone T84.84
      cardiac T82.847
      nervous system (brain) (peripheral
          nerve) (spinal) T85.840
      urinary T83.84
    fixation, internal (orthopedic) NEC T84.84
    gastrointestinal (bile duct) (esophagus)
        T85.848
    genital NEC T83.84
    heart NEC T82.847
    infusion NEC T85.848
    joint prosthesis T84.84
    ocular (corneal graft) (orbital implant)
        NEC T85.848
    orthopedic NEC T84.84
    specified NEC T85.848
    urinary NEC T83.84
    vascular NEC T82.848
    ventricular intracranial shunt T85.840
  due to malignancy (primary) (secondary) G89.3
  ear —*see* subcategory H92.0
  epigastric, epigastrium R10.13

Pain (*Continued*)
  eye —*see* Pain, ocular
  face, facial R51.9
    atypical G50.1
  female genital organs NEC N94.89
  finger —*see* Pain, limb, upper
  flank —*see* Pain, abdominal
  foot —*see* Pain, limb, lower
  gallbladder K82.9
  gas (intestinal) R14.1
  gastric —*see* Pain, abdominal
  generalized NOS R52
  genital organ
    female N94.89
    male N50.89
  groin —*see* Pain, abdominal, lower
  hand —*see* Pain, limb, upper
  head —*see* Headache
  heart —*see* Pain, precordial
  infra-orbital —*see* Neuralgia, trigeminal
  intercostal R07.82
  intermenstrual N94.0
  jaw R68.84
  joint M25.50
    ankle M25.57-•
    elbow M25.52-•
    finger M25.54-•
    foot M25.57-•
    hand M25.54-•
    hip M25.55-•
    knee M25.56-•
    shoulder M25.51-•
    specified site NEC M25.59
    toe M25.57-•
    wrist M25.53-•
  kidney N23
  laryngeal R07.0
  leg —*see* Pain, limb, lower
  limb M79.609
    lower M79.60-•
      foot M79.67-•
      lower leg M79.66-•
      thigh M79.65-•
      toe M79.67-•
    upper M79.60-•
      axilla M79.62-•
      finger M79.64-•
      forearm M79.63-•
      hand M79.64-•
      upper arm M79.62-•
  loin M54.50
  low back M54.50
    specified NEC M54.59
    vertebral end plate M54.51
    vertebrogenic M54.51
  lumbar region M54.50
    vertebral end plate M54.51
    vertebrogenic M54.51
  mandibular R68.84
  mastoid —*see* subcategory H92.0
  maxilla R68.84
  menstrual —*see also* Dysmenorrhea N94.6
  metacarpophalangeal (joint) —*see* Pain, joint,
      hand
  metatarsophalangeal (joint) —*see* Pain, joint,
      foot
  mouth K13.79
  muscle —*see* Myalgia
  musculoskeletal —*see also* Pain, by site M79.18
  myofascial M79.18
  nasal J34.89
  nasopharynx J39.2
  neck NEC M54.2
  nerve NEC —*see* Neuralgia
  neuromuscular —*see* Neuralgia
  nose J34.89
  ocular H57.1-•
  ophthalmic —*see* Pain, ocular
  orbital region —*see* Pain, ocular
  ovary N94.89
  over heart —*see* Pain, precordial
  ovulation N94.0

▶ New   ⇒ Revised   ~~deleted~~ Deleted   • Use Additional Character(s)

Pain *(Continued)*
  pelvic (female) R10.2
  penis N48.89
  pericardial —*see* Pain, precordial
  perineal, perineum R10.2
  pharynx J39.2
  pleura, pleural, pleuritic R07.81
  postoperative NOS G89.18
  postprocedural NOS G89.18
  post-thoracotomy G89.12
  precordial (region) R07.2
  premenstrual N94.3
  psychogenic (persistent) (any site) F45.41
  radicular (spinal) —*see* Radiculopathy
  rectum K62.89
  respiration R07.1
  retrosternal R07.2
  rheumatoid, muscular —*see* Myalgia
  rib R07.81
  root (spinal) —*see* Radiculopathy
  round ligament (stretch) R10.2
  sacroiliac M53.3
  sciatic —*see* Sciatica
  scrotum N50.82
  seminal vesicle N50.89
  shoulder M25.51-●
  spermatic cord N50.89
  spinal root —*see* Radiculopathy
  spine M54.9
    cervical M54.2
  ⇒ low back M54.50
      with sciatica M54.4-●
    ▶ vertebral end plate —*see* Pain,
        vertebrogenic
    thoracic M54.6
  stomach —*see* Pain, abdominal
  substernal R07.2
  temporomandibular (joint) M26.62-●
  testis N50.81-●
  thoracic spine M54.6
    with radicular and visceral pain M54.14
  throat R07.0
  tibia —*see* Pain, limb, lower
  toe —*see* Pain, limb, lower
  tongue K14.6
  tooth K08.89
  trigeminal —*see* Neuralgia, trigeminal
  tumor associated G89.3
  ureter N23
  urinary (organ) (system) N23
  uterus NEC N94.89
  vagina R10.2
  ⇒ vertebrogenic M54.89
    ▶ low back M54.51
    ▶ lumbar M54.51
    ▶ syndrome M54.89
  vesical R39.89
    associated with micturition —*see*
      Micturition, painful
  vulva R10.2
Painful —*see also* Pain
  coitus
    female N94.10
    male N53.12
    psychogenic F52.6
  ejaculation (semen) N53.12
    psychogenic F52.6
  erection —*see* Priapism
  feet syndrome E53.8
  joint replacement (hip) (knee) T84.84
  menstruation —*see* Dysmenorrhea
    psychogenic F45.8
  micturition —*see* Micturition, painful
  respiration R07.1
  scar NEC L90.5
  wire sutures T81.89
Painter's colic —*see* subcategory T56.0
Palate —*see* condition
Palatoplegia K13.79
Palatoschisis —*see* Cleft, palate
Palilalia R48.8
Palliative care Z51.5

Pallor R23.1
  optic disc, temporal —*see* Atrophy, optic
Palmar —*see also* condition
  fascia —*see* condition
Palpable
  cecum K63.89
  kidney N28.89
  ovary N83.8
  prostate N42.9
  spleen —*see* Splenomegaly
Palpitations (heart) R00.2
  psychogenic F45.8
Palsy —*see also* Paralysis G83.9
  atrophic diffuse (progressive) G12.22
  Bell's —*see also* Palsy, facial
    newborn P11.3
  brachial plexus NEC G54.0
    newborn (birth injury) P14.3
  brain —*see* Palsy, cerebral
  bulbar (progressive) (chronic) G12.22
    of childhood (Fazio-Londe) G12.1
    pseudo NEC G12.29
    supranuclear (progressive) G23.1
  cerebral (congenital) G80.9
    ataxic G80.4
    athetoid G80.3
    choreathetoid G80.3
    diplegic G80.8
      spastic G80.1
    dyskinetic G80.3
      athetoid G80.3
      choreathetoid G80.3
      distonic G80.3
    dystonic G80.3
    hemiplegic G80.8
      spastic G80.2
    mixed G80.8
    monoplegic G80.8
      spastic G80.1
    paraplegic G80.8
      spastic G80.1
    quadriplegic G80.8
      spastic G80.0
    spastic G80.1
      diplegic G80.1
      hemiplegic G80.2
      monoplegic G80.1
      quadriplegic G80.0
      specified NEC G80.1
      tetrapelgic G80.0
    specified NEC G80.8
    syphilitic A52.12
      congenital A50.49
    tetraplegic G80.8
      spastic G80.0
  cranial nerve —*see also* Disorder, nerve,
    cranial
    multiple G52.7
      in
        infectious disease B99 [G53]
        neoplastic disease —*see also* Neoplasm
          D49.9 [G53]
        parasitic disease B89 [G53]
        sarcoidosis D86.82
  creeping G12.22
  diver's T70.3
  Erb's P14.0
  facial G51.0
    newborn (birth injury) P11.3
  glossopharyngeal G52.1
  Klumpke (-Déjérine) P14.1
  lead —*see* subcategory T56.0
  median nerve (tardy) G56.1-●
  nerve G58.9
    specified NEC G58.8
  peroneal nerve (acute) (tardy) G57.3-●
  progressive supranuclear G23.1
  pseudobulbar NEC G12.29
  radial nerve (acute) G56.3-●
  seventh nerve —*see also* Palsy, facial
    newborn P11.3
  shaking —*see* Parkinsonism
  spastic (cerebral) (spinal) G80.1

Palsy *(Continued)*
  ulnar nerve (tardy) G56.2-●
  wasting G12.29
Paludism —*see* Malaria
Panangiitis M30.0
Panaris, panaritium —*see also* Cellulitis, digit
  with lymphangitis —*see* Lymphangitis, acute,
    digit
Panarteritis nodosa M30.0
  brain or cerebral I67.7
Pancake heart R93.1
  with cor pulmonale (chronic) I27.81
Pancarditis (acute) (chronic) I51.89
  rheumatic I09.89
    active or acute I01.8
Pancoast's syndrome or tumor C34.1-●
Pancolitis, ulcerative (chronic) K51.00
  with
    abscess K51.014
    complication K51.019
    fistula K51.013
    obstruction K51.012
    rectal bleeding K51.011
    specified complication NEC K51.018
Pancreas, pancreatic —*see* condition
Pancreatitis (annular) (apoplectic) (calcareous)
  (edematous) (hemorrhagic) (malignant)
  (subacute) (suppurative) K85.90
  with necrosis (uninfected) K85.91
    infected K85.92
  acute (without necrosis or infection)
    K85.90
    with necrosis (uninfected) K85.91
      infected K85.92
    alcohol induced (without necrosis or
      infection) K85.20
      with necrosis (uninfected) K85.21
        infected K85.22
    biliary (without necrosis or infection)
      K85.10
      with necrosis (uninfected) K85.11
        infected K85.12
    drug induced (without necrosis or
      infection) K85.30
      with necrosis (uninfected) K85.31
        infected K85.32
    gallstone (without necrosis or infection)
      K85.10
      with necrosis (uninfected) K85.11
        infected K85.12
    idiopathic (without necrosis or infection)
      K85.00
      with necrosis (uninfected) K85.01
        infected K85.02
    specified NEC (without necrosis or
      infection) K85.80
      with necrosis (uninfected) K85.81
        infected K85.82
  chronic (infectious) K86.1
    alcohol-induced K86.0
    recurrent K86.1
    relapsing K86.1
  cystic (chronic) K86.1
  cytomegaloviral B25.2
  fibrous (chronic) K86.1
  gallstone (without necrosis or infection)
    K85.10
    with necrosis (uninfected) K85.11
      infected K85.12
  gangrenous —*see* Pancreatitis, acute
  interstitial (chronic) K86.1
    acute —*see also* Pancreatitis, acute K85.80
  mumps B26.3
  recurrent
  ⇒ acute —*see* Pancreatitis, acute by type
    chronic
  relapsing, chronic K86.1
  syphilitic A52.74
Pancreatoblastoma —*see* Neoplasm, pancreas,
  malignant
Pancreolithiasis K86.89
Pancytolysis D75.89

Pancytopenia (acquired) D61.818
  with
    malformations D61.09
    myelodysplastic syndrome —see
      Syndrome, myelodysplastic
  antineoplastic chemotherapy induced
    D61.810
  congenital D61.09
  drug-induced NEC D61.811
PANDAS (pediatric autoimmune
  neuropsychiatric disorders associated with
  streptococcal infections syndrome) D89.89
Panencephalitis, subacute, sclerosing
  A81.1
Panhematopenia D61.9
  congenital D61.09
  constitutional D61.09
  splenic, primary D73.1
Panhemocytopenia D61.9
  congenital D61.09
  constitutional D61.09
Panhypogonadism E29.1
Panhypopituitarism E23.0
  prepubertal E23.0
Panic (attack) (state) F41.0
  reaction to exceptional stress (transient) F43.0
Panmyelopathy, familial, constitutional D61.09
Panmyelophthisis D61.82
  congenital D61.09
Panmyelosis (acute) (with myelofibrosis)
  C94.4-●
Panner's disease —see Osteochondrosis,
  juvenile, humerus
Panneuritis endemica E51.11
Panniculitis (nodular) (nonsuppurative) M79.3
  back M54.00
    cervical region M54.02
    cervicothoracic region M54.03
    lumbar region M54.06
    lumbosacral region M54.07
    multiple sites M54.09
    occipito-atlanto-axial region M54.01
    sacrococcygeal region M54.08
    thoracic region M54.04
    thoracolumbar region M54.05
  lupus L93.2
  mesenteric K65.4
  neck M54.02
    cervicothoracic region M54.03
    occipito-atlanto-axial region M54.01
  relapsing M35.6
Panniculus adiposus (abdominal) E65
Pannus (allergic) (cornea) (degenerativus)
  (keratic) H16.42-●
  abdominal (symptomatic) E65
  trachomatosus, trachomatous (active) A71.1
Panophthalmitis H44.01-●
Pansinusitis (chronic) (hyperplastic)
  (nonpurulent) (purulent) J32.4
  acute J01.40
    recurrent J01.41
  tuberculous A15.8
Panuveitis (sympathetic) H44.11-●
Panvalvular disease I08.9
  specified NEC I08.8
PAPA (pyogenic arthritis, pyoderma
  gangrenosum, and acne syndrome) M04.8
Papanicolaou smear, cervix Z12.4
  as part of routine gynecological examination
    Z01.419
    with abnormal findings Z01.411
  for suspected neoplasm Z12.4
  nonspecific abnormal finding R87.619
  routine Z01.419
    with abnormal findings Z01.411
Papilledema (choked disc) H47.10
  associated with
    decreased ocular pressure H47.12
    increased intracranial pressure H47.11
    retinal disorder H47.13
  Foster-Kennedy syndrome H47.14-●

Papillitis H46.00
  anus K62.89
  chronic lingual K14.4
  necrotizing, kidney N17.2
  optic H46.0-●
  rectum K62.89
  renal, necrotizing N17.2
  tongue K14.0
Papilloma —see also Neoplasm, benign,
    by site
  acuminatum (female) (male) (anogenital)
    A63.0
  basal cell L82.1
    inflamed L82.0
  benign pinta (primary) A67.0
  bladder (urinary) (transitional cell) D41.4
  choroid plexus (lateral ventricle) (third
      ventricle) D33.0
    anaplastic C71.5
    fourth ventricle D33.1
    malignant C71.5
  renal pelvis (transitional cell) D41.1-●
    benign D30.1-●
  Schneiderian
    specified site —see Neoplasm, benign, by
      site
    unspecified site D14.0
  serous surface
    borderline malignancy
      specified site —see Neoplasm, uncertain
        behavior, by site
      unspecified site D39.10
    specified site —see Neoplasm, benign, by
      site
    unspecified site D27.9
  transitional (cell)
    bladder (urinary) D41.4
    inverted type —see Neoplasm, uncertain
      behavior, by site
    renal pelvis D41.1-●
    ureter D41.2-●
  ureter (transitional cell) D41.2-●
    benign D30.2-●
  urothelial —see Neoplasm, uncertain
    behavior, by site
  villous —see Neoplasm, uncertain behavior,
    by site
    adenocarcinoma in —see Neoplasm,
      malignant, by site
    in situ —see Neoplasm, in situ
  yaws, plantar or palmar A66.1
Papillomata, multiple, of yaws A66.1
Papillomatosis —see also Neoplasm, benign,
    by site
  confluent and reticulated L83
  cystic, breast —see Mastopathy, cystic
  ductal, breast —see Mastopathy, cystic
  intraductal (diffuse) —see Neoplasm, benign,
    by site
  subareolar duct D24-●
Papillomavirus, as cause of disease classified
    elsewhere B97.7
Papillon-Léage and Psaume syndrome
    Q87.0
Papule(s) R23.8
  carate (primary) A67.0
  fibrous, of nose D22.39
  Gottron's L94.4
  pinta (primary) A67.0
Papulosis
  lymphomatoid C86.6
  malignant I77.89
Papyraceous fetus O31.0-●
Para-albuminemia E88.09
Paracephalus Q89.7
Parachute mitral valve Q23.2
Paracoccidioidomycosis B41.9
  disseminated B41.7
  generalized B41.7
  mucocutaneous-lymphangitic B41.8
  pulmonary B41.0

Paracoccidioidomycosis (Continued)
  specified NEC B41.8
  visceral B41.8
Paradentosis K05.4
Paraffinoma T88.8
Paraganglioma D44.7
  adrenal D35.0-●
    malignant C74.1-●
  aortic body D44.7
    malignant C75.5
  carotid body D44.6
    malignant C75.4
  chromaffin —see also Neoplasm, benign, by
    site
    malignant —see Neoplasm, malignant, by
      site
  extra-adrenal D44.7
    malignant C75.5
      specified site —see Neoplasm,
        malignant, by site
      unspecified site C75.5
    specified site —see Neoplasm, uncertain
      behavior, by site
    unspecified site D44.7
  gangliocytic D13.2
    specified site —see Neoplasm, benign, by
      site
    unspecified site D13.2
  glomus jugulare D44.7
    malignant C75.5
  jugular D44.7
  malignant C75.5
    specified site —see Neoplasm, malignant,
      by site
    unspecified site C75.5
  nonchromaffin D44.7
    malignant C75.5
      specified site —see Neoplasm,
        malignant, by site
      unspecified site C75.5
    specified site —see Neoplasm, uncertain
      behavior, by site
    unspecified site D44.7
  parasympathetic D44.7
    specified site —see Neoplasm, uncertain
      behavior, by site
    unspecified site D44.7
  specified site —see Neoplasm, uncertain
    behavior, by site
  sympathetic D44.7
    specified site —see Neoplasm, uncertain
      behavior, by site
    unspecified site D44.7
  unspecified site D44.7
Parageusia R43.2
  psychogenic F45.8
Paragonimiasis B66.4
Paragranuloma, Hodgkin —see Lymphoma,
  Hodgkin, specified NEC
Parahemophilia —see also Defect, coagulation
  D68.2
Parakeratosis R23.4
  variegata L41.0
Paralysis, paralytic (complete) (incomplete)
  G83.9
  with
    syphilis A52.17
  abducens, abducent (nerve) —see Strabismus,
    paralytic, sixth nerve
  abductor, lower extremity G57.9-●
  accessory nerve G52.8
  accommodation —see also Paresis, of
    accommodation
    hysterical F44.89
  acoustic nerve (except Deafness) —see
    subcategory H93.3
  agitans —see also Parkinsonism G20
    arteriosclerotic G21.4
  alternating (oculomotor) G83.89
  amyotrophic G12.21

▶ New   ⇒ Revised   ~~deleted~~ Deleted   ● Use Additional Character(s)

Paralysis, paralytic *(Continued)*
  ankle G57.9-●
  anus (sphincter) K62.89
  arm —*see* Monoplegia, upper limb
  ascending (spinal), acute G61.0
  association G12.29
  asthenic bulbar G70.00
    with exacerbation (acute) G70.01
    in crisis G70.01
  ataxic (hereditary) G11.9
    general (syphilitic) A52.17
  atrophic G58.9
    infantile, acute —*see* Poliomyelitis, paralytic
    progressive G12.22
    spinal (acute) —*see* Poliomyelitis, paralytic
  axillary G54.0
  Babinski-Nageotte's G83.89
  Bell's G51.0
    newborn P11.3
  Benedikt's G46.3
  birth injury P14.9
    spinal cord P11.5
  bladder (neurogenic) (sphincter)
      N31.2
  bowel, colon or intestine K56.0
  brachial plexus G54.0
    birth injury P14.3
    newborn (birth injury) P14.3
  brain G83.9
    diplegia G83.0
    triplegia G83.89
  bronchial J98.09
  Brown-Séquard G83.81
  bulbar (chronic) (progressive) G12.22
    infantile —*see* Poliomyelitis, paralytic
    poliomyelitic —*see* Poliomyelitis, paralytic
    pseudo G12.29
  bulbospinal G70.00
    with exacerbation (acute) G70.01
    in crisis G70.01
  cardiac —*see also* Failure, heart I50.9
  cerebrocerebellar, diplegic G80.1
  cervical
    plexus G54.2
    sympathetic G90.09
  Céstan-Chenais G46.3
  Charcot-Marie-Tooth type G60.0
  Clark's G80.9
  colon K56.0
  compressed air T70.3
  compression
    arm G56.9-●
    leg G57.9-●
    lower extremity G57.9-●
    upper extremity G56.9-●
  congenital (cerebral) —*see* Palsy, cerebral
  conjugate movement (gaze) (of eye) H51.0
    cortical (nuclear) (supranuclear) H51.0
  cordis —*see* Failure, heart
  cranial or cerebral nerve G52.9
  creeping G12.22
  crossed leg G83.89
  crutch —*see* Injury, brachial plexus
  deglutition R13.0
    hysterical F44.4
  dementia A52.17
  descending (spinal) NEC G12.29
  diaphragm (flaccid) J98.6
    due to accidental dissection of phrenic
        nerve during procedure —*see*
        Puncture, accidental complicating
        surgery
  digestive organs NEC K59.89
  diplegic —*see* Diplegia
  divergence (nuclear) H51.8
  diver's T70.3
  Duchenne's
    birth injury P14.0
    due to or associated with
        motor neuron disease G12.22
        muscular dystrophy G71.01

Paralysis, paralytic *(Continued)*
  due to intracranial or spinal birth injury —*see*
      Palsy, cerebral
  embolic (current episode) I63.4-●
  Erb (-Duchenne) (birth) (newborn) P14.0
  Erb's syphilitic spastic spinal A52.17
  esophagus K22.89
  eye muscle (extrinsic) H49.9
    intrinsic —*see also* Paresis, of
        accommodation
  facial (nerve) G51.0
    birth injury P11.3
    congenital P11.3
    following operation NEC —*see* Puncture,
        accidental complicating surgery
    newborn (birth injury) P11.3
  familial (recurrent) (periodic) G72.3
    spastic G11.4
  fauces J39.2
  finger G56.9-●
  gait R26.1
  gastric nerve (nondiabetic) G52.2
  gaze, conjugate H51.0
  general (progressive) (syphilitic) A52.17
    juvenile A50.45
  glottis J38.00
    bilateral J38.02
    unilateral J38.01
  gluteal G54.1
  Gubler (-Millard) G46.3
  hand —*see* Monoplegia, upper limb
  heart —*see* Arrest, cardiac
  hemiplegic —*see* Hemiplegia
  hyperkalemic periodic (familial) G72.3
  hypoglossal (nerve) G52.3
  hypokalemic periodic G72.3
  hysterical F44.4
  ileus K56.0
  infantile —*see also* Poliomyelitis, paralytic
      A80.30
    bulbar —*see* Poliomyelitis, paralytic
    cerebral —*see* Palsy, cerebral
    spastic —*see* Palsy, cerebral, spastic
  infective —*see* Poliomyelitis, paralytic
  inferior nuclear G83.9
  internuclear —*see* Ophthalmoplegia,
      internuclear
  intestine K56.0
  iris H57.09
    due to diphtheria (toxin) A36.89
  ischemic, Volkmann's (complicating trauma)
      T79.6
  Jackson's G83.89
  jake —*see* Poisoning, food, noxious, plant
  Jamaica ginger (jake) G62.2
  juvenile general A50.45
  Klumpke (-Déjérine) (birth) (newborn) P14.1
  labioglossal (laryngeal) (pharyngeal) G12.29
  Landry's G61.0
  laryngeal nerve (recurrent) (superior)
      (unilateral) J38.00
    bilateral J38.02
    unilateral J38.01
  larynx J38.00
    bilateral J38.02
    due to diphtheria (toxin) A36.2
    unilateral J38.01
  lateral G12.23
  lead —*see* subcategory T56.0
  left side —*see* Hemiplegia
  leg G83.1-●
    both —*see* Paraplegia
    crossed G83.89
    hysterical F44.4
    psychogenic F44.4
    transient or transitory R29.818
        traumatic NEC —*see* Injury, nerve, leg
  levator palpebrae superioris —*see*
      Blepharoptosis, paralytic
  limb —*see* Monoplegia
  lip K13.0

Paralysis, paralytic *(Continued)*
  Lissauer's A52.17
  lower limb —*see* Monoplegia, lower limb
    both —*see* Paraplegia
  lung J98.4
  median nerve G56.1-●
  medullary (tegmental) G83.89
  mesencephalic NEC G83.89
    tegmental G83.89
  middle alternating G83.89
  Millard-Gubler-Foville G46.3
  monoplegic —*see* Monoplegia
  motor G83.9
  muscle, muscular NEC G72.89
    due to nerve lesion G58.9
    eye (extrinsic) H49.9
        intrinsic —*see* Paresis, of accommodation
        oblique —*see* Strabismus, paralytic,
            fourth nerve
    iris sphincter H21.9
    ischemic (Volkmann's) (complicating
        trauma) T79.6
    progressive G12.21
    progressive, spinal G12.25
    pseudohypertrophic G71.02
    spinal progressive G12.25
  musculocutaneous nerve G56.9-●
  musculospiral G56.9-●
  nerve —*see also* Disorder, nerve
    abducent —*see* Strabismus, paralytic, sixth
        nerve
    accessory G52.8
    auditory (except Deafness) —*see*
        subcategory H93.3
    birth injury P14.9
    cranial or cerebral G52.9
    facial G51.0
        birth injury P11.3
        congenital P11.3
        newborn (birth injury) P11.3
    fourth or trochlear —*see* Strabismus,
        paralytic, fourth nerve
    newborn (birth injury) P14.9
    oculomotor —*see* Strabismus, paralytic,
        third nerve
    phrenic (birth injury) P14.2
    radial G56.3-●
    seventh or facial G51.0
        newborn (birth injury) P11.3
    sixth or abducent —*see* Strabismus,
        paralytic, sixth nerve
    syphilitic A52.15
    third or oculomotor —*see* Strabismus,
        paralytic, third nerve
    trigeminal G50.9
    trochlear —*see* Strabismus, paralytic,
        fourth nerve
    ulnar G56.2-●
  normokalemic periodic G72.3
  ocular H49.9
    alternating G83.89
  oculofacial, congenital (Moebius) Q87.0
  oculomotor (external bilateral) (nerve) —*see*
      Strabismus, paralytic, third nerve
  palate (soft) K13.79
  paratrigeminal G50.9
  periodic (familial) (hyperkalemic)
      (hypokalemic) (myotonic)
      (normokalemic) (potassium sensitive)
      (secondary) G72.3
  peripheral autonomic nervous system —*see*
      Neuropathy, peripheral, autonomic
  peroneal (nerve) G57.3-●
  pharynx J39.2
  phrenic nerve G56.8-●
  plantar nerve(s) G57.6-●
  pneumogastric nerve G52.2
  poliomyelitis (current) —*see* Poliomyelitis,
      paralytic
  popliteal nerve G57.3-●
  postepileptic transitory G83.84

Paralysis, paralytic (Continued)
progressive (atrophic) (bulbar) (spinal) G12.22
  general A52.17
  infantile acute —*see* Poliomyelitis, paralytic
  supranuclear G23.1
pseudobulbar G12.29
pseudohypertrophic (muscle) G71.09
psychogenic F44.4
quadriceps G57.9-●
quadriplegic —*see* Tetraplegia
radial nerve G56.3-●
rectus muscle (eye) H49.9
recurrent isolated sleep G47.53
respiratory (muscle) (system) (tract) R06.81
  center NEC G93.89
  congenital P28.89
  newborn P28.89
right side —*see* Hemiplegia
saturnine —*see* subcategory T56.0
sciatic nerve G57.0-●
senile G83.9
shaking —*see* Parkinsonism
shoulder G56.9-●
sleep, recurrent isolated G47.53
spastic G83.9
  cerebral —*see* Palsy, cerebral, spastic
  congenital (cerebral) —*see* Palsy, cerebral, spastic
  familial G11.4
  hereditary G11.4
  quadriplegic G80.0
  syphilitic (spinal) A52.17
sphincter, bladder —*see* Paralysis, bladder
spinal (cord) G83.9
  accessory nerve G52.8
  acute —*see* Poliomyelitis, paralytic
  ascending acute G61.0
  atrophic (acute) —*see also* Poliomyelitis, paralytic
    spastic, syphilitic A52.17
  congenital NEC —*see* Palsy, cerebral
  hereditary G95.89
  infantile —*see* Poliomyelitis, paralytic
  progressive G12.21
  muscle G12.25
  sequelae NEC G83.89
sternomastoid G52.8
stomach K31.84
  diabetic —*see* Diabetes, by type, with gastroparesis
  nerve G52.2
    diabetic —*see* Diabetes, by type, with gastroparesis
stroke —*see* Infarct, brain
subcapsularis G56.8-●
supranuclear (progressive) G23.1
sympathetic G90.8
  cervical G90.09
  nervous system —*see* Neuropathy, peripheral, autonomic
syndrome G83.9
  specified NEC G83.89
syphilitic spastic spinal (Erb's) A52.17
thigh G57.9-●
throat J39.2
  diphtheritic A36.0
  muscle J39.2
thrombotic (current episode) I63.3-●
thumb G56.9-●
tick —*see* Toxicity, venom, arthropod, specified NEC
Todd's (postepileptic transitory paralysis) G83.84
toe G57.6-●
tongue K14.8
transient R29.5
  arm or leg NEC R29.818
  traumatic NEC —*see* Injury, nerve
trapezius G52.8
traumatic, transient NEC —*see* Injury, nerve

Paralysis, paralytic (Continued)
trembling —*see* Parkinsonism
triceps brachii G56.9-●
trigeminal nerve G50.9
trochlear (nerve) —*see* Strabismus, paralytic, fourth nerve
ulnar nerve G56.2-●
upper limb —*see* Monoplegia, upper limb
uremic N18.9 [G99.8]
uveoparotitic D86.89
uvula K13.79
  postdiphtheritic A36.0
vagus nerve G52.2
vasomotor NEC G90.8
velum palati K13.79
vesical —*see* Paralysis, bladder
vestibular nerve (except Vertigo) —*see* subcategory H93.3
vocal cords J38.00
  bilateral J38.02
  unilateral J38.01
Volkmann's (complicating trauma) T79.6
wasting G12.29
Weber's G46.3
wrist G56.9-●
Paramedial urethrovesical orifice Q64.79
Paramenia N92.6
Parametritis —*see also* Disease, pelvis, inflammatory N73.2
acute N73.0
complicating abortion —*see* Abortion, by type, complicated by, parametritis
Parametrium, parametric —*see* condition
Paramnesia —*see* Amnesia
Paramolar K00.1
Paramyloidosis E85.89
Paramyoclonus multiplex G25.3
Paramyotonia (congenita) G71.19
Parangi —*see* Yaws
Paranoia (querulans) F22
senile F03
Paranoid
dementia (senile) F03
  praecox —*see* Schizophrenia
personality F60.0
psychosis (climacteric) (involutional) (menopausal) F22
  psychogenic (acute) F23
  senile F03
reaction (acute) F23
  chronic F22
schizophrenia F20.0
state (climacteric) (involutional) (menopausal) (simple) F22
  senile F03
tendencies F60.0
traits F60.0
trends F60.0
type, psychopathic personality F60.0
Paraparesis —*see* Paraplegia
Paraphasia R47.02
Paraphilia F65.9
Paraphimosis (congenital) N47.2
chancroidal A57
Paraphrenia, paraphrenic (late) F22
schizophrenia F20.0
Paraplegia (lower) G82.20
ataxic —*see* Degeneration, combined, spinal cord
complete G82.21
congenital (cerebral) G80.8
  spastic G80.1
familial spastic G11.4
functional (hysterical) F44.4
hereditary, spastic G11.4
hysterical F44.4
incomplete G82.22
Pott's A18.01
psychogenic F44.4

Paraplegia (Continued)
spastic
  Erb's spinal, syphilitic A52.17
  hereditary G11.4
  tropical G04.1
syphilitic (spastic) A52.17
traumatic
  current injury - code to injury with seventh character A
  sequela of previous injury - code to injury with seventh character S
tropical spastic G04.1
Parapoxvirus B08.60
specified NEC B08.69
Paraproteinemia D89.2
benign (familial) D89.2
monoclonal D47.2
secondary to malignant disease D47.2
Parapsoriasis L41.9
en plaques L41.4
guttata L41.1
large plaque L41.4
retiform, retiformis L41.5
small plaque L41.3
specified NEC L41.8
varioliformis (acuta) L41.0
Parasitic —*see also* condition
disease NEC B89
stomatitis B37.0
sycosis (beard) (scalp) B35.0
twin Q89.4
Parasitism B89
intestinal B82.9
skin B88.9
specified —*see* Infestation
Parasitophobia F40.218
Parasomnia G47.50
due to
  alcohol
    abuse F10.182
    dependence F10.282
    use F10.982
  amphetamines
    abuse F15.182
    dependence F15.282
    use F15.982
  caffeine
    abuse F15.182
    dependence F15.282
    use F15.982
  cocaine
    abuse F14.182
    dependence F14.282
    use F14.982
  drug NEC
    abuse F19.182
    dependence F19.282
    use F19.982
  opioid
    abuse F11.182
    dependence F11.282
    use F11.982
  psychoactive substance NEC
    abuse F19.182
    dependence F19.282
    use F19.982
  sedative, hypnotic, or anxiolytic
    abuse F13.182
    dependence F13.282
    use F13.982
  stimulant NEC
    abuse F15.182
    dependence F15.282
    use F15.982
in conditions classified elsewhere G47.54
nonorganic origin F51.8
organic G47.50
specified NEC G47.59
Paraspadias Q54.9
Paraspasmus facialis G51.8

▶ New   ⇒ Revised   ~~deleted~~ Deleted   ● Use Additional Character(s)

Parasuicide (attempt)
history of (personal) Z91.51
in family Z81.8
Parathyroid gland —see condition
Parathyroid tetany E20.9
Paratrachoma A74.0
Paratyphilitis —see Appendicitis
Paratyphoid (fever) —see Fever, paratyphoid
Paratyphus —see Fever, paratyphoid
Paraurethral duct Q64.79
Paraurethritis —see also Urethritis
gonococcal (acute) (chronic) (with abscess) A54.1
Paravaccinia NEC B08.04
Paravaginitis —see Vaginitis
Parencephalitis —see also Encephalitis
sequelae G09
Parent-child conflict —see Conflict, parent-child
estrangement NEC Z62.890
Paresis —see also Paralysis
accommodation —see Paresis, of accommodation
Bernhardt's G57.1-●
bladder (sphincter) —see also Paralysis, bladder
tabetic A52.17
bowel, colon or intestine K56.0
extrinsic muscle, eye H49.9
general (progressive) (syphilitic) A52.17
juvenile A50.45
heart —see Failure, heart
insane (syphilitic) A52.17
juvenile (general) A50.45
of accommodation H52.52-●
peripheral progressive (idiopathic) G60.3
pseudohypertrophic G71.09
senile G83.9
syphilitic (general) A52.17
congenital A50.45
vesical NEC N31.2
Paresthesia —see also Disturbance, sensation, skin R20.2
Bernhardt G57.1-●
Paretic —see condition
Parinaud's
conjunctivitis H10.89
oculoglandular syndrome H10.89
ophthalmoplegia H49.88
Parkinsonism (idiopathic) (primary) G20
with neurogenic orthostatic hypotension (symptomatic) G90.3
arteriosclerotic G21.4
dementia G31.83 [F02.80]
with behavioral disturbance G31.83 [F02.81]
due to
drugs NEC G21.19
neuroleptic G21.11
medication-induced NEC G21.19
neuroleptic induced G21.11
postencephalitic G21.3
secondary G21.9
due to
arteriosclerosis G21.4
drugs NEC G21.19
neuroleptic G21.11
encephalitis G21.3
external agents NEC G21.2
syphilis A52.19
specified NEC G21.8
syphilitic A52.19
treatment-induced NEC G21.19
vascular G21.4
Parkinson's disease, syndrome or tremor —see Parkinsonism
Parodontitis —see Periodontitis
Parodontosis K05.4
Paronychia —see also Cellulitis, digit
with lymphangitis —see Lymphangitis, acute, digit
candidal (chronic) B37.2
tuberculous (primary) A18.4
Parorexia (psychogenic) F50.89

Parosmia R43.1
psychogenic F45.8
Parotid gland —see condition
Parotitis, parotiditis (allergic) (nonspecific toxic) (purulent) (septic) (suppurative) — see also Sialoadenitis
epidemic —see Mumps
infectious —see Mumps
postoperative K91.89
surgical K91.89
Parrot fever A70
Parrot's disease (early congenital syphilitic pseudoparalysis) A50.02
Parry-Romberg syndrome G51.8
Parry's disease or syndrome E05.00
with thyroid storm E05.01
Pars planitis —see Cyclitis
Parsonage (-Aldren)-Turner syndrome G54.5
Parson's disease (exophthalmic goiter) E05.00
with thyroid storm E05.01
Particolored infant Q82.8
Parturition —see Delivery
Parulis K04.7
with sinus K04.6
Parvovirus, as cause of disease classified elsewhere B97.6
Pasini and Pierini's atrophoderma L90.3
Passage
false, urethra N36.5
meconium (newborn) during delivery P03.82
of sounds or bougies —see Attention to, artificial, opening
Passive —see condition
smoking Z77.22
▶ Past due on rent or mortgage Z59.81- ●
Pasteurella septica A28.0
Pasteurellosis —see Infection, Pasteurella
PAT (paroxysmal atrial tachycardia) I47.1
Patau's syndrome —see Trisomy, 13
Patches
mucous (syphilitic) A51.39
congenital A50.07
smokers' (mouth) K13.24
Patellar —see condition
Patent —see also Imperfect, closure
canal of Nuck Q52.4
cervix N88.3
ductus arteriosus or Botallo's Q25.0
foramen
botalli Q21.1
ovale Q21.1
interauricular septum Q21.1
interventricular septum Q21.0
omphalomesenteric duct Q43.0
os (uteri) —see Patent, cervix
ostium secundum Q21.1
urachus Q64.4
vitelline duct Q43.0
Paterson (-Brown)(-Kelly) syndrome or web D50.1
Pathologic, pathological —see also condition
asphyxia R09.01
fire-setting F63.1
gambling F63.0
ovum O02.0
resorption, tooth K03.3
stealing F63.2
Pathology (of) —see Disease
periradicular, associated with previous endodontic treatment NEC M27.59
Pattern, sleep-wake, irregular G47.23
Patulous —see also Imperfect, closure (congenital)
alimentary tract Q45.8
lower Q43.8
upper Q40.8
eustachian tube H69.0-●
Pause, sinoatrial I49.5
Paxton's disease B36.2
Pearl(s)
enamel K00.2
Epstein's K09.8

Pearl-worker's disease —see Osteomyelitis, specified type NEC
Pectenosis K62.4
Pectoral —see condition
Pectus
carinatum (congenital) Q67.7
acquired M95.4
rachitic sequelae (late effect) E64.3
excavatum (congenital) Q67.6
acquired M95.4
rachitic sequelae (late effect) E64.3
recurvatum (congenital) Q67.6
Pedatrophia E41
Pederosis F65.4
Pediatric inflammatory multisystem syndrome M35.81
Pediculosis (infestation) B85.2
capitis (head-louse) (any site) B85.0
corporis (body-louse) (any site) B85.1
eyelid B85.0
mixed (classifiable to more than one of the titles B85.0-B85.3) B85.4
pubis (pubic louse) (any site) B85.3
vestimenti B85.1
vulvae B85.3
Pediculus (infestation) —see Pediculosis
Pedophilia F65.4
Peg-shaped teeth K00.2
Pelade —see Alopecia, areata
Pelger-Huët anomaly or syndrome D72.0
Peliosis (rheumatica) D69.0
hepatis K76.4
with toxic liver disease K71.8
Pelizaeus-Merzbacher disease E75.29
Pellagra (alcoholic) (with polyneuropathy) E52
Pellagra-cerebellar-ataxia-renal aminoaciduria syndrome E72.02
Pellegrini (-Stieda) disease or syndrome —see Bursitis, tibial collateral
Pellizzi's syndrome E34.8
Pel's crisis A52.11
Pelvic — see also condition
examination (periodic) (routine) Z01.419
with abnormal findings Z01.411
kidney, congenital Q63.2
Pelviolithiasis —see Calculus, kidney
Pelviperitonitis —see also Peritonitis, pelvic
gonococcal A54.24
puerperal O85
Pelvis — see condition or type
Pemphigoid L12.9
benign, mucous membrane L12.1
bullous L12.0
cicatricial L12.1
juvenile L12.2
ocular L12.1
specified NEC L12.8
Pemphigus L10.9
benign familial (chronic) Q82.8
Brazilian L10.3
circinatus L13.0
conjunctiva L12.1
drug-induced L10.5
erythematosus L10.4
foliaceous L10.2
gangrenous —see Gangrene
neonatorum L01.03
ocular L12.1
paraneoplastic L10.81
specified NEC L10.89
syphilitic (congenital) A50.06
vegetans L10.1
vulgaris L10.0
wildfire L10.3
Pendred's syndrome E07.1
Pendulous
abdomen, in pregnancy —see Pregnancy, complicated by, abnormal, pelvic organs or tissues NEC
breast N64.89

Penetrating wound —see also Puncture
  with internal injury —see Injury, by site
  eyeball —see Puncture, eyeball
  orbit (with or without foreign body) —see
    Puncture, orbit
  uterus by instrument with or following
    ectopic or molar pregnancy O08.6
Penicillosis B48.4
Penis —see condition
Penitis N48.29
Pentalogy of Fallot Q21.8
Pentasomy X syndrome Q97.1
Pentosuria (essential) E74.89
Percreta placenta O43.23-•
Peregrinating patient —see Disorder, factitious
Perforation, perforated (nontraumatic) (of)
  accidental during procedure (blood vessel)
    (nerve) (organ) —see Complication,
    accidental puncture or laceration
  antrum —see Sinusitis, maxillary
  appendix K35.22
    with localized peritonitis K35.32
  atrial septum, multiple Q21.1
  attic, ear —see Perforation, tympanum, attic
  bile duct (common) (hepatic) K83.2
    cystic K82.2
  bladder (urinary)
    with or following ectopic or molar
      pregnancy O08.6
    obstetrical trauma O71.5
    traumatic S37.29
      at delivery O71.5
  bowel K63.1
    with or following ectopic or molar
      pregnancy O08.6
    newborn P78.0
    obstetrical trauma O71.5
    traumatic —see Laceration, intestine
  broad ligament N83.8
    with or following ectopic or molar
      pregnancy O08.6
    obstetrical trauma O71.6
  by
    device, implant or graft —see also
      Complications, by site and type,
      mechanical T85.628
      arterial graft NEC —see Complication,
        cardiovascular device, mechanical,
        vascular
      breast (implant) T85.49
      catheter NEC T85.698
        cystostomy T83.090
        dialysis (renal) T82.49
          intraperitoneal T85.691
        infusion NEC T82.594
          spinal (epidural) (subdural) T85.690
        urinary —see also Complications,
          catheter, urinary T83.098
      electronic (electrode) (pulse generator)
        (stimulator)
        bone T84.390
        cardiac T82.199
          electrode T82.190
          pulse generator T82.191
          specified type NEC T82.198
        nervous system —see Complication,
          prosthetic device, mechanical,
          electronic nervous system
          stimulator
        urinary —see Complication,
          genitourinary, device, urinary,
          mechanical
      fixation, internal (orthopedic) NEC —
        see Complication, fixation device,
        mechanical
      gastrointestinal —see Complications,
        prosthetic device, mechanical,
        gastrointestinal device
      genital NEC T83.498
        intrauterine contraceptive device
          T83.39
        penile prosthesis T83.490

Perforation, perforated (Continued)
  by (Continued)
    device, implant or graft (Continued)
      heart NEC —see Complication,
        cardiovascular device, mechanical
      joint prosthesis —see Complications,
        joint prosthesis, mechanical,
        specified NEC, by site
      ocular NEC —see Complications,
        prosthetic device, mechanical,
        ocular device
      orthopedic NEC —see Complication,
        orthopedic, device, mechanical
      specified NEC T85.628
      urinary NEC —see also Complication,
        genitourinary, device, urinary,
        mechanical
        graft T83.29
      vascular NEC —see Complication,
        cardiovascular device, mechanical
      ventricular intracranial shunt T85.09
    foreign body left accidentally in
      operative wound T81.539
    instrument (any) during a procedure,
      accidental —see Puncture, accidental
      complicating surgery
  cecum K35.22
    with localized peritonitis K35.32
  cervix (uteri) N88.8
    with or following ectopic or molar
      pregnancy O08.6
    obstetrical trauma O71.3
  colon K63.1
    newborn P78.0
    obstetrical trauma O71.5
    traumatic —see Laceration, intestine, large
  common duct (bile) K83.2
  cornea (due to ulceration) —see Ulcer,
    cornea, perforated
  cystic duct K82.2
  diverticulum (intestine) K57.80
    with bleeding K57.81
    large intestine K57.20
      with
        bleeding K57.21
        small intestine K57.40
          with bleeding K57.41
    small intestine K57.00
      with
        bleeding K57.01
        large intestine K57.40
          with bleeding K57.41
  ear drum —see Perforation, tympanum
  esophagus K22.3
  ethmoidal sinus —see Sinusitis, ethmoidal
  frontal sinus —see Sinusitis, frontal
  gallbladder K82.2
  heart valve —see Endocarditis
  ileum K63.1
    newborn P78.0
    obstetrical trauma O71.5
    traumatic —see Laceration, intestine, small
  instrumental, surgical (accidental) (blood
    vessel) (nerve) (organ) —see Puncture,
    accidental complicating surgery
  intestine NEC K63.1
    with ectopic or molar pregnancy O08.6
    newborn P78.0
    obstetrical trauma O71.5
    traumatic —see Laceration, intestine
    ulcerative NEC K63.1
      newborn P78.0
  jejunum, jejunal K63.1
    obstetrical trauma O71.5
    traumatic —see Laceration, intestine, small
    ulcer —see Ulcer, gastrojejunal, with
      perforation
  joint prosthesis —see Complications, joint
    prosthesis, mechanical, specified NEC,
    by site
  mastoid (antrum) (cell) —see Disorder,
    mastoid, specified NEC

Perforation, perforated (Continued)
  maxillary sinus —see Sinusitis, maxillary
  membrana tympani —see Perforation,
    tympanum
  nasal
    septum J34.89
      congenital Q30.3
      syphilitic A52.73
    sinus J34.89
      congenital Q30.8
      due to sinusitis —see Sinusitis
  palate —see also Cleft, palate Q35.9
    syphilitic A52.79
  palatine vault —see also Cleft, palate, hard Q35.1
    syphilitic A52.79
    congenital A50.59
  pars flaccida (ear drum) —see Perforation,
    tympanum, attic
  pelvic
    floor S31.030
      with
        ectopic or molar pregnancy O08.6
        penetration into retroperitoneal space
          S31.031
        retained foreign body S31.040
          with penetration into
            retroperitoneal space S31.041
      following ectopic or molar pregnancy
        O08.6
      obstetrical trauma O70.1
    organ S37.99
      adrenal gland S37.818
      bladder —see Perforation, bladder
      fallopian tube S37.599
        bilateral S37.592
        unilateral S37.591
      kidney S37.09-•
      obstetrical trauma O71.5
      ovary S37.499
        bilateral S37.492
        unilateral S37.491
      prostate S37.828
      specified organ NEC S37.898
      ureter —see Perforation, ureter
      urethra —see Perforation, urethra
      uterus —see Perforation, uterus
  perineum —see Laceration, perineum
  pharynx J39.2
  rectum K63.1
    newborn P78.0
    obstetrical trauma O71.5
    traumatic S36.63
  root canal space due to endodontic treatment
    M27.51
  sigmoid K63.1
    newborn P78.0
    obstetrical trauma O71.5
    traumatic S36.533
  sinus (accessory) (chronic) (nasal) J34.89
  sphenoidal sinus —see Sinusitis, sphenoidal
  surgical (accidental) (by instrument) (blood
    vessel) (nerve) (organ) —see Puncture,
    accidental complicating surgery
  traumatic
    external —see Puncture
    eye —see Puncture, eyeball
    internal organ —see Injury, by site
  tympanum, tympanic (membrane) (persistent
    post-traumatic) (postinflammatory)
    H72.9-•
    attic H72.1-•
      multiple —see Perforation, tympanum,
        multiple
      total —see Perforation, tympanum, total
    central H72.0-•
      multiple —see Perforation, tympanum,
        multiple
      total —see Perforation, tympanum, total
    marginal NEC —see subcategory H72.2
    multiple H72.81-•
    pars flaccida —see Perforation, tympanum,
      attic

▶ New   ⇒ Revised   ~~deleted~~ Deleted   • Use Additional Character(s)

Perforation, perforated (Continued)
tympanum, tympanic (Continued)
total H72.82-●
traumatic, current episode S09.2-●
typhoid, gastrointestinal —see Typhoid
ulcer —see Ulcer, by site, with perforation
ureter N28.89
traumatic S37.19
urethra N36.8
with ectopic or molar pregnancy O08.6
following ectopic or molar pregnancy O08.6
obstetrical trauma O71.5
traumatic S37.39
at delivery O71.5
uterus
with ectopic or molar pregnancy O08.6
by intrauterine contraceptive device T83.39
following ectopic or molar pregnancy O08.6
obstetrical trauma O71.1
traumatic S37.69
obstetric O71.1
uvula K13.79
syphilitic A52.79
vagina
obstetrical trauma O71.4
other trauma - see Puncture, vagina
Periadenitis mucosa necrotica recurrens K12.0
Periappendicitis (acute) —see Appendicitis
Periarteritis nodosa (disseminated) (infectious)
(necrotizing) M30.0
Periarthritis (joint) —see also Enthesopathy
Duplay's M75.0-●
gonococcal A54.42
humeroscapularis —see Capsulitis, adhesive
scapulohumeral —see Capsulitis, adhesive
shoulder —see Capsulitis, adhesive
wrist M77.2-●
Periarthrosis (angioneural) —see Enthesopathy
Pericapsulitis, adhesive (shoulder) —see
Capsulitis, adhesive
Pericarditis (with decompensation) (with
effusion) I31.9
with rheumatic fever (conditions in I00)
active —see Pericarditis, rheumatic
inactive or quiescent I09.2
acute (hemorrhagic) (nonrheumatic) (Sicca)
I30.9
with chorea (acute) (rheumatic)
(Sydenham's) I02.0
benign I30.8
nonspecific I30.0
rheumatic I01.0
with chorea (acute) (Sydenham's) I02.0
adhesive or adherent (chronic) (external)
(internal) I31.0
acute —see Pericarditis, acute
rheumatic I09.2
bacterial (acute) (subacute) (with serous or
seropurulent effusion) I30.1
calcareous I31.1
cholesterol (chronic) I31.8
acute I30.9
chronic (nonrheumatic) I31.9
rheumatic I09.2
constrictive (chronic) I31.1
coxsackie B33.23
fibrinocaseous (tuberculous) A18.84
fibrinopurulent I30.1
fibrinous I30.8
fibrous I31.0
gonococcal A54.83
idiopathic I30.0
in systemic lupus erythematosus M32.12
infective I30.1
meningococcal A39.53
neoplastic (chronic) I31.8
acute I30.9
obliterans, obliterating I31.0
plastic I31.0
pneumococcal I30.1

Pericarditis (Continued)
postinfarction I24.1
purulent I30.1
rheumatic (active) (acute) (with effusion)
(with pneumonia) I01.0
with chorea (acute) (rheumatic)
(Sydenham's) I02.0
chronic or inactive (with chorea) I09.2
rheumatoid —see Rheumatoid, carditis
septic I30.1
serofibrinous I30.8
staphylococcal I30.1
streptococcal I30.1
suppurative I30.1
syphilitic A52.06
tuberculous A18.84
uremic N18.9 [I32]
viral I30.1
Pericardium, pericardial —see condition
Pericellulitis —see Cellulitis
Pericementitis (chronic) (suppurative) —see also
Periodontitis
acute K05.20
generalized —see Periodontitis, aggressive,
generalized
localized —see Periodontitis, aggressive,
localized
Perichondritis
auricle —see Perichondritis, ear
bronchus J98.09
ear (external) H61.00-●
acute H61.01-●
chronic H61.02-●
external auditory canal —see Perichondritis,
ear
larynx J38.7
syphilitic A52.73
typhoid A01.09
nose J34.89
pinna —see Perichondritis, ear
trachea J39.8
Periclasia K05.4
Pericoronitis —see Periodontitis
Pericystitis N30.90
with hematuria N30.91
Peridiverticulitis (intestine) K57.92
cecum —see Diverticulitis, intestine, large
colon —see Diverticulitis, intestine, large
duodenum —see Diverticulitis, intestine,
small
intestine —see Diverticulitis, intestine
jejunum —see Diverticulitis, intestine, small
rectosigmoid —see Diverticulitis, intestine,
large
rectum —see Diverticulitis, intestine, large
sigmoid —see Diverticulitis, intestine, large
Periendocarditis —see Endocarditis
Periepididymitis N45.1
Perifolliculitis L01.02
abscedens, caput, scalp L66.3
capitis, abscedens (et suffodiens) L66.3
superficial pustular L01.02
Perihepatitis K65.8
Perilabyrinthitis (acute) —see subcategory H83.0
Perimeningitis —see Meningitis
Perimetritis —see Endometritis
Perimetrosalpingitis —see Salpingo-oophoritis
Perineocele N81.81
Perinephric, perinephritic —see condition
Perinephritis —see also Infection, kidney
purulent —see Abscess, kidney
Perineum, perineal —see condition
Perineuritis NEC —see Neuralgia
Periodic —see condition
Periodontitis (chronic) (complex) (compound)
(local) (simplex) K05.30
acute K05.20
generalized K05.229
moderate K05.222
severe K05.223
slight K05.221

Periodontitis (Continued)
acute (Continued)
localized K05.219
moderate K05.212
severe K05.213
slight K05.211
apical K04.5
acute (pulpal origin) K04.4
generalized K05.329
moderate K05.322
severe K05.323
slight K05.321
localized K05.319
moderate K05.312
severe K05.313
slight K05.311
Periodontoclasia K05.4
Periodontosis (juvenile) K05.4
Periods —see also Menstruation
heavy N92.0
irregular N92.6
shortened intervals (irregular) N92.1
Perionychia —see also Cellulitis, digit
with lymphangitis —see Lymphangitis, acute,
digit
Perioophoritis —see Salpingo-oophoritis
Periorchitis N45.2
Periosteum, periosteal —see condition
Periostitis (albuminosa) (circumscribed)
(diffuse) (infective) (monomelic) —see also
Osteomyelitis
alveolar M27.3
alveolodental M27.3
dental M27.3
gonorrheal A54.43
jaw (lower) (upper) M27.2
orbit H05.03-●
syphilitic A52.77
congenital (early) A50.02 [M90.80]
secondary A51.46
tuberculous —see Tuberculosis, bone
yaws (hypertrophic) (early) (late) A66.6
[M90.80]
Periostosis (hyperplastic) —see also Disorder,
bone, specified type NEC
with osteomyelitis —see Osteomyelitis,
specified type NEC
Peripartum
cardiomyopathy O90.3
Periphlebitis —see Phlebitis
Periproctitis K62.89
Periprostatitis —see Prostatitis
Perirectal —see condition
Perirenal —see condition
Perisalpingitis —see Salpingo-oophoritis
Perisplenitis (infectional) D73.89
Peristalsis, visible or reversed R19.2
Peritendinitis —see Enthesopathy
Peritoneum, peritoneal —see condition
Peritonitis (adhesive) (bacterial) (fibrinous)
(hemorrhagic) (idiopathic) (localized)
(perforative) (primary) (with adhesions)
(with effusion) K65.9
with or following
abscess K65.1
appendicitis
with perforation or rupture K35.32
generalized (see also Appendicitis) K35.20
localized (see also Appendicitis) K35.30
diverticular disease (intestine) K57.80
with bleeding K57.81
ectopic or molar pregnancy O08.0
large intestine K57.20
with
bleeding K57.21
small intestine K57.40
with bleeding K57.41
small intestine K57.00
with
bleeding K57.01
large intestine K57.40
with bleeding K57.41

Peritonitis (Continued)
  acute (generalized) K65.0
  aseptic T81.61
  bile, biliary K65.3
  chemical T81.61
  chlamydial A74.81
  chronic proliferative K65.8
  complicating abortion —see Abortion, by
    type, complicated by, pelvic peritonitis
  congenital P78.1
  diaphragmatic K65.0
  diffuse K65.0
  diphtheritic A36.89
  disseminated K65.0
  due to
    bile K65.3
    foreign
      body or object accidentally left during
        a procedure (instrument) (sponge)
        (swab) T81.599
      substance accidentally left during a
        procedure (chemical) (powder)
        (talc) T81.61
    talc T81.61
    urine K65.8
  eosinophilic K65.8
    acute K65.0
  fibrocaseous (tuberculous) A18.31
  fibropurulent K65.0
  following ectopic or molar pregnancy
    O08.0
  general (ized) K65.0
  gonococcal A54.85
  meconium (newborn) P78.0
  neonatal P78.1
    meconium P78.0
  pancreatic K65.0
  paroxysmal, familial E85.0
    benign E85.0
  pelvic
    female N73.5
      acute N73.3
      chronic N73.4
        with adhesions N73.6
    male K65.0
  periodic, familial E85.0
  proliferative, chronic K65.8
  puerperal, postpartum, childbirth O85
  purulent K65.0
  septic K65.0
  specified NEC K65.8
  spontaneous bacterial K65.2
  subdiaphragmatic K65.0
  subphrenic K65.0
  suppurative K65.0
  syphilitic A52.74
    congenital (early) A50.08 [K67]
  talc T81.61
  tuberculous A18.31
  urine K65.8
Peritonsillar —see condition
Peritonsillitis J36
Perityphlitis K37
Periureteritis N28.89
Periurethral —see condition
Periurethritis (gangrenous) —see Urethritis
Periuterine —see condition
Perivaginitis —see Vaginitis
Perivasculitis, retinal H35.06-●
Perivasitis (chronic) N49.1
Perivesiculitis (seminal) —see Vesiculitis
Perlèche NEC K13.0
  due to
    candidiasis B37.83
    moniliasis B37.83
    riboflavin deficiency E53.0
    vitamin B2 (riboflavin) deficiency E53.0
Pernicious —see condition
Pernio, perniosis T69.1
Perpetrator (of abuse) —see Index to External
  Causes of Injury, Perpetrator

Persecution
  delusion F22
  social Z60.5
Perseveration (tonic) R48.8
Persistence, persistent (congenital)
  anal membrane Q42.3
    with fistula Q42.2
  arteria stapedia Q16.3
  atrioventricular canal Q21.2
  branchial cleft NOS Q18.2
    cyst Q18.0
    fistula Q18.0
    sinus Q18.0
  bulbus cordis in left ventricle Q21.8
  canal of Cloquet Q14.0
  capsule (opaque) Q12.8
  cilioretinal artery or vein Q14.8
  cloaca Q43.7
  communication —see Fistula, congenital
  convolutions
    aortic arch Q25.46
    fallopian tube Q50.6
    oviduct Q50.6
    uterine tube Q50.6
  double aortic arch Q25.45
  ductus arteriosus (Botalli) Q25.0
  fetal
    circulation P29.38
    form of cervix (uteri) Q51.828
    hemoglobin, hereditary (HPFH) D56.4
  foramen
    Botalli Q21.1
    ovale Q21.1
  Gartner's duct Q52.4
  hemoglobin, fetal (hereditary) (HPFH)
    D56.4
  hyaloid
    artery (generally incomplete) Q14.0
    system Q14.8
  hymen, in pregnancy or childbirth —see
    Pregnancy, complicated by, abnormal,
    vulva
  lanugo Q84.2
  left
    posterior cardinal vein Q26.8
    root with right arch of aorta Q25.49
    superior vena cava Q26.1
  Meckel's diverticulum Q43.0
    malignant —see Table of Neoplasms, small
      intestine, malignant
  mucosal disease (middle ear) —see
    Otitis, media, suppurative, chronic,
    tubotympanic
  nail(s), anomalous Q84.6
  omphalomesenteric duct Q43.0
  organ or site not listed —see Anomaly, by site
  ostium
    atrioventriculare commune Q21.2
    primum Q21.2
    secundum Q21.1
  ovarian rests in fallopian tube Q50.6
  pancreatic tissue in intestinal tract Q43.8
  primary (deciduous)
    teeth K00.6
    vitreous hyperplasia Q14.0
  pupillary membrane Q13.89
  rhesus (Rh)titer —see Complication(s),
    transfusion, incompatibility reaction, Rh
    (factor)
  right aortic arch Q25.47
  sinus
    urogenitalis
      female Q52.8
      male Q55.8
    venosus with imperfect incorporation in
      right auricle Q26.8
  thymus (gland) (hyperplasia) E32.0
  thyroglossal duct Q89.2
  thyrolingual duct Q89.2
  truncus arteriosus or communis Q20.0
  tunica vasculosa lentis Q12.2

Persistence, persistent (Continued)
  umbilical sinus Q64.4
  urachus Q64.4
  vitelline duct Q43.0
Person (with)
  admitted for clinical research, as a
    control subject (normal comparison)
    (participant) Z00.6
  awaiting admission to adequate facility
    elsewhere Z75.1
  concern (normal) about sick person in family
    Z63.6
  consulting on behalf of another Z71.0
  feigning illness Z76.5
  living (in)
    without
      adequate housing (heating) (space) Z59.1
      ➡housing (permanent) (temporary) Z59.00
      person able to render necessary care
        Z74.2
    ➡shelter Z59.02
    alone Z60.2
    boarding school Z59.3
    residential institution Z59.3
  on waiting list Z75.1
  sick or handicapped in family Z63.6
Personality (disorder) F60.9
  accentuation of traits (type A pattern) Z73.1
  affective F34.0
  aggressive F60.3
  amoral F60.2
  anacastic, anankastic F60.5
  antisocial F60.2
  anxious F60.6
  asocial F60.2
  asthenic F60.7
  avoidant F60.6
  borderline F60.3
  change due to organic condition (enduring)
    F07.0
  compulsive F60.5
  cycloid F34.0
  cyclothymic F34.0
  dependent F60.7
  depressive F34.1
  dissocial F60.2
  dual F44.81
  eccentric F60.89
  emotionally unstable F60.3
  expansive paranoid F60.0
  explosive F60.3
  fanatic F60.0
  haltlose type F60.89
  histrionic F60.4
  hyperthymic F34.0
  hypothymic F34.1
  hysterical F60.4
  immature F60.89
  inadequate F60.7
  labile (emotional) F60.3
  mixed (nonspecific) F60.89
  morally defective F60.2
  multiple F44.81
  narcissistic F60.81
  obsessional F60.5
  obsessive (-compulsive) F60.5
  organic F07.0
  overconscientious F60.5
  paranoid F60.0
  passive (-dependent) F60.7
  passive-aggressive F60.89
  pathologic F60.9
  pattern defect or disturbance F60.9
  pseudopsychopathic (organic) F07.0
  pseudoretarded (organic) F07.0
  psychoinfantile F60.4
  psychoneurotic NEC F60.89
  psychopathic F60.2
  querulant F60.0
  sadistic F60.89
  schizoid F60.1

▶ New   ➡ Revised   ~~deleted~~ Deleted   ● Use Additional Character(s)

Personality (Continued)
self-defeating F60.89
sensitive paranoid F60.0
sociopathic (amoral) (antisocial) (asocial)
(dissocial) F60.2
specified NEC F60.89
type A Z73.1
unstable (emotional) F60.3
Perthes' disease —see Legg-Calvé-Perthes
disease
Pertussis (see also Whooping cough) A37.90
Perversion, perverted
appetite F50.89
psychogenic F50.89
function
pituitary gland E23.2
posterior lobe E22.2
sense of smell and taste R43.8
psychogenic F45.8
sexual —see Deviation, sexual
Pervious, congenital —see also Imperfect, closure
ductus arteriosus Q25.0
Pes (congenital) —see also Talipes
acquired —see also Deformity, limb, foot,
specified NEC
planus —see Deformity, limb, flat foot
adductus Q66.89
cavus Q66.7-●
deformity NEC, acquired —see Deformity,
limb, foot, specified NEC
planus (acquired) (any degree) —see also
Deformity, limb, flat foot
rachitic sequelae (late effect) E64.3
valgus Q66.6
Pest, pestis —see Plague
Petechia, petechiae R23.3
newborn P54.5
Petechial typhus A75.9
Peter's anomaly Q13.4
Petit mal seizure —see Epilepsy, childhood,
absence
Petit's hernia —see Hernia, abdomen, specified
site NEC
Petrellidosis B48.2
Petrositis H70.20-●
acute H70.21-●
chronic H70.22-●
Peutz-Jeghers disease or syndrome Q85.8
Peyronie's disease N48.6
PFAPA (periodic fever, aphthous stomatitis,
pharyngitis, and adenopathy syndrome)
M04.8
Pfeiffer's disease —see Mononucleosis,
infectious
Phagedena (dry) (moist) (sloughing) —see also
Gangrene
geometric L88
penis N48.29
tropical —see Ulcer, skin
vulva N76.6
Phagedenic —see condition
Phakoma H35.89
Phakomatosis —see also specific eponymous
syndromes Q85.9
Bourneville's Q85.1
specified NEC Q85.8
Phantom limb syndrome (without pain) G54.7
with pain G54.6
Pharyngeal pouch syndrome D82.1
Pharyngitis (acute) (catarrhal) (gangrenous)
(infective) (malignant) (membranous)
(phlegmonous) (pseudomembranous)
(simple) (subacute) (suppurative)
(ulcerative) (viral) J02.9
with influenza, flu, or grippe —see Influenza,
with, pharyngitis
aphthous B08.5
atrophic J31.2
chlamydial A56.4
chronic (atrophic) (granular) (hypertrophic)
J31.2

Pharyngitis (Continued)
coxsackievirus B08.5
diphtheritic A36.0
enteroviral vesicular B08.5
follicular (chronic) J31.2
fusospirochetal A69.1
gonococcal A54.5
granular (chronic) J31.2
herpesviral B00.2
hypertrophic J31.2
infectional, chronic J31.2
influenzal —see Influenza, with, respiratory
manifestations NEC
lymphonodular, acute (enteroviral) B08.8
pneumococcal J02.8
purulent J02.9
putrid J02.9
septic J02.0
sicca J31.2
specified organism NEC J02.8
staphylococcal J02.8
streptococcal J02.0
syphilitic, congenital (early) A50.03
tuberculous A15.8
vesicular, enteroviral B08.5
viral NEC J02.8
Pharyngoconjunctivitis, viral B30.2
Pharyngolaryngitis (acute) J06.0
chronic J37.0
Pharyngoplegia J39.2
Pharyngotonsillitis, herpesviral B00.2
Pharyngotracheitis, chronic J42
Pharynx, pharyngeal —see condition
Phencyclidine-induced
anxiety disorder F16.980
bipolar and related disorder F16.94
depressive disorder F16.94
psychotic disorder F16.959
Phenomenon
Arthus' —see Arthus' phenomenon
jaw winking Q07.8
lupus erythematosus (LE) cell M32.9
Raynaud's (secondary) I73.00
with gangrene I73.01
vasomotor R55
vasospastic I73.9
vasovagal R55
Wenckebach's I44.1
Phenylketonuria E70.1
classical E70.0
maternal E70.1
Pheochromoblastoma
specified site —see Neoplasm, malignant, by
site
unspecified site C74.10
Pheochromocytoma
malignant
specified site —see Neoplasm, malignant,
by site
unspecified site C74.10
specified site —see Neoplasm, benign, by site
unspecified site D35.00
Pheohyphomycosis —see Chromomycosis
Pheomycosis —see Chromomycosis
Phimosis (congenital) (due to infection) N47.1
chancroidal A57
Phlebectasia —see also Varix
congenital Q27.4
Phlebitis (infective) (pyemic) (septic)
(suppurative) I80.9
antepartum —see Thrombophlebitis,
antepartum
blue —see Phlebitis, leg, deep
breast, superficial I80.8
calf muscular vein (NOS) I80.25-●
cavernous (venous) sinus —see Phlebitis,
intracranial (venous) sinus
cerebral (venous) sinus —see Phlebitis,
intracranial (venous) sinus
chest wall, superficial I80.8
cranial (venous) sinus —see Phlebitis,
intracranial (venous) sinus

Phlebitis (Continued)
deep (vessels) —see Phlebitis, leg, deep
due to implanted device —see Complications,
by site and type, specified NEC
during or resulting from a procedure T81.72
femoral vein (superficial) I80.1-●
femoropopliteal vein I80.0-●
gastrocnemial vein I80.25-●
gestational —see Phlebopathy, gestational
hepatic veins I80.8
iliac vein (common) (external) (internal)
I80.21-●
iliofemoral —see Phlebitis, femoral vein
intracranial (venous) sinus (any) G08
nonpyogenic I67.6
intraspinal venous sinuses and veins G08
nonpyogenic G95.19
lateral (venous) sinus —see Phlebitis,
intracranial (venous) sinus
leg I80.3
antepartum —see Thrombophlebitis,
antepartum
deep (vessels) NEC I80.20-●
iliac I80.21-●
popliteal vein I80.22-●
specified vessel NEC I80.29-●
tibial vein (anterior) (posterior) I80.23-●
femoral vein (superficial) I80.1-●
superficial (vessels) I80.0-●
longitudinal sinus —see Phlebitis, intracranial
(venous) sinus
lower limb —see Phlebitis, leg
migrans, migrating (superficial) I82.1
pelvic
with ectopic or molar pregnancy O08.0
following ectopic or molar pregnancy O08.0
puerperal, postpartum O87.1
peroneal vein I80.24-●
popliteal vein —see Phlebitis, leg, deep,
popliteal
portal (vein) K75.1
postoperative T81.72
pregnancy —see Thrombophlebitis,
antepartum
puerperal, postpartum, childbirth O87.0
deep O87.1
pelvic O87.1
superficial O87.0
retina —see Vasculitis, retina
saphenous (accessory) (great) (long)
(small) —see Phlebitis, leg, superficial
sinus (meninges) —see Phlebitis, intracranial
(venous) sinus
soleal vein I80.25-●
specified site NEC I80.8
syphilitic A52.09
tibial vein —see Phlebitis, leg, deep, tibial
ulcerative I80.9
leg —see Phlebitis, leg
umbilicus I80.8
uterus (septic) —see Endometritis
varicose (leg) (lower limb) —see Varix, leg,
with, inflammation
Phlebofibrosis I87.8
Phleboliths I87.8
Phlebopathy
gestational O22.9-●
puerperal O87.9
Phlebosclerosis I87.8
Phlebothrombosis —see also Thrombosis
antepartum —see Thrombophlebitis,
antepartum
pregnancy —see Thrombophlebitis,
antepartum
puerperal —see Thrombophlebitis, puerperal
Phlebotomus fever A93.1
Phlegmasia
alba dolens O87.1
nonpuerperal —see Phlebitis, femoral vein
cerulea dolens —see Phlebitis, leg, deep
Phlegmon —see Abscess
Phlegmonous —see condition

Phlyctenulosis (allergic) (keratoconjunctivitis) (nontuberculous) —*see also* Keratoconjunctivitis
  cornea —*see* Keratoconjunctivitis
  tuberculous A18.52
Phobia, phobic F40.9
  animal F40.218
    spiders F40.210
  examination F40.298
  reaction F40.9
  simple F40.298
  social F40.10
    generalized F40.11
  specific (isolated) F40.298
    animal F40.218
      spiders F40.210
    blood F40.230
    injection F40.231
    injury F40.233
    men F40.290
    natural environment F40.228
      thunderstorms F40.220
    situational F40.248
      bridges F40.242
      closed in spaces F40.240
      flying F40.243
      heights F40.241
    specified focus NEC F40.298
    transfusion F40.231
    women F40.291
  specified NEC F40.8
    medical care NEC F40.232
  state F40.9
Phocas' disease —*see* Mastopathy, cystic
Phocomelia Q73.1
  lower limb —*see* Agenesis, leg, with foot present
  upper limb —*see* Agenesis, arm, with hand present
Phoria H50.50
Phosphate-losing tubular disorder N25.0
Phosphatemia E83.39
Phosphaturia E83.39
Photodermatitis (sun) L56.8
  chronic L57.8
  due to drug L56.8
  light other than sun L59.8
Photokeratitis H16.13-•
Photophobia H53.14-•
Photophthalmia —*see* Photokeratitis
Photopsia H53.19
Photoretinitis —*see* Retinopathy, solar
Photosensitivity, photosensitization (sun) skin L56.8
  light other than sun L59.8
Phrenitis —*see* Encephalitis
Phrynoderma (vitamin A deficiency) E50.8
Phthiriasis (pubis) B85.3
  with any infestation classifiable to B85.0-B85.2 B85.4
Phthirus infestation —*see* Phthiriasis
Phthisis —*see also* Tuberculosis
  bulbi (infectional) —*see* Disorder, globe, degenerated condition, atrophy
  eyeball (due to infection) —*see* Disorder, globe, degenerated condition, atrophy
Phycomycosis —*see* Zygomycosis
Physalopteriasis B81.8
Physical restraint status Z78.1
Phytobezoar T18.9
  intestine T18.3
  stomach T18.2
Pian —*see* Yaws
Pianoma A66.1
Pica F50.89
  in adults F50.89
  infant or child F98.3
Picking, nose F98.8
Pick-Niemann disease —*see* Niemann-Pick disease or syndrome

Pick's
  cerebral atrophy G31.01 [F02.80]
    with behavioral disturbance G31.01 [F02.81]
  disease or syndrome (brain) G31.01 [F02.80]
    with behavioral disturbance G31.01 [F02.81]
    brain G31.01 [F02.80]
      with behavioral disturbance G31.01 [F02.81]
    pericardium (pericardial pseudocirrhosis of liver) I31.1
  syndrome
    brain G31.01 [F02.80]
      with behavioral disturbance G31.01 [F02.81]
    of heart (pericardial pseudocirrhosis of liver) I31.1
Pickwickian syndrome E66.2
Piebaldism E70.39
Piedra (beard) (scalp) B36.8
  black B36.3
  white B36.2
Pierre Robin deformity or syndrome Q87.0
Pierson's disease or osteochondrosis M91.0
Pig-bel A05.2
Pigeon
  breast or chest (acquired) M95.4
    congenital Q67.7
      rachitic sequelae (late effect) E64.3
  breeder's disease or lung J67.2
  fancier's disease or lung J67.2
  toe —*see* Deformity, toe, specified NEC
Pigmentation (abnormal) (anomaly) L81.9
  conjunctiva H11.13-•
  cornea (anterior) H18.01-•
    posterior H18.05-•
    stromal H18.06-•
  diminished melanin formation NEC L81.6
  iron L81.8
  lids, congenital Q82.8
  limbus corneae —*see* Pigmentation, cornea
  metals L81.8
  optic papilla, congenital Q14.2
  retina, congenital (grouped) (nevoid) Q14.1
  scrotum, congenital Q82.8
  tattoo L81.8
Piles —*see also* Hemorrhoids K64.9
Pili
  annulati or torti (congenital) Q84.1
  incarnati L73.1
Pill roller hand (intrinsic) —*see* Parkinsonism
Pilomatrixoma —*see* Neoplasm, skin, benign
  malignant —*see* Neoplasm, skin, malignant
Pilonidal —*see* condition
Pimple R23.8
PIMS M35.81
PIN —*see* Neoplasia, intraepithelial, prostate
Pinched nerve —*see* Neuropathy, entrapment
Pindborg tumor —*see* Cyst, calcifying odontogenic
Pineal body or gland —*see* condition
Pinealoblastoma C75.3
Pinealoma D44.5
  malignant C75.3
Pineoblastoma C75.3
Pineocytoma D44.5
Pinguecula H11.15-•
Pingueculitis H10.81-•
Pinhole meatus —*see also* Stricture, urethra N35.919
Pink
  disease —*see* subcategory T56.1
  eye —*see* Conjunctivitis, acute, mucopurulent
Pinkus' disease (lichen nitidus) L44.1
Pinpoint
  meatus —*see* Stricture, urethra
  os (uteri) —*see* Stricture, cervix
Pins and needles R20.2
Pinta A67.9
  cardiovascular lesions A67.2
  chancre (primary) A67.0

Pinta (*Continued*)
  erythematous plaques A67.1
  hyperchromic lesions A67.1
  hyperkeratosis A67.1
  lesions A67.9
    cardiovascular A67.2
    hyperchromic A67.1
    intermediate A67.1
    late A67.2
    mixed A67.3
    primary A67.0
    skin (achromic) (cicatricial) (dyschromic) A67.2
      hyperchromic A67.1
      mixed (achromic and hyperchromic) A67.3
  papule (primary) A67.0
  skin lesions (achromic) (cicatricial) (dyschromic) A67.2
    hyperchromic A67.1
    mixed (achromic and hyperchromic) A67.3
  vitiligo A67.2
Pintids A67.1
Pinworm (disease) (infection) (infestation) B80
Piroplasmosis (*see also* Babesiosis) B60.00
  specified NEC B60.09
Pistol wound —*see* Gunshot wound
Pitchers' elbow —*see* Derangement, joint, specified type NEC, elbow
Pithecoid pelvis Q74.2
  with disproportion (fetopelvic) O33.0
    causing obstructed labor O65.0
Pithiatism F48.8
Pitted —*see* Pitting
Pitting —*see also* Edema R60.9
  lip R60.0
  nail L60.8
  teeth K00.4
Pituitary gland —*see* condition
Pituitary-snuff-taker's disease J67.8
Pityriasis (capitis) L21.0
  alba L30.5
  circinata (et maculata) L42
  furfuracea L21.0
  Hebra's L26
  lichenoides L41.0
    chronica L41.1
    et varioliformis (acuta) L41.0
  maculata (et circinata) L30.5
  nigra B36.1
  pilaris, Hebra's L44.0
  rosea L42
  rotunda L44.8
  rubra (Hebra) pilaris L44.0
  simplex L30.5
  specified type NEC L30.5
  streptogenes L30.5
  versicolor (scrotal) B36.0
Placenta, placental —*see* Pregnancy, complicated by (care of) (management affected by), specified condition
Placentitis O41.14-•
Plagiocephaly Q67.3
Plague A20.9
  abortive A20.8
  ambulatory A20.8
  asymptomatic A20.8
  bubonic A20.0
  cellulocutaneous A20.1
  cutaneobubonic A20.1
  lymphatic gland A20.0
  meningitis A20.3
  pharyngeal A20.8
  pneumonic (primary) (secondary) A20.2
  pulmonary, pulmonic A20.2
  septicemic A20.7
  tonsillar A20.8
    septicemic A20.7
Planning, family
  contraception Z30.9
  procreation Z31.69

Plaque(s)
  artery, arterial —*see* Arteriosclerosis
  calcareous —*see* Calcification
  coronary, lipid rich I25.83
  epicardial I31.8
  erythematous, of pinta A67.1
  Hollenhorst's —*see* Occlusion, artery, retina
  lipid rich, coronary I25.83
  pleural (without asbestos) J92.9
    with asbestos J92.0
  tongue K13.29
Plasmacytoma C90.3-●
  extramedullary C90.2-●
  medullary C90.0-●
  solitary C90.3-●
Plasmacytopenia D72.818
Plasmacytosis D72.822
Plaster ulcer —*see* Ulcer, pressure, by site
Plateau iris syndrome (post-iridectomy)
    (postprocedural) (without glaucoma)
    H21.82
  with glaucoma H40.22-●
Platybasia Q75.8
Platyonychia (congenital) Q84.6
  acquired L60.8
Platypelloid pelvis M95.5
  with disproportion (fetopelvic) O33.0
    causing obstructed labor O65.0
  congenital Q74.2
Platyspondylisis Q76.49
Plaut (-Vincent) disease —*see also* Vincent's
    A69.1
Plethora R23.2
  newborn P61.1
Pleura, pleural —*see* condition
Pleuralgia R07.81
Pleurisy (acute) (adhesive) (chronic) (costal)
    (diaphragmatic) (double) (dry) (fibrinous)
    (fibrous) (interlobar) (latent) (plastic)
    (primary) (residual) (sicca) (sterile)
    (subacute) (unresolved) R09.1
  with
    adherent pleura J86.0
    effusion J90
      chylous, chyliform J94.0
      tuberculous (non primary) A15.6
        primary (progressive) A15.7
      tuberculosis —*see* Pleurisy, tuberculous
        (non primary)
  encysted —*see* Pleurisy, with effusion
  exudative —*see* Pleurisy, with effusion
  fibrinopurulent, fibropurulent —*see*
    Pyothorax
  hemorrhagic —*see* Hemothorax
  pneumococcal J90
  purulent —*see* Pyothorax
  septic —*see* Pyothorax
  serofibrinous —*see* Pleurisy, with effusion
  seropurulent —*see* Pyothorax
  serous —*see* Pleurisy, with effusion
  staphylococcal J86.9
  streptococcal J90
  suppurative —*see* Pyothorax
  traumatic (post) (current) —*see* Injury,
    intrathoracic, pleura
  tuberculous (with effusion) (non primary)
    A15.6
    primary (progressive) A15.7
Pleuritis sicca —*see* Pleurisy
Pleurobronchopneumonia —*see* Pneumonia,
  broncho
Pleurodynia R07.81
  epidemic B33.0
  viral B33.0
Pleuropericarditis —*see also* Pericarditis
  acute I30.9
Pleuropneumonia (acute) (bilateral) (double)
    (septic) —*see also* Pneumonia J18.8
  chronic —*see* Fibrosis, lung
Pleuro-pneumonia-like-organism (PPLO), as
    cause of disease classified elsewhere B96.0

Pleurorrhea —*see* Pleurisy, with effusion
Plexitis, brachial G54.0
Plica
  polonica B85.0
  syndrome, knee M67.5
  tonsil J35.8
Plicated tongue K14.5
Plug
  bronchus NEC J98.09
  meconium (newborn) NEC syndrome
    P76.0
  mucus —*see* Asphyxia, mucus
Plumbism —*see* subcategory T56.0
Plummer's disease E05.20
  with thyroid storm E05.21
Plummer-Vinson syndrome D50.1
Pluricarential syndrome of infancy E40
Plus (and minus) hand (intrinsic) —*see*
    Deformity, limb, specified type NEC,
    forearm
PMEI (polymorphic epilepsy in infancy)
    G40.83-●
Pneumathemia —*see* Air, embolism
Pneumatic hammer (drill) syndrome T75.21
Pneumatocele (lung) J98.4
  intracranial G93.89
  tension J44.9
Pneumatosis
  cystoides intestinalis K63.89
  intestinalis K63.89
  peritonei K66.8
Pneumaturia R39.89
Pneumoblastoma —*see* Neoplasm, lung,
  malignant
Pneumocephalus G93.89
Pneumococcemia A40.3
Pneumococcus, pneumococcal —*see* condition
Pneumoconiosis (due to) (inhalation of) J64
  with tuberculosis (any type in A15) J65
  aluminum J63.0
  asbestos J61
  bagasse, bagassosis J67.1
  bauxite J63.1
  beryllium J63.2
  coal miners' (simple) J60
  coalworkers' (simple) J60
  collier's J60
  cotton dust J66.0
  diatomite (diatomaceous earth) J62.8
  dust
    inorganic NEC J63.6
    lime J62.8
    marble J62.8
    organic NEC J66.8
  fumes or vapors (from silo) J68.9
  graphite J63.3
  grinder's J62.8
  kaolin J62.8
  mica J62.8
  millstone maker's J62.8
  mineral fibers NEC J61
  miner's J60
  moldy hay J67.0
  potter's J62.8
  rheumatoid —*see* Rheumatoid, lung
  sandblaster's J62.8
  silica, silicate NEC J62.8
    with carbon J60
  stonemason's J62.8
  talc (dust) J62.0
Pneumocystis carinii pneumonia B59
Pneumocystis jiroveci (pneumonia) B59
Pneumocystosis (with pneumonia) B59
Pneumohemopericardium I31.2
Pneumohemothorax J94.2
  traumatic S27.2
Pneumohydropericardium —*see* Pericarditis
Pneumohydrothorax —*see* Hydrothorax
Pneumomediastinum J98.2
  congenital or perinatal P25.2
Pneumomycosis B49 [J99]

Pneumonia (acute) (double) (migratory)
    (purulent) (septic) (unresolved) J18.9
  with
    influenza —*see* Influenza, with, pneumonia
    lung abscess J85.1
      due to specified organism —*see*
        Pneumonia, in (due to)
  2019 (novel) coronavirus J12.82
  adenoviral J12.0
  adynamic J18.2
  alba A50.04
  allergic (*see also* Pneumonitis,
    hypersensitivity) J82.89
  alveolar —*see* Pneumonia, lobar
  anaerobes J15.8
  anthrax A22.1
  apex, apical —*see* Pneumonia, lobar
  Ascaris B77.81
  aspiration J69.0
    due to
      aspiration of microorganisms
        bacterial J15.9
        viral J12.9
      food (regurgitated) J69.0
      gastric secretions J69.0
      milk (regurgitated) J69.0
      oils, essences J69.1
      solids, liquids NEC J69.8
      vomitus J69.0
    newborn P24.81
      amniotic fluid (clear) P24.11
      blood P24.21
      food (regurgitated) P24.31
      liquor (amnii) P24.11
      meconium P24.01
      milk P24.31
      mucus P24.11
      specified NEC P24.81
      stomach contents P24.31
    postprocedural J95.4
  atypical NEC J18.9
  bacillus J15.9
    specified NEC J15.8
  bacterial J15.9
    specified NEC J15.8
  Bacteroides (fragilis) (oralis)
    (melaninogenicus) J15.8
  basal, basic, basilar —*see* Pneumonia, by type
  bronchiolitis obliterans organized (BOOP)
    J84.89
  broncho-, bronchial (confluent) (croupous)
    (diffuse) (disseminated) (hemorrhagic)
    (involving lobes) (lobar) (terminal) J18.0
    allergic (*see also* Pneumonitis,
      hypersensitivity) J82.89
    aspiration —*see* Pneumonia, aspiration
    bacterial J15.9
      specified NEC J15.8
    chronic —*see* Fibrosis, lung
    diplococcal J13
    Eaton's agent J15.7
    Escherichia coli (E. coli) J15.5
    Friedländer's bacillus J15.0
    Hemophilus influenzae J14
    hypostatic J18.2
    inhalation —*see also* Pneumonia, aspiration
      due to fumes or vapors (chemical) J68.0
      of oils or essences J69.1
    Klebsiella (pneumoniae) J15.0
    lipid, lipoid J69.1
      endogenous J84.89
    Mycoplasma (pneumoniae) J15.7
    pleuro-pneumonia-like-organisms (PPLO)
      J15.7
    pneumococcal J13
    Proteus J15.6
    Pseudomonas J15.1
    Serratia marcescens J15.6
    specified organism NEC J16.8
    staphylococcal —*see* Pneumonia,
      staphylococcal

Pneumonia *(Continued)*
  broncho-, bronchial *(Continued)*
    streptococcal NEC J15.4
      group B J15.3
      pneumoniae J13
    viral, virus —*see* Pneumonia, viral
  Butyrivibrio (fibriosolvens) J15.8
  Candida B37.1
  caseous —*see* Tuberculosis, pulmonary
  catarrhal —*see* Pneumonia, broncho
  chlamydial J16.0
    congenital P23.1
  cholesterol J84.89
  cirrhotic (chronic) —*see* Fibrosis, lung
  Clostridium (haemolyticum) (novyi) J15.8
  confluent —*see* Pneumonia, broncho
  congenital (infective) P23.9
    due to
      bacterium NEC P23.6
      Chlamydia P23.1
      Escherichia coli P23.4
      Haemophilus influenzae P23.6
      infective organism NEC P23.8
      Klebsiella pneumoniae P23.6
      Mycoplasma P23.6
      Pseudomonas P23.5
      Staphylococcus P23.2
      Streptococcus (except group B) P23.6
        group B P23.3
      viral agent P23.0
    specified NEC P23.8
  coronavirus (novel) (disease) 2019 J12.82
  COVID-19 J12.82
  croupous —*see* Pneumonia, lobar
  cryptogenic organizing J84.116
  cytomegalic inclusion B25.0
  cytomegaloviral B25.0
  deglutition —*see* Pneumonia, aspiration
  desquamative interstitial J84.117
  diffuse —*see* Pneumonia, broncho
  diplococcal, diplococcus (broncho-) (lobar) J13
  disseminated (focal) —*see* Pneumonia, broncho
  Eaton's agent J15.7
  embolic, embolism —*see* Embolism, pulmonary
  Enterobacter J15.6
  eosinophilic J82.81
    acute J82.82
    chronic J82.81
  Escherichia coli (E. coli) J15.5
  Eubacterium J15.8
  fibrinous —*see* Pneumonia, lobar
  fibroid, fibrous (chronic) —*see* Fibrosis, lung
  Friedländer's bacillus J15.0
  Fusobacterium (nucleatum) J15.8
  gangrenous J85.0
  giant cell (measles) B05.2
  gonococcal A54.84
  gram-negative bacteria NEC J15.6
    anaerobic J15.8
  Hemophilus influenzae (broncho) (lobar) J14
  human metapneumovirus J12.3
  hypostatic (broncho) (lobar) J18.2
  in (due to)
    actinomycosis A42.0
    adenovirus J12.0
    anthrax A22.1
    ascariasis B77.81
    aspergillosis B44.9
    Bacillus anthracis A22.1
    Bacterium anitratum J15.6
    candidiasis B37.1
    chickenpox B01.2
    Chlamydia J16.0
      neonatal P23.1
    coccidioidomycosis B38.2
      acute B38.0
      chronic B38.1
    cytomegalovirus disease B25.0
    Diplococcus (pneumoniae) J13
    Eaton's agent J15.7

Pneumonia *(Continued)*
  in *(Continued)*
    Enterobacter J15.6
    Escherichia coli (E. coli) J15.5
    Friedländer's bacillus J15.0
    fumes and vapors (chemical) (inhalation) J68.0
    gonorrhea A54.84
    Hemophilus influenzae (H. influenzae) J14
    Herellea J15.6
    histoplasmosis B39.2
      acute B39.0
      chronic B39.1
    human metapneumovirus J12.3
    Klebsiella (pneumoniae) J15.0
    measles B05.2
    Mycoplasma (pneumoniae) J15.7
    nocardiosis, nocardiasis A43.0
    ornithosis A70
    parainfluenza virus J12.2
    pleuro-pneumonia-like-organism (PPLO) J15.7
    pneumococcus J13
    pneumocystosis (Pneumocystis carinii) (Pneumocystis jiroveci) B59
    Proteus J15.6
    Pseudomonas NEC J15.1
      pseudomallei A24.1
    psittacosis A70
    Q fever A78
    respiratory syncytial virus (RSV) J12.1
    rheumatic fever I00 *[J17]*
    rubella B06.81
    Salmonella (infection) A02.22
      typhi A01.03
    schistosomiasis B65.9 *[J17]*
    Serratia marcescens J15.6
    specified
      bacterium NEC J15.8
      organism NEC J16.8
    spirochetal NEC A69.8
    Staphylococcus J15.20
      aureus (methicillin susceptible) (MSSA) J15.211
        methicillin resistant (MRSA) J15.212
      specified NEC J15.29
    Streptococcus J15.4
      group B J15.3
      pneumoniae J13
      specified NEC J15.4
    toxoplasmosis B58.3
    tularemia A21.2
    typhoid (fever) A01.03
    varicella B01.2
    virus —*see* Pneumonia, viral
    whooping cough A37.91
      due to
        Bordetella parapertussis A37.11
        Bordetella pertussis A37.01
        specified NEC A37.81
    Yersinia pestis A20.2
  inhalation of food or vomit —*see* Pneumonia, aspiration
  interstitial J84.9
    chronic J84.111
    desquamative J84.117
    due to
      collagen vascular disease J84.178
      known underlying cause J84.178
    idiopathic NOS J84.111
    in disease classified elsewhere J84.178
    lymphocytic (due to collagen vascular disease) (in diseases classified elsewhere) J84.178
    lymphoid J84.2
    non-specific J84.89
      due to
        collagen vascular disease J84.178
        known underlying cause J84.178
      idiopathic J84.113
      in diseases classified elsewhere J84.178

Pneumonia *(Continued)*
  interstitial *(Continued)*
    plasma cell B59
    pseudomonas J15.1
    usual J84.112
      due to collagen vascular disease J84.178
      idiopathic J84.112
      in diseases classified elsewhere J84.178
    Klebsiella (pneumoniae) J15.0
    lipid, lipoid (exogenous) J69.1
      endogenous J84.89
    lobar (disseminated) (double) (interstitial) J18.1
      bacterial J15.9
        specified NEC J15.8
      chronic —*see* Fibrosis, lung
      Escherichia coli (E. coli) J15.5
      Friedländer's bacillus J15.0
      Hemophilus influenzae J14
      hypostatic J18.2
      Klebsiella (pneumoniae) J15.0
      pneumococcal J13
      Proteus J15.6
      Pseudomonas J15.1
      specified organism NEC J16.8
      staphylococcal —*see* Pneumonia, staphylococcal
      streptococcal NEC J15.4
      Streptococcus pneumoniae J13
      viral, virus —*see* Pneumonia, viral
    lobular —*see* Pneumonia, broncho
    Löffler's J82.89
    lymphoid interstitial J84.2
    massive —*see* Pneumonia, lobar
    meconium P24.01
    MRSA (Methicillin resistant Staphylococcus aureus) J15.212
    MSSA (methicillin susceptible Staphylococcus aureus) J15.211
    multilobar —*see* Pneumonia, by type
    Mycoplasma (pneumoniae) J15.7
    necrotic J85.0
    neonatal P23.9
      aspiration —*see* Aspiration, by substance, with pneumonia
    nitrogen dioxide J68.0
    organizing J84.89
      due to
        collagen vascular disease J84.178
        known underlying cause J84.178
      in diseases classified elsewhere J84.178
    orthostatic J18.2
    parainfluenza virus J12.2
    parenchymatous —*see* Fibrosis, lung
    passive J18.2
    patchy —*see* Pneumonia, broncho
    Peptococcus J15.8
    Peptostreptococcus J15.8
    plasma cell (of infants) B59
    pleurolobar —*see* Pneumonia, lobar
    pleuro-pneumonia-like organism (PPLO) J15.7
    pneumococcal (broncho) (lobar) J13
    Pneumocystis (carinii) (jiroveci) B59
    postinfectional NEC B99 *[J17]*
    postmeasles B05.2
    Proteus J15.6
    Pseudomonas J15.1
    psittacosis A70
    radiation J70.0
      respiratory syncytial virus (RSV) J12.1
    resulting from a procedure J95.89
    rheumatic I00 *[J17]*
    Salmonella (arizonae) (cholerae-suis) (enteritidis) (typhimurium) A02.22
      typhi A01.03
      typhoid fever A01.03
    SARS-associated coronavirus J12.81
    SARS-CoV-2 J12.82
    segmented, segmental —*see* Pneumonia, broncho-●
    Serratia marcescens J15.6

▶ New   ➡ Revised   ~~deleted~~ Deleted   ● Use Additional Character(s)

Pneumonia *(Continued)*
　specified NEC J18.8
　　bacterium NEC J15.8
　　organism NEC J16.8
　　virus NEC J12.89
　spirochetal NEC A69.8
　staphylococcal (broncho) (lobar) J15.20
　　aureus (methicillin susceptible) (MSSA)
　　　J15.211
　　　methicillin resistant (MRSA) J15.212
　　specified NEC J15.29
　static, stasis J18.2
　streptococcal NEC (broncho) (lobar) J15.4
　　group
　　　A J15.4
　　　B J15.3
　　　specified NEC J15.4
　Streptococcus pneumoniae J13
　syphilitic, congenital (early) A50.04
　traumatic (complication) (early) (secondary)
　　T79.8
　tuberculous (any) —*see* Tuberculosis,
　　pulmonary
　tularemic A21.2
　varicella B01.2
　Veillonella J15.8
　ventilator associated J95.851
　viral, virus (broncho) (interstitial) (lobar) J12.9
　　adenoviral J12.0
　　congenital P23.0
　　human metapneumovirus J12.3
　　parainfluenza J12.2
　　respiratory syncytial (RSV) J12.1
　　SARS-associated coronavirus J12.81
　　specified NEC J12.89
　white (congenital) A50.04
Pneumonic —*see* condition
Pneumonitis (acute) (primary)　*see also*
　　Pneumonia
　air-conditioner J67.7
　allergic (due to) J67.9
　　organic dust NEC J67.8
　　red cedar dust J67.8
　　sequoiosis J67.8
　　wood dust J67.8
　aspiration J69.0
　　due to
　　　anesthesia J95.4
　　　　during
　　　　　labor and delivery O74.0
　　　　　pregnancy O29.01-●
　　　　　puerperium O89.01
　　　fumes or gases J68.0
　　　obstetric O74.0
　chemical (due to gases, fumes or vapors)
　　(inhalation) J68.0
　　due to anesthesia J95.4
　cholesterol J84.89
　chronic —*see* Fibrosis, lung
　congenital rubella P35.0
　crack (cocaine) J68.0
　due to
　　beryllium J68.0
　　cadmium J68.0
　　crack (cocaine) J68.0
　　detergent J69.8
　　fluorocarbon-polymer J68.0
　　food, vomit (aspiration) J69.0
　　fumes or vapors J68.0
　　gases, fumes or vapors (inhalation) J68.0
　　inhalation
　　　blood J69.8
　　　essences J69.1
　　　food (regurgitated), milk, vomit J69.0
　　　oils, essences J69.1
　　　saliva J69.0
　　　solids, liquids NEC J69.8
　　manganese J68.0
　　nitrogen dioxide J68.0
　　oils, essences J69.1
　　solids, liquids NEC J69.8

Pneumonitis *(Continued)*
　due to *(Continued)*
　　toxoplasmosis (acquired) B58.3
　　　congenital P37.1
　　vanadium J68.0
　　ventilator J95.851
　eosinophilic J82.81
　　acute J82.82
　　chronic J82.81
　hypersensitivity J67.9
　　air conditioner lung J67.7
　　bagassosis J67.1
　　bird fancier's lung J67.2
　　farmer's lung J67.0
　　maltworker's lung J67.4
　　maple bark-stripper's lung J67.6
　　mushroom worker's lung J67.5
　　specified organic dust NEC J67.8
　　suberosis J67.3
　interstitial (chronic) J84.89
　　acute J84.114
　　lymphoid J84.2
　　non-specific J84.89
　　　idiopathic J84.113
　lymphoid, interstitial J84.2
　meconium P24.01
　postanesthetic J95.4
　　correct substance properly administered —
　　　see Table of Drugs and Chemcials, by
　　　drug, adverse effect
　　in labor and delivery O74.0
　　in pregnancy O29.01-●
　　obstetric O74.0
　　overdose or wrong substance given or taken
　　　(by accident) —*see* Table of Drugs and
　　　Chemicals, by drug, poisoning
　　postpartum, puerperal O89.01
　postoperative J95.4
　　obstetric O74.0
　radiation J70.0
　rubella, congenital P35.0
　ventilation (air-conditioning) J67.7
　ventilator associated J95.851
　wood-dust J67.8
Pneumoconiosis —*see* Pneumoconiosis
Pneumoparotid K11.8
Pneumopathy NEC J98.4
　alveolar J84.09
　due to organic dust NEC J66.8
　parietoalveolar J84.09
Pneumopericarditis —*see also* Pericarditis
　acute I30.9
Pneumopericardium —*see also* Pericarditis
　congenital P25.3
　newborn P25.3
　traumatic (post) —*see* Injury, heart
Pneumophagia (psychogenic) F45.8
Pneumopleurisy, pneumopleuritis —*see also*
　　Pneumonia J18.8
Pneumopyopericardium I30.1
Pneumopyothorax —*see* Pyopneumothorax
　with fistula J86.0
Pneumorrhagia —*see also* Hemorrhage, lung
　tuberculous —*see* Tuberculosis, pulmonary
Pneumothorax NOS J93.9
　acute J93.83
　chronic J93.81
　congenital P25.1
　perinatal period P25.1
　postprocedural J95.811
　specified NEC J93.83
　spontaneous NOS J93.83
　　newborn P25.1
　　primary J93.11
　　secondary J93.12
　　tension J93.0
　tense valvular, infectional J93.0
　tension (spontaneous) J93.0
　traumatic S27.0
　　with hemothorax S27.2
　tuberculous —*see* Tuberculosis, pulmonary

Podagra —*see also* Gout M10.9
Podencephalus Q01.9
Poikilocytosis R71.8
Poikiloderma L81.6
　Civatte's L57.3
　congenital Q82.8
　vasculare atrophicans L94.5
Poikilodermatomyositis M33.10
　with
　　myopathy M33.12
　　respiratory involvement M33.11
　　specified organ involvement NEC M33.19
Pointed ear (congenital) Q17.3
Poison ivy, oak, sumac or other plant
　dermatitis (allergic) (contact) L23.7
Poisoning (acute) —*see also* Table of Drugs and
　　Chemicals
　algae and toxins T65.82-●
　Bacillus B (aertrycke) (cholerae (suis))
　　(paratyphosus) (suipestifer) A02.9
　　botulinus A05.1
　bacterial toxins A05.9
　berries, noxious —*see* Poisoning, food,
　　noxious, berries
　botulism A05.1
　ciguatera fish T61.0-●
　Clostridium botulinum A05.1
　death-cap (Amanita phalloides) (Amanita
　　verna) —*see* Poisoning, food, noxious,
　　mushrooms
　drug —*see* Table of Drugs and Chemicals, by
　　drug, poisoning
　epidemic, fish (noxious) —*see* Poisoning,
　　seafood
　　bacterial A05.9
　fava bean D55.0
　fish (noxious) T61.9-●
　　bacterial —*see* Intoxication, foodborne, by
　　　agent
　　ciguatera fish —*see* Poisoning, ciguatera
　　　fish
　　scombroid fish —*see* Poisoning, scombroid
　　　fish
　　specified type NEC T61.77-●
　food NEC A05.9
　　bacterial —*see* Intoxication, foodborne, by
　　　agent
　　due to
　　　Bacillus (aertrycke) (choleraesuis)
　　　　(paratyphosus) (suipestifer) A02.9
　　　　botulinus A05.1
　　　Clostridium (perfringens) (Welchii)
　　　　A05.2
　　　salmonella (aertrycke) (callinarum)
　　　　(choleraesuis) (enteritidis)
　　　　(paratyphi) (suipestifer) A02.9
　　　　with
　　　　　gastroenteritis A02.0
　　　　　sepsis A02.1
　　　staphylococcus A05.0
　　　Vibrio
　　　　parahaemolyticus A05.3
　　　　vulnificus A05.5
　　noxious or naturally toxic T62.9-●
　　　berries —*see* subcategory T62.1-●
　　　fish —*see* Poisoning, seafood
　　　mushrooms —*see* subcategory T62.0X-●
　　　plants NEC —*see* subcategory T62.2X-●
　　　seafood —*see* Poisoning, seafood
　　　specified NEC —*see* subcategory
　　　　T62.8X-●
　ichthyotoxism —*see* Poisoning, seafood
　kreotoxism, food A05.9
　latex T65.81-●
　lead T56.0-●
　mushroom —*see* Poisoning, food, noxious,
　　mushroom
　mussels —*see also* Poisoning, shellfish
　　bacterial —*see* Intoxication, foodborne, by
　　　agent
　nicotine (tobacco) T65.2-●

Poisoning (Continued)
  noxious foodstuffs —see Poisoning, food, noxious
  plants, noxious —see Poisoning, food, noxious, plants NEC
  ptomaine —see Poisoning, food
  radiation J70.0
  Salmonella (arizonae) (cholerae-suis) (enteritidis) (typhimurium) A02.9
  scombroid fish T61.1-●
  seafood (noxious) T61.9-●
    bacterial —see Intoxication, foodborne, by agent
    fish —see Poisoning, fish
    shellfish —see Poisoning, shellfish
    specified NEC —see subcategory T61.8X-●
  shellfish (amnesic) (azaspiracid) (diarrheic) (neurotoxic) (noxious) (paralytic) T61.78-●
    bacterial —see Intoxication, foodborne, by agent
    ciguatera mollusk —see Poisoning, ciguatera fish
  specified substance NEC T65.891
  Staphylococcus, food A05.0
  tobacco (nicotine) T65.2-●
  water E87.79
Poker spine —see Spondylitis, ankylosing
Poland syndrome Q79.8
Polioencephalitis (acute) (bulbar) A80.9
  inferior G12.22
  influenzal —see Influenza, with, encephalopathy
  superior hemorrhagic (acute) (Wernicke's) E51.2
  Wernicke's E51.2
Polioencephalomyelitis (acute) (anterior) A80.9
  with beriberi E51.2
Polioencephalopathy, superior hemorrhagic E51.2
  with
    beriberi E51.11
    pellagra E52
Poliomeningoencephalitis —see Meningoencephalitis
Poliomyelitis (acute) (anterior) (epidemic) A80.9
  with paralysis (bulbar) —see Poliomyelitis, paralytic
  abortive A80.4
  ascending (progressive) —see Poliomyelitis, paralytic
  bulbar (paralytic) —see Poliomyelitis, paralytic
  congenital P35.8
  nonepidemic A80.9
  nonparalytic A80.4
  paralytic A80.30
    specified NEC A80.39
    vaccine-associated A80.0
    wild virus
      imported A80.1
      indigenous A80.2
  spinal, acute A80.9
Poliosis (eyebrow) (eyelashes) L67.1
  circumscripta, acquired L67.1
Pollakiuria R35.0
  psychogenic F45.8
Pollinosis J30.1
Pollitzer's disease L73.2
Polyadenitis —see also Lymphadenitis
  malignant A20.0
Polyalgia M79.89
Polyangiitis M30.0
  microscopic M31.7
  overlap syndrome M30.8
Polyarteritis
  microscopic M31.7
  nodosa M30.0
    with lung involvement M30.1
    juvenile M30.2
    related condition NEC M30.8

Polyarthralgia —see Pain, joint
Polyarthritis, polyarthropathy —see also Arthritis M13.0
  due to or associated with other specified conditions —see Arthritis
  epidemic (Australian) (with exanthema) B33.1
  infective —see Arthritis, pyogenic or pyemic
  inflammatory M06.4
  juvenile (chronic) (seronegative) M08.3
  migratory M13.8-●
  rheumatic, acute —see Fever, rheumatic
Polyarthrosis M15.9
  post-traumatic M15.3
  primary M15.0
  specified NEC M15.8
Polycarential syndrome of infancy E40
Polychondritis (atrophic) (chronic) —see also Disorder, cartilage, specified type NEC
  relapsing M94.1
Polycoria Q13.2
Polycystic (disease)
  degeneration, kidney Q61.3
    autosomal dominant (adult type) Q61.2
    autosomal recessive (infantile type) NEC Q61.19
  kidney Q61.3
    autosomal
      dominant Q61.2
      recessive NEC Q61.19
    autosomal dominant (adult type) Q61.2
    autosomal recessive (childhood type) NEC Q61.19
    infantile type NEC Q61.19
  liver Q44.6
  lung J98.4
    congenital Q33.0
  ovary, ovaries E28.2
  spleen Q89.09
Polycythemia (secondary) D75.1
  acquired D75.1
  benign (familial) D75.0
  due to
    donor twin P61.1
    erythropoietin D75.1
    fall in plasma volume D75.1
    high altitude D75.1
    maternal-fetal transfusion P61.1
    stress D75.1
  emotional D75.1
  erythropoietin D75.1
  familial (benign) D75.0
  Gaisböck's (hypertonica) D75.1
  high altitude D75.1
  hypertonica D75.1
  hypoxemic D75.1
  neonatorum P61.1
  nephrogenous D75.1
  relative D75.1
  secondary D75.1
  spurious D75.1
  stress D75.1
  vera D45
Polycytosis cryptogenica D75.1
Polydactylism, polydactyly Q69.9
  toes Q69.2
Polydipsia R63.1
Polydystrophy, pseudo-Hurler E77.0
Polyembryoma —see Neoplasm, malignant, by site
Polyglandular
  deficiency E31.0
  dyscrasia E31.9
  dysfunction E31.9
  syndrome E31.8
Polyhydramnios O40.-●
Polymastia Q83.1
Polymenorrhea N92.0
Polymyalgia M35.3
  arteritica, giant cell M31.5
  rheumatica M35.3
    with giant cell arteritis M31.5

Polymyositis (acute) (chronic) (hemorrhagic) M33.20
  with
    myopathy M33.22
    respiratory involvement M33.21
    skin involvement —see Dermatopolymyositis
    specified organ involvement NEC M33.29
  ossificans (generalisata) (progressiva) —see Myositis, ossificans, progressiva
Polyneuritis, polyneuritic —see also Polyneuropathy
  acute (post-)infective G61.0
  alcoholic G62.1
  cranialis G52.7
  demyelinating, chronic inflammatory (CIDP) G61.81
  diabetic —see Diabetes, polyneuropathy
  diphtheritic A36.83
  due to lack of vitamin NEC E56.9 [G63]
  endemic E51.11
  erythredema —see subcategory T56.1
  febrile, acute G61.0
  hereditary ataxic G60.1
  idiopathic, acute G61.0
  infective (acute) G61.0
  inflammatory, chronic demyelinating (CIDP) G61.81
  nutritional E63.9 [G63]
  postinfective (acute) G61.0
  specified NEC G62.89
Polyneuropathy (peripheral) G62.9
  alcoholic G62.1
  amyloid (Portuguese) E85.1 [G63]
    transthyretin-related (ATTR) familial E85.1
  arsenical E85.1 [G63]
  critical illness G62.81
  demyelinating, chronic inflammatory (CIDP) G61.81
  diabetic —see Diabetes, polyneuropathy
  drug-induced G62.0
  hereditary G60.9
    specified NEC G60.8
  idiopathic G60.9
    progressive G60.3
  in (due to)
    alcohol G62.1
      sequelae G65.2
    amyloidosis, familial (Portuguese) E85.1 [G63]
    antitetanus serum G61.1
    arsenic G62.2
      sequelae G65.2
    avitaminosis NEC E56.9 [G63]
    beriberi E51.11
    collagen vascular disease NEC M35.9 [G63]
    deficiency (of)
      B (-complex) vitamins E53.9 [G63]
      vitamin B6 E53.1 [G63]
    diabetes —see Diabetes, polyneuropathy
    diphtheria A36.83
    drug or medicament G62.0
      correct substance properly administered —see Table of Drugs and Chemicals, by drug, adverse effect
      overdose or wrong substance given or taken —see Table of Drugs and Chemicals, by drug, poisoning
    endocrine disease NEC E34.9 [G63]
    herpes zoster B02.23
    hypoglycemia E16.2 [G63]
    infectious
      disease NEC B99 [G63]
      mononucleosis B27.91
    lack of vitamin NEC E56.9 [G63]
    lead G62.2
      sequelae G65.2
    leprosy A30.9 [G63]
    Lyme disease A69.22
    metabolic disease NEC E88.9 [G63]

▶ New   ⇒ Revised   ~~deleted~~ Deleted   ● Use Additional Character(s)

Polyneuropathy (*Continued*)
  in (*Continued*)
    microscopic polyangiitis M31.7 [G63]
    mumps B26.84
    neoplastic disease —*see also* Neoplasm
      D49.9 [G63]
    nutritional deficiency NEC E63.9 [G63]
    organophosphate compounds G62.2
      sequelae G65.2
    parasitic disease NEC B89 [G63]
    pellagra E52 [G63]
    polyarteritis nodosa M30.0
    porphyria E80.20 [G63]
    radiation G62.82
    rheumatoid arthritis —*see* Rheumatoid,
      polyneuropathy
    sarcoidosis D86.89
    serum G61.1
    syphilis (late) A52.15
      congenital A50.43
    systemic
      connective tissue disorder M35.9 [G63]
      lupus erythematosus M32.19
    toxic agent NEC G62.2
      sequelae G65.2
    transthyretin-related (ATTR) familial
      amyloid E85.1
    triorthocresyl phosphate G62.2
      sequelae G65.2
    tuberculosis A17.89
    uremia N18.9 [G63]
    vitamin B12 deficiency E53.8 [G63]
      with anemia (pernicious) D51.0 [G63]
        due to dietary deficiency D51.3 [G63]
    zoster B02.23
  inflammatory G61.9
    chronic demyelinating (CIDP) G61.81
    sequelae G65.1
    specified NEC G61.89
  lead G62.2
    sequelae G65.2
  nutritional NEC E63.9 [G63]
  postherpetic (zoster) B02.23
  progressive G60.3
  radiation-induced G62.82
  sensory (hereditary) (idiopathic) G60.8
  specified NEC G62.89
  syphilitic (late) A52.15
    congenital A50.43
Polyopia H53.8
Polyorchism, polyorchidism Q55.21
Polyosteoarthritis —*see also* Osteoarthritis,
  generalized M15.9-●
  post-traumatic M15.3
  specified NEC M15.8
Polyostotic fibrous dysplasia Q78.1
Polyotia Q17.0
Polyp, polypus
  accessory sinus J33.8
  adenocarcinoma in —*see* Neoplasm,
    malignant, by site
  adenocarcinoma in situ in —*see* Neoplasm, in
    situ, by site
  adenoid tissue J33.0
  adenomatous —*see also* Neoplasm, benign,
    by site
    adenocarcinoma in —*see* Neoplasm,
      malignant, by site
    adenocarcinoma in situ in —*see* Neoplasm,
      in situ, by site
    carcinoma in —*see* Neoplasm, malignant,
      by site
    carcinoma in situ in —*see* Neoplasm, in
      situ, by site
    multiple —*see* Neoplasm, benign
      adenocarcinoma in —*see* Neoplasm,
        malignant, by site
      adenocarcinoma in situ in —*see*
        Neoplasm, in situ, by site
  antrum J33.8
  anus, anal (canal) K62.0
  Bartholin's gland N84.3
  bladder D41.4

Polyp, polypus (*Continued*)
  carcinoma in —*see* Neoplasm, malignant, by
    site
  carcinoma in situ in —*see* Neoplasm, in situ,
    by site
  cecum D12.0
  cervix (uteri) N84.1
    in pregnancy or childbirth —*see* Pregnancy,
      complicated by, abnormal, cervix
    mucous N84.1
    nonneoplastic N84.1
  choanal J33.0
  cholesterol K82.4
  clitoris N84.3
  colon K63.5
    adenomatous D12.6
      ascending D12.6
      cecum D12.0
      descending D12.4
    ▶ ascending K63.5
      ▶ sigmoid D12.5
      ▶ transverse D12.3
    ▶ cecum K63.5
    ▶ descending K63.5
    inflammatory K51.40
      with
        abscess K51.414
        complication K51.419
          specified NEC K51.418
        fistula K51.413
        intestinal obstruction K51.412
        rectal bleeding K51.411
    sigmoid D12.5
    transverse D12.3
  corpus uteri N84.0
  dental K04.01
    irreversible K04.02
    reversible K04.01
  duodenum K31.7
  ear (middle) H74.4-●
  endometrium N84.0
  ▶ esophageal K22.81
  ▶ esophagogastric junction K22.82
  ethmoidal (sinus) J33.8
  fallopian tube N84.8
  female genital tract N84.9
    specified NEC N84.8
  frontal (sinus) J33.8
  gallbladder K82.4
  gingiva, gum K06.8
  hyperplastic, (any site) K63.5
  labia, labium (majus) (minus) N84.3
  larynx (mucous) J38.1
    adenomatous D14.1
  malignant —*see* Neoplasm, malignant, by site
  maxillary (sinus) J33.8
  middle ear —*see* Polyp, ear (middle)
  myometrium N84.0
  nares
    anterior J33.9
    posterior J33.0
  nasal (mucous) J33.9
    cavity J33.0
    septum J33.0
  nasopharyngeal J33.0
  nose (mucous) J33.9
  oviduct N84.8
  pharynx J39.2
  placenta O90.89
  prostate —*see* Enlargement, enlarged,
    prostate
  pudenda, pudendum N84.3
  pulpal (dental) K04.01
    irreversible K04.02
    reversible K04.01
  rectum (nonadenomatous) K62.1
    adenomatous —*see* Polyp, adenomatous
  septum (nasal) J33.0
  sinus (accessory) (ethmoidal) (frontal)
    (maxillary) (sphenoidal) J33.8
  sphenoidal (sinus) J33.8
  stomach K31.7
    adenomatous D13.1

Polyp, polypus (*Continued*)
  tube, fallopian N84.8
  turbinate, mucous membrane J33.8
  umbilical, newborn P83.6
  ureter N28.89
  urethra N36.2
  uterus (body) (corpus) (mucous) N84.0
    cervix N84.1
    in pregnancy or childbirth —*see* Pregnancy,
      complicated by, tumor, uterus
  vagina N84.2
  vocal cord (mucous) J38.1
  vulva N84.3
Polyphagia R63.2
Polyploidy Q92.7
Polypoid —*see* condition
Polyposis —*see also* Polyp
  coli (adenomatous) D12.6
    adenocarcinoma in C18.9
    adenocarcinoma in situ in —*see* Neoplasm,
      in situ, by site
    carcinoma in C18.9
  colon (adenomatous) D12.6
  familial D12.6
    adenocarcinoma in situ in —*see* Neoplasm,
      in situ, by site
  intestinal (adenomatous) D12.6
  malignant lymphomatous C83.1
  multiple, adenomatous —*see also* Neoplasm,
    benign D36.9
Polyradiculitis —*see* Polyneuropathy
Polyradiculoneuropathy (acute) (postinfective)
  (segmentally demyelinating) G61.0
Polyserositis
  due to pericarditis I31.1
  pericardial I31.1
  periodic, familial E85.0
  tuberculous A19.9
    acute A19.1
    chronic A19.8
Polysplenia syndrome Q89.09
Polysyndactyly —*see also* Syndactylism,
  syndactyly Q70.4
Polytrichia L68.3
Polyunguia Q84.6
Polyuria R35.89
  nocturnal R35.81
  psychogenic F45.8
  specified NEC R35.89
Pompe's disease (glycogen storage) E74.02
Pompholyx L30.1
Poncet's disease (tuberculous rheumatism)
  A18.09
Pond fracture —*see* Fracture, skull
Ponos B55.0
Pons, pontine —*see* condition
Poor
  aesthetic of existing restoration of tooth
    K08.56
  contractions, labor O62.2
  gingival margin to tooth restoration K08.51
  personal hygiene R46.0
  prenatal care, affecting management of
    pregnancy —*see* Pregnancy, complicated
    by, insufficient, prenatal care
  sucking reflex (newborn) R29.2
  urinary stream R39.12
  vision NEC H54.7
Poradenitis, nostras inguinalis or venerea
  A55
Porencephaly (congenital) (developmental)
  (true) Q04.6
  acquired G93.0
  nondevelopmental G93.0
  traumatic (post) F07.89
Porocephaliasis B88.8
Porokeratosis Q82.8
Poroma, eccrine —*see* Neoplasm, skin, benign
Porphyria (South African) E80.20
  acquired E80.20
  acute intermittent (hepatic) (Swedish)
    E80.21

Porphyria *(Continued)*
  cutanea tarda (hereditary) (symptomatic) E80.1
  due to drugs E80.20
    correct substance properly administered —
        see Table of Drugs and Chemicals, by
        drug, adverse effect
    overdose or wrong substance given
        or taken —*see* Table of Drugs and
        Chemicals, by drug, poisoning
  erythropoietic (congenital) (hereditary) E80.0
  hepatocutaneous type E80.1
  secondary E80.20
  toxic NEC E80.20
  variegata E80.20
Porphyrinuria —*see* Porphyria
Porphyruria —*see* Porphyria
Portal —*see* condition
Port wine nevus, mark, or stain Q82.5
Posadas-Wernicke disease B38.9
Positive
  culture (nonspecific)
    blood R78.81
    bronchial washings R84.5
    cerebrospinal fluid R83.5
    cervix uteri R87.5
    nasal secretions R84.5
    nipple discharge R89.5
    nose R84.5
      staphylococcus (Methicillin susceptible)
          Z22.321
        Methicillin resistant Z22.322
    peritoneal fluid R85.5
    pleural fluid R84.5
    prostatic secretions R86.5
    saliva R85.5
    seminal fluid R86.5
    sputum R84.5
    synovial fluid R89.5
    throat scrapings R84.5
    urine R82.79
    vagina R87.5
    vulva R87.5
    wound secretions R89.5
  PPD (skin test) R76.11
  serology for syphilis A53.0
    with signs or symptoms - code as Syphilis,
        by site and stage
    false R76.8
  skin test, tuberculin (without active
      tuberculosis) R76.11
  test, human immunodeficiency virus (HIV)
      R75
  VDRL A53.0
    with signs or symptoms - code by site and
        stage under Syphilis A53.9
  Wassermann reaction A53.0
▶ Post COVID-19 condition, unspecified U09.9
Postcardiotomy syndrome I97.0
Postcaval ureter Q62.62
Postcholecystectomy syndrome K91.5
Postclimacteric bleeding N95.0
Postcommissurotomy syndrome I97.0
Postconcussional syndrome F07.81
Postcontusional syndrome F07.81
Postcricoid region —*see* condition
Post-dates (40-42 weeks) (pregnancy) (mother)
      O48.0
    more than 42 weeks gestation O48.1
Postencephalitic syndrome F07.89
Posterior —*see* condition
Posterolateral sclerosis (spinal cord) —*see*
      Degeneration, combined
Postexanthematous —*see* condition
Postfebrile —*see* condition
Postgastrectomy dumping syndrome K91.1
Posthemiplegic chorea —*see* Monoplegia
Posthemorrhagic anemia (chronic) D50.0
  acute D62
  newborn P61.3
Postherpetic neuralgia (zoster) B02.29
  trigeminal B02.22

Posthitis N47.7
Postimmunization complication or reaction —
      see Complications, vaccination
Postinfectious —*see* condition
Postlaminectomy syndrome NEC M96.1
Postleukotomy syndrome F07.0
Postmastectomy lymphedema (syndrome) I97.2
Postmaturity, postmature (over 42 weeks)
  maternal (over 42 weeks gestation) O48.1
  newborn P08.22
Postmeasles complication NEC —*see also*
      condition B05.89
Postmenopausal
  endometrium (atrophic) N95.8
    suppurative —*see also* Endometritis N71.9
  osteoporosis —*see* Osteoporosis,
      postmenopausal
Postnasal drip R09.82
  due to
    allergic rhinitis —*see* Rhinitis, allergic
    common cold J00
    gastroesophageal reflux —*see* Reflux,
        gastroesophageal
    nasopharyngitis —*see* Nasopharyngitis
    other know condition — code to condition
    sinusitis —*see* Sinusitis
Postnatal —*see* condition
Postoperative (postprocedural) —*see*
      Complication, postoperative
  pneumothorax, therapeutic Z98.3
  state NEC Z98.890
Postpancreatectomy hyperglycemia E89.1
Postpartum —*see* Puerperal
Postphlebitic syndrome —*see* Syndrome,
      postthrombotic
Postpolio (myelitic) syndrome G14
Postpoliomyelitic —*see also* condition
  osteopathy —*see* Osteopathy, after
      poliomyelitis
Postprocedural —*see also* Postoperative
  hypoinsulinemia E89.1
Postschizophrenic depression F32.89
Postsurgery status —*see also* Status (post)
  pneumothorax, therapeutic Z98.3
Post-term (40-42 weeks) (pregnancy) (mother)
      O48.0
  infant P08.21
  more than 42 weeks gestation (mother) O48.1
Post-traumatic brain syndrome, nonpsychotic
      F07.81
Post-typhoid abscess A01.09
Postures, hysterical F44.2
Postvaccinal reaction or complication —*see*
      Complications, vaccination
Postvalvulotomy syndrome I97.0
Potain's
  disease (pulmonary edema) —*see* Edema, lung
  syndrome (gastrectasis with dyspepsia) K31.0
Potter's
  asthma J62.8
  facies Q60.6
  lung J62.8
  syndrome (with renal agenesis) Q60.6
Pott's
  curvature (spinal) A18.01
  disease or paraplegia A18.01
  spinal curvature A18.01
  tumor, puffy —*see* Osteomyelitis, specified
      type NEC
Pouch
  bronchus Q32.4
  Douglas' —*see* condition
  esophagus, esophageal, congenital Q39.6
    acquired K22.5
  gastric K31.4
  Hartmann's K82.8
  pharynx, pharyngeal (congenital) Q38.7
Pouchitis K91.850
Poultrymen's itch B88.0
Poverty NEC Z59.6
  extreme Z59.5

Poxvirus NEC B08.8
Prader-Willi syndrome Q87.11
Prader-Willi-like syndrome Q87.11
Preauricular appendage or tag Q17.0
Prebetalipoproteinemia (acquired) (essential)
      (familial) (hereditary) (primary)
      (secondary) E78.1
  with chylomicronemia E78.3
Precipitate labor or delivery O62.3
Preclimacteric bleeding (menorrhagia) N92.4
Precocious
  adrenarche E30.1
  menarche E30.1
  menstruation E30.1
  pubarche E30.1
  puberty E30.1
    central E22.8
  sexual development NEC E30.1
  thelarche E30.8
Precocity, sexual (constitutional) (cryptogenic)
      (female) (idiopathic) (male) E30.1
  with adrenal hyperplasia E25.9
    congenital E25.0
Precordial pain R07.2
Predeciduous teeth K00.2
Prediabetes, prediabetic R73.03
  complicating
    pregnancy —*see* Pregnancy, complicated
        by, diseases of, specified type or
        system NEC
    puerperium O99.893
Predislocation status of hip at birth Q65.6
Pre-eclampsia O14.9-●
  with pre-existing hypertension —*see*
      Hypertension, complicating pregnancy,
      pre-existing, with, pre-eclampsia
  complicating
    childbirth O14.94
    puerperium O14.95
  mild O14.0-●
    complicating
      childbirth O14.04
      puerperium O14.05
  moderate O14.0-●
    complicating
      childbirth O14.04
      puerperium O14.05
  severe O14.1-●
    with hemolysis, elevated liver enzymes
        and low platelet count (HELLP)
        O14.2-●
      complicating
        childbirth O14.24
        puerperium O14.25
    complicating
      childbirth O14.14
      puerperium O14.15
Pre-eruptive color change, teeth, tooth K00.8
Pre-excitation atrioventricular conduction I45.6
Preglaucoma H40.00-●
Pregnancy (single) (uterine) —*see also* Delivery
      and Puerperal Z33.1

Note: The Tabular must be reviewed for
assignment of the appropriate character
indicating the trimester of the pregnancy

Note: The Tabular must be reviewed for
assignment of appropriate seventh character
for multiple gestation codes in Chapter 15

  abdominal (ectopic) O00.00
    with intrauterine pregnancy O00.01
      with viable fetus O36.7-●
  ampullar O00.10-●
    with intrauterine pregnancy O00.11-●
  biochemical O02.81
  broad ligament O00.80
    with intrauterine pregnancy O00.81
  cervical O00.80
    with intrauterine pregnancy O00.81

▶ New   ⇒ Revised   ~~deleted~~ Deleted   ● Use Additional Character(s)

Pregnancy *(Continued)*
 chemical O02.81
 complicated NOS O26.9-●
 complicated by (care of) (management affected by)
  abnormal, abnormality
   cervix O34.4-●
    causing obstructed labor O65.5
   cord (umbilical) O69.9
   fetal heart rate or rhythm O36.83-●
   findings on antenatal screening of mother O28.9
    biochemical O28.1
    chromosomal O28.5
    cytological O28.2
    genetic O28.5
    hematological O28.0
    radiological O28.4
    specified NEC O28.8
    ultrasonic O28.3
   glucose (tolerance) NEC O99.810
   pelvic organs O34.9-●
    specified NEC O34.8-●
     causing obstructed labor O65.5
   pelvis (bony) (major) NEC O33.0
   perineum O34.7-●
   position
    placenta O44.0-●
     with hemorrhage O44.1-●
    uterus O34.59-●
   uterus O34.59-●
    causing obstructed labor O65.5
    congenital O34.0-●
   vagina O34.6-●
    causing obstructed labor O65.5
   vulva O34.7-●
    causing obstructed labor O65.5
  abruptio placentae —*see* Abruptio placentae
  abscess or cellulitis
   bladder O23.1-●
   breast O91.11-●
   genital organ or tract O23.9-●
  abuse
   physical O9A.31-●
   psychological O9A.51-●
   sexual O9A.41-●
  adverse effect anesthesia O29.9-●
   aspiration pneumonitis O29.01-●
   cardiac arrest O29.11-●
   cardiac complication NEC O29.19-●
   cardiac failure O29.12-●
   central nervous system complication NEC O29.29-●
   cerebral anoxia O29.21-●
   failed or difficult intubation O29.6-●
   inhalation of stomach contents or secretions NOS O29.01-●
   local, toxic reaction O29.3X
   Mendelson's syndrome O29.01-●
   pressure collapse of lung O29.02-●
   pulmonary complications NEC O29.09-●
   specified NEC O29.8X
   spinal and epidural type NEC O29.5X
    induced headache O29.4-●
  albuminuria —*see also* Proteinuria, gestational O12.1-●
  alcohol use O99.31-●
  amnionitis O41.12-●
  anaphylactoid syndrome of pregnancy O88.01-●
  anemia (conditions in D50-D64) (pre-existing) O99.01-●
   complicating the puerperium O99.03
  antepartum hemorrhage O46.9-●
   with coagulation defect —*see* Hemorrhage, antepartum, with coagulation defect
   specified NEC O46.8X-●
  appendicitis O99.61-●
  atrophy (yellow) (acute) liver (subacute) O26.61-●

Pregnancy *(Continued)*
 complicated by *(Continued)*
  bariatric surgery status O99.84-●
  bicornis or bicornuate uterus O34.0-●
  biliary tract problems O26.61-●
  breech presentation O32.1
  cardiovascular diseases (conditions in I00-I09, I20-I52, I70-I99) O99.41-●
  cerebrovascular disorders (conditions in I60-I69) O99.41-●
  cervical shortening O26.87-●
  cervicitis O23.51-●
  cesarean scar defect (isthmocele) O34.22
  chloasma (gravidarum) O26.89-●
  cholecystitis O99.61-●
  cholestasis (intrahepatic) O26.61-●
  chorioamnionitis O41.12-●
  circulatory system disorder (conditions in I00-I09, I20-I99, O99.41-●)
  compound presentation O32.6
  conjoined twins O30.02-●
  connective system disorders (conditions in M00-M99) O99.891
  contracted pelvis (general) O33.1
   inlet O33.2
   outlet O33.3
  convulsions (eclamptic) (uremic) —*see also* Eclampsia O15.9-●
  cracked nipple O92.11-●
  cystitis O23.1-●
  cystocele O34.8-●
  death of fetus (near term) O36.4
   early pregnancy O02.1
   of one fetus or more in multiple gestation O31.2-●
  deciduitis O41.14-●
  decreased fetal movement O36.81-●
  dental problems O99.61-●
  diabetes (mellitus) O24.91-●
   gestational (pregnancy induced) —*see* Diabetes, gestational
   pre-existing O24.31-●
    specified NEC O24.81-●
    type 1 O24.01-●
    type 2 O24.11-●
  digestive system disorders (conditions in K00-K93) O99.61-●
  diseases of —*see* Pregnancy, complicated by, specified body system disease
   biliary tract O26.61-●
   blood NEC (conditions in D65-D77) O99.11-●
   liver O26.61-●
   specified NEC O99.891
  disorders of —*see* Pregnancy, complicated by, specified body system disorder
   amniotic fluid and membranes O41.9-●
    specified NEC O41.8X-●
   biliary tract O26.61-●
   ear and mastoid process (conditions in H60-H95) O99.891
   eye and adnexa (conditions in H00-H59) O99.891
   liver O26.61-●
   skin (conditions in L00-L99) O99.71-●
   specified NEC O99.891
  displacement, uterus NEC O34.59-●
   causing obstructed labor O65.5
  disproportion (due to) O33.9
   fetal (ascites) (hydrops) (meningomyelocele) (sacral teratoma) (tumor) deformities NEC O33.7
   generally contracted pelvis O33.1
   hydrocephalic fetus O33.6
   inlet contraction of pelvis O33.2
   mixed maternal and fetal origin O33.4
   specified NEC O33.8
  double uterus O34.0-●
   causing obstructed labor O65.5
  drug use (conditions in F11-F19) O99.32-●

Pregnancy *(Continued)*
 complicated by *(Continued)*
  eclampsia, eclamptic (coma) (convulsions) (delirium) (nephritis) (uremia) (*see also* Eclampsia) O15-●
  ectopic pregnancy —*see* Pregnancy, ectopic
  edema O12.0-●
   with
    gestational hypertension, mild —*see also* Pre-eclampsia O14.0-●
    proteinuria O12.2-●
  effusion, amniotic fluid —*see* Pregnancy, complicated by, premature rupture of membranes
  elderly
   multigravida O09.52-●
   primigravida O09.51-●
  embolism —*see also* Embolism, obstetric, pregnancy O88.-●
  endocrine diseases NEC O99.28-●
  endometritis O86.12
  excessive weight gain O26.0-●
  exhaustion O26.81-●
   during labor and delivery O75.81
  face presentation O32.3
  failed induction of labor O61.9
  failed or difficult intubation for anesthesia O29.6-●
   instrumental O61.1
   mechanical O61.1
   medical O61.0
   specified NEC O61.8
   surgical O61.1
  false labor (pains) O47.9
   at or after 37 completed weeks of pregnancy O47.1
   before 37 completed weeks of pregnancy O47.0-●
  fatigue O26.81-●
   during labor and delivery O75.81
  fatty metamorphosis of liver O26.61-●
  female genital mutilation O34.8-● *[N90.81-●]*
  fetal (maternal care for)
   abnormality or damage O35.9
    acid-base balance O68
    specified type NEC O35.8
   acidemia O68
   acidosis O68
   alkalosis O68
   anemia and thrombocytopenia O36.82-●
   anencephaly O35.0
   bradycardia O36.83-●
   chromosomal abnormality (conditions in Q90-Q99) O35.1
   conjoined twins O30.02-●
   damage from
    amniocentesis O35.7
    biopsy procedures O35.7
    drug addiction O35.5
    hematological investigation O35.7
    intrauterine contraceptive device O35.7
    maternal
     alcohol addiction O35.4
     cytomegalovirus infection O35.3
     disease NEC O35.8
     drug addiction O35.5
     listeriosis O35.8
     rubella O35.3
     toxoplasmosis O35.8
     viral infection O35.3
    medical procedure NEC O35.7
    radiation O35.6
   death (near term) O36.4
    early pregnancy O02.1
   decreased movement O36.81-●
   depressed heart rate tones O36.83-●
   disproportion due to deformity (fetal) O33.7
   excessive growth (large for dates) O36.6-●
   growth retardation O36.59-●
    light for dates O36.59-●
    small for dates O36.59-●

Pregnancy *(Continued)*
  complicated by *(Continued)*
    fetal *(Continued)*
      heart rate irregularity (abnormal
          variability) (bradycardia)
          (decelerations) (tachycardia)
          O36.83-●
      hereditary disease O35.2
      hydrocephalus O35.0
      intrauterine death O36.4
      non-reassuring heart rate or rhythm
          O36.83-●
      poor growth O36.59-●
        light for dates O36.59-●
        small for dates O36.59-●
      problem O36.9-●
        specified NEC O36.89-●
      reduction (elective) O31.3-●
      selective termination O31.3-●
      spina bifida O35.0
      thrombocytopenia O36.82-●
    fibroid (tumor) (uterus) O34.1-●
    fissure of nipple O92.11-●
    gallstones O99.61-●
    gastric banding status O99.84-●
    gastric bypass status O99.84-●
    genital herpes (asymptomatic) (history of)
        (inactive) O98.3-●
    genital tract infection O23.9-●
    glomerular diseases (conditions in
        N00-N07) O26.83-●
      with hypertension, pre-existing —*see*
          Hypertension, complicating,
          pregnancy, pre-existing, with, renal
          disease
    gonorrhea O98.21-●
    grand multiparity O09.4
    habitual aborter —*see* Pregnancy,
        complicated by, recurrent pregnancy
        loss
    HELLP syndrome (hemolysis, elevated
        liver enzymes and low platelet count)
        O14.2-●
    hemorrhage
      antepartum —*see* Hemorrhage,
          antepartum
      before 20 completed weeks gestation
          O20.9
        specified NEC O20.8
      due to premature separation, placenta —
          see also Abruptio placentae O45.9-●
      early O20.9
        specified NEC O20.8
      threatened abortion O20.0
    hemorrhoids O22.4-●
    hepatitis (viral) O98.41-●
    herniation of uterus O34.59-●
    high
      head at term O32.4
      risk —*see* Supervision (of) (for),
          high-risk
    history of in utero procedure during
        previous pregnancy O09.82-●
    HIV O98.71-●
    human immunodeficiency virus (HIV)
        disease O98.71-●
    hydatidiform mole —*see also* Mole,
        hydatidiform O01.9-●
    hydramnios O40.-●
    hydrocephalic fetus (disproportion) O33.6
    hydrops
      amnii O40.-●
      fetalis O36.2-●
        associated with isoimmunization —*see
            also* Pregnancy, complicated by,
            isoimmunization O36.11-●
    hydrorrhea O42.90
    hyperemesis (gravidarum) (mild) —*see also*
        Hyperemesis, gravidarum O21.0-●
    hypertension —*see* Hypertension,
        complicating pregnancy

Pregnancy *(Continued)*
  complicated by *(Continued)*
    hypertensive
      heart and renal disease, pre-existing —
          see Hypertension, complicating,
          pregnancy, pre-existing, with, heart
          disease, with renal disease
      heart disease, pre-existing —*see*
          Hypertension, complicating,
          pregnancy, pre-existing, with, heart
          disease
      renal disease, pre-existing —*see*
          Hypertension, complicating,
          pregnancy, pre-existing, with, renal
          disease
    hypotension O26.5-●
    immune disorders NEC (conditions in
        D80-D89) O99.11-●
    incarceration, uterus O34.51-●
    incompetent cervix O34.3-●
    inconclusive fetal viability O36.80
    infection(s) O98.91-●
      amniotic fluid or sac O41.10-●
      bladder O23.1-●
      carrier state NEC O99.830
        streptococcus B O99.820
      genital organ or tract O23.9-●
        specified NEC O23.59-●
      genitourinary tract O23.9-●
      gonorrhea O98.21-●
      hepatitis (viral) O98.41-●
      HIV O98.71-●
      human immunodeficiency virus (HIV)
          O98.71-●
    ▶intrauterine O41.12
      kidney O23.0-●
      nipple O91.01-●
      parasitic disease O98.91-●
        specified NEC O98.81-●
      protozoal disease O98.61-●
      sexually transmitted NEC O98.31-●
      specified type NEC O98.81-●
      syphilis O98.11-●
      tuberculosis O98.01-●
      urethra O23.2-●
      urinary (tract) O23.4-●
        specified NEC O23.3-●
      viral disease O98.51-●
    ▶inflammation
    ▶intrauterine O41.12
    injury or poisoning (conditions in S00-T88)
        O9A.21-●
      due to abuse
        physical O9A.31-●
        psychological O9A.51-●
        sexual O9A.41-●
    insufficient
      prenatal care O09.3-●
      weight gain O26.1-●
    insulin resistance O26.89
    intrauterine fetal death (near term) O36.4
      early pregnancy O02.1
      multiple gestation (one fetus or more)
          O31.2-●
    isoimmunization O36.11-●
      anti-A sensitization O36.11-●
      anti-B sensitization O36.19-●
      Rh O36.09-●
        anti-D antibody O36.01-●
      specified NEC O36.19-●
    laceration of uterus NEC O71.81
    malformation
      placenta, placental (vessel) O43.10-●
        specified NEC O43.19-●
      uterus (congenital) O34.0-●
    malnutrition (conditions in E40-E46) O25.1-●
    maternal hypotension syndrome O26.5-●
    mental disorders (conditions in F01-F09,
        F20-F52 and F54-F99) O99.34-●
      alcohol use O99.31-●
      drug use O99.32-●
      smoking O99.33-●
    mentum presentation O32.3

Pregnancy *(Continued)*
  complicated by *(Continued)*
    metabolic disorders O99.28-●
    missed
      abortion O02.1
      delivery O36.4
    multiple gestations O30.9-●
      conjoined twins O30.02-●
      quadruplet —*see* Pregnancy, quadruplet
      specified complication NEC O31.8X-●
      specified number of multiples NEC —*see*
          Pregnancy, multiple (gestation),
          specified NEC
      triplet —*see* Pregnancy, triplet
      twin —*see* Pregnancy, twin
    musculoskeletal condition (conditions is
        M00-M99) O99.891
    necrosis, liver (conditions in K72) O26.61-●
    neoplasm
      benign
        cervix O34.4-●
        corpus uteri O34.1-●
        uterus O34.1-●
      malignant O9A.11-●
    nephropathy NEC O26.83-●
    nervous system condition (conditions in
        G00-G99) O99.35-●
    nutritional diseases NEC O99.28-●
    obesity (pre-existing) O99.21-●
    obesity surgery status O99.84-●
    oblique lie or presentation O32.2
    older mother —*see* Pregnancy, complicated
        by, elderly
    oligohydramnios O41.0-●
      with premature rupture of
          membranes —*see also* Pregnancy,
          complicated by, premature rupture
          of membranes O42-●
    onset (spontaneous) of labor after 37
        completed weeks of gestation but
        before 39 completed weeks gestation,
        with delivery by (planned) cesarean
        section O75.82
    oophoritis O23.52-●
    overdose, drug —*see also* Table of Drugs
        and Chemicals, by drug, poisoning
        O9A.21-●
    oversize fetus O33.5
    papyraceous fetus O31.0-●
    pelvic inflammatory disease O99.891
    periodontal disease O99.61-●
    peripheral neuritis O26.82-●
    peritoneal (pelvic) adhesions O99.891
    phlebitis O22.9-●
    phlebopathy O22.9-●
    phlebothrombosis (superficial) O22.2-●
      deep O22.3-●
    placenta accreta O43.21-●
    placenta increta O43.22-●
    placenta percreta O43.23-●
    placenta previa O44.0-●
      complete O44.0-●
        with hemorrhage O44.1-●
      marginal O44.2-●
        with hemorrhage O44.3-●
      partial O44.2-●
        with hemorrhage O44.3-●
    placental disorder O43.9-●
      specified NEC O43.89-●
    placental dysfunction O43.89-●
    placental infarction O43.81-●
    placental insufficiency O36.51-●
    placental transfusion syndromes
      fetomaternal O43.01-●
      fetus to fetus O43.02-●
      maternofetal O43.01-●
    placentitis O41.14-●
    pneumonia O99.51-●
    poisoning —*see also* Table of Drugs and
        Chemicals O9A.21-●
    polyhydramnios O40-●

▶ New   ⇒ Revised   ~~deleted~~ Deleted   ● Use Additional Character(s)

Pregnancy *(Continued)*
  complicated by *(Continued)*
    polymorphic eruption of pregnancy O26.86
    poor obstetric history NEC O09.29-●
    postmaturity (post-term) (40 to 42 weeks)
      O48.0
      more than 42 completed weeks gestation
        (prolonged) O48.1
    pre-eclampsia O14.9-●
      mild O14.0-●
      moderate O14.0-●
      severe O14.1-●
        with hemolysis, elevated liver
          enzymes and low platelet count
          (HELLP) O14.2-●
    premature labor —*see* Pregnancy,
      complicated by, preterm labor
    premature rupture of membranes O42.90
      full-term, unspecified as to length of
        time between rupture and onset of
        labor O42.92
      with onset of labor
        within 24 hours O42.00
          at or after 37 weeks gestation, onset
            of labor within 24 hours of
            rupture O42.02
          pre-term (before 37 completed
            weeks of gestation)
            O42.01-●
        after 24 hours O42.10
          at or after 37 weeks gestation,
            onset of labor more than
            24 hours following rupture
            O42.12
          pre-term (before 37 completed
            weeks of gestation) O42.11-●
      at or after 37 weeks gestation,
        unspecified as to length of time
        between rupture and onset of labor
        O42.92
      pre-term (before 37 completed weeks of
        gestation) O42.91-●
    premature separation of placenta —*see also*
      Abruptio placentae O45.9-●
    presentation, fetal —*see* Delivery,
      complicated by, malposition
    preterm delivery O60.10
    preterm labor
      with delivery O60.10
        preterm O60.10
        term O60.20
      second trimester
        with preterm delivery
          second trimester O60.12
          third trimester O60.13
        with term delivery O60.22
        without delivery O60.02
      third trimester
        with term delivery O60.23
        with third trimester preterm delivery
          O60.14
        without delivery O60.03
      without delivery O60.00
        second trimester O60.02
        third trimester O60.03
    previous history of —*see* Pregnancy,
      supervision of, high-risk
    prolapse, uterus O34.52-●
    proteinuria (gestational) —*see also*
      Proteinuria, gestational O12.1-●
      with edema O12.2-●
    pruritic urticarial papules and plaques of
      pregnancy (PUPPP) O26.86
    pruritus (neurogenic) O26.89-●
    psychosis or psychoneurosis (puerperal)
      F53.1
    ptyalism O26.89-●
    PUPPP (pruritic urticarial papules and
      plaques of pregnancy) O26.86
    pyelitis O23.0-●
    recurrent pregnancy loss O26.2-●

Pregnancy *(Continued)*
  complicated by *(Continued)*
    renal disease or failure NEC O26.83-●
      with secondary hypertension, pre-
        existing —*see* Hypertension,
        complicating, pregnancy, pre-
        existing, secondary
      hypertensive, pre-existing —*see*
        Hypertension, complicating,
        pregnancy, pre-existing, with, renal
        disease
    respiratory condition (conditions in
      J00-J99) O99.51-●
    retained, retention
      dead ovum O02.0
      intrauterine contraceptive device
        O26.3-●
    retroversion, uterus O34.53-●
    Rh immunization, incompatibility or
      sensitization NEC O36.09-●
      anti-D antibody O36.01-●
    rupture
      amnion (premature) —*see also*
        Pregnancy, complicated by,
        premature rupture of membranes
        O42-●
      membranes (premature) —*see also*
        Pregnancy, complicated by,
        premature rupture of membranes
        O42-●
      uterus (during labor) O71.1
        before onset of labor O71.0-●
    salivation (excessive) O26.89-●
    salpingitis O23.52-●
    salpingo-oophoritis O23.52-●
    sepsis (conditions in A40, A41) O98.81-●
    size date discrepancy (uterine) O26.84-●
    skin condition (conditions in L00-L99)
      O99.71-●
    smoking (tobacco) O99.33-●
    social problem O09.7-●
    specified condition NEC O26.89-●
    spotting O26.85-●
    streptococcus group B (GBS) carrier state
      O99.820
    subluxation of symphysis (pubis) O26.71-●
    syphilis (conditions in A50-A53) O98.11-●
    threatened
      abortion O20.0
      labor O47.9
        at or after 37 completed weeks of
          gestation O47.1
        before 37 completed weeks of
          gestation O47.0-●
    thrombophlebitis (superficial) O22.2-●
    thrombosis O22.9-●
      cerebral venous O22.5-●
      cerebrovenous sinus O22.5-●
      deep O22.3-●
    tobacco use disorder (smoking) O99.33-●
    torsion of uterus O34.59-●
    toxemia O14.9-●
    transverse lie or presentation O32.2
    tuberculosis (conditions in A15-A19)
      O98.01-●
    tumor (benign)
      cervix O34.4-●
      malignant O9A.11-●
      uterus O34.1-●
    unstable lie O32.0
    upper respiratory infection O99.51-●
    urethritis O23.2-●
    uterine size date discrepancy O26.84-●
    vaginitis or vulvitis O23.59-●
    varicose veins (lower extremities) O22.0-●
      genitals O22.1-●
      legs O22.0-●
      perineal O22.1-●
      vaginal or vulval O22.1-●
    venereal disease NEC (conditions in A63.8)
      O98.31-●

Pregnancy *(Continued)*
  complicated by *(Continued)*
    venous disorders O22.9-●
      specified NEC O22.8X-●
    very young mother —*see* Pregnancy,
      complicated by, young mother
    viral diseases (conditions in A80-B09,
      B25-B34) O98.51-●
    vomiting O21.9
      due to diseases classified elsewhere O21.8
      hyperemesis gravidarum (mild) —*see*
        also Hyperemesis, gravidarum
        O21.0-●
      late (occurring after 20 weeks of
        gestation) O21.2
    young mother
      multigravida O09.62-●
      primigravida O09.61-●
  concealed O09.3-●
  continuing following
    elective fetal reduction of one or more fetus
      O31.3-●
    intrauterine death of one or more fetus
      O31.2-●
    spontaneous abortion of one or more fetus
      O31.1-●
  cornual O00.80
    with intrauterine pregnancy O00.81
  ectopic (ruptured) O00.90
    with intrauterine pregnancy O00.91
    abdominal O00.00
      with
        intrauterine pregnancy O00.01
        viable fetus O36.7-●
    cervical O00.80
      with intrauterine pregnancy O00.81
    complicated (by) O08.9
      afibrinogenemia O08.1
      cardiac arrest O08.81
      chemical damage of pelvic organ(s)
        O08.6
      circulatory collapse O08.3
      defibrination syndrome O08.1
      electrolyte imbalance O08.5
      embolism (amniotic fluid) (blood clot)
        (pulmonary) (septic) O08.2
      endometritis O08.0
      genital tract and pelvic infection O08.0
      hemorrhage (delayed) (excessive) O08.1
      infection
        genital tract or pelvic O08.0
        kidney O08.83
        urinary tract O08.83
      intravascular coagulation O08.1
      laceration of pelvic organ(s)
        O08.6
      metabolic disorder O08.5
      oliguria O08.4
      oophoritis O08.0
      parametritis O08.0
      pelvic peritonitis O08.0
      perforation of pelvic organ(s)
        O08.6
      renal failure or shutdown O08.4
      salpingitis or salpingo-oophoritis
        O08.0
      sepsis O08.82
      shock O08.83
        septic O08.82
      specified condition NEC O08.89
      tubular necrosis (renal) O08.4
      uremia O08.4
      urinary infection O08.83
      venous complication NEC O08.7
        embolism O08.2
    cornual O00.80
      with intrauterine pregnancy
        O00.81
    intraligamentous O00.80
      with intrauterine pregnancy
        O00.81

Pregnancy *(Continued)*
  ectopic *(Continued)*
    mural O00.8Ø
      with intrauterine pregnancy O00.81
    ovarian O00.2Ø-●
      with intrauterine pregnancy O00.21-●
    specified site NEC O00.8Ø
      with intrauterine pregnancy O00.81
    tubal (ruptured) O00.1Ø-●
      with intrauterine pregnancy O00.11-●
  examination (normal) Z34.9-●
    first Z34.Ø-●
    high-risk —*see* Pregnancy, supervision of, high-risk
    specified Z34.8-●
  extrauterine —*see* Pregnancy, ectopic
  fallopian O00.1Ø-●
    with intrauterine pregnancy O00.11-●
  false F45.8
  gestational carrier Z33.3
  heptachorionic, hepta-amniotic (septuplets) O3Ø.83-●
  hexachorionic, hexa-amniotic (sextuplets) O3Ø.83-●
  hidden O09.3-●
  high-risk —*see* Pregnancy, supervision of, high-risk
  incidental finding Z33.1
  interstitial O00.8Ø
    with intrauterine pregnancy O00.81
  intraligamentous O00.8Ø
    with intrauterine pregnancy O00.81
  intramural O00.8Ø
    with intrauterine pregnancy O00.81
  intraperitoneal O00.ØØ
    with intrauterine pregnancy O00.Ø1
  isthmian O00.1Ø-●
    with intrauterine pregnancy O00.11-●
  mesometric (mural) O00.8Ø
    with intrauterine pregnancy O00.81
  molar NEC O02.Ø
    complicated (by) O08.9
      afibrinogenemia O08.1
      cardiac arrest O08.81
      chemical damage of pelvic organ(s) O08.6
      circulatory collapse O08.3
      defibrination syndrome O08.1
      electrolyte imbalance O08.5
      embolism (amniotic fluid) (blood clot) (pulmonary) (septic) O08.2
      endometritis O08.Ø
      genital tract and pelvic infection O08.Ø
      hemorrhage (delayed) (excessive) O08.1
      infection
        genital tract or pelvic O08.Ø
        kidney O08.83
        urinary tract O08.83
      intravascular coagulation O08.1
      laceration of pelvic organ(s) O08.6
      metabolic disorder O08.5
      oliguria O08.4
      oophoritis O08.Ø
      parametritis O08.Ø
      pelvic peritonitis O08.Ø
      perforation of pelvic organ(s) O08.6
      renal failure or shutdown O08.4
      salpingitis or salpingo-oophoritis O08.Ø
      sepsis O08.82
      shock O08.3
        septic O08.82
      specified condition NEC O08.89
      tubular necrosis (renal) O08.4
      uremia O08.4
      urinary infection O08.83
      venous complication NEC O08.7
        embolism O08.2
    hydatidiform —*see also* Mole, hydatidiform O01.9-●
  multiple (gestation) O3Ø.9-●
    greater than quadruplets —*see* Pregnancy, multiple (gestation), specified NEC

Pregnancy *(Continued)*
  multiple (gestation) *(Continued)*
    specified NEC O3Ø.8Ø-●
      with
        two or more monoamniotic fetuses O3Ø.82-●
        two or more monochorionic fetuses O3Ø.81-●
      number of chorions and amnions are both equal to the number of fetuses O3Ø.83-●
      two or more monoamniotic fetuses O3Ø.82-●
      two or more monochorionic fetuses O3Ø.81-●
      unable to determine number of placenta and number of amniotic sacs O3Ø.89-●
      unspecified number of placenta and unspecified number of amniotic sacs O3Ø.8Ø-●
  mural O00.8Ø
    with intrauterine pregnancy O00.81
  normal (supervision of) Z34.9-●
    first Z34.Ø-●
    high-risk —*see* Pregnancy, supervision of, high-risk
    specified Z34.8-●
  ovarian O00.2Ø-●
    with intrauterine pregnancy O00.21-●
  pentachorionic, penta-amniotic (quintuplets) O3Ø.83-●
  postmature (4Ø to 42 weeks) O48.Ø
    more than 42 weeks gestation O48.1
  post-term (4Ø to 42 weeks) O48.Ø
  prenatal care only Z34.9-●
    first Z34.Ø-●
    high-risk —*see* Pregnancy, supervision of, high-risk
    specified Z34.8-●
  prolonged (more than 42 weeks gestation) O48.1
  quadruplet O3Ø.2Ø-●
    with
      two or more monoamniotic fetuses O3Ø.22-●
      two or more monochorionic fetuses O3Ø.21-●
    quadrachorionic/quadra-amniotic O3Ø.23-●
    two or more monoamniotic fetuses O3Ø.22-●
    two or more monochorionic fetuses O3Ø.21-●
    unable to determine number of placenta and number of amniotic sacs O3Ø.29-●
    unspecified number of placenta and unspecified number of amniotic sacs O3Ø.2Ø-●
  quintuplet —*see* Pregnancy, multiple (gestation), specified NEC
  sextuplet —*see* Pregnancy, multiple (gestation), specified NEC
  supervision of
    concealed pregnancy O09.3-●
    elderly mother
      multigravida O09.52-●
      primigravida O09.51-●
    hidden pregnancy O09.3-●
    high-risk O09.9-●
      due to (history of)
        ectopic pregnancy O09.1-●
        elderly —*see* Pregnancy, supervision, elderly mother
        grand multiparity O09.4
        infertility O09.Ø-●
        insufficient prenatal care O09.3-●
        in utero procedure during previous pregnancy O09.82-●
        in vitro fertilization O09.81-●
        molar pregnancy O09.A-●
        multiple previous pregnancies O09.4-●
        older mother —*see* Pregnancy, supervision of, elderly mother

Pregnancy *(Continued)*
  supervision of *(Continued)*
    high-risk *(Continued)*
      due to *(Continued)*
        poor reproductive or obstetric history NEC O09.29-●
        pre-term labor O09.21-●
        previous
          neonatal death O09.29-●
        social problems O09.7-●
        specified NEC O09.89-●
        very young mother —*see* Pregnancy, supervision, young mother
      resulting from in vitro fertilization O09.81-●
    normal Z34.9-●
      first Z34.Ø-●
      specified NEC Z34.8-●
    young mother
      multigravida O09.62-●
      primigravida O09.61-●
  triplet O3Ø.1Ø-●
    with
      two or more monoamniotic fetuses O3Ø.12-●
      two or more monochorionic fetuses O3Ø.11-●
    trichorionic/triamniotic O3Ø.13-●
    two or more monoamniotic fetuses O3Ø.12-●
    two or more monochorionic fetuses O3Ø.11-●
    unable to determine number of placenta and number of amniotic sacs O3Ø.19-●
    unspecified number of placenta and unspecified number of amniotic sacs O3Ø.1Ø-●
  tubal (with abortion) (with rupture) O00.1Ø-●
    with intrauterine pregnancy O00.11-●
  twin O3Ø.ØØ-●
    conjoined O3Ø.Ø2-●
    dichorionic/diamniotic (two placenta, two amniotic sacs) O3Ø.Ø4-●
    monochorionic/diamniotic (one placenta, two amniotic sacs) O3Ø.Ø3-●
    monochorionic/monoamniotic (one placenta, one amniotic sac) O3Ø.Ø1-●
    unable to determine number of placenta and number of amniotic sacs O3Ø.Ø9-●
    unspecified number of placenta and unspecified number of amniotic sacs O3Ø.ØØ-●
  unwanted Z64.Ø
  weeks of gestation
    8 weeks Z3A.Ø8
    9 weeks Z3A.Ø9
    1Ø weeks Z3A.1Ø
    11 weeks Z3A.11
    12 weeks Z3A.12
    13 weeks Z3A.13
    14 weeks Z3A.14
    15 weeks Z3A.15
    16 weeks Z3A.16
    17 weeks Z3A.17
    18 weeks Z3A.18
    19 weeks Z3A.19
    2Ø weeks Z3A.2Ø
    21 weeks Z3A.21
    22 weeks Z3A.22
    23 weeks Z3A.23
    24 weeks Z3A.24
    25 weeks Z3A.25
    26 weeks Z3A.26
    27 weeks Z3A.27
    28 weeks Z3A.28
    29 weeks Z3A.29
    3Ø weeks Z3A.3Ø
    31 weeks Z3A.31
    32 weeks Z3A.32
    33 weeks Z3A.33
    34 weeks Z3A.34
    35 weeks Z3A.35
    36 weeks Z3A.36

P

▶ New   ⇒ Revised   ~~deleted~~ Deleted   ● Use Additional Character(s)

Pregnancy (*Continued*)
  weeks of gestation (*Continued*)
    37 weeks Z3A.37
    38 weeks Z3A.38
    39 weeks Z3A.39
    40 weeks Z3A.40
    41 weeks Z3A.41
    42 weeks Z3A.42
    greater than 42 weeks Z3A.49
    less than 8 weeks Z3A.01
    not specified Z3A.00
Preiser's disease —*see* Osteonecrosis,
    secondary, due to, trauma, metacarpus
Pre-kwashiorkor —*see* Malnutrition, severe
Preleukemia (syndrome) D46.9
Preluxation, hip, congenital Q65.6
Premature —*see also* condition
  adrenarche E27.0
  aging E34.8
  beats I49.40
    atrial I49.1
    auricular I49.1
    supraventricular I49.1
  birth NEC —*see* Preterm, newborn
  closure, foramen ovale Q21.8
  contraction
    atrial I49.1
    atrioventricular I49.49
    auricular I49.1
    auriculoventricular I49.2
    heart (extrasystole) I49.49
    junctional I49.2
    ventricular I49.3
  delivery —*see also* Pregnancy, complicated by,
    preterm labor O60.10
  ejaculation F52.4
  infant NEC —*see* Preterm, newborn
    light-for-dates —*see* Light for dates
  labor —*see* Pregnancy, complicated by,
    preterm labor
  lungs P28.0
  menopause E28.319
    asymptomatic E28.319
    symptomatic E28.310
  newborn
    extreme (less than 28 completed weeks) —
      see Immaturity, extreme
    less than 37 completed weeks —*see*
      Preterm, newborn
  puberty E30.1
  rupture membranes or amnion —*see*
    Pregnancy, complicated by, premature
    rupture of membranes
  senility E34.8
  thelarche E30.8
  ventricular systole I49.3
Prematurity NEC (less than 37 completed
    weeks) —*see* Preterm, newborn
  extreme (less than 28 completed weeks) —*see*
    Immaturity, extreme
Premenstrual
  dysphoric disorder (PMDD) F32.81
  tension (syndrome) N94.3
Premolarization, cuspids K00.2
Prenatal
  care, normal pregnancy —*see* Pregnancy,
    normal
  screening of mother —*see also* Encounter,
    antenatal Z36.9
  teeth K00.6
Preparatory care for subsequent treatment NEC
  for dialysis Z49.01
    peritoneal Z49.02
Prepartum —*see* condition
Preponderance, left or right ventricular I51.7
Prepuce —*see* condition
PRES (posterior reversible encephalopathy
    syndrome) I67.83
Presbycardia R54
Presbycusis, presbyacusia H91.1-●
▶**Presbyesophagus** K22.89

Presbyophrenia F03
Presbyopia H52.4
Prescription of contraceptives (initial) Z30.019
  barrier Z30.018
  diaphragm Z30.018
  emergency (postcoital) Z30.012
  implantable subdermal Z30.017
  injectable Z30.013
  intrauterine contraceptive device Z30.014
  pills Z30.011
  postcoital (emergency) Z30.012
  repeat Z30.40
    barrier Z30.49
    diaphragm Z30.49
    implantable subdermal Z30.46
    injectable Z30.42
    pills Z30.41
    specified type NEC Z30.49
    transdermal patch hormonal Z30.45
    vaginal ring hormonal Z30.44
  specified type NEC Z30.018
    transdermal patch hormonal Z30.016
    vaginal ring hormonal Z30.015
Presence (of)
  ankle-joint implant (functional) (prosthesis)
    Z96.66-●
  aortocoronary (bypass) graft Z95.1
  arterial-venous shunt (dialysis) Z99.2
  artificial
    eye (globe) Z97.0
    heart (fully implantable) (mechanical)
      Z95.812
      valve Z95.2
    larynx Z96.3
    lens (intraocular) Z96.1
    limb (complete) (partial) Z97.1-●
      arm Z97.1-●
        bilateral Z97.15
      leg Z97.1-●
        bilateral Z97.16
  audiological implant (functional) Z96.29
  bladder implant (functional) Z96.0
  bone
    conduction hearing device Z96.29
    implant (functional) NEC Z96.7
    joint (prosthesis) —*see* Presence, joint
      implant
  cardiac
    defibrillator (functional) (with synchronous
      cardiac pacemaker)Z95.810
    implant or graft Z95.9
      specified type NEC Z95.818
    pacemaker Z95.0
    resynchronization therapy
      defibrillator Z95.810
      pacemaker Z95.0
  cerebrospinal fluid drainage device Z98.2
  cochlear implant (functional) Z96.21
  contact lens (es) Z97.3
  coronary artery graft or prosthesis Z95.5
  CRT-D (cardiac resynchronization therapy
    defibrillator) Z95.810
  CRT-P (cardiac resynchronization therapy
    pacemaker) Z95.0
  cardioverter-defibrillator (ICD) Z95.810
  CSF shunt Z98.2
  dental prosthesis device Z97.2
  dentures Z97.2
  device (external) NEC Z97.8
    cardiac NEC Z95.818
    heart assist Z95.811
    implanted (functional) Z96.9
      specified NEC Z96.89
    prosthetic Z97.8
  ear implant Z96.20
    cochlear implant Z96.21
    myringotomy tube Z96.22
    specified type NEC Z96.29
  elbow-joint implant (functional) (prosthesis)
    Z96.62-●
  endocrine implant (functional) NEC Z96.49

Presence (*Continued*)
  eustachian tube stent or device (functional)
    Z96.29
  external hearing-aid or device Z97.4
  finger-joint implant (functional) (prosthetic)
    Z96.69-●
  functional implant Z96.9
    specified NEC Z96.89
  graft
    cardiac NEC Z95.818
    vascular NEC Z95.828
  hearing-aid or device (external) Z97.4
    implant (bone) (cochlear) (functional) Z96.21
  heart assist device Z95.811
  heart valve implant (functional) Z95.2
    prosthetic Z95.2
    specified type NEC Z95.4
    xenogenic Z95.3
  hip-joint implant (functional) (prosthesis)
    Z96.64-●
▶ICD (cardioverter-defibrillator) Z95.810
  implanted device (artificial) (functional)
    (prosthetic) Z96.9
    automatic cardiac defibrillator (with
      synchronous cardiac pacemaker)
      Z95.810
    cardiac pacemaker Z95.0
    cochlear Z96.21
    dental Z96.5
    heart Z95.812
    heart valve Z95.2
      prosthetic Z95.2
      specified NEC Z95.4
      xenogenic Z95.3
    insulin pump Z96.41
    intraocular lens Z96.1
    joint Z96.60
      ankle Z96.66-●
      elbow Z96.62-●
      finger Z96.69-●
      hip Z96.64-●
      knee Z96.65-●
      shoulder Z96.61-●
      specified NEC Z96.698
      wrist Z96.63-●
    larynx Z96.3
    myringotomy tube Z96.22
    otological Z96.20
      cochlear Z96.21
      eustachian stent Z96.29
      myringotomy Z96.22
      specified NEC Z96.29
      stapes Z96.29
    skin Z96.81
    skull plate Z96.7
    specified NEC Z96.89
    urogenital Z96.0
  insulin pump (functional) Z96.41
  intestinal bypass or anastomosis Z98.0
  intraocular lens (functional) Z96.1
  intrauterine contraceptive device (IUD) Z97.5
  intravascular implant (functional) (prosthetic)
    NEC Z95.9
    coronary artery Z95.5
    defibrillator (with synchronous cardiac
      pacemaker) Z95.810
    peripheral vessel (with angioplasty) Z95.820
  joint implant (prosthetic) (any) Z96.60
    ankle —*see* Presence, ankle joint implant
    elbow —*see* Presence, elbow joint implant
    finger —*see* Presence, finger joint implant
    hip —*see* Presence, hip joint implant
    knee —*see* Presence, knee joint implant
    shoulder —*see* Presence, shoulder joint
      implant
    specified joint NEC Z96.698
    wrist —*see* Presence, wrist joint implant
  knee-joint implant (functional) (prosthesis)
    Z96.65-●
  laryngeal implant (functional) Z96.3
  mandibular implant (dental) Z96.5

Presence *(Continued)*
  myringotomy tube(s) Z96.22
  neurostimulator (brain) (gastric) (peripheral
    nerve) (sacral nerve) (spinal cord) (vagus
    nerve) Z96.82
  orthopedic-joint implant (prosthetic) (any) —
    see Presence, joint implant
  otological implant (functional) Z96.29
  shoulder-joint implant (functional)
    (prosthesis) Z96.61-●
  skull-plate implant Z96.7
  spectacles Z97.3
  stapes implant (functional) Z96.29
  systemic lupus erythematosus [SLE] inhibitor
    D68.62
  tendon implant (functional) (graft) Z96.7
  tooth root(s) implant Z96.5
  ureteral stent Z96.0
  urethral stent Z96.0
  urogenital implant (functional) Z96.0
  vascular implant or device Z95.9
    access port device Z95.828
    specified type NEC Z95.828
  wrist-joint implant (functional) (prosthesis)
    Z96.63-●
Presenile —*see also* condition
  dementia F03
  premature aging E34.8
Presentation, fetal —*see* Delivery, complicated
  by, malposition
Prespondylolisthesis (congenital) Q76.2
Pressure
  area, skin —*see* Ulcer, pressure, by site
  brachial plexus G54.0
  brain G93.5
    injury at birth NEC P11.1
  cerebral —*see* Pressure, brain
  chest R07.89
  cone, tentorial G93.5
  hyposystolic —*see also* Hypotension
    incidental reading, without diagnosis of
      hypotension R03.1
  increased
    intracranial, benign G93.2
      injury at birth P11.0
    intraocular H40.05-●
  injury —*see* Ulcer, pressure, by site
  lumbosacral plexus G54.1
  mediastinum J98.59
  necrosis (chronic) —*see* Ulcer, pressure,
    by site
  parental, inappropriate (excessive) Z62.6
  sore (chronic) —*see* Ulcer, pressure, by site
  spinal cord G95.20
  ulcer (chronic) —*see* Ulcer, pressure, by site
  venous, increased I87.8
Pre-syncope R55
Preterm
  delivery (*see also* Pregnancy, complicated by,
    preterm labor) O60.10
  labor —*see* Pregnancy, complicated by,
    preterm labor
  newborn (infant) P07.30
    gestational age
      28 completed weeks (28 weeks, 0 days
        through 28 weeks, 6 days) P07.31
      29 completed weeks (29 weeks, 0 days
        through 29 weeks, 6 days) P07.32
      30 completed weeks (30 weeks, 0 days
        through 30 weeks, 6 days) P07.33
      31 completed weeks (31 weeks, 0 days
        through 31 weeks, 6 days) P07.34
      32 completed weeks (32 weeks, 0 days
        through 32 weeks, 6 days) P07.35
      33 completed weeks (33 weeks, 0 days
        through 33 weeks, 6 days) P07.36
      34 completed weeks (34 weeks, 0 days
        through 34 weeks, 6 days) P07.37
      35 completed weeks (35 weeks, 0 days
        through 35 weeks, 6 days) P07.38
      36 completed weeks (36 weeks, 0 days
        through 36 weeks, 6 days) P07.39

Previa
  placenta (total) (without hemorrhage)
    O44.0-●
    with hemorrhage O44.1-●
    complete O44.0-●
      with hemorrhage O44.1-●
    low —*see also* Delivery, complicated, by,
      placenta, low O44.4-●
      with hemorrhage O44.5-●
    marginal O44.2-●
      with hemorrhage O44.3-●
    partial O44.2-●
      with hemorrhage O44.3-●
  vasa O69.4
Priapism N48.30
  due to
    disease classified elsewhere N48.32
    drug N48.33
    specified cause NEC N48.39
    trauma N48.31
Prickling sensation (skin) R20.2
Prickly heat L74.0
Primary —*see* condition
Primigravida
  elderly, affecting management of pregnancy,
    labor and delivery (supervision only) —
    see Pregnancy, complicated by, elderly,
    primigravida
  older, affecting management of pregnancy,
    labor and delivery (supervision only) —
    see Pregnancy, complicated by, elderly,
    primigravida
  very young, affecting management
    of pregnancy, labor and delivery
    (supervision only) —*see* Pregnancy,
    complicated by, young mother,
    primigravida
Primipara
  elderly, affecting management of pregnancy,
    labor and delivery (supervision only) —
    see Pregnancy, complicated by, elderly,
    primigravida
  older, affecting management of pregnancy,
    labor and delivery (supervision only) —
    see Pregnancy, complicated by, elderly,
    primigravida
  very young, affecting management
    of pregnancy, labor and delivery
    (supervision only) —*see* Pregnancy,
    complicated by, young mother,
    primigravida
Primus varus (bilateral) Q66.21-●
PRIND (Prolonged reversible ischemic
  neurologic deficit) I63.9
Pringle's disease (tuberous sclerosis) Q85.1
Prinzmetal angina I20.1
Prizefighter ear —*see* Cauliflower ear
Problem (with) (related to)
  academic Z55.8
  acculturation Z60.3
  adjustment (to)
    change of job Z56.1
    life-cycle transition Z60.0
    pension Z60.0
    retirement Z60.0
  adopted child Z62.821
  alcoholism in family Z63.72
  ➡ bankruptcy Z59.89
  behavioral (adult) F69
    drug seeking Z76.5
  birth of sibling affecting child Z62.898
  care (of)
    provider dependency Z74.9
      specified NEC Z74.8
    sick or handicapped person in family or
      household Z63.6
  child
    abuse (affecting the child) —*see*
      Maltreatment, child
    custody or support proceedings Z65.3

Problem *(Continued)*
  child *(Continued)*
    in care of non-parental family member
      Z62.21
    in foster care Z62.21
    in welfare custody Z62.21
    living in orphanage or group home Z62.22
  child-rearing Z62.9
    specified NEC Z62.898
  communication (developmental) F80.9
  conflict or discord (with)
    boss Z56.4
    classmates Z55.4
    counselor Z64.4
    employer Z56.4
    family Z63.9
      specified NEC Z63.8
    probation officer Z64.4
    social worker Z64.4
    teachers Z55.4
    workmates Z56.4
  conviction in legal proceedings Z65.0
    with imprisonment Z65.1
  counselor Z64.4
  ➡ creditors Z59.89
  digestive K92.9
  drug addict in family Z63.72
  ear —*see* Disorder, ear
  economic Z59.9
    affecting care Z59.9
    ➡ specified NEC Z59.89
  education Z55.9
    specified NEC Z55.8
  employment Z56.9
    change of job Z56.1
    discord Z56.4
    environment Z56.5
    sexual harassment Z56.81
    specified NEC Z56.89
    stress NEC Z56.6
    stressful schedule Z56.3
    threat of job loss Z56.2
    unemployment Z56.0
  enuresis, child F98.0
  eye H57.9
  failed examinations (school) Z55.2
  falling Z91.81
  family —*see also* Disruption, family Z63.9-●
    specified NEC Z63.8
  ➡ feeding (elderly) (infant) R63.39
    newborn P92.9
      breast P92.5
      overfeeding P92.4
      slow P92.2
      specified NEC P92.8
      underfeeding P92.3
    nonorganic F50.89
  finance Z59.9
    ➡ specified NEC Z59.89
  ➡ foreclosure on loan Z59.89
  foster child Z62.822
  frightening experience(s) in childhood
    Z62.898
  genital NEC
    female N94.9
    male N50.9
  health care Z75.9
    specified NEC Z75.8
  hearing —*see* Deafness
  ➡ homelessness Z59.00
  housing Z59.9
    inadequate Z59.1
    ➡ isolated Z59.89
    ➡ specified NEC Z59.89
  identity (of childhood) F93.8
  illegitimate pregnancy (unwanted) Z64.0
  illiteracy Z55.0
  impaired mobility Z74.09
  imprisonment or incarceration Z65.1
  inadequate teaching affecting education
    Z55.8

▶ New   ➡ Revised   ~~deleted~~ Deleted   ● Use Additional Character(s)

Problem *(Continued)*
inappropriate (excessive) parental pressure Z62.6
influencing health status NEC Z78.9
in-law Z63.1
institutionalization, affecting child Z62.22
intrafamilial communication Z63.8
jealousy, child F93.8
landlord Z59.2
language (developmental) F80.9
learning (developmental) F81.9
legal Z65.3
  conviction without imprisonment Z65.0
  imprisonment Z65.1
  release from prison Z65.2
life-management Z73.9
  specified NEC Z73.89
life-style Z72.9
  gambling Z72.6
  high-risk sexual behavior (heterosexual) Z72.51
    bisexual Z72.53
    homosexual Z72.52
  inappropriate eating habits Z72.4
  self-damaging behavior NEC Z72.89
  specified NEC Z72.89
  tobacco use Z72.0
literacy Z55.9
  low level Z55.0
  specified NEC Z55.8
living alone Z60.2
lodgers Z59.2
loss of love relationship in childhood Z62.898
marital Z63.0
  involving
    divorce Z63.5
    estrangement Z63.5
    gender identity F66
mastication K08.89
medical
  care, within family Z63.6
  facilities Z75.9
    specified NEC Z75.8
mental F48.9
multiparity Z64.1
negative life events in childhood Z62.9
  altered pattern of family relationships Z62.898
  frightening experience Z62.898
  loss of
    love relationship Z62.898
    self-esteem Z62.898
  physical abuse (alleged) —*see* Maltreatment, child
  removal from home Z62.29
  specified event NEC Z62.898
neighbor Z59.2
neurological NEC R29.818
new step-parent affecting child Z62.898
none (feared complaint unfounded) Z71.1
occupational NEC Z56.89
parent-child —*see* Conflict, parent-child
personal hygiene Z91.89
personality F69
phase of life transition, adjustment Z60.0
presence of sick or disabled person in family or household Z63.79
  needing care Z63.6
primary support group (family) Z63.9
  specified NEC Z63.8
probation officer Z64.4
psychiatric F99
psychosexual (development) F66
psychosocial Z65.9
  religious or spiritual Z65.8
  specified NEC Z65.8
relationship Z63.9
  childhood F93.8
release from prison Z65.2
  religious or spiritual Z65.8

Problem *(Continued)*
removal from home affecting child Z62.29
seeking and accepting known hazardous and harmful
  behavioral or psychological interventions Z65.8
  chemical, nutritional or physical interventions Z65.8
sexual function (nonorganic) F52.9
sight H54.7
sleep disorder, child F51.9
smell —*see* Disturbance, sensation, smell
social
  environment Z60.9
    specified NEC Z60.8
  exclusion and rejection Z60.4
  worker Z64.4
speech R47.9
  developmental F80.9
  specified NEC R47.89
swallowing —*see* Dysphagia
taste —*see* Disturbance, sensation, taste
tic, child F95.0
underachievement in school Z55.3
unemployment Z56.0
  threatened Z56.2
unwanted pregnancy Z64.0
upbringing Z62.9
  specified NEC Z62.898
urinary N39.9
voice production R47.89
work schedule (stressful) Z56.3
Procedure (surgical)
converted
  arthroscopic to open Z53.33
  laparoscopic to open Z53.31
  specified procedure NEC to open Z53.39
  thoracoscopic to open Z53.32
for purpose other than remedying health state Z41.9
  specified NEC Z41.8
not done Z53.9
  because of
    administrative reasons Z53.8
    contraindication Z53.09
      smoking Z53.01
    patient's decision Z53.20
      for reasons of belief or group pressure Z53.1
      left against medical advice (AMA) Z53.29
    left without being seen Z53.21
    specified reason NEC Z53.29
    specified reason NEC Z53.8
Procidentia (uteri) N81.3
Proctalgia K62.89
  fugax K59.4
  spasmodic K59.4
Proctitis K62.89
  amebic (acute) A06.0
  chlamydial A56.3
  gonococcal A54.6
  granulomatous —*see* Enteritis, regional, large intestine
  herpetic A60.1
  radiation K62.7
  tuberculous A18.32
  ulcerative (chronic) K51.20
    with
      complication K51.219
        abscess K51.214
        fistula K51.213
        obstruction K51.212
        rectal bleeding K51.211
        specified NEC K51.218
Proctocele
female (without uterine prolapse) N81.6
  with uterine prolapse N81.2
    complete N81.3
male K62.3

Proctocolitis
allergic K52.29
food-induced eosinophilic K52.29
food protein-induced K52.29
milk protein-induced K52.29
mucosal —*see* Rectosigmoiditis, ulcerative
Proctoptosis K62.3
Proctorrhagia K62.5
Proctosigmoiditis K63.89
  ulcerative (chronic) —*see* Rectosigmoiditis, ulcerative
Proctospasm K59.4
  psychogenic F45.8
Profichet's disease —*see* Disorder, soft tissue, specified type NEC
Progeria E34.8
Prognathism (mandibular) (maxillary) M26.19
Progonoma (melanotic) —*see* Neoplasm, benign, by site
Progressive —*see* condition
Prolactinoma
specified site —*see* Neoplasm, benign, by site
unspecified site D35.2
Prolapse, prolapsed
anus, anal (canal) (sphincter) K62.2
arm or hand O32.2
  causing obstructed labor O64.4
bladder (mucosa) (sphincter) (acquired)
  congenital Q79.4
  female —*see* Cystocele
  male N32.89
breast implant (prosthetic) T85.49
cecostomy K94.09
cecum K63.4
cervix, cervical (hypertrophied) N81.2
  anterior lip, obstructing labor O65.5
  congenital Q51.828
  postpartal, old N81.2
  stump N81.85
ciliary body (traumatic) —*see* Laceration, eye(ball), with prolapse or loss of interocular tissue
colon (pedunculated) K63.4
colostomy K94.09
disc (intervertebral) —*see* Displacement, intervertebral disc
eye implant (orbital) T85.398
  lens (ocular) —*see* Complications, intraocular lens
fallopian tube N83.4-•
gastric (mucosa) K31.89
genital, female N81.9
  specified NEC N81.89
globe, nontraumatic —*see* Luxation, globe
ileostomy bud K94.19
intervertebral disc —*see* Displacement, intervertebral disc
intestine (small) K63.4
iris (traumatic) —*see* Laceration, eye(ball), with prolapse or loss of interocular tissue
  nontraumatic H21.89
kidney N28.83
  congenital Q63.2
laryngeal muscles or ventricle J38.7
liver K76.89
meatus urinarius N36.8
mitral (valve) I34.1
ocular lens implant —*see* Complications, intraocular lens
organ or site, congenital NEC —*see* Malposition, congenital
ovary N83.4-•
pelvic floor, female N81.89
perineum, female N81.89
rectum (mucosa) (sphincter) K62.3
  due to trichuris trichuria B79
spleen D73.89
stomach K31.89
umbilical cord
  complicating delivery O69.0

Prolapse, prolapsed (Continued)
  urachus, congenital Q64.4
  ureter N28.89
    with obstruction N13.5
      with infection N13.6
  ureterovesical orifice N28.89
  urethra (acquired) (infected) (mucosa)
      N36.8
    congenital Q64.71
  urinary meatus N36.8
    congenital Q64.72
  uterovaginal N81.4
    complete N81.3
    incomplete N81.2
  uterus (with prolapse of vagina) N81.4
    complete N81.3
    congenital Q51.818
    first degree N81.2
    in pregnancy or childbirth —see
        Pregnancy, complicated by,
        abnormal, uterus
    incomplete N81.2
    postpartal (old) N81.4
    second degree N81.2
    third degree N81.3
  uveal (traumatic) —see Laceration, eye(ball),
      with prolapse or loss of interocular
      tissue
  vagina (anterior) (wall) —see Cystocele
    with prolapse of uterus N81.4
      complete N81.3
      incomplete N81.2
    posterior wall N81.6
    posthysterectomy N99.3
  vitreous (humor) H43.0-•
    in wound —see Laceration, eye(ball),
        with prolapse or loss of interocular
        tissue
  womb —see Prolapse, uterus
Prolapsus, female N81.9
  specified NEC N81.89
Proliferation(s)
  primary cutaneous CD30-positive large T-cell
      C86.6
  prostate, atypical small acinar N42.32
Proliferative —see condition
Prolonged, prolongation (of)
  bleeding (time) (idiopathic) R79.1
  coagulation (time) R79.1
  gestation (over 42 completed weeks)
    mother O48.1
    newborn P08.22
  interval I44.0
  labor O63.9
    first stage O63.0
    second stage O63.1
  partial thromboplastin time (PTT) R79.1
  pregnancy (more than 42 weeks gestation)
      O48.1
  prothrombin time R79.1
  QT interval R94.31
  uterine contractions in labor O62.4
Prominence, prominent
  ischial spine or sacral promontory with
      disproportion (fetopelvic) O33.0
    causing obstructed labor O65.0
  auricle (congenital) (ear) Q17.5
  nose (congenital) acquired M95.0
Promiscuity —see High, risk, sexual behavior
Pronation
  ankle —see Deformity, limb, foot, specified
      NEC
  foot —see also Deformity, limb, foot, specified
      NEC
    congenital Q74.2
Prophylactic
  administration of
    antibiotics, long-term Z79.2
      short-term use - omit code

Prophylactic (Continued)
  antibiotics, long-term (Continued)
    drug —see also Long-term (current) drug
        therapy (use of) Z79.899-•
  medication Z79.899
  organ removal (for neoplasia management)
      Z40.00
    breast Z40.01
    fallopian tube(s) Z40.03
      with ovary(s) Z40.02
    ovary(s) Z40.02
    specified site NEC Z40.09
  surgery Z40.9
    for risk factors related to malignant
        neoplasm —see Prophylactic, organ
        removal
    specified NEC Z40.8
  vaccination Z23
Propionic acidemia E71.121
Proptosis (ocular) —see also Exophthalmos
  thyroid —see Hyperthyroidism, with goiter
Prosecution, anxiety concerning Z65.3
Prosopagnosia R48.3
Prostadynia N42.81
Prostate, prostatic —see condition
Prostatism —see Hyperplasia, prostate
Prostatitis (congestive) (suppurative) (with
    cystitis) N41.9
  acute N41.0
  cavitary N41.8
  chronic N41.1
  diverticular N41.8
  due to Trichomonas (vaginalis) A59.02
  fibrous N41.1
  gonococcal (acute) (chronic) A54.22
  granulomatous N41.4
  hypertrophic N41.1
  subacute N41.1
  trichomonal A59.02
  tuberculous A18.14
Prostatocystitis N41.3
Prostatorrhea N42.89
Prostatosis N42.82
Prostration R53.83
  heat —see also Heat, exhaustion
    anhydrotic T67.3
    due to
      salt (and water) depletion T67.4
      water depletion T67.3
  nervous F48.8
  senile R54
Protanomaly (anomalous trichromat) H53.54
Protanopia (complete) (incomplete) H53.54
Protection (against) (from) —see Prophylactic
Protein
  deficiency NEC —see Malnutrition
  malnutrition —see Malnutrition
  sickness —see also Reaction, serum T80.69
Proteinemia R77.9
Proteinosis
  alveolar (pulmonary) J84.01
  lipid or lipoid (of Urbach) E78.89
Proteinuria R80.9
  Bence Jones R80.3
  complicating pregnancy —see Proteinuria,
      gestational
  gestational
    complicating
      childbirth O12.14
      pregnancy O12.1-•
        with edema O12.2-•
      puerperium O12.15
  idiopathic R80.0
  isolated R80.0
    with glomerular lesion N06.9
      C3
        glomerulonephritis N06.A
        glomerulopathy N06.A
          with dense deposit disease
              N06.6
      dense deposit disease N06.6

Proteinuria (Continued)
  isolated (Continued)
    with glomerular lesion (Continued)
      diffuse
        crescentic glomerulonephritis N06.7
        endocapillary proliferative
            glomerulonephritis N06.4
        mesangiocapillary glomerulonephritis
            N06.5
      focal and segmental hyalinosis or
          sclerosis N06.1
      membranous (diffuse) N06.2
      mesangial proliferative (diffuse) N06.3
      minimal change N06.0
      specified pathology NEC N06.8
  orthostatic R80.2
    with glomerular lesion —see Proteinuria,
        isolated, with glomerular lesion
  persistent R80.1
    with glomerular lesion —see Proteinuria,
        isolated, with glomerular lesion
  postural R80.2
    with glomerular lesion —see Proteinuria,
        isolated, with glomerular lesion
  pre-eclamptic —see Pre-eclampsia
  puerperal O12.15
  specified type NEC R80.8
Proteolysis, pathologic D65
Proteus (mirabilis) (morganii), as cause of
    disease classified elsewhere B96.4
Prothrombin gene mutation D68.52
Protoporphyria, erythropoietic E80.0
Protozoal —see also condition
  disease B64
    specified NEC B60.8
Protrusion, protrusio
  acetabuli M24.7
  acetabulum (into pelvis) M24.7
  device, implant or graft —see also
      Complications, by site and type,
      mechanical T85.698
    arterial graft NEC —see Complication,
        cardiovascular device, mechanical,
        vascular
    breast (implant) T85.49
    catheter NEC T85.698
      cystostomy T83.090
      dialysis (renal) T82.49
        intraperitoneal T85.691
      infusion NEC T82.594
        spinal (epidural) (subdural) T85.690
      urinary —see also Complications,
          catheter, urinary T83.098
    electronic (electrode) (pulse generator)
        (stimulator)
      bone T84.390
      nervous system —see Complication,
          prosthetic device, mechanical,
          electronic nervous system
          stimulator
    fixation, internal (orthopedic) NEC —
        see Complication, fixation device,
        mechanical
    gastrointestinal —see Complications,
        prosthetic device, mechanical,
        gastrointestinal device
    genital NEC T83.498
      intrauterine contraceptive device T83.39
      penile prosthesis (cylinder) (implanted)
          (pump) (reservoir) T83.490
      testicular prosthesis T83.491
    heart NEC —see Complication,
        cardiovascular device, mechanical
    joint prosthesis —see Complications, joint
        prosthesis, mechanical, specified NEC,
        by site
    ocular NEC —see Complications, prosthetic
        device, mechanical, ocular device
    orthopedic NEC —see Complication,
        orthopedic, device, mechanical
    specified NEC T85.628

▶ New   ⇒ Revised   ~~deleted~~ Deleted   • Use Additional Character(s)

Protrusion, protrusio (Continued)
  device, implant or graft (Continued)
    urinary NEC —see also Complication,
      genitourinary, device, urinary,
      mechanical
      graft T83.29
    vascular NEC —see Complication,
      cardiovascular device, mechanical
    ventricular intracranial shunt T85.09
    intervertebral disc —see Displacement,
      intervertebral disc
    joint prosthesis —see Complications, joint
      prosthesis, mechanical, specified NEC,
      by site
    nucleus pulposus —see Displacement,
      intervertebral disc
Prune belly (syndrome) Q79.4
Prurigo (ferox) (gravis) (Hebrae) (Hebra's)
  (mitis) (simplex) L28.2
  Besnier's L20.0
  estivalis L56.4
  nodularis L28.1
  psychogenic F45.8
Pruritus, pruritic (essential) L29.9
  ani, anus L29.0
    psychogenic F45.8
  anogenital L29.3
    psychogenic F45.8
  due to onchocerca volvulus B73.1
  gravidarum —see Pregnancy, complicated by,
    specified pregnancy-related condition
    NEC
  hiemalis L29.8
  neurogenic (any site) F45.8
  perianal L29.0
  psychogenic (any site) F45.8
  scroti, scrotum L29.1
    psychogenic F45.8
  senile, senilis L29.8
  specified NEC L29.8
    psychogenic F45.8
  Trichomonas A59.9
  vulva, vulvae L29.2
    psychogenic F45.8
Pseudarthrosis, pseudoarthrosis (bone) —see
  Nonunion, fracture
  clavicle, congenital Q74.0
  joint, following fusion or arthrodesis M96.0
Pseudoaneurysm —see Aneurysm
Pseudoangina (pectoris) —see Angina
Pseudoangioma I81
Pseudoarteriosus Q28.8
Pseudoarthrosis —see Pseudarthrosis
Pseudobulbar affect (PBA) F48.2
Pseudochromhidrosis L67.8
Pseudocirrhosis, liver, pericardial I31.1
Pseudocowpox B08.03
Pseudocoxalgia M91.3-●
Pseudocroup J38.5
Pseudo-Cushing's syndrome, alcohol-induced
  E24.4
Pseudocyesis F45.8
Pseudocyst
  lung J98.4
  pancreas K86.3
  retina —see Cyst, retina
Pseudoelephantiasis neuroarthritica Q82.0
Pseudoexfoliation, capsule (lens) —see
  Cataract, specified NEC
Pseudofolliculitis barbae L73.1
Pseudoglioma H44.89
Pseudohemophilia (Bernuth's) (hereditary)
  (type B) D68.0
  Type A D69.8
  vascular D69.8
Pseudohermaphroditism Q56.3
  adrenal E25.8
  female Q56.2
    with adrenocortical disorder E25.8
    without adrenocortical disorder
      Q56.2

Pseudohermaphroditism (Continued)
  female (Continued)
    adrenal (congenital) E25.0
    unspecified E25.9
  male Q56.1
    with
      adrenocortical disorder E25.8
      androgen resistance E34.51
      cleft scrotum Q56.1
      feminizing testis E34.51
      5-alpha-reductase deficiency E29.1
    without gonadal disorder Q56.1
    adrenal E25.8
    unspecified E25.9
Pseudo-Hurler's polydystrophy E77.0
Pseudohydrocephalus G93.2
Pseudohypertrophic muscular dystrophy
  (Erb's) G71.02
Pseudohypertrophy, muscle G71.09
Pseudohypoparathyroidism E20.1
Pseudoinsomnia F51.03
Pseudoleukemia, infantile D64.89
Pseudomembranous —see condition
Pseudomeningocele (cerebral) (infective) (post-
  traumatic) G96.198
  postprocedural (spinal) G97.82
Pseudomenses (newborn) P54.6
Pseudomenstruation (newborn) P54.6
Pseudomonas
  aeruginosa, as cause of disease classified
    elsewhere B96.5
  mallei infection A24.0
    as cause of disease classified elsewhere
      B96.5
  pseudomallei, as cause of disease classified
    elsewhere B96.5
Pseudomyotonia G71.19
Pseudomyxoma peritonei C78.6
Pseudoneuritis, optic (nerve) (disc) (papilla),
  congenital Q14.2
Pseudo-obstruction intestine (acute) (chronic)
  (idiopathic) (intermittent secondary)
  (primary) K59.89
  colonic K59.81
Pseudopapilledema H47.33-●
  congenital Q14.2
Pseudoparalysis
  arm or leg R29.818
  atonic, congenital P94.2
Pseudopelade L66.0
Pseudophakia Z96.1
Pseudopolyarthritis, rhizomelic M35.3
Pseudopolycythemia D75.1
Pseudopseudohypoparathyroidism E20.1
Pseudopterygium H11.81-●
Pseudoptosis (eyelid) —see Blepharochalasis
Pseudopuberty, precocious
  female heterosexual E25.8
  male isosexual E25.8
Pseudorickets (renal) N25.0
Pseudorubella B08.20
Pseudosclerema, newborn P83.88
Pseudosclerosis (brain)
  Jakob's —see Creutzfeldt-Jakob disease or
    syndrome
  of Westphal (Strümpell) E83.01
  spastic —see Creutzfeldt-Jakob disease or
    syndrome
Pseudotetanus —see Convulsions
Pseudotetany R29.0
  hysterical F44.5
Pseudotruncus arteriosus Q25.49
Pseudotuberculosis A28.2
  enterocolitis A04.8
  pasteurella (infection) A28.0
Pseudotumor G93.2
  cerebri G93.2
  orbital H05.11-●
Pseudoxanthoma elasticum Q82.8
Psilosis (sprue) (tropical) K90.1
  nontropical K90.0

Psittacosis A70
Psoitis M60.88
Psoriasis L40.9
  arthropathic L40.50
    arthritis mutilans L40.52
    distal interphalangeal L40.51
    juvenile L40.54
    other specified L40.59
    spondylitis L40.53
  buccal K13.29
  flexural L40.8
  guttate L40.4
  mouth K13.29
  nummular L40.0
  plaque L40.0
  psychogenic F54
  pustular (generalized) L40.1
    palmaris et plantaris L40.3
  specified NEC L40.8
  vulgaris L40.0
Psychasthenia F48.8
Psychiatric disorder or problem F99
Psychogenic —see also condition
  factors associated with physical conditions
    F54
Psychological and behavioral factors affecting
  medical condition F59
Psychoneurosis, psychoneurotic —see also
  Neurosis
  anxiety (state) F41.1
  depersonalization F48.1
  hypochondriacal F45.21
  hysteria F44.9
  neurasthenic F48.8
  personality NEC F60.89
Psychopathy, psychopathic
  affectionless F94.2
  autistic F84.5
  constitution, post traumatic F07.81
  personality —see Disorder, personality
  sexual —see Deviation, sexual
  state F60.2
Psychosexual identity disorder of childhood
  F64.2
Psychosis, psychotic F29
  acute (transient) F23
    hysterical F44.9
  affective —see Disorder, mood
  alcoholic F10.959
    with
      abuse F10.159
      anxiety disorder F10.980
        with
          abuse F10.180
          dependence F10.280
      delirium tremens F10.231
      delusions F10.950
        with
          abuse F10.150
          dependence F10.250
      dementia F10.97
        with dependence F10.27
      dependence F10.259
      hallucinosis F10.951
        with
          abuse F10.151
          dependence F10.251
      mood disorder F10.94
        with
          abuse F10.14
          dependence F10.24
      paranoia F10.950
        with
          abuse F10.150
          dependence F10.250
      persisting amnesia F10.96
        with dependence F10.26
    amnestic confabulatory F10.96
      with dependence F10.26
    delirium tremens F10.231
    Korsakoff's, Korsakov's, Korsakow's F10.26

Psychosis, psychotic (Continued)
  alcoholic (Continued)
    paranoid type F10.950
      with
        abuse F10.150
        dependence F10.250
  anergastic —see Psychosis, organic
  arteriosclerotic (simple type) (uncomplicated)
    F01.50
    with behavioral disturbance F01.51
  childhood F84.0
    atypical F84.8
  climacteric —see Psychosis, involutional
  confusional F29
    acute or subacute F05
    reactive F23
  cycloid F23
  depressive —see Disorder, depressive
  disintegrative (childhood) F84.3
  drug-induced —see F11-F19 with .x59
    paranoid and hallucinatory states —see
      F11-F19 with .x50 or .x51
  due to or associated with
    addiction, drug —see F11-F19 with .X59
    dependence
      alcohol F10.259
      drug —see F11-F19 with .x59
    epilepsy F06.8
    Huntington's chorea F06.8
    ischemia, cerebrovascular (generalized)
      F06.8
    multiple sclerosis F06.8
    physical disease F06.8
    presenile dementia F03
    senile dementia F03
    vascular disease (arteriosclerotic) (cerebral)
      F01.50
      with behavioral disturbance F01.51
  epileptic F06.8
  episode F23
    due to or associated with physical
      condition F06.8
  exhaustive F43.0
  hallucinatory, chronic F28
  hypomanic F30.8
  hysterical (acute) F44.9
  induced F24
  infantile F84.0
    atypical F84.8
  infective (acute) (subacute) F05
  involutional F28
    depressive —see Disorder, depressive
    melancholic —see Disorder, depressive
    paranoid (state) F22
  Korsakoff's, Korsakov's, Korsakow's
    (nonalcoholic) F04
    alcoholic F10.96
      in dependence F10.26
    induced by other psychoactive
      substance —see categories F11-F19
      with .x5x
  mania, manic (single episode) F30.2
    recurrent type F31.89
  manic-depressive —see Disorder, bipolar
  menopausal —see Psychosis, involutional
  mixed schizophrenic and affective F25.8
  multi-infarct (cerebrovascular) F01.50
    with behavioral disturbance F01.51
  nonorganic F29
    specified NEC F28
  organic F09
    due to or associated with
      arteriosclerosis (cerebral) —see
        Psychosis, arteriosclerotic
      cerebrovascular disease,
        arteriosclerotic —see Psychosis,
        arteriosclerotic
      childbirth —see Psychosis, puerperal
      Creutzfeldt-Jakob disease or
        syndrome —see Creutzfeldt-Jakob
        disease or syndrome

Psychosis, psychotic (Continued)
  organic (Continued)
    due to or associated with (Continued)
      dependence, alcohol F10.259
      disease
        alcoholic liver F10.259
        brain, arteriosclerotic —see Psychosis,
          arteriosclerotic
        cerebrovascular F01.50
          with behavioral disturbance
            F01.51
        Creutzfeldt-Jakob —see Creutzfeldt-
          Jakob disease or syndrome
        endocrine or metabolic F06.8
          acute or subacute F05
        liver, alcoholic F10.259
      epilepsy transient (acute) F05
      infection
        brain (intracranial) F06.8
          acute or subacute F05
      intoxication
        alcoholic (acute) F10.259
        drug F11-F19 with .x59
      ischemia, cerebrovascular
        (generalized) —see Psychosis,
        arteriosclerotic
      puerperium —see Psychosis, puerperal
      trauma, brain (birth) (from electric
        current) (surgical) F06.8
        acute or subacute F05
    infective F06.8
      acute or subacute F05
    post-traumatic F06.8
      acute or subacute F05
  paranoiac F22
  paranoid (climacteric) (involutional)
    (menopausal) F22
    psychogenic (acute) F23
    schizophrenic F20.0
    senile F03
  postpartum F53.1
  presbyophrenic (type) F03
  presenile F03
  psychogenic (paranoid) F23
    depressive F32.3
  puerperal F53.1
    specified type —see Psychosis, by type
  reactive (brief) (transient) (emotional stress)
    (psychological trauma) F23
    depressive F32.3
      recurrent F33.3
    excitative type F30.8
  schizoaffective F25.9
    depressive type F25.1
    manic type F25.0
  schizophrenia, schizophrenic —see
    Schizophrenia
  schizophrenia-like, in epilepsy F06.2
  schizophreniform F20.81
    affective type F25.9
    brief F23
    confusional type F23
    mixed type F25.0
  senile NEC F03
    depressed or paranoid type F03
    simple deterioration F03
    specified type — code to condition
  shared F24
  situational (reactive) F23
  symbiotic (childhood) F84.3
  symptomatic F09
Psychosomatic —see Disorder,
  psychosomatic
Psychosyndrome, organic F07.9
Psychotic episode due to or associated with
  physical condition F06.8
Pterygium (eye) H11.00-●
  amyloid H11.01-●
  central H11.02-●
  colli Q18.3
  double H11.03-●

Psychosis, psychotic (Continued)
  peripheral
    progressive H11.05-●
    stationary H11.04-●
  recurrent H11.06-●
Ptilosis (eyelid) —see Madarosis
Ptomaine (poisoning) —see Poisoning, food
Ptosis —see also Blepharoptosis
  adiposa (false) —see Blepharoptosis
  breast N64.81
  brow H57.81-●
  cecum K63.4
  colon K63.4
  congenital (eyelid) Q10.0
    specified site NEC —see Anomaly, by site
  eyebrow H57.81-●
  eyelid —see Blepharoptosis
    congenital Q10.0
  gastric K31.89
  intestine K63.4
  kidney N28.83
  liver K76.89
  renal N28.83
  splanchnic K63.4
  spleen D73.89
  stomach K31.89
  viscera K63.4
PTP D69.51
Ptyalism (periodic) K11.7
  hysterical F45.8
  pregnancy —see Pregnancy, complicated by,
    specified pregnancy-related condition
    NEC
  psychogenic F45.8
Ptyalolithiasis K11.5
Pubarche, precocious E30.1
Pubertas praecox E30.1
Puberty (development state) Z00.3
  bleeding (excessive) N92.2
  delayed E30.0
  precocious (constitutional) (cryptogenic)
    (idiopathic) E30.1
    central E22.8
    due to
      ovarian hyperfunction E28.1
        estrogen E28.0
      testicular hyperfunction E29.0
    premature E30.1
    due to
      adrenal cortical hyperfunction E25.8
      pineal tumor E34.8
      pituitary (anterior) hyperfunction E22.8
Puckering, macula —see Degeneration, macula,
  puckering
Pudenda, pudendum —see condition
Puente's disease (simple glandular cheilitis)
  K13.0
Puerperal, puerperium (complicated by,
  complications)
  abnormal glucose (tolerance test) O99.815
  abscess
    areola O91.02
      associated with lactation O91.03
    Bartholin's gland O86.19
    breast O91.12
      associated with lactation O91.13
    cervix (uteri) O86.11
    genital organ NEC O86.19
    kidney O86.21
    mammary O91.12
      associated with lactation O91.13
    nipple O91.02
      associated with lactation O91.03
    peritoneum O85
    subareolar O91.12
      associated with lactation O91.13
    urinary tract —see Puerperal, infection,
      urinary
    uterus O86.12
    vagina (wall) O86.13
    vaginorectal O86.13
    vulvovaginal gland O86.13

▶ New   ⇒ Revised   ~~deleted~~ Deleted   ● Use Additional Character(s)

Puerperal, puerperium (Continued)
adnexitis O86.19
afibrinogenemia, or other coagulation defect
   O72.3
albuminuria (acute) (subacute) —see
   Proteinuria, gestational
alcohol use O99.315
anemia O90.81
   pre-existing (pre-pregnancy) O99.03
anesthetic death O89.8
apoplexy O99.43
bariatric surgery status O99.845
blood disorder NEC O99.13
blood dyscrasia O72.3
cardiomyopathy O90.3
cerebrovascular disorder (conditions in
   I60-I69) O99.43
cervicitis O86.11
circulatory system disorder O99.43
coagulopathy (any) O99.13
   with hemorrhage O72.3
complications O90.9
   specified NEC O90.89
convulsions —see Eclampsia
cystitis O86.22
cystopyelitis O86.29
delirium NEC F05
diabetes O24.93
   gestational —see Puerperal, gestational
      diabetes
   pre-existing O24.33
      specified NEC O24.83
      type 1 O24.03
      type 2 O24.13
digestive system disorder O99.63
disease O90.9
   breast NEC O92.29
   cerebrovascular (acute) O99.43
   nonobstetric NEC O99.893
   tubo-ovarian O86.19
   Valsuani's O99.03
disorder O90.9
   biliary tract O26.63
   lactation O92.70
   liver O26.63
   nonobstetric NEC O99.893
disruption
   cesarean wound O90.0
   episiotomy wound O90.1
   perineal laceration wound O90.1
drug use O99.325
eclampsia (with pre-existing hypertension)
   O15.2
embolism (pulmonary) (blood clot) —see
   Embolism, obstetric, puerperal
endocrine, nutritional or metabolic disease
   NEC O99.285
endophlebitis —see Puerperal, phlebitis
endotrachelitis O86.11
failure
   lactation (complete) O92.3
      partial O92.4
   renal, acute O90.4
fever (of unknown origin) O86.4
   septic O85
fissure, nipple O92.12
   associated with lactation O92.13
fistula
   breast (due to mastitis) O91.12
      associated with lactation O91.13
   nipple O91.02
      associated with lactation O91.03
galactophoritis O91.22
   associated with lactation O91.23
galactorrhea O92.6
gastric banding status O99.845
gastric bypass status O99.845
gastrointestinal disease NEC O99.63
gestational
   diabetes O24.439
      diet controlled O24.430
      insulin (and diet) controlled O24.434

Puerperal, puerperium (Continued)
gestational (Continued)
   diabetes (Continued)
      oral drug controlled (antidiabetic)
         (hypoglycemic) O24.435
   edema O12.05
      with proteinuria O12.25
   proteinuria O12.15
gonorrhea O98.23
hematoma, subdural O99.43
hemiplegia, cerebral O99.355-●
   due to cerebrovascular disorder O99.43
hemorrhage O72.1
   brain O99.43
   bulbar O99.43
   cerebellar O99.43
   cerebral O99.43
   cortical O99.43
   delayed or secondary O72.2
   extradural O99.43
   internal capsule O99.43
   intracranial O99.43
   intrapontine O99.43
   meningeal O99.43
   pontine O99.43
   retained placenta O72.0
   subarachnoid O99.43
   subcortical O99.43
   subdural O99.43
   third stage O72.0
   uterine, delayed O72.2
   ventricular O99.43
hemorrhoids O87.2
hepatorenal syndrome O90.4
hypertension —see Hypertension,
   complicating, puerperium
hypertrophy, breast O92.29
induration breast (fibrous) O92.29
infection O86.4
   cervix O86.11
   generalized O85
   genital tract NEC O86.19
      obstetric surgical wound O86.09
   kidney (bacillus coli) O86.21
   maternal O98.93
      carrier state NEC O99.835
      gonorrhea O98.23
      human immunodeficiency virus (HIV)
         O98.73
      protozoal O98.63
      sexually transmitted NEC O98.33
      specified NEC O98.83
      streptococcus group B (GBS) carrier state
         O99.825
      syphilis O98.13
      tuberculosis O98.03
      viral hepatitis O98.43
      viral NEC O98.53
   nipple O91.02
      associated with lactation O91.03
   peritoneum O85
   renal O86.21
   specified NEC O86.89
   urinary (asymptomatic) (tract) NEC O86.20
      bladder O86.22
      kidney O86.21
      specified site NEC O86.29
      urethra O86.22
   vagina O86.13
   vein —see Puerperal, phlebitis
ischemia, cerebral O99.43
lymphangitis O86.89
   breast O91.22
      associated with lactation O91.23
malignancy O9A.13
malnutrition O25.3
mammillitis O91.02
   associated with lactation O91.03
mammitis O91.22
   associated with lactation O91.23
mania F30.8

Puerperal, puerperium (Continued)
mastitis O91.22
   associated with lactation O91.23
   purulent O91.12
      associated with lactation O91.13
melancholia —see Disorder, depressive
mental disorder NEC O99.345
metroperitonitis O85
metrorrhagia —see Hemorrhage,
   postpartum
metrosalpingitis O86.19
metrovaginitis O86.13
milk leg O87.1
monoplegia, cerebral O99.43
mood disturbance O90.6
necrosis, liver (acute) (subacute)
   (conditions in subcategory K72.0) O26.63
   with renal failure O90.4
nervous system disorder O99.355
neuritis O90.89
obesity (pre-existing prior to pregnancy)
   O99.215
obesity surgery status O99.845
occlusion, precerebral artery O99.43
paralysis
   bladder (sphincter) O90.89
   cerebral O99.43
paralytic stroke O99.43
parametritis O85
paravaginitis O86.13
pelviperitonitis O85
perimetritis O86.12
perimetrosalpingitis O86.19
perinephritis O86.21
periphlebitis —see Puerperal phlebitis
peritoneal infection O85
peritonitis (pelvic) O85
perivaginitis O86.13
phlebitis O87.0
   deep O87.1
   pelvic O87.1
   superficial O87.0
phlebothrombosis, deep O87.1
phlegmasia alba dolens O87.1
placental polyp O90.89
pneumonia, embolic —see Embolism,
   obstetric, puerperal
pre-eclampsia —see Pre-eclampsia
psychosis F53.1
pyelitis O86.21
pyelocystitis O86.29
pyelonephritis O86.21
pyelonephrosis O86.21
pyemia O85
pyocystitis O86.29
pyohemia O85
pyometra O86.12
pyonephritis O86.21
pyosalpingitis O86.19
pyrexia (of unknown origin) O86.4
renal
   disease NEC O90.89
   failure O90.4
respiratory disease NEC O99.53
retention
   decidua —see Retention, decidua
   placenta O72.0
   secundines —see Retention,
      secundines
retracted nipple O92.02
salpingo-ovaritis O86.19
salpingoperitonitis O85
secondary perineal tear O90.1
sepsis O85
sepsis (pelvic) O85
septic thrombophlebitis O86.81
skin disorder NEC O99.73
specified condition NEC O99.893
stroke O99.43
subinvolution (uterus) O90.89
subluxation of symphysis (pubis) O26.73

Puerperal, puerperium *(Continued)*
  suppuration —*see* Puerperal, abscess
  tetanus A34
  thelitis O91.02
    associated with lactation O91.03
  thrombocytopenia O72.3
  thrombophlebitis (superficial) O87.0
    deep O87.1
    pelvic O87.1
    septic O86.81
  thrombosis (venous) —*see* Thrombosis,
    puerperal
  thyroiditis O90.5
  toxemia (eclamptic) (pre-eclamptic)
    (with convulsions) O15.2
  trauma, non-obstetric O9A.23
    caused by abuse (physical) (suspected)
      O9A.33
      confirmed O9A.33
      psychological (suspected) O9A.53
        confirmed O9A.53
      sexual (suspected) O9A.43
        confirmed O9A.43
  uremia (due to renal failure) O90.4
  urethritis O86.22
  vaginitis O86.13
  varicose veins (legs) O87.4
    vulva or perineum O87.8
  venous O87.9
  vulvitis O86.19
  vulvovaginitis O86.13
  white leg O87.1
Puerperium —*see* Puerperal
Pulmolithiasis J98.4
Pulmonary —*see* condition
Pulpitis (acute) (anachoretic) (chronic)
    (hyperplastic) (putrescent) (suppurative)
    (ulcerative) K04.01
  irreversible K04.02
  reversible K04.01
Pulpless tooth K04.99
Pulse
  alternating R00.8
  bigeminal R00.8
  fast R00.0
  feeble, rapid due to shock following injury
    T79.4
  rapid R00.0
  weak R09.89
Pulsus alternans or trigeminus R00.8
Punch drunk F07.81
Punctum lacrimale occlusion —*see* Obstruction,
    lacrimal
Puncture
  abdomen, abdominal
    wall S31.139
      with
        foreign body S31.149
        penetration into peritoneal cavity
          S31.639
          with foreign body S31.649
      epigastric region S31.132
        with
          foreign body S31.142
          penetration into peritoneal cavity
            S31.632
            with foreign body S31.642
      left
        lower quadrant S31.134
          with
            foreign body S31.144
            penetration into peritoneal cavity
              S31.634
              with foreign body S31.644
        upper quadrant S31.131
          with
            foreign body S31.141
            penetration into peritoneal cavity
              S31.631
              with foreign body S31.641

Puncture *(Continued)*
  abdomen, abdominal *(Continued)*
    wall *(Continued)*
      periumbilic region S31.135
        with
          foreign body S31.145
          penetration into peritoneal cavity
            S31.635
            with foreign body S31.645
      right
        lower quadrant S31.133
          with
            foreign body S31.143
            penetration into peritoneal cavity
              S31.633
              with foreign body S31.643
        upper quadrant S31.130
          with
            foreign body S31.140
            penetration into peritoneal cavity
              S31.630
              with foreign body S31.640
  accidental, complicating surgery —*see*
    Complication, accidental puncture or
    laceration
  alveolar (process) —*see* Puncture, oral cavity
  ankle S91.039
    with
      foreign body S91.049
    left S91.032
      with
        foreign body S91.042
    right S91.031
      with
        foreign body S91.041
  anus S31.833
    with foreign body S31.834
  arm (upper) S41.139
    with foreign body S41.149
    left S41.132
      with foreign body S41.142
    lower —*see* Puncture, forearm
    right S41.131
      with foreign body S41.141
  auditory canal (external) (meatus) —*see*
    Puncture, ear
  auricle, ear —*see* Puncture, ear
  axilla —*see* Puncture, arm
  back —*see also* Puncture, thorax, back
    lower S31.030
      with
        foreign body S31.040
          with penetration into
            retroperitoneal space S31.041
        penetration into retroperitoneal space
          S31.031
  bladder (traumatic) S37.29
    nontraumatic N32.89
  breast S21.039
    with foreign body S21.049
    left S21.032
      with foreign body S21.042
    right S21.031
      with foreign body S21.041
  buttock S31.803
    with foreign body S31.804
    left S31.823
      with foreign body S31.824
    right S31.813
      with foreign body S31.814
  by
    device, implant or graft —*see*
      Complications, by site and type,
      mechanical
    foreign body left accidentally in operative
      wound T81.539
    instrument (any) during a procedure,
      accidental —*see* Puncture, accidental
      complicating surgery
  calf —*see* Puncture, leg
  canaliculus lacrimalis —*see* Puncture, eyelid

Puncture *(Continued)*
  canthus, eye —*see* Puncture, eyelid
  cervical esophagus S11.23
    with foreign body S11.24
  cheek (external) S01.439
    with foreign body S01.449
    internal —*see* Puncture, oral cavity
    left S01.432
      with foreign body S01.442
    right S01.431
      with foreign body S01.441
  chest wall —*see* Puncture, thorax
  chin —*see* Puncture, head, specified site NEC
  clitoris —*see* Puncture, vulva
  costal region —*see* Puncture, thorax
  digit(s)
    foot —*see* Puncture, toe
    hand —*see* Puncture, finger
  ear (canal) (external) S01.339
    with foreign body S01.349
    drum S09.2-●
    left S01.332
      with foreign body S01.342
    right S01.331
      with foreign body S01.341
  elbow S51.039
    with
      foreign body S51.049
    left S51.032
      with
        foreign body S51.042
    right S51.031
      with
        foreign body S51.041
  epididymis —*see* Puncture, testis
  epigastric region —*see* Puncture, abdomen,
    wall, epigastric
  epiglottis S11.83
    with foreign body S11.84
  esophagus
    cervical S11.23
      with foreign body S11.24
    thoracic S27.818
  eyeball S05.6-●
    with foreign body S05.5-●
  eyebrow —*see* Puncture, eyelid
  eyelid S01.13-●
    with foreign body S01.14-●
    left S01.132
      with foreign body S01.142
    right S01.131
      with foreign body S01.141
  face NEC —*see* Puncture, head, specified site
    NEC
  finger(s) S61.239
    with
      damage to nail S61.339
        with
          foreign body S61.349
      foreign body S61.249
    index S61.238
      with
        damage to nail S61.338
          with
            foreign body S61.348
        foreign body S61.248
      left S61.231
        with
          damage to nail S61.331
            with
              foreign body S61.341
          foreign body S61.241
      right S61.230
        with
          damage to nail S61.330
            with
              foreign body S61.340
          foreign body S61.240
    little S61.238
      with
        damage to nail S61.338

▶ New   ⇒ Revised   ~~deleted~~ Deleted   ● Use Additional Character(s)

Puncture *(Continued)*
  finger *(Continued)*
    with *(Continued)*
      with *(Continued)*
        damage to nail *(Continued)*
          with
            foreign body S61.348
          foreign body S61.248
        left S61.237
          with
            damage to nail S61.337
              with
                foreign body S61.347
            foreign body S61.247
        right S61.236
          with
            damage to nail S61.336
              with
                foreign body S61.346
            foreign body S61.246
    middle S61.238
      with
        damage to nail S61.338
          with
            foreign body S61.348
        foreign body S61.248
      left S61.233
        with
          damage to nail S61.333
            with
              foreign body S61.343
           foreign body S61.243
      right S61.232
        with
          damage to nail S61.332
            with
              foreign body S61.342
           foreign body S61.242
    ring S61.238
      with
        damage to nail S61.338
          with
            foreign body S61.348
        foreign body S61.248
      left S61.235
        with
          damage to nail S61.335
            with
              foreign body S61.345
           foreign body S61.245
      right S61.234
        with
          damage to nail S61.334
            with
              foreign body S61.344
           foreign body S61.244
  flank S31.139
    with foreign body S31.149
  foot (except toe(s) alone) S91.339
    with foreign body S91.349
    left S91.332
      with foreign body S91.342
    right S91.331
      with foreign body S91.341
    toe —*see* Puncture, toe
  forearm S51.839
    with
      foreign body S51.849
    elbow only —*see* Puncture, elbow
    left S51.832
      with
        foreign body S51.842
    right S51.831
      with
        foreign body S51.841
  forehead —*see* Puncture, head, specified site NEC
  genital organs, external
    female S31.532
      with foreign body S31.542
      vagina —*see* Puncture, vagina
      vulva —*see* Puncture, vulva

Puncture *(Continued)*
  genital organs, external *(Continued)*
    male S31.531
      with foreign body S31.541
      penis —*see* Puncture, penis
      scrotum —*see* Puncture, scrotum
      testis —*see* Puncture, testis
  groin —*see* Puncture, abdomen, wall
  gum —*see* Puncture, oral cavity
  hand S61.439
    with
      foreign body S61.449
    finger —*see* Puncture, finger
    left S61.432
      with
        foreign body S61.442
    right S61.431
      with
        foreign body S61.441
    thumb —*see* Puncture, thumb
  head S01.93
    with foreign body S01.94
    cheek —*see* Puncture, cheek
    ear —*see* Puncture, ear
    eyelid —*see* Puncture, eyelid
    lip —*see* Puncture, oral cavity
    nose —*see* Puncture, nose
    oral cavity —*see* Puncture, oral cavity
    scalp S01.03
      with foreign body S01.04
    specified site NEC S01.83
      with foreign body S01.84
    temporomandibular area —*see* Puncture, cheek
  heart S26.99
    with hemopericardium S26.09
    without hemopericardium S26.19
  heel —*see* Puncture, foot
  hip S71.039
    with foreign body S71.049
    left S71.032
      with foreign body S71.042
    right S71.031
      with foreign body S71.041
  hymen —*see* Puncture, vagina
  hypochondrium —*see* Puncture, abdomen, wall
  hypogastric region —*see* Puncture, abdomen, wall
  inguinal region —*see* Puncture, abdomen, wall
  instep —*see* Puncture, foot
  internal organs —*see* Injury, by site
  interscapular region —*see* Puncture, thorax, back
  intestine
    large
      colon S36.599
        ascending S36.590
        descending S36.592
        sigmoid S36.593
        specified site NEC S36.598
        transverse S36.591
      rectum S36.69
    small S36.499
      duodenum S36.490
      specified site NEC S36.498
  intra-abdominal organ S36.99
    gallbladder S36.128
    intestine —*see* Puncture, intestine
    liver S36.118
    pancreas —*see* Puncture, pancreas
    peritoneum S36.81
    specified site NEC S36.898
    spleen S36.09
    stomach S36.39
  jaw —*see* Puncture, head, specified site NEC
  knee S81.039
    with foreign body S81.049
    left S81.032
      with foreign body S81.042

Puncture *(Continued)*
  knee *(Continued)*
    right S81.031
      with foreign body S81.041
  labium (majus) (minus) —*see* Puncture, vulva
  lacrimal duct —*see* Puncture, eyelid
  larynx S11.013
    with foreign body S11.014
  leg (lower) S81.839
    with foreign body S81.849
    foot —*see* Puncture, foot
    knee —*see* Puncture, knee
    left S81.832
      with foreign body S81.842
    right S81.831
      with foreign body S81.841
    upper —*see* Puncture, thigh
  lip S01.531
    with foreign body S01.541
  loin —*see* Puncture, abdomen, wall
  lower back —*see* Puncture, back, lower
  lumbar region —*see* Puncture, back, lower
  malar region —*see* Puncture, head, specified site NEC
  mammary —*see* Puncture, breast
  mastoid region —*see* Puncture, head, specified site NEC
  mouth —*see* Puncture, oral cavity
  nail
    finger —*see* Puncture, finger, with damage to nail
    toe —*see* Puncture, toe, with damage to nail
  nasal (septum) (sinus) —*see* Puncture, nose
  nasopharynx —*see* Puncture, head, specified site NEC
  neck S11.93
    with foreign body S11.94
    involving
      cervical esophagus —*see* Puncture, cervical esophagus
      larynx —*see* Puncture, larynx
      pharynx —*see* Puncture, pharynx
      thyroid gland —*see* Puncture, thyroid gland
      trachea —*see* Puncture, trachea
    specified site NEC S11.83
      with foreign body S11.84
  nose (septum) (sinus) S01.23
    with foreign body S01.24
  ocular —*see* Puncture, eyeball - oral cavity S01.532
    with foreign body S01.542
  orbit S05.4- ●
  palate —*see* Puncture, oral cavity
  palm —*see* Puncture, hand
  pancreas S36.299
    body S36.291
    head S36.290
    tail S36.292
  pelvis —*see* Puncture, back, lower
  penis S31.23
    with foreign body S31.24
  perineum
    female S31.43
      with foreign body S31.44
    male S31.139
      with foreign body S31.149
  periocular area (with or without lacrimal passages) —*see* Puncture, eyelid
  phalanges
    finger —*see* Puncture, finger
    toe —*see* Puncture, toe
  pharynx S11.23
    with foreign body S11.24
  pinna —*see* Puncture, ear
  popliteal space —*see* Puncture, knee
  prepuce —*see* Puncture, penis
  pubic region S31.139
    with foreign body S31.149

Puncture (*Continued*)
  pudendum —*see* Puncture, genital organs, external
  rectovaginal septum —*see* Puncture, vagina
  sacral region —*see* Puncture, back, lower
  sacroiliac region —*see* Puncture, back, lower
  salivary gland —*see* Puncture, oral cavity
  scalp S01.03
    with foreign body S01.04
  scapular region —*see* Puncture, shoulder
  scrotum S31.33
    with foreign body S31.34
  shin —*see* Puncture, leg
  shoulder S41.039
    with foreign body S41.049
    left S41.032
      with foreign body S41.042
    right S41.031
      with foreign body S41.041
  spermatic cord —*see* Puncture, testis
  sternal region —*see* Puncture, thorax, front
  submaxillary region —*see* Puncture, head, specified site NEC
  submental region —*see* Puncture, head, specified site NEC
  subungual
    finger(s) —*see* Puncture, finger, with damage to nail
    toe —*see* Puncture, toe, with damage to nail
  supraclavicular fossa —*see* Puncture, neck, specified site NEC
  temple, temporal region —*see* Puncture, head, specified site NEC
  temporomandibular area —*see* Puncture, cheek
  testis S31.33
    with foreign body S31.34
  thigh S71.139
    with foreign body S71.149
    left S71.132
      with foreign body S71.142
    right S71.131
      with foreign body S71.141
  thorax, thoracic (wall) S21.93
    with foreign body S21.94
    back S21.23-●
      with
        foreign body S21.24-●
          with penetration S21.44
        penetration S21.43
    breast —*see* Puncture, breast
    front S21.13-●
      with
        foreign body S21.14-●
          with penetration S21.34
        penetration S21.33
  throat —*see* Puncture, neck
  thumb S61.039
    with
      damage to nail S61.139
        with
          foreign body S61.149
      foreign body S61.049
    left S61.032
      with
        damage to nail S61.132
          with
            foreign body S61.142
        foreign body S61.042
    right S61.031
      with
        damage to nail S61.131
          with
            foreign body S61.141
        foreign body S61.041

Puncture (*Continued*)
  thyroid gland S11.13
    with foreign body S11.14
  toe(s) S91.139
    with
      damage to nail S91.239
        with
          foreign body S91.249
      foreign body S91.149
    great S91.133
      with
        damage to nail S91.233
          with
            foreign body S91.243
        foreign body S91.143
      left S91.132
        with
          damage to nail S91.232
            with
              foreign body S91.242
          foreign body S91.142
      right S91.131
        with
          damage to nail S91.231
            with
              foreign body S91.241
          foreign body S91.141
    lesser S91.136
      with
        damage to nail S91.236
          with
            foreign body S91.246
        foreign body S91.146
      left S91.135
        with
          damage to nail S91.235
            with
              foreign body S91.245
          foreign body S91.145
      right S91.134
        with
          damage to nail S91.234
            with
              foreign body S91.244
          foreign body S91.144
  tongue —*see* Puncture, oral cavity
  trachea S11.023
    with foreign body S11.024
  tunica vaginalis —*see* Puncture, testis
  tympanum, tympanic membrane S09.2-●
  umbilical region S31.135
    with foreign body S31.145
  uvula —*see* Puncture, oral cavity
  vagina S31.43
    with foreign body S31.44
  vocal cords S11.033
    with foreign body S11.034
  vulva S31.43
    with foreign body S31.44
  wrist S61.539
    with
      foreign body S61.549
    left S61.532
      with
        foreign body S61.542
    right S61.531
      with
        foreign body S61.541
PUO (pyrexia of unknown origin) R50.9
Pupillary membrane (persistent) Q13.89
Pupillotonia —*see* Anomaly, pupil, function, tonic pupil
Purpura D69.2
  abdominal D69.0
  allergic D69.0
  anaphylactoid D69.0
  annularis telangiectodes L81.7
  arthritic D69.0
  autoerythrocyte sensitization D69.2
  autoimmune D69.0

Purpura (*Continued*)
  bacterial D69.0
  Bateman's (senile) D69.2
  capillary fragility (hereditary) (idiopathic) D69.8
  cryoglobulinemic D89.1
  Devil's pinches D69.2
  fibrinolytic —*see* Fibrinolysis
  fulminans, fulminous D65
  gangrenous D65
  hemorrhagic, hemorrhagica D69.3
    not due to thrombocytopenia D69.0
  Henoch (-Schönlein) (allergic) D69.0
  hypergammaglobulinemic (benign) (Waldenström's) D89.0
  idiopathic (thrombocytopenic) D69.3
    nonthrombocytopenic D69.0
  immune thrombocytopenic D69.3
  infectious D69.0
  malignant D69.0
  neonatorum P54.5
  nervosa D69.0
  newborn P54.5
  nonthrombocytopenic D69.2
    hemorrhagic D69.0
    idiopathic D69.0
  nonthrombopenic D69.2
  peliosis rheumatica D69.0
  posttransfusion (post-transfusion) (from (fresh) whole blood or blood products) D69.51
  primary D69.49
  red cell membrane sensitivity D69.2
  rheumatica D69.0
  Schönlein (-Henoch) (allergic) D69.0
  scorbutic E54 [D77]
  senile D69.2
  simplex D69.2
  symptomatica D69.0
  telangiectasia annularis L81.7
  thrombocytopenic D69.49
    congenital D69.42
    hemorrhagic D69.3
    hereditary D69.42
    idiopathic D69.3
    immune D69.3
    neonatal, transitory P61.0
  ➡thrombotic M31.19
  thrombohemolytic —*see* Fibrinolysis
  thrombolytic —*see* Fibrinolysis
  thrombopenic D69.49
  ➡thrombotic, thrombocytopenic M31.19
  toxic D69.0
  vascular D69.0
  visceral symptoms D69.0
Purpuric spots R23.3
Purulent —*see* condition
Pus
  in
    stool R19.5
    urine N39.0
  tube (rupture) —*see* Salpingo-oophoritis
Pustular rash L08.0
Pustule (nonmalignant) L08.9
  malignant A22.0
Pustulosis palmaris et plantaris L40.3
Putnam (-Dana) **disease or syndrome** —*see* Degeneration, combined
Putrescent pulp (dental) K04.1
Pyarthritis, pyarthrosis —*see* Arthritis, pyogenic or pyemic
  tuberculous —*see* Tuberculosis, joint
Pyelectasis —*see* Hydronephrosis
Pyelitis (congenital) (uremic) —*see also* Pyelonephritis
  with
    calculus —*see* category N20
      with hydronephrosis N13.6
    contracted kidney N11.9

▶ New   ➡ Revised   ~~deleted~~ Deleted   ● Use Additional Character(s)

Pyelitis *(Continued)*
  acute N10
  chronic N11.9
    with calculus —*see* category N20
      with hydronephrosis N13.6
  cystica N28.84
  puerperal (postpartum) O86.21
  tuberculous A18.11
Pyelocystitis —*see* Pyelonephritis
Pyelonephritis —*see also* Nephritis,
    tubulo-interstitial
  with
    calculus —*see* category N20
      with hydronephrosis N13.6
    contracted kidney N11.9
  acute N10
  calculous —*see* category N20
    with hydronephrosis N13.6
  chronic N11.9
    with calculus —*see* category N20
      with hydronephrosis N13.6
    associated with ureteral obstruction or
      stricture N11.1
    nonobstructive N11.8
      with reflux (vesicoureteral) N11.0
    obstructive N11.1
    specified NEC N11.8
  in (due to)
    brucellosis A23.9 *[N16]*
    cryoglobulinemia (mixed) D89.1 *[N16]*
    cystinosis E72.04
    diphtheria A36.84
    glycogen storage disease E74.09 *[N16]*
    leukemia NEC C95.9-● *[N16]*
    lymphoma NEC C85.90 *[N16]*
    multiple myeloma C90.0-● *[N16]*
    obstruction N11.1
    Salmonella infection A02.25
    sarcoidosis D86.84
    sepsis A41.9 *[N16]*
    Sjögren's disease M35.04
    toxoplasmosis B58.83
    transplant rejection T86.91 *[N16]*
    Wilson's disease E83.01 *[N16]*
  nonobstructive N12
    with reflux (vesicoureteral) N11.0
    chronic N11.8
  syphilitic A52.75

Pyelonephrosis (obstructive) N11.1
  chronic N11.9
Pyelophlebitis I80.8
Pyeloureteritis cystica N28.85
Pyemia, pyemic (fever) (infection) (purulent) —
    see also Sepsis
  joint —*see* Arthritis, pyogenic or pyemic
  liver K75.1
  pneumococcal A40.3
  portal K75.1
  postvaccinal T88.0
  puerperal, postpartum, childbirth O85
  specified organism NEC A41.89
  tuberculous —*see* Tuberculosis, miliary
Pygopagus Q89.4
Pyknoepilepsy (idiopathic) —*see* Pyknolepsy
Pyknolepsy G40.A09
  intractable G40.A19
    with status epilepticus G40.A11
    without status epilepticus G40.A19
  not intractable G40.A09
    with status epilepticus G40.A01
    without status epilepticus G40.A09
Pylephlebitis K75.1
Pyle's syndrome Q78.5
Pylethrombophlebitis K75.1
Pylethrombosis K75.1
Pyloritis K29.90
  with bleeding K29.91
Pylorospasm (reflex) NEC K31.3
  congenital or infantile Q40.0
  neurotic F45.8
  newborn Q40.0
  psychogenic F45.8
Pylorus, pyloric —*see* condition
Pyoarthrosis —*see* Arthritis, pyogenic or
    pyemic
Pyocele
  mastoid —*see* Mastoiditis, acute
  sinus (accessory) —*see* Sinusitis
  turbinate (bone) J32.9
  urethra —*see also* Urethritis N34.0
Pyocolpos —*see* Vaginitis
Pyocystitis N30.80
  with hematuria N30.81
Pyoderma, pyodermia L08.0
  gangrenosum L88
  newborn P39.4

Pyoderma, pyodermia *(Continued)*
  phagedenic L88
  vegetans L08.81
Pyodermatitis L08.0
  vegetans L08.81
Pyogenic —*see* condition
Pyohydronephrosis N13.6
Pyometra, pyometrium, pyometritis —*see*
    Endometritis
Pyomyositis (tropical) —*see* Myositis,
    infective
Pyonephritis N12
Pyonephrosis N13.6
  tuberculous A18.11
Pyo-oophoritis —*see* Salpingo-oophoritis
Pyo-ovarium —*see* Salpingo-oophoritis
Pyopericarditis, pyopericardium
    I30.1
Pyophlebitis —*see* Phlebitis
Pyopneumopericardium I30.1
Pyopneumothorax (infective) J86.9
  with fistula J86.0
  tuberculous NEC A15.6
Pyosalpinx, pyosalpingitis —*see also*
    Salpingo-oophoritis
Pyothorax J86.9
  with fistula J86.0
  tuberculous NEC A15.6
Pyoureter N28.89
  tuberculous A18.11
Pyramidopallidonigral syndrome
    G20
Pyrexia (of unknown origin) R50.9
  atmospheric T67.01
  during labor NEC O75.2
  heat T67.01
  newborn P81.9
    environmentally-induced P81.0
  persistent R50.9
  puerperal O86.4
Pyroglobulinemia NEC E88.09
Pyromania F63.1
Pyrosis R12
Pyuria (bacterial) R82.81

Q

Q fever A78
  with pneumonia A78
Quadricuspid aortic valve Q23.8
Quadrilateral fever A78
Quadriparesis —*see* Quadriplegia
  meaning muscle weakness M62.81
Quadriplegia G82.50- •
  complete
    C1-C4 level G82.51
    C5-C7 level G82.53
  congenital (cerebral) (spinal) G80.8
    spastic G80.0

Quadriplegia *(Continued)*
  embolic (current episode) I63.4- •
  functional R53.2
  incomplete
    C1-C4 level G82.52
    C5-C7 level G82.54
  thrombotic (current episode) I63.3- •
  traumatic — code to injury with seventh
    character S
    current episode —*see* Injury, spinal (cord),
      cervical
Quadruplet, pregnancy —*see* Pregnancy,
  quadruplet
Quarrelsomeness F60.3

Queensland fever A77.3
Quervain's disease M65.4
  thyroid E06.1
Queyrat's erythroplasia D07.4
  penis D07.4
  specified site —*see* Neoplasm, skin,
    in situ
  unspecified site D07.4
Quincke's disease or edema T78.3
  hereditary D84.1
Quinsy (gangrenous) J36
Quintan fever A79.0
Quintuplet, pregnancy —*see* Pregnancy,
  quintuplet

▶ New   ⇒ Revised   ~~deleted~~ Deleted   • Use Additional Character(s)

R

Rabbit fever —*see* Tularemia
Rabies A82.9
  contact Z20.3
  exposure to Z20.3
  inoculation reaction —*see* Complications,
    vaccination
  sylvatic A82.0
  urban A82.1
Rachischisis —*see* Spina bifida
Rachitic —*see also* condition
  deformities of spine (late effect) (sequelae)
    E64.3
  pelvis (late effect) (sequelae) E64.3
    with disproportion (fetopelvic) O33.0
      causing obstructed labor O65.0
Rachitis, rachitism (acute) (tarda) —*see also*
  Rickets
  renalis N25.0
  sequelae E64.3
Radial nerve —*see* condition
Radiation
  burn —*see* Burn
  effects NOS T66
  sickness NOS T66
  therapy, encounter for Z51.0
Radiculitis (pressure) (vertebrogenic) —*see*
  Radiculopathy
Radiculomyelitis —*see also* Encephalitis
  toxic, due to
    Clostridium tetani A35
    Corynebacterium diphtheriae A36.82
Radiculopathy M54.10
  cervical region M54.12
  cervicothoracic region M54.13
  due to
    disc disorder
      C3 M50.11
      C4 M50.11
      C5 M50.121
      C6 M50.122
      C7 M50.123
      C8 M50.13
    displacement of intervertebral disc —*see*
      Disorder, disc, with, radiculopathy
  leg M54.1-●
  lumbar region M54.16
  lumbosacral region M54.17
  occipito-atlanto-axial region M54.11
  postherpetic B02.29
  sacrococcygeal region M54.18
  syphilitic A52.11
  thoracic region (with visceral pain)
    M54.14
  thoracolumbar region M54.15
Radiodermal burns (acute, chronic, or
  occupational) —*see* Burn
Radiodermatitis L58.9
  acute L58.0
  chronic L58.1
Radiotherapy session Z51.0
RAEB (refractory anemia with excess blasts)
  D46.2-●
Rage, meaning rabies —*see* Rabies
Ragpicker's disease A22.1
Ragsorter's disease A22.1
Raillietiniasis B71.8
Railroad neurosis F48.8
Railway spine F48.8
Raised —*see also* Elevated
  antibody titer R76.0
Rake teeth, tooth M26.39
Rales R09.89
Ramifying renal pelvis Q63.8
Ramsay-Hunt disease or syndrome —*see also*
  Hunt's disease B02.21
  meaning dyssynergia cerebellaris myoclonica
    G11.19
Ranula K11.6
  congenital Q38.4

Rape
  adult
    confirmed T74.21
    suspected T76.21
  alleged, observation or examination, ruled out
    adult Z04.41
    child Z04.42
  child
    confirmed T74.22
    suspected T76.22
Rapid
  feeble pulse, due to shock, following injury
    T79.4
  heart (beat) R00.0
    psychogenic F45.8
  second stage (delivery) O62.3
  time-zone change syndrome G47.25
Rarefaction, bone —*see* Disorder, bone, density
  and structure, specified NEC
Rash (toxic) R21
  canker A38.9
  diaper L22
  drug (internal use) L27.0
    contact —*see also* Dermatitis, due to, drugs,
      external L25.1
  following immunization T88.1
  food —*see* Dermatitis, due to, food
  heat L74.0
  napkin (psoriasiform) L22
  nettle —*see* Urticaria
  pustular L08.0
  rose R21
    epidemic B06.9
  scarlet A38.9
  serum —*see also* Reaction, serum T80.69
  wandering tongue K14.1
Rasmussen aneurysm —*see* Tuberculosis,
  pulmonary
Rasmussen encephalitis G04.81
Rat-bite fever A25.9
  due to Streptobacillus moniliformis A25.1
  spirochetal (morsus muris) A25.0
Rathke's pouch tumor D44.3
Raymond (-Céstan) syndrome I65.8
Raynaud's disease, phenomenon or syndrome
  (secondary) I73.00
  with gangrene (symmetric) I73.01
RDS (newborn) (type I) P22.0
  type II P22.1
Reaction —*see also* Disorder
  adaptation —*see* Disorder, adjustment
  adjustment (anxiety) (conduct disorder)
    (depressiveness) (distress) —*see*
    Disorder, adjustment
    with
      mutism, elective (child) (adolescent) F94.0
  adverse
    food (any) (ingested) NEC T78.1
      anaphylactic —*see* Shock, anaphylactic,
        due to food
  anaphylactoid —*see* Shock, anaphylactic
  affective —*see* Disorder, mood
  allergic —*see* Allergy
  anaphylactic —*see* Shock, anaphylactic
  anesthesia —*see* Anesthesia, complication
  antitoxin (prophylactic) (therapeutic) —*see*
    Complications, vaccination
  anxiety F41.1
  Arthus —*see* Arthus' phenomenon
  asthenic F48.8
  combat and operational stress F43.0
  compulsive F42.8
  conversion F44.9
  crisis, acute F43.0
  deoxyribonuclease (DNA) (DNase)
    hypersensitivity D69.2
  depressive (single episode) F32.9
    affective (single episode) F31.4
      recurrent episode F33.9
    neurotic F34.1
    psychoneurotic F34.1

Reaction (Continued)
  depressive (Continued)
    psychotic F32.3
    recurrent —*see* Disorder, depressive,
      recurrent
  dissociative F44.9
  drug NEC T88.7
    addictive —*see* Dependence, drug
      transmitted via placenta or breast
        milk —*see* Absorption, drug,
        addictive, through placenta
    allergic —*see* Allergy, drug
    lichenoid L43.2
    newborn P93.8
      gray baby syndrome P93.0
    overdose or poisoning (by accident) —*see*
      Table of Drugs and Chemicals, by
      drug, poisoning
    photoallergic L56.1
    phototoxic L56.0
    withdrawal —*see* Dependence, by drug,
      with, withdrawal
      infant of dependent mother P96.1
      newborn P96.1
    wrong substance given or taken (by
      accident) —*see* Table of Drugs and
      Chemicals, by drug, poisoning
  fear F40.9
    child (abnormal) F93.8
  febrile nonhemolytic transfusion (FNHTR)
    R50.84
  fluid loss, cerebrospinal G97.1
  foreign
    body NEC —*see* Granuloma, foreign body
      in operative wound (inadvertently
        left) —*see* Foreign body, accidentally
        left during a procedure
    substance accidentally left during a
      procedure (chemical) (powder) (talc)
      T81.60
      aseptic peritonitis T81.61
      body or object (instrument) (sponge)
        (swab) —*see* Foreign body,
        accidentally left during a
        procedure
      specified reaction NEC T81.69
  grief —*see* Disorder, adjustment
  Herxheimer's R68.89
  hyperkinetic —*see* Hyperkinesia
  hypochondriacal F45.20
  hypoglycemic, due to insulin E16.0
    with coma (diabetic) —*see* Diabetes, coma
      nondiabetic E15
    therapeutic misadventure —*see*
      subcategory T38.3
  hypomanic F30.8
  hysterical F44.9
  immunization —*see* Complications, vaccination
  incompatibility
    ABO blood group (infusion) (transfusion) —
      see Complication(s), transfusion,
      incompatibility reaction, ABO
      delayed serologic T80.39
    minor blood group (Duffy) (E) (K) (Kell)
      (Kidd) (Lewis) (M) (N) (P) (S)
      T80.89
    Rh (factor) (infusion) (transfusion) —
      see Complication(s), transfusion,
      incompatibility reaction, Rh (factor)
  inflammatory —*see* Infection
  infusion —*see* Complications, infusion
  inoculation (immune serum) —*see*
    Complications, vaccination
  insulin T38.3-●
  involutional psychotic —*see* Disorder,
    depressive
  leukemoid D72.823
    basophilic D72.823
    lymphocytic D72.823
    monocytic D72.823
    myelocytic D72.823
    neutrophilic D72.823

Reaction *(Continued)*
LSD (acute)
  due to drug abuse —*see* Abuse, drug,
    hallucinogen
  due to drug dependence —*see* Dependence,
    drug, hallucinogen
lumbar puncture G97.1
manic-depressive —*see* Disorder, bipolar
neurasthenic F48.8
neurogenic —*see* Neurosis
neurotic F48.9
neurotic-depressive F34.1
nitritoid —*see* Crisis, nitritoid - obsessive-
  compulsive F42
nonspecific
  to
    cell mediated immunity measurement
      of gamma interferon antigen
      response without active
      tuberculosis R76.12
    QuantiFERON-TB test (QFT) without
      active tuberculosis R76.12
    tuberculin test —*see also* Reaction,
      tuberculin skin test R76.11
obsessive-compulsive F42.8
organic, acute or subacute —*see* Delirium
paranoid (acute) F23
  chronic F22
  senile F03
passive dependency F60.7
phobic F40.9
post-traumatic stress, uncomplicated Z73.3
psychogenic F99
psychoneurotic —*see also* Neurosis
  compulsive F42.8
  depersonalization F48.1
  depressive F34.1
  hypochondriacal F45.20
  neurasthenic F48.8
  obsessive F42.8
psychophysiologic —*see* Disorder,
  somatoform
psychosomatic —*see* Disorder, somatoform
psychotic —*see* Psychosis
scarlet fever toxin —*see* Complications,
  vaccination
schizophrenic F23
  acute (brief) (undifferentiated) F23
  latent F21
  undifferentiated (acute) (brief) F23
serological for syphilis —*see* Serology for
  syphilis
serum T80.69
  anaphylactic (immediate) —*see also* Shock,
    anaphylactic T80.59
  specified reaction NEC
    due to
      administration of blood and blood
        products T80.61
      immunization T80.62
      serum specified NEC T80.69
      vaccination T80.62
situational —*see* Disorder, adjustment
somatization —*see* Disorder, somatoform
spinal puncture G97.1
  dural G97.1
stress (severe) F43.9
  acute (agitation) ("daze") (disorientation)
    (disturbance of consciousness) (flight
    reaction) (fugue) F43.0
  specified NEC F43.8
surgical procedure —*see* Complications,
  surgical procedure
tetanus antitoxin —*see* Complications,
  vaccination
toxic, to local anesthesia T81.59
  in labor and delivery O74.4
  in pregnancy O29.3X-●
  postpartum, puerperal O89.3
toxin-antitoxin —*see* Complications,
  vaccination

Reaction *(Continued)*
transfusion (blood) (bone marrow)
  (lymphocytes) (allergic) —*see*
  Complications, transfusion
tuberculin skin test, abnormal R76.11
vaccination (any) —*see* Complications,
  vaccination
withdrawing, child or adolescent F93.8
Reactive airway disease —*see* Asthma
Reactive depression —*see* Reaction, depressive
Rearrangement
chromosomal
  balanced (in) Q95.9
    abnormal individual (autosomal) Q95.2
      non-sex (autosomal) chromosomes
        Q95.2
      sex/non-sex chromosomes Q95.3
    specified NEC Q95.8
Recalcitrant patient —*see* Noncompliance
Recanalization, thrombus —*see* Thrombosis
Recession, receding
chamber angle (eye) H21.55-●
chin M26.09
gingival (postinfective) (postoperative)
  generalized K06.020
    minimal K06.021
    moderate K06.022
    severe K06.023
  localized K06.010
    minimal K06.011
    moderate K06.012
    severe K06.013
Recklinghausen's disease Q85.01
  bones E21.0
Reclus' disease (cystic) —*see* Mastopathy, cystic
Recrudescent typhus (fever) A75.1
Recruitment, auditory H93.21-●
Rectalgia K62.89
Rectitis K62.89
Rectocele
female (without uterine prolapse) N81.6
  with uterine prolapse N81.4
    incomplete N81.2
in pregnancy —*see* Pregnancy, complicated
  by, abnormal, pelvic organs or tissues
  NEC
male K62.3
Rectosigmoid junction —*see* condition
Rectosigmoiditis K63.89
ulcerative (chronic) K51.30
  with
    complication K51.319
      abscess K51.314
      fistula K51.313
      obstruction K51.312
      rectal bleeding K51.311
      specified NEC K51.318
Rectourethral —*see* condition
Rectovaginal —*see* condition
Rectovesical —*see* condition
Rectum, rectal —*see* condition
Recurrent —*see* condition
pregnancy loss —*see* Loss (of), pregnancy,
  recurrent
Red bugs B88.0
Red-cedar lung or pneumonitis J67.8
Red tide —*see also* Table of Drugs and
  Chemicals T65.82-●
Reduced
mobility Z74.09
ventilatory or vital capacity R94.2
Redundant, redundancy
anus (congenital) Q43.8
clitoris N90.89
colon (congenital) Q43.8
foreskin (congenital) N47.8
intestine (congenital) Q43.8
labia N90.69
organ or site, congenital NEC —*see* Accessory
panniculus (abdominal) E65
prepuce (congenital) N47.8

Redundant, redundancy *(Continued)*
pylorus K31.89
rectum (congenital) Q43.8
scrotum N50.89
sigmoid (congenital) Q43.8
skin L98.7
  and subcutaneous tissue L98.7
  of face L57.4
    eyelids —*see* Blepharochalasis
stomach K31.89
Reduplication —*see* Duplication
Reflex R29.2
hyperactive gag J39.2
pupillary, abnormal —*see* Anomaly, pupil,
  function
vasoconstriction I73.9
vasovagal R55
Reflux K21.9
acid K21.9
esophageal K21.9
  with esophagitis (without bleeding) K21.00
    with bleeding K21.01
  newborn P78.83
gastroesophageal K21.9
  with esophagitis (without bleeding) K21.00
    with bleeding K21.01
mitral —*see* Insufficiency, mitral
ureteral —*see* Reflux, vesicoureteral
vesicoureteral (with scarring) N13.70
  with
    nephropathy N13.729
      with hydroureter N13.739
        bilateral N13.732
        unilateral N13.731
      without hydroureter N13.729
        bilateral N13.722
        unilateral N13.721
      bilateral N13.722
      unilateral N13.721
    pyelonephritis (chronic) N11.0
  without nephropathy N13.71
  congenital Q62.7
Reforming, artificial openings —*see* Attention
  to, artificial, opening
Refractive error —*see* Disorder, refraction
Refsum's disease or syndrome G60.1
Refusal of
food, psychogenic F50.89
treatment (because of) Z53.20
  ▸‖left against medical advice (AMA) Z53.29
  ▶left without being seen Z53.21
  patient's decision NEC Z53.29
  reasons of belief or group pressure Z53.1
Regional —*see* condition
Regurgitation R11.10
aortic (valve) —*see* Insufficiency, aortic
food —*see also* Vomiting
  with reswallowing —*see* Rumination
  newborn P92.1
gastric contents —*see* Vomiting
heart —*see* Endocarditis
mitral (valve) —*see* Insufficiency, mitral
  congenital Q23.3
myocardial —*see* Endocarditis
pulmonary (valve) (heart) I37.1
  congenital Q22.2
  syphilitic A52.03
tricuspid —*see* Insufficiency, tricuspid
valve, valvular —*see* Endocarditis
  congenital Q24.8
vesicoureteral —*see* Reflux, vesicoureteral
Reichmann's disease or syndrome K31.89
Reifenstein syndrome E34.52
Reinsertion
implantable subdermal contraceptive Z30.46
intrauterine contraceptive device Z30.433
Reiter's disease, syndrome, or urethritis
  M02.30
ankle M02.37-●
elbow M02.32-●
foot joint M02.37-●
hand joint M02.34-●

▶ New   ⟹ Revised   ~~deleted~~ Deleted   ● Use Additional Character(s)

Reiter's disease, syndrome, or urethritis
 (Continued)
 hip M02.35-●
 knee M02.36-●
 multiple site M02.39
 shoulder M02.31-●
 vertebra M02.38
 wrist M02.33-●
Rejection
 food, psychogenic F50.89
 transplant T86.91
  bone T86.830
   marrow T86.01
  cornea T86.840-●
  heart T86.21
   with lung(s) T86.31
  intestine T86.850
  kidney T86.11
  liver T86.41
  lung(s) T86.810
   with heart T86.31
  organ (immune or nonimmune cause)
   T86.91
  pancreas T86.890
  skin (allograft) (autograft) T86.820
  specified NEC T86.890
  stem cell (peripheral blood) (umbilical
   cord) T86.5
Relapsing fever A68.9
 Carter's (Asiatic) A68.1
 Dutton's (West African) A68.1
 Koch's A68.9
 louse-borne (epidemic) A68.0
 Novy's (American) A68.1
 Obermeyers's (European) A68.0
 Spirillum A68.9
 tick borne (endemic) A68.1
Relationship
 occlusal
  open anterior M26.220
  open posterior M26.221
Relaxation
 anus (sphincter) K62.89
  psychogenic F45.8
 arch (foot) —*see also* Deformity, limb, flat foot
 back ligaments —*see* Instability, joint, spine
 bladder (sphincter) N31.2
 cardioesophageal K21.9
 cervix —*see* Incompetency, cervix
 diaphragm J98.6
 joint (capsule) (ligament) (paralytic) —*see*
  Flail, joint
  congenital NEC Q74.8
 lumbosacral (joint) —*see* subcategory M53.2
 pelvic floor N81.89
 perineum N81.89
 posture R29.3
 rectum (sphincter) K62.89
 sacroiliac (joint) —*see* subcategory M53.2
 scrotum N50.89
 urethra (sphincter) N36.44
 vesical N31.2
Release from prison, anxiety concerning Z65.2
Remains
 canal of Cloquet Q14.0
 capsule (opaque) Q14.8
Remittent fever (malarial) B54
Remnant
 canal of Cloquet Q14.0
 capsule (opaque) Q14.8
 cervix, cervical stump (acquired)
  (postoperative) N88.8
 cystic duct, postcholecystectomy K91.5
 fingernail L60.8
  congenital Q84.6
 meniscus, knee —*see* Derangement, knee,
  meniscus, specified NEC
 thyroglossal duct Q89.2
 tonsil J35.8
  infected (chronic) J35.01
 urachus Q64.4

Removal (from) (of)
 artificial
  arm Z44.00-●
   complete Z44.01-●
   partial Z44.02-●
  eye Z44.2-●
  leg Z44.10-●
   complete Z44.11-●
   partial Z44.12-●
 breast implant Z45.81
 cardiac pulse generator (battery) (end-of-life)
  Z45.010
 catheter (urinary) (indwelling) Z46.6
  from artificial opening —*see* Attention to,
   artificial, opening
  non-vascular Z46.82
  vascular NEC Z45.2
 device Z46.9
  contraceptive Z30.432
   implantable subdermal Z30.46
  implanted NEC Z45.89
  specified NEC Z46.89
 drains Z48.03
 dressing (nonsurgical) Z48.00
  surgical Z48.01
 external
  fixation device — code to fracture with
   seventh character D
  prosthesis, prosthetic device Z44.9
   breast Z44.3-●
   specified NEC Z44.8
 home in childhood (to foster home or
  institution) Z62.29
 ileostomy Z43.2
 insulin pump Z46.81
 myringotomy device (stent) (tube) Z45.82
 nervous system device NEC Z46.2
  brain neuropacemaker Z46.2
  visual substitution device Z16.2
   implanted Z45.31
 non-vascular catheter Z46.82
 organ, prophylactic (for neoplasia
  management) —*see* Prophylactic, organ
  removal
 orthodontic device Z46.4
 staples Z48.02
 stent
  ureteral Z46.6
 suture Z48.02
 urinary device Z46.6
 vascular access device or catheter Z45.2
Ren
 arcuatus Q63.1
 mobile, mobilis N28.89
  congenital Q63.8
 unguliformis Q63.1
Renal —*see* condition
Rendu-Osler-Weber disease or syndrome I78.0
Reninoma D41.0-●
Renon-Delille syndrome E23.3
Reovirus, as cause of disease classified
 elsewhere B97.5
Repeated falls NEC R29.6
Replaced chromosome by dicentric ring Q93.2
Replacement by artificial or mechanical device
 or prosthesis of
 bladder Z96.0
 blood vessel NEC Z95.828
 bone NEC Z96.7
 cochlea Z96.21
 coronary artery Z95.5
 eustachian tube Z96.29
 eye globe Z97.0
 heart Z95.812
  valve Z95.2
   prosthetic Z95.2
   specified NEC Z95.4
   xenogenic Z95.3
 intestine Z96.89
 joint Z96.60
  hip —*see* Presence, hip joint implant
  knee —*see* Presence, knee joint implant
  specified site NEC Z96.698

Replacement by artificial or mechanical device
 or prosthesis of *(Continued)*
 larynx Z96.3
 lens Z96.1
 limb(s) —*see* Presence, artificial, limb
 mandible NEC (for tooth root implant(s)) Z96.5
 organ NEC Z96.89
 peripheral vessel NEC Z95.828
 stapes Z96.29
 teeth Z97.2
 tendon Z96.7
 tissue NEC Z96.89
 tooth root(s) Z96.5
 vessel NEC Z95.828
  coronary (artery) Z95.5
Request for expert evidence Z04.89
Reserve, decreased or low
 cardiac —*see* Disease, heart
 kidney N28.89
▶**Residing**
 ▶in place not meant for human habitation
  (abandoned building) (car) (park)
  (sidewalk) Z59.02
 ▶on the street Z59.02
Residual —*see also* condition
 ovary syndrome N99.83
 state, schizophrenic F20.5
 urine R39.198
Resistance, resistant (to)
 activated protein C D68.51
 complicating pregnancy O26.89
 insulin E88.81
 organism(s)
  to
   drug Z16.30
    aminoglycosides Z16.29
    amoxicillin Z16.11
    ampicillin Z16.11
    antibiotic(s) Z16.20
     multiple Z16.24
     specified NEC Z16.29
    antifungal Z16.32
    antimicrobial (single) Z16.30
     multiple Z16.35
     specified NEC Z16.39
    antimycobacterial (single) Z16.341
     multiple Z16.342
    antiparasitic Z16.31
    antiviral Z16.33
    beta lactam antibiotics Z16.10
     specified NEC Z16.19
    cephalosporins Z16.19
    extended beta lactamase (ESBL) Z16.12
    fluoroquinolones Z16.23
    macrolides Z16.29
    methicillin —*see* MRSA
    multiple drugs (MDRO)
     antibiotics Z16.24
     antimicrobial Z16.35
     antimycobacterials Z16.342
    penicillins Z16.11
    quinine (and related compounds)
     Z16.31
    quinolones Z16.23
    sulfonamides Z16.29
    tetracyclines Z16.29
    tuberculostatics (single) Z16.341
     multiple Z16.342
    vancomycin Z16.21
     related antibiotics Z16.22
 thyroid hormone E07.89
Resorption
 dental (roots) K03.3
  alveoli M26.79
 teeth (external) (internal) (pathological)
  (roots) K03.3
Respiration
 Cheyne-Stokes R06.3
 decreased due to shock, following injury T79.4
 disorder of, psychogenic F45.8
 insufficient, or poor R06.89
  newborn P28.5

Respiration *(Continued)*
  painful R07.1
  sighing, psychogenic F45.8
Respiratory —*see also* condition
  distress syndrome (newborn) (type I) P22.0
    type II P22.1
  syncytial virus, as cause of disease classified
      elsewhere *(see also* Virus, respiratory
      syncytial (RSV)) B97.4
Respite care Z75.5
Response (drug)
  photoallergic L56.1
  phototoxic L56.0
Restenosis
  stent
    vascular
      end stent
        adjacent to stent —*see* Arteriosclerosis

        within the stent
          coronary T82.855
          peripheral T82.856
      in stent
        coronary vessel T82.855
        peripheral vessel T82.856
Restless legs (syndrome) G25.81
Restlessness R45.1
Restoration (of)
  dental
    aesthetically inadequate or displeasing
        K08.56
    defective K08.50
      specified NEC K08.59
    failure of marginal integrity K08.51
    failure of periodontal anatomical intergrity
        K08.54
  organ continuity from previous sterilization
      (tuboplasty) (vasoplasty) Z31.0
    aftercare Z31.42
  tooth (existing)
    contours biologically incompatible with
        oral health K08.54
    open margins K08.51
    overhanging K08.52
    poor aesthetic K08.56
    poor gingival margins K08.51
  unsatisfactory, of tooth K08.50
    specified NEC K08.59
Restorative material (dental)
  allergy to K08.55
  fractured K08.539
    with loss of material K08.531
    without loss of material K08.530
  unrepairable overhanging of K08.52
Restriction of housing space Z59.1
Rests, ovarian, in fallopian tube Q50.6
Restzustand (schizophrenic) F20.5
Retained —*see also* Retention
  cholelithiasis following cholecystectomy K91.86
  foreign body fragments (type of) Z18.9
    acrylics Z18.2
    animal quill(s) or spines Z18.31
    cement Z18.83
    concrete Z18.83
    crystalline Z18.83
    depleted isotope Z18.09
    depleted uranium Z18.01
    diethylhexyl phthalates Z18.2
    glass Z18.81
    isocyanate Z18.2
    magnetic metal Z18.11
    metal Z18.10
    nonmagnetic metal Z18.12
    nontherapeutic radioactive Z18.09
    organic NEC Z18.39
    plastic Z18.2
    quill(s) (animal) Z18.31
    radioactive (nontherapeutic) NEC Z18.09
    specified NEC Z18.89
    spine(s) (animal) Z18.31
    stone Z18.83
    tooth (teeth) Z18.32
    wood Z18.33

Retained *(Continued)*
  fragments (type of) Z18.9
    acrylics Z18.2
    animal quill(s) or spines Z18.31
    cement Z18.83
  fragments (type of) *(Continued)*
    concrete Z18.83
    crystalline Z18.83
    depleted isotope Z18.09
    depleted uranium Z18.01
    diethylhexyl phthalates Z18.2
    glass Z18.81
    isocyanate Z18.2
    magnetic metal Z18.11
    metal Z18.10
    nonmagnectic metal Z18.12
    nontherapeutic radioactive Z18.09
    organic NEC Z18.39
    plastic Z18.2
    quill(s) (animal) Z18.31
    radioactive (nontherapeutic) NEC Z18.09
    specified NEC Z18.89
    spine(s) (animal) Z18.31
    stone Z18.83
    tooth (teeth) Z18.32
    wood Z18.33
  gallstones, following cholecystectomy K91.86
Retardation
  development, developmental, specific —*see*
      Disorder, developmental
  endochondral bone growth —*see* Disorder,
      bone, development or growth
  growth R62.50
    due to malnutrition E45
  mental —*see* Disability, intellectual
  motor function, specific F82
  physical (child) R62.52
    due to malnutrition E45
  reading (specific) F81.0
  spelling (specific) (without reading disorder)
      F81.81
Retching —*see* Vomiting
Retention —*see also* Retained
  bladder —*see* Retention, urine
  carbon dioxide E87.2
  cholelithiasis following cholecystectomy K91.86
  cyst —*see* Cyst
  dead
    fetus (at or near term) (mother) O36.4
      early fetal death O02.1
    ovum O02.0
  decidua (fragments) (following delivery)
      (with hemorrhage) O72.2
    without hemorrhage O73.1
  deciduous tooth K00.6
  dental root K08.3
  fecal —*see* Constipation
  fetus
    dead O36.4
      early O02.1
  fluid R60.9
  foreign body —*see also* Foreign body, retained
    current trauma - code as Foreign body, by
        site or type
  gallstones, following cholecystectomy K91.86
  gastric K31.89
  intrauterine contraceptive device, in
      pregnancy —*see* Pregnancy, complicated
      by, retention, intrauterine device
  membranes (complicating delivery) (with
      hemorrhage) O72.2
    with abortion —*see* Abortion, by type
    without hemorrhage O73.1
  meniscus —*see* Derangement, meniscus
  menses N94.89
  milk (puerperal, postpartum) O92.79
  nitrogen, extrarenal R39.2
  ovary syndrome N99.83
  placenta (total) (with hemorrhage) O72.0
    without hemorrhage O73.0
    portions or fragments (with hemorrhage)
        O72.2
      without hemorrhage O73.1

Retention *(Continued)*
  products of conception
    early pregnancy (dead fetus) O02.1
    following
      delivery (with hemorrhage) O72.2
        without hemorrhage O73.1
    secundines (following delivery) (with
        hemorrhage) O72.0
      without hemorrhage O73.0
    complicating puerperium (delayed
        hemorrhage) O72.2
    partial O72.2
      without hemorrhage O73.1
  smegma, clitoris N90.89
  urine R33.9
    drug-induced R33.0
    due to hyperplasia (hypertrophy) of
        prostate —*see* Hyperplasia, prostate
    organic R33.8
      drug-induced R33.0
    psychogenic F45.8
    specified NEC R33.8
  water (in tissues) —*see* Edema
Reticular erythematous mucinosis L98.5
Reticulation, dust —*see* Pneumoconiosis
Reticulocytosis R70.1
Reticuloendotheliosis
  acute infantile C96.0
  leukemic C91.4-●
  nonlipid C96.0
Reticulohistiocytoma (giant-cell) D76.3
Reticuloid, actinic L57.1
Reticulosis (skin)
  acute of infancy C96.0
  hemophagocytic, familial D76.1
  histiocytic medullary C96.A
  lipomelanotic I89.8
  malignant (midline) C86.0
  polymorphic C86.0
  Sézary —*see* Sézary disease
Retina, retinal —*see also* condition
  dark area D49.81
Retinitis —*see also* Inflammation, chorioretinal
  albuminurica N18.9 *[H32]*
  diabetic —*see* Diabetes, retinitis
  disciformis —*see* Degeneration, macula
  focal —*see* Inflammation, chorioretinal, focal
  gravidarum —*see* Pregnancy, complicated by,
      specified pregnancy-related condition
      NEC
  juxtapapillaris —*see* Inflammation,
      chorioretinal, focal, juxtapapillary
  luetic —*see* Retinitis, syphilitic
  pigmentosa H35.52
  proliferans —*see* Disorder, globe,
      degenerative, specified type NEC
  proliferating —*see* Disorder, globe,
      degenerative, specified type NEC
  renal N18.9 *[H32]*
  syphilitic (early) (secondary) A51.43
    central, recurrent A52.71
    congenital (early) A50.01 *[H32]*
    late A52.71
  tuberculous A18.53
Retinoblastoma C69.2-●
  differentiated C69.2-●
  undifferentiated C69.2-●
Retinochoroiditis —*see also* Inflammation,
    chorioretinal
  disseminated —*see* Inflammation,
      chorioretinal, disseminated
    syphilitic A52.71
  focal —*see* Inflammation, chorioretinal
  juxtapapillaris —*see* Inflammation,
      chorioretinal, focal, juxtapapillary
Retinopathy (background) H35.00
  arteriosclerotic I70.8 *[H35.0-●]*
  atherosclerotic I70.8 *[H35.0-●]*
  central serous —*see* Chorioretinopathy,
      central serous
  Coats H35.02-●

▶ New   ⇒ Revised   ~~deleted~~ Deleted   ● Use Additional Character(s)

Retinopathy (Continued)
 diabetic —see Diabetes, retinopathy
 exudative H35.02-●
 hypertensive H35.03-●
 in (due to)
  diabetes —see Diabetes, retinopathy
 sickle-cell disorders D57.-● [H36]
 of prematurity H35.10-●
  stage 0 H35.11-●
  stage 1 H35.12-●
  stage 2 H35.13-●
  stage 3 H35.14-●
  stage 4 H35.15-●
  stage 5 H35.16-●
 pigmentary, congenital —see Dystrophy,
  retina
 proliferative NEC H35.2-●
  diabetic —see Diabetes, retinopathy,
   proliferative
  sickle-cell D57.-● [H36]
 solar H31.02-●
Retinoschisis H33.10-●
 congenital Q14.1
 specified type NEC H33.19-●
Retortamoniasis A07.8
Retractile testis Q55.22
Retraction
 cervix —see Retroversion, uterus
 drum (membrane) —see Disorder, tympanic
  membrane, specified NEC
 finger —see Deformity, finger
 lid H02.539
  left H02.536
   lower H02.535
   upper H02.534
  right H02.533
   lower H02.532
   upper H02.531
 lung J98.4
 mediastinum J98.59
 nipple N64.53
  associated with
   lactation O92.03
   pregnancy O92.01-●
   puerperium O92.02
  congenital Q83.8
 palmar fascia M72.0
 pleura —see Pleurisy
 ring, uterus (Bandl's) (pathological)
  O62.4
 sternum (congenital) Q76.7
  acquired M95.4
 uterus —see Retroversion, uterus
 valve (heart) —see Endocarditis
Retrobulbar —see condition
Retrocecal —see condition
Retrocession —see Retroversion
Retrodisplacement —see Retroversion
Retroflection, retroflexion —see Retroversion
Retrognathia, retrognathism (mandibular)
 (maxillary) M26.19
Retrograde menstruation N92.5
Retroperineal —see condition
Retroperitoneal —see condition
Retroperitonitis K68.9
Retropharyngeal —see condition
Retroplacental —see condition
Retroposition —see Retroversion
Retroprosthetic membrane T85.398
Retrosternal thyroid (congenital)
 Q89.2
Retroversion, retroverted
 cervix —see Retroversion, uterus
 female NEC —see Retroversion, uterus
 iris H21.89
 testis (congenital) Q55.29
 uterus (acquired) (acute) (any degree)
  (asymptomatic) (cervix) (postinfectional)
  (postpartal, old) N85.4
  congenital Q51.818
  in pregnancy O34.53-●

Retrovirus, as cause of disease classified
 elsewhere B97.30
 human
  immunodeficiency, type 2 (HIV 2) B97.35
  T-cell lymphotropic
   type I (HTLV-I) B97.33
   type II (HTLV-II) B97.34
 lentivirus B97.31
 oncovirus B97.32
 specified NEC B97.39
Retrusion, premaxilla (developmental) M26.09
Rett's disease or syndrome F84.2
Reverse peristalsis R19.2
Reye's syndrome G93.7
Rh (factor)
 hemolytic disease (newborn) P55.0
 incompatibility, immunization or sensitization
  affecting management of pregnancy NEC
   O36.09-●
   anti-D antibody O36.01-●
  newborn P55.0
  transfusion reaction —see Complication(s),
   transfusion, incompatibility reaction,
   Rh (factor)
 negative mother affecting newborn P55.0
 titer elevated —see Complication(s),
  transfusion, incompatibility reaction, Rh
  (factor)
 transfusion reaction —see Complication(s),
  transfusion, incompatibility reaction, Rh
  (factor)
Rhabdomyolysis (idiopathic) **NEC** M62.82
 traumatic T79.6
Rhabdomyoma —see also Neoplasm, connective
 tissue, benign
 adult —see Neoplasm, connective tissue, benign
 fetal —see Neoplasm, connective tissue, benign
 glycogenic —see Neoplasm, connective tissue,
  benign
Rhabdomyosarcoma (any type) —see
 Neoplasm, connective tissue, malignant
Rhabdosarcoma —see Rhabdomyosarcoma
Rhesus (factor) **incompatibility** —see Rh,
 incompatibility
Rheumatic (acute) (subacute)
 adherent pericardium I09.2
 chronic I09.89
 coronary arteritis I01.8
 degeneration, myocardium I09.0
 fever (acute) —see Fever, rheumatic
 heart —see Disease, heart, rheumatic
 myocardial degeneration —see Degeneration,
  myocardium
 myocarditis (chronic) (inactive) (with chorea)
  I09.0
  with chorea (acute) (rheumatic)
   (Sydenham's) I02.0
  active or acute I01.2
 pancarditis, acute I01.8
  with chorea (acute) (rheumatic)
   Sydenham's) I02.0
 pericarditis (active) (acute) (with effusion)
  (with pneumonia) I01.0
  with chorea (acute) (rheumatic)
   (Sydenham's) I02.0
  chronic or inactive I09.2
 pneumonia I00 [J17]
 torticollis M43.6
 typhoid fever A01.09
Rheumatism (articular) (neuralgic)
 (nonarticular) M79.0
 gout —see Arthritis, rheumatoid
 intercostal, meaning Tietze's disease M94.0
 palindromic (any site) M12.30
  ankle M12.37-●
  elbow M12.32-●
  foot joint M12.37-●
  hand joint M12.34-●
  hip M12.35-●
  knee M12.36-●
  multiple site M12.39

Rheumatism (Continued)
 palindromic (Continued)
  shoulder M12.31-●
  specified joint NEC M12.38
  vertebrae M12.38
  wrist M12.33-●
 sciatic M54.4-●
Rheumatoid —see also condition
 arthritis —see also Arthritis, rheumatoid
  with involvement of organs NEC M05.60
   ankle M05.67-●
   elbow M05.62-●
   foot joint M05.67-●
   hand joint M05.64-●
   hip M05.65-●
   knee M05.66-●
   multiple site M05.69
   shoulder M05.61-●
   vertebra —see Spondylitis, ankylosing
   wrist M05.63-●
  seronegative —see Arthritis, rheumatoid,
   seronegative
  seropositive —see Arthritis, rheumatoid,
   seropositive
 carditis M05.30
  ankle M05.37-●
  elbow M05.32-●
  foot joint M05.37-●
  hand joint M05.34-●
  hip M05.35-●
  knee M05.36-●
  multiple site M05.39
  shoulder M05.31-●
  vertebra —see Spondylitis, ankylosing
  wrist M05.33-●
 endocarditis —see Rheumatoid, carditis
 lung (disease) M05.10
  ankle M05.17-●
  elbow M05.12-●
  foot joint M05.17-●
  hand joint M05.14-●
  hip M05.15-●
  knee M05.16-●
  multiple site M05.19
  shoulder M05.11-●
  vertebra —see Spondylitis, ankylosing
  wrist M05.13 -●
 myocarditis —see Rheumatoid, carditis
 myopathy M05.40
  ankle M05.47-●
  elbow M05.42-●
  foot joint M05.47-●
  hand joint M05.44-●
  hip M05.45-●
  knee M05.46-●
  multiple site M05.49
  shoulder M05.41-●
  vertebra —see Spondylitis, ankylosing
  wrist M05.43-●
 pericarditis —see Rheumatoid, carditis
 polyarthritis —see Arthritis, rheumatoid
 polyneuropathy M05.50
  ankle M05.57-●
  elbow M05.52-●
  foot joint M05.57-●
  hand joint M05.54-●
  hip M05.55-●
  knee M05.56-●
  multiple site M05.59
  shoulder M05.51-●
  vertebra —see Spondylitis, ankylosing
  wrist M05.53-●
 vasculitis M05.20
  ankle M05.27-●
  elbow M05.22-●
  foot joint M05.27-●
  hand joint M05.24-●
  hip M05.25-●
  knee M05.26-●
  multiple site M05.29
  shoulder M05.21-●
  vertebra —see Spondylitis, ankylosing
  wrist M05.23-●

Rhinitis (atrophic) (catarrhal) (chronic)
  (croupous) (fibrinous) (granulomatous)
  (hyperplastic) (hypertrophic)
  (membranous) (obstructive) (purulent)
  (suppurative) (ulcerative) J31.0
  with
    sore throat —*see* Nasopharyngitis
  acute J00
  allergic J30.9
    with asthma J45.909
      with
        exacerbation (acute) J45.901
        status asthmaticus J45.902
      due to
        food J30.5
        pollen J30.1
      nonseasonal J30.89
      perennial J30.89
      seasonal NEC J30.2
      specified NEC J30.89
  infective J00
  pneumococcal J00
  syphilitic A52.73
    congenital A50.05 [J99]
  tuberculous A15.8
  vasomotor J30.0
Rhinoantritis (chronic) —*see* Sinusitis,
  maxillary
Rhinodacryolith —*see* Dacryolith
Rhinolith (nasal sinus) J34.89
Rhinomegaly J34.89
Rhinopharyngitis (acute) (subacute) —*see also*
  Nasopharyngitis
  chronic J31.1
  destructive ulcerating A66.5
  mutilans A66.5
Rhinophyma L71.1
Rhinorrhea J34.89
  cerebrospinal (fluid) G96.01
    postoperative G96.08
    specified NEC G96.08
    spontaneous G96.01
    traumatic G96.08
  paroxysmal —*see* Rhinitis, allergic
  spasmodic —*see* Rhinitis, allergic
Rhinosalpingitis —*see* Salpingitis, eustachian
Rhinoscleroma A48.8
Rhinosporidiosis B48.1
Rhinovirus infection NEC B34.8
Rhizomelic chondrodysplasia punctata E71.540
Rhythm
  atrioventricular nodal I49.8
  disorder I49.9
    coronary sinus I49.8
    ectopic I49.8
    nodal I49.8
  escape I49.9
  heart, abnormal I49.9
  idioventricular I44.2
  nodal I49.8
  sleep, inversion G47.2-●
    nonorganic origin —*see* Disorder, sleep,
      circadian rhythm, psychogenic
Rhytidosis facialis L98.8
Rib —*see also* condition
  cervical Q76.5
Riboflavin deficiency E53.0
Rice bodies —*see also* Loose, body, joint
  knee M23.4-●
Richter syndrome —*see* Leukemia, chronic
  lymphocytic, B-cell type
Richter's hernia —*see* Hernia, abdomen, with
  obstruction
Ricinism —*see* Poisoning, food, noxious, plant
Rickets (active) (acute) (adolescent) (chest wall)
  (congenital) (current) (infantile) (intestinal)
  E55.0
  adult —*see* Osteomalacia
  celiac K90.0
  hypophosphatemic with nephrotic-glycosuric
    dwarfism E72.09

Rickets *(Continued)*
  inactive E64.3
  kidney N25.0
  renal N25.0
  sequelae, any E64.3
  vitamin-D-resistant E83.31 [M90.80]
**Rickettsia 364D/R. philipii (Pacific Coast tick
  fever)** A77.8
Rickettsial disease A79.9
  specified type NEC A79.89
Rickettsialpox (Rickettsia akari) A79.1
Rickettsiosis A79.9
  due to
    Ehrlichia sennetsu A79.81
    Neorickettsia sennetsu A79.81
    Rickettsia akari (rickettsialpox) A79.1
  specified type NEC A79.89
  tick-borne A77.9
  vesicular A79.1
Rider's bone —*see* Ossification, muscle,
  specified NEC
Ridge, alveolus —*see also* condition
  flabby K06.8
Ridged ear, congenital Q17.3
Riedel's
  lobe, liver Q44.7
  struma, thyroiditis or disease E06.5
Rieger's anomaly or syndrome Q13.81
Riehl's melanosis L81.4
Rietti-Greppi-Micheli anemia D56.9
Rieux's hernia —*see* Hernia, abdomen, specified
  site NEC
Riga (-Fede) disease K14.0
Riggs' disease —*see* Periodontitis
Right aortic arch Q25.47
Right middle lobe syndrome J98.11
Rigid, rigidity —*see also* condition
  abdominal R19.30
    with severe abdominal pain R10.0
    epigastric R19.36
    generalized R19.37
    left lower quadrant R19.34
    left upper quadrant R19.32
    periumbilic R19.35
    right lower quadrant R19.33
    right upper quadrant R19.31
  articular, multiple, congenital Q68.8
  cervix (uteri) in pregnancy —*see* Pregnancy,
    complicated by, abnormal, cervix
  hymen (acquired) (congenital) N89.6
  nuchal R29.1
  pelvic floor in pregnancy —*see* Pregnancy,
    complicated by, abnormal, pelvic organs
    or tissues NEC
  perineum or vulva in pregnancy —*see*
    Pregnancy, complicated by, abnormal,
    vulva
  spine —*see* Dorsopathy, specified NEC
  vagina in pregnancy —*see* Pregnancy,
    complicated by, abnormal, vagina
Rigors R68.89
  with fever R50.9
Riley-Day syndrome G90.1
RIND (reversible ischemic neurologic deficit)
  I63.9
Ring(s)
  aorta (vascular) Q25.45
  Bandl's O62.4
  contraction, complicating delivery O62.4
  esophageal, lower (muscular) K22.2
  Fleischer's (cornea) H18.04-●
  hymenal, tight (acquired) (congenital)
    N89.6
  Kayser-Fleischer (cornea) H18.04-●
  retraction, uterus, pathological O62.4
  Schatzki's (esophagus) (lower) K22.2
    congenital Q39.3
  Soemmerring's —*see* Cataract, secondary
  vascular (congenital) Q25.8
    aorta Q25.45
Ringed hair (congenital) Q84.1

Ringworm B35.9
  beard B35.0
  black dot B35.0
  body B35.4
  Burmese B35.5
  corporeal B35.4
  foot B35.3
  groin B35.6
  hand B35.2
  honeycomb B35.0
  nails B35.1
  perianal (area) B35.6
  scalp B35.0
  specified NEC B35.8
  Tokelau B35.5
Rise, venous pressure I87.8
**Rising, PSA following treatment for malignant
  neoplasm of prostate** R97.21
Risk
  for
    dental caries Z91.849
      high Z91.843
      low Z91.841
      moderate Z91.842
    ►homelessness, imminent Z59.811
  suicidal
    ⇒meaning personal history of attempted
        suicide Z91.51
    meaning suicidal ideation —*see* Ideation,
        suicidal
Ritter's disease L00
Rivalry, sibling Z62.891
Rivalta's disease A42.2
River blindness B73.01
Robert's pelvis Q74.2
  with disproportion (fetopelvic) O33.0
    causing obstructed labor O65.0
Robin (-Pierre) syndrome Q87.0
Robinow-Silvermann-Smith syndrome Q87.19
Robinson's (hidrotic) ectodermal dysplasia or
  syndrome Q82.4
Robles' disease B73.01
Rocky Mountain (spotted) **fever** A77.0
Roetheln —*see* Rubella
Roger's disease Q21.0
Rokitansky-Aschoff sinuses (gallbladder) K82.8
Rolando's fracture (displaced) S62.22-●
  nondisplaced S62.22-●
Romano-Ward (prolonged QT interval)
  syndrome I45.81
Romberg's disease or syndrome G51.8
Roof, mouth —*see* condition
Rosacea L71.9
  acne L71.9
  keratitis L71.8
  specified NEC L71.8
Rosary, rachitic E55.0
Rose
  cold J30.1
  fever J30.1
  rash R21
    epidemic B06.9
Rosenbach's erysipeloid A26.0
Rosenthal's disease or syndrome D68.1
Roseola B09
  infantum B08.20
    due to human herpesvirus 6 B08.21
    due to human herpesvirus 7 B08.22
Ross River disease or fever B33.1
Rossbach's disease K31.89
  psychogenic F45.8
Rostan's asthma (cardiac) —*see* Failure,
  ventricular, left
Rotation
  anomalous, incomplete or insufficient,
    intestine Q43.3
  cecum (congenital) Q43.3
  colon (congenital) Q43.3
  spine, incomplete or insufficient —*see*
    Dorsopathy, deforming, specified NEC
  tooth, teeth, fully erupted M26.35
  vertebra, incomplete or insufficient —*see*
    Dorsopathy, deforming, specified NEC

▶ New   ⇒ Revised   ~~deleted~~ Deleted   ● Use Additional Character(s)

Rotes Quérol disease or syndrome —see
    Hyperostosis, ankylosing
Roth (-Bernhardt) disease or syndrome —see
    Meralgia paraesthetica
Rothmund (-Thomson) syndrome Q82.8
Rotor's disease or syndrome E80.6
Round
    back (with wedging of vertebrae) —see
        Kyphosis
    sequelae (late effect) of rickets E64.3
    worms (large) (infestation) NEC B82.0
        Ascariasis —see also Ascariasis B77.9
Roussy-Lévy syndrome G60.0
Rubella (German measles) B06.9
    complication NEC B06.09
        neurological B06.00
    congenital P35.0
    contact Z20.4
    exposure to Z20.4
    maternal
        care for (suspected) damage to fetus O35.3
        manifest rubella in infant P35.0
        suspected damage to fetus affecting
            management of pregnancy O35.3
    specified complications NEC B06.89
Rubeola (meaning measles) —see Measles
    meaning rubella —see Rubella
Rubeosis, iris —see Disorder, iris, vascular
Rubinstein-Taybi syndrome Q87.2
Rudimentary (congenital) —see also Agenesis
    arm —see Defect, reduction, upper limb
    bone Q79.9
    cervix uteri Q51.828
    eye Q11.2
    lobule of ear Q17.3
    patella Q74.1
    respiratory organs in thoracopagus Q89.4
    tracheal bronchus Q32.4
    uterus Q51.818
        in male Q56.1
    vagina Q52.0
Ruled out condition —see Observation,
    suspected
Rumination R11.10
    with nausea R11.2
    disorder of infancy F98.21
    neurotic F42.8
    newborn P92.1
    obsessional F42.8
    psychogenic F42.8
Runeberg's disease D51.0
Runny nose R09.89
Rupia (syphilitic) A51.39
    congenital A50.06
    tertiary A52.79
Rupture, ruptured
    abscess (spontaneous) - code by site under
        Abscess
    aneurysm —see Aneurysm
    anus (sphincter) —see Laceration, anus
    aorta, aortic I71.8
        abdominal I71.3
        arch I71.1
        ascending I71.1
        descending I71.8
            abdominal I71.3
            thoracic I71.1
        syphilitic A52.01
        thoracoabdominal I71.5
        thorax, thoracic I71.1
        transverse I71.1
        traumatic —see Injury, aorta, laceration,
            major
        valve or cusp —see also Endocarditis, aortic
            I35.8
    appendix (with peritonitis) (see also
        Appendicitis) K35.32
        with localized peritonitis (see also
            Appendicitis) K35.32
    arteriovenous fistula, brain —see Fistula,
        arteriovenous, brain, ruptured

Rupture, ruptured (Continued)
    artery I77.2
        brain —see Hemorrhage, intracranial,
            intracerebral
        coronary —see Infarct, myocardium
        heart —see Infarct, myocardium
        pulmonary I28.8
        traumatic (complication) —see Injury,
            blood vessel
    bile duct (common) (hepatic) K83.2
        cystic K82.2
    bladder (sphincter) (nontraumatic)
        (spontaneous) N32.89
        following ectopic or molar pregnancy
            O08.6
        obstetrical trauma O71.5
        traumatic S37.29
    blood vessel —see also Hemorrhage
        brain —see Hemorrhage, intracranial,
            intracerebral
        heart —see Infarct, myocardium
        traumatic (complication) —see Injury,
            blood vessel, laceration, major, by site
    bone —see Fracture
    bowel (nontraumatic) K63.1
    brain
        aneurysm (congenital) —see also
            Hemorrhage, intracranial,
            subarachnoid
            syphilitic A52.05
        hemorrhagic —see Hemorrhage,
            intracranial, intracerebral
    capillaries I78.8
    cardiac (auricle) (ventricle) (wall) I23.3
        with hemopericardium I23.0
        infectional I40.9
        traumatic —see Injury, heart
    cartilage (articular) (current) —see also Sprain
        knee S83.3-●
        semilunar —see Tear, meniscus
    cecum (with peritonitis) K65.0
        with peritoneal abscess K65.33
        traumatic S36.598
    celiac artery, traumatic —see Injury, blood
        vessel, celiac artery, laceration, major
    cerebral aneurysm (congenital) (see
        Hemorrhage, intracranial, subarachnoid)
    cervix (uteri)
        with ectopic or molar pregnancy O08.6
        following ectopic or molar pregnancy O08.6
        obstetrical trauma O71.3
        traumatic S37.69
    chordae tendineae NEC I51.1
        concurrent with acute myocardial
            infarction —see Infarct, myocardium
        following acute myocardial infarction
            (current complication) I23.4
    choroid (direct) (indirect) (traumatic) H31.32-●
    circle of Willis I60.6
    colon (nontraumatic) K63.1
        traumatic —see Injury, intestine, large
    cornea (traumatic) —see Injury, eye, laceration
    coronary (artery) (thrombotic) —see Infarct,
        myocardium
    corpus luteum (infected) (ovary) N83.1-●
    cyst —see Cyst
    cystic duct K82.2
    Descemet's membrane —see Change, corneal
        membrane, Descemet's, rupture
        traumatic —see Injury, eye, laceration
    diaphragm, traumatic —see Injury,
        intrathoracic, diaphragm
    disc —see Rupture, intervertebral disc
    diverticulum (intestine) K57.80
        with bleeding K57.81
        bladder N32.3
        large intestine K57.20
            with
                bleeding K57.21
                small intestine K57.40
                    with bleeding K57.41

Rupture, ruptured (Continued)
    diverticulum (Continued)
        small intestine K57.00
            with
                bleeding K57.01
                large intestine K57.40
                    with bleeding K57.41
    duodenal stump K31.89
    ear drum (nontraumatic) —see also
        Perforation, tympanum
        traumatic S09.2-●
            due to blast injury —see Injury, blast, ear
    esophagus K22.3
    eye (without prolapse or loss of intraocular
        tissue) —see Injury, eye, laceration
    fallopian tube NEC (nonobstetric)
        (nontraumatic) N83.8
        due to pregnancy O00.10-●
            with intrauterine pregnancy O00.11-●
    fontanel P13.1
    gallbladder K82.2
        traumatic S36.128
    gastric —see also Rupture, stomach
        vessel K92.2
    globe (eye) (traumatic) —see Injury, eye,
        laceration
    graafian follicle (hematoma) N83.0-●
    heart —see Rupture, cardiac
    hymen (nontraumatic) (nonintentional) N89.8
    internal organ, traumatic —see Injury, by site
    intervertebral disc —see Displacement,
        intervertebral disc
        traumatic —see Rupture, traumatic,
            intervertebral disc
    intestine NEC (nontraumatic) K63.1
        traumatic —see Injury, intestine
    iris —see also Abnormality, pupillary
        traumatic —see Injury, eye, laceration
    joint capsule, traumatic —see Sprain
    kidney (traumatic) S37.06-●
        birth injury P15.8
        nontraumatic N28.89
    lacrimal duct (traumatic) —see Injury, eye,
        specified site NEC
    lens (cataract) (traumatic) —see Cataract,
        traumatic
    ligament, traumatic —see Rupture, traumatic,
        ligament, by site
    liver S36.116
        birth injury P15.0
    lymphatic vessel I89.8
    marginal sinus (placental) (with
        hemorrhage) —see Hemorrhage,
        antepartum, specified cause NEC
    membrana tympani (nontraumatic) —see
        Perforation, tympanum
    membranes (spontaneous)
        artificial
            delayed delivery following O75.5
        delayed delivery following —see
            Pregnancy, complicated by, premature
            rupture of membranes
    meningeal artery I60.8
    meniscus (knee) —see also Tear, meniscus
        old —see Derangement, meniscus
        site other than knee - code as Sprain
    mesenteric artery, traumatic —see Injury,
        mesenteric, artery, laceration, major
    mesentery (nontraumatic) K66.8
        traumatic —see Injury, intra-abdominal,
            specified, site NEC
    mitral (valve) I34.8
    muscle (traumatic) —see also Strain
        diastasis —see Diastasis, muscle
        nontraumatic M62.10
            ankle M62.17-●
            foot M62.17-●
            forearm M62.13-●
            hand M62.14-●
            lower leg M62.16-●
            pelvic region M62.15-●

Rupture, ruptured *(Continued)*
 muscle *(Continued)*
  nontraumatic *(Continued)*
   shoulder region M62.11-●
   specified site NEC M62.18
   thigh M62.15-●
   upper arm M62.12-●
  traumatic —*see* Strain, by site
 musculotendinous junction NEC,
   nontraumatic —*see* Rupture, tendon,
   spontaneous
 mycotic aneurysm causing cerebral
   hemorrhage —*see* Hemorrhage,
   intracranial, subarachnoid
 myocardium, myocardial —*see* Rupture,
   cardiac
  traumatic —*see* Injury, heart
 nontraumatic, meaning hernia —*see* Hernia
 obstructed —*see* Hernia, by site, obstructed
 operation wound —*see* Disruption, wound,
   operation
 ovary, ovarian N83.8
  corpus luteum cyst N83.1-●
  follicle (graafian) N83.0-●
 oviduct (nonobstetric) (nontraumatic)
   N83.8
  due to pregnancy O00.10-●
   with intrauterine pregnancy
     O00.11-●
 pancreas (nontraumatic) K86.89
  traumatic S36.299
 papillary muscle NEC I51.2
  following acute myocardial infarction
     (current complication) I23.5
 pelvic
  floor, complicating delivery O70.1
  organ NEC, obstetrical trauma O71.5
 perineum (nonobstetric) (nontraumatic)
   N90.89
  complicating delivery —*see* Delivery,
     complicated, by, laceration, anus
     (sphincter)
 postoperative wound —*see* Disruption,
   wound, operation
 prostate (traumatic) S37.828
 pulmonary
  artery I28.8
  valve (heart) I37.8
  vein I28.8
  vessel I28.8
 pus tube —*see* Salpingitis
 pyosalpinx —*see* Salpingitis
 rectum (nontraumatic) K63.1
  traumatic S36.69
 retina, retinal (traumatic) (without
     detachment) —*see also* Break, retina
  with detachment —*see* Detachment,
     retina, with retinal, break
 rotator cuff (nontraumatic) M75.10-●
  complete M75.12-●
  incomplete M75.11-●
 sclera —*see* Injury, eye, laceration
 sigmoid (nontraumatic) K63.1
  traumatic S36.593
 spinal cord —*see also* Injury, spinal cord, by
   region
  due to injury at birth P11.5
  newborn (birth injury) P11.5
 spleen (traumatic) S36.09
  birth injury P15.1
  congenital (birth injury) P15.1
  due to P. vivax malaria B51.0
  nontraumatic D73.5
  spontaneous D73.5
 splenic vein R58
  traumatic —*see* Injury, blood vessel,
     splenic vein
 stomach (nontraumatic) (spontaneous)
   K31.89
  traumatic S36.39

 supraspinatus (complete) (incomplete)
     (nontraumatic) —*see* Tear, rotator cuff
 symphysis pubis
  obstetric O71.6
  traumatic S33.4
 synovium (cyst) M66.10
  ankle M66.17-●
  elbow M66.12-●
  finger M66.14-●
  foot M66.17-●
  forearm M66.13-●
  hand M66.14-●
  pelvic region M66.15-●
  shoulder region M66.11-●
  specified site NEC M66.18
  thigh M66.15-●
  toe M66.17-●
  upper arm M66.12-●
  wrist M66.13-●
 tendon (traumatic) —*see* Strain
  nontraumatic (spontaneous) M66.9
   ankle M66.87-●
   extensor M66.20
    ankle M66.27-●
    foot M66.27-●
    forearm M66.23-●
    hand M66.24-●
    lower leg M66.26-●
    multiple sites M66.29
    pelvic region M66.25-●
    shoulder region M66.21-●
    specified site NEC M66.28
    thigh M66.25-●
    upper arm M66.22-●
   flexor M66.30
    ankle M66.37-●
    foot M66.37-●
    forearm M66.33-●
    hand M66.34-●
    lower leg M66.36-●
    multiple sites M66.39
    pelvic region M66.35-●
    shoulder region M66.31-●
    specified site NEC M66.38
    thigh M66.35-●
    upper arm M66.32-●
   foot M66.87-●
   forearm M66.83-●
   hand M66.84-●
   lower leg M66.86-●
   multiple sites M66.89
   pelvic region M66.85-●
   shoulder region M66.81-●
   specified
    site NEC M66.88
    tendon M66.80
   thigh M66.85-●
   upper arm M66.82-●
 thoracic duct I89.8
 tonsil J35.8
 traumatic
  aorta —*see* Injury, aorta, laceration, major
  diaphragm —*see* Injury, intrathoracic,
     diaphragm
  external site —*see* Wound, open, by site
  eye —*see* Injury, eye, laceration
  internal organ —*see* Injury, by site
  intervertebral disc
   cervical S13.0
   lumbar S33.0
   thoracic S23.0
  kidney S37.06-●
  ligament —*see also* Sprain
   ankle —*see* Sprain, ankle
   carpus —*see* Rupture, traumatic,
     ligament, wrist
   collateral (hand) —*see* Rupture,
     traumatic, ligament, finger,
     collateral

 traumatic *(Continued)*
  ligament *(Continued)*
   finger (metacarpophalangeal)
       (interphalangeal) S63.40-●
    collateral S63.41-●
     index S63.41-●
     little S63.41-●
     middle S63.41-●
     ring S63.41-●
    index S63.40-●
    little S63.40-●
    middle S63.40-●
    palmar S63.42-●
     index S63.42-●
     little S63.42-●
     middle S63.42-●
     ring S63.42-●
    ring S63.40-●
    specified site NEC S63.499
     index S63.49-●
     little S63.49-●
     middle S63.49-●
     ring S63.49-●
    volar plate S63.43-●
     index S63.43-●
     little S63.43-●
     middle S63.43-●
     ring S63.43-●
   foot —*see* Sprain, foot
   radial collateral S53.2-●
   radiocarpal —*see* Rupture, traumatic,
     ligament, wrist, radiocarpal
   ulnar collateral S53.3-●
   ulnocarpal —*see* Rupture, traumatic,
     ligament, wrist, ulnocarpal
   wrist S63.30-●
    collateral S63.31-●
    radiocarpal S63.32-●
    specified site NEC S63.39-●
    ulnocarpal (palmar) S63.33-●
  liver S36.116
  membrana tympani —*see* Rupture, ear
     drum, traumatic
  muscle or tendon —*see* Strain
  myocardium —*see* Injury, heart
  pancreas S36.299
  rectum S36.69
  sigmoid S36.593
  spleen S36.09
  stomach S36.39
  symphysis pubis S33.4
  tympanum, tympanic (membrane) —*see*
     Rupture, ear drum, traumatic
  ureter S37.19
  uterus S37.69
  vagina —*see* Injury, vagina
  vena cava —*see* Injury, vena cava,
     laceration, major
 tricuspid (heart) (valve) I07.8
 tube, tubal (nonobstetric) (nontraumatic)
   N83.8
  abscess —*see* Salpingitis
  due to pregnancy O00.10-●
   with intrauterine pregnancy O00.11-●
 tympanum, tympanic (membrane)
     (nontraumatic) —*see also* Perforation,
     tympanic membrane H72.9-●
  traumatic —*see* Rupture, ear drum,
     traumatic
 umbilical cord, complicating delivery
   O69.89
 ureter (traumatic) S37.19
  nontraumatic N28.89
 urethra (nontraumatic) N36.8
  with ectopic or molar pregnancy O08.6
  following ectopic or molar pregnancy
   O08.6
  obstetrical trauma O71.5
  traumatic S37.39

▶ New　　⇒ Revised　　~~deleted~~ Deleted　　● Use Additional Character(s)

Rupture, ruptured (*Continued*)
  uterosacral ligament (nonobstetric)
      (nontraumatic) N83.8
  uterus (traumatic) S37.69
    before labor O71.0-•
    during or after labor O71.1
    nonpuerperal, nontraumatic N85.8
    pregnant (during labor) O71.1
      before labor O71.0-•
  vagina —*see* Injury, vagina
  valve, valvular (heart) —*see* Endocarditis
  varicose vein *see* Varix

Rupture, ruptured (*Continued*)
  varix —*see* Varix
  vena cava R58
    traumatic —*see* Injury, vena cava,
      laceration, major
  vesical (urinary) N32.89
  vessel (blood) R58
    pulmonary I28.8
    traumatic —*see* Injury, blood vessel
  viscus R19.8
  vulva complicating delivery O70.0

Russell-Silver syndrome Q87.19
Russian spring-summer type encephalitis A84.0
Rust's disease (tuberculous cervical spondylitis) A18.01
Ruvalcaba-Myhre-Smith syndrome E71.440
Rytand-Lipsitch syndrome I44.2

S

Saber, sabre shin or tibia (syphilitic) A50.56
  [M90.8-●]
Sac lacrimal —*see* condition
Saccharomyces infection B37.9
Saccharopinuria E72.3
Saccular —*see* condition
Sacculation
  aorta (nonsyphilitic) —*see* Aneurysm, aorta
  bladder N32.3
  intralaryngeal (congenital) (ventricular)
    Q31.3
  larynx (congenital) (ventricular) Q31.3
  organ or site, congenital —*see* Distortion
  pregnant uterus —*see* Pregnancy, complicated
    by, abnormal, uterus
  ureter N28.89
  urethra N36.1
  vesical N32.3
Sachs' amaurotic familial idiocy or disease
  E75.02
Sachs-Tay disease E75.02
Sacks-Libman disease M32.11
Sacralgia M53.3
Sacralization Q76.49
Sacrodynia M53.3
Sacroiliac joint —*see* condition
Sacroiliitis NEC M46.1
Sacrum —*see* condition
Saddle
  back —*see* Lordosis
  embolus
    abdominal aorta I74.01
    pulmonary artery I26.92
      with acute cor pulmonale I26.02
  injury — code to condition
  nose M95.0
    due to syphilis A50.57
Sadism (sexual) F65.52
Sadness, postpartal O90.6
Sadomasochism F65.50
Saemisch's ulcer (cornea) —*see* Ulcer, cornea,
    central
Sagging
  skin and subcutaneous tissue (following
    bariatric surgery weight loss) (following
    dietary weight loss) L98.7
Sahib disease B55.0
Sailors' skin L57.8
Saint
  Anthony's fire —*see* Erysipelas
  triad —*see* Hernia, diaphragm
  Vitus' dance —*see* Chorea, Sydenham's
Salaam
  attack(s) —*see* Epilepsy, spasms
  tic R25.8
Salicylism
  abuse F55.8
  overdose or wrong substance given —*see*
    Table of Drugs and Chemicals, by drug,
    poisoning
Salivary duct or gland —*see* condition
Salivation, excessive K11.7
Salmonella —*see* Infection, Salmonella
Salmonellosis A02.0
Salpingitis (catarrhal) (fallopian tube) (nodular)
    (pseudofollicular) (purulent) (septic)
    N70.91
  with oophoritis N70.93
  acute N70.01
    with oophoritis N70.03
  chlamydial A56.11
  chronic N70.11
    with oophoritis N70.13
  complicating abortion —*see* Abortion, by
    type, complicated by, salpingitis
  ear —*see* Salpingitis, eustachian
  eustachian (tube) H68.00-●
    acute H68.01-●
    chronic H68.02-●

Salpingitis *(Continued)*
  follicularis N70.11
    with oophoritis N70.13
  gonococcal (acute) (chronic) A54.24
  interstitial, chronic N70.11
    with oophoritis N70.13
  isthmica nodosa N70.11
    with oophoritis N70.13
  specific (gonococcal) (acute) (chronic) A54.24
  tuberculous (acute) (chronic) A18.17
  venereal (gonococcal) (acute) (chronic) A54.24
Salpingocele N83.4-●
Salpingo-oophoritis (catarrhal) (purulent)
    (ruptured) (septic) (suppurative) N70.93
  acute N70.03
    with ectopic or molar pregnancy O08.0
    following ectopic or molar pregnancy
      O08.0
    gonococcal A54.24
  chronic N70.13
  following ectopic or molar pregnancy O08.0
  gonococcal (acute) (chronic) A54.24
  puerperal O86.19
  specific (gonococcal) (acute) (chronic) A54.24
  subacute N70.03
  tuberculous (acute) (chronic) A18.17
  venereal (gonococcal) (acute) (chronic) A54.24
Salpingo-ovaritis —*see* Salpingo-oophoritis
Salpingoperitonitis —*see* Salpingo-oophoritis
Salzmann's nodular dystrophy —*see*
    Degeneration, cornea, nodular
Sampson's cyst or tumor N80.1
San Joaquin (Valley) **fever** B38.0
Sandblaster's asthma, lung or pneumoconiosis
    J62.8
Sander's disease (paranoia) F22
Sandfly fever A93.1
Sandhoff's disease E75.01
Sanfilippo (Type B) (Type C) (Type D)
    syndrome E76.22
Sanger-Brown ataxia G11.2
Sao Paulo fever or typhus A77.0
Saponification, mesenteric K65.8
Sarcocele (benign)
  syphilitic A52.76
    congenital A50.59
Sarcocystosis A07.8
Sarcoepiplocele —*see* Hernia
Sarcoepiplomphalocele Q79.2
Sarcoid —*see also* Sarcoidosis
  arthropathy D86.86
  Boeck's D86.9
  Darier-Roussy D86.3
  iridocyclitis D86.83
  meningitis D86.81
  myocarditis D86.85
  myositis D86.87
  pyelonephritis D86.84
  Spiegler-Fendt L08.89
Sarcoidosis D86.9
  with
    cranial nerve palsies D86.82
    hepatic granuloma D86.89
    polyarthritis D86.86
    tubulo-interstitial nephropathy D86.84
  combined sites NEC D86.89
  lung D86.0
    and lymph nodes D86.2
  lymph nodes D86.1
    and lung D86.2
  meninges D86.81
  skin D86.3
  specified type NEC D86.89
Sarcoma (of) —*see also* Neoplasm, connective
    tissue, malignant
  alveolar soft part —*see* Neoplasm, connective
    tissue, malignant
  ameloblastic C41.1
    upper jaw (bone) C41.0
  botryoid —*see* Neoplasm, connective tissue,
    malignant

Sarcoma *(Continued)*
  botryoides —*see* Neoplasm, connective tissue,
    malignant
  cerebellar C71.6
    circumscribed (arachnoidal) C71.6
  circumscribed (arachnoidal) cerebellar
    C71.6
  clear cell —*see also* Neoplasm, connective
    tissue, malignant
    kidney C64.-●
  dendritic cells (accessory cells) C96.4
  embryonal —*see* Neoplasm, connective tissue,
    malignant
  endometrial (stromal) C54.1
    isthmus C54.0
  epithelioid (cell) —*see* Neoplasm, connective
    tissue, malignant
  Ewing's —*see* Neoplasm, bone, malignant
  follicular dendritic cell C96.4
  germinoblastic (diffuse) —*see* Lymphoma,
    diffuse, large cell
    follicular —*see* Lymphoma, follicular,
      specified NEC
  giant cell (except of bone) —*see also*
    Neoplasm, connective tissue, malignant
    bone —*see* Neoplasm, bone, malignant
  glomoid —*see* Neoplasm, connective tissue,
    malignant
  granulocytic C92.3-●
  hemangioendothelial —*see* Neoplasm,
    connective tissue, malignant
  hemorrhagic, multiple —*see* Sarcoma,
    Kaposi's
  histiocytic C96.A
  Hodgkin —*see* Lymphoma, Hodgkin
  immunoblastic (diffuse) —*see* Lymphoma,
    diffuse large cell
  interdigitating dendritic cell C96.4
  Kaposi's
    colon C46.4
    connective tissue C46.1
    gastrointestinal organ C46.4
    lung C46.5-●
    lymph node(s) C46.3
    palate (hard) (soft) C46.2
    rectum C46.4
    skin C46.0
    specified site NEC C46.7
    stomach C46.4
    unspecified site C46.9
  Kupffer cell C22.3
  Langerhans cell C96.4
  leptomeningeal —*see* Neoplasm, meninges,
    malignant
  liver NEC C22.4
  lymphangioendothelial —*see* Neoplasm,
    connective tissue, malignant
  lymphoblastic —*see* Lymphoma,
    lymphoblastic (diffuse)
  lymphocytic —*see* Lymphoma, small cell
    B-cell
  mast cell C96.22
  melanotic —*see* Melanoma
  meningeal —*see* Neoplasm, meninges,
    malignant
  meningothelial —*see* Neoplasm, meninges,
    malignant
  mesenchymal —*see also* Neoplasm,
    connective tissue, malignant
    mixed —*see* Neoplasm, connective tissue,
      malignant
  mesothelial —*see* Mesothelioma
  monstrocellular
    specified site —*see* Neoplasm, malignant,
      by site
    unspecified site C71.9
  myeloid C92.3-●
  neurogenic —*see* Neoplasm, nerve,
    malignant
  odontogenic C41.1
    upper jaw (bone) C41.0

▶ New   ⇒ Revised   ~~deleted~~ Deleted   ● Use Additional Character(s)

Sarcoma *(Continued)*
   osteoblastic —*see* Neoplasm, bone, malignant
   osteogenic —*see also* Neoplasm, bone, malignant
      juxtacortical —*see* Neoplasm, bone, malignant
      periosteal —*see* Neoplasm, bone, malignant
   periosteal —*see also* Neoplasm, bone, malignant
      osteogenic —*see* Neoplasm, bone, malignant
   pleomorphic cell —*see* Neoplasm, connective tissue, malignant
   reticulum cell (diffuse) —*see* Lymphoma, diffuse large cell
      nodular —*see* Lymphoma, follicular
      pleomorphic cell type —*see* Lymphoma, diffuse large cell
   rhabdoid —*see* Neoplasm, malignant, by site
   round cell —*see* Neoplasm, connective tissue, malignant
   small cell —*see* Neoplasm, connective tissue, malignant
   soft tissue —*see* Neoplasm, connective tissue, malignant
   spindle cell —*see* Neoplasm, connective tissue, malignant
   stromal (endometrial) C54.1
      isthmus C54.0
   synovial —*see also* Neoplasm, connective tissue, malignant
      biphasic —*see* Neoplasm, connective tissue, malignant
      epithelioid cell —*see* Neoplasm, connective tissue, malignant
      spindle cell —*see* Neoplasm, connective tissue, malignant
Sarcomatosis
   meningeal —*see* Neoplasm, meninges, malignant
   specified site NEC —*see* Neoplasm, connective tissue, malignant
   unspecified site C80.1
Sarcopenia (age-related) M62.84
Sarcosinemia E72.59
Sarcosporidiosis (intestinal) A07.8
▶ SARS-CoV-2 —*see also* COVID-19
   ▶ sequelae (post acute) U09.9
Satiety, early R68.81
Saturnine —*see* condition
Saturnism
   overdose or wrong substance given or taken —*see* Table of Drugs and Chemicals, by drug, poisoning
Satyriasis F52.8
Sauriasis —*see* Ichthyosis
SBE (subacute bacterial endocarditis) I33.0
Scabies (any site) B86
Scabs R23.4
Scaglietti-Dagnini syndrome E22.0
Scald —*see* Burn
Scalenus anticus (anterior) syndrome G54.0
Scales R23.4
Scaling, skin R23.4
Scalp —*see* condition
Scapegoating affecting child Z62.3
Scaphocephaly Q75.0
Scapulalgia M89.8X1
Scapulohumeral myopathy G71.02
Scar, scarring —*see also* Cicatrix L90.5
   adherent L90.5
   atrophic L90.5
   cervix
      in pregnancy or childbirth —*see* Pregnancy, complicated by, abnormal cervix
   cheloid L91.0
   chorioretinal H31.00-●
      posterior pole macula H31.01-●
      postsurgical H59.81-●
      solar retinopathy H31.02-●
      specified type NEC H31.09-●

Scar, scarring *(Continued)*
   choroid —*see* Scar, chorioretinal
   conjunctiva H11.24-●
   cornea H17.9
      xerophthalmic —*see also* Opacity, cornea vitamin A deficiency E50.6
   defect (isthmocele) O34.22
   duodenum, obstructive K31.5
   hypertrophic L91.0
   keloid L91.0
   labia N90.89
   lung (base) J98.4
   macula —*see* Scar, chorioretinal, posterior pole
   muscle M62.89
   myocardium, myocardial I25.2
   painful L90.5
   posterior pole (eye) —*see* Scar, chorioretinal, posterior pole
   retina —*see* Scar, chorioretinal
   trachea J39.8
   transmural uterine, in pregnancy O34.29
   uterus N85.8
      in pregnancy O34.29
   vagina N89.8
      postoperative N99.2
   vulva N90.89
Scarabiasis B88.2
Scarlatina (anginosa) (maligna) A38.9
   myocarditis (acute) A38.1
      old —*see* Myocarditis
   otitis media A38.0
   ulcerosa A38.8
Scarlet fever (albuminuria) (angina) A38.9
Schamberg's disease (progressive pigmentary dermatosis) L81.7
Schatzki's ring (acquired) (esophagus) (lower) K22.2
   congenital Q39.3
Schaufenster krankheit I20.8
Schaumann's
   benign lymphogranulomatosis D86.1
   disease or syndrome —*see* Sarcoidosis
Scheie's syndrome E76.03
Schenck's disease B42.1
Scheuermann's disease or osteochondrosis — *see* Osteochondrosis, juvenile, spine
Schilder (-Flatau) disease G37.0
Schilling-type monocytic leukemia C93.0-●
Schimmelbusch's disease, cystic mastitis, or hyperplasia —*see* Mastopathy, cystic
Schistosoma infestation —*see* Infestation, Schistosoma
Schistosomiasis B65.9
   with muscle disorder B65.9 *[M63.80]*
      ankle B65.9 *[M63.87-●]*
      foot B65.9 *[M63.87-●]*
      forearm B65.9 *[M63.83-●]*
      hand B65.9 *[M63.84-●]*
      lower leg B65.9 *[M63.86-●]*
      multiple sites B65.9 *[M63.89]*
      pelvic region B65.9 *[M63.85-●]*
      shoulder region B65.9 *[M63.81-●]*
      specified site NEC B65.9 *[M63.88]*
      thigh B65.9 *[M63.85-●]*
      upper arm B65.9 *[M63.82-●]*
   Asiatic B65.2
   bladder B65.0
   chestermani B65.8
   colon B65.1
   cutaneous B65.3
   due to
      S. haematobium B65.0
      S. japonicum B65.2
      S. mansoni B65.1
      S. mattheii B65.8
   Eastern B65.2
   genitourinary tract B65.0
   intestinal B65.1
   lung NEC B65.9 *[J99]*
      pneumonia B65.9 *[J17]*
   Manson's (intestinal) B65.1

Schistosomiasis *(Continued)*
   oriental B65.2
   pulmonary NEC B65.9 *[J99]*
      pneumonia B65.9
   Schistosoma
      haematobium B65.0
      japonicum B65.2
      mansoni B65.1
   specified type NEC B65.8
   urinary B65.0
   vesical B65.0
Schizencephaly Q04.6
Schizoaffective psychosis F25.9
Schizodontia K00.2
Schizoid personality F60.1
Schizophrenia, schizophrenic F20.9
   acute (brief) (undifferentiated) F23
   atypical (form) F20.3
   borderline F21
   catalepsy F20.2
   catatonic (type) (excited) (withdrawn) F20.2
   cenesthopathic, cenesthesiopathic F20.89
   childhood type F84.5
   chronic undifferentiated F20.9
   cyclic F25.0
   disorganized (type) F20.1
   flexibilitas cerea F20.2
   hebephrenic (type) F20.1
   incipient F21
   latent F21
   negative type F20.5
   paranoid (type) F20.0
   paraphrenic F20.0
   post-psychotic depression F32.89
   prepsychotic F21
   prodromal F21
   pseudoneurotic F21
   pseudopsychopathic F21
   reaction F23
   residual (state) (type) F20.5
   restzustand F20.5
   schizoaffective (type) —*see* Psychosis, schizoaffective
   simple (type) F20.89
   simplex F20.89
   specified type NEC F20.89
   spectrum and other psychotic disorder F29
      specified NEC F28
   stupor F20.2
   syndrome of childhood F84.5
   undifferentiated (type) F20.3
      chronic F20.5
Schizothymia (persistent) F60.1
Schlatter-Osgood disease or osteochondrosis M92.52-●
Schlatter's tibia —*see* Osteochondrosis, juvenile, tibia
Schmidt's syndrome (polyglandular, autoimmune) E31.0
Schmincke's carcinoma or tumor —*see* Neoplasm, nasopharynx, malignant
Schmitz (-Stutzer) dysentery A03.0
Schmorl's disease or nodes
   lumbar region M51.46
   lumbosacral region M51.47
   sacrococcygeal region M53.3
   thoracic region M51.44
   thoracolumbar region M51.45
Schneiderian
   papilloma —*see* Neoplasm, nasopharynx benign
      specified site —*see* Neoplasm, benign, by site
      unspecified site D14.0
   specified site —*see* Neoplasm, malignant, by site
      unspecified site C30.0
Scholte's syndrome (malignant carcinoid) E34.0
Scholz (-Bielchowsky-Henneberg) disease or syndrome E75.25
Schönlein (-Henoch) disease or purpura (primary) (rheumatic) D69.0

Schottmuller's disease A01.4
Schroeder's syndrome (endocrine hypertensive) E27.0
Schüller-Christian disease or syndrome C96.5
Schultze's type acroparesthesia, simple I73.89
Schultz's disease or syndrome —*see* Agranulocytosis
Schwalbe-Ziehen-Oppenheim disease G24.1
Schwannoma —*see also* Neoplasm, nerve, benign
 malignant —*see also* Neoplasm, nerve, malignant
  with rhabdomyoblastic differentiation — *see* Neoplasm, nerve, malignant
 melanocytic —*see* Neoplasm, nerve, benign
 pigmented —*see* Neoplasm, nerve, benign
Schwannomatosis Q85.03
Schwartz (-Jampel) syndrome G71.13
Schwartz-Bartter syndrome E22.2
Schweniger-Buzzi anetoderma L90.1
Sciatic —*see* condition
➡ Sciatica (infective) M54.3
 with lumbago M54.4-●
  due to intervertebral disc disorder —*see* Disorder, disc, with, radiculopathy
 due to displacement of intervertebral disc (with lumbago) —*see* Disorder, disc, with, radiculopathy
 wallet M54.3-●
Scimitar syndrome Q26.8
Sclera —*see* condition
Sclerectasia H15.84-●
Scleredema
 adultorum —*see* Sclerosis, systemic
 Buschke's —*see* Sclerosis, systemic
 newborn P83.0
Sclerema (adiposum) (edematosum) (neonatorum) (newborn) P83.0
 adultorum —*see* Sclerosis, systemic
Scleriasis —*see* Scleroderma
Scleritis H15.00-●
 with corneal involvement H15.04-●
 anterior H15.01-●
 brawny H15.02-●
 in (due to) zoster B02.34
 posterior H15.03-●
 specified type NEC H15.09-●
 syphilitic A52.71
 tuberculous (nodular) A18.51
Sclerochoroiditis H31.8
Scleroconjunctivitis —*see* Scleritis
Sclerocystic ovary syndrome E28.2
Sclerodactyly, sclerodactylia L94.3
Scleroderma, sclerodermia (acrosclerotic) (diffuse) (generalized) (progressive) (pulmonary) —*see also* Sclerosis, systemic M34.9-●
 circumscribed L94.0
 linear L94.1
 localized L94.0
 newborn P83.88
 systemic M34.9
Sclerokeratitis H16.8
 tuberculous A18.52
Scleroma nasi A48.8
Scleromalacia (perforans) H15.05-●
Scleromyxedema L98.5
Sclérose en plaques G35
Sclerosis, sclerotic E27.8
 adrenal (gland) E27.8
 Alzheimer's —*see* Disease, Alzheimer's
 amyotrophic (lateral) G12.21
 aorta, aortic I70.0
  valve —*see* Endocarditis, aortic
 artery, arterial, arteriolar, arteriovascular — *see* Arteriosclerosis
 ascending multiple G35
 brain (generalized) (lobular) G37.9
  artery, arterial I67.2
  diffuse G37.0
  disseminated G35

Sclerosis, sclerotic (*Continued*)
 brain (*Continued*)
  insular G35
  Krabbe's E75.23
  miliary G35
  multiple G35
  presenile (Alzheimer's) —*see* Disease, Alzheimer's, early onset
  senile (arteriosclerotic) I67.2
  stem, multiple G35
  tuberous Q85.1
 bulbar, multiple G35
 bundle of His I44.39
 cardiac —*see* Disease, heart, ischemic, atherosclerotic
 cardiorenal —*see* Hypertension, cardiorenal
 cardiovascular —*see also* Disease, cardiovascular
  renal —*see* Hypertension, cardiorenal
 cerebellar —*see* Sclerosis, brain
 cerebral —*see* Sclerosis, brain
 cerebrospinal (disseminated) (multiple) G35
 cerebrovascular I67.2
 choroid —*see* Degeneration, choroid
 combined (spinal cord) —*see also* Degeneration, combined
  multiple G35
 concentric (Balo) G37.5
 cornea —*see* Opacity, cornea
 coronary (artery) I25.10
  with angina pectoris —*see* Arteriosclerosis, coronary (artery),
 corpus cavernosum
  female N90.89
  male N48.6
 diffuse (brain) (spinal cord) G37.0
 disseminated G35
 dorsal G35
 dorsolateral (spinal cord) —*see* Degeneration, combined
 endometrium N85.5
 extrapyramidal G25.9
 eye, nuclear (senile) —*see* Cataract, senile, nuclear
 focal and segmental (glomerular) —*see also* N00-N07 with fourth character .1 N05.1
 Friedreich's (spinal cord) G11.11
 funicular (spermatic cord) N50.89
 general (vascular) —*see* Arteriosclerosis
 gland (lymphatic) I89.8
 hepatic K74.1
  alcoholic K70.2
 hereditary
  cerebellar G11.9
  spinal (Friedreich's ataxia) G11.11
 hippocampal G93.81
 insular G35
 kidney —*see* Sclerosis, renal
 larynx J38.7
 lateral (amyotrophic) (descending) (spinal) G12.21
  primary G12.23
 lens, senile nuclear —*see* Cataract, senile, nuclear
 liver K74.1
  with fibrosis K74.2
   alcoholic K70.2
  alcoholic K70.2
  cardiac K76.1
 lung —*see* Fibrosis, lung
 mastoid —*see* Mastoiditis, chronic
 mesial temporal G93.81
 mitral I05.8
 Mönckeberg's (medial) —*see* Arteriosclerosis, extremities
 multiple (brain stem) (cerebral) (generalized) (spinal cord) G35
 myocardium, myocardial —*see* Disease, heart, ischemic, atherosclerotic
 nuclear (senile), eye —*see* Cataract, senile, nuclear

Sclerosis, sclerotic (*Continued*)
 ovary N83.8
 pancreas K86.89
 penis N48.6
 peripheral arteries —*see* Arteriosclerosis, extremities
 plaques G35
 pluriglandular E31.8
 polyglandular E31.8
 posterolateral (spinal cord) —*see* Degeneration, combined
 presenile (Alzheimer's) —*see* Disease, Alzheimer's, early onset
 primary, lateral G12.23
 progressive, systemic M34.0
 pulmonary —*see* Fibrosis, lung
  artery I27.0
  valve (heart) —*see* Endocarditis, pulmonary
 renal N26.9
  with
   cystine storage disease E72.09
   hypertensive heart disease (conditions in I11) —*see* Hypertension, cardiorenal
  arteriolar (hyaline) (hyperplastic) —*see* Hypertension, kidney
 retina (senile) (vascular) H35.00
 senile (vascular) —*see* Arteriosclerosis
 spinal (cord) (progressive) G95.89
  ascending G61.0
  combined —*see also* Degeneration, combined
   multiple G35
   syphilitic A52.11
  disseminated G35
  dorsolateral —*see* Degeneration, combined
  hereditary (Friedreich's) (mixed form) G11.11
  lateral (amyotrophic) G12.21
   progressive G12.23
  multiple G35
  posterior (syphilitic) A52.11
 stomach K31.89
 subendocardial, congenital I42.4
 systemic M34.9
  with
   lung involvement M34.81
   myopathy M34.82
   polyneuropathy M34.83
  drug-induced M34.2
  due to chemicals NEC M34.2
  progressive M34.0
  specified NEC M34.89
 temporal (mesial) G93.81
 tricuspid (heart) (valve) I07.8
 tuberous (brain) Q85.1
 tympanic membrane —*see* Disorder, tympanic membrane, specified NEC
 valve, valvular (heart) —*see* Endocarditis
 vascular —*see* Arteriosclerosis
 vein I87.8
Scoliosis (acquired) (postural) M41.9
 adolescent (idiopathic) —*see* Scoliosis, idiopathic, adolescent
 congenital Q67.5
  due to bony malformation Q76.3
  failure of segmentation (hemivertebra) Q76.3
  hemivertebra fusion Q76.3
  postural Q67.5
 degenerative M41.8-●
 idiopathic M41.20
  adolescent M41.129
   cervical region M41.122
   cervicothoracic region M41.123
   lumbar region M41.126
   lumbosacral region M41.127
   thoracic region M41.124
   thoracolumbar region M41.125
  cervical region M41.22
  cervicothoracic region M41.23

▶ New   ⇒ Revised   ~~deleted~~ Deleted   ● Use Additional Character(s)

Scoliosis *(Continued)*
  idiopathic *(Continued)*
    infantile M41.00
      cervical region M41.02
      cervicothoracic region M41.03
      lumbar region M41.06
      lumbosacral region M41.07
      sacrococcygeal region M41.08
      thoracic region M41.04
      thoracolumbar region M41.05
    juvenile M41.119
      cervical region M41.112
      cervicothoracic region M41.113
      lumbar region M41.116
      lumbosacral region M41.117
      thoracic region M41.114
      thoracolumbar region M41.115
    lumbar region M41.26
    lumbosacral region M41.27
    thoracic region M41.24
    thoracolumbar region M41.25
  infantile —*see* Scoliosis, idiopathic, infantile
  neuromuscular M41.40
    cervical region M41.42
    cervicothoracic region M41.43
    lumbar region M41.46
    lumbosacral region M41.47
    occipito-atlanto-axial region M41.41
    thoracic region M41.44
    thoracolumbar region M41.45
  paralytic —*see* Scoliosis, neuromuscular
  postradiation therapy M96.5
  rachitic (late effect or sequelae) E64.3 *[M49.80]*
    cervical region E64.3 *[M49.82]*
    cervicothoracic region E64.3 *[M49.83]*
    lumbar region E64.3 *[M49.86]*
    lumbosacral region E64.3 *[M49.87]*
    multiple sites E64.3 *[M49.89]*
    occipito-atlanto-axial region E64.3 *[M49.81]*
    sacrococcygeal region E64.3 *[M49.88]*
    thoracic region E64.3 *[M49.84]*
    thoracolumbar region E64.3 *[M49.85]*
  sciatic M54.4-●
  secondary (to) NEC M41.50
    cerebral palsy, Friedreich's ataxia,
      poliomyelitis, neuromuscular
      disorders —*see* Scoliosis,
      neuromuscular
    cervical region M41.52
    cervicothoracic region M41.53
    lumbar region M41.56
    lumbosacral region M41.57
    thoracic region M41.54
    thoracolumbar region M41.55
  specified form NEC M41.80
    cervical region M41.82
    cervicothoracic region M41.83
    lumbar region M41.86
    lumbosacral region M41.87
    thoracic region M41.84
    thoracolumbar region M41.85
  thoracogenic M41.30
    thoracic region M41.34
    thoracolumbar region M41.35
  tuberculous A18.01
Scoliotic pelvis
  with disproportion (fetopelvic) O33.0
    causing obstructed labor O65.0
Scorbutus, scorbutic —*see also* Scurvy
  anemia D53.2
Score, NIHSS (National Institutes of Health Stroke Scale) R29.7-●
Scotoma (arcuate) (Bjerrum) (central) (ring) — *see also* Defect, visual field, localized, scotoma
  scintillating H53.19
Scratch —*see* Abrasion
Scratchy throat R09.89
Screening (for) Z13.9
  alcoholism Z13.33
  anemia Z13.0
  anomaly, congenital Z13.89

Screening *(Continued)*
  antenatal, of mother —*see also* Encounter, antenatal Z36.9
  arterial hypertension Z13.6
  arthropod-borne viral disease NEC Z11.59
  autism Z13.41
  bacteriuria, asymptomatic Z13.89
    specified NEC Z13.39
  behavioral disorder Z13.30
  brain injury, traumatic Z13.850
  bronchitis, chronic Z13.83
  brucellosis Z11.2
  cardiovascular disorder Z13.6
  cataract Z13.5
  chlamydial diseases Z11.8
  cholera Z11.0
  chromosomal abnormalities (nonprocreative) NEC Z13.79
  colonoscopy Z12.11
  congenital
    dislocation of hip Z13.89
    eye disorder Z13.5
    malformation or deformation Z13.89
  contamination NEC Z13.88
  coronavirus (disease) (novel) 2019 Z11.52
  COVID-19 Z11.52
  cystic fibrosis Z13.228
  dengue fever Z11.59
  dental disorder Z13.84
  depression (adult) (adolescent) (child) Z13.31
    maternal Z13.32
    perinatal Z13.32
  developmental
    delays Z13.40
      global (milestones) Z13.42
      specified NEC Z13.49
    handicap Z13.42
    in early childhood Z13.42
  diabetes mellitus Z13.1
  diphtheria Z11.2
  disability, intellectual Z13.39
  disease or disorder Z13.9
    bacterial NEC Z11.2
      intestinal infectious Z11.0
      respiratory tuberculosis Z11.1
    behavioral Z13.30
      specified NEC Z13.39
    developmental delays Z13.40
      global (milestones) Z13.42
      specified NEC Z13.49
    mental health and behavioral Z13.30
      specified NEC Z13.39
    blood or blood-forming organ Z13.0
    cardiovascular Z13.6
    Chagas' Z11.6
    chlamydial Z11.8
    coronavirus (novel) 2019 Z11.52
    COVID-19 Z11.52
    dental Z13.89
    digestive tract NEC Z13.818
      lower GI Z13.811
      upper GI Z13.810
    ear Z13.5
    endocrine Z13.29
    eye Z13.5
    genitourinary Z13.89
    heart Z13.6
    human immunodeficiency virus (HIV) infection Z11.4
    immunity Z13.0
    infection
      intestinal Z11.0
      specified NEC Z11.6
    infectious Z11.9
    metabolic Z13.228
    neurological Z13.89
    nutritional Z13.21
      metabolic Z13.228
        lipoid disorders Z13.220
    protozoal Z11.6
      intestinal Z11.0

Screening *(Continued)*
  disease or disorder *(Continued)*
    respiratory Z13.83
    rheumatic Z13.828
    rickettsial Z11.8
    sexually-transmitted NEC Z11.3
      human immunodeficiency virus (HIV) Z11.4
    sickle-cell (trait) Z13.0
    skin Z13.89
    specified NEC Z13.89
    spirochetal Z11.8
    thyroid Z13.29
    vascular Z13.6
    venereal Z11.3
    viral NEC Z11.59
      coronavirus (disease) (novel) 2019 Z11.52
      COVID-19 Z11.52
      human immunodeficiency virus (HIV) Z11.4
      intestinal Z11.0
      SARS-CoV-2 Z11.52
  elevated titer Z13.89
  emphysema Z13.83
  encephalitis, viral (mosquito- or tick-borne) Z11.59
  exposure to contaminants (toxic) Z13.88
  fever
    dengue Z11.59
    hemorrhagic Z11.59
    yellow Z11.59
  filariasis Z11.6
  galactosemia Z13.228
  gastrointestinal condition Z13.818
  genetic (nonprocreative)- for procreative management —*see* Testing, genetic, for procreative management
    disease carrier status (nonprocreative) Z13.71
    specified NEC (nonprocreative) Z13.79
  genitourinary condition Z13.89
  glaucoma Z13.5
  gonorrhea Z11.3
  gout Z13.89
  helminthiasis (intestinal) Z11.6
  hematopoietic malignancy Z12.89
  hemoglobinopathies NEC Z13.0
  hemorrhagic fever Z11.59
  Hodgkin disease Z12.89
  human immunodeficiency virus (HIV) Z11.4
  human papillomavirus Z11.51
  hypertension Z13.6
  infant or child (over 28 days old) Z00.129
    with abnormal findings Z00.121
  immunity disorders Z13.0
  infection
    mycotic Z11.8
    parasitic Z11.8
  ingestion of radioactive substance Z13.88
  intellectual disability Z13.39
  intestinal
    helminthiasis Z11.6
    infectious disease Z11.0
  leishmaniasis Z11.6
  leprosy Z11.2
  leptospirosis Z11.8
  leukemia Z12.89
  lymphoma Z12.89
  malaria Z11.6
  malnutrition Z13.29
    metabolic Z13.228
    nutritional Z13.21
  measles Z11.59
  mental health disorder Z13.30
    specified NEC Z13.39
  metabolic errors, inborn Z13.228
  multiphasic Z13.89
  musculoskeletal disorder Z13.828
    osteoporosis Z13.820
  mycoses Z11.8

Screening (Continued)
  myocardial infarction (acute) Z13.6
  neoplasm (malignant) (of) Z12.9
    bladder Z12.6
    blood Z12.89
    breast Z12.39
      routine mammogram Z12.31
    cervix Z12.4
    colon Z12.11
    genitourinary organs NEC Z12.79
      bladder Z12.6
      cervix Z12.4
      ovary Z12.73
      prostate Z12.5
      testis Z12.71
      vagina Z12.72
    hematopoietic system Z12.89
    intestinal tract Z12.10
      colon Z12.11
      rectum Z12.12
      small intestine Z12.13
    lung Z12.2
    lymph (glands) Z12.89
    nervous system Z12.82
    oral cavity Z12.81
    prostate Z12.5
    rectum Z12.12
    respiratory organs Z12.2
    skin Z12.83
    small intestine Z12.13
    specified site NEC Z12.89
    stomach Z12.0
  nephropathy Z13.89
  nervous system disorders NEC Z13.858
  neurological condition Z13.89
  osteoporosis Z13.820
  parasitic infestation Z11.9
    specified NEC Z11.8
  phenylketonuria Z13.228
  plague Z11.2
  poisoning (chemical) (heavy metal) Z13.88
  poliomyelitis Z11.59
  postnatal, chromosomal abnormalities Z13.89
  prenatal, of mother —see also Encounter,
    antenatal Z36.9
  protozoal disease Z11.6
    intestinal Z11.0
  pulmonary tuberculosis Z11.1
  radiation exposure Z13.88
  respiratory condition Z13.83
  respiratory tuberculosis Z11.1
  rheumatoid arthritis Z13.828
  rubella Z11.59
  SARS-CoV-2 Z11.52
  schistosomiasis Z11.6
  sexually-transmitted disease NEC Z11.3
    human immunodeficiency virus (HIV) Z11.4
  sickle-cell disease or trait Z13.0
  skin condition Z13.89
  sleeping sickness Z11.6
  special Z13.9
    specified NEC Z13.89
  syphilis Z11.3
  tetanus Z11.2
  trachoma Z11.8
  traumatic brain injury Z13.850
  trypanosomiasis Z11.6
  tuberculosis, respiratory Z11.1
    active Z11.1
    latent Z11.7
  venereal disease Z11.3
  viral encephalitis (mosquito- or tick-borne)
    Z11.59
  whooping cough Z11.2
  worms, intestinal Z11.6
  yaws Z11.8
  yellow fever Z11.59
Scrofula, scrofulosis (tuberculosis of cervical
    lymph glands) A18.2
Scrofulide (primary) (tuberculous) A18.4
Scrofuloderma, scrofulodermia (any site)
    (primary) A18.4

Scrofulosus lichen (primary) (tuberculous) A18.4
Scrofulous —see condition
Scrotal tongue K14.5
Scrotum —see condition
Scurvy, scorbutic E54
  anemia D53.2
  gum E54
  infantile E54
  rickets E55.0 [M90.80]
Sealpox B08.62
Seasickness T75.3
Seatworm (infection) (infestation) B80
Sebaceous —see also condition
  cyst —see Cyst, sebaceous
Seborrhea, seborrheic L21.9
  capillitii R23.8
  capitis L21.0
  dermatitis L21.9
    infantile L21.1
  eczema L21.9
    infantile L21.1
  sicca L21.0
Seckel's syndrome Q87.19
Seclusion, pupil —see Membrane, pupillary
Second hand tobacco smoke exposure (acute)
    (chronic) Z77.22
  in the perinatal period P96.81
Secondary
  dentin (in pulp) K04.3
  neoplasm, secondaries —see Table of
    Neoplasms, secondary
Secretion
  antidiuretic hormone, inappropriate E22.2
  catecholamine, by pheochromocytoma E27.5
  hormone
    antidiuretic, inappropriate (syndrome)
      E22.2
    by
      carcinoid tumor E34.0
      pheochromocytoma E27.5
    ectopic NEC E34.2
  urinary
    excessive R35.89
    suppression R34
Section
  nerve, traumatic —see Injury, nerve
Sedative, hypnotic, or anxiolytic-induced
  anxiety disorder F13.980
  bipolar and related disorder F13.94
  delirium F13.921
  depressive disorder F13.94
  major neurocognitive disorder F13.97
  mild neurocognitive disorder F13.988
  psychotic disorder F13.959
  sexual dysfunction F13.981
  sleep disorder F13.982
Segmentation, incomplete (congenital) —see
    also Fusion
  bone NEC Q78.8
  lumbosacral (joint) (vertebra) Q76.49
Seitelberger's syndrome (infantile neuraxonal
    dystrophy) G31.89
Seizure(s) —see also Convulsions R56.9
  absence G40.A-●
  akinetic —see Epilepsy, generalized, specified
    NEC
  atonic —see Epilepsy, generalized, specified
    NEC
  autonomic (hysterical) F44.5
  convulsive —see Convulsions
  cortical (focal) (motor) —see Epilepsy,
    localization-related, symptomatic, with
    simple partial seizures
  disorder —see also Epilepsy G40.909
  due to stroke —see Sequelae (of), disease,
    cerebrovascular, by type, specified NEC
  epileptic —see Epilepsy
  febrile (simple) R56.00
    with status epilepticus G40.901
    complex (atypical) (complicated) R56.01
      with status epilepticus G40.901

Seizure (Continued)
  grand mal G40.409
    intractable G40.419
      with status epilepticus G40.411
      without status epilepticus G40.419
    not intractable G40.409
      with status epilepticus G40.401
      without status epilepticus G40.409
  heart —see Disease, heart
  hysterical F44.5
  intractable G40.919
    with status epilepticus G40.911
  Jacksonian (focal) (motor type) (sensory
    type) —see Epilepsy, localization-related,
    symptomatic, with simple partial seizures
  newborn P90
  nonspecific epileptic
    atonic —see Epilepsy, generalized, specified
      NEC
    clonic —see Epilepsy, generalized, specified
      NEC
    myoclonic —see Epilepsy, generalized,
      specified NEC
    tonic —see Epilepsy, generalized, specified
      NEC
    tonic-clonic —see Epilepsy, generalized,
      specified NEC
  partial, developing into secondarily
    generalized seizures
    complex —see Epilepsy, localization-
      related, symptomatic, with complex
      partial seizures
    simple —see Epilepsy, localization-related,
      symptomatic, with simple partial
      seizures
  petit mal G40.A-●
    intractable G40.A1-●
      with status epilepticus G40.A11
      without status epilepticus G40.A19
    not intractable G40.A0 -●
      with status epilepticus G40.A01
      without status epilepticus G40.A01
  post traumatic R56.1
  recurrent G40.909
  specified NEC G40.89
  uncinate —see Epilepsy, localization-related,
    symptomatic, with complex partial
    seizures
Selenium deficiency, dietary E59
Self-damaging behavior (life-style) Z72.89
Self-harm (attempted)
  history (personal)
    in family Z81.8
    nonsuicidal Z91.52
    suicidal Z91.51
  nonsuicidal R45.88
Self-injury, nonsuicidal R45.88
  personal history Z91.52
Self-mutilation (attempted)
  history (personal)
    in family Z81.8
    nonsuicidal Z91.52
    suicidal Z91.51
  nonsuicidal R45.88
Self-poisoning
  history (personal)
    in family Z81.8
  observation following (alleged) attempt Z03.6
Semicoma R40.1
Seminal vesiculitis N49.0
Seminoma C62.9-●
  specified site —see Neoplasm, malignant, by
    site
Senear-Usher disease or syndrome L10.4
Senectus R54
Senescence (without mention of psychosis) R54
Senile, senility —see also condition R41.81
  with
    acute confusional state F05
    mental changes NOS F03
    psychosis NEC —see Psychosis, senile
  asthenia R54
  cervix (atrophic) N88.8

▶ New   ⇒ Revised   ~~deleted~~ Deleted   ● Use Additional Character(s)

Senile, senility *(Continued)*
debility R54
endometrium (atrophic) N85.8
fallopian tube (atrophic) —*see* Atrophy,
 fallopian tube
heart (failure) R54
ovary (atrophic) —*see* Atrophy, ovary
premature E34.8
vagina, vaginitis (atrophic) N95.2
wart L82.1
Sensation
burning (skin) R20.8
 tongue K14.6
loss of R20.8
prickling (skin) R20.2
tingling (skin) R20.2
Sense loss
smell —*see* Disturbance, sensation, smell
taste —*see* Disturbance, sensation, taste
touch R20.8
Sensibility disturbance (cortical) (deep)
 (vibratory) R20.9
Sensitive, sensitivity —*see also* Allergy
carotid sinus G90.01
child (excessive) F93.8
cold, autoimmune D59.12
dentin K03.89
gluten (non-celiac) K90.41
latex Z91.040
methemoglobin D74.8
tuberculin, without clinical or radiological
 symptoms R76.11
visual
 glare H53.71
 impaired contrast H53.72
Sensitiver Beziehungswahn F22
Sensitization, auto-erythrocytic D69.2
Separation
anxiety, abnormal (of childhood) F93.0
apophysis, traumatic - code as Fracture, by site
choroid —*see* Detachment, choroid
epiphysis, epiphyseal
 nontraumatic —*see also* Osteochondropathy,
 specified type NEC
 upper femoral —*see* Slipped, epiphysis,
 upper femoral
 traumatic - code as Fracture, by site
fracture —*see* Fracture
infundibulum cardiac from right ventricle by
 a partition Q24.3
joint (traumatic) (current) - code by site under
 Dislocation
muscle (nontraumatic) —*see* Diastasis, muscle
pubic bone, obstetrical trauma O71.6
retina, retinal —*see* Detachment, retina
symphysis pubis, obstetrical trauma O71.6
tracheal ring, incomplete, congenital Q32.1
Sepsis (generalized) (unspecified organism)
 A41.9
with
 organ dysfunction (acute) (multiple) R65.20
 with septic shock R65.21
actinomycotic A42.7
adrenal hemorrhage syndrome
 (meningococcal) A39.1
anaerobic A41.4
Bacillus anthracis A22.7
Brucella —*see also* Brucellosis A23.9
candidal B37.7
cryptogenic A41.9
due to device, implant or graft T85.79
 arterial graft NEC T82.7
 breast (implant) T85.79
 catheter NEC T85.79
 dialysis (renal) T82.7
 intraperitoneal T85.71
 infusion NEC T82.7
 spinal (cranial) (epidural) (intrathecal)
 (spinal) (subarachnoid)
 (subdural) T85.735
 urethral indwelling T83.511
 urinary T83.518
 ectopic or molar pregnancy O08.82

Sepsis *(Continued)*
due to device, implant or graft*(Continued)*
 electronic (electrode) (pulse generator)
 (stimulator)
 bone T84.7
 cardiac T82.7
 nervous system T85.738
 brain T85.731
 neurostimulator generator T85.734
 peripheral nerve T85.732
 spinal cord T85.733
 urinary T83.590
 fixation, internal (orthopedic) —*see*
 Complication, fixation device,
 infection
 gastrointestinal (bile duct) (esophagus)
 T85.79
 neurostimulator electrode (lead) T85.732
 genital T83.69
 heart NEC T82.7
 valve (prosthesis) T82.6
 graft T82.7
 joint prosthesis —*see* Complication, joint
 prosthesis, infection
 ocular (corneal graft) (orbital implant) T85.79
 orthopedic NEC T84.7
 fixation device, internal —*see*
 Complication, fixation device,
 infection
 specified NEC T85.79
 vascular T82.7
 ventricular intracranial (communicating)
 shunt T85.730
during labor O75.3
Enterococcus A41.81
Erysipelothrix (rhusiopathiae) (erysipeloid)
 A26.7
Escherichia coli (E. coli) A41.5
extraintestinal yersiniosis A28.2
following
 abortion (subsequent episode) O08.0
 current episode —*see* Abortion
 ectopic or molar pregnancy O08.82
 immunization T88.0
 infusion, therapeutic injection or
 transfusion NEC T80.29
 obstetrical procedure O86.04
gangrenous A41.9
gonococcal A54.86
Gram-negative (organism) A41.5
 anaerobic A41.4
Haemophilus influenzae A41.3
herpesviral B00.7
intra-abdominal K65.1
intraocular —*see* Endophthalmitis, purulent
Listeria monocytogenes A32.7
localized — code to specific localized infection
 in operation wound T81.49
 skin —*see* Abscess
malleus A24.0
melioidosis A24.1
meningeal —*see* Meningitis
meningococcal A39.4
 acute A39.2
 chronic A39.3
MSSA (Methicillin susceptible
 Staphylococcus aureus) A41.01
newborn P36.9
 due to
 anaerobes NEC P36.5
 Escherichia coli P36.4
 Staphylococcus P36.30
 aureus P36.2
 specified NEC P36.39
 Streptococcus P36.10
 group B P36.0
 specified NEC P36.19
 specified NEC P36.8
Pasteurella multocida A28.0
pelvic, puerperal, postpartum, childbirth O85
pneumococcal A40.3
postprocedural T81.44

Sepsis *(Continued)*
puerperal, postpartum, childbirth (pelvic) O85
Salmonella (arizonae) (cholerae-suis)
 (enteritidis) (typhimurium) A02.1
severe R65.20
 with septic shock R65.21
Shigella (*see also* Dysentery, bacillary) A03.9
skin, localized —*see* Abscess
specified organism NEC A41.89
Staphylococcus, staphylococcal A41.2
 aureus (methicillin susceptible) (MSSA)
 A41.01
 methicillin resistant (MRSA) A41.02
 coagulase-negative A41.1
 specified NEC A41.1
Streptococcus, streptococcal A40.9
 agalactiae A40.1
 group
 A A40.0
 B A40.1
 D A41.81
 neonatal P36.10
 group B P36.0
 specified NEC P36.19
 pneumoniae A40.3
 pyogenes A40.0
 specified NEC A40.8
tracheostomy stoma J95.02
tularemic A21.7
umbilical, umbilical cord (newborn) —*see*
 Sepsis, newborn
Yersinia pestis A20.7
Septate —*see* Septum
Septic —*see* condition
arm —*see* Cellulitis, upper limb
 with lymphangitis —*see* Lymphangitis,
 acute, upper limb
embolus —*see* Embolism
finger —*see* Cellulitis, digit
 with lymphangitis —*see* Lymphangitis,
 acute, digit
foot —*see* Cellulitis, lower limb
 with lymphangitis —*see* Lymphangitis,
 acute, lower limb
gallbladder (acute) K81.0
hand —*see* Cellulitis, upper limb
 with lymphangitis —*see* Lymphangitis,
 acute, upper limb
joint —*see* Arthritis, pyogenic or pyemic
leg —*see* Cellulitis, lower limb
 with lymphangitis —*see* Lymphangitis,
 acute, lower limb
nail —*see also* Cellulitis, digit
 with lymphangitis —*see* Lymphangitis,
 acute, digit
sore —*see also* Abscess
 throat J02.0
 streptococcal J02.0
spleen (acute) D73.89
teeth, tooth (pulpal origin) K04.4
throat —*see* Pharyngitis
thrombus —*see* Thrombosis
toe —*see* Cellulitis, digit
 with lymphangitis —*see* Lymphangitis,
 acute, digit
tonsils, chronic J35.01
 with adenoiditis J35.03
uterus —*see* Endometritis
Septicemia A41.9
meaning sepsis —*see* Sepsis
Septum, septate (congenital) —*see also*
 Anomaly, by site
anal Q42.3
 with fistula Q42.2
aqueduct of Sylvius Q03.0
 with spina bifida —*see* Spina bifida, by site,
 with hydrocephalus
uterus (complete) (partial) Q51.28
 complete Q51.21
 partial Q51.22
 specified NEC Q51.28

Septum, septate (Continued)
  vagina Q52.10
    in pregnancy —see Pregnancy, complicated
        by, abnormal vagina
      causing obstructed labor O65.5
    longitudinal Q52.129
      microperforate
        left side Q52.124
        right side Q52.123
      nonobstruction Q52.120
      obstructing Q52.129
        left side Q52.122
        right side Q52.121
    transverse Q52.11
Sequelae (of) —see also condition
  abscess, intracranial or intraspinal (conditions
      in G06) G09
  amputation — code to injury with seventh
      character S
  burn and corrosion — code to injury with
      seventh character S
  calcium deficiency E64.8
  cerebrovascular disease —see Sequelae,
      disease, cerebrovascular
  childbirth O94
  contusion — code to injury with seventh
      character S
  corrosion —see Sequelae, burn and corrosion
  ▶ COVID-19 (post acute) U09.9
  crushing injury — code to injury with
      seventh character S
  disease
    cerebrovascular I69.90
      alteration of sensation I69.998
      aphasia I69.920
      apraxia I69.990
      ataxia I69.993
      cognitive deficits I69.91
      disturbance of vision I69.998
      dysarthria I69.922
      dysphagia I69.991
      dysphasia I69.921
      facial droop I69.992
      facial weakness I69.992
      fluency disorder I69.923
      hemiplegia I69.95-●
      hemorrhage
        intracerebral —see Sequelae,
            hemorrhage, intracerebral
        intracranial, nontraumatic NEC —
            see Sequelae, hemorrhage,
            intracranial, nontraumatic
        subarachnoid —see Sequelae,
            hemorrhage, subarachnoid
      language deficit I69.928
      monoplegia
        lower limb I69.94-●
        upper limb I69.93-●
      paralytic syndrome I69.96-●
      specified effect NEC I69.998
      specified type NEC I69.80
        alteration of sensation I69.898
        aphasia I69.820
        apraxia I69.890
        ataxia I69.893
        cognitive deficits I69.81
        disturbance of vision I69.898
        dysarthria I69.822
        dysphagia I69.891
        dysphasia I69.821
        facial droop I69.892
        facial weakness I69.892
        fluency disorder I69.823
        hemiplegia I69.85-●
        language deficit I69.828
        monoplegia
          lower limb I69.84-●
          upper limb I69.83-●
        paralytic syndrome I69.86-●
        specified effect NEC I69.898
      speech deficit I69.928
        speech deficit I69.828
      stroke NOS —see Sequelae, stroke NOS

Sequelae (Continued)
  dislocation — code to injury with seventh
      character S
  encephalitis or encephalomyelitis (conditions
      in G04) G09
    in infectious disease NEC B94.8
    viral B94.1
  external cause — code to injury with seventh
      character S
  foreign body entering natural orifice — code
      to injury with seventh character S
  fracture — code to injury with seventh
      character S
  frostbite — code to injury with seventh
      character S
  Hansen's disease B92
  hemorrhage
    intracerebral I69.10
      alteration of sensation I69.198
      aphasia I69.120
      apraxia I69.190
      ataxia I69.193
      cognitive deficits I69.11
      disturbance of vision I69.198
      dysarthria I69.122
      dysphagia I69.191
      dysphasia I69.121
      facial droop I69.192
      facial weakness I69.192
      fluency disorder I69.123
      hemiplegia I69.15-●
      language deficit NEC I69.128
      monoplegia
        lower limb I69.14-●
        upper limb I69.13-●
      paralytic syndrome I69.16-●
      specified effect NEC I69.198
      speech deficit NEC I69.128
    intracranial, nontraumatic NEC I69.20
      alteration of sensation I69.298
      aphasia I69.220
      apraxia I69.290
      ataxia I69.293
      cognitive deficits I69.21
      disturbance of vision I69.298
      dysarthria I69.222
      dysphagia I69.291
      dysphasia I69.221
      facial droop I69.292
      facial weakness I69.292
      fluency disorder I69.223
      hemiplegia I69.25-●
      language deficit NEC I69.228
      monoplegia
        lower limb I69.24-●
        upper limb I69.23-●
      paralytic syndrome I69.26-●
      specified effect NEC I69.298
      speech deficit NEC I69.228
    subarachnoid I69.00
      alteration of sensation I69.098
      aphasia I69.020
      apraxia I69.090
      ataxia I69.093
      cognitive deficits —see subcategory
          I69.01-●
      disturbance of vision I69.098
      dysarthria I69.022
      dysphagia I69.091
      dysphasia I69.021
      facial droop I69.092
      facial weakness I69.092
      fluency disorder I69.023
      hemiplegia I69.05-●
      language deficit NEC I69.028
      monoplegia
        lower limb I69.04-●
        upper limb I69.03-●
      paralytic syndrome I69.06-●
      specified effect NEC I69.098
      speech deficit NEC I69.028

Sequelae (Continued)
  hepatitis, viral B94.2
  hyperalimentation E68
  infarction
    cerebral I69.30
      alteration of sensation I69.398
      aphasia I69.320
      apraxia I69.390
      ataxia I69.393
      cognitive deficits I69.31
      disturbance of vision I69.398
      dysarthria I69.322
      dysphagia I69.391
      dysphasia I69.321
      facial droop I69.392
      facial weakness I69.392
      fluency disorder I69.323
      hemiplegia I69.35-●
      language deficit NEC I69.328
      monoplegia
        lower limb I69.34-●
        upper limb I69.33-●
      paralytic syndrome I69.36-●
      specified effect NEC I69.398
      speech deficit NEC I69.328
  infection, pyogenic, intracranial or intraspinal
      G09
  infectious disease B94.9
    specified NEC B94.8
  injury — code to injury with seventh
      character S
  leprosy B92
  meningitis
    bacterial (conditions in G00) G09
    other or unspecified cause (conditions in
        G03) G09
  muscle (and tendon) injury — code to injury
      with seventh character S
  myelitis —see Sequelae, encephalitis
  niacin deficiency E64.8
  nutritional deficiency E64.9
    specified NEC E64.8
  obstetrical condition O94
  parasitic disease B94.9
  phlebitis or thrombophlebitis of intracranial
      or intraspinal venous sinuses and veins
      (conditions in G08) G09
  poisoning — code to poisoning with seventh
      character S
    nonmedicinal substance —see Sequelae,
        toxic effect, nonmedicinal substance
  poliomyelitis (acute) B91
  pregnancy O94
  protein-energy malnutrition E64.0
  puerperium O94
  rickets E64.3
  ▶ SARS-CoV-2 (post acute) U09.9
  selenium deficiency E64.8
  sprain and strain — code to injury with
      seventh character S
  stroke NOS I69.30
    alteration in sensation I69.398
    aphasia I69.320
    apraxia I69.390
    ataxia I69.393
    cognitive deficits I69.31
    disturbance of vision I69.398
    dysarthria I69.322
    dysphagia I69.391
    dysphasia I69.321
    facial droop I69.392
    facial weakness I69.392
    hemiplegia I69.35-●
    language deficit NEC I69.328
    monoplegia
      lower limb I69.34-●
      upper limb I69.33-●
    paralytic syndrome I69.36-●
    specified effect NEC I69.398
    speech deficit NEC I69.328
  tendon and muscle injury — code to injury
      with seventh character S

▶ New   ⇒ Revised   ~~deleted~~ Deleted   ● Use Additional Character(s)

Sequelae *(Continued)*
  thiamine deficiency E64.8
  trachoma B94.0
  tuberculosis B90.9
    bones and joints B90.2
    central nervous system B90.0
    genitourinary B90.1
    pulmonary (respiratory) B90.9
    specified organs NEC B90.8
  viral
    encephalitis B94.1
    hepatitis B94.2
  vitamin deficiency NEC E64.8
    A E64.1
    B E64.8
    C E64.2
  wound, open — code to injury with seventh
      character S
Sequestration *—see also* Sequestrum
  disc *—see* Displacement, intervertebral
      disc
  lung, congenital Q33.2
Sequestrum
  bone *—see* Osteomyelitis, chronic
  dental M27.2
  jaw bone M27.2
  orbit *—see* Osteomyelitis, orbit
  sinus (accessory) (nasal) *—see* Sinusitis
Sequoiosis lung or pneumonitis J67.8
Serology for syphilis
  doubtful
    with signs or symptoms - code by site and
        stage under Syphilis
      follow-up of latent syphilis *—see* Syphilis,
          latent
  negative, with signs or symptoms — code by
      site and stage under Syphilis
  positive A53.0
    with signs or symptoms - code by site and
        stage under Syphilis
  reactivated A53.0
Seroma *—see also* Hematoma
  postprocedural *—see* Complication,
      postprocedural, seroma
  traumatic, secondary and recurrent
      T79.2
Seropurulent *—see* condition
Serositis, multiple K65.8
  pericardial I31.1
  peritoneal K65.8
Serous *—see* condition
Sertoli cell
  adenoma
    specified site *—see* Neoplasm, benign, by
        site
    unspecified site
      female D27.9
      male D29.20
  carcinoma
    specified site *—see* Neoplasm, malignant,
        by site
    unspecified site (male) C62.9-●
      female C56.9
  tumor
    with lipid storage
      specified site *—see* Neoplasm, benign,
          by site
      unspecified site
        female D27.9
        male D29.20
    specified site *—see* Neoplasm, benign, by
        site
    unspecified site
      female D27.9
      male D29.20
Sertoli-Leydig cell tumor *—see* Neoplasm,
    benign, by site
  specified site *—see* Neoplasm, benign, by site
  unspecified site
    female D27.9
    male D29.20

Serum
  allergy, allergic reaction *—see also* Reaction,
      serum T80.69
    shock *—see also* Shock, anaphylactic T80.59
  arthritis *—see also* Reaction, serum T80.69
  complication or reaction NEC *—see also*
      Reaction, serum T80.69
  disease NEC *—see also* Reaction, serum T80.69
  hepatitis *—see also* Hepatitis, viral, type B
    carrier (suspected) of B18.1
  intoxication *—see also* Reaction, serum T80.69
  neuritis *—see also* Reaction, serum T80.69
  neuropathy G61.1
  poisoning NEC *—see also* Reaction, serum
      T80.69
  rash NEC *—see also* Reaction, serum T80.69
  reaction NEC *—see also* Reaction, serum
      T80.69
  sickness NEC *—see also* Reaction, serum
      T80.69
  urticaria *—see also* Reaction, serum T80.69
Sesamoiditis M25.8-●
Sever's disease or osteochondrosis *—see*
    Osteochondrosis, juvenile, tarsus
Severe sepsis R65.20
  with septic shock R65.21
Sex
  chromosome mosaics Q97.8
    lines with various numbers of
        X chromosomes Q97.2
  education Z70.8
  reassignment surgery status Z87.890
Sextuplet pregnancy *—see* Pregnancy,
    sextuplet
Sexual
  function, disorder of (psychogenic) F52.9
  immaturity (female) (male) E30.0
  impotence (psychogenic) organic origin
      NEC *—see* Dysfunction, sexual, male
  precocity (constitutional) (cryptogenic)
      (female) (idiopathic) (male) E30.1
Sexuality, pathologic *—see* Deviation, sexual
Sézary disease C84.1-●
Shadow, lung R91.8
Shaking palsy or paralysis *—see* Parkinsonism
Shallowness, acetabulum *—see* Derangement,
    joint, specified type NEC, hip
Shaver's disease J63.1
Sheath (tendon) *—see* condition
Sheathing, retinal vessels H35.01-●
Shedding
  nail L60.8
  premature, primary (deciduous) teeth
      K00.6
Sheehan's disease or syndrome E23.0
Shelf, rectal K62.89
Shell teeth K00.5
Shellshock (current) F43.0
  lasting state *—see* Disorder, post-traumatic
      stress
Shield kidney Q63.1
Shift
  auditory threshold (temporary) H93.24-●
  mediastinal R93.89
Shifting sleep-work schedule (affecting sleep)
    G47.26
Shiga (-Kruse) dysentery A03.0
Shiga's bacillus A03.0
Shigella (dysentery) *—see* Dysentery,
    bacillary
Shigellosis A03.9
  Group A A03.0
  Group B A03.1
  Group C A03.2
  Group D A03.3
Shin splints S86.89
Shingles *—see* Herpes, zoster
Shipyard disease or eye B30.0
Shirodkar suture, in pregnancy *—see*
    Pregnancy, complicated by, incompetent
    cervix

Shock R57.9
  with ectopic or molar pregnancy O08.3
  adrenal (cortical) (Addisonian) E27.2
  adverse food reaction (anaphylactic) *—see*
      Shock, anaphylactic, due to food
  allergic *—see* Shock, anaphylactic
  anaphylactic T78.2
    chemical *—see* Table of Drugs and
        Chemicals
    due to drug or medicinal substance
      correct substance properly administered
          T88.6
      overdose or wrong substance given or
          taken (by accident) *—see* Table of
          Drugs and Chemicals, by drug,
          poisoning
    due to food (nonpoisonous) T78.00
      additives T78.06
      dairy products T78.07
      eggs T78.08
      fish T78.03
        shellfish T78.02
      fruit T78.04
      milk T78.07
      nuts T78.05
        multiple types T78.05
        peanuts T78.01
      peanuts T78.01
      seeds T78.05
      specified type NEC T78.09
      vegetable T78.04
    following sting(s) *—see* Venom
    immunization T80.52
    serum T80.59
      blood and blood products T80.51
      immunization T80.52
      specified NEC T80.59
      vaccination T80.52
  anaphylactoid *—see* Shock, anaphylactic
  anesthetic
    correct substance properly administered
        T88.2
    overdose or wrong substance given
        or taken *—see* Table of Drugs and
        Chemicals, by drug, poisoning
    specified anesthetic *—see* Table of
        Drugs and Chemicals, by drug,
        poisoning
  cardiogenic R57.0
  chemical substance *—see* Table of Drugs and
      Chemicals
  complicating ectopic or molar pregnancy O08.3
  culture *—see* Disorder, adjustment
  drug
    due to correct substance properly
        administered T88.6
    overdose or wrong substance given or
        taken (by accident) *—see* Table of
        Drugs and Chemicals, by drug,
        poisoning
  during or after labor and delivery O75.1
  electric T75.4
    (taser) T75.4
  endotoxic R65.21
    postprocedural (resulting from a procedure,
        not elsewhere classified) T81.12
  following
    ectopic or molar pregnancy O08.3
    injury (immediate) (delayed) T79.4
    labor and delivery O75.1
  food (anaphylactic) *—see* Shock, anaphylactic,
      due to food
  from electroshock gun (taser) T75.4
  gram-negative R65.21
    postprocedural (resulting from a procedure,
        not elsewhere classified) T81.12
  hematologic R57.8
  hemorrhagic R57.8
    surgery (intraoperative) (postoperative)
        T81.19
    trauma T79.4

Shock (Continued)
  hypovolemic R57.1
    surgical T81.19
    traumatic T79.4
  insulin E15
    therapeutic misadventure —*see*
        subcategory T38.3
  kidney N17.0
    traumatic (following crushing) T79.5
  lightning T75.01
  liver K72.00
  lung J80
  obstetric O75.1
    with ectopic or molar pregnancy O08.3
    following ectopic or molar pregnancy
        O08.3
  pleural (surgical) T81.19
    due to trauma T79.4
  postprocedural (postoperative) T81.10
    with ectopic or molar pregnancy O08.3
    cardiogenic T81.11
    endotoxic T81.12
    following ectopic or molar pregnancy
        O08.3
    gram-negative T81.12
    hypovolemic T81.19
    septic T81.12
    specified type NEC T81.19
  psychic F43.0
  septic (due to severe sepsis) R65.21
  specified NEC R57.8
  surgical T81.10
  taser gun (taser) T75.4
  therapeutic misadventure NEC T81.10
  thyroxin
    overdose or wrong substance given
        or taken —*see* Table of Drugs and
        Chemicals, by drug, poisoning
  toxic, syndrome A48.3
  transfusion —*see* Complications, transfusion
  traumatic (immediate) (delayed) T79.4
Shoemaker's chest M95.4
Short, shortening, shortness
  arm (acquired) —*see also* Deformity, limb,
      unequal length
    congenital Q71.81-•
    forearm —*see* Deformity, limb, unequal
        length
  bowel syndrome K91.2
  breath R06.02
  cervical (complicating pregnancy) O26.87-•
    non-gravid uterus N88.3
  common bile duct, congenital Q44.5
  cord (umbilical), complicating delivery O69.3
  cystic duct, congenital Q44.5
  esophagus (congenital) Q39.8
  femur (acquired) —*see* Deformity, limb,
      unequal length, femur
    congenital —*see* Defect, reduction, lower
        limb, longitudinal, femur
  frenum, frenulum, linguae (congenital) Q38.1
  hip (acquired) —*see also* Deformity, limb,
      unequal length
    congenital Q65.89
  leg (acquired) —*see also* Deformity, limb,
      unequal length
    congenital Q72.81-•
    lower leg —*see also* Deformity, limb,
        unequal length
  limbed stature, with immunodeficiency
      D82.2
  lower limb (acquired) —*see also* Deformity,
      limb, unequal length
    congenital Q72.81-•
  organ or site, congenital NEC —*see* Distortion
  palate, congenital Q38.5
  radius (acquired) —*see also* Deformity, limb,
      unequal length
    congenital —*see* Defect, reduction, upper
        limb, longitudinal, radius
  rib syndrome Q77.2

Short, shortening, shortness(Continued)
  stature (child) (hereditary) (idiopathic) NEC
      R62.52
    constitutional E34.3
    due to endocrine disorder E34.3
    Laron-type E34.3
Short, shortening, shortness (Continued)
  tendon —*see also* Contraction, tendon
    with contracture of joint —*see* Contraction,
        joint
    Achilles (acquired) M67.0-•
      congenital Q66.89
    congenital Q79.8
  thigh (acquired) —*see also* Deformity, limb,
      unequal length, femur
    congenital —*see* Defect, reduction, lower
        limb, longitudinal, femur
  tibialis anterior (tendon) —*see* Contraction,
      tendon
  umbilical cord
    complicating delivery O69.3
  upper limb, congenital —*see* Defect, reduction,
      upper limb, specified type NEC
  urethra N36.8
  uvula, congenital Q38.5
  vagina (congenital) Q52.4
Shortsightedness —*see* Myopia
Shoshin (acute fulminating beriberi) E51.11
Shoulder —*see* condition
Shovel-shaped incisors K00.2
Shower, thromboembolic —*see* Embolism
Shunt
  arterial-venous (dialysis) Z99.2
  arteriovenous, pulmonary (acquired) I28.0
    congenital Q25.72
  cerebral ventricle (communicating) in situ Z98.2
  surgical, prosthetic, with complications —*see*
      Complications, cardiovascular, device or
      implant Shutdown, renal N28.9
Shutdown, renal N28.9
Shy-Drager syndrome G90.3
Sialadenitis, sialadenosis (any gland) (chronic)
    (periodic) (suppurative) —*see* Sialoadenitis
Sialectasia K11.8
Sialidosis E77.1
Sialitis, silitis (any gland) (chronic)
    (suppurative) —*see* Sialoadenitis
Sialoadenitis (any gland) (periodic)
    (suppurative) K11.20
  acute K11.21
    recurrent K11.22
  chronic K11.23
Sialoadenopathy K11.9
Sialoangitis —*see* Sialoadenitis
Sialodochitis (fibrinosa) —*see* Sialoadenitis
Sialodocholithiasis K11.5
Sialolithiasis K11.5
Sialometaplasia, necrotizing K11.8
Sialorrhea —*see also* Ptyalism
  periodic —*see* Sialoadenitis
Sialosis K11.7
Siamese twin Q89.4
Sibling rivalry Z62.891
Sicard's syndrome G52.7
➡ **Sicca syndrome** —*see* Syndrome, Sjogren
  ~~with~~
    ~~keratoconjunctivitis M35.01~~
    ~~lung involvement M35.02~~
    ~~myopathy M35.03~~
    ~~renal tubulo-interstitial disorders M35.04~~
    ~~specified organ involvement NEC M35.09~~
Sick R69
  or handicapped person in family Z63.79
    needing care at home Z63.6
  sinus (syndrome) I49.5
Sick-euthyroid syndrome E07.81
Sickle-cell
  anemia —*see* Disease, sickle-cell
  beta plus —*see* Disease, sickle-cell,
      thalassemia, beta plus
  beta zero —*see* Disease, sickle-cell,
      thalassemia, beta zero
  trait D57.3

Sicklemia —*see also* Disease, sickle-cell
  trait D57.3
Sickness
  air (travel) T75.3
  airplane T75.3
  alpine T70.29
  altitude T70.20
  Andes T70.29
  aviator's T70.29
  balloon T70.29
  car T75.3
  compressed air T70.3
  decompression T70.3
  green D50.8
  milk —*see* Poisoning, food, noxious
  motion T75.3
  mountain T70.29
    acute D75.1
  protein —*see also* Reaction, serum T80.69
  radiation T66
  roundabout (motion) T75.3
  sea T75.3
  serum NEC —*see also* Reaction, serum T80.69
  sleeping (African) B56.9
    by Trypanosoma B56.9
      brucei
        gambiense B56.0
        rhodesiense B56.1
    East African B56.1
    Gambian B56.0
    Rhodesian B56.1
    West African B56.0
  swing (motion) T75.3
  train (railway) (travel) T75.3
  travel (any vehicle) T75.3
Sideropenia —*see* Anemia, iron deficiency
Siderosilicosis J62.8
Siderosis (lung) J63.4
  brain G93.89
  eye (globe) —*see* Disorder, globe,
      degenerative, siderosis
Siemens' syndrome (ectodermal dysplasia) Q82.8
Sighing R06.89
  psychogenic F45.8
Sigmoid —*see also* condition
  flexure —*see* condition
  kidney Q63.1
Sigmoiditis —*see also* Enteritis K52.9
  infectious A09
  noninfectious K52.9
Silfversköld's syndrome Q78.9
Silicosiderosis J62.8
Silicosis, silicotic (simple) (complicated) J62.8
  with tuberculosis J65
Silicotuberculosis J65
Silo-fillers' disease J68.8
  bronchitis J68.0
  pneumonitis J68.0
  pulmonary edema J68.1
Silver's syndrome Q87.19
Simian malaria B53.1
Simmonds' cachexia or disease E23.0
Simons' disease or syndrome (progressive
    lipodystrophy) E88.1
Simple, simplex —*see* condition
Simulation, conscious (of illness) Z76.5
Simultanagnosia (asimultagnosia) R48.3
Sin Nombre virus disease (Hantavirus)
    (cardio)-pulmonary syndrome) B33.4
Sinding-Larsen disease or osteochondrosis —
    see Osteochondrosis, juvenile, patella
Singapore hemorrhagic fever A91
Singer's node or nodule J38.2
Single
  atrium Q21.2
  coronary artery Q24.5
  umbilical artery Q27.0
  ventricle Q20.4
Singultus R06.6
  epidemicus B33.0
Sinus —*see also* Fistula
  abdominal K63.89
  arrest I45.5

▶ New   ➡ Revised   ~~deleted~~ Deleted   • Use Additional Character(s)

Sinus *(Continued)*
  arrhythmia I49.8
  bradycardia R00.1
  branchial cleft (internal) (external) Q18.0
  coccygeal —*see* Sinus, pilonidal
  dental K04.6
  dermal (congenital) Q06.8
    with abscess Q06.8
    coccygeal, pilonidal —*see* Sinus, coccygeal
  infected, skin NEC L08.89
  marginal, ruptured or bleeding —*see*
    Hemorrhage, antepartum, specified
    cause NEC
  medial, face and neck Q18.8
  pause I45.5
  pericranii Q01.9
  pilonidal (infected) (rectum) L05.92
    with abscess L05.02
  preauricular Q18.1
  rectovaginal N82.3
  Rokitansky-Aschoff (gallbladder) K82.8
  sacrococcygeal (dermoid) (infected) —*see*
    Sinus, pilonidal
  tachycardia R00.0
    paroxysmal I47.1
  tarsi syndrome M25.57- •
  testis N50.89
  tract (postinfective) —*see* Fistula
  urachus Q64.4
Sinusitis (accessory) (chronic) (hyperplastic)
  (nasal) (nonpurulent) (purulent) J32.9
  acute J01.90
    ethmoidal J01.20
      recurrent J01.21
    frontal J01.10
      recurrent J01.11
    involving more than one sinus, other than
      pansinusitis J01.80
      recurrent J01.81
    maxillary J01.00
      recurrent J01.01
    pansinusitis J01.40
      recurrent J01.41
    recurrent J01.91
    specified NEC J01.80
      recurrent J01.81
    sphenoidal J01.30
      recurrent J01.31
  allergic —*see* Rhinitis, allergic
  due to high altitude T70.1
  ethmoidal J32.2
    acute J01.20
      recurrent J01.21
  frontal J32.1
    acute J01.10
      recurrent J01.11
  influenzal —*see* Influenza, with, respiratory
    manifestations NEC
  involving more than one sinus but not
    pansinusitis J32.8
    acute J01.80
      recurrent J01.81
  maxillary J32.0
    acute J01.00
      recurrent J01.01
  sphenoidal J32.3
    acute J01.30
      recurrent J01.31
  tuberculous, any sinus A15.8
Sinusitis-bronchiectasis-situs inversus
  (syndrome) (triad) Q89.3
Sipple's syndrome E31.22
Sirenomelia (syndrome) Q87.2
Siriasis T67.01
Sirkari's disease B55.0
Siti A65
Situation, psychiatric F99
Situational
  disturbance (transient) —*see* Disorder,
    adjustment
    acute F43.0

Situational *(Continued)*
  maladjustment —*see* Disorder, adjustment
  reaction —*see* Disorder, adjustment
    acute F43.0
Situs inversus or transversus (abdominalis)
  (thoracis) Q89.3
Sixth disease B08.20
  due to human herpesvirus 6 B08.21
  due to human herpesvirus 7 B08.22
Sjögren-Larsson syndrome Q87.19
Sjögren's syndrome or disease —*see* Syndrome,
  Sjögren
Skeletal —*see* condition
Skene's gland —*see* condition
Skenitis —*see* Urethritis
Skerljevo A65
Skevas-Zerfus disease —*see* Toxicity, venom,
  marine animal, sea anemone
Skin —*see also* condition
  clammy R23.1
  donor —*see* Donor, skin
  dry L85.3
  hidebound M35.9
Slate-dressers' or slate-miners' lung J62.8
Sleep
  apnea —*see* Apnea, sleep
  deprivation Z72.820
  disorder or disturbance G47.9
    child F51.9
    nonorganic origin F51.9
    specified NEC G47.8
  disturbance G47.9
    nonorganic origin F51.9
  drunkenness F51.9
  rhythm inversion G47.2- •
  terrors F51.4
  walking F51.3
    hysterical F44.89
Sleep hygiene
  abuse Z72.821
  inadequate Z72.821
  poor Z72.821
Sleeping sickness —*see* Sickness, sleeping
Sleeplessness —*see* Insomnia
  menopausal N95.11
Sleep-wake schedule disorder G47.20
Slim disease (in HIV infection) B20
Slipped, slipping
  epiphysis (traumatic) —*see also*
    Osteochondropathy, specified type
    NEC
    capital femoral (traumatic)
      acute (on chronic) S79.01- •
    current traumatic - code as Fracture,
      by site
    upper femoral (nontraumatic) M93.00- •
      acute M93.01- •
      on chronic M93.03- •
      chronic M93.02- •
  intervertebral disc —*see* Displacement,
    intervertebral disc
  ligature, umbilical P51.8
  patella —*see* Disorder, patella, derangement
    NEC
  rib M89.8X8
  sacroiliac joint —*see* subcategory M53.2
  tendon —*see* Disorder, tendon
  ulnar nerve, nontraumatic —*see* Lesion,
    nerve, ulnar
  vertebra NEC —*see* Spondylolisthesis
Slocumb's syndrome E27.0
Sloughing (multiple) (phagedena) (skin) —*see
  also* Gangrene
  abscess —*see* Abscess
  appendix K38.8
  fascia —*see* Disorder, soft tissue, specified
    type NEC
  scrotum N50.89
  tendon —*see* Disorder, tendon
  transplanted organ —*see* Rejection, transplant
  ulcer —*see* Ulcer, skin

Slow
  feeding, newborn P92.2
  flow syndrome, coronary I20.8
  heart(beat) R00.1
Slowing, urinary stream R39.198
Sluder's neuralgia (syndrome) G44.89
Slurred, slurring speech R47.81
Small (ness)
  for gestational age —*see* Small for dates
  introitus, vagina N89.6
  kidney (unknown cause) N27.9
    bilateral N27.1
    unilateral N27.0
  ovary (congenital) Q50.39
  pelvis
    with disproportion (fetopelvic) O33.1
      causing obstructed labor O65.1
  uterus N85.8
  white kidney N03.9
Small-and-light-for-dates —*see* Small for
  dates
Small-for-dates (infant) P05.10
  with weight of
    499 grams or less P05.11
    500-749 grams P05.12
    750-999 grams P05.13
    1000-1249 grams P05.14
    1250-1499 grams P05.15
    1500-1749 grams P05.16
    1750-1999 grams P05.17
    2000-2499 grams P05.18
    2500 grams and over P05.19
  specified NEC P05.19
Smallpox B03
Smearing, fecal R15.1
SMEI (severe myoclonic epilepsy in infancy)
  G40.83- •
Smith-Lemli-Opitz syndrome E78.72
Smith's fracture S52.54- •
Smoker —*see* Dependence, drug, nicotine
Smoker's
  bronchitis J41.0
  cough J41.0
  palate K13.24
  throat J31.2
  tongue K13.24
Smoking
  passive Z77.22
Smothering spells R06.81
Snaggle teeth, tooth M26.39
Snapping
  finger —*see* Trigger finger
  hip —*see* Derangement, joint, specified type
    NEC, hip
    involving the iliotiblial band M76.3- •
  knee —*see* Derangement, knee
    involving the iliotiblial band M76.3- •
Sneddon-Wilkinson disease or syndrome
  (sub-corneal pustular dermatosis)
  L13.1
Sneezing (intractable) R06.7
Sniffing
  cocaine
    abuse —*see* Abuse, drug, cocaine
    dependence —*see* Dependence, drug,
      cocaine
  gasoline
    abuse —*see* Abuse, drug, inhalant
    dependence —*see* Dependence, drug,
      inhalant
  glue (airplane)
    abuse —*see* Abuse, drug, inhalant
    drug dependence —*see* Dependence, drug,
      inhalant
Sniffles
  newborn P28.89
Snoring R06.83
Snow blindness —*see* Photokeratitis
Snuffles (non-syphilitic) R06.5
  newborn P28.89
  syphilitic (infant) A50.05 *[J99]*

S

Social
  exclusion Z60.4
    due to discrimination or persecution
      (perceived) Z60.5
  ⇒migrant Z59.00
    acculturation difficulty Z60.3
  rejection Z60.4
    due to discrimination or persecution Z60.5
  role conflict NEC Z73.5
  skills inadequacy NEC Z73.4
  transplantation Z60.3
Sodoku A25.0
Soemmerring's ring —see Cataract, secondary
Soft —see also condition
  nails L60.3
Softening
  bone —see Osteomalacia
  brain (necrotic) (progressive) G93.89
    congenital Q04.8
    embolic I63.4-●
    hemorrhagic —see Hemorrhage,
      intracranial, intracerebral
    occlusive I63.5-●
    thrombotic I63.3-●
  cartilage M94.2-●
    patella M22.4-●
  cerebellar —see Softening, brain
  cerebral —see Softening, brain
  cerebrospinal —see Softening, brain
  myocardial, heart —see Degeneration,
    myocardial
  spinal cord G95.89
  stomach K31.89
Soldier's
  heart F45.8
  patches I31.0
Solitary
  cyst, kidney N28.1
  kidney, congenital Q60.0
Solvent abuse —see Abuse, drug, inhalant
  dependence —see Dependence, drug,
    inhalant
Somatization reaction, somatic reaction —see
  Disorder, somatoform
Somnambulism F51.3
  hysterical F44.89
Somnolence R40.0
  nonorganic origin F51.11
Sonne dysentery A03.3
Soor B37.0
Sore
  bed —see Ulcer, pressure, by site
  chiclero B55.1
  Delhi B55.1
  desert —see Ulcer, skin
  eye H57.1-●
  Lahore B55.1
  mouth K13.79
    canker K12.0
  muscle M79.10
  Naga —see Ulcer, skin
  of skin —see Ulcer, skin - oriental B55.1
  pressure —see Ulcer, pressure, by site
  skin L98.9
  soft A57
  throat (acute) —see also Pharyngitis
    with influenza, flu, or grippe —see
      Influenza, with, respiratory
      manifestations NEC
    chronic J31.2
    coxsackie (virus) B08.5
    diphtheritic A36.0
    herpesviral B00.2
    influenzal —see Influenza, with, respiratory
      manifestations NEC
    septic J02.0
    streptococcal (ulcerative) J02.0
    viral NEC J02.8
      coxsackie B08.5
  tropical —see Ulcer, skin
  veldt —see Ulcer, skin

Soto's syndrome (cerebral gigantism) Q87.3
South African cardiomyopathy syndrome I42.8
Southeast Asian hemorrhagic fever A91
Spacing
  abnormal, tooth, teeth, fully erupted M26.30
  excessive, tooth, fully erupted M26.32
Spade-like hand (congenital) Q68.1
Spading nail L60.8
  congenital Q84.6
Spanish collar N47.1
Sparganosis B70.1
Spasm(s), spastic, spasticity —see also condition
  R25.2
  accommodation —see Spasm, of
    accommodation
  ampulla of Vater K83.4
  anus, ani (sphincter) (reflex) K59.4
    psychogenic F45.8
  artery I73.9
    cerebral G45.9
  Bell's G51.3-●
  bladder (sphincter, external or internal)
    N32.89
    psychogenic F45.8
  bronchus, bronchiole J98.01
  cardia K22.0
  cardiac I20.1
  carpopedal —see Tetany
  cerebral (arteries) (vascular) G45.9
  cervix, complicating delivery O62.4
  ciliary body (of accommodation) —see Spasm,
    of accommodation
  colon —see also Irritable, bowel K58.9
    with diarrhea K58.0
    psychogenic F45.8
  common duct K83.8
  compulsive —see Tic
  conjugate H51.8
  coronary (artery) I20.1
  diaphragm (reflex) R06.6
    epidemic B33.0
    psychogenic F45.8
  duodenum K59.89
  epidemic diaphragmatic (transient) B33.0
  esophagus (diffuse) K22.4
    psychogenic F45.8
  facial G51.3-●
  fallopian tube N83.8
  gastrointestinal (tract) K31.89
    psychogenic F45.8
  glottis J38.5
    hysterical F44.4
    psychogenic F45.8
      conversion reaction F44.4
    reflex through recurrent laryngeal nerve
      J38.5
  habit —see Tic
  heart I20.1
  hemifacial (clonic) G51.3-●
  hourglass —see Contraction, hourglass
  hysterical F44.4
  infantile —see Epilepsy, spasms
  inferior oblique, eye H51.8
  intestinal —see also Syndrome, irritable bowel
    K58.9
    psychogenic F45.8
  larynx, laryngeal J38.5
    hysterical F44.4
    psychogenic F45.8
      conversion reaction F44.4
  levator palpebrae superioris —see Disorder,
    eyelid function
  muscle NEC M62.838
    back M62.830
  nerve, trigeminal G51.0
  nervous F45.8
  nodding F98.4
  occupational F48.8
  oculogyric H51.8
    psychogenic F45.8
  of accommodation H52.53-●

Spasm(s), spastic, spasticity (Continued)
  ophthalmic artery —see Occlusion, artery,
    retina
  perineal, female N94.89
  peroneo-extensor —see also Deformity, limb,
    flat foot
  pharynx (reflex) J39.2
    hysterical F45.8
    psychogenic F45.8
  psychogenic F45.8
  pylorus NEC K31.3
    adult hypertrophic K31.89
    congenital or infantile Q40.0
    psychogenic F45.8
  rectum (sphincter) K59.4
    psychogenic F45.8
  retinal (artery) —see Occlusion, artery, retina
  sigmoid —see also Syndrome, irritable bowel
    K58.9
    psychogenic F45.8
  sphincter of Oddi K83.4
  stomach K31.89
    neurotic F45.8
  throat J39.2
    hysterical F45.8
    psychogenic F45.8
  tic F95.9
    chronic F95.1
    transient of childhood F95.0
  tongue K14.8
  torsion (progressive) G24.1
  trigeminal nerve —see Neuralgia, trigeminal
  ureter N13.5
  urethra (sphincter) N35.919
  uterus N85.8
    complicating labor O62.4
  vagina N94.2
    psychogenic F52.5
  vascular I73.9
  vasomotor I73.9
  vein NEC I87.8
  viscera —see Pain, abdominal
Spasmodic —see condition
Spasmophilia —see Tetany
Spasmus nutans F98.4
Spastic, spasticity —see also Spasm
  child (cerebral) (congenital) (paralysis)
    G80.1
Speaker's throat R49.8
Specific, specified —see condition
Speech
  defect, disorder, disturbance, impediment —
    see Disorder, speech R47.9
    psychogenic, in childhood and adolescence
      F98.8
    slurring R47.81
    specified NEC R47.89
Spencer's disease A08.19
Spens' syndrome (syncope with heart block)
  I45.9
Sperm counts (fertility testing) Z31.41
  postvasectomy Z30.8
    reversal Z31.42
Spermatic cord —see condition
Spermatocele N43.40
  congenital Q55.4
  multiple N43.42
  single N43.41
Spermatocystitis N49.0
Spermatocytoma C62.9-●
  specified site —see Neoplasm, malignant, by
    site
Spermatorrhea N50.89
Sphacelus —see Gangrene
Sphenoidal —see condition
Sphenoiditis (chronic) —see Sinusitis,
  sphenoidal
Sphenopalatine ganglion neuralgia
  G90.09
Sphericity, increased, lens (congenital)
  Q12.4

▶ New   ⇒ Revised   ~~deleted~~ Deleted   ● Use Additional Character(s)

Spherocytosis (congenital) (familial) (hereditary) D58.0
  hemoglobin disease D58.0
  sickle-cell (disease) D57.8-●
Spherophakia Q12.4
Sphincter —see condition
Sphincteritis, sphincter of Oddi —see Cholangitis
Sphingolipidosis E75.3
  specified NEC E75.29
Sphingomyelinosis E75.3
Spicule tooth K00.2
Spider
  bite —see Toxicity, venom, spider
    nonvenomous —see Bite, by site, superficial, insect
  fingers —see Syndrome, Marfan's
  nevus I78.1
  toes —see Syndrome, Marfan's
  vascular I78.1
Spiegler-Fendt
  benign lymphocytoma L98.8
  sarcoid L08.89
Spielmeyer-Vogt disease E75.4
Spina bifida (aperta) Q05.9
  with hydrocephalus NEC Q05.4
  cervical Q05.5
    with hydrocephalus Q05.0
  dorsal Q05.6
    with hydrocephalus Q05.1
  lumbar Q05.7
    with hydrocephalus Q05.2
  lumbosacral Q05.7
    with hydrocephalus Q05.2
  occulta Q76.0
  sacral Q05.8
    with hydrocephalus Q05.3
  thoracic Q05.6
    with hydrocephalus Q05.1
  thoracolumbar Q05.6
    with hydrocephalus Q05.1
Spindle, Krukenberg's —see Pigmentation, cornea, posterior
Spine, spinal —see condition
Spiradenoma (eccrine) —see Neoplasm, skin, benign
Spirillosis A25.0
Spirillum
  minus A25.0
  obermeieri infection A68.0
Spirochetal —see condition
Spirochetosis A69.9
  arthritic, arthritica A69.9
  bronchopulmonary A69.8
  icterohemorrhagic A27.0
  lung A69.8
Spirometrosis B70.1
Spitting blood —see Hemoptysis
Splanchnoptosis K63.4
Spleen, splenic —see condition
Splenectasis —see Splenomegaly
Splenitis (interstitial) (malignant) (nonspecific) D73.89
  malarial —see also Malaria B54 [D77]
  tuberculous A18.85
Splenocele D73.89
Splenomegaly, splenomegalia (Bengal) (cryptogenic) (idiopathic) (tropical) R16.1
  with hepatomegaly R16.2
  cirrhotic D73.2
  congenital Q89.09
  congestive, chronic D73.2
  Egyptian B65.1
  Gaucher's E75.22
  malarial —see also Malaria B54 [D77]
  neutropenic D73.81
  Niemann-Pick —see Niemann-Pick disease or syndrome
  siderotic D73.2
  syphilitic A52.79
    congenital (early) A50.08 [D77]

Splenopathy D73.9
Splenoptosis D73.89
Splenosis D73.89
Splinter —see Foreign body, superficial, by site
Split, splitting
  foot Q72.7-●
  hand Q71.6
  heart sounds R01.2
  lip, congenital —see Cleft, lip
  nails L60.3
  urinary stream R39.13
Spondylarthrosis —see Spondylosis
Spondylitis (chronic) —see also Spondylopathy, inflammatory
  ankylopoietica —see Spondylitis, ankylosing
  ankylosing (chronic) M45.9
    with lung involvement M45.9 [J99]
    cervical region M45.2
    cervicothoracic region M45.3
    juvenile M08.1
    lumbar region M45.6
    lumbosacral region M45.7
    multiple sites M45.0
    occipito-atlanto-axial region M45.1
    sacrococcygeal region M45.8
    thoracic region M45.4
    thoracolumbar region M45.5
  atrophic (ligamentous) —see Spondylitis, ankylosing
  deformans (chronic) —see Spondylosis
  gonococcal A54.41
  gouty —see also Gout, by type, vertebrae M10.08
  in (due to)
    brucellosis A23.9 [M49.80]
      cervical region A23.9 [M49.82]
      cervicothoracic region A23.9 [M49.83]
      lumbar region A23.9 [M49.86]
      lumbosacral region A23.9 [M49.87]
      multiple sites A23.9 [M49.89]
      occipito-atlanto-axial region A23.9 [M49.81]
      sacrococcygeal region A23.9 [M49.88]
      thoracic region A23.9 [M49.84]
      thoracolumbar region A23.9 [M49.85]
    enterobacteria —see also subcategory M49.8 A04.9
    tuberculosis A18.01
  infectious NEC —see Spondylopathy, infective
  juvenile ankylosing (chronic) M08.1
  Kümmell's —see Spondylopathy, traumatic
  Marie-Strümpell —see Spondylitis, ankylosing
  muscularis —see Spondylopathy, specified NEC
  psoriatic L40.53
  rheumatoid —see Spondylitis, ankylosing
  rhizomelica —see Spondylitis, ankylosing
  sacroiliac NEC M46.1
  senescent, senile —see Spondylosis
  traumatic (chronic) or post-traumatic —see Spondylopathy, traumatic
  tuberculous A18.01
  typhosa A01.05
Spondyloarthritis
  axial —see also Spondlyitis, ankylosing
  ⇛non-radiographic M45.A0
    ⇛cervical M45.A2
    ⇛cervicothoracic M45.A3
    ⇛lumbar M45.A6
    ⇛lumbosacral M45.A7
    ⇛multiple sites M45.AB
    ⇛occipito-atlanto-axial region M45.A1
    ⇛sacral and sacrococcygeal M45.A8
    ⇛thoracic M45.A4
    ⇛thoracolumbar M45.A5
Spondylolisthesis (acquired) (degenerative) M43.10
  with disproportion (fetopelvic) O33.0
    causing obstructed labor O65.0

Spondylolisthesis (Continued)
  cervical region M43.12
  cervicothoracic region M43.13
  congenital Q76.2
  lumbar region M43.16
  lumbosacral region M43.17
  multiple sites M43.19
  occipito-atlanto-axial region M43.11
  sacrococcygeal region M43.18
  thoracic region M43.14
  thoracolumbar region M43.15
  traumatic (old) M43.10
    acute
      fifth cervical (displaced) S12.430
        nondisplaced S12.431
        specified type NEC (displaced) S12.450
          nondisplaced S12.451
        type III S12.44
      fourth cervical (displaced) S12.330
        nondisplaced S12.331
        specified type NEC (displaced) S12.350
          nondisplaced S12.351
        type III S12.34
      second cervical (displaced) S12.130
        nondisplaced S12.131
        specified type NEC (displaced) S12.150
          nondisplaced S12.151
        type III S12.14
      seventh cervical (displaced) S12.630
        nondisplaced S12.631
        specified type NEC (displaced) S12.650
          nondisplaced S12.651
        type III S12.64
      sixth cervical (displaced) S12.530
        nondisplaced S12.531
        specified type NEC (displaced) S12.550
          nondisplaced S12.551
        type III S12.54
      third cervical (displaced) S12.230
        nondisplaced S12.231
        specified type NEC (displaced) S12.250
          nondisplaced S12.251
        type III S12.24
Spondylolysis (acquired) M43.00
  cervical region M43.02
  cervicothoracic region M43.03
  congenital Q76.2
  lumbar region M43.06
  lumbosacral region M43.07
    with disproportion (fetopelvic) O33.0
      causing obstructed labor O65.8
  multiple sites M43.09
  occipito-atlanto-axial region M43.01
  sacrococcygeal region M43.08
  thoracic region M43.04
  thoracolumbar region M43.05
Spondylopathy M48.9
  infective NEC M46.50
    cervical region M46.52
    cervicothoracic region M46.53
    lumbar region M46.56
    lumbosacral region M46.57
    multiple sites M46.59
    occipito-atlanto-axial region M46.51
    sacrococcygeal region M46.58
    thoracic region M46.54
    thoracolumbar region M46.55
  inflammatory M46.90
    cervical region M46.92
    cervicothoracic region M46.93
    lumbar region M46.96
    lumbosacral region M46.97
    multiple sites M46.99
    occipito-atlanto-axial region M46.91
    sacrococcygeal region M46.98

Spondylopathy *(Continued)*
  inflammatory *(Continued)*
    specified type NEC M46.80
      cervical region M46.82
      cervicothoracic region M46.83
      lumbar region M46.86
      lumbosacral region M46.87
      multiple sites M46.89
      occipito-atlanto-axial region M46.81
      sacrococcygeal region M46.88
      thoracic region M46.84
      thoracolumbar region M46.85
    thoracic region M46.94
    thoracolumbar region M46.95
  neuropathic, in
    syringomyelia and syringobulbia G95.0
    tabes dorsalis A52.11
  specified NEC —*see* subcategory M48.8
  traumatic M48.30
    cervical region M48.32
    cervicothoracic region M48.33
    lumbar region M48.36
    lumbosacral region M48.37
    occipito-atlanto-axial region M48.31
    sacrococcygeal region M48.38
    thoracic region M48.34
    thoracolumbar region M48.35
Spondylosis M47.9
  with
    disproportion (fetopelvic) O33.0
      causing obstructed labor O65.0
    myelopathy NEC M47.10
      cervical region M47.12
      cervicothoracic region M47.13
      lumbar region M47.16
      occipito-atlanto-axial region M47.11
      thoracic region M47.14
      thoracolumbar region M47.15
    radiculopathy M47.20
      cervical region M47.22
      cervicothoracic region M47.23
      lumbar region M47.26
      lumbosacral region M47.27
      occipito-atlanto-axial region M47.21
      sacrococcygeal region M47.28
      thoracic region M47.24
      thoracolumbar region M47.25
  without myelopathy or radiculopathy
    M47.819
    cervical region M47.812
    cervicothoracic region M47.813
    lumbar region M47.816
    lumbosacral region M47.817
    occipito-atlanto-axial region M47.811
    sacrococcygeal region M47.818
    thoracic region M47.814
    thoracolumbar region M47.815
  specified NEC M47.899
    cervical region M47.892
    cervicothoracic region M47.893
    ▶facet joint (*see also* Spondylosis) M47.819
    lumbar region M47.896
    lumbosacral region M47.897
    occipito-atlanto-axial region M47.891
    sacrococcygeal region M47.898
    thoracic region M47.894
    thoracolumbar region M47.895
  traumatic —*see* Spondylopathy, traumatic
Sponge
  inadvertently left in operation wound —*see*
    Foreign body, accidentally left during a
    procedure
  kidney (medullary) Q61.5
Sponge-diver's disease —*see* Toxicity, venom,
    marine animal, sea anemone
Spongioblastoma (any type) —*see* Neoplasm,
    malignant, by site
  specified site —*see* Neoplasm, malignant, by
    site
  unspecified site C71.9
Spongioneuroblastoma —*see* Neoplasm,
    malignant, by site

Spontaneous —*see also* condition
  fracture (cause unknown) —*see* Fracture,
    pathological
Spoon nail L60.3
  congenital Q84.6
Sporadic —*see* condition
Sporothrix schenckii infection —*see*
    Sporotrichosis
Sporotrichosis B42.9
  arthritis B42.82
  disseminated B42.7
  generalized B42.7
  lymphocutaneous (fixed) (progressive)
    B42.1
  pulmonary B42.0
  specified NEC B42.89
Spots, spotting (in) (of)
  Bitot's —*see also* Pigmentation, conjunctiva
    in the young child E50.1
      vitamin A deficiency E50.1
  café, au lait L81.3
  Cayenne pepper I78.1
  cotton wool, retina —*see* Occlusion, artery,
    retina
  de Morgan's (senile angiomas) I78.1
  Fuchs' black (myopic) —*see also* Myopia,
    degenerative H44.2-●
  intermenstrual (regular) N92.0
    irregular N92.1
  Koplik's B05.9
  liver L81.4
  pregnancy O26.85-●
  purpuric R23.3
  ruby I78.1
Spotted fever —*see* Fever, spotted A77.9
Sprain (joint) (ligament)
  acromioclavicular joint or ligament S43.5-●
  ankle S93.40-●
    calcaneofibular ligament S93.41-●
    deltoid ligament S93.42-●
    internal collateral ligament —*see* Sprain,
      ankle, specified ligament NEC
    specified ligament NEC S93.49-●
    talofibular ligament —*see* Sprain, ankle,
      specified ligament NEC
    tibiofibular ligament S93.43-●
  anterior longitudinal, cervical S13.4
  atlas, atlanto-axial, atlanto-occipital S13.4
  breast bone —*see* Sprain, sternum
  calcaneofibular —*see* Sprain, ankle
  carpal —*see* Sprain, wrist
  carpometacarpal —*see* Sprain, hand, specified
    site NEC
  cartilage
    costal S23.41
    semilunar (knee) —*see* Sprain, knee,
      specified site NEC
      with current tear —*see* Tear, meniscus
    thyroid region S13.5
    xiphoid —*see* Sprain, sternum
  cervical, cervicodorsal, cervicothoracic S13.4
  chondrosternal S23.421
  coracoclavicular S43.8-●
  coracohumeral S43.41-●
  coronary, knee —*see* Sprain, knee, specified
    site NEC
  costal cartilage S23.41
  cricoarytenoid articulation or ligament S13.5
  cricothyroid articulation S13.5
  cruciate, knee —*see* Sprain, knee, cruciate
  deltoid, ankle —*see* Sprain, ankle
  dorsal (spine) S23.3
  elbow S53.40-●
    radial collateral ligament S53.43-●
    radiohumeral S53.41-●
    rupture
      radial collateral ligament —*see* Rupture,
        traumatic, ligament, radial
        collateral
      ulnar collateral ligament —*see* Rupture,
        traumatic, ligament, ulnar collateral

Sprain *(Continued)*
  elbow *(Continued)*
    specified type NEC S53.49-●
    ulnar collateral ligament S53.44-●
    ulnohumeral S53.42-●
  femur, head —*see* Sprain, hip
  fibular collateral, knee —*see* Sprain, knee,
    collateral
  fibulocalcaneal —*see* Sprain, ankle
  finger(s) S63.61-●
    index S63.61-●
    interphalangeal (joint) S63.63-●
      index S63.63-●
      little S63.63-●
      middle S63.63-●
      ring S63.63-●
    little S63.61-●
    metacarpophalangeal (joint) S63.65-●
    middle S63.61-●
    ring S63.61-●
    specified site NEC S63.69-●
      index S63.69-●
      little S63.69-●
      middle S63.69-●
      ring S63.69-●
  foot S93.60-●
    specified ligament NEC S93.69-●
    tarsal ligament S93.61-●
    tarsometatarsal ligament S93.62-●
    toe —*see* Sprain, toe
  hand S63.9-●
    finger —*see* Sprain, finger
    specified site NEC —*see* subcategory
      S63.8
    thumb —*see* Sprain, thumb
  head S03.9
  hip S73.10-●
    iliofemoral ligament S73.11-●
    ischiocapsular (ligament) S73.12-●
    specified NEC S73.19-●
  iliofemoral —*see* Sprain, hip
  innominate
    acetabulum —*see* Sprain, hip
    sacral junction S33.6
  internal
    collateral, ankle —*see* Sprain, ankle
    semilunar cartilage —*see* Sprain, knee,
      specified site NEC
  interphalangeal
    finger —*see* Sprain, finger, interphalangeal
      (joint)
    toe —*see* Sprain, toe, interphalangeal joint
  ischiocapsular —*see* Sprain, hip
  ischiofemoral —*see* Sprain, hip
  jaw (articular disc) (cartilage) (meniscus)
    S03.4-●
    old M26.69
  knee S83.9-●
    collateral ligament S83.40-●
      lateral (fibular) S83.42-●
      medial (tibial) S83.41-●
    cruciate ligament S83.50-●
      anterior S83.51-●
      posterior S83.52-●
    lateral (fibular) collateral ligament S83.42-●
    medial (tibial) collateral ligament S83.41-●
    patellar ligament S76.11-●
    specified site NEC S83.8X-●
    superior tibiofibular joint (ligament)
      S83.6-●
  lateral collateral, knee —*see* Sprain, knee,
    collateral
  lumbar (spine) S33.5
  lumbosacral S33.9
  mandible (articular disc) S03.4-●
    old M26.69
  medial collateral, knee —*see* Sprain, knee,
    collateral
  meniscus
    jaw S03.4-●
      old M26.69

▶ New   ⇒ Revised   ~~deleted~~ Deleted   ● Use Additional Character(s)

Sprain *(Continued)*
  meniscus *(Continued)*
    knee —*see* Sprain, knee, specified site NEC
      with current tear —*see* Tear, meniscus
      old —*see* Derangement, knee,
        meniscus, due to old tear
    mandible S03.4-●
      old M26.69
  metacarpal (distal) (proximal) —*see* Sprain,
    hand, specified site NEC
  metacarpophalangeal —*see* Sprain, finger,
    metacarpophalangeal (joint)
  metatarsophalangeal —*see* Sprain, toe,
    metatarsophalangeal joint
  midcarpal —*see* Sprain, hand, specified site
    NEC
  midtarsal —*see* Sprain, foot, specified site
    NEC
  neck S13.9
    anterior longitudinal cervical ligament
      S13.4
    atlanto-axial joint S13.4
    atlanto-occipital joint S13.4
    cervical spine S13.4
    cricoarytenoid ligament S13.5
    cricothyroid ligament S13.5
    specified site NEC S13.8
    thyroid region (cartilage) S13.5
  nose S03.8
  orbicular, hip —*see* Sprain, hip
  patella —*see* Sprain, knee, specified site
    NEC
  patellar ligament S76.11-●
  pelvis NEC S33.8
  phalanx
    finger —*see* Sprain, finger
    toe —*see* Sprain, toe
  pubofemoral —*see* Sprain, hip
  radiocarpal —*see* Sprain, wrist
  radiohumeral —*see* Sprain, elbow
  radius, collateral —*see* Rupture, traumatic,
    ligament, radial collateral
  rib (cage) S23.41
  rotator cuff (capsule) S43.42-●
  sacroiliac (region)
    chronic or old —*see* subcategory M53.2
    joint S33.6
  scaphoid (hand) —*see* Sprain, hand, specified
    site NEC
  scapula (r) —*see* Sprain, shoulder girdle,
    specified site NEC
  semilunar cartilage (knee) —*see* Sprain, knee,
    specified site NEC
    with current tear —*see* Tear, meniscus
    old —*see* Derangement, knee, meniscus,
      due to old tear
  shoulder joint S43.40-●
    acromioclavicular joint (ligament) —*see*
      Sprain, acromioclavicular joint
    blade —*see* Sprain, shoulder, girdle,
      specified site NEC
    coracoclavicular joint (ligament) —*see*
      Sprain, coracoclavicular joint
    coracohumeral ligament —*see* Sprain,
      coracohumeral joint
    girdle S43.9-●
      specified site NEC S43.8-●
    rotator cuff —*see* Sprain, rotator cuff
    specified site NEC S43.49-●
    sternoclavicular joint (ligament) —*see*
      Sprain, sternoclavicular joint
  spine
    cervical S13.4
    lumbar S33.5
    thoracic S23.3
  sternoclavicular joint S43.6-●
  sternum S23.429
    chondrosternal joint S23.421
    specified site NEC S23.428
    sternoclavicular (joint) (ligament)
      S23.420

Sprain *(Continued)*
  symphysis
    jaw S03.4-●
      old M26.69
    mandibular S03.4-●
      old M26.69
  talofibular —*see* Sprain, ankle
  tarsal —*see* Sprain, foot, specified site NEC
  tarsometatarsal —*see* Sprain, foot, specified
    site NEC
  temporomandibular S03.4-●
    old M26.69
  thorax S23.9
    ribs S23.41
    specified site NEC S23.8
    spine S23.3
    sternum —*see* Sprain, sternum
  thumb S63.60-●
    interphalangeal (joint) S63.62-●
    metacarpophalangeal (joint) S63.64-●
    specified site NEC S63.68-●
  thyroid cartilage or region S13.5
  tibia (proximal end) —*see* Sprain, knee,
    specified site NEC
  tibial collateral, knee —*see* Sprain, knee,
    collateral
  tibiofibular
    distal —*see* Sprain, ankle
    superior —*see* Sprain, knee, specified site
      NEC
  toe(s) S93.50-●
    great S93.50-●
    interphalangeal joint S93.51-●
      great S93.51-●
      lesser S93.51-●
    lesser S93.50-●
    metatarsophalangeal joint S93.52-●
      great S93.52-●
      lesser S93.52-●
  ulna, collateral —*see* Rupture, traumatic,
    ligament, ulnar collateral
  ulnohumeral —*see* Sprain, elbow
  wrist S63.50-●
    carpal S63.51-●
    radiocarpal S63.52-●
    specified site NEC S63.59-●
  xiphoid cartilage —*see* Sprain, sternum
Sprengel's deformity (congenital) Q74.0
Sprue (tropical) K90.1
  celiac K90.0
  idiopathic K90.49
  meaning thrush B37.0
  nontropical K90.0
Spur, bone —*see also* Enthesopathy
  calcaneal M77.3-●
  iliac crest M76.2-●
  nose (septum) J34.89
Spurway's syndrome Q78.0
Sputum
  abnormal (amount) (color) (odor) (purulent)
    R09.3
  blood-stained R04.2
  excessive (cause unknown) R09.3
Squamous —*see also* condition
  epithelium in
    cervical canal (congenital) Q51.828
    uterine mucosa (congenital) Q51.818
Squashed nose M95.0
  congenital Q67.4
Squeeze, diver's T70.3
Squint —*see also* Strabismus
  accommodative —*see* Strabismus, convergent
    concomitant
SSADHD (succinic semialdehyde
  dehydrogenase deficiency) E72.81
St. Hubert's disease A82.9
Stab —*see also* Laceration
  internal organs —*see* Injury, by site
Stafne's cyst or cavity M27.0
Staggering gait R26.0
  hysterical F44.4

Staghorn calculus —*see* Calculus, kidney
Stähli's line (cornea) (pigment) —*see*
  Pigmentation, cornea, anterior
Stain, staining
  meconium (newborn) P96.83
  port wine Q82.5
  tooth, teeth (hard tissues) (extrinsic) K03.6
    due to
      accretions K03.6
      deposits (betel) (black) (green) (materia
        alba) (orange) (soft) (tobacco) K03.6
      metals (copper) (silver) K03.7
      nicotine K03.6
      pulpal bleeding K03.7
      tobacco K03.6
    intrinsic K00.8
Stammering —*see also* Disorder, fluency
  F80.81
Standstill
  auricular I45.5
  cardiac —*see* Arrest, cardiac
  sinoatrial I45.5
  ventricular —*see* Arrest, cardiac
Stannosis J63.5
Stanton's disease —*see* Melioidosis
Staphylitis (acute) (catarrhal) (chronic)
  (gangrenous) (membranous) (suppurative)
  (ulcerative) K12.2
Staphylococcal scalded skin syndrome L00
Staphylococcemia A41.2
Staphylococcus, staphylococcal —*see also*
  condition
  as cause of disease classified elsewhere
    B95.8
    aureus (methicillin susceptible) (MSSA)
      B95.61
      methicillin resistant (MRSA) B95.62
    specified NEC, as cause of disease classified
      elsewhere B95.7
Staphyloma (sclera)
  cornea H18.72-●
  equatorial H15.81-●
  localized (anterior) H15.82-●
  posticum H15.83-●
  ring H15.85-●
Stargardt's disease —*see* Dystrophy, retina
Starvation (inanition) (due to lack of food)
  T73.0
  edema —*see* Malnutrition, severe
Stasis
  bile (noncalculous) K83.1
  bronchus J98.09
    with infection —*see* Bronchitis
  cardiac —*see* Failure, heart, congestive
  cecum K59.89
  colon K59.89
  dermatitis I87.2
    with
      varicose ulcer —*see* Varix, leg, with ulcer,
        with inflammation
      varicose veins —*see* Varix, leg, with,
        inflammation
    due to postthrombotic syndrome —*see*
      Syndrome, postthrombotic
  duodenal K31.5
  eczema —*see* Varix, leg, with, inflammation
  edema —*see* Hypertension, venous (chronic),
    idiopathic
  foot T69.0-●
  ileocecal coil K59.89
  ileum K59.89
  intestinal K59.89
  jejunum K59.89
  kidney N19
  liver (cirrhotic) K76.1
  lymphatic I89.8
  pneumonia J18.2
  pulmonary —*see* Edema, lung
  rectal K59.89
  renal N19
    tubular N17.0

Stasis *(Continued)*
 ulcer —*see* Varix, leg, with, ulcer
  without varicose veins I87.2
 urine —*see* Retention, urine
 venous I87.8
State *(of)*
 affective and paranoid, mixed, organic
   psychotic F06.8
 agitated R45.1
  acute reaction to stress F43.0
 anxiety (neurotic) F41.1
 apprehension F41.1
 burn-out Z73.0
 climacteric, female Z78.0
  symptomatic N95.1
 compulsive F42.8
  mixed with obsessional thoughts F42.2
 confusional (psychogenic) F44.89
  acute —*see also* Delirium
   with
     arteriosclerotic dementia F01.50
      with behavioral disturbance F01.51
     senility or dementia F05
    alcoholic F10.231
   epileptic F05
   reactive (from emotional stress,
     psychological trauma) F44.89
   subacute —*see* Delirium
 convulsive —*see* Convulsions
 crisis F43.0
 depressive F32.A
  neurotic F34.1
 dissociative F44.9
 emotional shock (stress) R45.7
 hypercoagulation —*see* Hypercoagulable
 locked-in G83.5
 menopausal Z78.0
  symptomatic N95.1
 neurotic F48.9
  with depersonalization F48.1
 obsessional F42.8
 oneiroid (schizophrenia-like) F23
 organic
  hallucinatory (nonalcoholic) F06.0
  paranoid (-hallucinatory) F06.2
 panic F41.0
 paranoid F22
  climacteric F22
  involutional F22
  menopausal F22
  organic F06.2
  senile F03
  simple F22
 persistent vegetative R40.3
 phobic F40.9
 postleukotomy F07.0
 pregnant
  gestational carrier Z33.3
  incidental Z33.1
 psychogenic, twilight F44.89
 psychopathic (constitutional) F60.2
 psychotic, organic —*see also* Psychosis,
   organic
  mixed paranoid and affective F06.8
  senile or presenile F03
  transient NEC F06.8
   with
     depression F06.31
     hallucinations F06.0
 residual schizophrenic F20.5
 restlessness R45.1
 stress (emotional) R45.7
 tension (mental) F48.9
  specified NEC F48.8
 transient organic psychotic NEC F06.8
  depressive type F06.31
  hallucinatory type F06.0
 twilight
  epileptic F05
  psychogenic F44.89
 vegetative, persistent R40.3

State *(Continued)*
 vital exhaustion Z73.0
 withdrawal —*see* Withdrawal, state
Status (post) —*see also* Presence (of)
 absence, epileptic —*see* Epilepsy, by type,
   with status epilepticus
 administration of tPA (rtPA) in a different
   facility within the last 24 hours prior to
   admission to the current facility
   Z92.82
 adrenalectomy (unilateral) (bilateral)
   E89.6
 anastomosis Z98.0
 anginosus I20.9
 angioplasty (peripheral) Z98.62
  with implant Z95.820
  coronary artery Z98.61
   with implant Z95.5
 aortocoronary bypass Z95.1
 arthrodesis Z98.1
 artificial opening (of) Z93.9
  gastrointestinal tract Z93.4
  specified NEC Z93.8
  urinary tract Z93.6
  vagina Z93.8
 asthmaticus —*see* Asthma, by type, with
   status asthmaticus
 awaiting organ transplant Z76.82
 bariatric surgery Z98.84
 bed confinement Z74.01
 bleb, filtering (vitreous), after glaucoma
   surgery Z98.83
 breast implant Z98.82
  removal Z98.86
 cataract extraction Z98.4- ●
 cholecystectomy Z90.49
 clitorectomy N90.811
  with excision of labia minora N90.812
 colectomy (complete) (partial) Z90.49
 colonization —*see* Carrier (suspected) of
 colostomy Z93.3
 convulsivus idiopathicus —*see* Epilepsy, by
   type, with status epilepticus
 coronary artery angioplasty —*see* Status,
   angioplasty, coronary artery
 coronary artery bypass graft Z95.1
 cystectomy (urinary bladder) Z90.6
 cystostomy Z93.50
  appendico-vesicostomy Z93.52
  cutaneous Z93.51
  specified NEC Z93.59
 delinquent immunization Z28.3
 dental Z98.818
  crown Z98.811
  fillings Z98.811
  restoration Z98.811
  sealant Z98.810
  specified NEC Z98.818
 deployment (current) (military) Z56.82
 dialysis (hemodialysis) (peritoneal) Z99.2
 do not resuscitate (DNR) Z66
 donor —*see* Donor
 embedded fragments —*see* Retained, foreign
   body fragments (type of)
 embedded splinter —*see* Retained, foreign
   body fragments (type of)
 enterostomy Z93.4
 epileptic, epilepticus —*see also* Epilepsy, by
   type, with status epilepticus G40.901
 estrogen receptor
  negative Z17.1
  positive Z17.0
 female genital cutting —*see* Female genital
   mutilation status
 female genital mutilation —*see* Female genital
   mutilation status
 filtering (vitreous) bleb after glaucoma
   surgery Z98.83
 gastrectomy (complete) (partial) Z90.3
 gastric banding Z98.84
 gastric bypass for obesity Z98.84

Status *(Continued)*
 gastrostomy Z93.1
 human immunodeficiency virus (HIV)
   infection, asymptomatic Z21
 hysterectomy (complete) (total) Z90.710
  partial (with remaining cervial stump)
   Z90.711
 ileostomy Z93.2
 implant
  breast Z98.82
 infibulation N90.813
 intestinal bypass Z98.0
 jejunostomy Z93.4
 lapsed immunization schedule Z28.3
 laryngectomy Z90.02
 lymphaticus E32.8
 malignancy
  castrate resistant prostate Z19.2
  hormone resistant Z19.2
  hormone sensitive Z19.1
 marmoratus G80.3
 mastectomy (unilateral) (bilateral) Z90.1- ●
 military deployment status (current) Z56.82
  in theater or in support of military war,
   peacekeeping and humanitarian
   operations Z56.82
 nephrectomy (unilateral) (bilateral) Z90.5
 nephrostomy Z93.6
 obesity surgery Z98.84
 oophorectomy
  bilateral Z90.722
  unilateral Z90.721
 organ replacement
  by artificial or mechanical device or
   prosthesis of
    artery Z95.828
    bladder Z96.0
    blood vessel Z95.828
    breast Z97.8
    eye globe Z97.0
    heart Z95.812
     valve Z95.2
    intestine Z97.8
    joint Z96.60
      hip —*see* Presence, hip joint implant
      knee —*see* Presence, knee joint
       implant
      specified site NEC Z96.698
    kidney Z97.8
    larynx Z96.3
    lens Z96.1
    limbs —*see* Presence, artificial, limb
    liver Z97.8
    lung Z97.8
    pancreas Z97.8
  by organ transplant (heterologous)
   (homologous) —*see* Transplant
 pacemaker
  brain Z96.89
  cardiac Z95.0
  specified NEC Z96.89
 pancreatectomy Z90.410
  complete Z90.410
  partial Z90.411
  total Z90.410
 pneumonectomy (complete) (partial) Z90.2
 pneumothorax, therapeutic Z98.3
 postcommotio cerebri F07.81
 postoperative (postprocedural) NEC
   Z98.890
  breast implant Z98.82
  dental Z98.818
   crown Z98.811
   fillings Z98.811
   restoration Z98.811
   sealant Z98.810
   specified NEC Z98.818
  pneumothorax, therapeutic Z98.3
  uterine scar Z98.891
 postpartum (routine follow-up) Z39.2
  care immediately after delivery Z39.0

▶ New   ⇛ Revised   ~~deleted~~ Deleted   ● Use Additional Character(s)

Status *(Continued)*
  postsurgical (postprocedural) NEC
    Z98.890
    pneumothorax, therapeutic Z98.3
  pregnancy, incidental Z33.1
  prosthesis coronary angioplasty Z95.5
  pseudophakia Z96.1
  renal dialysis (hemodialysis) (peritoneal) Z99.2
  retained foreign body —*see* Retained, foreign
    body fragments (type of)
  reversed jejunal transposition (for bypass)
    Z98.0
  salpingo-oophorectomy
    bilateral Z90.722
    unilateral Z90.721
  sex reassignment surgery status Z87.890
  shunt
    arteriovenous (for dialysis) Z99.2
    cerebrospinal fluid Z98.2
    ventricular (communicating) (for drainage)
      Z98.2
  splenectomy Z90.81
  thymicolymphaticus E32.8
  thymicus E32.8
  thymolymphaticus E32.8
  thyroidectomy (hypothyroidism) E89.0
  tooth (teeth) extraction —*see also* Absence,
    teeth, acquired K08.409
  tPA (rtPA) administration in a different
    facility within the last 24 hours prior to
    admission to current facility Z92.82
  tracheostomy Z93.0
  transplant —*see* Transplant
    organ removed Z98.85
  tubal ligation Z98.51
  underimmunization Z28.3
  ureterostomy Z93.6
  urethrostomy Z93.6
  vagina, artificial Z93.8
  vasectomy Z98.52
  wheelchair confinement Z99.3
Stealing
  child problem F91.8
    in company with others Z72.810
  pathological (compulsive) F63.2
Steam burn —*see* Burn
Steatocystoma multiplex L72.2
Steatohepatitis (nonalcoholic) (NASH) K75.81
Steatoma L72.3
  eyelid (cystic) —*see* Dermatosis, eyelid
    infected —*see* Hordeolum
Steatorrhea (chronic) K90.9
  with lacteal obstruction K90.2
  idiopathic (adult) (infantile) K90.9
  pancreatic K90.3
  primary K90.0
  tropical K90.1
Steatosis E88.89
  heart —*see* Degeneration, myocardial
  kidney N28.89
  liver NEC K76.0
Steele-Richardson-Olszewski disease or
  syndrome G23.1
Steinbrocker's syndrome G90.8
Steinert's disease G71.11
Stein-Leventhal syndrome E28.2
Stein's syndrome E28.2
STEMI —*see also* Infarct, myocardium, ST
  elevation I21.3
Stenocardia I20.8
Stenocephaly Q75.8
Stenosis, stenotic (cicatricial) —*see also*
  Stricture
  ampulla of Vater K83.1
  anus, anal (canal) (sphincter) K62.4
    and rectum K62.4
    congenital Q42.3
      with fistula Q42.2
  aorta (ascending) (supraventricular)
    (congenital) Q25.1
    arteriosclerotic I70.0

Stenosis, stenotic *(Continued)*
  aorta *(Continued)*
    calcified I70.0
    supravalvular Q25.3
  aortic (valve) I35.0
    with insufficiency I35.2
    congenital Q23.0
    rheumatic I06.0
      with
        incompetency, insufficiency or
          regurgitation I06.2
          with mitral (valve) disease I08.0
            with tricuspid (valve) disease
              I08.3
        mitral (valve) disease I08.0
          with tricuspid (valve) disease
            I08.3
        tricuspid (valve) disease I08.2
          with mitral (valve) disease I08.3
    specified cause NEC I35.0
    syphilitic A52.03
  aqueduct of Sylvius (congenital) Q03.0
    with spina bifida —*see* Spina bifida,
      by site, with hydrocephalus
    acquired G91.1
  artery NEC —*see also* Arteriosclerosis I77.1
    celiac I77.4
    cerebral —*see* Occlusion, artery, cerebral
    extremities —*see* Arteriosclerosis,
      extremities
    precerebral —*see* Occlusion, artery,
      precerebral
    pulmonary (congenital) Q25.6
      acquired I28.8
    renal I70.1
    stent
      coronary T82.855
      peripheral T82.856
  bile duct (common) (hepatic) K83.1
    congenital Q44.3
  bladder-neck (acquired) N32.0
    congenital Q64.31
  brain G93.89
  bronchus J98.09
    congenital Q32.3
    syphilitic A52.72
  cardia (stomach) K22.2
    congenital Q39.3
  cardiovascular —*see* Disease, cardiovascular
  caudal M48.08
  cervix, cervical (canal) N88.2
    congenital Q51.828
    in pregnancy or childbirth —*see*
      Pregnancy, complicated by, abnormal
      cervix
  colon —*see also* Obstruction, intestine
    congenital Q42.9
      specified NEC Q42.8
  colostomy K94.03
  common (bile) duct K83.1
    congenital Q44.3
  coronary (artery) —*see* Disease, heart,
    ischemic, atherosclerotic
  cystic duct —*see* Obstruction, gallbladder
  due to presence of device, implant or
    graft —*see also* Complications, by site
    and type, specified NEC T85.858
    arterial graft NEC T82.858
    breast (implant) T85.858
    catheter T85.858
      dialysis (renal) T82.858
        intraperitoneal T85.858
      infusion NEC T82.858
        spinal (epidural) (subdural)
          T85.850
      urinary (indwelling) T83.85
    fixation, internal (orthopedic) NEC
      T84.85
    gastrointestinal (bile duct) (esophagus)
      T85.858
    genital NEC T83.85

Stenosis, stenotic *(Continued)*
  due to presence of device, implant or graft
    (Continued)
    heart NEC T82.857
    joint prosthesis T84.85
    ocular (corneal graft) (orbital implant)
      NEC T85.858
    orthopedic NEC T84.85
    specified NEC T85.858
    urinary NEC T83.85
    vascular NEC T82.858
    ventricular intracranial shunt
      T85.850
  duodenum K31.5
    congenital Q41.0
  ejaculatory duct NEC N50.89
  endocervical os —*see* Stenosis, cervix
  enterostomy K94.13
  esophagus K22.2
    congenital Q39.3
    syphilitic A52.79
      congenital A50.59 *[K23]*
  eustachian tube —*see* Obstruction, eustachian
    tube
  external ear canal (acquired) H61.30-●
    congenital Q16.1
    due to
      inflammation H61.32-●
      trauma H61.31-●
    postprocedural H95.81-●
    specified cause NEC H61.39-●
  gallbladder —*see* Obstruction, gallbladder
  glottis J38.6
  heart valve (*see also* Endocarditis) I38
  aortic —*see* Stenosis, aortic
    congenital Q24.8
  mitral —*see* Stenosis, mitral
  pulmonary —*see* Stenosis, pulmonary,
    valve
  tricuspid —*see* Stenosis, tricuspid Q22.4
  hepatic duct K83.1
  hymen N89.6
  hypertrophic subaortic (idiopathic) I42.1
  ileum —*see also* Obstruction, intestine,
    specified NEC K56.699
    congenital Q41.2
  infundibulum cardia Q24.3
  intervertebral foramina —*see also* Lesion,
    biomechanical, specified NEC
    connective tissue M99.79
      abdomen M99.79
      cervical region M99.71
      cervicothoracic M99.71
      head region M99.70
      lumbar region M99.73
      lumbosacral M99.73
      occipitocervical M99.70
      sacral region M99.74
      sacrococcygeal M99.74
      sacroiliac M99.74
      specified NEC M99.79
      thoracic region M99.72
      thoracolumbar M99.72
    disc M99.79
      abdomen M99.79
      cervical region M99.71
      cervicothoracic M99.71
      head region M99.70
      lower extremity M99.76
      lumbar region M99.73
      lumbosacral M99.73
      occipitocervical M99.70
      pelvic M99.75
      rib cage M99.78
      sacral region M99.74
      sacrococcygeal M99.74
      sacroiliac M99.74
      specified NEC M99.79
      thoracic region M99.72
      thoracolumbar M99.72
      upper extremity M99.77

Stenosis, stenotic (Continued)
  intervertebral foramina (Continued)
    osseous M99.69
      abdomen M99.69
      cervical region M99.61
      cervicothoracic M99.61
      head region M99.60
      lower extremity M99.66
      lumbar region M99.63
      lumbosacral M99.63
      occipitocervical M99.60
      pelvic M99.65
      rib cage M99.68
      sacral region M99.64
      sacrococcygeal M99.64
      sacroiliac M99.64
      specified NEC M99.69
      thoracic region M99.62
      thoracolumbar M99.62
      upper extremity M99.67
    subluxation —see Stenosis, intervertebral
      foramina, osseous
  intestine —see also Obstruction, intestine
    congenital (small) Q41.9
      large Q42.9
        specified NEC Q42.8
      specified NEC Q41.8
  jejunum —see also Obstruction, intestine,
      specified NEC K56.699
    congenital Q41.1
  lacrimal (passage)
    canaliculi H04.54-●
    congenital Q10.5
    duct H04.55-●
    punctum H04.56-●
    sac H04.57-●
  lacrimonasal duct —see Stenosis, lacrimal,
      duct
    congenital Q10.5
  larynx J38.6
    congenital NEC Q31.8
      subglottic Q31.1
    syphilitic A52.73
      congenital A50.59 [J99]
  mitral (chronic) (inactive) (valve) I05.0
    with
      aortic valve disease I08.0
      incompetency, insufficiency or
        regurgitation I05.2
    active or acute I01.1
      with rheumatic or Sydenham's chorea
        I02.0
    congenital Q23.2
    specified cause, except rheumatic I34.2
    syphilitic A52.03
  myocardium, myocardial —see also
      Degeneration, myocardial
    hypertrophic subaortic (idiopathic) I42.1
  nares (anterior) (posterior) J34.89
    congenital Q30.0
  nasal duct —see also Stenosis, lacrimal, duct
    congenital Q10.5
  nasolacrimal duct —see also Stenosis, lacrimal,
      duct
    congenital Q10.5
  neural canal —see also Lesion, biomechanical,
      specified NEC
    connective tissue M99.49
      abdomen M99.49
      cervical region M99.41
      cervicothoracic M99.41
      head region M99.40
      lower extremity M99.46
      lumbar region M99.43
      lumbosacral M99.43
      occipitocervical M99.40
      pelvic M99.45
      rib cage M99.48
      sacral region M99.44
      sacrococcygeal M99.44
      sacroiliac M99.44

Stenosis, stenotic (Continued)
  neural canal (Continued)
    connective tissue (Continued)
      specified NEC M99.49
      thoracic region M99.42
      thoracolumbar M99.42
      upper extremity M99.47
    intervertebral disc M99.59
      abdomen M99.59
      cervical region M99.51
      cervicothoracic M99.51
      head region M99.50
      lower extremity M99.56
      lumbar region M99.53
      lumbosacral M99.53
      occipitocervical M99.50
      pelvic M99.55
      rib cage M99.58
      sacral region M99.54
      sacrococcygeal M99.54
      sacroiliac M99.54
      specified NEC M99.59
      thoracic region M99.52
      thoracolumbar M99.52
      upper extremity M99.57
    osseous M99.39
      abdomen M99.39
      cervical region M99.31
      cervicothoracic M99.31
      head region M99.30
      lower extremity M99.36
      lumbar region M99.33
      lumbosacral M99.33
      occipitocervical M99.30
      pelvic M99.35
      rib cage M99.38
      sacral region M99.34
      sacrococcygeal M99.34
      sacroiliac M99.34
      specified NEC M99.39
      thoracic region M99.32
      thoracolumbar M99.32
      upper extremity M99.37
    subluxation M99.29
      cervical region M99.21
      cervicothoracic M99.21
      head region M99.20
      lower extremity M99.26
      lumbar region M99.23
      lumbosacral M99.23
      occipitocervical M99.20
      pelvic M99.25
      rib cage M99.28
      sacral region M99.24
      sacrococcygeal M99.24
      sacroiliac M99.24
      specified NEC M99.29
      thoracic region M99.22
      thoracolumbar M99.22
      upper extremity M99.27
  organ or site, congenital NEC —see Atresia,
      by site
  papilla of Vater K83.1
  pulmonary (artery) (congenital) Q25.6
    with ventricular septal defect,
      transposition of aorta, and
      hypertrophy of right ventricle
      Q21.3
    acquired I28.8
    in tetralogy of Fallot Q21.3
    infundibular Q24.3
    subvalvular Q24.3
    supravalvular Q25.6
    valve I37.0
      with insufficiency I37.2
      congenital Q22.1
      rheumatic I09.89
        with aortic, mitral or tricuspid (valve)
          disease I08.8
    vein, acquired I28.8
    vessel NEC I28.8

Stenosis, stenotic (Continued)
  pulmonic (congenital) Q22.1
    infundibular Q24.3
    subvalvular Q24.3
  pylorus (hypertrophic) (acquired) K31.1
    adult K31.1
    congenital Q40.0
    infantile Q40.0
  rectum (sphincter) —see Stricture, rectum
  renal artery I70.1
    congenital Q27.1
  salivary duct (any) K11.8
  sphincter of Oddi K83.1
  spinal M48.00
    cervical region M48.02
    cervicothoracic region M48.03
    lumbar region (NOS) (without neurogenic
      claudication) M48.061
      with neurogenic claudication M48.062
    lumbosacral region M48.07
    occipito-atlanto-axial region M48.01
    sacrococcygeal region M48.08
    thoracic region M48.04
    thoracolumbar region M48.05
  stent
    vascular
      end stent
        adjacent to stent —see Arteriosclerosis
        within the stent
          coronary T82.855
          peripheral T82.856
      in stent
        coronary vessel T82.855
        peripheral vessel T82.856
  stomach, hourglass K31.2
  subaortic (congenital) Q24.4
    hypertrophic (idiopathic) I42.1
  subglottic J38.6
    congenital Q31.1
    postprocedural J95.5
  trachea J39.8
    congenital Q32.1
    syphilitic A52.73
    tuberculous NEC A15.5
  tracheostomy J95.03
  tricuspid (valve) I07.0
    with
      aortic (valve) disease I08.2
      incompetency, insufficiency or
        regurgitation I07.2
      with aortic (valve) disease I08.2
        with mitral (valve) disease I08.3
      mitral (valve) disease I08.1
        with aortic (valve) disease I08.3
    congenital Q22.4
    nonrheumatic I36.0
      with insufficiency I36.2
  tubal N97.1
  ureter —see Atresia, ureter
  ureteropelvic junction, congenital
      Q62.11
  ureterovesical orifice, congenital Q62.12
  urethra (valve) —see also Stricture, urethra
    congenital Q64.32
  urinary meatus, congenital Q64.33
  vagina N89.5
    congenital Q52.4
    in pregnancy —see Pregnancy, complicated
      by, abnormal vagina
    causing obstructed labor O65.5
  valve (cardiac) (heart) —see also Endocarditis
      I38
    congenital Q24.8
      aortic Q23.0
      mitral Q23.2
      pulmonary Q22.1
      tricuspid Q22.4
  vena cava (inferior) (superior) I87.1
    congenital Q26.0
  vesicourethral orifice Q64.31
  vulva N90.5

Strain (*Continued*)
physical NOS Z73.3
  work-related Z56.6
postural —*see also* Disorder, soft tissue, due
    to use
psychological NEC Z73.3
tendon —*see* Injury, muscle, by site, strain
Straining, on urination R39.16
Strand, vitreous —*see* Opacity, vitreous,
  membranes and strands
Strangulation, strangulated —*see also*
  Asphyxia, traumatic
appendix K38.8
bladder-neck N32.0
bowel or colon K56.2
food or foreign body —*see* Foreign body, by
    site
hemorrhoids —*see* Hemorrhoids, with
    complication
hernia —*see also* Hernia, by site, with
    obstruction
  with gangrene —*see* Hernia, by site, with
      gangrene
intestine (large) (small) K56.2
  with hernia —*see also* Hernia, by site, with
      obstruction
    with gangrene —*see* Hernia, by site, with
        gangrene
mesentery K56.2
mucus —*see* Asphyxia, mucus
omentum K56.2
organ or site, congenital NEC —*see* Atresia,
    by site
ovary —*see* Torsion, ovary
penis N48.89
  foreign body T19.4
rupture —*see* Hernia, by site, with obstruction
stomach due to hernia —*see also* Hernia, by
    site, with obstruction
  with gangrene —*see* Hernia, by site, with
      gangrene
vesicourethral orifice N32.0
Strangury R30.0
Straw itch B88.0
Strawberry
gallbladder K82.4
mark Q82.5
tongue (red) (white) K14.3
Streak(s)
macula, angioid H35.33
ovarian Q50.32
Strephosymbolia F81.0
secondary to organic lesion R48.8
Streptobacillary fever A25.1
Streptobacillosis A25.1
Streptobacillus moniliformis A25.1
Streptococcus, streptococcal —*see also*
  condition
as cause of disease classified elsewhere B95.5
group
  A, as cause of disease classified elsewhere
      B95.0
  B, as cause of disease classified elsewhere
      B95.1
  D, as cause of disease classified elsewhere
      B95.2
pneumoniae, as cause of disease classified
    elsewhere B95.3
specified NEC, as cause of disease classified
    elsewhere B95.4
Streptomycosis B47.1
Streptotrichosis A48.8
Stress F43.9
family —*see* Disruption, family
fetal P84
  complicating pregnancy O77.9
    due to drug administration O77.1
mental NEC Z73.3
  work-related Z56.6
physical NEC Z73.3
  work-related Z56.6

Stress (*Continued*)
polycythemia D75.1
reaction —*see also* Reaction, stress F43.9
work schedule Z56.3
Stretching, nerve —*see* Injury, nerve
Striae albicantes, atrophicae or distensae
  (cutis) L90.6
Stricture —*see also* Stenosis
ampulla of Vater K83.1
anus (sphincter) K62.4
  congenital Q42.3
    with fistula Q42.2
  infantile Q42.3
    with fistula Q42.2
aorta (ascending) (congenital) Q25.1
  arteriosclerotic I70.0
  calcified I70.0
  supravalvular, congenital Q25.3
aortic (valve) —*see* Stenosis, aortic
aqueduct of Sylvius (congenital) Q03.0
  with spina bifida —*see* Spina bifida, by site,
      with hydrocephalus
  acquired G91.1
artery I77.1
  basilar —*see* Occlusion, artery, basilar
  carotid —*see* Occlusion, artery, carotid
  celiac I77.4
  congenital (peripheral) Q27.8
    cerebral Q28.3
    coronary Q24.5
    digestive system Q27.8
    lower limb Q27.8
    retinal Q14.1
    specified site NEC Q27.8
    umbilical Q27.0
    upper limb Q27.8
  coronary —*see* Disease, heart, ischemic,
      atherosclerotic
    congenital Q24.5
  precerebral —*see* Occlusion, artery,
      precerebral
  pulmonary (congenital) Q25.6
    acquired I28.8
  renal I70.1
  vertebral —*see* Occlusion, artery, vertebral
auditory canal (external) (congenital)
  acquired —*see* Stenosis, external ear canal
bile duct (common) (hepatic) K83.1
  congenital Q44.3
  postoperative K91.89
bladder N32.89
  neck N32.0
bowel —*see* Obstruction, intestine
brain G93.89
bronchus J98.09
  congenital Q32.3
  syphilitic A52.72
cardia (stomach) K22.2
  congenital Q39.3
cardiac —*see also* Disease, heart
  orifice (stomach) K22.2
cecum —*see* Obstruction, intestine
cervix, cervical (canal) N88.2
  congenital Q51.828
  in pregnancy —*see* Pregnancy, complicated
      by, abnormal cervix
    causing obstructed labor O65.5
colon —*see also* Obstruction, intestine
  congenital Q42.9
    specified NEC Q42.8
colostomy K94.03
common (bile) duct K83.1
coronary (artery) —*see* Disease, heart,
    ischemic, atherosclerotic
cystic duct —*see* Obstruction, gallbladder
digestive organs NEC, congenital Q45.8
duodenum K31.5
  congenital Q41.0
ear canal (external) (congenital) Q16.1
  acquired —*see* Stricture, auditory canal,
      acquired

Stricture (*Continued*)
ejaculatory duct N50.89
enterostomy K94.13
esophagus K22.2
  congenital Q39.3
  syphilitic A52.79
    congenital A50.59 [K23]
eustachian tube —*see also* Obstruction,
    eustachian tube
  congenital Q17.8
fallopian tube N97.1
  gonococcal A54.24
  tuberculous A18.17
gallbladder —*see* Obstruction, gallbladder
glottis J38.6
heart —*see also* Disease, heart
  valve (*see also* Endocarditis) I38
    aortic Q23.0
    mitral Q23.2
    pulmonary Q22.1
    tricuspid Q22.4
hepatic duct K83.1
hourglass, of stomach K31.2
hymen N89.6
hypopharynx J39.2
ileum —*see also* Obstruction, intestine,
    specified NEC K56.699
  congenital Q41.2
intestine —*see also* Obstruction, intestine
  congenital (small) Q41.9
    large Q42.9
      specified NEC Q42.8
    specified NEC Q41.8
  ischemic K55.1
jejunum —*see also* Obstruction, intestine,
    specified NEC K56.699
  congenital Q41.1
lacrimal passages —*see also* Stenosis, lacrimal
  congenital Q10.5
larynx J38.6
  congenital NEC Q31.8
    subglottic Q31.1
  syphilitic A52.73
    congenital A50.59 [J99]
meatus
  ear (congenital) Q16.1
    acquired —*see* Stricture, auditory canal,
        acquired
    osseous (ear) (congenital) Q16.1
      acquired —*see* Stricture, auditory canal,
          acquired
  urinarius —*see also* Stricture, urethra
    congenital Q64.33
mitral (valve) —*see* Stenosis, mitral
myocardium, myocardial I51.5
  hypertrophic subaortic (idiopathic) I42.1
nares (anterior) (posterior) J34.89
  congenital Q30.0
nasal duct —*see also* Stenosis, lacrimal, duct
  congenital Q10.5
nasolacrimal duct —*see also* Stenosis, lacrimal,
    duct
  congenital Q10.5
nasopharynx J39.2
  syphilitic A52.73
nose J34.89
  congenital Q30.0
nostril (anterior) (posterior) J34.89
  congenital Q30.0
  syphilitic A52.73
    congenital A50.59 [J99]
organ or site, congenital NEC —*see* Atresia,
    by site
os uteri —*see* Stricture, cervix
osseous meatus (ear) (congenital) Q16.1
  acquired —*see* Stricture, auditory canal,
      acquired
oviduct —*see* Stricture, fallopian tube
pelviureteric junction (congenital) Q62.11
  acquired, with hydronephrosis N13.0
penis, by foreign body T19.4

▶ New ⇒ Revised ~~deleted~~ Deleted ● Use Additional Character(s)

Stricture *(Continued)*
  pharynx J39.2
  prostate N42.89
  pulmonary, pulmonic
    artery (congenital) Q25.6
      acquired I28.8
      noncongenital I28.8
    infundibulum (congenital) Q24.3
    valve I37.0
      congenital Q22.1
    vein, acquired I28.8
    vessel NEC I28.8
  punctum lacrimale —*see also* Stenosis,
      lacrimal, punctum
    congenital Q10.5
  pylorus (hypertrophic) K31.1
    adult K31.1
    congenital Q40.0
    infantile Q40.0
  rectosigmoid —*see also* Obstruction, intestine,
      specified NEC K56.699
  rectum (sphincter) K62.4
    congenital Q42.1
      with fistula Q42.0
    due to
      chlamydial lymphogranuloma A55
      irradiation K91.89
      lymphogranuloma venereum A55
    gonococcal A54.6
    inflammatory (chlamydial) A55
    syphilitic A52.74
    tuberculous A18.32
  renal artery I70.1
    congenital Q27.1
  salivary duct or gland (any) K11.8
  sigmoid (flexure) —*see* Obstruction, intestine
  spermatic cord N50.89
  stoma (following) (of)
    colostomy K94.03
    enterostomy K94.13
    gastrostomy K94.23
    ileostomy K94.13
    tracheostomy J95.03
  stomach K31.89
    congenital Q40.2
    hourglass K31.2
  subaortic Q24.4
    hypertrophic (acquired) (idiopathic) I42.1
  subglottic J38.6
  syphilitic NEC A52.79
  trachea J39.8
    congenital Q32.1
    syphilitic A52.73
    tuberculous NEC A15.5
  tracheostomy J95.03
  tricuspid (valve) —*see* Stenosis, tricuspid
  tunica vaginalis N50.89
  ureter (postoperative) N13.5
    with
      hydronephrosis N13.1
        with infection N13.6
      pyelonephritis (chronic) N11.1
    congenital —*see* Atresia, ureter
    tuberculous A18.11
  ureteropelvic junction (congenital) Q62.11
    acquired, with hydronephrosis N13.0
  ureterovesical orifice N13.5
    with infection N13.6
  urethra (organic) (spasmodic) *(see also*
      Stricture, urethra, male N35.919
    associated with schistosomiasis
        B65.0 *[N37]*
    congenital Q64.39
      valvular (posterior) Q64.2
    due to
      infection —*see* Stricture, urethra,
          postinfective
      trauma —*see* Stricture, urethra,
          post-traumatic
    female N35.92
    gonococcal, gonorrheal A54.01

Stricture *(Continued)*
  urethra (organic) (spasmodic) *(Continued)*
    infective NEC —*see* Stricture, urethra,
        postinfective
    late effect (sequelae) of injury —*see*
        Stricture, urethra, post-traumatic
    male N35.919
      anterior urethra N35.914
      bulbous urethra N35.912
      meatal N35.911
      membranous urethra N35.913
      overlapping sites N35.916
    postcatheterization —*see* Stricture, urethra,
        postprocedural
    postinfective NEC
      female N35.12
      male N35.119
        anterior urethra N35.114
        bulbous urethra N35.112
        meatal N35.111
        membranous urethra N35.113
        overlapping sites N35.116
    postobstetric N35.021
    postoperative —*see* Stricture, urethra,
        postprocedural
    postprocedural
      female N99.12
      male N99.114
        anterior bulbous urethra N99.113
        bulbous urethra N99.111
        fossa navicularis N99.115
        meatal N99.110
        membranous urethra N99.112
        overlapping sites N35.116
    post-traumatic
      female N35.028
        due to childbirth N35.021
      male N35.014
        anterior urethra N35.013
        bulbous urethra N35.011
        meatal N35.010
        membranous urethra N35.012
        overlapping sites N35.016
    sequela (late effect) of
      childbirth N35.021
      injury —*see* Stricture, urethra,
          post-traumatic
    specified cause NEC
      female N35.82
      male N35.819
        anterior urethra N35.814
        bulbous urethra N35.812
        meatal N35.811
        membranous urethra N35.813
        overlapping sites N35.816
    syphilitic A52.76
    traumatic —*see* Stricture, urethra,
        post-traumatic
    valvular (posterior), congenital Q64.2
  urinary meatus —*see* Stricture, urethra
  uterus, uterine (synechiae) N85.6
    os (external) (internal) —*see* Stricture,
        cervix
  vagina (outlet) —*see* Stenosis, vagina
  valve (cardiac) (heart) —*see also* Endocarditis
    congenital
      aortic Q23.0
      mitral Q23.2
      pulmonary Q22.1
      tricuspid Q22.4
  vas deferens N50.89
    congenital Q55.4
  vein I87.1
  vena cava (inferior) (superior) NEC I87.1
    congenital Q26.0
  vesicourethral orifice N32.0
    congenital Q64.31
  vulva (acquired) N90.5
Stridor R06.1
  congenital (larynx) P28.89
Stridulous —*see* condition

Stroke (apoplectic) (brain) (embolic) (ischemic)
    (paralytic) (thrombotic) I63.9
  cerebral, perinatal P91.82-●
  cryptogenic —*see also* infarction, cerebral
      I63.9
  epileptic —*see* Epilepsy
  heat T67.01
    exertional T67.02
    specified NEC T67.09
  in evolution I63.9
  intraoperative
    during cardiac surgery I97.810
    during other surgery I97.811
  ischemic, perinatal arterial P91.82-●
  lightning —*see* Lightning
  meaning
    cerebral hemorrhage — code to
        Hemorrhage, intracranial
    cerebral infarction — code to Infarction,
        cerebral
  neonatal P91.82-●
  postprocedural
    following cardiac surgery I97.820
    following other surgery I97.821
  sun T67.01
    specified NEC T67.09
  unspecified (NOS) I63.9
Stromatosis, endometrial D39.0
Strongyloidiasis, strongyloidosis B78.9
  cutaneous B78.1
  disseminated B78.7
  intestinal B78.0
Strophulus pruriginosus L28.2
Struck by lightning —*see* Lightning
Struma —*see also* Goiter
  Hashimoto E06.3
  lymphomatosa E06.3
  nodosa (simplex) E04.9
    endemic E01.2
      multinodular E01.1
    multinodular E04.2
      iodine-deficiency related E01.1
    toxic or with hyperthyroidism E05.20
      with thyroid storm E05.21
      multinodular E05.20
        with thyroid storm E05.21
      uninodular E05.10
        with thyroid storm E05.11
    toxicosa E05.20
      with thyroid storm E05.21
      multinodular E05.20
        with thyroid storm E05.21
      uninodular E05.10
        with thyroid storm E05.11
    uninodular E04.1
  ovarii D27.-●
  Riedel's E06.5
Strumipriva cachexia E03.4
Strümpell-Marie spine —*see* Spondylitis,
    ankylosing
Strümpell-Westphal pseudosclerosis E83.01
Stuart deficiency disease (factor X) D68.2
Stuart-Prower factor deficiency (factor X)
    D68.2
Student's elbow —*see* Bursitis, elbow,
    olecranon
Stump —*see* Amputation
Stunting, nutritional E45
Stupor (catatonic) R40.1
  depressive (single episode) F32.89
    recurrent episode F33.8
  dissociative F44.2
  manic F30.2
  manic-depressive F31.89
  psychogenic (anergic) F44.2
  reaction to exceptional stress (transient) F43.0
Sturge (-Weber) (-Dimitri) (-Kalischer) **disease
    or syndrome** Q85.8
Stuttering F80.81
  adult onset F98.5
  childhood onset F80.81

Stuttering *(Continued)*
  following cerebrovascular disease —
    see Disorder, fluency, following
    cerebrovascular disease
  in conditions classified elsewhere R47.82
Sty, stye (external) (internal) (meibomian)
    (zeisian) —*see* Hordeolum
Subacidity, gastric K31.89
  psychogenic F45.8
Subacute —*see* condition
Subarachnoid —*see* condition
Subcortical —*see* condition
Subcostal syndrome, nerve compression —*see*
    Mononeuropathy, upper limb, specified
    site NEC
Subcutaneous, subcuticular —*see* condition
Subdural —*see* condition
Subendocardium —*see* condition
Subependymoma
  specified site —*see* Neoplasm, uncertain
    behavior, by site
  unspecified site D43.2
Suberosis J67.3
Subglossitis —*see* Glossitis
Subhemophilia D66
Subinvolution
  breast (postlactational) (postpuerperal)
    N64.89
  puerperal O90.89
  uterus (chronic) (nonpuerperal) N85.3
    puerperal O90.89
Sublingual —*see* condition
Sublinguitis —*see* Sialoadenitis
Subluxatable hip Q65.6
Subluxation —*see also* Dislocation
  acromioclavicular S43.11-●
  ankle S93.0-●
  atlantoaxial, recurrent M43.4
    with myelopathy M43.3
  carpometacarpal (joint) NEC S63.05-●
    thumb S63.04-●
  complex, vertebral —*see* Complex,
    subluxation
  congenital —*see also* Malposition, congenital
    hip —*see* Dislocation, hip, congenital,
      partial
    joint (excluding hip)
      lower limb Q68.8
      shoulder Q68.8
      upper limb Q68.8
  elbow (traumatic) S53.10-●
    anterior S53.11-●
    lateral S53.14-●
    medial S53.13-●
    posterior S53.12-●
    specified type NEC S53.19-●
  finger S63.20-●
    index S63.20-●
    interphalangeal S63.22-●
      distal S63.24-●
        index S63.24-●
        little S63.24-●
        middle S63.24-●
        ring S63.24-●
      index S63.22-●
      little S63.22-●
      middle S63.22-●
      proximal S63.23-●
        index S63.23-●
        little S63.23-●
        middle S63.23-●
        ring S63.23-●
      ring S63.22-●
    little S63.20-●
    metacarpophalangeal S63.21-●
      index S63.21-●
      little S63.21-●
      middle S63.21-●
      ring S63.21-●
    middle S63.20-●
    ring S63.20-●

Subluxation *(Continued)*
  foot S93.30-●
    specified site NEC S93.33-●
    tarsal joint S93.31-●
    tarsometatarsal joint S93.32-●
    toe —*see* Subluxation, toe
  hip S73.00-●
    anterior S73.03-●
      obturator S73.02-●
    central S73.04-●
    posterior S73.01-●
  interphalangeal (joint)
    finger S63.22-●
      distal joint S63.24-●
        index S63.24-●
        little S63.24-●
        middle S63.24-●
        ring S63.24-●
      index S63.22-●
      little S63.22-●
      middle S63.22-●
      proximal joint S63.23-●
        index S63.23-●
        little S63.23-●
        middle S63.23-●
        ring S63.23-●
    thumb S63.12-●
    toe S93.13-●
      great S93.13-●
      lesser S93.13-●
  joint prosthesis —*see* Complications, joint
    prosthesis, mechanical, displacement,
    by site
  knee S83.10-●
    cap —*see* Subluxation, patella
    patella —*see* Subluxation, patella
    proximal tibia
      anteriorly S83.11-●
      laterally S83.14-●
      medially S83.13-●
      posteriorly S83.12-●
    specified type NEC S83.19-●
  lens —*see* Dislocation, lens, partial
  ligament, traumatic —*see* Sprain,
    by site
  metacarpal (bone)
    proximal end S63.06-●
  metacarpophalangeal (joint)
    finger S63.21-●
      index S63.21-●
      little S63.21-●
      middle S63.21-●
      ring S63.21-●
    thumb S63.11-●
  metatarsophalangeal joint S93.14-●
    great toe S93.14-●
    lesser toe S93.14-●
  midcarpal (joint) S63.03-●
  patella S83.00-●
    lateral S83.01-●
    recurrent (nontraumatic) —*see*
      Dislocation, patella, recurrent,
      incomplete
    specified type NEC S83.09-●
  pathological —*see* Dislocation,
    pathological
  radial head S53.00-●
    anterior S53.01-●
    nursemaid's elbow S53.03-●
    posterior S53.02-●
    specified type NEC S53.09-●
  radiocarpal (joint) S63.02-●
  radioulnar (joint)
    distal S63.01-●
    proximal —*see* Subluxation, elbow
  shoulder
    congenital Q68.8
    girdle S43.30-●
      scapula S43.31-●
      specified site NEC S43.39-●

Subluxation *(Continued)*
  shoulder *(Continued)*
    traumatic S43.00-●
      anterior S43.01-●
      inferior S43.03-●
      posterior S43.02-●
      specified type NEC S43.08-●
  sternoclavicular (joint) S43.20-●
    anterior S43.21-●
    posterior S43.22-●
  symphysis (pubis)
  thumb S63.103
    interphalangeal joint —*see* Subluxation,
      interphalangeal (joint), thumb
    metacarpophalangeal joint —*see*
      Subluxation, metacarpophalangeal
      (joint), thumb
  toe(s) S93.10-●
    great S93.10-●
      interphalangeal joint S93.13-●
      metatarsophalangeal joint S93.14-●
    interphalangeal joint S93.13-●
    lesser S93.10-●
      interphalangeal joint S93.13-●
      metatarsophalangeal joint S93.14-●
    metatarsophalangeal joint S93.149
  ulnohumeral joint —*see* Subluxation, elbow
  vertebral
    recurrent NEC —*see* subcategory M43.5
    traumatic
      cervical S13.100
        atlantoaxial joint S13.120
        atlantooccipital joint S13.110
        atloidooccipital joint S13.110
        joint between
          C0 and C1 S13.110
          C1 and C2 S13.120
          C2 and C3 S13.130
          C3 and C4 S13.140
          C4 and C5 S13.150
          C5 and C6 S13.160
          C6 and C7 S13.170
          C7 and T1 S13.180
        occipitoatloid joint S13.110
      lumbar S33.100
        joint between
          L1 and L2 S33.110
          L2 and L3 S33.120
          L3 and L4 S33.130
          L4 and L5 S33.140
      thoracic S23.100
        joint between
          T1 and T2 S23.110
          T2 and T3 S23.120
          T3 and T4 S23.122
          T4 and T5 S23.130
          T5 and T6 S23.132
          T6 and T7 S23.140
          T7 and T8 S23.142
          T8 and T9 S23.150
          T9 and T10 S23.152
          T10 and T11 S23.160
          T11 and T12 S23.162
          T12 and L1 S23.170
  ulna
    distal end S63.07-●
    proximal end —*see* Subluxation, elbow
  wrist (carpal bone) S63.00-●
    carpometacarpal joint —*see* Subluxation,
      carpometacarpal (joint)
    distal radioulnar joint —*see* Subluxation,
      radioulnar (joint), distal
    metacarpal bone, proximal —*see* Subluxation,
      metacarpal (bone), proximal
    midcarpal —*see* Subluxation, midcarpal
      (joint)
    radiocarpal joint —*see* Subluxation,
      radiocarpal (joint)
    recurrent —*see* Dislocation, recurrent, wrist
    specified site NEC S63.09-●
    ulna —*see* Subluxation, ulna, distal end

▶ New ⇒ Revised ~~deleted~~ Deleted ● Use Additional Character(s)

Submaxillary —see condition
Submersion (fatal) (nonfatal) T75.1
Submucous —see condition
Subnormal, subnormality
  accommodation (old age) H52.4
  mental —see Disability, intellectual
  temperature (accidental) T68
Subphrenic —see condition
Subscapular nerve —see condition
Subseptus uterus Q51.28
Subsiding appendicitis K36
Substance (other psychoactive) -induced
  anxiety disorder F19.980
  bipolar and related disorder F19.94
  delirium F19.921
  depressive disorder F19.94
  major neurocognitive disorder F19.97
  mild neurocognitive disorder F19.988
  obsessive-compulsive and related disorder
    F19.988
  psychotic disorder F19.959
  sexual dysfunction F19.981
  sleep disorder F19.982
Substernal thyroid E04.9
  congenital Q89.2
Substitution disorder F44.9
Subtentorial —see condition
Subthyroidism (acquired) —see also
  Hypothyroidism
  congenital E03.1
Succenturiate placenta O43.19-●
Sucking thumb, child (excessive) F98.8
Sudamen, sudamina L74.1
Sudanese kala-azar B55.0
Sudden
  hearing loss —see Deafness, sudden
  heart failure —see Failure, heart
Sudeck's atrophy, disease, or syndrome —see
  Algoneurodystrophy
Suffocation —see Asphyxia, traumatic
Sugar
  blood
    high (transient) R73.9
    low (transient) E16.2
  in urine R81
Suicide, suicidal (attempted) T14.91
  by poisoning —see Table of Drugs and
    Chemicals
  history of (personal) Z91.51
    in family Z81.8
  ideation —see Ideation, suicidal
  risk
    meaning personal history of attempted
      suicide Z91.51
    meaning suicidal ideation —see Ideation,
      suicidal
  tendencies
    meaning personal history of attempted
      suicide Z91.51
    meaning suicidal ideation —see Ideation,
      suicidal
  trauma —see nature of injury by site
Suipestifer infection —see Infection, salmonella
Sulfhemoglobinemia, sulphemoglobinemia
  (acquired) (with methemoglobinemia) D74.8
Sumatran mite fever A75.3
Summer —see condition
Sunburn L55.9
  due to
    tanning bed (acute) L56.8
      chronic L57.8
    ultraviolet radiation (acute) L56.8
      chronic L57.8
  first degree L55.0
  second degree L55.1
  third degree L55.2
SUNCT (short lasting unilateral neuralgiform
  headache with conjunctival injection and
  tearing) G44.059
  intractable G44.051
  not intractable G44.059

Sundowning F05
Sunken acetabulum —see Derangement, joint,
  specified type NEC, hip
Sunstroke T67.01
  specified NEC T67.09
Superfecundation —see Pregnancy, multiple
Superfetation —see Pregnancy, multiple
Superinvolution (uterus) N85.8
Supernumerary (congenital)
  aortic cusps Q23.8
  auditory ossicles Q16.3
  bone Q79.8
  breast Q83.1
  carpal bones Q74.0
  cusps, heart valve NEC Q24.8
    aortic Q23.8
    mitral Q23.2
    pulmonary Q22.3
  digit(s) Q69.9
  ear (lobule) Q17.0
  fallopian tube Q50.6
  finger Q69.0
  hymen Q52.4
  kidney Q63.0
  lacrimonasal duct Q10.6
  lobule (ear) Q17.0
  mitral cusps Q23.2
  muscle Q79.8
  nipple(s) Q83.3
  organ or site not listed —see Accessory
    ossicles, auditory Q16.3
  ovary Q50.31
  oviduct Q50.6
  pulmonary, pulmonic cusps Q22.3
  rib Q76.6
    cervical or first (syndrome) Q76.5
  roots (of teeth) K00.2
  spleen Q89.09
  tarsal bones Q74.2
  teeth K00.1
  testis Q55.29
  thumb Q69.1
  toe Q69.2
  uterus Q51.28
  vagina Q52.1
  vertebra Q76.49
Supervision (of)
  contraceptive —see Prescription,
    contraceptives
  dietary (for) Z71.3
    allergy (food) Z71.3
    colitis Z71.3
    diabetes mellitus Z71.3
    food allergy or intolerance Z71.3
    gastritis Z71.3
    hypercholesterolemia Z71.3
    hypoglycemia Z71.3
    intolerance (food) Z71.3
    obesity Z71.3
    specified NEC Z71.3
  healthy infant or child Z76.2
    foundling Z76.1
  high-risk pregnancy —see Pregnancy,
    complicated by, high, risk
  lactation Z39.1
  pregnancy —see Pregnancy, supervision of
Supplemental teeth K00.1
Suppression
  binocular vision H53.34
  lactation O92.5
  menstruation N94.89
  ovarian secretion E28.39
  renal N28.9
  urine, urinary secretion R34
Suppuration, suppurative —see also condition
  accessory sinus (chronic) —see Sinusitis
  adrenal gland
  antrum (chronic) —see Sinusitis, maxillary
  bladder —see Cystitis
  brain G06.0
    sequelae G09

Suppuration, suppurative (Continued)
  breast N61.1
    puerperal, postpartum or gestational —see
      Mastitis, obstetric, purulent
  dental periosteum M27.3
  ear (middle) —see also Otitis, media
    external NEC —see Otitis, externa, infective
    internal —see subcategory H83.0
  ethmoidal (chronic) (sinus) —see Sinusitis,
    ethmoidal
  fallopian tube —see Salpingo-oophoritis
  frontal (chronic) (sinus) —see Sinusitis, frontal
  gallbladder (acute) K81.0
  gum K05.20
    generalized —see Periodontitis, aggressive,
      generalized
    localized —see Periodontitis, aggressive,
      localized
  intracranial G06.0
  joint —see Arthritis, pyogenic or pyemic
  labyrinthine —see subcategory H83.0
  lung —see Abscess, lung
  mammary gland N61.1
    puerperal, postpartum O91.12
    associated with lactation O91.13
  maxilla, maxillary M27.2
    sinus (chronic) —see Sinusitis, maxillary
  muscle —see Myositis, infective
  nasal sinus (chronic) —see Sinusitis
  pancreas, acute —see also Pancreatitis, acute
    K85.80
  parotid gland —see Sialoadenitis
  pelvis, pelvic
    female —see Disease, pelvis, inflammatory
    male K65.0
  pericranial —see Osteomyelitis
  salivary duct or gland (any) —see
    Sialoadenitis
  sinus (accessory) (chronic) (nasal) —see
    Sinusitis
  sphenoidal sinus (chronic) —see Sinusitis,
    sphenoidal
  thymus (gland) E32.1
  thyroid (gland) E06.0
  tonsil —see Tonsillitis
  uterus —see Endometritis
Supraeruption of tooth (teeth) M26.34
Supraglottitis J04.30
  with obstruction J04.31
Suprarenal (gland) —see condition
Suprascapular nerve —see condition
Suprasellar —see condition
Surfer's knots or nodules S89.8-●
Surgical
  emphysema T81.82
  procedures, complication or misadventure —
    see Complications, surgical procedures
  shock T81.10
Surveillance (of) (for) —see also Observation
  alcohol abuse Z71.41
  contraceptive —see Prescription, contraceptives
  dietary Z71.3
  drug abuse Z71.51
Susceptibility to disease, genetic Z15.89
  malignant neoplasm Z15.09
    breast Z15.01
    endometrium Z15.04
    ovary Z15.02
    prostate Z15.03
    specified NEC Z15.09
  multiple endocrine neoplasia Z15.81
Suspected condition, ruled out —see also
  Observation, suspected
  amniotic cavity and membrane Z03.71
  cervical shortening Z03.75
  fetal anomaly Z03.73
  fetal growth Z03.74
  maternal and fetal conditions NEC Z03.79
  newborn —see also Observation, newborn,
    suspected condition ruled out Z05.9
  oligohydramnios Z03.71

Suspected condition, ruled out (*Continued*)
  placental problem Z03.72
  polyhydramnios Z03.71
Suspended uterus
  in pregnancy or childbirth —*see* Pregnancy,
    complicated by, abnormal uterus
Sutton's nevus D22.9
Suture
  burst (in operation wound) T81.31
    external operation wound T81.31
    internal operation wound T81.32
  inadvertently left in operation wound —*see*
    Foreign body, accidentally left during a
    procedure
  removal Z48.02
Swab inadvertently left in operation wound —
  see Foreign body, accidentally left during a
  procedure
Swallowed, swallowing
  difficulty —*see* Dysphagia
  foreign body —*see* Foreign body, alimentary
    tract
Swan-neck deformity (finger) —*see* Deformity,
  finger, swan-neck
Swearing, compulsive F42.8
  in Gilles de la Tourette's syndrome F95.2
Sweat, sweats
  fetid L75.0
  night R61
Sweating, excessive R61
Sweeley-Klionsky disease E75.21
Sweet's disease or dermatosis L98.2
Swelling (of) R60.9
  abdomen, abdominal (not referable to any
    particular organ) —*see* Mass,
    abdominal
  ankle —*see* Effusion, joint, ankle
  arm M79.89
    forearm M79.89
  breast —*see also* Lump, breast N63.0
  Calabar B74.3
  cervical gland R59.0
  chest, localized R22.2
  ear H93.8- ●
  extremity (lower) (upper) —*see* Disorder, soft
    tissue, specified type NEC
  finger M79.89
  foot M79.89
  glands R59.9
    generalized R59.1
    localized R59.0
  hand M79.89
  head (localized) R22.0
  inflammatory —*see* Inflammation
  intra-abdominal —*see* Mass, abdominal
  joint —*see* Effusion, joint
  leg M79.89
    lower M79.89
  limb —*see* Disorder, soft tissue, specified type
    NEC
  localized (skin) R22.9
    chest R22.2
    head R22.0
    limb
      lower —*see* Mass, localized, limb, lower
      upper —*see* Mass, localized, limb, upper
    neck R22.1
    trunk R22.2
  neck (localized) R22.1
  pelvic —*see* Mass, abdominal
  scrotum N50.89
  splenic —*see* Splenomegaly
  testis N50.89
  toe M79.89
  umbilical R19.09
  wandering, due to Gnathostoma
    (spinigerum) B83.1
  white —*see* Tuberculosis, arthritis
Swift (-Feer) disease
  overdose or wrong substance given
    or taken —*see* Table of Drugs and
    Chemicals, by drug, poisoning

Swimmer's
  cramp T75.1
  ear H60.33- ●
  itch B65.3
Swimming in the head R42
Swollen —*see* Swelling
Swyer syndrome Q99.1
Sycosis L73.8
  barbae (not parasitic) L73.8
  contagiosa (mycotic) B35.0
  lupoides L73.8
  mycotic B35.0
  parasitic B35.0
  vulgaris L73.8
Sydenham's chorea —*see* Chorea, Sydenham's
Sylvatic yellow fever A95.0
Sylvest's disease B33.0
Symblepharon H11.23- ●
  congenital Q10.3
Symond's syndrome G93.2
Sympathetic —*see* condition
Sympatheticotonia G90.8
Sympathicoblastoma
  specified site —*see* Neoplasm, malignant, by
    site
  unspecified site C74.90
Sympathogonioma —*see* Sympathicoblastoma
Symphalangy (fingers) (toes) Q70.9
Symptoms NEC R68.89
  breast NEC N64.59
  cold J00
  development NEC R63.8
  factitious, self-induced —*see* Disorder,
    factitious
  genital organs, female R10.2
  involving
    abdomen NEC R19.8
    appearance NEC R46.89
    awareness R41.9
      altered mental status R41.82
      amnesia —*see* Amnesia
      borderline intellectual functioning
        R41.83
      coma —*see* Coma
      disorientation R41.0
      neurologic neglect syndrome R41.4
      senile cognitive decline R41.81
      specified symptom NEC R41.89
    behavior NEC R46.89
    cardiovascular system NEC R09.89
    chest NEC R09.89
    circulatory system NEC R09.89
    cognitive functions R41.9
      altered mental status R41.82
      amnesia —*see* Amnesia
      borderline intellectual functioning
        R41.83
      coma —*see* Coma
      disorientation R41.0
      neurologic neglect syndrome
        R41.4
      senile cognitive decline R41.81
      specified symptom NEC R41.89
    development NEC R62.50
    digestive system NEC R19.8
    emotional state NEC R45.89
      emotional lability R45.86
    food and fluid intake R63.8
    general perceptions and sensations
      R44.9
      specified NEC R44.8
    musculoskeletal system R29.91
      specified NEC R29.898
    nervous system R29.90
      specified NEC R29.818
    pelvis NEC R19.8
    respiratory system NEC R09.89
    skin and integument R23.9
    urinary system R39.9
  menopausal N95.1
  metabolism NEC R63.8

Symptoms NEC (*Continued*)
  neurotic F48.8
  of infancy R68.19
  pelvis NEC, female R10.2
  skin and integument NEC R23.9
  subcutaneous tissue NEC R23.9
  viral cold J00
Sympus Q74.2
Syncephalus Q89.4
Synchondrosis
  abnormal (congenital) Q78.8
  ischiopubic M91.0
Synchysis (scintillans) (senile) (vitreous body)
  H43.89
Syncope (near) (pre-) R55
  anginosa I20.8
  bradycardia R00.1
  cardiac R55
  carotid sinus G90.01
  due to spinal (lumbar) puncture G97.1
  heart R55
  heat T67.1
 ⇒ laryngeal R05.4
  psychogenic F48.8
 ⇒ tussive R05.8
  vasoconstriction R55
  vasodepressor R55
  vasomotor R55
  vasovagal R55
Syndactylism, syndactyly Q70.9
  complex (with synostosis)
    fingers Q70.0- ●
    toes Q70.2- ●
  simple (without synostosis)
    fingers Q70.1- ●
    toes Q70.3- ●
Syndrome —*see also* Disease
  5q minus NOS D46.C
  48,XXXX Q97.1
  49,XXXXX Q97.1
  abdominal
    acute R10.0
    muscle deficiency Q79.4
  abnormal innervation H02.519
    left H02.516
      lower H02.515
      upper H02.514
    right H02.513
      lower H02.512
      upper H02.511
  abstinence, neonatal P96.1
  acid pulmonary aspiration, obstetric O74.0
  acquired immunodeficiency —*see* Human,
    immunodeficiency virus (HIV) disease
  acute abdominal R10.0
  acute respiratory distress (adult) (child) J80
    idiopathic J84.114
  Adair-Dighton Q78.0
  Adams-Stokes (-Morgagni) I45.9
  adiposogenital E23.6
  adrenal
    hemorrhage (meningococcal) A39.1
    meningococcic A39.1
  adrenocortical —*see* Cushing's, syndrome
  adrenogenital E25.9
    congenital, associated with enzyme
      deficiency E25.0
  afferent loop NEC K91.89
  Alagille's Q44.7
  alcohol withdrawal (without convulsions) —
    see Dependence, alcohol, with,
    withdrawal
  Alder's D72.0
  Aldrich (-Wiskott) D82.0
  alien hand R41.4
  Alport Q87.81
  alveolar hypoventilation E66.2
  alveolocapillary block J84.10
  amnesia, amnestic (confabulatory) (due to) —
    see Disorder, amnesic
  amyostatic (Wilson's disease) E83.01

▶ New   ⇒ Revised   ~~deleted~~ Deleted   ● Use Additional Character(s)

Syndrome *(Continued)*
  androgen insensitivity E34.50
    complete E34.51
    partial E34.52
  androgen resistance *(see also* Syndrome,
      androgen insensitivity) E34.50
  Angelman Q93.51
  anginal —*see* Angina
  ankyloglossia superior Q38.1
  anterior
    chest wall R07.89
    cord G83.82
    spinal artery G95.19
      compression M47.019
        cervical region M47.012
        cervicothoracic region M47.013
        lumbar region M47.016
        occipito-atlanto-axial region M47.011
        thoracic region M47.014
        thoracolumbar region M47.015
    tibial M76.81-●
  antibody deficiency D80.9
    agammaglobulinemic D80.1
      hereditary D80.0
    congenital D80.0
    hypogammaglobulinemic D80.1
      hereditary D80.0
  anticardiolipin (-antibody) D68.61
  antidepressant discontinuation T43.205
  antiphospholipid (-antibody) D68.61
  aortic
    arch M31.4
    bifurcation I74.09
  aortomesenteric duodenum occlusion K31.5
  apical ballooning (transient left ventricular)
      I51.81
  arcuate ligament I77.4
  argentaffin, argintaffinoma E34.0
  Arnold-Chiari —*see* Arnold-Chiari disease
  Arrillaga-Ayerza I27.0
  arterial tortuosity Q87.82
  arteriovenous steal T82.898-●
  Asherman's N85.6
  aspiration, of newborn —*see* Aspiration, by
      substance, with pneumonia
      meconium P24.01
  ataxia-telangiectasia G11.3
  auriculotemporal G50.8
  autoerythrocyte sensitization (Gardner-
      Diamond) D69.2
  autoimmune lymphoproliferative [ALPS]
      D89.82
  autoimmune polyglandular E31.0
  autoinflammatory M04.9
    specified type NEC M04.8
  autosomal —*see* Abnormal, autosomes
  Avellis' G46.8
  Ayerza (-Arrillaga) I27.0
  Babinski-Nageotte G83.89
  Bakwin-Krida Q78.5
  bare lymphocyte D81.6
  Barré-Guillain G61.0
  Barré-Liéou M53.0
  Barrett's —*see* Barrett's, esophagus
  Barsony-Polgar K22.4
  Barsony-Teschendorf K22.4
  Barth E78.71
  Bartter's E26.81
  basal cell nevus Q87.89
  Basedow's E05.00
    with thyroid storm E05.01
  basilar artery G45.0
  Batten-Steinert G71.11
  battered
    baby or child —*see* Maltreatment, child,
        physical abuse
    spouse —*see* Maltreatment, adult, physical
        abuse
  Beals Q87.40
  Beau's I51.5
  Beck's I65.8

Syndrome *(Continued)*
  Benedikt's G46.3
  Béquez César (-Steinbrinck-Chédiak-Higashi)
      D70.330
  Bernhardt-Roth —*see* Meralgia paresthetica
  Bernheim's —*see* Failure, heart, right
  big spleen D73.1
  bilateral polycystic ovarian E28.2
  Bing-Horton's —*see* Horton's headache
  Birt-Hogg-Dube syndrome Q87.89
  Björck (-Thorsen) E34.0
  black
    lung J60
    widow spider bite —*see* Toxicity, venom,
        spider, black widow
  Blackfan-Diamond D61.01
  Blau M04.8
  blind loop K90.2
    congenital Q43.8
    postsurgical K91.2
  blue sclera Q78.0
  blue toe I75.02-●
  Boder-Sedgewick G11.3
  Boerhaave's K22.3
  Borjeson Forssman Lehmann Q89.8
  Bouillaud's I01.9
  Bourneville (-Pringle) Q85.1
  Bouveret (-Hoffman) I47.9
  brachial plexus G54.0
  bradycardia-tachycardia I49.5
  brain (nonpsychotic) F09
    with psychosis, psychotic reaction F09
    acute or subacute —*see* Delirium
    congenital —*see* Disability, intellectual
    organic F09
      post-traumatic (nonpsychotic) F07.81
        psychotic F09
    personality change F07.0
    postcontusional F07.81
    post-traumatic, nonpsychotic F07.81
    psycho-organic F09
    psychotic F06.8
  brain stem stroke G46.3
  Brandt's (acrodermatitis enteropathica)
      E83.2
  broad ligament laceration N83.8
  Brock's J98.11
  bronze baby P83.88
  Brown-Sequard G83.81
  Brugada I49.8
  bubbly lung P27.0
  Buchem's M85.2
  Budd-Chiari I82.0
  bulbar (progressive) G12.22
  Bürger-Grütz E78.3
  Burke's K86.89
  Burnett's (milk-alkali) E83.52
  burning feet E53.9
  Bywaters' T79.5
  Call-Fleming I67.841
  carbohydrate-deficient glycoprotein (CDGS)
      E77.8
  carcinogenic thrombophlebitis I82.1
  carcinoid E34.0
  cardiac asthma I50.1
  cardiacos negros I27.0
  cardiofaciocutaneous Q87.89
  cardiopulmonary-obesity E66.2
  cardiorenal —*see* Hypertension, cardiorenal
  cardiorespiratory distress (idiopathic),
      newborn P22.0
  cardiovascular renal —*see* Hypertension,
      cardiorenal
  carotid
    artery (hemispheric) (internal)
        G45.1
    body G90.01
    sinus G90.01
  carpal tunnel G56.0-●
  Cassidy (-Scholte) E34.0
  cat-cry Q93.4

Syndrome *(Continued)*
  cat eye Q92.8
  cauda equina G83.4
  causalgia —*see* Causalgia
  celiac K90.0
    artery compression I77.4
    axis I77.4
  central pain G89.0
  cerebellar
    hereditary G11.9
    stroke G46.4
  cerebellomedullary malformation —*see* Spina
      bifida
  cerebral
    artery
      anterior G46.1
      middle G46.0
      posterior G46.2
    gigantism E22.0
  cervical (root) M53.1
    disc —*see* Disorder, disc, cervical, with
        neuritis
    fusion Q76.1
    posterior, sympathicus M53.0
    rib Q76.5
    sympathetic paralysis G90.2
  cervicobrachial (diffuse) M53.1
  cervicocranial M53.0
  cervicodorsal outlet G54.2
  cervicothoracic outlet G54.0
  Céstan (-Raymond) I65.8
  Charcot's (angina cruris) (intermittent
      claudication) I73.9
  Charcot-Weiss-Baker G90.09
  CHARGE Q89.8
  Chédiak-Higashi (-Steinbrinck) E70.330
  chest wall R07.1
  Chiari's (hepatic vein thrombosis) I82.0
  Chilaiditi's Q43.3
  child maltreatment —*see* Maltreatment,
      child
  chondrocostal junction M94.0
  chondroectodermal dysplasia Q77.6
  chromosome 4 short arm deletion Q93.3
  chromosome 5 short arm deletion Q93.4
  chronic
    infantile neurological, cutaneous and
        articular (CINCA) M04.2
    pain G89.4
      personality F68.8
  Churg-Strauss M30.1
  Clarke-Hadfield K86.89
  Clerambault's automatism G93.89
  Clouston's (hidrotic ectodermal dysplasia)
      Q82.4
  clumsiness, clumsy child F82
  cluster headache G44.009
    intractable G44.001
    not intractable G44.009
  Coffin-Lowry Q89.8
  cold injury (newborn) P80.0
  combined immunity deficiency D81.9
  compartment (deep) (posterior) (traumatic)
      T79.A0
    abdomen T79.A3
    lower extremity (hip, buttock, thigh, leg,
        foot, toes) T79.A2
    nontraumatic
      abdomen M79.A3
      lower extremity (hip, buttock, thigh, leg,
          foot, toes) M79.A2-●
      specified site NEC M79.A9
      upper extremity (shoulder, arm, forearm,
          wrist, hand, fingers) M79.A1-●
    postprocedural —*see* Syndrome
        compartment, nontraumatic
    specified site NEC T79.A9
    upper extremity (shoulder, arm, forearm,
        wrist, hand, fingers) T79.A1
  complex regional pain —*see* Syndrome, pain,
      complex regional

Syndrome *(Continued)*

compression T79.5
  anterior spinal —*see* Syndrome, anterior, spinal artery, compression
  cauda equina G83.4
  celiac artery I77.4
  vertebral artery M47.029
    cervical region M47.022
    occipito-atlanto-axial region M47.021
concussion F07.81
congenital
  affecting multiple systems NEC Q87.89
  central alveolar hypoventilation G47.35
  facial diplegia Q87.0
  muscular hypertrophy-cerebral Q87.89
  oculo-auriculovertebral Q87.0
  oculofacial diplegia (Moebius) Q87.0
  rubella (manifest) P35.0
congestion-fibrosis (pelvic), female N94.89
congestive dysmenorrhea N94.6
Conn's E26.01
connective tissue M35.9
  overlap NEC M35.1
conus medullaris G95.81
cord
  anterior G83.82
  posterior G83.83
coronary
  acute NEC I24.9
  insufficiency or intermediate I20.0
  slow flow I20.8
Costen's (complex) M26.69
costochondral junction M94.0
costoclavicular G54.0
costovertebral E22.0
Cowden Q85.8
craniovertebral M53.0
Creutzfeldt-Jakob —*see* Creutzfeldt-Jakob disease or syndrome
cri-du-chat Q93.4
crib death R99
cricopharyngeal —*see* Dysphagia
croup J05.0
CRPS I —*see* Syndrome, pain, complex regional I
crush T79.5
cubital tunnel —*see* Lesion, nerve, ulnar
Curschmann (-Batten) (-Steinert) G71.11
Cushing's E24.9
  alcohol-induced E24.4
  drug-induced E24.2
  due to
    alcohol
    drugs E24.2
    ectopic ACTH E24.3
    overproduction of pituitary ACTH E24.0
  overdose or wrong substance given or taken —*see* Table of Drugs and Chemicals, by drug, poisoning
  pituitary-dependent E24.0
  specified type NEC E24.8
cryopyrin-associated periodic M04.2
cryptophthalmos Q87.0
cystic duct stump K91.5
cytokine release D89.839
  grade 1 D89.831
  grade 2 D89.832
  grade 3 D89.833
  grade 4 D89.834
  grade 5 D89.835
Dana-Putnam D51.0
Danbolt (-Cross) (acrodermatitis enteropathica) E83.2
Dandy-Walker Q03.1
  with spina bifida Q07.01
Danlos' (*see also* Syndrome, Ehlers-Danlos) Q79.60

Syndrome *(Continued)*

defibrination —*see also* Fibrinolysis
  with
    antepartum hemorrhage —*see* Hemorrhage, antepartum, with coagulation defect
    intrapartum hemorrhage —*see* Hemorrhage, complicating, delivery
  newborn P60
  postpartum O72.3
Degos' I77.8
Déjérine-Roussy G89.0
delayed sleep phase G47.21
demyelinating G37.9
dependence —*see* F10-F19 with fourth character .2
depersonalization (-derealization) F48.1
De Quervain E34.51
de Toni-Fanconi (-Debré) E72.09
  with cystinosis E72.04
de Vivo syndrome E74.810
diabetes mellitus-hypertension-nephrosis —*see* Diabetes, nephrosis
diabetes mellitus in newborn infant P70.2
diabetes-nephrosis —*see* Diabetes, nephrosis
diabetic amyotrophy —*see* Diabetes, amyotrophy
dialysis associated steal T82.898-●
Diamond-Blackfan D61.01
Diamond-Gardener D69.2
DIC (diffuse or disseminated intravascular coagulopathy) D65
di George's D82.1
Dighton's Q78.0
disequilibrium E87.8
Döhle body-panmyelopathic D72.0
dorsolateral medullary G46.4
double athetosis G80.3
Down (*see also* Down syndrome) Q90.9
Dravet (intractable) G40.834
  with status epilepticus G40.833
  without status epilepticus G40.834
Dresbach's (elliptocytosis) D58.1
DRESS (drug rash with eosinophilia and systemic symptoms) D72.12
Dressler's (postmyocardial infarction) I24.1
  postcardiotomy I97.0
drug rash with eosinophilia and systemic symptoms (DRESS) D72.12
drug withdrawal, infant of dependent mother P96.1
dry eye H04.12-●
due to abnormality
  chromosomal Q99.9
  sex
    female phenotype Q97.9
    male phenotype Q98.9
  specified NEC Q99.8
dumping (postgastrectomy) K91.1
  nonsurgical K31.89
Dupré's (meningism) R29.1
dysmetabolic X E88.81
dyspraxia, developmental F82
Eagle-Barrett Q79.4
Eaton-Lambert —*see* Syndrome, Lambert-Eaton
Ebstein's Q22.5
ectopic ACTH E24.3
eczema-thrombocytopenia D82.0
Eddowes' Q78.0
effort (psychogenic) F45.8
Ehlers-Danlos Q79.60
  classical (cEDS) (classical EDS) Q79.61
  hypermobile (hEDS) (hypermobile EDS) Q79.62
  specified NEC Q79.69
  vascular (vascular EDS) (vEDS) Q79.63
Eisenmenger's I27.83
Ekman's Q78.0
electric feet E53.8
Ellis-van Creveld Q77.6

Syndrome *(Continued)*

empty nest Z60.0
endocrine-hypertensive E27.0
entrapment —*see* Neuropathy, entrapment
eosinophilia-myalgia M35.89
epileptic —*see also* Epilepsy, by type
  absence G40.A09
    intractable G40.A19
      with status epilepticus G40.A11
      without status epilepticus G40.A19
    not intractable G40.A09
      with status epilepticus G40.A01
      without status epilepticus G40.A09
Erdheim-Chester (ECD) E88.89
Erdheim's E22.0
erythrocyte fragmentation D59.4
Evans D69.41
exhaustion F48.8
extrapyramidal G25.9
  specified NEC G25.89
eye retraction —*see* Strabismus
eyelid-malar-mandible Q87.0
Faber's D50.9
facet M47.89-●
▶ facet joint (*see also* Spondylosis) M47.819
facial pain, paroxysmal G50.0
Fallot's Q21.3
familial cold autoinflammatory M04.2
familial eczema-thrombocytopenia (Wiskott-Aldrich) D82.0
Fanconi (-de Toni) (-Debré) E72.09
  with cystinosis E72.04
Fanconi's (anemia) (congenital pancytopenia) D61.09
fatigue
  chronic R53.82
  psychogenic F48.8
faulty bowel habit K59.39
Feil-Klippel (brevicollis) Q76.1
Felty's —*see* Felty's syndrome
fertile eunuch E23.0
fetal
  alcohol (dysmorphic) Q86.0
  hydantoin Q86.1
Fiedler's I40.1
first arch Q87.0
fish odor E72.89
Fisher's G61.0
Fitzhugh-Curtis
  due to
    Chlamydia trachomatis A74.81
    Neisseria gonorrhorea (gonococcal peritonitis) A54.85
Fitz's —*see also* Pancreatitis, acute K85.80
Flajani (-Basedow) E05.00
  with thyroid storm E05.01
flatback —*see* Flatback syndrome
floppy
  baby P94.2
  iris (intraoeprative) (IFIS) H21.81
  mitral valve I34.1
flush E34.0
Foix-Alajouanine G95.19
Fong's Q87.2
food protein-induced enterocolitis (FPIES) K52.21
foramen magnum G93.5
Foster-Kennedy H47.14-●
Foville's (peduncular) G46.3
fragile X Q99.2
Franceschetti Q75.4
Frey's
  auriculotemporal G50.8
  hyperhidrosis L74.52
Friderichsen-Waterhouse A39.1
Froin's G95.89
frontal lobe F07.0
Fukuhara E88.49
functional
  bowel K59.9
  prepubertal castrate E29.1
Gaisböck's D75.1

▶ New   ⇒ Revised   ~~deleted~~ Deleted   ● Use Additional Character(s)

Syndrome *(Continued)*
  ganglion (basal ganglia brain) G25.9
    geniculi G51.1
  Gardner-Diamond D69.2
  gastroesophageal
    junction K22.0
    laceration-hemorrhage K22.6
  gastrojejunal loop obstruction K91.89
  Gee-Herter-Heubner K90.0
  Gelineau's G47.419
    with cataplexy G47.411
  genito-anorectal A55
  Gerstmann-Sträussler-Scheinker (GSS) A81.82
  Gianotti-Crosti L44.4
  giant platelet (Bernard-Soulier) D69.1
  Gilles de la Tourette's F95.2
  Glass Q87.89
  Gleich's D72.118
  goiter-deafness E07.1
  Goldberg Q89.8
  Goldberg-Maxwell E34.51
  Good's D83.8
  Gopalan' (burning feet) E53.8
  Gorlin's Q87.89
  Gougerot-Blum L81.7
  Gouley's I31.1
  Gower's R55
  gray or grey (newborn) P93.0
    platelet D69.1
  Gubler-Millard G46.3
  Guillain-Barré (-Strohl) G61.0
  gustatory sweating G50.8
  Hadfield-Clarke K86.89
  hair tourniquet —*see* Constriction, external,
    by site
  Hamman's J98.19
  hand-foot L27.1
  hand-shoulder G90.8
  hantavirus (cardio)-pulmonary (HPS) (HCPS)
    B33.4
  happy puppet Q93.51
  Harada's H30.81-●
  Hayem-Faber D50.9
  headache NEC G44.89
    complicated NEC G44.59
  Heberden's I20.8
  Hedinger's E34.0
  Hegglin's D72.0
  HELLP (hemolysis, elevated liver enzymes
    and low platelet count) O14.2-●
    complicating
      childbirth O14.24
        puerperium O14.25
  hemolytic-uremic D59.3
  hemophagocytic, infection-associated D76.2
  Henoch-Schönlein D69.0
  hepatic flexure K59.89
  hepatopulmonary K76.81
  hepatorenal K76.7
    following delivery O90.4
    postoperative or postprocedural K91.83
    postpartum, puerperal O90.4
  hepatourologic K76.7
▶ hereditary alpha tryptasemia D89.44
  Herter (-Gee) (nontropical sprue) K90.0
  Heubner-Herter K90.0
  Heyd's K76.7
  Hilger's G90.09
  histamine-like (fish poisoning) —*see*
    Poisoning, fish
  histiocytic D76.3
  histiocytosis NEC D76.3
  HIV infection, acute B20
  Hoffmann-Werdnig G12.0
  Hollander-Simons E88.1
  Hoppe-Goldflam G70.00
    with exacerbation (acute) G70.01
    in crisis G70.01
  Horner's G90.2
  hungry bone E83.81
  hunterian glossitis D51.0
  Hutchinson's triad A50.53

Syndrome *(Continued)*
  hyperabduction G54.0
  hyperammonemia-hyperornithinemia-
    homocitrullinemia E72.4
  hypereosinophilic (HES) D72.119
    idiopathic (IHES) D72.110
    lymphocytic variant (LHES) D72.111
▶ myeloid D72.118
    specified NEC D72.118
  hyperimmunoglobulin D M04.1
  hyperimmunoglobulin E (IgE) D82.4
  hyperkalemic E87.5
  hyperkinetic —*see* Hyperkinesia
  hypermobility M35.7
  hypernatremia E87.0
  hyperosmolarity E87.0
  hyperperfusion G97.82
  hypersplenic D73.1
  hypertransfusion, newborn P61.1
  hyperventilation F45.8
  hyperviscosity (of serum)
    polycythemic D75.1
    sclerothymic D58.8
  hypoglycemic (familial) (neonatal) E16.2
  hypokalemic E87.6
  hyponatremic E87.1
  hypopituitarism E23.0
  hypoplastic left-heart Q23.4
  hypopotassemia E87.6
  hyposmolality E87.1
  hypotension, maternal O26.5-●
  hypothenar hammer I73.89
  hypoventilation, obesity (OHS) E66.2
  ICF (intravascular coagulation-fibrinolysis) D65
  idiopathic
    cardiorespiratory distress, newborn P22.0
    nephrotic (infantile) N04.9
  iliotibial band M76.3-●
  immobility, immobilization (paraplegic) M62.3
▶ immune effector cell-associated neurotoxicity
    (ICANS) G92.00
  ▶ grade
    ▶ 1 G92.01
    ▶ 2 G92.02
    ▶ 3 G92.03
    ▶ 4 G92.04
    ▶ 5 G92.05
    ▶ unspecified G92.00
  immune reconstitution D89.3
  immune reconstitution inflammatory [IRIS]
    D89.3
  immunity deficiency, combined D81.9
  immunodeficiency
    acquired —*see* Human, immunodeficiency
      virus (HIV) disease
    combined D81.9
  impending coronary I20.0
  impingement, shoulder M75.4-●
  inappropriate secretion of antidiuretic
    hormone E22.2
  infant
    gestational diabetes P70.0
    of diabetic mother P70.1
  infantilism (pituitary) E23.0
  inferior vena cava I87.1
  inspissated bile (newborn) P59.1
  institutional (childhood) F94.2
  insufficient sleep F51.12
  intermediate coronary (artery) I20.0
  interspinous ligament —*see* Spondylopathy,
    specified NEC
  intestinal
    carcinoid E34.0
    knot K56.2
  intravascular coagulation-fibrinolysis (ICF)
    D65
  iodine-deficiency, congenital E00.9
    type
      mixed E00.2
      myxedematous E00.1
      neurological E00.0
  IRDS (idiopathic respiratory distress,
    newborn) P22.0

Syndrome *(Continued)*
  irritable
    bowel K58.9
      with
        constipation K58.1
        diarrhea K58.0
      mixed K58.2
      psychogenic F45.8
      specified NEC K58.8
    heart (psychogenic) F45.8
    weakness F48.8
  ischemic
    bowel (transient) K55.9
      chronic K55.1
      due to mesenteric artery insufficiency
        K55.1
      steal T82.898
  IVC (intravascular coagulopathy) D65
  Ivemark's Q89.01
  Jaccoud's —*see* Arthropathy, postrheumatic,
    chronic
  Jackson's G83.89
  Jakob-Creutzfeldt —*see* Creutzfeldt-Jakob
    disease or syndrome
  jaw-winking Q07.8
  Jervell-Lange-Nielsen I45.81
  jet lag G47.25
  Job's D71
  Joseph-Diamond-Blackfan D61.01
  jugular foramen G52.7
  Kabuki Q89.8
  Kanner's (autism) F84.0
  Kartagener's Q89.3
  Kelly's D50.1
  Kimmelstiel Wilson —*see* Diabetes,specified
    type, with Kimmelstiel-Wilson disease
  Klein (e)-Levine G47.13
  Klippel-Feil (brevicollis) Q76.1
  Köhler-Pellegrini-Steida —*see* Bursitis, tibial
    collateral
  König's K59.89
  Korsakoff (-Wernicke) (nonalcoholic) F04
    alcoholic F10.26
  Kostmann's D70.0
  Krabbe's congenital muscle hypoplasia Q79.8
  labyrinthine —*see* subcategory H83.2
  lacunar NEC G46.7
  Lambert-Eaton G70.80
    in
      neoplastic disease G73.1
      specified disease NEC G70.81
  Landau-Kleffner —*see* Epilepsy, specified NEC
  Larsen's Q74.8
  lateral
    cutaneous nerve of thigh G57.1-●
    medullary G46.4
  Launois' E22.0
  lazy
    leukocyte D70.8
    posture M62.3
  Lemiere I80.8
  Lennox-Gastaut G40.812
    intractable G40.814
      with status epilepticus G40.813
      without status epilepticus G40.814
    not intractable G40.812
      with status epilepticus G40.811
      without status epilepticus G40.812
  lenticular, progressive E83.01
  Leopold-Levi's E05.90
  Lev's I44.2
  Li-Fraumeni Z15.01
  Lichtheim's D51.0
  Lightwood's N25.89
  Lignac (de Toni) (-Fanconi) (-Debré)
    E72.09
    with cystinosis E72.04
  Likoff's I20.8
  limbic epilepsy personality F07.0
  liver-kidney K76.7
  lobotomy F07.0
  Löffler's J82.89
  long arm 18 or 21 deletion Q93.89

Syndrome (Continued)

long QT I45.81

Louis-Barré G11.3

low

    atmospheric pressure T70.29

▶back M54.50

    output (cardiac) I50.9

lower radicular, newborn (birth injury) P14.8

Luetscher's (dehydration) E86.0

Lupus anticoagulant D68.62

Lutembacher's Q21.1

macrophage activation D76.1

    due to infection D76.2

magnesium-deficiency R29.0

Majeed M04.8

Mal de Debarquement R42

malabsorption K90.9

    postsurgical K91.2

malformation, congenital, due to

    alcohol Q86.0

    exogenous cause NEC Q86.8

    hydantoin Q86.1

    warfarin Q86.2

malignant

    carcinoid E34.0

    neuroleptic G21.0

Mallory-Weiss K22.6

mandibulofacial dysostosis Q75.4

manic-depressive —see Disorder, bipolar

maple-syrup-urine E71.0

Marable's I77.4

Marfan's Q87.40

    with

        cardiovascular manifestations Q87.418

          aortic dilation Q87.410

        ocular manifestations Q87.42

        skeletal manifestations Q87.43

Marie's (acromegaly) E22.0

mast cell activation —see Activation, mast cell

maternal hypotension —see Syndrome, hypotension, maternal

May (-Hegglin) D72.0

McArdle (-Schmidt) (-Pearson) E74.04

McQuarrie's E16.2

meconium plug (newborn) P76.0

median arcuate ligament I77.4

Meekeren-Ehlers-Danlos Q79.6

megavitamin-B6 E67.2

Meige G24.4

MELAS E88.41

Mendelson's O74.0

MERRF (myoclonic epilepsy associated with ragged-red fibers) E88.42

mesenteric

    artery (superior) K55.1

    vascular insufficiency K55.1

metabolic E88.81

metastatic carcinoid E34.0

micrognathia-glossoptosis Q87.0

midbrain NEC G93.89

middle lobe (lung) J98.19

middle radicular G54.0

migraine —see also Migraine G43.909- ●

Mikulicz' K11.8

milk-alkali E83.52

Millard-Gubler G46.3

Miller-Dieker Q93.88

Miller-Fisher G61.0

Minkowski-Chauffard D58.0

Mirizzi's K83.1

MNGIE (Mitochondrial Neurogastrointestinal Encephalopathy) E88.49

Möbius, ophthalmoplegic migraine —see Migraine, ophthalmoplegic

monofixation H50.42

Morel-Moore M85.2

Morel-Morgagni M85.2

Morgagni (-Morel) (-Stewart) M85.2

Morgagni-Adams-Stokes I45.9

Mounier-Kuhn Q32.4

    with bronchiectasis J47.9

Syndrome (Continued)

Mounier-Kuhn (Continued)

    with bronchiectasis(Continued)

        with

          exacerbation (acute) J47.1

          lower respiratory infection J47.0

    acquired J98.09

        with bronchiectasis J47.9

          with

            exacerbation (acute) J47.1

            lower respiratory infection J47.0

Muckle-Wells M04.2

mucocutaneous lymph node (acute febrile) (MCLS) M30.3

multiple endocrine neoplasia (MEN) —see Neoplasia, endocrine, multiple (MEN}

multiple operations —see Disorder, factitious

multisystem inflammatory (in adults) (in children) M35.81

myasthenic G70.9

    in

        diabetes mellitus —see Diabetes, amyotrophy

        endocrine disease NEC E34.9 [G73.3]

        neoplastic disease —see also Neoplasm D49.9 [G73.3]

        thyrotoxicosis (hyperthyroidism) E05.90 [G73.3]

          with thyroid storm E05.91 [G73.3]

myelodysplastic D46.9

    with

        5q deletion D46.C

        isolated del (5q) chromosomal abnormality D46.C

        multilineage dysplasia D46.A

          with ringed sideroblasts D46.B

    lesions, low grade D46.20

    specified NEC D46.Z

myeloid hypereosinophilic D72.118

myelopathic pain G89.0

myeloproliferative (chronic) D47.1

myofascial pain M79.18

Naffziger's G54.0

nail patella Q87.2

NARP (Neuropathy, Ataxia and Retinitis pigmentosa) E88.49

neonatal abstinence P96.1

nephritic —see also Nephritis

    with edema —see Nephrosis

    acute N00.9

    chronic N03.9

    rapidly progressive N01.9

nephrotic (congenital) —see also Nephrosis N04.9

    with

        C3

          glomerulonephritis N04.A

          glomerulopathy N04.A

            with dense deposit disease N04.6

        dense deposit disease N04.6

        diffuse

          crescentic glomerulonephritis N04.7

          endocapillary proliferative glomerulonephritis N04.4

          membranous glomerulonephritis N04.2

          mesangial proliferative glomerulonephritis N04.3

          mesangiocapillary glomerulonephritis N04.5

        focal and segmental glomerular lesions N04.1

        minor glomerular abnormality N04.0

        specified morphological changes NEC N04.8

    diabetic —see Diabetes, nephrosis

neurologic neglect R41.4

Nezelof's D81.4

Nonne-Milroy-Meige Q82.0

Nothnagel's vasomotor acroparesthesia I73.89

obesity hypoventilation (OHS) E66.2

oculomotor H51.9

Ogilvie K59.81

Syndrome (Continued)

ophthalmoplegia-cerebellar ataxia —see Strabismus, paralytic, third nerve

oral allergy T78.1

oral-facial-digital Q87.0

organic

    affective F06.30

    amnesic (not alcohol- or drug-induced) F04

    brain F09

    depressive F06.31

    hallucinosis F06.0

    personality F07.0

Ormond's N13.5

oro-facial-digital Q87.0

os trigonum Q68.8

Osler-Weber-Rendu I78.0

osteoporosis-osteomalacia M83.8

Osterreicher-Turner Q87.2

otolith —see subcategory H81.8

oto-palatal-digital Q87.0

outlet (thoracic) G54.0

ovary

    polycystic E28.2

    resistant E28.39

    sclerocystic E28.2

Owren's D68.2

Paget-Schroetter I82.890

pain —see also Pain

    complex regional I G90.50

        lower limb G90.52- ●

        specified site NEC G90.59

        upper limb G90.51- ●

    complex regional II —see Causalgia

painful

    bruising D69.2

    feet E53.8

    prostate N42.81

paralysis agitans —see Parkinsonism

paralytic G83.9

    specified NEC G83.89

Parinaud's H51.0

parkinsonian —see Parkinsonism

Parkinson's —see Parkinsonism

paroxysmal facial pain G50.0

Parry's E05.00

    with thyroid storm E05.01

Parsonage (-Aldren)-Turner G54.5

patella clunk M25.86- ●

Paterson (-Brown) (-Kelly) D50.1

pectoral girdle I77.89

pectoralis minor I77.89

pediatric autoimmune neuropsychiatric disorders associated with streptococcal infections (PANDAS) D89.89

pediatric inflammatory multisystem M35.81

Pelger-Huet D72.0

pellagra-cerebellar ataxia-renal aminoaciduria E72.02

pellagroid E52

Pellegrini-Stieda —see Bursitis, tibial collateral

pelvic congestion-fibrosis, female N94.89

penta X Q97.1

peptic ulcer —see Ulcer, peptic

perabduction I77.89

periodic fever M04.1

periodic fever, aphthous stomatitis, pharyngitis, and adenopathy [PFAPA] M04.8

periodic headache, in adults and children — see Headache, periodic syndromes in adults and children

periurethral fibrosis N13.5

phantom limb (without pain) G54.7

    with pain G54.6

pharyngeal pouch D82.1

Pick's —see Disease, Pick's

Pickwickian E66.2

PIE (pulmonary infiltration with eosinophilia) J82.89

pigmentary pallidal degeneration (progressive) G23.0

pineal E34.8

pituitary E22.0

▶ New   ⇒ Revised   ~~deleted~~ Deleted   ● Use Additional Character(s)

Syndrome *(Continued)*
  placental transfusion —*see* Pregnancy,
      complicated by, placental transfusion
      syndromes
  plantar fascia M72.2
  plateau iris (post-iridectomy)
      (postprocedural) H21.82
  Plummer-Vinson D50.1
  pluricarential of infancy E40
  plurideficiency E40
  pluriglandular (compensatory) E31.8
      autoimmune E31.0
  pneumatic hammer T75.21
  polyangiitis overlap M30.8
  polycarential of infancy E40
  polyglandular E31.8
      autoimmune E31.0
  polysplenia Q89.09
  pontine NEC G93.89
  popliteal
      artery entrapment I77.89
      web Q87.89
  postcardiac injury
      postcardiotomy I97.0
      postmyocardial infarction I24.1
  postcardiotomy I97.0
  post chemoembolization — code to
      associated conditions
  postcholecystectomy K91.5
  postcommissurotomy I97.0
  postconcussional F07.81
  postcontusional F07.81
  post-COVID (-19) U09.9
  postencephalitic F07.89
  post endometrial ablation N99.85
  posterior
      cervical sympathetic M53.0
      cord G83.83
      fossa compression G93.5
      reversible encephalopathy (PRES) I67.83
  postgastrectomy (dumping) K91.1
  postgastric surgery K91.1
  postinfarction I24.1
  postlaminectomy NEC M96.1
  postleukotomy F07.0
  postmastectomy lymphedema I97.2
  postmyocardial infarction I24.1
  postoperative NEC T81.9
      blind loop K90.2
  postpartum panhypopituitary (Sheehan) E23.0
  postpolio (myelitic) G14
  postthrombotic I87.009
      with
          inflammation I87.02-•
              with ulcer I87.03-•
          specified complication NEC I87.09-•
          ulcer I87.01-•
              with inflammation I87.03-•
      asymptomatic I87.00-•
  postvagotomy K91.1
  postvalvulotomy I97.0
  postviral NEC G93.3
      fatigue G93.3
  Potain's K31.0
  potassium intoxication E87.5
  Prader-Willi Q87.11
  Prader-Willi-like Q87.19
  precerebral artery (multiple) (bilateral) G45.2
  preinfarction I20.0
  preleukemic D46.9
  premature senility E34.8
  premenstrual dysphoric F32.81
  premenstrual tension N94.3
  Prinzmetal-Massumi R07.1
  prune belly Q79.4
  pseudocarpal tunnel (sublimis) —*see*
      Syndrome, carpal tunnel
  pseudoparalytica G70.00
      with exacerbation (acute) G70.01
      in crisis G70.01
  pseudo-Turner's Q87.19

Syndrome *(Continued)*
  psycho-organic (nonpsychotic severity) F07.9
      acute or subacute F05
      depressive type F06.31
      hallucinatory type F06.0
      nonpsychotic severity F07.0
      specified NEC F07.89
  pulmonary
      arteriosclerosis I27.0
      dysmaturity (Wilson-Mikity) P27.0
      hypoperfusion (idiopathic) P22.0
      renal (hemorrhagic) (Goodpasture's) M31.0
  pure
      motor lacunar G46.5
      sensory lacunar G46.6
  Putnam-Dana D51.0
  pyogenic arthritis, pyoderma gangrenosum,
      and acne [PAPA] M04.8
  pyramidopallidonigral G20
  pyriformis —*see* Lesion, nerve, sciatic
  QT interval prolongation I45.81
  radicular NEC —*see* Radiculopathy
      upper limbs, newborn (birth injury) P14.3
  rapid time-zone change G47.25
  Rasmussen G04.81
  Raymond (-Céstan) I65.8
  Raynaud's I73.00
      with gangrene I73.01
  RDS (respiratory distress syndrome,
      newborn) P22.0
  reactive airways dysfunction J68.3
  Refsum's G60.1
  Reifenstein E34.52
  renal glomerulohyalinosis-diabetic —*see*
      Diabetes, nephrosis
  Rendu-Osler-Weber I78.0
  residual ovary N99.83
  resistant ovary E28.39
  respiratory
      distress
          acute J80
              adult J80
              child J80
              idiopathic J84.114
          newborn (idiopathic) (type I) P22.0
              type II P22.1
  restless legs G25.81
  retinoblastoma (familial) C69.2
  retroperitoneal fibrosis N13.5
  retroviral seroconversion (acute) Z21
  Reye's G93.7
  Richter —*see* Leukemia, chronic lymphocytic,
      B-cell type
  Ridley's I50.1
  right
      heart, hypoplastic Q22.6
      ventricular obstruction —*see* Failure, heart,
          right
  Romano-Ward (prolonged QT interval) I45.81
  rotator cuff, shoulder —*see also* Tear, rotator
      cuff M75.10-•
  Rotes Quérol —*see* Hyperostosis, ankylosing
  Roth —*see* Meralgia paresthetica
  rubella (congenital) P35.0
  Ruvalcaba-Myhre-Smith E71.440
  Rytand-Lipsitch I44.2
  salt
      depletion E87.1
          due to heat NEC T67.8
              causing heat exhaustion or prostration
                  T67.4
      low E87.1
  salt-losing N28.89
  SATB2-associated Q87.89
  Scaglietti-Dagnini E22.0
  scalenus anticus (anterior) G54.0
  scapulocostal —*see* Mononeuropathy, upper
      limb, specified site NEC
  scapuloperoneal G71.09
  schizophrenic, of childhood NEC F84.5
  Schnitzler D47.2
  Scholte's E34.0

Syndrome *(Continued)*
  Schroeder's E27.0
  Schüller-Christian C96.5
  Schwachman's —*see* Syndrome, Shwachman's
  Schwartz (-Jampel) G71.13
  Schwartz-Bartter E22.2
  scimitar Q26.8
  sclerocystic ovary E28.2
  Seitelberger's G31.89
  septicemic adrenal hemorrhage A39.1
  seroconversion, retroviral (acute) Z21
  serous meningitis G93.2
  severe acute respiratory (SARS) J12.81
      coronavirus 2 -*see also* COVID-19 U07.1
          pneumonia J12.82
  shaken infant T74.4
  shock (traumatic) T79.4
      kidney N17.0
          following crush injury T79.5
      toxic A48.3
  shock-lung J80
  Shone's — code to specific anomalies
  short
      bowel K91.2
      rib Q77.2
  shoulder-hand —*see* Algoneurodystrophy
  Shwachman's D70.4
  sicca —*see* Syndrome, Sjögren
  sick
      cell E87.1
      sinus I49.5
  sick-euthyroid E07.81
  sideropenic D50.1
  Siemens' ectodermal dysplasia Q82.4
  Silfverskiöld's Q78.9
  Simons' E88.1
  sinus tarsi M25.57-•
  sinusitis-bronchiectasis-situs inversus Q89.3
  Sipple's E31.22
  sirenomelia Q87.2
  Sjögren M35.00
      with
          central nervous system involvement
              M35.07
          dental involvement M35.0C
          gastrointestinal involvement M35.08
          glomerular disease M35.0A
          inflammatory arthritis M35.05
          keratoconjunctivitis M35.01
          lung involvement M35.02
          myopathy M35.03
          peripheral nervous system involvement
              M35.06
          renal tubular acidosis M35.04
          specified organ involvement, NEC
              M35.09
          tubulo-interstitial nephropathy M35.04
          vasculitis M35.0B
  Slocumb's E27.0
  slow flow, coronary I20.8
  Sluder's G44.89
  Smith-Magenis Q93.88
  Sneddon-Wilkinson L13.1
  Sotos' Q87.3
  South African cardiomyopathy I42.8
  spasmodic
      upward movement, eyes H51.8
      winking F95.8
  Spen's I45.9
  splenic
      agenesis Q89.01
      flexure K59.89
      neutropenia D73.81
  Spurway's Q78.0
  staphylococcal scalded skin L00
  steal
      arteriovenous T82.898-•
      ischemic T82.898-•
      subclavian G45.8
  Stein-Leventhal E28.2
  Stein's E28.2
  Stevens-Johnson syndrome L51.1
      toxic epidermal necrolysis overlap L51.3

Syndrome *(Continued)*
  Stewart-Morel M85.2
  Stickler Q89.8
  stiff baby Q89.8
  stiff man G25.82
  Still-Felty —*see* Felty's syndrome
  Stokes (-Adams) I45.9
  stone heart I50.1
  straight back, congenital Q76.49
  subclavian steal G45.8
  subcoracoid-pectoralis minor G54.0
  subcostal nerve compression I77.89
  subphrenic interposition Q43.3
  superior
    cerebellar artery I63.89
    mesenteric artery K55.1
    semi-circular canal dehiscence H83.8X-•
    vena cava I87.1
  supine hypotensive (maternal) —*see*
      Syndrome, hypotension, maternal
  suprarenal cortical E27.0
  supraspinatus —*see also* Tear, rotator cuff
      M75.10-•
  Susac G93.49
  swallowed blood P78.2
  sweat retention L74.0
  Swyer Q99.1
  Symond's G93.2
  sympathetic
    cervical paralysis G90.2
    pelvic, female N94.89
  systemic inflammatory response (SIRS), of
      non-infectious origin (without organ
      dysfunction) R65.10
    with acute organ dysfunction R65.11
  tachycardia-bradycardia I49.5
  takotsubo I51.81
  TAR (thrombocytopenia with absent radius)
      Q87.2
  tarsal tunnel G57.5-•
  teething K00.7
  tegmental G93.89
  telangiectasic-pigmentation-cataract Q82.8
  temporal pyramidal apex —*see* Otitis, media,
      suppurative, acute
  temporomandibular joint-pain-dysfunction
      M26.62-•
  Terry's —*see also* Myopia, degenerative
      H44.2-•
  testicular feminization —*see also* Syndrome,
      androgen insensitivity E34.51
  thalamic pain (hyperesthetic) G89.0
  thoracic outlet (compression) G54.0
  Thorson-Björck E34.0
  thrombocytopenia with absent radius (TAR)
      Q87.2
  thyroid-adrenocortical insufficiency E31.0
  tibial
    anterior M76.81-•
    posterior M76.82-•
  Tietze's M94.0
  time-zone (rapid) G47.25
  Toni-Fanconi E72.09
    with cystinosis E72.04
  Touraine's Q79.8
  tourniquet —*see* Constriction, external, by site
  toxic shock A48.3
  transient left ventricular apical ballooning
      I51.81
  traumatic vasospastic T75.22
  Treacher Collins Q75.4
  triple X, female Q97.0
  trisomy Q92.9
    13 Q91.7
      meiotic nondisjunction Q91.4
      mitotic nondisjunction Q91.5
      mosaicism Q91.5
      translocation Q91.6
    18 Q91.3
      meiotic nondisjunction Q91.0
      mitotic nondisjunction Q91.1
      mosaicism Q91.1
      translocation Q91.2

Syndrome *(Continued)*
  trisomy Q92.9
    20 (q)(p) Q92.8
    21 Q90.9
      meiotic nondisjunction Q90.0
      mitotic nondisjunction Q90.1
      mosaicism Q90.1
      translocation Q90.2
    22 Q92.8
  tropical wet feet T69.0-•
  Trousseau's I82.1
  tumor lysis (following antineoplastic
      chemotherapy) (spontaneous) NEC E88.3
  tumor necrosis factor receptor associated
      periodic (TRAPS) M04.1
  Twiddler's (due to)
    automatic implantable defibrillator T82.198
    cardiac pacemaker T82.198
  Unverricht (-Lundborg) —*see* Epilepsy,
      generalized, idiopathic
  upward gaze H51.8
  uremia, chronic —*see also* Disease, kidney,
      chronic N18.9
  urethral N34.3
  urethro-oculo-articular —*see* Reiter's disease
  urohepatic K76.7
  vago-hypoglossal G52.7
  van Buchem's M85.2
  van der Hoeve's Q78.0
  vascular NEC in cerebrovascular disease G46.8
  vasoconstriction, reversible cerebrovascular
      I67.841
  vasomotor I73.9
  vasospastic (traumatic) T75.22
  vasovagal R55
  VATER Q87.2
  velo-cardio-facial Q93.81
  vena cava (inferior) (superior) (obstruction)
      I87.1
  vertebral
    artery G45.0
      compression —*see* Syndrome, anterior,
          spinal artery, compression
    steal G45.0
  vertebro-basilar artery G45.0
  ➥vertebrogenic (pain) (*see also* Pain,
      vertebrogenic) M54.89
  vertiginous —*see* Disorder, vestibular function
  Vinson-Plummer D50.1
  virus B34.9
  visceral larva migrans B83.0
  visual disorientation H53.8
  vitamin B6 deficiency E53.1
  vitreal corneal H59.01-•
  vitreous (touch) H59.01-•
  Vogt-Koyanagi H20.82-•
  Volkmann's T79.6
  von Schroetter's I82.890
  von Willebrand (-Jürgen) D68.0
  Waldenström-Kjellberg D50.1
  Wallenberg's G46.3
  water retention E87.79
  Waterhouse (-Friderichsen) A39.1
  Weber-Gubler G46.3
  Weber-Leyden G46.3
  Weber's G46.3
  Wegener's M31.30
    with
      kidney involvement M31.31
      lung involvement M31.30
        with kidney involvement M31.31
  Weingarten's (tropical eosinophilia) J82.89
  Weiss-Baker G90.09
  Werdnig-Hoffman G12.0
  Werner's E31.21
  Werner's E34.8
  Wernicke-Korsakoff (nonalcoholic) F04
    alcoholic F10.26
  West's —*see* Epilepsy, spasms
  Westphal-Strümpell E83.01
  wet
    feet (maceration) (tropical) T69.0-•
    lung, newborn P22.1

Syndrome *(Continued)*
  whiplash S13.4
  whistling face Q87.0
  Wilkie's K55.1
  Wilkinson-Sneddon L13.1
  Willebrand (-Jürgens) D68.0
  Williams Q93.82
  Wilson's (hepatolenticular degeneration) E83.01
  Wiskott-Aldrich D82.0
  withdrawal —*see* Withdrawal, state
    drug
      infant of dependent mother P96.1
      therapeutic use, newborn P96.2
  Woakes' (ethmoiditis) J33.1
  Wright's (hyperabduction) G54.0
  X I20.9
  XXXX Q97.1
  XXXXX Q97.1
  XXXXY Q98.1
  XXY Q98.0
  Yao M04.8
  yellow nail L60.5
  Zahorsky's B08.5
  Zellweger syndrome E71.510
  Zellweger-like syndrome E71.541
Synechia (anterior) (iris) (posterior) (pupil) —
    see also Adhesions, iris
  intra-uterine (traumatic) N85.6
Synesthesia R20.8
Syngamiasis, syngamosis B83.3
Synodontia K00.2
Synorchidism, synorchism Q55.1
Synostosis (congenital) Q78.8
  astragalo-scaphoid Q74.2
  radioulnar Q74.0
Synovial sarcoma —*see* Neoplasm, connective
    tissue, malignant
Synovioma (malignant) —*see also* Neoplasm,
    connective tissue, malignant
  benign —*see* Neoplasm, connective tissue,
      benign
Synoviosarcoma —*see* Neoplasm, connective
    tissue, malignant
Synovitis —*see also* Tenosynovitis M65.9
  crepitant
    hand M70.0-•
    wrist M70.03-•
  gonococcal A54.49
  gouty —*see* Gout
  in (due to)
    crystals M65.8-•
    gonorrhea A54.49
    syphilis (late) A52.78
    use, overuse, pressure —*see* Disorder, soft
        tissue, due to use
  infective NEC —*see* Tenosynovitis, infective
      NEC
  specified NEC —*see* Tenosynovitis, specified
      type NEC
  syphilitic A52.78
    congenital (early) A50.02
  toxic —*see* Synovitis, transient
  transient M67.3-•
    ankle M67.37-•
    elbow M67.32-•
    foot joint M67.37-•
    hand joint M67.34-•
    hip M67.35-•
    knee M67.36-•
    multiple site M67.39
    pelvic region M67.35-•
    shoulder M67.31-•
    specified joint NEC M67.38
    wrist M67.33-•
  traumatic, current —*see* Sprain
  tuberculous —*see* Tuberculosis, synovitis
  villonodular (pigmented) M12.2-•
    ankle M12.27-•
    elbow M12.22-•
    foot joint M12.27-•
    hand joint M12.24-•
    hip M12.25-•
    knee M12.26-•

▶ New   ➥ Revised   ~~deleted~~ Deleted   • Use Additional Character(s)

Synovitis *(Continued)*
  villonodular *(Continued)*
    multiple site M12.29
    pelvic region M12.25-●
    shoulder M12.21-●
    specified joint NEC M12.28
    vertebrae M12.28
    wrist M12.23-●
Syphilid A51.39
  congenital A50.06
  newborn A50.06
  tubercular (late) A52.79
Syphilis, syphilitic (acquired) A53.9
  abdomen (late) A52.79
  acoustic nerve A52.15
  adenopathy (secondary) A51.49
  adrenal (gland) (with cortical hypofunction) A52.79
  age under 2 years NOS —*see also* Syphilis, congenital, early
    acquired A51.9
  alopecia (secondary) A51.32
  anemia (late) A52.79 *[D63.8]*
  aneurysm (aorta) (ruptured) A52.01
    central nervous system A52.05
    congenital A50.54 *[I79.0]*
  anus (late) A52.74
    primary A51.1
    secondary A51.39
  aorta (arch) (abdominal) (thoracic) A52.02
    aneurysm A52.01
  aortic (insufficiency) (regurgitation) (stenosis) A52.03
    aneurysm A52.01
  arachnoid (adhesive) (cerebral) (spinal) A52.13
  asymptomatic —*see* Syphilis, latent
  ataxia (locomotor) A52.11
  atrophoderma maculatum A51.39
  auricular fibrillation A52.06
  bladder (late) A52.76
  bone A52.77
    secondary A51.46
  brain A52.17
  breast (late) A52.79
  bronchus (late) A52.72
  bubo (primary) A51.0
  bulbar palsy A52.19
  bursa (late) A52.78
  cardiac decompensation A52.06
  cardiovascular A52.00
  central nervous system (late) (recurrent) (relapse) (tertiary) A52.3
    with
      ataxia A52.11
      general paralysis A52.17
        juvenile A50.45
      paresis (general) A52.17
        juvenile A50.45
      tabes (dorsalis) A52.11
        juvenile A50.45
      taboparesis A52.17
        juvenile A50.45
    aneurysm A52.05
    congenital A50.40
    juvenile A50.40
    remission in (sustained) A52.3
    serology doubtful, negative, or positive A52.3
    specified nature or site NEC A52.19
    vascular A52.05
  cerebral A52.17
    meningovascular A52.13
    nerves (multiple palsies) A52.15
    sclerosis A52.17
    thrombosis A52.05
  cerebrospinal (tabetic type) A52.12
  cerebrovascular A52.05
  cervix (late) A52.76
  chancre (multiple) A51.0
    extragenital A51.2
    Rollet's A51.0
  Charcot's joint A52.16
  chorioretinitis A51.43
    congenital A50.01

Syphilis, syphilitic *(Continued)*
  chorioretinitis *(Continued)*
    late A52.71
    prenatal A50.01
  choroiditis —*see* Syphilitic chorioretinitis
  choroidoretinitis —*see* Syphilitic chorioretinitis
  ciliary body (secondary) A51.43
    late A52.71
  colon (late) A52.74
  combined spinal sclerosis A52.11
  condyloma (latum) A51.31
  congenital A50.9
    with
      paresis (general) A50.45
      tabes (dorsalis) A50.45
      taboparesis A50.45
    chorioretinitis, choroiditis A50.01 *[H32]*
    early, or less than 2 years after birth NEC A50.2
      with manifestations —*see* Syphilis, congenital, early, symptomatic
      latent (without manifestations) A50.1
        negative spinal fluid test A50.1
        serology positive A50.1
      symptomatic A50.09
        cutaneous A50.06
        mucocutaneous A50.07
        oculopathy A50.01
        osteochondropathy A50.02
        pharyngitis A50.03
        pneumonia A50.04
        rhinitis A50.05
        visceral A50.08
    interstitial keratitis A50.31
    juvenile neurosyphilis A50.45
    late, or 2 years or more after birth NEC A50.7
      chorioretinitis, choroiditis A50.32
      interstitial keratitis A50.31
      juvenile neurosyphilis A50.45
      latent (without manifestations) A50.6
        negative spinal fluid test A50.6
        serology positive A50.6
      symptomatic or with manifestations NEC A50.59
        arthropathy A50.55
        cardiovascular A50.54
        Clutton's joints A50.51
        Hutchinson's teeth A50.52
        Hutchinson's triad A50.53
        osteochondropathy A50.56
        saddle nose A50.57
  conjugal A53.9
    tabes A52.11
  conjunctiva (late) A52.71
  contact Z20.2
  cord bladder A52.19
  cornea, late A52.71
  coronary (artery) (sclerosis) A52.06
  coryza, congenital A50.05
  cranial nerve A52.15
    multiple palsies A52.15
  cutaneous —*see* Syphilis, skin
  dacryocystitis (late) A52.71
  degeneration, spinal cord A52.12
  dementia paralytica A52.17
    juvenilis A50.45
  destruction of bone A52.77
  dilatation, aorta A52.01
  due to blood transfusion A53.9
  dura mater A52.13
  ear A52.79
    inner A52.79
      nerve (eighth) A52.15
      neurorecurrence A52.15
  early A51.9
    cardiovascular A52.00
    central nervous system A52.3
    latent (without manifestations) (less than 2 years after infection) A51.5
      negative spinal fluid test A51.5
      serological relapse after treatment A51.5
      serology positive A51.5
    relapse (treated, untreated) A51.9

Syphilis, syphilitic *(Continued)*
  early *(Continued)*
    skin A51.39
    symptomatic A51.9
      extragenital chancre A51.2
      primary, except extragenital chancre A51.0
      secondary —*see also* Syphilis, secondary A51.39
      relapse (treated, untreated) A51.49
    ulcer A51.39
  eighth nerve (neuritis) A52.15
  endemic A65
  endocarditis A52.03
    aortic A52.03
    pulmonary A52.03
  epididymis (late) A52.76
  epiglottis (late) A52.73
  epiphysitis (congenital) (early) A50.02
  episcleritis (late) A52.71
  esophagus A52.79
  eustachian tube A52.73
  exposure to Z20.2
  eye A52.71
  eyelid (late) (with gumma) A52.71
  fallopian tube (late) A52.76
  fracture A52.77
  gallbladder (late) A52.74
  gastric (polyposis) (late) A52.74
  general A53.9
    paralysis A52.17
      juvenile A50.45
  genital (primary) A51.0
  glaucoma A52.71
  gumma NEC A52.79
    cardiovascular system A52.00
    central nervous system A52.3
    congenital A50.59
  heart (block) (decompensation) (disease) (failure) A52.06 *[I52]*
    valve NEC A52.03
  hemianesthesia A52.19
  hemianopsia A52.71
  hemiparesis A52.17
  hemiplegia A52.17
  hepatic artery A52.09
  hepatis A52.74
  hepatomegaly, congenital A50.08
  hereditaria tarda —*see* Syphilis, congenital, late
  hereditary —*see* Syphilis, congenital
  Hutchinson's teeth A50.52
  hyalitis A52.71
  inactive —*see* Syphilis, latent
  infantum —*see* Syphilis, congenital
  inherited —*see* Syphilis, congenital
  internal ear A52.79
  intestine (late) A52.74
  iris, iritis (secondary) A51.43
    late A52.71
  joint (late) A52.77
  keratitis (congenital) (interstitial) (late) A50.31
  kidney (late) A52.75
  lacrimal passages (late) A52.71
  larynx (late) A52.73
  late A52.9
    cardiovascular A52.00
    central nervous system A52.3
    kidney A52.75
    latent or 2 years or more after infection (without manifestations) A52.8
      negative spinal fluid test A52.8
      serology positive A52.8
    paresis A52.17
    specified site NEC A52.79
    symptomatic or with manifestations A52.79
    tabes A52.11
  latent A53.0
    with signs or symptoms - code by site and stage under Syphilis

Syphilis, syphilitic *(Continued)*
  latent *(Continued)*
    central nervous system A52.2
    date of infection unspecified A53.0
    early, or less than 2 years after infection A51.5
    follow-up of latent syphilis A53.0
      date of infection unspecified A53.0
      late, or 2 years or more after infection A52.8
    late, or 2 years or more after infection A52.8
    positive serology (only finding) A53.0
      date of infection unspecified A53.0
      early, or less than 2 years after infection A51.5
      late, or 2 years or more after infection A52.8
  lens (late) A52.71
  leukoderma A51.39
    late A52.79
  lienitis A52.79
  lip A51.39
    chancre (primary) A51.2
    late A52.79
  Lissauer's paralysis A52.17
  liver A52.74
  locomotor ataxia A52.11
  lung A52.72
  lymph gland (early) (secondary) A51.49
    late A52.79
  lymphadenitis (secondary) A51.49
  macular atrophy of skin A51.39
    striated A52.79
  mediastinum (late) A52.73
  meninges (adhesive) (brain) (spinal cord) A52.13
  meningitis A52.13
    acute (secondary) A51.41
    congenital A50.41
  meningoencephalitis A52.14
  meningovascular A52.13
    congenital A50.41
  mesarteritis A52.09
    brain A52.04
  middle ear A52.77
  mitral stenosis A52.03
  monoplegia A52.17
  mouth (secondary) A51.39
    late A52.79
  mucocutaneous (secondary) A51.39
    late A52.79
  mucous
    membrane (secondary) A51.39
      late A52.79
    patches A51.39
      congenital A50.07
  mulberry molars A50.52
  muscle A52.78
  myocardium A52.06
  nasal sinus (late) A52.73
  neonatorum —*see* Syphilis, congenital
  nephrotic syndrome (secondary) A51.44
  nerve palsy (any cranial nerve) A52.15
    multiple A52.15
  nervous system, central A52.3
  neuritis A52.15
    acoustic A52.15
  neurorecidive of retina A52.19
  neuroretinitis A52.19
  newborn —*see* Syphilis, congenital
  nodular superficial (late) A52.79
  nonvenereal A65
  nose (late) A52.73
    saddle back deformity A50.57
  occlusive arterial disease A52.09
  oculopathy A52.71
  ophthalmic (late) A52.71
  optic nerve (atrophy) (neuritis) (papilla) A52.15
  orbit (late) A52.71

Syphilis, syphilitic *(Continued)*
  organic A53.9
  osseous (late) A52.77
  osteochondritis (congenital) (early) A50.02 *[M90.80]*
  osteoporosis A52.77
  ovary (late) A52.76
  oviduct (late) A52.76
  palate (late) A52.79
  pancreas (late) A52.74
  paralysis A52.17
    general A52.17
      juvenile A50.45
  paresis (general) A52.17
    juvenile A50.45
  paresthesia A52.19
  Parkinson's disease or syndrome A52.19
  paroxysmal tachycardia A52.06
  pemphigus (congenital) A50.06
  penis (chancre) A51.0
    late A52.76
  pericardium A52.06
  perichondritis, larynx (late) A52.73
  periosteum (late) A52.77
    congenital (early) A50.02 *[M90.80]*
    early (secondary) A51.46
  peripheral nerve A52.79
  petrous bone (late) A52.77
  pharynx (late) A52.73
    secondary A51.39
  pituitary (gland) A52.79
  pleura (late) A52.73
  pneumonia, white A50.04
  pontine lesion A52.17
  portal vein A52.09
  primary A51.0
    anal A51.1
    and secondary —*see* Syphilis, secondary
    central nervous system A52.3
    extragenital chancre NEC A51.2
    fingers A51.2
    genital A51.0
    lip A51.2
    specified site NEC A51.2
    tonsils A51.2
  prostate (late) A52.76
  ptosis (eyelid) A52.71
  pulmonary (late) A52.72
    artery A52.09
  pyelonephritis (late) A52.75
  recently acquired, symptomatic A51.9
  rectum (late) A52.74
  respiratory tract (late) A52.73
  retina, late A52.71
  retrobulbar neuritis A52.15
  salpingitis A52.76
  sclera (late) A52.71
  sclerosis
    cerebral A52.17
    coronary A52.06
    multiple A52.11
  scotoma (central) A52.71
  scrotum (late) A52.76
  secondary (and primary) A51.49
    adenopathy A51.49
    anus A51.39
    bone A51.46
    chorioretinitis, choroiditis A51.43
    hepatitis A51.45
    liver A51.45
    lymphadenitis A51.49
    meningitis (acute) A51.41
    mouth A51.39
    mucous membranes A51.39
    periosteum, periostitis A51.46
    pharynx A51.39
    relapse (treated, untreated) A51.49
    skin A51.39
    specified form NEC A51.49
    tonsil A51.39

Syphilis, syphilitic *(Continued)*
  secondary *(Continued)*
    ulcer A51.39
    viscera NEC A51.49
    vulva A51.39
  seminal vesicle (late) A52.76
  seronegative with signs or symptoms - code by site and stage under Syphilis
  seropositive
    with signs or symptoms - code by site and stage under Syphilis
    follow-up of latent syphilis —*see* Syphilis, latent
    only finding —*see* Syphilis, latent
  seventh nerve (paralysis) A52.15
  sinus, sinusitis (late) A52.73
  skeletal system A52.77
  skin (with ulceration) (early) (secondary) A51.39
    late or tertiary A52.79
  small intestine A52.74
  spastic spinal paralysis A52.17
  spermatic cord (late) A52.76
  spinal (cord) A52.12
  spleen A52.79
  splenomegaly A52.79
  spondylitis A52.77
  staphyloma A52.71
  stigmata (congenital) A50.59
  stomach A52.74
  synovium A52.78
  tabes dorsalis (late) A52.11
    juvenile A50.45
  tabetic type A52.11
    juvenile A50.45
  taboparesis A52.17
    juvenile A50.45
  tachycardia A52.06
  tendon (late) A52.78
  tertiary A52.9
    with symptoms NEC A52.79
    cardiovascular A52.00
    central nervous system A52.3
    multiple NEC A52.79
    specified site NEC A52.79
  testis A52.76
  thorax A52.73
  throat A52.73
  thymus (gland) (late) A52.79
  thyroid (late) A52.79
  tongue (late) A52.79
  tonsil (lingual) (late) A52.73
    primary A51.2
    secondary A51.39
  trachea (late) A52.73
  tunica vaginalis (late) A52.76
  ulcer (any site) (early) (secondary) A51.39
    late A52.79
    perforating A52.79
      foot A52.11
  urethra (late) A52.76
  urogenital (late) A52.76
  uterus (late) A52.76
  uveal tract (secondary) A51.43
    late A52.71
  uveitis (secondary) A51.43
    late A52.71
  uvula (late) (perforated) A52.79
  vagina A51.0
    late A52.76
  valvulitis NEC A52.03
  vascular A52.00
    brain (cerebral) A52.05
  ventriculi A52.74
  vesicae urinariae (late) A52.76
  viscera (abdominal) (late) A52.74
    secondary A51.49
  vitreous (opacities) (late) A52.71
    hemorrhage A52.71

▶ New   ⇒ Revised   ~~deleted~~ Deleted   ● Use Additional Character(s)

Syphilis, syphilitic *(Continued)*
  vulva A51.0
    late A52.76
    secondary A51.39
Syphiloma A52.79
  cardiovascular system A52.00
  central nervous system A52.3
  circulatory system A52.00
  congenital A50.59
Syphilophobia F45.29
Syringadenoma —*see also* Neoplasm, skin,
    benign
  papillary —*see* Neoplasm, skin, benign

Syringobulbia G95.0
Syringocystadenoma —*see* Neoplasm, skin,
    benign
  papillary —*see* Neoplasm, skin, benign
Syringoma —*see also* Neoplasm, skin, benign
  chondroid —*see* Neoplasm, skin, benign
Syringomyelia G95.0
Syringomyelitis —*see* Encephalitis
Syringomyelocele —*see* Spina bifida
Syringopontia G95.0

System, systemic —*see also* condition
  disease, combined —*see* Degeneration,
    combined
  inflammatory response syndrome (SIRS) of
    non-infectious origin (without organ
    dysfunction) R65.10
    with acute organ dysfunction R65.11
  lupus erythematosus M32.9
    inhibitor present D68.62

T

▶ New ⇒ Revised ~~deleted~~ Deleted ● Use Additional Character(s)

Tear, torn *(Continued)*
  periurethral tissue, obstetrical trauma O71.82
    with ectopic or molar pregnancy O08.6
    following ectopic or molar pregnancy
      O08.6
  rectovaginal septum —*see* Laceration, vagina
  retina, retinal (without detachment)
    (horseshoe) —*see also* Break, retina,
    horseshoe
    with detachment —*see* Detachment, retina,
      with retinal, break
  rotator cuff (nontraumatic) M75.10-●
    complete M75.12-●
    incomplete M75.11-●
    traumatic S46.01-●
      capsule S43.42-●
  semilunar cartilage, knee —*see* Tear, meniscus
  supraspinatus (complete) (incomplete)
    (nontraumatic) —*see also* Tear, rotator
    cuff M75.10-●
  tendon —*see* Strain
  tentorial, at birth P10.4
  umbilical cord
    complicating delivery O69.89
  urethra
    with ectopic or molar pregnancy O08.6
    following ectopic or molar pregnancy
      O08.6
    obstetrical trauma O71.5
  uterus —*see* Injury, uterus
  vagina —*see* Laceration, vagina
  vessel, from catheter —*see* Puncture,
    accidental complicating surgery
  vulva, complicating delivery O70.0
Tear-stone —*see* Dacryolith
Teeth —*see also* condition
  grinding
    psychogenic F45.8
    sleep related G47.63
Teething (syndrome) K00.7
Telangiectasia, telangiectasis (verrucous) I78.1
  ataxic (cerebellar) (Louis-Bar) G11.3
  familial I78.0
  hemorrhagic, hereditary (congenital) (senile)
    I78.0
  hereditary, hemorrhagic (congenital) (senile)
    I78.0
  juxtafoveal H35.07-●
  macular H35.07-●
  macularis eruptiva perstans D47.01
  parafoveal H35.07-●
  retinal (idiopathic) (juxtafoveal) (macular)
    (parafoveal) H35.07-●
  spider I78.1
Telephone scatologia F65.89
Telescoped bowel or intestine K56.1
  congenital Q43.8
Temperature
  body, high (of unknown origin) R50.9
  cold, trauma from T69.9
    newborn P80.0
    specified effect NEC T69.8
Temple —*see* condition
Temporal —*see* condition
Temporomandibular joint pain-dysfunction
  syndrome M26.62-●
Temporosphenoidal —*see* condition
Tendency
  bleeding —*see* Defect, coagulation
  suicide
  ➪ meaning personal history of attempted
    suicide Z91.51
    meaning suicidal ideation —*see* Ideation,
      suicidal
  to fall R29.6
Tenderness, abdominal R10.819
  epigastric R10.816
  generalized R10.817
  left lower quadrant R10.814
  left upper quadrant R10.812
  periumbilic R10.815

Tenderness, abdominal *(Continued)*
  rebound R10.829
    epigastric R10.826
    generalized R10.827
    left lower quadrant R10.824
    left upper quadrant R10.822
    periumbilic R10.825
    right lower quadrant R10.823
    right upper quadrant R10.821
  right lower quadrant R10.813
  right upper quadrant R10.811
Tendinitis, tendonitis —*see also* Enthesopathy
  Achilles M76.6-●
  adhesive —*see* Tenosynovitis, specified type
    NEC
    shoulder —*see* Capsulitis, adhesive
  bicipital M75.2-●
  calcific M65.2-●
    ankle M65.27-●
    foot M65.27-●
    forearm M65.23-●
    hand M65.24-●
    lower leg M65.26-●
    multiple sites M65.29
    pelvic region M65.25-●
    shoulder M75.3-●
    specified site NEC M65.28
    thigh M65.25-●
    upper arm M65.22-●
  due to use, overuse, pressure —*see also*
    Disorder, soft tissue, due to use
    specified NEC —*see* Disorder, soft tissue,
      due to use, specified NEC
  gluteal M76.0-●
  patellar M76.5-●
  peroneal M76.7-●
  psoas M76.1-●
  tibial (posterior) M76.82-●
    anterior M76.81-●
  trochanteric —*see* Bursitis, hip, trochanteric
Tendon —*see* condition
Tendosynovitis —*see* Tenosynovitis
Tenesmus (rectal) R19.8
  vesical R30.1
Tennis elbow —*see* Epicondylitis, lateral
Tenonitis —*see also* Tenosynovitis
  eye (capsule) H05.04-●
Tenontosynovitis —*see* Tenosynovitis
Tenontothecitis —*see* Tenosynovitis
Tenophyte —*see* Disorder, synovium, specified
  type NEC
Tenosynovitis —*see also* Synovitis M65.9
  adhesive —*see* Tenosynovitis, specified type
    NEC
    shoulder —*see* Capsulitis, adhesive
  bicipital (calcifying) —*see* Tendinitis,
    bicipital
  gonococcal A54.49
  in (due to)
    crystals M65.8-●
    gonorrhea A54.49
    syphilis (late) A52.78
    use, overuse, pressure —*see also* Disorder,
      soft tissue, due to use
      specified NEC —*see* Disorder, soft tissue,
        due to use, specified NEC
  infective NEC M65.1-●
    ankle M65.17-●
    foot M65.17-●
    forearm M65.13-●
    hand M65.14-●
    lower leg M65.16-●
    multiple sites M65.19
    pelvic region M65.15-●
    shoulder region M65.11-●
    specified site NEC M65.18
    thigh M65.15-●
    upper arm M65.12-●
  radial styloid M65.4
  shoulder region M65.81-●
    adhesive —*see* Capsulitis, adhesive

Tenosynovitis *(Continued)*
  specified type NEC M65.88-●
    ankle M65.87-●
    foot M65.87-●
    forearm M65.83-●
    hand M65.84-●
    lower leg M65.86-●
    multiple sites M65.89
    pelvic region M65.85-●
    shoulder region M65.81-●
    specified site NEC M65.88
    thigh M65.85-●
    upper arm M65.82-●
  tuberculous —*see* Tuberculosis, tenosynovitis
Tenovaginitis —*see* Tenosynovitis
Tension
  arterial, high —*see also* Hypertension
    without diagnosis of hypertension R03.0
  headache G44.209
    intractable G44.201
    not intractable G44.209
  nervous R45.0
  pneumothorax J93.0
  premenstrual N94.3
  state (mental) F48.9
Tentorium —*see* condition
Teratencephalus Q89.8
Teratism Q89.7
Teratoblastoma (malignant) —*see* Neoplasm,
  malignant, by site
Teratocarcinoma —*see also* Neoplasm,
  malignant, by site
  liver C22.7
Teratoma (solid) —*see also* Neoplasm, uncertain
  behavior, by site
  with embryonal carcinoma, mixed —*see*
    Neoplasm, malignant, by site
  with malignant transformation —*see*
    Neoplasm, malignant, by site
  adult (cystic) —*see* Neoplasm, benign, by site
  benign —*see* Neoplasm, benign, by site
  combined with choriocarcinoma —*see*
    Neoplasm, malignant, by site
  cystic (adult) —*see* Neoplasm, benign, by site
  differentiated —*see* Neoplasm, benign, by site
  embryonal —*see also* Neoplasm, malignant,
    by site
    liver C22.7
  immature —*see* Neoplasm, malignant, by site
  liver C22.7
    adult, benign, cystic, differentiated type or
      mature D13.4
  malignant —*see also* Neoplasm, malignant,
    by site
    anaplastic —*see* Neoplasm, malignant, by
      site
    intermediate —*see* Neoplasm, malignant,
      by site
    specified site —*see* Neoplasm,
      malignant, by site
    unspecified site C62.90
    undifferentiated —*see* Neoplasm,
      malignant, by site
  mature —*see* Neoplasm, uncertain behavior,
    by site
    malignant —*see* Neoplasm, by site,
      malignant, by site
  ovary D27.-●
    embryonal, immature or malignant C56-●
  solid —*see* Neoplasm, uncertain behavior,
    by site
  testis C62.9-●
    adult, benign, cystic, differentiated type or
      mature D29.2-●
    scrotal C62.1-●
    undescended C62.0-●
Termination
  anomalous —*see also* Malposition, congenital
    right pulmonary vein Q26.3
  pregnancy, elective Z33.2
Ternidens diminutus infestation B81.8
Ternidensiasis B81.8

Threatened
    abortion O20.0
        with subsequent abortion O03.9
    job loss, anxiety concerning Z56.2
    labor (without delivery) O47.9
        at or after 37 completed weeks of gestation
            O47.1
        before 37 completed weeks of gestation
            O47.0-●
    loss of job, anxiety concerning Z56.2
    miscarriage O20.0
    unemployment, anxiety concerning Z56.2
Three-day fever A93.1
Threshers' lung J67.0
Thrix annulata (congenital) Q84.1
Throat —see condition
Thrombasthenia (Glanzmann) (hemorrhagic)
    (hereditary) D69.1
Thromboangiitis I73.1
    obliterans (general) I73.1
        cerebral I67.89
        vessels
            brain I67.89
            spinal cord I67.89
Thromboarteritis —see Arteritis
Thromboasthenia (Glanzmann) (hemorrhagic)
    (hereditary) D69.1
Thrombocytasthenia (Glanzmann) D69.1
Thrombocythemia (hemorrhagic) (see also
    Thrombocytosis) D75.839
▶ essential D47.3
▶ idiopathic D47.3
▶ primary D47.3
Thrombocytopathy (dystrophic) (granulopenic)
    D69.1
Thrombocytopenia, thrombocytopenic D69.6
    with absent radius (TAR) Q87.2
    congenital D69.42
    dilutional D69.59
    due to
        drugs D69.59
        extracorporeal circulation of blood D69.59
        (massive)blood transfusion D69.59
        platelet alloimmunization D69.59
    essential D69.3
    heparin induced (HIT) D75.82
    hereditary D69.42
    idiopathic D69.3
    neonatal, transitory P61.0
        due to
            exchange transfusion P61.0
            idiopathic maternal thrombocytopenia
                P61.0
            isoimmunization P61.0
    primary NEC D69.49
        idiopathic D69.3
    puerperal, postpartum O72.3
    secondary D69.59
    transient neonatal P61.0
Thrombocytosis, essential D47.3
    primary D47.3
▶ Thrombocytosis D75.839
▶ essential D47.3
▶ idiopathic D47.3
▶ primary D47.3
▶ reactive D75.838
▶ secondary D75.838
▶ specified NEC D75.838
Thromboembolism —see Embolism
Thrombopathy (Bernard-Soulier) D69.1
    constitutional D68.0
    Willebrand-Jurgens D68.0
Thrombopenia —see Thrombocytopenia
Thrombophilia D68.59
    primary NEC D68.59
    secondary NEC D68.69
    specified NEC D68.69
Thrombophlebitis I80.9
    antepartum O22.2-●
        deep O22.3-●
        superficial O22.2-●
    calf muscular vein (NOS) I80.25-●

Thrombophlebitis (Continued)
    cavernous (venous) sinus G08
        complicating pregnancy O22.5-●
        nonpyogenic I67.6
    cerebral (sinus) (vein) G08
        nonpyogenic I67.6
        sequelae G09
    due to implanted device —see Complications,
        by site and type, specified NEC
    during or resulting from a procedure NEC
        T81.72
    femoral vein (superficial) I80.1-●
    femoropopliteal vein I80.0-●
    gastrocnemial vein I80.25-●
    hepatic (vein) I80.8
    idiopathic, recurrent I82.1
    iliac vein (common) (external) (internal)
        I80.21-●
    iliofemoral I80.1-●
    intracranial venous sinus (any) G08
        nonpyogenic I67.6
        sequelae G09
    intraspinal venous sinuses and veins G08
        nonpyogenic G95.19
    lateral (venous) sinus G08
        nonpyogenic I67.6
    leg I80.3
        superficial I80.0-●
    longitudinal (venous) sinus G08
        nonpyogenic I67.6
    lower extremity I80.299
    migrans, migrating I82.1
    pelvic
        with ectopic or molar pregnancy O08.0
        following ectopic or molar pregnancy O08.0
        puerperal O87.1
    peroneal vein I80.24 ●
    popliteal vein —see Phlebitis, leg, deep,
        popliteal
    portal (vein) K75.1
    postoperative T81.72
    pregnancy —see Thrombophlebitis, antepartum
    puerperal, postpartum, childbirth O87.0
        deep O87.1
        pelvic O87.1
        septic O86.81
        superficial O87.0
    saphenous (greater) (lesser) I80.0-●
    sinus (intracranial) G08
        nonpyogenic I67.6
    soleal vein I80.25-●
    specified site NEC I80.8
    tibial vein (anterior) (posterior) I80.23-●
Thrombosis, thrombotic (bland) (multiple)
    (progressive) (silent) (vessel) I82.90
    anal K64.5
    antepartum —see Thrombophlebitis,
        antepartum
    aorta, aortic I74.10
        abdominal I74.09
            saddle I74.01
        bifurcation I74.09
            saddle I74.01
        specified site NEC I74.19
        terminal I74.09
        thoracic I74.11
        valve —see Endocarditis, aortic
    apoplexy I63.3-●
    artery, arteries (postinfectional) I74.9
        auditory, internal —see Occlusion, artery,
            precerebral, specified NEC
        basilar —see Occlusion, artery, basilar
        carotid (common) (internal) —see
            Occlusion, artery, carotid
        cerebellar (anterior inferior) (posterior
            inferior) (superior) —see Occlusion,
            artery, cerebellar
        cerebral —see Occlusion, artery, cerebral
        choroidal (anterior) —see Occlusion, artery,
            precerebral, specified NEC
        communicating, posterior —see Occlusion,
            artery, precerebral, specified NEC

Thrombosis, thrombotic (Continued)
    artery, arteries (Continued)
        coronary —see also Infarct, myocardium
            not resulting in infarction I24.0
        hepatic I74.8
        hypophyseal —see Occlusion, artery,
            precerebral, specified NEC
        iliac I74.5
        limb I74.4
            lower I74.3
            upper I74.2
        meningeal, anterior or posterior —see
            Occlusion, artery, cerebral, specified
            NEC
        mesenteric (with gangrene) —see also
            Infarct, intestine K55.069
        ophthalmic —see Occlusion, artery, retina
        pontine —see Occlusion, artery, precerebral,
            specified NEC
        precerebral —see Occlusion, artery,
            precerebral
        pulmonary (iatrogenic) —see Embolism,
            pulmonary
        renal N28.0
        retinal —see Occlusion, artery, retina
        spinal, anterior or posterior G95.11
        traumatic NEC T14.8
        vertebral —see Occlusion, artery, vertebral
    atrium, auricular —see also Infarct, myocardium
        following acute myocardial infarction
            (current complication) I23.6
        not resulting in infarction I51.3
        old I51.3
    basilar (artery) —see Occlusion, artery, basilar
    brain (artery) (stem) —see also Occlusion,
        artery, cerebral
        due to syphilis A52.05
        puerperal O99.43
        sinus —see Thrombosis, intracranial
            venous sinus
    capillary I78.8
    cardiac —see also Infarct, myocardium
        not resulting in infarction I51.3
        valve —see Endocarditis
        old I51.3
    carotid (artery) (common) (internal) —see
        Occlusion, artery, carotid
    cavernous (venous) sinus —see Thrombosis,
        intracranial venous sinus
    cerebellar artery (anterior inferior) (posterior
        inferior) (superior) I66.3
    cerebral (artery) —see Occlusion, artery, cerebral
    cerebrovenous sinus —see also Thrombosis,
        intracranial venous sinus
        puerperium O87.3
    chronic I82.91
    coronary (artery) (vein) —see also Infarct,
        myocardium
        not resulting in infarction I24.0
    corpus cavernosum N48.89
    cortical I66.9
    deep —see Embolism, vein, lower extremity
    due to device, implant or graft —see also
        Complications, by site and type,
        specified NEC T85.868
        arterial graft NEC T82.868
        breast (implant) T85.868
        catheter NEC T85.868
            dialysis (renal) T82.868
                intraperitoneal T85.868
            infusion NEC T82.868
                spinal (epidural) (subdural) T85.860
            urinary (indwelling) T83.86
        electronic (electrode) (pulse generator)
            (stimulator)
            bone T84.86
            cardiac T82.867
            nervous system (brain) (peripheral
                nerve) (spinal) T85.860
            urinary T83.86
        fixation, internal (orthopedic) NEC T84.86
        gastrointestinal (bile duct) (esophagus)
            T85.868

Thrombosis, thrombotic *(Continued)*
- due to device, implant or graft *(Continued)*
  - genital NEC T83.86
  - heart T82.867
  - joint prosthesis T84.86
  - ocular (corneal graft) (orbital implant) NEC T85.868
  - orthopedic NEC T84.86
  - specified NEC T85.868
  - urinary NEC T83.86
  - vascular NEC T82.868
  - ventricular intracranial shunt T85.860
- during the puerperium —*see* Thrombosis, puerperal
- endocardial —*see also* Infarct, myocardium
  - not resulting in infarction I51.3
- eye —*see* Occlusion, retina
- genital organ
  - female NEC N94.89
    - pregnancy —*see* Thrombophlebitis, antepartum
  - male N50.1
- gestational —*see* Phlebopathy, gestational
- heart (chamber) —*see also* Infarct, myocardium
  - not resulting in infarction I51.3
  - old I51.3
- hepatic (vein) I82.0
  - artery I74.8
- history (of) Z86.718
- intestine (with gangrene) —*see also* Infarct, intestine K55.069
- intracardiac NEC (apical) (atrial) (auricular) (ventricular) (old) I51.3
- intracranial (arterial) I66.9
  - venous sinus (any) G08
    - nonpyogenic origin I67.6
    - puerperium O87.3
- intramural —*see also* Infarct, myocardium
  - not resulting in infarction I51.3
  - old I51.3
- intraspinal venous sinuses and veins G08
  - nonpyogenic G95.19
- kidney (artery) N28.0
- lateral (venous) sinus —*see* Thrombosis, intracranial venous sinus
- leg —*see* Thrombosis, vein, lower extremity
  - arterial I74.3
- liver (venous) I82.0
  - artery I74.8
  - portal vein I81
- longitudinal (venous) sinus —*see* Thrombosis, intracranial venous sinus
- lower limb —*see* Thrombosis, vein, lower extremity
- lung (iatrogenic) (postoperative) —*see* Embolism, pulmonary
- meninges (brain) (arterial) I66.8
- mesenteric (artery) (with gangrene) —*see also* Infarct, intestine K55.069
  - vein (inferior) (superior) K55.0-●
- mitral I34.8
- mural —*see also* Infarct, myocardium
  - due to syphilis A52.06
  - not resulting in infarction I51.3
  - old I51.3
- omentum (with gangrene) —*see also* Infarct, intestine K55.069
- ophthalmic —*see* Occlusion, retina
- pampiniform plexus (male) N50.1
- parietal —*see also* Infarct, myocardium
  - not resulting in infarction I24.0
- penis, superficial vein N48.81
- perianal venous K64.5
- peripheral arteries I74.4
  - upper I74.2
- personal history (of) Z86.718
- portal I81
  - due to syphilis A52.09
- precerebral artery —*see* Occlusion, artery, precerebral
- puerperal, postpartum O87.0
  - brain (artery) O99.43
    - venous (sinus) O87.3

Thrombosis, thrombotic *(Continued)*
- puerperal, postpartum*(Continued)*
  - cardiac O99.43
  - cerebral (artery) O99.43
    - venous (sinus) O87.3
  - superficial O87.0
- pulmonary (artery) (iatrogenic) (postoperative) (vein) —*see* Embolism, pulmonary
- renal (artery) N28.0
  - vein I82.3
- resulting from presence of device, implant or graft —*see* Complications, by site and type, specified NEC
- retina, retinal —*see* Occlusion, retina
- scrotum N50.1
- seminal vesicle N50.1
- sigmoid (venous) sinus —*see* Thrombosis, intracranial venous sinus
- sinus, intracranial (any) —*see* Thrombosis, intracranial venous sinus
- specified site NEC I82.890
  - chronic I82.891
- spermatic cord N50.1
- spinal cord (arterial) G95.11
  - due to syphilis A52.09
  - pyogenic origin G06.1
- spleen, splenic D73.5
  - artery I74.8
- testis N50.1
- traumatic NEC T14.8
- tricuspid I07.8
- tumor —*see* Neoplasm, by site
- tunica vaginalis N50.1
- umbilical cord (vessels), complicating delivery O69.5
- vas deferens N50.1
- vein (acute) I82.90
  - antecubital I82.61-●
    - chronic I82.71-●
  - axillary I82.A1-●
    - chronic I82.A2-●
  - basilic I82.61-●
    - chronic I82.71-●
  - brachial I82.62-●
    - chronic I82.72-●
  - brachiocephalic (innominate) I82.290
    - chronic I82.291
  - cerebral, nonpyogenic I67.6
  - cephalic I82.61-●
    - chronic I82.71-●
  - chronic I82.91
  - deep (DVT) I82.40-●
    - calf I82.4Z-●
      - chronic I82.5Z-●
    - lower leg I82.4Z-●
      - chronic I82.5Z-●
    - thigh I82.4Y-●
      - chronic I82.5Y-●
    - ⇒upper leg I82.4Y ●
    - ⇒chronic I82.5Y-●
  - femoral I82.41-●
    - chronic I82.51-●
  - iliac (iliofemoral) I82.42-●
    - chronic I82.52-●
  - innominate I82.290
    - chronic I82.291
  - internal jugular I82.C1-●
    - chronic I82.C2-●
  - lower extremity
    - deep I82.40-●
      - chronic I82.50-●
      - specified NEC I82.49-●
        - chronic NEC I82.59-●
    - distal
      - deep I82.4Z-●
    - proximal
      - deep I82.4Y-●
        - chronic I82.5Y-●
    - superficial I82.81-●
  - perianal K64.5
  - popliteal I82.43-●
    - chronic I82.53-●

Thrombosis, thrombotic *(Continued)*
- vein *(Continued)*
  - radial I82.62-●
    - chronic I82.72-●
  - renal I82.3
  - saphenous (greater) (lesser) I82.81-●
  - specified NEC I82.890
    - chronic NEC I82.891
  - subclavian I82.B1-●
    - chronic I82.B2-●
  - thoracic NEC I82.290
    - chronic I82.291
  - tibial I82.44-●
    - chronic I82.54-●
  - ulnar I82.62-●
    - chronic I82.72-●
  - upper extremity I82.60-●
    - chronic I82.70-●
    - deep I82.62-●
      - chronic I82.72-●
    - superficial I82.61-●
      - chronic I82.71-●
- vena cava
  - inferior I82.220
    - chronic I82.221
  - superior I82.210
    - chronic I82.211
- venous, perianal K64.5
- ventricle —*see also* Infarct, myocardium
  - following acute myocardial infarction (current complication) I23.6
  - not resulting in infarction I24.0
  - old I51.3

Thrombus —*see* Thrombosis

Thrush —*see also* Candidiasis
- newborn P37.5
- oral B37.0
- vaginal B37.3

Thumb —*see also* condition
- sucking (child problem) F98.8

Thymitis E32.8

Thymoma —*see also* Neoplasm, thymus, by type
- malignant C37
- metaplastic C37
- microscopic D15.0
- sclerosing C37
- type A C37
- type AB C37
- type B1 C37
- type B2 C37
- type B3 C37

Thymus, thymic (gland) —*see* condition

Thyrocele —*see* Goiter

Thyroglossal —*see also* condition
- cyst Q89.2
- duct, persistent Q89.2

Thyroid (gland) (body) —*see also* condition
- hormone resistance E07.89
- lingual Q89.2
- nodule (cystic) (nontoxic) (single) E04.1

Thyroiditis E06.9
- acute (nonsuppurative) (pyogenic) (suppurative) E06.0
- autoimmune E06.3
- chronic (nonspecific) (sclerosing) E06.5
  - with thyrotoxicosis, transient E06.2
  - fibrous E06.5
  - lymphadenoid E06.3
  - lymphocytic E06.3
  - lymphoid E06.3
- de Quervain's E06.1
- drug-induced E06.4
- fibrous (chronic) E06.5
- giant-cell (follicular) E06.1
- granulomatous (de Quervain) (subacute) E06.1
- Hashimoto's (struma lymphomatosa) E06.3
- iatrogenic E06.4
- ligneous E06.5
- lymphocytic (chronic) E06.3
- lymphoid E06.3
- lymphomatous E06.3
- nonsuppurative E06.1
- postpartum, puerperal O90.5

▶ New   ⇒ Revised   ~~deleted~~ Deleted   ● Use Additional Character(s)

Thyroiditis *(Continued)*
  pseudotuberculous E06.1
  pyogenic E06.0
  radiation E06.4
  Riedel's E06.5
  subacute (granulomatous) E06.1
  suppurative E06.0
  tuberculous A18.81
  viral E06.1
  woody E06.5
Thyrolingual duct, persistent Q89.2
Thyromegaly E01.0
Thyrotoxic
  crisis —*see* Thyrotoxicosis
  heart disease or failure —*see also*
    Thyrotoxicosis E05.90 *[143]*
    with thyroid storm E05.91 *[143]*
  storm —*see* Thyrotoxicosis
Thyrotoxicosis (recurrent) E05.90
  with
    goiter (diffuse) E05.00
      with thyroid storm E05.01
      adenomatous uninodular E05.10
        with thyroid storm E05.11
      multinodular E05.20
        with thyroid storm E05.21
      nodular E05.20
        with thyroid storm E05.21
      uninodular E05.10
        with thyroid storm E05.11
    infiltrative
      dermopathy E05.00
        with thyroid storm E05.01
      ophthalmopathy E05.00
        with thyroid storm E05.01
    single thyroid nodule E05.10
      with thyroid storm E05.11
    thyroid storm E05.91
  due to
    ectopic thyroid nodule or tissue E05.30
      with thyroid storm E05.31
    ingestion of (excessive) thyroid material
      E05.40
      with thyroid storm E05.41
    overproduction of thyroid-stimulating
      hormone E05.80
      with thyroid storm E05.81
    specified cause NEC E05.80
      with thyroid storm E05.81
  factitia E05.40
    with thyroid storm E05.41
  heart —*see also* Failure, heart, high-output
    E05.90 *[143]*
    with thyroid storm —*see also* Failure, heart,
      high-output E05.91 *[143]*
    failure —*see also* Failure, heart, high-output
      E05.90 *[143]*
  neonatal (transient) P72.1
  transient with chronic thyroiditis E06.2
Tibia vara M92.51-●
Tic (disorder) F95.9
  breathing F95.8
  child problem F95.0
  compulsive F95.1
  de la Tourette F95.2
  degenerative (generalized) (localized) G25.69
    facial G25.69
  disorder
    chronic
      motor F95.1
      vocal F95.1
    combined vocal and multiple motor F95.2
    transient F95.0
  douloureux G50.0
    atypical G50.1
    postherpetic, postzoster B02.22
  drug-induced G25.61
  eyelid F95.8
  habit F95.9
    chronic F95.1
    transient of childhood F95.0
  lid, transient of childhood F95.0

Tic *(Continued)*
  motor-verbal F95.2
  occupational F48.8
  orbicularis F95.8
    transient of childhood F95.0
  organic origin G25.69
  postchoreic G25.69
  provisional F95.0
  psychogenic, compulsive F95.1
  salaam R25.8
  spasm (motor or vocal) F95.9
    chronic F95.1
    transient of childhood F95.0
  specified NEC F95.8
Tick-borne —*see* condition
Tietze's disease or syndrome M94.0
Tight, tightness
  anus K62.89
  chest R07.89
  fascia (lata) M62.89
  foreskin (congenital) N47.1
  hymen, hymenal ring N89.6
  introitus (acquired) (congenital) N89.6
  rectal sphincter K62.89
  tendon —*see* Short, tendon
  urethral sphincter N35.919
Tilting vertebra —*see* Dorsopathy, deforming,
  specified NEC
Timidity, child F93.8
Tin-miner's lung J63.5
Tinea (intersecta) (tarsi) B35.9
  amiantacea L44.8
  asbestina B35.0
  barbae B35.0
  beard B35.0
  black dot B35.0
  blanca B36.2
  capitis B35.0
  corporis B35.4
  cruris B35.6
  flava B36.0
  foot B35.3
  furfuracea B36.0
  imbricata (Tokelau) B35.5
  kerion B35.0
  manuum B35.2
  microsporic —*see* Dermatophytosis
  nigra B36.1
  nodosa —*see* Piedra
  pedis B35.3
  scalp B35.0
  specified NEC B35.8
  sycosis B35.0
  tonsurans B35.0
  trichophytic —*see* Dermatophytosis
  unguium B35.1
  versicolor B36.0
Tingling sensation (skin) R20.2
Tinnitus NOS H93.1-●
  audible H93.1-●
  aurium H93.1-●
  pulsatile H93.A-●
  subjective H93.1-●
Tipped tooth (teeth) M26.33
Tipping
  pelvis M95.5
    with disproportion (fetopelvic) O33.0
      causing obstructed labor O65.0
  tooth (teeth), fully erupted M26.33
Tiredness R53.83
Tissue —*see* condition
Tobacco (nicotine)
  abuse —*see* Tobacco, use
  dependence —*see* Dependence, drug, nicotine
  harmful use Z72.0
  heart —*see* Tobacco, toxic effect
  maternal use, affecting newborn P04.2
  toxic effect —*see* Table of Drugs and
    Chemicals, by substance, poisoning
    chewing tobacco —*see* Table of Drugs
      and Chemicals, by substance, poisoning

Tobacco *(Continued)*
  toxic effect *(Continued)*
    cigarettes —*see* Table of Drugs and
      Chemicals, by substance, poisoning
  use Z72.0
    complicating
      childbirth O99.334
      pregnancy O99.33-●
      puerperium O99.335
    counseling and surveillance Z71.6
    history Z87.891
  withdrawal state —*see also* Dependence,
    drug, nicotine F17.203
Tocopherol deficiency E56.0
Todd's
  cirrhosis K74.3
  paralysis (postepileptic) (transitory) G83.84
Toe —*see* condition
Toilet, artificial opening —*see* Attention to,
  artificial, opening
Tokelau (ringworm) B35.5
Tollwut —*see* Rabies
Tommaselli's disease R31.9
  correct substance properly administered —*see*
    Table of Drugs and Chemicals, by drug,
    adverse effect
  overdose or wrong substance given
    or taken —*see* Table of Drugs and
    Chemicals, by drug, poisoning
Tongue —*see also* condition
  tie Q38.1
Tonic pupil —*see* Anomaly, pupil, function,
  tonic pupil
Toni-Fanconi syndrome (cystinosis)
  E72.09
  with cystinosis E72.04
Tonsil —*see* condition
Tonsillitis (acute) (catarrhal) (croupous)
    (follicular) (gangrenous) (infective)
    (lacunar) (lingual) (malignant)
    (membranous) (parenchymatous)
    (phlegmonous) (pseudomembranous)
    (purulent) (septic) (subacute) (suppurative)
    (toxic) (ulcerative) (vesicular) (viral) J03.90
  chronic J35.01
    with adenoiditis J35.03
  diphtheritic A36.0
  hypertrophic J35.01
    with adenoiditis J35.03
  recurrent J03.91
  specified organism NEC J03.80
    recurrent J03.81
  staphylococcal J03.80
    recurrent J03.81
  streptococcal J03.00
    recurrent J03.01
  tuberculous A15.8
  Vincent's A69.1
Tooth, teeth —*see* condition
Toothache K08.89
Topagnosis R20.8
Tophi —*see* Gout, chronic
TORCH infection —*see* Infection, congenital
  without active infection P00.2
Torn —*see* Tear
Tornwaldt's cyst or disease J39.2
Torsion
  accessory tube —*see* Torsion, fallopian tube
  adnexa (female) —*see* Torsion, fallopian tube
  aorta, acquired I77.1
  appendix epididymis N44.04
  appendix testis N44.03
  bile duct (common) (hepatic) K83.8
    congenital Q44.5
  bowel, colon or intestine K56.2
  cervix —*see* Malposition, uterus
  cystic duct K82.8
  dystonia —*see* Dystonia, torsion
  epididymis (appendix) N44.04
  fallopian tube N83.52-●
    with ovary N83.53

Torsion *(Continued)*
gallbladder K82.8
congenital Q44.1
hydatid of Morgagni
female N83.52-●
male N44.03
kidney (pedicle) (leading to infarction)
N28.0
Meckel's diverticulum (congenital) Q43.0
malignant —*see* Table of Neoplasms, small
intestine, malignant
mesentery K56.2
omentum K56.2
organ or site, congenital NEC —*see* Anomaly,
by site
ovary (pedicle) N83.51-●
with fallopian tube N83.53
congenital Q50.2
oviduct —*see* Torsion, fallopian tube
penis (acquired) N48.82
congenital Q55.63
spasm —*see* Dystonia, torsion
spermatic cord N44.02
extravaginal N44.01
intravaginal N44.02
spleen D73.5
testis, testicle N44.00
appendix N44.03
tibia —*see* Deformity, limb, specified type
NEC, lower leg
uterus —*see* Malposition, uterus
Torticollis (intermittent) (spastic) M43.6
congenital (sternomastoid) Q68.0
due to birth injury P15.8
hysterical F44.4
ocular R29.891
psychogenic F45.8
conversion reaction F44.4
rheumatic M43.6
rheumatoid M06.88
spasmodic G24.3
traumatic, current S13.4
Tortipelvis G24.1
Tortuous
aortic arch Q25.46
artery I77.1
organ or site, congenital NEC —*see* Distortion
retinal vessel, congenital Q14.1
ureter N13.8
urethra N36.8
vein —*see* Varix
Torture, victim of Z65.4
Torula, torular (histolytica) (infection) —*see*
Cryptococcosis
Torulosis —*see* Cryptococcosis
Torus (mandibularis) (palatinus) M27.0
fracture —*see* Fracture, by site, torus
Touraine's syndrome Q79.8
Tourette's syndrome F95.2
Tourniquet syndrome —*see* Constriction,
external, by site
Tower skull Q75.0
with exophthalmos Q87.0
Toxemia R68.89
bacterial —*see* Sepsis
burn —*see* Burn
eclamptic (with pre-existing hypertension) —
see Eclampsia
erysipelatous —*see* Erysipelas
fatigue R68.89
food —*see* Poisoning, food
gastrointestinal K52.1
intestinal K52.1
kidney —*see* Uremia
malarial —*see* Malaria
myocardial —*see* Myocarditis, toxic
of pregnancy —*see* Pre-eclampsia
pre-eclamptic —*see* Pre-eclampsia
small intestine K52.1
staphylococcal, due to food A05.0
stasis R68.89

Toxemia *(Continued)*
uremic —*see* Uremia
urinary —*see* Uremia
Toxemica cerebropathia psychica
(nonalcoholic) F04
alcoholic —*see* Alcohol, amnestic disorder
Toxic (poisoning) —*see also* condition T65.91
effect —*see* Table of Drugs and Chemicals, by
substance, poisoning
shock syndrome A48.3
thyroid (gland) —*see* Thyrotoxicosis
Toxicemia —*see* Toxemia
Toxicity —*see* Table of Drugs and Chemicals, by
substance, poisoning
fava bean D55.0
food, noxious —*see* Poisoning, food
from drug or nonmedicinal substance —*see*
Table of Drugs and Chemicals, by drug
Toxicosis —*see also* Toxemia
capillary, hemorrhagic D69.0
Toxinfection, gastrointestinal K52.1
Toxocariasis B83.0
Toxoplasma, toxoplasmosis (acquired) B58.9
with
hepatitis B58.1
meningoencephalitis B58.2
ocular involvement B58.00
other organ involvement B58.89
pneumonia, pneumonitis B58.3
congenital (acute) (subacute) (chronic) P37.1
maternal, manifest toxoplasmosis in infant
(acute) (subacute) (chronic) P37.1
**tPA (rtPA) administation in a different facility
within the last 24 hours prior to admission
to current facility** Z92.82
Trabeculation, bladder N32.89
Trachea —*see* condition
Tracheitis (catarrhal) (infantile) (membranous)
(plastic) (septal) (suppurative) (viral) J04.10
with
bronchitis (15 years of age and above) J40
acute or subacute —*see* Bronchitis, acute
chronic J42
tuberculous NEC A15.5
under 15 years of age J20.9
laryngitis (acute) J04.2
chronic J37.1
tuberculous NEC A15.5
acute J04.10
with obstruction J04.11
chronic J42
with
bronchitis (chronic) J42
laryngitis (chronic) J37.1
diphtheritic (membranous) A36.89
due to external agent —*see* Inflammation,
respiratory, upper, due to
syphilitic A52.73
tuberculous A15.5
Trachelitis (nonvenereal) —*see* Cervicitis
Tracheobronchial —*see* condition
Tracheobronchitis (15 years of age and
above) —*see also* Bronchitis
due to
Bordetella bronchiseptica A37.80
with pneumonia A37.81
Francisella tularensis A21.8
Tracheobronchomegaly Q32.4
with bronchiectasis J47.9
with
exacerbation (acute) J47.1
lower respiratory infection J47.0
acquired J98.09
with bronchiectasis J47.9
with
exacerbation (acute) J47.1
lower respiratory infection J47.0
Tracheobronchopneumonitis —*see* Pneumonia,
broncho-●
Tracheocele (external) (internal) J39.8
congenital Q32.1

Tracheomalacia J39.8
congenital Q32.0
Tracheopharyngitis (acute) J06.9
chronic J42
due to external agent —*see* Inflammation,
respiratory, upper, due to
Tracheostenosis J39.8
Tracheostomy
complication —*see* Complication,
tracheostomy
status Z93.0
attention to Z43.0
malfunctioning J95.03
Trachoma, trachomatous A71.9
active (stage) A71.1
contraction of conjunctiva A71.1
dubium A71.0
healed or sequelae B94.0
initial (stage) A71.0
pannus A71.1
Türck's J37.0
Traction, vitreomacular H43.82-●
Train sickness T75.3
Trait(s)
Hb-S D57.3
hemoglobin
abnormal NEC D58.2
with thalassemia D56.3
C —*see* Disease, hemoglobin C
S (Hb-S) D57.3
Lepore D56.3
personality, accentuated Z73.1
sickle-cell D57.3
with elliptocytosis or spherocytosis
D57.3
type A personality Z73.1
⇒**Tramp** Z59.00
Trance R41.89
hysterical F44.89
Transaminasemia R74.01
Transection
abdomen (partial) S38.3
aorta (incomplete) —*see also* Injury, aorta
complete —*see* Injury, aorta, laceration,
major
carotid artery (incomplete) —*see also* Injury,
blood vessel, carotid, laceration
complete —*see* Injury, blood vessel, carotid,
laceration, major
celiac artery (incomplete) S35.211
branch (incomplete) S35.291
complete S35.292
complete S35.212
innominate
artery (incomplete) —*see also* Injury, blood
vessel, thoracic, innominate, artery,
laceration
complete —*see* Injury, blood vessel,
thoracic, innominate, artery,
laceration, major
vein (incomplete) —*see also* Injury, blood
vessel, thoracic, innominate, vein,
laceration
complete —*see* Injury, blood vessel,
thoracic, innominate, vein,
laceration, major
jugular vein (external) (incomplete) —*see
also* Injury, blood vessel, jugular vein,
laceration
complete —*see* Injury, blood vessel, jugular
vein, laceration, major
internal (incomplete) —*see also* Injury,
blood vessel, jugular vein, internal,
laceration
complete —*see* Injury, blood vessel,
jugular vein, internal, laceration,
major
mesenteric artery (incomplete) —*see also*
Injury, mesenteric, artery, laceration
complete —*see* Injury, mesenteric artery,
laceration, major

▶ New   ⇒ Revised   ~~deleted~~ Deleted   ● Use Additional Character(s)

Transection (*Continued*)
  pulmonary vessel (incomplete) —*see also*
    Injury, blood vessel, thoracic, pulmonary,
    laceration
    complete —*see* Injury, blood vessel,
      thoracic, pulmonary, laceration, major
  subclavian —*see* Transection, innominate
  vena cava (incomplete) —*see also* Injury, vena
    cava
    complete —*see* Injury, vena cava,
      laceration, major
  vertebral artery (incomplete) —*see also* Injury,
    blood vessel, vertebral, laceration
    complete —*see* Injury, blood vessel,
      vertebral, laceration, major
Transfusion
  associated (red blood cell) hemochromatosis
    E83.111
  blood
    ABO incompatible —*see* Complication(s),
      transfusion, incompatibility reaction,
      ABO
    minor blood group (Duffy) (E) (K) (Kell)
      (Kidd) (Lewis) (M) (N) (P) (S)
      T80.89
    reaction or complication —*see*
      Complications, transfusion
  fetomaternal (mother) —*see* Pregnancy,
    complicated by, placenta, transfusion
    syndrome
  maternofetal (mother) —*see* Pregnancy,
    complicated by, placenta, transfusion
    syndrome
  placental (syndrome) (mother) —*see*
    Pregnancy, complicated by, placenta,
    transfusion syndrome
  reaction (adverse) —*see* Complications,
    transfusion
  related acute lung injury (TRALI) J95.84
  twin-to-twin —*see* Pregnancy, complicated
    by, placenta, transfusion syndrome, fetus
    to fetus
Transient (meaning homeless) —*see also*
  condition Z59.00
Translocation
  balanced autosomal Q95.9
    in normal individual Q95.0
  chromosomes NEC Q99.8
    balanced and insertion in normal
      individual Q95.0
  Down's syndrome Q90.2
  trisomy
    13 Q91.6
    18 Q91.2
    21 Q90.2
Translucency, iris —*see* Degeneration, iris
**Transmission of chemical substances through
  the placenta** —*see* Absorption, chemical,
  through placenta
Transparency, lung, unilateral J43.0
Transplant (ed) (status) Z94.9
  awaiting organ Z76.82
  bone Z94.6
    marrow Z94.81
  candidate Z76.82
  complication —*see* Complication, transplant
  cornea Z94.7
  heart Z94.1
    and lung(s) Z94.3
    valve Z95.2
      prosthetic Z95.2
      specified NEC Z95.4
      xenogenic Z95.3
  intestine Z94.82
  kidney Z94.0
  liver Z94.4
  lung(s) Z94.2
    and heart Z94.3
  organ (failure) (infection) (rejection)Z94.9
    removal status Z98.85
  pancreas Z94.83

Transplant (*Continued*)
  skin Z94.5
  social Z60.3
  specified organ or tissue NEC Z94.89
  stem cells Z94.84
  tissue Z94.9
Transplants, ovarian, endometrial N80.1
Transposed —*see* Transposition
Transposition (congenital) —*see also*
  Malposition, congenital
  abdominal viscera Q89.3
  aorta (dextra) Q20.3
  appendix Q43.8
  colon Q43.8
  corrected Q20.5
  great vessels (complete) (partial) Q20.3
  heart Q24.0
    with complete transposition of viscera
      Q89.3
  intestine (large) (small) Q43.8
  reversed jejunal (for bypass) (status) Z98.0
  scrotum Q55.23
  stomach Q40.2
    with general transposition of viscera Q89.3
  tooth, teeth, fully erupted M26.30
  vessels, great (complete) (partial) Q20.3
  viscera (abdominal) (thoracic) Q89.3
Transsexualism F64.0
Transverse —*see also* condition
  arrest (deep), in labor O64.0
  lie (mother) O32.2
    causing obstructed labor O64.8
Transvestism, transvestitism (dual-role)
  F64.1
  fetishistic F65.1
Trapped placenta (with hemorrhage) O72.0
  without hemorrhage O73.0
TRAPS (tumor necrosis factor receptor
  associated periodic syndrome) M04.1
Trauma, traumatism —*see also* Injury
  acoustic —*see* subcategory H83.3
  birth —*see* Birth, injury
  complicating ectopic or molar pregnancy
    O08.6
  during delivery O71.9
  following ectopic or molar pregnancy O08.6
  obstetric O71.9
    specified NEC O71.89
  occlusal
    primary K08.81
    secondary K08.82
Traumatic —*see also* condition
  brain injury S06.9
Treacher Collins syndrome Q75.4
Treitz's hernia —*see* Hernia, abdomen, specified
  site NEC
Trematode infestation —*see* Infestation, fluke
Trematodiasis —*see* Infestation, fluke
Trembling paralysis —*see* Parkinsonism
Tremor(s) R25.1
  drug induced G25.1
  essential (benign) G25.0
  familial G25.0
  hereditary G25.0
  hysterical F44.4
  intention G25.2
  medication induced postural G25.1
  mercurial —*see* subcategory T56.1
  Parkinson's —*see* Parkinsonism
  psychogenic (conversion reaction) F44.4
  senilis R54
  specified type NEC G25.2
Trench
  fever A79.0
  foot —*see* Immersion, foot
  mouth A69.1
Treponema pallidum infection —*see* Syphilis
Treponematosis
  due to
    T. pallidum —*see* Syphilis
    T. pertenue —*see* Yaws

Triad
  Hutchinson's (congenital syphilis) A50.53
  Kartagener's Q89.3
  Saint's —*see* Hernia, diaphragm
Trichiasis (eyelid) H02.059
  with entropion —*see* Entropion
  left H02.056
    lower H02.055
    upper H02.054
  right H02.053
    lower H02.052
    upper H02.051
Trichinella spiralis (infection) (infestation) B75
**Trichinellosis, trichiniasis, trichinelliasis,
  trichinosis** B75
  with muscle disorder B75 [*M63.80*]
    ankle B75 [*M63.87-●*]
    foot B75 [*M63.87-●*]
    forearm B75 [*M63.83-●*]
    hand B75 [*M63.84-●*]
    lower leg B75 [*M63.86-●*]
    multiple sites B75 [*M63.89*]
    pelvic region B75 [*M63.85-●*]
    shoulder region B75 [*M63.81-●*]
    specified site NEC B75 [*M63.88*]
    thigh B75 [*M63.85-●*]
    upper arm B75 [*M63.82-●*]
Trichobezoar T18.9
  intestine T18.3
  stomach T18.2
Trichocephaliasis, trichocephalosis B79
Trichocephalus infestation B79
Trichoclasis L67.8
Trichoepithelioma —*see also* Neoplasm, skin,
  benign
  malignant —*see* Neoplasm, skin, malignant
Trichofolliculoma —*see* Neoplasm, skin,
  benign
Tricholemmoma —*see* Neoplasm, skin,
  benign
Trichomoniasis A59.9
  bladder A59.03
  cervix A59.09
  intestinal A07.8
  prostate A59.02
  seminal vesicles A59.09
  specified site NEC A59.8
  urethra A59.03
  urogenitalis A59.00
  vagina A59.01
  vulva A59.01
Trichomycosis
  axillaris A48.8
  nodosa, nodularis B36.8
Trichonodosis L67.8
Trichophytid, trichophyton infection —*see*
  Dermatophytosis
Trichophytobezoar T18.9
  intestine T18.3
  stomach T18.2
Trichophytosis —*see* Dermatophytosis
Trichoptilosis L67.8
Trichorrhexis (nodosa) (invaginata) L67.0
Trichosis axillaris A48.8
Trichosporosis nodosa B36.2
Trichostasis spinulosa (congenital) Q84.1
Trichostrongyliasis, trichostrongylosis (small
  intestine) B81.2
Trichostrongylus infection B81.2
Trichotillomania F63.3
Trichromat, trichromatopsia, anomalous
  (congenital) H53.55
Trichuriasis B79
Trichuris trichiura (infection) (infestation) (any
  site) B79
Tricuspid (valve) —*see* condition
Trifid —*see also* Accessory
  kidney (pelvis) Q63.8
  tongue Q38.3
Trigeminal neuralgia —*see* Neuralgia,
  trigeminal

Trigeminy R00.8
Trigger finger (acquired) M65.30
　congenital Q74.0
　index finger M65.32-●
　little finger M65.35-●
　middle finger M65.33-●
　ring finger M65.34-●
　thumb M65.31-●
Trigonitis (bladder) (chronic)
　　(pseudomembranous) N30.30
　with hematuria N30.31
Trigonocephaly Q75.0
Trilocular heart —see Cor triloculare
Trimethylaminuria E72.52
Tripartite placenta O43.19-●
Triphalangeal thumb Q74.0
Triple —see also Accessory
　kidneys Q63.0
　uteri Q51.818
　X, female Q97.0
Triple I O41.12-●
Triplegia G83.89
　congenital G80.8
Triplet (newborn) —see also Newborn, triplet
　complicating pregnancy —see Pregnancy, triplet
Triplication —see Accessory
Triploidy Q92.7
Trismus R25.2
　neonatorum A33
　newborn A33
Trisomy (syndrome) Q92.9
　13 (partial) Q91.7
　　meiotic nondisjunction Q91.4
　　mitotic nondisjunction Q91.5
　　mosaicism Q91.5
　　translocation Q91.6
　18 (partial) Q91.3
　　meiotic nondisjunction Q91.0
　　mitotic nondisjunction Q91.1
　　mosaicism Q91.1
　　translocation Q91.2
　20 Q92.8
　21 (partial) Q90.9
　　meiotic nondisjunction Q90.0
　　mitotic nondisjunction Q90.1
　　mosaicism Q90.1
　　translocation Q90.2
　22 Q92.8
　autosomes Q92.9
　chromosome specified NEC Q92.8
　　partial Q92.2
　　　due to unbalanced translocation Q92.5
　　specified NEC Q92.8
　　whole (nonsex chromosome)
　　　meiotic nondisjunction Q92.0
　　　mitotic nondisjunction Q92.1
　　　mosaicism Q92.1
　due to
　　dicentrics —see Extra, marker
　　　chromosomes
　　extra rings —see Extra, marker
　　　chromosomes
　　isochromosomes —see Extra, marker
　　　chromosomes
　specified NEC Q92.8
　whole chromosome Q92.9
　　meiotic nondisjunction Q92.0
　　mitotic nondisjunction Q92.1
　　mosaicism Q92.1
　　partial Q92.9
　　specified NEC Q92.8
Tritanomaly, tritanopia H53.55
Trombiculosis, trombiculiasis, trombidiosis
　B88.0
Trophedema (congenital) (hereditary) Q82.0
Trophoblastic disease —see also Mole,
　hydatidiform O01.9
Tropholymphedema Q82.0
Trophoneurosis NEC G96.89
　disseminated M34.9
Tropical —see condition

Trouble —see also Disease
　heart —see Disease, heart
　kidney —see Disease, renal
　nervous R45.0
　sinus —see Sinusitis
Trousseau's syndrome (thrombophlebitis
　migrans) I82.1
Truancy, childhood
　from school Z72.810
Truncus
　arteriosus (persistent) Q20.0
　communis Q20.0
Trunk —see condition
Trypanosomiasis
　African B56.9
　　by Trypanosoma brucei
　　　gambiense B56.0
　　　rhodesiense B56.1
　American —see Chagas' disease
　Brazilian —see Chagas' disease
　by Trypanosoma
　　brucei gambiense B56.0
　　brucei rhodesiense B56.1
　　cruzi —see Chagas' disease
　gambiensis, Gambian B56.0
　rhodesiensis, Rhodesian B56.1
　South American —see Chagas' disease
　where
　　African trypanosomiasis is prevalent
　　　B56.9
　　Chagas' disease is prevalent B57.2
▶ Tryptasemia, hereditary alpha D89.44
T-shaped incisors K00.2
Tsutsugamushi (disease) (fever) A75.3
Tube, tubal, tubular —see condition
Tubercle —see also Tuberculosis
　brain, solitary A17.81
　Darwin's Q17.8
　Ghon, primary infection A15.7
Tuberculid, tuberculide (indurating,
　subcutaneous) (lichenoid) (miliary)
　(papulonecrotic) (primary) (skin) A18.4
Tuberculoma —see also Tuberculosis
　brain A17.81
　meninges (cerebral) (spinal) A17.1
　spinal cord A17.81
Tuberculosis, tubercular, tuberculous
　　(calcification) (calcified) (caseous)
　　(chromogenic acid-fast bacilli)
　　(degeneration) (fibrocaseous) (fistula)
　　(interstitial) (isolated circumscribed
　　lesions) (necrosis) (parenchymatous)
　　(ulcerative) A15.9
　with pneumoconiosis (any condition in
　　J60-J64) J65
　abdomen (lymph gland) A18.39
　abscess (respiratory) A15.9
　　bone A18.03
　　　hip A18.02
　　　knee A18.02
　　　sacrum A18.01
　　　specified site NEC A18.03
　　　spinal A18.01
　　　vertebra A18.01
　　brain A17.81
　　breast A18.89
　　Cowper's gland A18.15
　　dura (mater) (cerebral) (spinal) A17.81
　　epidural (cerebral) (spinal) A17.81
　　female pelvis A18.17
　　frontal sinus A15.8
　　genital organs NEC A18.10
　　genitourinary A18.10
　　gland (lymphatic) —see Tuberculosis,
　　　lymph gland
　　hip A18.02
　　intestine A18.32
　　ischiorectal A18.32
　　joint NEC A18.02
　　　hip A18.02
　　　knee A18.02

Tuberculosis, tubercular, tuberculous
　(Continued)
　abscess (Continued)
　　joint NEC (Continued)
　　　specified NEC A18.02
　　　vertebral A18.01
　　kidney A18.11
　　knee A18.02
　　latent Z22.7
　　lumbar (spine) A18.01
　　lung —see Tuberculosis, pulmonary
　　meninges (cerebral) (spinal) A17.0
　　muscle A18.09
　　perianal (fistula) A18.32
　　perinephritic A18.11
　　perirectal A18.32
　　rectum A18.32
　　retropharyngeal A15.8
　　sacrum A18.01
　　scrofulous A18.2
　　scrotum A18.15
　　skin (primary) A18.4
　　spinal cord A17.81
　　spine or vertebra (column) A18.01
　　subdiaphragmatic A18.31
　　testis A18.15
　　urinary A18.13
　　uterus A18.17
　accessory sinus —see Tuberculosis, sinus
　Addison's disease A18.7
　adenitis —see Tuberculosis, lymph gland
　adenoids A15.8
　adenopathy —see Tuberculosis, lymph gland
　adherent pericardium A18.84
　adnexa (uteri) A18.17
　adrenal (capsule) (gland) A18.7
　alimentary canal A18.32
　anemia A18.89
　ankle (joint) (bone) A18.02
　anus A18.32
　apex, apical —see Tuberculosis, pulmonary
　appendicitis, appendix A18.32
　arachnoid A17.0
　artery, arteritis A18.89
　　cerebral A18.89
　arthritis (chronic) (synovial) A18.02
　　spine or vertebra (column) A18.01
　articular —see Tuberculosis, joint
　ascites A18.31
　asthma —see Tuberculosis, pulmonary
　axilla, axillary (gland) A18.2
　bladder A18.12
　bone A18.03
　　hip A18.02
　　knee A18.02
　　limb NEC A18.03
　　sacrum A18.01
　　spine or vertebral column A18.01
　bowel (miliary) A18.32
　brain A17.81
　breast A18.89
　broad ligament A18.17
　bronchi, bronchial, bronchus A15.5
　　ectasia, ectasis (bronchiectasis) —see
　　　Tuberculosis, pulmonary
　　fistula A15.5
　　　primary (progressive) A15.7
　　gland or node A15.4
　　　primary (progressive) A15.7
　　lymph gland or node A15.4
　　　primary (progressive) A15.7
　bronchiectasis —see Tuberculosis, pulmonary
　bronchitis A15.5
　bronchopleural A15.6
　bronchopneumonia, bronchopneumonic —see
　　Tuberculosis, pulmonary
　bronchorrhagia A15.5
　bronchotracheal A15.5
　bronze disease A18.7
　buccal cavity A18.83
　bulbourethral gland A18.15

▶ New　⇉ Revised　~~deleted~~ Deleted　● Use Additional Character(s)

Tuberculosis, tubercular, tuberculous
(Continued)
bursa A18.09
cachexia A15.9
cardiomyopathy A18.84
caries —*see* Tuberculosis, bone
cartilage A18.02
  intervertebral A18.01
catarrhal —*see* Tuberculosis, respiratory
cecum A18.32
cellulitis (primary) A18.4
cerebellum A17.81
cerebral, cerebrum A17.81
cerebrospinal A17.81
  meninges A17.0
cervical (lymph gland or node) A18.2
cervicitis, cervix (uteri) A18.16
chest —*see* Tuberculosis, respiratory
chorioretinitis A18.53
choroid, choroiditis A18.53
ciliary body A18.54
colitis A18.32
collier's J65
colliquativa (primary) A18.4
colon A18.32
complex, primary A15.7
congenital P37.0
conjunctiva A18.59
connective tissue (systemic) A18.89
contact Z20.1
cornea (ulcer) A18.52
Cowper's gland A18.15
coxae A18.02
coxalgia A18.02
cul de sac of Douglas A18.17
curvature, spine A18.01
cutis (colliquativa) (primary) A18.4
cyst, ovary A18.18
cystitis A18.12
dactylitis A18.03
diarrhea A18.32
diffuse —*see* Tuberculosis, miliary
digestive tract A18.32
disseminated —*see* Tuberculosis, miliary
duodenum A18.32
dura (mater) (cerebral) (spinal) A17.0
  abscess (cerebral) (spinal) A17.81
dysentery A18.32
ear (inner) (middle) A18.6
  bone A18.03
  external (primary) A18.4
  skin (primary) A18.4
elbow A18.02
emphysema —*see* Tuberculosis, pulmonary
empyema A15.6
encephalitis A17.82
endarteritis A18.89
endocarditis A18.84
  aortic A18.84
  mitral A18.84
  pulmonary A18.84
  tricuspid A18.84
endocrine glands NEC A18.82
endometrium A18.17
enteric, enterica, enteritis A18.32
enterocolitis A18.32
epididymis, epididymitis A18.15
epidural abscess (cerebral) (spinal) A17.81
epiglottis A15.5
episcleritis A18.51
erythema (induratum) (nodosum) (primary)
  A18.4
esophagus A18.83
eustachian tube A18.6
exposure (to) Z20.1
exudative —*see* Tuberculosis, pulmonary
eye A18.50
eyelid (primary) (lupus) A18.4
fallopian tube (acute) (chronic) A18.17
fascia A18.09
fauces A15.8

Tuberculosis, tubercular, tuberculous
(Continued)
female pelvic inflammatory disease
  A18.17
finger A18.03
first infection A15.7
gallbladder A18.83
ganglion A18.09
gastritis A18.83
gastrocolic fistula A18.32
gastroenteritis A18.32
gastrointestinal tract A18.32
general, generalized —*see* Tuberculosis,
  miliary
genital organs A18.10
genitourinary A18.10
genu A18.02
glandula suprarenalis A18.7
glandular, general A18.2
glottis A15.5
grinder's J65
gum A18.83
hand A18.03
heart A18.84
hematogenous —*see* Tuberculosis, miliary
hemoptysis —*see* Tuberculosis, pulmonary
hemorrhage NEC —*see* Tuberculosis,
  pulmonary
hemothorax A15.6
hepatitis A18.83
hilar lymph nodes A15.4
  primary (progressive) A15.7
hip (joint) (disease) (bone) A18.02
hydropneumothorax A15.6
hydrothorax A15.6
hypoadrenalism A18.7
hypopharynx A15.8
ileocecal (hyperplastic) A18.32
ileocolitis A18.32
ileum A18.32
iliac spine (superior) A18.03
immunological findings only A15.7
indurativa (primary) A18.4
infantile A15.7
infection A15.9
  without clinical manifestations A15.7
infraclavicular gland A18.2
inguinal gland A18.2
inguinalis A18.2
intestine (any part) A18.32
iridocyclitis A18.54
iris, iritis A18.54
ischiorectal A18.32
jaw A18.03
jejunum A18.32
joint A18.02
  vertebral A18.01
keratitis (interstitial) A18.52
keratoconjunctivitis A18.52
kidney A18.11
knee (joint) A18.02
kyphosis, kyphoscoliosis A18.01
laryngitis A15.5
larynx A15.5
latent Z22.7
leptomeninges, leptomeningitis (cerebral)
  (spinal) A17.0
lichenoides (primary) A18.4
linguae A18.83
lip A18.83
liver A18.83
lordosis A18.01
lung —*see* Tuberculosis, pulmonary
lupus vulgaris A18.4
lymph gland or node (peripheral) A18.2
  abdomen A18.39
  bronchial A15.4
    primary (progressive) A15.7
  cervical A18.2
  hilar A15.4
    primary (progressive) A15.7

Tuberculosis, tubercular, tuberculous
(Continued)
lymph gland or node *(Continued)*
  intrathoracic A15.4
    primary (progressive) A15.7
  mediastinal A15.4
    primary (progressive) A15.7
  mesenteric A18.39
  retroperitoneal A18.39
  tracheobronchial A15.4
    primary (progressive) A15.7
lymphadenitis —*see* Tuberculosis, lymph
  gland
lymphangitis —*see* Tuberculosis, lymph
  gland
lymphatic (gland) (vessel) —*see* Tuberculosis,
  lymph gland
mammary gland A18.89
marasmus A15.9
mastoiditis A18.03
mediastinal lymph gland or node
  A15.4
  primary (progressive) A15.7
mediastinitis A15.8
  primary (progressive) A15.7
mediastinum A15.8
  primary (progressive) A15.7
medulla A17.81
melanosis, Addisonian A18.7
meninges, meningitis (basilar) (cerebral)
  (cerebrospinal) (spinal) A17.0
meningoencephalitis A17.82
mesentery, mesenteric (gland or node)
  A18.39
miliary A19.9
  acute A19.2
    multiple sites A19.1
    single specified site A19.0
  chronic A19.8
  specified NEC A19.8
millstone makers' J65
miner's J65
molder's J65
mouth A18.83
multiple A19.9
  acute A19.1
  chronic A19.8
muscle A18.09
myelitis A17.82
myocardium, myocarditis A18.84
nasal (passage) (sinus) A15.8
nasopharynx A15.8
neck gland A18.2
nephritis A18.11
nerve (mononeuropathy) A17.83
nervous system A17.9
nose (septum) A15.8
ocular A18.50
omentum A18.31
oophoritis (acute) (chronic) A18.17
optic (nerve trunk) (papilla) A18.59
orbit A18.59
orchitis A18.15
organ, specified NEC A18.89
osseous —*see* Tuberculosis, bone
osteitis —*see* Tuberculosis, bone
osteomyelitis —*see* Tuberculosis, bone
otitis media A18.6
ovary, ovaritis (acute) (chronic) A18.17
oviduct (acute) (chronic) A18.17
pachymeningitis A17.0
palate (soft) A18.83
pancreas A18.83
papulonecrotic (a) (primary) A18.4
parathyroid glands A18.82
paronychia (primary) A18.4
parotid gland or region A18.83
pelvis (bony) A18.03
penis A18.15
peribronchitis A15.5
pericardium, pericarditis A18.84

Tuberculosis, tubercular, tuberculous
    (Continued)
    perichondritis, larynx A15.5
    periostitis —*see* Tuberculosis, bone
    perirectal fistula A18.32
    peritoneum NEC A18.31
    peritonitis A18.31
    pharynx, pharyngitis A15.8
    phlyctenulosis (keratoconjunctivitis) A18.52
    phthisis NEC —*see* Tuberculosis, pulmonary
    pituitary gland A18.82
    pleura, pleural, pleurisy, pleuritis (fibrinous)
        (obliterative) (purulent) (simple plastic)
        (with effusion) A15.6
        primary (progressive) A15.7
    pneumonia, pneumonic —*see* Tuberculosis,
        pulmonary
    pneumothorax (spontaneous) (tense
        valvular) —*see* Tuberculosis, pulmonary
    polyneuropathy A17.89
    polyserositis A19.9
        acute A19.1
        chronic A19.8
    potter's J65
    prepuce A18.15
    primary (complex) A15.7
    proctitis A18.32
    prostate, prostatitis A18.14
    pulmonalis —*see* Tuberculosis, pulmonary
    pulmonary (cavitated) (fibrotic) (infiltrative)
        (nodular) A15.0
        childhood type or first infection A15.7
        primary (complex) A15.7
    pyelitis A18.11
    pyelonephritis A18.11
    pyemia —*see* Tuberculosis, miliary
    pyonephrosis A18.11
    pyopneumothorax A15.6
    pyothorax A15.6
    rectum (fistula) (with abscess) A18.32
    reinfection stage —*see* Tuberculosis,
        pulmonary
    renal A18.11
    renis A18.11
    respiratory A15.9
        primary A15.7
        specified site NEC A15.8
    retina, retinitis A18.53
    retroperitoneal (lymph gland or node)
        A18.39
    rheumatism NEC A18.09
    rhinitis A15.8
    sacroiliac (joint) A18.01
    sacrum A18.01
    salivary gland A18.83
    salpingitis (acute) (chronic) A18.17
    sandblaster's J65
    sclera A18.51
    scoliosis A18.01
    scrofulous A18.2
    scrotum A18.15
    seminal tract or vesicle A18.15
    senile A15.9
    septic —*see* Tuberculosis, miliary
    shoulder (joint) A18.02
        blade A18.03
    sigmoid A18.32
    sinus (any nasal) A15.8
        bone A18.03
        epididymis A18.15
    skeletal NEC A18.03
    skin (any site) (primary) A18.4
    small intestine A18.32
    soft palate A18.83
    spermatic cord A18.15
    spine, spinal (column) A18.01
        cord A17.81
        medulla A17.81
        membrane A17.0
        meninges A17.0
    spleen, splenitis A18.85

Tuberculosis, tubercular, tuberculous
    (Continued)
    spondylitis A18.01
    sternoclavicular joint A18.02
    stomach A18.83
    stonemason's J65
    subcutaneous tissue (cellular) (primary)
        A18.4
    subcutis (primary) A18.4
    subdeltoid bursa A18.83
    submaxillary (region) A18.83
    supraclavicular gland A18.2
    suprarenal (capsule) (gland) A18.7
    swelling, joint —*see also* category M01 (*see also*
        Tuberculosis, joint) A18.02
    symphysis pubis A18.02
    synovitis A18.09
        articular A18.02
        spine or vertebra A18.01
    systemic —*see* Tuberculosis, miliary
    tarsitis A18.4
    tendon (sheath) —*see* Tuberculosis,
        tenosynovitis
    tenosynovitis A18.09
        spine or vertebra A18.01
    testis A18.15
    throat A15.8
    thymus gland A18.82
    thyroid gland A18.81
    tongue A18.83
    tonsil, tonsillitis A15.8
    trachea, tracheal A15.5
        lymph gland or node A15.4
            primary (progressive) A15.7
    tracheobronchial A15.5
        lymph gland or node A15.4
            primary (progressive) A15.7
    tubal (acute) (chronic) A18.17
    tunica vaginalis A18.15
    ulcer (skin) (primary) A18.4
        bowel or intestine A18.32
        specified NEC - code under Tuberculosis,
            by site
    unspecified site A15.9
    ureter A18.11
    urethra, urethral (gland) A18.13
    urinary organ or tract A18.13
    uterus A18.17
    uveal tract A18.54
    uvula A18.83
    vagina A18.18
    vas deferens A18.15
    verruca, verrucosa (cutis) (primary) A18.4
    vertebra (column) A18.01
    vesiculitis A18.15
    vulva A18.18
    wrist (joint) A18.02
Tuberculum
    Carabelli —*see* Note at K00.2
    occlusal —*see* Note at K00.2
    paramolare K00.2
Tuberosity, enitre maxillary M26.07
Tuberous sclerosis (brain) Q85.1
Tubo-ovarian —*see* condition
Tuboplasty, after previous sterilization
    Z31.0
    aftercare Z31.42
Tubotympanitis, catarrhal (chronic) —*see* Otitis,
    media, nonsuppurative, chronic, serous
Tularemia A21.9
    with
        conjunctivitis A21.1
        pneumonia A21.2
    abdominal A21.3
    bronchopneumonic A21.2
    conjunctivitis A21.1
    cryptogenic A21.3
    enteric A21.3
    gastrointestinal A21.3
    generalized A21.7
    ingestion A21.3

Tularemia *(Continued)*
    intestinal A21.3
    oculoglandular A21.1
    ophthalmic A21.1
    pneumonia (any), pneumonic A21.2
    pulmonary A21.2
    sepsis A21.7
    specified NEC A21.8
    typhoidal A21.7
    ulceroglandular A21.0
Tularensis conjunctivitis A21.1
Tumefaction —*see also* Swelling
    liver —*see* Hypertrophy, liver
Tumor —*see also* Neoplasm, unspecified
        behavior, by site
    acinar cell —*see* Neoplasm, uncertain
        behavior, by site
    acinic cell —*see* Neoplasm, uncertain
        behavior, by site
    adenocarcinoid —*see* Neoplasm, malignant,
        by site
    adenomatoid —*see also* Neoplasm, benign,
        by site
        odontogenic —*see* Cyst, calcifying
            odontogenic
    adnexal (skin) —*see* Neoplasm, skin, benign,
        by site
    adrenal
        cortical (benign) D35.0-●
            malignant C74.0-●
        rest —*see* Neoplasm, benign, by site
    alpha-cell
        malignant
            pancreas C25.4
            specified site NEC —*see* Neoplasm,
                malignant, by site
            unspecified site C25.4
        pancreas D13.7
        specified site NEC —*see* Neoplasm, benign,
            by site
        unspecified site D13.7
    aneurysmal —*see* Aneurysm
    aortic body D44.7
        malignant C75.5
    Askin's —*see* Neoplasm, connective tissue,
        malignant
    basal cell —*see also* Neoplasm, skin, uncertain
        behavior D48.5
    Bednar —*see* Neoplasm, skin, malignant
    benign (unclassified) —*see* Neoplasm, benign,
        by site
    beta-cell
        malignant
            pancreas C25.4
            specified site NEC —*see* Neoplasm,
                malignant, by site
            unspecified site C25.4
        pancreas D13.7
        specified site NEC —*see* Neoplasm, benign,
            by site
        unspecified site D13.7
    Brenner D27.9
        borderline malignancy D39.1-●
        malignant C56-●
        proliferating D39.1
    bronchial alveolar, intravascular D38.1
    Brooke's —*see* Neoplasm, skin, benign
    brown fat —*see* Lipoma
    Burkitt —*see* Lymphoma, Burkitt
    calcifying epithelial odontogenic —*see* Cyst,
        calcifying odontogenic
    carcinoid D3A.00
        benign D3A.00
            appendix D3A.020
            ascending colon D3A.022
            bronchus (lung) D3A.090
            cecum D3A.021
            colon D3A.029
            descending colon D3A.024
            duodenum D3A.010
            foregut NOS D3A.094

▶ New   ⇒ Revised   ~~deleted~~ Deleted   ● Use Additional Character(s)

Tumor *(Continued)*
  carcinoid *(Continued)*
    malignant *(Continued)*
      hindgut NOS D3A.096
      ileum D3A.012
      jejunum D3A.011
      kidney D3A.093
      large intestine D3A.029
      lung (bronchus) D3A.090
      midgut NOS D3A.095
      rectum D3A.026
      sigmoid colon D3A.025
      small intestine D3A.019
      specified NEC D3A.098
      stomach D3A.092
      thymus D3A.091
      transverse colon D3A.023
    malignant C7A.00
      appendix C7A.020
      ascending colon C7A.022
      bronchus (lung) C7A.090
      cecum C7A.021
      colon C7A.029
      descending colon C7A.024
      duodenum C7A.010
      foregut NOS C7A.094
      hindgut NOS C7A.096
      ileum C7A.012
      jejunum C7A.011
      kidney C7A.093
      large intestine C7A.029
      lung (bronchus) C7A.090
      midgut NOS C7A.095
      rectum C7A.026
      sigmoid colon C7A.025
      small intestine C7A.019
      specified NEC C7A.098
      stomach C7A.092
      thymus C7A.091
      transverse colon C7A.023
    mesentary metastasis C7B.04
    secondary C7B.00
      bone C7B.03
      distant lymph nodes C7B.01
      liver C7B.02
      peritoneum C7B.04
      specified NEC C7B.09
  carotid body D44.6
    malignant C75.4
  cells —*see also* Neoplasm, unspecified behavior, by site
    benign —*see* Neoplasm, benign, by site
    malignant —*see* Neoplasm, malignant, by site
    uncertain whether benign or malignant —*see* Neoplasm, uncertain behavior, by site
  cervix, in pregnancy or childbirth —*see* Pregnancy, complicated by, tumor, cervix
  chondromatous giant cell —*see* Neoplasm, bone, benign
  chromaffin —*see also* Neoplasm, benign, by site
    malignant —*see* Neoplasm, malignant, by site
  Cock's peculiar L72.3
  Codman's —*see* Neoplasm, bone, benign
  dentigerous, mixed —*see* Cyst, calcifying odontogenic
  dermoid —*see* Neoplasm, benign, by site
    with malignant transformation C56.-●
  desmoid (extra-abdominal) —*see also* Neoplasm, connective tissue, uncertain behavior
    abdominal —*see* Neoplasm, connective tissue, uncertain behavior
  embolus —*see* Neoplasm, secondary, by site

Tumor *(Continued)*
  embryonal (mixed) —*see also* Neoplasm, uncertain behavior, by site
    liver C22.7
  endodermal sinus
    specified site —*see* Neoplasm, malignant, by site
    unspecified site
      female C56.-●
      male C62.90
  epithelial
    benign —*see* Neoplasm, benign, by site
    malignant —*see* Neoplasm, malignant, by site
  Ewing's —*see* Neoplasm, bone, malignant, by site
  fatty —*see* Lipoma
  fibroid —*see* Leiomyoma
  G cell
    malignant
      pancreas C25.4
      specified site NEC —*see* Neoplasm, malignant, by site
      unspecified site C25.4
    specified site —*see* Neoplasm, uncertain behavior, by site
    unspecified site D37.8
  germ cell —*see also* Neoplasm, malignant, by site
    mixed —*see* Neoplasm, malignant, by site
  ghost cell, odontogenic —*see* Cyst, calcifying odontogenic
  giant cell —*see also* Neoplasm, uncertain behavior, by site
    bone D48.0
      malignant —*see* Neoplasm, bone, malignant
    chondromatous —*see* Neoplasm, bone, benign
    malignant —*see* Neoplasm, malignant, by site
    soft parts —*see* Neoplasm, connective tissue, uncertain behavior
      malignant —*see* Neoplasm, connective tissue, malignant
  glomus D18.00
    intra-abdominal D18.03
    intracranial D18.02
    jugulare D44.7
      malignant C75.5
    skin D18.01
    specified site NEC D18.09
  gonadal stromal —*see* Neoplasm, uncertain behavior, by site
  granular cell —*see also* Neoplasm, connective tissue, benign
    malignant —*see* Neoplasm, connective tissue, malignant
  granulosa cell D39.1-●
    juvenile D39.1-●
    malignant C56-●
  granulosa cell-theca cell D39.1-●
    malignant C56-●
  Grawitz's C64-●
  hemorrhoidal —*see* Hemorrhoids
  hilar cell D27-●
  hilus cell D27-●
  Hurthle cell (benign) D34
    malignant C73
  hydatid —*see* Echinococcus
  hypernephroid —*see also* Neoplasm, uncertain behavior, by site
  interstitial cell —*see also* Neoplasm, uncertain behavior, by site
    benign —*see* Neoplasm, benign, by site
    malignant —*see* Neoplasm, malignant, by site
  intravascular bronchial alveolar D38.1

Tumor *(Continued)*
  islet cell —*see* Neoplasm, benign, by site
    malignant —*see* Neoplasm, malignant, by site
      pancreas C25.4
      specified site NEC —*see* Neoplasm, malignant, by site
      unspecified site C25.4
    pancreas D13.7
    specified site NEC —*see* Neoplasm, benign, by site
    unspecified site D13.7
  juxtaglomerular D41.0-●
  Klatskin's C24.0
  Krukenberg's C79.6-●
  Leydig cell —*see* Neoplasm, uncertain behavior, by site
    benign —*see* Neoplasm, benign, by site
      specified site —*see* Neoplasm, benign, by site
      unspecified site
        female D27.9
        male D29.20
    malignant —*see* Neoplasm, malignant, by site
      specified site —*see* Neoplasm, malignant, by site
      unspecified site
        female C56.9
        male C62.90
    specified site —*see* Neoplasm, uncertain behavior, by site
    unspecified site
      female D39.10
      male D40.10
  lipid cell, ovary D27-●
  lipoid cell, ovary D27-●
  malignant —*see also* Neoplasm, malignant, by site C80.1
    fusiform cell (type) C80.1
    giant cell (type) C80.1
    localized, plasma cell —*see* Plasmacytoma, solitary
    mixed NEC C80.1
    small cell (type) C80.1
    spindle cell (type) C80.1
    unclassified C80.1
  mast cell D47.09
  melanotic, neuroectodermal —*see* Neoplasm, benign, by site
  Merkel cell —*see* Carcinoma, Merkel cell
  mesenchymal
    malignant —*see* Neoplasm, connective tissue, malignant
    mixed —*see* Neoplasm, connective tissue, uncertain behavior
  mesodermal, mixed —*see also* Neoplasm, malignant, by site
    liver C22.4
  mesonephric —*see also* Neoplasm, uncertain behavior, by site
    malignant —*see* Neoplasm, malignant, by site
  metastatic
    from specified site —*see* Neoplasm, malignant, by site
    of specified site —*see* Neoplasm, malignant, by site
    to specified site —*see* Neoplasm, secondary, by site
  mixed NEC —*see also* Neoplasm, benign, by site
    malignant —*see* Neoplasm, malignant, by site
  mucinous of low malignant potential
    specified site —*see* Neoplasm, malignant, by site
    unspecified site C56.9
  mucocarcinoid
    specified site —*see* Neoplasm, malignant, by site
    unspecified site C18.1

Tumor (*Continued*)
- mucoepidermoid —*see* Neoplasm, uncertain behavior, by site
- Müllerian, mixed
  - specified site —*see* Neoplasm, malignant, by site
  - unspecified site C54.9
- myoepithelial —*see* Neoplasm, benign, by site
- neuroectodermal (peripheral) —*see* Neoplasm, malignant, by site
  - primitive
    - specified site —*see* Neoplasm, malignant, by site
    - unspecified site C71.9
- neuroendocrine D3A.8
  - malignant poorly differentiated C7A.1
  - secondary NEC C7B.8
  - specified NEC C7A.8
- neurogenic olfactory C30.0
- nonencapsulated sclerosing C73
- odontogenic (adenomatoid) (benign) (calcifying epithelial) (keratocystic) (squamous) —*see* Cyst, calcifying odontogenic
  - malignant C41.1
    - upper jaw (bone) C41.0
- ovarian stromal D39.1-●
- ovary, in pregnancy —*see* Pregnancy, complicated by
- pacinian —*see* Neoplasm, skin, benign
- Pancoast's —*see* Pancoast's syndrome
- papillary —*see also* Papilloma
  - cystic D37.9
  - mucinous of low malignant potential C56-●
    - specified site —*see* Neoplasm, malignant, by site
    - unspecified site C56.9
  - serous of low malignant potential
    - specified site —*see* Neoplasm, malignant, by site
    - unspecified site C56.9
- pelvic, in pregnancy or childbirth —*see* Pregnancy, complicated by
- phantom F45.8
- phyllodes D48.6-●
  - benign D24-●
  - malignant —*see* Neoplasm, breast, malignant
- Pindborg —*see* Cyst, calcifying odontogenic
- placental site trophoblastic D39.2
- plasma cell (malignant) (localized) —*see* Plasmacytoma, solitary
- polyvesicular vitelline
  - specified site —*see* Neoplasm, malignant, by site
  - unspecified site
    - female C56.9
    - male C62.90
- Pott's puffy —*see* Osteomyelitis, specified NEC
- Rathke's pouch D44.3
- retinal anlage —*see* Neoplasm, benign, by site
- salivary gland type, mixed —*see* Neoplasm, salivary gland, benign
  - malignant —*see* Neoplasm, salivary gland, malignant
- Sampson's N80.1
- Schmincke's —*see* Neoplasm, nasopharynx, malignant
- sclerosing stromal D27-●
- sebaceous —*see* Cyst, sebaceous
- secondary —*see* Neoplasm, secondary, by site
  - carcinoid C7B.00
    - bone C7B.03
    - distant lymph nodes C7B.01
    - liver C7B.02
    - peritoneum C7B.04
    - specified NEC C7B.09
  - neuroendocrine NEC C7B.8

Tumor (*Continued*)
- serous of low malignant potential
  - specified site —*see* Neoplasm, malignant, by site
  - unspecified site C56.9
- Sertoli cell —*see* Neoplasm, benign, by site
  - with lipid storage
    - specified site —*see* Neoplasm, benign, by site
    - unspecified site
      - female D27.9
      - male D29.20
  - specified site —*see* Neoplasm, benign, by site
  - unspecified site
    - female D27.9
    - male D29.20
- Sertoli-Leydig cell —*see* Neoplasm, benign, by site
  - specified site —*see* Neoplasm, benign, by site
  - unspecified site
    - female D27.9
    - male D29.20
- sex cord(-stromal) —*see* Neoplasm, uncertain behavior, by site
  - with annular tubules D39.1-●
- skin appendage —*see* Neoplasm, skin, benign
- smooth muscle —*see* Neoplasm, connective tissue, uncertain behavior
- soft tissue
  - benign —*see* Neoplasm, connective tissue, benign
  - malignant —*see* Neoplasm, connective tissue, malignant
- sternomastoid (congenital) Q68.0
- stromal
  - endometrial D39.0
  - gastric D48.1
    - benign D21.4
    - malignant C16.9
    - uncertain behavior D48.1
  - gastrointestinal C49.A-●
    - benign D21.4
    - esophagus C49.A1
    - large intestine C49.A4
    - malignant C49.A0
      - colon C49.A4
      - duodenum C49.A3
      - esophagus C49.A1
      - ileum C49.A3
      - jejunum C49.A3
      - Meckel diverticulum C49.A3
      - large intestine C49.A4
      - omentum C49.A9
      - peritoneum C49.A9
      - rectum C49.A5
      - small intestine C49.A3
      - specified site NEC C49.A9
      - stomach C49.A2
    - rectum C49.A5
    - small intestine C49.A3
    - specified site NEC C49.A9
    - stomach C49.A2
    - uncertain behavior D48.1
  - intestine
    - benign D21.4
    - malignant
      - large C49.A4
      - small C49.A3
    - uncertain behavior D48.1
  - ovarian D39.1-●
  - stomach C49.A2
    - benign D21.4
    - malignant C49.A2
    - uncertain behavior D48.1
- sweat gland —*see also* Neoplasm, skin, uncertain behavior
  - benign —*see* Neoplasm, skin, benign
  - malignant —*see* Neoplasm, skin, malignant

Tumor (*Continued*)
- syphilitic, brain A52.17
- testicular D40.10
- testicular stromal D40.1-●
- theca cell D27.-●
- theca cell-granulosa cell D39.1-●
- Triton, malignant —*see* Neoplasm, nerve, malignant
- trophoblastic, placental site D39.2
- turban D23.4
- uterus (body), in pregnancy or childbirth —*see* Pregnancy, complicated by, tumor, uterus
- vagina, in pregnancy or childbirth —*see* Pregnancy, complicated by
- varicose —*see* Varix
- von Recklinghausen's —*see* Neurofibromatosis
- vulva or perineum, in pregnancy or childbirth —*see* Pregnancy, complicated by
  - causing obstructed labor O65.5
- Warthin's —*see* Neoplasm, salivary gland, benign
- Wilms' C64-●
- yolk sac —*see* Neoplasm, malignant, by site
  - specified site —*see* Neoplasm, malignant, by site
  - unspecified site
    - female C56.9
    - male C62.90

Tumor lysis syndrome (following antineoplastic chemotherapy) (spontaneous) NEC E88.3
Tumorlet —*see* Neoplasm, uncertain behavior, by site
Tungiasis B88.1
Tunica vasculosa lentis Q12.2
Turban tumor D23.4
Türck's trachoma J37.0
Turner-Kieser syndrome Q87.2
Turner-like syndrome Q87.19
Turner's
- hypoplasia (tooth) K00.4
- syndrome Q96.9
  - specified NEC Q96.8
- tooth K00.4
Turner-Ullrich syndrome Q96.9
Tussis convulsiva —*see* Whooping cough
Twiddler's syndrome (due to)
- automatic implantable defibrillator T82.198
- cardiac pacemaker T82.198
Twilight state
- epileptic F05
- psychogenic F44.89
Twin (newborn) —*see also* Newborn, twin
- conjoined Q89.4
- pregnancy —*see* Pregnancy, twin
Twinning, teeth K00.2
Twist, twisted
- bowel, colon or intestine K56.2
- hair (congenital) Q84.1
- mesentery K56.2
- omentum K56.2
- organ or site, congenital NEC —*see* Anomaly, by site
- ovarian pedicle —*see* Torsion, ovary
Twitching R25.3
Tylosis (acquired) L84
- buccalis K13.29
- linguae K13.29
- palmaris et plantaris (congenital) (inherited) Q82.8
  - acquired L85.1
Tympanism R14.0
Tympanites (abdominal) (intestinal) R14.0
Tympanitis —*see* Myringitis
Tympanosclerosis —*see* subcategory H74.0
Tympanum —*see* condition

▶ New ➡ Revised ~~deleted~~ Deleted ● Use Additional Character(s)

Tympany
abdomen R14.0
chest R09.89
Type A behavior pattern Z73.1
Typhlitis —*see* Appendicitis
Typhoenteritis —*see* Typhoid
Typhoid (abortive) (ambulant) (any site)
(clinical) (fever) (hemorrhagic) (infection)
(intermittent) (malignant) (rheumatic)
(Widal negative) A01.00
with pneumonia A01.03
abdominal A01.09
arthritis A01.04
carrier (suspected) of Z22.0
cholecystitis (current) A01.09
endocarditis A01.02
heart involvement A01.02
inoculation reaction —*see* Complications,
vaccination
meningitis A01.01
mesenteric lymph nodes A01.09
myocarditis A01.02
Orientia Tsutsugamushi (scrub typhus) A75.3
osteomyelitis A01.05
perichondritis, larynx A01.09
pneumonia A01.03

Typhoid (*Continued*)
specified NEC A01.09
spine A01.05
ulcer (perforating) A01.09
Typhomalaria (fever) —*see* Malaria
Typhomania A01.00
Typhoperitonitis A01.09
Typhus (fever) A75.9
abdominal, abdominalis —*see* Typhoid
African tick A77.1
amarillic A95.9
brain A75.9 *[G94]*
cerebral A75.9 *[G94]*
classical A75.0
due to Rickettsia
prowazekii A75.0
recrudescent A75.1
tsutsugamushi A75.3
typhi A75.2
endemic (flea-borne) A75.2
epidemic (louse-borne) A75.0
exanthematic NEC A75.0
exanthematicus SAI A75.0
brillii SAI A75.1
mexicanus SAI A75.2
typhus murinus A75.2

Typhus (*Continued*)
exanthematicus (*Continued*)
flea-borne A75.2
India tick A77.1
Kenya (tick) A77.1
louse-borne A75.0
Mexican A75.2
mite-borne A75.3
murine A75.2
North Asian tick-borne A77.2
petechial A75.9
Queensland tick A77.3
rat A75.2
recrudescent A75.1
recurrens —*see* Fever, relapsing
Sao Paulo A77.0
scrub (China) (India) (Malaysia) (New
Guinea) A75.3
shop (of Malaysia) A75.2
Siberian tick A77.2
tick-borne A77.9
tropical (mite-borne) A75.3
Tyrosinemia E70.21
newborn, transitory P74.5
Tyrosinosis E70.21
Tyrosinuria E70.29

U

Uhl's anomaly or disease Q24.8
Ulcer, ulcerated, ulcerating, ulceration,
    ulcerative
alveolar process M27.3
amebic (intestine) A06.1
    skin A06.7
anastomotic —see Ulcer, gastrojejunal
anorectal K62.6
antral —see Ulcer, stomach
anus (sphincter) (solitary) K62.6
aorta —see Aneurysm
aphthous (oral) (recurrent) K12.0
    genital organ(s)
        female N76.6
        male N50.89
artery I77.2
atrophic —see Ulcer, skin
    decubitus —see Ulcer, pressure, by site
back L98.429
    with
        bone involvement without evidence of
            necrosis L98.426
        bone necrosis L98.424
        exposed fat layer L98.422
        muscle involvement without evidence of
            necrosis L98.425
        muscle necrosis L98.423
        skin breakdown only L98.421
        specified severity NEC L98.428
Barrett's (esophagus) K22.10
    with bleeding K22.11
bile duct (common) (hepatic) K83.8
bladder (solitary) (sphincter) NEC N32.89
    bilharzial B65.9 [N33]
    in schistosomiasis (bilharzial) B65.9 [N33]
    submucosal —see Cystitis, interstitial
    tuberculous A18.12
bleeding K27.4
bone —see Osteomyelitis, specified type NEC
bowel —see Ulcer, intestine
breast N61.1
bronchus J98.09
buccal (cavity) (traumatic) K12.1
Buruli A31.1
buttock L98.419
    with
        bone involvement without evidence of
            necrosis L98.416
        bone necrosis L98.414
        exposed fat layer L98.412
        muscle involvement without evidence of
            necrosis L98.415
        muscle necrosis L98.413
        skin breakdown only L98.411
        specified severity NEC L98.418
cancerous —see Neoplasm, malignant, by site
cardia K22.10
    with bleeding K22.11
cardioesophageal (peptic) K22.10
    with bleeding K22.11
cecum —see Ulcer, intestine
cervix (uteri) (decubitus) (trophic) N86
    with cervicitis N72
chancroidal A57
chiclero B55.1
chronic (cause unknown) —see Ulcer, skin
Cochin-China B55.1
colon —see Ulcer, intestine
conjunctiva H10.89
cornea H16.00-●
    with hypopyon H16.03-●
    central H16.01-●
    dendritic (herpes simplex) B00.52
    marginal H16.04-●
    Mooren's H16.05-●
    mycotic H16.06-●
    perforated H16.07-●
    ring H16.02-●
    tuberculous (phlyctenular) A18.52

Ulcer, ulcerated, ulcerating, ulceration,
    ulcerative (Continued)
corpus cavernosum (chronic) N48.5
crural —see Ulcer, lower limb
Curling's —see Ulcer, peptic, acute
Cushing's —see Ulcer, peptic, acute
cystic duct K82.8
cystitis (interstitial) —see Cystitis,
    interstitial
decubitus —see Ulcer, pressure, by site
dendritic, cornea (herpes simplex) B00.52
diabetes, diabetic —see Diabetes, ulcer
Dieulafoy's K25.0
due to
    infection NEC —see Ulcer, skin
    radiation NEC L59.8
    trophic disturbance (any region) —see
        Ulcer, skin
    X-ray L58.1
duodenum, duodenal (eroded) (peptic)
    K26.9
    with
        hemorrhage K26.4
            and perforation K26.6
        perforation K26.5
        acute K26.3
            with
                hemorrhage K26.0
                    and perforation K26.2
                perforation K26.1
        chronic K26.7
            with
                hemorrhage K26.4
                    and perforation K26.6
                perforation K26.5
dysenteric A09
elusive —see Cystitis, interstitial
endocarditis (acute) (chronic) (subacute) I28.8
epiglottis J38.7
esophagus (peptic) K22.10
    with bleeding K22.11
    due to
        aspirin K22.10
            with bleeding K22.11
        gastrointestinal reflux disease (without
            bleeding) K21.00
            with bleeding K21.01
        ingestion of chemical or medicament
            K22.10
            with bleeding K22.11
        fungal K22.10
            with bleeding K22.11
        infective K22.10
            with bleeding K22.11
        varicose —see Varix, esophagus
eyelid (region) H01.8
fauces J39.2
Fenwick (-Hunner) (solitary) —see Cystitis,
    interstitial
fistulous —see Ulcer, skin
foot (indolent) (trophic) —see Ulcer, lower
    limb
frambesial, initial A66.0
frenum (tongue) K14.0
gallbladder or duct K82.8
gangrenous —see Gangrene
gastric —see Ulcer, stomach
gastrocolic —see Ulcer, gastrojejunal
gastroduodenal —see Ulcer, peptic
gastroesophageal —see Ulcer, stomach
gastrointestinal —see Ulcer, gastrojejunal
gastrojejunal (peptic) K28.9
    with
        hemorrhage K28.4
            and perforation K28.6
        perforation K28.5
        acute K28.3
            with
                hemorrhage K28.0
                    and perforation K28.2
                perforation K28.1

Ulcer, ulcerated, ulcerating, ulceration,
    ulcerative (Continued)
gastrojejunal (Continued)
    chronic K28.7
        with
            hemorrhage K28.4
                and perforation K28.6
            perforation K28.5
gastrojejunocolic —see Ulcer, gastrojejunal
gingiva K06.8
gingivitis K05.10
    nonplaque induced K05.11
    plaque induced K05.10
glottis J38.7
granuloma of pudenda A58
gum K06.8
gumma, due to yaws A66.4
heel —see Ulcer, lower limb
hemorrhoid —see also Hemorrhoids, by
    degree K64.8
Hunner's —see Cystitis, interstitial
hypopharynx J39.2
hypopyon (chronic) (subacute) —see Ulcer,
    cornea, with hypopyon
hypostaticum —see Ulcer, varicose
ileum —see Ulcer, intestine
intestine, intestinal K63.3
    with perforation K63.1
    amebic A06.1
    duodenal —see Ulcer, duodenum
    granulocytopenic (with hemorrhage) —see
        Neutropenia
    marginal —see Ulcer, gastrojejunal
    perforating K63.1
        newborn P78.0
    primary, small intestine K63.3
    rectum K62.6
    stercoraceous, stercoral K63.3
    tuberculous A18.32
    typhoid (fever) —see Typhoid
    varicose I86.8
jejunum, jejunal —see Ulcer, gastrojejunal
keratitis —see Ulcer, cornea
knee —see Ulcer, lower limb
labium (majus) (minus) N76.6
laryngitis —see Laryngitis
larynx (aphthous) (contact) J38.7
    diphtheritic A36.2
leg —see Ulcer, lower limb
lip K13.0
Lipschütz's N76.6
lower limb (atrophic) (chronic) (neurogenic)
    (perforating) (pyogenic) (trophic)
    (tropical) L97.909
    with
        bone involvement without evidence of
            necrosis L97.906
        bone necrosis L97.904
        exposed fat layer L97.902
        muscle involvement without evidence of
            necrosis L97.905
        muscle necrosis L97.903
        skin breakdown only L97.901
        specified severity NEC L97.908
    ankle L97.309
        with
            bone involvement without evidence of
                necrosis L97.306
            bone necrosis L97.304
            exposed fat layer L97.302
            muscle involvement without evidence
                of necrosis L97.305
            muscle necrosis L97.303
            skin breakdown only L97.301
            specified severity NEC L97.308
        left L97.329
            with
                bone involvement without evidence
                    of necrosis L97.326
                bone necrosis L97.324
                exposed fat layer L97.322

Ulcer, ulcerated, ulcerating, ulceration,
  ulcerative *(Continued)*
  lower limb *(Continued)*
    ankle *(Continued)*
      left *(Continued)*
        with *(Continued)*
          muscle involvement without
            evidence of necrosis
            L97.325
          muscle necrosis L97.323
          skin breakdown only L97.321
          specified severity NEC L97.328
      right L97.319
        with
          bone involvement without evidence
            of necrosis L97.316
          bone necrosis L97.314
          exposed fat layer L97.312
          muscle involvement without
            evidence of necrosis
            L97.315
          muscle necrosis L97.313
          skin breakdown only L97.311
          specified severity NEC L97.318
    calf L97.209
      with
        bone involvement without evidence of
          necrosis L97.206
        bone necrosis L97.204
        exposed fat layer L97.202
        muscle involvement without evidence
          of necrosis L97.205
        muscle necrosis L97.203
        skin breakdown only L97.201
        specified severity NEC L97.208
      left L97.229
        with
          bone involvement without evidence
            of necrosis L97.226
          bone necrosis L97.224
          exposed fat layer L97.222
          muscle involvement without
            evidence of necrosis
            L97.225
          muscle necrosis L97.223
          skin breakdown only L97.221
          specified severity NEC L97.228
      right L97.219
        with
          bone involvement without evidence
            of necrosis L97.216
          bone necrosis L97.214
          exposed fat layer L97.212
          muscle involvement without
            evidence of necrosis L97.215
          muscle necrosis L97.213
          skin breakdown only L97.211
          specified severity NEC L97.218
    decubitus —*see* Ulcer, pressure, by site
    foot specified NEC L97.509
      with
        bone involvement without evidence of
          necrosis L97.506
        bone necrosis L97.504
        exposed fat layer L97.502
        muscle involvement without evidence
          of necrosis L97.505
        muscle necrosis L97.503
        skin breakdown only L97.501
        specified severity NEC L97.508
      left L97.529
        with
          bone involvement without evidence
            of necrosis L97.526
          bone necrosis L97.524
          exposed fat layer L97.522
          muscle involvement without
            evidence of necrosis L97.525
          muscle necrosis L97.523
          skin breakdown only L97.521
          specified severity NEC L97.528

Ulcer, ulcerated, ulcerating, ulceration,
  ulcerative *(Continued)*
  lower limb *(Continued)*
    foot specified *(Continued)*
      right L97.519
        with
          bone involvement without evidence
            of necrosis L97.516
          bone necrosis L97.514
          exposed fat layer L97.512
          muscle involvement without
            evidence of necrosis L97.515
          muscle necrosis L97.513
          skin breakdown only L97.511
          specified severity NEC L97.518
    heel L97.409
      with
        bone involvement without evidence of
          necrosis L97.406
        bone necrosis L97.404
        exposed fat layer L97.402
        muscle involvement without evidence
          of necrosis L97.405
        muscle necrosis L97.403
        skin breakdown only L97.401
        specified severity NEC L97.408
      left L97.429
        with
          bone involvement without evidence
            of necrosis L97.426
          bone necrosis L97.424
          exposed fat layer L97.422
          muscle involvement without
            evidence of necrosis L97.425
          muscle necrosis L97.423
          skin breakdown only L97.421
          specified severity NEC L97.428
      right L97.419
        with
          bone involvement without evidence
            of necrosis L97.416
          bone necrosis L97.414
          exposed fat layer L97.412
          muscle involvement without
            evidence of necrosis L97.415
          muscle necrosis L97.413
          skin breakdown only L97.411
          specified severity NEC L97.418
    left L97.929
      with
        bone involvement without evidence of
          necrosis L97.926
        bone necrosis L97.924
        exposed fat layer L97.922
        muscle involvement without evidence
          of necrosis L97.925
        muscle necrosis L97.923
        skin breakdown only L97.921
        specified severity NEC L97.928
    lower leg NOS L97.909
      with
        bone involvement without evidence of
          necrosis L97.906
        bone necrosis L97.904
        exposed fat layer L97.902
        muscle involvement without evidence
          of necrosis L97.905
        muscle necrosis L97.903
        skin breakdown only L97.901
        specified severity NEC L97.908
      left L97.929
        with
          bone involvement without evidence
            of necrosis L97.926
          bone necrosis L97.924
          exposed fat layer L97.922
          muscle involvement without
            evidence of necrosis L97.925
          muscle necrosis L97.923
          skin breakdown only L97.921
          specified severity NEC L97.928

Ulcer, ulcerated, ulcerating, ulceration,
  ulcerative *(Continued)*
  lower limb *(Continued)*
    lower leg NOS *(Continued)*
      right L97.919
        with
          bone involvement without evidence
            of necrosis L97.916
          bone necrosis L97.914
          exposed fat layer L97.912
          muscle involvement without
            evidence of necrosis L97.915
          muscle necrosis L97.913
          skin breakdown only L97.911
          specified severity NEC L97.918
    specified site NEC L97.809
      with
        bone involvement without evidence
          of necrosis L97.806
        bone necrosis L97.804
        exposed fat layer L97.802
        muscle involvement without
          evidence of necrosis L97.805
        muscle necrosis L97.803
        skin breakdown only L97.801
        specified severity NEC L97.808
      left L97.829
        with
          bone involvement without
            evidence of necrosis L97.826
          bone necrosis L97.824
          exposed fat layer L97.822
          muscle involvement without
            evidence of necrosis L97.825
          muscle necrosis L97.823
          skin breakdown only L97.821
          specified severity NEC L97.828
      right L97.819
        with
          bone involvement without
            evidence of necrosis L97.816
          bone necrosis L97.814
          exposed fat layer L97.812
          muscle involvement without
            evidence of necrosis L97.815
          muscle necrosis L97.813
          skin breakdown only L97.811
          specified severity NEC L97.818
    midfoot L97.409
      with
        bone involvement without evidence of
          necrosis L97.406
        bone necrosis L97.404
        exposed fat layer L97.402
        muscle involvement without evidence
          of necrosis L97.405
        muscle necrosis L97.403
        skin breakdown only L97.401
        specified severity NEC L97.408
      left L97.429
        with
          bone involvement without evidence
            of necrosis L97.426
          bone necrosis L97.424
          exposed fat layer L97.422
          muscle involvement without
            evidence of necrosis L97.425
          muscle necrosis L97.423
          skin breakdown only L97.421
          specified severity NEC L97.428
      right L97.419
        with
          bone involvement without evidence
            of necrosis L97.416
          bone necrosis L97.414
          exposed fat layer L97.412
          muscle involvement without
            evidence of necrosis L97.415
          muscle necrosis L97.413
          skin breakdown only L97.411
          specified severity NEC L97.418

Ulcer, ulcerated, ulcerating, ulceration,
  ulcerative *(Continued)*
 lower limb *(Continued)*
  right L97.919
   with
    bone involvement without evidence of
      necrosis L97.916
    bone necrosis L97.914
    exposed fat layer L97.912
    muscle involvement without evidence
      of necrosis L97.915
    muscle necrosis L97.913
    skin breakdown only L97.911
    specified severity NEC L97.918
   thigh L97.109
    with
     bone involvement without evidence of
       necrosis L97.106
     bone necrosis L97.104
     exposed fat layer L97.102
     muscle involvement without evidence
       of necrosis L97.105
     muscle necrosis L97.103
     skin breakdown only L97.101
     specified severity NEC L97.108
    left L97.129
     with
      bone involvement without evidence
        of necrosis L97.126
      bone necrosis L97.124
      exposed fat layer L97.122
      muscle involvement without
        evidence of necrosis L97.125
      muscle necrosis L97.123
      skin breakdown only L97.121
      specified severity NEC L97.128
     right L97.119
      with
       bone involvement without evidence
         of necrosis L97.116
       bone necrosis L97.114
       exposed fat layer L97.112
       muscle involvement without
         evidence of necrosis L97.115
       muscle necrosis L97.113
       skin breakdown only L97.111
       specified severity NEC L97.118
    toe L97.509
     with
      bone involvement without evidence of
        necrosis L97.506
      bone necrosis L97.504
      exposed fat layer L97.502
      muscle involvement without evidence
        of necrosis L97.505
      muscle necrosis L97.503
      skin breakdown only L97.501
      specified severity NEC L97.508
     left L97.529
      with
       bone involvement without evidence
         of necrosis L97.526
       bone necrosis L97.524
       exposed fat layer L97.522
       muscle involvement without
         evidence of necrosis L97.525
       muscle necrosis L97.523
       skin breakdown only L97.521
       specified severity NEC L97.528
      right L97.519
       with
        bone involvement without evidence
          of necrosis L97.516
        bone necrosis L97.514
        exposed fat layer L97.512
        muscle involvement without
          evidence of necrosis L97.515
        muscle necrosis L97.513
        skin breakdown only L97.511
        specified severity NEC
          L97.518

Ulcer, ulcerated, ulcerating, ulceration,
  ulcerative *(Continued)*
 lower limb *(Continued)*
  leprous A30.1
  syphilitic A52.19
  varicose —*see* Varix, leg, with, ulcer
 luetic —*see* Ulcer, syphilitic
 lung J98.4
  tuberculous —*see* Tuberculosis, pulmonary
 malignant —*see* Neoplasm, malignant, by site
 marginal NEC —*see* Ulcer, gastrojejunal
 meatus (urinarius) N34.2
 Meckel's diverticulum Q43.0
  malignant —*see* Table of Neoplasms, small
    intestine, malignant
 Meleney's (chronic undermining) —*see* Ulcer,
   skin
 Mooren's (cornea) —*see* Ulcer, cornea,
   Mooren's
 mycobacterial (skin) A31.1
 nasopharynx J39.2
 neck, uterus N86
 neurogenic NEC —*see* Ulcer, skin
 nose, nasal (passage) (infective) (septum) J34.0
  skin —*see* Ulcer, skin
  spirochetal A69.8
  varicose (bleeding) I86.8
 oral mucosa (traumatic) K12.1
 palate (soft) K12.1
 penis (chronic) N48.5
 peptic (site unspecified) K27.9
  with
   hemorrhage K27.4
    and perforation K27.6
   perforation K27.5
  acute K27.3
   with
    hemorrhage K27.0
     and perforation K27.2
    perforation K27.1
  chronic K27.7
   with
    hemorrhage K27.4
     and perforation K27.6
    perforation K27.5
  esophagus K22.10
   with bleeding K22.11
  newborn P78.82
 perforating K27.5
  skin —*see* Ulcer, skin
 peritonsillar J35.8
 phagedenic (tropical) —*see* Ulcer, skin
 pharynx J39.2
 phlebitis —*see* Phlebitis
 plaster —*see* Ulcer, pressure, by site
 popliteal space —*see* Ulcer, lower limb
 postpyloric —*see* Ulcer, duodenum
 prepuce N47.7
 prepyloric —*see* Ulcer, stomach
 pressure (pressure area) L89.9-●
  ankle L89.5-●
  back L89.1-●
  buttock L89.3-●
  coccyx L89.15-●
  contiguous site of back, buttock, hip
    L89.4-●
  elbow L89.0-●
  face L89.81-●
  head L89.81-●
  heel L89.6-●
  hip L89.2-●
  sacral region (tailbone) L89.15-●
  specified site NEC L89.89-●
  stage 1 (healing) (pre-ulcer skin changes
    limited to persistent focal edema)
   ankle L89.5-●
   back L89.1-●
   buttock L89.3-●
   coccyx L89.15-●
   contiguous site of back, buttock, hip
     L89.4-●

Ulcer, ulcerated, ulcerating, ulceration,
  ulcerative *(Continued)*
 pressure *(Continued)*
  stage 1 *(Continued)*
   elbow L89.0-●
   face L89.81-●
   head L89.81-●
   heel L89.6-●
   hip L89.2-●
   sacral region (tailbone) L89.15-●
   specified site NEC L89.89-●
  stage 2 (healing) (abrasion, blister,
    partial thickness skin loss involving
    epidermis and/or dermis)
   ankle L89.5-●
   back L89.1-●
   buttock L89.3-●
   coccyx L89.15-●
   contiguous site of back, buttock, hip
     L89.4-●
   elbow L89.0-●
   face L89.81-●
   head L89.81-●
   heel L89.6-●
   hip L89.2-●
   sacral region (tailbone) L89.15-●
   specified site NEC L89.89-●
  stage 3 (healing) (full thickness skin loss
    involving damage or necrosis of
    subcutaneous tissue)
   ankle L89.5-●
   back L89.1-●
   buttock L89.3-●
   coccyx L89.15-●
   contiguous site of back, buttock, hip
     L89.4-●
   elbow L89.0-●
   face L89.81-●
   head L89.81-●
   heel L89.6-●
   hip L89.2-●
   sacral region (tailbone) L89.15-●
   specified site NEC L89.89-●
  stage 4 (healing) (necrosis of soft tissues
    through to underlying muscle,
    tendon, or bone)
   ankle L89.5-●
   back L89.1-●
   buttock L89.3-●
   coccyx L89.15-●
   contiguous site of back, buttock, hip
     L89.4-●
   elbow L89.0-●
   face L89.81-●
   head L89.81-●
   heel L89.6-●
   hip L89.2-●
   sacral region (tailbone) L89.15-●
   specified site NEC L89.89-●
  unspecified stage
   ankle L89.5-●
   back L89.1-●
   buttock L89.3-●
   coccyx L89.15-●
   contiguous site of back, buttock, hip
     L89.4-●
   elbow L89.0-●
   face L89.81-●
   head L89.81-●
   heel L89.6-●
   hip L89.2-●
   sacral region (tailbone) L89.15-●
   specified site NEC L89.89-●
  unstageable
   ankle L89.5-●
   back L89.1-●
   buttock L89.3-●
   coccyx L89.15-●
   contiguous site of back, buttock, hip
     L89.4-●
   elbow L89.0-●

▶ New   ⇒ Revised   ~~deleted~~ Deleted   ● Use Additional Character(s)

Ulcer, ulcerated, ulcerating, ulceration, ulcerative *(Continued)*
  pressure *(Continued)*
    unstageable *(Continued)*
      face L89.81-●
      head L89.81-●
      heel L89.6-●
      hip L89.2-●
      sacral region (tailbone) L89.15-●
      specified site NEC L89.89-●
  primary of intestine K63.3
    with perforation K63.1
  prostate N41.9
  pyloric —*see* Ulcer, stomach
  rectosigmoid K63.3
    with perforation K63.1
  rectum (sphincter) (solitary) K62.6
    stercoraceous, stercoral K62.6
  retina —*see* Inflammation, chorioretinal
  rodent —*see also* Neoplasm, skin, malignant
  sclera —*see* Scleritis
  scrofulous (tuberculous) A18.2
  scrotum N50.89
    tuberculous A18.15
    varicose I86.1
  seminal vesicle N50.89
  sigmoid —*see* Ulcer, intestine
  skin (atrophic) (chronic) (neurogenic) (non-healing) (perforating) (pyogenic) (trophic) (tropical) L98.499
    with gangrene —*see* Gangrene
    amebic A06.7
    back —*see* Ulcer, back
    buttock —*see* Ulcer, buttock
    decubitus —*see* Ulcer, pressure
    lower limb —*see* Ulcer, lower limb
    mycobacterial A31.1
    specified site NEC L98.499
      with
        bone involvement without evidence of necrosis L98.496
        bone necrosis L98.494
        exposed fat layer L98.492
        muscle involvement without evidence of necrosis L98.495
        muscle necrosis L98.493
        skin breakdown only L98.491
        specified severity NEC L98.498
    tuberculous (primary) A18.4
    varicose —*see* Ulcer, varicose
  sloughing —*see* Ulcer, skin
  solitary, anus or rectum (sphincter) K62.6
  sore throat J02.9
    streptococcal J02.0
  spermatic cord N50.89
  spine (tuberculous) A18.01
  stasis (venous) —*see* Varix, leg, with, ulcer
    without varicose veins I87.2
  stercoraceous, stercoral K63.3
    with perforation K63.1
    anus or rectum K62.6
  stoma, stomal —*see* Ulcer, gastrojejunal
  stomach (eroded) (peptic) (round) K25.9
    with
      hemorrhage K25.4
        and perforation K25.6
      perforation K25.5
    acute K25.3
      with
        hemorrhage K25.0
          and perforation K25.2
        perforation K25.1
    chronic K25.7
      with
        hemorrhage K25.4
          and perforation K25.6
        perforation K25.5
  stomal —*see* Ulcer, gastrojejunal
  stomatitis K12.1
  stress —*see* Ulcer, peptic

Ulcer, ulcerated, ulcerating, ulceration, ulcerative *(Continued)*
  strumous (tuberculous) A18.2
  submucosal, bladder —*see* Cystitis, interstitial
  syphilitic (any site) (early) (secondary) A51.39
    late A52.79
      perforating A52.79
        foot A52.11
  testis N50.89
  thigh —*see* Ulcer, lower limb
  throat J39.2
    diphtheritic A36.0
  toe —*see* Ulcer, lower limb
  tongue (traumatic) K14.0
  tonsil J35.8
    diphtheritic A36.0
  trachea J39.8
  trophic —*see* Ulcer, skin
  tropical —*see* Ulcer, skin
  tuberculous —*see* Tuberculosis, ulcer
  tunica vaginalis N50.89
  turbinate J34.89
  typhoid (perforating) —*see* Typhoid
  unspecified site —*see* Ulcer, skin
  urethra (meatus) —*see* Urethritis
  uterus N85.8
    cervix N86
      with cervicitis N72
    neck N86
      with cervicitis N72
  vagina N76.5
    in Behçet's disease M35.2 *[N77.0]*
    pessary N89.8
  valve, heart I33.0
  varicose (lower limb, any part) —*see also* Varix, leg, with, ulcer
    broad ligament I86.2
    esophagus —*see* Varix, esophagus
    inflamed or infected —*see* Varix, leg, with ulcer, with inflammation
    nasal septum I86.8
    perineum I86.3
    scrotum I86.1
    specified site NEC I86.8
    sublingual I86.0
    vulva I86.3
  vas deferens N50.89
  vulva (acute) (infectional) N76.6
    in (due to)
      Behçet's disease M35.2 *[N77.0]*
      herpesviral (herpes simplex) infection A60.04
      tuberculosis A18.18
  vulvobuccal, recurring N76.6
  X-ray L58.1
  yaws A66.4
Ulcerosa scarlatina A38.8
Ulcus —*see also* Ulcer
  cutis tuberculosum A18.4
  duodeni —*see* Ulcer, duodenum
  durum (syphilitic) A51.0
    extragenital A51.2
  gastrojejunale —*see* Ulcer, gastrojejunal
  hypostaticum —*see* Ulcer, varicose
  molle (cutis) (skin) A57
  serpens corneae —*see* Ulcer, cornea, central
  ventriculi —*see* Ulcer, stomach
Ulegyria Q04.8
Ulerythema
  ophryogenes, congenital Q84.2
  sycosiforme L73.8
Ullrich(-Bonnevie)(-Turner) syndrome —*see also* Turner's syndrome Q87.19
Ullrich-Feichtiger syndrome Q87.0
Ulnar —*see* condition
Ulorrhagia, ulorrhea K06.8
Umbilicus, umbilical —*see* condition
Unacceptable
  contours of tooth K08.54
  morphology of tooth K08.54

Unavailability (of)
  bed at medical facility Z75.1
  health service-related agencies Z75.4
  medical facilities (at) Z75.3
    due to
      investigation by social service agency Z75.2
      lack of services at home Z75.0
      remoteness from facility Z75.3
      waiting list Z75.1
    home Z75.0
    outpatient clinic Z75.3
  schooling Z55.1
  social service agencies Z75.4
Uncinaria americana infestation B76.1
Uncinariasis B76.9
Uncongenial work Z56.5
Unconscious (ness) —*see* Coma
Underachievement in school Z55.3
Underdevelopment —*see also* Undeveloped
  nose Q30.1
  sexual E30.0
Underdosing —*see also* Table of Drugs and Chemicals, categories T36-T50, with final character 6 Z91.14
  intentional NEC Z91.128
    due to financial hardship of patient Z91.120
  unintentional NEC Z91.138
    due to patient's age related debility Z91.130
Underfeeding, newborn P92.3
Underfill, endodontic M27.53
Underimmunization status Z28.3
Undernourishment —*see* Malnutrition
Undernutrition —*see* Malnutrition
Under observation —*see* Observation
Underweight R63.6
  for gestational age —*see* Light for dates
Underwood's disease P83.0
Undescended —*see also* Malposition, congenital
  cecum Q43.3
  colon Q43.3
  testicle —*see* Cryptorchid
Undeveloped, undevelopment —*see also* Hypoplasia
  brain (congenital) Q02
  cerebral (congenital) Q02
  heart Q24.8
  lung Q33.6
  testis E29.1
  uterus E30.0
Undiagnosed (disease) R69
Undulant fever —*see* Brucellosis
Unemployment, anxiety concerning Z56.0
  threatened Z56.2
Unequal length (acquired) (limb) —*see also* Deformity, limb, unequal length
  leg —*see also* Deformity, limb, unequal length
    congenital Q72.9-●
Unextracted dental root K08.3
Unguis incarnatus L60.0
Unhappiness R45.2
Unicornate uterus Q51.4
  in pregnancy or childbirth O34.00
Unilateral —*see also* condition
  development, breast N64.89
  organ or site, congenital NEC —*see* Agenesis, by site
Unilocular heart Q20.8
Union, abnormal —*see also* Fusion
  larynx and trachea Q34.8
Universal mesentery Q43.3
Unrepairable overhanging of dental restorative materials K08.52
Unsatisfactory
  restoration of tooth K08.50
    specified NEC K08.59
  sample of cytologic smear
    anus R85.615
    cervix R87.615
    vagina R87.625
  surroundings Z59.1
  work Z56.5

Unsoundness of mind —*see* Psychosis
Unstable
　back NEC —*see* Instability, joint, spine
　hip (congenital) Q65.6
　　acquired —*see* Derangement, joint,
　　　specified type NEC, hip
　joint —*see* Instability, joint
　　secondary to removal of joint prosthesis
　　　M96.89
　lie (mother) O32.0
　lumbosacral joint (congenital) —*see*
　　subcategory M53.2
　sacroiliac —*see* subcategory M53.2
　spine NEC —*see* Instability, joint, spine
Unsteadiness on feet R26.81
Untruthfulness, child problem F91.8
Unverricht(-Lundborg) disease or epilepsy —
　see Epilepsy, generalized, idiopathic
~~Unwanted pregnancy Z64.0~~
▶Unwanted
　▶multiple moves in the last 12 months
　　Z59.81- ●
　▶pregnancy Z64.0
Upbringing, institutional Z62.22
　away from parents NEC Z62.29
　in care of non-parental family member Z62.21
　in foster care Z62.21
　in orphanage or group home Z62.22
　in welfare custody Z62.21
Upper respiratory —*see* condition
Upset
　gastric K30
　gastrointestinal K30
　　psychogenic F45.8
　intestinal (large) (small) K59.9
　　psychogenic F45.8
　menstruation N93.9
　mental F48.9
　stomach K30
　　psychogenic F45.8
Urachus —*see also* condition
　patent or persistent Q64.4
Urbach-Oppenheim disease (necrobiosis
　　lipoidica diabeticorum) —*see* E08-E13 with
　　.620
Urbach's lipoid proteinosis E78.89
Urbach-Wiethe disease E78.89
Urban yellow fever A95.1
Urea
　blood, high —*see* Uremia
　cycle metabolism disorder —*see* Disorder,
　　urea cycle metabolism
Uremia, uremic N19
　with
　　ectopic or molar pregnancy O08.4
　　polyneuropathy N18.9 [G63]
　chronic NOS —*see also* Disease, kidney,
　　chronic N18.9
　　due to hypertension —*see* Hypertensive,
　　　kidney
　complicating
　ectopic or molar pregnancy O08.4
　congenital P96.0
　extrarenal R39.2
　following ectopic or molar pregnancy O08.4
　newborn P96.0
　prenatal R39.2
Ureter, ureteral —*see* condition
Ureteralgia N23
Ureterectasis —*see* Hydroureter
Ureteritis N28.89
　cystica N28.86
　due to calculus N20.1
　　with calculus, kidney N20.2
　　　with hydronephrosis N13.2
　gonococcal (acute) (chronic) A54.21
　nonspecific N28.89
Ureterocele N28.89
　congenital (orthotopic) Q62.31
　ectopic Q62.32
Ureterolith, ureterolithiasis —*see* Calculus, ureter
Ureterostomy
　attention to Z43.6

status Z93.6
Urethra, urethral —*see* condition
Urethralgia R39.89
Urethritis (anterior) (posterior) N34.2
　calculous N21.1
　candidal B37.41
　chlamydial A56.01
　diplococcal (gonococcal) A54.01
　　with abscess (accessory gland)
　　　(periurethral) A54.1
　gonococcal A54.01
　　with abscess (accessory gland)
　　　(periurethral) A54.1
　nongonococcal N34.1
　　Reiter's —*see* Reiter's disease
　nonspecific N34.1
　nonvenereal N34.1
　postmenopausal N34.2
　puerperal O86.22
　Reiter's —*see* Reiter's disease
　specified NEC N34.2
　trichomonal or due to Trichomonas
　　(vaginalis) A59.03
Urethrocele N81.0
　with
　　cystocele —*see* Cystocele
　　prolapse of uterus —*see* Prolapse, uterus
Urethrolithiasis (with colic or infection) N21.1
Urethrorectal —*see* condition
Urethrorrhagia N36.8
Urethrorrhea R36.9
Urethrostomy
　attention to Z43.6
　status Z93.6
Urethrotrigonitis —*see* Trigonitis
Urethrovaginal —*see* condition
Urgency
　fecal R15.2
　hypertensive —*see* Hypertension
　urinary N39.15
Urhidrosis, uridrosis L74.8
Uric acid in blood (increased) E79.0
Uricacidemia (asymptomatic) E79.0
Uricemia (asymptomatic) E79.0
Uricosuria R82.998
Urinary —*see* condition
Urination
　frequent R35.0
　painful R30.9
Urine
　blood in —*see* Hematuria
➡discharge, excessive R35.89
　enuresis, nonorganic origin F98.0
　extravasation R39.0
　frequency R35.0
　incontinence R32
　　nonorganic origin F98.0
　intermittent stream R39.198
　pus in N39.0
　retention or stasis R33.9
　　organic R33.8
　　　drug-induced R33.0
　　psychogenic F45.8
　secretion
　　deficient R34
➡　excessive R35.89
　　frequency R35.0
　stream
　　intermittent R39.198
　　slowing R39.198
　　splitting R39.13
　　weak R39.12
Urinemia —*see* Uremia
Urinoma, urethra N36.8
Uroarthritis, infectious (Reiter's) —*see* Reiter's
　disease
Urodialysis R34
Urolithiasis —*see* Calculus, urinary
Uronephrosis —*see* Hydronephrosis
Uropathy N39.9
　obstructive N13.9

　　specified NEC N13.8
Uropathy (Continued)
　reflux N13.9
　　specified NEC N13.8
　vesicoureteral reflux-associated —*see* Reflux,
　　vesicoureteral
Urosepsis — code to condition
Urticaria L50.9
　with angioneurotic edema T78.3
　　hereditary D84.1
　allergic L50.0
　cholinergic L50.5
　chronic L50.8
　cold, familial L50.2
　contact L50.6
　dermatographic L50.3
　due to
　　cold or heat L50.2
　　drugs L50.0
　　food L50.0
　　inhalants L50.0
　　plants L50.6
　　serum —*see also* Reaction, serum
　　　T80.69
　factitial L50.3
　familial cold M04.2
　giant T78.3
　　hereditary D84.1
　gigantea T78.3
　idiopathic L50.1
　larynx T78.3
　　hereditary D84.1
　neonatorum P83.88
　nonallergic L50.1
　papulosa (Hebra) L28.2
　pigmentosa D47.01
　　congenital Q82.2
　　of neonatal onset Q82.2
　　of newborn onset Q82.2
　recurrent periodic L50.8
　serum —*see also* Reaction, serum T80.69
　solar L56.3
　specified type NEC L50.8
　thermal (cold) (heat) L50.2
　vibratory L50.4
　xanthelasmoidea —*see* Urticaria pigmentosa
Use (of)
　alcohol Z72.89
　　with
　　　intoxication F10.929
　　　sleep disorder F10.982
　　　withdrawal F10.939
　　　　with
　　　　　perceptual disturbance F10.932
　　　　delirium F10.931
　　　　uncomplicated F10.930
　　harmful —*see* Abuse, alcohol
　amphetamines —*see* Use, stimulant NEC
　caffeine —*see* Use, stimulant NEC
　cannabis F12.90
　　with
　　　anxiety disorder F12.980
　　　intoxication F12.929
　　　　with
　　　　　delirium F12.921
　　　　　perceptual disturbance F12.922
　　　　uncomplicated F12.920
　　　other specified disorder F12.988
　　　psychosis F12.959
　　　　delusions F12.950
　　　　hallucinations F12.951
　　　unspecified disorder F12.99
　　　withdrawal F12.93
　cocaine F14.90
　　with
　　　anxiety disorder F14.980
　　　intoxication F14.929
　　　　with
　　　　　delirium F14.921
　　　　　perceptual disturbance F14.922
　　　　uncomplicated F14.920

▶ New　　⇛ Revised　　~~deleted~~ Deleted　　● Use Additional Character(s)

other specified disorder F14.988
Use *(Continued)*
  cocaine *(Continued)*
    with *(Continued)*
      psychosis F14.959
        delusions F14.950
        hallucinations F14.951
      sexual dysfunction F14.981
      sleep disorder F14.982
      unspecified disorder F14.99
      withdrawal F14.93
    harmful —*see* Abuse, drug, cocaine
  drug(s) NEC F19.90
    with sleep disorder F19.982
    harmful —*see* Abuse, drug, by type
  hallucinogen NEC F16.90
    with
      anxiety disorder F16.980
      intoxication F16.929
        with
          delirium F16.921
        uncomplicated F16.920
      mood disorder F16.94
      other specified disorder F16.988
      perception disorder (flashbacks) F16.983
      psychosis F16.959
        delusions F16.950
        hallucinations F16.951
      unspecified disorder F16.99
    harmful —*see* Abuse, drug, hallucinogen NEC
  inhalants F18.90
    with
      anxiety disorder F18.980
      intoxication F18.929
        with delirium F18.921
        uncomplicated F18.920
      mood disorder F18.94
      other specified disorder F18.988
      persisting dementia F18.97
      psychosis F18.959
        delusions F18.950
        hallucinations F18.951
      unspecified disorder F18.99
    harmful —*see* Abuse, drug, inhalant
  methadone —*see* Use, opioid
  nonprescribed drugs F19.90
    harmful —*see* Abuse, non-psychoactive substance
  opioid F11.90
    with
      disorder F11.99
        mood F11.94
        sleep F11.982
        specified type NEC F11.988
      intoxication F11.929
        with
          delirium F11.921
          perceptual disturbance F11.922
        uncomplicated F11.920
      withdrawal F11.93

harmful —*see* Abuse, drug, opioid
Use *(Continued)*
  patent medicines F19.90
    harmful —*see* Abuse, non-psychoactive substance
  psychoactive drug NEC F19.90
    with
      anxiety disorder F19.980
      intoxication F19.929
        with
          delirium F19.921
          perceptual disturbance F19.922
        uncomplicated F19.920
      mood disorder F19.94
      other specified disorder F19.988
      persisting
        amnestic disorder F19.96
        dementia F19.97
      psychosis F19.959
        delusions F19.950
        hallucinations F19.951
      sexual dysfunction F19.981
      sleep disorder F19.982
      unspecified disorder F19.99
      withdrawal F19.939
        with
          delirium F19.931
          perceptual disturbance F19.932
        uncomplicated F19.930
    harmful —*see* Abuse, drug NEC, psychoactive NEC
  sedative, hypnotic, or anxiolytic F13.90
    with
      anxiety disorder F13.980
      intoxication F13.929
        with
          delirium F13.921
        uncomplicated F13.920
      other specified disorder F13.988
      persisting
        amnestic disorder F13.96
        dementia F13.97
      psychosis F13.959
        delusions F13.950
        hallucinations F13.951
      sexual dysfunction F13.981
      sleep disorder F13.982
      unspecified disorder F13.99
    harmful —*see* Abuse, drug, sedative, hypnotic, or anxiolytic
  stimulant NEC F15.90
    with
      anxiety disorder F15.980
      intoxication F15.929
        with
          delirium F15.921
          perceptual disturbance F15.922

uncomplicated F15.920
Use *(Continued)*
  stimulant NEC *(Continued)*
    with *(Continued)*
      mood disorder F15.94
      other specified disorder F15.988
      psychosis F15.959
        delusions F15.950
        hallucinations F15.951
      sexual dysfunction F15.981
      sleep disorder F15.982
      unspecified disorder F15.99
      withdrawal F15.93
    harmful —*see* Abuse, drug, stimulant NEC
  tobacco Z72.0
    with dependence —*see* Dependence, drug, nicotine
  volatile solvents —*see also* Use, inhalant F18.90
    harmful —*see* Abuse, drug, inhalant
Usher-Senear disease or syndrome L10.4
Uta B55.1
Uteromegaly N85.2
Uterovaginal —*see* condition
Uterovesical —*see* condition
Uveal —*see* condition
Uveitis (anterior) —*see also* Iridocyclitis
  acute —*see* Iridocyclitis, acute
  chronic —*see* Iridocyclitis, chronic
  due to toxoplasmosis (acquired) B58.09
    congenital P37.1
  granulomatous —*see* Iridocyclitis, chronic
  heterochromic —*see* Cyclitis, Fuchs' heterochromic
  lens-induced —*see* Iridocyclitis, lens-induced
  posterior —*see* Chorioretinitis
  sympathetic H44.13- ●
  syphilitic (secondary) A51.43
    congenital (early) A50.01
    late A52.71
  tuberculous A18.54
Uveoencephalitis —*see* Inflammation, chorioretinal
Uveokeratitis —*see* Iridocyclitis
Uveoparotitis D86.89
Uvula —*see* condition
Uvulitis (acute) (catarrhal) (chronic) (membranous) (suppurative) (ulcerative) K12.2

V

Vaccination (prophylactic)
  complication or reaction —*see* Complications, vaccination
  delayed Z28.9
  encounter for Z23
  not done —*see* Immunization, not done, because (of)
Vaccinia (generalized) (localized) T88.1
  without vaccination B08.011
  congenital P35.8
Vacuum, in sinus (accessory) (nasal) J34.89
Vagabond, vagabondage Z59.00
Vagabond's disease B85.1
Vagina, vaginal —*see* condition
Vaginalitis (tunica) (testis) N49.1
Vaginismus (reflex) N94.2
  functional F52.5
  nonorganic F52.5
  psychogenic F52.5
  secondary N94.2
Vaginitis (acute) (circumscribed) (diffuse) (emphysematous) (nonvenereal) (ulcerative) N76.0
  with ectopic or molar pregnancy O08.0
  amebic A06.82
  atrophic, postmenopausal N95.2
  bacterial N76.0
  blennorrhagic (gonococcal) A54.02
  candidal B37.3
  chlamydial A56.02
  chronic N76.1
  due to Trichomonas (vaginalis) A59.01
  following ectopic or molar pregnancy O08.0
  gonococcal A54.02
    with abscess (accessory gland) (periurethral) A54.1
  granuloma A58
  in (due to)
    candidiasis B37.3
    herpesviral (herpes simplex) infection A60.04
    pinworm infection B80 [N77.1]
  monilial B37.3
  mycotic (candidal) B37.3
  postmenopausal atrophic N95.2
  puerperal (postpartum) O86.13
  senile (atrophic) N95.2
  subacute or chronic N76.1
  syphilitic (early) A51.0
    late A52.76
  trichomonal A59.01
  tuberculous A18.18
Vaginosis —*see* Vaginitis
Vagotonia G52.2
Vagrancy Z59.00
VAIN —*see* Neoplasia, intraepithelial, vagina
Vallecula —*see* condition
Valley fever B38.0
Valsuani's disease —*see* Anemia, obstetric
Valve, valvular (formation) —*see also* condition
  cerebral ventricle (communicating) in situ Z98.2
  cervix, internal os Q51.828
  congenital NEC —*see* Atresia, by site
  ureter (pelvic junction) (vesical orifice) Q62.39
  urethra (congenital) (posterior) Q64.2
Valvulitis (chronic) —*see* Endocarditis
Valvulopathy —*see* Endocarditis
Van Bogaert's leukoencephalopathy (sclerosing) (subacute) A81.1
Van Bogaert-Scherer-Epstein disease or syndrome E75.5
Van Buchem's syndrome M85.2
Van Creveld-von Gierke disease E74.01
Van der Hoeve (-de Kleyn) syndrome Q78.0
Van der Woude's syndrome Q38.0
Van Neck's disease or osteochondrosis M91.0
Vanishing lung J44.9

Vapor asphyxia or suffocation T59.9
  specified agent —*see* Table of Drugs and Chemicals
Variance, lethal ball, prosthetic heart valve T82.09
Variants, thalassemic D56.8
Variations in hair color L67.1
Varicella B01.9
  with
    complications NEC B01.89
    encephalitis B01.11
    encephalomyelitis B01.11
    meningitis B01.0
    myelitis B01.12
    pneumonia B01.2
  congenital P35.8
Varices —*see* Varix
Varicocele (scrotum) (thrombosed) I86.1
  ovary I86.2
  perineum I86.3
  spermatic cord (ulcerated) I86.1
Varicose
  aneurysm (ruptured) I77.0
  dermatitis —*see* Varix, leg, with, inflammation
  eczema —*see* Varix, leg, with, inflammation
  phlebitis —*see* Varix, with, inflammation
  tumor —*see* Varix
  ulcer (lower limb, any part) —*see also* Varix, leg, with, ulcer
    anus —*see also* Hemorrhoids K64.8
    esophagus —*see* Varix, esophagus
    inflamed or infected —*see* Varix, leg, with ulcer, with inflammation
    nasal septum I86.8
    perineum I86.3
    scrotum I86.1
    specified site NEC I86.8
  vein —*see* Varix
  vessel —*see* Varix, leg
Varicosis, varicosities, varicosity —*see* Varix
Variola (major) (minor) B03
Varioloid B03
Varix (lower limb) I83.90
  with
    bleeding I83.899
    edema I83.899
    inflammation I83.10
      with ulcer (venous) I83.209
    pain I83.819
    rupture I83.899
    specified complication NEC I83.899
    stasis dermatitis I83.10
      with ulcer (venous) I83.209
    swelling I83.899
    ulcer I83.009
      with inflammation I83.209
  aneurysmal I77.0
  asymptomatic I83.9-●
  bladder I86.2
  broad ligament I86.2
  complicating
    childbirth (lower extremity) O87.4
      anus or rectum O87.2
      genital (vagina, vulva or perineum) O87.8
    pregnancy (lower extremity) O22.0-●
      anus or rectum O22.4-●
      genital (vagina, vulva or perineum) O22.1-●
    puerperium (lower extremity) O87.4
      anus or rectum O87.2
      genital (vagina, vulva, perineum) O87.8
  congenital (any site) Q27.8
  esophagus (idiopathic) (primary) (ulcerated) I85.00
    bleeding I85.01
    congenital Q27.8
    in (due to)
      alcoholic liver disease I85.10
        bleeding I85.11
      cirrhosis of liver I85.10
        bleeding I85.11

Varix (*Continued*)
  esophagus (*Continued*)
    in (*Continued*)
      portal hypertension I85.10
        bleeding I85.11
      schistosomiasis I85.10
        bleeding I85.11
      toxic liver disease I85.10
        bleeding I85.11
    secondary I85.10
      bleeding I85.11
  gastric I86.4
  inflamed or infected I83.10
    ulcerated I83.209
  labia (majora) I86.3
  leg (asymptomatic) I83.9-●
    with
      edema I83.899
      inflammation I83.10
        with ulcer —*see* Varix, leg, with, ulcer, with inflammation by site
      pain I83.819
      specified complication NEC I83.899
      swelling I83.899
      ulcer I83.0-●
        with inflammation I83.2-●
          ankle I83.003
            with inflammation I83.203
          calf I83.002
            with inflammation I83.202
          foot NEC I83.005
            with inflammation I83.205
          heel I83.004
            with inflammation I83.204
          lower leg NEC I83.008
            with inflammation I83.208
          midfoot I83.004
            with inflammation I83.204
          thigh I83.001
            with inflammation I83.201
    bilateral (asymptomatic) I83.93
      with
        edema I83.893
        pain I83.813
        specified complication NEC I83.893
        swelling I83.893
        ulcer I83.0-●
          with inflammation I83.209
    left (asymptomatic) I83.92
      with
        edema I83.892
        inflammation I83.12
          with ulcer —*see* Varix, leg, with, ulcer, with inflammation by site
        pain I83.812
        specified complication NEC I83.892
        swelling I83.892
        ulcer I83.029
          with inflammation I83.229
          ankle I83.023
            with inflammation I83.223
          calf I83.022
            with inflammation I83.222
          foot NEC I83.025
            with inflammation I83.225
          heel I83.024
            with inflammation I83.224
          lower leg NEC I83.028
            with inflammation I83.228
          midfoot I83.024
            with inflammation I83.224
          thigh I83.021
            with inflammation I83.221
    right (asymptomatic) I83.91
      with
        edema I83.891
        inflammation I83.11
          with ulcer —*see* Varix, leg, with, ulcer, with inflammation by site

▶ New   ➡ Revised   ~~deleted~~ Deleted   ● Use Additional Character(s)

Varix *(Continued)*
  leg *(Continued)*
    right *(Continued)*
      with *(Continued)*
        pain I83.811
        specified complication NEC I83.891
        swelling I83.891
        ulcer I83.019
          with inflammation I83.219
          ankle I83.013
            with inflammation I83.213
          calf I83.012
            with inflammation I83.212
          foot NEC I83.015
            with inflammation I83.215
          heel I83.014
            with inflammation I83.214
          lower leg NEC I83.018
            with inflammation I83.218
          midfoot I83.014
            with inflammation I83.214
          thigh I83.011
            with inflammation I83.211
  nasal septum I86.8
  orbit I86.8
    congenital Q27.8
  ovary I86.2
  papillary I78.1
  pelvis I86.2
  perineum I86.3
  pharynx I86.8
  placenta O43.89-•
  renal papilla I86.8
  retina H35.09
  scrotum (ulcerated) I86.1
  sigmoid colon I86.8
  specified site NEC I86.8
  spinal (cord) (vessels) I86.8
  spleen, splenic (vein) (with phlebolith) I86.8
  stomach I86.4
  sublingual I86.0
  ulcerated I83.009
    inflamed or infected I83.209
  uterine ligament I86.2
  vagina I86.8
  vocal cord I86.8
  vulva I86.3
Vas deferens —*see* condition
Vas deferentitis N49.1
Vasa previa O69.4
  hemorrhage from, affecting newborn P50.0
Vascular —*see also* condition
  loop on optic papilla Q14.2
  spasm I73.9
  spider I78.1
Vascularization, cornea —*see*
  Neovascularization, cornea
Vasculitis I77.6
  allergic D69.0
  cryoglobulinemic D89.1
  disseminated I77.6
  hypocomplementemic M31.8
  kidney I77.89
▶leukocytoclastic M31.0
  livedoid L95.0
  nodular L95.8
  retina H35.06-•
  rheumatic —*see* Fever, rheumatic
  rheumatoid —*see* Rheumatoid, vasculitis
  skin (limited to) L95.9
    specified NEC L95.8
  systemic M31.8
Vasculopathy, necrotizing M31.9
  cardiac allograft T86.290
  specified NEC M31.8
Vasitis (nodosa) N49.1
  tuberculous A18.15
Vasodilation I73.9
Vasomotor —*see* condition
Vasoplasty, after previous sterilization Z31.0
  aftercare Z31.42

Vasospasm (vasoconstriction) I73.9
  cerebral (cerebrovascular) (artery) I67.848
    reversible I67.841
  coronary I20.1
  nerve
    arm —*see* Mononeuropathy, upper limb
    brachial plexus G54.0
    cervical plexus G54.2
    leg —*see* Mononeuropathy, lower limb
  peripheral NOS I73.9
  retina (artery) —*see* Occlusion, artery, retina
Vasospastic —*see* condition
Vasovagal attack (paroxysmal) R55
  psychogenic F45.8
VATER syndrome Q87.2
Vater's ampulla —*see* condition
Vegetation, vegetative
  adenoid (nasal fossa) J35.8
  endocarditis (acute) (any valve) (subacute) I33.0
  heart (mycotic) (valve) I33.0
Veil
  Jackson's Q43.3
Vein, venous —*see* condition
Veldt sore —*see* Ulcer, skin
Velpeau's hernia —*see* Hernia, femoral
Venereal
  bubo A55
  disease A64
  granuloma inguinale A58
  lymphogranuloma (Durand-Nicolas-Favre) A55
Venofibrosis I87.8
Venom, venomous —*see* Table of Drugs and Chemicals, by animal or substance, poisoning
Venous —*see* condition
Ventilator lung, newborn P27.8
Ventral —*see* condition
Ventricle, ventricular —*see also* condition
  escape I49.3
  inversion Q20.5
Ventriculitis (cerebral) —*see also* Encephalitis G04.90
Ventriculostomy status Z98.2
Vernet's syndrome G52.7
Verneuil's disease (syphilitic bursitis) A52.78
Verruca (due to HPV) (filiformis) (simplex) (viral) (vulgaris) B07.9
  acuminata A63.0
  necrogenica (primary) (tuberculosa) A18.4
  plana B07.8
  plantaris B07.0
  seborrheica L82.1
    inflamed L82.0
  senile (seborrheic) L82.1
    inflamed L82.0
  tuberculosa (primary) A18.4
  venereal A63.0
Verrucosities —*see* Verruca
Verruga peruana, peruviana A44.1
Version
  cervix —*see* Malposition, uterus
  uterus (postinfectional) (postpartal, old) —*see* Malposition, uterus
Vertebra, vertebral —*see* condition
Vertical talus (congenital) Q66.80
  left foot Q66.82
  right foot Q66.81
Vertigo R42
  auditory —*see* Vertigo, aural
  aural H81.31-•
  benign paroxysmal (positional) H81.1-•
  central (origin) H81.4
  cerebral H81.4
  Dix and Hallpike (epidemic) —*see* Neuronitis, vestibular
  due to infrasound T75.23

Vertigo *(Continued)*
  epidemic A88.1
    Dix and Hallpike —*see* Neuronitis, vestibular
    Pedersen's —*see* Neuronitis, vestibular
    vestibular neuronitis —*see* Neuronitis, vestibular
  hysterical F44.89
  infrasound T75.23
  labyrinthine —*see* subcategory H81.0
▶laryngeal R05.4
  malignant positional H81.4
  Ménière's —*see* subcategory H81.40
  menopausal N95.11
  otogenic —*see* Vertigo, aural
  paroxysmal positional, benign —*see* Vertigo, benign paroxysmal
  Pedersen's (epidemic) —*see* Neuronitis, vestibular
  peripheral NEC H81.39-•
  positional
    benign paroxysmal —*see* Vertigo, benign paroxysmal
    malignant H81.4
Very-low-density-lipoprotein-type (VLDL) hyperlipoproteinemia E78.1
Vesania —*see* Psychosis
Vesical —*see* condition
Vesicle
  cutaneous R23.8
  seminal —*see* condition
  skin R23.8
Vesicocolic —*see* condition
Vesicoperineal —*see* condition
Vesicorectal —*see* condition
Vesicourethrorectal —*see* condition
Vesicovaginal —*see* condition
Vesicular —*see* condition
Vesiculitis (seminal) N49.0
  amebic A06.82
  gonorrheal (acute) (chronic) A54.23
  trichomonal A59.09
  tuberculous A18.15
Vestibulitis (ear) —*see also* subcategory H83.0
  nose (external) J34.89
  vulvar N94.810
Vestibulopathy, acute peripheral (recurrent) —*see* Neuronitis, vestibular
Vestige, vestigial —*see also* Persistence
  branchial Q18.0
  structures in vitreous Q14.0
Vibration
  adverse effects T75.20
    pneumatic hammer syndrome T75.21
    specified effect NEC T75.29
    vasospastic syndrome T75.22
    vertigo from infrasound T75.23
  exposure (occupational) Z57.7
  vertigo T75.23
Vibriosis A28.9
Victim (of)
  crime Z65.4
  disaster Z65.5
  terrorism Z65.4
  torture Z65.4
  war Z65.5
Vidal's disease L28.0
Villaret's syndrome G52.7
Villous —*see* condition
VIN —*see* Neoplasia, intraepithelial, vulva
Vincent's infection (angina) (gingivitis) A69.1
  stomatitis NEC A69.1
Vinson-Plummer syndrome D50.1
Violence, physical R45.6
Viosterol deficiency —*see* Deficiency, calciferol
Vipoma —*see* Neoplasm, malignant, by site
Viremia B34.9
Virilism (adrenal) E25.9
  congenital E25.0
Virilization (female) (suprarenal) E25.9
  congenital E25.0
  isosexual E28.2

Virulent bubo A57
Virus, viral —*see also* condition
 as cause of disease classified elsewhere
  B97.89
  ⇒respiratory syncytial virus (RSV) —*see* Virus,
   infection, respiratory syncytial (RSV)
 cytomegalovirus B25.9
 human immunodeficiency (HIV) —*see*
  Human, immunodeficiency virus (HIV)
  disease
 infection —*see* Infection, virus
 respiratory syncytial (RSV)
  as cause of disease classified elsewhere
   B97.4
  bronchiolitis J21.0
  bronchitis J20.5
  bronchopneumonia J12.1
  otitis media H65-● [B97.4]
  pneumonia J12.1
  upper respiratory infection J06.9 [B97.4]
 specified NEC B34.8
 swine influenza (viruses that normally cause
   infections in pigs) —*see also* Influenza,
   due to, identified novel influenza A virus
   J09.X2
 West Nile (fever) A92.30
  with
   complications NEC A92.39
   cranial nerve disorders A92.32
   encephalitis A92.31
   encephalomyelitis A92.31
   neurologic manifestation NEC A92.32
   optic neuritis A92.32
   polyradiculitis A92.32
Viscera, visceral —*see* condition
Visceroptosis K63.4
Visible peristalsis R19.2
Vision, visual
 binocular, suppression H53.34
 blurred, blurring H53.8
  hysterical F44.6
 defect, defective NEC H54.7
 disorientation (syndrome) H53.8
 disturbance H53.9
  hysterical F44.6
 double H53.2
 examination Z01.00
  with abnormal findings Z01.01
  following failed vision screening Z01.020
   with abnormal findings Z01.021
 field, limitation (defect) —*see* Defect, visual
  field
 hallucinations R44.1
 halos H53.19
 loss —*see* Loss, vision
  sudden —*see* Disturbance, vision,
   subjective, loss, sudden
 low (both eyes) —*see* Low, vision
 perception, simultaneous without fusion
  H53.33
Vitality, lack or want of R53.83
 newborn P96.89
Vitamin deficiency —*see* Deficiency, vitamin

Vitelline duct, persistent Q43.0
Vitiligo L80
 eyelid H02.739
  left H02.736
   lower H02.735
   upper H02.734
  right H02.733
   lower H02.732
   upper H02.731
 pinta A67.2
 vulva N90.89
Vitreal corneal syndrome H59.01-●
Vitreoretinopathy, proliferative —*see also*
  Retinopathy, proliferative
 with retinal detachment —*see* Detachment,
  retina, traction
Vitreous —*see also* condition
 touch syndrome —*see* Complication,
  postprocedural, following cataract
  surgery
Vocal cord —*see* condition
Vogt-Koyanagi syndrome H20.82-●
Vogt's disease or syndrome G80.3
Vogt-Spielmeyer amaurotic idiocy or disease
  E75.4
Voice
 change R49.9
  specified NEC R49.8
 loss —*see* Aphonia
Volhynian fever A79.0
Volkmann's ischemic contracture or paralysis
  (complicating trauma) T79.6
Volvulus (bowel) (colon) (intestine) K56.2
 with perforation K56.2
 congenital Q43.8
 duodenum K31.5
 fallopian tube —*see* Torsion, fallopian tube
 oviduct —*see* Torsion, fallopian tube
 stomach (due to absence of gastrocolic
  ligament) K31.89
Vomiting R11.10
 with nausea R11.2
 without nausea R11.11
 asphyxia —*see* Foreign body, by site, causing
  asphyxia, gastric contents
 bilious (cause unknown) R11.14
  following gastro-intestinal surgery K91.0
  in newborn P92.01
 blood —*see* Hematemesis
 causing asphyxia, choking, or suffocation —
  see Foreign body, by site
 cyclical, in migraine G43.A0
  with refractory migraine G43.A1
  intractable G43.A1
  not intractable G43.A0
  psychogenic F50.89
  without refractory migraine G43.A0
 cyclical syndrome NOS (unrelated to
  migraine) R53.1
  persistent R11.15

Vomiting (Continued)
 fecal mater R11.13
 following gastrointestinal surgery K91.0
  psychogenic F50.89
 functional K31.89
 hysterical F50.89
 nervous F50.89
 neurotic F50.89
 newborn NEC P92.09
  bilious P92.01
 periodic R11.10
  psychogenic F50.89
 projectile R11.12
 psychogenic F50.89
 uremic —*see* Uremia
Vomito negro —*see* Fever, yellow
Von Bezold's abscess —*see* Mastoiditis, acute
Von Economo-Cruchet disease A85.8
Von Eulenburg's disease G71.19
Von Gierke's disease E74.01
Von Hippel (-Lindau) disease or syndrome
  Q85.8
Von Jaksch's anemia or disease D64.89
Von Recklinghausen
 disease (neurofibromatosis) Q85.01
 bones E21.0
Von Schroetter's syndrome I82.890
Von Willebrand (-Jurgens)(-Minot) disease or
  syndrome D68.0
Von Zumbusch's disease L40.1
Voyeurism F65.3
Vrolik's disease Q78.0
Vulva —*see* condition
Vulvismus N94.2
Vulvitis (acute) (allergic) (atrophic)
  (hypertrophic) (intertriginous) (senile)
  N76.2
 with ectopic or molar pregnancy O08.0
 adhesive, congenital Q52.79
 blennorrhagic (gonococcal) A54.02
 candidal B37.3
 chlamydial A56.02
 due to Haemophilus ducreyi A57
 following ectopic or molar pregnancy O08.0
 gonococcal A54.02
  with abscess (accessory gland)
   (periurethral) A54.1
 herpesviral A60.04
 leukoplakic N90.4
 monilial B37.3
 puerperal (postpartum) O86.19
 subacute or chronic N76.3
 syphilitic (early) A51.0
  late A52.76
 trichomonal A59.01
 tuberculous A18.18
Vulvodynia N94.819
 specified NEC N94.818
Vulvorectal —*see* condition
Vulvovaginitis (acute) —*see* Vaginitis

W

Waiting list, person on Z75.1
  for organ transplant Z76.82
  undergoing social agency investigation Z75.2
Waldenström
  hypergammaglobulinemia D89.0
  syndrome or macroglobulinemia C88.0
Waldenström-Kjellberg syndrome D50.1
Walking
  difficulty R26.2
    psychogenic F44.4
  sleep F51.3
    hysterical F44.89
Wall, abdominal —see condition
Wallenberg's disease or syndrome G46.3
Wallgren's disease I87.8
Wandering
  gallbladder, congenital Q44.1
  in diseases classified elsewhere Z91.83
  kidney, congenital Q63.8
  organ or site, congenital NEC —see
    Malposition, congenital, by site
  pacemaker (heart) I49.8
  spleen D73.89
War neurosis F48.8
Wart (due to HPV) (filiform) (infectious)
  (viral) B07.9
  anogenital region (venereal) A63.0
  common B07.8
  external genital organs (venereal)
    A63.0
  flat B07.8
  Hassal-Henle's (of cornea) H18.49
  Peruvian A44.1
  plantar B07.0
  prosector (tuberculous) A18.4
  seborrheic L82.1
    inflamed L82.0
  senile (seborrheic) L82.1
    inflamed L82.0
  tuberculous A18.4
  venereal A63.0
Warthin's tumor —see Neoplasm, salivary
  gland, benign
Wassilieff's disease A27.0
Wasting
  disease R64
  ➨due to malnutrition E43
  ▶with marasmus E41
  ➨extreme (due to malnutrition) E43
  ▶with marasmus E41
  muscle NEC —see Atrophy, muscle
Water
  clefts (senile cataract) —see Cataract, senile,
    incipient
  deprivation of T73.1
  intoxication E87.79
  itch B76.9
  lack of T73.1
  ▶safe drinking Z58.6
  loading E87.70
  on
    brain —see Hydrocephalus
    chest J94.8
  poisoning E87.79
Waterbrash R12
Waterhouse(-Friderichsen) syndrome or
  disease (meningococcal) A39.1
Water-losing nephritis N25.89
Watermelon stomach K31.819
  with hemorrhage K31.811
  without hemorrhage K31.819
Watsoniasis B66.8
Wax in ear —see Impaction, cerumen
Weak, weakening, weakness (generalized)
  R53.1
  arches (acquired) —see also Deformity, limb,
    flat foot
  bladder (sphincter) R32

Weak, weakening, weakness (Continued)
  facial R29.810
    following
      cerebrovascular disease I69.992
        cerebral infarction I69.392
        intracerebral hemorrhage I69.192
        nontraumatic intracranial hemorrhage
          NEC I69.292
        specified disease NEC I69.892
        stroke I69.392
        subarachnoid hemorrhage I69.092
  foot (double) —see also Weak, arches
  heart, cardiac —see Failure, heart
  mind F70
  muscle M62.81
  myocardium —see Failure, heart
  newborn P96.89
  pelvic fundus N81.89
  pubocervical tissue N81.82
  rectovaginal tissue N81.83
  senile R54
  urinary stream R39.12
  valvular —see Endocarditis
Wear, worn (with normal or routine use)
  articular bearing surface of internal joint
    prosthesis —see Complications, joint
    prosthesis, mechanical, wear of articular
    bearing surfaces, by site
  device, implant or graft —see Complications,
    by site, mechanical complication
  tooth, teeth (approximal) (hard tissues)
    (interproximal) (occlusal) K03.0
Weather, weathered
  effects of
    cold T69.9
      specified effect NEC T69.8
    hot —see Heat
  skin L57.8
Weaver's syndrome Q87.3
Web, webbed (congenital)
  duodenal Q43.8
  esophagus Q39.4
  fingers Q70.1
  larynx (glottic) (subglottic) Q31.0
  neck (pterygium colli) Q18.3
  Paterson-Kelly D50.1
  popliteal syndrome Q87.89
  toes Q70.3
Weber-Christian disease M35.6
Weber-Cockayne syndrome (epidermolysis
  bullosa) Q81.8
Weber-Gubler syndrome G46.3
Weber-Leyden syndrome G46.3
Weber-Osler syndrome I78.0
Weber's paralysis or syndrome G46.3
Wedge-shaped or wedging vertebra —see
  Collapse, vertebra NEC
Wegener's granulomatosis or syndrome
  M31.30
  with
    kidney involvement M31.31
    lung involvement M31.30
      with kidney involvement M31.31
Wegner's disease A50.02
Weight
  1000-2499 grams at birth (low) —see Low,
    birthweight
  999 grams or less at birth (extremely low) —
    see Low, birthweight, extreme
  and length below 10th percentile for
    gestational age P05.1-●
  below but length above 10th percentile for
    gestational age P05.0-●
  gain (abnormal) (excessive) R63.5
    in pregnancy —see Pregnancy, complicated
      by, excessive weight gain
    low —see Pregnancy, complicated by,
      insufficient, weight gain
  loss (abnormal) (cause unknown) R63.4
Weightlessness (effect of) T75.82

Weil (l)-Marchesani syndrome Q87.19
Weil's disease A27.0
Weingarten's syndrome J82.89
Weir Mitchell's disease I73.81
Weiss-Baker syndrome G90.09
Wells' disease L98.3
Wen —see Cyst, sebaceous
Wenckebach's block or phenomenon I44.1
Werdnig-Hoffmann syndrome (muscular
  atrophy) G12.0
Werlhof's disease D69.3
Werner-His disease A79.0
Wermer's disease or syndrome E31.21
Werner's disease or syndrome E34.8
Wernicke-Korsakoff's syndrome or psychosis
  (alcoholic) F10.96
  with dependence F10.26
  drug-induced
    due to drug abuse —see Abuse, drug, by
      type, with amnestic disorder
    due to drug dependence —see
      Dependence, drug, by type, with
      amnestic disorder
  nonalcoholic F04
Wernicke-Posadas disease B38.9
Wernicke's
  developmental aphasia F80.2
  disease or syndrome E51.2
  encephalopathy E51.2
  polioencephalitis, superior E51.2
West African fever B50.8
Westphal-Strümpell syndrome E83.01
West's syndrome —see Epilepsy, spasms
Wet
  feet, tropical (maceration) (syndrome) —see
    Immersion, foot
  lung (syndrome), newborn P22.1
Wharton's duct —see condition
Wheal —see Urticaria
Wheezing R06.2
Whiplash injury S13.4
Whipple's disease —see also subcategory
  M14.8-● K90.81
Whipworm (disease) (infection) (infestation)
  B79
Whistling face Q87.0
White —see also condition
  kidney, small N03.9
  leg, puerperal, postpartum, childbirth O87.1
  mouth B37.0
  patches of mouth K13.29
  spot lesions, teeth
    chewing surface K02.51
    pit and fissure surface K02.51
    smooth surface K02.61
Whitehead L70.0
Whitlow —see also Cellulitis, digit
  with lymphangitis —see Lymphangitis, acute,
    digit
  herpesviral B00.89
Whitmore's disease or fever —see Melioidosis
Whooping cough A37.90
  with pneumonia A37.91
  due to Bordetella
    bronchiseptica A37.81
    parapertussis A37.11
    pertussis A37.01
    specified organism NEC A37.81
  due to
    Bordetella
      bronchiseptica A37.80
        with pneumonia A37.81
      parapertussis A37.10
        with pneumonia A37.11
      pertussis A37.00
        with pneumonia A37.01
      specified NEC A37.80
        with pneumonia A37.81
Wichman's asthma J38.5
Wide cranial sutures, newborn P96.3

Widening aorta —*see* Ectasia, aorta
  with aneurysm —*see* Aneurysm, aorta
Wilkie's disease or syndrome K55.1
Wilkinson-Sneddon disease or syndrome
    L13.1
Willebrand (-Jürgens) thrombopathy D68.0
Williams syndrome Q93.82
Willige-Hunt disease or syndrome G23.1
Wilms' tumor C64-●
Wilson-Mikity syndrome P27.0
Wilson's
  disease or syndrome E83.01
  hepatolenticular degeneration E83.01
  lichen ruber L43.9
Window —*see also* Imperfect, closure
  aorticopulmonary Q21.4
Winter —*see* condition
Wiskott-Aldrich syndrome D82.0
Withdrawal state —*see also* Dependence, drug
    by type, with withdrawal
  alcohol
    with perceptual disturbances F10.232
    without perceptual disturbances F10.239
  caffeine F15.93
  cannabis F12.23
  newborn
    correct therapeutic substance properly
        administered P96.2
    infant of dependent mother P96.1
  therapeutic substance, neonatal P96.2
Witts' anemia D50.8
Witzelsucht F07.0
Woakes' ethmoiditis or syndrome J33.1
Wolff-Hirschorn syndrome Q93.3
Wolff-Parkinson-White syndrome I45.6
Wolhynian fever A79.0
Wolman's disease E75.5
Wood lung or pneumonitis J67.8
Woolly, wooly hair (congenital) (nevus) Q84.1
Woolsorter's disease A22.1
Word
  blindness (congenital) (developmental)
      F81.0
  deafness (congenital) (developmental)
      H93.25
Worm(s) (infection) (infestation) —*see also*
    Infestation, helminth
  guinea B72
  in intestine NEC B82.0
Worm-eaten soles A66.3
Worn out —*see* Exhaustion
  cardiac
    defibrillator (with synchronous cardiac
        pacemaker) Z45.02
    pacemaker
      battery Z45.010
      lead Z45.018
    device, implant or graft —*see* Complications,
        by site, mechanical
Worried well Z71.1
Worries R45.82
Wound check Z48.0-●
  due to injury - code to Injury, by site, using
      appropriate seventh character for
      subsequent encounter
Wound, open T14.8-●
  abdomen, abdominal
    wall S31.109
      with penetration into peritoneal cavity
          S31.609
      bite —*see* Bite, abdomen, wall
      epigastric region S31.102
        with penetration into peritoneal cavity
            S31.602
        bite —*see* Bite, abdomen, wall,
            epigastric region
        laceration —*see* Laceration, abdomen,
            wall, epigastric region
        puncture —*see* Puncture, abdomen,
            wall, epigastric region

Wound, open *(Continued)*
  abdomen, abdominal *(Continued)*
    wall *(Continued)*
      laceration —*see* Laceration, abdomen, wall
      left
        lower quadrant S31.104
          with penetration into peritoneal
              cavity S31.604
          bite —*see* Bite, abdomen, wall, left,
              lower quadrant
          laceration —*see* Laceration, abdomen,
              wall, left, lower quadrant
          puncture —*see* Puncture, abdomen,
              wall, left, lower quadrant
        upper quadrant S31.101
          with penetration into peritoneal
              cavity S31.601
          bite —*see* Bite, abdomen, wall, left,
              upper quadrant
          laceration —*see* Laceration,
              abdomen, wall, left, upper
              quadrant
          puncture —*see* Puncture, abdomen,
              wall, left, upper quadrant
      periumbilic region S31.105
        with penetration into peritoneal cavity
            S31.605
        bite —*see* Bite, abdomen, wall,
            periumbilic region
        laceration —*see* Laceration, abdomen,
            wall, periumbilic region
        puncture —*see* Puncture, abdomen,
            wall, periumbilic region
      puncture —*see* Puncture, abdomen,
          wall
      right
        lower quadrant S31.103
          with penetration into peritoneal
              cavity S31.603
          bite —*see* Bite, abdomen, wall, right,
              lower quadrant
          laceration —*see* Laceration,
              abdomen, wall, right, lower
              quadrant
          puncture —*see* Puncture, abdomen,
              wall, right, lower quadrant
        upper quadrant S31.100
          with penetration into peritoneal
              cavity S31.600
          bite —*see* Bite, abdomen, wall, right,
              upper quadrant
          laceration —*see* Laceration,
              abdomen, wall, right, upper
              quadrant
          puncture —*see* Puncture, abdomen,
              wall, right, upper quadrant
  alveolar (process) —*see* Wound, open, oral
      cavity
  ankle S91.00-●
    bite —*see* Bite, ankle
    laceration —*see* Laceration, ankle
    puncture —*see* Puncture, ankle
  antecubital space —*see* Wound, open, elbow
  anterior chamber, eye —*see* Wound, open,
      ocular
  anus S31.839
    bite S31.835
    laceration —*see* Laceration, anus
    puncture —*see* Puncture, anus
  arm (upper) S41.10-●
    with amputation —*see* Amputation,
        traumatic, arm
    bite —*see* Bite, arm
    forearm —*see* Wound, open, forearm
    laceration —*see* Laceration, arm
    puncture —*see* Puncture, arm
  auditory canal (external) (meatus) —*see*
      Wound, open, ear
  auricle, ear —*see* Wound, open, ear
  axilla —*see* Wound, open, arm

Wound, open *(Continued)*
  back —*see also* Wound, open, thorax, back
    lower S31.000
      with penetration into retroperitoneal
          space S31.001
      bite —*see* Bite, back, lower
      laceration —*see* Laceration, back, lower
      puncture —*see* Puncture, back, lower
  bite —*see* Bite
  blood vessel —*see* Injury, blood vessel
  breast S21.00-●
    with amputation —*see* Amputation,
        traumatic, breast
    bite —*see* Bite, breast
    laceration —*see* Laceration, breast
    puncture —*see* Puncture, breast
  buttock S31.809
    bite —*see* Bite, buttock
    laceration —*see* Laceration, buttock
    left S31.829
    puncture —*see* Puncture, buttock
    right S31.819
  calf —*see* Wound, open, leg
  canaliculus lacrimalis —*see* Wound, open,
      eyelid
  canthus, eye —*see* Wound, open, eyelid
  cervical esophagus S11.20
    bite S11.25
    laceration —*see* Laceration, esophagus,
        traumatic, cervical
    puncture —*see* Puncture, cervical
        esophagus
  cheek (external) S01.40-●
    bite —*see* Bite, cheek
    internal —*see* Wound, open, oral cavity
    laceration —*see* Laceration, cheek
    puncture —*see* Puncture, cheek
  chest wall —*see* Wound, open, thorax
  chin —*see* Wound, open, head, specified site
      NEC
  choroid —*see* Wound, open, ocular
  ciliary body (eye) —*see* Wound, open,
      ocular
  clitoris S31.40
    with amputation —*see* Amputation,
        traumatic, clitoris
    bite S31.45
    laceration —*see* Laceration, vulva
    puncture —*see* Puncture, vulva
  conjunctiva —*see* Wound, open, ocular
  cornea —*see* Wound, open, ocular
  costal region —*see* Wound, open, thorax
  Descemet's membrane —*see* Wound, open,
      ocular
  digit(s)
    foot —*see* Wound, open, toe
    hand —*see* Wound, open, finger
  ear (canal) (external) S01.30-●
    with amputation —*see* Amputation,
        traumatic, ear
    bite —*see* Bite, ear
    drum S09.2-●
    laceration —*see* Laceration, ear
    puncture —*see* Puncture, ear
  elbow S51.00-●
    bite —*see* Bite, elbow
    laceration —*see* Laceration, elbow
    puncture —*see* Puncture, elbow
  epididymis —*see* Wound, open, testis
  epigastric region S31.102
    with penetration into peritoneal cavity
        S31.602
    bite —*see* Bite, abdomen, wall, epigastric
        region
    laceration —*see* Laceration, abdomen, wall,
        epigastric region
    puncture —*see* Puncture, abdomen, wall,
        epigastric region
  epiglottis —*see* Wound, open, neck, specified
      site NEC

▶ New   ⇒ Revised   ~~deleted~~ Deleted   ● Use Additional Character(s)

Wound, open *(Continued)*
  esophagus (thoracic) S27.819
    cervical —*see* Wound, open, cervical
      esophagus
    laceration S27.813
    specified type NEC S27.818
  eye —*see* Wound, open, ocular
  eyeball —*see* Wound, open, ocular
  eyebrow —*see* Wound, open, eyelid
  eyelid S01.10-●
    bite —*see* Bite, eyelid
    laceration —*see* Laceration, eyelid
    puncture —*see* Puncture, eyelid
  face NEC —*see* Wound, open, head, specified
    site NEC
  finger(s) S61.209
    with
      amputation —*see* Amputation,
        traumatic, finger
      damage to nail S61.309
    bite —*see* Bite, finger
    index S61.208
      with
        damage to nail S61.308
      left S61.201
        with
          damage to nail S61.301
      right S61.200
        with
          damage to nail S61.300
    laceration —*see* Laceration, finger
    little S61.208
      with
        damage to nail S61.308
      left S61.207
        with damage to nail S61.307
      right S61.206
        with damage to nail S61.306
    middle S61.208
      with
        damage to nail S61.308
      left S61.203
        with damage to nail S61.303
      right S61.202
        with damage to nail S61.302
    puncture —*see* Puncture, finger
    ring S61.208
      with
        damage to nail S61.308
      left S61.205
        with damage to nail S61.305
      right S61.204
        with damage to nail S61.304
  flank —*see* Wound, open, abdomen, wall
  foot (except toe(s) alone) S91.30-●
    with amputation —*see* Amputation,
      traumatic, foot
    bite —*see* Bite, foot
    laceration —*see* Laceration, foot
    puncture —*see* Puncture, foot
    toe —*see* Wound, open, toe
  forearm S51.80-●
    with
      amputation —*see* Amputation,
        traumatic, forearm
    bite —*see* Bite, forearm
    elbow only —*see* Wound, open, elbow
    laceration —*see* Laceration, forearm
    puncture —*see* Puncture, forearm
  forehead —*see* Wound, open, head, specified
    site NEC
  genital organs, external
    with amputation —*see* Amputation,
      traumatic, genital organs
    bite —*see* Bite, genital organ
    female S31.502
      vagina S31.40
      vulva S31.40
    laceration —*see* Laceration, genital
      organ

Wound, open *(Continued)*
  genital organs, external *(Continued)*
    male S31.501
      penis S31.20
      scrotum S31.30
      testes S31.30
    puncture —*see* Puncture, genital organ
  globe (eye) —*see* Wound, open, ocular
  groin —*see* Wound, open, abdomen, wall
  gum —*see* Wound, open, oral cavity
  hand S61.40-●
    with
      amputation —*see* Amputation,
        traumatic, hand
    bite —*see* Bite, hand
    finger(s) —*see* Wound, open, finger
    laceration —*see* Laceration, hand
    puncture —*see* Puncture, hand
    thumb —*see* Wound, open, thumb
  head S01.90
    bite —*see* Bite, head
    cheek —*see* Wound, open, cheek
    ear —*see* Wound, open, ear
    eyelid —*see* Wound, open, eyelid
    laceration —*see* Laceration, head
    lip —*see* Wound, open, lip
    nose S01.20
    oral cavity —*see* Wound, open, oral
      cavity
    puncture —*see* Puncture, head
    scalp —*see* Wound, open, scalp
    specified site NEC S01.80
    temporomandibular area —*see* Wound,
      open, cheek
  heel —*see* Wound, open, foot
  hip S71.00-●
    with amputation —*see* Amputation,
      traumatic, hip
    bite —*see* Bite, hip
    laceration —*see* Laceration, hip
    puncture —*see* Puncture, hip
  hymen S31.40
    bite —*see* Bite, vulva
    laceration —*see* Laceration, vagina
    puncture —*see* Puncture, vagina
  hypochondrium S31.109
    bite —*see* Bite, hypochondrium
    laceration —*see* Laceration,
      hypochondrium
    puncture —*see* Puncture, hypochondrium
  hypogastric region S31.109
    bite —*see* Bite, hypogastric region
    laceration —*see* Laceration, hypogastric
      region
    puncture —*see* Puncture, hypogastric
      region
  iliac (region) —*see* Wound, open, inguinal
    region
  inguinal region S31.109
    bite —*see* Bite, abdomen, wall, lower
      quadrant
    laceration —*see* Laceration, inguinal
      region
    puncture —*see* Puncture, inguinal
      region
  instep —*see* Wound, open, foot
  interscapular region —*see* Wound, open,
    thorax, back
  intraocular —*see* Wound, open, ocular
  iris —*see* Wound, open, ocular
  jaw —*see* Wound, open, head, specified site
    NEC
  knee S81.00-●
    bite —*see* Bite, knee
    laceration —*see* Laceration, knee
    puncture —*see* Puncture, knee
  labium (majus) (minus) —*see* Wound, open,
    vulva
  laceration —*see* Laceration, by site
  lacrimal duct —*see* Wound, open, eyelid

Wound, open *(Continued)*
  larynx S11.019
    bite —*see* Bite, larynx
    laceration —*see* Laceration, larynx
    puncture —*see* Puncture, larynx
  left
    lower quadrant S31.104
      with penetration into peritoneal cavity
        S31.604
      bite —*see* Bite, abdomen, wall, left, lower
        quadrant
      laceration —*see* Laceration, abdomen,
        wall, left, lower quadrant
      puncture —*see* Puncture, abdomen, wall,
        left, lower quadrant
    upper quadrant S31.101
      with penetration into peritoneal cavity
        S31.601
      bite —*see* Bite, abdomen, wall, left,
        upper quadrant
      laceration —*see* Laceration, abdomen,
        wall, left, upper quadrant
      puncture —*see* Puncture, abdomen, wall,
        left, upper quadrant
  leg (lower) S81.80-●
    with amputation —*see* Amputation,
      traumatic, leg
    ankle —*see* Wound, open, ankle
    bite —*see* Bite, leg
    foot —*see* Wound, open, foot
    knee —*see* Wound, open, knee
    laceration —*see* Laceration, leg
    puncture —*see* Puncture, leg
    toe —*see* Wound, open, toe
    upper —*see* Wound, open, thigh
  lip S01.501
    bite —*see* Bite, lip
    laceration —*see* Laceration, lip
    puncture —*see* Puncture, lip
  loin S31.109
    bite —*see* Bite, abdomen, wall
    laceration —*see* Laceration, loin
    puncture —*see* Puncture, loin
  lower back —*see* Wound, open, back,
    lower
  lumbar region —*see* Wound, open, back,
    lower
  malar region —*see* Wound, open, head,
    specified site NEC
  mammary —*see* Wound, open, breast
  mastoid region —*see* Wound, open, head,
    specified site NEC
  mouth —*see* Wound, open, oral cavity
  nail
    finger —*see* Wound, open, finger, with
      damage to nail
    toe —*see* Wound, open, toe, with damage
      to nail
  nape (neck) —*see* Wound, open, neck
  nasal (septum) (sinus) —*see* Wound, open,
    nose
  nasopharynx —*see* Wound, open, head,
    specified site NEC
  neck S11.90
    bite —*see* Bite, neck
    involving
      cervical esophagus S11.20
      larynx —*see* Wound, open, larynx
      pharynx S11.20
      thyroid S11.10
      trachea (cervical) S11.029
        bite —*see* Bite, trachea
        laceration S11.021
          with foreign body S11.022
        puncture S11.023
          with foreign body S11.024
    laceration —*see* Laceration, neck
    puncture —*see* Puncture, neck
    specified site NEC S11.80
      specified type NEC S11.89

Wound, open (*Continued*)
  nose (septum) (sinus) S01.20
    with amputation —*see* Amputation,
      traumatic, nose
    bite —*see* Bite, nose
    laceration —*see* Laceration, nose
    puncture —*see* Puncture, nose
  ocular S05.90
    avulsion (traumatic enucleation) S05.7-●
    eyeball S05.6-●
      with foreign body S05.5-●
    eyelid —*see* Wound, open, eyelid
    laceration and rupture S05.3-●
      with prolapse or loss of intraocular
        tissue S05.2-●
    orbit (penetrating) (with or without foreign
      body) S05.4-●
    periocular area —*see* Wound, open, eyelid
    specified NEC S05.8X-●
  oral cavity S01.502
    bite S01.552
    laceration —*see* Laceration, oral cavity
    puncture —*see* Puncture, oral cavity
  orbit —*see* Wound, open, ocular, orbit
  palate —*see* Wound, open, oral cavity
  palm —*see* Wound, open, hand
  pelvis, pelvic —*see also* Wound, open, back,
    lower
    girdle —*see* Wound, open, hip
  penetrating —*see* Puncture, by site
  penis S31.20
    with amputation —*see* Amputation,
      traumatic, penis
    bite S31.25
    laceration —*see* Laceration, penis
    puncture —*see* Puncture, penis
  perineum
    bite —*see* Bite, perineum
    female S31.502
    laceration —*see* Laceration, perineum
    male S31.501
    puncture —*see* Puncture, perineum
  periocular area (with or without lacrimal
    passages) —*see* Wound, open, eyelid
  periumbilic region S31.105
    with penetration into peritoneal cavity
      S31.605
    bite —*see* Bite, abdomen, wall, periumbilic
      region
    laceration —*see* Laceration, abdomen, wall,
      periumbilic region
    puncture —*see* Puncture, abdomen, wall,
      periumbilic region
  phalanges
    finger —*see* Wound, open, finger
    toe —*see* Wound, open, toe
  pharynx S11.20
  pinna —*see* Wound, open, ear
  popliteal space —*see* Wound, open, knee
  prepuce —*see* Wound, open, penis
  pubic region —*see* Wound, open, back, lower
  pudendum —*see* Wound, open, genital
    organs, external
  puncture wound —*see* Puncture
  rectovaginal septum —*see* Wound, open,
    vagina
  right
    lower quadrant S31.103
      with penetration into peritoneal cavity
        S31.603
      bite —*see* Bite, abdomen, wall, right,
        lower quadrant
      laceration —*see* Laceration, abdomen,
        wall, right, lower quadrant
      puncture —*see* Puncture, abdomen, wall,
        right, lower quadrant
    upper quadrant S31.100
      with penetration into peritoneal cavity
        S31.600

Wound, open (*Continued*)
  right (*Continued*)
    upper quadrant (*Continued*)
      bite —*see* Bite, abdomen, wall, right,
        upper quadrant
      laceration —*see* Laceration, abdomen,
        wall, right, upper quadrant
      puncture —*see* Puncture, abdomen, wall,
        right, upper quadrant
  sacral region —*see* Wound, open, back, lower
  sacroiliac region —*see* Wound, open, back,
    lower
  salivary gland —*see* Wound, open, oral cavity
  scalp S01.00
    bite S01.05
    laceration —*see* Laceration, scalp
    puncture —*see* Puncture, scalp
  scalpel, newborn (birth injury) P15.8
  scapular region —*see* Wound, open, shoulder
  sclera —*see* Wound, open, ocular
  scrotum S31.30
    with amputation —*see* Amputation,
      traumatic, scrotum
    bite S31.35
    laceration —*see* Laceration, scrotum
    puncture —*see* Puncture, scrotum
  shin —*see* Wound, open, leg
  shoulder S41.00-●
    with amputation —*see* Amputation,
      traumatic, arm
    bite —*see* Bite, shoulder
    laceration —*see* Laceration, shoulder
    puncture —*see* Puncture, shoulder
  skin NOS T14.8
  spermatic cord —*see* Wound, open, testis
  sternal region —*see* Wound, open, thorax,
    front wall
  submaxillary region —*see* Wound, open,
    head, specified site NEC
  submental region —*see* Wound, open, head,
    specified site NEC
  subungual
    finger(s) —*see* Wound, open, finger
    toe(s) —*see* Wound, open, toe
  supraclavicular region —*see* Wound, open,
    neck, specified site NEC
  temple, temporal region —*see* Wound, open,
    head, specified site NEC
  temporomandibular area —*see* Wound, open,
    cheek
  testis S31.30
    with amputation —*see* Amputation,
      traumatic, testes
    bite S31.35
    laceration —*see* Laceration, testis
    puncture —*see* Puncture, testis
  thigh S71.10-●
    with amputation —*see* Amputation,
      traumatic, hip
    bite —*see* Bite, thigh
    laceration —*see* Laceration, thigh
    puncture —*see* Puncture, thigh
  thorax, thoracic (wall) S21.90
    back S21.20-●
      with penetration S21.40
    bite —*see* Bite, thorax
    breast —*see* Wound, open, breast
    front S21.10-●
      with penetration S21.30
    laceration —*see* Laceration, thorax
    puncture —*see* Puncture, thorax
  throat —*see* Wound, open, neck
  thumb S61.009
    with
      amputation —*see* Amputation,
        traumatic, thumb
      damage to nail S61.109
    bite —*see* Bite, thumb
    laceration —*see* Laceration, thumb

Wound, open (*Continued*)
  thumb (*Continued*)
    left S61.002
      with
        damage to nail S61.102
      puncture —*see* Puncture, thumb
    right S61.001
      with
        damage to nail S61.101
  thyroid (gland) —*see* Wound, open, neck,
    thyroid
  toe(s) S91.109
    with
      amputation —*see* Amputation,
        traumatic, toe
      damage to nail S91.209
    bite —*see* Bite, toe
    great S91.103
      with
        damage to nail S91.203
      left S91.102
        with
          damage to nail S91.202
      right S91.101
        with
          damage to nail S91.201
    laceration —*see* Laceration, toe
    lesser S91.106
      with
        damage to nail S91.206
      left S91.105
        with
          damage to nail S91.205
      right S91.104
        with
          damage to nail S91.204
    puncture —*see* Puncture, toe
  tongue —*see* Wound, open, oral cavity
  trachea (cervical region) —*see* Wound, open,
    neck, trachea
  tunica vaginalis —*see* Wound, open, testis
  tympanum, tympanic membrane S09.2-●
    laceration —*see* Laceration, ear, drum
    puncture —*see* Puncture, tympanum
  umbilical region —*see* Wound, open,
    abdomen, wall, periumbilic region
  uvula —*see* Wound, open, oral cavity
  vagina S31.40
    bite S31.45
    laceration —*see* Laceration, vagina
    puncture —*see* Puncture, vagina
  vitreous (humor) —*see* Wound, open, ocular
  vocal cord S11.039
    bite —*see* Bite, vocal cord
    laceration S11.031
      with foreign body S11.032
    puncture S11.033
      with foreign body S11.034
  vulva S31.40
    with amputation —*see* Amputation,
      traumatic, vulva
    bite S31.45
    laceration —*see* Laceration, vulva
    puncture —*see* Puncture, vulva
  wrist S61.50-●
    bite —*see* Bite, wrist
    laceration —*see* Laceration, wrist
    puncture —*see* Puncture, wrist
Wound, superficial —*see* Injury (*see also*
  specified injury type)
Wright's syndrome G54.0
Wrist —*see* condition
Wrong drug (by accident) (given in error) —
  see Table of Drugs and Chemicals, by
  drug, poisoning
Wry neck —*see* Torticollis
Wuchereria (bancrofti) **infestation** B74.0
Wuchereriasis B74.0
Wuchernde Struma Langhans C73

▶ New   ⇨ Revised   ~~deleted~~ Deleted   ● Use Additional Character(s)

X

Xanthelasma (eyelid) (palpebrarum) H02.60
  left H02.66
    lower H02.65
    upper H02.64
  right H02.63
    lower H02.62
    upper H02.61
Xanthelasmatosis (essential) E78.2
Xanthinuria, hereditary E79.8
Xanthoastrocytoma
  specified site —*see* Neoplasm, malignant, by
    site
  unspecified site C71.9
Xanthofibroma —*see* Neoplasm, connective
  tissue, benign
Xanthogranuloma D76.3
Xanthoma(s), xanthomatosis (primary)
  (familial) (hereditary) E75.5
  with
    hyperlipoproteinemia
      Type I E78.3
      Type III E78.2
      Type IV E78.1
      Type V E78.3
  bone (generalisata) C96.5
  cerebrotendinous E75.5
  cutaneotendinous E75.5

Xanthoma(s), xanthomatosis *(Continued)*
  disseminatum (skin) E78.2
  eruptive E78.2
  hypercholesterinemic E78.00
  hypercholesterolemic E78.00
  hyperlipidemic E78.5
  joint E75.5
  multiple (skin) E78.2
  tendon (sheath) E75.5
  tuberosum E78.2
  tuberous E78.2
  tubo-eruptive E78.2
  verrucous, oral mucosa K13.4
Xanthosis R23.8
Xenophobia F40.10
Xeroderma —*see also* Ichthyosis
  acquired L85.0
    eyelid H01.149
      left H01.146
        lower H01.145
        upper H01.144
      right H01.143
        lower H01.142
        upper H01.141
  pigmentosum Q82.1
  vitamin A deficiency E50.8
Xerophthalmia (vitamin A deficiency) E50.7
  unrelated to vitamin A deficiency —*see*
    Keratoconjunctivitis

Xerosis
  conjunctiva H11.14-●
    with Bitot's spots —*see also* Pigmentation,
      conjunctiva
      vitamin A deficiency E50.1
    vitamin A deficiency E50.0
  cornea H18.89-●
    with ulceration —*see* Ulcer, cornea
      vitamin A deficiency E50.3
    vitamin A deficiency E50.2
  ⮡cutis (dry skin) L85.3
  skin L85.3
Xerostomia K11.7
Xiphopagus Q89.4
XO syndrome Q96.9
X-ray (of)
  abnormal findings —*see* Abnormal,
    diagnostic imaging
  breast (mammogram) (routine) Z12.31
  chest
    routine (as part of a general medical
      examination) Z00.00
      with abnormal findings Z00.01
  routine (as part of a general medical
    examination) Z00.00
    with abnormal findings Z00.01
XXXXY syndrome Q98.1
XXY syndrome Q98.0

Y

Yaba pox virus disease B08.72
Yatapoxvirus B08.70
  specified NEC B08.79
Yawning R06.89
  psychogenic F45.8
Yaws A66.9
  bone lesions A66.6
  butter A66.1
  chancre A66.0
  cutaneous, less than five years after infection
    A66.2
  early (cutaneous) (macular) (maculopapular)
    (micropapular) (papular) A66.2
    frambeside A66.2
    skin lesions NEC A66.2
  eyelid A66.2
  ganglion A66.6
  gangosis, gangosa A66.5
  gumma, gummata A66.4
    bone A66.6
  gummatous
    frambeside A66.4
    osteitis A66.6
    periostitis A66.6
  hydrarthrosis —*see also* subcategory
    M14.8-• A66.6
  hyperkeratosis (early) (late) A66.3

Yaws *(Continued)*
  initial lesions A66.0
  joint lesions —*see also* subcategory
    M14.8-• A66.6
  juxta-articular nodules A66.7
  late nodular (ulcerated) A66.4
  latent (without clinical manifestations) (with
    positive serology) A66.8
  mother A66.0
  mucosal A66.7
  multiple papillomata A66.1
  nodular, late (ulcerated) A66.4
  osteitis A66.6
  papilloma, plantar or palmar A66.1
  periostitis (hypertrophic) A66.6
  specified NEC A66.7
  ulcers A66.4
  wet crab A66.1
Yeast infection —*see also* Candidiasis B37.9
Yellow
  atrophy (liver) —*see* Failure, hepatic
  fever —*see* Fever, yellow
  jack —*see* Fever, yellow
  jaundice —*see* Jaundice
  nail syndrome L60.5
Yersiniosis —*see also* Infection, Yersinia
  extraintestinal A28.2
  intestinal A04.6

Z

Zahorsky's syndrome (herpangina) B08.5
Zellweger's syndrome E71.510
Zenker's diverticulum (esophagus) K22.5
Ziehen-Oppenheim disease G24.1
Zieve's syndrome K70.0
Zika NOS A92.5
  congenital P35.4
Zinc
  deficiency, dietary E60
  metabolism disorder E83.2
Zollinger-Ellison syndrome E16.4
Zona —*see* Herpes, zoster
Zoophobia F40.218
Zoster (herpes) —*see* Herpes, zoster
Zygomycosis B46.9
  specified NEC B46.8
Zymotic —*see* condition

▶ New   ⇒ Revised   ~~deleted~~ Deleted   • Use Additional Character(s)

ICD-10-CM
Table of Neoplasms

The list below gives the code numbers for neoplasms by anatomical site. For each site there are six possible code numbers according to whether the neoplasm in question is malignant, benign, in situ, of uncertain behavior, or of unspecified nature. The description of the neoplasm will often indicate which of the six columns is appropriate; e.g., malignant melanoma of skin, benign fibroadenoma of breast, carcinoma in situ of cervix uteri.

Where such descriptors are not present, the remainder of the Index should be consulted where guidance is given to the appropriate column for each morphological (histological) variety listed; e.g., Mesonephroma — see Neoplasm, malignant; Embryoma — see also Neoplasm, uncertain behavior; Disease, Bowen's — see Neoplasm, skin, in situ. However, the guidance in the Index can be overridden if one of the descriptors mentioned above is present; e.g., malignant adenoma of colon is coded to C18.9 and not to D12.6 as the adjective "Malignant" overrides the Index entry 'Adenoma — see also Neoplasm, benign.'

Codes listed with a dash -, following the code have a required additional character for laterality. The Tabular must be reviewed for the complete code.

	Malignant Primary	Malignant Secondary	Ca in situ	Benign	Uncertain Behavior	Unspecified Behavior
Neoplasm, neoplastic	C80.1	C79.9	D09.9	D36.9	D48.9	D49.9
abdomen, abdominal	C76.2	C79.8-●	D09.8	D36.7	D48.7	D49.89
cavity	C76.2	C79.8-●	D09.8	D36.7	D48.7	D49.89
organ	C76.2	C79.8-●	D09.8	D36.7	D48.7	D49.89
viscera	C76.2	C79.8-●	D09.8	D36.7	D48.7	D49.89
wall — see also Neoplasm, abdomen, wall, skin	C44.509	C79.2-●	D04.5	D23.5	D48.5	D49.2
connective tissue	C49.4	C79.8-●	—	D21.4	D48.1	D49.2
skin	C44.509					
basal cell carcinoma	C44.519	—	—	—	—	—
specified type NEC	C44.599	—	—	—	—	—
squamous cell carcinoma	C44.529	—	—	—	—	—
abdominopelvic	C76.8	C79.8-●	—	D36.7	D48.7	D49.89
accessory sinus — see Neoplasm, sinus						
acoustic nerve	C72.4-●	C79.49	—	D33.3	D43.3	D49.7
adenoid (pharynx) (tissue)	C11.1	C79.89	D00.08	D10.6	D37.05	D49.0
adipose tissue — see also Neoplasm, connective tissue	C49.4	C79.89	—	D21.9	D48.1	D49.2
adnexa (uterine)	C57.4	C79.89	D07.39	D28.7	D39.8	D49.59
adrenal	C74.9-●	C79.7-●	D09.3	D35.0-●	D44.1-●	D49.7
capsule	C74.9-●	C79.7-●	D09.3	D35.0-●	D44.1-●	D49.7
cortex	C74.0-●	C79.7-●	D09.3	D35.0-●	D44.1-●	D49.7
gland	C74.9-●	C79.7-●	D09.3	D35.0-●	D44.1-●	D49.7
medulla	C74.1-●	C79.7-●	D09.3	D35.0-●	D44.1-●	D49.7
ala nasi (external) — see also Neoplasm, skin, nose	C44.301	C79.2	D04.39	D23.39	D48.5	D49.2

	Malignant Primary	Malignant Secondary	Ca in situ	Benign	Uncertain Behavior	Unspecified Behavior
alimentary canal or tract NEC	C26.9	C78.80	D01.9	D13.9	D37.9	D49.0
alveolar	C03.9	C79.89	D00.03	D10.39	D37.09	D49.0
mucosa	C03.9	C79.89	D00.03	D10.39	D37.09	D49.0
lower	C03.1	C79.89	D00.03	D10.39	D37.09	D49.0
upper	C03.0	C79.89	D00.03	D10.39	D37.09	D49.0
ridge or process	C41.1	C79.51	—	D16.5-●	D48.0	D49.2
carcinoma	C03.9	C79.8-●	—	—	—	—
lower	C03.1	C79.8-●	—	—	—	—
upper	C03.0	C79.8 ●	—	—	—	—
lower	C41.1	C79.51	—	D16.5-●	D48.0	D49.2
mucosa	C03.9	C79.89	D00.03	D10.39	D37.09	D49.0
lower	C03.1	C79.89	D00.03	D10.39	D37.09	D49.0
upper	C03.0	C79.89	D00.03	D10.39	D37.09	D49.0
upper	C41.0	C79.51	—	D16.4-●	D48.0	D49.2
sulcus	C06.1	C79.89	D00.02	D10.39	D37.09	D49.0
alveolus	C03.9	C79.89	D00.03	D10.39	D37.09	D49.0
lower	C03.1	C79.89	D00.03	D10.39	D37.09	D49.0
upper	C03.0	C79.89	D00.03	D10.39	D37.09	D49.0
ampulla of Vater	C24.1	C78.89	D01.5	D13.5	D37.6	D49.0
ankle NEC	C76.5-●	C79.89	D04.7-●	D36.7	D48.7	D49.89
anorectum, anorectal (junction)	C21.8	C78.5	D01.3	D12.9	D37.8	D49.0
antecubital fossa or space	C76.4-●	C79.89	D04.6-●	D36.7	D48.7	D49.89
antrum (Highmore) (maxillary)	C31.0	C78.39	D02.3	D14.0	D38.5	D49.1
pyloric	C16.3	C78.89	D00.2	D13.1	D37.1	D49.0
tympanicum	C30.1	C78.39	D02.3	D14.0	D38.5	D49.1
anus, anal	C21.0	C78.5	D01.3	D12.9	D37.8	D49.0
canal	C21.1	C78.5	D01.3	D12.9	D37.8	D49.0
cloacogenic zone	C21.2	C78.5	D01.3	D12.9	D37.8	D49.0
margin — see also Neoplasm, anus, skin	C44.500	C79.2	D04.5	D23.5	D48.5	D49.2
overlapping lesion with rectosigmoid junction or rectum	C21.8	—	—	—	—	—
skin	C44.500	C79.2	D04.5	D23.5	D48.5	D49.2
basal cell carcinoma	C44.510	—	—	—	—	—
specified type NEC	C44.590	—	—	—	—	—
squamous cell carcinoma	C44.520	—	—	—	—	—
sphincter	C21.1	C78.5	D01.3	D12.9	D37.8	D49.0
aorta (thoracic)	C49.3	C79.89	—	D21.3	D48.1	D49.2
abdominal	C49.4	C79.89	—	D21.4	D48.1	D49.2
aortic body	C75.5	C79.89	—	D35.6	D44.7	D49.7
aponeurosis	C49.9	C79.89	—	D21.9	D48.1	D49.2
palmar	C49.1-●	C79.89	—	D21.1-●	D48.1	D49.2
plantar	C49.2-●	C79.89	—	D21.2-●	D48.1	D49.2

TABLE OF NEOPLASMS

◀ New　◀▮ Revised　~~deleted~~ Deleted　● Use Additional Character(s)

TABLE OF NEOPLASMS

	Malignant Primary	Malignant Secondary	Ca in situ	Benign	Uncertain Behavior	Unspecified Behavior
appendix	C18.1	C78.5	D01.0	D12.1	D37.3	D49.0
arachnoid	C70.9	C79.49	—	D32.9	D42.9	D49.7
cerebral	C70.0	C79.32	—	D32.0	D42.0	D49.7
spinal	C70.1	C79.49	—	D32.1	D42.1	D49.7
areola	C50.0-●	C79.81	D05.-●	D24.-●	D48.6-●	D49.3
arm NEC	C76.4-●	C79.89	D04.6-●	D36.7	D48.7	D49.89
artery — see Neoplasm, connective tissue						
aryepiglottic fold	C13.1	C79.89	D00.08	D10.7	D37.05	D49.0
hypopharyngeal aspect	C13.1	C79.89	D00.08	D10.7	D37.05	D49.0
laryngeal aspect	C32.1	C78.39	D02.0	D14.1	D38.0	D49.1
marginal zone	C13.1	C79.89	D00.08	D10.7	D37.05	D49.0
arytenoid (cartilage)	C32.3	C78.39	D02.0	D14.1	D38.0	D49.1
fold — see Neoplasm, aryepiglottic						
associated with transplanted organ	C80.2	—	—	—	—	—
atlas	C41.2	C79.51	—	D16.6	D48.0	D49.2
atrium, cardiac	C38.0	C79.89	—	D15.1	D48.7	D49.89
auditory						
canal (external) (skin)	C44.20-●	C79.2	D04.2-●	D23.2-●	D48.5	D49.2
internal	C30.1	C78.39	D02.3	D14.0	D38.5	D49.1
nerve	C72.4-●	C79.49	—	D33.3	D43.3	D49.7
tube	C30.1	C78.39	D02.3	D14.0	D38.5	D49.1
opening	C11.2	C79.89	D00.08	D10.6	D37.05	D49.0
auricle, ear — see also Neoplasm, skin, ear	C44.20-●	C79.2	D04.2-●	D23.2-●	D48.5	D49.2
auricular canal (external) — see also Neoplasm, skin, ear	C44.20-●	C79.2	D04.2-●	D23.2-●	D48.5	D49.2
internal	C30.1	C78.39	D02.3	D14.0	D38.5	D49.2
autonomic nerve or nervous system NEC (see Neoplasm, nerve, peripheral)						
axilla, axillary	C76.1	C79.89	D09.8	D36.7	D48.7	D49.89
fold — see also Neoplasm, skin, trunk	C44.509	C79.2	D04.5	D23.5	D48.5	D49.2
back NEC	C76.8	C79.89	D04.5	D36.7	D48.7	D49.89
Bartholin's gland	C51.0	C79.82	D07.1	D28.0	D39.8	D49.59
basal ganglia	C71.0	C79.31	—	D33.0	D43.0	D49.6
basis pedunculi	C71.7	C79.31	—	D33.1	D43.1	D49.6
bile or biliary (tract)	C24.9	C78.89	D01.5	D13.5	D37.6	D49.0
canaliculi (biliferi) (intrahepatic)	C22.1	C78.7	D01.5	D13.4	D37.6	D49.0
canals, interlobular	C22.1	C78.89	D01.5	D13.4	D37.6	D49.0

	Malignant Primary	Malignant Secondary	Ca in situ	Benign	Uncertain Behavior	Unspecified Behavior
bile or biliary (Continued)						
duct or passage (common) (cystic) (extrahepatic)	C24.0	C78.89	D01.5	D13.5	D37.6	D49.0
interlobular	C22.1	C78.89	D01.5	D13.4	D37.6	D49.0
intrahepatic	C22.1	C78.7	D01.5	D13.4	D37.6	D49.0
and extrahepatic	C24.8	C78.89	D01.5	D13.5	D37.6	D49.0
bladder (urinary)	C67.9	C79.11	D09.0	D30.3	D41.4	D49.4
dome	C67.1	C79.11	D09.0	D30.3	D41.4	D49.4
neck	C67.5	C79.11	D09.0	D30.3	D41.4	D49.4
orifice	C67.9	C79.11	D09.0	D30.3	D41.4	D49.4
ureteric	C67.6	C79.11	D09.0	D30.3	D41.4	D49.4
urethral	C67.5	C79.11	D09.0	D30.3	D41.4	D49.4
overlapping lesion	C67.8	—	—	—	—	—
sphincter	C67.8	C79.11	D09.0	D30.3	D41.4	D49.4
trigone	C67.0	C79.11	D09.0	D30.3	D41.4	D49.4
urachus	C67.7	C79.11	D09.0	D30.3	D41.4	D49.4
wall	C67.9	C79.11	D09.0	D30.3	D41.4	D49.4
anterior	C67.3	C79.11	D09.0	D30.3	D41.4	D49.4
lateral	C67.2	C79.11	D09.0	D30.3	D41.4	D49.4
posterior	C67.4	C79.11	D09.0	D30.3	D41.4	D49.4
blood vessel — see Neoplasm, connective tissue						
bone (periosteum)	C41.9	C79.51	—	D16.9-●	D48.0	D49.2
acetabulum	C41.4	C79.51	—	D16.8-●	D48.0	D49.2
ankle	C40.3-●	C79.51	—	D16.3-●	—	—
arm NEC	C40.0-●	C79.51	—	D16.0-●	—	—
astragalus	C40.3-●	C79.51	—	D16.3-●	—	—
atlas	C41.2	C79.51	—	D16.6-●	D48.0	D49.2
axis	C41.2	C79.51	—	D16.6-●	D48.0	D49.2
back NEC	C41.2	C79.51	—	D16.6-●	D48.0	D49.2
calcaneus	C40.3-●	C79.51	—	D16.3-●	—	—
calvarium	C41.0	C79.51	—	D16.4-●	D48.0	D49.2
carpus (any)	C40.1-●	C79.51	—	D16.1-●	—	—
cartilage NEC	C41.9	C79.51	—	D16.9-●	D48.0	D49.2
clavicle	C41.3	C79.51	—	D16.7-●	D48.0	D49.2
clivus	C41.0	C79.51	—	D16.4-●	D48.0	D49.2
coccygeal vertebra	C41.4	C79.51	—	D16.8-●	D48.0	D49.2
coccyx	C41.4	C79.51	—	D16.8-●	D48.0	D49.2
costal cartilage	C41.3	C79.51	—	D16.7-●	D48.0	D49.2
costovertebral joint	C41.3	C79.51	—	D16.7-●	D48.0	D49.2
cranial	C41.0	C79.51	—	D16.4-●	D48.0	D49.2
cuboid	C40.3-●	C79.51	—	D16.3-●	—	—
cuneiform	C41.9	C79.51	—	D16.9-●	D48.0	D49.2
elbow	C40.0-●	C79.51	—	D16.0-●	—	—

◀ New   ◀◀ Revised   ~~deleted~~ Deleted   ● Use Additional Character(s)

TABLE OF NEOPLASMS

	Malignant Primary	Malignant Secondary	Ca in situ	Benign	Uncertain Behavior	Unspecified Behavior
bone *(Continued)*						
ethmoid (labyrinth)	C41.0	C79.51	—	D16.4-●	D48.0	D49.2
face	C41.0	C79.51	—	D16.4-●	D48.0	D49.2
femur (any part)	C40.2-●	C79.51	—	D16.2-●	—	—
fibula (any part)	C40.2-●	C79.51	—	D16.2-●	—	—
finger (any)	C40.1-●	C79.51	—	D16.1-●	—	—
foot	C40.3-●	C79.51	—	D16.3-●	—	—
forearm	C40.0-●	C79.51	—	D16.0-●	—	—
frontal	C41.0	C79.51	—	D16.4-●	D48.0	D49.2
hand	C40.1-●	C79.51	—	D16.1-●	—	—
heel	C40.3-●	C79.51	—	D16.3-●	—	—
hip	C41.4	C79.51	—	D16.8-●	D48.0	D49.2
humerus (any part)	C40.0-●	C79.51	—	D16.0-●	—	—
hyoid	C41.0	C79.51	—	D16.4-●	D48.0	D49.2
ilium	C41.4	C79.51	—	D16.8-●	D48.0	D49.2
innominate	C41.4	C79.51	—	D16.8-●	D48.0	D49.2
intervertebral cartilage or disc	C41.2	C79.51	—	D16.6-●	D48.0	D49.2
ischium	C41.4	C79.51	—	D16.8-●	D48.0	D49.2
jaw (lower)	C41.1	C79.51	—	D16.5-●	D48.0	D49.2
knee	C40.2-●	C79.51	—	D16.2-●	—	—
leg NEC	C40.2-●	C79.51	—	D16.2-●	—	—
limb NEC	C40.9-●	C79.51	—	D16.9-●	—	—
lower (long bones)	C40.2-●	C79.51	—	D16.2-●	—	—
short bones	C40.3-●	C79.51	—	D16.3-●	—	—
upper (long bones)	C40.0-●	C79.51	—	D16.0-●	—	—
short bones	C40.1-●	C79.51	—	D16.1-●	—	—
malar	C41.0	C79.51	—	D16.4-●	D48.0	D49.2
mandible	C41.1	C79.51	—	D16.5-●	D48.0	D49.2
marrow NEC (any bone)	C96.9	C79.52	—	—	D47.9	D49.89
mastoid	C41.0	C79.51	—	D16.4-●	D48.0	D49.2
maxilla, maxillary (superior)	C41.0	C79.51	—	D16.4-●	D48.0	D49.2
inferior	C41.1	C79.51	—	D16.5-●	D48.0	D49.2
metacarpus (any)	C40.1-●	C79.51	—	D16.1-●	—	—
metatarsus (any)	C40.3-●	C79.51	—	D16.3-●	—	—
overlapping sites	C40.8-●	—	—	—	—	—
navicular						
ankle	C40.3-●	C79.51	—	—	—	—
hand	C40.1-●	C79.51	—	—	—	—
nose, nasal	C41.0	C79.51	—	D16.4-●	D48.0	D49.2
occipital	C41.0	C79.51	—	D16.4-●	D48.0	D49.2
orbit	C41.0	C79.51	—	D16.4-●	D48.0	D49.2
parietal	C41.0	C79.51	—	D16.4-●	D48.0	D49.2
patella	C40.2-●	C79.51	—	—	—	—
pelvic	C41.4	C79.51	—	D16.8	D48.0	D49.2

	Malignant Primary	Malignant Secondary	Ca in situ	Benign	Uncertain Behavior	Unspecified Behavior
bone *(Continued)*						
phalanges						
foot	C40.3-●	C79.51	—	—	—	—
hand	C40.1-●	C79.51	—	—	—	—
pubic	C41.4	C79.51	—	D16.8	D48.0	D49.2
radius (any part)	C40.0-●	C79.51	—	D16.0-●	—	—
rib	C41.3	C79.51	—	D16.7	D48.0	D49.2
sacral vertebra	C41.4	C79.51	—	D16.8	D48.0	D49.2
sacrum	C41.4	C79.51	—	D16.8	D48.0	D49.2
scaphoid	—	—	—	—	—	—
of ankle	C40.3-●	C79.51	—	—	—	—
of hand	C40.1-●	C79.51	—	—	—	—
scapula (any part)	C40.0-●	C79.51	—	D16.0-●	—	—
sella turcica	C41.0	C79.51	—	D16.4-●	D48.0	D49.2
shoulder	C40.0-●	C79.51	—	D16.0-●	—	—
skull	C41.0	C79.51	—	D16.4-●	D48.0	D49.2
sphenoid	C41.0	C79.51	—	D16.4-●	D48.0	D49.2
spine, spinal (column)	C41.2	C79.51	—	D16.6	D48.0	D49.2
coccyx	C41.4	C79.51	—	D16.8	D48.0	D49.2
sacrum	C41.4	C79.51	—	D16.8	D48.0	D49.2
sternum	C41.3	C79.51	—	D16.7	D48.0	D49.2
tarsus (any)	C40.3-●	C79.51	—	—	—	—
temporal	C41.0	C79.51	—	D16.4-●	D48.0	D49.2
thumb	C40.1-●	C79.51	—	—	—	—
tibia (any part)	C40.2-●	C79.51	—	—	—	—
toe (any)	C40.3-●	C79.51	—	—	—	—
trapozium	C40.1-●	C79.51	—	—	—	—
trapezoid	C40.1-●	C79.51	—	—	—	—
turbinate	C41.0	C79.51	—	D16.4-●	D48.0	D49.2
ulna (any part)	C40.0-●	C79.51	—	D16.0-●	—	—
unciform	C40.1-●	C79.51	—	—	—	—
vertebra (column)	C41.2	C79.51	—	D16.6	D48.0	D49.2
coccyx	C41.4	C79.51	—	D16.8	D48.0	D49.2
sacrum	C41.4	C79.51	—	D16.8	D48.0	D49.2
vomer	C41.0	C79.51	—	D16.4-●	D48.0	D49.2
wrist	C40.1	C79.51	—	—	—	—
xiphoid process	C41.3	C79.51	—	D16.7	D48.0	D49.2
zygomatic	C41.0	C79.51	—	D16.4-●	D48.0	D49.2
book-leaf (mouth)	C06.89	C79.89	D00.00	D10.39	D37.09	D49.0
bowel—*see Neoplasm, intestine*						
brachial plexus	C47.1-●	C79.89	—	D36.12	D48.2	D49.2
brain NEC	C71.9	C79.31	—	D33.2	D43.2	D49.6
basal ganglia	C71.0	C79.31	—	D33.0	D43.0	D49.6
cerebellopontine angle	C71.6	C79.31	—	D33.1	D43.1	D49.6

◀ New　◀ Revised　~~deleted~~ Deleted　● Use Additional Character(s)

TABLE OF NEOPLASMS

TABLE OF NEOPLASMS

	Malignant Primary	Malignant Secondary	Ca in situ	Benign	Uncertain Behavior	Unspecified Behavior
brain NEC *(Continued)*						
cerebellum NOS	C71.6	C79.31	—	D33.1	D43.1	D49.6
cerebrum	C71.0	C79.31	—	D33.0	D43.0	D49.6
choroid plexus	C71.7	C79.31	—	D33.1	D43.1	D49.6
corpus callosum	C71.8	C79.31	—	D33.2	D43.2	D49.6
corpus striatum	C71.0	C79.31	—	D33.0	D43.0	D49.6
cortex (cerebral)	C71.0	C79.31	—	D33.0	D43.0	D49.6
frontal lobe	C71.1	C79.31	—	D33.0	D43.0	D49.6
globus pallidus	C71.0	C79.31	—	D33.0	D43.0	D49.6
hippocampus	C71.2	C79.31	—	D33.0	D43.0	D49.6
hypothalamus	C71.0	C79.31	—	D33.0	D43.0	D49.6
internal capsule	C71.0	C79.31	—	D33.0	D43.0	D49.6
medulla oblongata	C71.7	C79.31	—	D33.1	D43.1	D49.6
meninges	C70.0	C79.32	—	D32.0	D42.0	D49.7
midbrain	C71.7	C79.31	—	D33.1	D43.1	D49.6
occipital lobe	C71.4	C79.31	—	D33.0	D43.0	D49.6
overlapping lesion	C71.8	C79.31	—	—	—	—
parietal lobe	C71.3	C79.31	—	D33.0	D43.0	D49.6
peduncle	C71.7	C79.31	—	D33.1	D43.1	D49.6
pons	C71.7	C79.31	—	D33.1	D43.1	D49.6
stem	C71.7	C79.31	—	D33.1	D43.1	D49.6
tapetum	C71.8	C79.31	—	D33.2	D43.2	D49.6
temporal lobe	C71.2	C79.31	—	D33.0	D43.0	D49.6
thalamus	C71.0	C79.31	—	D33.0	D43.0	D49.6
uncus	C71.2	C79.31	—	D33.0	D43.0	D49.6
ventricle (floor)	C71.5	C79.31	—	D33.0	D43.0	D49.6
fourth	C71.7	C79.31	—	D33.1	D43.1	D49.6
branchial (cleft) (cyst) (vestiges)	C10.4	C79.89	D00.08	D10.5	D37.05	D49.0
breast (connective tissue) (glandular tissue) (soft parts)	C50.9-•	C79.81	D05.-•	D24.-•	D48.6-•	D49.3
areola	C50.0-•	C79.81	D05.-•	D24.-•	D48.6-•	D49.3
axillary tail	C50.6-•	C79.81	D05.-•	D24.-•	D48.6-•	D49.3
central portion	C50.1-•	C79.81	D05.-•	D24.-•	D48.6-•	D49.3
inner	C50.8-•	C79.81	D05.-•	D24.-•	D48.6-•	D49.3
lower	C50.8-•	C79.81	D05.-•	D24.-•	D48.6-•	D49.3
lower-inner quadrant	C50.3-•	C79.81	D05.-•	D24.-•	D48.6-•	D49.3
lower-outer quadrant	C50.5-•	C79.81	D05.-•	D24.-•	D48.6-•	D49.3
mastectomy site (skin) — *see also Neoplasm, breast, skin*	C44.501	C79.2	—	—	—	—
specified as breast tissue	C50.8-•	C79.81		—	—	—
midline	C50.8-•	C79.81	D05.-•	D24.-•	D48.6-•	D49.3
nipple	C50.0-•	C79.81	D05.-•	D24.-•	D48.6-•	D49.3
outer	C50.8-•	C79.81	D05.-•	D24.-•	D48.6-•	D49.3
overlapping lesion	C50.8-•	—				

	Malignant Primary	Malignant Secondary	Ca in situ	Benign	Uncertain Behavior	Unspecified Behavior
breast *(Continued)*						
skin	C44.501	C79.2	D04.5	D23.5	D48.5	D49.2
basal cell carcinoma	C44.511	—	—	—	—	—
specified type NEC	C44.591	—	—	—	—	—
squamous cell carcinoma	C44.521	—	—	—	—	—
tail (axillary)	C50.6-•	C79.81	D05.-•	D24.-•	D48.6-•	D49.3
upper	C50.8-•	C79.81	D05.-•	D24.-•	D48.6-•	D49.3
upper-inner quadrant	C50.2-•	C79.81	D05.-•	D24.-•	D48.6-•	D49.3
upper-outer quadrant	C50.4-•	C79.81	D05.-•	D24.-•	D48.6-•	D49.3
broad ligament	C57.1	C79.82	D07.39	D28.2	D39.8	D49.59
bronchiogenic, bronchogenic (lung)	C34.9-•	C78.0-•	D02.2-•	D14.3-•	D38.1	D49.1
bronchiole	C34.9-•	C78.0-•	D02.2-•	D14.3-•	D38.1	D49.1
bronchus	C34.9-•	C78.0-•	D02.2-•	D14.3-•	D38.1	D49.1
carina	C34.0-•	C78.0-•	D02.2-•	D14.3-•	D38.1	D49.1
lower lobe of lung	C34.3-•	C78.0-•	D02.2-•	D14.3-•	D38.1	D49.1
main	C34.0-•	C78.0-•	D02.2-•	D14.3-•	D38.1	D49.1
middle lobe of lung	C34.2	C78.0-•	D02.21	D14.31	D38.1	D49.1
overlapping lesion	C34.8-•	—	—	—	—	—
upper lobe of lung	C34.1-•	C78.0-•	D02.2-•	D14.3-•	D38.1	D49.1
brow	C44.309	C79.2	D04.39	D23.39	D48.5	D49.2
basal cell carcinoma	C44.319	—	—	—	—	—
specified type NEC	C44.399	—	—	—	—	—
squamous cell carcinoma	C44.329	—	—	—	—	—
buccal (cavity)	C06.9	C79.89	D00.00	D10.39	D37.09	D49.0
commissure	C06.0	C79.89	D00.02	D10.39	D37.09	D49.0
groove (lower) (upper)	C06.1	C79.89	D00.02	D10.39	D37.09	D49.0
mucosa	C06.0	C79.89	D00.02	D10.39	D37.09	D49.0
sulcus (lower) (upper)	C06.1	C79.89	D00.02	D10.39	D37.09	D49.0
bulbourethral gland	C68.0	C79.19	D09.19	D30.4	D41.3	D49.59
bursa — *see Neoplasm, connective tissue*						
buttock NEC	C76.3	C79.89	D04.5	D36.7	D48.7	D49.89
calf	C76.5-•	C79.89	D04.7-•	D36.7	D48.7	D49.89
calvarium	C41.0	C79.51	—	D16.4-•	D48.0	D49.2
calyx, renal	C65.-•	C79.0-•	D09.19	D30.1-•	D41.1-•	D49.51-•
canal						
anal	C21.1	C78.5	D01.3	D12.9	D37.8	D49.0
auditory (external) — *see also Neoplasm, skin, ear*	C44.20-•	C79.2	D04.2-•	D23.2-•	D48.5	D49.2
auricular (external) — *see also Neoplasm, skin, ear*	C44.20-•	C79.2	D04.2-•	D23.2-•	D48.5	D49.2
canaliculi, biliary (biliferi) (intrahepatic)	C22.1	C78.7	D01.5	D13.4	D37.6	D49.0

◀ New   ◀| Revised   ~~deleted~~ Deleted   • Use Additional Character(s)

	Malignant Primary	Malignant Secondary	Ca in situ	Benign	Uncertain Behavior	Unspecified Behavior
canthus (eye) (inner) (outer)	C44.10-●	C79.2	D04.1-●	D23.1-●	D48.5	D49.2
basal cell carcinoma	C44.11-●	—	—	—	—	—
sebaceous cell	C44.13-●	—	—	—	—	—
specified type NEC	C44.19-●	—	—	—	—	—
squamous cell carcinoma	C44.12-●	—	—	—	—	—
capillary — see Neoplasm, connective tissue						
caput coli	C18.0	C78.5	D01.0	D12.0	D37.4	D49.0
carcinoid — see Tumor, carcinoid						
cardia (gastric)	C16.0	C78.89	D00.2	D13.1	D37.1	D49.0
cardiac orifice (stomach)	C16.0	C78.89	D00.2	D13.1	D37.1	D49.0
cardio-esophageal junction	C16.0	C78.89	D00.2	D13.1	D37.1	D49.0
cardio-esophagus	C16.0	C78.89	D00.2	D13.1	D37.1	D49.0
carina (bronchus)	C34.0-●	C78.0-●	D02.2-●	D14.3-●	D38.1	D49.1
carotid (artery)	C49.0	C79.89	—	D21.0	D48.1	D49.2
body	C75.4	C79.89	—	D35.5	D44.6	D49.7
carpus (any bone)	C40.1-●	C79.51	—	D16.1-●	—	—
cartilage (articular) (joint) NEC — see also Neoplasm, bone	C41.9	C79.51	—	D16.9-●	D48.0	D49.2
arytenoid	C32.3	C78.39	D02.0	D14.1	D38.0	D49.1
auricular	C49.0	C79.89	—	D21.0	D48.1	D49.2
bronchi	C34.0-●	C78.39	—	D14.3-●	D38.1	D49.1
costal	C41.3	C79.51	—	D16.7	D48.0	D49.2
cricoid	C32.3	C78.39	D02.0	D14.1	D38.0	D49.1
cuneiform	C32.3	C78.39	D02.0	D14.1	D38.0	D49.1
ear (external)	C49.0	C79.89	—	D21.0	D48.1	D49.2
ensiform	C41.3	C79.51	—	D16.7	D48.0	D49.2
epiglottis	C32.1	C78.39	D02.0	D14.1	D38.0	D49.1
anterior surface	C10.1	C79.89	D00.08	D10.5	D37.05	D49.0
eyelid	C49.0	C79.89	—	D21.0	D48.1	D49.2
intervertebral	C41.2	C79.51	—	D16.6	D48.0	D49.2
larynx, laryngeal	C32.3	C78.39	D02.0	D14.1	D38.0	D49.1
nose, nasal	C30.0	C78.39	D02.3	D14.0	D38.5	D49.1
pinna	C49.0	C79.89	—	D21.0	D48.1	D49.2
rib	C41.3	C79.51	—	D16.7	D48.0	D49.2
semilunar (knee)	C40.2-●	C79.51	—	D16.2-●	D48.0	D49.2
thyroid	C32.3	C78.39	D02.0	D14.1	D38.0	D49.1
trachea	C33	C78.39	D02.1	D14.2	D38.1	D49.1
cauda equina	C72.1	C79.49	—	D33.4	D43.4	D49.7
cavity						
buccal	C06.9	C79.89	D00.00	D10.30	D37.09	D49.0
nasal	C30.0	C78.39	D02.3	D14.0	D38.5	D49.1
oral	C06.9	C79.89	D00.00	D10.30	D37.09	D49.0
cavity (Continued)						
peritoneal	C48.2	C78.6	—	D20.1	D48.4	D49.0
tympanic	C30.1	C78.39	D02.3	D14.0	D38.5	D49.1
cecum	C18.0	C78.5	D01.0	D12.0	D37.4	D49.0
central nervous system	C72.9	C79.40				
cerebellopontine (angle)	C71.6	C79.31	—	D33.1	D43.1	D49.6
cerebellum, cerebellar	C71.6	C79.31	—	D33.1	D43.1	D49.6
cerebrum, cerebra (cortex) (hemisphere) (white matter)	C71.0	C79.31	—	D33.0	D43.0	D49.6
meninges	C70.0	C79.32	—	D32.0	D42.0	D49.7
peduncle	C71.7	C79.31	—	D33.1	D43.1	D49.6
ventricle	C71.5	C79.31	—	D33.0	D43.0	D49.6
fourth	C71.7	C79.31	—	D33.1	D43.1	D49.6
cervical region	C76.0	C79.89	D09.8	D36.7	D48.7	D49.89
cervix (cervical) (uteri) (uterus)	C53.9	C79.82	D06.9	D26.0	D39.0	D49.59
canal	C53.0	C79.82	D06.0	D26.0	D39.0	D49.59
endocervix (canal) (gland)	C53.0	C79.82	D06.0	D26.0	D39.0	D49.59
exocervix	C53.1	C79.82	D06.1	D26.0	D39.0	D49.59
external os	C53.1	C79.82	D06.1	D26.0	D39.0	D49.59
internal os	C53.0	C79.82	D06.0	D26.0	D39.0	D49.59
nabothian gland	C53.0	C79.82	D06.0	D26.0	D39.0	D49.59
overlapping lesion	C53.8	—	—	—	—	—
squamocolumnar junction	C53.8	C79.82	D06.7	D26.0	D39.0	D49.59
stump	C53.8	C79.82	D06.7	D26.0	D39.0	D49.59
cheek	C76.0	C79.89	D09.8	D36.7	D48.7	D49.89
external	C44.309	C79.2	D04.39	D23.39	D48.5	D49.2
basal cell carcinoma	C44.319	—	—	—	—	—
specified type NEC	C44.399	—	—	—	—	—
squamous cell carcinoma	C44.329	—	—	—	—	—
inner aspect	C06.0	C79.89	D00.02	D10.39	D37.09	D49.0
internal	C06.0	C79.89	D00.02	D10.39	D37.09	D49.0
mucosa	C06.0	C79.89	D00.02	D10.39	D37.09	D49.0
chest (wall) NEC	C76.1	C79.89	D09.8	D36.7	D48.7	D49.89
chiasma opticum	C72.3-●	C79.49	—	D33.3	D43.3	D49.7
chin	C44.309	C79.2	D04.39	D23.39	D48.5	D49.2
basal cell carcinoma	C44.319	—	—	—	—	—
specified type NEC	C44.399	—	—	—	—	—
squamous cell carcinoma	C44.329	—	—	—	—	—
choana	C11.3	C79.89	D00.08	D10.6	D37.05	D49.0
cholangiole	C22.1	C78.89	D01.5	D13.4	D37.6	D49.0
choledochal duct	C24.0	C78.89	D01.5	D13.5	D37.6	D49.0
choroid	C69.3-●	C79.49	D09.2-●	D31.3-●	D48.7	D49.81
plexus	C71.5	C79.31	—	D33.0	D43.0	D49.6
ciliary body	C69.4-●	C79.49	D09.2-●	D31.4-●	D48.7	D49.89

◄ New ◖ Revised ~~deleted~~ Deleted ● Use Additional Character(s)

TABLE OF NEOPLASMS

	Malignant Primary	Malignant Secondary	Ca in situ	Benign	Uncertain Behavior	Unspecified Behavior
clavicle	C41.3	C79.51	—	D16.7	D48.0	D49.2
clitoris	C51.2	C79.82	D07.1	D28.0	D39.8	D49.59
clivus	C41.0	C79.51	—	D16.4-●	D48.0	D49.2
cloacogenic zone	C21.2	C78.5	D01.3	D12.9	D37.8	D49.0
coccygeal						
body or glomus	C49.5	C79.89	—	D21.5	D48.1	D49.2
vertebra	C41.4	C79.51	—	D16.8	D48.0	D49.2
coccyx	C41.4	C79.51	—	D16.8	D48.0	D49.2
colon — *see also Neoplasm, intestine, large*	C18.9	C78.5	—	—	—	—
with rectum	C19	C78.5	D01.1	D12.7	D37.5	D49.0
column, spinal — *see Neoplasm, spine*						
columnella — *see also Neoplasm, skin, face*	C44.390	C79.2	D04.39	D23.39	D48.5	D49.2
commissure						
labial, lip	C00.6	C79.89	D00.01	D10.39	D37.01	D49.0
laryngeal	C32.0	C78.39	D02.0	D14.1	D38.0	D49.1
common (bile) duct	C24.0	C78.89	D01.5	D13.5	D37.6	D49.0
concha — *see also Neoplasm, skin, ear*	C44.20-●	C79.2	D04.2-●	D23.2-●	D48.5	D49.2
nose	C30.0	C78.39	D02.3	D14.0	D38.5	D49.1
conjunctiva	C69.0-●	C79.49	D09.2-●	D31.0-●	D48.7	D49.89
connective tissue NEC	C49.9	C79.89	—	D21.9	D48.1	D49.2

Note: For neoplasms of connective tissue (blood vessel, bursa, fascia, ligament, muscle, peripheral nerves, sympathetic and parasympathetic nerves and ganglia, synovia, tendon, etc.) or of morphological types that indicate connective tissue, code according to the list under "Neoplasm, connective tissue." For sites that do not appear in this list, code to neoplasm of that site; e.g., fibrosarcoma, pancreas (C25.9)

Note: Morphological types that indicate connective tissue appear in their proper place in the alphabetic index with the instruction "*see Neoplasm, connective tissue ....*"

	Malignant Primary	Malignant Secondary	Ca in situ	Benign	Uncertain Behavior	Unspecified Behavior
abdomen	C49.4	C79.89	—	D21.4	D48.1	D49.2
abdominal wall	C49.4	C79.89	—	D21.4	D48.1	D49.2
ankle	C49.2-●	C79.89	—	D21.2-●	D48.1	D49.2
antecubital fossa or space	C49.1-●	C79.89	—	D21.1-●	D48.1	D49.2
arm	C49.1-●	C79.89	—	D21.1-●	D48.1	D49.2
auricle (ear)	C49.0	C79.89	—	D21.0	D48.1	D49.2
axilla	C49.3	C79.89	—	D21.3	D48.1	D49.2
back	C49.6	C79.89	—	D21.6	D48.1	D49.2
breast — *see Neoplasm, breast*						
buttock	C49.5	C79.89	—	D21.5	D48.1	D49.2
calf	C49.2-●	C79.89	—	D21.2-●	D48.1	D49.2
cervical region	C49.0	C79.89	—	D21.0	D48.1	D49.2

connective tissue NEC *(Continued)*	Malignant Primary	Malignant Secondary	Ca in situ	Benign	Uncertain Behavior	Unspecified Behavior
cheek	C49.0	C79.89	—	D21.0	D48.1	D49.2
chest (wall)	C49.3	C79.89	—	D21.3	D48.1	D49.2
chin	C49.0	C79.89	—	D21.0	D48.1	D49.2
diaphragm	C49.3	C79.89	—	D21.3	D48.1	D49.2
ear (external)	C49.0	C79.89	—	D21.0	D48.1	D49.2
elbow	C49.1-●	C79.89	—	D21.1-●	D48.1	D49.2
extrarectal	C49.5	C79.89	—	D21.5	D48.1	D49.2
extremity	C49.9	C79.89	—	D21.9	D48.1	D49.2
lower	C49.2-●	C79.89	—	D21.2-●	D48.1	D49.2
upper	C49.1-●	C79.89	—	D21.1-●	D48.1	D49.2
eyelid	C49.0	C79.89	—	D21.0	D48.1	D49.2
face	C49.0	C79.89	—	D21.0	D48.1	D49.2
finger	C49.1-●	C79.89	—	D21.1-●	D48.1	D49.2
flank	C49.6	C79.89	—	D21.6	D48.1	D49.2
foot	C49.2-●	C79.89	—	D21.2-●	D48.1	D49.2
forearm	C49.1-●	C79.89	—	D21.1-●	D48.1	D49.2
forehead	C49.0	C79.89	—	D21.0	D48.1	D49.2
gastric	C49.4	C79.89	—	D21.4	D48.1	D49.2
gastrointestinal	C49.4	C79.89	—	D21.4	D48.1	D49.2
gluteal region	C49.5	C79.89	—	D21.5	D48.1	D49.2
great vessels NEC	C49.3	C79.89	—	D21.3	D48.1	D49.2
groin	C49.5	C79.89	—	D21.5	D48.1	D49.2
hand	C49.1-●	C79.89	—	D21.1-●	D48.1	D49.2
head	C49.0	C79.89	—	D21.0	D48.1	D49.2
heel	C49.2-●	C79.89	—	D21.2-●	D48.1	D49.2
hip	C49.2-●	C79.89	—	D21.2-●	D48.1	D49.2
hypochondrium	C49.4	C79.89	—	D21.4	D48.1	D49.2
iliopsoas muscle	C49.5	C79.89	—	D21.5	D48.1	D49.2
infraclavicular region	C49.3	C79.89	—	D21.3	D48.1	D49.2
inguinal (canal) (region)	C49.5	C79.89	—	D21.5	D48.1	D49.2
intestinal	C49.4	C79.89	—	D21.4	D48.1	D49.2
intrathoracic	C49.3	C79.89	—	D21.3	D48.1	D49.2
ischiorectal fossa	C49.5	C79.89	—	D21.5	D48.1	D49.2
jaw	C03.9	C79.89	D00.03	D10.39	D48.1	D49.0
knee	C49.2-●	C79.89	—	D21.2-●	D48.1	D49.2
leg	C49.2-●	C79.89	—	D21.2-●	D48.1	D49.2
limb NEC	C49.9	C79.89	—	D21.9	D48.1	D49.2
lower	C49.2-●	C79.89	—	D21.2-●	D48.1	D49.2
upper	C49.1-●	C79.89	—	D21.1-●	D48.1	D49.2
nates	C49.5	C79.89	—	D21.5	D48.1	D49.2
neck	C49.0	C79.89	—	D21.0	D48.1	D49.2
orbit	C69.6-●	C79.49	D09.2-●	D31.6-●	D48.1	D49.89
overlapping lesion	C49.8	—	—	—	—	—

◀ New   ◀◀ Revised   ~~deleted~~ Deleted   ● Use Additional Character(s)

	Malignant Primary	Malignant Secondary	Ca in situ	Benign	Uncertain Behavior	Unspecified Behavior
connective tissue NEC *(Continued)*						
pararectal	C49.5	C79.89	—	D21.5	D48.1	D49.2
para-urethral	C49.5	C79.89	—	D21.5	D48.1	D49.2
paravaginal	C49.5	C79.89	—	D21.5	D48.1	D49.2
pelvis (floor)	C49.5	C79.89	—	D21.5	D48.1	D49.2
pelvo-abdominal	C49.8	C79.89	—	D21.6	D48.1	D49.2
perineum	C49.5	C79.89	—	D21.5	D48.1	D49.2
perirectal (tissue)	C49.5	C79.89	—	D21.5	D48.1	D49.2
periurethral (tissue)	C49.5	C79.89	—	D21.5	D48.1	D49.2
popliteal fossa or space	C49.2-●	C79.89	—	D21.2-●	D48.1	D49.2
presacral	C49.5	C79.89	—	D21.5	D48.1	D49.2
psoas muscle	C49.4	C79.89	—	D21.4	D48.1	D49.2
pterygoid fossa	C49.0	C79.89	—	D21.0	D48.1	D49.2
rectovaginal septum or wall	C49.5	C79.89	—	D21.5	D48.1	D49.2
rectovesical	C49.5	C79.89	—	D21.5	D48.1	D49.2
retroperitoneum	C48.0	C78.6	—	D20.0	D48.3	D49.0
sacrococcygeal region	C49.5	C79.89	—	D21.5	D48.1	D49.2
scalp	C49.0	C79.89	—	D21.0	D48.1	D49.2
scapular region	C49.3	C79.89	—	D21.3	D48.1	D49.2
shoulder	C49.1-●	C79.89	—	D21.1-●	D48.1	D49.2
skin (dermis) NEC — *see also Neoplasm, skin, by site*	C44.90	C79.2	D04.9	D23.9	D48.5	D49.2
stomach	C49.4	C79.89	—	D21.4	D48.1	D49.2
submental	C49.0	C79.89	—	D21.0	D48.1	D49.2
supraclavicular region	C49.0	C79.89	—	D21.0	D48.1	D49.2
temple	C49.0	C79.89	—	D21.0	D48.1	D49.2
temporal region	C49.0	C79.89	—	D21.0	D48.1	D49.2
thigh	C49.2-●	C79.89	—	D21.2-●	D48.1	D49.2
thoracic (duct) (wall)	C49.3	C79.89	—	D21.3	D48.1	D49.2
thorax	C49.3	C79.89	—	D21.3	D48.1	D49.2
thumb	C49.1-●	C79.89	—	D21.1-●	D48.1	D49.2
toe	C49.2-●	C79.89	—	D21.2-●	D48.1	D49.2
trunk	C49.6	C79.89	—	D21.6	D48.1	D49.2
umbilicus	C49.4	C79.89	—	D21.4	D48.1	D49.2
vesicorectal	C49.5	C79.89	—	D21.5	D48.1	D49.2
wrist	C49.1-●	C79.89	—	D21.1 ●	D48.1	D49.2
conus medullaris	C72.0	C79.49	—	D33.4	D43.4	D49.7
cord (true) (vocal)	C32.0	C78.39	D02.0	D14.1	D38.0	D49.1
false	C32.1	C78.39	D02.0	D14.1	D38.0	D49.1
spermatic	C63.1-●	C79.82	D07.69	D29.8	D40.8	D49.59
spinal (cervical) (lumbar) (thoracic)	C72.0	C79.49	—	D33.4	D43.4	D49.7
cornea (limbus)	C69.1-●	C79.49	D09.2-●	D31.1-●	D48.7	D49.89
corpus						
corpus *(Continued)*						
albicans	C56.-●	C79.6-●	D07.39	D27.-●	D39.1-●	D49.59
callosum, brain	C71.0	C79.31	—	D33.2	D43.2	D49.6
cavernosum	C60.2	C79.82	D07.4	D29.0	D40.8	D49.59
gastric	C16.2	C78.89	D00.2	D13.1	D37.1	D49.0
overlapping sites	C54.8	—	—	—	—	—
penis	C60.2	C79.82	D07.4	D29.0	D40.8	D49.59
striatum, cerebrum	C71.0	C79.31	—	D33.0	D43.0	D49.6
uteri	C54.9	C79.82	D07.0	D26.1	D39.0	D49.59
isthmus	C54.0	C79.82	D07.0	D26.1	D39.0	D49.59
cortex						
adrenal	C74.0-●	C79.7-●	D09.3	D35.0-●	D44.1-●	D49.7
cerebral	C71.0	C79.31	—	D33.0	D43.0	D49.6
costal cartilage	C41.3	C79.51	—	D16.7	D48.0	D49.2
costovertebral joint	C41.3	C79.51	—	D16.7	D48.0	D49.2
Cowper's gland	C68.0	C79.19	D09.19	D30.4	D41.3	D49.59
cranial (fossa, any)	C71.9	C79.31	—	D33.2	D43.2	D49.6
meninges	C70.0	C79.32	—	D32.0	D42.0	D49.7
nerve	C72.50	C79.49	—	D33.3	D43.3	D49.7
specified NEC	C72.59	C79.49	—	D33.3	D43.3	D49.7
craniobuccal pouch	C75.2	C79.89	D09.3	D35.2	D44.3	D49.7
craniopharyngeal (duct) (pouch)	C75.2	C79.89	D09.3	D35.3	D44.4	D49.7
cricoid	C13.0	C79.89	D00.08	D10.7	D37.05	D49.0
cartilage	C32.3	C78.39	D02.0	D14.1	D38.0	D49.1
cricopharynx	C13.0	C79.89	D00.08	D10.7	D37.05	D49.0
crypt of Morgagni	C21.8	C78.5	D01.3	D12.9	D37.8	D49.0
crystalline lens	C69.4-●	C79.49	D09.2-●	D31.4-●	D48.7	D49.89
cul-de-sac (Douglas')	C48.1	C78.6	—	D20.1	D48.4	D49.0
cuneiform cartilage	C32.3	C78.39	D02.0	D14.1	D38.0	D49.1
cutaneous — *see Neoplasm, skin*						
cutis — *see Neoplasm, skin*						
cystic (bile) duct (common)	C24.0	C78.89	D01.5	D13.5	D37.6	D49.0
dermis — *see Neoplasm, skin*						
diaphragm	C49.3	C79.89	—	D21.3	D48.1	D49.2
digestive organs, system, tube, or tract NEC	C26.9	C78.89	D01.9	D13.9	D37.9	D49.0
disc, intervertebral	C41.2	C79.51	—	D16.6	D48.0	D49.2
disease, generalized	C80.0	—	—	—	—	—
disseminated	C80.0	—	—	—	—	—
Douglas' cul-de-sac or pouch	C48.1	C78.6	—	D20.1	D48.4	D49.0
duodenojejunal junction	C17.8	C78.4	D01.49	D13.39	D37.2	D49.0
duodenum	C17.0	C78.4	D01.49	D13.2	D37.2	D49.0

◀ New ◀ Revised ~~deleted~~ Deleted ● Use Additional Character(s)

TABLE OF NEOPLASMS

	Malignant Primary	Malignant Secondary	Ca in situ	Benign	Uncertain Behavior	Unspecified Behavior
dura (cranial) (mater)	C70.9	C79.49	—	D32.9	D42.9	D49.7
cerebral	C70.0	C79.32	—	D32.0	D42.0	D49.7
spinal	C70.1	C79.49	—	D32.1	D42.1	D49.7
ear (external) — see also Neoplasm, skin, ear	C44.20-●	C79.2	D04.2-●	D23.2-●	D48.5	D49.2
auricle or auris — see also Neoplasm, skin, ear	C44.20-●	C79.2	D04.2-●	D23.2-●	D48.5	D49.2
canal, external — see also Neoplasm, skin, ear	C44.20-●	C79.2	D04.2-●	D23.2-●	D48.5	D49.2
cartilage	C49.0	C79.89	—	D21.0	D48.1	D49.2
external meatus — see also Neoplasm, skin, ear	C44.20-●	C79.2	D04.2-●	D23.2-●	D48.5	D49.2
inner	C30.1	C78.39	D02.3	D14.0	D38.5	D49.1
lobule — see also Neoplasm, skin, ear	C44.20-●	C79.2	D04.2-●	D23.2-●	D48.5	D49.2
middle	C30.1	C78.39	D02.3	D14.0	D38.5	D49.1
overlapping lesion with accessory sinuses	C31.8	—	—	—	—	—
skin	C44.20-●	C79.2	D04.2-●	D23.2-●	D48.5	D49.2
basal cell carcinoma	C44.21-●	—	—	—	—	—
specified type NEC	C44.29-●	—	—	—	—	—
squamous cell carcinoma	C44.22-●	—	—	—	—	—
earlobe	C44.20-●	C79.2	D04.2-●	D23.2-●	D48.5	D49.2
basal cell carcinoma	C44.21-●	—	—	—	—	—
specified type NEC	C44.29-●	—	—	—	—	—
squamous cell carcinoma	C44.22-●	—	—	—	—	—
ejaculatory duct	C63.7	C79.82	D07.69	D29.8	D40.8	D49.59
elbow NEC	C76.4-●	C79.89	D04.6-●	D36.7	D48.7	D49.89
endocardium	C38.0	C79.89	—	D15.1	D48.7	D49.89
endocervix (canal) (gland)	C53.0	C79.82	D06.0	D26.0	D39.0	D49.59
endocrine gland NEC	C75.9	C79.89	D09.3	D35.9	D44.9	D49.7
pluriglandular	C75.8	C79.89	D09.3	D35.7	D44.9	D49.7
endometrium (gland) (stroma)	C54.1	C79.82	D07.0	D26.1	D39.0	D49.59
ensiform cartilage	C41.3	C79.51	—	D16.7	D48.0	D49.2
enteric — see Neoplasm, intestine						
ependyma (brain)	C71.5	C79.31	—	D33.0	D43.0	D49.6
fourth ventricle	C71.7	C79.31	—	D33.1	D43.1	D49.6
epicardium	C38.0	C79.89	—	D15.1	D48.7	D49.89
epididymis	C63.0-●	C79.82	D07.69	D29.3-●	D40.8	D49.59
epidural	C72.9	C79.49	—	D33.9	D43.9	D49.7
epiglottis	C32.1	C78.39	D02.0	D14.1	D38.0	D49.1
anterior aspect or surface	C10.1	C79.89	D00.08	D10.5	D37.05	D49.0
cartilage	C32.3	C78.39	D02.0	D14.1	D38.0	D49.1
free border (margin)	C10.1	C79.89	D00.08	D10.5	D37.05	D49.0
junctional region	C10.8	C79.89	D00.08	D10.5	D37.05	D49.0
posterior (laryngeal) surface	C32.1	C78.39	D02.0	D14.1	D38.0	D49.1
suprahyoid portion	C32.1	C78.39	D02.0	D14.1	D38.0	D49.1
esophagogastric junction	C16.0	C78.89	D00.2	D13.1	D37.1	D49.0
esophagus	C15.9	C78.89	D00.1	D13.0	D37.8	D49.0
abdominal	C15.5	C78.89	D00.1	D13.0	D37.8	D49.0
cervical	C15.3	C78.89	D00.1	D13.0	D37.8	D49.0
distal (third)	C15.5	C78.89	D00.1	D13.0	D37.8	D49.0
lower (third)	C15.5	C78.89	D00.1	D13.0	D37.8	D49.0
middle (third)	C15.4	C78.89	D00.1	D13.0	D37.8	D49.0
overlapping lesion	C15.8	—	—	—	—	—
proximal (third)	C15.3	C78.89	D00.1	D13.0	D37.8	D49.0
thoracic	C15.4	C78.89	D00.1	D13.0	D37.8	D49.0
upper (third)	C15.3	C78.89	D00.1	D13.0	D37.8	D49.0
ethmoid (sinus)	C31.1	C78.39	D02.3	D14.0	D38.5	D49.1
bone or labyrinth	C41.0	C79.51	—	D16.4-●	D48.0	D49.2
eustachian tube	C30.1	C78.39	D02.3	D14.0	D38.5	D49.1
exocervix	C53.1	C79.82	D06.1	D26.0	D39.0	D49.59
external						
meatus (ear) — see also Neoplasm, skin, ear	C44.20-●	C79.2	D04.2-●	D23.2-●	D48.5	D49.2
os, cervix uteri	C53.1	C79.82	D06.1	D26.0	D39.0	D49.59
extradural	C72.9	C79.49	—	D33.9	D43.9	D49.7
extrahepatic (bile) duct	C24.0	C78.89	D01.5	D13.5	D37.6	D49.0
overlapping lesion with gallbladder	C24.8	—	—	—	—	—
extraocular muscle	C69.6-●	C79.49	D09.2-●	D31.6-●	D48.7	D49.89
extrarectal	C76.3	C79.89	D09.8	D36.7	D48.7	D49.89
extremity	C76.8	C79.89	D04.8	D36.7	D48.7	D49.89
lower	C76.5-●	C79.89	D04.7-●	D36.7	D48.7	D49.89
upper	C76.4-●	C79.89	D04.6-●	D36.7	D48.7	D49.89
eye NEC	C69.9-●	C79.49	D09.2	D31.9	D48.7	D49.89
overlapping sites	C69.8	—	—	—	—	—
eyeball	C69.9-●	C79.49	D09.2-●	D31.9-●	D48.7	D49.89
eyebrow	C44.309	C79.2	D04.39	D23.39	D48.5	D49.2
basal cell carcinoma	C44.319	—	—	—	—	—
specified type NEC	C44.399	—	—	—	—	—
squamous cell carcinoma	C44.329	—	—	—	—	—
eyelid (lower) (skin) (upper)	C44.10-●	—	—	—	—	—
basal cell carcinoma	C44.11-●	—	—	—	—	—
cartilage	C49.0	C79.89	—	D21.0	D48.1	D49.2
sebaceous cell	C44.13-●	—	—	—	—	—
specified type NEC	C44.19-●	—	—	—	—	—
squamous cell carcinoma	C44.12-●	—	—	—	—	—

◀ New   ◀ Revised   ~~deleted~~ Deleted   ● Use Additional Character(s)

	Malignant Primary	Malignant Secondary	Ca in situ	Benign	Uncertain Behavior	Unspecified Behavior
face NEC	C76.0	C79.89	D04.39	D36.7	D48.7	D49.89
fallopian tube (accessory)	C57.0-●	C79.82	D07.39	D28.2	D39.8	D49.59
falx (cerebella) (cerebri)	C70.0	C79.32	—	D32.0	D42.0	D49.7
fascia — see also Neoplasm, connective tissue						
palmar	C49.1-●	C79.89	—	D21.1-●	D48.1	D49.2
plantar	C49.2-●	C79.89	—	D21.2-●	D48.1	D49.2
fatty tissue — see Neoplasm, connective tissue						
fauces, faucial NEC	C10.9	C79.89	D00.08	D10.5	D37.05	D49.0
pillars	C09.1	C79.89	D00.08	D10.5	D37.05	D49.0
tonsil	C09.9	C79.89	D00.08	D10.4	D37.05	D49.0
femur (any part)	C40.2-●	—	—	D16.2-●	—	—
fetal membrane	C58	C79.82	D07.0	D26.7	D39.2	D49.59
fibrous tissue — see Neoplasm, connective tissue						
fibula (any part)	C40.2-●	C79.51	—	D16.2-●	—	—
filum terminale	C72.0	C79.49	—	D33.4	D43.4	D49.7
finger NEC	C76.4-●	C79.89	D04.6-●	D36.7	D48.7	D49.89
flank NEC	C76.8	C79.89	D04.5	D36.7	D48.7	D49.89
follicle, nabothian	C53.0	C79.82	D06.0	D26.0	D39.0	D49.59
foot NEC	C76.5-●	C79.89	D04.7-●	D36.7	D48.7	D49.89
forearm NEC	C76.4-●	C79.89	D04.6-●	D36.7	D48.7	D49.89
forehead (skin)	C44.309	C79.2	D04.39	D23.39	D48.5	D49.2
basal cell carcinoma	C44.319	—	—	—	—	—
specified type NEC	C44.399	—	—	—	—	—
squamous cell carcinoma	C44.329	—	—	—	—	—
foreskin	C60.0	C79.82	D07.4	D29.0	D40.8	D49.59
fornix						
pharyngeal	C11.3	C79.89	D00.08	D10.6	D37.05	D49.0
vagina	C52	C79.82	D07.2	D28.1	D39.8	D49.59
fossa (of)						
anterior (cranial)	C71.9	C79.31	—	D33.2	D43.2	D49.6
cranial	C71.9	C79.31	—	D33.2	D43.2	D49.6
ischiorectal	C76.3	C79.89	D09.8	D36.7	D48.7	D49.89
middle (cranial)	C71.9	C79.31	—	D33.2	D43.2	D49.6
piriform	C12	C79.89	D00.08	D10.7	D37.05	D49.0
pituitary	C75.1	C79.89	D09.3	D35.2	D44.3	D49.7
posterior (cranial)	C71.9	C79.31	—	D33.2	D43.2	D49.6
pterygoid	C49.0	C79.89	—	D21.0	D48.1	D49.2
pyriform	C12	C79.89	D00.08	D10.7	D37.05	D49.0
Rosenmuller	C11.2	C79.89	D00.08	D10.6	D37.05	D49.0
tonsillar	C09.0	C79.89	D00.08	D10.5	D37.05	D49.0
fourchette	C51.9	C79.82	D07.1	D28.0	D39.8	D49.59

	Malignant Primary	Malignant Secondary	Ca in situ	Benign	Uncertain Behavior	Unspecified Behavior
frenulum						
labii — see Neoplasm, lip, internal						
linguae	C02.2	C79.89	D00.07	D10.1	D37.02	D49.0
frontal						
bone	C41.0	C79.51	—	D16.4-●	D48.0	D49.2
lobe, brain	C71.1	C79.31	—	D33.0	D43.0	D49.6
pole	C71.1	C79.31	—	D33.0	D43.0	D49.6
sinus	C31.2	C78.39	D02.3	D14.0	D38.5	D49.1
fundus						
stomach	C16.1	C78.89	D00.2	D13.1	D37.1	D49.0
uterus	C54.3	C79.82	D07.0	D26.1	D39.0	D49.59
gall duct (extrahepatic)	C24.0	C78.89	D01.5	D13.5	D37.6	D49.0
intrahepatic	C22.1	C78.7	D01.5	D13.4	D37.6	D49.0
gallbladder	C23	C78.89	D01.5	D13.5	D37.6	D49.0
overlapping lesion with extrahepatic bile ducts	C24.8	—	—	—	—	—
ganglia — see also Neoplasm, nerve, peripheral	C47.9	C79.89	—	D36.10	D48.2	D49.2
basal	C71.0	C79.31	—	D33.0	D43.0	D49.6
cranial nerve	C72.50	C79.49	—	D33.3	D43.3	D49.7
Gartner's duct	C52	C79.82	D07.2	D28.1	D39.8	D49.59
gastric — see Neoplasm, stomach						
gastrocolic	C26.9	C78.89	D01.9	D13.9	D37.9	D49.0
gastroesophageal junction	C16.0	C78.89	D00.2	D13.1	D37.1	D49.0
gastrointestinal (tract) NEC	C26.9	C78.89	D01.9	D13.9	D37.9	D49.0
generalized	C80.0	—	—	—	—	—
genital organ or tract						
female NEC	C57.9	C79.82	D07.30	D28.9	D39.9	D49.59
overlapping lesion	C57.8	—	—	—	—	—
specified site NEC	C57.7	C79.82	D07.39	D28.7	D39.8	D49.59
male NEC	C63.9	C79.82	D07.60	D29.9	D40.9	D49.59
overlapping lesion	C63.8	—	—	—	—	—
specified site NEC	C63.7	C79.82	D07.69	D29.8	D40.8	D49.59
genitourinary tract						
female	C57.9	C79.82	D07.30	D28.9	D39.9	D49.59
male	C63.9	C79.82	D07.60	D29.9	D40.9	D49.59
gingiva (alveolar) (marginal)	C03.9	C79.89	D00.03	D10.39	D37.09	D49.0
lower	C03.1	C79.89	D00.03	D10.39	D37.09	D49.0
mandibular	C03.1	C79.89	D00.03	D10.39	D37.09	D49.0
maxillary	C03.0	C79.89	D00.03	D10.39	D37.09	D49.0
upper	C03.0	C79.89	D00.03	D10.39	D37.09	D49.0

◀ New   ◀ Revised   ~~deleted~~ Deleted   ● Use Additional Character(s)

TABLE OF NEOPLASMS

	Malignant Primary	Malignant Secondary	Ca in situ	Benign	Uncertain Behavior	Unspecified Behavior
gland, glandular (lymphatic) (system) — see also Neoplasm, lymph gland						
endocrine NEC	C75.9	C79.89	D09.3	D35.9	D44.9	D49.7
salivary — see Neoplasm, salivary gland						
glans penis	C60.1	C79.82	D07.4	D29.0	D40.8	D49.59
globus pallidus	C71.0	C79.31	—	D33.0	D43.0	D49.6
glomus						
coccygeal	C49.5	C79.89	—	D21.5	D48.1	D49.2
jugularis	C75.5	C79.89	—	D35.6	D44.7	D49.7
glosso-epiglottic fold(s)	C10.1	C79.89	D00.08	D10.5	D37.05	D49.0
glossopalatine fold	C09.1	C79.89	D00.08	D10.5	D37.05	D49.0
glossopharyngeal sulcus	C09.0	C79.89	D00.08	D10.5	D37.05	D49.0
glottis	C32.0	C78.39	D02.0	D14.1	D38.0	D49.1
gluteal region	C76.3	C79.89	D04.5	D36.7	D48.7	D49.89
great vessels NEC	C49.3	C79.89	—	D21.3	D48.1	D49.2
groin NEC	C76.3	C79.89	D04.5	D36.7	D48.7	D49.89
gum	C03.9	C79.89	D00.03	D10.39	D37.09	D49.0
lower	C03.1	C79.89	D00.03	D10.39	D37.09	D49.0
upper	C03.0	C79.89	D00.03	D10.39	D37.09	D49.0
hand NEC	C76.4-●	C79.89	D04.6-●	D36.7	D48.7	D49.89
head NEC	C76.0	C79.89	D04.4	D36.7	D48.7	D49.89
heart	C38.0	C79.89	—	D15.1	D48.7	D49.89
heel NEC	C76.5-●	C79.89	D04.7-●	D36.7	D48.7	D49.89
helix — see also Neoplasm, skin, ear	C44.20-●	C79.2	D04.2-●	D23.2-●	D48.5	D49.2
hematopoietic, hemopoietic tissue NEC	C96.9	—	—	—	—	—
specified NEC	C96.Z	—	—	—	—	—
hemisphere, cerebral	C71.0	C79.31	—	D33.0	D43.0	D49.6
hemorrhoidal zone	C21.1	C78.5	D01.3	D12.9	D37.8	D49.0
hepatic — see also Index to disease, by histology	C22.9	C78.7	D01.5	D13.4	D37.6	D49.0
duct (bile)	C24.0	C78.89	D01.5	D13.5	D37.6	D49.0
flexure (colon)	C18.3	C78.5	D01.0	D12.3	D37.4	D49.0
primary	C22.8	C78.7	D01.5	D13.4	D37.6	D49.0
hepatobiliary	C24.9	C79.89	D01.5	D13.5	D37.6	D49.0
hepatoblastoma	C22.2	C78.7	D01.5	D13.4	D37.6	D49.0
hepatoma	C22.0	C78.7	D01.5	D13.4	D37.6	D49.0
hilus of lung	C34.0-●	C78.0-●	D02.2-●	D14.3-●	D38.1	D49.1
hip NEC	C76.5-●	C79.89	D04.7-●	D36.7	D48.7	D49.89
hippocampus, brain	C71.2	C79.31	—	D33.0	D43.0	D49.6
humerus (any part)	C40.0-●	C79.51	—	D16.0-●	—	—
hymen	C52	C79.82	D07.2	D28.1	D39.8	D49.59

	Malignant Primary	Malignant Secondary	Ca in situ	Benign	Uncertain Behavior	Unspecified Behavior
hypopharynx, hypopharyngeal NEC	C13.9	C79.89	D00.08	D10.7	D37.05	D49.0
overlapping lesion	C13.8	—	—	—	—	—
postcricoid region	C13.0	C79.89	D00.08	D10.7	D37.05	D49.0
posterior wall	C13.2	C79.89	D00.08	D10.7	D37.05	D49.0
pyriform fossa (sinus)	C12	C79.89	D00.08	D10.7	D37.05	D49.0
hypophysis	C75.1	C79.89	D09.3	D35.2	D44.3	D49.7
hypothalamus	C71.0	C79.31	—	D33.0	D43.0	D49.6
ileocecum, ileocecal (coil) (junction) (valve)	C18.0	C78.5	D01.0	D12.0	D37.4	D49.0
ileum	C17.2	C78.4	D01.49	D13.39	D37.2	D49.0
ilium	C41.4	C79.51	—	D16.8	D48.0	D49.2
immunoproliferative NEC	C88.9	—	—	—	—	—
infraclavicular (region)	C76.1	C79.89	D04.5	D36.7	D48.7	D49.89
inguinal (region)	C76.3	C79.89	D04.5	D36.7	D48.7	D49.89
insula	C71.0	C79.31	—	D33.0	D43.0	D49.6
insular tissue (pancreas)	C25.4	C78.89	D01.7	D13.7	D37.8	D49.0
brain	C71.0	C79.31	—	D33.0	D43.0	D49.6
interarytenoid fold	C13.1	C79.89	D00.08	D10.7	D37.05	D49.0
hypopharyngeal aspect	C13.1	C79.89	D00.08	D10.7	D37.05	D49.0
laryngeal aspect	C32.1	C78.39	D02.0	D14.1	D38.0	D49.1
marginal zone	C13.1	C79.89	D00.08	D10.7	D37.05	D49.0
interdental papillae	C03.9	C79.89	D00.03	D10.39	D37.09	D49.0
lower	C03.1	C79.89	D00.03	D10.39	D37.09	D49.0
upper	C03.0	C79.89	D00.03	D10.39	D37.09	D49.0
internal						
capsule	C71.0	C79.31	—	D33.0	D43.0	D49.6
os (cervix)	C53.0	C79.82	D06.0	D26.0	D39.0	D49.59
intervertebral cartilage or disc	C41.2	C79.51	—	D16.6	D48.0	D49.2
intestine, intestinal	C26.0	C78.80	D01.40	D13.9	D37.8	D49.0
large	C18.9	C78.5	D01.0	D12.6	D37.4	D49.0
appendix	C18.1	C78.5	D01.0	D12.1	D37.3	D49.0
caput coli	C18.0	C78.5	D01.0	D12.0	D37.4	D49.0
cecum	C18.0	C78.5	D01.0	D12.0	D37.4	D49.0
colon	C18.9	C78.5	D01.0	D12.6	D37.4	D49.0
and rectum	C19	C78.5	D01.1	D12.7	D37.5	D49.0
ascending	C18.2	C78.5	D01.0	D12.2	D37.4	D49.0
caput	C18.0	C78.5	D01.0	D12.0	D37.4	D49.0
descending	C18.6	C78.5	D01.0	D12.4	D37.4	D49.0
distal	C18.6	C78.5	D01.0	D12.4	D37.4	D49.0
left	C18.6	C78.5	D01.0	D12.4	D37.4	D49.0
overlapping lesion	C18.8	—	—	—	—	—
pelvic	C18.7	C78.5	D01.0	D12.5	D37.4	D49.0
right	C18.2	C78.5	D01.0	D12.2	D37.4	D49.0

◀ New ◀ Revised ~~deleted~~ Deleted ● Use Additional Character(s)

	Malignant Primary	Malignant Secondary	Ca in situ	Benign	Uncertain Behavior	Unspecified Behavior
intestine, intestinal *(Continued)*						
large *(Continued)*						
colon *(Continued)*						
sigmoid (flexure)	C18.7	C78.5	D01.0	D12.5	D37.4	D49.0
transverse	C18.4	C78.5	D01.0	D12.3	D37.4	D49.0
hepatic flexure	C18.3	C78.5	D01.0	D12.3	D37.4	D49.0
ileocecum, ileocecal (coil) (valve)	C18.0	C78.5	D01.0	D12.0	D37.4	D49.0
overlapping lesion	C18.8	—	—	—	—	—
sigmoid flexure (lower) (upper)	C18.7	C78.5	D01.0	D12.5	D37.4	D49.0
splenic flexure	C18.5	C78.5	D01.0	D12.3	D37.4	D49.0
small	C17.9	C78.4	D01.40	D13.30	D37.2	D49.0
duodenum	C17.0	C78.4	D01.49	D13.2	D37.2	D49.0
ileum	C17.2	C78.4	D01.49	D13.39	D37.2	D49.0
jejunum	C17.1	C78.4	D01.49	D13.39	D37.2	D49.0
overlapping lesion	C17.8	—	—	—	—	—
tract NEC	C26.0	C78.89	D01.40	D13.9	D37.8	D49.0
intra-abdominal	C76.2	C79.89	D09.8	D36.7	D48.7	D49.89
intracranial NEC	C71.9	C79.31	—	D33.2	D43.2	D49.6
intrahepatic (bile) duct	C22.1	C78.7	D01.5	D13.4	D37.6	D49.0
intraocular	C69.9-●	C79.49	D09.2-●	D31.9-●	D48.7	D49.89
intraorbital	C69.6-●	C79.49	D09.2-●	D31.6-●	D48.7	D49.89
intrasellar	C75.1	C79.89	D09.3	D35.2	D44.3	D49.7
intrathoracic (cavity) (organs)	C76.1	C79.89	D09.8	D15.9	D48.7	D49.89
specified NEC	C76.1	C79.89	D09.8	D15.7	—	—
iris	C69.4-●	C79.49	D09.2-●	D31.4-●	D48.7	D49.89
ischiorectal (fossa)	C76.3	C79.89	D09.8	D36.7	D48.7	D49.89
ischium	C41.4	C79.51	—	D16.8	D48.0	D49.2
island of Reil	C71.0	C79.31	—	D33.0	D43.0	D49.6
islands or islets of Langerhans	C25.4	C78.89	D01.7	D13.7	D37.8	D49.0
isthmus uteri	C54.0	C79.82	D07.0	D26.1	D39.0	D49.59
jaw	C76.0	C79.89	D09.8	D36.7	D48.7	D49.89
bone	C41.1	C79.51	—	D16.5-●	D48.0	D49.2
lower	C41.1	C79.51	—	D16.5-●	—	—
upper	C41.0	C79.51	—	D16.4-●	—	—
carcinoma (any type) (lower) (upper)	C76.0	C79.89				
skin—*see also Neoplasm, skin, face*	C44.309	C79.2	D04.39	D23.39	D48.5	D49.2
soft tissues	C03.9	C79.89	D00.03	D10.39	D37.09	D49.0
lower	C03.1	C79.89	D00.03	D10.39	D37.09	D49.0
upper	C03.0	C79.89	D00.03	D10.39	D37.09	D49.0
jejunum	C17.1	C78.4	D01.49	D13.39	D37.2	D49.0

	Malignant Primary	Malignant Secondary	Ca in situ	Benign	Uncertain Behavior	Unspecified Behavior
joint NEC—*see also Neoplasm, bone*	C41.9	C79.51	—	D16.9-●	D48.0	D49.2
acromioclavicular	C40.0-●	C79.51	—	D16.0-●	—	—
bursa or synovial membrane—*see Neoplasm, connective tissue*						
costovertebral	C41.3	C79.51	—	D16.7	D48.0	D49.2
sternocostal	C41.3	C79.51	—	D16.7	D48.0	D49.2
temporomandibular	C41.1	C79.51	—	D16.5-●	D48.0	D49.2
junction						
anorectal	C21.8	C78.5	D01.3	D12.9	D37.8	D49.0
cardioesophageal	C16.0	C78.89	D00.2	D13.1	D37.1	D49.0
esophagogastric	C16.0	C78.89	D00.2	D13.1	D37.1	D49.0
gastroesophageal	C16.0	C78.89	D00.2	D13.1	D37.1	D49.0
hard and soft palate	C05.9	C79.89	D00.00	D10.39	D37.09	D49.0
ileocecal	C18.0	C78.5	D01.0	D12.0	D37.4	D49.0
pelvirectal	C19	C78.5	D01.1	D12.7	D37.5	D49.0
pelviureteric	C65.-●	C79.0-●	D09.19	D30.1-●	D41.1-●	D49.59
rectosigmoid	C19	C78.5	D01.1	D12.7	D37.5	D49.0
squamocolumnar, of cervix	C53.8	C79.82	D06.7	D26.0	D39.0	D49.59
Kaposi's sarcoma—*see Kaposi's, sarcoma*						
kidney (parenchymal)	C64.-●	C79.0-●	D09.19	D30.0-●	D41.0-●	D49.51-●
calyx	C65.-●	C79.0-●	D09.19	D30.1-●	D41.1-●	D49.51-●
hilus	C65.-●	C79.0-●	D09.19	D30.1-●	D41.1-●	D49.51-●
pelvis	C65.-●	C79.0-●	D09.19	D30.1-●	D41.1-●	D49.51-●
knee NEC	C76.5-●	C79.89	D04.7-●	D36.7	D48.7	D49.89
labia (skin)	C51.9	C79.82	D07.1	D28.0	D39.8	D49.59
majora	C51.0	C79.82	D07.1	D28.0	D39.8	D49.59
minora	C51.1	C79.82	D07.1	D28.0	D39.8	D49.59
labial—*see also Neoplasm, lip*	C00.9	C79.89	D00.01	D10.0	D37.01	D49.0
sulcus (lower) (upper)	C06.1	C79.89	D00.02	D10.39	D37.09	D49.0
labium (skin)	C51.9	C79.82	D07.1	D28.0	D39.8	D49.59
majus	C51.0	C79.82	D07.1	D28.0	D39.8	D49.59
minus	C51.1	C79.82	D07.1	D28.0	D39.8	D49.59
lacrimal						
canaliculi	C69.5-●	C79.49	D09.2-●	D31.5-●	D48.7	D49.89
duct (nasal)	C69.5-●	C79.49	D09.2-●	D31.5-●	D48.7	D49.89
gland	C69.5-●	C79.49	D09.2-●	D31.5-●	D48.7	D49.89
punctum	C69.5-●	C79.49	D09.2-●	D31.5-●	D48.7	D49.89
sac	C69.5-●	C79.49	D09.2-●	D31.5-●	D48.7	D49.89
Langerhans, islands or islets	C25.4	C78.89	D01.7	D13.7	D37.8	D49.0
laryngopharynx	C13.9	C79.89	D00.08	D10.7	D37.05	D49.0

◀ New ◀ Revised ~~deleted~~ Deleted ● Use Additional Character(s)

TABLE OF NEOPLASMS

TABLE OF NEOPLASMS

	Malignant Primary	Malignant Secondary	Ca in situ	Benign	Uncertain Behavior	Unspecified Behavior
larynx, laryngeal NEC	C32.9	C78.39	D02.0	D14.1	D38.0	D49.1
aryepiglottic fold	C32.1	C78.39	D02.0	D14.1	D38.0	D49.1
cartilage (arytenoid) (cricoid) (cuneiform) (thyroid)	C32.3	C78.39	D02.0	D14.1	D38.0	D49.1
commissure (anterior) (posterior)	C32.0	C78.39	D02.0	D14.1	D38.0	D49.1
extrinsic NEC	C32.1	C78.39	D02.0	D14.1	D38.0	D49.1
meaning hypopharynx	C13.9	C79.89	D00.08	D10.7	D37.05	D49.0
interarytenoid fold	C32.1	C78.39	D02.0	D14.1	D38.0	D49.1
intrinsic	C32.0	C78.39	D02.0	D14.1	D38.0	D49.1
overlapping lesion	C32.8	—	—	—	—	—
ventricular band	C32.1	C78.39	D02.0	D14.1	D38.0	D49.1
leg NEC	C76.5-●	C79.89	D04.7-●	D36.7	D48.7	D49.89
lens, crystalline	C69.4-●	C79.49	D09.2-●	D31.4-●	D48.7	D49.89
lid (lower) (upper)	C44.10-●	C79.2	D04.1-●	D23.1-●	D48.5	D49.2
basal cell carcinoma	C44.11-●	—	—	—	—	—
sebaceous cell	C44.13-●	—	—	—	—	—
specified type NEC	C44.19-●	—	—	—	—	—
squamous cell carcinoma	C44.12-●	—	—	—	—	—
ligament — *see also Neoplasm, connective tissue*						
broad	C57.1	C79.82	D07.39	D28.2	D39.8	D49.59
Mackenrodt's	C57.7	C79.82	D07.39	D28.7	D39.8	D49.59
non-uterine — *see Neoplasm, connective tissue*						
round	C57.2	C79.82	—	D28.2	D39.8	D49.59
sacro-uterine	C57.3	C79.82	—	D28.2	D39.8	D49.59
uterine	C57.3	C79.82	—	D28.2	D39.8	D49.59
utero-ovarian	C57.7	C79.82	D07.39	D28.2	D39.8	D49.59
uterosacral	C57.3	C79.82	—	D28.2	D39.8	D49.59
limb	C76.8	C79.89	D04.8	D36.7	D48.7	D49.89
lower	C76.5-●	C79.89	D04.7-●	D36.7	D48.7	D49.89
upper	C76.4-●	C79.89	D04.6-●	D36.7	D48.7	D49.89
limbus of cornea	C69.1-●	C79.49	D09.2-●	D31.1-●	D48.7	D49.89
lingual NEC — *see also Neoplasm, tongue*	C02.9	C79.89	D00.07	D10.1	D37.02	D49.0
lingula, lung	C34.1-●	C78.0-●	D02.2-●	D14.3-●	D38.1	D49.1
lip	C00.9	C79.89	D00.01	D10.0	D37.01	D49.0
buccal aspect — *see Neoplasm, lip, internal*						
commissure	C00.6	C79.89	D00.01	D10.0	D37.01	D49.0
external	C00.2	C79.89	D00.01	D10.0	D37.01	D49.0
lower	C00.1	C79.89	D00.01	D10.0	D37.01	D49.0
upper	C00.0	C79.89	D00.01	D10.0	D37.01	D49.0
frenulum — *see Neoplasm, lip, internal*						

	Malignant Primary	Malignant Secondary	Ca in situ	Benign	Uncertain Behavior	Unspecified Behavior
lip *(Continued)*						
inner aspect — *see Neoplasm, lip, internal*						
internal	C00.5	C79.89	D00.01	D10.0	D37.01	D49.0
lower	C00.4	C79.89	D00.01	D10.0	D37.01	D49.0
upper	C00.3	C79.89	D00.01	D10.0	D37.01	D49.0
lipstick area	C00.2	C79.89	D00.01	D10.0	D37.01	D49.0
lower	C00.1	C79.89	D00.01	D10.0	D37.01	D49.0
upper	C00.0	C79.89	D00.01	D10.0	D37.01	D49.0
lower	C00.1	C79.89	D00.01	D10.0	D37.01	D49.0
internal	C00.4	C79.89	D00.01	D10.0	D37.01	D49.0
mucosa — *see Neoplasm, lip, internal*						
oral aspect — *see Neoplasm, lip, internal*						
overlapping lesion	C00.8	—	—	—	—	—
with oral cavity or pharynx	C14.8	—	—	—	—	—
skin (commissure) (lower) (upper)	C44.00	C79.2	D04.0	D23.0	D48.5	D49.2
basal cell carcinoma	C44.01	—	—	—	—	—
specified type NEC	C44.09	—	—	—	—	—
squamous cell carcinoma	C44.02	—	—	—	—	—
upper	C00.0	C79.89	D00.01	D10.0	D37.01	D49.0
internal	C00.3	C79.89	D00.01	D10.0	D37.01	D49.0
vermilion border	C00.2	C79.89	D00.01	D10.0	D37.01	D49.0
lower	C00.1	C79.89	D00.01	D10.0	D37.01	D49.0
upper	C00.0	C79.89	D00.01	D10.0	D37.01	D49.0
lipomatous — *see Lipoma, by site*						
liver — *see also Index to disease, by histology*	C22.9	C78.7	D01.5	D13.4	D37.6	D49.0
primary	C22.8	C78.7	D01.5	D13.4	D37.6	D49.0
lumbosacral plexus	C47.5	C79.89	—	D36.16	D48.2	D49.2
lung	C34.9-●	C78.0-●	D02.2-●	D14.3-●	D38.1	D49.1
azygos lobe	C34.1-●	C78.0-●	D02.2-●	D14.3-●	D38.1	D49.1
carina	C34.0-●	C78.0-●	D02.2-●	D14.3-●	D38.1	D49.1
hilus	C34.0-●	C78.0-●	D02.2-●	D14.3-●	D38.1	D49.1
linqula	C34.1-●	C78.0-●	D02.2-●	D14.3-●	D38.1	D49.1
lobe NEC	C34.9-●	C78.0-●	D02.2-●	D14.3-●	D38.1	D49.1
lower lobe	C34.3-●	C78.0-●	D02.2-●	D14.3-●	D38.1	D49.1
main bronchus	C34.0-●	C78.0-●	D02.2-●	D14.3-●	D38.1	D49.1
mesothelioma — *see Mesothelioma*						
middle lobe	C34.2	C78.0-●	D02.21	D14.31	D38.1	D49.1
overlapping lesion	C34.8-●	—	—	—	—	—
upper lobe	C34.1-●	C78.0-●	D02.2-●	D14.3-●	D38.1	D49.1

◀ New ◀ Revised ~~deleted~~ Deleted ● Use Additional Character(s)

	Malignant Primary	Malignant Secondary	Ca in situ	Benign	Uncertain Behavior	Unspecified Behavior
lymph, lymphatic channel NEC	C49.9	C79.89	—	D21.9	D48.1	D49.2
gland (secondary)	—	C77.9	—	D36.0	D48.7	D49.89
abdominal	—	C77.2	—	D36.0	D48.7	D49.89
aortic	—	C77.2	—	D36.0	D48.7	D49.89
arm	—	C77.3	—	D36.0	D48.7	D49.89
auricular (anterior) (posterior)	—	C77.0	—	D36.0	D48.7	D49.89
axilla, axillary	—	C77.3	—	D36.0	D48.7	D49.89
brachial	—	C77.3	—	D36.0	D48.7	D49.89
bronchial	—	C77.1	—	D36.0	D48.7	D49.89
bronchopulmonary	—	C77.1	—	D36.0	D48.7	D49.89
celiac	—	C77.2	—	D36.0	D48.7	D49.89
cervical	—	C77.0	—	D36.0	D48.7	D49.89
cervicofacial	—	C77.0	—	D36.0	D48.7	D49.89
Cloquet	—	C77.4	—	D36.0	D48.7	D49.89
colic	—	C77.2	—	D36.0	D48.7	D49.89
common duct	—	C77.2	—	D36.0	D48.7	D49.89
cubital	—	C77.3	—	D36.0	D48.7	D49.89
diaphragmatic	—	C77.1	—	D36.0	D48.7	D49.89
epigastric, inferior	—	C77.1	—	D36.0	D48.7	D49.89
epitrochlear	—	C77.3	—	D36.0	D48.7	D49.89
esophageal	—	C77.1	—	D36.0	D48.7	D49.89
face	—	C77.0	—	D36.0	D48.7	D49.89
femoral	—	C77.4	—	D36.0	D48.7	D49.89
gastric	—	C77.2	—	D36.0	D48.7	D49.89
groin	—	C77.4	—	D36.0	D48.7	D49.89
head	—	C77.0	—	D36.0	D48.7	D49.89
hepatic	—	C77.2	—	D36.0	D48.7	D49.89
hilar (pulmonary)	—	C77.1	—	D36.0	D48.7	D49.89
splenic	—	C77.2	—	D36.0	D48.7	D49.89
hypogastric	—	C77.5	—	D36.0	D48.7	D49.89
ileocolic	—	C77.2	—	D36.0	D48.7	D49.89
iliac	—	C77.5	—	D36.0	D48.7	D49.89
infraclavicular	—	C77.3	—	D36.0	D48.7	D49.89
inguina, Inguinal	—	C77.4	—	D36.0	D48.7	D49.89
innominate	—	C77.1	—	D36.0	D48.7	D49.89
intercostal	—	C77.1	—	D36.0	D48.7	D49.89
intestinal	—	C77.2	—	D36.0	D48.7	D49.89
intrabdominal	—	C77.2	—	D36.0	D48.7	D49.89
intrapelvic	—	C77.5	—	D36.0	D48.7	D49.89
intrathoracic	—	C77.1	—	D36.0	D48.7	D49.89
jugular	—	C77.0	—	D36.0	D48.7	D49.89
leg	—	C77.4	—	D36.0	D48.7	D49.89
limb						
lower	—	C77.4	—	D36.0	D48.7	D49.89
upper	—	C77.3	—	D36.0	D48.7	D49.89
lymph, lymphatic channel NEC (Continued) gland (Continued)						
lower limb	—	C77.4	—	D36.0	D48.7	D49.89
lumbar	—	C77.2	—	D36.0	D48.7	D49.89
mandibular	—	C77.0	—	D36.0	D48.7	D49.89
mediastinal	—	C77.1	—	D36.0	D48.7	D49.89
mesenteric (inferior) (superior)	—	C77.2	—	D36.0	D48.7	D49.89
midcolic	—	C77.2	—	D36.0	D48.7	D49.89
multiple sites in categories C77.0 - C77.5	—	C77.8	—	D36.0	D48.7	D49.89
neck	—	C77.0	—	D36.0	D48.7	D49.89
obturator	—	C77.5	—	D36.0	D48.7	D49.89
occipital	—	C77.0	—	D36.0	D48.7	D49.89
pancreatic	—	C77.2	—	D36.0	D48.7	D49.89
para aortic	—	C77.2	—	D36.0	D48.7	D49.89
paracervical	—	C77.5	—	D36.0	D48.7	D49.89
parametrial	—	C77.5	—	D36.0	D48.7	D49.89
parasternal	—	C77.1	—	D36.0	D48.7	D49.89
parotid	—	C77.0	—	D36.0	D48.7	D49.89
pectoral	—	C77.3	—	D36.0	D48.7	D49.89
pelvic	—	C77.5	—	D36.0	D48.7	D49.89
peri-aortic	—	C77.2	—	D36.0	D48.7	D49.89
peripancreatic	—	C77.2	—	D36.0	D48.7	D49.89
popliteal	—	C77.4	—	D36.0	D48.7	D49.89
porta hepatis	—	C77.2	—	D36.0	D48.7	D49.89
portal	—	C77.2	—	D36.0	D48.7	D49.89
preauricular	—	C77.0	—	D36.0	D48.7	D49.89
prelaryngeal	—	C77.0	—	D36.0	D48.7	D49.89
presymphysial	—	C77.5	—	D36.0	D48.7	D49.89
pretracheal	—	C77.0	—	D36.0	D48.7	D49.89
primary (any site) NEC	C96.9	—	—	—	—	—
pulmonary (hiler)	—	C77.1	—	D36.0	D48.7	D49.89
pyloric	—	C77.2	—	D36.0	D48.7	D49.89
retroperitoneal	—	C77.2	—	D36.0	D48.7	D49.89
retropharyngeal	—	C77.0	—	D36.0	D48.7	D49.89
Rosenmuller's	—	C77.4	—	D36.0	D48.7	D49.89
sacral	—	C77.5	—	D36.0	D48.7	D49.89
scalene	—	C77.0	—	D36.0	D48.7	D49.89
site NEC	—	C77.9	—	D36.0	D48.7	D49.89
splenic (hilar)	—	C77.2	—	D36.0	D48.7	D49.89
subclavicular	—	C77.3	—	D36.0	D48.7	D49.89
subinguinal	—	C77.4	—	D36.0	D48.7	D49.89

◀ New ◀ Revised ~~deleted~~ Deleted ● Use Additional Character(s)

TABLE OF NEOPLASMS

	Malignant Primary	Malignant Secondary	Ca in situ	Benign	Uncertain Behavior	Unspecified Behavior
lymph, lymphatic channel NEC *(Continued)*						
gland *(Continued)*						
sublingual	—	C77.0	—	D36.0	D48.7	D49.89
submandibular	—	C77.0	—	D36.0	D48.7	D49.89
submaxillary	—	C77.0	—	D36.0	D48.7	D49.89
submental	—	C77.0	—	D36.0	D48.7	D49.89
subscapular	—	C77.3	—	D36.0	D48.7	D49.89
supraclavicular	—	C77.0	—	D36.0	D48.7	D49.89
thoracic	—	C77.1	—	D36.0	D48.7	D49.89
tibial	—	C77.4	—	D36.0	D48.7	D49.89
tracheal	—	C77.1	—	D36.0	D48.7	D49.89
tracheobronchial	—	C77.1	—	D36.0	D48.7	D49.89
upper limb	—	C77.3	—	D36.0	D48.7	D49.89
Virchow's	—	C77.0	—	D36.0	D48.7	D49.89
node — *see also Neoplasm, lymph gland*						
primary NEC	C96.9	—	—	—	—	—
vessel — *see also Neoplasm, connective tissue*	C49.9	C79.89	—	D21.9	D48.1	D49.2
Mackenrodt's ligament	C57.7	C79.82	D07.39	D28.7	D39.8	D49.59
malar	C41.0	C79.51	—	D16.4-●	D48.0	D49.2
region — *see Neoplasm, cheek*						
mammary gland — *see Neoplasm, breast*						
mandible	C41.1	C79.51	—	D16.5-●	D48.0	D49.2
alveolar						
mucosa (carcinoma)	C03.1	C79.89	D00.03	D10.39	D37.09	D49.0
ridge or process	C41.1	C79.51	—	D16.5-●	D48.0	D49.2
marrow (bone) NEC	C96.9	C79.52	—	—	D47.9	D49.89
mastectomy site (skin) — *see also Neoplasm, breast, skin*	C44.501	C79.2	—	—	—	—
specified as breast tissue	C50.8-●	C79.81	—	—	—	—
mastoid (air cells) (antrum) (cavity)	C30.1	C78.39	D02.3	D14.0	D38.5	D49.1
bone or process	C41.0	C79.51	—	D16.4-●	D48.0	D49.2
maxilla, maxillary (superior)	C41.0	C79.51	—	D16.4-●	D48.0	D49.2
alveolar						
mucosa	C03.0	C79.89	D00.03	D10.39	D37.09	D49.0
ridge or process (carcinoma)	C41.0	C79.51	—	D16.4-●	D48.0	D49.2
antrum	C31.0	C78.39	D02.3	D14.0	D38.5	D49.1
carcinoma	C03.0	C79.51				
inferior — *see Neoplasm, mandible*						
sinus	C31.0	C78.39	D02.3	D14.0	D38.5	D49.1

	Malignant Primary	Malignant Secondary	Ca in situ	Benign	Uncertain Behavior	Unspecified Behavior
meatus external (ear) — *see also Neoplasm, skin, ear*	C44.20-●	C79.2	D04.2-●	D23.2-●	D48.5	D49.2
Meckel diverticulum, malignant	C17.3	C78.4	D01.49	D13.39	D37.2	D49.0
mediastinum, mediastinal	C38.3	C78.1	—	D15.2	D38.3	D49.89
anterior	C38.1	C78.1	—	D15.2	D38.3	D49.89
posterior	C38.2	C78.1	—	D15.2	D38.3	D49.89
medulla						
adrenal	C74.1-●	C79.7-●	D09.3	D35.0-●	D44.1-●	D49.7
oblongata	C71.7	C79.31	—	D33.1	D43.1	D49.6
meibomian gland	C44.10-●	C79.2	D04.1-●	D23.1-●	D48.5	D49.2
basal cell carcinoma	C44.11-●	—	—	—	—	—
sebaceous cell	C44.13-●	—	—	—	—	—
specified type NEC	C44.19-●	—	—	—	—	—
squamous cell carcinoma	C44.12-●	—	—	—	—	—
melanoma — *see Melanoma*						
meninges	C70.9	C79.49	—	D32.9	D42.9	D49.7
brain	C70.0	C79.32	—	D32.0	D42.0	D49.7
cerebral	C70.0	C79.32	—	D32.0	D42.0	D49.7
crainial	C70.0	C79.32	—	D32.0	D42.0	D49.7
intracranial	C70.0	C79.32	—	D32.0	D42.0	D49.7
spinal (cord)	C70.1	C79.49	—	D32.1	D42.1	D49.7
meniscus, knee joint (lateral) (medial)	C40.2-●	C79.51	—	D16.2-●	D48.0	D49.2
Merkel cell — *see Carcinoma, Merkel cell*						
mesentery, mesenteric	C48.1	C78.6	—	D20.1	D48.4	D49.0
mesoappendix	C48.1	C78.6	—	D20.1	D48.4	D49.0
mesocolon	C48.1	C78.6	—	D20.1	D48.4	D49.0
mesopharynx — *see Neoplasm, oropharynx*						
mesosalpinx	C57.1	C79.82	D07.39	D28.2	D39.8	D49.59
mesothelial tissue — *see Mesothelioma*						
mesothelioma — *see Mesothelioma*						
mesovarium	C57.1	C79.82	D07.39	D28.2	D39.8	D49.59
metacarpus (any bone)	C40.1-●	C79.51	—	D16.1-●	—	—
metastatic NEC — *see also Neoplasm, by site, secondary*	—	C79.9	—	—	—	—
metatarsus (any bone)	C40.3-●	C79.51	—	D16.3-●	—	—
midbrain	C71.7	C79.31	—	D33.1	D43.1	D49.6
milk duct — *see Neoplasm, breast*						
mons						
pubis	C51.9	C79.82	D07.1	D28.0	D39.8	D49.59
veneris	C51.9	C79.82	D07.1	D28.0	D39.8	D49.59

◄ New ◄ Revised ~~deleted~~ Deleted ● Use Additional Character(s)

	Malignant Primary	Malignant Secondary	Ca in situ	Benign	Uncertain Behavior	Unspecified Behavior
motor tract	C72.9	C79.49	—	D33.9	D43.9	D49.7
brain	C71.9	C79.31	—	D33.2	D43.2	D49.6
cauda equina	C72.1	C79.49		D33.4	D43.4	D49.7
spinal	C72.0	C79.49		D33.4	D43.4	D49.7
mouth	C06.9	C79.89	D00.00	D10.30	D37.09	D49.0
book-leaf	C06.89	C79.89		—	—	—
floor	C04.9	C79.89	D00.06	D10.2	D37.09	D49.0
anterior portion	C04.0	C79.89	D00.06	D10.2	D37.09	D49.0
lateral portion	C04.1	C79.89	D00.06	D10.2	D37.09	D49.0
overlapping lesion	C04.8	—	—	—	—	—
overlapping NEC	C06.80	—	—	—	—	—
roof	C05.9	C79.89	D00.00	D10.39	D37.09	D49.0
specified part NEC	C06.89	C79.89	D00.00	D10.39	D37.09	D49.0
vestibule	C06.1	C79.89	D00.00	D10.39	D37.09	D49.0
mucosa						
alveolar (ridge or process)	C03.9	C79.89	D00.03	D10.39	D37.09	D49.0
lower	C03.1	C79.89	D00.03	D10.39	D37.09	D49.0
upper	C03.0	C79.89	D00.03	D10.39	D37.09	D49.0
buccal	C06.0	C79.89	D00.02	D10.39	D37.09	D49.0
cheek	C06.0	C79.89	D00.02	D10.39	D37.09	D49.0
lip — see Neoplasm, lip, internal						
nasal	C30.0	C78.39	D02.3	D14.0	D38.5	D49.1
oral	C06.0	C79.89	D00.02	D10.39	D37.09	D49.0
Mullerian duct						
female	C57.7	C79.82	D07.39	D28.7	D39.8	D49.59
male	C63.7	C79.82	D07.69	D29.8	D40.8	D49.59
muscle — see also Neoplasm, connective tissue						
extraocular	C69.6-●	C79.49	D09.2-●	D31.6-●	D48.7	D49.89
myocardium	C38.0	C79.89	—	D15.1	D48.7	D49.89
myometrium	C54.2	C79.82	D07.0	D26.1	D39.0	D49.59
myopericardium	C38.0	C79.89	—	D15.1	D48.7	D49.89
nabothian gland (follicle)	C53.0	C79.82	D06.0	D26.0	D39.0	D49.59
nail — see also Neoplasm, skin, limb	C44.90	C79.2	D04.9	D23.9	D48.5	D49.2
finger — see also Neoplasm, skin, limb, upper	C44.60-●	C79.2	D04.6-●	D23.6-●	D48.5	D49.2
toe — see also Neoplasm, skin, limb, lower	C44.70-●	C79.2	D04.7-●	D23.7-●	D48.5	D49.2
nares, naris (anterior) (posterior)	C30.0	C78.39	D02.3	D14.0	D38.5	D49.1
nasal — see Neoplasm, nose						
nasolabial groove — see also Neoplasm, skin, face	C44.309	C79.2	D04.39	D23.39	D48.5	D49.2
nasolacrimal duct	C69.5-●	C79.49	D09.2-●	D31.5-●	D48.7	D49.89

	Malignant Primary	Malignant Secondary	Ca in situ	Benign	Uncertain Behavior	Unspecified Behavior
nasopharynx, nasopharyngeal	C11.9	C79.89	D00.08	D10.6	D37.05	D49.0
floor	C11.3	C79.89	D00.08	D10.6	D37.05	D49.0
overlapping lesion	C11.8	—	—	—	—	—
roof	C11.0	C79.89	D00.08	D10.6	D37.05	D49.0
wall	C11.9	C79.89	D00.08	D10.6	D37.05	D49.0
anterior	C11.3	C79.89	D00.08	D10.6	D37.05	D49.0
lateral	C11.2	C79.89	D00.08	D10.6	D37.05	D49.0
posterior	C11.1	C79.89	D00.08	D10.6	D37.05	D49.0
superior	C11.0	C79.89	D00.08	D10.6	D37.05	D49.0
nates — see also Neoplasm, skin, trunk	C44.509	C79.2	D04.5	D23.5	D48.5	D49.2
neck NEC	C76.0	C79.89	D09.8	D36.7	D48.7	D49.89
skin	C44.40	—	—	—	—	—
basal cell carcinoma	C44.41	—	—	—	—	—
specified type NEC	C44.49	—	—	—	—	—
squamous cell carcinoma	C44.42	—	—	—	—	—
nerve (ganglion)	C47.9	C79.89	—	D36.10	D48.2	D49.89
abducens	C72.59	C79.49	—	D33.3	D43.3	D49.7
accessory (spinal)	C72.59	C79.49	—	D33.3	D43.3	D49.7
acoustic	C72.4-●	C79.49	—	D33.3	D43.3	D49.7
auditory	C72.4-●	C79.49	—	D33.3	D43.3	D49.7
autonomic NEC — see also Neoplasm, nerve, peripheral	C47.9	C79.89	—	D36.10	D48.2	D49.2
brachial	C47.1-●	C79.89	—	D36.12	D48.2	D49.2
cranial	C72.50	C79.49	—	D33.3	D43.3	D49.7
specified NEC	C72.59	C79.49	—	D33.3	D43.3	D49.7
facial	C72.59	C79.49	—	D33.3	D43.3	D49.7
femoral	C47.2-●	C79.89	—	D36.13	D48.2	D49.2
ganglion NEC — see also Neoplasm, nerve, peripheral	C47.9	C79.89	—	D36.10	D48.2	D49.2
glossopharyngeal	C72.59	C79.49	—	D33.3	D43.3	D49.7
hypoglossal	C72.59	C79.49	—	D33.3	D43.3	D49.7
intercostal	C47.3	C79.89	—	D36.14	D48.2	D49.2
lumbar	C47.6	C79.89	—	D36.17	D48.2	D49.2
median	C47.1-●	C79.89	—	D36.12	D48.2	D49.2
obturator	C47.2-●	C79.89	—	D36.13	D48.2	D49.2
oculomotor	C72.59	C79.49	—	D33.3	D43.3	D49.7
olfactory	C47.2-●	C79.49	—	D33.3	D43.3	D49.7
optic	C72.3-●	C79.49	—	D33.3	D43.3	D49.7
parasympathetic NEC	C47.9	C79.89	—	D36.10	D48.2	D49.2
peripheral NEC	C47.9	C79.89	—	D36.10	D48.2	D49.2
abdomen	C47.4	C79.89	—	D36.15	D48.2	D49.2
abdominal wall	C47.4	C79.89	—	D36.15	D48.2	D49.2

◀ New ◀ Revised ~~deleted~~ Deleted ● Use Additional Character(s)

	Malignant Primary	Malignant Secondary	Ca in situ	Benign	Uncertain Behavior	Unspecified Behavior
nerve *(Continued)*						
peripheral NEC *(Continued)*						
ankle	C47.2-●	C79.89	—	D36.13	D48.2	D49.2
antecubital fossa or space	C47.1-●	C79.89	—	D36.12	D48.2	D49.2
arm	C47.1-●	C79.89	—	D36.12	D48.2	D49.2
auricle (ear)	C47.0	C79.89	—	D36.11	D48.2	D49.2
axilla	C47.3	C79.89	—	D36.12	D48.2	D49.2
back	C47.6	C79.89	—	D36.17	D48.2	D49.2
buttock	C47.5	C79.89	—	D36.16	D48.2	D49.2
calf	C47.2-●	C79.89	—	D36.13	D48.2	D49.2
cervical region	C47.0	C79.89	—	D36.11	D48.2	D49.2
cheek	C47.0	C79.89	—	D36.11	D48.2	D49.2
chest (wall)	C47.3	C79.89	—	D36.14	D48.2	D49.2
chin	C47.0	C79.89	—	D36.11	D48.2	D49.2
ear (external)	C47.0	C79.89	—	D36.11	D48.2	D49.2
elbow	C47.1-●	C79.89	—	D36.12	D48.2	D49.2
extrarectal	C47.5	C79.89	—	D36.16	D48.2	D49.2
extremity	C47.9	C79.89	—	D36.10	D48.2	D49.2
lower	C47.2-●	C79.89	—	D36.13	D48.2	D49.2
upper	C47.1-●	C79.89	—	D36.12	D48.2	D49.2
eyelid	C47.0	C79.89	—	D36.11	D48.2	D49.2
face	C47.0	C79.89	—	D36.11	D48.2	D49.2
finger	C47.1-●	C79.89	—	D36.12	D48.2	D49.2
flank	C47.6	C79.89	—	D36.17	D48.2	D49.2
foot	C47.2-●	C79.89	—	D36.13	D48.2	D49.2
forearm	C47.1-●	C79.89	—	D36.12	D48.2	D49.2
forehead	C47.0	C79.89	—	D36.11	D48.2	D49.2
gluteal region	C47.5	C79.89	—	D36.16	D48.2	D49.2
groin	C47.5	C79.89	—	D36.16	D48.2	D49.2
hand	C47.1-●	C79.89	—	D36.12	D48.2	D49.2
head	C47.0	C79.89	—	D36.11	D48.2	D49.2
heel	C47.2-●	C79.89	—	D36.13	D48.2	D49.2
hip	C47.2-●	C79.89	—	D36.13	D48.2	D49.2
infraclavicular region	C47.3	C79.89	—	D36.14	D48.2	D49.2
inguinal (canal) (region)	C47.5	C79.89	—	D36.16	D48.2	D49.2
intrathoracic	C47.3	C79.89	—	D36.14	D48.2	D49.2
ischiorectal fossa	C47.5	C79.89	—	D36.16	D48.2	D49.2
knee	C47.2-●	C79.89	—	D36.13	D48.2	D49.2
leg	C47.2-●	C79.89	—	D36.13	D48.2	D49.2
limb NEC	C47.9	C79.89	—	D36.10	D48.2	D49.2
lower	C47.2-●	C79.89	—	D36.13	D48.2	D49.2
upper	C47.1-●	C79.89	—	D36.12	D48.2	D49.2
nates	C47.5	C79.89	—	D36.16	D48.2	D49.2
neck	C47.0	C79.89	—	D36.11	D48.2	D49.2

	Malignant Primary	Malignant Secondary	Ca in situ	Benign	Uncertain Behavior	Unspecified Behavior
nerve *(Continued)*						
peripheral NEC *(Continued)*						
orbit	C69.6-●	C79.49	—	D31.6-●	D48.7	D49.2
pararectal	C47.5	C79.89	—	D36.16	D48.2	D49.2
paraurethral	C47.5	C79.89	—	D36.16	D48.2	D49.2
paravaginal	C47.5	C79.89	—	D36.16	D48.2	D49.2
pelvis (floor)	C47.5	C79.89	—	D36.16	D48.2	D49.2
pelvoabdominal	C47.8	C79.89	—	D36.17	D48.2	D49.2
perineum	C47.5	C79.89	—	D36.16	D48.2	D49.2
perirectal (tissue)	C47.5	C79.89	—	D36.16	D48.2	D49.2
periurethral (tissue)	C47.5	C79.89	—	D36.16	D48.2	D49.2
popliteal fossa or space	C47.2-●	C79.89	—	D36.13	D48.2	D49.2
presacral	C47.5	C79.89	—	D36.16	D48.2	D49.2
pterygoid fossa	C47.0	C79.89	—	D36.11	D48.2	D49.2
rectovaginal septum or wall	C47.5	C79.89	—	D36.16	D48.2	D49.2
rectovesical	C47.5	C79.89	—	D36.16	D48.2	D49.2
sacrococcygeal region	C47.5	C79.89	—	D36.16	D48.2	D49.2
scalp	C47.0	C79.89	—	D36.11	D48.2	D49.2
scapular region	C47.3	C79.89	—	D36.14	D48.2	D49.2
shoulder	C47.1-●	C79.89	—	D36.12	D48.2	D49.2
submental	C47.0	C79.89	—	D36.11	D48.2	D49.2
supraclavicular region	C47.0	C79.89	—	D36.11	D48.2	D49.2
temple	C47.0	C79.89	—	D36.11	D48.2	D49.2
temporal region	C47.0	C79.89	—	D36.11	D48.2	D49.2
thigh	C47.2-●	C79.89	—	D36.13	D48.2	D49.2
thoracic (duct) (wall)	C47.3	C79.89	—	D36.14	D48.2	D49.2
thorax	C47.3	C79.89	—	D36.14	D48.2	D49.2
thumb	C47.1-●	C79.89	—	D36.12	D48.2	D49.2
toe	C47.2-●	C79.89	—	D36.13	D48.2	D49.2
trunk	C47.6	C79.89	—	D36.17	D48.2	D49.2
umbilicus	C47.4	C79.89	—	D36.15	D48.2	D49.2
vesicorectal	C47.5	C79.89	—	D36.16	D48.2	D49.2
wrist	C47.1-●	C79.89	—	D36.12	D48.2	D49.2
radial	C47.1-●	C79.89	—	D36.12	D48.2	D49.2
sacral	C47.5	C79.89	—	D36.16	D48.2	D49.2
sciatic	C47.2-●	C79.89	—	D36.13	D48.2	D49.2
spinal NEC	C47.9	C79.89	—	D36.10	D48.2	D49.2
accessory	C72.59	C79.49	—	D33.3	D43.3	D49.7
sympathetic NEC — *see also* *Neoplasm, nerve, peripheral*	C47.9	C79.89	—	D36.10	D48.2	D49.2
trigeminal	C72.59	C79.49	—	D33.3	D43.3	D49.7
trochlear	C72.59	C79.49	—	D33.3	D43.3	D49.7
ulnar	C47.1-●	C79.89	—	D36.12	D48.2	D49.2
vagus	C72.59	C79.49	—	D33.3	D43.3	D49.7

◀ New   ◀ Revised   ~~deleted~~ Deleted   ● Use Additional Character(s)

	Malignant Primary	Malignant Secondary	Ca in situ	Benign	Uncertain Behavior	Unspecified Behavior
nervous system (central)	C72.9	C79.40	—	D33.9	D43.9	D49.7
autonomic — see Neoplasm, nerve, peripheral						
parasympathetic — see Neoplasm, nerve, peripheral						
specified site NEC	—	C79.49	—	D33.7	D43.8	—
sympathetic — see Neoplasm, nerve, peripheral						
nevus — see Nevus						
nipple	C50.0-•	C79.81	D05.-•	D24.-•	—	—
nose, nasal	C76.0	C79.89	D09.8	D36.7	D48.7	D49.89
ala (external) (nasi) — see also Neoplasm, nose, skin	C44.301	C79.2	D04.39	D23.39	D48.5	D49.2
bone	C41.0	C79.51	—	D16.4-•	D48.0	D49.2
cartilage	C30.0	C78.39	D02.3	D14.0	D38.5	D49.1
cavity	C30.0	C78.39	D02.3	D14.0	D38.5	D49.1
choana	C11.3	C79.89	D00.08	D10.6	D37.05	D49.0
external (skin) — see also Neoplasm, nose, skin	C44.301	C79.2	D04.39	D23.39	D48.5	D49.2
fossa	C30.0	C78.39	D02.3	D14.0	D38.5	D49.1
internal	C30.0	C78.39	D02.3	D14.0	D38.5	D49.1
mucosa	C30.0	C78.39	D02.3	D14.0	D38.5	D49.1
septum	C30.0	C78.39	D02.3	D14.0	D38.5	D49.1
posterior margin	C11.3	C79.89	D00.08	D10.6	D37.05	D49.0
sinus — see Neoplasm, sinus						
skin	C44.301	C79.2	D04.39	D23.39	D48.5	D49.2
basal cell carcinoma	C44.311	—	—	—	—	—
specified type NEC	C44.391	—	—	—	—	—
squamous cell carcinoma	C44.321	—	—	—	—	—
turbinate (mucosa)	C30.0	C78.39	D02.3	D14.0	D38.5	D49.1
bone	C41.0	C79.51	—	D16.4-•	D48.0	D49.2
vestibule	C30.0	C78.39	D02.3	D14.0	D38.5	D49.1
nostril	C30.0	C78.39	D02.3	D14.0	D38.5	D49.1
nucleus pulposus	C41.2	C79.51	—	D16.6	D48.0	D49.2
occipital						
bone	C41.0	C79.51	—	D16.4-•	D48.0	D49.2
lobe or pole, brain	C71.4	C79.31	—	D33.0	D43.0	D49.6
odontogenic — see Neoplasm, jaw bone						
olfactory nerve or bulb	C72.2-•	C79.49	—	D33.3	D43.3	D49.7
olive (brain)	C71.7	C79.31	—	D33.1	D43.1	D49.6
omentum	C48.1	C78.6	—	D20.1	D48.4	D49.0
operculum (brain)	C71.0	C79.31	—	D33.0	D43.0	D49.6
optic nerve, chiasm, or tract	C72.3-•	C79.49	—	D33.3	D43.3	D49.7
oral (cavity)	C06.9	C79.89	D00.00	D10.30	D37.09	D49.0
ill-defined	C14.8	C79.89	D00.00	D10.30	D37.09	D49.0
mucosa	C06.0	C79.89	D00.02	D10.39	D37.09	D49.0
orbit	C69.6-•	C79.49	D09.2-•	D31.6-•	D48.7	D49.89
autonomic nerve	C69.6-•	C79.49	—	D31.6-•	D48.7	D49.2
bone	C41.0	C79.51	—	D16.4-•	D48.0	D49.2
eye	C69.6-•	C79.49	D09.2-•	D31.6-•	D48.7	D49.89
peripheral nerves	C69.6-•	C79.49	—	D31.6-•	D48.7	D49.2
soft parts	C69.6-•	C79.49	D09.2-•	D31.6-•	D48.7	D49.89
organ of Zuckerkandl	C75.5	C79.89	—	D35.6	D44.7	D49.7
oropharynx	C10.9	C79.89	D00.08	D10.5	D37.05	D49.0
branchial cleft (vestige)	C10.4	C79.89	D00.08	D10.5	D37.05	D49.0
junctional region	C10.8	C79.89	D00.08	D10.5	D37.05	D49.0
lateral wall	C10.2	C79.89	D00.08	D10.5	D37.05	D49.0
overlapping lesion	C10.8	—	—	—	—	—
pillars or fauces	C09.1	C79.89	D00.08	D10.5	D37.05	D49.0
posterior wall	C10.3	C79.89	D00.08	D10.5	D37.05	D49.0
vallecula	C10.0	C79.89	D00.08	D10.5	D37.05	D49.0
os						
external	C53.1	C79.82	D06.1	D26.0	D39.0	D49.59
internal	C53.0	C79.82	D06.0	D26.0	D39.0	D49.59
ovary	C56.-•	C79.6-•	D07.39	D27.-•	D39.1-•	D49.59
oviduct	C57.0-•	C79.82	D07.39	D28.2	D39.8	D49.59
palate	C05.9	C79.89	D00.00	D10.39	D37.09	D49.0
hard	C05.0	C79.89	D00.05	D10.39	D37.09	D49.0
junction of hard and soft palate	C05.9	C79.89	D00.00	D10.39	D37.09	D49.0
overlapping lesions	C05.8	—	—	—	—	—
soft	C05.1	C79.89	D00.04	D10.39	D37.09	D49.0
nasopharyngeal surface	C11.3	C79.89	D00.08	D10.6	D37.05	D49.0
posterior surface	C11.3	C79.89	D00.08	D10.6	D37.05	D49.0
superior surface	C11.3	C79.89	D00.08	D10.6	D37.05	D49.0
palatoglossal arch	C09.1	C79.89	D00.08	D10.5	D37.09	D49.0
palatopharyngeal arch	C09.1	C79.89	D00.00	D10.5	D37.09	D49.0
pallium	C71.0	C79.31	—	D33.0	D43.0	D49.6
palpebra	C44.10-•	C79.2	D04.1-•	D23.1-•	D48.5	D49.2
basal cell carcinoma	C44.11-•	—	—	—	—	—
sebaceous cell	C44.13-•	—	—	—	—	—
specified type NEC	C44.19-•	—	—	—	—	—
squamous cell carcinoma	C44.12-•	—	—	—	—	—
pancreas	C25.9	C78.89	D01.7	D13.6	D37.8	D49.0
body	C25.1	C78.89	D01.7	D13.6	D37.8	D49.0
duct (of Santorini) (of Wirsung)	C25.3	C78.89	D01.7	D13.6	D37.8	D49.0
ectopic tissue	C25.7	C78.89	—	D13.6	D37.8	D49.0
head	C25.0	C78.89	D01.7	D13.6	D37.8	D49.0

◀ New   ◀ Revised   ~~deleted~~ Deleted   • Use Additional Character(s)

TABLE OF NEOPLASMS

	Malignant Primary	Malignant Secondary	Ca in situ	Benign	Uncertain Behavior	Unspecified Behavior
pancreas *(Continued)*						
islet cells	C25.4	C78.89	D01.7	D13.7	D37.8	D49.0
neck	C25.7	C78.89	D01.7	D13.6	D37.8	D49.0
overlapping lesion	C25.8	—	—	—	—	—
tail	C25.2	C78.89	D01.7	D13.6	D37.8	D49.0
para-aortic body	C75.5	C79.89	—	D35.6	D44.7	D49.7
paraganglion NEC	C75.5	C79.89	—	D35.6	D44.7	D49.7
parametrium	C57.3	C79.82	—	D28.2	D39.8	D49.59
paranephric	C48.0	C78.6	—	D20.0	D48.3	D49.0
pararectal	C76.3	C79.89	—	D36.7	D48.7	D49.89
parasagittal (region)	C76.0	C79.89	D09.8	D36.7	D48.7	D49.89
parasellar	C72.9	C79.49	—	D33.9	D43.8	D49.7
parathyroid (gland)	C75.0	C79.89	D09.3	D35.1	D44.2	D49.7
paraurethral	C76.3	C79.89	—	D36.7	D48.7	D49.89
gland	C68.1	C79.19	D09.19	D30.8	D41.8	D49.59
paravaginal	C76.3	C79.89	—	D36.7	D48.7	D49.89
parenchyma, kidney	C64.-●	C79.0-●	D09.19	D30.0-●	D41.0-●	D49.51-●
parietal						
bone	C41.0	C79.51	—	D16.4-●	D48.0	D49.2
lobe, brain	C71.3	C79.31	—	D33.0	D43.0	D49.6
paroophoron	C57.1	C79.82	D07.39	D28.2	D39.8	D49.59
parotid (duct) (gland)	C07	C79.89	D00.00	D11.0	D37.030	D49.0
parovarium	C57.1	C79.82	D07.39	D28.2	D39.8	D49.59
patella	C40.20	C79.51		—	—	—
peduncle, cerebral	C71.7	C79.31	—	D33.1	D43.1	D49.6
pelvirectal junction	C19	C78.5	D01.1	D12.7	D37.5	D49.0
pelvis, pelvic	C76.3	C79.89	D09.8	D36.7	D48.7	D49.89
bone	C41.4	C79.51	—	D16.8	D48.0	D49.2
floor	C76.3	C79.89	D09.8	D36.7	D48.7	D49.89
renal	C65.-●	C79.0-●	D09.19	D30.1-●	D41.1-●	D49.51-●
viscera	C76.3	C79.89	D09.8	D36.7	D48.7	D49.89
wall	C76.3	C79.89	D09.8	D36.7	D48.7	D49.89
pelvo-abdominal	C76.8	C79.89	D09.8	D36.7	D48.7	D49.89
penis	C60.9	C79.82	D07.4	D29.0	D40.8	D49.59
body	C60.2	C79.82	D07.4	D29.0	D40.8	D49.59
corpus (cavernosum)	C60.2	C79.82	D07.4	D29.0	D40.8	D49.59
glans	C60.1	C79.82	D07.4	D29.0	D40.8	D49.59
overlapping sites	C60.8	—	—	—	—	—
skin NEC	C60.9	C79.82	D07.4	D29.0	D40.8	D49.59
periadrenal (tissue)	C48.0	C78.6	—	D20.0	D48.3	D49.0
perianal (skin) — *see also* Neoplasm, anus, skin	C44.500	C79.2	D04.5	D23.5	D48.5	D49.2
pericardium	C38.0	C79.89	—	D15.1	D48.7	D49.89
perinephric	C48.0	C78.6	—	D20.0	D48.3	D49.0
perineum	C76.3	C79.89	D09.8	D36.7	D48.7	D49.89
periodontal tissue NEC	C03.9	C79.89	D00.03	D10.39	D37.09	D49.0
periosteum — *see* Neoplasm, bone						
peripancreatic	C48.0	C78.6	—	D20.0	D48.3	D49.0
peripheral nerve NEC	C47.9	C79.89	—	D36.10	D48.2	D49.2
perirectal (tissue)	C76.3	C79.89	—	D36.7	D48.7	D49.89
perirenal (tissue)	C48.0	C78.6	—	D20.0	D48.3	D49.0
peritoneum, peritoneal (cavity)	C48.2	C78.6	—	D20.1	D48.4	D49.0
benign mesothelial tissue — *see* Mesothelioma, benign						
overlapping lesion	C48.8	—	—	—	—	—
with digestive organs	C26.9	—	—	—	—	—
parietal	C48.1	C78.6	—	D20.1	D48.4	D49.0
pelvic	C48.1	C78.6	—	D20.1	D48.4	D49.0
specified part NEC	C48.1	C78.6	—	D20.1	D48.4	D49.0
peritonsillar (tissue)	C76.0	C79.89	D09.8	D36.7	D48.7	D49.89
periurethral tissue	C76.3	C79.89	—	D36.7	D48.7	D49.89
phalanges						
foot	C40.3-●	C79.51		D16.3-●	—	—
hand	C40.1-●	C79.51		D16.1-●	—	—
pharynx, pharyngeal	C14.0	C79.89	D00.08	D10.9	D37.05	D49.0
bursa	C11.1	C79.89	D00.08	D10.6	D37.05	D49.0
fornix	C11.3	C79.89	D00.08	D10.6	D37.05	D49.0
recess	C11.2	C79.89	D00.08	D10.6	D37.05	D49.0
region	C14.0	C79.89	D00.08	D10.9	D37.05	D49.0
tonsil	C11.1	C79.89	D00.08	D10.6	D37.05	D49.0
wall (lateral) (posterior)	C14.0	C79.89	D00.08	D10.9	D37.05	D49.0
pia mater	C70.9	C79.40	—	D32.9	D42.9	D49.7
cerebral	C70.0	C79.32	—	D32.0	D42.0	D49.7
cranial	C70.0	C79.32	—	D32.0	D42.0	D49.7
spinal	C70.1	C79.49	—	D32.1	D42.1	D49.7
pillars of fauces	C09.1	C79.89	D00.08	D10.5	D37.05	D49.0
pineal (body) (gland)	C75.3	C79.89	D09.3	D35.4	D44.5	D49.7
pinna (ear) NEC — *see also* Neoplasm, skin, ear	C44.20-●	C79.2	D04.2-●	D23.2-●	D48.5	D49.2
piriform fossa or sinus	C12	C79.89	D00.08	D10.7	D37.05	D49.0
pituitary (body) (fossa) (gland) (lobe)	C75.1	C79.89	D09.3	D35.2	D44.3	D49.7
placenta	C58	C79.82	D07.0	D26.7	D39.2	D49.59
pleura, pleural (cavity)	C38.4	C78.2	—	D19.0	D38.2	D49.1
overlapping lesion with heart or mediastinum	C38.8	—	—	—	—	—
parietal	C38.4	C78.2	—	D19.0	D38.2	D49.1
visceral	C38.4	C78.2	—	D19.0	D38.2	D49.1

◀ New   ◀ Revised   ~~deleted~~ Deleted   ● Use Additional Character(s)

	Malignant Primary	Malignant Secondary	Ca in situ	Benign	Uncertain Behavior	Unspecified Behavior
plexus						
brachial	C47.1-●	C79.89	—	D36.12	D48.2	D49.2
cervical	C47.0	C79.89	—	D36.11	D48.2	D49.2
choroid	C71.5	C79.31	—	D33.0	D43.0	D49.6
lumbosacral	C47.5	C79.89	—	D36.16	D48.2	D49.2
sacral	C47.5	C79.89	—	D36.16	D48.2	D49.2
pluriendocrine	C75.8	C79.89	D09.3	D35.7	D44.9	D49.7
pole						
frontal	C71.1	C79.31	—	D33.0	D43.0	D49.6
occipital	C71.4	C79.31	—	D33.0	D43.0	D49.6
pons (varolii)	C71.7	C79.31	—	D33.1	D43.1	D49.6
popliteal fossa or space	C76.5-●	C79.89	D04.7-●	D36.7	D48.7	D49.89
postcricoid (region)	C13.0	C79.89	D00.08	D10.7	D37.05	D49.0
posterior fossa (cranial)	C71.9	C79.31	—	D33.2	D43.2	D49.6
postnasal space	C11.9	C79.89	D00.08	D10.6	D37.05	D49.0
prepuce	C60.0	C79.82	D07.4	D29.0	D40.8	D49.59
prepylorus	C16.4	C78.89	D00.2	D13.1	D37.1	D49.0
presacral (region)	C76.3	C79.89	—	D36.7	D48.7	D49.89
prostate (gland)	C61	C79.82	D07.5	D29.1	D40.0	D49.59
utricle	C68.0	C79.19	D09.19	D30.4	D41.3	D49.59
pterygoid fossa	C49.0	C79.89	—	D21.0	D48.1	D49.2
pubic bone	C41.4	C79.51	—	D16.8	D48.0	D49.2
pudenda, pudendum (female)	C51.9	C79.82	D07.1	D28.0	D39.8	D49.59
pulmonary—see also Neoplasm, lung	C34.9-●	C78.0-●	D02.2-●	D14.3-●	D38.1	D49.1
putamen	C71.0	C79.31	—	D33.0	D43.0	D49.6
pyloric						
antrum	C16.3	C78.89	D00.2	D13.1	D37.1	D49.0
canal	C16.4	C78.89	D00.2	D13.1	D37.1	D49.0
pylorus	C16.4	C78.89	D00.2	D13.1	D37.1	D49.0
pyramid (brain)	C71.7	C79.31	—	D33.1	D43.1	D49.6
pyriform fossa or sinus	C12	C79.89	D00.08	D10.7	D37.05	D49.0
radius (any part)	C40.0-●	C79.51		D16.0-●	—	—
Rathke's pouch	C75.1	C79.89	D09.3	D35.2	D44.3	D49.7
rectosigmoid (junction)	C19	C78.5	D01.1	D12.7	D37.5	D49.0
overlapping lesion with anus or rectum	C21.8	—				
rectouterine pouch	C48.1	C78.6	—	D20.1	D48.4	D49.0
rectovaginal septum or wall	C76.3	C79.89	D09.8	D36.7	D48.7	D49.89
rectovesical septum	C76.3	C79.89	D09.8	D36.7	D48.7	D49.89
rectum (ampulla)	C20	C78.5	D01.2	D12.8	D37.5	D49.0
and colon	C19	C78.5	D01.1	D12.7	D37.5	D49.0
overlapping lesion with anus or rectosigmoid junction	C21.8	—	—	—	—	—

	Malignant Primary	Malignant Secondary	Ca in situ	Benign	Uncertain Behavior	Unspecified Behavior
renal	C64.-●	C79.0-●	D09.19	D30.0-●	D41.0-●	D49.51-●
calyx	C65.-●	C79.0-●	D09.19	D30.1-●	D41.1-●	D49.51-●
hilus	C65.-●	C79.0-●	D09.19	D30.1-●	D41.1-●	D49.51-●
parenchyma	C64.-●	C79.0-●	D09.19	D30.0-●	D41.0-●	D49.51-●
pelvis	C65.-●	C79.0-●	D09.19	D30.1-●	D41.1-●	D49.51-●
respiratory						
organs or system NEC	C39.9	C78.30	D02.4	D14.4	D38.6	D49.1
tract NEC	C39.9	C78.30	D02.4	D14.4	D38.5	D49.1
upper	C39.0	C78.30	D02.4	D14.4	D38.5	D49.1
retina	C69.2-●	C79.49	D09.2-●	D31.2-●	D48.7	D49.81
retrobulbar	C69.6-●	C79.49	—	D31.6-●	D48.7	D49.89
retrocecal	C48.0	C78.6	—	D20.0	D48.3	D49.0
retromolar (area) (triangle) (trigone)	C06.2	C79.89	D00.00	D10.39	D37.09	D49.0
retro-orbital	C76.0	C79.89	D09.8	D36.7	D48.7	D49.89
retroperitoneal (space) (tissue)	C48.0	C78.6	—	D20.0	D48.3	D49.0
retroperitoneum	C48.0	C78.6	—	D20.0	D48.3	D49.0
retropharyngeal	C14.0	C79.89	D00.08	D10.9	D37.05	D49.0
retrovesical (septum)	C76.3	C79.89	D09.8	D36.7	D48.7	D49.89
rhinencephalon	C71.0	C79.31	—	D33.0	D43.0	D49.6
rib	C41.3	C79.51	—	D16.7	D48.0	D49.2
Rosenmuller's fossa	C11.2	C79.89	D00.08	D10.6	D37.05	D49.0
round ligament	C57.2	C79.82	—	D28.2	D39.8	D49.59
sacrococcyx, sacrococcygeal	C41.4	C79.51	—	D16.8	D48.0	D49.2
region	C76.3	C79.89	D09.8	D36.7	D48.7	D49.89
sacrouterine ligament	C57.3	C79.02	—	D28.2	D39.8	D49.59
sacrum, sacral (vertebra)	C41.4	C79.51	—	D16.8	D48.0	D49.2
salivary gland or duct (major)	C08.9	C79.89	D00.00	D11.9	D37.039	D49.0
minor NEC	C06.9	C79.89	D00.00	D10.39	D37.04	D49.0
overlapping lesion	C08.9	—	—	—	—	—
parotid	C07	C79.89	D00.00	D11.0	D37.030	D49.0
pluriglandular	C08.9	C79.89	D00.00	D11.9	D37.039	D49.0
sublingual	C08.1	C79.89	D00.00	D11.7	D37.031	D49.0
submandibular	C08.0	C79.89	D00.00	D11.7	D37.032	D49.0
submaxillary	C08.0	C79.89	D00.00	D11.7	D37.032	D49.0
salpinx (uterine)	C57.0-●	C79.82	D07.39	D28.2	D39.8	D49.59
Santorini's duct	C25.3	C78.89	D01.7	D13.6	D37.8	D49.0
scalp	C44.40	C79.2	D04.4	D23.4	D48.5	D49.2
basal cell carcinoma	C44.41	—	—	—	—	—
specified type NEC	C44.49	—	—	—	—	—
squamous cell carcinoma	C44.42	—	—	—	—	—
scapula (any part)	C40.0-●	C79.51	—	D16.0-●	—	—
scapular region	C76.1	C79.89	D09.8	D36.7	D48.7	D49.89

◀ New ◀ Revised ~~deleted~~ Deleted ● Use Additional Character(s)

TABLE OF NEOPLASMS

	Malignant Primary	Malignant Secondary	Ca in situ	Benign	Uncertain Behavior	Unspecified Behavior
scar NEC — see also Neoplasm, skin, by site	C44.90	C79.2	D04.9	D23.9	D48.5	D49.2
sciatic nerve	C47.2-●	C79.89	—	D36.13	D48.2	D49.2
sclera	C69.4-●	C79.49	D09.2-●	D31.4-●	D48.7	D49.89
scrotum (skin)	C63.2	C79.82	D07.61	D29.4	D40.8	D49.59
sebaceous gland — see Neoplasm, skin						
sella turcica	C75.1	C79.89	D09.3	D35.2	D44.3	D49.7
bone	C41.0	C79.51	—	D16.4-●	D48.0	D49.2
semilunar cartilage (knee)	C40.2-●	C79.51	—	D16.2-●	D48.0	D49.2
seminal vesicle	C63.7	C79.82	D07.69	D29.8	D40.8	D49.59
septum						
nasal	C30.0	C78.39	D02.3	D14.0	D38.5	D49.1
posterior margin	C11.3	C79.89	D00.08	D10.6	D37.05	D49.0
rectovaginal	C76.3	C79.89	D09.8	D36.7	D48.7	D49.89
rectovesical	C76.3	C79.89	D09.8	D36.7	D48.7	D49.89
urethrovaginal	C57.9	C79.82	D07.30	D28.9	D39.9	D49.59
vesicovaginal	C57.9	C79.82	D07.30	D28.9	D39.9	D49.59
shoulder NEC	C76.4-●	C79.89	D04.6-●	D36.7	D48.7	D49.89
sigmoid flexure (lower) (upper)	C18.7	C78.5	D01.0	D12.5	D37.4	D49.0
sinus (accessory)	C31.9	C78.39	D02.3	D14.0	D38.5	D49.1
bone (any)	C41.0	C79.51	—	D16.4-●	D48.0	D49.2
ethmoidal	C31.1	C78.39	D02.3	D14.0	D38.5	D49.1
frontal	C31.2	C78.39	D02.3	D14.0	D38.5	D49.1
maxillary	C31.0	C78.39	D02.3	D14.0	D38.5	D49.1
nasal, paranasal NEC	C31.9	C78.39	D02.3	D14.0	D38.5	D49.1
overlapping lesion	C31.8	—	—	—	—	—
pyriform	C12	C79.89	D00.08	D10.7	D37.05	D49.0
sphenoid	C31.3	C78.39	D02.3	D14.0	D38.5	D49.1
skeleton, skeletal NEC	C41.9	C79.51	—	D16.9-●	D48.0	D49.2
Skene's gland	C68.1	C79.19	D09.19	D30.8	D41.8	D49.59
skin NOS	C44.90	C79.2	D04.9	D23.9	D48.5	D49.2
abdominal wall	C44.509	C79.2	D04.5	D23.5	D48.5	D49.2
basal cell carcinoma	C44.519	—	—	—	—	—
specified type NEC	C44.599	—	—	—	—	—
squamous cell carcinoma	C44.529	—	—	—	—	—
ala nasi — see also Neoplasm, nose, skin	C44.301	C79.2	D04.39	D23.39	D48.5	D49.2
ankle — see also Neoplasm, skin, limb, lower	C44.70-●	C79.2	D04.7-●	D23.7-●	D48.5	D49.2
antecubital space — see also Neoplasm, skin, limb, upper	C44.60-●	C79.2	D04.6-●	D23.6-●	D48.5	D49.2
skin NOS *(Continued)*						
anus	C44.500	C79.2	D04.5	D23.5	D48.5	D49.2
basal cell carcinoma	C44.510	—	—	—	—	—
specified type NEC	C44.590	—	—	—	—	—
squamous cell carcinoma	C44.520	—	—	—	—	—
arm — see also Neoplasm, skin, limb, upper	C44.60-●	C79.2	D04.6-●	D23.6-●	D48.5	D49.2
auditory canal (external) — see also Neoplasm, skin, ear	C44.20-●	C79.2	D04.2-●	D23.2-●	D48.5	D49.2
auricle (ear) — see also Neoplasm, skin, ear	C44.20-●	C79.2	D04.2-●	D23.2-●	D48.5	D49.2
auricular canal (external) — see also Neoplasm, skin, ear	C44.20-●	C79.2	D04.2-●	D23.2-●	D48.5	D49.2
axilla, axillary fold — see also Neoplasm, skin, trunk	C44.509	C79.2	D04.5	D23.5	D48.5	D49.2
back — see also Neoplasm, skin, trunk	C44.509	C79.2	D04.5	D23.5	D48.5	D49.2
basal cell carcinoma	C44.91					
breast	C44.501	C79.2	D04.5	D23.5	D48.5	D49.2
basal cell carcinoma	C44.511	—	—	—	—	—
specified type NEC	C44.591	—	—	—	—	—
squamous cell carcinoma	C44.521	—	—	—	—	—
brow — see also Neoplasm, skin, face	C44.309	C79.2	D04.39	D23.39	D48.5	D49.2
buttock — see also Neoplasm, skin, trunk	C44.509	C79.2	D04.5	D23.5	D48.5	D49.2
calf — see also Neoplasm, skin, limb, lower	C44.70-●	C79.2	D04.7-●	D23.7-●	D48.5	D49.2
canthus (eye) (inner) (outer)	C44.10-●	C79.2	D04.1-●	D23.1-●	D48.5	D49.2
basal cell carcinoma	C44.11-●	—	—	—	—	—
sebaceous cell	C44.13-●	—	—	—	—	—
specified type NEC	C44.19-●	—	—	—	—	—
squamous cell carcinoma	C44.12-●	—	—	—	—	—
cervical region — see also Neoplasm, skin, neck	C44.40	C79.2	D04.4	D23.4	D48.5	D49.2
cheek (external) — see also Neoplasm, skin, face	C44.309	C79.2	D04.39	D23.39	D48.5	D49.2
chest (wall) — see also Neoplasm, skin, trunk	C44.509	C79.2	D04.5	D23.5	D48.5	D49.2
chin — see also Neoplasm, skin, face	C44.309	C79.2	D04.39	D23.39	D48.5	D49.2
clavicular area — see also Neoplasm, skin, trunk	C44.509	C79.2	D04.5	D23.5	D48.5	D49.2
clitoris	C51.2	C79.82	D07.1	D28.0	D39.8	D49.59

◀ New   ◀ Revised   ~~deleted~~ Deleted   ● Use Additional Character(s)

TABLE OF NEOPLASMS

	Malignant Primary	Malignant Secondary	Ca in situ	Benign	Uncertain Behavior	Unspecified Behavior
skin NOS *(Continued)*						
columnella — *see also Neoplasm, skin, face*	C44.309	C79.2	D04.39	D23.39	D48.5	D49.2
concha — *see also Neoplasm, skin, ear*	C44.20-●	C79.2	D04.2-●	D23.2-●	D48.5	D49.2
ear (external)	C44.20-●	C79.2	D04.2-●	D23.2-●	D48.5	D49.2
basal cell carcinoma	C44.21-●	—	—	—	—	—
specified type NEC	C44.29-●	—	—	—	—	—
squamous cell carcinoma	C44.22-●	—	—	—	—	—
elbow — *see also Neoplasm, skin, limb, upper*	C44.60-●	C79.2	D04.6-●	D23.6-●	D48.5	D49.2
eyebrow — *see also Neoplasm, skin, face*	C44.309	C79.2	D04.39	D23.39	D48.5	D49.2
eyelid	C44.10-●	C79.2	D04.1-●	D23.1-●	D48.5	D49.2
basal cell carcinoma	C44.11-●	—	—	—	—	—
sebaceous cell	C44.13-●	—	—	—	—	—
specified type NEC	C44.19-●	—	—	—	—	—
squamous cell carcinoma	C44.12-●	—	—	—	—	—
face NOS	C44.300	C79.2	D04.30	D23.30	D48.5	D49.2
basal cell carcinoma	C44.310	—	—	—	—	—
specified type NEC	C44.390	—	—	—	—	—
squamous cell carcinoma	C44.320	—	—	—	—	—
female genital organs (external)	C51.9	C79.82	D07.1	D28.0	D39.8	D49.59
clitoris	C51.2	C79.82	D07.1	D28.0	D39.8	D49.59
labium NEC	C51.9	C79.82	D07.1	D28.0	D39.8	D49.59
majus	C51.0	C79.82	D07.1	D28.0	D39.8	D49.59
minus	C51.1	C79.82	D07.1	D28.0	D39.8	D49.59
pudendum	C51.9	C79.82	D07.1	D28.0	D39.8	D49.59
vulva	C51.9	C79.82	D07.1	D28.0	D39.8	D49.59
finger — *see also Neoplasm, skin, limb, upper*	C44.60-●	C79.2	D04.6-●	D23.6-●	D48.5	D49.2
flank — *see also Neoplasm, skin, trunk*	C44.509	C79.2	D04.5	D23.5	D48.5	D49.2
foot — *see also Neoplasm, skin, limb, lower*	C44.70-●	C79.2	D04.7-●	D23.7-●	D48.5	D49.2
forearm — *see also Neoplasm, skin, limb, upper*	C44.60-●	C79.2	D04.6-●	D23.6-●	D48.5	D49.2
forehead — *see also Neoplasm, skin, face*	C44.309	C79.2	D04.39	D23.39	D48.5	D49.2
glabella — *see also Neoplasm, skin, face*	C44.309	C79.2	D04.39	D23.39	D48.5	D49.2
gluteal region — *see also Neoplasm, skin, trunk*	C44.509	C79.2	D04.5	D23.5	D48.5	D49.2
groin — *see also Neoplasm, skin, trunk*	C44.509	C79.2	D04.5	D23.5	D48.5	D49.2
skin NOS *(Continued)*						
hand — *see also Neoplasm, skin, limb, upper*	C44.60-●	C79.2	D04.6-●	D23.6-●	D48.5	D49.2
head NEC — *see also Neoplasm, skin, scalp*	C44.40	C79.2	D04.4	D23.4	D48.5	D49.2
heel — *see also Neoplasm, skin, limb, lower*	C44.70-●	C79.2	D04.7-●	D23.7-●	D48.5	D49.2
helix — *see also Neoplasm, skin, ear*	C44.20-●	C79.2	D04.2-●	D23.2-●	D48.5	D49.2
hip — *see also Neoplasm, skin, limb, lower*	C44.70-●	C79.2	D04.7-●	D23.7-●	D48.5	D49.2
infraclavicular region — *see also Neoplasm, skin, trunk*	C44.509	C79.2	D04.5	D23.5	D48.5	D49.2
inguinal region — *see also Neoplasm, skin, trunk*	C44.509	C79.2	D04.5	D23.5	D48.5	D49.2
jaw — *see also Neoplasm, skin, face*	C44.309	C79.2	D04.39	D23.39	D48.5	D49.2
Kaposi's sarcoma — *see Kaposi's, sarcoma, skin*						
knee — *see also Neoplasm, skin, limb, lower*	C44.70-●	C79.2	D04.7-●	D23.7-●	D48.5	D49.2
labia						
majora	C51.0	C79.82	D07.1	D28.0	D39.8	D49.59
minora	C51.1	C79.82	D07.1	D28.0	D39.8	D49.59
leg — *see also Neoplasm, skin, limb, lower*	C44.70-●	C79.2	D04.7-●	D23.7-●	D48.5	D49.2
lid (lower) (upper)	C44.10-●	C79.2	D04.1-●	D23.1-●	D48.5	D49.2
basal cell carcinoma	C44.11-●	—	—	—	—	—
sebaceous cell	C44.13-●	—	—	—	—	—
specified type NEC	C44.19-●	—	—	—	—	—
squamous cell carcinoma	C44.12-●	—	—	—	—	—
limb NEC	C44.90	C79.2	D04.9	D23.9	D48.5	D49.2
basal cell carcinoma	C44.91					
lower	C44.70-●	C79.2	D04.7-●	D23.7-●	D48.5	D49.2
basal cell carcinoma	C44.71-●	—	—	—	—	—
specified type NEC	C44.79-●	—	—	—	—	—
squamous cell carcinoma	C44.72-●	—	—	—	—	—
upper	C44.60-●	C79.2	D04.6-●	D23.6-●	D48.5	D49.2
basal cell carcinoma	C44.61-●	—	—	—	—	—
specified type NEC	C44.69-●	—	—	—	—	—
squamous cell carcinoma	C44.62-●	—	—	—	—	—
lip (lower) (upper)	C44.00	C79.2	D04.0	D23.0	D48.5	D49.2
basal cell carcinoma	C44.01	—	—	—	—	—
specified type NEC	C44.09	—	—	—	—	—
squamous cell carcinoma	C44.02					

◄ New   ◄◄ Revised   ~~deleted~~ Deleted   ● Use Additional Character(s)

TABLE OF NEOPLASMS (left margin, rotated)

skin NOS (Continued)	Malignant Primary	Malignant Secondary	Ca in situ	Benign	Uncertain Behavior	Unspecified Behavior
male genital organs	C63.9	C79.82	D07.60	D29.9	D40.8	D49.59
penis	C60.9	C79.82	D07.4	D29.0	D40.8	D49.59
prepuce	C60.0	C79.82	D07.4	D29.0	D40.8	D49.59
scrotum	C63.2	C79.82	D07.61	D29.4	D40.8	D49.59
mastectomy site (skin) — *see also Neoplasm, skin, breast*	C44.501	C79.2	—	—	—	—
specified as breast tissue	C50.8-●	C79.81	—	—	—	—
meatus, acoustic (external) — *see also Neoplasm, skin, ear*	C44.20-●	C79.2	D04.2-●	D23.2-●	D48.5	D49.2
melanotic — *see Melanoma*						
Merkel cell — *see Carcinoma, Merkel cell*						
nates — *see also Neoplasm, skin, trunk*	C44.509	C79.2	D04.5	D23.5	D48.5	D49.2
neck	C44.40	C79.2	D04.4	D23.4	D48.5	D49.2
basal cell carcinoma	C44.41	—	—	—	—	—
specified type NEC	C44.49	—	—	—	—	—
squamous cell carcinoma	C44.42	—	—	—	—	—
nevus — *see Nevus, skin*						
nose (external) — *see also Neoplasm, nose, skin*	C44.301	C79.2	D04.39	D23.39	D48.5	D49.2
overlapping lesion	C44.80	—	—	—	—	—
basal cell carcinoma	C44.81	—	—	—	—	—
specified type NEC	C44.89	—	—	—	—	—
squamous cell carcinoma	C44.82	—	—	—	—	—
palm — *see also Neoplasm, skin, limb, upper*	C44.60-●	C79.2	D04.6-●	D23.6-●	D48.5	D49.2
palpebra	C44.10-●	C79.2	D04.1-●	D23.1-●	D48.5	D49.2
basal cell carcinoma	C44.11-●	—	—	—	—	—
sebaceous cell	C44.13-●	—	—	—	—	—
specified type NEC	C44.19-●	—	—	—	—	—
squamous cell carcinoma	C44.12-●	—	—	—	—	—
penis NEC	C60.9	C79.82	D07.4	D29.0	D40.8	D49.59
perianal — *see also Neoplasm, skin, anus*	C44.500	C79.2	D04.5	D23.5	D48.5	D49.2
perineum — *see also Neoplasm, skin, anus*	C44.500	C79.2	D04.5	D23.5	D48.5	D49.2
pinna — *see also Neoplasm, skin, ear*	C44.20-●	C79.2	D04.2-●	D23.2-●	D48.5	D49.2
plantar — *see also Neoplasm, skin, limb, lower*	C44.70-●	C79.2	D04.7-●	D23.7-●	D48.5	D49.2
popliteal fossa or space — *see also Neoplasm, skin, limb, lower*	C44.70-●	C79.2	D04.7-●	D23.7-●	D48.5	D49.2

skin NOS (Continued)	Malignant Primary	Malignant Secondary	Ca in situ	Benign	Uncertain Behavior	Unspecified Behavior
prepuce	C60.0	C79.82	D07.4	D29.0	D40.8	D49.59
pubes — *see also Neoplasm, skin, trunk*	C44.509	C79.2	D04.5	D23.5	D48.5	D49.2
sacrococcygeal region — *see also Neoplasm, skin, trunk*	C44.509	C79.2	D04.5	D23.5	D48.5	D49.2
scalp	C44.40	C79.2	D04.4	D23.4	D48.5	D49.2
basal cell carcinoma	C44.41	—	—	—	—	—
specified type NEC	C44.49	—	—	—	—	—
squamous cell carcinoma	C44.42	—	—	—	—	—
scapular region — *see also Neoplasm, skin, trunk*	C44.509	C79.2	D04.5	D23.5	D48.5	D49.2
scrotum	C63.2	C79.82	D07.61	D29.4	D40.8	D49.59
shoulder — *see also Neoplasm, skin, limb, upper*	C44.60-●	C79.2	D04.6-●	D23.6-●	D48.5	D49.2
sole (foot) — *see also Neoplasm, skin, limb, lower*	C44.70-●	C79.2	D04.7-●	D23.7-●	D48.5	D49.2
specified sites NEC	C44.80	C79.2	D04.8	D23.9	D48.5	D49.2
basal cell carcinoma	C44.81	—	—	—	—	—
specified type NEC	C44.89	—	—	—	—	—
squamous cell carcinoma	C44.82	—	—	—	—	—
specified type NEC	C44.99	—	—	—	—	—
squamous cell carcinoma	C44.92	—	—	—	—	—
submammary fold — *see also Neoplasm, skin, trunk*	C44.509	C79.2	D04.5	D23.5	D48.5	D49.2
supraclavicular region — *see also Neoplasm, skin, neck*	C44.40	C79.2	D04.4	D23.4	D48.5	D49.2
temple — *see also Neoplasm, skin, face*	C44.309	C79.2	D04.39	D23.39	D48.5	D49.2
thigh — *see also Neoplasm, skin, limb, lower*	C44.70-●	C79.2	D04.7-●	D23.7-●	D48.5	D49.2
thoracic wall — *see also Neoplasm, skin, trunk*	C44.509	C79.2	D04.5	D23.5	D48.5	D49.2
thumb — *see also Neoplasm, skin, limb, upper*	C44.60-●	C79.2	D04.6-●	D23.6-●	D48.5	D49.2
toe — *see also Neoplasm, skin, limb, lower*	C44.70-●	C79.2	D04.7-●	D23.7-●	D48.5	D49.2
tragus — *see also Neoplasm, skin, ear*	C44.20-●	C79.2	D04.2-●	D23.2-●	D48.5	D49.2
trunk	C44.509	C79.2	D04.5	D23.5	D48.5	D49.2
basal cell carcinoma	C44.519	—	—	—	—	—
specified type NEC	C44.599	—	—	—	—	—
squamous cell carcinoma	C44.529	—	—	—	—	—
umbilicus — *see also Neoplasm, skin, trunk*	C44.509	C79.2	D04.5	D23.5	D48.5	D49.2

◀ New ◀ Revised ~~deleted~~ Deleted ● Use Additional Character(s)

	Malignant Primary	Malignant Secondary	Ca in situ	Benign	Uncertain Behavior	Unspecified Behavior
skin NOS *(Continued)*						
vulva	C51.9	C79.82	D07.1	D28.0	D39.8	D49.59
overlapping lesion	C51.8	—	—	—	—	—
wrist — *see also Neoplasm, skin, limb, upper*	C44.60-•	C79.2	D04.6-•	D23.6-•	D48.5	D49.2
skull	C41.0	C79.51	—	D16.4-•	D48.0	D49.2
soft parts or tissues — *see Neoplasm, connective tissue*						
specified site NEC	C76.8	C79.89	D09.8	D36.7	D48.7	D49.89
spermatic cord	C63.1-•	C79.82	D07.69	D29.8	D40.8	D49.59
sphenoid	C31.3	C78.39	D02.3	D14.0	D38.5	D49.1
bone	C41.0	C79.51	—	D16.4-•	D48.0	D49.2
sinus	C31.3	C78.39	D02.3	D14.0	D38.5	D49.1
sphincter						
anal	C21.1	C78.5	D01.3	D12.9	D37.8	D49.0
of Oddi	C24.0	C78.89	D01.5	D13.5	D37.6	D49.0
spine, spinal (column)	C41.2	C79.51	—	D16.6	D48.0	D49.2
bulb	C71.7	C79.31	—	D33.1	D43.1	D49.6
coccyx	C41.4	C79.51	—	D16.8	D48.0	D49.2
cord (cervical) (lumbar) (sacral) (thoracic)	C72.0	C79.49	—	D33.4	D43.4	D49.7
dura mater	C70.1	C79.49	—	D32.1	D42.1	D49.7
lumbosacral	C41.2	C79.51	—	D16.6	D48.0	D49.2
marrow NEC	C96.9	C79.52	—	—	D47.9	D49.89
membrane	C70.1	C79.49	—	D32.1	D42.1	D49.7
meninges	C70.1	C79.49	—	D32.1	D42.1	D49.7
nerve (root)	C47.9	C79.89	—	D36.10	D48.2	D49.2
pia mater	C70.1	C79.49	—	D32.1	D42.1	D49.7
root	C47.9	C79.89	—	D36.10	D48.2	D49.2
sacrum	C41.4	C79.51	—	D16.8	D48.0	D49.2
spleen, splenic NEC	C26.1	C78.89	D01.7	D13.9	D37.8	D49.0
flexure (colon)	C18.5	C78.5	D01.0	D12.3	D37.4	D49.0
stem, brain	C71.7	C79.31	—	D33.1	D43.1	D49.6
Stensen's duct	C07	C79.89	D00.00	D11.0	D37.030	D49.0
sternum	C41.3	C79.51	—	D16.7	D48.0	D49.2
stomach	C16.9	C78.89	D00.2	D13.1	D37.1	D49.0
antrum (pyloric)	C16.3	C78.89	D00.2	D13.1	D37.1	D49.0
body	C16.2	C78.89	D00.2	D13.1	D37.1	D49.0
cardia	C16.0	C78.89	D00.2	D13.1	D37.1	D49.0
cardiac orifice	C16.0	C78.89	D00.2	D13.1	D37.1	D49.0
corpus	C16.2	C78.89	D00.2	D13.1	D37.1	D49.0
fundus	C16.1	C78.89	D00.2	D13.1	D37.1	D49.0
greater curvature NEC	C16.6	C78.89	D00.2	D13.1	D37.1	D49.0
lesser curvature NEC	C16.5	C78.89	D00.2	D13.1	D37.1	D49.0

	Malignant Primary	Malignant Secondary	Ca in situ	Benign	Uncertain Behavior	Unspecified Behavior
stomach *(Continued)*						
overlapping lesion	C16.8	—	—	—	—	—
prepylorus	C16.4	C78.89	D00.2	D13.1	D37.1	D49.0
pylorus	C16.4	C78.89	D00.2	D13.1	D37.1	D49.0
wall NEC	C16.9	C78.89	D00.2	D13.1	D37.1	D49.0
anterior NEC	C16.8	C78.89	D00.2	D13.1	D37.1	D49.0
posterior NEC	C16.8	C78.89	D00.2	D13.1	D37.1	D49.0
stroma, endometrial	C54.1	C79.82	D07.0	D26.1	D39.0	D49.59
stump, cervical	C53.8	C79.82	D06.7	D26.0	D39.0	D49.59
subcutaneous (nodule) (tissue) NEC — *see Neoplasm, connective tissue*						
subdural	C70.9	C79.32	—	D32.9	D42.9	D49.7
subglottis, subglottic	C32.2	C78.39	D02.0	D14.1	D38.0	D49.1
sublingual	C04.9	C79.89	D00.06	D10.2	D37.09	D49.0
gland or duct	C08.1	C79.89	D00.00	D11.7	D37.031	D49.0
submandibular gland	C08.0	C79.89	D00.00	D11.7	D37.032	D49.0
submaxillary gland or duct	C08.0	C79.89	D00.00	D11.7	D37.032	D49.0
submental	C76.0	C79.89	D09.8	D36.7	D48.7	D49.89
subpleural	C34.9-•	C78.0-•	D02.2-•	D14.3-•	D38.1	D49.1
substernal	C38.1	C78.1	—	D15.2	D38.3	D49.89
sudoriferous, sudoriparous gland, site unspecified	C44.90	C79.2	D04.9	D23.9	D48.5	D49.2
specified site — *see Neoplasm, skin*						
supraclavicular region	C76.0	C79.89	D09.8	D36.7	D48.7	D49.89
supraglottis	C32.1	C78.39	D02.0	D14.1	D38.0	D49.1
suprarenal	C74.9-•	C79.7-•	D09.3	D35.0-•	D44.1-•	D49.7
capsule	C74.9-•	C79.7-•	D09.3	D35.0-•	D44.1-•	D49.7
cortex	C74.0-•	C79.7-•	D09.3	D35.0-•	D44.1-•	D49.7
gland	C74.9-•	C79.7-•	D09.3	D35.0-•	D44.1-•	D49.7
medulla	C74.1-•	C79.7-•	D09.3	D35.0-•	D44.1-•	D49.7
suprasellar (region)	C71.9	C79.31	—	D33.2	D43.2	D49.6
supratentorial (brain) NEC	C71.0	C79.31	—	D33.0	D43.0	D49.6
sweat gland (apocrine) (eccrine), site unspecified	C44.90	C79.2	D04.9	D23.9	D48.5	D49.2
specified site — *see Neoplasm, skin*						
sympathetic nerve or nervous system NEC	C47.9	C79.89	—	D36.10	D48.2	D49.2
symphysis pubis	C41.4	C79.51	—	D16.8	D48.0	D49.2
synovial membrane — *see Neoplasm, connective tissue*						
tapetum, brain	C71.8	C79.31	—	D33.2	D43.2	D49.6

TABLE OF NEOPLASMS

	Malignant Primary	Malignant Secondary	Ca in situ	Benign	Uncertain Behavior	Unspecified Behavior
tarsus (any bone)	C40.3-●	C79.51	—	D16.3-●	—	—
temple (skin) — *see also Neoplasm, skin, face*	C44.309	C79.2	D04.39	D23.39	D48.5	D49.2
temporal						
bone	C41.0	C79.51	—	D16.4-●	D48.0	D49.2
lobe or pole	C71.2	C79.31	—	D33.0	D43.0	D49.6
region	C76.0	C79.89	D09.8	D36.7	D48.7	D49.89
skin — *see also Neoplasm, skin, face*	C44.309	C79.2	D04.39	D23.39	D48.5	D49.2
tendon (sheath) — *see Neoplasm, connective tissue*						
tentorium (cerebelli)	C70.0	C79.32	—	D32.0	D42.0	D49.7
testis, testes	C62.9-●	C79.82	D07.69	D29.2-●	D40.1-●	D49.59
descended	C62.1-●	C79.82	D07.69	D29.2-●	D40.1-●	D49.59
ectopic	C62.0-●	C79.82	D07.69	D29.2-●	D40.1-●	D49.59
retained	C62.0-●	C79.82	D07.69	D29.2-●	D40.1-●	D49.59
scrotal	C62.1-●	C79.82	D07.69	D29.2-●	D40.1-●	D49.59
undescended	C62.0-●	C79.82	D07.69	D29.2-●	D40.1-●	D49.59
unspecified whether descended or undescended	C62.9-●	C79.82	D07.69	D29.2-●	D40.1-●	D49.59
thalamus	C71.0	C79.31	—	D33.0	D43.0	D49.6
thigh NEC	C76.5-●	C79.89	D04.7-●	D36.7	D48.7	D49.89
thorax, thoracic (cavity) (organs NEC)	C76.1	C79.89	D09.8	D36.7	D48.7	D49.89
duct	C49.3	C79.89	—	D21.3	D48.1	D49.2
wall NEC	C76.1	C79.89	D09.8	D36.7	D48.7	D49.89
throat	C14.0	C79.89	D00.08	D10.9	D37.05	D49.0
thumb NEC	C76.4-●	C79.89	D04.6-●	D36.7	D48.7	D49.89
thymus (gland)	C37	C79.89	D09.3	D15.0	D38.4	D49.89
thyroglossal duct	C73	C79.89	D09.3	D34	D44.0	D49.7
thyroid (gland)	C73	C79.89	D09.3	D34	D44.0	D49.7
cartilage	C32.3	C78.39	D02.0	D14.1	D38.0	D49.1
tibia (any part)	C40.2-●	C79.51	—	D16.2-●	—	—
toe NEC	C76.5-●	C79.89	D04.7-●	D36.7	D48.7	D49.89
tongue	C02.9	C79.89	D00.07	D10.0	D37.02	D49.0
anterior (two-thirds) NEC	C02.3	C79.89	D00.07	D10.1	D37.02	D49.0
dorsal surface	C02.0	C79.89	D00.07	D10.1	D37.02	D49.0
ventral surface	C02.2	C79.89	D00.07	D10.1	D37.02	D49.0
base (dorsal surface)	C01	C79.89	D00.07	D10.1	D37.02	D49.0
border (lateral)	C02.1	C79.89	D00.07	D10.1	D37.02	D49.0
dorsal surface NEC	C02.0	C79.89	D00.07	D10.1	D37.02	D49.0
fixed part NEC	C01	C79.89	D00.07	D10.1	D37.02	D49.0
foreamen cecum	C02.0	C79.89	D00.07	D10.1	D37.02	D49.0
frenulum linguae	C02.2	C79.89	D00.07	D10.1	D37.02	D49.0
tongue *(Continued)*						
junctional zone	C02.8	C79.89	D00.07	D10.1	D37.02	D49.0
margin (lateral)	C02.1	C79.89	D00.07	D10.1	D37.02	D49.0
midline NEC	C02.0	C79.89	D00.07	D10.1	D37.02	D49.0
mobile part NEC	C02.3	C79.89	D00.07	D10.1	D37.02	D49.0
overlapping lesion	C02.8	—	—	—	—	—
posterior (third)	C01	C79.89	D00.07	D10.1	D37.02	D49.0
root	C01	C79.89	D00.07	D10.1	D37.02	D49.0
surface (dorsal)	C02.0	C79.89	D00.07	D10.1	D37.02	D49.0
base	C01	C79.89	D00.07	D10.1	D37.02	D49.0
ventral	C02.2	C79.89	D00.07	D10.1	D37.02	D49.0
tip	C02.1	C79.89	D00.07	D10.1	D37.02	D49.0
tonsil	C02.4	C79.89	D00.07	D10.1	D37.02	D49.0
tonsil	C09.9	C79.89	D00.08	D10.4	D37.05	D49.0
fauces, faucial	C09.9	C79.89	D00.08	D10.4	D37.05	D49.0
lingual	C02.4	C79.89	D00.07	D10.1	D37.02	D49.0
overlapping sites	C09.8	—	—	—	—	—
palatine	C09.9	C79.89	D00.08	D10.4	D37.05	D49.0
pharyngeal	C11.1	C79.89	D00.08	D10.6	D37.05	D49.0
pillar (anterior) (posterior)	C09.1	C79.89	D00.08	D10.5	D37.05	D49.0
tonsillar fossa	C09.0	C79.89	D00.08	D10.5	D37.05	D49.0
tooth socket NEC	C03.9	C79.89	D00.03	D10.39	D37.09	D49.0
trachea (cartilage) (mucosa)	C33	C78.39	D02.1	D14.2	D38.1	D49.1
overlapping lesion with bronchus or lung	C34.8-●	—	—	—	—	—
tracheobronchial	C34.8-●	C78.39	D02.1	D14.2	D38.1	D49.1
overlapping lesion with lung	C34.8-●	—	—	—	—	—
tragus — *see also Neoplasm, skin, ear*	C44.20-●	C79.2	D04.2-●	D23.2-●	D48.5	D49.2
trunk NEC	C76.8	C79.89	D04.5	D36.7	D48.7	D49.89
tubo-ovarian	C57.8	C79.82	D07.39	D28.7	D39.8	D49.59
tunica vaginalis	C63.7	C79.82	D07.69	D29.8	D40.8	D49.59
turbinate (bone)	C41.0	C79.51	—	D16.4-●	D48.0	D49.2
nasal	C30.0	C78.39	D02.3	D14.0	D38.5	D49.1
tympanic cavity	C30.1	C78.39	D02.3	D14.0	D38.5	D49.1
ulna (any part)	C40.0-●	C79.51	—	D16.0-●	—	—
umbilicus, umbilical — *see also Neoplasm, skin, trunk*	C44.509	C79.2	D04.5	D23.5	D48.5	D49.2
uncus, brain	C71.2	C79.31	—	D33.0	D43.0	D49.6
unknown site or unspecified	C80.1	C79.9	D09.9	D36.9	D48.9	D49.9
urachus	C67.7	C79.11	D09.0	D30.3	D41.4	D49.4
ureter, ureteral	C66.-●	C79.19	D09.19	D30.2-●	D41.2-●	D49.59
orifice (bladder)	C67.6	C79.11	D09.0	D30.3	D41.4	D49.4
ureter-bladder (junction)	C67.6	C79.11	D09.0	D30.3	D41.4	D49.4

◀ New   ◀ Revised   ~~deleted~~ Deleted   ● Use Additional Character(s)

	Malignant Primary	Malignant Secondary	Ca in situ	Benign	Uncertain Behavior	Unspecified Behavior
urethra, urethral (gland)	C68.0	C79.19	D09.19	D30.4	D41.3	D49.59
orifice, internal	C67.5	C79.11	D09.0	D30.3	D41.4	D49.4
urethrovaginal (septum)	C57.9	C79.82	D07.30	D28.9	D39.8	D49.59
urinary organ or system	C68.9	C79.10	D09.10	D30.9	D41.9	D49.59
bladder — *see Neoplasm, bladder*						
overlapping lesion	C68.8	—	—	—	—	—
specified sites NEC	C68.8	C79.19	D09.19	D30.8	D41.8	D49.59
utero-ovarian	C57.8	C79.82	D07.39	D28.7	D39.8	D49.59
ligament	C57.1	C79.82	D07.39	D28.2	D39.8	D49.59
uterosacral ligament	C57.3	C79.82	—	D28.2	D39.8	D49.59
uterus, uteri, uterine	C55	C79.82	D07.0	D26.9	D39.0	D49.59
adnexa NEC	C57.4	C79.82	D07.39	D28.7	D39.8	D49.59
body	C54.9	C79.82	D07.0	D26.1	D39.0	D49.59
cervix	C53.9	C79.82	D06.9	D26.0	D39.0	D49.59
cornu	C54.9	C79.82	D07.0	D26.1	D39.0	D49.59
corpus	C54.9	C79.82	D07.0	D26.1	D39.0	D49.59
endocervix (canal) (gland)	C53.0	C79.82	D06.0	D26.0	D39.0	D49.59
endometrium	C54.1	C79.82	D07.0	D26.1	D39.0	D49.59
exocervix	C53.1	C79.82	D06.1	D26.0	D39.0	D49.59
external os	C53.1	C79.82	D06.1	D26.0	D39.0	D49.59
fundus	C54.3	C79.82	D07.0	D26.1	D39.0	D49.59
internal os	C53.0	C79.82	D06.0	D26.0	D39.0	D49.59
isthmus	C54.0	C79.82	D07.0	D26.1	D39.0	D49.59
ligament	C57.3	C79.82	—	D28.2	D39.8	D49.59
broad	C57.1	C79.82	D07.39	D28.2	D39.8	D49.59
round	C57.2	C79.82	—	D28.2	D39.8	D49.59
lower segment	C54.0	C79.82	D07.0	D26.1	D39.0	D49.59
myometrium	C54.2	C79.82	D07.0	D26.1	D39.0	D49.59
overlapping sites	C54.8	—	—	—	—	—
squamocolumnar junction	C53.8	C79.82	D06.7	D26.0	D39.0	D49.59
tube	C57.0-•	C79.82	D07.39	D28.2	D39.8	D49.59
utricle, prostatic	C68.0	C79.19	D09.19	D30.4	D41.3	D49.59
uveal tract	C69.4-•	C79.49	D09.2-•	D31.4-•	D48.7	D49.89
uvula	C05.2	C79.89	D00.04	D10.39	D37.09	D49.0
vagina, vaginal (fornix) (vault) (wall)	C52	C79.82	D07.2	D28.1	D39.8	D49.59
vaginovesical	C57.9	C79.82	D07.30	D28.9	D39.9	D49.59
septum	C57.9	C79.82	D07.30	D28.9	D39.9	D49.59
vallecula (epiglottis)	C10.0	C79.89	D00.08	D10.5	D37.05	D49.0
vas deferens	C63.1-•	C79.82	D07.69	D29.8	D40.8	D49.59
vascular — *see Neoplasm, connective tissue*						

	Malignant Primary	Malignant Secondary	Ca in situ	Benign	Uncertain Behavior	Unspecified Behavior
Vater's ampulla	C24.1	C78.89	D01.5	D13.5	D37.6	D49.0
vein, venous — *see Neoplasm, connective tissue*						
vena cava (abdominal) (inferior)	C49.4	C79.89	—	D21.4	D48.1	D49.2
superior	C49.3	C79.89	—	D21.3	D48.1	D49.2
ventricle (cerebral) (floor) (lateral) (third)	C71.5	C79.31	—	D33.0	D43.0	D49.6
cardiac (left) (right)	C38.0	C79.89	—	D15.1	D48.7	D49.89
fourth	C71.7	C79.31	—	D33.1	D43.1	D49.6
ventricular band of larynx	C32.1	C78.39	D02.0	D14.1	D38.0	D49.1
ventriculus — *see Neoplasm, stomach*						
vermillion border — *see Neoplasm, lip*						
vermis, cerebellum	C71.6	C79.31	—	D33.1	D43.1	D49.6
vertebra (column)	C41.2	C79.51	—	D16.6	D48.0	D49.2
coccyx	C41.4	C79.51	—	D16.8-•	D48.0	D49.2
marrow NEC	C96.9	C79.52	—	—	D47.9	D49.89
sacrum	C41.4	C79.51	—	D16.8 •	D48.0	D49.2
vesical — *see Neoplasm, bladder*						
vesicle, seminal	C63.7	C79.82	D07.69	D29.8	D40.8	D49.59
vesicocervical tissue	C57.9	C79.82	D07.30	D28.9	D39.9	D49.59
vesicorectal	C76.3	C79.82	D09.8	D36.7	D48.7	D49.89
vesicovaginal	C57.9	C79.82	D07.30	D28.9	D39.9	D49.59
septum	C57.9	C79.82	D07.30	D28.9	D39.8	D49.59
vessel (blood) — *see Neoplasm, connective tissue*						
vestibular gland, greater	C51.0	C79.82	D07.1	D28.0	D39.8	D49.59
vestibule						
mouth	C06.1	C79.89	D00.00	D10.39	D37.09	D49.0
nose	C30.0	C78.39	D02.3	D14.0	D38.5	D49.1
Virchow's gland	C77.0	C77.0	—	D36.0	D48.7	D49.89
viscera NEC	C76.8	C79.89	D09.8	D36.7	D48.7	D49.89
vocal cords (true)	C32.0	C78.39	D02.0	D14.1	D38.0	D49.1
false	C32.1	C78.39	D02.0	D14.1	D38.0	D49.1
vomer	C41.0	C79.51	—	D16.4-•	D48.0	D49.2
vulva	C51.9	C79.82	D07.1	D28.0	D39.8	D49.59
vulvovaginal gland	C51.0	C79.82	D07.1	D28.0	D39.8	D49.59
Waldeyer's ring	C14.2	C79.89	D00.08	D10.9	D37.05	D49.0
Wharton's duct	C08.0	C79.89	D00.00	D11.7	D37.032	D49.0
white matter (central) (cerebral)	C71.0	C79.31	—	D33.0	D43.0	D49.6
windpipe	C33	C78.39	D02.1	D14.2	D38.1	D49.1

TABLE OF NEOPLASMS

	Malignant Primary	Malignant Secondary	Ca in situ	Benign	Uncertain Behavior	Unspecified Behavior
Wirsung's duct	C25.3	C78.89	D01.7	D13.6	D37.8	D49.0
wolffian (body) (duct)						
female	C57.7	C79.82	D07.39	D28.7	D39.8	D49.59
male	C63.7	C79.82	D07.69	D29.8	D40.8	D49.59

	Malignant Primary	Malignant Secondary	Ca in situ	Benign	Uncertain Behavior	Unspecified Behavior
womb — *see Neoplasm, uterus*						
wrist NEC	C76.4-●	C79.89	D04.6-●	D36.7	D48.7	D49.89
xiphoid process	C41.3	C79.51	—	D16.7	D48.0	D49.2
Zuckerkandl organ	C75.5	C79.89	—	D35.6	D44.7	D49.7

TABLE OF NEOPLASMS

◄ New   ◖ Revised   ~~deleted~~ Deleted   ● Use Additional Character(s)

ICD-10-CM
Table of Drugs and Chemicals

Substance	Poisoning, Accidental (Unintentional)	Poisoning, Intentional Self-Harm	Poisoning, Assault	Poisoning, Undetermined	Adverse Effect	Underdosing
#						
1-propanol	T51.3X1	T51.3X2	T51.3X3	T51.3X4	—	—
2-propanol	T51.2X1	T51.2X2	T51.2X3	T51.2X4	—	—
2,4-D (dichlorophen-oxyacetic acid)	T60.3X1	T60.3X2	T60.3X3	T60.3X4	—	—
2,4-toluene diisocyanate	T65.0X1	T65.0X2	T65.0X3	T65.0X4	—	—
2,4,5-T (trichloro-phenoxyacetic acid)	T60.1X1	T60.1X2	T60.1X3	T60.1X4	—	—
3,4-methylenedioxy-methamphetamine	T43.641	T43.642	T43.643	T43.644	—	—
14-hydroxydihydro-morphinone	T40.2X1	T40.2X2	T40.2X3	T40.2X4	T40.2X5	T40.2X6
A						
ABOB	T37.5X1	T37.5X2	T37.5X3	T37.5X4	T37.5X5	T37.5X6
Abrine	T62.2X1	T62.2X2	T62.2X3	T62.2X4	—	—
Abrus (seed)	T62.2X1	T62.2X2	T62.2X3	T62.2X4	—	—
Absinthe	T51.0X1	T51.0X2	T51.0X3	T51.0X4	—	—
beverage	T51.0X1	T51.0X2	T51.0X3	T51.0X4	—	—
Acaricide	T60.8X1	T60.8X2	T60.8X3	T60.8X4	—	—
Acebutolol	T44.7X1	T44.7X2	T44.7X3	T44.7X4	T44.7X5	T44.7X6
Acecarbromal	T42.6X1	T42.6X2	T42.6X3	T42.6X4	T42.6X5	T42.6X6
Aceclidine	T44.1X1	T44.1X2	T44.1X3	T44.1X4	T44.1X5	T44.1X6
Acedapsone	T37.0X1	T37.0X2	T37.0X3	T37.0X4	T37.0X5	T37.0X6
Acefylline piperazine	T48.6X1	T48.6X2	T48.6X3	T48.6X4	T48.6X5	T48.6X6
Acemorphan	T40.2X1	T40.2X2	T40.2X3	T40.2X4	T40.2X5	T40.2X6
Acenocoumarin	T45.511	T45.512	T45.513	T45.514	T45.515	T45.516
Acenocoumarol	T45.511	T45.512	T45.513	T45.514	T45.515	T45.516
Acepifylline	T48.6X1	T48.6X2	T48.6X3	T48.6X4	T48.6X5	T48.6X6
Acepromazine	T43.3X1	T43.3X2	T43.3X3	T43.3X4	T43.3X5	T43.3X6
Acesulfamethoxypyridazine	T37.0X1	T37.0X2	T37.0X3	T37.0X4	T37.0X5	T37.0X6
Acetal	T52.8X1	T52.8X2	T52.8X3	T52.8X4	—	—
Acetaldehyde (vapor)	T52.8X1	T52.8X2	T52.8X3	T52.8X4	—	—
liquid	T65.891	T65.892	T65.893	T65.894	—	—
P-Acetamidophenol	T39.1X1	T39.1X2	T39.1X3	T39.1X4	T39.1X5	T39.1X6
Acetaminophen	T39.1X1	T39.1X2	T39.1X3	T39.1X4	T39.1X5	T39.1X6
Acetaminosalol	T39.1X1	T39.1X2	T39.1X3	T39.1X4	T39.1X5	T39.1X6
Acetanilide	T39.1X1	T39.1X2	T39.1X3	T39.1X4	T39.1X5	T39.1X6
Acetarsol	T37.3X1	T37.3X2	T37.3X3	T37.3X4	T37.3X5	T37.3X6
Acetazolamide	T50.2X1	T50.2X2	T50.2X3	T50.2X4	T50.2X5	T50.2X6
Acetiamine	T45.2X1	T45.2X2	T45.2X3	T45.2X4	T45.2X5	T45.2X6
Acetic						
acid	T54.2X1	T54.2X2	T54.2X3	T54.2X4	—	—
with sodium acetate (ointment)	T49.3X1	T49.3X2	T49.3X3	T49.3X4	T49.3X5	T49.3X6

Substance	Poisoning, Accidental (Unintentional)	Poisoning, Intentional Self-Harm	Poisoning, Assault	Poisoning, Undetermined	Adverse Effect	Underdosing
Acetic *(Continued)*						
acid *(Continued)*						
ester (solvent) (vapor)	T52.8X1	T52.8X2	T52.8X3	T52.8X4	—	—
irrigating solution	T50.3X1	T50.3X2	T50.3X3	T50.3X4	T50.3X5	T50.3X6
medicinal (lotion)	T49.2X1	T49.2X2	T49.2X3	T49.2X4	T49.2X5	T49.2X6
anhydride	T65.891	T65.892	T65.893	T65.894	—	—
ether (vapor)	T52.8X1	T52.8X2	T52.8X3	T52.8X4	—	—
Acetohexamide	T38.3X1	T38.3X2	T38.3X3	T38.3X4	T38.3X5	T38.3X6
Acetohydroxamic acid	T50.991	T50.992	T50.993	T50.994	T50.995	T50.996
Acetomenaphthone	T45.7X1	T45.7X2	T45.7X3	T45.7X4	T45.7X5	T45.7X6
Acetomorphine	T40.1X1	T40.1X2	T40.1X3	T40.1X4	—	—
Acetone (oils)	T52.4X1	T52.4X2	T52.4X3	T52.4X4	—	—
chlorinated	T52.4X1	T52.4X2	T52.4X3	T52.4X4	—	—
vapor	T52.4X1	T52.4X2	T52.4X3	T52.4X4	—	—
Acetonitrile	T52.8X1	T52.8X2	T52.8X3	T52.8X4	—	—
Acetophenazine	T43.3X1	T43.3X2	T43.3X3	T43.3X4	T43.3X5	T43.3X6
Acetophenetedin	T39.1X1	T39.1X2	T39.1X3	T39.1X4	T39.1X5	T39.1X6
Acetophenone	T52.4X1	T52.4X2	T52.4X3	T52.4X4	—	—
Acetorphine	T40.2X1	T40.2X2	T40.2X3	T40.2X4	—	—
Acetosulfone (sodium)	T37.1X1	T37.1X2	T37.1X3	T37.1X4	T37.1X5	T37.1X6
Acetrizoate (sodium)	T50.8X1	T50.8X2	T50.8X3	T50.8X4	T50.8X5	T50.8X6
Acetylcarbromal	T42.6X1	T42.6X2	T42.6X3	T42.6X4	T42.6X5	T42.6X6
Acetrizoic acid	T50.8X1	T50.8X2	T50.8X3	T50.8X4	T50.8X5	T50.8X6
Acetyl						
bromide	T53.6X1	T53.6X2	T53.6X3	T53.6X4	—	—
chloride	T53.6X1	T53.6X2	T53.6X3	T53.6X4	—	—
Acetylcholine						
chloride	T44.1X1	T44.1X2	T44.1X3	T44.1X4	T44.1X5	T44.1X6
derivative	T44.1X1	T44.1X2	T44.1X3	T44.1X4	T44.1X5	T44.1X6
Acetylcysteine	T48.4X1	T48.4X2	T48.4X3	T48.4X4	T48.4X5	T48.4X6
Acetyldigitoxin	T46.0X1	T46.0X2	T46.0X3	T46.0X4	T46.0X5	T46.0X6
Acetyldigoxin	T46.0X1	T46.0X2	T46.0X3	T46.0X4	T46.0X5	T46.0X6
Acetyldihydrocodeine	T40.2X1	T40.2X2	T40.2X3	T40.2X4	—	—
Acetyldihydrocodeinone	T40.2X1	T40.2X2	T40.2X3	T40.2X4	—	—
Acetylene (gas)	T59.891	T59.892	T59.893	T59.894	—	—
dichloride	T53.6X1	T53.6X2	T53.6X3	T53.6X4	—	—
incomplete combustion of	T58.11	T58.12	T58.13	T58.14	—	—
industrial	T59.891	T59.892	T59.893	T59.894	—	—
tetrachloride	T53.6X1	T53.6X2	T53.6X3	T53.6X4	—	—
vapor	T53.6X1	T53.6X2	T53.6X3	T53.6X4	—	—
Acetylphenylhydrazine	T39.8X1	T39.8X2	T39.8X3	T39.8X4	T39.8X5	T39.8X6
Acetylpheneturide	T42.6X1	T42.6X2	T42.6X3	T42.6X4	T42.6X5	T42.6X6

◀ New   ◀ Revised   ~~deleted~~ Deleted

TABLE OF DRUGS AND CHEMICALS

TABLE OF DRUGS AND CHEMICALS

	External Cause (T-Code)					
Substance	Poisoning, Accidental (Unintentional)	Poisoning, Intentional Self-Harm	Poisoning, Assault	Poisoning, Undetermined	Adverse Effect	Underdosing
Acetylsalicylic acid (salts)	T39.011	T39.012	T39.013	T39.014	T39.015	T39.016
enteric coated	T39.011	T39.012	T39.013	T39.014	T39.015	T39.016
Acetylsulfamethoxypyridazine	T37.0X1	T37.0X2	T37.0X3	T37.0X4	T37.0X5	T37.0X6
Achromycin	T36.4X1	T36.4X2	T36.4X3	T36.4X4	T36.4X5	T36.4X6
ophthalmic preparation	T49.5X1	T49.5X2	T49.5X3	T49.5X4	T49.5X5	T49.5X6
topical NEC	T49.0X1	T49.0X2	T49.0X3	T49.0X4	T49.0X5	T49.0X6
Aciclovir	T37.5X1	T37.5X2	T37.5X3	T37.5X4	T37.5X5	T37.5X6
Acid (corrosive) NEC	T54.2X1	T54.2X2	T54.2X3	T54.2X4	—	—
Acidifying agent NEC	T50.901	T50.902	T50.903	T50.904	T50.905	T50.906
Acipimox	T46.6X1	T46.6X2	T46.6X3	T46.6X4	T46.6X5	T46.6X6
Acitretin	T50.991	T50.992	T50.993	T50.994	T50.995	T50.996
Aclarubicin	T45.1X1	T45.1X2	T45.1X3	T45.1X4	T45.1X5	T45.1X6
Aclatonium napadisilate	T48.1X1	T48.1X2	T48.1X3	T48.1X4	T48.1X5	T48.1X6
Aconite (wild)	T46.991	T46.992	T46.993	T46.994	T46.995	T46.996
Aconitine	T46.991	T46.992	T46.993	T46.994	T46.995	T46.996
Aconitum ferox	T46.991	T46.992	T46.993	T46.994	T46.995	T46.996
Acridine	T65.6X1	T65.6X2	T65.6X3	T65.6X4	—	—
vapor	T59.891	T59.892	T59.893	T59.894	—	—
Acriflavine	T37.91	T37.92	T37.93	T37.94	T37.95	T37.96
Acriflavinium chloride	T49.0X1	T49.0X2	T49.0X3	T49.0X4	T49.0X5	T49.0X6
Acrinol	T49.0X1	T49.0X2	T49.0X3	T49.0X4	T49.0X5	T49.0X6
Acrisorcin	T49.0X1	T49.0X2	T49.0X3	T49.0X4	T49.0X5	T49.0X6
Acrivastine	T45.0X1	T45.0X2	T45.0X3	T45.0X4	T45.0X5	T45.0X6
Acrolein (gas)	T59.891	T59.892	T59.893	T59.894	—	—
liquid	T54.1X1	T54.1X2	T54.1X3	T54.1X4	—	—
Acrylamide	T65.891	T65.892	T65.893	T65.894	—	—
Acrylic resin	T49.3X1	T49.3X2	T49.3X3	T49.3X4	T49.3X5	T49.3X6
Acrylonitrile	T65.891	T65.892	T65.893	T65.894		
Actaea spicata	T62.2X1	T62.2X2	T62.2X3	T62.2X4	—	—
berry	T62.1X1	T62.1X2	T62.1X3	T62.1X4	—	—
Acterol	T37.3X1	T37.3X2	T37.3X3	T37.3X4	T37.3X5	T37.3X6
ACTH	T38.811	T38.812	T38.813	T38.814	T38.815	T38.816
Actinomycin C	T45.1X1	T45.1X2	T45.1X3	T45.1X4	T45.1X5	T45.1X6
Actinomycin D	T45.1X1	T45.1X2	T45.1X3	T45.1X4	T45.1X5	T45.1X6
Activated charcoal — *see also Charcoal, medicinal*	T47.6X1	T47.6X2	T47.6X3	T47.6X4	T47.6X5	T47.6X6
Acyclovir	T37.5X1	T37.5X2	T37.5X3	T37.5X4	T37.5X5	T37.5X6
Adenine	T45.2X1	T45.2X2	T45.2X3	T45.2X4	T45.2X5	T45.2X6
arabinoside	T37.5X1	T37.5X2	T37.5X3	T37.5X4	T37.5X5	T37.5X6
Adenosine (phosphate)	T46.2X1	T46.2X2	T46.2X3	T46.2X4	T46.2X5	T46.2X6
ADH	T38.891	T38.892	T38.893	T38.894	T38.895	T38.896
Adhesive NEC	T65.891	T65.892	T65.893	T65.894	—	—

	External Cause (T-Code)					
Substance	Poisoning, Accidental (Unintentional)	Poisoning, Intentional Self-Harm	Poisoning, Assault	Poisoning, Undetermined	Adverse Effect	Underdosing
Adicillin	T36.0X1	T36.0X2	T36.0X3	T36.0X4	T36.0X5	T36.0X6
Adiphenine	T44.3X1	T44.3X2	T44.3X3	T44.3X4	T44.3X5	T44.3X6
Adipiodone	T50.8X1	T50.8X2	T50.8X3	T50.8X4	T50.8X5	T50.8X6
Adjunct, pharmaceutical	T50.901	T50.902	T50.903	T50.904	T50.905	T50.906
Adrenal (extract, cortex or medulla) (glucocorticoids) (hormones) (mineralo corticoids)	T38.0X1	T38.0X2	T38.0X3	T38.0X4	T38.0X5	T38.0X6
ENT agent	T49.6X1	T49.6X2	T49.6X3	T49.6X4	T49.6X5	T49.6X6
ophthalmic preparation	T49.5X1	T49.5X2	T49.5X3	T49.5X4	T49.5X5	T49.5X6
topical NEC	T49.0X1	T49.0X2	T49.0X3	T49.0X4	T49.0X5	T49.0X6
Adrenaline	T44.5X1	T44.5X2	T44.5X3	T44.5X4	T44.5X5	T44.5X6
Adrenalin — *see Adrenaline*						
Adrenergic NEC	T44.901	T44.902	T44.903	T44.904	T44.905	T44.906
blocking agent NEC	T44.8X1	T44.8X2	T44.8X3	T44.8X4	T44.8X5	T44.8X6
beta, heart	T44.7X1	T44.7X2	T44.7X3	T44.7X4	T44.7X5	T44.7X6
specified NEC	T44.991	T44.992	T44.993	T44.994	T44.995	T44.996
Adrenochrome						
(mono) semicarbazone	T46.991	T46.992	T46.993	T46.994	T46.995	T46.996
derivative	T46.991	T46.992	T46.993	T46.994	T46.995	T46.996
Adrenocorticotrophic hormone	T38.811	T38.812	T38.813	T38.814	T38.815	T38.816
Adrenocorticotrophin	T38.811	T38.812	T38.813	T38.814	T38.815	T38.816
Adriamycin	T45.1X1	T45.1X2	T45.1X3	T45.1X4	T45.1X5	T45.1X6
Aerosol spray NEC	T65.91	T65.92	T65.93	T65.94	—	—
Aerosporin	T36.8X1	T36.8X2	T36.8X3	T36.8X4	T36.8X5	T36.8X6
ENT agent	T49.6X1	T49.6X2	T49.6X3	T49.6X4	T49.6X5	T49.6X6
ophthalmic preparation	T49.5X1	T49.5X2	T49.5X3	T49.5X4	T49.5X5	T49.5X6
topical NEC	T49.0X1	T49.0X2	T49.0X3	T49.0X4	T49.0X5	T49.0X6
Aethusa cynapium	T62.2X1	T62.2X2	T62.2X3	T62.2X4	—	—
Afghanistan black	T40.711	T40.712	T40.713	T40.714	T40.715	T40.716
Aflatoxin	T64.01	T64.02	T64.03	T64.04	—	—
Afloqualone	T42.8X1	T42.8X2	T42.8X3	T42.8X4	T42.8X5	T42.8X6
African boxwood	T62.2X1	T62.2X2	T62.2X3	T62.2X4	—	—
Agar	T47.4X1	T47.4X2	T47.4X3	T47.4X4	T47.4X5	T47.4X6
Agonist						
predominantly						
alpha-adrenoreceptor	T44.4X1	T44.4X2	T44.4X3	T44.4X4	T44.4X5	T44.4X6
beta-adrenoreceptor	T44.5X1	T44.5X2	T44.5X3	T44.5X4	T44.5X5	T44.5X6
Agricultural agent NEC	T65.91	T65.92	T65.93	T65.94	—	—
Agrypnal	T42.3X1	T42.3X2	T42.3X3	T42.3X4	T42.3X5	T42.3X6
AHLG	T50.Z11	T50.Z12	T50.Z13	T50.Z14	T50.Z15	T50.Z16
Air contaminant(s), source/type NOS	T65.91	T65.92	T65.93	T65.94	—	—

◀ New   ◀ Revised   ~~deleted~~ Deleted

	External Cause (T-Code)					
Substance	Poisoning, Accidental (Unintentional)	Poisoning, Intentional Self-Harm	Poisoning, Assault	Poisoning, Undetermined	Adverse Effect	Underdosing
Ajmaline	T46.2X1	T46.2X2	T46.2X3	T46.2X4	T46.2X5	T46.2X6
Akritoin	T37.8X1	T37.8X2	T37.8X3	T37.8X4	T37.8X5	T37.8X6
Akee	T62.1X1	T62.1X2	T62.1X3	T62.1X4	—	—
Akrinol	T49.0X1	T49.0X2	T49.0X3	T49.0X4	T49.0X5	T49.0X6
Alacepril	T46.4X1	T46.4X2	T46.4X3	T46.4X4	T46.4X5	T46.4X6
Alantolactone	T37.4X1	T37.4X2	T37.4X3	T37.4X4	T37.4X5	T37.4X6
Albamycin	T36.8X1	T36.8X2	T36.8X3	T36.8X4	T36.8X5	T36.8X6
Albendazole	T37.4X1	T37.4X2	T37.4X3	T37.4X4	T37.4X5	T37.4X6
Albumin						
bovine	T45.8X1	T45.8X2	T45.8X3	T45.8X4	T45.8X5	T45.8X6
human serum	T45.8X1	T45.8X2	T45.8X3	T45.8X4	T45.8X5	T45.8X6
salt-poor	T45.8X1	T45.8X2	T45.8X3	T45.8X4	T45.8X5	T45.8X6
normal human serum	T45.8X1	T45.8X2	T45.8X3	T45.8X4	T45.8X5	T45.8X6
Albuterol	T48.6X1	T48.6X2	T48.6X3	T48.6X4	T48.6X5	T48.6X6
Albutoin	T42.0X1	T42.0X2	T42.0X3	T42.0X4	T42.0X5	T42.0X6
Alclometasone	T49.0X1	T49.0X2	T49.0X3	T49.0X4	T49.0X5	T49.0X6
Alcohol	T51.91	T51.92	T51.93	T51.94	—	—
absolute	T51.0X1	T51.0X2	T51.0X3	T51.0X4	—	—
beverage	T51.0X1	T51.0X2	T51.0X3	T51.0X4	—	—
allyl	T51.8X1	T51.8X2	T51.8X3	T51.8X4	—	—
amyl	T51.3X1	T51.3X2	T51.3X3	T51.3X4	—	—
antifreeze	T51.1X1	T51.1X2	T51.1X3	T51.1X4	—	—
beverage	T51.0X1	T51.0X2	T51.0X3	T51.0X4	—	—
butyl	T51.3X1	T51.3X2	T51.3X3	T51.3X4	—	—
dehydrated	T51.0X1	T51.0X2	T51.0X3	T51.0X4	—	—
beverage	T51.0X1	T51.0X2	T51.0X3	T51.0X4	—	—
denatured	T51.0X1	T51.0X2	T51.0X3	T51.0X4	—	—
deterrent NEC	T50.6X1	T50.6X2	T50.6X3	T50.6X4	T50.6X5	T50.6X6
diagnostic (gastric function)	T50.8X1	T50.8X2	T50.8X3	T50.8X4	T50.8X5	T50.8X6
ethyl	T51.0X1	T51.0X2	T51.0X3	T51.0X4	—	—
beverage	T51.0X1	T51.0X2	T51.0X3	T51.0X4	—	—
grain	T51.0X1	T51.0X2	T51.0X3	T51.0X4	—	—
beverage	T51.0X1	T51.0X2	T51.0X3	T51.0X4	—	—
industrial	T51.0X1	T51.0X2	T51.0X3	T51.0X4	—	—
isopropyl	T51.2X1	T51.2X2	T51.2X3	T51.2X4	—	—
methyl	T51.1X1	T51.1X2	T51.1X3	T51.1X4	—	—
preparation for consumption	T51.0X1	T51.0X2	T51.0X3	T51.0X4	—	—
propyl	T51.3X1	T51.3X2	T51.3X3	T51.3X4	—	—
secondary	T51.2X1	T51.2X2	T51.2X3	T51.2X4	—	—
radiator	T51.1X1	T51.1X2	T51.1X3	T51.1X4	—	—
rubbing	T51.2X1	T51.2X2	T51.2X3	T51.2X4	—	—
specified type NEC	T51.8X1	T51.8X2	T51.8X3	T51.8X4	—	—

	External Cause (T-Code)					
Substance	Poisoning, Accidental (Unintentional)	Poisoning, Intentional Self-Harm	Poisoning, Assault	Poisoning, Undetermined	Adverse Effect	Underdosing
Alcohol *(Continued)*						
surgical	T51.0X1	T51.0X2	T51.0X3	T51.0X4	—	—
vapor (from any type of Alcohol)	T59.891	T59.892	T59.893	T59.894	—	—
wood	T51.1X1	T51.1X2	T51.1X3	T51.1X4	—	—
Alcuronium (chloride)	T48.1X1	T48.1X2	T48.1X3	T48.1X4	T48.1X5	T48.1X6
Aldactone	T50.0X1	T50.0X2	T50.0X3	T50.0X4	T50.0X5	T50.0X6
Aldesulfone sodium	T37.1X1	T37.1X2	T37.1X3	T37.1X4	T37.1X5	T37.1X6
Aldicarb	T60.0X1	T60.0X2	T60.0X3	T60.0X4	—	—
Aldomet	T46.5X1	T46.5X2	T46.5X3	T46.5X4	T46.5X5	T46.5X6
Aldosterone	T50.0X1	T50.0X2	T50.0X3	T50.0X4	T50.0X5	T50.0X6
Aldrin (dust)	T60.1X1	T60.1X2	T60.1X3	T60.1X4	—	—
Aleve — *see Naproxen*						
Alexitol sodium	T47.1X1	T47.1X2	T47.1X3	T47.1X4	T47.1X5	T47.1X6
Alfacalcidol	T45.2X1	T45.2X2	T45.2X3	T45.2X4	T45.2X5	T45.2X6
Alfadolone	T41.1X1	T41.1X2	T41.1X3	T41.1X4	T41.1X5	T41.1X6
Alfaxalone	T41.1X1	T41.1X2	T41.1X3	T41.1X4	T41.1X5	T41.1X6
Alfentanil	T40.411	T40.412	T40.413	T40.414	T40.415	T40.416
Alfuzosin (hydrochloride)	T44.8X1	T44.8X2	T44.8X3	T44.8X4	T44.8X5	T44.8X6
Algae (harmful) (toxin)	T65.821	T65.822	T65.823	T65.824	—	—
Algeldrate	T47.1X1	T47.1X2	T47.1X3	T47.1X4	T47.1X5	T47.1X6
Algin	T47.8X1	T47.8X2	T47.8X3	T47.8X4	T47.8X5	T47.8X6
Alglucerase	T45.3X1	T45.3X2	T45.3X3	T45.3X4	T45.3X5	T45.3X6
Alidase	T45.3X1	T45.3X2	T45.3X3	T45.3X4	T45.3X5	T45.3X6
Alimemazine	T43.3X1	T43.3X2	T43.3X3	T43.3X4	T43.3X5	T43.3X6
Aliphatic thiocyanates	T65.0X1	T65.0X2	T65.0X3	T65.0X4	—	—
Alizapride	T45.0X1	T45.0X2	T45.0X3	T45.0X4	T45.0X5	T45.0X6
Alkali (caustic)	T54.3X1	T54.3X2	T54.3X3	T54.3X4	—	—
Alkalizing agent NEC	T50.901	T50.902	T50.903	T50.904	T50.905	T50.906
Alkaline antiseptic solution (aromatic)	T49.6X1	T49.6X2	T49.6X3	T49.6X4	T49.6X5	T49.6X6
Alkalinizing agents (medicinal)	T50.901	T50.902	T50.903	T50.904	T50.905	T50.906
Alka-seltzer	T39.011	T39.012	T39.013	T39.014	T39.015	T39.016
Alkavervir	T46.5X1	T46.5X2	T46.5X3	T46.5X4	T46.5X5	T46.5X6
Alkonium (bromide)	T49.0X1	T49.0X2	T49.0X3	T49.0X4	T49.0X5	T49.0X6
Alkylating drug NEC	T45.1X1	T45.1X2	T45.1X3	T45.1X4	T45.1X5	T45.1X6
antimyeloproliferative	T45.1X1	T45.1X2	T45.1X3	T45.1X4	T45.1X5	T45.1X6
lymphatic	T45.1X1	T45.1X2	T45.1X3	T45.1X4	T45.1X5	T45.1X6
Alkylisocyanate	T65.0X1	T65.0X2	T65.0X3	T65.0X4	—	—
Allantoin	T49.411	T49.412	T49.413	T49.414	T49.415	T49.416
Allegron	T43.0X1	T43.0X2	T43.0X3	T43.0X4	T43.0X5	T43.0X6
Allethrin	T49.0X1	T49.0X2	T49.0X3	T49.0X4	T49.0X5	T49.0X6
Allobarbital	T42.3X1	T42.3X2	T42.3X3	T42.3X4	T42.3X5	T42.3X6

◀ New   ◀ Revised   ~~deleted~~ Deleted

Substance	External Cause (T-Code)					
	Poisoning, Accidental (Unintentional)	Poisoning, Intentional Self-Harm	Poisoning, Assault	Poisoning, Undetermined	Adverse Effect	Underdosing
Allopurinol	T50.4X1	T50.4X2	T50.4X3	T50.4X4	T50.4X5	T50.4X6
Allyl						
alcohol	T51.8X1	T51.8X2	T51.8X3	T51.8X4	—	—
disulfide	T46.6X1	T46.6X2	T46.6X3	T46.6X4	T46.6X5	T46.6X6
Allylestrenol	T38.5X1	T38.5X2	T38.5X3	T38.5X4	T38.5X5	T38.5X6
Allylisopropylacetylurea	T42.6X1	T42.6X2	T42.6X3	T42.6X4	T42.6X5	T42.6X6
Allylisopropylmalonylurea	T42.3X1	T42.3X2	T42.3X3	T42.3X4	T42.3X5	T42.3X6
Allylthiourea	T49.3X1	T49.3X2	T49.3X3	T49.3X4	T49.3X5	T49.3X6
Allyltribromide	T42.6X1	T42.6X2	T42.6X3	T42.6X4	T42.6X5	T42.6X6
Allypropymal	T42.3X1	T42.3X2	T42.3X3	T42.3X4	T42.3X5	T42.3X6
Almagate	T47.1X1	T47.1X2	T47.1X3	T47.1X4	T47.1X5	T47.1X6
Almasilate	T47.1X1	T47.1X2	T47.1X3	T47.1X4	T47.1X5	T47.1X6
Almitrine	T50.7X1	T50.7X2	T50.7X3	T50.7X4	T50.7X5	T50.7X6
Aloes	T47.2X1	T47.2X2	T47.2X3	T47.2X4	T47.2X5	T47.2X6
Aloglutamol	T47.1X1	T47.1X2	T47.1X3	T47.1X4	T47.1X5	T47.1X6
Aloin	T47.2X1	T47.2X2	T47.2X3	T47.2X4	T47.2X5	T47.2X6
Aloxidone	T42.2X1	T42.2X2	T42.2X3	T42.2X4	T42.2X5	T42.2X6
Alpha						
acetyldigoxin	T46.0X1	T46.0X2	T46.0X3	T46.0X4	T46.0X5	T46.0X6
adrenergic blocking drug	T44.6X1	T44.6X2	T44.6X3	T44.6X4	T44.6X5	T44.6X6
amylase	T45.3X1	T45.3X2	T45.3X3	T45.3X4	T45.3X5	T45.3X6
tocoferol (acetate)	T45.2X1	T45.2X2	T45.2X3	T45.2X4	T45.2X5	T45.2X6
tocopherol	T45.2X1	T45.2X2	T45.2X3	T45.2X4	T45.2X5	T45.2X6
Alphadolone	T41.1X1	T41.1X2	T41.1X3	T41.1X4	T41.1X5	T41.1X6
Alphaprodine	T40.491	T40.492	T40.493	T40.494	T40.495	T40.496
Alphaxalone	T41.1X1	T41.1X2	T41.1X3	T41.1X4	T41.1X5	T41.1X6
Alprazolam	T42.4X1	T42.4X2	T42.4X3	T42.4X4	T42.4X5	T42.4X6
Alprenolol	T44.7X1	T44.7X2	T44.7X3	T44.7X4	T44.7X5	T44.7X6
Alprostadil	T46.7X1	T46.7X2	T46.7X3	T46.7X4	T46.7X5	T46.7X6
Alsactide	T38.811	T38.812	T38.813	T38.814	T38.815	T38.816
Alseroxylon	T46.5X1	T46.5X2	T46.5X3	T46.5X4	T46.5X5	T46.5X6
Alteplase	T45.611	T45.612	T45.613	T45.614	T45.615	T45.616
Altizide	T50.2X1	T50.2X2	T50.2X3	T50.2X4	T50.2X5	T50.2X6
Altretamine	T45.1X1	T45.1X2	T45.1X3	T45.1X4	T45.1X5	T45.1X6
Alum (medicinal)	T49.4X1	T49.4X2	T49.4X3	T49.4X4	T49.4X5	T49.4X6
nonmedicinal (ammonium) (potassium)	T56.891	T56.892	T56.893	T56.894	—	—
Aluminium, aluminum						
acetate	T49.2X1	T49.2X2	T49.2X3	T49.2X4	T49.2X5	T49.2X6
solution	T49.0X1	T49.0X2	T49.0X3	T49.0X4	T49.0X5	T49.0X6
aspirin	T39.011	T39.012	T39.013	T39.014	T39.015	T39.016
bis (acetylsalicylate)	T39.011	T39.012	T39.013	T39.014	T39.015	T39.016

Substance	External Cause (T-Code)					
	Poisoning, Accidental (Unintentional)	Poisoning, Intentional Self-Harm	Poisoning, Assault	Poisoning, Undetermined	Adverse Effect	Underdosing
Aluminium, aluminum (Continued)						
carbonate (gel, basic)	T47.1X1	T47.1X2	T47.1X3	T47.1X4	T47.1X5	T47.1X6
chlorhydroxide-complex	T47.1X1	T47.1X2	T47.1X3	T47.1X4	T47.1X5	T47.1X6
chloride	T49.2X1	T49.2X2	T49.2X3	T49.2X4	T49.2X5	T49.2X6
clofibrate	T46.6X1	T46.6X2	T46.6X3	T46.6X4	T46.6X5	T46.6X6
diacetate	T49.2X1	T49.2X2	T49.2X3	T49.2X4	T49.2X5	T49.2X6
glycinate	T47.1X1	T47.1X2	T47.1X3	T47.1X4	T47.1X5	T47.1X6
hydroxide (gel)	T47.1X1	T47.1X2	T47.1X3	T47.1X4	T47.1X5	T47.1X6
hydroxide-magnesium carb. gel	T47.1X1	T47.1X2	T47.1X3	T47.1X4	T47.1X5	T47.1X6
magnesium silicate	T47.1X1	T47.1X2	T47.1X3	T47.1X4	T47.1X5	T47.1X6
nicotinate	T46.7X1	T46.7X2	T46.7X3	T46.7X4	T46.7X5	T46.7X6
ointment (surgical) (topical)	T49.3X1	T49.3X2	T49.3X3	T49.3X4	T49.3X5	T49.3X6
phosphate	T47.1X1	T47.1X2	T47.1X3	T47.1X4	T47.1X5	T47.1X6
salicylate	T39.091	T39.092	T39.093	T39.094	T39.095	T39.096
silicate	T47.1X1	T47.1X2	T47.1X3	T47.1X4	T47.1X5	T47.1X6
sodium silicate	T47.1X1	T47.1X2	T47.1X3	T47.1X4	T47.1X5	T47.1X6
subacetate	T49.2X1	T49.2X2	T49.2X3	T49.2X4	T49.2X5	T49.2X6
sulfate	T49.0X1	T49.0X2	T49.0X3	T49.0X4	T49.0X5	T49.0X6
tannate	T47.6X1	T47.6X2	T47.6X3	T47.6X4	T47.6X5	T47.6X6
topical NEC	T49.3X1	T49.3X2	T49.3X3	T49.3X4	T49.3X5	T49.3X6
Alurate	T42.3X1	T42.3X2	T42.3X3	T42.3X4	T42.3X5	T42.3X6
Alverine	T44.3X1	T44.3X2	T44.3X3	T44.3X4	T44.3X5	T44.3X6
Alvodine	T40.2X1	T40.2X2	T40.2X3	T40.2X4	T40.2X5	T40.2X6
Amanita phalloides	T62.0X1	T62.0X2	T62.0X3	T62.0X4	—	—
Amanitine	T62.0X1	T62.0X2	T62.0X3	T62.0X4	—	—
Amantadine	T42.8X1	T42.8X2	T42.8X3	T42.8X4	T42.8X5	T42.8X6
Ambazone	T49.6X1	T49.6X2	T49.6X3	T49.6X4	T49.6X5	T49.6X6
Ambenonium (chloride)	T44.0X1	T44.0X2	T44.0X3	T44.0X4	T44.0X5	T44.0X6
Ambroxol	T48.4X1	T48.4X2	T48.4X3	T48.4X4	T48.4X5	T48.4X6
Ambuphylline	T48.6X1	T48.6X2	T48.6X3	T48.6X4	T48.6X5	T48.6X6
Ambutonium bromide	T44.3X1	T44.3X2	T44.3X3	T44.3X4	T44.3X5	T44.3X6
Amcinonide	T49.0X1	T49.0X2	T49.0X3	T49.0X4	T49.0X5	T49.0X6
Amdinocilline	T36.0X1	T36.0X2	T36.0X3	T36.0X4	T36.0X5	T36.0X6
Ametazole	T50.8X1	T50.8X2	T50.8X3	T50.8X4	T50.8X5	T50.8X6
Amethocaine	T41.3X1	T41.3X2	T41.3X3	T41.3X4	T41.3X5	T41.3X6
regional	T41.3X1	T41.3X2	T41.3X3	T41.3X4	T41.3X5	T41.3X6
spinal	T41.3X1	T41.3X2	T41.3X3	T41.3X4	T41.3X5	T41.3X6
Amethopterin	T45.1X1	T45.1X2	T45.1X3	T45.1X4	T45.1X5	T45.1X6
Amezinium metilsulfate	T44.991	T44.992	T44.993	T44.994	T44.995	T44.996
Amfebutamone	T43.291	T43.292	T43.293	T43.294	T43.295	T43.296
Amfepramone	T50.5X1	T50.5X2	T50.5X3	T50.5X4	T50.5X5	T50.5X6

◀ New   ◀ Revised   ~~deleted~~ Deleted

Substance	Poisoning, Accidental (Unintentional)	Poisoning, Intentional Self-Harm	Poisoning, Assault	Poisoning, Undetermined	Adverse Effect	Underdosing
Amfetamine	T43.621	T43.622	T43.623	T43.624	T43.625	T43.626
Amfetaminil	T43.621	T43.622	T43.623	T43.624	T43.625	T43.626
Amfomycin	T36.8X1	T36.8X2	T36.8X3	T36.8X4	T36.8X5	T36.8X6
Amidefrine mesilate	T48.5X1	T48.5X2	T48.5X3	T48.5X4	T48.5X5	T48.5X6
Amidone	T40.3X1	T40.3X2	T40.3X3	T40.3X4	T40.3X5	T40.3X6
Amidopyrine	T39.2X1	T39.2X2	T39.2X3	T39.2X4	T39.2X5	T39.2X6
Amidotrizoate	T50.8X1	T50.8X2	T50.8X3	T50.8X4	T50.8X5	T50.8X6
Amiflamine	T43.1X1	T43.1X2	T43.1X3	T43.1X4	T43.1X5	T43.1X6
Amikacin	T36.5X1	T36.5X2	T36.5X3	T36.5X4	T36.5X5	T36.5X6
Amikhelline	T46.3X1	T46.3X2	T46.3X3	T46.3X4	T46.3X5	T46.3X6
Amiloride	T50.2X1	T50.2X2	T50.2X3	T50.2X4	T50.2X5	T50.2X6
Aminacrine	T49.0X1	T49.0X2	T49.0X3	T49.0X4	T49.0X5	T49.0X6
Amineptine	T43.011	T43.012	T43.013	T43.014	T43.015	T43.016
Aminitrozole	T37.3X1	T37.3X2	T37.3X3	T37.3X4	T37.3X5	T37.3X6
Aminoacetic acid (derivatives)	T50.3X1	T50.3X2	T50.3X3	150.3X4	T50.3X5	T50.3X6
Amino acids	T50.3X1	T50.3X2	T50.3X3	T50.3X4	T50.3X5	T50.3X6
Aminoacridine	T49.0X1	T49.0X2	T49.0X3	T49.0X4	T49.0X5	T49.0X6
Aminobenzoic acid (-p)	T49.3X1	T49.3X2	T49.3X3	T49.3X4	T49.3X5	T49.3X6
4-Aminobutyric acid	T43.8X1	T43.8X2	T43.8X3	T43.8X4	T43.8X5	T43.8X6
Aminocaproic acid	T45.621	T45.622	T45.623	T45.624	T45.625	T45.626
Aminofenazone	T39.2X1	T39.2X2	T39.2X3	T39.2X4	T39.2X5	T39.2X6
Aminoethylisothiourium	T45.8X1	T45.8X2	T45.8X3	T45.8X4	T45.8X5	T45.8X6
Aminoglutethimide	T45.1X1	T45.1X2	T45.1X3	T45.1X4	T45.1X5	T45.1X6
Aminohippuric acid	T50.8X1	T50.8X2	T50.8X3	T50.8X4	T50.8X5	T50.8X6
Aminomethylbenzoic acid	T45.691	T45.692	T45.693	T45.694	T45.695	T45.696
Aminometradine	T50.2X1	T50.2X2	T50.2X3	T50.2X4	T50.2X5	T50.2X6
Aminopentamide	T44.3X1	T44.3X2	T44.3X3	T44.3X4	T44.3X5	T44.3X6
Aminophenazone	T39.2X1	T39.2X2	T39.2X3	T39.2X4	T39.2X5	T39.2X6
Aminophenol	T54.0X1	T54.0X2	T54.0X3	T54.0X4	—	—
4-Aminophenol derivatives	T39.1X1	T39.1X2	T39.1X3	T39.1X4	T39.1X5	T39.1X6
Aminophenylpyridone	T43.591	T43.592	T43.593	T43.594	T43.595	T43.596
Aminophylline	T48.6X1	T48.6X2	T48.6X3	T48.6X4	T48.6X5	T48.6X6
Aminopterin sodium	T45.1X1	T45.1X2	T45.1X3	T45.1X4	T45.1X5	T45.1X6
Aminopyrine	T39.2X1	T39.2X2	T39.2X3	T39.2X4	T39.2X5	T39.2X6
8-Aminoquinoline drugs	T37.2X1	T37.2X2	T37.2X3	T37.2X4	T37.2X5	T37.2X6
Aminorex	T50.5X1	T50.5X2	T50.5X3	T50.5X4	T50.5X5	T50.5X6
Aminosalicylic acid	T37.1X1	T37.1X2	T37.1X3	T37.1X4	T37.1X5	T37.1X6
Aminosalylum	T37.1X1	T37.1X2	T37.1X3	T37.1X4	T37.1X5	T37.1X6
Amiodarone	T46.2X1	T46.2X2	T46.2X3	T46.2X4	T46.2X5	T46.2X6
Amiphenazole	T50.7X1	T50.7X2	T50.7X3	T50.7X4	T50.7X5	T50.7X6
Amiquinsin	T46.5X1	T46.5X2	T46.5X3	T46.5X4	T46.5X5	T46.5X6
Amisometradine	T50.2X1	T50.2X2	T50.2X3	T50.2X4	T50.2X5	T50.2X6
Amisulpride	T43.591	T43.592	T43.593	T43.594	T43.595	T43.596
Amitriptyline	T43.021	T43.022	T43.023	T43.024	T43.025	T43.026
Amitriptylinoxide	T43.021	T43.022	T43.023	T43.024	T43.025	T43.026
Amlexanox	T48.6X1	T48.6X2	T48.6X3	T48.6X4	T48.6X5	T48.6X6
Ammonia (fumes) (gas) (vapor)	T59.891	T59.892	T59.893	T59.894	—	—
aromatic spirit	T48.991	T48.992	T48.993	T48.994	T48.995	T48.996
liquid (household)	T54.3X1	T54.3X2	T54.3X3	T54.3X4	—	—
Ammoniated mercury	T49.0X1	T49.0X2	T49.0X3	T49.0X4	T49.0X5	T49.0X6
Ammonium						
acid tartrate	T49.5X1	T49.5X2	T49.5X3	T49.5X4	T49.5X5	T49.5X6
bromide	T42.6X1	T42.6X2	T42.6X3	T42.6X4	T42.6X5	T42.6X6
carbonate	T54.3X1	T54.3X2	T54.3X3	T54.3X4	—	—
chloride	T50.991	T50.992	T50.993	T50.994	T50.995	T50.996
expectorant	T48.4X1	T48.4X2	T48.4X3	T48.4X4	T48.4X5	T48.4X6
compounds (household) NEC	T54.3X1	T54.3X2	T54.3X3	T54.3X4	—	—
fumes (any usage)	T59.891	T59.892	T59.893	T59.894	—	—
industrial	T54.3X1	T54.3X2	T54.3X3	T54.3X4	—	—
ichthyosulronate	T49.4X1	T49.4X2	T49.4X3	T49.4X4	T49.4X5	T49.4X6
mandelate	T37.91	T37.92	T37.93	T37.94	T37.95	T37.96
sulfamate	T60.3X1	T60.3X2	T60.3X3	T60.3X4	—	—
sulfonate resin	T47.8X1	T47.8X2	T47.8X3	T47.8X4	T47.8X5	T47.8X6
Amobarbital (sodium)	T42.3X1	T42.3X2	T42.3X3	T42.3X4	T42.3X5	T42.3X6
Amodiaquine	T37.2X1	T37.2X2	T37.2X3	T37.2X4	T37.2X5	T37.2X6
Amopyroquin(e)	T37.2X1	T37.2X2	T37.2X3	T37.2X4	T37.2X5	T37.2X6
Amoxapine	T43.011	T43.012	T43.013	T43.014	T43.015	T43.016
Amoxicillin	T36.0X1	T36.0X2	T36.0X3	T36.0X4	T36.0X5	T36.0X6
Amperozide	T43.591	T43.592	T43.593	T43.594	T43.595	T43.596
Amphenidone	T43.591	T43.592	T43.593	T43.594	T43.595	T43.596
Amphetamine NEC	T43.621	T43.622	T43.623	T43.624	T43.625	T43.626
Amphomycin	T36.8X1	T36.8X2	T36.8X3	T36.8X4	T36.8X5	T36.8X6
Amphotalide	T37.4X1	T37.4X2	T37.4X3	T37.4X4	T37.4X5	T37.4X6
Amphotericin B	T36.7X1	T36.7X2	T36.7X3	T36.7X4	T36.7X5	T36.7X6
topical	T49.0X1	T49.0X2	T49.0X3	T49.0X4	T49.0X5	T49.0X6
Ampicillin	T36.0X1	T36.0X2	T36.0X3	T36.0X4	T36.0X5	T36.0X6
Amprotropine	T44.3X1	T44.3X2	T44.3X3	T44.3X4	T44.3X5	T44.3X6
Amsacrine	T45.1X1	T45.1X2	T45.1X3	T45.1X4	T45.1X5	T45.1X6
Amygdaline	T62.2X1	T62.2X2	T62.2X3	T62.2X4	—	—
Amyl						
acetate	T52.8X1	T52.8X2	T52.8X3	T52.8X4	—	—
vapor	T59.891	T59.892	T59.893	T59.894	—	—
alcohol	T51.3X1	T51.3X2	T51.3X3	T51.3X4	—	—
chloride	T53.6X1	T53.6X2	T53.6X3	T53.6X4	—	—

◀ New   ◀ Revised   ~~deleted~~ Deleted

Substance	Poisoning, Accidental (Unintentional)	Poisoning, Intentional Self-Harm	Poisoning, Assault	Poisoning, Undetermined	Adverse Effect	Underdosing
Amyl *(Continued)*						
formate	T52.8X1	T52.8X2	T52.8X3	T52.8X4	—	—
nitrite	T46.3X1	T46.3X2	T46.3X3	T46.3X4	T46.3X5	T46.3X6
propionate	T65.891	T65.892	T65.893	T65.894	—	—
Amylase	T47.5X1	T47.5X2	T47.5X3	T47.5X4	T47.5X5	T47.5X6
Amyleine, regional	T41.3X1	T41.3X2	T41.3X3	T41.3X4	T41.3X5	T41.3X6
Amylene						
dichloride	T53.6X1	T53.6X2	T53.6X3	T53.6X4	—	—
hydrate	T51.3X1	T51.3X2	T51.3X3	T51.3X4	—	—
Amylmetacresol	T49.6X1	T49.6X2	T49.6X3	T49.6X4	T49.6X5	T49.6X6
Amylobarbitone	T42.3X1	T42.3X2	T42.3X3	T42.3X4	T42.3X5	T42.3X6
Amylocaine, regional	T41.3X1	T41.3X2	T41.3X3	T41.3X4	T41.3X5	T41.3X6
infiltration (subcutaneous)	T41.3X1	T41.3X2	T41.3X3	T41.3X4	T41.3X5	T41.3X6
nerve block (peripheral) (plexus)	T41.3X1	T41.3X2	T41.3X3	T41.3X4	T41.3X5	T41.3X6
spinal	T41.3X1	T41.3X2	T41.3X3	T41.3X4	T41.3X5	T41.3X6
topical (surface)	T41.3X1	T41.3X2	T41.3X3	T41.3X4	T41.3X5	T41.3X6
Amylopectin	T47.6X1	T47.6X2	T47.6X3	T47.6X4	T47.6X5	T47.6X6
Amytal (sodium)	T42.3X1	T42.3X2	T42.3X3	T42.3X4	T42.3X5	T42.3X6
Anabolic steroid	T38.7X1	T38.7X2	T38.7X3	T38.7X4	T38.7X5	T38.7X6
Analeptic NEC	T50.7X1	T50.7X2	T50.7X3	T50.7X4	T50.7X5	T50.7X6
Analgesic	T39.91	T39.92	T39.93	T39.94	T39.95	T39.96
anti-inflammatory NEC	T39.91	T39.92	T39.93	T39.94	T39.95	T39.96
propionic acid derivative	T39.311	T39.312	T39.313	T39.314	T39.315	T39.316
antirheumatic NEC	T39.4X1	T39.4X2	T39.4X3	T39.4X4	T39.4X5	T39.4X6
aromatic NEC	T39.1X1	T39.1X2	T39.1X3	T39.1X4	T39.1X5	T39.1X6
narcotic NEC	T40.601	T40.602	T40.603	T40.604	T40.605	T40.606
combination	T40.601	T40.602	T40.603	T40.604	T40.605	T40.606
obstetric	T40.601	T40.602	T40.603	T40.604	T40.605	T40.606
non-narcotic NEC	T39.91	T39.92	T39.93	T39.94	T39.95	T39.96
combination	T39.91	T39.92	T39.93	T39.94	T39.95	T39.96
pyrazole	T39.2X1	T39.2X2	T39.2X3	T39.2X4	T39.2X5	T39.2X6
specified NEC	T39.8X1	T39.8X2	T39.8X3	T39.8X4	T39.8X5	T39.8X6
Analgin	T39.2X1	T39.2X2	T39.2X3	T39.2X4	T39.2X5	T39.2X6
Anamirta cocculus	T62.1X1	T62.1X2	T62.1X3	T62.1X4	—	—
Ancillin	T36.0X1	T36.0X2	T36.0X3	T36.0X4	T36.0X5	T36.0X6
Ancrod	T45.691	T45.692	T45.693	T45.694	T45.695	T45.696
Androgen	T38.7X1	T38.7X2	T38.7X3	T38.7X4	T38.7X5	T38.7X6
Androgen-estrogen mixture	T38.7X1	T38.7X2	T38.7X3	T38.7X4	T38.7X5	T38.7X6
Androstalone	T38.7X1	T38.7X2	T38.7X3	T38.7X4	T38.7X5	T38.7X6
Androstanolone	T38.7X1	T38.7X2	T38.7X3	T38.7X4	T38.7X5	T38.7X6
Androsterone	T38.7X1	T38.7X2	T38.7X3	T38.7X4	T38.7X5	T38.7X6

Substance	Poisoning, Accidental (Unintentional)	Poisoning, Intentional Self-Harm	Poisoning, Assault	Poisoning, Undetermined	Adverse Effect	Underdosing
Anemone pulsatilla	T62.2X1	T62.2X2	T62.2X3	T62.2X4	—	—
Anesthesia						
caudal	T41.3X1	T41.3X2	T41.3X3	T41.3X4	T41.3X5	T41.3X6
endotracheal	T41.0X1	T41.0X2	T41.0X3	T41.0X4	T41.0X5	T41.0X6
epidural	T41.3X1	T41.3X2	T41.3X3	T41.3X4	T41.3X5	T41.3X6
inhalation	T41.0X1	T41.0X2	T41.0X3	T41.0X4	T41.0X5	T41.0X6
local	T41.3X1	T41.3X2	T41.3X3	T41.3X4	T41.3X5	T41.3X6
mucosal	T41.3X1	T41.3X2	T41.3X3	T41.3X4	T41.3X5	T41.3X6
muscle relaxation	T48.1X1	T48.1X2	T48.1X3	T48.1X4	T48.1X5	T48.1X6
nerve blocking	T41.3X1	T41.3X2	T41.3X3	T41.3X4	T41.3X5	T41.3X6
plexus blocking	T41.3X1	T41.3X2	T41.3X3	T41.3X4	T41.3X5	T41.3X6
potentiated	T41.201	T41.202	T41.203	T41.204	T41.205	T41.206
rectal	T41.201	T41.202	T41.203	T41.204	T41.205	T41.206
general	T41.201	T41.202	T41.203	T41.204	T41.205	T41.206
local	T41.3X1	T41.3X2	T41.3X3	T41.3X4	T41.3X5	T41.3X6
regional	T41.3X1	T41.3X2	T41.3X3	T41.3X4	T41.3X5	T41.3X6
surface	T41.3X1	T41.3X2	T41.3X3	T41.3X4	T41.3X5	T41.3X6
Anesthetic NEC—*see also Anesthesia*	T41.41	T41.42	T41.43	T41.44	T41.45	T41.46
with muscle relaxant	T41.201	T41.202	T41.203	T41.204	T41.205	T41.206
general	T41.201	T41.202	T41.203	T41.204	T41.205	T41.206
local	T41.3X1	T41.3X2	T41.3X3	T41.3X4	T41.3X5	T41.3X6
gaseous NEC	T41.0X1	T41.0X2	T41.0X3	T41.0X4	T41.0X5	T41.0X6
general NEC	T41.201	T41.202	T41.203	T41.204	T41.205	T41.206
halogenated hydrocarbon derivatives NEC	T41.0X1	T41.0X2	T41.0X3	T41.0X4	T41.0X5	T41.0X6
infiltration NEC	T41.3X1	T41.3X2	T41.3X3	T41.3X4	T41.3X5	T41.3X6
intravenous NEC	T41.1X1	T41.1X2	T41.1X3	T41.1X4	T41.1X5	T41.1X6
local NEC	T41.3X1	T41.3X2	T41.3X3	T41.3X4	T41.3X5	T41.3X6
rectal	T41.201	T41.202	T41.203	T41.204	T41.205	T41.206
general	T41.201	T41.202	T41.203	T41.204	T41.205	T41.206
local	T41.3X1	T41.3X2	T41.3X3	T41.3X4	T41.3X5	T41.3X6
regional NEC	T41.3X1	T41.3X2	T41.3X3	T41.3X4	T41.3X5	T41.3X6
spinal NEC	T41.3X1	T41.3X2	T41.3X3	T41.3X4	T41.3X5	T41.3X6
thiobarbiturate	T41.1X1	T41.1X2	T41.1X3	T41.1X4	T41.1X5	T41.1X6
topical	T41.3X1	T41.3X2	T41.3X3	T41.3X4	T41.3X5	T41.3X6
Aneurine	T45.2X1	T45.2X2	T45.2X3	T45.2X4	T45.2X5	T45.2X6
Angio-Conray	T50.8X1	T50.8X2	T50.8X3	T50.8X4	T50.8X5	T50.8X6
Angiotensin	T44.5X1	T44.5X2	T44.5X3	T44.5X4	T44.5X5	T44.5X6
Angiotensinamide	T44.991	T44.992	T44.993	T44.994	T44.995	T44.996
Anhydrohydroxy-progesterone	T38.5X1	T38.5X2	T38.5X3	T38.5X4	T38.5X5	T38.5X6
Anhydron	T50.2X1	T50.2X2	T50.2X3	T50.2X4	T50.2X5	T50.2X6
Anileridine	T40.491	T40.492	T40.493	T40.494	T40.495	T40.496

◀ New ◀|| Revised ~~deleted~~ Deleted

Substance	External Cause (T-Code) Poisoning, Accidental (Unintentional)	Poisoning, Intentional Self-Harm	Poisoning, Assault	Poisoning, Undetermined	Adverse Effect	Underdosing
Aniline (dye) (liquid)	T65.3X1	T65.3X2	T65.3X3	T65.3X4	—	—
analgesic	T39.1X1	T39.1X2	T39.1X3	T39.1X4	T39.1X5	T39.1X6
derivatives, therapeutic NEC	T39.1X1	T39.1X2	T39.1X3	T39.1X4	T39.1X5	T39.1X6
vapor	T65.3X1	T65.3X2	T65.3X3	T65.3X4	—	—
Anise oil	T47.5X1	T47.5X2	T47.5X3	T47.5X4	T47.5X5	T47.5X6
Aniscoropine	T44.3X1	T44.3X2	T44.3X3	T44.3X4	T44.3X5	T44.3X6
Anisidine	T65.3X1	T65.3X2	T65.3X3	T65.3X4	—	—
Anisindione	T45.511	T45.512	T45.513	T45.514	T45.515	T45.516
Anisotropine methyl-bromide	T44.3X1	T44.3X2	T44.3X3	T44.3X4	T44.3X5	T44.3X6
Anistreplase	T45.611	T45.612	T45.613	T45.614	T45.615	T45.616
Anorexiant (central)	T50.5X1	T50.5X2	T50.5X3	T50.5X4	T50.5X5	T50.5X6
Anorexic agents	T50.5X1	T50.5X2	T50.5X3	T50.5X4	T50.5X5	T50.5X6
Ansamycin	T36.6X1	T36.6X2	T36.6X3	T36.6X4	T36.6X5	T36.6X6
Ant (bite) (sting)	T63.421	T63.422	T63.423	T63.424	—	—
Antabuse	T50.6X1	T50.6X2	T50.6X3	T50.6X4	T50.6X5	T50.6X6
Ant poison— see Insecticide						
Antacid NEC	T47.1X1	T47.1X2	T47.1X3	T47.1X4	T47.1X5	T47.1X6
Antagonist						
Aldosterone	T50.0X1	T50.0X2	T50.0X3	T50.0X4	T50.0X5	T50.0X6
alpha-adrenoreceptor	T44.6X1	T44.6X2	T44.6X3	T44.6X4	T44.6X5	T44.6X6
anticoagulant	T45.7X1	T45.7X2	T45.7X3	T45.7X4	T45.7X5	T45.7X6
beta-adrenoreceptor	T44.7X1	T44.7X2	T44.7X3	T44.7X4	T44.7X5	T44.7X6
extrapyramidal NEC	T44.3X1	T44.3X2	T44.3X3	T44.3X4	T44.3X5	T44.3X6
folic acid	T45.1X1	T45.1X2	T45.1X3	T45.1X4	T45.1X5	T45.1X6
H2 receptor	T47.0X1	T47.0X2	T47.0X3	T47.0X4	T47.0X5	T47.0X6
heavy metal	T45.8X1	T45.8X2	T45.8X3	T45.8X4	T45.8X5	T45.8X6
narcotic analgesic	T50.7X1	T50.7X2	T50.7X3	T50.7X4	T50.7X5	T50.7X6
opiate	T50.7X1	T50.7X2	T50.7X3	T50.7X4	T50.7X5	T50.7X6
pyrimidine	T45.1X1	T45.1X2	T45.1X3	T45.1X4	T45.1X5	T45.1X6
serotonin	T46.5X1	T46.5X2	T46.5X3	T46.5X4	T46.5X5	T46.5X6
Antazolin(e)	T45.0X1	T45.0X2	T45.0X3	T45.0X4	T45.0X5	T45.0X6
Anterior pituitary hormone NEC	T38.811	T38.812	T38.813	T38.814	T38.815	T38.816
Anthelmintic NEC	T37.4X1	T37.4X2	T37.4X3	T37.4X4	T37.4X5	T37.4X6
Anthiolimine	T37.4X1	T37.4X2	T37.4X3	T37.4X4	T37.4X5	T37.4X6
Anthralin	T49.4X1	T49.4X2	T49.4X3	T49.4X4	T49.4X5	T49.4X6
Anthramycin	T45.1X1	T45.1X2	T45.1X3	T45.1X4	T45.1X5	T45.1X6
Antiadrenergic NEC	T44.8X1	T44.8X2	T44.8X3	T44.8X4	T44.8X5	T44.8X6
Antiallergic NEC	T45.0X1	T45.0X2	T45.0X3	T45.0X4	T45.0X5	T45.0X6
Anti-anemic (drug) (preparation)	T45.8X1	T45.8X2	T45.8X3	T45.8X4	T45.8X5	T45.8X6
Antiandrogen NEC	T38.6X1	T38.6X2	T38.6X3	T38.6X4	T38.6X5	T38.6X6
Antianxiety drug NEC	T43.501	T43.502	T43.503	T43.504	T43.505	T43.506
Antiaris toxicaria	T65.891	T65.892	T65.893	T65.894	—	—

Substance	External Cause (T-Code) Poisoning, Accidental (Unintentional)	Poisoning, Intentional Self-Harm	Poisoning, Assault	Poisoning, Undetermined	Adverse Effect	Underdosing
Antiarteriosclerotic drug	T46.6X1	T46.6X2	T46.6X3	T46.6X4	T46.6X5	T46.6X6
Antiasthmatic drug NEC	T48.6X1	T48.6X2	T48.6X3	T48.6X4	T48.6X5	T48.6X6
Antibiotic NEC	T36.91	T36.92	T36.93	T36.94	T36.95	T36.96
aminoglycoside	T36.5X1	T36.5X2	T36.5X3	T36.5X4	T36.5X5	T36.5X6
anticancer	T45.1X1	T45.1X2	T45.1X3	T45.1X4	T45.1X5	T45.1X6
antifungal	T36.7X1	T36.7X2	T36.7X3	T36.7X4	T36.7X5	T36.7X6
antimycobacterial	T36.5X1	T36.5X2	T36.5X3	T36.5X4	T36.5X5	T36.5X6
antineoplastic	T45.1X1	T45.1X2	T45.1X3	T45.1X4	T45.1X5	T45.1X6
cephalosporin (group)	T36.1X1	T36.1X2	T36.1X3	T36.1X4	T36.1X5	T36.1X6
chloramphenicol (group)	T36.2X1	T36.2X2	T36.2X3	T36.2X4	T36.2X5	T36.2X6
ENT	T49.6X1	T49.6X2	T49.6X3	T49.6X4	T49.6X5	T49.6X6
eye	T49.5X1	T49.5X2	T49.5X3	T49.5X4	T49.5X5	T49.5X6
fungicidal (local)	T49.0X1	T49.0X2	T49.0X3	T49.0X4	T49.0X5	T49.0X6
Intestinal	T36.8X1	T36.8X2	T36.8X3	T36.8X4	T36.8X5	T36.8X6
b-lactam NEC	T36.1X1	T36.1X2	T36.1X3	T36.1X4	T36.1X5	T36.1X6
local	T49.0X1	T49.0X2	T49.0X3	T49.0X4	T49.0X5	T49.0X6
macrolides	T36.3X1	T36.3X2	T36.3X3	T36.3X4	T36.3X5	T36.3X6
polypeptide	T36.8X1	T36.8X2	T36.8X3	T36.8X4	T36.8X5	T36.8X6
specified NEC	T36.8X1	T36.8X2	T36.8X3	T36.8X4	T36.8X5	T36.8X6
tetracycline (group)	T36.4X1	T36.4X2	T36.4X3	T36.4X4	T36.4X5	T36.4X6
throat	T49.6X1	T49.6X2	T49.6X3	T49.6X4	T49.6X5	T49.6X6
Anticancer agents NEC	T45.1X1	T45.1X2	T45.1X3	T45.1X4	T45.1X5	T45.1X6
Anticholesterolemic drug NEC	T46.6X1	T46.6X2	T46.6X3	T46.6X4	T46.6X5	T46.6X6
Anticholinergic NEC	T44.3X1	T44.3X2	T44.3X3	T44.3X4	T44.3X5	T44.3X6
Anticholinesterase	T44.0X1	T44.0X2	T44.0X3	T44.0X4	T44.0X5	T44.0X6
organophosphorus	T44.0X1	T44.0X2	T44.0X3	T44.0X4	T44.0X5	T44.0X6
insecticide	T60.0X1	T60.0X2	T60.0X3	T60.0X4	—	—
nerve gas	T59.891	T59.892	T59.893	T59.894	—	—
reversible	T44.0X1	T44.0X2	T44.0X3	T44.0X4	T44.0X5	T44.0X6
ophthalmological	T49.5X1	T49.5X2	T49.5X3	T49.5X4	T49.5X5	T49.5X6
Anticoagulant NEC	T45.511	T45.512	T45.513	T45.514	T45.515	T45.516
Antagonist	T45.7X1	T45.7X2	T45.7X3	T45.7X4	T45.7X5	T45.7X6
Anti-common-cold drug NEC	T48.5X1	T48.5X2	T48.5X3	T48.5X4	T48.5X5	T48.5X6
Anticonvulsant	T42.71	T42.72	T42.73	T42.74	T42.75	T42.76
barbiturate	T42.3X1	T42.3X2	T42.3X3	T42.3X4	T42.3X5	T42.3X6
combination (with barbiturate)	T42.3X1	T42.3X2	T42.3X3	T42.3X4	T42.3X5	T42.3X6
hydantoin	T42.0X1	T42.0X2	T42.0X3	T42.0X4	T42.0X5	T42.0X6
hypnotic NEC	T42.6X1	T42.6X2	T42.6X3	T42.6X4	T42.6X5	T42.6X6
oxazolidinedione	T42.2X1	T42.2X2	T42.2X3	T42.2X4	T42.2X5	T42.2X6
pyrimidinedione	T42.6X1	T42.6X2	T42.6X3	T42.6X4	T42.6X5	T42.6X6
specified NEC	T42.6X1	T42.6X2	T42.6X3	T42.6X4	T42.6X5	T42.6X6
succinimide	T42.2X1	T42.2X2	T42.2X3	T42.2X4	T42.2X5	T42.2X6

TABLE OF DRUGS AND CHEMICALS

TABLE OF DRUGS AND CHEMICALS

Substance	External Cause (T-Code)					
	Poisoning, Accidental (Unintentional)	Poisoning, Intentional Self-Harm	Poisoning, Assault	Poisoning, Undetermined	Adverse Effect	Underdosing
Anti-D immunoglobulin (human)	T50.Z11	T50.Z12	T50.Z13	T50.Z14	T50.Z15	T50.Z16
Antidepressant NEC	T43.201	T43.202	T43.203	T43.204	T43.205	T43.206
monoamine oxidase inhibitor	T43.1X1	T43.1X2	T43.1X3	T43.1X4	T43.1X5	T43.1X6
selective serotonin norepinephrine reuptake inhibitor	T43.211	T43.212	T43.213	T43.214	T43.215	T43.216
selective serotonin reuptake inhibitor	T43.221	T43.222	T43.223	T43.224	T43.225	T43.226
specified NEC	T43.291	T43.292	T43.293	T43.294	T43.295	T43.296
tetracyclic	T43.021	T43.022	T43.023	T43.024	T43.025	T43.026
triazolopyridine	T43.221	T43.222	T43.223	T43.224	T43.225	T43.226
tricyclic	T43.011	T43.012	T43.013	T43.014	T43.015	T43.016
Antidiabetic NEC	T38.3X1	T38.3X2	T38.3X3	T38.3X4	T38.3X5	T38.3X6
biguanide	T38.3X1	T38.3X2	T38.3X3	T38.3X4	T38.3X5	T38.3X6
and sulfonyl combined	T38.3X1	T38.3X2	T38.3X3	T38.3X4	T38.3X5	T38.3X6
combined	T38.3X1	T38.3X2	T38.3X3	T38.3X4	T38.3X5	T38.3X6
sulfonylurea	T38.3X1	T38.3X2	T38.3X3	T38.3X4	T38.3X5	
Antidiarrheal drug NEC	T47.6X1	T47.6X2	T47.6X3	T47.6X4	T47.6X5	T47.6X6
absorbent	T47.6X1	T47.6X2	T47.6X3	T47.6X4	T47.6X5	T47.6X6
Antidiphtheria serum	T50.Z11	T50.Z12	T50.Z13	T50.Z14	T50.Z15	T50.Z16
Antidiuretic hormone	T38.891	T38.892	T38.893	T38.894	T38.895	T38.896
Antidote NEC	T50.6X1	T50.6X2	T50.6X3	T50.6X4	T50.6X5	T50.6X6
heavy metal	T45.8X1	T45.8X2	T45.8X3	T45.8X4	T45.8X5	T45.8X6
Antidysrhythmic NEC	T46.2X1	T46.2X2	T46.2X3	T46.2X4	T46.2X5	T46.2X6
Antiemetic drug	T45.0X1	T45.0X2	T45.0X3	T45.0X4	T45.0X5	T45.0X6
Antiepilepsy agent	T42.71	T42.72	T42.73	T42.74	T42.75	T42.76
combination	T42.5X1	T42.5X2	T42.5X3	T42.5X4	T42.5X5	T42.5X6
mixed	T42.5X1	T42.5X2	T42.5X3	T42.5X4	T42.5X5	T42.5X6
specified, NEC	T42.6X1	T42.6X2	T42.6X3	T42.6X4	T42.6X5	T42.6X6
Antiestrogen NEC	T38.6X1	T38.6X2	T38.6X3	T38.6X4	T38.6X5	T38.6X6
Antifertility pill	T38.4X1	T38.4X2	T38.4X3	T38.4X4	T38.4X5	T38.4X6
Antifibrinolytic drug	T45.621	T45.622	T45.623	T45.624	T45.625	T45.626
Antifilarial drug	T37.4X1	T37.4X2	T37.4X3	T37.4X4	T37.4X5	T37.4X6
Antiflatulent	T47.5X1	T47.5X2	T47.5X3	T47.5X4	T47.5X5	T47.5X6
Antifreeze	T65.91	T65.92	T65.93	T65.94	—	—
alcohol	T51.1X1	T51.1X2	T51.1X3	T51.1X4	—	—
ethylene glycol	T51.8X1	T51.8X2	T51.8X3	T51.8X4	—	—
Antifungal						
antibiotic (systemic)	T36.7X1	T36.7X2	T36.7X3	T36.7X4	T36.7X5	T36.7X6
anti-infective NEC	T37.91	T37.92	T37.93	T37.94	T37.95	T37.96
disinfectant, local	T49.0X1	T49.0X2	T49.0X3	T49.0X4	T49.0X5	T49.0X6
nonmedicinal (spray)	T60.3X1	T60.3X2	T60.3X3	T60.3X4	—	—
topical	T49.0X1	T49.0X2	T49.0X3	T49.0X4	T49.0X5	T49.0X6

Substance	External Cause (T-Code)					
	Poisoning, Accidental (Unintentional)	Poisoning, Intentional Self-Harm	Poisoning, Assault	Poisoning, Undetermined	Adverse Effect	Underdosing
Anti-gastric-secretion drug NEC	T47.1X1	T47.1X2	T47.1X3	T47.1X4	T47.1X5	T47.1X6
Antigonadotrophin NEC	T38.6X1	T38.6X2	T38.6X3	T38.6X4	T38.6X5	T38.6X6
Antihallucinogen	T43.501	T43.502	T43.503	T43.504	T43.505	T43.506
Antihelmintics	T37.4X1	T37.4X2	T37.4X3	T37.4X4	T37.4X5	T37.4X6
Antihemophilic						
factor	T45.8X1	T45.8X2	T45.8X3	T45.8X4	T45.8X5	T45.8X6
fraction	T45.8X1	T45.8X2	T45.8X3	T45.8X4	T45.8X5	T45.8X6
globulin concentrate	T45.7X1	T45.7X2	T45.7X3	T45.7X4	T45.7X5	T45.7X6
human plasma	T45.8X1	T45.8X2	T45.8X3	T45.8X4	T45.8X5	T45.8X6
plasma, dried	T45.7X1	T45.7X2	T45.7X3	T45.7X4	T45.7X5	T45.7X6
Antihemorrhoidal preparation	T49.2X1	T49.2X2	T49.2X3	T49.2X4	T49.2X5	T49.2X6
Antiheparin drug	T45.7X1	T45.7X2	T45.7X3	T45.7X4	T45.7X5	T45.7X6
Antihistamine	T45.0X1	T45.0X2	T45.0X3	T45.0X4	T45.0X5	T45.0X6
Antihookworm drug	T37.4X1	T37.4X2	T37.4X3	T37.4X4	T37.4X5	T37.4X6
Anti-human lymphocytic globulin	T50.Z11	T50.Z12	T50.Z13	T50.Z14	T50.Z15	T50.Z16
Antihyperlipidemic drug	T46.6X1	T46.6X2	T46.6X3	T46.6X4	T46.6X5	T46.6X6
Antihypertensive drug NEC	T46.5X1	T46.5X2	T46.5X3	T46.5X4	T46.5X5	T46.5X6
Anti-infective NEC	T37.91	T37.92	T37.93	T37.94	T37.95	T37.96
anthelmintic	T37.4X1	T37.4X2	T37.4X3	T37.4X4	T37.4X5	T37.4X6
antibiotics	T36.91	T36.92	T36.93	T36.94	T36.95	T36.96
specified NEC	T36.8X1	T36.8X2	T36.8X3	T36.8X4	T36.8X5	T36.8X6
antimalarial	T37.2X1	T37.2X2	T37.2X3	T37.2X4	T37.2X5	T37.2X6
antimycobacterial NEC	T37.1X1	T37.1X2	T37.1X3	T37.1X4	T37.1X5	T37.1X6
antibiotics	T36.5X1	T36.5X2	T36.5X3	T36.5X4	T36.5X5	T36.5X6
antiprotozoal NEC	T37.3X1	T37.3X2	T37.3X3	T37.3X4	T37.3X5	T37.3X6
blood	T37.2X1	T37.2X2	T37.2X3	T37.2X4	T37.2X5	T37.2X6
antiviral	T37.5X1	T37.5X2	T37.5X3	T37.5X4	T37.5X5	T37.5X6
arsenical	T37.8X1	T37.8X2	T37.8X3	T37.8X4	T37.8X5	T37.8X6
bismuth, local	T49.0X1	T49.0X2	T49.0X3	T49.0X4	T49.0X5	T49.0X6
ENT	T49.6X1	T49.6X2	T49.6X3	T49.6X4	T49.6X5	T49.6X6
eye NEC	T49.5X1	T49.5X2	T49.5X3	T49.5X4	T49.5X5	T49.5X6
heavy metals NEC	T37.8X1	T37.8X2	T37.8X3	T37.8X4	T37.8X5	T37.8X6
local NEC	T49.0X1	T49.0X2	T49.0X3	T49.0X4	T49.0X5	T49.0X6
specified NEC	T49.0X1	T49.0X2	T49.0X3	T49.0X4	T49.0X5	T49.0X6
mixed	T37.91	T37.92	T37.93	T37.94	T37.95	T37.96
ophthalmic preparation	T49.5X1	T49.5X2	T49.5X3	T49.5X4	T49.5X5	T49.5X6
topical NEC	T49.0X1	T49.0X2	T49.0X3	T49.0X4	T49.0X5	T49.0X6
Anti-inflammatory drug NEC	T49.0X1	T49.0X2	T49.0X3	T49.0X4	T49.0X5	T49.0X6
local	T49.0X1	T49.0X2	T49.0X3	T49.0X4	T49.0X5	T49.0X6
nonsteroidal NEC	T39.391	T39.392	T39.393	T39.394	T39.395	T39.396
propionic acid derivative	T39.311	T39.312	T39.313	T39.314	T39.315	T39.316
specified NEC	T39.391	T39.392	T39.393	T39.394	T39.395	T39.396

◀ New ◀ Revised ~~deleted~~ Deleted

Substance	External Cause (T-Code) Poisoning, Accidental (Unintentional)	Poisoning, Intentional Self-Harm	Poisoning, Assault	Poisoning, Undetermined	Adverse Effect	Underdosing
Antikaluretic	T50.3X1	T50.3X2	T50.3X3	T50.3X4	T50.3X5	T50.3X6
Antiknock (tetraethyl lead)	T56.0X1	T56.0X2	T56.0X3	T56.0X4	—	—
Antilipemic drug NEC	T46.6X1	T46.6X2	T46.6X3	T46.6X4	T46.6X5	T46.6X6
Antimalarial	T37.2X1	T37.2X2	T37.2X3	T37.2X4	T37.2X5	T37.2X6
prophylactic NEC	T37.2X1	T37.2X2	T37.2X3	T37.2X4	T37.2X5	T37.2X6
pyrimidine derivative	T37.2X1	T37.2X2	T37.2X3	T37.2X4	T37.2X5	T37.2X6
Antimetabolite	T45.1X1	T45.1X2	T45.1X3	T45.1X4	T45.1X5	T45.1X6
Antimitotic agent	T45.1X1	T45.1X2	T45.1X3	T45.1X4	T45.1X5	T45.1X6
Antimony (compounds) (vapor) NEC	T56.891	T56.892	T56.893	T56.894	—	—
anti-infectives	T37.8X1	T37.8X2	T37.8X3	T37.8X4	T37.8X5	T37.8X6
dimercaptosuccinate	T37.3X1	T37.3X2	T37.3X3	T37.3X4	T37.3X5	T37.3X6
hydride	T56.891	T56.892	T56.893	T56.894	—	—
pesticide (vapor)	T60.8X1	T60.8X2	T60.8X3	T60.8X4	—	—
potassium (sodium) tartrate	T37.8X1	T37.8X2	T37.8X3	T37.8X4	T37.8X5	T37.8X6
sodium dimercaptosuccinate	T37.3X1	T37.3X2	T37.3X3	T37.3X4	T37.3X5	T37.3X6
tartrated	T37.8X1	T37.8X2	T37.8X3	T37.8X4	T37.8X5	T37.8X6
Antimuscarinic NEC	T44.3X1	T44.3X2	T44.3X3	T44.3X4	T44.3X5	T44.3X6
Antimycobacterial drug NEC	T37.1X1	T37.1X2	T37.1X3	T37.1X4	T37.1X5	T37.1X6
antibiotics	T36.5X1	T36.5X2	T36.5X3	T36.5X4	T36.5X5	T36.5X6
combination	T37.1X1	T37.1X2	T37.1X3	T37.1X4	T37.1X5	T37.1X6
Antinausea drug	T45.0X1	T45.0X2	T45.0X3	T45.0X4	T45.0X5	T45.0X6
Antinematode drug	T37.4X1	T37.4X2	T37.4X3	T37.4X4	T37.4X5	T37.4X6
Antineoplastic NEC	T45.1X1	T45.1X2	T45.1X3	T45.1X4	T45.1X5	T45.1X6
alkaloidal	T45.1X1	T45.1X2	T45.1X3	T45.1X4	T45.1X5	T45.1X6
antibiotics	T45.1X1	T45.1X2	T45.1X3	T45.1X4	T45.1X5	T45.1X6
combination	T45.1X1	T45.1X2	T45.1X3	T45.1X4	T45.1X5	T45.1X6
estrogen	T38.5X1	T38.5X2	T38.5X3	T38.5X4	T38.5X5	T38.5X6
steroid	T38.7X1	T38.7X2	T38.7X3	T38.7X4	T38.7X5	T38.7X6
Antiparasitic drug (systemic)	T37.91	T37.92	T37.93	T37.94	T37.95	T37.96
local	T49.0X1	T49.0X2	T49.0X3	T49.0X4	T49.0X5	T49.0X6
specified NEC	T37.8X1	T37.8X2	T37.8X3	T37.8X4	T37.8X5	T37.8X6
Antiparkinsonism drug NEC	T42.8X1	T42.8X2	T42.8X3	T42.8X4	T42.8X5	T42.8X6
Antiperspirant NEC	T49.2X1	T49.2X2	T49.2X3	T49.2X4	T49.2X5	T49.2X6
Antiphlogistic NEC	T39.4X1	T39.4X2	T39.4X3	T39.4X4	T39.4X5	T39.4X6
Antiplatyhelmintic drug	T37.4X1	T37.4X2	T37.4X3	T37.4X4	T37.4X5	T37.4X6
Antiprotozoal drug NEC	T37.3X1	T37.3X2	T37.3X3	T37.3X4	T37.3X5	T37.3X6
blood	T37.2X1	T37.2X2	T37.2X3	T37.2X4	T37.2X5	T37.2X6
local	T49.0X1	T49.0X2	T49.0X3	T49.0X4	T49.0X5	T49.0X6
Antipruritic drug NEC	T49.1X1	T49.1X2	T49.1X3	T49.1X4	T49.1X5	T49.1X6
Antipsychotic drug	T43.501	T43.502	T43.503	T43.504	T43.505	T43.506
specified NEC	T43.591	T43.592	T43.593	T43.594	T43.595	T43.596

Substance	External Cause (T-Code) Poisoning, Accidental (Unintentional)	Poisoning, Intentional Self-Harm	Poisoning, Assault	Poisoning, Undetermined	Adverse Effect	Underdosing
Antipyretic	T39.91	T39.92	T39.93	T39.94	T39.95	T39.96
specified NEC	T39.8X1	T39.8X2	T39.8X3	T39.8X4	T39.8X5	T39.8X6
Antipyrine	T39.2X1	T39.2X2	T39.2X3	T39.2X4	T39.2X5	T39.2X6
Antirabies hyperimmune serum	T50.Z11	T50.Z12	T50.Z13	T50.Z14	T50.Z15	T50.Z16
Antirheumatic NEC	T39.4X1	T39.4X2	T39.4X3	T39.4X4	T39.4X5	T39.4X6
Antirigidity drug NEC	T42.8X1	T42.8X2	T42.8X3	T42.8X4	T42.8X5	T42.8X6
Antischistosomal drug	T37.4X1	T37.4X2	T37.4X3	T37.4X4	T37.4X5	T37.4X6
Antiscorpion sera	T50.Z11	T50.Z12	T50.Z13	T50.Z14	T50.Z15	T50.Z16
Antiseborrheics	T49.4X1	T49.4X2	T49.4X3	T49.4X4	T49.4X5	T49.4X6
Antiseptics (external) (medicinal)	T49.0X1	T49.0X2	T49.0X3	T49.0X4	T49.0X5	T49.0X6
Antistine	T45.0X1	T45.0X2	T45.0X3	T45.0X4	T45.0X5	T45.0X6
Antitapeworm drug	T37.4X1	T37.4X2	T37.4X3	T37.4X4	T37.4X5	T37.4X6
Antitetanus immunoglobulin	T50.Z11	T50.Z12	T50.Z13	T50.Z14	T50.Z15	T50.Z16
Antithrombotic	T45.521	T45.522	T45.523	T45.524	T45.525	T45.526
Antithyroid drug NEC	T38.2X1	T38.2X2	T38.2X3	T38.2X4	T38.2X5	T38.2X6
Antitoxin	T50.Z11	T50.Z12	T50.Z13	T50.Z14	T50.Z15	T50.Z16
diphtheria	T50.Z11	T50.Z12	T50.Z13	T50.Z14	T50.Z15	T50.Z16
gas gangrene	T50.Z11	T50.Z12	T50.Z13	T50.Z14	T50.Z15	T50.Z16
tetanus	T50.Z11	T50.Z12	T50.Z13	T50.Z14	T50.Z15	T50.Z16
Antitoxin, any	T50.901	T50.902	T50.903	T50.904	T50.905	T50.906
Antitrichomonal drug	T37.3X1	T37.3X2	T37.3X3	T37.3X4	T37.3X5	T37.3X6
Antituberculars	T37.1X1	T37.1X2	T37.1X3	T37.1X4	T37.1X5	T37.1X6
antibiotics	T36.5X1	T36.5X2	T36.5X3	T36.5X4	T36.5X5	T36.5X6
Antitussive NEC	T48.3X1	T48.3X2	T48.3X3	T48.3X4	T48.3X5	T48.3X6
codeine mixture	T40.2X1	T40.2X2	T40.2X3	T40.2X4	T40.2X5	T40.2X6
opiate	T40.2X1	T40.2X2	T40.2X3	T40.2X4	T40.2X5	T40.2X6
Antivaricose drug	T46.8X1	T46.8X2	T46.8X3	T46.8X4	T46.8X5	T46.8X6
Antivenin, antivenom (sera)	T50.Z11	T50.Z12	T50.Z13	T50.Z14	T50.Z15	T50.Z16
crotaline	T50.Z11	T50.Z12	T50.Z13	T50.Z14	T50.Z15	T50.Z16
spider bite	T50.Z11	T50.Z12	T50.Z13	T50.Z14	T50.Z15	T50.Z16
Antivertigo drug	T45.0X1	T45.0X2	T45.0X3	T45.0X4	T45.0X5	T45.0X6
Antiviral drug NEC	T37.5X1	T37.5X2	T37.5X3	T37.5X4	T37.5X5	T37.5X6
eye	T49.5X1	T49.5X2	T49.5X3	T49.5X4	T49.5X5	T49.5X6
Antiwhipworm drug	T37.4X1	T37.4X2	T37.4X3	T37.4X4	T37.4X5	T37.4X6
Ant poisons — see Pesticides						
Antrol — see also by specific chemical substance	T60.91	T60.92	T60.93	T60.94	—	—
fungicide	T60.91	T60.92	T60.93	T60.94	—	—
ANTU (alpha naphthylthiourea)	T60.4X1	T60.4X2	T60.4X3	T60.4X4	—	—
Apalcillin	T36.0X1	T36.0X2	T36.0X3	T36.0X4	T36.0X5	T36.0X6
APC	T48.5X1	T48.5X2	T48.5X3	T48.5X4	T48.5X5	T48.5X6
Aplonidine	T44.4X1	T44.4X2	T44.4X3	T44.4X4	T44.4X5	T44.4X6
Apomorphine	T47.7X1	T47.7X2	T47.7X3	T47.7X4	T47.7X5	T47.7X6

TABLE OF DRUGS AND CHEMICALS

	External Cause (T-Code)					
Substance	Poisoning, Accidental (Unintentional)	Poisoning, Intentional Self-Harm	Poisoning, Assault	Poisoning, Undetermined	Adverse Effect	Underdosing
Appetite depressants, central	T50.5X1	T50.5X2	T50.5X3	T50.5X4	T50.5X5	T50.5X6
Apraclonidine (hydrochloride)	T44.4X1	T44.4X2	T44.4X3	T44.4X4	T44.4X5	T44.4X6
Apresoline	T46.5X1	T46.5X2	T46.5X3	T46.5X4	T46.5X5	T46.5X6
Aprindine	T46.2X1	T46.2X2	T46.2X3	T46.2X4	T46.2X5	T46.2X6
Aprobarbital	T42.3X1	T42.3X2	T42.3X3	T42.3X4	T42.3X5	T42.3X6
Apronalide	T42.6X1	T42.6X2	T42.6X3	T42.6X4	T42.6X5	T42.6X6
Aprotinin	T45.621	T45.622	T45.623	T45.624	T45.625	T45.626
Aptocaine	T41.3X1	T41.3X2	T41.3X3	T41.3X4	T41.3X5	T41.3X6
Aqua fortis	T54.2X1	T54.2X2	T54.2X3	T54.2X4	—	—
Ara-A	T37.5X1	T37.5X2	T37.5X3	T37.5X4	T37.5X5	T37.5X6
Ara-C	T45.1X1	T45.1X2	T45.1X3	T45.1X4	T45.1X5	T45.1X6
Arachis oil	T49.3X1	T49.3X2	T49.3X3	T49.3X4	T49.3X5	T49.3X6
cathartic	T47.4X1	T47.4X2	T47.4X3	T47.4X4	T47.4X5	T47.4X6
Aralen	T37.2X1	T37.2X2	T37.2X3	T37.2X4	T37.2X5	T37.2X6
Arecoline	T44.1X1	T44.1X2	T44.1X3	T44.1X4	T44.1X5	T44.1X6
Arginine	T50.991	T50.992	T50.993	T50.994	T50.995	T50.996
glutamate	T50.991	T50.992	T50.993	T50.994	T50.995	T50.996
Argyrol	T49.0X1	T49.0X2	T49.0X3	T49.0X4	T49.0X5	T49.0X6
ENT agent	T49.6X1	T49.6X2	T49.6X3	T49.6X4	T49.6X5	T49.6X6
ophthalmic preparation	T49.5X1	T49.5X2	T49.5X3	T49.5X4	T49.5X5	T49.5X6
Aristocort	T38.0X1	T38.0X2	T38.0X3	T38.0X4	T38.0X5	T38.0X6
ENT agent	T49.6X1	T49.6X2	T49.6X3	T49.6X4	T49.6X5	T49.6X6
ophthalmic preparation	T49.5X1	T49.5X2	T49.5X3	T49.5X4	T49.5X5	T49.5X6
topical NEC	T49.0X1	T49.0X2	T49.0X3	T49.0X4	T49.0X5	T49.0X6
Aromatics, corrosive	T54.1X1	T54.1X2	T54.1X3	T54.1X4	—	—
disinfectants	T54.1X1	T54.1X2	T54.1X3	T54.1X4	—	—
Arsenate of lead	T57.0X1	T57.0X2	T57.0X3	T57.0X4	—	—
herbicide	T57.0X1	T57.0X2	T57.0X3	T57.0X4	—	—
Arsenic, arsenicals (compounds) (dust) (vapor) NEC	T57.0X1	T57.0X2	T57.0X3	T57.0X4	—	—
anti-infectives	T37.8X1	T37.8X2	T37.8X3	T37.8X4	T37.8X5	T37.8X6
pesticide (dust) (fumes)	T57.0X1	T57.0X2	T57.0X3	T57.0X4	—	—
Arsine (gas)	T57.0X1	T57.0X2	T57.0X3	T57.0X4	—	—
Arsphenamine (silver)	T37.8X1	T37.8X2	T37.8X3	T37.8X4	T37.8X5	T37.8X6
Arsthinol	T37.3X1	T37.3X2	T37.3X3	T37.3X4	T37.3X5	T37.3X6
Artane	T44.3X1	T44.3X2	T44.3X3	T44.3X4	T44.3X5	T44.3X6
Arthropod (venomous) NEC	T63.481	T63.482	T63.483	T63.484	—	—
Articaine	T41.3X1	T41.3X2	T41.3X3	T41.3X4	T41.3X5	T41.3X6
Asbestos	T57.8X1	T57.8X2	T57.8X3	T57.8X4	—	—
Ascaridole	T37.4X1	T37.4X2	T37.4X3	T37.4X4	T37.4X5	T37.4X6
Ascorbic acid	T45.2X1	T45.2X2	T45.2X3	T45.2X4	T45.2X5	T45.2X6
Asiaticoside	T49.0X1	T49.0X2	T49.0X3	T49.0X4	T49.0X5	T49.0X6

	External Cause (T-Code)					
Substance	Poisoning, Accidental (Unintentional)	Poisoning, Intentional Self-Harm	Poisoning, Assault	Poisoning, Undetermined	Adverse Effect	Underdosing
Asparaginase	T45.1X1	T45.1X2	T45.1X3	T45.1X4	T45.1X5	T45.1X6
Aspidium (oleoresin)	T37.4X1	T37.4X2	T37.4X3	T37.4X4	T37.4X5	T37.4X6
Aspirin (aluminum) (soluble)	T39.011	T39.012	T39.013	T39.014	T39.015	T39.016
Aspoxicillin	T36.0X1	T36.0X2	T36.0X3	T36.0X4	T36.0X5	T36.0X6
Astemizole	T45.0X1	T45.0X2	T45.0X3	T45.0X4	T45.0X5	T45.0X6
Astringent (local)	T49.2X1	T49.2X2	T49.2X3	T49.2X4	T49.2X5	T49.2X6
specified NEC	T49.2X1	T49.2X2	T49.2X3	T49.2X4	T49.2X5	T49.2X6
Astromicin	T36.5X1	T36.5X2	T36.5X3	T36.5X4	T36.5X5	T36.5X6
Ataractic drug NEC	T43.501	T43.502	T43.503	T43.504	T43.505	T43.506
Atenolol	T44.7X1	T44.7X2	T44.7X3	T44.7X4	T44.7X5	T44.7X6
Atonia drug, intestinal	T47.4X1	T47.4X2	T47.4X3	T47.4X4	T47.4X5	T47.4X6
Atophan	T50.4X1	T50.4X2	T50.4X3	T50.4X4	T50.4X5	T50.4X6
Atracurium besilate	T48.1X1	T48.1X2	T48.1X3	T48.1X4	T48.1X5	T48.1X6
Atropine	T44.3X1	T44.3X2	T44.3X3	T44.3X4	T44.3X5	T44.3X6
derivative	T44.3X1	T44.3X2	T44.3X3	T44.3X4	T44.3X5	T44.3X6
methonitrate	T44.3X1	T44.3X2	T44.3X3	T44.3X4	T44.3X5	T44.3X6
Attapulgite	T47.6X1	T47.6X2	T47.6X3	T47.6X4	T47.6X5	T47.6X6
Attenuvax	T50.991	T50.992	T50.993	T50.994	T50.995	T50.996
Auramine	T65.891	T65.892	T65.893	T65.894	—	—
dye	T65.6X1	T65.6X2	T65.6X3	T65.6X4	—	—
fungicide	T60.3X1	T60.3X2	T60.3X3	T60.3X4	—	—
Auranofin	T39.4X1	T39.4X2	T39.4X3	T39.4X4	T39.4X5	T39.4X6
Aurantiin	T46.991	T46.992	T46.993	T46.994	T46.995	T46.996
Aureomycin	T36.4X1	T36.4X2	T36.4X3	T36.4X4	T36.4X5	T36.4X6
ophthalmic preparation	T49.5X1	T49.5X2	T49.5X3	T49.5X4	T49.5X5	T49.5X6
topical NEC	T49.0X1	T49.0X2	T49.0X3	T49.0X4	T49.0X5	T49.0X6
Aurothioglucose	T39.4X1	T39.4X2	T39.4X3	T39.4X4	T39.4X5	T39.4X6
Aurothioglycanide	T39.4X1	T39.4X2	T39.4X3	T39.4X4	T39.4X5	T39.4X6
Aurothiomalate sodium	T39.4X1	T39.4X2	T39.4X3	T39.4X4	T39.4X5	T39.4X6
Aurotioprol	T39.4X1	T39.4X2	T39.4X3	T39.4X4	T39.4X5	T39.4X6
Automobile fuel	T52.0X1	T52.0X2	T52.0X3	T52.0X4	—	—
Autonomic nervous system agent NEC	T44.901	T44.902	T44.903	T44.904	T44.905	T44.906
Avlosulfon	T37.1X1	T37.1X2	T37.1X3	T37.1X4	T37.1X5	T37.1X6
Avomine	T42.6X1	T42.6X2	T42.6X3	T42.6X4	T42.6X5	T42.6X6
Axerophthol	T45.2X1	T45.2X2	T45.2X3	T45.2X4	T45.2X5	T45.2X6
Azacitidine	T45.1X1	T45.1X2	T45.1X3	T45.1X4	T45.1X5	T45.1X6
Azacyclonol	T43.591	T43.592	T43.593	T43.594	T43.595	T43.596
Azadirachta	T60.2X1	T60.2X2	T60.2X3	T60.2X4	—	—
Azanidazole	T37.3X1	T37.3X2	T37.3X3	T37.3X4	T37.3X5	T37.3X6
Azapetine	T46.7X1	T46.7X2	T46.7X3	T46.7X4	T46.7X5	T46.7X6
Azapropazone	T39.2X1	T39.2X2	T39.2X3	T39.2X4	T39.2X5	T39.2X6

◀ New   ◀ Revised   ~~deleted~~ Deleted

Substance	Poisoning, Accidental (Unintentional)	Poisoning, Intentional Self-Harm	Poisoning, Assault	Poisoning, Undetermined	Adverse Effect	Underdosing
Beryllium (compounds)	T56.7X1	T56.7X2	T56.7X3	T56.7X4	—	—
b-acetyldigoxin	T46.0X1	T46.0X2	T46.0X3	T46.0X4	T46.0X5	T46.0X6
beta adrenergic blocking agent, heart	T44.7X1	T44.7X2	T44.7X3	T44.7X4	T44.7X5	T44.7X6
b-benzalbutyramide	T46.6X1	T46.6X2	T46.6X3	T46.6X4	T46.6X5	T46.6X6
Betacarotene	T45.2X1	T45.2X2	T45.2X3	T45.2X4	T45.2X5	T45.2X6
b-eucaine	T49.1X1	T49.1X2	T49.1X3	T49.1X4	T49.1X5	T49.1X6
Beta-Chlor	T42.6X1	T42.6X2	T42.6X3	T42.6X4	T42.6X5	T42.6X6
b-galactosidase	T47.5X1	T47.5X2	T47.5X3	T47.5X4	T47.5X5	T47.5X6
Betahistine	T46.7X1	T46.7X2	T46.7X3	T46.7X4	T46.7X5	T46.7X6
Betaine	T47.5X1	T47.5X2	T47.5X3	T47.5X4	T47.5X5	T47.5X6
Betamethasone	T49.0X1	T49.0X2	T49.0X3	T49.0X4	T49.0X5	T49.0X6
topical	T49.0X1	T49.0X2	T49.0X3	T49.0X4	T49.0X5	T49.0X6
Betamicin	T36.8X1	T36.8X2	T36.8X3	T36.8X4	T36.8X5	T36.8X6
Betanidine	T46.5X1	T46.5X2	T46.5X3	T46.5X4	T46.5X5	T46.5X6
b-sitosterol(s)	T46.6X1	T46.6X2	T46.6X3	T46.6X4	T46.6X5	T46.6X6
Betaxolol	T44.7X1	T44.7X2	T44.7X3	T44.7X4	T44.7X5	T44.7X6
Betazole	T50.8X1	T50.8X2	T50.8X3	T50.8X4	T50.8X5	T50.8X6
Bethanechol	T44.1X1	T44.1X2	T44.1X3	T44.1X4	T44.1X5	T44.1X6
chloride	T44.1X1	T44.1X2	T44.1X3	T44.1X4	T44.1X5	T44.1X6
Bethanidine	T46.5X1	T46.5X2	T46.5X3	T46.5X4	T46.5X5	T46.5X6
Betoxycaine	T41.3X1	T41.3X2	T41.3X3	T41.3X4	T41.3X5	T41.3X6
Betula oil	T49.3X1	T49.3X2	T49.3X3	T49.3X4	T49.3X5	T49.3X6
Bevantolol	T44.7X1	T44.7X2	T44.7X3	T44.7X4	T44.7X5	T44.7X6
Bevonium metilsulfate	T44.3X1	T44.3X2	T44.3X3	T44.3X4	T44.3X5	T44.3X6
Bezafibrate	T46.6X1	T46.6X2	T46.6X3	T46.6X4	T46.6X5	T46.6X6
Bezitramide	T40.491	T40.492	T40.493	T40.494	T40.495	T40.496
BHA	T50.991	T50.992	T50.993	T50.994	T50.995	T50.996
Bhang	T40.711	T40.712	T40.713	T40.714	T40.715	T40.716
BHC (medicinal)	T49.0X1	T49.0X2	T49.0X3	T49.0X4	T49.0X5	T49.0X6
nonmedicinal (vapor)	T53.6X1	T53.6X2	T53.6X3	T53.6X4	—	—
Bialamicol	T37.3X1	T37.3X2	T37.3X3	T37.3X4	T37.3X5	T37.3X6
Bibenzonium bromide	T48.3X1	T48.3X2	T48.3X3	T48.3X4	T48.3X5	T48.3X6
Bibrocathol	T49.5X1	T49.5X2	T49.5X3	T49.5X4	T49.5X5	T49.5X6
Bichloride of mercury — see Mercury, chloride						
Bichromates (calcium) (potassium) (sodium) (crystals)	T57.8X1	T57.8X2	T57.8X3	T57.8X4	—	—
fumes	T56.2X1	T56.2X2	T56.2X3	T56.2X4	—	—
Biclotymol	T49.6X1	T49.6X2	T49.6X3	T49.6X4	T49.6X5	T49.6X6
Bicucculine	T50.7X1	T50.7X2	T50.7X3	T50.7X4	T50.7X5	T50.7X6
Bifemelane	T43.291	T43.292	T43.293	T43.294	T43.295	T43.296
Biguanide derivatives, oral	T38.3X1	T38.3X2	T38.3X3	T38.3X4	T38.3X5	T38.3X6

Substance	Poisoning, Accidental (Unintentional)	Poisoning, Intentional Self-Harm	Poisoning, Assault	Poisoning, Undetermined	Adverse Effect	Underdosing
Biligrafin	T50.8X1	T50.8X2	T50.8X3	T50.8X4	T50.8X5	T50.8X6
Bile salts	T47.5X1	T47.5X2	T47.5X3	T47.5X4	T47.5X5	T47.5X6
Bilopaque	T50.8X1	T50.8X2	T50.8X3	T50.8X4	T50.8X5	T50.8X6
Binifibrate	T46.6X1	T46.6X2	T46.6X3	T46.6X4	T46.6X5	T46.6X6
Binitrobenzol	T65.3X1	T65.3X2	T65.3X3	T65.3X4	—	—
Bioflavonoid(s)	T46.991	T46.992	T46.993	T46.994	T46.995	T46.996
Biological substance NEC	T50.901	T50.902	T50.903	T50.904	T50.905	T50.906
Biotin	T45.2X1	T45.2X2	T45.2X3	T45.2X4	T45.2X5	T45.2X6
Biperiden	T44.3X1	T44.3X2	T44.3X3	T44.3X4	T44.3X5	T44.3X6
Bisacodyl	T47.2X1	T47.2X2	T47.2X3	T47.2X4	T47.2X5	T47.2X6
Bisbentiamine	T45.2X1	T45.2X2	T45.2X3	T45.2X4	T45.2X5	T45.2X6
Bisbutiamine	T45.2X1	T45.2X2	T45.2X3	T45.2X4	T45.2X5	T45.2X6
Bisdequalinium (salts) (diacetate)	T49.6X1	T49.6X2	T49.6X3	T49.6X4	T49.6X5	T49.6X6
Bishydroxycoumarin	T45.511	T45.512	T45.513	T45.514	T45.515	T45.516
Bismarsen	T37.8X1	T37.8X2	T37.8X3	T37.8X4	T37.8X5	T37.8X6
Bismuth salts	T47.6X1	T47.6X2	T47.6X3	T47.6X4	T47.6X5	T47.6X6
aluminate	T47.1X1	T47.1X2	T47.1X3	T47.1X4	T47.1X5	T47.1X6
anti-infectives	T37.8X1	T37.8X2	T37.8X3	T37.8X4	T37.8X5	T37.8X6
formic iodide	T49.0X1	T49.0X2	T49.0X3	T49.0X4	T49.0X5	T49.0X6
glycolylarsenate	T49.0X1	T49.0X2	T49.0X3	T49.0X4	T49.0X5	T49.0X6
nonmedicinal (compounds) NEC	T65.91	T65.92	T65.93	T65.94	—	—
subcarbonate	T47.6X1	T47.6X2	T47.6X3	T47.6X4	T47.6X5	T47.6X6
subsalicylate	T37.8X1	T37.8X2	T37.8X3	T37.8X4	T37.8X5	T37.8X6
sulfarsphenamine	T37.8X1	T37.8X2	T37.8X3	T37.8X4	T37.8X5	T37.8X6
Bisoprolol	T44.7X1	T44.7X2	T44.7X3	T44.7X4	T44.7X5	T44.7X6
Bisoxatin	T47.2X1	T47.2X2	T47.2X3	T47.2X4	T47.2X5	T47.2X6
Bisulepin (hydrochloride)	T45.0X1	T45.0X2	T45.0X3	T45.0X4	T45.0X5	T45.0X6
Bithionol	T37.8X1	T37.8X2	T37.8X3	T37.8X4	T37.8X5	T37.8X6
anthelminthic	T37.4X1	T37.4X2	T37.4X3	T37.4X4	T37.4X5	T37.4X6
Bitolterol	T48.6X1	T48.6X2	T48.6X3	T48.6X4	T48.6X5	T48.6X6
Bitoscanate	T37.4X1	T37.4X2	T37.4X3	T37.4X4	T37.4X5	T37.4X6
Bitter almond oil	T62.8X1	T62.8X2	T62.8X3	T62.8X4	—	—
Bittersweet	T62.2X1	T62.2X2	T62.2X3	T62.2X4	—	—
Black						
flag	T60.91	T60.92	T60.93	T60.94	—	—
henbane	T62.2X1	T62.2X2	T62.2X3	T62.2X4	—	—
leaf (40)	T60.91	T60.92	T60.93	T60.94	—	—
widow spider (bite)	T63.311	T63.312	T63.313	T63.314	—	—
antivenin	T50.Z11	T50.Z12	T50.Z13	T50.Z14	T50.Z15	T50.Z16
Blast furnace gas (carbon monoxide from)	T58.8X1	T58.8X2	T58.8X3	T58.8X4	—	—
Bleach	T54.91	T54.92	T54.93	T54.94	—	—

◀ New ◀ Revised ~~deleted~~ Deleted

TABLE OF DRUGS AND CHEMICALS

TABLE OF DRUGS AND CHEMICALS

Substance	Poisoning, Accidental (Unintentional)	Poisoning, Intentional Self-Harm	Poisoning, Assault	Poisoning, Undetermined	Adverse Effect	Underdosing
	External Cause (T-Code)					
Bleaching agent (medicinal)	T49.4X1	T49.4X2	T49.4X3	T49.4X4	T49.4X5	T49.4X6
Bleomycin	T45.1X1	T45.1X2	T45.1X3	T45.1X4	T45.1X5	T45.1X6
Blockain	T41.3X1	T41.3X2	T41.3X3	T41.3X4	T41.3X5	T41.3X6
infiltration (subcutaneous)	T41.3X1	T41.3X2	T41.3X3	T41.3X4	T41.3X5	T41.3X6
nerve block (peripheral) (plexus)	T41.3X1	T41.3X2	T41.3X3	T41.3X4	T41.3X5	T41.3X6
topical (surface)	T41.3X1	T41.3X2	T41.3X3	T41.3X4	T41.3X5	T41.3X6
Blockers, calcium channel	T46.1X1	T46.1X2	T46.1X4	T46.1X4	T46.1X5	T46.1X6
Blood (derivatives) (natural) (plasma) (whole)	T45.8X1	T45.8X2	T45.8X3	T45.8X4	T45.8X5	T45.8X6
dried	T45.8X1	T45.8X2	T45.8X3	T45.8X4	T45.8X5	T45.8X6
drug affecting NEC	T45.91	T45.92	T45.93	T45.94	T45.95	T45.96
expander NEC	T45.8X1	T45.8X2	T45.8X3	T45.8X4	T45.8X5	T45.8X6
fraction NEC	T45.8X1	T45.8X2	T45.8X3	T45.8X4	T45.8X5	T45.8X6
substitute (macromolecular)	T45.8X1	T45.8X2	T45.8X3	T45.8X4	T45.8X5	T45.8X6
Blue velvet	T40.2X1	T40.2X2	T40.2X3	T40.2X4	—	—
Bone meal	T62.8X1	T62.8X2	T62.8X3	T62.8X4	—	—
Bonine	T45.0X1	T45.0X2	T45.0X3	T45.0X4	T45.0X5	T45.0X6
Bopindolol	T44.7X1	T44.7X2	T44.7X3	T44.7X4	T44.7X5	T44.7X6
Boracic acid	T49.0X1	T49.0X2	T49.0X3	T49.0X4	T49.0X5	T49.0X6
ENT agent	T49.6X1	T49.6X2	T49.6X3	T49.6X4	T49.6X5	T49.6X6
ophthalmic preparation	T49.5X1	T49.5X2	T49.5X3	T49.5X4	T49.5X5	T49.5X6
Borane complex	T57.8X1	T57.8X2	T57.8X3	T57.8X4	—	—
Borate(s)	T57.8X1	T57.8X2	T57.8X3	T57.8X4	—	—
buffer	T50.991	T50.992	T50.993	T50.994	T50.995	T50.996
cleanser	T54.91	T54.92	T54.93	T54.94	—	—
sodium	T57.8X1	T57.8X2	T57.8X3	T57.8X4	—	—
Borax (cleanser)	T54.91	T54.92	T54.93	T54.94	—	—
Bordeaux mixture	T60.3X1	T60.3X2	T60.3X3	T60.3X4	—	—
Boric acid	T49.0X1	T49.0X2	T49.0X3	T49.0X4	T49.0X5	T49.0X6
ENT agent	T49.6X1	T49.6X2	T49.6X3	T49.6X4	T49.6X5	T49.6X6
ophthalmic preparation	T49.5X1	T49.5X2	T49.5X3	T49.5X4	T49.5X5	T49.5X6
Bornaprine	T44.3X1	T44.3X2	T44.3X3	T44.3X4	T44.3X5	T44.3X6
Boron	T57.8X1	T57.8X2	T57.8X3	T57.8X4	—	—
hydride NEC	T57.8X1	T57.8X2	T57.8X3	T57.8X4	—	—
fumes or gas	T57.8X1	T57.8X2	T57.8X3	T57.8X4	—	—
trifluoride	T59.891	T59.892	T59.893	T59.894	—	—
Botox	T48.291	T48.292	T48.293	T48.294	T48.295	T48.296
Botulinus anti-toxin (type A, B)	T50.Z11	T50.Z12	T50.Z13	T50.Z14	T50.Z15	T50.Z16
Brake fluid vapor	T59.891	T59.892	T59.893	T59.894	—	—
Brallobarbital	T42.3X1	T42.3X2	T42.3X3	T42.3X4	T42.3X5	T42.3X6
Bran (wheat)	T47.4X1	T47.4X2	T47.4X3	T47.4X4	T47.4X5	T47.4X6
Brass (fumes)	T56.891	T56.892	T56.893	T56.894	—	—

Substance	Poisoning, Accidental (Unintentional)	Poisoning, Intentional Self-Harm	Poisoning, Assault	Poisoning, Undetermined	Adverse Effect	Underdosing
	External Cause (T-Code)					
Brasso	T52.0X1	T52.0X2	T52.0X3	T52.0X4	—	—
Bretylium tosilate	T46.2X1	T46.2X2	T46.2X3	T46.2X4	T46.2X5	T46.2X6
Brevital (sodium)	T41.1X1	T41.1X2	T41.1X3	T41.1X4	T41.1X5	T41.1X6
Brinase	T45.3X1	T45.3X2	T45.3X3	T45.3X4	T45.3X5	T45.3X6
British antilewisite	T45.8X1	T45.8X2	T45.8X3	T45.8X4	T45.8X5	T45.8X6
Brodifacoum	T60.4X1	T60.4X2	T60.4X3	T60.4X4	—	—
Bromal (hydrate)	T42.6X1	T42.6X2	T42.6X3	T42.6X4	T42.6X5	T42.6X6
Bromazepam	T42.4X1	T42.4X2	T42.4X3	T42.4X4	T42.4X5	T42.4X6
Bromazine	T45.0X1	T45.0X2	T45.0X3	T45.0X4	T45.0X5	T45.0X6
Brombenzylcyanide	T59.3X1	T59.3X2	T59.3X3	T59.3X4	—	—
Bromelains	T45.3X1	T45.3X2	T45.3X3	T45.3X4	T45.3X5	T45.3X6
Bromethalin	T60.4X1	T60.4X2	T60.4X3	T60.4X4	—	—
Bromhexine	T48.4X1	T48.4X2	T48.4X3	T48.4X4	T48.4X5	T48.4X6
Bromide salts	T42.6X1	T42.6X2	T42.6X3	T42.6X4	T42.6X5	T42.6X6
Bromindione	T45.511	T45.512	T45.513	T45.514	T45.515	T45.516
Bromine						
compounds (medicinal)	T42.6X1	T42.6X2	T42.6X3	T42.6X4	T42.6X5	T42.6X6
sedative	T42.6X1	T42.6X2	T42.6X3	T42.6X4	T42.6X5	T42.6X6
vapor	T59.891	T59.892	T59.893	T59.894	—	—
Bromisovalum	T42.6X1	T42.6X2	T42.6X3	T42.6X4	T42.6X5	T42.6X6
Bromisoval	T42.6X1	T42.6X2	T42.6X3	T42.6X4	T42.6X5	T42.6X6
Bromobenzylcyanide	T59.3X1	T59.3X2	T59.3X3	T59.3X4	—	—
Bromochlorosalicylani-lide	T49.0X1	T49.0X2	T49.0X3	T49.0X4	T49.0X5	T49.0X6
Bromocriptine	T42.8X1	T42.8X2	T42.8X3	T42.8X4	T42.8X5	T42.8X6
Bromodiphenhydramine	T45.0X1	T45.0X2	T45.0X3	T45.0X4	T45.0X5	T45.0X6
Bromoform	T42.6X1	T42.6X2	T42.6X3	T42.6X4	T42.6X5	T42.6X6
Bromophenol blue reagent	T50.991	T50.992	T50.993	T50.994	T50.995	T50.996
Bromopride	T47.8X1	T47.8X2	T47.8X3	T47.8X4	T47.8X5	T47.8X6
Bromosalicylchloranitide	T49.0X1	T49.0X2	T49.0X3	T49.0X4	T49.0X5	T49.0X6
Bromosalicylhydroxamic acid	T37.1X1	T37.1X2	T37.1X3	T37.1X4	T37.1X5	T37.1X6
Bromo-seltzer	T39.1X1	T39.1X2	T39.1X3	T39.1X4	T39.1X5	T39.1X6
Bromoxynil	T60.3X1	T60.3X2	T60.3X3	T60.3X4	—	—
Bromperidol	T43.4X1	T43.4X2	T43.4X3	T43.4X4	T43.4X5	T43.4X6
Brompheniramine	T45.0X1	T45.0X2	T45.0X3	T45.0X4	T45.0X5	T45.0X6
Bromsulfophthalein	T50.8X1	T50.8X2	T50.8X3	T50.8X4	T50.8X5	T50.8X6
Bromural	T42.6X1	T42.6X2	T42.6X3	T42.6X4	T42.6X5	T42.6X6
Bromvaletone	T42.6X1	T42.6X2	T42.6X3	T42.6X4	T42.6X5	T42.6X6
Bronchodilator NEC	T48.6X1	T48.6X2	T48.6X3	T48.6X4	T48.6X5	T48.6X6
Brotizolam	T42.4X1	T42.4X2	T42.4X3	T42.4X4	T42.4X5	T42.4X6
Brovincamine	T46.7X1	T46.7X2	T46.7X3	T46.7X4	T46.7X5	T46.7X6
Brown spider (bite) (venom)	T63.391	T63.392	T63.393	T63.394	—	—

◀ New   ◀ Revised   ~~deleted~~ Deleted

Substance	Poisoning, Accidental (Unintentional)	Poisoning, Intentional Self-Harm	Poisoning, Assault	Poisoning, Undetermined	Adverse Effect	Underdosing
Brown recluse spider (bite) (venom)	T63.331	T63.332	T63.333	T63.334	—	—
Broxaterol	T48.6X1	T48.6X2	T48.6X3	T48.6X4	T48.6X5	T48.6X6
Broxuridine	T45.1X1	T45.1X2	T45.1X3	T45.1X4	T45.1X5	T45.1X6
Broxyquinoline	T37.8X1	T37.8X2	T37.8X3	T37.8X4	T37.8X5	T37.8X6
Bruceine	T48.291	T48.292	T48.293	T48.294	T48.295	T48.296
Brucia	T62.2X1	T62.2X2	T62.2X3	T62.2X4	—	—
Brucine	T65.1X1	T65.1X2	T65.1X3	T65.1X4	—	—
Brunswick green — see Copper						
Bruten — see Ibuprofen						
Bryonia	T47.2X1	T47.2X2	T47.2X3	T47.2X4	T47.2X5	T47.2X6
Buclizine	T45.0X1	T45.0X2	T45.0X3	T45.0X4	T45.0X5	T45.0X6
Buclosamide	149.0X1	T49.0X2	T49.0X3	T49.0X4	T49.0X5	T49.0X6
Budesonide	T44.5X1	T44.5X2	T44.5X3	T44.5X4	T44.5X5	I44.5X6
Budralazine	T46.5X1	T46.5X2	T46.5X3	T46.5X4	T46.5X5	T46.5X6
Bufferln	T39.011	T39.012	T39.013	T39.014	T39.015	I39.016
Buflomedil	T46.7X1	T46.7X2	T46.7X3	T46.7X4	T46.7X5	T46.7X6
Buformin	T38.3X1	T38.3X2	T38.3X3	T38.3X4	T38.3X5	T38.3X6
Bufotenine	T40.991	T40.992	T40.993	T40.994	—	—
Bufrolin	148.6X1	T48.6X2	T48.6X3	T48.6X4	T48.6X5	T48.6X6
Bufylline	T48.6X1	T48.6X2	T48.6X3	T48.6X4	T48.6X5	T48.6X6
Bulk filler	T50.5X1	T50.5X2	T50.5X3	T50.5X4	T50.5X5	T50.5X6
cathartic	T47.4X1	T47.4X2	T47.4X3	T47.4X4	T47.4X5	T47.4X6
Bumetanide	T50.1X1	T50.1X2	T50.1X3	T50.1X4	T50.1X5	T50.1X6
Bunaftine	T46.2X1	T46.2X2	T46.2X3	T46.2X4	T46.2X5	T46.2X6
Bunamiodyl	T50.8X1	I50.8X2	T50.8X3	T50.8X4	T50.8X5	T50.8X6
Bunazosin	T44.6X1	T44.6X2	T44.6X3	T44.6X4	T44.6X5	T44.6X6
Bunitrolol	T44.7X1	T44.7X2	T44.7X3	T44.7X4	T44.7X5	T44.7X6
Buphenine	T46.7X1	T46.7X2	T46.7X3	T46.7X4	T46.7X5	T46.7X6
Bupivacaine	T41.3X1	T41.3X2	T41.3X3	T41.3X4	T41.3X5	T41.3X6
infiltration (subcutaneous)	T41.3X1	T41.3X2	T41.3X3	T41.3X4	T41.3X5	T41.3X6
nerve block (peripheral) (plexus)	T41.3X1	T41.3X2	T41.3X3	T41.3X4	T41.3X5	T41.3X6
spinal	T41.3X1	T41.3X2	T41.3X3	T41.3X4	T41.3X5	T41.3X6
Bupranolol	T44.7X1	T44.7X2	T44.7X3	T44.7X4	T44.7X5	T44.7X6
Buprenorphine	T40.491	T40.492	T40.493	T40.494	T40.495	T40.496
Bupropion	T43.291	I43.292	T43.293	T43.294	T43.295	T43.296
Burimamide	T47.1X1	T47.1X2	T47.1X3	T47.1X4	T47.1X5	T47.1X6
Buserelin	T38.891	T38.892	T38.893	T38.894	T38.895	T38.896
Buspirone	T43.591	I43.592	T43.593	T43.594	T43.595	T43.596
Busulfan, busulphan	T45.1X1	T45.1X2	T45.1X3	T45.1X4	T45.1X5	T45.1X6
Butabarbital (sodium)	T42.3X1	T42.3X2	T42.3X3	T42.3X4	T42.3X5	T42.3X6
Butabarbitone	T42.3X1	T42.3X2	T42.3X3	T42.3X4	T42.3X5	T42.3X6

Substance	Poisoning, Accidental (Unintentional)	Poisoning, Intentional Self-Harm	Poisoning, Assault	Poisoning, Undetermined	Adverse Effect	Underdosing
Butabarpal	T42.3X1	T42.3X2	T42.3X3	T42.3X4	T42.3X5	T42.3X6
Butacaine	T41.3X1	T41.3X2	T41.3X3	T41.3X4	T41.3X5	T41.3X6
Butalamine	T46.7X1	T46.7X2	T46.7X3	T46.7X4	T46.7X5	T46.7X6
Butalbital	T42.3X1	T42.3X2	T42.3X3	T42.3X4	T42.3X5	T42.3X6
Butallylonal	T42.3X1	T42.3X2	T42.3X3	T42.3X4	T42.3X5	T42.3X6
Butamben	T41.3X1	T41.3X2	T41.3X3	T41.3X4	T41.3X5	T41.3X6
Butamirate	T48.3X1	T48.3X2	T48.3X3	T48.3X4	T48.3X5	T48.3X6
Butane (distributed in mobile container)	T59.891	T59.892	T59.893	T59.894	—	—
distributed through pipes	T59.891	T59.892	T59.893	T59.894	—	—
incomplete combustion	T58.11	T58.12	T58.13	T58.14		
Butanilicaine	T41.3X1	T41.3X2	T41.3X3	T41.3X4	T41.3X5	T41.3X6
Butanol	T51.3X1	T51.3X2	T51.3X3	T51.3X4		
Butanone, 2-butanone	T52.4X1	T52.4X2	T52.4X3	T52.4X4	—	—
Butantrone	T49.4X1	T49.4X2	I49.4X3	T49.4X4	T49.4X5	T49.4X6
Butaperazine	T43.3X1	T43.3X2	T43.3X3	T43.3X4	T43.3X5	T43.3X6
Butazolidin	T39.2X1	T39.2X2	T39.2X3	T39.2X4	T39.2X5	T39.2X6
Butetamate	T48.6X1	T48.6X2	T48.6X3	T48.6X4	148.6X5	T48.6X6
Butethal	T42.3X1	T42.3X2	T42.3X3	T42.3X4	T42.3X5	T42.3X6
Butethamate	T44.3X1	T44.3X2	T44.3X3	T44.3X4	T44.3X5	T44.3X6
Buthalitone (sodium)	T41.1X1	T41.1X2	T41.1X3	T41.1X4	T41.1X5	T41.1X6
Butisol (sodium)	T42.3X1	T42.3X2	T42.3X3	T42.3X4	T42.3X5	T42.3X6
Butizide	T50.2X1	T50.2X2	T50.2X3	T50.2X4	T50.2X5	T50.2X6
Butobarbital	T42.3X1	T42.3X2	T42.3X3	T42.3X4	T42.3X5	T42.3X6
sodium	T42.3X1	T42.3X2	T42.3X3	T42.3X4	T42.3X5	T42.3X6
Butobarbitone	T42.3X1	T42.3X2	T42.3X3	T42.3X4	T42.3X5	T42.3X6
Butoconazole (nitrate)	T49.0X1	T49.0X2	T49.0X3	T49.0X4	T49.0X5	T49.0X6
Butorphanol	T40.491	T40.492	T40.493	T40.494	T40.495	T40.496
Butriptyline	T43.011	T43.012	T43.013	T43.014	T43.015	T43.016
Butropium bromide	T44.3X1	T44.3X2	T44.3X3	T44.3X4	T44.3X5	T44.3X6
Buttercups	T62.2X1	T62.2X2	T62.2X3	T62.2X4	—	—
Butter of antimony — see Antimony						
Butyl						
acetate (secondary)	T52.8X1	T52.8X2	T52.8X3	T52.8X4	—	—
alcohol	T51.3X1	T51.3X2	T51.3X3	T51.3X4	—	—
aminobenzoate	T41.3X1	T41.3X2	T41.3X3	T41.3X4	T41.3X5	T41.3X6
butyrate	T52.8X1	T52.8X2	T52.8X3	T52.8X4	—	—
carbinol	T51.3X1	T51.3X2	T51.3X3	T51.3X4	—	—
carbitol	T52.3X1	T52.3X2	T52.3X3	T52.3X4	—	—
cellosolve	T52.3X1	T52.3X2	T52.3X3	T52.3X4		—
chloral (hydrate)	T42.6X1	T42.6X2	T42.6X3	T42.6X4	T42.6X5	T42.6X6
formate	T52.8X1	T52.8X2	T52.8X3	T52.8X4	—	—

TABLE OF DRUGS AND CHEMICALS

Substance	Poisoning, Accidental (Unintentional)	Poisoning, Intentional Self-Harm	Poisoning, Assault	Poisoning, Undetermined	Adverse Effect	Underdosing
Butyl *(Continued)*						
lactate	T52.8X1	T52.8X2	T52.8X3	T52.8X4	—	—
propionate	T52.8X1	T52.8X2	T52.8X3	T52.8X4	—	—
scopolamine bromide	T44.3X1	T44.3X2	T44.3X3	T44.3X4	T44.3X5	T44.3X6
thiobarbital sodium	T41.1X1	T41.1X2	T41.1X3	T41.1X4	T41.1X5	T41.1X6
Butylated hydroxy-anisole	T50.991	T50.992	T50.993	T50.994	T50.995	T50.996
Butylchloral hydrate	T42.6X1	T42.6X2	T42.6X3	T42.6X4	T42.6X5	T42.6X6
Butyltoluene	T52.2X1	T52.2X2	T52.2X3	T52.2X4	—	—
Butyn	T41.3X1	T41.3X2	T41.3X3	T41.3X4	T41.3X5	T41.3X6
Butyrophenone (-based tranquilizers)	T43.4X1	T43.4X2	T43.4X3	T43.4X4	T43.4X5	T43.4X6
C						
Cabergoline	T42.8X1	T42.8X2	T42.8X3	T42.8X4	T42.8X5	T42.8X6
Cacodyl, cacodylic acid	T57.0X1	T57.0X2	T57.0X3	T57.0X4	—	—
Cactinomycin	T45.1X1	T45.1X2	T45.1X3	T45.1X4	T45.1X5	T45.1X6
Cade oil	T49.4X1	T49.4X2	T49.4X3	T49.4X4	T49.4X5	T49.4X6
Cadexomer iodine	T49.0X1	T49.0X2	T49.0X3	T49.0X4	T49.0X5	T49.0X6
Cadmium (chloride) (fumes) (oxide)	T56.3X1	T56.3X2	T56.3X3	T56.3X4	—	—
sulfide (medicinal) NEC	T49.4X1	T49.4X2	T49.4X3	T49.4X4	T49.4X5	T49.4X6
Cadralazine	T46.5X1	T46.5X2	T46.5X3	T46.5X4	T46.5X5	T46.5X6
Caffeine	T43.611	T43.612	T43.613	T43.614	T43.615	T43.616
Calabar bean	T62.2X1	T62.2X2	T62.2X3	T62.2X4	—	—
Caladium seguinum	T62.2X1	T62.2X2	T62.2X3	T62.2X4	—	—
Calamine (lotion)	T49.3X1	T49.3X2	T49.3X3	T49.3X4	T49.3X5	T49.3X6
Calcifediol	T45.2X1	T45.2X2	T45.2X3	T45.2X4	T45.2X5	T45.2X6
Calciferol	T45.2X1	T45.2X2	T45.2X3	T45.2X4	T45.2X5	T45.2X6
Calcitonin	T50.991	T50.992	T50.993	T50.994	T50.995	T50.996
Calcitriol	T45.2X1	T45.2X2	T45.2X3	T45.2X4	T45.2X5	T45.2X6
Calcium	T50.3X1	T50.3X2	T50.3X3	T50.3X4	T50.3X5	T50.3X6
actylsalicylate	T39.011	T39.012	T39.013	T39.014	T39.015	T39.016
benzamidosalicylate	T37.1X1	T37.1X2	T37.1X3	T37.1X4	T37.1X5	T37.1X6
bromide	T42.6X1	T42.6X2	T42.6X3	T42.6X4	T42.6X5	T42.6X6
bromolactobionate	T42.6X1	T42.6X2	T42.6X3	T42.6X4	T42.6X5	T42.6X6
carbaspirin	T39.011	T39.012	T39.013	T39.014	T39.015	T39.016
carbimide	T50.6X1	T50.6X2	T50.6X3	T50.6X4	T50.6X5	T50.6X6
carbonate	T47.1X1	T47.1X2	T47.1X3	T47.1X4	T47.1X5	T47.1X6
chloride	T50.991	T50.992	T50.993	T50.994	T50.995	T50.996
anhydrous	T50.991	T50.992	T50.993	T50.994	T50.995	T50.996
cyanide	T57.8X1	T57.8X2	T57.8X3	T57.8X4	—	—
dioctyl sulfosuccinate	T47.4X1	T47.4X2	T47.4X3	T47.4X4	T47.4X5	T47.4X6
disodium edathamil	T45.8X1	T45.8X2	T45.8X3	T45.8X4	T45.8X5	T45.8X6

Substance	Poisoning, Accidental (Unintentional)	Poisoning, Intentional Self-Harm	Poisoning, Assault	Poisoning, Undetermined	Adverse Effect	Underdosing
Calcium *(Continued)*						
disodium edetate	T45.8X1	T45.8X2	T45.8X3	T45.8X4	T45.8X5	T45.8X6
dobesilate	T46.991	T46.992	T46.993	T46.994	T46.995	T46.996
EDTA	T45.8X1	T45.8X2	T45.8X3	T45.8X4	T45.8X5	T45.8X6
ferrous citrate	T45.4X1	T45.4X2	T45.4X3	T45.4X4	T45.4X5	T45.4X6
folinate	T45.8X1	T45.8X2	T45.8X3	T45.8X4	T45.8X5	T45.8X6
glubionate	T50.3X1	T50.3X2	T50.3X3	T50.3X4	T50.3X5	T50.3X6
gluconate	T50.3X1	T50.3X2	T50.3X3	T50.3X4	T50.3X5	T50.3X6
gluconogalactogluconate	T50.3X1	T50.3X2	T50.3X3	T50.3X4	T50.3X5	T50.3X6
hydrate, hydroxide	T54.3X1	T54.3X2	T54.3X3	T54.3X4	—	—
hypochlorite	T54.3X1	T54.3X2	T54.3X3	T54.3X4	—	—
iodide	T48.4X1	T48.4X2	T48.4X3	T48.4X4	T48.4X5	T48.4X6
ipodate	T50.8X1	T50.8X2	T50.8X3	T50.8X4	T50.8X5	T50.8X6
lactate	T50.3X1	T50.3X2	T50.3X3	T50.3X4	T50.3X5	T50.3X6
leucovorin	T45.8X1	T45.8X2	T45.8X3	T45.8X4	T45.8X5	T45.8X6
mandelate	T37.91	T37.92	T37.93	T37.94	T37.95	T37.96
oxide	T54.3X1	T54.3X2	T54.3X3	T54.3X4	—	—
pantothenate	T45.2X1	T45.2X2	T45.2X3	T45.2X4	T45.2X5	T45.2X6
phosphate	T50.3X1	T50.3X2	T50.3X3	T50.3X4	T50.3X5	T50.3X6
salicylate	T39.091	T39.092	T39.093	T39.094	T39.095	T39.096
salts	T50.3X1	T50.3X2	T50.3X3	T50.3X4	T50.3X5	T50.3X6
Calculus-dissolving drug	T50.991	T50.992	T50.993	T50.994	T50.995	T50.996
Calomel	T49.0X1	T49.0X2	T49.0X3	T49.0X4	T49.0X5	T49.0X6
Caloric agent	T50.3X1	T50.3X2	T50.3X3	T50.3X4	T50.3X5	T50.3X6
Calusterone	T38.7X1	T38.7X2	T38.7X3	T38.7X4	T38.7X5	T38.7X6
Camazepam	T42.4X1	T42.4X2	T42.4X3	T42.4X4	T42.4X5	T42.4X6
Camomile	T49.0X1	T49.0X2	T49.0X3	T49.0X4	T49.0X5	T49.0X6
Camoquin	T37.2X1	T37.2X2	T37.2X3	T37.2X4	T37.2X5	T37.2X6
Camphor						
insecticide	T60.2X1	T60.2X2	T60.2X3	T60.2X4	—	—
medicinal	T49.8X1	T49.8X2	T49.8X3	T49.8X4	T49.8X5	T49.8X6
Camylofin	T44.3X1	T44.3X2	T44.3X3	T44.3X4	T44.3X5	T44.3X6
Cancer chemotherapy drug regimen	T45.1X1	T45.1X2	T45.1X3	T45.1X4	T45.1X5	T45.1X6
Candeptin	T49.0X1	T49.0X2	T49.0X3	T49.0X4	T49.0X5	T49.0X6
Candicidin	T49.0X1	T49.0X2	T49.0X3	T49.0X4	T49.0X5	T49.0X6
Cannabinoids, synthetic	T40.721	T40.722	T40.723	T40.724	T40.725	T40.726
Cannabinol	T40.711	T40.712	T40.713	T40.714	T40.715	T40.716
Cannabis (derivatives)	T40.711	T40.712	T40.713	T40.714	T40.715	T40.716
Canned heat	T51.1X1	T51.1X2	T51.1X3	T51.1X4	—	—
Canrenoic acid	T50.0X1	T50.0X2	T50.0X3	T50.0X4	T50.0X5	T50.0X6
Canrenone	T50.0X1	T50.0X2	T50.0X3	T50.0X4	T50.0X5	T50.0X6

◀ New   ◀ Revised   ~~deleted~~ Deleted

Substance	External Cause (T-Code)					
	Poisoning, Accidental (Unintentional)	Poisoning, Intentional Self-Harm	Poisoning, Assault	Poisoning, Undetermined	Adverse Effect	Underdosing
Cantharides, cantharidin, cantharis	T49.8X1	T49.8X2	T49.8X3	T49.8X4	T49.8X5	T49.8X6
Canthaxanthin	T50.991	T50.992	T50.993	T50.994	T50.995	T50.996
Capillary-active drug NEC	T46.901	T46.902	T46.903	T46.904	T46.905	T46.906
Capreomycin	T36.8X1	T36.8X2	T36.8X3	T36.8X4	T36.8X5	T36.8X6
Capsicum	T49.4X1	T49.4X2	T49.4X3	T49.4X4	T49.4X5	T49.4X6
Captafol	T60.3X1	T60.3X2	T60.3X3	T60.3X4	—	—
Captan	T60.3X1	T60.3X2	T60.3X3	T60.3X4	—	—
Captodiame, captodiamine	T43.591	T43.592	T43.593	T43.594	T43.595	T43.596
Captopril	T46.4X1	T46.4X2	T46.4X3	T46.4X4	T46.4X5	T46.4X6
Caramiphen	T44.3X1	T44.3X2	T44.3X3	T44.3X4	T44.3X5	T44.3X6
Carazolol	T44.7X1	T44.7X2	T44.7X3	T44.7X4	T44.7X5	T44.7X6
Carbachol	T44.1X1	T44.1X2	T44.1X3	T44.1X4	T44.1X5	T44.1X6
Carbacrylamine (resin)	T50.3X1	T50.3X2	T50.3X3	T50.3X4	T50.3X5	T50.3X6
Carbamate (insecticide)	T60.0X1	T60.0X2	T60.0X3	T60.0X4	—	—
Carbamate (sedative)	T42.6X1	T42.6X2	T42.6X3	T42.6X4	T42.6X5	T42.6X6
herbicide	T60.0X1	T60.0X2	T60.0X3	T60.0X4	—	—
insecticide	T60.0X1	T60.0X2	T60.0X3	T60.0X4	—	—
Carbamazepine	T42.1X1	T42.1X2	T42.1X3	T42.1X4	T42.1X5	T42.1X6
Carbamide	T47.3X1	T47.3X2	T47.3X3	T47.3X4	T47.3X5	T47.3X6
peroxide	T49.0X1	T49.0X2	T49.0X3	T49.0X4	T49.0X5	T49.0X6
topical	T49.8X1	T49.8X2	T49.8X3	T49.8X4	T49.8X5	T49.8X6
Carbamylcholine chloride	T44.1X1	T44.1X2	T44.1X3	T44.1X4	T44.1X5	T44.1X6
Carbaril	T60.0X1	T60.0X2	T60.0X3	T60.0X4	—	—
Carbarsone	T37.3X1	T37.3X2	T37.3X3	T37.3X4	T37.3X5	T37.3X6
Carbaryl	T60.0X1	T60.0X2	T60.0X3	T60.0X4	—	—
Carbaspirin	T39.011	T39.012	T39.013	T39.014	T39.015	T39.016
Carbazochrome (salicylate) (sodium sulfonate)	T49.4X1	T49.4X2	T49.4X3	T49.4X4	T49.4X5	T49.4X6
Carbenicillin	T36.0X1	T36.0X2	T36.0X3	T36.0X4	T36.0X5	T36.0X6
Carbenoxolone	T47.1X1	T47.1X2	T47.1X3	T47.1X4	T47.1X5	T47.1X6
Carbetapentane	T48.3X1	T48.3X2	T48.3X3	T48.3X4	T48.3X5	T48.3X6
Carbethyl salicylate	T39.091	T39.092	T39.093	T39.094	T39.095	T39.096
Carbidopa (with levodopa)	T42.8X1	T42.8X2	T42.8X3	T42.8X4	T42.8X5	T42.8X6
Carbimazole	T38.2X1	T38.2X2	T38.2X3	T38.2X4	T38.2X5	T38.2X6
Carbinol	T51.1X1	T51.1X2	T51.1X3	T51.1X4	—	—
Carbinoxamine	T45.0X1	T45.0X2	T45.0X3	T45.0X4	T45.0X5	T45.0X6
Carbiphene	T39.8X1	T39.8X2	T39.8X3	T39.8X4	T39.8X5	T39.8X6
Carbitol	T52.3X1	T52.3X2	T52.3X3	T52.3X4	—	—
Carbocaine	T41.3X1	T41.3X2	T41.3X3	T41.3X4	T41.3X5	T41.3X6
infiltration (subcutaneous)	T41.3X1	T41.3X2	T41.3X3	T41.3X4	T41.3X5	T41.3X6
nerve block (peripheral) (plexus)	T41.3X1	T41.3X2	T41.3X3	T41.3X4	T41.3X5	T41.3X6
topical (surface)	T41.3X1	T41.3X2	T41.3X3	T41.3X4	T41.3X5	T41.3X6

Substance	External Cause (T-Code)					
	Poisoning, Accidental (Unintentional)	Poisoning, Intentional Self-Harm	Poisoning, Assault	Poisoning, Undetermined	Adverse Effect	Underdosing
Carbo medicinalis	T47.6X1	T47.6X2	T47.6X3	T47.6X4	T47.6X5	T47.6X6
Carbomycin	T36.8X1	T36.8X2	T36.8X3	T36.8X4	T36.8X5	T36.8X6
Carbocisteine	T48.4X1	T48.4X2	T48.4X3	T48.4X4	T48.4X5	T48.4X6
Carbocromen	T46.3X1	T46.3X2	T46.3X3	T46.3X4	T46.3X5	T46.3X6
Carbol fuchsin	T49.0X1	T49.0X2	T49.0X3	T49.0X4	T49.0X5	T49.0X6
Carbolic acid — see also Phenol	T54.0X1	T54.0X2	T54.0X3	T54.0X4	—	—
Carbolonium (bromide)	T48.1X1	T48.1X2	T48.1X3	T48.1X4	T48.1X5	T48.1X6
Carbon						
bisulfide (liquid)	T65.4X1	T65.4X2	T65.4X3	T65.4X4	—	—
vapor	T65.4X1	T65.4X2	T65.4X3	T65.4X4	—	—
dioxide (gas)	T59.7X1	T59.7X2	T59.7X3	T59.7X4	—	—
medicinal	T41.5X1	T41.5X2	T41.5X3	T41.5X4	T41.5X5	T41.5X6
nonmedicinal	T59.7X1	T59.7X2	T59.7X3	T59.7X4	—	—
snow	T49.4X1	T49.4X2	T49.4X3	T49.4X4	T49.4X5	T49.4X6
disulfide (liquid)	T65.4X1	T65.4X2	T65.4X3	T65.4X4	—	—
vapor	T65.4X1	T65.4X2	T65.4X3	T65.4X4	—	—
monoxide (from incomplete combustion)	T58.91	T58.92	T58.93	T58.94	—	—
blast furnace gas	T58.8X1	T58.8X2	T58.8X3	T58.8X4	—	—
butane (distributed in mobile container)	T58.11	T58.12	T58.13	T58.14	—	—
distributed through pipes	T58.11	T58.12	T58.13	T58.14	—	—
charcoal fumes	T58.2X1	T58.2X2	T58.2X3	T58.2X4	—	—
coal	T58.2X1	T58.2X2	T58.2X3	T58.2X4	—	—
coke (in domestic stoves, fireplaces)	T58.2X1	T58.2X2	T58.2X3	T58.2X4	—	—
gas (piped)	T58.11	T58.12	T58.13	T58.14	—	—
solid (in domestic stoves, fireplaces)	T58.2X1	T58.2X2	T58.2X3	T58.2X4	—	—
exhaust gas (motor) not in transit	T58.01	T58.02	T58.03	T58.04	—	—
combustion engine, any not in watercraft	T58.01	T58.02	T58.03	T58.04	—	—
farm tractor, not in transit	T58.01	T58.02	T58.03	T58.04	—	—
gas engine	T58.01	T58.02	T58.03	T58.04	—	—
motor pump	T58.01	T58.02	T58.03	T58.04	—	—
motor vehicle, not in transit	T58.01	T58.02	T58.03	T58.04	—	—
fuel (in domestic use)	T58.2X1	T58.2X2	T58.2X3	T58.2X4	—	—
gas (piped)	T58.11	T58.12	T58.13	T58.14	—	—
in mobile container	T58.11	T58.12	T58.13	T58.14	—	—
utility	T58.11	T58.12	T58.13	T58.14	—	—
in mobile container	T58.11	T58.12	T58.13	T58.14	—	—
piped (natural)	T58.11	T58.12	T58.13	T58.14	—	—

Substance	External Cause (T-Code) Poisoning, Accidental (Unintentional)	Poisoning, Intentional Self-Harm	Poisoning, Assault	Poisoning, Undetermined	Adverse Effect	Underdosing
Carbon (Continued)						
monoxide (Continued)						
illuminating gas	T58.11	T58.12	T58.13	T58.14	—	—
industrial fuels or gases, any	T58.8X1	T58.8X2	T58.8X3	T58.8X4	—	—
kerosene (in domestic stoves, fireplaces)	T58.2X1	T58.2X2	T58.2X3	T58.2X4	—	—
kiln gas or vapor	T58.8X1	T58.8X2	T58.8X3	T58.8X4	—	—
motor exhaust gas, not in transit	T58.01	T58.02	T58.03	T58.04	—	—
piped gas (manufactured) (natural)	T58.11	T58.12	T58.13	T58.14	—	—
producer gas	T58.8X1	T58.8X2	T58.8X3	T58.8X4	—	—
propane (distributed in mobile container)	T58.11	T58.12	T58.13	T58.14	—	—
distributed through pipes	T58.11	T58.12	T58.13	T58.14	—	—
specified source NEC	T58.8X1	T58.8X2	T58.8X3	T58.8X4	—	—
stove gas	T58.11	T58.12	T58.13	T58.14	—	—
piped	T58.11	T58.12	T58.13	T58.14	—	—
utility gas	T58.11	T58.12	T58.13	T58.14	—	—
piped	T58.11	T58.12	T58.13	T58.14	—	—
water gas	T58.11	T58.12	T58.13	T58.14	—	—
wood (in domestic stoves, fireplaces)	T58.2X1	T58.2X2	T58.2X3	T58.2X4	—	—
tetrachloride (vapor) NEC	T53.0X1	T53.0X2	T53.0X3	T53.0X4	—	—
liquid (cleansing agent) NEC	T53.0X1	T53.0X2	T53.0X3	T53.0X4	—	—
solvent	T53.0X1	T53.0X2	T53.0X3	T53.0X4	—	—
Carbonic acid gas	T59.7X1	T59.7X2	T59.7X3	T59.7X4	—	—
anhydrase inhibitor NEC	T50.2X1	T50.2X2	T50.2X3	T50.2X4	T50.2X5	T50.2X6
Carbophenothion	T60.0X1	T60.0X2	T60.0X3	T60.0X4	—	—
Carboplatin	T45.1X1	T45.1X2	T45.1X3	T45.1X4	T45.1X5	T45.1X6
Carboprost	T48.0X1	T48.0X2	T48.0X3	T48.0X4	T48.0X5	T48.0X6
Carboquone	T45.1X1	T45.1X2	T45.1X3	T45.1X4	T45.1X5	T45.1X6
Carbowax	T49.3X1	T49.3X2	T49.3X3	T49.3X4	T49.3X5	T49.3X6
Carboxymethyl-cellulose	T47.4X1	T47.4X2	T47.4X3	T47.4X4	T47.4X5	T47.4X6
S-Carboxymethyl-cysteine	T48.4X1	T48.4X2	T48.4X3	T48.4X4	T48.4X5	T48.4X6
Carbrital	T42.3X1	T42.3X2	T42.3X3	T42.3X4	T42.3X5	T42.3X6
Carbromal	T42.6X1	T42.6X2	T42.6X3	T42.6X4	T42.6X5	T42.6X6
Carbutamide	T38.3X1	T38.3X2	T38.3X3	T38.3X4	T38.3X5	T38.3X6
Carbuterol	T48.6X1	T48.6X2	T48.6X3	T48.6X4	T48.6X5	T48.6X6
Cardiac						
depressants	T46.2X1	T46.2X2	T46.2X3	T46.2X4	T46.2X5	T46.2X6
rhythm regulator	T46.2X1	T46.2X2	T46.2X3	T46.2X4	T46.2X5	T46.2X6
specified NEC	T46.2X1	T46.2X2	T46.2X3	T46.2X4	T46.2X5	T46.2X6

Substance	External Cause (T-Code) Poisoning, Accidental (Unintentional)	Poisoning, Intentional Self-Harm	Poisoning, Assault	Poisoning, Undetermined	Adverse Effect	Underdosing
Cardiografin	T50.8X1	T50.8X2	T50.8X3	T50.8X4	T50.8X5	T50.8X6
Cardio-green	T50.8X1	T50.8X2	T50.8X3	T50.8X4	T50.8X5	T50.8X6
Cardiotonic (glycoside) NEC	T46.0X1	T46.0X2	T46.0X3	T46.0X4	T46.0X5	T46.0X6
Cardiovascular drug NEC	T46.901	T46.902	T46.903	T46.904	T46.905	T46.906
Cardrase	T50.2X1	T50.2X2	T50.2X3	T50.2X4	T50.2X5	T50.2X6
Carfusin	T49.0X1	T49.0X2	T49.0X3	T49.0X4	T49.0X5	T49.0X6
Carfecillin	T36.0X1	T36.0X2	T36.0X3	T36.0X4	T36.0X5	T36.0X6
Carfenazine	T43.3X1	T43.3X2	T43.3X3	T43.3X4	T43.3X5	T43.3X6
Carindacillin	T36.0X1	T36.0X2	T36.0X3	T36.0X4	T36.0X5	T36.0X6
Carisoprodol	T42.8X1	T42.8X2	T42.8X3	T42.8X4	T42.8X5	T42.8X6
Carmellose	T47.4X1	T47.4X2	T47.4X3	T47.4X4	T47.4X5	T47.4X6
Carminative	T47.5X1	T47.5X2	T47.5X3	T47.5X4	T47.5X5	T47.5X6
Carmofur	T45.1X1	T45.1X2	T45.1X3	T45.1X4	T45.1X5	T45.1X6
Carmustine	T45.1X1	T45.1X2	T45.1X3	T45.1X4	T45.1X5	T45.1X6
Carotene	T45.2X1	T45.2X2	T45.2X3	T45.2X4	T45.2X5	T45.2X6
Carphenazine	T43.3X1	T43.3X2	T43.3X3	T43.3X4	T43.3X5	T43.3X6
Carpipramine	T42.4X1	T42.4X2	T42.4X3	T42.4X4	T42.4X5	T42.4X6
Carprofen	T39.311	T39.312	T39.313	T39.314	T39.315	T39.316
Carpronium chloride	T44.3X1	T44.3X2	T44.3X3	T44.3X4	T44.3X5	T44.3X6
Carrageenan	T47.8X1	T47.8X2	T47.8X3	T47.8X4	T47.8X5	T47.8X6
Carteolol	T44.7X1	T44.7X2	T44.7X3	T44.7X4	T44.7X5	T44.7X6
Carter's Little Pills	T47.2X1	T47.2X2	T47.2X3	T47.2X4	T47.2X5	T47.2X6
Cascara (sagrada)	T47.2X1	T47.2X2	T47.2X3	T47.2X4	T47.2X5	T47.2X6
Cassava	T62.2X1	T62.2X2	T62.2X3	T62.2X4	—	—
Castellani's paint	T49.0X1	T49.0X2	T49.0X3	T49.0X4	T49.0X5	T49.0X6
Castor						
bean	T62.2X1	T62.2X2	T62.2X3	T62.2X4	—	—
oil	T47.2X1	T47.2X2	T47.2X3	T47.2X4	T47.2X5	T47.2X6
Catalase	T45.3X1	T45.3X2	T45.3X3	T45.3X4	T45.3X5	T45.3X6
Caterpillar (sting)	T63.431	T63.432	T63.433	T63.434	—	—
Catha (edulis) (tea)	T43.691	T43.692	T43.693	T43.694	—	—
Cathartic NEC	T47.4X1	T47.4X2	T47.4X3	T47.4X4	T47.4X5	T47.4X6
anthacene derivative	T47.2X1	T47.2X2	T47.2X3	T47.2X4	T47.2X5	T47.2X6
bulk	T47.4X1	T47.4X2	T47.4X3	T47.4X4	T47.4X5	T47.4X6
contact	T47.2X1	T47.2X2	T47.2X3	T47.2X4	T47.2X5	T47.2X6
emollient NEC	T47.4X1	T47.4X2	T47.4X3	T47.4X4	T47.4X5	T47.4X6
irritant NEC	T47.2X1	T47.2X2	T47.2X3	T47.2X4	T47.2X5	T47.2X6
mucilage	T47.4X1	T47.4X2	T47.4X3	T47.4X4	T47.4X5	T47.4X6
saline	T47.3X1	T47.3X2	T47.3X3	T47.3X4	T47.3X5	T47.3X6
vegetable	T47.2X1	T47.2X2	T47.2X3	T47.2X4	T47.2X5	T47.2X6
Cathine	T50.5X1	T50.5X2	T50.5X3	T50.5X4	T50.5X5	T50.5X6
Cathomycin	T36.8X1	T36.8X2	T36.8X3	T36.8X4	T36.8X5	T36.8X6

◄ New ◄ Revised ~~deleted~~ Deleted

Substance	Poisoning, Accidental (Unintentional)	Poisoning, Intentional Self-Harm	Poisoning, Assault	Poisoning, Undetermined	Adverse Effect	Underdosing
Cation exchange resin	T50.3X1	T50.3X2	T50.3X3	T50.3X4	T50.3X5	T50.3X6
Caustic(s) NEC	T54.91	T54.92	T54.93	T54.94	—	—
alkali	T54.3X1	T54.3X2	T54.3X3	T54.3X4	—	—
hydroxide	T54.3X1	T54.3X2	T54.3X3	T54.3X4	—	—
potash	T54.3X1	T54.3X2	T54.3X3	T54.3X4	—	—
soda	T54.3X1	T54.3X2	T54.3X3	T54.3X4	—	—
specified NEC	T54.91	T54.92	T54.93	T54.94	—	—
Ceepryn	T49.0X1	T49.0X2	T49.0X3	T49.0X4	T49.0X5	T49.0X6
ENT agent	T49.6X1	T49.6X2	T49.6X3	T49.6X4	T49.6X5	T49.6X6
lozenges	T49.6X1	T49.6X2	T49.6X3	T49.6X4	T49.6X5	T49.6X6
Cefacetrile	T36.1X1	T36.1X2	T36.1X3	T36.1X4	T36.1X5	T36.1X6
Cefaclor	T36.1X1	T36.1X2	T36.1X3	T36.1X4	T36.1X5	T36.1X6
Cefadroxil	T36.1X1	T36.1X2	T36.1X3	T36.1X4	T36.1X5	T36.1X6
Cefalexin	T36.1X1	T36.1X2	T36.1X3	T36.1X4	T36.1X5	T36.1X6
Cefaloglycin	T36.1X1	T36.1X2	T36.1X3	T36.1X4	T36.1X5	T36.1X6
Cefaloridine	T36.1X1	T36.1X2	T36.1X3	T36.1X4	T36.1X5	T36.1X6
Cefalosporins	T36.1X1	T36.1X2	T36.1X3	T36.1X4	T36.1X5	T36.1X6
Cefalotin	T36.1X1	T36.1X2	T36.1X3	T36.1X4	T36.1X5	T36.1X6
Cefamandole	T36.1X1	T36.1X2	T36.1X3	T36.1X4	T36.1X5	T36.1X6
Cefamycin antibiotic	T36.1X1	T36.1X2	T36.1X3	T36.1X4	T36.1X5	T36.1X6
Cefapirin	T36.1X1	T36.1X2	T36.1X3	T36.1X4	T36.1X5	T36.1X6
Cefatrizine	T36.1X1	T36.1X2	T36.1X3	T36.1X4	T36.1X5	T36.1X6
Cefazedone	T36.1X1	T36.1X2	T36.1X3	T36.1X4	T36.1X5	T36.1X6
Cefazolin	T36.1X1	T36.1X2	T36.1X3	T36.1X4	T36.1X5	T36.1X6
Cefbuperazone	T36.1X1	T36.1X2	T36.1X3	T36.1X4	T36.1X5	T36.1X6
Cefetamet	T36.1X1	T36.1X2	T36.1X3	T36.1X4	T36.1X5	T36.1X6
Cefixime	T36.1X1	T36.1X2	T36.1X3	T36.1X4	T36.1X5	T36.1X6
Cefmenoxime	T36.1X1	T36.1X2	T36.1X3	T36.1X4	T36.1X5	T36.1X6
Cefmetazole	T36.1X1	T36.1X2	T36.1X3	T36.1X4	T36.1X5	T36.1X6
Cefminox	T36.1X1	T36.1X2	T36.1X3	T36.1X4	T36.1X5	T36.1X6
Cefonicid	T36.1X1	T36.1X2	T36.1X3	T36.1X4	T36.1X5	T36.1X6
Cefoperazone	T36.1X1	T36.1X2	T36.1X3	T36.1X4	T36.1X5	T36.1X6
Cefor anide	T36.1X1	T36.1X2	T36.1X3	T36.1X4	T36.1X5	T36.1X6
Cefotaxime	T36.1X1	T36.1X2	T36.1X3	T36.1X4	T36.1X5	T36.1X6
Cefotetan	T36.1X1	T36.1X2	T36.1X3	T36.1X4	T36.1X5	T36.1X6
Cefotiam	T36.1X1	T36.1X2	T36.1X3	T36.1X4	T36.1X5	T36.1X6
Cefoxitin	T36.1X1	T36.1X2	T36.1X3	T36.1X4	T36.1X5	T36.1X6
Cefpimizole	T36.1X1	T36.1X2	T36.1X3	T36.1X4	T36.1X5	T36.1X6
Cefpiramide	T36.1X1	T36.1X2	T36.1X3	T36.1X4	T36.1X5	T36.1X6
Cefradine	T36.1X1	T36.1X2	T36.1X3	T36.1X4	T36.1X5	T36.1X6
Cefroxadine	T36.1X1	T36.1X2	T36.1X3	T36.1X4	T36.1X5	T36.1X6
Cefsulodin	T36.1X1	T36.1X2	T36.1X3	T36.1X4	T36.1X5	T36.1X6

Substance	Poisoning, Accidental (Unintentional)	Poisoning, Intentional Self-Harm	Poisoning, Assault	Poisoning, Undetermined	Adverse Effect	Underdosing
Ceftazidime	T36.1X1	T36.1X2	T36.1X3	T36.1X4	T36.1X5	T36.1X6
Cefteram	T36.1X1	T36.1X2	T36.1X3	T36.1X4	T36.1X5	T36.1X6
Ceftezole	T36.1X1	T36.1X2	T36.1X3	T36.1X4	T36.1X5	T36.1X6
Ceftizoxime	T36.1X1	T36.1X2	T36.1X3	T36.1X4	T36.1X5	T36.1X6
Ceftriaxone	T36.1X1	T36.1X2	T36.1X3	T36.1X4	T36.1X5	T36.1X6
Cefuroxime	T36.1X1	T36.1X2	T36.1X3	T36.1X4	T36.1X5	T36.1X6
Cefuzonam	T36.1X1	T36.1X2	T36.1X3	T36.1X4	T36.1X5	T36.1X6
Celestone	T38.0X1	T38.0X2	T38.0X3	T38.0X4	T38.0X5	T38.0X6
topical	T49.0X1	T49.0X2	T49.0X3	T49.0X4	T49.0X5	T49.0X6
Celiprolol	T44.7X1	T44.7X2	T44.7X3	T44.7X4	T44.7X5	T44.7X6
Cellosolve	T52.91	T52.92	T52.93	T52.94	—	—
Cell stimulants and proliferants	T49.8X1	T49.8X2	T49.8X3	T49.8X4	T49.8X5	T49.8X6
Celluloce						
cathartic	T47.4X1	T47.4X2	T47.4X3	T47.4X4	T47.4X5	T47.4X6
hydroxyethyl	T47.4X1	T47.4X2	T47.4X3	T47.4X4	T47.4X5	T47.4X6
nitrates (topical)	T49.3X1	T49.3X2	T49.3X3	T49.3X4	T49.3X5	T49.3X6
oxidized	T49.4X1	T49.4X2	T49.4X3	T49.4X4	T49.4X5	T49.4X6
Centipede (bite)	T63.411	T63.412	T63.413	T63.414	—	—
Central nervous system						
depressants	T42.71	T42.72	T42.73	T42.74	T42.75	T42.76
anesthetic (general) NEC	T41.201	T41.202	T41.203	T41.204	T41.205	T41.206
gases NEC	T41.0X1	T41.0X2	T41.0X3	T41.0X4	T41.0X5	T41.0X6
intravenous	T41.1X1	T41.1X2	T41.1X3	T41.1X4	T41.1X5	T41.1X6
barbiturates	T42.3X1	T42.3X2	T42.3X3	T42.3X4	T42.3X5	T42.3X6
benzodiazepines	T42.4X1	T42.4X2	T42.4X3	T42.4X4	T42.4X5	T42.4X6
bromides	T42.6X1	T42.6X2	T42.6X3	T42.6X4	T42.6X5	T42.6X6
cannabis sativa	T40.711	T40.712	T40.713	T40.714	T40.715	T40.716
chloral hydrate	T42.6X1	T42.6X2	T42.6X3	T42.6X4	T42.6X5	T42.6X6
ethanol	T51.0X1	T51.0X2	T51.0X3	T51.0X4	—	—
hallucinogenics	T40.901	T40.902	T40.903	T40.904	T40.905	T40.906
hypnotics	T42.71	T42.72	T42.73	T42.74	T42.75	T42.76
specified NEC	T42.6X1	T42.6X2	T42.6X3	T42.6X4	T42.6X5	T42.6X6
muscle relaxants	T42.8X1	T42.8X2	T42.8X3	T42.8X4	T42.8X5	T42.8X6
paraldehyde	T42.6X1	T42.6X2	T42.6X3	T42.6X4	T42.6X5	T42.6X6
sedatives; sedative-hypnotics	T42.71	T42.72	T42.73	T42.74	T42.75	T42.76
mixed NEC	T42.6X1	T42.6X2	T42.6X3	T42.6X4	T42.6X5	T42.6X6
specified NEC	T42.6X1	T42.6X2	T42.6X3	T42.6X4	T42.6X5	T42.6X6
muscle-tone depressants	T42.8X1	T42.8X2	T42.8X3	T42.8X4	T42.8X5	T42.8X6
stimulants	T43.601	T43.602	T43.603	T43.604	T43.605	T43.606
amphetamines	T43.621	T43.622	T43.623	T43.624	T43.625	T43.626
analeptics	T50.7X1	T50.7X2	T50.7X3	T50.7X4	T50.7X5	T50.7X6

◀ New   ◀ Revised   ~~deleted~~ Deleted

Substance	Poisoning, Accidental (Unintentional)	Poisoning, Intentional Self-Harm	Poisoning, Assault	Poisoning, Undetermined	Adverse Effect	Underdosing
Central nervous system *(Continued)*						
stimulants *(Continued)*						
antidepressants	T43.201	T43.202	T43.203	T43.204	T43.205	T43.206
opiate antagonists	T50.7X1	T50.7X2	T50.7X3	T50.7X4	T50.7X5	T50.7X6
specified NEC	T43.691	T43.692	T43.693	T43.694	T43.695	T43.696
Cephalexin	T36.1X1	T36.1X2	T36.1X3	T36.1X4	T36.1X5	T36.1X6
Cephaloglycin	T36.1X1	T36.1X2	T36.1X3	T36.1X4	T36.1X5	T36.1X6
Cephaloridine	T36.1X1	T36.1X2	T36.1X3	T36.1X4	T36.1X5	T36.1X6
Cephalosporins	T36.1X1	T36.1X2	T36.1X3	T36.1X4	T36.1X5	T36.1X6
N (adicillin)	T36.0X1	T36.0X2	T36.0X3	T36.0X4	T36.0X5	T36.0X6
Cephalothin	T36.1X1	T36.1X2	T36.1X3	T36.1X4	T36.1X5	T36.1X6
Cephalotin	T36.1X1	T36.1X2	T36.1X3	T36.1X4	T36.1X5	T36.1X6
Cephradine	T36.1X1	T36.1X2	T36.1X3	T36.1X4	T36.1X5	T36.1X6
Cerbera (odallam)	T62.2X1	T62.2X2	T62.2X3	T62.2X4	—	—
Cerberin	T46.0X1	T46.0X2	T46.0X3	T46.0X4	T46.0X5	T46.0X6
Cerebral stimulants	T43.601	T43.602	T43.603	T43.604	T43.605	T43.606
psychotherapeutic	T43.601	T43.602	T43.603	T43.604	T43.605	T43.606
specified NEC	T43.691	T43.692	T43.693	T43.694	T43.695	T43.696
Cerium oxalate	T45.0X1	T45.0X2	T45.0X3	T45.0X4	T45.0X5	T45.0X6
Cerous oxalate	T45.0X1	T45.0X2	T45.0X3	T45.0X4	T45.0X5	T45.0X6
Ceruletide	T50.8X1	T50.8X2	T50.8X3	T50.8X4	T50.8X5	T50.8X6
Cetalkonium (chloride)	T49.0X1	T49.0X2	T49.0X3	T49.0X4	T49.0X5	T49.0X6
Cethexonium chloride	T49.0X1	T49.0X2	T49.0X3	T49.0X4	T49.0X5	T49.0X6
Cetiedil	T46.7X1	T46.7X2	T46.7X3	T46.7X4	T46.7X5	T46.7X6
Cetirizine	T45.0X1	T45.0X2	T45.0X3	T45.0X4	T45.0X5	T45.0X6
Cetomacrogol	T50.991	T50.992	T50.993	T50.994	T50.995	T50.996
Cetotiamine	T45.2X1	T45.2X2	T45.2X3	T45.2X4	T45.2X5	T45.2X6
Cetoxime	T45.0X1	T45.0X2	T45.0X3	T45.0X4	T45.0X5	T45.0X6
Cetraxate	T47.1X1	T47.1X2	T47.1X3	T47.1X4	T47.1X5	T47.1X6
Cetrimide	T49.0X1	T49.0X2	T49.0X3	T49.0X4	T49.0X5	T49.0X6
Cetrimonium (bromide)	T49.0X1	T49.0X2	T49.0X3	T49.0X4	T49.0X5	T49.0X6
Cetylpyridinium chloride	T49.0X1	T49.0X2	T49.0X3	T49.0X4	T49.0X5	T49.0X6
ENT agent	T49.6X1	T49.6X2	T49.6X3	T49.6X4	T49.6X5	T49.6X6
lozenges	T49.6X1	T49.6X2	T49.6X3	T49.6X4	T49.6X5	T49.6X6
Cevadillasee Sabadilla						
Cevitamic acid	T45.2X1	T45.2X2	T45.2X3	T45.2X4	T45.2X5	T45.2X6
Chalk, precipitated	T47.1X1	T47.1X2	T47.1X3	T47.1X4	T47.1X5	T47.1X6
Chamomile	T49.0X1	T49.0X2	T49.0X3	T49.0X4	T49.0X5	T49.0X6
Ch'an su	T46.0X1	T46.0X2	T46.0X3	T46.0X4	T46.0X5	T46.0X6
Charcoal	T47.6X1	T47.6X2	T47.6X3	T47.6X4	T47.6X5	T47.6X6
activated — *see also Charcoal, medicinal*	T47.6X1	T47.6X2	T47.6X3	T47.6X4	T47.6X5	T47.6X6

Substance	Poisoning, Accidental (Unintentional)	Poisoning, Intentional Self-Harm	Poisoning, Assault	Poisoning, Undetermined	Adverse Effect	Underdosing
Charcoal *(Continued)*						
fumes (Carbon monoxide)	T58.2X1	T58.2X2	T58.2X3	T58.2X4	—	—
industrial	T58.8X1	T58.8X2	T58.8X3	T58.8X4	—	—
medicinal (activated)	T47.6X1	T47.6X2	T47.6X3	T47.6X4	T47.6X5	T47.6X6
antidiarrheal	T47.6X1	T47.6X2	T47.6X3	T47.6X4	T47.6X5	T47.6X6
poison control	T47.8X1	T47.8X2	T47.8X3	T47.8X4	T47.8X5	T47.8X6
specified use other than for diarrhea	T47.8X1	T47.8X2	T47.8X3	T47.8X4	T47.8X5	T47.8X6
topical	T49.8X1	T49.8X2	T49.8X3	T49.8X4	T49.8X5	T49.8X6
Chaulmosulfone	T37.1X1	T37.1X2	T37.1X3	T37.1X4	T37.1X5	T37.1X6
Chelating agent NEC	T50.6X1	T50.6X2	T50.6X3	T50.6X4	T50.6X5	T50.6X6
Chelidonium majus	T62.2X1	T62.2X2	T62.2X3	T62.2X4	—	—
Chemical substance NEC	T65.91	T65.92	T65.93	T65.94	—	—
Chenodeoxycholic acid	T47.5X1	T47.5X2	T47.5X3	T47.5X4	T47.5X5	T47.5X6
Chenodiol	T47.5X1	T47.5X2	T47.5X3	T47.5X4	T47.5X5	T47.5X6
Chenopodium	T37.4X1	T37.4X2	T37.4X3	T37.4X4	T37.4X5	T37.4X6
Cherry laurel	T62.2X1	T62.2X2	T62.2X3	T62.2X4	—	—
Chinidin(e)	T46.2X1	T46.2X2	T46.2X3	T46.2X4	T46.2X5	T46.2X6
Chiniofon	T37.8X1	T37.8X2	T37.8X3	T37.8X4	T37.8X5	T37.8X6
Chlophedianol	T48.3X1	T48.3X2	T48.3X3	T48.3X4	T48.3X5	T48.3X6
Chloral	T42.6X1	T42.6X2	T42.6X3	T42.6X4	T42.6X5	T42.6X6
derivative	T42.6X1	T42.6X2	T42.6X3	T42.6X4	T42.6X5	T42.6X6
hydrate	T42.6X1	T42.6X2	T42.6X3	T42.6X4	T42.6X5	T42.6X6
Chloralamide	T42.6X1	T42.6X2	T42.6X3	T42.6X4	T42.6X5	T42.6X6
Chloralodol	T42.6X1	T42.6X2	T42.6X3	T42.6X4	T42.6X5	T42.6X6
Chloralose	T60.4X1	T60.4X2	T60.4X3	T60.4X4	—	—
Chlorambucil	T45.1X1	T45.1X2	T45.1X3	T45.1X4	T45.1X5	T45.1X6
Chloramine	T57.8X1	T57.8X2	T57.8X3	T57.8X4	—	—
T	T49.0X1	T49.0X2	T49.0X3	T49.0X4	T49.0X5	T49.0X6
topical	T49.0X1	T49.0X2	T49.0X3	T49.0X4	T49.0X5	T49.0X6
Chloramphenicol	T36.2X1	T36.2X2	T36.2X3	T36.2X4	T36.2X5	T36.2X6
ENT agent	T49.6X1	T49.6X2	T49.6X3	T49.6X4	T49.6X5	T49.6X6
ophthalmic preparation	T49.5X1	T49.5X2	T49.5X3	T49.5X4	T49.5X5	T49.5X6
topical NEC	T49.0X1	T49.0X2	T49.0X3	T49.0X4	T49.0X5	T49.0X6
Chlorate (potassium) (sodium) NEC	T60.3X1	T60.3X2	T60.3X3	T60.3X4	—	—
herbicide	T60.3X1	T60.3X2	T60.3X3	T60.3X4	—	—
Chlorazanil	T50.2X1	T50.2X2	T50.2X3	T50.2X4	T50.2X5	T50.2X6
Chlorbenzene, chlorbenzol	T53.7X1	T53.7X2	T53.7X3	T53.7X4	—	—
Chlorbenzoxamine	T44.3X1	T44.3X2	T44.3X3	T44.3X4	T44.3X5	T44.3X6
Chlorbutol	T42.6X1	T42.6X2	T42.6X3	T42.6X4	T42.6X5	T42.6X6
Chlorcyclizine	T45.0X1	T45.0X2	T45.0X3	T45.0X4	T45.0X5	T45.0X6

New ◀ Revised ◀ ~~deleted~~ Deleted

Substance	Poisoning, Accidental (Unintentional)	Poisoning, Intentional Self-Harm	Poisoning, Assault	Poisoning, Undetermined	Adverse Effect	Underdosing
Chlordan(e) (dust)	T60.1X1	T60.1X2	T60.1X3	T60.1X4	—	—
Chlordantoin	T49.0X1	T49.0X2	T49.0X3	T49.0X4	T49.0X5	T49.0X6
Chlordiazepoxide	T42.4X1	T42.4X2	T42.4X3	T42.4X4	T42.4X5	T42.4X6
Chlordiethyl benzamide	T49.3X1	T49.3X2	T49.3X3	T49.3X4	T49.3X5	T49.3X6
Chloresium	T49.8X1	T49.8X2	T49.8X3	T49.8X4	T49.8X5	T49.8X6
Chlorethiazol	T42.6X1	T42.6X2	T42.6X3	T42.6X4	T42.6X5	T42.6X6
Chlorethyl — see Ethyl chloride						
Chloretone	T42.6X1	T42.6X2	T42.6X3	T42.6X4	T42.6X5	T42.6X6
Chlorex	T53.6X1	T53.6X2	T53.6X3	T53.6X4	—	—
insecticide	T60.1X1	T60.1X2	T60.1X3	T60.1X4	—	—
Chlorfenvinphos	T60.0X1	T60.0X2	T60.0X3	T60.0X4	—	—
Chlorhexadol	T42.6X1	T42.6X2	T42.6X3	T42.6X4	T42.6X5	T42.6X6
Chlorhexamide	T45.1X1	T45.1X2	T45.1X3	T45.1X4	T45.1X5	T45.1X6
Chlorhexidine	T49.0X1	T49.0X2	T49.0X3	T49.0X4	T49.0X5	T49.0X6
Chlorhydroxyquinolin	T49.0X1	T49.0X2	T49.0X3	T49.0X4	T49.0X5	T49.0X6
Chloride of lime (bleach)	T54.3X1	T54.3X2	T54.3X3	T54.3X4	—	—
Chlorimipramine	T43.011	T43.012	T43.013	T43.014	T43.015	T43.016
Chlorinated						
camphene	T53.6X1	T53.6X2	T53.6X3	T53.6X4	—	—
diphenyl	T53.7X1	T53.7X2	T53.7X3	T53.7X4	—	—
hydrocarbons NEC	T53.91	T53.92	T53.93	T53.94	—	—
solvents	T53.91	T53.92	T53.93	T53.94	—	—
lime (bleach)	T54.3X1	T54.3X2	T54.3X3	T54.3X4	—	—
and boric acid solution	T49.0X1	T49.0X2	T49.0X3	T49.0X4	T49.0X5	T49.0X6
naphthalene (insecticide)	T60.1X1	T60.1X2	T60.1X3	T60.1X4	—	—
industrial (non-pesticide)	T53.7X1	T53.7X2	T53.7X3	T53.7X4	—	—
pesticide NEC	T60.8X1	T60.8X2	T60.8X3	T60.8X4	—	—
soda — see also Sodium hypochlorite						
solution	T49.0X1	T49.0X2	T49.0X3	T49.0X4	T49.0X5	T49.0X6
Chlorine (fumes) (gas)	T59.4X1	T59.4X2	T59.4X3	T59.4X4	—	—
bleach	T54.3X1	T54.3X2	T54.3X3	T54.3X4	—	—
compound gas NEC	T59.4X1	T59.4X2	T59.4X3	T59.4X4	—	—
disinfectant	T59.4X1	T59.4X2	T59.4X3	T59.4X4	—	—
releasing agents NEC	T59.4X1	T59.4X2	T59.4X3	T59.4X4	—	—
Chlorisondamine chloride	T46.991	T46.992	T46.993	T46.994	T46.995	T46.996
Chlormadinone	T38.5X1	T38.5X2	T38.5X3	T38.5X4	T38.5X5	T38.5X6
Chlormephos	T60.0X1	T60.0X2	T60.0X3	T60.0X4	—	—
Chlormerodrin	T50.2X1	T50.2X2	T50.2X3	T50.2X4	T50.2X5	T50.2X6
Chlormethiazole	T42.6X1	T42.6X2	T42.6X3	T42.6X4	T42.6X5	T42.6X6
Chlormethine	T45.1X1	T45.1X2	T45.1X3	T45.1X4	T45.1X5	T45.1X6
Chlormethylenecycline	T36.4X1	T36.4X2	T36.4X3	T36.4X4	T36.4X5	T36.4X6

Substance	Poisoning, Accidental (Unintentional)	Poisoning, Intentional Self-Harm	Poisoning, Assault	Poisoning, Undetermined	Adverse Effect	Underdosing
Chlormezanone	T42.6X1	T42.6X2	T42.6X3	T42.6X4	T42.6X5	T42.6X6
Chloroacetic acid	T60.3X1	T60.3X2	T60.3X3	T60.3X4	—	—
Chloroacetone	T59.3X1	T59.3X2	T59.3X3	T59.3X4	—	—
Chloroacetophenone	T59.3X1	T59.3X2	T59.3X3	T59.3X4	—	—
Chloroaniline	T53.7X1	T53.7X2	T53.7X3	T53.7X4	—	—
Chlorobenzene, chlorobenzol	T53.7X1	T53.7X2	T53.7X3	T53.7X4	—	—
Chlorobromomethane (fire extinguisher)	T53.6X1	T53.6X2	T53.6X3	T53.6X4	—	—
Chlorobutanol	T49.0X1	T49.0X2	T49.0X3	T49.0X4	T49.0X5	T49.0X6
Chlorocresol	T49.0X1	T49.0X2	T49.0X3	T49.0X4	T49.0X5	T49.0X6
Chlorodehydro-methyltestosterone	T38.7X1	T38.7X2	T38.7X3	T38.7X4	T38.7X5	T38.7X6
Chlorodinitrobenzene	T53.7X1	T53.7X2	T53.7X3	T53.7X4	—	—
dust or vapor	T53.7X1	T53.7X2	T53.7X3	T53.7X4	—	—
Chlorodiphenyl	T53.7X1	T53.7X2	T53.7X3	T53.7X4	—	—
Chloroethane — see Ethyl chloride						
Chloroethylene	T53.6X1	T53.6X2	T53.6X3	T53.6X4	—	—
Chlorofluorocarbons	T53.5X1	T53.5X2	T53.5X3	T53.5X4	—	—
Chloroform (fumes) (vapor)	T53.1X1	T53.1X2	T53.1X3	T53.1X4	—	—
anesthetic	T41.0X1	T41.0X2	T41.0X3	T41.0X4	T41.0X5	T41.0X6
solvent	T53.1X1	T53.1X2	T53.1X3	T53.1X4	—	—
water, concentrated	T41.0X1	T41.0X2	T41.0X3	T41.0X4	T41.0X5	T41.0X6
Chloroguanide	T37.2X1	T37.2X2	T37.2X3	T37.2X4	T37.2X5	T37.2X6
Chloromycetin	T36.2X1	T36.2X2	T36.2X3	T36.2X4	T36.2X5	T36.2X6
ENT agent	T49.6X1	T49.6X2	T49.6X3	T49.6X4	T49.6X5	T49.6X6
ophthalmic preparation	T49.5X1	T49.5X2	T49.5X3	T49.5X4	T49.5X5	T49.5X6
otic solution	T49.6X1	T49.6X2	T49.6X3	T49.6X4	T49.6X5	T49.6X6
topical NEC	T49.0X1	T49.0X2	T49.0X3	T49.0X4	T49.0X5	T49.0X6
Chloronitrobenzene	T53.7X1	T53.7X2	T53.7X3	T53.7X4	—	—
dust or vapor	T53.7X1	T53.7X2	T53.7X3	T53.7X4	—	—
Chlorophacinone	T60.4X1	T60.4X2	T60.4X3	T60.4X4	—	—
Chlorophenol	T53.7X1	T53.7X2	T53.7X3	T53.7X4	—	—
Chlorophenothane	T60.1X1	T60.1X2	T60.1X3	T60.1X4	—	—
Chlorophyll	T50.991	T50.992	T50.993	T50.994	T50.995	T50.996
Chloropicrin (fumes)	T53.6X1	T53.6X2	T53.6X3	T53.6X4	—	—
fumigant	T60.8X1	T60.8X2	T60.8X3	T60.8X4	—	—
fungicide	T60.3X1	T60.3X2	T60.3X3	T60.3X4	—	—
pesticide	T60.8X1	T60.8X2	T60.8X3	T60.8X4	—	—
Chloroprocaine	T41.3X1	T41.3X2	T41.3X3	T41.3X4	T41.3X5	T41.3X6
infiltration (subcutaneous)	T41.3X1	T41.3X2	T41.3X3	T41.3X4	T41.3X5	T41.3X6
nerve block (peripheral) (plexus)	T41.3X1	T41.3X2	T41.3X3	T41.3X4	T41.3X5	T41.3X6
spinal	T41.3X1	T41.3X2	T41.3X3	T41.3X4	T41.3X5	T41.3X6

◀ New ◀ Revised deleted Deleted

	External Cause (T-Code)					
Substance	Poisoning, Accidental (Unintentional)	Poisoning, Intentional Self-Harm	Poisoning, Assault	Poisoning, Undetermined	Adverse Effect	Underdosing
Chloroptic	T49.5X1	T49.5X2	T49.5X3	T49.5X4	T49.5X5	T49.5X6
Chloropurine	T45.1X1	T45.1X2	T45.1X3	T45.1X4	T45.1X5	T45.1X6
Chloropyramine	T45.0X1	T45.0X2	T45.0X3	T45.0X4	T45.0X5	T45.0X6
Chloropyrifos	T60.0X1	T60.0X2	T60.0X3	T60.0X4	—	—
Chloropyrilene	T45.0X1	T45.0X2	T45.0X3	T45.0X4	T45.0X5	T45.0X6
Chloroquine	T37.2X1	T37.2X2	T37.2X3	T37.2X4	T37.2X5	T37.2X6
Chlorothalonil	T60.3X1	T60.3X2	T60.3X3	T60.3X4	—	—
Chlorothen	T45.0X1	T45.0X2	T45.0X3	T45.0X4	T45.0X5	T45.0X6
Chlorothiazide	T50.2X1	T50.2X2	T50.2X3	T50.2X4	T50.2X5	T50.2X6
Chlorothymol	T49.4X1	T49.4X2	T49.4X3	T49.4X4	T49.4X5	T49.4X6
Chlorotrianisene	T38.5X1	T38.5X2	T38.5X3	T38.5X4	T38.5X5	T38.5X6
Chlorovinyldichloro-arsine, not in war	T57.0X1	T57.0X2	T57.0X3	T57.0X4	—	—
Chloroxine	T49.4X1	T49.4X2	T49.4X3	T49.4X4	T49.4X5	T49.4X6
Chloroxylenol	T49.0X1	T49.0X2	T49.0X3	T49.0X4	T49.0X5	T49.0X6
Chlorphenamine	T45.0X1	T45.0X2	T45.0X3	T45.0X4	T45.0X5	T45.0X6
Chlorphenesin	T42.8X1	T42.8X2	T42.8X3	T42.8X4	T42.8X5	T42.8X6
topical (antifungal)	T49.0X1	T49.0X2	T49.0X3	T49.0X4	T49.0X5	T49.0X6
Chlorpheniramine	T45.0X1	T45.0X2	T45.0X3	T45.0X4	T45.0X5	T45.0X6
Chlorphenoxamine	T45.0X1	T45.0X2	T45.0X3	T45.0X4	T45.0X5	T45.0X6
Chlorphentermine	T50.5X1	T50.5X2	T50.5X3	T50.5X4	T50.5X5	T50.5X6
Chlorprocaine — see Chloroprocaine						
Chlorproguanil	T37.2X1	T37.2X2	T37.2X3	T37.2X4	T37.2X5	T37.2X6
Chlorpromazine	T43.3X1	T43.3X2	T43.3X3	T43.3X4	T43.3X5	T43.3X6
Chlorpropamide	T38.3X1	T38.3X2	T38.3X3	T38.3X4	T38.3X5	T38.3X6
Chlorprothixene	T43.4X1	T43.4X2	T43.4X3	T43.4X4	T43.4X5	T43.4X6
Chlorquinaldol	T49.0X1	T49.0X2	T49.0X3	T49.0X4	T49.0X5	T49.0X6
Chlorquinol	T49.0X1	T49.0X2	T49.0X3	T49.0X4	T49.0X5	T49.0X6
Chlortalidone	T50.2X1	T50.2X2	T50.2X3	T50.2X4	T50.2X5	T50.2X6
Chlortetracycline	T36.4X1	T36.4X2	T36.4X3	T36.4X4	T36.4X5	T36.4X6
Chlorthalidone	T50.2X1	T50.2X2	T50.2X3	T50.2X4	T50.2X5	T50.2X6
Chlorthiophos	T60.0X1	T60.0X2	T60.0X3	T60.0X4	—	—
Chlorotrianisene	T38.5X1	T38.5X2	T38.5X3	T38.5X4	T38.5X5	T38.5X6
Chlor-Trimeton	T45.0X1	T45.0X2	T45.0X3	T45.0X4	T45.0X5	T45.0X6
Chlorthion	T60.0X1	T60.0X2	T60.0X3	T60.0X4	—	—
Chlorzoxazone	T42.8X1	T42.8X2	T42.8X3	T42.8X4	T42.8X5	T42.8X6
Choke damp	T59.7X1	T59.7X2	T59.7X3	T59.7X4	—	—
Cholagogues	T47.5X1	T47.5X2	T47.5X3	T47.5X4	T47.5X5	T47.5X6
Cholebrine	T50.8X1	T50.8X2	T50.8X3	T50.8X4	T50.8X5	T50.8X6
Cholecalciferol	T45.2X1	T45.2X2	T45.2X3	T45.2X4	T45.2X5	T45.2X6
Cholecystokinin	T50.8X1	T50.8X2	T50.8X3	T50.8X4	T50.8X5	T50.8X6
Cholera vaccine	T50.A91	T50.A92	T50.A93	T50.A94	T50.A95	T50.A96

	External Cause (T-Code)					
Substance	Poisoning, Accidental (Unintentional)	Poisoning, Intentional Self-Harm	Poisoning, Assault	Poisoning, Undetermined	Adverse Effect	Underdosing
Choleretic	T47.5X1	T47.5X2	T47.5X3	T47.5X4	T47.5X5	T47.5X6
Cholesterol-lowering agents	T46.6X1	T46.6X2	T46.6X3	T46.6X4	T46.6X5	T46.6X6
Cholestyramine (resin)	T46.6X1	T46.6X2	T46.6X3	T46.6X4	T46.6X5	T46.6X6
Cholic acid	T47.5X1	T47.5X2	T47.5X3	T47.5X4	T47.5X5	T47.5X6
Choline	T48.6X1	T48.6X2	T48.6X3	T48.6X4	T48.6X5	T48.6X6
chloride	T50.991	T50.992	T50.993	T50.994	T50.995	T50.996
dihydrogen citrate	T50.991	T50.992	T50.993	T50.994	T50.995	T50.996
salicylate	T39.091	T39.092	T39.093	T39.094	T39.095	T39.096
theophyllinate	T48.6X1	T48.6X2	T48.6X3	T48.6X4	T48.6X5	T48.6X6
Cholinergic (drug) NEC	T44.1X1	T44.1X2	T44.1X3	T44.1X4	T44.1X5	T44.1X6
muscle tone enhancer	T44.1X1	T44.1X2	T44.1X3	T44.1X4	T44.1X5	T44.1X6
organophosphorus	T44.0X1	T44.0X2	T44.0X3	T44.0X4	T44.0X5	T44.0X6
insecticide	T60.0X1	T60.0X2	T60.0X3	T60.0X4	—	—
nerve gas	T59.891	T59.892	T59.893	T59.894	—	—
trimethyl ammonium propanediol	T44.1X1	T44.1X2	T44.1X3	T44.1X4	T44.1X5	T44.1X6
Cholinesterase reactivator	T50.6X1	T50.6X2	T50.6X3	T50.6X4	T50.6X5	T50.6X6
Cholografin	T50.8X1	T50.8X2	T50.8X3	T50.8X4	T50.8X5	T50.8X6
Chorionic gonadotropin	T38.891	T38.892	T38.893	T38.894	T38.895	T38.896
Chromate	T56.2X1	T56.2X2	T56.2X3	T56.2X4	—	—
dust or mist	T56.2X1	T56.2X2	T56.2X3	T56.2X4	—	—
lead — see also Lead	T56.0X1	T56.0X2	T56.0X3	T56.0X4	—	—
paint	T56.0X1	T56.0X2	T56.0X3	T56.0X4	—	—
Chromic						
acid	T56.2X1	T56.2X2	T56.2X3	T56.2X4	—	—
dust or mist	T56.2X1	T56.2X2	T56.2X3	T56.2X4	—	—
phosphate 32P	T45.1X1	T45.1X2	T45.1X3	T45.1X4	T45.1X5	T45.1X6
Chromium	T56.2X1	T56.2X2	T56.2X3	T56.2X4	—	—
compounds — see Chromate						
sesquioxide	T50.8X1	T50.8X2	T50.8X3	T50.8X4	T50.8X5	T50.8X6
Chromomycin A3	T45.1X1	T45.1X2	T45.1X3	T45.1X4	T45.1X5	T45.1X6
Chromonar	T46.3X1	T46.3X2	T46.3X3	T46.3X4	T46.3X5	T46.3X6
Chromyl chloride	T56.2X1	T56.2X2	T56.2X3	T56.2X4	—	—
Chrysarobin	T49.4X1	T49.4X2	T49.4X3	T49.4X4	T49.4X5	T49.4X6
Chrysazin	T47.2X1	T47.2X2	T47.2X3	T47.2X4	T47.2X5	T47.2X6
Chymar	T45.3X1	T45.3X2	T45.3X3	T45.3X4	T45.3X5	T45.3X6
ophthalmic preparation	T49.5X1	T49.5X2	T49.5X3	T49.5X4	T49.5X5	T49.5X6
Chymopapain	T45.3X1	T45.3X2	T45.3X3	T45.3X4	T45.3X5	T45.3X6
Chymotrypsin	T45.3X1	T45.3X2	T45.3X3	T45.3X4	T45.3X5	T45.3X6
ophthalmic preparation	T49.5X1	T49.5X2	T49.5X3	T49.5X4	T49.5X5	T49.5X6
Cianidanol	T50.991	T50.992	T50.993	T50.994	T50.995	T50.996
Cianopramine	T43.011	T43.012	T43.013	T43.014	T43.015	T43.016
Cibenzoline	T46.2X1	T46.2X2	T46.2X3	T46.2X4	T46.2X5	T46.2X6

◀ New   ◀ Revised   ~~deleted~~ Deleted

Substance	External Cause (T-Code)					
	Poisoning, Accidental (Unintentional)	Poisoning, Intentional Self-Harm	Poisoning, Assault	Poisoning, Undetermined	Adverse Effect	Underdosing
Ciclacillin	T36.0X1	T36.0X2	T36.0X3	T36.0X4	T36.0X5	T36.0X6
Ciclobarbital — see Hexobarbital						
Ciclonicate	T46.7X1	T46.7X2	T46.7X3	T46.7X4	T46.7X5	T46.7X6
Ciclopirox (olamine)	T49.0X1	T49.0X2	T49.0X3	T49.0X4	T49.0X5	T49.0X6
Ciclosporin	T45.1X1	T45.1X2	T45.1X3	T45.1X4	T45.1X5	T45.1X6
Cicuta maculata or virosa	T62.2X1	T62.2X2	T62.2X3	T62.2X4	—	—
Cicutoxin	T62.2X1	T62.2X2	T62.2X3	T62.2X4	—	—
Cigarette lighter fluid	T52.0X1	T52.0X2	T52.0X3	T52.0X4	—	—
Cigarettes (tobacco)	T65.221	T65.222	T65.223	T65.224	—	—
Ciguatoxin	T61.01	T61.02	T61.03	T61.04	—	—
Cilazapril	T46.4X1	T46.4X2	T46.4X3	T46.4X4	T46.4X5	T46.4X6
Cimetidine	T47.0X1	T47.0X2	T47.0X3	T47.0X4	T47.0X5	T47.0X6
Cimetropium bromide	T44.3X1	T44.3X2	T44.3X3	T44.3X4	T44.3X5	T44.3X6
Cinchocaine	T41.3X1	T41.3X2	T41.3X3	T41.3X4	T41.3X5	T41.3X6
topical (surface)	T41.3X1	T41.3X2	T41.3X3	T41.3X4	T41.3X5	T41.3X6
Cinchona	T37.2X1	T37.2X2	T37.2X3	T37.2X4	T37.2X5	T37.2X6
Cinchonine alkaloids	T37.2X1	T37.2X2	T37.2X3	T37.2X4	T37.2X5	T37.2X6
Cinchophen	T50.4X1	T50.4X2	T50.4X3	T50.4X4	T50.4X5	T50.4X6
Cinepazide	T46.7X1	T46.7X2	T46.7X3	T46.7X4	T46.7X5	T46.7X6
Cinnamedrine	T48.5X1	T48.5X2	T48.5X3	T48.5X4	T48.5X5	T48.5X6
Cinnarizine	T45.0X1	T45.0X2	T45.0X3	T45.0X4	T45.0X5	T45.0X6
Cinoxacin	T37.8X1	T37.8X2	T37.8X3	T37.8X4	T37.8X5	T37.8X6
Ciprofibrate	T46.6X1	T46.6X2	T46.6X3	T46.6X4	T46.6X5	T46.6X6
Ciprofloxacin	T36.8X1	T36.8X2	T36.8X3	T36.8X4	T36.8X5	T36.8X6
Cisapride	T47.8X1	T47.8X2	T47.8X3	T47.8X4	T47.8X5	T47.8X6
Cisplatin	T45.1X1	T45.1X2	T45.1X3	T45.1X4	T45.1X5	T45.1X6
Citalopram	T43.221	T43.222	T43.223	T43.224	T43.225	T43.226
Citanest	T41.3X1	T41.3X2	T41.3X3	T41.3X4	T41.3X5	T41.3X6
infiltration (subcutaneous)	T41.3X1	T41.3X2	T41.3X3	T41.3X4	T41.3X5	T41.3X6
nerve block (peripheral) (plexus)	T41.3X1	T41.3X2	T41.3X3	T41.3X4	T41.3X5	T41.3X6
Citric acid	T47.5X1	T47.5X2	T47.5X3	T47.5X4	T47.5X5	T47.5X6
Citrovorum (factor)	T45.8X1	T45.8X2	T45.8X3	T45.8X4	T45.8X5	T45.8X6
Claviceps purpurea	T62.2X1	T62.2X2	T62.2X3	T62.2X4	—	—
Clavulanic acid	T36.1X1	T36.1X2	T36.1X3	T36.1X4	T36.1X5	T36.1X6
Cleaner, cleansing agent, type not specified	T65.891	T65.892	T65.893	T65.894	—	—
of paint or varnish	T52.91	T52.92	T52.93	T52.94	—	—
specified type NEC	T65.891	T65.892	T65.893	T65.894	—	—
Clebopride	T47.8X1	T47.8X2	T47.8X3	T47.8X4	T47.8X5	T47.8X6
Clefamide	T37.3X1	T37.3X2	T37.3X3	T37.3X4	T37.3X5	T37.3X6
Clemastine	T45.0X1	T45.0X2	T45.0X3	T45.0X4	T45.0X5	T45.0X6
Clematis vitalba	T62.2X1	T62.2X2	T62.2X3	T62.2X4		

Substance	External Cause (T-Code)					
	Poisoning, Accidental (Unintentional)	Poisoning, Intentional Self-Harm	Poisoning, Assault	Poisoning, Undetermined	Adverse Effect	Underdosing
Clemizole	T45.0X1	T45.0X2	T45.0X3	T45.0X4	T45.0X5	T45.0X6
penicillin	T36.0X1	T36.0X2	T36.0X3	T36.0X4	T36.0X5	T36.0X6
Clenbuterol	T48.6X1	T48.6X2	T48.6X3	T48.6X4	T48.6X5	T48.6X6
Clidinium bromide	T44.3X1	T44.3X2	T44.3X3	T44.3X4	T44.3X5	T44.3X6
Clindamycin	T36.8X1	T36.8X2	T36.8X3	T36.8X4	T36.8X5	T36.8X6
Clinofibrate	T46.6X1	T46.6X2	T46.6X3	T46.6X4	T46.6X5	T46.6X6
Clioquinol	T37.8X1	T37.8X2	T37.8X3	T37.8X4	T37.8X5	T37.8X6
Cliradon	T40.2X1	T40.2X2	T40.2X3	T40.2X4	—	—
Clobazam	T42.4X1	T42.4X2	T42.4X3	T42.4X4	T42.4X5	T42.4X6
Clobenzorex	T50.5X1	T50.5X2	T50.5X3	T50.5X4	T50.5X5	T50.5X6
Clobetasol	T49.0X1	T49.0X2	T49.0X3	T49.0X4	T49.0X5	T49.0X6
Clobetasone	T49.0X1	T49.0X2	T49.0X3	T49.0X4	T49.0X5	T49.0X6
Clobutinol	T48.3X1	T48.3X2	T48.3X3	T48.3X4	T48.3X5	T48.3X6
Clocapramine	T43.0X1	T43.0X2	T43.0X3	T43.0X4	T43.0X5	T43.0X6
Clocortolone	T38.0X1	T38.0X2	T38.0X3	T38.0X4	T38.0X5	T38.0X6
Clodantoin	T49.0X1	T49.0X2	T49.0X3	T49.0X4	T49.0X5	T49.0X6
Clodronic acid	T50.991	T50.992	T50.993	T50.994	T50.995	T50.996
Clofazimine	T37.1X1	T37.1X2	T37.1X3	T37.1X4	T37.1X5	T37.1X6
Clofedanol	T48.3X1	T48.3X2	T48.3X3	T48.3X4	T48.3X5	T48.3X6
Clofenamide	T50.2X1	T50.2X2	T50.2X3	T50.2X4	T50.2X5	T50.2X6
Clofenotane	T49.0X1	T49.0X2	T49.0X3	T49.0X4	T49.0X5	T49.0X6
Clofezone	T39.2X1	T39.2X2	T39.2X3	T39.2X4	T39.2X5	T39.2X6
Clofibrate	T46.6X1	T46.6X2	T46.6X3	T46.6X4	T46.6X5	T46.6X6
Clofibride	T46.6X1	T46.6X2	T46.6X3	T46.6X4	T46.6X5	T46.6X6
Cloforex	T50.5X1	T50.5X2	T50.5X3	T50.5X4	T50.5X5	T50.5X6
Clomacran	T43.0X1	T43.0X2	T43.0X3	T43.0X4	T43.0X5	T43.0X6
Clomethiazole	T42.6X1	T42.6X2	T42.6X3	T42.6X4	T42.6X5	T42.6X6
Clometocillin	T36.0X1	T36.0X2	T36.0X3	T36.0X4	T36.0X5	T36.0X6
Clomifene	T38.5X1	T38.5X2	T38.5X3	T38.5X4	T38.5X5	T38.5X6
Clomiphene	T38.5X1	T38.5X2	T38.5X3	T38.5X4	T38.5X5	T38.5X6
Clomipramine	T43.011	T43.012	T43.013	T43.014	T43.015	T43.016
Clomocycline	T36.4X1	T36.4X2	T36.4X3	T36.4X4	T36.4X5	T36.4X6
Clonazepam	T42.4X1	T42.4X2	T42.4X3	T42.4X4	T42.4X5	T42.4X6
Clonidine	T46.5X1	T46.5X2	T46.5X3	T46.5X4	T46.5X5	T46.5X6
Clonixin	T39.8X1	T39.8X2	T39.8X3	T39.8X4	T39.8X5	T39.8X6
Clopamide	T50.2X1	T50.2X2	T50.2X3	T50.2X4	T50.2X5	T50.2X6
Clopenthixol	T43.4X1	T43.4X2	T43.4X3	T43.4X4	T43.4X5	T43.4X6
Cloperastine	T48.3X1	T48.3X2	T48.3X3	T48.3X4	T48.3X5	T48.3X6
Clophedianol	T48.3X1	T48.3X2	T48.3X3	T48.3X4	T48.3X5	T48.3X6
Cloponone	T36.2X1	T36.2X2	T36.2X3	T36.2X4	T36.2X5	T36.2X6
Cloprednol	T38.0X1	T38.0X2	T38.0X3	T38.0X4	T38.0X5	T38.0X6
Cloral betaine	T42.6X1	T42.6X2	T42.6X3	T42.6X4	T42.6X5	T42.6X6

◀ New ◀ Revised ~~deleted~~ Deleted

TABLE OF DRUGS AND CHEMICALS

Substance	External Cause (T-Code)					
	Poisoning, Accidental (Unintentional)	Poisoning, Intentional Self-Harm	Poisoning, Assault	Poisoning, Undetermined	Adverse Effect	Underdosing
Cloramfenicol	T36.2X1	T36.2X2	T36.2X3	T36.2X4	T36.2X5	T36.2X6
Clorazepate (dipotassium)	T42.4X1	T42.4X2	T42.4X3	T42.4X4	T42.4X5	T42.4X6
Clorexolone	T50.2X1	T50.2X2	T50.2X3	T50.2X4	T50.2X5	T50.2X6
Clorox (bleach)	T54.91	T54.92	T54.93	T54.94	—	—
Clorfenamine	T45.0X1	T45.0X2	T45.0X3	T45.0X4	T45.0X5	T45.0X6
Clorgiline	T43.1X1	T43.1X2	T43.1X3	T43.1X4	T43.1X5	T43.1X6
Clorotepine	T44.3X1	T44.3X2	T44.3X3	T44.3X4	T44.3X5	T44.3X6
Clorprenaline	T48.6X1	T48.6X2	T48.6X3	T48.6X4	T48.6X5	T48.6X6
Clortermine	T50.5X1	T50.5X2	T50.5X3	T50.5X4	T50.5X5	T50.5X6
Clotiapine	T43.591	T43.592	T43.593	T43.594	T43.595	T43.596
Clotiazepam	T42.4X1	T42.4X2	T42.4X3	T42.4X4	T42.4X5	T42.4X6
Clotibric acid	T46.6X1	T46.6X2	T46.6X3	T46.6X4	T46.6X5	T46.6X6
Clotrimazole	T49.0X1	T49.0X2	T49.0X3	T49.0X4	T49.0X5	T49.0X6
Cloxacillin	T36.0X1	T36.0X2	T36.0X3	T36.0X4	T36.0X5	T36.0X6
Cloxazolam	T42.4X1	T42.4X2	T42.4X3	T42.4X4	T42.4X5	T42.4X6
Cloxiquine	T49.0X1	T49.0X2	T49.0X3	T49.0X4	T49.0X5	T49.0X6
Clozapine	T42.4X1	T42.4X2	T42.4X3	T42.4X4	T42.4X5	T42.4X6
Coagulant NEC	T45.7X1	T45.7X2	T45.7X3	T45.7X4	T45.7X5	T45.7X6
Coal (carbon monoxide from) — see also Carbon, monoxide, coal	T58.2X1	T58.2X2	T58.2X3	T58.2X4	—	—
oil — see Kerosene						
tar	T49.1X1	T49.1X2	T49.1X3	T49.1X4	T49.1X5	T49.1X6
fumes	T59.891	T59.892	T59.893	T59.894	—	—
medicinal (ointment)	T49.4X1	T49.4X2	T49.4X3	T49.4X4	T49.4X5	T49.4X6
analgesics NEC	T39.2X1	T39.2X2	T39.2X3	T39.2X4	T39.2X5	T39.2X6
naphtha (solvent)	T52.0X1	T52.0X2	T52.0X3	T52.0X4		
Cobalamine	T45.2X1	T45.2X2	T45.2X3	T45.2X4	T45.2X5	T45.2X6
Cobalt (nonmedicinal) (fumes) (industrial)	T56.891	T56.892	T56.893	T56.894		
medicinal (trace) (chloride)	T45.8X1	T45.8X2	T45.8X3	T45.8X4	T45.8X5	T45.8X6
Cobra (venom)	T63.041	T63.042	T63.043	T63.044		
Coca (leaf)	T40.5X1	T40.5X2	T40.5X3	T40.5X4	T40.5X5	T40.5X6
Cocaine	T40.5X1	T40.5X2	T40.5X3	T40.5X4	T40.5X5	T40.5X6
topical anesthetic	T41.3X1	T41.3X2	T41.3X3	T41.3X4	T41.3X5	T41.3X6
Cocarboxylase	T45.3X1	T45.3X2	T45.3X3	T45.3X4	T45.3X5	T45.3X6
Coccidioidin	T50.8X1	T50.8X2	T50.8X3	T50.8X4	T50.8X5	T50.8X6
Cocculus indicus	T62.1X1	T62.1X2	T62.1X3	T62.1X4		
Cochineal	T65.6X1	T65.6X2	T65.6X3	T65.6X4		
medicinal products	T50.991	T50.992	T50.993	T50.994	T50.995	T50.996
Codeine	T40.2X1	T40.2X2	T40.2X3	T40.2X4	T40.2X5	T40.2X6
Cod-liver oil	T45.2X1	T45.2X2	T45.2X3	T45.2X4	T45.2X5	T45.2X6

Substance	External Cause (T-Code)					
	Poisoning, Accidental (Unintentional)	Poisoning, Intentional Self-Harm	Poisoning, Assault	Poisoning, Undetermined	Adverse Effect	Underdosing
Coenzyme A	T50.991	T50.992	T50.993	T50.994	T50.995	T50.996
Coffee	T62.8X1	T62.8X2	T62.8X3	T62.8X4	—	—
Cogalactoisomerase	T50.991	T50.992	T50.993	T50.994	T50.995	T50.996
Cogentin	T44.3X1	T44.3X2	T44.3X3	T44.3X4	T44.3X5	T44.3X6
Coke fumes or gas (carbon monoxide)	T58.2X1	T58.2X2	T58.2X3	T58.2X4	—	—
industrial use	T58.8X1	T58.8X2	T58.8X3	T58.8X4	—	—
Colace	T47.4X1	T47.4X2	T47.4X3	T47.4X4	T47.4X5	T47.4X6
Colaspase	T45.1X1	T45.1X2	T45.1X3	T45.1X4	T45.1X5	T45.1X6
Colchicine	T50.4X1	T50.4X2	T50.4X3	T50.4X4	T50.4X5	T50.4X6
Colchicum	T62.2X1	T62.2X2	T62.2X3	T62.2X4	—	—
Cold cream	T49.3X1	T49.3X2	T49.3X3	T49.3X4	T49.3X5	T49.3X6
Colecalciferol	T45.2X1	T45.2X2	T45.2X3	T45.2X4	T45.2X5	T45.2X6
Colestipol	T46.6X1	T46.6X2	T46.6X3	T46.6X4	T46.6X5	T46.6X6
Colestyramine	T46.6X1	T46.6X2	T46.6X3	T46.6X4	T46.6X5	T46.6X6
Colimycin	T36.8X1	T36.8X2	T36.8X3	T36.8X4	T36.8X5	T36.8X6
Colistimethate	T36.8X1	T36.8X2	T36.8X3	T36.8X4	T36.8X5	T36.8X6
Colistin	T36.8X1	T36.8X2	T36.8X3	T36.8X4	T36.8X5	T36.8X6
sulfate (eye preparation)	T49.5X1	T49.5X2	T49.5X3	T49.5X4	T49.5X5	T49.5X6
Collagen	T50.991	T50.992	T50.993	T50.994	T50.995	T50.996
Collagenase	T49.4X1	T49.4X2	T49.4X3	T49.4X4	T49.4X5	T49.4X6
Collodion	T49.3X1	T49.3X2	T49.3X3	T49.3X4	T49.3X5	T49.3X6
Colocynth	T47.2X1	T47.2X2	T47.2X3	T47.2X4	T47.2X5	T47.2X6
Colophony adhesive	T49.3X1	T49.3X2	T49.3X3	T49.3X4	T49.3X5	T49.3X6
Colorant — see also Dye	T50.991	T50.992	T50.993	T50.994	T50.995	T50.996
Coloring matter — see Dye(s)						
Combustion gas (after combustion) — see Carbon, monoxide						
prior to combustion	T59.891	T59.892	T59.893	T59.894	—	—
Compazine	T43.3X1	T43.3X2	T43.3X3	T43.3X4	T43.3X5	T43.3X6
Compound						
42 (warfarin)	T60.4X1	T60.4X2	T60.4X3	T60.4X4	—	—
269 (endrin)	T60.1X1	T60.1X2	T60.1X3	T60.1X4	—	—
497 (dieldrin)	T60.1X1	T60.1X2	T60.1X3	T60.1X4	—	—
1080 (sodium fluoroacetate)	T60.4X1	T60.4X2	T60.4X3	T60.4X4	—	—
3422 (parathion)	T60.0X1	T60.0X2	T60.0X3	T60.0X4	—	—
3911 (phorate)	T60.0X1	T60.0X2	T60.0X3	T60.0X4	—	—
3956 (toxaphene)	T60.1X1	T60.1X2	T60.1X3	T60.1X4	—	—
4049 (malathion)	T60.0X1	T60.0X2	T60.0X3	T60.0X4	—	—
4069 (malathion)	T60.0X1	T60.0X2	T60.0X3	T60.0X4	—	—
4124 (dicapthon)	T60.0X1	T60.0X2	T60.0X3	T60.0X4	—	—

◀ New ◀ Revised ~~deleted~~ Deleted

	External Cause (T-Code)					
Substance	Poisoning, Accidental (Unintentional)	Poisoning, Intentional Self-Harm	Poisoning, Assault	Poisoning, Undetermined	Adverse Effect	Underdosing
Compound *(Continued)*						
E (cortisone)	T38.0X1	T38.0X2	T38.0X3	T38.0X4	T38.0X5	T38.0X6
F (hydrocortisone)	T38.0X1	T38.0X2	T38.0X3	T38.0X4	T38.0X5	T38.0X6
Congener, anabolic	T38.7X1	T38.7X2	T38.7X3	T38.7X4	T38.7X5	T38.7X6
Congo red	T50.8X1	T50.8X2	T50.8X3	T50.8X4	T50.8X5	T50.8X6
Coniine, conine	T62.2X1	T62.2X2	T62.2X3	T62.2X4	—	—
Conium (maculatum)	T62.2X1	T62.2X2	T62.2X3	T62.2X4	—	—
Conjugated estrogenic substances	T38.5X1	T38.5X2	T38.5X3	T38.5X4	T38.5X5	T38.5X6
Contac	T48.5X1	T48.5X2	T48.5X3	T48.5X4	T48.5X5	T48.5X6
Contact lens solution	T49.5X1	T49.5X2	T49.5X3	T49.5X4	T49.5X5	T49.5X6
Contraceptive (oral)	T38.4X1	T38.4X2	T38.4X3	T38.4X4	T38.4X5	T38.4X6
vaginal	T49.8X1	T49.8X2	T49.8X3	T49.8X4	T49.8X5	T19.8X6
Contrast medium, radiography	T50.8X1	T50.8X2	T50.8X3	T50.8X4	T50.8X5	T50.8X6
Convallaria glycosides	T46.0X1	T46.0X2	T46.0X3	T46.0X4	T46.0X5	T46.0X6
Convallaria majalis	T62.2X1	T62.2X2	T62.2X3	T62.2X4		—
berry	T62.1X1	T62.1X2	T62.1X3	T62.1X4	—	—
Copper (dust) (fumes) (nonmedicinal) NEC	T56.4X1	T56.4X2	T56.4X3	T56.4X4	—	—
arsenate, arsenite	T57.0X1	T57.0X2	T57.0X3	T57.0X4	—	—
insecticide	T60.2X1	T60.2X2	T60.2X3	T60.2X4	—	—
emetic	T47.7X1	T47.7X2	T47.7X3	T47.7X4	147.7X5	T47.7X6
fungicide	T60.3X1	T60.3X2	T60.3X3	T60.3X4	—	—
gluconate	T49.0X1	T49.0X2	T49.0X3	T49.0X4	T49.0X5	T49.0X6
insecticide	T60.2X1	T60.2X2	T60.2X3	T60.2X4	—	—
medicinal (trace)	T45.8X1	T45.8X2	T45.8X3	T45.8X4	T45.8X5	T45.8X6
oleate	T49.0X1	T49.0X2	T49.0X3	T49.0X4	T49.0X5	T49.0X6
sulfate	T56.4X1	T56.4X2	T56.4X3	T56.4X4	—	—
cupric	T56.4X1	T56.4X2	T56.4X3	T56.4X4	—	—
fungicide	T60.3X1	T60.3X2	T60.3X3	T60.3X4	—	—
medicinal						
ear	T49.6X1	T49.6X2	T49.6X3	T49.6X4	T49.6X5	T49.6X6
emetic	T47.7X1	T47.7X2	T47.7X3	T47.7X4	T47.7X5	T47.7X6
eye	T49.5X1	T49.5X2	T49.5X3	T49.5X4	T49.5X5	T49.5X6
cuprous	T56.4X1	T56.4X2	T56.4X3	T56.4X4	—	—
fungicide	T60.3X1	T60.3X2	T60.3X3	T60.3X4	—	—
medicinal						
ear	T49.6X1	T49.6X2	T49.6X3	T49.6X4	T49.6X5	T49.6X6
emetic	T47.7X1	T47.7X2	T47.7X3	T47.7X4	T47.7X5	T47.7X6
eye	T49.5X1	T49.5X2	T49.5X3	T49.5X4	T49.5X5	T49.5X6
Copperhead snake (bite) (venom)	T63.061	T63.062	T63.063	T63.064	—	—
Coral (sting)	T63.691	T63.692	T63.693	T63.694	—	—
snake (bite) (venom)	T63.021	T63.022	T63.023	T63.024	—	—

	External Cause (T-Code)					
Substance	Poisoning, Accidental (Unintentional)	Poisoning, Intentional Self-Harm	Poisoning, Assault	Poisoning, Undetermined	Adverse Effect	Underdosing
Corbadrine	T49.6X1	T49.6X2	T49.6X3	T49.6X4	T49.6X5	T49.6X6
Cordran	T49.0X1	T49.0X2	T49.0X3	T49.0X4	T49.0X5	T49.0X6
Cordite	T65.891	T65.892	T65.893	T65.894	—	—
vapor	T59.891	T59.892	T59.893	T59.894	—	—
Corn cures	T49.4X1	T49.4X2	T49.4X3	T49.4X4	T49.4X5	T49.4X6
Cornhusker's lotion	T49.3X1	T49.3X2	T49.3X3	T49.3X4	T49.3X5	T49.3X6
Corn starch	T49.3X1	T49.3X2	T49.3X3	T49.3X4	T49.3X5	T49.3X6
Coronary vasodilator NEC	T46.3X1	T46.3X2	T46.3X3	T46.3X4	T46.3X5	T46.3X6
Corrosive NEC	T54.91	T54.92	T54.93	T54.94	—	—
acid NEC	T54.2X1	T54.2X2	T54.2X3	T54.2X4	—	—
aromatics	T54.1X1	T54.1X2	T54.1X3	T54.1X4		
disinfectant	T54.1X1	T54.1X2	T54.1X3	T54.1X4		
fumes NEC	T54.91	T54.92	T54.93	T54.94	—	—
specified NEC	T54.91	T54.92	T54.93	T54.94	—	—
sublimate	T56.1X1	T56.1X2	T56.1X3	T56.1X4	—	—
Cortate	T38.0X1	T38.0X2	T38.0X3	T38.0X4	T38.0X5	T38.0X6
Cort-Dome	T38.0X1	T38.0X2	T38.0X3	T38.0X4	T38.0X5	T38.0X6
ENT agent	T49.6X1	T49.6X2	T49.6X3	T49.6X4	T49.6X5	T49.6X6
ophthalmic preparation	T49.5X1	T49.5X2	T49.5X3	T49.5X4	T49.5X5	T49.5X6
topical NEC	T49.0X1	T49.0X2	T49.0X3	T49.0X4	T49.0X5	T49.0X6
Cortef	T38.0X1	T38.0X2	T38.0X3	T38.0X4	T38.0X5	T38.0X6
ENT agent	T49.6X1	T49.6X2	T49.6X3	T49.6X4	T49.6X5	T49.6X6
ophthalmic preparation	T49.5X1	T49.5X2	T49.5X3	T49.5X4	T49.5X5	T49.5X6
topical NEC	T49.0X1	T49.0X2	T49.0X3	T49.0X4	T49.0X5	T49.0X6
Corticosteroid	T38.0X1	T38.0X2	T38.0X3	T38.0X4	T38.0X5	T38.0X6
ENT agent	T49.6X1	T49.6X2	T49.6X3	T49.6X4	T49.6X5	T49.6X6
mineral	T50.0X1	T50.0X2	T50.0X3	T50.0X4	T50.0X5	T50.0X6
ophthalmic	T49.5X1	T49.5X2	T49.5X3	T49.5X4	T49.5X5	T49.5X6
topical NEC	T49.0X1	T49.0X2	T49.0X3	T49.0X4	T49.0X5	T49.0X6
Corticotropin	T38.811	T38.812	T38.813	T38.814	T38.815	T38.816
Cortisol	T49.0X1	T49.0X2	T49.0X3	T49.0X4	T49.0X5	T49.0X6
ENT agent	T49.6X1	T49.6X2	T49.6X3	T49.6X4	T49.6X5	T49.6X6
ophthalmic preparation	T49.5X1	T49.5X2	T49.5X3	T49.5X4	T49.5X5	T49.5X6
topical NEC	T49.0X1	T49.0X2	T49.0X3	T49.0X4	T49.0X5	T49.0X6
Cortisone (acetate)	T38.0X1	T38.0X2	T38.0X3	T38.0X4	T38.0X5	T38.0X6
ENT agent	T49.6X1	T49.6X2	T49.6X3	T49.6X4	T49.6X5	T49.6X6
ophthalmic preparation	T49.5X1	T49.5X2	T49.5X3	T49.5X4	T49.5X5	T49.5X6
topical NEC	T49.0X1	T49.0X2	T49.0X3	T49.0X4	T49.0X5	T49.0X6
Cortivazol	T38.0X1	T38.0X2	T38.0X3	T38.0X4	T38.0X5	T38.0X6
Cortogen	T38.0X1	T38.0X2	T38.0X3	T38.0X4	T38.0X5	T38.0X6
ENT agent	T49.6X1	T49.6X2	T49.6X3	T49.6X4	T49.6X5	T49.6X6
ophthalmic preparation	T49.5X1	T49.5X2	T49.5X3	T49.5X4	T49.5X5	T49.5X6

◀ New   ◀ Revised   ~~deleted~~ Deleted

TABLE OF DRUGS AND CHEMICALS

TABLE OF DRUGS AND CHEMICALS

Substance	External Cause (T-Code) Poisoning, Accidental (Unintentional)	Poisoning, Intentional Self-Harm	Poisoning, Assault	Poisoning, Undetermined	Adverse Effect	Underdosing
Cortone	T38.0X1	T38.0X2	T38.0X3	T38.0X4	T38.0X5	T38.0X6
ENT agent	T49.6X1	T49.6X2	T49.6X3	T49.6X4	T49.6X5	T49.6X6
ophthalmic preparation	T49.5X1	T49.5X2	T49.5X3	T49.5X4	T49.5X5	T49.5X6
Cortril	T38.0X1	T38.0X2	T38.0X3	T38.0X4	T38.0X5	T38.0X6
ENT agent	T49.6X1	T49.6X2	T49.6X3	T49.6X4	T49.6X5	T49.6X6
ophthalmic preparation	T49.5X1	T49.5X2	T49.5X3	T49.5X4	T49.5X5	T49.5X6
topical NEC	T49.0X1	T49.0X2	T49.0X3	T49.0X4	T49.0X5	T49.0X6
Corynebacterium parvum	T45.1X1	T45.1X2	T45.1X3	T45.1X4	T45.1X5	T45.1X6
Cosmetic preparation	T49.8X1	T49.8X2	T49.8X3	T49.8X4	T49.8X5	T49.8X6
Cosmetics	T49.8X1	T49.8X2	T49.8X3	T49.8X4	T49.8X5	T49.8X6
Cosyntropin	T38.811	T38.812	T38.813	T38.814	T38.815	T38.816
Cotarnine	T45.7X1	T45.7X2	T45.7X3	T45.7X4	T45.7X5	T45.7X6
Co-trimoxazole	T36.8X1	T36.8X2	T36.8X3	T36.8X4	T36.8X5	T36.8X6
Cottonseed oil	T49.3X1	T49.3X2	T49.3X3	T49.3X4	T49.3X5	T49.3X6
Cough mixture (syrup)	T48.4X1	T48.4X2	T48.4X3	T48.4X4	T48.4X5	T48.4X6
containing opiates	T40.2X1	T40.2X2	T40.2X3	T40.2X4	T40.2X5	T40.2X6
expectorants	T48.4X1	T48.4X2	T48.4X3	T48.4X4	T48.4X5	T48.4X6
Coumadin	T45.511	T45.512	T45.513	T45.514	T45.515	T45.516
rodenticide	T60.4X1	T60.4X2	T60.4X3	T60.4X4	—	—
Coumaphos	T60.0X1	T60.0X2	T60.0X3	T60.0X4	—	—
Coumarin	T45.511	T45.512	T45.513	T45.514	T45.515	T45.516
Coumetarol	T45.511	T45.512	T45.513	T45.514	T45.515	T45.516
Cowbane	T62.2X1	T62.2X2	T62.2X3	T62.2X4	—	—
Cozyme	T45.2X1	T45.2X2	T45.2X3	T45.2X4	T45.2X5	T45.2X6
Crack	T40.5X1	T40.5X2	T40.5X3	T40.5X4	—	—
Crataegus extract	T46.0X1	T46.0X2	T46.0X3	T46.0X4	T46.0X5	T46.0X6
Creolin	T54.1X1	T54.1X2	T54.1X3	T54.1X4	—	—
disinfectant	T54.1X1	T54.1X2	T54.1X3	T54.1X4	—	—
Creosol (compound)	T49.0X1	T49.0X2	T49.0X3	T49.0X4	T49.0X5	T49.0X6
Creosote (coal tar) (beechwood)	T49.0X1	T49.0X2	T49.0X3	T49.0X4	T49.0X5	T49.0X6
medicinal (expectorant)	T48.4X1	T48.4X2	T48.4X3	T48.4X4	T48.4X5	T48.4X6
syrup	T48.4X1	T48.4X2	T48.4X3	T48.4X4	T48.4X5	T48.4X6
Cresol(s)	T49.0X1	T49.0X2	T49.0X3	T49.0X4	T49.0X5	T49.0X6
and soap solution	T49.0X1	T49.0X2	T49.0X3	T49.0X4	T49.0X5	T49.0X6
Cresyl acetate	T49.0X1	T49.0X2	T49.0X3	T49.0X4	T49.0X5	T49.0X6
Cresylic acid	T49.0X1	T49.0X2	T49.0X3	T49.0X4	T49.0X5	T49.0X6
Crimidine	T60.4X1	T60.4X2	T60.4X3	T60.4X4	—	—
Croconazole	T37.8X1	T37.8X2	T37.8X3	T37.8X4	T37.8X5	T37.8X6
Cromoglicic acid	T48.6X1	T48.6X2	T48.6X3	T48.6X4	T48.6X5	T48.6X6
Cromolyn	T48.6X1	T48.6X2	T48.6X3	T48.6X4	T48.6X5	T48.6X6
Cromonar	T46.3X1	T46.3X2	T46.3X3	T46.3X4	T46.3X5	T46.3X6

Substance	External Cause (T-Code) Poisoning, Accidental (Unintentional)	Poisoning, Intentional Self-Harm	Poisoning, Assault	Poisoning, Undetermined	Adverse Effect	Underdosing
Cropropamide	T39.8X1	T39.8X2	T39.8X3	T39.8X4	T39.8X5	T39.8X6
with crotethamide	T50.7X1	T50.7X2	T50.7X3	T50.7X4	T50.7X5	T50.7X6
Crotamiton	T49.0X1	T49.0X2	T49.0X3	T49.0X4	T49.0X5	T49.0X6
Crotethamide	T39.8X1	T39.8X2	T39.8X3	T39.8X4	T39.8X5	T39.8X6
with cropropamide	T50.7X1	T50.7X2	T50.7X3	T50.7X4	T50.7X5	T50.7X6
Croton (oil)	T47.2X1	T47.2X2	T47.2X3	T47.2X4	T47.2X5	T47.2X6
chloral	T42.6X1	T42.6X2	T42.6X3	T42.6X4	T42.6X5	T42.6X6
Crude oil	T52.0X1	T52.0X2	T52.0X3	T52.0X4	—	—
Cryogenine	T39.8X1	T39.8X2	T39.8X3	T39.8X4	T39.8X5	T39.8X6
Cryolite (vapor)	T60.1X1	T60.1X2	T60.1X3	T60.1X4	—	—
insecticide	T60.1X1	T60.1X2	T60.1X3	T60.1X4	—	—
Cryptenamine (tannates)	T46.5X1	T46.5X2	T46.5X3	T46.5X4	T46.5X5	T46.5X6
Crystal violet	T49.0X1	T49.0X2	T49.0X3	T49.0X4	T49.0X5	T49.0X6
Cuckoopint	T62.2X1	T62.2X2	T62.2X3	T62.2X4	—	—
Cumetharol	T45.511	T45.512	T45.513	T45.514	T45.515	T45.516
Cupric						
acetate	T60.3X1	T60.3X2	T60.3X3	T60.3X4	—	—
acetoarsenite	T57.0X1	T57.0X2	T57.0X3	T57.0X4	—	—
arsenate	T57.0X1	T57.0X2	T57.0X3	T57.0X4	—	—
gluconate	T49.0X1	T49.0X2	T49.0X3	T49.0X4	T49.0X5	T49.0X6
oleate	T49.0X1	T49.0X2	T49.0X3	T49.0X4	T49.0X5	T49.0X6
sulfate	T56.4X1	T56.4X2	T56.4X3	T56.4X4	—	—
Cuprous sulfate — see also Copper sulfate	T56.4X1	T56.4X2	T56.4X3	T56.4X4	—	—
Curare, curarine	T48.1X1	T48.1X2	T48.1X3	T48.1X4	T48.1X5	T48.1X6
Cyamemazine	T43.3X1	T43.3X2	T43.3X3	T43.3X4	T43.3X5	T43.3X6
Cyamopsis tetragono-loba	T46.6X1	T46.6X2	T46.6X3	T46.6X4	T46.6X5	T46.6X6
Cyanacetyl hydrazide	T37.1X1	T37.1X2	T37.1X3	T37.1X4	T37.1X5	T37.1X6
Cyanic acid (gas)	T59.891	T59.892	T59.893	T59.894	—	—
Cyanide(s) (compounds) (potassium) (sodium) NEC	T65.0X1	T65.0X2	T65.0X3	T65.0X4	—	—
dust or gas (inhalation) NEC	T57.3X1	T57.3X2	T57.3X3	T57.3X4	—	—
fumigant	T65.0X1	T65.0X2	T65.0X3	T65.0X4	—	—
hydrogen	T57.3X1	T57.3X2	T57.3X3	T57.3X4	—	—
mercuric — see Mercury						
pesticide (dust) (fumes)	T65.0X1	T65.0X2	T65.0X3	T65.0X4	—	—
Cyanoacrylate adhesive	T49.3X1	T49.3X2	T49.3X3	T49.3X4	T49.3X5	T49.3X6
Cyanocobalamin	T45.8X1	T45.8X2	T45.8X3	T45.8X4	T45.8X5	T45.8X6
Cyanogen (chloride) (gas) NEC	T59.891	T59.892	T59.893	T59.894	—	—
Cyclacillin	T36.0X1	T36.0X2	T36.0X3	T36.0X4	T36.0X5	T36.0X6
Cyclaine	T41.3X1	T41.3X2	T41.3X3	T41.3X4	T41.3X5	T41.3X6
Cyclamate	T50.991	T50.992	T50.993	T50.994	T50.995	T50.996

◀ New ◀ Revised ~~deleted~~ Deleted

Substance	Poisoning, Accidental (Unintentional)	Poisoning, Intentional Self-Harm	Poisoning, Assault	Poisoning, Undetermined	Adverse Effect	Underdosing
Cyclamen europaeum	T62.2X1	T62.2X2	T62.2X3	T62.2X4	—	—
Cyclandelate	T46.7X1	T46.7X2	T46.7X3	T46.7X4	T46.7X5	T46.7X6
Cyclazocine	T50.7X1	T50.7X2	T50.7X3	T50.7X4	T50.7X5	T50.7X6
Cyclizine	T45.0X1	T45.0X2	T45.0X3	T45.0X4	T45.0X5	T45.0X6
Cyclobarbital	T42.3X1	T42.3X2	T42.3X3	T42.3X4	T42.3X5	T42.3X6
Cyclobarbitone	T42.3X1	T42.3X2	T42.3X3	T42.3X4	T42.3X5	T42.3X6
Cyclobenzaprine	T48.1X1	T48.1X2	T48.1X3	T48.1X4	T48.1X5	T48.1X6
Cyclodrine	T44.3X1	T44.3X2	T44.3X3	T44.3X4	T44.3X5	T44.3X6
Cycloguanil embonate	T37.2X1	T37.2X2	T37.2X3	T37.2X4	T37.2X5	T37.2X6
Cycloheptadiene	T43.291	T43.292	T43.293	T43.294	T43.295	T43.296
Cyclohexane	T52.8X1	T52.8X2	T52.8X3	T52.8X4	—	—
Cyclohexanol	T51.8X1	T51.8X2	T51.8X3	T51.8X4	—	—
Cyclohexanone	T52.4X1	T52.4X2	T52.4X3	T52.4X4	—	—
Cycloheximide	T60.3X1	T60.3X2	T60.3X3	T60.3X4	—	—
Cyclohexyl acetate	T52.8X1	T52.8X2	T52.8X3	T52.8X4	—	—
Cycloleucin	T45.1X1	T45.1X2	T45.1X3	T45.1X4	T45.1X5	T45.1X6
Cyclomethycaine	T41.3X1	T41.3X2	T41.3X3	T41.3X4	T41.3X5	T41.3X6
Cyclopentamine	T44.4X1	T44.4X2	T44.4X3	T44.4X4	T44.4X5	T44.4X6
Cyclopenthiazide	T50.2X1	T50.2X2	T50.2X3	T50.2X4	T50.2X5	T50.2X6
Cyclopentolate	T44.3X1	T44.3X2	T44.3X3	T44.3X4	T44.3X5	T44.3X6
Cyclophosphamide	T45.1X1	T45.1X2	T45.1X3	T45.1X4	T45.1X5	T45.1X6
Cycloplegic drug	T49.5X1	T49.5X2	T49.5X3	T49.5X4	T49.5X5	T49.5X6
Cyclopropane	T41.291	T41.292	T41.293	T41.294	T41.295	T41.296
Cyclopyrabital	T39.8X1	T39.8X2	T39.8X3	T39.8X4	T39.8X5	T39.8X6
Cycloserine	T37.1X1	T37.1X2	T37.1X3	T37.1X4	T37.1X5	T37.1X6
Cyclosporin	T45.1X1	T45.1X2	T45.1X3	T45.1X4	T45.1X5	T45.1X6
Cyclothiazide	T50.2X1	T50.2X2	T50.2X3	T50.2X4	T50.2X5	T50.2X6
Cycrimine	T44.3X1	T44.3X2	T44.3X3	T44.3X4	T44.3X5	T44.3X6
Cyhalothrin	T60.1X1	T60.1X2	T60.1X3	T60.1X4	—	—
Cymarin	T46.0X1	T46.0X2	T46.0X3	T46.0X4	T46.0X5	T46.0X6
Cypermethrin	T60.1X1	T60.1X2	T60.1X3	T60.1X4	—	—
Cyphenothrin	T60.2X1	T60.2X2	T60.2X3	T60.2X4	—	—
Cyproheptadine	T45.0X1	T45.0X2	T45.0X3	T45.0X4	T45.0X5	T45.0X6
Cyprolidol	T43.291	T43.292	T43.293	T43.294	T43.295	T43.296
Cyproterone	T38.6X1	T38.6X2	T38.6X3	T38.6X4	T38.6X5	T38.6X6
Cysteamine	T50.6X1	T50.6X2	T50.6X3	T50.6X4	T50.6X5	T50.6X6
Cytarabine	T45.1X1	T45.1X2	T45.1X3	T45.1X4	T45.1X5	T45.1X6
Cytisus						
laburnum	T62.2X1	T62.2X2	T62.2X3	T62.2X4	—	—
scoparius	T62.2X1	T62.2X2	T62.2X3	T62.2X4	—	—
Cytochrome C	T47.5X1	T47.5X2	T47.5X3	T47.5X4	T47.5X5	T47.5X6
Cytomel	T38.1X1	T38.1X2	T38.1X3	T38.1X4	T38.1X5	T38.1X6

Substance	Poisoning, Accidental (Unintentional)	Poisoning, Intentional Self-Harm	Poisoning, Assault	Poisoning, Undetermined	Adverse Effect	Underdosing
Cytosine arabinoside	T45.1X1	T45.1X2	T45.1X3	T45.1X4	T45.1X5	T45.1X6
Cytoxan	T45.1X1	T45.1X2	T45.1X3	T45.1X4	T45.1X5	T45.1X6
Cytozyme	T45.7X1	T45.7X2	T45.7X3	T45.7X4	T45.7X5	T45.7X6
2,4-D	T60.3X1	T60.3X2	T60.3X3	T60.3X4	—	—
D						
Dacarbazine	T45.1X1	T45.1X2	T45.1X3	T45.1X4	T45.1X5	T45.1X6
Dactinomycin	T45.1X1	T45.1X2	T45.1X3	T45.1X4	T45.1X5	T45.1X6
DADPS	T37.1X1	T37.1X2	T37.1X3	T37.1X4	T37.1X5	T37.1X6
Dakin's solution	T49.0X1	T49.0X2	T49.0X3	T49.0X4	T49.0X5	T49.0X6
Dalapon (sodium)	T60.3X1	T60.3X2	T60.3X3	T60.3X4	—	—
Dalmane	T42.4X1	T42.4X2	T42.4X3	T42.4X4	T42.4X5	T42.4X6
Danazol	T38.6X1	T38.6X2	T38.6X3	T38.6X4	T38.6X5	T38.6X6
Danilone	T45.511	T45.512	T45.513	T45.514	T45.515	T45.516
Danthron	T47.2X1	T47.2X2	T47.2X3	T47.2X4	T47.2X5	T47.2X6
Dantrolene	T42.8X1	T42.8X2	T42.8X3	T42.8X4	T42.8X5	T42.8X6
Dantron	T47.2X1	T47.2X2	T47.2X3	T47.2X4	T47.2X5	T47.2X6
Daphne (gnidium) (mezereum)	T62.2X1	T62.2X2	T62.2X3	T62.2X4	—	—
berry	T62.1X1	T62.1X2	T62.1X3	T62.1X4	—	—
Dapsone	T37.1X1	T37.1X2	T37.1X3	T37.1X4	T37.1X5	T37.1X6
Daraprim	T37.2X1	T37.2X2	T37.2X3	T37.2X4	T37.2X5	T37.2X6
Darnel	T62.2X1	T62.2X2	T62.2X3	T62.2X4	—	—
Darvon	T39.8X1	T39.8X2	T39.8X3	T39.8X4	T39.8X5	T39.8X6
Daunomycin	T45.1X1	T45.1X2	T45.1X3	T45.1X4	T45.1X5	T45.1X6
Daunorubicin	T45.1X1	T45.1X2	T45.1X3	T45.1X4	T45.1X5	T45.1X6
DBI	T38.3X1	T38.3X2	T38.3X3	T38.3X4	T38.3X5	T38.3X6
D-Con	T60.91	T60.92	T60.93	T60.94	—	—
insecticide	T60.2X1	T60.2X2	T60.2X3	T60.2X4	—	—
rodenticide	T60.4X1	T60.4X2	T60.4X3	T60.4X4	—	—
DDAVP	T38.891	T38.892	T38.893	T38.894	T38.895	T38.896
DDE (bis(chlorophenyl)-dichloroethylene)	T60.2X1	T60.2X2	T60.2X3	T60.2X4		
DDS	T37.1X1	T37.1X2	T37.1X3	T37.1X4	T37.1X5	T37.1X6
DDT (dust)	T60.1X1	T60.1X2	T60.1X3	T60.1X4	—	—
Deadly nightshade—see also Belladonna	T62.2X1	T62.2X2	T62.2X3	T62.2X4		
berry	T62.1X1	T62.1X2	T62.1X3	T62.1X4	—	—
Deamino-D-arginine vasopressin	T38.891	T38.892	T38.893	T38.894	T38.895	T38.896
Deanol (aceglumate)	T50.991	T50.992	T50.993	T50.994	T50.995	T50.996
Debrisoquine	T46.5X1	T46.5X2	T46.5X3	T46.5X4	T46.5X5	T46.5X6
Decaborane	T57.8X1	T57.8X2	T57.8X3	T57.8X4	—	—
fumes	T59.891	T59.892	T59.893	T59.894	—	—

◀ New   ◀ Revised   ~~deleted~~ Deleted

TABLE OF DRUGS AND CHEMICALS

Substance	Poisoning, Accidental (Unintentional)	Poisoning, Intentional Self-Harm	Poisoning, Assault	Poisoning, Undetermined	Adverse Effect	Underdosing
Decadron	T38.0X1	T38.0X2	T38.0X3	T38.0X4	T38.0X5	T38.0X6
ENT agent	T49.6X1	T49.6X2	T49.6X3	T49.6X4	T49.6X5	T49.6X6
ophthalmic preparation	T49.5X1	T49.5X2	T49.5X3	T49.5X4	T49.5X5	T49.5X6
topical NEC	T49.0X1	T49.0X2	T49.0X3	T49.0X4	T49.0X5	T49.0X6
Decahydronaphthalene	T52.8X1	T52.8X2	T52.8X3	T52.8X4	—	—
Decalin	T52.8X1	T52.8X2	T52.8X3	T52.8X4	—	—
Decamethonium (bromide)	T48.1X1	T48.1X2	T48.1X3	T48.1X4	T48.1X5	T48.1X6
Decholin	T47.5X1	T47.5X2	T47.5X3	T47.5X4	T47.5X5	T47.5X6
Declomycin	T36.4X1	T36.4X2	T36.4X3	T36.4X4	T36.4X5	T36.4X6
Decongestant, nasal (mucosa)	T48.5X1	T48.5X2	T48.5X3	T48.5X4	T48.5X5	T48.5X6
combination	T48.5X1	T48.5X2	T48.5X3	T48.5X4	T48.5X5	T48.5X6
Deet	T60.8X1	T60.8X2	T60.8X3	T60.8X4	—	—
Deferoxamine	T45.8X1	T45.8X2	T45.8X3	T45.8X4	T45.8X5	T45.8X6
Deflazacort	T38.0X1	T38.0X2	T38.0X3	T38.0X4	T38.0X5	T38.0X6
Deglycyrrhizinized extract of licorice	T48.4X1	T48.4X2	T48.4X3	T48.4X4	T48.4X5	T48.4X6
Dehydrocholic acid	T47.5X1	T47.5X2	T47.5X3	T47.5X4	T47.5X5	T47.5X6
Dehydroemetine	T37.3X1	T37.3X2	T37.3X3	T37.3X4	T37.3X5	T37.3X6
Dekalin	T52.8X1	T52.8X2	T52.8X3	T52.8X4	—	—
Delalutin	T38.5X1	T38.5X2	T38.5X3	T38.5X4	T38.5X5	T38.5X6
Delphinium	T62.2X1	T62.2X2	T62.2X3	T62.2X4	—	—
Deltasone	T38.0X1	T38.0X2	T38.0X3	T38.0X4	T38.0X5	T38.0X6
Deltra	T38.0X1	T38.0X2	T38.0X3	T38.0X4	T38.0X5	T38.0X6
Delvinal	T42.3X1	T42.3X2	T42.3X3	T42.3X4	T42.3X5	T42.3X6
Delorazepam	T42.4X1	T42.4X2	T42.4X3	T42.4X4	T42.4X5	T42.4X6
Deltamethrin	T60.1X1	T60.1X2	T60.1X3	T60.1X4	—	—
Demecarium (bromide)	T49.5X1	T49.5X2	T49.5X3	T49.5X4	T49.5X5	T49.5X6
Demeclocycline	T36.4X1	T36.4X2	T36.4X3	T36.4X4	T36.4X5	T36.4X6
Demecolcine	T45.1X1	T45.1X2	T45.1X3	T45.1X4	T45.1X5	T45.1X6
Demegestone	T38.5X1	T38.5X2	T38.5X3	T38.5X4	T38.5X5	T38.5X6
Demelanizing agents	T49.8X1	T49.8X2	T49.8X3	T49.8X4	T49.8X5	T49.8X6
Demephion -O and -S	T60.0X1	T60.0X2	T60.0X3	T60.0X4	—	—
Demerol	T40.2X1	T40.2X2	T40.2X3	T40.2X4	T40.2X5	T40.2X6
Demethylchlortetracycline	T36.4X1	T36.4X2	T36.4X3	T36.4X4	T36.4X5	T36.4X6
Demethyltetracycline	T36.4X1	T36.4X2	T36.4X3	T36.4X4	T36.4X5	T36.4X6
Demeton -O and -S	T60.0X1	T60.0X2	T60.0X3	T60.0X4	—	—
Demulcent (external)	T49.3X1	T49.3X2	T49.3X3	T49.3X4	T49.3X5	T49.3X6
specified NEC	T49.3X1	T49.3X2	T49.3X3	T49.3X4	T49.3X5	T49.3X6
Demulen	T38.4X1	T38.4X2	T38.4X3	T38.4X4	T38.4X5	T38.4X6
Denatured alcohol	T51.0X1	T51.0X2	T51.0X3	T51.0X4	—	—
Dendrid	T49.5X1	T49.5X2	T49.5X3	T49.5X4	T49.5X5	T49.5X6
Dental drug, topical application NEC	T49.7X1	T49.7X2	T49.7X3	T49.7X4	T49.7X5	T49.7X6

Substance	Poisoning, Accidental (Unintentional)	Poisoning, Intentional Self-Harm	Poisoning, Assault	Poisoning, Undetermined	Adverse Effect	Underdosing
Dentifrice	T49.7X1	T49.7X2	T49.7X3	T49.7X4	T49.7X5	T49.7X6
Deodorant spray (feminine hygiene)	T49.8X1	T49.8X2	T49.8X3	T49.8X4	T49.8X5	T49.8X6
Deoxycortone	T50.0X1	T50.0X2	T50.0X3	T50.0X4	T50.0X5	T50.0X6
2-Deoxy-5-fluorouridine	T45.1X1	T45.1X2	T45.1X3	T45.1X4	T45.1X5	T45.1X6
5-Deoxy-5-fluorouridine	T45.1X1	T45.1X2	T45.1X3	T45.1X4	T45.1X5	T45.1X6
Deoxyribonuclease (pancreatic)	T45.3X1	T45.3X2	T45.3X3	T45.3X4	T45.3X5	T45.3X6
Depilatory	T49.4X1	T49.4X2	T49.4X3	T49.4X4	T49.4X5	T49.4X6
Deprenalin	T42.8X1	T42.8X2	T42.8X3	T42.8X4	T42.8X5	T42.8X6
Deprenyl	T42.8X1	T42.8X2	T42.8X3	T42.8X4	T42.8X5	T42.8X6
Depressant, appetite	T50.5X1	T50.5X2	T50.5X3	T50.5X4	T50.5X5	T50.5X6
Depressant						
appetite, central	T50.5X1	T50.5X2	T50.5X3	T50.5X4	T50.5X5	T50.5X6
cardiac	T46.2X1	T46.2X2	T46.2X3	T46.2X4	T46.2X5	T46.2X6
central nervous system (anesthetic) — see also Central nervous system, depressants	T42.71	T42.72	T42.73	T42.74	T42.75	T42.76
general anesthetic	T41.201	T41.202	T41.203	T41.204	T41.205	T41.206
muscle tone	T42.8X1	T42.8X2	T42.8X3	T42.8X4	T42.8X5	T42.8X6
muscle tone, central	T42.8X1	T42.8X2	T42.8X3	T42.8X4	T42.8X5	T42.8X6
psychotherapeutic	T43.501	T43.502	T43.503	T43.504	T43.505	T43.506
Deptropine	T45.0X1	T45.0X2	T45.0X3	T45.0X4	T45.0X5	T45.0X6
Dequalinium (chloride)	T49.0X1	T49.0X2	T49.0X3	T49.0X4	T49.0X5	T49.0X6
Derris root	T60.2X1	T60.2X2	T60.2X3	T60.2X4	—	—
Deserpidine	T43.011	T43.012	T43.013	T43.014	T43.015	T43.016
Desferrioxamine	T45.8X1	T45.8X2	T45.8X3	T45.8X4	T45.8X5	T45.8X6
Desipramine	T43.0X1	T43.0X2	T43.0X3	T43.0X4	T43.0X5	T43.0X6
Deslanoside	T46.0X1	T46.0X2	T46.0X3	T46.0X4	T46.0X5	T46.0X6
Desloughing agent	T49.4X1	T49.4X2	T49.4X3	T49.4X4	T49.4X5	T49.4X6
Desmethylimipramine	T43.011	T43.012	T43.013	T43.014	T43.015	T43.016
Desmopressin	T38.891	T38.892	T38.893	T38.894	T38.895	T38.896
Desocodeine	T40.2X1	T40.2X2	T40.2X3	T40.2X4	T40.2X5	T40.2X6
Desogestrel	T38.5X1	T38.5X2	T38.5X3	T38.5X4	T38.5X5	T38.5X6
Desomorphine	T40.2X1	T40.2X2	T40.2X3	T40.2X4	—	—
Desonide	T49.0X1	T49.0X2	T49.0X3	T49.0X4	T49.0X5	T49.0X6
Desoximetasone	T49.0X1	T49.0X2	T49.0X3	T49.0X4	T49.0X5	T49.0X6
Desoxycorticosteroid	T50.0X1	T50.0X2	T50.0X3	T50.0X4	T50.0X5	T50.0X6
Desoxycortone	T50.0X1	T50.0X2	T50.0X3	T50.0X4	T50.0X5	T50.0X6
Desoxyephedrine	T43.621	T43.622	T43.623	T43.624	T43.625	T43.626
Detaxtran	T46.6X1	T46.6X2	T46.6X3	T46.6X4	T46.6X5	T46.6X6
Detergent	T49.2X1	T49.2X2	T49.2X3	T49.2X4	T49.2X5	T49.2X6
external medication	T49.2X1	T49.2X2	T49.2X3	T49.2X4	T49.2X5	T49.2X6
local	T49.2X1	T49.2X2	T49.2X3	T49.2X4	T49.2X5	T49.2X6

◀ New   ◀▌ Revised   ~~deleted~~ Deleted

Substance	External Cause (T-Code)					
	Poisoning, Accidental (Unintentional)	Poisoning, Intentional Self-Harm	Poisoning, Assault	Poisoning, Undetermined	Adverse Effect	Underdosing
Detergent *(Continued)*						
medicinal	T49.2X1	T49.2X2	T49.2X3	T49.2X4	T49.2X5	T49.2X6
nonmedicinal	T55.1X1	T55.1X2	T55.1X3	T55.1X4	—	—
specified NEC	T55.1X1	T55.1X2	T55.1X3	T55.1X4	T55.1X5	T55.1X6
Deterrent, alcohol	T50.6X1	T50.6X2	T50.6X3	T50.6X4	T50.6X5	T50.6X6
Detoxifying agent	T50.6X1	T50.6X2	T50.6X3	T50.6X4	T50.6X5	T50.6X6
Detrothyronine	T38.1X1	T38.1X2	T38.1X3	T38.1X4	T38.1X5	T38.1X6
Dettol (external medication)	T49.0X1	T49.0X2	T49.0X3	T49.0X4	T49.0X5	T49.0X6
Dexamethasone	T38.0X1	T38.0X2	T38.0X3	T38.0X4	T38.0X5	T38.0X6
ENT agent	T49.6X1	T49.6X2	T49.6X3	T49.6X4	T49.6X5	T49.6X6
ophthalmic preparation	T49.5X1	T49.5X2	T49.5X3	T49.5X4	T49.5X5	T49.5X6
topical NEC	T49.0X1	T49.0X2	T49.0X3	T49.0X4	T49.0X5	T49.0X6
Dexamfetamine	T43.621	T43.622	T43.623	T43.624	T43.625	T43.626
Dexamphetamine	T43.621	T43.622	T43.623	T43.624	T43.625	T43.626
Dexbrompheniramine	T45.0X1	T45.0X2	T45.0X3	T45.0X4	T45.0X5	T45.0X6
Dexchlorpheniramine	T45.0X1	T45.0X2	T45.0X3	T45.0X4	T45.0X5	T45.0X6
Dexedrine	T43.621	T43.622	T43.623	T43.624	T43.625	T43.626
Dexetimide	T44.3X1	T44.3X2	T44.3X3	T44.3X4	T44.3X5	T44.3X6
Dexfenfluramine	T50.5X1	T50.5X2	T50.5X3	T50.5X4	T50.5X5	T50.5X6
Dexpanthenol	T45.2X1	T45.2X2	T45.2X3	T45.2X4	T45.2X5	T45.2X6
Dextran (40) (70) (150)	T45.8X1	T45.8X2	T45.8X3	T45.8X4	T45.8X5	T45.8X6
Dextriferron	T45.4X1	T45.4X2	T45.4X3	T45.4X4	T45.4X5	T45.4X6
Dextroamphetamine	T43.621	T43.622	T43.623	T43.624	T43.625	T43.626
Dextro calcium pantothenate	T45.2X1	T45.2X2	T45.2X3	T45.2X4	T45.2X5	T45.2X6
Dextromethorphan	T48.3X1	T48.3X2	T48.3X3	T48.3X4	T48.3X5	T48.3X6
Dextromoramide	T40.491	T40.492	T40.493	T40.494	—	—
topical	T49.8X1	T49.8X2	T49.8X3	T49.8X4	T49.8X5	T49.8X6
Dextro pantothenyl alcohol	T45.2X1	T45.2X2	T45.2X3	T45.2X4	T45.2X5	T45.2X6
Dextropropoxyphene	T40.491	T40.492	T40.493	T40.494	T40.495	T40.496
Dextrorphan	T40.2X1	T40.2X2	T40.2X3	T40.2X4	T40.2X5	T40.2X6
Dextrose	T50.3X1	T50.3X2	T50.3X3	T50.3X4	T50.3X5	T50.3X6
concentrated solution, intravenous	T46.8X1	T46.8X2	T46.8X3	T46.8X4	T46.8X5	T46.8X6
Dextrothyroxin	T38.1X1	T38.1X2	T38.1X3	T38.1X4	T38.1X5	T38.1X6
Dextrothyroxine sodium	T38.1X1	T38.1X2	T38.1X3	T38.1X4	T38.1X5	T38.1X6
DFP	T44.0X1	T44.0X2	T44.0X3	T44.0X4	T44.0X5	T44.0X6
DHE	T37.3X1	T37.3X2	T37.3X3	T37.3X4	T37.3X5	T37.3X6
45	T46.5X1	T46.5X2	T46.5X3	T46.5X4	T46.5X5	T46.5X6
Diabinese	T38.3X1	T38.3X2	T38.3X3	T38.3X4	T38.3X5	T38.3X6
Diacetone alcohol	T52.4X1	T52.4X2	T52.4X3	T52.4X4	—	—
Diacetyl monoxime	T50.991	T50.992	T50.993	T50.994	—	—
Diacetylmorphine	T40.1X1	T40.1X2	T40.1X3	T40.1X4	—	—

Substance	External Cause (T-Code)					
	Poisoning, Accidental (Unintentional)	Poisoning, Intentional Self-Harm	Poisoning, Assault	Poisoning, Undetermined	Adverse Effect	Underdosing
Diachylon plaster	T49.4X1	T49.4X2	T49.4X3	T49.4X4	T49.4X5	T49.4X6
Diaethylstilboestrolum	T38.5X1	T38.5X2	T38.5X3	T38.5X4	T38.5X5	T38.5X6
Diagnostic agent NEC	T50.8X1	T50.8X2	T50.8X3	T50.8X4	T50.8X5	T50.8X6
Dial (soap)	T49.2X1	T49.2X2	T49.2X3	T49.2X4	T49.2X5	T49.2X6
sedative	T42.3X1	T42.3X2	T42.3X3	T42.3X4	T42.3X5	T42.3X6
Dialkyl carbonate	T52.91	T52.92	T52.93	T52.94	—	—
Diallylbarbituric acid	T42.3X1	T42.3X2	T42.3X3	T42.3X4	T42.3X5	T42.3X6
Diallymal	T42.3X1	T42.3X2	T42.3X3	T42.3X4	T42.3X5	T42.3X6
Dialysis solution (intraperitoneal)	T50.3X1	T50.3X2	T50.3X3	T50.3X4	T50.3X5	T50.3X6
Diaminodiphenylsulfone	T37.1X1	T37.1X2	T37.1X3	T37.1X4	T37.1X5	T37.1X6
Diamorphine	T40.1X1	T40.1X2	T40.1X3	T40.1X4	—	—
Diamox	T50.2X1	T50.2X2	T50.2X3	T50.2X4	T50.2X5	T50.2X6
Diamthazole	T49.0X1	T49.0X2	T49.0X3	T49.0X4	T49.0X5	T49.0X6
Dianthone	T47.2X1	T47.2X2	T47.2X3	T47.2X4	T47.2X5	T47.2X6
Diaphenylsulfone	T37.0X1	T37.0X2	T37.0X3	T37.0X4	T37.0X5	T37.0X6
Diasone (sodium)	T37.1X1	T37.1X2	T37.1X3	T37.1X4	T37.1X5	T37.1X6
Diastase	T47.5X1	T47.5X2	T47.5X3	T47.5X4	T47.5X5	T47.5X6
Diatrizoate	T50.8X1	T50.8X2	T50.8X3	T50.8X4	T50.8X5	T50.8X6
Diazepam	T42.4X1	T42.4X2	T42.4X3	T42.4X4	T42.4X5	T42.4X6
Diazinon	T60.0X1	T60.0X2	T60.0X3	T60.0X4	—	—
Diazomethane (gas)	T59.891	T59.892	T59.893	T59.894	—	—
Diazoxide	T46.5X1	T46.5X2	T46.5X3	T46.5X4	T46.5X5	T46.5X6
Dibekacin	T36.5X1	T36.5X2	T36.5X3	T36.5X4	T36.5X5	T36.5X6
Dibenamine	T44.6X1	T44.6X2	T44.6X3	T44.6X4	T44.6X5	T44.6X6
Dibenzepin	T43.011	T43.012	T43.013	T43.014	T43.015	T43.016
Dibenzheptropine	T45.0X1	T45.0X2	T45.0X3	T45.0X4	T45.0X5	T45.0X6
Dibenzyline	T44.6X1	T44.6X2	T44.6X3	T44.6X4	T44.6X5	T44.6X6
Diborane (gas)	T59.891	T59.892	T59.893	T59.894	—	—
Dibromochloropropane	T60.8X1	T60.8X2	T60.8X3	T60.8X4	—	—
Dibromodulcitol	T45.1X1	T45.1X2	T45.1X3	T45.1X4	T45.1X5	T45.1X6
Dibromoethane	T53.6X1	T53.6X2	T53.6X3	T53.6X4	—	—
Dibromomannitol	T45.1X1	T45.1X2	T45.1X3	T45.1X4	T45.1X5	T45.1X6
Dibromopropamidine isethionate	T49.0X1	T49.0X2	T49.0X3	T49.0X4	T49.0X5	T49.0X6
Dibrompropamidine	T49.0X1	T49.0X2	T49.0X3	T49.0X4	T49.0X5	T49.0X6
Dibucaine	T41.3X1	T41.3X2	T41.3X3	T41.3X4	T41.3X5	T41.3X6
topical (surface)	T41.3X1	T41.3X2	T41.3X3	T41.3X4	T41.3X5	T41.3X6
Dibunate sodium	T48.3X1	T48.3X2	T48.3X3	T48.3X4	T48.3X5	T48.3X6
Dibutoline sulfate	T44.3X1	T44.3X2	T44.3X3	T44.3X4	T44.3X5	T44.3X6
Dicamba	T60.3X1	T60.3X2	T60.3X3	T60.3X4	—	—
Dicapthon	T60.0X1	T60.0X2	T60.0X3	T60.0X4	—	—
Dichlobenil	T60.3X1	T60.3X2	T60.3X3	T60.3X4	—	—
Dichlone	T60.3X1	T60.3X2	T60.3X3	T60.3X4	—	—

◀ New   ◀ Revised   ~~deleted~~ Deleted

Substance	External Cause (T-Code)					
	Poisoning, Accidental (Unintentional)	Poisoning, Intentional Self-Harm	Poisoning, Assault	Poisoning, Undetermined	Adverse Effect	Underdosing
Dichloralphenozone	T42.6X1	T42.6X2	T42.6X3	T42.6X4	T42.6X5	T42.6X6
Dichlorbenzidine	T65.3X1	T65.3X2	T65.3X3	T65.3X4	—	—
Dichlorhydrin	T52.8X1	T52.8X2	T52.8X3	T52.8X4	—	—
Dichlorhydroxyquinoline	T37.8X1	T37.8X2	T37.8X3	T37.8X4	T37.8X5	T37.8X6
Dichlorobenzene	T53.7X1	T53.7X2	T53.7X3	T53.7X4	—	—
Dichlorobenzyl alcohol	T49.6X1	T49.6X2	T49.6X3	T49.6X4	T49.6X5	T49.6X6
Dichlorodifluoromethane	T53.5X1	T53.5X2	T53.5X3	T53.5X4	—	—
Dichloroethane	T52.8X1	T52.8X2	T52.8X3	T52.8X4	—	—
Sym-Dichloroethyl ether	T53.6X1	T53.6X2	T53.6X3	T53.6X4	—	—
Dichloroethyl sulfide, not in war	T59.891	T59.892	T59.893	T59.894	—	—
Dichloroethylene	T53.6X1	T53.6X2	T53.6X3	T53.6X4	—	—
Dichloroformoxine, not in war	T59.891	T59.892	T59.893	T59.894	—	—
Dichlorohydrin, alpha-dichlorohydrin	T52.8X1	T52.8X2	T52.8X3	T52.8X4	—	—
Dichloromethane (solvent)	T53.4X1	T53.4X2	T53.4X3	T53.4X4	—	—
vapor	T53.4X1	T53.4X2	T53.4X3	T53.4X4	—	—
Dichloronaphthoquinone	T60.3X1	T60.3X2	T60.3X3	T60.3X4	—	—
Dichlorophen	T37.4X1	T37.4X2	T37.4X3	T37.4X4	T37.4X5	T37.4X6
2,4-Dichlorophenoxy-acetic acid	T60.3X1	T60.3X2	T60.3X3	T60.3X4	—	—
Dichloropropene	T60.3X1	T60.3X2	T60.3X3	T60.3X4	—	—
Dichloropropionic acid	T60.3X1	T60.3X2	T60.3X3	T60.3X4	—	—
Dichlorphenamide	T50.2X1	T50.2X2	T50.2X3	T50.2X4	T50.2X5	T50.2X6
Dichlorvos	T60.0X1	T60.0X2	T60.0X3	T60.0X4	—	—
Diclofenac	T39.391	T39.392	T39.393	T39.394	T39.395	T39.396
Diclofenamide	T50.2X1	T50.2X2	T50.2X3	T50.2X4	T50.2X5	T50.2X6
Diclofensine	T43.291	T43.292	T43.293	T43.294	T43.295	T43.296
Diclonixine	T39.8X1	T39.8X2	T39.8X3	T39.8X4	T39.8X5	T39.8X6
Dicloxacillin	T36.0X1	T36.0X2	T36.0X3	T36.0X4	T36.0X5	T36.0X6
Dicophane	T49.0X1	T49.0X2	T49.0X3	T49.0X4	T49.0X5	T49.0X6
Dicoumarol, dicoumarin, dicumarol	T45.511	T45.512	T45.513	T45.514	T45.515	T45.516
Dicrotophos	T60.0X1	T60.0X2	T60.0X3	T60.0X4	—	—
Dicyanogen (gas)	T65.0X1	T65.0X2	T65.0X3	T65.0X4	—	—
Dicyclomine	T44.3X1	T44.3X2	T44.3X3	T44.3X4	T44.3X5	T44.3X6
Dicycloverine	T44.3X1	T44.3X2	T44.3X3	T44.3X4	T44.3X5	T44.3X6
Dideoxycytidine	T37.5X1	T37.5X2	T37.5X3	T37.5X4	T37.5X5	T37.5X6
Dideoxyinosine	T37.5X1	T37.5X2	T37.5X3	T37.5X4	T37.5X5	T37.5X6
Dieldrin (vapor)	T60.1X1	T60.1X2	T60.1X3	T60.1X4	—	—
Diemal	T42.3X1	T42.3X2	T42.3X3	T42.3X4	T42.3X5	T42.3X6
Dienestrol	T38.5X1	T38.5X2	T38.5X3	T38.5X4	T38.5X5	T38.5X6
Dienoestrol	T38.5X1	T38.5X2	T38.5X3	T38.5X4	T38.5X5	T38.5X6
Dietetic drug NEC	T50.901	T50.902	T50.903	T50.904	T50.905	T50.906
Diethazine	T42.8X1	T42.8X2	T42.8X3	T42.8X4	T42.8X5	T42.8X6

Substance	External Cause (T-Code)					
	Poisoning, Accidental (Unintentional)	Poisoning, Intentional Self-Harm	Poisoning, Assault	Poisoning, Undetermined	Adverse Effect	Underdosing
Diethyl						
barbituric acid	T42.3X1	T42.3X2	T42.3X3	T42.3X4	T42.3X5	T42.3X6
carbamazine	T37.4X1	T37.4X2	T37.4X3	T37.4X4	T37.4X5	T37.4X6
carbinol	T51.3X1	T51.3X2	T51.3X3	T51.3X4	—	—
carbonate	T52.8X1	T52.8X2	T52.8X3	T52.8X4	—	—
ether (vapor) — see also Ether	T41.0X1	T41.0X2	T41.0X3	T41.0X4	T41.0X5	T41.0X6
oxide	T52.8X1	T52.8X2	T52.8X3	T52.8X4	—	—
propion	T50.5X1	T50.5X2	T50.5X3	T50.5X4	T50.5X5	T50.5X6
stilbestrol	T38.5X1	T38.5X2	T38.5X3	T38.5X4	T38.5X5	T38.5X6
toluamide (nonmedicinal)	T60.8X1	T60.8X2	T60.8X3	T60.8X4	—	—
medicinal	T49.3X1	T49.3X2	T49.3X3	T49.3X4	T49.3X5	T49.3X6
Diethylcarbamazine	T37.4X1	T37.4X2	T37.4X3	T37.4X4	T37.4X5	T37.4X6
Diethylene						
dioxide	T52.8X1	T52.8X2	T52.8X3	T52.8X4	—	—
glycol (monoacetate) (monobutyl ether) (monoethyl ether)	T52.3X1	T52.3X2	T52.3X3	T52.3X4	—	—
Diethylhexylphthalate	T65.891	T65.892	T65.893	T65.894	—	—
Diethylpropion	T50.5X1	T50.5X2	T50.5X3	T50.5X4	T50.5X5	T50.5X6
Diethylstilbestrol	T38.5X1	T38.5X2	T38.5X3	T38.5X4	T38.5X5	T38.5X6
Diethylstilboestrol	T38.5X1	T38.5X2	T38.5X3	T38.5X4	T38.5X5	T38.5X6
Diethylsulfone-diethylmethane	T42.6X1	T42.6X2	T42.6X3	T42.6X4	T42.6X5	T42.6X6
Diethyltoluamide	T49.0X1	T49.0X2	T49.0X3	T49.0X4	T49.0X5	T49.0X6
Diethyltryptamine (DET)	T40.991	T40.992	T40.993	T40.994	—	—
Difebarbamate	T42.3X1	T42.3X2	T42.3X3	T42.3X4	T42.3X5	T42.3X6
Difencloxazine	T40.2X1	T40.2X2	T40.2X3	T40.2X4	T40.2X5	T40.2X6
Difenidol	T45.0X1	T45.0X2	T45.0X3	T45.0X4	T45.0X5	T45.0X6
Difenoxin	T47.6X1	T47.6X2	T47.6X3	T47.6X4	T47.6X5	T47.6X6
Difetarsone	T37.3X1	T37.3X2	T37.3X3	T37.3X4	T37.3X5	T37.3X6
Diffusin	T45.3X1	T45.3X2	T45.3X3	T45.3X4	T45.3X5	T45.3X6
Diflorasone	T49.0X1	T49.0X2	T49.0X3	T49.0X4	T49.0X5	T49.0X6
Diflubenzuron	T60.1X1	T60.1X2	T60.1X3	T60.1X4	—	—
Diflos	T44.0X1	T44.0X2	T44.0X3	T44.0X4	T44.0X5	T44.0X6
Diflucortolone	T49.0X1	T49.0X2	T49.0X3	T49.0X4	T49.0X5	T49.0X6
Diflunisal	T39.091	T39.092	T39.093	T39.094	T39.095	T39.096
Difluoromethyldopa	T42.8X1	T42.8X2	T42.8X3	T42.8X4	T42.8X5	T42.8X6
Difluorophate	T44.0X1	T44.0X2	T44.0X3	T44.0X4	T44.0X5	T44.0X6
Digestant NEC	T47.5X1	T47.5X2	T47.5X3	T47.5X4	T47.5X5	T47.5X6
Digitalin(e)	T46.0X1	T46.0X2	T46.0X3	T46.0X4	T46.0X5	T46.0X6
Digitalis (leaf) (glycoside)	T46.0X1	T46.0X2	T46.0X3	T46.0X4	T46.0X5	T46.0X6
lanata	T46.0X1	T46.0X2	T46.0X3	T46.0X4	T46.0X5	T46.0X6
purpurea	T46.0X1	T46.0X2	T46.0X3	T46.0X4	T46.0X5	T46.0X6
Digitoxin	T46.0X1	T46.0X2	T46.0X3	T46.0X4	T46.0X5	T46.0X6

◀ New ◀ Revised deleted Deleted

	External Cause (T-Code)					
Substance	Poisoning, Accidental (Unintentional)	Poisoning, Intentional Self-Harm	Poisoning, Assault	Poisoning, Undetermined	Adverse Effect	Underdosing
Digitoxose	T46.0X1	T46.0X2	T46.0X3	T46.0X4	T46.0X5	T46.0X6
Digoxin	T46.0X1	T46.0X2	T46.0X3	T46.0X4	T46.0X5	T46.0X6
Digoxine	T46.0X1	T46.0X2	T46.0X3	T46.0X4	T46.0X5	T46.0X6
Dihydralazine	T46.5X1	T46.5X2	T46.5X3	T46.5X4	T46.5X5	T46.5X6
Dihydrazine	T46.5X1	T46.5X2	T46.5X3	T46.5X4	T46.5X5	T46.5X6
Dihydrocodeinone	T40.2X1	T40.2X2	T40.2X3	T40.2X4	T40.2X5	T40.2X6
Dihydroergocornine	T46.7X1	T46.7X2	T46.7X3	T46.7X4	T46.7X5	T46.7X6
Dihydroergocristine (mesilate)	T46.7X1	T46.7X2	T46.7X3	T46.7X4	T46.7X5	T46.7X6
Dihydroergokryptine	T46.7X1	T46.7X2	T46.7X3	T46.7X4	T46.7X5	T46.7X6
Dihydroergotamine	T46.5X1	T46.5X2	T46.5X3	T46.5X4	T46.5X5	T46.5X6
Dihydroergotoxine	T46.7X1	T46.7X2	T46.7X3	T46.7X4	T46.7X5	T46.7X6
mesilate	T46.7X1	T46.7X2	T46.7X3	T46.7X4	T46.7X5	T46.7X6
Dihydrohydroxycodein-one	T40.2X1	T40.2X2	T40.2X3	T40.2X4	T40.2X5	T40.2X6
Dihydrohydroxymorphinone	T40.2X1	T40.2X2	T40.2X3	T40.2X4	T40.2X5	T40.2X6
Dihydroisocodeine	T40.2X1	T40.2X2	T40.2X3	T40.2X4	T40.2X5	T40.2X6
Dihydromorphine	T40.2X1	T40.2X2	T40.2X3	T40.2X4	—	—
Dihydromorphinone	T40.2X1	T40.2X2	T40.2X3	T40.2X4	T40.2X5	T40.2X6
Dihydrostreptomycin	T36.5X1	T36.5X2	T36.5X3	T36.5X4	T36.5X5	T36.5X6
Dihydrotachysterol	T45.2X1	T45.2X2	T45.2X3	T45.2X4	T45.2X5	T45.2X6
Dihydroxyaluminum aminoacetate	T47.1X1	T47.1X2	T47.1X3	T47.1X4	T47.1X5	T47.1X6
Dihydroxyaluminum sodium carbonate	T47.1X1	T47.1X2	T47.1X3	T47.1X4	T47.1X5	T47.1X6
Dihydroxyanthraquinone	T47.2X1	T47.2X2	T47.2X3	T47.2X4	T47.2X5	T47.2X6
Dihydroxycodeinone	T40.2X1	T40.2X2	T40.2X3	T40.2X4	T40.2X5	T40.2X6
Dihydroxypropyl theophylline	T50.2X1	T50.2X2	T50.2X3	T50.2X4	T50.2X5	T50.2X6
Diiodohydroxyquin	T37.8X1	T37.8X2	T37.8X3	T37.8X4	T37.8X5	T37.8X6
topical	T49.0X1	T49.0X2	T49.0X3	T49.0X4	T49.0X5	T49.0X6
Diiodohydroxyquinoline	T37.8X1	T37.8X2	T37.8X3	T37.8X4	T37.8X5	T37.8X6
Diiodotyrosine	T38.2X1	T38.2X2	T38.2X3	T38.2X4	T38.2X5	T38.2X6
Diisopromine	T44.3X1	T44.3X2	T44.3X3	T44.3X4	T44.3X5	T44.3X6
Diisopropylamine	T46.3X1	T46.3X2	T46.3X3	T46.3X4	T46.3X5	T46.3X6
Diisopropylfluorophosphonate	T44.0X1	T44.0X2	T44.0X3	T44.0X4	T44.0X5	T44.0X6
Dilantin	T42.0X1	T42.0X2	T42.0X3	T42.0X4	T42.0X5	T42.0X6
Dilaudid	T40.2X1	T40.2X2	T40.2X3	T40.2X4	T40.2X5	T40.2X6
Dilazep	T46.3X1	T46.3X2	T46.3X3	T46.3X4	T46.3X5	T46.3X6
Dill	T47.5X1	T47.5X2	T47.5X3	T47.5X4	T47.5X5	T47.5X6
Diloxanide	T37.3X1	T37.3X2	T37.3X3	T37.3X4	T37.3X5	T37.3X6
Diltiazem	T46.1X1	T46.1X2	T46.1X3	T46.1X4	T46.1X5	T46.1X6
Dimazole	T49.0X1	T49.0X2	T49.0X3	T49.0X4	T49.0X5	T49.0X6
Dimefline	T50.7X1	T50.7X2	T50.7X3	T50.7X4	T50.7X5	T50.7X6
Dimefox	T60.0X1	T60.0X2	T60.0X3	T60.0X4	—	—

	External Cause (T-Code)					
Substance	Poisoning, Accidental (Unintentional)	Poisoning, Intentional Self-Harm	Poisoning, Assault	Poisoning, Undetermined	Adverse Effect	Underdosing
Dimemorfan	T48.3X1	T48.3X2	T48.3X3	T48.3X4	T48.3X5	T48.3X6
Dimenhydrinate	T45.0X1	T45.0X2	T45.0X3	T45.0X4	T45.0X5	T45.0X6
Dimercaprol (British anti-lewisite)	T45.8X1	T45.8X2	T45.8X3	T45.8X4	T45.8X5	T45.8X6
Dimercaptopropanol	T45.8X1	T45.8X2	T45.8X3	T45.8X4	T45.8X5	T45.8X6
Dimestrol	T38.5X1	T38.5X2	T38.5X3	T38.5X4	T38.5X5	T38.5X6
Dimetane	T45.0X1	T45.0X2	T45.0X3	T45.0X4	T45.0X5	T45.0X6
Dimethicone	T47.1X1	T47.1X2	T47.1X3	T47.1X4	T47.1X5	T47.1X6
Dimethindene	T45.0X1	T45.0X2	T45.0X3	T45.0X4	T45.0X5	T45.0X6
Dimethisoquin	T49.1X1	T49.1X2	T49.1X3	T49.1X4	T49.1X5	T49.1X6
Dimethisterone	T38.5X1	T38.5X2	T38.5X3	T38.5X4	T38.5X5	T38.5X6
Dimethoate	T60.0X1	T60.0X2	T60.0X3	T60.0X4	—	—
Dimethocaine	T41.3X1	T41.3X2	T41.3X3	T41.3X4	T41.3X5	T41.3X6
Dimethoxanate	T48.3X1	T48.3X2	T48.3X3	T48.3X4	T48.3X5	T48.3X6
Dimethyl						
arsine, arsinic acid	T57.0X1	T57.0X2	T57.0X3	T57.0X4	—	—
carbinol	T51.2X1	T51.2X2	T51.2X3	T51.2X4	—	—
carbonate	T52.8X1	T52.8X2	T52.8X3	T52.8X4	—	—
diguanide	T38.3X1	T38.3X2	T38.3X3	T38.3X4	T38.3X5	T38.3X6
ketone	T52.4X1	T52.4X2	T52.4X3	T52.4X4	—	—
vapor	T52.4X1	T52.4X2	T52.4X3	T52.4X4	—	—
meperidine	T40.2X1	T40.2X2	T40.2X3	T40.2X4	T40.2X5	T40.2X6
parathion	T60.0X1	T60.0X2	T60.0X3	T60.0X4	—	—
phthlate	T49.3X1	T49.3X2	T49.3X3	T49.3X4	T49.3X5	T49.3X6
polysiloxane	T47.8X1	T47.8X2	T47.8X3	T47.8X4	T47.8X5	T47.8X6
sulfate (fumes)	T59.891	T59.892	T59.893	T59.894	—	—
liquid	T65.891	T65.892	T65.893	T65.894	—	—
sulfoxide (nonmedicinal)	T52.8X1	T52.8X2	T52.8X3	T52.8X4	—	—
medicinal	T49.4X1	T49.4X2	T49.4X3	T49.4X4	T49.4X5	T49.4X6
tryptamine	T40.991	T40.992	T40.993	T40.994	—	—
tubocurarine	T48.1X1	T48.1X2	T48.1X3	T48.1X4	T48.1X5	T48.1X6
Dimethylamine sulfate	T49.4X1	T49.4X2	T49.4X3	T49.4X4	T49.4X5	T49.4X6
Dimethylformamide	T52.8X1	T52.8X2	T52.8X3	T52.8X4	—	—
Dimethyltubocurarinium chloride	T48.1X1	T48.1X2	T48.1X3	T48.1X4	T48.1X5	T48.1X6
Dimeticone	T47.1X1	T47.1X2	T47.1X3	T47.1X4	T47.1X5	T47.1X6
Dimetilan	T60.0X1	T60.0X2	T60.0X3	T60.0X4	—	—
Dimetindene	T45.0X1	T45.0X2	T45.0X3	T45.0X4	T45.0X5	T45.0X6
Dimetotiazine	T43.3X1	T43.3X2	T43.3X3	T43.3X4	T43.3X5	T43.3X6
Dimorpholamine	T50.7X1	T50.7X2	T50.7X3	T50.7X4	T50.7X5	T50.7X6
Dimoxyline	T46.3X1	T46.3X2	T46.3X3	T46.3X4	T46.3X5	T46.3X6
Dinitrobenzene	T65.3X1	T65.3X2	T65.3X3	T65.3X4	—	—
vapor	T59.891	T59.892	T59.893	T59.894	—	—

◀ New ◀ Revised ~~deleted~~ Deleted

TABLE OF DRUGS AND CHEMICALS

Substance	Poisoning, Accidental (Unintentional)	Poisoning, Intentional Self-Harm	Poisoning, Assault	Poisoning, Undetermined	Adverse Effect	Underdosing
Dinitrobenzol	T65.3X1	T65.3X2	T65.3X3	T65.3X4	—	—
vapor	T59.891	T59.892	T59.893	T59.894	—	—
Dinitrobutylphenol	T65.3X1	T65.3X2	T65.3X3	T65.3X4	—	—
Dinitro (-ortho-)cresol (pesticide) (spray)	T65.3X1	T65.3X2	T65.3X3	T65.3X4	—	—
Dinitrocyclohexylphenol	T65.3X1	T65.3X2	T65.3X3	T65.3X4	—	—
Dinitrophenol	T65.3X1	T65.3X2	T65.3X3	T65.3X4	—	—
Dinoprost	T48.0X1	T48.0X2	T48.0X3	T48.0X4	T48.0X5	T48.0X6
Dinoprostone	T48.0X1	T48.0X2	T48.0X3	T48.0X4	T48.0X5	T48.0X6
Dinoseb	T60.3X1	T60.3X2	T60.3X3	T60.3X4	—	—
Dioctyl sulfosuccinate (calcium) (sodium)	T47.4X1	T47.4X2	T47.4X3	T47.4X4	T47.4X5	T47.4X6
Diodone	T50.8X1	T50.8X2	T50.8X3	T50.8X4	T50.8X5	T50.8X6
Diodoquin	T37.8X1	T37.8X2	T37.8X3	T37.8X4	T37.8X5	T37.8X6
Dionin	T40.2X1	T40.2X2	T40.2X3	T40.2X4	T40.2X5	T40.2X6
Diosmin	T46.991	T46.992	T46.993	T46.994	T46.995	T46.996
Dioxane	T52.8X1	T52.8X2	T52.8X3	T52.8X4	—	—
Dioxathion	T60.0X1	T60.0X2	T60.0X3	T60.0X4	—	—
Dioxin	T53.7X1	T53.7X2	T53.7X3	T53.7X4	—	—
Dioxopromethazine	T43.3X1	T43.3X2	T43.3X3	T43.3X4	T43.3X5	T43.3X6
Dioxyline	T46.3X1	T46.3X2	T46.3X3	T46.3X4	T46.3X5	T46.3X6
Dipentene	T52.8X1	T52.8X2	T52.8X3	T52.8X4	—	—
Diperodon	T41.3X1	T41.3X2	T41.3X3	T41.3X4	T41.3X5	T41.3X6
Diphacinone	T60.4X1	T60.4X2	T60.4X3	T60.4X4	—	—
Diphemanil	T44.3X1	T44.3X2	T44.3X3	T44.3X4	T44.3X5	T44.3X6
metilsulfate	T44.3X1	T44.3X2	T44.3X3	T44.3X4	T44.3X5	T44.3X6
Diphenadione	T45.511	T45.512	T45.513	T45.514	T45.515	T45.516
rodenticide	T60.4X1	T60.4X2	T60.4X3	T60.4X4	—	—
Diphenhydramine	T45.0X1	T45.0X2	T45.0X3	T45.0X4	T45.0X5	T45.0X6
Diphenidol	T45.0X1	T45.0X2	T45.0X3	T45.0X4	T45.0X5	T45.0X6
Diphenoxylate	T47.6X1	T47.6X2	T47.6X3	T47.6X4	T47.6X5	T47.6X6
Diphenylamine	T65.3X1	T65.3X2	T65.3X3	T65.3X4	—	—
Diphenylbutazone	T39.2X1	T39.2X2	T39.2X3	T39.2X4	T39.2X5	T39.2X6
Diphenylchloroarsine, not in war	T57.0X1	T57.0X2	T57.0X3	T57.0X4	—	—
Diphenylhydantoin	T42.0X1	T42.0X2	T42.0X3	T42.0X4	T42.0X5	T42.0X6
Diphenylmethane dye	T52.1X1	T52.1X2	T52.1X3	T52.1X4	—	—
Diphenylpyraline	T45.0X1	T45.0X2	T45.0X3	T45.0X4	T45.0X5	T45.0X6
Diphtheria						
antitoxin	T50.Z11	T50.Z12	T50.Z13	T50.Z14	T50.Z15	T50.Z16
toxoid	T50.A91	T50.A92	T50.A93	T50.A94	T50.A95	T50.A96
with tetanus toxoid	T50.A21	T50.A22	T50.A23	T50.A24	T50.A25	T50.A26
with pertussis component	T50.A11	T50.A12	T50.A13	T50.A14	T50.A15	T50.A16

Substance	Poisoning, Accidental (Unintentional)	Poisoning, Intentional Self-Harm	Poisoning, Assault	Poisoning, Undetermined	Adverse Effect	Underdosing
Diphtheria (Continued)						
vaccine (combination)	T50.A91	T50.A92	T50.A93	T50.A94	T50.A95	T50.A96
combination						
including pertussis	T50.A11	T50.A12	T50.A13	T50.A14	T50.A15	T50.A16
without pertussis	T50.A21	T50.A22	T50.A23	T50.A24	T50.A25	T50.A26
Diphylline	T50.2X1	T50.2X2	T50.2X3	T50.2X4	T50.2X5	T50.2X6
Dipipanone	T40.491	T40.492	T40.493	T40.494	—	—
Dipivefrine	T49.5X1	T49.5X2	T49.5X3	T49.5X4	T49.5X5	T49.5X6
Diplovax	T50.B91	T50.B92	T50.B93	T50.B94	T50.B95	T50.B96
Diprophylline	T50.2X1	T50.2X2	T50.2X3	T50.2X4	T50.2X5	T50.2X6
Dipropyline	T48.291	T48.292	T48.293	T48.294	T48.295	T48.296
Dipyridamole	T46.3X1	T46.3X2	T46.3X3	T46.3X4	T46.3X5	T46.3X6
Dipyrone	T39.2X1	T39.2X2	T39.2X3	T39.2X4	T39.2X5	T39.2X6
Diquat (dibromide)	T60.3X1	T60.3X2	T60.3X3	T60.3X4	—	—
Disinfectant	T65.891	T65.892	T65.893	T65.894	—	—
alkaline	T54.3X1	T54.3X2	T54.3X3	T54.3X4	—	—
aromatic	T54.1X1	T54.1X2	T54.1X3	T54.1X4	—	—
intestinal	T37.8X1	T37.8X2	T37.8X3	T37.8X4	T37.8X5	T37.8X6
Disipal	T42.8X1	T42.8X2	T42.8X3	T42.8X4	T42.8X5	T42.8X6
Disodium edetate	T50.6X1	T50.6X2	T50.6X3	T50.6X4	T50.6X5	T50.6X6
Disoprofol	T41.291	T41.292	T41.293	T41.294	T41.295	T41.296
Disopyramide	T46.2X1	T46.2X2	T46.2X3	T46.2X4	T46.2X5	T46.2X6
Distigmine (bromide)	T44.0X1	T44.0X2	T44.0X3	T44.0X4	T44.0X5	T44.0X6
Disulfamide	T50.2X1	T50.2X2	T50.2X3	T50.2X4	T50.2X5	T50.2X6
Disulfanilamide	T37.0X1	T37.0X2	T37.0X3	T37.0X4	T37.0X5	T37.0X6
Disulfiram	T50.6X1	T50.6X2	T50.6X3	T50.6X4	T50.6X5	T50.6X6
Disulfoton	T60.0X1	T60.0X2	T60.0X3	T60.0X4	—	—
Dithiazanine iodide	T37.4X1	T37.4X2	T37.4X3	T37.4X4	T37.4X5	T37.4X6
Dithiocarbamate	T60.0X1	T60.0X2	T60.0X3	T60.0X4	—	—
Dithranol	T49.4X1	T49.4X2	T49.4X3	T49.4X4	T49.4X5	T49.4X6
Diucardin	T50.2X1	T50.2X2	T50.2X3	T50.2X4	T50.2X5	T50.2X6
Diupres	T50.2X1	T50.2X2	T50.2X3	T50.2X4	T50.2X5	T50.2X6
Diuretic NEC	T50.2X1	T50.2X2	T50.2X3	T50.2X4	T50.2X5	T50.2X6
benzothiadiazine	T50.2X1	T50.2X2	T50.2X3	T50.2X4	T50.2X5	T50.2X6
carbonic acid anhydrase inhibitors	T50.2X1	T50.2X2	T50.2X3	T50.2X4	T50.2X5	T50.2X6
furfuryl NEC	T50.2X1	T50.2X2	T50.2X3	T50.2X4	T50.2X5	T50.2X6
loop (high-ceiling)	T50.1X1	T50.1X2	T50.1X3	T50.1X4	T50.1X5	T50.1X6
mercurial NEC	T50.2X1	T50.2X2	T50.2X3	T50.2X4	T50.2X5	T50.2X6
osmotic	T50.2X1	T50.2X2	T50.2X3	T50.2X4	T50.2X5	T50.2X6
purine NEC	T50.2X1	T50.2X2	T50.2X3	T50.2X4	T50.2X5	T50.2X6
saluretic NEC	T50.2X1	T50.2X2	T50.2X3	T50.2X4	T50.2X5	T50.2X6

◀ New ◀ Revised ~~deleted~~ Deleted

Substance	Poisoning, Accidental (Unintentional)	Poisoning, Intentional Self-Harm	Poisoning, Assault	Poisoning, Undetermined	Adverse Effect	Underdosing
Diuretic NEC *(Continued)*						
sulfonamide	T50.2X1	T50.2X2	T50.2X3	T50.2X4	T50.2X5	T50.2X6
thiazide NEC	T50.2X1	T50.2X2	T50.2X3	T50.2X4	T50.2X5	T50.2X6
xanthine	T50.2X1	T50.2X2	T50.2X3	T50.2X4	T50.2X5	T50.2X6
Diurgin	T50.2X1	T50.2X2	T50.2X3	T50.2X4	T50.2X5	T50.2X6
Diuril	T50.2X1	T50.2X2	T50.2X3	T50.2X4	T50.2X5	T50.2X6
Diuron	T60.3X1	T60.3X2	T60.3X3	T60.3X4	—	—
Divalproex	T42.6X1	T42.6X2	T42.6X3	T42.6X4	T42.6X5	T42.6X6
Divinyl ether	T41.0X1	T41.0X2	T41.0X3	T41.0X4	T41.0X5	T41.0X6
Dixanthogen	I49.0X1	I49.0X2	I49.0X3	I49.0X4	I49.0X5	I49.0X6
Dixyrazine	T43.3X1	T43.3X2	T43.3X3	T43.3X4	T43.3X5	T43.3X6
D-lysergic acid diethylamide	T40.8X1	T40.8X2	T40.8X3	T40.8X4	—	—
DMCT	T36.4X1	T36.4X2	T36.4X3	T36.4X4	T36.4X5	T36.4X6
DMSO — *see Dimethyl sulfoxide*						
DNBP	T60.3X1	T60.3X2	T60.3X3	T60.3X4	—	—
DNOC	T65.3X1	T65.3X2	T65.3X3	T65.3X4	—	—
DOCA	T38.0X1	T38.0X2	T38.0X3	T38.0X4	T38.0X5	T38.0X6
Dobutamine	T44.5X1	T44.5X2	T44.5X3	T44.5X4	T44.5X5	T44.5X6
Docusate sodium	T47.4X1	T47.4X2	T47.4X3	T47.4X4	T47.4X5	T47.4X6
Dodicin	T49.0X1	T49.0X2	T49.0X3	T49.0X4	T49.0X5	T49.0X6
Dofamium chloride	T49.0X1	T49.0X2	T49.0X3	T49.0X4	T49.0X5	T49.0X6
Dolophine	T40.3X1	T40.3X2	T40.3X3	T40.3X4	T40.3X5	T40.3X6
Doloxene	T39.8X1	T39.8X2	T39.8X3	T39.8X4	T39.8X5	T39.8X6
Domestic gas (after combustion) — *see Gas, utility*						
prior to combustion	T59.891	T59.892	T59.893	T59.894	—	—
Domiodol	T48.4X1	T48.4X2	T48.4X3	T48.4X4	T48.4X5	T48.4X6
Domiphen (bromide)	T49.0X1	T49.0X2	T49.0X3	T49.0X4	T49.0X5	T49.0X6
Domperidone	T45.0X1	T45.0X2	T45.0X3	T45.0X4	T45.0X5	T45.0X6
Dopa	T42.8X1	T42.8X2	T42.8X3	T42.8X4	T42.8X5	T42.8X6
Dopamine	T44.991	T44.992	T44.993	T44.994	T44.995	T44.996
Doriden	T42.6X1	T42.6X2	T42.6X3	T42.6X4	T42.6X5	T42.6X6
Dormiral	T42.3X1	T42.3X2	T42.3X3	T42.3X4	T42.3X5	T42.3X6
Dormison	T42.6X1	T42.6X2	T42.6X3	T42.6X4	T42.6X5	T42.6X6
Dornase	T48.4X1	T48.4X2	T48.4X3	T48.4X4	T48.4X5	T48.4X6
Dorsacaine	T41.3X1	T41.3X2	T41.3X3	T41.3X4	T41.3X5	T41.3X6
Dosulepin	T43.011	T43.012	T43.013	T43.014	T43.015	T43.016
Dothiepin	T43.011	T43.012	T43.013	T43.014	T43.015	T43.016
Doxantrazole	T48.6X1	T48.6X2	T48.6X3	T48.6X4	T48.6X5	T48.6X6
Doxapram	T50.7X1	T50.7X2	T50.7X3	T50.7X4	T50.7X5	T50.7X6
Doxazosin	T44.6X1	T44.6X2	T44.6X3	T44.6X4	T44.6X5	T44.6X6
Doxepin	T43.011	T43.012	T43.013	T43.014	T43.015	T43.016
Doxifluridine	T45.1X1	T45.1X2	T45.1X3	T45.1X4	T45.1X5	T45.1X6
Doxorubicin	T45.1X1	T45.1X2	T45.1X3	T45.1X4	T45.1X5	T45.1X6
Doxycycline	T36.4X1	T36.4X2	T36.4X3	T36.4X4	T36.4X5	T36.4X6
Doxylamine	T45.0X1	T45.0X2	T45.0X3	T45.0X4	T45.0X5	T45.0X6
Dramamine	T45.0X1	T45.0X2	T45.0X3	T45.0X4	T45.0X5	T45.0X6
Drano (drain cleaner)	T54.3X1	T54.3X2	T54.3X3	T54.3X4	—	—
Dressing, live pulp	T49.7X1	T49.7X2	T49.7X3	T49.7X4	T49.7X5	T49.7X6
Drocode	T40.2X1	T40.2X2	T40.2X3	T40.2X4	T40.2X5	T40.2X6
Dromoran	T40.2X1	T40.2X2	T40.2X3	T40.2X4	T40.2X5	T40.2X6
Dromostanolone	T38.7X1	T38.7X2	T38.7X3	T38.7X4	T38.7X5	T38.7X6
Dronabinol	T40.711	T40.712	T40.713	T40.714	T40.715	T40.716
Droperidol	T43.591	T43.592	T43.593	T43.594	T43.595	T43.596
Dropropizine	T48.3X1	T48.3X2	T48.3X3	T48.3X4	T48.3X5	T48.3X6
Drostanolone	T38.7X1	T38.7X2	T38.7X3	T38.7X4	T38.7X5	T38.7X6
Drotaverine	T44.3X1	T44.3X2	T44.3X3	T44.3X4	T44.3X5	I44.3X6
Drotrecogin alfa	T45.511	T45.512	T45.513	T45.514	T45.515	T45.516
Drug NEC	T50.901	T50.902	T50.903	T50.904	T50.905	T50.906
specified NEC	T50.991	T50.992	T50.993	T50.994	T50.995	T50.996
DTIC	T45.1X1	T45.1X2	T45.1X3	T45.1X4	T45.1X5	T45.1X6
Duboisine	T44.3X1	T44.3X2	T44.3X3	T44.3X4	T44.3X5	T44.3X6
Dulcolax	T47.2X1	T47.2X2	T47.2X3	T47.2X4	T47.2X5	T47.2X6
Duponol (C) (EP)	T49.2X1	T49.2X2	T49.2X3	T49.2X4	T49.2X5	T49.2X6
Durabolin	T38.7X1	T38.7X2	T38.7X3	T38.7X4	T38.7X5	T38.7X6
Dyclone	T41.3X1	T41.3X2	T41.3X3	T41.3X4	T41.3X5	T41.3X6
Dyclonine	T41.3X1	T41.3X2	T41.3X3	T41.3X4	T41.3X5	T41.3X6
Dydrogesterone	T38.5X1	T38.5X2	T38.5X3	T38.5X4	T38.5X5	T38.5X6
Dye NEC	T65.6X1	T65.6X2	T65.6X3	T65.6X4	—	—
antiseptic	T49.0X1	T49.0X2	T49.0X3	T49.0X4	T49.0X5	T49.0X6
diagnostic agents	T50.8X1	T50.8X2	T50.8X3	T50.8X4	T50.8X5	T50.8X6
pharmaceutical NEC	T50.901	T50.902	T50.903	T50.904	T50.905	T50.906
Dyflos	T44.0X1	T44.0X2	T44.0X3	T44.0X4	T44.0X5	T44.0X6
Dymelor	T38.3X1	T38.3X2	T38.3X3	T38.3X4	T38.3X5	T38.3X6
Dynamite	T65.3X1	T65.3X2	T65.3X3	T65.3X4	—	—
fumes	T59.891	T59.892	T59.893	T59.894	—	—
Dyphylline	T44.3X1	T44.3X2	T44.3X3	T44.3X4	T44.3X5	T44.3X6
E						
Ear drug NEC	T49.6X1	T49.6X2	T49.6X3	T49.6X4	T49.6X5	T49.6X6
Ear preparations	T49.6X1	T49.6X2	T49.6X3	T49.6X4	T49.6X5	T49.6X6
Econazole	T49.0X1	T49.0X2	T49.0X3	T49.0X4	T49.0X5	T49.0X6
Ecothiopate iodide	T49.5X1	T49.5X2	T49.5X3	T49.5X4	T49.5X5	T49.5X6
Echothiophate, echothiopate, ecothiopate	T49.5X1	T49.5X2	T49.5X3	T49.5X4	T49.5X5	T49.5X6

TABLE OF DRUGS AND CHEMICALS

	External Cause (T-Code)					
Substance	Poisoning, Accidental (Unintentional)	Poisoning, Intentional Self-Harm	Poisoning, Assault	Poisoning, Undetermined	Adverse Effect	Underdosing
Ecstasy	T43.641	T43.642	T43.643	T43.644	—	—
Ectylurea	T42.6X1	T42.6X2	T42.6X3	T42.6X4	T42.6X5	T42.6X6
Edathamil disodium	T45.8X1	T45.8X2	T45.8X3	T45.8X4	T45.8X5	T45.8X6
Edecrin	T50.1X1	T50.1X2	T50.1X3	T50.1X4	T50.1X5	T50.1X6
Edetate, disodium (calcium)	T45.8X1	T45.8X2	T45.8X3	T45.8X4	T45.8X5	T45.8X6
Edoxudine	T49.5X1	T49.5X2	T49.5X3	T49.5X4	T49.5X5	T49.5X6
Edrophonium	T44.0X1	T44.0X2	T44.0X3	T44.0X4	T44.0X5	T44.0X6
chloride	T44.0X1	T44.0X2	T44.0X3	T44.0X4	T44.0X5	T44.0X6
EDTA	T50.6X1	T50.6X2	T50.6X3	T50.6X4	T50.6X5	T50.6X6
Eflornithine	T37.2X1	T37.2X2	T37.2X3	T37.2X4	T37.2X5	T37.2X6
Efloxate	T46.3X1	T46.3X2	T46.3X3	T46.3X4	T46.3X5	T46.3X6
Elase	T49.8X1	T49.8X2	T49.8X3	T49.8X4	T49.8X5	T49.8X6
Elastase	T47.5X1	T47.5X2	T47.5X3	T47.5X4	T47.5X5	T47.5X6
Elaterium	T47.2X1	T47.2X2	T47.2X3	T47.2X4	T47.2X5	T47.2X6
Elcatonin	T50.991	T50.992	T50.993	T50.994	T50.995	T50.996
Elder	T62.2X1	T62.2X2	T62.2X3	T62.2X4	—	—
berry (unripe)	T62.1X1	T62.1X2	T62.1X3	T62.1X4	—	—
Electrolyte balance drug	T50.3X1	T50.3X2	T50.3X3	T50.3X4	T50.3X5	T50.3X6
Electrolytes NEC	T50.3X1	T50.3X2	T50.3X3	T50.3X4	T50.3X5	T50.3X6
Electrolytic agent NEC	T50.3X1	T50.3X2	T50.3X3	T50.3X4	T50.3X5	T50.3X6
Elemental diet	T50.901	T50.902	T50.903	T50.904	T50.905	T50.906
Elliptinium acetate	T45.1X1	T45.1X2	T45.1X3	T45.1X4	T45.1X5	T45.1X6
Embramine	T45.0X1	T45.0X2	T45.0X3	T45.0X4	T45.0X5	T45.0X6
Emepronium (salts)	T44.3X1	T44.3X2	T44.3X3	T44.3X4	T44.3X5	T44.3X6
bromide	T44.3X1	T44.3X2	T44.3X3	T44.3X4	T44.3X5	T44.3X6
Emetic NEC	T47.7X1	T47.7X2	T47.7X3	T47.7X4	T47.7X5	T47.7X6
Emetine	T37.3X1	T37.3X2	T37.3X3	T37.3X4	T37.3X5	T37.3X6
Emollient NEC	T49.3X1	T49.3X2	T49.3X3	T49.3X4	T49.3X5	T49.3X6
Emorfazone	T39.8X1	T39.8X2	T39.8X3	T39.8X4	T39.8X5	T39.8X6
Emylcamate	T43.591	T43.592	T43.593	T43.594	T43.595	T43.596
Enalapril	T46.4X1	T46.4X2	T46.4X3	T46.4X4	T46.4X5	T46.4X6
Enalaprilat	T46.4X1	T46.4X2	T46.4X3	T46.4X4	T46.4X5	T46.4X6
Encainide	T46.2X1	T46.2X2	T46.2X3	T46.2X4	T46.2X5	T46.2X6
Endocaine	T41.3X1	T41.3X2	T41.3X3	T41.3X4	T41.3X5	T41.3X6
Endosulfan	T60.2X1	T60.2X2	T60.2X3	T60.2X4	—	—
Endothall	T60.3X1	T60.3X2	T60.3X3	T60.3X4	—	—
Endralazine	T46.5X1	T46.5X2	T46.5X3	T46.5X4	T46.5X5	T46.5X6
Endrin	T60.1X1	T60.1X2	T60.1X3	T60.1X4	—	—
Enflurane	T41.0X1	T41.0X2	T41.0X3	T41.0X4	T41.0X5	T41.0X6
Enhexymal	T42.3X1	T42.3X2	T42.3X3	T42.3X4	T42.3X5	T42.3X6
Enocitabine	T45.1X1	T45.1X2	T45.1X3	T45.1X4	T45.1X5	T45.1X6
Enovid	T38.4X1	T38.4X2	T38.4X3	T38.4X4	T38.4X5	T38.4X6

	External Cause (T-Code)					
Substance	Poisoning, Accidental (Unintentional)	Poisoning, Intentional Self-Harm	Poisoning, Assault	Poisoning, Undetermined	Adverse Effect	Underdosing
Enoxacin	T36.8X1	T36.8X2	T36.8X3	T36.8X4	T36.8X5	T36.8X6
Enoxaparin (sodium)	T45.511	T45.512	T45.513	T45.514	T45.515	T45.516
Enpiprazole	T43.591	T43.592	T43.593	T43.594	T43.595	T43.596
Enprofylline	T48.6X1	T48.6X2	T48.6X3	T48.6X4	T48.6X5	T48.6X6
Enprostil	T47.1X1	T47.1X2	T47.1X3	T47.1X4	T47.1X5	T47.1X6
ENT preparations (anti-infectives)	T49.6X1	T49.6X2	T49.6X3	T49.6X4	T49.6X5	T49.6X6
Enviomycin	T36.8X1	T36.8X2	T36.8X3	T36.8X4	T36.8X5	T36.8X6
Enzodase	T45.3X1	T45.3X2	T45.3X3	T45.3X4	T45.3X5	T45.3X6
Enzyme NEC	T45.3X1	T45.3X2	T45.3X3	T45.3X4	T45.3X5	T45.3X6
depolymerizing	T49.8X1	T49.8X2	T49.8X3	T49.8X4	T49.8X5	T49.8X6
fibrolytic	T45.3X1	T45.3X2	T45.3X3	T45.3X4	T45.3X5	T45.3X6
gastric	T47.5X1	T47.5X2	T47.5X3	T47.5X4	T47.5X5	T47.5X6
intestinal	T47.5X1	T47.5X2	T47.5X3	T47.5X4	T47.5X5	T47.5X6
local action	T49.4X1	T49.4X2	T49.4X3	T49.4X4	T49.4X5	T49.4X6
proteolytic	T49.4X1	T49.4X2	T49.4X3	T49.4X4	T49.4X5	T49.4X6
thrombolytic	T45.3X1	T45.3X2	T45.3X3	T45.3X4	T45.3X5	T45.3X6
EPAB	T41.3X1	T41.3X2	T41.3X3	T41.3X4	T41.3X5	T41.3X6
Epanutin	T42.0X1	T42.0X2	T42.0X3	T42.0X4	T42.0X5	T42.0X6
Ephedra	T44.991	T44.992	T44.993	T44.994	T44.995	T44.996
Ephedrine	T44.991	T44.992	T44.993	T44.994	T44.995	T44.996
Epichlorhydrin, epichlorohydrin	T52.8X1	T52.8X2	T52.8X3	T52.8X4	—	—
Epicillin	T36.0X1	T36.0X2	T36.0X3	T36.0X4	T36.0X5	T36.0X6
Epiestriol	T38.5X1	T38.5X2	T38.5X3	T38.5X4	T38.5X5	T38.5X6
Epilim — see Sodium valproate						
Epimestrol	T38.5X1	T38.5X2	T38.5X3	T38.5X4	T38.5X5	T38.5X6
Epinephrine	T44.5X1	T44.5X2	T44.5X3	T44.5X4	T44.5X5	T44.5X6
Epirubicin	T45.1X1	T45.1X2	T45.1X3	T45.1X4	T45.1X5	T45.1X6
Epitiostanol	T38.7X1	T38.7X2	T38.7X3	T38.7X4	T38.7X5	T38.7X6
Epitizide	T50.2X1	T50.2X2	T50.2X3	T50.2X4	T50.2X5	T50.2X6
EPN	T60.0X1	T60.0X2	T60.0X3	T60.0X4	—	—
EPO	T45.8X1	T45.8X2	T45.8X3	T45.8X4	T45.8X5	T45.8X6
Epoetin alpha	T45.8X1	T45.8X2	T45.8X3	T45.8X4	T45.8X5	T45.8X6
Epomediol	T50.991	T50.992	T50.993	T50.994	T50.995	T50.996
Epoprostenol	T45.521	T45.522	T45.523	T45.524	T45.525	T45.526
Epoxy resin	T65.891	T65.892	T65.893	T65.894	—	—
Eprazinone	T48.4X1	T48.4X2	T48.4X3	T48.4X4	T48.4X5	T48.4X6
Epsilon amino-caproic acid	T45.621	T45.622	T45.623	T45.624	T45.625	T45.626
Epsom salt	T47.3X1	T47.3X2	T47.3X3	T47.3X4	T47.3X5	T47.3X6
Eptazocine	T40.491	T40.492	T40.493	T40.494	T40.495	T40.496
Equanil	T43.591	T43.592	T43.593	T43.594	T43.595	T43.596
Equisetum	T62.2X1	T62.2X2	T62.2X3	T62.2X4	—	—
diuretic	T50.2X1	T50.2X2	T50.2X3	T50.2X4	T50.2X5	T50.2X6

◀ New ◀ Revised ~~deleted~~ Deleted

Substance	External Cause (T-Code)					
	Poisoning, Accidental (Unintentional)	Poisoning, Intentional Self-Harm	Poisoning, Assault	Poisoning, Undetermined	Adverse Effect	Underdosing
Ergobasine	T48.0X1	T48.0X2	T48.0X3	T48.0X4	T48.0X5	T48.0X6
Ergocalciferol	T45.2X1	T45.2X2	T45.2X3	T45.2X4	T45.2X5	T45.2X6
Ergoloid mesylates	T46.7X1	T46.7X2	T46.7X3	T46.7X4	T46.7X5	T46.7X6
Ergometrine	T48.0X1	T48.0X2	T48.0X3	T48.0X4	T48.0X5	T48.0X6
Ergonovine	T48.0X1	T48.0X2	T48.0X3	T48.0X4	T48.0X5	T48.0X6
Ergot NEC	T64.81	T64.82	T64.83	T64.84	—	—
derivative	T48.0X1	T48.0X2	T48.0X3	T48.0X4	T48.0X5	T48.0X6
medicinal (alkaloids)	T48.0X1	T48.0X2	T48.0X3	T48.0X4	T48.0X5	T48.0X6
prepared	T48.0X1	T48.0X2	T48.0X3	T48.0X4	T48.0X5	T48.0X6
Ergotamine	T46.5X1	T46.5X2	T46.5X3	T46.5X4	T46.5X5	T46.5X6
Ergotocine	T48.0X1	T48.0X2	T48.0X3	T48.0X4	T48.0X5	T48.0X6
Ergotrate	T48.0X1	T48.0X2	T48.0X3	T48.0X4	T48.0X5	T48.0X6
Eritrityl tetranitrate	T46.3X1	T46.3X2	T46.3X3	T46.3X4	T46.3X5	T46.3X6
Erythrityl tetranitrate	T46.3X1	T46.3X2	T46.3X3	T46.3X4	T46.3X5	T46.3X6
Erythrol tetranitrate	T46.3X1	T46.3X2	T46.3X3	T46.3X4	T46.3X5	T46.3X6
Erythromycin (salts)	T36.3X1	T36.3X2	T36.3X3	T36.3X4	T36.3X5	T36.3X6
ophthalmic preparation	T49.5X1	T49.5X2	T49.5X3	T49.5X4	T49.5X5	T49.5X6
topical NEC	T49.0X1	T49.0X2	T49.0X3	T49.0X4	T49.0X5	T49.0X6
Erythropoietin	T45.8X1	T45.8X2	T45.8X3	T45.8X4	T45.8X5	T45.8X6
human	T45.8X1	T45.8X2	T45.8X3	T45.8X4	T45.8X5	T45.8X6
Escin	T46.991	T46.992	T46.993	T46.994	T46.995	T46.996
Esculin	T45.2X1	T45.2X2	T45.2X3	T45.2X4	T45.2X5	T45.2X6
Esculoside	T45.2X1	T45.2X2	T45.2X3	T45.2X4	T45.2X5	T45.2X6
ESDT (ether-soluble tar distillate)	T49.1X1	T49.1X2	T49.1X3	T49.1X4	T49.1X5	T49.1X6
Eserine	T49.5X1	T49.5X2	T49.5X3	T49.5X4	T49.5X5	T49.5X6
Esflurbiprofen	T39.311	T39.312	T39.313	T39.314	T39.315	T39.316
Eskabarb	T42.3X1	T42.3X2	T42.3X3	T42.3X4	T42.3X5	T42.3X6
Eskalith	T43.8X1	T43.8X2	T43.8X3	T43.8X4	T43.8X5	T43.8X6
Esmolol	T44.7X1	T44.7X2	T44.7X3	T44.7X4	T44.7X5	T44.7X6
Estanozolol	T38.7X1	T38.7X2	T38.7X3	T38.7X4	T38.7X5	T38.7X6
Estazolam	T42.4X1	T42.4X2	T42.4X3	T42.4X4	T42.4X5	T42.4X6
Estradiol	T38.5X1	T38.5X2	T38.5X3	T38.5X4	T38.5X5	T38.5X6
with testosterone	T38.7X1	T38.7X2	T38.7X3	T38.7X4	T38.7X5	T38.7X6
benzoate	T38.5X1	T38.5X2	T38.5X3	T38.5X4	T38.5X5	T38.5X6
Estramustine	T45.1X1	T45.1X2	T45.1X3	T45.1X4	T45.1X5	T45.1X6
Estriol	T38.5X1	T38.5X2	T38.5X3	T38.5X4	T38.5X5	T38.5X6
Estrogen	T38.5X1	T38.5X2	T38.5X3	T38.5X4	T38.5X5	T38.5X6
with progesterone	T38.5X1	T38.5X2	T38.5X3	T38.5X4	T38.5X5	T38.5X6
conjugated	T38.5X1	T38.5X2	T38.5X3	T38.5X4	T38.5X5	T38.5X6
Estrone	T38.5X1	T38.5X2	T38.5X3	T38.5X4	T38.5X5	T38.5X6
Estropipate	T38.5X1	T38.5X2	T38.5X3	T38.5X4	T38.5X5	T38.5X6

Substance	External Cause (T-Code)					
	Poisoning, Accidental (Unintentional)	Poisoning, Intentional Self-Harm	Poisoning, Assault	Poisoning, Undetermined	Adverse Effect	Underdosing
Etacrynate sodium	T50.1X1	T50.1X2	T50.1X3	T50.1X4	T50.1X5	T50.1X6
Etacrynic acid	T50.1X1	T50.1X2	T50.1X3	T50.1X4	T50.1X5	T50.1X6
Etafedrine	T48.6X1	T48.6X2	T48.6X3	T48.6X4	T48.6X5	T48.6X6
Etafenone	T46.3X1	T46.3X2	T46.3X3	T46.3X4	T46.3X5	T46.3X6
Etambutol	T37.1X1	T37.1X2	T37.1X3	T37.1X4	T37.1X5	T37.1X6
Etamiphyllin	T48.6X1	T48.6X2	T48.6X3	T48.6X4	T48.6X5	T48.6X6
Etamivan	T50.7X1	T50.7X2	T50.7X3	T50.7X4	T50.7X5	T50.7X6
Etamsylate	T45.7X1	T45.7X2	T45.7X3	T45.7X4	T45.7X5	T45.7X6
Etebenecid	T50.4X1	T50.4X2	T50.4X3	T50.4X4	T50.4X5	T50.4X6
Ethacridine	T49.0X1	T49.0X2	T49.0X3	T49.0X4	T49.0X5	T49.0X6
Ethacrynic acid	T50.1X1	T50.1X2	T50.1X3	T50.1X4	T50.1X5	T50.1X6
Ethadione	T42.2X1	T42.2X2	T42.2X3	T42.2X4	T42.2X5	T42.2X6
Ethambutol	T37.1X1	T37.1X2	T37.1X3	T37.1X4	T37.1X5	T37.1X6
Ethamide	T50.2X1	T50.2X2	T50.2X3	T50.2X4	T50.2X5	T50.2X6
Ethamivan	T50.7X1	T50.7X2	T50.7X3	T50.7X4	T50.7X5	T50.7X6
Ethamsylate	T45.7X1	T45.7X2	T45.7X3	T45.7X4	T45.7X5	T45.7X6
Ethanol	T51.0X1	T51.0X2	T51.0X3	T51.0X4	—	—
beverage	T51.0X1	T51.0X2	T51.0X3	T51.0X4	—	—
Ethanolamine oleate	T46.8X1	T46.8X2	T46.8X3	T46.8X4	T46.8X5	T46.8X6
Ethaverine	T44.3X1	T44.3X2	T44.3X3	T44.3X4	T44.3X5	T44.3X6
Ethchlorvynol	T42.6X1	T42.6X2	T42.6X3	T42.6X4	T42.6X5	T42.6X6
Ethebenecid	T50.4X1	T50.4X2	T50.4X3	T50.4X4	T50.4X5	T50.4X6
Ether (vapor)	T41.0X1	T41.0X2	T41.0X3	T41.0X4	T41.0X5	T41.0X6
anesthetic	T41.0X1	T41.0X2	T41.0X3	T41.0X4	T41.0X5	T41.0X6
divinyl	T41.0X1	T41.0X2	T41.0X3	T41.0X4	T41.0X5	T41.0X6
ethyl (medicinal)	T41.0X1	T41.0X2	T41.0X3	T41.0X4	T41.0X5	T41.0X6
nonmedicinal	T52.8X1	T52.8X2	T52.8X3	T52.8X4	—	—
petroleum—*see Ligroin*						
solvent	T52.8X1	T52.8X2	T52.8X3	T52.8X4	—	—
Ethiazide	T50.2X1	T50.2X2	T50.2X3	T50.2X4	T50.2X5	T50.2X6
Ethidium chloride (vapor)	T59.891	T59.892	T59.893	T59.894	—	—
Ethinamate	T42.6X1	T42.6X2	T42.6X3	T42.6X4	T42.6X5	T42.6X6
Ethinylestradiol, ethinyloestradiol	T38.5X1	T38.5X2	T38.5X3	T38.5X4	T38.5X5	T38.5X6
with						
levonorgestrel	T38.4X1	T38.4X2	T38.4X3	T38.4X4	T38.4X5	T38.4X6
norethisterone	T38.4X1	T38.4X2	T38.4X3	T38.4X4	T38.4X5	T38.4X6
Ethiodized oil (131 I)	T50.8X1	T50.8X2	T50.8X3	T50.8X4	T50.8X5	T50.8X6
Ethion	T60.0X1	T60.0X2	T60.0X3	T60.0X4	—	—
Ethionamide	T37.1X1	T37.1X2	T37.1X3	T37.1X4	T37.1X5	T37.1X6
Ethioniamide	T37.1X1	T37.1X2	T37.1X3	T37.1X4	T37.1X5	T37.1X6
Ethisterone	T38.5X1	T38.5X2	T38.5X3	T38.5X4	T38.5X5	T38.5X6
Ethobral	T42.3X1	T42.3X2	T42.3X3	T42.3X4	T42.3X5	T42.3X6

Substance	External Cause (T-Code)					
	Poisoning, Accidental (Unintentional)	Poisoning, Intentional Self-Harm	Poisoning, Assault	Poisoning, Undetermined	Adverse Effect	Underdosing
Ethocaine (infiltration) (topical)	T41.3X1	T41.3X2	T41.3X3	T41.3X4	T41.3X5	T41.3X6
nerve block (peripheral) (plexus)	T41.3X1	T41.3X2	T41.3X3	T41.3X4	T41.3X5	T41.3X6
spinal	T41.3X1	T41.3X2	T41.3X3	T41.3X4	T41.3X5	T41.3X6
Ethoheptazine	T40.491	T40.492	T40.493	T40.494	T40.495	T40.496
Ethopropazine	T44.3X1	T44.3X2	T44.3X3	T44.3X4	T44.3X5	T44.3X6
Ethosuximide	T42.2X1	T42.2X2	T42.2X3	T42.2X4	T42.2X5	T42.2X6
Ethotoin	T42.0X1	T42.0X2	T42.0X3	T42.0X4	T42.0X5	T42.0X6
Ethoxazene	T37.91	T37.92	T37.93	T37.94	T37.95	T37.96
Ethoxazorutoside	T46.991	T46.992	T46.993	T46.994	T46.995	T46.996
2-Ethoxyethanol	T52.3X1	T52.3X2	T52.3X3	T52.3X4	—	—
Ethoxzolamide	T50.2X1	T50.2X2	T50.2X3	T50.2X4	T50.2X5	T50.2X6
Ethyl						
acetate	T52.8X1	T52.8X2	T52.8X3	T52.8X4	—	—
alcohol	T51.0X1	T51.0X2	T51.0X3	T51.0X4	—	—
beverage	T51.0X1	T51.0X2	T51.0X3	T51.0X4	—	—
aldehyde (vapor)	T59.891	T59.892	T59.893	T59.894	—	—
liquid	T52.8X1	T52.8X2	T52.8X3	T52.8X4	—	—
aminobenzoate	T41.3X1	T41.3X2	T41.3X3	T41.3X4	T41.3X5	T41.3X6
aminophenothiazine	T43.3X1	T43.3X2	T43.3X3	T43.3X4	T43.3X5	T43.3X6
benzoate	T52.8X1	T52.8X2	T52.8X3	T52.8X4	—	—
biscoumacetate	T45.511	T45.512	T45.513	T45.514	T45.515	T45.516
bromide (anesthetic)	T41.0X1	T41.0X2	T41.0X3	T41.0X4	T41.0X5	T41.0X6
carbamate	T45.1X1	T45.1X2	T45.1X3	T45.1X4	T45.1X5	T45.1X6
carbinol	T51.3X1	T51.3X2	T51.3X3	T51.3X4	—	—
carbonate	T52.8X1	T52.8X2	T52.8X3	T52.8X4	—	—
chaulmoograte	T37.1X1	T37.1X2	T37.1X3	T37.1X4	T37.1X5	T37.1X6
chloride (anesthetic)	T41.0X1	T41.0X2	T41.0X3	T41.0X4	T41.0X5	T41.0X6
anesthetic (local)	T41.3X1	T41.3X2	T41.3X3	T41.3X4	T41.3X5	T41.3X6
inhaled	T41.0X1	T41.0X2	T41.0X3	T41.0X4	T41.0X5	T41.0X6
local	T49.4X1	T49.4X2	T49.4X3	T49.4X4	T49.4X5	T49.4X6
solvent	T53.6X1	T53.6X2	T53.6X3	T53.6X4	—	—
dibunate	T48.3X1	T48.3X2	T48.3X3	T48.3X4	T48.3X5	T48.3X6
dichloroarsine (vapor)	T57.0X1	T57.0X2	T57.0X3	T57.0X4	—	—
estranol	T38.7X1	T38.7X2	T38.7X3	T38.7X4	T38.7X5	T38.7X6
ether — see also Ether	T52.8X1	T52.8X2	T52.8X3	T52.8X4	—	—
formate NEC (solvent)	T52.0X1	T52.0X2	T52.0X3	T52.0X4	—	—
fumarate	T49.4X1	T49.4X2	T49.4X3	T49.4X4	T49.4X5	T49.4X6
hydroxyisobutyrate NEC (solvent)	T52.8X1	T52.8X2	T52.8X3	T52.8X4	—	—
iodoacetate	T59.3X1	T59.3X2	T59.3X3	T59.3X4	—	—
lactate NEC (solvent)	T52.8X1	T52.8X2	T52.8X3	T52.8X4	—	—
loflazepate	T42.4X1	T42.4X2	T42.4X3	T42.4X4	T42.4X5	T42.4X6

Substance	External Cause (T-Code)					
	Poisoning, Accidental (Unintentional)	Poisoning, Intentional Self-Harm	Poisoning, Assault	Poisoning, Undetermined	Adverse Effect	Underdosing
Ethyl (Continued)						
mercuric chloride	T56.1X1	T56.1X2	T56.1X3	T56.1X4	—	—
methylcarbinol	T51.8X1	T51.8X2	T51.8X3	T51.8X4	—	—
morphine	T40.2X1	T40.2X2	T40.2X3	T40.2X4	T40.2X5	T40.2X6
noradrenaline	T48.6X1	T48.6X2	T48.6X3	T48.6X4	T48.6X5	T48.6X6
oxybutyrate NEC (solvent)	T52.8X1	T52.8X2	T52.8X3	T52.8X4	—	—
Ethylene (gas)	T59.891	T59.892	T59.893	T59.894	—	—
anesthetic (general)	T41.0X1	T41.0X2	T41.0X3	T41.0X4	T41.0X5	T41.0X6
chlorohydrin	T52.8X1	T52.8X2	T52.8X3	T52.8X4	—	—
vapor	T53.6X1	T53.6X2	T53.6X3	T53.6X4	—	—
dichloride	T52.8X1	T52.8X2	T52.8X3	T52.8X4	—	—
vapor	T53.6X1	T53.6X2	T53.6X3	T53.6X4	—	—
dinitrate	T52.3X1	T52.3X2	T52.3X3	T52.3X4	—	—
glycol(s)	T52.8X1	T52.8X2	T52.8X3	T52.8X4	—	—
dinitrate	T52.3X1	T52.3X2	T52.3X3	T52.3X4	—	—
monobutyl ether	T52.3X1	T52.3X2	T52.3X3	T52.3X4	—	—
imine	T54.1X1	T54.1X2	T54.1X3	T54.1X4	—	—
oxide (fumigant) (nonmedicinal)	T59.891	T59.892	T59.893	T59.894	—	—
medicinal	T49.0X1	T49.0X2	T49.0X3	T49.0X4	T49.0X5	T49.0X6
Ethylenediamine theophylline	T48.6X1	T48.6X2	T48.6X3	T48.6X4	T48.6X5	T48.6X6
Ethylenediaminetetra-acetic acid	T50.6X1	T50.6X2	T50.6X3	T50.6X4	T50.6X5	T50.6X6
Ethylenedinitrilotetra-acetate	T50.6X1	T50.6X2	T50.6X3	T50.6X4	T50.6X5	T50.6X6
Ethylestrenol	T38.7X1	T38.7X2	T38.7X3	T38.7X4	T38.7X5	T38.7X6
Ethylhydroxycellulose	T47.4X1	T47.4X2	T47.4X3	T47.4X4	T47.4X5	T47.4X6
Ethylidene						
chloride NEC	T53.6X1	T53.6X2	T53.6X3	T53.6X4	—	—
diacetate	T60.3X1	T60.3X2	T60.3X3	T60.3X4	—	—
dicoumarin	T45.511	T45.512	T45.513	T45.514	T45.515	T45.516
dicoumarol	T45.511	T45.512	T45.513	T45.514	T45.515	T45.516
diethyl ether	T52.0X1	T52.0X2	T52.0X3	T52.0X4	—	—
Ethylmorphine	T40.2X1	T40.2X2	T40.2X3	T40.2X4	T40.2X5	T40.2X6
Ethylnorepinephrine	T48.6X1	T48.6X2	T48.6X3	T48.6X4	T48.6X5	T48.6X6
Ethylparachlorophen-oxyisobutyrate	T46.6X1	T46.6X2	T46.6X3	T46.6X4	T46.6X5	T46.6X6
Ethynodiol	T38.4X1	T38.4X2	T38.4X3	T38.4X4	T38.4X5	T38.4X6
with mestranol diacetate	T38.4X1	T38.4X2	T38.4X3	T38.4X4	T38.4X5	T38.4X6
Etidocaine	T41.3X1	T41.3X2	T41.3X3	T41.3X4	T41.3X5	T41.3X6
infiltration (subcutaneous)	T41.3X1	T41.3X2	T41.3X3	T41.3X4	T41.3X5	T41.3X6
nerve (peripheral) (plexus)	T41.3X1	T41.3X2	T41.3X3	T41.3X4	T41.3X5	T41.3X6
Etidronate	T50.991	T50.992	T50.993	T50.994	T50.995	T50.996
Etidronic acid (disodium salt)	T50.991	T50.992	T50.993	T50.994	T50.995	T50.996
Etifoxine	T42.6X1	T42.6X2	T42.6X3	T42.6X4	T42.6X5	T42.6X6

◀ New ◀ Revised ~~deleted~~ Deleted

Substance	Poisoning, Accidental (Unintentional)	Poisoning, Intentional Self-Harm	Poisoning, Assault	Poisoning, Undetermined	Adverse Effect	Underdosing
Etilefrine	T44.4X1	T44.4X2	T44.4X3	T44.4X4	T44.4X5	T44.4X6
Etilfen	T42.3X1	T42.3X2	T42.3X3	T42.3X4	T42.3X5	T42.3X6
Etinodiol	T38.4X1	T38.4X2	T38.4X3	T38.4X4	T38.4X5	T38.4X6
Etiroxate	T46.6X1	T46.6X2	T46.6X3	T46.6X4	T46.6X5	T46.6X6
Etizolam	T42.4X1	T42.4X2	T42.4X3	T42.4X4	T42.4X5	T42.4X6
Etodolac	T39.391	T39.392	T39.393	T39.394	T39.395	T39.396
Etofamide	T37.3X1	T37.3X2	T37.3X3	T37.3X4	T37.3X5	T37.3X6
Etofibrate	T46.6X1	T46.6X2	T46.6X3	T46.6X4	T46.6X5	T46.6X6
Etofylline	T46.7X1	T46.7X2	T46.7X3	T46.7X4	T46.7X5	T46.7X6
clofibrate	T46.6X1	T46.6X2	T46.6X3	T46.6X4	T46.6X5	T46.6X6
Etoglucid	T45.1X1	T45.1X2	T45.1X3	T45.1X4	T45.1X5	T45.1X6
Etomidate	T41.1X1	T41.1X2	T41.1X3	T41.1X4	T41.1X5	T41.1X6
Etomide	T39.8X1	T39.8X2	T39.8X3	T39.8X4	T39.8X5	T39.8X6
Etomidoline	T44.3X1	T44.3X2	T44.3X3	T44.3X4	T44.3X5	T44.3X6
Etoposide	T45.1X1	T45.1X2	T45.1X3	T45.1X4	T45.1X5	T45.1X6
Etorphine	T40.2X1	T40.2X2	T40.2X3	T40.2X4	T40.2X5	T40.2X6
Etoval	T42.3X1	T42.3X2	T42.3X3	T42.3X4	T42.3X5	T42.3X6
Etazolln	T50.1X1	T50.1X2	T50.1X3	T50.1X4	T50.1X5	T50.1X6
Etretinate	T50.991	T50.992	T50.993	T50.994	T50.995	T50.996
Etryptamine	T43.691	T43.692	T43.693	T43.694	T43.695	T43.696
Etybenzatropine	T44.3X1	T44.3X2	T44.3X3	T44.3X4	T44.3X5	T44.3X6
Etynodiol	T38.4X1	T38.4X2	T38.4X3	T38.4X4	T38.4X5	T38.4X6
Eucaine	T41.3X1	T41.3X2	T41.3X3	T41.3X4	T41.3X5	T41.3X6
Eucalyptus oil	T49.7X1	T49.7X2	T49.7X3	T49.7X4	T49.7X5	T49.7X6
Eucatropine	T49.5X1	T49.5X2	T49.5X3	T49.5X4	T49.5X5	T49.5X6
Eucodal	T40.2X1	T40.2X2	T40.2X3	T40.2X4	T40.2X5	T40.2X6
Euneryl	T42.3X1	T42.3X2	T42.3X3	T42.3X4	T42.3X5	T42.3X6
Euphthalmine	T44.3X1	T44.3X2	T44.3X3	T44.3X4	T44.3X5	T44.3X6
Eurax	T49.0X1	T49.0X2	T49.0X3	T49.0X4	T49.0X5	T49.0X6
Euresol	T49.4X1	T49.4X2	T49.4X3	T49.4X4	T49.4X5	T49.4X6
Euthroid	T38.1X1	T38.1X2	T38.1X3	T38.1X4	T38.1X5	T38.1X6
Evans blue	T50.8X1	T50.8X2	T50.8X3	T50.8X4	T50.8X5	T50.8X6
Evipal	T42.3X1	T42.3X2	T42.3X3	T42.3X4	T42.3X5	T42.3X6
sodium	T41.1X1	T41.1X2	T41.1X3	T41.1X4	T41.1X5	T41.1X6
Evipan	T42.3X1	T42.3X2	T42.3X3	T42.3X4	T42.3X5	T42.3X6
sodlum	T41.1X1	T41.1X2	T41.1X3	T41.1X4	T41.1X5	T41.1X6
Exalamide	T49.0X1	T49.0X2	T49.0X3	T49.0X4	T49.0X5	T49.0X6
Exalgin	T39.1X1	T39.1X2	T39.1X3	T39.1X4	T39.1X5	T39.1X6
Excipients, pharmaceutical	T50.901	T50.902	T50.903	T50.904	T50.905	T50.906
Exhaust gas (engine) (motor vehicle)	T58.01	T58.02	T58.03	T58.04	—	—
Ex-Lax (phenolphthalein)	T47.2X1	T47.2X2	T47.2X3	T47.2X4	T47.2X5	T47.2X6
Expectorant NEC	T48.4X1	T48.4X2	T48.4X3	T48.4X4	T48.4X5	T48.4X6

Substance	Poisoning, Accidental (Unintentional)	Poisoning, Intentional Self-Harm	Poisoning, Assault	Poisoning, Undetermined	Adverse Effect	Underdosing
Extended insulin zinc suspension	T38.3X1	T38.3X2	T38.3X3	T38.3X4	T38.3X5	T38.3X6
External medications (skin) (mucous membrane)	T49.91	T49.92	T49.93	T49.94	T49.95	T49.96
dental agent	T49.7X1	T49.7X2	T49.7X3	T49.7X4	T49.7X5	T49.7X6
ENT agent	T49.6X1	T49.6X2	T49.6X3	T49.6X4	T49.6X5	T49.6X6
ophthalmic preparation	T49.5X1	T49.5X2	T49.5X3	T49.5X4	T49.5X5	T49.5X6
specified NEC	T49.8X1	T49.8X2	T49.8X3	T49.8X4	T49.8X5	T49.8X6
Extrapyramidal antagonist NEC	T44.3X1	T44.3X2	T44.3X3	T44.3X4	T44.3X5	T44.3X6
Eye agents (anti-infective)	T49.5X1	T49.5X2	T49.5X3	T49.5X4	T49.5X5	T49.5X6
Eye drug NEC	T49.5X1	T49.5X2	T49.5X3	T49.5X4	T49.5X5	T49.5X6

F

Substance	Poisoning, Accidental (Unintentional)	Poisoning, Intentional Self-Harm	Poisoning, Assault	Poisoning, Undetermined	Adverse Effect	Underdosing
FAC (fluorouracil + doxorubicin + cyclophosphamide)	T45.1X1	T45.1X2	T45.1X3	T45.1X4	T45.1X5	T45.1X6
Factor						
I (fibrinogen)	T45.8X1	T45.8X2	T45.8X3	T45.8X4	T45.8X5	T45.8X6
III (thromboplastin)	T45.8X1	T45.8X2	T45.8X3	T45.8X4	T45.8X5	T45.8X6
VIII (antihemophilic Factor) (Concentrate)	T45.8X1	T45.8X2	T45.8X3	T45.8X4	T45.8X5	T45.8X6
IX complex	T45.7X1	T45.7X2	T45.7X3	T45.7X4	T45.7X5	T45.7X6
human	T45.8X1	T45.8X2	T45.8X3	T45.8X4	T45.8X5	T45.8X6
Famotidine	T47.0X1	T47.0X2	T47.0X3	T47.0X4	T47.0X5	T47.0X6
Fat suspension, intravenous	T50.991	T50.992	T50.993	T50.994	T50.995	T50.996
Fazadinium bromide	T48.1X1	T48.1X2	T48.1X3	T48.1X4	T48.1X5	T48.1X6
Febarbamate	T42.3X1	T42.3X2	T42.3X3	T42.3X4	T42.3X5	T42.3X6
Fecal softener	T47.4X1	T47.4X2	T47.4X3	T47.4X4	T47.4X5	T47.4X6
Fedrilate	T48.3X1	T48.3X2	T48.3X3	T48.3X4	T48.3X5	T48.3X6
Felodipine	T46.1X1	T46.1X2	T46.1X3	T46.1X4	T46.1X5	T46.1X6
Felypressin	T38.891	T38.892	T38.893	T38.894	T38.895	T38.896
Femoxetine	T43.221	T43.222	T43.223	T43.224	T43.225	T43.226
Fenalcomine	T46.3X1	T46.3X2	T46.3X3	T46.3X4	T46.3X5	T46.3X6
Fenamisal	T37.1X1	T37.1X2	T37.1X3	T37.1X4	T37.1X5	T37.1X6
Fenazone	T39.2X1	T39.2X2	T39.2X3	T39.2X4	T39.2X5	T39.2X6
Fenbendazole	T37.4X1	T37.4X2	T37.4X3	T37.4X4	T37.4X5	T37.4X6
Fenbutrazate	T50.5X1	T50.5X2	T50.5X3	T50.5X4	T50.5X5	T50.5X6
Fencamfamine	T43.691	T43.692	T43.693	T43.694	T43.695	T43.696
Fendiline	T46.1X1	T46.1X2	T46.1X3	T46.1X4	T46.1X5	T46.1X6
Fenetylline	T43.691	T43.692	T43.693	T43.694	T43.695	T43.696
Fenflumizole	T39.391	T39.392	T39.393	T39.394	T39.395	T39.396
Fenfluramine	T50.5X1	T50.5X2	T50.5X3	T50.5X4	T50.5X5	T50.5X6
Fenobarbital	T42.3X1	T42.3X2	T42.3X3	T42.3X4	T42.3X5	T42.3X6
Fenofibrate	T46.6X1	T46.6X2	T46.6X3	T46.6X4	T46.6X5	T46.6X6
Fenoprofen	T39.311	T39.312	T39.313	T39.314	T39.315	T39.316
Fenoterol	T48.6X1	T48.6X2	T48.6X3	T48.6X4	T48.6X5	T48.6X6

◀ New ◀ Revised ~~deleted~~ Deleted

TABLE OF DRUGS AND CHEMICALS

TABLE OF DRUGS AND CHEMICALS

Substance	External Cause (T-Code)					
	Poisoning, Accidental (Unintentional)	Poisoning, Intentional Self-Harm	Poisoning, Assault	Poisoning, Undetermined	Adverse Effect	Underdosing
Fenoverine	T44.3X1	T44.3X2	T44.3X3	T44.3X4	T44.3X5	T44.3X6
Fenoxazoline	T48.5X1	T48.5X2	T48.5X3	T48.5X4	T48.5X5	T48.5X6
Fenproporex	T50.5X1	T50.5X2	T50.5X3	T50.5X4	T50.5X5	T50.5X6
Fenquizone	T50.2X1	T50.2X2	T50.2X3	T50.2X4	T50.2X5	T50.2X6
Fentanyl (analogs)	T40.411	T40.412	T40.413	T40.414	T40.415	T40.416
Fentazin	T43.3X1	T43.3X2	T43.3X3	T43.3X4	T43.3X5	T43.3X6
Fenthion	T60.0X1	T60.0X2	T60.0X3	T60.0X4	—	—
Fenticlor	T49.0X1	T49.0X2	T49.0X3	T49.0X4	T49.0X5	T49.0X6
Fenylbutazone	T39.2X1	T39.2X2	T39.2X3	T39.2X4	T39.2X5	T39.2X6
Feprazone	T39.2X1	T39.2X2	T39.2X3	T39.2X4	T39.2X5	T39.2X6
Fer de lance (bite) (venom)	T63.061	T63.062	T63.063	T63.064	—	—
Ferric — see also Iron						
chloride	T45.4X1	T45.4X2	T45.4X3	T45.4X4	T45.4X5	T45.4X6
citrate	T45.4X1	T45.4X2	T45.4X3	T45.4X4	T45.4X5	T45.4X6
hydroxide						
colloidal	T45.4X1	T45.4X2	T45.4X3	T45.4X4	T45.4X5	T45.4X6
polymaltose	T45.4X1	T45.4X2	T45.4X3	T45.4X4	T45.4X5	T45.4X6
pyrophosphate	T45.4X1	T45.4X2	T45.4X3	T45.4X4	T45.4X5	T45.4X6
Ferritin	T45.4X1	T45.4X2	T45.4X3	T45.4X4	T45.4X5	T45.4X6
Ferrocholinate	T45.4X1	T45.4X2	T45.4X3	T45.4X4	T45.4X5	T45.4X6
Ferrodextrane	T45.4X1	T45.4X2	T45.4X3	T45.4X4	T45.4X5	T45.4X6
Ferropolimaler	T45.4X1	T45.4X2	T45.4X3	T45.4X4	T45.4X5	T45.4X6
Ferrous — see also Iron						
phosphate	T45.4X1	T45.4X2	T45.4X3	T45.4X4	T45.4X5	T45.4X6
salt	T45.4X1	T45.4X2	T45.4X3	T45.4X4	T45.4X5	T45.4X6
with folic acid	T45.4X1	T45.4X2	T45.4X3	T45.4X4	T45.4X5	T45.4X6
Ferrous fumarate, gluconate, lactate, salt NEC, sulfate (medicinal)	T45.4X1	T45.4X2	T45.4X3	T45.4X4	T45.4X5	T45.4X6
Ferrovanadium (fumes)	T59.891	T59.892	T59.893	T59.894	—	—
Ferrum — see Iron						
Fertilizers NEC	T65.891	T65.892	T65.893	T65.894	—	—
with herbicide mixture	T60.3X1	T60.3X2	T60.3X3	T60.3X4	—	—
Fetoxilate	T47.6X1	T47.6X2	T47.6X3	T47.6X4	T47.6X5	T47.6X6
Fiber, dietary	T47.4X1	T47.4X2	T47.4X3	T47.4X4	T47.4X5	T47.4X6
Fibrinogen (human)	T45.8X1	T45.8X2	T45.8X3	T45.8X4	T45.8X5	T45.8X6
Fibrinolysin (human)	T45.691	T45.692	T45.693	T45.694	T45.695	T45.696
Fibrinolysis						
affecting drug	T45.601	T45.602	T45.603	T45.604	T45.605	T45.606
inhibitor NEC	T45.621	T45.622	T45.623	T45.624	T45.625	T45.626
Fibrinolytic drug	T45.611	T45.612	T45.613	T45.614	T45.615	T45.616
Filix mas	T37.4X1	T37.4X2	T37.4X3	T37.4X4	T37.4X5	T37.4X6
Filtering cream	T49.3X1	T49.3X2	T49.3X3	T49.3X4	T49.3X5	T49.3X6

Substance	External Cause (T-Code)					
	Poisoning, Accidental (Unintentional)	Poisoning, Intentional Self-Harm	Poisoning, Assault	Poisoning, Undetermined	Adverse Effect	Underdosing
Fiorinal	T39.011	T39.012	T39.013	T39.014	T39.015	T39.016
Firedamp	T59.891	T59.892	T59.893	T59.894	—	—
Fish, noxious, nonbacterial	T61.91	T61.92	T61.93	T61.94	—	—
ciguatera	T61.01	T61.02	T61.03	T61.04	—	—
scombroid	T61.11	T61.12	T61.13	T61.14	—	—
shell	T61.781	T61.782	T61.783	T61.784	—	—
specified NEC	T61.771	T61.772	T61.773	T61.774	—	—
Flagyl	T37.3X1	T37.3X2	T37.3X3	T37.3X4	T37.3X5	T37.3X6
Flavine adenine dinucleotide	T45.2X1	T45.2X2	T45.2X3	T45.2X4	T45.2X5	T45.2X6
Flavodic acid	T46.991	T46.992	T46.993	T46.994	T46.995	T46.996
Flavoxate	T44.3X1	T44.3X2	T44.3X3	T44.3X4	T44.3X5	T44.3X6
Flaxedil	T48.1X1	T48.1X2	T48.1X3	T48.1X4	T48.1X5	T48.1X6
Flaxseed (medicinal)	T49.3X1	T49.3X2	T49.3X3	T49.3X4	T49.3X5	T49.3X6
Flecainide	T46.2X1	T46.2X2	T46.2X3	T46.2X4	T46.2X5	T46.2X6
Fleroxacin	T36.8X1	T36.8X2	T36.8X3	T36.8X4	T36.8X5	T36.8X6
Floctafenine	T39.8X1	T39.8X2	T39.8X3	T39.8X4	T39.8X5	T39.8X6
Flomax	T44.6X1	T44.6X2	T44.6X3	T44.6X4	T44.6X5	T44.6X6
Flomoxef	T36.1X1	T36.1X2	T36.1X3	T36.1X4	T36.1X5	T36.1X6
Flopropione	T44.3X1	T44.3X2	T44.3X3	T44.3X4	T44.3X5	T44.3X6
Florantyrone	T47.5X1	T47.5X2	T47.5X3	T47.5X4	T47.5X5	T47.5X6
Floraquin	T37.8X1	T37.8X2	T37.8X3	T37.8X4	T37.8X5	T37.8X6
Florinef	T38.0X1	T38.0X2	T38.0X3	T38.0X4	T38.0X5	T38.0X6
ENT agent	T49.6X1	T49.6X2	T49.6X3	T49.6X4	T49.6X5	T49.6X6
ophthalmic preparation	T49.5X1	T49.5X2	T49.5X3	T49.5X4	T49.5X5	T49.5X6
topical NEC	T49.0X1	T49.0X2	T49.0X3	T49.0X4	T49.0X5	T49.0X6
Flowers of sulfur	T49.4X1	T49.4X2	T49.4X3	T49.4X4	T49.4X5	T49.4X6
Floxuridine	T45.1X1	T45.1X2	T45.1X3	T45.1X4	T45.1X5	T45.1X6
Fluanisone	T43.4X1	T43.4X2	T43.4X3	T43.4X4	T43.4X5	T43.4X6
Flubendazole	T37.4X1	T37.4X2	T37.4X3	T37.4X4	T37.4X5	T37.4X6
Fluclorolone acetonide	T49.0X1	T49.0X2	T49.0X3	T49.0X4	T49.0X5	T49.0X6
Flucloxacillin	T36.0X1	T36.0X2	T36.0X3	T36.0X4	T36.0X5	T36.0X6
Fluconazole	T37.8X1	T37.8X2	T37.8X3	T37.8X4	T37.8X5	T37.8X6
Flucytosine	T37.8X1	T37.8X2	T37.8X3	T37.8X4	T37.8X5	T37.8X6
Fludeoxyglucose (18F)	T50.8X1	T50.8X2	T50.8X3	T50.8X4	T50.8X5	T50.8X6
Fludiazepam	T42.4X1	T42.4X2	T42.4X3	T42.4X4	T42.4X5	T42.4X6
Fludrocortisone	T50.0X1	T50.0X2	T50.0X3	T50.0X4	T50.0X5	T50.0X6
ENT agent	T49.6X1	T49.6X2	T49.6X3	T49.6X4	T49.6X5	T49.6X6
ophthalmic preparation	T49.5X1	T49.5X2	T49.5X3	T49.5X4	T49.5X5	T49.5X6
topical NEC	T49.0X1	T49.0X2	T49.0X3	T49.0X4	T49.0X5	T49.0X6
Fludroxycortide	T49.0X1	T49.0X2	T49.0X3	T49.0X4	T49.0X5	T49.0X6
Flufenamic acid	T39.391	T39.392	T39.393	T39.394	T39.395	T39.396
Fluindione	T45.511	T45.512	T45.513	T45.514	T45.515	T45.516

◀ New   ◀ Revised   ~~deleted~~ Deleted

Substance	Poisoning, Accidental (Unintentional)	Poisoning, Intentional Self-Harm	Poisoning, Assault	Poisoning, Undetermined	Adverse Effect	Underdosing
Flumequine	T37.8X1	T37.8X2	T37.8X3	T37.8X4	T37.8X5	T37.8X6
Flumethasone	T49.0X1	T49.0X2	T49.0X3	T49.0X4	T49.0X5	T49.0X6
Flumethiazide	T50.2X1	T50.2X2	T50.2X3	T50.2X4	T50.2X5	T50.2X6
Flumidin	T37.5X1	T37.5X2	T37.5X3	T37.5X4	T37.5X5	T37.5X6
Flunarizine	T46.7X1	T46.7X2	T46.7X3	T46.7X4	T46.7X5	T46.7X6
Flunidazole	T37.8X1	T37.8X2	T37.8X3	T37.8X4	T37.8X5	T37.8X6
Flunisolide	T48.6X1	T48.6X2	T48.6X3	T48.6X4	T48.6X5	T48.6X6
Flunitrazepam	T42.4X1	T42.4X2	T42.4X3	T42.4X4	T42.4X5	T42.4X6
Fluocinolone (acetonide)	T49.0X1	T49.0X2	T49.0X3	T49.0X4	T49.0X5	T49.0X6
Fluocinonide	T49.0X1	T49.0X2	T49.0X3	T49.0X4	T49.0X5	T49.0X6
Fluocortin (butyl)	T49.0X1	T49.0X2	T49.0X3	T49.0X4	T49.0X5	T49.0X6
Fluocortolone	T49.0X1	T49.0X2	T49.0X3	T49.0X4	T49.0X5	T49.0X6
Fluohydrocortisone	T38.0X1	T38.0X2	T38.0X3	T38.0X4	T38.0X5	T38.0X6
ENT agent	T49.6X1	T49.6X2	T49.6X3	T49.6X4	T49.6X5	T49.6X6
ophthalmic preparation	T49.5X1	T49.5X2	T49.5X3	T49.5X4	T49.5X5	T49.5X6
topical NEC	T49.0X1	T49.0X2	T49.0X3	T49.0X4	T49.0X5	T49.0X6
Fluonid	T49.0X1	T49.0X2	T49.0X3	T49.0X4	T49.0X5	T49.0X6
Fluopromazine	T43.3X1	T43.3X2	T43.3X3	T43.3X4	T43.3X5	T43.3X6
Fluoroacetate	T60.8X1	T60.8X2	T60.8X3	T60.8X4	—	—
Fluorescein	T50.8X1	T50.8X2	T50.8X3	T50.8X4	T50.8X5	T50.8X6
Fluorhydrocortisone	T50.0X1	T50.0X2	T50.0X3	T50.0X4	T50.0X5	T50.0X6
Fluoride (nonmedicinal) (pesticide) (sodium) NEC	T60.8X1	T60.8X2	T60.8X3	T60.8X4	—	—
hydrogen — *see Hydrofluoric acid*						
medicinal NEC	T50.991	T50.992	T50.993	T50.994	T50.995	T50.996
dental use	T49.7X1	T49.7X2	T49.7X3	T49.7X4	T49.7X5	T49.7X6
not pesticide NEC	T54.91	T54.92	T54.93	T54.94	—	—
stannous	T49.7X1	T49.7X2	T49.7X3	T49.7X4	T49.7X5	T49.7X6
Fluorinated corticosteroids	T38.0X1	T38.0X2	T38.0X3	T38.0X4	T38.0X5	T38.0X6
Fluorine (gas)	T59.5X1	T59.5X2	T59.5X3	T59.5X4	—	—
salt — *see Fluoride(s)*						
Fluoristan	T49.7X1	T49.7X2	T49.7X3	T49.7X4	T49.7X5	T49.7X6
Fluormetholone	T49.0X1	T49.0X2	T49.0X3	T49.0X4	T49.0X5	T49.0X6
Fluoroacetate	T60.8X1	T60.8X2	T60.8X3	T60.8X4	—	—
Fluorocarbon monomer	T53.6X1	T53.6X2	T53.6X3	T53.6X4	—	—
Fluorocytosine	T37.8X1	T37.8X2	T37.8X3	T37.8X4	T37.8X5	T37.8X6
Fluorodeoxyuridine	T45.1X1	T45.1X2	T45.1X3	T45.1X4	T45.1X5	T45.1X6
Fluorometholone	T49.0X1	T49.0X2	T49.0X3	T49.0X4	T49.0X5	T49.0X6
ophthalmic preparation	T49.5X1	T49.5X2	T49.5X3	T49.5X4	T49.5X5	T49.5X6
Fluorophosphate insecticide	T60.0X1	T60.0X2	T60.0X3	T60.0X4	—	—
Fluorosol	T46.3X1	T46.3X2	T46.3X3	T46.3X4	T46.3X5	T46.3X6
Fluorouracil	T45.1X1	T45.1X2	T45.1X3	T45.1X4	T45.1X5	T45.1X6

Substance	Poisoning, Accidental (Unintentional)	Poisoning, Intentional Self-Harm	Poisoning, Assault	Poisoning, Undetermined	Adverse Effect	Underdosing
Fluorphenylalanine	T49.5X1	T49.5X2	T49.5X3	T49.5X4	T49.5X5	T49.5X6
Fluothane	T41.0X1	T41.0X2	T41.0X3	T41.0X4	T41.0X5	T41.0X6
Fluoxetine	T43.221	T43.222	T43.223	T43.224	T43.225	T43.226
Fluoxymesterone	T38.7X1	T38.7X2	T38.7X3	T38.7X4	T38.7X5	T38.7X6
Flupenthixol	T43.4X1	T43.4X2	T43.4X3	T43.4X4	T43.4X5	T43.4X6
Flupentixol	T43.4X1	T43.4X2	T43.4X3	T43.4X4	T43.4X5	T43.4X6
Fluphenazine	T43.3X1	T43.3X2	T43.3X3	T43.3X4	T43.3X5	T43.3X6
Fluprednidene	T49.0X1	T49.0X2	T49.0X3	T49.0X4	T49.0X5	T49.0X6
Fluprednisolone	T38.0X1	T38.0X2	T38.0X3	T38.0X4	T38.0X5	T38.0X6
Fluradoline	T39.8X1	T39.8X2	T39.8X3	T39.8X4	T39.8X5	T39.8X6
Flurandrenolide	T49.0X1	T49.0X2	T49.0X3	T49.0X4	T49.0X5	T49.0X6
Flurandrenolone	I49.0X1	I49.0X2	I49.0X3	I49.0X4	I49.0X5	I49.0X6
Flurazepam	T42.4X1	T42.4X2	T42.4X3	T42.4X4	T42.4X5	T42.4X6
Flurbiprofen	T39.311	T39.312	T39.313	T39.314	T39.315	T39.316
Flurobate	T49.0X1	T49.0X2	T49.0X3	T49.0X4	T49.0X5	T49.0X6
Flurotyl	T43.291	T43.292	T43.293	T43.294	T43.295	T43.296
Fluroxene	T41.0X1	T41.0X2	T41.0X3	T41.0X4	T41.0X5	T41.0X6
Fluspirilene	T43.591	T43.592	T43.593	T43.594	T43.595	T43.596
Flutamide	T38.6X1	T38.6X2	T38.6X3	T38.6X4	T38.6X5	T38.6X6
Flutazolam	T42.4X1	T42.4X2	T42.4X3	T42.4X4	T42.4X5	T42.4X6
Fluticasone propionate	T38.0X1	T38.0X2	T38.0X3	T38.0X4	T38.0X5	T38.0X6
Flutoprazepam	T42.4X1	T42.4X2	T42.4X3	T42.4X4	T42.4X5	T42.4X6
Flutropium bromide	T48.6X1	T48.6X2	T48.6X3	T48.6X4	T48.6X5	T48.6X6
Fluvoxamine	T43.221	T43.222	T43.223	T43.224	T43.225	T43.226
Folacin	T45.8X1	T45.8X2	T45.8X3	T45.8X4	T45.8X5	T45.8X6
Folic acid	T45.8X1	T45.8X2	T45.8X3	T45.8X4	T45.8X5	T45.8X6
with ferrous salt	T45.2X1	T45.2X2	T45.2X3	T45.2X4	T45.2X5	T45.2X6
antagonist	T45.1X1	T45.1X2	T45.1X3	T45.1X4	T45.1X5	T45.1X6
Folinic acid	T45.8X1	T45.8X2	T45.8X3	T45.8X4	T45.8X5	T45.8X6
Folium stramoniae	T48.6X1	T48.6X2	T48.6X3	T48.6X4	T48.6X5	T48.6X6
Follicle-stimulating hormone, human	T38.811	T38.812	T38.813	T38.814	T38.815	T38.816
Folpet	T60.3X1	T60.3X2	T60.3X3	T60.3X4	—	—
Fominoben	T48.3X1	T48.3X2	T48.3X3	T48.3X4	T48.3X5	T48.3X6
Food, foodstuffs, noxious, nonbacterial, NEC	T62.91	T62.92	T62.93	T62.94	—	—
berries	T62.1X1	T62.1X2	T62.1X3	T62.1X4	—	—
fish — *see also Fish*	T61.91	T61.92	T61.93	T61.94	—	—
mushrooms	T62.0X1	T62.0X2	T62.0X3	T62.0X4	—	—
plants	T62.2X1	T62.2X2	T62.2X3	T62.2X4	—	—
seafood	T61.91	T61.92	T61.93	T61.94	—	—
specified NEC	T61.8X1	T61.8X2	T61.8X3	T61.8X4	—	—
seeds	T62.2X1	T62.2X2	T62.2X3	T62.2X4	—	—

◀ New   ◀ Revised   ~~deleted~~ Deleted

TABLE OF DRUGS AND CHEMICALS

Substance	Poisoning, Accidental (Unintentional)	Poisoning, Intentional Self-Harm	Poisoning, Assault	Poisoning, Undetermined	Adverse Effect	Underdosing
Food, foodstuffs, noxious, nonbacterial, NEC *(Continued)*						
shellfish	T61.781	T61.782	T61.783	T61.784	—	—
specified NEC	T62.8X1	T62.8X2	T62.8X3	T62.8X4	—	—
Fool's parsley	T62.2X1	T62.2X2	T62.2X3	T62.2X4	—	—
Formaldehyde (solution), gas or vapor	T59.2X1	T59.2X2	T59.2X3	T59.2X4	—	—
fungicide	T60.3X1	T60.3X2	T60.3X3	T60.3X4	—	—
Formalin	T59.2X1	T59.2X2	T59.2X3	T59.2X4	—	—
fungicide	T60.3X1	T60.3X2	T60.3X3	T60.3X4	—	—
vapor	T59.2X1	T59.2X2	T59.2X3	T59.2X4	—	—
Formic acid	T54.2X1	T54.2X2	T54.2X3	T54.2X4	—	—
vapor	T59.891	T59.892	T59.893	T59.894	—	—
Foscarnet sodium	T37.5X1	T37.5X2	T37.5X3	T37.5X4	T37.5X5	T37.5X6
Fosfestrol	T38.5X1	T38.5X2	T38.5X3	T38.5X4	T38.5X5	T38.5X6
Fosfomycin	T36.8X1	T36.8X2	T36.8X3	T36.8X4	T36.8X5	T36.8X6
Fosfonet sodium	T37.5X1	T37.5X2	T37.5X3	T37.5X4	T37.5X5	T37.5X6
Fosinopril	T46.4X1	T46.4X2	T46.4X3	T46.4X4	T46.4X5	T46.4X6
sodium	T46.4X1	T46.4X2	T46.4X3	T46.4X4	T46.4X5	T46.4X6
Fowler's solution	T57.0X1	T57.0X2	T57.0X3	T57.0X4	—	—
Foxglove	T62.2X1	T62.2X2	T62.2X3	T62.2X4	—	—
Framycetin	T36.5X1	T36.5X2	T36.5X3	T36.5X4	T36.5X5	T36.5X6
Frangula	T47.2X1	T47.2X2	T47.2X3	T47.2X4	T47.2X5	T47.2X6
extract	T47.2X1	T47.2X2	T47.2X3	T47.2X4	T47.2X5	T47.2X6
Frei antigen	T50.8X1	T50.8X2	T50.8X3	T50.8X4	T50.8X5	T50.8X6
Freon	T53.5X1	T53.5X2	T53.5X3	T53.5X4	—	—
Fructose	T50.3X1	T50.3X2	T50.3X3	T50.3X4	T50.3X5	T50.3X6
Frusemide	T50.1X1	T50.1X2	T50.1X3	T50.1X4	T50.1X5	T50.1X6
FSH	T38.811	T38.812	T38.813	T38.814	T38.815	T38.816
Ftorafur	T45.1X1	T45.1X2	T45.1X3	T45.1X4	T45.1X5	T45.1X6
Fuel						
automobile	T52.0X1	T52.0X2	T52.0X3	T52.0X4	—	—
exhaust gas, not in transit	T58.01	T58.02	T58.03	T58.04	—	—
vapor NEC	T52.0X1	T52.0X2	T52.0X3	T52.0X4	—	—
gas (domestic use) — *see also Carbon, monoxide, fuel, utility*	T59.891	T59.892	T59.893	T59.894	—	—
utility	T59.891	T59.892	T59.893	T59.894	—	—
in mobile container	T59.891	T59.892	T59.893	T59.894	—	—
incomplete combustion of — *see Carbon, monoxide, fuel, utility*						
piped (natural)	T59.891	T59.892	T59.893	T59.894	—	—
industrial, incomplete combustion	T58.8X1	T58.8X2	T58.8X3	T58.8X4	—	—

Substance	Poisoning, Accidental (Unintentional)	Poisoning, Intentional Self-Harm	Poisoning, Assault	Poisoning, Undetermined	Adverse Effect	Underdosing
Fugillin	T36.8X1	T36.8X2	T36.8X3	T36.8X4	T36.8X5	T36.8X6
Fulminate of mercury	T56.1X1	T56.1X2	T56.1X3	T56.1X4	—	—
Fulvicin	T36.7X1	T36.7X2	T36.7X3	T36.7X4	T36.7X5	T36.7X6
Fumadil	T36.8X1	T36.8X2	T36.8X3	T36.8X4	T36.8X5	T36.8X6
Fumagillin	T36.8X1	T36.8X2	T36.8X3	T36.8X4	T36.8X5	T36.8X6
Fumaric acid	T49.4X1	T49.4X2	T49.4X3	T49.4X4	T49.4X5	T49.4X6
Fumes (from)	T59.91	T59.92	T59.93	T59.94	—	—
carbon monoxide — *see Carbon, monoxide*						
charcoal (domestic use) — *see Charcoal, fumes*						
chloroform — *see Chloroform*						
coke (in domestic stoves, fireplaces) — *see Coke, fumes*						
corrosive NEC	T54.91	T54.92	T54.93	T54.94	—	—
ether — *see Ether*						
freons	T53.5X1	T53.5X2	T53.5X3	T53.5X4	—	—
hydrocarbons	T59.891	T59.892	T59.893	T59.894	—	—
petroleum (liquefied)	T59.891	T59.892	T59.893	T59.894	—	—
distributed through pipes (pure or mixed with air)	T59.891	T59.892	T59.893	T59.894	—	—
lead — *see Lead*						
metal — *see Metals, or the specified metal*						
nitrogen dioxide	T59.0X1	T59.0X2	T59.0X3	T59.0X4	—	—
pesticides — *see Pesticides*						
petroleum (liquefied)	T59.891	T59.892	T59.893	T59.894	—	—
distributed through pipes (pure or mixed with air)	T59.891	T59.892	T59.893	T59.894	—	—
polyester	T59.891	T59.892	T59.893	T59.894	—	—
specified source NEC — *see also substance specified*	T59.891	T59.892	T59.893	T59.894	—	—
sulfur dioxide	T59.1X1	T59.1X2	T59.1X3	T59.1X4	—	—
Fumigant NEC	T60.91	T60.92	T60.93	T60.94	—	—
Fungi, noxious, used as food	T62.0X1	T62.0X2	T62.0X3	T62.0X4	—	—
Fungicide NEC (nonmedicinal)	T60.3X1	T60.3X2	T60.3X3	T60.3X4	—	—
Fungizone	T36.7X1	T36.7X2	T36.7X3	T36.7X4	T36.7X5	T36.7X6
topical	T49.0X1	T49.0X2	T49.0X3	T49.0X4	T49.0X5	T49.0X6
Furacin	T49.0X1	T49.0X2	T49.0X3	T49.0X4	T49.0X5	T49.0X6
Furadantin	T37.91	T37.92	T37.93	T37.94	T37.95	T37.96
Furazolidone	T37.8X1	T37.8X2	T37.8X3	T37.8X4	T37.8X5	T37.8X6
Furazolium chloride	T49.0X1	T49.0X2	T49.0X3	T49.0X4	T49.0X5	T49.0X6
Furfural	T52.8X1	T52.8X2	T52.8X3	T52.8X4	—	—

◀ New ◀ Revised ~~deleted~~ Deleted

TABLE OF DRUGS AND CHEMICALS

Substance	Poisoning, Accidental (Unintentional)	Poisoning, Intentional Self-Harm	Poisoning, Assault	Poisoning, Undetermined	Adverse Effect	Underdosing
Furnace (coal burning) (domestic), gas from industrial	T58.2X1	T58.2X2	T58.2X3	T58.2X4	—	—
industrial	T58.8X1	T58.8X2	T58.8X3	T58.8X4	—	—
Furniture polish	T65.891	T65.892	T65.893	T65.894	—	—
Furosemide	T50.1X1	T50.1X2	T50.1X3	T50.1X4	T50.1X5	T50.1X6
Furoxone	T37.91	T37.92	T37.93	T37.94	T37.95	T37.96
Fursultiamine	T45.2X1	T45.2X2	T45.2X3	T45.2X4	T45.2X5	T45.2X6
Fusafungine	T36.8X1	T36.8X2	T36.8X3	T36.8X4	T36.8X5	T36.8X6
Fusel oil (any) (amyl) (butyl) (propyl), vapor	T51.3X1	T51.3X2	T51.3X3	T51.3X4	—	—
Fusidate (ethanolamine) (sodium)	T36.8X1	T36.8X2	T36.8X3	T36.8X4	T36.8X5	T36.8X6
Fusidic acid	T36.8X1	T36.8X2	T36.8X3	T36.0X4	T36.0X5	T36.0X6
Fytic acid, nonasodium	T50.6X1	T50.6X2	T50.6X3	T50.6X4	T50.6X5	T50.6X6

G

Substance	Poisoning, Accidental (Unintentional)	Poisoning, Intentional Self-Harm	Poisoning, Assault	Poisoning, Undetermined	Adverse Effect	Underdosing
GABA	T43.8X1	T43.8X2	T43.8X3	T43.8X4	T43.8X5	T43.8X6
Gadopentetic acid	T50.8X1	T50.8X2	T50.8X3	T50.8X4	T50.8X5	T50.8X6
Galactose	T50.3X1	T50.3X2	T50.3X3	T50.3X4	T50.3X5	T50.3X6
b-Galactosidase	T47.5X1	T47.5X2	T47.5X3	T47.5X4	T47.5X5	T47.5X6
Galantamine	T44.0X1	T44.0X2	T44.0X3	T44.0X4	T44.0X5	T44.0X6
Gallamine (triethiodide)	T48.1X1	T48.1X2	T48.1X3	T48.1X4	T48.1X5	T48.1X6
Gallium citrate	T50.991	T50.992	T50.993	T50.994	T50.995	T50.996
Gallopamil	T46.1X1	T46.1X2	T46.1X3	T46.1X4	T46.1X5	T46.1X6
Gamboge	T47.2X1	T47.2X2	T47.2X3	T47.2X4	T47.2X5	T47.2X6
Gamimune	T50.Z11	T50.Z12	T50.Z13	T50.Z14	T50.Z15	T50.Z16
Gamma-aminobutyric acid	T43.8X1	T43.8X2	T43.8X3	T43.8X4	T43.8X5	T43.8X6
Gamma-benzene hexachloride (medicinal)	T49.0X1	T49.0X2	T49.0X3	T49.0X4	T49.0X5	T49.0X6
nonmedicinal, vapor	T53.6X1	T53.6X2	T53.6X3	T53.6X4	—	—
Gamma-BHC (medicinal) — see also Gamma-benzene hexachloride	T49.0X1	T49.0X2	T49.0X3	T49.0X4	T49.0X5	T49.0X6
Gamma globulin	T50.Z11	T50.Z12	T50.Z13	T50.Z14	T50.Z15	T50.Z16
Gamulin	T50.Z11	T50.Z12	T50.Z13	T50.Z14	T50.Z15	T50.Z16
Ganciclovir (sodium)	T37.5X1	T37.5X2	T37.5X3	T37.5X4	T37.5X5	T37.5X6
Ganglionic blocking drug NEC	T44.2X1	T44.2X2	T44.2X3	T44.2X4	T44.2X5	T44.2X6
specified NEC	T44.2X1	T44.2X2	T44.2X3	T44.2X4	T44.2X5	T44.2X6
Ganja	T40.711	T40.712	T40.713	T40.714	T40.715	T40.716 ◀
Garamycin	T36.5X1	T36.5X2	T36.5X3	T36.5X4	T36.5X5	T36.5X6
ophthalmic preparation	T49.5X1	T49.5X2	T49.5X3	T49.5X4	T49.5X5	T49.5X6
topical NEC	T49.0X1	T49.0X2	T49.0X3	T49.0X4	T49.0X5	T49.0X6
Gardenal	T42.3X1	T42.3X2	T42.3X3	T42.3X4	T42.3X5	T42.3X6
Gardepanyl	T42.3X1	T42.3X2	T42.3X3	T42.3X4	T42.3X5	T42.3X6

Substance	Poisoning, Accidental (Unintentional)	Poisoning, Intentional Self-Harm	Poisoning, Assault	Poisoning, Undetermined	Adverse Effect	Underdosing
Gas NEC	T59.91	T59.92	T59.93	T59.94	—	—
acetylene	T59.891	T59.892	T59.893	T59.894	—	—
incomplete combustion of	T58.11	T58.12	T58.13	T58.14		
air contaminants, source or type not specified	T59.91	T59.92	T59.93	T59.94	—	—
anesthetic	T41.0X1	T41.0X2	T41.0X3	T41.0X4	T41.0X5	T41.0X6
blast furnace	T58.8X1	T58.8X2	T58.8X3	T58.8X4		
butane — see Butane						
carbon monoxide — see Carbon, monoxide						
chlorine	T59.4X1	T59.4X2	T59.4X3	T59.4X4	—	—
coal	T58.2X1	T58.2X2	T58.2X3	T58.2X4		
cyanide	T57.3X1	T57.3X2	T57.3X3	T57.3X4	—	—
dicyanogen	T65.0X1	T65.0X2	T65.0X3	T65.0X4	—	—
domestic — see Domestic gas	T57.91	T57.92	T57.93	T57.94		
exhaust	T57.91	T57.92	T57.93	T57.94	—	—
from utility (for cooking, heating, or lighting) (after combustion) see Carbon, monoxide, fuel, utility						
prior to combustion	T59.891	T59.892	T59.893	T59.894	—	—
from wood or coal-burning stove or fireplace	T57.91	T57.92	T57.93	T57.94	—	—
fuel (domestic use) (after combustion) — see also Carbon, monoxide, fuel	T57.91	T57.92	T57.93	T57.94	—	—
industrial use	T58.8X1	T58.8X2	T58.8X3	T58.8X4		
prior to combustion	T59.891	T59.892	T59.893	T59.894	—	—
utility	T59.891	T59.892	T59.893	T59.894	—	—
in mobile container	T59.891	T59.892	T59.893	T59.894	—	—
incomplete combustion of — see Carbon, monoxide, fuel, utility						
piped (natural)	T59.891	T59.892	T59.893	T59.894	—	—
garage	T58.01	T58.02	T58.03	T58.04		
hydrocarbon NEC	T59.891	T59.892	T59.893	T59.894	—	—
incomplete combustion of — see Carbon, monoxide, fuel, utility						
liquefied — see Butane						
piped	T59.891	T59.892	T59.893	T59.894	—	—
hydrocyanic acid	T65.0X1	T65.0X2	T65.0X3	T65.0X4	—	—

TABLE OF DRUGS AND CHEMICALS

Substance	External Cause (T-Code)					
	Poisoning, Accidental (Unintentional)	Poisoning, Intentional Self-Harm	Poisoning, Assault	Poisoning, Undetermined	Adverse Effect	Underdosing
Gas NEC (Continued)						
illuminating (after combustion)	T58.11	T58.12	T58.13	T58.14	—	—
prior to combustion	T59.891	T59.892	T59.893	T59.894	—	—
incomplete combustion, any—see Carbon, monoxide						
kiln	T58.8X1	T58.8X2	T58.8X3	T58.8X4	—	—
lacrimogenic	T59.3X1	T59.3X2	T59.3X3	T59.3X4	—	—
liquefied petroleum—see Butane						
marsh	T59.891	T59.892	T59.893	T59.894	—	—
motor exhaust, not in transit	T58.01	T58.02	T58.03	T58.04	—	—
mustard, not in war	T59.891	T59.892	T59.893	T59.894	—	—
natural	T59.891	T59.892	T59.893	T59.894	—	—
nerve, not in war	T59.91	T59.92	T59.93	T59.94	—	—
oil	T52.0X1	T52.0X2	T52.0X3	T52.0X4	—	—
petroleum (liquefied) (distributed in mobile containers)	T59.891	T59.892	T59.893	T59.894		
piped (pure or mixed with air)	T59.891	T59.892	T59.893	T59.894		
piped (manufactured) (natural) NEC	T59.891	T59.892	T59.893	T59.894	—	—
producer	T58.8X1	T58.8X2	T58.8X3	T58.8X4	—	—
propane—see Propane						
refrigerant (chlorofluoro-carbon)	T53.5X1	T53.5X2	T53.5X3	T53.5X4	—	—
not chlorofluoro-carbon	T59.891	T59.892	T59.893	T59.894	—	—
sewer	T59.91	T59.92	T59.93	T59.94	—	—
specified source NEC	T59.91	T59.92	T59.93	T59.94	—	—
stove (after combustion)	T58.11	T58.12	T58.13	T58.14	—	—
tear	T59.3X1	T59.3X2	T59.3X3	T59.3X4	—	—
therapeutic	T41.5X1	T41.5X2	T41.5X3	T41.5X4	T41.5X5	T41.5X6
utility (for cooking, heating, or lighting) (piped) NEC	T59.891	T59.892	T59.893	T59.894	—	—
in mobile container	T59.891	T59.892	T59.893	T59.894	—	—
incomplete combustion of—see Carbon, monoxide, fuel, utilty						
piped (natural)	T59.891	T59.892	T59.893	T59.894	—	—
water	T58.11	T58.12	T58.13	T58.14	—	—
incomplete combustion of—see Carbon, monoxide, fuel, utility						

Substance	External Cause (T-Code)					
	Poisoning, Accidental (Unintentional)	Poisoning, Intentional Self-Harm	Poisoning, Assault	Poisoning, Undetermined	Adverse Effect	Underdosing
Gaseous substance—see Gas						
Gasoline	T52.0X1	T52.0X2	T52.0X3	T52.0X4	—	—
vapor	T52.0X1	T52.0X2	T52.0X3	T52.0X4	—	—
Gastric enzymes	T47.5X1	T47.5X2	T47.5X3	T47.5X4	T47.5X5	T47.5X6
Gastrografin	T50.8X1	T50.8X2	T50.8X3	T50.8X4	T50.8X5	T50.8X6
Gastrointestinal drug	T47.91	T47.92	T47.93	T47.94	T47.95	T47.96
biological	T47.8X1	T47.8X2	T47.8X3	T47.8X4	T47.8X5	T47.8X6
specified NEC	T47.8X1	T47.8X2	T47.8X3	T47.8X4	T47.8X5	T47.8X6
Gaultheria procumbens	T62.2X1	T62.2X2	T62.2X3	T62.2X4	—	—
Gelatin (intravenous)	T45.8X1	T45.8X2	T45.8X3	T45.8X4	T45.8X5	T45.8X6
absorbable (sponge)	T45.7X1	T45.7X2	T45.7X3	T45.7X4	T45.7X5	T45.7X6
Gefarnate	T44.3X1	T44.3X2	T44.3X3	T44.3X4	T44.3X5	T44.3X6
Gelfilm	T49.8X1	T49.8X2	T49.8X3	T49.8X4	T49.8X5	T49.8X6
Gelfoam	T45.7X1	T45.7X2	T45.7X3	T45.7X4	T45.7X5	T45.7X6
Gelsemine	T50.991	T50.992	T50.993	T50.994	T50.995	T50.996
Gelsemium (sempervirens)	T62.2X1	T62.2X2	T62.2X3	T62.2X4	—	—
Gemeprost	T48.0X1	T48.0X2	T48.0X3	T48.0X4	T48.0X5	T48.0X6
Gemfibrozil	T46.6X1	T46.6X2	T46.6X3	T46.6X4	T46.6X5	T46.6X6
Gemonil	T42.3X1	T42.3X2	T42.3X3	T42.3X4	T42.3X5	T42.3X6
Gentamicin	T36.5X1	T36.5X2	T36.5X3	T36.5X4	T36.5X5	T36.5X6
ophthalmic preparation	T49.5X1	T49.5X2	T49.5X3	T49.5X4	T49.5X5	T49.5X6
topical NEC	T49.0X1	T49.0X2	T49.0X3	T49.0X4	T49.0X5	T49.0X6
Gentian	T47.5X1	T47.5X2	T47.5X3	T47.5X4	T47.5X5	T47.5X6
violet	T49.0X1	T49.0X2	T49.0X3	T49.0X4	T49.0X5	T49.0X6
Gepefrine	T44.4X1	T44.4X2	T44.4X3	T44.4X4	T44.4X5	T44.4X6
Gestonorone caproate	T38.5X1	T38.5X2	T38.5X3	T38.5X4	T38.5X5	T38.5X6
Gexane	T49.0X1	T49.0X2	T49.0X3	T49.0X4	T49.0X5	T49.0X6
Gila monster (venom)	T63.111	T63.112	T63.113	T63.114	—	—
Ginger	T47.5X1	T47.5X2	T47.5X3	T47.5X4	T47.5X5	T47.5X6
Jamaica—see Jamaica, ginger						
Gitalin	T46.0X1	T46.0X2	T46.0X3	T46.0X4	T46.0X5	T46.0X6
amorphous	T46.0X1	T46.0X2	T46.0X3	T46.0X4	T46.0X5	T46.0X6
Gitaloxin	T46.0X1	T46.0X2	T46.0X3	T46.0X4	T46.0X5	T46.0X6
Gitoxin	T46.0X1	T46.0X2	T46.0X3	T46.0X4	T46.0X5	T46.0X6
Glafenine	T39.8X1	T39.8X2	T39.8X3	T39.8X4	T39.8X5	T39.8X6
Glandular extract (medicinal) NEC	T50.Z91	T50.Z92	T50.Z93	T50.Z94	T50.Z95	T50.Z96
Glaucarubin	T37.3X1	T37.3X2	T37.3X3	T37.3X4	T37.3X5	T37.3X6
Glibenclamide	T38.3X1	T38.3X2	T38.3X3	T38.3X4	T38.3X5	T38.3X6
Glibornuride	T38.3X1	T38.3X2	T38.3X3	T38.3X4	T38.3X5	T38.3X6
Gliclazide	T38.3X1	T38.3X2	T38.3X3	T38.3X4	T38.3X5	T38.3X6
Glimidine	T38.3X1	T38.3X2	T38.3X3	T38.3X4	T38.3X5	T38.3X6

◄ New ◄ Revised ~~deleted~~ Deleted

Substance	Poisoning, Accidental (Unintentional)	Poisoning, Intentional Self-Harm	Poisoning, Assault	Poisoning, Undetermined	Adverse Effect	Underdosing
Glipizide	T38.3X1	T38.3X2	T38.3X3	T38.3X4	T38.3X5	T38.3X6
Gliquidone	T38.3X1	T38.3X2	T38.3X3	T38.3X4	T38.3X5	T38.3X6
Glisolamide	T38.3X1	T38.3X2	T38.3X3	T38.3X4	T38.3X5	T38.3X6
Glisoxepide	T38.3X1	T38.3X2	T38.3X3	T38.3X4	T38.3X5	T38.3X6
Globin zinc insulin	T38.3X1	T38.3X2	T38.3X3	T38.3X4	T38.3X5	T38.3X6
Globulin						
antilymphocytic	T50.Z11	T50.Z12	T50.Z13	T50.Z14	T50.Z15	T50.Z16
antirhesus	T50.Z11	T50.Z12	T50.Z13	T50.Z14	T50.Z15	T50.Z16
antivenin	T50.Z11	T50.Z12	T50.Z13	T50.Z14	T50.Z15	T50.Z16
antiviral	T50.Z11	T50.Z12	T50.Z13	T50.Z14	T50.Z15	T50.Z16
Glucagon	T38.3X1	T38.3X2	T38.3X3	T38.3X4	T38.3X5	T38.3X6
Glucocorticoids	T38.0X1	T38.0X2	T38.0X3	T38.0X4	T38.0X5	T38.0X6
Glucocorticosteroid	T38.0X1	T38.0X2	T38.0X3	T38.0X4	T38.0X5	T38.0X6
Gluconic acid	T50.991	T50.992	T50.993	T50.994	T50.995	T50.996
Glucosamine sulfate	T39.4X1	T39.4X2	T39.4X3	T39.4X4	T39.4X5	T39.4X6
Glucose	T50.3X1	T50.3X2	T50.3X3	T50.3X4	T50.3X5	T50.3X6
with sodium chloride	T50.3X1	T50.3X2	T50.3X3	T50.3X4	T50.3X5	T50.3X6
Glucosulfone sodium	T37.1X1	T37.1X2	T37.1X3	T37.1X4	T37.1X5	T37.1X6
Glucurolactone	T47.8X1	T47.8X2	T47.8X3	T47.8X4	T47.8X5	T47.8X6
Glue NEC	T52.8X1	T52.8X2	T52.8X3	T52.8X4	—	—
Glutamic acid	T47.5X1	T47.5X2	T47.5X3	T47.5X4	T47.5X5	T47.5X6
Glutaral (medicinal)	T49.0X1	T49.0X2	T49.0X3	T49.0X4	T49.0X5	T49.0X6
nonmedicinal	T65.891	T65.892	T65.893	T65.894	—	—
Glutaraldehyde (nonmedicinal)	T65.891	T65.892	T65.893	T65.894	—	—
medicinal	T49.0X1	T49.0X2	T49.0X3	T49.0X4	T49.0X5	T49.0X6
Glutathione	T50.6X1	T50.6X2	T50.6X3	T50.6X4	T50.6X5	T50.6X6
Glutethimide	T42.6X1	T42.6X2	T42.6X3	T42.6X4	T42.6X5	T42.6X6
Glyburide	T38.3X1	T38.3X2	T38.3X3	T38.3X4	T38.3X5	T38.3X6
Glycerin	T47.4X1	T47.4X2	T47.4X3	T47.4X4	T47.4X5	T47.4X6
Glycerol	T47.4X1	T47.4X2	T47.4X3	T47.4X4	T47.4X5	T47.4X6
borax	T49.6X1	T49.6X2	T49.6X3	T49.6X4	T49.6X5	T49.6X6
intravenous	T50.3X1	T50.3X2	T50.3X3	T50.3X4	T50.3X5	T50.3X6
iodinated	T48.4X1	T48.4X2	T48.4X3	T48.4X4	T48.4X5	T48.4X6
Glycerophosphate	T50.991	T50.992	T50.993	T50.994	T50.995	T50.996
Glyceryl						
gualacolate	T48.4X1	T48.4X2	T48.4X3	T48.4X4	T48.4X5	T48.4X6
nitrate	T46.3X1	T46.3X2	T46.3X3	T46.3X4	T46.3X5	T46.3X6
triacetate (topical)	T49.0X1	T49.0X2	T49.0X3	T49.0X4	T49.0X5	T49.0X6
trinitrate	T46.3X1	T46.3X2	T46.3X3	T46.3X4	T46.3X5	T46.3X6
Glycine	T50.3X1	T50.3X2	T50.3X3	T50.3X4	T50.3X5	T50.3X6
Glyclopyramide	T38.3X1	T38.3X2	T38.3X3	T38.3X4	T38.3X5	T38.3X6
Glycobiarsol	T37.3X1	T37.3X2	T37.3X3	T37.3X4	T37.3X5	T37.3X6

Substance	Poisoning, Accidental (Unintentional)	Poisoning, Intentional Self-Harm	Poisoning, Assault	Poisoning, Undetermined	Adverse Effect	Underdosing
Glycols (ether)	T52.3X1	T52.3X2	T52.3X3	T52.3X4	—	—
Glyconiazide	T37.1X1	T37.1X2	T37.1X3	T37.1X4	T37.1X5	T37.1X6
Glycopyrrolate	T44.3X1	T44.3X2	T44.3X3	T44.3X4	T44.3X5	T44.3X6
Glycopyrronium	T44.3X1	T44.3X2	T44.3X3	T44.3X4	T44.3X5	T44.3X6
bromide	T44.3X1	T44.3X2	T44.3X3	T44.3X4	T44.3X5	T44.3X6
Glycoside, cardiac (stimulant)	T46.0X1	T46.0X2	T46.0X3	T46.0X4	T46.0X5	T46.0X6
Glycyclamide	T38.3X1	T38.3X2	T38.3X3	T38.3X4	T38.3X5	T38.3X6
Glycyrrhiza extract	T48.4X1	T48.4X2	T48.4X3	T48.4X4	T48.4X5	T48.4X6
Glycyrrhizic acid	T48.4X1	T48.4X2	T48.4X3	T48.4X4	T48.4X5	T48.4X6
Glycyrrhizinate potassium	T48.4X1	T48.4X2	T48.4X3	T48.4X4	T48.4X5	T48.4X6
Glymidine sodium	T38.3X1	T38.3X2	T38.3X3	T38.3X4	T38.3X5	T38.3X6
Glyphosate	T60.3X1	T60.3X2	T60.3X3	T60.3X4	—	—
Glyphylline	T48.6X1	T48.6X2	T48.6X3	T48.6X4	T48.6X5	T48.6X6
Gold						
colloidal (I98Au)	T45.1X1	T45.1X2	T45.1X3	T45.1X4	T45.1X5	T45.1X6
salts	T39.4X1	T39.4X2	T39.4X3	T39.4X4	T39.4X5	T39.4X6
Golden sulfide of antimony	T56.891	T56.892	T56.893	T56.894	—	—
Goldylocks	T62.2X1	T62.2X2	T62.2X3	T62.2X4	—	—
Gonadal tissue extract	T38.901	T38.902	T38.903	T38.904	T38.905	T38.906
female	T38.5X1	T38.5X2	T38.5X3	T38.5X4	T38.5X5	T38.5X6
male	T38.7X1	T38.7X2	T38.7X3	T38.7X4	T38.7X5	T38.7X6
Gonadorelin	T38.891	T38.892	T38.893	T38.894	T38.895	T38.896
Gonadotropin	T38.891	T38.892	T38.893	T38.894	T38.895	T38.896
chorionic	T38.891	T38.892	T38.893	T38.894	T38.895	T38.896
pituitary	T38.811	T38.812	T38.813	T38.814	T38.815	T38.816
Goserelin	T45.1X1	T45.1X2	T45.1X3	T45.1X4	T45.1X5	T45.1X6
Grain alcohol	T51.0X1	T51.0X2	T51.0X3	T51.0X4	—	—
Gramicidin	T49.0X1	T49.0X2	T49.0X3	T49.0X4	T49.0X5	T49.0X6
Granisetron	T45.0X1	T45.0X2	T45.0X3	T45.0X4	T45.0X5	T45.0X6
Gratiola officinalis	T62.2X1	T62.2X2	T62.2X3	T62.2X4	—	—
Grease	T65.891	T65.892	T65.893	T65.894	—	—
Green hellebore	T62.2X1	T62.2X2	T62.2X3	T62.2X4	—	—
Green soap	T49.2X1	T49.2X2	T49.2X3	T49.2X4	T49.2X5	T49.2X6
Grifulvin	T36.7X1	T36.7X2	T36.7X3	T36.7X4	T36.7X5	T36.7X6
Griseofulvin	T36.7X1	T36.7X2	T36.7X3	T36.7X4	T36.7X5	T36.7X6
Growth hormone	T38.811	T38.812	T38.813	T38.814	T38.815	T38.816
Guaiacol derivatives	T48.4X1	T48.4X2	T48.4X3	T48.4X4	T48.4X5	T48.4X6
Guaiac reagent	T50.991	T50.992	T50.993	T50.994	T50.995	T50.996
Guaifenesin	T48.4X1	T48.4X2	T48.4X3	T48.4X4	T48.4X5	T48.4X6
Guaimesal	T48.4X1	T48.4X2	T48.4X3	T48.4X4	T48.4X5	T48.4X6
Guaiphenesin	T48.4X1	T48.4X2	T48.4X3	T48.4X4	T48.4X5	T48.4X6
Guamecycline	T36.4X1	T36.4X2	T36.4X3	T36.4X4	T36.4X5	T36.4X6

◀ New ◀ Revised ~~deleted~~ Deleted

	External Cause (T-Code)					
Substance	Poisoning, Accidental (Unintentional)	Poisoning, Intentional Self-Harm	Poisoning, Assault	Poisoning, Undetermined	Adverse Effect	Underdosing
Guanabenz	T46.5X1	T46.5X2	T46.5X3	T46.5X4	T46.5X5	T46.5X6
Guanacline	T46.5X1	T46.5X2	T46.5X3	T46.5X4	T46.5X5	T46.5X6
Guanadrel	T46.5X1	T46.5X2	T46.5X3	T46.5X4	T46.5X5	T46.5X6
Guanatol	T37.2X1	T37.2X2	T37.2X3	T37.2X4	T37.2X5	T37.2X6
Guanethidine	T46.5X1	T46.5X2	T46.5X3	T46.5X4	T46.5X5	T46.5X6
Guanfacine	T46.5X1	T46.5X2	T46.5X3	T46.5X4	T46.5X5	T46.5X6
Guano	T65.891	T65.892	T65.893	T65.894	—	—
Guanochlor	T46.5X1	T46.5X2	T46.5X3	T46.5X4	T46.5X5	T46.5X6
Guanoclor	T46.5X1	T46.5X2	T46.5X3	T46.5X4	T46.5X5	T46.5X6
Guanoctine	T46.5X1	T46.5X2	T46.5X3	T46.5X4	T46.5X5	T46.5X6
Guanoxabenz	T46.5X1	T46.5X2	T46.5X3	T46.5X4	T46.5X5	T46.5X6
Guanoxan	T46.5X1	T46.5X2	T46.5X3	T46.5X4	T46.5X5	T46.5X6
Guar gum (medicinal)	T46.6X1	T46.6X2	T46.6X3	T46.6X4	T46.6X5	T46.6X6
H						
Hachimycin	T36.7X1	T36.7X2	T36.7X3	T36.7X4	T36.7X5	T36.7X6
Hair						
dye	T49.4X1	T49.4X2	T49.4X3	T49.4X4	T49.4X5	T49.4X6
preparation NEC	T49.4X1	T49.4X2	T49.4X3	T49.4X4	T49.4X5	T49.4X6
Halazepam	T42.4X1	T42.4X2	T42.4X3	T42.4X4	T42.4X5	T42.4X6
Halcinolone	T49.0X1	T49.0X2	T49.0X3	T49.0X4	T49.0X5	T49.0X6
Halcinonide	T49.0X1	T49.0X2	T49.0X3	T49.0X4	T49.0X5	T49.0X6
Halethazole	T49.0X1	T49.0X2	T49.0X3	T49.0X4	T49.0X5	T49.0X6
Hallucinogen NOS	T40.901	T40.902	T40.903	T40.904	T40.905	T40.906
specified NEC	T40.991	T40.992	T40.993	T40.994	T40.995	T40.996
Halofantrine	T37.2X1	T37.2X2	T37.2X3	T37.2X4	T37.2X5	T37.2X6
Halofenate	T46.6X1	T46.6X2	T46.6X3	T46.6X4	T46.6X5	T46.6X6
Halometasone	T49.0X1	T49.0X2	T49.0X3	T49.0X4	T49.0X5	T49.0X6
Haloperidol	T43.4X1	T43.4X2	T43.4X3	T43.4X4	T43.4X5	T43.4X6
Haloprogin	T49.0X1	T49.0X2	T49.0X3	T49.0X4	T49.0X5	T49.0X6
Halotex	T49.0X1	T49.0X2	T49.0X3	T49.0X4	T49.0X5	T49.0X6
Halothane	T41.0X1	T41.0X2	T41.0X3	T41.0X4	T41.0X5	T41.0X6
Haloxazolam	T42.4X1	T42.4X2	T42.4X3	T42.4X4	T42.4X5	T42.4X6
Halquinols	T49.0X1	T49.0X2	T49.0X3	T49.0X4	T49.0X5	T49.0X6
Hamamelis	T49.2X1	T49.2X2	T49.2X3	T49.2X4	T49.2X5	T49.2X6
Haptendextran	T45.8X1	T45.8X2	T45.8X3	T45.8X4	T45.8X5	T45.8X6
Harmonyl	T46.5X1	T46.5X2	T46.5X3	T46.5X4	T46.5X5	T46.5X6
Hartmann's solution	T50.3X1	T50.3X2	T50.3X3	T50.3X4	T50.3X5	T50.3X6
Hashish	T40.711	T40.712	T40.713	T40.714	T40.715	T40.716
Hawaiian Woodrose seeds	T40.991	T40.992	T40.993	T40.994	—	—
HCB	T60.3X1	T60.3X2	T60.3X3	T60.3X4	—	—
HCH	T53.6X1	T53.6X2	T53.6X3	T53.6X4	—	—
medicinal	T49.0X1	T49.0X2	T49.0X3	T49.0X4	T49.0X5	T49.0X6

	External Cause (T-Code)					
Substance	Poisoning, Accidental (Unintentional)	Poisoning, Intentional Self-Harm	Poisoning, Assault	Poisoning, Undetermined	Adverse Effect	Underdosing
HCN	T57.3X1	T57.3X2	T57.3X3	T57.3X4	—	—
Headache cures, drugs, powders NEC	T50.901	T50.902	T50.903	T50.904	T50.905	T50.906
Heavenly Blue (morning glory)	T40.991	T40.992	T40.993	T40.994	—	—
Heavy metal antidote	T45.8X1	T45.8X2	T45.8X3	T45.8X4	T45.8X5	T45.8X6
Hedaquinium	T49.0X1	T49.0X2	T49.0X3	T49.0X4	T49.0X5	T49.0X6
Hedge hyssop	T62.2X1	T62.2X2	T62.2X3	T62.2X4	—	—
Heet	T49.8X1	T49.8X2	T49.8X3	T49.8X4	T49.8X5	T49.8X6
Helium	T48.991	T48.992	T48.993	T48.994	T48.995	T48.996
Helenin	T37.4X1	T37.4X2	T37.4X3	T37.4X4	T37.4X5	T37.4X6
Hellebore (black) (green) (white)	T62.2X1	T62.2X2	T62.2X3	T62.2X4	—	—
Helium (nonmedicinal) NEC	T59.891	T59.892	T59.893	T59.894	—	—
medicinal	T48.991	T48.992	T48.993	T48.994	T48.995	T48.996
Hematin	T45.8X1	T45.8X2	T45.8X3	T45.8X4	T45.8X5	T45.8X6
Hematinic preparation	T45.8X1	T45.8X2	T45.8X3	T45.8X4	T45.8X5	T45.8X6
Hemlock	T62.2X1	T62.2X2	T62.2X3	T62.2X4	—	—
Hemostatic	T45.621	T45.622	T45.623	T45.624	T45.625	T45.626
drug, systemic	T45.621	T45.622	T45.623	T45.624	T45.625	T45.626
Hemostyptic	T49.4X1	T49.4X2	T49.4X3	T49.4X4	T49.4X5	T49.4X6
Henbane	T62.2X1	T62.2X2	T62.2X3	T62.2X4	—	—
Heparin (sodium)	T45.511	T45.512	T45.513	T45.514	T45.515	T45.516
action reverser	T45.7X1	T45.7X2	T45.7X3	T45.7X4	T45.7X5	T45.7X6
Heparin-fraction	T45.511	T45.512	T45.513	T45.514	T45.515	T45.516
Heparinoid (systemic)	T45.511	T45.512	T45.513	T45.514	T45.515	T45.516
Hepatic secretion stimulant	T47.8X1	T47.8X2	T47.8X3	T47.8X4	T47.8X5	T47.8X6
Hepatitis B						
immune globulin	T50.Z11	T50.Z12	T50.Z13	T50.Z14	T50.Z15	T50.Z16
vaccine	T50.B91	T50.B92	T50.B93	T50.B94	T50.B95	T50.B96
Hepronicate	T46.7X1	T46.7X2	T46.7X3	T46.7X4	T46.7X5	T46.7X6
Heptabarb	T42.3X1	T42.3X2	T42.3X3	T42.3X4	T42.3X5	T42.3X6
Heptabarbitone	T42.3X1	T42.3X2	T42.3X3	T42.3X4	T42.3X5	T42.3X6
Heptabarbital	T42.3X1	T42.3X2	T42.3X3	T42.3X4	T42.3X5	T42.3X6
Heptachlor	T60.1X1	T60.1X2	T60.1X3	T60.1X4	—	—
Heptalgin	T40.2X1	T40.2X2	T40.2X3	T40.2X4	T40.2X5	T40.2X6
Heptaminol	T46.3X1	T46.3X2	T46.3X3	T46.3X4	T46.3X5	T46.3X6
Herbicide NEC	T60.3X1	T60.3X2	T60.3X3	T60.3X4	—	—
Heroin	T40.1X1	T40.1X2	T40.1X3	T40.1X4	—	—
Herplex	T49.5X1	T49.5X2	T49.5X3	T49.5X4	T49.5X5	T49.5X6
HES	T45.8X1	T45.8X2	T45.8X3	T45.8X4	T45.8X5	T45.8X6
Hesperidin	T46.991	T46.992	T46.993	T46.994	T46.995	T46.996
Hetacillin	T36.0X1	T36.0X2	T36.0X3	T36.0X4	T36.0X5	T36.0X6

◄ New   ◄ Revised   ~~deleted~~ Deleted

Substance	Poisoning, Accidental (Unintentional)	Poisoning, Intentional Self-Harm	Poisoning, Assault	Poisoning, Undetermined	Adverse Effect	Underdosing
Hetastarch	T45.8X1	T45.8X2	T45.8X3	T45.8X4	T45.8X5	T45.8X6
HETP	T60.0X1	T60.0X2	T60.0X3	T60.0X4	—	—
Hexachlorobenzene (vapor)	T60.3X1	T60.3X2	T60.3X3	T60.3X4	—	—
Hexachlorocyclohexane	T53.6X1	T53.6X2	T53.6X3	T53.6X4	—	—
Hexachlorophene	T49.0X1	T49.0X2	T49.0X3	T49.0X4	T49.0X5	T49.0X6
Hexadiline	T46.3X1	T46.3X2	T46.3X3	T46.3X4	T46.3X5	T46.3X6
Hexadimethrine (bromide)	T45.7X1	T45.7X2	T45.7X3	T45.7X4	T45.7X5	T45.7X6
Hexadylamine	T46.3X1	T46.3X2	T46.3X3	T46.3X4	T46.3X5	T46.3X6
Hexaethyl tetraphosphate	T60.0X1	T60.0X2	T60.0X3	T60.0X4	—	—
Hexafluorenium bromide	T48.1X1	T48.1X2	T48.1X3	T48.1X4	T48.1X5	T48.1X6
Hexafluorodiethyl ether	T43.291	T43.292	T43.293	T43.294	T43.295	T43.296
Hexafluronium (bromide)	T48.1X1	T48.1X2	T48.1X3	T48.1X4	T48.1X5	T48.1X6
Hexahydrobenzol	T52.8X1	T52.8X2	T52.8X3	T52.8X4	—	—
Hexahydrocresol(s)	T51.8X1	T51.8X2	T51.8X3	T51.8X4	—	—
arsenide	T57.0X1	T57.0X2	T57.0X3	T57.0X4	—	—
arseniurated	T57.0X1	T57.0X2	T57.0X3	T57.0X4	—	—
cyanide	T57.3X1	T57.3X2	T57.3X3	T57.3X4	—	—
gas	T59.891	T59.892	T59.893	T59.894	—	—
Fluoride (liquid)	T57.8X1	T57.8X2	T57.8X3	T57.8X4	—	—
vapor	T59.891	T59.892	T59.893	T59.894	—	—
phophorated	T60.0X1	T60.0X2	T60.0X3	T60.0X4	—	—
sulfate	T57.8X1	T57.8X2	T57.8X3	T57.8X4	—	—
sulfide (gas)	T59.6X1	T59.6X2	T59.6X3	T59.6X4	—	—
arseniurated	T57.0X1	T57.0X2	T57.0X3	T57.0X4	—	—
sulfurated	T57.8X1	T57.8X2	T57.8X3	T57.8X4	—	—
Hexahydrophenol	T51.8X1	T51.8X2	T51.8X3	T51.8X4	—	—
Hexa-germ	T49.2X1	T49.2X2	T49.2X3	T49.2X4	T49.2X5	T49.2X6
Hexalen	T51.8X1	T51.8X2	T51.8X3	T51.8X4	—	—
Hexamethonium bromide	T44.2X1	T44.2X2	T44.2X3	T44.2X4	T44.2X5	T44.2X6
Hexamethylene	T52.8X1	T52.8X2	T52.8X3	T52.8X4	—	—
Hexamethylmelamine	T45.1X1	T45.1X2	T45.1X3	T45.1X4	T45.1X5	T45.1X6
Hexamidine	T49.0X1	T49.0X2	T49.0X3	T49.0X4	T49.0X5	T49.0X6
Hexamine (mandelate)	T37.8X1	T37.8X2	T37.8X3	T37.8X4	T37.8X5	T37.8X6
Hexanone, 2-hexanone	T52.4X1	T52.4X2	T52.4X3	T52.4X4	—	—
Hexanuorenium	T48.1X1	T48.1X2	T48.1X3	T48.1X4	T48.1X5	T48.1X6
Hexapropymate	T42.6X1	T42.6X2	T42.6X3	T42.6X4	T42.6X5	T42.6X6
Hexasonium iodide	T44.3X1	T44.3X2	T44.3X3	T44.3X4	T44.3X5	T44.3X6
Hexcarbacholine bromide	T48.1X1	T48.1X2	T48.1X3	T48.1X4	T48.1X5	T48.1X6
Hexemal	T42.3X1	T42.3X2	T42.3X3	T42.3X4	T42.3X5	T42.3X6
Hexestrol	T38.5X1	T38.5X2	T38.5X3	T38.5X4	T38.5X5	T38.5X6
Hexethal (sodium)	T42.3X1	T42.3X2	T42.3X3	T42.3X4	T42.3X5	T42.3X6
Hexetidine	T37.8X1	T37.8X2	T37.8X3	T37.8X4	T37.8X5	T37.8X6

Substance	Poisoning, Accidental (Unintentional)	Poisoning, Intentional Self-Harm	Poisoning, Assault	Poisoning, Undetermined	Adverse Effect	Underdosing
Hexobarbital	T42.3X1	T42.3X2	T42.3X3	T42.3X4	T42.3X5	T42.3X6
rectal	T41.291	T41.292	T41.293	T41.294	T41.295	T41.296
sodium	T41.1X1	T41.1X2	T41.1X3	T41.1X4	T41.1X5	T41.1X6
Hexobendine	T46.3X1	T46.3X2	T46.3X3	T46.3X4	T46.3X5	T46.3X6
Hexocyclium	T44.3X1	T44.3X2	T44.3X3	T44.3X4	T44.3X5	T44.3X6
metilsulfate	T44.3X1	T44.3X2	T44.3X3	T44.3X4	T44.3X5	T44.3X6
Hexoestrol	T38.5X1	T38.5X2	T38.5X3	T38.5X4	T38.5X5	T38.5X6
Hexone	T52.4X1	T52.4X2	T52.4X3	T52.4X4	—	—
Hexoprenaline	T48.6X1	T48.6X2	T48.6X3	T48.6X4	T48.6X5	T48.6X6
Hexylcaine	T41.3X1	T41.3X2	T41.3X3	T41.3X4	T41.3X5	T41.3X6
Hexylresorcinol	T52.2X1	T52.2X2	T52.2X3	T52.2X4	—	—
HGH (human growth hormone)	T38.811	T38.812	T38.813	T38.814	T38.815	T38.816
Hinkle's pills	T47.2X1	T47.2X2	T47.2X3	T47.2X4	T47.2X5	T47.2X6
Histalog	T50.8X1	T50.8X2	T50.8X3	T50.8X4	T50.8X5	T50.8X6
Histamine (phosphate)	T50.8X1	T50.8X2	T50.8X3	T50.8X4	T50.8X5	T50.8X6
Histoplasmin	T50.8X1	T50.8X2	T50.8X3	T50.8X4	T50.8X5	T50.8X6
Holly berries	T62.2X1	T62.2X2	T62.2X3	T62.2X4	—	—
Homatropine	T44.3X1	T44.3X2	T44.3X3	T44.3X4	T44.3X5	T44.3X6
methylbromide	T44.3X1	T44.3X2	T44.3X3	T44.3X4	T44.3X5	T44.3X6
Homochlorcyclizine	T45.0X1	T45.0X2	T45.0X3	T45.0X4	T45.0X5	T45.0X6
Homosalate	T49.3X1	T49.3X2	T49.3X3	T49.3X4	T49.3X5	T49.3X6
Homo-tet	T50.Z11	T50.Z12	T50.Z13	T50.Z14	T50.Z15	T50.Z16
Hormone	T38.801	T38.802	T38.803	T38.804	T38.805	T38.806
adrenal cortical steroids	T38.0X1	T38.0X2	T38.0X3	T38.0X4	T38.0X5	T38.0X6
androgenic	T38.7X1	T38.7X2	T38.7X3	T38.7X4	T38.7X5	T38.7X6
anterior pituitary NEC	T38.811	T38.812	T38.813	T38.814	T38.815	T38.816
antidiabetic agents	T38.3X1	T38.3X2	T38.3X3	T38.3X4	T38.3X5	T38.3X6
antidiuretic	T38.891	T38.892	T38.893	T38.894	T38.895	T38.896
cancer therapy	T45.1X1	T45.1X2	T45.1X3	T45.1X4	T45.1X5	T45.1X6
follicle stimulating	T38.811	T38.812	T38.813	T38.814	T38.815	T38.816
gonadotropic	T38.891	T38.892	T38.893	T38.894	T38.895	T38.896
pituitary	T38.811	T38.812	T38.813	T38.814	T38.815	T38.816
growth	T38.811	T38.812	T38.813	T38.814	T38.815	T38.816
luteinizing	T38.811	T38.812	T38.813	T38.814	T38.815	T38.816
ovarian	T38.5X1	T38.5X2	T38.5X3	T38.5X4	T38.5X5	T38.5X6
oxytocic	T48.0X1	T48.0X2	T48.0X3	T48.0X4	T48.0X5	T48.0X6
parathyroid (derivatives)	T50.991	T50.992	T50.993	T50.994	T50.995	T50.996
pituitary (posterior) NEC	T38.891	T38.892	T38.893	T38.894	T38.895	T38.896
anterior	T38.811	T38.812	T38.813	T38.814	T38.815	T38.816
specified, NEC	T38.891	T38.892	T38.893	T38.894	T38.895	T38.896
thyroid	T38.1X1	T38.1X2	T38.1X3	T38.1X4	T38.1X5	T38.1X6
Hornet (sting)	T63.451	T63.452	T63.453	T63.454	—	—

◀ New ◀ Revised ~~deleted~~ Deleted

TABLE OF DRUGS AND CHEMICALS

TABLE OF DRUGS AND CHEMICALS

	External Cause (T-Code)					
Substance	Poisoning, Accidental (Unintentional)	Poisoning, Intentional Self-Harm	Poisoning, Assault	Poisoning, Undetermined	Adverse Effect	Underdosing
Horse anti-human lymphocytic serum	T50.Z11	T50.Z12	T50.Z13	T50.Z14	T50.Z15	T50.Z16
Horticulture agent NEC	T65.91	T65.92	T65.93	T65.94	—	—
with pesticide	T60.91	T60.92	T60.93	T60.94	—	—
Human						
albumin	T45.8X1	T45.8X2	T45.8X3	T45.8X4	T45.8X5	T45.8X6
growth hormone (HGH)	T38.811	T38.812	T38.813	T38.814	T38.815	T38.816
immune serum	T50.Z11	T50.Z12	T50.Z13	T50.Z14	T50.Z15	T50.Z16
Hyaluronidase	T45.3X1	T45.3X2	T45.3X3	T45.3X4	T45.3X5	T45.3X6
Hyazyme	T45.3X1	T45.3X2	T45.3X3	T45.3X4	T45.3X5	T45.3X6
Hycodan	T40.2X1	T40.2X2	T40.2X3	T40.2X4	T40.2X5	T40.2X6
Hydantoin derivative NEC	T42.0X1	T42.0X2	T42.0X3	T42.0X4	T42.0X5	T42.0X6
Hydeltra	T38.0X1	T38.0X2	T38.0X3	T38.0X4	T38.0X5	T38.0X6
Hydergine	T44.6X1	T44.6X2	T44.6X3	T44.6X4	T44.6X5	T44.6X6
Hydrabamine penicillin	T36.0X1	T36.0X2	T36.0X3	T36.0X4	T36.0X5	T36.0X6
Hydralazine	T46.5X1	T46.5X2	T46.5X3	T46.5X4	T46.5X5	T46.5X6
Hydrargaphen	T49.0X1	T49.0X2	T49.0X3	T49.0X4	T49.0X5	T49.0X6
Hydrargyri amino-chloridum	T49.0X1	T49.0X2	T49.0X3	T49.0X4	T49.0X5	T49.0X6
Hydrastine	T48.291	T48.292	T48.293	T48.294	T48.295	T48.296
Hydrazine	T54.1X1	T54.1X2	T54.1X3	T54.1X4	—	—
monoamine oxidase inhibitors	T43.1X1	T43.1X2	T43.1X3	T43.1X4	T43.1X5	T43.1X6
Hydrazoic acid, azides	T54.2X1	T54.2X2	T54.2X3	T54.2X4	—	—
Hydriodic acid	T48.4X1	T48.4X2	T48.4X3	T48.4X4	T48.4X5	T48.4X6
Hydrocarbon gas	T59.891	T59.892	T59.893	T59.894	—	—
incomplete combustion of — see Carbon, monoxide, fuel, utility						
liquefied (mobile container)	T59.891	T59.892	T59.893	T59.894	—	—
piped (natural)	T59.891	T59.892	T59.893	T59.894	—	—
Hydrochloric acid (liquid)	T54.2X1	T54.2X2	T54.2X3	T54.2X4	—	—
medicinal (digestant)	T47.5X1	T47.5X2	T47.5X3	T47.5X4	T47.5X5	T47.5X6
vapor	T59.891	T59.892	T59.893	T59.894	—	—
Hydrochlorothiazide	T50.2X1	T50.2X2	T50.2X3	T50.2X4	T50.2X5	T50.2X6
Hydrocodone	T40.2X1	T40.2X2	T40.2X3	T40.2X4	T40.2X5	T40.2X6
Hydrocortisone (derivatives)	T38.0X1	T38.0X2	T38.0X3	T38.0X4	T38.0X5	T38.0X6
aceponate	T49.0X1	T49.0X2	T49.0X3	T49.0X4	T49.0X5	T49.0X6
ENT agent	T49.6X1	T49.6X2	T49.6X3	T49.6X4	T49.6X5	T49.6X6
ophthalmic preparation	T49.5X1	T49.5X2	T49.5X3	T49.5X4	T49.5X5	T49.5X6
topical NEC	T49.0X1	T49.0X2	T49.0X3	T49.0X4	T49.0X5	T49.0X6
Hydrocortone	T38.0X1	T38.0X2	T38.0X3	T38.0X4	T38.0X5	T38.0X6
ENT agent	T49.6X1	T49.6X2	T49.6X3	T49.6X4	T49.6X5	T49.6X6
ophthalmic preparation	T49.5X1	T49.5X2	T49.5X3	T49.5X4	T49.5X5	T49.5X6
topical NEC	T49.0X1	T49.0X2	T49.0X3	T49.0X4	T49.0X5	T49.0X6

	External Cause (T-Code)					
Substance	Poisoning, Accidental (Unintentional)	Poisoning, Intentional Self-Harm	Poisoning, Assault	Poisoning, Undetermined	Adverse Effect	Underdosing
Hydrocyanic acid (liquid)	T57.3X1	T57.3X2	T57.3X3	T57.3X4	—	—
gas	T65.0X1	T65.0X2	T65.0X3	T65.0X4	—	—
Hydroflumethiazide	T50.2X1	T50.2X2	T50.2X3	T50.2X4	T50.2X5	T50.2X6
Hydrofluoric acid (liquid)	T54.2X1	T54.2X2	T54.2X3	T54.2X4	—	—
vapor	T59.891	T59.892	T59.893	T59.894	—	—
Hydrogen	T59.891	T59.892	T59.893	T59.894	—	—
arsenide	T57.0X1	T57.0X2	T57.0X3	T57.0X4	—	—
arseniureted	T57.0X1	T57.0X2	T57.0X3	T57.0X4	—	—
chloride	T57.8X1	T57.8X2	T57.8X3	T57.8X4	—	—
cyanide (salts)	T57.3X1	T57.3X2	T57.3X3	T57.3X4	—	—
gas	T57.3X1	T57.3X2	T57.3X3	T57.3X4	—	—
Fluoride	T59.5X1	T59.5X2	T59.5X3	T59.5X4	—	—
vapor	T59.5X1	T59.5X2	T59.5X3	T59.5X4	—	—
peroxide	T49.0X1	T49.0X2	T49.0X3	T49.0X4	T49.0X5	T49.0X6
phosphureted	T57.1X1	T57.1X2	T57.1X3	T57.1X4	—	—
sulfide	T59.6X1	T59.6X2	T59.6X3	T59.6X4	—	—
arseniureted	T57.0X1	T57.0X2	T57.0X3	T57.0X4	—	—
sulfureted	T59.6X1	T59.6X2	T59.6X3	T59.6X4	—	—
Hydromethylpyridine	T46.7X1	T46.7X2	T46.7X3	T46.7X4	T46.7X5	T46.7X6
Hydromorphinol	T40.2X1	T40.2X2	T40.2X3	T40.2X4	—	—
Hydromorphinone	T40.2X1	T40.2X2	T40.2X3	T40.2X4	T40.2X5	T40.2X6
Hydromorphone	T40.2X1	T40.2X2	T40.2X3	T40.2X4	T40.2X5	T40.2X6
Hydromox	T50.2X1	T50.2X2	T50.2X3	T50.2X4	T50.2X5	T50.2X6
Hydrophilic lotion	T49.3X1	T49.3X2	T49.3X3	T49.3X4	T49.3X5	T49.3X6
Hydroquinidine	T46.2X1	T46.2X2	T46.2X3	T46.2X4	T46.2X5	T46.2X6
Hydroquinone	T52.2X1	T52.2X2	T52.2X3	T52.2X4	—	—
vapor	T59.891	T59.892	T59.893	T59.894	—	—
Hydrosulfuric acid (gas)	T59.6X1	T59.6X2	T59.6X3	T59.6X4	—	—
Hydrotalcite	T47.1X1	T47.1X2	T47.1X3	T47.1X4	T47.1X5	T47.1X6
Hydrous wool fat	T49.3X1	T49.3X2	T49.3X3	T49.3X4	T49.3X5	T49.3X6
Hydroxide, caustic	T54.3X1	T54.3X2	T54.3X3	T54.3X4	—	—
Hydroxocobalamin	T45.8X1	T45.8X2	T45.8X3	T45.8X4	T45.8X5	T45.8X6
Hydroxyamphetamine	T49.5X1	T49.5X2	T49.5X3	T49.5X4	T49.5X5	T49.5X6
Hydroxycarbamide	T45.1X1	T45.1X2	T45.1X3	T45.1X4	T45.1X5	T45.1X6
Hydroxychloroquine	T37.8X1	T37.8X2	T37.8X3	T37.8X4	T37.8X5	T37.8X6
Hydroxydihydrocodeinone	T40.2X1	T40.2X2	T40.2X3	T40.2X4	T40.2X5	T40.2X6
Hydroxyestrone	T38.5X1	T38.5X2	T38.5X3	T38.5X4	T38.5X5	T38.5X6
Hydroxyethyl starch	T45.8X1	T45.8X2	T45.8X3	T45.8X4	T45.8X5	T45.8X6
Hydroxymethylpentanone	T52.4X1	T52.4X2	T52.4X3	T52.4X4	—	—
Hydroxyphenamate	T43.591	T43.592	T43.593	T43.594	T43.595	T43.596
Hydroxyphenylbutazone	T39.2X1	T39.2X2	T39.2X3	T39.2X4	T39.2X5	T39.2X6

◀ New ◀ Revised ~~deleted~~ Deleted

Substance	Poisoning, Accidental (Unintentional)	Poisoning, Intentional Self-Harm	Poisoning, Assault	Poisoning, Undetermined	Adverse Effect	Underdosing
Hydroxyprogesterone	T38.5X1	T38.5X2	T38.5X3	T38.5X4	T38.5X5	T38.5X6
caproate	T38.5X1	T38.5X2	T38.5X3	T38.5X4	T38.5X5	T38.5X6
Hydroxyquinoline (derivatives) NEC	T37.8X1	T37.8X2	T37.8X3	T37.8X4	T37.8X5	T37.8X6
Hydroxystilbamidine	T37.3X1	T37.3X2	T37.3X3	T37.3X4	T37.3X5	T37.3X6
Hydroxytoluene (nonmedicinal)	T54.0X1	T54.0X2	T54.0X3	T54.0X4	—	—
medicinal	T49.0X1	T49.0X2	T49.0X3	T49.0X4	T49.0X5	T49.0X6
Hydroxyurea	T45.1X1	T45.1X2	T45.1X3	T45.1X4	T45.1X5	T45.1X6
Hydroxyzine	T43.591	T43.592	T43.593	T43.594	T43.595	T43.596
Hyoscine	T44.3X1	T44.3X2	T44.3X3	T44.3X4	T44.3X5	T44.3X6
Hyoscyamine	T44.3X1	T44.3X2	T44.3X3	T44.3X4	T44.3X5	T44.3X6
Hyoscyamus	T44.3X1	T44.3X2	T44.3X3	T44.3X4	T44.3X5	T44.3X6
dry extract	T44.3X1	T44.3X2	T44.3X3	T44.3X4	T44.3X5	T44.3X6
Hypaque	T50.8X1	T50.8X2	T50.8X3	T50.8X4	T50.8X5	T50.8X6
Hypertussis	T50.Z11	T50.Z12	T50.Z13	T50.Z14	T50.Z15	T50.Z16
Hypnotic	T42.71	T42.72	T42.73	T42.74	T42.75	T42.76
anticonvulsant	T42.71	T42.72	T42.73	T42.74	T42.75	T42.76
specified NEC	T42.6X1	T42.6X2	T42.6X3	T42.6X4	T42.6X5	T42.6X6
Hypochlorite	T49.0X1	T49.0X2	T49.0X3	T49.0X4	T49.0X5	T49.0X6
Hypophysis, posterior	T38.891	T38.892	T38.893	T38.894	T38.895	T38.896
Hypotensive NEC	T46.5X1	T46.5X2	T46.5X3	T46.5X4	T46.5X5	T46.5X6
Hypromellose	T49.5X1	T49.5X2	T49.5X3	T49.5X4	T49.5X5	T49.5X6

I

Substance	Poisoning, Accidental (Unintentional)	Poisoning, Intentional Self-Harm	Poisoning, Assault	Poisoning, Undetermined	Adverse Effect	Underdosing
Ibacitabine	T37.5X1	T37.5X2	T37.5X3	T37.5X4	T37.5X5	T37.5X6
Ibopamine	T44.991	T44.992	T44.993	T44.994	T44.995	T44.996
Ibufenac	T39.311	T39.312	T39.313	T39.314	T39.315	T39.316
Ibuprofen	T39.311	T39.312	T39.313	T39.314	T39.315	T39.316
Ibuproxam	T39.311	T39.312	T39.313	T39.314	T39.315	T39.316
Ibuterol	T48.6X1	T48.6X2	T48.6X3	T48.6X4	T48.6X5	T48.6X6
Ichthammol	T49.0X1	T49.0X2	T49.0X3	T49.0X4	T49.0X5	T49.0X6
Ichthyol	T49.4X1	T49.4X2	T49.4X3	T49.4X4	T49.4X5	T49.4X6
Idarubicin	T45.1X1	T45.1X2	T45.1X3	T45.1X4	T45.1X5	T45.1X6
Idrocilamide	T42.8X1	T42.8X2	T42.8X3	T42.8X4	T42.8X5	T42.8X6
Ifenprodil	T46.7X1	T46.7X2	T46.7X3	T46.7X4	T46.7X5	T46.7X6
Ifosfamide	T45.1X1	T45.1X2	T45.1X3	T45.1X4	T45.1X5	T45.1X6
Iletin	T38.3X1	T38.3X2	T38.3X3	T38.3X4	T38.3X5	T38.3X6
Ilex	T62.2X1	T62.2X2	T62.2X3	T62.2X4	—	—
Illuminating gas (after combustion)	T58.11	T58.12	T58.13	T58.14	—	—
prior to combustion	T59.891	T59.892	T59.893	T59.894	—	—
Ilopan	T45.2X1	T45.2X2	T45.2X3	T45.2X4	T45.2X5	T45.2X6
Iloprost	T46.7X1	T46.7X2	T46.7X3	T46.7X4	T46.7X5	T46.7X6

Substance	Poisoning, Accidental (Unintentional)	Poisoning, Intentional Self-Harm	Poisoning, Assault	Poisoning, Undetermined	Adverse Effect	Underdosing
Ilotycin	T36.3X1	T36.3X2	T36.3X3	T36.3X4	T36.3X5	T36.3X6
ophthalmic preparation	T49.5X1	T49.5X2	T49.5X3	T49.5X4	T49.5X5	T49.5X6
topical NEC	T49.0X1	T49.0X2	T49.0X3	T49.0X4	T49.0X5	T49.0X6
Imidazole-4-carboxamide	T45.1X1	T45.1X2	T45.1X3	T45.1X4	T45.1X5	T45.1X6
Imipenem	T36.0X1	T36.0X2	T36.0X3	T36.0X4	T36.0X5	T36.0X6
Imipramine	T43.011	T43.012	T43.013	T43.014	T43.015	T43.016
Iminostilbene	T42.1X1	T42.1X2	T42.1X3	T42.1X4	T42.1X5	T42.1X6
Immu-G	T50.Z11	T50.Z12	T50.Z13	T50.Z14	T50.Z15	T50.Z16
Immuglobin	T50.Z11	T50.Z12	T50.Z13	T50.Z14	T50.Z15	T50.Z16
Immune						
globulin	T50.Z11	T50.Z12	T50.Z13	T50.Z14	T50.Z15	T50.Z16
serum globulin	T50.Z11	T50.Z12	T50.Z13	T50.Z14	T50.Z15	T50.Z16
Immunoglobin human (intravenous) (normal)	T50.Z11	T50.Z12	T50.Z13	T50.Z14	T50.Z15	T50.Z16
unmodified	T50.Z11	T50.Z12	T50.Z13	T50.Z14	T50.Z15	T50.Z16
Immunosuppressive drug	T45.1X1	T45.1X2	T45.1X3	T45.1X4	T45.1X5	T45.1X6
Immu-tetanus	T50.Z11	T50.Z12	T50.Z13	T50.Z14	T50.Z15	T50.Z16
Indalpine	T43.221	T43.222	T43.223	T43.224	T43.225	T43.226
Indanazoline	T48.5X1	T48.5X2	T48.5X3	T48.5X4	T48.5X5	T48.5X6
Indandione (derivatives)	T45.511	T45.512	T45.513	T45.514	T45.515	T45.516
Indapamide	T46.5X1	T46.5X2	T46.5X3	T46.5X4	T46.5X5	T46.5X6
Indendione (derivatives)	T45.511	T45.512	T45.513	T45.514	T45.515	T45.516
Indenolol	T44.7X1	T44.7X2	T44.7X3	T44.7X4	T44.7X5	T44.7X6
Inderal	T44.7X1	T44.7X2	T44.7X3	T44.7X4	T44.7X5	T44.7X6
Indian						
hemp	T40.711	T40.712	T40.713	T40.714	T40.715	T40.716
tobacco	T62.2X1	T62.2X2	T62.2X3	T62.2X4	—	—
Indigo carmine	T50.8X1	T50.8X2	T50.8X3	T50.8X4	T50.8X5	T50.8X6
Indobufen	T45.521	T45.522	T45.523	T45.524	T45.525	T45.526
Indocin	T39.2X1	T39.2X2	T39.2X3	T39.2X4	T39.2X5	T39.2X6
Indocyanine green	T50.8X1	T50.8X2	T50.8X3	T50.8X4	T50.8X5	T50.8X6
Indometacin	T39.391	T39.392	T39.393	T39.394	T39.395	T39.396
Indomethacin	T39.391	T39.392	T39.393	T39.394	T39.395	T39.396
farnesil	T39.4X1	T39.4X2	T39.4X3	T39.4X4	T39.4X5	T39.4X6
Indoramin	T44.6X1	T44.6X2	T44.6X3	T44.6X4	T44.6X5	T44.6X6
Industrial						
alcohol	T51.0X1	T51.0X2	T51.0X3	T51.0X4	—	—
fumes	T59.891	T59.892	T59.893	T59.894	—	—
solvents (fumes) (vapors)	T52.91	T52.92	T52.93	T52.94	—	—
Influenza vaccine	T50.B91	T50.B92	T50.B93	T50.B94	T50.B95	T50.B96
Ingested substance NEC	T65.91	T65.92	T65.93	T65.94	—	—
INH	T37.1X1	T37.1X2	T37.1X3	T37.1X4	T37.1X5	T37.1X6

TABLE OF DRUGS AND CHEMICALS

Substance	External Cause (T-Code) Poisoning, Accidental (Unintentional)	Poisoning, Intentional Self-Harm	Poisoning, Assault	Poisoning, Undetermined	Adverse Effect	Underdosing
Inhalation, gas (noxious) — *see Gas*						
Inhibitor						
angiotensin-converting enzyme	T46.4X1	T46.4X2	T46.4X3	T46.4X4	T46.4X5	T46.4X6
carbonic anhydrase	T50.2X1	T50.2X2	T50.2X3	T50.2X4	T50.2X5	T50.2X6
fibrinolysis	T45.621	T45.622	T45.623	T45.624	T45.625	T45.626
monoamine oxidase NEC	T43.1X1	T43.1X2	T43.1X3	T43.1X4	T43.1X5	T43.1X6
hydrazine	T43.1X1	T43.1X2	T43.1X3	T43.1X4	T43.1X5	T43.1X6
postsynaptic	T43.8X1	T43.8X2	T43.8X3	T43.8X4	T43.8X5	T43.8X6
prothrombin synthesis	T45.511	T45.512	T45.513	T45.514	T45.515	T45.516
Ink	T65.891	T65.892	T65.893	T65.894	—	—
Inorganic substance NEC	T57.91	T57.92	T57.93	T57.94	—	—
Inosine pranobex	T37.5X1	T37.5X2	T37.5X3	T37.5X4	T37.5X5	T37.5X6
Inositol	T50.991	T50.992	T50.993	T50.994	T50.995	T50.996
nicotinate	T46.7X1	T46.7X2	T46.7X3	T46.7X4	T46.7X5	T46.7X6
Inproquone	T45.1X1	T45.1X2	T45.1X3	T45.1X4	T45.1X5	T45.1X6
Insect (sting), venomous	T63.481	T63.482	T63.483	T63.484	—	—
ant	T63.421	T63.422	T63.423	T63.424	—	—
bee	T63.441	T63.442	T63.443	T63.444	—	—
caterpillar	T63.431	T63.432	T63.433	T63.434	—	—
hornet	T63.451	T63.452	T63.453	T63.454	—	—
wasp	T63.461	T63.462	T63.463	T63.464	—	—
Insecticide NEC	T60.91	T60.92	T60.93	T60.94	—	—
carbamate	T60.0X1	T60.0X2	T60.0X3	T60.0X4	—	—
chlorinated	T60.1X1	T60.1X2	T60.1X3	T60.1X4	—	—
mixed	T60.91	T60.92	T60.93	T60.94	—	—
organochlorine	T60.1X1	T60.1X2	T60.1X3	T60.1X4	—	—
organophosphorus	T60.0X1	T60.0X2	T60.0X3	T60.0X4	—	—
Insular tissue extract	T38.3X1	T38.3X2	T38.3X3	T38.3X4	T38.3X5	T38.3X6
Insulin (amorphous) (globin) (isophane) (Lente) (NPH) (Semilente) (Ultralente)	T38.3X1	T38.3X2	T38.3X3	T38.3X4	T38.3X5	T38.3X6
defalan	T38.3X1	T38.3X2	T38.3X3	T38.3X4	T38.3X5	T38.3X6
human	T38.3X1	T38.3X2	T38.3X3	T38.3X4	T38.3X5	T38.3X6
injection, soluble	T38.3X1	T38.3X2	T38.3X3	T38.3X4	T38.3X5	T38.3X6
biphasic	T38.3X1	T38.3X2	T38.3X3	T38.3X4	T38.3X5	T38.3X6
intermediate acting	T38.3X1	T38.3X2	T38.3X3	T38.3X4	T38.3X5	T38.3X6
protamine zinc	T38.3X1	T38.3X2	T38.3X3	T38.3X4	T38.3X5	T38.3X6
slow acting	T38.3X1	T38.3X2	T38.3X3	T38.3X4	T38.3X5	T38.3X6
zinc						
protamine injection	T38.3X1	T38.3X2	T38.3X3	T38.3X4	T38.3X5	T38.3X6
suspension (amorphous) (crystalline)	T38.3X1	T38.3X2	T38.3X3	T38.3X4	T38.3X5	T38.3X6

Substance	External Cause (T-Code) Poisoning, Accidental (Unintentional)	Poisoning, Intentional Self-Harm	Poisoning, Assault	Poisoning, Undetermined	Adverse Effect	Underdosing
Interferon (alpha) (beta) (gamma)	T37.5X1	T37.5X2	T37.5X3	T37.5X4	T37.5X5	T37.5X6
Intestinal motility control drug	T47.6X1	T47.6X2	T47.6X3	T47.6X4	T47.6X5	T47.6X6
biological	T47.8X1	T47.8X2	T47.8X3	T47.8X4	T47.8X5	T47.8X6
Intranarcon	T41.1X1	T41.1X2	T41.1X3	T41.1X4	T41.1X5	T41.1X6
Intravenous						
amino acids	T50.991	T50.992	T50.993	T50.994	T50.995	T50.996
fat suspension	T50.991	T50.992	T50.993	T50.994	T50.995	T50.996
Inulin	T50.8X1	T50.8X2	T50.8X3	T50.8X4	T50.8X5	T50.8X6
Invert sugar	T50.3X1	T50.3X2	T50.3X3	T50.3X4	T50.3X5	T50.3X6
Inza — *see Naproxen*						
Iobenzamic acid	T50.8X1	T50.8X2	T50.8X3	T50.8X4	T50.8X5	T50.8X6
Iocarmic acid	T50.8X1	T50.8X2	T50.8X3	T50.8X4	T50.8X5	T50.8X6
Iocetamic acid	T50.8X1	T50.8X2	T50.8X3	T50.8X4	T50.8X5	T50.8X6
Iodamide	T50.8X1	T50.8X2	T50.8X3	T50.8X4	T50.8X5	T50.8X6
Iodide NEC — *see also Iodine*	T49.0X1	T49.0X2	T49.0X3	T49.0X4	T49.0X5	T49.0X6
mercury (ointment)	T49.0X1	T49.0X2	T49.0X3	T49.0X4	T49.0X5	T49.0X6
methylate	T49.0X1	T49.0X2	T49.0X3	T49.0X4	T49.0X5	T49.0X6
potassium (expectorant) NEC	T48.4X1	T48.4X2	T48.4X3	T48.4X4	T48.4X5	T48.4X6
Iodinated						
contrast medium	T50.8X1	T50.8X2	T50.8X3	T50.8X4	T50.8X5	T50.8X6
glycerol	T48.4X1	T48.4X2	T48.4X3	T48.4X4	T48.4X5	T48.4X6
human serum albumin (131I)	T50.8X1	T50.8X2	T50.8X3	T50.8X4	T50.8X5	T50.8X6
Iodine (antiseptic, external) (tincture) NEC	T49.0X1	T49.0X2	T49.0X3	T49.0X4	T49.0X5	T49.0X6
125 — *see also Radiation sickness, and Exposure to radioactivce isotopes*	T50.8X1	T50.8X2	T50.8X3	T50.8X4	T50.8X5	T50.8X6
therapeutic	T50.991	T50.992	T50.993	T50.994	T50.995	T50.996
131 — *see also Radiation sickness, and Exposure to radioactivce isotopes*	T50.8X1	T50.8X2	T50.8X3	T50.8X4	T50.8X5	T50.8X6
therapeutic	T38.2X1	T38.2X2	T38.2X3	T38.2X4	T38.2X5	T38.2X6
diagnostic	T50.8X1	T50.8X2	T50.8X3	T50.8X4	T50.8X5	T50.8X6
for thyroid conditions (antithyroid)	T38.2X1	T38.2X2	T38.2X3	T38.2X4	T38.2X5	T38.2X6
solution	T49.0X1	T49.0X2	T49.0X3	T49.0X4	T49.0X5	T49.0X6
vapor	T59.891	T59.892	T59.893	T59.894	—	—
Iodipamide	T50.8X1	T50.8X2	T50.8X3	T50.8X4	T50.8X5	T50.8X6
Iodized (poppy seed) oil	T50.8X1	T50.8X2	T50.8X3	T50.8X4	T50.8X5	T50.8X6
Iodobismitol	T37.8X1	T37.8X2	T37.8X3	T37.8X4	T37.8X5	T37.8X6
Iodochlorhydroxyquin	T37.8X1	T37.8X2	T37.8X3	T37.8X4	T37.8X5	T37.8X6
topical	T49.0X1	T49.0X2	T49.0X3	T49.0X4	T49.0X5	T49.0X6
Iodochlorhydroxyquino-line	T37.8X1	T37.8X2	T37.8X3	T37.8X4	T37.8X5	T37.8X6
Iodocholesterol (131I)	T50.8X1	T50.8X2	T50.8X3	T50.8X4	T50.8X5	T50.8X6

◀ New ◀ Revised ~~deleted~~ Deleted

Substance	External Cause (T-Code)					
	Poisoning, Accidental (Unintentional)	Poisoning, Intentional Self-Harm	Poisoning, Assault	Poisoning, Undetermined	Adverse Effect	Underdosing
Iodoform	T49.0X1	T49.0X2	T49.0X3	T49.0X4	T49.0X5	T49.0X6
Iodohippuric acid	T50.8X1	T50.8X2	T50.8X3	T50.8X4	T50.8X5	T50.8X6
Iodopanoic acid	T50.8X1	T50.8X2	T50.8X3	T50.8X4	T50.8X5	T50.8X6
Iodophthalein (sodium)	T50.8X1	T50.8X2	T50.8X3	T50.8X4	T50.8X5	T50.8X6
Iodopyracet	T50.8X1	T50.8X2	T50.8X3	T50.8X4	T50.8X5	T50.8X6
Iodoquinol	T37.8X1	T37.8X2	T37.8X3	T37.8X4	T37.8X5	T37.8X6
Iodoxamic acid	T50.8X1	T50.8X2	T50.8X3	T50.8X4	T50.8X5	T50.8X6
Iofendylate	T50.8X1	T50.8X2	T50.8X3	T50.8X4	T50.8X5	T50.8X6
Ioglycamic acid	T50.8X1	T50.8X2	T50.8X3	T50.8X4	T50.8X5	T50.8X6
Iohexol	T50.8X1	T50.8X2	T50.8X3	T50.8X4	T50.8X5	T50.8X6
Ion exchange resin						
anion	T47.8X1	T47.8X2	T47.8X3	T47.8X4	T47.8X5	T47.8X6
cation	T50.3X1	T50.3X2	T50.3X3	T50.3X4	T50.3X5	T50.3X6
cholestyramine	T46.6X1	T46.6X2	T46.6X3	T46.6X4	T46.6X5	T46.6X6
intestinal	T47.8X1	T47.8X2	T47.8X3	T47.8X4	T47.8X5	T47.8X6
Iopamidol	T50.8X1	T50.8X2	T50.8X3	T50.8X4	T50.8X5	T50.8X6
Iopanoic acid	T50.8X1	T50.8X2	T50.8X3	T50.8X4	T50.8X5	T50.8X6
Iophenoic acid	T50.8X1	T50.8X2	T50.8X3	T50.8X4	T50.8X5	T50.8X6
Iopodate, sodium	T50.8X1	T50.8X2	T50.8X3	T50.8X4	T50.8X5	T50.8X6
Iopodic acid	T50.8X1	T50.8X2	T50.8X3	T50.8X4	T50.8X5	T50.8X6
Iopromide	T50.8X1	T50.8X2	T50.8X3	T50.8X4	T50.8X5	T50.8X6
Iopydol	T50.8X1	T50.8X2	T50.8X3	T50.8X4	T50.8X5	T50.8X6
Iotalamic acid	T50.8X1	T50.8X2	T50.8X3	T50.8X4	T50.8X5	T50.8X6
Iothalamate	T50.8X1	T50.8X2	T50.8X3	T50.8X4	T50.8X5	T50.8X6
Iothiouracil	T38.2X1	T38.2X2	T38.2X3	T38.2X4	T38.2X5	T38.2X6
Iotrol	T50.8X1	T50.8X2	T50.8X3	T50.8X4	T50.8X5	T50.8X6
Iotrolan	T50.8X1	T50.8X2	T50.8X3	T50.8X4	T50.8X5	T50.8X6
Iotroxate	T50.8X1	T50.8X2	T50.8X3	T50.8X4	T50.8X5	T50.8X6
Iotroxic acid	T50.8X1	T50.8X2	T50.8X3	T50.8X4	T50.8X5	T50.8X6
Ioversol	T50.8X1	T50.8X2	T50.8X3	T50.8X4	T50.8X5	T50.8X6
Ioxaglate	T50.8X1	T50.8X2	T50.8X3	T50.8X4	T50.8X5	T50.8X6
Ioxaglic acid	T50.8X1	T50.8X2	T50.8X3	T50.8X4	T50.8X5	T50.8X6
Ioxitalamic acid	T50.8X1	T50.8X2	T50.8X3	T50.8X4	T50.8X5	T50.8X6
Ipecac	T47.7X1	T47.7X2	T47.7X3	T47.7X4	T47.7X5	T47.7X6
Ipecacuanha	T48.4X1	T48.4X2	T48.4X3	T48.4X4	T48.4X5	T48.4X6
Ipodate, calcium	T50.8X1	T50.8X2	T50.8X3	T50.8X4	T50.8X5	T50.8X6
Ipral	T42.3X1	T42.3X2	T42.3X3	T42.3X4	T42.3X5	T42.3X6
Ipratropium (bromide)	T48.6X1	T48.6X2	T48.6X3	T48.6X4	T48.6X5	T48.6X6
Ipriflavone	T46.3X1	T46.3X2	T46.3X3	T46.3X4	T46.3X5	T46.3X6
Iprindole	T43.011	T43.012	T43.013	T43.014	T43.015	T43.016
Iproclozide	T43.1X1	T43.1X2	T43.1X3	T43.1X4	T43.1X5	T43.1X6
Iprofenin	T50.8X1	T50.8X2	T50.8X3	T50.8X4	T50.8X5	T50.8X6
Iproheptine	T49.2X1	T49.2X2	T49.2X3	T49.2X4	T49.2X5	T49.2X6
Iproniazid	T43.1X1	T43.1X2	T43.1X3	T43.1X4	T43.1X5	T43.1X6
Iproplatin	T45.1X1	T45.1X2	T45.1X3	T45.1X4	T45.1X5	T45.1X6
Iproveratril	T46.1X1	T46.1X2	T46.1X3	T46.1X4	T46.1X5	T46.1X6
Iron (compounds) (medicinal) NEC	T45.4X1	T45.4X2	T45.4X3	T45.4X4	T45.4X5	T45.4X6
ammonium	T45.4X1	T45.4X2	T45.4X3	T45.4X4	T45.4X5	T45.4X6
dextran injection	T45.4X1	T45.4X2	T45.4X3	T45.4X4	T45.4X5	T45.4X6
nonmedicinal	T56.891	T56.892	T56.893	T56.894	—	—
salts	T45.4X1	T45.4X2	T45.4X3	T45.4X4	T45.4X5	T45.4X6
sorbitex	T45.4X1	T45.4X2	T45.4X3	T45.4X4	T45.4X5	T45.4X6
sorbitol citric acid complex	T45.4X1	T45.4X2	T45.4X3	T45.4X4	T45.4X5	T45.4X6
Irrigating fluid (vaginal)	T49.8X1	T49.8X2	T49.8X3	T49.8X4	T49.8X5	T49.8X6
eye	T49.5X1	T49.5X2	T49.5X3	T49.5X4	T49.5X5	T49.5X6
Isepamicin	T36.5X1	T36.5X2	T36.5X3	T36.5X4	T36.5X5	T36.5X6
Isoaminile (citrate)	T48.3X1	T48.3X2	T48.3X3	T48.3X4	T48.3X5	T48.3X6
Isoamyl nitrite	T46.3X1	T46.3X2	T46.3X3	T46.3X4	T46.3X5	T46.3X6
Isobenzan	T60.1X1	T60.1X2	T60.1X3	T60.1X4	—	—
Isobutyl acetate	T52.8X1	T52.8X2	T52.8X3	T52.8X4	—	—
Isocarboxazid	T43.1X1	T43.1X2	T43.1X3	T43.1X4	T43.1X5	T43.1X6
Isoconazole	T49.0X1	T49.0X2	T49.0X3	T49.0X4	T49.0X5	T49.0X6
Isocyanate	T65.0X1	T65.0X2	T65.0X3	T65.0X4	—	—
Isoephedrine	T44.991	T44.992	T44.993	T44.994	T44.995	T44.996
Isoetarine	T48.6X1	T48.6X2	T48.6X3	T48.6X4	T48.6X5	T48.6X6
Isoethadione	T42.2X1	T42.2X2	T42.2X3	T42.2X4	T42.2X5	T42.2X6
Isoetharine	T44.5X1	T44.5X2	T44.5X3	T44.5X4	T44.5X5	T44.5X6
Isoflurane	T41.0X1	T41.0X2	T41.0X3	T41.0X4	T41.0X5	T41.0X6
Isoflurophate	T44.0X1	T44.0X2	T44.0X3	T44.0X4	T44.0X5	T44.0X6
Isomaltose, ferric complex	T45.4X1	T45.4X2	T45.4X3	T45.4X4	T45.4X5	T45.4X6
Isometheptene	T44.3X1	T44.3X2	T44.3X3	T44.3X4	T44.3X5	T44.3X6
Isoniazid	T37.1X1	T37.1X2	T37.1X3	T37.1X4	T37.1X5	T37.1X6
with						
rifampicin	T36.6X1	T36.6X2	T36.6X3	T36.6X4	T36.6X5	T36.6X6
thioacetazone	T37.1X1	T37.1X2	T37.1X3	T37.1X4	T37.1X5	T37.1X6
Isonicotinic acid hydrazide	T37.1X1	T37.1X2	T37.1X3	T37.1X4	T37.1X5	T37.1X6
Isonipecaine	T40.491	T40.492	T40.493	T40.494	T40.495	T40.496
Isopentaquine	T37.2X1	T37.2X2	T37.2X3	T37.2X4	T37.2X5	T37.2X6
Isophane insulin	T38.3X1	T38.3X2	T38.3X3	T38.3X4	T38.3X5	T38.3X6
Isophorone	T65.891	T65.892	T65.893	T65.894	—	—
Isophosphamide	T45.1X1	T45.1X2	T45.1X3	T45.1X4	T45.1X5	T45.1X6
Isopregnenone	T38.5X1	T38.5X2	T38.5X3	T38.5X4	T38.5X5	T38.5X6
Isoprenaline	T48.6X1	T48.6X2	T48.6X3	T48.6X4	T48.6X5	T48.6X6
Isopromethazine	T43.3X1	T43.3X2	T43.3X3	T43.3X4	T43.3X5	T43.3X6

◀ New   ◀ Revised   ~~deleted~~ Deleted

Substance	Poisoning, Accidental (Unintentional)	Poisoning, Intentional Self-Harm	Poisoning, Assault	Poisoning, Undetermined	Adverse Effect	Underdosing
Isopropamide	T44.3X1	T44.3X2	T44.3X3	T44.3X4	T44.3X5	T44.3X6
iodide	T44.3X1	T44.3X2	T44.3X3	T44.3X4	T44.3X5	T44.3X6
Isopropanol	T51.2X1	T51.2X2	T51.2X3	T51.2X4	—	—
Isopropyl						
acetate	T52.8X1	T52.8X2	T52.8X3	T52.8X4	—	—
alcohol	T51.2X1	T51.2X2	T51.2X3	T51.2X4	—	—
medicinal	T49.4X1	T49.4X2	T49.4X3	T49.4X4	T49.4X5	T49.4X6
ether	T52.8X1	T52.8X2	T52.8X3	T52.8X4	—	—
Isopropylaminophena-zone	T39.2X1	T39.2X2	T39.2X3	T39.2X4	T39.2X5	T39.2X6
Isoproterenol	T48.6X1	T48.6X2	T48.6X3	T48.6X4	T48.6X5	T48.6X6
Isosorbide dinitrate	T46.3X1	T46.3X2	T46.3X3	T46.3X4	T46.3X5	T46.3X6
Isothipendyl	T45.0X1	T45.0X2	T45.0X3	T45.0X4	T45.0X5	T45.0X6
Isotretinoin	T50.991	T50.992	T50.993	T50.994	T50.995	T50.996
Isoxazolyl penicillin	T36.0X1	T36.0X2	T36.0X3	T36.0X4	T36.0X5	T36.0X6
Isoxicam	T39.391	T39.392	T39.393	T39.394	T39.395	T39.396
Isoxsuprine	T46.7X1	T46.7X2	T46.7X3	T46.7X4	T46.7X5	T46.7X6
Ispagula	T47.4X1	T47.4X2	T47.4X3	T47.4X4	T47.4X5	T47.4X6
husk	T47.4X1	T47.4X2	T47.4X3	T47.4X4	T47.4X5	T47.4X6
Isradipine	T46.1X1	T46.1X2	T46.1X3	T46.1X4	T46.1X5	T46.1X6
I-thyroxine sodium	T38.1X1	T38.1X2	T38.1X3	T38.1X4	T38.1X5	T38.1X6
Itraconazole	T37.8X1	T37.8X2	T37.8X3	T37.8X4	T37.8X5	T37.8X6
Itramin tosilate	T46.3X1	T46.3X2	T46.3X3	T46.3X4	T46.3X5	T46.3X6
Ivermectin	T37.4X1	T37.4X2	T37.4X3	T37.4X4	T37.4X5	T37.4X6
Izoniazid	T37.1X1	T37.1X2	T37.1X3	T37.1X4	T37.1X5	T37.1X6
with thioacetazone	T37.1X1	T37.1X2	T37.1X3	T37.1X4	T37.1X5	T37.1X6
J						
Jalap	T47.2X1	T47.2X2	T47.2X3	T47.2X4	T47.2X5	T47.2X6
Jamaica						
dogwood (bark)	T39.8X1	T39.8X2	T39.8X3	T39.8X4	T39.8X5	T39.8X6
ginger	T65.891	T65.892	T65.893	T65.894	—	—
root	T62.2X1	T62.2X2	T62.2X3	T62.2X4	—	—
Jatropha	T62.2X1	T62.2X2	T62.2X3	T62.2X4	—	—
curcas	T62.2X1	T62.2X2	T62.2X3	T62.2X4	—	—
Jectofer	T45.4X1	T45.4X2	T45.4X3	T45.4X4	T45.4X5	T45.4X6
Jellyfish (sting)	T63.621	T63.622	T63.623	T63.624		
Jequirity (bean)	T62.2X1	T62.2X2	T62.2X3	T62.2X4		
Jimson weed (stramonium)	T62.2X1	T62.2X2	T62.2X3	T62.2X4	—	—
seeds	T62.2X1	T62.2X2	T62.2X3	T62.2X4	—	—
Josamycin	T36.3X1	T36.3X2	T36.3X3	T36.3X4	T36.3X5	T36.3X6
Juniper tar	T49.1X1	T49.1X2	T49.1X3	T49.1X4	T49.1X5	T49.1X6

Substance	Poisoning, Accidental (Unintentional)	Poisoning, Intentional Self-Harm	Poisoning, Assault	Poisoning, Undetermined	Adverse Effect	Underdosing
K						
Kallidinogenase	T46.7X1	T46.7X2	T46.7X3	T46.7X4	T46.7X5	T46.7X6
Kallikrein	T46.7X1	T46.7X2	T46.7X3	T46.7X4	T46.7X5	T46.7X6
Kanamycin	T36.5X1	T36.5X2	T36.5X3	T36.5X4	T36.5X5	T36.5X6
Kantrex	T36.5X1	T36.5X2	T36.5X3	T36.5X4	T36.5X5	T36.5X6
Kaolin	T47.6X1	T47.6X2	T47.6X3	T47.6X4	T47.6X5	T47.6X6
light	T47.6X1	T47.6X2	T47.6X3	T47.6X4	T47.6X5	T47.6X6
Karaya (gum)	T47.4X1	T47.4X2	T47.4X3	T47.4X4	T47.4X5	T47.4X6
Kebuzone	T39.2X1	T39.2X2	T39.2X3	T39.2X4	T39.2X5	T39.2X6
Kelevan	T60.1X1	T60.1X2	T60.1X3	T60.1X4	—	—
Kemithal	T41.1X1	T41.1X2	T41.1X3	T41.1X4	T41.1X5	T41.1X6
Kenacort	T38.0X1	T38.0X2	T38.0X3	T38.0X4	T38.0X5	T38.0X6
Keratolytic drug NEC	T49.4X1	T49.4X2	T49.4X3	T49.4X4	T49.4X5	T49.4X6
anthracene	T49.4X1	T49.4X2	T49.4X3	T49.4X4	T49.4X5	T49.4X6
Keratoplastic NEC	T49.4X1	T49.4X2	T49.4X3	T49.4X4	T49.4X5	T49.4X6
Kerosene, kerosine (fuel) (solvent) NEC	T52.0X1	T52.0X2	T52.0X3	T52.0X4	—	—
insecticide	T52.0X1	T52.0X2	T52.0X3	T52.0X4	—	—
vapor	T52.0X1	T52.0X2	T52.0X3	T52.0X4	—	—
Ketamine	T41.291	T41.292	T41.293	T41.294	T41.295	T41.296
Ketazolam	T42.4X1	T42.4X2	T42.4X3	T42.4X4	T42.4X5	T42.4X6
Ketazon	T39.2X1	T39.2X2	T39.2X3	T39.2X4	T39.2X5	T39.2X6
Ketobemidone	T40.491	T40.492	T40.493	T40.494	—	—
Ketoconazole	T49.0X1	T49.0X2	T49.0X3	T49.0X4	T49.0X5	T49.0X6
Ketols	T52.4X1	T52.4X2	T52.4X3	T52.4X4	—	—
Ketone oils	T52.4X1	T52.4X2	T52.4X3	T52.4X4	—	—
Ketoprofen	T39.311	T39.312	T39.313	T39.314	T39.315	T39.316
Ketorolac	T39.8X1	T39.8X2	T39.8X3	T39.8X4	T39.8X5	T39.8X6
Ketotifen	T45.0X1	T45.0X2	T45.0X3	T45.0X4	T45.0X5	T45.0X6
Khat	T43.691	T43.692	T43.693	T43.694	—	—
Khellin	T46.3X1	T46.3X2	T46.3X3	T46.3X4	T46.3X5	T46.3X6
Khelloside	T46.3X1	T46.3X2	T46.3X3	T46.3X4	T46.3X5	T46.3X6
Kiln gas or vapor (carbon monoxide)	T58.8X1	T58.8X2	T58.8X3	T58.8X4	—	—
Kitasamycin	T36.3X1	T36.3X2	T36.3X3	T36.3X4	T36.3X5	T36.3X6
Konsyl	T47.4X1	T47.4X2	T47.4X3	T47.4X4	T47.4X5	T47.4X6
Kosam seed	T62.2X1	T62.2X2	T62.2X3	T62.2X4	—	—
Krait (venom)	T63.091	T63.092	T63.093	T63.094	—	—
Kwell (insecticide)	T60.1X1	T60.1X2	T60.1X3	T60.1X4	—	—
anti-infective (topical)	T49.0X1	T49.0X2	T49.0X3	T49.0X4	T49.0X5	T49.0X6

◄ New ◄ Revised ~~deleted~~ Deleted

Substance	Poisoning, Accidental (Unintentional)	Poisoning, Intentional Self-Harm	Poisoning, Assault	Poisoning, Undetermined	Adverse Effect	Underdosing
L						
Labetalol	T44.8X1	T44.8X2	T44.8X3	T44.8X4	T44.8X5	T44.8X6
Laburnum (seeds)	T62.2X1	T62.2X2	T62.2X3	T62.2X4	—	—
leaves	T62.2X1	T62.2X2	T62.2X3	T62.2X4	—	—
Lachesine	T49.5X1	T49.5X2	T49.5X3	T49.5X4	T49.5X5	T49.5X6
Lacidipine	T46.5X1	T46.5X2	T46.5X3	T46.5X4	T46.5X5	T46.5X6
Lacquer	T65.6X1	T65.6X2	T65.6X3	T65.6X4	—	—
Lacrimogenic gas	T59.3X1	T59.3X2	T59.3X3	T59.3X4	—	—
Lactated potassic saline	T50.3X1	T50.3X2	T50.3X3	T50.3X4	T50.3X5	T50.3X6
Lactic acid	T49.8X1	T49.8X2	T49.8X3	T49.8X4	T49.8X5	T49.8X6
Lactobacillus						
acidophilus	T47.6X1	T47.6X2	T47.6X3	T47.6X4	T47.6X5	T47.6X6
compound	T47.6X1	T47.6X2	T47.6X3	T47.6X4	T47.6X5	T47.6X6
bifidus, lyophilized	T47.6X1	T47.6X2	T47.6X3	T47.6X4	T47.6X5	T47.6X6
bulgaricus	T47.6X1	T47.6X2	T47.6X3	T47.6X4	T47.6X5	T47.6X6
sporogenes	T47.6X1	T47.6X2	T47.6X3	T47.6X4	T47.6X5	T47.6X6
Lactoflavin	T45.2X1	T45.2X2	T45.2X3	T45.2X4	T45.2X5	T45.2X6
Lactose (as excipient)	T50.901	T50.902	T50.903	T50.904	T50.905	T50.906
Lactuca (virosa) (extract)	T42.6X1	T42.6X2	T42.6X3	T42.6X4	T42.6X5	T42.6X6
Lactucarium	T42.6X1	T42.6X2	T42.6X3	T42.6X4	T42.6X5	T42.6X6
Lactulose	T47.3X1	T47.3X2	T47.3X3	T47.3X4	T47.3X5	T47.3X6
Laevo — see Levo-						
Lanatosides	T46.0X1	T46.0X2	T46.0X3	T46.0X4	T46.0X5	T46.0X6
Lanolin	T49.3X1	T49.3X2	T49.3X3	T49.3X4	T49.3X5	T49.3X6
Largactil	T43.3X1	T43.3X2	T43.3X3	T43.3X4	T43.3X5	T43.3X6
Larkspur	T62.2X1	T62.2X2	T62.2X3	T62.2X4	—	—
Laroxyl	T43.011	T43.012	T43.013	T43.014	T43.015	T43.016
Lassar's paste	T49.4X1	T49.4X2	T49.4X3	T49.4X4	T49.4X5	T49.4X6
Lasix	T50.1X1	T50.1X2	T50.1X3	T50.1X4	T50.1X5	T50.1X6
Latamoxef	T36.1X1	T36.1X2	T36.1X3	T36.1X4	T36.1X5	T36.1X6
Latex	T65.811	T65.812	T65.813	T65.814	—	—
Lathyrus (seed)	T62.2X1	T62.2X2	T62.2X3	T62.2X4	—	—
Laudanum	T40.0X1	T40.0X2	T40.0X3	T40.0X4	T40.0X5	T40.0X6
Laudexium	T48.1X1	T48.1X2	T48.1X3	T48.1X4	T48.1X5	T48.1X6
Laughing gas	T41.0X1	T41.0X2	T41.0X3	T41.0X4	T41.0X5	T41.0X6
Laurel, black or cherry	T62.2X1	T62.2X2	T62.2X3	T62.2X4	—	—
Laurolinium	T49.0X1	T49.0X2	T49.0X3	T49.0X4	T49.0X5	T49.0X6
Lauryl sulfoacetate	T49.2X1	T49.2X2	T49.2X3	T49.2X4	T49.2X5	T49.2X6

Substance	Poisoning, Accidental (Unintentional)	Poisoning, Intentional Self-Harm	Poisoning, Assault	Poisoning, Undetermined	Adverse Effect	Underdosing
Laxative NEC	T47.4X1	T47.4X2	T47.4X3	T47.4X4	T47.4X5	T47.4X6
osmotic	T47.3X1	T47.3X2	T47.3X3	T47.3X4	T47.3X5	T47.3X6
saline	T47.3X1	T47.3X2	T47.3X3	T47.3X4	T47.3X5	T47.3X6
stimulant	T47.2X1	T47.2X2	T47.2X3	T47.2X4	T47.2X5	T47.2X6
L-dopa	T42.8X1	T42.8X2	T42.8X3	T42.8X4	T42.8X5	T42.8X6
Lead (dust) (fumes) (vapor) NEC	T56.0X1	T56.0X2	T56.0X3	T56.0X4	—	—
acetate	T49.2X1	T49.2X2	T49.2X3	T49.2X4	T49.2X5	T49.2X6
alkyl (fuel additive)	T56.0X1	T56.0X2	T56.0X3	T56.0X4	—	—
anti-infectives	T37.8X1	T37.8X2	T37.8X3	T37.8X4	T37.8X5	T37.8X6
antiknock compound (tetraethyl)	T56.0X1	T56.0X2	T56.0X3	T56.0X4	—	—
arsenate, arsenite (dust) (herbicide) (insecticide) (vapor)	T57.0X1	T57.0X2	T57.0X3	T57.0X4		
carbonate	T56.0X1	T56.0X2	T56.0X3	T56.0X4	—	—
paint	T56.0X1	T56.0X2	T56.0X3	T56.0X4	—	—
chromate	T56.0X1	T56.0X2	T56.0X3	T56.0X4	—	—
paint	T56.0X1	T56.0X2	T56.0X3	T56.0X4	—	—
dioxide	T56.0X1	T56.0X2	T56.0X3	T56.0X4	—	—
inorganic	T56.0X1	T56.0X2	T56.0X3	T56.0X4	—	—
iodide	T56.0X1	T56.0X2	T56.0X3	T56.0X4		
pigment (paint)	T56.0X1	T56.0X2	T56.0X3	T56.0X4	—	—
monoxide (dust)	T56.0X1	T56.0X2	T56.0X3	T56.0X4		
paint	T56.0X1	T56.0X2	T56.0X3	T56.0X4		
organic	T56.0X1	T56.0X2	T56.0X3	T56.0X4		
oxide	T56.0X1	T56.0X2	T56.0X3	T56.0X4		
paint	T56.0X1	T56.0X2	T56.0X3	T56.0X4		
paint	T56.0X1	T56.0X2	T56.0X3	T56.0X4	—	—
salts	T56.0X1	T56.0X2	T56.0X3	T56.0X4		
specified compound NEC	T56.0X1	T56.0X2	T56.0X3	T56.0X4		
tetra-ethyl	T56.0X1	T56.0X2	T56.0X3	T56.0X4	—	—
Lebanese red	T40.711	T40.712	T40.713	T40.714	T40.715	T40.716
Lefetamine	T39.8X1	T39.8X2	T39.8X3	T39.8X4	T39.8X5	T39.8X6
Lenperone	T43.4X1	T43.4X2	T43.4X3	T43.4X4	T43.4X5	T43.4X6
Lente lietin (insulin)	T38.3X1	T38.3X2	T38.3X3	T38.3X4	T38.3X5	T38.3X6
Leptazol	T50.7X1	T50.7X2	T50.7X3	T50.7X4	T50.7X5	T50.7X6
Leptophos	T60.0X1	T60.0X2	T60.0X3	T60.0X4	—	—
Leritine	T40.2X1	T40.2X2	T40.2X3	T40.2X4	T40.2X5	T40.2X6
Letosteine	T48.4X1	T48.4X2	T48.4X3	T48.4X4	T48.4X5	T48.4X6
Letter	T38.1X1	T38.1X2	T38.1X3	T38.1X4	T38.1X5	T38.1X6
Lettuce opium	T42.6X1	T42.6X2	T42.6X3	T42.6X4	T42.6X5	T42.6X6
Leucinocaine	T41.3X1	T41.3X2	T41.3X3	T41.3X4	T41.3X5	T41.3X6

◀ New ◀ Revised ~~deleted~~ Deleted

TABLE OF DRUGS AND CHEMICALS

Substance	External Cause (T-Code)					
	Poisoning, Accidental (Unintentional)	Poisoning, Intentional Self-Harm	Poisoning, Assault	Poisoning, Undetermined	Adverse Effect	Underdosing
Leucocianidol	T46.991	T46.992	T46.993	T46.994	T46.995	T46.996
Leucovorin (factor)	T45.8X1	T45.8X2	T45.8X3	T45.8X4	T45.8X5	T45.8X6
Leukeran	T45.1X1	T45.1X2	T45.1X3	T45.1X4	T45.1X5	T45.1X6
Leuprolide	T38.891	T38.892	T38.893	T38.894	T38.895	T38.896
Levalbuterol	T48.6X1	T48.6X2	T48.6X3	T48.6X4	T48.6X5	T48.6X6
Levallorphan	T50.7X1	T50.7X2	T50.7X3	T50.7X4	T50.7X5	T50.7X6
Levamisole	T37.4X1	T37.4X2	T37.4X3	T37.4X4	T37.4X5	T37.4X6
Levanil	T42.6X1	T42.6X2	T42.6X3	T42.6X4	T42.6X5	T42.6X6
Levarterenol	T44.4X1	T44.4X2	T44.4X3	T44.4X4	T44.4X5	T44.4X6
Levdropropizine	T48.3X1	T48.3X2	T48.3X3	T48.3X4	T48.3X5	T48.3X6
Levobunolol	T49.5X1	T49.5X2	T49.5X3	T49.5X4	T49.5X5	T49.5X6
Levocabastine (hydrochloride)	T45.0X1	T45.0X2	T45.0X3	T45.0X4	T45.0X5	T45.0X6
Levocarnitine	T50.991	T50.992	T50.993	T50.994	T50.995	T50.996
Levodopa	T42.8X1	T42.8X2	T42.8X3	T42.8X4	T42.8X5	T42.8X6
with carbidopa	T42.8X1	T42.8X2	T42.8X3	T42.8X4	T42.8X5	T42.8X6
Levo-dromoran	T40.2X1	T40.2X2	T40.2X3	T40.2X4	T40.2X5	T40.2X6
Levoglutamide	T50.991	T50.992	T50.993	T50.994	T50.995	T50.996
Levoid	T38.1X1	T38.1X2	T38.1X3	T38.1X4	T38.1X5	T38.1X6
Levo-iso-methadone	T40.3X1	T40.3X2	T40.3X3	T40.3X4	T40.3X5	T40.3X6
Levomepromazine	T43.3X1	T43.3X2	T43.3X3	T43.3X4	T43.3X5	T43.3X6
Levonordefrin	T49.6X1	T49.6X2	T49.6X3	T49.6X4	T49.6X5	T49.6X6
Levonorgestrel	T38.4X1	T38.4X2	T38.4X3	T38.4X4	T38.4X5	T38.4X6
with ethinylestradiol	T38.5X1	T38.5X2	T38.5X3	T38.5X4	T38.5X5	T38.5X6
Levopromazine	T43.3X1	T43.3X2	T43.3X3	T43.3X4	T43.3X5	T43.3X6
Levoprome	T42.6X1	T42.6X2	T42.6X3	T42.6X4	T42.6X5	T42.6X6
Levopropoxyphene	T40.491	T40.492	T40.493	T40.494	T40.495	T40.496
Levopropylhexedrine	T50.5X1	T50.5X2	T50.5X3	T50.5X4	T50.5X5	T50.5X6
Levoproxyphylline	T48.6X1	T48.6X2	T48.6X3	T48.6X4	T48.6X5	T48.6X6
Levorphanol	T40.491	T40.492	T40.493	T40.494	T40.495	T40.496
Levothyroxine	T38.1X1	T38.1X2	T38.1X3	T38.1X4	T38.1X5	T38.1X6
sodium	T38.1X1	T38.1X2	T38.1X3	T38.1X4	T38.1X5	T38.1X6
Levsin	T44.3X1	T44.3X2	T44.3X3	T44.3X4	T44.3X5	T44.3X6
Levulose	T50.3X1	T50.3X2	T50.3X3	T50.3X4	T50.3X5	T50.3X6
Lewisite (gas), not in war	T57.0X1	T57.0X2	T57.0X3	T57.0X4	—	—
Librium	T42.4X1	T42.4X2	T42.4X3	T42.4X4	T42.4X5	T42.4X6
Lidex	T49.0X1	T49.0X2	T49.0X3	T49.0X4	T49.0X5	T49.0X6
Lidocaine	T41.3X1	T41.3X2	T41.3X3	T41.3X4	T41.3X5	T41.3X6
regional	T41.3X1	T41.3X2	T41.3X3	T41.3X4	T41.3X5	T41.3X6
spinal	T41.3X1	T41.3X2	T41.3X3	T41.3X4	T41.3X5	T41.3X6
Lidofenin	T50.8X1	T50.8X2	T50.8X3	T50.8X4	T50.8X5	T50.8X6
Lidoflazine	T46.1X1	T46.1X2	T46.1X3	T46.1X4	T46.1X5	T46.1X6
Lighter fluid	T52.0X1	T52.0X2	T52.0X3	T52.0X4	—	—

Substance	External Cause (T-Code)					
	Poisoning, Accidental (Unintentional)	Poisoning, Intentional Self-Harm	Poisoning, Assault	Poisoning, Undetermined	Adverse Effect	Underdosing
Lignin hemicellulose	T47.6X1	T47.6X2	T47.6X3	T47.6X4	T47.6X5	T47.6X6
Lignocaine	T41.3X1	T41.3X2	T41.3X3	T41.3X4	T41.3X5	T41.3X6
regional	T41.3X1	T41.3X2	T41.3X3	T41.3X4	T41.3X5	T41.3X6
spinal	T41.3X1	T41.3X2	T41.3X3	T41.3X4	T41.3X5	T41.3X6
Ligroin(e) (solvent)	T52.0X1	T52.0X2	T52.0X3	T52.0X4	—	—
vapor	T59.891	T59.892	T59.893	T59.894	—	—
Ligustrum vulgare	T62.2X1	T62.2X2	T62.2X3	T62.2X4	—	—
Lily of the valley	T62.2X1	T62.2X2	T62.2X3	T62.2X4	—	—
Lime (chloride)	T54.3X1	T54.3X2	T54.3X3	T54.3X4	—	—
Limonene	T52.8X1	T52.8X2	T52.8X3	T52.8X4	—	—
Lincomycin	T36.8X1	T36.8X2	T36.8X3	T36.8X4	T36.8X5	T36.8X6
Lindane (insecticide) (nonmedicinal) (vapor)	T53.6X1	T53.6X2	T53.6X3	T53.6X4	—	—
medicinal	T49.0X1	T49.0X2	T49.0X3	T49.0X4	T49.0X5	T49.0X6
Liniments NEC	T49.91	T49.92	T49.93	T49.94	T49.95	T49.96
Linoleic acid	T46.6X1	T46.6X2	T46.6X3	T46.6X4	T46.6X5	T46.6X6
Linolenic acid	T46.6X1	T46.6X2	T46.6X3	T46.6X4	T46.6X5	T46.6X6
Linseed	T47.4X1	T47.4X2	T47.4X3	T47.4X4	T47.4X5	T47.4X6
Liothyronine	T38.1X1	T38.1X2	T38.1X3	T38.1X4	T38.1X5	T38.1X6
Liotrix	T38.1X1	T38.1X2	T38.1X3	T38.1X4	T38.1X5	T38.1X6
Lipancreatin	T47.5X1	T47.5X2	T47.5X3	T47.5X4	T47.5X5	T47.5X6
Lipo-alprostadil	T46.7X1	T46.7X2	T46.7X3	T46.7X4	T46.7X5	T46.7X6
Lipo-Lutin	T38.5X1	T38.5X2	T38.5X3	T38.5X4	T38.5X5	T38.5X6
Lipotropic drug NEC	T50.901	T50.902	T50.903	T50.904	T50.905	T50.906
Liquefied petroleum gases	T59.891	T59.892	T59.893	T59.894	—	—
piped (pure or mixed with air)	T59.891	T59.892	T59.893	T59.894	—	—
Liquid						
paraffin	T47.4X1	T47.4X2	T47.4X3	T47.4X4	T47.4X5	T47.4X6
petrolatum	T47.4X1	T47.4X2	T47.4X3	T47.4X4	T47.4X5	T47.4X6
topical	T49.3X1	T49.3X2	T49.3X3	T49.3X4	T49.3X5	T49.3X6
specified NEC	T65.891	T65.892	T65.893	T65.894	—	—
substance	T65.91	T65.92	T65.93	T65.94	—	—
Liquor creosolis compositus	T65.891	T65.892	T65.893	T65.894	—	—
Liquorice	T48.4X1	T48.4X2	T48.4X3	T48.4X4	T48.4X5	T48.4X6
extract	T47.8X1	T47.8X2	T47.8X3	T47.8X4	T47.8X5	T47.8X6
Lirugen	T50.991	T50.992	T50.993	T50.994	T50.995	T50.996
Lisinopril	T46.4X1	T46.4X2	T46.4X3	T46.4X4	T46.4X5	T46.4X6
Lisuride	T42.8X1	T42.8X2	T42.8X3	T42.8X4	T42.8X5	T42.8X6
Lithane	T43.8X1	T43.8X2	T43.8X3	T43.8X4	T43.8X5	T43.8X6
Lithium	T56.891	T56.892	T56.893	T56.894	—	—
gluconate	T43.591	T43.592	T43.593	T43.594	T43.595	T43.596
salts (carbonate)	T43.591	T43.592	T43.593	T43.594	T43.595	T43.596

◀ New ◀ Revised ~~deleted~~ Deleted

Substance	External Cause (T-Code)					
	Poisoning, Accidental (Unintentional)	Poisoning, Intentional Self-Harm	Poisoning, Assault	Poisoning, Undetermined	Adverse Effect	Underdosing
Lithonate	T43.8X1	T43.8X2	T43.8X3	T43.8X4	T43.8X5	T43.8X6
Liver						
extract	T45.8X1	T45.8X2	T45.8X3	T45.8X4	T45.8X5	T45.8X6
for parenteral use	T45.8X1	T45.8X2	T45.8X3	T45.8X4	T45.8X5	T45.8X6
fraction 1	T45.8X1	T45.8X2	T45.8X3	T45.8X4	T45.8X5	T45.8X6
hydrolysate	T45.8X1	T45.8X2	T45.8X3	T45.8X4	T45.8X5	T45.8X6
Lizard (bite) (venom)	T63.121	T63.122	T63.123	T63.124	—	—
LMD	T45.8X1	T45.8X2	T45.8X3	T45.8X4	T45.8X5	T45.8X6
Lobelia	T62.2X1	T62.2X2	T62.2X3	T62.2X4	—	—
Lobeline	T50.7X1	T50.7X2	T50.7X3	T50.7X4	T50.7X5	T50.7X6
Local action drug NEC	T49.8X1	T49.8X2	T49.8X3	T49.8X4	T49.8X5	T49.8X6
Locorten	T49.0X1	T49.0X2	T49.0X3	T49.0X4	T49.0X5	T49.0X6
Lofepramine	T43.011	T43.012	T43.013	T43.014	T43.015	T43.016
Lolium temulentum	T62.2X1	T62.2X2	T62.2X3	T62.2X4	—	—
Lomotil	T47.6X1	T47.6X2	T47.6X3	T47.6X4	T47.6X5	T47.6X6
Lomustine	T45.1X1	T45.1X2	T45.1X3	T45.1X4	T45.1X5	T45.1X6
Lonidamine	T45.1X1	T45.1X2	T45.1X3	T45.1X4	T45.1X5	T45.1X6
Loperamide	T47.6X1	T47.6X2	T47.6X3	T47.6X4	T47.6X5	T47.6X6
Loprazolam	T42.4X1	T42.4X2	T42.4X3	T42.4X4	T42.4X5	T42.4X6
Lorajmine	T46.2X1	T46.2X2	T46.2X3	T46.2X4	T46.2X5	T46.2X6
Loratidine	T45.0X1	T45.0X2	T45.0X3	T45.0X4	T45.0X5	T45.0X6
Lorazepam	T42.4X1	T42.4X2	T42.4X3	T42.4X4	T42.4X5	T42.4X6
Lorcainide	T46.2X1	T46.2X2	T46.2X3	T46.2X4	T46.2X5	T46.2X6
Lormetazepam	T42.4X1	T42.4X2	T42.4X3	T42.4X4	T42.4X5	T42.4X6
Lotions NEC	T49.91	T49.92	T49.93	T49.94	T49.95	T49.96
Lotusate	T42.3X1	T42.3X2	T42.3X3	T42.3X4	T42.3X5	T42.3X6
Lovastatin	T46.6X1	T46.6X2	T46.6X3	T46.6X4	T46.6X5	T46.6X6
Loxapine	T43.591	T43.592	T43.593	T43.594	T43.595	T43.596
Lowila	T49.2X1	T49.2X2	T49.2X3	T49.2X4	T49.2X5	T49.2X6
Lozenges (throat)	T49.6X1	T49.6X2	T49.6X3	T49.6X4	T49.6X5	T49.6X6
LSD	T40.8X1	T40.8X2	T40.8X3	T40.8X4	—	—
L-Tryptophan — see Amino acid						
Lubricant, eye	T49.5X1	T49.5X2	T49.5X3	T49.5X4	T49.5X5	T49.5X6
Lubricating oil NEC	T52.0X1	T52.0X2	T52.0X3	T52.0X4	—	—
Lucanthone	T37.4X1	T37.4X2	T37.4X3	T37.4X4	T37.4X5	T37.4X6
Luminal	T42.3X1	T42.3X2	T42.3X3	T42.3X4	T42.3X5	T42.3X6
Lung irritant (gas) NEC	T59.91	T59.92	T59.93	T59.94	—	—
Luteinizing hormone	T38.811	T38.812	T38.813	T38.814	T38.815	T38.816
Lutocylol	T38.5X1	T38.5X2	T38.5X3	T38.5X4	T38.5X5	T38.5X6
Lutromone	T38.5X1	T38.5X2	T38.5X3	T38.5X4	T38.5X5	T38.5X6
Lututrin	T48.291	T48.292	T48.293	T48.294	T48.295	T48.296
Lye (Concentrated)	T54.3X1	T54.3X2	T54.3X3	T54.3X4	—	—

Substance	External Cause (T-Code)					
	Poisoning, Accidental (Unintentional)	Poisoning, Intentional Self-Harm	Poisoning, Assault	Poisoning, Undetermined	Adverse Effect	Underdosing
Lygranum (skin test)	T50.8X1	T50.8X2	T50.8X3	T50.8X4	T50.8X5	T50.8X6
Lymecycline	T36.4X1	T36.4X2	T36.4X3	T36.4X4	T36.4X5	T36.4X6
Lymphogranuloma venereum antigen	T50.8X1	T50.8X2	T50.8X3	T50.8X4	T50.8X5	T50.8X6
Lynestrenol	T38.4X1	T38.4X2	T38.4X3	T38.4X4	T38.4X5	T38.4X6
Lypressin	T38.891	T38.892	T38.893	T38.894	T38.895	T38.896
Lyovac Sodium Edecrin	T50.1X1	T50.1X2	T50.1X3	T50.1X4	T50.1X5	T50.1X6
Lysergic acid diethylamide	T40.8X1	T40.8X2	T40.8X3	T40.8X4	—	—
Lysergide	T40.8X1	T40.8X2	T40.8X3	T40.8X4	—	—
Lysine vasopressin	T38.891	T38.892	T38.893	T38.894	T38.895	T38.896
Lysol	T54.1X1	T54.1X2	T54.1X3	T54.1X4		
Lysozyme	T49.0X1	T49.0X2	T49.0X3	T49.0X4	T49.0X5	T49.0X6
Lytta (vitatta)	T49.8X1	T49.8X2	T49.8X3	T49.8X4	T49.8X5	T49.8X6
M						
Mace	T59.3X1	T59.3X2	T59.3X3	T59.3X4	—	—
Macrogol	T50.991	T50.992	T50.993	T50.994	T50.995	T50.996
Macrolide						
anabolic drug	T38.7X1	T38.7X2	T38.7X3	T38.7X4	T38.7X5	T38.7X6
antibiotic	T36.3X1	T36.3X2	T36.3X3	T36.3X4	T36.3X5	T36.3X6
Mafenide	T49.0X1	T49.0X2	T49.0X3	T49.0X4	T49.0X5	T49.0X6
Magaldrate	T47.1X1	T47.1X2	T47.1X3	T47.1X4	T47.1X5	T47.1X6
Magic mushroom	T40.991	T40.992	T40.993	T40.994	—	—
Magnamycin	T36.8X1	T36.8X2	T36.8X3	T36.8X4	T36.8X5	T36.8X6
Magnesia magma	T47.1X1	T47.1X2	T47.1X3	T47.1X4	T47.1X5	T47.1X6
Magnesium NEC	T56.891	T56.892	T56.893	T56.894	—	—
carbonate	T47.1X1	T47.1X2	T47.1X3	T47.1X4	T47.1X5	T47.1X6
citrate	T47.4X1	T47.4X2	T47.4X3	T47.4X4	T47.4X5	T47.4X6
hydroxide	T47.1X1	T47.1X2	T47.1X3	T47.1X4	T47.1X5	T47.1X6
oxide	T47.1X1	T47.1X2	T47.1X3	T47.1X4	T47.1X5	T47.1X6
peroxide	T49.0X1	T49.0X2	T49.0X3	T49.0X4	T49.0X5	T49.0X6
salicylate	T39.091	T39.092	T39.093	T39.094	T39.095	T39.096
silicofluoride	T50.3X1	T50.3X2	T50.3X3	T50.3X4	T50.3X5	T50.3X6
sulfate	T47.4X1	T47.4X2	T47.4X3	T47.4X4	T47.4X5	T47.4X6
thiosulfate	T45.0X1	T45.0X2	T45.0X3	T45.0X4	T45.0X5	T45.0X6
trisilicate	T47.1X1	T47.1X2	T47.1X3	T47.1X4	T47.1X5	T47.1X6
Malathion (medicinal)	T49.0X1	T49.0X2	T49.0X3	T49.0X4	T49.0X5	T49.0X6
insecticide	T60.0X1	T60.0X2	T60.0X3	T60.0X4	—	—
Male fern extract	T37.4X1	T37.4X2	T37.4X3	T37.4X4	T37.4X5	T37.4X6
M-AMSA	T45.1X1	T45.1X2	T45.1X3	T45.1X4	T45.1X5	T45.1X6
Mandelic acid	T37.8X1	T37.8X2	T37.8X3	T37.8X4	T37.8X5	T37.8X6
Manganese (dioxide) (salts)	T57.2X1	T57.2X2	T57.2X3	T57.2X4	—	—
medicinal	T50.991	T50.992	T50.993	T50.994	T50.995	T50.996

◀ New   ◀ Revised   ~~deleted~~ Deleted

Substance	External Cause (T-Code)					
	Poisoning, Accidental (Unintentional)	Poisoning, Intentional Self-Harm	Poisoning, Assault	Poisoning, Undetermined	Adverse Effect	Underdosing
Mannitol	T47.3X1	T47.3X2	T47.3X3	T47.3X4	T47.3X5	T47.3X6
hexanitrate	T46.3X1	T46.3X2	T46.3X3	T46.3X4	T46.3X5	T46.3X6
Mannomustine	T45.1X1	T45.1X2	T45.1X3	T45.1X4	T45.1X5	T45.1X6
MAO inhibitors	T43.1X1	T43.1X2	T43.1X3	T43.1X4	T43.1X5	T43.1X6
Mapharsen	T37.8X1	T37.8X2	T37.8X3	T37.8X4	T37.8X5	T37.8X6
Maphenide	T49.0X1	T49.0X2	T49.0X3	T49.0X4	T49.0X5	T49.0X6
Maprotiline	T43.021	T43.022	T43.023	T43.024	T43.025	T43.026
Marcaine	T41.3X1	T41.3X2	T41.3X3	T41.3X4	T41.3X5	T41.3X6
infiltration (subcutaneous)	T41.3X1	T41.3X2	T41.3X3	T41.3X4	T41.3X5	T41.3X6
nerve block (peripheral) (plexus)	T41.3X1	T41.3X2	T41.3X3	T41.3X4	T41.3X5	T41.3X6
Marezine	T45.0X1	T45.0X2	T45.0X3	T45.0X4	T45.0X5	T45.0X6
Marihuana	T40.711	T40.712	T40.713	T40.714	T40.715	T40.716 ◀
Marijuana	T40.711	T40.712	T40.713	T40.714	T40.715	T40.716 ◀
Marine (sting)	T63.691	T63.692	T63.693	T63.694	—	—
animals (sting)	T63.691	T63.692	T63.693	T63.694	—	—
plants (sting)	T63.711	T63.712	T63.713	T63.714	—	—
Marplan	T43.1X1	T43.1X2	T43.1X3	T43.1X4	T43.1X5	T43.1X6
Marsh gas	T59.891	T59.892	T59.893	T59.894	—	—
Marsilid	T43.1X1	T43.1X2	T43.1X3	T43.1X4	T43.1X5	T43.1X6
Matulane	T45.1X1	T45.1X2	T45.1X3	T45.1X4	T45.1X5	T45.1X6
Mazindol	T50.5X1	T50.5X2	T50.5X3	T50.5X4	T50.5X5	T50.5X6
MCPA	T60.3X1	T60.3X2	T60.3X3	T60.3X4	—	—
MDMA	T43.641	T43.642	T43.643	T43.644	—	—
Meadow saffron	T62.2X1	T62.2X2	T62.2X3	T62.2X4	—	—
Measles virus vaccine (attenuated)	T50.B91	T50.B92	T50.B93	T50.B94	T50.B95	T50.B96
Meat, noxious	T62.8X1	T62.8X2	T62.8X3	T62.8X4	—	—
Meballymal	T42.3X1	T42.3X2	T42.3X3	T42.3X4	T42.3X5	T42.3X6
Mebanazine	T43.1X1	T43.1X2	T43.1X3	T43.1X4	T43.1X5	T43.1X6
Mebaral	T42.3X1	T42.3X2	T42.3X3	T42.3X4	T42.3X5	T42.3X6
Mebendazole	T37.4X1	T37.4X2	T37.4X3	T37.4X4	T37.4X5	T37.4X6
Mebeverine	T44.3X1	T44.3X2	T44.3X3	T44.3X4	T44.3X5	T44.3X6
Mebhydrolin	T45.0X1	T45.0X2	T45.0X3	T45.0X4	T45.0X5	T45.0X6
Mebumal	T42.3X1	T42.3X2	T42.3X3	T42.3X4	T42.3X5	T42.3X6
Mebutamate	T43.591	T43.592	T43.593	T43.594	T43.595	T43.596
Mecamylamine	T44.2X1	T44.2X2	T44.2X3	T44.2X4	T44.2X5	T44.2X6
Mechlorethamine	T45.1X1	T45.1X2	T45.1X3	T45.1X4	T45.1X5	T45.1X6
Mecillinam	T36.0X1	T36.0X2	T36.0X3	T36.0X4	T36.0X5	T36.0X6
Meclizine (hydrochloride)	T45.0X1	T45.0X2	T45.0X3	T45.0X4	T45.0X5	T45.0X6
Meclocycline	T36.4X1	T36.4X2	T36.4X3	T36.4X4	T36.4X5	T36.4X6
Meclofenamate	T39.391	T39.392	T39.393	T39.394	T39.395	T39.396
Meclofenamic acid	T39.391	T39.392	T39.393	T39.394	T39.395	T39.396

Substance	External Cause (T-Code)					
	Poisoning, Accidental (Unintentional)	Poisoning, Intentional Self-Harm	Poisoning, Assault	Poisoning, Undetermined	Adverse Effect	Underdosing
Meclofenoxate	T43.691	T43.692	T43.693	T43.694	T43.695	T43.696
Meclozine	T45.0X1	T45.0X2	T45.0X3	T45.0X4	T45.0X5	T45.0X6
Mecobalamin	T45.8X1	T45.8X2	T45.8X3	T45.8X4	T45.8X5	T45.8X6
Mecoprop	T60.3X1	T60.3X2	T60.3X3	T60.3X4	—	—
Mecrilate	T49.3X1	T49.3X2	T49.3X3	T49.3X4	T49.3X5	T49.3X6
Mecysteine	T48.4X1	T48.4X2	T48.4X3	T48.4X4	T48.4X5	T48.4X6
Medazepam	T42.4X1	T42.4X2	T42.4X3	T42.4X4	T42.4X5	T42.4X6
Medicament NEC	T50.901	T50.902	T50.903	T50.904	T50.905	T50.906
Medinal	T42.3X1	T42.3X2	T42.3X3	T42.3X4	T42.3X5	T42.3X6
Medomin	T42.3X1	T42.3X2	T42.3X3	T42.3X4	T42.3X5	T42.3X6
Medrogestone	T38.5X1	T38.5X2	T38.5X3	T38.5X4	T38.5X5	T38.5X6
Medroxalol	T44.8X1	T44.8X2	T44.8X3	T44.8X4	T44.8X5	T44.8X6
Medroxyprogesterone acetate (depot)	T38.5X1	T38.5X2	T38.5X3	T38.5X4	T38.5X5	T38.5X6
Medrysone	T49.0X1	T49.0X2	T49.0X3	T49.0X4	T49.0X5	T49.0X6
Mefenamic acid	T39.391	T39.392	T39.393	T39.394	T39.395	T39.396
Mefenorex	T50.5X1	T50.5X2	T50.5X3	T50.5X4	T50.5X5	T50.5X6
Mefloquine	T37.2X1	T37.2X2	T37.2X3	T37.2X4	T37.2X5	T37.2X6
Mefruside	T50.2X1	T50.2X2	T50.2X3	T50.2X4	T50.2X5	T50.2X6
Megahallucinogen	T40.901	T40.902	T40.903	T40.904	T40.905	T40.906
Megestrol	T38.5X1	T38.5X2	T38.5X3	T38.5X4	T38.5X5	T38.5X6
Meglumine						
antimoniate	T37.8X1	T37.8X2	T37.8X3	T37.8X4	T37.8X5	T37.8X6
diatrizoate	T50.8X1	T50.8X2	T50.8X3	T50.8X4	T50.8X5	T50.8X6
iodipamide	T50.8X1	T50.8X2	T50.8X3	T50.8X4	T50.8X5	T50.8X6
iotroxate	T50.8X1	T50.8X2	T50.8X3	T50.8X4	T50.8X5	T50.8X6
MEK (methyl ethyl ketone)	T52.4X1	T52.4X2	T52.4X3	T52.4X4	—	—
Meladrazine	T44.3X1	T44.3X2	T44.3X3	T44.3X4	T44.3X5	T44.3X6
Meladinin	T49.3X1	T49.3X2	T49.3X3	T49.3X4	T49.3X5	T49.3X6
Melaleuca alternifolia oil	T49.0X1	T49.0X2	T49.0X3	T49.0X4	T49.0X5	T49.0X6
Melanizing agents	T49.3X1	T49.3X2	T49.3X3	T49.3X4	T49.3X5	T49.3X6
Melanocyte-stimulating hormone	T38.891	T38.892	T38.893	T38.894	T38.895	T38.896
Melarsonyl potassium	T37.3X1	T37.3X2	T37.3X3	T37.3X4	T37.3X5	T37.3X6
Melarsoprol	T37.3X1	T37.3X2	T37.3X3	T37.3X4	T37.3X5	T37.3X6
Melia azedarach	T62.2X1	T62.2X2	T62.2X3	T62.2X4	—	—
Melitracen	T43.011	T43.012	T43.013	T43.014	T43.015	T43.016
Mellaril	T43.3X1	T43.3X2	T43.3X3	T43.3X4	T43.3X5	T43.3X6
Meloxine	T49.3X1	T49.3X2	T49.3X3	T49.3X4	T49.3X5	T49.3X6
Melperone	T43.4X1	T43.4X2	T43.4X3	T43.4X4	T43.4X5	T43.4X6
Melphalan	T45.1X1	T45.1X2	T45.1X3	T45.1X4	T45.1X5	T45.1X6
Memantine	T43.8X1	T43.8X2	T43.8X3	T43.8X4	T43.8X5	T43.8X6

◀ New   ◀ Revised   ~~deleted~~ Deleted

TABLE OF DRUGS AND CHEMICALS

Substance	Poisoning, Accidental (Unintentional)	Poisoning, Intentional Self-Harm	Poisoning, Assault	Poisoning, Undetermined	Adverse Effect	Underdosing
Menadiol	T45.7X1	T45.7X2	T45.7X3	T45.7X4	T45.7X5	T45.7X6
sodium sulfate	T45.7X1	T45.7X2	T45.7X3	T45.7X4	T45.7X5	T45.7X6
Menadione	T45.7X1	T45.7X2	T45.7X3	T45.7X4	T45.7X5	T45.7X6
sodium bisulfite	T45.7X1	T45.7X2	T45.7X3	T45.7X4	T45.7X5	T45.7X6
Menaphthone	T45.7X1	T45.7X2	T45.7X3	T45.7X4	T45.7X5	T45.7X6
Menaquinone	T45.7X1	T45.7X2	T45.7X3	T45.7X4	T45.7X5	T45.7X6
Menatetrenone	T45.7X1	T45.7X2	T45.7X3	T45.7X4	T45.7X5	T45.7X6
Meningococcal vaccine	T50.A91	T50.A92	T50.A93	T50.A94	T50.A95	T50.A96
Menningovax (-AC) (-C)	T50.A91	T50.A92	T50.A93	T50.A94	T50.A95	T50.A96
Menotropins	T38.811	T38.812	T38.813	T38.814	T38.815	T38.816
Menthol	T48.5X1	T48.5X2	T48.5X3	T48.5X4	T48.5X5	T48.5X6
Mepacrine	T37.2X1	T37.2X2	T37.2X3	T37.2X4	T37.2X5	T37.2X6
Meparfynol	T42.6X1	T42.6X2	T42.6X3	T42.6X4	T42.6X5	T42.6X6
Mepartricin	T36.7X1	T36.7X2	T36.7X3	T36.7X4	T36.7X5	T36.7X6
Mepazine	T43.3X1	T43.3X2	T43.3X3	T43.3X4	T43.3X5	T43.3X6
Mepenzolate	T44.3X1	T44.3X2	T44.3X3	T44.3X4	T44.3X5	T44.3X6
bromide	T44.3X1	T44.3X2	T44.3X3	T44.3X4	T44.3X5	T44.3X6
Meperidine	T40.491	T40.492	T40.493	T40.494	T40.495	T40.496
Mephebarbital	T42.3X1	T42.3X2	T42.3X3	T42.3X4	T42.3X5	T42.3X6
Mephenamin(e)	T42.8X1	T42.8X2	T42.8X3	T42.8X4	T42.8X5	T42.8X6
Mephenesin	T42.8X1	T42.8X2	T42.8X3	T42.8X4	T42.8X5	T42.8X6
Mephenhydramine	T45.0X1	T45.0X2	T45.0X3	T45.0X4	T45.0X5	T45.0X6
Mephenoxalone	T42.8X1	T42.8X2	T42.8X3	T42.8X4	T42.8X5	T42.8X6
Mephentermine	T44.991	T44.992	T44.993	T44.994	T44.995	T44.996
Mephenytoin	T42.0X1	T42.0X2	T42.0X3	T42.0X4	T42.0X5	T42.0X6
with phenobarbital	T42.3X1	T42.3X2	T42.3X3	T42.3X4	T42.3X5	T42.3X6
Mephobarbital	T42.3X1	T42.3X2	T42.3X3	T42.3X4	T42.3X5	T42.3X6
Mephosfolan	T60.0X1	T60.0X2	T60.0X3	T60.0X4	—	—
Mepindolol	T44.7X1	T44.7X2	T44.7X3	T44.7X4	T44.7X5	T44.7X6
Mepiperphenidol	T44.3X1	T44.3X2	T44.3X3	T44.3X4	T44.3X5	T44.3X6
Mepitiostane	T38.7X1	T38.7X2	T38.7X3	T38.7X4	T38.7X5	T38.7X6
Mepivacaine	T41.3X1	T41.3X2	T41.3X3	T41.3X4	T41.3X5	T41.3X6
epidural	T41.3X1	T41.3X2	T41.3X3	T41.3X4	T41.3X5	T41.3X6
Meprednisone	T38.0X1	T38.0X2	T38.0X3	T38.0X4	T38.0X5	T38.0X6
Meprobam	T43.591	T43.592	T43.593	T43.594	T43.595	T43.596
Meprobamate	T43.591	T43.592	T43.593	T43.594	T43.595	T43.596
Meproscillarin	T46.0X1	T46.0X2	T46.0X3	T46.0X4	T46.0X5	T46.0X6
Meprylcaine	T41.3X1	T41.3X2	T41.3X3	T41.3X4	T41.3X5	T41.3X6
Meptazinol	T39.8X1	T39.8X2	T39.8X3	T39.8X4	T39.8X5	T39.8X6
Mepyramine	T45.0X1	T45.0X2	T45.0X3	T45.0X4	T45.0X5	T45.0X6
Mequitazine	T43.3X1	T43.3X2	T43.3X3	T43.3X4	T43.3X5	T43.3X6
Meralluride	T50.2X1	T50.2X2	T50.2X3	T50.2X4	T50.2X5	T50.2X6

Substance	Poisoning, Accidental (Unintentional)	Poisoning, Intentional Self-Harm	Poisoning, Assault	Poisoning, Undetermined	Adverse Effect	Underdosing
Merbaphen	T50.2X1	T50.2X2	T50.2X3	T50.2X4	T50.2X5	T50.2X6
Merbromin	T49.0X1	T49.0X2	T49.0X3	T49.0X4	T49.0X5	T49.0X6
Mercaptobenzothiazole salts	T49.0X1	T49.0X2	T49.0X3	T49.0X4	T49.0X5	T49.0X6
Mercaptomerin	T50.2X1	T50.2X2	T50.2X3	T50.2X4	T50.2X5	T50.2X6
Mercaptopurine	T45.1X1	T45.1X2	T45.1X3	T45.1X4	T45.1X5	T45.1X6
Mercumatilin	T50.2X1	T50.2X2	T50.2X3	T50.2X4	T50.2X5	T50.2X6
Mercuramide	T50.2X1	T50.2X2	T50.2X3	T50.2X4	T50.2X5	T50.2X6
Mercurochrome	T49.0X1	T49.0X2	T49.0X3	T49.0X4	T49.0X5	T49.0X6
Mercurophylline	T50.2X1	T50.2X2	T50.2X3	T50.2X4	T50.2X5	T50.2X6
Mercury, mercurial, mercuric, mercurous (compounds) (cyanide) (fumes) (nonmedicinal) (vapor) NEC	T56.1X1	T56.1X2	T56.1X3	T56.1X4	—	—
ammoniated	T49.0X1	T49.0X2	T49.0X3	T49.0X4	T49.0X5	T49.0X6
anti-infective						
local	T49.0X1	T49.0X2	T49.0X3	T49.0X4	T49.0X5	T49.0X6
systemic	T37.8X1	T37.8X2	T37.8X3	T37.8X4	T37.8X5	T37.8X6
topical	T49.0X1	T49.0X2	T49.0X3	T49.0X4	T49.0X5	T49.0X6
chloride (ammoniated)	T49.0X1	T49.0X2	T49.0X3	T49.0X4	T49.0X5	T49.0X6
fungicide	T56.1X1	T56.1X2	T56.1X3	T56.1X4	—	—
diuretic NEC	T50.2X1	T50.2X2	T50.2X3	T50.2X4	T50.2X5	T50.2X6
fungicide	T56.1X1	T56.1X2	T56.1X3	T56.1X4	—	—
organic (fungicide)	T56.1X1	T56.1X2	T56.1X3	T56.1X4	—	—
oxide, yellow	T49.0X1	T49.0X2	T49.0X3	T49.0X4	T49.0X5	T49.0X6
Mersalyl	T50.2X1	T50.2X2	T50.2X3	T50.2X4	T50.2X5	T50.2X6
Merthiolate	T49.0X1	T49.0X2	T49.0X3	T49.0X4	T49.0X5	T49.0X6
ophthalmic preparation	T49.5X1	T49.5X2	T49.5X3	T49.5X4	T49.5X5	T49.5X6
Meruvax	T50.B91	T50.B92	T50.B93	T50.B94	T50.B95	T50.B96
Mesalazine	T47.8X1	T47.8X2	T47.8X3	T47.8X4	T47.8X5	T47.8X6
Mescal buttons	T40.991	T40.992	T40.993	T40.994	—	—
Mescaline	T40.991	T40.992	T40.993	T40.994	—	—
Mesna	T48.4X1	T48.4X2	T48.4X3	T48.4X4	T48.4X5	T48.4X6
Mesoglycan	T46.6X1	T46.6X2	T46.6X3	T46.6X4	T46.6X5	T46.6X6
Mesoridazine	T43.3X1	T43.3X2	T43.3X3	T43.3X4	T43.3X5	T43.3X6
Mestanolone	T38.7X1	T38.7X2	T38.7X3	T38.7X4	T38.7X5	T38.7X6
Mesterolone	T38.7X1	T38.7X2	T38.7X3	T38.7X4	T38.7X5	T38.7X6
Mestranol	T38.5X1	T38.5X2	T38.5X3	T38.5X4	T38.5X5	T38.5X6
Mesulergine	T42.8X1	T42.8X2	T42.8X3	T42.8X4	T42.8X5	T42.8X6
Mesulfen	T49.0X1	T49.0X2	T49.0X3	T49.0X4	T49.0X5	T49.0X6
Mesuximide	T42.2X1	T42.2X2	T42.2X3	T42.2X4	T42.2X5	T42.2X6
Metabutethamine	T41.3X1	T41.3X2	T41.3X3	T41.3X4	T41.3X5	T41.3X6
Metactesylacetate	T49.0X1	T49.0X2	T49.0X3	T49.0X4	T49.0X5	T49.0X6

◀ New   ◀ Revised   deleted Deleted

	External Cause (T-Code)					
Substance	Poisoning, Accidental (Unintentional)	Poisoning, Intentional Self-Harm	Poisoning, Assault	Poisoning, Undetermined	Adverse Effect	Underdosing
Metacycline	T36.4X1	T36.4X2	T36.4X3	T36.4X4	T36.4X5	T36.4X6
Metaldehyde (snail killer) NEC	T60.8X1	T60.8X2	T60.8X3	T60.8X4	—	—
Metals (heavy) (nonmedicinal)	T56.91	T56.92	T56.93	T56.94	—	—
dust, fumes, or vapor NEC	T56.91	T56.92	T56.93	T56.94	—	—
light NEC	T56.91	T56.92	T56.93	T56.94	—	—
dust, fumes, or vapor NEC	T56.91	T56.92	T56.93	T56.94	—	—
specified NEC	T56.891	T56.892	T56.893	T56.894	—	—
thallium	T56.811	T56.812	T56.813	T56.814	—	—
Metamfetamine	T43.621	T43.622	T43.623	T43.624	T43.625	T43.626
Metamizole sodium	T39.2X1	T39.2X2	T39.2X3	T39.2X4	T39.2X5	T39.2X6
Metampicillin	T36.0X1	T36.0X2	T36.0X3	T36.0X4	T36.0X5	T36.0X6
Metamucil	T47.4X1	T47.4X2	T47.4X3	T47.4X4	T47.4X5	T47.4X6
Metaphen	T49.0X1	T49.0X2	T49.0X3	T49.0X4	T49.0X5	T49.0X6
Metandienone	T38.7X1	T38.7X2	T38.7X3	T38.7X4	T38.7X5	T38.7X6
Metandrostenolone	T38.7X1	T38.7X2	T38.7X3	T38.7X4	T38.7X5	T38.7X6
Metaphos	T60.0X1	T60.0X2	T60.0X3	T60.0X4	—	—
Metapramine	T43.011	T43.012	T43.013	T43.014	T43.015	T43.016
Metaproterenol	T48.291	T48.292	T48.293	T48.294	T48.295	T48.296
Metaraminol	T44.4X1	T44.4X2	T44.4X3	T44.4X4	T44.4X5	T44.4X6
Metaxalone	T42.8X1	T42.8X2	T42.8X3	T42.8X4	T42.8X5	T42.8X6
Metenolone	T38.7X1	T38.7X2	T38.7X3	T38.7X4	T38.7X5	T38.7X6
Metergoline	T42.8X1	T42.8X2	T42.8X3	T42.8X4	T42.8X5	T42.8X6
Metescufylline	T46.991	T46.992	T46.993	T46.994	T46.995	T46.996
Metetoin	T42.0X1	T42.0X2	T42.0X3	T42.0X4	T42.0X5	T42.0X6
Metformin	T38.3X1	T38.3X2	T38.3X3	T38.3X4	T38.3X5	T38.3X6
Methacholine	T44.1X1	T44.1X2	T44.1X3	T44.1X4	T44.1X5	T44.1X6
Methacycline	T36.4X1	T36.4X2	T36.4X3	T36.4X4	T36.4X5	T36.4X6
Methadone	T40.3X1	T40.3X2	T40.3X3	T40.3X4	T40.3X5	T40.3X6
Methallenestril	T38.5X1	T38.5X2	T38.5X3	T38.5X4	T38.5X5	T38.5X6
Methallenoestril	T38.5X1	T38.5X2	T38.5X3	T38.5X4	T38.5X5	T38.5X6
Methamphetamine	T43.621	T43.622	T43.623	T43.624	T43.625	T43.626
Methampyrone	T39.2X1	T39.2X2	T39.2X3	T39.2X4	T39.2X5	T39.2X6
Methandienone	T38.7X1	T38.7X2	T38.7X3	T38.7X4	T38.7X5	T38.7X6
Methandriol	T38.7X1	T38.7X2	T38.7X3	T38.7X4	T38.7X5	T38.7X6
Methandrostenolone	T38.7X1	T38.7X2	T38.7X3	T38.7X4	T38.7X5	T38.7X6
Methane	T59.891	T59.892	T59.893	T59.894	—	—
Methanethiol	T59.891	T59.892	T59.893	T59.894	—	—
Methaniazide	T37.1X1	T37.1X2	T37.1X3	T37.1X4	T37.1X5	T37.1X6
Methanol (vapor)	T51.1X1	T51.1X2	T51.1X3	T51.1X4	—	—
Methantheline	T44.3X1	T44.3X2	T44.3X3	T44.3X4	T44.3X5	T44.3X6
Methanthelinium bromide	T44.3X1	T44.3X2	T44.3X3	T44.3X4	T44.3X5	T44.3X6
Methaphenilene	T45.0X1	T45.0X2	T45.0X3	T45.0X4	T45.0X5	T45.0X6

	External Cause (T-Code)					
Substance	Poisoning, Accidental (Unintentional)	Poisoning, Intentional Self-Harm	Poisoning, Assault	Poisoning, Undetermined	Adverse Effect	Underdosing
Methapyrilene	T45.0X1	T45.0X2	T45.0X3	T45.0X4	T45.0X5	T45.0X6
Methaqualone (compound)	T42.6X1	T42.6X2	T42.6X3	T42.6X4	T42.6X5	T42.6X6
Metharbital	T42.3X1	T42.3X2	T42.3X3	T42.3X4	T42.3X5	T42.3X6
Methazolamide	T50.2X1	T50.2X2	T50.2X3	T50.2X4	T50.2X5	T50.2X6
Methdilazine	T43.3X1	T43.3X2	T43.3X3	T43.3X4	T43.3X5	T43.3X6
Methedrine	T43.621	T43.622	T43.623	T43.624	T43.625	T43.626
Methenamine (mandelate)	T37.8X1	T37.8X2	T37.8X3	T37.8X4	T37.8X5	T37.8X6
Methenolone	T38.7X1	T38.7X2	T38.7X3	T38.7X4	T38.7X5	T38.7X6
Methergine	T48.0X1	T48.0X2	T48.0X3	T48.0X4	T48.0X5	T48.0X6
Methetoin	T42.0X1	T42.0X2	T42.0X3	T42.0X4	T42.0X5	T42.0X6
Methiacil	T38.2X1	T38.2X2	T38.2X3	T38.2X4	T38.2X5	T38.2X6
Methicillin	T36.0X1	T36.0X2	T36.0X3	T36.0X4	T36.0X5	T36.0X6
Methimazole	T38.2X1	T38.2X2	T38.2X3	T38.2X4	T38.2X5	T38.2X6
Methiodal sodium	T50.8X1	T50.8X2	T50.8X3	T50.8X4	T50.8X5	T50.8X6
Methionine	T50.991	T50.992	T50.993	T50.994	T50.995	T50.996
Methisazone	T37.5X1	T37.5X2	T37.5X3	T37.5X4	T37.5X5	T37.5X6
Methisoprinol	T37.5X1	T37.5X2	T37.5X3	T37.5X4	T37.5X5	T37.5X6
Methitural	T42.3X1	T42.3X2	T42.3X3	T42.3X4	T42.3X5	T42.3X6
Methixene	T44.3X1	T44.3X2	T44.3X3	T44.3X4	T44.3X5	T44.3X6
Methobarbital, methobarbitone	T42.3X1	T42.3X2	T42.3X3	T42.3X4	T42.3X5	T42.3X6
Methocarbamol	T42.8X1	T42.8X2	T42.8X3	T42.8X4	T42.8X5	T42.8X6
skeletal muscle relaxant	T48.1X1	T48.1X2	T48.1X3	T48.1X4	T48.1X5	T48.1X6
Methohexital	T41.1X1	T41.1X2	T41.1X3	T41.1X4	T41.1X5	T41.1X6
Methohexitone	T41.1X1	T41.1X2	T41.1X3	T41.1X4	T41.1X5	T41.1X6
Methoin	T42.0X1	T42.0X2	T42.0X3	T42.0X4	T42.0X5	T42.0X6
Methopholine	T39.8X1	T39.8X2	T39.8X3	T39.8X4	T39.8X5	T39.8X6
Methopromazine	T43.3X1	T43.3X2	T43.3X3	T43.3X4	T43.3X5	T43.3X6
Methorate	T48.3X1	T48.3X2	T48.3X3	T48.3X4	T48.3X5	T48.3X6
Methoserpidine	T46.5X1	T46.5X2	T46.5X3	T46.5X4	T46.5X5	T46.5X6
Methotrexate	T45.1X1	T45.1X2	T45.1X3	T45.1X4	T45.1X5	T45.1X6
Methotrimeprazine	T43.3X1	T43.3X2	T43.3X3	T43.3X4	T43.3X5	T43.3X6
Methoxa-Dome	T49.3X1	T49.3X2	T49.3X3	T49.3X4	T49.3X5	T49.3X6
Methoxamine	T44.4X1	T44.4X2	T44.4X3	T44.4X4	T44.4X5	T44.4X6
Methoxsalen	T50.991	T50.992	T50.993	T50.994	T50.995	T50.996
Methoxyaniline	T65.3X1	T65.3X2	T65.3X3	T65.3X4	—	—
Methoxybenzyl penicillin	T36.0X1	T36.0X2	T36.0X3	T36.0X4	T36.0X5	T36.0X6
Methoxychlor	T53.7X1	T53.7X2	T53.7X3	T53.7X4	—	—
Methoxy-DDT	T53.7X1	T53.7X2	T53.7X3	T53.7X4	—	—
2-Methoxyethanol	T52.3X1	T52.3X2	T52.3X3	T52.3X4	—	—
Methoxyflurane	T41.0X1	T41.0X2	T41.0X3	T41.0X4	T41.0X5	T41.0X6
Methoxyphenamine	T48.6X1	T48.6X2	T48.6X3	T48.6X4	T48.6X5	T48.6X6
Methoxypromazine	T43.3X1	T43.3X2	T43.3X3	T43.3X4	T43.3X5	T43.3X6

◄ New   ◄ Revised   ~~deleted~~ Deleted

Substance	External Cause (T-Code)					
	Poisoning, Accidental (Unintentional)	Poisoning, Intentional Self-Harm	Poisoning, Assault	Poisoning, Undetermined	Adverse Effect	Underdosing
5-Methoxypsoralen (5-MOP)	T50.991	T50.992	T50.993	T50.994	T50.995	T50.996
8-Methoxypsoralen (8-MOP)	T50.991	T50.992	T50.993	T50.994	T50.995	T50.996
Methscopolamine bromide	T44.3X1	T44.3X2	T44.3X3	T44.3X4	T44.3X5	T44.3X6
Methsuximide	T42.2X1	T42.2X2	T42.2X3	T42.2X4	T42.2X5	T42.2X6
Methyclothiazide	T50.2X1	T50.2X2	T50.2X3	T50.2X4	T50.2X5	T50.2X6
Methyl						
acetate	T52.4X1	T52.4X2	T52.4X3	T52.4X4	—	—
acetone	T52.4X1	T52.4X2	T52.4X3	T52.4X4	—	—
acrylate	T65.891	T65.892	T65.893	T65.894	—	—
alcohol	T51.1X1	T51.1X2	T51.1X3	T51.1X4	—	—
aminophenol	T65.3X1	T65.3X2	T65.3X3	T65.3X4	—	—
amphetamine	T43.621	T43.622	T43.623	T43.624	T43.625	T43.626
androstanolone	T38.7X1	T38.7X2	T38.7X3	T38.7X4	T38.7X5	T38.7X6
atropine	T44.3X1	T44.3X2	T44.3X3	T44.3X4	T44.3X5	T44.3X6
benzene	152.2X1	T52.2X2	T52.2X3	T52.2X4	—	—
benzoate	T52.8X1	T52.8X2	T52.8X3	T52.8X4	—	—
benzol	T52.2X1	T52.2X2	T52.2X3	T52.2X4	—	—
bromide (gas)	T59.891	T59.892	T59.893	T59.894	—	—
fumigant	T60.8X1	T60.8X2	T60.8X3	T60.8X4	—	—
butanol	T51.3X1	T51.3X2	T51.3X3	T51.3X4	—	—
carbinol	T51.1X1	T51.1X2	T51.1X3	T51.1X4	—	—
carbonate	T52.8X1	T52.8X2	T52.8X3	T52.8X4	—	—
CCNU	T45.1X1	T45.1X2	T45.1X3	T45.1X4	T45.1X5	T45.1X6
cellosolve	T52.91	T52.92	T52.93	T52.94	—	—
cellulose	T47.4X1	T47.4X2	T47.4X3	T47.4X4	T47.4X5	T47.4X6
chloride (gas)	T59.891	T59.892	T59.893	T59.894	—	—
chloroformate	T59.3X1	T59.3X2	T59.3X3	T59.3X4	—	—
cyclohexane	T52.8X1	T52.8X2	T52.8X3	T52.8X4	—	—
cyclohexanol	T51.8X1	T51.8X2	T51.8X3	T51.8X4	—	—
cyclohexanone	T52.8X1	T52.8X2	T52.8X3	T52.8X4	—	—
cyclohexyl acetate	T52.8X1	T52.8X2	T52.8X3	T52.8X4	—	—
demeton	T60.0X1	T60.0X2	T60.0X3	T60.0X4	—	—
dihydromorphinone	T40.2X1	T40.2X2	T40.2X3	T40.2X4	T40.2X5	T40.2X6
ergometrine	T48.0X1	T48.0X2	T48.0X3	T48.0X4	T48.0X5	T48.0X6
ergonovine	T48.0X1	T48.0X2	T48.0X3	T48.0X4	T48.0X5	T48.0X6
ethyl ketone	T52.4X1	T52.4X2	T52.4X3	T52.4X4	—	—
glucamine antimonate	T37.8X1	T37.8X2	T37.8X3	T37.8X4	T37.8X5	T37.8X6
hydrazine	T65.891	T65.892	T65.893	T65.894	—	—
iodide	T65.891	T65.892	T65.893	T65.894	—	—
isobutyl ketone	T52.4X1	T52.4X2	T52.4X3	T52.4X4	—	—
isothiocyanate	T60.3X1	T60.3X2	T60.3X3	T60.3X4	—	—
mercaptan	T59.891	T59.892	T59.893	T59.894	—	—

Substance	External Cause (T-Code)					
	Poisoning, Accidental (Unintentional)	Poisoning, Intentional Self-Harm	Poisoning, Assault	Poisoning, Undetermined	Adverse Effect	Underdosing
Methyl *(Continued)*						
morphine NEC	T40.2X1	T40.2X2	T40.2X3	T40.2X4	T40.2X5	T40.2X6
nicotinate	T49.4X1	T49.4X2	T49.4X3	T49.4X4	T49.4X5	T49.4X6
paraben	T49.0X1	T49.0X2	T49.0X3	T49.0X4	T49.0X5	T49.0X6
parafynol	T42.6X1	T42.6X2	T42.6X3	T42.6X4	T42.6X5	T42.6X6
parathion	T60.0X1	T60.0X2	T60.0X3	T60.0X4	—	—
peridol	T43.4X1	T43.4X2	T43.4X3	T43.4X4	T43.4X5	T43.4X6
phenidate	T43.631	T43.632	T43.633	T43.634	T43.635	T43.636
prednisolone	T38.0X1	T38.0X2	T38.0X3	T38.0X4	T38.0X5	T38.0X6
ENT agent	T49.6X1	T49.6X2	T49.6X3	T49.6X4	T49.6X5	T49.6X6
ophthalmic preparation	T49.5X1	T49.5X2	T49.5X3	T49.5X4	T49.5X5	T49.5X6
topical NEC	T49.0X1	T49.0X2	T49.0X3	T49.0X4	T49.0X5	T49.0X6
propylcarbinol	T51.3X1	T51.3X2	T51.3X3	T51.3X4	—	—
rosaniline NEC	T49.0X1	T49.0X2	T49.0X3	T49.0X4	T49.0X5	T49.0X6
salicylate	T49.2X1	T49.2X2	T49.2X3	T49.2X4	T49.2X5	T49.2X6
sulfate (fumes)	T59.891	T59.892	T59.893	T59.894	—	—
liquid	T52.8X1	T52.8X2	T52.8X3	T52.8X4	—	—
sulfonal	T42.6X1	T42.6X2	T42.6X3	T42.6X4	T42.6X5	T42.6X6
testosterone	T38.7X1	T38.7X2	T38.7X3	T38.7X4	T38.7X5	T38.7X6
thiouracil	T38.2X1	T38.2X2	T38.2X3	T38.2X4	T38.2X5	T38.2X6
Methylamphetamine	T43.621	T43.622	T43.623	T43.624	T43.625	T43.626
Methylated spirit	T51.1X1	T51.1X2	T51.1X3	T51.1X4	—	—
Methylatropine nitrate	T44.3X1	T44.3X2	T44.3X3	T44.3X4	T44.3X5	T44.3X6
Methylbenactyzium bromide	T44.3X1	T44.3X2	T44.3X3	T44.3X4	T44.3X5	T44.3X6
Methylbenzethonium chloride	T49.0X1	T49.0X2	T49.0X3	T49.0X4	T49.0X5	T49.0X6
Methylcellulose	T47.4X1	T47.4X2	T47.4X3	T47.4X4	T47.4X5	T47.4X6
laxative	T47.4X1	T47.4X2	T47.4X3	T47.4X4	T47.4X5	T47.4X6
Methylchlorophenoxy-acetic acid	T60.3X1	T60.3X2	T60.3X3	T60.3X4	—	—
Methyldopa	T46.5X1	T46.5X2	T46.5X3	T46.5X4	T46.5X5	T46.5X6
Methyldopate	T46.5X1	T46.5X2	T46.5X3	T46.5X4	T46.5X5	T46.5X6
Methylene						
blue	T50.6X1	T50.6X2	T50.6X3	T50.6X4	T50.6X5	T50.6X6
chloride or dichloride (solvent) NEC	T53.4X1	T53.4X2	T53.4X3	T53.4X4	—	—
Methylenedioxyamphet-amine	T43.621	T43.622	T43.623	T43.624	T43.625	T43.626
Methylenedioxymethamphetamine	T43.641	T43.642	T43.643	T43.644	—	—
Methylergometrine	T48.0X1	T48.0X2	T48.0X3	T48.0X4	T48.0X5	T48.0X6
Methylergonovine	T48.0X1	T48.0X2	T48.0X3	T48.0X4	T48.0X5	T48.0X6
Methylestrenolone	T38.5X1	T38.5X2	T38.5X3	T38.5X4	T38.5X5	T38.5X6
Methylethyl cellulose	T50.991	T50.992	T50.993	T50.994	T50.995	T50.996
Methylhexabital	T42.3X1	T42.3X2	T42.3X3	T42.3X4	T42.3X5	T42.3X6
Methylmorphine	T40.2X1	T40.2X2	T40.2X3	T40.2X4	T40.2X5	T40.2X6

TABLE OF DRUGS AND CHEMICALS

TABLE OF DRUGS AND CHEMICALS

Substance	Poisoning, Accidental (Unintentional)	Poisoning, Intentional Self-Harm	Poisoning, Assault	Poisoning, Undetermined	Adverse Effect	Underdosing
Methylparaben (ophthalmic)	T49.5X1	T49.5X2	T49.5X3	T49.5X4	T49.5X5	T49.5X6
Methylparafynol	T42.6X1	T42.6X2	T42.6X3	T42.6X4	T42.6X5	T42.6X6
Methylpentynol, methylpenthynol	T42.6X1	T42.6X2	T42.6X3	T42.6X4	T42.6X5	T42.6X6
Methylphenidate	T43.631	T43.632	T43.633	T43.634	T43.635	T43.636
Methylphenobarbital	T42.3X1	T42.3X2	T42.3X3	T42.3X4	T42.3X5	T42.3X6
Methylpolysiloxane	T47.1X1	T47.1X2	T47.1X3	T47.1X4	T47.1X5	T47.1X6
Methylprednisolone — see Methyl, prednisolone						
Methylrosaniline	T49.0X1	T49.0X2	T49.0X3	T49.0X4	T49.0X5	T49.0X6
Methylrosanilinium chloride	T49.0X1	T49.0X2	T49.0X3	T49.0X4	T49.0X5	T49.0X6
Methyltestosterone	T38.7X1	T38.7X2	T38.7X3	T38.7X4	T38.7X5	T38.7X6
Methylthionine chloride	T50.6X1	T50.6X2	T50.6X3	T50.6X4	T50.6X5	T50.6X6
Methylthioninium chloride	T50.6X1	T50.6X2	T50.6X3	T50.6X4	T50.6X5	T50.6X6
Methylthiouracil	T38.2X1	T38.2X2	T38.2X3	T38.2X4	T38.2X5	T38.2X6
Methyprylon	T42.6X1	T42.6X2	T42.6X3	T42.6X4	T42.6X5	T42.6X6
Methysergide	T46.5X1	T46.5X2	T46.5X3	T46.5X4	T46.5X5	T46.5X6
Metiamide	T47.1X1	T47.1X2	T47.1X3	T47.1X4	T47.1X5	T47.1X6
Meticillin	T36.0X1	T36.0X2	T36.0X3	T36.0X4	T36.0X5	T36.0X6
Meticrane	T50.2X1	T50.2X2	T50.2X3	T50.2X4	T50.2X5	T50.2X6
Metildigoxin	T46.0X1	T46.0X2	T46.0X3	T46.0X4	T46.0X5	T46.0X6
Metipranolol	T49.5X1	T49.5X2	T49.5X3	T49.5X4	T49.5X5	T49.5X6
Metirosine	T46.5X1	T46.5X2	T46.5X3	T46.5X4	T46.5X5	T46.5X6
Metisazone	T37.5X1	T37.5X2	T37.5X3	T37.5X4	T37.5X5	T37.5X6
Metixene	T44.3X1	T44.3X2	T44.3X3	T44.3X4	T44.3X5	T44.3X6
Metizoline	T48.5X1	T48.5X2	T48.5X3	T48.5X4	T48.5X5	T48.5X6
Metoclopramide	T45.0X1	T45.0X2	T45.0X3	T45.0X4	T45.0X5	T45.0X6
Metofenazate	T43.3X1	T43.3X2	T43.3X3	T43.3X4	T43.3X5	T43.3X6
Metofoline	T39.8X1	T39.8X2	T39.8X3	T39.8X4	T39.8X5	T39.8X6
Metolazone	T50.2X1	T50.2X2	T50.2X3	T50.2X4	T50.2X5	T50.2X6
Metopon	T40.2X1	T40.2X2	T40.2X3	T40.2X4	T40.2X5	T40.2X6
Metoprine	T45.1X1	T45.1X2	T45.1X3	T45.1X4	T45.1X5	T45.1X6
Metoprolol	T44.7X1	T44.7X2	T44.7X3	T44.7X4	T44.7X5	T44.7X6
Metrifonate	T60.0X1	T60.0X2	T60.0X3	T60.0X4	—	—
Metrizamide	T50.8X1	T50.8X2	T50.8X3	T50.8X4	T50.8X5	T50.8X6
Metrizoic acid	T50.8X1	T50.8X2	T50.8X3	T50.8X4	T50.8X5	T50.8X6
Metronidazole	T37.8X1	T37.8X2	T37.8X3	T37.8X4	T37.8X5	T37.8X6
Metycaine	T41.3X1	T41.3X2	T41.3X3	T41.3X4	T41.3X5	T41.3X6
infiltration (subcutaneous)	T41.3X1	T41.3X2	T41.3X3	T41.3X4	T41.3X5	T41.3X6
nerve block (peripheral) (plexus)	T41.3X1	T41.3X2	T41.3X3	T41.3X4	T41.3X5	T41.3X6
topical (surface)	T41.3X1	T41.3X2	T41.3X3	T41.3X4	T41.3X5	T41.3X6
Metyrapone	T50.8X1	T50.8X2	T50.8X3	T50.8X4	T50.8X5	T50.8X6
Mevinphos	T60.0X1	T60.0X2	T60.0X3	T60.0X4	—	—

Substance	Poisoning, Accidental (Unintentional)	Poisoning, Intentional Self-Harm	Poisoning, Assault	Poisoning, Undetermined	Adverse Effect	Underdosing
Mexazolam	T42.4X1	T42.4X2	T42.4X3	T42.4X4	T42.4X5	T42.4X6
Mexenone	T49.3X1	T49.3X2	T49.3X3	T49.3X4	T49.3X5	T49.3X6
Mexiletine	T46.2X1	T46.2X2	T46.2X3	T46.2X4	T46.2X5	T46.2X6
Mezereon	T62.2X1	T62.2X2	T62.2X3	T62.2X4	—	—
berries	T62.1X1	T62.1X2	T62.1X3	T62.1X4	—	—
Mezlocillin	T36.0X1	T36.0X2	T36.0X3	T36.0X4	T36.0X5	T36.0X6
Mianserin	T43.021	T43.022	T43.023	T43.024	T43.025	T43.026
Micatin	T49.0X1	T49.0X2	T49.0X3	T49.0X4	T49.0X5	T49.0X6
Miconazole	T49.0X1	T49.0X2	T49.0X3	T49.0X4	T49.0X5	T49.0X6
Micronomicin	T36.5X1	T36.5X2	T36.5X3	T36.5X4	T36.5X5	T36.5X6
Midazolam	T42.4X1	T42.4X2	T42.4X3	T42.4X4	T42.4X5	T42.4X6
Midecamycin	T36.3X1	T36.3X2	T36.3X3	T36.3X4	T36.3X5	T36.3X6
Mifepristone	T38.6X1	T38.6X2	T38.6X3	T38.6X4	T38.6X5	T38.6X6
Milk of magnesia	T47.1X1	T47.1X2	T47.1X3	T47.1X4	T47.1X5	T47.1X6
Millipede (tropical) (venomous)	T63.411	T63.412	T63.413	T63.414	—	—
Miltown	T43.591	T43.592	T43.593	T43.594	T43.595	T43.596
Milverine	T44.3X1	T44.3X2	T44.3X3	T44.3X4	T44.3X5	T44.3X6
Minaprine	T43.291	T43.292	T43.293	T43.294	T43.295	T43.296
Minaxolone	T41.291	T41.292	T41.293	T41.294	T41.295	T41.296
Mineral						
acids	T54.2X1	T54.2X2	T54.2X3	T54.2X4	—	—
oil (laxative) (medicinal)	T47.4X1	T47.4X2	T47.4X3	T47.4X4	T47.4X5	T47.4X6
emulsion	T47.2X1	T47.2X2	T47.2X3	T47.2X4	T47.2X5	T47.2X6
nonmedicinal	T52.0X1	T52.0X2	T52.0X3	T52.0X4	—	—
topical	T49.3X1	T49.3X2	T49.3X3	T49.3X4	T49.3X5	T49.3X6
salt NEC	T50.3X1	T50.3X2	T50.3X3	T50.3X4	T50.3X5	T50.3X6
spirits	T52.0X1	T52.0X2	T52.0X3	T52.0X4	—	—
Mineralocorticosteroid	T50.0X1	T50.0X2	T50.0X3	T50.0X4	T50.0X5	T50.0X6
Minocycline	T36.4X1	T36.4X2	T36.4X3	T36.4X4	T36.4X5	T36.4X6
Minoxidil	T46.7X1	T46.7X2	T46.7X3	T46.7X4	T46.7X5	T46.7X6
Miokamycin	T36.3X1	T36.3X2	T36.3X3	T36.3X4	T36.3X5	T36.3X6
Miotic drug	T49.5X1	T49.5X2	T49.5X3	T49.5X4	T49.5X5	T49.5X6
Mipafox	T60.0X1	T60.0X2	T60.0X3	T60.0X4	—	—
Mirex	T60.1X1	T60.1X2	T60.1X3	T60.1X4	—	—
Mirtazapine	T43.021	T43.022	T43.023	T43.024	T43.025	T43.026
Misonidazole	T37.3X1	T37.3X2	T37.3X3	T37.3X4	T37.3X5	T37.3X6
Misoprostol	T47.1X1	T47.1X2	T47.1X3	T47.1X4	T47.1X5	T47.1X6
Mithramycin	T45.1X1	T45.1X2	T45.1X3	T45.1X4	T45.1X5	T45.1X6
Mitobronitol	T45.1X1	T45.1X2	T45.1X3	T45.1X4	T45.1X5	T45.1X6
Mitoguazone	T45.1X1	T45.1X2	T45.1X3	T45.1X4	T45.1X5	T45.1X6
Mitolactol	T45.1X1	T45.1X2	T45.1X3	T45.1X4	T45.1X5	T45.1X6
Mitomycin	T45.1X1	T45.1X2	T45.1X3	T45.1X4	T45.1X5	T45.1X6

◀ New   ◀ Revised   deleted Deleted

Substance	Poisoning, Accidental (Unintentional)	Poisoning, Intentional Self-Harm	Poisoning, Assault	Poisoning, Undetermined	Adverse Effect	Underdosing
Mitopodozide	T45.1X1	T45.1X2	T45.1X3	T45.1X4	T45.1X5	T45.1X6
Mitotane	T45.1X1	T45.1X2	T45.1X3	T45.1X4	T45.1X5	T45.1X6
Mitoxantrone	T45.1X1	T45.1X2	T45.1X3	T45.1X4	T45.1X5	T45.1X6
Mivacurium chloride	T48.1X1	T48.1X2	T48.1X3	T48.1X4	T48.1X5	T48.1X6
Miyari bacteria	T47.6X1	T47.6X2	T47.6X3	T47.6X4	T47.6X5	T47.6X6
Moclobemide	T43.1X1	T43.1X2	T43.1X3	T43.1X4	T43.1X5	T43.1X6
Moderil	T46.5X1	T46.5X2	T46.5X3	T46.5X4	T46.5X5	T46.5X6
Mofebutazone	T39.2X1	T39.2X2	T39.2X3	T39.2X4	T39.2X5	T39.2X6
Mogadon — see Nitrazepam						
Molindone	T43.591	T43.592	T43.593	T43.594	T43.595	T43.596
Molsidomine	T46.3X1	T46.3X2	T46.3X3	T46.3X4	T46.3X5	T46.3X6
Mometasone	T49.0X1	T49.0X2	T49.0X3	T49.0X4	T49.0X5	T49.0X6
Monistat	T49.0X1	T49.0X2	T49.0X3	T49.0X4	T49.0X5	T49.0X6
Monkshood	T62.2X1	T62.2X2	T62.2X3	T62.2X4	—	—
Monoamine oxidase inhibitor NEC	T43.1X1	T43.1X2	T43.1X3	T43.1X4	T43.1X5	T43.1X6
hydrazine	T43.1X1	T43.1X2	T43.1X3	T43.1X4	T43.1X5	T43.1X6
Monobenzone	T49.4X1	T49.4X2	T49.4X3	T49.4X4	T49.4X5	T49.4X6
Monochloroacetic acid	T60.3X1	T60.3X2	T60.3X3	T60.3X4	—	—
Monochlorobenzene	T53.7X1	T53.7X2	T53.7X3	T53.7X4		
Monoethanolamine	T46.8X1	T46.8X2	T46.8X3	T46.8X4	T46.8X5	T46.8X6
oleate	T46.8X1	T46.8X2	T46.8X3	T46.8X4	T46.8X5	T46.8X6
Monooctanoin	T50.991	T50.992	T50.993	T50.994	T50.995	T50.996
Monophenylbutazone	T39.2X1	T39.2X2	T39.2X3	T39.2X4	T39.2X5	T39.2X6
Monosodium glutamate	T65.891	T65.892	T65.893	T65.894	—	—
Monosulfiram	T49.0X1	T49.0X2	T49.0X3	T49.0X4	T49.0X5	T49.0X6
Monoxide, carbon — see Carbon, monoxide	T57.91	T57.92	T57.93	T57.94	—	—
Monoxidine hydrochloride	T46.1X1	T46.1X2	T46.1X3	T46.1X4	T46.1X5	T46.1X6
Monuron	T60.3X1	T60.3X2	T60.3X3	T60.3X4	—	—
Moperone	T43.4X1	T43.4X2	T43.4X3	T43.4X4	T43.4X5	T43.4X6
Mopidamol	T45.1X1	T45.1X2	T45.1X3	T45.1X4	T45.1X5	T45.1X6
MOPP (mechlorethamine + vincristine + prednisone + procarbazine)	T45.1X1	T45.1X2	T45.1X3	T45.1X4	T45.1X5	T45.1X6
Morfin	T40.2X1	T40.2X2	T40.2X3	T40.2X4	T40.2X5	T40.2X6
Morinamide	T37.1X1	T37.1X2	T37.1X3	T37.1X4	T37.1X5	T37.1X6
Morning glory seeds	T40.991	T40.992	T40.993	T40.994	—	—
Moroxydine	T37.5X1	T37.5X2	T37.5X3	T37.5X4	T37.5X5	T37.5X6
Morphazinamide	T37.1X1	T37.1X2	T37.1X3	T37.1X4	T37.1X5	T37.1X6
Morphine	T40.2X1	T40.2X2	T40.2X3	T40.2X4	T40.2X5	T40.2X6
antagonist	T50.7X1	T50.7X2	T50.7X3	T50.7X4	T50.7X5	T50.7X6
Morpholinylethylmorphine	T40.2X1	T40.2X2	T40.2X3	T40.2X4	—	—
Morsuximide	T42.2X1	T42.2X2	T42.2X3	T42.2X4	T42.2X5	T42.2X6

Substance	Poisoning, Accidental (Unintentional)	Poisoning, Intentional Self-Harm	Poisoning, Assault	Poisoning, Undetermined	Adverse Effect	Underdosing
Mosapramine	T43.591	T43.592	T43.593	T43.594	T43.595	T43.596
Moth balls — see also Pesticides	T60.2X1	T60.2X2	T60.2X3	T60.2X4	—	—
naphthalene	T60.2X1	T60.2X2	T60.2X3	T60.2X4	—	—
paradichlorobenzene	T60.1X1	T60.1X2	T60.1X3	T60.1X4	—	—
Motor exhaust gas	T58.01	T58.02	T58.03	T58.04		
Mouthwash (antiseptic) (zinc chloride)	T49.6X1	T49.6X2	T49.6X3	T49.6X4	T49.6X5	T49.6X6
Moxastine	T45.0X1	T45.0X2	T45.0X3	T45.0X4	T45.0X5	T45.0X6
Moxaverine	T44.3X1	T44.3X2	T44.3X3	T44.3X4	T44.3X5	T44.3X6
Moxifensine	T43.291	T43.292	T43.293	T43.294	T43.295	T43.296
Moxisylyte	T46.7X1	T46.7X2	T46.7X3	T46.7X4	T46.7X5	T46.7X6
Mucilage, plant	T47.4X1	T47.4X2	T47.4X3	T47.4X4	T47.4X5	T47.4X6
Mucolytic drug	T48.4X1	T48.4X2	T48.4X3	T48.4X4	T48.4X5	T48.4X6
Mucomyst	T48.4X1	T48.4X2	T48.4X3	T48.4X4	T48.4X5	T48.4X6
Mucous membrane agents (external)	T49.91	T49.92	T49.93	T49.94	T49.95	T49.96
specified NEC	T49.8X1	T49.8X2	T49.8X3	T49.8X4	T49.8X5	T49.8X6
Multiple unspecified drugs, medicaments and biological substances	T50.911	T50.912	T50.913	T50.914	T50.915	T50.916
Mumps						
immune globulin (human)	T50.Z11	T50.Z12	T50.Z13	T50.Z14	T50.Z15	T50.Z16
skin test antigen	T50.8X1	T50.8X2	T50.8X3	T50.8X4	T50.8X5	T50.8X6
vaccine	T50.B91	T50.B92	T50.B93	T50.B94	T50.B95	T50.B96
Mumpsvax	T50.B91	T50.B92	T50.B93	T50.B94	T50.B95	T50.B96
Mupirocin	T49.0X1	T49.0X2	T49.0X3	T49.0X4	T49.0X5	T49.0X6
Muriatic acid — see Hydrochloric acid						
Muromonab-CD3	T45.1X1	T45.1X2	T45.1X3	T45.1X4	T45.1X5	T45.1X6
Muscle relaxant — see Relaxant, muscle						
Muscle-action drug NEC	T48.201	T48.202	T48.203	T48.204	T48.205	T48.206
Muscle affecting agents NEC	T48.201	T48.202	T48.203	T48.204	T48.205	T48.206
oxytocic	T48.0X1	T48.0X2	T48.0X3	T48.0X4	T48.0X5	T48.0X6
relaxants	T48.201	T48.202	T48.203	T48.204	T48.205	T48.206
central nervous system	T42.8X1	T42.8X2	T42.8X3	T42.8X4	T42.8X5	T42.8X6
skeletal	T48.1X1	T48.1X2	T48.1X3	T48.1X4	T48.1X5	T48.1X6
smooth	T44.3X1	T44.3X2	T44.3X3	T44.3X4	T44.3X5	T44.3X6
Muscle-tone depressant, central NEC	T42.8X1	T42.8X2	T42.8X3	T42.8X4	T42.8X5	T42.8X6
specified NEC	T42.8X1	T42.8X2	T42.8X3	T42.8X4	T42.8X5	T42.8X6
Mushroom, noxious	T62.0X1	T62.0X2	T62.0X3	T62.0X4	—	—
Mussel, noxious	T61.781	T61.782	T61.783	T61.784	—	—

◀ New ◀ Revised deleted Deleted

TABLE OF DRUGS AND CHEMICALS

Substance	Poisoning, Accidental (Unintentional)	Poisoning, Intentional Self-Harm	Poisoning, Assault	Poisoning, Undetermined	Adverse Effect	Underdosing
Mustard (emetic)	T47.7X1	T47.7X2	T47.7X3	T47.7X4	T47.7X5	T47.7X6
black	T47.7X1	T47.7X2	T47.7X3	T47.7X4	T47.7X5	T47.7X6
gas, not in war	T59.91	T59.92	T59.93	T59.94	—	—
nitrogen	T45.1X1	T45.1X2	T45.1X3	T45.1X4	T45.1X5	T45.1X6
Mustine	T45.1X1	T45.1X2	T45.1X3	T45.1X4	T45.1X5	T45.1X6
M-vac	T45.1X1	T45.1X2	T45.1X3	T45.1X4	T45.1X5	T45.1X6
Mycifradin	T36.5X1	T36.5X2	T36.5X3	T36.5X4	T36.5X5	T36.5X6
topical	T49.0X1	T49.0X2	T49.0X3	T49.0X4	T49.0X5	T49.0X6
Mycitracin	T36.8X1	T36.8X2	T36.8X3	T36.8X4	T36.8X5	T36.8X6
ophthalmic preparation	T49.5X1	T49.5X2	T49.5X3	T49.5X4	T49.5X5	T49.5X6
Mycostatin	T36.7X1	T36.7X2	T36.7X3	T36.7X4	T36.7X5	T36.7X6
topical	T49.0X1	T49.0X2	T49.0X3	T49.0X4	T49.0X5	T49.0X6
Mycotoxins	T64.81	T64.82	T64.83	T64.84	—	—
aflatoxin	T64.01	T64.02	T64.03	T64.04	—	—
specified NEC	T64.81	T64.82	T64.83	T64.84	—	—
Mydriacyl	T44.3X1	T44.3X2	T44.3X3	T44.3X4	T44.3X5	T44.3X6
Mydriatic drug	T49.5X1	T49.5X2	T49.5X3	T49.5X4	T49.5X5	T49.5X6
Myelobromal	T45.1X1	T45.1X2	T45.1X3	T45.1X4	T45.1X5	T45.1X6
Myleran	T45.1X1	T45.1X2	T45.1X3	T45.1X4	T45.1X5	T45.1X6
Myochrysin(e)	T39.2X1	T39.2X2	T39.2X3	T39.2X4	T39.2X5	T39.2X6
Myoneural blocking agents	T48.1X1	T48.1X2	T48.1X3	T48.1X4	T48.1X5	T48.1X6
Myralact	T49.0X1	T49.0X2	T49.0X3	T49.0X4	T49.0X5	T49.0X6
Myristica fragrans	T62.2X1	T62.2X2	T62.2X3	T62.2X4	—	—
Myristicin	T65.891	T65.892	T65.893	T65.894	—	—
Mysoline	T42.3X1	T42.3X2	T42.3X3	T42.3X4	T42.3X5	T42.3X6
N						
Nabilone	T40.711	T40.712	T40.713	T40.714	T40.715	T40.716
Nabumetone	T39.391	T39.392	T39.393	T39.394	T39.395	T39.396
Nadolol	T44.7X1	T44.7X2	T44.7X3	T44.7X4	T44.7X5	T44.7X6
Nafcillin	T36.0X1	T36.0X2	T36.0X3	T36.0X4	T36.0X5	T36.0X6
Nafoxidine	T38.6X1	T38.6X2	T38.6X3	T38.6X4	T38.6X5	T38.6X6
Naftazone	T46.991	T46.992	T46.993	T46.994	T46.995	T46.996
Naftidrofuryl (oxalate)	T46.7X1	T46.7X2	T46.7X3	T46.7X4	T46.7X5	T46.7X6
Naftifine	T49.0X1	T49.0X2	T49.0X3	T49.0X4	T49.0X5	T49.0X6
Nail polish remover	T52.91	T52.92	T52.93	T52.94	—	—
Nalbuphine	T40.491	T40.492	T40.493	T40.494	T40.495	T40.496
Naled	T60.0X1	T60.0X2	T60.0X3	T60.0X4	—	—
Nalidixic acid	T37.8X1	T37.8X2	T37.8X3	T37.8X4	T37.8X5	T37.8X6
Nalorphine	T50.7X1	T50.7X2	T50.7X3	T50.7X4	T50.7X5	T50.7X6
Naloxone	T50.7X1	T50.7X2	T50.7X3	T50.7X4	T50.7X5	T50.7X6
Naltrexone	T50.7X1	T50.7X2	T50.7X3	T50.7X4	T50.7X5	T50.7X6
Namenda	T43.8X1	T43.8X2	T43.8X3	T43.8X4	T43.8X5	T43.8X6

Substance	Poisoning, Accidental (Unintentional)	Poisoning, Intentional Self-Harm	Poisoning, Assault	Poisoning, Undetermined	Adverse Effect	Underdosing
Nandrolone	T38.7X1	T38.7X2	T38.7X3	T38.7X4	T38.7X5	T38.7X6
Naphazoline	T48.5X1	T48.5X2	T48.5X3	T48.5X4	T48.5X5	T48.5X6
Naphtha (painters') (petroleum)	T52.0X1	T52.0X2	T52.0X3	T52.0X4	—	—
solvent	T52.0X1	T52.0X2	T52.0X3	T52.0X4	—	—
vapor	T52.0X1	T52.0X2	T52.0X3	T52.0X4	—	—
Naphthalene (non-chlorinated)	T60.2X1	T60.2X2	T60.2X3	T60.2X4	—	—
chlorinated	T60.1X1	T60.1X2	T60.1X3	T60.1X4	—	—
vapor	T60.1X1	T60.1X2	T60.1X3	T60.1X4	—	—
insecticide or moth repellent	T60.2X1	T60.2X2	T60.2X3	T60.2X4	—	—
chlorinated	T60.1X1	T60.1X2	T60.1X3	T60.1X4	—	—
vapor	T60.2X1	T60.2X2	T60.2X3	T60.2X4	—	—
chlorinated	T60.1X1	T60.1X2	T60.1X3	T60.1X4	—	—
Naphthol	T65.891	T65.892	T65.893	T65.894	—	—
Naphthylamine	T65.891	T65.892	T65.893	T65.894	—	—
Naphthylthiourea (ANTU)	T60.4X1	T60.4X2	T60.4X3	T60.4X4	—	—
Naprosyn — *see Naproxen*						
Naproxen	T39.311	T39.312	T39.313	T39.314	T39.315	T39.316
Narcotic (drug)	T40.601	T40.602	T40.603	T40.604	T40.605	T40.606
analgesic NEC	T40.601	T40.602	T40.603	T40.604	T40.605	T40.606
antagonist	T50.7X1	T50.7X2	T50.7X3	T50.7X4	T50.7X5	T50.7X6
specified NEC	T40.691	T40.692	T40.693	T40.694	T40.695	T40.696
synthetic	T40.491	T40.492	T40.493	T40.494	T40.495	T40.496
Narcotine	T48.3X1	T48.3X2	T48.3X3	T48.3X4	T48.3X5	T48.3X6
Nardil	T43.1X1	T43.1X2	T43.1X3	T43.1X4	T43.1X5	T43.1X6
Nasal drug NEC	T49.6X1	T49.6X2	T49.6X3	T49.6X4	T49.6X5	T49.6X6
Natamycin	T49.0X1	T49.0X2	T49.0X3	T49.0X4	T49.0X5	T49.0X6
Natrium cyanide — *see Cyanide(s)*						
Natural gas	T59.891	T59.892	T59.893	T59.894	—	—
incomplete combustion	T57.91	T57.92	T57.93	T57.94	—	—
Natural						
blood (product)	T45.8X1	T45.8X2	T45.8X3	T45.8X4	T45.8X5	T45.8X6
gas (piped)	T59.891	T59.892	T59.893	T59.894	—	—
incomplete combustion	T58.11	T58.12	T58.13	T58.14	—	—
Nealbarbital	T42.3X1	T42.3X2	T42.3X3	T42.3X4	T42.3X5	T42.3X6
Nectadon	T48.3X1	T48.3X2	T48.3X3	T48.3X4	T48.3X5	T48.3X6
Nedocromil	T48.6X1	T48.6X2	T48.6X3	T48.6X4	T48.6X5	T48.6X6
Nefopam	T39.8X1	T39.8X2	T39.8X3	T39.8X4	T39.8X5	T39.8X6
Nematocyst (sting)	T63.691	T63.692	T63.693	T63.694	—	—
Nembutal	T42.3X1	T42.3X2	T42.3X3	T42.3X4	T42.3X5	T42.3X6
Nemonapride	T43.591	T43.592	T43.593	T43.594	T43.595	T43.596
Neoarsphenamine	T37.8X1	T37.8X2	T37.8X3	T37.8X4	T37.8X5	T37.8X6

◀ New ◀ Revised ~~deleted~~ Deleted

Substance	Poisoning, Accidental (Unintentional)	Poisoning, Intentional Self-Harm	Poisoning, Assault	Poisoning, Undetermined	Adverse Effect	Underdosing
Neocinchophen	T50.4X1	T50.4X2	T50.4X3	T50.4X4	T50.4X5	T50.4X6
Neomycin (derivatives)	T36.5X1	T36.5X2	T36.5X3	T36.5X4	T36.5X5	T36.5X6
with						
bacitracin	T49.0X1	T49.0X2	T49.0X3	T49.0X4	T49.0X5	T49.0X6
neostigmine	T44.0X1	T44.0X2	T44.0X3	T44.0X4	T44.0X5	T44.0X6
ENT agent	T49.6X1	T49.6X2	T49.6X3	T49.6X4	T49.6X5	T49.6X6
ophthalmic preparation	T49.5X1	T49.5X2	T49.5X3	T49.5X4	T49.5X5	T49.5X6
topical NEC	T49.0X1	T49.0X2	T49.0X3	T49.0X4	T49.0X5	T49.0X6
Neonal	T42.3X1	T42.3X2	T42.3X3	T42.3X4	T42.3X5	T42.3X6
Neoprontosil	T37.0X1	T37.0X2	T37.0X3	T37.0X4	T37.0X5	T37.0X6
Neosalvarsan	T37.8X1	T37.8X2	T37.8X3	T37.8X4	T37.8X5	T37.8X6
Neosilversalvarsan	T37.8X1	T37.8X2	T37.8X3	T37.8X4	T37.8X5	T37.8X6
Neosporin	T36.8X1	T36.8X2	T36.8X3	T36.8X4	T36.8X5	T36.8X6
ENT agent	T49.6X1	T49.6X2	T49.6X3	T49.6X4	T49.6X5	T49.6X6
opthalmic preparation	T49.5X1	T49.5X2	T49.5X3	T49.5X4	T49.5X5	T49.5X6
topical NEC	T49.0X1	T49.0X2	T49.0X3	T49.0X4	T49.0X5	T49.0X6
Neostigmine bromide	T44.0X1	T44.0X2	T44.0X3	T44.0X4	T44.0X5	T44.0X6
Neraval	T42.3X1	T42.3X2	T42.3X3	T42.3X4	T42.3X5	T42.3X6
Neravan	T42.3X1	T42.3X2	T42.3X3	T42.3X4	T42.3X5	T42.3X6
Nerium oleander	T62.2X1	T62.2X2	T62.2X3	T62.2X4	—	—
Nerve gas, not in war	T59.91	T59.92	T59.93	T59.94	—	—
Nesacaine	T41.3X1	T41.3X2	T41.3X3	T41.3X4	T41.3X5	T41.3X6
infiltration (subcutaneous)	T41.3X1	T41.3X2	T41.3X3	T41.3X4	T41.3X5	T41.3X6
nerve block (peripheral) (plexus)	T41.3X1	T41.3X2	T41.3X3	T41.3X4	T41.3X5	T41.3X6
Netilmicin	T36.5X1	T36.5X2	T36.5X3	T36.5X4	T36.5X5	T36.5X6
Neurobarb	T42.3X1	T42.3X2	T42.3X3	T42.3X4	T42.3X5	T42.3X6
Neuroleptic drug NEC	T43.501	T43.502	T43.503	T43.504	T43.505	T43.506
Neuromuscular blocking drug	T48.1X1	T48.1X2	T48.1X3	T48.1X4	T48.1X5	T48.1X6
Neutral insulin injection	T38.3X1	T38.3X2	T38.3X3	T38.3X4	T38.3X5	T38.3X6
Neutral spirits	T51.0X1	T51.0X2	T51.0X3	T51.0X4	—	—
beverage	T51.0X1	T51.0X2	T51.0X3	T51.0X4	—	—
Niacin	T46.7X1	T46.7X2	T46.7X3	T46.7X4	T46.7X5	T46.7X6
Niacinamide	T45.2X1	T45.2X2	T45.2X3	T45.2X4	T45.2X5	T45.2X6
Nialamide	T43.1X1	T43.1X2	T43.1X3	T43.1X4	T43.1X5	T43.1X6
Niaprazine	T42.6X1	T42.6X2	T42.6X3	T42.6X4	T42.6X5	T42.6X6
Nicametate	T46.7X1	T46.7X2	T46.7X3	T46.7X4	T46.7X5	T46.7X6
Nicardipine	T46.1X1	T46.1X2	T46.1X3	T46.1X4	T46.1X5	T46.1X6
Nicergoline	T46.7X1	T46.7X2	T46.7X3	T46.7X4	T46.7X5	T46.7X6
Nickel (carbonyl) (tetra-carbonyl) (fumes) (vapor)	T56.891	T56.892	T56.893	T56.894	—	—

Substance	Poisoning, Accidental (Unintentional)	Poisoning, Intentional Self-Harm	Poisoning, Assault	Poisoning, Undetermined	Adverse Effect	Underdosing
Nickelocene	T56.891	T56.892	T56.893	T56.894	—	—
Niclosamide	T37.4X1	T37.4X2	T37.4X3	T37.4X4	T37.4X5	T37.4X6
Nicofuranose	T46.7X1	T46.7X2	T46.7X3	T46.7X4	T46.7X5	T46.7X6
Nicomorphine	T40.2X1	T40.2X2	T40.2X3	T40.2X4	—	—
Nicorandil	T46.3X1	T46.3X2	T46.3X3	T46.3X4	T46.3X5	T46.3X6
Nicotiana (plant)	T62.2X1	T62.2X2	T62.2X3	T62.2X4	—	—
Nicotinamide	T45.2X1	T45.2X2	T45.2X3	T45.2X4	T45.2X5	T45.2X6
Nicotine (insecticide) (spray) (sulfate) NEC	T60.2X1	T60.2X2	T60.2X3	T60.2X4	—	—
from tobacco	T65.291	T65.292	T65.293	T65.294	—	—
cigarettes	T65.221	T65.222	T65.223	T65.224	—	—
not insecticide	T65.291	T65.292	T65.293	T65.294		—
Nicotinic acid	T46.7X1	T46.7X2	T46.7X3	T46.7X4	T46.7X5	T46.7X6
Nicotinyl alcohol	T46.7X1	T46.7X2	T46.7X3	T46.7X4	T46.7X5	T46.7X6
Nicoumalone	T45.511	T45.512	T45.513	T45.514	T45.515	T45.516
Nifedipine	T46.1X1	T46.1X2	T46.1X3	T46.1X4	T46.1X5	T46.1X6
Nifenazone	T39.2X1	T39.2X2	T39.2X3	T39.2X4	T39.2X5	T39.2X6
Nifuraldezone	T37.91	T37.92	T37.93	T37.94	T37.95	T37.96
Nifuratel	T37.8X1	T37.8X2	T37.8X3	T37.8X4	T37.8X5	T37.8X6
Nifurtimox	T37.3X1	T37.3X2	T37.3X3	T37.3X4	T37.3X5	T37.3X6
Nifurtoinol	T37.8X1	T37.8X2	T37.8X3	T37.8X4	T37.8X5	T37.8X6
Nightshade, deadly (solanum) — see also Belladonna	T62.2X1	T62.2X2	T62.2X3	T62.2X4	—	—
berry	T62.1X1	T62.1X2	T62.1X3	T62.1X4	—	—
Nikethamide	T50.7X1	T50.7X2	T50.7X3	T50.7X4	T50.7X5	T50.7X6
Nilstat	T36.7X1	T36.7X2	T36.7X3	T36.7X4	T36.7X5	T36.7X6
topical	T49.0X1	T49.0X2	T49.0X3	T49.0X4	T49.0X5	T49.0X6
Nilutamide	T38.6X1	T38.6X2	T38.6X3	T38.6X4	T38.6X5	T38.6X6
Nimesulide	T39.391	T39.392	T39.393	T39.394	T39.395	T39.396
Nimetazepam	T42.4X1	T42.4X2	T42.4X3	T42.4X4	T42.4X5	T42.4X6
Nimodipine	T46.1X1	T46.1X2	T46.1X3	T46.1X4	T46.1X5	T46.1X6
Nimorazole	T37.3X1	T37.3X2	T37.3X3	T37.3X4	T37.3X5	T37.3X6
Nimustine	T45.1X1	T45.1X2	T45.1X3	T45.1X4	T45.1X5	T45.1X6
Niridazole	T37.4X1	T37.4X2	T37.4X3	T37.4X4	T37.4X5	T37.4X6
Nisentil	T40.2X1	T40.2X2	T40.2X3	T40.2X4	T40.2X5	T40.2X6
Nisoldipine	T46.1X1	T46.1X2	T46.1X3	T46.1X4	T46.1X5	T46.1X6
Nitramine	T65.3X1	T65.3X2	T65.3X3	T65.3X4	—	—
Nitrate, organic	T46.3X1	T46.3X2	T46.3X3	T46.3X4	T46.3X5	T46.3X6
Nitrazepam	T42.4X1	T42.4X2	T42.4X3	T42.4X4	T42.4X5	T42.4X6
Nitrefazole	T50.6X1	T50.6X2	T50.6X3	T50.6X4	T50.6X5	T50.6X6
Nitrendipine	T46.1X1	T46.1X2	T46.1X3	T46.1X4	T46.1X5	T46.1X6

◀ New ◀◀ Revised ~~deleted~~ Deleted

	External Cause (T-Code)					
Substance	Poisoning, Accidental (Unintentional)	Poisoning, Intentional Self-Harm	Poisoning, Assault	Poisoning, Undetermined	Adverse Effect	Underdosing
Nitric						
acid (liquid)	T54.2X1	T54.2X2	T54.2X3	T54.2X4	—	—
vapor	T59.891	T59.892	T59.893	T59.894	—	—
oxide (gas)	T59.0X1	T59.0X2	T59.0X3	T59.0X4	—	—
Nitrimidazine	T37.3X1	T37.3X2	T37.3X3	T37.3X4	T37.3X5	T37.3X6
Nitrite, amyl (medicinal) (vapor)	T46.3X1	T46.3X2	T46.3X3	T46.3X4	T46.3X5	T46.3X6
Nitroaniline	T65.3X1	T65.3X2	T65.3X3	T65.3X4	—	—
vapor	T59.891	T59.892	T59.893	T59.894	—	—
Nitrobenzene, nitrobenzol	T65.3X1	T65.3X2	T65.3X3	T65.3X4	—	—
vapor	T65.3X1	T65.3X2	T65.3X3	T65.3X4	—	—
Nitrocellulose	T65.891	T65.892	T65.893	T65.894	—	—
lacquer	T65.891	T65.892	T65.893	T65.894	—	—
Nitrodiphenyl	T65.3X1	T65.3X2	T65.3X3	T65.3X4	—	—
Nitrofural	T49.0X1	T49.0X2	T49.0X3	T49.0X4	T49.0X5	T49.0X6
Nitrofurantoin	T37.8X1	T37.8X2	T37.8X3	T37.8X4	T37.8X5	T37.8X6
Nitrofurazone	T49.0X1	T49.0X2	T49.0X3	T49.0X4	T49.0X5	T49.0X6
Nitrogen	T59.0X1	T59.0X2	T59.0X3	T59.0X4	—	—
mustard	T45.1X1	T45.1X2	T45.1X3	T45.1X4	T45.1X5	T45.1X6
Nitroglycerin, nitro-glycerol (medicinal)	T46.3X1	T46.3X2	T46.3X3	T46.3X4	T46.3X5	T46.3X6
nonmedicinal	T65.5X1	T65.5X2	T65.5X3	T65.5X4	—	—
fumes	T65.5X1	T65.5X2	T65.5X3	T65.5X4	—	—
Nitroglycol	T52.3X1	T52.3X2	T52.3X3	T52.3X4	—	—
Nitrohydrochloric acid	T54.2X1	T54.2X2	T54.2X3	T54.2X4	—	—
Nitromersol	T49.0X1	T49.0X2	T49.0X3	T49.0X4	T49.0X5	T49.0X6
Nitronaphthalene	T65.891	T65.892	T65.893	T65.894	—	—
Nitrophenol	T54.0X1	T54.0X2	T54.0X3	T54.0X4	—	—
Nitropropane	T52.8X1	T52.8X2	T52.8X3	T52.8X4	—	—
Nitroprusside	T46.5X1	T46.5X2	T46.5X3	T46.5X4	T46.5X5	T46.5X6
Nitrosodimethylamine	T65.3X1	T65.3X2	T65.3X3	T65.3X4	—	—
Nitrothiazol	T37.4X1	T37.4X2	T37.4X3	T37.4X4	T37.4X5	T37.4X6
Nitrotoluene, nitrotoluol	T65.3X1	T65.3X2	T65.3X3	T65.3X4	—	—
vapor	T65.3X1	T65.3X2	T65.3X3	T65.3X4	—	—
Nitrous						
acid (liquid)	T54.2X1	T54.2X2	T54.2X3	T54.2X4	—	—
fumes	T59.891	T59.892	T59.893	T59.894	—	—
ether spirit	T46.3X1	T46.3X2	T46.3X3	T46.3X4	T46.3X5	T46.3X6
oxide	T41.0X1	T41.0X2	T41.0X3	T41.0X4	T41.0X5	T41.0X6
Nitroxoline	T37.8X1	T37.8X2	T37.8X3	T37.8X4	T37.8X5	T37.8X6
Nitrozone	T49.0X1	T49.0X2	T49.0X3	T49.0X4	T49.0X5	T49.0X6
Nizatidine	T47.0X1	T47.0X2		T47.0X4	T47.0X5	T47.0X6

	External Cause (T-Code)					
Substance	Poisoning, Accidental (Unintentional)	Poisoning, Intentional Self-Harm	Poisoning, Assault	Poisoning, Undetermined	Adverse Effect	Underdosing
Nizofenone	T43.8X1	T43.8X2	T43.8X3	T43.8X4	T43.8X5	T43.8X6
Noctec	T42.6X1	T42.6X2	T42.6X3	T42.6X4	T42.6X5	T42.6X6
Noludar	T42.6X1	T42.6X2	T42.6X3	T42.6X4	T42.6X5	T42.6X6
Noptil	T42.3X1	T42.3X2	T42.3X3	T42.3X4	T42.3X5	T42.3X6
Nomegestrol	T38.5X1	T38.5X2	T38.5X3	T38.5X4	T38.5X5	T38.5X6
Nomifensine	T43.291	T43.292	T43.293	T43.294	T43.295	T43.296
Nonoxinol	T49.8X1	T49.8X2	T49.8X3	T49.8X4	T49.8X5	T49.8X6
Nonylphenoxy (polyethoxy-ethanol)	T49.8X1	T49.8X2	T49.8X3	T49.8X4	T49.8X5	T49.8X6
Noptil	T42.3X1	T42.3X2	T42.3X3	T42.3X4	T42.3X5	T42.3X6
Noradrenaline	T44.4X1	T44.4X2	T44.4X3	T44.4X4	T44.4X5	T44.4X6
Noramidopyrine	T39.2X1	T39.2X2	T39.2X3	T39.2X4	T39.2X5	T39.2X6
methanesulfonate sodium	T39.2X1	T39.2X2	T39.2X3	T39.2X4	T39.2X5	T39.2X6
Norbormide	T60.4X1	T60.4X2	T60.4X3	T60.4X4	—	—
Nordazepam	T42.4X1	T42.4X2	T42.4X3	T42.4X4	T42.4X5	T42.4X6
Norepinephrine	T44.4X1	T44.4X2	T44.4X3	T44.4X4	T44.4X5	T44.4X6
Norethandrolone	T38.7X1	T38.7X2	T38.7X3	T38.7X4	T38.7X5	T38.7X6
Norethindrone	T38.4X1	T38.4X2	T38.4X3	T38.4X4	T38.4X5	T38.4X6
Norethisterone (acetate) (enantate)	T38.4X1	T38.4X2	T38.4X3	T38.4X4	T38.4X5	T38.4X6
with ethinylestradiol	T38.5X1	T38.5X2	T38.5X3	T38.5X4	T38.5X5	T38.5X6
Noretynodrel	T38.5X1	T38.5X2	T38.5X3	T38.5X4	T38.5X5	T38.5X6
Norfenefrine	T44.4X1	T44.4X2	T44.4X3	T44.4X4	T44.4X5	T44.4X6
Norfloxacin	T36.8X1	T36.8X2	T36.8X3	T36.8X4	T36.8X5	T36.8X6
Norgestrel	T38.4X1	T38.4X2	T38.4X3	T38.4X4	T38.4X5	T38.4X6
Norgestrienone	T38.4X1	T38.4X2	T38.4X3	T38.4X4	T38.4X5	T38.4X6
Norlestrin	T38.4X1	T38.4X2	T38.4X3	T38.4X4	T38.4X5	T38.4X6
Norlutin	T38.4X1	T38.4X2	T38.4X3	T38.4X4	T38.4X5	T38.4X6
Normal serum albumin (human), salt-poor	T45.8X1	T45.8X2	T45.8X3	T45.8X4	T45.8X5	T45.8X6
Normethandrone	T38.5X1	T38.5X2	T38.5X3	T38.5X4	T38.5X5	T38.5X6
Normison — see Benzodiazepines						
Normorphine	T40.2X1	T40.2X2	T40.2X3	T40.2X4	—	—
Norpseudoephedrine	T50.5X1	T50.5X2	T50.5X3	T50.5X4	T50.5X5	T50.5X6
Nortestosterone (furanpropionate)	T38.7X1	T38.7X2	T38.7X3	T38.7X4	T38.7X5	T38.7X6
Nortriptyline	T43.011	T43.012	T43.013	T43.014	T43.015	T43.016
Noscapine	T48.3X1	T48.3X2	T48.3X3	T48.3X4	T48.3X5	T48.3X6
Nose preparations	T49.6X1	T49.6X2	T49.6X3	T49.6X4	T49.6X5	T49.6X6
Novobiocin	T36.5X1	T36.5X2	T36.5X3	T36.5X4	T36.5X5	T36.5X6
Novocain (infiltration) (topical)	T41.3X1	T41.3X2	T41.3X3	T41.3X4	T41.3X5	T41.3X6
nerve block (peripheral) (plexus)	T41.3X1	T41.3X2	T41.3X3	T41.3X4	T41.3X5	T41.3X6
spinal	T41.3X1	T41.3X2	T41.3X3	T41.3X4	T41.3X5	T41.3X6

◀ New   ◀ Revised   ~~deleted~~ Deleted

Substance	Poisoning, Accidental (Unintentional)	Poisoning, Intentional Self-Harm	Poisoning, Assault	Poisoning, Undetermined	Adverse Effect	Underdosing
Noxious foodstuff	T62.91	T62.92	T62.93	T62.94	—	—
specified NEC	T62.8X1	T62.8X2	T62.8X3	T62.8X4	—	—
Noxiptiline	T43.011	T43.012	T43.013	T43.014	T43.015	T43.016
Noxytiolin	T49.0X1	T49.0X2	T49.0X3	T49.0X4	T49.0X5	T49.0X6
NPH Iletin (insulin)	T38.3X1	T38.3X2	T38.3X3	T38.3X4	T38.3X5	T38.3X6
Numorphan	T40.2X1	T40.2X2	T40.2X3	T40.2X4	T40.2X5	T40.2X6
Nunol	T42.3X1	T42.3X2	T42.3X3	T42.3X4	T42.3X5	T42.3X6
Nupercaine (spinal anesthetic)	T41.3X1	T41.3X2	T41.3X3	T41.3X4	T41.3X5	T41.3X6
topical (surface)	T41.3X1	T41.3X2	T41.3X3	T41.3X4	T41.3X5	T41.3X6
Nutmeg oil (liniment)	T49.3X1	T49.3X2	T49.3X3	T49.3X4	T49.3X5	I49.3X6
Nutritional supplement	T50.901	T50.902	T50.903	T50.904	T50.905	T50.906
Nux vomica	T65.1X1	T65.1X2	T65.1X3	T65.1X4	—	—
Nydrazid	T37.1X1	T37.1X2	T37.1X3	T37.1X4	T37.1X5	T37.1X6
Nylidrin	T46.7X1	T46.7X2	T46.7X3	T46.7X4	T46.7X5	T46.7X6
Nystatin	T36.7X1	T36.7X2	T36.7X3	T36.7X4	T36.7X5	T36.7X6
topical	T49.0X1	T49.0X2	T49.0X3	T49.0X4	T49.0X5	T49.0X6
Nytol	T45.0X1	T45.0X2	T45.0X3	T45.0X4	T45.0X5	T45.0X6

O

Substance	Poisoning, Accidental (Unintentional)	Poisoning, Intentional Self-Harm	Poisoning, Assault	Poisoning, Undetermined	Adverse Effect	Underdosing
Obidoxime chloride	T50.6X1	T50.6X2	T50.6X3	T50.6X4	T50.6X5	T50.6X6
Octafonium (chloride)	T49.3X1	T49.3X2	T49.3X3	T49.3X4	T49.3X5	T49.3X6
Octamethyl pyrophosphoramide	T60.0X1	T60.0X2	T60.0X3	T60.0X4	—	—
Octanoin	T50.991	T50.992	T50.993	T50.994	T50.995	T50.996
Octatropine methylbromide	T44.3X1	T44.3X2	T44.3X3	T44.3X4	T44.3X5	T44.3X6
Octotiamine	T45.2X1	T45.2X2	T45.2X3	T45.2X4	T45.2X5	T45.2X6
Octoxinol (9)	T49.8X1	T49.8X2	T49.8X3	T49.8X4	T49.8X5	T49.8X6
Octreotide	T38.991	T38.992	T38.993	T38.994	T38.995	T38.996
Octyl nitrite	T46.3X1	T46.3X2	T46.3X3	T46.3X4	T46.3X5	T46.3X6
Oestradiol	T38.5X1	T38.5X2	T38.5X3	T38.5X4	T38.5X5	T38.5X6
Oestriol	T38.5X1	T38.5X2	T38.5X3	T38.5X4	T38.5X5	T38.5X6
Oestrogen	T38.5X1	T38.5X2	T38.5X3	T38.5X4	T38.5X5	T38.5X6
Oestrone	T38.5X1	T38.5X2	T38.5X3	T38.5X4	T38.5X5	T38.5X6
Ofloxacin	T36.8X1	T36.8X2	T36.8X3	T36.8X4	T36.8X5	T36.8X6
Oil (of)	T65.891	T65.892	T65.893	T65.894	—	—
bitter almond	T62.8X1	T62.8X2	T62.8X3	T62.8X4	—	—
cloves	T49.7X1	T49.7X2	T49.7X3	T49.7X4	T49.7X5	T49.7X6
colors	T65.6X1	T65.6X2	T65.6X3	T65.6X4	—	—
fumes	T59.891	T59.892	T59.893	T59.894	—	—
lubricating	T52.0X1	T52.0X2	T52.0X3	T52.0X4	—	—
Niobe	T52.8X1	T52.8X2	T52.8X3	T52.8X4	—	—

Substance	Poisoning, Accidental (Unintentional)	Poisoning, Intentional Self-Harm	Poisoning, Assault	Poisoning, Undetermined	Adverse Effect	Underdosing
Oil (of) (Continued)						
vitriol (liquid)	T54.2X1	T54.2X2	T54.2X3	T54.2X4	—	—
fumes	T54.2X1	T54.2X2	T54.2X3	T54.2X4	—	—
wintergreen (bitter) NEC	T49.3X1	T49.3X2	T49.3X3	T49.3X4	T49.3X5	T49.3X6
Oily preparation (for skin)	T49.3X1	T49.3X2	T49.3X3	T49.3X4	T49.3X5	T49.3X6
Ointment NEC	T49.3X1	T49.3X2	T49.3X3	T49.3X4	T49.3X5	T49.3X6
Olanzapine	T43.591	T43.592	T43.593	T43.594	T43.595	T43.596
Oleander	T62.2X1	T62.2X2	T62.2X3	T62.2X4	—	—
Oleandomycin	T36.3X1	T36.3X2	T36.3X3	T36.3X4	T36.3X5	T36.3X6
Oleandrin	T46.0X1	T46.0X2	T46.0X3	T46.0X4	T46.0X5	T46.0X6
Oleic acid	T46.6X1	T46.6X2	T46.6X3	T46.6X4	T46.6X5	T46.6X6
Oleovitamin A	T45.2X1	T45.2X2	T45.2X3	T45.2X4	T45.2X5	T45.2X6
Oleum ricini	T47.2X1	T47.2X2	T47.2X3	T47.2X4	T47.2X5	T47.2X6
Olive oil (medicinal) NEC	T47.4X1	T47.4X2	T47.4X3	T47.4X4	T47.4X5	T47.4X6
Olivomycin	T45.1X1	T45.1X2	T45.1X3	T45.1X4	T45.1X5	T45.1X6
Olsalazine	T47.8X1	T47.8X2	T47.8X3	T47.8X4	T47.8X5	T47.8X6
Omeprazole	T47.1X1	T47.1X2	T47.1X3	T47.1X4	T47.1X5	T47.1X6
OMPA	T60.0X1	T60.0X2	T60.0X3	I60.0X4	—	—
Ondansetron	T45.0X1	T45.0X2	T45.0X3	T45.0X4	T45.0X5	T45.0X6
Oncovin	T45.1X1	T45.1X2	T45.1X3	T45.1X4	T45.1X5	T45.1X6
Ophthaine	T41.3X1	T41.3X2	T41.3X3	T41.3X4	T41.3X5	T41.3X6
Ophthetic	T41.3X1	T41.3X2	T41.3X3	T41.3X4	T41.3X5	T41.3X6
Opiate NEC	T40.601	T40.602	T40.603	T40.604	T40.605	T40.606
antagonists	T50.7X1	T50.7X2	T50.7X3	T50.7X4	T50.7X5	T50.7X6
Opioid NEC	T40.2X1	T40.2X2	T40.2X3	T40.2X4	T40.2X5	T40.2X6
Opipramol	T43.011	T43.012	T43.013	T43.014	T43.015	T43.016
Opium alkaloids (total)	T40.0X1	T40.0X2	T40.0X3	T40.0X4	T40.0X5	T40.0X6
standardized powdered	T40.0X1	T40.0X2	T40.0X3	T40.0X4	T40.0X5	T40.0X6
tincture (camphorated)	T40.0X1	T40.0X2	T40.0X3	T40.0X4	T40.0X5	T40.0X6
Oracon	T38.4X1	T38.4X2	T38.4X3	T38.4X4	T38.4X5	T38.4X6
Oragrafin	T50.8X1	T50.8X2	T50.8X3	T50.8X4	T50.8X5	T50.8X6
Oral contraceptives	T38.4X1	I38.4X2	T38.4X3	T38.4X4	T38.4X5	T38.4X6
Oral rehydration salts	T50.3X1	T50.3X2	T50.3X3	T50.3X4	T50.3X5	T50.3X6
Orazamide	T50.991	T50.992	T50.993	T50.994	T50.995	T50.996
Orciprenaline	T48.291	T48.292	T48.293	T48.294	T48.295	T48.296
Organidin	T48.4X1	T48.4X2	T48.4X3	T48.4X4	T48.4X5	T48.4X6
Organonitrate NEC	T46.3X1	T46.3X2	T46.3X3	T46.3X4	T46.3X5	T46.3X6
Organophosphates	T60.0X1	T60.0X2	T60.0X3	T60.0X4	—	—
Orimune	T50.B91	T50.B92	T50.B93	T50.B94	T50.B95	T50.B96
Orinase	T38.3X1	T38.3X2	T38.3X3	T38.3X4	T38.3X5	T38.3X6
Ormeloxifene	T38.6X1	T38.6X2	T38.6X3	T38.6X4	T38.6X5	T38.6X6

◀ New ◀ Revised ~~deleted~~ Deleted

TABLE OF DRUGS AND CHEMICALS

Substance	External Cause (T-Code)					
	Poisoning, Accidental (Unintentional)	Poisoning, Intentional Self-Harm	Poisoning, Assault	Poisoning, Undetermined	Adverse Effect	Underdosing
Ornidazole	T37.3X1	T37.3X2	T37.3X3	T37.3X4	T37.3X5	T37.3X6
Ornithine aspartate	T50.991	T50.992	T50.993	T50.994	T50.995	T50.996
Ornoprostil	T47.1X1	T47.1X2	T47.1X3	T47.1X4	T47.1X5	T47.1X6
Orphenadrine (hydrochloride)	T42.8X1	T42.8X2	T42.8X3	T42.8X4	T42.8X5	T42.8X6
Ortal (sodium)	T42.3X1	T42.3X2	T42.3X3	T42.3X4	T42.3X5	T42.3X6
Orthoboric acid	T49.0X1	T49.0X2	T49.0X3	T49.0X4	T49.0X5	T49.0X6
ENT agent	T49.6X1	T49.6X2	T49.6X3	T49.6X4	T49.6X5	T49.6X6
ophthalmic preparation	T49.5X1	T49.5X2	T49.5X3	T49.5X4	T49.5X5	T49.5X6
Orthocaine	T41.3X1	T41.3X2	T41.3X3	T41.3X4	T41.3X5	T41.3X6
Orthodichlorobenzene	T53.7X1	T53.7X2	T53.7X3	T53.7X4	—	—
Ortho-Novum	T38.4X1	T38.4X2	T38.4X3	T38.4X4	T38.4X5	T38.4X6
Orthotolidine (reagent)	T54.2X1	T54.2X2	T54.2X3	T54.2X4	—	—
Osmic acid (liquid)	T54.2X1	T54.2X2	T54.2X3	T54.2X4	—	—
fumes	T54.2X1	T54.2X2	T54.2X3	T54.2X4	—	—
Osmotic diuretics	T50.2X1	T50.2X2	T50.2X3	T50.2X4	T50.2X5	T50.2X6
Otilonium bromide	T44.3X1	T44.3X2	T44.3X3	T44.3X4	T44.3X5	T44.3X6
Otorhinolaryngological drug NEC	T49.6X1	T49.6X2	T49.6X3	T49.6X4	T49.6X5	T49.6X6
Ouabain(e)	T46.0X1	T46.0X2	T46.0X3	T46.0X4	T46.0X5	T46.0X6
Ovarian						
hormone	T38.5X1	T38.5X2	T38.5X3	T38.5X4	T38.5X5	T38.5X6
stimulant	T38.5X1	T38.5X2	T38.5X3	T38.5X4	T38.5X5	T38.5X6
Ovral	T38.4X1	T38.4X2	T38.4X3	T38.4X4	T38.4X5	T38.4X6
Ovulen	T38.4X1	T38.4X2	T38.4X3	T38.4X4	T38.4X5	T38.4X6
Oxacillin	T36.0X1	T36.0X2	T36.0X3	T36.0X4	T36.0X5	T36.0X6
Oxalic acid	T54.2X1	T54.2X2	T54.2X3	T54.2X4	—	—
ammonium salt	T50.991	T50.992	T50.993	T50.994	T50.995	T50.996
Oxamniquine	T37.4X1	T37.4X2	T37.4X3	T37.4X4	T37.4X5	T37.4X6
Oxanamide	T43.591	T43.592	T43.593	T43.594	T43.595	T43.596
Oxandrolone	T38.7X1	T38.7X2	T38.7X3	T38.7X4	T38.7X5	T38.7X6
Oxantel	T37.4X1	T37.4X2	T37.4X3	T37.4X4	T37.4X5	T37.4X6
Oxapium iodide	T44.3X1	T44.3X2	T44.3X3	T44.3X4	T44.3X5	T44.3X6
Oxaprotiline	T43.021	T43.022	T43.023	T43.024	T43.025	T43.026
Oxaprozin	T39.311	T39.312	T39.313	T39.314	T39.315	T39.316
Oxatomide	T45.0X1	T45.0X2	T45.0X3	T45.0X4	T45.0X5	T45.0X6
Oxazepam	T42.4X1	T42.4X2	T42.4X3	T42.4X4	T42.4X5	T42.4X6
Oxazimedrine	T50.5X1	T50.5X2	T50.5X3	T50.5X4	T50.5X5	T50.5X6
Oxazolam	T42.4X1	T42.4X2	T42.4X3	T42.4X4	T42.4X5	T42.4X6
Oxazolidine derivatives	T42.2X1	T42.2X2	T42.2X3	T42.2X4	T42.2X5	T42.2X6
Oxazolidinedione (derivative)	T42.2X1	T42.2X2	T42.2X3	T42.2X4	T42.2X5	T42.2X6
Ox bile extract	T47.5X1	T47.5X2	T47.5X3	T47.5X4	T47.5X5	T47.5X6
Oxcarbazepine	T42.1X1	T42.1X2	T42.1X3	T42.1X4	T42.1X5	T42.1X6
Oxedrine	T44.4X1	T44.4X2	T44.4X3	T44.4X4	T44.4X5	T44.4X6

Substance	External Cause (T-Code)					
	Poisoning, Accidental (Unintentional)	Poisoning, Intentional Self-Harm	Poisoning, Assault	Poisoning, Undetermined	Adverse Effect	Underdosing
Oxeladin (citrate)	T48.3X1	T48.3X2	T48.3X3	T48.3X4	T48.3X5	T48.3X6
Oxendolone	T38.5X1	T38.5X2	T38.5X3	T38.5X4	T38.5X5	T38.5X6
Oxetacaine	T41.3X1	T41.3X2	T41.3X3	T41.3X4	T41.3X5	T41.3X6
Oxethazine	T41.3X1	T41.3X2	T41.3X3	T41.3X4	T41.3X5	T41.3X6
Oxetorone	T39.8X1	T39.8X2	T39.8X3	T39.8X4	T39.8X5	T39.8X6
Oxiconazole	T49.0X1	T49.0X2	T49.0X3	T49.0X4	T49.0X5	T49.0X6
Oxidizing agent NEC	T54.91	T54.92	T54.93	T54.94	—	—
Oxipurinol	T50.4X1	T50.4X2	T50.4X3	T50.4X4	T50.4X5	T50.4X6
Oxitriptan	T43.291	T43.292	T43.293	T43.294	T43.295	T43.296
Oxitropium bromide	T48.6X1	T48.6X2	T48.6X3	T48.6X4	T48.6X5	T48.6X6
Oxodipine	T46.1X1	T46.1X2	T46.1X3	T46.1X4	T46.1X5	T46.1X6
Oxolamine	T48.3X1	T48.3X2	T48.3X3	T48.3X4	T48.3X5	T48.3X6
Oxolinic acid	T37.8X1	T37.8X2	T37.8X3	T37.8X4	T37.8X5	T37.8X6
Oxomemazine	T43.3X1	T43.3X2	T43.3X3	T43.3X4	T43.3X5	T43.3X6
Oxophenarsine	T37.3X1	T37.3X2	T37.3X3	T37.3X4	T37.3X5	T37.3X6
Oxprenolol	T44.7X1	T44.7X2	T44.7X3	T44.7X4	T44.7X5	T44.7X6
Oxsoralen	T49.3X1	T49.3X2	T49.3X3	T49.3X4	T49.3X5	T49.3X6
Oxtriphylline	T48.6X1	T48.6X2	T48.6X3	T48.6X4	T48.6X5	T48.6X6
Oxybate sodium	T41.291	T41.292	T41.293	T41.294	T41.295	T41.296
Oxybuprocaine	T41.3X1	T41.3X2	T41.3X3	T41.3X4	T41.3X5	T41.3X6
Oxybutynin	T44.3X1	T44.3X2	T44.3X3	T44.3X4	T44.3X5	T44.3X6
Oxychlorosene	T49.0X1	T49.0X2	T49.0X3	T49.0X4	T49.0X5	T49.0X6
Oxycodone	T40.2X1	T40.2X2	T40.2X3	T40.2X4	T40.2X5	T40.2X6
Oxyfedrine	T46.3X1	T46.3X2	T46.3X3	T46.3X4	T46.3X5	T46.3X6
Oxygen	T41.5X1	T41.5X2	T41.5X3	T41.5X4	T41.5X5	T41.5X6
Oxylone	T49.0X1	T49.0X2	T49.0X3	T49.0X4	T49.0X5	T49.0X6
ophthalmic preparation	T49.5X1	T49.5X2	T49.5X3	T49.5X4	T49.5X5	T49.5X6
Oxymesterone	T38.7X1	T38.7X2	T38.7X3	T38.7X4	T38.7X5	T38.7X6
Oxymetazoline	T48.5X1	T48.5X2	T48.5X3	T48.5X4	T48.5X5	T48.5X6
Oxymetholone	T38.7X1	T38.7X2	T38.7X3	T38.7X4	T38.7X5	T38.7X6
Oxymorphone	T40.2X1	T40.2X2	T40.2X3	T40.2X4	T40.2X5	T40.2X6
Oxypertine	T43.591	T43.592	T43.593	T43.594	T43.595	T43.596
Oxyphenbutazone	T39.2X1	T39.2X2	T39.2X3	T39.2X4	T39.2X5	T39.2X6
Oxyphencyclimine	T44.3X1	T44.3X2	T44.3X3	T44.3X4	T44.3X5	T44.3X6
Oxyphenisatine	T47.2X1	T47.2X2	T47.2X3	T47.2X4	T47.2X5	T47.2X6
Oxyphenonium bromide	T44.3X1	T44.3X2	T44.3X3	T44.3X4	T44.3X5	T44.3X6
Oxypolygelatin	T45.8X1	T45.8X2	T45.8X3	T45.8X4	T45.8X5	T45.8X6
Oxyquinoline (derivatives)	T37.8X1	T37.8X2	T37.8X3	T37.8X4	T37.8X5	T37.8X6
Oxytetracycline	T36.4X1	T36.4X2	T36.4X3	T36.4X4	T36.4X5	T36.4X6
Oxytocic drug NEC	T48.0X1	T48.0X2	T48.0X3	T48.0X4	T48.0X5	T48.0X6
Oxytocin (synthetic)	T48.0X1	T48.0X2	T48.0X3	T48.0X4	T48.0X5	T48.0X6
Ozone	T59.891	T59.892	T59.893	T59.894	—	—

◀ New   ◀ Revised   ~~deleted~~ Deleted

Substance	Poisoning, Accidental (Unintentional)	Poisoning, Intentional Self-Harm	Poisoning, Assault	Poisoning, Undetermined	Adverse Effect	Underdosing
P						
PABA	T49.3X1	T49.3X2	T49.3X3	T49.3X4	T49.3X5	T49.3X6
Packed red cells	T45.8X1	T45.8X2	T45.8X3	T45.8X4	T45.8X5	T45.8X6
Padimate	T49.3X1	T49.3X2	T49.3X3	T49.3X4	T49.3X5	T49.3X6
Paint NEC	T65.6X1	T65.6X2	T65.6X3	T65.6X4	—	—
cleaner	T52.91	T52.92	T52.93	T52.94	—	—
fumes NEC	T59.891	T59.892	T59.893	T59.894	—	—
lead (fumes)	T56.0X1	T56.0X2	T56.0X3	T56.0X4	—	—
solvent NEC	T52.8X1	T52.8X2	T52.8X3	T52.8X4	—	—
stripper	T52.8X1	T52.8X2	T52.8X3	T52.8X4	—	—
Palfium	T40.2X1	T40.2X2	T40.2X3	T40.2X4	—	—
Palm kernel oil	T50.991	T50.992	T50.993	T50.994	T50.995	T50.996
Paludrine	T37.2X1	T37.2X2	T37.2X3	T37.2X4	T37.2X5	T37.2X6
PAM (pralidoxime)	T50.6X1	T50.6X2	T50.6X3	T50.6X4	T50.6X5	T50.6X6
Pamaquine (naphthoate)	T37.2X1	T37.2X2	T37.2X3	T37.2X4	T37.2X5	T37.2X6
Panadol	T39.1X1	T39.1X2	T39.1X3	T39.1X4	T39.1X5	T39.1X6
Pancreatic						
digestive secretion stimulant	T47.8X1	T47.8X2	T47.8X3	T47.8X4	T47.8X5	T47.8X6
dornase	T45.3X1	T45.3X2	T45.3X3	T45.3X4	T45.3X5	T45.3X6
Pancreatin	T47.5X1	T47.5X2	T47.5X3	T47.5X4	T47.5X5	T47.5X6
Pancrelipase	T47.5X1	T47.5X2	T47.5X3	T47.5X4	T47.5X5	T47.5X6
Pancuronium (bromide)	T48.1X1	T48.1X2	T48.1X3	T48.1X4	T48.1X5	T48.1X6
Pangamic acid	T45.2X1	T45.2X2	T45.2X3	T45.2X4	T45.2X5	T45.2X6
Panthenol	T45.2X1	T45.2X2	T45.2X3	T45.2X4	T45.2X5	T45.2X6
topical	T49.8X1	T49.8X2	T49.8X3	T49.8X4	T49.8X5	T49.8X6
Pantopon	T40.0X1	T40.0X2	T40.0X3	T40.0X4	T40.0X5	T40.0X6
Pantothenic acid	T45.2X1	T45.2X2	T45.2X3	T45.2X4	T45.2X5	T45.2X6
Panwarfin	T45.511	T45.512	T45.513	T45.514	T45.515	T45.516
Papain	T47.5X1	T47.5X2	T47.5X3	T47.5X4	T47.5X5	T47.5X6
digestant	T47.5X1	T47.5X2	T47.5X3	T47.5X4	T47.5X5	T47.5X6
Papaveretum	T40.0X1	T40.0X2	T40.0X3	T40.0X4	T40.0X5	T40.0X6
Papaverine	T44.3X1	T44.3X2	T44.3X3	T44.3X4	T44.3X5	T44.3X6
Para-acetamidophenol	T39.1X1	T39.1X2	T39.1X3	T39.1X4	T39.1X5	T39.1X6
Para-aminobenzoic acid	T49.3X1	T49.3X2	T49.3X3	T49.3X4	T49.3X5	T49.3X6
Para-aminophenol derivatives	T39.1X1	T39.1X2	T39.1X3	T39.1X4	T39.1X5	T39.1X6
Para-aminosalicylic acid	T37.1X1	T37.1X2	T37.1X3	T37.1X4	T37.1X5	T37.1X6
Paracetaldehyde	T42.6X1	T42.6X2	T42.6X3	T42.6X4	T42.6X5	T42.6X6
Paracetamol	T39.1X1	T39.1X2	T39.1X3	T39.1X4	T39.1X5	T39.1X6
Parachlorophenol (camphorated)	T49.0X1	T49.0X2	T49.0X3	T49.0X4	T49.0X5	T49.0X6
Paracodin	T40.2X1	T40.2X2	T40.2X3	T40.2X4	T40.2X5	T40.2X6
Paradione	T42.2X1	T42.2X2	T42.2X3	T42.2X4	T42.2X5	T42.2X6

Substance	Poisoning, Accidental (Unintentional)	Poisoning, Intentional Self-Harm	Poisoning, Assault	Poisoning, Undetermined	Adverse Effect	Underdosing
Paraffin(s) (wax)	T52.0X1	T52.0X2	T52.0X3	T52.0X4	—	—
liquid (medicinal)	T47.4X1	T47.4X2	T47.4X3	T47.4X4	T47.4X5	T47.4X6
nonmedicinal	T52.0X1	T52.0X2	T52.0X3	T52.0X4	—	—
Paraformaldehyde	T60.3X1	T60.3X2	T60.3X3	T60.3X4	—	—
Paraldehyde	T42.6X1	T42.6X2	T42.6X3	T42.6X4	T42.6X5	T42.6X6
Paramethadione	T42.2X1	T42.2X2	T42.2X3	T42.2X4	T42.2X5	T42.2X6
Paramethasone	T38.0X1	T38.0X2	T38.0X3	T38.0X4	T38.0X5	T38.0X6
acetate	T49.0X1	T49.0X2	T49.0X3	T49.0X4	T49.0X5	T49.0X6
Paraoxon	T60.0X1	T60.0X2	T60.0X3	T60.0X4	—	—
Paraquat	T60.3X1	T60.3X2	T60.3X3	T60.3X4	—	—
Parasympatholytic NEC	T44.3X1	T44.3X2	T44.3X3	T44.3X4	T44.3X5	T44.3X6
Parasympathomimetic drug NEC	T44.1X1	T44.1X2	T44.1X3	T44.1X4	T44.1X5	T44.1X6
Parathion	T60.0X1	T60.0X2	T60.0X3	T60.0X4	—	—
Parathormone	T50.991	T50.992	T50.993	T50.994	T50.995	T50.996
Parathyroid extract	T50.991	T50.992	T50.993	T50.994	T50.995	T50.996
Paratyphoid vaccine	T50.A91	T50.A92	T50.A93	T50.A94	T50.A95	T50.A96
Paredrine	T44.4X1	T44.4X2	T44.4X3	T44.4X4	T44.4X5	T44.4X6
Paregoric	T40.0X1	T40.0X2	T40.0X3	T40.0X4	T40.0X5	T40.0X6
Pargyline	T46.5X1	T46.5X2	T46.5X3	T46.5X4	T46.5X5	T46.5X6
Paris green	T57.0X1	T57.0X2	T57.0X3	T57.0X4	—	—
insecticide	T57.0X1	T57.0X2	T57.0X3	T57.0X4	—	—
Parnate	T43.1X1	T43.1X2	T43.1X3	T43.1X4	T43.1X5	T43.1X6
Paromomycin	T36.5X1	T36.5X2	T36.5X3	T36.5X4	T36.5X5	T36.5X6
Paroxypropione	T45.1X1	T45.1X2	T45.1X3	T45.1X4	T45.1X5	T45.1X6
Parzone	T40.2X1	T40.2X2	T40.2X3	T40.2X4	T40.2X5	T40.2X6
PAS	T37.1X1	T37.1X2	T37.1X3	T37.1X4	T37.1X5	T37.1X6
Pasiniazid	T37.1X1	T37.1X2	T37.1X3	T37.1X4	T37.1X5	T37.1X6
PBB (polybrominated biphenyls)	T65.891	T65.892	T65.893	T65.894	—	—
PCB	T65.891	T65.892	T65.893	T65.894	—	—
PCP						
meaning pentachlorophenol	T60.1X1	T60.1X2	T60.1X3	T60.1X4	—	—
fungicide	T60.3X1	T60.3X2	T60.3X3	T60.3X4	—	—
herbicide	T60.3X1	T60.3X2	T60.3X3	T60.3X4	—	—
insecticide	T60.1X1	T60.1X2	T60.1X3	T60.1X4	—	—
meaning phencyclidine	T40.991	T40.992	T40.993	T40.994	—	—
Peach kernel oil (emulsion)	T47.4X1	T47.4X2	T47.4X3	T47.4X4	T47.4X5	T47.4X6
Peanut oil (emulsion) NEC	T47.4X1	T47.4X2	T47.4X3	T47.4X4	T47.4X5	T47.4X6
topical	T49.3X1	T49.3X2	T49.3X3	T49.3X4	T49.3X5	T49.3X6
Pearly Gates (morning glory seeds)	T40.991	T40.992	T40.993	T40.994	—	—
Pecazine	T43.3X1	T43.3X2	T43.3X3	T43.3X4	T43.3X5	T43.3X6
Pectin	T47.6X1	T47.6X2	T47.6X3	T47.6X4	T47.6X5	T47.6X6

◀ New ◀ Revised deleted Deleted

TABLE OF DRUGS AND CHEMICALS

Substance	Poisoning, Accidental (Unintentional)	Poisoning, Intentional Self-Harm	Poisoning, Assault	Poisoning, Undetermined	Adverse Effect	Underdosing
Pefloxacin	T37.8X1	T37.8X2	T37.8X3	T37.8X4	T37.8X5	T37.8X6
Pegademase, bovine	T50.Z91	T50.Z92	T50.Z93	T50.Z94	T50.Z95	T50.Z96
Pelletierine tannate	T37.4X1	T37.4X2	T37.4X3	T37.4X4	T37.4X5	T37.4X6
Pemirolast (potassium)	T48.6X1	T48.6X2	T48.6X3	T48.6X4	T48.6X5	T48.6X6
Pemoline	T50.7X1	T50.7X2	T50.7X3	T50.7X4	T50.7X5	T50.7X6
Pempidine	T44.2X1	T44.2X2	T44.2X3	T44.2X4	T44.2X5	T44.2X6
Penamecillin	T36.0X1	T36.0X2	T36.0X3	T36.0X4	T36.0X5	T36.0X6
Penbutolol	T44.7X1	T44.7X2	T44.7X3	T44.7X4	T44.7X5	T44.7X6
Penethamate	T36.0X1	T36.0X2	T36.0X3	T36.0X4	T36.0X5	T36.0X6
Penfluridol	T43.591	T43.592	T43.593	T43.594	T43.595	T43.596
Penflutizide	T50.2X1	T50.2X2	T50.2X3	T50.2X4	T50.2X5	T50.2X6
Pengitoxin	T46.0X1	T46.0X2	T46.0X3	T46.0X4	T46.0X5	T46.0X6
Penicillamine	T50.6X1	T50.6X2	T50.6X3	T50.6X4	T50.6X5	T50.6X6
Penicillin (any)	T36.0X1	T36.0X2	T36.0X3	T36.0X4	T36.0X5	T36.0X6
Penicillinase	T45.3X1	T45.3X2	T45.3X3	T45.3X4	T45.3X5	T45.3X6
Penicilloyl polylysine	T50.8X1	T50.8X2	T50.8X3	T50.8X4	T50.8X5	T50.8X6
Penimepicycline	T36.4X1	T36.4X2	T36.4X3	T36.4X4	T36.4X5	T36.4X6
Pentachloroethane	T53.6X1	T53.6X2	T53.6X3	T53.6X4	—	—
Pentachloronaphthalene	T53.7X1	T53.7X2	T53.7X3	T53.7X4	—	—
Pentachlorophenol (pesticide)	T60.1X1	T60.1X2	T60.1X3	T60.1X4	—	—
fungicide	T60.3X1	T60.3X2	T60.3X3	T60.3X4	—	—
herbicide	T60.3X1	T60.3X2	T60.3X3	T60.3X4	—	—
insecticide	T60.1X1	T60.1X2	T60.1X3	T60.1X4	—	—
Pentaerythritol tetranitrate	T46.3X1	T46.3X2	T46.3X3	T46.3X4	T46.3X5	T46.3X6
Pentaerythritol	T46.3X1	T46.3X2	T46.3X3	T46.3X4	T46.3X5	T46.3X6
chloral	T42.6X1	T42.6X2	T42.6X3	T42.6X4	T42.6X5	T42.6X6
tetranitrate NEC	T46.3X1	T46.3X2	T46.3X3	T46.3X4	T46.3X5	T46.3X6
Pentagastrin	T50.8X1	T50.8X2	T50.8X3	T50.8X4	T50.8X5	T50.8X6
Pentalin	T53.6X1	T53.6X2	T53.6X3	T53.6X4	—	—
Pentamethonium bromide	T44.2X1	T44.2X2	T44.2X3	T44.2X4	T44.2X5	T44.2X6
Pentamidine	T37.3X1	T37.3X2	T37.3X3	T37.3X4	T37.3X5	T37.3X6
Pentanol	T51.3X1	T51.3X2	T51.3X3	T51.3X4	—	—
Pentapyrrolinium (bitartrate)	T44.2X1	T44.2X2	T44.2X3	T44.2X4	T44.2X5	T44.2X6
Pentaquine	T37.2X1	T37.2X2	T37.2X3	T37.2X4	T37.2X5	T37.2X6
Pentazocine	T40.491	T40.492	T40.493	T40.494	T40.495	T40.496
Pentetrazole	T50.7X1	T50.7X2	T50.7X3	T50.7X4	T50.7X5	T50.7X6
Penthienate bromide	T44.3X1	T44.3X2	T44.3X3	T44.3X4	T44.3X5	T44.3X6
Pentifylline	T46.7X1	T46.7X2	T46.7X3	T46.7X4	T46.7X5	T46.7X6
Pentobarbital	T42.3X1	T42.3X2	T42.3X3	T42.3X4	T42.3X5	T42.3X6
sodium	T42.3X1	T42.3X2	T42.3X3	T42.3X4	T42.3X5	T42.3X6
Pentobarbitone	T42.3X1	T42.3X2	T42.3X3	T42.3X4	T42.3X5	T42.3X6
Pentolonium tartrate	T44.2X1	T44.2X2	T44.2X3	T44.2X4	T44.2X5	T44.2X6

Substance	Poisoning, Accidental (Unintentional)	Poisoning, Intentional Self-Harm	Poisoning, Assault	Poisoning, Undetermined	Adverse Effect	Underdosing
Pentosan polysulfate (sodium)	T39.8X1	T39.8X2	T39.8X3	T39.8X4	T39.8X5	T39.8X6
Pentostatin	T45.1X1	T45.1X2	T45.1X3	T45.1X4	T45.1X5	T45.1X6
Pentothal	T41.1X1	T41.1X2	T41.1X3	T41.1X4	T41.1X5	T41.1X6
Pentoxifylline	T46.7X1	T46.7X2	T46.7X3	T46.7X4	T46.7X5	T46.7X6
Pentoxyverine	T48.3X1	T48.3X2	T48.3X3	T48.3X4	T48.3X5	T48.3X6
Pentrinat	T46.3X1	T46.3X2	T46.3X3	T46.3X4	T46.3X5	T46.3X6
Pentylenetetrazole	T50.7X1	T50.7X2	T50.7X3	T50.7X4	T50.7X5	T50.7X6
Pentylsalicylamide	T37.1X1	T37.1X2	T37.1X3	T37.1X4	T37.1X5	T37.1X6
Pentymal	T42.3X1	T42.3X2	T42.3X3	T42.3X4	T42.3X5	T42.3X6
Peplomycin	T45.1X1	T45.1X2	T45.1X3	T45.1X4	T45.1X5	T45.1X6
Peppermint (oil)	T47.5X1	T47.5X2	T47.5X3	T47.5X4	T47.5X5	T47.5X6
Pepsin	T47.5X1	T47.5X2	T47.5X3	T47.5X4	T47.5X5	T47.5X6
digestant	T47.5X1	T47.5X2	T47.5X3	T47.5X4	T47.5X5	T47.5X6
Pepstatin	T47.1X1	T47.1X2	T47.1X3	T47.1X4	T47.1X5	T47.1X6
Peptavlon	T50.8X1	T50.8X2	T50.8X3	T50.8X4	T50.8X5	T50.8X6
Perazine	T43.3X1	T43.3X2	T43.3X3	T43.3X4	T43.3X5	T43.3X6
Percaine (spinal)	T41.3X1	T41.3X2	T41.3X3	T41.3X4	T41.3X5	T41.3X6
topical (surface)	T41.3X1	T41.3X2	T41.3X3	T41.3X4	T41.3X5	T41.3X6
Perchloroethylene	T53.3X1	T53.3X2	T53.3X3	T53.3X4	—	—
medicinal	T37.4X1	T37.4X2	T37.4X3	T37.4X4	T37.4X5	T37.4X6
vapor	T53.3X1	T53.3X2	T53.3X3	T53.3X4	—	—
Percodan	T40.2X1	T40.2X2	T40.2X3	T40.2X4	T40.2X5	T40.2X6
Percogesic — see also Acetaminophen	T45.0X1	T45.0X2	T45.0X3	T45.0X4	T45.0X5	T45.0X6
Percorten	T38.0X1	T38.0X2	T38.0X3	T38.0X4	T38.0X5	T38.0X6
Pergolide	T42.8X1	T42.8X2	T42.8X3	T42.8X4	T42.8X5	T42.8X6
Pergonal	T38.811	T38.812	T38.813	T38.814	T38.815	T38.816
Perhexilene	T46.3X1	T46.3X2	T46.3X3	T46.3X4	T46.3X5	T46.3X6
Perhexiline (maleate)	T46.3X1	T46.3X2	T46.3X3	T46.3X4	T46.3X5	T46.3X6
Periactin	T45.0X1	T45.0X2	T45.0X3	T45.0X4	T45.0X5	T45.0X6
Periciazine	T43.3X1	T43.3X2	T43.3X3	T43.3X4	T43.3X5	T43.3X6
Periclor	T42.6X1	T42.6X2	T42.6X3	T42.6X4	T42.6X5	T42.6X6
Perindopril	T46.4X1	T46.4X2	T46.4X3	T46.4X4	T46.4X5	T46.4X6
Perisoxal	T39.8X1	T39.8X2	T39.8X3	T39.8X4	T39.8X5	T39.8X6
Peritrate	T46.3X1	T46.3X2	T46.3X3	T46.3X4	T46.3X5	T46.3X6
Peritoneal dialysis solution	T50.3X1	T50.3X2	T50.3X3	T50.3X4	T50.3X5	T50.3X6
Perlapine	T42.4X1	T42.4X2	T42.4X3	T42.4X4	T42.4X5	T42.4X6
Permanganate	T65.891	T65.892	T65.893	T65.894	—	—
Permethrin	T60.1X1	T60.1X2	T60.1X3	T60.1X4	—	—
Pernocton	T42.3X1	T42.3X2	T42.3X3	T42.3X4	T42.3X5	T42.3X6
Pernoston	T42.3X1	T42.3X2	T42.3X3	T42.3X4	T42.3X5	T42.3X6
Peronine	T40.2X1	T40.2X2	T40.2X3	T40.2X4	—	—
Perphenazine	T43.3X1	T43.3X2	T43.3X3	T43.3X4	T43.3X5	T43.3X6

◄ New   ◄| Revised   ~~deleted~~ Deleted

Substance	External Cause (T-Code)					
	Poisoning, Accidental (Unintentional)	Poisoning, Intentional Self-Harm	Poisoning, Assault	Poisoning, Undetermined	Adverse Effect	Underdosing
Pertofrane	T43.Ø11	T43.Ø12	T43.Ø13	T43.Ø14	T43.Ø15	T43.Ø16
Pertussis						
immune serum (human)	T5Ø.Z11	T5Ø.Z12	T5Ø.Z13	T5Ø.Z14	T5Ø.Z15	T5Ø.Z16
vaccine (with diphtheria toxoid) (with tetanus toxoid)	T5Ø.A11	T5Ø.A12	T5Ø.A13	T5Ø.A14	T5Ø.A15	T5Ø.A16
Peruvian balsam	T49.ØX1	T49.ØX2	T49.ØX3	T49.ØX4	T49.ØX5	T49.ØX6
Peruvoside	T46.ØX1	T46.ØX2	T46.ØX3	T46.ØX4	T46.ØX5	T46.ØX6
Pesticide (dust) (fumes) (vapor) NEC	T6Ø.91	T6Ø.92	T6Ø.93	T6Ø.94	—	—
arsenic	T57.ØX1	T57.ØX2	T57.ØX3	T57.ØX4	—	—
chlorinated	T6Ø.1X1	T6Ø.1X2	T6Ø.1X3	T6Ø.1X4	—	—
cyanide	T65.ØX1	T65.ØX2	T65.ØX3	T65.ØX4	—	—
kerosene	T52.ØX1	T52.ØX2	T52.ØX3	T52.ØX4	—	—
mixture (of compounds)	T6Ø.91	T6Ø.92	T6Ø.93	T6Ø.94	—	—
naphthalene	T6Ø.2X1	T6Ø.2X2	T6Ø.2X3	T6Ø.2X4	—	—
organochlorine (compounds)	T6Ø.1X1	T6Ø.1X2	T6Ø.1X3	T6Ø.1X4	—	—
petroleum (distillate) (products) NEC	T6Ø.8X1	T6Ø.8X2	T6Ø.8X3	T6Ø.8X1		
specified ingredient NEC	T6Ø.8X1	T6Ø.8X2	T6Ø.8X3	T6Ø.8X4	—	—
strychnine	T65.1X1	T65.1X2	T65.1X3	T65.1X4	—	—
thallium	T6Ø.4X1	T6Ø.4X2	T6Ø.4X3	T6Ø.4X4	—	—
Pethidine	T4Ø.491	T4Ø.492	T4Ø.493	T4Ø.494	T4Ø.495	T4Ø.496
Petrichloral	T42.6X1	T42.6X2	T42.6X3	T42.6X4	T42.6X5	T42.6X6
Petrol	T52.ØX1	T52.ØX2	T52.ØX3	T52.ØX4	—	—
vapor	T52.ØX1	T52.ØX2	T52.ØX3	T52.ØX4	—	—
Petrolatum	T49.3X1	T49.3X2	T49.3X3	T49.3X4	T49.3X5	T49.3X6
hydrophilic	T49.3X1	T49.3X2	T49.3X3	T49.3X4	T49.3X5	T49.3X6
liquid	T47.4X1	T47.4X2	T47.4X3	T47.4X4	T47.4X5	T47.4X6
topical	T49.3X1	T49.3X2	T49.3X3	T49.3X4	T49.3X5	T49.3X6
nonmedicinal	T52.ØX1	T52.ØX2	T52.ØX3	T52.ØX4	—	—
red veterinary	T49.3X1	T49.3X2	T49.3X3	T49.3X4	T49.3X5	T49.3X6
white	T49.3X1	T49.3X2	T49.3X3	T49.3X4	T49.3X5	T49.3X6
Petroleum (products) NEC	T52.ØX1	T52.ØX2	T52.ØX3	T52.ØX4	—	—
benzine(s) — see Ligroin						
ether — see Ligroin						
jelly — see Petrolatum						
naphtha — see Ligroin						
pesticide	T6Ø.8X1	T6Ø.8X2	T6Ø.8X3	T6Ø.8X4	—	—
solids	T52.ØX1	T52.ØX2	T52.ØX3	T52.ØX4	—	—
solvents	T52.ØX1	T52.ØX2	T52.ØX3	T52.ØX4	—	—
vapor	T52.ØX1	T52.ØX2	T52.ØX3	T52.ØX4	—	—
Peyote	T4Ø.991	T4Ø.992	T4Ø.993	T4Ø.994	—	—
Phanodorm, phanodorn	T42.3X1	T42.3X2	T42.3X3	T42.3X4	T42.3X5	T42.3X6

Substance	External Cause (T-Code)					
	Poisoning, Accidental (Unintentional)	Poisoning, Intentional Self-Harm	Poisoning, Assault	Poisoning, Undetermined	Adverse Effect	Underdosing
Phanquinone	T37.3X1	T37.3X2	T37.3X3	T37.3X4	T37.3X5	T37.3X6
Phanquone	T37.3X1	T37.3X2	T37.3X3	T37.3X4	T37.3X5	T37.3X6
Pharmaceutical						
adjunct NEC	T5Ø.9Ø1	T5Ø.9Ø2	T5Ø.9Ø3	T5Ø.9Ø4	T5Ø.9Ø5	T5Ø.9Ø6
excipient NEC	T5Ø.9Ø1	T5Ø.9Ø2	T5Ø.9Ø3	T5Ø.9Ø4	T5Ø.9Ø5	T5Ø.9Ø6
sweetener	T5Ø.9Ø1	T5Ø.9Ø2	T5Ø.9Ø3	T5Ø.9Ø4	T5Ø.9Ø5	T5Ø.9Ø6
viscous agent	T5Ø.9Ø1	T5Ø.9Ø2	T5Ø.9Ø3	T5Ø.9Ø4	T5Ø.9Ø5	T5Ø.9Ø6
Phemitone	T42.3X1	T42.3X2	T42.3X3	T42.3X4	T42.3X5	T42.3X6
Phenacaine	T41.3X1	T41.3X2	T41.3X3	T41.3X4	T41.3X5	T41.3X6
Phenacemide	T42.6X1	T42.6X2	T42.6X3	T42.6X4	T42.6X5	T42.6X6
Phenacetin	T39.1X1	T39.1X2	T39.1X3	T39.1X4	T39.1X5	T39.1X6
Phenadoxone	T4Ø.2X1	T4Ø.2X2	T4Ø.2X3	T4Ø.2X4	—	—
Phenaglycodol	T43.591	T43.592	T43.593	T43.594	T43.595	T43.596
Phenantoin	T42.ØX1	T42.ØX2	T42.ØX3	T42.ØX4	T42.ØX5	T42.ØX6
Phenaphthazine reagent	T5Ø.991	T5Ø.992	T5Ø.993	T5Ø.994	T5Ø.995	T5Ø.996
Phenazocine	T4Ø.491	T4Ø.492	T4Ø.493	T4Ø.494	T4Ø.495	T4Ø.496
Phenazone	T39.2X1	T39.2X2	T39.2X3	T39.2X4	T39.2X5	T39.2X6
Phenazopyridine	T39.8X1	T39.8X2	T39.8X3	T39.8X4	T39.8X5	T39.8X6
Phenbenicillin	T36.ØX1	T36.ØX2	T36.ØX3	T36.ØX4	T36.ØX5	T36.ØX6
Phenbutrazate	T5Ø.5X1	T5Ø.5X2	T5Ø.5X3	T5Ø.5X4	T5Ø.5X5	T5Ø.5X6
Phencyclidine	T4Ø.991	T4Ø.992	T4Ø.993	T4Ø.994	T4Ø.995	T4Ø.996
Phendimetrazine	T5Ø.5X1	T5Ø.5X2	T5Ø.5X3	T5Ø.5X4	T5Ø.5X5	T5Ø.5X6
Phenelzine	T43.1X1	T43.1X2	T43.1X3	T43.1X4	T43.1X5	T43.1X6
Phenemal	T42.3X1	T42.3X2	T42.3X3	T42.3X4	T42.3X5	T42.3X6
Phenergan	T42.6X1	T42.6X2	T42.6X3	T42.6X4	T42.6X5	T42.6X6
Pheneticillin	T36.ØX1	T36.ØX2	T36.ØX3	T36.ØX4	T36.ØX5	T36.ØX6
Pheneturide	T42.6X1	T42.6X2	T42.6X3	T42.6X4	T42.6X5	T42.6X6
Phenformin	T38.3X1	T38.3X2	T38.3X3	T38.3X4	T38.3X5	T38.3X6
Phenglutarimide	T44.3X1	T44.3X2	T44.3X3	T44.3X4	T44.3X5	T44.3X6
Phenicarbazide	T39.8X1	T39.8X2	T39.8X3	T39.8X4	T39.8X5	T39.8X6
Phenindamine	T45.ØX1	T45.ØX2	T45.ØX3	T45.ØX4	T45.ØX5	T45.ØX6
Phenindione	T45.511	T45.512	T45.513	T45.514	T45.515	T45.516
Pheniprazine	T43.1X1	T43.1X2	T43.1X3	T43.1X4	T43.1X5	T43.1X6
Pheniramine	T45.ØX1	T45.ØX2	T45.ØX3	T45.ØX4	T45.ØX5	T45.ØX6
Phenisatin	T47.2X1	T47.2X2	T47.2X3	T47.2X4	T47.2X5	T47.2X6
Phenmetrazine	T5Ø.5X1	T5Ø.5X2	T5Ø.5X3	T5Ø.5X4	T5Ø.5X5	T5Ø.5X6
Phenobal	T42.3X1	T42.3X2	T42.3X3	T42.3X4	T42.3X5	
Phenobarbital	T42.3X1	T42.3X2	T42.3X3	T42.3X4	T42.3X5	T42.3X6
with						
mephenytoin	T42.3X1	T42.3X2	T42.3X3	T42.3X4	T42.3X5	T42.3X6
phenytoin	T42.3X1	T42.3X2	T42.3X3	T42.3X4	T42.3X5	T42.3X6
sodium	T42.3X1	T42.3X2	T42.3X3	T42.3X4	T42.3X5	T42.3X6

◀ New　　◀ Revised　　deleted Deleted

TABLE OF DRUGS AND CHEMICALS

TABLE OF DRUGS AND CHEMICALS

Substance	External Cause (T-Code) Poisoning, Accidental (Unintentional)	Poisoning, Intentional Self-Harm	Poisoning, Assault	Poisoning, Undetermined	Adverse Effect	Underdosing
Phenobarbitone	T42.3X1	T42.3X2	T42.3X3	T42.3X4	T42.3X5	T42.3X6
Phenobutiodil	T50.8X1	T50.8X2	T50.8X3	T50.8X4	T50.8X5	T50.8X6
Phenoctide	T49.0X1	T49.0X2	T49.0X3	T49.0X4	T49.0X5	T49.0X6
Phenol	T49.0X1	T49.0X2	T49.0X3	T49.0X4	T49.0X5	T49.0X6
disinfectant	T54.0X1	T54.0X2	T54.0X3	T54.0X4	—	—
in oil injection	T46.8X1	T46.8X2	T46.8X3	T46.8X4	T46.8X5	T46.8X6
medicinal	T49.1X1	T49.1X2	T49.1X3	T49.1X4	T49.1X5	T49.1X6
nonmedicinal NEC	T54.0X1	T54.0X2	T54.0X3	T54.0X4	—	—
pesticide	T60.8X1	T60.8X2	T60.8X3	T60.8X4	—	—
red	T50.8X1	T50.8X2	T50.8X3	T50.8X4	T50.8X5	T50.8X6
Phenolic preparation	T49.1X1	T49.1X2	T49.1X3	T49.1X4	T49.1X5	T49.1X6
Phenolphthalein	T47.2X1	T47.2X2	T47.2X3	T47.2X4	T47.2X5	T47.2X6
Phenolsulfonphthalein	T50.8X1	T50.8X2	T50.8X3	T50.8X4	T50.8X5	T50.8X6
Phenomorphan	T40.2X1	T40.2X2	T40.2X3	T40.2X4	—	—
Phenonyl	T42.3X1	T42.3X2	T42.3X3	T42.3X4	T42.3X5	T42.3X6
Phenoperidine	T40.491	T40.492	T40.493	T40.494	—	—
Phenopyrazone	T46.991	T46.992	T46.993	T46.994	T46.995	T46.996
Phenoquin	T50.4X1	T50.4X2	T50.4X3	T50.4X4	T50.4X5	T50.4X6
Phenothiazine (psychotropic) NEC	T43.3X1	T43.3X2	T43.3X3	T43.3X4	T43.3X5	T43.3X6
insecticide	T60.2X1	T60.2X2	T60.2X3	T60.2X4	—	—
Phenothrin	T49.0X1	T49.0X2	T49.0X3	T49.0X4	T49.0X5	T49.0X6
Phenoxybenzamine	T46.7X1	T46.7X2	T46.7X3	T46.7X4	T46.7X5	T46.7X6
Phenoxyethanol	T49.0X1	T49.0X2	T49.0X3	T49.0X4	T49.0X5	T49.0X6
Phenoxymethyl penicillin	T36.0X1	T36.0X2	T36.0X3	T36.0X4	T36.0X5	T36.0X6
Phenprobamate	T42.8X1	T42.8X2	T42.8X3	T42.8X4	T42.8X5	T42.8X6
Phenprocoumon	T45.511	T45.512	T45.513	T45.514	T45.515	T45.516
Phensuximide	T42.2X1	T42.2X2	T42.2X3	T42.2X4	T42.2X5	T42.2X6
Phentermine	T50.5X1	T50.5X2	T50.5X3	T50.5X4	T50.5X5	T50.5X6
Phenthicillin	T36.0X1	T36.0X2	T36.0X3	T36.0X4	T36.0X5	T36.0X6
Phentolamine	T46.7X1	T46.7X2	T46.7X3	T46.7X4	T46.7X5	T46.7X6
Phenyl						
butazone	T39.2X1	T39.2X2	T39.2X3	T39.2X4	T39.2X5	T39.2X6
enediamine	T65.3X1	T65.3X2	T65.3X3	T65.3X4	—	—
hydrazine	T65.3X1	T65.3X2	T65.3X3	T65.3X4	—	—
antineoplastic	T45.1X1	T45.1X2	T45.1X3	T45.1X4	T45.1X5	T45.1X6
mercuric compounds—see Mercury						
salicylate	T49.3X1	T49.3X2	T49.3X3	T49.3X4	T49.3X5	T49.3X6
Phenylalanine mustard	T45.1X1	T45.1X2	T45.1X3	T45.1X4	T45.1X5	T45.1X6
Phenylbutazone	T39.2X1	T39.2X2	T39.2X3	T39.2X4	T39.2X5	T39.2X6
Phenylenediamine	T65.3X1	T65.3X2	T65.3X3	T65.3X4	—	—
Phenylephrine	T44.4X1	T44.4X2	T44.4X3	T44.4X4	T44.4X5	T44.4X6

Substance	External Cause (T-Code) Poisoning, Accidental (Unintentional)	Poisoning, Intentional Self-Harm	Poisoning, Assault	Poisoning, Undetermined	Adverse Effect	Underdosing
Phenylethylbiguanide	T38.3X1	T38.3X2	T38.3X3	T38.3X4	T38.3X5	T38.3X6
Phenylmercuric						
acetate	T49.0X1	T49.0X2	T49.0X3	T49.0X4	T49.0X5	T49.0X6
borate	T49.0X1	T49.0X2	T49.0X3	T49.0X4	T49.0X5	T49.0X6
nitrate	T49.0X1	T49.0X2	T49.0X3	T49.0X4	T49.0X5	T49.0X6
Phenylmethylbarbitone	T42.3X1	T42.3X2	T42.3X3	T42.3X4	T42.3X5	T42.3X6
Phenylpropanol	T47.5X1	T47.5X2	T47.5X3	T47.5X4	T47.5X5	T47.5X6
Phenylpropanolamine	T44.991	T44.992	T44.993	T44.994	T44.995	T44.996
Phenylsulfthion	T60.0X1	T60.0X2	T60.0X3	T60.0X4	—	—
Phenyltoloxamine	T45.0X1	T45.0X2	T45.0X3	T45.0X4	T45.0X5	T45.0X6
Phenyramidol, phenyramidon	T39.8X1	T39.8X2	T39.8X3	T39.8X4	T39.8X5	T39.8X6
Phenytoin	T42.0X1	T42.0X2	T42.0X3	T42.0X4	T42.0X5	T42.0X6
with Phenobarbital	T42.3X1	T42.3X2	T42.3X3	T42.3X4	T42.3X5	T42.3X6
pHisoHex	T49.2X1	T49.2X2	T49.2X3	T49.2X4	T49.2X5	T49.2X6
Pholcodine	T48.3X1	T48.3X2	T48.3X3	T48.3X4	T48.3X5	T48.3X6
Pholedrine	T46.991	T46.992	T46.993	T46.994	T46.995	T46.996
Phorate	T60.0X1	T60.0X2	T60.0X3	T60.0X4	—	—
Phosdrin	T60.0X1	T60.0X2	T60.0X3	T60.0X4	—	—
Phosfolan	T60.0X1	T60.0X2	T60.0X3	T60.0X4	—	—
Phosgene (gas)	T59.891	T59.892	T59.893	T59.894	—	—
Phosphamidon	T60.0X1	T60.0X2	T60.0X3	T60.0X4	—	—
Phosphate	T65.891	T65.892	T65.893	T65.894	—	—
laxative	T47.4X1	T47.4X2	T47.4X3	T47.4X4	T47.4X5	T47.4X6
organic	T60.0X1	T60.0X2	T60.0X3	T60.0X4	—	—
solvent	T52.91	T52.92	T52.93	T52.94	—	—
tricresyl	T65.891	T65.892	T65.893	T65.894	—	—
Phosphine	T57.1X1	T57.1X2	T57.1X3	T57.1X4	—	—
fumigant	T57.1X1	T57.1X2	T57.1X3	T57.1X4	—	—
Phospholine	T49.5X1	T49.5X2	T49.5X3	T49.5X4	T49.5X5	T49.5X6
Phosphoric acid	T54.2X1	T54.2X2	T54.2X3	T54.2X4	—	—
Phosphorus (compound) NEC	T57.1X1	T57.1X2	T57.1X3	T57.1X4	—	—
pesticide	T60.0X1	T60.0X2	T60.0X3	T60.0X4	—	—
Phthalates	T65.891	T65.892	T65.893	T65.894	—	—
Phthalic anhydride	T65.891	T65.892	T65.893	T65.894	—	—
Phthalimidoglutarimide	T42.6X1	T42.6X2	T42.6X3	T42.6X4	T42.6X5	T42.6X6
Phthalylsulfathiazole	T37.0X1	T37.0X2	T37.0X3	T37.0X4	T37.0X5	T37.0X6
Phylloquinone	T45.7X1	T45.7X2	T45.7X3	T45.7X4	T45.7X5	T45.7X6
Physeptone	T40.3X1	T40.3X2	T40.3X3	T40.3X4	T40.3X5	T40.3X6
Physostigma venenosum	T62.2X1	T62.2X2	T62.2X3	T62.2X4	—	—
Physostigmine	T49.5X1	T49.5X2	T49.5X3	T49.5X4	T49.5X5	T49.5X6
Phytolacca decandra	T62.2X1	T62.2X2	T62.2X3	T62.2X4	—	—
berries	T62.1X1	T62.1X2	T62.1X3	T62.1X4	—	—

◀ New ◀ Revised ~~deleted~~ Deleted

Substance	Poisoning, Accidental (Unintentional)	Poisoning, Intentional Self-Harm	Poisoning, Assault	Poisoning, Undetermined	Adverse Effect	Underdosing
	External Cause (T-Code)					
Phytomenadione	T45.7X1	T45.7X2	T45.7X3	T45.7X4	T45.7X5	T45.7X6
Phytonadione	T45.7X1	T45.7X2	T45.7X3	T45.7X4	T45.7X5	T45.7X6
Picoperine	T48.3X1	T48.3X2	T48.3X3	T48.3X4	T48.3X5	T48.3X6
Picosulfate (sodium)	T47.2X1	T47.2X2	T47.2X3	T47.2X4	T47.2X5	T47.2X6
Picric (acid)	T54.2X1	T54.2X2	T54.2X3	T54.2X4	—	—
Picrotoxin	T50.7X1	T50.7X2	T50.7X3	T50.7X4	T50.7X5	T50.7X6
Piketoprofen	T49.0X1	T49.0X2	T49.0X3	T49.0X4	T49.0X5	T49.0X6
Pilocarpine	T44.1X1	T44.1X2	T44.1X3	T44.1X4	T44.1X5	T44.1X6
Pilocarpus (jaborandi) extract	T44.1X1	T44.1X2	T44.1X3	T44.1X4	T44.1X5	T44.1X6
Pilsicainide (hydrochloride)	T46.2X1	T46.2X2	T46.2X3	T46.2X4	T46.2X5	T46.2X6
Pimaricin	T36.7X1	T36.7X2	T36.7X3	T36.7X4	T36.7X5	T36.7X6
Pimeclone	T50.7X1	T50.7X2	T50.7X3	T50.7X4	T50.7X5	T50.7X6
Pimelic ketone	T52.8X1	T52.8X2	T52.8X3	T52.8X4	—	—
Pimethixene	T45.0X1	T45.0X2	T45.0X3	T45.0X4	T45.0X5	T45.0X6
Piminodine	T40.2X1	T40.2X2	T40.2X3	T40.2X4	T40.2X5	T40.2X6
Pimozide	T43.591	T43.592	T43.593	T43.594	T43.595	T43.596
Pinacidil	T46.5X1	T46.5X2	T46.5X3	T46.5X4	T46.5X5	T46.5X6
Pinaverium bromide	T44.3X1	T44.3X2	T44.3X3	T44.3X4	T44.3X5	T44.3X6
Pinazepam	T42.4X1	T42.4X2	T42.4X3	T42.4X4	T42.4X5	T42.4X6
Pindolol	T44.7X1	T44.7X2	T44.7X3	T44.7X4	T44.7X5	T44.7X6
Pindone	T60.4X1	T60.4X2	T60.4X3	T60.4X4	—	—
Pine oil (disinfectant)	T65.891	T65.892	T65.893	T65.894	—	—
Pinkroot	T37.4X1	T37.4X2	T37.4X3	T37.4X4	T37.4X5	T37.4X6
Pipadone	T40.2X1	T40.2X2	T40.2X3	T40.2X4	—	—
Pipamazine	T45.0X1	T45.0X2	T45.0X3	T45.0X4	T45.0X5	T45.0X6
Pipamperone	T43.4X1	T43.4X2	T43.4X3	T43.4X4	T43.4X5	T43.4X6
Pipazetate	T48.3X1	T48.3X2	T48.3X3	T48.3X4	T48.3X5	T48.3X6
Pipemidic acid	T37.8X1	T37.8X2	T37.8X3	T37.8X4	T37.8X5	T37.8X6
Pipenzolate bromide	T44.3X1	T44.3X2	T44.3X3	T44.3X4	T44.3X5	T44.3X6
Piperacetazine	T43.3X1	T43.3X2	T43.3X3	T43.3X4	T43.3X5	T43.3X6
Piperacillin	T36.0X1	T36.0X2	T36.0X3	T36.0X4	T36.0X5	T36.0X6
Piperazine	T37.4X1	T37.4X2	T37.4X3	T37.4X4	T37.4X5	T37.4X6
estrone sulfate	T38.5X1	T38.5X2	T38.5X3	T38.5X4	T38.5X5	T38.5X6
Piper cubeba	T62.2X1	T62.2X2	T62.2X3	T62.2X4	—	—
Piperidione	T48.3X1	T48.3X2	T48.3X3	T48.3X4	—	—
Piperidolate	T44.3X1	T44.3X2	T44.3X3	T44.3X4	T44.3X5	T44.3X6
Piperocaine	T41.3X1	T41.3X2	T41.3X3	T41.3X4	T41.3X5	T41.3X6
infiltration (subcutaneous)	T41.3X1	T41.3X2	T41.3X3	T41.3X4	T41.3X5	T41.3X6
nerve block (peripheral) (plexus)	T41.3X1	T41.3X2	T41.3X3	T41.3X4	T41.3X5	T41.3X6
topical (surface)	T41.3X1	T41.3X2	T41.3X3	T41.3X4	T41.3X5	T41.3X6
Piperonyl butoxide	T60.8X1	T60.8X2	T60.8X3	T60.8X4	—	—
Pipethanate	T44.3X1	T44.3X2	T44.3X3	T44.3X4	T44.3X5	T44.3X6

Substance	Poisoning, Accidental (Unintentional)	Poisoning, Intentional Self-Harm	Poisoning, Assault	Poisoning, Undetermined	Adverse Effect	Underdosing
	External Cause (T-Code)					
Pipobroman	T45.1X1	T45.1X2	T45.1X3	T45.1X4	T45.1X5	T45.1X6
Pipofezine	T43.0X1	T43.0X2	T43.0X3	T43.0X4	T43.0X5	T43.0X6
Pipotiazine	T43.3X1	T43.3X2	T43.3X3	T43.3X4	T43.3X5	T43.3X6
Pipoxizine	T45.0X1	T45.0X2	T45.0X3	T45.0X4	T45.0X5	T45.0X6
Pipradrol	T43.691	T43.692	T43.693	T43.694	T43.695	T43.696
Piprinhydrinate	T45.0X1	T45.0X2	T45.0X3	T45.0X4	T45.0X5	T45.0X6
Pirarubicin	T45.1X1	T45.1X2	T45.1X3	T45.1X4	T45.1X5	T45.1X6
Pirazinamide	T37.1X1	T37.1X2	T37.1X3	T37.1X4	T37.1X5	T37.1X6
Pirbuterol	T48.6X1	T48.6X2	T48.6X3	T48.6X4	T48.6X5	T48.6X6
Pirenzepine	T47.1X1	T47.1X2	T47.1X3	T47.1X4	T47.1X5	T47.1X6
Piretanide	T50.1X1	T50.1X2	T50.1X3	T50.1X4	T50.1X5	T50.1X6
Piribedil	T42.8X1	T42.8X2	T42.8X3	T42.8X4	T42.8X5	T42.8X6
Piridoxilate	T46.3X1	T46.3X2	T46.3X3	T46.3X4	T46.3X5	T46.3X6
Piritramide	T40.491	T40.492	T40.493	T40.494	—	—
Pirlindole	T43.0X1	T43.0X2	T43.0X3	T43.0X4	T43.0X5	T43.0X6
Piromidic acid	T37.8X1	T37.8X2	T37.8X3	T37.8X4	T37.8X5	T37.8X6
Piroxicam	T39.391	T39.392	T39.393	T39.394	T39.395	T39.396
beta-cyclodextrin complex	T39.8X1	T39.8X2	T39.8X3	T39.8X4	T39.8X5	T39.8X6
Pirozadil	T46.6X1	T46.6X2	T46.6X3	T46.6X4	T46.6X5	T46.6X6
Piscidia (bark) (erythrina)	T39.8X1	T39.8X2	T39.8X3	T39.8X4	T39.8X5	T39.8X6
Pitch	T65.891	T65.892	T65.893	T65.894	—	—
Pitkin's solution	T41.3X1	T41.3X2	T41.3X3	T41.3X4	T41.3X5	T41.3X6
Pitocin	T48.0X1	T48.0X2	T48.0X3	T48.0X4	T48.0X5	T48.0X6
Pitressin (tannate)	T38.891	T38.892	T38.893	T38.894	T38.895	T38.896
Pituitary extracts (posterior)	T38.891	T38.892	T38.893	T38.894	T38.895	T38.896
anterior	T38.811	T38.812	T38.813	T38.814	T38.815	T38.816
Pituitrin	T38.891	T38.892	T38.893	T38.894	T38.895	T38.896
Pivampicillin	T36.0X1	T36.0X2	T36.0X3	T36.0X4	T36.0X5	T36.0X6
Pivmecillinam	T36.0X1	T36.0X2	T36.0X3	T36.0X4	T36.0X5	T36.0X6
Placental hormone	T38.891	T38.892	T38.893	T38.894	T38.895	T38.896
Placidyl	T42.6X1	T42.6X2	T42.6X3	T42.6X4	T42.6X5	T42.6X6
Plague vaccine	T50.A91	T50.A92	T50.A93	T50.A94	T50.A95	T50.A96
Plant						
food or fertilizer NEC	T65.891	T65.892	T65.893	T65.894	—	—
containing herbicide	T60.3X1	T60.3X2	T60.3X3	T60.3X4	—	—
noxious, used as food	T62.2X1	T62.2X2	T62.2X3	T62.2X4	—	—
berries	T62.1X1	T62.1X2	T62.1X3	T62.1X4	—	—
seeds	T62.2X1	T62.2X2	T62.2X3	T62.2X4	—	—
specified type NEC	T62.2X1	T62.2X2	T62.2X3	T62.2X4	—	—
Plasma	T45.8X1	T45.8X2	T45.8X3	T45.8X4	T45.8X5	T45.8X6
expander NEC	T45.8X1	T45.8X2	T45.8X3	T45.8X4	T45.8X5	T45.8X6
protein fraction (human)	T45.8X1	T45.8X2	T45.8X3	T45.8X4	T45.8X5	T45.8X6

◀ New ◀ Revised ~~deleted~~ Deleted

TABLE OF DRUGS AND CHEMICALS

TABLE OF DRUGS AND CHEMICALS

Substance	External Cause (T-Code)					
	Poisoning, Accidental (Unintentional)	Poisoning, Intentional Self-Harm	Poisoning, Assault	Poisoning, Undetermined	Adverse Effect	Underdosing
Plasmanate	T45.8X1	T45.8X2	T45.8X3	T45.8X4	T45.8X5	T45.8X6
Plasminogen (tissue) activator	T45.611	T45.612	T45.613	T45.614	T45.615	T45.616
Plaster dressing	T49.3X1	T49.3X2	T49.3X3	T49.3X4	T49.3X5	T49.3X6
Plastic dressing	T49.3X1	T49.3X2	T49.3X3	T49.3X4	T49.3X5	T49.3X6
Plegicil	T43.3X1	T43.3X2	T43.3X3	T43.3X4	T43.3X5	T43.3X6
Plicamycin	T45.1X1	T45.1X2	T45.1X3	T45.1X4	T45.1X5	T45.1X6
Podophyllotoxin	T49.8X1	T49.8X2	T49.8X3	T49.8X4	T49.8X5	T49.8X6
Podophyllum (resin)	T49.4X1	T49.4X2	T49.4X3	T49.4X4	T49.4X5	T49.4X6
Poison NEC	T65.91	T65.92	T65.93	T65.94	—	—
Poisonous berries	T62.1X1	T62.1X2	T62.1X3	T62.1X4	—	—
Pokeweed (any part)	T62.2X1	T62.2X2	T62.2X3	T62.2X4	—	—
Poldine metilsulfate	T44.3X1	T44.3X2	T44.3X3	T44.3X4	T44.3X5	T44.3X6
Polidexide (sulfate)	T46.6X1	T46.6X2	T46.6X3	T46.6X4	T46.6X5	T46.6X6
Polidocanol	T46.8X1	T46.8X2	T46.8X3	T46.8X4	T46.8X5	T46.8X6
Poliomyelitis vaccine	T50.B91	T50.B92	T50.B93	T50.B94	T50.B95	T50.B96
Polish (car) (floor) (furniture) (metal) (porcelain) (silver)	T65.891	T65.892	T65.893	T65.894	—	—
abrasive	T65.891	T65.892	T65.893	T65.894	—	—
porcelain	T65.891	T65.892	T65.893	T65.894	—	—
Poloxalkol	T47.4X1	T47.4X2	T47.4X3	T47.4X4	T47.4X5	T47.4X6
Poloxamer	T47.4X1	T47.4X2	T47.4X3	T47.4X4	T47.4X5	T47.4X6
Polyaminostyrene resins	T50.3X1	T50.3X2	T50.3X3	T50.3X4	T50.3X5	T50.3X6
Polycarbophil	T47.4X1	T47.4X2	T47.4X3	T47.4X4	T47.4X5	T47.4X6
Polychlorinated biphenyl	T65.891	T65.892	T65.893	T65.894	—	—
Polycycline	T36.4X1	T36.4X2	T36.4X3	T36.4X4	T36.4X5	T36.4X6
Polyester fumes	T59.891	T59.892	T59.893	T59.894	—	—
Polyester resin hardener	T52.91	T52.92	T52.93	T52.94	—	—
fumes	T59.891	T59.892	T59.893	T59.894	—	—
Polyestradiol phosphate	T38.5X1	T38.5X2	T38.5X3	T38.5X4	T38.5X5	T38.5X6
Polyethanolamine alkyl sulfate	T49.2X1	T49.2X2	T49.2X3	T49.2X4	T49.2X5	T49.2X6
Polyethylene adhesive	T49.3X1	T49.3X2	T49.3X3	T49.3X4	T49.3X5	T49.3X6
Polyferose	T45.4X1	T45.4X2	T45.4X3	T45.4X4	T45.4X5	T45.4X6
Polygeline	T45.8X1	T45.8X2	T45.8X3	T45.8X4	T45.8X5	T45.8X6
Polymyxin	T36.8X1	T36.8X2	T36.8X3	T36.8X4	T36.8X5	T36.8X6
B	T36.8X1	T36.8X2	T36.8X3	T36.8X4	T36.8X5	T36.8X6
ENT agent	T49.6X1	T49.6X2	T49.6X3	T49.6X4	T49.6X5	T49.6X6
ophthalmic preparation	T49.5X1	T49.5X2	T49.5X3	T49.5X4	T49.5X5	T49.5X6
topical NEC	T49.0X1	T49.0X2	T49.0X3	T49.0X4	T49.0X5	T49.0X6
E sulfate (eye preparation)	T49.5X1	T49.5X2	T49.5X3	T49.5X4	T49.5X5	T49.5X6
Polynoxylin	T49.0X1	T49.0X2	T49.0X3	T49.0X4	T49.0X5	T49.0X6
Polyoestradiol phosphate	T38.5X1	T38.5X2	T38.5X3	T38.5X4	T38.5X5	T38.5X6
Polyoxymethyleneurea	T49.0X1	T49.0X2	T49.0X3	T49.0X4	T49.0X5	T49.0X6

Substance	External Cause (T-Code)					
	Poisoning, Accidental (Unintentional)	Poisoning, Intentional Self-Harm	Poisoning, Assault	Poisoning, Undetermined	Adverse Effect	Underdosing
Polysilane	T47.8X1	T47.8X2	T47.8X3	T47.8X4	T47.8X5	T47.8X6
Polytetrafluoroethylene (inhaled)	T59.891	T59.892	T59.893	T59.894	—	—
Polythiazide	T50.2X1	T50.2X2	T50.2X3	T50.2X4	T50.2X5	T50.2X6
Polyvidone	T45.8X1	T45.8X2	T45.8X3	T45.8X4	T45.8X5	T45.8X6
Polyvinylpyrrolidone	T45.8X1	T45.8X2	T45.8X3	T45.8X4	T45.8X5	T45.8X6
Pontocaine (hydrochloride) (infiltration) (topical)	T41.3X1	T41.3X2	T41.3X3	T41.3X4	T41.3X5	T41.3X6
nerve block (peripheral) (plexus)	T41.3X1	T41.3X2	T41.3X3	T41.3X4	T41.3X5	T41.3X6
spinal	T41.3X1	T41.3X2	T41.3X3	T41.3X4	T41.3X5	T41.3X6
Porfiromycin	T45.1X1	T45.1X2	T45.1X3	T45.1X4	T45.1X5	T45.1X6
Posterior pituitary hormone NEC	T38.891	T38.892	T38.893	T38.894	T38.895	T38.896
Pot	T40.711	T40.712	T40.713	T40.714	T40.715	T40.716
Potash (caustic)	T54.3X1	T54.3X2	T54.3X3	T54.3X4	—	—
Potassic saline injection (lactated)	T50.3X1	T50.3X2	T50.3X3	T50.3X4	T50.3X5	T50.3X6
Potassium (salts) NEC	T50.3X1	T50.3X2	T50.3X3	T50.3X4	T50.3X5	T50.3X6
aminobenzoate	T45.8X1	T45.8X2	T45.8X3	T45.8X4	T45.8X5	T45.8X6
aminosalicylate	T37.1X1	T37.1X2	T37.1X3	T37.1X4	T37.1X5	T37.1X6
antimony 'tartrate'	T37.8X1	T37.8X2	T37.8X3	T37.8X4	T37.8X5	T37.8X6
arsenite (solution)	T57.0X1	T57.0X2	T57.0X3	T57.0X4	—	—
bichromate	T56.2X1	T56.2X2	T56.2X3	T56.2X4	—	—
bisulfate	T47.3X1	T47.3X2	T47.3X3	T47.3X4	T47.3X5	T47.3X6
bromide	T42.6X1	T42.6X2	T42.6X3	T42.6X4	T42.6X5	T42.6X6
canrenoate	T50.0X1	T50.0X2	T50.0X3	T50.0X4	T50.0X5	T50.0X6
carbonate	T54.3X1	T54.3X2	T54.3X3	T54.3X4	—	—
chlorate NEC	T65.891	T65.892	T65.893	T65.894	—	—
chloride	T50.3X1	T50.3X2	T50.3X3	T50.3X4	T50.3X5	T50.3X6
citrate	T50.991	T50.992	T50.993	T50.994	T50.995	T50.996
cyanide	T65.0X1	T65.0X2	T65.0X3	T65.0X4	—	—
ferric hexacyanoferrate (medicinal)	T50.6X1	T50.6X2	T50.6X3	T50.6X4	T50.6X5	T50.6X6
nonmedicinal	T65.891	T65.892	T65.893	T65.894	—	—
Fluoride	T57.8X1	T57.8X2	T57.8X3	T57.8X4	—	—
glucaldrate	T47.1X1	T47.1X2	T47.1X3	T47.1X4	T47.1X5	T47.1X6
hydroxide	T54.3X1	T54.3X2	T54.3X3	T54.3X4	—	—
iodate	T49.0X1	T49.0X2	T49.0X3	T49.0X4	T49.0X5	T49.0X6
iodide	T48.4X1	T48.4X2	T48.4X3	T48.4X4	T48.4X5	T48.4X6
nitrate	T57.8X1	T57.8X2	T57.8X3	T57.8X4	—	—
oxalate	T65.891	T65.892	T65.893	T65.894	—	—
perchlorate (nonmedicinal) NEC	T65.891	T65.892	T65.893	T65.894	—	—
antithyroid	T38.2X1	T38.2X2	T38.2X3	T38.2X4	T38.2X5	T38.2X6
medicinal	T38.2X1	T38.2X2	T38.2X3	T38.2X4	T38.2X5	T38.2X6

◀ New ◀ Revised ~~deleted~~ Deleted

Substance	Poisoning, Accidental (Unintentional)	Poisoning, Intentional Self-Harm	Poisoning, Assault	Poisoning, Undetermined	Adverse Effect	Underdosing
Permanganate (nonmedicinal)	T65.891	T65.892	T65.893	T65.894	—	—
medicinal	T49.0X1	T49.0X2	T49.0X3	T49.0X4	T49.0X5	T49.0X6
sulfate	T47.2X1	T47.2X2	T47.2X3	T47.2X4	T47.2X5	T47.2X6
Potassium-removing resin	T50.3X1	T50.3X2	T50.3X3	T50.3X4	T50.3X5	T50.3X6
Potassium-retaining drug	T50.3X1	T50.3X2	T50.3X3	T50.3X4	T50.3X5	T50.3X6
Povidone	T45.8X1	T45.8X2	T45.8X3	T45.8X4	T45.8X5	T45.8X6
iodine	T49.0X1	T49.0X2	T49.0X3	T49.0X4	T49.0X5	T49.0X6
Practolol	T44.7X1	T44.7X2	T44.7X3	T44.7X4	T44.7X5	T44.7X6
Prajmalium bitartrate	T46.2X1	T46.2X2	T46.2X3	T46.2X4	T46.2X5	T46.2X6
Pralidoxime (iodide)	T50.6X1	T50.6X2	T50.6X3	T50.6X4	T50.6X5	T50.6X6
chloride	T50.6X1	T50.6X2	T50.6X3	T50.6X4	T50.6X5	T50.6X6
Pramiverine	T44.3X1	T44.3X2	T44.3X3	T44.3X4	T44.3X5	T44.3X6
Pramocaine	T49.1X1	T49.1X2	T49.1X3	T49.1X4	T49.1X5	T49.1X6
Pramoxine	T49.1X1	T49.1X2	T49.1X3	T49.1X4	T49.1X5	T49.1X6
Prasterone	T38.7X1	T38.7X2	T38.7X3	T38.7X4	T38.7X5	T38.7X6
Pravastatin	T46.6X1	T46.6X2	T46.6X3	T46.6X4	T46.6X5	T46.6X6
Prazepam	T42.4X1	T42.4X2	T42.4X3	T42.4X4	T42.4X5	T42.4X6
Praziquantel	T37.4X1	T37.4X2	T37.4X3	T37.4X4	T37.4X5	T37.4X6
Prazitone	T43.291	T43.292	T43.293	T43.294	T43.295	T43.296
Prazosin	T44.6X1	T44.6X2	T44.6X3	T44.6X4	T44.6X5	T44.6X6
Prednicarbate	T49.0X1	T49.0X2	T49.0X3	T49.0X4	T49.0X5	T49.0X6
Prednimustine	T45.1X1	T45.1X2	T45.1X3	T45.1X4	T45.1X5	T45.1X6
Prednisolone	T38.0X1	T38.0X2	T38.0X3	T38.0X4	T38.0X5	T38.0X6
ENT agent	T49.6X1	T49.6X2	T49.6X3	T49.6X4	T49.6X5	T49.6X6
ophthalmic preparation	T49.5X1	T49.5X2	T49.5X3	T49.5X4	T49.5X5	T49.5X6
steaglate	T49.0X1	T49.0X2	T49.0X3	T49.0X4	T49.0X5	T49.0X6
topical NEC	T49.0X1	T49.0X2	T49.0X3	T49.0X4	T49.0X5	T49.0X6
Prednisone	T38.0X1	T38.0X2	T38.0X3	T38.0X4	T38.0X5	T38.0X6
Prednylidene	T38.0X1	T38.0X2	T38.0X3	T38.0X4	T38.0X5	T38.0X6
Pregnandiol	T38.5X1	T38.5X2	T38.5X3	T38.5X4	T38.5X5	T38.5X6
Pregneninolone	T38.5X1	T38.5X2	T38.5X3	T38.5X4	T38.5X5	T38.5X6
Preludin	T43.691	T43.692	T43.693	T43.694	T43.695	T43.696
Premarin	T38.5X1	T38.5X2	T38.5X3	T38.5X4	T38.5X5	T38.5X6
Premedication anesthetic	T41.201	T41.202	T41.203	T41.204	T41.205	T41.206
Prenalterol	T44.5X1	T44.5X2	T44.5X3	T44.5X4	T44.5X5	T44.5X6
Prenoxdiazine	T48.3X1	T48.3X2	T48.3X3	T48.3X4	T48.3X5	T48.3X6
Prenylamine	T46.3X1	T46.3X2	T46.3X3	T46.3X4	T46.3X5	T46.3X6
Preparation, local	T49.4X1	T49.4X2	T49.4X3	T49.4X4	T49.4X5	T49.4X6
Preparation H	T49.8X1	T49.8X2	T49.8X3	T49.8X4	T49.8X5	T49.8X6
Preservative (nonmedicinal)	T65.891	T65.892	T65.893	T65.894	—	—
medicinal	T50.901	T50.902	T50.903	T50.904	T50.905	T50.906
wood	T60.91	T60.92	T60.93	T60.94	—	—

Substance	Poisoning, Accidental (Unintentional)	Poisoning, Intentional Self-Harm	Poisoning, Assault	Poisoning, Undetermined	Adverse Effect	Underdosing
Prethcamide	T50.7X1	T50.7X2	T50.7X3	T50.7X4	T50.7X5	T50.7X6
Pride of China	T62.2X1	T62.2X2	T62.2X3	T62.2X4	—	—
Pridinol	T44.3X1	T44.3X2	T44.3X3	T44.3X4	T44.3X5	T44.3X6
Prifinium bromide	T44.3X1	T44.3X2	T44.3X3	T44.3X4	T44.3X5	T44.3X6
Prilocaine	T41.3X1	T41.3X2	T41.3X3	T41.3X4	T41.3X5	T41.3X6
infiltration (subcutaneous)	T41.3X1	T41.3X2	T41.3X3	T41.3X4	T41.3X5	T41.3X6
nerve block (peripheral) (plexus)	T41.3X1	T41.3X2	T41.3X3	T41.3X4	T41.3X5	T41.3X6
regional	T41.3X1	T41.3X2	T41.3X3	T41.3X4	T41.3X5	T41.3X6
Primaquine	T37.2X1	T37.2X2	T37.2X3	T37.2X4	T37.2X5	T37.2X6
Primidone	T42.6X1	T42.6X2	T42.6X3	T42.6X4	T42.6X5	T42.6X6
Primula (veris)	T62.2X1	T62.2X2	T62.2X3	T62.2X4	—	—
Prinadol	T40.2X1	T40.2X2	T40.2X3	T40.2X4	T40.2X5	T40.2X6
Priscol, Priscoline	T44.6X1	T44.6X2	T44.6X3	T44.6X4	T44.6X5	T44.6X6
Pristinamycin	T36.3X1	T36.3X2	T36.3X3	T36.3X4	T36.3X5	T36.3X6
Privet	T62.2X1	T62.2X2	T62.2X3	T62.2X4	—	—
berries	T62.1X1	T62.1X2	T62.1X3	T62.1X4	—	—
Privine	T44.4X1	T44.4X2	T44.4X3	T44.4X4	T44.4X5	T44.4X6
Pro-Banthine	T44.3X1	T44.3X2	T44.3X3	T44.3X4	T44.3X5	T44.3X6
Probarbital	T42.3X1	T42.3X2	T42.3X3	T42.3X4	T42.3X5	T42.3X6
Probenecid	T50.4X1	T50.4X2	T50.4X3	T50.4X4	T50.4X5	T50.4X6
Probucol	T46.6X1	T46.6X2	T46.6X3	T46.6X4	T46.6X5	T46.6X6
Procainamide	T46.2X1	T46.2X2	T46.2X3	T46.2X4	T46.2X5	T46.2X6
Procaine	T41.3X1	T41.3X2	T41.3X3	T41.3X4	T41.3X5	T41.3X6
benzylpenicillin	T36.0X1	T36.0X2	T36.0X3	T36.0X4	T36.0X5	T36.0X6
nerve block (peripheral) (plexus)	T41.3X1	T41.3X2	T41.3X3	T41.3X4	T41.3X5	T41.3X6
penicillin G	T36.0X1	T36.0X2	T36.0X3	T36.0X4	T36.0X5	T36.0X6
regional	T41.3X1	T41.3X2	T41.3X3	T41.3X4	T41.3X5	T41.3X6
spinal	T41.3X1	T41.3X2	T41.3X3	T41.3X4	T41.3X5	T41.3X6
Procalmidol	T43.591	T43.592	T43.593	T43.594	T43.595	T43.596
Procarbazine	T45.1X1	T45.1X2	T45.1X3	T45.1X4	T45.1X5	T45.1X6
Procaterol	T44.5X1	T44.5X2	T44.5X3	T44.5X4	T44.5X5	T44.5X6
Prochlorperazine	T43.3X1	T43.3X2	T43.3X3	T43.3X4	T43.3X5	T43.3X6
Procyclidine	T44.3X1	T44.3X2	T44.3X3	T44.3X4	T44.3X5	T44.3X6
Producer gas	T58.8X1	T58.8X2	T58.8X3	T58.8X4	—	—
Profadol	T40.491	T40.492	T40.493	T40.494	T40.495	T40.496
Profenamine	T44.3X1	T44.3X2	T44.3X3	T44.3X4	T44.3X5	T44.3X6
Profenil	T44.3X1	T44.3X2	T44.3X3	T44.3X4	T44.3X5	T44.3X6
Proflavine	T49.0X1	T49.0X2	T49.0X3	T49.0X4	T49.0X5	T49.0X6
Progabide	T42.6X1	T42.6X2	T42.6X3	T42.6X4	T42.6X5	T42.6X6
Progestin	T38.5X1	T38.5X2	T38.5X3	T38.5X4	T38.5X5	T38.5X6
oral contraceptive	T38.4X1	T38.4X2	T38.4X3	T38.4X4	T38.4X5	T38.4X6

◀ New   ◀ Revised   ~~deleted~~ Deleted

	External Cause (T-Code)					
Substance	Poisoning, Accidental (Unintentional)	Poisoning, Intentional Self-Harm	Poisoning, Assault	Poisoning, Undetermined	Adverse Effect	Underdosing
Progesterone	T38.5X1	T38.5X2	T38.5X3	T38.5X4	T38.5X5	T38.5X6
Progestogen NEC	T38.5X1	T38.5X2	T38.5X3	T38.5X4	T38.5X5	T38.5X6
Progestone	T38.5X1	T38.5X2	T38.5X3	T38.5X4	T38.5X5	T38.5X6
Proglumide	T47.1X1	T47.1X2	T47.1X3	T47.1X4	T47.1X5	T47.1X6
Proguanil	T37.2X1	T37.2X2	T37.2X3	T37.2X4	T37.2X5	T37.2X6
Prolactin	T38.811	T38.812	T38.813	T38.814	T38.815	T38.816
Prolintane	T43.691	T43.692	T43.693	T43.694	T43.695	T43.696
Proloid	T38.1X1	T38.1X2	T38.1X3	T38.1X4	T38.1X5	T38.1X6
Proluton	T38.5X1	T38.5X2	T38.5X3	T38.5X4	T38.5X5	T38.5X6
Promacetin	T37.1X1	T37.1X2	T37.1X3	T37.1X4	T37.1X5	T37.1X6
Promazine	T43.3X1	T43.3X2	T43.3X3	T43.3X4	T43.3X5	T43.3X6
Promedol	T40.2X1	T40.2X2	T40.2X3	T40.2X4	—	—
Promegestone	T38.5X1	T38.5X2	T38.5X3	T38.5X4	T38.5X5	T38.5X6
Promethazine (teoclate)	T43.3X1	T43.3X2	T43.3X3	T43.3X4	T43.3X5	T43.3X6
Promin	T37.1X1	T37.1X2	T37.1X3	T37.1X4	T37.1X5	T37.1X6
Pronase	T45.3X1	T45.3X2	T45.3X3	T45.3X4	T45.3X5	T45.3X6
Pronestyl (hydrochloride)	T46.2X1	T46.2X2	T46.2X3	T46.2X4	T46.2X5	T46.2X6
Pronetalol	T44.7X1	T44.7X2	T44.7X3	T44.7X4	T44.7X5	T44.7X6
Prontosil	T37.0X1	T37.0X2	T37.0X3	T37.0X4	T37.0X5	T37.0X6
Propachlor	T60.3X1	T60.3X2	T60.3X3	T60.3X4	—	—
Propafenone	T46.2X1	T46.2X2	T46.2X3	T46.2X4	T46.2X5	T46.2X6
Propallylonal	T42.3X1	T42.3X2	T42.3X3	T42.3X4	T42.3X5	T42.3X6
Propamidine	T49.0X1	T49.0X2	T49.0X3	T49.0X4	T49.0X5	T49.0X6
Propane (distributed in mobile container)	T59.891	T59.892	T59.893	T59.894	—	—
distributed through pipes	T59.891	T59.892	T59.893	T59.894	—	—
incomplete combustion	T57.11	T57.12	T57.13	T57.14	—	—
Propanidid	T41.291	T41.292	T41.293	T41.294	T41.295	T41.296
Propanil	T60.3X1	T60.3X2	T60.3X3	T60.3X4	—	—
1-Propanol	T51.3X1	T51.3X2	T51.3X3	T51.3X4	—	—
2-Propanol	T51.2X1	T51.2X2	T51.2X3	T51.2X4	—	—
Propantheline	T44.3X1	T44.3X2	T44.3X3	T44.3X4	T44.3X5	T44.3X6
bromide	T44.3X1	T44.3X2	T44.3X3	T44.3X4	T44.3X5	T44.3X6
Proparacaine	T41.3X1	T41.3X2	T41.3X3	T41.3X4	T41.3X5	T41.3X6
Propatylnitrate	T46.3X1	T46.3X2	T46.3X3	T46.3X4	T46.3X5	T46.3X6
Propicillin	T36.0X1	T36.0X2	T36.0X3	T36.0X4	T36.0X5	T36.0X6
Propiolactone	T49.0X1	T49.0X2	T49.0X3	T49.0X4	T49.0X5	T49.0X6
Propiomazine	T45.0X1	T45.0X2	T45.0X3	T45.0X4	T45.0X5	T45.0X6
Propionaldehyde (medicinal)	T42.6X1	T42.6X2	T42.6X3	T42.6X4	T42.6X5	T42.6X6
Propionate (calcium) (sodium)	T49.0X1	T49.0X2	T49.0X3	T49.0X4	T49.0X5	T49.0X6
Propion gel	T49.0X1	T49.0X2	T49.0X3	T49.0X4	T49.0X5	T49.0X6

	External Cause (T-Code)					
Substance	Poisoning, Accidental (Unintentional)	Poisoning, Intentional Self-Harm	Poisoning, Assault	Poisoning, Undetermined	Adverse Effect	Underdosing
Propitocaine	T41.3X1	T41.3X2	T41.3X3	T41.3X4	T41.3X5	T41.3X6
infiltration (subcutaneous)	T41.3X1	T41.3X2	T41.3X3	T41.3X4	T41.3X5	T41.3X6
nerve block (peripheral) (plexus)	T41.3X1	T41.3X2	T41.3X3	T41.3X4	T41.3X5	T41.3X6
Propofol	T41.291	T41.292	T41.293	T41.294	T41.295	T41.296
Propoxur	T60.0X1	T60.0X2	T60.0X3	T60.0X4	—	—
Propoxycaine	T41.3X1	T41.3X2	T41.3X3	T41.3X4	T41.3X5	T41.3X6
infiltration (subcutaneous)	T41.3X1	T41.3X2	T41.3X3	T41.3X4	T41.3X5	T41.3X6
nerve block (peripheral) (plexus)	T41.3X1	T41.3X2	T41.3X3	T41.3X4	T41.3X5	T41.3X6
topical (surface)	T41.3X1	T41.3X2	T41.3X3	T41.3X4	T41.3X5	T41.3X6
Propoxyphene	T40.491	T40.492	T40.493	T40.494	T40.495	T40.496
Propranolol	T44.7X1	T44.7X2	T44.7X3	T44.7X4	T44.7X5	T44.7X6
Propyl						
alcohol	T51.3X1	T51.3X2	T51.3X3	T51.3X4	—	—
carbinol	T51.3X1	T51.3X2	T51.3X3	T51.3X4	—	—
hexadrine	T44.4X1	T44.4X2	T44.4X3	T44.4X4	T44.4X5	T44.4X6
iodone	T50.8X1	T50.8X2	T50.8X3	T50.8X4	T50.8X5	T50.8X6
thiouracil	T38.2X1	T38.2X2	T38.2X3	T38.2X4	T38.2X5	T38.2X6
Propylaminophenothiazine	T43.3X1	T43.3X2	T43.3X3	T43.3X4	T43.3X5	T43.3X6
Propylene	T59.891	T59.892	T59.893	T59.894	—	—
Propylhexedrine	T48.5X1	T48.5X2	T48.5X3	T48.5X4	T48.5X5	T48.5X6
Propyliodone	T50.8X1	T50.8X2	T50.8X3	T50.8X4	T50.8X5	T50.8X6
Propylthiouracil	T38.2X1	T38.2X2	T38.2X3	T38.2X4	T38.2X5	T38.2X6
Propylparaben (ophthalmic)	T49.5X1	T49.5X2	T49.5X3	T49.5X4	T49.5X5	T49.5X6
Propyphenazone	T39.2X1	T39.2X2	T39.2X3	T39.2X4	T39.2X5	T39.2X6
Proquazone	T39.391	T39.392	T39.393	T39.394	T39.395	T39.396
Proscillaridin	T46.0X1	T46.0X2	T46.0X3	T46.0X4	T46.0X5	T46.0X6
Prostacyclin	T45.521	T45.522	T45.523	T45.524	T45.525	T45.526
Prostaglandin (I2)	T45.521	T45.522	T45.523	T45.524	T45.525	T45.526
E1	T46.7X1	T46.7X2	T46.7X3	T46.7X4	T46.7X5	T46.7X6
E2	T48.0X1	T48.0X2	T48.0X3	T48.0X4	T48.0X5	T48.0X6
F2 alpha	T48.0X1	T48.0X2	T48.0X3	T48.0X4	T48.0X5	T48.0X6
Prostigmin	T44.0X1	T44.0X2	T44.0X3	T44.0X4	T44.0X5	T44.0X6
Prosultiamine	T45.2X1	T45.2X2	T45.2X3	T45.2X4	T45.2X5	T45.2X6
Protamine sulfate	T45.7X1	T45.7X2	T45.7X3	T45.7X4	T45.7X5	T45.7X6
zinc insulin	T38.3X1	T38.3X2	T38.3X3	T38.3X4	T38.3X5	T38.3X6
Protease	T47.5X1	T47.5X2	T47.5X3	T47.5X4	T47.5X5	T47.5X6
Protectant, skin NEC	T49.3X1	T49.3X2	T49.3X3	T49.3X4	T49.3X5	T49.3X6
Protein hydrolysate	T50.991	T50.992	T50.993	T50.994	T50.995	T50.996
Prothiaden — *see Dothiepin hydrochloride*						
Prothionamide	T37.1X1	T37.1X2	T37.1X3	T37.1X4	T37.1X5	T37.1X6

◄ New   ◀ Revised   ~~deleted~~ Deleted

Substance	External Cause (T-Code)					
	Poisoning, Accidental (Unintentional)	Poisoning, Intentional Self-Harm	Poisoning, Assault	Poisoning, Undetermined	Adverse Effect	Underdosing
Prothipendyl	T43.591	T43.592	T43.593	T43.594	T43.595	T43.596
Prothoate	T60.0X1	T60.0X2	T60.0X3	T60.0X4	—	—
Prothrombin						
activator	T45.7X1	T45.7X2	T45.7X3	T45.7X4	T45.7X5	T45.7X6
synthesis inhibitor	T45.511	T45.512	T45.513	T45.514	T45.515	T45.516
Protionamide	T37.1X1	T37.1X2	T37.1X3	T37.1X4	T37.1X5	T37.1X6
Protirelin	T38.891	T38.892	T38.893	T38.894	T38.895	T38.896
Protokylol	T48.6X1	T48.6X2	T48.6X3	T48.6X4	T48.6X5	T48.6X6
Protopam	T50.6X1	T50.6X2	T50.6X3	T50.6X4	T50.6X5	T50.6X6
Protoveratrine(s) (A) (B)	T46.5X1	T46.5X2	T46.5X3	T46.5X4	T46.5X5	T46.5X6
Protriptyline	T43.011	T43.012	T43.013	T43.014	T43.015	T43.016
Provera	T38.5X1	T38.5X2	T38.5X3	T38.5X4	T38.5X5	T38.5X6
Provitamin A	T45.2X1	T45.2X2	T45.2X3	T45.2X4	T45.2X5	T45.2X6
Proxibarbal	T42.3X1	T42.3X2	T42.3X3	T42.3X4	T42.3X5	T42.3X6
Proxymetacaine	T41.3X1	T41.3X2	T41.3X3	T41.3X4	T41.3X5	T41.3X6
Proxyphylline	T48.6X1	T48.6X2	T48.6X3	T48.6X4	T48.6X5	T48.6X6
Prozac — see Fluoxetine hydrochloride						
Prunus						
laurocerasus	T62.2X1	T62.2X2	T62.2X3	T62.2X4	—	—
virginiana	T62.2X1	T62.2X2	T62.2X3	T62.2X4	—	—
Prussian blue						
commercial	T65.891	T65.892	T65.893	T65.894	—	—
therapeutic	T50.6X1	T50.6X2	T50.6X3	T50.6X4	T50.6X5	T50.6X6
Prussic acid	T65.0X1	T65.0X2	T65.0X3	T65.0X4	—	—
vapor	T57.3X1	T57.3X2	T57.3X3	T57.3X4	—	—
Pseudoephedrine	T44.991	T44.992	T44.993	T44.994	T44.995	T44.996
Psilocin	T40.991	T40.992	T40.993	T40.994	—	—
Psilocybin	T40.991	T40.992	T40.993	T40.994	—	—
Psilocybine	T40.991	T40.992	T40.993	T40.994	—	—
Psoralene (nonmedicinal)	T65.891	T65.892	T65.893	T65.894	—	—
Psoralens (medicinal)	T50.991	T50.992	T50.993	T50.994	T50.995	T50.996
PSP (phenolsulfonphthalein)	T50.8X1	T50.8X2	T50.8X3	T50.8X4	T50.8X5	T50.8X6
Psychodysleptic drug NOS	T40.901	T40.902	T40.903	T40.904	T40.905	T40.906
specified NEC	T40.991	T40.992	T40.993	T40.994	T40.995	T40.996
Psychostimulant	T43.601	T43.602	T43.603	T43.604	T43.605	T43.606
amphetamine	T43.621	T43.622	T43.623	T43.624	T43.625	T43.626
caffeine	T43.611	T43.612	T43.613	T43.614	T43.615	T43.616
methylphenidate	T43.631	T43.632	T43.633	T43.634	T43.635	T43.636
specified NEC	T43.691	T43.692	T43.693	T43.694	T43.695	T43.696
Psychotherapeutic drug NEC	T43.91	T43.92	T43.93	T43.94	T43.95	T43.96
antidepressants — see also Antidepressant	T43.201	T43.202	T43.203	T43.204	T43.205	T43.206

Substance	External Cause (T-Code)					
	Poisoning, Accidental (Unintentional)	Poisoning, Intentional Self-Harm	Poisoning, Assault	Poisoning, Undetermined	Adverse Effect	Underdosing
Psychotherapeutic drug NEC (Continued)						
specified NEC	T43.8X1	T43.8X2	T43.8X3	T43.8X4	T43.8X5	T43.8X6
tranquilizers NEC	T43.501	T43.502	T43.503	T43.504	T43.505	T43.506
Psychotomimetic agents	T40.901	T40.902	T40.903	T40.904	T40.905	T40.906
Psychotropic drug NEC	T43.91	T43.92	T43.93	T43.94	T43.95	T43.96
specified NEC	T43.8X1	T43.8X2	T43.8X3	T43.8X4	T43.8X5	T43.8X6
Psyllium hydrophilic mucilloid	T47.4X1	T47.4X2	T47.4X3	T47.4X4	T47.4X5	T47.4X6
Pteroylglutamic acid	T45.8X1	T45.8X2	T45.8X3	T45.8X4	T45.8X5	T45.8X6
Pteroyltriglutamate	T45.1X1	T45.1X2	T45.1X3	T45.1X4	T45.1X5	T45.1X6
PTFE — see Polytetrafluoroethylene						
Pulp						
devitalizing paste	T49.7X1	T49.7X2	T49.7X3	T49.7X4	T49.7X5	T49.7X6
dressing	T49.7X1	T49.7X2	T49.7X3	T49.7X4	T49.7X5	T49.7X6
Pulsatilla	T62.2X1	T62.2X2	T62.2X3	T62.2X4	—	—
Pumpkin seed extract	T37.4X1	T37.4X2	T37.4X3	T37.4X4	T37.4X5	T37.4X6
Purex (bleach)	T54.91	T54.92	T54.93	T54.94	—	—
Purgative NEC — see also Cathartic	T47.4X1	T47.4X2	T47.4X3	T47.4X4	T47.4X5	T47.4X6
Purine analogue (antineoplastic)	T45.1X1	T45.1X2	T45.1X3	T45.1X4	T45.1X5	T45.1X6
Purine diuretics	T50.2X1	T50.2X2	T50.2X3	T50.2X4	T50.2X5	T50.2X6
Purinethol	T45.1X1	T45.1X2	T45.1X3	T45.1X4	T45.1X5	T45.1X6
PVP	T45.8X1	T45.8X2	T45.8X3	T45.8X4	T45.8X5	T45.8X6
Pyrabital	T39.8X1	T39.8X2	T39.8X3	T39.8X4	T39.8X5	T39.8X6
Pyramidon	T39.2X1	T39.2X2	T39.2X3	T39.2X4	T39.2X5	T39.2X6
Pyrantel	T37.4X1	T37.4X2	T37.4X3	T37.4X4	T37.4X5	T37.4X6
Pyrathiazine	T45.0X1	T45.0X2	T45.0X3	T45.0X4	T45.0X5	T45.0X6
Pyrazinamide	T37.1X1	T37.1X2	T37.1X3	T37.1X4	T37.1X5	T37.1X6
Pyrazinoic acid (amide)	T37.1X1	T37.1X2	T37.1X3	T37.1X4	T37.1X5	T37.1X6
Pyrazole (derivatives)	T39.2X1	T39.2X2	T39.2X3	T39.2X4	T39.2X5	T39.2X6
Pyrazolone analgesic NEC	T39.2X1	T39.2X2	T39.2X3	T39.2X4	T39.2X5	T39.2X6
Pyrethrin, pyrethrum (nonmedicinal)	T60.2X1	T60.2X2	T60.2X3	T60.2X4	—	—
Pyrethrum extract	T49.0X1	T49.0X2	T49.0X3	T49.0X4	T49.0X5	T49.0X6
Pyribenzamine	T45.0X1	T45.0X2	T45.0X3	T45.0X4	T45.0X5	T45.0X6
Pyridine	T52.8X1	T52.8X2	T52.8X3	T52.8X4	—	—
aldoxime methiodide	T50.6X1	T50.6X2	T50.6X3	T50.6X4	T50.6X5	T50.6X6
aldoxime methyl chloride	T50.6X1	T50.6X2	T50.6X3	T50.6X4	T50.6X5	T50.6X6
vapor	T59.891	T59.892	T59.893	T59.894	—	—
Pyridium	T39.8X1	T39.8X2	T39.8X3	T39.8X4	T39.8X5	T39.8X6
Pyridostigmine bromide	T44.0X1	T44.0X2	T44.0X3	T44.0X4	T44.0X5	T44.0X6
Pyridoxal phosphate	T45.2X1	T45.2X2	T45.2X3	T45.2X4	T45.2X5	T45.2X6

TABLE OF DRUGS AND CHEMICALS

Substance	Poisoning, Accidental (Unintentional)	Poisoning, Intentional Self-Harm	Poisoning, Assault	Poisoning, Undetermined	Adverse Effect	Underdosing
Pyridoxine	T45.2X1	T45.2X2	T45.2X3	T45.2X4	T45.2X5	T45.2X6
Pyrilamine	T45.0X1	T45.0X2	T45.0X3	T45.0X4	T45.0X5	T45.0X6
Pyrimethamine	T37.2X1	T37.2X2	T37.2X3	T37.2X4	T37.2X5	T37.2X6
with sulfadoxine	T37.2X1	T37.2X2	T37.2X3	T37.2X4	T37.2X5	T37.2X6
Pyrimidine antagonist	T45.1X1	T45.1X2	T45.1X3	T45.1X4	T45.1X5	T45.1X6
Pyriminil	T60.4X1	T60.4X2	T60.4X3	T60.4X4	—	—
Pyrithione zinc	T49.4X1	T49.4X2	T49.4X3	T49.4X4	T49.4X5	T49.4X6
Pyrithyldione	T42.6X1	T42.6X2	T42.6X3	T42.6X4	T42.6X5	T42.6X6
Pyrogallic acid	T49.0X1	T49.0X2	T49.0X3	T49.0X4	T49.0X5	T49.0X6
Pyrogallol	T49.0X1	T49.0X2	T49.0X3	T49.0X4	T49.0X5	T49.0X6
Pyroxylin	T49.3X1	T49.3X2	T49.3X3	T49.3X4	T49.3X5	T49.3X6
Pyrrobutamine	T45.0X1	T45.0X2	T45.0X3	T45.0X4	T45.0X5	T45.0X6
Pyrrolizidine alkaloids	T62.8X1	T62.8X2	T62.8X3	T62.8X4	—	—
Pyrvinium chloride	T37.4X1	T37.4X2	T37.4X3	T37.4X4	T37.4X5	T37.4X6
PZI	T38.3X1	T38.3X2	T38.3X3	T38.3X4	T38.3X5	T38.3X6
Q						
Quaalude	T42.6X1	T42.6X2	T42.6X3	T42.6X4	T42.6X5	T42.6X6
Quarternary ammonium						
anti-infective	T49.0X1	T49.0X2	T49.0X3	T49.0X4	T49.0X5	T49.0X6
ganglion blocking	T44.2X1	T44.2X2	T44.2X3	T44.2X4	T44.2X5	T44.2X6
parasympatholytic	T44.3X1	T44.3X2	T44.3X3	T44.3X4	T44.3X5	T44.3X6
Quazepam	T42.4X1	T42.4X2	T42.4X3	T42.4X4	T42.4X5	T42.4X6
Quicklime	T54.3X1	T54.3X2	T54.3X3	T54.3X4	—	—
Quillaja extract	T48.4X1	T48.4X2	T48.4X3	T48.4X4	T48.4X5	T48.4X6
Quinacrine	T37.2X1	T37.2X2	T37.2X3	T37.2X4	T37.2X5	T37.2X6
Quinaglute	T46.2X1	T46.2X2	T46.2X3	T46.2X4	T46.2X5	T46.2X6
Quinalbarbital	T42.3X1	T42.3X2	T42.3X3	T42.3X4	T42.3X5	T42.3X6
Quinalbarbitone sodium	T42.3X1	T42.3X2	T42.3X3	T42.3X4	T42.3X5	T42.3X6
Quinalphos	T60.0X1	T60.0X2	T60.0X3	T60.0X4	—	—
Quinapril	T46.4X1	T46.4X2	T46.4X3	T46.4X4	T46.4X5	T46.4X6
Quinestradiol	T38.5X1	T38.5X2	T38.5X3	T38.5X4	T38.5X5	T38.5X6
Quinestradol	T38.5X1	T38.5X2	T38.5X3	T38.5X4	T38.5X5	T38.5X6
Quinestrol	T38.5X1	T38.5X2	T38.5X3	T38.5X4	T38.5X5	T38.5X6
Quinethazone	T50.2X1	T50.2X2	T50.2X3	T50.2X4	T50.2X5	T50.2X6
Quingestanol	T38.4X1	T38.4X2	T38.4X3	T38.4X4	T38.4X5	T38.4X6
Quinidine	T46.2X1	T46.2X2	T46.2X3	T46.2X4	T46.2X5	T46.2X6
Quinine	T37.2X1	T37.2X2	T37.2X3	T37.2X4	T37.2X5	T37.2X6
Quiniobine	T37.8X1	T37.8X2	T37.8X3	T37.8X4	T37.8X5	T37.8X6
Quinisocaine	T49.1X1	T49.1X2	T49.1X3	T49.1X4	T49.1X5	T49.1X6
Quinocide	T37.2X1	T37.2X2	T37.2X3	T37.2X4	T37.2X5	T37.2X6
Quinoline (derivatives) NEC	T37.8X1	T37.8X2	T37.8X3	T37.8X4	T37.8X5	T37.8X6

Substance	Poisoning, Accidental (Unintentional)	Poisoning, Intentional Self-Harm	Poisoning, Assault	Poisoning, Undetermined	Adverse Effect	Underdosing
Quinupramine	T43.011	T43.012	T43.013	T43.014	T43.015	T43.016
Quotane	T41.3X1	T41.3X2	T41.3X3	T41.3X4	T41.3X5	T41.3X6
R						
Rabies						
immune globulin (human)	T50.Z11	T50.Z12	T50.Z13	T50.Z14	T50.Z15	T50.Z16
vaccine	T50.B91	T50.B92	T50.B93	T50.B94	T50.B95	T50.B96
Racemoramide	T40.2X1	T40.2X2	T40.2X3	T40.2X4	—	—
Racemorphan	T40.2X1	T40.2X2	T40.2X3	T40.2X4	T40.2X5	T40.2X6
Racepinefrin	T44.5X1	T44.5X2	T44.5X3	T44.5X4	T44.5X5	T44.5X6
Raclopride	T43.591	T43.592	T43.593	T43.594	T43.595	T43.596
Radiator alcohol	T51.1X1	T51.1X2	T51.1X3	T51.1X4	—	—
Radioactive drug NEC	T50.8X1	T50.8X2	T50.8X3	T50.8X4	T50.8X5	T50.8X6
Radio-opaque (drugs) (materials)	T50.8X1	T50.8X2	T50.8X3	T50.8X4	T50.8X5	T50.8X6
Ramifenazone	T39.2X1	T39.2X2	T39.2X3	T39.2X4	T39.2X5	T39.2X6
Ramipril	T46.4X1	T46.4X2	T46.4X3	T46.4X4	T46.4X5	T46.4X6
Ranitidine	T47.0X1	T47.0X2	T47.0X3	T47.0X4	T47.0X5	T47.0X6
Ranunculus	T62.2X1	T62.2X2	T62.2X3	T62.2X4	—	—
Rat poison NEC	T60.4X1	T60.4X2	T60.4X3	T60.4X4	—	—
Rattlesnake (venom)	T63.011	T63.012	T63.013	T63.014	—	—
Raubasine	T46.7X1	T46.7X2	T46.7X3	T46.7X4	T46.7X5	T46.7X6
Raudixin	T46.5X1	T46.5X2	T46.5X3	T46.5X4	T46.5X5	T46.5X6
Rautensin	T46.5X1	T46.5X2	T46.5X3	T46.5X4	T46.5X5	T46.5X6
Rautina	T46.5X1	T46.5X2	T46.5X3	T46.5X4	T46.5X5	T46.5X6
Rautotal	T46.5X1	T46.5X2	T46.5X3	T46.5X4	T46.5X5	T46.5X6
Rauwiloid	T46.5X1	T46.5X2	T46.5X3	T46.5X4	T46.5X5	T46.5X6
Rauwoldin	T46.5X1	T46.5X2	T46.5X3	T46.5X4	T46.5X5	T46.5X6
Rauwolfia (alkaloids)	T46.5X1	T46.5X2	T46.5X3	T46.5X4	T46.5X5	T46.5X6
Razoxane	T45.1X1	T45.1X2	T45.1X3	T45.1X4	T45.1X5	T45.1X6
Realgar	T57.0X1	T57.0X2	T57.0X3	T57.0X4	—	—
Recombinant (R) — see specific protein						
Red blood cells, packed	T45.8X1	T45.8X2	T45.8X3	T45.8X4	T45.8X5	T45.8X6
Red squill (scilliroside)	T60.4X1	T60.4X2	T60.4X3	T60.4X4	—	—
Reducing agent, industrial NEC	T65.891	T65.892	T65.893	T65.894	—	—
Refrigerant gas (chlorofluoro-carbon)	T53.5X1	T53.5X2	T53.5X3	T53.5X4	—	—
not chlorofluoro-carbon	T59.891	T59.892	T59.893	T59.894	—	—
Regroton	T50.2X1	T50.2X2	T50.2X3	T50.2X4	T50.2X5	T50.2X6
Rehydration salts (oral)	T50.3X1	T50.3X2	T50.3X3	T50.3X4	T50.3X5	T50.3X6
Rela	T42.8X1	T42.8X2	T42.8X3	T42.8X4	T42.8X5	T42.8X6

◀ New ◀◀ Revised ~~deleted~~ Deleted

Substance	Poisoning, Accidental (Unintentional)	Poisoning, Intentional Self-Harm	Poisoning, Assault	Poisoning, Undetermined	Adverse Effect	Underdosing
Relaxant, muscle						
anesthetic	T48.1X1	T48.1X2	T48.1X3	T48.1X4	T48.1X5	T48.1X6
central nervous system	T42.8X1	T42.8X2	T42.8X3	T42.8X4	T42.8X5	T42.8X6
skeletal NEC	T48.1X1	T48.1X2	T48.1X3	T48.1X4	T48.1X5	T48.1X6
smooth NEC	T44.3X1	T44.3X2	T44.3X3	T44.3X4	T44.3X5	T44.3X6
Remoxipride	T43.591	T43.592	T43.593	T43.594	T43.595	T43.596
Renese	T50.2X1	T50.2X2	T50.2X3	T50.2X4	T50.2X5	T50.2X6
Renografin	T50.8X1	T50.8X2	T50.8X3	T50.8X4	T50.8X5	T50.8X6
Replacement solution	T50.3X1	T50.3X2	T50.3X3	T50.3X4	T50.3X5	T50.3X6
Reproterol	T48.6X1	T48.6X2	T48.6X3	T48.6X4	T48.6X5	T48.6X6
Rescinnamine	T46.5X1	T46.5X2	T46.5X3	T46.5X4	T46.5X5	T46.5X6
Reserpin(e)	T46.5X1	T46.5X2	T46.5X3	T46.5X4	T46.5X5	T46.5X6
Resorcin, resorcinol (nonmedicinal)	T65.891	T65.892	T65.893	T65.894	—	—
medicinal	T49.4X1	T49.4X2	T49.4X3	T49.4X4	T49.4X5	T49.4X6
Respaire	T48.4X1	T48.4X2	T48.4X3	T48.4X4	T48.4X5	T48.4X6
Respiratory drug NEC	T48.901	T48.902	T48.903	T48.904	T48.905	T48.906
antiasthmatic NEC	T48.6X1	T48.6X2	T48.6X3	T48.6X4	T48.6X5	T48.6X6
anti-common-cold NEC	T48.5X1	T48.5X2	T48.5X3	T48.5X4	T48.5X5	T48.5X6
expectorant NEC	T48.4X1	T48.4X2	T48.4X3	T48.4X4	T48.4X5	T48.4X6
stimulant	T48.901	T48.902	T48.903	T48.904	T48.905	T48.906
Retinoic acid	T49.0X1	T49.0X2	T49.0X3	T49.0X4	T49.0X5	T49.0X6
Retinol	T45.2X1	T45.2X2	T45.2X3	T45.2X4	T45.2X5	T45.2X6
Rh (D) immune globulin (human)	T50.Z11	T50.Z12	T50.Z13	T50.Z14	T50.Z15	T50.Z16
Rhodine	T39.011	T39.012	T39.013	T39.014	T39.015	T39.016
RhoGAM	T50.Z11	T50.Z12	T50.Z13	T50.Z14	T50.Z15	T50.Z16
Rhubarb						
dry extract	T47.2X1	T47.2X2	T47.2X3	T47.2X4	T47.2X5	T47.2X6
tincture, compound	T47.2X1	T47.2X2	T47.2X3	T47.2X4	T47.2X5	T47.2X6
Ribavirin	T37.5X1	T37.5X2	T37.5X3	T37.5X4	T37.5X5	T37.5X6
Riboflavin	T45.2X1	T45.2X2	T45.2X3	T45.2X4	T45.2X5	T45.2X6
Ribostamycin	T36.5X1	T36.5X2	T36.5X3	T36.5X4	T36.5X5	T36.5X6
Ricin	T62.2X1	T62.2X2	T62.2X3	T62.2X4	—	—
Ricinus communis	T62.2X1	T62.2X2	T62.2X3	T62.2X4	—	—
Rickettsial vaccine NEC	T50.A91	T50.A92	T50.A93	T50.A94	T50.A95	T50.A96
Rifabutin	T36.6X1	T36.6X2	T36.6X3	T36.6X4	T36.6X5	T36.6X6
Rifamide	T36.6X1	T36.6X2	T36.6X3	T36.6X4	T36.6X5	T36.6X6
Rifampicin	T36.6X1	T36.6X2	T36.6X3	T36.6X4	T36.6X5	T36.6X6
with isoniazid	T37.1X1	T37.1X2	T37.1X3	T37.1X4	T37.1X5	T37.1X6
Rifampin	T36.6X1	T36.6X2	T36.6X3	T36.6X4	T36.6X5	T36.6X6
Rifamycin	T36.6X1	T36.6X2	T36.6X3	T36.6X4	T36.6X5	T36.6X6
Rifaximin	T36.6X1	T36.6X2	T36.6X3	T36.6X4	T36.6X5	T36.6X6

Substance	Poisoning, Accidental (Unintentional)	Poisoning, Intentional Self-Harm	Poisoning, Assault	Poisoning, Undetermined	Adverse Effect	Underdosing
Rimantadine	T37.5X1	T37.5X2	T37.5X3	T37.5X4	T37.5X5	T37.5X6
Rimazolium metilsulfate	T39.8X1	T39.8X2	T39.8X3	T39.8X4	T39.8X5	T39.8X6
Rimifon	T37.1X1	T37.1X2	T37.1X3	T37.1X4	T37.1X5	T37.1X6
Rimiterol	T48.6X1	T48.6X2	T48.6X3	T48.6X4	T48.6X5	T48.6X6
Ringer (lactate) solution	T50.3X1	T50.3X2	T50.3X3	T50.3X4	T50.3X5	T50.3X6
Ristocetin	T36.8X1	T36.8X2	T36.8X3	T36.8X4	T36.8X5	T36.8X6
Ritalin	T43.631	T43.632	T43.633	T43.634	T43.635	T43.636
Ritodrine	T44.5X1	T44.5X2	T44.5X3	T44.5X4	T44.5X5	T44.5X6
Roach killer — *see Insecticide*						
Rociverine	T44.3X1	T44.3X2	T44.3X3	T44.3X4	T44.3X5	T44.3X6
Rocky Mountain spotted fever vaccine	T50.A91	T50.A92	T50.A93	T50.A94	T50.A95	T50.A96
Rodenticide NEC	T60.4X1	T60.4X2	T60.4X3	T60.4X4	—	—
Rohypnol	T42.4X1	T42.4X2	T42.4X3	T42.4X4	T42.4X5	T42.4X6
Rokitamycin	T36.3X1	T36.3X2	T36.3X3	T36.3X4	T36.3X5	T36.3X6
Rolaids	T47.1X1	T47.1X2	T47.1X3	T47.1X4	T47.1X5	T47.1X6
Rolitetracycline	T36.4X1	T36.4X2	T36.4X3	T36.4X4	T36.4X5	T36.4X6
Romilar	T48.3X1	T48.3X2	T48.3X3	T48.3X4	T48.3X5	T48.3X6
Ronifibrate	T46.6X1	T46.6X2	T46.6X3	T46.6X4	T46.6X5	T46.6X6
Rosaprostol	T47.1X1	T47.1X2	T47.1X3	T47.1X4	T47.1X5	T47.1X6
Rose bengal sodium (131I)	T50.8X1	T50.8X2	T50.8X3	T50.8X4	T50.8X5	T50.8X6
Rose water ointment	T49.3X1	T49.3X2	T49.3X3	T49.3X4	T49.3X5	T49.3X6
Rosoxacin	T37.8X1	T37.8X2	T37.8X3	T37.8X4	T37.8X5	T37.8X6
Rotenone	T60.2X1	T60.2X2	T60.2X3	T60.2X4	—	—
Rotoxamine	T45.0X1	T45.0X2	T45.0X3	T45.0X4	T45.0X5	T45.0X6
Rough-on-rats	T60.4X1	T60.4X2	T60.4X3	T60.4X4	—	—
Roxatidine	T47.0X1	T47.0X2	T47.0X3	T47.0X4	T47.0X5	T47.0X6
Roxithromycin	T36.3X1	T36.3X2	T36.3X3	T36.3X4	T36.3X5	T36.3X6
Rt-PA	T45.611	T45.612	T45.613	T45.614	T45.615	T45.616
Rubbing alcohol	T51.2X1	T51.2X2	T51.2X3	T51.2X4	—	—
Rubefacient	T49.4X1	T49.4X2	T49.4X3	T49.4X4	T49.4X5	T49.4X6
Rubella vaccine	T50.B91	T50.B92	T50.B93	T50.B94	T50.B95	T50.B96
Rubelogen	T50.B91	T50.B92	T50.B93	T50.B94	T50.B95	T50.B96
Rubeovax	T50.991	T50.992	T50.993	T50.994	T50.995	T50.996
Rubidium chloride Rb82	T50.8X1	T50.8X2	T50.8X3	T50.8X4	T50.8X5	T50.8X6
Rubidomycin	T45.1X1	T45.1X2	T45.1X3	T45.1X4	T45.1X5	T45.1X6
Rue	T62.2X1	T62.2X2	T62.2X3	T62.2X4	—	—
Rufocromomycin	T45.1X1	T45.1X2	T45.1X3	T45.1X4	T45.1X5	T45.1X6
Russel's viper venin	T45.7X1	T45.7X2	T45.7X3	T45.7X4	T45.7X5	T45.7X6
Ruta (graveolens)	T62.2X1	T62.2X2	T62.2X3	T62.2X4	—	—
Rutinum	T46.991	T46.992	T46.993	T46.994	T46.995	T46.996
Rutoside	T46.991	T46.992	T46.993	T46.994	T46.995	T46.996

◀ New   ◀ Revised   ~~deleted~~ Deleted

TABLE OF DRUGS AND CHEMICALS

Substance	Poisoning, Accidental (Unintentional)	Poisoning, Intentional Self-Harm	Poisoning, Assault	Poisoning, Undetermined	Adverse Effect	Underdosing
S						
Sabadilla (plant)	T62.2X1	T62.2X2	T62.2X3	T62.2X4	—	—
pesticide	T60.2X1	T60.2X2	T60.2X3	T60.2X4	—	—
Saccharated iron oxide	T45.8X1	T45.8X2	T45.8X3	T45.8X4	T45.8X5	T45.8X6
Saccharin	T50.901	T50.902	T50.903	T50.904	T50.905	T50.906
Saccharomyces boulardii	T47.6X1	T47.6X2	T47.6X3	T47.6X4	T47.6X5	T47.6X6
Safflower oil	T46.6X1	T46.6X2	T46.6X3	T46.6X4	T46.6X5	T46.6X6
Safrazine	T43.1X1	T43.1X2	T43.1X3	T43.1X4	T43.1X5	T43.1X6
Salazosulfapyridine	T37.0X1	T37.0X2	T37.0X3	T37.0X4	T37.0X5	T37.0X6
Salbutamol	T48.6X1	T48.6X2	T48.6X3	T48.6X4	T48.6X5	T48.6X6
Salicylamide	T39.091	T39.092	T39.093	T39.094	T39.095	T39.096
Salicylate NEC	T39.091	T39.092	T39.093	T39.094	T39.095	T39.096
methyl	T49.3X1	T49.3X2	T49.3X3	T49.3X4	T49.3X5	T49.3X6
theobromine calcium	T50.2X1	T50.2X2	T50.2X3	T50.2X4	T50.2X5	T50.2X6
Salicylazosulfapyridine	T37.0X1	T37.0X2	T37.0X3	T37.0X4	T37.0X5	T37.0X6
Salicylhydroxamic acid	T49.0X1	T49.0X2	T49.0X3	T49.0X4	T49.0X5	T49.0X6
Salicylic acid	T49.4X1	T49.4X2	T49.4X3	T49.4X4	T49.4X5	T49.4X6
with benzoic acid	T49.4X1	T49.4X2	T49.4X3	T49.4X4	T49.4X5	T49.4X6
congeners	T39.091	T39.092	T39.093	T39.094	T39.095	T39.096
derivative	T39.091	T39.092	T39.093	T39.094	T39.095	T39.096
salts	T39.091	T39.092	T39.093	T39.094	T39.095	T39.096
Salinazid	T37.1X1	T37.1X2	T37.1X3	T37.1X4	T37.1X5	T37.1X6
Salmeterol	T48.6X1	T48.6X2	T48.6X3	T48.6X4	T48.6X5	T48.6X6
Salol	T49.3X1	T49.3X2	T49.3X3	T49.3X4	T49.3X5	T49.3X6
Salsalate	T39.091	T39.092	T39.093	T39.094	T39.095	T39.096
Salt substitute	T50.901	T50.902	T50.903	T50.904	T50.905	T50.906
Salt-replacing drug	T50.901	T50.902	T50.903	T50.904	T50.905	T50.906
Salt-retaining mineralocorticoid	T50.0X1	T50.0X2	T50.0X3	T50.0X4	T50.0X5	T50.0X6
Saluretic NEC	T50.2X1	T50.2X2	T50.2X3	T50.2X4	T50.2X5	T50.2X6
Saluron	T50.2X1	T50.2X2	T50.2X3	T50.2X4	T50.2X5	T50.2X6
Salvarsan 606 (neosilver) (silver)	T37.8X1	T37.8X2	T37.8X3	T37.8X4	T37.8X5	T37.8X6
Sambucus canadensis	T62.2X1	T62.2X2	T62.2X3	T62.2X4	—	—
berry	T62.1X1	T62.1X2	T62.1X3	T62.1X4	—	—
Sandril	T46.5X1	T46.5X2	T46.5X3	T46.5X4	T46.5X5	T46.5X6
Sanguinaria canadensis	T62.2X1	T62.2X2	T62.2X3	T62.2X4	—	—
Saniflush (cleaner)	T54.2X1	T54.2X2	T54.2X3	T54.2X4	—	—
Santonin	T37.4X1	T37.4X2	T37.4X3	T37.4X4	T37.4X5	T37.4X6
Santyl	T49.8X1	T49.8X2	T49.8X3	T49.8X4	T49.8X5	T49.8X6
Saralasin	T46.5X1	T46.5X2	T46.5X3	T46.5X4	T46.5X5	T46.5X6
Sarcolysin	T45.1X1	T45.1X2	T45.1X3	T45.1X4	T45.1X5	T45.1X6
Sarkomycin	T45.1X1	T45.1X2	T45.1X3	T45.1X4	T45.1X5	T45.1X6
Saroten	T43.011	T43.012	T43.013	T43.014	T43.015	T43.016

Substance	Poisoning, Accidental (Unintentional)	Poisoning, Intentional Self-Harm	Poisoning, Assault	Poisoning, Undetermined	Adverse Effect	Underdosing
Saturnine — see Lead						
Savin (oil)	T49.4X1	T49.4X2	T49.4X3	T49.4X4	T49.4X5	T49.4X6
Scammony	T47.2X1	T47.2X2	T47.2X3	T47.2X4	T47.2X5	T47.2X6
Scarlet red	T49.8X1	T49.8X2	T49.8X3	T49.8X4	T49.8X5	T49.8X6
Scheele's green	T57.0X1	T57.0X2	T57.0X3	T57.0X4	—	—
insecticide	T57.0X1	T57.0X2	T57.0X3	T57.0X4	—	—
Schizontozide (blood) (tissue)	T37.2X1	T37.2X2	T37.2X3	T37.2X4	T37.2X5	T37.2X6
Schradan	T60.0X1	T60.0X2	T60.0X3	T60.0X4	—	—
Schweinfurth green	T57.0X1	T57.0X2	T57.0X3	T57.0X4	—	—
insecticide	T57.0X1	T57.0X2	T57.0X3	T57.0X4	—	—
Scilla, rat poison	T60.4X1	T60.4X2	T60.4X3	T60.4X4	—	—
Scillaren	T60.4X1	T60.4X2	T60.4X3	T60.4X4	—	—
Sclerosing agent	T46.8X1	T46.8X2	T46.8X3	T46.8X4	T46.8X5	T46.8X6
Scombrotoxin	T61.11	T61.12	T61.13	T61.14	—	—
Scopolamine	T44.3X1	T44.3X2	T44.3X3	T44.3X4	T44.3X5	T44.3X6
Scopolia extract	T44.3X1	T44.3X2	T44.3X3	T44.3X4	T44.3X5	T44.3X6
Scouring powder	T65.891	T65.892	T65.893	T65.894	—	—
Sea						
anemone (sting)	T63.631	T63.632	T63.633	T63.634	—	—
cucumber (sting)	T63.691	T63.692	T63.693	T63.694	—	—
snake (bite) (venom)	T63.091	T63.092	T63.093	T63.094	—	—
urchin spine (puncture)	T63.691	T63.692	T63.693	T63.694	—	—
Seafood	T61.91	T61.92	T61.93	T61.94	—	—
specified NEC	T61.8X1	T61.8X2	T61.8X3	T61.8X4	—	—
Secbutabarbital	T42.3X1	T42.3X2	T42.3X3	T42.3X4	T42.3X5	T42.3X6
Secbutabarbitone	T42.3X1	T42.3X2	T42.3X3	T42.3X4	T42.3X5	T42.3X6
Secnidazole	T37.3X1	T37.3X2	T37.3X3	T37.3X4	T37.3X5	T37.3X6
Secobarbital	T42.3X1	T42.3X2	T42.3X3	T42.3X4	T42.3X5	T42.3X6
Seconal	T42.3X1	T42.3X2	T42.3X3	T42.3X4	T42.3X5	T42.3X6
Secretin	T50.8X1	T50.8X2	T50.8X3	T50.8X4	T50.8X5	T50.8X6
Sedative NEC	T42.71	T42.72	T42.73	T42.74	T42.75	T42.76
mixed NEC	T42.6X1	T42.6X2	T42.6X3	T42.6X4	T42.6X5	T42.6X6
Sedormid	T42.6X1	T42.6X2	T42.6X3	T42.6X4	T42.6X5	T42.6X6
Seed disinfectant or dressing	T60.8X1	T60.8X2	T60.8X3	T60.8X4	—	—
Seeds (poisonous)	T62.2X1	T62.2X2	T62.2X3	T62.2X4	—	—
Selegiline	T42.8X1	T42.8X2	T42.8X3	T42.8X4	T42.8X5	T42.8X6
Selenium NEC	T56.891	T56.892	T56.893	T56.894		
disulfide or sulfide	T49.4X1	T49.4X2	T49.4X3	T49.4X4	T49.4X5	T49.4X6
fumes	T59.891	T59.892	T59.893	T59.894	—	—
sulfide	T49.4X1	T49.4X2	T49.4X3	T49.4X4	T49.4X5	T49.4X6
Selenomethionine (75Se)	T50.8X1	T50.8X2	T50.8X3	T50.8X4	T50.8X5	T50.8X6
Selsun	T49.4X1	T49.4X2	T49.4X3	T49.4X4	T49.4X5	T49.4X6

◀ New ◀ Revised ~~deleted~~ Deleted

Substance	Poisoning, Accidental (Unintentional)	Poisoning, Intentional Self-Harm	Poisoning, Assault	Poisoning, Undetermined	Adverse Effect	Underdosing
Semustine	T45.1X1	T45.1X2	T45.1X3	T45.1X4	T45.1X5	T45.1X6
Senega syrup	T48.4X1	T48.4X2	T48.4X3	T48.4X4	T48.4X5	T48.4X6
Senna	T47.2X1	T47.2X2	T47.2X3	T47.2X4	T47.2X5	T47.2X6
Sennoside A+B	T47.2X1	T47.2X2	T47.2X3	T47.2X4	T47.2X5	T47.2X6
Septisol	T49.2X1	T49.2X2	T49.2X3	T49.2X4	T49.2X5	T49.2X6
Seractide	T38.811	T38.812	T38.813	T38.814	T38.815	T38.816
Serax	T42.4X1	T42.4X2	T42.4X3	T42.4X4	T42.4X5	T42.4X6
Serenesil	T42.6X1	T42.6X2	T42.6X3	T42.6X4	T42.6X5	T42.6X6
Serenium (hydrochloride)	T37.91	T37.92	T37.93	T37.94	T37.95	T37.96
Serepax — see Oxazepam						
Sermorelin	T38.891	T38.892	T38.893	T38.894	T38.895	T38.896
Sernyl	T41.1X1	T41.1X2	T41.1X3	T41.1X4	T41.1X5	T41.1X6
Serotonin	T50.991	T50.992	T50.993	T50.994	T50.995	T50.996
Serpasil	T46.5X1	T46.5X2	T46.5X3	T46.5X4	T46.5X5	T46.5X6
Serrapeptase	T45.3X1	T45.3X2	T45.3X3	T45.3X4	T45.3X5	T45.3X6
Serum						
antibotulinus	T50.Z11	T50.Z12	T50.Z13	T50.Z14	T50.Z15	T50.Z16
anticytotoxic	T50.Z11	T50.Z12	T50.Z13	T50.Z14	T50.Z15	T50.Z16
antidiphtheria	T50.Z11	T50.Z12	T50.Z13	T50.Z14	T50.Z15	T50.Z16
antimeningococcus	T50.Z11	T50.Z12	T50.Z13	T50.Z14	T50.Z15	T50.Z16
anti-Rh	T50.Z11	T50.Z12	T50.Z13	T50.Z14	T50.Z15	T50.Z16
anti-snake-bite	T50.Z11	T50.Z12	T50.Z13	T50.Z14	T50.Z15	T50.Z16
antitetanic	T50.Z11	T50.Z12	T50.Z13	T50.Z14	T50.Z15	T50.Z16
antitoxic	T50.Z11	T50.Z12	T50.Z13	T50.Z14	T50.Z15	T50.Z16
complement (inhibitor)	T45.8X1	T45.8X2	T45.8X3	T45.8X4	T45.8X5	T45.8X6
convalescent	T50.Z11	T50.Z12	T50.Z13	T50.Z14	T50.Z15	T50.Z16
hemolytic complement	T45.8X1	T45.8X2	T45.8X3	T45.8X4	T45.8X5	T45.8X6
immune (human)	T50.Z11	T50.Z12	T50.Z13	T50.Z14	T50.Z15	T50.Z16
protective NEC	T50.Z11	T50.Z12	T50.Z13	T50.Z14	T50.Z15	T50.Z16
Setastine	T45.0X1	T45.0X2	T45.0X3	T45.0X4	T45.0X5	T45.0X6
Setoperone	T43.591	T43.592	T43.593	T43.594	T43.595	T43.596
Sewer gas	T59.91	T59.92	T59.93	T59.94	—	—
Shampoo	T55.0X1	T55.0X2	T55.0X3	T55.0X4	—	—
Shellfish, noxious, nonbacterial	T61.781	T61.782	T61.783	T61.784	—	—
Sildenafil	T46.7X1	T46.7X2	T46.7X3	T46.7X4	T46.7X5	T46.7X6
Silibinin	T50.991	T50.992	T50.993	T50.994	T50.995	T50.996
Silicone NEC	T65.891	T65.892	T65.893	T65.894	—	—
medicinal	T49.3X1	T49.3X2	T49.3X3	T49.3X4	T49.3X5	T49.3X6
Silvadene	T49.0X1	T49.0X2	T49.0X3	T49.0X4	T49.0X5	T49.0X6
Silver	T49.0X1	T49.0X2	T49.0X3	T49.0X4	T49.0X5	T49.0X6
anti-infectives	T49.0X1	T49.0X2	T49.0X3	T49.0X4	T49.0X5	T49.0X6
arsphenamine	T37.8X1	T37.8X2	T37.8X3	T37.8X4	T37.8X5	T37.8X6

Substance	Poisoning, Accidental (Unintentional)	Poisoning, Intentional Self-Harm	Poisoning, Assault	Poisoning, Undetermined	Adverse Effect	Underdosing
Silver (Continued)						
colloidal	T49.0X1	T49.0X2	T49.0X3	T49.0X4	T49.0X5	T49.0X6
nitrate	T49.0X1	T49.0X2	T49.0X3	T49.0X4	T49.0X5	T49.0X6
ophthalmic preparation	T49.5X1	T49.5X2	T49.5X3	T49.5X4	T49.5X5	T49.5X6
toughened (keratolytic)	T49.4X1	T49.4X2	T49.4X3	T49.4X4	T49.4X5	T49.4X6
nonmedicinal (dust)	T56.891	T56.892	T56.893	T56.894	—	—
protein	T49.5X1	T49.5X2	T49.5X3	T49.5X4	T49.5X5	T49.5X6
salvarsan	T37.8X1	T37.8X2	T37.8X3	T37.8X4	T37.8X5	T37.8X6
sulfadiazine	T49.4X1	T49.4X2	T49.4X3	T49.4X4	T49.4X5	T49.4X6
Silymarin	T50.991	T50.992	T50.993	T50.994	T50.995	T50.996
Simaldrate	T47.1X1	T47.1X2	T47.1X3	T47.1X4	T47.1X5	T47.1X6
Simazine	T60.3X1	T60.3X2	T60.3X3	T60.3X4	—	—
Simethicone	T47.1X1	T47.1X2	T47.1X3	T47.1X4	T47.1X5	T47.1X6
Simfibrate	T46.6X1	T46.6X2	T46.6X3	T46.6X4	T46.6X5	T46.6X6
Simvastatin	T46.6X1	T46.6X2	T46.6X3	T46.6X4	T46.6X5	146.6X6
Sincalide	T50.8X1	T50.8X2	T50.8X3	T50.8X4	T50.8X5	T50.8X6
Sinequan	T43.011	T43.012	T43.013	T43.014	T43.015	T43.016
Singoserp	T46.5X1	T46.5X2	T46.5X3	T46.5X4	T46.5X5	T46.5X6
Sintrom	T45.511	T45.512	T45.513	T45.514	T45.515	T45.516
Sisomicin	T36.5X1	T36.5X2	T36.5X3	T36.5X4	T36.5X5	T36.5X6
Sitosterols	T46.6X1	T46.6X2	T46.6X3	T46.6X4	T46.6X5	T46.6X6
Skeletal muscle relaxants	T48.1X1	T48.1X2	T48.1X3	T48.1X4	T48.1X5	T48.1X6
Skin						
agents (external)	T49.91	T49.92	T49.93	T49.94	T49.95	T49.96
specified NEC	T49.8X1	T49.8X2	T49.8X3	T49.8X4	T49.8X5	T49.8X6
test antigen	T50.8X1	T50.8X2	T50.8X3	T50.8X4	T50.8X5	T50.8X6
Sleep-eze	T45.0X1	T45.0X2	T45.0X3	T45.0X4	T45.0X5	T45.0X6
Sleeping draught, pill	T42.71	T42.72	T42.73	T42.74	T42.75	T42.76
Smallpox vaccine	T50.B11	T50.B12	T50.B13	T50.B14	T50.B15	T50.B16
Smelter fumes NEC	T56.91	T56.92	T56.93	T56.94	—	—
Smog	T59.1X1	T59.1X2	T59.1X3	T59.1X4	—	—
Smoke NEC	T59.811	T59.812	T59.813	T59.814	—	—
Smooth muscle relaxant	T44.3X1	T44.3X2	T44.3X3	T44.3X4	T44.3X5	T44.3X6
Snail killer NEC	T60.8X1	T60.8X2	T60.8X3	T60.8X4	—	—
Snake venom or bite	T63.001	T63.002	T63.003	T63.004	—	—
hemocoagulase	T45.7X1	T45.7X2	T45.7X3	T45.7X4	T45.7X5	T45.7X6
Snuff	T65.211	T65.212	T65.213	T65.214	—	—
Soap (powder) (product)	T55.0X1	T55.0X2	T55.0X3	T55.0X4	—	—
enema	T47.4X1	T47.4X2	T47.4X3	T47.4X4	T47.4X5	T47.4X6
medicinal, soft	T49.2X1	T49.2X2	T49.2X3	T49.2X4	T49.2X5	T49.2X6
superfatted	T49.2X1	T49.2X2	T49.2X3	T49.2X4	T49.2X5	T49.2X6
Sobrerol	T48.4X1	T48.4X2	T48.4X3	T48.4X4	T48.4X5	T48.4X6

◀ New   ◀ Revised   ~~deleted~~ Deleted

TABLE OF DRUGS AND CHEMICALS

TABLE OF DRUGS AND CHEMICALS

Substance	External Cause (T-Code)					
	Poisoning, Accidental (Unintentional)	Poisoning, Intentional Self-Harm	Poisoning, Assault	Poisoning, Undetermined	Adverse Effect	Underdosing
Soda (caustic)	T54.3X1	T54.3X2	T54.3X3	T54.3X4	—	—
bicarb	T47.1X1	T47.1X2	T47.1X3	T47.1X4	T47.1X5	T47.1X6
chlorinated — see Sodium, hypochlorite						
Sodium						
acetosulfone	T37.1X1	T37.1X2	T37.1X3	T37.1X4	T37.1X5	T37.1X6
acetrizoate	T50.8X1	T50.8X2	T50.8X3	T50.8X4	T50.8X5	T50.8X6
acid phosphate	T50.3X1	T50.3X2	T50.3X3	T50.3X4	T50.3X5	T50.3X6
alginate	T47.8X1	T47.8X2	T47.8X3	T47.8X4	T47.8X5	T47.8X6
amidotrizoate	T50.8X1	T50.8X2	T50.8X3	T50.8X4	T50.8X5	T50.8X6
aminopterin	T45.1X1	T45.1X2	T45.1X3	T45.1X4	T45.1X5	T45.1X6
amylosulfate	T47.8X1	T47.8X2	T47.8X3	T47.8X4	T47.8X5	T47.8X6
amytal	T42.3X1	T42.3X2	T42.3X3	T42.3X4	T42.3X5	T42.3X6
antimony gluconate	T37.3X1	T37.3X2	T37.3X3	T37.3X4	T37.3X5	T37.3X6
arsenate	T57.0X1	T57.0X2	T57.0X3	T57.0X4	—	—
aurothiomalate	T39.4X1	T39.4X2	T39.4X3	T39.4X4	T39.4X5	T39.4X6
aurothiosulfate	T39.4X1	T39.4X2	T39.4X3	T39.4X4	T39.4X5	T39.4X6
barbiturate	T42.3X1	T42.3X2	T42.3X3	T42.3X4	T42.3X5	T42.3X6
basic phosphate	T47.4X1	T47.4X2	T47.4X3	T47.4X4	T47.4X5	T47.4X6
bicarbonate	T47.1X1	T47.1X2	T47.1X3	T47.1X4	T47.1X5	T47.1X6
bichromate	T57.8X1	T57.8X2	T57.8X3	T57.8X4	—	—
biphosphate	T50.3X1	T50.3X2	T50.3X3	T50.3X4	T50.3X5	T50.3X6
bisulfate	T65.891	T65.892	T65.893	T65.894	—	—
borate						
cleanser	T57.8X1	T57.8X2	T57.8X3	T57.8X4	—	—
eye	T49.5X1	T49.5X2	T49.5X3	T49.5X4	T49.5X5	T49.5X6
therapeutic	T49.8X1	T49.8X2	T49.8X3	T49.8X4	T49.8X5	T49.8X6
bromide	T42.6X1	T42.6X2	T42.6X3	T42.6X4	T42.6X5	T42.6X6
cacodylate (nonmedicinal) NEC	T50.8X1	T50.8X2	T50.8X3	T50.8X4	T50.8X5	T50.8X6
anti-infective	T37.8X1	T37.8X2	T37.8X3	T37.8X4	T37.8X5	T37.8X6
herbicide	T60.3X1	T60.3X2	T60.3X3	T60.3X4	—	—
calcium edetate	T45.8X1	T45.8X2	T45.8X3	T45.8X4	T45.8X5	T45.8X6
carbonate NEC	T54.3X1	T54.3X2	T54.3X3	T54.3X4	—	—
chlorate NEC	T65.891	T65.892	T65.893	T65.894	—	—
herbicide	T54.91	T54.92	T54.93	T54.94	—	—
chloride	T50.3X1	T50.3X2	T50.3X3	T50.3X4	T50.3X5	T50.3X6
with glucose	T50.3X1	T50.3X2	T50.3X3	T50.3X4	T50.3X5	T50.3X6
chromate	T65.891	T65.892	T65.893	T65.894	—	—
citrate	T50.991	T50.992	T50.993	T50.994	T50.995	T50.996
cromoglicate	T48.6X1	T48.6X2	T48.6X3	T48.6X4	T48.6X5	T48.6X6
cyanide	T65.0X1	T65.0X2	T65.0X3	T65.0X4	—	—
cyclamate	T50.3X1	T50.3X2	T50.3X3	T50.3X4	T50.3X5	T50.3X6

Substance	External Cause (T-Code)					
	Poisoning, Accidental (Unintentional)	Poisoning, Intentional Self-Harm	Poisoning, Assault	Poisoning, Undetermined	Adverse Effect	Underdosing
Sodium (Continued)						
dehydrocholate	T45.8X1	T45.8X2	T45.8X3	T45.8X4	T45.8X5	T45.8X6
diatrizoate	T50.8X1	T50.8X2	T50.8X3	T50.8X4	T50.8X5	T50.8X6
dibunate	T48.4X1	T48.4X2	T48.4X3	T48.4X4	T48.4X5	T48.4X6
dioctyl sulfosuccinate	T47.4X1	T47.4X2	T47.4X3	T47.4X4	T47.4X5	T47.4X6
dipantoyl ferrate	T45.8X1	T45.8X2	T45.8X3	T45.8X4	T45.8X5	T45.8X6
edetate	T45.8X1	T45.8X2	T45.8X3	T45.8X4	T45.8X5	T45.8X6
ethacrynate	T50.1X1	T50.1X2	T50.1X3	T50.1X4	T50.1X5	T50.1X6
feredetate	T45.8X1	T45.8X2	T45.8X3	T45.8X4	T45.8X5	T45.8X6
Fluoride — see Fluoride						
fluoroacetate (dust) (pesticide)	T60.4X1	T60.4X2	T60.4X3	T60.4X4	—	—
free salt	T50.3X1	T50.3X2	T50.3X3	T50.3X4	T50.3X5	T50.3X6
fusidate	T36.8X1	T36.8X2	T36.8X3	T36.8X4	T36.8X5	T36.8X6
glucaldrate	T47.1X1	T47.1X2	T47.1X3	T47.1X4	T47.1X5	T47.1X6
glucosulfone	T37.1X1	T37.1X2	T37.1X3	T37.1X4	T37.1X5	T37.1X6
glutamate	T45.8X1	T45.8X2	T45.8X3	T45.8X4	T45.8X5	T45.8X6
hydrogen carbonate	T50.3X1	T50.3X2	T50.3X3	T50.3X4	T50.3X5	T50.3X6
hydroxide	T54.3X1	T54.3X2	T54.3X3	T54.3X4	—	—
hypochlorite (bleach) NEC	T54.3X1	T54.3X2	T54.3X3	T54.3X4	—	—
disinfectant	T54.3X1	T54.3X2	T54.3X3	T54.3X4	—	—
medicinal (anti-infective) (external)	T49.0X1	T49.0X2	T49.0X3	T49.0X4	T49.0X5	T49.0X6
vapor	T54.3X1	T54.3X2	T54.3X3	T54.3X4	—	—
hyposulfite	T49.0X1	T49.0X2	T49.0X3	T49.0X4	T49.0X5	T49.0X6
indigotin disulfonate	T50.8X1	T50.8X2	T50.8X3	T50.8X4	T50.8X5	T50.8X6
iodide	T50.991	T50.992	T50.993	T50.994	T50.995	T50.996
I-131	T50.8X1	T50.8X2	T50.8X3	T50.8X4	T50.8X5	T50.8X6
therapeutic	T38.2X1	T38.2X2	T38.2X3	T38.2X4	T38.2X5	T38.2X6
iodohippurate (131I)	T50.8X1	T50.8X2	T50.8X3	T50.8X4	T50.8X5	T50.8X6
iopodate	T50.8X1	T50.8X2	T50.8X3	T50.8X4	T50.8X5	T50.8X6
iothalamate	T50.8X1	T50.8X2	T50.8X3	T50.8X4	T50.8X5	T50.8X6
iron edetate	T45.4X1	T45.4X2	T45.4X3	T45.4X4	T45.4X5	T45.4X6
lactate (compound solution)	T45.8X1	T45.8X2	T45.8X3	T45.8X4	T45.8X5	T45.8X6
lauryl (sulfate)	T49.2X1	T49.2X2	T49.2X3	T49.2X4	T49.2X5	T49.2X6
(L)-triiodothyronine	T38.1X1	T38.1X2	T38.1X3	T38.1X4	T38.1X5	T38.1X6
magnesium citrate	T50.991	T50.992	T50.993	T50.994	T50.995	T50.996
mersalate	T50.2X1	T50.2X2	T50.2X3	T50.2X4	T50.2X5	T50.2X6
metasilicate	T65.891	T65.892	T65.893	T65.894	—	—
metrizoate	T50.8X1	T50.8X2	T50.8X3	T50.8X4	T50.8X5	T50.8X6
monofluoroacetate (pesticide)	T60.1X1	T60.1X2	T60.1X3	T60.1X4	—	—
morrhuate	T46.8X1	T46.8X2	T46.8X3	T46.8X4	T46.8X5	T46.8X6
nafcillin	T36.0X1	T36.0X2	T36.0X3	T36.0X4	T36.0X5	T36.0X6

◀ New ◀ Revised ~~deleted~~ Deleted

Substance	External Cause (T-Code)					
	Poisoning, Accidental (Unintentional)	Poisoning, Intentional Self-Harm	Poisoning, Assault	Poisoning, Undetermined	Adverse Effect	Underdosing
Sodium *(Continued)*						
nitrate (oxidizing agent)	T65.891	T65.892	T65.893	T65.894	—	—
nitrite	T50.6X1	T50.6X2	T50.6X3	T50.6X4	T50.6X5	T50.6X6
nitroferricyanide	T46.5X1	T46.5X2	T46.5X3	T46.5X4	T46.5X5	T46.5X6
nitroprusside	T46.5X1	T46.5X2	T46.5X3	T46.5X4	T46.5X5	T46.5X6
oxalate	T65.891	T65.892	T65.893	T65.894	—	—
oxide/peroxide	T65.891	T65.892	T65.893	T65.894	—	—
oxybate	T41.291	T41.292	T41.293	T41.294	T41.295	T41.296
para-aminohippurate	T50.8X1	T50.8X2	T50.8X3	T50.8X4	T50.8X5	T50.8X6
perborate (nonmedicinal) NEC	T65.891	T65.892	T65.893	T65.894	—	—
medicinal	T49.0X1	T49.0X2	T49.0X3	T49.0X4	T49.0X5	T49.0X6
soap	T55.0X1	T55.0X2	T55.0X3	T55.0X4	—	—
percarbonate — *see Sodium, perborate*						
pertechnetate Tc99m	T50.8X1	T50.8X2	T50.8X3	T50.8X4	T50.8X5	T50.8X6
phosphate						
cellulose	T45.8X1	T45.8X2	T45.8X3	T45.8X4	T45.8X5	T45.8X6
dibasic	T47.2X1	T47.2X2	T47.2X3	T47.2X4	T47.2X5	T47.2X6
monobasic	T47.2X1	T47.2X2	T47.2X3	T47.2X4	T47.2X5	T47.2X6
phytate	T50.6X1	T50.6X2	T50.6X3	T50.6X4	T50.6X5	T50.6X6
picosulfate	T47.2X1	T47.2X2	T47.2X3	T47.2X4	T47.2X5	T47.2X6
polyhydroxyaluminium monocarbonate	T47.1X1	T47.1X2	T47.1X3	T47.1X4	T47.1X5	T47.1X6
polystyrene sulfonate	T50.3X1	T50.3X2	T50.3X3	T50.3X4	T50.3X5	T50.3X6
propionate	T49.0X1	T49.0X2	T49.0X3	T49.0X4	T49.0X5	T49.0X6
propyl hydroxybenzoate	T50.991	T50.992	T50.993	T50.994	T50.995	T50.996
psylliate	T46.8X1	T46.8X2	T46.8X3	T46.8X4	T46.8X5	T46.8X6
removing resins	T50.3X1	T50.3X2	T50.3X3	T50.3X4	T50.3X5	T50.3X6
salicylate	T39.091	T39.092	T39.093	T39.094	T39.095	T39.096
salt NEC	T50.3X1	T50.3X2	T50.3X3	T50.3X4	T50.3X5	T50.3X6
selenate	T60.2X1	T60.2X2	T60.2X3	T60.2X4	—	—
stibogluconate	T37.3X1	T37.3X2	T37.3X3	T37.3X4	T37.3X5	T37.3X6
sulfate	T47.4X1	T47.4X2	T47.4X3	T47.4X4	T47.4X5	T47.4X6
sulfoxone	T37.1X1	T37.1X2	T37.1X3	T37.1X4	T37.1X5	T37.1X6
tetradecyl sulfate	T46.8X1	T46.8X2	T46.8X3	T46.8X4	T46.8X5	T46.8X6
thiopental	T41.1X1	T41.1X2	T41.1X3	T41.1X4	T41.1X5	T41.1X6
thiosalicylate	T39.091	T39.092	T39.093	T39.094	T39.095	T39.096
thiosulfate	T50.6X1	T50.6X2	T50.6X3	T50.6X4	T50.6X5	T50.6X6
tolbutamide	T38.3X1	T38.3X2	T38.3X3	T38.3X4	T38.3X5	T38.3X6
l-triiodothyronine	T38.1X1	T38.1X2	T38.1X3	T38.1X4	T38.1X5	T38.1X6
tyropanoate	T50.8X1	T50.8X2	T50.8X3	T50.8X4	T50.8X5	T50.8X6
valproate	T42.6X1	T42.6X2	T42.6X3	T42.6X4	T42.6X5	T42.6X6
versenate	T50.6X1	T50.6X2	T50.6X3	T50.6X4	T50.6X5	T50.6X6

Substance	External Cause (T-Code)					
	Poisoning, Accidental (Unintentional)	Poisoning, Intentional Self-Harm	Poisoning, Assault	Poisoning, Undetermined	Adverse Effect	Underdosing
Sodium-free salt	T50.901	T50.902	T50.903	T50.904	T50.905	T50.906
Sodium-removing resin	T50.3X1	T50.3X2	T50.3X3	T50.3X4	T50.3X5	T50.3X6
Soft soap	T55.0X1	T55.0X2	T55.0X3	T55.0X4	—	—
Solanine	T62.2X1	T62.2X2	T62.2X3	T62.2X4	—	—
berries	T62.1X1	T62.1X2	T62.1X3	T62.1X4	—	—
Solanum dulcamara	T62.2X1	T62.2X2	T62.2X3	T62.2X4	—	—
berries	T62.1X1	T62.1X2	T62.1X3	T62.1X4	—	—
Solapsone	T37.1X1	T37.1X2	T37.1X3	T37.1X4	T37.1X5	T37.1X6
Solar lotion	T49.3X1	T49.3X2	T49.3X3	T49.3X4	T49.3X5	T49.3X6
Solasulfone	T37.1X1	T37.1X2	T37.1X3	T37.1X4	T37.1X5	T37.1X6
Soldering fluid	T65.891	T65.892	T65.893	T65.894		
Solid substance	T65.91	T65.92	T65.93	T65.94	—	—
specified NEC	T65.891	T65.892	T65.893	T65.894	—	—
Solvent, industrial NEC	T52.91	T52.92	T52.93	T52.94		
naphtha	T52.0X1	T52.0X2	T52.0X3	T52.0X4	—	—
petroleum	T52.0X1	T52.0X2	T52.0X3	T52.0X4	—	—
specified NEC	T52.8X1	T52.8X2	T52.8X3	T52.8X4	—	—
Soma	T42.8X1	T42.8X2	T42.8X3	T42.8X4	T42.8X5	T42.8X6
Somatorelin	T38.891	T38.892	T38.893	T38.894	T38.895	T38.896
Somatostatin	T38.991	T38.992	T38.993	T38.994	T38.995	T38.996
Somatotropin	T38.811	T38.812	T38.813	T38.814	T38.815	T38.816
Somatrem	T38.811	T38.812	T38.813	T38.814	T38.815	T38.816
Somatropin	T38.811	T38.812	T38.813	T38.814	T38.815	T38.816
Sominex	T45.0X1	T45.0X2	T45.0X3	T45.0X4	T45.0X5	T45.0X6
Somnos	T42.6X1	T42.6X2	T42.6X3	T42.6X4	T42.6X5	T42.6X6
Somonal	T42.3X1	T42.3X2	T42.3X3	T42.3X4	T42.3X5	T42.3X6
Soneryl	T42.3X1	T42.3X2	T42.3X3	T42.3X4	T42.3X5	T42.3X6
Soothing syrup	T50.901	T50.902	T50.903	T50.904	T50.905	T50.906
Sopor	T42.6X1	T42.6X2	T42.6X3	T42.6X4	T42.6X5	T42.6X6
Soporific	T42.71	T42.72	T42.73	T42.74	T42.75	T42.76
Soporific drug	T42.71	T42.72	T42.73	T42.74	T42.75	T42.76
specified type NEC	T42.6X1	T42.6X2	T42.6X3	T42.6X4	T42.6X5	T42.6X6
Sorbide nitrate	T46.3X1	T46.3X2	T46.3X3	T46.3X4	T46.3X5	T46.3X6
Sorbitol	T47.4X1	T47.4X2	T47.4X3	T47.4X4	T47.4X5	T47.4X6
Sotalol	T44.7X1	T44.7X2	T44.7X3	T44.7X4	T44.7X5	T44.7X6
Sotradecol	T46.8X1	T46.8X2	T46.8X3	T46.8X4	T46.8X5	T46.8X6
Soysterol	T46.6X1	T46.6X2	T46.6X3	T46.6X4	T46.6X5	T46.6X6
Spacoline	T44.3X1	T44.3X2	T44.3X3	T44.3X4	T44.3X5	T44.3X6
Spanish fly	T49.8X1	T49.8X2	T49.8X3	T49.8X4	T49.8X5	T49.8X6
Sparine	T43.3X1	T43.3X2	T43.3X3	T43.3X4	T43.3X5	T43.3X6
Sparteine	T48.0X1	T48.0X2	T48.0X3	T48.0X4	T48.0X5	T48.0X6

◀ New ◀ Revised ~~deleted~~ Deleted

TABLE OF DRUGS AND CHEMICALS

TABLE OF DRUGS AND CHEMICALS

| | External Cause (T-Code) | | | | | |
Substance	Poisoning, Accidental (Unintentional)	Poisoning, Intentional Self-Harm	Poisoning, Assault	Poisoning, Undetermined	Adverse Effect	Underdosing
Spasmolytic						
anticholinergics	T44.3X1	T44.3X2	T44.3X3	T44.3X4	T44.3X5	T44.3X6
autonomic	T44.3X1	T44.3X2	T44.3X3	T44.3X4	T44.3X5	T44.3X6
bronchial NEC	T48.6X1	T48.6X2	T48.6X3	T48.6X4	T48.6X5	T48.6X6
quaternary ammonium	T44.3X1	T44.3X2	T44.3X3	T44.3X4	T44.3X5	T44.3X6
skeletal muscle NEC	T48.1X1	T48.1X2	T48.1X3	T48.1X4	T48.1X5	T48.1X6
Spectinomycin	T36.5X1	T36.5X2	T36.5X3	T36.5X4	T36.5X5	T36.5X6
Speed	T43.621	T43.622	T43.623	T43.624	T43.625	T43.626
Spermicide	T49.8X1	T49.8X2	T49.8X3	T49.8X4	T49.8X5	T49.8X6
Spider (bite) (venom)	T63.391	T63.392	T63.393	T63.394	—	—
antivenin	T50.Z11	T50.Z12	T50.Z13	T50.Z14	T50.Z15	T50.Z16
Spigelia (root)	T37.4X1	T37.4X2	T37.4X3	T37.4X4	T37.4X5	T37.4X6
Spindle inactivator	T50.4X1	T50.4X2	T50.4X3	T50.4X4	T50.4X5	T50.4X6
Spiperone	T43.4X1	T43.4X2	T43.4X3	T43.4X4	T43.4X5	T43.4X6
Spiramycin	T36.3X1	T36.3X2	T36.3X3	T36.3X4	T36.3X5	T36.3X6
Spirapril	T46.4X1	T46.4X2	T46.4X3	T46.4X4	T46.4X5	T46.4X6
Spirilene	T43.591	T43.592	T43.593	T43.594	T43.595	T43.596
Spirit(s) (neutral) NEC	T51.0X1	T51.0X2	T51.0X3	T51.0X4	—	—
beverage	T51.0X1	T51.0X2	T51.0X3	T51.0X4	—	—
industrial	T51.0X1	T51.0X2	T51.0X3	T51.0X4	—	—
mineral	T52.0X1	T52.0X2	T52.0X3	T52.0X4	—	—
of salt — see Hydrochloric acid						
surgical	T51.0X1	T51.0X2	T51.0X3	T51.0X4	—	—
Spironolactone	T50.0X1	T50.0X2	T50.0X3	T50.0X4	T50.0X5	T50.0X6
Spiroperidol	T43.4X1	T43.4X2	T43.4X3	T43.4X4	T43.4X5	T43.4X6
Sponge, absorbable (gelatin)	T45.7X1	T45.7X2	T45.7X3	T45.7X4	T45.7X5	T45.7X6
Sporostacin	T49.0X1	T49.0X2	T49.0X3	T49.0X4	T49.0X5	T49.0X6
Spray (aerosol)	T65.91	T65.92	T65.93	T65.94	—	—
cosmetic	T65.891	T65.892	T65.893	T65.894	—	—
medicinal NEC	T50.901	T50.902	T50.903	T50.904	T50.905	T50.906
pesticides — see Pesticides						
specified content — see specific substance						
Spurge flax	T62.2X1	T62.2X2	T62.2X3	T62.2X4	—	—
Spurges	T62.2X1	T62.2X2	T62.2X3	T62.2X4	—	—
Sputum viscosity-lowering drug	T48.4X1	T48.4X2	T48.4X3	T48.4X4	T48.4X5	T48.4X6
Squill	T46.0X1	T46.0X2	T46.0X3	T46.0X4	T46.0X5	T46.0X6
rat poison	T60.4X1	T60.4X2	T60.4X3	T60.4X4	—	—
Squirting cucumber (cathartic)	T47.2X1	T47.2X2	T47.2X3	T47.2X4	T47.2X5	T47.2X6
Stains	T65.6X1	T65.6X2	T65.6X3	T65.6X4	—	—
Stannous fluoride	T49.7X1	T49.7X2	T49.7X3	T49.7X4	T49.7X5	T49.7X6
Stanolone	T38.7X1	T38.7X2	T38.7X3	T38.7X4	T38.7X5	T38.7X6

| | External Cause (T-Code) | | | | | |
Substance	Poisoning, Accidental (Unintentional)	Poisoning, Intentional Self-Harm	Poisoning, Assault	Poisoning, Undetermined	Adverse Effect	Underdosing
Stanozolol	T38.7X1	T38.7X2	T38.7X3	T38.7X4	T38.7X5	T38.7X6
Staphisagria or stavesacre (pediculicide)	T49.0X1	T49.0X2	T49.0X3	T49.0X4	T49.0X5	T49.0X6
Starch	T50.901	T50.902	T50.903	T50.904	T50.905	T50.906
Stelazine	T43.3X1	T43.3X2	T43.3X3	T43.3X4	T43.3X5	T43.3X6
Stemetil	T43.3X1	T43.3X2	T43.3X3	T43.3X4	T43.3X5	T43.3X6
Stepronin	T48.4X1	T48.4X2	T48.4X3	T48.4X4	T48.4X5	T48.4X6
Sterculia	T47.4X1	T47.4X2	T47.4X3	T47.4X4	T47.4X5	T47.4X6
Sternutator gas	T59.891	T59.892	T59.893	T59.894	—	—
Steroid	T38.0X1	T38.0X2	T38.0X3	T38.0X4	T38.0X5	T38.0X6
anabolic	T38.7X1	T38.7X2	T38.7X3	T38.7X4	T38.7X5	T38.7X6
androgenic	T38.7X1	T38.7X2	T38.7X3	T38.7X4	T38.7X5	T38.7X6
antineoplastic, hormone	T38.7X1	T38.7X2	T38.7X3	T38.7X4	T38.7X5	T38.7X6
estrogen	T38.5X1	T38.5X2	T38.5X3	T38.5X4	T38.5X5	T38.5X6
ENT agent	T49.6X1	T49.6X2	T49.6X3	T49.6X4	T49.6X5	T49.6X6
ophthalmic preparation	T49.5X1	T49.5X2	T49.5X3	T49.5X4	T49.5X5	T49.5X6
topical NEC	T49.0X1	T49.0X2	T49.0X3	T49.0X4	T49.0X5	T49.0X6
Stibine	T56.891	T56.892	T56.893	T56.894	—	—
Stibogluconate	T37.3X1	T37.3X2	T37.3X3	T37.3X4	T37.3X5	T37.3X6
Stibophen	T37.4X1	T37.4X2	T37.4X3	T37.4X4	T37.4X5	T37.4X6
Stilbamidine (isetionate)	T37.3X1	T37.3X2	T37.3X3	T37.3X4	T37.3X5	T37.3X6
Stilbestrol	T38.5X1	T38.5X2	T38.5X3	T38.5X4	T38.5X5	T38.5X6
Stilboestrol	T38.5X1	T38.5X2	T38.5X3	T38.5X4	T38.5X5	T38.5X6
Stimulant						
central nervous system — see also Psychostimulant	T43.601	T43.602	T43.603	T43.604	T43.605	T43.606
analeptics	T50.7X1	T50.7X2	T50.7X3	T50.7X4	T50.7X5	T50.7X6
opiate antagonist	T50.7X1	T50.7X2	T50.7X3	T50.7X4	T50.7X5	T50.7X6
psychotherapeutic NEC — see also Psychotherapeutic drug	T43.601	T43.602	T43.603	T43.604	T43.605	T43.606
specified NEC	T43.691	T43.692	T43.693	T43.694	T43.695	T43.696
respiratory	T48.901	T48.902	T48.903	T48.904	T48.905	T48.906
Stone-dissolving drug	T50.901	T50.902	T50.903	T50.904	T50.905	T50.906
Storage battery (cells) (acid)	T54.2X1	T54.2X2	T54.2X3	T54.2X4	—	—
Stovaine	T41.3X1	T41.3X2	T41.3X3	T41.3X4	T41.3X5	T41.3X6
infiltration (subcutaneous)	T41.3X1	T41.3X2	T41.3X3	T41.3X4	T41.3X5	T41.3X6
nerve block (peripheral) (plexus)	T41.3X1	T41.3X2	T41.3X3	T41.3X4	T41.3X5	T41.3X6
spinal	T41.3X1	T41.3X2	T41.3X3	T41.3X4	T41.3X5	T41.3X6
topical (surface)	T41.3X1	T41.3X2	T41.3X3	T41.3X4	T41.3X5	T41.3X6
Stovarsal	T37.8X1	T37.8X2	T37.8X3	T37.8X4	T37.8X5	T37.8X6
Stove gas — see Gas, stove	T57.91	T57.92	T57.93	T57.94	—	—

◄ New   ◄ Revised   ~~deleted~~ Deleted

Substance	Poisoning, Accidental (Unintentional)	Poisoning, Intentional Self-Harm	Poisoning, Assault	Poisoning, Undetermined	Adverse Effect	Underdosing
Stoxil	T49.5X1	T49.5X2	T49.5X3	T49.5X4	T49.5X5	T49.5X6
Stramonium	T48.6X1	T48.6X2	T48.6X3	T48.6X4	T48.6X5	T48.6X6
natural state	T62.2X1	T62.2X2	T62.2X3	T62.2X4	—	—
Streptodornase	T45.3X1	T45.3X2	T45.3X3	T45.3X4	T45.3X5	T45.3X6
Streptoduocin	T36.5X1	T36.5X2	T36.5X3	T36.5X4	T36.5X5	T36.5X6
Streptokinase	T45.611	T45.612	T45.613	T45.614	T45.615	T45.616
Streptomycin (derivative)	T36.5X1	T36.5X2	T36.5X3	T36.5X4	T36.5X5	T36.5X6
Streptonivicin	T36.5X1	T36.5X2	T36.5X3	T36.5X4	T36.5X5	T36.5X6
Streptovarycin	T36.5X1	T36.5X2	T36.5X3	T36.5X4	T36.5X5	T36.5X6
Streptozocin	T45.1X1	T45.1X2	T45.1X3	T45.1X4	T45.1X5	T45.1X6
Streptozotocin	T45.1X1	T45.1X2	T45.1X3	T45.1X4	T45.1X5	T45.1X6
Stripper (paint) (solvent)	T52.8X1	T52.8X2	T52.8X3	T52.8X4	—	—
Strobane	T60.1X1	T60.1X2	T60.1X3	T60.1X4	—	—
Strofantina	T46.0X1	T46.0X2	T46.0X3	T46.0X4	T46.0X5	T46.0X6
Strophanthin (g) (k)	T46.0X1	T46.0X2	T46.0X3	T46.0X4	T46.0X5	T46.0X6
Strophanthus	T46.0X1	T46.0X2	T46.0X3	T46.0X4	T46.0X5	T46.0X6
Strophantin	T46.0X1	T46.0X2	T46.0X3	T46.0X4	T46.0X5	T46.0X6
Strophantin-g	T46.0X1	T46.0X2	T46.0X3	T46.0X4	T46.0X5	T46.0X6
Strychnine (nonmedicinal) (pesticide) (salts)	T65.1X1	T65.1X2	T65.1X3	T65.1X4	—	—
medicinal	T48.291	T48.292	T48.293	T48.294	T48.295	T48.296
Strychnos (ignatii) — see Strychnine						
Styramate	T42.8X1	T42.8X2	T42.8X3	T42.8X4	T42.8X5	T42.8X6
Styrene	T65.891	T65.892	T65.893	T65.894	—	—
Succinimide, antiepileptic or anticonvulsant	T42.2X1	T42.2X2	T42.2X3	T42.2X4	T42.2X5	T42.2X6
mercuric — see Mercury						
Succinylcholine	T48.1X1	T48.1X2	T48.1X3	T48.1X4	T48.1X5	T48.1X6
Succinylsulfathiazole	T37.0X1	T37.0X2	T37.0X3	T37.0X4	T37.0X5	T37.0X6
Sucralfate	T47.1X1	T47.1X2	T47.1X3	T47.1X4	T47.1X5	T47.1X6
Sucrose	T50.3X1	T50.3X2	T50.3X3	T50.3X4	T50.3X5	T50.3X6
Sufentanil	T40.411	T40.412	T40.413	T40.414	T40.415	T40.416
Sulbactam	T36.0X1	T36.0X2	T36.0X3	T36.0X4	T36.0X5	T36.0X6
Sulbenicillin	T36.0X1	T36.0X2	T36.0X3	T36.0X4	T36.0X5	T36.0X6
Sulbentine	T49.0X1	T49.0X2	T49.0X3	T49.0X4	T49.0X5	T49.0X6
Sulfacetamide	T49.0X1	T49.0X2	T49.0X3	T49.0X4	T49.0X5	T49.0X6
ophthalmic preparation	T49.5X1	T49.5X2	T49.5X3	T49.5X4	T49.5X5	T49.5X6
Sulfachlorpyridazine	T37.0X1	T37.0X2	T37.0X3	T37.0X4	T37.0X5	T37.0X6
Sulfacitine	T37.0X1	T37.0X2	T37.0X3	T37.0X4	T37.0X5	T37.0X6
Sulfadiasulfone sodium	T37.0X1	T37.0X2	T37.0X3	T37.0X4	T37.0X5	T37.0X6
Sulfadiazine	T37.0X1	T37.0X2	T37.0X3	T37.0X4	T37.0X5	T37.0X6
silver (topical)	T49.0X1	T49.0X2	T49.0X3	T49.0X4	T49.0X5	T49.0X6

Substance	Poisoning, Accidental (Unintentional)	Poisoning, Intentional Self-Harm	Poisoning, Assault	Poisoning, Undetermined	Adverse Effect	Underdosing
Sulfadimethoxine	T37.0X1	T37.0X2	T37.0X3	T37.0X4	T37.0X5	T37.0X6
Sulfadimidine	T37.0X1	T37.0X2	T37.0X3	T37.0X4	T37.0X5	T37.0X6
Sulfadoxine	T37.0X1	T37.0X2	T37.0X3	T37.0X4	T37.0X5	T37.0X6
with pyrimethamine	T37.2X1	T37.2X2	T37.2X3	T37.2X4	T37.2X5	T37.2X6
Sulfaethidole	T37.0X1	T37.0X2	T37.0X3	T37.0X4	T37.0X5	T37.0X6
Sulfafurazole	T37.0X1	T37.0X2	T37.0X3	T37.0X4	T37.0X5	T37.0X6
Sulfaguanidine	T37.0X1	T37.0X2	T37.0X3	T37.0X4	T37.0X5	T37.0X6
Sulfalene	T37.0X1	T37.0X2	T37.0X3	T37.0X4	T37.0X5	T37.0X6
Sulfaloxate	T37.0X1	T37.0X2	T37.0X3	T37.0X4	T37.0X5	T37.0X6
Sulfaloxic acid	T37.0X1	T37.0X2	T37.0X3	T37.0X4	T37.0X5	T37.0X6
Sulfamazone	T39.2X1	T39.2X2	T39.2X3	T39.2X4	T39.2X5	T39.2X6
Sulfamerazine	T37.0X1	T37.0X2	T37.0X3	T37.0X4	T37.0X5	T37.0X6
Sulfameter	T37.0X1	T37.0X2	T37.0X3	T37.0X4	T37.0X5	T37.0X6
Sulfamethazine	T37.0X1	T37.0X2	T37.0X3	T37.0X4	T37.0X5	T37.0X6
Sulfamethizole	T37.0X1	T37.0X2	T37.0X3	T37.0X4	T37.0X5	T37.0X6
Sulfamethoxazole	T37.0X1	T37.0X2	T37.0X3	T37.0X4	T37.0X5	T37.0X6
with trimethoprim	T36.8X1	T36.8X2	T36.8X3	T36.8X4	T36.8X5	T36.8X6
Sulfamethoxydiazine	T37.0X1	T37.0X2	T37.0X3	T37.0X4	T37.0X5	T37.0X6
Sulfamethoxypyridazine	T37.0X1	T37.0X2	T37.0X3	T37.0X4	T37.0X5	T37.0X6
Sulfamethylthiazole	T37.0X1	T37.0X2	T37.0X3	T37.0X4	T37.0X5	T37.0X6
Sulfametoxydiazine	T37.0X1	T37.0X2	T37.0X3	T37.0X4	T37.0X5	T37.0X6
Sulfamidopyrine	T39.2X1	T39.2X2	T39.2X3	T39.2X4	T39.2X5	T39.2X6
Sulfamonomethoxine	T37.0X1	T37.0X2	T37.0X3	T37.0X4	T37.0X5	T37.0X6
Sulfamoxole	T37.0X1	T37.0X2	T37.0X3	T37.0X4	T37.0X5	T37.0X6
Sulfamylon	T49.0X1	T49.0X2	T49.0X3	T49.0X4	T49.0X5	T49.0X6
Sulfan blue (diagnostic dye)	T50.8X1	T50.8X2	T50.8X3	T50.8X4	T50.8X5	T50.8X6
Sulfanilamide	T37.0X1	T37.0X2	T37.0X3	T37.0X4	T37.0X5	T37.0X6
Sulfanilylguanidine	T37.0X1	T37.0X2	T37.0X3	T37.0X4	T37.0X5	T37.0X6
Sulfaperin	T37.0X1	T37.0X2	T37.0X3	T37.0X4	T37.0X5	T37.0X6
Sulfaphenazole	T37.0X1	T37.0X2	T37.0X3	T37.0X4	T37.0X5	T37.0X6
Sulfaphenylthiazole	T37.0X1	T37.0X2	T37.0X3	T37.0X4	T37.0X5	T37.0X6
Sulfaproxyline	T37.0X1	T37.0X2	T37.0X3	T37.0X4	T37.0X5	T37.0X6
Sulfapyridine	T37.0X1	T37.0X2	T37.0X3	T37.0X4	T37.0X5	T37.0X6
Sulfapyrimidine	T37.0X1	T37.0X2	T37.0X3	T37.0X4	T37.0X5	T37.0X6
Sulfarsphenamine	T37.8X1	T37.8X2	T37.8X3	T37.8X4	T37.8X5	T37.8X6
Sulfasalazine	T37.0X1	T37.0X2	T37.0X3	T37.0X4	T37.0X5	T37.0X6
Sulfasuxidine	T37.0X1	T37.0X2	T37.0X3	T37.0X4	T37.0X5	T37.0X6
Sulfasymazine	T37.0X1	T37.0X2	T37.0X3	T37.0X4	T37.0X5	T37.0X6
Sulfated amylopectin	T47.8X1	T47.8X2	T47.8X3	T47.8X4	T47.8X5	T47.8X6
Sulfathiazole	T37.0X1	T37.0X2	T37.0X3	T37.0X4	T37.0X5	T37.0X6
Sulfatostearate	T49.2X1	T49.2X2	T49.2X3	T49.2X4	T49.2X5	T49.2X6
Sulfinpyrazone	T50.4X1	T50.4X2	T50.4X3	T50.4X4	T50.4X5	T50.4X6

◀ New   ◀ Revised   ~~deleted~~ Deleted

	External Cause (T-Code)					
Substance	Poisoning, Accidental (Unintentional)	Poisoning, Intentional Self-Harm	Poisoning, Assault	Poisoning, Undetermined	Adverse Effect	Underdosing
Sulfiram	T49.0X1	T49.0X2	T49.0X3	T49.0X4	T49.0X5	T49.0X6
Sulfisomidine	T37.0X1	T37.0X2	T37.0X3	T37.0X4	T37.0X5	T37.0X6
Sulfisoxazole	T37.0X1	T37.0X2	T37.0X3	T37.0X4	T37.0X5	T37.0X6
ophthalmic preparation	T49.5X1	T49.5X2	T49.5X3	T49.5X4	T49.5X5	T49.5X6
Sulfobromophthalein (sodium)	T50.8X1	T50.8X2	T50.8X3	T50.8X4	T50.8X5	T50.8X6
Sulfobromphthalein	T50.8X1	T50.8X2	T50.8X3	T50.8X4	T50.8X5	T50.8X6
Sulfogaiacol	T48.4X1	T48.4X2	T48.4X3	T48.4X4	T48.4X5	T48.4X6
Sulfomyxin	T36.8X1	T36.8X2	T36.8X3	T36.8X4	T36.8X5	T36.8X6
Sulfonal	T42.6X1	T42.6X2	T42.6X3	T42.6X4	T42.6X5	T42.6X6
Sulfonamide NEC	T37.0X1	T37.0X2	T37.0X3	T37.0X4	T37.0X5	T37.0X6
eye	T49.5X1	T49.5X2	T49.5X3	T49.5X4	T49.5X5	T49.5X6
Sulfonazide	T37.1X1	T37.1X2	T37.1X3	T37.1X4	T37.1X5	T37.1X6
Sulfones	T37.1X1	T37.1X2	T37.1X3	T37.1X4	T37.1X5	T37.1X6
Sulfonethylmethane	T42.6X1	T42.6X2	T42.6X3	T42.6X4	T42.6X5	T42.6X6
Sulfonmethane	T42.6X1	T42.6X2	T42.6X3	T42.6X4	T42.6X5	T42.6X6
Sulfonphthal, sulfonphthol	T50.8X1	T50.8X2	T50.8X3	T50.8X4	T50.8X5	T50.8X6
Sulfonylurea derivatives, oral	T38.3X1	T38.3X2	T38.3X3	T38.3X4	T38.3X5	T38.3X6
Sulforidazine	T43.3X1	T43.3X2	T43.3X3	T43.3X4	T43.3X5	T43.3X6
Sulfoxone	T37.1X1	T37.1X2	T37.1X3	T37.1X4	T37.1X5	T37.1X6
Sulfur, sulfurated, sulfuric, sulfurous, sulfuryl (compounds NEC) (medicinal)	T49.4X1	T49.4X2	T49.4X3	T49.4X4	T49.4X5	T49.4X6
acid	T54.2X1	T54.2X2	T54.2X3	T54.2X4	—	—
dioxide (gas)	T59.1X1	T59.1X2	T59.1X3	T59.1X4	—	—
ether — see Ether(s)						
hydrogen	T59.6X1	T59.6X2	T59.6X3	T59.6X4	—	—
medicinal (keratolytic) (ointment) NEC	T49.4X1	T49.4X2	T49.4X3	T49.4X4	T49.4X5	T49.4X6
ointment	T49.0X1	T49.0X2	T49.0X3	T49.0X4	T49.0X5	T49.0X6
pesticide (vapor)	T60.91	T60.92	T60.93	T60.94	—	—
vapor NEC	T59.891	T59.892	T59.893	T59.894	—	—
Sulfuric acid	T54.2X1	T54.2X2	T54.2X3	T54.2X4	—	—
Sulglicotide	T47.1X1	T47.1X2	T47.1X3	T47.1X4	T47.1X5	T47.1X6
Sulindac	T39.391	T39.392	T39.393	T39.394	T39.395	T39.396
Sulisatin	T47.2X1	T47.2X2	T47.2X3	T47.2X4	T47.2X5	T47.2X6
Sulisobenzone	T49.3X1	T49.3X2	T49.3X3	T49.3X4	T49.3X5	T49.3X6
Sulkowitch's reagent	T50.8X1	T50.8X2	T50.8X3	T50.8X4	T50.8X5	T50.8X6
Sulmetozine	T44.3X1	T44.3X2	T44.3X3	T44.3X4	T44.3X5	T44.3X6
Suloctidil	T46.7X1	T46.7X2	T46.7X3	T46.7X4	T46.7X5	T46.7X6
Sulph — see also Sulf-						
Sulphadiazine	T37.0X1	T37.0X2	T37.0X3	T37.0X4	T37.0X5	T37.0X6
Sulphadimethoxine	T37.0X1	T37.0X2	T37.0X3	T37.0X4	T37.0X5	T37.0X6

	External Cause (T-Code)					
Substance	Poisoning, Accidental (Unintentional)	Poisoning, Intentional Self-Harm	Poisoning, Assault	Poisoning, Undetermined	Adverse Effect	Underdosing
Sulphadimidine	T37.0X1	T37.0X2	T37.0X3	T37.0X4	T37.0X5	T37.0X6
Sulphadione	T37.1X1	T37.1X2	T37.1X3	T37.1X4	T37.1X5	T37.1X6
Sulphafurazole	T37.0X1	T37.0X2	T37.0X3	T37.0X4	T37.0X5	T37.0X6
Sulphamethizole	T37.0X1	T37.0X2	T37.0X3	T37.0X4	T37.0X5	T37.0X6
Sulphamethoxazole	T37.0X1	T37.0X2	T37.0X3	T37.0X4	T37.0X5	T37.0X6
Sulphan blue	T50.8X1	T50.8X2	T50.8X3	T50.8X4	T50.8X5	T50.8X6
Sulphaphenazole	T37.0X1	T37.0X2	T37.0X3	T37.0X4	T37.0X5	T37.0X6
Sulphapyridine	T37.0X1	T37.0X2	T37.0X3	T37.0X4	T37.0X5	T37.0X6
Sulphasalazine	T37.0X1	T37.0X2	T37.0X3	T37.0X4	T37.0X5	T37.0X6
Sulphinpyrazone	T50.4X1	T50.4X2	T50.4X3	T50.4X4	T50.4X5	T50.4X6
Sulpiride	T43.591	T43.592	T43.593	T43.594	T43.595	T43.596
Sulprostone	T48.0X1	T48.0X2	T48.0X3	T48.0X4	T48.0X5	T48.0X6
Sulpyrine	T39.2X1	T39.2X2	T39.2X3	T39.2X4	T39.2X5	T39.2X6
Sultamicillin	T36.0X1	T36.0X2	T36.0X3	T36.0X4	T36.0X5	T36.0X6
Sulthiame	T42.6X1	T42.6X2	T42.6X3	T42.6X4	T42.6X5	T42.6X6
Sultiame	T42.6X1	T42.6X2	T42.6X3	T42.6X4	T42.6X5	T42.6X6
Sultopride	T43.591	T43.592	T43.593	T43.594	T43.595	T43.596
Sumatriptan	T39.8X1	T39.8X2	T39.8X3	T39.8X4	T39.8X5	T39.8X6
Sunflower seed oil	T46.6X1	T46.6X2	T46.6X3	T46.6X4	T46.6X5	T46.6X6
Superinone	T48.4X1	T48.4X2	T48.4X3	T48.4X4	T48.4X5	T48.4X6
Suprofen	T39.311	T39.312	T39.313	T39.314	T39.315	T39.316
Suramin (sodium)	T37.4X1	T37.4X2	T37.4X3	T37.4X4	T37.4X5	T37.4X6
Surfacaine	T41.3X1	T41.3X2	T41.3X3	T41.3X4	T41.3X5	T41.3X6
Surital	T41.1X1	T41.1X2	T41.1X3	T41.1X4	T41.1X5	T41.1X6
Sutilains	T45.3X1	T45.3X2	T45.3X3	T45.3X4	T45.3X5	T45.3X6
Suxamethonium (chloride)	T48.1X1	T48.1X2	T48.1X3	T48.1X4	T48.1X5	T48.1X6
Suxethonium (chloride)	T48.1X1	T48.1X2	T48.1X3	T48.1X4	T48.1X5	T48.1X6
Suxibuzone	T39.2X1	T39.2X2	T39.2X3	T39.2X4	T39.2X5	T39.2X6
Sweet oil (birch)	T49.3X1	T49.3X2	T49.3X3	T49.3X4	T49.3X5	T49.3X6
Sweet niter spirit	T46.3X1	T46.3X2	T46.3X3	T46.3X4	T46.3X5	T46.3X6
Sweetener	T50.901	T50.902	T50.903	T50.904	T50.905	T50.906
Sym-dichloroethyl ether	T53.6X1	T53.6X2	T53.6X3	T53.6X4	—	—
Sympatholytic NEC	T44.8X1	T44.8X2	T44.8X3	T44.8X4	T44.8X5	T44.8X6
haloalkylamine	T44.8X1	T44.8X2	T44.8X3	T44.8X4	T44.8X5	T44.8X6
Sympathomimetic NEC	T44.901	T44.902	T44.903	T44.904	T44.905	T44.906
anti-common-cold	T48.5X1	T48.5X2	T48.5X3	T48.5X4	T48.5X5	T48.5X6
bronchodilator	T48.6X1	T48.6X2	T48.6X3	T48.6X4	T48.6X5	T48.6X6
specified NEC	T44.991	T44.992	T44.993	T44.994	T44.995	T44.996
Synagis	T50.B91	T50.B92	T50.B93	T50.B94	T50.B95	T50.B96
Synalar	T49.0X1	T49.0X2	T49.0X3	T49.0X4	T49.0X5	T49.0X6
Synthetic cannabinoids	T40.721	T40.722	T40.723	T40.724	T40.725	T40.726
Synthroid	T38.1X1	T38.1X2	T38.1X3	T38.1X4	T38.1X5	T38.1X6

◀ New   ◀ Revised   ~~deleted~~ Deleted

Substance	External Cause (T-Code) Poisoning, Accidental (Unintentional)	Poisoning, Intentional Self-Harm	Poisoning, Assault	Poisoning, Undetermined	Adverse Effect	Underdosing
Syntocinon	T48.0X1	T48.0X2	T48.0X3	T48.0X4	T48.0X5	T48.0X6
Syrosingopine	T46.5X1	T46.5X2	T46.5X3	T46.5X4	T46.5X5	T46.5X6
Systemic drug	T45.91	T45.92	T45.93	T45.94	T45.95	T45.96
specified NEC	T45.8X1	T45.8X2	T45.8X3	T45.8X4	T45.8X5	T45.8X6
2,4,5-T	T60.3X1	T60.3X2	T60.3X3	T60.3X4	—	—
T						
Tablets — see also specified substance	T50.901	T50.902	T50.903	T50.904	T50.905	T50.906
Tace	T38.5X1	T38.5X2	T38.5X3	T38.5X4	T38.5X5	T38.5X6
Tacrine	T44.0X1	T44.0X2	T44.0X3	T44.0X4	T44.0X5	T44.0X6
Tadalafil	T46.7X1	T46.7X2	T46.7X3	T46.7X4	T46.7X5	T46.7X6
Talampicillin	T36.0X1	T36.0X2	T36.0X3	T36.0X4	T36.0X5	T36.0X6
Talbutal	T42.3X1	T42.3X2	T42.3X3	T42.3X4	T42.3X5	T42.3X6
Talc powder	I49.3X1	T49.3X2	T49.3X3	T49.3X4	T49.3X5	T49.3X6
Talcum	T49.3X1	T49.3X2	T49.3X3	T49.3X4	T49.3X5	T49.3X6
Taleranol	T38.6X1	T38.6X2	T38.6X3	T38.6X4	T38.6X5	T38.6X6
Tamoxifen	T38.6X1	T38.6X2	T38.6X3	T38.6X4	T38.6X5	T38.6X6
Tamsulosin	T44.6X1	T44.6X2	T44.6X3	T44.6X4	T44.6X5	T44.6X6
Tandearil, tanderil	T39.2X1	T39.2X2	T39.2X3	T39.2X4	T39.2X5	T39.2X6
Tannic acid	T49.2X1	T49.2X2	T49.2X3	T49.2X4	T49.2X5	T49.2X6
medicinal (astringent)	T49.2X1	T49.2X2	T49.2X3	T49.2X4	T49.2X5	T49.2X6
Tannin — see Tannic acid						
Tansy	T62.2X1	T62.2X2	T62.2X3	T62.2X4	—	—
TAO	T36.3X1	T36.3X2	T36.3X3	T36.3X4	T36.3X5	T36.3X6
Tapazole	T38.2X1	T38.2X2	T38.2X3	T38.2X4	T38.2X5	T38.2X6
Tar NEC	T52.0X1	T52.0X2	T52.0X3	T52.0X4	—	—
camphor	T60.1X1	T60.1X2	T60.1X3	T60.1X4	—	—
distillate	T49.1X1	T49.1X2	T49.1X3	T49.1X4	T49.1X5	T49.1X6
fumes	T59.891	T59.892	T59.893	T59.894	—	—
medicinal	T49.1X1	T49.1X2	T49.1X3	T49.1X4	T49.1X5	T49.1X6
ointment	T49.1X1	T49.1X2	T49.1X3	T49.1X4	T49.1X5	T49.1X6
Taractan	T43.591	T43.592	T43.593	T43.594	T43.595	T43.596
Tarantula (venomous)	T63.321	T63.322	T63.323	T63.324	—	—
Tartar emetic	T37.8X1	T37.8X2	T37.8X3	T37.8X4	T37.8X5	T37.8X6
Tartaric acid	T65.891	T65.892	T65.893	T65.894	—	—
Tartrated antimony (anti-infective)	T37.8X1	T37.8X2	T37.8X3	T37.8X4	T37.8X5	T37.8X6
Tartrate, laxative	T47.4X1	T47.4X2	T47.4X3	T47.4X4	T47.4X5	T47.4X6
Tauromustine	T45.1X1	T45.1X2	T45.1X3	T45.1X4	T45.1X5	T45.1X6
TCA — see Trichloroacetic acid						
TCDD	T53.7X1	T53.7X2	T53.7X3	T53.7X4	—	—
TDI (vapor)	T65.0X1	T65.0X2	T65.0X3	T65.0X4	—	—
Tear						
gas	T59.3X1	T59.3X2	T59.3X3	T59.3X4	—	—
solution	T49.5X1	T49.5X2	T49.5X3	T49.5X4	T49.5X5	T49.5X6
Teclothiazide	T50.2X1	T50.2X2	T50.2X3	T50.2X4	T50.2X5	T50.2X6
Teclozan	T37.3X1	T37.3X2	T37.3X3	T37.3X4	T37.3X5	T37.3X6
Tegafur	T45.1X1	T45.1X2	T45.1X3	T45.1X4	T45.1X5	T45.1X6
Tegretol	T42.1X1	T42.1X2	T42.1X3	T42.1X4	T42.1X5	T42.1X6
Teicoplanin	T36.8X1	T36.8X2	T36.8X3	T36.8X4	T36.8X5	T36.8X6
Telepaque	T50.8X1	T50.8X2	T50.8X3	T50.8X4	T50.8X5	T50.8X6
Tellurium	T56.891	T56.892	T56.893	T56.894	—	—
fumes	T56.891	T56.892	T56.893	T56.894	—	—
TEM	T45.1X1	T45.1X2	T45.1X3	T45.1X4	T45.1X5	T45.1X6
Temazepam	T42.4X1	T42.4X2	T42.4X3	T42.4X4	T42.4X5	T42.4X6
Temocillin	T36.0X1	T36.0X2	T36.0X3	T36.0X4	T36.0X5	T36.0X6
Tenamfetamine	T43.621	T43.622	T43.623	T43.624	T43.625	T43.626
Teniposide	T45.1X1	T45.1X2	T45.1X3	T45.1X4	T45.1X5	T45.1X6
Tenitramine	T46.3X1	T46.3X2	T46.3X3	T46.3X4	T46.3X5	T46.3X6
Tenoglicin	T48.4X1	T48.4X2	T48.4X3	T48.4X4	T48.4X5	T48.4X6
Tenonitrozole	T37.3X1	T37.3X2	T37.3X3	T37.3X4	T37.3X5	T37.3X6
Tenoxicam	T39.391	T39.392	T39.393	T39.394	T39.395	T39.396
TEPA	T45.1X1	T45.1X2	T45.1X3	T45.1X4	T45.1X5	T45.1X6
TEPP	T60.0X1	T60.0X2	T60.0X3	T60.0X4	—	—
Teprotide	T46.5X1	T46.5X2	T46.5X3	T46.5X4	T46.5X5	T46.5X6
Terazosin	T44.6X1	T44.6X2	T44.6X3	T44.6X4	T44.6X5	T44.6X6
Terbufos	T60.0X1	T60.0X2	T60.0X3	T60.0X4	—	—
Terbutaline	T48.6X1	T48.6X2	T48.6X3	T48.6X4	T48.6X5	T48.6X6
Terconazole	T49.0X1	T49.0X2	T49.0X3	T49.0X4	T49.0X5	T49.0X6
Terfenadine	T45.0X1	T45.0X2	T45.0X3	T45.0X4	T45.0X5	T45.0X6
Teriparatide (acetate)	T50.991	T50.992	T50.993	T50.994	T50.995	T50.996
Terizidone	T37.1X1	T37.1X2	T37.1X3	T37.1X4	T37.1X5	T37.1X6
Terlipressin	T38.891	T38.892	T38.893	T38.894	T38.895	T38.896
Terodiline	T46.3X1	T46.3X2	T46.3X3	T46.3X4	T46.3X5	T46.3X6
Teroxalene	T37.4X1	T37.4X2	T37.4X3	T37.4X4	T37.4X5	T37.4X6
Terpin(cis) hydrate	T48.4X1	T48.4X2	T48.4X3	T48.4X4	T48.4X5	T48.4X6
Terramycin	T36.4X1	T36.4X2	T36.4X3	T36.4X4	T36.4X5	T36.4X6
Tertatolol	T44.7X1	T44.7X2	T44.7X3	T44.7X4	T44.7X5	T44.7X6
Tessalon	T48.3X1	T48.3X2	T48.3X3	T48.3X4	T48.3X5	T48.3X6
Testolactone	T38.7X1	T38.7X2	T38.7X3	T38.7X4	T38.7X5	T38.7X6
Testosterone	T38.7X1	T38.7X2	T38.7X3	T38.7X4	T38.7X5	T38.7X6
Tetanus toxoid or vaccine	T50.A91	T50.A92	T50.A93	T50.A94	T50.A95	T50.A96
antitoxin	T50.Z11	T50.Z12	T50.Z13	T50.Z14	T50.Z15	T50.Z16
immune globulin (human)	T50.Z11	T50.Z12	T50.Z13	T50.Z14	T50.Z15	T50.Z16

◄ New   ◄ Revised   ~~deleted~~ Deleted

	External Cause (T-Code)					
Substance	Poisoning, Accidental (Unintentional)	Poisoning, Intentional Self-Harm	Poisoning, Assault	Poisoning, Undetermined	Adverse Effect	Underdosing
Tetanus toxoid or vaccine (Continued)						
toxoid	T50.A91	T50.A92	T50.A93	T50.A94	T50.A95	T50.A96
with diphtheria toxoid	T50.A21	T50.A22	T50.A23	T50.A24	T50.A25	T50.A26
with pertussis	T50.A11	T50.A12	T50.A13	T50.A14	T50.A15	T50.A16
Tetrabenazine	T43.591	T43.592	T43.593	T43.594	T43.595	T43.596
Tetracaine	T41.3X1	T41.3X2	T41.3X3	T41.3X4	T41.3X5	T41.3X6
nerve block (peripheral) (plexus)	T41.3X1	T41.3X2	T41.3X3	T41.3X4	T41.3X5	T41.3X6
regional	T41.3X1	T41.3X2	T41.3X3	T41.3X4	T41.3X5	T41.3X6
spinal	T41.3X1	T41.3X2	T41.3X3	T41.3X4	T41.3X5	T41.3X6
Tetrachlorethylene — see Tetrachloroethylene						
Tetrachlormethiazide	T50.2X1	T50.2X2	T50.2X3	T50.2X4	T50.2X5	T50.2X6
2,3,7,8-Tetrachlorodibenzo-p-dioxin	T53.7X1	T53.7X2	T53.7X3	T53.7X4	—	—
Tetrachloroethane	T53.6X1	T53.6X2	T53.6X3	T53.6X4	—	—
vapor	T53.6X1	T53.6X2	T53.6X3	T53.6X4	—	—
paint or varnish	T53.6X1	T53.6X2	T53.6X3	T53.6X4	—	—
Tetrachloroethylene (liquid)	T53.3X1	T53.3X2	T53.3X3	T53.3X4	—	—
medicinal	T37.4X1	T37.4X2	T37.4X3	T37.4X4	T37.4X5	T37.4X6
vapor	T53.3X1	T53.3X2	T53.3X3	T53.3X4	—	—
Tetrachloromethane — see Carbon tetrachloride						
Tetracosactide	T38.811	T38.812	T38.813	T38.814	T38.815	T38.816
Tetracosactrin	T38.811	T38.812	T38.813	T38.814	T38.815	T38.816
Tetracycline	T36.4X1	T36.4X2	T36.4X3	T36.4X4	T36.4X5	T36.4X6
ophthalmic preparation	T49.5X1	T49.5X2	T49.5X3	T49.5X4	T49.5X5	T49.5X6
topical NEC	T49.0X1	T49.0X2	T49.0X3	T49.0X4	T49.0X5	T49.0X6
Tetradifon	T60.8X1	T60.8X2	T60.8X3	T60.8X4	—	—
Tetradotoxin	T61.771	T61.772	T61.773	T61.774	—	—
Tetraethyl						
lead	T56.0X1	T56.0X2	T56.0X3	T56.0X4	—	—
pyrophosphate	T60.0X1	T60.0X2	T60.0X3	T60.0X4	—	—
Tetraethylammonium chloride	T44.2X1	T44.2X2	T44.2X3	T44.2X4	T44.2X5	T44.2X6
Tetraethylthiuram disulfide	T50.6X1	T50.6X2	T50.6X3	T50.6X4	T50.6X5	T50.6X6
Tetrahydroaminoacridine	T44.0X1	T44.0X2	T44.0X3	T44.0X4	T44.0X5	T44.0X6
Tetrahydrocannabinol	T40.711	T40.712	T40.713	T40.714	T40.715	T40.716
Tetrahydrofuran	T52.8X1	T52.8X2	T52.8X3	T52.8X4	—	—
Tetrahydronaphthalene	T52.8X1	T52.8X2	T52.8X3	T52.8X4	—	—
Tetrahydrozoline	T49.5X1	T49.5X2	T49.5X3	T49.5X4	T49.5X5	T49.5X6
Tetralin	T52.8X1	T52.8X2	T52.8X3	T52.8X4	—	—
Tetramethrin	T60.2X1	T60.2X2	T60.2X3	T60.2X4	—	—

	External Cause (T-Code)					
Substance	Poisoning, Accidental (Unintentional)	Poisoning, Intentional Self-Harm	Poisoning, Assault	Poisoning, Undetermined	Adverse Effect	Underdosing
Tetramethylthiuram (disulfide) NEC	T60.3X1	T60.3X2	T60.3X3	T60.3X4	—	—
medicinal	T49.0X1	T49.0X2	T49.0X3	T49.0X4	T49.0X5	T49.0X6
Tetramisole	T37.4X1	T37.4X2	T37.4X3	T37.4X4	T37.4X5	T37.4X6
Tetranicotinoyl fructose	T46.7X1	T46.7X2	T46.7X3	T46.7X4	T46.7X5	T46.7X6
Tetronal	T42.6X1	T42.6X2	T42.6X3	T42.6X4	T42.6X5	T42.6X6
Tetrazepam	T42.4X1	T42.4X2	T42.4X3	T42.4X4	T42.4X5	T42.4X6
Tetryl	T65.3X1	T65.3X2	T65.3X3	T65.3X4	—	—
Tetrylammonium chloride	T44.2X1	T44.2X2	T44.2X3	T44.2X4	T44.2X5	T44.2X6
Tetryzoline	T49.5X1	T49.5X2	T49.5X3	T49.5X4	T49.5X5	T49.5X6
Thalidomide	T45.1X1	T45.1X2	T45.1X3	T45.1X4	T45.1X5	T45.1X6
Thallium (compounds) (dust) NEC	T56.811	T56.812	T56.813	T56.814	—	—
pesticide	T60.4X1	T60.4X2	T60.4X3	T60.4X4	—	—
THC	T40.711	T40.712	T40.713	T40.714	T40.715	T40.716
Thebacon	T48.3X1	T48.3X2	T48.3X3	T48.3X4	T48.3X5	T48.3X6
Thebaine	T40.2X1	T40.2X2	T40.2X3	T40.2X4	T40.2X5	T40.2X6
Thenoic acid	T49.6X1	T49.6X2	T49.6X3	T49.6X4	T49.6X5	T49.6X6
Thenyldiamine	T45.0X1	T45.0X2	T45.0X3	T45.0X4	T45.0X5	T45.0X6
Theobromine (calcium salicylate)	T48.6X1	T48.6X2	T48.6X3	T48.6X4	T48.6X5	T48.6X6
sodium salicylate	T48.6X1	T48.6X2	T48.6X3	T48.6X4	T48.6X5	T48.6X6
Theophyllamine	T48.6X1	T48.6X2	T48.6X3	T48.6X4	T48.6X5	T48.6X6
Theophylline	T48.6X1	T48.6X2	T48.6X3	T48.6X4	T48.6X5	T48.6X6
aminobenzoic acid	T48.6X1	T48.6X2	T48.6X3	T48.6X4	T48.6X5	T48.6X6
ethylenediamine	T48.6X1	T48.6X2	T48.6X3	T48.6X4	T48.6X5	T48.6X6
piperazine p-amino-benzoate	T48.6X1	T48.6X2	T48.6X3	T48.6X4	T48.6X5	T48.6X6
Thiabendazole	T37.4X1	T37.4X2	T37.4X3	T37.4X4	T37.4X5	T37.4X6
Thialbarbital	T41.1X1	T41.1X2	T41.1X3	T41.1X4	T41.1X5	T41.1X6
Thiamazole	T38.2X1	T38.2X2	T38.2X3	T38.2X4	T38.2X5	T38.2X6
Thiambutosine	T37.1X1	T37.1X2	T37.1X3	T37.1X4	T37.1X5	T37.1X6
Thiamine	T45.2X1	T45.2X2	T45.2X3	T45.2X4	T45.2X5	T45.2X6
Thiamphenicol	T36.2X1	T36.2X2	T36.2X3	T36.2X4	T36.2X5	T36.2X6
Thiamylal	T41.1X1	T41.1X2	T41.1X3	T41.1X4	T41.1X5	T41.1X6
sodium	T41.1X1	T41.1X2	T41.1X3	T41.1X4	T41.1X5	T41.1X6
Thiazesim	T43.291	T43.292	T43.293	T43.294	T43.295	T43.296
Thiazides (diuretics)	T50.2X1	T50.2X2	T50.2X3	T50.2X4	T50.2X5	T50.2X6
Thiazinamium metilsulfate	T43.3X1	T43.3X2	T43.3X3	T43.3X4	T43.3X5	T43.3X6
Thiethylperazine	T43.3X1	T43.3X2	T43.3X3	T43.3X4	T43.3X5	T43.3X6
Thimerosal	T49.0X1	T49.0X2	T49.0X3	T49.0X4	T49.0X5	T49.0X6
ophthalmic preparation	T49.5X1	T49.5X2	T49.5X3	T49.5X4	T49.5X5	T49.5X6
Thioacetazone	T37.1X1	T37.1X2	T37.1X3	T37.1X4	T37.1X5	T37.1X6
with isoniazid	T37.1X1	T37.1X2	T37.1X3	T37.1X4	T37.1X5	T37.1X6
Thiobarbital sodium	T41.1X1	T41.1X2	T41.1X3	T41.1X4	T41.1X5	T41.1X6

◀ New ◀ Revised ~~deleted~~ Deleted

Substance	External Cause (T-Code)					
	Poisoning, Accidental (Unintentional)	Poisoning, Intentional Self-Harm	Poisoning, Assault	Poisoning, Undetermined	Adverse Effect	Underdosing
Thiobarbiturate anesthetic	T41.1X1	T41.1X2	T41.1X3	T41.1X4	T41.1X5	T41.1X6
Thiobismol	T37.8X1	T37.8X2	T37.8X3	T37.8X4	T37.8X5	T37.8X6
Thiobutabarbital sodium	T41.1X1	T41.1X2	T41.1X3	T41.1X4	T41.1X5	T41.1X6
Thiocarbamate (insecticide)	T60.0X1	T60.0X2	T60.0X3	T60.0X4	—	—
Thiocarbamide	T38.2X1	T38.2X2	T38.2X3	T38.2X4	T38.2X5	T38.2X6
Thiocarbarsone	T37.8X1	T37.8X2	T37.8X3	T37.8X4	T37.8X5	T37.8X6
Thiocarlide	T37.1X1	T37.1X2	T37.1X3	T37.1X4	T37.1X5	T37.1X6
Thioctamide	T50.991	T50.992	T50.993	T50.994	T50.995	T50.996
Thioctic acid	T50.991	T50.992	T50.993	T50.994	T50.995	T50.996
Thiofos	T60.0X1	T60.0X2	T60.0X3	T60.0X4	—	—
Thioglycolate	T49.4X1	T49.4X2	T49.4X3	T49.4X4	T49.4X5	T49.4X6
Thioglycolic acid	T65.891	T65.892	T65.893	T65.894	—	—
Thioguanine	T45.1X1	T45.1X2	T45.1X3	T45.1X4	T45.1X5	T45.1X6
Thiomercaptomerin	T50.2X1	T50.2X2	T50.2X3	T50.2X4	T50.2X5	T50.2X6
Thiomerin	T50.2X1	T50.2X2	T50.2X3	T50.2X4	T50.2X5	T50.2X6
Thiomersal	T49.0X1	T49.0X2	T49.0X3	T49.0X4	T49.0X5	T49.0X6
Thionazin	T60.0X1	T60.0X2	T60.0X3	T60.0X4	—	—
Thiopental (sodium)	T41.1X1	T41.1X2	T41.1X3	T41.1X4	T41.1X5	T41.1X6
Thiopentone (sodium)	T41.1X1	T41.1X2	T41.1X3	T41.1X4	T41.1X5	T41.1X6
Thiopropazate	T43.3X1	T43.3X2	T43.3X3	T43.3X4	T43.3X5	T43.3X6
Thioproperazine	T43.3X1	T43.3X2	T43.3X3	T43.3X4	T43.3X5	T43.3X6
Thioridazine	T43.3X1	T43.3X2	T43.3X3	T43.3X4	T43.3X5	T43.3X6
Thiosinamine	T49.3X1	T49.3X2	T49.3X3	T49.3X4	T49.3X5	T49.3X6
Thiotepa	T45.1X1	T45.1X2	T45.1X3	T45.1X4	T45.1X5	T45.1X6
Thiothixene	T43.4X1	T43.4X2	T43.4X3	T43.4X4	T43.4X5	T43.4X6
Thiouracil (benzyl) (methyl) (propyl)	T38.2X1	T38.2X2	T38.2X3	T38.2X4	T38.2X5	T38.2X6
Thiourea	T38.2X1	T38.2X2	T38.2X3	T38.2X4	T38.2X5	T38.2X6
Thiphenamil	T44.3X1	T44.3X2	T44.3X3	T44.3X4	T44.3X5	T44.3X6
Thiram	T60.3X1	T60.3X2	T60.3X3	T60.3X4	—	—
medicinal	T49.2X1	T49.2X2	T49.2X3	T49.2X4	T49.2X5	T49.2X6
Thonzylamine (systemic)	T45.0X1	T45.0X2	T45.0X3	T45.0X4	T45.0X5	T45.0X6
mucosal decongestant	T48.5X1	T48.5X2	T48.5X3	T48.5X4	T48.5X5	T48.5X6
Thorazine	T43.3X1	T43.3X2	T43.3X3	T43.3X4	T43.3X5	T43.3X6
Thorium dioxide suspension	T50.8X1	T50.8X2	T50.8X3	T50.8X4	T50.8X5	T50.8X6
Thornapple	T62.2X1	T62.2X2	T62.2X3	T62.2X4		
Throat drug NEC	T49.6X1	T49.6X2	T49.6X3	T49.6X4	T49.6X5	T49.6X6
Thrombin	T45.7X1	T45.7X2	T45.7X3	T45.7X4	T45.7X5	T45.7X6
Thrombolysin	T45.611	T45.612	T45.613	T45.614	T45.615	T45.616
Thromboplastin	T45.7X1	T45.7X2	T45.7X3	T45.7X4	T45.7X5	T45.7X6
Thurfyl nicotinate	T46.7X1	T46.7X2	T46.7X3	T46.7X4	T46.7X5	T46.7X6
Thymol	T49.0X1	T49.0X2	T49.0X3	T49.0X4	T49.0X5	T49.0X6

Substance	External Cause (T-Code)					
	Poisoning, Accidental (Unintentional)	Poisoning, Intentional Self-Harm	Poisoning, Assault	Poisoning, Undetermined	Adverse Effect	Underdosing
Thymopentin	T37.5X1	T37.5X2	T37.5X3	T37.5X4	T37.5X5	T37.5X6
Thymoxamine	T46.7X1	T46.7X2	T46.7X3	T46.7X4	T46.7X5	T46.7X6
Thymus extract	T38.891	T38.892	T38.893	T38.894	T38.895	T38.896
Thyreotrophic hormone	T38.811	T38.812	T38.813	T38.814	T38.815	T38.816
Thyroglobulin	T38.1X1	T38.1X2	T38.1X3	T38.1X4	T38.1X5	T38.1X6
Thyroid (hormone)	T38.1X1	T38.1X2	T38.1X3	T38.1X4	T38.1X5	T38.1X6
Thyrolar	T38.1X1	T38.1X2	T38.1X3	T38.1X4	T38.1X5	T38.1X6
Thyrotrophin	T38.811	T38.812	T38.813	T38.814	T38.815	T38.816
Thyrotropic hormone	T38.811	T38.812	T38.813	T38.814	T38.815	T38.816
Thyroxine	T38.1X1	T38.1X2	T38.1X3	T38.1X4	T38.1X5	T38.1X6
Tiabendazole	T37.4X1	T37.4X2	T37.4X3	T37.4X4	T37.4X5	T37.4X6
Tiamizide	T50.2X1	T50.2X2	T50.2X3	T50.2X4	T50.2X5	T50.2X6
Tianeptine	T43.291	T43.292	T43.293	T43.294	T43.295	T43.296
Tiapamil	T46.1X1	T46.1X2	T46.1X3	T46.1X4	T46.1X5	T46.1X6
Tiapride	T43.591	T43.592	T43.593	T43.594	T43.595	T43.596
Tiaprofenic acid	T39.311	T39.312	T39.313	T39.314	T39.315	T39.316
Tiaramide	T39.8X1	T39.8X2	T39.8X3	T39.8X4	T39.8X5	T39.8X6
Ticarcillin	T36.0X1	T36.0X2	T36.0X3	T36.0X4	T36.0X5	T36.0X6
Ticlatone	T49.0X1	T49.0X2	T49.0X3	T49.0X4	T49.0X5	T49.0X6
Ticlopidine	T45.521	T45.522	T45.523	T45.524	T45.525	T45.526
Ticrynafen	T50.1X1	T50.1X2	T50.1X3	T50.1X4	T50.1X5	T50.1X6
Tidiacic	T50.991	T50.992	T50.993	T50.994	T50.995	T50.996
Tiemonium	T44.3X1	T44.3X2	T44.3X3	T44.3X4	T44.3X5	T44.3X6
iodide	T44.3X1	T44.3X2	T44.3X3	T44.3X4	T44.3X5	T44.3X6
Tienilic acid	T50.1X1	T50.1X2	T50.1X3	T50.1X4	T50.1X5	T50.1X6
Tifenamil	T44.3X1	T44.3X2	T44.3X3	T44.3X4	T44.3X5	T44.3X6
Tigan	T45.0X1	T45.0X2	T45.0X3	T45.0X4	T45.0X5	T45.0X6
Tigloidine	T44.3X1	T44.3X2	T44.3X3	T44.3X4	T44.3X5	T44.3X6
Tilactase	T47.5X1	T47.5X2	T47.5X3	T47.5X4	T47.5X5	T47.5X6
Tiletamine	T41.291	T41.292	T41.293	T41.294	T41.295	T41.296
Tilidine	T40.441	T40.442	T40.443	T40.444	—	—
Timepidium bromide	T44.3X1	T44.3X2	T44.3X3	T44.3X4	T44.3X5	T44.3X6
Timiperone	T43.4X1	T43.4X2	T43.4X3	T43.4X4	T43.4X5	T43.4X6
Timolol	T44.7X1	T44.7X2	T44.7X3	T44.7X4	T44.7X5	T44.7X6
Tin (chloride) (dust) (oxide) NEC	T56.6X1	T56.6X2	T56.6X3	T56.6X4	—	—
anti-infectives	T37.8X1	T37.8X2	T37.8X3	T37.8X4	T37.8X5	T37.8X6
Tincture, iodine — see Iodine						
Tindal	T43.3X1	T43.3X2	T43.3X3	T43.3X4	T43.3X5	T43.3X6
Tinidazole	T37.3X1	T37.3X2	T37.3X3	T37.3X4	T37.3X5	T37.3X6
Tinoridine	T39.8X1	T39.8X2	T39.8X3	T39.8X4	T39.8X5	T39.8X6
Tiocarlide	T37.1X1	T37.1X2	T37.1X3	T37.1X4	T37.1X5	T37.1X6
Tioclomarol	T45.511	T45.512	T45.513	T45.514	T45.515	T45.516

◄ New ◄ Revised ~~deleted~~ Deleted

TABLE OF DRUGS AND CHEMICALS

Substance	Poisoning, Accidental (Unintentional)	Poisoning, Intentional Self-Harm	Poisoning, Assault	Poisoning, Undetermined	Adverse Effect	Underdosing
Tioconazole	T49.0X1	T49.0X2	T49.0X3	T49.0X4	T49.0X5	T49.0X6
Tioguanine	T45.1X1	T45.1X2	T45.1X3	T45.1X4	T45.1X5	T45.1X6
Tiopronin	T50.991	T50.992	T50.993	T50.994	T50.995	T50.996
Tiotixene	T43.4X1	T43.4X2	T43.4X3	T43.4X4	T43.4X5	T43.4X6
Tioxolone	T49.4X1	T49.4X2	T49.4X3	T49.4X4	T49.4X5	T49.4X6
Tipepidine	T48.3X1	T48.3X2	T48.3X3	T48.3X4	T48.3X5	T48.3X6
Tiquizium bromide	T44.3X1	T44.3X2	T44.3X3	T44.3X4	T44.3X5	T44.3X6
Tiratricol	T38.1X1	T38.1X2	T38.1X3	T38.1X4	T38.1X5	T38.1X6
Tisopurine	T50.4X1	T50.4X2	T50.4X3	T50.4X4	T50.4X5	T50.4X6
Titanium (compounds) (vapor)	T56.891	T56.892	T56.893	T56.894	—	—
dioxide	T49.3X1	T49.3X2	T49.3X3	T49.3X4	T49.3X5	T49.3X6
ointment	T49.3X1	T49.3X2	T49.3X3	T49.3X4	T49.3X5	T49.3X6
oxide	T49.3X1	T49.3X2	T49.3X3	T49.3X4	T49.3X5	T49.3X6
tetrachloride	T56.891	T56.892	T56.893	T56.894	—	—
Titanocene	T56.891	T56.892	T56.893	T56.894	—	—
Titroid	T38.1X1	T38.1X2	T38.1X3	T38.1X4	T38.1X5	T38.1X6
Tizanidine	T42.8X1	T42.8X2	T42.8X3	T42.8X4	T42.8X5	T42.8X6
TMTD	T60.3X1	T60.3X2	T60.3X3	T60.3X4		
TNT (fumes)	T65.3X1	T65.3X2	T65.3X3	T65.3X4	—	—
Toadstool	T62.0X1	T62.0X2	T62.0X3	T62.0X4		
Tobacco NEC	T65.291	T65.292	T65.293	T65.294	—	
cigarettes	T65.221	T65.222	T65.223	T65.224	—	
Indian	T62.2X1	T62.2X2	T62.2X3	T62.2X4	—	
smoke, second-hand	T65.221	T65.222	T65.223	T65.224	—	
Tobramycin	T36.5X1	T36.5X2	T36.5X3	T36.5X4	T36.5X5	T36.5X6
Tocainide	T46.2X1	T46.2X2	T46.2X3	T46.2X4	T46.2X5	T46.2X6
Tocoferol	T45.2X1	T45.2X2	T45.2X3	T45.2X4	T45.2X5	T45.2X6
Tocopherol	T45.2X1	T45.2X2	T45.2X3	T45.2X4	T45.2X5	T45.2X6
acetate	T45.2X1	T45.2X2	T45.2X3	T45.2X4	T45.2X5	T45.2X6
Tocosamine	T48.0X1	T48.0X2	T48.0X3	T48.0X4	T48.0X5	T48.0X6
Todralazine	T46.5X1	T46.5X2	T46.5X3	T46.5X4	T46.5X5	T46.5X6
Tofisopam	T42.4X1	T42.4X2	T42.4X3	T42.4X4	T42.4X5	T42.4X6
Tofranil	T43.011	T43.012	T43.013	T43.014	T43.015	T43.016
Toilet deodorizer	T65.891	T65.892	T65.893	T65.894	—	—
Tolamolol	T44.7X1	T44.7X2	T44.7X3	T44.7X4	T44.7X5	T44.7X6
Tolazamide	T38.3X1	T38.3X2	T38.3X3	T38.3X4	T38.3X5	T38.3X6
Tolazoline	T46.7X1	T46.7X2	T46.7X3	T46.7X4	T46.7X5	T46.7X6
Tolbutamide (sodium)	T38.3X1	T38.3X2	T38.3X3	T38.3X4	T38.3X5	T38.3X6
Tolciclate	T49.0X1	T49.0X2	T49.0X3	T49.0X4	T49.0X5	T49.0X6
Tolmetin	T39.391	T39.392	T39.393	T39.394	T39.395	T39.396
Tolnaftate	T49.0X1	T49.0X2	T49.0X3	T49.0X4	T49.0X5	T49.0X6
Tolonidine	T46.5X1	T46.5X2	T46.5X3	T46.5X4	T46.5X5	T46.5X6

Substance	Poisoning, Accidental (Unintentional)	Poisoning, Intentional Self-Harm	Poisoning, Assault	Poisoning, Undetermined	Adverse Effect	Underdosing
Toloxatone	T42.6X1	T42.6X2	T42.6X3	T42.6X4	T42.6X5	T42.6X6
Tolperisone	T44.3X1	T44.3X2	T44.3X3	T44.3X4	T44.3X5	T44.3X6
Tolserol	T42.8X1	T42.8X2	T42.8X3	T42.8X4	T42.8X5	T42.8X6
Toluene (liquid)	T52.2X1	T52.2X2	T52.2X3	T52.2X4	—	—
diisocyanate	T65.0X1	T65.0X2	T65.0X3	T65.0X4	—	—
Toluidine	T65.891	T65.892	T65.893	T65.894	—	—
vapor	T59.891	T59.892	T59.893	T59.894	—	—
Toluol (liquid)	T52.2X1	T52.2X2	T52.2X3	T52.2X4	—	—
vapor	T52.2X1	T52.2X2	T52.2X3	T52.2X4	—	—
Toluylenediamine	T65.3X1	T65.3X2	T65.3X3	T65.3X4	—	—
Tolylene-2,4-diisocyanate	T65.0X1	T65.0X2	T65.0X3	T65.0X4	—	—
Tonic NEC	T50.901	T50.902	T50.903	T50.904	T50.905	T50.906
Topical action drug NEC	T49.91	T49.92	T49.93	T49.94	T49.95	T49.96
ear, nose or throat	T49.6X1	T49.6X2	T49.6X3	T49.6X4	T49.6X5	T49.6X6
eye	T49.5X1	T49.5X2	T49.5X3	T49.5X4	T49.5X5	T49.5X6
skin	T49.91	T49.92	T49.93	T49.94	T49.95	T49.96
specified NEC	T49.8X1	T49.8X2	T49.8X3	T49.8X4	T49.8X5	T49.8X6
Toquizine	T44.3X1	T44.3X2	T44.3X3	T44.3X4	T44.3X5	T44.3X6
Toremifene	T38.6X1	T38.6X2	T38.6X3	T38.6X4	T38.6X5	T38.6X6
Tosylchloramide sodium	T49.8X1	T49.8X2	T49.8X3	T49.8X4	T49.8X5	T49.8X6
Toxaphene (dust) (spray)	T60.1X1	T60.1X2	T60.1X3	T60.1X4	—	—
Toxin, diphtheria (Schick Test)	T50.8X1	T50.8X2	T50.8X3	T50.8X4	T50.8X5	T50.8X6
Toxoid						
combined	T50.A21	T50.A22	T50.A23	T50.A24	T50.A25	T50.A26
diphtheria	T50.A91	T50.A92	T50.A93	T50.A94	T50.A95	T50.A96
tetanus	T50.A91	T50.A92	T50.A93	T50.A94	T50.A95	T50.A96
Trace element NEC	T45.8X1	T45.8X2	T45.8X3	T45.8X4	T45.8X5	T45.8X6
Tractor fuel NEC	T52.0X1	T52.0X2	T52.0X3	T52.0X4	—	—
Tragacanth	T50.991	T50.992	T50.993	T50.994	T50.995	T50.996
Tramadol	T40.421	T40.422	T40.423	T40.424	T40.425	T40.426
Tramazoline	T48.5X1	T48.5X2	T48.5X3	T48.5X4	T48.5X5	T48.5X6
Tranexamic acid	T45.621	T45.622	T45.623	T45.624	T45.625	T45.626
Tranilast	T45.0X1	T45.0X2	T45.0X3	T45.0X4	T45.0X5	T45.0X6
Tranquilizer NEC	T43.501	T43.502	T43.503	T43.504	T43.505	T43.506
with hypnotic or sedative	T42.6X1	T42.6X2	T42.6X3	T42.6X4	T42.6X5	T42.6X6
benzodiazepine NEC	T42.4X1	T42.4X2	T42.4X3	T42.4X4	T42.4X5	T42.4X6
butyrophenone NEC	T43.4X1	T43.4X2	T43.4X3	T43.4X4	T43.4X5	T43.4X6
carbamate	T43.591	T43.592	T43.593	T43.594	T43.595	T43.596
dimethylamine	T43.3X1	T43.3X2	T43.3X3	T43.3X4	T43.3X5	T43.3X6
ethylamine	T43.3X1	T43.3X2	T43.3X3	T43.3X4	T43.3X5	T43.3X6
hydroxyzine	T43.591	T43.592	T43.593	T43.594	T43.595	T43.596
major NEC	T43.501	T43.502	T43.503	T43.504	T43.505	T43.506

◀ New   ◀ Revised   ~~deleted~~ Deleted

Substance	Poisoning, Accidental (Unintentional)	Poisoning, Intentional Self-Harm	Poisoning, Assault	Poisoning, Undetermined	Adverse Effect	Underdosing
Tranquilizer NEC *(Continued)*						
penothiazine NEC	T43.3X1	T43.3X2	T43.3X3	T43.3X4	T43.3X5	T43.3X6
phenothiazine-based	T43.3X1	T43.3X2	T43.3X3	T43.3X4	T43.3X5	T43.3X6
piperazine NEC	T43.3X1	T43.3X2	T43.3X3	T43.3X4	T43.3X5	T43.3X6
piperidine	T43.3X1	T43.3X2	T43.3X3	T43.3X4	T43.3X5	T43.3X6
propylamine	T43.3X1	T43.3X2	T43.3X3	T43.3X4	T43.3X5	T43.3X6
specified NEC	T43.591	T43.592	T43.593	T43.594	T43.595	T43.596
thioxanthene NEC	T43.591	T43.592	T43.593	T43.594	T43.595	T43.596
Tranxene	T42.4X1	T42.4X2	T42.4X3	T42.4X4	T42.4X5	T42.4X6
Tranylcypromine	T43.1X1	T43.1X2	T43.1X3	T43.1X4	T43.1X5	T43.1X6
Trapidil	T46.3X1	T46.3X2	T46.3X3	T46.3X4	T46.3X5	T46.3X6
Trasentine	T44.3X1	T44.3X2	T44.3X3	T44.3X4	T44.3X5	T44.3X6
Travert	T50.3X1	T50.3X2	T50.3X3	T50.3X4	T50.3X5	T50.3X6
Trazodone	T43.211	T43.212	T43.213	T43.214	T43.215	T43.216
Trecator	T37.1X1	T37.1X2	T37.1X3	T37.1X4	T37.1X5	T37.1X6
Treosulfan	T45.1X1	T45.1X2	T45.1X3	T45.1X4	T45.1X5	T45.1X6
Tretamine	T45.1X1	T45.1X2	T45.1X3	T45.1X4	T45.1X5	T45.1X6
Tretinoin	T49.0X1	T49.0X2	T49.0X3	T49.0X4	T49.0X5	T49.0X6
Tretoquinol	T48.6X1	T48.6X2	T48.6X3	T48.6X4	T48.6X5	T48.6X6
Triacetin	T49.0X1	T49.0X2	T49.0X3	T49.0X4	T49.0X5	T49.0X6
Triacetoxyanthracene	T49.4X1	T49.4X2	T49.4X3	T49.4X4	T49.4X5	T49.4X6
Triacetyloleandomycin	T36.3X1	T36.3X2	T36.3X3	T36.3X4	T36.3X5	T36.3X6
Triamcinolone	T38.0X1	T38.0X2	T38.0X3	T38.0X4	T38.0X5	T38.0X6
ENT agent	T49.6X1	T49.6X2	T49.6X3	T49.6X4	T49.6X5	T49.6X6
hexacetonide	T49.0X1	T49.0X2	T49.0X3	T49.0X4	T49.0X5	T49.0X6
ophthalmic preparation	T49.5X1	T49.5X2	T49.5X3	T49.5X4	T49.5X5	T49.5X6
topical NEC	T49.0X1	T49.0X2	T49.0X3	T49.0X4	T49.0X5	T49.0X6
Triampyzine	T44.3X1	T44.3X2	T44.3X3	T44.3X4	T44.3X5	T44.3X6
Triamterene	T50.2X1	T50.2X2	T50.2X3	T50.2X4	T50.2X5	T50.2X6
Triazine (herbicide)	T60.3X1	T60.3X2	T60.3X3	T60.3X4		—
Triaziquone	T45.1X1	T45.1X2	T45.1X3	T45.1X4	T45.1X5	T45.1X6
Triazolam	T42.4X1	T42.4X2	T42.4X3	T42.4X4	T42.4X5	T42.4X6
Triazole (herbicide)	T60.3X1	T60.3X2	T60.3X3	T60.3X4	—	—
Tribenoside	T46.991	T46.992	T46.993	T46.994	T46.995	T46.996
Tribromacetaldehyde	T42.6X1	T42.6X2	T42.6X3	T42.6X4	T42.6X5	T42.6X6
Tribromoethanol, rectal	T41.291	T41.292	T41.293	T41.294	T41.295	T41.296
Tribromomethane	T42.6X1	T42.6X2	T42.6X3	T42.6X4	T42.6X5	T42.6X6
Trichlorethane	T53.2X1	T53.2X2	T53.2X3	T53.2X4	—	—
Trichlorethylene	T53.2X1	T53.2X2	T53.2X3	T53.2X4	—	—
Trichlorfon	T60.0X1	T60.0X2	T60.0X3	T60.0X4	—	—
Trichlormethiazide	T50.2X1	T50.2X2	T50.2X3	T50.2X4	T50.2X5	T50.2X6
Trichlormethine	T45.1X1	T45.1X2	T45.1X3	T45.1X4	T45.1X5	T45.1X6

Substance	Poisoning, Accidental (Unintentional)	Poisoning, Intentional Self-Harm	Poisoning, Assault	Poisoning, Undetermined	Adverse Effect	Underdosing
Trichloroacetic acid, Trichloracetic acid	T54.2X1	T54.2X2	T54.2X3	T54.2X4	—	—
medicinal	T49.4X1	T49.4X2	T49.4X3	T49.4X4	T49.4X5	T49.4X6
Trichloroethane	T53.2X1	T53.2X2	T53.2X3	T53.2X4	—	—
Trichloroethanol	T42.6X1	T42.6X2	T42.6X3	T42.6X4	T42.6X5	T42.6X6
Trichloroethylene (liquid) (vapor)	T53.2X1	T53.2X2	T53.2X3	T53.2X4	—	—
anesthetic (gas)	T41.0X1	T41.0X2	T41.0X3	T41.0X4	T41.0X5	T41.0X6
vapor NEC	T53.2X1	T53.2X2	T53.2X3	T53.2X4	—	—
Trichloroethyl phosphate	T42.6X1	T42.6X2	T42.6X3	T42.6X4	T42.6X5	T42.6X6
Trichlorofluoromethane NEC	T53.5X1	T53.5X2	T53.5X3	T53.5X4	—	—
Trichloronate	T60.0X1	T60.0X2	T60.0X3	T60.0X4	—	—
2,4,5-Trichlorophen oxyacetic acid	T60.3X1	T60.3X2	T60.3X3	T60.3X4	—	—
Trichloropropane	T53.6X1	T53.6X2	T53.6X3	T53.6X4	—	—
Trichlorotriethylamine	T45.1X1	T45.1X2	T45.1X3	T45.1X4	T45.1X5	T45.1X6
Trichomonacides NEC	T37.3X1	T37.3X2	T37.3X3	T37.3X4	T37.3X5	T37.3X6
Trichomycin	T36.7X1	T36.7X2	T36.7X3	T36.7X4	T36.7X5	T36.7X6
Triclobisonium chloride	T49.0X1	T49.0X2	T49.0X3	T49.0X4	T49.0X5	T49.0X6
Triclocarban	T49.0X1	T49.0X2	T49.0X3	T49.0X4	T49.0X5	T49.0X6
Triclofos	T42.6X1	T42.6X2	T42.6X3	T42.6X4	T42.6X5	T42.6X6
Triclosan	T49.0X1	T49.0X2	T49.0X3	T49.0X4	T49.0X5	T49.0X6
Tricresyl phosphate	T65.891	T65.892	T65.893	T65.894	—	—
solvent	T52.91	T52.92	T52.93	T52.94		
Tricyclamol chloride	T44.3X1	T44.3X2	T44.3X3	T44.3X4	T44.3X5	T44.3X6
Tridesilon	T49.0X1	T49.0X2	T49.0X3	T49.0X4	T49.0X5	T49.0X6
Tridihexethyl iodide	T44.3X1	T44.3X2	T44.3X3	T44.3X4	T44.3X5	T44.3X6
Tridione	T42.2X1	T42.2X2	T42.2X3	T42.2X4	T42.2X5	T42.2X6
Trientine	T45.8X1	T45.8X2	T45.8X3	T45.8X4	T45.8X5	T45.8X6
Triethanolamine NEC	T54.3X1	T54.3X2	T54.3X3	T54.3X4	—	—
detergent	T54.3X1	T54.3X2	T54.3X3	T54.3X4	—	—
trinitrate (biphosphate)	T46.3X1	T46.3X2	T46.3X3	T46.3X4	T46.3X5	T46.3X6
Triethanomelamine	T45.1X1	T45.1X2	T45.1X3	T45.1X4	T45.1X5	T45.1X6
Triethylenemelamine	T45.1X1	T45.1X2	T45.1X3	T45.1X4	T45.1X5	T45.1X6
Triethylenephosphoramide	T45.1X1	T45.1X2	T45.1X3	T45.1X4	T45.1X5	T45.1X6
Triethylenethiophosphoramide	T45.1X1	T45.1X2	T45.1X3	T45.1X4	T45.1X5	T45.1X6
Trifluoperazine	T43.3X1	T43.3X2	T43.3X3	T43.3X4	T43.3X5	T43.3X6
Trifluoroethyl vinyl ether	T41.0X1	T41.0X2	T41.0X3	T41.0X4	T41.0X5	T41.0X6
Trifluperidol	T43.4X1	T43.4X2	T43.4X3	T43.4X4	T43.4X5	T43.4X6
Triflupromazine	T43.3X1	T43.3X2	T43.3X3	T43.3X4	T43.3X5	T43.3X6
Trifluridine	T37.5X1	T37.5X2	T37.5X3	T37.5X4	T37.5X5	T37.5X6
Triflusal	T45.521	T45.522	T45.523	T45.524	T45.525	T45.526
Trihexyphenidyl	T44.3X1	T44.3X2	T44.3X3	T44.3X4	T44.3X5	T44.3X6
Triiodothyronine	T38.1X1	T38.1X2	T38.1X3	T38.1X4	T38.1X5	T38.1X6

◀ New ◀ Revised ~~deleted~~ Deleted

TABLE OF DRUGS AND CHEMICALS

Substance	Poisoning, Accidental (Unintentional)	Poisoning, Intentional Self-Harm	Poisoning, Assault	Poisoning, Undetermined	Adverse Effect	Underdosing
Trilene	T41.0X1	T41.0X2	T41.0X3	T41.0X4	T41.0X5	T41.0X6
Trilostane	T38.991	T38.992	T38.993	T38.994	T38.995	T38.996
Trimebutine	T44.3X1	T44.3X2	T44.3X3	T44.3X4	T44.3X5	T44.3X6
Trimecaine	T41.3X1	T41.3X2	T41.3X3	T41.3X4	T41.3X5	T41.3X6
Trimeprazine (tartrate)	T44.3X1	T44.3X2	T44.3X3	T44.3X4	T44.3X5	T44.3X6
Trimetaphan camsilate	T44.2X1	T44.2X2	T44.2X3	T44.2X4	T44.2X5	T44.2X6
Trimetazidine	T46.7X1	T46.7X2	T46.7X3	T46.7X4	T46.7X5	T46.7X6
Trimethadione	T42.2X1	T42.2X2	T42.2X3	T42.2X4	T42.2X5	T42.2X6
Trimethaphan	T44.2X1	T44.2X2	T44.2X3	T44.2X4	T44.2X5	T44.2X6
Trimethidinium	T44.2X1	T44.2X2	T44.2X3	T44.2X4	T44.2X5	T44.2X6
Trimethobenzamide	T45.0X1	T45.0X2	T45.0X3	T45.0X4	T45.0X5	T45.0X6
Trimethoprim	T37.8X1	T37.8X2	T37.8X3	T37.8X4	T37.8X5	T37.8X6
with sulfamethoxazole	T36.8X1	T36.8X2	T36.8X3	T36.8X4	T36.8X5	T36.8X6
Trimethylcarbinol	T51.3X1	T51.3X2	T51.3X3	T51.3X4	—	—
Trimethylpsoralen	T49.3X1	T49.3X2	T49.3X3	T49.3X4	T49.3X5	T49.3X6
Trimeton	T45.0X1	T45.0X2	T45.0X3	T45.0X4	T45.0X5	T45.0X6
Trimetrexate	T45.1X1	T45.1X2	T45.1X3	T45.1X4	T45.1X5	T45.1X6
Trimipramine	T43.011	T43.012	T43.013	T43.014	T43.015	T43.016
Trimustine	T45.1X1	T45.1X2	T45.1X3	T45.1X4	T45.1X5	T45.1X6
Trinitrine	T46.3X1	T46.3X2	T46.3X3	T46.3X4	T46.3X5	T46.3X6
Trinitrobenzol	T65.3X1	T65.3X2	T65.3X3	T65.3X4	—	—
Trinitrophenol	T65.3X1	T65.3X2	T65.3X3	T65.3X4	—	—
Trinitrotoluene (fumes)	T65.3X1	T65.3X2	T65.3X3	T65.3X4	—	—
Trional	T42.6X1	T42.6X2	T42.6X3	T42.6X4	T42.6X5	T42.6X6
Triorthocresyl phosphate	T65.891	T65.892	T65.893	T65.894	—	—
Trioxide of arsenic	T57.0X1	T57.0X2	T57.0X3	T57.0X4	—	—
Trioxysalen	T49.4X1	T49.4X2	T49.4X3	T49.4X4	T49.4X5	T49.4X6
Tripamide	T50.2X1	T50.2X2	T50.2X3	T50.2X4	T50.2X5	T50.2X6
Triparanol	T46.6X1	T46.6X2	T46.6X3	T46.6X4	T46.6X5	T46.6X6
Tripelennamine	T45.0X1	T45.0X2	T45.0X3	T45.0X4	T45.0X5	T45.0X6
Triperiden	T44.3X1	T44.3X2	T44.3X3	T44.3X4	T44.3X5	T44.3X6
Triperidol	T43.4X1	T43.4X2	T43.4X3	T43.4X4	T43.4X5	T43.4X6
Triphenylphosphate	T65.891	T65.892	T65.893	T65.894	—	—
Triple						
bromides	T42.6X1	T42.6X2	T42.6X3	T42.6X4	T42.6X5	T42.6X6
carbonate	T47.1X1	T47.1X2	T47.1X3	T47.1X4	T47.1X5	T47.1X6
vaccine						
DPT	T50.A11	T50.A12	T50.A13	T50.A14	T50.A15	T50.A16
including pertussis	T50.A11	T50.A12	T50.A13	T50.A14	T50.A15	T50.A16
MMR	T50.B91	T50.B92	—	—	—	—
Triprolidine	T45.0X1	T45.0X2	T45.0X3	T45.0X4	T45.0X5	T45.0X6
Trisodium hydrogen edetate	T50.6X1	T50.6X2	T50.6X3	T50.6X4	T50.6X5	T50.6X6

Substance	Poisoning, Accidental (Unintentional)	Poisoning, Intentional Self-Harm	Poisoning, Assault	Poisoning, Undetermined	Adverse Effect	Underdosing
Trisoralen	T49.3X1	T49.3X2	T49.3X3	T49.3X4	T49.3X5	T49.3X6
Trisulfapyrimidines	T37.0X1	T37.0X2	T37.0X3	T37.0X4	T37.0X5	T37.0X6
Trithiozine	T44.3X1	T44.3X2	T44.3X3	T44.3X4	T44.3X5	T44.3X6
Tritiozine	T44.3X1	T44.3X2	T44.3X3	T44.3X4	T44.3X5	T44.3X6
Tritoqualine	T45.0X1	T45.0X2	T45.0X3	T45.0X4	T45.0X5	T45.0X6
Trofosfamide	T45.1X1	T45.1X2	T45.1X3	T45.1X4	T45.1X5	T45.1X6
Troleandomycin	T36.3X1	T36.3X2	T36.3X3	T36.3X4	T36.3X5	T36.3X6
Trolnitrate (phosphate)	T46.3X1	T46.3X2	T46.3X3	T46.3X4	T46.3X5	T46.3X6
Tromantadine	T37.5X1	T37.5X2	T37.5X3	T37.5X4	T37.5X5	T37.5X6
Trometamol	T50.2X1	T50.2X2	T50.2X3	T50.2X4	T50.2X5	T50.2X6
Tromethamine	T50.2X1	T50.2X2	T50.2X3	T50.2X4	T50.2X5	T50.2X6
Tronothane	T41.3X1	T41.3X2	T41.3X3	T41.3X4	T41.3X5	T41.3X6
Tropacine	T44.3X1	T44.3X2	T44.3X3	T44.3X4	T44.3X5	T44.3X6
Tropatepine	T44.3X1	T44.3X2	T44.3X3	T44.3X4	T44.3X5	T44.3X6
Tropicamide	T44.3X1	T44.3X2	T44.3X3	T44.3X4	T44.3X5	T44.3X6
Trospium chloride	T44.3X1	T44.3X2	T44.3X3	T44.3X4	T44.3X5	T44.3X6
Troxerutin	T46.991	T46.992	T46.993	T46.994	T46.995	T46.996
Troxidone	T42.2X1	T42.2X2	T42.2X3	T42.2X4	T42.2X5	T42.2X6
Tryparsamide	T37.3X1	T37.3X2	T37.3X3	T37.3X4	T37.3X5	T37.3X6
Trypsin	T45.3X1	T45.3X2	T45.3X3	T45.3X4	T45.3X5	T45.3X6
Tryptizol	T43.011	T43.012	T43.013	T43.014	T43.015	T43.016
TSH	T38.811	T38.812	T38.813	T38.814	T38.815	T38.816
Tuaminoheptane	T48.5X1	T48.5X2	T48.5X3	T48.5X4	T48.5X5	T48.5X6
Tuberculin, purified protein derivative (PPD)	T50.8X1	T50.8X2	T50.8X3	T50.8X4	T50.8X5	T50.8X6
Tubocurare	T48.1X1	T48.1X2	T48.1X3	T48.1X4	T48.1X5	T48.1X6
Tubocurarine (chloride)	T48.1X1	T48.1X2	T48.1X3	T48.1X4	T48.1X5	T48.1X6
Tulobuterol	T48.6X1	T48.6X2	T48.6X3	T48.6X4	T48.6X5	T48.6X6
Turpentine (spirits of)	T52.8X1	T52.8X2	T52.8X3	T52.8X4	—	—
vapor	T52.8X1	T52.8X2	T52.8X3	T52.8X4	—	—
Tybamate	T43.591	T43.592	T43.593	T43.594	T43.595	T43.596
Tyloxapol	T48.4X1	T48.4X2	T48.4X3	T48.4X4	T48.4X5	T48.4X6
Tymazoline	T48.5X1	T48.5X2	T48.5X3	T48.5X4	T48.5X5	T48.5X6
Typhoid-paratyphoid vaccine	T50.A91	T50.A92	T50.A93	T50.A94	T50.A95	T50.A96
Typhus vaccine	T50.A91	T50.A92	T50.A93	T50.A94	T50.A95	T50.A96
Tyropanoate	T50.8X1	T50.8X2	T50.8X3	T50.8X4	T50.8X5	T50.8X6
Tyrothricin	T49.6X1	T49.6X2	T49.6X3	T49.6X4	T49.6X5	T49.6X6
ENT agent	T49.6X1	T49.6X2	T49.6X3	T49.6X4	T49.6X5	T49.6X6
ophthalmic preparation	T49.5X1	T49.5X2	T49.5X3	T49.5X4	T49.5X5	T49.5X6
U						
Ufenamate	T39.391	T39.392	T39.393	T39.394	T39.395	T39.396
Ultraviolet light protectant	T49.3X1	T49.3X2	T49.3X3	T49.3X4	T49.3X5	T49.3X6

◀ New ◀ Revised deleted Deleted

Substance	External Cause (T-Code) Poisoning, Accidental (Unintentional)	Poisoning, Intentional Self-Harm	Poisoning, Assault	Poisoning, Undetermined	Adverse Effect	Underdosing
Undecenoic acid	T49.0X1	T49.0X2	T49.0X3	T49.0X4	T49.0X5	T49.0X6
Undecoylium	T49.0X1	T49.0X2	T49.0X3	T49.0X4	T49.0X5	T49.0X6
Undecylenic acid (derivatives)	T49.0X1	T49.0X2	T49.0X3	T49.0X4	T49.0X5	T49.0X6
Unna's boot	T49.3X1	T49.3X2	T49.3X3	T49.3X4	T49.3X5	T49.3X6
Unsaturated fatty acid	T46.6X1	T46.6X2	T46.6X3	T46.6X4	T46.6X5	T46.6X6
Uracil mustard	T45.1X1	T45.1X2	T45.1X3	T45.1X4	T45.1X5	T45.1X6
Uramustine	T45.1X1	T45.1X2	T45.1X3	T45.1X4	T45.1X5	T45.1X6
Urapidil	T46.5X1	T46.5X2	T46.5X3	T46.5X4	T46.5X5	T46.5X6
Urari	T48.1X1	T48.1X2	T48.1X3	T48.1X4	T48.1X5	T48.1X6
Urate oxidase	T50.4X1	T50.4X2	T50.4X3	T50.4X4	T50.4X5	T50.4X6
Urea	T47.3X1	T47.3X2	T47.3X3	T47.3X4	T47.3X5	T47.3X6
peroxide	T49.0X1	T49.0X2	T49.0X3	T49.0X4	T49.0X5	T49.0X6
stibamine	T37.4X1	T37.4X2	T37.4X3	T37.4X4	T37.4X5	T37.4X6
topical	T49.8X1	T49.8X2	T49.8X3	T49.8X4	T49.8X5	T49.8X6
Urethane	T45.1X1	T45.1X2	T45.1X3	T45.1X4	T45.1X5	T45.1X6
Urginea (maritima) (scilla) — see Squill						
Uric acid metabolism drug NEC	T50.4X1	T50.4X2	T50.4X3	T50.4X4	T50.4X5	T50.4X6
Uricosuric agent	T50.4X1	T50.4X2	T50.4X3	T50.4X4	T50.4X5	T50.4X6
Urinary anti-infective	T37.8X1	T37.8X2	T37.8X3	T37.8X4	T37.8X5	T37.8X6
Urofollitropin	T38.811	T38.812	T38.813	T38.814	T38.815	T38.816
Urokinase	T45.611	T45.612	T45.613	T45.614	T45.615	T45.616
Urokon	T50.8X1	T50.8X2	T50.8X3	T50.8X4	T50.8X5	T50.8X6
Ursodeoxycholic acid	T50.991	T50.992	T50.993	T50.994	T50.995	T50.996
Ursodiol	T50.991	T50.992	T50.993	T50.994	T50.995	T50.996
Urtica	T62.2X1	T62.2X2	T62.2X3	T62.2X4	—	—
Utility gas — see Gas, utility						
V						
Vaccine NEC	T50.Z91	T50.Z92	T50.Z93	T50.Z94	T50.Z95	T50.Z96
antineoplastic	T50.Z91	T50.Z92	T50.Z93	T50.Z94	T50.Z95	T50.Z96
bacterial NEC	T50.A91	T50.A92	T50.A93	T50.A94	T50.A95	T50.A96
with						
other bacterial component	T50.A91	T50.A92	T50.A93	T50.A94	T50.A95	T50.A96
pertussis component	T50.A91	T50.A92	T50.A93	T50.A94	T50.A95	T50.A96
viral-rickettsial component	T50.A91	T50.A92	T50.A93	T50.A94	T50.A95	T50.A96
mixed NEC	T50.A91	T50.A92	T50.A93	T50.A94	T50.A95	T50.A96
BCG	T50.A91	T50.A92	T50.A93	T50.A94	T50.A95	T50.A96
cholera	T50.A91	T50.A92	T50.A93	T50.A94	T50.A95	T50.A96
diphtheria	T50.A91	T50.A92	T50.A93	T50.A94	T50.A95	T50.A96
with tetanus	T50.A21	T50.A22	T50.A23	T50.A24	T50.A25	T50.A26
and pertussis	T50.A11	T50.A12	T50.A13	T50.A14	T50.A15	T50.A16

Substance	External Cause (T-Code) Poisoning, Accidental (Unintentional)	Poisoning, Intentional Self-Harm	Poisoning, Assault	Poisoning, Undetermined	Adverse Effect	Underdosing
Vaccine NEC *(Continued)*						
influenza	T50.B91	T50.B92	T50.B93	T50.B94	T50.B95	T50.B96
measles	T50.B91	T50.B92	T50.B93	T50.B94	T50.B95	T50.B96
with mumps and rubella	T50.B91	T50.B92	T50.B93	T50.B94	T50.B95	T50.B96
meningococcal	T50.A91	T50.A92	T50.A93	T50.A94	T50.A95	T50.A96
mumps	T50.B91	T50.B92	T50.B93	T50.B94	T50.B95	T50.B96
paratyphoid	T50.A91	T50.A92	T50.A93	T50.A94	T50.A95	T50.A96
pertussis	T50.A11	T50.A12	T50.A13	T50.A14	T50.A15	T50.A16
with diphtheria	T50.A11	T50.A12	T50.A13	T50.A14	T50.A15	T50.A16
and tetanus	T50.A11	T50.A12	T50.A13	T50.A14	T50.A15	T50.A16
plague	T50.A91	T50.A92	T50.A93	T50.A94	T50.A95	T50.A96
poliomyelitis	T50.B91	T50.B92	T50.B93	T50.B94	T50.B95	T50.B96
poliovirus	T50.B91	T50.B92	T50.B93	T50.B94	T50.B95	T50.B96
rabies	T50.B91	T50.B92	T50.B93	T50.B94	T50.B95	T50.B96
respiratory syncytial virus	T50.B91	T50.B92	T50.B93	T50.B94	T50.B95	T50.B96
rickettsial NEC	T50.A91	T50.A92	T50.A93	T50.A94	T50.A95	T50.A96
with						
bacterial component	T50.A21	T50.A22	T50.A23	T50.A24	T50.A25	T50.A26
Rocky Mountain spotted fever	T50.A91	T50.A92	T50.A93	T50.A94	T50.A95	T50.A96
rubella	T50.B91	T50.B92	T50.B93	T50.B94	T50.B95	T50.B96
sabin oral	T50.B91	T50.B92	T50.B93	T50.B94	T50.B95	T50.B96
smallpox	T50.B11	T50.B12	T50.B13	T50.B14	T50.B15	T50.B16
TAB	T50.A91	T50.A92	T50.A93	T50.A94	T50.A95	T50.A96
tetanus	T50.A91	T50.A92	T50.A93	T50.A94	T50.A95	T50.A96
typhoid	T50.A91	T50.A92	T50.A93	T50.A94	T50.A95	T50.A96
typhus	T50.A91	T50.A92	T50.A93	T50.A94	T50.A95	T50.A96
viral NEC	T50.B91	T50.B92	T50.B93	T50.B94	T50.B95	T50.B96
yellow fever	T50.B91	T50.B92	T50.B93	T50.B94	T50.B95	T50.B96
Vaccinia immune globulin	T50.Z11	T50.Z12	T50.Z13	T50.Z14	T50.Z15	T50.Z16
Vaginal contraceptives	T49.8X1	T49.8X2	T49.8X3	T49.8X4	T49.8X5	T49.8X6
Valerian						
root	T42.6X1	T42.6X2	T42.6X3	T42.6X4	T42.6X5	T42.6X6
tincture	T42.6X1	T42.6X2	T42.6X3	T42.6X4	T42.6X5	T42.6X6
Valethamate bromide	T44.3X1	T44.3X2	T44.3X3	T44.3X4	T44.3X5	T44.3X6
Valisone	T49.0X1	T49.0X2	T49.0X3	T49.0X4	T49.0X5	T49.0X6
Valium	T42.4X1	T42.4X2	T42.4X3	T42.4X4	T42.4X5	T42.4X6
Valmid	T42.6X1	T42.6X2	T42.6X3	T42.6X4	T42.6X5	T42.6X6
Valnoctamide	T42.6X1	T42.6X2	T42.6X3	T42.6X4	T42.6X5	T42.6X6
Valproate (sodium)	T42.6X1	T42.6X2	T42.6X3	T42.6X4	T42.6X5	T42.6X6
Valproic acid	T42.6X1	T42.6X2	T42.6X3	T42.6X4	T42.6X5	T42.6X6
Valpromide	T42.6X1	T42.6X2	T42.6X3	T42.6X4	T42.6X5	T42.6X6
Vanadium	T56.891	T56.892	T56.893	T56.894	—	—

◀ New ◀ Revised ~~deleted~~ Deleted

TABLE OF DRUGS AND CHEMICALS

	External Cause (T-Code)					
Substance	Poisoning, Accidental (Unintentional)	Poisoning, Intentional Self-Harm	Poisoning, Assault	Poisoning, Undetermined	Adverse Effect	Underdosing
Vancomycin	T36.8X1	T36.8X2	T36.8X3	T36.8X4	T36.8X5	T36.8X6
Vapor — *see also Gas*	T59.91	T59.92	T59.93	T59.94	—	—
kiln (carbon monoxide)	T58.8X1	T58.8X2	T58.8X3	T58.8X4	—	—
lead — *see Lead*						
specified source NEC	T59.891	T59.892	T59.893	T59.894	—	—
Vardenafil	T46.7X1	T46.7X2	T46.7X3	T46.7X4	T46.7X5	T46.7X6
Varicose reduction drug	T46.8X1	T46.8X2	T46.8X3	T46.8X4	T46.8X5	T46.8X6
Varnish	T65.4X1	T65.4X2	T65.4X3	T65.4X4		
cleaner	T52.91	T52.92	T52.93	T52.94	—	—
Vaseline	T49.3X1	T49.3X2	T49.3X3	T49.3X4	T49.3X5	T49.3X6
Vasodilan	T46.7X1	T46.7X2	T46.7X3	T46.7X4	T46.7X5	T46.7X6
Vasodilator						
coronary NEC	T46.3X1	T46.3X2	T46.3X3	T46.3X4	T46.3X5	T46.3X6
peripheral NEC	T46.7X1	T46.7X2	T46.7X3	T46.7X4	T46.7X5	T46.7X6
Vasopressin	T38.891	T38.892	T38.893	T38.894	T38.895	T38.896
Vasopressor drugs	T38.891	T38.892	T38.893	T38.894	T38.895	T38.896
Vecuronium bromide	T48.1X1	T48.1X2	T48.1X3	T48.1X4	T48.1X5	T48.1X6
Vegetable extract, astringent	T49.2X1	T49.2X2	T49.2X3	T49.2X4	T49.2X5	T49.2X6
Venlafaxine	T43.211	T43.212	T43.213	T43.214	T43.215	T43.216
Venom, venomous (bite) (sting)	T63.91	T63.92	T63.93	T63.94	—	—
amphibian NEC	T63.831	T63.832	T63.833	T63.834	—	—
animal NEC	T63.891	T63.892	T63.893	T63.894	—	—
ant	T63.421	T63.422	T63.423	T63.424	—	—
arthropod NEC	T63.481	T63.482	T63.483	T63.484	—	—
bee	T63.441	T63.442	T63.443	T63.444	—	—
centipede	T63.411	T63.412	T63.413	T63.414	—	—
fish	T63.591	T63.592	T63.593	T63.594	—	—
frog	T63.811	T63.812	T63.813	T63.814	—	—
hornet	T63.451	T63.452	T63.453	T63.454	—	—
insect NEC	T63.481	T63.482	T63.483	T63.484	—	—
lizard	T63.121	T63.122	T63.123	T63.124	—	—
marine						
animals	T63.691	T63.692	T63.693	T63.694	—	—
bluebottle	T63.611	T63.612	T63.613	T63.614	—	—
jellyfish NEC	T63.621	T63.622	T63.623	T63.624	—	—
Portuguese Man-o-war	T63.611	T63.612	T63.613	T63.614	—	—
sea anemone	T63.631	T63.632	T63.633	T63.634	—	—
specified NEC	T63.691	T63.692	T63.693	T63.694	—	—
fish	T63.591	T63.592	T63.593	T63.594	—	—
plants	T63.711	T63.712	T63.713	T63.714	—	—
sting ray	T63.511	T63.512	T63.513	T63.514	—	—

	External Cause (T-Code)					
Substance	Poisoning, Accidental (Unintentional)	Poisoning, Intentional Self-Harm	Poisoning, Assault	Poisoning, Undetermined	Adverse Effect	Underdosing
Venom, venomous *(Continued)*						
millipede (tropical)	T63.411	T63.412	T63.413	T63.414	—	—
plant NEC	T63.791	T63.792	T63.793	T63.794	—	—
marine	T63.711	T63.712	T63.713	T63.714	—	—
reptile	T63.191	T63.192	T63.193	T63.194	—	—
gila monster	T63.111	T63.112	T63.113	T63.114	—	—
lizard NEC	T63.121	T63.122	T63.123	T63.124	—	—
scorpion	T63.2X1	T63.2X2	T63.2X3	T63.2X4	—	—
snake	T63.001	T63.002	T63.003	T63.004	—	—
African NEC	T63.081	T63.082	T63.083	T63.084	—	—
American (North) (South) NEC	T63.061	T63.062	T63.063	T63.064	—	—
Asian	T63.081	T63.082	T63.083	T63.084	—	—
Australian	T63.071	T63.072	T63.073	T63.074	—	—
cobra	T63.041	T63.042	T63.043	T63.044	—	—
coral snake	T63.021	T63.022	T63.023	T63.024	—	—
rattlesnake	T63.011	T63.012	T63.013	T63.014	—	—
specified NEC	T63.091	T63.092	T63.093	T63.094	—	—
taipan	T63.031	T63.032	T63.033	T63.034	—	—
specified NEC	T63.891	T63.892	T63.893	T63.894	—	—
spider	T63.301	T63.302	T63.303	T63.304	—	—
black widow	T63.311	T63.312	T63.313	T63.314	—	—
brown recluse	T63.331	T63.332	T63.333	T63.334	—	—
specified NEC	T63.391	T63.392	T63.393	T63.394	—	—
tarantula	T63.321	T63.322	T63.323	T63.324	—	—
sting ray	T63.511	T63.512	T63.513	T63.514	—	—
toad	T63.821	T63.822	T63.823	T63.824	—	—
wasp	T63.461	T63.462	T63.463	T63.464	—	—
Venous sclerosing drug NEC	T46.8X1	T46.8X2	T46.8X3	T46.8X4	T46.8X5	T46.8X6
Ventolin — *see Albuterol*						
Verapamil	T46.1X1	T46.1X2	T46.1X3	T46.1X4	T46.1X5	T46.1X6
Veramon	T42.3X1	T42.3X2	T42.3X3	T42.3X4	T42.3X5	T42.3X6
Veratrine	T46.5X1	T46.5X2	T46.5X3	T46.5X4	T46.5X5	T46.5X6
Veratrum						
album	T62.2X1	T62.2X2	T62.2X3	T62.2X4	—	—
alkaloids	T46.5X1	T46.5X2	T46.5X3	T46.5X4	T46.5X5	T46.5X6
viride	T62.2X1	T62.2X2	T62.2X3	T62.2X4	—	—
Verdigris	T60.3X1	T60.3X2	T60.3X3	T60.3X4	—	—
Veronal	T42.3X1	T42.3X2	T42.3X3	T42.3X4	T42.3X5	T42.3X6
Veroxil	T37.4X1	T37.4X2	T37.4X3	T37.4X4	T37.4X5	T37.4X6
Versenate	T50.6X1	T50.6X2	T50.6X3	T50.6X4	T50.6X5	T50.6X6

◀ New ◀◀ Revised ~~deleted~~ Deleted

Substance	Poisoning, Accidental (Unintentional)	Poisoning, Intentional Self-Harm	Poisoning, Assault	Poisoning, Undetermined	Adverse Effect	Underdosing
Versidyne	T39.8X1	T39.8X2	T39.8X3	T39.8X4	T39.8X5	T39.8X6
Vetrabutine	T48.0X1	T48.0X2	T48.0X3	T48.0X4	T48.0X5	T48.0X6
Vidarabine	T37.5X1	T37.5X2	T37.5X3	T37.5X4	T37.5X5	T37.5X6
Vienna						
green	T57.0X1	T57.0X2	T57.0X3	T57.0X4	—	—
insecticide	T60.2X1	T60.2X2	T60.2X3	T60.2X4	—	—
red	T57.0X1	T57.0X2	T57.0X3	T57.0X4	—	—
pharmaceutical dye	T50.991	T50.992	T50.993	T50.994	T50.995	T50.996
Vigabatrin	T42.6X1	T42.6X2	T42.6X3	T42.6X4	T42.6X5	T42.6X6
Viloxazine	T43.291	T43.292	T43.293	T43.294	T43.295	T43.296
Viminol	T39.8X1	T39.8X2	T39.8X3	T39.8X4	T39.8X5	T39.8X6
Vinbarbital, vinbarbitone	T42.3X1	T42.3X2	T42.3X3	T42.3X4	T42.3X5	T42.3X6
Vinblastine	T45.1X1	T45.1X2	T45.1X3	T45.1X4	T45.1X5	T45.1X6
Vinburnine	T46.7X1	T46.7X2	T46.7X3	T46.7X4	T46.7X5	T46.7X6
Vincamine	T45.1X1	T45.1X2	T45.1X3	T45.1X4	T45.1X5	T45.1X6
Vincristine	T45.1X1	T45.1X2	T45.1X3	T45.1X4	T45.1X5	T45.1X6
Vindesine	T45.1X1	T45.1X2	T45.1X3	T45.1X4	T45.1X5	T45.1X6
Vinesthene, vinethene	T41.0X1	T41.0X2	T41.0X3	T41.0X4	T41.0X5	T41.0X6
Vinorelbine tartrate	T45.1X1	T45.1X2	T45.1X3	T45.1X4	T45.1X5	T45.1X6
Vinpocetine	T46.7X1	T46.7X2	T46.7X3	T46.7X4	T46.7X5	T46.7X6
Vinyl						
acetate	T65.891	T65.892	T65.893	T65.894	—	—
bital	T42.3X1	T42.3X2	T42.3X3	T42.3X4	T42.3X5	T42.3X6
bromide	T65.891	T65.892	T65.893	T65.894	—	—
chloride	T59.891	T59.892	T59.893	T59.894	—	—
ether	T41.0X1	T41.0X2	T41.0X3	T41.0X4	T41.0X5	T41.0X6
Vinylbital	T42.3X1	T42.3X2	T42.3X3	T42.3X4	T42.3X5	T42.3X6
Vinylidene chloride	T65.891	T65.892	T65.893	T65.894	—	—
Vioform	T37.8X1	T37.8X2	T37.8X3	T37.8X4	T37.8X5	T37.8X6
topical	T49.0X1	T49.0X2	T49.0X3	T49.0X4	T49.0X5	T49.0X6
Viomycin	T36.8X1	T36.8X2	T36.8X3	T36.8X4	T36.8X5	T36.8X6
Viosterol	T45.2X1	T45.2X2	T45.2X3	T45.2X4	T45.2X5	T45.2X6
Viper (venom)	T63.091	T63.092	T63.093	T63.094	—	—
Viprynium	T37.4X1	T37.4X2	T37.4X3	T37.4X4	T37.4X5	T37.4X6
Viquidil	T46.7X1	T46.7X2	T46.7X3	T46.7X4	T46.7X5	T46.7X6
Viral vaccine NEC	T50.B91	T50.B92	T50.B93	T50.B94	T50.B95	T50.B96
Virginiamycin	T36.8X1	T36.8X2	T36.8X3	T36.8X4	T36.8X5	T36.8X6
Virugon	T37.5X1	T37.5X2	T37.5X3	T37.5X4	T37.5X5	T37.5X6
Viscous agent	T50.901	T50.902	T50.903	T50.904	T50.905	T50.906
Visine	T49.5X1	T49.5X2	T49.5X3	T49.5X4	T49.5X5	T49.5X6
Visnadine	T46.3X1	T46.3X2	T46.3X3	T46.3X4	T46.3X5	T46.3X6

Substance	Poisoning, Accidental (Unintentional)	Poisoning, Intentional Self-Harm	Poisoning, Assault	Poisoning, Undetermined	Adverse Effect	Underdosing
Vitamin NEC	T45.2X1	T45.2X2	T45.2X3	T45.2X4	T45.2X5	T45.2X6
A	T45.2X1	T45.2X2	T45.2X3	T45.2X4	T45.2X5	T45.2X6
B NEC	T45.2X1	T45.2X2	T45.2X3	T45.2X4	T45.2X5	T45.2X6
nicotinic acid	T46.7X1	T46.7X2	T46.7X3	T46.7X4	T46.7X5	T46.7X6
B1	T45.2X1	T45.2X2	T45.2X3	T45.2X4	T45.2X5	T45.2X6
B2	T45.2X1	T45.2X2	T45.2X3	T45.2X4	T45.2X5	T45.2X6
B6	T45.2X1	T45.2X2	T45.2X3	T45.2X4	T45.2X5	T45.2X6
B12	T45.2X1	T45.2X2	T45.2X3	T45.2X4	T45.2X5	T45.2X6
B15	T45.2X1	T45.2X2	T45.2X3	T45.2X4	T45.2X5	T45.2X6
C	T45.2X1	T45.2X2	T45.2X3	T45.2X4	T45.2X5	T45.2X6
D	T45.2X1	T45.2X2	T45.2X3	T45.2X4	T45.2X5	T45.2X6
D2	T45.2X1	T45.2X2	T45.2X3	T45.2X4	T45.2X5	T45.2X6
D3	T45.2X1	T45.2X2	T45.2X3	T45.2X4	T45.2X5	T45.2X6
E	T45.2X1	T45.2X2	T45.2X3	T45.2X4	T45.2X5	T45.2X6
E acetate	T45.2X1	T45.2X2	T45.2X3	T45.2X4	T45.2X5	T45.2X6
hematopoietic	T45.8X1	T45.8X2	T45.8X3	T45.8X4	T45.8X5	T45.8X6
K NEC	T45.7X1	T45.7X2	T45.7X3	T45.7X4	T45.7X5	T45.7X6
K1	T45.7X1	T45.7X2	T45.7X3	T45.7X4	T45.7X5	T45.7X6
K2	T45.7X1	T45.7X2	T45.7X3	T45.7X4	T45.7X5	T45.7X6
PP	T45.2X1	T45.2X2	T45.2X3	T45.2X4	T45.2X5	T45.2X6
ulceroprotectant	T47.1X1	T47.1X2	T47.1X3	T47.1X4	T47.1X5	T47.1X6
Vleminckx's solution	T49.4X1	T49.4X2	T49.4X3	T49.4X4	T49.4X5	T49.4X6
Voltaren — see Diclofenac sodium						
W						
Warfarin	T45.511	T45.512	T45.513	T45.514	T45.515	T45.516
rodenticide	T60.4X1	T60.4X2	T60.4X3	T60.4X4	—	—
sodium	T45.511	T45.512	T45.513	T45.514	T45.515	T45.516
Wasp (sting)	T63.461	T63.462	T63.463	T63.464	—	—
Water						
balance drug	T50.3X1	T50.3X2	T50.3X3	T50.3X4	T50.3X5	T50.3X6
distilled	T50.3X1	T50.3X2	T50.3X3	T50.3X4	T50.3X5	T50.3X6
gas — see Gas, water						
incomplete combustion of — see Carbon, monoxide, fuel, utility						
hemlock	T62.2X1	T62.2X2	T62.2X3	T62.2X4	—	—
moccasin (venom)	T63.061	T63.062	T63.063	T63.064	—	—
purified	T50.3X1	T50.3X2	T50.3X3	T50.3X4	T50.3X5	T50.3X6
Wax (paraffin) (petroleum)	T52.0X1	T52.0X2	T52.0X3	T52.0X4	—	—
automobile	T65.891	T65.892	T65.893	T65.894	—	—
floor	T52.0X1	T52.0X2	T52.0X3	T52.0X4	—	—

◄ New   ◄ Revised   ~~deleted~~ Deleted

TABLE OF DRUGS AND CHEMICALS

Substance	External Cause (T-Code)					
	Poisoning, Accidental (Unintentional)	Poisoning, Intentional Self-Harm	Poisoning, Assault	Poisoning, Undetermined	Adverse Effect	Underdosing
Weed killers NEC	T60.3X1	T60.3X2	T60.3X3	T60.3X4	—	—
Welldorm	T42.6X1	T42.6X2	T42.6X3	T42.6X4	T42.6X5	T42.6X6
White						
arsenic	T57.0X1	T57.0X2	T57.0X3	T57.0X4	—	—
hellebore	T62.2X1	T62.2X2	T62.2X3	T62.2X4	—	—
lotion (keratolytic)	T49.4X1	T49.4X2	T49.4X3	T49.4X4	T49.4X5	T49.4X6
spirit	T52.0X1	T52.0X2	T52.0X3	T52.0X4	—	—
Whitewash	T65.891	T65.892	T65.893	T65.894	—	—
Whole blood (human)	T45.8X1	T45.8X2	T45.8X3	T45.8X4	T45.8X5	T45.8X6
Wild						
black cherry	T62.2X1	T62.2X2	T62.2X3	T62.2X4	—	—
poisonous plants NEC	T62.2X1	T62.2X2	T62.2X3	T62.2X4	—	—
Window cleaning fluid	T65.891	T65.892	T65.893	T65.894	—	—
Wintergreen (oil)	T49.3X1	T49.3X2	T49.3X3	T49.3X4	T49.3X5	T49.3X6
Wisterine	T62.2X1	T62.2X2	T62.2X3	T62.2X4	—	—
Witch hazel	T49.2X1	T49.2X2	T49.2X3	T49.2X4	T49.2X5	T49.2X6
Wood alcohol or spirit	T51.1X1	T51.1X2	T51.1X3	T51.1X4	—	—
Wool fat (hydrous)	T49.3X1	T49.3X2	T49.3X3	T49.3X4	T49.3X5	T49.3X6
Woorali	T48.1X1	T48.1X2	T48.1X3	T48.1X4	T48.1X5	T48.1X6
Wormseed, American	T37.4X1	T37.4X2	T37.4X3	T37.4X4	T37.4X5	T37.4X6
X						
Xamoterol	T44.5X1	T44.5X2	T44.5X3	T44.5X4	T44.5X5	T44.5X6
Xanthine diuretics	T50.2X1	T50.2X2	T50.2X3	T50.2X4	T50.2X5	T50.2X6
Xanthinol nicotinate	T46.7X1	T46.7X2	T46.7X3	T46.7X4	T46.7X5	T46.7X6
Xanthotoxin	T49.3X1	T49.3X2	T49.3X3	T49.3X4	T49.3X5	T49.3X6
Xantinol nicotinate	T46.7X1	T46.7X2	T46.7X3	T46.7X4	T46.7X5	T46.7X6
Xantocillin	T36.0X1	T36.0X2	T36.0X3	T36.0X4	T36.0X5	T36.0X6
Xenon (127Xe) (133Xe)	T50.8X1	T50.8X2	T50.8X3	T50.8X4	T50.8X5	T50.8X6
Xenysalate	T49.4X1	T49.4X2	T49.4X3	T49.4X4	T49.4X5	T49.4X6
Xibornol	T37.8X1	T37.8X2	T37.8X3	T37.8X4	T37.8X5	T37.8X6
Xigris	T45.511	T45.512	T45.513	T45.514	T45.515	T45.516
Xipamide	T50.2X1	T50.2X2	T50.2X3	T50.2X4	T50.2X5	T50.2X6
Xylene (vapor)	T52.2X1	T52.2X2	T52.2X3	T52.2X4	—	—
Xylocaine (infiltration) (topical)	T41.3X1	T41.3X2	T41.3X3	T41.3X4	T41.3X5	T41.3X6
nerve block (peripheral) (plexus)	T41.3X1	T41.3X2	T41.3X3	T41.3X4	T41.3X5	T41.3X6
spinal	T41.3X1	T41.3X2	T41.3X3	T41.3X4	T41.3X5	T41.3X6
Xylol (vapor)	T52.2X1	T52.2X2	T52.2X3	T52.2X4	—	—
Xylometazoline	T48.5X1	T48.5X2	T48.5X3	T48.5X4	T48.5X5	T48.5X6

Substance	External Cause (T-Code)					
	Poisoning, Accidental (Unintentional)	Poisoning, Intentional Self-Harm	Poisoning, Assault	Poisoning, Undetermined	Adverse Effect	Underdosing
Y						
Yeast	T45.2X1	T45.2X2	T45.2X3	T45.2X4	T45.2X5	T45.2X6
dried	T45.2X1	T45.2X2	T45.2X3	T45.2X4	T45.2X5	T45.2X6
Yellow						
fever vaccine	T50.B91	T50.B92	T50.B93	T50.B94	T50.B95	T50.B96
jasmine	T62.2X1	T62.2X2	T62.2X3	T62.2X4	—	—
phenolphthalein	T47.2X1	T47.2X2	T47.2X3	T47.2X4	T47.2X5	T47.2X6
Yew	T62.2X1	T62.2X2	T62.2X3	T62.2X4	—	—
Yohimbic acid	T40.991	T40.992	T40.993	T40.994	T40.995	T40.996
Z						
Zactane	T39.8X1	T39.8X2	T39.8X3	T39.8X4	T39.8X5	T39.8X6
Zalcitabine	T37.5X1	T37.5X2	T37.5X3	T37.5X4	T37.5X5	T37.5X6
Zaroxolyn	T50.2X1	T50.2X2	T50.2X3	T50.2X4	T50.2X5	T50.2X6
Zephiran (topical)	T49.0X1	T49.0X2	T49.0X3	T49.0X4	T49.0X5	T49.0X6
ophthalmic preparation	T49.5X1	T49.5X2	T49.5X3	T49.5X4	T49.5X5	T49.5X6
Zeranol	T38.7X1	T38.7X2	T38.7X3	T38.7X4	T38.7X5	T38.7X6
Zerone	T51.1X1	T51.1X2	T51.1X3	T51.1X4	—	—
Zidovudine	T37.5X1	T37.5X2	T37.5X3	T37.5X4	T37.5X5	T37.5X6
Zimeldine	T43.221	T43.222	T43.223	T43.224	T43.225	T43.226
Zinc (compounds) (fumes) (vapor) NEC	T56.5X1	T56.5X2	T56.5X3	T56.5X4	—	—
anti-infectives	T49.0X1	T49.0X2	T49.0X3	T49.0X4	T49.0X5	T49.0X6
antivaricose	T46.8X1	T46.8X2	T46.8X3	T46.8X4	T46.8X5	T46.8X6
bacitracin	T49.0X1	T49.0X2	T49.0X3	T49.0X4	T49.0X5	T49.0X6
chloride (mouthwash)	T49.6X1	T49.6X2	T49.6X3	T49.6X4	T49.6X5	T49.6X6
chromate	T56.5X1	T56.5X2	T56.5X3	T56.5X4	—	—
gelatin	T49.3X1	T49.3X2	T49.3X3	T49.3X4	T49.3X5	T49.3X6
oxide	T49.3X1	T49.3X2	T49.3X3	T49.3X4	T49.3X5	T49.3X6
plaster	T49.3X1	T49.3X2	T49.3X3	T49.3X4	T49.3X5	T49.3X6
peroxide	T49.0X1	T49.0X2	T49.0X3	T49.0X4	T49.0X5	T49.0X6
pesticides	T56.5X1	T56.5X2	T56.5X3	T56.5X4	—	—
phosphide	T60.4X1	T60.4X2	T60.4X3	T60.4X4	—	—
pyrithionate	T49.4X1	T49.4X2	T49.4X3	T49.4X4	T49.4X5	T49.4X6
stearate	T49.3X1	T49.3X2	T49.3X3	T49.3X4	T49.3X5	T49.3X6
sulfate	T49.5X1	T49.5X2	T49.5X3	T49.5X4	T49.5X5	T49.5X6
ENT agent	T49.6X1	T49.6X2	T49.6X3	T49.6X4	T49.6X5	T49.6X6
ophthalmic solution	T49.5X1	T49.5X2	T49.5X3	T49.5X4	T49.5X5	T49.5X6
topical NEC	T49.0X1	T49.0X2	T49.0X3	T49.0X4	T49.0X5	T49.0X6
undecylenate	T49.0X1	T49.0X2	T49.0X3	T49.0X4	T49.0X5	T49.0X6

◀ New ◀ Revised ~~deleted~~ Deleted

	External Cause (T-Code)					
Substance	Poisoning, Accidental (Unintentional)	Poisoning, Intentional Self-Harm	Poisoning, Assault	Poisoning, Undetermined	Adverse Effect	Underdosing
Zineb	T60.0X1	T60.0X2	T60.0X3	T60.0X4	—	—
Zinostatin	T45.1X1	T45.1X2	T45.1X3	T45.1X4	T45.1X5	T45.1X6
Zipeprol	T48.3X1	T48.3X2	T48.3X3	T48.3X4	T48.3X5	T48.3X6
Zofenopril	T46.4X1	T46.4X2	T46.4X3	T46.4X4	T46.4X5	T46.4X6
Zolpidem	T42.6X1	T42.6X2	T42.6X3	T42.6X4	T42.6X5	T42.6X6
Zomepirac	T39.391	T39.392	T39.393	T39.394	T39.395	T39.396
Zopiclone	T42.6X1	T42.6X2	T42.6X3	T42.6X4	T42.6X5	T42.6X6

	External Cause (T-Code)					
Substance	Poisoning, Accidental (Unintentional)	Poisoning, Intentional Self-Harm	Poisoning, Assault	Poisoning, Undetermined	Adverse Effect	Underdosing
Zorubicin	T45.1X1	T45.1X2	T45.1X3	T45.1X4	T45.1X5	T45.1X6
Zotepine	T43.591	T43.592	T43.593	T43.594	T43.595	T43.596
Zovant	T45.511	T45.512	T45.513	T45.514	T45.515	T45.516
Zoxazolamine	T42.8X1	T42.8X2	T42.8X3	T42.8X4	T42.8X5	T42.8X6
Zuclopenthixol	T43.4X1	T43.4X2	T43.4X3	T43.4X4	T43.4X5	T43.4X6
Zygadenus (venenosus)	T62.2X1	T62.2X2	T62.2X3	T62.2X4	—	—
Zyprexa	T43.591	T43.592	T43.593	T43.594	T43.595	T43.596

◀ New ◀ Revised deleted Deleted

TABLE OF DRUGS AND CHEMICALS

External Cause
of Injuries Index

A

Abandonment (causing exposure to weather conditions) (with intent to injure or kill) NEC X58

Abuse (adult) (child) (mental) (physical) (sexual) X58

Accident (to) X58

aircraft (in transit) (powered) —*see also* Accident, transport, aircraft

due to, caused by cataclysm —*see* Forces of nature, by type

animal-drawn vehicle —*see* Accident, transport, animal-drawn vehicle occupant

animal-rider —*see* Accident, transport, animal-rider

automobile —*see* Accident, transport, car occupant

bare foot water skiier V94.4

boat, boating —*see also* Accident, watercraft

striking swimmer

powered V94.11

unpowered V94.12

bus —*see* Accident, transport, bus occupant

cable car, not on rails V98.0

on rails —*see* Accident, transport, streetcar occupant

car —*see* Accident, transport, car occupant

caused by, due to

animal NEC W64

chain hoist W24.0

cold (excessive) —*see* Exposure, cold

corrosive liquid, substance —*see* Table of Drugs and Chemicals

cutting or piercing instrument —*see* Contact, with, by type of instrument

drive belt W24.0

electric

current —*see* Exposure, electric current

motor —*see also* Contact, with, by type of machine W31.3

current (of) W86.8

environmental factor NEC X58

explosive material —*see* Explosion

fire, flames —*see* Exposure, fire

firearm missile —*see* Discharge, firearm by type

heat (excessive) —*see* Heat

hot —*see* Contact, with, hot

ignition —*see* Ignition

lifting device W24.0

lightning —*see* subcategory T75.0

causing fire —*see* Exposure, fire

machine, machinery —*see* Contact, with, by type of machine

natural factor NEC X58

pulley (block) W24.0

radiation —*see* Radiation

steam X13.1

inhalation X13.0

pipe X16

thunderbolt —*see* subcategory T75.0

causing fire —*see* Exposure, fire

transmission device W24.1

coach —*see* Accident, transport, bus occupant

coal car —*see* Accident, transport, industrial vehicle occupant

diving —*see also* Fall, into, water

with

drowning or submersion —*see* Drowning

forklift —*see* Accident, transport, industrial vehicle occupant

heavy transport vehicle NOS —*see* Accident, transport, truck occupant

ice yacht V98.2

Accident *(Continued)*

in

medical, surgical procedure

as, or due to misadventure —*see* Misadventure

causing an abnormal reaction or later complication without mention of misadventure —*see also* Complication of or following, by type of procedure Y84.9

land yacht V98.1

late effect of —*see* W00-X58 with 7th character S

logging car —*see* Accident, transport, industrial vehicle occupant

machine, machinery —*see also* Contact, with, by type of machine

on board watercraft V93.69

explosion —*see* Explosion, in, watercraft

fire —*see* Burn, on board watercraft

powered craft V93.63

ferry boat V93.61

fishing boat V93.62

jet ski V93.63

liner V93.61

merchant ship V93.60

passenger ship V93.61

sailboat V93.64

mine tram —*see* Accident, transport, industrial vehicle occupant

mobility scooter (motorized) —*see* Accident, transport, pedestrian, conveyance, specified type NEC

motor scooter —*see* Accident, transport, motorcyclist

motor vehicle NOS (traffic) —*see also* Accident, transport V89.2

nontraffic V89.0

three-wheeled NOS —*see* Accident, transport, three-wheeled motor vehicle occupant

motorcycle NOS —*see* Accident, transport, motorcyclist

nonmotor vehicle NOS (nontraffic) —*see also* Accident, transport V89.1

traffic NOS V89.3

nontraffic (victim's mode of transport NOS) V88.9

collision (between) V88.7

bus and truck V88.5

car and:

bus V88.3

pickup V88.2

three-wheeled motor vehicle V88.0

train V88.6

truck V88.4

two-wheeled motor vehicle V88.0

van V88.2

specified vehicle NEC and:

three-wheeled motor vehicle V88.1

two-wheeled motor vehicle V88.1

known mode of transport —*see* Accident, transport, by type of vehicle

noncollision V88.8

on board watercraft V93.89

powered craft V93.83

ferry boat V93.81

fishing boat V93.82

jet ski V93.83

liner V93.81

merchant ship V93.80

passenger ship V93.81

unpowered craft V93.88

canoe V93.85

inflatable V93.86

in tow

recreational V94.31

specified NEC V94.32

kayak V93.85

Accident *(Continued)*

on board watercraft *(Continued)*

unpowered craft *(Continued)*

sailboat V93.84

surf-board V93.88

water skis V93.87

windsurfer V93.88

parachutist V97.29

entangled in object V97.21

injured on landing V97.22

pedal cycle —*see* Accident, transport, pedal cyclist

pedestrian (on foot)

with

another pedestrian W51

with fall W03

due to ice or snow W00.0

on pedestrian conveyance NEC V00.09

rider of

hoverboard V00.038

Segway V00.038

standing

electric scooter V00.031

micro-mobility pedestrian conveyance NEC V00.038

roller skater (in-line) V00.01

skate boarder V00.02

transport vehicle —*see* Accident, transport

on pedestrian conveyance —*see* Accident, transport, pedestrian, conveyance

pick-up truck or van —*see* Accident, transport, pickup truck occupant

quarry truck —*see* Accident, transport, industrial vehicle occupant

railway vehicle (any) (in motion) —*see* Accident, transport, railway vehicle occupant

due to cataclysm —*see* Forces of nature, by type

scooter (non-motorized) —*see* Accident, transport, pedestrian, conveyance, scooter

sequelae of —*see* W00-X58 with 7th character S

skateboard —*see* Accident, transport, pedestrian, conveyance, skateboard

ski (ing) —*see* Accident, transport, pedestrian, conveyance

lift V98.3

specified cause NEC X58

streetcar —*see* Accident, transport, streetcar occupant

traffic (victim's mode of transport NOS) V87.9

collision (between) V87.7

bus and truck V87.5

car and:

bus V87.3

pickup V87.2

three-wheeled motor vehicle V87.0

train V87.6

truck V87.4

two-wheeled motor vehicle V87.0

van V87.2

specified vehicle NEC V86.39

and

three-wheeled motor vehicle V87.1

two-wheeled motor vehicle V87.1

driver V86.09

person on outside V86.29

passenger V86.19

while boarding or alighting V86.49

known mode of transport —*see* Accident, transport, by type of vehicle

noncollision V87.8

▶ New   ➠ Revised   ~~deleted~~ Deleted   ● Use Additional Character(s)

Accident *(Continued)*
transport (involving injury to) V99
18 wheeler —*see* Accident, transport, truck
occupant
agricultural vehicle occupant (nontraffic)
V84.9
driver V84.5
hanger-on V84.7
passenger V84.6
traffic V84.3
driver V84.0
hanger-on V84.2
passenger V84.1
while boarding or alighting
V84.4
aircraft NEC V97.89
military NEC V97.818
with civilian aircraft V97.810
civilian injured by V97.811
occupant injured (in)
nonpowered craft accident V96.9
balloon V96.00
collision V96.03
crash V96.01
explosion V96.05
fire V96.04
forced landing V96.02
specified type NEC V96.09
glider V96.20
collision V96.23
crash V96.21
explosion V96.25
fire V96.24
forced landing V96.22
specified type NEC V96.29
hang glider V96.10
collision V96.13
crash V96.11
explosion V96.15
fire V96.14
forced landing V96.12
specified type NEC V96.19
specified craft NEC V96.8
powered craft accident V95.9
fixed wing NEC
commercial V95.30
collision V95.33
crash V95.31
explosion V95.35
fire V95.34
forced landing V95.32
specified type NEC V95.39
private V95.20
collision V95.23
crash V95.21
explosion V95.25
fire V95.24
forced landing V95.22
specified type NEC V95.29
glider V95.10
collision V95.13
crash V95.11
explosion V95.15
fire V95.14
forced landing V95.12
specified type NEC V95.19
helicopter V95.00
collision V95.03
crash V95.01
explosion V95.05
fire V95.04
forced landing V95.02
specified type NEC V95.09
spacecraft V95.40
collision V95.43
crash V95.41
explosion V95.45
fire V95.44
forced landing V95.42
specified type NEC V95.49
specified craft NEC V95.8

Accident *(Continued)*
transport *(Continued)*
aircraft NEC *(Continued)*
occupant injured *(Continued)*
powered craft accident *(Continued)*
ultralight V95.10
collision V95.13
crash V95.11
explosion V95.15
fire V95.14
forced landing V95.12
specified type NEC V95.19
specified accident NEC V97.0
while boarding or alighting V97.1
person (injured by)
falling from, in or on aircraft V97.0
machinery on aircraft V97.89
on ground with aircraft involvement
V97.39
rotating propeller V97.32
struck by object falling from aircraft
V97.31
sucked into aircraft jet V97.33
while boarding or alighting aircraft
V97.1
airport (battery-powered) passenger
vehicle —*see* Accident, transport,
industrial vehicle occupant
all-terrain vehicle occupant (nontraffic)
V86.95
driver V86.55
dune buggy —*see* Accident, transport,
dune buggy occupant
hanger-on V86.75
passenger V86.65
snowmobile —*see* Accident, transport,
snowmobile occupant
specified type NEC V86.99
driver V86.59
passenger V86.69
person on outside V86.79
traffic V86.35
driver V86.05
hanger-on V86.25
passenger V86.15
while boarding or alighting V86.45
ambulance occupant (traffic) V86.31
driver V86.01
hanger-on V86.21
nontraffic V86.91
driver V86.51
hanger-on V86.71
passenger V86.61
passenger V86.11
while boarding or alighting V86.41
animal-drawn vehicle occupant (in) V80.929
collision (with)
animal V80.12
being ridden V80.711
animal-drawn vehicle V80.721
bus V80.42
car V80.42
fixed or stationary object V80.82
military vehicle V80.920
nonmotor vehicle V80.791
pedal cycle V80.22
pedestrian V80.12
pickup V80.42
railway train or vehicle V80.62
specified motor vehicle NEC V80.52
streetcar V80.731
truck V80.42
two-or three-wheeled motor vehicle
V80.32
van V80.42
noncollision V80.02
specified circumstance NEC V80.928
animal-rider V80.919
collision (with)
animal V80.11
being ridden V80.710

Accident *(Continued)*
transport *(Continued)*
animal-rider *(Continued)*
collision *(Continued)*
animal-drawn vehicle V80.720
bus V80.41
car V80.41
fixed or stationary object V80.81
military vehicle V80.910
nonmotor vehicle V80.790
pedal cycle V80.21
pedestrian V80.11
pickup V80.41
railway train or vehicle V80.61
specified motor vehicle NEC V80.51
streetcar V80.730
truck V80.41
two- or three-wheeled motor vehicle
V80.31
van V80.41
noncollision V80.018
specified as horse rider V80.010
specified circumstance NEC V80.918
armored car —*see* Accident, transport,
truck occupant
battery-powered truck (baggage) (mail) —
see Accident, transport, industrial
vehicle occupant
bus occupant V79.9
collision (with)
animal (traffic) V70.9
being ridden (traffic) V76.9
nontraffic V76.3
while boarding or alighting V76.4
nontraffic V70.3
while boarding or alighting V70.4
animal-drawn vehicle (traffic) V76.9
nontraffic V76.3
while boarding or alighting V76.4
bus (traffic) V74.9
nontraffic V74.3
while boarding or alighting V74.4
car (traffic) V73.9
nontraffic V73.3
while boarding or alighting V73.4
motor vehicle NOS (traffic) V79.60
nontraffic V79.20
specified type NEC (traffic) V79.69
nontraffic V79.29
pedal cycle (traffic) V71.9
nontraffic V71.3
while boarding or alighting V71.4
pickup truck (traffic) V73.9
nontraffic V73.3
while boarding or alighting V73.4
railway vehicle (traffic) V75.9
nontraffic V75.3
while boarding or alighting V75.4
specified vehicle NEC (traffic) V76.9
nontraffic V76.3
while boarding or alighting V76.4
stationary object (traffic) V77.9
nontraffic V77.3
while boarding or alighting V77.4
streetcar (traffic) V76.9
nontraffic V76.3
while boarding or alighting V76.4
three wheeled motor vehicle (traffic)
V72.9
nontraffic V72.3
while boarding or alighting V72.4
truck (traffic) V74.9
nontraffic V74.3
while boarding or alighting V74.4
two wheeled motor vehicle (traffic)
V72.9
nontraffic V72.3
while boarding or alighting V72.4
van (traffic) V73.9
nontraffic V73.3
while boarding or alighting V73.4

Accident *(Continued)*
  transport *(Continued)*
    bus occupant *(Continued)*
      driver
        collision (with)
          animal (traffic) V70.5
            being ridden (traffic) V76.5
              nontraffic V76.0
            nontraffic V70.0
          animal-drawn vehicle (traffic) V76.5
            nontraffic V76.0
          bus (traffic) V74.5
            nontraffic V74.0
          car (traffic) V73.5
            nontraffic V73.0
          motor vehicle NOS (traffic) V79.40
            nontraffic V79.00
            specified type NEC (traffic) V79.49
              nontraffic V79.09
          pedal cycle (traffic) V71.5
            nontraffic V71.0
          pickup truck (traffic) V73.5
            nontraffic V73.0
          railway vehicle (traffic) V75.5
            nontraffic V75.0
          specified vehicle NEC (traffic) V76.5
            nontraffic V76.0
          stationary object (traffic) V77.5
            nontraffic V77.0
          streetcar (traffic) V76.5
            nontraffic V76.0
          three wheeled motor vehicle (traffic) V72.5
            nontraffic V72.0
          truck (traffic) V74.5
            nontraffic V74.0
          two wheeled motor vehicle (traffic) V72.5
            nontraffic V72.0
          van (traffic) V73.5
            nontraffic V73.0
        noncollision accident (traffic) V78.5
          nontraffic V78.0
      hanger-on
        collision (with)
          animal (traffic) V70.7
            being ridden (traffic) V76.7
              nontraffic V76.2
            nontraffic V70.2
          animal-drawn vehicle (traffic) V76.7
            nontraffic V76.2
          bus (traffic) V74.7
            nontraffic V74.2
          car (traffic) V73.7
            nontraffic V73.2
          pedal cycle (traffic) V71.7
            nontraffic V71.2
          pickup truck (traffic) V73.7
            nontraffic V73.2
          railway vehicle (traffic) V75.7
            nontraffic V75.2
          specified vehicle NEC (traffic) V76.7
            nontraffic V76.2
          stationary object (traffic) V77.7
            nontraffic V77.2
          streetcar (traffic) V76.7
            nontraffic V76.2
          three wheeled motor vehicle (traffic) V72.7
            nontraffic V72.2
          truck (traffic) V74.7
            nontraffic V74.2
          two wheeled motor vehicle (traffic) V72.7
            nontraffic V72.2
          van (traffic) V73.7
            nontraffic V73.2
        noncollision accident (traffic) V78.7
          nontraffic V78.2

Accident *(Continued)*
  transport *(Continued)*
    bus occupant *(Continued)*
      noncollision accident (traffic) V78.9
        nontraffic V78.3
        while boarding or alighting V78.4
      nontraffic V79.3
      passenger
        collision (with)
          animal (traffic) V70.6
            being ridden (traffic) V76.6
              nontraffic V76.1
            nontraffic V70.1
          animal-drawn vehicle (traffic) V76.6
            nontraffic V76.1
          bus (traffic) V74.6
            nontraffic V74.1
          car (traffic) V73.6
            nontraffic V73.1
          motor vehicle NOS (traffic) V79.50
            nontraffic V79.10
            specified type NEC (traffic) V79.59
              nontraffic V79.19
          pedal cycle (traffic) V71.6
            nontraffic V71.1
          pickup truck (traffic) V73.6
            nontraffic V73.1
          railway vehicle (traffic) V75.6
            nontraffic V75.1
          specified vehicle NEC (traffic) V76.6
            nontraffic V76.1
          stationary object (traffic) V77.6
            nontraffic V77.1
          streetcar (traffic) V76.6
            nontraffic V76.1
          three wheeled motor vehicle (traffic) V72.6
            nontraffic V72.1
          truck (traffic) V74.6
            nontraffic V74.1
          two wheeled motor vehicle (traffic) V72.6
            nontraffic V72.1
          van (traffic) V73.6
            nontraffic V73.1
        noncollision accident (traffic) V78.6
          nontraffic V78.1
      specified type NEC V79.88
      military vehicle V79.81
    cable car, not on rails V98.0
      on rails —*see* Accident, transport, streetcar occupant
    car occupant V49.9
      ambulance occupant —*see* Accident, transport, ambulance occupant
      collision (with)
        animal (traffic) V40.9
          being ridden (traffic) V46.9
            nontraffic V46.3
            while boarding or alighting V46.4
          nontraffic V40.3
          while boarding or alighting V40.4
        animal-drawn vehicle (traffic) V46.9
          nontraffic V46.3
          while boarding or alighting V46.4
        bus (traffic) V44.9
          nontraffic V44.3
          while boarding or alighting V44.4
        car (traffic) V43.92
          nontraffic V43.32
          while boarding or alighting V43.42
        motor vehicle NOS (traffic) V49.60
          nontraffic V49.20
          specified type NEC (traffic) V49.69
            nontraffic V49.29
        pedal cycle (traffic) V41.9
          nontraffic V41.3
          while boarding or alighting V41.4

Accident *(Continued)*
  transport *(Continued)*
    car occupant *(Continued)*
      collision *(Continued)*
        pickup truck (traffic) V43.93
          nontraffic V43.33
          while boarding or alighting V43.43
        railway vehicle (traffic) V45.9
          nontraffic V45.3
          while boarding or alighting V45.4
        specified vehicle NEC (traffic) V46.9
          nontraffic V46.3
          while boarding or alighting V46.4
        sport utility vehicle (traffic) V43.91
          nontraffic V43.31
          while boarding or alighting V43.41
        stationary object (traffic) V47.9
          nontraffic V47.3
          while boarding or alighting V47.4
        streetcar (traffic) V46.9
          nontraffic V46.3
          while boarding or alighting V46.4
        three wheeled motor vehicle (traffic) V42.9
          nontraffic V42.3
          while boarding or alighting V42.4
        truck (traffic) V44.9
          nontraffic V44.3
          while boarding or alighting V44.4
        two wheeled motor vehicle (traffic) V42.9
          nontraffic V42.3
          while boarding or alighting V42.4
        van (traffic) V43.94
          nontraffic V43.34
          while boarding or alighting V43.44
      driver
        collision (with)
          animal (traffic) V40.5
            being ridden (traffic) V46.5
              nontraffic V46.0
            nontraffic V40.0
          animal-drawn vehicle (traffic) V46.5
            nontraffic V46.0
          bus (traffic) V44.5
            nontraffic V44.0
          car (traffic) V43.52
            nontraffic V43.02
          motor vehicle NOS (traffic) V49.40
            nontraffic V49.00
            specified type NEC (traffic) V49.49
              nontraffic V49.09
          pedal cycle (traffic) V41.5
            nontraffic V41.0
          pickup truck (traffic) V43.53
            nontraffic V43.03
          railway vehicle (traffic) V45.5
            nontraffic V45.0
          specified vehicle NEC (traffic) V46.5
            nontraffic V46.0
          sport utility vehicle (traffic) V43.51
            nontraffic V43.01
          stationary object (traffic) V47.5
            nontraffic V47.0
          streetcar (traffic) V46.5
            nontraffic V46.0
          three wheeled motor vehicle (traffic) V42.5
            nontraffic V42.0
          truck (traffic) V44.5
            nontraffic V44.0
          two wheeled motor vehicle (traffic) V42.5
            nontraffic V42.0
          van (traffic) V43.54
            nontraffic V43.04
        noncollision accident (traffic) V48.5
          nontraffic V48.0

▶ New   ⇒ Revised   ~~deleted~~ Deleted   ● Use Additional Character(s)

Accident *(Continued)*
  transport *(Continued)*
    car occupant *(Continued)*
      hanger-on
        collision (with)
          animal (traffic) V40.7
            being ridden (traffic) V46.7
              nontraffic V46.2
            nontraffic V40.2
          animal-drawn vehicle (traffic)
              V46.7
            nontraffic V46.2
          bus (traffic) V44.7
            nontraffic V44.2
          car (traffic) V43.72
            nontraffic V43.22
          pedal cycle (traffic) V41.7
            nontraffic V41.2
          pickup truck (traffic) V43.73
            nontraffic V43.23
          railway vehicle (traffic) V45.7
            nontraffic V45.2
          specified vehicle NEC (traffic) V46.7
            nontraffic V46.2
          sport utility vehicle (traffic) V43.71
            nontraffic V43.21
          stationary object (traffic) V47.7
            nontraffic V47.2
          streetcar (traffic) V46.7
            nontraffic V46.2
          three wheeled motor vehicle
              (traffic) V42.7
            nontraffic V42.2
          truck (traffic) V44.7
            nontraffic V44.2
          two wheeled motor vehicle (traffic)
              V42.7
            nontraffic V42.2
          van (traffic) V43.74
            nontraffic V43.24
        noncollision accident (traffic) V48.7
          nontraffic V48.2
      noncollision accident (traffic) V48.9
        nontraffic V48.3
      while boarding or alighting V48.4
      nontraffic V49.3
      passenger
        collision (with)
          animal (traffic) V40.6
            being ridden (traffic) V46.6
              nontraffic V46.1
            nontraffic V40.1
          animal-drawn vehicle (traffic) V46.6
            nontraffic V46.1
          bus (traffic) V44.6
            nontraffic V44.1
          car (traffic) V43.62
            nontraffic V43.12
          motor vehicle NOS (traffic) V49.50
            nontraffic V49.10
            specified type NEC (traffic) V49.59
              nontraffic V49.19
          pedal cycle (traffic) V41.6
            nontraffic V41.1
          pickup truck (traffic) V43.63
            nontraffic V43.13
          railway vehicle (traffic) V45.6
            nontraffic V45.1
          specified vehicle NEC (traffic) V46.6
            nontraffic V46.1
          sport utility vehicle (traffic) V43.61
            nontraffic V43.11
          stationary object (traffic) V47.6
            nontraffic V47.1
          streetcar (traffic) V46.6
            nontraffic V46.1
          three wheeled motor vehicle
              (traffic) V42.6
            nontraffic V42.1
          truck (traffic) V44.6
            nontraffic V44.1

Accident *(Continued)*
  transport *(Continued)*
    car occupant *(Continued)*
      passenger *(Continued)*
        collision *(Continued)*
          two wheeled motor vehicle (traffic)
              V42.6
            nontraffic V42.1
          van (traffic) V43.64
            nontraffic V43.14
        noncollision accident (traffic) V48.6
          nontraffic V48.1
        specified type NEC V49.88
        military vehicle V49.81
    coal car —*see* Accident, transport,
        industrial vehicle occupant
    construction vehicle occupant (nontraffic)
        V85.9
      driver V85.5
      hanger-on V85.7
      passenger V85.6
      traffic V85.3
        driver V85.0
        hanger-on V85.2
        passenger V85.1
      while boarding or alighting V85.4
    dirt bike rider (nontraffic) V86.96
      driver V86.56
      hanger-on V86.76
      passenger V86.66
      traffic V86.36
        driver V86.06
        hanger-on V86.26
        passenger V86.16
      while boarding or alighting V86.46
    due to cataclysm —*see* Forces of nature,
        by type
    dune buggy occupant (nontraffic) V86.93
      driver V86.53
      hanger-on V86.73
      passenger V86.63
      traffic V86.33
        driver V86.03
        hanger-on V86.23
        passenger V86.13
      while boarding or alighting V86.43
    forklift —*see* Accident, transport,
        industrial vehicle occupant
    go cart —*see* Accident, transport, all-terrain
        vehicle occupant
    golf cart —*see* Accident, transport,
        all-terrain vehicle occupant
    heavy transport vehicle occupant —
        see Accident, transport, truck occupant
    hoverboard V00.848
    ice yacht V98.2
    industrial vehicle occupant (nontraffic)
        V83.9
      driver V83.5
      hanger-on V83.7
      passenger V83.6
      traffic V83.3
        driver V83.0
        hanger-on V83.2
        passenger V83.1
      while boarding or alighting V83.4
    interurban electric car —*see* Accident,
        transport, streetcar
    land yacht V98.1
    logging car —*see* Accident, transport,
        industrial vehicle occupant
    military vehicle occupant (traffic)
        V86.34
      driver V86.04
      hanger-on V86.24
      nontraffic V86.94
        driver V86.54
        hanger-on V86.74
        passenger V86.64
      passenger V86.14
      while boarding or alighting V86.44

Accident *(Continued)*
  transport *(Continued)*
    mine tram —*see* Accident, transport,
        industrial vehicle occupant
    motor vehicle NEC occupant (traffic) V89.2
    motorcoach —*see* Accident, transport,
        bus occupant
    motor/cross bike rider —*see also* Accident,
        transport, dirt bike rider V86.96
    motorcyclist V29.9
      collision (with)
        animal (traffic) V20.9
          being ridden (traffic) V26.9
            nontraffic V26.2
            while boarding or alighting V26.3
          nontraffic V20.2
          while boarding or alighting V20.3
        animal-drawn vehicle (traffic) V26.9
          nontraffic V26.2
          while boarding or alighting V26.3
        bus (traffic) V24.9
          nontraffic V24.2
          while boarding or alighting V24.3
        car (traffic) V23.9
          nontraffic V23.2
          while boarding or alighting V23.3
        motor vehicle NOS (traffic) V29.60
          nontraffic V29.20
          specified type NEC (traffic) V29.69
            nontraffic V29.29
        pedal cycle (traffic) V21.9
          nontraffic V21.2
          while boarding or alighting V21.3
        pickup truck (traffic) V23.9
          nontraffic V23.2
          while boarding or alighting V23.3
        railway vehicle (traffic) V25.9
          nontraffic V25.2
          while boarding or alighting V25.3
        specified vehicle NEC (traffic) V26.9
          nontraffic V26.2
          while boarding or alighting V26.3
        stationary object (traffic) V27.9
          nontraffic V27.2
          while boarding or alighting V27.3
        streetcar (traffic) V26.9
          nontraffic V26.2
          while boarding or alighting V26.3
        three wheeled motor vehicle (traffic)
            V22.9
          nontraffic V22.2
          while boarding or alighting V22.3
        truck (traffic) V24.9
          nontraffic V24.2
          while boarding or alighting V24.3
        two wheeled motor vehicle (traffic)
            V22.9
          nontraffic V22.2
          while boarding or alighting V22.3
        van (traffic) V23.9
          nontraffic V23.2
          while boarding or alighting V23.3
      driver
        collision (with)
          animal (traffic) V20.4
            being ridden (traffic) V26.4
              nontraffic V26.0
            nontraffic V20.0
          animal-drawn vehicle (traffic) V26.4
            nontraffic V26.0
          bus (traffic) V24.4
            nontraffic V24.0
          car (traffic) V23.4
            nontraffic V23.0
          motor vehicle NOS (traffic) V29.40
            nontraffic V29.00
            specified type NEC (traffic)
                V29.49
              nontraffic V29.09
          pedal cycle (traffic) V21.4
            nontraffic V21.0

Accident *(Continued)*
  transport *(Continued)*
    motorcyclist *(Continued)*
      driver *(Continued)*
        collision *(Continued)*
          pickup truck (traffic) V23.4
            nontraffic V23.0
          railway vehicle (traffic) V25.4
            nontraffic V25.0
          specified vehicle NEC (traffic) V26.4
            nontraffic V26.0
          stationary object (traffic) V27.4
            nontraffic V27.0
          streetcar (traffic) V26.4
            nontraffic V26.0
          three wheeled motor vehicle (traffic) V22.4
            nontraffic V22.0
          truck (traffic) V24.4
            nontraffic V24.0
          two wheeled motor vehicle (traffic) V22.4
            nontraffic V22.0
          van (traffic) V23.4
            nontraffic V23.0
        noncollision accident (traffic) V28.4
          nontraffic V28.0
       noncollision accident (traffic) V28.9
        nontraffic V28.2
       while boarding or alighting V28.3
      nontraffic V29.3
      passenger
        collision (with)
          animal (traffic) V20.5
            being ridden (traffic) V26.5
              nontraffic V26.1
            nontraffic V20.1
          animal-drawn vehicle (traffic) V26.5
            nontraffic V26.1
          bus (traffic) V24.5
            nontraffic V24.1
          car (traffic) V23.5
            nontraffic V23.1
          motor vehicle NOS (traffic) V29.50
            nontraffic V29.10
             specified type NEC (traffic) V29.59
              nontraffic V29.19
          pedal cycle (traffic) V21.5
            nontraffic V21.1
          pickup truck (traffic) V23.5
            nontraffic V23.1
          railway vehicle (traffic) V25.5
            nontraffic V25.1
          specified vehicle NEC (traffic) V26.5
            nontraffic V26.1
          stationary object (traffic) V27.5
            nontraffic V27.1
          streetcar (traffic) V26.5
            nontraffic V26.1
          three wheeled motor vehicle (traffic) V22.5
            nontraffic V22.1
          truck (traffic) V24.5
            nontraffic V24.1
          two wheeled motor vehicle (traffic) V22.5
            nontraffic V22.1
          van (traffic) V23.5
            nontraffic V23.1
        noncollision accident (traffic) V28.5
          nontraffic V28.1
      specified type NEC V29.88
        military vehicle V29.81
    occupant (of)
      aircraft (powered) V95.9
        fixed wing
          commercial —*see* Accident, transport, aircraft, occupant, powered, fixed wing, commercial

Accident *(Continued)*
  transport *(Continued)*
    occupant *(Continued)*
      aircraft *(Continued)*
        fixed wing *(Continued)*
          private —*see* Accident, transport, aircraft, occupant, powered, fixed wing, private
        nonpowered V96.9
        specified NEC V95.8
      airport battery-powered vehicle —*see* Accident, transport, industrial vehicle occupant
      all-terrain vehicle (ATV) —*see* Accident, transport, all-terrain vehicle occupant
      animal-drawn vehicle —*see* Accident, transport, animal-drawn vehicle occupant
      automobile —*see* Accident, transport, car occupant
      balloon V96.00
      battery-powered vehicle —*see* Accident, transport, industrial vehicle occupant
      bicycle —*see* Accident, transport, pedal cyclist
        motorized —*see* Accident, transport, motorcycle rider
      boat NEC —*see* Accident, watercraft
      bulldozer —*see* Accident, transport, construction vehicle occupant
      bus —*see* Accident, transport, bus occupant
      cable car (on rails) —*see also* Accident, transport, streetcar occupant
        not on rails V98.0
      car —*see also* Accident, transport, car occupant
        cable (on rails) —*see also* Accident, transport, streetcar occupant
          not on rails V98.0
      coach —*see* Accident, transport, bus occupant
      coal-car —*see* Accident, transport, industrial vehicle occupant
      digger —*see* Accident, transport, construction vehicle occupant
      dump truck —*see* Accident, transport, construction vehicle occupant
      earth-leveler —*see* Accident, transport, construction vehicle occupant
      farm machinery (self-propelled) —*see* Accident, transport, agricultural vehicle occupant
      forklift —*see* Accident, transport, industrial vehicle occupant
      glider (unpowered) V96.20
        hang V96.10
        powered (microlight) (ultralight) —*see* Accident, transport, aircraft, occupant, powered, glider
      glider (unpowered) NEC V96.20
      hang-glider V96.10
      harvester —*see* Accident, transport, agricultural vehicle occupant
      heavy (transport) vehicle —*see* Accident, transport, truck occupant
      helicopter —*see* Accident, transport, aircraft, occupant, helicopter
      ice-yacht V98.2
      kite (carrying person) V96.8
      land-yacht V98.1
      logging car —*see* Accident, transport, industrial vehicle occupant
      mechanical shovel —*see* Accident, transport, construction vehicle occupant
      microlight —*see* Accident, transport, aircraft, occupant, powered, glider

Accident *(Continued)*
  transport *(Continued)*
    occupant *(Continued)*
      minibus —*see* Accident, transport, pickup truck occupant
      minivan —*see* Accident, transport, pickup truck occupant
      moped —*see* Accident, transport, motorcycle
      motor scooter —*see* Accident, transport, motorcycle
      motorcycle (with sidecar) —*see* Accident, transport, motorcycle
      off-road motor-vehicle —*see also* Accident, transport, all-terrain vehicle occupant V86.99
      pedal cycle —*see also* Accident, transport, pedal cyclist
      pick-up (truck) —*see* Accident, transport, pickup truck occupant
      railway (train) (vehicle) (subterranean) (elevated) —*see* Accident, transport, railway vehicle occupant
      rickshaw —*see* Accident, transport, pedal cycle
        pedal driven —*see* Accident, transport, pedal cyclist
      road-roller —*see* Accident, transport, construction vehicle occupant
      ship NOS V94.9
      ski-lift (chair) (gondola) V98.3
      snowmobile —*see* Accident, transport, snowmobile occupant
      spacecraft, spaceship —*see* Accident, transport, aircraft, occupant, spacecraft
      sport utility vehicle —*see* Accident, transport, pickup truck occupant
      streetcar (interurban) (operating on public street or highway) —*see* Accident, transport, streetcar occupant
      SUV —*see* Accident, transport, pickup truck occupant
      téléférique V98.0
      three-wheeled vehicle (motorized) —*see also* Accident, transport, three-wheeled motor vehicle occupant
        nonmotorized —*see* Accident, transport, pedal cycle
      tractor (farm) (and trailer) —*see* Accident, transport, agricultural vehicle occupant
      train —*see* Accident, transport, railway vehicle occupant
      tram —*see* Accident, transport, streetcar occupant
        in mine or quarry —*see* Accident, transport, industrial vehicle occupant
      tricycle —*see* Accident, transport, pedal cycle
        motorized —*see* Accident, transport, three-wheeled motor vehicle
      trolley —*see* Accident, transport, streetcar occupant
        in mine or quarry —*see* Accident, transport, industrial vehicle occupant
      tub, in mine or quarry —*see* Accident, transport, industrial vehicle occupant
      ultralight —*see* Accident, transport, aircraft, occupant, powered, glider
      van —*see* Accident, transport, van occupant
      vehicle NEC V89.9
        heavy transport —*see* Accident, transport, truck occupant
        motor (traffic) NEC V89.2
          nontraffic NEC V89.0

▶ New   ⇒ Revised   ~~deleted~~ Deleted   ● Use Additional Character(s)

Accident (Continued)
  transport (Continued)
    occupant (Continued)
      watercraft NOS V94.9
        causing drowning —see Drowning,
          resulting from accident to boat
      off-road motor-vehicle —see also Accident,
        transport, all-terrain vehicle occupant
        V86.99
    parachutist V97.29
      after accident to aircraft —see Accident,
        transport, aircraft
      entangled in object V97.21
      injured on landing V97.22
    pedal cyclist V19.9
      collision (with)
        animal (traffic) V10.9
          being ridden (traffic) V16.9
            nontraffic V16.2
              while boarding or alighting
                V16.3
          nontraffic V10.2
        while boarding or alighting V10.3
        animal-drawn vehicle (traffic) V16.9
          nontraffic V16.2
          while boarding or alighting V16.3
        bus (traffic) V14.9
          nontraffic V14.2
          while boarding or alighting V14.3
        car (traffic) V13.9
          nontraffic V13.2
          while boarding or alighting V13.3
        motor vehicle NOS (traffic) V19.60
          nontraffic V19.20
          specified type NEC (traffic) V19.69
            nontraffic V19.29
        pedal cycle (traffic) V11.9
          nontraffic V11.2
          while boarding or alighting V11.3
        pickup truck (traffic) V13.9
          nontraffic V13.2
          while boarding or alighting V13.3
        railway vehicle (traffic) V15.9
          nontraffic V15.2
          while boarding or alighting V15.3
        specified vehicle NEC (traffic) V16.9
          nontraffic V16.2
          while boarding or alighting V16.3
        stationary object (traffic) V17.9
          nontraffic V17.2
          while boarding or alighting V17.3
        streetcar (traffic) V16.9
          nontraffic V16.2
          while boarding or alighting V16.3
        three wheeled motor vehicle (traffic)
          V12.9
          nontraffic V12.2
          while boarding or alighting V12.3
        truck (traffic) V14.9
          nontraffic V14.2
          while boarding or alighting V14.3
        two wheeled motor vehicle (traffic)
          V12.9
          nontraffic V12.2
          while boarding or alighting V12.3
        van (traffic) V13.9
          nontraffic V13.2
          while boarding or alighting V13.3
      driver
        collision (with)
          animal (traffic) V10.4
            being ridden (traffic) V16.4
              nontraffic V16.0
            nontraffic V10.0
          animal-drawn vehicle (traffic)
            V16.4
            nontraffic V16.0
          bus (traffic) V14.4
            nontraffic V14.0
          car (traffic) V13.4
            nontraffic V13.0

Accident (Continued)
  transport (Continued)
    pedal cyclist (Continued)
      driver (Continued)
        collision (Continued)
          motor vehicle NOS (traffic) V19.40
            nontraffic V19.00
            specified type NEC (traffic) V19.49
              nontraffic V19.09
          pedal cycle (traffic) V11.4
            nontraffic V11.0
          pickup truck (traffic) V13.4
            nontraffic V13.0
          railway vehicle (traffic) V15.4
            nontraffic V15.0
          specified vehicle NEC (traffic) V16.4
            nontraffic V16.0
          stationary object (traffic) V17.4
            nontraffic V17.0
          streetcar (traffic) V16.4
            nontraffic V16.0
          three wheeled motor vehicle
            (traffic) V12.4
            nontraffic V12.0
          truck (traffic) V14.4
            nontraffic V14.0
          two wheeled motor vehicle (traffic)
            V12.4
            nontraffic V12.0
          van (traffic) V13.4
            nontraffic V13.0
        noncollision accident (traffic) V18.4
          nontraffic V18.0
      noncollision accident (traffic) V18.9
        nontraffic V18.2
        while boarding or alighting V18.3
      nontraffic V19.3
      passenger
        collision (with)
          animal (traffic) V10.5
            being ridden (traffic) V16.5
              nontraffic V16.1
            nontraffic V10.1
          animal-drawn vehicle (traffic) V16.5
            nontraffic V16.1
          bus (traffic) V14.5
            nontraffic V14.1
          car (traffic) V13.5
            nontraffic V13.1
          motor vehicle NOS (traffic) V19.50
            nontraffic V19.10
            specified type NEC (traffic)
              V19.59
              nontraffic V19.19
          pedal cycle (traffic) V11.5
            nontraffic V11.1
          pickup truck (traffic) V13.5
            nontraffic V13.1
          railway vehicle (traffic) V15.5
            nontraffic V15.1
          specified vehicle NEC (traffic) V16.5
            nontraffic V16.1
          stationary object (traffic) V17.5
            nontraffic V17.1
          streetcar (traffic) V16.5
            nontraffic V16.1
          three wheeled motor vehicle
            (traffic) V12.5
            nontraffic V12.1
          truck (traffic) V14.5
            nontraffic V14.1
          two wheeled motor vehicle (traffic)
            V12.5
            nontraffic V12.1
          van (traffic) V13.5
            nontraffic V13.1
        noncollision accident (traffic) V18.5
          nontraffic V18.1
      specified type NEC V19.88
        military vehicle V19.81
    pedestrian

Accident (Continued)
  transport (Continued)
    pedestrian (Continued)
      conveyance (occupant) V09.9
      baby stroller V00.828
        collision (with) V09.9
          animal being ridden or animal
            drawn vehicle V06.99
            nontraffic V06.09
            traffic V06.19
          bus or heavy transport V04.99
            nontraffic V04.09
            traffic V04.19
          car V03.99
            nontraffic V03.09
            traffic V03.19
          pedal cycle V01.99
            nontraffic V01.09
            traffic V01.19
          pick-up truck or van V03.99
            nontraffic V03.09
            traffic V03.19
          railway (train) (vehicle)
            V05.99
            nontraffic V05.09
            traffic V05.19
          stationary object V00.822
          streetcar V06.99
            nontraffic V06.09
            traffic V06.19
          two- or three-wheeled motor
            vehicle V02.99
            nontraffic V02.09
            traffic V02.19
          vehicle V09.9
            animal-drawn V06.99
              nontraffic V06.09
              traffic V06.19
            motor
              nontraffic V09.00
              traffic V09.20
        fall V00.821
        nontraffic V09.1
          involving motor vehicle NEC
            V09.00
        traffic V09.3
          involving motor vehicle NEC
            V09.20
      flat-bottomed NEC V00.388
        collision (with) V09.9
          animal being ridden or animal
            drawn vehicle V06.99
            nontraffic V06.09
            traffic V06.19
          bus or heavy transport V04.99
            nontraffic V04.09
            traffic V04.19
          car V03.99
            nontraffic V03.09
            traffic V03.19
          pedal cycle V01.99
            nontraffic V01.09
            traffic V01.19
          pick-up truck or van V03.99
            nontraffic V03.09
            traffic V03.19
          railway (train) (vehicle) V05.99
            nontraffic V05.09
            traffic V05.19
          stationary object V00.382
          streetcar V06.99
            nontraffic V06.09
            traffic V06.19
          two-or three-wheeled motor
            vehicle V02.99
            nontraffic V02.09
            traffic V02.19
          vehicle V09.9
            animal-drawn V06.99
              nontraffic V06.09
              traffic V06.19

Accident (Continued)
  transport (Continued)
    pedestrian (Continued)
      conveyance (Continued)
        flat-bottomed NEC (Continued)
          collision (Continued)
            vehicle (Continued)
              motor
                nontraffic V09.00
                traffic V09.20
          fall V00.381
          nontraffic V09.1
            involving motor vehicle NEC
              V09.00
          snow
            board —see Accident, transport,
              pedestrian, conveyance,
              snow board
            ski —see Accident, transport,
              pedestrian, conveyance, skis
              (snow)
          traffic V09.3
            involving motor vehicle NEC
              V09.20
        gliding type NEC V00.288
          collision (with) V09.9
            animal being ridden or animal
              drawn vehicle V06.99
              nontraffic V06.09
              traffic V06.19
            bus or heavy transport
              V04.99
              nontraffic V04.09
              traffic V04.19
            car V03.99
              nontraffic V03.09
              traffic V03.19
            pedal cycle V01.99
              nontraffic V01.09
              traffic V01.19
            pick-up truck or van V03.99
              nontraffic V03.09
              traffic V03.19
            railway (train) (vehicle) V05.99
              nontraffic V05.09
              traffic V05.19
            stationary object V00.282
            streetcar V06.99
              nontraffic V06.09
              traffic V06.19
            two- or three-wheeled motor
              vehicle V02.99
              nontraffic V02.09
              traffic V02.19
            vehicle V09.9
              animal-drawn V06.99
                nontraffic V06.09
                traffic V06.19
              motor
                nontraffic V09.00
                traffic V09.20
        fall V00.281
        heelies —see Accident, transport,
          pedestrian, conveyance,
          heelies
        hoverboard
          collision with
            animal being ridden or animal
              drawn vehicle V06.938
              nontraffic V06.038
              traffic V06.138
            bus or heavy transport
              V04.938
              nontraffic V04.038
              traffic V04.138
            car V03.938
              nontraffic V03.038
              traffic V03.138
            pedal cycle V01.938
              nontraffic V01.038
              traffic V01.138

Accident (Continued)
  transport (Continued)
    pedestrian (Continued)
      conveyance (Continued)
        gliding type NEC (Continued)
          hoverboard (Continued)
            collision with (Continued)
              pick-up or van V03.938
                nontraffic V03.038
                traffic V03.138
              railway (train) (vehicle) V05.938
                nontraffic V05.038
                traffic V05.138
              streetcar V06.938
                nontraffic V06.038
                traffic V06.138
              three-wheeled motor vehicle
                V02.938
                nontraffic V02.038
                traffic V02.138
              two-wheeled motor vehicle
                V02.938
                nontraffic V02.038
                traffic V02.138
              vehicle, nonmotor, specified
                NEC V06.938
                nontraffic V06.038
                traffic V06.138
            fall V00.848
        ice skate —see Accident, transport,
          pedestrian, conveyance, ice
          skate
        nontraffic V09.1
          involving motor vehicle NEC
            V09.00
        Segway
          collision with
            animal being ridden or animal
              drawn vehicle V06.938
              nontraffic V06.038
              traffic V06.138
            bus or heavy transport V04.938
              nontraffic V04.038
              traffic V04.138
            car V03.938
              nontraffic V03.038
              traffic V03.138
            pedal cycle V01.938
              nontraffic V01.038
              traffic V01.138
            pick-up or van V03.038
              nontraffic V01.038
              traffic V03.138
            railway (train) (vehicle) V05.938
              nontraffic V05.038
              traffic V05.138
            streetcar V06.938
              nontraffic V06.038
              traffic V06.138
            three-wheeled motor vehicle
              V02.938
              nontraffic V02.038
              traffic V02.138
            two-wheeled motor vehicle
              V02.938
              nontraffic V02.038
              traffic V02.138
            vehicle, nonmotor, specified
              NEC V06.938
              nontraffic V06.038
              traffic V06.138
          fall V00.848
        sled —see Accident, transport,
          pedestrian, conveyance, sled
        standing
          electric scooter
            collision with
              animal being ridden or
                animal drawn vehicle
                V06.931
                nontraffic V06.031
                traffic V06.131

Accident (Continued)
  transport (Continued)
    pedestrian (Continued)
      conveyance (Continued)
        gliding type NEC (Continued)
          standing (Continued)
            electric scooter (Continued)
              collision with (Continued)
                bus or heavy transport
                  V04.931
                  nontraffic V04.031
                  traffic V04.131
                car V03.931
                  nontraffic V03.031
                  traffic V03.131
                pedal cycle V01.931
                  nontraffic V01.031
                  traffic V01.131
                pick-up or van V03.931
                  nontraffic V03.031
                  traffic V03.131
                railway (train) (vehicle)
                  V05.931
                  nontraffic V05.031
                  traffic V05.131
                streetcar V06.931
                  nontraffic V06.031
                  traffic V06.131
                three-wheeled motor vehicle
                  V02.931
                  nontraffic V02.031
                  traffic V02.131
                two-wheeled motor vehicle
                  V02.931
                  nontraffic V02.031
                  traffic V02.131
                vehicle, nonmotor, specified
                NEC V06.931
                nontraffic V06.031
                traffic V06.131
            fall V00.841
        micro-mobility pedestrian
          conveyance
        collision with
          animal being ridden or
            animal drawn vehicle
            V06.938
            nontraffic V06.038
            traffic V06.138
          bus or heavy transport
            V04.938
            nontraffic V04.038
            traffic V04.138
          car V03.938
            nontraffic V03.038
            traffic V03.138
          pedal cycle V01.938
            nontraffic V01.038
            traffic V01.138
          pick-up or van V03.938
            nontraffic V03.038
            traffic V03.138
          railway (train) (vehicle)
            V05.938
            nontraffic V05.038
            traffic V05.138
          stationary object V00.842
          streetcar V06.938
            nontraffic V06.038
            traffic V06.138
          three-wheeled motor vehicle
            V02.938
            nontraffic V02.038
            traffic V02.138
          two-wheeled motor vehicle
            V02.938
            nontraffic V02.038
            traffic V02.138
          vehicle, nonmotor, specified
            NEC V06.938
            nontraffic V06.038
            traffic V06.138
        fall V00.848

▶ New   ⇒ Revised   ~~deleted~~ Deleted   ● Use Additional Character(s)

Accident *(Continued)*
  transport *(Continued)*
    pedestrian *(Continued)*
      conveyance *(Continued)*
        gliding type NEC *(Continued)*
          traffic V09.3
            involving motor vehicle NEC V09.20
          wheelies —*see* Accident, transport, pedestrian, conveyance, heelies
        heelies V00.158
          colliding with stationary object V00.152
          fall V00.151
        ice skates V00.218
          collision (with) V09.9
            animal being ridden or animal drawn vehicle V06.99
              nontraffic V06.09
              traffic V06.19
            bus or heavy transport V04.99
              nontraffic V04.09
              traffic V04.19
            car V03.99
              nontraffic V03.09
              traffic V03.19
            pedal cycle V01.99
              nontraffic V01.09
              traffic V01.19
            pick-up truck or van V03.99
              nontraffic V03.09
              traffic V03.19
            railway (train) (vehicle) V05.99
              nontraffic V05.09
              traffic V05.19
            stationary object V00.212
            streetcar V06.99
              nontraffic V06.09
              traffic V06.19
            two- or three-wheeled motor vehicle V02.99
              nontraffic V02.09
              traffic V02.19
            vehicle V09.9
              animal-drawn V06.99
                nontraffic V06.09
                traffic V06.19
              motor
                nontraffic V09.00
                traffic V09.20
          fall V00.211
          nontraffic V09.1
            involving motor vehicle NEC V09.00
          traffic V09.3
            involving motor vehicle NEC V09.20
        motorized mobility scooter V00.838
          collision with stationary object V00.832
          fall from V00.831
          nontraffic V09.1
            involving motor vehicle V09.00
              military V09.01
              specified type NEC V09.09
        roller skates (non in-line) V00.128
          collision (with) V09.9
            animal being ridden or animal drawn vehicle V06.91
              nontraffic V06.01
              traffic V06.11
            bus or heavy transport V04.91
              nontraffic V04.01
              traffic V04.11
            car V03.91
              nontraffic V03.01
              traffic V03.11

Accident *(Continued)*
  transport *(Continued)*
    pedestrian *(Continued)*
      conveyance *(Continued)*
        roller skates *(Continued)*
          collision *(Continued)*
            pedal cycle V01.91
              nontraffic V01.01
              traffic V01.11
            pick-up truck or van V03.91
              nontraffic V03.01
              traffic V03.11
            railway (train) (vehicle) V05.91
              nontraffic V05.01
              traffic V05.11
            stationary object V00.122
            streetcar V06.91
              nontraffic V06.01
              traffic V06.11
            two- or three-wheeled motor vehicle V02.91
              nontraffic V02.01
              traffic V02.11
            vehicle V09.9
              animal-drawn V06.91
                nontraffic V06.01
                traffic V06.11
              motor
                nontraffic V09.00
                traffic V09.20
          fall V00.121
          in-line V00.118
            collision —*see also* Accident, transport, pedestrian, conveyance occupant, roller skates, collision
              with stationary object V00.112
            fall V00.111
            nontraffic V09.1
              involving motor vehicle NEC V09.00
            traffic V09.3
              involving motor vehicle NEC V09.20
        rolling shoes V00.158
          colliding with stationary object V00.152
          fall V00.151
        rolling type NEC V00.188
          collision (with) V09.9
            animal being ridden or animal drawn vehicle V06.99
              nontraffic V06.09
              traffic V06.19
            bus or heavy transport V04.99
              nontraffic V04.09
              traffic V04.19
            car V03.99
              nontraffic V03.09
              traffic V03.19
            pedal cycle V01.99
              nontraffic V01.09
              traffic V01.19
            pick-up truck or van V03.99
              nontraffic V03.09
              traffic V03.19
            railway (train) (vehicle) V05.99
              nontraffic V05.09
              traffic V05.19
            stationary object V00.182
            streetcar V06.99
              nontraffic V06.09
              traffic V06.19
            two- or three-wheeled motor vehicle V02.99
              nontraffic V02.09
              traffic V02.19

Accident *(Continued)*
  transport *(Continued)*
    pedestrian *(Continued)*
      conveyance *(Continued)*
        rolling type NEC *(Continued)*
          collision *(Continued)*
            vehicle V09.9
              animal-drawn V06.99
                nontraffic V06.09
                traffic V06.19
              motor
                nontraffic V09.00
                traffic V09.20
          fall V00.181
          in-line roller skate —*see* Accident, transport, pedestrian, conveyance, roller skate, in-line
          nontraffic V09.1
            involving motor vehicle NEC V09.00
          roller skate —*see* Accident, transport, pedestrian, conveyance, roller skate
          scooter (non-motorized) — *see* Accident, transport, pedestrian, conveyance, scooter
          skateboard —*see* Accident, transport, pedestrian, conveyance, skateboard
          traffic V09.3
            involving motor vehicle NEC V09.20
        scooter (non-motorized) V00.148
          collision (with) V09.9
            animal being ridden or animal drawn vehicle V06.99
              nontraffic V06.09
              traffic V06.19
            bus or heavy transport V04.99
              nontraffic V04.09
              traffic V04.19
            car V03.99
              nontraffic V03.09
              traffic V03.19
            pedal cycle V01.99
              nontraffic V01.09
              traffic V01.19
            pick-up truck or van V03.99
              nontraffic V03.09
              traffic V03.19
            railway (train) (vehicle) V05.99
              nontraffic V05.09
              traffic V05.19
            stationary object V00.142
            streetcar V06.99
              nontraffic V06.09
              traffic V06.19
            two- or three-wheeled motor vehicle V02.99
              nontraffic V02.09
              traffic V02.19
            vehicle V09.9
              animal-drawn V06.99
                nontraffic V06.09
                traffic V06.19
              motor
                nontraffic V09.00
                traffic V09.20
          fall V00.141
          nontraffic V09.1
            involving motor vehicle NEC V09.00
          traffic V09.3
            involving motor vehicle NEC V09.20

Accident (Continued)
  transport (Continued)
    pedestrian (Continued)
      conveyance (Continued)
        skate board V00.138
          collision (with) V09.9
            animal being ridden or animal
              drawn vehicle V06.92
              nontraffic V06.02
              traffic V06.12
            bus or heavy transport
              V04.92
              nontraffic V04.02
              traffic V04.12
            car V03.92
              nontraffic V03.02
              traffic V03.12
            pedal cycle V01.92
              nontraffic V01.02
              traffic V01.12
            pick-up truck or van V03.92
              nontraffic V03.02
              traffic V03.12
            railway (train) (vehicle) V05.92
              nontraffic V05.02
              traffic V05.12
            stationary object V00.132
            streetcar V06.92
              nontraffic V06.02
              traffic V06.12
            two- or three-wheeled motor
              vehicle V02.92
              nontraffic V02.02
              traffic V02.12
            vehicle V09.9
              animal-drawn V06.92
                nontraffic V06.02
                traffic V06.12
              motor
                nontraffic V09.00
                traffic V09.20
        fall V00.131
        nontraffic V09.1
          involving motor vehicle NEC
            V09.00
        traffic V09.3
          involving motor vehicle NEC
            V09.20
        skis (snow) V00.328
          collision (with) V09.9
            animal being ridden or animal
              drawn vehicle V06.99
              nontraffic V06.09
              traffic V06.19
            bus or heavy transport V04.99
              nontraffic V04.09
              traffic V04.19
            car V03.99
              nontraffic V03.09
              traffic V03.19
            pedal cycle V01.99
              nontraffic V01.09
              traffic V01.19
            pick-up truck or van V03.99
              nontraffic V03.09
              traffic V03.19
            railway (train) (vehicle) V05.99
              nontraffic V05.09
              traffic V05.19
            stationary object V00.322
            streetcar V06.99
              nontraffic V06.09
              traffic V06.19
            two- or three-wheeled motor
              vehicle V02.99
              nontraffic V02.09
              traffic V02.19
            vehicle V09.9
              animal-drawn V06.99
                nontraffic V06.09
                traffic V06.19

Accident (Continued)
  transport (Continued)
    pedestrian (Continued)
      conveyance (Continued)
        sled (Continued)
          collision (Continued)
            vehicle (Continued)
              motor
                nontraffic V09.00
                traffic V09.20
          fall V00.321
          nontraffic V09.1
            involving motor vehicle NEC
              V09.00
          traffic V09.3
            involving motor vehicle NEC
              V09.20
        sled V00.228
          collision (with) V09.9
            animal being ridden or animal
              drawn vehicle V06.99
              nontraffic V06.09
              traffic V06.19
            bus or heavy transport V04.99
              nontraffic V04.09
              traffic V04.19
            car V03.99
              nontraffic V03.09
              traffic V03.19
            pedal cycle V01.99
              nontraffic V01.09
              traffic V01.19
            pick-up truck or van V03.99
              nontraffic V03.09
              traffic V03.19
            railway (train) (vehicle) V05.99
              nontraffic V05.09
              traffic V05.19
            stationary object V00.222
            streetcar V06.99
              nontraffic V06.09
              traffic V06.19
            two- or three-wheeled motor
              vehicle V02.99
              nontraffic V02.09
              traffic V02.19
            vehicle V09.9
              animal-drawn V06.99
                nontraffic V06.09
                traffic V06.19
              motor
                nontraffic V09.00
                traffic V09.20
          fall V00.221
          nontraffic V09.1
            involving motor vehicle NEC
              V09.00
          traffic V09.3
            involving motor vehicle NEC
              V09.20
        snow board V00.318
          collision (with) V09.9
            animal being ridden or animal
              drawn vehicle V06.99
              nontraffic V06.09
              traffic V06.19
            bus or heavy transport V04.99
              nontraffic V04.09
              traffic V04.19
            car V03.99
              nontraffic V03.09
              traffic V03.19
            pedal cycle V01.99
              nontraffic V01.09
              traffic V01.19
            pick-up truck or van V03.99
              nontraffic V03.09
              traffic V03.19
            railway (train) (vehicle) V05.99
              nontraffic V05.09
              traffic V05.19

Accident (Continued)
  transport (Continued)
    pedestrian (Continued)
      conveyance (Continued)
        snow board (Continued)
          collision (Continued)
            stationary object V00.312
            streetcar V06.99
              nontraffic V06.09
              traffic V06.19
            two- or three-wheeled motor
              vehicle V02.99
              nontraffic V02.09
              traffic V02.19
            vehicle V09.9
              animal-drawn V06.99
                nontraffic V06.09
                traffic V06.19
              motor
                nontraffic V09.00
                traffic V09.20
          fall V00.311
          nontraffic V09.1
            involving motor vehicle NEC
              V09.00
          traffic V09.3
            involving motor vehicle NEC
              V09.20
        specified type NEC V00.898
          collision (with) V09.9
            animal being ridden or animal
              drawn vehicle V06.99
              nontraffic V06.09
              traffic V06.19
            bus or heavy transport V04.99
              nontraffic V04.09
              traffic V04.19
            car V03.99
              nontraffic V03.09
              traffic V03.19
            pedal cycle V01.99
              nontraffic V01.09
              traffic V01.19
            pick-up truck or van V03.99
              nontraffic V03.09
              traffic V03.19
            railway (train) (vehicle) V05.99
              nontraffic V05.09
              traffic V05.19
            stationary object V00.892
            streetcar V06.99
              nontraffic V06.09
              traffic V06.19
            two- or three-wheeled motor
              vehicle V02.99
              nontraffic V02.09
              traffic V02.19
            vehicle V09.9
              animal-drawn V06.99
                nontraffic V06.09
                traffic V06.19
              motor
                nontraffic V09.00
                traffic V09.20
          fall V00.891
          nontraffic V09.1
            involving motor vehicle NEC
              V09.00
          traffic V09.3
            involving motor vehicle NEC
              V09.20
        traffic V09.3
          involving motor vehicle V09.20
            military V09.21
            specified type NEC V09.29
        wheelchair (powered) V00.818
          collision (with) V09.9
            animal being ridden or animal
              drawn vehicle V06.99
              nontraffic V06.09
              traffic V06.19

▶ New   ⇒ Revised   ~~deleted~~ Deleted   ● Use Additional Character(s)

Accident *(Continued)*
  transport *(Continued)*
    pedestrian *(Continued)*
      conveyance *(Continued)*
        wheelchair *(Continued)*
          collision *(Continued)*
            bus or heavy transport V04.99
              nontraffic V04.09
              traffic V04.19
            car V03.99
              nontraffic V03.09
              traffic V03.19
            pedal cycle V01.99
              nontraffic V01.09
              traffic V01.19
            pick-up truck or van V03.99
              nontraffic V03.09
              traffic V03.19
            railway (train) (vehicle) V05.99
              nontraffic V05.09
              traffic V05.19
            stationary object V00.812
            streetcar V06.99
              nontraffic V06.09
              traffic V06.19
            two- or three-wheeled motor
              vehicle V02.99
              nontraffic V02.09
              traffic V02.19
            vehicle V09.9
              animal-drawn V06.99
                nontraffic V06.09
                traffic V06.19
              motor
                nontraffic V09.00
                traffic V09.20
          fall V00.811
          nontraffic V09.1
            involving motor vehicle NEC
              V09.00
          traffic V09.3
            involving motor vehicle NEC
              V09.20
        wheeled shoe V00.158
          colliding with stationary object
            V00.152
          fall V00.151
      on foot —*see also* Accident, pedestrian
        collision (with)
          animal being ridden or animal
            drawn vehicle V06.90
            nontraffic V06.00
            traffic V06.10
          bus or heavy transport V04.90
            nontraffic V04.00
            traffic V04.10
          car V03.90
            nontraffic V03.00
            traffic V03.10
          pedal cycle V01.90
            nontraffic V01.00
            traffic V01.10
          pick-up truck or van V03.90
            nontraffic V03.00
            traffic V03.10
          railway (train) (vehicle) V05.90
            nontraffic V05.00
            traffic V05.10
          streetcar V06.90
            nontraffic V06.00
            traffic V06.10
          two- or three-wheeled motor
            vehicle V02.90
            nontraffic V02.00
            traffic V02.10
          vehicle V09.9
            animal-drawn V06.90
              nontraffic V06.00
              traffic V06.10
            motor
              nontraffic V09.00
              traffic V09.20

Accident *(Continued)*
  transport *(Continued)*
    pedestrian *(Continued)*
      on foot *(Continued)*
        nontraffic V09.1
          involving motor vehicle V09.00
            military V09.01
            specified type NEC V09.09
        traffic V09.3
          involving motor vehicle V09.20
            military V09.21
            specified type NEC V09.29
      person NEC (unknown way or
        transportation) V99
        collision (between)
          bus (with)
            heavy transport vehicle (traffic)
              V87.5
            nontraffic V88.5
          car (with)
            nontraffic V88.5
            bus (traffic) V87.3
              nontraffic V88.3
            heavy transport vehicle (traffic)
              V87.4
              nontraffic V88.4
            pick-up truck or van (traffic)
              V87.2
              nontraffic V88.2
            train or railway vehicle (traffic)
              V87.6
              nontraffic V88.6
            two- or three-wheeled motor
              vehicle (traffic) V87.0
              nontraffic V88.0
          motor vehicle (traffic) NEC V87.7
            nontraffic V88.7
          two- or three-wheeled vehicle (with)
           (traffic)
            motor vehicle NEC V87.1
            nontraffic V88.1
         nonmotor vehicle (collision)
          (noncollision) (traffic) V87.9
          nontraffic V88.9
      pickup truck occupant V59.9
        collision (with)
          animal (traffic) V50.9
            being ridden (traffic) V56.9
              nontraffic V56.3
              while boarding or alighting
                V56.4
            nontraffic V50.3
            while boarding or alighting V50.4
          animal-drawn vehicle (traffic) V56.9
            nontraffic V56.3
            while boarding or alighting V56.4
          bus (traffic) V54.9
            nontraffic V54.3
            while boarding or alighting V54.4
          car (traffic) V53.9
            nontraffic V53.3
            while boarding or alighting V53.4
          motor vehicle NOS (traffic) V59.60
            nontraffic V59.20
            specified type NEC (traffic) V59.69
              nontraffic V59.29
          pedal cycle (traffic) V51.9
            nontraffic V51.3
            while boarding or alighting V51.4
          pickup truck (traffic) V53.9
            nontraffic V53.3
            while boarding or alighting V53.4
          railway vehicle (traffic) V55.9
            nontraffic V55.3
            while boarding or alighting V55.4
          specified vehicle NEC (traffic) V56.9
            nontraffic V56.3
            while boarding or alighting V56.4
          stationary object (traffic) V57.9
            nontraffic V57.3
            while boarding or alighting V57.4

Accident *(Continued)*
  transport *(Continued)*
    pickup truck occupant *(Continued)*
      collision (with) *(Continued)*
        streetcar (traffic) V56.9
          nontraffic V56.3
          while boarding or alighting V56.4
        three wheeled motor vehicle (traffic)
          V52.9
          nontraffic V52.3
          while boarding or alighting V52.4
        truck (traffic) V54.9
          nontraffic V54.3
          while boarding or alighting V54.4
        two wheeled motor vehicle (traffic)
          V52.9
          nontraffic V52.3
          while boarding or alighting V52.4
        van (traffic) V53.9
          nontraffic V53.3
          while boarding or alighting V53.4
      driver
        collision (with)
          animal (traffic) V50.5
            being ridden (traffic) V56.5
              nontraffic V56.0
            nontraffic V50.0
          animal-drawn vehicle (traffic)
            V56.5
            nontraffic V56.0
          bus (traffic) V54.5
            nontraffic V54.0
          car (traffic) V53.5
            nontraffic V53.0
          motor vehicle NOS (traffic) V59.40
            nontraffic V59.00
            specified type NEC (traffic)
              V59.49
              nontraffic V59.09
          pedal cycle (traffic) V51.5
            nontraffic V51.0
          pickup truck (traffic) V53.5
            nontraffic V53.0
          railway vehicle (traffic) V55.5
            nontraffic V55.0
          specified vehicle NEC (traffic) V56.5
            nontraffic V56.0
          stationary object (traffic) V57.5
            nontraffic V57.0
          streetcar (traffic) V56.5
            nontraffic V56.0
          three wheeled motor vehicle
            (traffic) V52.5
            nontraffic V52.0
          truck (traffic) V54.5
            nontraffic V54.0
          two wheeled motor vehicle (traffic)
            V52.5
            nontraffic V52.0
          van (traffic) V53.5
            nontraffic V53.0
        noncollision accident (traffic) V58.5
          nontraffic V58.0
      hanger-on
        collision (with)
          animal (traffic) V50.7
            being ridden (traffic) V56.7
              nontraffic V56.2
            nontraffic V50.2
          animal-drawn vehicle (traffic) V56.7
            nontraffic V56.2
          bus (traffic) V54.7
            nontraffic V54.2
          car (traffic) V53.7
            nontraffic V53.2
          pedal cycle (traffic) V51.7
            nontraffic V51.2
          pickup truck (traffic) V53.7
            nontraffic V53.2
          railway vehicle (traffic) V55.7
            nontraffic V55.2

Accident *(Continued)*
  transport *(Continued)*
    pickup truck occupant *(Continued)*
      hanger-on *(Continued)*
        collision *(Continued)*
          specified vehicle NEC (traffic) V56.7
            nontraffic V56.2
          stationary object (traffic) V57.7
            nontraffic V57.2
          streetcar (traffic) V56.7
            nontraffic V56.2
          three wheeled motor vehicle
            (traffic) V52.7
            nontraffic V52.2
          truck (traffic) V54.7
            nontraffic V54.2
          two wheeled motor vehicle (traffic)
            V52.7
            nontraffic V52.2
          van (traffic) V53.7
            nontraffic V53.2
        noncollision accident (traffic) V58.7
          nontraffic V58.2
      noncollision accident (traffic) V58.9
        nontraffic V58.3
        while boarding or alighting V58.4
      nontraffic V59.3
      passenger
        collision (with)
          animal (traffic) V50.6
            being ridden (traffic) V56.6
              nontraffic V56.1
            nontraffic V50.1
          animal-drawn vehicle (traffic) V56.6
            nontraffic V56.1
          bus (traffic) V54.6
            nontraffic V54.1
          car (traffic) V53.6
            nontraffic V53.1
          motor vehicle NOS (traffic) V59.50
            nontraffic V59.10
            specified type NEC (traffic) V59.59
              nontraffic V59.19
          pedal cycle (traffic) V51.6
            nontraffic V51.1
          pickup truck (traffic) V53.6
            nontraffic V53.1
          railway vehicle (traffic) V55.6
            nontraffic V55.1
          specified vehicle NEC (traffic) V56.6
            nontraffic V56.1
          stationary object (traffic) V57.6
            nontraffic V57.1
          streetcar (traffic) V56.6
            nontraffic V56.1
          three wheeled motor vehicle
            (traffic) V52.6
            nontraffic V52.1
          truck (traffic) V54.6
            nontraffic V54.1
          two wheeled motor vehicle (traffic)
            V52.6
            nontraffic V52.1
          van (traffic) V53.6
            nontraffic V53.1
        noncollision accident (traffic) V58.6
          nontraffic V58.1
      specified type NEC V59.88
        military vehicle V59.81
    quarry truck —*see* Accident, transport,
      industrial vehicle occupant
    race car —*see* Accident, transport, motor
      vehicle NEC occupant
    railway vehicle occupant V81.9
      collision (with) V81.3
        motor vehicle (non-military) (traffic)
          V81.1
          military V81.83
          nontraffic V81.0
        rolling stock V81.2
        specified object NEC V81.3

Accident *(Continued)*
  transport *(Continued)*
    railway vehicle occupant *(Continued)*
      during derailment V81.7
        with antecedent collision —*see*
          Accident, transport, railway
          vehicle occupant, collision
      explosion V81.81
      fall (in railway vehicle) V81.5
        during derailment V81.7
          with antecedent collision —*see*
            Accident, transport, railway
            vehicle occupant, collision
        from railway vehicle V81.6
          during derailment V81.7
            with antecedent collision —*see*
              Accident, transport,
              railway vehicle occupant,
              collision
        while boarding or alighting V81.4
      fire V81.81
      object falling onto train V81.82
      specified type NEC V81.89
      while boarding or alighting V81.4
    Segway V00.848
    ski lift V98.3
    snowmobile occupant (nontraffic) V86.92
      driver V86.52
      hanger-on V86.72
      passenger V86.62
      traffic V86.32
        driver V86.02
        hanger-on V86.22
        passenger V86.12
      while boarding or alighting V86.42
    specified NEC V98.8
    sport utility vehicle occupant —*see also*
      Accident, transport, pickup truck
      occupant
    streetcar occupant V82.9
      collision (with) V82.3
        motor vehicle (traffic) V82.1
          nontraffic V82.0
        rolling stock V82.2
      during derailment V82.7
        with antecedent collision —*see*
          Accident, transport, streetcar
          occupant, collision
      fall (in streetcar) V82.5
        during derailment V82.7
          with antecedent collision —*see*
            Accident, transport, streetcar
            occupant, collision
        from streetcar V82.6
          during derailment V82.7
            with antecedent collision —*see*
              Accident, transport, streetcar
              occupant, collision
          while boarding or alighting
            V82.4
        while boarding or alighting V82.4
      specified type NEC V82.8
      while boarding or alighting V82.4
    three-wheeled motor vehicle occupant
      V39.9
      collision (with)
        animal (traffic) V30.9
          being ridden (traffic) V36.9
            nontraffic V36.3
            while boarding or alighting V36.4
          nontraffic V30.3
          while boarding or alighting V30.4
        animal-drawn vehicle (traffic) V36.9
          nontraffic V36.3
          while boarding or alighting V36.4
        bus (traffic) V34.9
          nontraffic V34.3
          while boarding or alighting V34.4
        car (traffic) V33.9
          nontraffic V33.3
          while boarding or alighting V33.4

Accident *(Continued)*
  transport *(Continued)*
    three-wheeled motor vehicle occupant
      (Continued)
      collision *(Continued)*
        motor vehicle NOS (traffic) V39.60
          nontraffic V39.20
          specified type NEC (traffic)
            V39.69
            nontraffic V39.29
        pedal cycle (traffic) V31.9
          nontraffic V31.3
          while boarding or alighting
            V31.4
        pickup truck (traffic) V33.9
          nontraffic V33.3
          while boarding or alighting
            V33.4
        railway vehicle (traffic) V35.9
          nontraffic V35.3
          while boarding or alighting
            V35.4
        specified vehicle NEC (traffic) V36.9
          nontraffic V36.3
          while boarding or alighting V36.4
        stationary object (traffic) V37.9
          nontraffic V37.3
          while boarding or alighting V37.4
        streetcar (traffic) V36.9
          nontraffic V36.3
          while boarding or alighting V36.4
        three wheeled motor vehicle (traffic)
          V32.9
          nontraffic V32.3
          while boarding or alighting V32.4
        truck (traffic) V34.9
          nontraffic V34.3
          while boarding or alighting V34.4
        two wheeled motor vehicle (traffic)
          V32.9
          nontraffic V32.3
          while boarding or alighting V32.4
        van (traffic) V33.9
          nontraffic V33.3
          while boarding or alighting V33.4
      driver
        collision (with)
          animal (traffic) V30.5
            being ridden (traffic) V36.5
              nontraffic V36.0
            nontraffic V30.0
          animal-drawn vehicle (traffic) V36.5
            nontraffic V36.0
          bus (traffic) V34.5
            nontraffic V34.0
          car (traffic) V33.5
            nontraffic V33.0
          motor vehicle NOS (traffic)
            V39.40
            nontraffic V39.00
            specified type NEC (traffic)
              V39.49
              nontraffic V39.09
          pedal cycle (traffic) V31.5
            nontraffic V31.0
          pickup truck (traffic) V33.5
            nontraffic V33.0
          railway vehicle (traffic) V35.5
            nontraffic V35.0
          specified vehicle NEC (traffic)
            V36.5
            nontraffic V36.0
          stationary object (traffic) V37.5
            nontraffic V37.0
          streetcar (traffic) V36.5
            nontraffic V36.0
          three wheeled motor vehicle
            (traffic) V32.5
            nontraffic V32.0
          truck (traffic) V34.5
            nontraffic V34.0

▶ New   ⇒ Revised   ~~deleted~~ Deleted   ● Use Additional Character(s)

Accident *(Continued)*
 transport *(Continued)*
  three-wheeled motor vehicle occupant
   (Continued)
   driver *(Continued)*
    collision *(Continued)*
     two wheeled motor vehicle (traffic)
      V32.5
      nontraffic V32.0
     van (traffic) V33.5
      nontraffic V33.0
    noncollision accident (traffic) V38.5
     nontraffic V38.0
   hanger-on
    collision (with)
     animal (traffic) V30.7
      being ridden (traffic) V36.7
       nontraffic V36.2
      nontraffic V30.2
     animal-drawn vehicle (traffic) V36.7
      nontraffic V36.2
     bus (traffic) V34.7
      nontraffic V34.2
     car (traffic) V33.7
      nontraffic V33.2
     pedal cycle (traffic) V31.7
      nontraffic V31.2
     pickup truck (traffic) V33.7
      nontraffic V33.2
     railway vehicle (traffic) V35.7
      nontraffic V35.2
     specified vehicle NEC (traffic) V36.7
      nontraffic V36.2
     stationary object (traffic) V37.7
      nontraffic V37.2
     streetcar (traffic) V36.7
      nontraffic V36.2
     three wheeled motor vehicle
      (traffic) V32.7
      nontraffic V32.2
     truck (traffic) V34.7
      nontraffic V34.2
     two wheeled motor vehicle (traffic)
      V32.7
      nontraffic V32.2
     van (traffic) V33.7
      nontraffic V33.2
    noncollision accident (traffic) V38.7
     nontraffic V38.2
   noncollision accident (traffic) V38.9
    nontraffic V38.3
    while boarding or alighting V38.4
   nontraffic V39.3
   passenger
    collision (with)
     animal (traffic) V30.6
      being ridden (traffic) V36.6
       nontraffic V36.1
      nontraffic V30.1
     animal-drawn vehicle (traffic) V36.6
      nontraffic V36.1
     bus (traffic) V34.6
      nontraffic V34.1
     car (traffic) V33.6
      nontraffic V33.1
     motor vehicle NOS (traffic) V39.50
      nontraffic V39.10
      specified type NEC (traffic)
       V39.59
       nontraffic V39.19
     pedal cycle (traffic) V31.6
      nontraffic V31.1
     pickup truck (traffic) V33.6
      nontraffic V33.1
     railway vehicle (traffic) V35.6
      nontraffic V35.1
     specified vehicle NEC (traffic)
      V36.6
      nontraffic V36.1
     stationary object (traffic) V37.6
      nontraffic V37.1

Accident *(Continued)*
 transport *(Continued)*
  three-wheeled motor vehicle occupant
   (Continued)
   passenger *(Continued)*
    collision *(Continued)*
     streetcar (traffic) V36.6
      nontraffic V36.1
     three wheeled motor vehicle
      (traffic) V32.6
      nontraffic V32.1
     truck (traffic) V34.6
      nontraffic V34.1
     two wheeled motor vehicle (traffic)
      V32.6
      nontraffic V32.1
     van (traffic) V33.6
      nontraffic V33.1
    noncollision accident (traffic)
     V38.6
     nontraffic V38.1
   specified type NEC V39.89
    military vehicle V39.81
  tractor (farm) (and trailer) —*see* Accident,
   transport, agricultural vehicle
   occupant
  tram —*see* Accident, transport, streetcar
   in mine or quarry —*see* Accident,
    transport, industrial vehicle
    occupant
  trolley —*see* Accident, transport, streetcar
   in mine or quarry —*see* Accident,
    transport, industrial vehicle
    occupant
  truck (heavy) occupant V69.9
   collision (with)
    animal (traffic) V60.9
     being ridden (traffic) V66.9
      nontraffic V66.3
       while boarding or alighting
        V66.4
     nontraffic V60.3
     while boarding or alighting V60.4
    animal-drawn vehicle (traffic) V66.9
     nontraffic V66.3
     while boarding or alighting V66.4
    bus (traffic) V64.9
     nontraffic V64.3
     while boarding or alighting V64.4
    car (traffic) V63.9
     nontraffic V63.3
     while boarding or alighting V63.4
    motor vehicle NOS (traffic) V69.60
     nontraffic V69.20
     specified type NEC (traffic) V69.69
      nontraffic V69.29
    pedal cycle (traffic) V61.9
     nontraffic V61.3
     while boarding or alighting V61.4
    pickup truck (traffic) V63.9
     nontraffic V63.3
     while boarding or alighting V63.4
    railway vehicle (traffic) V65.9
     nontraffic V65.3
     while boarding or alighting V65.4
    specified vehicle NEC (traffic) V66.9
     nontraffic V66.3
     while boarding or alighting V66.4
    stationary object (traffic) V67.9
     nontraffic V67.3
     while boarding or alighting V67.4
    streetcar (traffic) V66.9
     nontraffic V66.3
     while boarding or alighting V66.4
    three wheeled motor vehicle (traffic)
     V62.9
     nontraffic V62.3
     while boarding or alighting V62.4
    truck (traffic) V64.9
     nontraffic V64.3
     while boarding or alighting V64.4

Accident *(Continued)*
 transport *(Continued)*
  truck occupant *(Continued)*
   collision *(Continued)*
    two wheeled motor vehicle (traffic)
     V62.9
     nontraffic V62.3
     while boarding or alighting V62.4
    van (traffic) V63.9
     nontraffic V63.3
     while boarding or alighting V63.4
   driver
    collision (with)
     animal (traffic) V60.5
      being ridden (traffic) V66.5
       nontraffic V66.0
      nontraffic V60.0
     animal-drawn vehicle (traffic) V66.5
      nontraffic V66.0
     bus (traffic) V64.5
      nontraffic V64.0
     car (traffic) V63.5
      nontraffic V63.0
     motor vehicle NOS (traffic) V69.40
      nontraffic V69.00
      specified type NEC (traffic)
       V69.49
       nontraffic V69.09
     pedal cycle (traffic) V61.5
      nontraffic V61.0
     pickup truck (traffic) V63.5
      nontraffic V63.0
     railway vehicle (traffic) V65.5
      nontraffic V65.0
     specified vehicle NEC (traffic) V66.5
      nontraffic V66.0
     stationary object (traffic) V67.5
      nontraffic V67.0
     streetcar (traffic) V66.5
      nontraffic V66.0
     three wheeled motor vehicle
      (traffic) V62.5
      nontraffic V62.0
     truck (traffic) V64.5
      nontraffic V64.0
     two wheeled motor vehicle (traffic)
      V62.5
      nontraffic V62.0
     van (traffic) V63.5
      nontraffic V63.0
    noncollision accident (traffic) V68.5
     nontraffic V68.0
   dump —*see* Accident, transport,
    construction vehicle occupant
   hanger-on
    collision (with)
     animal (traffic) V60.7
      being ridden (traffic) V66.7
       nontraffic V66.2
      nontraffic V60.2
     animal-drawn vehicle (traffic) V66.7
      nontraffic V66.2
     bus (traffic) V64.7
      nontraffic V64.2
     car (traffic) V63.7
      nontraffic V63.2
     pedal cycle (traffic) V61.7
      nontraffic V61.2
     pickup truck (traffic) V63.7
      nontraffic V63.2
     railway vehicle (traffic) V65.7
      nontraffic V65.2
     specified vehicle NEC (traffic) V66.7
      nontraffic V66.2
     stationary object (traffic) V67.7
      nontraffic V67.2
     streetcar (traffic) V66.7
      nontraffic V66.2
     three wheeled motor vehicle
      (traffic) V62.7
      nontraffic V62.2

Accident *(Continued)*
 transport *(Continued)*
  truck occupant *(Continued)*
   hanger-on *(Continued)*
    collision *(Continued)*
     truck (traffic) V64.7
      nontraffic V64.2
     two wheeled motor vehicle (traffic)
       V62.7
      nontraffic V62.2
     van (traffic) V63.7
      nontraffic V63.2
    noncollision accident (traffic) V68.7
     nontraffic V68.2
   noncollision accident (traffic) V68.9
    nontraffic V68.3
    while boarding or alighting V68.4
   nontraffic V69.3
   passenger
    collision (with)
     animal (traffic) V60.6
      being ridden (traffic) V66.6
       nontraffic V66.1
      nontraffic V60.1
     animal-drawn vehicle (traffic) V66.6
      nontraffic V66.1
     bus (traffic) V64.6
      nontraffic V64.1
     car (traffic) V63.6
      nontraffic V63.1
     motor vehicle NOS (traffic) V69.50
      nontraffic V69.10
      specified type NEC (traffic)
        V69.59
       nontraffic V69.19
     pedal cycle (traffic) V61.6
      nontraffic V61.1
     pickup truck (traffic) V63.6
      nontraffic V63.1
     railway vehicle (traffic) V65.6
      nontraffic V65.1
     specified vehicle NEC (traffic) V66.6
      nontraffic V66.1
     stationary object (traffic) V67.6
      nontraffic V67.1
     streetcar (traffic) V66.6
      nontraffic V66.1
     three wheeled motor vehicle
        (traffic) V62.6
      nontraffic V62.1
     truck (traffic) V64.6
      nontraffic V64.1
     two wheeled motor vehicle (traffic)
        V62.6
      nontraffic V62.1
     van (traffic) V63.6
      nontraffic V63.1
    noncollision accident (traffic) V68.6
     nontraffic V68.1
   pickup —*see* Accident, transport, pickup
     truck occupant
   specified type NEC V69.88
    military vehicle V69.81
  van occupant V59.9
   collision (with)
    animal (traffic) V50.9
     being ridden (traffic) V56.9
      nontraffic V56.3
      while boarding or alighting
        V56.4
     nontraffic V50.3
     while boarding or alighting V50.4
    animal-drawn vehicle (traffic) V56.9
     nontraffic V56.3
     while boarding or alighting V56.4
    bus (traffic) V54.9
     nontraffic V54.3
     while boarding or alighting V54.4
    car (traffic) V53.9
     nontraffic V53.3
     while boarding or alighting V53.4

Accident *(Continued)*
 transport *(Continued)*
  van occupant *(Continued)*
   collision *(Continued)*
    motor vehicle NOS (traffic) V59.60
     nontraffic V59.20
     specified type NEC (traffic) V59.69
      nontraffic V59.29
    pedal cycle (traffic) V51.9
     nontraffic V51.3
     while boarding or alighting V51.4
    pickup truck (traffic) V53.9
     nontraffic V53.3
     while boarding or alighting V53.4
    railway vehicle (traffic) V55.9
     nontraffic V55.3
     while boarding or alighting V55.4
    specified vehicle NEC (traffic) V56.9
     nontraffic V56.3
     while boarding or alighting V56.4
    stationary object (traffic) V57.9
     nontraffic V57.3
     while boarding or alighting V57.4
    streetcar (traffic) V56.9
     nontraffic V56.3
     while boarding or alighting V56.4
    three wheeled motor vehicle (traffic)
       V52.9
     nontraffic V52.3
     while boarding or alighting V52.4
    truck (traffic) V54.9
     nontraffic V54.3
     while boarding or alighting V54.4
    two wheeled motor vehicle (traffic)
       V52.9
     nontraffic V52.3
     while boarding or alighting V52.4
    van (traffic) V53.9
     nontraffic V53.3
     while boarding or alighting V53.4
   driver
    collision (with)
     animal (traffic) V50.5
      being ridden (traffic) V56.5
       nontraffic V56.0
      nontraffic V50.0
     animal-drawn vehicle (traffic) V56.5
      nontraffic V56.0
     bus (traffic) V54.5
      nontraffic V54.0
     car (traffic) V53.5
      nontraffic V53.0
     motor vehicle NOS (traffic) V59.40
      nontraffic V59.00
      specified type NEC (traffic)
        V59.49
       nontraffic V59.09
     pedal cycle (traffic) V51.5
      nontraffic V51.0
     pickup truck (traffic) V53.5
      nontraffic V53.0
     railway vehicle (traffic) V55.5
      nontraffic V55.0
     specified vehicle NEC (traffic) V56.5
      nontraffic V56.0
     stationary object (traffic) V57.5
      nontraffic V57.0
     streetcar (traffic) V56.5
      nontraffic V56.0
     three wheeled motor vehicle
        (traffic) V52.5
      nontraffic V52.0
     truck (traffic) V54.5
      nontraffic V54.0
     two wheeled motor vehicle (traffic)
        V52.5
      nontraffic V52.0
     van (traffic) V53.5
      nontraffic V53.0
    noncollision accident (traffic) V58.5
     nontraffic V58.0

Accident *(Continued)*
 transport *(Continued)*
  van occupant *(Continued)*
   hanger-on
    collision (with)
     animal (traffic) V50.7
      being ridden (traffic) V56.7
       nontraffic V56.2
      nontraffic V50.2
     animal-drawn vehicle (traffic) V56.7
      nontraffic V56.2
     bus (traffic) V54.7
      nontraffic V54.2
     car (traffic) V53.7
      nontraffic V53.2
     pedal cycle (traffic) V51.7
      nontraffic V51.2
     pickup truck (traffic) V53.7
      nontraffic V53.2
     railway vehicle (traffic) V55.7
      nontraffic V55.2
     specified vehicle NEC (traffic) V56.7
      nontraffic V56.2
     stationary object (traffic) V57.7
      nontraffic V57.2
     streetcar (traffic) V56.7
      nontraffic V56.2
     three wheeled motor vehicle
        (traffic) V52.7
      nontraffic V52.2
     truck (traffic) V54.7
      nontraffic V54.2
     two wheeled motor vehicle (traffic)
        V52.7
      nontraffic V52.2
     van (traffic) V53.7
      nontraffic V53.2
    noncollision accident (traffic) V58.7
     nontraffic V58.2
   noncollision accident (traffic) V58.9
    nontraffic V58.3
    while boarding or alighting V58.4
   nontraffic V59.3
   passenger
    collision (with)
     animal (traffic) V50.6
      being ridden (traffic) V56.6
       nontraffic V56.1
      nontraffic V50.1
     animal-drawn vehicle (traffic) V56.6
      nontraffic V56.1
     bus (traffic) V54.6
      nontraffic V54.1
     car (traffic) V53.6
      nontraffic V53.1
     motor vehicle NOS (traffic) V59.50
      nontraffic V59.10
      specified type NEC (traffic) V59.59
       nontraffic V59.19
     pedal cycle (traffic) V51.6
      nontraffic V51.1
     pickup truck (traffic) V53.6
      nontraffic V53.1
     railway vehicle (traffic) V55.6
      nontraffic V55.1
     specified vehicle NEC (traffic) V56.6
      nontraffic V56.1
     stationary object (traffic) V57.6
      nontraffic V57.1
     streetcar (traffic) V56.6
      nontraffic V56.1
     three wheeled motor vehicle
        (traffic) V52.6
      nontraffic V52.1
     truck (traffic) V54.6
      nontraffic V54.1
     two wheeled motor vehicle (traffic)
        V52.6
      nontraffic V52.1
     van (traffic) V53.6
      nontraffic V53.1

▶ New   ⇒ Revised   ~~deleted~~ Deleted   ● Use Additional Character(s)

▶ New   ⇒ Revised   ~~deleted~~ Deleted   ● Use Additional Character(s)

Activity *(Continued)*
 hockey (ice) Y93.22
  field Y93.65
 horseback riding Y93.52
 household (interior) maintenance NEC Y93. E9
 ice NEC Y93.29
  dancing Y93.21
  hockey Y93.22
  skating Y93.21
 inline roller skating Y93.51
 ironing Y93.E4
 judo Y93.75
 jumping (off) NEC Y93.39
  BASE (Building, Antenna, Span, Earth) Y93.33
  bungee Y93.34
  jacks Y93.A2
  rope Y93.56
 jumping jacks Y93.A2
 jumping rope Y93.56
 karate Y93.75
 kayaking (in calm and turbulent water) Y93.16
 keyboarding (computer) Y93.C1
 kickball Y93.6A
 knitting Y93.D1
 lacrosse Y93.65
 land maintenance NEC Y93.H9
 landscaping Y93.H2
 laundry Y93.E2
 machines (exercise)
  primarily for cardiorespiratory conditioning Y93.A1
  primarily for muscle strengthening Y93.B1
 maintenance
  exterior building NEC Y93.H9
  household (interior) NEC Y93.E9
  land Y93.H9
  property Y93.H9
 marching (on level or elevated terrain) Y93.Ø1
 martial arts Y93.75
 microwave oven Y93.G3
 milking an animal Y93.K2
 mopping (floor) Y93.E5
 mountain climbing Y93.31
 muscle strengthening
  exercises (non-machine) NEC Y93.B9
  machines Y93.B1
 musical keyboard (electronic) playing Y93.J1
 nordic skiing Y93.24
 obstacle course Y93.A5
 oven (microwave) Y93.G3
 packing up and unpacking in moving to a new residence Y93.E6
 parasailing Y93.19
 pass out game Y93.85
 percussion instrument playing NEC Y93.J2
 personal
  bathing and showering Y93.E1
  hygiene NEC Y93.E8
  showering Y93.E1
 physical games generally associated with school recess, summer camp and children Y93.6A
 physical training NEC Y93.A9
 piano playing Y93.J1
 pilates Y93.B4
 platform diving Y93.12
 playing musical instrument
  brass instrument Y93.J4
  drum Y93.J2
  musical keyboard (electronic) Y93.J1
  percussion instrument NEC Y93.J2
  piano Y93.J1
  string instrument Y93.J3
  winds instrument Y93.J4
 property maintenance
  exterior NEC Y93.H9
  interior NEC Y93.E9
 pruning (garden and lawn) Y93.H2

Activity *(Continued)*
 pull-ups Y93.B2
 push-ups Y93.B2
 racquetball Y93.73
 rafting (in calm and turbulent water) Y93.16
 raking (leaves) Y93.H1
 rappelling Y93.32
 refereeing a sports activity Y93.81
 residential relocation Y93.E6
 rhythmic gymnastics Y93.43
 rhythmic movement NEC Y93.49
 riding
  horseback Y93.52
  rollercoaster Y93.I1
 rock climbing Y93.31
 roller skating (inline) Y93.51
 rollercoaster riding Y93.I1
 rough housing and horseplay Y93.83
 rowing (in calm and turbulent water) Y93.16
 rugby Y93.63
 SCUBA diving Y93.15
 sewing Y93.D2
 shoveling Y93.H1
  dirt Y93.H1
  snow Y93.H1
 showering (personal) Y93.E1
 sit-ups Y93.B2
 skateboarding Y93.51
 skating (ice) Y93.21
  roller Y93.51
 skiing (alpine) (downhill) Y93.23
  cross country Y93.24
  nordic Y93.24
  water Y93.17
 sledding (snow) Y93.23
 sleeping (sleep) Y93.84
 smoking and grilling food Y93.G2
 snorkeling Y93.15
 snow NEC Y93.29
  boarding Y93.23
  shoveling Y93.H1
  sledding Y93.23
  tubing Y93.23
 soccer Y93.66
 softball Y93.64
 specified NEC Y93.89
 spectator at an event Y93.82
 sports NEC Y93.79
  sports played as a team or group NEC Y93.69
  sports played individually NEC Y93.59
 springboard diving Y93.12
 squash Y93.73
 stationary bike Y93.A1
 step (stepping) exercise (class) Y93.A3
 stepper machine Y93.A1
 stove Y93.G3
 string instrument playing Y93.J3
 surfing Y93.18
  wind Y93.18
 swimming Y93.11
 tackle football Y93.61
 tap dancing Y93.41
 tennis Y93.73
 tobogganing Y93.23
 touch football Y93.62
 track and field events (non-running) Y93.57
  running Y93.Ø2
 trampoline Y93.44
 treadmill Y93.A1
 trimming shrubs Y93.H2
 tubing (in calm and turbulent water) Y93.16
  snow Y93.23
 ultimate frisbee Y93.74
 underwater diving Y93.15
 unpacking in moving to a new residence Y93.E6
 use of stove, oven and microwave oven Y93. G3

Activity *(Continued)*
 vacuuming Y93.E3
 volleyball (beach) (court) Y93.68
 wake boarding Y93.17
 walking (on level or elevated terrain) Y93.Ø1
  an animal Y93.K1
 walking an animal Y93.K1
 wall climbing Y93.31
 warm up and cool down exercises Y93.A2
 water NEC Y93.19
  aerobics Y93.14
  craft NEC Y93.19
  exercise Y93.14
  polo Y93.13
  skiing Y93.17
  sliding Y93.18
  survival training and testing Y93.19
 weeding (garden and lawn) Y93.H2
 wind instrument playing Y93.J4
 windsurfing Y93.18
 wrestling Y93.72
 yoga Y93.42
Adverse effect of drugs —*see* Table of Drugs and Chemicals
Aerosinusitis —*see* Air, pressure
After-effect, late —*see* Sequelae
Air
 blast in war operations —*see* War operations, air blast
 pressure
  change, rapid
   during
    ascent W94.29
     while (in) (surfacing from)
      aircraft W94.23
      deep water diving W94.21
      underground W94.22
    descent W94.39
     in
      aircraft W94.31
      water W94.32
  high, prolonged W94.Ø
  low, prolonged W94.12
   due to residence or long visit at high altitude W94.11
Alpine sickness W94.11
Altitude sickness W94.11
Anaphylactic shock, anaphylaxis —*see* Table of Drugs and Chemicals
Andes disease W94.11
Arachnidism, arachnoidism X58
Arson (with intent to injure or kill) X97
Asphyxia, asphyxiation
 by
  food (bone) (seed) —*see* categories T17 and T18
  gas —*see also* Table of Drugs and Chemicals
  legal
   execution —*see* Legal, intervention, gas
   intervention —*see* Legal, intervention, gas
 from
  fire —*see also* Exposure, fire
   in war operations —*see* War operations, fire
  ignition —*see* Ignition
  vomitus T17.81
 in war operations —*see* War operations, restriction of airway
Aspiration
 food (any type) (into respiratory tract) (with asphyxia, obstruction respiratory tract, suffocation) —*see* categories T17 and T18
 foreign body —*see* Foreign body, aspiration
 vomitus (with asphyxia, obstruction respiratory tract, suffocation) T17.81
Assassination (attempt) —*see* Assault

A

▶ New   ⇒ Revised   ~~deleted~~ Deleted   ● Use Additional Character(s)

Assault (homicidal) (by) (in) Y09
  arson X97
  bite (of human being) Y04.1
  bodily force Y04.8
    bite Y04.1
    bumping into Y04.2
    sexual —*see* subcategories T74.0, T76.0
    unarmed fight Y04.0
  bomb X96.9
    antipersonnel X96.0
    fertilizer X96.3
    gasoline X96.1
    letter X96.2
    petrol X96.1
    pipe X96.3
    specified NEC X96.8
  brawl (hand) (fists) (foot) (unarmed)
      Y04.0
  burning, burns (by fire) NEC X97
    acid Y08.89
    caustic, corrosive substance Y08.89
    chemical from swallowing caustic,
        corrosive substance —*see* Table of
        Drugs and Chemicals
    cigarette(s) X97
    hot object X98.9
      fluid NEC X98.2
      household appliance X98.3
      specified NEC X98.8
      steam X98.0
      tap water X98.1
      vapors X98.0
    scalding —*see* Assault, burning
    steam X98.0
    vitriol Y08.89
  caustic, corrosive substance (gas) Y08.89
  crashing of
    aircraft Y08.81
    motor vehicle Y03.8
      pushed in front of Y02.0
      run over Y03.0
      specified NEC Y03.8
  cutting or piercing instrument X99.9
    dagger X99.2
    glass X99.0

Assault *(Continued)*
  cutting or piercing instrument *(Continued)*
    knife X99.1
    specified NEC X99.8
    sword X99.2
  dagger X99.2
  drowning (in) X92.9
    bathtub X92.0
    natural water X92.3
    specified NEC X92.8
    swimming pool X92.1
      following fall X92.2
  dynamite X96.8
  explosive(s) (material) X96.9
  fight (hand) (fists) (foot) (unarmed)
      Y04.0
    with weapon —*see* Assault, by type of
        weapon
  fire X97
  firearm X95.9
    airgun X95.01
    handgun X93
    hunting rifle X94.1
    larger X94.9
      specified NEC X94.8
    machine gun X94.2
    shotgun X94.0
    specified NEC X95.8
  from high place Y01
  gunshot (wound) NEC —*see* Assault, firearm,
      by type
  incendiary device X97
  injury Y09
    to child due to criminal abortion attempt
        NEC Y08.89
  knife X99.1
  late effect of —*see* X92-Y08 with 7th
      character S
  placing before moving object NEC
      Y02.8
    motor vehicle Y02.0
  poisoning —*see* categories T36-T65 with 7th
      character S
  puncture, any part of body —*see* Assault,
      cutting or piercing instrument

Assault *(Continued)*
  pushing
    before moving object NEC Y02.8
      motor vehicle Y02.0
      subway train Y02.1
      train Y02.1
  rape T74.2-●
  scalding —*see* Assault, burning
  sequelae of —*see* X92-Y08 with 7th character S
  sexual (by bodily force) T74.2-●
  shooting —*see* Assault, firearm
  specified means NEC Y08.89
  stab, any part of body —*see* Assault, cutting
      or piercing instrument
  steam X98.0
  striking against
    other person Y04.2
    sports equipment Y08.09
      baseball bat Y08.02
      hockey stick Y08.01
  struck by
    sports equipment Y08.09
      baseball bat Y08.02
      hockey stick Y08.01
  submersion —*see* Assault, drowning
  violence Y09
  weapon Y09
    blunt Y00
    cutting or piercing —*see* Assault, cutting or
        piercing instrument
    firearm —*see* Assault, firearm
  wound Y09
    cutting —*see* Assault, cutting or piercing
        instrument
    gunshot —*see* Assault, firearm
    knife X99.1
    piercing —*see* Assault, cutting or piercing
        instrument
    puncture —*see* Assault, cutting or piercing
        instrument
    stab —*see* Assault, cutting or piercing
        instrument
Attack by mammals NEC W55.89
Avalanche —*see* Landslide
Aviator's disease —*see* Air, pressure

B

▶ New   ⇒ Revised   ~~deleted~~ Deleted   ● Use Additional Character(s)

Burn, burned, burning (*Continued*)
local application of externally applied
  substance in medical or surgical care
  Y63.5
machinery (hot) X17
matches X08.8
  with ignition of clothing NEC X06.2
    nightwear X05
mattress —*see* Exposure, fire, uncontrolled,
  building, bed
medicament, externally applied Y63.5
metal (hot) (liquid) (molten) NEC X18
nightwear (nightclothes, nightdress, gown,
  pajamas, robe) X05
object (hot) NEC X19
on board watercraft
  due to
    accident to watercraft V91.09
      powered craft V91.03
        ferry boat V91.01
        fishing boat V91.02
        jet ski V91.03
        liner V91.01
        merchant ship V91.00
        passenger ship V91.01
      unpowered craft V91.08
        canoe V91.05
        inflatable V91.06
        kayak V91.05
        sailboat V91.04
        surf-board V91.08
        water skis V91.07
        windsurfer V91.08
    fire on board V93.09
      ferry boat V93.01
      fishing boat V93.02
      jet ski V93.03
      liner V93.01
      merchant ship V93.00
      passenger ship V93.01
      powered craft NEC V93.03
      sailboat V93.04

Burn, burned, burning (*Continued*)
on board watercraft (*Continued*)
  due to (*Continued*)
    specified heat source NEC on board
      V93.19
      ferry boat V93.11
      fishing boat V93.12
      jet ski V93.13
      liner V93.11
      merchant ship V93.10
      passenger ship V93.11
      powered craft NEC V93.13
      sailboat V93.14
pipe (hot) X16
  smoking X08.8
    with ignition of clothing NEC X06.2
      nightwear X05
powder —*see* Powder burn
radiator (hot) X16
saucepan (hot) (glass) (metal) X15.3
  stated as undetermined whether
    accidental or intentional
    Y27.3
  suicide (attempt) X77.3
self-inflicted X76
  stated as undetermined whether
    accidental or intentional
    Y26
stated as undetermined whether
  accidental or intentional Y27.0
steam X13.1
  pipe X16
    stated as undetermined whether
      accidental or intentional
      Y27.8
  stated as undetermined whether
    accidental or intentional Y27.0
  suicide (attempt) X77.0
stove (hot) (kitchen) X15.0
  stated as undetermined whether
    accidental or intentional Y27.3
  suicide (attempt) X77.3

Burn, burned, burning (*Continued*)
substance (hot) NEC X19
  boiling X12
    stated as undetermined whether
      accidental or intentional Y27.2
    suicide (attempt) X77.2
  molten (metal) X18
suicide (attempt) NEC X76
  hot
    household appliance X77.3
    object X77.9
  stated as undetermined whether accidental or
    intentional Y27.0
therapeutic misadventure
  heat in local application or packing during
    medical or surgical procedure Y63.5
  overdose of radiation Y63.2
toaster (hot) X15.1
  stated as undetermined whether accidental
    or intentional Y27.3
  suicide (attempt) X77.3
tool (hot) X17
torch, welding X08.8
  with ignition of clothing NEC X06.2
    nightwear X05
trash fire (controlled) —*see* Exposure, fire,
  controlled, not in building
  uncontrolled —*see* Exposure, fire,
    uncontrolled, not in building
vapor (hot) X13.1
  stated as undetermined whether accidental
    or intentional Y27.0
  suicide (attempt) X77.0
Very pistol —*see* Discharge, firearm NEC
Butted by animal W55.82
  bull W55.22
  cow W55.22
  goat W55.32
  horse W55.12
  pig W55.42
  sheep W55.32

C

Caisson disease —*see* Air, pressure, change

Campfire (exposure to) (controlled) —*see also* Exposure, fire, controlled, not in building

uncontrolled —*see* Exposure, fire, uncontrolled, not in building

Capital punishment (any means) —*see* Legal, intervention

Car sickness T75.3

Casualty (not due to war) NEC X58

war —*see* War operations

Cat

bite W55.01

scratch W55.03

Cataclysm, cataclysmic (any injury) NEC —*see* Forces of nature

Catching fire —*see* Exposure, fire

Caught

between

folding object W23.0

objects (moving) (stationary and moving) W23.0

and machinery —*see* Contact, with, by type of machine

stationary W23.1

sliding door and door frame W23.0

by, in

machinery (moving parts of) —*see* Contact, with, by type of machine

washing-machine wringer W23.0

under packing crate (due to losing grip) W23.1

Cave-in caused by cataclysmic earth surface movement or eruption —*see* Landslide

Change(s) in air pressure —*see* Air, pressure, change

Choked, choking (on) (any object except food or vomitus)

food (bone) (seed) —*see* categories T17 and T18

vomitus T17.81-●

Civil insurrection —*see* War operations

Cloudburst (any injury) X37.8

Cold, exposure to (accidental) (excessive) (extreme) (natural) (place) NEC —*see* Exposure, cold

Collapse

building W20.1

burning (uncontrolled fire) X00.2

dam or man-made structure (causing earth movement) X36.0

machinery —*see* Contact, with, by type of machine

structure W20.1

burning (uncontrolled fire) X00.2

Collision (accidental) NEC —*see also* Accident, transport V89.9

pedestrian W51

with fall W03

due to ice or snow W00.0

involving pedestrian conveyance —*see* Accident, transport, pedestrian, conveyance

and

crowd or human stampede (with fall) W52

object W22.8

with fall —*see* Fall, due to, bumping against, object

person(s) —*see* Collision, pedestrian

transport vehicle NEC V89.9

and

avalanche, fallen or not moving —*see* Accident, transport

falling or moving —*see* Landslide

landslide, fallen or not moving —*see* Accident, transport

falling or moving —*see* Landslide

Collision NEC (*Continued*)

transport vehicle NEC (*Continued*)

due to cataclysm —*see* Forces of nature, by type

intentional, purposeful suicide (attempt) —*see* Suicide, collision

Combustion, spontaneous —*see* Ignition

Complication (delayed) of or following (medical or surgical procedure) Y84.9

with misadventure —*see* Misadventure

amputation of limb(s) Y83.5

anastomosis (arteriovenous) (blood vessel) (gastrojejunal) (tendon) (natural or artificial material) Y83.2

aspiration (of fluid) Y84.4

tissue Y84.8

biopsy Y84.8

blood

sampling Y84.7

transfusion

procedure Y84.8

bypass Y83.2

catheterization (urinary) Y84.6

cardiac Y84.0

colostomy Y83.3

cystostomy Y83.3

dialysis (kidney) Y84.1

drug —*see* Table of Drugs and Chemicals

due to misadventure —*see* Misadventure

duodenostomy Y83.3

electroshock therapy Y84.3

external stoma, creation of Y83.3

formation of external stoma Y83.3

gastrostomy Y83.3

graft Y83.2

hypothermia (medically-induced) Y84.8

implant, implantation (of)

artificial

internal device (cardiac pacemaker) (electrodes in brain) (heart valve prosthesis) (orthopedic) Y83.1

material or tissue (for anastomosis or bypass) Y83.2

with creation of external stoma Y83.3

natural tissues (for anastomosis or bypass) Y83.2

with creation of external stoma Y83.3

infusion

procedure Y84.8

injection —*see* Table of Drugs and Chemicals

procedure Y84.8

insertion of gastric or duodenal sound Y84.5

insulin-shock therapy Y84.3

paracentesis (abdominal) (thoracic) (aspirative) Y84.4

procedures other than surgical operation —*see* Complication of or following, by type of procedure

radiological procedure or therapy Y84.2

removal of organ (partial) (total) NEC Y83.6

sampling

blood Y84.7

fluid NEC Y84.4

tissue Y84.8

shock therapy Y84.3

surgical operation NEC —*see also* Complication of or following, by type of operation Y83.9

reconstructive NEC Y83.4

with

anastomosis, bypass or graft Y83.2

formation of external stoma Y83.3

specified NEC Y83.8

transfusion —*see also* Table of Drugs and Chemicals

procedure Y84.8

transplant, transplantation (heart) (kidney) (liver) (whole organ, any) Y83.0

partial organ Y83.4

ureterostomy Y83.3

Complication of or following (*Continued*)

vaccination —*see also* Table of Drugs and Chemicals

procedure Y84.8

Compression

divers' squeeze —*see* Air, pressure, change

trachea by

food (lodged in esophagus) —*see* categories T17 and T18

vomitus (lodged in esophagus) T17.81-●

Conflagration —*see* Exposure, fire, uncontrolled

Constriction (external)

hair W49.01

jewelry W49.04

ring W49.04

rubber band W49.03

specified item NEC W49.09

string W49.02

thread W49.02

Contact (accidental)

with

abrasive wheel (metalworking) W31.1

alligator W58.09

bite W58.01

crushing W58.03

strike W58.02

amphibian W62.9

frog W62.0

toad W62.1

animal (nonvenomous) NEC W64

marine W56.89

bite W56.81

dolphin —*see* Contact, with, dolphin

fish NEC —*see* Contact, with, fish

mammal —*see* Contact, with, mammal, marine

orca —*see* Contact, with, orca

sea lion —*see* Contact, with, sea lion

shark —*see* Contact, with, shark

strike W56.82

animate mechanical force NEC W64

arrow W21.89

not thrown, projected or falling W45.8

arthropods (nonvenomous) W57

axe W27.0

band-saw (industrial) W31.2

bayonet —*see* Bayonet wound

bee(s) X58

bench-saw (industrial) W31.2

bird W61.99

bite W61.91

chicken —*see* Contact, with, chicken

duck —*see* Contact, with, duck

goose —*see* Contact, with, goose

macaw —*see* Contact, with, macaw

parrot —*see* Contact, with, parrot

psittacine —*see* Contact, with, psittacine

strike W61.92

turkey —*see* Contact, with, turkey

blender W29.0

boiling water X12

stated as undetermined whether accidental or intentional Y27.2

suicide (attempt) X77.2

bore, earth-drilling or mining (land) (seabed) W31.0

buffalo —*see* Contact, with, hoof stock NEC

bull W55.29

bite W55.21

gored W55.22

strike W55.22

bumper cars W31.81

camel —*see* Contact, with, hoof stock NEC

can

lid W26.8

opener W27.4

powered W29.0

cat W55.09

bite W55.01

scratch W55.03

caterpillar (venomous) X58

▶ New   ⟾ Revised   ~~deleted~~ Deleted   ● Use Additional Character(s)

Contact *(Continued)*
  with *(Continued)*
    centipede (venomous) X58
    chain
      hoist W24.0
        agricultural operations W30.89
      saw W29.3
    chicken W61.39
      peck W61.33
      strike W61.32
    chisel W27.0
    circular saw W31.2
    cobra X58
    combine (harvester) W30.0
    conveyer belt W24.1
    cooker (hot) X15.8
      stated as undetermined whether
        accidental or intentional Y27.3
      suicide (attempt) X77.3
    coral X58
    cotton gin W31.82
    cow W55.29
      bite W55.21
      strike W55.22
    crane W24.0
      agricultural operations W30.89
    crocodile W58.19
      bite W58.11
      crushing W58.13
      strike W58.12
    dagger W26.1
      stated as undetermined whether
        accidental or intentional Y28.2
      suicide (attempt) X78.2
    dairy equipment W31.82
    dart W21.89
      not thrown, projected or falling W45.8
    deer —*see* Contact, with, hoof stock
      NEC
    derrick W24.0
      agricultural operations W30.89
        hay W30.2
    dog W54.8
      bite W54.0
      strike W54.1
    dolphin W56.09
      bite W56.01
      strike W56.02
    donkey —*see* Contact, with, hoof stock
      NEC
    drill (powered) W29.8
      earth (land) (seabed) W31.0
      nonpowered W27.8
    drive belt W24.0
      agricultural operations W30.89
    dry ice —*see* Exposure, cold, man-made
    dryer (clothes) (powered) (spin) W29.2
    duck W61.69
      bite W61.61
      strike W61.62
    earth(-)
      drilling machine (industrial) W31.0
      scraping machine in stationary use
        W31.83
    edge of stiff paper W26.2
    electric
      beater W29.0
      blanket X16
      fan W29.2
        commercial W31.82
      knife W29.1
      mixer W29.0
    elevator (building) W24.0
      agricultural operations W30.89
        grain W30.3
    engine(s), hot NEC X17
    excavating machine W31.0
    farm machine W30.9
    feces —*see* Contact, with, by type of
      animal
    fer de lance X58

Contact *(Continued)*
  with *(Continued)*
    fish W56.59
      bite W56.51
      shark —*see* Contact, with, shark
      strike W56.52
    flying horses W31.81
    forging (metalworking) machine
      W31.1
    fork W27.4
    forklift (truck) W24.0
      agricultural operations W30.89
    frog W62.0
    garden
      cultivator (powered) W29.3
        riding W30.89
      fork W27.1
    gas turbine W31.3
    Gila monster X58
    giraffe —*see* Contact, with, hoof stock
      NEC
    glass (sharp) (broken) W25
      with subsequent fall W18.02
      assault X99.0
      due to fall —*see* Fall, by type
      stated as undetermined whether
        accidental or intentional Y28. 0
      suicide (attempt) X78.0
    goat W55.39
      bite W55.31
      strike W55.32
    goose W61.59
      bite W61.51
      strike W61.52
    hand
      saw W27.0
      tool (not powered) NEC W27.8
        powered W29.8
    harvester W30.0
    hay-derrick W30.2
    heat NEC X19
      from appliance (electrical)
        (household) —*see* Contact, with,
        hot, household appliance
      heating appliance X16
    heating
      appliance (hot) X16
      pad (electric) X16
    hedge-trimmer (powered) W29.3
    hoe W27.1
    hoist (chain) (shaft) NEC W24.0
      agricultural W30.89
    hoof stock NEC W55.39
      bite W55.31
      strike W55.32
    hornet(s) X58
    horse W55.19
      bite W55.11
      strike W55.12
    hot
      air X14.1
        inhalation X14.0
      cooker X15.8
      drinks X10.0
      engine X17
      fats X10.2
      fluids NEC X12
        assault X98.2
        suicide (attempt) X77.2
        undetermined whether accidental or
          intentional Y27.2
      food X10.1
      gases X14.1
        inhalation X14.0
      heating appliance X16
      household appliance X15.8
        assault X98.3
        cooker X15.8
        hotplate X15.2
        kettle X15.8
        light bulb X15.8

Contact *(Continued)*
  with *(Continued)*
    hot *(Continued)*
      household appliance *(Continued)*
        object NEC X19
          assault X98.8
          stated as undetermined whether
            accidental or intentional Y27.9
          suicide (attempt) X77.8
        saucepan X15.3
        skillet X15.3
        stated as undetermined whether
          accidental or intentional Y27.3
        stove X15.0
        suicide (attempt) X77.3
        toaster X15.1
      kettle X15.8
      light bulb X15.8
      liquid NEC —*see also* Burn X12
        drinks X10.0
        stated as undetermined whether
          accidental or intentional Y27.2
        suicide (attempt) X77.2
        tap water X11.8
          stated as undetermined whether
            accidental or intentional Y27.1
          suicide (attempt) X77.1
      machinery X17
      metal (molten) (liquid) NEC X18
      object (not producing fire or flames)
        NEC X19
      oil (cooking) X10.2
      pipe X16
      plate X15.2
      radiator X16
      saucepan (glass) (metal) X15.3
      skillet X15.3
      stove (kitchen) X15.0
      substance NEC X19
      tap-water X11.8
        assault X98.1
        heated on stove X12
          stated as undetermined whether
            accidental or intentional Y27.2
          suicide (attempt) X77.2
        in bathtub X11.0
        running X11.1
        stated as undetermined whether
          accidental or intentional Y27.1
        suicide (attempt) X77.1
      toaster X15.1
      tool X17
      vapors X13.1
        inhalation X13.0
      water (tap) X11.8
        boiling X12
          stated as undetermined whether
            accidental or intentional Y27.2
          suicide (attempt) X77.2
        heated on stove X12
          stated as undetermined whether
            accidental or intentional Y27.2
          suicide (attempt) X77.2
        in bathtub X11.0
        running X11.1
        stated as undetermined whether
          accidental or intentional Y27.1
        suicide (attempt) X77.1
    hotplate X15.2
    ice-pick W27.4
    insect (nonvenomous) NEC W57
    kettle (hot) X15.8
    knife W26.0
      assault X99.1
      electric W29.1
      stated as undetermined whether
        accidental or intentional Y28.1
      suicide (attempt) X78.1
    lathe (metalworking) W31.1
      turnings W45.8
      woodworking W31.2

Contact *(Continued)*
  with *(Continued)*
    lawnmower (powered) (ridden) W28
      causing electrocution W86.8
        suicide (attempt) X83.1
      unpowered W27.1
    lift, lifting (devices) W24.0
      agricultural operations W30.89
      shaft W24.0
    liquefied gas —*see* Exposure, cold,
        man-made
    liquid air, hydrogen, nitrogen —*see*
        Exposure, cold, man-made
    lizard (nonvenomous) W59.09
      bite W59.01
      strike W59.02
    llama —*see* Contact, with, hoof stock NEC
    macaw W61.19
      bite W61.11
      strike W61.12
    machine, machinery W31.9
      abrasive wheel W31.1
      agricultural including animal-powered
          W30.9
        combine harvester W30.0
        grain storage elevator W30.3
        hay derrick W30.2
        power take-off device W30.1
        reaper W30.0
        specified NEC W30.89
        thresher W30.0
        transport vehicle, stationary W30.81
      band saw W31.2
      bench saw W31.2
      circular saw W31.2
      commercial NEC W31.82
      drilling, metal (industrial) W31.1
      earth-drilling W31.0
      earthmoving or scraping W31.89
      excavating W31.89
      forging machine W31.1
      gas turbine W31.3
      hot X17
      internal combustion engine W31.3
      land drill W31.0
      lathe W31.1
      lifting (devices) W24.0
      metal drill W31.1
      metalworking (industrial) W31.1
      milling, metal W31.1
      mining W31.0
      molding W31.2
      overhead plane W31.2
      power press, metal W31.1
      prime mover W31.3
      printing W31.89
      radial saw W31.2
      recreational W31.81
      roller-coaster W31.81
      rolling mill, metal W31.1
      sander W31.2
      seabed drill W31.0
      shaft
        hoist W31.0
        lift W31.0
      specified NEC W31.89
      spinning W31.89
      steam engine W31.3
      transmission W24.1
      undercutter W31.0
      water driven turbine W31.3
      weaving W31.89
      woodworking or forming (industrial)
          W31.2
    mammal (feces) (urine) W55.89
      bull —*see* Contact, with, bull
      cat —*see* Contact, with, cat
      cow —*see* Contact, with, cow
      goat —*see* Contact, with, goat
      hoof stock —*see* Contact, with, hoof
          stock

Contact *(Continued)*
  with *(Continued)*
    mammal *(Continued)*
      horse —*see* Contact, with, horse
      marine W56.39
        dolphin —*see* Contact, with, dolphin
        orca —*see* Contact, with, orca
        sea lion —*see* Contact, with, sea lion
        specified NEC W56.39
          bite W56.31
          strike W56.32
      pig —*see* Contact, with, pig
      raccoon —*see* Contact, with, raccoon
      rodent —*see* Contact, with, rodent
      sheep —*see* Contact, with, sheep
      specified NEC W55.89
        bite W55.81
        strike W55.82
    marine
      animal W56.89
        bite W56.81
        dolphin —*see* Contact, with, dolphin
        fish NEC —*see* Contact, with, fish
        mammal —*see* Contact, with,
            mammal, marine
        orca —*see* Contact, with, orca
        sea lion —*see* Contact, with, sea lion
        shark —*see* Contact, with, shark
        strike W56.82
    meat
      grinder (domestic) W29.0
        industrial W31.82
        nonpowered W27.4
      slicer (domestic) W29.0
        industrial W31.82
    merry go round W31.81
    metal, (hot) (liquid) (molten) NEC X18
    millipede W57
    nail W45.0
      gun W29.4
    needle (sewing) W27.3
      hypodermic W46.0
        contaminated W46.1
    object (blunt) NEC
      hot NEC X19
      legal intervention —*see* Legal,
          intervention, blunt object
      sharp NEC W45.8
        inflicted by other person NEC W45.8
          stated as
            intentional homicide (attempt) —
                see Assault, cutting or
                piercing instrument
        legal intervention —*see* Legal,
            intervention, sharp object
        self-inflicted X78.9
    orca W56.29
      bite W56.21
      strike W56.22
    overhead plane W31.2
    paper (as sharp object) W26.2
    paper-cutter W27.5
    parrot W61.09
      bite W61.01
      strike W61.02
    pig W55.49
      bite W55.41
      strike W55.42
    pipe, hot X16
    pitchfork W27.1
    plane (metal) (wood) W27.0
      overhead W31.2
    plant thorns, spines, sharp leaves or other
        mechanisms W60
    powered
      garden cultivator W29.3
      household appliance, implement, or
          machine W29.8
      saw (industrial) W31.2
        hand W29.8
      printing machine W31.89

Contact *(Continued)*
  with *(Continued)*
    psittacine bird W61.29
      bite W61.21
      macaw —*see* Contact, with, macaw
      parrot —*see* Contact, with, parrot
      strike W61.22
    pulley (block) (transmission) W24.0
      agricultural operations W30.89
    raccoon W55.59
      bite W55.51
      strike W55.52
    radial-saw (industrial) W31.2
    radiator (hot) X16
    rake W27.1
    rattlesnake X58
    reaper W30.0
    reptile W59.89
      lizard —*see* Contact, with, lizard
      snake —*see* Contact, with, snake
      specified NEC W59.89
        bite W59.81
        crushing W59.83
        strike W59.82
      turtle —*see* Contact, with, turtle
    rivet gun (powered) W29.4
    road scraper —*see* Accident, transport,
        construction vehicle
    rodent (feces) (urine) W53.89
      bite W53.81
      mouse W53.09
        bite W53.01
      rat W53.19
        bite W53.11
      specified NEC W53.89
        bite W53.81
      squirrel W53.29
        bite W53.21
    roller coaster W31.81
    rope NEC W24.0
      agricultural operations W30.89
    saliva —*see* Contact, with, by type of
        animal
    sander W29.8
      industrial W31.2
    saucepan (hot) (glass) (metal) X15.3
    saw W27.0
      band (industrial) W31.2
      bench (industrial) W31.2
      chain W29.3
      hand W27.0
    sawing machine, metal W31.1
    scissors W27.2
    scorpion X58
    screwdriver W27.0
      powered W29.8
    sea
      anemone, cucumber or urchin (spine)
          X58
      lion W56.19
        bite W56.11
        strike W56.12
    serpent —*see* Contact, with, snake, by type
    sewing-machine (electric) (powered) W29.2
      not powered W27.8
    shaft (hoist) (lift) (transmission) NEC W24.0
      agricultural W30.89
    shark W56.49
      bite W56.41
      strike W56.42
    sharp object(s) W26.9
      specified NEC W26.8
    shears (hand) W27.2
      powered (industrial) W31.1
        domestic W29.2
    sheep W55.39
      bite W55.31
      strike W55.32
    shovel W27.8
      steam —*see* Accident, transport,
          construction vehicle

▶ New   ⇒ Revised   ~~deleted~~ Deleted   • Use Additional Character(s)

Contact *(Continued)*
  with *(Continued)*
    snake (nonvenomous) W59.19
      bite W59.11
      crushing W59.13
      strike W59.12
    spade W27.1
    spider (venomous) X58
    spin-drier W29.2
    spinning machine W31.89
    splinter W45.8
    sports equipment W21.9
    staple gun (powered) W29.8
    steam X13.1
      engine W31.3
      inhalation X13.0
      pipe X16
      shovel W31.89
    stove (hot) (kitchen) X15.0
    substance, hot NEC X19
      molten (metal) X18
    sword W26.1
      assault X99.2
      stated as undetermined whether
        accidental or intentional
        Y28.2
      suicide (attempt) X78.2
    tarantula X58
    thresher W30.0
    tin can lid W26.8
    toad W62.1
    toaster (hot) X15.1
    tool W27.8
      hand (not powered) W27.8
        auger W27.0
        axe W27.0
        can opener W27.4
        chisel W27.0
        fork W27.4
        garden W27.1
        handsaw W27.0
        hoe W27.1
        ice-pick W27.4
        kitchen utensil W27.4
        manual
          lawn mower W27.1
          sewing machine W27.8
        meat grinder W27.4
        needle (sewing) W27.3
          hypodermic W46.0
            contaminated W46.1
        paper cutter W27.5
        pitchfork W27.1
        rake W27.1
        scissors W27.2
        screwdriver W27.0
        specified NEC W27.8
        workbench W27.0
      hot X17
      powered W29.8
        blender W29.0
          commercial W31.82
        can opener W29.0
          commercial W31.82
        chainsaw W29.3
        clothes dryer W29.2
          commercial W31.82
        dishwasher W29.2
          commercial W31.82
        edger W29.3
        electric fan W29.2
          commercial W31.82
        electric knife W29.1
        food processor W29.0
          commercial W31.82
        garbage disposal W29.0
          commercial W31.82

Contact *(Continued)*
  with *(Continued)*
    tool *(Continued)*
      powered *(Continued)*
        garden tool W29.3
        hedge trimmer W29.3
        ice maker W29.0
          commercial W31.82
        kitchen appliance W29.0
          commercial W31.82
        lawn mower W28
        meat grinder W29.0
          commercial W31.82
        mixer W29.0
          commercial W31.82
        rototiller W29.3
        sewing machine W29.2
          commercial W31.82
        washing machine W29.2
          commercial W31.82
    transmission device (belt, cable, chain,
      gear, pinion, shaft) W24.1
      agricultural operations W30.89
    turbine (gas) (water-driven) W31.3
    turkey W61.49
      peck W61.43
      strike W61.42
    turtle (nonvenomous) W59.29
      bite W59.21
      strike W59.22
      terrestrial W59.89
        bite W59.81
        crushing W59.83
        strike W59.82
    under-cutter W31.0
    urine —*see* Contact, with, by type of animal
    vehicle
      agricultural use (transport) —*see*
        Accident, transport, agricultural
        vehicle
        not on public highway W30.81
      industrial use (transport) —*see*
        Accident, transport, industrial
        vehicle
        not on public highway W31.83
      off-road use (transport) —*see* Accident,
        transport, all-terrain or off-road
        vehicle
        not on public highway W31.83
      special construction use (transport) —*see*
        Accident, transport, construction
        vehicle
        not on public highway W31.83
    venomous
      animal X58
      arthropods X58
      lizard X58
      marine animal NEC X58
      marine plant NEC X58
      millipedes (tropical) X58
      plant(s) X58
      snake X58
      spider X58
      viper X58
    washing-machine (powered) W29.2
    wasp X58
    weaving-machine W31.89
    winch W24.0
      agricultural operations W30.89
    wire NEC W24.0
      agricultural operations W30.89
    wood slivers W45.8
    yellow jacket X58
    zebra —*see* Contact, with, hoof stock NEC
  pressure X50.9
  stress X50.9
Coup de soleil X32

Crash
  aircraft (in transit) (powered) V95.9
    balloon V96.01
    fixed wing NEC (private) V95.21
      commercial V95.31
    glider V96.21
      hang V96.11
      powered V95.11
    helicopter V95.01
    in war operations —*see* War operations,
      destruction of aircraft
    microlight V95.11
    nonpowered V96.9
      specified NEC V96.8
    powered NEC V95.8
    stated as
      homicide (attempt) Y08.81
      suicide (attempt) X83.0
    ultralight V95.11
  spacecraft V95.41
  transport vehicle NEC —*see also* Accident,
    transport V89.9
    homicide (attempt) Y03.8
    motor NEC (traffic) V89.2
      homicide (attempt) Y03.8
      suicide (attempt) —*see* Suicide, collision
Cruelty (mental) (physical) (sexual) X58
Crushed (accidentally) X58
  between objects (moving) (stationary and
    moving) W23.0
    stationary W23.1
  by
    alligator W58.03
    avalanche NEC —*see* Landslide
    cave-in W20.0
      caused by cataclysmic earth surface
        movement —*see* Landslide
    crocodile W58.13
    crowd or human stampede W52
    falling
      aircraft V97.39
        in war operations —*see* War
          operations, destruction of aircraft
      earth, material W20.0
        caused by cataclysmic earth surface
          movement —*see* Landslide
      object NEC W20.8
    landslide NEC —*see* Landslide
    lizard (nonvenomous) W59.09
    machinery —*see* Contact, with, by type of
      machine
    reptile NEC W59.89
    snake (nonvenomous) W59.13
  in
    machinery —*see* Contact, with, by type of
      machine
Cut, cutting (any part of body) (accidental) —
  see also Contact, with, by object or machine
  during medical or surgical treatment as
    misadventure —*see* Index to Diseases
    and Injuries, Complications
  homicide (attempt) —*see* Assault, cutting or
    piercing instrument
  inflicted by other person —*see* Assault,
    cutting or piercing instrument
  legal
    execution —*see* Legal, intervention
    intervention —*see* Legal, intervention,
      sharp object
  machine NEC —*see also* Contact, with, by
    type of machine W31.9
  self-inflicted —*see* Suicide, cutting or piercing
    instrument
  suicide (attempt) —*see* Suicide, cutting or
    piercing instrument
Cyclone (any injury) X37.1

D

Decapitation (accidental circumstances)
  NEC X58
  homicide X99.9
  legal execution —*see* Legal, intervention
Dehydration from lack of water X58
Deprivation X58
Derailment (accidental)
  railway (rolling stock) (train) (vehicle)
    (without antecedent collision) V81.7
    with antecedent collision —*see* Accident,
      transport, railway vehicle occupant
  streetcar (without antecedent collision) V82.7
    with antecedent collision —*see* Accident,
      transport, streetcar occupant
Descent
  parachute (voluntary) (without accident to
    aircraft) V97.29
    due to accident to aircraft —*see* Accident,
      transport, aircraft
Desertion X58
Destitution X58
Disability, late effect or sequela of injury —*see*
  Sequelae
Discharge (accidental)
  airgun W34.010
    assault X95.01
    homicide (attempt) X95.01
    stated as undetermined whether accidental
      or intentional Y24.0
    suicide (attempt) X74.01
  BB gun —*see* Discharge, airgun
  firearm (accidental) W34.00
    assault X95.9
    handgun (pistol) (revolver) W32.0
      assault X93
      homicide (attempt) X93
      legal intervention —*see* Legal,
        intervention, firearm, handgun
      stated as undetermined whether
        accidental or intentional Y22
      suicide (attempt) X72
    homicide (attempt) X95.9
    hunting rifle W33.02
      assault X94.1
      homicide (attempt) X94.1
      legal intervention
        injuring
          bystander Y35.032
          law enforcement personnel Y35.031
          suspect Y35.033
          unspecified person Y35.039
      stated as undetermined whether
        accidental or intentional Y23.1
      suicide (attempt) X73.1
    larger W33.00
      assault X94.9
      homicide (attempt) X94.9
      hunting rifle —*see* Discharge, firearm,
        hunting rifle
      legal intervention —*see* Legal,
        intervention, firearm by type of
        firearm
      machine gun —*see* Discharge, firearm,
        machine gun
      shotgun —*see* Discharge, firearm,
        shotgun
      specified NEC W33.09
        assault X94.8
        homicide (attempt) X94.8
        legal intervention
          injuring
            bystander Y35.092
            law enforcement personnel
              Y35.091
            suspect Y35.093
            unspecified person Y35.099
        stated as undetermined whether
          accidental or intentional Y23.8
        suicide (attempt) X73.8

Discharge *(Continued)*
  firearm *(Continued)*
    larger *(Continued)*
      stated as undetermined whether
        accidental or intentional Y23.9
      suicide (attempt) X73.9
    legal intervention
      injuring
        bystander Y35.002
        law enforcement personnel Y35.001
        suspect Y35.03
        unspecified person Y35.009
      using rubber bullet
        injuring
          bystander Y35.042
          law enforcement personnel Y35.041
          suspect Y35.043
          unspecified person Y35.049
    machine gun W33.03
      assault X94.2
      homicide (attempt) X94.2
      legal intervention —*see* Legal,
        intervention, firearm, machine gun
      stated as undetermined whether
        accidental or intentional Y23.3
      suicide (attempt) X73.2
    pellet gun —*see* Discharge, airgun
    shotgun W33.01
      assault X94.0
      homicide (attempt) X94.0
      legal intervention —*see* Legal,
        intervention, firearm, specified NEC
      stated as undetermined whether
        accidental or intentional Y23.0
      suicide (attempt) X73.0
    specified NEC W34.09
      assault X95.8
      homicide (attempt) X95.8
      legal intervention —*see* Legal,
        intervention, firearm, specified NEC
      stated as undetermined whether
        accidental or intentional Y24.8
      suicide (attempt) X74.8
    stated as undetermined whether accidental
      or intentional Y24.9
    suicide (attempt) X74.9
    Very pistol W34.09
      assault X95.8
      homicide (attempt) X95.8
      stated as undetermined whether
        accidental or intentional Y24.8
      suicide (attempt) X74.8
  firework(s) W39
    stated as undetermined whether accidental
      or intentional Y25
  gas-operated gun NEC W34.018
    airgun —*see* Discharge, airgun
    assault X95.09
    homicide (attempt) X95.09
    paintball gun —*see* Discharge, paintball gun
    stated as undetermined whether accidental
      or intentional Y24.8
    suicide (attempt) X74.09
  gun NEC —*see also* Discharge, firearm NEC
    air —*see* Discharge, airgun
    BB —*see* Discharge, airgun
    for single hand use —*see* Discharge,
      firearm, handgun
    hand —*see* Discharge, firearm, handgun
    machine —*see* Discharge, firearm, machine
      gun
    other specified —*see* Discharge, firearm
      NEC
    paintball —*see* Discharge, paintball gun
    pellet —*see* Discharge, airgun
  handgun —*see* Discharge, firearm, handgun
  machine gun —*see* Discharge, firearm,
    machine gun
  paintball gun W34.011
    assault X95.02
    homicide (attempt) X95.02

Discharge *(Continued)*
  paintball gun *(Continued)*
    stated as undetermined whether accidental
      or intentional Y24.8
    suicide (attempt) X74.02
  pistol —*see* Discharge, firearm, handgun
    flare —*see* Discharge, firearm, Very pistol
    pellet —*see* Discharge, airgun
    Very —*see* Discharge, firearm, Very pistol
  revolver —*see* Discharge, firearm, handgun
  rifle (hunting) —*see* Discharge, firearm,
    hunting rifle
  shotgun —*see* Discharge, firearm, shotgun
  spring-operated gun NEC W34.018
    assault X95.09
    homicide (attempt) X95.09
    stated as undetermined whether accidental
      or intentional Y24.8
    suicide (attempt) X74.09
Disease
  Andes W94.11
  aviator's —*see* Air, pressure
  range W94.11
Diver's disease, palsy, paralysis, squeeze —*see*
  Air, pressure
Diving (into water) —*see* Accident, diving
Dog bite W54.0
Dragged by transport vehicle NEC —*see also*
  Accident, transport V09.9
Drinking poison (accidental) —*see* Table of
  Drugs and Chemicals
Dropped (accidentally) **while being carried or
  supported by other person** W04
Drowning (accidental) W74
  assault X92.9
  due to
    accident (to)
      machinery —*see* Contact, with, by type
        of machine
      watercraft V90.89
        burning V90.29
          powered V90.23
            fishing boat V90.22
            jet ski V90.23
            merchant ship V90.20
            passenger ship V90.21
          unpowered V90.28
            canoe V90.25
            inflatable V90.26
            kayak V90.25
            sailboat V90.24
            water skis V90.27
        crushed V90.39
          powered V90.33
            fishing boat V90.32
            jet ski V90.33
            merchant ship V90.30
            passenger ship V90.31
          unpowered V90.38
            canoe V90.35
            inflatable V90.36
            kayak V90.35
            sailboat V90.34
            water skis V90.37
        overturning V90.09
          powered V90.03
            fishing boat V90.02
            jet ski V90.03
            merchant ship V90.00
            passenger ship V90.01
          unpowered V90.08
            canoe V90.05
            inflatable V90.06
            kayak V90.05
            sailboat V90.04
        sinking V90.19
          powered V90.13
            fishing boat V90.12
            jet ski V90.13
            merchant ship V90.10
            passenger ship V90.11

▶ New   ➡ Revised   ~~deleted~~ Deleted   ● Use Additional Character(s)

Drowning *(Continued)*
  due to *(Continued)*
    accident *(Continued)*
      watercraft *(Continued)*
        sinking *(Continued)*
          unpowered V90.18
            canoe V90.15
            inflatable V90.16
            kayak V90.15
            sailboat V90.14
        specified type NEC V90.89
          powered V90.83
            fishing boat V90.82
            jet ski V90.83
            merchant ship V90.80
            passenger ship V90.81
          unpowered V90.88
            canoe V90.85
            inflatable V90.86
            kayak V90.85
            sailboat V90.84
            water skis V90.87
    avalanche —*see* Landslide
    cataclysmic
      earth surface movement NEC —*see*
        Forces of nature, earth movement
      storm —*see* Forces of nature, cataclysmic
        storm
    cloudburst X37.8
    cyclone X37.1
    fall overboard (from) V92.09
      powered craft V92.03
        ferry boat V92.01
        fishing boat V92.02
        jet ski V92.03
        liner V92.01
        merchant ship V92.00
        passenger ship V92.01
      resulting from
        accident to watercraft —*see* Drowning,
          due to, accident to, watercraft
        being washed overboard (from)
          V92.29
          powered craft V92.23
            ferry boat V92.21
            fishing boat V92.22
            jet ski V92.23
            liner V92.21
            merchant ship V92.20
            passenger ship V92.21
          unpowered craft V92.28
            canoe V92.25
            inflatable V92.26
            kayak V92.25
            sailboat V92.24
            surf-board V92.28
            water skis V92.27
            windsurfer V92.28
        motion of watercraft V92.19
          powered craft V92.13
            ferry boat V92.11
            fishing boat V92.12
            jet ski V92.13
            liner V92.11
            merchant ship V92.10
            passenger ship V92.11
          unpowered craft
            canoe V92.15
            inflatable V92.16
            kayak V92.15
            sailboat V92.14
      unpowered craft V92.08
        canoe V92.05
        inflatable V92.06
        kayak V92.05

Drowning *(Continued)*
  due to *(Continued)*
    fall overboard *(Continued)*
      unpowered craft *(Continued)*
        sailboat V92.04
        surf-board V92.08
        water skis V92.07
        windsurfer V92.08
    hurricane X37.0
    jumping into water from watercraft
      (involved in accident) —*see also*
      Drowning, due to, accident to,
      watercraft
      without accident to or on watercraft
        W16.711
    tidal wave NEC —*see* Forces of nature,
      tidal wave
    torrential rain X37.8
  following
    fall
      into
        bathtub W16.211
        bucket W16.221
        fountain —*see* Drowning, following,
          fall, into, water, specified NEC
        quarry —*see* Drowning, following,
          fall, into, water, specified NEC
        reservoir —*see* Drowning, following,
          fall, into, water, specified NEC
        swimming-pool W16.011
          stated as undetermined whether
            accidental or intentional
            Y21.3
          striking
            bottom W16.021
            wall W16.031
          suicide (attempt) X71.2
        water NOS W16.41
          natural (lake) (open sea) (river)
            (stream) (pond) W16.111
            striking
              bottom W16.121
              side W16.131
          specified NEC W16.311
            striking
              bottom W16.321
              wall W16.331
      overboard NEC —*see* Drowning, due to,
        fall overboard
    jump or dive
      from boat W16.711
        striking bottom W16.721
      into
        fountain —*see* Drowning, following,
          jump or dive, into, water,
          specified NEC
        quarry —*see* Drowning, following,
          jump or dive, into, water,
          specified NEC
        reservoir —*see* Drowning, following,
          jump or dive, into, water,
          specified NEC
        swimming-pool W16.511
          striking
            bottom W16.521
            wall W16.531
          suicide (attempt) X71.2
        water NOS W16.91
          natural (lake) (open sea) (river)
            (stream) (pond) W16.611
          specified NEC W16.811
            striking
              bottom W16.821
              wall W16.831
          striking bottom W16.621

Drowning *(Continued)*
  homicide (attempt) X92.9
  in
    bathtub (accidental) W65
      assault X92.0
      following fall W16.211
        stated as undetermined whether
          accidental or intentional
          Y21.1
      stated as undetermined whether
        accidental or intentional Y21.0
      suicide (attempt) X71.0
    lake —*see* Drowning, in, natural water
    natural water (lake) (open sea) (river)
      (stream) (pond) W69
      assault X92.3
      following
        dive or jump W16.611
          striking bottom W16.621
        fall W16.111
          striking
            bottom W16.121
            side W16.131
      stated as undetermined whether
        accidental or intentional Y21.4
      suicide (attempt) X71.3
    quarry —*see* Drowning, in, specified place
      NEC
    quenching tank —*see* Drowning, in,
      specified place NEC
    reservoir —*see* Drowning, in, specified
      place NEC
    river —*see* Drowning, in, natural water
    sea —*see* Drowning, in, natural water
    specified place NEC W73
      assault X92.8
      following
        dive or jump W16.811
          striking
            bottom W16.821
            wall W16.831
        fall W16.311
          striking
            bottom W16.321
            wall W16.331
      stated as undetermined whether
        accidental or intentional Y21.8
      suicide (attempt) X71.8
    stream —*see* Drowning, in, natural water
    swimming-pool W67
      assault X92.1
        following fall X92.2
      following
        dive or jump W16.511
          striking
            bottom W16.521
            wall W16.531
        fall W16.011
          striking
            bottom W16.021
            wall W16.031
      stated as undetermined whether
        accidental or intentional Y21.2
        following fall Y21.3
      suicide (attempt) X71.1
        following fall X71.2
    war operations —*see* War operations,
      restriction of airway
  resulting from accident to watercraft —*see*
    Drowning, due to, accident, watercraft
  self-inflicted X71.9
  stated as undetermined whether accidental or
    intentional Y21.9
  suicide (attempt) X71.9

E

Earth (surface) movement NEC —see Forces of nature, earth movement
Earth falling (on) W20.0
  caused by cataclysmic earth surface movement or eruption —see Landslide
Earthquake (any injury) X34
Effect(s) (adverse) of
  air pressure (any) —see Air, pressure
  cold, excessive (exposure to) —see Exposure, cold
  heat (excessive) —see Heat
  hot place (weather) —see Heat
  insolation X30
  late —see Sequelae
  motion —see Motion
  nuclear explosion or weapon in war operations —see War operations, nuclear weapon
  radiation —see Radiation
  travel —see Travel
Electric shock (accidental) (by) (in) —see Exposure, electric current
Electrocution (accidental) —see Exposure, electric current
Endotracheal tube wrongly placed during anesthetic procedure Y65.3
Entanglement
  in
    bed linen, causing suffocation —see category T71
    wheel of pedal cycle V19.88
Entry of foreign body or material —see Foreign body
Environmental pollution related condition — see Z57
Execution, legal (any method) —see Legal, intervention
Exhaustion
  cold —see Exposure, cold
  due to excessive exertion —see also Overexertion X50.9
  heat —see Heat
Explosion (accidental) (of) (with secondary fire) W40.9
  acetylene W40.1
  aerosol can W36.1
  air tank (compressed) (in machinery) W36.2
  aircraft (in transit) (powered) NEC V95.9
    balloon V96.05
    fixed wing NEC (private) V95.25
      commercial V95.35
    glider V96.25
      hang V96.15
      powered V95.15
    helicopter V95.05
    in war operations —see War operations, destruction of aircraft
    microlight V95.15
    nonpowered V96.9
      specified NEC V96.8
    powered NEC V95.8
    stated as
      homicide (attempt) Y03.8
      suicide (attempt) X83.0
    ultralight V95.15
  anesthetic gas in operating room W40.1
  antipersonnel bomb W40.8
    assault X96.0
    homicide (attempt) X96.0
    suicide (attempt) X75
  assault X96.9
  bicycle tire W37.0
  blasting (cap) (materials) W40.0
  boiler (machinery), not on transport vehicle W35
    on watercraft —see Explosion, in, watercraft
  butane W40.1
  caused by other person X96.9
  coal gas W40.1

Explosion (Continued)
  detonator W40.0
  dump (munitions) W40.8
  dynamite W40.0
    in
      assault X96.8
      homicide (attempt) X96.8
      legal intervention
        injuring
          bystander Y35.112
          law enforcement personnel Y35.111
          suspect Y35.113
          unspecified person Y35.119
      suicide (attempt) X75
  explosive (material) W40.9
    gas W40.1
    in blasting operation W40.0
    specified NEC W40.8
      in
        assault X96.8
        homicide (attempt) X96.8
        legal intervention
          injuring
            bystander Y35.192
            law enforcement personnel Y35.191
            suspect Y35.193
            unspecified person Y35.199
        suicide (attempt) X75
  factory (munitions) W40.8
  fertilizer bomb W40.8
    assault X96.3
    homicide (attempt) X96.3
    suicide (attempt) X75
  fire-damp W40.1
  firearm (parts) NEC W34.19
    airgun W34.110
    BB gun W34.110
    gas, air or spring-operated gun NEC W34.118
    handgun W32.1
    hunting rifle W33.12
    larger firearm W33.10
      specified NEC W33.19
    machine gun W33.13
    paintball gun W34.111
    pellet gun W34.110
    shotgun W33.11
    Very pistol [flare] W34.19
  fireworks W39
  gas (coal) (explosive) W40.1
    cylinder W36.9
      aerosol can W36.1
      air tank W36.2
      pressurized W36.3
      specified NEC W36.8
  gasoline (fumes) (tank) not in moving motor vehicle W40.1
    bomb W40.8
      assault X96.1
      homicide (attempt) X96.1
      suicide (attempt) X75
    in motor vehicle —see Accident, transport, by type of vehicle
  grain store W40.8
  grenade W40.8
    in
      assault X96.8
      homicide (attempt) X96.8
      legal intervention
        injuring
          bystander Y35.192
          law enforcement personnel Y35.191
          suspect Y35.193
          unspecified person Y35.199
      suicide (attempt) X75
  handgun (parts) —see Explosion, firearm, handgun (parts)
  homicide (attempt) X96.9
    antipersonnel bomb —see Explosion, antipersonnel bomb
    fertilizer bomb —see Explosion, fertilizer bomb

Explosion (Continued)
  homicide (Continued)
    gasoline bomb —see Explosion, gasoline bomb
    letter bomb —see Explosion, letter bomb
    pipe bomb —see Explosion, pipe bomb
    specified NEC X96.8
  hose, pressurized W37.8
  hot water heater, tank (in machinery) W35
    on watercraft —see Explosion, in, watercraft
  in, on
    dump W40.8
    factory W40.8
    mine (of explosive gases) NEC W40.1
    watercraft V93.59
      powered craft V93.53
        ferry boat V93.51
        fishing boat V93.52
        jet ski V93.53
        liner V93.51
        merchant ship V93.50
        passenger ship V93.51
        sailboat V93.54
  letter bomb W40.8
    assault X96.2
    homicide (attempt) X96.2
    suicide (attempt) X75
  machinery —see also Contact, with, by type of machine
    on board watercraft —see Explosion, in, watercraft
    pressure vessel —see Explosion, by type of vessel
  methane W40.1
  mine W40.1
  missile NEC W40.8
  mortar bomb W40.8
    in
      assault X96.8
      homicide (attempt) X96.8
      legal intervention
        injuring
          bystander Y35.192
          law enforcement personnel Y35.191
          suspect Y35.193
          unspecified person Y35.199
      suicide (attempt) X75
  munitions (dump) (factory) W40.8
  pipe, pressurized W37.8
    bomb W40.8
      assault X96.4
      homicide (attempt) X96.4
      suicide (attempt) X75
  pressure, pressurized
    cooker W38
    gas tank (in machinery) W36.3
    hose W37.8
    pipe W37.8
    specified device NEC W38
    tire W37.8
      bicycle W37.0
    vessel (in machinery) W38
  propane W40.1
  self-inflicted X75
  shell (artillery) NEC W40.8
    during war operations —see War operations, explosion
    in
      legal intervention
        injuring
          bystander Y35.122
          law enforcement personnel Y35.121
          suspect Y35.123
          unspecified person Y35.129
    war —see War operations, explosion
  spacecraft V95.45
  stated as undetermined whether accidental or intentional Y25
  steam or water lines (in machinery) W37.8
  stove W40.9
  suicide (attempt) X75

▶ New   ⇨ Revised   ~~deleted~~ Deleted   ● Use Additional Character(s)

Explosion *(Continued)*
  tire, pressurized W37.8
    bicycle W37.0
  undetermined whether accidental or
    intentional Y25
  vehicle tire NEC W37.8
    bicycle W37.0
  war operations —*see* War operations,
    explosion
Exposure (to) X58
  air pressure change —*see* Air, pressure
  cold (accidental) (excessive) (extreme)
    (natural) (place) X31
    assault Y08.89
    due to
      man-made conditions W93.8
        dry ice (contact) W93.01
          inhalation W93.02
        liquid air (contact) (hydrogen)
          (nitrogen) W93.11
          inhalation W93.12
        refrigeration unit (deep freeze)
          W93.2
        suicide (attempt) X83.2
      weather (conditions) X31
    homicide (attempt) Y08.89
    self-inflicted X83.2
  due to abandonment or neglect X58
  electric current W86.8
    appliance (faulty) W86.8
      domestic W86.0
    caused by other person Y08.89
    conductor (faulty) W86.1
    control apparatus (faulty) W86.1
    electric power generating plant,
      distribution station W86.1
    electroshock gun —*see* Exposure, electric
      current, taser
    high-voltage cable W85
    homicide (attempt) Y08.89
    legal execution —*see* Legal, intervention,
      specified means NEC
    lightning —*see* subcategory T75.0
    live rail W86.8
    misadventure in medical or surgical
      procedure in electroshock therapy
      Y63.4
    motor (electric) (faulty) W86.8
      domestic W86.0
    self-inflicted X83.1
    specified NEC W86.8
      domestic W86.0
    stun gun —*see* Exposure, electric current,
      taser
    suicide (attempt) X83.1
    taser W86.8
      assault Y08.89
      legal intervention —*see* category Y35
      self-harm (intentional) X83.8
      undetermined intent Y33
    third rail W86.8
    transformer (faulty) W86.1
    transmission lines W85
  environmental tobacco smoke X58
  excessive
    cold —*see* Exposure, cold
    heat (natural) NEC X30
      man-made W92
  factor(s) NOS X58
    environmental NEC X58
    man-made NEC W99
    natural NEC —*see* Forces of nature
    specified NEC X58
  fire, flames (accidental) X08.8
    assault X97
    campfire —*see* Exposure, fire, controlled,
      not in building
    controlled (in)
      with ignition (of) clothing —*see also*
        Ignition, clothes X06.2
        nightwear X05

Exposure *(Continued)*
  fire, flames *(Continued)*
    controlled *(Continued)*
      bonfire —*see* Exposure, fire, controlled,
        not in building
      brazier (in building or structure) —*see*
        also Exposure, fire, controlled,
        building
        not in building or structure —*see*
          Exposure, fire, controlled, not in
          building
      building or structure X02.0
        with
          fall from building X02.3
          from building X02.5
          injury due to building collapse
            X02.2
          smoke inhalation X02.1
        hit by object from building X02.4
        specified mode of injury NEC X02.8
      fireplace, furnace or stove —*see*
        Exposure, fire, controlled, building
      not in building or structure X03.0
        with
          fall X03.3
          smoke inhalation X03.1
        hit by object X03.4
        specified mode of injury NEC X03.8
      trash —*see* Exposure, fire, controlled, not
        in building
      fireplace —*see* Exposure, fire, controlled,
        building
      fittings or furniture (in building or
        structure) (uncontrolled) —*see*
        Exposure, fire, uncontrolled, building
      forest (uncontrolled) —*see* Exposure, fire,
        uncontrolled, not in building
      grass (uncontrolled) —*see* Exposure, fire,
        uncontrolled, not in building
      hay (uncontrolled) —*see* Exposure, fire,
        uncontrolled, not in building
      homicide (attempt) X97
      ignition of highly flammable material X04
      in, of, on, starting in
        machinery —*see* Contact, with, by type
          of machine
        motor vehicle (in motion) —*see also*
          Accident, transport, occupant by
          type of vehicle V87.8
          with collision —*see* Collision
        railway rolling stock, train, vehicle
          V81.81
          with collision —*see* Accident,
            transport, railway vehicle
            occupant
        street car (in motion) V82.8
          with collision —*see* Accident,
            transport, streetcar occupant
        transport vehicle NEC —*see also*
          Accident, transport
          with collision —*see* Collision
        war operations —*see also* War operations,
          fire
          from nuclear explosion —*see* War
            operations, nuclear weapons
        watercraft (in transit) (not in transit)
          V91.09
          localized —*see* Burn, on board
            watercraft, due to, fire on board
          powered craft V91.03
            ferry boat V91.01
            fishing boat V91.02
            jet skis V91.03
            liner V91.01
            merchant ship V91.00
            passenger ship V91.01
          unpowered craft V91.08
            canoe V91.05
            inflatable V91.06
            kayak V91.05
            sailboat V91.04

Exposure *(Continued)*
  fire, flames *(Continued)*
    in, of, on, starting in *(Continued)*
      watercraft *(Continued)*
        unpowered craft *(Continued)*
          surf-board V91.08
          waterskis V91.07
          windsurfer V91.08
    lumber (uncontrolled) —*see* Exposure, fire,
      uncontrolled, not in building
    mine (uncontrolled) —*see* Exposure, fire,
      uncontrolled, not in building
    prairie (uncontrolled) —*see* Exposure, fire,
      uncontrolled, not in building
    resulting from
      explosion —*see* Explosion
      lightning X08.8
    self-inflicted X76
    specified NEC X08.8
    started by other person X97
    stated as undetermined whether accidental
      or intentional Y26
    stove —*see* Exposure, fire, controlled,
      building
    suicide (attempt) X76
    tunnel (uncontrolled) —*see* Exposure, fire,
      uncontrolled, not in building
    uncontrolled
      in building or structure X00.0
        with
          fall from building X00.3
          injury due to building collapse
            X00.2
          jump from building X00.5
          smoke inhalation X00.1
        bed X08.00
          due to
            cigarette X08.01
            specified material NEC X08.09
        furniture NEC X08.20
          due to
            cigarette X08.21
            specified material NEC X08.29
        hit by object from building X00.4
        sofa X08.10
          due to
            cigarette X08.11
            specified material NEC
              X08.19
        specified mode of injury NEC
          X00.8
      not in building or structure (any)
        X01.0
        with
          fall X01.3
          smoke inhalation X01.1
        hit by object X01.4
        specified mode of injury NEC
          X01.8
    undetermined whether accidental or
      intentional Y26
  forces of nature NEC —*see* Forces of nature
  G-forces (abnormal) W49.9
  gravitational forces (abnormal) W49.9
  heat (natural) NEC —*see* Heat
  high-pressure jet (hydraulic) (pneumatic)
    W49.9
  hydraulic jet W49.9
  inanimate mechanical force W49.9
  jet, high-pressure (hydraulic) (pneumatic)
    W49.9
  lightning —*see* subcategory T75.0
    causing fire —*see* Exposure, fire
  mechanical forces NEC W49.9
    animate NEC W64
    inanimate NEC W49.9
  noise W42.9
    supersonic W42.0
  noxious substance —*see* Table of Drugs and
    Chemicals
  pneumatic jet W49.9

Exposure *(Continued)*
prolonged in deep-freeze unit or refrigerator
  W93.2
radiation —*see* Radiation
smoke —*see also* Exposure, fire
  tobacco, second hand Z77.22
specified factors NEC X58
sunlight X32
  man-made (sun lamp) W89.8
    tanning bed W89.1
supersonic waves W42.Ø
transmission line(s), electric W85
vibration W49.9

Exposure *(Continued)*
waves
  infrasound W49.9
  sound W42.9
  supersonic W42.Ø
weather NEC —*see* Forces of nature
External cause status Y99.9
child assisting in compensated work for
  family Y99.8
civilian activity done for financial or other
  compensation Y99.Ø
civilian activity done for income or pay
  Y99.Ø

External cause status *(Continued)*
family member assisting in compensated
  work for other family member Y99.8
hobby not done for income Y99.8
leisure activity Y99.8
military activity Y99.1
off-duty activity of military personnel Y99.8
recreation or sport not for income or while a
  student Y99.8
specified NEC Y99.8
student activity Y99.8
volunteer activity Y99.2

▶ New　⇒ Revised　deleted Deleted　● Use Additional Character(s)

F

Factors, supplemental
  alcohol
    blood level
      less than 20mg/100ml Y90.0
      presence in blood, level not specified
          Y90.9
      20-39mg/100ml Y90.1
      40-59mg/100ml Y90.2
      60-79mg/100ml Y90.3
      80-99mg/100ml Y90.4
      100-119mg/100ml Y90.5
      120-199mg/100ml Y90.6
      200-239mg/100ml Y90.7
      240mg/100ml or more Y90.8
      presence in blood, but level not specified
          Y90.9
  environmental-pollution-related condition —
      see Z57
  nosocomial condition Y95
  work-related condition Y99.0
Failure
  in suture or ligature during surgical
      procedure Y65.2
  mechanical, of instrument or apparatus
      (any) (during any medical or surgical
      procedure) Y65.8
  sterile precautions (during medical and
      surgical care) —see Misadventure,
      failure, sterile precautions, by type of
      procedure
  to
    introduce tube or instrument Y65.4
      endotracheal tube during anesthesia Y65.3
    make curve (transport vehicle) NEC —see
        Accident, transport
    remove tube or instrument Y65.4
Fall, falling (accidental) W19
  building W20.1
    burning (uncontrolled fire) X00.3
  down
    embankment W17.81
    escalator W10.0
    hill W17.81
    ladder W11
    ramp W10.2
    stairs, steps W10.9
  due to
    bumping against
      object W18.00
        sharp glass W18.02
        specified NEC W18.09
        sports equipment W18.01
      person W03
        due to ice or snow W00.0
        on pedestrian conveyance —see
            Accident, transport, pedestrian,
            conveyance
    collision with another person W03
      due to ice or snow W00.0
      involving pedestrian conveyance —see
          Accident, transport, pedestrian,
          conveyance
    grocery cart tipping over W17.82
    ice or snow W00.9
      from one level to another W00.2
        on stairs or steps W00.1
      involving pedestrian conveyance —see
          Accident, transport, pedestrian,
          conveyance
      on same level W00.0
    slipping (on moving sidewalk) W01.0
      with subsequent striking against object
          W01.10
        furniture W01.190
        sharp object W01.119
          glass W01.110
          power tool or machine W01.111
          specified NEC W01.118
        specified NEC W01.198

Fall, falling (Continued)
  due to (Continued)
    striking against
      object W18.00
        sharp glass W18.02
        specified NEC W18.09
        sports equipment W18.01
      person W03
        due to ice or snow W00.0
        on pedestrian conveyance —see
            Accident, transport, pedestrian,
            conveyance
  earth (with asphyxia or suffocation (by
      pressure)) —see Earth, falling
  from, off, out of
    aircraft NEC (with accident to aircraft
        NEC) V97.0
      while boarding or alighting V97.1
    balcony W13.0
    bed W06
    boat, ship, watercraft NEC (with drowning
        or submersion) —see Drowning, due
        to, fall overboard
      with hitting bottom or object V94.0
    bridge W13.1
    building W13.9
      burning (uncontrolled fire) X00.3
    cavity W17.2
    chair W07
    cherry picker W17.89
    cliff W15
    dock W17.4
    embankment W17.81
    escalator W10.0
    flagpole W13.8
    furniture NEC W08
    grocery cart W17.82
    haystack W17.89
    high place NEC W17.89
      stated as undetermined whether
          accidental or intentional Y30
    hole W17.2
    incline W10.2
    ladder W11
    lifting device W17.89
    machine, machinery —see also Contact,
        with, by type of machine
      not in operation W17.89
    manhole W17.1
    mobile elevated work platform [MEWP]
        W17.89
    motorized mobility scooter W05.2
    one level to another NEC W17.89
      intentional, purposeful, suicide
          (attempt) X80
      stated as undetermined whether
          accidental or intentional Y30
    pit W17.2
    playground equipment W09.8
      jungle gym W09.2
      slide W09.0
      swing W09.1
    quarry W17.89
    railing W13.9
    ramp W10.2
    roof W13.2
    scaffolding W12
    scooter (nonmotorized) W05.1
      motorized mobility W05.2
    sky lift W17.89
    stairs, steps W10.9
      curb W10.1
        due to ice or snow W00.1
      escalator W10.0
      incline W10.2
      ramp W10.2
      sidewalk curb W10.1
      specified NEC W10.8
    Standing
      electric scooter V00.841
      micro-mobility pedestrian conveyance
          V00.848

Fall, falling (Continued)
  from, off, out of (Continued)
    stepladder W11
    storm drain W17.1
    streetcar NEC V82.6
      with antecedent collision —see
          Accident, transport, streetcar
          occupant
      while boarding or alighting V82.4
    structure NEC W13.8
      burning (uncontrolled fire) X00.3
    table W08
    toilet W18.11
      with subsequent striking against object
          W18.12
    train NEC V81.6
      during derailment (without antecedent
          collision) V81.7
      with antecedent collision —see
          Accident, transport, railway
          vehicle occupant
      while boarding or alighting V81.4
    transport vehicle after collision —see
        Accident, transport, by type of
        vehicle, collision
    tree W14
    vehicle (in motion) NEC —see also
        Accident, transport V89.9
      motor NEC —see also Accident,
          transport, occupant, by type of
          vehicle V87.8
      stationary W17.89
        while boarding or alighting —see
            Accident, transport, by type of
            vehicle, while boarding or
            alighting
    viaduct W13.8
    wall W13.8
    watercraft —see also Drowning, due to, fall
        overboard
      with hitting bottom or object V94.0
    well W17.0
    wheelchair, non-moving W05.0
      powered —see Accident, transport,
          pedestrian, conveyance occupant,
          specified type NEC
    window W13.4
  in, on
    aircraft NEC V97.0
      with accident to aircraft V97.0
      while boarding or alighting V97.1
    bathtub (empty) W18.2
      filled W16.212
        causing drowning W16.211
    escalator W10.0
    incline W10.2
    ladder W11
    machine, machinery —see Contact, with,
        by type of machine
    object, edged, pointed or sharp (with
        cut) —see Fall, by type
    playground equipment W09.8
      jungle gym W09.2
      slide W09.0
      swing W09.1
    ramp W10.2
    scaffolding W12
    shower W18.2
      causing drowning W16.211
    staircase, stairs, steps W10.9
      curb W10.1
      due to ice or snow W00.1
      escalator W10.0
      incline W10.2
      specified NEC W10.8
    streetcar (without antecedent collision)
        V82.5
      with antecedent collision —see
          Accident, transport, streetcar
          occupant
      while boarding or alighting V82.4

Fall, falling (Continued)
  in, on (Continued)
    train (without antecedent collision) V81.5
      with antecedent collision —see Accident, transport, railway vehicle occupant
      during derailment (without antecedent collision) V81.7
        with antecedent collision —see Accident, transport, railway vehicle occupant
      while boarding or alighting V81.4
    transport vehicle after collision —see Accident, transport, by type of vehicle, collision
    watercraft V93.39
      due to
        accident to craft V91.29
          powered craft V91.23
            ferry boat V91.21
            fishing boat V91.22
            jet ski V91.23
            liner V91.21
            merchant ship V91.20
            passenger ship V91.21
          unpowered craft
            canoe V91.25
            inflatable V91.26
            kayak V91.25
            sailboat V91.24
        powered craft V93.33
          ferry boat V93.31
          fishing boat V93.32
          jet ski V93.33
          liner V93.31
          merchant ship V93.30
          passenger ship V93.31
        unpowered craft V93.38
          canoe V93.35
          inflatable V93.36
          kayak V93.35
          sailboat V93.34
          surf-board V93.38
          windsurfer V93.38
  into
    cavity W17.2
    dock W17.4
    fire —see Exposure, fire, by type
    haystack W17.89
    hole W17.2
    manhole W17.1
    moving part of machinery —see Contact, with, by type of machine
    ocean —see Fall, into, water
    opening in surface NEC W17.89
    pit W17.2
    pond —see Fall, into, water
    quarry W17.89
    river —see Fall, into, water
    shaft W17.89
    storm drain W17.1
    stream —see Fall, into, water
    swimming pool —see also Fall, into, water, in, swimming pool
      empty W17.3
    tank W17.89
    water W16.42
      causing drowning W16.41
      from watercraft —see Drowning, due to, fall overboard
      hitting diving board W21.4
      in
        bathtub W16.212
          causing drowning W16.211
        bucket W16.222
          causing drowning W16.221
        natural body of water W16.112
          causing drowning W16.111
          striking
            bottom W16.122
              causing drowning W16.121

Fall, falling (Continued)
  into (Continued)
    water (Continued)
      in (Continued)
        natural body of water (Continued)
          striking (Continued)
            side W16.132
              causing drowning W16.131
        specified water NEC W16.312
          causing drowning W16.311
          striking
            bottom W16.322
              causing drowning W16.321
            wall W16.332
              causing drowning W16.331
        swimming pool W16.012
          causing drowning W16.011
          striking
            bottom W16.022
              causing drowning W16.021
            wall W16.032
              causing drowning W16.031
        utility bucket W16.222
          causing drowning W16.221
    well W17.0
  involving
    bed W06
    chair W07
    furniture NEC W08
    glass —see Fall, by type
    playground equipment W09.8
      jungle gym W09.2
      slide W09.0
      swing W09.1
    roller blades —see Accident, transport, pedestrian, conveyance
    skateboard(s) —see Accident, transport, pedestrian, conveyance
    skates (ice) (in line) (roller) —see Accident, transport, pedestrian, conveyance
    skis —see Accident, transport, pedestrian, conveyance
    table W08
    wheelchair, non-moving W05.0
      powered —see Accident, transport, pedestrian, conveyance, specified type NEC
  object —see Struck by, object, falling
  off
    toilet W18.11
      with subsequent striking against object W18.12
  on same level W18.30
    due to
      specified NEC W18.39
      stepping on an object W18.31
  out of
    bed W06
    building NEC W13.8
    chair W07
    furniture NEC W08
    wheelchair, non-moving W05.0
      powered —see Accident, transport, pedestrian, conveyance, specified type NEC
    window W13.4
  over
    animal W01.0
    cliff W15
    embankment W17.81
    small object W01.0
  rock W20.8
  same level W18.30
    from
      being crushed, pushed, or stepped on by a crowd or human stampede W52
      collision, pushing, shoving, by or with other person W03
      slipping, stumbling, tripping W01.0

Fall, falling (Continued)
  same level (Continued)
    involving ice or snow W00.0
      involving skates (ice) (roller), skateboard, skis —see Accident, transport, pedestrian, conveyance
    snowslide (avalanche) —see Landslide
    stone W20.8
    structure W20.1
      burning (uncontrolled fire) X00.3
    through
      bridge W13.1
      floor W13.3
      roof W13.2
      wall W13.8
      window W13.4
    timber W20.8
    tree (caused by lightning) W20.8
    while being carried or supported by other person(s) W04

Fallen on by
  animal (not being ridden) NEC W55.89
Felo-de-se —see Suicide
Fight (hand) (fists) (foot) —see Assault, fight
Fire (accidental) —see Exposure, fire
Firearm discharge —see Discharge, firearm
Fireball effects from nuclear explosion in war operations —see War operations, nuclear weapons
Fireworks (explosion) W39
Flash burns from explosion —see Explosion
Flood (any injury) (caused by) X38
  collapse of man-made structure causing earth movement X36.0
  tidal wave —see Forces of nature, tidal wave
Food (any type) in
  air passages (with asphyxia, obstruction, or suffocation) —see categories T17 and T18
  alimentary tract causing asphyxia (due to compression of trachea) —see categories T17 and T18
Forces of nature X39.8
  avalanche X36.1
    causing transport accident —see Accident, transport, by type of vehicle
  blizzard X37.2
  cataclysmic storm X37.9
    with flood X38
    blizzard X37.2
    cloudburst X37.8
    cyclone X37.1
    dust storm X37.3
    hurricane X37.0
    specified storm NEC X37.8
    storm surge X37.0
    tornado X37.1
    twister X37.1
    typhoon X37.0
  cloudburst X37.8
  cold (natural) X31
  cyclone X37.1
  dam collapse causing earth movement X36.0
  dust storm X37.3
  earth movement X36.1
    caused by dam or structure collapse X36.0
    earthquake X34
  earthquake X34
  flood (caused by) X38
    dam collapse X36.0
    tidal wave —see Forces of nature, tidal wave
  heat (natural) X30
  hurricane X37.0
  landslide X36.1
    causing transport accident —see Accident, transport, by type of vehicle
  lightning —see subcategory T75.0
    causing fire —see Exposure, fire
  mudslide X36.1
    causing transport accident —see Accident, transport, by type of vehicle

▶ New   ⇒ Revised   ~~deleted~~ Deleted   ● Use Additional Character(s)

Forces of nature *(Continued)*
   radiation (natural) X39.Ø8
      radon X39.Ø1
   radon X39.Ø1
   specified force NEC X39.8
   storm surge X37.Ø
   structure collapse causing
      earth movement
      X36.Ø
   sunlight X32
   tidal wave X37.41
      due to
         earthquake X37.41
         landslide X37.43
         storm X37.42
         volcanic eruption X37.41
   tornado X37.1

Forces of nature *(Continued)*
   tsunami X37.41
   twister X37.1
   typhoon X37.Ø
   volcanic eruption X35
Foreign body
   aspiration —*see* Index to Diseases and
      Injuries, Foreign body, respiratory
      tract
   embedded in skin W45
   entering through skin W45.8
      can lid W26.2
      nail W45.Ø
      paper W26.2
      specified NEC 45.8
      splinter W45.8

Forest fire (exposure to) —*see* Exposure, fire,
   uncontrolled, not in building
Found injured X58
   from exposure (to) —*see* Exposure
   on
      highway, road(way), street V89.9
      railway right of way V81.9
Fracture (circumstances unknown or
   unspecified) X58
   due to specified cause NEC X58
Freezing —*see* Exposure, cold
Frostbite X31
   due to man-made conditions —*see* Exposure,
      cold, man-made
Frozen —*see* Exposure, cold

G

Gored by bull W55.22
Gunshot wound W34.ØØ

H

Hailstones, injured by X39.8
Hanged herself or himself —*see* Hanging,
   self-inflicted
Hanging (accidental) —*see also* category T71
   legal execution —*see* Legal, intervention,
      specified means NEC
Heat (effects of) (excessive) X3Ø
   due to
      man-made conditions W92
         on board watercraft V93.29
            fishing boat V93.22
            merchant ship V93.2Ø
            passenger ship V93.21
            sailboat V93.24
            specified powered craft NEC V93.23
      weather (conditions) X3Ø

Heat *(Continued)*
   from
      electric heating apparatus causing
         burning X16
      nuclear explosion in war operations —
         see War operations, nuclear
         weapons
      inappropriate in local application or
         packing in medical or surgical
         procedure Y63.5
Hemorrhage
   delayed following medical or surgical
      treatment without mention of
      misadventure —*see* Index to Diseases
      and Injuries, Complication(s)
   during medical or surgical treatment as
      misadventure —*see* Index to Diseases
      and Injuries, Complication(s)

High
   altitude (effects) —*see* Air, pressure, low
   level of radioactivity, effects —*see* Radiation
   pressure (effects) —*see* Air, pressure, high
   temperature, effects —*see* Heat
Hit, hitting (accidental) by —*see* Struck by
Hitting against —*see* Striking against
Homicide (attempt) (justifiable) —*see* Assault
Hot
   place, effects —*see also* Heat
   weather, effects X3Ø
House fire (uncontrolled) —*see* Exposure, fire,
   uncontrolled, building
Humidity, causing problem X39.8
Hunger X58
Hurricane (any injury) X37.Ø
Hypobarism, hypobaropathy —*see* Air,
   pressure, low

I

Ictus
  caloris —*see also* Heat
  solaris X30
Ignition (accidental) —*see also* Exposure, fire
      X08.8
  anesthetic gas in operating room W40.1
  apparel X06.2
    from highly flammable material X04
    nightwear X05
  bed linen (sheets) (spreads) (pillows)
      (mattress) —*see* Exposure, fire,
      uncontrolled, building, bed
  benzine X04
  clothes, clothing NEC (from controlled fire)
      X06.2
    from
      highly flammable material X04
  ether X04
    in operating room W40.1
  explosive material —*see* Explosion
  gasoline X04
  jewelry (plastic) (any) X06.0
  kerosene X04
  material
    explosive —*see* Explosion
    highly flammable with secondary
        explosion X04
  nightwear X05
  paraffin X04
  petrol X04
Immersion (accidental) —*see also* Drowning
  hand or foot due to cold (excessive) X31
Implantation of quills of porcupine W55.89
Inanition (from) (hunger) X58
  thirst X58.8
Inappropriate operation performed
  correct operation on wrong side or body part
      (wrong side) (wrong site) Y65.53
  operation intended for another patient done
      on wrong patient Y65.52
  wrong operation performed on correct
      patient Y65.51
Inattention after, at birth (homicidal intent)
      (infanticidal intent) X58
Incident, adverse
  device
    anesthesiology Y70.8
      accessory Y70.2
      diagnostic Y70.0
      miscellaneous Y70.8
      monitoring Y70.0
      prosthetic Y70.2
      rehabilitative Y70.1
      surgical Y70.3
      therapeutic Y70.1
    cardiovascular Y71.8
      accessory Y71.2
      diagnostic Y71.0
      miscellaneous Y71.8
      monitoring Y71.0
      prosthetic Y71.2
      rehabilitative Y71.1
      surgical Y71.3
      therapeutic Y71.1
    gastroenterology Y73.8
      accessory Y73.2
      diagnostic Y73.0
      miscellaneous Y73.8
      monitoring Y73.0
      prosthetic Y73.2
      rehabilitative Y73.1
      surgical Y73.3
      therapeutic Y73.1
    general
      hospital Y74.8
        accessory Y74.2
        diagnostic Y74.0
        miscellaneous Y74.8
        monitoring Y74.0

Incident, adverse *(Continued)*
  device *(Continued)*
    general *(Continued)*
      hospital *(Continued)*
        prosthetic Y74.2
        rehabilitative Y74.1
        surgical Y74.3
        therapeutic Y74.1
      surgical Y81.8
        accessory Y81.2
        diagnostic Y81.0
        miscellaneous Y81.8
        monitoring Y81.0
        prosthetic Y81.2
        rehabilitative Y81.1
        surgical Y81.3
        therapeutic Y81.1
    gynecological Y76.8
      accessory Y76.2
      diagnostic Y76.0
      miscellaneous Y76.8
      monitoring Y76.0
      prosthetic Y76.2
      rehabilitative Y76.1
      surgical Y76.3
      therapeutic Y76.1
    medical Y82.9
      specified type NEC Y82.8
    neurological Y75.8
      accessory Y75.2
      diagnostic Y75.0
      miscellaneous Y75.8
      monitoring Y75.0
      prosthetic Y75.2
      rehabilitative Y75.1
      surgical Y75.3
      therapeutic Y75.1
    obstetrical Y76.8
      accessory Y76.2
      diagnostic Y76.0
      miscellaneous Y76.8
      monitoring Y76.0
      prosthetic Y76.2
      rehabilitative Y76.1
      surgical Y76.3
      therapeutic Y76.1
    ophthalmic Y77.8
      accessory Y77.2
      contact lens (rigid gas permeable)
          (soft) (hydrophilic)) Y77.11
      diagnostic Y77.0
      miscellaneous Y77.8
      monitoring Y77.0
      prosthetic Y77.2
      rehabilitative Y77.19
      surgical Y77.3
      therapeutic Y77.19
    orthopedic Y79.8
      accessory Y79.2
      diagnostic Y79.0
      miscellaneous Y79.8
      monitoring Y79.0
      prosthetic Y79.2
      rehabilitative Y79.1
      surgical Y79.3
      therapeutic Y79.1
    otorhinolaryngological Y72.8
      accessory Y72.2
      diagnostic Y72.0
      miscellaneous Y72.8
      monitoring Y72.0
      prosthetic Y72.2
      rehabilitative Y72.1
      surgical Y72.3
      therapeutic Y72.1
    personal use Y74.8
      accessory Y74.2
      diagnostic Y74.0
      miscellaneous Y74.8
      monitoring Y74.0
      prosthetic Y74.2

Incident, adverse *(Continued)*
  device *(Continued)*
    personal use *(Continued)*
      rehabilitative Y74.1
      surgical Y74.3
      therapeutic Y74.1
    physical medicine Y80.8
      accessory Y80.2
      diagnostic Y80.0
      miscellaneous Y80.8
      monitoring Y80.0
      prosthetic Y80.2
      rehabilitative Y80.1
      surgical Y80.3
      therapeutic Y80.1
    plastic surgical Y81.8
      accessory Y81.2
      diagnostic Y81.0
      miscellaneous Y81.8
      monitoring Y81.0
      prosthetic Y81.2
      rehabilitative Y81.1
      surgical Y81.3
      therapeutic Y81.1
    radiological Y78.8
      accessory Y78.2
      diagnostic Y78.0
      miscellaneous Y78.8
      monitoring Y78.0
      prosthetic Y78.2
      rehabilitative Y78.1
      surgical Y78.3
      therapeutic Y78.1
    urology Y73.8
      accessory Y73.2
      diagnostic Y73.0
      miscellaneous Y73.8
      monitoring Y73.0
      prosthetic Y73.2
      rehabilitative Y73.1
      surgical Y73.3
      therapeutic Y73.1
Incineration (accidental) —*see* Exposure, fire
Infanticide —*see* Assault
Infrasound waves (causing injury) W49.9
Ingestion
  foreign body (causing injury) (with
      obstruction) —*see* Foreign body,
      alimentary canal
  poisonous
    plant(s) X58
    substance NEC —*see* Table of Drugs and
        Chemicals
Inhalation
  excessively cold substance, man-made —*see*
      Exposure, cold, man-made
  food (any type) (into respiratory tract) (with
      asphyxia, obstruction respiratory tract,
      suffocation) —*see* categories T17 and T18
  foreign body —*see* Foreign body, aspiration
  gastric contents (with asphyxia, obstruction
      respiratory passage, suffocation) T17.81-●
  hot air or gases X14.0
  liquid air, hydrogen, nitrogen W93.12
    suicide (attempt) X83.2
  steam X13.0
    assault X98.0
    stated as undetermined whether accidental
        or intentional Y27.0
    suicide (attempt) X77.0
  toxic gas —*see* Table of Drugs and
      Chemicals
  vomitus (with asphyxia, obstruction
      respiratory passage, suffocation) T17.81-●
Injury, injured (accidental(ly)) **NOS** X58
  by, caused by, from
    assault —*see* Assault
    law-enforcing agent, police, in course
        of legal intervention —*see* Legal
        intervention
    suicide (attempt) X83.8

▶ New   ⇒ Revised   ~~deleted~~ Deleted   ● Use Additional Character(s)

Injury, injured NOS *(Continued)*
    due to, in
        civil insurrection —*see* War
            operations
        fight —*see also* Assault, fight
            Y04.0
        war operations —*see* War
            operations
    homicide —*see also* Assault Y09
    inflicted (by)
        in course of arrest (attempted), suppression
            of disturbance, maintenance of order,
            by law-enforcing agents —*see* Legal
            intervention

Injury, injured NOS *(Continued)*
    inflicted *(Continued)*
        other person
            stated as
                accidental X58
                intentional, homicide (attempt) —*see*
                    Assault
                undetermined whether accidental or
                    intentional Y33
        purposely (inflicted) by other person(s) —*see*
            Assault
        self-inflicted X83.8
            stated as accidental X58
        specified cause NEC X58

Injury, injured NOS *(Continued)*
    undetermined whether accidental or
        intentional Y33
Insolation, effects X30
Insufficient nourishment X58
Interruption of respiration (by)
    food (lodged in esophagus) —*see* categories
        T17 and T18
    vomitus (lodged in esophagus) T17.81-●
Intervention, legal —*see* Legal intervention
Intoxication
    drug —*see* Table of Drugs and Chemicals
    poison —*see* Table of Drugs and
        Chemicals

J

Jammed (accidentally)
    between objects (moving) (stationary and
        moving) W23.0
    stationary W23.1
Jumped, Jumping
    before moving object NEC X81.8
        motor vehicle X81.0
        subway train X81.1
        train X81.1
        undetermined whether accidental or
            intentional Y31
    from
        boat (into water) voluntarily,
            without accident (to or on boat)
            W16.712
            with
                accident to or on boat —*see* Accident,
                    watercraft
                drowning or submersion W16.711
                    suicide (attempt) X71.3

Jumped, jumping *(Continued)*
    from *(Continued)*
        boat voluntarily, without accident
            (Continued)
            striking bottom W16.722
                causing drowning W16.721
        building —*see also* Jumped, from,
            high place W13.9
            burning (uncontrolled fire)
                X00.5
        high place NEC W17.89
            suicide (attempt) X80
            undetermined whether accidental or
                intentional Y30
        structure —*see also* Jumped, from, high
            place W13.9
            burning (uncontrolled fire)
                X00.5
    into water W16.92
        causing drowning W16.91
        from, off watercraft —*see* Jumped, from,
            boat

Jumped, jumping *(Continued)*
    into water *(Continued)*
        in
            natural body W16.612
                causing drowning W16.611
                striking bottom W16.622
                    causing drowning W16.621
            specified place NEC W16.812
                causing drowning W16.811
                striking
                    bottom W16.822
                        causing drowning W16.821
                    wall W16.832
                        causing drowning W16.831
            swimming pool W16.512
                causing drowning W16.511
                striking
                    bottom W16.522
                        causing drowning W16.521
                    wall W16.532
                        causing drowning W16.531
        suicide (attempt) X71.3

I, J, & K

K

Kicked by
    animal NEC W55.82
    person(s) (accidentally) W50.1
        with intent to injure or kill Y04.0
        as, or caused by, a crowd or human
            stampede (with fall) W52
        assault Y04.0
        homicide (attempt) Y04.0
        in
            fight Y04.0
            legal intervention
                injuring
                    bystander Y35.812
                    law enforcement personnel
                        Y35.811
                    suspect Y35.813
                    unspecified person Y35.819

Kicking
    against
        object W22.8
            sports equipment W21.9
            stationary W22.09
                sports equipment W21.89
        person —*see* Striking against, person
        sports equipment W21.9
    carpet stretcher with knee X50.3
Killed, killing (accidentally) **NOS** —*see also*
    Injury X58
    in
        action —*see* War operations
        brawl, fight (hand) (fists) (foot) Y04.0
            by weapon —*see also* Assault
                cutting, piercing —*see* Assault, cutting
                    or piercing instrument
                firearm —*see* Discharge, firearm, by
                    type, homicide

Killed, killing NOS *(Continued)*
    self
        stated as
            accident NOS X58
            suicide —*see* Suicide
            undetermined whether accidental or
                intentional Y33
Kneeling (prolonged) (static) X50.1
Knocked down (accidentally) (by) **NOS** X58
    animal (not being ridden) NEC —*see also*
        Struck by, by type of animal
    crowd or human stampede W52
    person W51
        in brawl, fight Y04.0
    transport vehicle NEC —*see also* Accident,
        transport V09.9

L

Laceration NEC —*see* Injury
Lack of
  care (helpless person) (infant) (newborn) X58
  food except as result of abandonment or neglect X58
    due to abandonment or neglect X58
  water except as result of transport accident X58
    due to transport accident —*see* Accident, transport, by type
  helpless person, infant, newborn X58
Landslide (falling on transport vehicle) X36.1
  caused by collapse of man-made structure X36.0
Late effect —*see* Sequelae
Legal
  execution (any method) —*see* Legal, intervention
  intervention (by)
    baton —*see* Legal, intervention, blunt object, baton
    bayonet —*see* Legal, intervention, sharp object, bayonet
    blow —*see* Legal, intervention, manhandling
    blunt object
      baton
        injuring
          bystander Y35.312
          law enforcement personnel Y35.311
          suspect Y35.313
          unspecified person Y35.319
      injuring
        bystander Y35.302
        law enforcement personnel Y35.301
        suspect Y35.303
        unspecified person Y35.309
      specified NEC
        injuring
          bystander Y35.392
          law enforcement personnel Y35.391
          suspect Y35.393
          unspecified person Y35.399
      stave
        injuring
          bystander Y35.392
          law enforcement personnel Y35.391
          suspect Y35.393
          unspecified person Y35.399
    bomb —*see* Legal, intervention, explosive
    conducted energy device
      injuring
        bystander Y35.832
        law enforcement personnel Y35.831
        suspect Y35.833
        unspecified person Y35.839
    cutting or piercing instrument —*see* Legal, intervention, sharp object
    dynamite —*see* Legal, intervention, explosive, dynamite
    electroshock device (taser)
      injuring
        bystander Y35.832
        law enforcement personnel Y35.831
        suspect Y35.833
        unspecified person Y35.839
    explosive(s)
      dynamite
        injuring
          bystander Y35.112
          law enforcement personnel Y35.111
          suspect Y35.113
          unspecified person Y35.119
      grenade
        injuring
          bystander Y35.192
          law enforcement personnel Y35.191
          suspect Y35.193
          unspecified person Y35.199

Legal *(Continued)*
  intervention *(Continued)*
    explosive *(Continued)*
      injuring
        bystander Y35.102
        law enforcement personnel Y35.101
        suspect Y35.103
        unspecified person Y35.109
      mortar bomb
        injuring
          bystander Y35.192
          law enforcement personnel Y35.191
          suspect Y35.193
          unspecified person Y35.199
      shell
        injuring
          bystander Y35.122
          law enforcement personnel Y35.121
          suspect Y35.123
          unspecified person Y35.129
      specified NEC
        injuring
          bystander Y35.192
          law enforcement personnel Y35.191
          suspect Y35.193
          unspecified person Y35.199
    firearm(s) (discharge)
      handgun
        injuring
          bystander Y35.022
          law enforcement personnel Y35.021
          suspect Y35.023
          unspecified person Y35.029
      injuring
        bystander Y35.002
        law enforcement personnel Y35.001
        suspect Y35.003
        unspecified person Y35.009
      machine gun
        injuring
          bystander Y35.012
          law enforcement personnel Y35.011
          suspect Y35.013
          unspecified person Y35.019
      rifle pellet
        injuring
          bystander Y35.032
          law enforcement personnel Y35.031
          suspect Y35.033
          unspecified person Y35.039
      rubber bullet
        injuring
          bystander Y35.042
          law enforcement personnel Y35.041
          suspect Y35.043
          unspecified person Y35.049
      shotgun —*see* Legal, intervention, firearm, specified NEC
      specified NEC
        injuring
          bystander Y35.092
          law enforcement personnel Y35.091
          suspect Y35.093
          unspecified person Y35.099
    gas (asphyxiation) (poisoning)
      injuring
        bystander Y35.202
        law enforcement personnel Y35.201
        suspect Y35.203
        unspecified person Y35.209
      specified NEC
        injuring
          bystander Y35.292
          law enforcement personnel Y35.291
          suspect Y35.293
          unspecified person Y35.299
      tear gas
        injuring
          bystander Y35.212
          law enforcement personnel Y35.211
          suspect Y35.213
          unspecified person Y35.219

Legal *(Continued)*
  intervention *(Continued)*
    grenade —*see* Legal, intervention, explosive, grenade
    injuring
      bystander Y35.92
      law enforcement personnel Y35.91
      suspect Y35.93
      unspecified person Y35.99
    late effect (of) —*see* with 7th character S Y35
    manhandling
      injuring
        bystander Y35.812
        law enforcement personnel Y35.811
        suspect Y35.813
        unspecified person Y35.819
    sequelae (of) —*see* with 7th character S Y35
    sharp objects
      bayonet
        injuring
          bystander Y35.412
          law enforcement personnel Y35.411
          suspect Y35.413
          unspecified person Y35.419
      injuring
        bystander Y35.402
        law enforcement personnel Y35.401
        suspect Y35.403
        unspecified person Y35.409
      specified NEC
        injuring
          bystander Y35.492
          law enforcement personnel Y35.491
          suspect Y35.493
          unspecified person Y35.499
    specified means NEC
      injuring
        bystander Y35.892
        law enforcement personnel Y35.891
        suspect Y35.893
      ▶ unspecified person Y35.899
    stabbing —*see* Legal, intervention, sharp object
    stave —*see* Legal, intervention, blunt object, stave
    stun gun
      injuring
        bystander Y35.832
        law enforcement personnel Y35.831
        suspect Y35.833
        unspecified person Y35.839
    taser
      injuring
        bystander Y35.832
        law enforcement personnel Y35.831
        suspect Y35.833
        unspecified person Y35.839
    tear gas —*see* Legal, intervention, gas, tear gas
    truncheon —*see* Legal, intervention, blunt object, stave
Lifting —*see also* Overexertion
  heavy objects X50.0
  weights X50.0
Lightning (shock) (stroke) (struck by) —*see* subcategory T75.0
  causing fire —*see* Exposure, fire
Loss of control (transport vehicle) NEC —*see* Accident, transport
Lost at sea NOS —*see* Drowning, due to, fall overboard
Low
  pressure (effects) —*see* Air, pressure, low
  temperature (effects) —*see* Exposure, cold
Lying before train, vehicle or other moving object X81.8
  subway train X81.1
  train X81.1
  undetermined whether accidental or intentional Y31
Lynching —*see* Assault

▶ New   ⇒ Revised   ~~deleted~~ Deleted   ● Use Additional Character(s)

M

Malfunction (mechanism or component) (of)
  firearm
    airgun W34.10
    BB gun W34.110
    gas, air or spring-operated gun NEC
      W34.118
    handgun W32.1
    hunting rifle W33.12
    larger firearm W33.10
      specified NEC W33.19
    machine gun W33.13
    paintball gun W34.111
    pellet gun W34.110
    shotgun W33.11
    specified NEC W34.19
    Very pistol [flare] W34.19
  handgun —see Malfunction, firearm,
    handgun
Maltreatment —see Perpetrator
Mangled (accidentally) NOS X58
Manhandling (in brawl, fight) Y04.0
  legal intervention —see Legal, intervention,
    manhandling
Manslaughter (nonaccidental) —see Assault
Mauled by animal NEC W55.89
Medical procedure, complication of
  (delayed or as an abnormal reaction
    without mention of misadventure) —see
    Complication of or following, by specified
    type of procedure
  due to or as a result of misadventure —see
    Misadventure
Melting (due to fire) —see also Exposure, fire
  apparel NEC X06.3
  clothes, clothing NEC X06.3
    nightwear X05
  fittings or furniture (burning building)
    (uncontrolled fire) X00.8
  nightwear X05
  plastic jewelry X06.1
Mental cruelty X58
Military operations (injuries to military and
  civilians occuring during peacetime on
  military property and during routine
  military exercises and operations) (by)
  (from) (involving) Y37.90-●
  air blast Y37.20-●
  aircraft
    destruction —see Military operations,
      destruction of aircraft
  airway restriction —see Military operations,
    restriction of airways
  asphyxiation —see Military operations,
    restriction of airways
  biological weapons Y37.6X-●
  blast Y37.20-●
  blast fragments Y37.20-●
  blast wave Y37.20-●
  blast wind Y37.20-●
  bomb Y37.20-●
    dirty Y37.50-●
    gasoline Y37.31-●
    incendiary Y37.31-●
    petrol Y37.31-●
  bullet Y37.43-●
    incendiary Y37.32-●
    rubber Y37.41-●
  chemical weapons Y37.7X-●
  combat
    hand to hand (unarmed) combat
      Y37.44-●
    using blunt or piercing object Y37.45-●
  conflagration —see Military operations, fire
  conventional warfare NEC Y37.49-●
  depth-charge Y37.01-●
  destruction of aircraft Y37.10-●
    due to
      air to air missile Y37.11-●
      collision with other aircraft Y37.12-●

Military operations (Continued)
  destruction of aircraft (Continued)
    due to (Continued)
      detonation (accidental) of onboard
        munitions and explosives Y37.14-●
      enemy fire or explosives Y37.11-●
      explosive placed on aircraft Y37.11-●
      onboard fire Y37.13-●
      rocket propelled grenade [RPG] Y37.11-●
      small arms fire Y37.11-●
      surface to air missile Y37.11-●
    specified NEC Y37.19-●
  detonation (accidental) of
    onboard marine weapons Y37.05-●
    own munitions or munitions launch device
      Y37.24-●
  dirty bomb Y37.50-●
  explosion (of) Y37.20-●
    aerial bomb Y37.21-●
    bomb NOS —see also Military operations,
      bomb(s) Y37.20-●
    fragments Y37.20-●
    grenade Y37.29-●
    guided missile Y37.22-●
    improvised explosive device [IED]
      (person-borne) (roadside) (vehicle-
      borne) Y37.23-●
    land mine Y37.29-●
    marine mine (at sea) (in harbor) Y37.02-●
    marine weapon Y37.00-●
      specified NEC Y37.09-●
    own munitions or munitions launch device
      (accidental) Y37.24-●
    sea-based artillery shell Y37.03-●
    specified NEC Y37.29-●
    torpedo Y37.04-●
  fire Y37.30-●
    specified NEC Y37.39-●
  firearms
    discharge Y37.43-●
    pellets Y37.42-●
  flamethrower Y37.33-●
  fragments (from) (of)
    improvised explosive device [IED]
      (person-borne) (roadside) (vehicle-
      borne) Y37.26-●
    munitions Y37.25-●
    specified NEC Y37.29-●
    weapons Y37.27-●
  friendly fire Y37.92-●
  hand to hand (unarmed) combat Y37.44-●
  hot substances —see Military operations, fire
  incendiary bullet Y37.32-●
  nuclear weapon (effects of) Y37.50-●
    acute radiation exposure Y37.54-●
    blast pressure Y37.51-●
    direct blast Y37.51-●
    direct heat Y37.53-●
    fallout exposure Y37.54-●
    fireball Y37.53-●
    indirect blast (struck or crushed by blast
      debris) (being thrown by blast)
      Y37.52-●
    ionizing radiation (immediate exposure)
      Y37.54-●
    nuclear radiation Y37.54-●
    radiation
      ionizing (immediate exposure) Y37.54-●
      nuclear Y37.54-●
      thermal Y37.53-●
    secondary effects Y37.54-●
    specified NEC Y37.59-●
    thermal radiation Y37.53-●
  restriction of air (airway)
    intentional Y37.46-●
    unintentional Y37.47-●
  rubber bullets Y37.41-●
  shrapnel NOS Y37.29-●
  suffocation —see Military operations,
    restriction of airways
  unconventional warfare NEC Y37.7X-●

Military operations (Continued)
  underwater blast NOS Y37.00-●
  warfare
    conventional NEC Y37.49-●
    unconventional NEC Y37.7X-●
  weapon of mass destruction [WMD]
    Y37.91-●
  weapons
    biological weapons Y37.6X-●
    chemical Y37.7X-●
    nuclear (effects of) Y37.50-●
      acute radiation exposure Y37.54-●
      blast pressure Y37.51-●
      direct blast Y37.51-●
      direct heat Y37.53-●
      fallout exposure Y37.54-●
      fireball Y37.53-●
      radiation
        ionizing (immediate exposure)
          Y37.54-●
        nuclear Y37.54-●
        thermal Y37.53-●
      secondary effects Y37.54-●
      specified NEC Y37.59-●
    of mass destruction [WMD] Y37.91-●
Misadventure(s) to patient(s) during surgical
or medical care Y69
  contaminated medical or biological substance
    (blood, drug, fluid) Y64.9
    administered (by) NEC Y64.9
      immunization Y64.1
      infusion Y64.0
      injection Y64.1
      specified means NEC Y64.8
      transfusion Y64.0
      vaccination Y64.1
  excessive amount of blood or other fluid
    during transfusion or infusion Y63.0
  failure
    in dosage Y63.9
      electroshock therapy Y63.4
      inappropriate temperature (too hot or
        too cold) in local application and
        packing Y63.5
      infusion
        excessive amount of fluid Y63.0
        incorrect dilution of fluid Y63.1
      insulin-shock therapy Y63.4
      nonadministration of necessary drug or
        biological substance Y63.6
      overdose —see Table of Drugs and
        Chemicals
      radiation, in therapy Y63.2
      radiation
        overdose Y63.2
      specified procedure NEC Y63.8
      transfusion
        excessive amount of blood Y63.0
    mechanical, of instrument or apparatus
      (any) (during any procedure) Y65.8
    sterile precautions (during procedure)
      Y62.9
      aspiration of fluid or tissue (by puncture
        or catheterization, except heart)
        Y62.6
      biopsy (except needle aspiration)
        Y62.8
        needle (aspirating) Y62.6
      blood sampling Y62.6
      catheterization Y62.6
        heart Y62.5
      dialysis (kidney) Y62.2
      endoscopic examination Y62.4
      enema Y62.8
      immunization Y62.3
      infusion Y62.1
      injection Y62.3
      needle biopsy Y62.6
      paracentesis (abdominal) (thoracic)
        Y62.6
      perfusion Y62.2

Misadventure(s) to patient(s) during surgical
    or medical care *(Continued)*
failure *(Continued)*
    sterile precautions *(Continued)*
        puncture (lumbar) Y62.6
        removal of catheter or packing
            Y62.8
        specified procedure NEC Y62.8
        surgical operation Y62.0
        transfusion Y62.1
        vaccination Y62.3
    suture or ligature during surgical
        procedure Y65.2
    to introduce or to remove tube or
        instrument —*see* Failure, to
hemorrhage —*see* Index to Diseases and
    Injuries, Complication(s)
inadvertent exposure of patient to radiation
    Y63.3
inappropriate
    operation performed —*see*
        Inappropriate operation
        performed
    temperature (too hot or too cold) in
        local application or packing
        Y63.5

Misadventure(s) to patient(s) during surgical
    or medical care *(Continued)*
infusion —*see also* Misadventure, by type,
    infusion Y69
    excessive amount of fluid Y63.0
    incorrect dilution of fluid Y63.1
    wrong fluid Y65.1
mismatched blood in transfusion Y65.0
nonadministration of necessary drug or
    biological substance Y63.6
overdose —*see* Table of Drugs and
    Chemicals
    radiation (in therapy) Y63.2
perforation —*see* Index to Diseases and
    Injuries, Complication(s)
performance of inappropriate operation —*see*
    Inappropriate operation performed
puncture —*see* Index to Diseases and Injuries,
    Complication(s)
specified type NEC Y65.8
    failure
        suture or ligature during surgical
            operation Y65.2
        to introduce or to remove tube or
            instrument —*see* Failure, to
    infusion of wrong fluid Y65.1

Misadventure(s) to patient(s) during surgical
    or medical care *(Continued)*
specified type NEC *(Continued)*
    performance of inappropriate operation —
        see Inappropriate operation performed
    transfusion of mismatched blood Y65.0
    wrong
        fluid in infusion Y65.1
        placement of endotracheal tube during
            anesthetic procedure Y65.3
transfusion —*see* Misadventure, by type,
    transfusion
    excessive amount of blood Y63.0
    mismatched blood Y65.0
wrong
    drug given in error —*see* Table of Drugs
        and Chemicals
    fluid in infusion Y65.1
    placement of endotracheal tube during
        anesthetic procedure Y65.3
Mismatched blood in transfusion Y65.0
Motion sickness T75.3
Mountain sickness W94.11
Mudslide (of cataclysmic nature) —*see*
    Landslide
Murder (attempt) —*see* Assault

N

Nail
    contact with W45.0
        gun W29.4
    embedded in skin W45.0
Neglect (criminal) (homicidal intent) X58

Noise (causing injury) (pollution) W42.9
    supersonic W42.0
Nonadministration (of)
    drug or biological substance (necessary)
        Y63.6
    surgical and medical care Y66
Nosocomial condition Y95

O

Object
    falling
        from, in, on, hitting
            machinery —*see* Contact, with, by type
                of machine
    set in motion by
        accidental explosion or rupture of pressure
            vessel W38
        firearm —*see* Discharge, firearm, by type
        machine (ry) —*see* Contact, with, by type
            of machine
Overdose (drug) —*see* Table of Drugs and
    Chemicals
    radiation Y63.2

Overexertion X50.9
    from
        prolonged static or awkward postures
            X50.1
        repetitive movements X50.3
        specified strenuous movements or postures
            NEC X50.9
        strenuous movement or load X50.0
Overexposure (accidental) (to)
    cold —*see also* Exposure, cold X31
        due to man-made conditions —*see*
            Exposure, cold, man-made
    heat —*see also* Heat X30
    radiation —*see* Radiation
    radioactivity W88.0
    sun (sunburn) X32

Overexposure *(Continued)*
    weather NEC —*see* Forces of nature
    wind NEC —*see* Forces of nature
Overheated —*see* Heat
Overturning (accidental)
    machinery —*see* Contact, with, by type of
        machine
    transport vehicle NEC —*see also* Accident,
        transport V89.9
    watercraft (causing drowning,
        submersion) —*see also* Drowning, due to,
        accident to, watercraft, overturning
        causing injury except drowning or
            submersion —*see* Accident, watercraft,
            causing, injury NEC

▶ New   ⇒ Revised   ~~deleted~~ Deleted   ● Use Additional Character(s)

M, N, & O

P

Parachute descent (voluntary) (without
  accident to aircraft) V97.29
  due to accident to aircraft —see Accident,
    transport, aircraft
Pecked by bird W61.99
Perforation during medical or surgical
  treatment as misadventure —see Index to
  Diseases and Injuries, Complication(s)
Perpetrator, perpetration, of assault,
  maltreatment and neglect (by) Y07.9
  boyfriend Y07.03
  brother Y07.410
    stepbrother Y07.435
  coach Y07.53
  cousin
    female Y07.491
    male Y07.490
  daycare provider Y07.519
    at-home
      adult care Y07.512
      childcare Y07.510
    care center
      adult care Y07.513
      childcare Y07.511
  family member NEC Y07.499
  father Y07.11
    adoptive Y07.13
    foster Y07.420
    stepfather Y07.430
  foster father Y07.420
  foster mother Y07.421
  girl friend Y07.04
  healthcare provider Y07.529
    mental health Y07.521
    specified NEC Y07.528
  husband Y07.01
  instructor Y07.53
  mother Y07.12
    adoptive Y07.14
    foster Y07.421
    stepmother Y07.433
  nonfamily member Y07.50
    specified NEC Y07.59
  nurse Y07.528
  occupational therapist Y07.528
  partner of parent
    female Y07.434
    male Y07.432
  physical therapist Y07.528
  sister Y07.411
  speech therapist Y07.528
  stepbrother Y07.435
  stepfather Y07.430
  stepmother Y07.433
  stepsister Y07.436
  teacher Y07.53
  wife Y07.02
Piercing —see Contact, with, by type of object
  or machine
Pinched
  between objects (moving) (stationary and
    moving) W23.0
    stationary W23.1
Pinned under machine (ry) —see Contact, with,
  by type of machine
Place of occurrence Y92.9
  abandoned house Y92.89
  airplane Y92.813
  airport Y92.520
  ambulatory health services establishment
    NEC Y92.538
  ambulatory surgery center Y92.530
  amusement park Y92.831
  apartment (co-op) —see Place of occurrence,
    residence, apartment
  assembly hall Y92.29
  bank Y92.510
  barn Y92.71
  baseball field Y92.320

Place of occurrence (Continued)
  basketball court Y92.310
  beach Y92.832
  boarding house —see Place of occurrence,
    residence, boarding house
  boat Y92.814
  bowling alley Y92.39
  bridge Y92.89
  building under construction Y92.61
  bus Y92.811
    station Y92.521
  cafe Y92.511
  campsite Y92.833
  campus —see Place of occurrence, school
  canal Y92.89
  car Y92.810
  casino Y92.59
  children's home —see Place of occurrence,
    residence, institutional, orphanage
  church Y92.22
  cinema Y92.26
  clubhouse Y92.29
  coal pit Y92.64
  college (community) Y92.214
  condominium —see Place of occurrence,
    residence, apartment
  construction area —see Place of occurrence,
    industrial and construction area
  convalescent home —see Place of occurrence,
    residence, institutional, nursing home
  court-house Y92.240
  cricket ground Y92.328
  cultural building Y92.258
    art gallery Y92.250
    museum Y92.251
    music hall Y92.252
    opera house Y92.253
    specified NEC Y92.258
    theater Y92.254
  dancehall Y92.252
  day nursery Y92.210
  dentist office Y92.531
  derelict house Y92.89
  desert Y92.820
  dock NOS Y92.89
  dockyard Y92.62
  doctor's office Y92.531
  dormitory —see Place of occurrence,
    residence, institutional, school dormitory
  dry dock Y92.62
  factory (building) (premises) Y92.63
  farm (land under cultivation) (outbuildings)
    Y92.79
    barn Y92.71
    chicken coop Y92.72
    field Y92.73
    hen house Y92.72
    house —see Place of occurrence, residence,
      house
    orchard Y92.74
    specified NEC Y92.79
  football field Y92.321
  forest Y92.821
  freeway Y92.411
  gallery Y92.250
  garage (commercial) Y92.59
    boarding house Y92.044
    military base Y92.135
    mobile home Y92.025
    nursing home Y92.124
    orphanage Y92.114
    private house Y92.015
    reform school Y92.155
  gas station Y92.524
  gasworks Y92.69
  golf course Y92.39
  gravel pit Y92.64
  grocery Y92.512
  gymnasium Y92.39
  handball court Y92.318
  harbor Y92.89

Place of occurrence (Continued)
  harness racing course Y92.39
  healthcare provider office Y92.531
  highway (interstate) Y92.411
  hill Y92.828
  hockey rink Y92.330
  home —see Place of occurrence, residence
  hospice —see Place of occurrence, residence,
    institutional, nursing home
  hospital Y92.239
    cafeteria Y92.233
    corridor Y92.232
    operating room Y92.234
    patient
      bathroom Y92.231
      room Y92.230
    specified NEC Y92.238
  hotel Y92.59
  house —see also Place of occurrence, residence
    abandoned Y92.89
    under construction Y92.61
  industrial and construction area (yard)
    Y92.69
    building under construction Y92.61
    dock Y92.62
    dry dock Y92.62
    factory Y92.63
    gasworks Y92.69
    mine Y92.64
    oil rig Y92.65
    pit Y92.64
    power station Y92.69
    shipyard Y92.62
    specified NEC Y92.69
    tunnel under construction Y92.69
    workshop Y92.69
  kindergarten Y92.211
  lacrosse field Y92.328
  lake Y92.828
  library Y92.241
  mall Y92.59
  market Y92.512
  marsh Y92.828
  military
    base —see Place of occurrence, residence,
      institutional, military base
    training ground Y92.84
  mine Y92.64
  mosque Y92.22
  motel Y92.59
  motorway (interstate) Y92.411
  mountain Y92.828
  movie-house Y92.26
  museum Y92.251
  music-hall Y92.252
  not applicable Y92.9
  nuclear power station Y92.69
  nursing home —see Place of occurrence,
    residence, institutional, nursing home
  office building Y92.59
  offshore installation Y92.65
  oil rig Y92.65
  old people's home —see Place of occurrence,
    residence, institutional, specified NEC
  opera-house Y92.253
  orphanage —see Place of occurrence,
    residence, institutional, orphanage
  outpatient surgery center Y92.530
  park (public) Y92.830
    amusement Y92.831
  parking garage Y92.89
    lot Y92.481
  pavement Y92.480
  physician office Y92.531
  polo field Y92.328
  pond Y92.828
  post office Y92.242
  power station Y92.69
  prairie Y92.828
  prison —see Place of occurrence, residence,
    institutional, prison

► New   ⇒ Revised   ~~deleted~~ Deleted   ● Use Additional Character(s)

Place of occurrence *(Continued)*
  swimming pool *(Continued)*
    private *(Continued)*
      prison Y92.146
      reform school Y92.156
      single family residence Y92.016
  synagogue Y92.22
  television station Y92.59
  tennis court Y92.312
  theater Y92.254
  trade area Y92.59
    bank Y92.510
    cafe Y92.511
    casino Y92.59
    garage Y92.59
    hotel Y92.59
    market Y92.512
    office building Y92.59
    radio station Y92.59
    restaurant Y92.511
    shop Y92.513
    shopping mall Y92.59
    store Y92.512
    supermarket Y92.512
    television station Y92.59
    warehouse Y92.59
  trailer park, residential —*see* Place of occurrence, residence, mobile home
  trailer site NOS Y92.89
  train Y92.815
    station Y92.522
  truck Y92.812
  tunnel under construction Y92. 69
  university Y92.214
  urgent (health) care center Y92.532
  vehicle (transport) Y92.818
    airplane Y92.813
    boat Y92.814
    bus Y92.811
    car Y92.810
    specified NEC Y92.818
    subway car Y92.816
    train Y92.815
    truck Y92.812
  warehouse Y92.59
  water reservoir Y92.89
  wilderness area Y92.828
    desert Y92.820
    forest Y92.821
    marsh Y92.828
    mountain Y92.828
    prairie Y92.828
    specified NEC Y92.828
    swamp Y92.828
  workshop Y92.69
  yard, private Y92.096
    boarding house Y92.046
    mobile home Y92.027
    single family house Y92.017

Place of occurrence *(Continued)*
  youth center Y92.29
  zoo (zoological garden) Y92.834
Plumbism —*see* Table of Drugs and Chemicals, lead
Poisoning (accidental) (by) —*see also* Table of Drugs and Chemicals
  by plant, thorns, spines, sharp leaves or other mechanisms NEC X58
  carbon monoxide
    generated by
      motor vehicle —*see* Accident, transport
      watercraft (in transit) (not in transit) V93.89
        ferry boat V93.81
        fishing boat V93.82
        jet skis V93.83
        liner V93.81
        merchant ship V93.80
        passenger ship V93.81
        powered craft NEC V93.83
  caused by injection of poisons into skin by plant thorns, spines, sharp leaves X58
  marine or sea plants (venomous) X58
  exhaust gas
    generated by
      motor vehicle —*see* Accident, transport
      watercraft (in transit) (not in transit) V93.89
        ferry boat V93.81
        fishing boat V93.82
        jet skis V93.83
        liner V93.81
        merchant ship V93.80
        passenger ship V93.81
        powered craft NEC V93.83
  fumes or smoke due to
    explosion —*see also* Explosion W40.9
    fire —*see* Exposure, fire
    ignition —*see* Ignition
  gas
    in legal intervention —*see* Legal, intervention, gas
    legal execution —*see* Legal, intervention, gas
  in war operations —*see* War operations
  legal
    execution —*see* Legal, intervention, gas
    intervention
      by gas —*see* Legal, intervention, gas
      other specified means —*see* Legal, intervention, specified means NEC
Powder burn (by) (from)
  airgun W34.110
  BB gun W34.110
  firearm NEC W34.19
  gas, air or spring-operated gun NEC W34.118
  handgun W32.1
  hunting rifle W33.12

Powder burn *(Continued)*
  larger firearm W33.10
    specified NEC W33.19
  machine gun W33.13
  paintball gun W34.111
  pellet gun W34.110
  shotgun W33.11
  Very pistol [flare] W34.19
Premature cessation (of) surgical and medical care Y66
Privation (food) (water) X58
Procedure (operation)
  correct, on wrong side or body part (wrong side) (wrong site) Y65.53
  intended for another patient done on wrong patient Y65.52
  performed on patient not scheduled for surgery Y65.52
  performed on wrong patient Y65.52
  wrong, performed on correct patient Y65.51
Prolonged
  sitting in transport vehicle —*see* Travel, by type of vehicle
  stay in
    high altitude as cause of anoxia, barodontalgia, barotitis or hypoxia W94.11
    weightless environment X52
Pulling, excessive —*see also* Overexertion X50.9
Puncture, puncturing —*see also* Contact, with, by type of object or machine
  by
    plant thorns, spines, sharp leaves or other mechanisms NEC W60
  during medical or surgical treatment as misadventure —*see* Index to Diseases and Injuries, Complication(s)
Pushed, pushing (accidental) (injury in)
  by other person(s) (accidental) W51
    with fall W03
      due to ice or snow W00.0
    as, or caused by, a crowd or human stampede (with fall) W52
    before moving object NEC Y02.8
      motor vehicle Y02.0
      subway train Y02.1
      train Y02.1
    from
      high place NEC
        in accidental circumstances W17.89
        stated as
          intentional, homicide (attempt) Y01
          undetermined whether accidental or intentional Y30
      transport vehicle NEC —*see also* Accident, transport V89.9
        stated as
          intentional, homicide (attempt) Y08.89
  overexertion X50.9

R

Radiation (exposure to)
- arc lamps W89.0
- atomic power plant (malfunction) NEC W88.1
- complication of or abnormal reaction to medical radiotherapy Y84.2
- electromagnetic, ionizing W88.0
- gamma rays W88.1
- in
  - war operations (from or following nuclear explosion) —see also War operations
- inadvertent exposure of patient (receiving test or therapy) Y63.3
- infrared (heaters and lamps) W90.1
  - excessive heat from W92
- ionized, ionizing (particles, artificially accelerated)
  - radioisotopes W88.1
  - specified NEC W88.8
  - x-rays W88.0
- isotopes, radioactive —see Radiation, radioactive isotopes
- laser(s) W90.2
  - in war operations —see War operations
  - misadventure in medical care Y63.2
- light sources (man-made visible and ultraviolet) W89.9
  - natural X32
  - specified NEC W89.8
  - tanning bed W89.1
  - welding light W89.0
- man-made visible light W89.9
  - specified NEC W89.8
  - tanning bed W89.1
  - welding light W89.0
- microwave W90.8
- misadventure in medical or surgical procedure Y63.2

Radiation (Continued)
- natural NEC X39.08
  - radon X39.01
- overdose (in medical or surgical procedure) Y63.2
- radar W90.0
- radioactive isotopes (any) W88.1
  - atomic power plant malfunction W88.1
  - misadventure in medical or surgical treatment Y63.2
- radiofrequency W90.0
- radium NEC W88.1
- sun X32
- ultraviolet (light) (man-made) W89.9
  - natural X32
  - specified NEC W89.8
  - tanning bed W89.1
  - welding light W89.0
- welding arc, torch, or light W89.0
  - excessive heat from W92
- x-rays (hard) (soft) W88.0

Range disease W94.11
Rape (attempted) T74.2-●
Rat bite W53.11
Reaching (prolonged) (static) X50.1
Reaction, abnormal to medical procedure —see also Complication of or following, by type of procedure Y84.9
- with misadventure —see Misadventure
- biologicals —see Table of Drugs and Chemicals
- drugs —see Table of Drugs and Chemicals
- vaccine —see Table of Drugs and Chemicals

Recoil
- airgun W34.110
- BB gun W34.110
- firearm NEC W34.19
- gas, air or spring-operated gun NEC W34.118

Recoil (Continued)
- handgun W32.1
- hunting rifle W33.12
- larger firearm W33.10
  - specified NEC W33.19
- machine gun W33.13
- paintball gun W34.111
- pellet W34.110
- shotgun W33.11
- Very pistol [flare] W34.19
Reduction in
- atmospheric pressure —see Air, pressure, change
Rock falling on or hitting (accidentally) (person) W20.8
- in cave-in W20.0
Run over (accidentally) (by)
- animal (not being ridden) NEC W55.89
- machinery —see Contact, with, by specified type of machine
- transport vehicle NEC —see also Accident, transport V09.9
  - intentional homicide (attempt) Y03.0
  - motor NEC V09.20
    - intentional homicide (attempt) Y03.0
Running
- before moving object X81.8
  - motor vehicle X81.0
Running off, away
- animal (being ridden) —see also Accident, transport V80.918
  - not being ridden W55.89
- animal-drawn vehicle NEC —see also Accident, transport V80.928
- highway, road(way), street
  - transport vehicle NEC —see also Accident, transport V89.9
Rupture pressurized devices —see Explosion, by type of device

▶ New   ⇒ Revised   ~~deleted~~ Deleted   ● Use Additional Character(s)

S

Saturnism —*see* Table of Drugs and Chemicals, lead
Scald, scalding (accidental) (by) (from) (in) X19
  air (hot) X14.1
  gases (hot) X14.1
  homicide (attempt) —*see* Assault, burning, hot object
  inflicted by other person
    stated as intentional, homicide (attempt) — *see* Assault, burning, hot object
  liquid (boiling) (hot) NEC X12
    stated as undetermined whether accidental or intentional Y27.2
    suicide (attempt) X77.2
  local application of externally applied substance in medical or surgical care Y63.5
  metal (molten) (liquid) (hot) NEC X18
  self-inflicted X77.9
  stated as undetermined whether accidental or intentional Y27.8
  steam X13.1
    assault X98.0
    stated as undetermined whether accidental or intentional Y27.0
    suicide (attempt) X77.0
  suicide (attempt) X77.9
  vapor (hot) X13.1
    assault X98.0
    stated as undetermined whether accidental or intentional Y27.0
    suicide (attempt) X77.0
Scratched by
  cat W55.03
  person(s) (accidentally) W50.4
    with intent to injure or kill Y04.0
    as, or caused by, a crowd or human stampede (with fall) W52
    assault Y04.0
    homicide (attempt) Y04.0
    in
      fight Y04.0
      legal intervention
        injuring
          bystander Y35.892
          law enforcement personnel Y35.891
          suspect Y35.893
          ▶ unspecified person Y35.899
Seasickness T75.3
Self-harm NEC —*see also* External cause by type, undetermined whether accidental or intentional
  intentional —*see* Suicide
  poisoning NEC —*see* Table of drugs and biologicals, accident
Self-inflicted (injury) NEC —*see also* External cause by type, undetermined whether accidental or intentional
  intentional —*see* Suicide
  poisoning NEC —*see* Table of drugs and biologicals, accident
Sequelae (of)
  accident NEC —*see* W00-X58 with 7th character S
  assault (homicidal) (any means) —*see* X92-Y08 with 7th character S
  homicide, attempt (any means) —*see* X92-Y08 with 7th character S
  injury undetermined whether accidentally or purposely inflicted —*see* Y21-Y33 with 7th character S
  intentional self-harm (classifiable to X71-X83) —*see* X71-X83 with 7th character S
  legal intervention (*see* with 7th character S Y35)
  motor vehicle accident —*see* V00-V99 with 7th character S
  suicide, attempt (any means) —*see* X71-X83 with 7th character S

Sequelae (*Continued*)
  transport accident —*see* V00-V99 with 7th character S
  war operations —*see* War operations
Shock
  electric —*see* Exposure, electric current
  from electric appliance (any) (faulty) W86.8
    domestic W86.0
    suicide (attempt) X83.1
Shooting, shot (accidental (ly)) —*see also* Discharge, firearm, by type
  herself or himself —*see* Discharge, firearm by type, self-inflicted
  homicide (attempt) —*see* Discharge, firearm by type, homicide
  in war operations —*see* War operations
  inflicted by other person —*see* Discharge, firearm by type, homicide
    accidental —*see* Discharge, firearm, by type of firearm
  legal
    execution —*see* Legal, intervention, firearm
    intervention —*see* Legal, intervention, firearm
  self-inflicted —*see* Discharge, firearm by type, suicide
    accidental —*see* Discharge, firearm, by type of firearm
  suicide (attempt) —*see* Discharge, firearm by type, suicide
Shoving (accidentally) **by other person** —*see* Pushed, by other person
Sickness
  alpine W94.11
  motion —*see* Motion
  mountain W94.11
Sinking (accidental)
  watercraft (causing drowning, submersion) —*see also* Drowning, due to, accident to, watercraft, sinking
    causing injury except drowning or submersion —*see* Accident, watercraft, causing, injury NEC
Siriasis X32
Sitting (prolonged) (static) X50.1
Slashed wrists —*see* Cut, self-inflicted
Slipping (accidental) (on same level) (with fall) W01.0
  without fall W18.40
    due to
      specified NEC W18.49
      stepping from one level to another W18.43
      stepping into hole or opening W18.42
      stepping on object W18.41
  on
    ice W00.0
      with skates —*see* Accident, transport, pedestrian, conveyance
    mud W01.0
    oil W01.0
    snow W00.0
      with skis —*see* Accident, transport, pedestrian, conveyance
    surface (slippery) (wet) NEC W01.0
Sliver, wood, contact with W45.8
Smoldering (due to fire) —*see* Exposure, fire
Sodomy (attempted) **by force** T74.2-●
Sound waves (causing injury) W42.9
  supersonic W42.0
Splinter, contact with W45.8
Stab, stabbing —*see* Cut
Standing (prolonged) (static) X50.1
Starvation X58
Status of external cause Y99.9
  child assisting in compensated work for family Y99.8
  civilian activity done for financial or other compensation Y99.0
  civilian activity done for income or pay Y99.0

Status of external cause (*Continued*)
  family member assisting in compensated work for other family member Y99.8
  hobby not done for income Y99.8
  leisure activity Y99.8
  military activity Y99.1
  off-duty activity of military personnel Y99.8
  recreation or sport not for income or while a student Y99.8
  specified NEC Y99.8
  student activity Y99.8
  volunteer activity Y99.2
Stepped on
  by
    animal (not being ridden) NEC W55.89
    crowd or human stampede W52
    person W50.0
Stepping on
  object W22.8
    with fall W18.31
    sports equipment W21.9
    stationary W22.09
      sports equipment W21.89
  person W51
    by crowd or human stampede W52
  sports equipment W21.9
Sting
  arthropod, nonvenomous W57
  insect, nonvenomous W57
Storm (cataclysmic) —*see* Forces of nature, cataclysmic storm
Straining, excessive —*see also* Overexertion X50.9
Strangling —*see* Strangulation
Strangulation (accidental) —*see* category T71
Strenuous movements —*see also* Overexertion X50.9
Striking against
  airbag (automobile) W22.10
    driver side W22.11
    front passenger side W22.12
    specified NEC W22.19
  bottom when
    diving or jumping into water (in) W16.822
      causing drowning W16.821
      from boat W16.722
        causing drowning W16.721
      natural body W16.622
        causing drowning W16.821
      swimming pool W16.522
        causing drowning W16.521
    falling into water (in) W16.322
      causing drowning W16.321
      fountain —*see* Striking against, bottom when, falling into water, specified NEC
      natural body W16.122
        causing drowning W16.121
      reservoir —*see* Striking against, bottom when, falling into water, specified NEC
      specified NEC W16.322
        causing drowning W16.321
      swimming pool W16.022
        causing drowning W16.021
  diving board (swimming-pool) W21.4
  object W22.8
    with
      drowning or submersion —*see* Drowning
      fall —*see* Fall, due to, bumping against, object
    caused by crowd or human stampede (with fall) W52
    furniture W22.03
    lamppost W22.02
    sports equipment W21.9
    stationary W22.09
      sports equipment W21.89
    wall W22.01

Striking against *(Continued)*
  person(s) W51
    with fall W03
      due to ice or snow W00.0
    as, or caused by, a crowd or human
      stampede (with fall) W52
    assault Y04.2
    homicide (attempt) Y04.2
  sports equipment W21.9
  wall (when) W22.01
    diving or jumping into water (in) W16.832
      causing drowning W16.831
      swimming pool W16.532
        causing drowning W16.531
    falling into water (in) W16.332
      causing drowning W16.331
      fountain —*see* Striking against, wall
        when, falling into water, specified
        NEC
      natural body W16.132
        causing drowning W16.131
      reservoir —*see* Striking against, wall
        when, falling into water, specified
        NEC
      specified NEC W16.332
        causing drowning W16.331
      swimming pool W16.032
        causing drowning W16.031
    swimming pool (when) W22.042
      causing drowning W22.041
      diving or jumping into water W16.532
        causing drowning W16.531
      falling into water W16.032
        causing drowning W16.031
Struck (accidentally) by
  airbag (automobile) W22.10
    driver side W22.11
    front passenger side W22.12
    specified NEC W22.19
  alligator W58.02
  animal (not being ridden) NEC W55.89
  avalanche —*see* Landslide
  ball (hit) (thrown) W21.00
    assault Y08.09
    baseball W21.03
    basketball W21.05
    football W21.01
    golf ball W21.04
    football W21.01
    soccer W21.02
    softball W21.07
    specified NEC W21.09
    volleyball W21.06
  bat or racquet
    baseball bat W21.11
      assault Y08.02
    golf club W21.13
      assault Y08.09
    specified NEC W21.19
      assault Y08.09
    tennis racquet W21.12
      assault Y08.09
  bullet —*see also* Discharge, firearm by type
    in war operations —*see* War operations
  crocodile W58.12
  dog W54.1
  flare, Very pistol —*see* Discharge, firearm
    NEC
  hailstones X39.8
  hockey (ice)
    field
      puck W21.221
      stick W21.211
    puck W21.220
    stick W21.210
      assault Y08.01
  landslide —*see* Landslide
  law-enforcement agent (on duty) —*see* Legal,
    intervention, manhandling
    with blunt object —*see* Legal, intervention,
      blunt object

Struck by *(Continued)*
  lightning —*see* subcategory T75.0
    causing fire —*see* Exposure, fire
  machine —*see* Contact, with, by type of
    machine
  mammal NEC W55.89
    marine W56.32
  marine animal W56.82
  missile
    firearm —*see* Discharge, firearm by type
    in war operations —*see* War operations,
      missile
  object W22.8
    blunt W22.8
      assault Y00
      suicide (attempt) X79
      undetermined whether accidental or
        intentional Y29
    falling W20.8
      from, in, on
        building W20.1
          burning (uncontrolled fire) X00.4
        cataclysmic
          earth surface movement NEC —*see*
            Landslide
          storm —*see* Forces of nature,
            cataclysmic storm
        cave-in W20.0
        earthquake X34
        machine (in operation) —*see* Contact,
          with, by type of machine
        structure W20.1
          burning X00.4
        transport vehicle (in motion) —*see*
          Accident, transport, by type of
          vehicle
        watercraft V93.49
          due to
            accident to craft V91.39
              powered craft V91.33
                ferry boat V91.31
                fishing boat V91.32
                jet ski V91.33
                liner V91.31
                merchant ship V91.30
                passenger ship V91.31
              unpowered craft V91.38
                canoe V91.35
                inflatable V91.36
                kayak V91.35
                sailboat V91.34
                surf-board V91.38
                windsurfer V91.38
            powered craft V93.43
              ferry boat V93.41
              fishing boat V93.42
              jet ski V93.43
              liner V93.41
              merchant ship V93.40
              passenger ship V93.41
            unpowered craft V93.48
              sailboat V93.44
              surf-board V93.48
              windsurfer V93.48
    moving NEC W20.8
    projected W20.8
      assault Y00
      in sports W21.9
        assault Y08.09
        ball W21.00
          baseball W21.03
          basketball W21.05
          football W21.01
          golf ball W21.04
          soccer W21.02
          softball W21.07
          specified NEC W21.09
          volleyball W21.06
        bat or racquet
          baseball bat W21.11
            assault Y08.02

Struck by *(Continued)*
  object *(Continued)*
    projected *(Continued)*
      in sports *(Continued)*
        bat or racquet *(Continued)*
          golf club W21.13
            assault Y08.09-●
          specified NEC W21.19
            assault Y08.09
          tennis racquet W21.12
            assault Y08.09
        hockey (ice)
          field
            puck W21.221
            stick W21.211
          puck W21.220
          stick W21.210
            assault Y08.01
        specified NEC W21.89
    set in motion by explosion —*see* Explosion
    thrown W20.8
      assault Y00
      in sports W21.9
        assault Y08.09
        ball W21.00
          baseball W21.03
          basketball W21.05
          football W21.01
          golf ball W21.04
          soccer W21.02
          soft ball W21.07
          specified NEC W21.09
          volleyball W21.06
        bat or racquet
          baseball bat W21.11
            assault Y08.02
          golf club W21.13
            assault Y08.09
          specified NEC W21.19
            assault Y08.09
          tennis racquet W21.12
            assault Y08.09
        hockey (ice)
          field
            puck W21.221
            stick W21.211
          puck W21.220
          stick W21.210
            assault Y08.01
        specified NEC W21.89
  other person(s) W50.0
    with
      blunt object W22.8
        intentional, homicide (attempt) Y00
        sports equipment W21.9
        undetermined whether accidental or
          intentional Y29
      fall W03
        due to ice or snow W00.0
    as, or caused by, a crowd or human
      stampede (with fall) W52
    assault Y04.2
    homicide (attempt) Y04.2
    in legal intervention
      injuring
        bystander Y35.812
        law enforcement personnel Y35.811
        suspect Y35.813
        unspecified person Y35.819
    sports equipment W21.9
  police (on duty) —*see* Legal, intervention,
    manhandling
    with blunt object —*see* Legal, intervention,
      blunt object
  sports equipment W21.9
    assault Y08.09
    ball W21.00
      baseball W21.03
      basketball W21.05
      football W21.01
      golf ball W21.04
      soccer W21.02

▶ New   ⇒ Revised   ~~deleted~~ Deleted   ● Use Additional Character(s)

Struck by (Continued)
  sports equipment (Continued)
    ball (Continued)
      soft ball W21.07
      specified NEC W21.09
      volleyball W21.06
    bat or racquet
      baseball bat W21.11
        assault Y08.02
      golf club W21.13
        assault Y08.09
      specified NEC W21.19
      tennis racquet W21.12
        assault Y08.09
    cleats (shoe) W21.31
    foot wear NEC W21.39
    football helmet W21.81
    hockey (ice)
      field
        puck W21.221
        stick W21.211
      puck W21.220
      stick W21.210
        assault Y08.01
    skate blades W21.32
    specified NEC W21.89
      assault Y08.09
  thunderbolt —see subcategory
    T75.0
  causing fire —see Exposure, fire
  transport vehicle NEC —see also Accident,
    transport V09.9
    intentional, homicide (attempt) Y03.0
    motor NEC —see also Accident, transport
      V09.20
      homicide Y03.0
  vehicle (transport) NEC —see Accident,
    transport, by type of vehicle
    stationary (falling from jack,
      hydraulic lift, ramp)
      W20.8
Stumbling
  without fall W18.40
    due to
      specified NEC W18.49
      stepping from one level to another
        W18.43
      stepping into hole or opening W18.42
      stepping on object W18.41
  over
    animal NEC W01.0
      with fall W18.09
    carpet, rug or (small) object W22.8
      with fall W18.09
    person W51
      with fall W03
        due to ice or snow W00.0

Submersion (accidental) —see Drowning
Suffocation (accidental) (by external means)
  (by pressure) (mechanical) —see also
    category T71
  due to, by
    avalanche —see Landslide
    explosion —see Explosion
    fire —see Exposure, fire
    food, any type (aspiration) (ingestion)
      (inhalation) —see categories T17 and
      T18
    ignition —see Ignition
    landslide —see Landslide
    machine (ry) —see Contact, with, by type
      of machine
    vomitus (aspiration) (inhalation)
      T17.81-●
  in
    burning building X00.8
Suicide, suicidal (attempted) (by) X83.8
  blunt object X79
  burning, burns X76
    hot object X77.9
      fluid NEC X77.2
      household appliance X77.3
      specified NEC X77.8
      steam X77.0
      tap water X77.1
      vapors X77.0
  caustic substance —see Table of Drugs and
    Chemicals
  cold, extreme X83.2
  collision of motor vehicle with
    motor vehicle X82.0
    specified NEC X82.8
    train X82.1
    tree X82.2
  crashing of aircraft X83.0
  cut (any part of body) X78.9
  cutting or piercing instrument X78.9
    dagger X78.2
    glass X78.0
    knife X78.1
    specified NEC X78.8
    sword X78.2
  drowning (in) X71.9
    bathtub X71.0
    natural water X71.3
    specified NEC X71.8
    swimming pool X71.1
      following fall X71.2
  electrocution X83.1
  explosive(s) (material) X75
  fire, flames X76
  firearm X74.9
    airgun X74.01
    handgun X72

Suicide, suicidal (Continued)
  firearm (Continued)
    hunting rifle X73.1
    larger X73.9
      specified NEC X73.8
    machine gun X73.2
    shotgun X73.0
    specified NEC X74.8
  hanging X83.8
  hot object —see Suicide, burning, hot object
  jumping
    before moving object X81.8
      motor vehicle X81.0
      subway train X81.1
      train X81.1
    from high place X80
  late effect of attempt —see X71-X83 with 7th
    character S
  lying before moving object, train, vehicle X81.8
  poisoning —see Table of Drugs and
    Chemicals
  puncture (any part of body) —see Suicide,
    cutting or piercing instrument
  scald —see Suicide, burning, hot object
  sequelae of attempt —see X71-X83 with 7th
    character S
  sharp object (any) —see Suicide, cutting or
    piercing instrument
  shooting —see Suicide, firearm
  specified means NEC X83.8
  stab (any part of body) —see Suicide, cutting
    or piercing instrument
  steam, hot vapors X77.0
  strangulation X83.8
  submersion —see Suicide, drowning
  suffocation X83.8
  wound NEC X83.8
Sunstroke X32
Supersonic waves (causing injury) W42.0
Surgical procedure, complication of (delayed
  or as an abnormal reaction without
  mention of misadventure) —see also
  Complication of or following, by type of
  procedure
  due to or as a result of misadventure —see
    Misadventure
Swallowed, swallowing
  foreign body —see Foreign body, alimentary
    canal
  poison —see Table of Drugs and Chemicals
  substance
    caustic or corrosive —see Table of Drugs
      and Chemicals
    poisonous —see Table of Drugs and
      Chemicals

S

T

Tackle in sport W03
Terrorism (involving) Y38.80
  biological weapons Y38.6X-●
  chemical weapons Y38.7X-●
  conflagration Y38.3X-●
  drowning and submersion Y38.89-●
  explosion Y38.2X-●
    destruction of aircraft Y38.1X-●
    marine weapons Y38.0X-●
  fire Y38.3X-●
  firearms Y38.4X-●
  hot substances Y38.3X-●
  lasers Y38.89-●
  nuclear weapons Y38.5X-●
  piercing or stabbing instruments
    Y38.89-●
  secondary effects Y38.9X-●
  specified method NEC Y38.89-●
  suicide bomber Y38.81-●
Thirst X58
Threat to breathing
  aspiration —*see* Aspiration
  due to cave-in, falling earth or substance
    NEC —*see* category T71
Thrown (accidentally)
  against part (any) of or object in transport
    vehicle (in motion) NEC —*see also*
    Accident, transport

Thrown (*Continued*)
  from
    high place, homicide (attempt) Y01
    machinery —*see* Contact, with, by type of
      machine
    transport vehicle NEC —*see also* Accident,
      transport V89.9
  off —*see* Thrown, from
Thunderbolt —*see* subcategory T75.0
  causing fire —*see* Exposure, fire
Tidal wave (any injury) NEC —*see* Forces of
  nature, tidal wave
Took
  overdose (drug) —*see* Table of Drugs and
    Chemicals
  poison —*see* Table of Drugs and
    Chemicals
Tornado (any injury) X37.1
Torrential rain (any injury) X37.8
Torture X58
Trampled by animal NEC W55.89
Trapped (accidentally)
  between objects (moving) (stationary and
    moving) —*see* Caught
  by part (any) of
    motorcycle V29.88
    pedal cycle V19.88
    transport vehicle NEC —*see also* Accident,
      transport V89.9
Travel (effects) (sickness) T75.3

Tree falling on or hitting (accidentally)
  (person) W20.8
Tripping
  without fall W18.40
    due to
      specified NEC W18.49
      stepping from one level to another
        W18.43
      stepping into hole or opening
        W18.42
      stepping on object W18.41
  over
    animal W01.0
      with fall W01.0
    carpet, rug or (small) object W22.8
      with fall W18.09
    person W51
      with fall W03
        due to ice or snow W00.0
Twisted by person(s) (accidentally) W50.2
  with intent to injure or kill Y04.0
  as, or caused by, a crowd or human stampede
    (with fall) W52
  assault Y04.0
  homicide (attempt) Y04.0
  in
    fight Y04.0
    legal intervention —*see* Legal, intervention,
      manhandling
Twisting (prolonged) (static) X50.1

U

**Underdosing of necessary drugs, medicaments
  or biological substances** Y63.6
Undetermined intent (contact)
  (exposure)
  automobile collision Y32
  blunt object Y29
  drowning (submersion) (in) Y21.9
    bathtub Y21.0
      after fall Y21.1
    natural water (lake) (ocean) (pond) (river)
      (stream) Y21.4
    specified place NEC Y21.8
    swimming pool Y21.2
      after fall Y21.3
  explosive material Y25
  fall, jump or push from high place Y30
  falling, lying or running before moving object
    Y31
  fire Y26

Undetermined intent (*Continued*)
  firearm discharge Y24.9
    airgun (BB) (pellet) Y24.0
    handgun (pistol) (revolver)
      Y22
    hunting rifle Y23.1
    larger Y23.9
      hunting rifle Y23.1
      machine gun Y23.3
      military Y23.2
      shotgun Y23.0
      specified type NEC Y23.8
    machine gun Y23.3
    military Y23.2
    shotgun Y23.0
    specified type NEC Y24.8
    Very pistol Y24.8
  hot object Y27.9
    fluid NEC Y27.2
    household appliance Y27.3
    specified object NEC Y27.8

Undetermined intent (*Continued*)
  hot object (*Continued*)
    steam Y27.0
    tap water Y27.1
    vapor Y27.0
  jump, fall or push from high place Y30
  lying, falling or running before moving object
    Y31
  motor vehicle crash Y32
  push, fall or jump from high place Y30
  running, falling or lying before moving object
    Y31
  sharp object Y28.9
    dagger Y28.2
    glass Y28.0
    knife Y28.1
    specified object NEC Y28.8
    sword Y28.2
  smoke Y26
  specified event NEC Y33
Use of hand as hammer X50.3

V

Vibration (causing injury) W49.9
Victim (of)
  avalanche —*see* Landslide
  earth movements NEC —*see* Forces of nature,
    earth movement
  earthquake X34

Victim (*Continued*)
  flood —*see* Flood
  landslide —*see* Landslide
  lightning —*see* subcategory T75.0
    causing fire —*see* Exposure, fire
  storm (cataclysmic) NEC —*see* Forces of
    nature, cataclysmic storm
  volcanic eruption X35

Volcanic eruption (any injury) X35
Vomitus, gastric contents in air passages (with
  asphyxia, obstruction or
  suffocation) T17.81-●

▶ New   ⟹ Revised   ~~deleted~~ Deleted   ● Use Additional Character(s)

PART III

ICD-10-CM Tabular List of Diseases and Injuries

CHAPTER 1

CERTAIN INFECTIOUS AND PARASITIC DISEASES (A00-B99)

OGCR Chapter-Specific Coding Guidelines

1. **Chapter 1: Certain Infectious and Parasitic Diseases (A00-B99)**

   a. **Human Immunodeficiency Virus (HIV) Infections**

      1) **Code only confirmed cases**

      Code only confirmed cases of HIV infection/illness. This is an exception to the hospital inpatient guideline Section II, H.

      In this context, "confirmation" does not require documentation of positive serology or culture for HIV; the provider's diagnostic statement that the patient is HIV positive, or has an HIV-related illness is sufficient.

      2) **Selection and sequencing of HIV codes**

         (a) **Patient admitted for HIV-related condition**

         If a patient is admitted for an HIV-related condition, the principal diagnosis should be B20, Human immunodeficiency virus [HIV] disease followed by additional diagnosis codes for all reported HIV-related conditions.

         (b) **Patient with HIV disease admitted for unrelated condition**

         If a patient with HIV disease is admitted for an unrelated condition (such as a traumatic injury), the code for the unrelated condition (e.g., the nature of injury code) should be the principal diagnosis. Other diagnoses would be B20 followed by additional diagnosis codes for all reported HIV-related conditions.

         (c) **Whether the patient is newly diagnosed**

         Whether the patient is newly diagnosed or has had previous admissions/encounters for HIV conditions is irrelevant to the sequencing decision.

         (d) **Asymptomatic human immunodeficiency virus**

         Z21, Asymptomatic human immunodeficiency virus [HIV] infection status, is to be applied when the patient without any documentation of symptoms is listed as being "HIV positive," "known HIV," "HIV test positive," or similar terminology. Do not use this code if the term "AIDS" is used or if the patient is treated for any HIV-related illness or is described as having any condition(s) resulting from his/her HIV positive status; use B20 in these cases.

         (e) **Patients with inconclusive HIV serology**

         Patients with inconclusive HIV serology, but no definitive diagnosis or manifestations of the illness, may be assigned code R75, Inconclusive laboratory evidence of human immunodeficiency virus [HIV].

         (f) **Previously diagnosed HIV-related illness**

         Patients with any known prior diagnosis of an HIV-related illness should be coded to B20. Once a patient has developed an HIV-related illness, the patient should always be assigned code B20 on every subsequent admission/encounter. Patients previously diagnosed with any HIV illness (B20) should never be assigned to R75 or Z21, Asymptomatic human immunodeficiency virus [HIV] infection status.

         (g) **HIV Infection in Pregnancy, Childbirth and the Puerperium**

         During pregnancy, childbirth or the puerperium, a patient admitted (or presenting for a health care encounter) because of an HIV-related illness should receive a principal diagnosis code of O98.7-, Human immunodeficiency virus [HIV] disease complicating pregnancy, childbirth and the puerperium, followed by B20 and the code(s) for the HIV-related illness(es). Codes from Chapter 15 always take sequencing priority.

         Patients with asymptomatic HIV infection status admitted (or presenting for a health care encounter) during pregnancy, childbirth, or the puerperium should receive codes of O98.7- and Z21.

         (h) **Encounters for testing for HIV**

         If a patient is being seen to determine his/her HIV status, use code Z11.4, Encounter for screening for human immunodeficiency virus [HIV]. Use additional codes for any associated high-risk behavior.

         If a patient with signs or symptoms is being seen for HIV testing, code the signs and symptoms. An additional counseling code Z71.7, Human immunodeficiency virus [HIV] counseling, may be used if counseling is provided during the encounter for the test.

         When a patient returns to be informed of his/her HIV test results and the test result is negative, use code Z71.7, Human immunodeficiency virus [HIV] counseling.

If the results are positive, see previous guidelines and assign codes as appropriate.

   b. **Infectious agents as the cause of diseases classified to other chapters**

   Certain infections are classified in chapters other than Chapter 1 and no organism is identified as part of the infection code. In these instances, it is necessary to use an additional code from Chapter 1 to identify the organism. A code from category B95, Streptococcus, Staphylococcus, and Enterococcus as the cause of diseases classified to other chapters, B96, Other bacterial agents as the cause of diseases classified to other chapters, or B97, Viral agents as the cause of diseases classified to other chapters, is to be used as an additional code to identify the organism. An instructional note will be found at the infection code advising that an additional organism code is required.

   c. **Infections resistant to antibiotics**

   Many bacterial infections are resistant to current antibiotics. It is necessary to identify all infections documented as antibiotic resistant. Assign a code from category Z16, Resistance to antimicrobial drugs, following the infection code only if the infection code does not identify drug resistance.

   d. **Sepsis, Severe Sepsis, and Septic Shock**

      1) **Coding of Sepsis and Severe Sepsis**

         (a) **Sepsis**

         For a diagnosis of sepsis, assign the appropriate code for the underlying systemic infection. If the type of infection or causal organism is not further specified, assign code A41.9, Sepsis, unspecified organism.

         A code from subcategory R65.2, Severe sepsis, should not be assigned unless severe sepsis or an associated acute organ dysfunction is documented.

            (i) Negative or inconclusive blood cultures and sepsis

            Negative or inconclusive blood cultures do not preclude a diagnosis of sepsis in patients with clinical evidence of the condition, however, the provider should be queried.

            (ii) Urosepsis

            The term urosepsis is a nonspecific term. It is not to be considered synonymous with sepsis. It has no default code in the Alphabetic Index. Should a provider use this term, he/she must be queried for clarification.

            (iii) Sepsis with organ dysfunction

            If a patient has sepsis and associated acute organ dysfunction or multiple organ dysfunction (MOD), follow the instructions for coding severe sepsis.

            (iv) Acute organ dysfunction that is not clearly associated with the sepsis

            If a patient has sepsis and an acute organ dysfunction, but the medical record documentation indicates that the acute organ dysfunction is related to a medical condition other than the sepsis, do not assign a code from subcategory R65.2, Severe sepsis. An acute organ dysfunction must be associated with the sepsis in order to assign the severe sepsis code. If the documentation is not clear as to whether an acute organ dysfunction is related to the sepsis or another medical condition, query the provider.

         (b) **Severe sepsis**

         The coding of severe sepsis requires a minimum of 2 codes: first a code for the underlying systemic infection, followed by a code from subcategory R65.2, Severe sepsis. If the causal organism is not documented, assign code A41.9, Sepsis, unspecified organism, for the infection. Additional code(s) for the associated acute organ dysfunction are also required.

         Due to the complex nature of severe sepsis, some cases may require querying the provider prior to assignment of the codes.

      2) **Septic shock**

         (a) Septic shock generally refers to circulatory failure associated with severe sepsis, and therefore, it represents a type of acute organ dysfunction.

         For all cases of septic shock, the code for the systemic infection should be sequenced first, followed by code R65.21, Severe sepsis with septic shock or code T81.12, Postprocedural septic shock.

Any additional codes for the other acute organ dysfunctions should also be assigned. As noted in the sequencing instructions in the Tabular List, the code for septic shock cannot be assigned as a principal diagnosis.

3) Sequencing of severe sepsis

If severe sepsis is present on admission, and meets the definition of principal diagnosis, the underlying systemic infection should be assigned as principal diagnosis followed by the appropriate code from subcategory R65.2 as required by the sequencing rules in the Tabular List. A code from subcategory R65.2 can never be assigned as a principal diagnosis.

When severe sepsis develops during an encounter (it was not present on admission) the underlying systemic infection and the appropriate code from subcategory R65.2 should be assigned as secondary diagnoses.

Severe sepsis may be present on admission but the diagnosis may not be confirmed until sometime after admission. If the documentation is not clear whether severe sepsis was present on admission, the provider should be queried.

4) Sepsis and severe sepsis with a localized infection

If the reason for admission is both sepsis or severe sepsis and a localized infection, such as pneumonia or cellulitis, a code(s) for the underlying systemic infection should be assigned first and the code for the localized infection should be assigned as a secondary diagnosis. If the patient has severe sepsis, a code from subcategory R65.2 should also be assigned as a secondary diagnosis. If the patient is admitted with a localized infection, such as pneumonia, and sepsis/severe sepsis doesn't develop until after admission, the localized infection should be assigned first, followed by the appropriate sepsis/severe sepsis codes.

5) Sepsis due to a postprocedural infection

(a) Documentation of causal relationship

As with all postprocedural complications, code assignment is based on the provider's documentation of the relationship between the infection and the procedure.

(b) Sepsis due to a postprocedural infection

For infections following a procedure, a code from T81.40, to T81.43, Infection following a procedure, or O86.00 to O86.03, Infection of obstetric surgical wound, that identifies the site of the infection should be coded first, if known. Assign an additional code for sepsis following a procedure (T81.44) or sepsis following an obstetrical procedure (O86.04). Use an additional code to identify the infectious agent. If the patient has severe sepsis the appropriate code from subcategory R65.2 should also be assigned with the additional code(s) for any acute organ dysfunction.

For infections following infusion, transfusion, therapeutic injection, or immunization, a code from subcategory T80.2, Infections following infusion, transfusion, and therapeutic injection, or code T88.0-, Infection following immunization, should be coded first, followed by the code for the specific Infection. If the patient has severe sepsis, the appropriate code from subcategory R65.2 should also be assigned, with the additional codes(s) for any acute organ dysfunction.

(c) Postprocedural infection and postprocedural septic shock

If a postprocedural infection has resulted in postprocedural septic shock, assign the codes indicated above for sepsis due to a postprocedural infection, followed by code T81.12-, Postprocedural septic shock. Do not assign code R65.21, Severe sepsis with septic shock. Additional code(s) should be assigned for any acute organ dysfunction.

6) Sepsis and severe sepsis associated with a noninfectious process (condition)

In some cases a noninfectious process (condition), such as trauma, may lead to an infection which can result in sepsis or severe sepsis. If sepsis or severe sepsis is documented as associated with a noninfectious condition, such as a burn or serious injury, and this condition meets the definition for principal diagnosis, the code for the noninfectious condition should be sequenced first, followed by the code for the resulting infection. If severe sepsis is present, a code from subcategory R65.2 should also be assigned with any associated organ dysfunction(s) codes. It is not necessary to assign a code from subcategory R65.1, Systemic inflammatory response syndrome (SIRS) of noninfectious origin, for these cases.

If the infection meets the definition of principal diagnosis it should be sequenced before the noninfectious condition. When both the associated noninfectious condition and the infection meet the definition of principal diagnosis either may be assigned as principal diagnosis.

Only one code from category R65, Symptoms and signs specifically associated with systemic inflammation and infection, should be assigned. Therefore, when a noninfectious condition leads to an infection resulting in severe sepsis, assign the appropriate code from subcategory R65.2, Severe sepsis. Do not additionally assign a code from subcategory R65.1, Systemic inflammatory response syndrome (SIRS) of noninfectious origin.
See Section I.C.18. SIRS due to non-infectious process

7) Sepsis and septic shock complicating abortion, pregnancy, childbirth, and the puerperium

See Section I.C.15. Sepsis and septic shock complicating abortion, pregnancy, childbirth and the puerperium

8) Newborn sepsis

See Section I.C.16. f. Bacterial sepsis of Newborn

e. Methicillin Resistant Staphylococcus aureus (MRSA) Conditions

1) Selection and sequencing of MRSA codes

(a) Combination codes for MRSA infection

When a patient is diagnosed with an infection that is due to methicillin resistant *Staphylococcus aureus* (MRSA), and that infection has a combination code that includes the causal organism (e.g., sepsis, pneumonia) assign the appropriate combination code for the condition (e.g., A41.02, Sepsis due to Methicillin resistant Staphylococcus aureus or code J15.212, Pneumonia due to Methicillin resistant Staphylococcus aureus). Do not assign code B95.62, Methicillin resistant Staphylococcus aureus infection as the cause of diseases classified elsewhere, as an additional code because the combination code includes the type of infection and the MRSA organism. Do not assign a code from subcategory Z16.11, Resistance to penicillins, as an additional diagnosis.
See Section C.1. for instructions on coding and sequencing of sepsis and severe sepsis.

(b) Other codes for MRSA infection

When there is documentation of a current infection (e.g., wound infection, stitch abscess, urinary tract infection) due to MRSA, and that infection does not have a combination code that includes the causal organism, assign the appropriate code to identify the condition along with code B95.62, Methicillin resistant Staphylococcus aureus infection as the cause of diseases classified elsewhere for the MRSA infection. Do not assign a code from subcategory Z16.11, Resistance to penicillins.

(c) Methicillin susceptible Staphylococcus aureus (MSSA) and MRSA colonization

The condition or state of being colonized or carrying MSSA or MRSA is called colonization or carriage, while an individual person is described as being colonized or being a carrier. Colonization means that MSSA or MSRA is present on or in the body without necessarily causing illness. A positive MRSA colonization test might be documented by the provider as "MRSA screen positive" or "MRSA nasal swab positive".

Assign code Z22.322, Carrier or suspected carrier of Methicillin resistant Staphylococcus aureus, for patients documented as having MRSA colonization. Assign code Z22.321, Carrier or suspected carrier of Methicillin susceptible Staphylococcus aureus, for patient documented as having MSSA colonization. Colonization is not necessarily indicative of a disease process or as the cause of a specific condition the patient may have unless documented as such by the provider.

(d) MRSA colonization and infection

If a patient is documented as having both MRSA colonization and infection during a hospital admission, code Z22.322, Carrier or suspected carrier of Methicillin resistant Staphylococcus aureus, and a code for the MRSA infection may both be assigned.

f. Zika virus infections

1) Code only confirmed cases

Code only a confirmed diagnosis of Zika virus (A92.5, Zika virus disease) as documented by the provider. This is an exception to the hospital inpatient guideline Section II, H.

In this context, "confirmation" does not require documentation of the type of test performed; the physician's diagnostic statement that the condition is confirmed is sufficient. This code should be assigned regardless of the stated mode of transmission.

If the provider documents "suspected", "possible" or "probable" Zika, do not assign code A92.5. Assign a code(s) explaining the reason for encounter (such as fever, rash, or joint pain) or Z20.821, Contact with and (suspected) exposure to Zika virus.

CHAPTER 1

CERTAIN INFECTIOUS AND PARASITIC DISEASES (A00-B99)

Includes diseases generally recognized as communicable or transmissible

Use additional code to identify resistance to antimicrobial drugs (Z16.-)

Excludes1 certain localized infections - see body system-related chapters

Excludes2 carrier or suspected carrier of infectious disease (Z22.-)

infectious and parasitic diseases complicating pregnancy, childbirth and the puerperium (O98.-)

infectious and parasitic diseases specific to the perinatal period (P35-P39)

influenza and other acute respiratory infections (J00-J22)

This chapter contains the following blocks:

A00-A09	Intestinal infectious diseases
A15-A19	Tuberculosis
A20-A28	Certain zoonotic bacterial diseases
A30-A49	Other bacterial diseases
A50-A64	Infections with a predominantly sexual mode of transmission
A65-A69	Other spirochetal diseases
A70-A74	Other diseases caused by chlamydiae
A75-A79	Rickettsioses
A80-A89	Viral and prion infections of the central nervous system
A90-A99	Arthropod-borne viral fevers and viral hemorrhagic fevers
B00-B09	Viral infections characterized by skin and mucous membrane lesions
B10	Other human herpesviruses
B15-B19	Viral hepatitis
B20	Human immunodeficiency virus [HIV] disease
B25-B34	Other viral diseases
B35-B49	Mycoses
B50-B64	Protozoal diseases
B65-B83	Helminthiases
B85-B89	Pediculosis, acariasis and other infestations
B90-B94	Sequelae of infectious and parasitic diseases
B95-B97	Bacterial and viral infectious agents
B99	Other infectious diseases

INTESTINAL INFECTIOUS DISEASES (A00-A09)

● **A00 Cholera**
A serious, often deadly, infectious disease of the small intestine
Ex: **For category A00 CC codes:** See PDX Collection 2

　A00.0 Cholera due to Vibrio cholerae 01, biovar cholerae
　　Classical cholera

　A00.1 Cholera due to Vibrio cholerae 01, biovar eltor
　　Cholera eltor

　A00.9 Cholera, unspecified

● **A01 Typhoid and paratyphoid fevers**
Caused by Salmonella typhi and Salmonella paratyphi A, B, and C bacteria
Ex: **For category A01 CC codes:** See PDX Collection 3

　● **A01.0 Typhoid fever**
　　Infection due to Salmonella typhi

　　A01.00 Typhoid fever, unspecified

　　A01.01 Typhoid meningitis

　　A01.02 Typhoid fever with heart involvement
　　　Typhoid endocarditis
　　　Typhoid myocarditis

　　A01.03 Typhoid pneumonia

　　A01.04 Typhoid arthritis

　　A01.05 Typhoid osteomyelitis

　　A01.09 Typhoid fever with other complications

　A01.1 Paratyphoid fever A

　A01.2 Paratyphoid fever B

　A01.3 Paratyphoid fever C

　A01.4 Paratyphoid fever, unspecified
　　Infection due to Salmonella paratyphi NOS

● **A02 Other salmonella infections**
　Includes infection or foodborne intoxication due to any Salmonella species other than S. typhi and S. paratyphi

　A02.0 Salmonella enteritis
　　Salmonellosis
　　Ex: See PDX Collection 4

　A02.1 Salmonella sepsis
　　Ex: See PDX Collection 5

　● **A02.2 Localized salmonella infections**

　　A02.20 Localized salmonella infection, unspecified
　　　Specified in the documentation as localized, but unspecified as to type

　　A02.21 Salmonella meningitis
　　　Specified as localized in the meninges
　　　Ex: See PDX Collection 6

　　A02.22 Salmonella pneumonia
　　　Specified as localized in the lungs
　　　Ex: See PDX Collection 7

　　A02.23 Salmonella arthritis
　　　Specified as localized in the joints
　　　Ex: See PDX Collection 8

　　A02.24 Salmonella osteomyelitis
　　　Specified as localized in bone
　　　Ex: See PDX Collection 9

　　A02.25 Salmonella pyelonephritis
　　　Salmonella tubulo-interstitial nephropathy
　　　Ex: See PDX Collection 10

　　A02.29 Salmonella with other localized infection
　　　Specified as localized (because it is still under localized heading) but does not assign into any of the above codes
　　　Ex: See PDX Collection 10

　A02.8 Other specified salmonella infections
　　Any specified salmonella infection which does NOT assign into any of the above codes (not specified as localized)
　　Ex: See PDX Collection 11

　A02.9 Salmonella infection, unspecified
　　Unspecified in the documentation as to specific type of salmonella
　　Ex: See PDX Collection 12

Item 1-1 Salmonella is a bacterium that lives in the intestines of fowl and mammals and can spread to humans through improper food preparation and cooking. Salmonellosis is an infection with the bacterium. Symptoms include diarrhea, fever, and abdominal cramps 12 to 72 hours after infection. The illness usually lasts 4 to 7 days, and most persons recover without treatment. The diarrhea may be so severe that the patient needs to be hospitalized. Patients with immunocompromised systems in chronic, ill health are more likely to have the infection invade their bloodstream with life-threatening results. For example, patients with sickle cell disease are more prone to salmonella osteomyelitis than others.

CHAPTER 1 (A00-B99)

652

▶ New　⇒ Revised　~~deleted~~ Deleted　Excludes 1　Excludes 2　Includes　Use additional　Code first　Code also　Key words
OGCR Official Guidelines　● Unacceptable Principal Diagnosis　X Assign placeholder X　● Use Additional Character(s)　▷ Manifestation Code　Coding Clinic

● **A03   Shigellosis**
An infectious disease caused by bacteria (Shigella)

A03.0   Shigellosis due to Shigella dysenteriae 🐾
Group A shigellosis [Shiga-Kruse dysentery]
(Ex:) See PDX Collection 13

A03.1   Shigellosis due to Shigella flexneri
Group B shigellosis

A03.2   Shigellosis due to Shigella boydii
Group C shigellosis

A03.3   Shigellosis due to Shigella sonnei
Group D shigellosis

A03.8   Other shigellosis

A03.9   Shigellosis, unspecified
Bacillary dysentery NOS

● **A04   Other bacterial intestinal infections**

Excludes1   bacterial foodborne intoxications, NEC (A05.-)
tuberculous enteritis (A18.32)
(Ex:) **For category A04 CC codes A04.0-A04.4:** See PDX Collection 14
For category A04 CC codes A04.5-A04.8: See PDX Collection 15

A04.0   Enteropathogenic Escherichia coli infection 🐾
Pertaining to or producing intestinal disease

A04.1   Enterotoxigenic Escherichia coli infection 🐾
Producing or containing intestinal toxin

A04.2   Enteroinvasive Escherichia coli infection 🐾
*Capable of penetrating and spreading through intestinal
mucosal epithelium*

A04.3   Enterohemorrhagic Escherichia coli infection 🐾
Causing bloody diarrhea, resulting from microorganisms

A04.4   Other intestinal Escherichia coli infections 🐾
Escherichia coli enteritis NOS

A04.5   Campylobacter enteritis 🐾
Spiral shaped bacterium

A04.6   Enteritis due to Yersinia enterocolitica 🐾
Excludes1   extraintestinal yersiniosis (A28.2)
*Transmitted by infected food/water and person-to-person
contact, affecting intestinal tract*

● **A04.7   Enterocolitis due to Clostridium difficile**
Foodborne intoxication by Clostridium difficile
Pseudomembraneous colitis
*Marked by fibrinous deposit (false membrane) with enmeshed
necrotic cells*

**A04.71   Enterocolitis due to Clostridium difficile,
recurrent** 🐾
Coding Clinic: 2020, Q1, P18

**A04.72   Enterocolitis due to Clostridium difficile, not
specified as recurrent** 🐾

A04.8   Other specified bacterial intestinal infections 🐾

A04.9   Bacterial intestinal infection, unspecified 🐾
Bacterial enteritis NOS
(Ex:) See PDX Collection 16

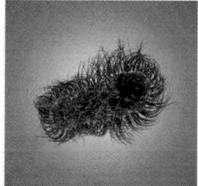

Figure 1-1   Electron micrograph of escherichia coli (E. coli) expressing
P fimbriae. (Getty Image)

Item 1-2   *Escherichia coli [E. coli]* is a Gram-negative bacterium found
in the intestinal tracts of humans and animals and is usually nonpathogenic.
Pathogenic strains can cause diarrhea or pyogenic (pus-producing) infections.
Can be a threat to food safety.

● **A05   Other bacterial foodborne intoxications, not elsewhere classified**
Excludes1   Clostridium difficile foodborne intoxication and
infection (A04.7-)
Escherichia coli infection (A04.0-A04.4)
listeriosis (A32.-)
salmonella foodborne intoxication and infection
(A02.-)
toxic effect of noxious foodstuffs (T61-T62)
(Ex:) **For category A05 CC codes unless otherwise indicated:** See PDX Collection 17

A05.0   Foodborne staphylococcal intoxication 🐾

A05.1   Botulism food poisoning 🐾
Botulism NOS
Classical foodborne intoxication due to Clostridium
botulinum
Excludes1   infant botulism (A48.51)
wound botulism (A48.52)
(Ex:) See PDX Collection 18

**A05.2   Foodborne Clostridium perfringens [Clostridium
welchii] intoxication** 🐾
*Type A causes gas gangrene and necrotizing colitis; major
cause of food poisoning in humans*
Enteritis necroticans
Pig-bel
(Ex:) See PDX Collection 19

A05.3   Foodborne Vibrio parahaemolyticus intoxication 🐾
*Organism that survives only in high salt environment
(halophilic), major cause of gastroenteritis due to
consumption of raw or improperly cooked fish/seafood*

A05.4   Foodborne Bacillus cereus intoxication 🐾
*Spore-forming species commonly found in soil, causes
food poisoning from formation of intestinal toxins in
contaminated foods*

A05.5   Foodborne Vibrio vulnificus intoxication 🐾
*Species that survives in high salt environment (halophilic)
with infection by eating raw seafood causes septicemia
and cellulitis*

A05.8   Other specified bacterial foodborne intoxications 🐾

A05.9   Bacterial foodborne intoxication, unspecified

● **A06   Amebiasis**
*An intestinal illness caused by the microscopic parasite Entamoeba
histolytica*
Includes   infection due to Entamoeba histolytica
Excludes1   other protozoal intestinal diseases (A07.-)
Excludes2   acanthamebiasis (B60.1-)
Naegleriasis (B60.2)

A06.0   Acute amebic dysentery 🐾
Acute amebiasis
Intestinal amebiasis NOS
(Ex:) See PDX Collection 20

A06.1   Chronic intestinal amebiasis 🐾
(Ex:) See PDX Collection 20

A06.2   Amebic nondysenteric colitis 🐾
Pertaining to single cell microorganism
(Ex:) See PDX Collection 21

A06.3   Ameboma of intestine 🐾
*Tumorlike mass produced by localized inflammation often in
intestine*
Ameboma NOS
(Ex:) See PDX Collection 22

A06.4   Amebic liver abscess 🐾
Hepatic amebiasis
(Ex:) See PDX Collection 23

CHAPTER 1 (A00-B99)

N   Newborn Age: 0   P   Pediatric Age: 0-17   M   Maternity DX: 9-64   A   Adult Age: 15-124   ♀   Females Only   ♂   Males Only
🐾 Complication\Comorbidity   🐾 Major C\C   (Ex:) CC/MCC Exclusions   🐾 Hospital-Acquired Condition   🐾 Hierarchical Condition Category

653

A06.5   **Amebic lung abscess** 🅒🅗🅒
     Amebic abscess of lung (and liver)
     (Ex:) See PDX Collection 24

A06.6   **Amebic brain abscess** 🅒
     Amebic abscess of brain (and liver) (and lung)
     (Ex:) See PDX Collection 25

A06.7   **Cutaneous amebiasis**

● **A06.8**   **Amebic infection of other sites**
     (Ex:) **For category A06.8 CC codes: See PDX Collection 22**

     A06.81   **Amebic cystitis** 🅒

     A06.82   **Other amebic genitourinary infections** 🅒
         Amebic balanitis
         Amebic vesiculitis
         Amebic vulvovaginitis

     A06.89   **Other amebic infections** 🅒
         Amebic appendicitis
         Amebic splenic abscess

A06.9   **Amebiasis, unspecified**

● **A07**   **Other protozoal intestinal diseases**
     (Ex:) **For category A07 CC codes unless otherwise indicated: See PDX Collection 26**

     A07.0   **Balantidiasis**
         Balantidial dysentery
         Infection by protozoa that may cause diarrhea and dysentery, with ulceration of colonic mucous membranes

     A07.1   **Giardiasis [lambliasis]** 🅒
         Common infection in small intestine spread by contaminated food, water, or direct person-to-person contact

     A07.2   **Cryptosporidiosis** 🅒🅒
         Human infection with protozoa usually seen as self-limited diarrhea in those who work with cattle

     A07.3   **Isosporiasis** 🅒
         Human intestinal disease caused by protozoa
         Infection due to Isospora belli and Isospora hominis
         Intestinal coccidiosis
         Isosporosis

     A07.4   **Cyclosporiasis** 🅒
         Infection by protozoa with most common species infecting humans being C cayetanensis
         (Ex:) See PDX Collection 27

     A07.8   **Other specified protozoal intestinal diseases** 🅒
         Intestinal microsporidiosis
         Intestinal trichomoniasis
         Sarcocystosis
         Sarcosporidiosis

     A07.9   **Protozoal intestinal disease, unspecified** 🅒
         Flagellate diarrhea
         Protozoal colitis
         Protozoal diarrhea
         Protozoal dysentery

● **A08**   **Viral and other specified intestinal infections**
     Excludes1   influenza with involvement of gastrointestinal tract (J09.X3, J10.2, J11.2)
     (Ex:) **For category A08 CC codes: See PDX Collection 28**

     A08.0   **Rotaviral enteritis** 🅒

●   **A08.1**   **Acute gastroenteropathy due to Norwalk agent and other small round viruses**

     A08.11   **Acute gastroenteropathy due to Norwalk agent** 🅒
         Acute gastroenteropathy due to Norovirus
         Acute gastroenteropathy due to Norwalk-like agent

     A08.19   **Acute gastroenteropathy due to other small round viruses** 🅒
         Acute gastroenteropathy due to small round virus [SRV] NOS

     A08.2   **Adenoviral enteritis** 🅒

● **A08.3**   **Other viral enteritis**

     A08.31   **Calicivirus enteritis** 🅒

     A08.32   **Astrovirus enteritis** 🅒

     A08.39   **Other viral enteritis** 🅒
         Coxsackie virus enteritis
         Echovirus enteritis
         Enterovirus enteritis NEC
         Torovirus enteritis

     A08.4   **Viral intestinal infection, unspecified**
         Viral enteritis NOS
         Viral gastroenteritis NOS
         Viral gastroenteropathy NOS
         Coding Clinic: 2016, Q3, P12

     A08.8   **Other specified intestinal infections**

A09   **Infectious gastroenteritis and colitis, unspecified** 🅒
     Infectious colitis NOS
     Infectious enteritis NOS
     Infectious gastroenteritis NOS

     Excludes1   colitis NOS (K52.9)
         diarrhea NOS (R19.7)
         enteritis NOS (K52.9)
         gastroenteritis NOS (K52.9)
         noninfective gastroenteritis and colitis, unspecified (K52.9)

     (Ex:) See PDX Collection 17

TUBERCULOSIS (A15-A19)

Includes	infections due to Mycobacterium tuberculosis and Mycobacterium bovis
Excludes1	congenital tuberculosis (P37.0) nonspecific reaction to test for tuberculosis without active tuberculosis (R76.1-) pneumoconiosis associated with tuberculosis, any type in A15 (J65) positive PPD (R76.11) positive tuberculin skin test without active tuberculosis (R76.11) sequelae of tuberculosis (B90.-) silicotuberculosis (J65)

● **A15**   **Respiratory tuberculosis**
     (Ex:) **For category A15 CC codes unless otherwise indicated: See PDX Collection 29**

     A15.0   **Tuberculosis of lung** 🅒
         Tuberculous bronchiectasis
         Chronic dilatation of bronchi
         Tuberculous fibrosis of lung
         Tuberculous pneumonia
         Tuberculous pneumothorax

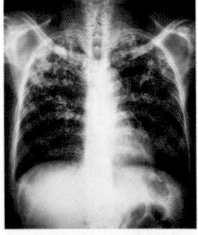

Figure 1-2   Far advanced bilateral pulmonary tuberculosis before and after 8 months of treatment with streptomycin, PAS, and isoniazid. (Getty Image)

Item 1-3 Tuberculosis is a common and deadly infectious disease caused by the *Mycobacterium tuberculosis* organism. The first tuberculosis infection is called the **primary infection** and most commonly attacks the lungs but can affect the central nervous system, lymphatic system, circulatory system, genitourinary system, bones, joints, and even the skin. A **Ghon** lesion is the **initial lesion.** A **secondary lesion** occurs when the tubercle bacilli are carried to other areas.

CHAPTER 1 (A00-B99)

654

▶ New   ⇒ Revised   ~~deleted~~ Deleted   Excludes 1   Excludes 2   Includes   Use additional   Code first   Code also   Key words

OGCR Official Guidelines   ● Unacceptable Principal Diagnosis   X Assign placeholder X   ● Use Additional Character(s)   ▶ Manifestation Code   **Coding Clinic**

Item 1–4 Although it primarily affects the lungs, the bacteria *Mycobacterium tuberculosis* can travel from the pulmonary circulation to virtually any organ in the body, much as a cancer metastasizes to a secondary site. If the immune system becomes compromised by age or disease, what would otherwise be a self-limiting primary tuberculosis in the lungs will develop in other organs. These are known as extrapulmonary sites.

A15.4 Tuberculosis of intrathoracic lymph nodes 🅗
  Tuberculosis of hilar lymph nodes
  Tuberculosis of mediastinal lymph nodes
  Tuberculosis of tracheobronchial lymph nodes
    Excludes1 tuberculosis specified as primary (A15.7)

A15.5 Tuberculosis of larynx, trachea and bronchus 🅗
  Tuberculosis of bronchus
  Tuberculosis of glottis
  Tuberculosis of larynx
  Tuberculosis of trachea

A15.6 Tuberculous pleurisy 🅗
  Tuberculosis of pleura
  Tuberculous empyema
    Excludes1 primary respiratory tuberculosis (A15.7)

A15.7 Primary respiratory tuberculosis 🅗
  (Ex:) See PDX Collection 30

A15.8 Other respiratory tuberculosis 🅗
  Mediastinal tuberculosis
  Nasopharyngeal tuberculosis
  Tuberculosis of nose
  Tuberculosis of sinus [any nasal]
  (Ex:) See PDX Collection 31

A15.9 Respiratory tuberculosis unspecified 🅗
  (Ex:) See PDX Collection 31

●**A17 Tuberculosis of nervous system**
  A17.0 Tuberculous meningitis 🅗
    Tuberculosis of meninges (cerebral) (spinal)
    Tuberculous leptomeningitis
      Excludes1 tuberculous meningoencephalitis
                    (A17.82)
    (Ex:) See PDX Collection 32

  A17.1 Meningeal tuberculoma 🅗
    Tuberculoma of meninges (cerebral) (spinal)
      Excludes2 tuberculoma of brain and spinal cord
                    (A17.81)
    (Ex:) See PDX Collection 32

  ●**A17.8 Other tuberculosis of nervous system**
    A17.81 Tuberculoma of brain and spinal cord 🅗
      Tuberculous abscess of brain and spinal cord
      (Ex:) See PDX Collection 33

    A17.82 Tuberculous meningoencephalitis 🅗
      Inflammation of brain and meninges; AKA
        cerebromeningitis and encephalomeningitis
      Tuberculous myelitis
      (Ex:) See PDX Collection 33

    A17.83 Tuberculous neuritis 🅗
      Tuberculous mononeuropathy
      (Ex:) See PDX Collection 3209

    A17.89 Other tuberculosis of nervous system 🅗
      Tuberculous polyneuropathy
      (Ex:) See PDX Collection 34

  A17.9 Tuberculosis of nervous system, unspecified 🅗
    (Ex:) See PDX Collection 35

●**A18 Tuberculosis of other organs**
  ●**A18.0 Tuberculosis of bones and joints**
    A18.01 Tuberculosis of spine 🅗
      Pott's disease or curvature of spine
      Tuberculous arthritis
      Tuberculous osteomyelitis of spine
      Tuberculous spondylitis
      (Ex:) See PDX Collection 36

    A18.02 Tuberculous arthritis of other joints 🅗
      Tuberculosis of hip (joint)
      Tuberculosis of knee (joint)
      (Ex:) See PDX Collection 37

    A18.03 Tuberculosis of other bones 🅗
      Tuberculous mastoiditis
      Tuberculous osteomyelitis
      (Ex:) See PDX Collection 38

    A18.09 Other musculoskeletal tuberculosis 🅗
      Tuberculous myositis
      Tuberculous synovitis
      Tuberculous tenosynovitis
      (Ex:) See PDX Collection 39

  ●**A18.1 Tuberculosis of genitourinary system**
    A18.10 Tuberculosis of genitourinary system, unspecified 🅗
      (Ex:) See PDX Collection 40

    A18.11 Tuberculosis of kidney and ureter 🅗
      (Ex:) See PDX Collection 41

    A18.12 Tuberculosis of bladder 🅗
      (Ex:) See PDX Collection 41

    A18.13 Tuberculosis of other urinary organs 🅗
      Tuberculous urethritis
      (Ex:) See PDX Collection 41

    A18.14 Tuberculosis of prostate ♂ 🅗   **A**
      (Ex:) See PDX Collection 42

    A18.15 Tuberculosis of other male genital organs ♂ 🅗
      (Ex:) See PDX Collection 42

    A18.16 Tuberculosis of cervix ♀ 🅗
      (Ex:) See PDX Collection 43

    A18.17 Tuberculous female pelvic inflammatory disease ♀ 🅗
      Tuberculous endometritis
      Tuberculous oophoritis and salpingitis
        Oophoritis = inflammation of ovary
        Salpingitis = inflammation of fallopian tube
      (Ex:) See PDX Collection 43

    A18.18 Tuberculosis of other female genital organs ♀ 🅗
      Tuberculous ulceration of vulva
      (Ex:) See PDX Collection 43

  A18.2 Tuberculous peripheral lymphadenopathy 🅗
    Tuberculous adenitis
      Excludes2 tuberculosis of bronchial and mediastinal
                    lymph nodes (A15.4)
                    tuberculosis of mesenteric and
                    retroperitoneal lymph nodes
                    (A18.39)
                    tuberculous tracheobronchial adenopathy
                    (A15.4)
    (Ex:) See PDX Collection 44

  ●**A18.3 Tuberculosis of intestines, peritoneum and mesenteric glands**
    (Ex:) **For category A18.3 CC codes:** See PDX Collection 45

    A18.31 Tuberculous peritonitis 🅗
      Tuberculous ascites

    A18.32 Tuberculous enteritis 🅗
      Tuberculosis of anus and rectum
      Tuberculosis of intestine (large) (small)

    A18.39 Retroperitoneal tuberculosis 🅗
      Tuberculosis of mesenteric glands
      Tuberculosis of retroperitoneal (lymph glands)

CHAPTER 1 (A00-B99)

N Newborn Age: 0   **P** Pediatric Age: 0–17   **M** Maternity DX: 9–64   **A** Adult Age: 15–124   ♀ Females Only   ♂ Males Only
🅗 Complication\Comorbidity   🅗 Major C\C   (Ex:) CC/MCC Exclusions   🅗 Hospital-Acquired Condition   🅗 Hierarchical Condition Category

A18.4   **Tuberculosis of** `skin and subcutaneous tissue` 🔎
    Erythema induratum, tuberculous
    Lupus excedens
    Lupus vulgaris NOS
    Lupus vulgaris of eyelid
       Cutaneous tuberculosis characterized by reddish brown
        plaque on skin surrounded by papules and nodules
    Scrofuloderma
       Type of cutaneous tuberculosis, with direct extension of
        tuberculosis into skin from underlying structures;
        AKA tuberculosis colliquativa
    Tuberculosis of external ear
    Excludes2 lupus erythematosus (L93.-)
               systemic lupus erythematosus (M32.-)
    (Ex:) See PDX Collection 30

● A18.5   **Tuberculosis of** `eye`
    Excludes2 lupus vulgaris of eyelid (A18.4)
    (Ex:) For category A18.5 CC codes: See PDX Collection 46

    A18.50   **Tuberculosis of eye,** `unspecified` 🔎

    A18.51   **Tuberculous** `episcleritis` 🔎
        Inflammation of episclera and adjacent tissues

    A18.52   **Tuberculous** `keratitis` 🔎
        Tuberculous interstitial keratitis
        Tuberculous keratoconjunctivitis (interstitial)
          (phlyctenular)
        Inflammation of cornea and conjunctiva

    A18.53   **Tuberculous** `chorioretinitis` 🔎
        Inflammation of choroid and retina;
         retinochoroiditis

    A18.54   **Tuberculous** `iridocyclitis` 🔎
        Inflammation of iris and ciliary body

    A18.59   **Other tuberculosis of eye** 🔎
        Tuberculous conjunctivitis

A18.6   **Tuberculosis of (inner) (middle)** `ear` 🔎
    Tuberculous otitis media
    Excludes2 tuberculosis of external ear (A18.4)
               tuberculous mastoiditis (A18.03)
    (Ex:) See PDX Collection 47

A18.7   **Tuberculosis of** `adrenal glands` 🔎
    Tuberculous Addison's disease
    (Ex:) See PDX Collection 48

● A18.8   **Tuberculosis of** `other` **specified organs**

    A18.81   **Tuberculosis of** `thyroid gland` 🔎
        (Ex:) See PDX Collection 49

    A18.82   **Tuberculosis of other** `endocrine glands` 🔎
        Tuberculosis of pituitary gland
        Tuberculosis of thymus gland
        (Ex:) See PDX Collection 35

    A18.83   **Tuberculosis of** `digestive tract organs`, **not**
        elsewhere classified 🔎
        Excludes1 tuberculosis of intestine (A18.32)
        (Ex:) See PDX Collection 45

    A18.84   **Tuberculosis of** `heart` 🔎
        Tuberculous cardiomyopathy
        Tuberculous endocarditis
        Tuberculous myocarditis
        Tuberculous pericarditis
        (Ex:) See PDX Collection 35

    A18.85   **Tuberculosis of** `spleen` 🔎
        (Ex:) See PDX Collection 50

    A18.89   **Tuberculosis of** `other sites` 🔎
        Tuberculosis of muscle
        Tuberculous cerebral arteritis
        (Ex:) See PDX Collection 35

Item 1–5   Miliary tuberculosis can be a life-threatening condition. If a tuberculous lesion enters a blood vessel, immense dissemination of tuberculous organisms can occur if the immune system is weak. High-risk populations—children under 4 years of age, the elderly, or the immunocompromised—are particularly prone to this type of infection. The lesions will have a millet seedlike appearance on chest x-ray. Bronchial washings and biopsy may aid in diagnosis.

● A19   **Miliary tuberculosis**
    Includes   disseminated tuberculosis
                generalized tuberculosis
                tuberculous polyserositis
    (Ex:) For category A19 CC codes: See PDX Collection 51

    A19.0   Acute miliary tuberculosis of a `single` specified site 🔎
    A19.1   Acute miliary tuberculosis of `multiple sites` 🔎
    A19.2   Acute miliary tuberculosis, `unspecified` 🔎
    A19.8   `Other` miliary tuberculosis 🔎
    A19.9   Miliary tuberculosis, `unspecified` 🔎

CERTAIN ZOONOTIC BACTERIAL DISEASES (A20-A28)

● A20   **Plague**
    Infectious disease caused by a Yersinia pestis bacterium, transmitted
    by a rodent flea bite or handling of infected animal
    Includes   infection due to Yersinia pestis

    A20.0   **Bubonic plague** 🔎
        (Ex:) See PDX Collection 52

    A20.1   **Cellulocutaneous plague** 🔎
        Skin and subcutaneous tissue plague
        (Ex:) See PDX Collection 52

    A20.2   **Pneumonic plague** 🔎 🔎
        (Ex:) See PDX Collection 53

    A20.3   **Plague** `meningitis` 🔎
        (Ex:) See PDX Collection 54

    A20.7   **Septicemic plague** 🔎 🔎
        (Ex:) See PDX Collection 55

    A20.8   **Other forms of plague** 🔎
        Abortive plague
        Asymptomatic plague
        Pestis minor
        Systemic bacterial disease
        (Ex:) See PDX Collection 54

    A20.9   **Plague,** `unspecified` 🔎
        (Ex:) See PDX Collection 56

● A21   **Tularemia**
    Caused by Francisella tularensis bacterium found in rodents, rabbits,
    and hares and transmitted to humans by contact with infected
    animal tissues or by ticks, biting flies, or mosquitoes
    Includes   deer-fly fever
                infection due to Francisella tularensis
                rabbit fever
    Coding Clinic: 2016, Q4, P25

    A21.0   **Ulceroglandular tularemia** 🔎
        Most common form of tularemia in humans is painful,
         swollen, erythematous papule at point of inoculation
         that ruptures to form shallow ulcer
        (Ex:) See PDX Collection 57

    A21.1   **Oculoglandular tularemia** 🔎
        Primary site of entry is conjunctival sac, results in
         granulomatous corneal lesions
        Ophthalmic tularemia
        (Ex:) See PDX Collection 58

    A21.2   **Pulmonary tularemia** 🔎 🔎
        (Ex:) See PDX Collection 59

A21.3   **Gastrointestinal tularemia** 🦠
     Abdominal tularemia
     (Ex:) See PDX Collection 60

A21.7   **Generalized tularemia** 🦠
     (Ex:) See PDX Collection 61

A21.8   **Other forms of tularemia** 🦠
     (Ex:) See PDX Collection 61

A21.9   **Tularemia, unspecified** 🦠
     (Ex:) See PDX Collection 61

● **A22**   **Anthrax**
     An acute infectious disease caused by the spore-forming Bacillus
     anthracis; occurs in humans exposed to infected animals or
     tissue from infected animals
     Includes   infection due to Bacillus anthracis

A22.0   **Cutaneous anthrax** 🦠
     Malignant carbuncle
     Malignant pustule
     (Ex:) See PDX Collection 62

A22.1   **Pulmonary anthrax** 🦠🦠
     Inhalation anthrax
     Ragpicker's disease
     Woolsorter's disease
     (Ex:) See PDX Collection 63

A22.2   **Gastrointestinal anthrax** 🦠
     (Ex:) See PDX Collection 64

A22.7   **Anthrax sepsis** 🦠🦠
     Infectious bacterial disease
     MCC when PDx is its own MCC
     (Ex:) See PDX Collection 5

A22.8   **Other forms of anthrax** 🦠
     Anthrax meningitis
     (Ex:) See PDX Collection 65

A22.9   **Anthrax, unspecified** 🦠
     (Ex:) See PDX Collection 66

● **A23**   **Brucellosis**
     Includes   Malta fever
                Mediterranean fever
                undulant fever

A23.0   **Brucellosis due to Brucella melitensis**
     Resulting in flu-like symptoms that may lead to chronic
     symptoms that include recurrent fevers, joint pain, and
     fatigue

A23.1   **Brucellosis due to Brucella abortus**
     Most common cause of brucellosis in humans; AKA Bang
     bacillus

A23.2   **Brucellosis due to Brucella suis**
     Species found primarily in pigs, rabbits, and reindeer

A23.3   **Brucellosis due to Brucella canis**
     Species that causes respiratory tract infection in humans

A23.8   **Other brucellosis** 🦠
     (Ex:) See PDX Collection 67

A23.9   **Brucellosis, unspecified** 🦠
     (Ex:) See PDX Collection 67

● **A24**   **Glanders and melioidosis**
     Infection, usually of rodents, which spreads to other animals and
     humans, caused by Burkholderia pseudomallei through break
     in skin contaminated with infested soil or water
     (Ex:) **For category A24 CC codes unless otherwise indicated:** See PDX Collection 69

A24.0   **Glanders** 🦠
     Infection due to Pseudomonas mallei
     Malleus
     (Ex:) See PDX Collection 68

A24.1   **Acute and fulminating melioidosis** 🦠
     Melioidosis pneumonia
     Melioidosis sepsis

A24.2   **Subacute and chronic melioidosis** 🦠

A24.3   **Other melioidosis** 🦠

A24.9   **Melioidosis, unspecified** 🦠
     Infection due to Pseudomonas pseudomallei NOS
     Whitmore's disease

● **A25**   **Rat-bite fevers**
     RBF, infectious disease caused by Streptobacillus moniliformis or
     Spirillum minus.
     (Ex:) **For category A25 CC codes:** See PDX Collection 70

A25.0   **Spirillosis** 🦠
     Any disease condition caused by spirilla
     Sodoku

A25.1   **Streptobacillosis** 🦠
     Acute, febrile human illness caused by bacteria transmitted
     by rats in most cases, passed from rodent to human via
     rodent's urine or mucous secretions; AKA rat fever
     Epidemic arthritic erythema
     Haverhill fever
     Streptobacillary rat-bite fever

A25.9   **Rat-bite fever, unspecified** 🦠

● **A26**   **Erysipeloid**
     Infection with Erysipelothrix rhusiopathiae, occurring often as
     occupational disease resulting from handling infected fish,
     shellfish, meat, or poultry

A26.0   **Cutaneous erysipeloid**
     Erythema migrans

A26.7   **Erysipelothrix sepsis** 🦠🦠
     MCC when PDx is its own MCC
     (Ex:) See PDX Collection 71

A26.8   **Other forms of erysipeloid**

A26.9   **Erysipeloid, unspecified**

● **A27**   **Leptospirosis**
     Occurs most commonly in the tropics
     (Ex:) **For category A27 CC codes unless otherwise indicated:** See PDX Collection 72

A27.0   **Leptospirosis icterohemorrhagica** 🦠
     Leptospiral or spirochetal jaundice (hemorrhagic)
     Weil's disease

● **A27.8**   **Other forms of leptospirosis**

     A27.81   **Aseptic meningitis in leptospirosis** 🦠
              (Ex:) See PDX Collection 73

     A27.89   **Other forms of leptospirosis** 🦠

A27.9   **Leptospirosis, unspecified** 🦠

● **A28**   **Other zoonotic bacterial diseases, not elsewhere classified**
     (Ex:) **For category A28 CC codes unless otherwise indicated:** See PDX Collection 74

A28.0   **Pasteurellosis** 🦠
     Infection of humans or other animals by species of
     Pasteurella

A28.1   **Cat-scratch disease** 🦠
     Cat-scratch fever
     (Ex:) See PDX Collection 75

A28.2   **Extraintestinal yersiniosis** 🦠
     Infection from Yersinia enterocolitica; AKA enteric
     yersiniosis, intestinal yersiniosis, Yersinia enteritis
     Excludes1   enteritis due to Yersinia enterocolitica
                      (A04.6)
                      plague (A20.-)

A28.8   **Other specified zoonotic bacterial diseases, not elsewhere classified** 🦠

A28.9   **Zoonotic bacterial disease, unspecified** 🦠

Item 1-6 Brucellosis: An infectious disease caused by the bacterium Brucella. Humans are infected by contact with contaminated animals or animal products. In humans brucellosis symptoms that are similar to the flu include fever, sweats, headaches, back pains, and physical weakness. Severe infections of the central nervous system or lining of the heart may occur. Brucellosis can also cause chronic symptoms that include recurrent fevers, joint pain, and fatigue.

N   Newborn Age: 0   **P**   Pediatric Age: 0–17   **M**   Maternity DX: 9–64   **A**   Adult Age: 15–124   ♀   Females Only   ♂   Males Only

🦠   Complication\Comorbidity   🦠   Major C\C   (Ex:)   CC/MCC Exclusions   🦠   Hospital-Acquired Condition   🦠   Hierarchical Condition Category

CHAPTER 1 (A00-B99)

OTHER BACTERIAL DISEASES (A30-A49)

● **A30 Leprosy [Hansen's disease]**
Chronic infectious disease attacking the skin, peripheral nerves, and mucous membranes

> **Includes**   infection due to Mycobacterium leprae
> **Excludes1**   sequelae of leprosy (B92)

A30.0 Indeterminate leprosy 🔖
I leprosy
(Ex:) See PDX Collection 76

A30.1 Tuberculoid leprosy 🔖
TT leprosy
(Ex:) See PDX Collection 77

A30.2 Borderline tuberculoid leprosy 🔖
BT leprosy
(Ex:) See PDX Collection 78

A30.3 Borderline leprosy 🔖
BB leprosy
(Ex:) See PDX Collection 78

A30.4 Borderline lepromatous leprosy 🔖
BL leprosy
(Ex:) See PDX Collection 78

A30.5 Lepromatous leprosy 🔖
LL leprosy
(Ex:) See PDX Collection 79

A30.8 Other forms of leprosy 🔖
(Ex:) See PDX Collection 80

A30.9 Leprosy, unspecified 🔖
(Ex:) See PDX Collection 81

● **A31 Infection due to other mycobacteria**

> **Excludes2**   leprosy (A30.-)
>   tuberculosis (A15-A19)

(Ex:) **For category A31 CC codes unless otherwise indicated:** See PDX Collection 83

A31.0 Pulmonary mycobacterial infection 🔖 🅡🅒🅒
Infection due to Mycobacterium avium
Infection due to Mycobacterium intracellulare [Battey bacillus]
Infection due to Mycobacterium kansasii
(Ex:) See PDX Collection 82

A31.1 Cutaneous mycobacterial infection 🔖
Buruli ulcer
Infection due to Mycobacterium marinum
Infection due to Mycobacterium ulcerans

A31.2 Disseminated mycobacterium avium-intracellulare complex (DMAC) 🔖 🅡🅒🅒
MAC sepsis

A31.8 Other mycobacterial infections 🔖

A31.9 Mycobacterial infection, unspecified 🔖
Atypical mycobacterial infection NOS
Mycobacteriosis NOS

● **A32 Listeriosis**
Infection caused by Listeria monocytogenes

> **Includes**   listerial foodborne infection
> **Excludes1**   neonatal (disseminated) listeriosis (P37.2)

(Ex:) **For category A32 CC codes unless otherwise indicated:** See PDX Collection 74

A32.0 Cutaneous listeriosis 🔖

● **A32.1 Listerial meningitis and meningoencephalitis**

A32.11 Listerial meningitis 🔖

A32.12 Listerial meningoencephalitis 🔖

A32.7 Listerial sepsis 🔖 🅡🅒🅒
MCC when PDx is its own MCC
(Ex:) See PDX Collection 71

A32.8 Other forms of listeriosis

A32.81 Oculoglandular listeriosis 🔖
Primary infection site is conjunctival sac, which if untreated may result in perforation of cornea and optic atrophy

A32.82 Listerial endocarditis 🔖
Exudative and proliferative inflammatory condition of endocardium caused by listeria bacteria

A32.89 Other forms of listeriosis 🔖
Listerial cerebral arteritis

A32.9 Listeriosis, unspecified 🔖

A33 Tetanus neonatorum 🔖   N
Neonate = newborn
(Ex:) See PDX Collection 84

A34 Obstetrical tetanus ♀ 🔖   M
(Ex:) See PDX Collection 85

A35 Other tetanus 🔖
Tetanus NOS

> **Excludes1**   tetanus neonatorum (A33)
>   obstetrical tetanus (A34)

(Ex:) See PDX Collection 86

● **A36 Diphtheria**
(Ex:) **For category A36 CC codes unless otherwise indicated:** See PDX Collection 87

A36.0 Pharyngeal diphtheria 🔖
Diphtheritic membranous angina
Tonsillar diphtheria

A36.1 Nasopharyngeal diphtheria 🔖

A36.2 Laryngeal diphtheria 🔖
Diphtheritic laryngotracheitis

A36.3 Cutaneous diphtheria 🔖

> **Excludes2**   erythrasma (L08.1)

● **A36.8 Other diphtheria**

A36.81 Diphtheritic cardiomyopathy 🔖 🅡🅒🅒
Diphtheritic myocarditis
(Ex:) See PDX Collection 88

A36.82 Diphtheritic radiculomyelitis 🔖

A36.83 Diphtheritic polyneuritis 🔖

A36.84 Diphtheritic tubulo-interstitial nephropathy 🔖

A36.85 Diphtheritic cystitis 🔖

A36.86 Diphtheritic conjunctivitis 🔖

A36.89 Other diphtheritic complications 🔖
Diphtheritic peritonitis

A36.9 Diphtheria, unspecified 🔖

● **A37 Whooping cough**
Pertussis is a highly contagious disease caused by the bacterium Bordetella pertussis and results in a whooping sounding cough.
(Ex:) **For category A37 CC codes A37.00, A37.10, A37.80, A37.90:** See PDX Collection 89
For category A37 CC codes A37.01, A37.11, A37.81, A37.91: See PDX Collection 90

● **A37.0 Whooping cough due to Bordetella pertussis**

A37.00 Whooping cough due to Bordetella pertussis without pneumonia 🔖
▶ Paroxysmal cough due to Bordetella pertussis without pneumonia

A37.01 Whooping cough due to Bordetella pertussis with pneumonia 🔖
▶ Paroxysmal cough due to Bordetella pertussis without pneumonia

MCC when PDx is its own MCC

> **Item 1-7 Diphtheria:** A highly contagious bacterial disease that results in the formation of an adherent membrane in the throat that may lead to suffocation. In its most poisonous form, it attacks the heart and lungs. It is spread by direct physical contact or breathing the aerosolized secretions of infected individuals. The exact location is specified in the codes.

▶ New   ⟹ Revised   ~~deleted~~ Deleted   Excludes 1   Excludes 2   Includes   Use additional   Code first   Code also   Key words

OGCR Official Guidelines   ● Unacceptable Principal Diagnosis   X Assign placeholder X   ● Use Additional Character(s)   ▶ Manifestation Code   **Coding Clinic**

658

● **A37.1 Whooping cough due to Bordetella parapertussis**
     A37.10 Whooping cough due to Bordetella parapertussis without pneumonia 🦠
     A37.11 Whooping cough due to Bordetella parapertussis with pneumonia 🦠
         MCC when PDx is its own MCC

● **A37.8 Whooping cough due to other Bordetella species**
     A37.80 Whooping cough due to other Bordetella species without pneumonia 🦠
     A37.81 Whooping cough due to other Bordetella species with pneumonia 🦠
         MCC when PDx is its own MCC

● **A37.9 Whooping cough, unspecified species**
     A37.90 Whooping cough, unspecified species without pneumonia 🦠
     A37.91 Whooping cough, unspecified species with pneumonia 🦠
         MCC when PDx is its own MCC

● **A38 Scarlet fever**
     Most commonly caused by the bacteria Streptococcus pneumoniae and Neisseria meningitides
     Includes   scarlatina
     Excludes2   streptococcal sore throat (J02.0)
     Ⓔⓧ **For category A38 CC codes:** See PDX Collection 91
     A38.0 Scarlet fever with otitis media 🦠
     A38.1 Scarlet fever with myocarditis 🦠
     A38.8 Scarlet fever with other complications 🦠
     A38.9 Scarlet fever, uncomplicated 🦠
         Scarlet fever, NOS

● **A39 Meningococcal infection**
     Most commonly caused by the bacteria Streptococcus pneumoniae and Neisseria meningitides
     A39.0 Meningococcal meningitis 🦠
         Ⓔⓧ See PDX Collection 92
     A39.1 Waterhouse-Friderichsen syndrome 🦠🦠
         Fulminating complication of meningococcemia
         Meningococcal hemorrhagic adrenalitis
         Meningococcic adrenal syndrome
         Ⓔⓧ See PDX Collection 93
     A39.2 Acute meningococcemia 🦠🦠
         Ⓔⓧ See PDX Collection 94
     A39.3 Chronic meningococcemia 🦠🦠
         Ⓔⓧ See PDX Collection 94
     A39.4 Meningococcemia, unspecified 🦠🦠
         Ⓔⓧ See PDX Collection 94

● **A39.5 Meningococcal heart disease**
     A39.50 Meningococcal carditis, unspecified 🦠
         Ⓔⓧ See PDX Collection 95
     A39.51 Meningococcal endocarditis 🦠
         Ⓔⓧ See PDX Collection 96
     A39.52 Meningococcal myocarditis 🦠
         Ⓔⓧ See PDX Collection 97
     A39.53 Meningococcal pericarditis 🦠
         Ⓔⓧ See PDX Collection 98

● **A39.8 Other meningococcal infections**
     A39.81 Meningococcal encephalitis 🦠
         Ⓔⓧ See PDX Collection 99
     A39.82 Meningococcal retrobulbar neuritis 🦠
         Optic neuritis in portion of optic nerve posterior to eyeball; AKA postocular optic neuritis
         Ⓔⓧ See PDX Collection 100
     A39.83 Meningococcal arthritis 🦠🦠
         Ⓔⓧ See PDX Collection 101

     A39.84 Postmeningococcal arthritis 🦠🦠
         Ⓔⓧ See PDX Collection 101
     A39.89 Other meningococcal infections 🦠
         Meningococcal conjunctivitis
         Ⓔⓧ See PDX Collection 102
   A39.9 Meningococcal infection, unspecified 🦠
         Meningococcal disease NOS
         Ⓔⓧ See PDX Collection 102

● **A40 Streptococcal sepsis**
     Code first
         postprocedural streptococcal sepsis (T81.44)
         streptococcal sepsis during labor (O75.3)
         streptococcal sepsis following abortion or ectopic or molar pregnancy (O03-O07, O08.0)
         streptococcal sepsis following immunization (T88.0)
         streptococcal sepsis following infusion, transfusion or therapeutic injection (T80.2-)
     Excludes1   neonatal (P36.0-P36.1)
         puerperal sepsis (O85)
         sepsis due to Streptococcus, group D (A41.81)
     Ⓔⓧ **For category A40 CC codes unless otherwise indicated:** See PDX Collection 71
   A40.0 Sepsis due to streptococcus, group A 🦠🦠
   A40.1 Sepsis due to streptococcus, group B 🦠🦠
         Coding Clinic: 2019, Q1, P14
   A40.3 Sepsis due to Streptococcus pneumoniae 🦠🦠
         Pneumococcal sepsis
         Ⓔⓧ See PDX Collection 3210
   A40.8 Other streptococcal sepsis 🦠🦠
   A40.9 Streptococcal sepsis, unspecified 🦠🦠

● **A41 Other sepsis**
     Code first
         postprocedural sepsis (T81.44)
         sepsis during labor (O75.3)
         sepsis following abortion, ectopic or molar pregnancy (O03-O07, O08.0)
         sepsis following immunization (T88.0)
         sepsis following infusion, transfusion or therapeutic injection (T80.2-)
     Excludes1   bacteremia NOS (R78.81)
         neonatal (P36.-)
         puerperal sepsis (O85)
         streptococcal sepsis (A40.-)
     Excludes2   sepsis (due to) (in) actinomycotic (A42.7)
         sepsis (due to) (in) anthrax (A22.7)
         sepsis (due to) (in) candidal (B37.7)
         sepsis (due to) (in) Erysipelothrix (A26.7)
         sepsis (due to) (in) extraintestinal yersiniosis (A28.2)
         sepsis (due to) (in) gonococcal (A54.86)
         sepsis (due to) (in) herpesviral (B00.7)
         sepsis (due to) (in) listerial (A32.7)
         sepsis (due to) (in) melioidosis (A24.1)
         sepsis (due to) (in) meningococcal (A39.2-A39.4)
         sepsis (due to) (in) plague (A20.7)
         sepsis (due to) (in) tularemia (A21.7)
         toxic shock syndrome (A48.3)
     Ⓔⓧ **For category A41 CC codes:** See PDX Collection 71
     Coding Clinic: 2016, Q1, P39

● **A41.0 Sepsis due to Staphylococcus aureus**
     A41.01 Sepsis due to Methicillin susceptible Staphylococcus aureus 🦠🦠
         MSSA sepsis
         Staphylococcus aureus sepsis NOS
     A41.02 Sepsis due to Methicillin resistant Staphylococcus aureus 🦠🦠
   A41.1 Sepsis due to other specified staphylococcus 🦠🦠
         Coagulase negative staphylococcus sepsis

N Newborn Age: 0   **P** Pediatric Age: 0–17   **M** Maternity DX: 9–64   **A** Adult Age: 15–124   ♀ Females Only   ♂ Males Only

🦠 Complication\Comorbidity   🦠 Major C\C   Ⓔⓧ CC/MCC Exclusions   🦠 Hospital-Acquired Condition   🦠 Hierarchical Condition Category   **659**

CHAPTER 1 (A00-B99)

A41.2   Sepsis due to unspecified staphylococcus 🦠🦠

A41.3   Sepsis due to Hemophilus influenzae 🦠🦠

A41.4   Sepsis due to anaerobes 🦠🦠

       Excludes1   gas gangrene (A48.0)

● A41.5   Sepsis due to other Gram-negative organisms

     A41.50   Gram-negative sepsis, unspecified 🦠🦠

         Gram-negative sepsis NOS

     A41.51   Sepsis due to Escherichia coli [E. coli] 🦠🦠

         Coding Clinic: 2018, Q1, P16

     A41.52   Sepsis due to Pseudomonas 🦠🦠

         Pseudomonas aeroginosa

     A41.53   Sepsis due to Serratia 🦠🦠

     A41.59   Other Gram-negative sepsis 🦠🦠

         Coding Clinic: 2019, Q1, P13

● A41.8   Other specified sepsis

     A41.81   Sepsis due to Enterococcus 🦠🦠

     A41.89   Other specified sepsis 🦠🦠

         Coding Clinic: 2021, Q1, P33; 2016, Q3, P8-14

A41.9   Sepsis, unspecified organism 🦠🦠

     Septicemia NOS

     Coding Clinic: 2018, Q4, P18

● A42   Actinomycosis

     Excludes1   actinomycetoma (B47.1)

A42.0   Pulmonary actinomycosis 🦠🦠

     (Ex:) See PDX Collection 103

A42.1   Abdominal actinomycosis 🦠

     (Ex:) See PDX Collection 104

A42.2   Cervicofacial actinomycosis 🦠

     (Ex:) See PDX Collection 105

A42.7   Actinomycotic sepsis 🦠🦠

     (Ex:) See PDX Collection 71

● A42.8   Other forms of actinomycosis

     (Ex:) For category A42.8 CC codes: See PDX Collection 106

     A42.81   Actinomycotic meningitis 🦠

     A42.82   Actinomycotic encephalitis 🦠

     A42.89   Other forms of actinomycosis 🦠

A42.9   Actinomycosis, unspecified 🦠

     (Ex:) See PDX Collection 106

● A43   Nocardiosis

A43.0   Pulmonary nocardiosis 🦠🦠

     (Ex:) See PDX Collection 103

A43.1   Cutaneous nocardiosis 🦠

     (Ex:) See PDX Collection 107

A43.8   Other forms of nocardiosis 🦠

     (Ex:) See PDX Collection 106

A43.9   Nocardiosis, unspecified 🦠

     (Ex:) See PDX Collection 106

● A44   Bartonellosis

     (Ex:) For category A44 CC codes: See PDX Collection 108

A44.0   Systemic bartonellosis 🦠

     Oroya fever

A44.1   Cutaneous and mucocutaneous bartonellosis 🦠

     Verruga peruana

A44.8   Other forms of bartonellosis 🦠

A44.9   Bartonellosis, unspecified 🦠

A46   Erysipelas

     Excludes1   postpartum or puerperal erysipelas (O86.89)

Item 1–8   **Gas gangrene** is a necrotizing subcutaneous infection that will cause tissue death. Patients with poor circulation (e.g., diabetes, peripheral nephropathy) will have low oxygen content in their tissues (hypoxia), which allows the Clostridium bacteria to flourish. Gas gangrene often occurs at the site of a surgical wound or trauma. Onset is sudden and dramatic. Treatment can include debridement, amputation, and/or hyperbaric oxygen treatments.

● A48   Other bacterial diseases, not elsewhere classified

     Excludes1   actinomycetoma (B47.1)

A48.0   Gas gangrene 🦠🦠

     Clostridial cellulitis

     Clostridial myonecrosis

     (Ex:) See PDX Collection 109

     Coding Clinic: 2017, Q4, P102

A48.1   Legionnaires' disease 🦠🦠

     (Ex:) See PDX Collection 110

A48.2   Nonpneumonic Legionnaires' disease [Pontiac fever]

A48.3   Toxic shock syndrome 🦠🦠

     Use additional code to identify the organism (B95, B96)

     Excludes1   endotoxic shock NOS (R57.8)

         sepsis NOS (A41.9)

     (Ex:) See PDX Collection 111

A48.4   Brazilian purpuric fever

     Systemic Hemophilus aegyptius infection

● A48.5   Other specified botulism

     Non-foodborne intoxication due to toxins of Clostridium botulinum [C. botulinum]

     Excludes1   food poisoning due to toxins of Clostridium botulinum (A05.1)

     A48.51   Infant botulism 🦠   P

         (Ex:) See PDX Collection 18

     A48.52   Wound botulism 🦠

         Non-foodborne botulism NOS

         Use additional code for associated wound

         (Ex:) See PDX Collection 18

A48.8   Other specified bacterial diseases

● A49   Bacterial infection of unspecified site

     Excludes1   bacterial agents as the cause of diseases classified elsewhere (B95-B96)

         chlamydial infection NOS (A74.9)

         meningococcal infection NOS (A39.9)

         rickettsial infection NOS (A79.9)

         spirochetal infection NOS (A69.9)

● A49.0   Staphylococcal infection, unspecified site

     A49.01   Methicillin susceptible Staphylococcus aureus infection, unspecified site

         Methicillin susceptible Staphylococcus aureus (MSSA) infection

         Staphylococcus aureus infection NOS

     A49.02   Methicillin resistant Staphylococcus aureus infection, unspecified site

         Methicillin resistant Staphylococcus aureus (MRSA) infection

A49.1   Streptococcal infection, unspecified site

A49.2   Hemophilus influenzae infection, unspecified site

     Any of seven bacterium of genus Haemophilus

A49.3   Mycoplasma infection, unspecified site

     Bacterium of class Mollicutes, unusual group of bacteria distinguished by absence of cell wall

A49.8   Other bacterial infections of unspecified site

A49.9   Bacterial infection, unspecified

     Excludes1   bacteremia NOS (R78.81)

▶ New   ⟹ Revised   ~~deleted~~ Deleted   Excludes 1   Excludes 2   Includes   Use additional   Code first   Code also   Key words

OGCR Official Guidelines   ● Unacceptable Principal Diagnosis   X Assign placeholder X   ● Use Additional Character(s)   ▌ Manifestation Code   Coding Clinic

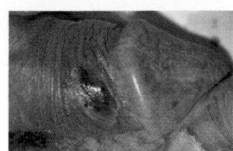

Figure 1-3 Chancre of primary syphilis. (From James WD, Berger TG, Elston DM: Andrews' Diseases of the Skin: Clinical Dermatology, Philadelphia, Saunders Elsevier, 2006)

Item 1–9 Syphilis, also known as lues, is the most serious of the venereal diseases caused by *Treponema pallidum*. The **primary** stage is characterized by an ulceration known as **chancre,** which usually appears on the genitals but can also develop on the anus, lips, tonsils, breasts, or fingers. Syphilis is easy to cure in its early stages. A single intramuscular injection of penicillin will usually cure a person who has had syphilis for less than a year.

The **secondary** stage is characterized by a rash that can affect any area of the body. **Latent** syphilis is divided into **early,** which is diagnosed within two years of infection, and **late,** which is diagnosed two years or more after infection. Additional doses of penicillin or another antibiotic are needed to treat someone who has had syphilis for longer than a year. For those allergic to penicillin, there are other antibiotic treatments. **Congenital** syphilis is also labeled **early** or **late** based on the time of diagnosis.

INFECTIONS WITH A PREDOMINANTLY SEXUAL MODE OF TRANSMISSION (A50-A64)

> **Excludes1**　human immunodeficiency virus [HIV] disease (B20)
> nonspecific and nongonococcal urethritis (N34.1)
> Reiter's disease (M02.3-)

● **A50　Congenital syphilis**
　● **A50.0　Early congenital syphilis, symptomatic**
　　　　Any congenital syphilitic condition specified as early or manifest less than two years after birth
　　　　(Ex:) **For category A50.0 CC codes:** See PDX Collection 112
　　　A50.01　Early congenital syphilitic oculopathy
　　　A50.02　Early congenital syphilitic osteochondropathy
　　　A50.03　Early congenital syphilitic pharyngitis
　　　　　　Early congenital syphilitic laryngitis
　　　A50.04　Early congenital syphilitic pneumonia
　　　A50.05　Early congenital syphilitic rhinitis
　　　A50.06　Early cutaneous congenital syphilis
　　　A50.07　Early mucocutaneous congenital syphilis
　　　A50.08　Early visceral congenital syphilis
　　　A50.09　Other early congenital syphilis, symptomatic
　　A50.1　Early congenital syphilis, latent
　　　　Congenital syphilis without clinical manifestations, with positive serological reaction and negative spinal fluid test, less than two years after birth
　　A50.2　Early congenital syphilis, unspecified
　　　　Congenital syphilis NOS less than two years after birth
　　　　(Ex:) See PDX Collection 113
　● **A50.3　Late congenital syphilitic oculopathy**
　　　Excludes1　Hutchinson's triad (A50.53)
　　　　(Ex:) **For category A50.3 CC codes:** See PDX Collection 112
　　　A50.30　Late congenital syphilitic oculopathy, unspecified
　　　A50.31　Late congenital syphilitic interstitial keratitis
　　　A50.32　Late congenital syphilitic chorioretinitis
　　　A50.39　Other late congenital syphilitic oculopathy

● **A50.4　Late congenital neurosyphilis [juvenile neurosyphilis]**
　　　Use additional code to identify any associated mental disorder
　　　Excludes1　Hutchinson's triad (A50.53)
　　　(Ex:) **For category A50.4 CC codes unless otherwise indicated:** See PDX Collection 114
　　　A50.40　Late congenital neurosyphilis, unspecified
　　　　　　Juvenile neurosyphilis NOS
　　　A50.41　Late congenital syphilitic meningitis
　　　　　　(Ex:) See PDX Collection 115
　　　A50.42　Late congenital syphilitic encephalitis
　　　A50.43　Late congenital syphilitic polyneuropathy
　　　A50.44　Late congenital syphilitic optic nerve atrophy
　　　　　　(Ex:) See PDX Collection 112
　　　A50.45　Juvenile general paresis
　　　　　　Dementia paralytica juvenilis
　　　　　　Juvenile tabetoparetic neurosyphilis
　　　A50.49　Other late congenital neurosyphilis
　　　　　　Juvenile tabes dorsalis
　● **A50.5　Other late congenital syphilis, symptomatic**
　　　　Any congenital syphilitic condition specified as late or manifest two years or more after birth
　　　　(Ex:) **For category A50.5 CC codes:** See PDX Collection 112
　　　A50.51　Clutton's joints
　　　A50.52　Hutchinson's teeth
　　　A50.53　Hutchinson's triad
　　　A50.54　Late congenital cardiovascular syphilis
　　　A50.55　Late congenital syphilitic arthropathy
　　　A50.56　Late congenital syphilitic osteochondropathy
　　　A50.57　Syphilitic saddle nose
　　　A50.59　Other late congenital syphilis, symptomatic
　　A50.6　Late congenital syphilis, latent
　　　　Congenital syphilis without clinical manifestations, with positive serological reaction and negative spinal fluid test, two years or more after birth.
　　A50.7　Late congenital syphilis, unspecified
　　　　Congenital syphilis NOS two years or more after birth.
　　A50.9　Congenital syphilis, unspecified

● **A51　Early syphilis**
　　A51.0　Primary genital syphilis
　　　　Syphilitic chancre NOS
　　A51.1　Primary anal syphilis
　　A51.2　Primary syphilis of other sites
　● **A51.3　Secondary syphilis of skin and mucous membranes**
　　　A51.31　Condyloma latum
　　　　　　(Ex:) See PDX Collection 112
　　　A51.32　Syphilitic alopecia
　　　　　　(Ex:) See PDX Collection 116
　　　A51.39　Other secondary syphilis of skin
　　　　　　Syphilitic leukoderma
　　　　　　Syphilitic mucous patch
　　　　　Excludes1　late syphilitic leukoderma (A52.79)
　　　　　　(Ex:) See PDX Collection 112
　● **A51.4　Other secondary syphilis**
　　　A51.41　Secondary syphilitic meningitis
　　　　　　(Ex:) See PDX Collection 117
　　　A51.42　Secondary syphilitic female pelvic disease ♀
　　　　　　(Ex:) See PDX Collection 113
　　　A51.43　Secondary syphilitic oculopathy
　　　　　　Secondary syphilitic chorioretinitis
　　　　　　Secondary syphilitic iridocyclitis, iritis
　　　　　　Secondary syphilitic uveitis
　　　　　　(Ex:) See PDX Collection 112

N Newborn Age: 0　　**P** Pediatric Age: 0–17　　**M** Maternity DX: 9–64　　**A** Adult Age: 15–124　　♀ Females Only　　♂ Males Only

 Complication\Comorbidity　　 Major C\C　　(Ex:) CC/MCC Exclusions　　 Hospital-Acquired Condition　　 Hierarchical Condition Category

A51.44 Secondary syphilitic nephritis 🔍
Ex: See PDX Collection 113

A51.45 Secondary syphilitic hepatitis 🔍
Ex: See PDX Collection 118

A51.46 Secondary syphilitic osteopathy 🔍
Ex: See PDX Collection 119

A51.49 Other secondary syphilitic conditions 🔍
Secondary syphilitic lymphadenopathy
Secondary syphilitic myositis
Ex: See PDX Collection 3211

A51.5 Early syphilis, latent
Syphilis (acquired) without clinical manifestations, with positive serological reaction and negative spinal fluid test, less than two years after infection.

A51.9 Early syphilis, unspecified

● **A52 Late syphilis**

● **A52.0 Cardiovascular and cerebrovascular syphilis**
Ex: For category A52.0 CC codes: See PDX Collection 114

A52.00 Cardiovascular syphilis, unspecified 🔍

A52.01 Syphilitic aneurysm of aorta 🔍

A52.02 Syphilitic aortitis 🔍

A52.03 Syphilitic endocarditis 🔍
Syphilitic aortic valve incompetence or stenosis
Syphilitic mitral valve stenosis
Syphilitic pulmonary valve regurgitation

A52.04 Syphilitic cerebral arteritis 🔍

A52.05 Other cerebrovascular syphilis 🔍
Syphilitic cerebral aneurysm (ruptured) (non-ruptured)
Syphilitic cerebral thrombosis

A52.06 Other syphilitic heart involvement 🔍
Syphilitic coronary artery disease
Syphilitic myocarditis
Syphilitic pericarditis

A52.09 Other cardiovascular syphilis 🔍

● **A52.1 Symptomatic neurosyphilis**
Ex: For category A52.1 CC codes unless otherwise indicated: See PDX Collection 114

A52.10 Symptomatic neurosyphilis, unspecified 🔍

A52.11 Tabes dorsalis 🔍
Cognitive decline with progressive degeneration of posterior columns, roots, and ganglia of spinal cord, occur 15-20 years after initial infection of syphilis; AKA Duchenne disease
Locomotor ataxia (progressive)
Tabetic neurosyphilis

A52.12 Other cerebrospinal syphilis 🔍

A52.13 Late syphilitic meningitis 🔍
Ex: See PDX Collection 115

A52.14 Late syphilitic encephalitis 🔍

A52.15 Late syphilitic neuropathy 🔍
Late syphilitic acoustic neuritis
Late syphilitic optic (nerve) atrophy
Late syphilitic polyneuropathy
Late syphilitic retrobulbar neuritis

A52.16 Charcôt's arthropathy (tabetic) 🔍
Progressive musculoskeletal condition characterized by joint dislocation, fractures, and deformities, results in progressive destruction of bone and soft tissue of weight-bearing joints

A52.17 General paresis 🔍
Chronic meningoencephalitis results in loss of cortical function, or progressive dementia and generalized paralysis, occurring 10-20 years after initial infection of syphilis; AKA Bayle disease, dementia paralytica, paralytic dementiaparetic neurosyphilis, syphilitic meningoencephalitis
Dementia paralytica

A52.19 Other symptomatic neurosyphilis 🔍
Syphilitic parkinsonism

A52.2 Asymptomatic neurosyphilis 🔍
Ex: See PDX Collection 114

A52.3 Neurosyphilis, unspecified 🔍
Gumma (syphilitic)
Destructive lesions of syphilis
Syphilis (late)
Syphiloma
Ex: See PDX Collection 114
Coding Clinic: 2021, Q2, P6

● **A52.7 Other symptomatic late syphilis**
Ex: For category A52.7 CC codes unless otherwise indicated: See PDX Collection 116

A52.71 Late syphilitic oculopathy 🔍
Late syphilitic chorioretinitis
Late syphilitic episcleritis
Ex: See PDX Collection 120

A52.72 Syphilis of lung and bronchus 🔍

A52.73 Symptomatic late syphilis of other respiratory organs 🔍

A52.74 Syphilis of liver and other viscera 🔍
Late syphilitic peritonitis

A52.75 Syphilis of kidney and ureter 🔍
Syphilitic glomerular disease

A52.76 Other genitourinary symptomatic late syphilis ♀
Late syphilitic female pelvic inflammatory disease

A52.77 Syphilis of bone and joint 🔍

A52.78 Syphilis of other musculoskeletal tissue 🔍
Late syphilitic bursitis
Syphilis [stage unspecified] of bursa
Syphilis [stage unspecified] of muscle
Syphilis [stage unspecified] of synovium
Syphilis [stage unspecified] of tendon

A52.79 Other symptomatic late syphilis 🔍
Late syphilitic leukoderma
Syphilis of adrenal gland
Syphilis of pituitary gland
Syphilis of thyroid gland
Syphilitic splenomegaly
Excludes1 syphilitic leukoderma (secondary) (A51.39)

A52.8 Late syphilis, latent
Syphilis (acquired) without clinical manifestations, with positive serological reaction and negative spinal fluid test, two years or more after infection

A52.9 Late syphilis, unspecified

● **A53 Other and unspecified syphilis**

A53.0 Latent syphilis, unspecified as early or late
Latent syphilis NOS
Positive serological reaction for syphilis

A53.9 Syphilis, unspecified
Infection due to Treponema pallidum NOS
Syphilis (acquired) NOS
Excludes1 syphilis NOS under two years of age (A50.2)

● **A54 Gonococcal infection**

● **A54.0 Gonococcal infection of lower genitourinary tract without periurethral or accessory gland abscess**
Excludes1 gonococcal infection with genitourinary gland abscess (A54.1)
gonococcal infection with periurethral abscess (A54.1)
Ex: For category A54.0 CC codes: See PDX Collection 121

A54.00 Gonococcal infection of lower genitourinary tract, unspecified 🔍

A54.01 Gonococcal cystitis and urethritis, unspecified 🔍

A54.02 Gonococcal vulvovaginitis, unspecified ♀ 🔍

A54.03 Gonococcal cervicitis, unspecified ♀ 🔍

A54.09 Other gonococcal infection of lower genitourinary tract 🔍

Item 1-10 An STD (sexually transmitted disease) caused by **Neisseria gonorrhoeae** that flourishes in the warm, moist areas of the reproductive tract. Untreated gonorrhea spreads to other parts of the body, causing inflammation of the testes or prostate or pelvic inflammatory disease (PID).

A54.1 Gonococcal infection of lower genitourinary tract with periurethral and accessory gland abscess 🅒
    Gonococcal Bartholin's gland abscess

● **A54.2** Gonococcal pelviperitonitis and other gonococcal genitourinary infection
    (Ex) For category A54.2 CC codes: See PDX Collection 121

    A54.21 Gonococcal infection of kidney and ureter 🅒

    A54.22 Gonococcal prostatitis ♂ 🅒

    A54.23 Gonococcal infection of other male genital organs ♂ 🅒
        Gonococcal epididymitis
        Gonococcal orchitis

    A54.24 Gonococcal female pelvic inflammatory disease ♀ 🅒
        Gonococcal pelviperitonitis
        Excludes1 gonococcal peritonitis (A54.85)

    A54.29 Other gonococcal genitourinary infections 🅒

● **A54.3** Gonococcal infection of eye
    (Ex) For category A54.3 CC codes: See PDX Collection 116

    A54.30 Gonococcal infection of eye, unspecified 🅒

    A54.31 Gonococcal conjunctivitis 🅒
        Form of bacterial conjunctivitis contracted by newborns during delivery; AKA neonatal conjunctivitis
        Ophthalmia neonatorum due to gonococcus

    A54.32 Gonococcal iridocyclitis 🅒
        Inflammation of iris and of ciliary body due to gonococcal infection

    A54.33 Gonococcal keratitis 🅒
        Inflammation of cornea due to gonococcal infection; AKA keratoconjunctivitis, keratopathy

    A54.39 Other gonococcal eye infection 🅒
        Gonococcal endophthalmia

● **A54.4** Gonococcal infection of musculoskeletal system
    (Ex) For category A54.4 CC codes: See PDX Collection 122

    A54.40 Gonococcal infection of musculoskeletal system, unspecified 🅒 🅒

    A54.41 Gonococcal spondylopathy 🅒 🅒
        Disorder of vertebrae due to gonococcal infection; AKA rachiopathy

    A54.42 Gonococcal arthritis 🅒 🅒
        Excludes2 gonococcal infection of spine (A54.41)

    A54.43 Gonococcal osteomyelitis 🅒 🅒
        Excludes2 gonococcal infection of spine (A54.41)

    A54.49 Gonococcal infection of other musculoskeletal tissue 🅒 🅒
        Gonococcal bursitis
        Gonococcal myositis
        Gonococcal synovitis
        Gonococcal tenosynovitis

A54.5 Gonococcal pharyngitis

A54.6 Gonococcal infection of anus and rectum

● **A54.8** Other gonococcal infections

    A54.81 Gonococcal meningitis 🅒
        (Ex) See PDX Collection 117

    A54.82 Gonococcal brain abscess 🅒
        (Ex) See PDX Collection 123

    A54.83 Gonococcal heart infection 🅒
        Gonococcal endocarditis
        Gonococcal myocarditis
        Gonococcal pericarditis
        (Ex) See PDX Collection 124

    A54.84 Gonococcal pneumonia 🅒 🅒
        (Ex) See PDX Collection 123

    A54.85 Gonococcal peritonitis 🅒 🅒
        Excludes1 gonococcal pelviperitonitis (A54.24)
        (Ex) See PDX Collection 125

    A54.86 Gonococcal sepsis 🅒 🅒
        MCC when PDx is its own MCC
        (Ex) See PDX Collection 71

    A54.89 Other gonococcal infections 🅒
        Gonococcal keratoderma
        Gonococcal lymphadenitis
        (Ex) See PDX Collection 123

A54.9 Gonococcal infection, unspecified 🅒
    (Ex) See PDX Collection 123

A55 Chlamydial lymphogranuloma (venereum)
    Climatic or tropical bubo
    Durand-Nicolas-Favre disease
    Esthiomene
    Lymphogranuloma inguinale

● **A56** Other sexually transmitted chlamydial diseases
    Includes sexually transmitted diseases due to Chlamydia trachomatis
    Excludes1 neonatal chlamydial conjunctivitis (P39.1)
        neonatal chlamydial pneumonia (P23.1)
    Excludes2 chlamydial lymphogranuloma (A55)
        conditions classified to A74.-

  ● **A56.0** Chlamydial infection of lower genitourinary tract

    A56.00 Chlamydial infection of lower genitourinary tract, unspecified

    A56.01 Chlamydial cystitis and urethritis

    A56.02 Chlamydial vulvovaginitis ♀

    A56.09 Other chlamydial infection of lower genitourinary tract
        Chlamydial cervicitis

  ● **A56.1** Chlamydial infection of pelviperitoneum and other genitourinary organs

    A56.11 Chlamydial female pelvic inflammatory disease ♀

    A56.19 Other chlamydial genitourinary infection
        Chlamydial epididymitis
        Chlamydial orchitis

  A56.2 Chlamydial infection of genitourinary tract, unspecified

  A56.3 Chlamydial infection of anus and rectum

  A56.4 Chlamydial infection of pharynx

  A56.8 Sexually transmitted chlamydial infection of other sites

A57 Chancroid
    Ulcus molle
    Sexually transmitted infection caused by bacteria, Haemophilus ducreyi

A58 Granuloma inguinale
    Chronic, progressive, ulcerative granulomatous disease
    Donovanosis

CHAPTER 1 (A00-B99)

N Newborn Age: 0   **P** Pediatric Age: 0–17   **M** Maternity DX: 9–64   **A** Adult Age: 15–124   ♀ Females Only   ♂ Males Only

🅒 Complication\Comorbidity   🅒 Major C\C   (Ex) CC/MCC Exclusions   🅒 Hospital-Acquired Condition   🅒 Hierarchical Condition Category

● **A59**   **Trichomoniasis**
     Excludes2   intestinal trichomoniasis (A07.8)
     A common STD caused by a parasite, Trichomonas vaginalis
   ● **A59.0**   **Urogenital trichomoniasis**
     A59.00   **Urogenital trichomoniasis, unspecified**
         Fluor (vaginalis) due to Trichomonas
         Leukorrhea (vaginalis) due to Trichomonas
     A59.01   **Trichomonal vulvovaginitis ♀**
     A59.02   **Trichomonal prostatitis ♂**
     A59.03   **Trichomonal cystitis and urethritis**
     A59.09   **Other urogenital trichomoniasis**
         Common sexually transmitted disease (STD)
         caused by single-celled protozoan parasite;
         AKA trich
         Trichomonas cervicitis
   A59.8   **Trichomoniasis of other sites**
   A59.9   **Trichomoniasis, unspecified**

● **A60**   **Anogenital herpesviral [herpes simplex] infections**
   ● **A60.0**   **Herpesviral infection of genitalia and urogenital tract**
     A60.00   **Herpesviral infection of urogenital system, unspecified**
     A60.01   **Herpesviral infection of penis ♂**
     A60.02   **Herpesviral infection of other male genital organs ♂**
     A60.03   **Herpesviral cervicitis ♀**
     A60.04   **Herpesviral vulvovaginitis ♀**
         Herpesviral [herpes simplex] ulceration
         Herpesviral [herpes simplex] vaginitis
         Herpesviral [herpes simplex] vulvitis
     A60.09   **Herpesviral infection of other urogenital tract**
         Coding Clinic: 2020, Q1, P20
   A60.1   **Herpesviral infection of perianal skin and rectum**
   A60.9   **Anogenital herpesviral infection, unspecified**

● **A63**   **Other predominantly sexually transmitted diseases, not elsewhere classified**
     Excludes2   molluscum contagiosum (B08.1)
                 papilloma of cervix (D26.0)
   A63.0   **Anogenital (venereal) warts**
         Anogenital warts due to (human) papillomavirus [HPV]
         Condyloma acuminatum
   A63.8   **Other specified predominantly sexually transmitted diseases**

   A64   **Unspecified sexually transmitted disease**

OTHER SPIROCHETAL DISEASES (A65-A69)

     Excludes2   leptospirosis (A27.-)
                 syphilis (A50-A53)

   A65   **Nonvenereal syphilis**
     Bejel
     Endemic syphilis
     Njovera

● **A66**   **Yaws**
     Endemic, infectious, tropical disease caused by spirochete, spread by direct contact; AKA frambesia, framboesia, frambesia tropica
     Includes   bouba
               frambesia (tropica)
               pian
   A66.0   **Initial lesions of yaws**
     Chancre of yaws
     Frambesia, initial or primary
     Initial frambesial ulcer
     Mother yaw
   A66.1   **Multiple papillomata and wet crab yaws**
     Frambesioma
     Pianoma
     Plantar or palmar papilloma of yaws

   A66.2   **Other early skin lesions of yaws**
     Cutaneous yaws, less than five years after infection
     Early yaws (cutaneous)(macular)(maculopapular) (micropapular)(papular)
     Frambeside of early yaws
   A66.3   **Hyperkeratosis of yaws**
     Hypertrophy of stratum corneum of skin in which there are small, hard, verrucous scales
     Ghoul hand
     Hyperkeratosis, palmar or plantar (early) (late) due to yaws
     Worm-eaten soles
   A66.4   **Gummata and ulcers of yaws**
     Small, rubbery granuloma with necrotic center and inflamed characteristic of advanced stage of syphilis; AKA syphiloma
     Gummatous frambeside
     Nodular late yaws (ulcerated)
   A66.5   **Gangosa**
     Manifestation of yaws that develops in the soft palate and spreads eroding bone, cartilage, and soft tissue
     Rhinopharyngitis mutilans
   A66.6   **Bone and joint lesions of yaws** 📝
     Yaws ganglion
     Yaws goundou
     Yaws gumma, bone
     Yaws gummatous osteitis or periostitis
     Yaws hydrarthrosis
     Yaws osteitis
     Yaws periostitis (hypertrophic)
   A66.7   **Other manifestations of yaws**
     Juxta-articular nodules of yaws
     Mucosal yaws
   A66.8   **Latent yaws**
     Yaws without clinical manifestations, with positive serology
   A66.9   **Yaws, unspecified**

● **A67**   **Pinta [carate]**
     Group of nonvenereal diseases caused by Treponema species
   A67.0   **Primary lesions of pinta**
     Chancre (primary) of pinta
     Papule (primary) of pinta
   A67.1   **Intermediate lesions of pinta**
     Erythematous plaques of pinta
     Hyperchromic lesions of pinta
     Hyperkeratosis of pinta
     Pintids
   A67.2   **Late lesions of pinta**
     Achromic skin lesions of pinta
     Cicatricial skin lesions of pinta
     Dyschromic skin lesions of pinta
   A67.3   **Mixed lesions of pinta**
     Achromic with hyperchromic skin lesions of pinta [carate]
   A67.9   **Pinta, unspecified**

● **A68**   **Relapsing fevers**
     Includes   recurrent fever
     Excludes2   Lyme disease (A69.2-)
     (Ex) **For category A68 CC codes:** See PDX Collection 108
   A68.0   **Louse-borne relapsing fever** 📝
     Relapsing fever due to Borrelia recurrentis
   A68.1   **Tick-borne relapsing fever** 📝
     Relapsing fever due to any Borrelia species other than Borrelia recurrentis
   A68.9   **Relapsing fever, unspecified** 📝

▶ New   ⇒ Revised   ~~deleted~~ Deleted   Excludes 1   Excludes 2   Includes   Use additional   Code first   Code also   Key words
OGCR Official Guidelines   ● Unacceptable Principal Diagnosis   X Assign placeholder X   ● Use Additional Character(s)   ▶ Manifestation Code   Coding Clinic

Item 1-11 Cancrum oris, also known as **noma** or **gangrenous stomatitis,** begins as an ulcer of the gingiva and results in a progressive gangrenous process.

● **A69 Other spirochetal infections**

　A69.0 Necrotizing ulcerative stomatitis
　　Cancrum oris
　　Fusospirochetal gangrene
　　Noma
　　Stomatitis gangrenosa

　A69.1 Other Vincent's infections 🅗
　　Fusospirochetal pharyngitis
　　Necrotizing ulcerative (acute) gingivitis
　　Necrotizing ulcerative (acute) gingivostomatitis
　　Spirochetal stomatitis
　　Trench mouth
　　Vincent's angina
　　Vincent's gingivitis
　　Ⓔⓧ See PDX Collection 126

● **A69.2 Lyme disease**
　　Erythema chronicum migrans due to Borrelia
　　　burgdorferi
　　Ⓔⓧ **For category A69.2 CC codes:** See PDX Collection 108

　A69.20 Lyme disease, unspecified 🅗
　A69.21 Meningitis due to Lyme disease 🅗
　A69.22 Other neurologic disorders in Lyme disease 🅗
　　　Cranial neuritis
　　　Meningoencephalitis
　　　Polyneuropathy
　A69.23 Arthritis due to Lyme disease 🅗🅜
　A69.29 Other conditions associated with Lyme disease 🅗
　　　Myopericarditis due to Lyme disease
　　　Coding Clinic: 2016, Q3, P12

　A69.8 Other specified spirochetal infections

　A69.9 Spirochetal infection, unspecified

OTHER DISEASES CAUSED BY CHLAMYDIAE (A70-A74)

　Excludes1　sexually transmitted chlamydial diseases
　　　(A55-A56)

A70 Chlamydia psittaci infections 🅗
　　Ornithosis
　　Parrot fever
　　Psittacosis
　　Ⓔⓧ See PDX Collection 127

● **A71 Trachoma**
　Excludes1　sequelae of trachoma (B94.0)

　A71.0 Initial stage of trachoma
　　Trachoma dubium

　A71.1 Active stage of trachoma
　　Granular conjunctivitis (trachomatous)
　　Trachomatous follicular conjunctivitis
　　Trachomatous pannus

　A71.9 Trachoma, unspecified

● **A74 Other diseases caused by chlamydiae**
　Excludes1　neonatal chlamydial conjunctivitis (P39.1)
　　　neonatal chlamydial pneumonia (P23.1)
　　　Reiter's disease (M02.3-)
　　　sexually transmitted chlamydial diseases
　　　(A55-A56)
　Excludes2　chlamydial pneumonia (J16.0)

　A74.0 Chlamydial conjunctivitis
　　Paratrachoma

● **A74.8 Other chlamydial diseases**
　A74.81 Chlamydial peritonitis
　A74.89 Other chlamydial diseases

　A74.9 Chlamydial infection, unspecified
　　Chlamydiosis NOS

Item 1-12 Rickettsioses are diseases spread from ticks, lice, fleas, or mites to humans.
　Typhus is spread to humans chiefly by the fleas of rats.
　Endemic identifies a disease as being present in low numbers of humans at all times, whereas **epidemic** identifies a disease as being present in high numbers of humans at a specific time. Morbidity (death) is higher in epidemic diseases.
　Brill's disease, also known as **Brill-Zinsser disease,** is spread from human to human by body lice and also from the lice of flying squirrels. **Scrub typhus** is spread in the same ways as Brill's disease.
　Malaria is spread to humans by mosquitoes.

RICKETTSIOSES (A75-A79)

● **A75 Typhus fever**
　Excludes1　rickettsiosis due to Ehrlichia sennetsu (A79.81)
　　Ⓔⓧ For category A75 CC codes unless otherwise indicated: See PDX Collection 108

　A75.0 Epidemic louse-borne typhus fever due to Rickettsia prowazekii 🅗
　　Organisms transmitted between humans via louse
　　Classical typhus (fever)
　　Epidemic (louse-borne) typhus

　A75.1 Recrudescent typhus [Brill's disease] 🅗
　　Brill-Zinsser disease

　A75.2 Typhus fever due to Rickettsia typhi 🅗
　　Murine (flea-borne) typhus

　A75.3 Typhus fever due to Rickettsia tsutsugamushi 🅗
　　Scrub (mite-borne) typhus
　　Tsutsugamushi fever
　　Typhus fever due to Orientia Tsutsugamushi (scrub typhus)

　A75.9 Typhus fever, unspecified 🅗
　　Typhus (fever) NOS
　　Ⓔⓧ See PDX Collection 128

● **A77 Spotted fever [tick-borne rickettsioses]**
　　Ⓔⓧ For category A77 CC codes: See PDX Collection 108

　A77.0 Spotted fever due to Rickettsia rickettsii 🅗
　　Rocky Mountain spotted fever
　　Sao Paulo fever

　A77.1 Spotted fever due to Rickettsia conorii 🅗
　　African tick typhus
　　Boutonneuse fever
　　India tick typhus
　　Kenya tick typhus
　　Marseilles fever
　　Mediterranean tick fever

　A77.2 Spotted fever due to Rickettsia siberica 🅗
　　North Asian tick fever
　　Siberian tick typhus

　A77.3 Spotted fever due to Rickettsia australis 🅗
　　Queensland tick typhus

● **A77.4 Ehrlichiosis**
　　Type of tick-borne fever caused by bacteria infection
　Excludes1　~~Rickettsiosis due to Ehrlichia sennetsu (A79.81)~~
　　▶anaplasmosis [A. phagocytophilum] (A79.82)
　　▶rickettsiosis due to Ehrlichia sennetsu (A79.81)
　A77.40 Ehrlichiosis, unspecified 🅗
　A77.41 Ehrlichiosis chafeensis [E. chafeensis] 🅗
　A77.49 Other ehrlichiosis 🅗
　　　Ehrlichiosis due to E. ewingii
　　　Ehrlichiosis due to E. muris euclairensis

　A77.8 Other spotted fevers 🅗
　　Rickettsia 364D/R. philipii (Pacific Coast tick fever)
　　Spotted fever due to Rickettsia africae (African tick bite fever)
　　Spotted fever due to Rickettsia parkeri]

　A77.9 Spotted fever, unspecified 🅗
　　Tick-borne typhus NOS

A78   Q fever 🔑
     Infection due to Coxiella burnetii
     Nine Mile fever
     Quadrilateral fever
     Ⓔⓧ See PDX Collection 108

● **A79   Other rickettsioses**
     Ⓔⓧ **For category A79 CC codes unless otherwise indicated:** See PDX Collection 129

     A79.0   Trench fever 🔑
        Quintan fever
        Wolhynian fever
        Ⓔⓧ See PDX Collection 108

     A79.1   Rickettsialpox due to Rickettsia akari 🔑
        Kew Garden fever
        Vesicular rickettsiosis

     ● **A79.8   Other specified rickettsioses**
        A79.81   Rickettsiosis due to Ehrlichia sennetsu 🔑
           Rickettsiosis due to Neorickettsia sennetsu
       ▶ **A79.82 Anaplasmosis [A. phagocytophilum]**
           ▶ Transfusion transmitted A. phagocytophilum
        A79.89   Other specified rickettsioses 🔑

     A79.9   Rickettsiosis, unspecified 🔑
        Rickettsial infection NOS

VIRAL AND PRION INFECTIONS OF THE CENTRAL NERVOUS SYSTEM (A80-A89)

     Excludes1   postpolio syndrome (G14)
                 sequelae of poliomyelitis (B91)
                 sequelae of viral encephalitis (B94.1)

● **A80   Acute poliomyelitis**
     ▶ **Excludes1**   acute flaccid myelitis (G04.82)
     Ⓔⓧ **For category A80 CC codes:** See PDX Collection 130

     A80.0   Acute paralytic poliomyelitis, vaccine-associated 🔑
     A80.1   Acute paralytic poliomyelitis, wild virus, imported 🔑
     A80.2   Acute paralytic poliomyelitis, wild virus, indigenous 🔑
     ● **A80.3   Acute paralytic poliomyelitis, other and unspecified**
        A80.30   Acute paralytic poliomyelitis, unspecified 🔑
        A80.39   Other acute paralytic poliomyelitis 🔑
     A80.4   Acute nonparalytic poliomyelitis
     A80.9   Acute poliomyelitis, unspecified

● **A81   Atypical virus infections of central nervous system**
     Includes   diseases of the central nervous system caused by prions
     Use additional code to identify:
       dementia with behavioral disturbance (F02.81)
       dementia without behavioral disturbance (F02.80)

     ● **A81.0   Creutzfeldt-Jakob disease**
       Ⓔⓧ **For category A81.0 CC codes:** See PDX Collection 131

        A81.00   Creutzfeldt-Jakob disease, unspecified 🔑
           Jakob-Creutzfeldt disease, unspecified
        A81.01   Variant Creutzfeldt-Jakob disease 🔑
           vCJD
        A81.09   Other Creutzfeldt-Jakob disease 🔑
           CJD
           Familial Creutzfeldt-Jakob disease
           Iatrogenic Creutzfeldt-Jakob disease
           Sporadic Creutzfeldt-Jakob disease
           Subacute spongiform encephalopathy (with dementia)

     A81.1   Subacute sclerosing panencephalitis 🔑
        Type of viral encephalitis that causes parenchymatous lesions in gray and white matter of brain
        Dawson's inclusion body encephalitis
        Van Bogaert's sclerosing leukoencephalopathy
        Ⓔⓧ See PDX Collection 132

     A81.2   Progressive multifocal leukoencephalopathy 🔑
        Group of diseases affecting white matter of brain
        Multifocal leukoencephalopathy NOS
        Ⓔⓧ See PDX Collection 133

Item 1-13   Acute Poliomyelitis: Also called infantile paralysis and is caused by the poliovirus, which enters the body orally and infects the intestinal wall and then enters the blood stream and central nervous system, causing muscle weakness and paralysis. This disease has been nearly eradicated with the polio vaccine.

     ● **A81.8   Other atypical virus infections of central nervous system**
       Ⓔⓧ **For category A81.8 CC codes unless otherwise indicated:** See PDX Collection 135

        A81.81   Kuru 🔑
           Ⓔⓧ See PDX Collection 134
        A81.82   Gerstmann-Sträussler-Scheinker syndrome 🔑
           GSS syndrome
        A81.83   Fatal familial insomnia 🔑
           FFI
        A81.89   Other atypical virus infections of central nervous system 🔑

     A81.9   Atypical virus infection of central nervous system, unspecified 🔑
        Prion diseases of the central nervous system NOS
        Ⓔⓧ See PDX Collection 134

● **A82   Rabies**
     Viral disease affecting the central nervous system and transmitted from infected mammals to man
     Ⓔⓧ **For category A82 CC codes:** See PDX Collection 136

     A82.0   Sylvatic rabies 🔑
     A82.1   Urban rabies 🔑
     A82.9   Rabies, unspecified 🔑

● **A83   Mosquito-borne viral encephalitis**
     Inflammation of the brain caused most commonly by Herpes Simplex virus
     Includes   mosquito-borne viral meningoencephalitis
     Excludes2   Venezuelan equine encephalitis (A92.2)
                 West Nile fever (A92.3-)
                 West Nile virus (A92.3-)
     Ⓔⓧ **For category A83 CC codes:** See PDX Collection 137

     A83.0   Japanese encephalitis 🔑
     A83.1   Western equine encephalitis 🔑
     A83.2   Eastern equine encephalitis 🔑
     A83.3   St. Louis encephalitis 🔑
     A83.4   Australian encephalitis 🔑
        Kunjin virus disease
     A83.5   California encephalitis 🔑
        California meningoencephalitis
        La Crosse encephalitis
     A83.6   Rocio virus disease 🔑
        Mosquito-borne virus
     A83.8   Other mosquito-borne viral encephalitis 🔑
     A83.9   Mosquito-borne viral encephalitis, unspecified 🔑

● **A84   Tick-borne viral encephalitis**
     Includes   tick-borne viral meningoencephalitis
     Ⓔⓧ **For category A84 CC codes:** See PDX Collection 137

     A84.0   Far Eastern tick-borne encephalitis [Russian spring-summer encephalitis] 🔑
     A84.1   Central European tick-borne encephalitis 🔑
     A84.8   Other tick-borne viral encephalitis 🔑
        A84.81   Powassan virus disease 🔑
           Ⓔⓧ See PDX Collection 4057
        A84.89   Other tick-borne viral encephalitis 🔑
           Louping ill
           Code first, if applicable, transfusion related infection (T80.22-)
           Ⓔⓧ See PDX Collection 4073
     A84.9   Tick-borne viral encephalitis, unspecified 🔑

CHAPTER 1 (A00-B99)

▶ New   ⇒ Revised   ~~deleted~~ Deleted   Excludes 1   Excludes 2   Includes   Use additional   Code first   Code also   Key words

OGCR Official Guidelines   ● Unacceptable Principal Diagnosis   X Assign placeholder X   ● Use Additional Character(s)   ▶ Manifestation Code   **Coding Clinic**

Item 1-14 Encephalitis is an inflammation of the brain most often caused by a virus but may also be caused by a bacteria and most commonly transmitted by a mosquito. **Myelitis** is an inflammation of the spinal cord that may disrupt CNS function. Untreated myelitis may rapidly lead to permanent damage to the spinal cord. **Encephalomyelitis** is a general term for an inflammation of the brain and spinal cord.

● **A85   Other viral encephalitis, not elsewhere classified**

| **Includes** | specified viral encephalomyelitis NEC |
| | specified viral meningoencephalitis NEC |

Excludes1	benign myalgic encephalomyelitis (G93.3)
	encephalitis due to cytomegalovirus (B25.8)
	encephalitis due to herpesvirus NEC (B10.0-)
	encephalitis due to herpesvirus [herpes simplex] (B00.4)
	encephalitis due to measles virus (B05.0)
	encephalitis due to mumps virus (B26.2)
	encephalitis due to poliomyelitis virus (A80.-)
	encephalitis due to zoster (B02.0)
	lymphocytic choriomeningitis (A87.2)

ⒺⓍ **For category A85 CC codes unless otherwise indicated: See PDX Collection 138**

A85.0   Enteroviral encephalitis 🅒
Enteroviral encephalomyelitis

A85.1   Adenoviral encephalitis 🅒
Adenoviral meningoencephalitis

A85.2   Arthropod-borne viral encephalitis, unspecified 🅒
    Excludes1   West nile virus with encephalitis (A92.31)
    ⒺⓍ See PDX Collection 137

A85.8   Other specified viral encephalitis 🅒
Encephalitis lethargica
Von Economo-Cruchet disease

A86   Unspecified viral encephalitis 🅒
Viral encephalomyelitis NOS
Viral meningoencephalitis NOS
ⒺⓍ See PDX Collection 139

● **A87   Viral meningitis**

Excludes1	meningitis due to herpesvirus [herpes simplex] (B00.3)
	meningitis due to measles virus (B05.1)
	meningitis due to mumps virus (B26.1)
	meningitis due to poliomyelitis virus (A80.-)
	meningitis due to zoster (B02.1)

ⒺⓍ **For category A87 CC codes unless otherwise indicated: See PDX Collection 140**

A87.0   Enteroviral meningitis 🅒
Group of common viruses responsible for the majority of viral meningitis
Coxsackievirus meningitis
Echovirus meningitis

A87.1   Adenoviral meningitis 🅒

A87.2   Lymphocytic choriomeningitis 🅒
Lymphocytic meningoencephalitis
ⒺⓍ See PDX Collection 141

A87.8   Other viral meningitis 🅒

A87.9   Viral meningitis, unspecified 🅒

● **A88   Other viral infections of central nervous system, not elsewhere classified**

| **Excludes1** | viral encephalitis NOS (A86) |
| | viral meningitis NOS (A87.9) |

A88.0   Enteroviral exanthematous fever [Boston exanthem] 🅒
Infectious skin eruption
ⒺⓍ See PDX Collection 137

A88.1   Epidemic vertigo

A88.8   Other specified viral infections of central nervous system 🅒
ⒺⓍ See PDX Collection 138

A89   Unspecified viral infection of central nervous system 🅒
ⒺⓍ See PDX Collection 139

OGCR Section I. C.1.f.

Certain Infectious and Parasitic Diseases (A00-B99)

Zika virus infections

Code only confirmed cases

Code only a confirmed diagnosis of Zika virus (A92.5, Zika virus disease) as documented by the provider. This is an exception to the hospital inpatient guideline Section II, H.

In this context, "confirmation" does not require documentation of the type of test performed; the physician's diagnostic statement that the condition is confirmed is sufficient. This code should be assigned regardless of the stated mode of transmission.

If the provider documents "suspected", "possible" or "probable" Zika, do not assign code A92.5. Assign a code(s) explaining the reason for encounter (such as fever, rash, or joint pain) or Z20.828, Contact with and (suspected) exposure to other viral communicable diseases.

ARTHROPOD-BORNE VIRAL FEVERS AND VIRAL HEMORRHAGIC FEVERS (A90-A99)

A90   Dengue fever [classical dengue] 🅒
Acute, self-limited disease, characterized by fever, prostration, severe muscle pains, headache, rash, lymphadenopathy, and leukopenia, caused by dengue virus; AKA breakbone, dandy
    Excludes1   dengue hemorrhagic fever (A91)
    ⒺⓍ See PDX Collection 142
    Coding Clinic: 2016, Q3, P13

A91   Dengue hemorrhagic fever 🅒
Serious follow-up to regular dengue, with symptoms of hemorrhage
ⒺⓍ See PDX Collection 143

● **A92   Other mosquito-borne viral fevers**
    Excludes1   Ross River disease (B33.1)

A92.0   Chikungunya virus disease 🅒
Transmitted by mosquitoes
Chikungunya (hemorrhagic) fever
ⒺⓍ See PDX Collection 143

A92.1   O'nyong-nyong fever 🅒
Acute, nonfatal febrile disease transmitted by mosquitoes, which clinically resembles dengue and chikungunya
ⒺⓍ See PDX Collection 144

A92.2   Venezuelan equine fever 🅒
Venezuelan equine encephalitis
Venezuelan equine encephalomyelitis virus disease
ⒺⓍ See PDX Collection 144

● **A92.3   West Nile virus infection**
West Nile fever

    A92.30   West Nile virus infection, unspecified 🅒
       West Nile fever NOS
       West Nile fever without complications
       West Nile virus NOS
       ⒺⓍ See PDX Collection 3610

    A92.31   West Nile virus infection with encephalitis 🅒
       West Nile encephalitis
       West Nile encephalomyelitis
       Coding Clinic: 2016, Q3, P13
       ⒺⓍ See PDX Collection 3612

    A92.32   West Nile virus infection with other neurologic manifestation 🅒
       Use additional code to specify the neurologic manifestation
       ⒺⓍ See PDX Collection 3614

    A92.39   West Nile virus infection with other complications 🅒
       Use additional code to specify the other conditions

A92.4   Rift Valley fever 🅒
    ⒺⓍ See PDX Collection 144

A92.5   Zika virus disease 🅒
Zika virus fever
Zika virus infection
Zika NOS
    Excludes1   congenital Zika virus disease (P35.4)
    ⒺⓍ See PDX Collection 144
    Coding Clinic: 2016, Q4, P4-7, 121

A92.8   Other specified mosquito-borne viral fevers 🅒
    ⒺⓍ See PDX Collection 144

A92.9   Mosquito-borne viral fever, unspecified 🅒
    ⒺⓍ See PDX Collection 143

N   Newborn Age: 0   **P**   Pediatric Age: 0–17   **M**   Maternity DX: 9–64   **A**   Adult Age: 15–124   ♀   Females Only   ♂   Males Only

🅒 Complication\Comorbidity   🅒 Major C\C   ⒺⓍ CC/MCC Exclusions   Hospital-Acquired Condition   Hierarchical Condition Category

● **A93** **Other arthropod-borne viral fevers, not elsewhere classified**

   A93.0 **Oropouche virus disease** 🔊
Tropical viral infection
Oropouche fever
(Ex:) See PDX Collection 144

   A93.1 **Sandfly fever** 🔊
Pappataci fever
Phlebotomus fever
(Ex:) See PDX Collection 143

   A93.2 **Colorado tick fever** 🔊
(Ex:) See PDX Collection 143

   A93.8 **Other specified arthropod-borne viral fevers** 🔊
Piry virus disease
Vesicular stomatitis virus disease [Indiana fever]
(Ex:) See PDX Collection 143

● **A94** **Unspecified arthropod-borne viral fever** 🔊
Arboviral fever NOS
Arbovirus infection NOS
(Ex:) See PDX Collection 143

● **A95** **Yellow fever**
Acute infectious disease transmitted by mosquitoes
(Ex:) **For category A95 CC codes:** See PDX Collection 146

   A95.0 **Sylvatic yellow fever** 🔊
Jungle yellow fever

   A95.1 **Urban yellow fever** 🔊

   A95.9 **Yellow fever, unspecified** 🔊

● **A96** **Arenaviral hemorrhagic fever**
Virus that causes various hemorrhagic fevers
(Ex:) **For category A96 CC codes:** See PDX Collection 147

   A96.0 **Junin hemorrhagic fever** 🔊
Argentinian hemorrhagic fever

   A96.1 **Machupo hemorrhagic fever** 🔊
Transmitted by contact with infected rodents
Bolivian hemorrhagic fever

   A96.2 **Lassa fever**
Acute type of hemorrhagic fever caused by contact with disease carrying mouse or person

   A96.8 **Other arenaviral hemorrhagic fevers** 🔊

   A96.9 **Arenaviral hemorrhagic fever, unspecified** 🔊

● **A98** **Other viral hemorrhagic fevers, not elsewhere classified**
   Excludes1   chikungunya hemorrhagic fever (A92.0)
             dengue hemorrhagic fever (A91)
(Ex:) **For category A98 CC codes unless otherwise indicated:** See PDX Collection 143

   A98.0 **Crimean-Congo hemorrhagic fever** 🔊
Virus transmitted by ticks and contact with blood, secretions, or fluids from infected humans or animals
Central Asian hemorrhagic fever

   A98.1 **Omsk hemorrhagic fever** 🔊
Transmitted to humans by bites of infected ticks or contact with infected muskrats

   A98.2 **Kyasanur Forest disease** 🔊
Transmitted via infected monkeys, voles, ticks

   A98.3 **Marburg virus disease**
Rare, acute, often fatal type of hemorrhagic fever

   A98.4 **Ebola virus disease**

   A98.5 **Hemorrhagic fever with renal syndrome** 🔊
Epidemic hemorrhagic fever
Korean hemorrhagic fever
Russian hemorrhagic fever
Hantaan virus disease
Hantavirus disease with renal manifestations
Nephropathia epidemica
Songo fever
    Excludes1   hantavirus (cardio)-pulmonary syndrome
               (B33.4)
    (Ex:) See PDX Collection 148

   A98.8 **Other specified viral hemorrhagic fevers** 🔊

● **A99** **Unspecified viral hemorrhagic fever** 🔊
(Ex:) See PDX Collection 143

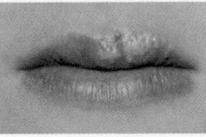

Figure 1-4   Primary herpes simplex in and around the mouth. The infection is usually acquired from siblings or parents and is readily transmitted to other direct contacts. (Getty Image)

Item 1–15   **Herpes** is a viral disease for which there is no cure. There are two types of the herpes simplex virus: **Type I** causes **cold sores** or **fever blisters,** and **Type II** causes **genital herpes.** The virus can be spread from a sore on the lips to the genitals or from the genitals to the lips.

VIRAL INFECTIONS CHARACTERIZED BY SKIN AND MUCOUS MEMBRANE LESIONS (B00-B09)

● **B00** **Herpesviral [herpes simplex] infections**
   Excludes1   congenital herpesviral infections (P35.2)
   Excludes2   anogenital herpesviral infection (A60.-)
               gammaherpesviral mononucleosis (B27.0-)
               herpangina (B08.5)

   B00.0 **Eczema herpeticum**
Cutaneous eruption caused by herpes simplex virus (HSV) type 1, HSV-2, coxsackievirus A16, or vaccinia virus
Kaposi's varicelliform eruption

   B00.1 **Herpesviral vesicular dermatitis**
Vesicle formation; characteristics include formation of blisters and scabs on feet and legs
Herpes simplex facialis
Herpes simplex labialis
Herpes simplex otitis externa
Vesicular dermatitis of ear
Vesicular dermatitis of lip

   B00.2 **Herpesviral gingivostomatitis and pharyngotonsillitis** 🔊
Inflammation involving both gingivae and oral mucosa
Herpesviral pharyngitis
Inflammation of pharynx and tonsils; AKA tonsillopharyngitis
(Ex:) See PDX Collection 149

   B00.3 **Herpesviral meningitis** 🔊
(Ex:) See PDX Collection 150

   B00.4 **Herpesviral encephalitis** 🔊
Herpesviral meningoencephalitis
Simian B disease
    Excludes1   herpesviral encephalitis due to herpesvirus 6 and 7 (B10.01, B10.09)
               non-simplex herpesviral encephalitis (B10.0-)
    (Ex:) See PDX Collection 151

● **B00.5** **Herpesviral ocular disease**
    (Ex:) **For category B00.5 CC codes:** See PDX Collection 152

    B00.50 **Herpesviral ocular disease, unspecified** 🔊

    B00.51 **Herpesviral iridocyclitis** 🔊
Herpesviral iritis
Herpesviral uveitis, anterior

    B00.52 **Herpesviral keratitis** 🔊
Herpesviral keratoconjunctivitis

    B00.53 **Herpesviral conjunctivitis** 🔊

    B00.59 **Other herpesviral disease of eye** 🔊
Herpesviral dermatitis of eyelid

   B00.7 **Disseminated herpesviral disease** 🔊🔊
Herpesviral sepsis
(Ex:) See PDX Collection 153

▶ New   ⇒ Revised   ~~deleted~~ Deleted   Excludes 1   Excludes 2   Includes   Use additional   Code first   Code also   Key words
OGCR Official Guidelines   ● Unacceptable Principal Diagnosis   X Assign placeholder X   ● Use Additional Character(s)   ▶ Manifestation Code   Coding Clinic

● **B00.8**   **Other forms of herpesviral infections**

     B00.81   Herpesviral hepatitis 🅒
         (Ex:) See PDX Collection 154

     B00.82   Herpes simplex myelitis 🅒 🅡🅒
         (Ex:) See PDX Collection 155

     B00.89   Other herpesviral infection 🅒
         Herpesviral whitlow
         (Ex:) See PDX Collection 156

   B00.9   **Herpesviral infection, unspecified**
       Herpes simplex infection NOS

● **B01**   **Varicella [chickenpox]**
     Very contagious disease caused by the varicella zoster virus that
     results in an itchy outbreak of skin blisters (varicella). The same
     virus causes shingles (zoster).

   B01.0   **Varicella meningitis** 🅒
       (Ex:) See PDX Collection 157

● **B01.1**   **Varicella encephalitis, myelitis and encephalomyelitis**
       Postchickenpox encephalitis, myelitis and
       encephalomyelitis

     B01.11   Varicella encephalitis and encephalomyelitis 🅒
         Postchickenpox encephalitis and
         encephalomyelitis
         (Ex:) See PDX Collection 158

     B01.12   Varicella myelitis 🅒 🅡🅒
         Postchickenpox myelitis
         (Ex:) See PDX Collection 159

   B01.2   **Varicella pneumonia** 🅒
       (Ex:) See PDX Collection 160

● **B01.8**   **Varicella with other complications**
       (Ex:) **For category B01.8 CC codes:** See PDX Collection 157

     B01.81   Varicella keratitis 🅒

     B01.89   Other varicella complications 🅒

   B01.9   **Varicella without complication** 🅒
       Varicella NOS
       (Ex:) See PDX Collection 157

● **B02**   **Zoster [herpes zoster]**

     Includes   shingles
              zona

   B02.0   **Zoster encephalitis** 🅒
       Zoster meningoencephalitis
       (Ex:) See PDX Collection 161

   B02.1   **Zoster meningitis** 🅒
       (Ex:) See PDX Collection 162

● **B02.2**   **Zoster with other nervous system involvement**
       (Ex:) **For category B02.2 CC codes unless otherwise indicated:** See PDX
       Collection 161
       Coding Clinic: 2019, Q1, P18

     B02.21   Postherpetic geniculate ganglionitis 🅒

     B02.22   Postherpetic trigeminal neuralgia 🅒

     B02.23   Postherpetic polyneuropathy 🅒

     B02.24   Postherpetic myelitis 🅒 🅡🅒
         Herpes zoster myelitis
         (Ex:) See PDX Collection 163

     B02.29   Other postherpetic nervous system
         involvement 🅒
         Postherpetic radiculopathy

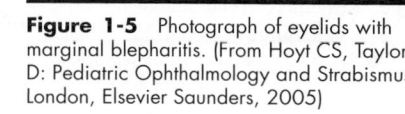

Figure 1-5 Photograph of eyelids with marginal blepharitis. (From Hoyt CS, Taylor D: Pediatric Ophthalmology and Strabismus, London, Elsevier Saunders, 2005)

Item 1–17 Blepharitis is a common condition in which the eyelid is swollen and yellow scaling and conjunctivitis develop. Usually the hair on the scalp and brow is involved.

● **B02.3**   **Zoster ocular disease**
       (Ex:) **For category B02.3 CC codes:** See PDX Collection 164

     B02.30   Zoster ocular disease, unspecified 🅒

     B02.31   Zoster conjunctivitis 🅒

     B02.32   Zoster iridocyclitis 🅒

     B02.33   Zoster keratitis 🅒
         Herpes zoster keratoconjunctivitis

     B02.34   Zoster scleritis 🅒

     B02.39   Other herpes zoster eye disease 🅒
         Zoster blepharitis

   B02.7   **Disseminated zoster** 🅒
       (Ex:) See PDX Collection 165

   B02.8   **Zoster with other complications** 🅒
       Herpes zoster otitis externa
       (Ex:) See PDX Collection 165

   B02.9   **Zoster without complications** 🅒
       Zoster NOS

   B03   **Smallpox** 🅒
     Note: In 1980 the 33rd World Health Assembly declared
     that smallpox had been eradicated. The classification is
     maintained for surveillance purposes.
     (Ex:) See PDX Collection 166

   B04   **Monkeypox** 🅒
     Disease occurring in captive monkeys and other mammals that may
     be transmitted to humans, clinically similar to smallpox
     (Ex:) See PDX Collection 167

● **B05**   **Measles**

     Includes   morbilli

     Excludes1   subacute sclerosing panencephalitis (A81.1)

   B05.0   **Measles complicated by encephalitis** 🅒
       Postmeasles encephalitis
       (Ex:) See PDX Collection 168

   B05.1   **Measles complicated by meningitis** 🅒
       Postmeasles meningitis
       (Ex:) See PDX Collection 169

   B05.2   **Measles complicated by pneumonia** 🅒
       Postmeasles pneumonia
       (Ex:) See PDX Collection 170

   B05.3   **Measles complicated by otitis media**
       Postmeasles otitis media

   B05.4   **Measles with intestinal complications** 🅒
       (Ex:) See PDX Collection 169

● **B05.8**   **Measles with other complications**

     B05.81   Measles keratitis and keratoconjunctivitis 🅒
         (Ex:) See PDX Collection 171

     B05.89   Other measles complications 🅒
         (Ex:) See PDX Collection 169

   B05.9   **Measles without complication**
       Measles NOS

CHAPTER 1 (A00-B99)

Item 1-16 Zoster: Also known as **_shingles_** and is caused by the same virus as chickenpox. After exposure, the virus lies dormant in nerve tissue and is activated by factors including aging, stress, suppression of the immune system, and certain medication. It begins as a unilateral rash that leads to blisters and sores on the skin. It may involve the nerve pathways of the eye, forehead, nose, and eyelids and may be very painful with long-term systemic effects.

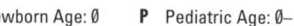

N Newborn Age: 0   **P** Pediatric Age: 0–17   **M** Maternity DX: 9–64   **A** Adult Age: 15–124   ♀ Females Only   ♂ Males Only

🅒 Complication\Comorbidity   🅜 Major C\C   (Ex:) CC/MCC Exclusions   🅡🅒 Hospital-Acquired Condition   🅒 Hierarchical Condition Category

● **B06   Rubella [German measles]**
Excludes1   congenital rubella (P35.0)

● **B06.0   Rubella with neurological complications**
(Ex:) For category B06.0 CC codes: See PDX Collection 172

B06.00   Rubella with neurological complication, unspecified 🔖

B06.01   Rubella encephalitis 🔖
Rubella meningoencephalitis

B06.02   Rubella meningitis 🔖

B06.09   Other neurological complications of rubella 🔖

● **B06.8   Rubella with other complications**

B06.81   Rubella pneumonia 🔖
(Ex:) See PDX Collection 172

B06.82   Rubella arthritis 🔖🔖
(Ex:) See PDX Collection 173

B06.89   Other rubella complications 🔖
(Ex:) See PDX Collection 172

B06.9   Rubella without complication
Rubella NOS

● **B07   Viral warts**
Includes   verruca simplex
verruca vulgaris
viral warts due to human papillomavirus

Excludes2   anogenital (venereal) warts (A63.0)
papilloma of bladder (D41.4)
papilloma of cervix (D26.0)
papilloma larynx (D14.1)

B07.0   Plantar wart
Verruca plantaris

B07.8   Other viral warts
Common wart
Flat wart
Verruca plana

B07.9   Viral wart, unspecified

● **B08   Other viral infections characterized by skin and mucous membrane lesions, not elsewhere classified**
Excludes1   vesicular stomatitis virus disease (A93.8)

● **B08.0   Other orthopoxvirus infections**
Excludes2   monkeypox (B04)

● **B08.01   Cowpox and vaccinia not from vaccine**

B08.010   Cowpox

B08.011   Vaccinia not from vaccine
Excludes1   vaccinia (from vaccination) (generalized) (T88.1)

B08.02   Orf virus disease
Contagious pustular dermatitis
Ecthyma contagiosum

B08.03   Pseudocowpox [milker's node]

B08.04   Paravaccinia, unspecified

B08.09   Other orthopoxvirus infections
Orthopoxvirus infection NOS

B08.1   Molluscum contagiosum
Various skin diseases characterized by soft, rounded, cutaneous lesions

● **B08.2   Exanthema subitum [sixth disease] Roseola infantum**
Acute, short-lived high fever in infants and young children followed by a rash mainly on the trunk, caused by human herpesvirus 6

B08.20   Exanthema subitum [sixth disease], unspecified Roseola infantum, unspecified   P

B08.21   Exanthema subitum [sixth disease] due to human herpesvirus 6 Roseola infantum due to human herpesvirus 6   P
Virus results in sudden rash; infection results in lifelong persistence

B08.22   Exanthema subitum [sixth disease] due to human herpesvirus 7 Roseola infantum due to human herpesvirus 7   P

B08.3   Erythema infectiosum [fifth disease] 🔖
Moderately contagious, epidemic disease in children caused by B19 virus; onset of rash that begins as redness of cheeks, later there is rash on trunk and limbs; when this fades, there may be central clearing that leaves lacelike pattern
(Ex:) See PDX Collection 174

B08.4   Enteroviral vesicular stomatitis with exanthem
Hand, foot and mouth disease
Check your documentation—this code is HAND, foot, and mouth disease. Code B08.8 is foot and mouth disease.

B08.5   Enteroviral vesicular pharyngitis
Herpangina

● **B08.6   Parapoxvirus infections**

B08.60   Parapoxvirus infection, unspecified

B08.61   Bovine stomatitis

B08.62   Sealpox

B08.69   Other parapoxvirus infections

● **B08.7   Yatapoxvirus infections**

B08.70   Yatapoxvirus infection, unspecified

B08.71   Tanapox virus disease 🔖
(Ex:) See PDX Collection 167

B08.72   Yaba pox virus disease
Yaba monkey tumor disease

B08.79   Other yatapoxvirus infections

B08.8   Other specified viral infections characterized by skin and mucous membrane lesions
Enteroviral lymphonodular pharyngitis
Foot-and-mouth disease
Check your documentation. Code B08.4 is for HAND, foot, and mouth disease.
Poxvirus NEC

● **B09   Unspecified viral infection characterized by skin and mucous membrane lesions**
Viral enanthema NOS
Viral exanthema NOS

OTHER HUMAN HERPESVIRUSES (B10)

● **B10   Other human herpesviruses**
Excludes2   cytomegalovirus (B25.9)
Epstein-Barr virus (B27.0-)
herpes NOS (B00.9)
herpes simplex (B00.-)
herpes zoster (B02.-)
human herpesvirus NOS (B00.-)
human herpesvirus 1 and 2 (B00.-)
human herpesvirus 3 (B01.-, B02.-)
human herpesvirus 4 (B27.0-)
human herpesvirus 5 (B25.-)
varicella (B01.-)
zoster (B02.-)

● **B10.0   Other human herpesvirus encephalitis**
Excludes2   herpes encephalitis NOS (B00.4)
herpes simplex encephalitis (B00.4)
human herpesvirus encephalitis (B00.4)
simian B herpes virus encephalitis (B00.4)
(Ex:) For category B10.0 CC codes: See PDX Collection 151

B10.01   Human herpesvirus 6 encephalitis 🔖
Sudden rash or roseola

B10.09   Other human herpesvirus encephalitis 🔖
Human herpesvirus 7 encephalitis
Virus closely related to human herpesvirus 6, but not known to cause any disease

---

▶ New   ⇒ Revised   ~~deleted~~ Deleted   Excludes 1   Excludes 2   Includes   Use additional   Code first   Code also   Key words

OGCR Official Guidelines   ● Unacceptable Principal Diagnosis   X Assign placeholder X   ● Use Additional Character(s)   ▶ Manifestation Code   Coding Clinic

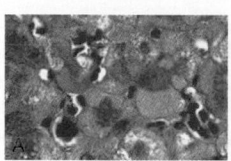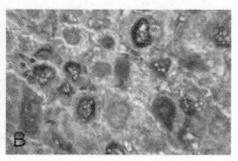

Figure 1-6 Hepatitis B viral infection. **A.** Liver parenchyma showing hepatocytes with diffuse granular cytoplasm, so-called ground glass hepatocytes (H&E). **B.** Immunoperoxidase stains from the same case, showing cytoplasmic inclusions of viral particles. (From Kumar: Robbins and Cotran: Pathologic Basis of Disease, ed 8, Saunders, An Imprint of Elsevier, 2009)

Item 1–18 Hepatitis A (HAV) was formerly called epidemic, infectious, short-incubation, or acute catarrhal jaundice hepatitis. The primary transmission mode is the oral–fecal route. **Hepatitis B (HBV)** was formerly called long-incubation period, serum, or homologous serum hepatitis. Transmission modes are through blood from infected persons and from body fluids of infected mother to neonate. **Hepatitis C (HCV),** caused by the hepatitis C virus, is primarily transfusion associated. **Hepatitis D (HDV),** also called delta hepatitis, is caused by the hepatitis D virus in patients formerly or currently infected with hepatitis B. **Hepatitis E (HEV)** is also called enterically transmitted non-A, non-B hepatitis. The primary transmission mode is the oral–fecal route, usually through contaminated water.

● **B10.8   Other human herpesvirus infection**

 B10.81   Human herpesvirus 6 infection
  Causative agent of exanthema subitum that results in sudden rash

 B10.82   Human herpesvirus 7 infection
  Closely related to human herpesvirus 6, but not known cause any disease

 B10.89   Other human herpesvirus infection
  Human herpesvirus 8 infection
  May be the cause of Kaposi sarcoma, a malignant tumor
  Kaposi's sarcoma-associated herpesvirus infection

VIRAL HEPATITIS (B15-B19)

Excludes1	sequelae of viral hepatitis (B94.2)
Excludes2	cytomegaloviral hepatitis (B25.1)
	herpesviral [herpes simplex] hepatitis (B00.81)

● **B15   Acute hepatitis A**
 (Ex:) **For category B15 CC codes:** See PDX Collection 175

 B15.0   Hepatitis A with hepatic coma 🔖

 B15.9   Hepatitis A without hepatic coma 🔖
  Hepatitis A (acute) (viral) NOS

● **B16   Acute hepatitis B**
 (Ex:) **For category B16 CC codes:** See PDX Collection 175

 B16.0   Acute hepatitis B with delta-agent with hepatic coma 🔖

 B16.1   Acute hepatitis B with delta-agent without hepatic coma 🔖

 B16.2   Acute hepatitis B without delta-agent with hepatic coma 🔖

 B16.9   Acute hepatitis B without delta-agent and without hepatic coma 🔖
  Hepatitis B (acute) (viral) NOS
  Coding Clinic: 2016, Q3, P13

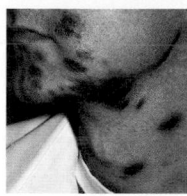

Figure 1-7 Kaposi's sarcoma. There are large confluent hyperpigmented patch-stage lesions with lymphedema. (From Kanski, JJ: Clinical Diagnosis in Ophthalmology, London, Elsevier Mosby, 2006)

Item 1–19 AIDS (acquired immune deficiency syndrome) is caused by **HIV** (human immunodeficiency virus). HIV affects certain white blood cells (T-4 lymphocytes) and destroys the ability of the cells to fight infections, making patients susceptible to a host of infectious diseases (e.g., ***Pneumocystis carinii* pneumonia [PCP], Kaposi's sarcoma,** and **lymphoma). AIDS-related complex (ARC)** is an early stage of AIDS in which tests for HIV are positive but the symptoms are mild.

● **B17   Other acute viral hepatitis**
 (Ex:) **For category B17 CC codes:** See PDX Collection 175

 B17.0   Acute delta-(super) infection of hepatitis B carrier 🔖

● **B17.1   Acute hepatitis C**

  B17.10   Acute hepatitis C without hepatic coma 🔖
   Acute hepatitis C NOS

  B17.11   Acute hepatitis C with hepatic coma 🔖

 B17.2   Acute hepatitis E 🔖

 B17.8   Other specified acute viral hepatitis 🔖
  Hepatitis non-A non-B (acute) (viral) NEC

 B17.9   Acute viral hepatitis, unspecified 🔖
  Acute hepatitis NOS
  Acute infectious hepatitis NOS

● **B18   Chronic viral hepatitis**

 Includes   Carrier of viral hepatitis
 (Ex:) **For category B18 CC codes:** See PDX Collection 175

 B18.0   Chronic viral hepatitis B with delta-agent 🔖 🔖

 B18.1   Chronic viral hepatitis B without delta-agent 🔖 🔖
  Carrier of viral hepatitis B
  Chronic (viral) hepatitis B

 B18.2   Chronic viral hepatitis C 🔖 🔖
  Carrier of viral hepatitis C
  Coding Clinic: 2018, Q1, P4; 2017, Q1, P41

 B18.8   Other chronic viral hepatitis 🔖 🔖
  Carrier of other viral hepatitis

 B18.9   Chronic viral hepatitis, unspecified 🔖 🔖
  Carrier of unspecified viral hepatitis

● **B19   Unspecified viral hepatitis**
 (Ex:) **For category B19 CC codes:** See PDX Collection 175

 B19.0   Unspecified viral hepatitis with hepatic coma 🔖

● **B19.1   Unspecified viral hepatitis B**

  B19.10   Unspecified viral hepatitis B without hepatic coma 🔖
   Unspecified viral hepatitis B NOS

  B19.11   Unspecified viral hepatitis B with hepatic coma 🔖

● **B19.2   Unspecified viral hepatitis C**

  B19.20   Unspecified viral hepatitis C without hepatic coma 🔖
   Viral hepatitis C NOS

  B19.21   Unspecified viral hepatitis C with hepatic coma 🔖

 B19.9   Unspecified viral hepatitis without hepatic coma 🔖
  Viral hepatitis NOS

CHAPTER 1 (A00-B99)

N Newborn Age: 0   **P** Pediatric Age: 0–17   **M** Maternity DX: 9–64   **A** Adult Age: 15–124   ♀ Females Only   ♂ Males Only

🔖 Complication\Comorbidity   Major C\C   (Ex:) CC/MCC Exclusions   Hospital-Acquired Condition   🔖 Hierarchical Condition Category

OGCR   Section I. C.1.a.

Certain Infectious and Parasitic Diseases (A00-B99)

a.   Human Immunodeficiency Virus (HIV) Infections

1)   Code only confirmed cases

Code only confirmed cases of HIV infection illness. This is an exception to the hospital inpatient guideline Section II, H.

In this context, "confirmation" does not require documentation of positive serology or culture for HIV; the provider's diagnostic statement that the patient is HIV positive or has an HIV-related illness is sufficient.

HUMAN IMMUNODEFICIENCY VIRUS [HIV] DISEASE (B20)

B20   **Human immunodeficiency virus [HIV] disease** 🔑 🔑

     Includes   acquired immune deficiency syndrome [AIDS]
                AIDS-related complex [ARC]
                HIV infection, symptomatic

     Code first Human immunodeficiency virus [HIV] disease complicating pregnancy, childbirth and the puerperium, if applicable (O98.7-)

     Use additional code(s) to identify all manifestations of HIV infection

     Excludes1   asymptomatic human immunodeficiency virus [HIV] infection status (Z21)
                exposure to HIV virus (Z20.6)
                inconclusive serologic evidence of HIV (R75)

     (Ex.) See PDX Collection 176

     Coding Clinic: 2021, Q2, P6; 2019, Q1, P9-11

OTHER VIRAL DISEASES (B25-B34)

● **B25**   **Cytomegaloviral disease**

     AKA: HCMV or Human Herpesvirus 5 (HHV-5)

     Excludes1   congenital cytomegalovirus infection (P35.1)
                cytomegaloviral mononucleosis (B27.1-)

     B25.0   **Cytomegaloviral pneumonitis** 🔑 🔑
         MCC when PDx is its own MCC
         (Ex.) See PDX Collection 110

     B25.1   **Cytomegaloviral hepatitis** 🔑 🔑
         CC when PDx is its own CC
         (Ex.) See PDX Collection 3212

     B25.2   **Cytomegaloviral pancreatitis** 🔑 🔑
         MCC when PDx is its own MCC
         (Ex.) See PDX Collection 177

     B25.8   **Other cytomegaloviral diseases** 🔑 🔑
         Cytomegaloviral encephalitis
         (Ex.) See PDX Collection 178

     B25.9   **Cytomegaloviral disease, unspecified** 🔑 🔑
         (Ex.) See PDX Collection 178

● **B26**   **Mumps**

     Includes   epidemic parotitis
                infectious parotitis
     Acute, contagious, viral disease

     B26.0   **Mumps orchitis** ♂ 🔑
         (Ex.) See PDX Collection 179

     B26.1   **Mumps meningitis** 🔑
         (Ex.) See PDX Collection 180

     B26.2   **Mumps encephalitis** 🔑
         (Ex.) See PDX Collection 181

     B26.3   **Mumps pancreatitis** 🔑
         (Ex.) See PDX Collection 182

● **B26.8**   **Mumps with other complications**

     (Ex.) **For category B26.8 CC codes unless otherwise indicated:** See PDX Collection 184

     B26.81   **Mumps hepatitis** 🔑
         (Ex.) See PDX Collection 183

     B26.82   **Mumps myocarditis** 🔑

     B26.83   **Mumps nephritis** 🔑

     B26.84   **Mumps polyneuropathy** 🔑
         (Ex.) See PDX Collection 185

     B26.85   **Mumps arthritis** 🔑 🔑

     B26.89   **Other mumps complications** 🔑

     B26.9   **Mumps without complication**
         Mumps NOS
         Mumps parotitis NOS

● **B27**   **Infectious mononucleosis**

     Includes   glandular fever
                monocytic angina
                Pfeiffer's disease

● **B27.0**   **Gammaherpesviral mononucleosis**

     AKA: Pfeiffer's disease, infective mononucleosis
     Mononucleosis due to Epstein-Barr virus

     B27.00   **Gammaherpesviral mononucleosis without complication**
         Infective mononucleosis

     B27.01   **Gammaherpesviral mononucleosis with polyneuropathy**

     B27.02   **Gammaherpesviral mononucleosis with meningitis**

     B27.09   **Gammaherpesviral mononucleosis with other complications**
         Hepatomegaly in gammaherpesviral mononucleosis

● **B27.1**   **Cytomegaloviral mononucleosis**

     Infectious disease resembling infectious mononucleosis

     B27.10   **Cytomegaloviral mononucleosis without complications**

     B27.11   **Cytomegaloviral mononucleosis with polyneuropathy**

     B27.12   **Cytomegaloviral mononucleosis with meningitis**

     B27.19   **Cytomegaloviral mononucleosis with other complication**
         Hepatomegaly in cytomegaloviral mononucleosis

● **B27.8**   **Other infectious mononucleosis**

     B27.80   **Other infectious mononucleosis without complication**

     B27.81   **Other infectious mononucleosis with polyneuropathy**

     B27.82   **Other infectious mononucleosis with meningitis**

     B27.89   **Other infectious mononucleosis with other complication**
         Hepatomegaly in other infectious mononucleosis

● **B27.9**   **Infectious mononucleosis, unspecified**

     B27.90   **Infectious mononucleosis, unspecified without complication**

     B27.91   **Infectious mononucleosis, unspecified with polyneuropathy**

     B27.92   **Infectious mononucleosis, unspecified with meningitis**

     B27.99   **Infectious mononucleosis, unspecified with other complication**
         Hepatomegaly in unspecified infectious mononucleosis

▶ New   ⇒ Revised   ~~deleted~~ Deleted   Excludes 1   Excludes 2   Includes   Use additional   Code first   Code also   Key words

OGCR Official Guidelines   ● Unacceptable Principal Diagnosis   X Assign placeholder X   ● Use Additional Character(s)   ▶ Manifestation Code   Coding Clinic

● **B30**   **Viral conjunctivitis**

> **Excludes1**   herpesviral [herpes simplex] ocular disease (B00.5)
> ocular zoster (B02.3)

     B30.0   **Keratoconjunctivitis due to adenovirus**
         Epidemic keratoconjunctivitis
         Shipyard eye

     B30.1   **Conjunctivitis due to adenovirus**
         Acute adenoviral follicular conjunctivitis
         Swimming-pool conjunctivitis

     B30.2   **Viral pharyngoconjunctivitis**

     B30.3   **Acute epidemic hemorrhagic conjunctivitis (enteroviral)**
         Conjunctivitis due to coxsackievirus 24
         Conjunctivitis due to enterovirus 70
         Hemorrhagic conjunctivitis (acute)(epidemic)

     B30.8   **Other viral conjunctivitis**
         Newcastle conjunctivitis

     B30.9   **Viral conjunctivitis, unspecified**

● **B33**   **Other viral diseases, not elsewhere classified**

     B33.0   **Epidemic myalgia**
         Acute infectious disease, caused by group A coxsackie viruses or other enteroviruses with symptoms that include sudden pain in chest or upper abdomen with fever
         Bornholm disease

     B33.1   **Ross River disease** 🔖
         Epidemic polyarthritis and exanthema
         Ross River fever
         (Ex:) See PDX Collection 144

     ● **B33.2**   **Viral carditis**
         Coxsackie (virus) carditis

         B33.20   **Viral carditis, unspecified** 🔖
             (Ex:) See PDX Collection 186

         B33.21   **Viral endocarditis** 🔖
             (Ex:) See PDX Collection 187

         B33.22   **Viral myocarditis** 🔖
             (Ex:) See PDX Collection 186

         B33.23   **Viral pericarditis** 🔖
             (Ex:) See PDX Collection 188

         B33.24   **Viral cardiomyopathy** 🔖

     B33.3   **Retrovirus infections, not elsewhere classified**
         Retrovirus infection NOS

     B33.4   **Hantavirus (cardio)-pulmonary syndrome [HPS] [HCPS]** 🔖
         Hantavirus disease with pulmonary manifestations
         Sin nombre virus disease

         Use additional code to identify any associated acute kidney failure (N17.9)

         > **Excludes1**   hantavirus disease with renal manifestations (A98.5)
                     hemorrhagic fever with renal manifestations (A98.5)
         (Ex:) See PDX Collection 189

     B33.8   **Other specified viral diseases**

         > **Excludes1**   anogenital human papillomavirus infection (A63.0)
                     viral warts due to human papillomavirus infection (B07)

● **B34**   **Viral infection of unspecified site**

> **Excludes1**   anogenital human papillomavirus infection (A63.0)
> cytomegaloviral disease NOS (B25.9)
> herpesvirus [herpes simplex] infection NOS (B00.9)
> retrovirus infection NOS (B33.3)
> viral agents as the cause of diseases classified elsewhere (B97.-)
> viral warts due to human papillomavirus infection (B07)

     B34.0   **Adenovirus infection, unspecified**

     B34.1   **Enterovirus infection, unspecified**
         Intestinal tract infection
         Coxsackievirus infection NOS
         Echovirus infection NOS

     B34.2   **Coronavirus infection, unspecified**

         > **Excludes1**   COVID-19 (U07.1)
                     pneumonia due to SARS-associated coronavirus (J12.81)

     B34.3   **Parvovirus infection, unspecified** 🔖
         (Ex:) See PDX Collection 174

     B34.4   **Papovavirus infection, unspecified**

     B34.8   **Other viral infections of unspecified site**

     B34.9   **Viral infection, unspecified**
         Viremia NOS
         Coding Clinic: 2016, Q3, P10

MYCOSES (B35-B49)

> **Excludes2**   hypersensitivity pneumonitis due to organic dust (J67.-)
> mycosis fungoides (C84.0-)

● **B35**   **Dermatophytosis**
     AKA tinea or ringworm

> **Includes**   favus
> infections due to species of Epidermophyton, Micro-sporum and Trichophyton
> tinea, any type except those in B36.-

     B35.0   **Tinea barbae and tinea capitis**
         Beard ringworm
         Kerion
         Scalp ringworm
         Sycosis, mycotic

     B35.1   **Tinea unguium**
         White patches or pits on surface or edges of nails, followed by infection under nail plate
         Dermatophytic onychia
         Dermatophytosis of nail
         Onychomycosis
         Ringworm of nails

     B35.2   **Tinea manuum**
         Tinea of hands
         Dermatophytosis of hand
         Hand ringworm

     B35.3   **Tinea pedis**
         Tinea affecting feet
         Athlete's foot
         Dermatophytosis of foot
         Foot ringworm

     B35.4   **Tinea corporis**
         Infecting skin areas other than hands
         Ringworm of the body

N Newborn Age: 0   **P** Pediatric Age: 0–17   **M** Maternity DX: 9–64   **A** Adult Age: 15–124   ♀ Females Only   ♂ Males Only

🔖 Complication\Comorbidity   🔖 Major C\C   (Ex:) CC/MCC Exclusions   🔖 Hospital-Acquired Condition   🔖 Hierarchical Condition Category

673

CHAPTER 1 (A00-B99)

CHAPTER 1 (A00–B99)

B35.5   Tinea imbricata
Chronic tropical tinea corporis; AKA Oriental ringworm, tinea inguinalis, tinea cruris
Tokelau

B35.6   Tinea cruris
In groin or perineal area, spreading to adjacent regions; AKA jock itch, eczema marginatum, ringworm of groin, or tinea inguinalis
Dhobi itch
Groin ringworm
Jock itch

B35.8   Other dermatophytoses
Disseminated dermatophytosis
Granulomatous dermatophytosis

B35.9   Dermatophytosis, unspecified
Ringworm NOS

● **B36   Other superficial mycoses**

B36.0   Pityriasis versicolor
Common, chronic, symptomless disorder that includes macular patches of various sizes and shapes; AKA liver spots
Tinea flava
Tinea versicolor

B36.1   Tinea nigra
Minor fungal infection, with dark lesions, usually on skin of hands
Keratomycosis nigricans palmaris
Microsporosis nigra
Pityriasis nigra

B36.2   White piedra
White to light brown nodules on hair of beard, axilla, or groin; AKA trichosporosis
Tinea blanca

B36.3   Black piedra
Characterized by small black or brown nodules on shafts of scalp hair

B36.8   Other specified superficial mycoses

B36.9   Superficial mycosis, unspecified

● **B37   Candidiasis**

   Includes   candidosis
                 moniliasis

   Excludes1   neonatal candidiasis (P37.5)

B37.0   Candidal stomatitis 🔧
Oral thrush
(Ex:) See PDX Collection 190

B37.1   Pulmonary candidiasis 🔧🔧
Candidal bronchitis
Candidal pneumonia
(Ex:) See PDX Collection 190

B37.2   Candidiasis of skin and nail
Candidal onychia
Candidal paronychia

   Excludes2   diaper dermatitis (L22)

B37.3   Candidiasis of vulva and vagina ♀
Candidal vulvovaginitis
Monilial vulvovaginitis
Vaginal thrush

● **B37.4   Candidiasis of other urogenital sites**
(Ex:) For category B37.4 CC codes: See PDX Collection 191

   B37.41   Candidal cystitis and urethritis 🔧🔧

   B37.42   Candidal balanitis ♂
Male condition only

   B37.49   Other urogenital candidiasis 🔧🔧
Candidal pyelonephritis

B37.5   Candidal meningitis 🔧
(Ex:) See PDX Collection 192

B37.6   Candidal endocarditis 🔧
(Ex:) See PDX Collection 190

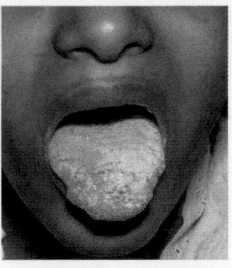

Figure 1-8   Oral candidiasis (thrush). (From James WD, Berger T, Elston D: Andrews' Diseases of the Skin: Clinical Dermatology, 11e, Saunders, 2011)

Item 1–20 Candidiasis, also called oidiomycosis or moniliasis, is a fungal infection. It most often appears on moist cutaneous areas of the body but can also be responsible for a variety of systemic infections such as endocarditis, meningitis, arthritis, and myositis. Antifungal medications cure most yeast infections.

B37.7   Candidal sepsis 🔧🔧
Disseminated candidiasis systemic candidiasis
MCC when PDx is its own MCC
(Ex:) See PDX Collection 193

● **B37.8   Candidiasis of other sites**
(Ex:) For category B37.8 CC codes unless otherwise indicated: See PDX Collection 190

   B37.81   Candidal esophagitis 🔧🔧

   B37.82   Candidal enteritis 🔧
Candidal proctitis

   B37.83   Candidal cheilitis 🔧
Inflammation affecting lip

   B37.84   Candidal otitis externa 🔧
Inflammation of external auditory canal

   B37.89   Other sites of candidiasis 🔧
Infection manifested by invasive candidiasis
Candidal osteomyelitis
(Ex:) See PDX Collection 194

B37.9   Candidiasis, unspecified
Thrush NOS

● **B38   Coccidioidomycosis**
Fungal disease; AKA coccidioidosis, coccidioidal granuloma, Posadas, or Posadas-Wernicke disease

B38.0   Acute pulmonary coccidioidomycosis 🔧🔧
(Ex:) See PDX Collection 195

B38.1   Chronic pulmonary coccidioidomycosis 🔧🔧
(Ex:) See PDX Collection 196

B38.2   Pulmonary coccidioidomycosis, unspecified 🔧🔧
(Ex:) See PDX Collection 196

B38.3   Cutaneous coccidioidomycosis 🔧
(Ex:) See PDX Collection 197

B38.4   Coccidioidomycosis meningitis 🔧
(Ex:) See PDX Collection 198

B38.7   Disseminated coccidioidomycosis 🔧
Generalized coccidioidomycosis
(Ex:) See PDX Collection 199

● **B38.8   Other forms of coccidioidomycosis**

   B38.81   Prostatic coccidioidomycosis ♂ 🔧
(Ex:) See PDX Collection 197

   B38.89   Other forms of coccidioidomycosis 🔧
(Ex:) See PDX Collection 199

B38.9   Coccidioidomycosis, unspecified 🔧
(Ex:) See PDX Collection 199

▶ New   ⇒ Revised   ~~deleted~~ Deleted   Excludes 1   Excludes 2   Includes   Use additional   Code first   Code also   Key words

OGCR Official Guidelines   ● Unacceptable Principal Diagnosis   X Assign placeholder X   ● Use Additional Character(s)   ▶ Manifestation Code   **Coding Clinic**

Item 1–21 Bird and bat droppings that fall into the soil give rise to a fungus that can spread airborne spores. When inhaled into the lungs, these spores divide and multiply into lesions. Histoplasmosis capsulatum takes three forms: primary (lodged in the lungs only), chronic (resembles TB), and disseminated (infection has moved to other organs). This is an opportunistic infection in immunosuppressed patients.

● **B39   Histoplasmosis**
   Infection resulting from inhalation or ingestion of spores; AKA Darling disease
   Code first associated AIDS (B20)
   Use additional code for any associated manifestations, such as:
      endocarditis (I39)
      meningitis (G02)
      pericarditis (I32)
      retinitis (H32)

   B39.0   Acute pulmonary histoplasmosis capsulati 🔖🔖
      (Ex:) See PDX Collection 200

   B39.1   Chronic pulmonary histoplasmosis capsulati 🔖🔖
      (Ex:) See PDX Collection 200

   B39.2   Pulmonary histoplasmosis capsulati, unspecified 🔖🔖
      (Ex:) See PDX Collection 200

   B39.3   Disseminated histoplasmosis capsulati 🔖
      Generalized histoplasmosis capsulati
      (Ex:) See PDX Collection 201

   B39.4   Histoplasmosis capsulati, unspecified
      American histoplasmosis

   B39.5   Histoplasmosis duboisii
      African histoplasmosis

   B39.9   Histoplasmosis, unspecified

● **B40   Blastomycosis**
   Rare and potentially fatal infection caused by inhaling fungus found in moist soil in temperate climates.

   Excludes1   Brazilian blastomycosis (B41.-)
                  keloidal blastomycosis (B48.0)
   (Ex:) **For category B40 CC codes:** See PDX Collection 202

   B40.0   Acute pulmonary blastomycosis 🔖🔖
   B40.1   Chronic pulmonary blastomycosis 🔖🔖
   B40.2   Pulmonary blastomycosis, unspecified 🔖🔖
   B40.3   Cutaneous blastomycosis 🔖
   B40.7   Disseminated blastomycosis 🔖
      Generalized blastomycosis

   ● **B40.8   Other forms of blastomycosis**
      B40.81   Blastomycotic meningoencephalitis 🔖
         Meningomyelitis due to blastomycosis
      B40.89   Other forms of blastomycosis 🔖

   B40.9   Blastomycosis, unspecified 🔖

● **B41   Paracoccidioidomycosis**
   Fungal infection usually chronic that begins in lungs, spreads to mucocutaneous areas which may extend to skin, tonsils, gastrointestinal lymphatics, liver, and spleen; AKA Almeida or Lutz-Splendore-Almeida disease, Brazilian or South American blastomycosis, or paracoccidioidal granuloma

   Includes   Brazilian blastomycosis
                Lutz' disease
   (Ex:) **For category B41 CC codes:** See PDX Collection 203

   B41.0   Pulmonary paracoccidioidomycosis 🔖🔖
   B41.7   Disseminated paracoccidioidomycosis 🔖
      Generalized paracoccidioidomycosis
   B41.8   Other forms of paracoccidioidomycosis 🔖
   B41.9   Paracoccidioidomycosis, unspecified 🔖

● **B42   Sporotrichosis**
   Chronic fungal infection with nodular lesions

   B42.0   Pulmonary sporotrichosis
   B42.1   Lymphocutaneous sporotrichosis
   B42.7   Disseminated sporotrichosis
      Generalized sporotrichosis

   ● **B42.8   Other forms of sporotrichosis**
      B42.81   Cerebral sporotrichosis
         Meningitis due to sporotrichosis
      B42.82   Sporotrichosis arthritis 🔖
      B42.89   Other forms of sporotrichosis

   B42.9   Sporotrichosis, unspecified

● **B43   Chromomycosis and pheomycotic abscess**
   Chronic fungal infection of skin, initiated at site of puncture affecting lower limb or foot (mossy foot)

   B43.0   Cutaneous chromomycosis
      Dermatitis verrucosa
   B43.1   Pheomycotic brain abscess
      Cerebral chromomycosis
   B43.2   Subcutaneous pheomycotic abscess and cyst
   B43.8   Other forms of chromomycosis
   B43.9   Chromomycosis, unspecified

● **B44   Aspergillosis**
   Infection marked by inflammatory lesions in skin, ear, orbit, nasal sinuses, lungs, and occasionally bones and meninges

   Includes   aspergilloma
   (Ex:) **For category B44 CC codes unless otherwise indicated:** See PDX Collection 204

   B44.0   Invasive pulmonary aspergillosis 🔖🔖
      MCC when PDx is its own MCC
      (Ex:) See PDX Collection 110
   B44.1   Other pulmonary aspergillosis 🔖🔖
   B44.2   Tonsillar aspergillosis 🔖🔖
   B44.7   Disseminated aspergillosis 🔖🔖
      Generalized aspergillosis

   ● **B44.8   Other forms of aspergillosis**
      B44.81   Allergic bronchopulmonary aspergillosis 🔖🔖
         (Ex:) See PDX Collection 205
      B44.89   Other forms of aspergillosis 🔖🔖

   B44.9   Aspergillosis, unspecified 🔖🔖

● **B45   Cryptococcosis**
   Infection in the immunocompromised and fatal if left untreated; AKA torulosis, Buschke, or Busse-Buschke disease
   (Ex:) **For category B45 CC codes unless otherwise indicated:** See PDX Collection 206

   B45.0   Pulmonary cryptococcosis 🔖🔖
   B45.1   Cerebral cryptococcosis 🔖🔖
      Cryptococcal meningitis
      Cryptococcosis meningocerebralis
      MCC when PDx is its own MCC
      (Ex:) See PDX Collection 207
   B45.2   Cutaneous cryptococcosis 🔖🔖
   B45.3   Osseous cryptococcosis 🔖🔖
   B45.7   Disseminated cryptococcosis 🔖🔖
      Generalized cryptococcosis
   B45.8   Other forms of cryptococcosis 🔖🔖
   B45.9   Cryptococcosis, unspecified 🔖🔖

N Newborn Age: 0   **P** Pediatric Age: 0–17   **M** Maternity DX: 9–64   **A** Adult Age: 15–124   ♀ Females Only   ♂ Males Only
🔖 Complication\Comorbidity   🔖 Major C\C   (Ex:) CC/MCC Exclusions   🔖 Hospital-Acquired Condition   🔖 Hierarchical Condition Category

CHAPTER 1 (A00-B99)

675

CHAPTER 1 (A00-B99)

● **B46**   **Zygomycosis**
    Fungal infections including subcutaneous lesions and infection of sinuses, brain, or lungs
    (Ex) **For category B46 CC codes:** See PDX Collection 208

    B46.0   **Pulmonary mucormycosis** 🐾🐾
          Fungal infection affecting lung

    B46.1   **Rhinocerebral mucormycosis** 🐾🐾

    B46.2   **Gastrointestinal mucormycosis** 🐾🐾

    B46.3   **Cutaneous mucormycosis** 🐾🐾
          Subcutaneous mucormycosis

    B46.4   **Disseminated mucormycosis** 🐾🐾
          Generalized mucormycosis

    B46.5   **Mucormycosis, unspecified** 🐾🐾

    B46.8   **Other zygomycoses** 🐾🐾
          Entomophthoromycosis

    B46.9   **Zygomycosis, unspecified** 🐾🐾
          Phycomycosis NOS

● **B47**   **Mycetoma**
    Slow progressive, destructive fungal infection of cutaneous and subcutaneous tissues, fascia, and bone, primarily seen in foot (Madura foot) or leg

    B47.0   **Eumycetoma** 🐾
          Madura foot, mycotic Maduromycosis
          (Ex) See PDX Collection 209

    B47.1   **Actinomycetoma** 🐾
          (Ex) See PDX Collection 106

    B47.9   **Mycetoma, unspecified** 🐾
          Madura foot NOS
          (Ex) See PDX Collection 210

● **B48**   **Other mycoses, not elsewhere classified**

    B48.0   **Lobomycosis**
          Infection with symptoms of red, smooth, hard cutaneous nodules resembling keloids
          Keloidal blastomycosis
          Lobo's disease

    B48.1   **Rhinosporidiosis**
          Chronic, localized granulomatous fungal infection, affecting mucocutaneous tissues, usually of nose characterized by polyps, papillomas, and wartlike lesions

    B48.2   **Allescheriasis** 🐾
          Fungal infection
          Infection due to Pseudallescheria boydii
          Excludes1   eumycetoma (B47.0)
          (Ex) See PDX Collection 211

    B48.3   **Geotrichosis** 🐾
          Fungal infection usually of bronchi, lungs, mouth, or intestinal tract
          Geotrichum stomatitis
          (Ex) See PDX Collection 212

    B48.4   **Penicillosis** 🐾🐾
          Fungal infection
          Talaromycosis
          (Ex) See PDX Collection 204

    B48.8   **Other specified mycoses** 🐾🐾
          Adiaspiromycosis
          Infection of tissue and organs by Alternaria
          Infection of tissue and organs by Drechslera
          Infection of tissue and organs by Fusarium
          Infection of tissue and organs by saprophytic fungi NEC
          (Ex) See PDX Collection 213

  B49   **Unspecified mycosis** 🐾
          Fungemia NOS
          (Ex) See PDX Collection 212

PROTOZOAL DISEASES (B50-B64)

    Excludes1   amebiasis (A06.-)
          other protozoal intestinal diseases (A07.-)

● **B50**   **Plasmodium falciparum malaria**
    Severe form of malaria that can be fatal
    Includes   mixed infections of Plasmodium falciparum with any other Plasmodium species
    (Ex) **For category B50 CC codes:** See PDX Collection 214

    B50.0   **Plasmodium falciparum malaria with cerebral complications** 🐾
          Cerebral malaria NOS

    B50.8   **Other severe and complicated Plasmodium falciparum malaria** 🐾
          Severe or complicated Plasmodium falciparum malaria NOS

    B50.9   **Plasmodium falciparum malaria, unspecified** 🐾

● **B51**   **Plasmodium vivax malaria**
    Includes   mixed infections of Plasmodium vivax with other Plasmodium species, except Plasmodium falciparum
    Excludes1   plasmodium vivax with Plasmodium falciparum (B50.-)
    (Ex) **For category B51 CC codes unless otherwise indicated:** See PDX Collection 214

    B51.0   **Plasmodium vivax malaria with rupture of spleen** 🐾

    B51.8   **Plasmodium vivax malaria with other complications** 🐾

    B51.9   **Plasmodium vivax malaria without complication** 🐾
          Plasmodium vivax malaria NOS
          (Ex) See PDX Collection 215

● **B52**   **Plasmodium malariae malaria**
    Causes fever that recurs at approximately three-day intervals (quartan fever), longer than two-day (tertian) intervals of other malarial parasites
    Includes   mixed infections of Plasmodium malariae with other Plasmodium species, except Plasmodium falciparum and Plasmodium vivax
    Excludes1   plasmodium falciparum (B50.-)
          plasmodium vivax (B51.-)
    (Ex) **For category B52 CC codes unless otherwise indicated:** See PDX Collection 214

    B52.0   **Plasmodium malariae malaria with nephropathy** 🐾
          CC when PDx is its own CC
          (Ex) See PDX Collection 216

    B52.8   **Plasmodium malariae malaria with other complications** 🐾

    B52.9   **Plasmodium malariae malaria without complication** 🐾
          Plasmodium malariae malaria NOS

● **B53**   **Other specified malaria**
    (Ex) **For category B53 CC codes unless otherwise indicated:** See PDX Collection 214

    B53.0   **Plasmodium ovale malaria** 🐾
          Least diagnosed type of malaria spread by female mosquitoes of rare species
          Excludes1   plasmodium ovale with Plasmodium falciparum (B50.-)
                plasmodium ovale with Plasmodium malariae (B52.-)
                plasmodium ovale with Plasmodium vivax (B51.-)

    B53.1   **Malaria due to simian plasmodia** 🐾
          Malaria-like disease (parasite infection)
          Excludes1   malaria due to simian plasmodia with Plasmodium falciparum (B50.-)
                malaria due to simian plasmodia with Plasmodium malariae (B52.-)
                malaria due to simian plasmodia with Plasmodium ovale (B53.0)
                malaria due to simian plasmodia with Plasmodium vivax (B51.-)

    B53.8   **Other malaria, not elsewhere classified** 🐾

▶ New   ⇒ Revised   ~~deleted~~ Deleted   Excludes 1   Excludes 2   Includes   Use additional   Code first   Code also   Key words

OGCR Official Guidelines   ● Unacceptable Principal Diagnosis   X Assign placeholder X   ● Use Additional Character(s)   ▷ Manifestation Code   **Coding Clinic**

B54   Unspecified malaria 🅒
     (Ex:) See PDX Collection 217

● B55   Leishmaniasis
     Protozoal infection
     (Ex:) **For category B55 CC codes:** See PDX Collection 218

     B55.0   Visceral leishmaniasis 🅒
           Kala-azar
           Post-kala-azar dermal leishmaniasis

     B55.1   Cutaneous leishmaniasis 🅒

     B55.2   Mucocutaneous leishmaniasis 🅒

     B55.9   Leishmaniasis, unspecified 🅒

● B56   African trypanosomiasis
     Human African trypanosomiasis (HAT) is transmitted by fly bites
     (Ex:) **For category B56 CC codes:** See PDX Collection 218

     B56.0   Gambiense trypanosomiasis 🅒
           Infection due to Trypanosoma brucei gambiense
           West African sleeping sickness

     B56.1   Rhodesiense trypanosomiasis 🅒
           East African sleeping sickness
           Infection due to Trypanosoma brucei rhodesiense

     B56.9   African trypanosomiasis, unspecified 🅒
           Sleeping sickness NOS

● B57   Chagas' disease
     Tropical parasitic disease
     Includes   American trypanosomiasis
                    infection due to Trypanosoma cruzi

     B57.0   Acute Chagas' disease with heart involvement 🅒
           Acute Chagas' disease with myocarditis
           (Ex:) See PDX Collection 219

     B57.1   Acute Chagas' disease without heart involvement 🅒
           Acute Chagas' disease NOS
           (Ex:) See PDX Collection 218

     B57.2   Chagas' disease (chronic) with heart involvement 🅒
           American trypanosomiasis NOS
           Chagas' disease (chronic) NOS
           Chagas' disease (chronic) with myocarditis
           Trypanosomiasis NOS
           (Ex:) See PDX Collection 219

●   B57.3   Chagas' disease (chronic) with digestive system involvement
           (Ex:) **For category B57.3 CC codes:** See PDX Collection 218

         B57.30   Chagas' disease with digestive system involvement, unspecified 🅒

         B57.31   Megaesophagus in Chagas' disease 🅒

         B57.32   Megacolon in Chagas' disease 🅒

         B57.39   Other digestive system involvement in Chagas' disease

●   B57.4   Chagas' disease (chronic) with nervous system involvement
           (Ex:) **For category B57.4 CC codes:** See PDX Collection 218

         B57.40   Chagas' disease with nervous system involvement, unspecified 🅒

         B57.41   Meningitis in Chagas' disease 🅒

         B57.42   Meningoencephalitis in Chagas' disease 🅒

         B57.49   Other nervous system involvement in Chagas' disease 🅒

     B57.5   Chagas' disease (chronic) with other organ involvement 🅒
           (Ex:) See PDX Collection 218

● B58   Toxoplasmosis
     Infection by protozoon transmitted in cysts in feces of cats
     Includes   infection due to Toxoplasma gondii
     Excludes1   congenital toxoplasmosis (P37.1)

●   B58.0   Toxoplasma oculopathy

         B58.00   Toxoplasma oculopathy, unspecified 🅒
              (Ex:) See PDX Collection 220

         B58.01   Toxoplasma chorioretinitis 🅒
              (Ex:) See PDX Collection 221

         B58.09   Other toxoplasma oculopathy 🅒
              Toxoplasma uveitis
              (Ex:) See PDX Collection 222

Item 1–22   **Toxoplasmosis** is caused by the protozoa **Toxoplasma gondii,** of which the house cat can be a host. Human infection occurs when contact is made with materials containing the pathogen, such as feces, contaminated soil, or ingestion of infected lamb, goat, or pork. Of the infected, very few have symptoms because a healthy person's immune system keeps the parasite from causing illness. When the immune system is compromised, symptoms may occur. Clinical symptoms include flu-like symptoms, but the disease progresses to include the eyes and the brain in babies.

     B58.1   Toxoplasma hepatitis 🅒
           (Ex:) See PDX Collection 223

     B58.2   Toxoplasma meningoencephalitis 🅒🅒
           (Ex:) See PDX Collection 224

     B58.3   Pulmonary toxoplasmosis 🅒🅒
           (Ex:) See PDX Collection 225

●   B58.8   Toxoplasmosis with other organ involvement
           (Ex:) **For category B58.8 CC codes unless otherwise indicated:** See PDX Collection 220

         B58.81   Toxoplasma myocarditis 🅒
              (Ex:) See PDX Collection 226

         B58.82   Toxoplasma myositis 🅒

         B58.83   Toxoplasma tubulo-interstitial nephropathy 🅒
              Toxoplasma pyelonephritis

         B58.89   Toxoplasmosis with other organ involvement 🅒

     B58.9   Toxoplasmosis, unspecified 🅒
           (Ex:) See PDX Collection 227

  B59   Pneumocystosis 🅒🅒
     Caused by fungus
     Pneumonia due to Pneumocystis carinii
     Pneumonia due to Pneumocystis jiroveci
     (Ex:) See PDX Collection 228

● B60   Other protozoal diseases, not elsewhere classified
     Excludes1   cryptosporidiosis (A07.2)
                  intestinal microsporidiosis (A07.8)
                  isosporiasis (A07.3)

     B60.0   Babesiosis 🅒
           Tickborne disease caused by microscopic organisms
           (Ex:) See PDX Collection 4064

         B60.00   Babesiosis, unspecified 🅒
              Babesiosis due to unspecified Babesia species
              Piroplasmosis, unspecified

         B60.01   Babesiosis due to Babesia microti 🅒
              Infection due to B. microti

         B60.02   Babesiosis due to Babesia duncani 🅒
              Infection due to B. duncani and B. duncani-type species

         B60.03   Babesiosis due to Babesia divergens 🅒
              Babesiosis due to Babesia MO-1
              Infection due to B. divergens and B. divergens-like strains

         B60.09   Other babesiosis 🅒
              Babesiosis due to Babesia KO-1
              Babesiosis due to Babesia venatorum
              Infection due to other Babesia species
              Infection due to other protozoa of the order Piroplasmida
              Other piroplasmosis

●   B60.1   Acanthamebiasis
           (Ex:) **For category B60.1 CC codes:** See PDX Collection 229

         B60.10   Acanthamebiasis, unspecified 🅒

         B60.11   Meningoencephalitis due to Acanthamoeba (culbertsoni)

         B60.12   Conjunctivitis due to Acanthamoeba

         B60.13   Keratoconjunctivitis due to Acanthamoeba

         B60.19   Other acanthamebic disease 🅒

N Newborn Age: 0   **P** Pediatric Age: 0–17   **M** Maternity DX: 9–64   **A** Adult Age: 15–124   ♀ Females Only   ♂ Males Only

🅒 Complication\Comorbidity   🅒 Major C\C   (Ex:) CC/MCC Exclusions   🅒 Hospital-Acquired Condition   🅒 Hierarchical Condition Category

677

CHAPTER 1 (A00–B99)

B60.2   **Naegleriasis** 🔑
Infection with microscopic organisms
Primary amebic meningoencephalitis
Ⓔ See PDX Collection 229

B60.8   **Other specified protozoal diseases**
Microsporidiosis

B64   **Unspecified protozoal disease**

HELMINTHIASES (B65-B83)

Diseases or infestations caused by parasitic worms

● **B65**   **Schistosomiasis [bilharziasis]**
Infection with flukes (flat parasitic worms)
Includes   snail fever
Ⓔ **For category B65 CC codes:** See PDX Collection 230

B65.0   **Schistosomiasis due to Schistosoma haematobium [urinary schistosomiasis]** 🔑

B65.1   **Schistosomiasis due to Schistosoma mansoni [intestinal schistosomiasis]** 🔑

B65.2   **Schistosomiasis due to Schistosoma japonicum** 🔑
Asiatic schistosomiasis

B65.3   **Cercarial dermatitis** 🔑
Swimmer's itch

B65.8   **Other schistosomiasis** 🔑
Infection due to Schistosoma intercalatum
Infection due to Schistosoma mattheei
Infection due to Schistosoma mekongi

B65.9   **Schistosomiasis, unspecified** 🔑

● **B66**   **Other fluke infections**
Trematode (parasitic worms)
Ⓔ **For category B66 CC codes:** See PDX Collection 231

B66.0   **Opisthorchiasis** 🔑
Infection due to cat liver fluke
Infection due to Opisthorchis (felineus)(viverrini)

B66.1   **Clonorchiasis** 🔑
Chinese liver fluke disease
Infection due to Clonorchis sinensis
Oriental liver fluke disease

B66.2   **Dicroceliasis** 🔑
Liver fluke
Infection due to Dicrocoelium dendriticum
Lancet fluke infection

B66.3   **Fascioliasis** 🔑
Infection due to Fasciola gigantica
Infection due to Fasciola hepatica
Infection due to Fasciola indica
Sheep liver fluke disease

B66.4   **Paragonimiasis** 🔑🔑
Infection due to Paragonimus species
Lung fluke disease
Pulmonary distomiasis

B66.5   **Fasciolopsiasis** 🔑
Largest intestinal fluke in humans
Infection due to Fasciolopsis buski
Intestinal distomiasis

B66.8   **Other specified fluke infections** 🔑
Echinostomiasis
Heterophyiasis
Metagonimiasis
Nanophyetiasis
Watsoniasis

B66.9   **Fluke infection, unspecified**

● **B67**   **Echinococcosis**
Larval forms of tapeworms usually of liver or lungs
Includes   hydatidosis

B67.0   **Echinococcus granulosus infection of liver** 🔑
Ⓔ See PDX Collection 232

B67.1   **Echinococcus granulosus infection of lung** 🔑🔑
Ⓔ See PDX Collection 233

B67.2   **Echinococcus granulosus infection of bone** 🔑
Ⓔ See PDX Collection 234

Item 1-23 Echinococcosis: Also known as hydatid disease; is caused by Echinococcus granulosus, E. multilocularis, and E. vogeli tapeworms; and is contracted from infected food. Found in southern South America, the Mediterranean, the Middle East, central Asia, and Africa and uncommon in the United States but has been reported in California, New Mexico, Arizona and Utah. The disease is treated with medication over a long course, as it is resistive.

● **B67.3**   **Echinococcus granulosus infection, other and multiple sites**

B67.31   **Echinococcus granulosus infection, thyroid gland** 🔑
Ⓔ See PDX Collection 235

B67.32   **Echinococcus granulosus infection, multiple sites** 🔑
Ⓔ See PDX Collection 234

B67.39   **Echinococcus granulosus infection, other sites** 🔑
Ⓔ See PDX Collection 234

B67.4   **Echinococcus granulosus infection, unspecified** 🔑
Dog tapeworm (infection)
Ⓔ See PDX Collection 236

B67.5   **Echinococcus multilocularis infection of liver** 🔑
Ⓔ See PDX Collection 237

● **B67.6**   **Echinococcus multilocularis infection, other and multiple sites**
Ⓔ **For category B67.6 CC codes:** See PDX Collection 238

B67.61   **Echinococcus multilocularis infection, multiple sites** 🔑

B67.69   **Echinococcus multilocularis infection, other sites** 🔑

B67.7   **Echinococcus multilocularis infection, unspecified** 🔑
Ⓔ See PDX Collection 239

B67.8   **Echinococcosis, unspecified, of liver** 🔑
Ⓔ See PDX Collection 240

● **B67.9**   **Echinococcosis, other and unspecified**
Ⓔ **For category B67.9 CC codes:** See PDX Collection 240

B67.90   **Echinococcosis, unspecified** 🔑
Echinococcosis NOS

B67.99   **Other echinococcosis** 🔑

● **B68**   **Taeniasis**
Intestinal tapeworm (cestode) infection from raw or undercooked meat of infected animal
Excludes1   cysticercosis (B69.-)

B68.0   **Taenia solium taeniasis** 🔑
Pork tapeworm (infection)
Ⓔ See PDX Collection 241

B68.1   **Taenia saginata taeniasis** 🔑
Beef tapeworm (infection)
Infection due to adult tapeworm Taenia saginata
Ⓔ See PDX Collection 242

B68.9   **Taeniasis, unspecified** 🔑
Ⓔ See PDX Collection 242

● **B69**   **Cysticercosis**
Systemic illness caused by the larvae of pork tapeworm
Includes   cysticerciasis infection due to larval form of Taenia solium
Ⓔ **For category B69 CC codes:** See PDX Collection 242

B69.0   **Cysticercosis of central nervous system** 🔑

B69.1   **Cysticercosis of eye** 🔑

● **B69.8**   **Cysticercosis of other sites**

B69.81   **Myositis in cysticercosis** 🔑

B69.89   **Cysticercosis of other sites** 🔑

B69.9   **Cysticercosis, unspecified** 🔑

▶ New   ⇒ Revised   ~~deleted~~ Deleted   Excludes 1   Excludes 2   Includes   Use additional   Code first   Code also   Key words
OGCR Official Guidelines   ● Unacceptable Principal Diagnosis   X Assign placeholder X   ● Use Additional Character(s)   ▶ Manifestation Code   Coding Clinic

● **B70   Diphyllobothriasis and sparganosis**
     Infection with tapeworms seen most often from inadequately cooked fish
     (Ex:) **For category B70 CC codes:** See PDX Collection 242

     B70.0   Diphyllobothriasis 🦠
         Diphyllobothrium (adult) (latum) (pacificum) infection
         Fish tapeworm (infection)
         Excludes2   larval diphyllobothriasis (B70.1)

     B70.1   Sparganosis 🦠
         Infection with migrating tapeworm larvae, which invade subcutaneous tissues, causing inflammation and fibrosis that resembles cellulitis
         Infection due to Sparganum (mansoni) (proliferum)
         Infection due to Spirometra larva
         Larval diphyllobothriasis
         Spirometrosis

● **B71   Other cestode infections**
     (Ex:) **For category B71 CC codes:** See PDX Collection 242

     B71.0   Hymenolepiasis 🦠
         Intestinal infestation with tapeworms
         Dwarf tapeworm infection
         Rat tapeworm (infection)

     B71.1   Dipylidiasis 🦠
         Infection with tapeworm common to dogs and cats and seen in children having close contact with infected pets

     B71.8   Other specified cestode infections 🦠
         Infection by the larval stage of a tapeworm, usually through fruit or vegetables
         Coenurosis

     B71.9   Cestode infection, unspecified
         Tapeworm (infection) NOS

● **B72   Dracunculiasis** 🦠
     Infection with roundworms
     Includes   guinea worm infection
         Infection due to Dracunculus medinensis
     (Ex:) See PDX Collection 243

● **B73   Onchocerciasis**
     Infection with parasitic worm
     Includes   onchocerca volvulus infection
         onchocercosis
         river blindness

     ● **B73.0   Onchocerciasis with eye disease**
         (Ex:) **For category B73 CC codes:** See PDX Collection 243

         B73.00   Onchocerciasis with eye involvement, unspecified 🦠

         B73.01   Onchocerciasis with endophthalmitis 🦠

         B73.02   Onchocerciasis with glaucoma 🦠

         B73.09   Onchocerciasis with other eye involvement 🦠
             Infestation of eyelid due to onchocerciasis

     B73.1   Onchocerciasis without eye disease 🦠

● **B74   Filariasis**
     Infestation with slender threadlike worms
     ⇒**Excludes2**   onchocerciasis (B73)
         tropical (pulmonary) eosinophilia NOS (J82.89)
     (Ex:) **For category B74 CC codes:** See PDX Collection 243

     B74.0   Filariasis due to Wuchereria bancrofti 🦠
         Bancroftian elephantiasis
         Bancroftian filariasis

     B74.1   Filariasis due to Brugia malayi 🦠

     B74.2   Filariasis due to Brugia timori 🦠

     B74.3   Loiasis 🦠
         Infection with round worms growing in subcutaneous connective tissue
         Calabar swelling
         Eyeworm disease of Africa
         Loa loa infection

     B74.4   Mansonelliasis 🦠
         Infection with filarial parasite
         Infection due to Mansonella ozzardi
         Infection due to Mansonella perstans
         Infection due to Mansonella streptocerca

     B74.8   Other filariases 🦠
         Dirofilariasis

     B74.9   Filariasis, unspecified 🦠

● **B75   Trichinellosis** 🦠
     Infestation with parasitic roundworms ingested in undercooked contaminated meat
     Includes   infection due to Trichinella species trichiniasis
     (Ex:) See PDX Collection 244

● **B76   Hookworm diseases**
     Occurs in hot, humid parts of world where larvae are soil borne, enter digestive tract through skin of feet/legs or in contaminated food/water; AKA ground itch
     Includes   uncinariasis
     (Ex:) **For category B76 CC codes:** See PDX Collection 245

     B76.0   Ancylostomiasis 🦠
         Infection due to Ancylostoma species

     B76.1   Necatoriasis 🦠
         Infection due to Necator americanus

     B76.8   Other hookworm diseases 🦠

     B76.9   Hookworm disease, unspecified 🦠
         Cutaneous larva migrans NOS

● **B77   Ascariasis**
     Infection by roundworm in small intestine
     Includes   ascaridiasis
         roundworm infection

     B77.0   Ascariasis with intestinal complications 🦠
         (Ex:) See PDX Collection 246

     ● **B77.8   Ascariasis with other complications**
         B77.81   Ascariasis pneumonia 🦠
             MCC when PDx is its own MCC
             (Ex:) See PDX Collection 247

         B77.89   Ascariasis with other complications 🦠
             (Ex:) See PDX Collection 246

     B77.9   Ascariasis, unspecified 🦠
         (Ex:) See PDX Collection 246

● **B78   Strongyloidiasis**
     Infection with adult female roundworms
     Excludes1   trichostrongyliasis (B81.2)
     (Ex:) **For category B78 CC codes:** See PDX Collection 246

     B78.0   Intestinal strongyloidiasis 🦠

     B78.1   Cutaneous strongyloidiasis 🦠

     B78.7   Disseminated strongyloidiasis 🦠

     B78.9   Strongyloidiasis, unspecified 🦠

● **B79   Trichuriasis** 🦠
     Intestinal infection with roundworms
     Includes   trichocephaliasis
         whipworm (disease)(infection)
     (Ex:) See PDX Collection 246

● **B80   Enterobiasis** 🦠
     Intestinal infection with pinworms
     Includes   oxyuriasis
         pinworm infection
         threadworm infection
     (Ex:) See PDX Collection 246

CHAPTER 1 (A00-B99)

N Newborn Age: 0   **P** Pediatric Age: 0–17   **M** Maternity DX: 9–64   **A** Adult Age: 15–124   ♀ Females Only   ♂ Males Only

🦠 Complication\Comorbidity   🦠 Major C\C   (Ex:) CC/MCC Exclusions   🦠 Hospital-Acquired Condition   🦠 Hierarchical Condition Category

679

CHAPTER 1 (A00-B99)

● **B81   Other intestinal helminthiases, not elsewhere classified**
Diseases or infestations caused by parasitic worms

> **Excludes1**   angiostrongyliasis due to:
> Angiostrongylus cantonensis (B83.2)
> Parastrongylus cantonensis (B83.2)
> (Ex:) For category B81 CC codes B81.0-B81.2: See PDX Collection 246
> For category B81 CC codes B81.3-B81.8: See PDX Collection 248

B81.0   Anisakiasis 🔗
Roundworm infection via contaminated undercooked infected fish or marine mammals
Infection due to Anisakis larva

B81.1   Intestinal capillariasis 🔗
Infestation with of parasites (nematodes)
Capillariasis NOS
Infection due to Capillaria philippinensis

> **Excludes2**   hepatic capillariasis (B83.8)

B81.2   Trichostrongyliasis 🔗

B81.3   Intestinal angiostrongyliasis 🔗
Angiostrongyliasis due to:
Angiostrongylus costaricensis (B83.2)
Parastrongylus costaricensis (B83.2)

B81.4   Mixed intestinal helminthiases 🔗
Infection due to intestinal helminths classified to more than one of the categories B65.0-B81.3 and B81.8
Mixed helminthiasis NOS

B81.8   Other specified intestinal helminthiases 🔗
Infection due to Oesophagostomum species [esophagostomiasis]
Infection due to Ternidens diminutus [ternidensiasis]

● **B82   Unspecified intestinal parasitism**

B82.0   Intestinal helminthiasis, unspecified 🔗
Infected with worms
(Ex:) See PDX Collection 248

B82.9   Intestinal parasitism, unspecified

● **B83   Other helminthiases**
Caused by parasitic worms

> **Excludes1**   capillariasis NOS (B81.1)
> **Excludes2**   intestinal capillariasis (B81.1)

B83.0   Visceral larva migrans
Prolonged migration of nematode larvae
Toxocariasis

B83.1   Gnathostomiasis
Infection with nematode occurring from ingested undercooked fish contaminated with larvae; larvae migrate to subcutaneous tissue or deeper tissues, results are abscesses
Wandering swelling

B83.2   Angiostrongyliasis due to Parastrongylus cantonensis
Nematode infection caused by eating contaminated raw snails, slugs, or paratenic hosts such as prawns or crabs; larval worms migrate to central nervous system resulting in eosinophilic meningitis
Eosinophilic meningoencephalitis due to Parastrongylus cantonensis

> **Excludes2**   intestinal angiostrongyliasis (B81.3)

B83.3   Syngamiasis
Infestation with gapeworm from turkey, pheasant, guinea fowl, goose, and wild birds
Syngamosis

B83.4   Internal hirudiniasis
Infestation by leeches

> **Excludes2**   external hirudiniasis (B88.3)

B83.8   Other specified helminthiases
Parasitic worm infestation
Acanthocephaliasis
Gongylonemiasis
Hepatic capillariasis
Metastrongyliasis
Thelaziasis

B83.9   Helminthiasis, unspecified
Worms NOS

> **Excludes1**   intestinal helminthiasis NOS (B82.0)

PEDICULOSIS, ACARIASIS AND OTHER INFESTATIONS (B85-B89)

● **B85   Pediculosis and phthiriasis**
Infestation of lice

B85.0   Pediculosis due to Pediculus humanus capitis
Head-louse infestation

B85.1   Pediculosis due to Pediculus humanus corporis
Body-louse infestation

B85.2   Pediculosis, unspecified

B85.3   Phthiriasis
Crab or pubic lice
Infestation by crab-louse
Infestation by Phthirus pubis

B85.4   Mixed pediculosis and phthiriasis
Infestation classifiable to more than one of the categories B85.0-B85.3

B86   Scabies
Contagious dermatitis caused by mites
Sarcoptic itch

● **B87   Myiasis**
Infestation by fly maggots

> **Includes**   infestation by larva of flies

B87.0   Cutaneous myiasis
Creeping myiasis

B87.1   Wound myiasis
Traumatic myiasis

B87.2   Ocular myiasis

B87.3   Nasopharyngeal myiasis
Laryngeal myiasis

B87.4   Aural myiasis

● **B87.8   Myiasis of other sites**

B87.81   Genitourinary myiasis

B87.82   Intestinal myiasis

B87.89   Myiasis of other sites

B87.9   Myiasis, unspecified

● **B88   Other infestations**

B88.0   Other acariasis
Acarine dermatitis
Dermatitis due to Demodex species
Dermatitis due to Dermanyssus gallinae
Dermatitis due to Liponyssoides sanguineus
Trombiculosis

> **Excludes2**   scabies (B86)

B88.1   Tungiasis [sandflea infestation]
Inflammatory skin disease caused by infestation of fleas

B88.2   Other arthropod infestations
Scarabiasis

B88.3   External hirudiniasis
Leech infestation NOS

> **Excludes2**   internal hirudiniasis (B83.4)

B88.8   Other specified infestations
Infection of topical fresh water fish parasite
Ichthyoparasitism due to Vandellia cirrhosa
Linguatulosis
Porocephaliasis

B88.9   Infestation, unspecified
Infestation (skin) NOS
Infestation by mites NOS
Skin parasites NOS

B89   Unspecified parasitic disease

▶ New   ⇒ Revised   ~~deleted~~ Deleted   Excludes 1   Excludes 2   Includes   Use additional   Code first   Code also   Key words

OGCR Official Guidelines   ● Unacceptable Principal Diagnosis   X Assign placeholder X   ● Use Additional Character(s)   ▌ Manifestation Code   Coding Clinic

SEQUELAE OF INFECTIOUS AND PARASITIC DISEASES (B90-B94)

Note: Categories B90-B94 are to be used to indicate conditions in categories A00-B89 as the cause of sequelae, which are themselves classified elsewhere. The 'sequelae' include conditions specified as such; they also include residuals of diseases classifiable to the above categories if there is evidence that the disease itself is no longer present. Codes from these categories are not to be used for chronic infections. Code chronic current infections to active infectious disease as appropriate.

Code first condition resulting from (sequela) the infectious or parasitic disease

● **B90   Sequelae of tuberculosis**
Condition resulting from tuberculosis

B90.0   Sequelae of central nervous system tuberculosis

B90.1   Sequelae of genitourinary tuberculosis

B90.2   Sequelae of tuberculosis of bones and joints

B90.8   Sequelae of tuberculosis of other organs
   Excludes2   sequelae of respiratory tuberculosis (B90.9)

B90.9   Sequelae of respiratory and unspecified tuberculosis
Sequelae of tuberculosis NOS

B91   Sequelae of poliomyelitis
   Excludes1   postpolio syndrome (G14)

B92   Sequelae of leprosy

● **B94   Sequelae of other and unspecified infectious and parasitic diseases**

B94.0   Sequelae of trachoma

B94.1   Sequelae of viral encephalitis

B94.2   Sequelae of viral hepatitis

B94.8   Sequelae of other specified infectious and parasitic diseases
Coding Clinic: 2021, Q1, P34,37,41,44,46,48

B94.9   Sequelae of unspecified infectious and parasitic disease
   ▶**Excludes2**   post COVID-19 condition (U09.9)
   Coding Clinic: 2017, Q4, P109

OGCR Section I.C.1.b.

Certain infectious and parasitic diseases

Infectious agents as the cause of diseases classified to other chapters

Certain infections are classified in chapters other than Chapter 1 and no organism is identified as part of the infection code. In these instances, it is necessary to use an additional code from Chapter 1 to identify the organism. A code from category B95, Streptococcus, Staphylococcus, and Enterococcus as the cause of diseases classified to other chapters, B96, Other bacterial agents as the cause of diseases classified to other chapters, or B97, Viral agents as the cause of diseases classified to other chapters, is to be used as an additional code to identify the organism. An instructional note will be found at the infection code advising that an additional organism code is required.

BACTERIAL AND VIRAL INFECTIOUS AGENTS (B95-B97)

Note: These categories are provided for use as supplementary or additional codes to identify the infectious agent(s) in diseases classified elsewhere.
Code the disease first, then the bacterium. Do not report codes from B95-B97 for sepsis.

● **B95   Streptococcus, Staphylococcus, and Enterococcus as the cause of diseases classified elsewhere**

● **B95.0   Streptococcus, group A, as the cause of diseases classified elsewhere**

● **B95.1   Streptococcus, group B, as the cause of diseases classified elsewhere**
Coding Clinic: 2020, Q1, P10; 2019, Q2, P9-10; 2018, Q4, P23

● **B95.2   Enterococcus as the cause of diseases classified elsewhere**

● **B95.3   Streptococcus pneumoniae as the cause of diseases classified elsewhere**

● **B95.4   Other streptococcus as the cause of diseases classified elsewhere**

● **B95.5   Unspecified streptococcus as the cause of diseases classified elsewhere**

● **B95.6   Staphylococcus aureus as the cause of diseases classified elsewhere**

● **B95.61   Methicillin susceptible Staphylococcus aureus infection as the cause of diseases classified elsewhere**
Methicillin susceptible Staphylococcus aureus (MSSA) infection as the cause of diseases classified elsewhere
Staphylococcus aureus infection NOS as the cause of diseases classified elsewhere

● **B95.62   Methicillin resistant Staphylococcus aureus infection as the cause of diseases classified elsewhere**
Methicillin resistant staphylococcus aureus (MRSA) infection as the cause of diseases classified elsewhere
Coding Clinic: 2016, Q1, P13

● **B95.7   Other staphylococcus as the cause of diseases classified elsewhere**

● **B95.8   Unspecified staphylococcus as the cause of diseases classified elsewhere**

● **B96   Other bacterial agents as the cause of diseases classified elsewhere**

● **B96.0   Mycoplasma pneumoniae [M. pneumoniae] as the cause of diseases classified elsewhere**
Pleuro-pneumonia-like-organism [PPLO]

● **B96.1   Klebsiella pneumoniae [K. pneumoniae] as the cause of diseases classified elsewhere**

● **B96.2   Escherichia coli [E. coli] as the cause of diseases classified elsewhere**

● **B96.20   Unspecified Escherichia coli [E. coli] as the cause of diseases classified elsewhere**
Escherichia coli [E. coli] NOS
Coding Clinic: 2018, Q4, P34; 2018, Q1, P10

● **B96.21   Shiga toxin-producing Escherichia coli [E. coli] [STEC] O157 as the cause of diseases classified elsewhere**
E. coli O157:H- (nonmotile) with confirmation of Shiga toxin
E. coli O157 with confirmation of Shiga toxin when H antigen is unknown, or is not H7
O157:H7 Escherichia coli [E.coli] with or without confirmation of Shiga toxin-production
Shiga toxin-producing Escherichia coli [E.coli] O157:H7 with or without confirmation of Shiga toxin-production
STEC O157:H7 with or without confirmation of Shiga toxin-production

● **B96.22   Other specified Shiga toxin-producing Escherichia coli [E. coli] [STEC] as the cause of diseases classified elsewhere**
Non-O157 Shiga toxin-producing Escherichia coli [E.coli]
Non-O157 Shiga toxin-producing Escherichia coli [E.coli] with known O group

● **B96.23   Unspecified Shiga toxin-producing Escherichia coli [E. coli] [STEC] as the cause of diseases classified elsewhere**
Shiga toxin-producing Escherichia coli [E. coli] with unspecified O group
STEC NOS

● **B96.29   Other Escherichia coli [E. coli] as the cause of diseases classified elsewhere**
Non-Shiga toxin-producing E. coli

N Newborn Age: 0   **P** Pediatric Age: 0–17   **M** Maternity DX: 9–64   **A** Adult Age: 15–124   ♀ Females Only   ♂ Males Only

🅒 Complication\Comorbidity   🅜 Major C\C   (Ex) CC/MCC Exclusions   🅗 Hospital-Acquired Condition   🅗 Hierarchical Condition Category

● B96.3   Hemophilus influenzae [H. influenzae] as the cause of diseases classified elsewhere

● B96.4   Proteus (mirabilis) (morganii) as the cause of diseases classified elsewhere

● B96.5   Pseudomonas (aeruginosa) (mallei) (pseudomallei) as the cause of diseases classified elsewhere
            Coding Clinic: 2015, Q1, P18

● B96.6   Bacteroides fragilis [B. fragilis] as the cause of diseases classified elsewhere

● B96.7   Clostridium perfringens [C. perfringens] as the cause of diseases classified elsewhere

● B96.8   Other specified bacterial agents as the cause of diseases classified elsewhere

    ● B96.81   Helicobacter pylori [H. pylori] as the cause of diseases classified elsewhere

    ● B96.82   Vibrio vulnificus as the cause of diseases classified elsewhere

    ● B96.89   Other specified bacterial agents as the cause of diseases classified elsewhere

● B97   Viral agents as the cause of diseases classified elsewhere

    ● B97.0   Adenovirus as the cause of diseases classified elsewhere

    ● B97.1   Enterovirus as the cause of diseases classified elsewhere

        ● B97.10   Unspecified enterovirus as the cause of diseases classified elsewhere

        ● B97.11   Coxsackievirus as the cause of diseases classified elsewhere

        ● B97.12   Echovirus as the cause of diseases classified elsewhere

        ● B97.19   Other enterovirus as the cause of diseases classified elsewhere

    ● B97.2   Coronavirus as the cause of diseases classified elsewhere

        ● B97.21   SARS-associated coronavirus as the cause of diseases classified elsewhere 🦠

            Excludes1   pneumonia due to SARS-associated coronavirus (J12.81)

                    (Ex:) See PDX Collection 249

        ● B97.29   Other coronavirus as the cause of diseases classified elsewhere

Item 1–24   Retrovirus develops by copying its RNA, genetic materials, into the DNA, which then produces new virus particles. It is from the Retroviridae virus family. **Human T-cell lymphotropic virus, Type I (HTLV-I),** is also called human T-cell leukemia virus, Type I, and is a retrovirus thought to cause T-cell leukemia/lymphoma. **Human T-cell lymphotropic virus, Type II (HTLV-II),** is also called human T-cell leukemia virus, Type II, and is a retrovirus associated with hematologic disorders.

HIV-2 is one of the serotypes of HIV and is usually confined to West Africa, whereas **HIV-1** is found worldwide.

● B97.3   Retrovirus as the cause of diseases classified elsewhere

        Excludes1   human immunodeficiency virus [HIV] disease (B20)

    ● B97.30   Unspecified retrovirus as the cause of diseases classified elsewhere

    ● B97.31   Lentivirus as the cause of diseases classified elsewhere

    ● B97.32   Oncovirus as the cause of diseases classified elsewhere

    ● B97.33   Human T-cell lymphotrophic virus, type I [HTLV-I] as the cause of diseases classified elsewhere 🦠
                (Ex:) See PDX Collection 250

    ● B97.34   Human T-cell lymphotrophic virus, type II [HTLV-II] as the cause of diseases classified elsewhere 🦠
                (Ex:) See PDX Collection 251

    ● B97.35   Human immunodeficiency virus, type 2 [HIV 2] as the cause of diseases classified elsewhere 🦠🦠
                (Ex:) See PDX Collection 252

    ● B97.39   Other retrovirus as the cause of diseases classified elsewhere

● B97.4   Respiratory syncytial virus as the cause of diseases classified elsewhere

        RSV as the cause of diseases classified elsewhere

        Code first related disorders, such as:
            otitis media (H65.-)
            upper respiratory infection (J06.9)

        ▶ Excludes1   acute bronchiolitis due to respiratory syncytial virus (RSV) (J21.0)
                        acute bronchitis due to respiratory syncytial virus (RSV) (J20.5)
                        respiratory syncytial virus (RSV) pneumonia (J12.1)

● B97.5   Reovirus as the cause of diseases classified elsewhere

● B97.6   Parvovirus as the cause of diseases classified elsewhere

● B97.7   Papillomavirus as the cause of diseases classified elsewhere

● B97.8   Other viral agents as the cause of diseases classified elsewhere

    ● B97.81   Human metapneumovirus as the cause of diseases classified elsewhere

    ● B97.89   Other viral agents as the cause of diseases classified elsewhere
                Coding Clinic: 2016, Q3, P8-10, 14

OTHER INFECTIOUS DISEASES (B99)

● B99   Other and unspecified infectious diseases

    B99.8   Other infectious disease

    B99.9   Unspecified infectious disease

CHAPTER 1 (A00-B99)

▶ New   ⇒ Revised   ~~deleted~~ Deleted   Excludes 1   Excludes 2   Includes   Use additional   Code first   Code also   Key words

OGCR Official Guidelines   ● Unacceptable Principal Diagnosis   X Assign placeholder X   ● Use Additional Character(s)   ⫸ Manifestation Code   Coding Clinic

CHAPTER 2

NEOPLASMS (C00-D49)

Chapter-Specific Coding Guidelines

2. **Chapter 2: Neoplasms (C00-D49)**
   General guidelines
   Chapter 2 of the ICD-10-CM contains the codes for most benign and all malignant neoplasms. Certain benign neoplasms, such as prostatic adenomas, may be found in the specific body system chapters. To properly code a neoplasm it is necessary to determine from the record if the neoplasm is benign, in-situ, malignant, or of uncertain histologic behavior. If malignant, any secondary (metastatic) sites should also be determined.

   Primary malignant neoplasms overlapping site boundaries
   A primary malignant neoplasm that overlaps two or more contiguous (next to each other) sites should be classified to the subcategory/code .8 ('overlapping lesion'), unless the combination is specifically indexed elsewhere. For multiple neoplasms of the same site that are not contiguous such as tumors in different quadrants of the same breast, codes for each site should be assigned.

   Malignant neoplasm of ectopic tissue
   Malignant neoplasms of ectopic tissue are to be coded to the site of origin mentioned, e.g., ectopic pancreatic malignant neoplasms involving the stomach are coded to malignant neoplasm of pancreas, unspecified (C25.9).

   The neoplasm table in the Alphabetic Index should be referenced first. However, if the histological term is documented, that term should be referenced first, rather than going immediately to the Neoplasm Table, in order to determine which column in the Neoplasm Table is appropriate. For example, if the documentation indicates "adenoma," refer to the term in the Alphabetic Index to review the entries under this term and the instructional note to "see also neoplasm, by site, benign." The table provides the proper code based on the type of neoplasm and the site. It is important to select the proper column in the table that corresponds to the type of neoplasm. The Tabular List should then be referenced to verify that the correct code has been selected from the table and that a more specific site code does not exist.

   See Section I.C.21, Factors influencing health status and contact with health services, Status, for information regarding Z15.0, codes for genetic susceptibility to cancer.

   a. **Treatment directed at the malignancy**
   If the treatment is directed at the malignancy, designate the malignancy as the principal diagnosis.

   The only exception to this guideline is if a patient admission/encounter is solely for the administration of chemotherapy, immunotherapy or external beam radiation therapy, assign the appropriate Z51.— code as the first-listed or principal diagnosis, and the diagnosis or problem for which the service is being performed as a secondary diagnosis.

   b. **Treatment of secondary site**
   When a patient is admitted because of a primary neoplasm with metastasis and treatment is directed toward the secondary site only, the secondary neoplasm is designated as the principal diagnosis even though the primary malignancy is still present.

   c. **Coding and sequencing of complications**
   Coding and sequencing of complications associated with the malignancies or with the therapy thereof are subject to the following guidelines:

   1) **Anemia associated with malignancy**
   When admission/encounter is for management of an anemia associated with the malignancy, and the treatment is only for anemia, the appropriate code for the malignancy is sequenced as the principal or first-listed diagnosis followed by the appropriate code for the anemia (such as code D63.0, Anemia in neoplastic disease).

   2) **Anemia associated with chemotherapy, immunotherapy and radiation therapy**
   When the admission/encounter is for management of an anemia associated with an adverse effect of the administration of chemotherapy or immunotherapy and the only treatment is for the anemia, the anemia code is sequenced first followed by

the appropriate codes for the neoplasm and the adverse effect (T45.1X5, Adverse effect of antineoplastic and immunosuppressive drugs).

When the admission/encounter is for management of an anemia associated with an adverse effect of radiotherapy, the anemia code should be sequenced first, followed by the appropriate neoplasm code and code Y84.2, Radiological procedure and radiotherapy as the cause of abnormal reaction of the patient, or of later complication, without mention of misadventure at the time of the procedure.

   3) **Management of dehydration due to the malignancy**
   When the admission/encounter is for management of dehydration due to the malignancy and only the dehydration is being treated (intravenous rehydration), the dehydration is sequenced first, followed by the code(s) for the malignancy.

   4) **Treatment of a complication resulting from a surgical procedure**
   When the admission/encounter is for treatment of a complication resulting from a surgical procedure, designate the complication as the principal or first-listed diagnosis if treatment is directed at resolving the complication.

   d. **Primary malignancy previously excised**
   When a primary malignancy has been previously excised or eradicated from its site and there is no further treatment directed to that site and there is no evidence of any existing primary malignancy at that site, a code from category Z85, Personal history of malignant neoplasm, should be used to indicate the former site of the malignancy. Any mention of extension, invasion, or metastasis to another site is coded as a secondary malignant neoplasm to that site. The secondary site may be the principal or first-listed with the Z85 code used as a secondary code.

   e. **Admissions/Encounters involving chemotherapy, immunotherapy and radiation therapy**

   1) **Episode of care involves surgical removal of neoplasm**
   When an episode of care involves the surgical removal of a neoplasm, primary or secondary site, followed by adjunct chemotherapy or radiation treatment during the same episode of care, the code for the neoplasm should be assigned as principal or first-listed diagnosis.

   2) **Patient admission/encounter solely for administration of chemotherapy, immunotherapy and radiation therapy**
   If a patient admission/encounter is solely for the administration of chemotherapy, immunotherapy or external beam radiation therapy assign code Z51.0, Encounter for antineoplastic radiation therapy, or Z51.11, Encounter for antineoplastic chemotherapy, or Z51.12, Encounter for antineoplastic immunotherapy as the first-listed or principal diagnosis. If a patient receives more than one of these therapies during the same admission more than one of these codes may be assigned, in any sequence.

   The malignancy for which the therapy is being administered should be assigned as a secondary diagnosis.

   If a patient admission/encounter is for the insertion or implantation of radioactive elements (e.g., brachytherapy) the appropriate code for the malignancy is sequenced as the principal or first-listed diagnosis. Code Z51.0 should not be assigned.

   3) **Patient admitted for radiation therapy, chemotherapy or immunotherapy and develops complications**
   When a patient is admitted for the purpose of external beam radiotherapy, immunotherapy or chemotherapy and develops complications such as uncontrolled nausea and vomiting or dehydration, the principal or first-listed diagnosis is Z51.0, Encounter for antineoplastic radiation therapy, or Z51.11, Encounter for antineoplastic chemotherapy, or Z51.12, Encounter for antineoplastic immunotherapy followed by any codes for the complications.

   When a patient is admitted for the purpose of insertion or implantation of radioactive elements (e.g., brachytherapy) and develops complications such as uncontrolled nausea and vomiting or dehydration, the principal or first-listed diagnosis is the appropriate code for the malignancy followed by any codes for the complications.

   f. **Admission/encounter to determine extent of malignancy**
   When the reason for admission/encounter is to determine the extent of the malignancy, or for a procedure such as paracentesis

or thoracentesis, the primary malignancy or appropriate metastatic site is designated as the principal or first-listed diagnosis, even though chemotherapy or radiotherapy is administered.

g. Symptoms, signs, and abnormal findings listed in Chapter 18 associated with neoplasms

Symptoms, signs, and ill-defined conditions listed in Chapter 18 characteristic of, or associated with, an existing primary or secondary site malignancy cannot be used to replace the malignancy as principal or first-listed diagnosis, regardless of the number of admissions or encounters for treatment and care of the neoplasm.

See Section I.C.21. Factors influencing health status and contact with health services, Encounter for prophylactic organ removal.

h. Admission/encounter for pain control/management

See Section I.C.6. for information on coding admission/encounter for pain control/management.

i. Malignancy in two or more noncontiguous sites

A patient may have more than one malignant tumor in the same organ. These tumors may represent different primaries or metastatic disease, depending on the site. Should the documentation be unclear, the provider should be queried as to the status of each tumor so that the correct codes can be assigned.

j. Disseminated malignant neoplasm, unspecified

Code C80.0, Disseminated malignant neoplasm, unspecified, is for use only in those cases where the patient has advanced metastatic disease and no known primary or secondary sites are specified. It should not be used in place of assigning codes for the primary site and all known secondary sites.

k. Malignant neoplasm without specification of site

Code C80.1, Malignant (primary) neoplasm, unspecified, equates to Cancer, unspecified. This code should only be used when no determination can be made as to the primary site of a malignancy. This code should rarely be used in the inpatient setting.

l. Sequencing of neoplasm codes

1) Encounter for treatment of primary malignancy

If the reason for the encounter is for treatment of a primary malignancy, assign the malignancy as the principal/first-listed diagnosis. The primary site is to be sequenced first, followed by any metastatic sites.

2) Encounter for treatment of secondary malignancy

When an encounter is for a primary malignancy with metastasis and treatment is directed toward the metastatic (secondary) site(s) only, the metastatic site(s) is designated as the principal/first-listed diagnosis. The primary malignancy is coded as an additional code.

3) Malignant neoplasm in a pregnant patient

When a pregnant woman has a malignant neoplasm, a code from subcategory O9A.1-, Malignant neoplasm complicating pregnancy, childbirth, and the puerperium, should be sequenced first, followed by the appropriate code from Chapter 2 to indicate the type of neoplasm.

4) Encounter for complication associated with a neoplasm

When an encounter is for management of a complication associated with a neoplasm, such as dehydration, and the treatment is only for the complication, the complication is coded first, followed by the appropriate code(s) for the neoplasm.

The exception to this guideline is anemia. When the admission/encounter is for management of an anemia associated with the malignancy, and the treatment is only for anemia, the appropriate code for the malignancy is sequenced as the principal or first-listed diagnosis followed by code D63.0, Anemia in neoplastic disease.

5) Complication from surgical procedure for treatment of a neoplasm

When an encounter is for treatment of a complication resulting from a surgical procedure performed for the treatment of the neoplasm, designate the complication as the principal/first-listed diagnosis. See guideline regarding the coding of a current malignancy versus personal history to determine if the code for the neoplasm should also be assigned.

6) Pathologic fracture due to a neoplasm

When an encounter is for a pathological fracture due to a neoplasm, and the focus of treatment is the fracture, a code from subcategory M84.5, Pathological fracture in neoplastic disease, should be sequenced first, followed by the code for the neoplasm.

If the focus of treatment is the neoplasm with an associated pathological fracture, the neoplasm code should be sequenced first, followed by a code from M84.5 for the pathological fracture.

m. Current malignancy versus personal history of malignancy

When a primary malignancy has been excised but further treatment, such as an additional surgery for the malignancy, radiation therapy or chemotherapy is directed to that site, the primary malignancy code should be used until treatment is completed.

When a primary malignancy has been previously excised or eradicated from its site, there is no further treatment (of the malignancy) directed to that site, and there is no evidence of any existing primary malignancy at that site, a code from category Z85, Personal history of malignant neoplasm, should be used to indicate the former site of the malignancy.

Subcategories Z85.0–Z85.7 should only be assigned for the former site of a primary malignancy, not the site of a secondary malignancy. Codes from subcategory Z85.8-, may be assigned for the former site(s) of either a primary or secondary malignancy included in this subcategory.

See Section I.C.21. Factors influencing health status and contact with health services, History (of)

n. Leukemia, Multiple Myeloma, and Malignant Plasma Cell Neoplasms in remission versus personal history

The categories for leukemia, and category C90, Multiple myeloma and malignant plasma cell neoplasms, have codes indicating whether or not the leukemia has achieved remission. There are also codes Z85.6, Personal history of leukemia, and Z85.79, Personal history of other malignant neoplasms of lymphoid, hematopoietic and related tissues. If the documentation is unclear, as to whether the leukemia has achieved remission, the provider should be queried.

See Section I.C.21. Factors influencing health status and contact with health services, History (of)

o. Aftercare following surgery for neoplasm

See Section I.C.21. Factors influencing health status and contact with health services, Aftercare

p. Follow-up care for completed treatment of a malignancy

See Section I.C.21. Factors influencing health status and contact with health services, Follow-up

q. Prophylactic organ removal for prevention of malignancy

See Section I.C. 21, Factors influencing health status and contact with health services, Prophylactic organ removal

r. Malignant neoplasm associated with transplanted organ

A malignant neoplasm of a transplanted organ should be coded as a transplant complication. Assign first the appropriate code from category T86.-, Complications of transplanted organs and tissue, followed by code C80.2, Malignant neoplasm associated with transplanted organ. Use an additional code for the specific malignancy.

Item 2–1 Neoplasm: Neo = new, plasm = growth, development, formation. This new growth (mass, tumor) can be malignant or benign, which is confirmed by the pathology report. Do not assign a code to a neoplasm until you review the pathology report. Certain CPT codes will specify benign or malignant lesion, so be certain the diagnosis code supports the procedure code.

CHAPTER 2

NEOPLASMS (C00-D49)

This chapter contains the following blocks:

C00-C14	Malignant neoplasms of lip, oral cavity and pharynx
C15-C26	Malignant neoplasms of digestive organs
C30-C39	Malignant neoplasms of respiratory and intrathoracic organs
C40-C41	Malignant neoplasms of bone and articular cartilage
C43-C44	Melanoma and other malignant neoplasms of skin
C45-C49	Malignant neoplasms of mesothelial and soft tissue
C50	Malignant neoplasms of breast
C51-C58	Malignant neoplasms of female genital organs
C60-C63	Malignant neoplasms of male genital organs
C64-C68	Malignant neoplasms of urinary tract
C69-C72	Malignant neoplasms of eye, brain and other parts of central nervous system
C73-C75	Malignant neoplasms of thyroid and other endocrine glands
C7A	Malignant neuroendocrine tumors
C7B	Secondary neuroendocrine tumors
C76-C80	Malignant neoplasms of ill-defined, other secondary and unspecified sites
C81-C96	Malignant neoplasms of lymphoid, hematopoietic and related tissue
D00-D09	In situ neoplasms
D10-D36	Benign neoplasms, except benign neuroendocrine tumors
D3A	Benign neuroendocrine tumors
D37-D48	Neoplasms of uncertain behavior, polycythemia vera and myelodysplastic syndromes
D49	Neoplasms of unspecified behavior

Notes: Functional activity

All neoplasms are classified in this chapter, whether they are functionally active or not. An additional code from Chapter 4 may be used, to identify functional activity associated with any neoplasm.

Morphology [Histology]

Chapter 2 classifies neoplasms primarily by site (topography), with broad groupings for behavior, malignant, in situ, benign, etc. The Table of Neoplasms should be used to identify the correct topography code. In a few cases, such as for malignant melanoma and certain neuroendocrine tumors, the morphology (histologic type) is included in the category and codes.

Primary malignant neoplasms overlapping site boundaries

A primary malignant neoplasm that overlaps two or more contiguous (next to each other) sites should be classified to the subcategory/code .8 ("overlapping lesion"), unless the combination is specifically indexed elsewhere. For multiple neoplasms of the same site that are not contiguous, such as tumors in different quadrants of the same breast, codes for each site should be assigned.

Malignant neoplasm of ectopic tissue

Malignant neoplasms of ectopic tissue are to be coded to the site mentioned, e.g., ectopic pancreatic malignant neoplasms are coded to pancreas, unspecified (C25.9).

MALIGNANT NEOPLASMS (C00-C96)

MALIGNANT NEOPLASMS, STATED OR PRESUMED TO BE PRIMARY (OF SPECIFIED SITES), AND CERTAIN SPECIFIED HISTOLOGIES, EXCEPT NEUROENDOCRINE, AND OF LYMPHOID, HEMATOPOIETIC AND RELATED TISSUE (C00-C75)

MALIGNANT NEOPLASMS OF LIP, ORAL CAVITY AND PHARYNX (C00-C14)

● **C00   Malignant neoplasm of lip**
    Use additional code to identify:
        alcohol abuse and dependence (F10.-)
        history of tobacco dependence (Z87.891)
        tobacco dependence (F17.-)
        tobacco use (Z72.0)

    Excludes1   malignant melanoma of lip (C43.0)
                    Merkel cell carcinoma of lip (C4A.0)
                    other and unspecified malignant neoplasm of skin of lip (C44.0-)

C00.0   **Malignant neoplasm of external upper lip**
        Malignant neoplasm of lipstick area of upper lip
        Malignant neoplasm of upper lip NOS
        Malignant neoplasm of vermilion border of upper lip

C00.1   **Malignant neoplasm of external lower lip**
        Malignant neoplasm of lower lip NOS
        Malignant neoplasm of lipstick area of lower lip
        Malignant neoplasm of vermilion border of lower lip

C00.2   **Malignant neoplasm of external lip, unspecified**
        Malignant neoplasm of vermilion border of lip NOS

C00.3   **Malignant neoplasm of upper lip, inner aspect**
        Malignant neoplasm of buccal aspect of upper lip
        Malignant neoplasm of frenulum of upper lip
        Malignant neoplasm of mucosa of upper lip
        Malignant neoplasm of oral aspect of upper lip

C00.4   **Malignant neoplasm of lower lip, inner aspect**
        Malignant neoplasm of buccal aspect of lower lip
        Malignant neoplasm of frenulum of lower lip
        Malignant neoplasm of mucosa of lower lip
        Malignant neoplasm of oral aspect of lower lip

C00.5   **Malignant neoplasm of lip, unspecified, inner aspect**
        Malignant neoplasm of buccal aspect of lip, unspecified
        Malignant neoplasm of frenulum of lip, unspecified
        Malignant neoplasm of mucosa of lip, unspecified
        Malignant neoplasm of oral aspect of lip, unspecified

C00.6   **Malignant neoplasm of commissure of lip, unspecified**
        Commissure: Site of union of corresponding parts

C00.8   **Malignant neoplasm of overlapping sites of lip**

C00.9   **Malignant neoplasm of lip, unspecified**

N Newborn Age: 0   **P** Pediatric Age: 0–17   **M** Maternity DX: 9–64   **A** Adult Age: 15–124   ♀ Females Only   ♂ Males Only

🐾 Complication\Comorbidity   🐾 Major C\C   (Ex:) CC/MCC Exclusions   🐾 Hospital-Acquired Condition   🐾 Hierarchical Condition Category   **685**

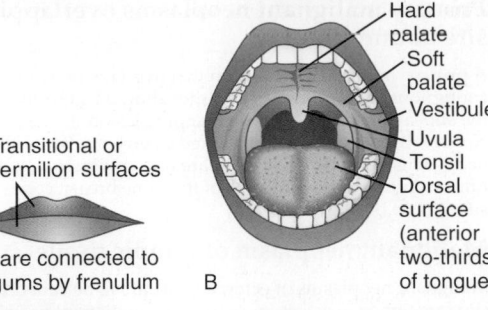

Figure 2-1 Anatomical structures of the mouth and lips. **A.** Transitional or vermilion borders. Lips are connected to the gums by frenulum. **B.** Dorsal surface. **C.** Ventral surface.

C01   Malignant neoplasm of base of tongue
> Malignant neoplasm of dorsal surface of base of tongue
> Malignant neoplasm of fixed part of tongue NOS
> Malignant neoplasm of posterior third of tongue
>
> Use additional code to identify:
>> alcohol abuse and dependence (F10.-)
>> history of tobacco dependence (Z87.891)
>> tobacco dependence (F17.-)
>> tobacco use (Z72.0)

C02   Malignant neoplasm of other and unspecified parts of tongue
> Use additional code to identify:
>> alcohol abuse and dependence (F10.-)
>> history of tobacco dependence (Z87.891)
>> tobacco dependence (F17.-)
>> tobacco use (Z72.0)

   C02.0   Malignant neoplasm of dorsal surface of tongue
> Malignant neoplasm of anterior two-thirds of tongue, dorsal surface
>
> **Excludes2**   malignant neoplasm of dorsal surface of base of tongue (C01)

   C02.1   Malignant neoplasm of border of tongue
> Malignant neoplasm of tip of tongue

   C02.2   Malignant neoplasm of ventral surface of tongue
> Malignant neoplasm of anterior two-thirds of tongue, ventral surface
> Malignant neoplasm of frenulum linguae

   C02.3   Malignant neoplasm of anterior two-thirds of tongue, part unspecified
> Malignant neoplasm of middle third of tongue NOS
> Malignant neoplasm of mobile part of tongue NOS

   C02.4   Malignant neoplasm of lingual tonsil
> *Lingual tonsil: Aggregation of lymph follicles at root of tongue*
>
> **Excludes2**   malignant neoplasm of tonsil NOS (C09.9)

   C02.8   Malignant neoplasm of overlapping sites of tongue
> Malignant neoplasm of two or more contiguous sites of tongue

   C02.9   Malignant neoplasm of tongue, unspecified

C03   Malignant neoplasm of gum
> **Includes**   malignant neoplasm of alveolar (ridge) mucosa
> malignant neoplasm of gingiva
>
> Use additional code to identify:
>> alcohol abuse and dependence (F10.-)
>> history of tobacco dependence (Z87.891)
>> tobacco dependence (F17.-)
>> tobacco use (Z72.0)
>
> **Excludes2**   malignant odontogenic neoplasms (C41.0-C41.1)

   C03.0   Malignant neoplasm of upper gum
   C03.1   Malignant neoplasm of lower gum
   C03.9   Malignant neoplasm of gum, unspecified

C04   Malignant neoplasm of floor of mouth
> Use additional code to identify:
>> alcohol abuse and dependence (F10.-)
>> history of tobacco dependence (Z87.891)
>> tobacco dependence (F17.-)
>> tobacco use (Z72.0)

   C04.0   Malignant neoplasm of anterior floor of mouth
> Malignant neoplasm of anterior to the premolar-canine junction

   C04.1   Malignant neoplasm of lateral floor of mouth
   C04.8   Malignant neoplasm of overlapping sites of floor of mouth
   C04.9   Malignant neoplasm of floor of mouth, unspecified

C05   Malignant neoplasm of palate
> Use additional code to identify:
>> alcohol abuse and dependence (F10.-)
>> history of tobacco dependence (Z87.891)
>> tobacco dependence (F17.-)
>> tobacco use (Z72.0)
>
> **Excludes1**   Kaposi's sarcoma of palate (C46.2)

   C05.0   Malignant neoplasm of hard palate
   C05.1   Malignant neoplasm of soft palate
> **Excludes2**   malignant neoplasm of nasopharyngeal surface of soft palate (C11.3)

   C05.2   Malignant neoplasm of uvula
   C05.8   Malignant neoplasm of overlapping sites of palate
   C05.9   Malignant neoplasm of palate, unspecified
> Malignant neoplasm of roof of mouth

C06   Malignant neoplasm of other and unspecified parts of mouth
> Use additional code to identify:
>> alcohol abuse and dependence (F10.-)
>> history of tobacco dependence (Z87.891)
>> tobacco dependence (F17.-)
>> tobacco use (Z72.0)

   C06.0   Malignant neoplasm of cheek mucosa
> Malignant neoplasm of buccal mucosa NOS
> Malignant neoplasm of internal cheek

   C06.1   Malignant neoplasm of vestibule of mouth
> Malignant neoplasm of buccal sulcus (upper) (lower)
> Malignant neoplasm of labial sulcus (upper) (lower)

   C06.2   Malignant neoplasm of retromolar area
   C06.8   Malignant neoplasm of overlapping sites of other and unspecified parts of mouth

     C06.80   Malignant neoplasm of overlapping sites of unspecified parts of mouth
     C06.89   Malignant neoplasm of overlapping sites of other parts of mouth
> 'book leaf' neoplasm [ventral surface of tongue and floor of mouth]

   C06.9   Malignant neoplasm of mouth, unspecified
> Malignant neoplasm of minor salivary gland, unspecified site
> Malignant neoplasm of oral cavity NOS

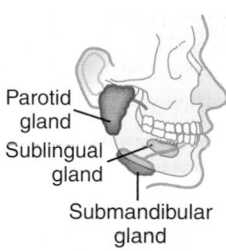

Figure 2-2 Major salivary glands.

C07 Malignant neoplasm of parotid gland 🅗
    Use additional code to identify:
        alcohol abuse and dependence (F10.-)
        exposure to environmental tobacco smoke (Z77.22)
        exposure to tobacco smoke in the perinatal period (P96.81)
        history of tobacco dependence (Z87.891)
        occupational exposure to environmental tobacco smoke
            (Z57.31)
        tobacco dependence (F17.-)
        tobacco use (Z72.0)

● **C08 Malignant neoplasm of other and unspecified major salivary glands**
    Includes   malignant neoplasm of salivary ducts
    Use additional code to identify:
        alcohol abuse and dependence (F10.-)
        exposure to environmental tobacco smoke (Z77.22)
        exposure to tobacco smoke in the perinatal period (P96.81)
        history of tobacco dependence (Z87.891)
        occupational exposure to environmental tobacco smoke
            (Z57.31)
        tobacco dependence (F17.-)
        tobacco use (Z72.0)
    Excludes1   malignant neoplasms of specified minor salivary
               glands which are classified according to their
               anatomical location
    Excludes2   malignant neoplasms of minor salivary glands
               NOS (C06.9)
               malignant neoplasm of parotid gland (C07)

C08.0 Malignant neoplasm of submandibular gland 🅗
    Malignant neoplasm of submaxillary gland

C08.1 Malignant neoplasm of sublingual gland 🅗

C08.9 Malignant neoplasm of major salivary gland, unspecified 🅗
    Malignant neoplasm of salivary gland (major) NOS

★ **(See Plate 28 of the Anatomy Illustrations.)**

● **C09 Malignant neoplasm of tonsil**
    Use additional code to identify:
        alcohol abuse and dependence (F10.-)
        exposure to environmental tobacco smoke (Z77.22)
        exposure to tobacco smoke in the perinatal period (P96.81)
        history of tobacco dependence (Z87.891)
        occupational exposure to environmental tobacco smoke
            (Z57.31)
        tobacco dependence (F17.-)
        tobacco use (Z72.0)
    Excludes2   malignant neoplasm of lingual tonsil (C02.4)
               malignant neoplasm of pharyngeal tonsil (C11.1)

C09.0 Malignant neoplasm of tonsillar fossa 🅗
    Surface of palatine (two masses of lymphatic tissue on sides of throat) tonsils

C09.1 Malignant neoplasm of tonsillar pillar (anterior) (posterior) 🅗
    Extension from palatine (two masses of lymphatic tissue on sides of throat) tonsils

C09.8 Malignant neoplasm of overlapping sites of tonsil 🅗

C09.9 Malignant neoplasm of tonsil, unspecified 🅗
    Malignant neoplasm of tonsil NOS
    Malignant neoplasm of faucial tonsils
    Malignant neoplasm of palatine tonsils

● **C10 Malignant neoplasm of oropharynx**
    Area of throat at back of mouth
    Use additional code to identify:
        alcohol abuse and dependence (F10.-)
        exposure to environmental tobacco smoke (Z77.22)
        exposure to tobacco smoke in the perinatal period (P96.81)
        history of tobacco dependence (Z87.891)
        occupational exposure to environmental tobacco smoke
            (Z57.31)
        tobacco dependence (F17.-)
        tobacco use (Z72.0)
    Excludes2   malignant neoplasm of tonsil (C09.-)

C10.0 Malignant neoplasm of vallecula 🅗
    Vallecula, depression or furrow

C10.1 Malignant neoplasm of anterior surface of epiglottis 🅗
    Malignant neoplasm of epiglottis, free border [margin]
    Malignant neoplasm of glossoepiglottic fold(s)
    Excludes2   malignant neoplasm of epiglottis
               (suprahyoid portion) NOS (C32.1)

C10.2 Malignant neoplasm of lateral wall of oropharynx 🅗

C10.3 Malignant neoplasm of posterior wall of oropharynx 🅗

C10.4 Malignant neoplasm of branchial cleft 🅗
    Congenital slitlike openings formed between branchial arches pharyngeal groove
    Malignant neoplasm of branchial cyst [site of neoplasm]

C10.8 Malignant neoplasm of overlapping sites of oropharynx 🅗
    Malignant neoplasm of junctional region of oropharynx

C10.9 Malignant neoplasm of oropharynx, unspecified 🅗

● **C11 Malignant neoplasm of nasopharynx**
    Use additional code to identify:
        exposure to environmental tobacco smoke (Z77.22)
        exposure to tobacco smoke in the perinatal period (P96.81)
        history of tobacco dependence (Z87.891)
        occupational exposure to environmental tobacco smoke
            (Z57.31)
        tobacco dependence (F17.-)
        tobacco use (Z72.0)

C11.0 Malignant neoplasm of superior wall of nasopharynx 🅗
    Part of pharynx that lies above soft palate
    Malignant neoplasm of roof of nasopharynx

C11.1 Malignant neoplasm of posterior wall of nasopharynx 🅗
    Malignant neoplasm of adenoid
    Malignant neoplasm of pharyngeal tonsil

C11.2 Malignant neoplasm of lateral wall of nasopharynx 🅗
    Malignant neoplasm of fossa of Rosenmüller
    Malignant neoplasm of opening of auditory tube
    Malignant neoplasm of pharyngeal recess

C11.3 Malignant neoplasm of anterior wall of nasopharynx 🅗
    Malignant neoplasm of floor of nasopharynx
    Malignant neoplasm of nasopharyngeal (anterior) (posterior) surface of soft palate
    Malignant neoplasm of posterior margin of nasal choana
    Malignant neoplasm of posterior margin of nasal septum

C11.8 Malignant neoplasm of overlapping sites of nasopharynx 🅗

C11.9 Malignant neoplasm of nasopharynx, unspecified 🅗
    Malignant neoplasm of nasopharyngeal wall NOS

C12 Malignant neoplasm of pyriform sinus 🅗
    Malignant neoplasm of pyriform fossa
    Use additional code to identify:
        exposure to environmental tobacco smoke (Z77.22)
        exposure to tobacco smoke in the perinatal period (P96.81)
        history of tobacco dependence (Z87.891)
        occupational exposure to environmental tobacco smoke
            (Z57.31)
        tobacco dependence (F17.-)
        tobacco use (Z72.0)

CHAPTER 2 (C00-D49)

N Newborn Age: 0   **P** Pediatric Age: 0–17   **M** Maternity DX: 9–64   **A** Adult Age: 15–124   ♀ Females Only   ♂ Males Only

🅒 Complication\Comorbidity   🅒 Major C\C   (Ex) CC/MCC Exclusions   🅗 Hospital-Acquired Condition   🅗 Hierarchical Condition Category   **687**

CHAPTER 2 (C00–D49)

● **C13**   **Malignant neoplasm of hypopharynx**

Use additional code to identify:
exposure to environmental tobacco smoke (Z77.22)
exposure to tobacco smoke in the perinatal period (P96.81)
history of tobacco dependence (Z87.891)
occupational exposure to environmental tobacco smoke (Z57.31)
tobacco dependence (F17.-)
tobacco use (Z72.0)

Excludes2   malignant neoplasm of pyriform sinus (C12)

   C13.0   **Malignant neoplasm of postcricoid region** 🔵
Behind the cricoid cartilage of neck

   C13.1   **Malignant neoplasm of aryepiglottic fold, hypopharyngeal aspect** 🔵
Arytenoepiglottic fold, triangular opening between side of epiglottis and apex of arytenoid cartilage
Malignant neoplasm of aryepiglottic fold, marginal zone
Malignant neoplasm of aryepiglottic fold NOS
Malignant neoplasm of interarytenoid fold, marginal zone
Malignant neoplasm of interarytenoid fold NOS

       Excludes2   malignant neoplasm of aryepiglottic fold or interarytenoid fold, laryngeal aspect (C32.1)

   C13.2   **Malignant neoplasm of posterior wall of hypopharynx** 🔵

   C13.8   **Malignant neoplasm of overlapping sites of hypopharynx** 🔵

   C13.9   **Malignant neoplasm of hypopharynx, unspecified** 🔵
Malignant neoplasm of hypopharyngeal wall NOS

● **C14**   **Malignant neoplasm of other and ill-defined sites in the lip, oral cavity and pharynx**

Use additional code to identify:
alcohol abuse and dependence (F10.-)
exposure to environmental tobacco smoke (Z77.22)
exposure to tobacco smoke in the perinatal period (P96.81)
history of tobacco dependence (Z87.891)
occupational exposure to environmental tobacco smoke (Z57.31)
tobacco dependence (F17.-)
tobacco use (Z72.0)

Excludes1   malignant neoplasm of oral cavity NOS (C06.9)

   C14.0   **Malignant neoplasm of pharynx, unspecified** 🔵

   C14.2   **Malignant neoplasm of Waldeyer's ring** 🔵

   C14.8   **Malignant neoplasm of overlapping sites of lip, oral cavity and pharynx** 🔵
Primary malignant neoplasm of two or more contiguous sites of lip, oral cavity and pharynx

       Excludes1   'book leaf' neoplasm [ventral surface of tongue and floor of mouth] (C06.89)

MALIGNANT NEOPLASM OF DIGESTIVE ORGANS (C15-C26)

Excludes1   Kaposi's sarcoma of gastrointestinal sites (C46.4)

Excludes2   gastrointestinal stromal tumors (C49.A-)

● **C15**   **Malignant neoplasms of esophagus**

Use additional code to identify:
alcohol abuse and dependence (F10.-)

(Ex:) **For category C15 CC codes:** See PDX Collection 253

   C15.3   **Malignant neoplasm of upper third of esophagus** 🔵🔵

   C15.4   **Malignant neoplasm of middle third of esophagus** 🔵🔵

   C15.5   **Malignant neoplasm of lower third of esophagus** 🔵🔵

       Excludes1   malignant neoplasm of cardio-esophageal junction (C16.0)

   C15.8   **Malignant neoplasm of overlapping sites of esophagus** 🔵🔵

   C15.9   **Malignant neoplasm of esophagus, unspecified** 🔵🔵

● **C16**   **Malignant neoplasm of stomach**

Use additional code to identify:
alcohol abuse and dependence (F10.-)

Excludes2   malignant carcinoid tumor of the stomach (C7A.092)

(Ex:) **For category C16 CC codes:** See PDX Collection 254

   C16.0   **Malignant neoplasm of cardia** 🔵🔵
Malignant neoplasm of cardiac orifice
Malignant neoplasm of cardio-esophageal junction
Malignant neoplasm of esophagus and stomach
Malignant neoplasm of gastro-esophageal junction

   C16.1   **Malignant neoplasm of fundus of stomach** 🔵🔵

   C16.2   **Malignant neoplasm of body of stomach** 🔵🔵

   C16.3   **Malignant neoplasm of pyloric antrum** 🔵🔵
Malignant neoplasm of gastric antrum

   C16.4   **Malignant neoplasm of pylorus** 🔵🔵
Malignant neoplasm of prepylorus
Malignant neoplasm of pyloric canal

   C16.5   **Malignant neoplasm of lesser curvature of stomach, unspecified** 🔵🔵
Malignant neoplasm of lesser curvature of stomach, not classifiable to C16.1-C16.4

   C16.6   **Malignant neoplasm of greater curvature of stomach, unspecified** 🔵🔵
Malignant neoplasm of greater curvature of stomach, not classifiable to C16.0-C16.4

   C16.8   **Malignant neoplasm of overlapping sites of stomach** 🔵🔵

   C16.9   **Malignant neoplasm of stomach, unspecified** 🔵🔵
Gastric cancer NOS

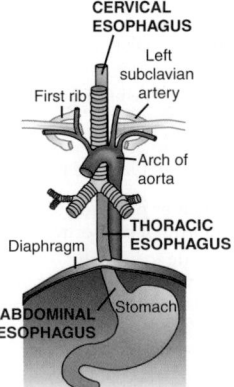

Figure 2-3   The esophagus is the muscular tube that connects the pharynx and the stomach. The 10 inch (25 cm) long esophagus is divided into three parts: **cervical, thoracic,** and **abdominal.**

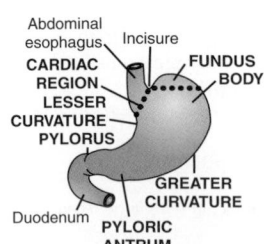

Figure 2-4   Parts of the stomach.

Item 2–2   The esophagus opens into the stomach through the **cardiac orifice,** also called the **cardioesophageal junction.** The **cardia** is adjacent to the cardiac orifice. The stomach widens into the **greater** and **lesser curvatures.** The **pyloric antrum** precedes the **pylorus,** which opens to the duodenum.

▶ New   ⇒ Revised   ~~deleted~~ Deleted   Excludes 1   Excludes 2   Includes   Use additional   Code first   Code also   Key words

688   OGCR Official Guidelines   ● Unacceptable Principal Diagnosis   X Assign placeholder X   ● Use Additional Character(s)   ▶ Manifestation Code   **Coding Clinic**

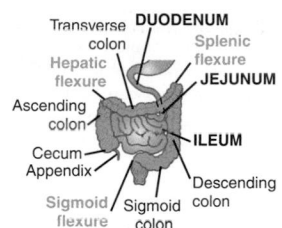

Transverse colon　DUODENUM　Splenic flexure
Hepatic flexure　JEJUNUM
Ascending colon
ILEUM
Cecum
Appendix
Descending colon
Sigmoid flexure　Sigmoid colon

Figure 2-5 Small intestine and colon.

● **C17** Malignant neoplasm of small intestine

> **Excludes1** malignant carcinoid tumor of the small intestine (C7A.Ø1)

C17.Ø Malignant neoplasm of duodenum 🔹🔹
> *First or proximal portion of small intestine, extending from pylorus to jejunum*
> (Ex) See PDX Collection 255

C17.1 Malignant neoplasm of jejunum 🔹🔹
> *Second section of small intestine, extending from duodenum to ileum*
> (Ex) See PDX Collection 256

C17.2 Malignant neoplasm of ileum 🔹🔹
> *Distal and longest portion of small intestine, extending from jejunum to cecum*
>> **Excludes1** malignant neoplasm of ileocecal valve (C18.Ø)
> (Ex) See PDX Collection 257

C17.3 Meckel's diverticulum, malignant 🔹🔹
> *Appendage of ileum*
>> **Excludes1** Meckel's diverticulum, congenital (Q43.Ø)
> (Ex) See PDX Collection 258

C17.8 Malignant neoplasm of overlapping sites of small intestine 🔹🔹
> (Ex) See PDX Collection 259

C17.9 Malignant neoplasm of small intestine, unspecified 🔹🔹
> (Ex) See PDX Collection 259

● **C18** Malignant neoplasm of colon

> **Excludes1** malignant carcinoid tumors of the colon (C7A.Ø2)

C18.Ø Malignant neoplasm of cecum 🔹🔹
> *First section of large intestine*
> Malignant neoplasm of ileocecal valve
> (Ex) See PDX Collection 260

C18.1 Malignant neoplasm of appendix 🔹🔹
> *Blind ended tube connected to the cecum; AKA vermiform appendix*
> (Ex) See PDX Collection 261

C18.2 Malignant neoplasm of ascending colon 🔹🔹
> *Ascending colon is between cecum and right colic flexure*
> (Ex) See PDX Collection 262

C18.3 Malignant neoplasm of hepatic flexure 🔹🔹
> *A flexure is a bending in a structure or organ. Note the three flexures illustrated in Figure 2–5.*
> (Ex) See PDX Collection 263

C18.4 Malignant neoplasm of transverse colon 🔹🔹
> *Portion of colon that runs transversely across upper part of abdomen, between right and left colic flexures*
> (Ex) See PDX Collection 264

C18.5 Malignant neoplasm of splenic flexure 🔹🔹
> *Bend at junction of transverse and descending colon*
> (Ex) See PDX Collection 265

C18.6 Malignant neoplasm of descending colon 🔹🔹
> *Portion between left colic flexure and sigmoid colon at pelvic brim; AKA iliac colon*
> (Ex) See PDX Collection 266

C18.7 Malignant neoplasm of sigmoid colon 🔹🔹
> *S-shaped part of colon extending from pelvic brim to third segment of sacrum*
> Malignant neoplasm of sigmoid (flexure)
>> **Excludes1** malignant neoplasm of rectosigmoid junction (C19)
> (Ex) See PDX Collection 267

C18.8 Malignant neoplasm of overlapping sites of colon 🔹🔹
> (Ex) See PDX Collection 268

C18.9 Malignant neoplasm of colon, unspecified 🔹🔹
> Malignant neoplasm of large intestine NOS
> (Ex) See PDX Collection 268

C19 Malignant neoplasm of rectosigmoid junction 🔹🔹
> Malignant neoplasm of colon with rectum
> Malignant neoplasm of rectosigmoid (colon)
>> **Excludes1** malignant carcinoid tumors of the colon (C7A.Ø2-)
> (Ex) See PDX Collection 269

C20 Malignant neoplasm of rectum 🔹🔹
> Malignant neoplasm of rectal ampulla
>> **Excludes1** malignant carcinoid tumor of the rectum (C7A.Ø26)
> (Ex) See PDX Collection 270

● **C21** Malignant neoplasm of anus and anal canal
> **Excludes2** malignant carcinoid tumors of the colon (C7A.Ø2-)
> malignant melanoma of anal margin (C43.51)
> malignant melanoma of anal skin (C43.51)
> malignant melanoma of perianal skin (C43.51)
> other and unspecified malignant neoplasm of anal margin (C44.5ØØ, C44.51Ø, C44.52Ø, C44.59Ø)
> other and unspecified malignant neoplasm of anal skin (C44.5ØØ, C44.51Ø, C44.52Ø, C44.59Ø)
> other and unspecified malignant neoplasm of perianal skin (C44.5ØØ, C44.51Ø, C44.52Ø, C44.59Ø)
> (Ex) For category C21 CC codes C21.Ø C21.1: See PDX Collection 271
> For category C21 CC codes C21.2-C21.8: See PDX Collection 272

C21.Ø Malignant neoplasm of anus, unspecified 🔹🔹

C21.1 Malignant neoplasm of anal canal 🔹🔹
> *Terminal part of large intestine*
> Malignant neoplasm of anal sphincter

C21.2 Malignant neoplasm of cloacogenic zone 🔹🔹

C21.8 Malignant neoplasm of overlapping sites of rectum, anus and anal canal 🔹🔹
> Malignant neoplasm of anorectal junction
> Malignant neoplasm of anorectum
> Primary malignant neoplasm of two or more contiguous sites of rectum, anus and anal canal

CHAPTER 2 (CØØ-D49)

N Newborn Age: Ø　　P Pediatric Age: Ø–17　　M Maternity DX: 9–64　　A Adult Age: 15–124　　♀ Females Only　　♂ Males Only

🔹 Complication\Comorbidity　　🔹 Major C\C　　(Ex) CC/MCC Exclusions　　🔹 Hospital-Acquired Condition　　🔹 Hierarchical Condition Category

689

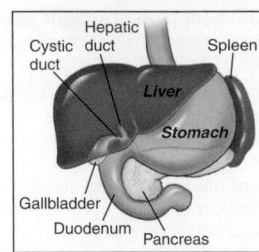

Figure 2-6 Diagram of liver, gallbladder, hepatic duct, pancreas, and spleen. (From Thibodeau and Patton: Anatomy and Physiology, ed 7, Mosby, 2010)

Item 2–3 Islets of Langerhans (endocrine producing cells comprising 1% to 2% of the pancreatic mass) make and secrete hormones that regulate the body's production of insulin, glucagon, and stomach acid. Breakdown of the insulin-producing cells can cause diabetes mellitus. Islet cell tumors can be benign or malignant and include glucagonomas, insulinomas, gastrinomas, and neuroendocrine tumor. The neoplasm table must be consulted for the correct neoplasm code.

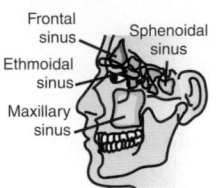

Figure 2-7 Paranasal sinuses. (From Buck CJ: Step-by-Step Medical Coding, ed 2016, St. Louis, Elsevier, 2016)

● **C22 Malignant neoplasm of liver and intrahepatic bile ducts**
Intrahepatic: Within liver
Use additional code to identify:
   alcohol abuse and dependence (F10.-)
   hepatitis B (B16.-, B18.0-B18.1) hepatitis C (B17.1-, B18.2)
> **Excludes1** malignant neoplasm of biliary tract NOS (C24.9)
>   secondary malignant neoplasm of liver and intrahepatic bile duct (C78.7)
(Ex:) **For category C22 CC codes:** See PDX Collection 273

C22.0 Liver cell carcinoma
   Hepatocellular carcinoma
   Hepatoma
C22.1 Intrahepatic bile duct carcinoma
   Cholangiocarcinoma
   Adenocarcinoma (cancer that originates in glandular tissue) arising from epithelium of intrahepatic bile ducts
> **Excludes1** malignant neoplasm of hepatic duct (C24.0)
C22.2 Hepatoblastoma
   Malignant intrahepatic tumor
C22.3 Angiosarcoma of liver
   Kupffer cell sarcoma
C22.4 Other sarcomas of liver
C22.7 Other specified carcinomas of liver
C22.8 Malignant neoplasm of liver, primary, unspecified as to type
C22.9 Malignant neoplasm of liver, not specified as primary or secondary

C23 Malignant neoplasm of gallbladder
(Ex:) See PDX Collection 274

● **C24 Malignant neoplasm of other and unspecified parts of biliary tract**
> **Excludes1** malignant neoplasm of intrahepatic bile duct (C22.1)
C24.0 Malignant neoplasm of extrahepatic bile duct
   Extrahepatic = outside the liver
   Malignant neoplasm of biliary duct or passage NOS
   Malignant neoplasm of common bile duct
   Malignant neoplasm of cystic duct
   Malignant neoplasm of hepatic duct
   (Ex:) See PDX Collection 275
C24.1 Malignant neoplasm of ampulla of Vater
   Union of pancreatic duct and common bile duct
   (Ex:) See PDX Collection 276
C24.8 Malignant neoplasm of overlapping sites of biliary tract
   Malignant neoplasm involving both intrahepatic and extrahepatic bile ducts
   Primary malignant neoplasm of two or more contiguous sites of biliary tract
   (Ex:) See PDX Collection 277
C24.9 Malignant neoplasm of biliary tract, unspecified
   (Ex:) See PDX Collection 277

● **C25 Malignant neoplasm of pancreas**
Check documentation for specific site.
➡ Code also if applicable exocrine pancreatic insufficiency (K86.81)
   Use additional code to identify:
      alcohol abuse and dependence (F10.-)
   (Ex:) **For category C25 CC codes:** See PDX Collection 278
C25.0 Malignant neoplasm of head of pancreas
C25.1 Malignant neoplasm of body of pancreas
   Coding Clinic: 2018, Q4, P40
C25.2 Malignant neoplasm of tail of pancreas
C25.3 Malignant neoplasm of pancreatic duct
C25.4 Malignant neoplasm of endocrine pancreas
   Malignant neoplasm of islets of Langerhans
   That part of the pancreas that acts as endocrine gland and consists of islets of Langerhans
   Use additional code to identify any functional activity.
C25.7 Malignant neoplasm of other parts of pancreas
   Malignant neoplasm of neck of pancreas
C25.8 Malignant neoplasm of overlapping sites of pancreas
C25.9 Malignant neoplasm of pancreas, unspecified

● **C26 Malignant neoplasm of other and ill-defined digestive organs**
> **Excludes1** malignant neoplasm of peritoneum and retroperitoneum (C48.-)
C26.0 Malignant neoplasm of intestinal tract, part unspecified
   Malignant neoplasm of intestine NOS
C26.1 Malignant neoplasm of spleen
> **Excludes1** Hodgkin lymphoma (C81.-)
>   non-Hodgkin lymphoma (C82-C85)
C26.9 Malignant neoplasm of ill-defined sites within the digestive system
   Malignant neoplasm of alimentary canal or tract NOS
   Malignant neoplasm of gastrointestinal tract NOS
> **Excludes1** malignant neoplasm of abdominal NOS (C76.2)
>   malignant neoplasm of intra-abdominal NOS (C76.2)

CHAPTER 2 (C00-D49)

▶ New ➡ Revised ~~deleted~~ Deleted Excludes 1 Excludes 2 Includes Use additional Code first Code also Key words
OGCR Official Guidelines ● Unacceptable Principal Diagnosis X Assign placeholder X ● Use Additional Character(s) ▷ Manifestation Code Coding Clinic

MALIGNANT NEOPLASMS OF RESPIRATORY AND INTRATHORACIC ORGANS (C30-C39)

Includes	malignant neoplasm of middle ear
Excludes1	mesothelioma (C45.-)

● C30   **Malignant neoplasm of nasal cavity and middle ear**

     C30.0   **Malignant neoplasm of nasal cavity** 🐾

         Malignant neoplasm of cartilage of nose
         Malignant neoplasm of nasal concha
         Malignant neoplasm of internal nose
         Malignant neoplasm of septum of nose
         Malignant neoplasm of vestibule of nose
           Anterior part of nasal cavity

         Excludes1   malignant neoplasm of nasal bone (C41.0)
                     malignant neoplasm of nose NOS (C76.0)
                     malignant neoplasm of olfactory bulb (C72.2-)
                     malignant neoplasm of posterior margin of nasal septum and choana (C11.3)
                     malignant melanoma of skin of nose (C43.31)
                     ⟶ malignant neoplasm of turbinates (C41.0)
                     other and unspecified malignant neoplasm of skin of nose (C44.301, C44.311, C44.321, C44.391)

     C30.1   **Malignant neoplasm of middle ear** 🐾

         Malignant neoplasm of antrum tympanicum
           Boney cavity or chamber
         Malignant neoplasm of auditory tube
         Malignant neoplasm of eustachian tube
         Malignant neoplasm of inner ear
         Malignant neoplasm of mastoid air cells
         Malignant neoplasm of tympanic cavity

         Excludes1   malignant neoplasm of auricular canal (external) (C43.2-, C44.2-)
                     malignant neoplasm of bone of ear (meatus) (C41.0)
                     malignant neoplasm of cartilage of ear (C49.0)
                     malignant melanoma of skin of (external) ear (C43.2-)
                     other and unspecified malignant neoplasm of skin of (external) ear (C44.2-)

● C31   **Malignant neoplasm of accessory sinuses**
       Paired sinuses in bones of face

     C31.0   **Malignant neoplasm of maxillary sinus** 🐾
         Malignant neoplasm of antrum (Highmore) (maxillary)

     C31.1   **Malignant neoplasm of ethmoidal sinus** 🐾

     C31.2   **Malignant neoplasm of frontal sinus** 🐾

     C31.3   **Malignant neoplasm of sphenoid sinus** 🐾

     C31.8   **Malignant neoplasm of overlapping sites of accessory sinuses** 🐾

     C31.9   **Malignant neoplasm of accessory sinus, unspecified** 🐾

● C32   **Malignant neoplasm of larynx**
       Use additional code to identify:
         alcohol abuse and dependence (F10.-)
         exposure to environmental tobacco smoke (Z77.22)
         exposure to tobacco smoke in the perinatal period (P96.81)
         history of tobacco dependence (Z87.891)
         occupational exposure to environmental tobacco smoke (Z57.31)
         tobacco dependence (F17.-)
         tobacco use (Z72.0)

     C32.0   **Malignant neoplasm of glottis** 🐾
         Vocal apparatus of larynx, consisting of true vocal cords (plicae vocales) and opening between them (rima glottidis)
         Malignant neoplasm of intrinsic larynx
         Malignant neoplasm of laryngeal commissure (anterior) (posterior)
         Malignant neoplasm of vocal cord (true) NOS
           *True vocal cords ("lower vocal folds") produce vocalization when air from the lungs passes between them. Check your documentation. Code C32.1 is for malignant neoplasm of the **false** vocal cords.*

     C32.1   **Malignant neoplasm of supraglottis** 🐾
         Area of pharynx above glottis
         Malignant neoplasm of aryepiglottic fold or interarytenoid fold, laryngeal aspect
         Malignant neoplasm of epiglottis (suprahyoid portion) NOS
         Malignant neoplasm of extrinsic larynx
         Malignant neoplasm of false vocal cord
           False vocal cords ("upper vocal folds") are not involved in vocalization. Check your documentation. Code C32.0 is for true vocal cords.
         Malignant neoplasm of posterior (laryngeal) surface of epiglottis
         Malignant neoplasm of ventricular bands

         Excludes2   malignant neoplasm of anterior surface of epiglottis (C10.1)
                     malignant neoplasm of aryepiglottic fold or interarytenoid fold, hypopharyngeal aspect (C13.1)
                     malignant neoplasm of aryepiglottic fold or interarytenoid fold, marginal zone (C13.1)
                     malignant neoplasm of aryepiglottic fold or interarytenoid fold NOS (C13.1)

     C32.2   **Malignant neoplasm of subglottis** 🐾
         Lowest part of larynx from just below vocal cords down to top of trachea

     C32.3   **Malignant neoplasm of laryngeal cartilage** 🐾
         Cartilages of larynx, including cricoid, thyroid, and epiglottic, and two each of arytenoid, corniculate, and cuneiform

     C32.8   **Malignant neoplasm of overlapping sites of larynx** 🐾

     C32.9   **Malignant neoplasm of larynx, unspecified** 🐾

C33   **Malignant neoplasm of trachea** 🐾🐾
       Use additional code to identify:
         exposure to environmental tobacco smoke (Z77.22)
         exposure to tobacco smoke in the perinatal period (P96.81)
         history of tobacco dependence (Z87.891)
         occupational exposure to environmental tobacco smoke (Z57.31)
         tobacco dependence (F17.-)
         tobacco use (Z72.0)
       (Ex.) See PDX Collection 279

N Newborn Age: 0   **P** Pediatric Age: 0–17   **M** Maternity DX: 9–64   **A** Adult Age: 15–124   ♀ Females Only   ♂ Males Only

🐾 Complication\Comorbidity   🐾 Major C\C   (Ex.) CC/MCC Exclusions   🐾 Hospital-Acquired Condition   🐾 Hierarchical Condition Category

691

CHAPTER 2 (C00–D49)

● **C34**   **Malignant neoplasm of bronchus and lung**
Use additional code to identify:
     exposure to environmental tobacco smoke (Z77.22)
     exposure to tobacco smoke in the perinatal period (P96.81)
     history of tobacco dependence (Z87.891)
     occupational exposure to environmental tobacco smoke
        (Z57.31)
     tobacco dependence (F17.-)
     tobacco use (Z72.0)

     Excludes1   Kaposi's sarcoma of lung (C46.5-)
                  malignant carcinoid tumor of the bronchus and
                  lung (C7A.090)

  ● **C34.0**   **Malignant neoplasm of main bronchus**
       Malignant neoplasm of carina
         Ridgelike structure
       Malignant neoplasm of hilus (of lung)
         Anatomic depression or pit
       (Ex:) **For category C34.0 CC codes:** See PDX Collection 280

       C34.00   Malignant neoplasm of unspecified main
                bronchus

       C34.01   Malignant neoplasm of right main
                bronchus

       C34.02   Malignant neoplasm of left main bronchus

  ● **C34.1**   **Malignant neoplasm of upper lobe, bronchus or lung**
       (Ex:) **For category C34.1 CC codes:** See PDX Collection 281

       C34.10   Malignant neoplasm of unspecified bronchus
                or lung

       C34.11   Malignant neoplasm of upper lobe, right
                bronchus or lung

       C34.12   Malignant neoplasm of upper lobe, left
                bronchus or lung

    C34.2   **Malignant neoplasm of middle lobe, bronchus or
        lung**
       (Ex:) See PDX Collection 282

  ● **C34.3**   **Malignant neoplasm of lower lobe, bronchus or lung**
       (Ex:) **For category C34.4 CC codes:** See PDX Collection 283

       C34.30   Malignant neoplasm of lower lobe, unspecified
                bronchus or lung

       C34.31   Malignant neoplasm of lower lobe, right
                bronchus or lung

       C34.32   Malignant neoplasm of lower lobe, left
                bronchus or lung

  ● **C34.8**   **Malignant neoplasm of overlapping sites of bronchus
       and lung**
       (Ex:) **For category C34.8 CC codes:** See PDX Collection 284

       C34.80   Malignant neoplasm of overlapping sites
                of unspecified bronchus and lung

       C34.81   Malignant neoplasm of overlapping sites of
                right bronchus and lung

       C34.82   Malignant neoplasm of overlapping sites of left
                bronchus and lung

  ● **C34.9**   **Malignant neoplasm of unspecified part of bronchus or
       lung**
       (Ex:) **For category C34.9 CC codes:** See PDX Collection 284

       C34.90   Malignant neoplasm of unspecified part of
                unspecified bronchus or lung
                Lung cancer NOS

       C34.91   Malignant neoplasm of unspecified part of
                right bronchus or lung

       C34.92   Malignant neoplasm of unspecified part of left
                bronchus or lung

● **C37**   **Malignant neoplasm of thymus**
     Excludes1   malignant carcinoid tumor of the thymus
                   (C7A.091)
     (Ex:) See PDX Collection 285

● **C38**   **Malignant neoplasm of heart, mediastinum and pleura**
     Excludes1   mesothelioma (C45.-)
     (Ex:) **For category C38 CC codes unless otherwise indicated:** See PDX Collection 287

    C38.0   **Malignant neoplasm of heart**
       Malignant neoplasm of pericardium
       Excludes1   malignant neoplasm of great vessels
                     (C49.3)
       (Ex:) See PDX Collection 286

    C38.1   **Malignant neoplasm of anterior mediastinum**

    C38.2   **Malignant neoplasm of posterior mediastinum**

    C38.3   **Malignant neoplasm of mediastinum,
        part unspecified**

    C38.4   **Malignant neoplasm of pleura**
       (Ex:) See PDX Collection 288

    C38.8   **Malignant neoplasm of overlapping sites of heart,
        mediastinum and pleura**
         *Pleura are comprised of serous membrane that lines the
            thoracic cavity (parietal) and covers the lungs (visceral).*

● **C39**   **Malignant neoplasm of other and ill-defined sites in the
     respiratory system and intrathoracic organs**
     Intrathoracic: within thorax/chest
     Use additional code to identify:
        exposure to environmental tobacco smoke (Z77.22)
        exposure to tobacco smoke in the perinatal period (P96.81)
        history of tobacco dependence (Z87.891)
        occupational exposure to environmental tobacco smoke
          (Z57.31)
        tobacco dependence (F17.-)
        tobacco use (Z72.0)

     Excludes1   intrathoracic malignant neoplasm NOS (C76.1)
                  thoracic malignant neoplasm NOS (C76.1)

    C39.0   **Malignant neoplasm of upper respiratory tract,
        part unspecified**

    C39.9   **Malignant neoplasm of lower respiratory tract,
        part unspecified**
       Malignant neoplasm of respiratory tract NOS

MALIGNANT NEOPLASMS OF BONE AND ARTICULAR CARTILAGE (C40-C41)

     Includes   malignant neoplasm of cartilage (articular) (joint)
              malignant neoplasm of periosteum

     Excludes1   malignant neoplasm of bone marrow NOS (C96.9)
              malignant neoplasm of synovia (C49.-)

● **C40**   **Malignant neoplasm of bone and articular cartilage of limbs**
     Use additional code to identify major osseous defect, if
     applicable (M89.7-)

  ● **C40.0**   **Malignant neoplasm of scapula and long bones of upper
       limb**
       (Ex:) **For category C40.0 CC codes:** See PDX Collection 289

       C40.00   Malignant neoplasm of scapula and long bones
                of unspecified upper limb

       C40.01   Malignant neoplasm of scapula and long bones
                of right upper limb

       C40.02   Malignant neoplasm of scapula and long bones
                of left upper limb

  ● **C40.1**   **Malignant neoplasm of short bones of upper limb**
       (Ex:) **For category C40.1 CC codes:** See PDX Collection 290

       C40.10   Malignant neoplasm of short bones
                of unspecified upper limb

       C40.11   Malignant neoplasm of short bones of right
                upper limb

       C40.12   Malignant neoplasm of short bones of left
                upper limb

▶ New   ⇒ Revised   ~~deleted~~ Deleted   Excludes 1   Excludes 2   Includes   Use additional   Code first   Code also   Key words
OGCR Official Guidelines   ● Unacceptable Principal Diagnosis   X Assign placeholder X   ● Use Additional Character(s)   ▶ Manifestation Code   Coding Clinic

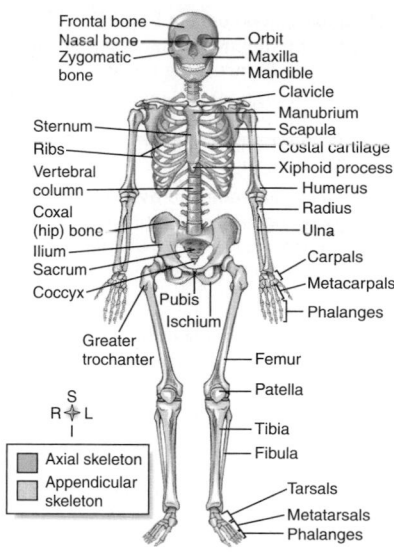

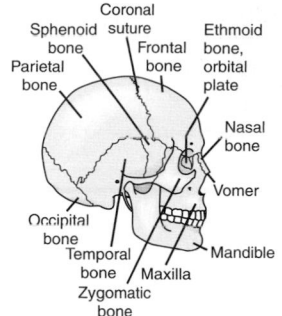

Figure 2-9 Bones of the skull.

Figure 2-8 Diagram of skeleton of trunk and limbs with bones labeled. (From Thibodeau and Patton: Anatomy and Physiology, ed 7, Mosby, 2010)

● C40.2   Malignant neoplasm of long bones of lower limb
  (Ex:) **For category C40.2 CC codes:** See PDX Collection 291

  C40.20   Malignant neoplasm of long bones of unspecified lower limb 🖊️🖊️

  C40.21   Malignant neoplasm of long bones of right lower limb 🖊️🖊️

  C40.22   Malignant neoplasm of long bones of left lower limb 🖊️🖊️

● C40.3   Malignant neoplasm of short bones of lower limb
  (Ex:) **For category C40.3 CC codes:** See PDX Collection 292

  C40.30   Malignant neoplasm of short bones of unspecified lower limb 🖊️🖊️

  C40.31   Malignant neoplasm of short bones of right lower limb 🖊️🖊️

  C40.32   Malignant neoplasm of short bones of left lower limb 🖊️🖊️

● C40.8   Malignant neoplasm of overlapping sites of bone and articular cartilage of limb
  (Ex:) **For category C40.8 CC codes:** See PDX Collection 293

  C40.80   Malignant neoplasm of overlapping sites of bone and articular cartilage of unspecified limb 🖊️🖊️

  C40.81   Malignant neoplasm of overlapping sites of bone and articular cartilage of right limb 🖊️🖊️

  C40.82   Malignant neoplasm of overlapping sites of bone and articular cartilage of left limb 🖊️🖊️

● C40.9   Malignant neoplasm of unspecified bones and articular cartilage of limb
  (Ex:) **For category C40.9 CC codes:** See PDX Collection 293

  C40.90   Malignant neoplasm of unspecified bones and articular cartilage of unspecified limb 🖊️🖊️

  C40.91   Malignant neoplasm of unspecified bones and articular cartilage of right limb 🖊️🖊️

  C40.92   Malignant neoplasm of unspecified bones and articular cartilage of left limb 🖊️🖊️

● C41   **Malignant neoplasm of bone and articular cartilage of other and unspecified sites**
  Excludes1   malignant neoplasm of bones of limbs (C40.-)
  malignant neoplasm of cartilage of ear (C49.0)
  malignant neoplasm of cartilage of eyelid (C49.0)
  malignant neoplasm of cartilage of larynx (C32.3)
  malignant neoplasm of cartilage of limbs (C40.-)
  malignant neoplasm of cartilage of nose (C30.0)

  C41.0   **Malignant neoplasm of bones of skull and face** 🖊️🖊️
  Malignant neoplasm of maxilla (superior)
  Malignant neoplasm of orbital bone

  Excludes2   carcinoma, any type except intraosseous or odontogenic of:
  maxillary sinus (C31.0)
  upper jaw (C03.0)
  malignant neoplasm of jaw bone (lower) (C41.1)
  (Ex:) See PDX Collection 294

  C41.1   **Malignant neoplasm of mandible** 🖊️🖊️
  Malignant neoplasm of inferior maxilla
  Malignant neoplasm of lower jaw bone

  Excludes2   carcinoma, any type except intraosseous or odontogenic of:
  jaw NOS (C03.9)
  lower (C03.1)
  malignant neoplasm of upper jaw bone (C41.0)
  (Ex:) See PDX Collection 295

  C41.2   **Malignant neoplasm of vertebral column** 🖊️🖊️
  Excludes1   malignant neoplasm of sacrum and coccyx (C41.4)
  (Ex:) See PDX Collection 296

  C41.3   **Malignant neoplasm of ribs, sternum and clavicle** 🖊️🖊️
  (Ex:) See PDX Collection 297

  C41.4   **Malignant neoplasm of pelvic bones, sacrum and coccyx** 🖊️🖊️
  (Ex:) See PDX Collection 298

  C41.9   **Malignant neoplasm of bone and articular cartilage, unspecified** 🖊️🖊️
  (Ex:) See PDX Collection 293

MELANOMA AND OTHER MALIGNANT NEOPLASMS OF SKIN (C43-C44)

● C43   Malignant melanoma of skin
  Excludes1   melanoma in situ (D03.-)
  Excludes2   malignant melanoma of skin of genital organs (C51-C52, C60.-, C63.-)
  Merkel cell carcinoma (C4A.-)
  sites other than skin-code to malignant neoplasm of the site

  C43.0   Malignant melanoma of lip 🖊️
  Excludes1   malignant neoplasm of vermilion border of lip (C00.0-C00.2)

N Newborn Age: 0   P Pediatric Age: 0–17   M Maternity DX: 9–64   A Adult Age: 15–124   ♀ Females Only   ♂ Males Only

🖊️ Complication\Comorbidity   🖊️ Major C\C   (Ex:) CC/MCC Exclusions   🖊️ Hospital-Acquired Condition   🖊️ Hierarchical Condition Category

693

CHAPTER 2 (C00–D49)

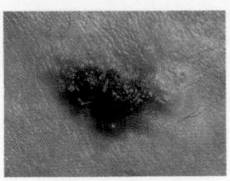

Figure 2-10   Malignant melanoma of skin. (Getty Image)

Item 2–4   Malignant melanoma is a serious form of skin cancer that affects the melanocytes (pigment-forming cells) and is caused by ultraviolet (UV) rays from the sun that damage skin. It is most commonly seen in the 40- to 60-year-olds with fair skin, blue or green eyes, and red or blond hair who sunburn easily.

Melanoma can spread very rapidly and is the most deadly form of skin cancer. It is less common than other types of skin cancer. The rate of melanoma is increasing and currently is the leading cause of death from skin disease.

● **C43.1**   **Malignant melanoma of eyelid, including canthus**
     Canthus: Either corner of eye where upper and lower eyelids meet
     C43.10   Malignant melanoma of unspecified eyelid, including canthus 🐾
●   **C43.11**   Malignant melanoma of right eyelid, including canthus 🐾
         C43.111   Malignant melanoma of right upper eyelid, including canthus 🐾
         C43.112   Malignant melanoma of right lower eyelid, including canthus 🐾
●   **C43.12**   Malignant melanoma of left eyelid, including canthus 🐾
         C43.121   Malignant melanoma of left upper eyelid, including canthus 🐾
         C43.122   Malignant melanoma of left lower eyelid, including canthus 🐾
● **C43.2**   **Malignant melanoma of ear and external auricular canal**
     C43.20   Malignant melanoma of unspecified ear and external auricular canal 🐾
     C43.21   Malignant melanoma of right ear and external auricular canal 🐾
     C43.22   Malignant melanoma of left ear and external auricular canal 🐾
● **C43.3**   **Malignant melanoma of other and unspecified parts of face**
     C43.30   Malignant melanoma of unspecified part of face 🐾
     C43.31   Malignant melanoma of nose 🐾
     C43.39   Malignant melanoma of other parts of face 🐾
   C43.4   Malignant melanoma of scalp and neck 🐾
● **C43.5**   **Malignant melanoma of trunk**
     Excludes2   malignant neoplasm of anus NOS (C21.0)
                malignant neoplasm of scrotum (C63.2)
     C43.51   Malignant melanoma of anal skin 🐾
         Malignant melanoma of anal margin
         Malignant melanoma of perianal skin
     C43.52   Malignant melanoma of skin of breast 🐾
     C43.59   Malignant melanoma of other part of trunk 🐾
● **C43.6**   **Malignant melanoma of upper limb, including shoulder**
     C43.60   Malignant melanoma of upper limb, including shoulder, unspecified side 🐾
     C43.61   Malignant melanoma of right upper limb, including shoulder 🐾
     C43.62   Malignant melanoma of left upper limb, including shoulder 🐾

● **C43.7**   **Malignant melanoma of lower limb, including hip**
     C43.70   Malignant melanoma of unspecified lower limb, including hip 🐾
     C43.71   Malignant melanoma of right lower limb, including hip 🐾
     C43.72   Malignant melanoma of left lower limb, including hip 🐾
   C43.8   Malignant melanoma of overlapping sites of skin 🐾
   C43.9   Malignant melanoma of skin, unspecified 🐾
     Malignant melanoma of unspecified site of skin
     Melanoma (malignant) NOS
●**C4A**   **Merkel cell carcinoma**
   C4A.0   **Merkel cell carcinoma of lip** 🐾
     Excludes1   malignant neoplasm of vermilion border of lip (C00.0-C00.2)
● **C4A.1**   **Merkel cell carcinoma of eyelid, including canthus**
     C4A.10   Merkel cell carcinoma of unspecified eyelid, including canthus 🐾
●   **C4A.11**   Merkel cell carcinoma of right eyelid, including canthus 🐾
         C4A.111   Merkel cell carcinoma of right upper eyelid, including canthus 🐾
         C4A.112   Merkel cell carcinoma of right lower eyelid, including canthus 🐾
●   **C4A.12**   Merkel cell carcinoma of left eyelid, including canthus 🐾
         C4A.121   Merkel cell carcinoma of left upper eyelid, including canthus 🐾
         C4A.122   Merkel cell carcinoma of left lower eyelid, including canthus 🐾
● **C4A.2**   **Merkel cell carcinoma of ear and external auricular canal**
     C4A.20   Merkel cell carcinoma of unspecified ear and external auricular canal 🐾
     C4A.21   Merkel cell carcinoma of right ear and external auricular canal 🐾
     C4A.22   Merkel cell carcinoma of left ear and external auricular canal 🐾
● **C4A.3**   **Merkel cell carcinoma of other and unspecified parts of face**
     C4A.30   Merkel cell carcinoma of unspecified part of face 🐾
     C4A.31   Merkel cell carcinoma of nose 🐾
     C4A.39   Merkel cell carcinoma of other parts of face 🐾
   C4A.4   Merkel cell carcinoma of scalp and neck 🐾
● **C4A.5**   **Merkel cell carcinoma of trunk**
     Excludes2   malignant neoplasm of anus NOS (C21.0)
                malignant neoplasm of scrotum (C63.2)
     C4A.51   Merkel cell carcinoma of anal skin 🐾
         Merkel cell carcinoma of anal margin
         Merkel cell carcinoma of perianal skin
     C4A.52   Merkel cell carcinoma of skin of breast 🐾
     C4A.59   Merkel cell carcinoma of other part of trunk 🐾
● **C4A.6**   **Merkel cell carcinoma of upper limb, including shoulder**
     C4A.60   Merkel cell carcinoma of unspecified upper limb, including shoulder 🐾
     C4A.61   Merkel cell carcinoma of right upper limb, including shoulder 🐾
     C4A.62   Merkel cell carcinoma of left upper limb, including shoulder 🐾
● **C4A.7**   **Merkel cell carcinoma of lower limb, including hip**
     C4A.70   Merkel cell carcinoma of unspecified lower limb, including hip 🐾
     C4A.71   Merkel cell carcinoma of right lower limb, including hip 🐾
     C4A.72   Merkel cell carcinoma of left lower limb, including hip 🐾
   C4A.8   Merkel cell carcinoma of overlapping sites 🐾
   C4A.9   Merkel cell carcinoma, unspecified 🐾
     Merkel cell carcinoma of unspecified site
     Merkel cell carcinoma NOS

▶ New   ⇒ Revised   ~~deleted~~ Deleted   Excludes 1   Excludes 2   Includes   Use additional   Code first   Code also   Key words
OGCR Official Guidelines   ● Unacceptable Principal Diagnosis   X Assign placeholder X   ● Use Additional Character(s)   ▶ Manifestation Code   **Coding Clinic**

● **C44**   **Other and unspecified malignant neoplasm of skin**

     Includes   malignant neoplasm of sebaceous glands
                     malignant neoplasm of sweat glands

     Excludes1   Kaposi's sarcoma of skin (C46.0)
                     malignant melanoma of skin (C43.-)
                     malignant neoplasm of skin of genital organs
                         (C51-C52, C60.-, C63.2)
                     Merkel cell carcinoma (C4A.-)

● **C44.0**   Other and unspecified malignant neoplasm of skin of lip

     Excludes1   malignant neoplasm of lip (C00.-)

   C44.00   Unspecified malignant neoplasm of skin of lip

   C44.01   Basal cell carcinoma of skin of lip

   C44.02   Squamous cell carcinoma of skin of lip

   C44.09   Other specified malignant neoplasm of skin of lip

● **C44.1**   Other and unspecified malignant neoplasm of skin of eyelid, including canthus

     Excludes1   connective tissue of eyelid (C49.0)

   ● C44.10   Unspecified malignant neoplasm of skin of eyelid, including canthus

     C44.101   Unspecified malignant neoplasm of skin of unspecified eyelid, including canthus

     ● C44.102   Unspecified malignant neoplasm of skin of right eyelid, including canthus

         C44.1021   Unspecified malignant neoplasm of skin of right upper eyelid, including canthus

         C44.1022   Unspecified malignant neoplasm of skin of right lower eyelid, including canthus

     ● C44.109   Unspecified malignant neoplasm of skin of left eyelid, including canthus

         C44.1091   Unspecified malignant neoplasm of skin of left upper eyelid, including canthus

         C44.1092   Unspecified malignant neoplasm of skin of left lower eyelid, including canthus

   ● C44.11   Basal cell carcinoma of skin of eyelid, including canthus

     C44.111   Basal cell carcinoma of skin of unspecified eyelid, including canthus

     ● C44.112   Basal cell carcinoma of skin of right eyelid, including canthus

         C44.1121   Basal cell carcinoma of skin of right upper eyelid, including canthus

         C44.1122   Basal cell carcinoma of skin of right lower eyelid, including canthus

     ● C44.119   Basal cell carcinoma of skin of left eyelid, including canthus

         C44.1191   Basal cell carcinoma of skin of left upper eyelid, including canthus

         C44.1192   Basal cell carcinoma of skin of left lower eyelid, including canthus

   ● C44.12   Squamous cell carcinoma of skin of eyelid, including canthus

     C44.121   Squamous cell carcinoma of skin of unspecified eyelid, including canthus

● C44.122   Squamous cell carcinoma of skin of right eyelid, including canthus

   C44.1221   Squamous cell carcinoma of skin of right upper eyelid, including canthus

   C44.1222   Squamous cell carcinoma of skin of right lower eyelid, including canthus

● C44.129   Squamous cell carcinoma of skin of left eyelid, including canthus

   C44.1291   Squamous cell carcinoma of skin of left upper eyelid, including canthus

   C44.1292   Squamous cell carcinoma of skin of left lower eyelid, including canthus

● C44.13   Sebaceous cell carcinoma of skin of eyelid, including canthus

   C44.131   Sebaceous cell carcinoma of skin of unspecified eyelid, including canthus

● C44.132   Sebaceous cell carcinoma of skin of right eyelid, including canthus

   C44.1321   Sebaceous cell carcinoma of skin of right upper eyelid, including canthus

   C44.1322   Sebaceous cell carcinoma of skin of right lower eyelid, including canthus

● C44.139   Sebaceous cell carcinoma of skin of left eyelid, including canthus

   C44.1391   Sebaceous cell carcinoma of skin of left upper eyelid, including canthus

   C44.1392   Sebaceous cell carcinoma of skin of left lower eyelid, including canthus

● C44.19   Other specified malignant neoplasm of skin of eyelid, including canthus

   C44.191   Other specified malignant neoplasm of skin of unspecified eyelid, including canthus

● C44.192   Other specified malignant neoplasm of skin of right eyelid, including canthus

   C44.1921   Other specified malignant neoplasm of skin of right upper eyelid, including canthus

   C44.1922   Other specified malignant neoplasm of skin of right lower eyelid, including canthus

● C44.199   Other specified malignant neoplasm of skin of left eyelid, including canthus

   C44.1991   Other specified malignant neoplasm of skin of left upper eyelid, including canthus

   C44.1992   Other specified malignant neoplasm of skin of left lower eyelid, including canthus

● **C44.2**   Other and unspecified malignant neoplasm of skin of ear and external auricular canal

     Excludes1   connective tissue of ear (C49.0)

● C44.20   Unspecified malignant neoplasm of skin of ear and external auricular canal

   C44.201   Unspecified malignant neoplasm of skin of unspecified ear and external auricular canal

N Newborn Age: 0   **P** Pediatric Age: 0–17   **M** Maternity DX: 9–64   **A** Adult Age: 15–124   ♀ Females Only   ♂ Males Only

🅒 Complication\Comorbidity   🅒 Major C\C   (Ex) CC/MCC Exclusions   🅒 Hospital-Acquired Condition   🅒 Hierarchical Condition Category

695

      C44.202   Unspecified malignant neoplasm of skin of right ear and external auricular canal

      C44.209   Unspecified malignant neoplasm of skin of left ear and external auricular canal

● C44.21   Basal cell carcinoma of skin of ear and external auricular canal

      C44.211   Basal cell carcinoma of skin of unspecified ear and external auricular canal

      C44.212   Basal cell carcinoma of skin of right ear and external auricular canal

      C44.219   Basal cell carcinoma of skin of left ear and external auricular canal

● C44.22   Squamous cell carcinoma of skin of ear and external auricular canal

      C44.221   Squamous cell carcinoma of skin of unspecified ear and external auricular canal

      C44.222   Squamous cell carcinoma of skin of right ear and external auricular canal

      C44.229   Squamous cell carcinoma of skin of left ear and external auricular canal

● C44.29   Other specified malignant neoplasm of skin of ear and external auricular canal

      C44.291   Other specified malignant neoplasm of skin of unspecified ear and external auricular canal

      C44.292   Other specified malignant neoplasm of skin of right ear and external auricular canal

      C44.299   Other specified malignant neoplasm of skin of left ear and external auricular canal

● C44.3   Other and unspecified malignant neoplasm of skin of other and unspecified parts of face

● C44.30   Unspecified malignant neoplasm of skin of other and unspecified parts of face

      C44.300   Unspecified malignant neoplasm of skin of unspecified part of face

      C44.301   Unspecified malignant neoplasm of skin of nose

      C44.309   Unspecified malignant neoplasm of skin of other parts of face

● C44.31   Basal cell carcinoma of skin of other and unspecified parts of face

      C44.310   Basal cell carcinoma of skin of unspecified parts of face

      C44.311   Basal cell carcinoma of skin of nose

      C44.319   Basal cell carcinoma of skin of other parts of face

         Coding Clinic: 2017, Q1, P4

● C44.32   Squamous cell carcinoma of skin of other and unspecified parts of face

      C44.320   Squamous cell carcinoma of skin of unspecified parts of face

      C44.321   Squamous cell carcinoma of skin of nose

      C44.329   Squamous cell carcinoma of skin of other parts of face

● C44.39   Other specified malignant neoplasm of skin of other and unspecified parts of face

      C44.390   Other specified malignant neoplasm of skin of unspecified parts of face

      C44.391   Other specified malignant neoplasm of skin of nose

      C44.399   Other specified malignant neoplasm of skin of other parts of face

● C44.4   Other and unspecified malignant neoplasm of skin of scalp and neck

      C44.40   Unspecified malignant neoplasm of skin of scalp and neck

      C44.41   Basal cell carcinoma of skin of scalp and neck

      C44.42   Squamous cell carcinoma of skin of scalp and neck

      C44.49   Other specified malignant neoplasm of skin of scalp and neck

● C44.5   Other and unspecified malignant neoplasm of skin of trunk

     Excludes1   anus NOS (C21.0)
                 scrotum (C63.2)

● C44.50   Unspecified malignant neoplasm of skin of trunk

      C44.500   Unspecified malignant neoplasm of anal skin
          Unspecified malignant neoplasm of anal margin
          Unspecified malignant neoplasm of perianal skin

      C44.501   Unspecified malignant neoplasm of skin of breast

      C44.509   Unspecified malignant neoplasm of skin of other part of trunk

● C44.51   Basal cell carcinoma of skin of trunk

      C44.510   Basal cell carcinoma of anal skin
          Basal cell carcinoma of anal margin
          Basal cell carcinoma of perianal skin

      C44.511   Basal cell carcinoma of skin of breast

      C44.519   Basal cell carcinoma of skin of other part of trunk

● C44.52   Squamous cell carcinoma of skin of trunk

      C44.520   Squamous cell carcinoma of anal skin
          Squamous cell carcinoma of anal margin
          Squamous cell carcinoma of perianal skin

      C44.521   Squamous cell carcinoma of skin of breast

      C44.529   Squamous cell carcinoma of skin of other part of trunk

● C44.59   Other specified malignant neoplasm of skin of trunk

      C44.590   Other specified malignant neoplasm of anal skin
          Other specified malignant neoplasm of anal margin
          Other specified malignant neoplasm of perianal skin

      C44.591   Other specified malignant neoplasm of skin of breast

      C44.599   Other specified malignant neoplasm of skin of other part of trunk

● C44.6   Other and unspecified malignant neoplasm of skin of upper limb, including shoulder

● C44.60   Unspecified malignant neoplasm of skin of upper limb, including shoulder

      C44.601   Unspecified malignant neoplasm of skin of unspecified upper limb, including shoulder

      C44.602   Unspecified malignant neoplasm of skin of right upper limb, including shoulder

      C44.609   Unspecified malignant neoplasm of skin of left upper limb, including shoulder

● C44.61   Basal cell carcinoma of skin of upper limb, including shoulder

      C44.611   Basal cell carcinoma of skin of unspecified upper limb, including shoulder

▶ New   ⇒ Revised   ~~deleted~~ Deleted   Excludes 1   Excludes 2   Includes   Use additional   Code first   Code also   Key words

OGCR Official Guidelines   ● Unacceptable Principal Diagnosis   X Assign placeholder X   ● Use Additional Character(s)   ▸ Manifestation Code   Coding Clinic

　　　　C44.612　Basal cell carcinoma of skin of right upper limb, including shoulder

　　　　C44.619　Basal cell carcinoma of skin of left upper limb, including shoulder

　●C44.62　Squamous cell carcinoma of skin of upper limb, including shoulder

　　　　C44.621　Squamous cell carcinoma of skin of unspecified upper limb, including shoulder

　　　　C44.622　Squamous cell carcinoma of skin of right upper limb, including shoulder

　　　　C44.629　Squamous cell carcinoma of skin of left upper limb, including shoulder

　●C44.69　Other specified malignant neoplasm of skin of upper limb, including shoulder

　　　　C44.691　Other specified malignant neoplasm of skin of unspecified upper limb, including shoulder

　　　　C44.692　Other specified malignant neoplasm of skin of right upper limb, including shoulder

　　　　C44.699　Other specified malignant neoplasm of skin of left upper limb, including shoulder

●C44.7　Other and unspecified malignant neoplasm of skin of lower limb, including hip

　●C44.70　Unspecified malignant neoplasm of skin of lower limb, including hip

　　　　C44.701　Unspecified malignant neoplasm of skin of unspecified lower limb, including hip

　　　　C44.702　Unspecified malignant neoplasm of skin of right lower limb, including hip

　　　　C44.709　Unspecified malignant neoplasm of skin of left lower limb, including hip

　●C44.71　Basal cell carcinoma of skin of lower limb, including hip

　　　　C44.711　Basal cell carcinoma of skin of unspecified lower limb, including hip

　　　　C44.712　Basal cell carcinoma of skin of right lower limb, including hip

　　　　C44.719　Basal cell carcinoma of skin of left lower limb, including hip

　●C44.72　Squamous cell carcinoma of skin of lower limb, including hip

　　　　C44.721　Squamous cell carcinoma of skin of unspecified lower limb, including hip

　　　　C44.722　Squamous cell carcinoma of skin of right lower limb, including hip

　　　　C44.729　Squamous cell carcinoma of skin of left lower limb, including hip

　●C44.79　Other specified malignant neoplasm of skin of lower limb, including hip

　　　　C44.791　Other specified malignant neoplasm of skin of unspecified lower limb, including hip

　　　　C44.792　Other specified malignant neoplasm of skin of right lower limb, including hip

　　　　C44.799　Other specified malignant neoplasm of skin of left lower limb, including hip

●C44.8　Other and unspecified malignant neoplasm of overlapping sites of skin

　　　　C44.80　Unspecified malignant neoplasm of overlapping sites of skin

　　　　C44.81　Basal cell carcinoma of overlapping sites of skin

　　　　C44.82　Squamous cell carcinoma of overlapping sites of skin

　　　　C44.89　Other specified malignant neoplasm of overlapping sites of skin

●C44.9　Other and unspecified malignant neoplasm of skin, unspecified

　　　　C44.90　Unspecified malignant neoplasm of skin, unspecified
　　　　　　　　Malignant neoplasm of unspecified site of skin

　　　　C44.91　Basal cell carcinoma of skin, unspecified

　　　　C44.92　Squamous cell carcinoma of skin, unspecified

　　　　C44.99　Other specified malignant neoplasm of skin, unspecified

---

MALIGNANT NEOPLASMS OF MESOTHELIAL AND SOFT TISSUE (C45-C49)

●C45　Mesothelioma
Malignant cells develop in protective lining that covers internal organs (mesothelium) caused by exposure to asbestos

　　C45.0　Mesothelioma of pleura
　　　　Excludes1　other malignant neoplasm of pleura (C38.4)
　　　　Ex: See PDX Collection 288
　　　　Coding Clinic: 2017, Q2, P11

　　C45.1　Mesothelioma of peritoneum
　　　　Mesothelioma of cul-de-sac
　　　　Mesothelioma of mesentery
　　　　Mesothelioma of mesocolon
　　　　Mesothelioma of omentum
　　　　Mesothelioma of peritoneum (parietal) (pelvic)
　　　　Excludes1　other malignant neoplasm of soft tissue of peritoneum (C48.-)
　　　　Ex: See PDX Collection 299

　　C45.2　Mesothelioma of pericardium
　　　　Excludes1　other malignant neoplasm of pericardium (C38.0)
　　　　Ex: See PDX Collection 286

　　C45.7　Mesothelioma of other sites

　　C45.9　Mesothelioma, unspecified

●C46　Kaposi's sarcoma
Code first any human immunodeficiency virus [HIV] disease (B20)

　　C46.0　Kaposi's sarcoma of skin
　　　　Ex: See PDX Collection 300

　　C46.1　Kaposi's sarcoma of soft tissue
　　　　Kaposi's sarcoma of blood vessel
　　　　Kaposi's sarcoma of connective tissue
　　　　Kaposi's sarcoma of fascia
　　　　Kaposi's sarcoma of ligament
　　　　Kaposi's sarcoma of lymphatic(s) NEC
　　　　Kaposi's sarcoma of muscle
　　　　Excludes2　Kaposi's sarcoma of lymph glands and nodes (C46.3)
　　　　Ex: See PDX Collection 301

　　C46.2　Kaposi's sarcoma of palate
　　　　Ex: See PDX Collection 302

　　C46.3　Kaposi's sarcoma of lymph nodes
　　　　Ex: See PDX Collection 303

　　C46.4　Kaposi's sarcoma of gastrointestinal sites
　　　　Ex: See PDX Collection 304

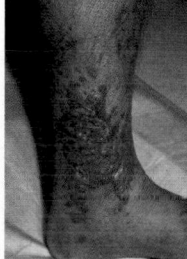

Figure 2-11 Kaposi's sarcoma. There are large confluent hyperpigmented patch-stage lesions with lymphedema. (From Goldman L, Ausiello D, Arend W, Armitage J, Clemmons D, Drazen J, Griggs R, et al: Cecil Medicine: Expert Consult, 23e, Saunders, 2007)

Item 2–5　Kaposi's sarcoma is a cancer that causes patches of abnormal tissue to grow under the skin; in the lining of the mouth, nose, and throat; or in other organs, often beginning and spreading to other organs. Patients who have had organ transplants or patients with AIDS are at high risk for this malignancy.

N Newborn Age: 0　**P** Pediatric Age: 0–17　**M** Maternity DX: 9–64　**A** Adult Age: 15–124　♀ Females Only　♂ Males Only

Complication\Comorbidity　　Major C\C　　Ex: CC/MCC Exclusions　　Hospital-Acquired Condition　　Hierarchical Condition Category

● **C46.5** **Kaposi's sarcoma of lung**
    (Ex:) **For category C46.5 CC codes:** See PDX Collection 284

    C46.50   Kaposi's sarcoma of unspecified lung
    C46.51   Kaposi's sarcoma of right lung
    C46.52   Kaposi's sarcoma of left lung

C46.7   **Kaposi's sarcoma of other sites**
    (Ex:) See PDX Collection 305

C46.9   **Kaposi's sarcoma, unspecified**
    Kaposi's sarcoma of unspecified site
    (Ex:) See PDX Collection 306

● **C47**   **Malignant neoplasm of peripheral nerves and autonomic nervous system**

    Includes   malignant neoplasm of sympathetic and parasympathetic nerves and ganglia

    Excludes1   Kaposi's sarcoma of soft tissue (C46.1)

C47.0   **Malignant neoplasm of peripheral nerves of head, face and neck**
    Excludes1   malignant neoplasm of peripheral nerves of orbit (C69.6-)
    (Ex:) See PDX Collection 3244

● **C47.1**   **Malignant neoplasm of peripheral nerves of upper limb, including shoulder**
    C47.10   Malignant neoplasm of peripheral nerves of unspecified upper limb, including shoulder
       (Ex:) See PDX Collection 3245
    C47.11   Malignant neoplasm of peripheral nerves of right upper limb, including shoulder
       (Ex:) See PDX Collection 3246
    C47.12   Malignant neoplasm of peripheral nerves of left upper limb, including shoulder
       (Ex:) See PDX Collection 3247

● **C47.2**   **Malignant neoplasm of peripheral nerves of lower limb, including hip**
    C47.20   Malignant neoplasm of peripheral nerves of unspecified lower limb, including hip
       (Ex:) See PDX Collection 3248
    C47.21   Malignant neoplasm of peripheral nerves of right lower limb, including hip
       (Ex:) See PDX Collection 3249
    C47.22   Malignant neoplasm of peripheral nerves of left lower limb, including hip
       (Ex:) See PDX Collection 3250

C47.3   **Malignant neoplasm of peripheral nerves of thorax**
    (Ex:) See PDX Collection 3251

C47.4   **Malignant neoplasm of peripheral nerves of abdomen**
    (Ex:) See PDX Collection 3252

C47.5   **Malignant neoplasm of peripheral nerves of pelvis**
    (Ex:) See PDX Collection 3253

C47.6   **Malignant neoplasm of peripheral nerves of trunk, unspecified**
    Malignant neoplasm of peripheral nerves of unspecified part of trunk
    (Ex:) See PDX Collection 3254

C47.8   **Malignant neoplasm of overlapping sites of peripheral nerves and autonomic nervous system**
    (Ex:) See PDX Collection 3255

C47.9   **Malignant neoplasm of peripheral nerves and autonomic nervous system, unspecified**
    Malignant neoplasm of unspecified site of peripheral nerves and autonomic nervous system
    (Ex:) See PDX Collection 3256

● **C48**   **Malignant neoplasm of retroperitoneum and peritoneum**
    Excludes1   Kaposi's sarcoma of connective tissue (C46.1)
       mesothelioma (C45.-)
    (Ex:) **For category C48 unless otherwise indicated:** See PDX Collection 299

C48.0   **Malignant neoplasm of retroperitoneum**
    Behind/outside of peritoneum
    (Ex:) See PDX Collection 308

C48.1   **Malignant neoplasm of specified parts of peritoneum**
    Serous membrane lining abdominopelvic walls and covering viscera
    Malignant neoplasm of cul-de-sac
    Malignant neoplasm of mesentery
    Malignant neoplasm of mesocolon
    Malignant neoplasm of omentum
    Malignant neoplasm of parietal peritoneum
    Malignant neoplasm of pelvic peritoneum

C48.2   **Malignant neoplasm of peritoneum, unspecified**

C48.8   **Malignant neoplasm of overlapping sites of retroperitoneum and peritoneum**

● **C49**   **Malignant neoplasm of other connective and soft tissue**

    Includes   malignant neoplasm of blood vessel
       malignant neoplasm of bursa
       malignant neoplasm of cartilage
       malignant neoplasm of fascia
       malignant neoplasm of fat
       malignant neoplasm of ligament, except uterine
       malignant neoplasm of lymphatic vessel
       malignant neoplasm of muscle
       malignant neoplasm of synovia
       malignant neoplasm of tendon (sheath)

    Excludes1   malignant neoplasm of cartilage (of):
       articular (C40-C41)
       larynx (C32.3)
       nose (C30.0)
       malignant neoplasm of connective tissue of breast (C50.-)

    Excludes2   Kaposi's sarcoma of soft tissue (C46.1)
       malignant neoplasm of heart (C38.0)
       malignant neoplasm of peripheral nerves and autonomic nervous system (C47.-)
       malignant neoplasm of peritoneum (C48.2)
       malignant neoplasm of retroperitoneum (C48.0)
       malignant neoplasm of uterine ligament (C57.3)
       mesothelioma (C45.-)

C49.0   **Malignant neoplasm of connective and soft tissue of head, face and neck**
    Malignant neoplasm of connective tissue of ear
    Malignant neoplasm of connective tissue of eyelid
    Excludes1   connective tissue of orbit (C69.6-)
    (Ex:) See PDX Collection 3257

● **C49.1**   **Malignant neoplasm of connective and soft tissue of upper limb, including shoulder**
    C49.10   Malignant neoplasm of connective and soft tissue of unspecified upper limb, including shoulder
       (Ex:) See PDX Collection 3258
    C49.11   Malignant neoplasm of connective and soft tissue of right upper limb, including shoulder
       (Ex:) See PDX Collection 3259
    C49.12   Malignant neoplasm of connective and soft tissue of left upper limb, including shoulder
       (Ex:) See PDX Collection 3260

● **C49.2**   **Malignant neoplasm of connective and soft tissue of lower limb, including hip**
    C49.20   Malignant neoplasm of connective and soft tissue of unspecified lower limb, including hip
       (Ex:) See PDX Collection 3261
    C49.21   Malignant neoplasm of connective and soft tissue of right lower limb, including hip
       (Ex:) See PDX Collection 3262
    C49.22   Malignant neoplasm of connective and soft tissue of left lower limb, including hip
       (Ex:) See PDX Collection 3263

▶ New   ⇒ Revised   ~~deleted~~ Deleted   Excludes 1   Excludes 2   Includes   Use additional   Code first   Code also   Key words

698

OGCR Official Guidelines   ● Unacceptable Principal Diagnosis   X Assign placeholder X   ● Use Additional Character(s)   ▸ Manifestation Code   **Coding Clinic**

C49.3 **Malignant neoplasm of connective and soft tissue of thorax**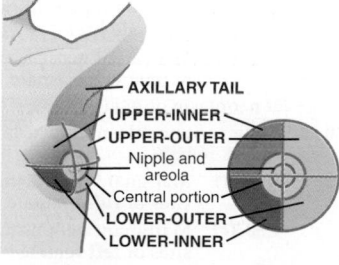
  Malignant neoplasm of axilla
  Malignant neoplasm of diaphragm
  Malignant neoplasm of great vessels
  Excludes1 malignant neoplasm of breast (C50.-)
    malignant neoplasm of heart (C38.0)
    malignant neoplasm of mediastinum (C38.1-C38.3)
    malignant neoplasm of thymus (C37)
  (Ex:) See PDX Collection 3264
  Coding Clinic: 2015, Q3, P19

C49.4 **Malignant neoplasm of connective and soft tissue of abdomen**
  Malignant neoplasm of abdominal wall
  Malignant neoplasm of hypochondrium
  (Ex:) See PDX Collection 3265
  Coding Clinic: 2019, Q4, P44

C49.5 **Malignant neoplasm of connective and soft tissue of pelvis**
  Malignant neoplasm of buttock
  Malignant neoplasm of groin
  Malignant neoplasm of perineum
  (Ex:) See PDX Collection 3266

C49.6 **Malignant neoplasm of connective and soft tissue of trunk, unspecified**
  Malignant neoplasm of back NOS
  (Ex:) See PDX Collection 3267

C49.8 **Malignant neoplasm of overlapping sites of connective and soft tissue**
  Primary malignant neoplasm of two or more contiguous sites of connective and soft tissue
  (Ex:) See PDX Collection 3268

C49.9 **Malignant neoplasm of connective and soft tissue, unspecified**
  (Ex:) See PDX Collection 3269

● C49.A **Gastrointestinal stromal tumor**
  Coding Clinic: 2016, Q4, P8

  C49.A0 **Gastrointestinal stromal tumor, unspecified site**
    (Ex:) See PDX Collection 3270

  C49.A1 **Gastrointestinal stromal tumor of esophagus**
    (Ex:) See PDX Collection 3271

  C49.A2 **Gastrointestinal stromal tumor of stomach**
    (Ex:) See PDX Collection 254

  C49.A3 **Gastrointestinal stromal tumor of small intestine**
    (Ex:) See PDX Collection 3272

  C49.A4 **Gastrointestinal stromal tumor of large intestine**
    (Ex:) See PDX Collection 3273

  C49.A5 **Gastrointestinal stromal tumor of rectum**
    (Ex:) See PDX Collection 3275

  C49.A9 **Gastrointestinal stromal tumor of other sites**
    (Ex:) See PDX Collection 3276

MALIGNANT NEOPLASMS OF BREAST (C50)

● C50 **Malignant neoplasm of breast**
  Includes connective tissue of breast
    Paget's disease of breast
    Paget's disease of nipple
    Intraductal carcinoma of breast characterized by eczema-like inflammatory skin changes
  Use additional code to identify estrogen receptor status (Z17.0, Z17.1)
  Excludes1 skin of breast (C44.501, C44.511, C44.521, C44.591)
  ● C50.0 **Malignant neoplasm of nipple and areola**
    ● C50.01 **Malignant neoplasm of nipple and areola, female**
      C50.011 **Malignant neoplasm of nipple and areola, right female breast** ♀

      C50.012 **Malignant neoplasm of nipple and areola, left female breast** ♀
      C50.019 **Malignant neoplasm of nipple and areola, unspecified female breast** ♀
    ● C50.02 **Malignant neoplasm of nipple and areola, male**
      C50.021 **Malignant neoplasm of nipple and areola, right male breast** ♂
      C50.022 **Malignant neoplasm of nipple and areola, left male breast** ♂
      C50.029 **Malignant neoplasm of nipple and areola, unspecified male breast** ♂
  ● C50.1 **Malignant neoplasm of central portion of breast**
    ● C50.11 **Malignant neoplasm of central portion of breast, female**
      C50.111 **Malignant neoplasm of central portion of right female breast** ♀
      C50.112 **Malignant neoplasm of central portion of left female breast** ♀
      C50.119 **Malignant neoplasm of central portion of unspecified female breast** ♀
    ● C50.12 **Malignant neoplasm of central portion of breast, male**
      C50.121 **Malignant neoplasm of central portion of right male breast** ♂
      C50.122 **Malignant neoplasm of central portion of left male breast** ♂
      C50.129 **Malignant neoplasm of central portion of unspecified male breast** ♂
  ● C50.2 **Malignant neoplasm of upper-inner quadrant of breast**
    ● C50.21 **Malignant neoplasm of upper-inner quadrant of breast, female**
      C50.211 **Malignant neoplasm of upper-inner quadrant of right female breast** ♀
      C50.212 **Malignant neoplasm of upper-inner quadrant of left female breast** ♀
      C50.219 **Malignant neoplasm of upper-inner quadrant of unspecified female breast** ♀
    ● C50.22 **Malignant neoplasm of upper-inner quadrant of breast, male**
      C50.221 **Malignant neoplasm of upper-inner quadrant of right male breast** ♂
      C50.222 **Malignant neoplasm of upper-inner quadrant of left male breast** ♂
      C50.229 **Malignant neoplasm of upper-inner quadrant of unspecified male breast** ♂
  ● C50.3 **Malignant neoplasm of lower-inner quadrant of breast**
    ● C50.31 **Malignant neoplasm of lower-inner quadrant of breast, female**
      C50.311 **Malignant neoplasm of lower-inner quadrant of right female breast** ♀
      C50.312 **Malignant neoplasm of lower-inner quadrant of left female breast** ♀
      C50.319 **Malignant neoplasm of lower-inner quadrant of unspecified female breast** ♀

AXILLARY TAIL
UPPER-INNER
UPPER-OUTER
Nipple and areola
Central portion
LOWER-OUTER
LOWER-INNER

Figure 2-12 Female breast quadrants and axillary tail.

N Newborn Age: 0   **P** Pediatric Age: 0–17   **M** Maternity DX: 9–64   **A** Adult Age: 15–124   ♀ Females Only   ♂ Males Only

Complication\Comorbidity   Major C\C   (Ex:) CC/MCC Exclusions   Hospital-Acquired Condition   Hierarchical Condition Category

● C50.32   Malignant neoplasm of lower-inner quadrant of breast, male

     C50.321   Malignant neoplasm of lower-inner quadrant of right male breast ♂ 🔬

     C50.322   Malignant neoplasm of lower-inner quadrant of left male breast ♂ 🔬

     C50.329   Malignant neoplasm of lower-inner quadrant of unspecified male breast ♂ 🔬

● C50.4   Malignant neoplasm of upper-outer quadrant of breast

   ● C50.41   Malignant neoplasm of upper-outer quadrant of breast, female

     C50.411   Malignant neoplasm of upper-outer quadrant of right female breast ♀ 🔬

     C50.412   Malignant neoplasm of upper-outer quadrant of left female breast ♀ 🔬

     C50.419   Malignant neoplasm of upper-outer quadrant of unspecified female breast ♀ 🔬

   ● C50.42   Malignant neoplasm of upper-outer quadrant of breast, male

     C50.421   Malignant neoplasm of upper-outer quadrant of right male breast ♂ 🔬

     C50.422   Malignant neoplasm of upper-outer quadrant of left male breast ♂ 🔬

     C50.429   Malignant neoplasm of upper-outer quadrant of unspecified male breast ♂ 🔬

● C50.5   Malignant neoplasm of lower-outer quadrant of breast

   ● C50.51   Malignant neoplasm of lower-outer quadrant of breast, female

     C50.511   Malignant neoplasm of lower-outer quadrant of right female breast ♀ 🔬

     C50.512   Malignant neoplasm of lower-outer quadrant of left female breast ♀ 🔬

     C50.519   Malignant neoplasm of lower-outer quadrant of unspecified female breast ♀ 🔬

   ● C50.52   Malignant neoplasm of lower-outer quadrant of breast, male

     C50.521   Malignant neoplasm of lower-outer quadrant of right male breast ♂ 🔬

     C50.522   Malignant neoplasm of lower-outer quadrant of left male breast ♂ 🔬

     C50.529   Malignant neoplasm of lower-outer quadrant of unspecified male breast ♂ 🔬

● C50.6   Malignant neoplasm of axillary tail of breast

   ● C50.61   Malignant neoplasm of axillary tail of breast, female

     C50.611   Malignant neoplasm of axillary tail of right female breast ♀ 🔬

     C50.612   Malignant neoplasm of axillary tail of left female breast ♀ 🔬

     C50.619   Malignant neoplasm of axillary tail of unspecified female breast ♀ 🔬

   ● C50.62   Malignant neoplasm of axillary tail of breast, male

     C50.621   Malignant neoplasm of axillary tail of right male breast ♂ 🔬

     C50.622   Malignant neoplasm of axillary tail of left male breast ♂ 🔬

     C50.629   Malignant neoplasm of axillary tail of unspecified male breast ♂ 🔬

● C50.8   Malignant neoplasm of overlapping sites of breast

   ● C50.81   Malignant neoplasm of overlapping sites of breast, female

     C50.811   Malignant neoplasm of overlapping sites of right female breast ♀ 🔬

     C50.812   Malignant neoplasm of overlapping sites of left female breast ♀ 🔬

     C50.819   Malignant neoplasm of overlapping sites of unspecified female breast ♀ 🔬

● C50.82   Malignant neoplasm of overlapping sites of breast, male

     C50.821   Malignant neoplasm of overlapping sites of right male breast ♂ 🔬

     C50.822   Malignant neoplasm of overlapping sites of left male breast ♂ 🔬

     C50.829   Malignant neoplasm of overlapping sites of unspecified male breast ♂ 🔬

● C50.9   Malignant neoplasm of breast of unspecified site

   ● C50.91   Malignant neoplasm of breast of unspecified site, female

     C50.911   Malignant neoplasm of unspecified site of right female breast ♀ 🔬

     C50.912   Malignant neoplasm of unspecified site of left female breast ♀ 🔬

     C50.919   Malignant neoplasm of unspecified site of unspecified female breast ♀ 🔬

   ● C50.92   Malignant neoplasm of breast of unspecified site, male

     C50.921   Malignant neoplasm of unspecified site of right male breast ♂ 🔬

     C50.922   Malignant neoplasm of unspecified site of left male breast ♂ 🔬

     C50.929   Malignant neoplasm of unspecified site of unspecified male breast ♂ 🔬

MALIGNANT NEOPLASMS OF FEMALE GENITAL ORGANS (C51-C58)

Includes   malignant neoplasm of skin of female genital organs

● C51   Malignant neoplasm of vulva

   Excludes1   carcinoma in situ of vulva (D07.1)

   C51.0   Malignant neoplasm of labium majus ♀ 🔬
     Outer folds of skin external female genitalia
     Malignant neoplasm of Bartholin's [greater vestibular] gland

   C51.1   Malignant neoplasm of labium minus ♀ 🔬
     Two inner folds surrounding vulva in female genitalia

   C51.2   Malignant neoplasm of clitoris ♀ 🔬

   C51.8   Malignant neoplasm of overlapping sites of vulva ♀ 🔬

   C51.9   Malignant neoplasm of vulva, unspecified ♀ 🔬
     Malignant neoplasm of external female genitalia NOS
     Malignant neoplasm of pudendum

● C52   Malignant neoplasm of vagina ♀ 🔬

   Excludes1   carcinoma in situ of vagina (D07.2)

● C53   Malignant neoplasm of cervix uteri

   Excludes1   carcinoma in situ of cervix uteri (D06.-)

   C53.0   Malignant neoplasm of endocervix ♀ 🔬
     Inside the cervix

   C53.1   Malignant neoplasm of exocervix ♀ 🔬
     Outside the cervix

   C53.8   Malignant neoplasm of overlapping sites of cervix uteri ♀ 🔬

   C53.9   Malignant neoplasm of cervix uteri, unspecified ♀ 🔬
     Coding Clinic: 2017, Q4, P103

● C54   Malignant neoplasm of corpus uteri

   C54.0   Malignant neoplasm of isthmus uteri ♀ 🔬
     Constricted part of uterus between cervix and body
     Malignant neoplasm of lower uterine segment

   C54.1   Malignant neoplasm of endometrium ♀ 🔬
     Lining of uterus

   C54.2   Malignant neoplasm of myometrium ♀ 🔬
     Middle layer of uterine wall consisting of smooth muscle supporting stromal and vascular tissue

   C54.3   Malignant neoplasm of fundus uteri ♀ 🔬
     Top rounded portion of uterus

   C54.8   Malignant neoplasm of overlapping sites of corpus uteri ♀ 🔬
     Main body of uterus

   C54.9   Malignant neoplasm of corpus uteri, unspecified ♀ 🔬

▶ New   ⇒ Revised   ~~deleted~~ Deleted   Excludes 1   Excludes 2   Includes   Use additional   Code first   Code also   Key words

OGCR Official Guidelines   ● Unacceptable Principal Diagnosis   X Assign placeholder X   ● Use Additional Character(s)   ▶ Manifestation Code   **Coding Clinic**

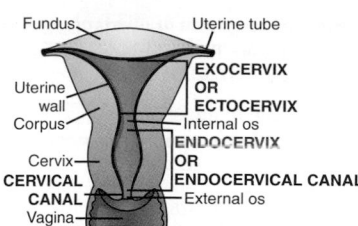

Figure 2-13   Cervix uteri.

C55   Malignant neoplasm of uterus, part unspecified ♀ 🐙

● C56   Malignant neoplasm of ovary
     Use additional code to identify any functional activity
     (Ex) **For category C56 CC Codes:** See PDX Collection 309
     C56.1   Malignant neoplasm of right ovary ♀ 🐙🐙
     C56.2   Malignant neoplasm of left ovary ♀ 🐙🐙
   ▶ C56.3   Malignant neoplasm of bilateral ovaries
     C56.9   Malignant neoplasm of unspecified ovary ♀ 🐙🐙

● C57   Malignant neoplasm of other and unspecified female genital organs
   ● C57.0   Malignant neoplasm of fallopian tube
       Malignant neoplasm of oviduct
       Malignant neoplasm of uterine tube
       C57.00   Malignant neoplasm of unspecified fallopian tube ♀ 🐙
       C57.01   Malignant neoplasm of right fallopian tube ♀ 🐙
       C57.02   Malignant neoplasm of left fallopian tube ♀ 🐙
   ● C57.1   Malignant neoplasm of broad ligament
       C57.10   Malignant neoplasm of unspecified broad ligament ♀ 🐙
       C57.11   Malignant neoplasm of right broad ligament ♀ 🐙
       C57.12   Malignant neoplasm of left broad ligament ♀ 🐙
   ● C57.2   Malignant neoplasm of round ligament
       C57.20   Malignant neoplasm of unspecified round ligament ♀ 🐙
       C57.21   Malignant neoplasm of right round ligament ♀ 🐙
       C57.22   Malignant neoplasm of left round ligament ♀ 🐙
     C57.3   Malignant neoplasm of parametrium ♀ 🐙
       Malignant neoplasm of uterine ligament NOS
     C57.4   Malignant neoplasm of uterine adnexa, unspecified ♀ 🐙
     C57.7   Malignant neoplasm of other specified female genital organs ♀ 🐙
       Malignant neoplasm of wolffian body or duct
     C57.8   Malignant neoplasm of overlapping sites of female genital organs ♀ 🐙
       Primary malignant neoplasm of two or more contiguous sites of the female genital organs whose point of origin cannot be determined
       Primary tubo-ovarian malignant neoplasm whose point of origin cannot be determined
       Primary utero-ovarian malignant neoplasm whose point of origin cannot be determined
     C57.9   Malignant neoplasm of female genital organ, unspecified ♀ 🐙
       Malignant neoplasm of female genitourinary tract NOS

C58   Malignant neoplasm of placenta ♀ 🐙   **M**
   Includes   choriocarcinoma NOS
       chorionepithelioma NOS
   Excludes1   chorioadenoma (destruens) (D39.2)
       hydatidiform mole NOS (O01.9)
       invasive hydatidiform mole (D39.2)
       male choriocarcinoma NOS (C62.9-)
       malignant hydatidiform mole (D39.2)

Figure 2-14   Penis and other male genital organs.

MALIGNANT NEOPLASMS OF MALE GENITAL ORGANS (C60-C63)

   Includes   malignant neoplasm of skin of male genital organs

● C60   Malignant neoplasm of penis
     C60.0   Malignant neoplasm of prepuce ♂ 🐙
       Malignant neoplasm of foreskin
     C60.1   Malignant neoplasm of glans penis ♂ 🐙
     C60.2   Malignant neoplasm of body of penis ♂ 🐙
       Malignant neoplasm of corpus cavernosum
     C60.8   Malignant neoplasm of overlapping sites of penis ♂ 🐙
     C60.9   Malignant neoplasm of penis, unspecified ♂ 🐙
       Malignant neoplasm of skin of penis NOS

C61   Malignant neoplasm of prostate ♂ 🐙
     Use additional code to identify:
     hormone sensitivity status (Z19.1-Z19.2)
     rising PSA following treatment for malignant neoplasm of prostate (R97.21)
   Excludes1   malignant neoplasm of seminal vesicle (C63.7)

● C62   Malignant neoplasm of testis
     Use additional code to identify any functional activity.
   ● C62.0   Malignant neoplasm of undescended testis
       Malignant neoplasm of ectopic testis
       Malignant neoplasm of retained testis
       C62.00   Malignant neoplasm of unspecified undescended testis ♂ 🐙
       C62.01   Malignant neoplasm of undescended right testis ♂ 🐙
       C62.02   Malignant neoplasm of undescended left testis ♂ 🐙
   ● C62.1   Malignant neoplasm of descended testis
       Malignant neoplasm of scrotal testis
       C62.10   Malignant neoplasm of unspecified descended testis, unspecified side ♂ 🐙
       C62.11   Malignant neoplasm of descended right testis ♂ 🐙
       C62.12   Malignant neoplasm of descended left testis ♂ 🐙
   ● C62.9   Malignant neoplasm of testis, unspecified whether descended or undescended
       C62.90   Malignant neoplasm of unspecified testis, unspecified whether descended or undescended ♂ 🐙
        Malignant neoplasm of testis NOS
       C62.91   Malignant neoplasm of right testis, unspecified whether descended or undescended ♂ 🐙
       C62.92   Malignant neoplasm of left testis, unspecified whether descended or undescended ♂ 🐙

● C63   Malignant neoplasm of other and unspecified male genital organs
   ● C63.0   Malignant neoplasm of epididymis
       C63.00   Malignant neoplasm of unspecified epididymis ♂ 🐙
       C63.01   Malignant neoplasm of right epididymis ♂ 🐙
       C63.02   Malignant neoplasm of left epididymis ♂ 🐙

CHAPTER 2 (C00-D49)

N Newborn Age: 0   **P** Pediatric Age: 0–17   **M** Maternity DX: 9–64   **A** Adult Age: 15–124   ♀ Females Only   ♂ Males Only

🐙 Complication\Comorbidity   🐙 Major C\C   (Ex) CC/MCC Exclusions   🐙 Hospital-Acquired Condition   🐙 Hierarchical Condition Category

701

● **C63.1** Malignant neoplasm of spermatic cord
    C63.10 Malignant neoplasm of unspecified spermatic cord ♂
    C63.11 Malignant neoplasm of right spermatic cord ♂
    C63.12 Malignant neoplasm of left spermatic cord ♂
  C63.2 Malignant neoplasm of scrotum ♂
    Malignant neoplasm of skin of scrotum
  C63.7 Malignant neoplasm of other specified male genital organs ♂
    Malignant neoplasm of seminal vesicle
    Malignant neoplasm of tunica vaginalis
  C63.8 Malignant neoplasm of overlapping sites of male genital organs ♂
    Primary malignant neoplasm of two or more contiguous sites of male genital organs whose point of origin cannot be determined
  C63.9 Malignant neoplasm of male genital organ, unspecified ♂
    Malignant neoplasm of male genitourinary tract NOS

MALIGNANT NEOPLASMS OF URINARY TRACT (C64-C68)

● **C64** Malignant neoplasm of kidney, except renal pelvis
    Excludes1 malignant carcinoid tumor of the kidney (C7A.093)
        malignant neoplasm of renal calyces (C65.-)
        malignant neoplasm of renal pelvis (C65.-)
    (Ex) **For category C64 CC Codes:** See PDX Collection 310
  C64.1 Malignant neoplasm of right kidney, except renal pelvis
  C64.2 Malignant neoplasm of left kidney, except renal pelvis
  C64.9 Malignant neoplasm of unspecified kidney, except renal pelvis

● **C65** Malignant neoplasm of renal pelvis
    Includes malignant neoplasm of pelviureteric junction
        malignant neoplasm of renal calyces
    (Ex) **For category C65 CC Codes:** See PDX Collection 310
  C65.1 Malignant neoplasm of right renal pelvis
  C65.2 Malignant neoplasm of left renal pelvis
  C65.9 Malignant neoplasm of unspecified renal pelvis

● **C66** Malignant neoplasm of ureter
    Excludes1 malignant neoplasm of ureteric orifice of bladder (C67.6)
    (Ex) **For category C66 CC Codes:** See PDX Collection 311
  C66.1 Malignant neoplasm of right ureter
  C66.2 Malignant neoplasm of left ureter
  C66.9 Malignant neoplasm of unspecified ureter

● **C67** Malignant neoplasm of bladder
  C67.0 Malignant neoplasm of trigone of bladder
    Triangular area formed by three openings in the floor of urinary bladder
  C67.1 Malignant neoplasm of dome of bladder
    Vaulted roof
  C67.2 Malignant neoplasm of lateral wall of bladder
    Side walls
  C67.3 Malignant neoplasm of anterior wall of bladder
    Front wall
  C67.4 Malignant neoplasm of posterior wall of bladder
    Back wall
  C67.5 Malignant neoplasm of bladder neck
    Joining of bladder and urethra
    Malignant neoplasm of internal urethral orifice
  C67.6 Malignant neoplasm of ureteric orifice
    Opening from bladder to ureters
  C67.7 Malignant neoplasm of urachus
    Embryonic canal that connects the urinary bladder with the structure that forms the umbilical cord (allantois)

  C67.8 Malignant neoplasm of overlapping sites of bladder
  C67.9 Malignant neoplasm of bladder, unspecified
    Coding Clinic: 2017, Q1, P6; 2016, Q1, P19

● **C68** Malignant neoplasm of other and unspecified urinary organs
    Excludes1 malignant neoplasm of female genitourinary tract NOS (C57.9)
        malignant neoplasm of male genitourinary tract NOS (C63.9)
    (Ex) **For category C68 CC codes C68.0-C68.1:** See PDX Collection 312
    For category C68 CC codes C68.8-C68.9: See PDX Collection 313
  C68.0 Malignant neoplasm of urethra
    Excludes1 malignant neoplasm of urethral orifice of bladder (C67.5)
  C68.1 Malignant neoplasm of paraurethral glands
    Group of glands of female urethra drained by paraurethral ducts; AKA Skene glands, female prostate
  C68.8 Malignant neoplasm of overlapping sites of urinary organs
    Primary malignant neoplasm of two or more contiguous sites of urinary organs whose point of origin cannot be determined
  C68.9 Malignant neoplasm of urinary organ, unspecified
    Malignant neoplasm of urinary system NOS

MALIGNANT NEOPLASMS OF EYE, BRAIN AND OTHER PARTS OF CENTRAL NERVOUS SYSTEM (C69-C72)

● **C69** Malignant neoplasm of eye and adnexa
    Excludes1 malignant neoplasm of connective tissue of eyelid (C49.0)
        malignant neoplasm of eyelid (skin) (C43.1-, C44.1-)
        malignant neoplasm of optic nerve (C72.3-)
● **C69.0** Malignant neoplasm of conjunctiva
    C69.00 Malignant neoplasm of unspecified conjunctiva
    C69.01 Malignant neoplasm of right conjunctiva
    C69.02 Malignant neoplasm of left conjunctiva
● **C69.1** Malignant neoplasm of cornea
    C69.10 Malignant neoplasm of unspecified cornea
    C69.11 Malignant neoplasm of right cornea
    C69.12 Malignant neoplasm of left cornea
● **C69.2** Malignant neoplasm of retina
    Excludes1 dark area on retina (D49.81)
        neoplasm of unspecified behavior of retina and choroid (D49.81)
        retinal freckle (D49.81)
    C69.20 Malignant neoplasm of unspecified retina
    C69.21 Malignant neoplasm of right retina
    C69.22 Malignant neoplasm of left retina
● **C69.3** Malignant neoplasm of choroid
    C69.30 Malignant neoplasm of unspecified choroid
    C69.31 Malignant neoplasm of right choroid
    C69.32 Malignant neoplasm of left choroid
● **C69.4** Malignant neoplasm of ciliary body
    C69.40 Malignant neoplasm of unspecified ciliary body
    C69.41 Malignant neoplasm of right ciliary body
    C69.42 Malignant neoplasm of left ciliary body
● **C69.5** Malignant neoplasm of lacrimal gland and duct
    Malignant neoplasm of lacrimal sac
    Malignant neoplasm of nasolacrimal duct
    C69.50 Malignant neoplasm of unspecified lacrimal gland and duct
    C69.51 Malignant neoplasm of right lacrimal gland and duct
    C69.52 Malignant neoplasm of left lacrimal gland and duct

▶ New   ⇒ Revised   ~~deleted~~ Deleted   Excludes 1   Excludes 2   Includes   Use additional   Code first   Code also   Key words
OGCR Official Guidelines   ● Unacceptable Principal Diagnosis   X Assign placeholder X   ● Use Additional Character(s)   ▶ Manifestation Code   Coding Clinic

● **C69.6** **Malignant neoplasm of orbit**
     Malignant neoplasm of connective tissue of orbit
     Malignant neoplasm of extraocular muscle
     Malignant neoplasm of peripheral nerves of orbit
     Malignant neoplasm of retrobulbar tissue
     Malignant neoplasm of retro-ocular tissue
     Excludes1   malignant neoplasm of orbital bone (C41.0)

     C69.60   Malignant neoplasm of unspecified orbit
     C69.61   Malignant neoplasm of right orbit
     C69.62   Malignant neoplasm of left orbit

● **C69.8** **Malignant neoplasm of overlapping sites of eye and adnexa**
     C69.80   Malignant neoplasm of overlapping sites of unspecified eye and adnexa
     C69.81   Malignant neoplasm of overlapping sites of right eye and adnexa
     C69.82   Malignant neoplasm of overlapping sites of left eye and adnexa

● **C69.9** **Malignant neoplasm of unspecified site of eye**
     Malignant neoplasm of eyeball
     C69.90   Malignant neoplasm of unspecified site of unspecified eye
     C69.91   Malignant neoplasm of unspecified site of right eye
     C69.92   Malignant neoplasm of unspecified site of left eye

● **C70** **Malignant neoplasm of meninges**
     C70.0   Malignant neoplasm of cerebral meninges
     Ex: See PDX Collection 314
     C70.1   Malignant neoplasm of spinal meninges
     Ex: See PDX Collection 315
     C70.9   Malignant neoplasm of meninges, unspecified
     Ex: See PDX Collection 314

● **C71** **Malignant neoplasm of brain**
     Excludes1   malignant neoplasm of cranial nerves (C72.2-C72.5)
           retrobulbar malignant neoplasm (C69.6-)
     Ex: For category C71 CC codes: See PDX Collection 316
     C71.0   Malignant neoplasm of cerebrum, except lobes and ventricles
     Malignant neoplasm of supratentorial NOS
     C71.1   Malignant neoplasm of frontal lobe
     C71.2   Malignant neoplasm of temporal lobe
     C71.3   Malignant neoplasm of parietal lobe
     C71.4   Malignant neoplasm of occipital lobe
     C71.5   Malignant neoplasm of cerebral ventricle
         Excludes1   malignant neoplasm of fourth cerebral ventricle (C71.7)
     C71.6   Malignant neoplasm of cerebellum
     C71.7   Malignant neoplasm of brain stem
     Malignant neoplasm of fourth cerebral ventricle
     Infratentorial malignant neoplasm NOS
     C71.8   Malignant neoplasm of overlapping sites of brain
     C71.9   Malignant neoplasm of brain, unspecified

● **C72** **Malignant neoplasm of spinal cord, cranial nerves and other parts of central nervous system**
     Excludes1   malignant neoplasm of meninges (C70.-)
           malignant neoplasm of peripheral nerves and autonomic nervous system (C47.-)
     Ex: For category C72 unless otherwise indicated: See PDX Collection 318
     C72.0   Malignant neoplasm of spinal cord
     Ex: See PDX Collection 317
     C72.1   Malignant neoplasm of cauda equina
     Lower end of spinal column
     Ex: See PDX Collection 317
     ● C72.2   Malignant neoplasm of olfactory nerve
     Malignant neoplasm of olfactory bulb
     C72.20   Malignant neoplasm of unspecified olfactory nerve
     C72.21   Malignant neoplasm of right olfactory nerve
     C72.22   Malignant neoplasm of left olfactory nerve

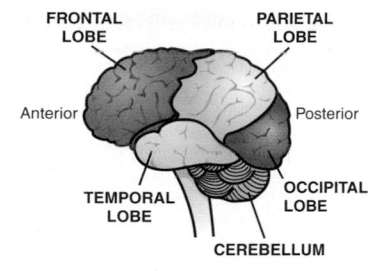

Figure 2-15   The brain.

● **C72.3** **Malignant neoplasm of optic nerve**
     C72.30   Malignant neoplasm of unspecified optic nerve
     C72.31   Malignant neoplasm of right optic nerve
     C72.32   Malignant neoplasm of left optic nerve

● **C72.4** **Malignant neoplasm of acoustic nerve**
     C72.40   Malignant neoplasm of unspecified acoustic nerve
     C72.41   Malignant neoplasm of right acoustic nerve
     C72.42   Malignant neoplasm of left acoustic nerve

● **C72.5** **Malignant neoplasm of other and unspecified cranial nerves**
     C72.50   Malignant neoplasm of unspecified cranial nerve
     Malignant neoplasm of cranial nerve NOS
     C72.59   Malignant neoplasm of other cranial nerves

     C72.9   Malignant neoplasm of central nervous system, unspecified
     Malignant neoplasm of unspecified site of central nervous system
     Malignant neoplasm of nervous system NOS
     Ex: See PDX Collection 319

MALIGNANT NEOPLASMS OF THYROID AND OTHER ENDOCRINE GLANDS (C73-C75)

C73 **Malignant neoplasm of thyroid gland**
     Use additional code to identify any functional activity

● **C74** **Malignant neoplasm of adrenal gland**
     Ex: For category C74 CC codes: See PDX Collection 320
     ● C74.0   Malignant neoplasm of cortex of adrenal gland
     C74.00   Malignant neoplasm of cortex of unspecified adrenal gland
     C74.01   Malignant neoplasm of cortex of right adrenal gland
     C74.02   Malignant neoplasm of cortex of left adrenal gland
     ● C74.1   Malignant neoplasm of medulla of adrenal gland
     Pair of glands situated on top of or above each kidney ("suprarenal")
     C74.10   Malignant neoplasm of medulla of unspecified adrenal gland
     C74.11   Malignant neoplasm of medulla of right adrenal gland
     C74.12   Malignant neoplasm of medulla of left adrenal gland
     ● C74.9   Malignant neoplasm of unspecified part of adrenal gland
     C74.90   Malignant neoplasm of unspecified part of unspecified adrenal gland
     C74.91   Malignant neoplasm of unspecified part of right adrenal gland
     C74.92   Malignant neoplasm of unspecified part of left adrenal gland

N Newborn Age: 0   **P** Pediatric Age: 0–17   **M** Maternity DX: 9–64   **A** Adult Age: 15–124   ♀ Females Only   ♂ Males Only

Complication\Comorbidity   Major C\C   Ex: CC/MCC Exclusions   Hospital-Acquired Condition   Hierarchical Condition Category

703

CHAPTER 2 (C00-D49)

CHAPTER 2 (C00–D49)

● **C75 Malignant neoplasm of other endocrine glands and related structures**

> **Excludes1**   malignant carcinoid tumors (C7A.0-)
> malignant neoplasm of adrenal gland (C74.-)
> malignant neoplasm of endocrine pancreas (C25.4)
> malignant neoplasm of islets of Langerhans (C25.4)
> malignant neoplasm of ovary (C56.-)
> malignant neoplasm of testis (C62.-)
> malignant neoplasm of thymus (C37)
> malignant neoplasm of thyroid gland (C73)
> malignant neuroendocrine tumors (C7A.-)

  C75.0 Malignant neoplasm of parathyroid gland 🔒🔒
> (Ex:) See PDX Collection 321

  C75.1 Malignant neoplasm of pituitary gland 🔒🔒
> (Ex:) See PDX Collection 322

  C75.2 Malignant neoplasm of craniopharyngeal duct 🔒🔒
> (Ex:) See PDX Collection 322

  C75.3 Malignant neoplasm of pineal gland 🔒🔒
> (Ex:) See PDX Collection 323

  C75.4 Malignant neoplasm of carotid body 🔒🔒
> (Ex:) See PDX Collection 324

  C75.5 Malignant neoplasm of aortic body and other paraganglia 🔒🔒
> (Ex:) See PDX Collection 325

  C75.8 Malignant neoplasm with pluriglandular involvement, unspecified 🔒🔒
> (Ex:) See PDX Collection 326

  C75.9 Malignant neoplasm of endocrine gland, unspecified 🔒🔒
> (Ex:) See PDX Collection 326

MALIGNANT NEUROENDOCRINE TUMORS (C7A)

● **C7A Malignant neuroendocrine tumors**
> Code also any associated multiple endocrine neoplasia [MEN] syndromes (E31.2-)
> Use additional code to identify any associated endocrine syndrome, such as:
> carcinoid syndrome (E34.0)
> **Excludes2**   malignant pancreatic islet cell tumors (C25.4)
> Merkel cell carcinoma (C4A.-)

  ● **C7A.0 Malignant carcinoid tumors**

    C7A.00 Malignant carcinoid tumor of unspecified site 🔒🔒
> (Ex:) See PDX Collection 346

    ● **C7A.01 Malignant carcinoid tumors of the small intestine**

      C7A.010 Malignant carcinoid tumor of the duodenum 🔒🔒
> (Ex:) See PDX Collection 347

      C7A.011 Malignant carcinoid tumor of the jejunum 🔒🔒
> (Ex:) See PDX Collection 348

      C7A.012 Malignant carcinoid tumor of the ileum 🔒🔒
> (Ex:) See PDX Collection 349

      C7A.019 Malignant carcinoid tumor of the small intestine, unspecified portion 🔒🔒
> (Ex:) See PDX Collection 350

    ● **C7A.02 Malignant carcinoid tumors of the appendix, large intestine, and rectum**

      C7A.020 Malignant carcinoid tumor of the appendix 🔒🔒
> (Ex:) See PDX Collection 351

      C7A.021 Malignant carcinoid tumor of the cecum 🔒🔒
> (Ex:) See PDX Collection 352

      C7A.022 Malignant carcinoid tumor of the ascending colon 🔒🔒
> (Ex:) See PDX Collection 353

      C7A.023 Malignant carcinoid tumor of the transverse colon 🔒🔒
> (Ex:) See PDX Collection 354

      C7A.024 Malignant carcinoid tumor of the descending colon 🔒🔒
> (Ex:) See PDX Collection 355

      C7A.025 Malignant carcinoid tumor of the sigmoid colon 🔒🔒
> (Ex:) See PDX Collection 356

      C7A.026 Malignant carcinoid tumor of the rectum 🔒🔒
> (Ex:) See PDX Collection 357

      C7A.029 Malignant carcinoid tumor of the large intestine, unspecified portion 🔒🔒
> Malignant carcinoid tumor of the colon NOS
> (Ex:) See PDX Collection 358

    ● **C7A.09 Malignant carcinoid tumors of other sites**
> (Ex:) ▸ For category C7A.09 CC codes unless otherwise indicated: See PDX Collection 361

      C7A.090 Malignant carcinoid tumor of the bronchus and lung 🔒🔒
> (Ex:) See PDX Collection 359

      C7A.091 Malignant carcinoid tumor of the thymus 🔒🔒
> (Ex:) See PDX Collection 360

      C7A.092 Malignant carcinoid tumor of the stomach 🔒🔒

      C7A.093 Malignant carcinoid tumor of the kidney 🔒🔒
> (Ex:) See PDX Collection 362

      C7A.094 Malignant carcinoid tumor of the foregut, unspecified 🔒🔒

      C7A.095 Malignant carcinoid tumor of the midgut, unspecified 🔒🔒

      C7A.096 Malignant carcinoid tumor of the hindgut, unspecified 🔒🔒

      C7A.098 Malignant carcinoid tumors of other sites 🔒🔒
> (Ex:) See PDX Collection 346

  C7A.1 Malignant poorly differentiated neuroendocrine tumors 🔒🔒
> Malignant poorly differentiated neuroendocrine tumor NOS
> Malignant poorly differentiated neuroendocrine carcinoma, any site
> High grade neuroendocrine carcinoma, any site
> (Ex:) See PDX Collection 346

  C7A.8 Other malignant neuroendocrine tumors 🔒🔒
> Secondary neuroendocrine tumors (C7B)
> (Ex:) See PDX Collection 346
> **Coding Clinic: 2019, Q3, P7**

SECONDARY NEUROENDOCRINE TUMORS (C7B)

● **C7B Secondary neuroendocrine tumors**
> Use additional code to identify any functional activity

  ● **C7B.0 Secondary carcinoid tumors**

    C7B.00 Secondary carcinoid tumors, unspecified site 🔒

    C7B.01 Secondary carcinoid tumors of distant lymph nodes 🔒🔒
> (Ex:) See PDX Collection 363

    C7B.02 Secondary carcinoid tumors of liver 🔒🔒
> (Ex:) See PDX Collection 364

    C7B.03 Secondary carcinoid tumors of bone 🔒🔒
> (Ex:) See PDX Collection 365

    C7B.04 Secondary carcinoid tumors of peritoneum 🔒🔒
> Mesentary metastasis of carcinoid tumor
> (Ex:) See PDX Collection 366

    C7B.09 Secondary carcinoid tumors of other sites 🔒🔒
> (Ex:) See PDX Collection 367

  C7B.1 Secondary Merkel cell carcinoma 🔒
> Merkel cell carcinoma nodal presentation
> Merkel cell carcinoma visceral metastatic presentation

  C7B.8 Other secondary neuroendocrine tumors 🔒🔒
> (Ex:) See PDX Collection 367
> **Coding Clinic: 2019, Q3, P7**

▶ New   ⇒ Revised   ~~deleted~~ Deleted   Excludes 1   Excludes 2   Includes   Use additional   Code first   Code also   Key words

OGCR Official Guidelines   ● Unacceptable Principal Diagnosis   X Assign placeholder X   ● Use Additional Character(s)   ▸ Manifestation Code   Coding Clinic

MALIGNANT NEOPLASMS OF ILL-DEFINED, OTHER SECONDARY AND UNSPECIFIED SITES (C76-C80)

● C76   Malignant neoplasm of other and ill-defined sites

     Excludes1   malignant neoplasm of female genitourinary tract NOS (C57.9)
                malignant neoplasm of male genitourinary tract NOS (C63.9)
                malignant neoplasm of lymphoid, hematopoietic and related tissue (C81-C96)
                malignant neoplasm of skin (C44.-)
                malignant neoplasm of unspecified site NOS (C80.1)

     C76.0   Malignant neoplasm of head, face and neck
           Malignant neoplasm of cheek NOS
           Malignant neoplasm of nose NOS

     C76.1   Malignant neoplasm of thorax
           Intrathoracic malignant neoplasm NOS
           Malignant neoplasm of axilla NOS
           Thoracic malignant neoplasm NOS

     C76.2   Malignant neoplasm of abdomen

     C76.3   Malignant neoplasm of pelvis
           Malignant neoplasm of groin NOS
           Malignant neoplasm of sites overlapping systems within the pelvis
           Rectovaginal (septum) malignant neoplasm
             Between rectum and vagina
           Rectovesical (septum) malignant neoplasm
             Between rectum and urinary bladder; AKA vesicorectal

● C76.4   Malignant neoplasm of upper limb

         C76.40   Malignant neoplasm of unspecified upper limb

         C76.41   Malignant neoplasm of right upper limb

         C76.42   Malignant neoplasm of left upper limb

● C76.5   Malignant neoplasm of lower limb

         C76.50   Malignant neoplasm of unspecified lower limb

         C76.51   Malignant neoplasm of right lower limb

         C76.52   Malignant neoplasm of left lower limb

     C76.8   Malignant neoplasm of other specified ill-defined sites
           Malignant neoplasm of overlapping ill-defined sites

● C77   Secondary and unspecified malignant neoplasm of lymph nodes

     Excludes1   malignant neoplasm of lymph nodes, specified as primary (C81-C86, C88, C96.-)
                mesentary metastasis of carcinoid tumor (C7B.04)
                secondary carcinoid tumors of distant lymph nodes (C7B.01)

     (Ex:) **For category C77 CC codes:** See PDX Collection 303

     C77.0   Secondary and unspecified malignant neoplasm of lymph nodes of head, face and neck
           Secondary and unspecified malignant neoplasm of supraclavicular lymph nodes

     C77.1   Secondary and unspecified malignant neoplasm of intrathoracic lymph nodes

     C77.2   Secondary and unspecified malignant neoplasm of intra-abdominal lymph nodes

     C77.3   Secondary and unspecified malignant neoplasm of axilla and upper limb lymph nodes
           Secondary and unspecified malignant neoplasm of pectoral lymph nodes

     C77.4   Secondary and unspecified malignant neoplasm of inguinal and lower limb lymph nodes

     C77.5   Secondary and unspecified malignant neoplasm of intrapelvic lymph nodes

     C77.8   Secondary and unspecified malignant neoplasm of lymph nodes of multiple regions

     C77.9   Secondary and unspecified malignant neoplasm of lymph node, unspecified

---

Item 2–6 The adrenal glands are a pair of glands situated on top of or above each kidney ("suprarenal") and chiefly responsible for regulating the stress response through the synthesis of corticosteroids and catecholamines, including cortisol and adrenaline.

● C78   Secondary malignant neoplasm of respiratory and digestive organs

     Excludes1   secondary carcinoid tumors of liver (C7B.02)
                secondary carcinoid tumors of peritoneum (C7B.04)

     Excludes2   lymph node metastases (C77.0)

● C78.0   Secondary malignant neoplasm of lung
         (Ex:) **For category C78.0 CC Codes:** See PDX Collection 327

         C78.00   Secondary malignant neoplasm of unspecified lung

         C78.01   Secondary malignant neoplasm of right lung

         C78.02   Secondary malignant neoplasm of left lung

     C78.1   Secondary malignant neoplasm of mediastinum
           Thoracic cavity between pleural cavities
           (Ex:) See PDX Collection 328

     C78.2   Secondary malignant neoplasm of pleura
           Serous membrane covering lungs and lining thoracic cavity
           (Ex:) See PDX Collection 329

● C78.3   Secondary malignant neoplasm of other and unspecified respiratory organs
         (Ex:) **For category C78.3 CC Codes:** See PDX Collection 330

         C78.30   Secondary malignant neoplasm of unspecified respiratory organ

         C78.39   Secondary malignant neoplasm of other respiratory organs

     C78.4   Secondary malignant neoplasm of small intestine
           (Ex:) See PDX Collection 331

     C78.5   Secondary malignant neoplasm of large intestine and rectum
           (Ex:) See PDX Collection 332

     C78.6   Secondary malignant neoplasm of retroperitoneum and peritoneum
           (Ex:) See PDX Collection 333
           Coding Clinic: 2017, Q2, P12

     C78.7   Secondary malignant neoplasm of liver and intrahepatic bile duct
           (Ex:) See PDX Collection 334

● C78.8   Secondary malignant neoplasm of other and unspecified digestive organs
         (Ex:) **For category C78.8 CC Codes:** See PDX Collection 335

         C78.80   Secondary malignant neoplasm of unspecified digestive organ

         C78.89   Secondary malignant neoplasm of other digestive organs
           Code also exocrine pancreatic insufficiency (K86.81)

● C79   Secondary malignant neoplasm of other and unspecified sites

     Excludes1   secondary carcinoid tumors (C7B.-)
                secondary neuroendocrine tumors (C7B.-)

● C79.0   Secondary malignant neoplasm of kidney and renal pelvis
         (Ex:) **For category C79.0 CC Codes:** See PDX Collection 336

         C79.00   Secondary malignant neoplasm of unspecified kidney and renal pelvis

         C79.01   Secondary malignant neoplasm of right kidney and renal pelvis

         C79.02   Secondary malignant neoplasm of left kidney and renal pelvis

● C79.1   Secondary malignant neoplasm of bladder and other and unspecified urinary organs
         (Ex:) **For category C79.1 CC Codes:** See PDX Collection 336

         C79.10   Secondary malignant neoplasm of unspecified urinary organs

         C79.11   Secondary malignant neoplasm of bladder
            Excludes2   lymph node metastases (C77.0)

         C79.19   Secondary malignant neoplasm of other urinary organs

---

N Newborn Age: 0   **P** Pediatric Age: 0–17   **M** Maternity DX: 9–64   **A** Adult Age: 15–124   ♀ Females Only   ♂ Males Only

Complication\Comorbidity   Major C\C   (Ex:) CC/MCC Exclusions   Hospital-Acquired Condition   Hierarchical Condition Category

CHAPTER 2 (C00-D49)

C79.2 Secondary malignant neoplasm of skin 🔴🔴
      Excludes1 secondary Merkel cell carcinoma (C7B.1)
      (Ex) See PDX Collection 337

● **C79.3** Secondary malignant neoplasm of brain and cerebral meninges
      C79.31 Secondary malignant neoplasm of brain 🔴🔴
            (Ex) See PDX Collection 338

      C79.32 Secondary malignant neoplasm of cerebral meninges 🔴🔴
            (Ex) See PDX Collection 339
            Coding Clinic: 2020, Q1, P13

● **C79.4** Secondary malignant neoplasm of other and unspecified parts of nervous system
      (Ex) For category C79.4 CC codes: See PDX Collection 339
      C79.40 Secondary malignant neoplasm of unspecified part of nervous system 🔴🔴

      C79.49 Secondary malignant neoplasm of other parts of nervous system 🔴🔴

● **C79.5** Secondary malignant neoplasm of bone and bone marrow
      Excludes1 secondary carcinoid tumors of bone (C7B.03)
      (Ex) For category C79.5 CC codes: See PDX Collection 340
      C79.51 Secondary malignant neoplasm of bone 🔴🔴
      C79.52 Secondary malignant neoplasm of bone marrow 🔴🔴

● **C79.6** Secondary malignant neoplasm of ovary
      (Ex) For category C79.6 CC codes: See PDX Collection 341
      C79.60 Secondary malignant neoplasm of unspecified ovary ♀ 🔴🔴

      C79.61 Secondary malignant neoplasm of right ovary ♀ 🔴🔴

      C79.62 Secondary malignant neoplasm of left ovary ♀ 🔴🔴

  ▶**C79.63** Secondary malignant neoplasm of bilateral ovaries

● **C79.7** Secondary malignant neoplasm of adrenal gland
      (Ex) For category C79.7 CC codes: See PDX Collection 342
      C79.70 Secondary malignant neoplasm of unspecified adrenal gland 🔴🔴

      C79.71 Secondary malignant neoplasm of right adrenal gland 🔴🔴

      C79.72 Secondary malignant neoplasm of left adrenal gland 🔴🔴

● **C79.8** Secondary malignant neoplasm of other specified sites
      C79.81 Secondary malignant neoplasm of breast 🔴🔴
            (Ex) See PDX Collection 343

      C79.82 Secondary malignant neoplasm of genital organs 🔴🔴
            (Ex) See PDX Collection 344

      C79.89 Secondary malignant neoplasm of other specified sites 🔴🔴
            (Ex) See PDX Collection 345
            Coding Clinic: 2017, Q2, P11

C79.9 Secondary malignant neoplasm of unspecified site 🔴🔴
      Metastatic cancer NOS
      Metastatic disease NOS
      Excludes1 carcinomatosis NOS (C80.0)
              generalized cancer NOS (C80.0)
              malignant (primary) neoplasm of unspecified site (C80.1)
      (Ex) See PDX Collection 345

Disseminated malignant neoplasm, unspecified
j. Code C80.0, Disseminated malignant neoplasm, unspecified, is for use only in those cases where the patient has advanced metastatic disease and no known primary or secondary sites are specified. It should not be used in place of assigning codes for the primary site and all known secondary sites.
Malignant neoplasm without specification of site
k. Code C80.1, Malignant (primary) neoplasm, unspecified, equates to Cancer, unspecified. This code should only be used when no determination can be made as to the primary site of a malignancy. This code should rarely be used in the inpatient setting.

● **C80** Malignant neoplasm without specification of site
      Excludes1 malignant carcinoid tumor of unspecified site (C7A.00)
              malignant neoplasm of specified multiple sites- code to each site

      C80.0 Disseminated malignant neoplasm, unspecified 🔴🔴
            Carcinomatosis NOS
            Generalized cancer, unspecified site (primary) (secondary)
            Generalized malignancy, unspecified site (primary) (secondary)
            (Ex) See PDX Collection 345

      C80.1 Malignant (primary) neoplasm, unspecified 🔴
            Cancer NOS
            Cancer unspecified site (primary)
            Carcinoma unspecified site (primary)
            Malignancy unspecified site (primary)
            Excludes1 secondary malignant neoplasm of unspecified site (C79.9)

●   **C80.2** Malignant neoplasm associated with transplanted organ 🔴🔴
            Code first complication of transplanted organ (T86.-)
            Use additional code to identify the specific malignancy
            (Ex) See PDX Collection 345

★ **(See Plate 1 of the Anatomy Illustrations.)**

MALIGNANT NEOPLASMS OF LYMPHOID, HEMATOPOIETIC AND RELATED TISSUE (C81-C96)

      Excludes2 Kaposi's sarcoma of lymph nodes (C46.3)
              secondary and unspecified neoplasm of lymph nodes (C77.-)
              secondary neoplasm of bone marrow (C79.52)
              secondary neoplasm of spleen (C78.89)

● **C81** Hodgkin lymphoma
      Form of malignant lymphoma with four types, nodular sclerosis, mixed cellularity, lymphocyte depleted, and lymphocyte predominant
      Excludes1 personal history of Hodgkin lymphoma (Z85.71)

● **C81.0** Nodular lymphocyte predominant Hodgkin lymphoma
      Least aggressive, least common, typically no symptoms
      Lymphocytic-histiocytic predominance Hodgkin's disease
      C81.00 Nodular lymphocyte predominant Hodgkin lymphoma, unspecified site 🔴🔴
            (Ex) See PDX Collection 368

      C81.01 Nodular lymphocyte predominant Hodgkin lymphoma, lymph nodes of head, face, and neck 🔴🔴
            (Ex) See PDX Collection 369

      C81.02 Nodular lymphocyte predominant Hodgkin lymphoma, intrathoracic lymph nodes 🔴🔴
            (Ex) See PDX Collection 370

      C81.03 Nodular lymphocyte predominant Hodgkin lymphoma, intra-abdominal lymph nodes 🔴🔴
            (Ex) See PDX Collection 371

      C81.04 Nodular lymphocyte predominant Hodgkin lymphoma, lymph nodes of axilla and upper limb 🔴🔴
            (Ex) See PDX Collection 372

C81.05   Nodular lymphocyte predominant Hodgkin lymphoma, lymph nodes of inguinal region and lower limb 🔹🔹
   (Ex:) See PDX Collection 373

C81.06   Nodular lymphocyte predominant Hodgkin lymphoma, intrapelvic lymph nodes 🔹🔹
   (Ex:) See PDX Collection 374

C81.07   Nodular lymphocyte predominant Hodgkin lymphoma, spleen 🔹🔹
   (Ex:) See PDX Collection 375

C81.08   Nodular lymphocyte predominant Hodgkin lymphoma, lymph nodes of multiple sites 🔹🔹
   (Ex:) See PDX Collection 368

C81.09   Nodular lymphocyte predominant Hodgkin lymphoma, extranodal and solid organ sites 🔹🔹
   (Ex:) See PDX Collection 368

● C81.1   Nodular sclerosis Hodgkin lymphoma
   Nodular sclerosis classical Hodgkin lymphoma
   Moderately aggressive; most common in young adults

C81.10   Nodular sclerosis Hodgkin lymphoma, unspecified site 🔹🔹
   (Ex:) See PDX Collection 376

C81.11   Nodular sclerosis Hodgkin lymphoma, lymph nodes of head, face, and neck 🔹🔹
   (Ex:) See PDX Collection 377

C81.12   Nodular sclerosis Hodgkin lymphoma, intrathoracic lymph nodes 🔹🔹
   (Ex:) See PDX Collection 378

C81.13   Nodular sclerosis Hodgkin lymphoma, intra-abdominal lymph nodes 🔹🔹
   (Ex:) See PDX Collection 379

C81.14   Nodular sclerosis Hodgkin lymphoma, lymph nodes of axilla and upper limb 🔹🔹
   (Ex:) See PDX Collection 380

C81.15   Nodular sclerosis Hodgkin lymphoma, lymph nodes of inguinal region and lower limb 🔹🔹
   (Ex:) See PDX Collection 381

C81.16   Nodular sclerosis Hodgkin lymphoma, intrapelvic lymph nodes 🔹🔹
   (Ex:) See PDX Collection 382

C81.17   Nodular sclerosis Hodgkin lymphoma, spleen 🔹🔹
   (Ex:) See PDX Collection 383

C81.18   Nodular sclerosis Hodgkin lymphoma, lymph nodes of multiple sites 🔹🔹
   (Ex:) See PDX Collection 376

C81.19   Nodular sclerosis Hodgkin lymphoma, extranodal and solid organ sites 🔹🔹
   (Ex:) See PDX Collection 376

● C81.2   Mixed cellularity Hodgkin lymphoma
   Mixed cellularity classical Hodgkin lymphoma
   A type of Hodgkin's that is moderately aggressive with mixed cell types

C81.20   Mixed cellularity Hodgkin lymphoma, unspecified site 🔹🔹
   (Ex:) See PDX Collection 384

C81.21   Mixed cellularity Hodgkin lymphoma, lymph nodes of head, face, and neck 🔹🔹
   (Ex:) See PDX Collection 385

C81.22   Mixed cellularity Hodgkin lymphoma, intrathoracic lymph nodes 🔹🔹
   (Ex:) See PDX Collection 386

C81.23   Mixed cellularity Hodgkin lymphoma, intra-abdominal lymph nodes 🔹🔹
   (Ex:) See PDX Collection 387

C81.24   Mixed cellularity Hodgkin lymphoma, lymph nodes of axilla and upper limb 🔹🔹
   (Ex:) See PDX Collection 388

C81.25   Mixed cellularity Hodgkin lymphoma, lymph nodes of inguinal region and lower limb 🔹🔹
   (Ex:) See PDX Collection 389

C81.26   Mixed cellularity Hodgkin lymphoma, intrapelvic lymph nodes 🔹🔹
   (Ex:) See PDX Collection 390

C81.27   Mixed cellularity Hodgkin lymphoma, spleen 🔹🔹
   (Ex:) See PDX Collection 391

C81.28   Mixed cellularity Hodgkin lymphoma, lymph nodes of multiple sites 🔹🔹
   (Ex:) See PDX Collection 384

C81.29   Mixed cellularity Hodgkin lymphoma, extranodal and solid organ sites 🔹🔹
   (Ex:) See PDX Collection 384

● C81.3   Lymphocyte depleted Hodgkin lymphoma
   Lymphocyte depleted classical Hodgkin lymphoma
   Most aggressive type with poor prognosis

C81.30   Lymphocyte depleted Hodgkin lymphoma, unspecified site 🔹🔹
   (Ex:) See PDX Collection 392

C81.31   Lymphocyte depleted Hodgkin lymphoma, lymph nodes of head, face, and neck 🔹🔹
   (Ex:) See PDX Collection 393

C81.32   Lymphocyte depleted Hodgkin lymphoma, intrathoracic lymph nodes 🔹🔹
   (Ex:) See PDX Collection 394

C81.33   Lymphocyte depleted Hodgkin lymphoma, intra-abdominal lymph nodes 🔹🔹
   (Ex:) See PDX Collection 395

C81.34   Lymphocyte depleted Hodgkin lymphoma, lymph nodes of axilla and upper limb 🔹🔹
   (Ex:) See PDX Collection 396

C81.35   Lymphocyte depleted Hodgkin lymphoma, lymph nodes of inguinal region and lower limb 🔹🔹
   (Ex:) See PDX Collection 397

C81.36   Lymphocyte depleted Hodgkin lymphoma, intrapelvic lymph nodes 🔹🔹
   (Ex:) See PDX Collection 398

C81.37   Lymphocyte depleted Hodgkin lymphoma, spleen 🔹🔹
   (Ex:) See PDX Collection 399

C81.38   Lymphocyte depleted Hodgkin lymphoma, lymph nodes of multiple sites 🔹🔹
   (Ex:) See PDX Collection 400

C81.39   Lymphocyte depleted Hodgkin lymphoma, extranodal and solid organ sites 🔹🔹
   (Ex:) See PDX Collection 392

● C81.4   Lymphocyte-rich Hodgkin lymphoma
   Lymphocyte-rich classical Hodgkin lymphoma
   Excludes1 nodular lymphocyte predominant Hodgkin lymphoma (C81.0-)

C81.40   Lymphocyte-rich Hodgkin lymphoma, unspecified site 🔹🔹
   (Ex:) See PDX Collection 368

C81.41   Lymphocyte-rich Hodgkin lymphoma, lymph nodes of head, face, and neck 🔹🔹
   (Ex:) See PDX Collection 369

C81.42   Lymphocyte-rich Hodgkin lymphoma, intrathoracic lymph nodes 🔹🔹
   (Ex:) See PDX Collection 370

C81.43   Lymphocyte-rich Hodgkin lymphoma, intra-abdominal lymph nodes 🔹🔹
   (Ex:) See PDX Collection 371

C81.44   Lymphocyte-rich Hodgkin lymphoma, lymph nodes of axilla and upper limb 🔹🔹
   (Ex:) See PDX Collection 372

C81.45   Lymphocyte-rich Hodgkin lymphoma, lymph nodes of inguinal region and lower limb 🔹🔹
   (Ex:) See PDX Collection 373

C81.46   Lymphocyte-rich Hodgkin lymphoma, intrapelvic lymph nodes 🔹🔹
   (Ex:) See PDX Collection 374

C81.47   Lymphocyte-rich Hodgkin lymphoma, spleen 🔹🔹
   (Ex:) See PDX Collection 375

N Newborn Age: 0 **P** Pediatric Age: 0–17 **M** Maternity DX: 9–64 **A** Adult Age: 15–124 ♀ Females Only ♂ Males Only

🔹 Complication\Comorbidity 🔹 Major C\C (Ex:) CC/MCC Exclusions 🔹 Hospital-Acquired Condition 🔹 Hierarchical Condition Category

707

CHAPTER 2 (C00-D49)

C81.48   Lymphocyte-rich Hodgkin lymphoma, lymph nodes of multiple sites
    (Ex:) See PDX Collection 368

C81.49   Lymphocyte-rich Hodgkin lymphoma, extranodal and solid organ sites
    (Ex:) See PDX Collection 368

● C81.7   Other Hodgkin lymphoma
    Classical Hodgkin lymphoma NOS
    Other classical Hodgkin lymphoma

C81.70   Other Hodgkin lymphoma, unspecified site
    (Ex:) See PDX Collection 401

C81.71   Other Hodgkin lymphoma, lymph nodes of head, face, and neck
    (Ex:) See PDX Collection 402

C81.72   Other Hodgkin lymphoma, intrathoracic lymph nodes
    (Ex:) See PDX Collection 403

C81.73   Other Hodgkin lymphoma, intra-abdominal lymph nodes
    (Ex:) See PDX Collection 404

C81.74   Other Hodgkin lymphoma, lymph nodes of axilla and upper limb
    (Ex:) See PDX Collection 405

C81.75   Other Hodgkin lymphoma, lymph nodes of inguinal region and lower limb
    (Ex:) See PDX Collection 406

C81.76   Other Hodgkin lymphoma, intrapelvic lymph nodes
    (Ex:) See PDX Collection 407

C81.77   Other Hodgkin lymphoma, spleen
    (Ex:) See PDX Collection 408

C81.78   Other Hodgkin lymphoma, lymph nodes of multiple sites
    (Ex:) See PDX Collection 401

C81.79   Other Hodgkin lymphoma, extranodal and solid organ sites
    (Ex:) See PDX Collection 401

● C81.9   Hodgkin lymphoma, unspecified

C81.90   Hodgkin lymphoma, unspecified, unspecified site
    (Ex:) See PDX Collection 409

C81.91   Hodgkin lymphoma, unspecified, lymph nodes of head, face, and neck
    (Ex:) See PDX Collection 410

C81.92   Hodgkin lymphoma, unspecified, intrathoracic lymph nodes
    (Ex:) See PDX Collection 411

C81.93   Hodgkin lymphoma, unspecified, intra-abdominal lymph nodes
    (Ex:) See PDX Collection 412

C81.94   Hodgkin lymphoma, unspecified, lymph nodes of axilla and upper limb
    (Ex:) See PDX Collection 413

C81.95   Hodgkin lymphoma, unspecified, lymph nodes of inguinal region and lower limb
    (Ex:) See PDX Collection 414

C81.96   Hodgkin lymphoma, unspecified, intrapelvic lymph nodes
    (Ex:) See PDX Collection 415

C81.97   Hodgkin lymphoma, unspecified, spleen
    (Ex:) See PDX Collection 416

C81.98   Hodgkin lymphoma, unspecified, lymph nodes of multiple sites
    (Ex:) See PDX Collection 409

C81.99   Hodgkin lymphoma, unspecified, extranodal and solid organ sites
    (Ex:) See PDX Collection 3213

● C82   Follicular lymphoma
    Group of malignant lymphomas

Includes   follicular lymphoma with or without diffuse areas

Excludes1   mature T/NK-cell lymphomas (C84.-)
    personal history of non-Hodgkin lymphoma (Z85.72)

● C82.0   Follicular lymphoma grade I

C82.00   Follicular lymphoma grade I, unspecified site
    (Ex:) See PDX Collection 417

C82.01   Follicular lymphoma grade I, lymph nodes of head, face, and neck
    (Ex:) See PDX Collection 418

C82.02   Follicular lymphoma grade I, intrathoracic lymph nodes
    (Ex:) See PDX Collection 419

C82.03   Follicular lymphoma grade I, intra-abdominal lymph nodes
    (Ex:) See PDX Collection 420

C82.04   Follicular lymphoma grade I, lymph nodes of axilla and upper limb
    (Ex:) See PDX Collection 421

C82.05   Follicular lymphoma grade I, lymph nodes of inguinal region and lower limb
    (Ex:) See PDX Collection 422

C82.06   Follicular lymphoma grade I, intrapelvic lymph nodes
    (Ex:) See PDX Collection 423

C82.07   Follicular lymphoma grade I, spleen
    (Ex:) See PDX Collection 424

C82.08   Follicular lymphoma grade I, lymph nodes of multiple sites
    (Ex:) See PDX Collection 425

C82.09   Follicular lymphoma grade I, extranodal and solid organ sites
    (Ex:) See PDX Collection 417

● C82.1   Follicular lymphoma grade II

C82.10   Follicular lymphoma grade II, unspecified site
    (Ex:) See PDX Collection 417

C82.11   Follicular lymphoma grade II, lymph nodes of head, face, and neck
    (Ex:) See PDX Collection 418

C82.12   Follicular lymphoma grade II, intrathoracic lymph nodes
    (Ex:) See PDX Collection 419

C82.13   Follicular lymphoma grade II, intra-abdominal lymph nodes
    (Ex:) See PDX Collection 420

C82.14   Follicular lymphoma grade II, lymph nodes of axilla and upper limb
    (Ex:) See PDX Collection 421

C82.15   Follicular lymphoma grade II, lymph nodes of inguinal region and lower limb
    (Ex:) See PDX Collection 422

C82.16   Follicular lymphoma grade II, intrapelvic lymph nodes
    (Ex:) See PDX Collection 423

C82.17   Follicular lymphoma grade II, spleen
    (Ex:) See PDX Collection 424

C82.18   Follicular lymphoma grade II, lymph nodes of multiple sites
    (Ex:) See PDX Collection 425

C82.19   Follicular lymphoma grade II, extranodal and solid organ sites
    (Ex:) See PDX Collection 417

▶ New   ⇒ Revised   ~~deleted~~ Deleted   Excludes 1   Excludes 2   Includes   Use additional   Code first   Code also   Key words

OGCR Official Guidelines   ● Unacceptable Principal Diagnosis   X Assign placeholder X   ● Use Additional Character(s)   ▸ Manifestation Code   **Coding Clinic**

● C82.2　Follicular lymphoma grade III, unspecified

　　C82.20　Follicular lymphoma grade III, unspecified, unspecified site 🔹🔹
　　　　　　Ex: See PDX Collection 417

　　C82.21　Follicular lymphoma grade III, unspecified, lymph nodes of head, face, and neck 🔹🔹
　　　　　　Ex: See PDX Collection 418

　　C82.22　Follicular lymphoma grade III, unspecified, intrathoracic lymph nodes 🔹🔹
　　　　　　Ex: See PDX Collection 419

　　C82.23　Follicular lymphoma grade III, unspecified, intra-abdominal lymph nodes 🔹🔹
　　　　　　Ex: See PDX Collection 420

　　C82.24　Follicular lymphoma grade III, unspecified, lymph nodes of axilla and upper limb 🔹🔹
　　　　　　Ex: See PDX Collection 421

　　C82.25　Follicular lymphoma grade III, unspecified, lymph nodes of inguinal region and lower limb 🔹🔹
　　　　　　Ex: See PDX Collection 422

　　C82.26　Follicular lymphoma grade III, unspecified, intrapelvic lymph nodes 🔹🔹
　　　　　　Ex: See PDX Collection 423

　　C82.27　Follicular lymphoma grade III, unspecified, spleen 🔹🔹
　　　　　　Ex: See PDX Collection 424

　　C82.28　Follicular lymphoma grade III, unspecified, lymph nodes of multiple sites 🔹🔹
　　　　　　Ex: See PDX Collection 425

　　C82.29　Follicular lymphoma grade III, unspecified, extranodal and solid organ sites 🔹🔹
　　　　　　Ex: See PDX Collection 417

● C82.3　Follicular lymphoma grade IIIa

　　C82.30　Follicular lymphoma grade IIIa, unspecified site 🔹🔹
　　　　　　Ex: See PDX Collection 417

　　C82.31　Follicular lymphoma grade IIIa, lymph nodes of head, face, and neck 🔹🔹
　　　　　　Ex: See PDX Collection 418

　　C82.32　Follicular lymphoma grade IIIa, intrathoracic lymph nodes 🔹🔹
　　　　　　Ex: See PDX Collection 419

　　C82.33　Follicular lymphoma grade IIIa, intra-abdominal lymph nodes 🔹🔹
　　　　　　Ex: See PDX Collection 420

　　C82.34　Follicular lymphoma grade IIIa, lymph nodes of axilla and upper limb 🔹🔹
　　　　　　Ex: See PDX Collection 421

　　C82.35　Follicular lymphoma grade IIIa, lymph nodes of inguinal region and lower limb 🔹🔹
　　　　　　Ex: See PDX Collection 422

　　C82.36　Follicular lymphoma grade IIIa, intrapelvic lymph nodes 🔹🔹
　　　　　　Ex: See PDX Collection 423

　　C82.37　Follicular lymphoma grade IIIa, spleen 🔹🔹
　　　　　　Ex: See PDX Collection 424

　　C82.38　Follicular lymphoma grade IIIa, lymph nodes of multiple sites 🔹🔹
　　　　　　Ex: See PDX Collection 425

　　C82.39　Follicular lymphoma grade IIIa, extranodal and solid organ sites 🔹🔹
　　　　　　Ex: See PDX Collection 417

● C82.4　Follicular lymphoma grade IIIb

　　C82.40　Follicular lymphoma grade IIIb, unspecified site 🔹🔹
　　　　　　Ex: See PDX Collection 417

　　C82.41　Follicular lymphoma grade IIIb, lymph nodes of head, face, and neck 🔹🔹
　　　　　　Ex: See PDX Collection 418

　　C82.42　Follicular lymphoma grade IIIb, intrathoracic lymph nodes 🔹🔹
　　　　　　Ex: See PDX Collection 419

　　C82.43　Follicular lymphoma grade IIIb, intra-abdominal lymph nodes 🔹🔹
　　　　　　Ex: See PDX Collection 420

　　C82.44　Follicular lymphoma grade IIIb, lymph nodes of axilla and upper limb 🔹🔹
　　　　　　Ex: See PDX Collection 421

　　C82.45　Follicular lymphoma grade IIIb, lymph nodes of inguinal region and lower limb 🔹🔹
　　　　　　Ex: See PDX Collection 422

　　C82.46　Follicular lymphoma grade IIIb, intrapelvic lymph nodes 🔹🔹
　　　　　　Ex: See PDX Collection 423

　　C82.47　Follicular lymphoma grade IIIb, spleen 🔹🔹
　　　　　　Ex: See PDX Collection 424

　　C82.48　Follicular lymphoma grade IIIb, lymph nodes of multiple sites 🔹🔹
　　　　　　Ex: See PDX Collection 425

　　C82.49　Follicular lymphoma grade IIIb, extranodal and solid organ sites 🔹🔹
　　　　　　Ex: See PDX Collection 417

● C82.5　Diffuse follicle center lymphoma

　　C82.50　Diffuse follicle center lymphoma, unspecified site 🔹🔹
　　　　　　Ex: See PDX Collection 426

　　C82.51　Diffuse follicle center lymphoma, lymph nodes of head, face, and neck 🔹🔹
　　　　　　Ex: See PDX Collection 427

　　C82.52　Diffuse follicle center lymphoma, intrathoracic lymph nodes 🔹🔹
　　　　　　Ex: See PDX Collection 428

　　C82.53　Diffuse follicle center lymphoma, intra-abdominal lymph nodes 🔹🔹
　　　　　　Ex: See PDX Collection 429

　　C82.54　Diffuse follicle center lymphoma, lymph nodes of axilla and upper limb 🔹🔹
　　　　　　Ex: See PDX Collection 430

　　C82.55　Diffuse follicle center lymphoma, lymph nodes of inguinal region and lower limb 🔹🔹
　　　　　　Ex: See PDX Collection 431

　　C82.56　Diffuse follicle center lymphoma, intrapelvic lymph nodes 🔹🔹
　　　　　　Ex: See PDX Collection 432

　　C82.57　Diffuse follicle center lymphoma, spleen 🔹🔹
　　　　　　Ex: See PDX Collection 433

　　C82.58　Diffuse follicle center lymphoma, lymph nodes of multiple sites 🔹🔹
　　　　　　Ex: See PDX Collection 434

　　C82.59　Diffuse follicle center lymphoma, extranodal and solid organ sites 🔹🔹
　　　　　　Ex: See PDX Collection 426

CHAPTER 2 (C00–D49)

N　Newborn Age: 0　　P　Pediatric Age: 0–17　　M　Maternity DX: 9–64　　A　Adult Age: 15–124　　♀　Females Only　　♂　Males Only

🔹 Complication\Comorbidity　　🔹 Major C\C　　Ex: CC/MCC Exclusions　　🔹 Hospital-Acquired Condition　　🔹 Hierarchical Condition Category

709

● **C82.6   Cutaneous follicle center lymphoma**

    C82.60   **Cutaneous follicle center lymphoma, unspecified site**
       (Ex:) See PDX Collection 417

    C82.61   **Cutaneous follicle center lymphoma, lymph nodes of head, face, and neck**
       (Ex:) See PDX Collection 418

    C82.62   **Cutaneous follicle center lymphoma, intrathoracic lymph nodes**
       (Ex:) See PDX Collection 419

    C82.63   **Cutaneous follicle center lymphoma, intra-abdominal lymph nodes**
       (Ex:) See PDX Collection 420

    C82.64   **Cutaneous follicle center lymphoma, lymph nodes of axilla and upper limb**
       (Ex:) See PDX Collection 421

    C82.65   **Cutaneous follicle center lymphoma, lymph nodes of inguinal region and lower limb**
       (Ex:) See PDX Collection 422

    C82.66   **Cutaneous follicle center lymphoma, intrapelvic lymph nodes**
       (Ex:) See PDX Collection 423

    C82.67   **Cutaneous follicle center lymphoma, spleen**
       (Ex:) See PDX Collection 424

    C82.68   **Cutaneous follicle center lymphoma, lymph nodes of multiple sites**
       (Ex:) See PDX Collection 425

    C82.69   **Cutaneous follicle center lymphoma, extranodal and solid organ sites**
       (Ex:) See PDX Collection 417

● **C82.8   Other types of follicular lymphoma**

    C82.80   **Other types of follicular lymphoma, unspecified site**
       (Ex:) See PDX Collection 417

    C82.81   **Other types of follicular lymphoma, lymph nodes of head, face, and neck**
       (Ex:) See PDX Collection 418

    C82.82   **Other types of follicular lymphoma, intrathoracic lymph nodes**
       (Ex:) See PDX Collection 419

    C82.83   **Other types of follicular lymphoma, intra-abdominal lymph nodes**
       (Ex:) See PDX Collection 420

    C82.84   **Other types of follicular lymphoma, lymph nodes of axilla and upper limb**
       (Ex:) See PDX Collection 421

    C82.85   **Other types of follicular lymphoma, lymph nodes of inguinal region and lower limb**
       (Ex:) See PDX Collection 422

    C82.86   **Other types of follicular lymphoma, intrapelvic lymph nodes**
       (Ex:) See PDX Collection 423

    C82.87   **Other types of follicular lymphoma, spleen**
       (Ex:) See PDX Collection 424

    C82.88   **Other types of follicular lymphoma, lymph nodes of multiple sites**
       (Ex:) See PDX Collection 425

    C82.89   **Other types of follicular lymphoma, extranodal and solid organ sites**
       (Ex:) See PDX Collection 417

● **C82.9   Follicular lymphoma, unspecified**

    C82.90   **Follicular lymphoma, unspecified, unspecified site**
       (Ex:) See PDX Collection 417

    C82.91   **Follicular lymphoma, unspecified, lymph nodes of head, face, and neck**
       (Ex:) See PDX Collection 418

    C82.92   **Follicular lymphoma, unspecified, intrathoracic lymph nodes**
       (Ex:) See PDX Collection 419

    C82.93   **Follicular lymphoma, unspecified, intra-abdominal lymph nodes**
       (Ex:) See PDX Collection 420

    C82.94   **Follicular lymphoma, unspecified, lymph nodes of axilla and upper limb**
       (Ex:) See PDX Collection 421

    C82.95   **Follicular lymphoma, unspecified, lymph nodes of inguinal region and lower limb**
       (Ex:) See PDX Collection 422

    C82.96   **Follicular lymphoma, unspecified, intrapelvic lymph nodes**
       (Ex:) See PDX Collection 423

    C82.97   **Follicular lymphoma, unspecified, spleen**
       (Ex:) See PDX Collection 424

    C82.98   **Follicular lymphoma, unspecified, lymph nodes of multiple sites**
       (Ex:) See PDX Collection 425

    C82.99   **Follicular lymphoma, unspecified, extranodal and solid organ sites**
       (Ex:) See PDX Collection 417

● **C83   Non-follicular lymphoma**

    Excludes1   personal history of non-Hodgkin lymphoma (Z85.72)

● **C83.0   Small cell B-cell lymphoma**
       Lymphoplasmacytic lymphoma
       Nodal marginal zone lymphoma
       Non-leukemic variant of B-CLL
       Splenic marginal zone lymphoma

       Excludes1   chronic lymphocytic leukemia (C91.1)
                     mature T/NK-cell lymphomas (C84.-)
                     Waldenström macroglobulinemia (C88.0)

    C83.00   **Small cell B-cell lymphoma, unspecified site**
       (Ex:) See PDX Collection 435

    C83.01   **Small cell B-cell lymphoma, lymph nodes of head, face, and neck**
       (Ex:) See PDX Collection 436

    C83.02   **Small cell B-cell lymphoma, intrathoracic lymph nodes**
       (Ex:) See PDX Collection 437

    C83.03   **Small cell B-cell lymphoma, intra-abdominal lymph nodes**
       (Ex:) See PDX Collection 438

    C83.04   **Small cell B-cell lymphoma, lymph nodes of axilla and upper limb**
       (Ex:) See PDX Collection 439

    C83.05   **Small cell B-cell lymphoma, lymph nodes of inguinal region and lower limb**
       (Ex:) See PDX Collection 440

    C83.06   **Small cell B-cell lymphoma, intrapelvic lymph nodes**
       (Ex:) See PDX Collection 441

    C83.07   **Small cell B-cell lymphoma, spleen**
       (Ex:) See PDX Collection 442

    C83.08   **Small cell B-cell lymphoma, lymph nodes of multiple sites**
       (Ex:) See PDX Collection 435

    C83.09   **Small cell B-cell lymphoma, extranodal and solid organ sites**
       (Ex:) See PDX Collection 435

▶ New   ⇒ Revised   ~~deleted~~ Deleted   Excludes 1   Excludes 2   Includes   Use additional   Code first   Code also   Key words

OGCR Official Guidelines   ● Unacceptable Principal Diagnosis   X Assign placeholder X   ● Use Additional Character(s)   ▶ Manifestation Code   **Coding Clinic**

● **C83.1** **Mantle cell lymphoma**
　　　　Centrocytic lymphoma
　　　　Malignant lymphomatous polyposis

　　C83.10 Mantle cell lymphoma, unspecified site 🔵🔴
　　　　　　(Ex:) See PDX Collection 426

　　C83.11 Mantle cell lymphoma, lymph nodes of head, face, and neck 🔵🔴
　　　　　　(Ex:) See PDX Collection 427

　　C83.12 Mantle cell lymphoma, intrathoracic lymph nodes 🔵🔴
　　　　　　(Ex:) See PDX Collection 428

　　C83.13 Mantle cell lymphoma, intra-abdominal lymph nodes 🔵🔴
　　　　　　(Ex:) See PDX Collection 429

　　C83.14 Mantle cell lymphoma, lymph nodes of axilla and upper limb 🔵🔴
　　　　　　(Ex:) See PDX Collection 430

　　C83.15 Mantle cell lymphoma, lymph nodes of inguinal region and lower limb 🔵🔴
　　　　　　(Ex:) See PDX Collection 431

　　C83.16 Mantle cell lymphoma, intrapelvic lymph nodes 🔵🔴
　　　　　　(Ex:) See PDX Collection 432

　　C83.17 Mantle cell lymphoma, spleen 🔵🔴
　　　　　　(Ex:) See PDX Collection 433

　　C83.18 Mantle cell lymphoma, lymph nodes of multiple sites 🔵🔴
　　　　　　(Ex:) See PDX Collection 434

　　C83.19 Mantle cell lymphoma, extranodal and solid organ sites 🔵🔴
　　　　　　(Ex:) See PDX Collection 426

● **C83.3** **Diffuse large B-cell lymphoma**
　　　　Anaplastic diffuse large B-cell lymphoma
　　　　CD30-positive diffuse large B-cell lymphoma
　　　　Centroblastic diffuse large B-cell lymphoma
　　　　Diffuse large B-cell lymphoma, subtype not specified
　　　　Immunoblastic diffuse large B-cell lymphoma
　　　　Plasmablastic diffuse large B-cell lymphoma
　　　　Diffuse large B-cell lymphoma, subtype not specified
　　　　T-cell rich diffuse large B-cell lymphoma

　　　　Excludes1　mediastinal (thymic) large B-cell lymphoma (C85.2-)
　　　　　　　　　　mature T/NK-cell lymphomas (C84.-)

　　C83.30 Diffuse large B-cell lymphoma, unspecified site 🔵🔴
　　　　　　(Ex:) See PDX Collection 443

　　C83.31 Diffuse large B-cell lymphoma, lymph nodes of head, face, and neck 🔵🔴
　　　　　　(Ex:) See PDX Collection 444

　　C83.32 Diffuse large B-cell lymphoma, intrathoracic lymph nodes 🔵🔴
　　　　　　(Ex:) See PDX Collection 445

　　C83.33 Diffuse large B-cell lymphoma, intra-abdominal lymph nodes 🔵🔴
　　　　　　(Ex:) See PDX Collection 446

　　C83.34 Diffuse large B-cell lymphoma, lymph nodes of axilla and upper limb 🔵🔴
　　　　　　(Ex:) See PDX Collection 447

　　C83.35 Diffuse large B-cell lymphoma, lymph nodes of inguinal region and lower limb 🔵🔴
　　　　　　(Ex:) See PDX Collection 448

　　C83.36 Diffuse large B-cell lymphoma, intrapelvic lymph nodes 🔵🔴
　　　　　　(Ex:) See PDX Collection 449

　　C83.37 Diffuse large B-cell lymphoma, spleen 🔵🔴
　　　　　　(Ex:) See PDX Collection 450

　　C83.38 Diffuse large B-cell lymphoma, lymph nodes of multiple sites 🔵🔴
　　　　　　(Ex:) See PDX Collection 443

　　C83.39 Diffuse large B-cell lymphoma, extranodal and solid organ sites 🔵🔴
　　　　　　(Ex:) See PDX Collection 443

● **C83.5** **Lymphoblastic (diffuse) lymphoma**
　　　　Highly malignant type of non-Hodgkin lymphoma with diffuse infiltration
　　　　B-precursor lymphoma
　　　　Lymphoblastic B-cell lymphoma
　　　　Lymphoblastic lymphoma NOS
　　　　Lymphoblastic T-cell lymphoma
　　　　T-precursor lymphoma

　　C83.50 Lymphoblastic (diffuse) lymphoma, unspecified site 🔵🔴
　　　　　　(Ex:) See PDX Collection 451

　　C83.51 Lymphoblastic (diffuse) lymphoma, lymph nodes of head, face, and neck 🔵🔴
　　　　　　(Ex:) See PDX Collection 452

　　C83.52 Lymphoblastic (diffuse) lymphoma, intrathoracic lymph nodes 🔵🔴
　　　　　　(Ex:) See PDX Collection 453

　　C83.53 Lymphoblastic (diffuse) lymphoma, intra-abdominal lymph nodes 🔵🔴
　　　　　　(Ex:) See PDX Collection 454

　　C83.54 Lymphoblastic (diffuse) lymphoma, lymph nodes of axilla and upper limb 🔵🔴
　　　　　　(Ex:) See PDX Collection 455

　　C83.55 Lymphoblastic (diffuse) lymphoma, lymph nodes of inguinal region and lower limb 🔵🔴
　　　　　　(Ex:) See PDX Collection 456

　　C83.56 Lymphoblastic (diffuse) lymphoma, intrapelvic lymph nodes 🔵🔴
　　　　　　(Ex:) See PDX Collection 457

　　C83.57 Lymphoblastic (diffuse) lymphoma, spleen 🔵🔴
　　　　　　(Ex:) See PDX Collection 458

　　C83.58 Lymphoblastic (diffuse) lymphoma, lymph nodes of multiple sites 🔵🔴
　　　　　　(Ex:) See PDX Collection 451

　　C83.59 Lymphoblastic (diffuse) lymphoma, extranodal and solid organ sites 🔵🔴
　　　　　　(Ex:) See PDX Collection 451

● **C83.7** **Burkitt lymphoma**
　　　　Form of small cell lymphoma
　　　　Atypical Burkitt lymphoma
　　　　Burkitt-like lymphoma

　　　　Excludes1　mature B-cell leukemia Burkitt type (C91.A-)

　　C83.70 Burkitt lymphoma, unspecified site 🔵🔴
　　　　　　(Ex:) See PDX Collection 459

　　C83.71 Burkitt lymphoma, lymph nodes of head, face, and neck 🔵🔴
　　　　　　(Ex:) See PDX Collection 460

　　C83.72 Burkitt lymphoma, intrathoracic lymph nodes 🔵🔴
　　　　　　(Ex:) See PDX Collection 461

　　C83.73 Burkitt lymphoma, intra-abdominal lymph nodes 🔵🔴
　　　　　　(Ex:) See PDX Collection 462

　　C83.74 Burkitt lymphoma, lymph nodes of axilla and upper limb 🔵🔴
　　　　　　(Ex:) See PDX Collection 463

　　C83.75 Burkitt lymphoma, lymph nodes of inguinal region and lower limb 🔵🔴
　　　　　　(Ex:) See PDX Collection 464

　　C83.76 Burkitt lymphoma, intrapelvic lymph nodes 🔵🔴
　　　　　　(Ex:) See PDX Collection 465

　　C83.77 Burkitt lymphoma, spleen 🔵🔴
　　　　　　(Ex:) See PDX Collection 466

　　C83.78 Burkitt lymphoma, lymph nodes of multiple sites 🔵🔴
　　　　　　(Ex:) See PDX Collection 459

　　C83.79 Burkitt lymphoma, extranodal and solid organ sites 🔵🔴
　　　　　　(Ex:) See PDX Collection 459

CHAPTER 2 (C00–D49)

N Newborn Age: 0　　**P** Pediatric Age: 0–17　　**M** Maternity DX: 9–64　　**A** Adult Age: 15–124　　♀ Females Only　　♂ Males Only

🔵 Complication\Comorbidity　　🔴 Major C\C　　(Ex:) CC/MCC Exclusions　　🔵 Hospital-Acquired Condition　　🔴 Hierarchical Condition Category

711

● **C83.8** Other non-follicular lymphoma
Intravascular large B-cell lymphoma
Lymphoid granulomatosis
Primary effusion B-cell lymphoma

Excludes1 mediastinal (thymic) large B-cell
lymphoma (C85.2-)
T-cell rich B-cell lymphoma (C83.3-)

C83.80 Other non-follicular lymphoma, unspecified
site 🔒🔒
(Ex:) See PDX Collection 435

C83.81 Other non-follicular lymphoma, lymph nodes
of head, face, and neck 🔒🔒
(Ex:) See PDX Collection 436

C83.82 Other non-follicular lymphoma, intrathoracic
lymph nodes 🔒🔒
(Ex:) See PDX Collection 437

C83.83 Other non-follicular lymphoma, intra-
abdominal lymph nodes 🔒🔒
(Ex:) See PDX Collection 438

C83.84 Other non-follicular lymphoma, lymph nodes
of axilla and upper limb 🔒🔒
(Ex:) See PDX Collection 439

C83.85 Other non-follicular lymphoma, lymph nodes
of inguinal region and lower limb 🔒🔒
(Ex:) See PDX Collection 440

C83.86 Other non-follicular lymphoma, intrapelvic
lymph nodes 🔒🔒
(Ex:) See PDX Collection 441

C83.87 Other non-follicular lymphoma, spleen 🔒🔒
(Ex:) See PDX Collection 442

C83.88 Other non-follicular lymphoma, lymph nodes
of multiple sites 🔒🔒
(Ex:) See PDX Collection 435

C83.89 Other non-follicular lymphoma, extranodal and
solid organ sites 🔒🔒
(Ex:) See PDX Collection 435

● **C83.9** Non-follicular (diffuse) lymphoma, unspecified

C83.90 Non-follicular (diffuse) lymphoma, unspecified,
unspecified site 🔒🔒
(Ex:) See PDX Collection 435

C83.91 Non-follicular (diffuse) lymphoma, unspecified,
lymph nodes of head, face, and neck 🔒🔒
(Ex:) See PDX Collection 436

C83.92 Non-follicular (diffuse) lymphoma, unspecified,
intrathoracic lymph nodes 🔒🔒
(Ex:) See PDX Collection 437

C83.93 Non-follicular (diffuse) lymphoma, unspecified,
intra-abdominal lymph nodes 🔒🔒
(Ex:) See PDX Collection 438

C83.94 Non-follicular (diffuse) lymphoma, unspecified,
lymph nodes of axilla and upper limb 🔒🔒
(Ex:) See PDX Collection 439

C83.95 Non-follicular (diffuse) lymphoma, unspecified,
lymph nodes of inguinal region and lower
limb 🔒🔒
(Ex:) See PDX Collection 440

C83.96 Non-follicular (diffuse) lymphoma, unspecified,
intrapelvic lymph nodes 🔒🔒
(Ex:) See PDX Collection 441

C83.97 Non-follicular (diffuse) lymphoma, unspecified,
spleen 🔒🔒
(Ex:) See PDX Collection 442

C83.98 Non-follicular (diffuse) lymphoma, unspecified,
lymph nodes of multiple sites 🔒🔒
(Ex:) See PDX Collection 435

C83.99 Non-follicular (diffuse) lymphoma, unspecified,
extranodal and solid organ sites 🔒🔒
(Ex:) See PDX Collection 435

● **C84** Mature T/NK-cell lymphomas

Excludes1 personal history of non-Hodgkin lymphoma
(Z85.72)

● **C84.0** Mycosis fungoides
*Chronic or rapidly progressive form of cutaneous T-cell
lymphoma; AKA granuloma fungoides*

Excludes1 peripheral T-cell lymphoma, not classified
(C84.4-)

C84.00 Mycosis fungoides, unspecified site 🔒🔒
(Ex:) See PDX Collection 467

C84.01 Mycosis fungoides, lymph nodes of head, face,
and neck 🔒🔒
(Ex:) See PDX Collection 468

C84.02 Mycosis fungoides, intrathoracic lymph
nodes 🔒🔒
(Ex:) See PDX Collection 469

C84.03 Mycosis fungoides, intra-abdominal lymph
nodes 🔒🔒
(Ex:) See PDX Collection 470

C84.04 Mycosis fungoides, lymph nodes of axilla and
upper limb 🔒🔒
(Ex:) See PDX Collection 471

C84.05 Mycosis fungoides, lymph nodes of inguinal
region and lower limb 🔒🔒
(Ex:) See PDX Collection 472

C84.06 Mycosis fungoides, intrapelvic lymph
nodes 🔒🔒
(Ex:) See PDX Collection 473

C84.07 Mycosis fungoides, spleen 🔒🔒
(Ex:) See PDX Collection 474

C84.08 Mycosis fungoides, lymph nodes of multiple
sites 🔒🔒
(Ex:) See PDX Collection 475

C84.09 Mycosis fungoides, extranodal and solid organ
sites 🔒🔒
(Ex:) See PDX Collection 467

● **C84.1** Sézary disease
Type of cutaneous lymphoma affecting T-cells

C84.10 Sézary disease, unspecified site 🔒🔒
(Ex:) See PDX Collection 476

C84.11 Sézary disease, lymph nodes of head, face, and
neck 🔒🔒
(Ex:) See PDX Collection 477

C84.12 Sézary disease, intrathoracic lymph nodes 🔒🔒
(Ex:) See PDX Collection 478

C84.13 Sézary disease, intra-abdominal lymph
nodes 🔒🔒
(Ex:) See PDX Collection 479

C84.14 Sézary disease, lymph nodes of axilla and
upper limb 🔒🔒
(Ex:) See PDX Collection 480

C84.15 Sézary disease, lymph nodes of inguinal region
and lower limb 🔒🔒
(Ex:) See PDX Collection 481

C84.16 Sézary disease, intrapelvic lymph nodes 🔒🔒
(Ex:) See PDX Collection 482

C84.17 Sézary disease, spleen 🔒🔒
(Ex:) See PDX Collection 483

C84.18 Sézary disease, lymph nodes of multiple
sites 🔒🔒
(Ex:) See PDX Collection 484

C84.19 Sézary disease, extranodal and solid organ
sites 🔒🔒
(Ex:) See PDX Collection 476

▶ New   ⇒ Revised   ~~deleted~~ Deleted   Excludes 1   Excludes 2   Includes   Use additional   Code first   Code also   Key words
OGCR Official Guidelines   ● Unacceptable Principal Diagnosis   X Assign placeholder X   ● Use Additional Character(s)   ▶ Manifestation Code   **Coding Clinic**

● **C84.4   Peripheral T-cell lymphoma, not classified**
Diverse group of blood carcinomas originating from T-cells, requiring aggressive chemotherapy
Lennert's lymphoma
Lymphoepithelioid lymphoma
Mature T-cell lymphoma, not elsewhere classified

     C84.40   Peripheral T-cell lymphoma, not classified, unspecified site 🔵🔵
         (Ex:) See PDX Collection 426

     C84.41   Peripheral T-cell lymphoma, not classified, lymph nodes of head, face, and neck 🔵🔵
         (Ex:) See PDX Collection 427

     C84.42   Peripheral T-cell lymphoma, not classified, intrathoracic lymph nodes 🔵🔵
         (Ex:) See PDX Collection 428

     C84.43   Peripheral T-cell lymphoma, not classified, intra-abdominal lymph nodes 🔵🔵
         (Ex:) See PDX Collection 429

     C84.44   Peripheral T-cell lymphoma, not classified, lymph nodes of axilla and upper limb 🔵🔵
         (Ex:) See PDX Collection 430

     C84.45   Peripheral T-cell lymphoma, not classified, lymph nodes of inguinal region and lower limb 🔵🔵
         (Ex:) See PDX Collection 431

     C84.46   Peripheral T-cell lymphoma, not classified, intrapelvic lymph nodes 🔵🔵
         (Ex:) See PDX Collection 432

     C84.47   Peripheral T-cell lymphoma, not classified, spleen 🔵🔵
         (Ex:) See PDX Collection 433

     C84.48   Peripheral T-cell lymphoma, not classified, lymph nodes of multiple sites 🔵🔵
         (Ex:) See PDX Collection 434

     C84.49   Peripheral T-cell lymphoma, not classified, extranodal and solid organ sites 🔵🔵
         (Ex:) See PDX Collection 426

● **C84.6   Anaplastic large cell lymphoma, ALK-positive**
Anaplastic large cell lymphoma, CD30-positive

     C84.60   Anaplastic large cell lymphoma, ALK-positive, unspecified site 🔵🔵
         (Ex:) See PDX Collection 426

     C84.61   Anaplastic large cell lymphoma, ALK-positive, lymph nodes of head, face, and neck 🔵🔵
         (Ex:) See PDX Collection 427

     C84.62   Anaplastic large cell lymphoma, ALK-positive, intrathoracic lymph nodes 🔵🔵
         (Ex:) See PDX Collection 428

     C84.63   Anaplastic large cell lymphoma, ALK-positive, intra-abdominal lymph nodes 🔵🔵
         (Ex:) See PDX Collection 429

     C84.64   Anaplastic large cell lymphoma, ALK-positive, lymph nodes of axilla and upper limb 🔵🔵
         (Ex:) See PDX Collection 430

     C84.65   Anaplastic large cell lymphoma, ALK-positive, lymph nodes of inguinal region and lower limb 🔵🔵
         (Ex:) See PDX Collection 431

     C84.66   Anaplastic large cell lymphoma, ALK-positive, intrapelvic lymph nodes 🔵🔵
         (Ex:) See PDX Collection 432

     C84.67   Anaplastic large cell lymphoma, ALK-positive, spleen 🔵🔵
         (Ex:) See PDX Collection 433

     C84.68   Anaplastic large cell lymphoma, ALK-positive, lymph nodes of multiple sites 🔵🔵
         (Ex:) See PDX Collection 434

     C84.69   Anaplastic large cell lymphoma, ALK-positive, extranodal and solid organ sites 🔵🔵
         (Ex:) See PDX Collection 426

Item 2-7   Lymphosarcoma, also known as malignant lymphoma, is a cancer of the lymph system exhibiting abnormal cells encompassing an entire lymph node creating a diffuse pattern without any definite organization. Diffuse pattern lymphoma has a more unfavorable survival outlook than those with a follicular or nodular pattern. Reticulosarcoma is the most common aggressive form of non-Hodgkin lymphoma.

● **C84.7   Anaplastic large cell lymphoma, ALK-negative**
     Excludes1   primary cutaneous CD30-positive T-cell proliferations (C86.6-)

     C84.70   Anaplastic large cell lymphoma, ALK-negative, unspecified site 🔵🔵
         (Ex:) See PDX Collection 426

     C84.71   Anaplastic large cell lymphoma, ALK-negative, lymph nodes of head, face, and neck 🔵🔵
         (Ex:) See PDX Collection 427

     C84.72   Anaplastic large cell lymphoma, ALK-negative, intrathoracic lymph nodes 🔵🔵
         (Ex:) See PDX Collection 428

     C84.73   Anaplastic large cell lymphoma, ALK-negative, intra-abdominal lymph nodes 🔵🔵
         (Ex:) See PDX Collection 429

     C84.74   Anaplastic large cell lymphoma, ALK-negative, lymph nodes of axilla and upper limb 🔵🔵
         (Ex:) See PDX Collection 430

     C84.75   Anaplastic large cell lymphoma, ALK-negative, lymph nodes of inguinal region and lower limb 🔵🔵
         (Ex:) See PDX Collection 431

     C84.76   Anaplastic large cell lymphoma, ALK-negative, intrapelvic lymph nodes 🔵🔵
         (Ex:) See PDX Collection 432

     C84.77   Anaplastic large cell lymphoma, ALK-negative, spleen 🔵🔵
         (Ex:) See PDX Collection 433

     C84.78   Anaplastic large cell lymphoma, ALK-negative, lymph nodes of multiple sites 🔵🔵
         (Ex:) See PDX Collection 434

     C84.79   Anaplastic large cell lymphoma, ALK-negative, extranodal and solid organ sites 🔵🔵
         (Ex:) See PDX Collection 426

   ▶ **C84.7A   Anaplastic large cell lymphoma, ALK-negative, breast**
     ▶ Breast implant associated anaplastic large cell lymphoma (BIA-ALCL)
   ▶ Use additional code to identify:
     ▶ breast implant status (Z98.82)
     ▶ personal history of breast implant removal (Z98.86)

● **C84.A   Cutaneous T-cell lymphoma, unspecified**

     C84.A0   Cutaneous T-cell lymphoma, unspecified, unspecified site 🔵🔵
         (Ex:) See PDX Collection 426

     C84.A1   Cutaneous T-cell lymphoma, unspecified lymph nodes of head, face, and neck 🔵🔵
         (Ex:) See PDX Collection 427

     C84.A2   Cutaneous T-cell lymphoma, unspecified, intrathoracic lymph nodes 🔵🔵
         (Ex:) See PDX Collection 428

     C84.A3   Cutaneous T-cell lymphoma, unspecified, intra-abdominal lymph nodes 🔵🔵
         (Ex:) See PDX Collection 429

     C84.A4   Cutaneous T-cell lymphoma, unspecified, lymph nodes of axilla and upper limb 🔵🔵
         (Ex:) See PDX Collection 430

     C84.A5   Cutaneous T-cell lymphoma, unspecified, lymph nodes of inguinal region and lower limb 🔵🔵
         (Ex:) See PDX Collection 431

     C84.A6   Cutaneous T-cell lymphoma, unspecified, intrapelvic lymph nodes 🔵🔵
         (Ex:) See PDX Collection 432

N Newborn Age: 0   **P** Pediatric Age: 0-17   **M** Maternity DX: 9-64   **A** Adult Age: 15-124   ♀ Females Only   ♂ Males Only
🔵 Complication\Comorbidity   🔵 Major C\C   (Ex:) CC/MCC Exclusions   🔵 Hospital-Acquired Condition   🔵 Hierarchical Condition Category

713

C84.A7 Cutaneous T-cell lymphoma, unspecified, spleen 🔖🔖
 (Ex:) See PDX Collection 433
 ▶ Coding Clinic: 2021, Q2, P7

C84.A8 Cutaneous T-cell lymphoma, unspecified, lymph nodes of multiple sites 🔖🔖
 (Ex:) See PDX Collection 434
 ▶ Coding Clinic: 2021, Q2, P7

C84.A9 Cutaneous T-cell lymphoma, unspecified, extranodal and solid organ sites 🔖🔖
 (Ex:) See PDX Collection 426

● C84.Z Other mature T/NK-cell lymphomas
Note: If T-cell lineage or involvement is mentioned in conjunction with a specific lymphoma, code to the more specific description.
Excludes1 angioimmunoblastic T-cell lymphoma (C86.5)
blastic NK-cell lymphoma (C86.4)
enteropathy-type T-cell lymphoma (C86.2)
extranodal NK-cell lymphoma, nasal type (C86.0)
hepatosplenic T-cell lymphoma (C86.1)
primary cutaneous CD30-positive T-cell proliferations (C86.6)
subcutaneous panniculitis-like T-cell lymphoma (C86.3)
T-cell leukemia (C91.1-)

C84.Z0 Other mature T/NK-cell lymphomas, unspecified site 🔖🔖
 (Ex:) See PDX Collection 426

C84.Z1 Other mature T/NK-cell lymphomas, lymph nodes of head, face, and neck 🔖🔖
 (Ex:) See PDX Collection 427

C84.Z2 Other mature T/NK-cell lymphomas, intrathoracic lymph nodes 🔖🔖
 (Ex:) See PDX Collection 428

C84.Z3 Other mature T/NK-cell lymphomas, intra-abdominal lymph nodes 🔖🔖
 (Ex:) See PDX Collection 429

C84.Z4 Other mature T/NK-cell lymphomas, lymph nodes of axilla and upper limb 🔖🔖
 (Ex:) See PDX Collection 430

C84.Z5 Other mature T/NK-cell lymphomas, lymph nodes of inguinal region and lower limb 🔖🔖
 (Ex:) See PDX Collection 431

C84.Z6 Other mature T/NK-cell lymphomas, intrapelvic lymph nodes 🔖🔖
 (Ex:) See PDX Collection 432

C84.Z7 Other mature T/NK-cell lymphomas, spleen 🔖🔖
 (Ex:) See PDX Collection 433

C84.Z8 Other mature T/NK-cell lymphomas, lymph nodes of multiple sites 🔖🔖
 (Ex:) See PDX Collection 434

C84.Z9 Other mature T/NK-cell lymphomas, extranodal and solid organ sites 🔖🔖
 (Ex:) See PDX Collection 426

● C84.9 Mature T/NK-cell lymphomas, unspecified
NK/T cell lymphoma NOS
Excludes1 mature T-cell lymphoma, not elsewhere classified (C84.4-)

C84.90 Mature T/NK-cell lymphomas, unspecified, unspecified site 🔖🔖
 (Ex:) See PDX Collection 426

C84.91 Mature T/NK-cell lymphomas, unspecified, lymph nodes of head, face, and neck 🔖🔖
 (Ex:) See PDX Collection 427

C84.92 Mature T/NK-cell lymphomas, unspecified, intrathoracic lymph nodes 🔖🔖
 (Ex:) See PDX Collection 428

C84.93 Mature T/NK-cell lymphomas, unspecified, intra-abdominal lymph nodes 🔖🔖
 (Ex:) See PDX Collection 429

C84.94 Mature T/NK-cell lymphomas, unspecified, lymph nodes of axilla and upper limb 🔖🔖
 (Ex:) See PDX Collection 430

C84.95 Mature T/NK-cell lymphomas, unspecified, lymph nodes of inguinal region and lower limb 🔖🔖
 (Ex:) See PDX Collection 431

C84.96 Mature T/NK-cell lymphomas, unspecified, intrapelvic lymph nodes 🔖🔖
 (Ex:) See PDX Collection 432

C84.97 Mature T/NK-cell lymphomas, unspecified, spleen 🔖🔖
 (Ex:) See PDX Collection 433

C84.98 Mature T/NK-cell lymphomas, unspecified, lymph nodes of multiple sites 🔖🔖
 (Ex:) See PDX Collection 434

C84.99 Mature T/NK-cell lymphomas, unspecified, extranodal and solid organ sites 🔖🔖
 (Ex:) See PDX Collection 426

● C85 Other specified and unspecified types of non-Hodgkin lymphoma
Excludes1 other specified types of T/NK-cell lymphoma (C86.-)
personal history of non-Hodgkin lymphoma (Z85.72)

● C85.1 Unspecified B-cell lymphoma
Note: If B-cell lineage or involvement is mentioned in conjunction with a specific lymphoma, code to the more specific description.

C85.10 Unspecified B-cell lymphoma, unspecified site 🔖🔖
 (Ex:) See PDX Collection 426

C85.11 Unspecified B-cell lymphoma, lymph nodes of head, face, and neck 🔖🔖
 (Ex:) See PDX Collection 427

C85.12 Unspecified B-cell lymphoma, intrathoracic lymph nodes 🔖🔖
 (Ex:) See PDX Collection 428

C85.13 Unspecified B-cell lymphoma, intra-abdominal lymph nodes 🔖🔖
 (Ex:) See PDX Collection 429

C85.14 Unspecified B-cell lymphoma, lymph nodes of axilla and upper limb 🔖🔖
 (Ex:) See PDX Collection 430

C85.15 Unspecified B-cell lymphoma, lymph nodes of inguinal region and lower limb 🔖🔖
 (Ex:) See PDX Collection 431

C85.16 Unspecified B-cell lymphoma, intrapelvic lymph nodes 🔖🔖
 (Ex:) See PDX Collection 432

C85.17 Unspecified B-cell lymphoma, spleen 🔖🔖
 (Ex:) See PDX Collection 433

C85.18 Unspecified B-cell lymphoma, lymph nodes of multiple sites 🔖🔖
 (Ex:) See PDX Collection 434

C85.19 Unspecified B-cell lymphoma, extranodal and solid organ sites 🔖🔖
 (Ex:) See PDX Collection 426

● C85.2 Mediastinal (thymic) large B-cell lymphoma

C85.20 Mediastinal (thymic) large B-cell lymphoma, unspecified site 🔖🔖
 (Ex:) See PDX Collection 426

C85.21 Mediastinal (thymic) large B-cell lymphoma, lymph nodes of head, face, and neck 🔖🔖
 (Ex:) See PDX Collection 427

C85.22 Mediastinal (thymic) large B-cell lymphoma, intrathoracic lymph nodes 🔖🔖
 (Ex:) See PDX Collection 428

C85.23 Mediastinal (thymic) large B-cell lymphoma, intra-abdominal lymph nodes 🔖🔖
 (Ex:) See PDX Collection 429

C85.24 Mediastinal (thymic) large B-cell lymphoma, lymph nodes of axilla and upper limb 🔖🔖
 (Ex:) See PDX Collection 430

C85.25 Mediastinal (thymic) large B-cell lymphoma, lymph nodes of inguinal region and lower limb
        (Ex:) See PDX Collection 431

C85.26 Mediastinal (thymic) large B-cell lymphoma, intrapelvic lymph nodes
        (Ex:) See PDX Collection 432

C85.27 Mediastinal (thymic) large B-cell lymphoma, spleen
        (Ex:) See PDX Collection 433

C85.28 Mediastinal (thymic) large B-cell lymphoma, lymph nodes of multiple sites
        (Ex:) See PDX Collection 434

C85.29 Mediastinal (thymic) large B-cell lymphoma, extranodal and solid organ sites
        (Ex:) See PDX Collection 426

● C85.8 Other specified types of non-Hodgkin lymphoma

C85.80 Other specified types of non-Hodgkin lymphoma, unspecified site
        (Ex:) See PDX Collection 426

C85.81 Other specified types of non-Hodgkin lymphoma, lymph nodes of head, face, and neck
        (Ex:) See PDX Collection 427

C85.82 Other specified types of non-Hodgkin lymphoma, intrathoracic lymph nodes
        (Ex:) See PDX Collection 428

C85.83 Other specified types of non-Hodgkin lymphoma, intra-abdominal lymph nodes
        (Ex:) See PDX Collection 429

C85.84 Other specified types of non-Hodgkin lymphoma, lymph nodes of axilla and upper limb
        (Ex:) See PDX Collection 430

C85.85 Other specified types of non-Hodgkin lymphoma, lymph nodes of inguinal region and lower limb
        (Ex:) See PDX Collection 431

C85.86 Other specified types of non-Hodgkin lymphoma, intrapelvic lymph nodes
        (Ex:) See PDX Collection 432

C85.87 Other specified types of non-Hodgkin lymphoma, spleen
        (Ex:) See PDX Collection 433

C85.88 Other specified types of non-Hodgkin lymphoma, lymph nodes of multiple sites
        (Ex:) See PDX Collection 434

C85.89 Other specified types of non-Hodgkin lymphoma, extranodal and solid organ sites
        (Ex:) See PDX Collection 426

● C85.9 Non-Hodgkin lymphoma, unspecified
        Lymphoma NOS
        Malignant lymphoma NOS
        Non-Hodgkin lymphoma NOS

C85.90 Non-Hodgkin lymphoma, unspecified, unspecified site
        (Ex:) See PDX Collection 426

C85.91 Non-Hodgkin lymphoma, unspecified, lymph nodes of head, face, and neck
        (Ex:) See PDX Collection 427

C85.92 Non-Hodgkin lymphoma, unspecified, intrathoracic lymph nodes
        (Ex:) See PDX Collection 428

C85.93 Non-Hodgkin lymphoma, unspecified, intra-abdominal lymph nodes
        (Ex:) See PDX Collection 429

C85.94 Non-Hodgkin lymphoma, unspecified, lymph nodes of axilla and upper limb
        (Ex:) See PDX Collection 430

C85.95 Non-Hodgkin lymphoma, unspecified, lymph nodes of inguinal region and lower limb
        (Ex:) See PDX Collection 431

C85.96 Non-Hodgkin lymphoma, unspecified, intrapelvic lymph nodes
        (Ex:) See PDX Collection 432

C85.97 Non-Hodgkin lymphoma, unspecified, spleen
        (Ex:) See PDX Collection 433

C85.98 Non-Hodgkin lymphoma, unspecified, lymph nodes of multiple sites
        (Ex:) See PDX Collection 434

C85.99 Non-Hodgkin lymphoma, unspecified, extranodal and solid organ sites
        (Ex:) See PDX Collection 426

● C86 Other specified types of T/NK-cell lymphoma
        Excludes1   anaplastic large cell lymphoma, ALK negative (C84.7-)
                    anaplastic large cell lymphoma, ALK positive (C84.6-)
                    mature T/NK-cell lymphomas (C84.-)
                    other specified types of non-Hodgkin lymphoma (C85.8-)

C86.0 Extranodal NK/T-cell lymphoma, nasal type
        (Ex:) See PDX Collection 427

C86.1 Hepatosplenic T-cell lymphoma
        Alpha-beta and gamma delta types
        (Ex:) See PDX Collection 433

C86.2 Enteropathy-type (intestinal) T-cell lymphoma
        Enteropathy associated T-cell lymphoma
        (Ex:) See PDX Collection 429

C86.3 Subcutaneous panniculitis-like T-cell lymphoma
        (Ex:) See PDX Collection 429

C86.4 Blastic NK-cell lymphoma
        Blastic plasmacytoid dendritic cell neoplasm (BPDCN)
        (Ex:) See PDX Collection 426

C86.5 Angioimmunoblastic T-cell lymphoma
        Angioimmunoblastic lymphadenopathy with dysproteinemia (AILD)
        (Ex:) See PDX Collection 435

C86.6 Primary cutaneous CD30-positive T-cell proliferations
        Lymphomatoid papulosis
        Primary cutaneous anaplastic large cell lymphoma
        Primary cutaneous CD30-positive large T-cell lymphoma
        (Ex:) See PDX Collection 435

● C88 Malignant immunoproliferative diseases and certain other B-cell lymphomas
        Diseases involving immune system
        Excludes1   B-cell lymphoma, unspecified (C85.1-)
                    personal history of other malignant neoplasms of lymphoid, hematopoietic and related tissues (Z85.79)

C88.0 Waldenström's macroglobulinemia
        Lymphoplasmacytic lymphoma with IgM-production
        Macroglobulinemia (idiopathic) (primary)
        Excludes1   small cell B cell lymphoma (C83.0)

C88.2 Heavy chain disease
        Franklin disease
        Gamma heavy chain disease
        Mu heavy chain disease
        (Ex:) See PDX Collection 485

C88.3 Immunoproliferative small intestinal disease
        Alpha heavy chain disease
        Mediterranean lymphoma
        (Ex:) See PDX Collection 485

C88.4 Extranodal marginal zone B-cell lymphoma of mucosa-associated lymphoid tissue [MALT-lymphoma]
        Lymphoma of skin-associated lymphoid tissue [SALT-lymphoma]
        Lymphoma of bronchial-associated lymphoid tissue [BALT-lymphoma]
        Excludes1   high malignant (diffuse large B-cell) lymphoma (C83.3-)
        (Ex:) See PDX Collection 426

C88.8 Other malignant immunoproliferative diseases
        (Ex:) See PDX Collection 486

C88.9 Malignant immunoproliferative disease, unspecified
        Immunoproliferative disease NOS
        (Ex:) See PDX Collection 485

CHAPTER 2 (C00-D49)

Item 2–8 **Multiple myeloma** is a cancer of a plasma cell (a type of white blood cell) and is an incurable but treatable disease. Immunoproliferative neoplasm is a term for diseases (mostly cancers) in which the immune system cells proliferate.

● **C90** **Multiple myeloma and malignant plasma cell neoplasms**
    Excludes1   personal history of other malignant neoplasms of lymphoid, hematopoietic and related tissues (Z85.79)
    (Ex:) **For category C90 CC codes:** See PDX Collection 485

  ● **C90.0** **Multiple myeloma**
      Kahler's disease
      Medullary plasmacytoma
      Myelomatosis
      Plasma cell myeloma
      Excludes1   solitary myeloma (C90.3-)
                 solitary plasmacytoma (C90.3-)

      C90.00 **Multiple myeloma not having achieved remission** 🔲🔲
          Multiple myeloma with failed remission
          Multiple myeloma NOS

      C90.01 **Multiple myeloma in remission** 🔲🔲
      C90.02 **Multiple myeloma in relapse** 🔲🔲

  ● **C90.1** **Plasma cell leukemia**
      Rare type of acute leukemia
      Plasmacytic leukemia
      Coding Clinic: 2019, Q2, P30

      C90.10 **Plasma cell leukemia not having achieved remission** 🔲🔲
          Plasma cell leukemia with failed remission
          Plasma cell leukemia NOS
          Coding Clinic: 2019, Q2, P30

      C90.11 **Plasma cell leukemia in remission** 🔲🔲
      C90.12 **Plasma cell leukemia in relapse** 🔲🔲

  ● **C90.2** **Extramedullary plasmacytoma**
      Malignant monoclonal plasma cell tumor growing in soft tissue; AKA plasma cell dyscrasias

      C90.20 **Extramedullary plasmacytoma not having achieved remission** 🔲🔲
          Extramedullary plasmacytoma with failed remission
          Extramedullary plasmacytoma NOS

      C90.21 **Extramedullary plasmacytoma in remission** 🔲🔲
      C90.22 **Extramedullary plasmacytoma in relapse** 🔲🔲

  ● **C90.3** **Solitary plasmacytoma**
      Localized malignant plasma cell tumor NOS
      Plasmacytoma NOS
      Solitary myeloma

      C90.30 **Solitary plasmacytoma not having achieved remission** 🔲🔲
          Solitary plasmacytoma with failed remission
          Solitary plasmacytoma NOS

      C90.31 **Solitary plasmacytoma in remission** 🔲🔲
      C90.32 **Solitary plasmacytoma in relapse** 🔲🔲

● **C91** **Lymphoid leukemia**
    Type of leukemia affecting circulating cells of lymphoid origin
    Excludes1   personal history of leukemia (Z85.6)
    (Ex:) **For category C91 CC codes unless otherwise indicated:** See PDX Collection 485

  ● **C91.0** **Acute lymphoblastic leukemia [ALL]**
      Note: Codes in subcategory C91.0 should only be used for T-cell and B-cell precursor leukemia

      C91.00 **Acute lymphoblastic leukemia not having achieved remission** 🔲🔲
          Acute lymphoblastic leukemia with failed remission
          Acute lymphoblastic leukemia NOS

      C91.01 **Acute lymphoblastic leukemia, in remission** 🔲🔲
      C91.02 **Acute lymphoblastic leukemia, in relapse** 🔲🔲

Item 2–9 Leukemia is a cancer (acute or chronic) of the blood-forming tissues of the bone marrow. Blood cells all start out as stem cells. They mature and become red cells, white cells, or platelets. There are three main types of leukocytes (white cells that fight infection): monocytes, lymphocytes, and granulocytes. **Acute monocytic leukemia** (AML) affects monocytes. **Acute lymphoid leukemia** (ALL) affects lymphocytes, and **acute myeloid leukemia** (AML) affects cells that typically develop into white blood cells (not lymphocytes), though it may develop in other blood cells.

  ● **C91.1** **Chronic lymphocytic leukemia of B-cell type**
      Lymphoplasmacytic leukemia
      Richter syndrome
      Excludes1   lymphoplasmacytic lymphoma (C83.0-)

      C91.10 **Chronic lymphocytic leukemia of B-cell type not having achieved remission** 🔲🔲
          Chronic lymphocytic leukemia of B-cell type with failed remission
          Chronic lymphocytic leukemia of B-cell type NOS

      C91.11 **Chronic lymphocytic leukemia of B-cell type in remission** 🔲🔲
      C91.12 **Chronic lymphocytic leukemia of B-cell type in relapse** 🔲🔲

  ● **C91.3** **Prolymphocytic leukemia of B-cell type**
      Chronic leukemia with symptoms of large number of circulating lymphocytes

      C91.30 **Prolymphocytic leukemia of B-cell type not having achieved remission** 🔲🔲
          Prolymphocytic leukemia of B-cell type with failed remission
          Prolymphocytic leukemia of B-cell type NOS

      C91.31 **Prolymphocytic leukemia of B-cell type, in remission** 🔲🔲
      C91.32 **Prolymphocytic leukemia of B-cell type, in relapse** 🔲🔲

  ● **C91.4** **Hairy cell leukemia**
      Chronic leukemia with splenomegaly and excessive number of abnormal large mononuclear cells covered by hairlike villi
      Leukemic reticuloendotheliosis
      (Ex:) **For category C91.4 CC codes:** See PDX Collection 487

      C91.40 **Hairy cell leukemia not having achieved remission** 🔲🔲
          Hairy cell leukemia with failed remission
          Hairy cell leukemia NOS

      C91.41 **Hairy cell leukemia, in remission** 🔲🔲
      C91.42 **Hairy cell leukemia, in relapse** 🔲🔲

  ● **C91.5** **Adult T-cell lymphoma/leukemia (HTLV-1-associated)**
      Acute variant of adult T-cell lymphoma/leukemia (HTLV-1-associated)
      Chronic variant of adult T-cell lymphoma/leukemia (HTLV-1-associated)
      Lymphomatoid variant of adult T-cell lymphoma/leukemia (HTLV-1-associated)
      Smouldering variant of adult T-cell lymphoma/leukemia (HTLV-1-associated)

      C91.50 **Adult T-cell lymphoma/leukemia (HTLV-1-associated) not having achieved remission** 🔲🔲   A
          Adult T-cell lymphoma/leukemia (HTLV-1-associated) with failed remission
          Adult T-cell lymphoma/leukemia (HTLV-1-associated) NOS

      C91.51 **Adult T-cell lymphoma/leukemia (HTLV-1-associated), in remission** 🔲🔲   A
      C91.52 **Adult T-cell lymphoma/leukemia (HTLV-1-associated), in relapse** 🔲🔲   A

▶ New   ⇒ Revised   ~~deleted~~ Deleted   Excludes 1   Excludes 2   Includes   Use additional   Code first   Code also   Key words
OGCR Official Guidelines   ● Unacceptable Principal Diagnosis   X Assign placeholder X   ● Use Additional Character(s)   ▶ Manifestation Code   Coding Clinic

● **C91.6   Prolymphocytic leukemia of T-cell type**

    C91.60   Prolymphocytic leukemia of T-cell type not having achieved remission 🅒🅡🅒

        Prolymphocytic leukemia of T-cell type with failed remission

        Prolymphocytic leukemia of T-cell type NOS

    C91.61   Prolymphocytic leukemia of T-cell type, in remission 🅒🅡🅒

    C91.62   Prolymphocytic leukemia of T-cell type, in relapse 🅒🅡🅒

● **C91.A   Mature B-cell leukemia Burkitt-type**

    Excludes1   Burkitt lymphoma (C83.7-)

    C91.A0   Mature B-cell leukemia Burkitt-type not having achieved remission 🅒🅡🅒

        Mature B-cell leukemia Burkitt-type with failed remission

        Mature B-cell leukemia Burkitt-type NOS

    C91.A1   Mature B-cell leukemia Burkitt-type, in remission 🅒🅡🅒

    C91.A2   Mature B-cell leukemia Burkitt-type, in relapse 🅒🅡🅒

● **C91.Z   Other lymphoid leukemia**

    T-cell large granular lymphocytic leukemia (associated with rheumatoid arthritis)

    C91.Z0   Other lymphoid leukemia not having achieved remission 🅒🅡🅒

        Other lymphoid leukemia with failed remission

        Other lymphoid leukemia NOS

        Coding Clinic: 2019, Q2, P25

    C91.Z1   Other lymphoid leukemia, in remission 🅒🅡🅒

    C91.Z2   Other lymphoid leukemia, in relapse 🅒🅡🅒

● **C91.9   Lymphoid leukemia, unspecified**

    C91.90   Lymphoid leukemia, unspecified not having achieved remission 🅒🅡🅒

        Lymphoid leukemia with failed remission

        Lymphoid leukemia NOS

    C91.91   Lymphoid leukemia, unspecified, in remission 🅒🅡🅒

    C91.92   Lymphoid leukemia, unspecified, in relapse 🅒🅡🅒

● **C92   Myeloid leukemia**

    Includes   granulocytic leukemia

        myelogenous leukemia

    Excludes1   personal history of leukemia (Z85.6)

    Ⓔⓧ **For category C92 CC codes: See PDX Collection 485**

    Coding Clinic: 2019, Q1, P16

● **C92.0   Acute myeloblastic leukemia**

    Acute myeloblastic leukemia, minimal differentiation

    Acute myeloblastic leukemia (with maturation)

    Acute myeloblastic leukemia 1/ETO

    Acute myeloblastic leukemia M0

    Acute myeloblastic leukemia M1

    Acute myeloblastic leukemia M2

    Acute myeloblastic leukemia with t(8;21)

    Acute myeloblastic leukemia (without a FAB classification) NOS

    Refractory anemia with excess blasts in transformation [RAEB T]

    Excludes1   acute exacerbation of chronic myeloid leukemia (C92.10)

        refractory anemia with excess of blasts not in transformation (D46.2-)

    Coding Clinic: 2018, Q4, P87

    C92.00   Acute myeloblastic leukemia, not having achieved remission 🅒🅡🅒

        Acute myeloblastic leukemia with failed remission

        Acute myeloblastic leukemia NOS

    C92.01   Acute myeloblastic leukemia, in remission 🅒🅡🅒

    C92.02   Acute myeloblastic leukemia, in relapse 🅒🅡🅒

● **C92.1   Chronic myeloid leukemia, BCR/ABL-positive**

    Chronic myelogenous leukemia, Philadelphia chromosome (Ph1) positive

    Chronic myelogenous leukemia, t(9;22) (q34;q11)

    Chronic myelogenous leukemia with crisis of blast cells

    Excludes1   atypical chronic myeloid leukemia BCR/ABL-negative (C92.2-)

        chronic myelomonocytic leukemia (C93.1-)

        chronic myeloproliferative disease (D47.1)

    C92.10   Chronic myeloid leukemia, BCR/ABL-positive, not having achieved remission 🅒🅡🅒

        Chronic myeloid leukemia, BCR/ABL-positive with failed remission

        Chronic myeloid leukemia, BCR/ABL-positive NOS

        Coding Clinic: 2017, Q1, P7

    C92.11   Chronic myeloid leukemia, BCR/ABL-positive, in remission 🅒🅡🅒

    C92.12   Chronic myeloid leukemia, BCR/ABL-positive, in relapse 🅒🅡🅒

● **C92.2   Atypical chronic myeloid leukemia, BCR/ABL-negative**

    C92.20   Atypical chronic myeloid leukemia, BCR/ABL-negative, not having achieved remission 🅒🅡🅒

        Atypical chronic myeloid leukemia, BCR/ABL-negative with failed remission

        Atypical chronic myeloid leukemia, BCR/ABL-negative NOS

    C92.21   Atypical chronic myeloid leukemia, BCR/ABL-negative, in remission 🅒🅡🅒

    C92.22   Atypical chronic myeloid leukemia, BCR/ABL-negative, in relapse 🅒🅡🅒

● **C92.3   Myeloid sarcoma**

    A malignant tumor of immature myeloid cells

    Chloroma

    Granulocytic sarcoma

    C92.30   Myeloid sarcoma, not having achieved remission 🅒🅡🅒

        Myeloid sarcoma with failed remission

        Myeloid sarcoma NOS

    C92.31   Myeloid sarcoma, in remission 🅒🅡🅒

    C92.32   Myeloid sarcoma, in relapse 🅒🅡🅒

● **C92.4   Acute promyelocytic leukemia**

    AML M3

    AML Me with t(15;17) and variants

    C92.40   Acute promyelocytic leukemia, not having achieved remission 🅒🅡🅒

        Acute promyelocytic leukemia with failed remission

        Acute promyelocytic leukemia NOS

    C92.41   Acute promyelocytic leukemia, in remission 🅒🅡🅒

    C92.42   Acute promyelocytic leukemia, in relapse 🅒🅡🅒

● **C92.5   Acute myelomonocytic leukemia**

    AML M4

    AML M4 Eo with inv(16) or t(16;16)

    C92.50   Acute myelomonocytic leukemia, not having achieved remission 🅒🅡🅒

        Acute myelomonocytic leukemia with failed remission

        Acute myelomonocytic leukemia NOS

    C92.51   Acute myelomonocytic leukemia, in remission 🅒🅡🅒

    C92.52   Acute myelomonocytic leukemia, in relapse 🅒🅡🅒

CHAPTER 2 (C00-D49)

N Newborn Age: 0   **P** Pediatric Age: 0–17   **M** Maternity DX: 9–64   **A** Adult Age: 15–124   ♀ Females Only   ♂ Males Only

🅒 Complication\Comorbidity   🅜 Major C\C   Ⓔⓧ CC/MCC Exclusions   🅗 Hospital-Acquired Condition   🅡🅒 Hierarchical Condition Category

717

CHAPTER 2 (C00-D49)

● **C92.6**   **Acute myeloid leukemia with 11q23-abnormality**
    Acute myeloid leukemia with variation of MLL-gene

    C92.60   **Acute myeloid leukemia with 11q23-abnormality not having achieved remission** 🔹🔹
       Acute myeloid leukemia with 11q23-abnormality with failed remission
       Acute myeloid leukemia with 11q23-abnormality NOS

    C92.61   **Acute myeloid leukemia with 11q23-abnormality in remission** 🔹🔹

    C92.62   **Acute myeloid leukemia with 11q23-abnormality in relapse** 🔹🔹

● **C92.A**   **Acute myeloid leukemia with multilineage dysplasia**
    Acute myeloid leukemia with dysplasia of remaining hematopoesis and/or myelodysplastic disease in its history

    C92.A0   **Acute myeloid leukemia with multilineage dysplasia, not having achieved remission** 🔹🔹
       Acute myeloid leukemia with multilineage dysplasia with failed remission
       Acute myeloid leukemia with multilineage dysplasia NOS

    C92.A1   **Acute myeloid leukemia with multilineage dysplasia, in remission** 🔹🔹

    C92.A2   **Acute myeloid leukemia with multilineage dysplasia, in relapse** 🔹🔹

● **C92.Z**   **Other myeloid leukemia**

    C92.Z0   **Other myeloid leukemia not having achieved remission** 🔹🔹
       Myeloid leukemia NEC with failed remission
       Myeloid leukemia NEC

    C92.Z1   **Other myeloid leukemia, in remission** 🔹🔹

    C92.Z2   **Other myeloid leukemia, in relapse** 🔹🔹

● **C92.9**   **Myeloid leukemia, unspecified**

    C92.90   **Myeloid leukemia, unspecified, not having achieved remission** 🔹🔹
       Myeloid leukemia, unspecified with failed remission
       Myeloid leukemia, unspecified NOS

    C92.91   **Myeloid leukemia, unspecified in remission** 🔹🔹

    C92.92   **Myeloid leukemia, unspecified in relapse** 🔹🔹

●● **C93**   **Monocytic leukemia**

    Includes   monocytoid leukemia

    Excludes1   personal history of leukemia (Z85.6)

    Ex: **For category C93 CC codes:** See PDX Collection 485

● **C93.0**   **Acute monoblastic/monocytic leukemia**
    AML M5
    AML M5a
    AML M5b

    C93.00   **Acute monoblastic/monocytic leukemia, not having achieved remission** 🔹🔹
       Acute monoblastic/monocytic leukemia with failed remission
       Acute monoblastic/monocytic leukemia NOS

    C93.01   **Acute monoblastic/monocytic leukemia, in remission** 🔹🔹

    C93.02   **Acute monoblastic/monocytic leukemia, in relapse** 🔹🔹

● **C93.1**   **Chronic myelomonocytic leukemia**
    Chronic monocytic leukemia
    CMML-1
    CMML-2
    CMML with eosinophilia
    Code also, if applicable, eosinophilia (D72.18)

    C93.10   **Chronic myelomonocytic leukemia not having achieved remission** 🔹🔹
       Chronic myelomonocytic leukemia with failed remission
       Chronic myelomonocytic leukemia NOS

    C93.11   **Chronic myelomonocytic leukemia, in remission** 🔹🔹

    C93.12   **Chronic myelomonocytic leukemia, in relapse** 🔹🔹

● **C93.3**   **Juvenile myelomonocytic leukemia**

    C93.30   **Juvenile myelomonocytic leukemia, not having achieved remission** 🔹🔹   P
       Juvenile myelomonocytic leukemia with failed remission
       Juvenile myelomonocytic leukemia NOS

    C93.31   **Juvenile myelomonocytic leukemia, in remission** 🔹🔹   P

    C93.32   **Juvenile myelomonocytic leukemia, in relapse** 🔹🔹   P

● **C93.Z**   **Other monocytic leukemia**

    C93.Z0   **Other monocytic leukemia, not having achieved remission** 🔹🔹
       Other monocytic leukemia NOS

    C93.Z1   **Other monocytic leukemia, in remission** 🔹🔹

    C93.Z2   **Other monocytic leukemia, in relapse** 🔹🔹

● **C93.9**   **Monocytic leukemia, unspecified**

    C93.90   **Monocytic leukemia, unspecified, not having achieved remission** 🔹🔹
       Monocytic leukemia, unspecified with failed remission
       Monocytic leukemia, unspecified NOS

    C93.91   **Monocytic leukemia, unspecified in remission** 🔹🔹

    C93.92   **Monocytic leukemia, unspecified in relapse** 🔹🔹

●● **C94**   **Other leukemias of specified cell type**

    Excludes1   leukemic reticuloendotheliosis (C91.4-)
       myelodysplastic syndromes (D46.-)
       personal history of leukemia (Z85.6)
       plasma cell leukemia (C90.1-)

    Ex: **For category C94 CC codes unless otherwise indicated:** See PDX Collection 485

● **C94.0**   **Acute erythroid leukemia**
    Acute myeloid leukemia M6(a)(b)
    Erythroleukemia

    C94.00   **Acute erythroid leukemia, not having achieved remission** 🔹🔹
       Acute erythroid leukemia with failed remission
       Acute erythroid leukemia NOS

    C94.01   **Acute erythroid leukemia, in remission** 🔹🔹

    C94.02   **Acute erythroid leukemia, in relapse** 🔹🔹

● **C94.2**   **Acute megakaryoblastic leukemia**
    Acute myeloid leukemia M7
    Acute megakaryocytic leukemia

    C94.20   **Acute megakaryoblastic leukemia not having achieved remission** 🔹🔹
       Acute megakaryoblastic leukemia with failed remission
       Acute megakaryoblastic leukemia NOS

    C94.21   **Acute megakaryoblastic leukemia, in remission** 🔹🔹

    C94.22   **Acute megakaryoblastic leukemia, in relapse** 🔹🔹

▶ New   ⟹ Revised   ~~deleted~~ Deleted   Excludes 1   Excludes 2   Includes   Use additional   Code first   Code also   Key words

OGCR Official Guidelines   ● Unacceptable Principal Diagnosis   X Assign placeholder X   ● Use Additional Character(s)   ⟩ Manifestation Code   **Coding Clinic**

● **C94.3 Mast cell leukemia**

  C94.30 Mast cell leukemia not having achieved remission 🔹🔹
    Mast cell leukemia with failed remission
    Mast cell leukemia NOS

  C94.31 Mast cell leukemia, in remission 🔹🔹

  C94.32 Mast cell leukemia, in relapse 🔹🔹

● **C94.4 Acute panmyelosis with myelofibrosis**
  Acute myelofibrosis

  Excludes1 myelofibrosis NOS (D75.81)
    secondary myelofibrosis NOS (D75.81)

  (Ex:) **For category C94.4 CC codes:** See PDX Collection 488

  C94.40 Acute panmyelosis with myelofibrosis not having achieved remission 🔹🔹
    Acute myelofibrosis NOS
    Acute panmyelosis with myelofibrosis with failed remission
    Acute panmyelosis NOS

  C94.41 Acute panmyelosis with myelofibrosis, in remission 🔹🔹

  C94.42 Acute panmyelosis with myelofibrosis, in relapse 🔹🔹

C94.6 Myelodysplastic disease, not classified 🔹🔹
  Myeloproliferative disease, not classified
  (Ex:) See PDX Collection 488

● **C94.8 Other specified leukemias**
  Aggressive NK-cell leukemia
  Acute basophilic leukemia

  C94.80 Other specified leukemias not having achieved remission 🔹🔹
    Other specified leukemia with failed remission
    Other specified leukemias NOS

  C94.81 Other specified leukemias, in remission 🔹🔹

  C94.82 Other specified leukemias, in relapse 🔹🔹

● **C95 Leukemia of unspecified cell type**

  Excludes1 personal history of leukemia (Z85.6)

  (Ex:) **For category C95 CC codes:** See PDX Collection 485

● **C95.0 Acute leukemia of unspecified cell type**
  Acute bilineal leukemia
  Acute mixed lineage leukemia
  Biphenotypic acute leukemia
  Stem cell leukemia of unclear lineage

  Excludes1 acute exacerbation of unspecified chronic leukemia (C95.10)

  C95.00 Acute leukemia of unspecified cell type not having achieved remission 🔹🔹
    Acute leukemia of unspecified cell type with failed remission
    Acute leukemia NOS

  C95.01 Acute leukemia of unspecified cell type, in remission 🔹🔹

  C95.02 Acute leukemia of unspecified cell type, in relapse 🔹🔹

● **C95.1 Chronic leukemia of unspecified cell type**

  C95.10 Chronic leukemia of unspecified cell type not having achieved remission 🔹🔹
    Chronic leukemia of unspecified cell type with failed remission
    Chronic leukemia NOS

  C95.11 Chronic leukemia of unspecified cell type, in remission 🔹🔹

  C95.12 Chronic leukemia of unspecified cell type, in relapse 🔹🔹

● **C95.9 Leukemia, unspecified**

  C95.90 Leukemia, unspecified not having achieved remission 🔹🔹
    Leukemia, unspecified with failed remission
    Leukemia NOS

  C95.91 Leukemia, unspecified, in remission 🔹🔹

  C95.92 Leukemia, unspecified, in relapse 🔹🔹

● **C96 Other and unspecified malignant neoplasms of lymphoid, hematopoietic and related tissue**

  Excludes1 personal history of other malignant neoplasms of lymphoid, hematopoietic and related tissues (Z85.79)

C96.0 Multifocal and multisystemic (disseminated) Langerhans-cell histiocytosis 🔹🔹
  Histiocytosis X, multisystemic
  Letterer-Siwe disease

  Excludes1 adult pulmonary Langerhans cell histiocytosis (J84.82)
    multifocal and unisystemic Langerhans-cell histiocytosis (C96.5)
    unifocal Langerhans-cell histiocytosis (C96.6)

  (Ex:) See PDX Collection 489

● **C96.2 Malignant mast cell neoplasm**

  Excludes1 indolent mastocytosis (D47.02)
    mast cell leukemia (C94.30)
    mastocytosis (congenital) (cutaneous) (Q82.2)

  (Ex:) **For category C96.2 CC codes:** See PDX Collection 490

  C96.20 Malignant mast cell neoplasm, unspecified 🔹🔹

  C96.21 Aggressive systemic mastocytosis 🔹🔹

  C96.22 Mast cell sarcoma 🔹🔹

  C96.29 Other malignant mast cell neoplasm 🔹🔹

C96.4 Sarcoma of dendritic cells (accessory cells) 🔹🔹
  Follicular dendritic cell sarcoma
  Interdigitating dendritic cell sarcoma
  Langerhans cell sarcoma
  (Ex:) See PDX Collection 491

C96.5 Multifocal and unisystemic Langerhans-cell histiocytosis 🔹🔹
  Hand-Schüller-Christian disease
  Histiocytosis X, multifocal

  Excludes1 multifocal and multisystemic (disseminated) Langerhans-cell histiocytosis (C96.0)
    unifocal Langerhans-cell histiocytosis (C96.6)

  (Ex:) See PDX Collection 492

C96.6 Unifocal Langerhans-cell histiocytosis 🔹🔹
  Eosinophilic granuloma
  Histiocytosis X, unifocal
  Histiocytosis X NOS
  Langerhans-cell histiocytosis NOS

  Excludes1 multifocal and multisysemic (disseminated) Langerhans-cell histiocytosis (C96.0)
    multifocal and unisystemic Langerhans-cell histiocytosis (C96.5)

  (Ex:) See PDX Collection 492

C96.A Histiocytic sarcoma 🔹🔹
  Malignant histiocytosis
  (Ex:) See PDX Collection 493

C96.Z Other specified malignant neoplasms of lymphoid, hematopoietic and related tissue 🔹🔹
  (Ex:) See PDX Collection 491

C96.9 Malignant neoplasm of lymphoid, hematopoietic and related tissue, unspecified 🔹🔹
  (Ex:) See PDX Collection 491

CHAPTER 2 (C00-D49)

N Newborn Age: 0   **P** Pediatric Age: 0–17   **M** Maternity DX: 9–64   **A** Adult Age: 15–124   ♀ Females Only   ♂ Males Only
🔹 Complication\Comorbidity   🔹 Major C\C   (Ex:) CC/MCC Exclusions   🔹 Hospital-Acquired Condition   🔹 Hierarchical Condition Category
719

IN SITU NEOPLASMS (D00-D09)

In situ is carcinoma involving cells in localized tissues that has not spread to nearby tissues

Includes   Bowen's disease
erythroplasia
grade III intraepithelial neoplasia
Queyrat's erythroplasia

● **D00   Carcinoma in situ of oral cavity, esophagus and stomach**
Excludes1   melanoma in situ (D03.-)

● **D00.0   Carcinoma in situ of lip, oral cavity and pharynx**
Use additional code to identify:
exposure to environmental tobacco smoke (Z77.22)
exposure to tobacco smoke in the perinatal period (P96.81)
history of tobacco dependence (Z87.891)
occupational exposure to environmental tobacco smoke (Z57.31)
tobacco dependence (F17.-)
tobacco use (Z72.0)
Excludes1   carcinoma in situ of aryepiglottic fold or interarytenoid fold, laryngeal aspect (D02.0)
carcinoma in situ of epiglottis NOS (D02.0)
carcinoma in situ of epiglottis suprahyoid portion (D02.0)
carcinoma in situ of skin of lip (D03.0, D04.0)

D00.00   Carcinoma in situ of oral cavity, unspecified site
D00.01   Carcinoma in situ of labial mucosa and vermilion border
D00.02   Carcinoma in situ of buccal mucosa
D00.03   Carcinoma in situ of gingiva and edentulous alveolar ridge
D00.04   Carcinoma in situ of soft palate
D00.05   Carcinoma in situ of hard palate
D00.06   Carcinoma in situ of floor of mouth
D00.07   Carcinoma in situ of tongue
D00.08   Carcinoma in situ of pharynx
Carcinoma in situ of aryepiglottic fold NOS
Carcinoma in situ of hypopharyngeal aspect of aryepiglottic fold
Carcinoma in situ of marginal zone of aryepiglottic fold

D00.1   Carcinoma in situ of esophagus
D00.2   Carcinoma in situ of stomach

● **D01   Carcinoma in situ of other and unspecified digestive organs**
Excludes1   melanoma in situ (D03.-)

D01.0   Carcinoma in situ of colon
Excludes1   carcinoma in situ of rectosigmoid junction (D01.1)

D01.1   Carcinoma in situ of rectosigmoid junction
D01.2   Carcinoma in situ of rectum
D01.3   Carcinoma in situ of anus and anal canal
Anal intraepithelial neoplasia III [AIN III]
Severe dysplasia of anus
Excludes1   anal intraepithelial neoplasia I and II [AIN I and AIN II] (K62.82)
carcinoma in situ of anal margin (D04.5)
carcinoma in situ of anal skin (D04.5)
carcinoma in situ of perianal skin (D04.5)

● **D01.4   Carcinoma in situ of other and unspecified parts of intestine**
Excludes1   carcinoma in situ of ampulla of Vater (D01.5)

D01.40   Carcinoma in situ of unspecified part of intestine
D01.49   Carcinoma in situ of other parts of intestine

D01.5   Carcinoma in situ of liver, gallbladder and bile ducts
Carcinoma in situ of ampulla of Vater
D01.7   Carcinoma in situ of other specified digestive organs
Carcinoma in situ of pancreas
D01.9   Carcinoma in situ of digestive organ, unspecified

● **D02   Carcinoma in situ of middle ear and respiratory system**
Use additional code to identify:
exposure to environmental tobacco smoke (Z77.22)
exposure to tobacco smoke in the perinatal period (P96.81)
history of tobacco dependence (Z87.891)
occupational exposure to environmental tobacco smoke (Z57.31)
tobacco dependence (F17.-)
tobacco use (Z72.0)
Excludes1   melanoma in situ (D03.-)

D02.0   Carcinoma in situ of larynx
Carcinoma in situ of aryepiglottic fold or interarytenoid fold, laryngeal aspect
Carcinoma in situ of epiglottis (suprahyoid portion)
Excludes1   carcinoma in situ of aryepiglottic fold or interarytenoid fold NOS (D00.08)
carcinoma in situ of hypopharyngeal aspect (D00.08)
carcinoma in situ of marginal zone (D00.08)

D02.1   Carcinoma in situ of trachea
● **D02.2   Carcinoma in situ of bronchus and lung**
D02.20   Carcinoma in situ of unspecified bronchus and lung
D02.21   Carcinoma in situ of right bronchus and lung
D02.22   Carcinoma in situ of left bronchus and lung

D02.3   Carcinoma in situ of other parts of respiratory system
Carcinoma in situ of accessory sinuses
Carcinoma in situ of middle ear
Carcinoma in situ of nasal cavities
Excludes1   carcinoma in situ of ear (external) (skin) (D04.2-)
carcinoma in situ of nose NOS (D09.8)
carcinoma in situ of skin of nose (D04.3)

D02.4   Carcinoma in situ of respiratory system, unspecified

● **D03   Melanoma in situ**
D03.0   Melanoma in situ of lip 🐾
● **D03.1   Melanoma in situ of eyelid, including canthus**
D03.10   Melanoma in situ of unspecified eyelid, including canthus 🐾
● **D03.11   Melanoma in situ of right eyelid, including canthus 🐾**
D03.111   Melanoma in situ of right upper eyelid, including canthus 🐾
D03.112   Melanoma in situ of right lower eyelid, including canthus 🐾
● **D03.12   Melanoma in situ of left eyelid, including canthus 🐾**
D03.121   Melanoma in situ of left upper eyelid, including canthus 🐾
D03.122   Melanoma in situ of left lower eyelid, including canthus 🐾

● **D03.2   Melanoma in situ of ear and external auricular canal**
D03.20   Melanoma in situ of unspecified ear and external auricular canal 🐾
D03.21   Melanoma in situ of right ear and external auricular canal 🐾
D03.22   Melanoma in situ of left ear and external auricular canal 🐾

▶ New   ⟹ Revised   ~~deleted~~ Deleted   Excludes 1   Excludes 2   Includes   Use additional   Code first   Code also   Key words
OGCR Official Guidelines   ● Unacceptable Principal Diagnosis   X Assign placeholder X   ● Use Additional Character(s)   ▶ Manifestation Code   **Coding Clinic**

● **D03.3**   Melanoma in situ of other and unspecified parts of face
     D03.30   Melanoma in situ of unspecified part of face 🐾
     D03.39   Melanoma in situ of other parts of face 🐾
   D03.4   Melanoma in situ of scalp and neck 🐾
● **D03.5**   Melanoma in situ of trunk
     D03.51   Melanoma in situ of anal skin 🐾
          Melanoma in situ of anal margin
          Melanoma in situ of perianal skin
     D03.52   Melanoma in situ of breast (skin) (soft tissue) 🐾
     D03.59   Melanoma in situ of other part of trunk 🐾
● **D03.6**   Melanoma in situ of upper limb, including shoulder
     D03.60   Melanoma in situ of unspecified upper limb, including shoulder 🐾
     D03.61   Melanoma in situ of right upper limb, including shoulder 🐾
     D03.62   Melanoma in situ of left upper limb, including shoulder 🐾
● **D03.7**   Melanoma in situ of lower limb, including hip
     D03.70   Melanoma in situ of unspecified lower limb, including hip 🐾
     D03.71   Melanoma in situ of right lower limb, including hip 🐾
     D03.72   Melanoma in situ of left lower limb, including hip 🐾
   D03.8   Melanoma in situ of other sites 🐾
          Melanoma in situ of scrotum
     Excludes1   carcinoma in situ of scrotum (D07.61)
   D03.9   Melanoma in situ, unspecified 🐾

● **D04**   Carcinoma in situ of skin
   Excludes1   erythroplasia of Queyrat (penis) NOS (D07.4)
          melanoma in situ (D03.-)
   D04.0   Carcinoma in situ of skin of lip
   Excludes2   carcinoma in situ of vermilion border of lip (D00.01)
● **D04.1**   Carcinoma in situ of skin of eyelid, including canthus
     D04.10   Carcinoma in situ of skin of unspecified eyelid, including canthus
     ● **D04.11**   Carcinoma in situ of skin of right eyelid, including canthus
         D04.111   Carcinoma in situ of skin of right upper eyelid, including canthus
         D04.112   Carcinoma in situ of skin of right lower eyelid, including canthus
     ● **D04.12**   Carcinoma in situ of skin of left eyelid, including canthus
         D04.121   Carcinoma in situ of skin of left upper eyelid, including canthus
           ⓔ **For category C16 CC codes:** See PDX Collection 306
         D04.122   Carcinoma in situ of skin of left lower eyelid, including canthus
           ⓔ **For category C16 CC codes:** See PDX Collection 306
● **D04.2**   Carcinoma in situ of skin of ear and external auricular canal
     D04.20   Carcinoma in situ of skin of unspecified ear and external auricular canal
     D04.21   Carcinoma in situ of skin of right ear and external auricular canal
     D04.22   Carcinoma in situ of skin of left ear and external auricular canal
● **D04.3**   Carcinoma in situ of skin of other and unspecified parts of face
     D04.30   Carcinoma in situ of skin of unspecified part of face
     D04.39   Carcinoma in situ of skin of other parts of face
   D04.4   Carcinoma in situ of skin of scalp and neck

● **D04.5**   Carcinoma in situ of skin of trunk
          Carcinoma in situ of anal margin
          Carcinoma in situ of anal skin
          Carcinoma in situ of perianal skin
          Carcinoma in situ of skin of breast
     Excludes1   carcinoma in situ of anus NOS (D01.3)
          carcinoma in situ of scrotum (D07.61)
          carcinoma in situ of skin of genital organs (D07.-)
● **D04.6**   Carcinoma in situ of skin of upper limb, including shoulder
     D04.60   Carcinoma in situ of skin of unspecified upper limb, including shoulder
     D04.61   Carcinoma in situ of skin of right upper limb, including shoulder
     D04.62   Carcinoma in situ of skin of left upper limb, including shoulder
● **D04.7**   Carcinoma in situ of skin of lower limb, including hip
     D04.70   Carcinoma in situ of skin of unspecified lower limb, including hip
     D04.71   Carcinoma in situ of skin of right lower limb, including hip
     D04.72   Carcinoma in situ of skin of left lower limb, including hip
   D04.8   Carcinoma in situ of skin of other sites
   D04.9   Carcinoma in situ of skin, unspecified

● **D05**   Carcinoma in situ of breast
   Excludes1   carcinoma in situ of skin of breast (D04.5)
          melanoma in situ of breast (skin) (D03.5)
          Paget's disease of breast or nipple (C50.-)
● **D05.0**   Lobular carcinoma in situ of breast
     D05.00   Lobular carcinoma in situ of unspecified breast
     D05.01   Lobular carcinoma in situ of right breast
     D05.02   Lobular carcinoma in situ of left breast
● **D05.1**   Intraductal carcinoma in situ of breast
     D05.10   Intraductal carcinoma in situ of unspecified breast
     D05.11   Intraductal carcinoma in situ of right breast
     D05.12   Intraductal carcinoma in situ of left breast
● **D05.8**   Other specified type of carcinoma in situ of breast
     D05.80   Other specified type of carcinoma in situ of unspecified breast
     D05.81   Other specified type of carcinoma in situ of right breast
     D05.82   Other specified type of carcinoma in situ of left breast
● **D05.9**   Unspecified type of carcinoma in situ of breast
     D05.90   Unspecified type of carcinoma in situ of unspecified breast
     D05.91   Unspecified type of carcinoma in situ of right breast
     D05.92   Unspecified type of carcinoma in situ of left breast

● **D06**   Carcinoma in situ of cervix uteri
   Includes   cervical adenocarcinoma in situ
          cervical intraepithelial glandular neoplasia
          cervical intraepithelial neoplasia III [CIN III]
          severe dysplasia of cervix uteri
   Excludes1   cervical intraepithelial neoplasia II [CIN II] (N87.1)
          cytologic evidence of malignancy of cervix without histologic confirmation (R87.614)
          high grade squamous intraepithelial lesion (HGSIL) of cervix (R87.613)
          melanoma in situ of cervix (D03.5)
          moderate cervical dysplasia (N87.1)
   D06.0   Carcinoma in situ of endocervix ♀
   D06.1   Carcinoma in situ of exocervix ♀
   D06.7   Carcinoma in situ of other parts of cervix ♀
   D06.9   Carcinoma in situ of cervix, unspecified ♀

N Newborn Age: 0   **P** Pediatric Age: 0–17   **M** Maternity DX: 9–64   **A** Adult Age: 15–124   ♀ Females Only   ♂ Males Only

🐾 Complication\Comorbidity   🐾 Major C\C   ⓔ CC/MCC Exclusions   🐾 Hospital-Acquired Condition   🐾 Hierarchical Condition Category

721

CHAPTER 2 (C00-D49)

● **D07   Carcinoma in situ of other and unspecified genital organs**
     Excludes1   melanoma in situ of trunk (D03.5)

   D07.0   Carcinoma in situ of endometrium ♀

   D07.1   Carcinoma in situ of vulva ♀
      Severe dysplasia of vulva
      Vulvar intraepithelial neoplasia III [VIN III]
      Excludes1   moderate dysplasia of vulva (N90.1)
                 vulvar intraepithelial neoplasia II [VIN II] (N90.1)

   D07.2   Carcinoma in situ of vagina ♀
      Severe dysplasia of vagina
      Vaginal intraepithelial neoplasia III [VIN III]
      Excludes1   moderate dysplasia of vagina (N89.1)
                 vaginal intraepithelial neoplasia II [VIN II] (N89.1)

● **D07.3   Carcinoma in situ of other and unspecified female genital organs**
     D07.30   Carcinoma in situ of unspecified female genital organs ♀
     D07.39   Carcinoma in situ of other female genital organs ♀

   D07.4   Carcinoma in situ of penis ♂
      Erythroplasia of Queyrat NOS

   D07.5   Carcinoma in situ of prostate ♂
      Prostatic intraepithelial neoplasia III (PIN III)
      Severe dysplasia of prostate
      Excludes1   dysplasia (mild) (moderate) of prostate (N42.3-)
                 prostatic intraepithelial neoplasia II [PIN II] (N42.3-)

● **D07.6   Carcinoma in situ of other and unspecified male genital organs**
     D07.60   Carcinoma in situ of unspecified male genital organs ♂
     D07.61   Carcinoma in situ of scrotum ♂
     D07.69   Carcinoma in situ of other male genital organs ♂

● **D09   Carcinoma in situ of other and unspecified sites**
     Excludes1   melanoma in situ (D03.-)

   D09.0   Carcinoma in situ of bladder

● **D09.1   Carcinoma in situ of other and unspecified urinary organs**
     D09.10   Carcinoma in situ of unspecified urinary organ
     D09.19   Carcinoma in situ of other urinary organs

● **D09.2   Carcinoma in situ of eye**
     Excludes1   carcinoma in situ of skin of eyelid (D04.1-)
     D09.20   Carcinoma in situ of unspecified eye
     D09.21   Carcinoma in situ of right eye
     D09.22   Carcinoma in situ of left eye

   D09.3   Carcinoma in situ of thyroid and other endocrine glands
     Excludes1   carcinoma in situ of endocrine pancreas (D01.7)
                 carcinoma in situ of ovary (D07.39)
                 carcinoma in situ of testis (D07.69)

   D09.8   Carcinoma in situ of other specified sites

   D09.9   Carcinoma in situ, unspecified

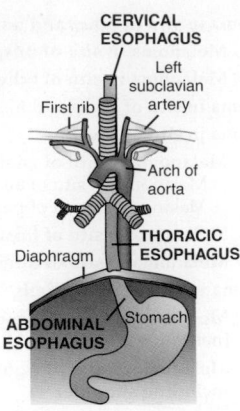

Figure 2-16   The esophagus is the muscular tube that connects the pharynx and the stomach. The 10 inch (25 cm) long esophagus is divided into three parts: **cervical, thoracic,** and **abdominal.**

BENIGN NEOPLASMS, EXCEPT BENIGN NEUROENDOCRINE TUMORS (D10-D36)

● **D10   Benign neoplasm of mouth and pharynx**

   D10.0   Benign neoplasm of lip
      Benign neoplasm of lip (frenulum) (inner aspect) (mucosa) (vermilion border)
      Excludes1   benign neoplasm of skin of lip (D22.0, D23.0)

   D10.1   Benign neoplasm of tongue
      Benign neoplasm of lingual tonsil

   D10.2   Benign neoplasm of floor of mouth

● **D10.3   Benign neoplasm of other and unspecified parts of mouth**
     D10.30   Benign neoplasm of unspecified part of mouth
     D10.39   Benign neoplasm of other parts of mouth
       Benign neoplasm of minor salivary gland NOS
       Excludes1   benign odontogenic neoplasms (D16.4-D16.5)
                 benign neoplasm of mucosa of lip (D10.0)
                 benign neoplasm of nasopharyngeal surface of soft palate (D10.6)

   D10.4   Benign neoplasm of tonsil
      Benign neoplasm of tonsil (faucial) (palatine)
      Excludes1   benign neoplasm of lingual tonsil (D10.1)
                 benign neoplasm of pharyngeal tonsil (D10.6)
                 benign neoplasm of tonsillar fossa (D10.5)
                 benign neoplasm of tonsillar pillars (D10.5)

   D10.5   Benign neoplasm of other parts of oropharynx
      Division of pharynx lying between soft palate and upper edge of epiglottis
      Benign neoplasm of epiglottis, anterior aspect
      Benign neoplasm of tonsillar fossa
      Benign neoplasm of tonsillar pillars
      Benign neoplasm of vallecula
      Excludes1   benign neoplasm of epiglottis NOS (D14.1)
                 benign neoplasm of epiglottis, suprahyoid portion (D14.1)

▶ New   ⇒ Revised   ~~deleted~~ Deleted   Excludes 1   Excludes 2   Includes   Use additional   Code first   Code also   Key words
OGCR Official Guidelines   ● Unacceptable Principal Diagnosis   X Assign placeholder X   ● Use Additional Character(s)   ▶ Manifestation Code   Coding Clinic

D10.6   Benign neoplasm of nasopharynx
        Segment of pharynx that lies above soft palate
        Benign neoplasm of pharyngeal tonsil
        Benign neoplasm of posterior margin of septum and
        choanae

D10.7   Benign neoplasm of hypopharynx
        *Segment of pharynx that lies below upper edge of epiglottis
        and opens into larynx and esophagus*

D10.9   Benign neoplasm of pharynx, unspecified

● D11   Benign neoplasm of major salivary glands
        Excludes1   benign neoplasms of specified minor salivary
                        glands which are classified according to their
                        anatomical location
                        benign neoplasms of minor salivary glands NOS
                        (D10.39)

D11.0   Benign neoplasm of parotid gland

D11.7   Benign neoplasm of other major salivary glands
        Benign neoplasm of sublingual salivary gland
        Benign neoplasm of submandibular salivary gland

D11.9   Benign neoplasm of major salivary gland, unspecified

● D12   Benign neoplasm of colon, rectum, anus and anal canal
        Excludes1   benign carcinoid tumors of the large intestine,
                        and rectum (D3A.02-)
                        polyp of colon NOS (K63.5)
        Coding Clinic: 2017, Q1, P15; 2015, Q2, P14

D12.0   Benign neoplasm of cecum
        Benign neoplasm of ileocecal valve

D12.1   Benign neoplasm of appendix
        Excludes1   benign carcinoid tumor of the appendix
                        (D3A.020)

D12.2   Benign neoplasm of ascending colon
        Coding Clinic: 2018, Q2, P14; 2017, Q1, P15

D12.3   Benign neoplasm of transverse colon
        Benign neoplasm of hepatic flexure
        Benign neoplasm of splenic flexure
           *Flexure is a bending in a structure or organ. Note the
           three flexures illustrated in Figure 2–17. Hepatic =
           liver, sigmoid = colon, splenic = spleen.*
        Coding Clinic: 2017, Q1, P16

D12.4   Benign neoplasm of descending colon
        Coding Clinic: 2015, Q2, P14

D12.5   Benign neoplasm of sigmoid colon

D12.6   Benign neoplasm of colon, unspecified
        Adenomatosis of colon
        Benign neoplasm of large intestine NOS
        Polyposis (hereditary) of colon
        Excludes1   inflammatory polyp of colon (K51.4-)
        Coding Clinic: 2017, Q1, P8-9

D12.7   Benign neoplasm of rectosigmoid junction
        Angle where sigmoid colon becomes rectum

D12.8   Benign neoplasm of rectum
        Excludes1   benign carcinoid tumor of the rectum
                        (D3A.026)
        Coding Clinic: 2018, Q1, P7

D12.9   Benign neoplasm of anus and anal canal
        Benign neoplasm of anus NOS
        Excludes1   benign neoplasm of anal margin (D22.5,
                        D23.5)
                        benign neoplasm of anal skin (D22.5,
                        D23.5)
                        benign neoplasm of perianal skin (D22.5,
                        D23.5)

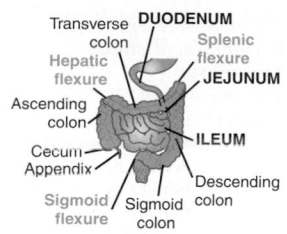

Figure 2-17   Small intestine and colon.

● D13   Benign neoplasm of other and ill-defined parts of digestive
        system
        Excludes1   benign stromal tumors of digestive system
                        (D21.4)

D13.0   Benign neoplasm of esophagus

D13.1   Benign neoplasm of stomach
        Excludes1   benign carcinoid tumor of the stomach
                        (D3A.092)

D13.2   Benign neoplasm of duodenum
        Excludes1   benign carcinoid tumor of the duodenum
                        (D3A.010)

● D13.3 Benign neoplasm of other and unspecified parts of small
        intestine
        Excludes1   benign carcinoid tumors of the small
                        intestine (D3A.01-)
                        benign neoplasm of ileocecal valve
                        (D12.0)

   D13.30   Benign neoplasm of unspecified part of small
            intestine

   D13.39   Benign neoplasm of other parts of small
            intestine

D13.4   Benign neoplasm of liver
        Benign neoplasm of intrahepatic bile ducts

D13.5   Benign neoplasm of extrahepatic bile ducts
        *Extensions of common hepatic bile duct (tube that collects
        bile from liver)*

D13.6   Benign neoplasm of pancreas
        Excludes1   benign neoplasm of endocrine pancreas
                        (D13.7)

D13.7   Benign neoplasm of endocrine pancreas
        Pancreatic islets: Cells scattered throughout pancreas
        Islet cell tumor
        Benign neoplasm of islets of Langerhans
        Use additional code to identify any functional activity.

D13.9   Benign neoplasm of ill-defined sites within the digestive
        system
        Benign neoplasm of digestive system NOS
        Benign neoplasm of intestine NOS
        Benign neoplasm of spleen

CHAPTER 2 (C00–D49)

N Newborn Age: 0   **P** Pediatric Age: 0–17   **M** Maternity DX: 9–64   **A** Adult Age: 15–124   ♀ Females Only   ♂ Males Only

🔹 Complication\Comorbidity   🔹 Major C\C   Ⓔⓧ CC/MCC Exclusions   🔹 Hospital-Acquired Condition   🔹 Hierarchical Condition Category   723

● **D14**   **Benign neoplasm of middle ear and respiratory system**

     D14.0   **Benign neoplasm of middle ear, nasal cavity and accessory sinuses**

         Benign neoplasm of cartilage of nose

           Excludes1   benign neoplasm of auricular canal (external) (D22.2-, D23.2-)

                       benign neoplasm of bone of ear (D16.4)

                       benign neoplasm of bone of nose (D16.4)

                       benign neoplasm of cartilage of ear (D21.0)

                       benign neoplasm of ear (external) (skin) (D22.2-, D23.2-)

                       benign neoplasm of nose NOS (D36.7)

                       benign neoplasm of skin of nose (D22.39, D23.39)

                       benign neoplasm of olfactory bulb (D33.3)

                       benign neoplasm of posterior margin of septum and choanae (D10.6)

                       polyp of accessory sinus (J33.8)

                       polyp of ear (middle) (H74.4)

                       polyp of nasal (cavity) (J33.-)

     D14.1   **Benign neoplasm of larynx**

         Adenomatous polyp of larynx

         Benign neoplasm of epiglottis (suprahyoid portion)

         Horseshoe-shaped bone in anterior midline of neck between chin and thyroid cartilage

           Excludes1   benign neoplasm of epiglottis, anterior aspect (D10.5)

                       polyp (nonadenomatous) of vocal cord or larynx (J38.1)

     D14.2   **Benign neoplasm of trachea**

     ● **D14.3**   **Benign neoplasm of bronchus and lung**

           Excludes1   benign carcinoid tumor of the bronchus and lung (D3A.090)

         D14.30   **Benign neoplasm of unspecified bronchus and lung**

         D14.31   **Benign neoplasm of right bronchus and lung**

         D14.32   **Benign neoplasm of left bronchus and lung**

     D14.4   **Benign neoplasm of respiratory system, unspecified**

● **D15**   **Benign neoplasm of other and unspecified intrathoracic organs**

       Excludes1   benign neoplasm of mesothelial tissue (D19.-)

     D15.0   **Benign neoplasm of thymus**

           Excludes1   benign carcinoid tumor of the thymus (D3A.091)

     D15.1   **Benign neoplasm of heart**

           Excludes1   benign neoplasm of great vessels (D21.3)

     D15.2   **Benign neoplasm of mediastinum**

     D15.7   **Benign neoplasm of other specified intrathoracic organs**

     D15.9   **Benign neoplasm of intrathoracic organ, unspecified**

● **D16**   **Benign neoplasm of bone and articular cartilage**

       Excludes1   benign neoplasm of connective tissue of ear (D21.0)

                     benign neoplasm of connective tissue of eyelid (D21.0)

                     benign neoplasm of connective tissue of larynx (D14.1)

                     benign neoplasm of connective tissue of nose (D14.0)

                     benign neoplasm of synovia (D21.-)

     ● **D16.0**   **Benign neoplasm of scapula and long bones of upper limb**

         D16.00   **Benign neoplasm of scapula and long bones of unspecified upper limb**

         D16.01   **Benign neoplasm of scapula and long bones of right upper limb**

         D16.02   **Benign neoplasm of scapula and long bones of left upper limb**

● **D16.1**   **Benign neoplasm of short bones of upper limb**

         D16.10   **Benign neoplasm of short bones of unspecified upper limb**

         D16.11   **Benign neoplasm of short bones of right upper limb**

         D16.12   **Benign neoplasm of short bones of left upper limb**

● **D16.2**   **Benign neoplasm of long bones of lower limb**

         D16.20   **Benign neoplasm of long bones of unspecified lower limb**

         D16.21   **Benign neoplasm of long bones of right lower limb**

         D16.22   **Benign neoplasm of long bones of left lower limb**

● **D16.3**   **Benign neoplasm of short bones of lower limb**

         D16.30   **Benign neoplasm of short bones of unspecified lower limb**

         D16.31   **Benign neoplasm of short bones of right lower limb**

         D16.32   **Benign neoplasm of short bones of left lower limb**

     D16.4   **Benign neoplasm of bones of skull and face**

         Benign neoplasm of maxilla (superior)

         Benign neoplasm of orbital bone

         Cavity or socket of skull in which eye and its appendages are located

         Keratocyst of maxilla

         Keratocystic odontogenic tumor of maxilla

           Excludes2   benign neoplasm of lower jaw bone (D16.5)

     D16.5   **Benign neoplasm of lower jaw bone**

         Keratocyst of mandible

         Keratocystic odontogenic tumor of mandible

     D16.6   **Benign neoplasm of vertebral column**

           Excludes1   benign neoplasm of sacrum and coccyx (D16.8)

     D16.7   **Benign neoplasm of ribs, sternum and clavicle**

     D16.8   **Benign neoplasm of pelvic bones, sacrum and coccyx**

     D16.9   **Benign neoplasm of bone and articular cartilage, unspecified**

● **D17**   **Benign lipomatous neoplasm**

     Slow-growing benign tumors (rubbery masses) of mature fat cells enclosed in a thin fibrous capsule

     D17.0   **Benign lipomatous neoplasm of skin and subcutaneous tissue of head, face and neck**

     D17.1   **Benign lipomatous neoplasm of skin and subcutaneous tissue of trunk**

     ● **D17.2**   **Benign lipomatous neoplasm of skin and subcutaneous tissue of limb**

         D17.20   **Benign lipomatous neoplasm of skin and subcutaneous tissue of unspecified limb**

         D17.21   **Benign lipomatous neoplasm of skin and subcutaneous tissue of right arm**

         D17.22   **Benign lipomatous neoplasm of skin and subcutaneous tissue of left arm**

         D17.23   **Benign lipomatous neoplasm of skin and subcutaneous tissue of right leg**

         D17.24   **Benign lipomatous neoplasm of skin and subcutaneous tissue of left leg**

     ● **D17.3**   **Benign lipomatous neoplasm of skin and subcutaneous tissue of other and unspecified sites**

         D17.30   **Benign lipomatous neoplasm of skin and subcutaneous tissue of unspecified sites**

         D17.39   **Benign lipomatous neoplasm of skin and subcutaneous tissue of other sites**

     D17.4   **Benign lipomatous neoplasm of intrathoracic organs**

▶ New   ⇒ Revised   ~~deleted~~ Deleted   Excludes 1   Excludes 2   Includes   Use additional   Code first   Code also   Key words

OGCR Official Guidelines   ● Unacceptable Principal Diagnosis   X Assign placeholder X   ● Use Additional Character(s)   ▶ Manifestation Code   **Coding Clinic**

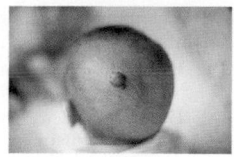

Figure 2-18   Hemangioma of skin and subcutaneous tissue. (Getty Image)

Item 2–10 Hemangiomas are abnormally dense collections of dilated capillaries that occur on the skin or in internal organs. Hemangiomas are both deep and superficial and undergo a rapid growth phase when the size increases rapidly, followed by a rest phase, in which the tumor changes very little, followed by an involutional phase in which the tumor begins to and can disappear altogether. **Lymphangiomas** or cystic hygroma are benign collections of overgrown lymph vessels and, although rare, may occur anywhere but most commonly on the head and neck of children and infants. Visceral organs, lungs, and gastrointestinal tract may also be involved.

D17.5   **Benign lipomatous neoplasm of intra-abdominal organs**

     Excludes1   benign lipomatous neoplasm of peritoneum and retroperitoneum (D17.79)

D17.6   **Benign lipomatous neoplasm of spermatic cord** ♂

● **D17.7**   **Benign lipomatous neoplasm of other sites**

     D17.71   **Benign lipomatous neoplasm of kidney**

     D17.72   **Benign lipomatous neoplasm of other genitourinary organ**

     D17.79   **Benign lipomatous neoplasm of other sites**
         Benign lipomatous neoplasm of peritoneum
         Benign lipomatous neoplasm of retroperitoneum

D17.9   **Benign lipomatous neoplasm, unspecified**
     Lipoma NOS

● **D18**   **Hemangioma and lymphangioma, any site**

     Excludes1   benign neoplasm of glomus jugulare (D35.6)
         blue or pigmented nevus (D22.-)
         nevus NOS (D22.-)
         vascular nevus (Q82.5)

● **D18.0**   **Hemangioma**
     Common type of vascular malformation
     Angioma NOS
     Cavernous nevus

     D18.00   **Hemangioma unspecified site**

     D18.01   **Hemangioma of skin and subcutaneous tissue**

     D18.02   **Hemangioma of intracranial structures** 🔵

     D18.03   **Hemangioma of intra-abdominal structures**

     D18.09   **Hemangioma of other sites**

D18.1   **Lymphangioma, any site**
     Coding Clinic: 2018, Q2, P13

● **D19**   **Benign neoplasm of mesothelial tissue**
     Mesothelial tissue is the membrane lining several body cavities

     D19.0   **Benign neoplasm of mesothelial tissue of pleura**

     D19.1   **Benign neoplasm of mesothelial tissue of peritoneum**

     D19.7   **Benign neoplasm of mesothelial tissue of other sites**

     D19.9   **Benign neoplasm of mesothelial tissue, unspecified**
         Benign mesothelioma NOS

● **D20**   **Benign neoplasm of soft tissue of retroperitoneum and peritoneum**

     Excludes1   benign lipomatous neoplasm of peritoneum and retroperitoneum (D17.79)
         benign neoplasm of mesothelial tissue (D19.-)

     D20.0   **Benign neoplasm of soft tissue of retroperitoneum**

     D20.1   **Benign neoplasm of soft tissue of peritoneum**

● **D21**   **Other benign neoplasms of connective and other soft tissue**

     Includes   benign neoplasm of blood vessel
         benign neoplasm of bursa
         benign neoplasm of cartilage
         benign neoplasm of fascia
         benign neoplasm of fat
         benign neoplasm of ligament, except uterine
         benign neoplasm of lymphatic channel
         benign neoplasm of muscle
         benign neoplasm of synovia
         benign neoplasm of tendon (sheath)
         benign stromal tumors

     Excludes1   benign neoplasm of articular cartilage (D16.-)
         benign neoplasm of cartilage of larynx (D14.1)
         benign neoplasm of cartilage of nose (D14.0)
         benign neoplasm of connective tissue of breast (D24.-)
         benign neoplasm of peripheral nerves and autonomic nervous system (D36.1-)
         benign neoplasm of peritoneum (D20.1)
         benign neoplasm of retroperitoneum (D20.0)
         benign neoplasm of uterine ligament, any (D28.2)
         benign neoplasm of vascular tissue (D18.-)
         hemangioma (D18.0-)
         lipomatous neoplasm (D17.-)
         lymphangioma (D18.1)
         uterine leiomyoma (D25.-)

     D21.0   **Benign neoplasm of connective and other soft tissue of head, face and neck**
         Benign neoplasm of connective tissue of ear
         Benign neoplasm of connective tissue of eyelid

         Excludes1   benign neoplasm of connective tissue of orbit (D31.6-)

●   **D21.1**   **Benign neoplasm of connective and other soft tissue of upper limb, including shoulder**

     D21.10   **Benign neoplasm of connective and other soft tissue of unspecified upper limb, including shoulder**

     D21.11   **Benign neoplasm of connective and other soft tissue of right upper limb, including shoulder**

     D21.12   **Benign neoplasm of connective and other soft tissue of left upper limb, including shoulder**

●   **D21.2**   **Benign neoplasm of connective and other soft tissue of lower limb, including hip**

     D21.20   **Benign neoplasm of connective and other soft tissue of unspecified lower limb, including hip**

     D21.21   **Benign neoplasm of connective and other soft tissue of right lower limb, including hip**

     D21.22   **Benign neoplasm of connective and other soft tissue of left lower limb, including hip**

     D21.3   **Benign neoplasm of connective and other soft tissue of thorax**
         Benign neoplasm of axilla
         Benign neoplasm of diaphragm
         Benign neoplasm of great vessels

         Excludes1   benign neoplasm of heart (D15.1)
         benign neoplasm of mediastinum (D15.2)
         benign neoplasm of thymus (D15.0)

     D21.4   **Benign neoplasm of connective and other soft tissue of abdomen**
         Benign stromal tumors of abdomen

     D21.5   **Benign neoplasm of connective and other soft tissue of pelvis**

         Excludes1   benign neoplasm of any uterine ligament (D28.2)
         uterine leiomyoma (D25.-)

     D21.6   **Benign neoplasm of connective and other soft tissue of trunk, unspecified**
         Benign neoplasm of connective and other soft tissue of back NOS

     D21.9   **Benign neoplasm of connective and other soft tissue, unspecified**

N Newborn Age: 0   **P** Pediatric Age: 0–17   **M** Maternity DX: 9–64   **A** Adult Age: 15–124   ♀ Females Only   ♂ Males Only

🔵 Complication\Comorbidity   🔵 Major C\C   (Ex) CC/MCC Exclusions   🔵 Hospital-Acquired Condition   🔵 Hierarchical Condition Category

● **D22 Melanocytic nevi**

Includes   atypical nevus
blue hairy pigmented nevus
nevus NOS

D22.0 Melanocytic nevi of lip
Skin lesions composed of nests of nevus cells with macules/papules

● **D22.1 Melanocytic nevi of eyelid, including canthus**

D22.10   Melanocytic nevi of unspecified eyelid, including canthus

● D22.11   Melanocytic nevi of right eyelid, including canthus

D22.111   Melanocytic nevi of right upper eyelid, including canthus

D22.112   Melanocytic nevi of right lower eyelid, including canthus

● D22.12   Melanocytic nevi of left eyelid, including canthus

D22.121   Melanocytic nevi of left upper eyelid, including canthus

D22.122   Melanocytic nevi of left lower eyelid, including canthus

● **D22.2 Melanocytic nevi of ear and external auricular canal**

D22.20   Melanocytic nevi of unspecified ear and external auricular canal

D22.21   Melanocytic nevi of right ear and external auricular canal

D22.22   Melanocytic nevi of left ear and external auricular canal

● **D22.3 Melanocytic nevi of other and unspecified parts of face**

D22.30   Melanocytic nevi of unspecified part of face

D22.39   Melanocytic nevi of other parts of face

D22.4 Melanocytic nevi of scalp and neck

D22.5 Melanocytic nevi of trunk
Melanocytic nevi of anal margin
Melanocytic nevi of anal skin
Melanocytic nevi of perianal skin
Melanocytic nevi of skin of breast

● **D22.6 Melanocytic nevi of upper limb, including shoulder**

D22.60   Melanocytic nevi of unspecified upper limb, including shoulder

D22.61   Melanocytic nevi of right upper limb, including shoulder

D22.62   Melanocytic nevi of left upper limb, including shoulder

● **D22.7 Melanocytic nevi of lower limb, including hip**

D22.70   Melanocytic nevi of unspecified lower limb, including hip

D22.71   Melanocytic nevi of right lower limb, including hip

D22.72   Melanocytic nevi of left lower limb, including hip

D22.9 Melanocytic nevi, unspecified

● **D23 Other benign neoplasms of skin**

Includes   benign neoplasm of hair follicles
benign neoplasm of sebaceous glands
benign neoplasm of sweat glands

Excludes1   benign lipomatous neoplasms of skin (D17.0-D17.3)

Excludes2   melanocytic nevi (D22.-)

D23.0 Other benign neoplasm of skin of lip

Excludes1   benign neoplasm of vermilion border of lip (D10.0)

● **D23.1 Other benign neoplasm of skin of eyelid, including canthus**

D23.10   Other benign neoplasm of skin unspecified of eyelid, including canthus

● D23.11   Other benign neoplasm of skin of right eyelid, including canthus

D23.111   Other benign neoplasm of skin of right upper eyelid, including canthus

D23.112   Other benign neoplasm of skin of right lower eyelid, including canthus

● D23.12   Other benign neoplasm of skin of left eyelid, including canthus

D23.121   Other benign neoplasm of skin of left upper eyelid, including canthus

D23.122   Other benign neoplasm of skin of left lower eyelid, including canthus

● **D23.2 Other benign neoplasm of skin of ear and external auricular canal**

D23.20   Other benign neoplasm of skin of unspecified ear and external auricular canal

D23.21   Other benign neoplasm of skin of right ear and external auricular canal

D23.22   Other benign neoplasm of skin of left ear and external auricular canal

● **D23.3 Other benign neoplasm of skin of other and unspecified parts of face**

D23.30   Other benign neoplasm of skin of unspecified part of face

D23.39   Other benign neoplasm of skin of other parts of face

D23.4 Other benign neoplasm of skin of scalp and neck

D23.5 Other benign neoplasm of skin of trunk
Other benign neoplasm of anal margin
Other benign neoplasm of anal skin
Other benign neoplasm of perianal skin
Other benign neoplasm of skin of breast

Excludes1   benign neoplasm of anus NOS (D12.9)

● **D23.6 Other benign neoplasm of skin of upper limb, including shoulder**

D23.60   Other benign neoplasm of skin of unspecified upper limb, including shoulder

D23.61   Other benign neoplasm of skin of right upper limb, including shoulder

D23.62   Other benign neoplasm of skin of left upper limb, including shoulder

● **D23.7 Other benign neoplasm of skin of lower limb, including hip**

D23.70   Other benign neoplasm of skin of unspecified lower limb, including hip

D23.71   Other benign neoplasm of skin of right lower limb, including hip

D23.72   Other benign neoplasm of skin of left lower limb, including hip

D23.9 Other benign neoplasm of skin, unspecified

● **D24 Benign neoplasm of breast**

Includes   benign neoplasm of connective tissue of breast
benign neoplasm of soft parts of breast
fibroadenoma of breast

Excludes2   adenofibrosis of breast (N60.2)
benign cyst of breast (N60.-)
benign mammary dysplasia (N60.-)
benign neoplasm of skin of breast (D22.5, D23.5)
fibrocystic disease of breast (N60.-)

D24.1 Benign neoplasm of right breast
Coding Clinic: 2017, Q1, P5

D24.2 Benign neoplasm of left breast

D24.9 Benign neoplasm of unspecified breast

▶ New   ➡ Revised   deleted Deleted   Excludes 1   Excludes 2   Includes   Use additional   Code first   Code also   Key words
OGCR Official Guidelines   ● Unacceptable Principal Diagnosis   X Assign placeholder X   ● Use Additional Character(s)   ▶ Manifestation Code   Coding Clinic

Item 2-11 Teratoma: terat = monster, oma = mass, tumor. Alternate terms: dermoid cyst of the ovary, ovarian teratoma. Teratomas are neoplasms and arise from germ cells (ovaries in female and testes in male) and can be benign or malignant. Teratomas have been known to contain hair, nails, and teeth, giving them a bizarre ("monster") appearance.

● **D25   Leiomyoma of uterus**
  Benign tumors or nodules of the uterine wall
  Includes   uterine fibroid
                uterine fibromyoma
                uterine myoma
  D25.0   Submucous leiomyoma of uterus ♀
  D25.1   Intramural leiomyoma of uterus ♀
          Interstitial leiomyoma of uterus
  D25.2   Subserosal leiomyoma of uterus ♀
          Subperitoneal leiomyoma of uterus
  D25.9   Leiomyoma of uterus, unspecified ♀

● **D26   Other benign neoplasms of uterus**
  D26.0   Other benign neoplasm of cervix uteri ♀
  D26.1   Other benign neoplasm of corpus uteri ♀
  D26.7   Other benign neoplasm of other parts of uterus ♀
  D26.9   Other benign neoplasm of uterus, unspecified ♀

● **D27   Benign neoplasm of ovary**
  Use additional code to identify any functional activity.
  Excludes2   corpus albicans cyst (N83.2-)
                corpus luteum cyst (N83.1-)
                endometrial cyst (N80.1)
                follicular (atretic) cyst (N83.0-)
                graafian follicle cyst (N83.0-)
                ovarian cyst NEC (N83.2-)
                ovarian retention cyst (N83.2-)
  D27.0   Benign neoplasm of right ovary ♀
  D27.1   Benign neoplasm of left ovary ♀
  D27.9   Benign neoplasm of unspecified ovary ♀
          Ovarian teratoma

● **D28   Benign neoplasm of other and unspecified female genital organs**
  Includes   adenomatous polyp
                benign neoplasm of skin of female genital organs
                benign teratoma
  Excludes1   epoophoron cyst (Q50.5)
                fimbrial cyst (Q50.4)
                Gartner's duct cyst (Q52.4)
                parovarian cyst (Q50.5)
  D28.0   Benign neoplasm of vulva ♀
  D28.1   Benign neoplasm of vagina ♀
  D28.2   Benign neoplasm of uterine tubes and ligaments ♀
          Benign neoplasm of fallopian tube
          Benign neoplasm of uterine ligament (broad) (round)
  D28.7   Benign neoplasm of other specified female genital organs ♀
  D28.9   Benign neoplasm of female genital organ, unspecified ♀

● **D29   Benign neoplasm of male genital organs**
  Includes   benign neoplasm of skin of male genital organs
  D29.0   Benign neoplasm of penis ♂
  D29.1   Benign neoplasm of prostate ♂
          Excludes1   enlarged prostate (N40.-)
  ● **D29.2   Benign neoplasm of testis**
          Use additional code to identify any functional activity.
          D29.20   Benign neoplasm of unspecified testis ♂
          D29.21   Benign neoplasm of right testis ♂
          D29.22   Benign neoplasm of left testis ♂
  ● **D29.3   Benign neoplasm of epididymis**
          D29.30   Benign neoplasm of unspecified epididymis ♂
          D29.31   Benign neoplasm of right epididymis ♂
          D29.32   Benign neoplasm of left epididymis ♂

D29.4   Benign neoplasm of scrotum ♂
        Benign neoplasm of skin of scrotum
D29.8   Benign neoplasm of other specified male genital organs ♂
        Benign neoplasm of seminal vesicle
        Benign neoplasm of spermatic cord
        Benign neoplasm of tunica vaginalis
D29.9   Benign neoplasm of male genital organ, unspecified ♂

● **D30   Benign neoplasm of urinary organs**
  ● **D30.0   Benign neoplasm of kidney**
          Excludes1   benign carcinoid tumor of the kidney (D3A.093)
                   benign neoplasm of renal calyces (D30.1-)
                   benign neoplasm of renal pelvis (D30.1-)
          D30.00   Benign neoplasm of unspecified kidney
          D30.01   Benign neoplasm of right kidney
          D30.02   Benign neoplasm of left kidney
  ● **D30.1   Benign neoplasm of renal pelvis**
          D30.10   Benign neoplasm of unspecified renal pelvis
          D30.11   Benign neoplasm of right renal pelvis
          D30.12   Benign neoplasm of left renal pelvis
  ● **D30.2   Benign neoplasm of ureter**
          Excludes1   benign neoplasm of ureteric orifice of bladder (D30.3)
          D30.20   Benign neoplasm of unspecified ureter
          D30.21   Benign neoplasm of right ureter
          D30.22   Benign neoplasm of left ureter
  D30.3   Benign neoplasm of bladder
          Benign neoplasm of ureteric orifice of bladder
          Benign neoplasm of urethral orifice of bladder
  D30.4   Benign neoplasm of urethra
          Excludes1   benign neoplasm of urethral orifice of bladder (D30.3)
  D30.8   Benign neoplasm of other specified urinary organs
          Benign neoplasm of paraurethral glands
  D30.9   Benign neoplasm of urinary organ, unspecified
          Benign neoplasm of urinary system NOS

● **D31   Benign neoplasm of eye and adnexa**
  Excludes1   benign neoplasm of connective tissue of eyelid (D21.0)
                benign neoplasm of optic nerve (D33.3)
                benign neoplasm of skin of eyelid (D22.1-, D23.1-)
  ● **D31.0   Benign neoplasm of conjunctiva**
          D31.00   Benign neoplasm of unspecified conjunctiva
          D31.01   Benign neoplasm of right conjunctiva
          D31.02   Benign neoplasm of left conjunctiva
  ● **D31.1   Benign neoplasm of cornea**
          D31.10   Benign neoplasm of unspecified cornea
          D31.11   Benign neoplasm of right cornea
          D31.12   Benign neoplasm of left cornea
  ● **D31.2   Benign neoplasm of retina**
          Excludes1   dark area on retina (D49.81)
                   hemangioma of retina (D49.81)
                   neoplasm of unspecified behavior of retina and choroid (D49.81)
                   retinal freckle (D49.81)
          D31.20   Benign neoplasm of unspecified retina
          D31.21   Benign neoplasm of right retina
          D31.22   Benign neoplasm of left retina
  ● **D31.3   Benign neoplasm of choroid**
          D31.30   Benign neoplasm of unspecified choroid
          D31.31   Benign neoplasm of right choroid
          D31.32   Benign neoplasm of left choroid
  ● **D31.4   Benign neoplasm of ciliary body**
          D31.40   Benign neoplasm of unspecified ciliary body
          D31.41   Benign neoplasm of right ciliary body
          D31.42   Benign neoplasm of left ciliary body

CHAPTER 2 (C00-D49)

N Newborn Age: 0   **P** Pediatric Age: 0–17   **M** Maternity DX: 9–64   **A** Adult Age: 15–124   ♀ Females Only   ♂ Males Only

Complication\Comorbidity   Major C\C   (Ex) CC/MCC Exclusions   Hospital-Acquired Condition   Hierarchical Condition Category

727

● **D31.5 Benign neoplasm of lacrimal gland and duct**
     Benign neoplasm of lacrimal sac
     Benign neoplasm of nasolacrimal duct
     D31.50 Benign neoplasm of unspecified lacrimal gland and duct
     D31.51 Benign neoplasm of right lacrimal gland and duct
     D31.52 Benign neoplasm of left lacrimal gland and duct

● **D31.6 Benign neoplasm of unspecified site of orbit**
     Benign neoplasm of connective tissue of orbit
     Benign neoplasm of extraocular muscle
     Benign neoplasm of peripheral nerves of orbit
     Benign neoplasm of retrobulbar tissue
     Benign neoplasm of retro-ocular tissue
     Excludes1   benign neoplasm of orbital bone (D16.4)
     D31.60 Benign neoplasm of unspecified site of unspecified orbit
     D31.61 Benign neoplasm of unspecified site of right orbit
     D31.62 Benign neoplasm of unspecified site of left orbit

● **D31.9 Benign neoplasm of unspecified part of eye**
     Benign neoplasm of eyeball
     D31.90 Benign neoplasm of unspecified part of unspecified eye
     D31.91 Benign neoplasm of unspecified part of right eye
     D31.92 Benign neoplasm of unspecified part of left eye

● **D32 Benign neoplasm of meninges**
     D32.0 Benign neoplasm of cerebral meninges 🔑
     D32.1 Benign neoplasm of spinal meninges 🔑
     D32.9 Benign neoplasm of meninges, unspecified 🔑
       Meningioma NOS

● **D33 Benign neoplasm of brain and other parts of central nervous system**
     Excludes1   angioma (D18.0-)
         benign neoplasm of meninges (D32.-)
         benign neoplasm of peripheral nerves and autonomic nervous system (D36.1-)
         hemangioma (D18.0-)
         neurofibromatosis (Q85.0-)
         retro-ocular benign neoplasm (D31.6-)
     D33.0 Benign neoplasm of brain, supratentorial 🔑
       Benign neoplasm of cerebral ventricle
       Benign neoplasm of cerebrum
       Benign neoplasm of frontal lobe
       Benign neoplasm of occipital lobe
       Benign neoplasm of parietal lobe
       Benign neoplasm of temporal lobe
       Excludes1   benign neoplasm of fourth ventricle (D33.1)
     D33.1 Benign neoplasm of brain, infratentorial 🔑
       Benign neoplasm of brain stem
       Benign neoplasm of cerebellum
       Benign neoplasm of fourth ventricle
     D33.2 Benign neoplasm of brain, unspecified 🔑
     D33.3 Benign neoplasm of cranial nerves 🔑
       Benign neoplasm of olfactory bulb
     D33.4 Benign neoplasm of spinal cord 🔑

     D33.7 Benign neoplasm of other specified parts of central nervous system 🔑
     D33.9 Benign neoplasm of central nervous system, unspecified 🔑
       Benign neoplasm of nervous system (central) NOS

D34 Benign neoplasm of thyroid gland
     Use additional code to identify any functional activity.

● **D35 Benign neoplasm of other and unspecified endocrine glands**
     Use additional code to identify any functional activity.
     Excludes1   benign neoplasm of endocrine pancreas (D13.7)
         benign neoplasm of ovary (D27.-)
         benign neoplasm of testis (D29.2.-)
         benign neoplasm of thymus (D15.0)
     ● **D35.0 Benign neoplasm of adrenal gland**
       D35.00 Benign neoplasm of unspecified adrenal gland
       D35.01 Benign neoplasm of right adrenal gland
       D35.02 Benign neoplasm of left adrenal gland
     D35.1 Benign neoplasm of parathyroid gland
     D35.2 Benign neoplasm of pituitary gland 🔑
     D35.3 Benign neoplasm of craniopharyngeal duct 🔑
     D35.4 Benign neoplasm of pineal gland 🔑
     D35.5 Benign neoplasm of carotid body
     D35.6 Benign neoplasm of aortic body and other paraganglia
       Benign tumor of glomus jugulare
     D35.7 Benign neoplasm of other specified endocrine glands
     D35.9 Benign neoplasm of endocrine gland, unspecified
       Benign neoplasm of unspecified endocrine gland

● **D36 Benign neoplasm of other and unspecified sites**
     D36.0 Benign neoplasm of lymph nodes
       Excludes1   lymphangioma (D18.1)
     ● **D36.1 Benign neoplasm of peripheral nerves and autonomic nervous system**
       Excludes1   benign neoplasm of peripheral nerves of orbit (D31.6-)
         neurofibromatosis (Q85.0-)
       D36.10 Benign neoplasm of peripheral nerves and autonomic nervous system, unspecified
       D36.11 Benign neoplasm of peripheral nerves and autonomic nervous system of face, head, and neck
       D36.12 Benign neoplasm of peripheral nerves and autonomic nervous system, upper limb, including shoulder
       D36.13 Benign neoplasm of peripheral nerves and autonomic nervous system of lower limb, including hip
       D36.14 Benign neoplasm of peripheral nerves and autonomic nervous system of thorax
       D36.15 Benign neoplasm of peripheral nerves and autonomic nervous system of abdomen
       D36.16 Benign neoplasm of peripheral nerves and autonomic nervous system of pelvis
       D36.17 Benign neoplasm of peripheral nerves and autonomic nervous system of trunk, unspecified
     D36.7 Benign neoplasm of other specified sites
       Benign neoplasm of nose NOS
       Benign neoplasm of back NOS
     D36.9 Benign neoplasm, unspecified site

▶ New   ⇛ Revised   ~~deleted~~ Deleted   Excludes 1   Excludes 2   Includes   Use additional   Code first   Code also   Key words
OGCR Official Guidelines   ● Unacceptable Principal Diagnosis   X Assign placeholder X   ● Use Additional Character(s)   ▷ Manifestation Code   **Coding Clinic**

BENIGN NEUROENDOCRINE TUMORS (D3A)

● **D3A Benign neuroendocrine tumors**

Code also any associated multiple endocrine neoplasia [MEN] syndromes (E31.2-)

Use additional code to identify any associated endocrine syndrome, such as:
carcinoid syndrome (E34.0)

Excludes2   benign pancreatic islet cell tumors (D13.7)

● **D3A.0 Benign carcinoid tumors**

  D3A.00 Benign carcinoid tumor of unspecified site
      Carcinoid tumor NOS

● **D3A.01 Benign carcinoid tumors of the small intestine**

  D3A.010 Benign carcinoid tumor of the duodenum

  D3A.011 Benign carcinoid tumor of the jejunum

  D3A.012 Benign carcinoid tumor of the ileum

  D3A.019 Benign carcinoid tumor of the small intestine, unspecified portion

● **D3A.02 Benign carcinoid tumors of the appendix, large intestine, and rectum**

  D3A.020 Benign carcinoid tumor of the appendix

  D3A.021 Benign carcinoid tumor of the cecum

  D3A.022 Benign carcinoid tumor of the ascending colon

  D3A.023 Benign carcinoid tumor of the transverse colon

  D3A.024 Benign carcinoid tumor of the descending colon

  D3A.025 Benign carcinoid tumor of the sigmoid colon

  D3A.026 Benign carcinoid tumor of the rectum

  D3A.029 Benign carcinoid tumor of the large intestine, unspecified portion
      Benign carcinoid tumor of the colon NOS

● **D3A.09 Benign carcinoid tumors of other sites**

  D3A.090 Benign carcinoid tumor of the bronchus and lung

  D3A.091 Benign carcinoid tumor of the thymus

  D3A.092 Benign carcinoid tumor of the stomach

  D3A.093 Benign carcinoid tumor of the kidney

  D3A.094 Benign carcinoid tumor of the foregut, unspecified

  D3A.095 Benign carcinoid tumor of the midgut, unspecified

  D3A.096 Benign carcinoid tumor of the hindgut, unspecified

  D3A.098 Benign carcinoid tumors of other sites

D3A.8 Other benign neuroendocrine tumors
  Neuroendocrine tumor NOS

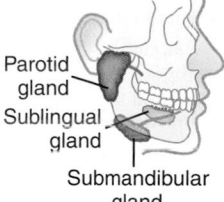

Figure 2-19 Major salivary glands.

NEOPLASMS OF UNCERTAIN BEHAVIOR, POLYCYTHEMIA VERA AND MYELODYSPLASTIC SYNDROMES (D37-D48)

Note: Categories D37-D44, and D48 classify by site neoplasms of uncertain behavior, i.e., histologic confirmation whether the neoplasm is malignant or benign cannot be made.

Excludes1   neoplasms of unspecified behavior (D49.-)

● **D37 Neoplasm of uncertain behavior of oral cavity and digestive organs**

Excludes1   stromal tumors of uncertain behavior of digestive system (D48.1)

● **D37.0 Neoplasm of uncertain behavior of lip, oral cavity and pharynx**

Excludes1   neoplasm of uncertain behavior of aryepiglottic fold or interarytenoid fold, laryngeal aspect (D38.0)
neoplasm of uncertain behavior of epiglottis NOS (D38.0)
neoplasm of uncertain behavior of skin of lip (D48.5)
neoplasm of uncertain behavior of suprahyoid portion of epiglottis (D38.0)

  D37.01 Neoplasm of uncertain behavior of lip
      Neoplasm of uncertain behavior of vermilion border of lip

  D37.02 Neoplasm of uncertain behavior of tongue

● **D37.03** Neoplasm of uncertain behavior of the major salivary glands

  D37.030 Neoplasm of uncertain behavior of the parotid salivary glands

  D37.031 Neoplasm of uncertain behavior of the sublingual salivary glands

  D37.032 Neoplasm of uncertain behavior of the submandibular salivary glands

  D37.039 Neoplasm of uncertain behavior of the major salivary glands, unspecified

  D37.04 Neoplasm of uncertain behavior of the minor salivary glands
      Neoplasm of uncertain behavior of submucosal salivary glands of lip
      Neoplasm of uncertain behavior of submucosal salivary glands of cheek
      Neoplasm of uncertain behavior of submucosal salivary glands of hard palate
      Neoplasm of uncertain behavior of submucosal salivary glands of soft palate

  D37.05 Neoplasm of uncertain behavior of pharynx
      Neoplasm of uncertain behavior of aryepiglottic fold of pharynx NOS
      Neoplasm of uncertain behavior of hypopharyngeal aspect of aryepiglottic fold of pharynx
      Neoplasm of uncertain behavior of marginal zone of aryepiglottic fold of pharynx

  D37.09 Neoplasm of uncertain behavior of other specified sites of the oral cavity

N Newborn Age: 0   **P** Pediatric Age: 0–17   **M** Maternity DX: 9–64   **A** Adult Age: 15–124   ♀ Females Only   ♂ Males Only

Complication\Comorbidity   Major C\C   (Ex) CC/MCC Exclusions   Hospital-Acquired Condition   Hierarchical Condition Category   **729**

CHAPTER 2 (C00-D49)

D37.1   Neoplasm of uncertain behavior of stomach

D37.2   Neoplasm of uncertain behavior of small intestine

D37.3   Neoplasm of uncertain behavior of appendix

D37.4   Neoplasm of uncertain behavior of colon

D37.5   Neoplasm of uncertain behavior of rectum
   Neoplasm of uncertain behavior of rectosigmoid junction
   Rectosigmoid junction: Angle where sigmoid colon becomes rectum

D37.6   Neoplasm of uncertain behavior of liver, gallbladder and bile ducts
   Neoplasm of uncertain behavior of ampulla of Vater
   Ampulla of Vater: Enlarged segment of ducts from liver and pancreas at entry point to small intestine

D37.8   Neoplasm of uncertain behavior of other specified digestive organs
   Neoplasm of uncertain behavior of anal canal
   Neoplasm of uncertain behavior of anal sphincter
   Neoplasm of uncertain behavior of anus NOS
   Neoplasm of uncertain behavior of esophagus
   Neoplasm of uncertain behavior of intestine NOS
   Neoplasm of uncertain behavior of pancreas
   Excludes1   neoplasm of uncertain behavior of anal margin (D48.5)
      neoplasm of uncertain behavior of anal skin (D48.5)
      neoplasm of uncertain behavior of perianal skin (D48.5)

D37.9   Neoplasm of uncertain behavior of digestive organ, unspecified

● D38   Neoplasm of uncertain behavior of middle ear and respiratory and intrathoracic organs
   Excludes1   neoplasm of uncertain behavior of heart (D48.7)

D38.0   Neoplasm of uncertain behavior of larynx
   Neoplasm of uncertain behavior of aryepiglottic fold or interarytenoid fold, laryngeal aspect
   Neoplasm of uncertain behavior of epiglottis (suprahyoid portion)
   Excludes1   neoplasm of uncertain behavior of aryepiglottic fold or interarytenoid fold NOS (D37.05)
      neoplasm of uncertain behavior of hypopharyngeal aspect of aryepiglottic fold (D37.05)
      neoplasm of uncertain behavior of marginal zone of aryepiglottic fold (D37.05)

D38.1   Neoplasm of uncertain behavior of trachea, bronchus and lung

D38.2   Neoplasm of uncertain behavior of pleura

D38.3   Neoplasm of uncertain behavior of mediastinum

D38.4   Neoplasm of uncertain behavior of thymus

D38.5   Neoplasm of uncertain behavior of other respiratory organs
   Neoplasm of uncertain behavior of accessory sinuses
   Neoplasm of uncertain behavior of cartilage of nose
   Neoplasm of uncertain behavior of middle ear
   Neoplasm of uncertain behavior of nasal cavities
   Excludes1   neoplasm of uncertain behavior of ear (external) (skin) (D48.5)
      neoplasm of uncertain behavior of nose NOS (D48.7)
      neoplasm of uncertain behavior of skin of nose (D48.5)

D38.6   Neoplasm of uncertain behavior of respiratory organ, unspecified

● D39   Neoplasm of uncertain behavior of female genital organs

D39.0   Neoplasm of uncertain behavior of uterus ♀

● D39.1   Neoplasm of uncertain behavior of ovary
   Use additional code to identify any functional activity.

D39.10   Neoplasm of uncertain behavior of unspecified ovary ♀

D39.11   Neoplasm of uncertain behavior of right ovary ♀

D39.12   Neoplasm of uncertain behavior of left ovary ♀

D39.2   Neoplasm of uncertain behavior of placenta ♀M
   Chorioadenoma destruens
   Invasive hydatidiform mole
   Malignant hydatidiform mole
   Excludes1   hydatidiform mole NOS (O01.9)

D39.8   Neoplasm of uncertain behavior of other specified female genital organs ♀
   Neoplasm of uncertain behavior of skin of female genital organs

D39.9   Neoplasm of uncertain behavior of female genital organ, unspecified ♀

● D40   Neoplasm of uncertain behavior of male genital organs

D40.0   Neoplasm of uncertain behavior of prostate ♂

● D40.1   Neoplasm of uncertain behavior of testis

D40.10   Neoplasm of uncertain behavior of unspecified testis ♂

D40.11   Neoplasm of uncertain behavior of right testis ♂

D40.12   Neoplasm of uncertain behavior of left testis ♂

D40.8   Neoplasm of uncertain behavior of other specified male genital organs ♂
   Neoplasm of uncertain behavior of skin of male genital organs

D40.9   Neoplasm of uncertain behavior of male genital organ, unspecified ♂

● D41   Neoplasm of uncertain behavior of urinary organs

● D41.0   Neoplasm of uncertain behavior of kidney
   Excludes1   neoplasm of uncertain behavior of renal pelvis (D41.1-)

D41.00   Neoplasm of uncertain behavior of unspecified kidney

D41.01   Neoplasm of uncertain behavior of right kidney

D41.02   Neoplasm of uncertain behavior of left kidney

● D41.1   Neoplasm of uncertain behavior of renal pelvis

D41.10   Neoplasm of uncertain behavior of unspecified renal pelvis

D41.11   Neoplasm of uncertain behavior of right renal pelvis

D41.12   Neoplasm of uncertain behavior of left renal pelvis

● D41.2   Neoplasm of uncertain behavior of ureter

D41.20   Neoplasm of uncertain behavior of unspecified ureter

D41.21   Neoplasm of uncertain behavior of right ureter

D41.22   Neoplasm of uncertain behavior of left ureter

D41.3   Neoplasm of uncertain behavior of urethra

D41.4   Neoplasm of uncertain behavior of bladder

D41.8   Neoplasm of uncertain behavior of other specified urinary organs

D41.9   Neoplasm of uncertain behavior of unspecified urinary organ

▶ New   ⇒ Revised   ~~deleted~~ Deleted   Excludes 1   Excludes 2   Includes   Use additional   Code first   Code also   Key words
OGCR Official Guidelines   ● Unacceptable Principal Diagnosis   X Assign placeholder X   ● Use Additional Character(s)   ▶ Manifestation Code   **Coding Clinic**

● **D42** Neoplasm of uncertain behavior of meninges
     D42.0 Neoplasm of uncertain behavior of cerebral meninges 🩺
     D42.1 Neoplasm of uncertain behavior of spinal meninges 🩺
     D42.9 Neoplasm of uncertain behavior of meninges, unspecified 🩺

● **D43** Neoplasm of uncertain behavior of brain and central nervous system
     Excludes1   neoplasm of uncertain behavior of peripheral nerves and autonomic nervous system (D48.2)

     D43.0 Neoplasm of uncertain behavior of brain, supratentorial 🩺
         Superior to tentorium of cerebellum
         Neoplasm of uncertain behavior of cerebral ventricle
         Neoplasm of uncertain behavior of cerebrum
         Neoplasm of uncertain behavior of frontal lobe
         Neoplasm of uncertain behavior of occipital lobe
         Neoplasm of uncertain behavior of parietal lobe
         Neoplasm of uncertain behavior of temporal lobe
         Excludes1   neoplasm of uncertain behavior of fourth ventricle (D43.1)

     D43.1 Neoplasm of uncertain behavior of brain, infratentorial 🩺
         Beneath the tentorium of cerebellum
         Neoplasm of uncertain behavior of brain stem
         Neoplasm of uncertain behavior of cerebellum
         Neoplasm of uncertain behavior of fourth ventricle

     D43.2 Neoplasm of uncertain behavior of brain, unspecified 🩺
     D43.3 Neoplasm of uncertain behavior of cranial nerves 🩺
     D43.4 Neoplasm of uncertain behavior of spinal cord 🩺
     D43.8 Neoplasm of uncertain behavior of other specified parts of central nervous system 🩺
     D43.9 Neoplasm of uncertain behavior of central nervous system, unspecified 🩺
         Neoplasm of uncertain behavior of nervous system (central) NOS

● **D44** Neoplasm of uncertain behavior of endocrine glands
     Excludes1   multiple endocrine adenomatosis (E31.2-)
         multiple endocrine neoplasia (E31.2-)
         neoplasm of uncertain behavior of endocrine pancreas (D37.8)
         neoplasm of uncertain behavior of ovary (D39.1)
         neoplasm of uncertain behavior of testis (D40.1-)
         neoplasm of uncertain behavior of thymus (D38.4)

     D44.0 Neoplasm of uncertain behavior of thyroid gland
● **D44.1** Neoplasm of uncertain behavior of adrenal gland
         Use additional code to identify any functional activity.
         D44.10 Neoplasm of uncertain behavior of unspecified adrenal gland
         D44.11 Neoplasm of uncertain behavior of right adrenal gland
         D44.12 Neoplasm of uncertain behavior of left adrenal gland

     D44.2 Neoplasm of uncertain behavior of parathyroid gland
     D44.3 Neoplasm of uncertain behavior of pituitary gland 🩺
         Use additional code to identify any functional activity.
     D44.4 Neoplasm of uncertain behavior of craniopharyngeal duct 🩺
     D44.5 Neoplasm of uncertain behavior of pineal gland 🩺
     D44.6 Neoplasm of uncertain behavior of carotid body 🩺
     D44.7 Neoplasm of uncertain behavior of aortic body and other paraganglia 🩺
         Coding Clinic: 2016, Q4, P26
     D44.9 Neoplasm of uncertain behavior of unspecified endocrine gland

● **D45** Polycythemia vera 🩺
     Excludes1   familial polycythemia (D75.0)
         secondary polycythemia (D75.1)
     Primary polycythemia. Secondary polycythemia is D75.1. Check your documentation. Polycythemia is caused by too many red blood cells, which increase the thickness of blood (viscosity). This can cause engorgement of the spleen (splenomegaly) with extra RBCs and potential clot formation.

● **D46** Myelodysplastic syndromes
     Use additional code for adverse effect, if applicable, to identify drug (T36-T50 with fifth or sixth character 5)
     Excludes2   drug-induced aplastic anemia (D61.1)
     D46.0 Refractory anemia without ring sideroblasts, so stated 🩺
         Refractory anemia without sideroblasts, without excess of blasts
     D46.1 Refractory anemia with ring sideroblasts RARS 🩺
● **D46.2** Refractory anemia with excess of blasts [RAEB]
         Form of myelodysplasia with increased immature white blood cells (blasts) in bone marrow
         D46.20 Refractory anemia with excess of blasts, unspecified RAEB NOS 🩺
         D46.21 Refractory anemia with excess of blasts 1 RAEB 1 🩺
             Bone marrow disease which results in insufficient RBCs (anemia) in which level of blasts is less than 10%
         D46.22 Refractory anemia with excess of blasts 2 RAEB 2 🩺 🩺
             Bone marrow disease manifested by insufficient numbers of RBCs (anemia) with level of blasts 10-20%
         (Ex) See PDX Collection 488
     D46.A Refractory cytopenia with multilineage dysplasia 🩺
     D46.B Refractory cytopenia with multilineage dysplasia and ring sideroblasts 🩺
         RCMD RS
     D46.C Myelodysplastic syndrome with isolated del(5q) chromosomal abnormality 🩺 🩺
         Myelodysplastic syndrome with 5q deletion
         5q minus syndrome NOS
         (Ex) See PDX Collection 488
     D46.4 Refractory anemia, unspecified 🩺
     D46.Z Other myelodysplastic syndromes 🩺
         Excludes1   chronic myelomonocytic leukemia (C93.1-)
     D46.9 Myelodysplastic syndrome, unspecified 🩺
         Myelodysplasia NOS

● **D47** Other neoplasms of uncertain behavior of lymphoid, hematopoietic and related tissue
● **D47.0** Mast cell neoplasms of uncertain behavior
     Excludes1   congenital cutaneous mastocytosis (Q82.2)
         histiocytic neoplasms of uncertain behavior (D47.Z9)
         malignant mast cell neoplasm (C96.2-)
     (Ex) **For category D47.0 CC codes:** See PDX Collection 494
     D47.01 Cutaneous mastocytosis 🩺
         Diffuse cutaneous mastocytosis
         Maculopapular cutaneous mastocytosis
         Solitary mastocytoma
         Telangiectasia macularis eruptiva perstans
         Urticaria pigmentosa
         Excludes1   congenital (diffuse) (maculopapular) cutaneous mastocytosis (Q82.2)
             congenital urticaria pigmentosa (Q82.2)
             extracutaneous mastocytoma (D47.09)

CHAPTER 2 (C00-D49)

N Newborn Age: 0   **P** Pediatric Age: 0–17   **M** Maternity DX: 9–64   **A** Adult Age: 15–124   ♀ Females Only   ♂ Males Only

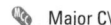 Complication\Comorbidity   🩺 Major C\C   (Ex) CC/MCC Exclusions   🩺 Hospital-Acquired Condition   🩺 Hierarchical Condition Category

731

D47.02 **Systemic mastocytosis**
Indolent systemic mastocytosis
Isolated bone marrow mastocytosis
Smoldering systemic mastocytosis
Systemic mastocytosis, with an associated hematological non-mast cell lineage disease (SM-AHNMD)
Code also if applicable, any associated hematological non-mast cell lineage disease, such as:
acute myeloid leukemia (C92.6-, C92.A-)
chronic myelomonocytic leukemia (C93.1-)
essential thrombocytosis (D47.3)
hypereosinophilic syndrome (D72.1)
myelodysplastic syndrome (D46.9)
myeloproliferative syndrome (D47.1)
non-Hodgkin lymphoma (C82-C85)
plasma cell myeloma (C90.0-)
polycythemia vera (D45)
Excludes1   aggressive systemic mastocytosis (C96.21)
mast cell leukemia (C94.3-)

D47.09 **Other mast cell neoplasms of uncertain behavior**
Extracutaneous mastocytoma
Mast cell tumor NOS
Mastocytoma NOS
Mastocytosis NOS

D47.1 **Chronic myeloproliferative disease**
Chronic neutrophilic leukemia
Myeloproliferative disease, unspecified
Excludes1   atypical chronic myeloid leukemia BCR/ABL-negative (C92.2-)
chronic myeloid leukemia BCR/ABL-positive (C92.1-)
myelofibrosis NOS (D75.81)
myelophthisic anemia (D61.82)
myelophthisis (D61.82)
secondary myelofibrosis NOS (D75.81)
(Ex:) See PDX Collection 488

D47.2 **Monoclonal gammopathy**
Monoclonal gammopathy of undetermined significance [MGUS]

D47.3 **Essential (hemorrhagic) thrombocythemia**
Essential thrombocytosis
Idiopathic hemorrhagic thrombocythemia
▶Primary thrombocytosis
Excludes2   reactive thrombocytosis (D75.838)
▶secondary thrombocytosis (D75.838)
▶thrombocythemia NOS (D75.839)
▶thrombocytosis NOS (D75.839)

D47.4 **Osteomyelofibrosis**
Chronic idiopathic myelofibrosis
Myelofibrosis (idiopathic) (with myeloid metaplasia)
Myelosclerosis (megakaryocytic) with myeloid metaplasia
Secondary myelofibrosis in myeloproliferative disease
Excludes1   acute myelofibrosis (C94.4-)

●D47.Z **Other specified neoplasms of uncertain behavior of lymphoid, hematopoietic and related tissue**
●D47.Z1 **Post-transplant lymphoproliferative disorder (PTLD)**
Code first complications of transplanted organs and tissue (T86.-)
(Ex:) See PDX Collection 495

D47.Z2 **Castleman disease**
➡Code also if applicable, human herpesvirus 8 infection (B10.89)
Excludes2   Kaposi's sarcoma (C46.-)
(Ex:) See PDX Collection 488
Coding Clinic: 2016, Q4, P8

D47.Z9 **Other specified neoplasms of uncertain behavior of lymphoid, hematopoietic and related tissue**
Histiocytic tumors of uncertain behavior
(Ex:) See PDX Collection 488

D47.9 **Neoplasm of uncertain behavior of lymphoid, hematopoietic and related tissue, unspecified**
Lymphoproliferative disease NOS
(Ex:) See PDX Collection 488

●D48 **Neoplasm of uncertain behavior of other and unspecified sites**
Excludes1   neurofibromatosis (nonmalignant) (Q85.0-)

D48.0 **Neoplasm of uncertain behavior of bone and articular cartilage**
Excludes1   neoplasm of uncertain behavior of cartilage of ear (D48.1)
neoplasm of uncertain behavior of cartilage of larynx (D38.0)
neoplasm of uncertain behavior of cartilage of nose (D38.5)
neoplasm of uncertain behavior of connective tissue of eyelid (D48.1)
neoplasm of uncertain behavior of synovia (D48.1)

D48.1 **Neoplasm of uncertain behavior of connective and other soft tissue**
Neoplasm of uncertain behavior of connective tissue of ear
Neoplasm of uncertain behavior of connective tissue of eyelid
Stromal tumors of uncertain behavior of digestive system
Excludes1   neoplasm of uncertain behavior of articular cartilage (D48.0)
neoplasm of uncertain behavior of cartilage of larynx (D38.0)
neoplasm of uncertain behavior of cartilage of nose (D38.5)
neoplasm of uncertain behavior of connective tissue of breast (D48.6-)

D48.2 **Neoplasm of uncertain behavior of peripheral nerves and autonomic nervous system**
Excludes1   neoplasm of uncertain behavior of peripheral nerves of orbit (D48.7)

D48.3 **Neoplasm of uncertain behavior of retroperitoneum**

D48.4 **Neoplasm of uncertain behavior of peritoneum**

D48.5 **Neoplasm of uncertain behavior of skin**
Neoplasm of uncertain behavior of anal margin
Neoplasm of uncertain behavior of anal skin
Neoplasm of uncertain behavior of perianal skin
Neoplasm of uncertain behavior of skin of breast
Excludes1   neoplasm of uncertain behavior of anus NOS (D37.8)
neoplasm of uncertain behavior of skin of genital organs (D39.8, D40.8)
neoplasm of uncertain behavior of vermilion border of lip (D37.0)

●D48.6 **Neoplasm of uncertain behavior of breast**
Neoplasm of uncertain behavior of connective tissue of breast
Cystosarcoma phyllodes
Excludes1   neoplasm of uncertain behavior of skin of breast (D48.5)

D48.60 **Neoplasm of uncertain behavior of unspecified breast**

D48.61 **Neoplasm of uncertain behavior of right breast**

D48.62 **Neoplasm of uncertain behavior of left breast**

D48.7 **Neoplasm of uncertain behavior of** other specified sites
 Neoplasm of uncertain behavior of eye
 Neoplasm of uncertain behavior of heart
 Neoplasm of uncertain behavior of peripheral nerves
  of orbit
 Excludes1 neoplasm of uncertain behavior of
   connective tissue (D48.1)
  neoplasm of uncertain behavior of skin of
   eyelid (D48.5)

D48.9 **Neoplasm of uncertain behavior,** unspecified

● D49 **Neoplasms of** unspecified behavior
 Note: Category D49 classifies by site neoplasms of unspecified
  morphology and behavior. The term "mass," unless
  otherwise stated, is not to be regarded as a neoplastic growth.
 Includes 'growth' NOS
   neoplasm NOS
   new growth NOS
   tumor NOS
 Excludes1 neoplasms of uncertain behavior (D37-D44, D48)

D49.0 **Neoplasm of unspecified behavior of** digestive system
 Excludes1 neoplasm of unspecified behavior of
   margin of anus (D49.2)
  neoplasm of unspecified behavior of
   perianal skin (D49.2)
  neoplasm of unspecified behavior of skin
   of anus (D49.2)

D49.1 **Neoplasm of unspecified behavior of** respiratory system

D49.2 **Neoplasm of unspecified behavior of** bone, soft tissue,
 and skin
 Excludes1 neoplasm of unspecified behavior of anal
   canal (D49.0)
  neoplasm of unspecified behavior of anus
   NOS (D49.0)
  neoplasm of unspecified behavior of bone
   marrow (D49.89)
  neoplasm of unspecified behavior of
   cartilage of larynx (D49.1)
  neoplasm of unspecified behavior of
   cartilage of nose (D49.1)
  neoplasm of unspecified behavior of
   connective tissue of breast (D49.3)
  neoplasm of unspecified behavior of skin
   of genital organs (D49.59)
  neoplasm of unspecified behavior of
   vermilion border of lip (D49.0)

D49.3 **Neoplasm of unspecified behavior of** breast
 Excludes1 neoplasm of unspecified behavior of skin
   of breast (D49.2)

D49.4 **Neoplasm of unspecified behavior of** bladder

● D49.5 **Neoplasm of unspecified behavior of** other
 genitourinary organs
 ● D49.51 **Neoplasm of unspecified behavior of** kidney
  D49.511 **Neoplasm of unspecified behavior of**
    right kidney
    Coding Clinic: 2016, Q4, P9
  D49.512 **Neoplasm of unspecified behavior of**
    left kidney
    Coding Clinic: 2016, Q4, P9
  D49.519 **Neoplasm of unspecified behavior of**
    unspecified kidney
    Coding Clinic: 2016, Q4, P9
 D49.59 **Neoplasm of unspecified behavior of** other
   genitourinary organ
   Coding Clinic: 2016, Q4, P9

D49.6 **Neoplasm of unspecified behavior of** brain 🐾
 Excludes1 neoplasm of unspecified behavior of
   cerebral meninges (D49.7)
  neoplasm of unspecified behavior of
   cranial nerves (D49.7)

D49.7 **Neoplasm of unspecified behavior of** endocrine glands
 and other parts of nervous system
 Excludes1 neoplasm of unspecified behavior
   of peripheral, sympathetic, and
   parasympathetic nerves and ganglia
   (D49.2)

● D49.8 **Neoplasm of unspecified behavior of** other specified
 sites
 Excludes1 neoplasm of unspecified behavior of
   eyelid (skin) (D49.2)
  neoplasm of unspecified behavior of
   eyelid cartilage (D49.2)
  neoplasm of unspecified behavior of great
   vessels (D49.2)
  neoplasm of unspecified behavior of optic
   nerve (D49.7)
 D49.81 **Neoplasm of unspecified behavior of** retina and
   choroid
   Dark area on retina
   Retinal freckle
 D49.89 **Neoplasm of unspecified behavior of** other
   specified sites

D49.9 **Neoplasm of unspecified behavior of** unspecified site

CHAPTER 2 (C00-D49)

3. Chapter 3: Disease of the blood and blood-forming organs and certain disorders involving the immune mechanism (D50-D89)
Reserved for future guideline expansion

CHAPTER 3

DISEASES OF THE BLOOD AND BLOOD-FORMING ORGANS AND CERTAIN DISORDERS INVOLVING THE IMMUNE MECHANISM (D50-D89)

Excludes2   autoimmune disease (systemic) NOS (M35.9)
certain conditions originating in the perinatal period (P00-P96)
complications of pregnancy, childbirth and the puerperium (O00-O9A)
congenital malformations, deformations and chromosomal abnormalities (Q00-Q99)
endocrine, nutritional and metabolic diseases (E00-E88)
human immunodeficiency virus [HIV] disease (B20)
injury, poisoning and certain other consequences of external causes (S00-T88)
neoplasms (C00-D49)
symptoms, signs and abnormal clinical and laboratory findings, not elsewhere classified (R00-R94)

This chapter contains the following blocks:

D50-D53	Nutritional anemias
D55-D59	Hemolytic anemias
D60-D64	Aplastic and other anemias and other bone marrow failure syndromes
D65-D69	Coagulation defects, purpura and other hemorrhagic conditions
D70-D77	Other disorders of blood and blood-forming organs
D78	Intraoperative and postprocedural complications of the spleen
D80-D89	Certain disorders involving the immune mechanism

NUTRITIONAL ANEMIAS (D50-D53)

● **D50   Iron deficiency anemia**
A disease characterized by a decrease in the number of red cells (hemoglobin) in the blood.

Includes   asiderotic anemia
hypochromic anemia

D50.0   Iron deficiency anemia secondary to blood loss (chronic)
Posthemorrhagic anemia (chronic)

Excludes1   acute posthemorrhagic anemia (D62)
congenital anemia from fetal blood loss (P61.3)
Coding Clinic: 2019, Q3, P17

D50.1   Sideropenic dysphagia
Weblike growth of membranes in throat that makes swallowing difficult
Kelly-Paterson syndrome
Plummer-Vinson syndrome

D50.8   Other iron deficiency anemias
Iron deficiency anemia due to inadequate dietary iron intake

D50.9   Iron deficiency anemia, unspecified

● **D51   Vitamin B12 deficiency anemia**
Excludes1   vitamin B12 deficiency (E53.8)

D51.0   Vitamin B12 deficiency anemia due to intrinsic factor deficiency
Addison anemia
Biermer anemia
Pernicious (congenital) anemia
Congenital intrinsic factor deficiency

D51.1   Vitamin B12 deficiency anemia due to selective vitamin B12 malabsorption with proteinuria
Imerslund (Gräsbeck) syndrome
Megaloblastic hereditary anemia

D51.2   Transcobalamin II deficiency

D51.3   Other dietary vitamin B12 deficiency anemia
Vegan anemia

D51.8   Other vitamin B12 deficiency anemias

D51.9   Vitamin B12 deficiency anemia, unspecified

● **D52   Folate deficiency anemia**
Excludes1   folate deficiency without anemia (E53.8)

D52.0   Dietary folate deficiency anemia
Nutritional megaloblastic anemia

D52.1   Drug-induced folate deficiency anemia
Use additional code for adverse effect, if applicable, to identify drug (T36-T50 with fifth or sixth character 5)

D52.8   Other folate deficiency anemias

D52.9   Folate deficiency anemia, unspecified
Folic acid deficiency anemia NOS

● **D53   Other nutritional anemias**
Includes   megaloblastic anemia unresponsive to vitamin B12 or folate therapy

D53.0   Protein deficiency anemia
Amino-acid deficiency anemia
Orotaciduric anemia
Excludes1   Lesch-Nyhan syndrome (E79.1)

D53.1   Other megaloblastic anemias, not elsewhere classified
Megaloblastic anemia NOS
Excludes1   Di Guglielmo's disease (C94.0)

D53.2   Scorbutic anemia
Anemia resulting from deficiency of ascorbic acid (vitamin C)
Excludes1   scurvy (E54)

D53.8   Other specified nutritional anemias
Anemia associated with deficiency of copper
Anemia associated with deficiency of molybdenum
Anemia associated with deficiency of zinc
Excludes1   nutritional deficiencies without anemia, such as:
copper deficiency NOS (E61.0)
molybdenum deficiency NOS (E61.5)
zinc deficiency NOS (E60)

D53.9   Nutritional anemia, unspecified
Simple chronic anemia
Excludes1   anemia NOS (D64.9)
Coding Clinic: 2018, Q4, P88

HEMOLYTIC ANEMIAS (D55-D59)

● **D55   Anemia due to enzyme disorders**
Excludes1   drug-induced enzyme deficiency anemia (D59.2)

D55.0   Anemia due to glucose-6-phosphate dehydrogenase [G6PD] deficiency 🔗
Favism
G6PD deficiency anemia
Excludes1   glucose-6-phosphate dehydrogenase (G6PD) deficiency without anemia (D75.A)

D55.1   Anemia due to other disorders of glutathione metabolism 🔗
Anemia (due to) enzyme deficiencies, except G6PD, related to the hexose monophosphate [HMP] shunt pathway
Anemia (due to) hemolytic nonspherocytic (hereditary), type I

▶ New   ◀ Revised   deleted Deleted   Excludes 1   Excludes 2   Includes   Use additional   Code first   Code also   Key words
OGCR Official Guidelines   ● Unacceptable Principal Diagnosis   X Assign placeholder X   ● Use Additional Character(s)   ▶ Manifestation Code   Coding Clinic

● **D55.2   Anemia due to disorders of glycolytic enzymes** 🅗
    ~~Hemolytic nonspherocytic (hereditary) anemia, type II~~
    ~~Hexokinase deficiency anemia~~
    ~~Pyruvate kinase [PK] deficiency anemia~~
    ~~Triose-phosphate isomerase deficiency anemia~~

   ▶ **D55.21 Anemia due to pyruvate kinase deficiency**
      ▶ PK deficiency anemia
      ▶ Pyruvate kinase deficiency anemia

   ▶ **D55.29 Anemia due to other disorders of glycolytic enzymes**
      ▶ Hexokinase deficiency anemia
      ▶ Triose-phosphate isomerase deficiency anemia

     Excludes1   disorders of glycolysis not associated with anemia (E74.81-)

● **D55.3   Anemia due to disorders of nucleotide metabolism** 🅗

● **D55.8   Other anemias due to enzyme disorders** 🅗

● **D55.9   Anemia due to enzyme disorder, unspecified** 🅗

● **D56   Thalassemia**
Hereditary disorders characterized by low production of hemoglobin or excessive destruction of red blood cells

     Excludes1   sickle-cell thalassemia (D57.4-)

D56.0   Alpha thalassemia 🅗
    Alpha thalassemia major
    Hemoglobin H Constant Spring
    Hemoglobin H disease
    Hydrops fetalis due to alpha thalassemia
    Severe alpha thalassemia
    Triple gene defect alpha thalassemia

    Use additional code, if applicable, for hydrops fetalis due to alpha thalassemia (P56.99)

     Excludes1   alpha thalassemia trait or minor (D56.3)
         asymptomatic alpha thalassemia (D56.3)
         hydrops fetalis due to isoimmunization (P56.0)
         hydrops fetalis not due to immune hemolysis (P83.2)

D56.1   Beta thalassemia 🅗
    Beta thalassemia major
    Cooley's anemia
    Homozygous beta thalassemia
    Severe beta thalassemia
    Thalassemia intermedia
    Thalassemia major

     Excludes1   beta thalassemia minor (D56.3)
         beta thalassemia trait (D56.3)
         delta-beta thalassemia (D56.2)
         hemoglobin E-beta thalassemia (D56.5)
         sickle-cell beta thalassemia (D57.4-)

D56.2   Delta-beta thalassemia 🅗
    Homozygous delta-beta thalassemia

     Excludes1   delta-beta thalassemia minor (D56.3)
         delta-beta thalassemia trait (D56.3)

D56.3   Thalassemia minor
Genetic disorders that have in common defective production of hemoglobin
    Alpha thalassemia minor
    Alpha thalassemia silent carrier
    Alpha thalassemia trait
    Beta thalassemia minor
    Beta thalassemia trait
    Delta-beta thalassemia minor
    Delta-beta thalassemia trait
    Thalassemia trait NOS

     Excludes1   alpha thalassemia (D56.0)
         beta thalassemia (D56.1)
         delta-beta thalassemia (D56.2)
         hemoglobin E-beta thalassemia (D56.5)
         sickle-cell trait (D57.3)

D56.4   Hereditary persistence of fetal hemoglobin [HPFH] 🅗
Persistent production of hemoglobin

D56.5   Hemoglobin E-beta thalassemia 🅗
     Excludes1   beta thalassemia (D56.1)
         beta thalassemia minor (D56.3)
         beta thalassemia trait (D56.3)
         delta-beta thalassemia (D56.2)
         delta-beta thalassemia trait (D56.3)
         hemoglobin E disease (D58.2)
         other hemoglobinopathies (D58.2)
         sickle-cell beta thalassemia (D57.4-)

D56.8   Other thalassemias 🅗
    Dominant thalassemia
    Hemoglobin C thalassemia
    Mixed thalassemia
    Thalassemia with other hemoglobinopathy

     Excludes1   hemoglobin C disease (D58.2)
         hemoglobin E disease (D58.2)
         other hemoglobinopathies (D58.2)
         sickle cell anemia (D57.-)
         sickle cell thalassemia (D57.4)

D56.9   Thalassemia, unspecified
    Mediterranean anemia (with other hemoglobinopathy)

● **D57   Sickle-cell disorders**
Inherited disease in which red blood cells, normally disc-shaped, become crescent shaped

    Use additional code for any associated fever (R50.81)

     Excludes1   other hemoglobinopathies (D58.-)

● **D57.0   Hb-SS disease with crisis**
    Sickle-cell disease with crisis
    Hb-SS disease with vasoocclusive pain

   D57.00   Hb-SS disease with crisis, unspecified 🅗🅗
     Hb-SS disease with (painful) crisis NOS
     Hb-SS disease with vasoocclusive pain NOS
     Ⓔⓧ See PDX Collection 4027

   D57.01   Hb-SS disease with acute chest syndrome 🅗🅗
     Ⓔⓧ See PDX Collection 4027

   D57.02   Hb-SS disease with splenic sequestration 🅗🅗
     Ⓔⓧ See PDX Collection 4027

   D57.03   Hb-SS disease with cerebral vascular involvement 🅗
     Code also, if applicable, cerebral infarction (I63.-)
     Ⓔⓧ See PDX Collection 4028

   D57.09   Hb-SS disease with crisis with other specified complication 🅗
     Use additional code to identify complications, such as:
      cholelithiasis (K80.-)
      priapism (N48.32)
     Ⓔⓧ See PDX Collection 4028

D57.1   Sickle-cell disease without crisis Hb-SS disease without crisis 🅗
    Sickle-cell anemia NOS
    Sickle-cell disease NOS
    Sickle-cell disorder NOS

● **D57.2   Sickle-cell/Hb-C disease**
    Hb-SC disease
    Hb-S/Hb-C disease

   D57.20   Sickle-cell/Hb-C disease without crisis 🅗

●   **D57.21   Sickle-cell/Hb-C disease with crisis**

   D57.211   Sickle-cell/Hb-C disease with acute chest syndrome 🅗 🅗🅗
     CC when PDX is its own CC
     Ⓔⓧ See PDX Collection 4027

   D57.212   Sickle-cell/Hb-C disease with splenic sequestration 🅗🅗
     Ⓔⓧ See PDX Collection 4027

   D57.213   Sickle-cell/Hb-C disease with cerebral vascular involvement 🅗
     Code also, if applicable, cerebral infarction (I63.-)
     Ⓔⓧ See PDX Collection 4074

N Newborn Age: 0   **P** Pediatric Age: 0–17   **M** Maternity DX: 9–64   **A** Adult Age: 15–124   ♀ Females Only   ♂ Males Only

🅗 Complication\Comorbidity   🅗 Major C\C   Ⓔⓧ CC/MCC Exclusions   🅗 Hospital-Acquired Condition   🅗 Hierarchical Condition Category

735

D57.218 Sickle-cell/Hb-C disease with crisis with other specified complication 🔑
Use additional code to identify complications, such as:
cholelithiasis (K80.-)
priapism (N48.32)
Ex: See PDX Collection 4074

D57.219 Sickle-cell/Hb-C disease with crisis, unspecified 🔑🔑
Sickle-cell/Hb-C disease with crisis NOS
Sickle-cell/Hb-C disease with vasoocclusive pain NOS
Ex: See PDX Collection 4027

D57.3 Sickle-cell trait 🔑
Hb-S trait
Heterozygous hemoglobin S

● **D57.4 Sickle-cell thalassemia**
Sickle-cell beta thalassemia
Thalassemia Hb-S disease

D57.40 Sickle-cell thalassemia without crisis 🔑
Microdrepanocytosis
Sickle-cell thalassemia NOS

● **D57.41 Sickle-cell thalassemia, unspecified, with crisis**
Sickle-cell "crisis" is precipitated when abnormally crescent-shaped red blood cells form clots and interrupt blood flow to major organs, causing severe pain and organ damage.
Sickle-cell thalassemia with (painful) crisis NOS
Sickle-cell thalassemia with vasoocclusive pain NOS

D57.411 Sickle-cell thalassemia, unspecified, with acute chest syndrome 🔑🔑🔑
CC when PDX is its own CC
Ex: See PDX Collection 4027

D57.412 Sickle-cell thalassemia with, unspecified, splenic sequestration 🔑🔑
Ex: See PDX Collection 4027

D57.413 Sickle-cell thalassemia, unspecified, with cerebral vascular involvement 🔑
Code also, if applicable cerebral infarction (I63.-)
Ex: See PDX Collection 4058

D57.418 Sickle-cell thalassemia, unspecified, with crisis with other specified complication 🔑
Use additional code to identify complications, such as:
cholelithiasis (K80.-)
priapism (N48.32)
Ex: See PDX Collection 4058

D57.419 Sickle-cell thalassemia with, unspecified, crisis 🔑🔑
Sickle-cell thalassemia with (painful) crisis NOS
⟹ Sickle-cell thalassemia with vasoocclusive pain NOS
Ex: See PDX Collection 4027

D57.42 Sickle-cell thalassemia beta zero without crisis
HbS-beta zero without crisis
Sickle-cell beta zero without crisis

● **D57.43 Sickle-cell thalassemia beta zero with crisis**
HbS-beta zero with crisis
Sickle-cell beta zero with crisis

D57.431 Sickle-cell thalassemia beta zero with acute chest syndrome 🔑
HbS-beta zero with acute chest syndrome
Sickle-cell beta zero with acute chest syndrome
Ex: See PDX Collection 4058

D57.432 Sickle-cell thalassemia beta zero with splenic sequestration 🔑
HbS-beta zero with splenic sequestration
Sickle-cell beta zero with splenic sequestration
Ex: See PDX Collection 4058

D57.433 Sickle-cell thalassemia beta zero with cerebral vascular involvement 🔑
HbS-beta zero with cerebral vascular involvement
Sickle-cell beta zero with cerebral vascular involvement
Code also, if applicable cerebral infarction (I63.-)
Ex: See PDX Collection 4058

D57.438 Sickle-cell thalassemia beta zero with crisis with other specified complication 🔑
HbS-beta zero with other specified complication
Sickle-cell beta zero with other specified complication
Use additional code to identify complications, such as:
cholelithiasis (K80.-)
priapism (N48.32)
Ex: See PDX Collection 4058

D57.439 Sickle-cell thalassemia beta zero with crisis, unspecified 🔑
HbS-beta zero with other specified complication
Sickle-cell beta zero with crisis unspecified
Sickle-cell thalassemia beta zero with (painful) crisis NOS
⟹ Sickle-cell thalassemia beta zero with vasoocclusive pain NOS
Ex: See PDX Collection 4058

D57.44 Sickle-cell thalassemia beta plus without crisis
HbS-beta plus without crisis
Sickle-cell beta plus without crisis

● **D57.45 Sickle-cell thalassemia beta plus with crisis**
HbS-beta plus with crisis
Sickle-cell beta plus with crisis

D57.451 Sickle-cell thalassemia beta plus with acute chest syndrome 🔑
HbS-beta plus with acute chest syndrome
Sickle-cell beta plus with acute chest syndrome
Ex: See PDX Collection 4058

D57.452 Sickle-cell thalassemia beta plus with splenic sequestration 🔑
HbS-beta plus with splenic sequestration
Sickle-cell beta plus with splenic sequestration
Ex: See PDX Collection 4058

D57.453 Sickle-cell thalassemia beta plus with cerebral vascular involvement 🔑
HbS-beta plus with cerebral vascular involvement
Sickle-cell beta plus with cerebral vascular involvement
Code also, if applicable cerebral infarction (I63.-)
Ex: See PDX Collection 4058

▶ New   ⟹ Revised   ~~deleted~~ Deleted   Excludes 1   Excludes 2   Includes   Use additional   Code first   Code also   Key words
OGCR Official Guidelines   ● Unacceptable Principal Diagnosis   X Assign placeholder X   ● Use Additional Character(s)   ▶ Manifestation Code   **Coding Clinic**

D57.458 **Sickle-cell thalassemia beta plus with crisis with other specified complication**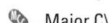
    HbS-beta plus with crisis with other specified complication
    Sickle-cell beta plus with crisis with other specified complication

    Use additional code to identify complications, such as:
        cholelithiasis (K80.-)
        priapism (N48.32)
    (Ex:) See PDX Collection 4058

D57.459 **Sickle-cell thalassemia beta plus with crisis, unspecified**
    HbS-beta plus with crisis with unspecified complication
    Sickle-cell beta plus with crisis with unspecified complication
    Sickle-cell thalassemia beta plus with (painful) crisis NOS
    ⟶Sickle-cell thalassemia beta plus with vasoocclusive pain NOS
    (Ex:) See PDX Collection 4058

● **D57.8 Other sickle-cell disorders**
    Hb-SD disease
    Hb-SE disease

    D57.80 **Other sickle-cell disorders without crisis**
    ● D57.81 **Other sickle-cell disorders with crisis**
        D57.811 **Other sickle-cell disorders with acute chest syndrome**
            (Ex:) See PDX Collection 4027
        D57.812 **Other sickle-cell disorders with splenic sequestration**
            (Ex:) See PDX Collection 4027
        D57.813 **Other sickle-cell disorders with cerebral vascular involvement**
            Code also, if applicable: cerebral infarction (I63.-)
            (Ex:) See PDX Collection 4028
        D57.818 **Other sickle-cell disorders with crisis with other specified complication**
            Use additional code to identify complications, such as:
                cholelithiasis (K80.-)
                priapism (N48.32)
            (Ex:) See PDX Collection 4028
        D57.819 **Other sickle-cell disorders with crisis, unspecified**
            Other sickle-cell disorders with crisis NOS
            Other sickle-cell disorders with vasoocclusive pain NOS
            (Ex:) See PDX Collection 4027

● **D58 Other hereditary hemolytic anemias**
    Genetic condition in which bone marrow is unable to compensate for premature destruction of red blood cells

    Excludes1   hemolytic anemia of the newborn (P55.-)

    D58.0 **Hereditary spherocytosis**
        Presence of spherocytes (spherically shaped red blood cells)
        Acholuric (familial) jaundice
        Congenital (spherocytic) hemolytic icterus
        Minkowski-Chauffard syndrome
    D58.1 **Hereditary elliptocytosis**
        Presence of large numbers of elliptocytes in blood
        Elliptocytosis (congenital)
        Ovalocytosis (congenital) (hereditary)

D58.2 **Other hemoglobinopathies**
    Abnormal hemoglobin NOS
    Congenital Heinz body anemia
    Hb-C disease
    Hb-D disease
    Hb-E disease
    Hemoglobinopathy NOS
    Unstable hemoglobin hemolytic disease

    Excludes1   familial polycythemia (D75.0)
                Hb-M disease (D74.0)
                hemoglobin E-beta thalassemia (D56.5)
                hereditary persistence of fetal hemoglobin [HPFH] (D56.4)
                high-altitude polycythemia (D75.1)
                methemoglobinemia (D74.-)
                other hemoglobinopathies with thalassemia (D56.8)

D58.8 **Other specified hereditary hemolytic anemias**
    Stomatocytosis
    (Ex:) See PDX Collection 497

D58.9 **Hereditary hemolytic anemia, unspecified**
    (Ex:) See PDX Collection 497

● **D59 Acquired hemolytic anemia**

    D59.0 **Drug-induced autoimmune hemolytic anemia**
        Use additional code for adverse effect, if applicable, to identify drug (T36-T50 with fifth or sixth character 5)
        (Ex:) See PDX Collection 4029

    D59.1 **Other autoimmune hemolytic anemias**
        Excludes2   Evans syndrome (D69.41)
                    hemolytic disease of newborn (P55.-)
                    paroxysmal cold hemoglobinuria (D59.6)

        D59.10 **Autoimmune hemolytic anemia, unspecified**
            (Ex:) See PDX Collection 4029
        D59.11 **Warm autoimmune hemolytic anemia**
            Warm type (primary) (secondary) (symptomatic) autoimmune hemolytic anemia
            Warm type autoimmune hemolytic disease
            (Ex:) See PDX Collection 4029
        D59.12 **Cold autoimmune hemolytic anemia**
            Chronic cold hemagglutinin disease
            Cold agglutinin disease
            Cold agglutinin hemoglobinuria
            Cold type (primary) (secondary) (symptomatic) autoimmune hemolytic anemia
            Cold type autoimmune hemolytic disease
            (Ex:) See PDX Collection 4029
        D59.13 **Mixed type autoimmune hemolytic anemia**
            Mixed type autoimmune hemolytic disease
            Mixed type, cold and warm, (primary) (secondary) (symptomatic) autoimmune hemolyticanemia
            (Ex:) See PDX Collection 4029
        D59.19 **Other autoimmune hemolytic anemia**
            (Ex:) See PDX Collection 4029

    D59.2 **Drug-induced nonautoimmune hemolytic anemia**
        Drug-induced enzyme deficiency anemia
        Use additional code for adverse effect, if applicable, to identify drug (T36-T50 with fifth or sixth character 5)
        (Ex:) See PDX Collection 4032

    D59.3 **Hemolytic-uremic syndrome**
        Use additional code to identify associated:
            E. coli infection (B96.2-)
            Pneumococcal pneumonia (J13)
            Shigella dysenteriae (A03.9)
        (Ex:) See PDX Collection 4032

    D59.4 **Other nonautoimmune hemolytic anemias**
        Mechanical hemolytic anemia
        Microangiopathic hemolytic anemia
        Toxic hemolytic anemia
        (Ex:) See PDX Collection 4032

CHAPTER 3 (D50-D89)

N Newborn Age: 0   P Pediatric Age: 0–17   M Maternity DX: 9–64   A Adult Age: 15–124   ♀ Females Only   ♂ Males Only

🗨 Complication\Comorbidity   🗨 Major C\C   (Ex:) CC/MCC Exclusions   🗨 Hospital-Acquired Condition   🗨 Hierarchical Condition Category

D59.5 Paroxysmal nocturnal hemoglobinuria [Marchiafava-Micheli] 🔹

    Excludes1   hemoglobinuria NOS (R82.3)

D59.6 Hemoglobinuria due to hemolysis from other external causes 🔹

    Hemoglobinuria from exertion

    March hemoglobinuria

    Paroxysmal cold hemoglobinuria

    Use additional code (Chapter 20) to identify external cause

    Excludes1   hemoglobinuria NOS (R82.3)

D59.8 Other acquired hemolytic anemias 🔹

D59.9 Acquired hemolytic anemia, unspecified 🔹🔹

    Idiopathic hemolytic anemia, chronic

    (Ex:) See PDX Collection 4032

APLASTIC AND OTHER ANEMIAS AND OTHER BONE MARROW FAILURE SYNDROMES (D60-D64)

● **D60 Acquired pure red cell aplasia [erythroblastopenia]**

    Deficiency of erythroblasts

    Includes   red cell aplasia (acquired) (adult) (with thymoma)

    Excludes1   congenital red cell aplasia (D61.01)

    (Ex:) **For category D60 MCC codes:** See PDX Collection 4032

  D60.0 Chronic acquired pure red cell aplasia 🔹🔹

    Lack of development of blood cell

  D60.1 Transient acquired pure red cell aplasia 🔹🔹

  D60.8 Other acquired pure red cell aplasias 🔹🔹

  D60.9 Acquired pure red cell aplasia, unspecified 🔹🔹

● **D61 Other aplastic anemias and other bone marrow failure syndromes**

    Excludes2   neutropenia (D70.-)

  ● **D61.0 Constitutional aplastic anemia**

    Condition where bone marrow is unable to produce blood cells

    D61.01 Constitutional (pure) red blood cell aplasia 🔹🔹

        Blackfan-Diamond syndrome

        Congenital (pure) red cell aplasia

        Familial hypoplastic anemia

        Primary (pure) red cell aplasia

        Red cell (pure) aplasia of infants

        Excludes1   acquired red cell aplasia (D60.9)

        (Ex:) See PDX Collection 498

    D61.09 Other constitutional aplastic anemia 🔹🔹

        Fanconi's anemia

        Pancytopenia with malformations

        (Ex:) See PDX Collection 499

  D61.1 Drug-induced aplastic anemia 🔹🔹

    Use additional code for adverse effect, if applicable, to identify drug (T36-T50 with fifth or sixth character 5)

    (Ex:) See PDX Collection 4032

  D61.2 Aplastic anemia due to other external agents 🔹🔹

    Code first, if applicable, toxic effects of substances chiefly nonmedicinal as to source (T51-T65)

    (Ex:) See PDX Collection 4032

  D61.3 Idiopathic aplastic anemia 🔹🔹

    (Ex:) See PDX Collection 4032

  ● **D61.8 Other specified aplastic anemias and other bone marrow failure syndromes**

    (Ex:) **For category D61.8 CC codes unless otherwise indicated:** See PDX Collection 500

  ● **D61.81 Pancytopenia**

    Marked deficiency of all the blood elements: Red blood cells (erythrocytes), white blood cells (leukocytes), and platelets (thrombocytes). Check laboratory results.

    Excludes1   pancytopenia (due to) (with) aplastic anemia (D61.9)

              pancytopenia (due to) (with) bone marrow infiltration (D61.82)

              pancytopenia (due to) (with) congenital (pure) red cell aplasia (D61.01)

              pancytopenia (due to) (with) hairy cell leukemia (C91.4-)

              pancytopenia (due to) (with) human immunodeficiency virus disease (B20.-)

              pancytopenia (due to) (with) leukoerythroblastic anemia (D61.82)

              pancytopenia (due to) (with) myeloproliferative disease (D47.1)

    Excludes2   pancytopenia (due to) (with) myelodysplastic syndromes (D46.-)

    D61.810 Antineoplastic chemotherapy induced pancytopenia 🔹🔹

        Excludes2   aplastic anemia due to antineoplastic chemotherapy (D61.1)

    D61.811 Other drug-induced pancytopenia 🔹🔹

        Excludes2   aplastic anemia due to drugs (D61.1)

    D61.818 Other pancytopenia 🔹🔹

        Coding Clinic: 2019, Q1, P16

    D61.82 Myelophthisis 🔹🔹

        Leukoerythroblastic anemia

        Myelophthisic anemia

        Panmyelophthisis

        Code also the underlying disorder, such as: malignant neoplasm of breast (C50.-) tuberculosis (A15.-)

        Excludes1   idiopathic myelofibrosis (D47.1) myelofibrosis NOS (D75.81)

              myelofibrosis with myeloid metaplasia (D47.4)

              primary myelofibrosis (D47.1)

              secondary myelofibrosis (D75.81)

    D61.89 Other specified aplastic anemias and other bone marrow failure syndromes 🔹🔹

        (Ex:) See PDX Collection 496

  D61.9 Aplastic anemia, unspecified 🔹🔹

    Hypoplastic anemia NOS

    Medullary hypoplasia

    (Ex:) See PDX Collection 496

D62 Acute posthemorrhagic anemia 🔹

    Excludes1   anemia due to chronic blood loss (D50.0) blood loss anemia NOS (D50.0) congenital anemia from fetal blood loss (P61.3)

    (Ex:) See PDX Collection 501

    Coding Clinic: 2019, Q3, P13,17

▶ New   ⟱ Revised   ~~deleted~~ Deleted   Excludes 1   Excludes 2   Includes   Use additional   Code first   Code also   Key words

OGCR Official Guidelines   ● Unacceptable Principal Diagnosis   X Assign placeholder X   ● Use Additional Character(s)   ▶ Manifestation Code   **Coding Clinic**

● D63 **Anemia in chronic diseases classified elsewhere**
  ▸ *D63.0 Anemia in neoplastic disease*
          Code first neoplasm (C00-D49)
          Excludes1 aplastic anemia due to antineoplastic
                          chemotherapy (D61.1)
          Excludes2 anemia due to antineoplastic
                          chemotherapy (D64.81)

          OGCR Section I.C.2.e.2.

          2) Anemia associated with chemotherapy,
          immunotherapy and radiation therapy
          When the admission/encounter is for management
          of an anemia associated with an adverse effect of the
          administration of chemotherapy or immunotherapy
          and the only treatment is for the anemia, the anemia
          code is sequenced first followed by the appropriate
          codes for the neoplasm and the adverse effect
          (T45.1X5, Adverse effect of antineoplastic and
          immunosuppressive drugs).

  ▸ *D63.1 Anemia in chronic kidney disease*
          Erythropoietin resistant anemia (EPO resistant anemia)
          Code first underlying chronic kidney disease (CKD) (N18.-)
  ▸ *D63.8 Anemia in other chronic diseases classified elsewhere*
          Code first underlying disease, such as:
              diphyllobothriasis (B70.0)
              hookworm disease (B76.0-B76.9)
              hypothyroidism (E00.0-E03.9)
              malaria (B50.0-B54)
              symptomatic late syphilis (A52.79)
              tuberculosis (A18.89)

● D64 **Other anemias**
      Excludes1 refractory anemia (D46.-)
                      refractory anemia with excess blasts in
                          transformation [RAEB T] (C92.0-)
  D64.0 **Hereditary** sideroblastic anemia 🅒
          Abnormal production RBCs (erythrocytes)
          Sex-linked hypochromic sideroblastic anemia
  ▸ *D64.1 Secondary sideroblastic anemia due to disease* 🅒
          Code first underlying disease
  D64.2 Secondary sideroblastic anemia due to drugs and toxins 🅒
          Code first poisoning due to drug or toxin, if applicable
              (T36-T65 with fifth or sixth character 1-4 or 6)
          Use additional code for adverse effect, if applicable, to
              identify drug (T36-T50 with fifth or sixth character 5)
  D64.3 **Other sideroblastic anemias** 🅒
          Sideroblastic anemia NOS
          Pyridoxine-responsive sideroblastic anemia NEC
  D64.4 **Congenital dyserythropoietic anemia**
          Any of several rare hereditary anemias, mostly types of
              macrocytic anemia
          Dyshematopoietic anemia (congenital)
          Excludes1 Blackfan-Diamond syndrome (D61.01)
                          Di Guglielmo's disease (C94.0)
● D64.8 **Other specified anemias**
      D64.81 **Anemia due to antineoplastic chemotherapy**
              Antineoplastic chemotherapy induced anemia
              ~~Excludes1   aplastic anemia due~~
                          ~~to antineoplastic~~
                          ~~chemotherapy (D61.1)~~
              ▸aplastic anemia due to antineoplastic
                  chemotherapy (D61.1)
              Excludes2 anemia in neoplastic disease
                              (D63.0)
      D64.89 **Other specified anemias**
              Infantile pseudoleukemia
  D64.9 **Anemia, unspecified**
          Coding Clinic: 2018, Q4, P88; 2017, Q1, P7

D65 **Disseminated intravascular coagulation [defibrination
      syndrome]** 🅒 🅡
      *Blood clots form and consume all coagulation proteins and platelets
          and disrupt normal coagulation, resulting in abnormal bleeding*
      Afibrinogenemia, acquired
      Consumption coagulopathy
      Diffuse or disseminated intravascular coagulation [DIC]
      Fibrinolytic hemorrhage, acquired
      Fibrinolytic purpura
      Purpura fulminans
      Excludes1 disseminated intravascular coagulation
                      (complicating):
                          abortion or ectopic or molar pregnancy
                              (O00-O07, O08.1)
                          in newborn (P60)
                          pregnancy, childbirth and the puerperium
                              (O45.0, O46.0, O67.0, O72.3)
      (Ex:) See PDX Collection 502
      Coding Clinic: 2021, Q1, P39; 2019, Q2, P25
D66 **Hereditary factor VIII deficiency** 🅒 🅡
      *Inherited coagulation disorder carried by females but most often
          affecting males*
      Classical hemophilia
      Deficiency factor VIII (with functional defect)
      Hemophilia NOS
      Hemophilia A
      Excludes1 factor VIII deficiency with vascular defect (D68.0)
      (Ex:) See PDX Collection 502
D67 **Hereditary factor IX deficiency** 🅒 🅡
      Christmas disease
      Factor IX deficiency (with functional defect)
      Hemophilia B
      Plasma thromboplastin component [PTC] deficiency
      (Ex:) See PDX Collection 502
● D68 **Other coagulation defects**
      Excludes1 abnormal coagulation profile (R79.1)
                      coagulation defects complicating abortion or
                          ectopic or molar pregnancy (O00-O07, O08.1)
                      coagulation defects complicating pregnancy,
                          childbirth and the puerperium (O45.0, O46.0,
                          O67.0, O72.3)
      Coding Clinic: 2016, Q1, P14
      D68.0 **Von Willebrand's disease** 🅒 🅡
              Congenital bleeding disorder
              Angiohemophilia
              Factor VIII deficiency with vascular defect
              Vascular hemophilia
              Excludes1 capillary fragility (hereditary) (D69.8)
                              factor VIII deficiency NOS (D66)
                              factor VIII deficiency with functional
                                  defect (D66)
              (Ex:) See PDX Collection 502
      D68.1 **Hereditary factor XI deficiency** 🅒 🅡
              *Deficiency of blood coagulation resulting in systemic blood-
                  clotting defect*
              Hemophilia C
              Plasma thromboplastin antecedent [PTA] deficiency
              Rosenthal's disease
              (Ex:) See PDX Collection 502
      D68.2 **Hereditary deficiency of other clotting factors** 🅒 🅡
              *Blood clotting disorders caused by hereditary deficiencies of
                  one or more clotting factors*
              AC globulin deficiency
              Congenital afibrinogenemia
              Deficiency of factor I [fibrinogen]
              Deficiency of factor II [prothrombin]
              Deficiency of factor V [labile]
              Deficiency of factor VII [stable]
              Deficiency of factor X [Stuart-Prower]
              Deficiency of factor XII [Hageman]
              Deficiency of factor XIII [fibrin stabilizing]
              Dysfibrinogenemia (congenital)
              Hypoproconvertinemia
              Owren's disease
              Proaccelerin deficiency
              (Ex:) See PDX Collection 502

N Newborn Age: 0   **P** Pediatric Age: 0–17   **M** Maternity DX: 9–64   **A** Adult Age: 15–124   ♀ Females Only   ♂ Males Only

🅒 Complication\Comorbidity   🅜 Major C\C   (Ex:) CC/MCC Exclusions   🅗 Hospital-Acquired Condition   🅡 Hierarchical Condition Category

739

● **D68.3**   **Hemorrhagic disorder due to circulating anticoagulants**
Blood clotting disorders caused by anticoagulants (warfarin and heparin)

● **D68.31**   **Hemorrhagic disorder due to intrinsic circulating anticoagulants, antibodies, or inhibitors**

      D68.311   **Acquired hemophilia** 🔹🔹
Autoimmune hemophilia
Autoimmune inhibitors to clotting factors
Secondary hemophilia
Ⓔ See PDX Collection 503

      D68.312   **Antiphospholipid antibody with hemorrhagic disorder** 🔹🔹
Lupus anticoagulant (LAC) with hemorrhagic disorder
Systemic lupus erythematosus [SLE] inhibitor with hemorrhagic disorder

          Excludes1   antiphospholipid antibody, finding without diagnosis (R76.0)
antiphospholipid antibody syndrome (D68.61)
antiphospholipid antibody with hypercoagulable state (D68.61)
lupus anticoagulant (LAC) finding without diagnosis (R76.0)
lupus anticoagulant (LAC) with hypercoagulable state (D68.62)
systemic lupus erythematosus [SLE] inhibitor finding without diagnosis (R76.0)
systemic lupus erythematosus [SLE] inhibitor with hypercoagulable state (D68.62)
Ⓔ See PDX Collection 504

      D68.318   **Other hemorrhagic disorder due to intrinsic circulating anticoagulants, antibodies, or inhibitors** 🔹🔹
Antithromboplastinemia
Antithromboplastinogenemia
Hemorrhagic disorder due to intrinsic increase in antithrombin
Hemorrhagic disorder due to intrinsic increase in anti-VIIIa
Hemorrhagic disorder due to intrinsic increase in anti-IXa
Hemorrhagic disorder due to intrinsic increase in anti-XIa
Ⓔ See PDX Collection 503

D68.32   **Hemorrhagic disorder due to extrinsic circulating anticoagulants** 🔹🔹
Drug-induced hemorrhagic disorder
Hemorrhagic disorder due to increase in anti-IIa
Hemorrhagic disorder due to increase in anti-Xa
Hyperheparinemia
Use additional code for adverse effect, if applicable, to identify drug (T45.515, T45.525)
Ⓔ See PDX Collection 502
Coding Clinic: 2021, Q1, P5; 2016, Q1, P14-15

D68.4   **Acquired coagulation factor deficiency** 🔹🔹
Deficiency of coagulation factor due to liver disease
Deficiency of coagulation factor due to vitamin K deficiency

    Excludes1   vitamin K deficiency of newborn (P53)
Ⓔ See PDX Collection 502

● **D68.5**   **Primary thrombophilia**
AKA idiopathic thrombocytopenia, may be acquired or congenital and is a common cause of coagulation disorders.
Primary hypercoagulable states

    Excludes1   antiphospholipid syndrome (D68.61)
lupus anticoagulant (D68.62)
secondary activated protein C resistance (D68.69)
secondary antiphospholipid antibody syndrome (D68.69)
secondary lupus anticoagulant with hypercoagulable state (D68.69)
secondary systemic lupus erythematosus [SLE] inhibitor with hypercoagulable state (D68.69)
systemic lupus erythematosus [SLE] inhibitor finding without diagnosis (R76.0)
systemic lupus erythematosus [SLE] inhibitor with hemorrhagic disorder (D68.312)
➠ thrombotic thrombocytopenic purpura (M31.19)
Ⓔ For category D68.5 CC codes: See PDX Collection 505

D68.51   **Activated protein C resistance** 🔹🔹
Factor V Leiden mutation

D68.52   **Prothrombin gene mutation** 🔹🔹

D68.59   **Other primary thrombophilia** 🔹🔹
Antithrombin III deficiency
Hypercoagulable state NOS
Primary hypercoagulable state NEC
Primary thrombophilia NEC
Protein C deficiency
Protein S deficiency
Thrombophilia NOS
▶ **Coding Clinic: 2021, Q2, P8-9**

● **D68.6**   **Other thrombophilia**
Other hypercoagulable states

    Excludes1   diffuse or disseminated intravascular coagulation [DIC] (D65)
heparin induced thrombocytopenia (HIT) (D75.82)
hyperhomocysteinemia (E72.11)
Ⓔ For category D68.6 CC codes: See PDX Collection 505

D68.61   **Antiphospholipid syndrome** 🔹🔹
Anticardiolipin syndrome
Antiphospholipid antibody syndrome

    Excludes1   anti-phospholipid antibody, finding without diagnosis (R76.0)
anti-phospholipid antibody with hemorrhagic disorder (D68.312)
lupus anticoagulant syndrome (D68.62)

▶ New   ➠ Revised   ~~deleted~~ Deleted   Excludes 1   Excludes 2   Includes   Use additional   Code first   Code also   Key words
OGCR Official Guidelines   ● Unacceptable Principal Diagnosis   X Assign placeholder X   ● Use Additional Character(s)   ▶ Manifestation Code   Coding Clinic

D68.62   Lupus anticoagulant syndrome 🔹🔹
    Lupus anticoagulant
    Presence of systemic lupus erythematosus [SLE] inhibitor
> **Excludes1**   anticardiolipin syndrome (D68.61)
>   antiphospholipid syndrome (D68.61)
>   lupus anticoagulant (LAC) finding without diagnosis (R76.0)
>   lupus anticoagulant (LAC) with hemorrhagic disorder (D68.312)

D68.69   Other thrombophilia 🔹🔹
    Hypercoagulable states NEC
    Secondary hypercoagulable state NOS
> ▶ Coding Clinic: 2021, Q2, P8

D68.8   Other specified coagulation defects 🔹🔹
> **Excludes1**   hemorrhagic disease of newborn (P53)

> (Ex:) See PDX Collection 502
> **Coding Clinic: 2021, Q1, P39-40**

D68.9   Coagulation defect, unspecified 🔹🔹
> (Ex:) See PDX Collection 502

● **D69   Purpura and other hemorrhagic conditions**
Group of conditions characterized by small hemorrhages in skin, mucous membranes, or serosal surfaces
> **Excludes1**   benign hypergammaglobulinemic purpura (D89.0)
>   cryoglobulinemic purpura (D89.1)
>   essential (hemorrhagic) thrombocythemia (D47.3)
>   hemorrhagic thrombocythemia (D47.3)
>   purpura fulminans (D65)
>   ⟹ thrombotic thrombocytopenic purpura (M31.19)
>   Waldenström hypergammaglobulinemic purpura (D89.0)

D69.0   Allergic purpura 🔹🔹
    Allergic vasculitis
    Nonthrombocytopenic hemorrhagic purpura
    Nonthrombocytopenic idiopathic purpura
    Purpura anaphylactoid
    Purpura Henoch(-Schönlein)
    Purpura rheumatica
    Vascular purpura
> **Excludes1**   thrombocytopenic hemorrhagic purpura (D69.3)
> (Ex:) See PDX Collection 502

D69.1   Qualitative platelet defects 🔹
    Bernard-Soulier [giant platelet] syndrome
    Glanzmann's disease
    Grey platelet syndrome
    Thromboasthenia (hemorrhagic) (hereditary)
    Thrombocytopathy
> **Excludes1**   von Willebrand's disease (D68.0)

D69.2   Other nonthrombocytopenic purpura 🔹
    Purpura NOS
    Purpura simplex
    Senile purpura

D69.3   Immune thrombocytopenic purpura 🔹🔹
    Hemorrhagic (thrombocytopenic) purpura
    Idiopathic thrombocytopenic purpura
    Tidal platelet dysgenesis
> (Ex:) See PDX Collection 502

● **D69.4   Other primary thrombocytopenia**
> **Excludes1**   transient neonatal thrombocytopenia (P61.0)
>   Wiskott-Aldrich syndrome (D82.0)

D69.41   Evans syndrome 🔹🔹
Acquired hemolytic anemia and thrombocytopenia
> (Ex:) See PDX Collection 502

D69.42   Congenital and hereditary thrombocytopenia purpura 🔹🔹
    Congenital thrombocytopenia
    Hereditary thrombocytopenia
Code first congenital or hereditary disorder, such as:
    thrombocytopenia with absent radius (TAR syndrome) (Q87.2)
> (Ex:) See PDX Collection 502

D69.49   Other primary thrombocytopenia 🔹
    Megakaryocytic hypoplasia
    Primary thrombocytopenia NOS

● **D69.5   Secondary thrombocytopenia**
Acquired reduction of number of platelets required for blood clotting
> **Excludes1**   heparin induced thrombocytopenia (HIT) (D75.82)
>   transient thrombocytopenia of newborn (P61.0)

D69.51   Posttransfusion purpura
    Posttransfusion purpura from whole blood (fresh) or blood products PTP

D69.59   Other secondary thrombocytopenia

D69.6   Thrombocytopenia, unspecified 🔹

D69.8   Other specified hemorrhagic conditions 🔹
    Capillary fragility (hereditary)
    Vascular pseudohemophilia

D69.9   Hemorrhagic condition, unspecified 🔹

OTHER DISORDERS OF BLOOD AND BLOOD-FORMING ORGANS (D70-D77)

● **D70   Neutropenia**
Decrease in number of neutrophils (type of white blood cell)
> **Includes**   agranulocytosis
>   decreased absolute neurophile count (ANC)

Use additional code for any associated:
    fever (R50.81)
    mucositis (J34.81, K12.3-, K92.81, N76.81)
> **Excludes1**   neutropenic splenomegaly (D73.81)
>   transient neonatal neutropenia (P61.5)

D70.0   Congenital agranulocytosis 🔹
Reduced numbers of neutrophils (type of white blood cell)
    Congenital neutropenia
    Infantile genetic agranulocytosis
    Kostmann's disease

D70.1   Agranulocytosis secondary to cancer chemotherapy 🔹
Decreased numbers of granulocytes (type of white blood cell)
Code also underlying neoplasm
Use additional code for adverse effect, if applicable, to identify drug (T45.1X5)

D70.2   Other drug-induced agranulocytosis 🔹
Use additional code for adverse effect, if applicable, to identify drug (T36-T50 with fifth or sixth character 5)

D70.3   Neutropenia due to infection 🔹

D70.4   Cyclic neutropenia 🔹
Chronic neutropenia (low number of type of white blood cell)
    Cyclic hematopoiesis
    Periodic neutropenia

D70.8   Other neutropenia 🔹

D70.9   Neutropenia, unspecified 🔹
> **Coding Clinic: 2019, Q2, P25**

D71   Functional disorders of polymorphonuclear neutrophils 🔹
Polymorphonuclear: varying shapes of nucleus; AKA PMNs
    Cell membrane receptor complex [CR3] defect
    Chronic (childhood) granulomatous disease
    Congenital dysphagocytosis
    Progressive septic granulomatosis

N Newborn Age: 0   **P** Pediatric Age: 0–17   **M** Maternity DX: 9–64   **A** Adult Age: 15–124   ♀ Females Only   ♂ Males Only

🔹 Complication\Comorbidity   🔹 Major C\C   (Ex:) CC/MCC Exclusions   🔹 Hospital-Acquired Condition   🔹 Hierarchical Condition Category   741

CHAPTER 3 (D50-D89)

CHAPTER 3 (D50-D89)

● D72   Other disorders of white blood cells
         Excludes1   basophilia (D72.824)
                     immunity disorders (D80-D89)
                     neutropenia (D70)
                     preleukemia (syndrome) (D46.9)
     D72.0   Genetic anomalies of leukocytes 🔖
             Alder (granulation) (granulocyte) anomaly
             Alder syndrome
             Hereditary leukocytic hypersegmentation
             Hereditary leukocytic hyposegmentation
             Hereditary leukomelanopathy
             May-Hegglin (granulation) (granulocyte) anomaly
             May-Hegglin syndrome
             Pelger-Huët (granulation) (granulocyte) anomaly
             Pelger-Huët syndrome
                 Excludes1   Chédiak (-Steinbrinck)-Higashi syndrome
                             (E70.330)
● D72.1   Eosinophilia
           *Formation and accumulation of high number of white cells in
           blood/tissue*
               Excludes2   Löffler's syndrome (J82.89)
                           pulmonary eosinophilia (J82.-)
       D72.10   Eosinophilia, unspecified
   ● D72.11   Hypereosinophilic syndrome [HES]
           D72.110   Idiopathic hypereosinophilic
                     syndrome [IHES]
           D72.111   Lymphocytic Variant
                     Hypereosinophilic Syndrome [LHES]
                     Lymphocyte variant
                         hypereosinophilia
                     Code also, if applicable, any
                         associated lymphocytic
                         neoplastic disorder
           D72.118   Other hypereosinophilic syndrome
                     Episodic angioedema with
                         eosinophilia
                     Gleich's syndrome
           D72.119   Hypereosinophilic syndrome [HES],
                     unspecified
       D72.12   Drug rash with eosinophilia and systemic
                symptoms syndrome
                DRESS syndrome
                Use additional code for adverse effect, if
                    applicable, to identify drug (T36-T50 with
                    fifth or sixth character 5)
     ▷ D72.18   *Eosinophilia in diseases classified elsewhere*
                Code first underlying disease, such as:
                    chronic myelomonocytic leukemia (C93.1-)
       D72.19   Other eosinophilia
                Familial eosinophilia
                Hereditary eosinophilia
● D72.8   Other specified disorders of white blood cells
           Excludes1   leukemia (C91-C95)
   ● D72.81   Decreased white blood cell count
                 Excludes1   neutropenia (D70.-)
           D72.810   Lymphocytopenia
                     Decreased lymphocytes
                     *Reduction in number of lympho cytes
                         in blood*
           D72.818   Other decreased white blood cell
                     count
                     Basophilic leukopenia
                     Eosinophilic leukopenia
                     Monocytopenia
                     Other decreased leukocytes
                     Plasmacytopenia
           D72.819   Decreased white blood cell
                     count, unspecified
                     Decreased leukocytes, unspecified
                     Leukocytopenia, unspecified
                     Leukopenia
                         Excludes1   malignant leukopenia
                                     (D70.9)

● D72.82   Elevated white blood cell count
             Excludes1   eosinophilia (D72.1)
         D72.820   Lymphocytosis (symptomatic)
                   Elevated lymphocytes
                   Excess of normal lymphocytes
         D72.821   Monocytosis (symptomatic)
                       Excludes1   infectious
                                   mononucleosis
                                   (B27.-)
         D72.822   Plasmacytosis
                   Presence of excess plasma cells
         D72.823   Leukemoid reaction
                   Basophilic leukemoid reaction
                   Leukemoid reaction NOS
                   Lymphocytic leukemoid reaction
                   Monocytic leukemoid reaction
                   Myelocytic leukemoid reaction
                   Neutrophilic leukemoid reaction
         D72.824   Basophilia
                   Increase of basophils in blood
         D72.825   Bandemia
                   Bandemia without diagnosis of
                       specific infection
                   *Excess number of band cells (immature
                       white blood cells) released by bone
                       marrow*
                       Excludes1   confirmed infection
                                   -code to infection
                                   leukemia (C91.-,
                                   C92.-, C93.-,
                                   C94.-, C95.-)
         D72.828   Other elevated white blood cell count
         D72.829   Elevated white blood cell
                   count, unspecified
                   Elevated leukocytes, unspecified
                   Leukocytosis, unspecified
       D72.89   Other specified disorders of white blood cells
                Abnormality of white blood cells NEC
     D72.9   Disorder of white blood cells, unspecified
              Abnormal leukocyte differential NOS

● D73   Diseases of spleen
     D73.0   Hyposplenism
              Diminished functioning of spleen
              Atrophy of spleen
                 Excludes1   asplenia (congenital) (Q89.01)
                             postsurgical absence of spleen (Z90.81)
     D73.1   Hypersplenism
              Accelerated function of spleen
                 Excludes1   neutropenic splenomegaly (D73.81)
                             primary splenic neutropenia (D73.81)
                             splenitis, splenomegaly in late syphilis
                                 (A52.79)
                             splenitis, splenomegaly in tuberculosis
                                 (A18.85)
                             splenomegaly NOS (R16.1)
                             splenomegaly congenital (Q89.0)
     D73.2   Chronic congestive splenomegaly
              Enlargement of spleen
     D73.3   Abscess of spleen
     D73.4   Cyst of spleen
     D73.5   Infarction of spleen
              Splenic rupture, nontraumatic
              Torsion of spleen
                 Excludes1   rupture of spleen due to Plasmodium
                                 vivax malaria (B51.0)
                             traumatic rupture of spleen (S36.03-)

▶ New   ⇒ Revised   ~~deleted~~ Deleted   Excludes 1   Excludes 2   Includes   Use additional   Code first   Code also   Key words
OGCR Official Guidelines   ● Unacceptable Principal Diagnosis   X Assign placeholder X   ● Use Additional Character(s)   ▷ Manifestation Code   Coding Clinic

● **D73.8 Other diseases of spleen**

    D73.81 Neutropenic splenomegaly
        Werner-Schultz disease
        Enlarged spleen responding to inadequate number
        of neutrophils

    D73.89 Other diseases of spleen
        Fibrosis of spleen NOS
        Perisplenitis
        Splenitis NOS

  D73.9 Disease of spleen, unspecified

● **D74 Methemoglobinemia**
  Excessive methemoglobin (form of hemoglobin)
  (Ex:) **For category D74 CC codes:** See PDX Collection 506

  D74.0 Congenital methemoglobinemia 🔵
      Congenital NADH-methemoglobin reductase
        deficiency
      Hemoglobin-M [Hb-M] disease
      Methemoglobinemia, hereditary

  D74.8 Other methemoglobinemias 🔵
      Acquired methemoglobinemia (with
        sulfhemoglobinemia)
      Toxic methemoglobinemia

  D74.9 Methemoglobinemia, unspecified 🔵

● **D75 Other and unspecified diseases of blood and blood-forming**
  organs

    Excludes2   acute lymphadenitis (L04.-)
             chronic lymphadenitis (I88.1)
             enlarged lymph nodes (R59.-)
             hypergammaglobulinemia NOS (D89.2)
             lymphadenitis NOS (I88.9)
             mesenteric lymphadenitis (acute) (chronic) (I88.0)

  D75.A Glucose-6-phosphate dehydrogenase (G6PD) deficiency
  without anemia

    Excludes1   glucose-6-phosphate dehydrogenase
             (G6PD) deficiency with anemia
             (D55.0)

  D75.0 Familial erythrocytosis
    Genetic mutation of gene that results in increased circulating
    RBCs
    Benign polycythemia
    Familial polycythemia

    Excludes1   hereditary ovalocytosis (D58.1)

  D75.1 Secondary polycythemia
    Increase in total red cell mass
    Acquired polycythemia
    Emotional polycythemia
    Erythrocytosis NOS
    Hypoxemic polycythemia
    Nephrogenous polycythemia
    Polycythemia due to erythropoietin
    Polycythemia due to fall in plasma volume
    Polycythemia due to high altitude
    Polycythemia due to stress
    Polycythemia NOS
    Relative polycythemia

    Excludes1   polycythemia neonatorum (P61.1)
             polycythemia vera (D45)

● **D75.8 Other specified diseases of blood and blood-forming**
  organs

 ▶ **D75.81 Myelofibrosis** 🔵🔵
      Replacing bone marrow by fibrous tissue
      Myelofibrosis NOS
      Secondary myelofibrosis NOS

      Code first the underlying disorder, such as:
        malignant neoplasm of breast (C50.-)

      Use additional code, if applicable,
        for associated therapy-related
        myelodysplastic syndrome (D46.-)

      Use additional code for adverse effect, if
        applicable, to identify drug (T45.1X5)

      Excludes1   acute myelofibrosis (C94.4-)
             idiopathic myelofibrosis (D47.1)
             leukoerythroblastic anemia
               (D61.82)
             myelofibrosis with myeloid
               metaplasia (D47.4)
             myelophthisic anemia (D61.82)
             myelophthisis (D61.82)
             primary myelofibrosis (D47.1)

    (Ex:) See PDX Collection 3619

  D75.82 Heparin induced thrombocytopenia (HIT) 🔵

 ▶● **D75.83 Thrombocytosis**

    ▶**Excludes2**   essential thrombocythemia (D47.3)

    ▶**D75.838 Other thrombocytosis**
      ▶Reactive thrombocytosis
      ▶Secondary thrombocytosis
      ▶Code also, underlying condition, if
        known and applicable

    ▶**D75.839 Thrombocytosis, unspecified**
      ▶Thrombocythemia NOS
      ▶Thrombocytosis NOS

  D75.89 Other specified diseases of blood and blood-
      forming organs

  D75.9 Disease of blood and blood-forming organs, unspecified

● **D76 Other specified diseases with participation of lymphoreticular**
  and reticulohistiocytic tissue

    Excludes1   (Abt-) Letterer-Siwe disease (C96.0)
             eosinophilic granuloma (C96.6)
             Hand-Schüller-Christian disease (C96.5)
             histiocytic medullary reticulosis (C96.9)
             histiocytic sarcoma (C96.A)
             histiocytosis X, multifocal (C96.5)
             histiocytosis X, unifocal (C96.6)
             Langerhans-cell histiocytosis, multifocal (C96.5)
             Langerhans-cell histiocytosis NOS (C96.6)
             Langerhans-cell histiocytosis, unifocal (C96.6)
             leukemic reticuloendotheliosis (C91.4-)
             lipomelanotic reticulosis (I89.8)
             malignant histiocytosis (C96.A)
             malignant reticulosis (C86.0)
             nonlipid reticuloendotheliosis (C96.0)

  D76.1 Hemophagocytic lymphohistiocytosis 🔵🔵
    Familial hemophagocytic reticulosis
    Histiocytoses of mononuclear phagocytes
    (Ex:) See PDX Collection 3621

  D76.2 Hemophagocytic syndrome, infection-associated 🔵🔵
    Use additional code to identify infectious agent or
      disease.
    (Ex:) See PDX Collection 3623

  D76.3 Other histiocytosis syndromes 🔵🔵
    Reticulohistiocytoma (giant-cell)
    Sinus histiocytosis with massive lymphadenopathy
    Xanthogranuloma
    (Ex:) See PDX Collection 507

CHAPTER 3 (D50-D89)

N Newborn Age: 0   **P** Pediatric Age: 0-17   **M** Maternity DX: 9-64   **A** Adult Age: 15-124   ♀ Females Only   ♂ Males Only

🔵 Complication\Comorbidity   🔵 Major C\C   (Ex:) CC/MCC Exclusions   🔵 Hospital-Acquired Condition   🔵 Hierarchical Condition Category

743

▶ D77 *Other disorders of blood and blood-forming organs in diseases classified elsewhere*

    Code first underlying disease, such as:
      amyloidosis (E85.-)
      congenital early syphilis (A50.0)
      echinococcosis (B67.0-B67.9)
      malaria (B50.0-B54)
      schistosomiasis [bilharziasis] (B65.0-B65.9)
      vitamin C deficiency (E54)

    Excludes 1   rupture of spleen due to Plasmodium vivax malaria (B51.0)
                    splenitis, splenomegaly in late syphilis (A52.79)
                    splenitis, splenomegaly in tuberculosis (A18.85)

INTRAOPERATIVE AND POSTPROCEDURAL COMPLICATIONS OF THE SPLEEN (D78)

● D78 Intraoperative and postprocedural complications of the spleen
    Coding Clinic: 2016, Q4, P9

  ● D78.0 Intraoperative hemorrhage and hematoma of the spleen complicating a procedure

      Excludes 1   intraoperative hemorrhage and hematoma of the spleen due to accidental puncture or laceration during a procedure (D78.1-)
      Ⓔⓧ For category D78.0 CC codes: See PDX Collection 508

    D78.01 Intraoperative hemorrhage and hematoma of the spleen complicating a procedure on the spleen 🔒

    D78.02 Intraoperative hemorrhage and hematoma of the spleen complicating other procedure 🔒

  ● D78.1 Accidental puncture and laceration of the spleen during a procedure
      Ⓔⓧ For category D78.1 CC codes: See PDX Collection 509

    D78.11 Accidental puncture and laceration of the spleen during a procedure on the spleen 🔒

    D78.12 Accidental puncture and laceration of the spleen during other procedure 🔒

  ● D78.2 Postprocedural hemorrhage of the spleen following a procedure
      Ⓔⓧ For category D78.2 CC codes: See PDX Collection 508

    D78.21 Postprocedural hemorrhage of the spleen following a procedure on the spleen 🔒

    D78.22 Postprocedural hemorrhage of the spleen following other procedure 🔒

  ● D78.3 Postprocedural hematoma and seroma of the spleen following a procedure
      Ⓔⓧ For category D78.3 CC codes: See PDX Collection 508

    D78.31 Postprocedural hematoma of the spleen following a procedure on the spleen 🔒

    D78.32 Postprocedural hematoma of the spleen following other procedure 🔒

    D78.33 Postprocedural seroma of the spleen following a procedure on the spleen 🔒

    D78.34 Postprocedural seroma of the spleen following other procedure 🔒

  ● D78.8 Other intraoperative and postprocedural complications of the spleen
      Use additional code, if applicable, to further specify disorder
      Ⓔⓧ For category D78.8 CC codes: See PDX Collection 510

    D78.81 Other intraoperative complications of the spleen 🔒

    D78.89 Other postprocedural complications of the spleen 🔒

CERTAIN DISORDERS INVOLVING THE IMMUNE MECHANISM (D80-D89)

  Includes   defects in the complement system
          immunodeficiency disorders, except human immunodeficiency virus [HIV] disease
          sarcoidosis

  Excludes 1   autoimmune disease (systemic) NOS (M35.9)
          functional disorders of polymorphonuclear neutrophils (D71)
          human immunodeficiency virus [HIV] disease (B20)

● D80 Immunodeficiency with predominantly antibody defects
    Ⓔⓧ For category D80 CC codes unless otherwise indicated: See PDX Collection 511

  D80.0 Hereditary hypogammaglobulinemia 🔒 🔒
      Autosomal recessive agammaglobulinemia (Swiss type)
      X-linked agammaglobulinemia [Bruton] (with growth hormone deficiency)

  D80.1 Nonfamilial hypogammaglobulinemia 🔒 🔒
      Abnormally low levels of all classes of immunoglobulins
      Agammaglobulinemia with immunoglobulin-bearing B-lymphocytes
      Common variable agammaglobulinemia [CVAgamma]
      Hypogammaglobulinemia NOS
      Ⓔⓧ See PDX Collection 512

  D80.2 Selective deficiency of immunoglobulin A [IgA] 🔒 🔒
      Ⓔⓧ See PDX Collection 512

  D80.3 Selective deficiency of immunoglobulin G [IgG] subclasses 🔒 🔒

  D80.4 Selective deficiency of immunoglobulin M [IgM] 🔒 🔒

  D80.5 Immunodeficiency with increased immunoglobulin M [IgM] 🔒 🔒

  D80.6 Antibody deficiency with near-normal immunoglobulins or with hyperimmunoglobulinemia 🔒 🔒
      Abnormally high levels of immunoglobulins in serum

  D80.7 Transient hypogammaglobulinemia of infancy 🔒 🔒

  D80.8 Other immunodeficiencies with predominantly antibody defects 🔒 🔒
      Kappa light chain deficiency

  D80.9 Immunodeficiency with predominantly antibody defects, unspecified 🔒 🔒

● D81 Combined immunodeficiencies
    Excludes 1   autosomal recessive agammaglobulinemia (Swiss type) (D80.0)
    Ⓔⓧ For category D81 CC codes unless otherwise indicated: See PDX Collection 511

  D81.0 Severe combined immunodeficiency [SCID] with reticular dysgenesis 🔒 🔒

  D81.1 Severe combined immunodeficiency [SCID] with low T- and B-cell numbers 🔒 🔒

  D81.2 Severe combined immunodeficiency [SCID] with low or normal B-cell numbers 🔒 🔒

  ● D81.3 Adenosine deaminase [ADA] deficiency 🔒
      Ⓔⓧ See PDX Collection 513

    D81.30 Adenosine deaminase deficiency, unspecified 🔒
        ADA deficiency NOS

    D81.31 Severe combined immunodeficiency due to adenosine deaminase deficiency 🔒
        ADA deficiency with SCID
        Adenosine deaminase [ADA] deficiency with severe combined immunodeficiency

    D81.32 Adenosine deaminase 2 deficiency 🔒
        ADA2 deficiency
        Adenosine deaminase deficiency type 2
        Code also, if applicable, any associated manifestations, such as:
        polyarteritis nodosa (M30.0)
        stroke (I63.-)

▶ New   ⟹ Revised   ~~deleted~~ Deleted   Excludes 1   Excludes 2   Includes   Use additional   Code first   Code also   Key words

OGCR Official Guidelines   ● Unacceptable Principal Diagnosis   X Assign placeholder X   ● Use Additional Character(s)   ▶ Manifestation Code   **Coding Clinic**

D81.39   Other adenosine deaminase deficiency 🐾
Adenosine deaminase [ADA] deficiency
type 1, NOS
Adenosine deaminase [ADA] deficiency
type 1, without SCID
Adenosine deaminase [ADA] deficiency
type 1, without severe combined
immunodeficiency
Partial ADA deficiency (type 1)
Partial adenosine deaminase deficiency (type 1)

D81.4   Nezelof's syndrome 🐾🐾

D81.5   Purine nucleoside phosphorylase [PNP] deficiency 🐾🐾
(Ex) See PDX Collection 513

D81.6   Major histocompatibility complex class I deficiency 🐾🐾
Bare lymphocyte syndrome

**D81.7   Major histocompatibility complex class II
deficiency** 🐾🐾

● **D81.8   Other combined immunodeficiencies**

● **D81.81   Biotin-dependent carboxylase deficiency**
Multiple carboxylase deficiency

> **Excludes1**   biotin-dependent carboxylase
> deficiency due to dietary
> deficiency of biotin (E53.8)

D81.810   Biotinidase deficiency

**D81.818   Other biotin-dependent carboxylase
deficiency**
Holocarboxylase synthetase
deficiency
Other multiple carboxylase
deficiency

**D81.819   Biotin-dependent carboxylase
deficiency, unspecified**
Multiple carboxylase deficiency,
unspecified

D81.89   Other combined immunodeficiencies 🐾🐾

D81.9   Combined immunodeficiency, unspecified 🐾🐾
Severe combined immunodeficiency disorder [SCID]
NOS

● **D82   Immunodeficiency associated with other major defects**

> **Excludes1**   ataxia telangiectasia [Louis-Bar] (G11.3)

D82.0   Wiskott-Aldrich syndrome 🐾🐾
X-linked immunodeficiency
Immunodeficiency with thrombocytopenia and eczema
(Ex) See PDX Collection 511

D82.1   Di George's syndrome 🐾🐾
*Congenital disorder with defective development of third and
fourth pharyngeal pouches*
Pharyngeal pouch syndrome
Thymic alymphoplasia
Thymic aplasia or hypoplasia with immunodeficiency
(Ex) See PDX Collection 511
Coding Clinic: 2019, Q3, P14

D82.2   Immunodeficiency with short-limbed stature 🐾

**D82.3   Immunodeficiency following hereditary defective
response to Epstein-Barr virus** 🐾
X-linked lymphoproliferative disease

D82.4   Hyperimmunoglobulin E [IgE] syndrome 🐾
*Suspected genetic defect that produces high levels of antibody
immunoglobulin (IgE) that causes skin and lung
infections and eczema*

**D82.8   Immunodeficiency associated with other specified major
defects** 🐾

**D82.9   Immunodeficiency associated with major
defect, unspecified** 🐾

Item 3-1 Sarcoidosis: A symptom of an inflammation producing tiny lumps
of cells (granulomas) in various organs, most commonly the lungs and lymph
nodes, that affect organ function. Cause is unknown occurring primarily in
20- to 40-year-olds, African-American, especially women, and those of Asian,
German, Irish, Scandinavian, and Puerto Rican heritage.

● **D83   Common variable immunodeficiency**
(Ex) **For category D83 CC codes:** See PDX Collection 511

**D83.0   Common variable immunodeficiency with predominant
abnormalities of B-cell numbers and function** 🐾🐾

**D83.1   Common variable immunodeficiency with predominant
immunoregulatory T-cell disorders** 🐾🐾

**D83.2   Common variable immunodeficiency with
autoantibodies to B- or T-cells** 🐾🐾

D83.8   Other common variable immunodeficiencies 🐾🐾

D83.9   Common variable immunodeficiency, unspecified 🐾🐾

● **D84   Other immunodeficiencies**

D84.0   Lymphocyte function antigen-1 [LFA-1] defect 🐾

● **D84.1   Defects in the complement system** 🐾
C1 esterase inhibitor [C1-INH] deficiency

D84.8   Other specified immunodeficiencies 🐾🐾
(Ex) See PDX Collection 4056

▷ *D84.81   Immunodeficiency due to conditions classified
elsewhere* 🐾

> *Code first underlying condition, such as:
> chromosomal abnormalities (Q90-Q99)
> diabetes mellitus (E08-E13)
> malignant neoplasms (C00-C96)*

> **Excludes1**   *certain disorders involving
> the immune mechanism
> (D80-D83, D84.0, D84.1,
> D84.9)
> human immunodeficiency virus
> [HIV] disease (B20)*

● *D84.82   Immunodeficiency due to drugs and external
causes*

D84.821   Immunodeficiency due to drugs 🐾
Immunodeficiency due to (current
or past) medication

Use additional code for adverse
effect if applicable, to identify
adverse effect of drug (T36-T50
with fifth or six character 5)

Use additional code, if applicable,
for associated long term
(current) drug therapy drug or
medication such as:
long term (current) drug therapy
systemic steroids (Z79.52)
other long term (current) drug
therapy (Z79.899)

*D84.822   Immunodeficiency due to external
causes* 🐾

Code also, if applicable, radiological
procedure and radiotherapy
(Y84.2)

Use additional code for external
cause such as:
exposure to ionizing radiation
(W88)

D84.89   Other immunodeficiencies 🐾

D84.9   Immunodeficiency, unspecified 🐾🐾
Immunocompromised NOS
Immunodeficient NOS
Immunosuppressed NOS]
(Ex) See PDX Collection 511

● **D86   Sarcoidosis**

D86.0   Sarcoidosis of lung 🐾

D86.1   Sarcoidosis of lymph nodes 🐾

D86.2   Sarcoidosis of lung with sarcoidosis of lymph nodes 🐾

D86.3   Sarcoidosis of skin

N Newborn Age: 0   **P** Pediatric Age: 0–17   **M** Maternity DX: 9–64   **A** Adult Age: 15–124   ♀ Females Only   ♂ Males Only

🐾 Complication\Comorbidity   🐾 Major C\C   (Ex) CC/MCC Exclusions   🐾 Hospital-Acquired Condition   🐾 Hierarchical Condition Category

CHAPTER 3 (D50-D89)

● D86.8   **Sarcoidosis of** other **sites**

     D86.81   **Sarcoid** meningitis

     D86.82   **Multiple cranial nerve palsies in sarcoidosis** 🔖

     D86.83   **Sarcoid** iridocyclitis
           Rare large tumor with irregular surface of iris

     D86.84   **Sarcoid** pyelonephritis
           Systemic disease of unknown etiology characterized by chronic granulomatous inflammation with tissue destruction of pelvis kidney
           Tubulo-interstitial nephropathy in sarcoidosis

     D86.85   **Sarcoid** myocarditis

     D86.86   **Sarcoid** arthropathy
           Polyarthritis in sarcoidosis

     D86.87   **Sarcoid** myositis
           Granumloma of muscle

     D86.89   **Sarcoidosis of** other **sites**
           Hepatic granuloma
           Uveoparotid fever [Heerfordt]

   D86.9   **Sarcoidosis,** unspecified

● **D89   Other disorders involving the immune mechanism, not elsewhere classified**

     Excludes1   hyperglobulinemia NOS (R77.1)
           monoclonal gammopathy (of undetermined significance) (D47.2)

     Excludes2   transplant failure and rejection (T86.-)

   D89.0   **Polyclonal hypergammaglobulinemia**
           Benign hypergammaglobulinemic purpura
           Polyclonal gammopathy NOS

   D89.1   **Cryoglobulinemia** 🔖
           Cryoglobulin (proteins) in blood that precipitate temperatures below 98.6° F; usually symptomatic of underlying disease
           Cryoglobulinemic purpura
           Cryoglobulinemic vasculitis
           Essential cryoglobulinemia
           Idiopathic cryoglobulinemia
           Mixed cryoglobulinemia
           Primary cryoglobulinemia
           Secondary cryoglobulinemia

   D89.2   **Hypergammaglobulinemia,** unspecified

   D89.3   **Immune reconstitution syndrome** 🔖
           Immune reconstitution inflammatory syndrome [IRIS]

     Use additional code for adverse effect, if applicable, to identify drug (T36-T50 with fifth or sixth character 5)

●   D89.4   **Mast cell activation syndrome and related disorders**

     Excludes1   aggressive systemic mastocytosis (C96.21)
           congenital cutaneous mastocytosis (Q82.2)
           (non-congenital) cutaneous mastocytosis (D47.01)
           (indolent) systemic mastocytosis (D47.02)
           malignant mast cell neoplasm (C96.2-)
           malignant mastocytoma (C96.29)
           mast cell leukemia (C94.3-)
           mast cell sarcoma (C96.22)
           mastocytoma NOS (D47.09)
           other mast cell neoplasms of uncertain behavior (D47.09)
           systemic mastocytosis associated with a clonal hematologic non-mast cell lineage disease (SM-AHNMD) (D47.02)
       Coding Clinic: 2016, Q4, P11

     D89.40   **Mast cell activation,** unspecified 🔖
           Mast cell activation disorder, unspecified
           Mast cell activation syndrome, NOS

     D89.41   **Monoclonal mast cell activation syndrome** 🔖
           Coding Clinic: 2016, Q4, P11

     D89.42   **Idiopathic mast cell activation syndrome** 🔖
           Coding Clinic: 2016, Q4, P11

▷ D89.44   **Hereditary alpha tryptasemia**
     ▷ Use additional code, if applicable, for:
       ▷ allergy status, other than to drugs and biological substances (Z91.0-)
       ▷ personal history of anaphylaxis (Z87.892)

   D89.43   **Secondary mast cell activation** 🔖
           Secondary mast cell activation syndrome
     Code also underlying etiology, if known
     Coding Clinic: 2016, Q4, P11

   D89.49   **Other mast cell activation disorder** 🔖
           Other mast cell activation syndrome
     Coding Clinic: 2016, Q4, P11

● D89.8   **Other specified disorders involving the immune mechanism, not elsewhere classified**

●   D89.81   **Graft-versus-host disease**
           Code first underlying cause, such as:
           complications of transplanted organs and tissue (T86.-)
           complications of blood transfusion (T80.89)
     Use additional code to identify associated manifestations, such as:
       desquamative dermatitis (L30.8)
       diarrhea (R19.7)
       elevated bilirubin (R17)
       hair loss (L65.9)
     (Ex:) **For category D89.81 CC codes:** See PDX Collection 514

     ● D89.810   **Acute graft-versus-host disease** 🔖🔖

     ● D89.811   **Chronic graft-versus-host disease** 🔖🔖

     ● D89.812   **Acute on chronic graft-versus-host disease** 🔖🔖

     ● D89.813   **Graft-versus-host disease, unspecified** 🔖🔖

   D89.82   **Autoimmune lymphoproliferative syndrome [ALPS]** 🔖

●   D89.83   **Cytokine release syndrome**
           Code first underlying cause, such as:
           complications following infusion, transfusion and therapeutic injection (T80.89-)
           complications of transplanted organs and tissue (T86.-)
     Use additional code to identify associated manifestations

     ● D89.831   **Cytokine release syndrome, grade 1**

     ● D89.832   **Cytokine release syndrome, grade 2**

     ● D89.833   **Cytokine release syndrome, grade 3** 🔖
           (Ex:) See PDX Collection 4123

     ● D89.834   **Cytokine release syndrome, grade 4** 🔖
           (Ex:) See PDX Collection 4123

     ● D89.835   **Cytokine release syndrome, grade 5** 🔖
           (Ex:) See PDX Collection 4123

     ● D89.839   **Cytokine release syndrome, grade unspecified**

   D89.89   **Other specified disorders involving the immune mechanism, not elsewhere classified** 🔖
         Excludes1   human immunodeficiency virus disease (B20)
       Coding Clinic: 2017, Q4, P109

   D89.9   **Disorder involving the immune mechanism,** unspecified 🔖
       Immune disease NOS
       Coding Clinic: 2015, Q3, P22

▶ New   ⇒ Revised   ~~deleted~~ Deleted   Excludes 1   Excludes 2   Includes   Use additional   Code first   Code also   Key words

746   OGCR Official Guidelines   ● Unacceptable Principal Diagnosis   X Assign placeholder X   ● Use Additional Character(s)   ▷ Manifestation Code   Coding Clinic

CHAPTER 4

ENDOCRINE, NUTRITIONAL AND METABOLIC DISEASES (E00-E89)

OGCR Chapter-Specific Coding Guidelines

4. **Chapter 4: Endocrine, Nutritional, and Metabolic Diseases (E00-E89)**

   a. **Diabetes mellitus**

   The diabetes mellitus codes are combination codes that include the type of diabetes mellitus, the body system affected, and the complications affecting that body system. As many codes within a particular category as are necessary to describe all of the complications of the disease may be used. They should be sequenced based on the reason for a particular encounter. Assign as many codes from categories E08 – E13 as needed to identify all of the associated conditions that the patient has.

   1) **Type of diabetes**

   The age of a patient is not the sole determining factor, though most type 1 diabetics develop the condition before reaching puberty. For this reason type 1 diabetes mellitus is also referred to as juvenile diabetes.

   2) **Type of diabetes mellitus not documented**

   If the type of diabetes mellitus is not documented in the medical record the default is E11.-, Type 2 diabetes mellitus.

   3) **Diabetes mellitus and the use of insulin oral hypoglycemics**

   If the documentation in a medical record does not indicate the type of diabetes but does indicate that the patient uses insulin, code E11, Type 2 diabetes mellitus, should be assigned. An additional code should be assigned from category Z79 to identify the long-term (current) use of insulin or oral hypoglycemic drugs. If the patient is treated with both oral medications and insulin, only the code for long-term (current) use of insulin should be assigned. Code Z79.4 should not be assigned if insulin is given temporarily to bring a type 2 patient's blood sugar under control during an encounter.

   4) **Diabetes mellitus in pregnancy and gestational diabetes**

   See Section I.C.15, *Diabetes mellitus in pregnancy.*
   See Section I.C.15. *Gestational (pregnancy induced) diabetes*

   5) **Complications due to insulin pump malfunction**

   (a) **Underdose of insulin due to insulin pump failure**

   An underdose of insulin due to an insulin pump failure should be assigned to a code from subcategory T85.6, Mechanical complication of other specified internal and external prosthetic devices, implants and grafts, that specifies the type of pump malfunction, as the principal or first-listed code, followed by code T38.3X6-, Underdosing of insulin and oral hypoglycemic [antidiabetic] drugs. Additional codes for the type of diabetes mellitus and any associated complications due to the underdosing should also be assigned.

   (b) **Overdose of insulin due to insulin pump failure**

   The principal or first-listed code for an encounter due to an insulin pump malfunction resulting in an overdose of insulin, should also be 185.6-, Mechanical complication of other specified internal and external prosthetic devices, implants and grafts, followed by code T38.3X1-, Poisoning by insulin and oral hypoglycemic [antidiabetic] drugs, accidental (unintentional).

   6) **Secondary diabetes mellitus**

   Codes under categories E08, Diabetes mellitus due to underlying condition, E09, Drug or chemical induced diabetes mellitus and E13, Other specified diabetes mellitus, identify complications/manifestations associated with secondary diabetes mellitus. Secondary diabetes is always caused by another condition or event (e.g., cystic fibrosis, malignant neoplasm of pancreas, pancreatectomy, adverse effect of drug, or poisoning).

   (a) **Secondary diabetes mellitus and the use of insulin or hypoglycemic drugs**

   For patients with secondary diabetes mellitus who routinely use insulin or oral hypoglycemic drugs, an additional code from category Z79 should be assigned to identify the long-term (current) use of insulin or oral hypoglycemic drugs. If the patient is treated with both oral medications and insulin, only the code for long-term (current) use of insulin should be assigned. Code Z79.4 should not be assigned if insulin is given temporarily to bring a type 2 patient's blood sugar under control during an encounter.

   (b) **Assigning and sequencing secondary diabetes codes and its causes**

   The sequencing of the secondary diabetes codes in relationship to codes for the cause of the diabetes is based on the Tabular List instructions for categories E08, E09 and E13.

   (i) **Secondary diabetes mellitus due to pancreatectomy** For postpancreatectomy diabetes mellitus (lack of insulin due to the surgical removal of all or part of the pancreas), assign code E89.1, Postprocedural hypoinsulinemia. Assign a code from category E13 and a code from subcategory Z90.41-, Acquired absence of pancreas, as additional codes.

   (ii) **Secondary diabetes due to drugs** Secondary diabetes may be caused by an adverse effect of correctly administered medications, poisoning or sequela of poisoning.

   See Section I.C.19.e for coding of adverse effects and poisoning, and Section I.C.20 for external cause code reporting.

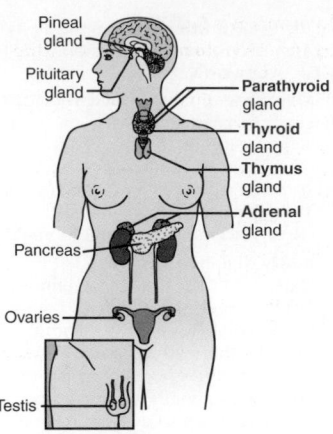

Figure 4-1 The endocrine system. (From Buck CJ: Step-by-Step Medical Coding, ed 2016, St. Louis, Elsevier, 2016)

CHAPTER 4

ENDOCRINE, NUTRITIONAL AND METABOLIC DISEASES (EØØ-E89)

All neoplasms, whether functionally active or not, are classified in Chapter 2. Appropriate codes in this chapter (i.e., E05.8, E07.0, E16-E31, E34.-) may be used as additional codes to indicate either functional activity by neoplasms and ectopic endocrine tissue or hyperfunction and hypofunction of endocrine glands associated with neoplasms and other conditions classified elsewhere.

> **Excludes1** transitory endocrine and metabolic disorders specific to newborn (P70-P74)

This chapter contains the following blocks:

EØØ-E07	Disorders of thyroid gland
E08-E13	Diabetes mellitus
E15-E16	Other disorders of glucose regulation and pancreatic internal secretion
E20-E35	Disorders of other endocrine glands
E36	Intraoperative complications of endocrine system
E40-E46	Malnutrition
E50-E64	Other nutritional deficiencies
E65-E68	Overweight, obesity and other hyperalimentation
E70-E88	Metabolic disorders
E89	Postprocedural endocrine and metabolic complications and disorders, not elsewhere classified

DISORDERS OF THYROID GLAND (EØØ-E07)

● **EØØ Congenital iodine-deficiency syndrome**

Use additional code (F70-F79) to identify associated intellectual disabilities.

> **Excludes1** subclinical iodine-deficiency hypothyroidism (E02)

EØØ.Ø Congenital iodine-deficiency syndrome, neurological type
Endemic cretinism, neurological type

EØØ.1 Congenital iodine-deficiency syndrome, myxedematous type
Dry, waxy type of swelling (nonpitting edema) with abnormal deposits of mucin in skin (mucinosis) and other tissues
Endemic hypothyroid cretinism
Endemic cretinism, myxedematous type

EØØ.2 Congenital iodine-deficiency syndrome, mixed type
Endemic cretinism, mixed type

EØØ.9 Congenital iodine-deficiency syndrome, unspecified
Congenital iodine-deficiency hypothyroidism NOS
Endemic cretinism NOS

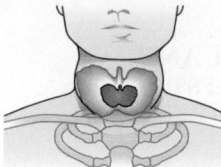

Figure 4-2 Goiter is an enlargement of the thyroid gland.

Item 4-1 Simple goiter indicates no nodules are present. The most common type of goiter is a **diffuse colloidal,** also called a **nontoxic** or **endemic** goiter.

● **E01 Iodine-deficiency related thyroid disorders and allied conditions**

> **Excludes1** congenital iodine-deficiency syndrome (EØØ.-)
> subclinical iodine-deficiency hypothyroidism (E02)

E01.Ø Iodine-deficiency related diffuse (endemic) goiter
Thyroid gland is enlarged

E01.1 Iodine-deficiency related multinodular (endemic) goiter
Iodine-deficiency related nodular goiter

E01.2 Iodine-deficiency related (endemic) goiter, unspecified
Endemic goiter NOS

E01.8 Other iodine-deficiency related thyroid disorders and allied conditions
Acquired iodine-deficiency hypothyroidism NOS

E02 Subclinical iodine-deficiency hypothyroidism
Coding Clinic: 2021, Q1, P8-9

● **E03 Other hypothyroidism**

> **Excludes1** iodine-deficiency related hypothyroidism (EØØ-E02)
> postprocedural hypothyroidism (E89.0)

E03.Ø Congenital hypothyroidism with diffuse goiter
Congenital parenchymatous goiter (nontoxic)
Congenital goiter (nontoxic) NOS

> **Excludes1** transitory congenital goiter with normal function (P72.0)

E03.1 Congenital hypothyroidism without goiter
Aplasia of thyroid (with myxedema)
Congenital atrophy of thyroid
Congenital hypothyroidism NOS

E03.2 Hypothyroidism due to medicaments and other exogenous substances

Code first poisoning due to drug or toxin, if applicable (T36-T65 with fifth or sixth character 1-4 or 6)

Use additional code for adverse effect, if applicable, to identify drug (T36-T50 with fifth or sixth character 5)

E03.3 Postinfectious hypothyroidism

E03.4 Atrophy of thyroid (acquired)

> **Excludes1** congenital atrophy of thyroid (E03.1)

E03.5 Myxedema coma 🔧🔧
Often fatal complication of long-term hypothyroidism
(Ex) See PDX Collection 515

E03.8 Other specified hypothyroidism

E03.9 Hypothyroidism, unspecified
Myxedema NOS
Coding Clinic: 2021, Q1, P9

Item 4-2 Hypothyroidism is a condition in which there are insufficient levels of thyroxine. **Cretinism** is congenital hypothyroidism, which can result in mental and physical retardation.

▶ New ⇒ Revised ~~deleted~~ Deleted Excludes 1 Excludes 2 Includes Use additional Code first Code also Key words
OGCR Official Guidelines ● Unacceptable Principal Diagnosis X Assign placeholder X ● Use Additional Character(s) ▮ Manifestation Code **Coding Clinic**

● **E04   Other nontoxic goiter**

    Excludes1   congenital goiter (NOS) (diffuse)
                       (parenchymatous) (E03.0)
                iodine-deficiency related goiter (E00-E02)

    E04.0   Nontoxic diffuse goiter
        Thyroid gland is enlarged
        Diffuse (colloid) nontoxic goiter
        Simple nontoxic goiter

    E04.1   Nontoxic single thyroid nodule
        Colloid nodule (cystic) (thyroid)
        Nontoxic uninodular goiter
        Thyroid (cystic) nodule NOS

    E04.2   Nontoxic multinodular goiter
        Enlarged thyroid gland with multiple nodules
        Cystic goiter NOS
        Multinodular (cystic) goiter NOS

    E04.8   Other specified nontoxic goiter

    E04.9   Nontoxic goiter, unspecified
        Goiter NOS
        Nodular goiter (nontoxic) NOS

● **E05   Thyrotoxicosis [hyperthyroidism]**
    Enlarged thyroid gland with multiple nodules

    Excludes1   chronic thyroiditis with transient thyrotoxicosis
                (E06.2)
                neonatal thyrotoxicosis (P72.1)

    (Ex:) **For category E05 CC codes:** See PDX Collection 516

●   **E05.0   Thyrotoxicosis with diffuse goiter**
        Exophthalmic or toxic goiter NOS
        Graves' disease
        Toxic diffuse goiter

    **E05.00   Thyrotoxicosis with diffuse goiter without
           thyrotoxic crisis or storm**

    **E05.01   Thyrotoxicosis with diffuse goiter with
           thyrotoxic crisis or storm** 🦠

●   **E05.1   Thyrotoxicosis with toxic single thyroid nodule**
        Thyrotoxicosis with toxic uninodular goiter

    **E05.10   Thyrotoxicosis with toxic single thyroid nodule
           without thyrotoxic crisis or storm**

    **E05.11   Thyrotoxicosis with toxic single thyroid nodule
           with thyrotoxic crisis or storm** 🦠

●   **E05.2   Thyrotoxicosis with toxic multinodular goiter**
        Toxic nodular goiter NOS

    **E05.20   Thyrotoxicosis with toxic multinodular goiter
           without thyrotoxic crisis or storm**

    **E05.21   Thyrotoxicosis with toxic multinodular goiter
           with thyrotoxic crisis or storm** 🦠

●   **E05.3   Thyrotoxicosis from ectopic thyroid tissue**

    **E05.30   Thyrotoxicosis from ectopic thyroid tissue
           without thyrotoxic crisis or storm**

    **E05.31   Thyrotoxicosis from ectopic thyroid tissue with
           thyrotoxic crisis or storm** 🦠

● **E05.4   Thyrotoxicosis factitia**

    **E05.40   Thyrotoxicosis factitia without thyrotoxic crisis
           or storm**

    **E05.41   Thyrotoxicosis factitia with thyrotoxic crisis or
           storm** 🦠

● **E05.8   Other thyrotoxicosis**
        Overproduction of thyroid-stimulating hormone

    **E05.80   Other thyrotoxicosis without thyrotoxic crisis or
           storm**

    **E05.81   Other thyrotoxicosis with thyrotoxic crisis or
           storm** 🦠

● **E05.9   Thyrotoxicosis, unspecified**
        Hyperthyroidism NOS

    **E05.90   Thyrotoxicosis, unspecified without thyrotoxic
           crisis or storm**

    **E05.91   Thyrotoxicosis, unspecified with thyrotoxic
           crisis or storm** 🦠

● **E06   Thyroiditis**
    *An inflammation of the thyroid gland which results in an inability to
    convert iodine into thyroid hormone*

    Excludes1   postpartum thyroiditis (O90.5)

    E06.0   Acute thyroiditis 🦠
        Abscess of thyroid
        Pyogenic thyroiditis
        Suppurative thyroiditis
        Use additional code (B95-B97) to identify infectious
           agent.
        (Ex:) See PDX Collection 517

    E06.1   Subacute thyroiditis
        *Inflammation of thyroid gland following viral upper
           respiratory infection*
        de Quervain thyroiditis
        Giant-cell thyroiditis
        Granulomatous thyroiditis
        Nonsuppurative thyroiditis
        Viral thyroiditis
        Excludes1   autoimmune thyroiditis (E06.3)

    E06.2   Chronic thyroiditis with transient thyrotoxicosis
        *Chronic inflammation of thyroid gland with intermittent
           overproduction of thyroid hormone*
        Excludes1   autoimmune thyroiditis (E06.3)

    E06.3   Autoimmune thyroiditis
        Hashimoto's thyroiditis
        Hashitoxicosis (transient)
        Lymphadenoid goiter
        Lymphocytic thyroiditis
        Struma lymphomatosa

    E06.4   Drug-induced thyroiditis
        Use additional code for adverse effect, if applicable,
           to identify drug (T36-T50 with fifth or sixth
           character 5)

    E06.5   Other chronic thyroiditis
        Chronic fibrous thyroiditis
        Chronic thyroiditis NOS
        Ligneous thyroiditis
        Riedel thyroiditis

    E06.9   Thyroiditis, unspecified

CHAPTER 4 (E00-E89)

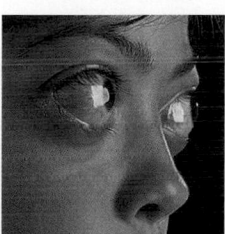

Figure 4-3   Graves' disease. In Graves' disease, exophthalmos often looks more pronounced than it actually is because of the extreme lid retraction that may occur. This patient, for instance, had minimal proptosis of the left eye but marked lid retraction. (From Lissauer T, Clayden G, and Craft A: Illustrated Textbook of Paediatrics, Edinburgh, Mosby, 2015)

Item 4–3   Thyrotoxicosis is a condition caused by excessive amounts of the thyroid hormone thyroxine production or hyperthyroidism. **Graves' disease is associated with hyperthyroidism** (known as **Basedow's disease** in Europe).

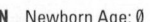

N Newborn Age: Ø   **P** Pediatric Age: Ø–17   **M** Maternity DX: 9–64   **A** Adult Age: 15–124   ♀ Females Only   ♂ Males Only

🦠 Complication\Comorbidity   🦠 Major C\C   (Ex:) CC/MCC Exclusions   🦠 Hospital-Acquired Condition   🦠 Hierarchical Condition Category

749

● **E07**   **Other disorders of thyroid**

   E07.0   **Hypersecretion of calcitonin**
         C-cell hyperplasia of thyroid
         Hypersecretion of thyrocalcitonin

   E07.1   **Dyshormogenetic goiter**
         Group of several types of goiter resulting from enzyme defects
           in hormone synthesis
         Familial dyshormogenetic goiter
         Pendred's syndrome
        | **Excludes1** | transitory congenital goiter with normal function (P72.0) |

  ● **E07.8**   **Other specified disorders of thyroid**

     E07.81   **Sick-euthyroid syndrome**
           Euthyroid sick-syndrome

     E07.89   **Other specified disorders of thyroid**
           Abnormality of thyroid-binding globulin
           Hemorrhage of thyroid
           Infarction of thyroid

   E07.9   **Disorder of thyroid, unspecified**

OGCR Section I.C.4.a.

> Diabetes mellitus
>
> The diabetes mellitus codes are combination codes that include the type of diabetes mellitus, body system affected, and the complications affecting that body system. As many codes within a particular category as are necessary to describe all of the complications of the disease may be used. They should be sequenced based on the reason for a particular visit. Assign as many codes from categories E08–E13 as needed to identify all of the associated conditions that the patient has.

DIABETES MELLITUS (E08-E13)

A metabolic disease that results in persistent hyperglycemia
Coding Clinic: 2016, Q4, P142

● **E08**   **Diabetes mellitus due to underlying condition**

   Code first the underlying condition, such as:
     congenital rubella (P35.0)
     Cushing's syndrome (E24.-)
     cystic fibrosis (E84.-)
     malignant neoplasm (C00-C96)
     malnutrition (E40-E46)
     pancreatitis and other diseases of the pancreas (K85-K86.-)

   Use additional code to identify control using:
     insulin (Z79.4)
     oral antidiabetic drugs (Z79.84)
     oral hypoglycemic drugs (Z79.84)

Excludes1	drug or chemical induced diabetes mellitus (E09.-)
	gestational diabetes (O24.4-)
	neonatal diabetes mellitus (P70.2)
	postpancreatectomy diabetes mellitus (E13.-)
	postprocedural diabetes mellitus (E13.-)
	secondary diabetes mellitus NEC (E13.-)
	type 1 diabetes mellitus (E10.-)
	type 2 diabetes mellitus (E11.-)

  ● **E08.0**   **Diabetes mellitus due to underlying condition with hyperosmolarity**
      (Ex:) **For category E08.0 CC codes:** See PDX Collection 518

    ▷ *E08.00*   *Diabetes mellitus due to underlying condition with hyperosmolarity without nonketotic hyperglycemic-hyperosmolar coma (NKHHC)* 🔖 🔖 🔖

    ▷ *E08.01*   *Diabetes mellitus due to underlying condition with hyperosmolarity with coma* 🔖 🔖 🔖

  ● **E08.1**   **Diabetes mellitus due to underlying condition with ketoacidosis**
      (Ex:) **For category E08.1 CC codes:** See PDX Collection 518

    ▷ *E08.10*   *Diabetes mellitus due to underlying condition with ketoacidosis without coma* 🔖 🔖 🔖

    ▷ *E08.11*   *Diabetes mellitus due to underlying condition with ketoacidosis with coma* 🔖 🔖

● **E08.2**   **Diabetes mellitus due to underlying condition with kidney complications**

    ▷ *E08.21*   *Diabetes mellitus due to underlying condition with diabetic nephropathy* 🔖
       Diabetes mellitus due to underlying condition with intercapillary glomerulosclerosis
       Diabetes mellitus due to underlying condition with intracapillary glomerulonephrosis
       Diabetes mellitus due to underlying condition with Kimmelstiel-Wilson disease

    ▷ *E08.22*   *Diabetes mellitus due to underlying condition with diabetic chronic kidney disease* 🔖
       Use additional code to identify stage of chronic kidney disease (N18.1-N18.6)

    ▷ *E08.29*   *Diabetes mellitus due to underlying condition with other diabetic kidney complication* 🔖
       Renal tubular degeneration in diabetes mellitus due to underlying condition

● **E08.3**   **Diabetes mellitus due to underlying condition with ophthalmic complications**
   Changes in blood vessels of retina in which blood vessels swell and leak fluid into retinal surface.
   Coding Clinic: 2016, Q4, P11

  ● **E08.31**   **Diabetes mellitus due to underlying condition with unspecified diabetic retinopathy**

    ▷ *E08.311*   *Diabetes mellitus due to underlying condition with unspecified diabetic retinopathy with macular edema* 🔖

    ▷ *E08.319*   *Diabetes mellitus due to underlying condition with unspecified diabetic retinopathy without macular edema* 🔖

  ● **E08.32**   **Diabetes mellitus due to underlying condition with mild nonproliferative diabetic retinopathy**
      Diabetes mellitus due to underlying condition with nonproliferative diabetic retinopathy NOS

      One of the following 7th characters is to be assigned to codes in subcategory E08.32 to designate laterality of the disease:

      | 1 | right eye |
2	left eye
3	bilateral
9	unspecified eye

    ● ▷ *E08.321*   *Diabetes mellitus due to underlying condition with mild nonproliferative diabetic retinopathy with macular edema* 🔖

    ● ▷ *E08.329*   *Diabetes mellitus due to underlying condition with mild nonproliferative diabetic retinopathy without macular edema* 🔖

  ● **E08.33**   **Diabetes mellitus due to underlying condition with moderate nonproliferative diabetic retinopathy**

      One of the following 7th characters is to be assigned to codes in subcategory E08.33 to designate laterality of the disease:

      | 1 | right eye |
2	left eye
3	bilateral
9	unspecified eye

    ● ▷ *E08.331*   *Diabetes mellitus due to underlying condition with moderate nonproliferative diabetic retinopathy with macular edema* 🔖

    ● ▷ *E08.339*   *Diabetes mellitus due to underlying condition with moderate nonproliferative diabetic retinopathy without macular edema* 🔖

▶ New   ⇒ Revised   ~~deleted~~ Deleted   Excludes 1   Excludes 2   Includes   Use additional   Code first   Code also   Key words

OGCR Official Guidelines   ● Unacceptable Principal Diagnosis   X Assign placeholder X   ● Use Additional Character(s)   ▷ Manifestation Code   **Coding Clinic**

● E08.34   **Diabetes mellitus due to underlying condition with severe nonproliferative diabetic retinopathy**

     One of the following 7th characters is to be assigned to codes in subcategory E08.34 to designate laterality of the disease:

     1   right eye
     2   left eye
     3   bilateral
     9   unspecified eye

●▶ *E08.341*   *Diabetes mellitus due to underlying condition with severe nonproliferative diabetic retinopathy with macular edema* 🔵

●▶ *E08.349*   *Diabetes mellitus due to underlying condition with severe nonproliferative diabetic retinopathy without macular edema* 🔵

● E08.35   **Diabetes mellitus due to underlying condition with proliferative diabetic retinopathy**

     One of the following 7th characters is to be assigned to codes in subcategory E08.35 to designate laterality of the disease:

     1   right eye
     2   left eye
     3   bilateral
     9   unspecified eye

●▶ *E08.351*   *Diabetes mellitus due to underlying condition with proliferative diabetic retinopathy with macular edema* 🔵

●▶ *E08.352*   *Diabetes mellitus due to underlying condition with proliferative diabetic retinopathy with traction retinal detachment involving the macula* 🔵

●▶ *E08.353*   *Diabetes mellitus due to underlying condition with proliferative diabetic retinopathy with traction retinal detachment not involving the macula* 🔵

●▶ *E08.354*   *Diabetes mellitus due to underlying condition with proliferative diabetic retinopathy with combined traction retinal detachment and rhegmatogenous retinal detachment* 🔵

●▶ *E08.355*   *Diabetes mellitus due to underlying condition with stable proliferative diabetic retinopathy* 🔵

●▶ *E08.359*   *Diabetes mellitus due to underlying condition with proliferative diabetic retinopathy without macular edema* 🔵

▶ *E08.36*   *Diabetes mellitus due to underlying condition with diabetic cataract* 🔵

X ●▶ *E08.37*   *Diabetes mellitus due to underlying condition with diabetic macular edema, resolved following treatment* 🔵

     One of the following 7th characters is to be assigned to code E08.37 to designate laterality of the disease:

     1   right eye
     2   left eye
     3   bilateral
     9   unspecified eye

▶ *E08.39*   *Diabetes mellitus due to underlying condition with other diabetic ophthalmic complication* 🔵
     Use additional code to identify manifestation, such as:
       diabetic glaucoma (H40-H42)

● E08.4   **Diabetes mellitus due to underlying condition with neurological complications**

▶ *E08.40*   *Diabetes mellitus due to underlying condition with diabetic neuropathy, unspecified* 🔵

▶ *E08.41*   *Diabetes mellitus due to underlying condition with diabetic mononeuropathy* 🔵

▶ *E08.42*   *Diabetes mellitus due to underlying condition with diabetic polyneuropathy* 🔵
     Diabetes mellitus due to underlying condition with diabetic neuralgia

▶ *E08.43*   *Diabetes mellitus due to underlying condition with diabetic autonomic (poly)neuropathy* 🔵
     Diabetes mellitus due to underlying condition with diabetic gastroparesis

▶ *E08.44*   *Diabetes mellitus due to underlying condition with diabetic amyotrophy* 🔵

▶ *E08.49*   *Diabetes mellitus due to underlying condition with other diabetic neurological complication* 🔵

● E08.5   **Diabetes mellitus due to underlying condition with circulatory complications**

▶ *E08.51*   *Diabetes mellitus due to underlying condition with diabetic peripheral angiopathy without gangrene* 🔵

▶ *E08.52*   *Diabetes mellitus due to underlying condition with diabetic peripheral angiopathy with gangrene* 🔵🔵

     Diabetes mellitus due to underlying condition with diabetic gangrene
     CC when PDx is its own CC
     (Ex:) See PDX Collection 3626

▶ *E08.59*   *Diabetes mellitus due to underlying condition with other circulatory complications* 🔵

● E08.6   **Diabetes mellitus due to underlying condition with other specified complications**

●▶ E08.61   **Diabetes mellitus due to underlying condition with diabetic arthropathy**

▶ *E08.610*   *Diabetes mellitus due to underlying condition with diabetic neuropathic arthropathy* 🔵
     Diabetes mellitus due to underlying condition with Charcôt's joints

▶ *E08.618*   *Diabetes mellitus due to underlying condition with other diabetic arthropathy* 🔵

● E08.62   **Diabetes mellitus due to underlying condition with skin complications**

▶ *E08.620*   *Diabetes mellitus due to underlying condition with diabetic dermatitis* 🔵
     Diabetes mellitus due to underlying condition with diabetic necrobiosis lipoidica

▶ *E08.621*   *Diabetes mellitus due to underlying condition with foot ulcer* 🔵
     Use additional code to identify site of ulcer (L97.4-, L97.5-)

▶ *E08.622*   *Diabetes mellitus due to underlying condition with other skin ulcer* 🔵
     Use additional code to identify site of ulcer (L97.1-L97.9, L98.41-L98.49)

▶ *E08.628*   *Diabetes mellitus due to underlying condition with other skin complications* 🔵

● E08.63   **Diabetes mellitus due to underlying condition with oral complications**

▶ *E08.630*   *Diabetes mellitus due to underlying condition with periodontal disease* 🔵

▶ *E08.638*   *Diabetes mellitus due to underlying condition with other oral complications* 🔵

N Newborn Age: 0   **P** Pediatric Age: 0–17   **M** Maternity DX: 9–64   **A** Adult Age: 15–124   ♀ Females Only   ♂ Males Only

🔵 Complication\Comorbidity   🔵 Major C\C   (Ex:) CC/MCC Exclusions   🔵 Hospital-Acquired Condition   🔵 Hierarchical Condition Category

751

CHAPTER 4 (E00-E89)

● **E08.64**   **Diabetes mellitus due to underlying condition with hypoglycemia**

    ▶ *E08.641*   *Diabetes mellitus due to underlying condition with hypoglycemia with coma* 🔖
         (Ex:)   See PDX Collection 518

    ▶ *E08.649*   *Diabetes mellitus due to underlying condition with hypoglycemia without coma* 🔖

   ▶ *E08.65*   *Diabetes mellitus due to underlying condition with hyperglycemia* 🔖

   ▶ *E08.69*   *Diabetes mellitus due to underlying condition with other specified complication* 🔖
       Use additional code to identify complication

▶ *E08.8*   *Diabetes mellitus due to underlying condition with unspecified complications* 🔖

▶ *E08.9*   *Diabetes mellitus due to underlying condition without complications* 🔖

● **E09**   **Drug or chemical induced diabetes mellitus**

   Code first poisoning due to drug or toxin, if applicable (T36-T65 with fifth or sixth character 1-4 or 6)

   Use additional code for adverse effect, if applicable, to identify drug (T36-T50 with fifth or sixth character 5)

   Use additional code to identify control using:
     insulin (Z79.4)
     oral antidiabetic drugs (Z79.84)
     oral hypoglycemic drugs (Z79.84)

   Excludes1   diabetes mellitus due to underlying condition (E08.-)
         gestational diabetes (O24.4-)
         neonatal diabetes mellitus (P70.2)
         postpancreatectomy diabetes mellitus (E13.-)
         postprocedural diabetes mellitus (E13.-)
         secondary diabetes mellitus NEC (E13.-)
         type 1 diabetes mellitus (E10.-)
         type 2 diabetes mellitus (E11.-)

● **E09.0**   **Drug or chemical induced diabetes mellitus with hyperosmolarity**
    (Ex:) **For category E09.0 CC codes:** See PDX Collection 518

   E09.00   **Drug or chemical induced diabetes mellitus with hyperosmolarity without nonketotic hyperglycemic-hyperosmolar coma (NKHHC)** 🔖 🔖 🔖

   E09.01   **Drug or chemical induced diabetes mellitus with hyperosmolarity with coma** 🔖 🔖 🔖

● **E09.1**   **Drug or chemical induced diabetes mellitus with ketoacidosis**
    (Ex:) **For category E09.1 CC codes:** See PDX Collection 518

   E09.10   **Drug or chemical induced diabetes mellitus with ketoacidosis without coma** 🔖 🔖 🔖

   E09.11   **Drug or chemical induced diabetes mellitus with ketoacidosis with coma** 🔖 🔖 🔖

● **E09.2**   **Drug or chemical induced diabetes mellitus with kidney complications**

   E09.21   **Drug or chemical induced diabetes mellitus with diabetic nephropathy** 🔖
      Drug or chemical induced diabetes mellitus with intercapillary glomerulosclerosis
      Drug or chemical induced diabetes mellitus with intracapillary glomerulonephrosis
      Drug or chemical induced diabetes mellitus with Kimmelstiel-Wilson disease

   E09.22   **Drug or chemical induced diabetes mellitus with diabetic chronic kidney disease** 🔖
      Use additional code to identify stage of chronic kidney disease (N18.1-N18.6)

   E09.29   **Drug or chemical induced diabetes mellitus with other diabetic kidney complication** 🔖
      Drug or chemical induced diabetes mellitus with renal tubular degeneration

● **E09.3**   **Drug or chemical induced diabetes mellitus with ophthalmic complications**
    Coding Clinic: 2016, Q4, P11

● **E09.31**   **Drug or chemical induced diabetes mellitus with unspecified diabetic retinopathy**

   E09.311   **Drug or chemical induced diabetes mellitus with unspecified diabetic retinopathy with macular edema** 🔖

   E09.319   **Drug or chemical induced diabetes mellitus with unspecified diabetic retinopathy without macular edema** 🔖

● **E09.32**   **Drug or chemical induced diabetes mellitus with mild nonproliferative diabetic retinopathy**
    Drug or chemical induced diabetes mellitus with nonproliferative diabetic retinopathy NOS

    One of the following 7th characters is to be assigned to codes in subcategory E09.32 to designate laterality of the disease:

1	right eye
2	left eye
3	bilateral
9	unspecified eye

   ● **E09.321**   **Drug or chemical induced diabetes mellitus with mild nonproliferative diabetic retinopathy with macular edema** 🔖

   ● **E09.329**   **Drug or chemical induced diabetes mellitus with mild nonproliferative diabetic retinopathy without macular edema** 🔖

● **E09.33**   **Drug or chemical induced diabetes mellitus with moderate nonproliferative diabetic retinopathy**

    One of the following 7th characters is to be assigned to codes in subcategory E09.33 to designate laterality of the disease:

1	right eye
2	left eye
3	bilateral
9	unspecified eye

   ● **E09.331**   **Drug or chemical induced diabetes mellitus with moderate nonproliferative diabetic retinopathy with macular edema** 🔖

   ● **E09.339**   **Drug or chemical induced diabetes mellitus with moderate nonproliferative diabetic retinopathy without macular edema** 🔖

● **E09.34**   **Drug or chemical induced diabetes mellitus with severe nonproliferative diabetic retinopathy**

    One of the following 7th characters is to be assigned to codes in subcategory E09.34 to designate laterality of the disease:

1	right eye
2	left eye
3	bilateral
9	unspecified eye

   ● **E09.341**   **Drug or chemical induced diabetes mellitus with severe nonproliferative diabetic retinopathy with macular edema** 🔖

   ● **E09.349**   **Drug or chemical induced diabetes mellitus with severe nonproliferative diabetic retinopathy without macular edema** 🔖

CHAPTER 4 (E00-E89)

752

▶ New   ⇒ Revised   ~~deleted~~ Deleted   Excludes 1   Excludes 2   Includes   Use additional   Code first   Code also   Key words
OGCR Official Guidelines   ● Unacceptable Principal Diagnosis   X Assign placeholder X   ● Use Additional Character(s)   ▶ Manifestation Code   Coding Clinic

● **E09.35** Drug or chemical induced diabetes mellitus with proliferative diabetic retinopathy

One of the following 7th characters is to be assigned to codes in subcategory E09.35 to designate laterality of the disease:

1   right eye
2   left eye
3   bilateral
9   unspecified eye

● **E09.351** Drug or chemical induced diabetes mellitus with proliferative diabetic retinopathy with macular edema 🩸

● **E09.352** Drug or chemical induced diabetes mellitus with proliferative diabetic retinopathy with traction retinal detachment involving the macula 🩸

● **E09.353** Drug or chemical induced diabetes mellitus with proliferative diabetic retinopathy with traction retinal detachment not involving the macula 🩸

● **E09.354** Drug or chemical induced diabetes mellitus with proliferative diabetic retinopathy with combined traction retinal detachment and rhegmatogenous retinal detachment 🩸

● **E09.355** Drug or chemical induced diabetes mellitus with stable proliferative diabetic retinopathy 🩸

● **E09.359** Drug or chemical induced diabetes mellitus with proliferative diabetic retinopathy without macular edema 🩸

E09.36 Drug or chemical induced diabetes mellitus with diabetic cataract 🩸

X ● **E09.37** Drug or chemical induced diabetes mellitus with diabetic macular edema, resolved following treatment 🩸

One of the following 7th characters is to be assigned to code E09.37 to designate laterality of the disease:

1   right eye
2   left eye
3   bilateral
9   unspecified eye

E09.39 Drug or chemical induced diabetes mellitus with other diabetic ophthalmic complication 🩸

Use additional code to identify manifestation, such as:
diabetic glaucoma (H40-H42)

● **E09.4** Drug or chemical induced diabetes mellitus with neurological complications

E09.40 Drug or chemical induced diabetes mellitus with neurological complications with diabetic neuropathy, unspecified 🩸

E09.41 Drug or chemical induced diabetes mellitus with neurological complications with diabetic mononeuropathy 🩸

E09.42 Drug or chemical induced diabetes mellitus with neurological complications with diabetic polyneuropathy 🩸
Drug or chemical induced diabetes mellitus with diabetic neuralgia

E09.43 Drug or chemical induced diabetes mellitus with neurological complications with diabetic autonomic (poly)neuropathy 🩸
Drug or chemical induced diabetes mellitus with diabetic gastroparesis

E09.44 Drug or chemical induced diabetes mellitus with neurological complications with diabetic amyotrophy 🩸

E09.49 Drug or chemical induced diabetes mellitus with neurological complications with other diabetic neurological complication 🩸

● **E09.5** Drug or chemical induced diabetes mellitus with circulatory complications

E09.51 Drug or chemical induced diabetes mellitus with diabetic peripheral angiopathy without gangrene 🩸

E09.52 Drug or chemical induced diabetes mellitus with diabetic peripheral angiopathy with gangrene 🩸🩸
Drug or chemical induced diabetes mellitus with diabetic gangrene
CC when PDx is its own CC
(Ex) See PDX Collection 3628

E09.59 Drug or chemical induced diabetes mellitus with other circulatory complications 🩸

● **E09.6** Drug or chemical induced diabetes mellitus with other specified complications

● **E09.61** Drug or chemical induced diabetes mellitus with diabetic arthropathy

E09.610 Drug or chemical induced diabetes mellitus with diabetic neuropathic arthropathy 🩸
Drug or chemical induced diabetes mellitus with Charcôt's joints
Progressive degeneration of weight-bearing joint

E09.618 Drug or chemical induced diabetes mellitus with other diabetic arthropathy 🩸

● **E09.62** Drug or chemical induced diabetes mellitus with skin complications

E09.620 Drug or chemical induced diabetes mellitus with diabetic dermatitis 🩸
Drug or chemical induced diabetes mellitus with diabetic necrobiosis lipoidica
Necrotizing skin condition

E09.621 Drug or chemical induced diabetes mellitus with foot ulcer 🩸
Use additional code to identify site of ulcer (L97.4-, L97.5-)

E09.622 Drug or chemical induced diabetes mellitus with other skin ulcer 🩸
Use additional code to identify site of ulcer (L97.1-L97.9, L98.41-L98.49)

E09.628 Drug or chemical induced diabetes mellitus with other skin complications 🩸

● **E09.63** Drug or chemical induced diabetes mellitus with oral complications

E09.630 Drug or chemical induced diabetes mellitus with periodontal disease 🩸

E09.638 Drug or chemical induced diabetes mellitus with other oral complications 🩸

● **E09.64** Drug or chemical induced diabetes mellitus with hypoglycemia

E09.641 Drug or chemical induced diabetes mellitus with hypoglycemia with coma 🩸🩸
(Ex) See PDX Collection 518

E09.649 Drug or chemical induced diabetes mellitus with hypoglycemia without coma 🩸

E09.65 Drug or chemical induced diabetes mellitus with hyperglycemia 🩸

E09.69 Drug or chemical induced diabetes mellitus with other specified complication 🩸
Use additional code to identify complication

E09.8 Drug or chemical induced diabetes mellitus with unspecified complications 🩸

E09.9 Drug or chemical induced diabetes mellitus without complications 🩸

CHAPTER 4 (E00-E89)

CHAPTER 4 (E00-E89)

● **E10   Type 1 diabetes mellitus**

Includes	brittle diabetes (mellitus)
	diabetes (mellitus) due to autoimmune process
	diabetes (mellitus) due to immune mediated pancreatic islet beta-cell destruction
	idiopathic diabetes (mellitus)
	juvenile onset diabetes (mellitus)
	ketosis-prone diabetes (mellitus)

Excludes1	diabetes mellitus due to underlying condition (E08.-)
	drug or chemical induced diabetes mellitus (E09.-)
	gestational diabetes (O24.4-)
	hyperglycemia NOS (R73.9)
	neonatal diabetes mellitus (P70.2)
	postpancreatectomy diabetes mellitus (E13.-)
	postprocedural diabetes mellitus (E13.-)
	secondary diabetes mellitus NEC (E13.-)
	type 2 diabetes mellitus (E11.-)

● **E10.1   Type 1 diabetes mellitus with ketoacidosis**

Acidosis accompanied by accumulation of ketone bodies (ketosis) in body tissues and fluids

Ex: For category E.10.1 CC codes: See PDX Collection 520

E10.10   Type 1 diabetes mellitus with ketoacidosis without coma 🔖🔖🔖
Coding Clinic: 2013, Q3, P20

E10.11   Type 1 diabetes mellitus with ketoacidosis with coma 🔖🔖🔖

● **E10.2   Type 1 diabetes mellitus with kidney complications**

E10.21   Type 1 diabetes mellitus with diabetic nephropathy 🔖
Type 1 diabetes mellitus with intercapillary glomerulosclerosis
Type 1 diabetes mellitus with intracapillary glomerulonephrosis
Type 1 diabetes mellitus with Kimmelstiel-Wilson disease

E10.22   Type 1 diabetes mellitus with diabetic chronic kidney disease 🔖
Use additional code to identify stage of chronic kidney disease (N18.1-N18.6)

E10.29   Type 1 diabetes mellitus with other diabetic kidney complication 🔖
Type 1 diabetes mellitus with renal tubular degeneration
Coding Clinic: 2016, Q1, P13

● **E10.3   Type 1 diabetes mellitus with ophthalmic complications**
Coding Clinic: 2016, Q4, P11

● **E10.31   Type 1 diabetes mellitus with unspecified diabetic retinopathy**

E10.311   Type 1 diabetes mellitus with unspecified diabetic retinopathy with macular edema 🔖

E10.319   Type 1 diabetes mellitus with unspecified diabetic retinopathy without macular edema 🔖

● **E10.32   Type 1 diabetes mellitus with mild nonproliferative diabetic retinopathy**
Type 1 diabetes mellitus with nonproliferative diabetic retinopathy NOS

One of the following 7th characters is to be assigned to codes in subcategory E10.32 to designate laterality of the disease:

1	right eye
2	left eye
3	bilateral
9	unspecified eye

● **E10.321   Type 1 diabetes mellitus with mild nonproliferative diabetic retinopathy with macular edema** 🔖

● **E10.329   Type 1 diabetes mellitus with mild nonproliferative diabetic retinopathy without macular edema** 🔖

● **E10.33   Type 1 diabetes mellitus with moderate nonproliferative diabetic retinopathy**

One of the following 7th characters is to be assigned to codes in subcategory E10.33 to designate laterality of the disease:

1	right eye
2	left eye
3	bilateral
9	unspecified eye

● **E10.331   Type 1 diabetes mellitus with moderate nonproliferative diabetic retinopathy with macular edema** 🔖

● **E10.339   Type 1 diabetes mellitus with moderate nonproliferative diabetic retinopathy without macular edema** 🔖

● **E10.34   Type 1 diabetes mellitus with severe nonproliferative diabetic retinopathy**

One of the following 7th characters is to be assigned to codes in subcategory E10.34 to designate laterality of the disease:

1	right eye
2	left eye
3	bilateral
9	unspecified eye

● **E10.341   Type 1 diabetes mellitus with severe nonproliferative diabetic retinopathy with macular edema** 🔖

● **E10.349   Type 1 diabetes mellitus with severe nonproliferative diabetic retinopathy without macular edema** 🔖

● **E10.35   Type 1 diabetes mellitus with proliferative diabetic retinopathy**

One of the following 7th characters is to be assigned to codes in subcategory E10.35 to designate laterality of the disease:

1	right eye
2	left eye
3	bilateral
9	unspecified eye

● **E10.351   Type 1 diabetes mellitus with proliferative diabetic retinopathy with macular edema** 🔖

● **E10.352   Type 1 diabetes mellitus with proliferative diabetic retinopathy with traction retinal detachment involving the macula** 🔖

● **E10.353   Type 1 diabetes mellitus with proliferative diabetic retinopathy with traction retinal detachment not involving the macula** 🔖

● **E10.354   Type 1 diabetes mellitus with proliferative diabetic retinopathy with combined traction retinal detachment and rhegmatogenous retinal detachment** 🔖

● **E10.355   Type 1 diabetes mellitus with stable proliferative diabetic retinopathy** 🔖

● **E10.359   Type 1 diabetes mellitus with proliferative diabetic retinopathy without macular edema** 🔖

E10.36   Type 1 diabetes mellitus with diabetic cataract 🔖

▶ New   ⇒ Revised   ~~deleted~~ Deleted   Excludes 1   Excludes 2   Includes   Use additional   Code first   Code also   Key words

OGCR Official Guidelines   ● Unacceptable Principal Diagnosis   X Assign placeholder X   ● Use Additional Character(s)   ▷ Manifestation Code   Coding Clinic

X ● **E10.37**   **Type 1 diabetes mellitus with diabetic macular edema, resolved following treatment** 🦠

One of the following 7th characters is to be assigned to code E10.37 to designate laterality of the disease:

1	right eye
2	left eye
3	bilateral
9	unspecified eye

     E10.39   **Type 1 diabetes mellitus with other diabetic ophthalmic complication** 🦠

Use additional code to identify manifestation, such as:
diabetic glaucoma (H40-H42)

● **E10.4**   **Type 1 diabetes mellitus with neurological complications**

     E10.40   **Type 1 diabetes mellitus with diabetic neuropathy, unspecified** 🦠

     E10.41   **Type 1 diabetes mellitus with diabetic mononeuropathy** 🦠

     E10.42   **Type 1 diabetes mellitus with diabetic polyneuropathy** 🦠

Type 1 diabetes mellitus with diabetic neuralgia

     E10.43   **Type 1 diabetes mellitus with diabetic autonomic (poly)neuropathy** 🦠

Type 1 diabetes mellitus with diabetic gastroparesis

     E10.44   **Type 1 diabetes mellitus with diabetic amyotrophy** 🦠

     E10.49   **Type 1 diabetes mellitus with other diabetic neurological complication** 🦠

● **E10.5**   **Type 1 diabetes mellitus with circulatory complications**

     E10.51   **Type 1 diabetes mellitus with diabetic peripheral angiopathy without gangrene** 🦠

     E10.52   **Type 1 diabetes mellitus with diabetic peripheral angiopathy with gangrene** 🦠 🦠

Type 1 diabetes mellitus with diabetic gangrene

CC when PDx is its own CC

Ⓔⓧ See PDX Collection 3630

     E10.59   **Type 1 diabetes mellitus with other circulatory complications** 🦠

● **E10.6**   **Type 1 diabetes mellitus with other specified complications**

●   **E10.61**   **Type 1 diabetes mellitus with diabetic arthropathy**

         E10.610   **Type 1 diabetes mellitus with diabetic neuropathic arthropathy** 🦠

Type 1 diabetes mellitus with Charcôt's joints

         E10.618   **Type 1 diabetes mellitus with other diabetic arthropathy** 🦠

●   **E10.62**   **Type 1 diabetes mellitus with skin complications**

         E10.620   **Type 1 diabetes mellitus with diabetic dermatitis** 🦠

Type 1 diabetes mellitus with diabetic necrobiosis lipoidica

         E10.621   **Type 1 diabetes mellitus with foot ulcer** 🦠

Use additional code to identify site of ulcer (L97.4-, L97.5-)

         E10.622   **Type 1 diabetes mellitus with other skin ulcer** 🦠

Use additional code to identify site of ulcer (L97.1-L97.9, L98.41-L98.49)

         E10.628   **Type 1 diabetes mellitus with other skin complications** 🦠

● **E10.63**   **Type 1 diabetes mellitus with oral complications**

     E10.630   **Type 1 diabetes mellitus with periodontal disease** 🦠

     E10.638   **Type 1 diabetes mellitus with other oral complications** 🦠

● **E10.64**   **Type 1 diabetes mellitus with hypoglycemia**

     E10.641   **Type 1 diabetes mellitus with hypoglycemia with coma** 🦠 🦠

Ⓔⓧ See PDX Collection 520

     E10.649   **Type 1 diabetes mellitus with hypoglycemia without coma** 🦠

Coding Clinic: 2016, Q1, P13

     E10.65   **Type 1 diabetes mellitus with hyperglycemia** 🦠

Coding Clinic: 2013, Q3, P20

     E10.69   **Type 1 diabetes mellitus with other specified complication** 🦠

Use additional code to identify complication

E10.8   **Type 1 diabetes mellitus with unspecified complications** 🦠

E10.9   **Type 1 diabetes mellitus without complications** 🦠

● **E11**   **Type 2 diabetes mellitus**

Includes   diabetes (mellitus) due to insulin secretory defect
diabetes NOS
insulin resistant diabetes (mellitus)

Use additional code to identify control using:
insulin (Z79.4)
oral antidiabetic drugs (Z79.84)
oral hypoglycemic drugs (Z79.84)

Excludes1   diabetes mellitus due to underlying condition (E08.-)
drug or chemical induced diabetes mellitus (E09.)
gestational diabetes (O24.4-)
neonatal diabetes mellitus (P70.2)
postpancreatectomy diabetes mellitus (E13.-)
postprocedural diabetes mellitus (E13.-)
secondary diabetes mellitus NEC (E13.-)
type 1 diabetes mellitus (E10.-)

Coding Clinic: 2020, Q1, P12; 2016, Q4, P121, Q2, P10

● **E11.0**   **Type 2 diabetes mellitus with hyperosmolarity**

Ⓔⓧ For category E11.0 CC codes: See PDX Collection 518

     E11.00   **Type 2 diabetes mellitus with hyperosmolarity without nonketotic hyperglycemic-hyperosmolar coma (NKHHC)** 🦠 🦠

     E11.01   **Type 2 diabetes mellitus with hyperosmolarity with coma** 🦠 🦠

● **E11.1**   **Type 2 diabetes mellitus with ketoacidosis**

Ⓔⓧ For category E11.1 CC codes: See PDX Collection 518

     E11.10   **Type 2 diabetes mellitus with ketoacidosis without coma** 🦠 🦠

Coding Clinic: 2017, Q4, P6

     E11.11   **Type 2 diabetes mellitus with ketoacidosis with coma** 🦠 🦠

● **E11.2**   **Type 2 diabetes mellitus with kidney complications**

     E11.21   **Type 2 diabetes mellitus with diabetic nephropathy** 🦠

Type 2 diabetes mellitus with intercapillary glomerulosclerosis
Type 2 diabetes mellitus with intracapillary glomerulonephrosis
Type 2 diabetes mellitus with Kimmelstiel-Wilson disease

Coding Clinic: 2019, Q3, P3

     E11.22   **Type 2 diabetes mellitus with diabetic chronic kidney disease** 🦠

Use additional code to identify stage of chronic kidney disease (N18.1-N18.6)

Coding Clinic: 2019, Q3, P3; 2018, Q4, P88; 2016, Q2, P36, Q1, P13

     E11.29   **Type 2 diabetes mellitus with other diabetic kidney complication** 🦠

Type 2 diabetes mellitus with renal tubular degeneration

N Newborn Age: 0   **P** Pediatric Age: 0–17   **M** Maternity DX: 9–64   **A** Adult Age: 15–124   ♀ Females Only   ♂ Males Only

🦠 Complication\Comorbidity   🦠 Major C\C   Ⓔⓧ CC/MCC Exclusions   🦠 Hospital-Acquired Condition   🦠 Hierarchical Condition Category

755

CHAPTER 4 (E00-E89)

● **E11.3**   **Type 2 diabetes mellitus with ophthalmic complications**
      Coding Clinic: 2016, Q4, P11

● **E11.31**   **Type 2 diabetes mellitus with unspecified diabetic retinopathy**

     E11.311   **Type 2 diabetes mellitus with unspecified diabetic retinopathy with macular edema** 🐾

     E11.319   **Type 2 diabetes mellitus with unspecified diabetic retinopathy without macular edema** 🐾
            Coding Clinic: 2013, Q3, P20

● **E11.32**   **Type 2 diabetes mellitus with mild nonproliferative diabetic retinopathy**

     Type 2 diabetes mellitus with nonproliferative diabetic retinopathy NOS

     One of the following 7th characters is to be assigned to codes in subcategory E11.32 to designate laterality of the disease:

1	right eye
2	left eye
3	bilateral
9	unspecified eye

    ● **E11.321**   **Type 2 diabetes mellitus with mild nonproliferative diabetic retinopathy with macular edema** 🐾

    ● **E11.329**   **Type 2 diabetes mellitus with mild nonproliferative diabetic retinopathy without macular edema** 🐾

● **E11.33**   **Type 2 diabetes mellitus with moderate nonproliferative diabetic retinopathy**

     One of the following 7th characters is to be assigned to codes in subcategory E11.33 to designate laterality of the disease:

1	right eye
2	left eye
3	bilateral
9	unspecified eye

    ● **E11.331**   **Type 2 diabetes mellitus with moderate nonproliferative diabetic retinopathy with macular edema** 🐾

    ● **E11.339**   **Type 2 diabetes mellitus with moderate nonproliferative diabetic retinopathy without macular edema** 🐾

● **E11.34**   **Type 2 diabetes mellitus with severe nonproliferative diabetic retinopathy**

     One of the following 7th characters is to be assigned to codes in subcategory E11.34 to designate laterality of the disease:

1	right eye
2	left eye
3	bilateral
9	unspecified eye

    ● **E11.341**   **Type 2 diabetes mellitus with severe nonproliferative diabetic retinopathy with macular edema** 🐾

    ● **E11.349**   **Type 2 diabetes mellitus with severe nonproliferative diabetic retinopathy without macular edema** 🐾

● **E11.35**   **Type 2 diabetes mellitus with proliferative diabetic retinopathy**

     One of the following 7th characters is to be assigned to codes in subcategory E11.35 to designate laterality of the disease:

1	right eye
2	left eye
3	bilateral
9	unspecified eye

    ● **E11.351**   **Type 2 diabetes mellitus with proliferative diabetic retinopathy with macular edema** 🐾

    ● **E11.352**   **Type 2 diabetes mellitus with proliferative diabetic retinopathy with traction retinal detachment involving the macula** 🐾

    ● **E11.353**   **Type 2 diabetes mellitus with proliferative diabetic retinopathy with traction retinal detachment not involving the macula** 🐾

    ● **E11.354**   **Type 2 diabetes mellitus with proliferative diabetic retinopathy with combined traction retinal detachment and rhegmatogenous retinal detachment** 🐾

    ● **E11.355**   **Type 2 diabetes mellitus with stable proliferative diabetic retinopathy** 🐾

    ● **E11.359**   **Type 2 diabetes mellitus with proliferative diabetic retinopathy without macular edema** 🐾

   E11.36   **Type 2 diabetes mellitus with diabetic cataract** 🐾
         Coding Clinic: 2019, Q2, P30-31; 2016, Q2, P36

X ● **E11.37**   **Type 2 diabetes mellitus with diabetic macular edema, resolved following treatment** 🐾

     One of the following 7th characters is to be assigned to code E11.37 to designate laterality of the disease:

1	right eye
2	left eye
3	bilateral
9	unspecified eye

   E11.39   **Type 2 diabetes mellitus with other diabetic ophthalmic complication** 🐾

     Use additional code to identify manifestation, such as:
        diabetic glaucoma (H40-H42)

● **E11.4**   **Type 2 diabetes mellitus with neurological complications**

   E11.40   **Type 2 diabetes mellitus with diabetic neuropathy, unspecified** 🐾

   E11.41   **Type 2 diabetes mellitus with diabetic mononeuropathy** 🐾

   E11.42   **Type 2 diabetes mellitus with diabetic polyneuropathy** 🐾
     Type 2 diabetes mellitus with diabetic neuralgia
       Coding Clinic: 2020, Q1, P12; 2016, Q1, P13

   E11.43   **Type 2 diabetes mellitus with diabetic autonomic (poly)neuropathy** 🐾
     Type 2 diabetes mellitus with diabetic gastroparesis
       Coding Clinic: 2016, Q2, P36

   E11.44   **Type 2 diabetes mellitus with diabetic amyotrophy** 🐾
       Coding Clinic: 2016, Q2, P36

   E11.49   **Type 2 diabetes mellitus with other diabetic neurological complication** 🐾

▶ New   ⇒ Revised   ~~deleted~~ Deleted   Excludes 1   Excludes 2   Includes   Use additional   Code first   Code also   Key words

756   OGCR Official Guidelines   ● Unacceptable Principal Diagnosis   X Assign placeholder X   ● Use Additional Character(s)   ▶ Manifestation Code   **Coding Clinic**

CHAPTER 4 (E00-E89)

● **E11.5**   **Type 2 diabetes mellitus with circulatory complications**

     E11.51   **Type 2 diabetes mellitus with diabetic peripheral angiopathy without gangrene** 🔹

     E11.52   **Type 2 diabetes mellitus with diabetic peripheral angiopathy with gangrene** 🔹
           Type 2 diabetes mellitus with diabetic gangrene 🔹
           CC when PDx is its own CC
           (Ex) See PDX Collection 3634
           Coding Clinic: 2017, Q4, P102

     E11.59   **Type 2 diabetes mellitus with other circulatory complications** 🔹

● **E11.6**   **Type 2 diabetes mellitus with other specified complications**

   ● **E11.61**   **Type 2 diabetes mellitus with diabetic arthropathy**

     E11.610   **Type 2 diabetes mellitus with diabetic neuropathic arthropathy** 🔹
           Type 2 diabetes mellitus with Charcôt's joints
           Coding Clinic: 2016, Q2, P36

     E11.618   **Type 2 diabetes mellitus with other diabetic arthropathy** 🔹
           Coding Clinic: 2018, Q2, P7; 2016, Q2, P36

   ● **E11.62**   **Type 2 diabetes mellitus with skin complications**

     E11.620   **Type 2 diabetes mellitus with diabetic dermatitis** 🔹
           Type 2 diabetes mellitus with diabetic necrobiosis lipoidica

     E11.621   **Type 2 diabetes mellitus with foot ulcer** 🔹
           Use additional code to identify site of ulcer (L97.4-, L97.5-)
           Coding Clinic: 2020, Q1, P12; 2016, Q1, P12

     E11.622   **Type 2 diabetes mellitus with other skin ulcer** 🔹
           Use additional code to identify site of ulcer (L97.1-L97.9, L98.41-L98.49)
           Coding Clinic: 2021, Q1, P8; 2017, Q4, P17

     E11.628   **Type 2 diabetes mellitus with other skin complications** 🔹

   ● **E11.63**   **Type 2 diabetes mellitus with oral complications**

     E11.630   **Type 2 diabetes mellitus with periodontal disease** 🔹

     E11.638   **Type 2 diabetes mellitus with other oral complications** 🔹

   ● **E11.64**   **Type 2 diabetes mellitus with hypoglycemia**

     E11.641   **Type 2 diabetes mellitus with hypoglycemia with coma** 🔹🔹
           (Ex) See PDX Collection 518

     E11.649   **Type 2 diabetes mellitus with hypoglycemia without coma** 🔹
           Coding Clinic: 2016, Q3, P42; 2015, Q3, P21

     E11.65   **Type 2 diabetes mellitus with hyperglycemia** 🔹
           Coding Clinic: 2013, Q3, P20

     E11.69   **Type 2 diabetes mellitus with other specified complication** 🔹
           Use additional code to identify complication
           Coding Clinic: 2020, Q1, P12; 2016, Q4, P142

   E11.8   **Type 2 diabetes mellitus with unspecified complications** 🔹

   E11.9   **Type 2 diabetes mellitus without complications** 🔹
     MCE: Questionable admission when principal dx
     Coding Clinic: 2016, Q4, P142, Q2, P36

● **E13**   **Other specified diabetes mellitus**

   Includes   diabetes mellitus due to genetic defects of beta-cell function
           diabetes mellitus due to genetic defects in insulin action
           postpancreatectomy diabetes mellitus
           postprocedural diabetes mellitus
           secondary diabetes mellitus NEC

     Use additional code to identify control using:
       insulin (Z79.4)
       oral antidiabetic drugs (Z79.84)
       oral hypoglycemic drugs (Z79.84)

   Excludes1   diabetes (mellitus) due to autoimmune process (E10.-)
           diabetes (mellitus) due to immune mediated pancreatic islet beta-cell destruction (E10.-)
           diabetes mellitus due to underlying condition (E08.-)
           drug or chemical induced diabetes mellitus (E09.-)
           gestational diabetes (O24.4-)
           neonatal diabetes mellitus (P70.2)
           type 1 diabetes mellitus (E10.-)

● **E13.0**   **Other specified diabetes mellitus with hyperosmolarity**
     (Ex) For category E13.0 CC codes: See PDX Collection 518

     E13.00   **Other specified diabetes mellitus with hyperosmolarity without nonketotic hyperglycemic-hyperosmolar coma (NKHHC)** 🔹 🔹🔹
         Excludes2   type 2 diabetes mellitus (E11.-)

     E13.01   **Other specified diabetes mellitus with hyperosmolarity with coma** 🔹 🔹🔹

● **E13.1**   **Other specified diabetes mellitus with ketoacidosis**
     (Ex) For category E13.1 CC codes: See PDX Collection 518

     E13.10   **Other specified diabetes mellitus with ketoacidosis without coma** 🔹 🔹🔹
           Coding Clinic: 2016, Q2, P10; 2013, Q1, P26

     E13.11   **Other specified diabetes mellitus with ketoacidosis with coma** 🔹 🔹🔹

● **E13.2**   **Other specified diabetes mellitus with kidney complications**

     E13.21   **Other specified diabetes mellitus with diabetic nephropathy** 🔹
           Other specified diabetes mellitus with intercapillary glomerulosclerosis
           Other specified diabetes mellitus with intracapillary glomerulonephrosis
           Other specified diabetes mellitus with Kimmelstiel-Wilson disease

     E13.22   **Other specified diabetes mellitus with diabetic chronic kidney disease** 🔹
           Use additional code to identify stage of chronic kidney disease (N18.1-N18.6)

     E13.29   **Other specified diabetes mellitus with other diabetic kidney complication** 🔹
           Other specified diabetes mellitus with renal tubular degeneration

● **E13.3**   **Other specified diabetes mellitus with ophthalmic complications**
     Coding Clinic: 2016, Q4, P11

   ● **E13.31**   **Other specified diabetes mellitus with unspecified diabetic retinopathy**

     E13.311   **Other specified diabetes mellitus with unspecified diabetic retinopathy with macular edema** 🔹

     E13.319   **Other specified diabetes mellitus with unspecified diabetic retinopathy without macular edema** 🔹

N   Newborn Age: 0   **P**   Pediatric Age: 0–17   **M**   Maternity DX: 9–64   **A**   Adult Age: 15–124   ♀   Females Only   ♂   Males Only

🔹   Complication\Comorbidity   🔹   Major C\C   (Ex)   CC/MCC Exclusions   🔹   Hospital-Acquired Condition   🔹   Hierarchical Condition Category

● **E13.32**   **Other specified diabetes mellitus with mild nonproliferative diabetic retinopathy**

     Other specified diabetes mellitus with nonproliferative diabetic retinopathy NOS

     One of the following 7th characters is to be assigned to codes in subcategory E13.32 to designate laterality of the disease:

1	right eye
2	left eye
3	bilateral
9	unspecified eye

● **E13.321**   Other specified diabetes mellitus with mild nonproliferative diabetic retinopathy **with macular edema** 🔖

● **E13.329**   Other specified diabetes mellitus with mild nonproliferative diabetic retinopathy **without macular edema** 🔖

● **E13.33**   Other specified diabetes mellitus with **moderate nonproliferative** diabetic retinopathy

     One of the following 7th characters is to be assigned to codes in subcategory E13.33 to designate laterality of the disease:

1	right eye
2	left eye
3	bilateral
9	unspecified eye

● **E13.331**   Other specified diabetes mellitus with moderate nonproliferative diabetic retinopathy **with macular edema** 🔖

● **E13.339**   Other specified diabetes mellitus with moderate nonproliferative diabetic retinopathy **without macular edema** 🔖

● **E13.34**   Other specified diabetes mellitus with **severe nonproliferative** diabetic retinopathy

     One of the following 7th characters is to be assigned to codes in subcategory E13.34 to designate laterality of the disease:

1	right eye
2	left eye
3	bilateral
9	unspecified eye

● **E13.341**   Other specified diabetes mellitus with severe nonproliferative diabetic retinopathy **with macular edema** 🔖

● **E13.349**   Other specified diabetes mellitus with severe nonproliferative diabetic retinopathy **without macular edema** 🔖

● **E13.35**   Other specified diabetes mellitus with **proliferative** diabetic retinopathy

     One of the following 7th characters is to be assigned to codes in subcategory E13.35 to designate laterality of the disease:

1	right eye
2	left eye
3	bilateral
9	unspecified eye

● **E13.351**   Other specified diabetes mellitus with proliferative diabetic retinopathy **with macular edema** 🔖

● **E13.352**   Other specified diabetes mellitus with proliferative diabetic retinopathy **with traction retinal detachment involving the macula** 🔖

● **E13.353**   Other specified diabetes mellitus with proliferative diabetic retinopathy **with traction retinal detachment not involving the macula** 🔖

● **E13.354**   Other specified diabetes mellitus with proliferative diabetic retinopathy **with combined traction retinal detachment and rhegmatogenous retinal detachment** 🔖

● **E13.355**   Other specified diabetes mellitus with **stable proliferative diabetic retinopathy** 🔖

● **E13.359**   Other specified diabetes mellitus with proliferative diabetic retinopathy **without macular edema** 🔖

   E13.36   Other specified diabetes mellitus with diabetic **cataract** 🔖

X ● **E13.37**   Other specified diabetes mellitus with diabetic macular edema, **resolved following treatment** 🔖

     One of the following 7th characters is to be assigned to code E13.37 to designate laterality of the disease:

1	right eye
2	left eye
3	bilateral
9	unspecified eye

   E13.39   Other specified diabetes mellitus with **other diabetic ophthalmic complication** 🔖

     Use additional code to identify manifestation, such as:

        diabetic glaucoma (H40-H42)

● **E13.4**   Other specified diabetes mellitus **with neurological complications**

   E13.40   Other specified diabetes mellitus with diabetic **neuropathy, unspecified** 🔖

   E13.41   Other specified diabetes mellitus with diabetic **mononeuropathy** 🔖

   E13.42   Other specified diabetes mellitus with diabetic **polyneuropathy** 🔖

     Other specified diabetes mellitus with diabetic neuralgia

   E13.43   Other specified diabetes mellitus with diabetic **autonomic (poly)neuropathy** 🔖

     Other specified diabetes mellitus with diabetic gastroparesis

   E13.44   Other specified diabetes mellitus with diabetic **amyotrophy** 🔖

   E13.49   Other specified diabetes mellitus with **other diabetic neurological complication** 🔖

● **E13.5**   Other specified diabetes mellitus **with circulatory complications**

   E13.51   Other specified diabetes mellitus with diabetic **peripheral angiopathy without gangrene** 🔖

   E13.52   Other specified diabetes mellitus with diabetic **peripheral angiopathy with gangrene** 🔖 🔖

     Other specified diabetes mellitus with diabetic gangrene

     CC when PDx is its own CC

     (Ex:) See PDX Collection 3634

   E13.59   Other specified diabetes mellitus with other circulatory complications 🔖

● **E13.6**   Other specified diabetes mellitus with **other specified complications**

● **E13.61**   Other specified diabetes mellitus with diabetic arthropathy

   E13.610   Other specified diabetes mellitus with diabetic **neuropathic** arthropathy 🔖

     Other specified diabetes mellitus with Charcôt's joints

   E13.618   Other specified diabetes mellitus with **other** diabetic arthropathy 🔖

▶ New   ⇒ Revised   ~~deleted~~ Deleted   Excludes 1   Excludes 2   Includes   Use additional   Code first   Code also   Key words

OGCR Official Guidelines   ● Unacceptable Principal Diagnosis   X Assign placeholder X   ● Use Additional Character(s)   ▶ Manifestation Code   **Coding Clinic**

● **E13.62 Other specified diabetes mellitus with skin complications**

     E13.620 Other specified diabetes mellitus with diabetic dermatitis 🐾
         Other specified diabetes mellitus with diabetic necrobiosis lipoidica

     E13.621 Other specified diabetes mellitus with foot ulcer 🐾
         Use additional code to identify site of ulcer (L97.4-, L97.5-)

     E13.622 Other specified diabetes mellitus with other skin ulcer 🐾
         Use additional code to identify site of ulcer (L97.1-L97.9, L98.41-L98.49)

     E13.628 Other specified diabetes mellitus with other skin complications 🐾

● **E13.63 Other specified diabetes mellitus with oral complications**

     E13.630 Other specified diabetes mellitus with periodontal disease 🐾

     E13.638 Other specified diabetes mellitus with other oral complications 🐾

● **E13.64 Other specified diabetes mellitus with hypoglycemia**

     E13.641 Other specified diabetes mellitus with hypoglycemia with coma 🐾🐾
         Ex: See PDX Collection 518

     E13.649 Other specified diabetes mellitus with hypoglycemia without coma 🐾

     E13.65 Other specified diabetes mellitus with hyperglycemia 🐾

     E13.69 Other specified diabetes mellitus with other specified complication 🐾
         Use additional code to identify complication

E13.8 Other specified diabetes mellitus with unspecified complications 🐾

E13.9 Other specified diabetes mellitus without complications 🐾
     MCE: Questionable admission when principal dx

OTHER DISORDERS OF GLUCOSE REGULATION AND PANCREATIC INTERNAL SECRETION (E15-E16)

E15 Nondiabetic hypoglycemic coma 🐾 🐾🐾
     Includes drug-induced insulin coma in nondiabetic
         hyperinsulinism with hypoglycemic coma
         hypoglycemic coma NOS
     Ex: See PDX Collection 520

● **E16 Other disorders of pancreatic internal secretion**

     E16.0 Drug-induced hypoglycemia without coma
         Excludes1 diabetes with hypoglycemia without coma (E09.649)
         Use additional code for adverse effect, if applicable, to identify drug (T36-T50 with fifth or sixth character 5)

     E16.1 Other hypoglycemia
         Functional hyperinsulinism
         Functional nonhyperinsulinemic hypoglycemia
         Hyperinsulinism NOS
         Hyperplasia of pancreatic islet beta cells NOS
         Excludes1 diabetes with hypoglycemia (E08.649, E10.649, E11.649, E13.649)
         hypoglycemia in infant of diabetic mother (P70.1)
         neonatal hypoglycemia (P70.4)

E16.2 Hypoglycemia, unspecified
     Excludes1 diabetes with hypoglycemia (E08.649, E10.649, E11.649, E13.649)
     Coding Clinic: 2016, Q3, P42

E16.3 Increased secretion of glucagon
     Hyperplasia of pancreatic endocrine cells with glucagon excess

E16.4 Increased secretion of gastrin
     Hypergastrinemia
     Hyperplasia of pancreatic endocrine cells with gastrin excess
     Zollinger-Ellison syndrome

E16.8 Other specified disorders of pancreatic internal secretion
     Increased secretion from endocrine pancreas of growth hormone-releasing hormone
     Increased secretion from endocrine pancreas of pancreatic polypeptide
     Increased secretion from endocrine pancreas of somatostatin
     Increased secretion from endocrine pancreas of vasoactive-intestinal polypeptide

E16.9 Disorder of pancreatic internal secretion, unspecified
     Islet-cell hyperplasia NOS
     Pancreatic endocrine cell hyperplasia NOS

DISORDERS OF OTHER ENDOCRINE GLANDS (E20-E35)

     Excludes1 galactorrhea (N64.3)
         gynecomastia (N62)

● **E20 Hypoparathyroidism**
     Greatly reduced function of parathyroid glands; AKA parathyroid insufficiency
     Excludes1 Di George's syndrome (D82.1)
         postprocedural hypoparathyroidism (E89.2)
         tetany NOS (R29.0)
         transitory neonatal hypoparathyroidism (P71.4)

     E20.0 Idiopathic hypoparathyroidism 🐾
         Rare condition, unknown cause; short dwarf-like with round face

     E20.1 Pseudohypoparathyroidism
         Hereditary condition resembling hypoparathyroidism, but caused by inability to respond to parathyroid hormone

     E20.8 Other hypoparathyroidism 🐾

     E20.9 Hypoparathyroidism, unspecified 🐾
         Parathyroid tetany

● **E21 Hyperparathyroidism and other disorders of parathyroid gland**
     Excludes1 adult osteomalacia (M83.-)
         ectopic hyperparathyroidism (E34.2)
         ~~familial hypocalciuric hypercalcemia (E83.52)~~
         hungry bone syndrome (E83.81)
         infantile and juvenile osteomalacia (E55.0)
     ▶ **Excludes2** familial hypocalciuric hypercalcemia (E83.52)

     E21.0 Primary hyperparathyroidism 🐾
         Hyperplasia of parathyroid
         Osteitis fibrosa cystica generalisata [von Recklinghausen's disease of bone]

     E21.1 Secondary hyperparathyroidism, not elsewhere classified 🐾
         Excludes1 secondary hyperparathyroidism of renal origin (N25.81)

Item 4-4 Hyperparathyroidism is an overactive parathyroid gland that secretes excessive parathormone, causing increased levels of circulating calcium. This results in a loss of calcium in the bone (osteoporosis).

     Hypoparathyroidism is an underactive parathyroid gland that results in decreased levels of circulating calcium. The primary manifestation is **tetany,** a continuous muscle spasm.

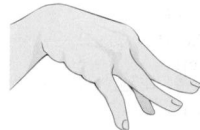

Figure 4-4 Tetany caused by hypoparathyroidism.

N Newborn Age: 0   P Pediatric Age: 0–17   M Maternity DX: 9–64   A Adult Age: 15–124   ♀ Females Only   ♂ Males Only

🐾 Complication\Comorbidity   🐾 Major C\C   **Ex:** CC/MCC Exclusions   🐾 Hospital-Acquired Condition   🐾 Hierarchical Condition Category

759

CHAPTER 4 (E00-E89)

Item 4–5   Hyperadrenalism is overactivity of the adrenal cortex, which secretes corticosteroid hormones. Excessive glucocorticoid hormone results in hyperglycemia (**Cushing's syndrome**), and excessive aldosterone results in **Conn's syndrome. Adrenogenital syndrome** is the result of excessive secretion of androgens, male hormones, which stimulates premature sexual development. **Hypoadrenalism, Addison's disease,** is a condition in which the adrenal glands atrophy.

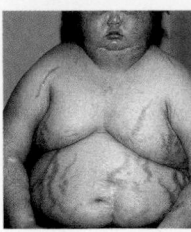

Figure 4-5   Centripetal and generalized obesity and dorsal kyphosis in a woman with Cushing's disease. (From Salvo SG: Mosby's Pathology for Massage Therapists, St. Louis, MO: Mosby/Elsevier, 2009)

E21.2   **Other hyperparathyroidism** 🔖🔖
  Tertiary hyperparathyroidism
  Excludes1   familial hypocalciuric hypercalcemia (E83.52)

E21.3   **Hyperparathyroidism, unspecified** 🔖

E21.4   **Other specified disorders of parathyroid gland** 🔖

E21.5   **Disorder of parathyroid gland, unspecified** 🔖

● E22   **Hyperfunction of pituitary gland**
  Excludes1   Cushing's syndrome (E24.-)
    Nelson's syndrome (E24.1)
    overproduction of ACTH not associated with Cushing's disease (E27.0)
    overproduction of pituitary ACTH (E24.0)
    overproduction of thyroid-stimulating hormone (E05.8-)
  (Ex) **For category E22 CC codes unless otherwise indicated:** See PDX Collection 521

E22.0   **Acromegaly and pituitary gigantism** 🔖
  Chronic disease caused by hypersecretion of growth hormone
  Overproduction of growth hormone
  Excludes1   constitutional gigantism (E34.4)
    constitutional tall stature (E34.4)
    increased secretion from endocrine pancreas of growth hormone-releasing hormone (E16.8)

E22.1   **Hyperprolactinemia** 🔖🔖
  Increased levels of prolactin
  Use additional code for adverse effect, if applicable, to identify drug (T36-T50 with fifth or sixth character 5)

E22.2   **Syndrome of inappropriate secretion of antidiuretic hormone** 🔖🔖
  (Ex) See PDX Collection 522

E22.8   **Other hyperfunction of pituitary gland** 🔖🔖
  Central precocious puberty

E22.9   **Hyperfunction of pituitary gland, unspecified** 🔖🔖

● E23   **Hypofunction and other disorders of the pituitary gland**
  Includes   the listed conditions whether the disorder is in the pituitary or the hypothalamus
  Excludes1   postprocedural hypopituitarism (E89.3)

E23.0   **Hypopituitarism** 🔖🔖
  Fertile eunuch syndrome
  Hypogonadotropic hypogonadism
  Idiopathic growth hormone deficiency
  Isolated deficiency of gonadotropin
  Isolated deficiency of growth hormone
  Isolated deficiency of pituitary hormone
  Kallmann's syndrome
  Lorain-Levi short stature
  Necrosis of pituitary gland (postpartum)
  Panhypopituitarism
  Pituitary cachexia
  Pituitary insufficiency NOS
  Pituitary short stature
  Sheehan's syndrome
  Simmonds' disease
  (Ex) See PDX Collection 523

E23.1   **Drug-induced hypopituitarism** 🔖
  Use additional code for adverse effect, if applicable, to identify drug (T36-T50 with fifth or sixth character 5)

E23.2   **Diabetes insipidus** 🔖🔖
  Excludes1   nephrogenic diabetes insipidus (N25.1)
  (Ex) See PDX Collection 524

E23.3   **Hypothalamic dysfunction, not elsewhere classified** 🔖
  Excludes1   Prader-Willi syndrome (Q87.11)
    Russell-Silver syndrome (Q87.19)

E23.6   **Other disorders of pituitary gland** 🔖
  Abscess of pituitary
  Adiposogenital dystrophy

E23.7   **Disorder of pituitary gland, unspecified** 🔖

● E24   **Cushing's syndrome**
  Excludes1   congenital adrenal hyperplasia (E25.0)
  (Ex) **For category E24 CC codes:** See PDX Collection 525

E24.0   **Pituitary-dependent Cushing's disease** 🔖🔖
  Overproduction of pituitary ACTH
  Pituitary-dependent hypercorticalism

E24.1   **Nelson's syndrome** 🔖

E24.2   **Drug-induced Cushing's syndrome** 🔖🔖
  Use additional code for adverse effect, if applicable, to identify drug (T36-T50 with fifth or sixth character 5)

E24.3   **Ectopic ACTH syndrome** 🔖🔖

E24.4   **Alcohol-induced pseudo-Cushing's syndrome** 🔖🔖

E24.8   **Other Cushing's syndrome** 🔖🔖

E24.9   **Cushing's syndrome, unspecified** 🔖🔖

● E25   **Adrenogenital disorders**
  Disorder of production of steroid hormone in adrenal gland
  Includes   adrenogenital syndromes, virilizing or feminizing, whether acquired or due to adrenal hyperplasia consequent on inborn enzyme defects in hormone synthesis
    female adrenal pseudohermaphroditism
    female heterosexual precocious pseudopuberty
    male isosexual precocious pseudopuberty
    male macrogenitosomia praecox
    male sexual precocity with adrenal hyperplasia
    male virilization (female)
  Excludes1   indeterminate sex and pseudohermaphroditism (Q56)
    chromosomal abnormalities (Q90-Q99)

E25.0   **Congenital adrenogenital disorders associated with enzyme deficiency** 🔖
  Congenital adrenal hyperplasia
  21-Hydroxylase deficiency
  Salt-losing congenital adrenal hyperplasia

E25.8   **Other adrenogenital disorders** 🔖
  Idiopathic adrenogenital disorder
  Use additional code for adverse effect, if applicable, to identify drug (T36-T50 with fifth or sixth character 5)

E25.9   **Adrenogenital disorder, unspecified** 🔖
  Adrenogenital syndrome NOS

▶ New   ⇒ Revised   ~~deleted~~ Deleted   Excludes 1   Excludes 2   Includes   Use additional   Code first   Code also   Key words
OGCR Official Guidelines   ● Unacceptable Principal Diagnosis   X Assign placeholder X   ● Use Additional Character(s)   ) Manifestation Code   **Coding Clinic**

CHAPTER 4 (E00-E89)

● **E26**   **Hyperaldosteronism**
Abnormality of electrolyte metabolism caused by excessive secretion of aldosterone

● **E26.0**   **Primary hyperaldosteronism**

     E26.01   **Conn's syndrome** 🔶
         Code also adrenal adenoma (D35.0-)

     E26.02   **Glucocorticoid-remediable aldosteronism** 🔶
         Familial aldosteronism type I

     E26.09   **Other primary hyperaldosteronism** 🔶
         Primary aldosteronism due to adrenal hyperplasia (bilateral)

E26.1   Secondary hyperaldosteronism 🔶

● **E26.8**   Other hyperaldosteronism

     E26.81   Bartter's syndrome 🔶

     E26.89   Other hyperaldosteronism 🔶

E26.9   Hyperaldosteronism, unspecified 🔶
     Aldosteronism NOS
     Hyperaldosteronism NOS

● **E27**   **Other disorders of adrenal gland**
     (Ex) **For category E27 CC codes:** See PDX Collection 526

E27.0   **Other adrenocortical overactivity** 🔶🔶
     Overproduction of ACTH, not associated with Cushing's disease
     Premature adrenarche
     Excludes1   Cushing's syndrome (E24.-)

E27.1   **Primary adrenocortical insufficiency** 🔶🔶
     Addison's disease
     Autoimmune adrenalitis
     Excludes1   Addison only phenotype adrenoleukodystrophy (E71.528)
         amyloidosis (E85.-)
         tuberculous Addison's disease (A18.7)
         Waterhouse-Friderichsen syndrome (A39.1)

E27.2   **Addisonian crisis** 🔶🔶
     Acute onset of adrenocortical insufficiency
     Adrenal crisis
     Adrenocortical crisis

E27.3   **Drug-induced adrenocortical insufficiency** 🔶🔶
     Use additional code for adverse effect, if applicable, to identify drug (T36-T50 with fifth or sixth character 5)

● **E27.4**   **Other and unspecified adrenocortical insufficiency**
     Excludes1   adrenoleukodystrophy [Addison-Schilder] (E71.528)
         Waterhouse-Friderichsen syndrome (A39.1)

     E27.40   Unspecified adrenocortical insufficiency 🔶🔶
         Adrenocortical insufficiency NOS
         Hypoaldosteronism

     E27.49   Other adrenocortical insufficiency 🔶🔶
         Adrenal hemorrhage
         Adrenal infarction

E27.5   **Adrenomedullary hyperfunction** 🔶🔶
     Adrenomedullary hyperplasia
     Catecholamine hypersecretion

E27.8   **Other specified disorders of adrenal gland** 🔶
     Abnormality of cortisol-binding globulin

E27.9   **Disorder of adrenal gland, unspecified** 🔶

● **E28**   **Ovarian dysfunction**
     Excludes1   isolated gonadotropin deficiency (E23.0)
         postprocedural ovarian failure (E89.4-)

E28.0   **Estrogen excess** ♀
     Use additional code for adverse effect, if applicable, to identify drug (T36-T50 with fifth or sixth character 5)

E28.1   **Androgen excess** ♀
     Hypersecretion of ovarian androgens
     Use additional code for adverse effect, if applicable, to identify drug (T36-T50 with fifth or sixth character 5)

E28.2   **Polycystic ovarian syndrome** ♀
     Sclerocystic ovary syndrome
     Stein-Leventhal syndrome

● **E28.3**   **Primary ovarian failure**
     Excludes1   pure gonadal dysgenesis (Q99.1)
         Turner's syndrome (Q96.-)

   ● **E28.31**   Premature menopause

     E28.310   Symptomatic premature menopause ♀   A
         Symptoms such as flushing, sleeplessness, headache, lack of concentration, associated with premature menopause

     E28.319   Asymptomatic premature menopause ♀   A
         Premature menopause NOS

     E28.39   Other primary ovarian failure ♀
         Decreased estrogen
         Resistant ovary syndrome

E28.8   **Other ovarian dysfunction** ♀
     Ovarian hyperfunction NOS
     Excludes1   postprocedural ovarian failure (E89.4-)

E28.9   **Ovarian dysfunction, unspecified** ♀

● **E29**   **Testicular dysfunction**
     Excludes1   androgen insensitivity syndrome (E34.5-)
         azoospermia or oligospermia NOS (N46.0-N46.1)
         isolated gonadotropin deficiency (E23.0)
         Klinefelter's syndrome (Q98.0-Q98.1, Q98.4)

E29.0   **Testicular hyperfunction** ♂
     Hypersecretion of testicular hormones

E29.1   **Testicular hypofunction** ♂
     Defective biosynthesis of testicular androgen NOS
     5-delta-Reductase deficiency (with male pseudohermaphroditism)
     Testicular hypogonadism NOS
     Use additional code for adverse effect, if applicable, to identify drug (T36-T50 with fifth or sixth character 5)
     Excludes1   postprocedural testicular hypofunction (E89.5)

E29.8   **Other testicular dysfunction** ♂

E29.9   **Testicular dysfunction, unspecified** ♂

● **E30**   **Disorders of puberty, not elsewhere classified**

E30.0   **Delayed puberty**
     Constitutional delay of puberty
     Delayed sexual development

E30.1   **Precocious puberty**   P
     Sexual maturation at earlier age than normal, or before age 8 in girls and 9 in boys, usually hormonal; AKA sexual precocity or pubertas praecox
     Precocious menstruation
     Excludes1   Albright (-McCune) (-Sternberg) syndrome (Q78.1)
         central precocious puberty (E22.8)
         congenital adrenal hyperplasia (E25.0)
         female heterosexual precocious pseudopuberty (E25.-)
         male isosexual precocious pseudopuberty (E25.-)

E30.8   **Other disorders of puberty**   P
     Premature thelarche

E30.9   **Disorder of puberty, unspecified**

N   Newborn Age: 0   **P**   Pediatric Age: 0–17   **M**   Maternity DX: 9–64   **A**   Adult Age: 15–124   ♀   Females Only   ♂   Males Only

🔶 Complication\Comorbidity   🔶 Major C\C   (Ex) CC/MCC Exclusions   🔶 Hospital-Acquired Condition   🔶 Hierarchical Condition Category

761

● **E31**   **Polyglandular dysfunction**

> **Excludes1**   ataxia telangiectasia [Louis-Bar] (G11.3)
> dystrophia myotonica [Steinert] (G71.11)
> pseudohypoparathyroidism (E20.1)

E31.0   **Autoimmune polyglandular failure** 🦠
Schmidt's syndrome

E31.1   **Polyglandular hyperfunction** 🦠

> **Excludes1**   multiple endocrine adenomatosis (E31.2-)
> multiple endocrine neoplasia (E31.2-)

● **E31.2**   **Multiple endocrine neoplasia [MEN] syndromes**
Adenomatous hyperplasia and malignant tumors in endocrine glands
Multiple endocrine adenomatosis

Code also any associated malignancies and other conditions associated with the syndromes

E31.20   **Multiple endocrine neoplasia [MEN] syndrome, unspecified** 🦠
Multiple endocrine adenomatosis NOS
Multiple endocrine neoplasia [MEN] syndrome NOS

E31.21   **Multiple endocrine neoplasia [MEN] type I** 🦠
Wermer's syndrome

E31.22   **Multiple endocrine neoplasia [MEN] type IIA** 🦠
Sipple's syndrome

E31.23   **Multiple endocrine neoplasia [MEN] type IIB** 🦠

E31.8   **Other polyglandular dysfunction** 🦠

E31.9   **Polyglandular dysfunction, unspecified** 🦠

● **E32**   **Diseases of thymus**

> **Excludes1**   aplasia or hypoplasia of thymus with immunodeficiency (D82.1)
> myasthenia gravis (G70.0)

E32.0   **Persistent hyperplasia of thymus** 🦠
Hypertrophy of thymus

E32.1   **Abscess of thymus** 🦠 🦠
(Ex:) See PDX Collection 527

E32.8   **Other diseases of thymus** 🦠

> **Excludes1**   aplasia or hypoplasia with immunodeficiency (D82.1)
> thymoma (D15.0)

E32.9   **Disease of thymus, unspecified** 🦠

● **E34**   **Other endocrine disorders**

> **Excludes1**   pseudohypoparathyroidism (E20.1)

E34.0   **Carcinoid syndrome** 🦠 🦠

> **Note:** May be used as an additional code to identify functional activity associated with a carcinoid tumor.
> (Ex:) See PDX Collection 528

E34.1   **Other hypersecretion of intestinal hormones**

E34.2   **Ectopic hormone secretion, not elsewhere classified**

> **Excludes1**   ectopic ACTH syndrome (E24.3)

E34.3   **Short stature due to endocrine disorder**
Constitutional short stature
Laron-type short stature

> **Excludes1**   achondroplastic short stature (Q77.4)
> hypochondroplastic short stature (Q77.4)
> nutritional short stature (E45)
> pituitary short stature (E23.0)
> progeria (E34.8)
> renal short stature (N25.0)
> Russell-Silver syndrome (Q87.19)
> short-limbed stature with immunodeficiency (D82.2)
> short stature in specific dysmorphic syndromes - code to syndrome - see Alphabetical Index
> short stature NOS (R62.52)

E34.4   **Constitutional tall stature** 🦠
Constitutional gigantism

E34.5   **Androgen insensitivity syndrome**

E34.50   **Androgen insensitivity syndrome, unspecified**
Androgen insensitivity NOS

E34.51   **Complete androgen insensitivity syndrome**
Complete androgen insensitivity
de Quervain syndrome
Goldberg-Maxwell syndrome

E34.52   **Partial androgen insensitivity syndrome**
Partial androgen insensitivity
Reifenstein syndrome

E34.8   **Other specified endocrine disorders**
Pineal gland dysfunction
Progeria

> **Excludes2**   pseudohypoparathyroidism (E20.1)

E34.9   **Endocrine disorder, unspecified**
Endocrine disturbance NOS
Hormone disturbance NOS

▷ **E35**   *Disorders of endocrine glands in diseases classified elsewhere*

> *Code first underlying disease, such as:*
> late congenital syphilis of thymus gland [Dubois disease] (A50.5)

> Use additional code, if applicable, to identify:
> sequelae of tuberculosis of other organs (B90.8)

> **Excludes1**   Echinococcus granulosus infection of thyroid gland (B67.3)
> meningococcal hemorrhagic adrenalitis (A39.1)
> syphilis of endocrine gland (A52.79)
> tuberculosis of adrenal gland, except calcification (A18.7)
> tuberculosis of endocrine gland NEC (A18.82)
> tuberculosis of thyroid gland (A18.81)
> Waterhouse-Friderichsen syndrome (A39.1)

INTRAOPERATIVE COMPLICATIONS OF ENDOCRINE SYSTEM (E36)

● **E36**   **Intraoperative complications of endocrine system**

> **Excludes2**   postprocedural endocrine and metabolic complications and disorders, not elsewhere classified (E89.-)

● **E36.0**   **Intraoperative hemorrhage and hematoma of an endocrine system organ or structure complicating a procedure**

> **Excludes1**   intraoperative hemorrhage and hematoma of an endocrine system organ or structure due to accidental puncture or laceration during a procedure (E36.1-)
> (Ex:) For category E36.0 CC codes: See PDX Collection 529

E36.01   **Intraoperative hemorrhage and hematoma of an endocrine system organ or structure complicating an endocrine system procedure** 🦠
Coding Clinic: 2020, Q1, P19

E36.02   **Intraoperative hemorrhage and hematoma of an endocrine system organ or structure complicating other procedure** 🦠

● **E36.1**   **Accidental puncture and laceration of an endocrine system organ or structure during a procedure**
(Ex:) For category E36.1 CC codes: See PDX Collection 509

E36.11   **Accidental puncture and laceration of an endocrine system organ or structure during an endocrine system procedure** 🦠

E36.12   **Accidental puncture and laceration of an endocrine system organ or structure during other procedure** 🦠

E36.8   **Other intraoperative complications of endocrine system**
Use additional code, if applicable, to further specify disorder

---

▶ New   ⟹ Revised   ~~deleted~~ Deleted   Excludes 1   Excludes 2   Includes   Use additional   Code first   Code also   Key words
OGCR Official Guidelines   ● Unacceptable Principal Diagnosis   X Assign placeholder X   ● Use Additional Character(s)   ▷ Manifestation Code   Coding Clinic

MALNUTRITION (E40-E46)

| **Excludes1** | intestinal malabsorption (K90.) |
| | sequelae of protein-calorie malnutrition (E64.0) |

| **Excludes2** | nutritional anemias (D50-D53) |
| | starvation (T73.0) |

E40   Kwashiorkor 🩸🩸
Malnutrition produced by severe protein deficiency
Severe malnutrition with nutritional edema with
dyspigmentation of skin and hair

> **Excludes1**   marasmic kwashiorkor (E42)

(Ex:) See PDX Collection 530
Coding Clinic: 22017, Q3, P25

E41   Nutritional marasmus 🩸🩸
Severe malnutrition with marasmus

> **Excludes1**   marasmic kwashiorkor (E42)

(Ex:) See PDX Collection 530
Coding Clinic: 2017, Q3, P24-25

E42   Marasmic kwashiorkor 🩸🩸
Severe protein malnutrition
Intermediate form severe protein-calorie malnutrition
Severe protein-calorie malnutrition with signs of both
      kwashiorkor and marasmus
(Ex:) See PDX Collection 530
Coding Clinic: 2017, Q3, P25

F43   Unspecified severe protein-calorie malnutrition 🩸🩸
Starvation edema
(Ex:) See PDX Collection 530
Coding Clinic: 2020, Q1, P5-6; 2017, Q4, P108-109; 2017, Q3, P25

● E44   Protein-calorie malnutrition of moderate and mild degree
(Ex:) For category E44 CC codes: See PDX Collection 530

| E44.0 | **Moderate** protein-calorie malnutrition 🩸🩸 |
| E44.1 | **Mild** protein-calorie malnutrition 🩸🩸 |

**E45   Retarded development following protein-calorie
        malnutrition** 🩸🩸
Nutritional short stature
Nutritional stunting
Physical retardation due to malnutrition
(Ex:) See PDX Collection 530

E46   Unspecified protein-calorie malnutrition 🩸🩸
Malnutrition NOS
Protein-calorie imbalance NOS

> **Excludes1**   nutritional deficiency NOS (E63.9)

(Ex:) See PDX Collection 530
Coding Clinic: 2017, Q3, P25

OTHER NUTRITIONAL DEFICIENCIES (E50-E64)

| **Excludes2** | nutritional anemias (D50-D53) |

● E50   Vitamin A deficiency

> **Excludes1**   sequelae of vitamin A deficiency (E64.1)

E50.0	**Vitamin A deficiency with conjunctival xerosis**
E50.1	**Vitamin A deficiency with Bitot's spot and conjunctival xerosis**
	Bitot's spot in the young child
E50.2	**Vitamin A deficiency with corneal xerosis**
E50.3	**Vitamin A deficiency with corneal ulceration and xerosis**
E50.4	**Vitamin A deficiency with keratomalacia**
	Eye disorder that results in dry cornea caused by vitamin A deficiency
E50.5	**Vitamin A deficiency with night blindness**
E50.6	**Vitamin A deficiency with xerophthalmic scars of cornea**
	Abnormal dryness and thickening of conjunctiva and cornea due to vitamin A deficiency
E50.7	**Other ocular manifestations** of vitamin A deficiency
	Xerophthalmia NOS

Item 4-6 Bitot's spots are the result of a buildup of keratin debris found on the superficial surface the conjunctiva; oval, triangular, or irregular in shape; and a sign of vitamin A deficiency and associated with night blindness. The disease may progress to **keratomalacia,** which can result in eventual prolapse of the iris and loss of the lens.

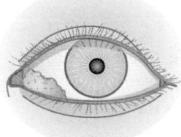

Figure 4-6   Bitot's spot on the conjunctiva.

E50.8	**Other manifestations** of vitamin A deficiency
	Follicular keratosis
	Xeroderma
E50.9	**Vitamin A deficiency, unspecified**
	Hypovitaminosis A NOS

● E51   Thiamine deficiency

> **Excludes1**   sequelae of thiamine deficiency (E64.8)

● E51.1   Beriberi
(Ex:) **For category E51.1 CC codes:** See PDX Collection 531

> **E51.11   Dry beriberi** 🩸
> *Thiamine deficiency with nervous system manifestation most often caused by excessive alcohol consumption*
> Beriberi NOS
> Beriberi with polyneuropathy

> **E51.12   Wet beriberi** 🩸
> *Thiamine deficiency with cardiovascular manifestation most often caused by excessive alcohol consumption*
> Beriberi with cardiovascular manifestations
> Cardiovascular beriberi
> Shoshin disease

E51.2	**Wernicke's encephalopathy** 🩸
	Acute disease of brain due to thiamine deficiency most often associated with excessive alcohol consumption
	(Ex:) See PDX Collection 531
E51.8	**Other manifestations of thiamine deficiency** 🩸
	(Ex:) See PDX Collection 531
E51.9	**Thiamine deficiency, unspecified** 🩸
	(Ex:) See PDX Collection 531

E52   Niacin deficiency [pellagra]
Niacin (-tryptophan) deficiency
Nicotinamide deficiency
Pellagra (alcoholic)

> **Excludes1**   sequelae of niacin deficiency (E64.8)

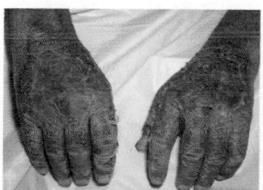

Figure 4-7   The sharply demarcated, characteristic scaling dermatitis of pellagra. (From James WD, Berger TG, Elston DM: Andrews' Diseases of the Skin: Clinical Dermatology, Philadelphia, Saunders Elsevier, 2006)

Item 4-7 Pellagra is associated with a deficiency of niacin and its precursor, **tryptophan.** Characteristics of the condition include diarrhea, dermatitis on exposed skin surfaces, dementia, and death. It is prevalent in developing countries where nutrition is inadequate. **Beriberi** is associated with thiamine deficiency.

N Newborn Age: 0   **P** Pediatric Age: 0–17   **M** Maternity DX: 9–64   **A** Adult Age: 15–124   ♀ Females Only   ♂ Males Only

🩸 Complication\Comorbidity   🩸 Major C\C   (Ex:) CC/MCC Exclusions   🩸 Hospital-Acquired Condition   🩸 Hierarchical Condition Category

763

CHAPTER 4 (E00-E89)

CHAPTER 4 (E00-E89)

● E53   **Deficiency of other B group vitamins**
     Excludes1   sequelae of vitamin B deficiency (E64.8)

     E53.0   **Riboflavin deficiency** 🔧
         Ariboflavinosis
         Vitamin B2 deficiency
         (Ex:) See PDX Collection 531

     E53.1   **Pyridoxine deficiency**
         Vitamin B6 deficiency
         Excludes1   pyridoxine-responsive sideroblastic anemia (D64.3)

     E53.8   **Deficiency of other specified B group vitamins**
         Biotin deficiency
         Cyanocobalamin deficiency
         Folate deficiency
         Folic acid deficiency
         Pantothenic acid deficiency
         Vitamin B12 deficiency
         Excludes1   folate deficiency anemia (D52.-)
                  vitamin B12 deficiency anemia (D51.-)

     E53.9   **Vitamin B deficiency, unspecified**

● E54   **Ascorbic acid deficiency**
     Deficiency of vitamin C
     Scurvy
     Excludes1   scorbutic anemia (D53.2)
               sequelae of vitamin C deficiency (E64.2)

● E55   **Vitamin D deficiency**
     Excludes1   adult osteomalacia (M83.-)
               osteoporosis (M80.-)
               sequelae of rickets (E64.3)

     E55.0   **Rickets, active** 🔧
         Infantile osteomalacia
         Juvenile osteomalacia
            Softening of bone
         Excludes1   celiac rickets (K90.0)
                  Crohn's rickets (K50.-)
                  hereditary vitamin D-dependent rickets (E83.32)
                  inactive rickets (E64.3)
                  renal rickets (N25.0)
                  sequelae of rickets (E64.3)
                  vitamin D-resistant rickets (E83.31)
         (Ex:) See PDX Collection 532

     E55.9   **Vitamin D deficiency, unspecified**
         Avitaminosis D

● E56   **Other vitamin deficiencies**
     Excludes1   sequelae of other vitamin deficiencies (E64.8)

     E56.0   **Deficiency of vitamin E**
     E56.1   **Deficiency of vitamin K**
         Excludes1   deficiency of coagulation factor due to vitamin K deficiency (D68.4)
                  vitamin K deficiency of newborn (P53)

     E56.8   **Deficiency of other vitamins**
     E56.9   **Vitamin deficiency, unspecified**

● E58   **Dietary calcium deficiency**
     Excludes1   disorders of calcium metabolism (E83.5-)
               sequelae of calcium deficiency (E64.8)

● E59   **Dietary selenium deficiency**
     Keshan disease
     Excludes1   sequelae of selenium deficiency (E64.8)

● E60   **Dietary zinc deficiency**

● E61   **Deficiency of other nutrient elements**
     Use additional code for adverse effect, if applicable, to identify drug (T36-T50 with fifth or sixth character 5)
     Excludes1   disorders of mineral metabolism (E83.-)
               iodine deficiency related thyroid disorders (E00-E02)
               sequelae of malnutrition and other nutritional deficiencies (E64.-)

     E61.0   **Copper deficiency**
     E61.1   **Iron deficiency**
         Excludes1   iron deficiency anemia (D50.-)
     E61.2   **Magnesium deficiency**
     E61.3   **Manganese deficiency**
     E61.4   **Chromium deficiency**
     E61.5   **Molybdenum deficiency**
     E61.6   **Vanadium deficiency**
     E61.7   **Deficiency of multiple nutrient elements**
     E61.8   **Deficiency of other specified nutrient elements**
     E61.9   **Deficiency of nutrient element, unspecified**

● E63   **Other nutritional deficiencies**
     ~~Excludes1~~
     ▶ **Excludes2**   dehydration (E86.0)
               failure to thrive, adult (R62.7)
               failure to thrive, child (R62.51)
               feeding problems in newborn (P92.-)
               sequelae of malnutrition and other nutritional deficiencies (E64.-)

     E63.0   **Essential fatty acid [EFA] deficiency**
     E63.1   **Imbalance of constituents of food intake**
     E63.8   **Other specified nutritional deficiencies**
     E63.9   **Nutritional deficiency, unspecified**

● E64   **Sequelae of malnutrition and other nutritional deficiencies**
     Pathological condition resulting from disease, injury, or other trauma
     Note: This category is to be used to indicate conditions in categories E43, E44, E46, E50-E63 as the cause of sequelae, which are themselves classified elsewhere. The "sequelae" include conditions specified as such; they also include the late effects of diseases classifiable to the above categories if the disease itself is no longer present
     Code first condition resulting from (sequela) of malnutrition and other nutritional deficiencies

     E64.0   **Sequelae of protein-calorie malnutrition** 🔧🔧
         Excludes2   retarded development following protein-calorie malnutrition (E45)
         (Ex:) See PDX Collection 530

     E64.1   **Sequelae of vitamin A deficiency**
     E64.2   **Sequelae of vitamin C deficiency**
     E64.3   **Sequelae of rickets**
     E64.8   **Sequelae of other nutritional deficiencies**
     E64.9   **Sequelae of unspecified nutritional deficiency**

▶ New   ⇒ Revised   ~~deleted~~ Deleted   Excludes 1   Excludes 2   Includes   Use additional   Code first   Code also   Key words

764   OGCR Official Guidelines   ● Unacceptable Principal Diagnosis   X Assign placeholder X   ● Use Additional Character(s)   ▶ Manifestation Code   Coding Clinic

OVERWEIGHT, OBESITY AND OTHER HYPERALIMENTATION (E65-E68)

E65   **Localized adiposity**
       Fat pad

● **E66**   **Overweight and obesity**
       Code first obesity complicating pregnancy, childbirth and the puerperium, if applicable (O99.21-)
       Use additional code to identify body mass index (BMI), if known (Z68.-)

       Excludes1   adiposogenital dystrophy (E23.6)
                      lipomatosis NOS (E88.2)
                      lipomatosis dolorosa [Dercum] (E88.2)
                      Prader-Willi syndrome (Q87.11)
       Coding Clinic: 2018, Q4, P80

●   **E66.0**   **Obesity due to excess calories**
       E66.01   **Morbid (severe) obesity due to excess calories**

                   Excludes1   morbid (severe) obesity with alveolar hypoventilation (E66.2)
                   Coding Clinic: 2018, Q4, P79

       E66.09   **Other obesity due to excess calories**
                   MCE: Questionable admission when principal dx

  E66.1   **Drug-induced obesity**
       MCE: Questionable admission when principal dx
       Use additional code for adverse effect, if applicable, to identify drug (T36-T50 with fifth or sixth character 5)

  E66.2   **Morbid (severe) obesity with alveolar hypoventilation**
       Uncommon condition of unknown cause leading to inadequate ventilation in lungs, even though lungs and airways are normal
       Obesity hypoventilation syndrome (OHS)
       Pickwickian syndrome
       (Ex) See PDX Collection 533

  E66.3   **Overweight**

  E66.8   **Other obesity**
       MCE: Questionable admission when principal dx

  E66.9   **Obesity, unspecified**
       Obesity NOS
       MCE: Questionable admission when principal dx
       Coding Clinic: 2021, Q2, P10-11

● **E67**   **Other hyperalimentation**
       Ingestion of more than optimal amount of nutrients

       Excludes1   hyperalimentation NOS (R63.2)
                      sequelae of hyperalimentation (E68)

  E67.0   **Hypervitaminosis A**

  E67.1   **Hypercarotenemia**

  E67.2   **Megavitamin-B6 syndrome**

  E67.3   **Hypervitaminosis D**

  E67.8   **Other specified hyperalimentation**

E68   **Sequelae of hyperalimentation**
       Code first condition resulting from (sequela) of hyperalimentation

METABOLIC DISORDERS (E70-E88)

  Excludes1   androgen insensitivity syndrome (E34.5-)
               congenital adrenal hyperplasia (E25.0)
               ~~Ehlers-Danlos syndromes (Q79.6-)~~
               hemolytic anemias attributable to enzyme disorders (D55.-)
               Marfan's syndrome (Q87.4)
               5-alpha-reductase deficiency (E29.1)

▶ **Excludes2**   Ehlers-Danlos syndromes (Q79.6-)

● **E70**   **Disorders of aromatic amino-acid metabolism**
       (Ex) For category E70 CC codes: See PDX Collection 534

  E70.0   **Classical phenylketonuria**
       Inherited disorder that increases to harmful levels amino acid phenylalanine

  E70.1   **Other hyperphenylalaninemias**

● **E70.2**   **Disorders of tyrosine metabolism**

       Excludes1   transitory tyrosinemia of newborn (P74.5)

       E70.20   **Disorder of tyrosine metabolism, unspecified**
                   Tyrosine: Nonessential amino acid occurring in most proteins

       E70.21   **Tyrosinemia**
                   Congenital amino acid metabolism
                   Hypertyrosinemia

       E70.29   **Other disorders of tyrosine metabolism**
                   Alkaptonuria
                   Ochronosis

● **E70.3**   **Albinism**
       Congenital condition of reduced or absent pigment in eyes, skin, and hair

       E70.30   **Albinism, unspecified**

●   **E70.31**   **Ocular albinism**

       E70.310   **X-linked ocular albinism**

       E70.311   **Autosomal recessive ocular albinism**

       E70.318   **Other ocular albinism**

       E70.319   **Ocular albinism, unspecified**

●   **E70.32**   **Oculocutaneous albinism**
       Partial or total lack of melanin pigment in eyes

       Excludes1   Chediak-Higashi syndrome (E70.330)
                   Hermansky-Pudlak syndrome (E70.331)

       E70.320   **Tyrosinase negative oculocutaneous albinism**
                   Albinism I
                   Oculocutaneous albinism ty-neg

       E70.321   **Tyrosinase positive oculocutaneous albinism**
                   Albinism II
                   Oculocutaneous albinism ty-pos

       E70.328   **Other oculocutaneous albinism**
                   Cross syndrome

       E70.329   **Oculocutaneous albinism, unspecified**

●   **E70.33**   **Albinism with hematologic abnormality**

       E70.330   **Chediak-Higashi syndrome**

       E70.331   **Hermansky-Pudlak syndrome**

       E70.338   **Other albinism with hematologic abnormality**

       E70.339   **Albinism with hematologic abnormality, unspecified**

       E70.39   **Other specified albinism**
                   Piebaldism

● **E70.4**   **Disorders of histidine metabolism**

       E70.40   **Disorders of histidine metabolism, unspecified**

       E70.41   **Histidinemia**

       E70.49   **Other disorders of histidine metabolism**

  E70.5   **Disorders of tryptophan metabolism**

● **E70.8**   **Other disorders of aromatic amino-acid metabolism**

       E70.81   **Aromatic L-amino acid decarboxylase deficiency**
                   AADC deficiency
                   (Ex) See PDX Collection 4045

       E70.89   **Other disorders of aromatic amino-acid metabolism**
                   (Ex) See PDX Collection 4045

  E70.9   **Disorder of aromatic amino-acid metabolism, unspecified**

N Newborn Age: 0   **P** Pediatric Age: 0–17   **M** Maternity DX: 9–64   **A** Adult Age: 15–124   ♀ Females Only   ♂ Males Only

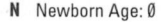 Complication\Comorbidity   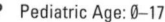 Major C\C   (Ex) CC/MCC Exclusions   Hospital-Acquired Condition   Hierarchical Condition Category

765

CHAPTER 4 (E00-E89)

CHAPTER 4 (E00–E89)

● **E71**   Disorders of branched-chain amino-acid metabolism and fatty-acid metabolism

     E71.0   Maple-syrup-urine disease 🔹🔹
         Due to defect in amino acid catabolism, causing severe ketoacidosis with smell of maple syrup in urine and on body
         Ⓔ See PDX Collection 534

   ● E71.1   Other disorders of branched-chain amino-acid metabolism
         Ⓔ For category E71.1 CC codes: See PDX Collection 534

     ● E71.11   Branched-chain organic acidurias
         E71.110   Isovaleric acidemia 🔹🔹
         E71.111   3-methylglutaconic aciduria 🔹🔹
         E71.118   Other branched-chain organic acidurias 🔹🔹

     ● E71.12   Disorders of propionate metabolism
         E71.120   Methylmalonic acidemia 🔹🔹
         E71.121   Propionic acidemia 🔹🔹
         E71.128   Other disorders of propionate metabolism 🔹🔹

     E71.19   Other disorders of branched-chain amino-acid metabolism 🔹🔹
         Hyperleucine-isoleucinemia
         Hypervalinemia

     E71.2   Disorder of branched-chain amino-acid metabolism, unspecified 🔹🔹
         Ⓔ See PDX Collection 534

   ● E71.3   Disorders of fatty-acid metabolism

     Excludes1   peroxisomal disorders (E71.5)
         Refsum's disease (G60.1)
         Schilder's disease (G37.0)

     Excludes2   carnitine deficiency due to inborn error of metabolism (E71.42)

     E71.30   Disorder of fatty-acid metabolism, unspecified

     ● E71.31   Disorders of fatty-acid oxidation
         E71.310   Long chain/very long chain acyl CoA dehydrogenase deficiency 🔹🔹
             LCAD
             VLCAD
             Ⓔ See PDX Collection 3636

         E71.311   Medium chain acyl CoA dehydrogenase deficiency 🔹🔹
             MCAD
             Ⓔ See PDX Collection 3638

         E71.312   Short chain acyl CoA dehydrogenase deficiency 🔹🔹
             SCAD
             Ⓔ See PDX Collection 3640

         E71.313   Glutaric aciduria type II 🔹🔹
             Glutaric aciduria type II A
             Glutaric aciduria type II B
             Glutaric aciduria type II C

             Excludes1   glutaric aciduria (type 1) NOS (E72.3)
             Ⓔ See PDX Collection 3642

         E71.314   Muscle carnitine palmitoyltransferase deficiency 🔹🔹
             Ⓔ See PDX Collection 3644

         E71.318   Other disorders of fatty-acid oxidation 🔹🔹
             Ⓔ See PDX Collection 3646

     E71.32   Disorders of ketone metabolism 🔹🔹
         Ⓔ See PDX Collection 535

     E71.39   Other disorders of fatty-acid metabolism 🔹🔹
         Ⓔ See PDX Collection 3648

   ● E71.4   Disorders of carnitine metabolism

     Excludes1   muscle carnitine palmitoyltransferase deficiency (E71.314)

     E71.40   Disorder of carnitine metabolism, unspecified 🔹

     E71.41   Primary carnitine deficiency 🔹

     E71.42   Carnitine deficiency due to inborn errors of metabolism 🔹
         Code also associated inborn error or metabolism

     E71.43   Iatrogenic carnitine deficiency 🔹
         Iatrogenic: Outcomes from activity of physicians
         Carnitine deficiency due to hemodialysis
         Carnitine deficiency due to Valproic acid therapy

   ● E71.44   Other secondary carnitine deficiency
         E71.440   Ruvalcaba-Myhre-Smith syndrome 🔹
         E71.448   Other secondary carnitine deficiency 🔹

   ● E71.5   Peroxisomal disorders
     Class of conditions which lead to disorders of lipid metabolism

     Excludes1   Schilder's disease (G37.0)

     E71.50   Peroxisomal disorder, unspecified 🔹🔹
         Ⓔ See PDX Collection 3650

   ● E71.51   Disorders of peroxisome biogenesis
     Group 1 peroxisomal disorders

     Excludes1   Refsum's disease (G60.1)

     E71.510   Zellweger syndrome 🔹🔹
         Ⓔ See PDX Collection 3652

     E71.511   Neonatal adrenoleukodystrophy 🔹🔹

         Excludes1   X-linked adrenoleuko-dystrophy (E71.42-)
         Ⓔ See PDX Collection 3654

     E71.518   Other disorders of peroxisome biogenesis 🔹🔹
         Ⓔ See PDX Collection 3656

   ● E71.52   X-linked adrenoleukodystrophy
     E71.520   Childhood cerebral X-linked adrenoleukodystrophy 🔹🔹
         Ⓔ See PDX Collection 3658

     E71.521   Adolescent X-linked adrenoleukodystrophy 🔹🔹
         Ⓔ See PDX Collection 3660

     E71.522   Adrenomyeloneuropathy 🔹🔹
         Ⓔ See PDX Collection 3662

     E71.528   Other X-linked adrenoleukodystrophy 🔹🔹
         Addison only phenotype adrenoleukodystrophy
         Addison-Schilder adrenoleukodystrophy
         Ⓔ See PDX Collection 3664

     E71.529   X-linked adrenoleukodystrophy, unspecified type 🔹🔹
         Ⓔ See PDX Collection 3666

     E71.53   Other group 2 peroxisomal disorders 🔹🔹
         Ⓔ See PDX Collection 3668

   ● E71.54   Other peroxisomal disorders
     E71.540   Rhizomelic chondrodysplasia punctata 🔹🔹
         Rare, severe, inherited disorder with limb shortening, bone and cartilage abnormalities, abnormal facial appearance, severe mental retardation, psychomotor retardation, and cataracts

         Excludes1   chondrodysplasia punctata NOS (Q77.3)
         Ⓔ See PDX Collection 3670

     E71.541   Zellweger-like syndrome 🔹🔹
         Ⓔ See PDX Collection 3672

     E71.542   Other group 3 peroxisomal disorders 🔹🔹
         Ⓔ See PDX Collection 3674

     E71.548   Other peroxisomal disorders 🔹🔹
         Ⓔ See PDX Collection 536

▶ New   ⇒ Revised   ~~deleted~~ Deleted   Excludes 1   Excludes 2   Includes   Use additional   Code first   Code also   Key words

OGCR Official Guidelines   ● Unacceptable Principal Diagnosis   X Assign placeholder X   ● Use Additional Character(s)   ▶ Manifestation Code   **Coding Clinic**

● **E72   Other disorders of amino-acid metabolism**

> Excludes1   disorders of:
> aromatic amino-acid metabolism (E70.-)
> branched-chain amino-acid metabolism
> (E71.0-E71.2)
> fatty-acid metabolism (E71.3)
> purine and pyrimidine metabolism (E79.-)
> gout (M1A.-, M10.-)
>
> (Ex) **For category E72 CC codes unless otherwise noted:** See PDX Collection 534

● **E72.0   Disorders of amino-acid transport**

> Excludes1   disorders of tryptophan metabolism
> (E70.5)

E72.00   Disorders of amino-acid transport, unspecified 🔹🔹

E72.01   Cystinuria 🔹🔹
Hereditary aminoaciduria due to impairment of renal transport with predominant symptom of urinary cystine calculi

E72.02   Hartnup's disease 🔹🔹
Inborn error of metabolism

E72.03   Lowe's syndrome 🔹🔹
X-linked disorder with rickets, hydrophthalmia, congenital glaucoma, cataracts, mental retardation, and renal tubule dysfunction
Use additional code for associated glaucoma (H42)
(Ex) See PDX Collection 3214

E72.04   Cystinosis 🔹🔹
Genetic disease with excessive deposits of amino acid cystine in cells
Fanconi (-de Toni) (-Debré) syndrome with cystinosis

> Excludes1   Fanconi (-de Toni) (-Debré) syndrome without cystinosis (E72.09)

E72.09   Other disorders of amino-acid transport 🔹🔹
Fanconi (-de Toni) (-Debré) syndrome, unspecified

● **E72.1   Disorders of sulfur-bearing amino-acid metabolism**

> Excludes1   cystinosis (E72.04)
> cystinuria (E72.01)
> transcobalamin II deficiency (D51.2)

E72.10   Disorders of sulfur-bearing amino-acid metabolism, unspecified 🔹🔹

E72.11   Homocystinuria 🔹🔹
Cystathionine synthase deficiency

E72.12   Methylenetetrahydrofolate reductase deficiency 🔹🔹

E72.19   Other disorders of sulfur-bearing amino-acid metabolism 🔹🔹
Cystathioninuria
Methioninemia
Sulfite oxidase deficiency

● **E72.2   Disorders of urea cycle metabolism**

> Excludes1   disorders of ornithine metabolism (E72.4)

E72.20   Disorder of urea cycle metabolism, unspecified 🔹🔹
Hyperammonemia
Elevated levels of ammonia

> Excludes1   hyperammonemia-hyperornithinemia-homocitrullinemia syndrome E72.4
> transient hyperammonemia of newborn (P74.6)

E72.21   Argininemia 🔹🔹
Disorder in which deficiency of enzyme arginase causes build-up of arginine and ammonia in blood

E72.22   Arginosuccinic aciduria 🔹🔹
Gene disorder of urea cycle resulting accumulation of ammonia

E72.23   Citrullinemia 🔹🔹
Urea cycle disorder that causes ammonia and other toxic substances to accumulate in blood

E72.29   Other disorders of urea cycle metabolism 🔹🔹

E72.3   Disorders of lysine and hydroxylysine metabolism 🔹🔹
Glutaric aciduria NOS
Glutaric aciduria (type I)
Hydroxylysinemia
Hyperlysinemia

> Excludes1   glutaric aciduria type II (E71.313)
> Refsum's disease (G60.1)
> Zellweger syndrome (E71.510)

E72.4   Disorders of ornithine metabolism 🔹🔹
Hyperammonemia-Hyperornithinemia-Homocitrullinemia syndrome
Ornithinemia (types I, II)
Ornithine transcarbamylase deficiency

> Excludes1   hereditary choroidal dystrophy (H31.2-)

● **E72.5   Disorders of glycine metabolism**

E72.50   Disorder of glycine metabolism, unspecified 🔹🔹

E72.51   Non-ketotic hyperglycinemia 🔹🔹

E72.52   Trimethylaminuria 🔹🔹

E72.53   Primary hyperoxaluria 🔹🔹
Oxalosis
Oxaluria

E72.59   Other disorders of glycine metabolism 🔹🔹
D-glycericacidemia
Hyperhydroxyprolinemia
Hyperprolinemia (types I, II)
Sarcosinemia

● **E72.8   Other specified disorders of amino-acid metabolism** 🔹

E72.81   Disorders of gamma aminobutyric acid metabolism 🔹🔹
4-hydroxybutyric aciduria
Disorders of GABA metabolism
GABA metabolic defect
GABA transaminase deficiency
GABA-T deficiency
Gamma-hydroxybutyric aciduria
SSADHD
Succinic semialdehyde dehydrogenase deficiency
(Ex) See PDX Collection 534

E72.89   Other specified disorders of amino-acid metabolism 🔹🔹
Disorders of beta-amino-acid metabolism
Disorders of gamma-glutamyl cycle
(Ex) See PDX Collection 534

E72.9   Disorder of amino-acid metabolism, unspecified 🔹🔹

● **E73   Lactose intolerance**
Intolerance for lactose, due to inherited deficiency of lactase activity in intestinal mucosa

E73.0   Congenital lactase deficiency

E73.1   Secondary lactase deficiency

E73.8   Other lactose intolerance

E73.9   Lactose intolerance, unspecified

● **E74   Other disorders of carbohydrate metabolism**

> Excludes1   diabetes mellitus (E08-E13)
> hypoglycemia NOS (E16.2)
> increased secretion of glucagon (E16.3)
> mucopolysaccharidosis (E76.0-E76.3)
>
> (Ex) **For category E74 CC codes:** See PDX Collection 534

● **E74.0   Glycogen storage disease**

E74.00   Glycogen storage disease, unspecified 🔹🔹

E74.01   von Gierke's disease 🔹🔹
Type I glycogen storage disease

E74.02   Pompe disease 🔹🔹
Cardiac glycogenosis
Type II glycogen storage disease

E74.03   Cori disease 🔹🔹
Forbes' disease
Type III glycogen storage disease

E74.04   McArdle disease 🔹🔹
Type V glycogen storage disease

N Newborn Age: 0   **P** Pediatric Age: 0–17   **M** Maternity DX: 9–64   **A** Adult Age: 15–124   ♀ Females Only   ♂ Males Only

🔹 Complication\Comorbidity   🔹 Major C\C   (Ex) CC/MCC Exclusions   🔹 Hospital-Acquired Condition   🔹 Hierarchical Condition Category

767

E74.09   Other glycogen storage disease
    Andersen disease
    Hers disease
    Tauri disease
    Glycogen storage disease, types Ø, IV, VI-XI
    Liver phosphorylase deficiency
    Muscle phosphofructokinase deficiency

E74.1   Disorders of fructose metabolism
    Excludes1   muscle phosphofructokinase deficiency (E74.09)

E74.10   Disorder of fructose metabolism, unspecified

E74.11   Essential fructosuria
    Fructokinase deficiency

E74.12   Hereditary fructose intolerance
    Fructosemia

E74.19   Other disorders of fructose metabolism
    Fructose-1, 6-diphosphatase deficiency

E74.2   Disorders of galactose metabolism

E74.20   Disorders of galactose metabolism, unspecified

E74.21   Galactosemia
    Genetic disorders resulting from defective simple sugar (galactose) metabolism

E74.29   Other disorders of galactose metabolism
    Galactokinase deficiency

E74.3   Other disorders of intestinal carbohydrate absorption
    Excludes2   lactose intolerance (E73.-)

E74.31   Sucrase-isomaltase deficiency
    Deficiency in metabolism in intestinal mucosa results in malabsorption of sucrose and starch

E74.39   Other disorders of intestinal carbohydrate absorption
    Disorder of intestinal carbohydrate absorption NOS
    Glucose-galactose malabsorption
    Sucrase deficiency

E74.4   Disorders of pyruvate metabolism and gluconeogenesis
    Deficiency of phosphoenolpyruvate carboxykinase
    Deficiency of pyruvate carboxylase
    Deficiency of pyruvate dehydrogenase
    Excludes1   disorders of pyruvate metabolism and gluconeogenesis with anemia (D55.-)
         Leigh's syndrome (G31.82)

E74.8   Other specified disorders of carbohydrate metabolism

E74.81   Disorders of glucose transport, not elsewhere classified

E74.810   Glucose transporter protein type 1 deficiency
    De Vivo syndrome
    Glucose transport defect, blood-brain barrier
    GLUT1 deficiency
    GLUT1 deficiency syndrome 1, infantile onset
    GLUT1 deficiency syndrome 2, childhood onset
    (Ex:) See PDX Collection 4089

E74.818   Other disorders of glucose transport
    (Familial) renal glycosuria
    (Ex:) See PDX Collection 4087

E74.819   Disorders of glucose transport, unspecified
    (Ex:) See PDX Collection 4088

E74.89   Other specified disorders of carbohydrate metabolism
    Essential pentosuria
    (Ex:) See PDX Collection 4082

E74.9   Disorder of carbohydrate metabolism, unspecified

Item 4–8   **Leukodystrophy** is characterized by degeneration and/or failure of the myelin formation of the central nervous system and sometimes of the peripheral nervous system. The disease is inherited and progressive.

E75   Disorders of sphingolipid metabolism and other lipid storage disorders
    Excludes1   mucolipidosis, types I-III (E77.0-E77.1)
         Refsum's disease (G60.1)

E75.0   GM2 gangliosidosis
    Rare metabolic disorder that causes destruction of nerve cells of brain and spinal cord
    (Ex:) **For category E75.0 CC codes:** See PDX Collection 537

E75.00   GM2 gangliosidosis, unspecified

E75.01   Sandhoff disease

E75.02   Tay-Sachs disease

E75.09   Other GM2 gangliosidosis
    Adult GM2 gangliosidosis
    Juvenile GM2 gangliosidosis

E75.1   Other and unspecified gangliosidosis
    (Ex:) **For category E75.1 CC codes:** See PDX Collection 537

E75.10   Unspecified gangliosidosis
    Gangliosidosis NOS

E75.11   Mucolipidosis IV
    Disorder with symptoms of psychomotor retardation and severe visual impairment

E75.19   Other gangliosidosis
    GM1 gangliosidosis
    GM3 gangliosidosis

E75.2   Other sphingolipidosis
    Lysosomal (a particle in a cytoplasm cell that contains digestive enzymes) storage diseases with symptoms of abnormal storage of amino acids
    Excludes1   adrenoleukodystrophy [Addison-Schilder] (E71.528)

E75.21   Fabry (-Anderson) disease

E75.22   Gaucher disease

E75.23   Krabbe disease
    (Ex:) See PDX Collection 538

E75.24   Niemann-Pick disease
    ▶Acid sphingomyelinase deficiency (ASMD)

E75.240   Niemann-Pick disease type A
    ▶Acid sphingomyelinase deficiency type A (ASMD type A)
    ▶Infantile neurovisceral acid sphingomyelinase deficiency

E75.241   Niemann-Pick disease type B
    ▶Acid sphingomyelinase deficiency type B (ASMD type B)
    ▶Chronic visceral acid sphingomyelinase deficiency

E75.242   Niemann-Pick disease type C

E75.243   Niemann-Pick disease type D

▶**E75.244**   Niemann-Pick disease type A/B
    ▶Acid sphingomyelinase deficiency type A/B (ASMD type A/B)
    ▶Chronic neurovisceral acid sphingomyelinase deficiency

E75.248   Other Niemann-Pick disease

E75.249   Niemann-Pick disease, unspecified
    ▶Acid sphingomyelinase deficiency (ASMD) NOS

E75.25   Metachromatic leukodystrophy
    (Ex:) See PDX Collection 538

E75.26   Sulfatase deficiency
    Multiple sulfatase deficiency (MSD)
    (Ex:) See PDX Collection 538

E75.29   Other sphingolipidosis
    Farber's syndrome
    Sulfatide lipidosis
    (Ex:) See PDX Collection 538

E75.3   Sphingolipidosis, unspecified

E75.4   Neuronal ceroid lipofuscinosis
    Batten disease
    Bielschowsky-Jansky disease
    Kufs disease
    Spielmeyer-Vogt disease
    (Ex:) See PDX Collection 537

▶ New   ⇒ Revised   ~~deleted~~ Deleted   Excludes 1   Excludes 2   Includes   Use additional   Code first   Code also   Key words

OGCR Official Guidelines   ● Unacceptable Principal Diagnosis   X Assign placeholder X   ● Use Additional Character(s)   ▷ Manifestation Code   Coding Clinic

E75.5   **Other lipid storage disorders**
     Cerebrotendinous cholesterosis [van Bogaert-Scherer-Epstein]
     Wolman's disease

E75.6   **Lipid storage disorder, unspecified**

● **E76**   **Disorders of glycosaminoglycan metabolism**
    (Ex) **For category E76 CC codes:** See PDX Collection 539

● **E76.0**   **Mucopolysaccharidosis, type I**
     Inborn metabolic disorder of enzymes that break down carbohydrates

     E76.01   **Hurler's syndrome**

     E76.02   **Hurler-Scheie syndrome**

     E76.03   **Scheie's syndrome**

E76.1   **Mucopolysaccharidosis, type II**
     Inborn metabolic disorder of enzymes that break down carbohydrates occurs in 2-4 year old males
     Hunter's syndrome

● **E76.2**   **Other mucopolysaccharidoses**

  ● **E76.21**   **Morquio mucopolysaccharidoses**

     E76.210   **Morquio A mucopolysaccharidoses**
       Classic Morquio syndrome
       Morquio syndrome A, type IVA
       Mucopolysaccharidosis, type IVA

     E76.211   **Morquio B mucopolysaccharidoses**
       Morquio-like mucopolysaccharidoses
       Morquio-like syndrome
       Morquio syndrome B
       Mucopolysaccharidosis, type IVB

     E76.219   **Morquio mucopolysaccharidoses, unspecified**
       Morquio syndrome
       Mucopolysaccharidosis, type IV

     E76.22   **Sanfilippo mucopolysaccharidoses**
       Mucopolysaccharidosis, type III (A) (B) (C) (D)
       Sanfilippo A syndrome
       Sanfilippo B syndrome
       Sanfilippo C syndrome
       Sanfilippo D syndrome

     E76.29   **Other mucopolysaccharidoses**
       beta-Glucuronidase deficiency
       Maroteaux-Lamy (mild) (severe) syndrome
       Mucopolysaccharidosis, types VI, VII

E76.3   **Mucopolysaccharidosis, unspecified**

E76.8   **Other disorders of glucosaminoglycan metabolism**

E76.9   **Glucosaminoglycan metabolism disorder, unspecified**

● **E77**   **Disorders of glycoprotein metabolism**

   E77.0   **Defects in post-translational modification of lysosomal enzymes**
     Mucolipidosis II [I-cell disease]
     Mucolipidosis III [pseudo-Hurler polydystrophy]

   E77.1   **Defects in glycoprotein degradation**
     Aspartylglucosaminuria
     Fucosidosis
     Mannosidosis
     Sialidosis [mucolipidosis I]

   E77.8   **Other disorders of glycoprotein metabolism**

   E77.9   **Disorder of glycoprotein metabolism, unspecified**

● **E78**   **Disorders of lipoprotein metabolism and other lipidemias**
    Excludes1   sphingolipidosis (E75.0-E75.3)

  ● **E78.0**   **Pure hypercholesterolemia**
     Coding Clinic: 2016, Q4, P13

     E78.00   **Pure hypercholesterolemia, unspecified**
       Fredrickson's hyperlipoproteinemia, type IIa
       Hyperbetalipoproteinemia
       Low-density-lipoprotein-type [LDL] hyperlipoproteinemia
       (Pure) hypercholesterolemia NOS
       Coding Clinic: 2016, Q4, P13

     E78.01   **Familial hypercholesterolemia**
       Coding Clinic: 2016, Q4, P13

E78.1   **Pure hyperglyceridemia**
     Elevated fasting triglycerides
     Endogenous hyperglyceridemia
     Fredrickson's hyperlipoproteinemia, type IV
     Hyperlipidemia, group B
     Hyperprebetalipoproteinemia
     Very-low-density-lipoprotein-type [VLDL] hyperlipoproteinemia

E78.2   **Mixed hyperlipidemia**
     Broad- or floating-betalipoproteinemia
     Combined hyperlipidemia NOS
     Elevated cholesterol with elevated triglycerides NEC
     Fredrickson's hyperlipoproteinemia, type IIb or III
     Hyperbetalipoproteinemia with prebetalipoproteinemia
     Hypercholesteremia with endogenous hyperglyceridemia
     Hyperlipidemia, group C
     Tubo-eruptive xanthoma
     Xanthoma tuberosum

    Excludes1   cerebrotendinous cholesterosis [van Bogaert-Scherer-Epstein] (E75.5)
       familial combined hyperlipidemia (E78.49)

E78.3   **Hyperchylomicronemia**
     Chylomicron retention disease
     Fredrickson's hyperlipoproteinemia, type I or V
     Hyperlipidemia, group D
     Mixed hyperglyceridemia

● **E78.4**   **Other hyperlipidemia**

     E78.41   **Elevated Lipoprotein(a)**
       Elevated Lp(a)
       (Ex) See PDX Collection 534

     E78.49   **Other hyperlipidemia**
       Familial combined hyperlipidemia
       (Ex) See PDX Collection 534

E78.5   **Hyperlipidemia, unspecified**

E78.6   **Lipoprotein deficiency**
     Abetalipoproteinemia
     Depressed HDL cholesterol
     High-density lipoprotein deficiency
     Hypoalphalipoproteinemia
     Hypobetalipoproteinemia (familial)
     Lecithin cholesterol acyltransferase deficiency
     Tangier disease

● **E78.7**   **Disorders of bile acid and cholesterol metabolism**
    Excludes1   Niemann-Pick disease type C (E75.242)
    (Ex) **For category E78.7 CC codes:** See PDX Collection 540

     E78.70   **Disorder of bile acid and cholesterol metabolism, unspecified**

     E78.71   **Barth syndrome**
       (Ex) See PDX Collection 3499

     E78.72   **Smith-Lemli-Opitz syndrome**
       (Ex) See PDX Collection 3499

     E78.79   **Other disorders of bile acid and cholesterol metabolism**

● **E78.8**   **Other disorders of lipoprotein metabolism**

     E78.81   **Lipoid dermatoarthritis**

     E78.89   **Other lipoprotein metabolism disorders**

E78.9   **Disorder of lipoprotein metabolism, unspecified**

● **E79**   **Disorders of purine and pyrimidine metabolism**
     Purines, along with pyrimidines, signal RNA and DNA production
    Excludes1   Ataxia-telangiectasia (Q87.19)
       Bloom's syndrome (Q82.8)
       Cockayne's syndrome (Q87.19)
       calculus of kidney (N20.0)
       combined immunodeficiency disorders (D81.-)
       Fanconi's anemia (D61.09)
       gout (M1A.-, M10.-)
       orotaciduric anemia (D53.0)
       progeria (E34.8)
       Werner's syndrome (E34.8)
       xeroderma pigmentosum (Q82.1)
    (Ex) **For category E79 CC codes:** See PDX Collection 513

E79.0   **Hyperuricemia without signs of inflammatory arthritis and tophaceous disease**
     Asymptomatic hyperuricemia

CHAPTER 4 (E00-E89)

N Newborn Age: 0   **P** Pediatric Age: 0–17   **M** Maternity DX: 9–64   **A** Adult Age: 15–124   ♀ Females Only   ♂ Males Only

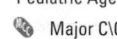 Complication\Comorbidity   Major C\C   (Ex) CC/MCC Exclusions   Hospital-Acquired Condition   Hierarchical Condition Category

E79.1   Lesch-Nyhan syndrome
> HGPRT deficiency

E79.2   Myoadenylate deaminase deficiency

E79.8   Other disorders of purine and pyrimidine metabolism
> Hereditary xanthinuria

E79.9   Disorder of purine and pyrimidine metabolism, unspecified

● **E80**   Disorders of porphyrin and bilirubin metabolism
> *Group of chemical compounds in RBCs that combine with iron to form heme*
>
> **Includes**   defects of catalase and peroxidase
>
> (Ex) For category E80 CC codes unless otherwise indicated: See PDX Collection 513

E80.0   Hereditary erythropoietic porphyria
> Congenital erythropoietic porphyria
> Erythropoietic protoporphyria

E80.1   Porphyria cutanea tarda

● **E80.2**   Other and unspecified porphyria

     E80.20   Unspecified porphyria
> Porphyria NOS

     E80.21   Acute intermittent (hepatic) porphyria

     E80.29   Other porphyria
> Hereditary coproporphyria

E80.3   Defects of catalase and peroxidase
> Acatalasia [Takahara]
> (Ex) See PDX Collection 492

E80.4   Gilbert syndrome

E80.5   Crigler-Najjar syndrome

E80.6   Other disorders of bilirubin metabolism
> Dubin-Johnson syndrome
> Rotor's syndrome

E80.7   Disorder of bilirubin metabolism, unspecified

● **E83**   Disorders of mineral metabolism
> **Excludes1**   dietary mineral deficiency (E58-E61)
> parathyroid disorders (E20-E21)
> vitamin D deficiency (E55.-)

● **E83.0**   Disorders of copper metabolism

     E83.00   Disorder of copper metabolism, unspecified

     E83.01   Wilson's disease
> Code also associated Kayser Fleischer ring (H18.04-)

     E83.09   Other disorders of copper metabolism
> Menkes' (kinky hair) (steely hair) disease

● **E83.1**   Disorders of iron metabolism
> **Excludes1**   iron deficiency anemia (D50.-)
> sideroblastic anemia (D64.0-D64.3)

     E83.10   Disorder of iron metabolism, unspecified

  ● **E83.11**   Hemochromatosis
> **Excludes1**   GALD (P78.84)
> Gestational alloimmune liver disease (P78.84)
> Neonatal hemochromatosis (P78.84)

     E83.110   Hereditary hemochromatosis
> Bronzed diabetes
> Pigmentary cirrhosis (of liver)
> Primary (hereditary) hemochromatosis

     E83.111   Hemochromatosis due to repeated red blood cell transfusions
> Iron overload due to repeated red blood cell transfusions
> Transfusion (red blood cell) associated hemochromatosis

     E83.118   Other hemochromatosis

     E83.119   Hemochromatosis, unspecified

     E83.19   Other disorders of iron metabolism
> Use additional code, if applicable, for idiopathic pulmonary hemosiderosis (J84.03)

E83.2   Disorders of zinc metabolism
> Acrodermatitis enteropathica

● **E83.3**   Disorders of phosphorus metabolism and phosphatases
> **Excludes1**   adult osteomalacia (M83.-)
> osteoporosis (M80.-)

     E83.30   Disorder of phosphorus metabolism, unspecified

     E83.31   Familial hypophosphatemia
> Vitamin D-resistant osteomalacia
> Vitamin D-resistant rickets
>
> **Excludes1**   vitamin D-deficiency rickets (E55.0)

     E83.32   Hereditary vitamin D-dependent rickets (type 1) (type 2)
> 25-hydroxyvitamin D 1-alpha-hydroxylase deficiency
> Pseudovitamin D deficiency
> Vitamin D receptor defect

     E83.39   Other disorders of phosphorus metabolism
> Acid phosphatase deficiency
> Hypophosphatasia

● **E83.4**   Disorders of magnesium metabolism

     E83.40   Disorders of magnesium metabolism, unspecified

     E83.41   Hypermagnesemia
> **Coding Clinic: 2016, Q4, P55**

     E83.42   Hypomagnesemia

     E83.49   Other disorders of magnesium metabolism

● **E83.5**   Disorders of calcium metabolism
> **Excludes1**   chondrocalcinosis (M11.1-M11.2)
> hungry bone syndrome (E83.81)
> hyperparathyroidism (E21.0-E21.3)

     E83.50   Unspecified disorder of calcium metabolism

     E83.51   Hypocalcemia

     E83.52   Hypercalcemia
> Familial hypocalciuric hypercalcemia

     E83.59   Other disorders of calcium metabolism
> Idiopathic hypercalciuria

● **E83.8**   Other disorders of mineral metabolism

     E83.81   Hungry bone syndrome

     E83.89   Other disorders of mineral metabolism

E83.9   Disorder of mineral metabolism, unspecified

● **E84**   Cystic fibrosis
> **Includes**   mucoviscidosis
>
> Code also exocrine pancreatic insufficiency (K86.81)
> (Ex) For category E84 CC codes: See PDX Collection 541

● **E84.0**   Cystic fibrosis with pulmonary manifestations
> Use additional code to identify any infectious organism present, such as:
> Pseudomonas (B96.5)
> **Coding Clinic: 2021, Q1, P24**

● **E84.1**   Cystic fibrosis with intestinal manifestations

     E84.11   Meconium ileus in cystic fibrosis   **N**
> **Excludes1**   meconium ileus not due to cystic fibrosis (P76.0)

     E84.19   Cystic fibrosis with other intestinal manifestations
> Distal intestinal obstruction syndrome

E84.8   Cystic fibrosis with other manifestations

E84.9   Cystic fibrosis, unspecified

● **E85**   Amyloidosis
> *A disorder resulting from the abnormal deposition of a particular protein (amyloid) into tissues of the body*
>
> **Excludes2**   Alzheimer's disease (G30.0-)
>
> (Ex) For category E85CC codes: See PDX Collection 542

E85.0   Non-neuropathic heredofamilial amyloidosis
> Hereditary amyloid nephropathy
> Code also associated disorders, such as:
> autoinflammatory syndromes (M04.-)
>
> **Excludes2**   Transthyretin-related (ATTR) familial amyloid cardiomyopathy (E85.4)

▶ New   ⇒ Revised   ~~deleted~~ Deleted   Excludes 1   Excludes 2   Includes   Use additional   Code first   Code also   Key words

OGCR Official Guidelines   ● Unacceptable Principal Diagnosis   X Assign placeholder X   ● Use Additional Character(s)   ▶ Manifestation Code   Coding Clinic

E85.1 Neuropathic heredofamilial amyloidosis 🅒 🅜
     Amyloid polyneuropathy (Portuguese)
     Transthyretin-related (ATTR) familial amyloid
       polyneuropathy
     Coding Clinic: 2012, Q4, P100

E85.2 Heredofamilial amyloidosis, unspecified 🅒 🅜

E85.3 Secondary systemic amyloidosis 🅒 🅜
     Hemodialysis-associated amyloidosis

E85.4 Organ-limited amyloidosis 🅒 🅜
     Localized amyloidosis
     Transthyretin-related (ATTR) familial amyloid
       cardiomyopathy

● **E85.8 Other amyloidosis**

     E85.81 Light chain (AL) amyloidosis 🅒 🅜

     **E85.82 Wild-type transthyretin-related (ATTR)
           amyloidosis** 🅒 🅜
           Senile systemic amyloidosis (SSA)

     E85.89 Other amyloidosis 🅒 🅜

E85.9 Amyloidosis, unspecified 🅒 🅜

● **E86 Volume depletion**

     Excludes1   dehydration of newborn (P74.1)
                 postprocedural hypovolemic shock (T81.19)
                 traumatic hypovolemic shock (T79.4)

     Excludes2   hypovolemic shock NOS (R57.1)

     Use additional code(s) for any associated disorders of
     electrolyte and acid-base balance (E87.-)
     Coding Clinic: 2019, Q2, P7

     E86.0 Dehydration
         Excessive loss of body water
         Coding Clinic: 2019, Q2, P7-8

     E86.1 Hypovolemia
         Diminished volume of circulating blood
         Depletion of volume of plasma

     E86.9 Volume depletion, unspecified
         Coding Clinic: 2019, Q2, P7-8

● **E87 Other disorders of fluid, electrolyte and acid-base balance**

     Excludes1   diabetes insipidus (E23.2)
                 electrolyte imbalance associated with
                     hyperemesis gravidarum (O21.1)
                 electrolyte imbalance following ectopic or molar
                     pregnancy (O08.5)
                 familial periodic paralysis (G72.3)

     Ⓔⓧ **For category E87 CC codes:** See PDX Collection 543

     E87.0 Hyperosmolality and hypernatremia 🅒
         Sodium [Na] excess
         Sodium [Na] overload
         Coding Clinic: 2018, Q2, P6

     E87.1 Hypo-osmolality and hyponatremia 🅒
         Sodium [Na] deficiency

         Excludes1   syndrome of inappropriate secretion of
                     antidiuretic hormone (E22.2)
         Coding Clinic: 2018, Q2, P6

     E87.2 Acidosis 🅒
         Acidosis NOS
         Lactic acidosis
         Metabolic acidosis
         Respiratory acidosis

         ⇒ **Excludes1**   diabetic acidosis - see categories E08-E10,
                     E11, E13 with ketoacidosis

Item 4–9   Circulating fluid volume is regulated by the amount of water and sodium ingested, excreted by the kidneys into the urine, and lost through the gastrointestinal tract, lungs, and skin. To maintain blood volume within a normal range, the kidneys regulate the amount of water and sodium lost into the urine. Too much (**fluid overload**) or too little fluid volume (**volume depletion**) will affect blood pressure. Severe cases of vomiting, diarrhea, bleeding, and burns (fluid loss through exposed burn surface area) can contribute to fluid loss. Internal body environment must maintain a precise balance (homeostasis) between too much fluid and too little fluid. This complex balancing mechanism is critical to good health.

E87.3 Alkalosis 🅒
     Alkalosis NOS
     Metabolic alkalosis
     Respiratory alkalosis

E87.4 Mixed disorder of acid-base balance 🅜

E87.5 Hyperkalemia
     Potassium [K] excess
     Potassium [K] overload

E87.6 Hypokalemia
     Potassium [K] deficiency

● **E87.7 Fluid overload**

     Excludes1   edema NOS (R60.9)
                 fluid retention (R60.9)

     E87.70 Fluid overload, unspecified

     E87.71 Transfusion associated circulatory overload
           Fluid overload due to transfusion (blood)
           (blood components) TACO

     E87.79 Other fluid overload

**E87.8 Other disorders of electrolyte and fluid balance, not
        elsewhere classified**
     Electrolyte imbalance NOS
     Hyperchloremia
     Hypochloremia

● **E88 Other and unspecified metabolic disorders**

     Use additional codes for associated conditions

     Excludes1   histiocytosis X (chronic) (C96.6)

● **E88.0 Disorders of plasma-protein metabolism, not elsewhere
         classified**

     Excludes1   monoclonal gammopathy (of
                     undetermined significance) (D47.2)
                 polyclonal hypergammaglobulinemia
                     (D89.0)
                 Waldenström macroglobulinemia (C88.0)

     Excludes2   disorder of lipoprotein metabolism (E78.-)

     **E88.01 Alpha-1-antitrypsin deficiency AAT
           deficiency** 🅜

     E88.02 Plasminogen deficiency 🅜
           Dysplasminogenemia
           Hypoplasminogenemia
           Type 1 plasminogen deficiency
           Type 2 plasminogen deficiency

           Code also, if applicable, ligneous conjunctivitis
              (H10.51)

           Use additional code for associated findings,
              such as:
              hydrocephalus (G91.4)
              otitis media (H67.-)
              respiratory disorder related to plasminogen
                 deficiency (J99)
           Ⓔⓧ See PDX Collection 534

     **E88.09 Other disorders of plasma-protein metabolism,
           not elsewhere classified**
           Bisalbuminemia

E88.1 Lipodystrophy, not elsewhere classified
     *Defective fat metabolism resulting in absence of subcutaneous
       fat*
     Lipodystrophy NOS

     Excludes1   Whipple's disease (K90.81)

E88.2 Lipomatosis, not elsewhere classified
     Abnormal tumorlike accumulations of fat in tissue
     Lipomatosis NOS
     Lipomatosis (Check) dolorosa [Dercum]

E88.3 Tumor lysis syndrome 🅜
     Tumor lysis syndrome (spontaneous)
     Tumor lysis syndrome following antineoplastic drug
       chemotherapy

     Use additional code for adverse effect, if applicable, to
       identify drug (T45.1X5)
     Ⓔⓧ See PDX Collection 544
     Coding Clinic: 2019, Q2, P25

CHAPTER 4 (E00-E89)

N   Newborn Age: 0   P   Pediatric Age: 0–17   M   Maternity DX: 9–64   A   Adult Age: 15–124   ♀ Females Only   ♂ Males Only

🅒 Complication\Comorbidity   🅜 Major C\C   Ⓔⓧ CC/MCC Exclusions   🅗 Hospital-Acquired Condition   🅗 Hierarchical Condition Category

771

● **E88.4 Mitochondrial metabolism disorders**
Congenital disorder of metabolism

> **Excludes1**   disorders of pyruvate metabolism (E74.4)
> Kearns-Sayre syndrome (H49.81)
> Leber's disease (H47.22)
> Leigh's encephalopathy (G31.82)
> Mitochondrial myopathy, NEC (G71.3)
> Reye's syndrome (G93.7)

   (Ex:) **For category E88.4 CC codes:** See PDX Collection 545

  E88.40 Mitochondrial metabolism disorder, unspecified 🔾🔾

  E88.41 MELAS syndrome 🔾🔾
Mitochondrial myopathy, encephalopathy, lactic acidosis and stroke-like episodes

  E88.42 MERRF syndrome 🔾🔾
Myoclonic epilepsy associated with ragged-red fibers

     Code also progressive myoclonic epilepsy (G40.3-)

  E88.49 Other mitochondrial metabolism disorders 🔾🔾

● **E88.8 Other specified metabolic disorders**

  E88.81 Metabolic syndrome
Dysmetabolic syndrome X

     Use additional codes for associated manifestations, such as:
     obesity (E66.-)

  E88.89 Other specified metabolic disorders 🔾
Launois-Bensaude adenolipomatosis

> **Excludes1**   adult pulmonary Langerhans cell histiocytosis (J84.82)

  E88.9 Metabolic disorder, unspecified

POSTPROCEDURAL ENDOCRINE AND METABOLIC COMPLICATIONS AND DISORDERS, NOT ELSEWHERE CLASSIFIED (E89)

● **E89 Postprocedural endocrine and metabolic complications and disorders, not elsewhere classified**

> **Excludes2**   intraoperative complications of endocrine system organ or structure (E36.0-, E36.1-, E36.8)

E89.0 Postprocedural hypothyroidism
Postirradiation hypothyroidism
Postsurgical hypothyroidism

E89.1 Postprocedural hypoinsulinemia 🔾
Postpancreatectomy hyperglycemia
Postsurgical hypoinsulinemia

  Use additional code, if applicable, to identify:
  acquired absence of pancreas (Z90.41-)
  diabetes mellitus (postpancreatectomy) (postprocedural) (E13.-)
  insulin use (Z79.4)

> **Excludes1**   transient postprocedural hyperglycemia (R73.9)
> transient postprocedural hypoglycemia (E16.2)

   (Ex:) See PDX Collection 520

E89.2 Postprocedural hypoparathyroidism 🔾
Parathyroprival tetany

E89.3 Postprocedural hypopituitarism 🔾
Postirradiation hypopituitarism

● **E89.4 Postprocedural ovarian failure**

  E89.40 Asymptomatic postprocedural ovarian failure ♀
Postprocedural ovarian failure NOS

  E89.41 Symptomatic postprocedural ovarian failure ♀
Symptoms such as flushing, sleeplessness, headache, lack of concentration, associated with postprocedural menopause

E89.5 Postprocedural testicular hypofunction ♂

E89.6 Postprocedural adrenocortical (-medullary) hypofunction 🔾🔾
   (Ex:) See PDX Collection 526

● **E89.8 Other postprocedural endocrine and metabolic complications and disorders**
   (Ex:) **For category E89.8 CC codes:** See PDX Collection 546
   Coding Clinic: 2016, Q4, P9

  ● **E89.81 Postprocedural hemorrhage of an endocrine system organ or structure following a procedure**

    E89.810 Postprocedural hemorrhage of an endocrine system organ or structure following an endocrine system procedure 🔾

    E89.811 Postprocedural hemorrhage of an endocrine system organ or structure following other procedure 🔾

  ● **E89.82 Postprocedural hematoma and seroma of an endocrine system organ or structure**

    E89.820 Postprocedural hematoma of an endocrine system organ or structure following an endocrine system procedure 🔾

    E89.821 Postprocedural hematoma of an endocrine system organ or structure following other procedure 🔾

    E89.822 Postprocedural seroma of an endocrine system organ or structure following an endocrine system procedure 🔾

    E89.823 Postprocedural seroma of an endocrine system organ or structure following other procedure 🔾

  E89.89 Other postprocedural endocrine and metabolic complications and disorders 🔾

     Use additional code, if applicable, to further specify disorder

CHAPTER 5

MENTAL, BEHAVIORAL AND NEURODEVELOPMENTAL DISORDERS (F01-F99)

OGCR Chapter-Specific Coding Guidelines

5. **Chapter 5: Mental, Behavioral and Neurodevelopmental disorders (F01 – F99)**

   a. **Pain disorders related to psychological factors**

   Assign code F45.41, for pain that is exclusively related to psychological disorders. As indicated by the Excludes 1 note under category G89, a code from category G89 should not be assigned with code F45.41

   Code F45.42, Pain disorders with related psychological factors, should be used with a code from category G89, Pain, not elsewhere classified, if there is documentation of a psychological component for a patient with acute or chronic pain.

   See Section I.C.6. Pain

   b. **Mental and behavioral disorders due to psychoactive substance use**

   1) **In Remission**

   Selection of codes for "in remission" for categories F10-F19, Mental and behavioral disorders due to psychoactive substance use (categories F10-F19 with -11, -.21) requires the provider's clinical judgment. The appropriate codes for "in remission" are assigned only on the basis of provider documentation (as defined in the Official Guidelines for Coding and Reporting), unless otherwise instructed by the classification.

   Mild substance use disorders in early or sustained remission are classified to the appropriate codes for substance abuse in remission, and moderate or severe substance use disorders in early or sustained remission are classified to the appropriate codes for substance dependence in remission.

   2) **Psychoactive Substance Use, Abuse and Dependence**

   When the provider documentation refers to use, abuse and dependence of the same substance (e.g., alcohol, opioid, cannabis, etc.), only one code should be assigned to identify the pattern of use based on the following hierarchy:

   - If both use and abuse are documented, assign only the code for abuse
   - If both abuse and dependence are documented, assign only the code for dependence
   - If use, abuse and dependence are all documented, assign only the code for dependence
   - If both use and dependence are documented, assign only the code for dependence

   3) **Psychoactive Substance Use, Unspecified**

   As with all other unspecified diagnoses, the codes for unspecified psychoactive substance use disorders (F10.9-, F11.9-, F12.9-, F13.9-, F14.9-, F15.9-, F16.9-, F19.9-, F19.9-) should only be assigned based on provider documentation and when they meet the definition of a reportable diagnosis (see Section III, Reporting Additional Diagnoses). These codes are to be used only when the psychoactive substance use is associated with a physical, mental or behavioral disorder, and such a relationship is documented by the provider.

   c. **Factitious Disorder**

   Factitious disorder imposed on self or Munchausen's syndrome is a disorder in which a person falsely reports or causes his or her own physical or psychological signs or symptoms. For patients with documented factitious disorder on self or Munchausen's syndrome, assign the appropriate code from subcategory F68.1-, Factitious disorder imposed on self.

   Munchausen's syndrome by proxy (MSBP) is a disorder in which a caregiver (perpetrator) falsely reports or causes an illness or injury in another person (victim) under his or her care, such as a child, an elderly adult, or a person who has a disability. The condition is also referred to as "factitious disorder imposed on another" or "factitious disorder by proxy." The perpetrator, not the victim, receives this diagnosis. Assign code F68.A, Factitious disorder imposed on another, to the perpetrator's record. For the victim of a patient suffering from MSBP, assign the appropriate code from categories T74, Adult and child abuse, neglect and other maltreatment, confirmed, or T76, Adult and child abuse, neglect and other maltreatment, suspected.

   See Section I.C.19.f. Adult and child abuse, neglect and other maltreatment

CHAPTER 5

MENTAL, BEHAVIORAL AND NEURODEVELOPMENTAL DISORDERS (F01-F99)

| Includes | disorders of psychological development |
| Excludes2 | symptoms, signs and abnormal clinical laboratory findings, not elsewhere classified (R00-R99) |

This chapter contains the following blocks:

F01-F09	Mental disorders due to known physiological conditions
F10-F19	Mental and behavioral disorders due to psychoactive substance use
F20-F29	Schizophrenia, schizotypal, delusional, and other non-mood psychotic disorders
F30-F39	Mood [affective] disorders
F40-F48	Anxiety, dissociative, stress-related, somatoform and other nonpsychotic mental disorders
F50-F59	Behavioral syndromes associated with physiological disturbances and physical factors
F60-F69	Disorders of adult personality and behavior
F70-F79	Intellectual disabilities
F80-F89	Pervasive and specific developmental disorders
F90-F98	Behavioral and emotional disorders with onset usually occurring in childhood and adolescence
F99	Unspecified mental disorder

MENTAL DISORDERS DUE TO KNOWN PHYSIOLOGICAL CONDITIONS (F01-F09)

This block comprises a range of mental disorders grouped together on the basis of their having in common a demonstrable etiology in cerebral disease, brain injury, or other insult leading to cerebral dysfunction. The dysfunction may be primary, as in diseases, injuries, and insults that affect the brain directly and selectively; or secondary, as in systemic diseases and disorders that attack the brain only as one of the multiple organs or systems of the body that are involved.

● **F01**   **Vascular dementia**

Vascular dementia as a result of infarction of the brain due to vascular disease, including hypertensive cerebrovascular disease.

| Includes | arteriosclerotic dementia |

Code first the underlying physiological condition or sequelae of cerebrovascular disease.

● **F01.5**   **Vascular dementia**

   ● **F01.50**   **Vascular dementia without behavioral disturbance**   A

       Major neurocognitive disorder without behavioral disturbance

       Coding Clinic: 2021, Q2, P4

   ● **F01.51**   **Vascular dementia with behavioral disturbance** 🔶   A

       Major neurocognitive disorder due to vascular disease, with behavioral disturbance

       Major neurocognitive disorder with aggressive behavior

       Major neurocognitive disorder with combative behavior

       Major neurocognitive disorder with violent behavior

       Vascular dementia with aggressive behavior

       Vascular dementia with combative behavior

       Vascular dementia with violent behavior

       Use additional code, if applicable, to identify wandering in vascular dementia (Z91.83)

       (Ex) See PDX Collection 547

N Newborn Age: 0   **P** Pediatric Age: 0–17   **M** Maternity DX: 9–64   **A** Adult Age: 15–124   ♀ Females Only   ♂ Males Only

🔵 Complication\Comorbidity   🔶 Major C\C   (Ex) CC/MCC Exclusions   🔵 Hospital-Acquired Condition   🔴 Hierarchical Condition Category

● **F02** **Dementia in other diseases classified elsewhere**

Code first the underlying physiological condition, such as:
Alzheimer's (G30.-)
cerebral lipidosis (E75.4)
Creutzfeldt-Jakob disease (A81.0-)
dementia with Lewy bodies (G31.83)
dementia with Parkinsonism (G31.83)
epilepsy and recurrent seizures (G40.-)
frontotemporal dementia (G31.09)
hepatolenticular degeneration (E83.0)
human immunodeficiency virus [HIV] disease (B20)
Huntington's disease (G10)
hypercalcemia (E83.52)
hypothyroidism, acquired (E00-E03.-)
intoxications (T36-T65)
Jakob-Creutzfeldt disease (A81.0-)
multiple sclerosis (G35)
neurosyphilis (A52.17)
niacin deficiency [pellagra] (E52)
Parkinson's disease (G20)
Pick's disease (G31.01)
polyarteritis nodosa (M30.0)
prion disease (A81.9)
systemic lupus erythematosus (M32.-)
traumatic brain injury (S06.-)
trypanosomiasis (B56.-, B57.-)
vitamin B deficiency (E53.8)

Includes Major neurocognitive disorder in other diseases classified elsewhere

Excludes2 dementia in alcohol and psychoactive substance disorders (F10-F19, with .17, .27, .97)
vascular dementia (F01.5-)
Coding Clinic: 2016, Q4, P141

● **F02.8** **Dementia in other diseases classified elsewhere**

▷ **F02.80** *Dementia in other diseases classified elsewhere without behavioral disturbance*
Dementia in other diseases classified elsewhere NOS
Major neurocognitive disorder in other diseases classified elsewhere
Coding Clinic: 2017, Q1, P43; 2016, Q2, P6

▷ **F02.81** *Dementia in other diseases classified elsewhere with behavioral disturbance*
Dementia in other diseases classified elsewhere with aggressive behavior
Dementia in other diseases classified elsewhere with combative behavior
Dementia in other diseases classified elsewhere with violent behavior
Major neurocognitive disorder in other diseases classified elsewhere with aggressive behavior
Major neurocognitive disorder in other diseases classified elsewhere with combative behavior
Major neurocognitive disorder in other diseases classified elsewhere with violent behavior

Use additional code, if applicable, to identify wandering in dementia in conditions classified elsewhere (Z91.83)
(Ex:) See PDX Collection 548
Coding Clinic: 2017, Q2, P8, Q1, P43

Item 5-1 Psychosis was a term formerly applied to any mental disorder but is now restricted to disturbances of a great magnitude in which there is a personality disintegration and loss of contact with reality.

● **F03** **Unspecified dementia**
Presenile dementia NOS
Presenile psychosis NOS
Primary degenerative dementia NOS
Senile dementia NOS
Senile dementia depressed or paranoid type
Senile psychosis NOS

Excludes1 senility NOS (R41.81)

Excludes2 mild memory disturbance due to known physiological condition (F06.8)
senile dementia with delirium or acute confusional state (F05)

● **F03.9** **Unspecified dementia**

F03.90 **Unspecified dementia without behavioral disturbance** A
Dementia NOS
Coding Clinic: 2021, Q2, P4; 2012, Q4, P92

F03.91 **Unspecified dementia with behavioral disturbance** A
Unspecified dementia with aggressive behavior
Unspecified dementia with combative behavior
Unspecified dementia with violent behavior

Use additional code, if applicable, to identify wandering in unspecified dementia (Z91.83)
(Ex:) See PDX Collection 548

● **F04** **Amnestic disorder due to known physiological condition**
Korsakov's psychosis or syndrome, nonalcoholic

Code first the underlying physiological condition

Excludes1 amnesia NOS (R41.3)
anterograde amnesia (R41.1)
dissociative amnesia (F44.0)
retrograde amnesia (R41.2)

Excludes2 alcohol-induced or unspecified Korsakov's syndrome (F10.26, F10.96)
Korsakov's syndrome induced by other psychoactive substances (F13.26, F13.96, F19.16, F19.26, F19.96)

● **F05** **Delirium due to known physiological condition**
Acute or subacute brain syndrome
Acute or subacute confusional state (nonalcoholic)
Acute or subacute infective psychosis
Acute or subacute organic reaction
Acute or subacute psycho-organic syndrome
Delirium of mixed etiology
Delirium superimposed on dementia
Sundowning

Code first the underlying physiological condition

Excludes1 delirium NOS (R41.0)

Excludes2 delirium tremens alcohol-induced or unspecified (F10.231, F10.921)
(Ex:) See PDX Collection 549
Coding Clinic: 2019, Q2, P34

● **F06** **Other mental disorders due to known physiological condition**
Includes mental disorders due to endocrine disorder
mental disorders due to exogenous hormone
mental disorders due to exogenous toxic substance
mental disorders due to primary cerebral disease
mental disorders due to somatic illness
mental disorders due to systemic disease affecting the brain

Code first the underlying physiological condition

Excludes1 unspecified dementia (F03)

Excludes2 delirium due to known physiological condition (F05)
dementia as classified in F01-F02
other mental disorders associated with alcohol and other psychoactive substances (F10-F19)
(Ex:) For category F06 CC codes: See PDX Collection 550

CHAPTER 5 (F01-F99)

● **F06.0** **Psychotic disorder with hallucinations** due to known **physiological condition** 🅗
    Organic hallucinatory state (nonalcoholic)
    Excludes2 hallucinations and perceptual disturbance induced by alcohol and other psychoactive substances (F10-F19 with .151, .251, .951)
               schizophrenia (F20.-)

● **F06.1** **Catatonic disorder** due to known physiological condition
    Catatonia associated with another mental disorder
    Catatonia NOS
    Excludes1 catatonic stupor (R40.1)
               stupor NOS (R40.1)
    Excludes2 catatonic schizophrenia (F20.2)
               dissociative stupor (F44.2)

● **F06.2** **Psychotic disorder with delusions** due to known **physiological condition** 🅗
    Paranoid and paranoid-hallucinatory organic states
    Schizophrenia-like psychosis in epilepsy
    Excludes2 alcohol and drug-induced psychotic disorder (F10-F19 with .150, .250, .950)
               brief psychotic disorder (F23)
               delusional disorder (F22)
               schizophrenia (F20.-)

● **F06.3** **Mood disorder** due to known physiological condition
    Excludes2 mood disorders due to alcohol and other psychoactive substances (F10-F19 with .14, .24, .94)
               mood disorders, not due to known physiological condition or unspecified (F30-F39)

  ● **F06.30** Mood disorder due to known physiological condition, **unspecified**

  ● **F06.31** Mood disorder due to known physiological condition **with depressive features**
    Depressive disorder due to known physiological condition, with depressive features

  ● **F06.32** Mood disorder due to known physiological condition **with major depressive-like episode**
    Depressive disorder due to known physiological condition, with major depressive-like episode

  ● **F06.33** Mood disorder due to known physiological condition **with manic features**
    Bipolar and related disorder due to a known physiological condition, with manic features
    Bipolar and related disorder due to known physiological condition, with manic- or hypomanic-like episodes

  ● **F06.34** Mood disorder due to known physiological condition **with mixed features**
    Bipolar and related disorder due to known physiological condition, with mixed features
    Depressive disorder due to known physiological condition, with mixed features

● **F06.4** **Anxiety disorder** due to known physiological condition
    Excludes2 anxiety disorders due to alcohol and other psychoactive substances (F10-F19 with .180, .280, .980)
               anxiety disorders, not due to known physiological condition or unspecified (F40.-, F41.-)

● **F06.8** **Other specified mental disorders** due to known physiological condition
    Epileptic psychosis NOS
    Obsessive-compulsive and related disorder due to a known physiological condition
    Organic dissociative disorder
    Organic emotionally labile [asthenic] disorder

● **F07** **Personality and behavioral disorders** due to known **physiological condition**
    Code first the underlying physiological condition

  ● **F07.0** **Personality change** due to known physiological condition
    Frontal lobe syndrome
    Limbic epilepsy personality syndrome
    Lobotomy syndrome
    Organic personality disorder
    Organic pseudopsychopathic personality
    Organic pseudoretarded personality
    Postleucotomy syndrome
    Code first underlying physiological condition
    Excludes1 mild cognitive impairment (G31.84)
               postconcussional syndrome (F07.81)
               postencephalitic syndrome (F07.89)
               signs and symptoms involving emotional state (R45.-)
    Excludes2 specific personality disorder (F60.-)

  ● **F07.8** **Other personality and behavioral disorders** due to known physiological condition

    ● **F07.81** **Postconcussional** syndrome
      Postcontusional syndrome (encephalopathy)
      Post-traumatic brain syndrome, nonpsychotic
      Use additional code to identify associated post-traumatic headache, if applicable (G44.3-)
      Excludes1 current concussion (brain) (S06.0-)
                 postencephalitic syndrome (F07.89)

    ● **F07.89** **Other personality and behavioral disorders** due to known **physiological condition**
      Postencephalitic syndrome
      Damage to temporal brain lobes with memory loss and abnormal behavior
      Right hemispheric organic affective disorder

  ● **F07.9** **Unspecified** personality and behavioral disorder due to known physiological condition
    Organic psychosyndrome
    Due to exposure to organic solvents

● **F09** **Unspecified mental disorder** due to known physiological condition
    Mental disorder NOS due to known physiological condition
    Organic brain syndrome NOS
    Organic mental disorder NOS
    Organic psychosis NOS
    Symptomatic psychosis NOS
    Code first the underlying physiological condition
    Excludes1 psychosis NOS (F29)

MENTAL AND BEHAVIORAL DISORDERS DUE TO PSYCHOACTIVE SUBSTANCE USE (F10-F19)

● **F10** **Alcohol related disorders**
    Use additional code for blood alcohol level, if applicable (Y90.-)
    (Ex:) **For category F10 CC codes:** See PDX Collection 3998
    Coding Clinic: 2019, Q3, P8

  ● **F10.1** **Alcohol abuse**
    Excludes1 alcohol dependence (F10.2-)
               alcohol use, unspecified (F10.9-)

    F10.10 **Alcohol abuse, uncomplicated**
      Alcohol use disorder, mild

    F10.11 **Alcohol abuse, in remission**
      Alcohol use disorder, mild, in early remission
      Alcohol use disorder, mild, in sustained remission

  ● **F10.12** **Alcohol abuse with intoxication**

    F10.120 **Alcohol abuse with intoxication, uncomplicated** 🅗

    F10.121 **Alcohol abuse with intoxication, delirium** 🅒 🅗

    F10.129 **Alcohol abuse with intoxication, unspecified** 🅗

N Newborn Age: 0   **P** Pediatric Age: 0–17   **M** Maternity DX: 9–64   **A** Adult Age: 15–124   ♀ Females Only   ♂ Males Only

🅒 Complication\Comorbidity   🅜 Major C\C   (Ex:) CC/MCC Exclusions   🅗 Hospital-Acquired Condition   🅗 Hierarchical Condition Category

775

CHAPTER 5 (F01-F99)

● F10.13   Alcohol abuse, with withdrawal
            F10.130   Alcohol abuse with withdrawal,
                       uncomplicated 🔖
                       (Ex) See PDX Collection 4080
            F10.131   Alcohol abuse with withdrawal
                       delirium 🔖
                       (Ex) See PDX Collection 4019
            F10.132   Alcohol abuse with withdrawal with
                       perceptual disturbance 🔖
                       (Ex) See PDX Collection 4081
            F10.139   Alcohol abuse with withdrawal,
                       unspecified 🔖
                       (Ex) See PDX Collection 4077

   F10.14   Alcohol abuse with alcohol-induced mood
            disorder 🔖🔖
            Alcohol use disorder, mild, with alcohol-
              induced bipolar or related disorder
            Alcohol use disorder, mild, with alcohol-
              induced depressive disorder

● F10.15   Alcohol abuse with alcohol-induced psychotic
           disorder
            F10.150   Alcohol abuse with alcohol-induced
                       psychotic disorder with delusions 🔖
            F10.151   Alcohol abuse with alcohol-induced
                       psychotic disorder with
                       hallucinations 🔖🔖
            F10.159   Alcohol abuse with alcohol-induced
                       psychotic disorder, unspecified 🔖🔖

● F10.18   Alcohol abuse with other alcohol-induced
           disorders
            F10.180   Alcohol abuse with alcohol-induced
                       anxiety disorder 🔖🔖
            F10.181   Alcohol abuse with alcohol-induced
                       sexual dysfunction 🔖🔖
            F10.182   Alcohol abuse with alcohol-induced
                       sleep disorder 🔖🔖
            F10.188   Alcohol abuse with other alcohol-
                       induced disorder 🔖🔖

   F10.19   Alcohol abuse with unspecified alcohol-
            induced disorder 🔖🔖

● F10.2   Alcohol dependence
            Excludes1   alcohol abuse (F10.1-)
                         alcohol use, unspecified (F10.9-)
            Excludes2   toxic effect of alcohol (T51.0-)
            Coding Clinic: 2019, Q3, P8

   F10.20   Alcohol dependence, uncomplicated 🔖
            Alcohol use disorder, moderate
            Alcohol use disorder, severe
            Coding Clinic: 2020, Q1, P9

   F10.21   Alcohol dependence, in remission 🔖
            Alcohol use disorder, moderate, in early
              remission
            Alcohol use disorder, moderate, in sustained
              remission
            Alcohol use disorder, severe, in early remission
            Alcohol use disorder, severe, in sustained
              remission

● F10.22   Alcohol dependence with intoxication
            Acute drunkenness (in alcoholism)
            Excludes2   alcohol dependence with
                         withdrawal (F10.23-)
            F10.220   Alcohol dependence with
                       intoxication, uncomplicated 🔖
            F10.221   Alcohol dependence with intoxication
                       delirium 🔖🔖
            F10.229   Alcohol dependence with
                       intoxication, unspecified 🔖

● F10.23   Alcohol dependence with withdrawal
            Excludes2   alcohol dependence with
                         intoxication (F10.22-)
            F10.230   Alcohol dependence with
                       withdrawal, uncomplicated 🔖🔖

            F10.231   Alcohol dependence with withdrawal
                       delirium 🔖🔖
            F10.232   Alcohol dependence with withdrawal
                       with perceptual disturbance 🔖🔖
            F10.239   Alcohol dependence with
                       withdrawal, unspecified 🔖🔖
                       Coding Clinic: 2015, Q2, P15

   F10.24   Alcohol dependence with alcohol-induced
            mood disorder 🔖🔖
            Alcohol use disorder, moderate, with alcohol-
              induced bipolar or related disorder
            Alcohol use disorder, moderate, with alcohol-
              induced depressive disorder
            Alcohol use disorder, severe, with alcohol-
              induced bipolar or related disorder
            Alcohol use disorder, severe, with alcohol-
              induced depressive disorder

● F10.25   Alcohol dependence with alcohol-induced
           psychotic disorder
            F10.250   Alcohol dependence with alcohol-
                       induced psychotic disorder with
                       delusions 🔖
            F10.251   Alcohol dependence with alcohol-
                       induced psychotic disorder with
                       hallucinations 🔖🔖
            F10.259   Alcohol dependence with alcohol-
                       induced psychotic
                       disorder, unspecified 🔖🔖

   F10.26   Alcohol dependence with alcohol-induced
            persisting amnestic disorder 🔖
            Alcohol use disorder, moderate, with alcohol-
              induced major neurocognitive disorder,
              amnestic-confabulatory type
            Alcohol use disorder, severe, with alcohol-
              induced major neurocognitive disorder,
              amnestic-confabulatory type

   F10.27   Alcohol dependence with alcohol-induced
            persisting dementia 🔖🔖
            Alcohol use disorder, moderate, with alcohol-
              induced major neurocognitive disorder,
              nonamnestic-confabulatory type
            Alcohol use disorder, severe, with alcohol-
              induced major neurocognitive disorder,
              nonamnestic-confabulatory type

● F10.28   Alcohol dependence with other alcohol-
           induced disorders
            F10.280   Alcohol dependence with alcohol-
                       induced anxiety disorder 🔖🔖
            F10.281   Alcohol dependence with alcohol-
                       induced sexual dysfunction 🔖🔖
            F10.282   Alcohol dependence with alcohol-
                       induced sleep disorder 🔖🔖
            F10.288   Alcohol dependence with other
                       alcohol-induced disorder 🔖🔖
                       Alcohol use disorder, moderate,
                         with alcohol-induced mild
                         neurocognitive disorder
                       Alcohol use disorder, severe,
                         with alcohol-induced mild
                         neurocognitive disorder
                       Coding Clinic: 2020, Q1, P9

   F10.29   Alcohol dependence with unspecified
            alcohol-induced disorder 🔖🔖

● F10.9   Alcohol use, unspecified
            Excludes1   alcohol abuse (F10.1-)
                         alcohol dependence (F10.2-)

● F10.92   Alcohol use, unspecified with intoxication
            F10.920   Alcohol use, unspecified with
                       intoxication, uncomplicated 🔖
            F10.921   Alcohol use, unspecified with
                       intoxication delirium 🔖🔖
            F10.929   Alcohol use, unspecified with
                       intoxication, unspecified 🔖

▶ New   ⇒ Revised   d̶e̶l̶e̶t̶e̶d̶ Deleted   Excludes 1   Excludes 2   Includes   Use additional   Code first   Code also   Key words

OGCR Official Guidelines   ● Unacceptable Principal Diagnosis   X Assign placeholder X   ● Use Additional Character(s)   ▶ Manifestation Code   Coding Clinic

● **F10.93**   **Alcohol use, unspecified with withdrawal**

     F10.930   Alcohol use, unspecified with withdrawal, uncomplicated 🔹
         Ⓔⓧ See PDX Collection 4076

     F10.931   Alcohol use, unspecified with withdrawal delirium 🔹
         Ⓔⓧ See PDX Collection 4019

     F10.932   Alcohol use, unspecified with withdrawal with perceptual disturbance 🔹
         Ⓔⓧ See PDX Collection 4078

     F10.939   Alcohol use, unspecified with withdrawal, unspecified 🔹
         Ⓔⓧ See PDX Collection 4079

   F10.94   **Alcohol use, unspecified with alcohol-induced mood disorder** 🔹🔹
        Alcohol-induced bipolar or related disorder, without use disorder
        Alcohol-induced depressive disorder, without use disorder

● **F10.95**   **Alcohol use, unspecified with alcohol-induced psychotic disorder**

     F10.950   Alcohol use, unspecified with alcohol-induced psychotic disorder with delusions 🔹

     F10.951   Alcohol use, unspecified with alcohol-induced psychotic disorder with hallucinations 🔹🔹

     F10.959   Alcohol use, unspecified with alcohol-induced psychotic disorder, unspecified 🔹🔹
         Alcohol-induced psychotic disorder without use disorder

   F10.96   **Alcohol use, unspecified with alcohol-induced persisting amnestic disorder** 🔹
        Alcohol-induced major neurocognitive disorder, amnestic-confabulatory type, without use disorder

   F10.97   **Alcohol use, unspecified with alcohol-induced persisting dementia** 🔹
        Alcohol-induced major neurocognitive disorder, nonamnestic-confabulatory type, without use disorder

● **F10.98**   **Alcohol use, unspecified with other alcohol-induced disorders**

     F10.980   Alcohol use, unspecified with alcohol-induced anxiety disorder 🔹🔹
         Alcohol-induced anxiety disorder, without use disorder

     F10.981   Alcohol use, unspecified with alcohol-induced sexual dysfunction 🔹🔹
         Alcohol-induced sexual dysfunction, without use disorder

     F10.982   Alcohol use, unspecified with alcohol-induced sleep disorder 🔹
         Alcohol-induced sleep disorder, without use disorder

     F10.988   Alcohol use, unspecified with other alcohol-induced disorder 🔹🔹
         Alcohol-induced mild neurocognitive disorder, without use disorder
         Coding Clinic: 2019, Q3, P8

   F10.99   **Alcohol use, unspecified with unspecified alcohol-induced disorder** 🔹🔹

● **F11**   **Opioid related disorders**
     Ⓔⓧ **For category F11 CC codes unless otherwise indicated:** See PDX Collection 3998

● **F11.1**   **Opioid abuse**
     Excludes1   opioid dependence (F11.2-)
              opioid use, unspecified (F11.9-)

   F11.10   **Opioid abuse, uncomplicated**
        Opioid use disorder, mild

   F11.11   **Opioid abuse, in remission**
        Opioid use disorder, mild, in early remission
        Opioid use disorder, mild, in sustained remission

● **F11.12**   **Opioid abuse with intoxication**

     F11.120   Opioid abuse with intoxication, uncomplicated 🔹

     F11.121   Opioid abuse with intoxication delirium 🔹🔹

     F11.122   Opioid abuse with intoxication with perceptual disturbance 🔹🔹

     F11.129   Opioid abuse with intoxication, unspecified 🔹

   F11.13   **Opioid abuse with withdrawal** 🔹
     Ⓔⓧ See PDX Collection 4009

   F11.14   **Opioid abuse with opioid-induced mood disorder** 🔹
        Opioid use disorder, mild, with opioid-induced depressive disorder

● **F11.15**   **Opioid abuse with opioid-induced psychotic disorder**

     F11.150   Opioid abuse with opioid-induced psychotic disorder with delusions 🔹🔹

     F11.151   Opioid abuse with opioid-induced psychotic disorder with hallucinations 🔹🔹

     F11.159   Opioid abuse with opioid-induced psychotic disorder, unspecified 🔹

● **F11.18**   **Opioid abuse with other opioid-induced disorder**

     F11.181   Opioid abuse with opioid-induced sexual dysfunction 🔹

     F11.182   Opioid abuse with opioid-induced sleep disorder 🔹

     F11.188   Opioid abuse with other opioid-induced disorder 🔹

   F11.19   **Opioid abuse with unspecified opioid-induced disorder** 🔹

● **F11.2**   **Opioid dependence**
     Excludes1   opioid abuse (F11.1-)
              opioid use, unspecified (F11.9-)
     Excludes2   opioid poisoning (T40.0—T40.2-)

   F11.20   **Opioid dependence, uncomplicated** 🔹🔹
        Opioid use disorder, moderate
        Opioid use disorder, severe
     Ⓔⓧ See PDX Collection 3215

   F11.21   **Opioid dependence, in remission** 🔹
        Opioid use disorder, moderate, in early remission
        Opioid use disorder, moderate, in sustained remission
        Opioid use disorder, severe, in early remission
        Opioid use disorder, severe, in sustained remission

● **F11.22**   **Opioid dependence with intoxication**
     Excludes1   opioid dependence with withdrawal (F11.23)

     F11.220   Opioid dependence with intoxication, uncomplicated 🔹

     F11.221   Opioid dependence with intoxication delirium 🔹🔹

     F11.222   Opioid dependence with intoxication with perceptual disturbance 🔹🔹
         Ⓔⓧ See PDX Collection 3556

     F11.229   Opioid dependence with intoxication, unspecified 🔹

   F11.23   **Opioid dependence with withdrawal** 🔹🔹
     Excludes1   opioid dependence with intoxication (F11.22-)

   F11.24   **Opioid dependence with opioid-induced mood disorder** 🔹
        Opioid use disorder, moderate, with opioid-induced depressive disorder

CHAPTER 5 (F01-F99)

N   Newborn Age: 0   P   Pediatric Age: 0–17   M   Maternity DX: 9–64   A   Adult Age: 15–124   ♀   Females Only   ♂   Males Only

🔹   Complication\Comorbidity   🔹   Major C\C   Ⓔⓧ   CC/MCC Exclusions   🔹   Hospital-Acquired Condition   🔹   Hierarchical Condition Category

777

● **F11.25   Opioid dependence with opioid-induced psychotic disorder**

    F11.250   Opioid dependence with opioid-induced psychotic disorder with delusions 🪙 🪙

    F11.251   Opioid dependence with opioid-induced psychotic disorder with hallucinations 🪙 🪙

    F11.259   Opioid dependence with opioid-induced psychotic disorder, unspecified 🪙 🪙
        (Ex:) See PDX Collection 3557

● **F11.28   Opioid dependence with other opioid-induced disorder**
    (Ex:) For category F11.28 CC codes: No exclusions

    F11.281   Opioid dependence with opioid-induced sexual dysfunction 🪙 🪙
        (Ex:) See PDX Collection 3558

    F11.282   Opioid dependence with opioid-induced sleep disorder 🪙 🪙
        (Ex:) See PDX Collection 3559

    F11.288   Opioid dependence with other opioid-induced disorder 🪙 🪙
        (Ex:) See PDX Collection 3560

    F11.29   Opioid dependence with unspecified opioid-induced disorder 🪙

● **F11.9   Opioid use, unspecified**

    Excludes1   opioid abuse (F11.1-)
             opioid dependence (F11.2-)

    F11.90   Opioid use, unspecified, uncomplicated

●   F11.92   Opioid use, unspecified with intoxication

        Excludes1   opioid use, unspecified with withdrawal (F11.93)

    F11.920   Opioid use, unspecified with intoxication, uncomplicated 🪙

    F11.921   Opioid use, unspecified with intoxication delirium 🪙 🪙
        Opioid-induced delirium

    F11.922   Opioid use, unspecified with intoxication with perceptual disturbance 🪙

    F11.929   Opioid use, unspecified with intoxication, unspecified 🪙

    F11.93   Opioid use, unspecified with withdrawal 🪙 🪙

        Excludes1   opioid use, unspecified with intoxication (F11.92-)

    F11.94   Opioid use, unspecified with opioid-induced mood disorder 🪙
        Opioid-induced depressive disorder, without use disorder

●   F11.95   Opioid use, unspecified with opioid-induced psychotic disorder

    F11.950   Opioid use, unspecified with opioid-induced psychotic disorder with delusions 🪙 🪙

    F11.951   Opioid use, unspecified with opioid-induced psychotic disorder with hallucinations 🪙 🪙

    F11.959   Opioid use, unspecified with opioid-induced psychotic disorder, unspecified 🪙

●   F11.98   Opioid use, unspecified with other specified opioid-induced disorder

    F11.981   Opioid use, unspecified with opioid-induced sexual dysfunction 🪙
        Opioid-induced sexual dysfunction, without use disorder

    F11.982   Opioid use, unspecified with opioid-induced sleep disorder 🪙
        Opioid-induced sleep disorder, without use disorder

    F11.988   Opioid use, unspecified with other opioid-induced disorder 🪙
        Opioid-induced anxiety disorder, without use disorder

    F11.99   Opioid use, unspecified with unspecified opioid-induced disorder 🪙

● **F12   Cannabis related disorders**

    Includes   marijuana

    (Ex:) For category F12 CC codes: See PDX Collection 3998

    Coding Clinic: 2020, Q1, P8

● **F12.1   Cannabis abuse**

    Excludes1   cannabis dependence (F12.2-)
             cannabis use, unspecified (F12.9-)

    F12.10   Cannabis abuse, uncomplicated
        Cannabis use disorder, mild

    F12.11   Cannabis abuse, in remission
        Cannabis use disorder, mild, in early remission
        Cannabis use disorder, mild, in sustained remission

●   F12.12   Cannabis abuse with intoxication

    F12.120   Cannabis abuse with intoxication, uncomplicated 🪙

    F12.121   Cannabis abuse with intoxication delirium 🪙 🪙

    F12.122   Cannabis abuse with intoxication with perceptual disturbance 🪙

    F12.129   Cannabis abuse with intoxication, unspecified 🪙

    F12.13   Cannabis abuse with withdrawal

●   F12.15   Cannabis abuse with psychotic disorder

    F12.150   Cannabis abuse with psychotic disorder with delusions 🪙 🪙

    F12.151   Cannabis abuse with psychotic disorder with hallucinations 🪙 🪙

    F12.159   Cannabis abuse with psychotic disorder, unspecified 🪙

●   F12.18   Cannabis abuse with other cannabis-induced disorder

    F12.180   Cannabis abuse with cannabis-induced anxiety disorder 🪙

    F12.188   Cannabis abuse with other cannabis-induced disorder 🪙
        Cannabis use disorder, mild, with cannabis-induced sleep disorder

    F12.19   Cannabis abuse with unspecified cannabis-induced disorder 🪙

● **F12.2   Cannabis dependence**

    Excludes1   cannabis abuse (F12.1-)
             cannabis use, unspecified (F12.9-)

    Excludes2   cannabis poisoning (T40.7-)

    F12.20   Cannabis dependence, uncomplicated 🪙
        Cannabis use disorder, moderate
        Cannabis use disorder, severe

    F12.21   Cannabis dependence, in remission 🪙
        Cannabis use disorder, moderate, in early remission
        Cannabis use disorder, moderate, in sustained remission
        Cannabis use disorder, severe, in early remission
        Cannabis use disorder, severe, in sustained remission

▶ New   ⇨ Revised   ~~deleted~~ Deleted   Excludes 1   Excludes 2   Includes   Use additional   Code first   Code also   Key words
OGCR Official Guidelines   ● Unacceptable Principal Diagnosis   X Assign placeholder X   ● Use Additional Character(s)   ▶ Manifestation Code   Coding Clinic

● **F12.22**   Cannabis dependence with intoxication

     F12.220   **Cannabis dependence with intoxication, uncomplicated** 🦠

     F12.221   **Cannabis dependence with intoxication delirium** 🦠🦠

     F12.222   **Cannabis dependence with intoxication with perceptual disturbance** 🦠

     F12.229   **Cannabis dependence with intoxication, unspecified** 🦠

   F12.23   **Cannabis dependence with withdrawal** 🦠🦠

● **F12.25**   Cannabis dependence with psychotic disorder

     F12.250   **Cannabis dependence with psychotic disorder with delusions** 🦠🦠

     F12.251   **Cannabis dependence with psychotic disorder with hallucinations** 🦠🦠

     F12.259   **Cannabis dependence with psychotic disorder, unspecified** 🦠

● **F12.28**   Cannabis dependence with other cannabis-induced disorder

     F12.280   **Cannabis dependence with cannabis-induced anxiety disorder** 🦠

     F12.288   **Cannabis dependence with other cannabis-induced disorder** 🦠
        Cannabis use disorder, moderate, with cannabis-induced sleep disorder
        Cannabis use disorder, severe, with cannabis-induced sleep disorder

   F12.29   **Cannabis dependence with unspecified cannabis-induced disorder** 🦠🦠

● **F12.9**   Cannabis use, unspecified

     Excludes1   cannabis abuse (F12.1-)
               cannabis dependence (F12.2-)

   F12.90   **Cannabis use, unspecified, uncomplicated**

● **F12.92**   Cannabis use, unspecified with intoxication

     F12.920   **Cannabis use, unspecified with intoxication, uncomplicated** 🦠

     F12.921   **Cannabis use, unspecified with intoxication delirium** 🦠🦠

     F12.922   **Cannabis use, unspecified with intoxication with perceptual disturbance** 🦠

     F12.929   **Cannabis use, unspecified with intoxication, unspecified** 🦠

   F12.93   **Cannabis use, unspecified with withdrawal** 🦠

● **F12.95**   Cannabis use, unspecified with psychotic disorder

     F12.950   **Cannabis use, unspecified with psychotic disorder with delusions** 🦠🦠

     F12.951   **Cannabis use, unspecified with psychotic disorder with hallucinations** 🦠🦠

     F12.959   **Cannabis use, unspecified with psychotic disorder, unspecified** 🦠
        Cannabis-induced psychotic disorder, without use disorder

● **F12.98**   Cannabis use, unspecified with other cannabis-induced disorder

     F12.980   **Cannabis use, unspecified with anxiety disorder** 🦠
        Cannabis-induced anxiety disorder, without use disorder

     F12.988   **Cannabis use, unspecified with other cannabis-induced disorder** 🦠
        Cannabis-induced sleep disorder, without use disorder

   F12.99   **Cannabis use, unspecified with unspecified cannabis-induced disorder** 🦠

● **F13**   Sedative, hypnotic, or anxiolytic related disorders
     (Ex:) **For category F13 CC codes unless otherwise indicated:** See PDX Collection 3998

● **F13.1**   Sedative, hypnotic or anxiolytic-related abuse

     Excludes1   sedative, hypnotic or anxiolytic-related dependence (F13.2-)
               sedative, hypnotic, or anxiolytic use, unspecified (F13.9-)

   F13.10   **Sedative, hypnotic or anxiolytic abuse, uncomplicated**
        Sedative, hypnotic, or anxiolytic use disorder, mild

   F13.11   **Sedative, hypnotic or anxiolytic abuse, in remission**
        Sedative, hypnotic or anxiolytic use disorder, mild, in early remission
        Sedative, hypnotic or anxiolytic use disorder, mild, in sustained remission

● **F13.12**   Sedative, hypnotic or anxiolytic abuse with intoxication

     F13.120   **Sedative, hypnotic or anxiolytic abuse with intoxication, uncomplicated** 🦠

     F13.121   **Sedative, hypnotic or anxiolytic abuse with intoxication delirium** 🦠🦠

     F13.129   **Sedative, hypnotic or anxiolytic abuse with intoxication, unspecified** 🦠

● **F13.13**   Sedative, hypnotic or anxiolytic abuse with withdrawal

     F13.130   **Sedative, hypnotic or anxiolytic abuse with withdrawal, uncomplicated** 🦠
        (Ex:) See PDX Collection 4009

     F13.131   **Sedative, hypnotic or anxiolytic abuse with withdrawal delirium** 🦠
        (Ex:) See PDX Collection 4009

     F13.132   **Sedative, hypnotic or anxiolytic abuse with withdrawal with perceptual disturbance** 🦠
        (Ex:) See PDX Collection 4009

     F13.139   **Sedative, hypnotic or anxiolytic abuse with withdrawal, unspecified** 🦠
        (Ex:) See PDX Collection 4009

   F13.14   **Sedative, hypnotic or anxiolytic abuse with sedative, hypnotic or anxiolytic-induced mood disorder** 🦠
        Sedative, hypnotic, or anxiolytic use disorder, mild, with sedative, hypnotic, or anxiolytic-induced bipolar or related disorder
        Sedative, hypnotic, or anxiolytic use disorder, mild, with sedative, hypnotic, or anxiolytic-induced depressive disorder

● **F13.15**   Sedative, hypnotic or anxiolytic abuse with sedative, hypnotic or anxiolytic-induced psychotic disorder

     F13.150   **Sedative, hypnotic or anxiolytic abuse with sedative, hypnotic or anxiolytic-induced psychotic disorder with delusions** 🦠🦠

     F13.151   **Sedative, hypnotic or anxiolytic abuse with sedative, hypnotic or anxiolytic-induced psychotic disorder with hallucinations** 🦠🦠

     F13.159   **Sedative, hypnotic or anxiolytic abuse with sedative, hypnotic or anxiolytic-induced psychotic disorder, unspecified** 🦠

● **F13.18**   Sedative, hypnotic or anxiolytic abuse with other sedative, hypnotic or anxiolytic-induced disorders

     F13.180   **Sedative, hypnotic or anxiolytic abuse with sedative, hypnotic or anxiolytic-induced anxiety disorder** 🦠

     F13.181   **Sedative, hypnotic or anxiolytic abuse with sedative, hypnotic or anxiolytic-induced sexual dysfunction** 🦠

CHAPTER 5 (F01-F99)

N   Newborn Age: 0   P   Pediatric Age: 0–17   M   Maternity DX: 9–64   A   Adult Age: 15–124   ♀   Females Only   ♂   Males Only

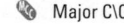   Complication\Comorbidity   🦠   Major C\C   (Ex:)   CC/MCC Exclusions   🦠   Hospital-Acquired Condition   🦠   Hierarchical Condition Category

779

CHAPTER 5 (F01-F99)

F13.182   Sedative, hypnotic or anxiolytic abuse with sedative, hypnotic or anxiolytic-induced sleep disorder

F13.188   Sedative, hypnotic or anxiolytic abuse with other sedative, hypnotic or anxiolytic-induced disorder

F13.19   Sedative, hypnotic or anxiolytic abuse with unspecified sedative, hypnotic or anxiolytic-induced disorder

● F13.2   Sedative, hypnotic or anxiolytic-related dependence

    Excludes1   sedative, hypnotic or anxiolytic-related abuse (F13.1-)
                sedative, hypnotic, or anxiolytic use, unspecified (F13.9-)

    Excludes2   sedative, hypnotic, or anxiolytic poisoning (T42.-)

F13.20   Sedative, hypnotic or anxiolytic dependence, uncomplicated
      (Ex:) See PDX Collection 3216

F13.21   Sedative, hypnotic or anxiolytic dependence, in remission
      Sedative, hypnotic or anxiolytic use disorder, moderate, in early remission
      Sedative, hypnotic or anxiolytic use disorder, moderate, in sustained remission
      Sedative, hypnotic or anxiolytic use disorder, severe, in early remission
      Sedative, hypnotic or anxiolytic use disorder, severe, in sustained remission

● F13.22   Sedative, hypnotic or anxiolytic dependence with intoxication

    Excludes1   sedative, hypnotic or anxiolytic dependence with withdrawal (F13.23-)

F13.220   Sedative, hypnotic or anxiolytic dependence with intoxication, uncomplicated

F13.221   Sedative, hypnotic or anxiolytic dependence with intoxication delirium

F13.229   Sedative, hypnotic or anxiolytic dependence with intoxication, unspecified

● F13.23   Sedative, hypnotic or anxiolytic dependence with withdrawal
      Sedative, hypnotic, or anxiolytic use disorder, moderate
      Sedative, hypnotic, or anxiolytic use disorder, severe

    Excludes1   sedative, hypnotic or anxiolytic dependence with intoxication (F13.22-)

F13.230   Sedative, hypnotic or anxiolytic dependence with withdrawal, uncomplicated

F13.231   Sedative, hypnotic or anxiolytic dependence with withdrawal delirium

F13.232   Sedative, hypnotic or anxiolytic dependence with withdrawal with perceptual disturbance
      Sedative, hypnotic, or anxiolytic withdrawal with perceptual disturbances

F13.239   Sedative, hypnotic or anxiolytic dependence with withdrawal, unspecified
      Sedative, hypnotic, or anxiolytic withdrawal without perceptual disturbances

F13.24   Sedative, hypnotic or anxiolytic dependence with sedative, hypnotic or anxiolytic-induced mood disorder
      Sedative, hypnotic, or anxiolytic use disorder, moderate, with sedative, hypnotic, or anxiolytic-induced bipolar or related disorder
      Sedative, hypnotic, or anxiolytic use disorder, moderate, with sedative, hypnotic, or anxiolytic-induced depressive disorder
      Sedative, hypnotic, or anxiolytic use disorder, severe, with sedative, hypnotic, or anxiolytic-induced bipolar or related disorder
      Sedative, hypnotic, or anxiolytic use disorder, severe, with sedative, hypnotic, or anxiolytic-induced depressive disorder

● F13.25   Sedative, hypnotic or anxiolytic dependence with sedative, hypnotic or anxiolytic-induced psychotic disorder

F13.250   Sedative, hypnotic or anxiolytic dependence with sedative, hypnotic or anxiolytic-induced psychotic disorder with delusions

F13.251   Sedative, hypnotic or anxiolytic dependence with sedative, hypnotic or anxiolytic-induced psychotic disorder with hallucinations

F13.259   Sedative, hypnotic or anxiolytic dependence with sedative, hypnotic or anxiolytic-induced psychotic disorder, unspecified
      (Ex:) See PDX Collection 3561

F13.26   Sedative, hypnotic or anxiolytic dependence with sedative, hypnotic or anxiolytic-induced persisting amnestic disorder
      (Ex:) See PDX Collection 3562

F13.27   Sedative, hypnotic or anxiolytic dependence with sedative, hypnotic or anxiolytic-induced persisting dementia
      Sedative, hypnotic, or anxiolytic use disorder, moderate, with sedative, hypnotic, or anxiolytic-induced major neurocognitive disorder
      Sedative, hypnotic, or anxiolytic use disorder, severe, with sedative, hypnotic, or anxiolytic-induced major neurocognitive disorder

● F13.28   Sedative, hypnotic or anxiolytic dependence with other sedative, hypnotic or anxiolytic-induced disorders
      (Ex:) For category F13.28 CC codes: See PDX Collection 3563-3566

F13.280   Sedative, hypnotic or anxiolytic dependence with sedative, hypnotic or anxiolytic-induced anxiety disorder

F13.281   Sedative, hypnotic or anxiolytic dependence with sedative, hypnotic or anxiolytic-induced sexual dysfunction

F13.282   Sedative, hypnotic or anxiolytic dependence with sedative, hypnotic or anxiolytic-induced sleep disorder

F13.288   Sedative, hypnotic or anxiolytic dependence with other sedative, hypnotic or anxiolytic-induced disorder 🪙 🪙
     Sedative, hypnotic, or anxiolytic use disorder, moderate, with sedative, hypnotic, or anxiolytic-induced mild neurocognitive disorder
     Sedative, hypnotic, or anxiolytic use disorder, severe, with sedative, hypnotic, or anxiolytic-induced mild neurocognitive disorder

F13.29   Sedative, hypnotic or anxiolytic dependence with unspecified sedative, hypnotic or anxiolytic-induced disorder 🪙

● F13.9   Sedative, hypnotic or anxiolytic-related use, unspecified
     Excludes1   sedative, hypnotic or anxiolytic-related abuse (F13.1-)
           sedative, hypnotic or anxiolytic-related dependence (F13.2-)

F13.90   Sedative, hypnotic, or anxiolytic use, unspecified, uncomplicated

● F13.92   Sedative, hypnotic or anxiolytic use, unspecified with intoxication
     Excludes1   sedative, hypnotic or anxiolytic use, unspecified with withdrawal (F13.93-)

     F13.920   Sedative, hypnotic or anxiolytic use, unspecified with intoxication, uncomplicated 🪙

     F13.921   Sedative, hypnotic or anxiolytic use, unspecified with intoxication delirium 🪙 🪙
           Sedative, hypnotic, or anxiolytic-induced delirium

     F13.929   Sedative, hypnotic or anxiolytic use, unspecified with intoxication, unspecified 🪙

● F13.93   Sedative, hypnotic or anxiolytic use, unspecified with withdrawal
     Excludes1   sedative, hypnotic or anxiolytic use, unspecified with intoxication (F13.92-)

     F13.930   Sedative, hypnotic or anxiolytic use, unspecified with withdrawal, uncomplicated 🪙 🪙

     F13.931   Sedative, hypnotic or anxiolytic use, unspecified with withdrawal delirium 🪙 🪙

     F13.932   Sedative, hypnotic or anxiolytic use, unspecified with withdrawal with perceptual disturbances 🪙 🪙

     F13.939   Sedative, hypnotic or anxiolytic use, unspecified with withdrawal, unspecified 🪙 🪙

F13.94   Sedative, hypnotic or anxiolytic use, unspecified with sedative, hypnotic or anxiolytic-induced mood disorder 🪙
     Sedative, hypnotic, or anxiolytic-induced bipolar or related disorder, without use disorder
     Sedative, hypnotic, or anxiolytic-induced depressive disorder, without use disorder

● F13.95   Sedative, hypnotic or anxiolytic use, unspecified with sedative, hypnotic or anxiolytic-induced psychotic disorder

     F13.950   Sedative, hypnotic or anxiolytic use, unspecified with sedative, hypnotic or anxiolytic-induced psychotic disorder with delusions 🪙 🪙

     F13.951   Sedative, hypnotic or anxiolytic use, unspecified with sedative, hypnotic or anxiolytic-induced psychotic disorder with hallucinations 🪙 🪙

     F13.959   Sedative, hypnotic or anxiolytic use, unspecified with sedative, hypnotic or anxiolytic-induced psychotic disorder, unspecified 🪙
           Sedative, hypnotic, or anxiolytic-induced psychotic disorder, without use disorder

F13.96   Sedative, hypnotic or anxiolytic use, unspecified with sedative, hypnotic or anxiolytic-induced persisting amnestic disorder 🪙

F13.97   Sedative, hypnotic or anxiolytic use, unspecified with sedative, hypnotic or anxiolytic-induced persisting dementia 🪙 🪙
     Sedative, hypnotic, or anxiolytic-induced major neurocognitive disorder, without use disorder

● F13.98   Sedative, hypnotic or anxiolytic use, unspecified with other sedative, hypnotic or anxiolytic-induced disorders

     F13.980   Sedative, hypnotic or anxiolytic use, unspecified with sedative, hypnotic or anxiolytic-induced anxiety disorder 🪙
           Sedative, hypnotic, or anxiolytic-induced anxiety disorder, without use disorder

     F13.981   Sedative, hypnotic or anxiolytic use, unspecified with sedative, hypnotic or anxiolytic-induced sexual dysfunction 🪙
           Sedative, hypnotic, or anxiolytic-induced sexual dysfunction disorder, without use disorder

     F13.982   Sedative, hypnotic or anxiolytic use, unspecified with sedative, hypnotic or anxiolytic-induced sleep disorder 🪙
           Sedative, hypnotic, or anxiolytic-induced sleep disorder, without use disorder

     F13.988   Sedative, hypnotic or anxiolytic use, unspecified with other sedative, hypnotic or anxiolytic-induced disorder 🪙
           Sedative, hypnotic, or anxiolytic-induced mild neurocognitive disorder

F13.99   Sedative, hypnotic or anxiolytic use, unspecified with unspecified sedative, hypnotic or anxiolytic-induced disorder 🪙

● F14   Cocaine related disorders
     Excludes2   other stimulant-related disorders (F15.-)
     (Ex:) **For category F14 CC codes unless otherwise indicated:** See PDX Collection 3998

● F14.1   Cocaine abuse
     Excludes1   cocaine dependence (F14.2-)
           cocaine use, unspecified (F14.9-)

     F14.10   Cocaine abuse, uncomplicated
           Cocaine use disorder, mild

     F14.11   Cocaine abuse, in remission
           Cocaine use disorder, mild, in early remission
           Cocaine use disorder, mild, in sustained remission

---

N Newborn Age: 0   **P** Pediatric Age: 0–17   **M** Maternity DX: 9–64   **A** Adult Age: 15–124   ♀ Females Only   ♂ Males Only

🪙 Complication\Comorbidity   🪙 Major C\C   (Ex:) CC/MCC Exclusions   🪙 Hospital-Acquired Condition   🪙 Hierarchical Condition Category

(side tab) CHAPTER 5 (F01-F99)

● **F14.12**   Cocaine abuse with intoxication

     F14.120   Cocaine abuse with intoxication, uncomplicated 🔧

     F14.121   Cocaine abuse with intoxication with delirium 🔧🔧

     F14.122   Cocaine abuse with intoxication with perceptual disturbance 🔧

     F14.129   Cocaine abuse with intoxication, unspecified 🔧

F14.13   Cocaine abuse, unspecified with withdrawal 🔧
     (Ex:) See PDX Collection 4009

F14.14   Cocaine abuse with cocaine-induced mood disorder 🔧
     Cocaine use disorder, mild, with cocaine-induced bipolar or related disorder
     Cocaine use disorder, mild, with cocaine-induced depressive disorder

● **F14.15**   Cocaine abuse with cocaine-induced psychotic disorder

     F14.150   Cocaine abuse with cocaine-induced psychotic disorder with delusions 🔧🔧

     F14.151   Cocaine abuse with cocaine-induced psychotic disorder with hallucinations 🔧🔧

     F14.159   Cocaine abuse with cocaine-induced psychotic disorder, unspecified 🔧

● **F14.18**   Cocaine abuse with other cocaine-induced disorder

     F14.180   Cocaine abuse with cocaine-induced anxiety disorder 🔧

     F14.181   Cocaine abuse with cocaine-induced sexual dysfunction 🔧

     F14.182   Cocaine abuse with cocaine-induced sleep disorder 🔧

     F14.188   Cocaine abuse with other cocaine-induced disorder 🔧
         Cocaine use disorder, mild, with cocaine-induced obsessive-compulsive or related disorder

F14.19   Cocaine abuse with unspecified cocaine-induced disorder 🔧

● **F14.2**   **Cocaine dependence**

     Excludes1   cocaine abuse (F14.1-)
               cocaine use, unspecified (F14.9-)

     Excludes2   cocaine poisoning (T40.5-)

     F14.20   Cocaine dependence, uncomplicated 🔧🔧
         Cocaine use disorder, moderate
         Cocaine use disorder, severe
         (Ex:) See PDX Collection 3217

     F14.21   Cocaine dependence, in remission 🔧
         Cocaine use disorder, moderate, in early remission
         Cocaine use disorder, moderate, in sustained remission
         Cocaine use disorder, severe, in early remission
         Cocaine use disorder, severe, in sustained remission
         Coding Clinic: 2017, Q2, P27

● **F14.22**   Cocaine dependence with intoxication

     Excludes1   cocaine dependence with withdrawal (F14.23)

     F14.220   Cocaine dependence with intoxication, uncomplicated 🔧

     F14.221   Cocaine dependence with intoxication delirium 🔧🔧

     F14.222   Cocaine dependence with intoxication with perceptual disturbance 🔧🔧
         (Ex:) See PDX Collection 3567

     F14.229   Cocaine dependence with intoxication, unspecified 🔧🔧
         (Ex:) See PDX Collection 3568

F14.23   Cocaine dependence with withdrawal 🔧🔧

     Excludes1   cocaine dependence with intoxication (F14.22-)

F14.24   Cocaine dependence with cocaine-induced mood disorder 🔧
     Cocaine use disorder, moderate, with cocaine-induced bipolar or related disorder
     Cocaine use disorder, moderate, with cocaine-induced depressive disorder
     Cocaine use disorder, severe, with cocaine-induced bipolar or related disorder
     Cocaine use disorder, severe, with cocaine-induced depressive disorder

● **F14.25**   Cocaine dependence with cocaine-induced psychotic disorder

     F14.250   Cocaine dependence with cocaine-induced psychotic disorder with delusions 🔧🔧

     F14.251   Cocaine dependence with cocaine-induced psychotic disorder with hallucinations 🔧🔧

     F14.259   Cocaine dependence with cocaine-induced psychotic disorder, unspecified 🔧🔧
         (Ex:) See PDX Collection 3569

● **F14.28**   Cocaine dependence with other cocaine-induced disorder

     F14.280   Cocaine dependence with cocaine-induced anxiety disorder 🔧🔧
         (Ex:) See PDX Collection 3570

     F14.281   Cocaine dependence with cocaine-induced sexual dysfunction 🔧🔧
         (Ex:) See PDX Collection 3571

     F14.282   Cocaine dependence with cocaine-induced sleep disorder 🔧🔧
         (Ex:) See PDX Collection 3572

     F14.288   Cocaine dependence with other cocaine-induced disorder 🔧🔧
         Cocaine use disorder, moderate, with cocaine-induced obsessive-compulsive or related disorder
         Cocaine use disorder, severe, with cocaine-induced obsessive-compulsive or related disorder
         (Ex:) See PDX Collection 3573

F14.29   Cocaine dependence with unspecified cocaine-induced disorder 🔧

● **F14.9**   Cocaine use, unspecified

     Excludes1   cocaine abuse (F14.1-)
               cocaine dependence (F14.2-)

     F14.90   Cocaine use, unspecified, uncomplicated
         Coding Clinic: 2018, Q2, P11

● **F14.92**   Cocaine use, unspecified with intoxication

     F14.920   Cocaine use, unspecified with intoxication, uncomplicated 🔧

     F14.921   Cocaine use, unspecified with intoxication delirium 🔧🔧

     F14.922   Cocaine use, unspecified with intoxication with perceptual disturbance 🔧

     F14.929   Cocaine use, unspecified with intoxication, unspecified 🔧

F14.93   Cocaine use, unspecified with withdrawal 🔧
     (Ex:) See PDX Collection 4009

▶ New   ⇒ Revised   ~~deleted~~ Deleted   Excludes 1   Excludes 2   Includes   Use additional   Code first   Code also   Key words

782   OGCR Official Guidelines   ● Unacceptable Principal Diagnosis   X Assign placeholder X   ● Use Additional Character(s)   ▶ Manifestation Code   Coding Clinic

F14.94   Cocaine use, unspecified with cocaine-induced mood disorder 🐾
     Cocaine-induced bipolar or related disorder, without use disorder
     Cocaine-induced depressive disorder, without use disorder

● **F14.95**   Cocaine use, unspecified with cocaine-induced psychotic disorder

     F14.950   Cocaine use, unspecified with cocaine-induced psychotic disorder with delusions 🐾🐾

     F14.951   Cocaine use, unspecified with cocaine-induced psychotic disorder with hallucinations 🐾🐾

     F14.959   Cocaine use, unspecified with cocaine-induced psychotic disorder, unspecified 🐾
        Cocaine-induced psychotic disorder, without use disorder

● **F14.98**   Cocaine use, unspecified with other specified cocaine-induced disorder

     F14.980   Cocaine use, unspecified with cocaine-induced anxiety disorder 🐾
        Cocaine-induced anxiety disorder, without use disorder

     F14.981   Cocaine use, unspecified with cocaine-induced sexual dysfunction 🐾
        Cocaine-induced sexual dysfunction, without use disorder

     F14.982   Cocaine use, unspecified with cocaine-induced sleep disorder 🐾
        Cocaine-induced sleep disorder, without use disorder

     F14.988   Cocaine use, unspecified with other cocaine-induced disorder 🐾
        Cocaine-induced obsessive-compulsive or related disorder

F14.99   Cocaine use, unspecified with unspecified cocaine-induced disorder 🐾

● **F15**   **Other stimulant related disorders**

     Includes   amphetamine-related disorders
                 caffeine

     Excludes2   cocaine-related disorders (F14.-)

     (Ex:) **For category F15 CC codes unless otherwise indicated:** See PDX Collection 3998

● **F15.1**   Other stimulant abuse

     Excludes1   other stimulant dependence (F15.2-)
                 other stimulant use, unspecified (F15.9-)

     F15.10   Other stimulant abuse, uncomplicated
        Amphetamine type substance use disorder, mild
        Other or unspecified stimulant use disorder, mild

     F15.11   Other stimulant abuse, in remission
        Amphetamine type substance use disorder, mild, in early remission
        Amphetamine type substance use disorder, mild, in sustained remission
        Other or unspecified stimulant use disorder, mild, in early remission
        Other or unspecified stimulant use disorder, mild, in sustained remission

● **F15.12**   Other stimulant abuse with intoxication

     F15.120   Other stimulant abuse with intoxication, uncomplicated 🐾

     F15.121   Other stimulant abuse with intoxication delirium 🐾🐾

     F15.122   Other stimulant abuse with intoxication with perceptual disturbance 🐾
        Amphetamine or other stimulant use disorder, mild, with amphetamine or other stimulant intoxication, with perceptual disturbances

     F15.129   Other stimulant abuse with intoxication, unspecified 🐾
        Amphetamine or other stimulant use disorder, mild, with amphetamine or other stimulant intoxication, without perceptual disturbances

F15.13   Other stimulant abuse with withdrawal 🐾
     (Ex:) See PDX Collection 4009

F15.14   Other stimulant abuse with stimulant-induced mood disorder 🐾
     Amphetamine or other stimulant use disorder, mild, with amphetamine or other stimulant-induced bipolar or related disorder
     Amphetamine or other stimulant use disorder, mild, with amphetamine or other stimulant-induced depressive disorder

● **F15.15**   Other stimulant abuse with stimulant-induced psychotic disorder

     F15.150   Other stimulant abuse with stimulant-induced psychotic disorder with delusions 🐾🐾

     F15.151   Other stimulant abuse with stimulant-induced psychotic disorder with hallucinations 🐾🐾

     F15.159   Other stimulant abuse with stimulant-induced psychotic disorder, unspecified 🐾

● **F15.18**   Other stimulant abuse with other stimulant-induced disorder

     F15.180   Other stimulant abuse with stimulant-induced anxiety disorder 🐾

     F15.181   Other stimulant abuse with stimulant-induced sexual dysfunction 🐾

     F15.182   Other stimulant abuse with stimulant-induced sleep disorder 🐾

     F15.188   Other stimulant abuse with other stimulant-induced disorder 🐾
        Amphetamine or other stimulant use disorder, mild, with amphetamine or other stimulant-induced obsessive-compulsive or related disorder

F15.19   Other stimulant abuse with unspecified stimulant-induced disorder 🐾

● **F15.2**   Other stimulant dependence

     Excludes1   other stimulant abuse (F15.1-)
                 other stimulant use, unspecified (F15.9-)

     F15.20   Other stimulant dependence, uncomplicated 🐾🐾
        Amphetamine type substance use disorder, moderate
        Amphetamine type substance use disorder, severe
        Other or unspecified stimulant use disorder, moderate
        Other or unspecified stimulant use disorder, severe
        (Ex:) See PDX Collection 3218

N Newborn Age: 0   **P** Pediatric Age: 0–17   **M** Maternity DX: 9–64   **A** Adult Age: 15–124   ♀ Females Only   ♂ Males Only

🐾 Complication\Comorbidity   🐾 Major C\C   (Ex:) CC/MCC Exclusions   Hospital-Acquired Condition   🐾 Hierarchical Condition Category

783

F15.21   Other stimulant dependence, in remission 🏷️

Amphetamine type substance use disorder, moderate, in early remission

Amphetamine type substance use disorder, moderate, in sustained remission

Amphetamine type substance use disorder, severe, in early remission

Amphetamine type substance use disorder, severe, in sustained remission

Other or unspecified stimulant use disorder, moderate, in early remission

Other or unspecified stimulant use disorder, moderate, in sustained remission

Other or unspecified stimulant use disorder, severe, in early remission

Other or unspecified stimulant use disorder, severe, in sustained remission

● **F15.22**   Other stimulant dependence with intoxication

> **Excludes1**   other stimulant dependence with withdrawal (F15.23)

     F15.220   Other stimulant dependence with intoxication, uncomplicated 🏷️

     F15.221   Other stimulant dependence with intoxication delirium 🏷️🏷️

     F15.222   Other stimulant dependence with intoxication with perceptual disturbance 🏷️🏷️

         Amphetamine or other stimulant use disorder, moderate, with amphetamine or other stimulant intoxication, with perceptual disturbances

         Amphetamine or other stimulant use disorder, severe, with amphetamine or other stimulant intoxication, with perceptual disturbances

         (Ex:) See PDX Collection 3574

     F15.229   Other stimulant dependence with intoxication, unspecified 🏷️

         Amphetamine or other stimulant use disorder, moderate, with amphetamine or other stimulant intoxication, without perceptual disturbances

         Amphetamine or other stimulant use disorder, severe, with amphetamine or other stimulant intoxication, without perceptual disturbances

F15.23   Other stimulant dependence with withdrawal 🏷️🏷️

     Amphetamine or other stimulant withdrawal

> **Excludes1**   other stimulant dependence with intoxication (F15.22-)

F15.24   Other stimulant dependence with stimulant-induced mood disorder 🏷️

     Amphetamine or other stimulant use disorder, moderate, with amphetamine or other stimulant-induced bipolar or related disorder

     Amphetamine or other stimulant use disorder, moderate, with amphetamine or other stimulant-induced depressive disorder

     Amphetamine or other stimulant use disorder, severe, with amphetamine or other stimulant-induced bipolar or related disorder

     Amphetamine or other stimulant use disorder, severe, with amphetamine or other stimulant-induced depressive disorder

● **F15.25**   Other stimulant dependence with stimulant-induced psychotic disorder

     F15.250   Other stimulant dependence with stimulant-induced psychotic disorder with delusions 🏷️🏷️

     F15.251   Other stimulant dependence with stimulant-induced psychotic disorder with hallucinations 🏷️🏷️

     F15.259   Other stimulant dependence with stimulant-induced psychotic disorder, unspecified 🏷️🏷️

         (Ex:) See PDX Collection 3575

● **F15.28**   Other stimulant dependence with other stimulant-induced disorder

     F15.280   Other stimulant dependence with stimulant-induced anxiety disorder 🏷️🏷️

         (Ex:) See PDX Collection 3576

     F15.281   Other stimulant dependence with stimulant-induced sexual dysfunction 🏷️🏷️

         (Ex:) See PDX Collection 3577

     F15.282   Other stimulant dependence with stimulant-induced sleep disorder 🏷️🏷️

         (Ex:) See PDX Collection 3578

     F15.288   Other stimulant dependence with other stimulant-induced disorder 🏷️🏷️

         Amphetamine or other stimulant use disorder, moderate, with amphetamine or other stimulant-induced obsessive-compulsive or related disorder

         Amphetamine or other stimulant use disorder, severe, with amphetamine or other stimulant-induced obsessive-compulsive or related disorder

         (Ex:) See PDX Collection 3579

F15.29   Other stimulant dependence with unspecified stimulant-induced disorder 🏷️

● **F15.9**   Other stimulant use, unspecified

> **Excludes1**   other stimulant abuse (F15.1-)
> other stimulant dependence (F15.2-)

F15.90   Other stimulant use, unspecified, uncomplicated

● **F15.92**   Other stimulant use, unspecified with intoxication

> **Excludes1**   other stimulant use, unspecified with withdrawal (F15.93)

     F15.920   Other stimulant use, unspecified with intoxication, uncomplicated 🏷️

     F15.921   Other stimulant use, unspecified with intoxication delirium 🏷️🏷️

         Amphetamine or other stimulant-induced delirium

     F15.922   Other stimulant use, unspecified with intoxication with perceptual disturbance 🏷️

     F15.929   Other stimulant use, unspecified with intoxication, unspecified 🏷️

         Caffeine intoxication

F15.93   Other stimulant use, unspecified with withdrawal 🏷️🏷️

     Caffeine withdrawal

> **Excludes1**   other stimulant use, unspecified with intoxication (F15.92-)

F15.94   Other stimulant use, unspecified with stimulant-induced mood disorder 🏷️

     Amphetamine or other stimulant-induced bipolar or related disorder, without use disorder

     Amphetamine or other stimulant-induced depressive disorder, without use disorder

● **F15.95** Other stimulant use, unspecified with stimulant-induced psychotic disorder

   F15.950 Other stimulant use, unspecified with stimulant-induced psychotic disorder with delusions 🦠🦠

   F15.951 Other stimulant use, unspecified with stimulant-induced psychotic disorder with hallucinations 🦠🦠

   F15.959 Other stimulant use, unspecified with stimulant-induced psychotic disorder, unspecified 🦠
       Amphetamine or other stimulant-induced psychotic disorder, without use disorder

● **F15.98** Other stimulant use, unspecified with other stimulant-induced disorder

   F15.980 Other stimulant use, unspecified with stimulant-induced anxiety disorder 🦠
       Amphetamine or other stimulant-induced anxiety disorder, without use disorder
       Caffeine-induced anxiety disorder, without use disorder

   F15.981 Other stimulant use, unspecified with stimulant-induced sexual dysfunction 🦠
       Amphetamine or other stimulant-induced sexual dysfunction, without use disorder

   F15.982 Other stimulant use, unspecified with stimulant-induced sleep disorder 🦠
       Amphetamine or other stimulant-induced sleep disorder, without use disorder
       Caffeine-induced sleep disorder, without use disorder

   F15.988 Other stimulant use, unspecified with other stimulant-induced disorder 🦠
       Amphetamine or other stimulant-induced obsessive-compulsive or related disorder, without use disorder

   F15.99 Other stimulant use, unspecified with unspecified stimulant-induced disorder 🦠

● **F16** Hallucinogen related disorders

   Includes ecstasy
             PCP
             phencyclidine

   (Ex:) **For category F16 CC codes unless otherwise indicated:** See PDX Collection 3998

● **F16.1** Hallucinogen abuse

   Excludes1 hallucinogen dependence (F16.2-)
            hallucinogen use, unspecified (F16.9-)

   F16.10 Hallucinogen abuse, uncomplicated
       Other hallucinogen use disorder, mild
       Phencyclidine use disorder, mild
       Coding Clinic: 2018, Q4, P31

   F16.11 Hallucinogen abuse, in remission
       Other hallucinogen use disorder, mild, in early remission
       Other hallucinogen use disorder, mild, in sustained remission
       Phencyclidine use disorder, mild, in early remission
       Phencyclidine use disorder, mild, in sustained remission

● **F16.12** Hallucinogen abuse with intoxication

   F16.120 Hallucinogen abuse with intoxication, uncomplicated 🦠

   F16.121 Hallucinogen abuse with intoxication with delirium 🦠🦠

   F16.122 Hallucinogen abuse with intoxication with perceptual disturbance 🦠

   F16.129 Hallucinogen abuse with intoxication, unspecified 🦠

F16.14 Hallucinogen abuse with hallucinogen-induced mood disorder 🦠
       Other hallucinogen use disorder, mild, with other hallucinogen-induced bipolar or related disorder
       Other hallucinogen use disorder, mild, with other hallucinogen-induced depressive disorder
       Phencyclidine use disorder, mild, with phencyclidine-induced bipolar or related disorder
       Phencyclidine use disorder, mild, with phencyclidine-induced depressive disorder

● **F16.15** Hallucinogen abuse with hallucinogen-induced psychotic disorder

   F16.150 Hallucinogen abuse with hallucinogen-induced psychotic disorder with delusions 🦠🦠

   F16.151 Hallucinogen abuse with hallucinogen-induced psychotic disorder with hallucinations 🦠🦠

   F16.159 Hallucinogen abuse with hallucinogen-induced psychotic disorder, unspecified 🦠

● **F16.18** Hallucinogen abuse with other hallucinogen-induced disorder

   F16.180 Hallucinogen abuse with hallucinogen-induced anxiety disorder 🦠

   F16.183 Hallucinogen abuse with hallucinogen persisting perception disorder (flashbacks) 🦠

   F16.188 Hallucinogen abuse with other hallucinogen-induced disorder 🦠

   F16.19 Hallucinogen abuse with unspecified hallucinogen-induced disorder 🦠

● **F16.2** Hallucinogen dependence

   Excludes1 hallucinogen abuse (F16.1-)
            hallucinogen use, unspecified (F16.9-)

   F16.20 Hallucinogen dependence, uncomplicated 🦠🦠
       Other hallucinogen use disorder, moderate
       Other hallucinogen use disorder, severe
       Phencyclidine use disorder, moderate
       Phencyclidine use disorder, severe
       (Ex:) See PDX Collection 3219

   F16.21 Hallucinogen dependence, in remission 🦠
       Other hallucinogen use disorder, moderate, in early remission
       Other hallucinogen use disorder, moderate, in sustained remission
       Other hallucinogen use disorder, severe, in early remission
       Other hallucinogen use disorder, severe, in sustained remission
       Phencyclidine use disorder, moderate, in early remission
       Phencyclidine use disorder, moderate, in sustained remission
       Phencyclidine use disorder, severe, in early remission
       Phencyclidine use disorder, severe, in sustained remission

● **F16.22** Hallucinogen dependence with intoxication

   F16.220 Hallucinogen dependence with intoxication, uncomplicated 🦠

   F16.221 Hallucinogen dependence with intoxication with delirium 🦠🦠

   F16.229 Hallucinogen dependence with intoxication, unspecified 🦠

N Newborn Age: 0   **P** Pediatric Age: 0–17   **M** Maternity DX: 9–64   **A** Adult Age: 15–124   ♀ Females Only   ♂ Males Only

🦠 Complication\Comorbidity   🦠 Major C\C   (Ex:) CC/MCC Exclusions   🦠 Hospital-Acquired Condition   🦠 Hierarchical Condition Category   785

CHAPTER 5 (F01-F99)

F16.24 Hallucinogen dependence with hallucinogen-induced mood disorder 🔑
Other hallucinogen use disorder, moderate, with other hallucinogen-induced bipolar or related disorder
Other hallucinogen use disorder, moderate, with other hallucinogen-induced depressive disorder
Other hallucinogen use disorder, severe, with other hallucinogen-induced bipolar or related disorder
Other hallucinogen use disorder, severe, with other hallucinogen-induced depressive disorder
Phencyclidine use disorder, moderate, with phencyclidine-induced bipolar or related disorder
Phencyclidine use disorder, moderate, with phencyclidine-induced depressive disorder
Phencyclidine use disorder, severe, with phencyclidine-induced bipolar or related disorder
Phencyclidine use disorder, severe, with phencyclidine-induced depressive disorder

● **F16.25 Hallucinogen dependence with hallucinogen-induced psychotic disorder**

     F16.250 Hallucinogen dependence with hallucinogen-induced psychotic disorder with delusions 🔒🔑

     F16.251 Hallucinogen dependence with hallucinogen-induced psychotic disorder with hallucinations 🔒🔑

     F16.259 Hallucinogen dependence with hallucinogen-induced psychotic disorder, unspecified 🔒🔑
(Ex:) See PDX Collection 3580

● **F16.28 Hallucinogen dependence with other hallucinogen-induced disorder**

     F16.280 Hallucinogen dependence with hallucinogen-induced anxiety disorder 🔒🔑
(Ex:) See PDX Collection 3581

     F16.283 Hallucinogen dependence with hallucinogen persisting perception disorder (flashbacks) 🔒🔑
(Ex:) See PDX Collection 3582

     F16.288 Hallucinogen dependence with other hallucinogen-induced disorder 🔒🔑
(Ex:) See PDX Collection 3583

     F16.29 Hallucinogen dependence with unspecified hallucinogen-induced disorder 🔑

● **F16.9 Hallucinogen use, unspecified**

     Excludes1   hallucinogen abuse (F16.1-)
hallucinogen dependence (F16.2-)

     F16.90 Hallucinogen use, unspecified, uncomplicated

● **F16.92 Hallucinogen use, unspecified with intoxication**

     F16.920 Hallucinogen use, unspecified with intoxication, uncomplicated 🔑

     F16.921 Hallucinogen use, unspecified with intoxication with delirium 🔒🔑
Other hallucinogen intoxication delirium

     F16.929 Hallucinogen use, unspecified with intoxication, unspecified 🔑

     F16.94 Hallucinogen use, unspecified with hallucinogen-induced mood disorder 🔑
Other hallucinogen-induced bipolar or related disorder, without use disorder
Other hallucinogen-induced depressive disorder, without use disorder
Phencyclidine-induced bipolar or related disorder, without use disorder
Phencyclidine-induced depressive disorder, without use disorder

● **F16.95 Hallucinogen use, unspecified with hallucinogen-induced psychotic disorder**

     F16.950 Hallucinogen use, unspecified with hallucinogen-induced psychotic disorder with delusions 🔒🔑

     F16.951 Hallucinogen use, unspecified with hallucinogen-induced psychotic disorder with hallucinations 🔒🔑

     F16.959 Hallucinogen use, unspecified with hallucinogen-induced psychotic disorder, unspecified 🔑
Other hallucinogen-induced psychotic disorder, without use disorder
Phencyclidine-induced psychotic disorder, without use disorder

● **F16.98 Hallucinogen use, unspecified with other specified hallucinogen-induced disorder**

     F16.980 Hallucinogen use, unspecified with hallucinogen-induced anxiety disorder 🔑
Other hallucinogen-induced anxiety disorder, without use disorder
Phencyclidine-induced anxiety disorder, without use disorder

     F16.983 Hallucinogen use, unspecified with hallucinogen persisting perception disorder (flashbacks) 🔑

     F16.988 Hallucinogen use, unspecified with other hallucinogen-induced disorder 🔑

     F16.99 Hallucinogen use, unspecified with unspecified hallucinogen-induced disorder 🔑

● **F17 Nicotine dependence**

     Excludes1   history of tobacco dependence (Z87.891)
tobacco use NOS (Z72.0)

     Excludes2   tobacco use (smoking) during pregnancy, childbirth and the puerperium (O99.33-)
toxic effect of nicotine (T65.2-)

(Ex:) **For category F17 CC codes:** See PDX Collection 3998

● **F17.2 Nicotine dependence**

     ● **F17.20 Nicotine dependence, unspecified**

       ● **F17.200 Nicotine dependence, unspecified, uncomplicated**
Tobacco use disorder, mild
Tobacco use disorder, moderate
Tobacco use disorder, severe
Coding Clinic: 2016, Q1, P37

       ● **F17.201 Nicotine dependence, unspecified, in remission**
Tobacco use disorder, mild, in early remission
Tobacco use disorder, mild, in sustained remission
Tobacco use disorder, moderate, in early remission
Tobacco use disorder, moderate, in sustained remission
Tobacco use disorder, severe, in early remission
Tobacco use disorder, severe, in sustained remission

▶ New   ➡ Revised   ~~deleted~~ Deleted   Excludes 1   Excludes 2   Includes   Use additional   Code first   Code also   Key words
OGCR Official Guidelines   ● Unacceptable Principal Diagnosis   X Assign placeholder X   ● Use Additional Character(s)   ▶ Manifestation Code   **Coding Clinic**

F17.203   Nicotine dependence unspecified, with withdrawal 🅒
Tobacco withdrawal

F17.208   Nicotine dependence, unspecified, with other nicotine-induced disorders

F17.209   Nicotine dependence, unspecified, with unspecified nicotine-induced disorders

● F17.21   Nicotine dependence, cigarettes

● F17.210   Nicotine dependence, cigarettes, uncomplicated
Coding Clinic: 2017, Q2, P28-29

● F17.211   Nicotine dependence, cigarettes, in remission
Tobacco use disorder, cigarettes, mild, in early remission
Tobacco use disorder, cigarettes, mild, in sustained remission
Tobacco use disorder, cigarettes, moderate, in early remission
Tobacco use disorder, cigarettes, moderate, in sustained remission
Tobacco use disorder, cigarettes, severe, in early remission
Tobacco use disorder, cigarettes, severe, in sustained remission

F17.213   Nicotine dependence, cigarettes, with withdrawal 🅒

F17.218   Nicotine dependence, cigarettes, with other nicotine-induced disorders

F17.219   Nicotine dependence, cigarettes, with unspecified nicotine-induced disorders

● F17.22   Nicotine dependence, chewing tobacco

● F17.220   Nicotine dependence, chewing tobacco, uncomplicated

● F17.221   Nicotine dependence, chewing tobacco, in remission
Tobacco use disorder, chewing tobacco, mild, in early remission
Tobacco use disorder, chewing tobacco, mild, in sustained remission
Tobacco use disorder, chewing tobacco, moderate, in early remission
Tobacco use disorder, chewing tobacco, moderate, in sustained remission
Tobacco use disorder, chewing tobacco, severe, in early remission
Tobacco use disorder, chewing tobacco, severe, in sustained remission

F17.223   Nicotine dependence, chewing tobacco, with withdrawal 🅒

F17.228   Nicotine dependence, chewing tobacco, with other nicotine-induced disorders

F17.229   Nicotine dependence, chewing tobacco, with unspecified nicotine-induced disorders

● F17.29   Nicotine dependence, other tobacco product

● F17.290   Nicotine dependence, other tobacco product, uncomplicated
Coding Clinic: 2017, Q2, P28-29

● F17.291   Nicotine dependence, other tobacco product, in remission
Tobacco use disorder, other tobacco product, mild, in early remission
Tobacco use disorder, other tobacco product, mild, in sustained remission
Tobacco use disorder, other tobacco product, moderate, in early remission
Tobacco use disorder, other tobacco product, moderate, in sustained remission
Tobacco use disorder, other tobacco product, severe, in early remission
Tobacco use disorder, other tobacco product, severe, in sustained remission

F17.293   Nicotine dependence, other tobacco product, with withdrawal 🅒

F17.298   Nicotine dependence, other tobacco product, with other nicotine-induced disorders

F17.299   Nicotine dependence, other tobacco product, with unspecified nicotine-induced disorders

● F18   Inhalant related disorders
Includes   volatile solvents
Ⓔ For category F18 CC codes unless otherwise indicated: See PDX Collection 3998

● F18.1   Inhalant abuse
Excludes1   inhalant dependence (F18.2-)
inhalant use, unspecified (F18.9-)

F18.10   Inhalant abuse, uncomplicated
Inhalant use disorder, mild

F18.11   Inhalant abuse, in remission
Inhalant use disorder, mild, in early remission
Inhalant use disorder, mild, in sustained remission

● F18.12   Inhalant abuse with intoxication

F18.120   Inhalant abuse with intoxication, uncomplicated 🅒

F18.121   Inhalant abuse with intoxication delirium 🅒🅒

F18.129   Inhalant abuse with intoxication, unspecified 🅒

F18.14   Inhalant abuse with inhalant-induced mood disorder 🅒
Inhalant use disorder, mild, with inhalant-induced depressive disorder

● F18.15   Inhalant abuse with inhalant-induced psychotic disorder

F18.150   Inhalant abuse with inhalant-induced psychotic disorder with delusions 🅒🅒

F18.151   Inhalant abuse with inhalant-induced psychotic disorder with hallucinations 🅒🅒

F18.159   Inhalant abuse with inhalant-induced psychotic disorder, unspecified 🅒

F18.17   Inhalant abuse with inhalant-induced dementia 🅒🅒
Inhalant use disorder, mild, with inhalant-induced major neurocognitive disorder

CHAPTER 5 (F01-F99)

● **F18.18** **Inhalant abuse with other inhalant-induced disorders**

    F18.180 **Inhalant abuse with inhalant-induced anxiety disorder** 🪙

    F18.188 **Inhalant abuse with other inhalant-induced disorder** 🪙

        Inhalant use disorder, mild, with inhalant-induced mild neurocognitive disorder

    F18.19 **Inhalant abuse with unspecified inhalant-induced disorder** 🪙

● **F18.2** **Inhalant dependence**

    Excludes1   inhalant abuse (F18.1-)
                 inhalant use, unspecified (F18.9-)

    F18.20 **Inhalant dependence, uncomplicated** 🪙🪙
        Inhalant use disorder, moderate
        Inhalant use disorder, severe
        (Ex:) See PDX Collection 3220

    F18.21 **Inhalant dependence, in remission** 🪙
        Inhalant use disorder, moderate, in early remission
        Inhalant use disorder, moderate, in sustained remission
        Inhalant use disorder, severe, in early remission
        Inhalant use disorder, severe, in sustained remission

● **F18.22** **Inhalant dependence with intoxication**

    F18.220 **Inhalant dependence with intoxication, uncomplicated** 🪙

    F18.221 **Inhalant dependence with intoxication delirium** 🪙🪙

    F18.229 **Inhalant dependence with intoxication, unspecified** 🪙

    F18.24 **Inhalant dependence with inhalant-induced mood disorder** 🪙
        Inhalant use disorder, moderate, with inhalant-induced depressive disorder
        Inhalant use disorder, severe, with inhalant-induced depressive disorder

● **F18.25** **Inhalant dependence with inhalant-induced psychotic disorder**

    F18.250 **Inhalant dependence with inhalant-induced psychotic disorder with delusions** 🪙🪙

    F18.251 **Inhalant dependence with inhalant-induced psychotic disorder with hallucinations** 🪙🪙

    F18.259 **Inhalant dependence with inhalant-induced psychotic disorder, unspecified** 🪙🪙
        (Ex:) See PDX Collection 3584

    F18.27 **Inhalant dependence with inhalant-induced dementia** 🪙🪙
        Inhalant use disorder, moderate, with inhalant-induced major neurocognitive disorder
        Inhalant use disorder, severe, with inhalant-induced major neurocognitive disorder

● **F18.28** **Inhalant dependence with other inhalant-induced disorders**

    F18.280 **Inhalant dependence with inhalant-induced anxiety disorder** 🪙🪙🪙
        (Ex:) See PDX Collection 3585

    F18.288 **Inhalant dependence with other inhalant-induced disorder** 🪙🪙
        Inhalant use disorder, moderate, with inhalant-induced mild neurocognitive disorder
        Inhalant use disorder, severe, with inhalant-induced mild neurocognitive disorder
        (Ex:) See PDX Collection 3586

    F18.29 **Inhalant dependence with unspecified inhalant-induced disorder** 🪙

● **F18.9** **Inhalant use, unspecified**

    Excludes1   inhalant abuse (F18.1-)
                 inhalant dependence (F18.2-)

    F18.90 **Inhalant use, unspecified, uncomplicated**

● **F18.92** **Inhalant use, unspecified with intoxication**

    F18.920 **Inhalant use, unspecified with intoxication, uncomplicated** 🪙

    F18.921 **Inhalant use, unspecified with intoxication with delirium** 🪙🪙

    F18.929 **Inhalant use, unspecified with intoxication, unspecified** 🪙

    F18.94 **Inhalant use, unspecified with inhalant-induced mood disorder** 🪙
        Inhalant-induced depressive disorder

● **F18.95** **Inhalant use, unspecified with inhalant-induced psychotic disorder**

    F18.950 **Inhalant use, unspecified with inhalant-induced psychotic disorder with delusions** 🪙🪙

    F18.951 **Inhalant use, unspecified with inhalant-induced psychotic disorder with hallucinations** 🪙🪙

    F18.959 **Inhalant use, unspecified with inhalant-induced psychotic disorder, unspecified** 🪙

    F18.97 **Inhalant use, unspecified with inhalant-induced persisting dementia** 🪙🪙
        Inhalant-induced major neurocognitive disorder

● **F18.98** **Inhalant use, unspecified with other inhalant-induced disorders**

    F18.980 **Inhalant use, unspecified with inhalant-induced anxiety disorder** 🪙

    F18.988 **Inhalant use, unspecified with other inhalant-induced disorder** 🪙
        Inhalant-induced mild neurocognitive disorder

    F18.99 **Inhalant use, unspecified with unspecified inhalant-induced disorder** 🪙

● **F19** **Other psychoactive substance related disorders**

    Includes   polysubstance drug use (indiscriminate drug use)

    (Ex:) **For category F19 CC codes unless otherwise indicated:** See PDX Collection 3998

● **F19.1** **Other psychoactive substance abuse**

    Excludes1   other psychoactive substance dependence (F19.2-)
                 other psychoactive substance use, unspecified (F19.9-)

    F19.10 **Other psychoactive substance abuse, uncomplicated**
        Other (or unknown) substance use disorder, mild

    F19.11 **Other psychoactive substance abuse, in remission**
        Other (or unknown) substance use disorder, mild, in early remission
        Other (or unknown) substance use disorder, mild, in sustained remission

● **F19.12** **Other psychoactive substance abuse with intoxication**

    F19.120 **Other psychoactive substance abuse with intoxication, uncomplicated** 🪙

    F19.121 **Other psychoactive substance abuse with intoxication delirium** 🪙🪙

    F19.122 **Other psychoactive substance abuse with intoxication with perceptual disturbances** 🪙

    F19.129 **Other psychoactive substance abuse with intoxication, unspecified** 🪙

▶ New   ⇒ Revised   ~~deleted~~ Deleted   Excludes 1   Excludes 2   Includes   Use additional   Code first   Code also   Key words

OGCR Official Guidelines   ● Unacceptable Principal Diagnosis   X Assign placeholder X   ● Use Additional Character(s)   ▶ Manifestation Code   **Coding Clinic**

● F19.13   Other psychoactive substance abuse with withdrawal

   F19.130   Other psychoactive substance abuse with withdrawal, uncomplicated 🕸
      (Ex:) See PDX Collection 4009

   F19.131   Other psychoactive substance abuse with withdrawal delirium 🕸
      (Ex:) See PDX Collection 4009

   F19.132   Other psychoactive substance abuse with withdrawal with perceptual disturbance 🕸
      (Ex:) See PDX Collection 4009

   F19.139   Other psychoactive substance abuse with withdrawal, unspecified 🕸
      (Ex:) See PDX Collection 4009

   F19.14   Other psychoactive substance abuse with psychoactive substance-induced mood disorder 🕸
      Other (or unknown) substance use disorder, mild, with other (or unknown) substance-induced bipolar or related disorder
      Other (or unknown) substance use disorder, mild, with other (or unknown) substance-induced depressive disorder

● F19.15   Other psychoactive substance abuse with psychoactive substance-induced psychotic disorder

   F19.150   Other psychoactive substance abuse with psychoactive substance-induced psychotic disorder with delusions 🕸🕸

   F19.151   Other psychoactive substance abuse with psychoactive substance-induced psychotic disorder with hallucinations 🕸🕸

   F19.159   Other psychoactive substance abuse with psychoactive substance-induced psychotic disorder, unspecified 🕸

   F19.16   Other psychoactive substance abuse with psychoactive substance-induced persisting amnestic disorder 🕸

   F19.17   Other psychoactive substance abuse with psychoactive substance-induced persisting dementia 🕸🕸
      Other (or unknown) substance use disorder, mild, with other (or unknown) substance-induced major neurocognitive disorder

● F19.18   Other psychoactive substance abuse with other psychoactive substance-induced disorders

   F19.180   Other psychoactive substance abuse with psychoactive substance-induced anxiety disorder 🕸

   F19.181   Other psychoactive substance abuse with psychoactive substance-induced sexual dysfunction 🕸

   F19.182   Other psychoactive substance abuse with psychoactive substance-induced sleep disorder 🕸

   F19.188   Other psychoactive substance abuse with other psychoactive substance-induced disorder 🕸
      Other (or unknown) substance use disorder, mild, with other (or unknown) substance-induced mild neurocognitive disorder
      Other (or unknown) substance use disorder, mild, with other (or unknown) substance-induced obsessive-compulsive or related disorder

   F19.19   Other psychoactive substance abuse with unspecified psychoactive substance-induced disorder 🕸

● F19.2   Other psychoactive substance dependence

   Excludes1   other psychoactive substance abuse (F19.1-)
               other psychoactive substance use, unspecified (F19.9-)

   F19.20   Other psychoactive substance dependence, uncomplicated 🕸🕸
      Other (or unknown) substance use disorder, moderate
      Other (or unknown) substance use disorder, severe
      (Ex:) See PDX Collection 3221

   F19.21   Other psychoactive substance dependence, in remission 🕸
      Other (or unknown) substance use disorder, moderate, in early remission
      Other (or unknown) substance use disorder, moderate, in sustained remission
      Other (or unknown) substance use disorder, severe, in early remission
      Other (or unknown) substance use disorder, severe, in sustained remission

● F19.22   Other psychoactive substance dependence with intoxication

   Excludes1   other psychoactive substance dependence with withdrawal (F19.23-)

   F19.220   Other psychoactive substance dependence with intoxication, uncomplicated 🕸

   F19.221   Other psychoactive substance dependence with intoxication delirium 🕸🕸

   F19.222   Other psychoactive substance dependence with intoxication with perceptual disturbance 🕸🕸
      (Ex:) See PDX Collection 3587

   F19.229   Other psychoactive substance dependence with intoxication, unspecified 🕸

● F19.23   Other psychoactive substance dependence with withdrawal

   Excludes1   other psychoactive substance dependence with intoxication (F19.22-)

   F19.230   Other psychoactive substance dependence with withdrawal, uncomplicated 🕸🕸

   F19.231   Other psychoactive substance dependence with withdrawal delirium 🕸🕸

   F19.232   Other psychoactive substance dependence with withdrawal with perceptual disturbance 🕸🕸

   F19.239   Other psychoactive substance dependence with withdrawal, unspecified 🕸🕸

   F19.24   Other psychoactive substance dependence with psychoactive substance-induced mood disorder 🕸
      Other (or unknown) substance use disorder, moderate, with other (or unknown) substance-induced bipolar or related disorder
      Other (or unknown) substance use disorder, moderate, with other (or unknown) substance-induced depressive disorder
      Other (or unknown) substance use disorder, severe, with other (or unknown) substance-induced bipolar or related disorder
      Other (or unknown) substance use disorder, severe, with other (or unknown) substance-induced depressive disorder

---

N Newborn Age: 0   P Pediatric Age: 0–17   M Maternity DX: 9–64   A Adult Age: 15–124   ♀ Females Only   ♂ Males Only
🕸 Complication\Comorbidity   🕸 Major C\C   (Ex:) CC/MCC Exclusions   🕸 Hospital-Acquired Condition   🕸 Hierarchical Condition Category

789

CHAPTER 5 (F01-F99)

● **F19.25 Other psychoactive substance dependence with psychoactive substance-induced psychotic disorder**

     F19.250 Other psychoactive substance dependence with psychoactive substance-induced psychotic disorder with delusions 🔒 🔒

     F19.251 Other psychoactive substance dependence with psychoactive substance-induced psychotic disorder with hallucinations 🔒 🔒

     F19.259 Other psychoactive substance dependence with psychoactive substance-induced psychotic disorder, unspecified 🔒 🔒
         (Ex:) See PDX Collection 3588

F19.26 Other psychoactive substance dependence with psychoactive substance-induced persisting amnestic disorder 🔒 🔒
     (Ex:) See PDX Collection 3589

F19.27 Other psychoactive substance dependence with psychoactive substance-induced persisting dementia 🔒 🔒
     Other (or unknown) substance use disorder, moderate, with other (or unknown) substance-induced major neurocognitive disorder
     Other (or unknown) substance use disorder, severe, with other (or unknown) substance-induced major neurocognitive disorder

● **F19.28 Other psychoactive substance dependence with other psychoactive substance-induced disorders**

     F19.280 Other psychoactive substance dependence with psychoactive substance-induced anxiety disorder 🔒 🔒
         (Ex:) See PDX Collection 3590

     F19.281 Other psychoactive substance dependence with psychoactive substance-induced sexual dysfunction 🔒 🔒
         (Ex:) See PDX Collection 3591

     F19.282 Other psychoactive substance dependence with psychoactive substance-induced sleep disorder 🔒 🔒
         (Ex:) See PDX Collection 3592

     F19.288 Other psychoactive substance dependence with other psychoactive substance-induced disorder 🔒 🔒
     Other (or unknown) substance use disorder, moderate, with other (or unknown) substance-induced mild neurocognitive disorder
     Other (or unknown) substance use disorder, severe, with other (or unknown) substance-induced mild neurocognitive disorder
     Other (or unknown) substance use disorder, moderate, with other (or unknown) substance-induced obsessive-compulsive or related disorder
     Other (or unknown) substance use disorder, severe, with other (or unknown) substance-induced obsessive-compulsive or related disorder
         (Ex:) See PDX Collection 3593

F19.29 Other psychoactive substance dependence with unspecified psychoactive substance-induced disorder 🔒

● **F19.9 Other psychoactive substance use, unspecified**
     Excludes1   other psychoactive substance abuse (F19.1-)
         other psychoactive substance dependence (F19.2-)

     F19.90 Other psychoactive substance use, unspecified, uncomplicated

● **F19.92 Other psychoactive substance use, unspecified with intoxication**
     Excludes1   other psychoactive substance use, unspecified with withdrawal (F19.93)

     F19.920 Other psychoactive substance use, unspecified with intoxication, uncomplicated 🔒

     F19.921 Other psychoactive substance use, unspecified with intoxication with delirium 🔒 🔒
     Other (or unknown) substance-induced delirium

     F19.922 Other psychoactive substance use, unspecified with intoxication with perceptual disturbance 🔒

     F19.929 Other psychoactive substance use, unspecified with intoxication, unspecified 🔒

● **F19.93 Other psychoactive substance use, unspecified with withdrawal**
     Excludes1   other psychoactive substance use, unspecified with intoxication (F19.92-)

     F19.930 Other psychoactive substance use, unspecified with withdrawal, uncomplicated 🔒 🔒

     F19.931 Other psychoactive substance use, unspecified with withdrawal delirium 🔒 🔒

     F19.932 Other psychoactive substance use, unspecified with withdrawal with perceptual disturbance 🔒 🔒

     F19.939 Other psychoactive substance use, unspecified with withdrawal, unspecified 🔒 🔒

F19.94 Other psychoactive substance use, unspecified with psychoactive substance-induced mood disorder 🔒
     Other (or unknown) substance-induced bipolar or related disorder, without use disorder
     Other (or unknown) substance-induced depressive disorder, without use disorder

● **F19.95 Other psychoactive substance use, unspecified with psychoactive substance-induced psychotic disorder**

     F19.950 Other psychoactive substance use, unspecified with psychoactive substance-induced psychotic disorder with delusions 🔒 🔒

     F19.951 Other psychoactive substance use, unspecified with psychoactive substance-induced psychotic disorder with hallucinations 🔒 🔒

     F19.959 Other psychoactive substance use, unspecified with psychoactive substance-induced psychotic disorder, unspecified 🔒
     Other or unknown substance-induced psychotic disorder, without use disorder

▶ New   ⏩ Revised   ~~deleted~~ Deleted   Excludes 1   Excludes 2   Includes   Use additional   Code first   Code also   Key words
OGCR Official Guidelines   ● Unacceptable Principal Diagnosis   X Assign placeholder X   ● Use Additional Character(s)   ▶ Manifestation Code   **Coding Clinic**

F19.96   Other psychoactive substance use, unspecified with psychoactive substance-induced persisting amnestic disorder 🖥

F19.97   Other psychoactive substance use, unspecified with psychoactive substance-induced persisting dementia 🖥🖥
    Other (or unknown) substance-induced major neurocognitive disorder, without use disorder

● **F19.98**   Other psychoactive substance use, unspecified with other psychoactive substance-induced disorders

    F19.980   Other psychoactive substance use, unspecified with psychoactive substance-induced anxiety disorder 🖥
       Other (or unknown) substance-induced anxiety disorder, without use disorder

    F19.981   Other psychoactive substance use, unspecified with psychoactive substance-induced sexual dysfunction 🖥
       Other (or unknown) substance-induced sexual dysfunction, without use disorder

    F19.982   Other psychoactive substance use, unspecified with psychoactive substance-induced sleep disorder 🖥
       Other (or unknown) substance-induced sleep disorder, without use disorder

    F19.988   Other psychoactive substance use, unspecified with other psychoactive substance-induced disorder 🖥
       Other (or unknown) substance-induced mild neurocognitive disorder, without use disorder
       Other (or unknown) substance-induced obsessive-compulsive or related disorder, without use disorder

F19.99   Other psychoactive substance use, unspecified with unspecified psychoactive substance-induced disorder 🖥

SCHIZOPHRENIA, SCHIZOTYPAL, DELUSIONAL, AND OTHER NON-MOOD PSYCHOTIC DISORDERS (F20-F29)

● **F20**   **Schizophrenia**
Personality disorders characterized by multiple mental and behavioral irregularities (may exhibit disorganized thinking, delusions, and auditory hallucinations)

   Excludes1   brief psychotic disorder (F23)
       cyclic schizophrenia (F25.0)
       mood [affective] disorders with psychotic symptoms (F30.2, F31.2, F31.5, F31.64, F32.3, F33.3)
       schizoaffective disorder (F25.-)
       schizophrenic reaction NOS (F23)

   Excludes2   schizophrenic reaction in:
       alcoholism (F10.15-, F10.25-, F10.95-)
       brain disease (F06.2)
       epilepsy (F06.2)
       psychoactive drug use (F11-F19 with .15, .25, .95)
       schizotypal disorder (F21)

   (Ex) **For category F20 CC codes:** See PDX Collection 551
   Coding Clinic: 2019, Q2, P32

F20.0   **Paranoid schizophrenia** 🖥🖥
    Paraphrenic schizophrenia
   Excludes1   involutional paranoid state (F22)
       paranoia (F22)

F20.1   **Disorganized schizophrenia** 🖥🖥
    Hebephrenic schizophrenia
    Hebephrenia

F20.2   **Catatonic schizophrenia** 🖥🖥
    Schizophrenic catalepsy
    Schizophrenic catatonia
    Schizophrenic flexibilitas cerea
   Excludes1   catatonic stupor (R40.1)

F20.3   **Undifferentiated schizophrenia** 🖥
    Atypical schizophrenia
   Excludes1   acute schizophrenia-like psychotic disorder (F23)
   Excludes2   post-schizophrenic depression (F32.89)

F20.5   **Residual schizophrenia** 🖥🖥
    Restzustand (schizophrenic)
    Schizophrenic residual state

● **F20.8**   **Other schizophrenia**
    F20.81   **Schizophreniform disorder** 🖥🖥
       Schizophreniform psychosis NOS
    F20.89   **Other schizophrenia** 🖥🖥
       Cenesthopathic schizophrenia
       Simple schizophrenia

F20.9   **Schizophrenia, unspecified** 🖥
   Coding Clinic: 2019, Q2, P32

F21   **Schizotypal disorder**
Personality disorder characterized by need for social isolation, odd behavior and thinking, and often unconventional beliefs
    Borderline schizophrenia
    Latent schizophrenia
    Latent schizophrenic reaction
    Prepsychotic schizophrenia
    Prodromal schizophrenia
    Pseudoneurotic schizophrenia
    Pseudopsychopathic schizophrenia
    Schizotypal personality disorder
   Excludes2   Asperger's syndrome (F84.5)
       schizoid personality disorder (F60.1)

F22   **Delusional disorders** 🖥
    Delusional dysmorphophobia
    Involutional paranoid state
    Paranoia
    Paranoia querulans
    Paranoid psychosis
    Paranoid state
    Paraphrenia (late)
    Sensitiver Beziehungswahn
   Excludes1   mood [affective] disorders with psychotic symptoms (F30.2, F31.2, F31.5, F31.64, F32.3, F33.3)
       paranoid schizophrenia (F20.0)
   Excludes2   paranoid personality disorder (F60.0)
       paranoid psychosis, psychogenic (F23)
       paranoid reaction (F23)

F23   **Brief psychotic disorder** 🖥
    Paranoid reaction
    Psychogenic paranoid psychosis
   Excludes2   mood [affective] disorders with psychotic symptoms (F30.2, F31.2, F31.5, F31.64, F32.3, F33.3)
   (Ex) See PDX Collection 3594
   Coding Clinic: 2019, Q2, P32

F24   **Shared psychotic disorder** 🖥
    Folie à deux
    Induced paranoid disorder
    Induced psychotic disorder

CHAPTER 5 (F01-F99)

N   Newborn Age: 0   **P**   Pediatric Age: 0–17   **M**   Maternity DX: 9–64   **A**   Adult Age: 15–124   ♀   Females Only   ♂   Males Only

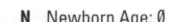 Complication\Comorbidity   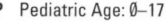 Major C\C   (Ex) CC/MCC Exclusions   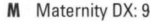 Hospital-Acquired Condition   🖥 Hierarchical Condition Category

CHAPTER 5 (F01-F99)

● **F25** **Schizoaffective disorders**
Mental disorder exhibiting major depressive episode, manic episode, or mixed episode occurs with symptoms of schizophrenia, and mood disorder

> **Excludes1**　mood [affective] disorders with psychotic symptoms (F30.2, F31.2, F31.5, F31.64, F32.3, F33.3)
> schizophrenia (F20.-)

F25.0 **Schizoaffective disorder, bipolar type** 🔹
Cyclic schizophrenia
Schizoaffective disorder, manic type
Schizoaffective disorder, mixed type
Schizoaffective psychosis, bipolar type

F25.1 **Schizoaffective disorder, depressive type** 🔹
Schizoaffective psychosis, depressive type

F25.8 **Other schizoaffective disorders** 🔹

F25.9 **Schizoaffective disorder, unspecified** 🔹
Schizoaffective psychosis NOS

F28 **Other psychotic disorder not due to a substance or known physiological condition**
Chronic hallucinatory psychosis
Other specified schizophrenia spectrum and other psychotic disorder

F29 **Unspecified psychosis not due to a substance or known physiological condition**
Psychosis NOS
Unspecified schizophrenia spectrum and other psychotic disorder

> **Excludes1**　mental disorder NOS (F99)
> unspecified mental disorder due to known physiological condition (F09)

MOOD [AFFECTIVE] DISORDERS (F30-F39)

● **F30** **Manic episode**
Elevated, expansive, or irritable mood

> **Includes**　bipolar disorder, single manic episode
> mixed affective episode

> **Excludes1**　bipolar disorder (F31.-)
> major depressive disorder, single episode (F32.-)
> major depressive disorder, recurrent (F33.-)

(Ex:) **For category F30 CC codes unless otherwise indicated:** See PDX Collection 551

● **F30.1** **Manic episode without psychotic symptoms**

F30.10 **Manic episode without psychotic symptoms, unspecified** 🔹

F30.11 **Manic episode without psychotic symptoms, mild** 🔹

F30.12 **Manic episode without psychotic symptoms, moderate** 🔹

F30.13 **Manic episode, severe, without psychotic symptoms** 🔹
(Ex:) See PDX Collection 552

F30.2 **Manic episode, severe with psychotic symptoms** 🔹
Manic stupor
Mania with mood-congruent psychotic symptoms
Mania with mood-incongruent psychotic symptoms

F30.3 **Manic episode in partial remission** 🔹

F30.4 **Manic episode in full remission** 🔹

F30.8 **Other manic episodes** 🔹
Abnormality of mood resembling mania but less intense
Hypomania

F30.9 **Manic episode, unspecified** 🔹
Mania NOS

● **F31** **Bipolar disorder**
Mood disorders with history of manic, mixed, or hypomanic episodes

> **Includes**　bipolar I disorder
> bipolar type I disorder
> manic-depressive illness
> manic-depressive psychosis
> manic-depressive reaction

> **Excludes1**　bipolar disorder, single manic episode (F30.-)
> major depressive disorder, single episode (F32.-)
> major depressive disorder, recurrent (F33.-)

> **Excludes2**　cyclothymia (F34.0)

(Ex:) **For category F31 CC codes unless otherwise indicated:** See PDX Collection 551
Coding Clinic: 2020, Q1, P23

F31.0 **Bipolar disorder, current episode hypomanic** 🔹

● **F31.1** **Bipolar disorder, current episode manic without psychotic features**

F31.10 **Bipolar disorder, current episode manic without psychotic features, unspecified** 🔹

F31.11 **Bipolar disorder, current episode manic without psychotic features, mild** 🔹

F31.12 **Bipolar disorder, current episode manic without psychotic features, moderate** 🔹

F31.13 **Bipolar disorder, current episode manic without psychotic features, severe** 🔹
(Ex:) See PDX Collection 553

F31.2 **Bipolar disorder, current episode manic severe with psychotic features** 🔹
Bipolar disorder, current episode manic with mood-congruent psychotic symptoms
Bipolar disorder, current episode manic with mood-incongruent psychotic symptoms
Bipolar I disorder, current or most recent episode manic with psychotic features

● **F31.3** **Bipolar disorder, current episode depressed, mild or moderate severity**

F31.30 **Bipolar disorder, current episode depressed, mild or moderate severity, unspecified** 🔹

F31.31 **Bipolar disorder, current episode depressed, mild** 🔹

F31.32 **Bipolar disorder, current episode depressed, moderate** 🔹

F31.4 **Bipolar disorder, current episode depressed, severe, without psychotic features** 🔹
(Ex:) See PDX Collection 554

F31.5 **Bipolar disorder, current episode depressed, severe, with psychotic features** 🔹
Bipolar disorder, current episode depressed with mood-incongruent psychotic symptoms
Bipolar disorder, current episode depressed with mood-congruent psychotic symptoms
Bipolar I disorder, current or most recent episode depressed, with psychotic features

● **F31.6** **Bipolar disorder, current episode mixed**

F31.60 **Bipolar disorder, current episode mixed, unspecified** 🔹

F31.61 **Bipolar disorder, current episode mixed, mild** 🔹

F31.62 **Bipolar disorder, current episode mixed, moderate** 🔹

F31.63 **Bipolar disorder, current episode mixed, severe, without psychotic features** 🔹
(Ex:) See PDX Collection 554

F31.64 **Bipolar disorder, current episode mixed, severe, with psychotic features** 🔹
Bipolar disorder, current episode mixed with mood-congruent psychotic symptoms
Bipolar disorder, current episode mixed with mood-incongruent psychotic symptoms

▶ New　⇒ Revised　~~deleted~~ Deleted　Excludes 1　Excludes 2　Includes　Use additional　Code first　Code also　Key words
OGCR Official Guidelines　● Unacceptable Principal Diagnosis　X Assign placeholder X　● Use Additional Character(s)　▷ Manifestation Code　**Coding Clinic**

● **F31.7** Bipolar disorder, currently in remission
  F31.70 Bipolar disorder, currently in remission, most recent episode unspecified 🔖
  F31.71 Bipolar disorder, in partial remission, most recent episode hypomanic 🔖
  F31.72 Bipolar disorder, in full remission, most recent episode hypomanic 🔖
  F31.73 Bipolar disorder, in partial remission, most recent episode manic 🔖
  F31.74 Bipolar disorder, in full remission, most recent episode manic 🔖
  F31.75 Bipolar disorder, in partial remission, most recent episode depressed 🔖
  F31.76 Bipolar disorder, in full remission, most recent episode depressed 🔖
  F31.77 Bipolar disorder, in partial remission, most recent episode mixed 🔖
  F31.78 Bipolar disorder, in full remission, most recent episode mixed 🔖

● **F31.8** Other bipolar disorders
  F31.81 Bipolar II disorder 🔖🔖
    Bipolar disorder, type 2
  F31.89 Other bipolar disorder 🔖🔖
    Recurrent manic episodes NOS

  F31.9 Bipolar disorder, unspecified 🔖
    Manic depression
    Coding Clinic: 2020, Q1, P23

➡● **F32** Depressive episode
  Includes single episode of agitated depression
          single episode of depressive reaction
          single episode of major depression
          single episode of psychogenic depression
          single episode of reactive depression
          single episode of vital depression

  Excludes1 bipolar disorder (F31.-)
          manic episode (F30.-)
          recurrent depressive disorder (F33.-)

  Excludes2 adjustment disorder (F43.2)

  F32.0 Major depressive disorder, single episode, mild 🔖🔖
    (Ex:) See PDX Collection 555

  F32.1 Major depressive disorder, single episode, moderate 🔖🔖
    (Ex:) See PDX Collection 555

  F32.2 Major depressive disorder, single episode, severe without psychotic features 🔖🔖
    (Ex:) See PDX Collection 555

  F32.3 Major depressive disorder, single episode, severe with psychotic features 🔖🔖
    Single episode of major depression with mood-congruent psychotic symptoms
    Single episode of major depression with mood-incongruent psychotic symptoms
    Single episode of major depression with psychotic symptoms
    Single episode of psychogenic depressive psychosis
    Single episode of psychotic depression
    Single episode of reactive depressive psychosis
    (Ex:) See PDX Collection 555

  F32.4 Major depressive disorder, single episode, in partial remission 🔖

  F32.5 Major depressive disorder, single episode, in full remission 🔖

● **F32.8** Other depressive episodes
  F32.81 Premenstrual dysphoric disorder ♀
    Excludes1 premenstrual tension syndrome (N94.3)
    Coding Clinic: 2016, Q4, P14

  F32.89 Other specified depressive episodes
    Atypical depression
    Post-schizophrenic depression
    Single episode of 'masked' depression NOS
    Coding Clinic: 2016, Q4, P14

  F32.9 Major depressive disorder, single episode, unspecified
    ~~Depression NOS~~
    ~~Depressive disorder NOS~~
    Major depression NOS
    Coding Clinic: 2021, Q1, P10

▶ **F32.A** Depression, unspecified
  ▶Depression NOS
  ▶Depressive disorder NOS

● **F33** Major depressive disorder, recurrent
  Includes recurrent episodes of depressive reaction
          recurrent episodes of endogenous depression
          recurrent episodes of major depression
          recurrent episodes of psychogenic depression
          recurrent episodes of reactive depression
          recurrent episodes of seasonal depressive disorder
          recurrent episodes of vital depression

  Excludes1 bipolar disorder (F31.-)
          manic episode (F30.-)

  (Ex:) For category F33 CC codes unless otherwise indicated: See PDX Collection 555
  Coding Clinic: 2020, Q1, P23

  F33.0 Major depressive disorder, recurrent, mild 🔖🔖
  F33.1 Major depressive disorder, recurrent, moderate 🔖🔖
  F33.2 Major depressive disorder, recurrent severe without psychotic features 🔖🔖
  F33.3 Major depressive disorder, recurrent, severe with psychotic symptoms 🔖🔖
    Endogenous depression with psychotic symptoms
    Major depressive disorder, recurrent, with psychotic features
    Recurrent severe episodes of major depression with mood-congruent psychotic symptoms
    Recurrent severe episodes of major depression with mood-incongruent psychotic symptoms
    Recurrent severe episodes of major depression with psychotic symptoms
    Recurrent severe episodes of psychogenic depressive psychosis
    Recurrent severe episodes of psychotic depression
    Recurrent severe episodes of reactive depressive psychosis
    (Ex:) See PDX Collection 551

● **F33.4** Major depressive disorder, recurrent, in remission
  F33.40 Major depressive disorder, recurrent, in remission, unspecified 🔖🔖
  F33.41 Major depressive disorder, recurrent, in partial remission 🔖
  F33.42 Major depressive disorder, recurrent, in full remission 🔖

  F33.8 Other recurrent depressive disorders 🔖🔖
    Recurrent brief depressive episodes
    (Ex:) See PDX Collection 551

  F33.9 Major depressive disorder, recurrent, unspecified 🔖🔖
    Monopolar depression NOS

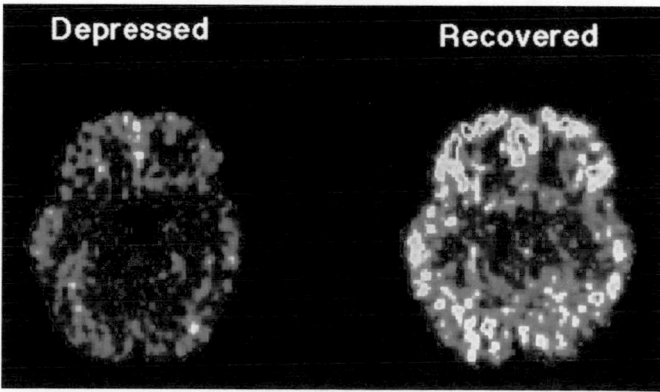

Figure 5-1 PET scan of depressed individual's brain before and after recovery. (From Fortinash KM: Psychiatric Mental Health Nursing, ed 4, St. Louis, Mosby, 2008)

N Newborn Age: 0   **P** Pediatric Age: 0–17   **M** Maternity DX: 9–64   **A** Adult Age: 15–124   ♀ Females Only   ♂ Males Only

🔖 Complication\Comorbidity   🔖 Major C\C   (Ex:) CC/MCC Exclusions   🔖 Hospital-Acquired Condition   🔖 Hierarchical Condition Category

793

CHAPTER 5 (F01–F99)

F34   Persistent mood [affective] disorders

    F34.0   Cyclothymic disorder
           Affective personality disorder
           Cycloid personality
           Cyclothymia
           Cyclothymic personality

    F34.1   Dysthymic disorder
           Depressive neurosis
           Depressive personality disorder
           Dysthymia
           Neurotic depression
           Persistent anxiety depression
           Persistent depressive disorder

        Excludes2   anxiety depression (mild or not persistent) (F41.8)

    ● F34.8   Other persistent mood [affective] disorders
        (Ex) For category F34.8 CC codes: See PDX Collection 551

        F34.81   Disruptive mood dysregulation disorder
           Coding Clinic: 2016, Q4, P14

        F34.89   Other specified persistent mood disorders
           Coding Clinic: 2016, Q4, P14

    F34.9   Persistent mood [affective] disorder, unspecified
        (Ex) See PDX Collection 551

  F39   Unspecified mood [affective] disorder
      Affective psychosis NOS

ANXIETY, DISSOCIATIVE, STRESS-RELATED, SOMATOFORM AND OTHER NONPSYCHOTIC MENTAL DISORDERS (F40-F48)

● F40   Phobic anxiety disorders
    Irrational fear with avoidance of the feared subject, activity, or situation even though the individual knows that the reaction is excessive

    ● F40.0   Agoraphobia
        Intense, irrational fear of open spaces

        F40.00   Agoraphobia, unspecified

        F40.01   Agoraphobia with panic disorder
           Panic disorder with agoraphobia
           Excludes1   panic disorder without agoraphobia (F41.0)

        F40.02   Agoraphobia without panic disorder

    ● F40.1   Social phobias
        Anthropophobia
        Social anxiety disorder
        Social anxiety disorder of childhood
        Social neurosis

        F40.10   Social phobia, unspecified

        F40.11   Social phobia, generalized

    ● F40.2   Specific (isolated) phobias
        Excludes2   dysmorphophobia (nondelusional) (F45.22)
                nosophobia (F45.22)

      ● F40.21   Animal type phobia
          F40.210   Arachnophobia
              Fear of spiders

          F40.218   Other animal type phobia

      ● F40.22   Natural environment type phobia
          F40.220   Fear of thunderstorms

          F40.228   Other natural environment type phobia

      ● F40.23   Blood, injection, injury type phobia
          F40.230   Fear of blood

          F40.231   Fear of injections and transfusions

          F40.232   Fear of other medical care

          F40.233   Fear of injury

      ● F40.24   Situational type phobia
          F40.240   Claustrophobia
              Fear of closed spaces

          F40.241   Acrophobia
              Fear of heights

          F40.242   Fear of bridges

          F40.243   Fear of flying

          F40.248   Other situational type phobia

      ● F40.29   Other specified phobia
          F40.290   Androphobia
              Fear of men

          F40.291   Gynephobia
              Fear of women

          F40.298   Other specified phobia

    F40.8   Other phobic anxiety disorders
        Phobic anxiety disorder of childhood

    F40.9   Phobic anxiety disorder, unspecified
        Phobia NOS
        Phobic state NOS

● F41   Other anxiety disorders
    Excludes2   anxiety in:
           acute stress reaction (F43.0)
           transient adjustment reaction (F43.2)
           neurasthenia (F48.8)
           psychophysiologic disorders (F45.-)
           separation anxiety (F93.0)

    F41.0   Panic disorder [episodic paroxysmal anxiety]
        Panic attack
        Panic state
        Excludes1   panic disorder with agoraphobia (F40.01)

    F41.1   Generalized anxiety disorder
        Anxiety neurosis
        Anxiety reaction
        Anxiety state
        Overanxious disorder
        Excludes2   neurasthenia (F48.8)

    F41.3   Other mixed anxiety disorders

    F41.8   Other specified anxiety disorders
        Anxiety depression (mild or not persistent)
        Anxiety hysteria
        Mixed anxiety and depressive disorder
        Coding Clinic: 2021, Q1, P11

    F41.9   Anxiety disorder, unspecified
        Anxiety NOS
        Coding Clinic: 2021, Q1, P11

● F42   Obsessive-compulsive disorder
    Anxiety disorder with recurrent obsessions or compulsions

    Excludes2   obsessive-compulsive personality (disorder) (F60.5)
           obsessive-compulsive symptoms occurring in depression (F32-F33)
           obsessive-compulsive symptoms occurring in schizophrenia (F20.-)

    F42.2   Mixed obsessional thoughts and acts
        Coding Clinic: 2016, Q4, P15

    F42.3   Hoarding disorder
        Coding Clinic: 2016, Q4, P14-15

    F42.4   Excoriation (skin-picking) disorder
        Excludes1   factitial dermatitis (L98.1)
            other specified behavioral and emotional disorders with onset usually occurring in early childhood and adolescence (F98.8)
        Coding Clinic: 2016, Q4, P14-15

    F42.8   Other obsessive-compulsive disorder
        Anancastic neurosis
        Obsessive-compulsive neurosis
        Coding Clinic: 2016, Q4, P15

    F42.9   Obsessive-compulsive disorder, unspecified
        Coding Clinic: 2016, Q4, P15

● F43   Reaction to severe stress and adjustment disorders
    F43.0   Acute stress reaction
        Acute crisis reaction
        Acute reaction to stress
        Combat and operational stress reaction
        Combat fatigue
        Crisis state
        Psychic shock

▶ New   ⟹ Revised   ~~deleted~~ Deleted   Excludes 1   Excludes 2   Includes   Use additional   Code first   Code also   Key words

OGCR Official Guidelines   ● Unacceptable Principal Diagnosis   X Assign placeholder X   ● Use Additional Character(s)   ▶ Manifestation Code   Coding Clinic

● **F43.1**   **Post-traumatic stress disorder (PTSD)**
     Traumatic neurosis

     F43.10   **Post-traumatic stress disorder, unspecified**

     F43.11   **Post-traumatic stress disorder, acute**

     F43.12   **Post-traumatic stress disorder, chronic**

● **F43.2**   **Adjustment disorders**
     Culture shock
     Grief reaction
     Hospitalism in children

     Excludes2   separation anxiety disorder of childhood (F93.0)

     F43.20   **Adjustment disorder, unspecified**

     F43.21   **Adjustment disorder with depressed mood**

     F43.22   **Adjustment disorder with anxiety**

     F43.23   **Adjustment disorder with mixed anxiety and depressed mood**

     F43.24   **Adjustment disorder with disturbance of conduct**

     F43.25   **Adjustment disorder with mixed disturbance of emotions and conduct**

     F43.29   **Adjustment disorder with other symptoms**

   F43.8   **Other reactions to severe stress**
     Other specified trauma and stressor-related disorder

   F43.9   **Reaction to severe stress, unspecified**
     Trauma and stressor-related disorder, NOS

● **F44**   **Dissociative and conversion disorders**

     Includes   conversion hysteria
                 conversion reaction
                 hysteria
                 hysterical psychosis

     Excludes2   malingering [conscious simulation] (Z76.5)

   F44.0   **Dissociative amnesia**
     Sudden loss of memory for personal information

     Excludes1   amnesia NOS (R41.3)
                 anterograde amnesia (R41.1)
                 dissociative amnesia with dissociative fugue (F44.1)
                 retrograde amnesia (R41.2)

     Excludes2   alcohol or other psychoactive substance-induced amnestic disorder (F10, F13, F19 with .26, .96)
                 amnestic disorder due to known physiological condition (F04)
                 postictal amnesia in epilepsy (G40.-)

   F44.1   **Dissociative fugue**
     Characterized by episode of sudden, unexpected travel with amnesia for past and partial to total confusion about identity or assumption of new identity
     Dissociative amnesia with dissociative fugue

     Excludes2   postictal fugue in epilepsy (G40.-)

   F44.2   **Dissociative stupor**
     Profound diminution or absence of voluntary movement and responsiveness to external stimuli

     Excludes1   catatonic stupor (R40.1)
                 stupor NOS (R40.1)

     Excludes2   catatonic disorder due to known physiological condition (F06.1)
                 depressive stupor (F32, F33)
                 manic stupor (F30, F31)

   F44.4   **Conversion disorder with motor symptom or deficit**
     Conversion disorder with abnormal movement
     Conversion disorder with speech symptoms
     Conversion disorder with swallowing symptoms
     Conversion disorder with weakness/paralysis
     Dissociative motor disorders
     Psychogenic aphonia
     Psychogenic dysphonia

   F44.5   **Conversion disorder with seizures or convulsions**
     Conversion disorder with attacks or seizures
     Dissociative convulsions
     Coding Clinic: 2019, Q1, P19

   F44.6   **Conversion disorder with sensory symptom or deficit**
     Conversion disorder with anesthesia or sensory loss
     Conversion disorder with special sensory symptoms
     Dissociative anesthesia and sensory loss
     Psychogenic deafness

   F44.7   **Conversion disorder with mixed symptom presentation**

● **F44.8**   **Other dissociative and conversion disorders**

     F44.81   **Dissociative identity disorder**
            Multiple personality disorder

     F44.89   **Other dissociative and conversion disorders**
            Ganser's syndrome
            Psychogenic confusion
            Psychogenic twilight state
            Trance and possession disorders

   F44.9   **Dissociative and conversion disorder, unspecified**
     Dissociative disorder NOS

OGCR Section I.C.5.a.

Pain disorders related to psychological factors
Assign code F45.41, for pain that is exclusively related to psychological disorders. As indicated by the Excludes 1 note under category G89, a code from category G89 should not be assigned with code F45.41 Code F45.42, Pain disorders with related psychological factors, should be used with a code from category G89, Pain, not elsewhere classified, if there is documentation of a psychological component for a patient with acute or chronic pain.
See Section I.C.6. Pain

● **F45**   **Somatoform disorders**
     Mental disorders characterized by symptoms suggesting general medical condition

     Excludes2   dissociative and conversion disorders (F44.-)
                 factitious disorders (F68.1-, F68.A)
                 hair-plucking (F63.3)
                 lalling (F80.0)
                 lisping (F80.0)
                 malingering [conscious simulation] (Z76.5)
                 nail-biting (F98.8)
                 psychological or behavioral factors associated with disorders or diseases classified elsewhere (F54)
                 sexual dysfunction, not due to a substance or known physiological condition (F52.-)
                 thumb-sucking (F98.8)
                 tic disorders (in childhood and adolescence) (F95.-)
                 Tourette's syndrome (F95.2)
                 trichotillomania (F63.3)

   F45.0   **Somatization disorder**
     Briquet's disorder
     Multiple psychosomatic disorder

   F45.1   **Undifferentiated somatoform disorder**
     Somatic symptom disorder
     Undifferentiated psychosomatic disorder

● **F45.2**   **Hypochondriacal disorders**
     Persistent, unrealistic preoccupation with possibility of having serious disease

     Excludes2   delusional dysmorphophobia (F22)
                 fixed delusions about bodily functions or shape (F22)

     F45.20   **Hypochondriacal disorder, unspecified**

     F45.21   **Hypochondriasis**
            Hypochondriacal neurosis
            Illness anxiety disorder

     F45.22   **Body dysmorphic disorder**
            Dysmorphophobia (nondelusional)
            Nosophobia

     F45.29   **Other hypochondriacal disorders**

● **F45.4**   **Pain disorders related to psychological factors**

     Excludes1   pain NOS (R52)

     F45.41   **Pain disorder exclusively related to psychological factors**
            Somatoform pain disorder (persistent)

     F45.42   **Pain disorder with related psychological factors**
            Code also associated acute or chronic pain (G89.-)

CHAPTER 5 (F01-F99)

F45.8   **Other somatoform disorders**
   Psychogenic dysmenorrhea
   Psychogenic dysphagia, including 'globus hystericus'
   Psychogenic pruritus
   Psychogenic torticollis
   Somatoform autonomic dysfunction
   Teeth grinding
   Excludes1   sleep related teeth grinding (G47.63)
   Coding Clinic: 2016, Q4, P118

F45.9   **Somatoform disorder, unspecified**
   Psychosomatic disorder NOS

● **F48**   **Other nonpsychotic mental disorders**

F48.1   **Depersonalization-derealization syndrome**

F48.2   **Pseudobulbar affect**
   Involuntary emotional expression disorder
   Code first underlying cause, if known, such as:
      amyotrophic lateral sclerosis (G12.21)
      multiple sclerosis (G35)
      sequelae of cerebrovascular disease (I69.-)
      sequelae of traumatic intracranial injury (S06.-)

F48.8   **Other specified nonpsychotic mental disorders**
   Dhat syndrome
   Neurasthenia
   Occupational neurosis, including writer's cramp
   Psychasthenia
   Psychasthenic neurosis
   Psychogenic syncope

F48.9   **Nonpsychotic mental disorder, unspecified**
   Neurosis NOS

BEHAVIORAL SYNDROMES ASSOCIATED WITH PHYSIOLOGICAL DISTURBANCES AND PHYSICAL FACTORS (F50-F59)

● **F50**   **Eating disorders**
   Excludes1   anorexia NOS (R63.0)
      ~~feeding difficulties (R63.3)~~
      feeding problems of newborn (P92.-)
      polyphagia (R63.2)
   Excludes2 ▶ feeding difficulties (R63.3)
      feeding disorder in infancy or childhood (F98.2-)

● **F50.0**   **Anorexia nervosa**
   Excludes1   loss of appetite (R63.0)
      psychogenic loss of appetite (F50.89)
   (Ex) For category F50.0 CC codes: See PDX Collection 556

   F50.00   **Anorexia nervosa, unspecified** 🔖

   F50.01   **Anorexia nervosa, restricting type** 🔖

   F50.02   **Anorexia nervosa, binge eating/purging type** 🔖
      Excludes1   bulimia nervosa (F50.2)

F50.2   **Bulimia nervosa** 🔖
   Bulimia NOS
   Hyperorexia nervosa
   Excludes1   anorexia nervosa, binge eating/purging
      type (F50.02)
   (Ex) See PDX Collection 557

● **F50.8**   **Other eating disorders**
   Excludes2   pica of infancy and childhood (F98.3)

   F50.81   **Binge eating disorder**
      Coding Clinic: 2016, Q4, P15

   F50.82   **Avoidant/restrictive food intake disorder**

   F50.89   **Other specified eating disorder**
      Pica in adults
      Psychogenic loss of appetite
      Coding Clinic: 2016, Q4, P16

F50.9   **Eating disorder, unspecified**
   Atypical anorexia nervosa
   Atypical bulimia nervosa
   Feeding or eating disorder, unspecified
   Other specified feeding disorder

● **F51**   **Sleep disorders not due to a substance or known physiological condition**
   Excludes2   organic sleep disorders (G47.-)

● **F51.0**   **Insomnia not due to a substance or known physiological condition**
   Excludes2   alcohol related insomnia (F10.182,
         F10.282, F10.982)
      drug-related insomnia (F11.182, F11.282,
         F11.982, F13.182, F13.282, F13.982,
         F14.182, F14.282, F14.982, F15.182,
         F15.282, F15.982, F19.182, F19.282,
         F19.982)
      insomnia NOS (G47.0-)
      insomnia due to known physiological
         condition (G47.0-)
      organic insomnia (G47.0-)
      sleep deprivation (Z72.820)

   F51.01   **Primary insomnia**
      Idiopathic insomnia

   F51.02   **Adjustment insomnia**

   F51.03   **Paradoxical insomnia**

   F51.04   **Psychophysiologic insomnia**

   F51.05   **Insomnia due to other mental disorder**
      Code also associated mental disorder

   F51.09   **Other insomnia not due to a substance or known physiological condition**

● **F51.1**   **Hypersomnia not due to a substance or known physiological condition**
   Hypersomnia: Excessive sleeping/sleepiness
   Excludes2   alcohol related hypersomnia (F10.182,
         F10.282, F10.982)
      drug-related hypersomnia (F11.182,
         F11.282, F11.982, F13.182, F13.282,
         F13.982, F14.182, F14.282, F14.982,
         F15.182, F15.282, F15.982, F19.182,
         F19.282, F19.982)
      hypersomnia NOS (G47.10)
      hypersomnia due to known physiological
         condition (G47.10)
      idiopathic hypersomnia (G47.11, G47.12)
      narcolepsy (G47.4-)

   F51.11   **Primary hypersomnia**

   F51.12   **Insufficient sleep syndrome**
      Excludes1   sleep deprivation (Z72.820)

   F51.13   **Hypersomnia due to other mental disorder**
      Code also associated mental disorder

   F51.19   **Other hypersomnia not due to a substance or known physiological condition**

F51.3   **Sleepwalking [somnambulism]**
   Non-rapid eye movement sleep arousal disorders,
      sleepwalking type

F51.4   **Sleep terrors [night terrors]**
   Non-rapid eye movement sleep arousal disorders, sleep
      terror type

F51.5   **Nightmare disorder**
   Dream anxiety disorder

F51.8   **Other sleep disorders not due to a substance or known physiological condition**

F51.9   **Sleep disorder not due to a substance or known physiological condition, unspecified**
   Emotional sleep disorder NOS

● **F52**   **Sexual dysfunction not due to a substance or known physiological condition**
   Excludes2   Dhat syndrome (F48.8)

F52.0   **Hypoactive sexual desire disorder**
   Total loss of feeling of sexual pleasure
   Lack or loss of sexual desire
   Male hypoactive sexual desire disorder
   Sexual anhedonia
   Excludes1   decreased libido (R68.82)

▶ New   ⟹ Revised   ~~deleted~~ Deleted   Excludes 1   Excludes 2   Includes   Use additional   Code first   Code also   Key words
OGCR Official Guidelines   ● Unacceptable Principal Diagnosis   X Assign placeholder X   ● Use Additional Character(s)   ▌ Manifestation Code   **Coding Clinic**

F52.1   Sexual aversion disorder
Sexual aversion and lack of sexual enjoyment

● **F52.2   Sexual arousal disorders**
Failure of genital response

F52.21   Male erectile disorder ♂
Erectile disorder
Psychogenic impotence
Excludes1   impotence of organic origin
(N52.-)
impotence NOS (N52.-)

F52.22   Female sexual arousal disorder ♀
Female sexual interest/arousal disorder

● **F52.3   Orgasmic disorder**
Inhibited orgasm
Psychogenic anorgasmy

F52.31   Female orgasmic disorder ♀

F52.32   Male orgasmic disorder ♂
Delayed ejaculation

F52.4   Premature ejaculation ♂

**F52.5   Vaginismus not due to a substance or known
physiological condition ♀**
Psychogenic vaginismus
Excludes2   vaginismus (due to a known
physiological condition) (N94.2)

**F52.6   Dyspareunia not due to a substance or known
physiological condition**
Dyspareunia: Difficult or painful sexual intercourse
Genito-pelvic pain penetration disorder
Psychogenic dyspareunia
Excludes2   dyspareunia (due to a known
physiological condition) (N94.1-)

**F52.8   Other sexual dysfunction not due to a substance or
known physiological condition**
Excessive sexual drive
Nymphomania
Satyriasis

● **F52.9   Unspecified sexual dysfunction not due to a substance or
known physiological condition**
Sexual dysfunction NOS

● **F53   Mental and behavioral disorders associated with the
puerperium, not elsewhere classified**
*Acute mental illness with sudden onset following childbirth with
symptoms of affective psychosis, disorientation, and confusion
are prevalent*
Excludes1   mood disorders with psychotic features (F30.2,
F31.2, F31.5, F31.64, F32.3, F33.3)
postpartum dysphoria (O90.6)
psychosis in schizophrenia, schizotypal,
delusional, and other psychotic disorders
(F20-F29)

F53.0   Postpartum depression ♀   **M**
Postnatal depression, NOS
Postpartum depression, NOS
Ⓔ See PDX Collection 550
Coding Clinic: 2018, Q4, P8

F53.1   Puerperal psychosis ♀   **M**
Postpartum psychosis
Puerperal psychosis, NOS
Ⓔ See PDX Collection 550
Coding Clinic: 2018, Q4, P9

▷ *F54   Psychological and behavioral factors associated with disorders
or diseases classified elsewhere*
Psychological factors affecting physical conditions
Code first the associated physical disorder, such as:
asthma (J45.-)
dermatitis (L23-L25)
gastric ulcer (K25.-)
mucous colitis (K58.-)
ulcerative colitis (K51.-)
urticaria (L50.-)
Excludes2   tension-type headache (G44.2)

● **F55   Abuse of non-psychoactive substances**
Excludes2   abuse of psychoactive substances (F10-F19)

F55.0   Abuse of antacids
F55.1   Abuse of herbal or folk remedies
F55.2   Abuse of laxatives
F55.3   Abuse of steroids or hormones
F55.4   Abuse of vitamins
F55.8   Abuse of other non-psychoactive substances

**F59   Unspecified behavioral syndromes associated with
physiological disturbances and physical factors**
Psychogenic physiological dysfunction NOS

DISORDERS OF ADULT PERSONALITY AND BEHAVIOR (F60-F69)

● **F60   Specific personality disorders**
*Long-term patterns of thoughts and behaviors causing serious
problems with relationships and work*

F60.0   Paranoid personality disorder
Hostile, devious, and combative response to disappointments
Expansive paranoid personality (disorder)
Fanatic personality (disorder)
Querulant personality (disorder)
Paranoid personality (disorder)
Sensitive paranoid personality (disorder)
Excludes2   paranoia (F22)
paranoia querulans (F22)
paranoid psychosis (F22)
paranoid schizophrenia (F20.0)
paranoid state (F22)

F60.1   Schizoid personality disorder
*Detachment from social relationships with minimal emotional
experiences and expressions*
Excludes2   Asperger's syndrome (F84.5)
delusional disorder (F22)
schizoid disorder of childhood (F84.5)
schizophrenia (F20.-)
schizotypal disorder (F21)

F60.2   Antisocial personality disorder
Continuous and chronic antisocial behavior
Amoral personality (disorder)
Asocial personality (disorder)
Dissocial personality disorder
Psychopathic personality (disorder)
Sociopathic personality (disorder)
Excludes1   conduct disorders (F91.-)
Excludes2   borderline personality disorder (F60.3)

F60.3   Borderline personality disorder
*Instability of mood, self-image or sense of self, and
interpersonal relationships*
Aggressive personality (disorder)
Emotionally unstable personality disorder
Explosive personality (disorder)
Excludes2   antisocial personality disorder (F60.2)

F60.4   Histrionic personality disorder
*Personality disorder with excessive emotional and attention-
seeking behavior*
Hysterical personality (disorder)
Psychoinfantile personality (disorder)

F60.5   Obsessive-compulsive personality disorder
Anankastic personality (disorder)
Compulsive personality (disorder)
Obsessional personality (disorder)
Excludes2   obsessive-compulsive disorder (F42.-)

F60.6   Avoidant personality disorder
Anxious personality disorder

F60.7   Dependent personality disorder
Asthenic personality (disorder)
Inadequate personality (disorder)
Passive personality (disorder)

N Newborn Age: 0   **P** Pediatric Age: 0–17   **M** Maternity DX: 9–64   **A** Adult Age: 15–124   ♀ Females Only   ♂ Males Only

Ⓒ Complication\Comorbidity   Ⓜ Major C\C   Ⓔ CC/MCC Exclusions   Ⓗ Hospital-Acquired Condition   Ⓗ Hierarchical Condition Category

CHAPTER 5 (F01-F99)

● F60.8   **Other specific personality disorders**
     F60.81   **Narcissistic personality disorder**
         Vanity, conceit, egotism or indifference to plight
         of others

     F60.89   **Other specific personality disorders**
         Eccentric personality disorder
         'Haltlose' type personality disorder
         Immature personality disorder
         Passive-aggressive personality disorder
         Psychoneurotic personality disorder
         Self-defeating personality disorder

     F60.9   **Personality disorder, unspecified**
         Character disorder NOS
         Character neurosis NOS
         Pathological personality NOS

● F63   **Impulse disorders**
     Excludes2   habitual excessive use of alcohol or psychoactive
         substances (F10-F19)
         impulse disorders involving sexual behavior (F65.-)

     F63.0   **Pathological gambling**
         Compulsive gambling
         Gambling disorder
         Excludes1   gambling and betting NOS (Z72.6)
         Excludes2   excessive gambling by manic patients
             (F30, F31)
             gambling in antisocial personality
             disorder (F60.2)

     F63.1   **Pyromania**
         Pathological fire-setting
         Excludes2   fire-setting (by) (in):
             adult with antisocial personality
             disorder (F60.2)
             alcohol or psychoactive substance
             intoxication (F10-F19)
             conduct disorders (F91.-)
             mental disorders due to known
             physiological condition (F01-F09)
             schizophrenia (F20.-)

     F63.2   **Kleptomania**
         Pathological stealing
         Excludes1   shoplifting as the reason for observation
             for suspected mental disorder
             (Z03.8)
         Excludes2   depressive disorder with stealing
             (F31-F33)
             stealing due to underlying mental
             condition-code to mental condition
             stealing in mental disorders due to known
             physiological condition (F01-F09)

     F63.3   **Trichotillomania**
         Hair plucking
         Excludes2   other stereotyped movement disorder
             (F98.4)

  ● F63.8   **Other impulse disorders**
         F63.81   **Intermittent explosive disorder**
         F63.89   **Other impulse disorders**

     F63.9   **Impulse disorder, unspecified**
         Impulse control disorder NOS

● F64   **Gender identity disorders**
     F64.0   **Transsexualism**
         Gender identity disorder in adolescence and adulthood
         Gender dysphoria in adolescents and adults
         Coding Clinic: 2016, Q4, P16

     F64.1   **Dual role transvestism**
         Use additional code to identify sex reassignment status
         (Z87.890)
         Excludes1   gender identity disorder in childhood
             (F64.2)
         Excludes2   fetishistic transvestism (F65.1)
         Coding Clinic: 2016, Q4, P16

     F64.2   **Gender identity disorder of childhood**   P
         Gender dysphoria in children
         Excludes1   gender identity disorder in adolescence
             and adulthood (F64.0)
         Excludes2   sexual maturation disorder (F66)

     F64.8   **Other gender identity disorders**
         Other specified gender dysphoria

     F64.9   **Gender identity disorder, unspecified**
         Gender dysphoria, unspecified
         Gender-role disorder NOS

● F65   **Paraphilias**
     F65.0   **Fetishism**
         Intense sexual urges and arousing fantasies using inanimate
         objects
         Fetishistic disorder

     F65.1   **Transvestic fetishism**
         Intense sexual urges, arousal, or orgasm associated with
         fantasized/actual cross-dressing
         Fetishistic transvestism
         Transvestic disorder

     F65.2   **Exhibitionism**
         Exhibitionistic disorder

     F65.3   **Voyeurism**
         Sexual urges or arousal involving real or fantasized
         observation of unsuspecting people who are naked,
         disrobing, or engaging in sexual activity
         Voyeuristic disorder

     F65.4   **Pedophilia**
         Pedophilic disorder

  ● F65.5   **Sadomasochism**
         F65.50   **Sadomasochism, unspecified**
         F65.51   **Sexual masochism**
             Sexual masochism disorder
         F65.52   **Sexual sadism**
             Sexual sadism disorder

  ● F65.8   **Other paraphilias**
         F65.81   **Frotteurism**
             Sexual arousal or orgasm is achieved by rubbing
             up against another person (or fantasies of), in
             crowded place with unsuspecting victim
             Frotteuristic disorder
         F65.89   **Other paraphilias**
             Necrophilia
             Other specified paraphilic disorder

     F65.9   **Paraphilia, unspecified**
         Paraphilic disorder, unspecified
         Sexual deviation NOS

  F66   **Other sexual disorders**
     Sexual maturation disorder
     Sexual relationship disorder

● F68   **Other disorders of adult personality and behavior**
  ● F68.1   **Factitious disorder imposed on self**
         Compensation neurosis
         Elaboration of physical symptoms for psychological
         reasons
         Hospital hopper syndrome
         Münchhausen's syndrome
         Peregrinating patient
         Excludes2   factitial dermatitis (L98.1)
             person feigning illness (with obvious
             motivation) (Z76.5)
         (Ex) **For category F68.1 CC codes: See PDX Collection 551**
         F68.10   **Factitious disorder imposed on self,**
             unspecified 🔖
         F68.11   **Factitious disorder imposed on self with**
             predominantly psychological signs and
             symptoms
         F68.12   **Factitious disorder imposed on self with**
             predominantly physical signs and symptoms 🔖
         F68.13   **Factitious disorder imposed on self with**
             combined psychological and physical signs and
             symptoms

▶ New   ⇒ Revised   ~~deleted~~ Deleted   Excludes 1   Excludes 2   Includes   Use additional   Code first   Code also   Key words

798   OGCR Official Guidelines   ● Unacceptable Principal Diagnosis   X Assign placeholder X   ● Use Additional Character(s)   ▶ Manifestation Code   **Coding Clinic**

F68.8   **Other** specified disorders of adult personality and behavior

F68.A   **Factitious** disorder imposed on another 🅒
     Factitious disorder by proxy
     Münchausen's by proxy
     (Ex:) See PDX Collection 551

F69   **Unspecified** disorder of adult personality and behavior   A

INTELLECTUAL DISABILITIES (F70-F79)

Code first any associated physical or developmental disorders

     Excludes1   borderline intellectual functioning, IQ above 70 to 84 (R41.83)

F70   **Mild** intellectual disabilities
     IQ level 50-55 to approximately 70
     Mild mental subnormality

F71   **Moderate** intellectual disabilities
     IQ level 35-40 to 50-55
     Moderate mental subnormality

F72   **Severe** intellectual disabilities 🅒
     IQ 20-25 to 35-40
     Severe mental subnormality
     (Ex:) See PDX Collection 558

F73   **Profound** intellectual disabilities 🅒
     IQ level below 20-25
     Profound mental subnormality
     (Ex:) See PDX Collection 558

● F78   **Other** intellectual disabilities

  ▶● F78.A   **Other** genetic related intellectual disabilities

    ▶ F78.A1   **SYNGAP1-related** intellectual disability
      ▶ *Code also, if applicable, any associated:*
      ▶ autism spectrum disorder (F84.0)
      ▶ autistic disorder (F84.0)
      ▶ encephalopathy (G93.4-)
      ▶ epilepsy and recurrent seizures (G40.-)
      ▶ other pervasive developmental disorders (F84.8)
      ▶ pervasive developmental disorder, NOS (F84.9)

    ▶ F78.A9   **Other** genetic related intellectual disability
       Code also, if applicable, any associated disorders

F79   **Unspecified** intellectual disabilities
     Mental deficiency NOS
     Mental subnormality NOS

PERVASIVE AND SPECIFIC DEVELOPMENTAL DISORDERS (F80-F89)

● F80   **Specific** developmental disorders of speech and language

   F80.0   **Phonological** disorder
     Communication disorder of unknown cause, characterized by failure to use age-appropriate sounds
     Dyslalia
     Functional speech articulation disorder
     Lalling
     Lisping
     Phonological developmental disorder
     Speech articulation developmental disorder
     Speech-sound disorder

     Excludes1   speech articulation impairment due to aphasia NOS (R47.01)
          speech articulation impairment due to apraxia (R48.2)

     Excludes2   speech articulation impairment due to hearing loss (F80.4)
          speech articulation impairment due to intellectual disabilities (F70-F79)
          speech articulation impairment with expressive language developmental disorder (F80.1)

speech articulation impairment with mixed receptive expressive language developmental disorder (F80.2)

   F80.1   **Expressive language** disorder
     Developmental dysphasia or aphasia, expressive type

     Excludes1   mixed receptive-expressive language disorder (F80.2)
          dysphasia and aphasia NOS (R47.-)

     Excludes2   acquired aphasia with epilepsy [Landau-Kleffner] (G40.80-)
          intellectual disabilities (F70-F79)
          pervasive developmental disorders (F84.-)
          selective mutism (F94.0)

   F80.2   **Mixed receptive-expressive language disorder**
     Developmental dysphasia or aphasia, receptive type
     Developmental Wernicke's aphasia

     Excludes1   central auditory processing disorder (H93.25)
          dysphasia or aphasia NOS (R47.-)
          expressive language disorder (F80.1)
          expressive type dysphasia or aphasia (F80.1)
          word deafness (H93.25)

     Excludes2   acquired aphasia with epilepsy [Landau-Kleffner] (G40.80-)
          intellectual disabilities (F70-F79)
          pervasive developmental disorders (F84.-)
          selective mutism (F94.0)

   F80.4   **Speech and language development delay due to hearing loss**
     Code also type of hearing loss (H90.-, H91.-)

● F80.8   **Other** developmental disorders of speech or language

   F80.81   **Childhood onset fluency disorder**
     Cluttering NOS
     Stuttering NOS

     Excludes1   adult onset fluency disorder (F98.5)
          fluency disorder in conditions classified elsewhere (R47.82)
          fluency disorder (stuttering) following cerebrovascular disease (I69. with final characters -23)

   F80.82   **Social pragmatic communication disorder**
     Excludes1   Asperger's syndrome (F84.5)
          autistic disorder (F84.0)
     Coding Clinic: 2016, Q4, P16

   F80.89   **Other** developmental disorders of speech and language
     Coding Clinic: 2017, Q1, P27

   F80.9   **Developmental disorder of speech and language, unspecified**
     Communication disorder NOS
     Language disorder NOS

● F81   **Specific** developmental disorders of scholastic skills

   F81.0   **Specific reading disorder**
     'Backward reading'
     Developmental dyslexia
     Specific learning disorder, with impairment in reading
     Specific reading retardation

     Excludes1   alexia NOS (R48.0)
          dyslexia NOS (R48.0)

   F81.2   **Mathematics disorder**
     Developmental acalculia
     Developmental arithmetical disorder
     Developmental Gerstmann's syndrome
     Specific learning disorder, with impairment in mathematics

     Excludes1   acalculia NOS (R48.8)

     Excludes2   arithmetic difficulties associated with a reading disorder (F81.0)

CHAPTER 5 (F01-F99)

N Newborn Age: 0   **P** Pediatric Age: 0–17   **M** Maternity DX: 9–64   **A** Adult Age: 15–124   ♀ Females Only   ♂ Males Only
🅒 Complication\Comorbidity   Major C\C   (Ex:) CC/MCC Exclusions   Hospital-Acquired Condition   Hierarchical Condition Category
799

arithmetical difficulties associated with a
spelling disorder (F81.81)
arithmetical difficulties due to inadequate
teaching (Z55.8)

● **F81.8   Other developmental disorders of scholastic skills**

    F81.81   Disorder of written expression
Specific learning disorder, with impairment in
written expression
Specific spelling disorder

    **F81.89   Other developmental disorders of scholastic
skills**

● **F81.9   Developmental disorder of scholastic skills, unspecified**
Knowledge acquisition disability NOS
Learning disability NOS
Learning disorder NOS

F82   Specific developmental disorder of motor function
Clumsy child syndrome
Developmental coordination disorder
Developmental dyspraxia

    Excludes1   abnormalities of gait and mobility (R26.-)
lack of coordination (R27.-)

    Excludes2   lack of coordination secondary to intellectual
disabilities (F70-F79)

● **F84   Pervasive developmental disorders**
~~Use additional code to identify any associated medical
condition and intellectual disabilities.~~

    ▶Code also any associated medical condition and
intellectual disabilities

    Ex: **For category F84 CC codes unless otherwise indicated:** See PDX Collection 551

    F84.0   Autistic disorder 🔄
Autism spectrum disorder
Infantile autism
Infantile psychosis
Kanner's syndrome

        Excludes1   Asperger's syndrome (F84.5)
Coding Clinic: 2017, Q1, P27

    F84.2   Rett's syndrome 🔄
Neurodevelopmental disorder

        Excludes1   Asperger's syndrome (F84.5)
Autistic disorder (F84.0)
other childhood disintegrative disorder
(F84.3)

        Ex: See PDX Collection 537

    F84.3   Other childhood disintegrative disorder 🔄   P
Dementia infantilis
*At least two years of normal development followed by
significant loss of language abilities, social skills,
bowel/bladder control, motor skills*
Disintegrative psychosis
Heller's syndrome
*At least two years of normal development followed by
significant loss of language abilities, social skills,
bowel/bladder control, motor skills*
Symbiotic psychosis
*Abnormal relationship to mothering figure, characterized
by intense separation anxiety, severe regression,
giving up of useful speech, and autism*

        Use additional code to identify any associated
neurological condition.

        Excludes1   Asperger's syndrome (F84.5)
Autistic disorder (F84.0)
Rett's syndrome (F84.2)

    F84.5   Asperger's syndrome 🔄
Developmental disorder
Asperger's disorder
Autistic psychopathy
Schizoid disorder of childhood

    F84.8   Other pervasive developmental disorders 🔄
Overactive disorder associated with intellectual
disabilities and stereotyped movements

    F84.9   Pervasive developmental disorder, unspecified 🔄
Atypical autism

F88   Other disorders of psychological development
Developmental agnosia
Global developmental delay
Other specified neurodevelopmental disorder

F89   Unspecified disorder of psychological development
Developmental disorder NOS
Neurodevelopmental disorder NOS

BEHAVIORAL AND EMOTIONAL DISORDERS WITH ONSET USUALLY OCCURRING IN CHILDHOOD AND ADOLESCENCE (F90-F98)

Note: Codes within categories F90-F98 may be used regardless
of the age of a patient. These disorders generally have onset
within the childhood or adolescent years, but may continue
throughout life or not be diagnosed until adulthood.

● **F90   Attention-deficit hyperactivity disorders**
Attention deficit disorder with hyperactivity=ADHD

    Includes   attention deficit disorder with hyperactivity
attention deficit syndrome with hyperactivity

    Excludes2   anxiety disorders (F40.-, F41.-)
mood [affective] disorders (F30-F39)
pervasive developmental disorders (F84.-)
schizophrenia (F20.-)

    **F90.0   Attention-deficit hyperactivity disorder, predominantly
inattentive type**
Attention-deficit/hyperactivity disorder, predominantly
inattentive presentation

    **F90.1   Attention-deficit hyperactivity disorder, predominantly
hyperactive type**
Attention-deficit/hyperactivity disorder, predominantly
hyperactive impulsive presentation

    F90.2   Attention-deficit hyperactivity disorder, combined type
Attention-deficit/hyperactivity disorder, combined
presentation

    F90.8   Attention-deficit hyperactivity disorder, other type

    F90.9   Attention-deficit hyperactivity disorder, unspecified type
Attention-deficit hyperactivity disorder of childhood or
adolescence NOS
Attention-deficit hyperactivity disorder NOS

● **F91   Conduct disorders**
Childhood/adolescence disruptive behavior disorder

    Excludes1   antisocial behavior (Z72.81-)
antisocial personality disorder (F60.2)

    Excludes2   conduct problems associated with attention-
deficit hyperactivity disorder (F90.-)
mood [affective] disorders (F30-F39)
pervasive developmental disorders (F84.-)
schizophrenia (F20.-)

    F91.0   Conduct disorder confined to family context

    F91.1   Conduct disorder, childhood-onset type
Unsocialized conduct disorder
Conduct disorder, solitary aggressive type
Unsocialized aggressive disorder

    F91.2   Conduct disorder, adolescent-onset type
Socialized conduct disorder
Conduct disorder, group type

    F91.3   Oppositional defiant disorder

    F91.8   Other conduct disorders
Other specified conduct disorder
Other specified disruptive disorder

    F91.9   Conduct disorder, unspecified
Behavioral disorder NOS
Conduct disorder NOS
Disruptive behavior disorder NOS
Disruptive disorder NOS

● **F93   Emotional disorders with onset specific to childhood**

    F93.0   Separation anxiety disorder of childhood

        Excludes2   mood [affective] disorders (F30-F39)
nonpsychotic mental disorders (F40-F48)
phobic anxiety disorder of childhood
(F40.8)
social phobia (F40.1)

▶ New   ⇒ Revised   ~~deleted~~ Deleted   Excludes 1   Excludes 2   Includes   Use additional   Code first   Code also   Key words

OGCR Official Guidelines   ● Unacceptable Principal Diagnosis   X Assign placeholder X   ● Use Additional Character(s)   ▷ Manifestation Code   Coding Clinic

CHAPTER 5 (F01-F99)

F93.8   **Other childhood emotional disorders**
     Identity disorder
     Excludes2   gender identity disorder of childhood
             (F64.2)

F93.9   **Childhood emotional disorder, unspecified**

● **F94**   **Disorders of social functioning with onset specific to childhood and adolescence**

F94.0   **Selective mutism**
     Elective mutism
     Excludes2   pervasive developmental disorders
             (F84.-)
             schizophrenia (F20.-)
             specific developmental disorders of
                speech and language (F80.-)
             transient mutism as part of separation
                anxiety in young children (F93.0)

F94.1   **Reactive attachment disorder of childhood**
     Use additional code to identify any associated failure to thrive or growth retardation
     Excludes1   disinhibited attachment disorder of
             childhood (F94.2)
             normal variation in pattern of selective
                attachment
     Excludes2   Asperger's syndrome (F84.5)
             maltreatment syndromes (T74.-)
             sexual or physical abuse in childhood,
                resulting in psychosocial problems
                (Z62.81-)

F94.2   **Disinhibited attachment disorder of childhood**
     Affectionless psychopathy
     Institutional syndrome
     Excludes1   reactive attachment disorder of childhood
             (F94.1)
     Excludes2   Asperger's syndrome (F84.5)
             attention-deficit hyperactivity disorders
                (F90.-)
             hospitalism in children (F43.2-)

F94.8   **Other childhood disorders of social functioning**

F94.9   **Childhood disorder of social functioning, unspecified**

● **F95**   **Tic disorder**
     Involuntary twitch

F95.0   **Transient tic disorder**
     Provisional tic disorder

F95.1   **Chronic motor or vocal tic disorder**

F95.2   **Tourette's disorder**
     Combined vocal and multiple motor tic disorder [de la Tourette]
     Tourette's syndrome

F95.8   **Other tic disorders**

F95.9   **Tic disorder, unspecified**
     Tic NOS

● **F98**   **Other behavioral and emotional disorders with onset usually occurring in childhood and adolescence**
     Excludes2   breath-holding spells (R06.89)
             gender identity disorder of childhood (F64.2)
             Kleine-Levin syndrome (G47.13)
             obsessive-compulsive disorder (F42.3-)
             sleep disorders not due to a substance or known
                physiological condition (F51.-)

F98.0   **Enuresis not due to a substance or known physiological condition**
     Enuresis: Urinary incontinence
     Enuresis (primary) (secondary) of nonorganic origin
     Functional enuresis
     Psychogenic enuresis
     Urinary incontinence of nonorganic origin
     Excludes1   enuresis NOS (R32)

Item 5–2 Enuresis: Bed wetting by children at night. Causes can be either psychological or medical (diabetes, urinary tract infections, or abnormalities). **Encopresis:** Overflow incontinence of bowels sometimes resulting from chronic constipation or fecal impaction. Check the documentation for additional diagnoses.

F98.1   **Encopresis not due to a substance or known physiological condition**
     Encopresis: Fecal incontinence
     Functional encopresis
     Incontinence of feces of nonorganic origin
     Psychogenic encopresis
     Use additional code to identify the cause of any coexisting constipation.
     Excludes1   encopresis NOS (R15.-)

● F98.2   **Other feeding disorders of infancy and childhood**
     ~~**Excludes1**   feeding difficulties (R63.3)~~
     Excludes2   anorexia nervosa and other eating
             disorders (F50.-)
             ▶ feeding difficulties (R63.3)
             feeding problems of newborn (P92.-)
             pica of infancy or childhood (F98.3)

F98.21   **Rumination disorder of infancy**

F98.29   **Other feeding disorders of infancy and early childhood**

F98.3   **Pica of infancy and childhood**
     Craving and eating substances such as paint, clay, or dirt to replace a nutritional deficit in the body.

F98.4   **Stereotyped movement disorders**
     Stereotype/habit disorder
     Excludes1   abnormal involuntary movements (R25.-)
     Excludes2   compulsions in obsessive-compulsive
             disorder (F42.-)
             hair plucking (F63.3)
             movement disorders of organic origin
                (G20-G25)
             nail-biting (F98.8)
             nose-picking (F98.8)
             stereotypies that are part of a broader
                psychiatric condition (F01-F95)
             thumb-sucking (F98.8)
             tic disorders (F95.-)
             trichotillomania (F63.3)

F98.5   **Adult onset fluency disorder**
     Excludes1   childhood onset fluency disorder (F80.81)
             dysphasia (R47.02)
             fluency disorder in conditions classified
                elsewhere (R47.82)
             fluency disorder (stuttering) following
                cerebrovascular disease (I69. with
                final characters -23)
             tic disorders (F95.-)

F98.8   **Other specified behavioral and emotional disorders with onset usually occurring in childhood and adolescence**
     Excessive masturbation
     Nail-biting
     Nose-picking
     Thumb-sucking

F98.9   **Unspecified behavioral and emotional disorders with onset usually occurring in childhood and adolescence**

UNSPECIFIED MENTAL DISORDER (F99)

F99   **Mental disorder, not otherwise specified**
     Mental illness NOS
     Excludes1   unspecified mental disorder due to known
             physiological condition (F09)

CHAPTER 5 (F01-F99)

N Newborn Age: 0   **P** Pediatric Age: 0–17   **M** Maternity DX: 9–64   **A** Adult Age: 15–124   ♀ Females Only   ♂ Males Only

Complication\Comorbidity   Major C\C   (Ex) CC/MCC Exclusions   Hospital-Acquired Condition   Hierarchical Condition Category

801

CHAPTER 6

DISEASES OF THE NERVOUS SYSTEM (G00-G99)

OGCR Chapter-Specific Coding Guidelines

6. Chapter 6: Diseases of the Nervous System (G00-G99)

a. Dominant/nondominant side

Codes from category G81, Hemiplegia and hemiparesis, and subcategories, G83.1, Monoplegia of lower limb, G83.2, Monoplegia of upper limb, and G83.3, Monoplegia, unspecified, identify whether the dominant or nondominant side is affected. Should the affected side be documented, but not specified as dominant or nondominant, and the classification system does not indicate a default, code selection is as follows:

- For ambidextrous patients, the default should be dominant.
- If the left side is affected, the default is nondominant.
- If the right side is affected, the default is dominant.

b. Pain - Category G89

1) General coding information

Codes in category G89, Pain, not elsewhere classified, may be used in conjunction with codes from other categories and chapters to provide more detail about acute or chronic pain and neoplasm-related pain, unless otherwise indicated below.

If the pain is not specified as acute or chronic, post-thoracotomy, postprocedural, or neoplasm-related, do not assign codes from category G89.

A code from category G89 should not be assigned if the underlying (definitive) diagnosis is known, unless the reason for the encounter is pain control/management and not management of the underlying condition.

When an admission or encounter is for a procedure aimed at treating the underlying condition (e.g., spinal fusion, kyphoplasty), a code for the underlying condition (e.g., vertebral fracture, spinal stenosis) should be assigned as the principal diagnosis. No code from category G89 should be assigned.

(a) Category G89 Codes as Principal or First-Listed Diagnosis

Category G89 codes are acceptable as principal diagnosis or the first-listed code:

- When pain control or pain management is the reason for the admission/encounter (e.g., a patient with displaced intervertebral disc, nerve impingement and severe back pain presents for injection of steroid into the spinal canal). The underlying cause of the pain should be reported as an additional diagnosis, if known.
- When a patient is admitted for the insertion of a neurostimulator for pain control, assign the appropriate pain code as the principal or first-listed diagnosis. When an admission or encounter is for a procedure aimed at treating the underlying condition and a neurostimulator is inserted for pain control during the same admission/encounter, a code for the underlying condition should be assigned as the principal diagnosis and the appropriate pain code should be assigned as a secondary diagnosis.

(b) Use of Category G89 Codes in Conjunction with Site Specific Pain Codes

(i) Assigning Category G89 and Site-Specific Pain Codes

Codes from category G89 may be used in conjunction with codes that identify the site of pain (including codes from Chapter 18) if the category G89 code provides additional information. For example, if the code describes the site of the pain, but does not fully describe whether the pain is acute or chronic, then both codes should be assigned.

(ii) Sequencing of Category G89 Codes with Site-Specific Pain Codes

The sequencing of category G89 codes with site-specific pain codes (including Chapter 18 codes), is dependent on the circumstances of the encounter/admission as follows:

- If the encounter is for pain control or pain management, assign the code from category G89 followed by the code identifying the specific site of pain (e.g., encounter for pain management for acute neck pain from trauma is assigned code G89.11, Acute pain due to trauma, followed by code M54.2, Cervicalgia, to identify the site of pain).
- If the encounter is for any other reason except pain control or pain management, and a related definitive diagnosis has not been established (confirmed) by the provider, assign the code for the specific site of pain first, followed by the appropriate code from category G89.

2) Pain due to devices, implants and grafts

See Section I.C.19. Pain due to medical devices

3) Postoperative Pain

The provider's documentation should be used to guide the coding of postoperative pain, as well as Section III. Reporting Additional Diagnoses and Section IV. Diagnostic Coding and Reporting in the Outpatient Setting.

The default for post-thoracotomy and other postoperative pain not specified as acute or chronic is the code for the acute form.

Routine or expected postoperative pain immediately after surgery should not be coded.

(a) Postoperative pain not associated with specific postoperative complication

Postoperative pain not associated with a specific postoperative complication is assigned to the appropriate postoperative pain code in category G89.

(b) Postoperative pain associated with specific postoperative complication

Postoperative pain associated with a specific postoperative complication (such as painful wire sutures) is assigned to the appropriate code(s) found in Chapter 19, Injury, poisoning, and certain other consequences of external causes. If appropriate, use additional code(s) from category G89 to identify acute or chronic pain (G89.18 or G89.28).

4) Chronic pain

Chronic pain is classified to subcategory G89.2. There is no time frame defining when pain becomes chronic pain. The provider's documentation should be used to guide use of these codes.

5) Neoplasm Related Pain

Code G89.3 is assigned to pain documented as being related, associated or due to cancer, primary or secondary malignancy, or tumor. This code is assigned regardless of whether the pain is acute or chronic.

This code may be assigned as the principal or first-listed code when the stated reason for the admission/encounter is documented as pain control/pain management. The underlying neoplasm should be reported as an additional diagnosis.

When the reason for the admission/encounter is management of the neoplasm and the pain associated with the neoplasm is also documented, code G89.3 may be assigned as an additional diagnosis. It is not necessary to assign an additional code for the site of the pain.

See Section I.C.2 for instructions on the sequencing of neoplasms for all other stated reasons for the admission/encounter (except for pain control/pain management).

6) Chronic pain syndrome

Central pain syndrome (G89.0) and chronic pain syndrome (G89.4) are different than the term "chronic pain," and therefore codes should only be used when the provider has specifically documented this condition.

See Section I.C.5. Pain disorders related to psychological factors

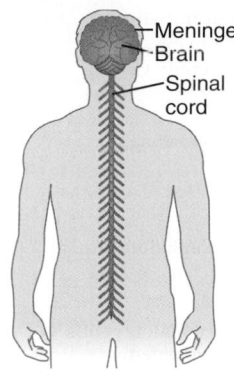

Meninges
Brain
Spinal cord

Figure 6-1 The brain and spinal cord make up the central nervous system.

Item 6–1 The two major classifications of the nervous system are the peripheral nervous system and the central nervous system (CNS). The central nervous system is composed of the brain and the spinal cord. The peripheral nervous system is composed of the parasympathetic and sympathetic systems. **Encephalitis** is the swelling of the brain. **Meningitis** is swelling of the covering of the brain, the meninges. Types and causes of brain infections are:

Type	Cause
purulent	bacterial
aseptic/abacterial	viral
chronic meningitis	mycobacterial and fungal

CHAPTER 6

DISEASES OF THE NERVOUS SYSTEM (G00-G99)

Excludes2   certain conditions originating in the perinatal period (P01-P96)
certain infectious and parasitic diseases (A00-B99)
complications of pregnancy, childbirth and the puerperium (O00-O9A)
congenital malformations, deformations, and chromosomal abnormalities (Q00-Q99)
endocrine, nutritional and metabolic diseases (E00-E88)
injury, poisoning and certain other consequences of external causes (S00-T88)
neoplasms (C00-D49)
symptoms, signs and abnormal clinical and laboratory findings, not elsewhere classified (R00-R94)

This chapter contains the following blocks:

G00-G09	Inflammatory diseases of the central nervous system
G10-G14	Systemic atrophies primarily affecting the central nervous system
G20-G26	Extrapyramidal and movement disorders
G30-G32	Other degenerative diseases of the nervous system
G35-G37	Demyelinating diseases of the central nervous system
G40-G47	Episodic and paroxysmal disorders
G50-G59	Nerve, nerve root and plexus disorders
G60-G65	Polyneuropathies and other disorders of the peripheral nervous system
G70-G73	Diseases of myoneural junction and muscle
G80-G83	Cerebral palsy and other paralytic syndromes
G89-G99	Other disorders of the nervous system

INFLAMMATORY DISEASES OF THE CENTRAL NERVOUS SYSTEM (G00-G09)

● **G00**   **Bacterial meningitis, not elsewhere classified**
An infection of the cerebrospinal fluid surrounding the spinal cord and brain.

Includes   bacterial arachnoiditis
bacterial leptomeningitis
bacterial meningitis
bacterial pachymeningitis

Excludes1   bacterial meningoencephalitis (G04.2)
bacterial meningomyelitis (G04.2)

(Ex:) **For category G00 CC codes:** See PDX Collection 207

G00.0   **Hemophilus meningitis** 🦠
Meningitis due to Hemophilus influenzae

G00.1   **Pneumococcal meningitis** 🦠
Meningitis due to Streptococcal pneumoniae

G00.2   **Streptococcal meningitis** 🦠
Use additional code to further identify organism (B95.0-B95.5)

G00.3   **Staphylococcal meningitis** 🦠
Use additional code to further identify organism (B95.61-B95.8)

G00.8   **Other bacterial meningitis** 🦠
Meningitis due to Escherichia coli
Meningitis due to Friedländer bacillus
Meningitis due to Klebsiella
Use additional code to further identify organism (B96.-)

G00.9   **Bacterial meningitis, unspecified** 🦠
Meningitis due to gram-negative bacteria, unspecified
Purulent meningitis NOS
Pyogenic meningitis NOS
Suppurative meningitis NOS

▷ **G01**   *Meningitis in bacterial diseases classified elsewhere* 🦠
Code first underlying disease

Excludes1   meningitis (in):
gonococcal (A54.81)
leptospirosis (A27.81)
listeriosis (A32.11)
Lyme disease (A69.21)
meningococcal (A39.0)
neurosyphilis (A52.13)
tuberculosis (A17.0)
meningoencephalitis and meningomyelitis in bacterial diseases classified elsewhere (G05)

(Ex:) See PDX Collection 207

▷ **G02**   *Meningitis in other infectious and parasitic diseases classified elsewhere* 🦠
Code first underlying disease, such as:
African trypanosomiasis (B56.-)
poliovirus infection (A80.-)

Excludes1   candidal meningitis (B37.5)
coccidioidomycosis meningitis (B38.4)
cryptococcal meningitis (B45.1)
herpesviral [herpes simplex] meningitis (B00.3)
infectious mononucleosis complicated by meningitis (B27.- with fourth character 2)
measles complicated by meningitis (B05.1)
meningoencephalitis and meningomyelitis in other infectious and parasitic diseases classified elsewhere (G05)
mumps meningitis (B26.1)
rubella meningitis (B06.02)
varicella [chickenpox] meningitis (B01.0)
zoster meningitis (B02.1)

(Ex:) See PDX Collection 559

N Newborn Age: 0   **P** Pediatric Age: 0–17   **M** Maternity DX: 9–64   **A** Adult Age: 15–124   ♀ Females Only   ♂ Males Only

🦠 Complication\Comorbidity   🦠 Major C\C   (Ex:) CC/MCC Exclusions   🦠 Hospital-Acquired Condition   🦠 Hierarchical Condition Category

803

CHAPTER 6 (G00-G99)

● **G03   Meningitis due to other and unspecified causes**

Includes   arachnoiditis NOS
leptomeningitis NOS
meningitis NOS
pachymeningitis NOS

Excludes1   meningoencephalitis (G04.-)
meningomyelitis (G04.-)

(Ex:) **For category G03 CC codes unless otherwise indicated:** See PDX Collection 207

G03.0   Nonpyogenic meningitis 🔹
Aseptic meningitis
Nonbacterial meningitis

G03.1   Chronic meningitis 🔹

G03.2   Benign recurrent meningitis [Mollaret] 🔹
(Ex:) See PDX Collection 140

G03.8   Meningitis due to other specified causes 🔹

G03.9   Meningitis, unspecified 🔹
Arachnoiditis (spinal) NOS

● **G04   Encephalitis, myelitis and encephalomyelitis**

Includes   acute ascending myelitis
meningoencephalitis
meningomyelitis

Excludes1   encephalopathy NOS (G93.40)
other noninfectious acute disseminated
encephalomyelitis (noninfectious ADEM)
(G04.81)

Excludes2   acute transverse myelitis (G37.3-)
alcoholic encephalopathy (G31.2)
benign myalgic encephalomyelitis (G93.3)
multiple sclerosis (G35)
subacute necrotizing myelitis (G37.4)
➠toxic encephalitis (G92.8)
➠toxic encephalopathy (G92.8)

● **G04.0   Acute disseminated encephalitis and encephalomyelitis (ADEM)**

Excludes1   acute necrotizing hemorrhagic
encephalopathy (G04.3-)

(Ex:) **For category G04.0 CC codes unless otherwise indicated:** See PDX Collection 560

G04.00   Acute disseminated encephalitis and encephalomyelitis, unspecified 🔹

▹ *G04.01   Postinfectious acute disseminated encephalitis and encephalomyelitis (postinfectious ADEM)* 🔹

Excludes1   post chickenpox encephalitis
(B01.1)
post measles encephalitis (B05.0)
post measles myelitis (B05.1)

G04.02   Postimmunization acute disseminated encephalitis, myelitis and encephalomyelitis 🔹
Encephalitis, post immunization
Encephalomyelitis, post immunization
Use additional code to identify the vaccine
(T50.A-, T50.B-, T50.Z-)
(Ex:) See PDX Collection 3222

G04.1   Tropical spastic paraplegia 🔹🔹
(Ex:) See PDX Collection 561

G04.2   Bacterial meningoencephalitis and meningomyelitis, not elsewhere classified 🔹
(Ex:) See PDX Collection 207

● **G04.3   Acute necrotizing hemorrhagic encephalopathy**
Sudden and severe CNS disease with pathology of hemorrhages and necrosis of white matter

Excludes1   acute disseminated encephalitis and
encephalomyelitis (G04.0-)

G04.30   Acute necrotizing hemorrhagic encephalopathy, unspecified 🔹
(Ex:) See PDX Collection 3223

G04.31   Postinfectious acute necrotizing hemorrhagic encephalopathy 🔹
(Ex:) See PDX Collection 560

G04.32   Postimmunization acute necrotizing hemorrhagic encephalopathy 🔹
Use additional code to identify vaccine
(T50.A-, T50.B-, T50.Z-)
(Ex:) See PDX Collection 3224

G04.39   Other acute necrotizing hemorrhagic encephalopathy 🔹
Code also underlying etiology, if applicable
(Ex:) See PDX Collection 3225

● **G04.8   Other encephalitis, myelitis and encephalomyelitis**
Code also any associated seizure (G40.-, R56.9)
(Ex:) **For category G04.8 CC codes:** See PDX Collection 560

G04.81   Other encephalitis and encephalomyelitis 🔹
Noninfectious acute disseminated
encephalomyelitis (noninfectious ADEM)

▹ **G04.82   Acute flaccid myelitis**
▹ **Excludes1**   transverse myelitis (G37.3)

G04.89   Other myelitis 🔹🔹
Coding Clinic: 2020, Q1, P14

● **G04.9   Encephalitis, myelitis and encephalomyelitis, unspecified**
(Ex:) **For category G04.9 CC codes:** See PDX Collection 4049

G04.90   Encephalitis and encephalomyelitis, unspecified 🔹
Ventriculitis (cerebral) NOS

G04.91   Myelitis, unspecified 🔹🔹

● **G05   Encephalitis, myelitis and encephalomyelitis in diseases classified elsewhere**
Code first underlying disease, such as:
▸congenital toxoplasmosis encephalitis, myelitis and
encephalomyelitis (P37.1)
▸cytomegaloviral encephalitis, myelitis and encephalomyelitis
(B25.8)
▸encephalitis, myelitis and encephalomyelitis (in) systemic
lupus erythematosus (M32.19)
▸eosinophilic meningoencephalitis (B83.2)
human immunodeficiency virus [HIV] disease (B20)
poliovirus (A80.-)
suppurative otitis media (H66.01-H66.4)
trichinellosis (B75)

Excludes1   adenoviral encephalitis, myelitis and
encephalomyelitis (A85.1)
~~congenital toxoplasmosis encephalitis, myelitis~~
~~and encephalomyelitis (P37.1)~~
~~cytomegaloviral encephalitis, myelitis and~~
~~encephalomyelitis (B25.8)~~
encephalitis, myelitis and encephalomyelitis (in)
measles (B05.0)
~~encephalitis, myelitis and encephalomyelitis (in)~~
~~systemic lupus erythematosus (M32.19)~~
enteroviral encephalitis, myelitis and
encephalomyelitis (A85.0)
~~eosinophilic meningoencephalitis (B83.2)~~
herpesviral [herpes simplex] encephalitis,
myelitis and encephalomyelitis (B00.4)
listerial encephalitis, myelitis and
encephalomyelitis (A32.12)
meningococcal encephalitis, myelitis and
encephalomyelitis (A39.81)
mumps encephalitis, myelitis and
encephalomyelitis (B26.2)
postchickenpox encephalitis, myelitis and
encephalomyelitis (B01.1-)
rubella encephalitis, myelitis and
encephalomyelitis (B06.01)
toxoplasmosis encephalitis, myelitis and
encephalomyelitis (B58.2)
zoster encephalitis, myelitis and
encephalomyelitis (B02.0)

(Ex:) **For category G05 CC codes:** See PDX Collection 560

▹ *G05.3   Encephalitis and encephalomyelitis in diseases classified elsewhere* 🔹
Meningoencephalitis in diseases classified elsewhere

▸ New   ➠ Revised   ~~deleted~~ Deleted   Excludes 1   Excludes 2   Includes   Use additional   Code first   Code also   Key words

OGCR Official Guidelines   ● Unacceptable Principal Diagnosis   X Assign placeholder X   ● Use Additional Character(s)   ▹ Manifestation Code   **Coding Clinic**

▶ *G05.4*   *Myelitis in diseases classified elsewhere* 🏷️🏷️
     Meningomyelitis in diseases classified elsewhere

● **G06**   **Intracranial and intraspinal abscess and granuloma**
     An accumulation of pus in either the brain or spinal cord
     Use additional code (B95-B97) to identify infectious agent.

     G06.0   **Intracranial abscess and granuloma** 🏷️
        Brain [any part] abscess (embolic)
        Cerebellar abscess (embolic)
        Cerebral abscess (embolic)
        Intracranial epidural abscess or granuloma
        Intracranial extradural abscess or granuloma
        Intracranial subdural abscess or granuloma
        Otogenic abscess (embolic)

        Excludes1   tuberculous intracranial abscess and
                    granuloma (A17.81)
        (Ex) See PDX Collection 563

     G06.1   **Intraspinal abscess and granuloma** 🏷️
        Abscess (embolic) of spinal cord [any part]
        Intraspinal epidural abscess or granuloma
        Intraspinal extradural abscess or granuloma
        Intraspinal subdural abscess or granuloma

        Excludes1   tuberculous intraspinal abscess and
                    granuloma (A17.81)
        (Ex) See PDX Collection 564

     G06.2   **Extradural and subdural abscess, unspecified** 🏷️
        (Ex) See PDX Collection 565

▶ *G07*   *Intracranial and intraspinal abscess and granuloma in diseases classified elsewhere* 🏷️

     Code first underlying disease, such as:
        schistosomiasis granuloma of brain (B65.-)
     Excludes1   abscess of brain:
             amebic (A06.6)
             chromomycotic (B43.1)
             gonococcal (A54.82)
             tuberculous (A17.81)
             tuberculoma of meninges (A17.1)
     (Ex) See PDX Collection 565

G08   **Intracranial and intraspinal phlebitis and thrombophlebitis** 🏷️
     Septic embolism of intracranial or intraspinal venous sinuses and veins
     Septic endophlebitis of intracranial or intraspinal venous sinuses and veins
     Septic phlebitis of intracranial or intraspinal venous sinuses and veins
     Septic thrombophlebitis of intracranial or intraspinal venous sinuses and veins
     Septic thrombosis of intracranial or intraspinal venous sinuses and veins

     Excludes1   intracranial phlebitis and thrombophlebitis
                complicating:
                abortion, ectopic or molar pregnancy
                    (O00-O07, O08.7)
                pregnancy, childbirth and the puerperium
                    (O22.5, O87.3)
                nonpyogenic intracranial phlebitis and
                    thrombophlebitis (I67.6)

     Excludes2   intracranial phlebitis and thrombophlebitis
                complicating nonpyogenic intraspinal
                phlebitis and thrombophlebitis (G95.1)
     (Ex) See PDX Collection 565

G09   **Sequelae of inflammatory diseases of central nervous system**
     Note: Category G09 is to be used to indicate conditions
           whose primary classification is to G00-G08 as the cause of
           sequelae, themselves classifiable elsewhere. The 'sequelae'
           include conditions specified as residuals.

     Code first condition resulting from (sequela) of inflammatory diseases of central nervous system

---

Item 6–2 Huntington's chorea is an inherited degenerative disorder of the central nervous system and is characterized by ceaseless, jerky movements and progressive cognitive and behavioral deterioration.

SYSTEMIC ATROPHIES PRIMARILY AFFECTING THE CENTRAL NERVOUS SYSTEM (G10-G14)

G10   **Huntington's disease** 🏷️🏷️
     Genetic disease with degeneration of cells of the nervous system, including brain
     Huntington's chorea
     Huntington's dementia

     Code also dementia in other diseases classified elsewhere
        without behavioral disturbance (F02.80)
     (Ex) See PDX Collection 566

● **G11**   **Hereditary ataxia**
     Genetic neurological disorder affecting coordination
     Excludes2   cerebral palsy (G80.-)
                hereditary and idiopathic neuropathy (G60.-)
                metabolic disorders (E70-E88)
     (Ex) **For category G11 CC codes unless otherwise indicated: See PDX Collection 569**

     G11.0   **Congenital nonprogressive ataxia** 🏷️🏷️

●   **G11.1**   **Early-onset cerebellar ataxia** 🏷️🏷️

        G11.10 Early-onset cerebellar ataxia, unspecified 🏷️
           (Ex) See PDX Collection 4048

        G11.11 Friedreich ataxia 🏷️
           Autosomal recessive Friedreich ataxia
           Friedreich ataxia with retained reflexes
           (Ex) See PDX Collection 4048

        G11.19 Other early-onset cerebellar ataxia 🏷️
           Early-onset cerebellar ataxia with essential tremor
           Early-onset cerebellar ataxia with myoclonus [Hunt's ataxia]
           Early-onset cerebellar ataxia with retained tendon reflexes
           X-linked recessive spinocerebellar ataxia
           (Ex) See PDX Collection 4048

     G11.2   **Late-onset cerebellar ataxia** 🏷️🏷️   **A**

     G11.3   **Cerebellar ataxia with defective DNA repair** 🏷️🏷️
        Ataxia telangiectasia [Louis-Bar]

        Excludes2   Cockayne's syndrome (Q87.19)
                   other disorders of purine and pyrimidine
                      metabolism (E79.-)
                   xeroderma pigmentosum (Q82.1)

     G11.4   **Hereditary spastic paraplegia** 🏷️🏷️
        (Ex) See PDX Collection 568

     G11.8   **Other hereditary ataxias** 🏷️🏷️

     G11.9   **Hereditary ataxia, unspecified** 🏷️🏷️
        Hereditary cerebellar ataxia NOS
        Hereditary cerebellar degeneration
        Hereditary cerebellar disease
        Hereditary cerebellar syndrome
        (Ex) See PDX Collection 569

● **G12**   **Spinal muscular atrophy and related syndromes**
     (Ex) **For category G12 CC codes: See PDX Collection 570**

     G12.0   **Infantile spinal muscular atrophy, type I [Werdnig-Hoffman]** 🏷️🏷️

     G12.1   **Other inherited spinal muscular atrophy** 🏷️🏷️
        Adult form spinal muscular atrophy
        Childhood form, type II spinal muscular atrophy
        Distal spinal muscular atrophy
        Juvenile form, type III spinal muscular atrophy [Kugelberg-Welander]
        Progressive bulbar palsy of childhood [Fazio-Londe]
        Scapuloperoneal form spinal muscular atrophy

CHAPTER 6 (G00-G99)

N Newborn Age: 0   **P** Pediatric Age: 0–17   **M** Maternity DX: 9–64   **A** Adult Age: 15–124   ♀ Females Only   ♂ Males Only

🏷️ Complication\Comorbidity   🏷️ Major C\C   (Ex) CC/MCC Exclusions   🏷️ Hospital-Acquired Condition   🏷️ Hierarchical Condition Category

805

● G12.2 **Motor neuron disease**
  Progressive disease of motor neurons that carry impulses to muscles to move
    G12.20 Motor neuron disease, unspecified 🦴🦴
    G12.21 Amyotrophic lateral sclerosis 🦴🦴   **A**
        Lou Gehrig's disease (ALS)
    G12.22 Progressive bulbar palsy 🦴🦴
    G12.23 Primary lateral sclerosis 🦴🦴
    G12.24 Familial motor neuron disease 🦴🦴
    G12.25 Progressive spinal muscle atrophy 🦴🦴
    G12.29 Other motor neuron disease 🦴🦴
  G12.8 **Other spinal muscular atrophies and related syndromes** 🦴🦴
  G12.9 Spinal muscular atrophy, **unspecified** 🦴🦴

● G13 **Systemic atrophies primarily affecting central nervous system in diseases classified elsewhere**
  ▶ *G13.0 Paraneoplastic neuromyopathy and neuropathy* 🦴
        Carcinomatous neuromyopathy
        Sensorial paraneoplastic neuropathy [Denny Brown]
        Code first underlying neoplasm (C00-D49)
  ▶ *G13.1 Other systemic atrophy primarily affecting central nervous system in neoplastic disease* 🦴
        Paraneoplastic limbic encephalopathy
        Code first underlying neoplasm (C00-D49)
  ▶ *G13.2 Systemic atrophy primarily affecting the central nervous system in myxedema*
        Code first underlying disease, such as:
            hypothyroidism (E03.-)
            myxedematous congenital iodine deficiency (E00.1)
  ▶ *G13.8 Systemic atrophy primarily affecting central nervous system in other diseases classified elsewhere*
        Code first underlying disease

  G14 **Postpolio syndrome**
    Includes Postpolio myelitic syndrome
    Excludes1 sequelae of poliomyelitis (B91)

EXTRAPYRAMIDAL AND MOVEMENT DISORDERS (G20-G26)

  G20 **Parkinson's disease** 🦴
  Progressive disease of the nervous system that affects muscle coordination
        Hemiparkinsonism
        Idiopathic Parkinsonism or Parkinson's disease
        Paralysis agitans
        Parkinsonism or Parkinson's disease NOS
        Primary Parkinsonism or Parkinson's disease
        Use additional code to identify:
            dementia with behavioral disturbance (F02.81)
            dementia without behavioral disturbance (F02.80)
    Excludes1 dementia with Parkinsonism (G31.83)
    Coding Clinic: 2017, Q2, P7-8; 2016, Q2, P7

● G21 **Secondary parkinsonism**
  Symptoms of Parkinson's caused by medicines, illness, or other nervous system disorder
    Excludes1 dementia with Parkinsonism (G31.83)
                Huntington's disease (G10)
                Shy-Drager syndrome (G90.3)
                syphilitic Parkinsonism (A52.19)
  G21.0 **Malignant neuroleptic syndrome** 🦴
        Use additional code for adverse effect, if applicable, to identify drug (T43.3X5, T43.4X5, T43.505, T43.595)
    Excludes1 neuroleptic induced parkinsonism (G21.11)
        (Ex:) See PDX Collection 571

● G21.1 **Other drug-induced secondary parkinsonism**
    (Ex:) For category G21.1 CC codes: See PDX Collection 572
    G21.11 **Neuroleptic induced parkinsonism** 🦴🦴
        Use additional code for adverse effect, if applicable, to identify drug (T43.3X5, T43.4X5, T43.505, T43.595)
        Excludes1 malignant neuroleptic syndrome (G21.0)
    G21.19 **Other drug induced secondary parkinsonism** 🦴🦴
        Other medication-induced parkinsonism
        Use additional code for adverse effect, if applicable, to identify drug (T36-T50 with fifth or sixth character 5)
  G21.2 **Secondary parkinsonism due to other external agents** 🦴🦴
        Code first (T51-T65) to identify external agent
  G21.3 **Postencephalitic parkinsonism** 🦴🦴
  G21.4 **Vascular parkinsonism** 🦴
  G21.8 **Other secondary parkinsonism** 🦴🦴
  G21.9 **Secondary parkinsonism, unspecified** 🦴🦴

● G23 **Other degenerative diseases of basal ganglia**
    Excludes2 multi-system degeneration of the autonomic nervous system (G90.3)
    (Ex:) For category G23 CC codes: See PDX Collection 3685-3693
  G23.0 **Hallervorden-Spatz disease** 🦴🦴
        Pigmentary pallidal degeneration
  G23.1 **Progressive supranuclear ophthalmoplegia [Steele-Richardson-Olszewski]** 🦴🦴
        Progressive supranuclear palsy
  G23.2 **Striatonigral degeneration** 🦴🦴
  G23.8 **Other specified degenerative diseases of basal ganglia** 🦴🦴
        Calcification of basal ganglia
  G23.9 **Degenerative disease of basal ganglia, unspecified** 🦴🦴

● G24 **Dystonia**
  Involuntary movements
    Includes dyskinesia
    Excludes2 athetoid cerebral palsy (G80.3)
● G24.0 **Drug induced dystonia**
        Use additional code for adverse effect, if applicable, to identify drug (T36-T50 with fifth or sixth character 5)
    G24.01 **Drug induced subacute dyskinesia**
        Drug induced blepharospasm
        Drug induced orofacial dyskinesia
        Neuroleptic induced tardive dyskinesia
        Tardive dyskinesia
    G24.02 **Drug induced acute dystonia** 🦴
        Acute dystonic reaction to drugs
        Neuroleptic induced acute dystonia
        (Ex:) See PDX Collection 3695
    G24.09 **Other drug induced dystonia** 🦴
        (Ex:) See PDX Collection 3697
  G24.1 **Genetic torsion dystonia**
        Dystonia deformans progressiva
        Dystonia musculorum deformans
        Familial torsion dystonia
        Idiopathic familial dystonia
        Idiopathic (torsion) dystonia NOS
        (Schwalbe-) Ziehen-Oppenheim disease
  G24.2 **Idiopathic nonfamilial dystonia** 🦴
        (Ex:) See PDX Collection 3699

G24.3　**Spasmodic torticollis**
　　　　Head tilts toward one side and chin is elevated and turned
　　　　toward opposite side (wry neck)
　　　　Excludes1　　congenital torticollis (Q68.0)
　　　　　　　　　　　　hysterical torticollis (F44.4)
　　　　　　　　　　　　ocular torticollis (R29.891)
　　　　　　　　　　　　psychogenic torticollis (F45.8)
　　　　　　　　　　　　torticollis NOS (M43.6)
　　　　　　　　　　　　traumatic recurrent torticollis (S13.4)

G24.4　**Idiopathic orofacial dystonia**
　　　　Orofacial dyskinesia
　　　　Excludes1　　drug induced orofacial dyskinesia
　　　　　　　　　　　　(G24.01)

G24.5　**Blepharospasm**
　　　　Tonic spasm of orbicularis oculi muscle, producing closure
　　　　of eyelids
　　　　Excludes1　　drug induced blepharospasm (G24.01)

G24.8　**Other dystonia** 🅗
　　　　Acquired torsion dystonia NOS
　　　　Ⓔⓧ See PDX Collection 574

G24.9　**Dystonia, unspecified**
　　　　Dyskinesia NOS

● **G25**　**Other extrapyramidal and movement disorders**
　　　　Extrapyramidal: Other than pyramidal tracts
　　　　Excludes2　　sleep related movement disorders (G47.6-)

G25.0　**Essential tremor**
　　　　Familial tremor
　　　　Excludes1　　tremor NOS (R25.1)

G25.1　**Drug-induced tremor**
　　　　Use additional code for adverse effect, if applicable,
　　　　　　to identify drug (T36-T50 with fifth or sixth
　　　　　　character 5)

G25.2　**Other specified forms of tremor**
　　　　Intention tremor

G25.3　**Myoclonus**
　　　　Shocklike contractions muscle(s)
　　　　Drug-induced myoclonus
　　　　Palatal myoclonus
　　　　Use additional code for adverse effect, if applicable,
　　　　　　to identify drug (T36-T50 with fifth or sixth
　　　　　　character 5)
　　　　Excludes1　　facial myokymia (G51.4)
　　　　　　　　　　　　myoclonic epilepsy (G40.-)

G25.4　**Drug-induced chorea**
　　　　Use additional code for adverse effect, if applicable,
　　　　　　to identify drug (T36-T50 with fifth or sixth
　　　　　　character 5)

G25.5　**Other chorea**
　　　　Continual, involuntary, jerky, movements
　　　　Chorea NOS
　　　　Excludes1　　chorea NOS with heart involvement
　　　　　　　　　　　　(I02.0)
　　　　　　　　　　　　Huntington's chorea (G10)
　　　　　　　　　　　　rheumatic chorea (I02.-)
　　　　　　　　　　　　Sydenham's chorea (I02.-)

● G25.6　**Drug induced tics and other tics of organic origin**
　　　　G25.61　**Drug induced tics**
　　　　　　　　Use additional code for adverse effect, if
　　　　　　　　　　applicable, to identify drug (T36-T50 with
　　　　　　　　　　fifth or sixth character 5)
　　　　G25.69　**Other tics of organic origin**
　　　　　　　　Excludes1　　habit spasm (F95.9)
　　　　　　　　　　　　　　　tic NOS (F95.9)
　　　　　　　　　　　　　　　Tourette's syndrome (F95.2)

● G25.7　**Other and unspecified drug induced movement**
　　　　disorders
　　　　　　Use additional code for adverse effect, if applicable,
　　　　　　　　to identify drug (T36-T50 with fifth or sixth
　　　　　　　　character 5)
　　　　G25.70　**Drug induced movement disorder, unspecified**
　　　　G25.71　**Drug induced akathisia**
　　　　　　　　Drug induced acathisia
　　　　　　　　Neuroleptic induced acute akathisia
　　　　　　　　Tardive akathisia
　　　　G25.79　**Other drug induced movement disorders**

● G25.8　**Other specified extrapyramidal and movement disorders**
　　　　G25.81　**Restless legs syndrome**
　　　　G25.82　**Stiff-man syndrome** 🅗
　　　　　　　　Ⓔⓧ See PDX Collection 575
　　　　G25.83　**Benign shuddering attacks**
　　　　G25.89　**Other specified extrapyramidal and movement**
　　　　　　　　disorders

G25.9　**Extrapyramidal and movement disorder, unspecified** 🅗
　　　　Ⓔⓧ See PDX Collection 575

▷ **G26**　*Extrapyramidal and movement disorders in diseases classified*
　　　　elsewhere
　　　　　Code first underlying disease

OTHER DEGENERATIVE DISEASES OF THE NERVOUS SYSTEM (G30-G32)

● **G30**　**Alzheimer's disease**
　　　　Progressive central neurodegenerative disorder
　　　　Includes　　Alzheimer's dementia senile and presenile forms
　　　　Use additional code to identify:
　　　　　delirium, if applicable (F05)
　　　　　dementia with behavioral disturbance (F02.81)
　　　　　dementia without behavioral disturbance (F02.80)
　　　　Excludes1　　senile degeneration of brain NEC (G31.1)
　　　　　　　　　　　　senile dementia NOS (F03)
　　　　　　　　　　　　senility NOS (R41.81)

G30.0　**Alzheimer's disease with early onset**
G30.1　**Alzheimer's disease with late onset**　　　　　　**A**
G30.8　**Other Alzheimer's disease**
G30.9　**Alzheimer's disease, unspecified**
　　　　Coding Clinic: 2017, Q1, P43; 2016, Q2, P6; 2012, Q4, P95

● **G31**　**Other degenerative diseases of nervous system, not elsewhere**
　　　　classified
　　　　For codes G31.0-G31.83, G31.85-G31.9, use additional code to
　　　　　identify:
　　　　　dementia with behavioral disturbance (F02.81)
　　　　　dementia without behavioral disturbance (F02.80)
　　　　Excludes2　　Reye's syndrome (G93.7)

● G31.0　**Frontotemporal dementia**
　　　　G31.01　**Pick's disease**
　　　　　　　　Primary progressive aphasia
　　　　　　　　Progressive isolated aphasia
　　　　G31.09　**Other frontotemporal dementia**
　　　　　　　　Frontal dementia

G31.1　**Senile degeneration of brain, not elsewhere classified**
　　　　Excludes1　　Alzheimer's disease (G30.-)
　　　　　　　　　　　　senility NOS (R41.81)

CHAPTER 6 (G00-G99)

N Newborn Age: 0　　**P** Pediatric Age: 0–17　　**M** Maternity DX: 9–64　　**A** Adult Age: 15–124　　♀ Females Only　　♂ Males Only

🅒 Complication\Comorbidity　　🅜 Major C\C　　Ⓔⓧ CC/MCC Exclusions　　🅗 Hospital-Acquired Condition　　🅗 Hierarchical Condition Category　　　　807

G31.2   **Degeneration of nervous system due to alcohol**
Alcoholic cerebellar ataxia
Alcoholic cerebellar degeneration
Alcoholic cerebral degeneration
Alcoholic encephalopathy
Dysfunction of the autonomic nervous system due to alcohol
Code also associated alcoholism (F10.-)

● G31.8   **Other specified degenerative diseases of nervous system**

G31.81   **Alpers' disease** 🕮
Rare neuronal degeneration of cerebral cortex disease of young children
Grey-matter degeneration
(Ex:) See PDX Collection 537
Coding Clinic: 2017, Q2, P7

G31.82   **Leigh's disease** 🕮
Rare neurometabolic disorder that affects central nervous system
Subacute necrotizing encephalopathy
(Ex:) See PDX Collection 537

G31.83   **Dementia with Lewy bodies**
Closely allied to Parkinson's Disease
Dementia with Parkinsonism
Lewy body dementia
Lewy body disease
Coding Clinic: 2017, Q2, P7; 2016, Q4, P141

G31.84   **Mild cognitive impairment, so stated**
Mild neurocognitive disorder

| **Excludes1** | age related cognitive decline (R41.81)
altered mental status (R41.82)
cerebral degeneration (G31.9)
change in mental status (R41.82)
cognitive deficits following (sequelae of) cerebral hemorrhage or infarction (I69.01-, I69.11-, I69.21-, I69.31-, I69.81-, I69.91-)
cognitive impairment due to intracranial or head injury (S06.-)
dementia (F01.-, F02.-, F03)
mild memory disturbance (F06.8)
neurologic neglect syndrome (R41.4)
personality change, nonpsychotic (F68.8) |

G31.85   **Corticobasal degeneration**

G31.89   **Other specified degenerative diseases of nervous system**

G31.9   **Degenerative disease of nervous system, unspecified**

● G32   **Other degenerative disorders of nervous system in diseases classified elsewhere**

▷ G32.0   *Subacute combined degeneration of spinal cord in diseases classified elsewhere* 🕮 🕮
Dana-Putnam syndrome
Sclerosis of spinal cord (combined) (dorsolateral) (posterolateral)
Code first underlying disease, such as:
anemia (D51.9)
dietary (D51.3)
pernicious (D51.0)
vitamin B12 deficiency (E53.8)

| **Excludes1** | syphilitic combined degeneration of spinal cord (A52.11) |

(Ex:) See PDX Collection 576

● G32.8   **Other specified degenerative disorders of nervous system in diseases classified elsewhere**
Code first underlying disease, such as:
amyloidosis cerebral degeneration (E85.-)
cerebral degeneration (due to) hypothyroidism (E00.0-E03.9)
cerebral degeneration (due to) neoplasm (C00-D49)
cerebral degeneration (due to) vitamin B deficiency, except thiamine (E52-E53.-)

| **Excludes1** | superior hemorrhagic polioencephalitis [Wernicke's encephalopathy] (E51.2) |

▷ G32.81   *Cerebellar ataxia in diseases classified elsewhere* 🕮 🕮
Code first underlying disease, such as:
celiac disease (with gluten ataxia) (K90.0)
cerebellar ataxia (in) neoplastic disease (paraneoplastic cerebellar degeneration) (C00-D49)
non-celiac gluten ataxia (M35.9)

| **Excludes1** | systemic atrophy primarily affecting the central nervous system in alcoholic cerebellar ataxia (G31.2)
systemic atrophy primarily affecting the central nervous system in myxedema (G13.2) |

(Ex:) See PDX Collection 567

▷ G32.89   *Other specified degenerative disorders of nervous system in diseases classified elsewhere*
Degenerative encephalopathy in diseases classified elsewhere

Item 6–3   Multiple sclerosis (MS) is a nervous system disease affecting the brain and spinal cord by damaging the myelin sheath surrounding and protecting nerve cells. The damage slows down/blocks messages between the brain and body. Symptoms are visual disturbances, muscle weakness, coordination and balance issues, numbness, prickling, thinking and memory problems. The cause is unknown, though it is thought that it may be an autoimmune disease. It affects women more than men, between 20 and 40 years of age. MS can be mild, but it may cause the loss of ability to write, walk, and speak. There is no cure, but medication may slow or control symptoms.

DEMYELINATING DISEASES OF THE CENTRAL NERVOUS SYSTEM (G35-G37)

G35   **Multiple sclerosis** 🕮
Destruction of central nervous system; four types: relapsing remitting, secondary progressive, primary progressive, and progressive relapsing
Disseminated multiple sclerosis
Generalized multiple sclerosis
Multiple sclerosis NOS
Multiple sclerosis of brain stem
Multiple sclerosis of cord
Coding Clinic: 2021, Q1, P7

● G36   **Other acute disseminated demyelination**

| **Excludes1** | postinfectious encephalitis and encephalomyelitis NOS (G04.01) |

(Ex:) For category G36 CC codes unless otherwise indicated: See PDX Collection 578

G36.0   **Neuromyelitis optica [Devic]** 🕮 🕮
Inflammatory disorder in which immune system attacks optic nerves and spinal cord producing inflammation of optic nerve (optic neuritis) and spinal cord (myelitis)
Demyelination in optic neuritis

| **Excludes1** | optic neuritis NOS (H46) |

(Ex:) See PDX Collection 577

G36.1   **Acute and subacute hemorrhagic leukoencephalitis [Hurst]** 🕮 🕮

G36.8   **Other specified acute disseminated demyelination** 🕮 🕮

G36.9   **Acute disseminated demyelination, unspecified** 🕮 🕮

▶ New   ⇒ Revised   ~~deleted~~ Deleted | Excludes 1 | | Excludes 2 | | Includes | | Use additional | | Code first | Code also | Key words |
OGCR Official Guidelines   ● Unacceptable Principal Diagnosis   X Assign placeholder X   🕮 Use Additional Character(s)   ▷ Manifestation Code   **Coding Clinic**

- **G37   Other demyelinating diseases of central nervous system**
  Destruction of central nervous system
  - **G37.0   Diffuse sclerosis of central nervous system** 🔹🔹
    Periaxial encephalitis
    Schilder's disease
    - **Excludes1**   X linked adrenoleukodystrophy (E71.52-)
    - (Ex:) See PDX Collection 3702
  - **G37.1   Central demyelination of corpus callosum** 🔹🔹
    - (Ex:) See PDX Collection 578
  - **G37.2   Central pontine myelinolysis** 🔹🔹
    - (Ex:) See PDX Collection 578
  - **G37.3   Acute transverse myelitis in demyelinating disease of central nervous system** 🔹🔹
    Acute transverse myelitis NOS
    Acute transverse myelopathy
    - **Excludes1**   acute flaccid myelitis (G04.82)
      multiple sclerosis (G35)
      neuromyelitis optica [Devic] (G36.0)
    - (Ex:) See PDX Collection 580
  - **G37.4   Subacute necrotizing myelitis of central nervous system** 🔹🔹
    - (Ex:) See PDX Collection 4049
  - **G37.5   Concentric sclerosis [Baló] of central nervous system** 🔹🔹
    - (Ex:) See PDX Collection 579
  - **G37.8   Other specified demyelinating diseases of central nervous system** 🔹🔹
    - (Ex:) See PDX Collection 578
  - **G37.9   Demyelinating disease of central nervous system, unspecified** 🔹🔹
    - (Ex:) See PDX Collection 578

EPISODIC AND PAROXYSMAL DISORDERS (G40-G47)

- **G40   Epilepsy and recurrent seizures**
  Note: The following terms are to be considered equivalent to intractable: pharmacoresistant (pharmacologically resistant), treatment resistant, refractory (medically) and poorly controlled
  - **Excludes1**   conversion disorder with seizures (F44.5)
    convulsions NOS (R56.9)
    post traumatic seizures (R56.1)
    seizure (convulsive) NOS (R56.9)
    seizure of newborn (P90)
  - **Excludes2**   hippocampal sclerosis (G93.81)
    mesial temporal sclerosis (G93.81)
    temporal sclerosis (G93.81)
    Todd's paralysis (G83.84)
  - **G40.0   Localization-related (focal) (partial) idiopathic epilepsy and epileptic syndromes with seizures of localized onset**
    Benign childhood epilepsy with centrotemporal EEG spikes
    Childhood epilepsy with occipital EEG paroxysms
    - **Excludes1**   adult onset localization-related epilepsy (G40.1-, G40.2-)
    - **G40.00   Localization-related (focal) (partial) idiopathic epilepsy and epileptic syndromes with seizures of localized onset, not intractable**
      Localization-related (focal) (partial) idiopathic epilepsy and epileptic syndromes with seizures of localized onset without intractability
      - **G40.001   Localization-related (focal) (partial) idiopathic epilepsy and epileptic syndromes with seizures of localized onset, not intractable, with status epilepticus** 🔹🔹
        - (Ex:) See PDX Collection 581
      - **G40.009   Localization-related (focal) (partial) idiopathic epilepsy and epileptic syndromes with seizures of localized onset, not intractable, without status epilepticus** 🔹🔹
        Localization-related (focal) (partial) idiopathic epilepsy and epileptic syndromes with seizures of localized onset NOS
        - (Ex:) See PDX Collection 581
    - **G40.01   Localization-related (focal) (partial) idiopathic epilepsy and epileptic syndromes with seizures of localized onset, intractable**
      - **G40.011   Localization-related (focal) (partial) idiopathic epilepsy and epileptic syndromes with seizures of localized onset, intractable, with status epilepticus** 🔹🔹
        - (Ex:) See PDX Collection 582
      - **G40.019   Localization-related (focal) (partial) idiopathic epilepsy and epileptic syndromes with seizures of localized onset, intractable, without status epilepticus** 🔹🔹
        - (Ex:) See PDX Collection 582
  - **G40.1   Localization-related (focal) (partial) symptomatic epilepsy and epileptic syndromes with simple partial seizures**
    Attacks without alteration of consciousness
    Epilepsia partialis continua [Kozhevnikof]
    Simple partial seizures developing into secondarily generalized seizures
    - **G40.10   Localization-related (focal) (partial) symptomatic epilepsy and epileptic syndromes with simple partial seizures, not intractable**
      Localization-related (focal) (partial) symptomatic epilepsy and epileptic syndromes with simple partial seizures without intractability
      - **G40.101   Localization-related (focal) (partial) symptomatic epilepsy and epileptic syndromes with simple partial seizures, not intractable, with status epilepticus** 🔹🔹
        - (Ex:) See PDX Collection 581
      - **G40.109   Localization-related (focal) (partial) symptomatic epilepsy and epileptic syndromes with simple partial seizures, not intractable, without status epilepticus** 🔹🔹
        Localization-related (focal) (partial) symptomatic epilepsy and epileptic syndromes with simple partial seizures NOS
        - (Ex:) See PDX Collection 581
    - **G40.11   Localization-related (focal) (partial) symptomatic epilepsy and epileptic syndromes with simple partial seizures, intractable**
      - **G40.111   Localization-related (focal) (partial) symptomatic epilepsy and epileptic syndromes with simple partial seizures, intractable, with status epilepticus** 🔹🔹
        - (Ex:) See PDX Collection 582
      - **G40.119   Localization-related (focal) (partial) symptomatic epilepsy and epileptic syndromes with simple partial seizures, intractable, without status epilepticus** 🔹🔹
        - (Ex:) See PDX Collection 582

N Newborn Age: 0   **P** Pediatric Age: 0–17   **M** Maternity DX: 9–64   **A** Adult Age: 15–124   ♀ Females Only   ♂ Males Only
🔹 Complication\Comorbidity   🔹 Major C\C   (Ex:) CC/MCC Exclusions   🔹 Hospital-Acquired Condition   🔹 Hierarchical Condition Category
809

CHAPTER 6 (G00-G99)

CHAPTER 6 (G00-G99)

● **G40.2**   **Localization-related (focal) (partial) symptomatic epilepsy and epileptic syndromes with complex partial seizures**

    Attacks with alteration of consciousness, often with automatisms

    Complex partial seizures developing into secondarily generalized seizures

  ● **G40.20**   **Localization-related (focal) (partial) symptomatic epilepsy and epileptic syndromes with complex partial seizures, not intractable**

      Localization-related (focal) (partial) symptomatic epilepsy and epileptic syndromes with complex partial seizures without intractability

      G40.201   **Localization-related (focal) (partial) symptomatic epilepsy and epileptic syndromes with complex partial seizures, not intractable, with status epilepticus** 🖋️ ℞

          (Ex:) See PDX Collection 581

      G40.209   **Localization-related (focal) (partial) symptomatic epilepsy and epileptic syndromes with complex partial seizures, not intractable, without status epilepticus** 🖋️ ℞

          Localization-related (focal) (partial) symptomatic epilepsy and epileptic syndromes with complex partial seizures NOS

          (Ex:) See PDX Collection 581

  ● **G40.21**   **Localization-related (focal) (partial) symptomatic epilepsy and epileptic syndromes with complex partial seizures, intractable**

      G40.211   **Localization-related (focal) (partial) symptomatic epilepsy and epileptic syndromes with complex partial seizures, intractable, with status epilepticus** 🖋️ ℞

          (Ex:) See PDX Collection 582

      G40.219   **Localization-related (focal) (partial) symptomatic epilepsy and epileptic syndromes with complex partial seizures, intractable, without status epilepticus** 🖋️ ℞

          (Ex:) See PDX Collection 582

● **G40.3**   **Generalized idiopathic epilepsy and epileptic syndromes**

    Code also MERRF syndrome, if applicable (E88.42)

  ● **G40.30**   **Generalized idiopathic epilepsy and epileptic syndromes, not intractable**

      Generalized idiopathic epilepsy and epileptic syndromes without intractability

      G40.301   **Generalized idiopathic epilepsy and epileptic syndromes, not intractable, with status epilepticus** 🖋️ ℞

          (Ex:) See PDX Collection 583

      G40.309   **Generalized idiopathic epilepsy and epileptic syndromes, not intractable, without status epilepticus** 🖋️

          Generalized idiopathic epilepsy and epileptic syndromes NOS

  ● **G40.31**   **Generalized idiopathic epilepsy and epileptic syndromes, intractable**

      G40.311   **Generalized idiopathic epilepsy and epileptic syndromes, intractable, with status epilepticus** 🖋️ ℞

          (Ex:) See PDX Collection 583

      G40.319   **Generalized idiopathic epilepsy and epileptic syndromes, intractable, without status epilepticus** 🖋️ ℞

          (Ex:) See PDX Collection 583

● **G40.4**   **Other generalized epilepsy and epileptic syndromes**

    Epilepsy with grand mal seizures on awakening
    Epilepsy with myoclonic absences
    Epilepsy with myoclonic-astatic seizures
    Grand mal seizure NOS
    Nonspecific atonic epileptic seizures
    Nonspecific clonic epileptic seizures
    Nonspecific myoclonic epileptic seizures
    Nonspecific tonic epileptic seizures
    Nonspecific tonic-clonic epileptic seizures
    Symptomatic early myoclonic encephalopathy

  ● **G40.40**   **Other generalized epilepsy and epileptic syndromes, not intractable**

      Other generalized epilepsy and epileptic syndromes without intractability
      Other generalized epilepsy and epileptic syndromes NOS

      G40.401   **Other generalized epilepsy and epileptic syndromes, not intractable, with status epilepticus** ℞

      G40.409   **Other generalized epilepsy and epileptic syndromes, not intractable, without status epilepticus** ℞

  ● **G40.41**   **Other generalized epilepsy and epileptic syndromes, intractable**

      G40.411   **Other generalized epilepsy and epileptic syndromes, intractable, with status epilepticus** 🖋️ ℞

          (Ex:) See PDX Collection 582

      G40.419   **Other generalized epilepsy and epileptic syndromes, intractable, without status epilepticus** 🖋️ ℞

          (Ex:) See PDX Collection 582

    G40.42   **Cyclin-Dependent Kinase-Like 5 Deficiency Disorder**

      CDKL5

      Use additional code, if known, to identify associated manifestations, such as:
        cortical blindness (H47.61-)
        global developmental delay (F88)

● **G40.5**   **Epileptic seizures related to external causes**

    Epileptic seizures related to alcohol
    Epileptic seizures related to drugs
    Epileptic seizures related to hormonal changes
    Epileptic seizures related to sleep deprivation
    Epileptic seizures related to stress

    Code also, if applicable, associated epilepsy and recurrent seizures (G40.-)

    Use additional code for adverse effect, if applicable, to identify drug (T36-T50 with fifth or sixth character 5)

    (Ex:) For category G40.5 CC codes: See PDX Collection 582

  ● **G40.50**   **Epileptic seizures related to external causes, not intractable**

      G40.501   **Epileptic seizures related to external causes, not intractable, with status epilepticus** 🖋️ ℞

      G40.509   **Epileptic seizures related to external causes, not intractable, without status epilepticus** 🖋️ ℞

          Epileptic seizures related to external causes, NOS

● **G40.8**   **Other epilepsy and recurrent seizures**

    Epilepsies and epileptic syndromes undetermined as to whether they are focal or generalized
    Landau-Kleffner syndrome

    (Ex:) For category G40.8 CC codes unless otherwise indicated: See PDX Collection 582

  ● **G40.80**   **Other epilepsy**

      G40.801   **Other epilepsy, not intractable, with status epilepticus** 🖋️ ℞

          Other epilepsy without intractability with status epilepticus

▶ New   ➡ Revised   ~~deleted~~ Deleted   Excludes 1   Excludes 2   Includes   Use additional   Code first   Code also   Key words

OGCR Official Guidelines   ● Unacceptable Principal Diagnosis   X Assign placeholder X   ● Use Additional Character(s)   ▸ Manifestation Code   **Coding Clinic**

G40.802 **Other epilepsy, not intractable, without status epilepticus** 🔹🔹
    Other epilepsy NOS
    Other epilepsy without intractability without status epilepticus

G40.803 **Other epilepsy, intractable, with status epilepticus** 🔹🔹

G40.804 **Other epilepsy, intractable, without status epilepticus** 🔹🔹

● G40.81 **Lennox-Gastaut syndrome**

G40.811 **Lennox-Gastaut syndrome, not intractable, with status epilepticus** 🔹🔹

G40.812 **Lennox-Gastaut syndrome, not intractable, without status epilepticus** 🔹🔹

G40.813 **Lennox-Gastaut syndrome, intractable, with status epilepticus** 🔹🔹

G40.814 **Lennox-Gastaut syndrome, intractable, without status epilepticus** 🔹🔹

● G40.82 **Epileptic spasms**
    Infantile spasms
    Salaam attacks
    West's syndrome

G40.821 **Epileptic spasms, not intractable, with status epilepticus** 🔹🔹
    (Ex:) See PDX Collection 581

G40.822 **Epileptic spasms, not intractable, without status epilepticus** 🔹🔹
    (Ex:) See PDX Collection 581

G40.823 **Epileptic spasms, intractable, with status epilepticus** 🔹🔹

G40.824 **Epileptic spasms, intractable, without status epilepticus** 🔹🔹

● G40.83 **Dravet syndrome**
    Polymorphic epilepsy in infancy (PMEI)
    Severe myoclonic epilepsy in infancy (SMEI)

G40.833 **Dravet syndrome, intractable, with status epilepticus** 🔹
    (Ex:) See PDX Collection 4007

G40.834 **Dravet syndrome, intractable, without status epilepticus** 🔹
    Dravet syndrome NOS
    (Ex:) See PDX Collection 4007

G40.89 **Other seizures** 🔹🔹
    Excludes1 post traumatic seizures (R56.1)
                 recurrent seizures NOS (G40.909)
                 seizure NOS (R56.9)

● G40.9 **Epilepsy, unspecified**

● G40.90 **Epilepsy, unspecified, not intractable**
    Epilepsy, unspecified, without intractability

G40.901 **Epilepsy, unspecified, not intractable, with status epilepticus** 🔹

G40.909 **Epilepsy, unspecified, not intractable, without status epilepticus** 🔹
    Epilepsy NOS
    Epileptic convulsions NOS
    Epileptic fits NOS
    Epileptic seizures NOS
    Recurrent seizures NOS
    Seizure disorder NOS
    Coding Clinic: 2021, Q2, P3

● G40.91 **Epilepsy, unspecified, intractable**
    Intractable seizure disorder NOS
    (Ex:) For category G40.91 CC codes: See PDX Collection 582

G40.911 **Epilepsy, unspecified, intractable, with status epilepticus** 🔹🔹

G40.919 **Epilepsy, unspecified, intractable, without status epilepticus** 🔹🔹

● G40.A **Absence epileptic syndrome**
    Childhood absence epilepsy [pyknolepsy]
    Juvenile absence epilepsy
    Absence epileptic syndrome, NOS

● G40.A0 **Absence epileptic syndrome, not intractable**

G40.A01 **Absence epileptic syndrome, not intractable, with status epilepticus** 🔹

G40.A09 **Absence epileptic syndrome, not intractable, without status epilepticus** 🔹

● G40.A1 **Absence epileptic syndrome, intractable**

G40.A11 **Absence epileptic syndrome, intractable, with status epilepticus** 🔹🔹
    (Ex:) See PDX Collection 582

G40.A19 **Absence epileptic syndrome, intractable, without status epilepticus** 🔹🔹
    (Ex:) See PDX Collection 582

● G40.B **Juvenile myoclonic epilepsy [impulsive petit mal]**
    (Ex:) For category G40.B CC codes: See PDX Collection 582

● G40.B0 **Juvenile myoclonic epilepsy, not intractable**

G40.B01 **Juvenile myoclonic epilepsy, not intractable, with status epilepticus** 🔹🔹

G40.B09 **Juvenile myoclonic epilepsy, not intractable, without status epilepticus** 🔹🔹

● G40.B1 **Juvenile myoclonic epilepsy, intractable**

G40.B11 **Juvenile myoclonic epilepsy, intractable, with status epilepticus** 🔹🔹

G40.B19 **Juvenile myoclonic epilepsy, intractable, without status epilepticus** 🔹🔹

● G43 **Migraine**
    Note: The following terms are to be considered equivalent to intractable: pharmacoresistant (pharmacologically resistant), treatment resistant, refractory (medically) and poorly controlled
    Use additional code for adverse effect, if applicable, to identify drug (T36-T50 with fifth or sixth character 5)
    Excludes1 headache NOS (R51.9)
                 lower half migraine (G44.00)
    Excludes2 headache syndromes (G44.-)

● G43.0 **Migraine without aura**
    Neurological disorder, generally recurring headaches without early symptom (aura)
    Common migraine
    Excludes1 chronic migraine without aura (G43.7-)

● G43.00 **Migraine without aura, not intractable**
    Neurological disorder, generally recurring headaches without early symptom (aura); resistant to cure, relief, or control
    Migraine without aura without mention of refractory migraine

G43.001 **Migraine without aura, not intractable, with status migrainosus**

G43.009 **Migraine without aura, not intractable, without status migrainosus**
    Migraine without aura NOS

● G43.01 **Migraine without aura, intractable**
    Intractable migraine: Not easily cured or managed; relentless pain from a migraine
    Migraine without aura with refractory migraine

G43.011 **Migraine without aura, intractable, with status migrainosus**

G43.019 **Migraine without aura, intractable, without status migrainosus**

N Newborn Age: 0   **P** Pediatric Age: 0–17   **M** Maternity DX: 9–64   **A** Adult Age: 15–124   ♀ Females Only   ♂ Males Only

🔹 Complication\Comorbidity   🔹 Major C\C   (Ex:) CC/MCC Exclusions   🔹 Hospital-Acquired Condition   🔹 Hierarchical Condition Category

811

CHAPTER 6 (G00–G99)

Item 6–4   Migraine headache is described as an intense pulsing or throbbing pain in one area of the head. It can be accompanied by extreme sensitivity to light (photophobic) and sound and is three times more common in women than in men. Symptoms include nausea and vomiting. Research indicates migraine headaches are caused by inherited abnormalities in genes that control the activities of certain cell populations in the brain.

● **G43.1**   **Migraine with aura**
     Basilar migraine
     Classical migraine
     Migraine equivalents
     Migraine preceded or accompanied by transient focal
         neurological phenomena
     Migraine triggered seizures
     Migraine with acute-onset aura
     Migraine with aura without headache (migraine
         equivalents)
     Migraine with prolonged aura
     Migraine with typical aura
     Retinal migraine
     Code also any associated seizure (G40.-, R56.9)
     Excludes1   persistent migraine aura (G43.5-, G43.6-)

● **G43.10**   **Migraine with aura, not intractable**
     Migraine with aura without mention of
         refractory migraine

     G43.101   **Migraine with aura, not intractable, with status migrainosus**

     G43.109   **Migraine with aura, not intractable, without status migrainosus**
         Migraine with aura NOS

● **G43.11**   **Migraine with aura, intractable**
     Migraine with aura with refractory migraine

     G43.111   **Migraine with aura, intractable, with status migrainosus**

     G43.119   **Migraine with aura, intractable, without status migrainosus**

● **G43.4**   **Hemiplegic migraine**
     Inherited migraine disorder causing temporary paralysis of
         one side of body followed by severe headache and nausea
     Familial migraine
     Sporadic migraine

   ● **G43.40**   **Hemiplegic migraine, not intractable**
     Hemiplegic migraine without refractory
         migraine

     G43.401   **Hemiplegic migraine, not intractable, with status migrainosus**

     G43.409   **Hemiplegic migraine, not intractable, without status migrainosus**
         Hemiplegic migraine NOS

   ● **G43.41**   **Hemiplegic migraine, intractable**
     Hemiplegic migraine with refractory migraine

     G43.411   **Hemiplegic migraine, intractable, with status migrainosus**

     G43.419   **Hemiplegic migraine, intractable, without status migrainosus**

● **G43.5**   **Persistent migraine aura without cerebral infarction**

   ● **G43.50**   **Persistent migraine aura without cerebral infarction, not intractable**
     Persistent migraine aura without cerebral
         infarction, without refractory migraine

     G43.501   **Persistent migraine aura without cerebral infarction, not intractable, with status migrainosus**

     G43.509   **Persistent migraine aura without cerebral infarction, not intractable, without status migrainosus**
         Persistent migraine aura NOS

   ● **G43.51**   **Persistent migraine aura without cerebral infarction, intractable**
     Persistent migraine aura without cerebral
         infarction, with refractory migraine

     G43.511   **Persistent migraine aura without cerebral infarction, intractable, with status migrainosus**

     G43.519   **Persistent migraine aura without cerebral infarction, intractable, without status migrainosus**

● **G43.6**   **Persistent migraine aura with cerebral infarction**
     Visual, motor, or psychic disturbances, paresthesias, and
         related neurologic abnormalities accompanying
         migraine
     Code also the type of cerebral infarction (I63.-)

   ● **G43.60**   **Persistent migraine aura with cerebral infarction, not intractable**
     Persistent migraine aura with cerebral
         infarction, without refractory migraine
     Ⓔ⨯ **For category G43.6 CC codes unless otherwise indicated:**
     See PDX Collection 584

     G43.601   **Persistent migraine aura with cerebral infarction, not intractable, with status migrainosus** 🗲

     G43.609   **Persistent migraine aura with cerebral infarction, not intractable, without status migrainosus** 🗲
         Ⓔ⨯ See PDX Collection 585

   ● **G43.61**   **Persistent migraine aura with cerebral infarction, intractable**
     Persistent migraine aura with cerebral
         infarction, with refractory migraine

     G43.611   **Persistent migraine aura with cerebral infarction, intractable, with status migrainosus** 🗲

     G43.619   **Persistent migraine aura with cerebral infarction, intractable, without status migrainosus** 🗲

● **G43.7**   **Chronic migraine without aura**
     Transformed migraine
     Excludes1   migraine without aura (G43.0-)

   ● **G43.70**   **Chronic migraine without aura, not intractable**
     Chronic migraine without aura, without
         refractory migraine

     G43.701   **Chronic migraine without aura, not intractable, with status migrainosus**

     G43.709   **Chronic migraine without aura, not intractable, without status migrainosus**
         Chronic migraine without aura NOS

   ● **G43.71**   **Chronic migraine without aura, intractable**
     Chronic migraine without aura, with refractory
         migraine

     G43.711   **Chronic migraine without aura, intractable, with status migrainosus**

     G43.719   **Chronic migraine without aura, intractable, without status migrainosus**

● **G43.A**   **Cyclical vomiting**
     Excludes1   cyclical vomiting syndrome unrelated to migraine
         (R11.15)

     G43.A0   **Cyclical vomiting, in migraine, not intractable**
         Cyclical vomiting, without refractory migraine

     G43.A1   **Cyclical vomiting, in migraine, intractable**
         Cyclical vomiting, with refractory migraine

● **G43.B**   **Ophthalmoplegic migraine**

     G43.B0   **Ophthalmoplegic migraine, not intractable**
         Ophthalmoplegic migraine, without refractory
            migraine

     G43.B1   **Ophthalmoplegic migraine, intractable**
         Ophthalmoplegic migraine, with refractory
            migraine

▶ New   ⇒ Revised   ~~deleted~~ Deleted   Excludes 1   Excludes 2   Includes   Use additional   Code first   Code also   Key words
OGCR Official Guidelines   ● Unacceptable Principal Diagnosis   X Assign placeholder X   ● Use Additional Character(s)   ▶ Manifestation Code   Coding Clinic

● **G43.C** Periodic headache syndromes in child or adult

   G43.C0 Periodic headache syndromes in child or adult, not intractable

      Periodic headache syndromes in child or adult, without refractory migraine

   G43.C1 Periodic headache syndromes in child or adult, intractable

      Periodic headache syndromes in child or adult, with refractory migraine

● **G43.D** Abdominal migraine

   G43.D0 Abdominal migraine, not intractable

      Abdominal migraine, without refractory migraine

   G43.D1 Abdominal migraine, intractable

      Abdominal migraine, with refractory migraine

● **G43.8** Other migraine

  ● **G43.80** Other migraine, not intractable

     Other migraine, without refractory migraine

    G43.801 Other migraine, not intractable, with status migrainosus

    G43.809 Other migraine, not intractable, without status migrainosus

  ● **G43.81** Other migraine, intractable

     Other migraine, with refractory migraine

    G43.811 Other migraine, intractable, with status migrainosus

    G43.819 Other migraine, intractable, without status migrainosus

  ● **G43.82** Menstrual migraine, not intractable

     Menstrual headache, not intractable

     Menstrual migraine, without refractory migraine

     Menstrually related migraine, not intractable

     Pre-menstrual headache, not intractable

     Pre-menstrual migraine, not intractable

     Pure menstrual migraine, not intractable

     Code also associated premenstrual tension syndrome (N94.3)

    G43.821 Menstrual migraine, not intractable, with status migrainosus ♀

    G43.829 Menstrual migraine, not intractable, without status migrainosus ♀

      Menstrual migraine NOS

  ● **G43.83** Menstrual migraine, intractable

     Menstrual headache, intractable

     Menstrual migraine, with refractory migraine

     Menstrually related migraine, intractable

     Pre-menstrual headache, intractable

     Pre-menstrual migraine, intractable

     Pure menstrual migraine, intractable

     Code also associated premenstrual tension syndrome (N94.3)

    G43.831 Menstrual migraine, intractable, with status migrainosus ♀

    G43.839 Menstrual migraine, intractable, without status migrainosus ♀

● **G43.9** Migraine, unspecified

  ● **G43.90** Migraine, unspecified, not intractable

     Migraine, unspecified, without refractory migraine

    G43.901 Migraine, unspecified, not intractable, with status migrainosus

      Status migrainosus NOS

    G43.909 Migraine, unspecified, not intractable, without status migrainosus

      Migraine NOS

● **G43.91** Migraine, unspecified, intractable

     Migraine, unspecified, with refractory migraine

    G43.911 Migraine, unspecified, intractable, with status migrainosus

    G43.919 Migraine, unspecified, intractable, without status migrainosus

● **G44** Other headache syndromes

  Excludes1 headache NOS (R51.9)

  Excludes2 atypical facial pain (G50.1)

     headache due to lumbar puncture (G97.1)

     migraines (G43.-)

     trigeminal neuralgia (G50.0)

● **G44.0** Cluster headaches and other trigeminal autonomic cephalgias (TAC)

  ● **G44.00** Cluster headache syndrome, unspecified

     Ciliary neuralgia

     Cluster headache NOS

     Histamine cephalgia

     Lower half migraine

     Migrainous neuralgia

    G44.001 Cluster headache syndrome, unspecified, intractable

    G44.009 Cluster headache syndrome, unspecified, not intractable

      Cluster headache syndrome NOS

  ● **G44.01** Episodic cluster headache

    G44.011 Episodic cluster headache, intractable

    G44.019 Episodic cluster headache, not intractable

      Episodic cluster headache NOS

  ● **G44.02** Chronic cluster headache

    G44.021 Chronic cluster headache, intractable

    G44.029 Chronic cluster headache, not intractable

      Chronic cluster headache NOS

  ● **G44.03** Episodic paroxysmal hemicrania

     Paroxysmal hemicrania NOS

    G44.031 Episodic paroxysmal hemicrania, intractable

    G44.039 Episodic paroxysmal hemicrania, not intractable

      Episodic paroxysmal hemicrania NOS

  ● **G44.04** Chronic paroxysmal hemicrania

     Unilateral headache

    G44.041 Chronic paroxysmal hemicrania, intractable

    G44.049 Chronic paroxysmal hemicrania, not intractable

      Chronic paroxysmal hemicrania NOS

  ● **G44.05** Short lasting unilateral neuralgiform headache with conjunctival injection and tearing (SUNCT)

    G44.051 Short lasting unilateral neuralgiform headache with conjunctival injection and tearing (SUNCT), intractable

    G44.059 Short lasting unilateral neuralgiform headache with conjunctival injection and tearing (SUNCT), not intractable

      Short lasting unilateral neuralgiform headache with conjunctival injection and tearing (SUNCT) NOS

  ● **G44.09** Other trigeminal autonomic cephalgias (TAC)

     Cluster headaches

    G44.091 Other trigeminal autonomic cephalgias (TAC), intractable

    G44.099 Other trigeminal autonomic cephalgias (TAC), not intractable

---

N Newborn Age: 0   **P** Pediatric Age: 0–17   **M** Maternity DX: 9–64   **A** Adult Age: 15–124   ♀ Females Only   ♂ Males Only

Complication\Comorbidity   Major C\C   (Ex) CC/MCC Exclusions   Hospital-Acquired Condition   Hierarchical Condition Category

G44.1   Vascular headache, not elsewhere classified
> **Excludes2**   cluster headache (G44.0)
> complicated headache syndromes (G44.5-)
> drug-induced headache (G44.4-)
> migraine (G43.-)
> other specified headache syndromes (G44.8-)
> post-traumatic headache (G44.3-)
> tension-type headache (G44.2-)

● **G44.2   Tension-type headache**
  ● **G44.20   Tension-type headache, unspecified**
    G44.201   Tension-type headache, unspecified, intractable
    G44.209   Tension-type headache, unspecified, not intractable
      Tension headache NOS
  ● **G44.21   Episodic tension-type headache**
    G44.211   Episodic tension-type headache, intractable
    G44.219   Episodic tension-type headache, not intractable
      Episodic tension-type headache NOS
  ● **G44.22   Chronic tension-type headache**
    G44.221   Chronic tension-type headache, intractable
    G44.229   Chronic tension-type headache, not intractable
      Chronic tension-type headache NOS

● **G44.3   Post-traumatic headache**
  ● **G44.30   Post-traumatic headache, unspecified**
    G44.301   Post-traumatic headache, unspecified, intractable
    G44.309   Post-traumatic headache, unspecified, not intractable
      Post-traumatic headache NOS
  ● **G44.31   Acute post-traumatic headache**
    G44.311   Acute post-traumatic headache, intractable
    G44.319   Acute post-traumatic headache, not intractable
      Acute post-traumatic headache NOS
  ● **G44.32   Chronic post-traumatic headache**
    G44.321   Chronic post-traumatic headache, intractable
    G44.329   Chronic post-traumatic headache, not intractable
      Chronic post-traumatic headache NOS

● **G44.4   Drug-induced headache, not elsewhere classified**
  Medication overuse headache
  Use additional code for adverse effect, if applicable, to identify drug (T36-T50 with fifth or sixth character 5)
  G44.40   Drug-induced headache, not elsewhere classified, not intractable
  G44.41   Drug-induced headache, not elsewhere classified, intractable

● **G44.5   Complicated headache syndromes**
  G44.51   Hemicrania continua
    Persistent unilateral headache
  G44.52   New daily persistent headache (NDPH)
  G44.53   Primary thunderclap headache
  G44.59   Other complicated headache syndrome

● **G44.8   Other specified headache syndromes**
> **Excludes2**   headache with orthostatic or positional component, not elsewhere classified (R51.0)

  G44.81   Hypnic headache
    Benign primary headaches
  G44.82   Headache associated with sexual activity
    Orgasmic headache
    Preorgasmic headache
  G44.83   Primary cough headache
  G44.84   Primary exertional headache
  G44.85   Primary stabbing headache
▶   **G44.86   Cervicogenic headache**
    Code also associated cervical spinal condition, if known
  G44.89   Other headache syndrome

● **G45   Transient cerebral ischemic attacks and related syndromes**
> **Excludes1**   neonatal cerebral ischemia (P91.0)
> transient retinal artery occlusion (H34.0-)

(Ex) **For category G45 CC codes unless otherwise indicated:** See PDX Collection 586
Coding Clinic: 2018, Q2, P9

  G45.0   Vertebro-basilar artery syndrome 🔍
  G45.1   Carotid artery syndrome (hemispheric) 🔍
  G45.2   Multiple and bilateral precerebral artery syndromes 🔍
  G45.3   Amaurosis fugax 🔍
    Transient visual loss in one eye
    (Ex) See PDX Collection 587
  G45.4   Transient global amnesia
    Episode of short-term memory loss, nonrecurrent, lasting few hours
> **Excludes1**   amnesia NOS (R41.3)

  G45.8   Other transient cerebral ischemic attacks and related syndromes 🔍
  G45.9   Transient cerebral ischemic attack, unspecified 🔍
    Spasm of cerebral artery
    TIA
    Transient cerebral ischemia NOS

● **G46   Vascular syndromes of brain in cerebrovascular diseases**
  Code first underlying cerebrovascular disease (I60-I69)
  G46.0   Middle cerebral artery syndrome 🔍
    (Ex) See PDX Collection 586
  G46.1   Anterior cerebral artery syndrome 🔍
    (Ex) See PDX Collection 586
  G46.2   Posterior cerebral artery syndrome 🔍
    (Ex) See PDX Collection 586
  G46.3   Brain stem stroke syndrome
    Benedikt syndrome
    Claude syndrome
    Foville syndrome
    Millard-Gubler syndrome
    Wallenberg syndrome
    Weber syndrome
  G46.4   Cerebellar stroke syndrome
  G46.5   Pure motor lacunar syndrome
    Occlusion of single deep penetrating artery
  G46.6   Pure sensory lacunar syndrome
  G46.7   Other lacunar syndromes
  G46.8   Other vascular syndromes of brain in cerebrovascular diseases

▶ New   ➠ Revised   ~~deleted~~ Deleted   Excludes 1   Excludes 2   Includes   Use additional   Code first   Code also   Key words
OGCR Official Guidelines   ● Unacceptable Principal Diagnosis   X Assign placeholder X   ● Use Additional Character(s)   ▌ Manifestation Code   Coding Clinic

● G47   **Sleep disorders**
     Excludes2   nightmares (F51.5)
                 nonorganic sleep disorders (F51.-)
                 sleep terrors (F51.4)
                 sleepwalking (F51.3)

   ● G47.0   **Insomnia**
       Excludes2   alcohol related insomnia (F10.182,
                       F10.282, F10.982)
                  drug-related insomnia (F11.182, F11.282,
                       F11.982, F13.182, F13.282, F13.982,
                       F14.182, F14.282, F14.982, F15.182,
                       F15.282, F15.982, F19.182, F19.282,
                       F19.982)
                  idiopathic insomnia (F51.01)
                  insomnia due to a mental disorder
                       (F51.05)
                  insomnia not due to a substance or
                       known physiological condition
                       (F51.0-)
                  nonorganic insomnia (F51.0-)
                  primary insomnia (F51.01)
                  sleep apnea (G47.3-)

       G47.00   **Insomnia, unspecified**
            Insomnia NOS

       G47.01   **Insomnia due to medical condition**
            Code also associated medical condition

       G47.09   **Other insomnia**

   ● G47.1   **Hypersomnia**
       Excludes2   alcohol-related hypersomnia (F10.182,
                       F10.282, F10.982)
                  drug-related hypersomnia (F11.182,
                       F11.282, F11.982, F13.182, F13.282,
                       F13.982, F14.182, F14.282, F14.982,
                       F15.182, F15.282, F15.982, F19.182,
                       F19.282, F19.982)
                  hypersomnia due to a mental disorder
                       (F51.13)
                  hypersomnia not due to a substance
                       or known physiological condition
                       (F51.1-)
                  primary hypersomnia (F51.11)
                  sleep apnea (G47.3-)

       G47.10   **Hypersomnia, unspecified**
            Hypersomnia NOS

       G47.11   **Idiopathic hypersomnia with long sleep time**
            Idiopathic hypersomnia NOS

       G47.12   **Idiopathic hypersomnia without long sleep time**

       G47.13   **Recurrent hypersomnia**
            Kleine-Levin syndrome
            Menstrual related hypersomnia

       G47.14   **Hypersomnia due to medical condition**
            Code also associated medical condition

       G47.19   **Other hypersomnia**

   ● G47.2   **Circadian rhythm sleep disorders**
       Disorders of the sleep wake schedule
       Inversion of nyctohemeral rhythm
       Inversion of sleep rhythm

       G47.20   **Circadian rhythm sleep disorder, unspecified type**
            Sleep wake schedule disorder NOS

       G47.21   **Circadian rhythm sleep disorder, delayed sleep phase type**
            Delayed sleep phase syndrome

       G47.22   **Circadian rhythm sleep disorder, advanced sleep phase type**

       G47.23   **Circadian rhythm sleep disorder, irregular sleep wake type**
            Irregular sleep-wake pattern

       G47.24   **Circadian rhythm sleep disorder, free running type**
            Circadian rhythm sleep disorder, non-24-hour
            sleep-wake type

       G47.25   **Circadian rhythm sleep disorder, jet lag type**

       G47.26   **Circadian rhythm sleep disorder, shift work type**

     ▶ **G47.27**   *Circadian rhythm sleep disorder in conditions classified elsewhere*
            Code first underlying condition

       G47.29   **Other circadian rhythm sleep disorder**

   ● G47.3   **Sleep apnea**
       Characterized by episodes in which breathing stops during sleep
       Code also any associated underlying condition
       Excludes1   apnea NOS (R06.81)
                  Cheyne-Stokes breathing (R06.3)
                  pickwickian syndrome (E66.2)
                  sleep apnea of newborn (P28.3)

       G47.30   **Sleep apnea, unspecified**
            Sleep apnea NOS

       G47.31   **Primary central sleep apnea**
            Idiopathic central sleep apnea

       G47.32   **High altitude periodic breathing**

       G47.33   **Obstructive sleep apnea (adult) (pediatric)**
            Obstructive sleep apnea hypopnea
            Excludes1   obstructive sleep apnea of
                       newborn (P28.3)

       G47.34   **Idiopathic sleep related nonobstructive alveolar hypoventilation**
            Sleep related hypoxia

       G47.35   **Congenital central alveolar hypoventilation syndrome**

     ▶ **G47.36**   *Sleep related hypoventilation in conditions classified elsewhere*
            Sleep related hypoxemia in conditions
            classified elsewhere
            Code first underlying condition

     ▶ **G47.37**   **Central** *sleep apnea in conditions classified elsewhere*
            Code first underlying condition

       G47.39   **Other sleep apnea**

   ● G47.4   **Narcolepsy and cataplexy**
       *Cataplexy is a disorder evidenced by seizures including minor slacking of the facial muscles to complete collapse and often affects people who have **narcolepsy**, a disorder in which there is great difficulty remaining awake during the daytime.*

   ● G47.41   **Narcolepsy**
       G47.411   **Narcolepsy with cataplexy**
       G47.419   **Narcolepsy without cataplexy**
            Narcolepsy NOS

   ● G47.42   **Narcolepsy in conditions classified elsewhere**
       Code first underlying condition
     ▶ **G47.421**   *Narcolepsy in conditions classified elsewhere with cataplexy*
     ▶ **G47.429**   *Narcolepsy in conditions classified elsewhere without cataplexy*

CHAPTER 6 (G00-G99)

N   Newborn Age: 0   P   Pediatric Age: 0–17   M   Maternity DX: 9–64   A   Adult Age: 15–124   ♀   Females Only   ♂   Males Only

🔵 Complication\Comorbidity   🔵 Major C\C   (Ex:) CC/MCC Exclusions   🔵 Hospital-Acquired Condition   🔵 Hierarchical Condition Category

815

● **G47.5 Parasomnia**
    Excludes1 alcohol induced parasomnia (F10.182, F10.282, F10.982)
        drug induced parasomnia (F11.182, F11.282, F11.982, F13.182, F13.282, F13.982, F14.182, F14.282, F14.982, F15.182, F15.282, F15.982, F19.182, F19.282, F19.982)
        parasomnia not due to a substance or known physiological condition (F51.8)

G47.50 Parasomnia, unspecified
    Parasomnia NOS
G47.51 Confusional arousals
G47.52 REM sleep behavior disorder
G47.53 Recurrent isolated sleep paralysis
▸ *G47.54 Parasomnia in conditions classified elsewhere*
    Code first underlying condition
G47.59 Other parasomnia

● **G47.6 Sleep related movement disorders**
    Excludes2 restless legs syndrome (G25.81)
G47.61 Periodic limb movement disorder
G47.62 Sleep related leg cramps
G47.63 Sleep related bruxism
    Excludes1 psychogenic bruxism (F45.8)
    Coding Clinic: 2016, Q4, P118
G47.69 Other sleep related movement disorders

G47.8 Other sleep disorders
    Other specified sleep-wake disorder
G47.9 Sleep disorder, unspecified
    Sleep disorder NOS
    Unspecified sleep-wake disorder

★**(See Plate 6 of the Anatomy Illustrations.)**

NERVE, NERVE ROOT AND PLEXUS DISORDERS (G50-G59)

Excludes1 current traumatic nerve, nerve root and plexus disorders - see Injury, nerve by body region
    neuralgia NOS (M79.2)
    neuritis NOS (M79.2)
    peripheral neuritis in pregnancy (O26.82-)
    radiculitis NOS (M54.1-)

● **G50 Disorders of trigeminal nerve**
    Includes disorders of 5th cranial nerve
G50.0 Trigeminal neuralgia
    Syndrome of paroxysmal facial pain
    Tic douloureux
G50.1 Atypical facial pain
G50.8 Other disorders of trigeminal nerve
G50.9 Disorder of trigeminal nerve, unspecified

● **G51 Facial nerve disorders**
    Includes disorders of 7th cranial nerve
G51.0 Bell's palsy
    Facial palsy
G51.1 Geniculate ganglionitis
    Rare disorder with symptoms of severe pain deep in ear, spreading to ear canal, outer ear, mastoid or eye regions
    Excludes1 postherpetic geniculate ganglionitis (B02.21)
G51.2 Melkersson's syndrome
    Melkersson-Rosenthal syndrome
● **G51.3 Clonic hemifacial spasm**
G51.31 Clonic hemifacial spasm, right
    (Ex) See PDX Collection 588, 589, 590
G51.32 Clonic hemifacial spasm, left
    (Ex) See PDX Collection 588, 589, 590
    Coding Clinic: 2018, Q4, P10
G51.33 Clonic hemifacial spasm, bilateral
    (Ex) See PDX Collection 588, 589, 590
G51.39 Clonic hemifacial spasm, unspecified
    (Ex) See PDX Collection 588, 589, 590
G51.4 Facial myokymia
    Involuntary facial muscle movement
G51.8 Other disorders of facial nerve
G51.9 Disorder of facial nerve, unspecified

● **G52 Disorders of other cranial nerves**
    Excludes2 disorders of acoustic [8th] nerve (H93.3)
    disorders of optic [2nd] nerve (H46, H47.0)
    paralytic strabismus due to nerve palsy (H49.0-H49.2)
G52.0 Disorders of olfactory nerve
    Disorders of 1st cranial nerve
G52.1 Disorders of glossopharyngeal nerve
    Disorder of 9th cranial nerve
    Glossopharyngeal neuralgia
G52.2 Disorders of vagus nerve
    Disorders of pneumogastric [10th] nerve
G52.3 Disorders of hypoglossal nerve
    Disorders of 12th cranial nerve
G52.7 Disorders of multiple cranial nerves
    Polyneuritis cranialis
G52.8 Disorders of other specified cranial nerves
G52.9 Cranial nerve disorder, unspecified

▸ *G53 Cranial nerve disorders in diseases classified elsewhere*
    Code first underlying disease, such as:
    neoplasm (C00-D49)
    Excludes1 multiple cranial nerve palsy in sarcoidosis (D86.82)
    multiple cranial nerve palsy in syphilis (A52.15)
    postherpetic geniculate ganglionitis (B02.21)
    postherpetic trigeminal neuralgia (B02.22)

● **G54 Nerve root and plexus disorders**
    Raiculopathy (nerve root disorder) caused by pressure on nerve root, most common cause is herniation of intervertebral disk. Plexus disorders (plexopathies) are due to compression or injury.
    Excludes1 current traumatic nerve root and plexus disorders - see nerve injury by body region
    intervertebral disc disorders (M50-M51)
    neuralgia or neuritis NOS (M79.2)
    neuritis or radiculitis brachial NOS (M54.13)
    neuritis or radiculitis lumbar NOS (M54.16)
    neuritis or radiculitis lumbosacral NOS (M54.17)
    neuritis or radiculitis thoracic NOS (M54.14)
    radiculitis NOS (M54.10)
    radiculopathy NOS (M54.10)
    spondylosis (M47.-)
G54.0 Brachial plexus disorders
    Thoracic outlet syndrome
G54.1 Lumbosacral plexus disorders

Item 6–5 Trigeminal neuralgia, tic douloureux, is a pain syndrome diagnosed from the patient's history alone. The condition is characterized by pain and a brief facial spasm or tic. Pain is unilateral and follows the sensory distribution of cranial nerve V, typically radiating to the maxillary (V2) or mandibular (V3) area.

Item 6–6 The most common facial nerve disorder is **Bell's Palsy,** which occurs suddenly and results in facial drooping unilaterally. This disorder is the result of a reaction to a virus that causes the facial nerve in the ear to swell, resulting in pressure in the bony canal.

▶ New ⇒ Revised ~~deleted~~ Deleted | Excludes 1 | Excludes 2 | Includes | Use additional | Code first | Code also | Key words
OGCR Official Guidelines ● Unacceptable Principal Diagnosis X Assign placeholder X ● Use Additional Character(s) ▸ Manifestation Code **Coding Clinic**

G54.2   **Cervical root** disorders, not elsewhere classified

G54.3   **Thoracic root** disorders, not elsewhere classified

G54.4   **Lumbosacral root** disorders, not elsewhere classified

G54.5   **Neuralgic amyotrophy**
     Parsonage-Aldren-Turner syndrome
     Shoulder-girdle neuritis
     Excludes1   neuralgic amyotrophy in diabetes mellitus (E08-E13 with .44)

G54.6   **Phantom limb syndrome with pain** 🅗
     Sensations (cramping, itching) in a limb that no longer exists

G54.7   **Phantom limb syndrome without pain** 🅗
     Phantom limb syndrome NOS

G54.8   **Other** nerve root and plexus disorders

G54.9   Nerve root and plexus disorder, **unspecified**

▶ *G55*   *Nerve root and plexus compressions in diseases classified elsewhere*
     Code first underlying disease, such as:
     neoplasm (C00-D49)
     Excludes1   nerve root compression (due to) (in) ankylosing spondylitis (M45.-)
           nerve root compression (due to) (in)dorsopathies (M53.-, M54.-)
           nerve root compression (due to) (in)intervertebral disc disorders (M50.1.-, M51.1.-)
           nerve root compression (due to) (in) spondylopathies (M46.-, M48.-)
           ▶nerve root compression (due to) (in) spondylosis (M47.0-, M47.2.-)

★ **(See Plates 472 and 473 on pages 56 and 57.)**

● G56   Mononeuropathies of **upper limb**
     Excludes1   current traumatic nerve disorder - see nerve injury by body region

 ● G56.0   **Carpal tunnel syndrome**
     G56.00   Carpal tunnel syndrome, **unspecified** upper limb
     G56.01   Carpal tunnel syndrome, **right** upper limb
     G56.02   Carpal tunnel syndrome, **left** upper limb
     G56.03   Carpal tunnel syndrome, **bilateral** upper limbs
         Coding Clinic: 2016, Q4, P17

 ● G56.1   Other lesions of **median nerve**
     G56.10   Other lesions of median nerve, **unspecified** side
     G56.11   Other lesions of median nerve, **right** upper limb
     G56.12   Other lesions of median nerve, **left** upper limb
     G56.13   Other lesions of median nerve, **bilateral** upper limbs
         Coding Clinic: 2016, Q4, P17

 ● G56.2   Lesion of **ulnar nerve**
     Tardy ulnar nerve palsy
     G56.20   Lesion of ulnar nerve, **unspecified** upper limb
     G56.21   Lesion of ulnar nerve, **right** upper limb
     G56.22   Lesion of ulnar nerve, **left** upper limb
     G56.23   Lesion of ulnar nerve, **bilateral** upper limbs
         Coding Clinic: 2016, Q4, P17

 ● G56.3   Lesion of **radial nerve**
     G56.30   Lesion of radial nerve, **unspecified** upper limb
     G56.31   Lesion of radial nerve, **right** upper limb
     G56.32   Lesion of radial nerve, **left** upper limb
     G56.33   Lesion of radial nerve, **bilateral** upper limbs
         Coding Clinic: 2016, Q4, P17

 ● G56.4   **Causalgia** of upper limb
     Intense burning pain and sensitivity to slight touch
     Complex regional pain syndrome II of upper limb
     Excludes1   complex regional pain syndrome I of lower limb (G90.52-)
           complex regional pain syndrome I of upper limb (G90.51-)
           complex regional pain syndrome II of lower limb (G57.7-)
           reflex sympathetic dystrophy of lower limb (G90.52-)
           reflex sympathetic dystrophy (G90.51-)
     G56.40   Causalgia of **unspecified** upper limb
     G56.41   Causalgia of **right** upper limb
     G56.42   Causalgia of **left** upper limb
     G56.43   Causalgia of **bilateral** upper limbs
         Coding Clinic: 2016, Q4, P17

 ● G56.8   **Other** specified mononeuropathies of upper limb
     Disease of a single nerve
     Interdigital neuroma of upper limb
     G56.80   Other specified mononeuropathies of **unspecified** upper limb
     G56.81   Other specified mononeuropathies of **right** upper limb
     G56.82   Other specified mononeuropathies of **left** upper limb
     G56.83   Other specified mononeuropathies of **bilateral** upper limbs
         Coding Clinic: 2016, Q4, P17

 ● G56.9   **Unspecified** mononeuropathy of upper limb
     Disease of a single nerve
     G56.90   Unspecified mononeuropathy of **unspecified** upper limb
     G56.91   Unspecified mononeuropathy of **right** upper limb
     G56.92   Unspecified mononeuropathy of **left** upper limb
     G56.93   Unspecified mononeuropathy of **bilateral** upper limbs
         Coding Clinic: 2016, Q4, P17

● G57   Mononeuropathies of **lower limb**
     Excludes1   current traumatic nerve disorder - see nerve injury by body region

★ **(See Plates 544 and 545 on pages 58 and 59.)**

 ● G57.0   Lesion of **sciatic nerve**
     Excludes1   sciatica NOS (M54.3-)
     Excludes2   sciatica attributed to intervertebral disc disorder (M51.1.-)
     G57.00   Lesion of sciatic nerve, **unspecified** lower limb
     G57.01   Lesion of sciatic nerve, **right** lower limb
     G57.02   Lesion of sciatic nerve, **left** lower limb
     G57.03   Lesion of sciatic nerve, **bilateral** lower limbs
         Coding Clinic: 2016, Q4, P1

 ● G57.1   **Meralgia paresthetica**
     Numbness or pain in outer thigh caused by injury to nerve
     Lateral cutaneous nerve of thigh syndrome
     G57.10   Meralgia paresthetica, **unspecified** lower limb
     G57.11   Meralgia paresthetica, **right** lower limb
     G57.12   Meralgia paresthetica, **left** lower limb
     G57.13   Meralgia paresthetica, **bilateral** lower limbs
         Coding Clinic: 2016, Q4, P1

 ● G57.2   Lesion of **femoral nerve**
     G57.20   Lesion of femoral nerve, **unspecified** lower limb
     G57.21   Lesion of femoral nerve, **right** lower limb
     G57.22   Lesion of femoral nerve, **left** lower limb
     G57.23   Lesion of femoral nerve, **bilateral** lower limbs
         Coding Clinic: 2016, Q4, P1

CHAPTER 6 (G00-G99)

N Newborn Age: 0   **P** Pediatric Age: 0–17   **M** Maternity DX: 9–64   **A** Adult Age: 15–124   ♀ Females Only   ♂ Males Only

🅒 Complication\Comorbidity   🅜 Major C\C   Ⓔ CC/MCC Exclusions   🅗 Hospital-Acquired Condition   🅗 Hierarchical Condition Category

817

● G57.3   Lesion of lateral popliteal nerve
           Peroneal nerve palsy
    G57.30   Lesion of lateral popliteal nerve, unspecified
             lower limb
    G57.31   Lesion of lateral popliteal nerve, right lower
             limb
    G57.32   Lesion of lateral popliteal nerve, left lower limb
    G57.33   Lesion of lateral popliteal nerve, bilateral lower
             limbs
             Coding Clinic: 2016, Q4, P1

● G57.4   Lesion of medial popliteal nerve
    G57.40   Lesion of medial popliteal nerve, unspecified
             lower limb
    G57.41   Lesion of medial popliteal nerve, right lower
             limb
    G57.42   Lesion of medial popliteal nerve, left lower
             limb
    G57.43   Lesion of medial popliteal nerve, bilateral
             lower limbs
             Coding Clinic: 2016, Q4, P1

● G57.5   Tarsal tunnel syndrome
    G57.50   Tarsal tunnel syndrome, unspecified lower limb
    G57.51   Tarsal tunnel syndrome, right lower limb
    G57.52   Tarsal tunnel syndrome, left lower limb
    G57.53   Tarsal tunnel syndrome, bilateral lower limbs
             Coding Clinic: 2016, Q4, P1

● G57.6   Lesion of plantar nerve
           Morton's metatarsalgia
    G57.60   Lesion of plantar nerve, unspecified lower limb
    G57.61   Lesion of plantar nerve, right lower limb
    G57.62   Lesion of plantar nerve, left lower limb
    G57.63   Lesion of plantar nerve, bilateral lower limbs
             Coding Clinic: 2016, Q4, P1

● G57.7   Causalgia of lower limb
           Complex regional pain syndrome II of lower limb
           Excludes1   complex regional pain syndrome I of
                       lower limb (G90.52-)
                       complex regional pain syndrome I of
                       upper limb (G90.51-)
                       complex regional pain syndrome II of
                       upper limb (G56.4-)
                       reflex sympathetic dystrophy of lower
                       limb (G90.52-)
                       reflex sympathetic dystrophy of upper
                       limb (G90.51-)
    G57.70   Causalgia of unspecified lower limb
    G57.71   Causalgia of right lower limb
    G57.72   Causalgia of left lower limb
    G57.73   Causalgia of bilateral lower limbs
             Coding Clinic: 2016, Q4, P1

● G57.8   Other specified mononeuropathies of lower limb
           Interdigital neuroma of lower limb
    G57.80   Other specified mononeuropathies
             of unspecified lower limb
    G57.81   Other specified mononeuropathies of right
             lower limb
    G57.82   Other specified mononeuropathies of left lower
             limb
    G57.83   Other specified mononeuropathies of bilateral
             lower limbs
             Coding Clinic: 2016, Q4, P17

● G57.9   Unspecified mononeuropathy of lower limb
    G57.90   Unspecified mononeuropathy of unspecified
             lower limb
    G57.91   Unspecified mononeuropathy of right lower
             limb
    G57.92   Unspecified mononeuropathy of left lower limb
    G57.93   Unspecified mononeuropathy of bilateral lower
             limbs
             Coding Clinic: 2016, Q4, P17

● G58   Other mononeuropathies
    G58.0   Intercostal neuropathy
    G58.7   Mononeuritis multiplex
    G58.8   Other specified mononeuropathies
    G58.9   Mononeuropathy, unspecified

▶ G59   *Mononeuropathy in diseases classified elsewhere*
          Code first underlying disease
          Excludes1   diabetic mononeuropathy (E08-E13 with .41)
                      syphilitic nerve paralysis (A52.19)
                      syphilitic neuritis (A52.15)
                      tuberculous mononeuropathy (A17.83)

**POLYNEUROPATHIES AND OTHER DISORDERS OF
THE PERIPHERAL NERVOUS SYSTEM (G60-G65)**

Excludes1   neuralgia NOS (M79.2)
            neuritis NOS (M79.2)
            peripheral neuritis in pregnancy (O26.82-)
            radiculitis NOS (M54.10)

● G60   Hereditary and idiopathic neuropathy
    G60.0   **Hereditary motor and sensory neuropathy**
             Charcot-Marie-Tooth disease
             Déjerine-Sottas disease
             Hereditary motor and sensory neuropathy, types I-IV
             Hypertrophic neuropathy of infancy
             Peroneal muscular atrophy (axonal type) (hypertrophic
                type)
             Roussy-Lévy syndrome
    G60.1   **Refsum's disease** 🔗
             Genetic disorder affecting fatty acid metabolism
             Infantile Refsum disease
             (Ex:) See PDX Collection 588
    G60.2   Neuropathy in association with hereditary ataxia
    G60.3   Idiopathic progressive neuropathy
    G60.8   **Other hereditary and idiopathic neuropathies**
             Dominantly inherited sensory neuropathy
             Morvan's disease
             Nelaton's syndrome
             Recessively inherited sensory neuropathy
    G60.9   Hereditary and idiopathic neuropathy, unspecified

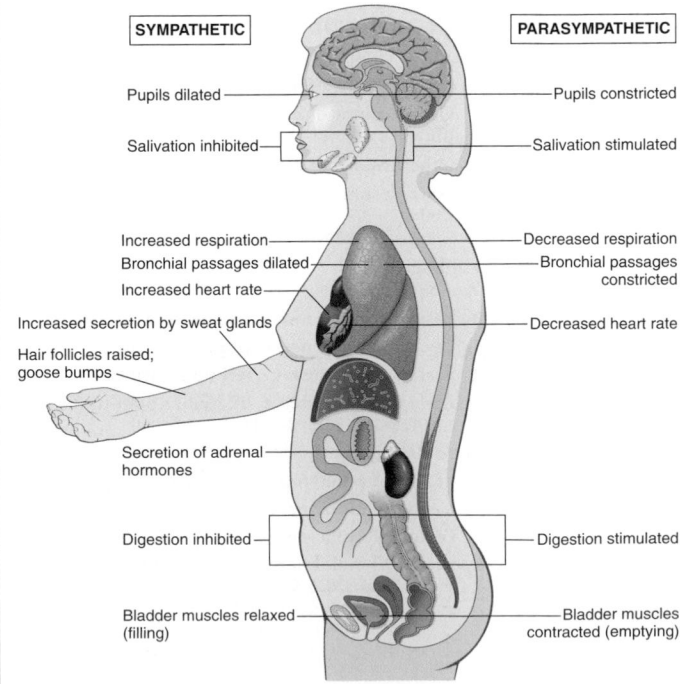

Figure 6-2 Actions of parasympathetic and sympathetic nerves. (From
Chabner: The Language of Medicine, ed 9, St. Louis, Saunders, 2011)

▶ New   ⇒ Revised   ~~deleted~~ Deleted   Excludes 1   Excludes 2   Includes   Use additional   Code first   Code also   Key words
OGCR Official Guidelines   ● Unacceptable Principal Diagnosis   X Assign placeholder X   ● Use Additional Character(s)   ▶ Manifestation Code   Coding Clinic

CHAPTER 6 (G00-G99)

Item 6–7 The **peripheral nervous system** consists of 31 pairs of spinal nerves, 12 pairs of cranial nerves, and the autonomic nerves, which are divided into the parasympathetic and sympathetic nerves. The cranial nerves are: olfactory (I), optic (II), oculomotor (III), trochlear (IV), trigeminal (V), abducens (VI), facial (VII), vestibulocochlear (VIII), glossopharyngeal (IX), vagus (X), accessory (XI), and hypoglossal (XII).

● **G61**   Inflammatory polyneuropathy
    G61.0   **Guillain-Barré syndrome** 🔖🔖
       Autoimmune disease affecting peripheral nervous system
       Acute (post-)infective polyneuritis
       Miller Fisher Syndrome
       (Ex:) See PDX Collection 92
    G61.1   **Serum neuropathy** 🔖
       Use additional code for adverse effect, if applicable, to identify serum (T50.-)
   ● **G61.8**   Other inflammatory polyneuropathies
       G61.81   **Chronic inflammatory demyelinating polyneuritis** 🔖🔖
          (Ex:) See PDX Collection 589
       G61.82   **Multifocal motor neuropathy** 🔖
          MMN
       G61.89   **Other inflammatory polyneuropathies** 🔖
    G61.9   Inflammatory polyneuropathy, unspecified 🔖

● **G62**   Other and unspecified polyneuropathies
    G62.0   Drug-induced polyneuropathy 🔖
       Use additional code for adverse effect, if applicable, to identify drug (T36-T50 with fifth or sixth character 5)
    G62.1   Alcoholic polyneuropathy 🔖
       Malfunction of many peripheral nerves throughout the body
       Coding Clinic: 2019, Q3, P8
    G62.2   Polyneuropathy due to other toxic agents 🔖
       Code first (T51-T65) to identify toxic agent
   ● **G62.8**   Other specified polyneuropathies
       G62.81   **Critical illness polyneuropathy** 🔖🔖
          Acute motor neuropathy
          (Ex:) See PDX Collection 590
       G62.82   **Radiation-induced polyneuropathy** 🔖
          Use additional external cause code (W88-W90, X39.0-) to identify cause
          Coding Clinic: 2016, Q4, P18
       G62.89   **Other specified polyneuropathies**
          Coding Clinic: 2016, Q2, P11
    G62.9   Polyneuropathy, unspecified
       Neuropathy NOS

▷ **G63**   *Polyneuropathy in diseases classified elsewhere* 🔖
    Code first underlying disease, such as:
       amyloidosis (E85.-)
       endocrine disease, except diabetes (E00-E07, E15-E16, E20-E34)
       metabolic diseases (E70-E88)
       neoplasm (C00-D49)
       nutritional deficiency (E40-E64)
    Excludes1   polyneuropathy (in):
       diabetes mellitus (E08-E13 with .42)
       diphtheria (A36.83)
       ~~infectious mononucleosis (B27.0-B27.9 with 1)~~
       infectious mononucleosis complicated by polyneuropathy (B27.0-B27.9 with fifth character 1)
       Lyme disease (A69.22)
       mumps (B26.84)
       postherpetic (B02.23)
       rheumatoid arthritis (M05.5-)
       scleroderma (M34.83)
       systemic lupus erythematosus (M32.19)
    Coding Clinic: 2021, Q1, P7; 2012, Q4, P100

   G64   Other disorders of peripheral nervous system
       Disorder of peripheral nervous system NOS

● **G65**   Sequelae of inflammatory and toxic polyneuropathies
    Code first condition resulting from (sequela) of inflammatory and toxic polyneuropathies
    G65.0   Sequelae of Guillain-Barré syndrome 🔖
    G65.1   Sequelae of other inflammatory polyneuropathy 🔖
    G65.2   Sequelae of toxic polyneuropathy 🔖

DISEASES OF MYONEURAL JUNCTION AND MUSCLE (G70-G73)

● **G70**   Myasthenia gravis and other myoneural disorders
    Excludes1   botulism (A05.1, A48.51-A48.52)
          transient neonatal myasthenia gravis (P94.0)
   ● **G70.0**   Myasthenia gravis
       Acquired and results in fatigable muscle weakness exacerbated by activity and improved with rest
       G70.00   **Myasthenia gravis without (acute) exacerbation** 🔖
          Myasthenia gravis NOS
       G70.01   **Myasthenia gravis with (acute) exacerbation** 🔖🔖
          Myasthenia gravis in crisis
          (Ex:) See PDX Collection 591
    G70.1   Toxic myoneural disorders 🔖
       Dysfunction at junction of muscle and motor nerve (myoneural junction)
       Code first (T51-T65) to identify toxic agent
    G70.2   Congenital and developmental myasthenia 🔖
   ● **G70.8**   Other specified myoneural disorders
       G70.80   **Lambert-Eaton syndrome, unspecified** 🔖🔖
          Lambert-Eaton syndrome NOS
          (Ex:) See PDX Collection 591
       ▷ **G70.81**   *Lambert-Eaton syndrome in disease classified elsewhere* 🔖🔖
          Code first underlying disease
          Excludes1   Lambert-Eaton syndrome in neoplastic disease (G73.1)
          (Ex:) See PDX Collection 591
       G70.89   **Other specified myoneural disorders** 🔖
    G70.9   Myoneural disorder, unspecified 🔖

● **G71**   Primary disorders of muscles
    Excludes2   arthrogryposis multiplex congenita (Q74.3)
          metabolic disorders (E70-E88)
          myositis (M60.-)
   ● **G71.0**   Muscular dystrophy 🔖🔖
       G71.00   **Muscular dystrophy, unspecified** 🔖
       G71.01   **Duchenne or Becker muscular dystrophy** 🔖
          Autosomal recessive, childhood type, muscular dystrophy resembling Duchenne or Becker muscular dystrophy
          Benign [Becker] muscular dystrophy
          Severe [Duchenne] muscular dystrophy
       G71.02   **Facioscapulohumeral muscular dystrophy** 🔖
          Scapulohumeral muscular dystrophy
          Coding Clinic: 2018, Q4, P12
       G71.09   **Other specified muscular dystrophies** 🔖
          Benign scapuloperoneal muscular dystrophy with early contractures [Emery-Dreifuss]
          Congenital muscular dystrophy NOS
          Congenital muscular dystrophy with specific morphological abnormalities of the muscle fiber
          Distal muscular dystrophy
          Limb-girdle muscular dystrophy
          Ocular muscular dystrophy
          Oculopharyngeal muscular dystrophy
          Scapuloperoneal muscular dystrophy
       (Ex:) See PDX Collection 592

N Newborn Age: 0   **P** Pediatric Age: 0–17   **M** Maternity DX: 9–64   **A** Adult Age: 15–124   ♀ Females Only   ♂ Males Only

🔖 Complication\Comorbidity   🔖 Major C\C   (Ex:) CC/MCC Exclusions   🔖 Hospital-Acquired Condition   🔖 Hierarchical Condition Category

819

CHAPTER 6 (G00-G99)

● G71.1 **Myotonic disorders**
    Inherited disorder that affects muscles tone
    G71.11 **Myotonic muscular dystrophy** 🐾
        Dystrophia myotonica [Steinert]
        Myotonia atrophica
        Myotonic dystrophy
        Proximal myotonic myopathy (PROMM)
        Steinert disease
    G71.12 **Myotonia congenita**
        Acetazolamide responsive myotonia congenita
        Dominant myotonia congenita [Thomsen
           disease]
        Myotonia levior
        Recessive myotonia congenita [Becker disease]
    G71.13 **Myotonic chondrodystrophy**
        Chondrodystrophic myotonia
        Congenital myotonic chondrodystrophy
        Schwartz-Jampel disease
    G71.14 **Drug induced myotonia**
        Use additional code for adverse effect, if
           applicable, to identify drug (T36-T50 with
           fifth or sixth character 5)
    G71.19 **Other specified myotonic disorders**
        Myotonia fluctuans
        Myotonia permanens
        Neuromyotonia [Isaacs]
        Paramyotonia congenita (of von Eulenburg)
        Pseudomyotonia
        Symptomatic myotonia

G71.2 **Congenital myopathies** 🐾🐾
    Excludes2 arthrogryposis multiplex congenita
          (Q74.3)
    (Ex:) **For category G71.2 CC codes:** See PDX Collection 4055
➡ G71.20 **Congenital myopathy, unspecified** 🐾
➡ G71.21 **Nemaline myopathy** 🐾
● G71.22 **Centronuclear myopathy**
    G71.220 **X-linked myotubular myopathy** 🐾
        Myotubular (centronuclear)
          myopathy
    G71.228 **Other centronuclear myopathy** 🐾
        Autosomal centronuclear myopathy
        Autosomal dominant centronuclear
          myopathy
        Autosomal recessive centronuclear
          myopathy
        Centronuclear myopathy, NOS
    G71.29 **Other congenital myopathy** 🐾
        Central core disease
        Minicore disease
        Multicore disease
        Multiminicore disease
    (Ex:) See PDX Collection 592

G71.3 **Mitochondrial myopathy, not elsewhere classified**
    Myopathies associated with increased number of enlarged,
    often abnormal, mitochondria in muscle fibers
    Excludes1 Kearns-Sayre syndrome (H49.81)
          Leber's disease (H47.21)
          Leigh's encephalopathy (G31.82)
          mitochondrial metabolism disorders
            (E88.4.-)
          Reye's syndrome (G93.7)

G71.8 **Other primary disorders of muscles**
G71.9 **Primary disorder of muscle, unspecified**
    Hereditary myopathy NOS

Item 6–8 Muscular dystrophies (MD) are a group of rare inherited muscle diseases. Voluntary muscles become progressively weaker. In the late stages of MD, fat and connective tissue replace muscle fibers. In some types of muscular dystrophy, heart muscles, other involuntary muscles, and other organs are affected. **Myopathies** is a general term for neuromuscular diseases in which the muscle fibers dysfunction for any one of many reasons, resulting in muscular weakness.

● G72 **Other and unspecified myopathies**
    Excludes1 arthrogryposis multiplex congenita (Q74.3)
          dermatopolymyositis (M33.-)
          ischemic infarction of muscle (M62.2-)
          myositis (M60.-)
          polymyositis (M33.2.-)
    G72.0 **Drug-induced myopathy** 🐾
        Use additional code for adverse effect, if applicable,
          to identify drug (T36-T50 with fifth or sixth
          character 5)
        (Ex:) See PDX Collection 593
    G72.1 **Alcoholic myopathy** 🐾
        Use additional code to identify alcoholism (F10.-)
        (Ex:) See PDX Collection 593
    G72.2 **Myopathy due to other toxic agents** 🐾
        Code first (T51-T65) to identify toxic agent
        (Ex:) See PDX Collection 593
    G72.3 **Periodic paralysis**
        Familial periodic paralysis
        Hyperkalemic periodic paralysis (familial)
        Hypokalemic periodic paralysis (familial)
        Myotonic periodic paralysis (familial)
        Normokalemic paralysis (familial)
        Potassium sensitive periodic paralysis
        Excludes1 paramyotonia congenita (of von
             Eulenburg) (G71.19)
● G72.4 **Inflammatory and immune myopathies, not elsewhere classified**
    G72.41 **Inclusion body myositis [IBM]**
    G72.49 **Other inflammatory and immune myopathies, not elsewhere classified**
        Inflammatory myopathy NOS
● G72.8 **Other specified myopathies**
    G72.81 **Critical illness myopathy** 🐾
        Acute necrotizing myopathy
        Acute quadriplegic myopathy
        Intensive care (ICU) myopathy
        Myopathy of critical illness
        (Ex:) See PDX Collection 594
    G72.89 **Other specified myopathies**
    G72.9 **Myopathy, unspecified**

● G73 **Disorders of myoneural junction and muscle in diseases classified elsewhere**
    (Ex:) **For category G73 CC codes:** See PDX Collection 591
● ▸ G73.1 *Lambert-Eaton syndrome in neoplastic disease* 🐾🐾
    Rare autoimmune disorder affecting calcium channels of
    nerve-muscle (neuromuscular) junction
    Code first underlying neoplasm (C00-D49)
    Excludes1 Lambert-Eaton syndrome not associated
          with neoplasm (G70.80-G70.81)
▸ G73.3 *Myasthenic syndromes in other diseases classified elsewhere* 🐾🐾
    Code first underlying disease, such as:
        neoplasm (C00-D49)
        thyrotoxicosis (E05.-)

▶ New   ⇛ Revised   ~~deleted~~ Deleted   Excludes 1   Excludes 2   Includes   Use additional   Code first   Code also   Key words

820   OGCR Official Guidelines   ● Unacceptable Principal Diagnosis   X Assign placeholder X   🐾 Use Additional Character(s)   ▸ Manifestation Code   Coding Clinic

▶ **G73.7** *Myopathy in diseases classified elsewhere*
    Code first underlying disease, such as:
       hyperparathyroidism (E21.0, E21.3)
       hypoparathyroidism (E20.-)
       glycogen storage disease (E74.0)
       lipid storage disorders (E75.-)

    Excludes1   myopathy in:
       rheumatoid arthritis (M05.32)
       sarcoidosis (D86.87)
       scleroderma (M34.82)
      ⇒ Sjögren syndrome (M35.03)
       systemic lupus erythematosus (M32.19)

CEREBRAL PALSY AND OTHER PARALYTIC SYNDROMES (G80-G83)

● **G80**   Cerebral palsy
    Excludes1   hereditary spastic paraplegia (G11.4)

    G80.0   **Spastic quadriplegic cerebral palsy** 🔹🔹
       Congenital spastic paralysis (cerebral)
       (Ex:) See PDX Collection 595

    G80.1   **Spastic diplegic cerebral palsy** 🔹🔹
       Spastic cerebral palsy NOS
       (Ex:) See PDX Collection 596

    G80.2   **Spastic hemiplegic cerebral palsy** 🔹🔹
       (Ex:) See PDX Collection 597

    G80.3   **Athetoid cerebral palsy** 🔹🔹
       Result of damage to cerebellum or basal ganglia responsible
       for processing neuromuscular signals
       Double athetosis (syndrome)
       Dyskinetic cerebral palsy
       Dystonic cerebral palsy
       Vogt disease
       (Ex:) See PDX Collection 598

    G80.4   **Ataxic cerebral palsy** 🔹
       Poor muscle tone and coordination

    G80.8   **Other cerebral palsy** 🔹
       Mixed cerebral palsy syndromes

    G80.9   **Cerebral palsy, unspecified** 🔹
       Cerebral palsy NOS

OGCR Section I.C.6.a.

Dominant/nondominant side

Codes from category G81, Hemiplegia and hemiparesis, and subcategories, G83.1, Monoplegia of lower limb, G83.2, Monoplegia of upper limb, and G83.3, Monoplegia, unspecified, identify whether the dominant and nondominant side is affected. Should the affected side be documented, but not specified as dominant or nondominant, and the classification system does not indicate a default, code selection is as follows:

- For ambidextrous patients, the default should be dominant.
- If the left side is affected, the default is nondominant.
- If the right side is affected, the default is dominant.

● **G81**   Hemiplegia and hemiparesis
    Note: This category is to be used only when hemiplegia (complete)(incomplete) is reported without further specification, or is stated to be old or longstanding but of unspecified cause. The category is also for use in multiple coding to identify these types of hemiplegia resulting from any cause.

    Excludes1   congenital cerebral palsy (G80.-)
       hemiplegia and hemiparesis due to sequela of cerebrovascular disease (I69.05-, I69.15-, I69.25-, I69.35-, I69.85-, I69.95-)
    (Ex:) **For category G81 CC codes:** See PDX Collection 561
    Coding Clinic: 2012, Q4, P106

● **G81.0**   **Flaccid hemiplegia**
    Paralysis of half of body with loss of tone of muscles of
    paralyzed part and absence of tendon reflexes

    G81.00   **Flaccid hemiplegia affecting** unspecified **side** 🔹🔹

    G81.01   **Flaccid hemiplegia affecting** right dominant **side** 🔹🔹

Item 6–9   **Hemiplegia** is complete paralysis of one side of the body—arm, leg, and trunk. **Hemiparesis** is a generalized weakness or incomplete paralysis of one side of the body. If most activities (eating, writing) are performed with the right hand, the right is the dominant side, and the left is the nondominant side. **Quadriplegia,** also called tetraplegia, is the complete paralysis of all four limbs. **Quadriparesis** is the incomplete paralysis of all four limbs. Nerve damage in C1–C4 is associated with lower limb paralysis, and C5–C7 damage is associated with upper limb paralysis. **Diplegia** is the paralysis of the upper limbs. **Monoplegia** is the complete paralysis of one limb.

    G81.02   **Flaccid hemiplegia affecting** left dominant **side** 🔹🔹

    G81.03   **Flaccid hemiplegia affecting** right nondominant **side** 🔹🔹

    G81.04   **Flaccid hemiplegia affecting** left nondominant **side** 🔹🔹

● **G81.1**   **Spastic hemiplegia**
    Paralysis of half of body with spasticity of muscles of
    paralyzed part and increased tendon reflexes

    G81.10   **Spastic hemiplegia affecting** unspecified **side** 🔹🔹

    G81.11   **Spastic hemiplegia affecting** right dominant **side** 🔹🔹

    G81.12   **Spastic hemiplegia affecting** left dominant **side** 🔹🔹

    G81.13   **Spastic hemiplegia affecting** right nondominant **side** 🔹🔹

    G81.14   **Spastic hemiplegia affecting** left nondominant **side** 🔹🔹

● **G81.9**   **Hemiplegia,** unspecified

    G81.90   **Hemiplegia, unspecified affecting** unspecified **side** 🔹🔹

    G81.91   **Hemiplegia, unspecified affecting** right dominant **side** 🔹🔹

    G81.92   **Hemiplegia, unspecified affecting** left dominant **side** 🔹🔹

    G81.93   **Hemiplegia, unspecified affecting** right nondominant **side** 🔹🔹

    G81.94   **Hemiplegia, unspecified affecting** left nondominant **side** 🔹🔹
       Coding Clinic: 2015, Q1, P26

● **G82**   Paraplegia (paraparesis) and quadriplegia (quadriparesis)
    Note: This category is to be used only when the listed conditions are reported without further specification, or are stated to be old or longstanding but of unspecified cause. The category is also for use in multiple coding to identify these conditions resulting from any cause.

    Excludes1   congenital cerebral palsy (G80.-)
       functional quadriplegia (R53.2)
       hysterical paralysis (F44.4)

● **G82.2**   **Paraplegia**
    Paralysis of both lower limbs NOS
    Paraparesis (lower) NOS
    Paraplegia (lower) NOS
    (Ex:) **For category G82.2 CC codes:** See PDX Collection 561

    G82.20   **Paraplegia,** unspecified 🔹🔹
       Coding Clinic: 2017, Q3, P3

    G82.21   **Paraplegia,** complete 🔹🔹

    G82.22   **Paraplegia,** incomplete 🔹🔹

● **G82.5**   **Quadriplegia**
    Paralysis of all limbs; AKA tetraplegia
    (Ex:) **For category G82.5 CC codes:** See PDX Collection 595

    G82.50   **Quadriplegia,** unspecified 🔹🔹

    G82.51   **Quadriplegia, C1-C4 complete** 🔹🔹

    G82.52   **Quadriplegia, C1-C4 incomplete** 🔹🔹

    G82.53   **Quadriplegia, C5-C7 complete** 🔹🔹

    G82.54   **Quadriplegia, C5-C7 incomplete** 🔹🔹

N Newborn Age: 0	**P** Pediatric Age: 0–17	**M** Maternity DX: 9–64	**A** Adult Age: 15–124	♀ Females Only	♂ Males Only

🔹 Complication\Comorbidity   🔹 Major C\C   (Ex:) CC/MCC Exclusions   🔹 Hospital-Acquired Condition   🔹 Hierarchical Condition Category

CHAPTER 6 (G00-G99)

● G83   **Other paralytic syndromes**

Note: This category is to be used only when the listed conditions are reported without further specification, or are stated to be old or longstanding but of unspecified cause. The category is also for use in multiple coding to identify these conditions resulting from any cause.

Includes   paralysis (complete) (incomplete), except as in G80-G82

G83.0   **Diplegia of upper limbs** 🔖🔖

Paralysis affecting limbs on both sides; AKA bilateral paralysis

Diplegia (upper)

Paralysis of both upper limbs

(Ex) See PDX Collection 599

● G83.1   **Monoplegia of lower limb**

Paralysis of limb on one side

Paralysis of lower limb

Excludes1   monoplegia of lower limbs due to sequela of cerebrovascular disease (I69.04-, I69.14-, I69.24-, I69.34-, I69.84-, I69.94-)

Coding Clinic: 2012, Q4, P106

G83.10   **Monoplegia of lower limb affecting unspecified side** 🔖

G83.11   **Monoplegia of lower limb affecting right dominant side** 🔖

G83.12   **Monoplegia of lower limb affecting left dominant side** 🔖

G83.13   **Monoplegia of lower limb affecting right nondominant side** 🔖

G83.14   **Monoplegia of lower limb affecting left nondominant side** 🔖

● G83.2   **Monoplegia of upper limb**

Paralysis of upper limb

Excludes1   monoplegia of upper limbs due to sequela of cerebrovascular disease (I69.03-, I69.13-, I69.23-, I69.33-, I69.83-, I69.93-)

Coding Clinic: 2012, Q4, P106

G83.20   **Monoplegia of upper limb affecting unspecified side** 🔖

G83.21   **Monoplegia of upper limb affecting right dominant side** 🔖

G83.22   **Monoplegia of upper limb affecting left dominant side** 🔖

G83.23   **Monoplegia of upper limb affecting right nondominant side** 🔖

G83.24   **Monoplegia of upper limb affecting left nondominant side** 🔖

● G83.3   **Monoplegia, unspecified**

Coding Clinic: 2012, Q4, P106

G83.30   **Monoplegia, unspecified affecting unspecified side** 🔖

G83.31   **Monoplegia, unspecified affecting right dominant side** 🔖

G83.32   **Monoplegia, unspecified affecting left dominant side** 🔖

G83.33   **Monoplegia, unspecified affecting right nondominant side** 🔖

G83.34   **Monoplegia, unspecified affecting left nondominant side** 🔖

G83.4   **Cauda equina syndrome** 🔖🔖

Aching pain due to compression of spinal nerve roots

Neurogenic bladder due to cauda equina syndrome

Excludes1   cord bladder NOS (G95.89)

neurogenic bladder NOS (N31.9)

(Ex) See PDX Collection 600

G83.5   **Locked-in state** 🔖🔖

(Ex) See PDX Collection 601

● G83.8   **Other specified paralytic syndromes**

Excludes1   paralytic syndromes due to current spinal cord injury-code to spinal cord injury (S14, S24, S34)

G83.81   **Brown-Séquard syndrome** 🔖

G83.82   **Anterior cord syndrome** 🔖

G83.83   **Posterior cord syndrome** 🔖

G83.84   **Todd's paralysis (postepileptic)** 🔖

G83.89   **Other specified paralytic syndromes** 🔖

G83.9   **Paralytic syndrome, unspecified** 🔖

OTHER DISORDERS OF THE NERVOUS SYSTEM (G89-G99)

● G89   **Pain, not elsewhere classified**

Code also related psychological factors associated with pain (F45.42)

Excludes1   generalized pain NOS (R52)

pain disorders exclusively related to psychological factors (F45.41)

pain NOS (R52)

Excludes2   atypical face pain (G50.1)

headache syndromes (G44.-)

localized pain, unspecified type - code to pain by site, such as:

    abdomen pain (R10.-)

    back pain (M54.9)

    breast pain (N64.4)

    chest pain (R07.1-R07.9)

    ear pain (H92.0-)

    eye pain (H57.1)

    headache (R51.9)

    joint pain (M25.5-)

    limb pain (M79.6-)

➥   lumbar region pain (M54.5-)

    painful urination (R30.9)

    pelvic and perineal pain (R10.2)

    shoulder pain (M25.51-)

    spine pain (M54.-)

    throat pain (R07.0)

    tongue pain (K14.6)

    tooth pain (K08.8)

renal colic (N23)

migraines (G43.-)

myalgia (M79.1-)

pain from prosthetic devices, implants, and grafts (T82.84, T83.84, T84.84, T85.84-)

phantom limb syndrome with pain (G54.6)

vulvar vestibulitis (N94.810)

vulvodynia (N94.81-)

G89.0   **Central pain syndrome**

Neurological condition causing intractable pain resulting from damage to CNS

Déjérine-Roussy syndrome

Myelopathic pain syndrome

Thalamic pain syndrome (hyperesthetic)

● G89.1   **Acute pain, not elsewhere classified**

G89.11   **Acute pain due to trauma**

G89.12   **Acute post-thoracotomy pain**

Post-thoracotomy pain NOS

G89.18   **Other acute postprocedural pain**

Postoperative pain NOS

Postprocedural pain NOS

● G89.2   **Chronic pain, not elsewhere classified**

Excludes1   causalgia, lower limb (G57.7-)

causalgia, upper limb (G56.4-)

central pain syndrome (G89.0)

chronic pain syndrome (G89.4)

complex regional pain syndrome II, lower limb (G57.7-)

complex regional pain syndrome II, upper limb (G56.4-)

neoplasm related chronic pain (G89.3)

reflex sympathetic dystrophy (G90.5-)

G89.21   **Chronic pain due to trauma**

G89.22   **Chronic post-thoracotomy pain**

G89.28   **Other chronic postprocedural pain**

Other chronic postoperative pain

G89.29   **Other chronic pain**

▶ New   ⇒ Revised   ~~deleted~~ Deleted   Excludes 1   Excludes 2   Includes   Use additional   Code first   Code also   Key words

OGCR Official Guidelines   ● Unacceptable Principal Diagnosis   X Assign placeholder X   ● Use Additional Character(s)   ▶ Manifestation Code   Coding Clinic

G89.3   **Neoplasm related pain (acute) (chronic)**
     Cancer associated pain
     Pain due to malignancy (primary) (secondary)
     Tumor associated pain

G89.4   Chronic pain syndrome
     Chronic pain associated with significant psychosocial
     dysfunction

● **G90**   **Disorders of autonomic nervous system**
     Excludes1   dysfunction of the autonomic nervous system
              due to alcohol (G31.2)

● **G90.0**   **Idiopathic peripheral autonomic neuropathy**

     G90.01   **Carotid sinus syncope**
            Carotid sinus syndrome

     G90.09   **Other idiopathic peripheral autonomic
             neuropathy**
            Idiopathic peripheral autonomic neuropathy
            NOS

G90.1   **Familial dysautonomia [Riley-Day]** 🧬
     Inherited disorder that affects nerve function

G90.2   **Horner's syndrome**
     Due to damage of the sympathetic nervous system
     Bernard(-Horner) syndrome
     Cervical sympathetic dystrophy or paralysis

G90.3   **Multi-system degeneration of the autonomic nervous
     system** 🧬🧬
     Neurogenic orthostatic hypotension [Shy-Drager]
     Excludes1   orthostatic hypotension NOS (I95.1)
     (Ex:) See PDX Collection 573

G90.4   **Autonomic dysreflexia**
     Syndrome resulting from lesions of spinal cord
     Use additional code to identify the cause, such as:
         fecal impaction (K56.41)
         pressure ulcer (pressure area) (L89.-)
         urinary tract infection (N39.0)

● **G90.5**   **Complex regional pain syndrome I (CRPS I)**
     Reflex sympathetic dystrophy
     Excludes1   causalgia of lower limb (G57.7-)
              causalgia of upper limb (G56.4-)
              complex regional pain syndrome II of
                 lower limb (G57.7-)
              complex regional pain syndrome II of
                 upper limb (G56.4-)
     (Ex:) **For category G90.5 CC codes unless otherwise indicated:** See PDX
     Collection 603

     G90.50   **Complex regional pain syndrome I,
             unspecified** 🧬
            (Ex:) See PDX Collection 602

     ● **G90.51**   **Complex regional pain syndrome I of upper
             limb**

         G90.511   **Complex regional pain syndrome I of
                right upper limb** 🧬

         G90.512   **Complex regional pain syndrome I of
                left upper limb** 🧬

         G90.513   **Complex regional pain syndrome I of
                upper limb, bilateral** 🧬

         G90.519   **Complex regional pain syndrome I
                of unspecified upper limb** 🧬

     ● **G90.52**   **Complex regional pain syndrome I of lower
             limb**

         G90.521   **Complex regional pain syndrome I of
                right lower limb** 🧬

         G90.522   **Complex regional pain syndrome I of
                left lower limb** 🧬

         G90.523   **Complex regional pain syndrome I of
                lower limb, bilateral** 🧬

         G90.529   **Complex regional pain syndrome I
                of unspecified lower limb** 🧬

     G90.59   **Complex regional pain syndrome I of other
             specified site** 🧬

G90.8   **Other disorders of autonomic nervous system**

G90.9   **Disorder of the autonomic nervous system, unspecified**

● **G91**   **Hydrocephalus**
     *Dilatation of cerebral ventricles, accompanied by accumulation of
     cerebrospinal fluid*
     Includes   acquired hydrocephalus
     Excludes1   Arnold-Chiari syndrome with hydrocephalus
              (Q07.-)
              congenital hydrocephalus (Q03.-)
              spina bifida with hydrocephalus (Q05.-)
     (Ex:) **For category G91 CC codes unless otherwise indicated:** See PDX Collection 605

G91.0   **Communicating hydrocephalus** 🧬
     Secondary normal pressure hydrocephalus
     (Ex:) See PDX Collection 604

G91.1   **Obstructive hydrocephalus** 🧬

G91.2   **(Idiopathic) normal pressure hydrocephalus** 🧬
     Normal pressure hydrocephalus NOS
     (Ex:) See PDX Collection 604

G91.3   **Post-traumatic hydrocephalus, unspecified** 🧬

◗ G91.4   *Hydrocephalus in diseases classified elsewhere*
     Code first underlying condition, such as:
         congenital syphilis (A50.4-)
         neoplasm (C00-D49)
         plasminogen deficiency (E88.02)
     Excludes1   hydrocephalus due to congenital
              toxoplasmosis (P37.1)

G91.8   **Other hydrocephalus** 🧬

G91.9   **Hydrocephalus, unspecified** 🧬

G92   **Toxic encephalopathy** 🧬

▶● **G92.0**   **Immune effector cell-associated neurotoxicity syndrome**
     ▶*Code first underlying cause such as:*
         ▶complications of immune effector cellular therapy
            (T80.82)
     ▶Code also associated signs and symptoms, such as
         seizures and cerebral edema
     ▶Code also, if applicable:
         ▶cerebral edema (G93.6)
         ▶unspecified convulsions (R56.9)

     ▶ **G92.00**   **Immune effector cell-associated neurotoxicity
             syndrome, grade unspecified**
            ▶ICANS, grade unspecified

     ▶ **G92.01**   **Immune effector cell-associated neurotoxicity
             syndrome, grade 1**
            ▶ICANS, grade 1

     ▶ **G92.02**   **Immune effector cell-associated neurotoxicity
             syndrome, grade 2**
            ▶ICANS, grade 2

     ▶ **G92.03**   **Immune effector cell-associated neurotoxicity
             syndrome, grade 3**
            ▶ICANS, grade 3

     ▶ **G92.04**   **Immune effector cell-associated neurotoxicity
             syndrome, grade 4**
            ▶ICANS, grade 4

     ▶ **G92.05**   **Immune effector cell-associated neurotoxicity
             syndrome, grade 5**
            ▶ICANS, grade 5

▶ **G92.8**   **Other toxic encephalopathy**
     ▶Toxic encephalitis
     ▶Toxic metabolic encephalopathy
     ▶*Code first poisoning due to drug or toxin, if applicable,
         (T36-T65 with fifth or sixth character 1-4 or 6)*
     ▶Use Additional code for adverse effect, if applicable,
         to identify drug (T36-T50 with fifth or sixth
         character 5)

N   Newborn Age: 0   **P**   Pediatric Age: 0–17   **M**   Maternity DX: 9–64   **A**   Adult Age: 15–124   ♀   Females Only   ♂   Males Only

🧬   Complication\Comorbidity   🧬   Major C\C   (Ex:)   CC/MCC Exclusions   🧬   Hospital-Acquired Condition   🧬   Hierarchical Condition Category

823

▶ G92.9   **Unspecified toxic encephalopathy**
   ▶ *Code first poisoning due to drug or toxin, if applicable,*
     (T36-T65 with fifth or sixth character 1-4 or 6)
   ▶ Use Additional code for adverse effect, if applicable,
     to identify drug (T36-T50 with fifth or sixth
     character 5)
   Disorder or disease of brain caused by chemicals
   ~~Toxic encephalitis~~
   ~~Toxic metabolic encephalopathy~~
   ~~Code first if applicable, drug-induced (T36-T50) or use (T51-T65) to~~
   ~~identify toxic agent~~
   (Ex:) See PDX Collection 606
   Coding Clinic: 2021, Q1, P13; 2017, Q1, P39-40

● G93   **Other disorders of brain**

   G93.0   **Cerebral cysts**
      Arachnoid cyst
      Porencephalic cyst, acquired
      Excludes1   acquired periventricular cysts of newborn
                      (P91.1)
                      congenital cerebral cysts (Q04.6)

   G93.1   **Anoxic brain damage, not elsewhere classified** 🔓🔓
      Permanent brain damage by lack of oxygen perfusion
      through brain tissues.
      Excludes1   cerebral anoxia due to anesthesia during
                      labor and delivery (O74.3)
                      cerebral anoxia due to anesthesia during
                      the puerperium (O89.2)
                      neonatal anoxia (P84)
      (Ex:) See PDX Collection 607

   G93.2   **Benign intracranial hypertension**
      Pseudotumor
      Excludes1   hypertensive encephalopathy (I67.4)
                      obstructive hydrocephalus (G91.1)

   G93.3   **Postviral fatigue syndrome**
      Benign myalgic encephalomyelitis
      Excludes1   chronic fatigue syndrome NOS (R53.82)

● G93.4   **Other and unspecified encephalopathy**
      Excludes1   alcoholic encephalopathy (G31.2)
                      encephalopathy in diseases classified
                      elsewhere (G94)
                      hypertensive encephalopathy (I67.4)
   ⇒ **Excludes2**   toxic (metabolic) encephalopathy (G92.8)
      Coding Clinic: 2017, Q2, P9

      G93.40   **Encephalopathy, unspecified** 🔓
               (Ex:) See PDX Collection 608

      G93.41   **Metabolic encephalopathy** 🔓
               Septic encephalopathy
               (Ex:) See PDX Collection 609
               Coding Clinic: 2017, Q2, P8; 2016, Q3, P42; 2015, Q3, P21

      G93.49   **Other encephalopathy** 🔓
               Encephalopathy NEC
               (Ex:) See PDX Collection 610
               **Coding Clinic: 2021, Q2, P3; 2018, Q4, P16; 2018, Q2, P22;
               2017, Q2, P9**

   G93.5   **Compression of brain** 🔓🔓
      Arnold-Chiari type 1 compression of brain
      Compression of brain (stem)
      Herniation of brain (stem)
      Excludes1   ~~diffuse traumatic compression of brain~~
                      ~~(S06.2-)~~
                      ~~focal traumatic compression of brain~~
                      ~~(S06.3-)~~
                   ▶ traumatic compression of brain (S06.A-)
      (Ex:) See PDX Collection 611

   G93.6   **Cerebral edema** 🔓🔓
      Excludes1   cerebral edema due to birth injury (P11.0)
                      traumatic cerebral edema (S06.1-)
      (Ex:) See PDX Collection 612

   G93.7   **Reye's syndrome** 🔓   P
      Life-threatening neurological condition, usually follows viral
      illness
      Code first (poisoning due to salicylates, if applicable
      (T39.0-, with sixth character 1-4)
      Use additional code for adverse effect due to salicylates,
      if applicable (T39.0-, with sixth character 5)
      (Ex:) See PDX Collection 613

● G93.8   **Other specified disorders of brain**
      G93.81   **Temporal sclerosis**
               Hippocampal sclerosis
               Mesial temporal sclerosis

      G93.82   **Brain death** 🔓
               (Ex:) See PDX Collection 515

      G93.89   **Other specified disorders of brain**
               Postradiation encephalopathy
               Coding Clinic: 2019, Q3, P9; 2016, Q4, P7

   G93.9   **Disorder of brain, unspecified**

▶ G94   *Other disorders of brain in diseases classified elsewhere*
      Code first underlying disease
      Excludes1   encephalopathy in congenital syphilis (A50.49)
                      encephalopathy in influenza (J09.X9, J10.81,
                      J11.81)
                      encephalopathy in syphilis (A52.19)
                      hydrocephalus in diseases classified elsewhere
                      (G91.4)
      Coding Clinic: 2018, Q2, P22; 2017, Q2, P8

● G95   **Other and unspecified diseases of spinal cord**
      Excludes2   myelitis (G04.-)

   G95.0   **Syringomyelia and syringobulbia** 🔓🔓
               (Ex:) See PDX Collection 614

● G95.1   **Vascular myelopathies**
      Excludes2   intraspinal phlebitis and
                      thrombophlebitis, except non-
                      pyogenic (G08)
      (Ex:) **For category G95.1 CC codes: See PDX Collection 603**

      G95.11   **Acute infarction of spinal cord (embolic)
               (nonembolic)** 🔓🔓
               Anoxia of spinal cord
               Arterial thrombosis of spinal cord

      G95.19   **Other vascular myelopathies** 🔓🔓
               Edema of spinal cord
               Hematomyelia
               Nonpyogenic intraspinal phlebitis and
               thrombophlebitis
               Subacute necrotic myelopathy

● G95.2   **Other and unspecified cord compression**
               (Ex:) **For category G95.2 CC codes: See PDX Collection 615**

      G95.20   **Unspecified cord compression** 🔓🔓

      G95.29   **Other cord compression** 🔓🔓

● G95.8   **Other specified diseases of spinal cord**
      Excludes1   neurogenic bladder NOS (N31.9)
                      neurogenic bladder due to cauda equina
                      syndrome (G83.4)
                      neuromuscular dysfunction of bladder
                      without spinal cord lesion (N31.-)
      (Ex:) **For category G95.8 CC codes: See PDX Collection 603**

      G95.81   **Conus medullaris syndrome** 🔓🔓
               Damage to gray matter and/or nerve roots in lower
               end of spinal cord

      G95.89   **Other specified diseases of spinal cord** 🔓🔓
               Cord bladder NOS
               Drug-induced myelopathy
               Radiation-induced myelopathy
               Excludes1   myelopathy NOS (G95.9)

   G95.9   **Disease of spinal cord, unspecified** 🔓🔓
      Myelopathy NOS
      (Ex:) See PDX Collection 615

● **G96**   **Other disorders of central nervous system**
   ● **G96.0**   **Cerebrospinal fluid leak** 🔗

> Code also if applicable:
> intracranial hypotension (G96.81-)
>> **Excludes1**   cerebrospinal fluid leak from spinal puncture (G97.0)
>
> (Ex:) For category G96.0 CC codes: See PDX Collection 4055
> Coding Clinic: 2018, Q2, P13

     G96.00   **Cerebrospinal fluid leak, unspecified** 🔗
> Code also if applicable:
> head injury (S00.- to S09.-)

     G96.01   **Cranial cerebrospinal fluid leak, spontaneous** 🔗
> Otorrhea due to spontaneous cerebrospinal fluid CSF leak
> Rhinorrhea due to spontaneous cerebrospinal fluid CSF leak
> Spontaneous cerebrospinal fluid leak from skull base

     G96.02   **Spinal cerebrospinal fluid leak, spontaneous** 🔗
> Spontaneous cerebrospinal fluid leak from spine

     G96.08   **Other cranial cerebrospinal fluid leak** 🔗
> Postoperative cranial cerebrospinal fluid leak
> Traumatic cranial cerebrospinal fluid leak
> Code also if applicable:
> head injury (S00.- to S09.-)

     G96.09   **Other spinal cerebrospinal fluid leak** 🔗
> Other spinal CSF leak
> Postoperative spinal cerebrospinal fluid leak
> Traumatic spinal cerebrospinal fluid leak
> Code also if applicable:
> head injury (S00.- to S09.-)

   ● **G96.1**   **Disorders of meninges, not elsewhere classified**
     G96.11   **Dural tear** 🔗
> Code also intracranial hypotension, if applicable (G96.81-)
>> **Excludes1**   accidental puncture or laceration of dura during a procedure (G97.41)
>
> (Ex:) See PDX Collection 509

     G96.12   **Meningeal adhesions (cerebral) (spinal)**
   ● **G96.19**   **Other disorders of meninges, not elsewhere classified**
     G96.191   **Perineural cyst**
> Cervical nerve root cyst
> Lumbar nerve root cyst
> Sacral nerve root cyst
> Tarlov cyst
> Thoracic nerve root cyst

     G96.198   **Other disorders of meninges, not elsewhere classified**

   ● **G96.8**   **Other specified disorders of central nervous system**
   ● **G96.81**   **Intracranial hypotension**
> Code also any associated diagnoses, such as:
> Brachial amyotrophy (G54.5)
> Cerebrospinal fluid leak from spine (G96.02)
> Cranial nerve disorders in diseases classified elsewhere (G53)
> Nerve root and compressions in diseases classified elsewhere (G55)
> Nonpyogenic thrombosis of intracranial venous system (I67.6)
> Nontraumatic intracerebral hemorrhage (I61.-)
> Nontraumatic subdural hemorrhage (I62.0-)
> Other and unspecified cord compression (G95.2-)
> Other secondary parkinsonism (G21.8)
> Reversible cerebrovascular vasoconstriction syndrome (I67.841)
> Spinal cord herniation (G95.89)
> Stroke (I63.-)
> Syringomyelia (G95.0)

     G96.810   **Intracranial hypotension, unspecified**
     G96.811   **Intracranial hypotension, spontaneous**
     G96.819   **Other intracranial hypotension**
     G96.89   **Other specified disorders of central nervous system**
   G96.9   **Disorder of central nervous system, unspecified**

● **G97**   **Intraoperative and postprocedural complications and disorders of nervous system, not elsewhere classified**
>> **Excludes2**   intraoperative and postprocedural cerebrovascular infarction (I97.81-, I97.82-)
>
> Coding Clinic: 2016, Q4, P9

   G97.0   **Cerebrospinal fluid leak from spinal puncture** 🔗
> Code also any associated diagnoses or complications, such as:
> intracranial hypotension following a procedure (G97.83-G97.84)
> (Ex:) See PDX Collection 617

   G97.1   **Other reaction to spinal and lumbar puncture**
> Headache due to lumbar puncture
> Other reaction to spinal dural puncture
> Code also, if applicable, any associated headache with orthostatic component (R51.0)

   G97.2   **Intracranial hypotension following ventricular shunting** 🔗
> Code also any associated diagnoses or complications
> (Ex:) See PDX Collection 617

   ● **G97.3**   **Intraoperative hemorrhage and hematoma of a nervous system organ or structure complicating a procedure**
>> **Excludes1**   intraoperative hemorrhage and hematoma of a nervous system organ or structure due to accidental puncture and laceration during a procedure (G97.4-)
>
> (Ex:) For category G97.3 CC codes: See PDX Collection 618

     G97.31   **Intraoperative hemorrhage and hematoma of a nervous system organ or structure complicating a nervous system procedure** 🔗
     G97.32   **Intraoperative hemorrhage and hematoma of a nervous system organ or structure complicating other procedure** 🔗

   ● **G97.4**   **Accidental puncture and laceration of a nervous system organ or structure during a procedure**
> (Ex:) For category G97.4 CC codes: See PDX Collection 509

     G97.41   **Accidental puncture or laceration of dura during a procedure** 🔗
> Incidental (inadvertent) durotomy
> Code also any associated diagnoses or complications

     G97.48   **Accidental puncture and laceration of other nervous system organ or structure during a nervous system procedure** 🔗
     G97.49   **Accidental puncture and laceration of other nervous system organ or structure during other procedure** 🔗

   ● **G97.5**   **Postprocedural hemorrhage of a nervous system organ or structure following a procedure**
> (Ex:) For category G97.5 CC codes: See PDX Collection 619

     G97.51   **Postprocedural hemorrhage of a nervous system organ or structure following a nervous system procedure** 🔗
     G97.52   **Postprocedural hemorrhage of a nervous system organ or structure following other procedure** 🔗

   ● **G97.6**   **Postprocedural hematoma and seroma of a nervous system organ or structure following a procedure**
> (Ex:) For category G97.6 CC codes: See PDX Collection 619

     G97.61   **Postprocedural hematoma of a nervous system organ or structure following a nervous system procedure** 🔗
     G97.62   **Postprocedural hematoma of a nervous system organ or structure following other procedure** 🔗

N Newborn Age: 0   **P** Pediatric Age: 0–17   **M** Maternity DX: 9–64   **A** Adult Age: 15–124   ♀ Females Only   ♂ Males Only

🔗 Complication\Comorbidity   🔗 Major C\C   (Ex:) CC/MCC Exclusions   🔗 Hospital-Acquired Condition   🔗 Hierarchical Condition Category

CHAPTER 6 (G00-G99)

G97.63   Postprocedural seroma of a nervous system organ or structure following a nervous system procedure 🔖

G97.64   Postprocedural seroma of a nervous system organ or structure following other procedure 🔖

● G97.8   Other intraoperative and postprocedural complications and disorders of nervous system

Use additional code to further specify disorder

(Ex:) For category G97.8 CC codes: See PDX Collection 617

G97.81   Other intraoperative complications of nervous system 🔖

G97.82   Other postprocedural complications and disorders of nervous system 🔖

G97.83   Intracranial hypotension following lumbar cerebrospinal fluid shunting 🔖

(Ex:) See PDX Collection 4072

Code also any associated diagnoses or complications

G97.84   Intracranial hypotension following other procedure 🔖

Code also, if applicable:
accidental puncture or laceration of dura during a procedure (G97.41)
cerebrospinal fluid leak from spinal puncture (G97.0)

(Ex:) See PDX Collection 4072

● G98   Other disorders of nervous system not elsewhere classified

Includes   nervous system disorder NOS

G98.0   Neurogenic arthritis, not elsewhere classified
Nonsyphilitic neurogenic arthropathy NEC
Nonsyphilitic neurogenic spondylopathy NEC

Excludes1   spondylopathy (in):
syringomyelia and syringobulbia (G95.0)
tabes dorsalis (A52.11)

G98.8   Other disorders of nervous system
Nervous system disorder NOS

● G99   Other disorders of nervous system in diseases classified elsewhere

▶ G99.0   Autonomic neuropathy in diseases classified elsewhere 🔖

Code first underlying disease, such as:
amyloidosis (E85.-)
gout (M1A.-, M10.-)
hyperthyroidism (E05.-)

Excludes1   diabetic autonomic neuropathy (E08-E13 with .43)

(Ex:) See PDX Collection 620

▶ G99.2   Myelopathy in diseases classified elsewhere 🔖🔖

Code first underlying disease, such as:
neoplasm (C00-D49)

Excludes1   myelopathy in:
intervertebral disease (M50.0-, M51.0-)
spondylosis (M47.0-, M47.1-)

(Ex:) See PDX Collection 603

▶ G99.8   Other specified disorders of nervous system in diseases classified elsewhere

Code first underlying disorder, such as:
amyloidosis (E85.-)
avitaminosis (E56.9)

Excludes1   nervous system involvement in:
cysticercosis (B69.0)
rubella (B06.0-)
syphilis (A52.1-)

CHAPTER 7

DISEASES OF THE EYE AND ADNEXA (H00–H59)

OGCR Chapter-Specific Coding Guidelines

> 7. Chapter 7: Diseases of the Eye and Adnexa (H00-H59)
>
>   a. Glaucoma
>
>   1) Assigning Glaucoma Codes
> Assign as many codes from category H40, Glaucoma, as needed to identify the type of glaucoma, the affected eye, and the glaucoma stage.
>
>   2) Bilateral glaucoma with same type and stage
> When a patient has bilateral glaucoma and both eyes are documented as being the same type and stage, and there is a code for bilateral glaucoma, report only the code for the type of glaucoma, bilateral, with the seventh character for the stage.
>
>   When a patient has bilateral glaucoma and both eyes are documented as being the same type and stage, and the classification does not provide a code for bilateral glaucoma (i.e., subcategories H40.10, H40.11, and H40.20) report only one code for the type of glaucoma with the appropriate seventh character for the stage.
>
>   3) Bilateral glaucoma stage with different types or stages
> When a patient has bilateral glaucoma and each eye is documented as having a different type or stage, and the classification distinguishes laterality, assign the appropriate code for each eye rather than the code for bilateral glaucoma.
>
>   When a patient has bilateral glaucoma and each eye is documented as having a different type, and the classification does not distinguish laterality (i.e., subcategories H40.10, H40.11 and H40.20), assign one code for each type of glaucoma with the appropriate seventh character for the stage.
>
>   When a patient has bilateral glaucoma and each eye is documented as having the same type, but different stage, and the classification does not distinguish laterality (i.e., subcategories H40.10, H40.11, and H40.20), assign a code for the type of glaucoma for each eye with the seventh character for the specific glaucoma stage documented for each eye.
>
>   4) Patient admitted with glaucoma and stage evolves during the admission
> If a patient is admitted with glaucoma and the stage progresses during the admission, assign the code for highest stage documented.
>
>   5) Indeterminate stage glaucoma
> Assignment of the seventh character "4" for "indeterminate stage" should be based on the clinical documentation. The seventh character "4" is used for glaucomas whose stage cannot be clinically determined. This seventh character should not be confused with the seventh character "0", unspecified, which should be assigned when there is no documentation regarding the stage of the glaucoma.
>
>   b. Blindness
> If "blindness" or "low vision" of both eyes is documented but the visual impairment category is not documented, assign code H54.3, Unqualified visual loss, both eyes. If "blindness" or "low vision" in one eye is documented but the visual impairment category is not documented, assign a code from H54.6-, Unqualified visual loss, one eye. If "blindness" or "visual loss" is documented without any information about whether one or both eyes are affected, assign code H54.7, Unspecified visual loss.

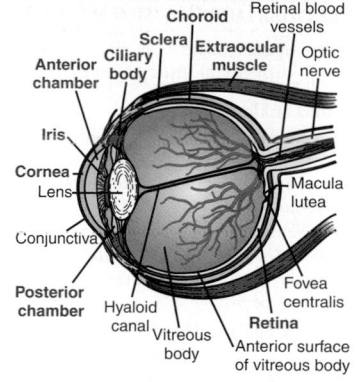

Figure 7–1 Eye and ocular adnexa. (From Buck CJ: Step-by-Step Medical Coding, ed 2016, St. Louis, Elsevier, 2016)

★ **(See Plate 15 of the Anatomy Illustrations.)**

CHAPTER 7

DISEASES OF THE EYE AND ADNEXA (H00–H59)

Note: Use an external cause code following the code for the eye condition, if applicable, to identify the cause of the eye condition

Excludes2 certain conditions originating in the perinatal period (P04-P96)

certain infectious and parasitic diseases (A00-B99)

complications of pregnancy, childbirth and the puerperium (O00-O9A)

congenital malformations, deformations, and chromosomal abnormalities (Q00-Q99)

diabetes mellitus related eye conditions (E09.3-, E10.3-, E11.3-, E13.3-)

endocrine, nutritional and metabolic diseases (E00-E88)

injury (trauma) of eye and orbit (S05.-)

injury, poisoning and certain other consequences of external causes (S00-T88)

neoplasms (C00-D49)

symptoms, signs and abnormal clinical and laboratory findings, not elsewhere classified (R00-R94)

syphilis related eye disorders (A50.01, A50.3-, A51.43, A52.71)

This chapter contains the following blocks:

H00-H05	Disorders of eyelid, lacrimal system and orbit
H10-H11	Disorders of conjunctiva
H15-H22	Disorders of sclera, cornea, iris and ciliary body
H25-H28	Disorders of lens
H30-H36	Disorders of choroid and retina
H40-H42	Glaucoma
H43-H44	Disorders of vitreous body and globe
H46-H47	Disorders of optic nerve and visual pathways
H49-H52	Disorders of ocular muscles, binocular movement, accommodation and refraction
H53-H54	Visual disturbances and blindness
H55-H57	Other disorders of eye and adnexa
H59	Intraoperative and postprocedural complications and disorders of eye and adnexa, not elsewhere classified

N Newborn Age: 0   **P** Pediatric Age: 0–17   **M** Maternity DX: 9–64   **A** Adult Age: 15–124   ♀ Females Only   ♂ Males Only

Complication\Comorbidity   Major C\C   (Ex) CC/MCC Exclusions   Hospital-Acquired Condition   Hierarchical Condition Category   827

DISORDERS OF EYELID, LACRIMAL SYSTEM AND ORBIT (H00-H05)

Excludes2　open wound of eyelid (S01.1-)
　　　　　　　superficial injury of eyelid (S00.1-, S00.2-)

● **H00　Hordeolum and chalazion**
　　Hordeolum: inflammatory staphylococcal infection of sebaceous glands of eyelids; AKA stye. Chalazion: eyelid mass

　● **H00.0　Hordeolum (externum) (internum) of eyelid**
　　　Bacterial infection (staphylococcus) of the sebaceous gland of the eyelid (stye)

　　● **H00.01　Hordeolum externum**
　　　　　Hordeolum NOS
　　　　　Stye

　　　　H00.011　Hordeolum externum right upper eyelid

　　　　H00.012　Hordeolum externum right lower eyelid

　　　　H00.013　Hordeolum externum right eye, unspecified eyelid

　　　　H00.014　Hordeolum externum left upper eyelid

　　　　H00.015　Hordeolum externum left lower eyelid

　　　　H00.016　Hordeolum externum left eye, unspecified eyelid

　　　　H00.019　Hordeolum externum unspecified eye, unspecified eyelid

　　● **H00.02　Hordeolum internum**
　　　　　Infection of meibomian gland

　　　　H00.021　Hordeolum internum right upper eyelid

　　　　H00.022　Hordeolum internum right lower eyelid

　　　　H00.023　Hordeolum internum right eye, unspecified eyelid

　　　　H00.024　Hordeolum internum left upper eyelid

　　　　H00.025　Hordeolum internum left lower eyelid

　　　　H00.026　Hordeolum internum left eye, unspecified eyelid

　　　　H00.029　Hordeolum internum unspecified eye, unspecified eyelid

　　● **H00.03　Abscess of eyelid**
　　　　　Furuncle of eyelid

　　　　H00.031　Abscess of right upper eyelid

　　　　H00.032　Abscess of right lower eyelid

　　　　H00.033　Abscess of eyelid right eye, unspecified eyelid

　　　　H00.034　Abscess of left upper eyelid

　　　　H00.035　Abscess of left lower eyelid

　　　　H00.036　Abscess of eyelid left eye, unspecified eyelid

　　　　H00.039　Abscess of eyelid unspecified eye, unspecified eyelid

　● **H00.1　Chalazion**
　　　Often caused by accumulation of meibomian gland secretions resulting from a blockage of duct.
　　　Meibomian (gland) cyst

　　　Excludes2　infected meibomian gland (H00.02-)

　　　H00.11　Chalazion right upper eyelid

　　　H00.12　Chalazion right lower eyelid

　　　H00.13　Chalazion right eye, unspecified eyelid

　　　H00.14　Chalazion left upper eyelid

　　　H00.15　Chalazion left lower eyelid

　　　H00.16　Chalazion left eye, unspecified eyelid

　　　H00.19　Chalazion unspecified eye, unspecified eyelid

● **H01　Other inflammation of eyelid**

　● **H01.0　Blepharitis**
　　　Inflammation of eyelids

　　　Excludes1　blepharoconjunctivitis (H10.5-)

　　● **H01.00　Unspecified blepharitis**

　　　　H01.001　Unspecified blepharitis right upper eyelid

　　　　H01.002　Unspecified blepharitis right lower eyelid

　　　　H01.003　Unspecified blepharitis right eye, unspecified eyelid

　　　　H01.004　Unspecified blepharitis left upper eyelid

　　　　H01.005　Unspecified blepharitis left lower eyelid

　　　　H01.006　Unspecified blepharitis left eye, unspecified eyelid

　　　　H01.009　Unspecified blepharitis unspecified eye, unspecified eyelid

　　　　H01.00A　Unspecified blepharitis right eye, upper and lower eyelids

　　　　H01.00B　Unspecified blepharitis left eye, upper and lower eyelids

　　● **H01.01　Ulcerative blepharitis**

　　　　H01.011　Ulcerative blepharitis right upper eyelid

　　　　H01.012　Ulcerative blepharitis right lower eyelid

　　　　H01.013　Ulcerative blepharitis right eye, unspecified eyelid

　　　　H01.014　Ulcerative blepharitis left upper eyelid

　　　　H01.015　Ulcerative blepharitis left lower eyelid

　　　　H01.016　Ulcerative blepharitis left eye, unspecified eyelid

　　　　H01.019　Ulcerative blepharitis unspecified eye, unspecified eyelid

　　　　H01.01A　Ulcerative blepharitis right eye, upper and lower eyelids

　　　　H01.01B　Ulcerative blepharitis left eye, upper and lower eyelids

　　● **H01.02　Squamous blepharitis**

　　　　H01.021　Squamous blepharitis right upper eyelid

　　　　H01.022　Squamous blepharitis right lower eyelid

　　　　H01.023　Squamous blepharitis right eye, unspecified eyelid

　　　　H01.024　Squamous blepharitis left upper eyelid

　　　　H01.025　Squamous blepharitis left lower eyelid

　　　　H01.026　Squamous blepharitis left eye, unspecified eyelid

　　　　H01.029　Squamous blepharitis unspecified eye, unspecified eyelid

　　　　H01.02A　Squamous blepharitis right eye, upper and lower eyelids

　　　　H01.02B　Squamous blepharitis left eye, upper and lower eyelids

　● **H01.1　Noninfectious dermatoses of eyelid**

　　● **H01.11　Allergic dermatitis of eyelid**
　　　　　Contact dermatitis of eyelid

　　　　H01.111　Allergic dermatitis of right upper eyelid

　　　　H01.112　Allergic dermatitis of right lower eyelid

　　　　H01.113　Allergic dermatitis of right eye, unspecified eyelid

---

▶ New　　⇒ Revised　　~~deleted~~ Deleted　　Excludes 1　　Excludes 2　　Includes　　Use additional　　Code first　　Code also　　Key words

OGCR Official Guidelines　　● Unacceptable Principal Diagnosis　　X Assign placeholder X　　● Use Additional Character(s)　　▷ Manifestation Code　　**Coding Clinic**

H01.114   Allergic dermatitis of left upper eyelid

H01.115   Allergic dermatitis of left lower eyelid

H01.116   Allergic dermatitis of left eye, unspecified eyelid

H01.119   Allergic dermatitis of unspecified eye, unspecified eyelid

● H01.12   Discoid lupus erythematosus of eyelid

H01.121   Discoid lupus erythematosus of right upper eyelid

H01.122   Discoid lupus erythematosus of right lower eyelid

H01.123   Discoid lupus erythematosus of right eye, unspecified eyelid

H01.124   Discoid lupus erythematosus of left upper eyelid

H01.125   Discoid lupus erythematosus of left lower eyelid

H01.126   Discoid lupus erythematosus of left eye, unspecified eyelid

H01.129   Discoid lupus erythematosus of unspecified eye, unspecified eyelid

● H01.13   Eczematous dermatitis of eyelid

H01.131   Eczematous dermatitis of right upper eyelid

H01.132   Eczematous dermatitis of right lower eyelid

H01.133   Eczematous dermatitis of right eye, unspecified eyelid

H01.134   Eczematous dermatitis of left upper eyelid

H01.135   Eczematous dermatitis of left lower eyelid

H01.136   Eczematous dermatitis of left eye, unspecified eyelid

H01.139   Eczematous dermatitis of unspecified eye, unspecified eyelid

● H01.14   Xeroderma of eyelid
Abnormally dry

H01.141   Xeroderma of right upper eyelid

H01.142   Xeroderma of right lower eyelid

H01.143   Xeroderma of right eye, unspecified eyelid

H01.144   Xeroderma of left upper eyelid

H01.145   Xeroderma of left lower eyelid

H01.146   Xeroderma of left eye, unspecified eyelid

H01.149   Xeroderma of unspecified eye, unspecified eyelid

H01.8   Other specified inflammations of eyelid

H01.9   Unspecified inflammation of eyelid
Inflammation of eyelid NOS

● H02   Other disorders of eyelid
Turning inward (inversion) of eyelid margin and ingrowing eyelashes
Excludes1   congenital malformations of eyelid (Q10.0-Q10.3)

● H02.0   Entropion and trichiasis of eyelid

● H02.00   Unspecified entropion of eyelid

H02.001   Unspecified entropion of right upper eyelid

H02.002   Unspecified entropion of right lower eyelid

H02.003   Unspecified entropion of right eye, unspecified eyelid

H02.004   Unspecified entropion of left upper eyelid

H02.005   Unspecified entropion of left lower eyelid

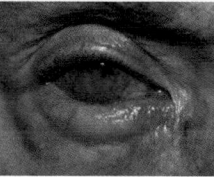

Figure 7-2   Right lower eyelid entropion. Note the inward rotation of the tarsal plate about the horizontal axis and the resultant contact between the mucocutaneous junction and ocular surface. (From Glynn M, Drake WM, Hutchison R: Hutchison's Clinical Methods: An Integrated Approach to Clinical Practice, Edinburgh, Saunders/Elsevier, 2012)

H02.006   Unspecified entropion of left eye, unspecified eyelid

H02.009   Unspecified entropion of unspecified eye, unspecified eyelid

● H02.01   Cicatricial entropion of eyelid
Scar

H02.011   Cicatricial entropion of right upper eyelid

H02.012   Cicatricial entropion of right lower eyelid

H02.013   Cicatricial entropion of right eye, unspecified eyelid

H02.014   Cicatricial entropion of left upper eyelid

H02.015   Cicatricial entropion of left lower eyelid

H02.016   Cicatricial entropion of left eye, unspecified eyelid

H02.019   Cicatricial entropion of unspecified eye, unspecified eyelid

● H02.02   Mechanical entropion of eyelid
Turning inward (inversion) of eyelid margin due to lack of support

H02.021   Mechanical entropion of right upper eyelid

H02.022   Mechanical entropion of right lower eyelid

H02.023   Mechanical entropion of right eye, unspecified eyelid

H02.024   Mechanical entropion of left upper eyelid

H02.025   Mechanical entropion of left lower eyelid

H02.026   Mechanical entropion of left eye, unspecified eyelid

H02.029   Mechanical entropion of unspecified eye, unspecified eyelid

● H02.03   Senile entropion of eyelid
Turning inward (inversion) of eyelid margin due to aging

H02.031   Senile entropion of right upper eyelid   A

H02.032   Senile entropion of right lower eyelid   A

H02.033   Senile entropion of right eye, unspecified eyelid   A

H02.034   Senile entropion of left upper eyelid   A

H02.035   Senile entropion of left lower eyelid   A

H02.036   Senile entropion of left eye, unspecified eyelid   A

H02.039   Senile entropion of unspecified eye, unspecified eyelid   A

● H02.04   Spastic entropion of eyelid
Turning inward (inversion) of eyelid margin caused by spasm of muscle

H02.041   Spastic entropion of right upper eyelid

H02.042   Spastic entropion of right lower eyelid

H02.043   Spastic entropion of right eye, unspecified eyelid

N   Newborn Age: 0   **P**   Pediatric Age: 0–17   **M**   Maternity DX: 9–64   **A**   Adult Age: 15–124   ♀   Females Only   ♂   Males Only

🅒🅒   Complication\Comorbidity   🅜   Major C\C   (Ex)   CC/MCC Exclusions   🅗   Hospital-Acquired Condition   🅗🅒   Hierarchical Condition Category

829

H02.044 Spastic entropion of left upper eyelid
H02.045 Spastic entropion of left lower eyelid
H02.046 Spastic entropion of left eye, unspecified eyelid
H02.049 Spastic entropion of unspecified eye, unspecified eyelid

● H02.05 Trichiasis without entropion
         Ingrowing hairs of eyelashes
H02.051 Trichiasis without entropion right upper eyelid
H02.052 Trichiasis without entropion right lower eyelid
H02.053 Trichiasis without entropion right eye, unspecified eyelid
H02.054 Trichiasis without entropion left upper eyelid
H02.055 Trichiasis without entropion left lower eyelid
H02.056 Trichiasis without entropion left eye, unspecified eyelid
H02.059 Trichiasis without entropion unspecified eye, unspecified eyelid

● H02.1 Ectropion of eyelid
        Eversion (pulling away) of eyelid
● H02.10 Unspecified ectropion of eyelid
H02.101 Unspecified ectropion of right upper eyelid
H02.102 Unspecified ectropion of right lower eyelid
H02.103 Unspecified ectropion of right eye, unspecified eyelid
H02.104 Unspecified ectropion of left upper eyelid
H02.105 Unspecified ectropion of left lower eyelid
H02.106 Unspecified ectropion of left eye, unspecified eyelid
H02.109 Unspecified ectropion of unspecified eye, unspecified eyelid

● H02.11 Cicatricial ectropion of eyelid
        Pulling of eyelid down and away from eye due to scar or tightening
H02.111 Cicatricial ectropion of right upper eyelid
H02.112 Cicatricial ectropion of right lower eyelid
H02.113 Cicatricial ectropion of right eye, unspecified eyelid
H02.114 Cicatricial ectropion of left upper eyelid
H02.115 Cicatricial ectropion of left lower eyelid
H02.116 Cicatricial ectropion of left eye, unspecified eyelid
H02.119 Cicatricial ectropion of unspecified eye, unspecified eyelid

● H02.12 Mechanical ectropion of eyelid
        Eversion (pulling away) of eyelid due to lack of support
H02.121 Mechanical ectropion of right upper eyelid
H02.122 Mechanical ectropion of right lower eyelid
H02.123 Mechanical ectropion of right eye, unspecified eyelid
H02.124 Mechanical ectropion of left upper eyelid
H02.125 Mechanical ectropion of left lower eyelid

H02.126 Mechanical ectropion of left eye, unspecified eyelid
H02.129 Mechanical ectropion of unspecified eye, unspecified eyelid

● H02.13 Senile ectropion of eyelid
        Eversion (pulling away) of eyelid due to age
H02.131 Senile ectropion of right upper eyelid   A
H02.132 Senile ectropion of right lower eyelid   A
H02.133 Senile ectropion of right eye, unspecified eyelid   A
H02.134 Senile ectropion of left upper eyelid   A
H02.135 Senile ectropion of left lower eyelid   A
H02.136 Senile ectropion of left eye, unspecified eyelid   A
H02.139 Senile ectropion of unspecified eye, unspecified eyelid   A

● H02.14 Spastic ectropion of eyelid
        Eversion (pulling away) of eyelid due to tonic muscle spasm
H02.141 Spastic ectropion of right upper eyelid
H02.142 Spastic ectropion of right lower eyelid
H02.143 Spastic ectropion of right eye, unspecified eyelid
H02.144 Spastic ectropion of left upper eyelid
H02.145 Spastic ectropion of left lower eyelid
H02.146 Spastic ectropion of left eye, unspecified eyelid
H02.149 Spastic ectropion of unspecified eye, unspecified eyelid

● H02.15 Paralytic ectropion of eyelid
H02.151 Paralytic ectropion of right upper eyelid
H02.152 Paralytic ectropion of right lower eyelid
H02.153 Paralytic ectropion of right eye, unspecified eyelid
H02.154 Paralytic ectropion of left upper eyelid
H02.155 Paralytic ectropion of left lower eyelid
H02.156 Paralytic ectropion of left eye, unspecified eyelid
H02.159 Paralytic ectropion of unspecified eye, unspecified eyelid

● H02.2 Lagophthalmos
        Condition in which eye cannot completely close
● H02.20 Unspecified lagophthalmos
H02.201 Unspecified lagophthalmos right upper eyelid
H02.202 Unspecified lagophthalmos right lower eyelid
H02.203 Unspecified lagophthalmos right eye, unspecified eyelid
H02.204 Unspecified lagophthalmos left upper eyelid
H02.205 Unspecified lagophthalmos left lower eyelid
H02.206 Unspecified lagophthalmos left eye, unspecified eyelid
H02.209 Unspecified lagophthalmos unspecified eye, unspecified eyelid
H02.20A Unspecified lagophthalmos right eye, upper and lower eyelids
H02.20B Unspecified lagophthalmos left eye, upper and lower eyelids
H02.20C Unspecified lagophthalmos, bilateral, upper and lower eyelids

▶ New   ⇒ Revised   ~~deleted~~ Deleted   Excludes 1   Excludes 2   Includes   Use additional   Code first   Code also   Key words
OGCR Official Guidelines   ● Unacceptable Principal Diagnosis   X Assign placeholder X   ● Use Additional Character(s)   ▶ Manifestation Code   Coding Clinic

● H02.21 Cicatricial lagophthalmos
    Upper or lower eyelid does not close due to scar or tightening
    H02.211 Cicatricial lagophthalmos right upper eyelid
    H02.212 Cicatricial lagophthalmos right lower eyelid
    H02.213 Cicatricial lagophthalmos right eye, unspecified eyelid
    H02.214 Cicatricial lagophthalmos left upper eyelid
    H02.215 Cicatricial lagophthalmos left lower eyelid
    H02.216 Cicatricial lagophthalmos left eye, unspecified eyelid
    H02.219 Cicatricial lagophthalmos unspecified eye, unspecified eyelid
    H02.21A Cicatricial lagophthalmos right eye, upper and lower eyelids
    H02.21B Cicatricial lagophthalmos left eye, upper and lower eyelids
    H02.21C Cicatricial lagophthalmos, bilateral, upper and lower eyelids

● H02.22 Mechanical lagophthalmos
    Inability to close lids due to structural disorder
    H02.221 Mechanical lagophthalmos right upper eyelid
    H02.222 Mechanical lagophthalmos right lower eyelid
    H02.223 Mechanical lagophthalmos right eye, unspecified eyelid
    H02.224 Mechanical lagophthalmos left upper eyelid
    H02.225 Mechanical lagophthalmos left lower eyelid
    H02.226 Mechanical lagophthalmos left eye, unspecified eyelid
    H02.229 Mechanical lagophthalmos unspecified eye, unspecified eyelid
    H02.22A Mechanical lagophthalmos right eye, upper and lower eyelids
    H02.22B Mechanical lagophthalmos left eye, upper and lower eyelids
    H02.22C Mechanical lagophthalmos, bilateral, upper and lower eyelids

● H02.23 Paralytic lagophthalmos
    Eyelids do not close due to paralysis
    H02.231 Paralytic lagophthalmos right upper eyelid
    H02.232 Paralytic lagophthalmos right lower eyelid
    H02.233 Paralytic lagophthalmos right eye, unspecified eyelid
    H02.234 Paralytic lagophthalmos left upper eyelid
    H02.235 Paralytic lagophthalmos left lower eyelid
    H02.236 Paralytic lagophthalmos left eye, unspecified eyelid
    H02.239 Paralytic lagophthalmos unspecified eye, unspecified eyelid
    H02.23A Paralytic lagophthalmos right eye, upper and lower eyelids
    H02.23B Paralytic lagophthalmos left eye, upper and lower eyelids
    H02.23C Paralytic lagophthalmos, bilateral, upper and lower eyelids

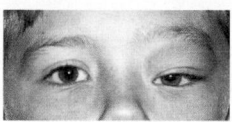

Figure 7-3 Ptosis of eyelid. (From Kanski JJ: Clinical Diagnosis in Ophthalmology, London, Elsevier Mosby, 2006)

Item 7-1 Ptosis of eyelid is drooping of the upper eyelid over the pupil when the eyes are fully opened resulting from nerve or muscle damage, which may require surgical correction.

★ **(See Plate 17 of the Anatomy Illustrations.)**

● H02.3 Blepharochalasis
    Relaxation of skin of eyelid, due to atrophy of intercellular tissue
    Pseudoptosis
    H02.30 Blepharochalasis unspecified eye, unspecified eyelid
    H02.31 Blepharochalasis right upper eyelid
    H02.32 Blepharochalasis right lower eyelid
    H02.33 Blepharochalasis right eye, unspecified eyelid
    H02.34 Blepharochalasis left upper eyelid
    H02.35 Blepharochalasis left lower eyelid
    H02.36 Blepharochalasis left eye, unspecified eyelid

● H02.4 Ptosis of eyelid
    Falling forward, drooping, sagging of eyelid
    ● H02.40 Unspecified ptosis of eyelid
        H02.401 Unspecified ptosis of right eyelid
        H02.402 Unspecified ptosis of left eyelid
        H02.403 Unspecified ptosis of bilateral eyelids
        H02.409 Unspecified ptosis of unspecified eyelid
    ● H02.41 Mechanical ptosis of eyelid
        H02.411 Mechanical ptosis of right eyelid
        H02.412 Mechanical ptosis of left eyelid
        H02.413 Mechanical ptosis of bilateral eyelids
        H02.419 Mechanical ptosis of unspecified eyelid
    ● H02.42 Myogenic ptosis of eyelid
        H02.421 Myogenic ptosis of right eyelid
        H02.422 Myogenic ptosis of left eyelid
        H02.423 Myogenic ptosis of bilateral eyelids
        H02.429 Myogenic ptosis of unspecified eyelid
    ● H02.43 Paralytic ptosis of eyelid
        Neurogenic ptosis of eyelid
        H02.431 Paralytic ptosis of right eyelid
        H02.432 Paralytic ptosis of left eyelid
        H02.433 Paralytic ptosis of bilateral eyelids
        H02.439 Paralytic ptosis unspecified eyelid

● H02.5 Other disorders affecting eyelid function
    Excludes2 blepharospasm (G24.5)
                   organic tic (G25.69)
                   psychogenic tic (F95.-)
    ● H02.51 Abnormal innervation syndrome
        H02.511 Abnormal innervation syndrome right upper eyelid
        H02.512 Abnormal innervation syndrome right lower eyelid
        H02.513 Abnormal innervation syndrome right eye, unspecified eyelid
        H02.514 Abnormal innervation syndrome left upper eyelid
        H02.515 Abnormal innervation syndrome left lower eyelid
        H02.516 Abnormal innervation syndrome left eye, unspecified eyelid
        H02.519 Abnormal innervation syndrome unspecified eye, unspecified eyelid

CHAPTER 7 (H00-H59)

N Newborn Age: 0   P Pediatric Age: 0–17   M Maternity DX: 9–64   A Adult Age: 15–124   ♀ Females Only   ♂ Males Only

🦠 Complication\Comorbidity   🦠 Major C\C   (Ex:) CC/MCC Exclusions   🦠 Hospital-Acquired Condition   🦠 Hierarchical Condition Category

831

● **H02.52   Blepharophimosis**
Drooping of eyelid with reduced lid size
Ankyloblepharon

   H02.521   Blepharophimosis right upper eyelid

   H02.522   Blepharophimosis right lower eyelid

   H02.523   Blepharophimosis right eye, unspecified eyelid

   H02.524   Blepharophimosis left upper eyelid

   H02.525   Blepharophimosis left lower eyelid

   H02.526   Blepharophimosis left eye, unspecified eyelid

   H02.529   Blepharophimosis unspecified eye, unspecified lid

● **H02.53   Eyelid retraction**
Eyelid lag

   H02.531   Eyelid retraction right upper eyelid

   H02.532   Eyelid retraction right lower eyelid

   H02.533   Eyelid retraction right eye, unspecified eyelid

   H02.534   Eyelid retraction left upper eyelid

   H02.535   Eyelid retraction left lower eyelid

   H02.536   Eyelid retraction left eye, unspecified eyelid

   H02.539   Eyelid retraction unspecified eye, unspecified lid

   H02.59   **Other disorders affecting eyelid function**
Deficient blink reflex
Sensory disorders

● **H02.6   Xanthelasma of eyelid**
Yellow-to-orange patches or pimples clustered together on eyelid

   H02.60   Xanthelasma of unspecified eye, unspecified eyelid

   H02.61   Xanthelasma of right upper eyelid

   H02.62   Xanthelasma of right lower eyelid

   H02.63   Xanthelasma of right eye, unspecified eyelid

   H02.64   Xanthelasma of left upper eyelid

   H02.65   Xanthelasma of left lower eyelid

   H02.66   Xanthelasma of left eye, unspecified eyelid

● **H02.7   Other and unspecified degenerative disorders of eyelid and periocular area**

   H02.70   Unspecified degenerative disorders of eyelid and periocular area

● **H02.71   Chloasma of eyelid and periocular area**
Dyspigmentation of eyelid
Hyperpigmentation of eyelid

   H02.711   Chloasma of right upper eyelid and periocular area

   H02.712   Chloasma of right lower eyelid and periocular area

   H02.713   Chloasma of right eye, unspecified eyelid and periocular area

   H02.714   Chloasma of left upper eyelid and periocular area

   H02.715   Chloasma of left lower eyelid and periocular area

   H02.716   Chloasma of left eye, unspecified eyelid and periocular area

   H02.719   Chloasma of unspecified eye, unspecified eyelid and periocular area

● **H02.72   Madarosis of eyelid and periocular area**
Loss of eyelashes and/or eyebrows
Hypotrichosis of eyelid

   H02.721   Madarosis of right upper eyelid and periocular area

   H02.722   Madarosis of right lower eyelid and periocular area

   H02.723   Madarosis of right eye, unspecified eyelid and periocular area

   H02.724   Madarosis of left upper eyelid and periocular area

   H02.725   Madarosis of left lower eyelid and periocular area

   H02.726   Madarosis of left eye, unspecified eyelid and periocular area

   H02.729   Madarosis of unspecified eye, unspecified eyelid and periocular area

● **H02.73   Vitiligo of eyelid and periocular area**
Skin pigmentation disease characterized by white patches
Hypopigmentation of eyelid

   H02.731   Vitiligo of right upper eyelid and periocular area

   H02.732   Vitiligo of right lower eyelid and periocular area

   H02.733   Vitiligo of right eye, unspecified eyelid and periocular area

   H02.734   Vitiligo of left upper eyelid and periocular area

   H02.735   Vitiligo of left lower eyelid and periocular area

   H02.736   Vitiligo of left eye, unspecified eyelid and periocular area

   H02.739   Vitiligo of unspecified eye, unspecified eyelid and periocular area

   H02.79   **Other degenerative disorders of eyelid and periocular area**

● **H02.8   Other specified disorders of eyelid**

● **H02.81   Retained foreign body in eyelid**
Use additional code to identify the type of retained foreign body (Z18.-)

     Excludes1   laceration of eyelid with foreign body (S01.12-)
retained intraocular foreign body (H44.6-, H44.7-)
superficial foreign body of eyelid and periocular area (S00.25-)

   H02.811   Retained foreign body in right upper eyelid

   H02.812   Retained foreign body in right lower eyelid

   H02.813   Retained foreign body in right eye, unspecified eyelid

   H02.814   Retained foreign body in left upper eyelid

   H02.815   Retained foreign body in left lower eyelid

   H02.816   Retained foreign body in left eye, unspecified eyelid

   H02.819   Retained foreign body in unspecified eye, unspecified eyelid

● **H02.82   Cysts of eyelid**
Sebaceous cyst of eyelid

   H02.821   Cysts of right upper eyelid

   H02.822   Cysts of right lower eyelid

   H02.823   Cysts of right eye, unspecified eyelid

   H02.824   Cysts of left upper eyelid

   H02.825   Cysts of left lower eyelid

   H02.826   Cysts of left eye, unspecified eyelid

   H02.829   Cysts of unspecified eye, unspecified eyelid

● **H02.83   Dermatochalasis of eyelid**
Skin is inelastic and hangs loosely in folds

   H02.831   Dermatochalasis of right upper eyelid

   H02.832   Dermatochalasis of right lower eyelid

   H02.833   Dermatochalasis of right eye, unspecified eyelid

   H02.834   Dermatochalasis of left upper eyelid

▶ New   ⇒ Revised   ~~deleted~~ Deleted   Excludes 1   Excludes 2   Includes   Use additional   Code first   Code also   Key words
OGCR Official Guidelines   ● Unacceptable Principal Diagnosis   X Assign placeholder X   ● Use Additional Character(s)   ▶ Manifestation Code   **Coding Clinic**

H02.835   Dermatochalasis of left lower eyelid

H02.836   Dermatochalasis of left eye, unspecified eyelid

H02.839   Dermatochalasis of unspecified eye, unspecified eyelid

● H02.84   Edema of eyelid
     Hyperemia of eyelid

H02.841   Edema of right upper eyelid

H02.842   Edema of right lower eyelid

H02.843   Edema of right eye, unspecified eyelid

H02.844   Edema of left upper eyelid

H02.845   Edema of left lower eyelid

H02.846   Edema of left eye, unspecified eyelid

H02.849   Edema of unspecified eye, unspecified eyelid

● H02.85   Elephantiasis of eyelid
     Massive secondary lymphedema with hypertrophy of skin and subcutaneous tissues (pachyderma)

H02.851   Elephantiasis of right upper eyelid

H02.852   Elephantiasis of right lower eyelid

H02.853   Elephantiasis of right eye, unspecified eyelid

H02.854   Elephantiasis of left upper eyelid

H02.855   Elephantiasis of left lower eyelid

H02.856   Elephantiasis of left eye, unspecified eyelid

H02.859   Elephantiasis of unspecified eye, unspecified eyelid

● H02.86   Hypertrichosis of eyelid
     Excessive growth of hair

H02.861   Hypertrichosis of right upper eyelid

H02.862   Hypertrichosis of right lower eyelid

H02.863   Hypertrichosis of right eye, unspecified eyelid

H02.864   Hypertrichosis of left upper eyelid

H02.865   Hypertrichosis of left lower eyelid

H02.866   Hypertrichosis of left eye, unspecified eyelid

H02.869   Hypertrichosis of unspecified eye, unspecified eyelid

● H02.87   Vascular anomalies of eyelid

H02.871   Vascular anomalies of right upper eyelid

H02.872   Vascular anomalies of right lower eyelid

H02.873   Vascular anomalies of right eye, unspecified eyelid

H02.874   Vascular anomalies of left upper eyelid

H02.875   Vascular anomalies of left lower eyelid

H02.876   Vascular anomalies of left eye, unspecified eyelid

H02.879   Vascular anomalies of unspecified eye, unspecified eyelid

● H02.88   Meibomian gland dysfunction of eyelid

H02.881   Meibomian gland dysfunction right upper eyelid

H02.882   Meibomian gland dysfunction right lower eyelid

H02.883   Meibomian gland dysfunction of right eye, unspecified eyelid

H02.884   Meibomian gland dysfunction left upper eyelid

H02.885   Meibomian gland dysfunction left lower eyelid

H02.886   Meibomian gland dysfunction of left eye, unspecified eyelid

H02.889   Meibomian gland dysfunction of unspecified eye, unspecified eyelid

H02.88A   Meibomian gland dysfunction right eye, upper and lower eyelids

H02.88B   Meibomian gland dysfunction left eye, upper and lower eyelids

H02.89   Other specified disorders of eyelid
     Hemorrhage of eyelid

H02.9   Unspecified disorder of eyelid
     Disorder of eyelid NOS

● H04   Disorders of lacrimal system

     Excludes 1   congenital malformations of lacrimal system (Q10.4-Q10.6)

● H04.0   Dacryoadenitis
     Inflammation of lacrimal gland

● H04.00   Unspecified dacryoadenitis

H04.001   Unspecified dacryoadenitis, right lacrimal gland

H04.002   Unspecified dacryoadenitis, left lacrimal gland

H04.003   Unspecified dacryoadenitis, bilateral lacrimal glands

H04.009   Unspecified dacryoadenitis, unspecified lacrimal gland

● H04.01   Acute dacryoadenitis

H04.011   Acute dacryoadenitis, right lacrimal gland

H04.012   Acute dacryoadenitis, left lacrimal gland

H04.013   Acute dacryoadenitis, bilateral lacrimal glands

H04.019   Acute dacryoadenitis, unspecified lacrimal gland

★ **(See Plate 19 of the Anatomy Illustrations.)**

● H04.02   Chronic dacryoadenitis

H04.021   Chronic dacryoadenitis, right lacrimal gland

H04.022   Chronic dacryoadenitis, left lacrimal gland

H04.023   Chronic dacryoadenitis, bilateral lacrimal gland

H04.029   Chronic dacryoadenitis, unspecified lacrimal gland

● H04.03   Chronic enlargement of lacrimal gland

H04.031   Chronic enlargement of right lacrimal gland

H04.032   Chronic enlargement of left lacrimal gland

H04.033   Chronic enlargement of bilateral lacrimal glands

H04.039   Chronic enlargement of unspecified lacrimal gland

● H04.1   Other disorders of lacrimal gland

● H04.11   Dacryops
     Watery eye or distention of lacrimal duct due to fluid

H04.111   Dacryops of right lacrimal gland

H04.112   Dacryops of left lacrimal gland

H04.113   Dacryops of bilateral lacrimal glands

H04.119   Dacryops of unspecified lacrimal gland

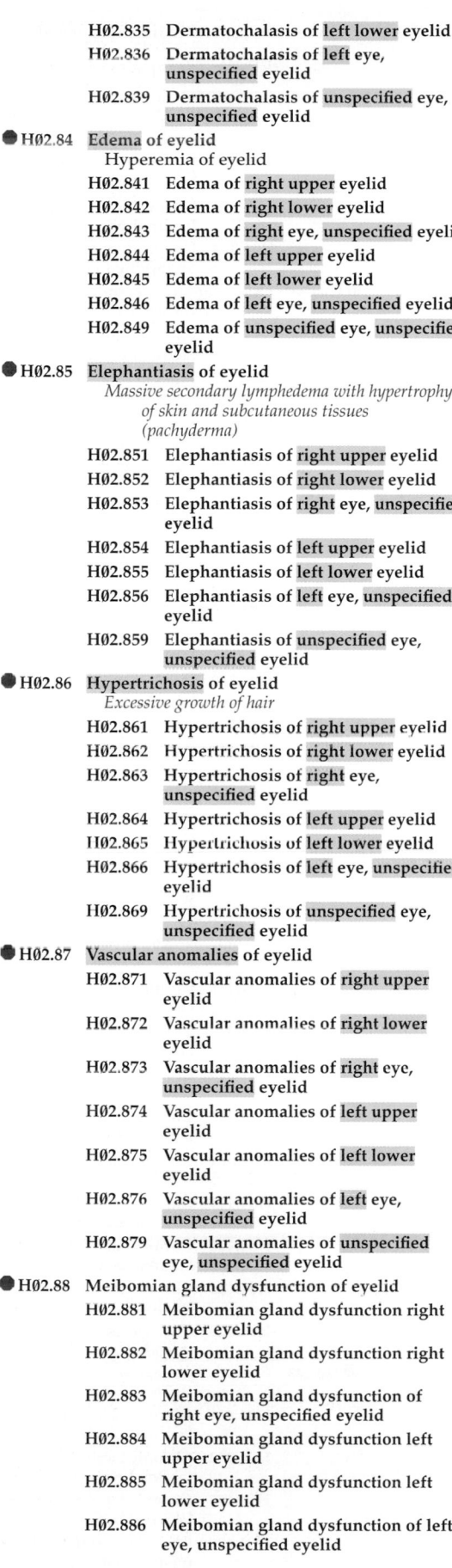

Figure 7-4   Lacrimal apparatus. (From Buck CJ: Step-by-Step Medical Coding, 2016, St. Louis, Elsevier, 2016)

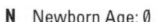 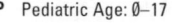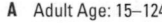
CHAPTER 7 (H00-H59)

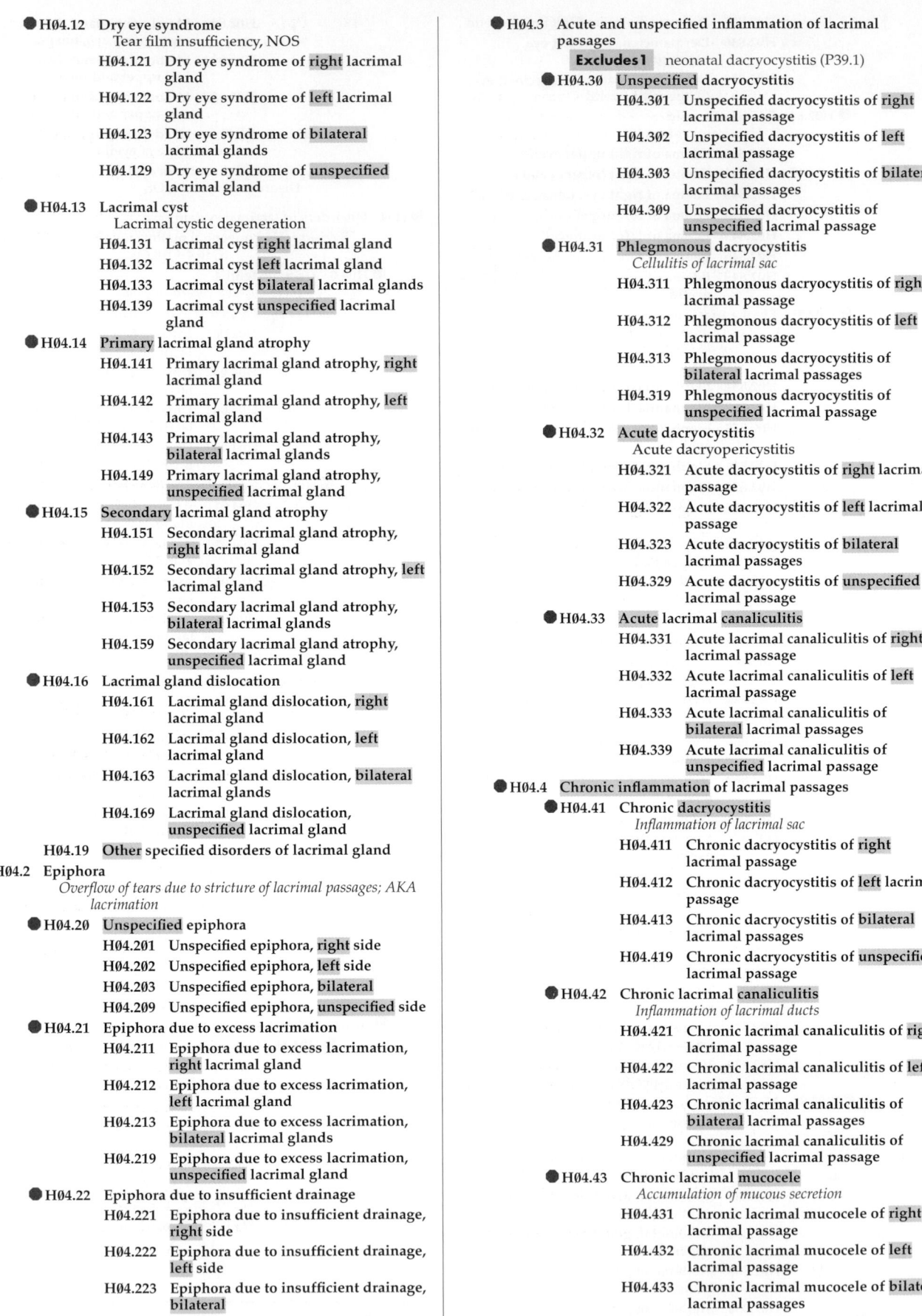

● **H04.12**   **Dry eye syndrome**
    Tear film insufficiency, NOS
    H04.121   Dry eye syndrome of right lacrimal gland
    H04.122   Dry eye syndrome of left lacrimal gland
    H04.123   Dry eye syndrome of bilateral lacrimal glands
    H04.129   Dry eye syndrome of unspecified lacrimal gland

● **H04.13**   **Lacrimal cyst**
    Lacrimal cystic degeneration
    H04.131   Lacrimal cyst right lacrimal gland
    H04.132   Lacrimal cyst left lacrimal gland
    H04.133   Lacrimal cyst bilateral lacrimal glands
    H04.139   Lacrimal cyst unspecified lacrimal gland

● **H04.14**   **Primary lacrimal gland atrophy**
    H04.141   Primary lacrimal gland atrophy, right lacrimal gland
    H04.142   Primary lacrimal gland atrophy, left lacrimal gland
    H04.143   Primary lacrimal gland atrophy, bilateral lacrimal glands
    H04.149   Primary lacrimal gland atrophy, unspecified lacrimal gland

● **H04.15**   **Secondary lacrimal gland atrophy**
    H04.151   Secondary lacrimal gland atrophy, right lacrimal gland
    H04.152   Secondary lacrimal gland atrophy, left lacrimal gland
    H04.153   Secondary lacrimal gland atrophy, bilateral lacrimal glands
    H04.159   Secondary lacrimal gland atrophy, unspecified lacrimal gland

● **H04.16**   **Lacrimal gland dislocation**
    H04.161   Lacrimal gland dislocation, right lacrimal gland
    H04.162   Lacrimal gland dislocation, left lacrimal gland
    H04.163   Lacrimal gland dislocation, bilateral lacrimal glands
    H04.169   Lacrimal gland dislocation, unspecified lacrimal gland

    H04.19   Other specified disorders of lacrimal gland

● **H04.2**   **Epiphora**
    Overflow of tears due to stricture of lacrimal passages; AKA lacrimation

● **H04.20**   **Unspecified epiphora**
    H04.201   Unspecified epiphora, right side
    H04.202   Unspecified epiphora, left side
    H04.203   Unspecified epiphora, bilateral
    H04.209   Unspecified epiphora, unspecified side

● **H04.21**   **Epiphora due to excess lacrimation**
    H04.211   Epiphora due to excess lacrimation, right lacrimal gland
    H04.212   Epiphora due to excess lacrimation, left lacrimal gland
    H04.213   Epiphora due to excess lacrimation, bilateral lacrimal glands
    H04.219   Epiphora due to excess lacrimation, unspecified lacrimal gland

● **H04.22**   **Epiphora due to insufficient drainage**
    H04.221   Epiphora due to insufficient drainage, right side
    H04.222   Epiphora due to insufficient drainage, left side
    H04.223   Epiphora due to insufficient drainage, bilateral
    H04.229   Epiphora due to insufficient drainage, unspecified side

● **H04.3**   **Acute and unspecified inflammation of lacrimal passages**
    Excludes1   neonatal dacryocystitis (P39.1)

● **H04.30**   **Unspecified dacryocystitis**
    H04.301   Unspecified dacryocystitis of right lacrimal passage
    H04.302   Unspecified dacryocystitis of left lacrimal passage
    H04.303   Unspecified dacryocystitis of bilateral lacrimal passages
    H04.309   Unspecified dacryocystitis of unspecified lacrimal passage

● **H04.31**   **Phlegmonous dacryocystitis**
    Cellulitis of lacrimal sac
    H04.311   Phlegmonous dacryocystitis of right lacrimal passage
    H04.312   Phlegmonous dacryocystitis of left lacrimal passage
    H04.313   Phlegmonous dacryocystitis of bilateral lacrimal passages
    H04.319   Phlegmonous dacryocystitis of unspecified lacrimal passage

● **H04.32**   **Acute dacryocystitis**
    Acute dacryopericystitis
    H04.321   Acute dacryocystitis of right lacrimal passage
    H04.322   Acute dacryocystitis of left lacrimal passage
    H04.323   Acute dacryocystitis of bilateral lacrimal passages
    H04.329   Acute dacryocystitis of unspecified lacrimal passage

● **H04.33**   **Acute lacrimal canaliculitis**
    H04.331   Acute lacrimal canaliculitis of right lacrimal passage
    H04.332   Acute lacrimal canaliculitis of left lacrimal passage
    H04.333   Acute lacrimal canaliculitis of bilateral lacrimal passages
    H04.339   Acute lacrimal canaliculitis of unspecified lacrimal passage

● **H04.4**   **Chronic inflammation of lacrimal passages**

● **H04.41**   **Chronic dacryocystitis**
    Inflammation of lacrimal sac
    H04.411   Chronic dacryocystitis of right lacrimal passage
    H04.412   Chronic dacryocystitis of left lacrimal passage
    H04.413   Chronic dacryocystitis of bilateral lacrimal passages
    H04.419   Chronic dacryocystitis of unspecified lacrimal passage

● **H04.42**   **Chronic lacrimal canaliculitis**
    Inflammation of lacrimal ducts
    H04.421   Chronic lacrimal canaliculitis of right lacrimal passage
    H04.422   Chronic lacrimal canaliculitis of left lacrimal passage
    H04.423   Chronic lacrimal canaliculitis of bilateral lacrimal passages
    H04.429   Chronic lacrimal canaliculitis of unspecified lacrimal passage

● **H04.43**   **Chronic lacrimal mucocele**
    Accumulation of mucous secretion
    H04.431   Chronic lacrimal mucocele of right lacrimal passage
    H04.432   Chronic lacrimal mucocele of left lacrimal passage
    H04.433   Chronic lacrimal mucocele of bilateral lacrimal passages
    H04.439   Chronic lacrimal mucocele of unspecified lacrimal passage

▶ New   ⇒ Revised   ~~deleted~~ Deleted   Excludes 1   Excludes 2   Includes   Use additional   Code first   Code also   Key words

OGCR Official Guidelines   ● Unacceptable Principal Diagnosis   X Assign placeholder X   ● Use Additional Character(s)   ▷ Manifestation Code   **Coding Clinic**

- **H04.5**   **Stenosis and insufficiency of lacrimal passages**
  - **H04.51**   Dacryolith
    - *Concretion in lacrimal sac/duct; AKA lacrimal calculus*
    - H04.511   Dacryolith of right lacrimal passage
    - H04.512   Dacryolith of left lacrimal passage
    - H04.513   Dacryolith of bilateral lacrimal passages
    - H04.519   Dacryolith of unspecified lacrimal passage
  - **H04.52**   Eversion of lacrimal punctum
    - *Turning out of lacrimal drainage opening*
    - H04.521   Eversion of right lacrimal punctum
    - H04.522   Eversion of left lacrimal punctum
    - H04.523   Eversion of bilateral lacrimal punctum
    - H04.529   Eversion of unspecified lacrimal punctum
  - **H04.53**   Neonatal obstruction of nasolacrimal duct
    - **Excludes1**   congenital stenosis and stricture of lacrimal duct (Q10.5)
    - H04.531   Neonatal obstruction of right nasolacrimal duct   **N**
    - H04.532   Neonatal obstruction of left nasolacrimal duct   **N**
    - H04.533   Neonatal obstruction of bilateral nasolacrimal duct   **N**
    - H04.539   Neonatal obstruction of unspecified nasolacrimal duct   **N**
  - **H04.54**   Stenosis of lacrimal canaliculi
    - H04.541   Stenosis of right lacrimal canaliculi
    - H04.542   Stenosis of left lacrimal canaliculi
    - H04.543   Stenosis of bilateral lacrimal canaliculi
    - H04.549   Stenosis of unspecified lacrimal canaliculi
  - **H04.55**   Acquired stenosis of nasolacrimal duct
    - H04.551   Acquired stenosis of right nasolacrimal duct
    - H04.552   Acquired stenosis of left nasolacrimal duct
    - H04.553   Acquired stenosis of bilateral nasolacrimal duct
    - H04.559   Acquired stenosis of unspecified nasolacrimal duct
  - **H04.56**   Stenosis of lacrimal punctum
    - H04.561   Stenosis of right lacrimal punctum
    - H04.562   Stenosis of left lacrimal punctum
    - H04.563   Stenosis of bilateral lacrimal punctum
    - H04.569   Stenosis of unspecified lacrimal punctum
  - **H04.57**   Stenosis of lacrimal sac
    - H04.571   Stenosis of right lacrimal sac
    - H04.572   Stenosis of left lacrimal sac
    - H04.573   Stenosis of bilateral lacrimal sac
    - H04.579   Stenosis of unspecified lacrimal sac
- **H04.6**   Other changes of lacrimal passages
  - **H04.61**   Lacrimal fistula
    - H04.611   Lacrimal fistula right lacrimal passage
    - H04.612   Lacrimal fistula left lacrimal passage
    - H04.613   Lacrimal fistula bilateral lacrimal passages
    - H04.619   Lacrimal fistula unspecified lacrimal passage
  - **H04.69**   Other changes of lacrimal passages

- **H04.8**   **Other disorders of lacrimal system**
  - **H04.81**   Granuloma of lacrimal passages
    - *Inflammatory response due to infectious or noninfectious agents*
    - H04.811   Granuloma of right lacrimal passage
    - H04.812   Granuloma of left lacrimal passage
    - H04.813   Granuloma of bilateral lacrimal passages
    - H04.819   Granuloma of unspecified lacrimal passage
  - H04.89   Other disorders of lacrimal system
  - H04.9   Disorder of lacrimal system, unspecified
- **H05**   **Disorders of orbit**
  - **Excludes1**   congenital malformation of orbit (Q10.7)
  - **H05.0**   Acute inflammation of orbit
    - H05.00   Unspecified acute inflammation of orbit
    - **H05.01**   Cellulitis of orbit
      - *Infection of soft tissue of orbit*
      - Abscess of orbit
      - (Ex) **For category H05.01 CC codes:** See PDX Collection 621
      - H05.011   Cellulitis of right orbit 🔧
      - H05.012   Cellulitis of left orbit 🔧
      - H05.013   Cellulitis of bilateral orbits 🔧
      - H05.019   Cellulitis of unspecified orbit 🔧
    - **H05.02**   Osteomyelitis of orbit
      - *Infection of boney orbit of eye*
      - (Ex) **For category H05.02 CC codes:** See PDX Collection 622
      - H05.021   Osteomyelitis of right orbit 🔧
      - H05.022   Osteomyelitis of left orbit 🔧
      - H05.023   Osteomyelitis of bilateral orbits 🔧
      - H05.029   Osteomyelitis of unspecified orbit 🔧
    - **H05.03**   Periostitis of orbit
      - *Inflammation of periosteum (membrane covering bone surface)*
      - (Ex) **For category H05.03 CC codes:** See PDX Collection 623
      - H05.031   Periostitis of right orbit 🔧
      - H05.032   Periostitis of left orbit 🔧
      - H05.033   Periostitis of bilateral orbits 🔧
      - H05.039   Periostitis of unspecified orbit 🔧
    - **H05.04**   Tenonitis of orbit
      - *Inflammation of tenon capsule (space enclosing fascia of Tenon between eyeball and fat of orbit)*
      - H05.041   Tenonitis of right orbit
      - H05.042   Tenonitis of left orbit
      - H05.043   Tenonitis of bilateral orbits
      - H05.049   Tenonitis of unspecified orbit
  - **H05.1**   Chronic inflammatory disorders of orbit
    - H05.10   Unspecified chronic inflammatory disorders of orbit
    - **H05.11**   Granuloma of orbit
      - *Pseudotumor (inflammatory) of orbit*
      - H05.111   Granuloma of right orbit
      - H05.112   Granuloma of left orbit
      - H05.113   Granuloma of bilateral orbits
      - H05.119   Granuloma of unspecified orbit
    - **H05.12**   Orbital myositis
      - *Inflammation of extraocular muscles of orbit*
      - H05.121   Orbital myositis, right orbit
      - H05.122   Orbital myositis, left orbit
      - H05.123   Orbital myositis, bilateral
      - H05.129   Orbital myositis, unspecified orbit

CHAPTER 7 (H00-H59)

N   Newborn Age: 0   **P**   Pediatric Age: 0–17   **M**   Maternity DX: 9–64   **A**   Adult Age: 15–124   ♀   Females Only   ♂   Males Only

🔧   Complication\Comorbidity   🔧   Major C\C   (Ex)   CC/MCC Exclusions   🔧   Hospital-Acquired Condition   🔧   Hierarchical Condition Category

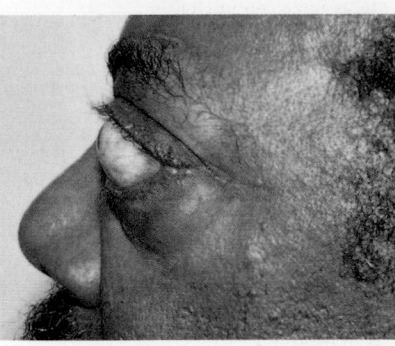

Figure 7-5 Exophthalmos. (From Black JM, Hokanson JH: Medical-Surgical Nursing: Clinical Management for Positive Outcomes, St. Louis, Saunders Elsevier, 2009)

● H05.2　Exophthalmic conditions
　　　　Bulging eyes
　　H05.20　Unspecified exophthalmos
● H05.21　Displacement (lateral) of globe
　　　　H05.211　Displacement (lateral) of globe, right eye
　　　　H05.212　Displacement (lateral) of globe, left eye
　　　　H05.213　Displacement (lateral) of globe, bilateral
　　　　H05.219　Displacement (lateral) of globe, unspecified eye
● H05.22　Edema of orbit
　　　　Orbital congestion
　　　　H05.221　Edema of right orbit
　　　　H05.222　Edema of left orbit
　　　　H05.223　Edema of bilateral orbit
　　　　H05.229　Edema of unspecified orbit
● H05.23　Hemorrhage of orbit
　　　　H05.231　Hemorrhage of right orbit
　　　　H05.232　Hemorrhage of left orbit
　　　　H05.233　Hemorrhage of bilateral orbit
　　　　H05.239　Hemorrhage of unspecified orbit
● H05.24　Constant exophthalmos
　　　　Constant bulging eyes, often symptom of Graves disease
　　　　H05.241　Constant exophthalmos, right eye
　　　　H05.242　Constant exophthalmos, left eye
　　　　H05.243　Constant exophthalmos, bilateral
　　　　H05.249　Constant exophthalmos, unspecified eye
● H05.25　Intermittent exophthalmos
　　　　Intermittent bulging eye occurring with bending forward or sharp turning of head
　　　　H05.251　Intermittent exophthalmos, right eye
　　　　H05.252　Intermittent exophthalmos, left eye
　　　　H05.253　Intermittent exophthalmos, bilateral
　　　　H05.259　Intermittent exophthalmos, unspecified eye
● H05.26　Pulsating exophthalmos
　　　　Bulging eyes with pulsation and bruit, often due to aneurysm pushing eye forward
　　　　H05.261　Pulsating exophthalmos, right eye
　　　　H05.262　Pulsating exophthalmos, left eye
　　　　H05.263　Pulsating exophthalmos, bilateral
　　　　H05.269　Pulsating exophthalmos, unspecified eye

● H05.3　Deformity of orbit
　　　Excludes1　congenital deformity of orbit (Q10.7)
　　　　　　　　hypertelorism (Q75.2)
　　H05.30　Unspecified deformity of orbit
● H05.31　Atrophy of orbit
　　　　H05.311　Atrophy of right orbit
　　　　H05.312　Atrophy of left orbit
　　　　H05.313　Atrophy of bilateral orbit
　　　　H05.319　Atrophy of unspecified orbit
● H05.32　Deformity of orbit due to bone disease
　　　　Code also associated bone disease
　　　　H05.321　Deformity of right orbit due to bone disease
　　　　H05.322　Deformity of left orbit due to bone disease
　　　　H05.323　Deformity of bilateral orbits due to bone disease
　　　　H05.329　Deformity of unspecified orbit due to bone disease
● H05.33　Deformity of orbit due to trauma or surgery
　　　　H05.331　Deformity of right orbit due to trauma or surgery
　　　　H05.332　Deformity of left orbit due to trauma or surgery
　　　　H05.333　Deformity of bilateral orbits due to trauma or surgery
　　　　H05.339　Deformity of unspecified orbit due to trauma or surgery
● H05.34　Enlargement of orbit
　　　　H05.341　Enlargement of right orbit
　　　　H05.342　Enlargement of left orbit
　　　　H05.343　Enlargement of bilateral orbits
　　　　H05.349　Enlargement of unspecified orbit
● H05.35　Exostosis of orbit
　　　　H05.351　Exostosis of right orbit
　　　　H05.352　Exostosis of left orbit
　　　　H05.353　Exostosis of bilateral orbits
　　　　H05.359　Exostosis of unspecified orbit
● H05.4　Enophthalmos
　　　　Recessed eyeball into orbit
● H05.40　Unspecified enophthalmos
　　　　H05.401　Unspecified enophthalmos, right eye
　　　　H05.402　Unspecified enophthalmos, left eye
　　　　H05.403　Unspecified enophthalmos, bilateral
　　　　H05.409　Unspecified enophthalmos, unspecified eye
● H05.41　Enophthalmos due to atrophy of orbital tissue
　　　　H05.411　Enophthalmos due to atrophy of orbital tissue, right eye
　　　　H05.412　Enophthalmos due to atrophy of orbital tissue, left eye
　　　　H05.413　Enophthalmos due to atrophy of orbital tissue, bilateral
　　　　H05.419　Enophthalmos due to atrophy of orbital tissue, unspecified eye
● H05.42　Enophthalmos due to trauma or surgery
　　　　H05.421　Enophthalmos due to trauma or surgery, right eye
　　　　H05.422　Enophthalmos due to trauma or surgery, left eye
　　　　H05.423　Enophthalmos due to trauma or surgery, bilateral
　　　　H05.429　Enophthalmos due to trauma or surgery, unspecified eye

▶ New　　▶ Revised　　~~deleted~~ Deleted　　Excludes 1　　Excludes 2　　Includes　　Use additional　　Code first　　Code also　　Key words
OGCR Official Guidelines　　● Unacceptable Principal Diagnosis　　X Assign placeholder X　　● Use Additional Character(s)　　▶ Manifestation Code　　**Coding Clinic**

● **H05.5**   **Retained (old) foreign body following penetrating wound of orbit**
    Retrobulbar foreign body
    Use additional code to identify the type of retained foreign body (Z18.-)
    Excludes1   current penetrating wound of orbit (S05.4-)
    Excludes2   retained foreign body of eyelid (H02.81-)
                 retained intraocular foreign body (H44.6-, H44.7-)
    H05.50   Retained (old) foreign body following penetrating wound of unspecified orbit
    H05.51   Retained (old) foreign body following penetrating wound of right orbit
    H05.52   Retained (old) foreign body following penetrating wound of left orbit
    H05.53   Retained (old) foreign body following penetrating wound of bilateral orbits

● **H05.8**   Other disorders of orbit
    ● **H05.81**   Cyst of orbit
       Encephalocele of orbit
       H05.811   Cyst of right orbit
       H05.812   Cyst of left orbit
       H05.813   Cyst of bilateral orbits
       H05.819   Cyst of unspecified orbit
    ● **H05.82**   Myopathy of extraocular muscles
       Weakness of muscles of eye
       H05.821   Myopathy of extraocular muscles, right orbit
       H05.822   Myopathy of extraocular muscles, left orbit
       H05.823   Myopathy of extraocular muscles, bilateral
       H05.829   Myopathy of extraocular muscles, unspecified orbit
    H05.89   Other disorders of orbit
● **H05.9**   Unspecified disorder of orbit

DISORDERS OF CONJUNCTIVA (H10-H11)

★ **(See Plate 18 of the Anatomy Illustrations.)**

● **H10**   Conjunctivitis
    Inflammation of membrane of the inside of the eyelid or on surface of eye (conjunctiva)
    Excludes1   keratoconjunctivitis (H16.2-)
    ● **H10.0**   Mucopurulent conjunctivitis
       ● **H10.01**   Acute follicular conjunctivitis
          H10.011   Acute follicular conjunctivitis, right eye
          H10.012   Acute follicular conjunctivitis, left eye
          H10.013   Acute follicular conjunctivitis, bilateral
          H10.019   Acute follicular conjunctivitis, unspecified eye
       ● **H10.02**   Other mucopurulent conjunctivitis
          H10.021   Other mucopurulent conjunctivitis, right eye
          H10.022   Other mucopurulent conjunctivitis, left eye
          H10.023   Other mucopurulent conjunctivitis, bilateral
          H10.029   Other mucopurulent conjunctivitis, unspecified eye
    ● **H10.1**   Acute atopic conjunctivitis
       Acute papillary conjunctivitis
       H10.10   Acute atopic conjunctivitis, unspecified eye
       H10.11   Acute atopic conjunctivitis, right eye
       H10.12   Acute atopic conjunctivitis, left eye
       H10.13   Acute atopic conjunctivitis, bilateral

● **H10.2**   Other acute conjunctivitis
    ● **H10.21**   Acute toxic conjunctivitis
       Acute chemical conjunctivitis
       Code first (T51-T65) to identify chemical and intent
       Excludes1   burn and corrosion of eye and adnexa (T26.-)
       H10.211   Acute toxic conjunctivitis, right eye
       H10.212   Acute toxic conjunctivitis, left eye
       H10.213   Acute toxic conjunctivitis, bilateral
       H10.219   Acute toxic conjunctivitis, unspecified eye
    ● **H10.22**   Pseudomembranous conjunctivitis
       H10.221   Pseudomembranous conjunctivitis, right eye
       H10.222   Pseudomembranous conjunctivitis, left eye
       H10.223   Pseudomembranous conjunctivitis, bilateral
       H10.229   Pseudomembranous conjunctivitis, unspecified eye
    ● **H10.23**   Serous conjunctivitis, except viral
       Excludes1   viral conjunctivitis (B30.-)
       H10.231   Serous conjunctivitis, except viral, right eye
       H10.232   Serous conjunctivitis, except viral, left eye
       H10.233   Serous conjunctivitis, except viral, bilateral
       H10.239   Serous conjunctivitis, except viral, unspecified eye
● **H10.3**   Unspecified acute conjunctivitis
    Excludes1   ophthalmia neonatorum NOS (P39.1)
    H10.30   Unspecified acute conjunctivitis, unspecified eye
    H10.31   Unspecified acute conjunctivitis, right eye
    H10.32   Unspecified acute conjunctivitis, left eye
    H10.33   Unspecified acute conjunctivitis, bilateral
● **H10.4**   Chronic conjunctivitis
    ● **H10.40**   Unspecified chronic conjunctivitis
       H10.401   Unspecified chronic conjunctivitis, right eye
       H10.402   Unspecified chronic conjunctivitis, left eye
       H10.403   Unspecified chronic conjunctivitis, bilateral
       H10.409   Unspecified chronic conjunctivitis, unspecified eye
    ● **H10.41**   Chronic giant papillary conjunctivitis
       Inflammation of membrane of the inside of the eyelid or on surface of eye often associated with contact lens wear
       H10.411   Chronic giant papillary conjunctivitis, right eye
       H10.412   Chronic giant papillary conjunctivitis, left eye
       H10.413   Chronic giant papillary conjunctivitis, bilateral
       H10.419   Chronic giant papillary conjunctivitis, unspecified eye
    ● **H10.42**   Simple chronic conjunctivitis
       H10.421   Simple chronic conjunctivitis, right eye
       H10.422   Simple chronic conjunctivitis, left eye
       H10.423   Simple chronic conjunctivitis, bilateral
       H10.429   Simple chronic conjunctivitis, unspecified eye

N Newborn Age: 0   **P** Pediatric Age: 0–17   **M** Maternity DX: 9–64   **A** Adult Age: 15–124   ♀ Females Only   ♂ Males Only
Complication\Comorbidity   Major C\C   (Ex) CC/MCC Exclusions   Hospital-Acquired Condition   Hierarchical Condition Category

● **H10.43 Chronic follicular conjunctivitis**
Inflammation of membrane of the inside of the eyelid or on surface of eye due to topical medications or infection

H10.431 Chronic follicular conjunctivitis, right eye

H10.432 Chronic follicular conjunctivitis, left eye

H10.433 Chronic follicular conjunctivitis, bilateral

H10.439 Chronic follicular conjunctivitis, unspecified eye

H10.44 Vernal conjunctivitis
Affecting children, especially boys in which there are flattened papules with thick, gelatinous exudate on conjunctivae on inside of upper lid

Excludes1   vernal keratoconjunctivitis with limbar and corneal involvement (H16.26-)

H10.45 Other chronic allergic conjunctivitis

● **H10.5 Blepharoconjunctivitis**
Inflammation of eyelids and conjunctiva

● **H10.50 Unspecified blepharoconjunctivitis**

H10.501 Unspecified blepharoconjunctivitis, right eye

H10.502 Unspecified blepharoconjunctivitis, left eye

H10.503 Unspecified blepharoconjunctivitis, bilateral

H10.509 Unspecified blepharoconjunctivitis, unspecified eye

● **H10.51 Ligneous conjunctivitis**
Code also underlying condition if known, such as:
plasminogen deficiency (E88.02)

H10.511 Ligneous conjunctivitis, right eye

H10.512 Ligneous conjunctivitis, left eye

H10.513 Ligneous conjunctivitis, bilateral

H10.519 Ligneous conjunctivitis, unspecified eye

● **H10.52 Angular blepharoconjunctivitis**

H10.521 Angular blepharoconjunctivitis, right eye

H10.522 Angular blepharoconjunctivitis, left eye

H10.523 Angular blepharoconjunctivitis, bilateral

H10.529 Angular blepharoconjunctivitis, unspecified eye

● **H10.53 Contact blepharoconjunctivitis**

H10.531 Contact blepharoconjunctivitis, right eye

H10.532 Contact blepharoconjunctivitis, left eye

H10.533 Contact blepharoconjunctivitis, bilateral

H10.539 Contact blepharoconjunctivitis, unspecified eye

● **H10.8 Other conjunctivitis**

● **H10.81 Pingueculitis**
Inflammation of a yellow, raised thickening on the white of the eye associated with chronic dry eyes

Excludes1   pinguecula (H11.15-)

H10.811 Pingueculitis, right eye

H10.812 Pingueculitis, left eye

H10.813 Pingueculitis, bilateral

H10.819 Pingueculitis, unspecified eye

● **H10.82 Rosacea conjunctivitis**
Code first underlying rosacea dermatitis (L71.-)

H10.821 Rosacea conjunctivitis, right eye

H10.822 Rosacea conjunctivitis, left eye

H10.823 Rosacea conjunctivitis, bilateral
Coding Clinic: 2018, Q4, P15

H10.829 Rosacea conjunctivitis, unspecified eye

H10.89 Other conjunctivitis

H10.9 Unspecified conjunctivitis

● **H11 Other disorders of conjunctiva**

Excludes1   keratoconjunctivitis (H16.2-)

● **H11.0 Pterygium of eye**

Excludes1   pseudopterygium (H11.81-)

● **H11.00 Unspecified pterygium of eye**

H11.001 Unspecified pterygium of right eye

H11.002 Unspecified pterygium of left eye

H11.003 Unspecified pterygium of eye, bilateral

H11.009 Unspecified pterygium of unspecified eye

● **H11.01 Amyloid pterygium**

H11.011 Amyloid pterygium of right eye

H11.012 Amyloid pterygium of left eye

H11.013 Amyloid pterygium of eye, bilateral

H11.019 Amyloid pterygium of unspecified eye

● **H11.02 Central pterygium of eye**

H11.021 Central pterygium of right eye

H11.022 Central pterygium of left eye

H11.023 Central pterygium of eye, bilateral

H11.029 Central pterygium of unspecified eye

● **H11.03 Double pterygium of eye**

H11.031 Double pterygium of right eye

H11.032 Double pterygium of left eye

H11.033 Double pterygium of eye, bilateral

H11.039 Double pterygium of unspecified eye

● **H11.04 Peripheral pterygium of eye, stationary**

H11.041 Peripheral pterygium, stationary, right eye

H11.042 Peripheral pterygium, stationary, left eye

H11.043 Peripheral pterygium, stationary, bilateral

H11.049 Peripheral pterygium, stationary, unspecified eye

● **H11.05 Peripheral pterygium of eye, progressive**

H11.051 Peripheral pterygium, progressive, right eye

H11.052 Peripheral pterygium, progressive, left eye

H11.053 Peripheral pterygium, progressive, bilateral

H11.059 Peripheral pterygium, progressive, unspecified eye

● **H11.06 Recurrent pterygium of eye**

H11.061 Recurrent pterygium of right eye

H11.062 Recurrent pterygium of left eye

H11.063 Recurrent pterygium of eye, bilateral

H11.069 Recurrent pterygium of unspecified eye

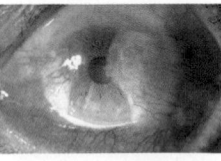

Figure 7-6   Double pterygium. Note both nasal and temporal pterygia in a 57-year-old farmer. (From Brightbill FS, McDonnell PJ: Corneal Surgery: Theory, Technique and Tissue, S.l., Mosby Elsevier, 2009)

Item 7–2 Pterygium is Greek for batlike. The condition is characterized by a membrane that extends from the limbus to the center of the cornea and resembles a wing.

▶ New   ⟹ Revised   ~~deleted~~ Deleted   Excludes 1   Excludes 2   Includes   Use additional   Code first   Code also   Key words

OGCR Official Guidelines   ● Unacceptable Principal Diagnosis   X Assign placeholder X   ▶ Use Additional Character(s)   ▶ Manifestation Code   **Coding Clinic**

● **H11.1**   **Conjunctival degenerations and deposits**
    Excludes2   pseudopterygium (H11.81)
   H11.10   Unspecified conjunctival degenerations
● H11.11   Conjunctival deposits
    H11.111   Conjunctival deposits, right eye
    H11.112   Conjunctival deposits, left eye
    H11.113   Conjunctival deposits, bilateral
    H11.119   Conjunctival deposits, unspecified eye
● H11.12   Conjunctival concretions
     White to yellow nodules within or beneath
     conjunctiva
    H11.121   Conjunctival concretions, right eye
    H11.122   Conjunctival concretions, left eye
    H11.123   Conjunctival concretions, bilateral
    H11.129   Conjunctival concretions, unspecified
          eye
● H11.13   Conjunctival pigmentations
     Conjunctival argyrosis [argyria]
    H11.131   Conjunctival pigmentations, right eye
    H11.132   Conjunctival pigmentations, left eye
    H11.133   Conjunctival pigmentations, bilateral
    H11.139   Conjunctival pigmentations,
          unspecified eye
● H11.14   Conjunctival xerosis, unspecified
    Excludes1   xerosis of conjunctiva due to
          vitamin A deficiency (E50.0,
          E50.1)
    H11.141   Conjunctival xerosis, unspecified,
          right eye
    H11.142   Conjunctival xerosis, unspecified, left
          eye
    H11.143   Conjunctival xerosis, unspecified,
          bilateral
    H11.149   Conjunctival xerosis, unspecified,
          unspecified eye
● H11.15   Pinguecula
     Yellowish spot near sclerocorneal junction, usually
     on nasal side; associated with aging
    Excludes1   pingueculitis (H10.81-)
    H11.151   Pinguecula, right eye
    H11.152   Pinguecula, left eye
    II11.153   Pinguecula, bilateral
    H11.159   Pinguecula, unspecified eye
● **H11.2**   **Conjunctival scars**
   ● H11.21   Conjunctival adhesions and strands (localized)
    H11.211   Conjunctival adhesions and strands
          (localized), right eye
    H11.212   Conjunctival adhesions and strands
          (localized), left eye
    H11.213   Conjunctival adhesions and strands
          (localized), bilateral
    H11.219   Conjunctival adhesions and strands
          (localized), unspecified eye
   ● H11.22   Conjunctival granuloma
    H11.221   Conjunctival granuloma, right eye
    H11.222   Conjunctival granuloma, left eye
    H11.223   Conjunctival granuloma, bilateral
    H11.229   Conjunctival granuloma, unspecified
   ● H11.23   Symblepharon
     Adhesion between tarsal conjunctiva and bulbar
     conjunctiva
    H11.231   Symblepharon, right eye
    H11.232   Symblepharon, left eye
    H11.233   Symblepharon, bilateral
    H11.239   Symblepharon, unspecified eye

● H11.24   Scarring of conjunctiva
    H11.241   Scarring of conjunctiva, right eye
    H11.242   Scarring of conjunctiva, left eye
    H11.243   Scarring of conjunctiva, bilateral
    H11.249   Scarring of conjunctiva, unspecified
          eye
● **H11.3**   **Conjunctival hemorrhage**
     Subconjunctival hemorrhage
   H11.30   Conjunctival hemorrhage, unspecified eye
   H11.31   Conjunctival hemorrhage, right eye
   H11.32   Conjunctival hemorrhage, left eye
   H11.33   Conjunctival hemorrhage, bilateral
● **H11.4**   **Other conjunctival vascular disorders and cysts**
   ● H11.41   Vascular abnormalities of conjunctiva
     Conjunctival aneurysm
    H11.411   Vascular abnormalities of
          conjunctiva, right eye
    H11.412   Vascular abnormalities of
          conjunctiva, left eye
    H11.413   Vascular abnormalities of
          conjunctiva, bilateral
    H11.419   Vascular abnormalities of
          conjunctiva, unspecified eye
   ● H11.42   Conjunctival edema
    H11.421   Conjunctival edema, right eye
    H11.422   Conjunctival edema, left eye
    H11.423   Conjunctival edema, bilateral
    H11.429   Conjunctival edema, unspecified eye
   ● H11.43   Conjunctival hyperemia
    H11.431   Conjunctival hyperemia, right eye
    H11.432   Conjunctival hyperemia, left eye
    H11.433   Conjunctival hyperemia, bilateral
    H11.439   Conjunctival hyperemia, unspecified
          eye
   ● H11.44   Conjunctival cysts
    H11.441   Conjunctival cysts, right eye
    H11.442   Conjunctival cysts, left eye
    H11.443   Conjunctival cysts, bilateral
    H11.449   Conjunctival cysts, unspecified eye
● **H11.8**   **Other specified disorders of conjunctiva**
   ● H11.81   Pseudopterygium of conjunctiva
     Conjunctival scar attached to cornea
    H11.811   Pseudopterygium of conjunctiva,
          right eye
    H11.812   Pseudopterygium of conjunctiva, left
          eye
    H11.813   Pseudopterygium of conjunctiva,
          bilateral
    H11.819   Pseudopterygium of conjunctiva,
          unspecified eye
   ● H11.82   Conjunctivochalasis
     Conjunctiva bulges over eyelid margin or covers
     lower punctum
    H11.821   Conjunctivochalasis, right eye
    H11.822   Conjunctivochalasis, left eye
    H11.823   Conjunctivochalasis, bilateral
    H11.829   Conjunctivochalasis, unspecified eye
   H11.89   Other specified disorders of conjunctiva
  H11.9   Unspecified disorder of conjunctiva

CHAPTER 7 (H00-H59)

CHAPTER 7 (H00-H59)

DISORDERS OF SCLERA, CORNEA, IRIS AND CILIARY BODY (H15-H22)

- ● **H15** Disorders of sclera
  - ● **H15.0** Scleritis
    - *Inflammation of the white (sclera and episclera) of the eye.*
    - ● **H15.00** Unspecified scleritis
      - H15.001 Unspecified scleritis, right eye
      - H15.002 Unspecified scleritis, left eye
      - H15.003 Unspecified scleritis, bilateral
      - H15.009 Unspecified scleritis, unspecified eye
    - ● **H15.01** Anterior scleritis
      - H15.011 Anterior scleritis, right eye
      - H15.012 Anterior scleritis, left eye
      - H15.013 Anterior scleritis, bilateral
      - H15.019 Anterior scleritis, unspecified eye
    - ● **H15.02** Brawny scleritis
      - *Swelling around the cornea that is gelantinous in appearance*
      - H15.021 Brawny scleritis, right eye
      - H15.022 Brawny scleritis, left eye
      - H15.023 Brawny scleritis, bilateral
      - H15.029 Brawny scleritis, unspecified eye
    - ● **H15.03** Posterior scleritis
      - Sclerotenonitis
      - H15.031 Posterior scleritis, right eye
      - H15.032 Posterior scleritis, left eye
      - H15.033 Posterior scleritis, bilateral
      - H15.039 Posterior scleritis, unspecified eye
    - ● **H15.04** Scleritis with corneal involvement
      - H15.041 Scleritis with corneal involvement, right eye
      - H15.042 Scleritis with corneal involvement, left eye
      - H15.043 Scleritis with corneal involvement, bilateral
      - H15.049 Scleritis with corneal involvement, unspecified eye
    - ● **H15.05** Scleromalacia perforans
      - *Necrotic without inflammation; usually associated with rheumatoid arthritis*
      - H15.051 Scleromalacia perforans, right eye
      - H15.052 Scleromalacia perforans, left eye
      - H15.053 Scleromalacia perforans, bilateral
      - H15.059 Scleromalacia perforans, unspecified eye
    - ● **H15.09** Other scleritis
      - Scleral abscess
      - H15.091 Other scleritis, right eye
      - H15.092 Other scleritis, left eye
      - H15.093 Other scleritis, bilateral
      - H15.099 Other scleritis, unspecified eye
  - ● **H15.1** Episcleritis
    - *Inflammation of the white (sclera and episclera) of the eye.*
    - ● **H15.10** Unspecified episcleritis
      - H15.101 Unspecified episcleritis, right eye
      - H15.102 Unspecified episcleritis, left eye
      - H15.103 Unspecified episcleritis, bilateral
      - H15.109 Unspecified episcleritis, unspecified eye
    - ● **H15.11** Episcleritis periodica fugax
      - *Transient, recurrent inflammation of portion of episclera (connective tissue on the surface of the sclera)*
      - H15.111 Episcleritis periodica fugax, right eye
      - H15.112 Episcleritis periodica fugax, left eye
      - H15.113 Episcleritis periodica fugax, bilateral
      - H15.119 Episcleritis periodica fugax, unspecified eye

- ● **H15.12** Nodular episcleritis
  - *Characterized by tender, localized, moveable nodule within inflamed area*
  - H15.121 Nodular episcleritis, right eye
  - H15.122 Nodular episcleritis, left eye
  - H15.123 Nodular episcleritis, bilateral
  - H15.129 Nodular episcleritis, unspecified eye
- ● **H15.8** Other disorders of sclera
  - **Excludes2** blue sclera (Q13.5)
    - degenerative myopia (H44.2-)
  - ● **H15.81** Equatorial staphyloma
    - H15.811 Equatorial staphyloma, right eye
    - H15.812 Equatorial staphyloma, left eye
    - H15.813 Equatorial staphyloma, bilateral
    - H15.819 Equatorial staphyloma, unspecified eye
  - ● **H15.82** Localized anterior staphyloma
    - H15.821 Localized anterior staphyloma, right eye
    - H15.822 Localized anterior staphyloma, left eye
    - H15.823 Localized anterior staphyloma, bilateral
    - H15.829 Localized anterior staphyloma, unspecified eye
  - ● **H15.83** Staphyloma posticum
    - H15.831 Staphyloma posticum, right eye
    - H15.832 Staphyloma posticum, left eye
    - H15.833 Staphyloma posticum, bilateral
    - H15.839 Staphyloma posticum, unspecified eye
  - ● **H15.84** Scleral ectasia
    - H15.841 Scleral ectasia, right eye
    - H15.842 Scleral ectasia, left eye
    - H15.843 Scleral ectasia, bilateral
    - H15.849 Scleral ectasia, unspecified eye
  - ● **H15.85** Ring staphyloma
    - H15.851 Ring staphyloma, right eye
    - H15.852 Ring staphyloma, left eye
    - H15.853 Ring staphyloma, bilateral
    - H15.859 Ring staphyloma, unspecified eye
  - H15.89 Other disorders of sclera
- H15.9 Unspecified disorder of sclera

- ● **H16** Keratitis
  - ● **H16.0** Corneal ulcer
    - ● **H16.00** Unspecified corneal ulcer
      - H16.001 Unspecified corneal ulcer, right eye
      - H16.002 Unspecified corneal ulcer, left eye
      - H16.003 Unspecified corneal ulcer, bilateral
      - H16.009 Unspecified corneal ulcer, unspecified eye
    - ● **H16.01** Central corneal ulcer
      - H16.011 Central corneal ulcer, right eye
      - H16.012 Central corneal ulcer, left eye
      - H16.013 Central corneal ulcer, bilateral
      - H16.019 Central corneal ulcer, unspecified eye
    - ● **H16.02** Ring corneal ulcer
      - H16.021 Ring corneal ulcer, right eye
      - H16.022 Ring corneal ulcer, left eye
      - H16.023 Ring corneal ulcer, bilateral
      - H16.029 Ring corneal ulcer, unspecified eye
    - ● **H16.03** Corneal ulcer with hypopyon
      - H16.031 Corneal ulcer with hypopyon, right eye
      - H16.032 Corneal ulcer with hypopyon, left eye
      - H16.033 Corneal ulcer with hypopyon, bilateral
      - H16.039 Corneal ulcer with hypopyon, unspecified eye

▶ New   ⇒ Revised   ~~deleted~~ Deleted   Excludes 1   Excludes 2   Includes   Use additional   Code first   Code also   Key words

OGCR Official Guidelines   ● Unacceptable Principal Diagnosis   **X** Assign placeholder X   ● Use Additional Character(s)   》 Manifestation Code   **Coding Clinic**

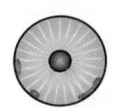 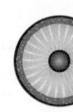 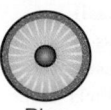 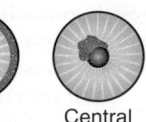 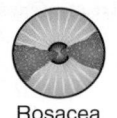 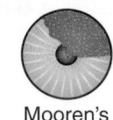

| Marginal (catarrhal) ulcer | Ring ulcer | Central corneal ulcer | Rosacea ulcer | Mooren's (rodent) ulcer |

Figure 7-7 Corneal ulcers: marginal, ring, central corneal, rosacea, and Mooren's.

Item 7–3 An infected ulcer is usually called a **serpiginous** or **hypopyon** ulcer, which is a pus sac in the anterior chamber of the eye. **Marginal** ulcers are usually asymptomatic, not primary, and are often superficial and simple. More severe marginal ulcers spread to form a ring ulcer. **Ring** ulcers can extend around the entire corneal periphery. **Central corneal** ulcers develop when there is an abrasion to the epithelium and an infection develops in the eroded area. The **pyocyaneal** ulcer is the most serious corneal infection, which, if left untreated, can lead to loss of the eye.

● **H16.04**   Marginal corneal ulcer
     H16.041   Marginal corneal ulcer, right eye
     H16.042   Marginal corneal ulcer, left eye
     H16.043   Marginal corneal ulcer, bilateral
     H16.049   Marginal corneal ulcer, unspecified eye

● **H16.05**   Mooren's corneal ulcer
     H16.051   Mooren's corneal ulcer, right eye
     H16.052   Mooren's corneal ulcer, left eye
     H16.053   Mooren's corneal ulcer, bilateral
     H16.059   Mooren's corneal ulcer, unspecified eye

● **H16.06**   Mycotic corneal ulcer
     H16.061   Mycotic corneal ulcer, right eye
     H16.062   Mycotic corneal ulcer, left eye
     H16.063   Mycotic corneal ulcer, bilateral
     H16.069   Mycotic corneal ulcer, unspecified eye

● **H16.07**   Perforated corneal ulcer
     H16.071   Perforated corneal ulcer, right eye
     H16.072   Perforated corneal ulcer, left eye
     H16.073   Perforated corneal ulcer, bilateral
     H16.079   Perforated corneal ulcer, unspecified eye

● **H16.1**   Other and unspecified superficial keratitis without conjunctivitis
   ● **H16.10**   Unspecified superficial keratitis
     H16.101   Unspecified superficial keratitis, right eye
     H16.102   Unspecified superficial keratitis, left eye
     H16.103   Unspecified superficial keratitis, bilateral
     H16.109   Unspecified superficial keratitis, unspecified eye

   ● **H16.11**   Macular keratitis
     Areolar keratitis
     Nummular keratitis
     Stellate keratitis
     Striate keratitis
     H16.111   Macular keratitis, right eye
     H16.112   Macular keratitis, left eye
     H16.113   Macular keratitis, bilateral
     H16.119   Macular keratitis, unspecified eye

   ● **H16.12**   Filamentary keratitis
     H16.121   Filamentary keratitis, right eye
     H16.122   Filamentary keratitis, left eye
     H16.123   Filamentary keratitis, bilateral
     H16.129   Filamentary keratitis, unspecified eye

   ● **H16.13**   Photokeratitis
     Snow blindness
     Welders' keratitis
     H16.131   Photokeratitis, right eye
     H16.132   Photokeratitis, left eye
     H16.133   Photokeratitis, bilateral
     H16.139   Photokeratitis, unspecified eye

   ● **H16.14**   Punctate keratitis
     H16.141   Punctate keratitis, right eye
     H16.142   Punctate keratitis, left eye
     H16.143   Punctate keratitis, bilateral
     H16.149   Punctate keratitis, unspecified eye

● **H16.2**   Keratoconjunctivitis
   ● **H16.20**   Unspecified keratoconjunctivitis
     Superficial keratitis with conjunctivitis NOS
     H16.201   Unspecified keratoconjunctivitis, right eye
     H16.202   Unspecified keratoconjunctivitis, left eye
     H16.203   Unspecified keratoconjunctivitis, bilateral
     H16.209   Unspecified keratoconjunctivitis, unspecified eye

   ● **H16.21**   Exposure keratoconjunctivitis
     H16.211   Exposure keratoconjunctivitis, right eye
     H16.212   Exposure keratoconjunctivitis, left eye
     H16.213   Exposure keratoconjunctivitis, bilateral
     H16.219   Exposure keratoconjunctivitis, unspecified eye

   ● **H16.22**   Keratoconjunctivitis sicca, not specified as Sjögren's
     Excludes 1   Sjogren's syndrome (M35.01)
     H16.221   Keratoconjunctivitis sicca, not specified as Sjögren's, right eye
     H16.222   Keratoconjunctivitis sicca, not specified as Sjögren's, left eye
     H16.223   Keratoconjunctivitis sicca, not specified as Sjögren's, bilateral
     H16.229   Keratoconjunctivitis sicca, not specified as Sjögren's, unspecified eye

   ● **H16.23**   Neurotrophic keratoconjunctivitis
     H16.231   Neurotrophic keratoconjunctivitis, right eye
     H16.232   Neurotrophic keratoconjunctivitis, left eye
     H16.233   Neurotrophic keratoconjunctivitis, bilateral
     H16.239   Neurotrophic keratoconjunctivitis, unspecified eye

   ● **H16.24**   Ophthalmia nodosa
     H16.241   Ophthalmia nodosa, right eye
     H16.242   Ophthalmia nodosa, left eye
     H16.243   Ophthalmia nodosa, bilateral
     H16.249   Ophthalmia nodosa, unspecified eye

   ● **H16.25**   Phlyctenular keratoconjunctivitis
     H16.251   Phlyctenular keratoconjunctivitis, right eye
     H16.252   Phlyctenular keratoconjunctivitis, left eye
     H16.253   Phlyctenular keratoconjunctivitis, bilateral
     H16.259   Phlyctenular keratoconjunctivitis, unspecified eye

CHAPTER 7 (H00-H59)

N Newborn Age: 0   **P** Pediatric Age: 0–17   **M** Maternity DX: 9–64   **A** Adult Age: 15–124   ♀ Females Only   ♂ Males Only

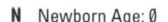 Complication\Comorbidity   Major C\C   (Ex) CC/MCC Exclusions   Hospital-Acquired Condition   Hierarchical Condition Category

841

- ● H16.26   Vernal keratoconjunctivitis, with limbar and corneal involvement
  - **Excludes1**   vernal conjunctivitis without limbar and corneal involvement (H10.44)
  - H16.261   Vernal keratoconjunctivitis, with limbar and corneal involvement, right eye
  - H16.262   Vernal keratoconjunctivitis, with limbar and corneal involvement, left eye
  - H16.263   Vernal keratoconjunctivitis, with limbar and corneal involvement, bilateral
  - H16.269   Vernal keratoconjunctivitis, with limbar and corneal involvement, unspecified eye
- ● H16.29   Other keratoconjunctivitis
  - H16.291   Other keratoconjunctivitis, right eye
  - H16.292   Other keratoconjunctivitis, left eye
  - H16.293   Other keratoconjunctivitis, bilateral
  - H16.299   Other keratoconjunctivitis, unspecified eye
- ● H16.3   Interstitial and deep keratitis
  - ● H16.30   Unspecified interstitial keratitis
    - H16.301   Unspecified interstitial keratitis, right eye
    - H16.302   Unspecified interstitial keratitis, left eye
    - H16.303   Unspecified interstitial keratitis, bilateral
    - H16.309   Unspecified interstitial keratitis, unspecified eye
  - ● H16.31   Corneal abscess
    - H16.311   Corneal abscess, right eye
    - H16.312   Corneal abscess, left eye
    - H16.313   Corneal abscess, bilateral
    - H16.319   Corneal abscess, unspecified eye
  - ● H16.32   Diffuse interstitial keratitis
    - Cogan's syndrome
    - H16.321   Diffuse interstitial keratitis, right eye
    - H16.322   Diffuse interstitial keratitis, left eye
    - H16.323   Diffuse interstitial keratitis, bilateral
    - H16.329   Diffuse interstitial keratitis, unspecified eye
  - ● H16.33   Sclerosing keratitis
    - H16.331   Sclerosing keratitis, right eye
    - H16.332   Sclerosing keratitis, left eye
    - H16.333   Sclerosing keratitis, bilateral
    - H16.339   Sclerosing keratitis, unspecified eye
  - ● H16.39   Other interstitial and deep keratitis
    - H16.391   Other interstitial and deep keratitis, right eye
    - H16.392   Other interstitial and deep keratitis, left eye
    - H16.393   Other interstitial and deep keratitis, bilateral
    - H16.399   Other interstitial and deep keratitis, unspecified eye
- ● H16.4   Corneal neovascularization
  - ● H16.40   Unspecified corneal neovascularization
    - H16.401   Unspecified corneal neovascularization, right eye
    - H16.402   Unspecified corneal neovascularization, left eye
    - H16.403   Unspecified corneal neovascularization, bilateral
    - H16.409   Unspecified corneal neovascularization, unspecified eye

- ● H16.41   Ghost vessels (corneal)
  - H16.411   Ghost vessels (corneal), right eye
  - H16.412   Ghost vessels (corneal), left eye
  - H16.413   Ghost vessels (corneal), bilateral
  - H16.419   Ghost vessels (corneal), unspecified eye
- ● H16.42   Pannus (corneal)
  - H16.421   Pannus (corneal), right eye
  - H16.422   Pannus (corneal), left eye
  - H16.423   Pannus (corneal), bilateral
  - H16.429   Pannus (corneal), unspecified eye
- ● H16.43   Localized vascularization of cornea
  - H16.431   Localized vascularization of cornea, right eye
  - H16.432   Localized vascularization of cornea, left eye
  - H16.433   Localized vascularization of cornea, bilateral
  - H16.439   Localized vascularization of cornea, unspecified eye
- ● H16.44   Deep vascularization of cornea
  - H16.441   Deep vascularization of cornea, right eye
  - H16.442   Deep vascularization of cornea, left eye
  - H16.443   Deep vascularization of cornea, bilateral
  - H16.449   Deep vascularization of cornea, unspecified eye
- ● H16.8   Other keratitis
- H16.9   Unspecified keratitis
- ● H17   Corneal scars and opacities
  - ● H17.0   Adherent leukoma
    - H17.00   Adherent leukoma, unspecified eye
    - H17.01   Adherent leukoma, right eye
    - H17.02   Adherent leukoma, left eye
    - H17.03   Adherent leukoma, bilateral
  - ● H17.1   Central corneal opacity
    - H17.10   Central corneal opacity, unspecified eye
    - H17.11   Central corneal opacity, right eye
    - H17.12   Central corneal opacity, left eye
    - H17.13   Central corneal opacity, bilateral
  - ● H17.8   Other corneal scars and opacities
    - ● H17.81   Minor opacity of cornea
      - Corneal nebula
      - H17.811   Minor opacity of cornea, right eye
      - H17.812   Minor opacity of cornea, left eye
      - H17.813   Minor opacity of cornea, bilateral
      - H17.819   Minor opacity of cornea, unspecified eye
    - ● H17.82   Peripheral opacity of cornea
      - H17.821   Peripheral opacity of cornea, right eye
      - H17.822   Peripheral opacity of cornea, left eye
      - H17.823   Peripheral opacity of cornea, bilateral
      - H17.829   Peripheral opacity of cornea, unspecified eye
    - H17.89   Other corneal scars and opacities
  - H17.9   Unspecified corneal scar and opacity
- ● H18   Other disorders of cornea
  - ● H18.0   Corneal pigmentations and deposits
    - ● H18.00   Unspecified corneal deposit
      - H18.001   Unspecified corneal deposit, right eye
      - H18.002   Unspecified corneal deposit, left eye
      - H18.003   Unspecified corneal deposit, bilateral
      - H18.009   Unspecified corneal deposit, unspecified eye

▶ New   ⇒ Revised   ~~deleted~~ Deleted   Excludes 1   Excludes 2   Includes   Use additional   Code first   Code also   Key words
OGCR Official Guidelines   ● Unacceptable Principal Diagnosis   X Assign placeholder X   ● Use Additional Character(s)   ▶ Manifestation Code   **Coding Clinic**

● **H18.01**   **Anterior corneal pigmentations**
     Staehli's line
   H18.011   Anterior corneal pigmentations, right eye
   H18.012   Anterior corneal pigmentations, left eye
   H18.013   Anterior corneal pigmentations, bilateral
   H18.019   Anterior corneal pigmentations, unspecified eye

● **H18.02**   **Argentous corneal deposits**
   H18.021   Argentous corneal deposits, right eye
   H18.022   Argentous corneal deposits, left eye
   H18.023   Argentous corneal deposits, bilateral
   H18.029   Argentous corneal deposits, unspecified eye

● **H18.03**   **Corneal deposits in metabolic disorders**
     Code also associated metabolic disorder
   H18.031   Corneal deposits in metabolic disorders, right eye
   H18.032   Corneal deposits in metabolic disorders, left eye
   H18.033   Corneal deposits in metabolic disorders, bilateral
   H18.039   Corneal deposits in metabolic disorders, unspecified eye

● **H18.04**   **Kayser-Fleischer ring**
     Code also associated Wilson's disease (E83.01)
   H18.041   Kayser-Fleischer ring, right eye
   H18.042   Kayser-Fleischer ring, left eye
   H18.043   Kayser-Fleischer ring, bilateral
   H18.049   Kayser-Fleischer ring, unspecified eye

● **H18.05**   **Posterior corneal pigmentations**
     Krukenberg's spindle
   H18.051   Posterior corneal pigmentations, right eye
   H18.052   Posterior corneal pigmentations, left eye
   H18.053   Posterior corneal pigmentations, bilateral
   H18.059   Posterior corneal pigmentations, unspecified eye

● **H18.06**   **Stromal corneal pigmentations**
     Hematocornea
   H18.061   Stromal corneal pigmentations, right eye
   H18.062   Stromal corneal pigmentations, left eye
   H18.063   Stromal corneal pigmentations, bilateral
   H18.069   Stromal corneal pigmentations, unspecified eye

● **H18.1**   **Bullous keratopathy**
   H18.10   Bullous keratopathy, unspecified eye
   H18.11   Bullous keratopathy, right eye
   H18.12   Bullous keratopathy, left eye
   H18.13   Bullous keratopathy, bilateral

● **H18.2**   **Other and unspecified corneal edema**
   H18.20   Unspecified corneal edema
   ● **H18.21**   Corneal edema secondary to contact lens
      Excludes2   other corneal disorders due to contact lens (H18.82-)
     H18.211   Corneal edema secondary to contact lens, right eye
     H18.212   Corneal edema secondary to contact lens, left eye
     H18.213   Corneal edema secondary to contact lens, bilateral
     H18.219   Corneal edema secondary to contact lens, unspecified eye

● **H18.22**   **Idiopathic corneal edema**
   H18.221   Idiopathic corneal edema, right eye
   H18.222   Idiopathic corneal edema, left eye
   H18.223   Idiopathic corneal edema, bilateral
   H18.229   Idiopathic corneal edema, unspecified eye

● **H18.23**   **Secondary corneal edema**
   H18.231   Secondary corneal edema, right eye
   H18.232   Secondary corneal edema, left eye
   H18.233   Secondary corneal edema, bilateral
   H18.239   Secondary corneal edema, unspecified eye

● **H18.3**   **Changes of corneal membranes**
   H18.30   Unspecified corneal membrane change
   ● **H18.31**   Folds and rupture in Bowman's membrane
     H18.311   Folds and rupture in Bowman's membrane, right eye
     H18.312   Folds and rupture in Bowman's membrane, left eye
     H18.313   Folds and rupture in Bowman's membrane, bilateral
     H18.319   Folds and rupture in Bowman's membrane, unspecified eye
   ● **H18.32**   Folds in Descemet's membrane
     H18.321   Folds in Descemet's membrane, right eye
     H18.322   Folds in Descemet's membrane, left eye
     H18.323   Folds in Descemet's membrane, bilateral
     H18.329   Folds in Descemet's membrane, unspecified eye
   ● **H18.33**   Rupture in Descemet's membrane
     H18.331   Rupture in Descemet's membrane, right eye
     H18.332   Rupture in Descemet's membrane, left eye
     H18.333   Rupture in Descemet's membrane, bilateral
     H18.339   Rupture in Descemet's membrane, unspecified eye

● **H18.4**   **Corneal degeneration**
     Excludes1   Mooren's ulcer (H16.0-)
          recurrent erosion of cornea (H18.83-)
   H18.40   Unspecified corneal degeneration
   ● **H18.41**   Arcus senilis
     Senile corneal changes
     H18.411   Arcus senilis, right eye
     H18.412   Arcus senilis, left eye
     H18.413   Arcus senilis, bilateral
     H18.419   Arcus senilis, unspecified eye
   ● **H18.42**   Band keratopathy
     H18.421   Band keratopathy, right eye
     H18.422   Band keratopathy, left eye
     H18.423   Band keratopathy, bilateral
     H18.429   Band keratopathy, unspecified eye
   H18.43   Other calcerous corneal degeneration
   ● **H18.44**   Keratomalacia
     Excludes1   keratomalacia due to vitamin A deficiency (E50.4)
     H18.441   Keratomalacia, right eye
     H18.442   Keratomalacia, left eye
     H18.443   Keratomalacia, bilateral
     H18.449   Keratomalacia, unspecified eye

CHAPTER 7 (H00-H59)

N Newborn Age: 0   **P** Pediatric Age: 0–17   **M** Maternity DX: 9–64   **A** Adult Age: 15–124   ♀ Females Only   ♂ Males Only

Complication\Comorbidity   Major C\C   (Ex) CC/MCC Exclusions   Hospital-Acquired Condition   Hierarchical Condition Category

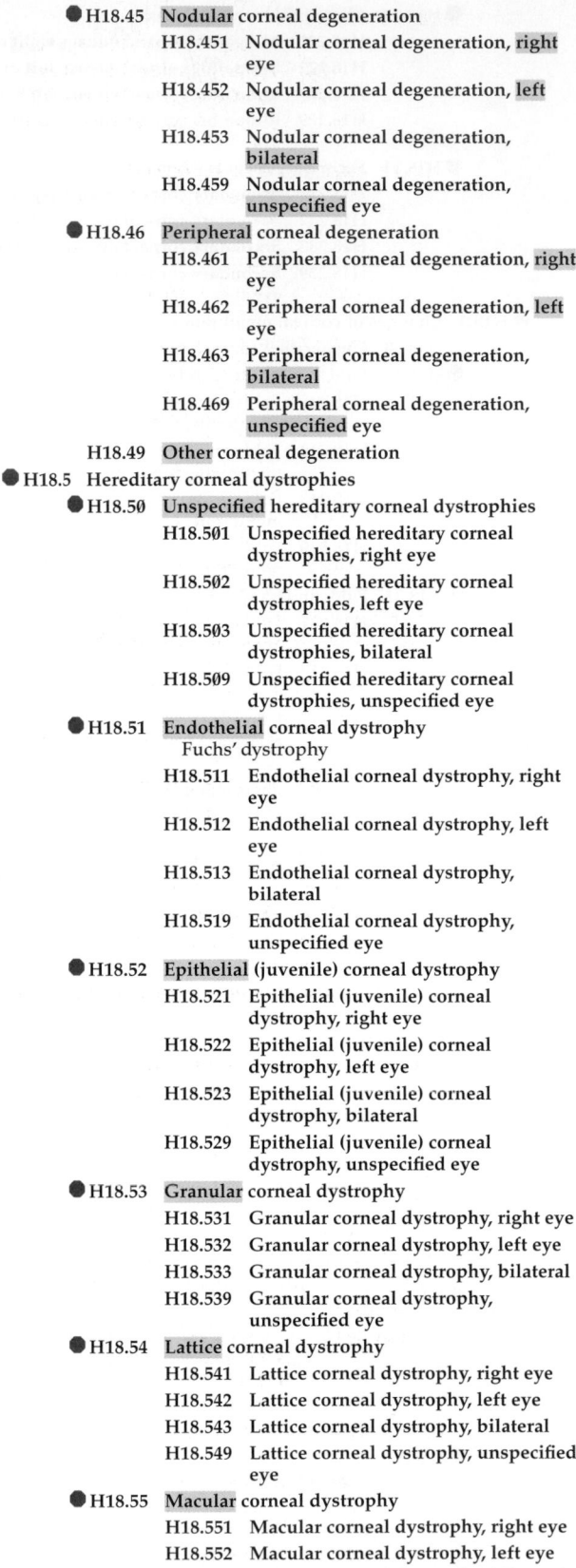

- ● H18.45   Nodular corneal degeneration
  - H18.451   Nodular corneal degeneration, right eye
  - H18.452   Nodular corneal degeneration, left eye
  - H18.453   Nodular corneal degeneration, bilateral
  - H18.459   Nodular corneal degeneration, unspecified eye
- ● H18.46   Peripheral corneal degeneration
  - H18.461   Peripheral corneal degeneration, right eye
  - H18.462   Peripheral corneal degeneration, left eye
  - H18.463   Peripheral corneal degeneration, bilateral
  - H18.469   Peripheral corneal degeneration, unspecified eye
  - H18.49   Other corneal degeneration
- ● H18.5   Hereditary corneal dystrophies
  - ● H18.50   Unspecified hereditary corneal dystrophies
    - H18.501   Unspecified hereditary corneal dystrophies, right eye
    - H18.502   Unspecified hereditary corneal dystrophies, left eye
    - H18.503   Unspecified hereditary corneal dystrophies, bilateral
    - H18.509   Unspecified hereditary corneal dystrophies, unspecified eye
  - ● H18.51   Endothelial corneal dystrophy
    Fuchs' dystrophy
    - H18.511   Endothelial corneal dystrophy, right eye
    - H18.512   Endothelial corneal dystrophy, left eye
    - H18.513   Endothelial corneal dystrophy, bilateral
    - H18.519   Endothelial corneal dystrophy, unspecified eye
  - ● H18.52   Epithelial (juvenile) corneal dystrophy
    - H18.521   Epithelial (juvenile) corneal dystrophy, right eye
    - H18.522   Epithelial (juvenile) corneal dystrophy, left eye
    - H18.523   Epithelial (juvenile) corneal dystrophy, bilateral
    - H18.529   Epithelial (juvenile) corneal dystrophy, unspecified eye
  - ● H18.53   Granular corneal dystrophy
    - H18.531   Granular corneal dystrophy, right eye
    - H18.532   Granular corneal dystrophy, left eye
    - H18.533   Granular corneal dystrophy, bilateral
    - H18.539   Granular corneal dystrophy, unspecified eye
  - ● H18.54   Lattice corneal dystrophy
    - H18.541   Lattice corneal dystrophy, right eye
    - H18.542   Lattice corneal dystrophy, left eye
    - H18.543   Lattice corneal dystrophy, bilateral
    - H18.549   Lattice corneal dystrophy, unspecified eye
  - ● H18.55   Macular corneal dystrophy
    - H18.551   Macular corneal dystrophy, right eye
    - H18.552   Macular corneal dystrophy, left eye
    - H18.553   Macular corneal dystrophy, bilateral
    - H18.559   Macular corneal dystrophy, unspecified eye

- ● H18.59   Other hereditary corneal dystrophies
  - H18.591   Other hereditary corneal dystrophies, right eye
  - H18.592   Other hereditary corneal dystrophies, left eye
  - H18.593   Other hereditary corneal dystrophies, bilateral
  - H18.599   Other hereditary corneal dystrophies, unspecified eye
- ● H18.6   Keratoconus
  - ● H18.60   Keratoconus, unspecified
    - H18.601   Keratoconus, unspecified, right eye
    - H18.602   Keratoconus, unspecified, left eye
    - H18.603   Keratoconus, unspecified, bilateral
    - H18.609   Keratoconus, unspecified, unspecified eye
  - ● H18.61   Keratoconus, stable
    - H18.611   Keratoconus, stable, right eye
    - H18.612   Keratoconus, stable, left eye
    - H18.613   Keratoconus, stable, bilateral
    - H18.619   Keratoconus, stable, unspecified eye
  - ● H18.62   Keratoconus, unstable
    Acute hydrops
    - H18.621   Keratoconus, unstable, right eye
    - H18.622   Keratoconus, unstable, left eye
    - H18.623   Keratoconus, unstable, bilateral
    - H18.629   Keratoconus, unstable, unspecified eye
- ● H18.7   Other and unspecified corneal deformities
  - **Excludes1**   congenital malformations of cornea (Q13.3-Q13.4)
  - H18.70   Unspecified corneal deformity
  - ● H18.71   Corneal ectasia
    - H18.711   Corneal ectasia, right eye
    - H18.712   Corneal ectasia, left eye
    - H18.713   Corneal ectasia, bilateral
    - H18.719   Corneal ectasia, unspecified eye
  - ● H18.72   Corneal staphyloma
    - H18.721   Corneal staphyloma, right eye
    - H18.722   Corneal staphyloma, left eye
    - H18.723   Corneal staphyloma, bilateral
    - H18.729   Corneal staphyloma, unspecified eye
  - ● H18.73   Descemetocele
    - H18.731   Descemetocele, right eye
    - H18.732   Descemetocele, left eye
    - H18.733   Descemetocele, bilateral
    - H18.739   Descemetocele, unspecified eye
  - ● H18.79   Other corneal deformities
    - H18.791   Other corneal deformities, right eye
    - H18.792   Other corneal deformities, left eye
    - H18.793   Other corneal deformities, bilateral
    - H18.799   Other corneal deformities, unspecified eye

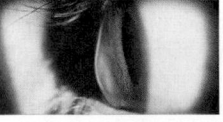

Figure 7-8   Lateral view of the displacement of the cone apex in keratoconus. (From Yanoff: Ophthalmology, ed 3, Mosby, Inc., 2008)

Item 7–4 Keratoconus results in corneal degeneration that begins in childhood, gradually changes the cornea from a round to cone shape, decreasing visual acuity. Treatment includes contact lenses. In severe cases the need for corneal transplant may be the treatment of choice; however, newer technologies may use high-frequency radio energy to shrink the edges of the cornea, pulling the central area back to a more normal shape. It can help delay or avoid the need for a corneal transplantation.

▶ New   ⇒ Revised   ~~deleted~~ Deleted   Excludes 1   Excludes 2   Includes   Use additional   Code first   Code also   Key words
OGCR Official Guidelines   ● Unacceptable Principal Diagnosis   X Assign placeholder X   ● Use Additional Character(s)   ▎ Manifestation Code   **Coding Clinic**

- **H18.8**   Other specified disorders of cornea
  - **H18.81**   Anesthesia and hypoesthesia of cornea
    - H18.811   Anesthesia and hypoesthesia of cornea, right eye
    - H18.812   Anesthesia and hypoesthesia of cornea, left eye
    - H18.813   Anesthesia and hypoesthesia of cornea, bilateral
    - H18.819   Anesthesia and hypoesthesia of cornea, unspecified eye
  - **H18.82**   Corneal disorder due to contact lens
    - **Excludes2**   corneal edema due to contact lens (H18.21-)
    - H18.821   Corneal disorder due to contact lens, right eye
    - H18.822   Corneal disorder due to contact lens, left eye
    - H18.823   Corneal disorder due to contact lens, bilateral
    - H18.829   Corneal disorder due to contact lens, unspecified eye
  - **H18.83**   Recurrent erosion of cornea
    - H18.831   Recurrent erosion of cornea, right eye
    - H18.832   Recurrent erosion of cornea, left eye
    - H18.833   Recurrent erosion of cornea, bilateral
    - H18.839   Recurrent erosion of cornea, unspecified eye
  - **H18.89**   Other specified disorders of cornea
    - H18.891   Other specified disorders of cornea, right eye
    - H18.892   Other specified disorders of cornea, left eye
    - H18.893   Other specified disorders of cornea, bilateral
    - H18.899   Other specified disorders of cornea, unspecified eye
  - **H18.9**   Unspecified disorder of cornea

- **H20**   Iridocyclitis
  - **H20.0**   Acute and subacute iridocyclitis
    - Acute anterior uveitis
    - Acute cyclitis
    - Acute iritis
    - Subacute anterior uveitis
    - Subacute cyclitis
    - Subacute iritis
    - **Excludes1**   iridocyclitis, iritis, uveitis (due to) (in) diabetes mellitus (E08-E13 with .39)
      - iridocyclitis, iritis, uveitis (due to) (in) diphtheria (A36.89)
      - iridocyclitis, iritis, uveitis (due to) (in) gonococcal (A54.32)
      - iridocyclitis, iritis, uveitis (due to) (in) herpes (simplex) (B00.51)
      - iridocyclitis, iritis, uveitis (due to) (in) herpes zoster (B02.32)
      - iridocyclitis, iritis, uveitis (due to) (in) late congenital syphilis (A50.39)
      - iridocyclitis, iritis, uveitis (due to) (in) late syphilis (A52.71)
      - iridocyclitis, iritis, uveitis (due to) (in) sarcoidosis (D86.83)
      - iridocyclitis, iritis, uveitis (due to) (in) syphilis (A51.43)
      - iridocyclitis, iritis, uveitis (due to) (in) toxoplasmosis (B58.09)
      - iridocyclitis, iritis, uveitis (due to) (in) tuberculosis (A18.54)
    - (Ex:) **For category H20 CC codes: See PDX Collection 624**
    - **H20.00**   Unspecified acute and subacute iridocyclitis

- **H20.01**   Primary iridocyclitis
  - H20.011   Primary iridocyclitis, right eye
  - H20.012   Primary iridocyclitis, left eye
  - H20.013   Primary iridocyclitis, bilateral
  - H20.019   Primary iridocyclitis, unspecified eye
- **H20.02**   Recurrent acute iridocyclitis
  - H20.021   Recurrent acute iridocyclitis, right eye
  - H20.022   Recurrent acute iridocyclitis, left eye
  - H20.023   Recurrent acute iridocyclitis, bilateral
  - H20.029   Recurrent acute iridocyclitis, unspecified eye
- **H20.03**   Secondary infectious iridocyclitis
  - H20.031   Secondary infectious iridocyclitis, right eye
  - H20.032   Secondary infectious iridocyclitis, left eye
  - H20.033   Secondary infectious iridocyclitis, bilateral
  - H20.039   Secondary infectious iridocyclitis, unspecified eye
- **H20.04**   Secondary noninfectious iridocyclitis
  - H20.041   Secondary noninfectious iridocyclitis, right eye
  - H20.042   Secondary noninfectious iridocyclitis, left eye
  - H20.043   Secondary noninfectious iridocyclitis, bilateral
  - H20.049   Secondary noninfectious iridocyclitis, unspecified eye
- **H20.05**   Hypopyon
  - H20.051   Hypopyon, right eye
  - H20.052   Hypopyon, left eye
  - H20.053   Hypopyon, bilateral
  - H20.059   Hypopyon, unspecified eye
- **H20.1**   Chronic iridocyclitis
  - Use additional code for any associated cataract (H26.21-)
  - **Excludes2**   posterior cyclitis (H30.2-)
  - H20.10   Chronic iridocyclitis, unspecified eye
  - H20.11   Chronic iridocyclitis, right eye
  - H20.12   Chronic iridocyclitis, left eye
  - H20.13   Chronic iridocyclitis, bilateral
- **H20.2**   Lens-induced iridocyclitis
  - H20.20   Lens-induced iridocyclitis, unspecified eye
  - H20.21   Lens-induced iridocyclitis, right eye
  - H20.22   Lens-induced iridocyclitis, left eye
  - H20.23   Lens-induced iridocyclitis, bilateral
- **H20.8**   Other iridocyclitis
  - **Excludes2**   glaucomatocyclitis crises (H40.4-)
    - posterior cyclitis (H30.2-)
    - sympathetic uveitis (H44.13-)
  - **H20.81**   Fuchs' heterochromic cyclitis
    - H20.811   Fuchs' heterochromic cyclitis, right eye
    - H20.812   Fuchs' heterochromic cyclitis, left eye
    - H20.813   Fuchs' heterochromic cyclitis, bilateral
    - H20.819   Fuchs' heterochromic cyclitis, unspecified eye

N Newborn Age: 0   **P** Pediatric Age: 0-17   **M** Maternity DX: 9-64   **A** Adult Age: 15-124   ♀ Females Only   ♂ Males Only

Complication\Comorbidity   Major C\C   (Ex:) CC/MCC Exclusions   Hospital-Acquired Condition   Hierarchical Condition Category

845

● H20.82   Vogt-Koyanagi syndrome
     H20.821   Vogt-Koyanagi syndrome, right eye
     H20.822   Vogt-Koyanagi syndrome, left eye
     H20.823   Vogt-Koyanagi syndrome, bilateral
     H20.829   Vogt-Koyanagi syndrome, unspecified eye

H20.9   Unspecified iridocyclitis 🔖
     Uveitis NOS

● H21   Other disorders of iris and ciliary body
     Excludes2   sympathetic uveitis (H44.1-)

● H21.0   Hyphema
     Excludes1   traumatic hyphema (S05.1-)
     H21.00   Hyphema, unspecified eye
     H21.01   Hyphema, right eye
     H21.02   Hyphema, left eye
     H21.03   Hyphema, bilateral

● H21.1   Other vascular disorders of iris and ciliary body
     Neovascularization of iris or ciliary body
     Rubeosis iridis
     Rubeosis of iris

   ● H21.1X   Other vascular disorders of iris and ciliary body
     H21.1X1   Other vascular disorders of iris and ciliary body, right eye
     H21.1X2   Other vascular disorders of iris and ciliary body, left eye
     H21.1X3   Other vascular disorders of iris and ciliary body, bilateral
     H21.1X9   Other vascular disorders of iris and ciliary body, unspecified eye

● H21.2   Degeneration of iris and ciliary body
   ● H21.21   Degeneration of chamber angle
     H21.211   Degeneration of chamber angle, right eye
     H21.212   Degeneration of chamber angle, left eye
     H21.213   Degeneration of chamber angle, bilateral
     H21.219   Degeneration of chamber angle, unspecified eye

   ● H21.22   Degeneration of ciliary body
     H21.221   Degeneration of ciliary body, right eye
     H21.222   Degeneration of ciliary body, left eye
     H21.223   Degeneration of ciliary body, bilateral
     H21.229   Degeneration of ciliary body, unspecified eye

   ● H21.23   Degeneration of iris (pigmentary)
     Translucency of iris
     H21.231   Degeneration of iris (pigmentary), right eye
     H21.232   Degeneration of iris (pigmentary), left eye
     H21.233   Degeneration of iris (pigmentary), bilateral
     H21.239   Degeneration of iris (pigmentary), unspecified eye

   ● H21.24   Degeneration of pupillary margin
     H21.241   Degeneration of pupillary margin, right eye
     H21.242   Degeneration of pupillary margin, left eye
     H21.243   Degeneration of pupillary margin, bilateral
     H21.249   Degeneration of pupillary margin, unspecified eye

● H21.25   Iridoschisis
     H21.251   Iridoschisis, right eye
     H21.252   Iridoschisis, left eye
     H21.253   Iridoschisis, bilateral
     H21.259   Iridoschisis, unspecified eye

● H21.26   Iris atrophy (essential) (progressive)
     H21.261   Iris atrophy (essential) (progressive), right eye
     H21.262   Iris atrophy (essential) (progressive), left eye
     H21.263   Iris atrophy (essential) (progressive), bilateral
     H21.269   Iris atrophy (essential) (progressive), unspecified eye

● H21.27   Miotic pupillary cyst
     H21.271   Miotic pupillary cyst, right eye
     H21.272   Miotic pupillary cyst, left eye
     H21.273   Miotic pupillary cyst, bilateral
     H21.279   Miotic pupillary cyst, unspecified eye

H21.29   Other iris atrophy

● H21.3   Cyst of iris, ciliary body and anterior chamber
     Excludes2   miotic pupillary cyst (H21.27-)

● H21.30   Idiopathic cysts of iris, ciliary body or anterior chamber
     Cyst of iris, ciliary body or anterior chamber NOS
     H21.301   Idiopathic cysts of iris, ciliary body or anterior chamber, right eye
     H21.302   Idiopathic cysts of iris, ciliary body or anterior chamber, left eye
     H21.303   Idiopathic cysts of iris, ciliary body or anterior chamber, bilateral
     H21.309   Idiopathic cysts of iris, ciliary body or anterior chamber, unspecified eye

● H21.31   Exudative cysts of iris or anterior chamber
     H21.311   Exudative cysts of iris or anterior chamber, right eye
     H21.312   Exudative cysts of iris or anterior chamber, left eye
     H21.313   Exudative cysts of iris or anterior chamber, bilateral
     H21.319   Exudative cysts of iris or anterior chamber, unspecified eye

● H21.32   Implantation cysts of iris, ciliary body or anterior chamber
     H21.321   Implantation cysts of iris, ciliary body or anterior chamber, right eye
     H21.322   Implantation cysts of iris, ciliary body or anterior chamber, left eye
     H21.323   Implantation cysts of iris, ciliary body or anterior chamber, bilateral
     H21.329   Implantation cysts of iris, ciliary body or anterior chamber, unspecified eye

● H21.33   Parasitic cyst of iris, ciliary body or anterior chamber
     (Ex:) **For category H21.33 CC codes:** See PDX Collection 625
     H21.331   Parasitic cyst of iris, ciliary body or anterior chamber, right eye 🔖
     H21.332   Parasitic cyst of iris, ciliary body or anterior chamber, left eye 🔖
     H21.333   Parasitic cyst of iris, ciliary body or anterior chamber, bilateral 🔖
     H21.339   Parasitic cyst of iris, ciliary body or anterior chamber, unspecified eye 🔖

▶ New   ⇒ Revised   deleted Deleted   Excludes 1   Excludes 2   Includes   Use additional   Code first   Code also   Key words
OGCR Official Guidelines   ● Unacceptable Principal Diagnosis   X Assign placeholder X   ● Use Additional Character(s)   ▌ Manifestation Code   **Coding Clinic**

● H21.34   Primary cyst of pars plana
     H21.341   Primary cyst of pars plana, right eye
     H21.342   Primary cyst of pars plana, left eye
     H21.343   Primary cyst of pars plana, bilateral
     H21.349   Primary cyst of pars plana, unspecified eye

● H21.35   Exudative cyst of pars plana
     H21.351   Exudative cyst of pars plana, right eye
     H21.352   Exudative cyst of pars plana, left eye
     H21.353   Exudative cyst of pars plana, bilateral
     H21.359   Exudative cyst of pars plana, unspecified eye

● H21.4   Pupillary membranes
     Iris bombé
     Pupillary occlusion
     Pupillary seclusion
     Excludes1   congenital pupillary membranes (Q13.8)
     H21.40   Pupillary membranes, unspecified eye
     H21.41   Pupillary membranes, right eye
     H21.42   Pupillary membranes, left eye
     H21.43   Pupillary membranes, bilateral

● H21.5   Other and unspecified adhesions and disruptions of iris and ciliary body
     Excludes1   corectopia (Q13.2)
     ● H21.50   Unspecified adhesions of iris
         Synechia (iris) NOS
         H21.501   Unspecified adhesions of iris, right eye
         H21.502   Unspecified adhesions of iris, left eye
         H21.503   Unspecified adhesions of iris, bilateral
         H21.509   Unspecified adhesions of iris and ciliary body, unspecified eye
     ● H21.51   Anterior synechiae (iris)
         H21.511   Anterior synechiae (iris), right eye
         H21.512   Anterior synechiae (iris), left eye
         H21.513   Anterior synechiae (iris), bilateral
         H21.519   Anterior synechiae (iris), unspecified eye
     ● H21.52   Goniosynechiae
         H21.521   Goniosynechiae, right eye
         H21.522   Goniosynechiae, left eye
         H21.523   Goniosynechiae, bilateral
         H21.529   Goniosynechiae, unspecified eye
     ● H21.53   Iridodialysis
         H21.531   Iridodialysis, right eye
         H21.532   Iridodialysis, left eye
         H21.533   Iridodialysis, bilateral
         H21.539   Iridodialysis, unspecified eye
     ● H21.54   Posterior synechiae (iris)
         H21.541   Posterior synechiae (iris), right eye
         H21.542   Posterior synechiae (iris), left eye
         H21.543   Posterior synechiae (iris), bilateral
         H21.549   Posterior synechiae (iris), unspecified eye
     ● H21.55   Recession of chamber angle
         H21.551   Recession of chamber angle, right eye
         H21.552   Recession of chamber angle, left eye
         H21.553   Recession of chamber angle, bilateral
         H21.559   Recession of chamber angle, unspecified eye

● H21.56   Pupillary abnormalities
     Deformed pupil
     Ectopic pupil
     Rupture of sphincter, pupil
     Excludes1   congenital deformity of pupil (Q13.2-)
     H21.561   Pupillary abnormality, right eye
     H21.562   Pupillary abnormality, left eye
     H21.563   Pupillary abnormality, bilateral
     H21.569   Pupillary abnormality, unspecified eye

● H21.8   Other specified disorders of iris and ciliary body
     H21.81   Floppy iris syndrome
         Intraoperative floppy iris syndrome (IFIS)
         Use additional code for adverse effect, if applicable, to identify drug (T36-T50 with fifth or sixth character 5)
     H21.82   Plateau iris syndrome (post-iridectomy) (postprocedural)
     H21.89   Other specified disorders of iris and ciliary body
● H21.9   Unspecified disorder of iris and ciliary body

◗ H22   *Disorders of iris and ciliary body in diseases classified elsewhere*
     Code first underlying disease, such as:
         gout (M1A.-, M10.-)
         leprosy (A30.-)
         parasitic disease (B89)

DISORDERS OF LENS (H25-H28)

● H25   Age-related cataract
     Senile cataract
     Excludes2   capsular glaucoma with pseudoexfoliation of lens (H40.1-)
     ● H25.0   Age-related incipient cataract
         ● H25.01   Cortical age-related cataract
             H25.011   Cortical age-related cataract, right eye   **A**
             H25.012   Cortical age-related cataract, left eye   **A**
             H25.013   Cortical age-related cataract, bilateral   **A**
             H25.019   Cortical age-related cataract, unspecified eye   **A**
         ● H25.03   Anterior subcapsular polar age-related cataract
             H25.031   Anterior subcapsular polar age-related cataract, right eye   **A**
             H25.032   Anterior subcapsular polar age-related cataract, left eye   **A**
             H25.033   Anterior subcapsular polar age-related cataract, bilateral   **A**
             H25.039   Anterior subcapsular polar age-related cataract, unspecified eye   **A**

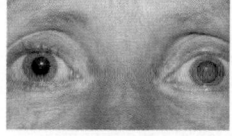

Figure 7-9   Age-related cataract. Nuclear sclerosis and cortical lens opacities are present. (From Ignatavicius DD, Workman ML: Medical-Surgical Nursing: Patient-Centered Collaborative Care, St. Louis, MO, Saunders/Elsevier, 2010)

Item 7-5   **Senile** cataracts are linked to the aging process. The most common area for the formation of a cataract is the cortical area of the lens. **Polar cataracts** can be either anterior or posterior. **Anterior polar cataracts** are more common and are small, white, capsular cataracts located on the anterior portion of the lens. **Total cataracts,** also called **complete** or **mature,** cause an opacity of all fibers of the lens. **Hypermature** describes a mature cataract with a swollen, milky cortex that covers the entire lens. **Immature,** also called **incipient,** cataracts have a clear cortex and are only slightly opaque. Treatment for all cataracts is the removal of the lens.

N Newborn Age: 0   **P** Pediatric Age: 0–17   **M** Maternity DX: 9–64   **A** Adult Age: 15–124   ♀ Females Only   ♂ Males Only
🦠 Complication\Comorbidity   🦠 Major C\C   (Ex) CC/MCC Exclusions   🦠 Hospital-Acquired Condition   🦠 Hierarchical Condition Category
847

CHAPTER 7 (H00-H59)

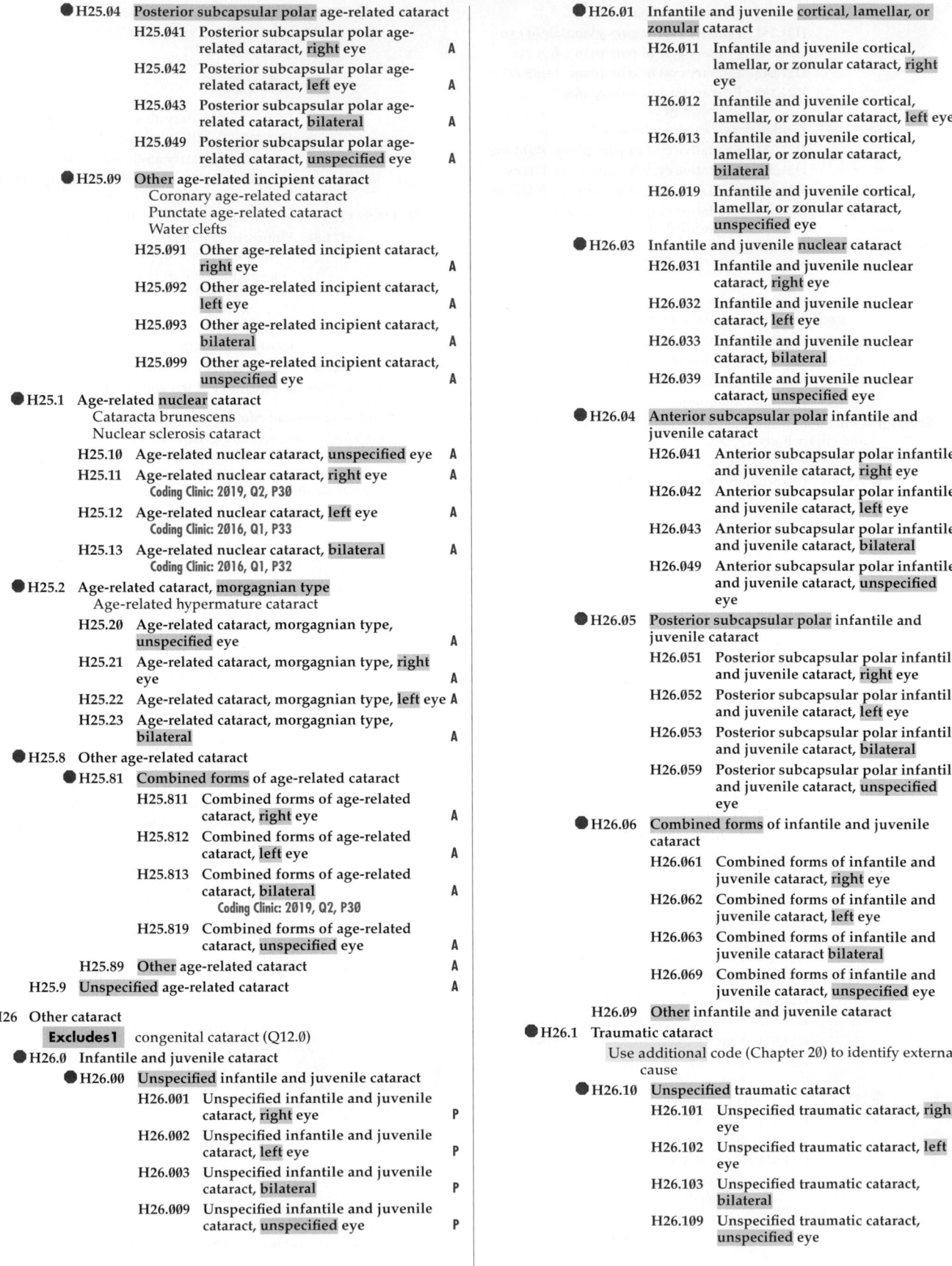

CHAPTER 7 (H00-H59)

● **H25.04** Posterior subcapsular polar age-related cataract
  - H25.041 Posterior subcapsular polar age-related cataract, right eye   A
  - H25.042 Posterior subcapsular polar age-related cataract, left eye   A
  - H25.043 Posterior subcapsular polar age-related cataract, bilateral   A
  - H25.049 Posterior subcapsular polar age-related cataract, unspecified eye   A

● **H25.09** Other age-related incipient cataract
  Coronary age-related cataract
  Punctate age-related cataract
  Water clefts
  - H25.091 Other age-related incipient cataract, right eye   A
  - H25.092 Other age-related incipient cataract, left eye   A
  - H25.093 Other age-related incipient cataract, bilateral   A
  - H25.099 Other age-related incipient cataract, unspecified eye   A

● **H25.1** Age-related nuclear cataract
  Cataracta brunescens
  Nuclear sclerosis cataract
  - H25.10 Age-related nuclear cataract, unspecified eye   A
  - H25.11 Age-related nuclear cataract, right eye   A
    Coding Clinic: 2019, Q2, P30
  - H25.12 Age-related nuclear cataract, left eye   A
    Coding Clinic: 2016, Q1, P33
  - H25.13 Age-related nuclear cataract, bilateral   A
    Coding Clinic: 2016, Q1, P32

● **H25.2** Age-related cataract, morgagnian type
  Age-related hypermature cataract
  - H25.20 Age-related cataract, morgagnian type, unspecified eye   A
  - H25.21 Age-related cataract, morgagnian type, right eye   A
  - H25.22 Age-related cataract, morgagnian type, left eye   A
  - H25.23 Age-related cataract, morgagnian type, bilateral   A

● **H25.8** Other age-related cataract
  ● H25.81 Combined forms of age-related cataract
    - H25.811 Combined forms of age-related cataract, right eye   A
    - H25.812 Combined forms of age-related cataract, left eye   A
    - H25.813 Combined forms of age-related cataract, bilateral   A
      Coding Clinic: 2019, Q2, P30
    - H25.819 Combined forms of age-related cataract, unspecified eye   A
  - H25.89 Other age-related cataract   A
- **H25.9** Unspecified age-related cataract   A

● **H26** Other cataract
  Excludes1 congenital cataract (Q12.0)
  ● **H26.0** Infantile and juvenile cataract
    ● H26.00 Unspecified infantile and juvenile cataract
      - H26.001 Unspecified infantile and juvenile cataract, right eye   P
      - H26.002 Unspecified infantile and juvenile cataract, left eye   P
      - H26.003 Unspecified infantile and juvenile cataract, bilateral   P
      - H26.009 Unspecified infantile and juvenile cataract, unspecified eye   P

● H26.01 Infantile and juvenile cortical, lamellar, or zonular cataract
  - H26.011 Infantile and juvenile cortical, lamellar, or zonular cataract, right eye   P
  - H26.012 Infantile and juvenile cortical, lamellar, or zonular cataract, left eye   P
  - H26.013 Infantile and juvenile cortical, lamellar, or zonular cataract, bilateral   P
  - H26.019 Infantile and juvenile cortical, lamellar, or zonular cataract, unspecified eye   P

● H26.03 Infantile and juvenile nuclear cataract
  - H26.031 Infantile and juvenile nuclear cataract, right eye   P
  - H26.032 Infantile and juvenile nuclear cataract, left eye   P
  - H26.033 Infantile and juvenile nuclear cataract, bilateral   P
  - H26.039 Infantile and juvenile nuclear cataract, unspecified eye   P

● H26.04 Anterior subcapsular polar infantile and juvenile cataract
  - H26.041 Anterior subcapsular polar infantile and juvenile cataract, right eye   P
  - H26.042 Anterior subcapsular polar infantile and juvenile cataract, left eye   P
  - H26.043 Anterior subcapsular polar infantile and juvenile cataract, bilateral   P
  - H26.049 Anterior subcapsular polar infantile and juvenile cataract, unspecified eye   P

● H26.05 Posterior subcapsular polar infantile and juvenile cataract
  - H26.051 Posterior subcapsular polar infantile and juvenile cataract, right eye   P
  - H26.052 Posterior subcapsular polar infantile and juvenile cataract, left eye   P
  - H26.053 Posterior subcapsular polar infantile and juvenile cataract, bilateral   P
  - H26.059 Posterior subcapsular polar infantile and juvenile cataract, unspecified eye   P

● H26.06 Combined forms of infantile and juvenile cataract
  - H26.061 Combined forms of infantile and juvenile cataract, right eye   P
  - H26.062 Combined forms of infantile and juvenile cataract, left eye   P
  - H26.063 Combined forms of infantile and juvenile cataract bilateral   P
  - H26.069 Combined forms of infantile and juvenile cataract, unspecified eye   P
  - H26.09 Other infantile and juvenile cataract   P

● **H26.1** Traumatic cataract
  Use additional code (Chapter 20) to identify external cause
  ● H26.10 Unspecified traumatic cataract
    - H26.101 Unspecified traumatic cataract, right eye
    - H26.102 Unspecified traumatic cataract, left eye
    - H26.103 Unspecified traumatic cataract, bilateral
    - H26.109 Unspecified traumatic cataract, unspecified eye

▶ New   ⇒ Revised   ~~deleted~~ Deleted   Excludes 1   Excludes 2   Includes   Use additional   Code first   Code also   Key words
OGCR Official Guidelines   ● Unacceptable Principal Diagnosis   X Assign placeholder X   ● Use Additional Character(s)   ▶ Manifestation Code   Coding Clinic

● H26.11   Localized traumatic opacities
- H26.111   Localized traumatic opacities, right eye
- H26.112   Localized traumatic opacities, left eye
- H26.113   Localized traumatic opacities, bilateral
- H26.119   Localized traumatic opacities, unspecified eye

● H26.12   Partially resolved traumatic cataract
- H26.121   Partially resolved traumatic cataract, right eye
- H26.122   Partially resolved traumatic cataract, left eye
- H26.123   Partially resolved traumatic cataract, bilateral
- H26.129   Partially resolved traumatic cataract, unspecified eye

● H26.13   Total traumatic cataract
- H26.131   Total traumatic cataract, right eye
- H26.132   Total traumatic cataract, left eye
- H26.133   Total traumatic cataract, bilateral
- H26.139   Total traumatic cataract, unspecified eye

● H26.2   Complicated cataract
- H26.20   Unspecified complicated cataract
  - Cataracta complicata NOS

● H26.21   Cataract with neovascularization

  Code also associated condition, such as: chronic iridocyclitis (H20.1-)

- H26.211   Cataract with neovascularization, right eye
- H26.212   Cataract with neovascularization, left eye
- H26.213   Cataract with neovascularization, bilateral
- H26.219   Cataract with neovascularization, unspecified eye

● H26.22   Cataract secondary to ocular disorders (degenerative) (inflammatory)

  Code also associated ocular disorder

- H26.221   Cataract secondary to ocular disorders (degenerative) (inflammatory), right eye
- H26.222   Cataract secondary to ocular disorders (degenerative) (inflammatory), left eye
- H26.223   Cataract secondary to ocular disorders (degenerative) (inflammatory), bilateral
- H26.229   Cataract secondary to ocular disorders (degenerative) (inflammatory), unspecified eye

● H26.23   Glaucomatous flecks (subcapsular)

  Code first underlying glaucoma (H40-H42)

- H26.231   Glaucomatous flecks (subcapsular), right eye
- H26.232   Glaucomatous flecks (subcapsular), left eye
- H26.233   Glaucomatous flecks (subcapsular), bilateral
- H26.239   Glaucomatous flecks (subcapsular), unspecified eye

● H26.3   Drug-induced cataract
  - Toxic cataract

  Use additional code for adverse effect, if applicable, to identify drug (T36-T50 with fifth or sixth character 5)

- H26.30   Drug-induced cataract, unspecified eye
- H26.31   Drug-induced cataract, right eye

H26.32   Drug-induced cataract, left eye
H26.33   Drug-induced cataract, bilateral

● H26.4   Secondary cataract
  Coding Clinic: 2018, Q2, P14
- H26.40   Unspecified secondary cataract

● H26.41   Soemmering's ring
- H26.411   Soemmering's ring, right eye
- H26.412   Soemmering's ring, left eye
- H26.413   Soemmering's ring, bilateral
- H26.419   Soemmering's ring, unspecified eye

● H26.49   Other secondary cataract
- H26.491   Other secondary cataract, right eye
- H26.492   Other secondary cataract, left eye
  - Coding Clinic: 2018, Q2, P13
- H26.493   Other secondary cataract, bilateral
- H26.499   Other secondary cataract, unspecified eye

H26.8   Other specified cataract
H26.9   Unspecified cataract

● H27   Other disorders of lens

  Excludes1   congenital lens malformations (Q12.-)
  mechanical complications of intraocular lens implant (T85.2)
  pseudophakia (Z96.1)

● H27.0   Aphakia
  Acquired absence of lens
  Acquired aphakia
  Aphakia due to trauma

  Excludes1   cataract extraction status (Z98.4-)
  congenital absence of lens (Q12.3)
  congenital aphakia (Q12.3)

- H27.00   Aphakia, unspecified eye
- H27.01   Aphakia, right eye
- H27.02   Aphakia, left eye
- H27.03   Aphakia, bilateral

● H27.1   Dislocation of lens
- H27.10   Unspecified dislocation of lens

● H27.11   Subluxation of lens
- H27.111   Subluxation of lens, right eye
- H27.112   Subluxation of lens, left eye
- H27.113   Subluxation of lens, bilateral
- H27.119   Subluxation of lens, unspecified eye

● H27.12   Anterior dislocation of lens
- H27.121   Anterior dislocation of lens, right eye
- H27.122   Anterior dislocation of lens, left eye
- H27.123   Anterior dislocation of lens, bilateral
- H27.129   Anterior dislocation of lens, unspecified eye

● H27.13   Posterior dislocation of lens
- H27.131   Posterior dislocation of lens, right eye
- H27.132   Posterior dislocation of lens, left eye
- H27.133   Posterior dislocation of lens, bilateral
- H27.139   Posterior dislocation of lens, unspecified eye

H27.8   Other specified disorders of lens
H27.9   Unspecified disorder of lens

▷ *H28   Cataract in diseases classified elsewhere*

  Code first underlying disease, such as:
  hypoparathyroidism (E20.-)
  myotonia (G71.1-)
  myxedema (E03.-)
  protein-calorie malnutrition (E40-E46)

  Excludes1   cataract in diabetes mellitus (E08.36, E09.36, E10.36, E11.36, E13.36)

CHAPTER 7 (H00-H59)

DISORDERS OF CHOROID AND RETINA (H30-H36)

★ **(See Plate 16 of the Anatomy Illustrations.)**

● H30   Chorioretinal inflammation

  ● H30.0   Focal chorioretinal inflammation
      Focal chorioretinitis
      Focal choroiditis
      Focal retinitis
      Focal retinochoroiditis

    ● H30.00   Unspecified focal chorioretinal inflammation
        Focal chorioretinitis NOS
        Focal choroiditis NOS
        Focal retinitis NOS
        Focal retinochoroiditis NOS

      H30.001   Unspecified focal chorioretinal inflammation, right eye

      H30.002   Unspecified focal chorioretinal inflammation, left eye

      H30.003   Unspecified focal chorioretinal inflammation, bilateral

      H30.009   Unspecified focal chorioretinal inflammation, unspecified eye

    ● H30.01   Focal chorioretinal inflammation, juxtapapillary

      H30.011   Focal chorioretinal inflammation, juxtapapillary, right eye

      H30.012   Focal chorioretinal inflammation, juxtapapillary, left eye

      H30.013   Focal chorioretinal inflammation, juxtapapillary, bilateral

      H30.019   Focal chorioretinal inflammation, juxtapapillary, unspecified eye

    ● H30.02   Focal chorioretinal inflammation of posterior pole

      H30.021   Focal chorioretinal inflammation of posterior pole, right eye

      H30.022   Focal chorioretinal inflammation of posterior pole, left eye

      H30.023   Focal chorioretinal inflammation of posterior pole, bilateral

      H30.029   Focal chorioretinal inflammation of posterior pole, unspecified eye

    ● H30.03   Focal chorioretinal inflammation, peripheral

      H30.031   Focal chorioretinal inflammation, peripheral, right eye

      H30.032   Focal chorioretinal inflammation, peripheral, left eye

      H30.033   Focal chorioretinal inflammation, peripheral, bilateral

      H30.039   Focal chorioretinal inflammation, peripheral, unspecified eye

    ● H30.04   Focal chorioretinal inflammation, macular or paramacular

      H30.041   Focal chorioretinal inflammation, macular or paramacular, right eye

      H30.042   Focal chorioretinal inflammation, macular or paramacular, left eye

      H30.043   Focal chorioretinal inflammation, macular or paramacular, bilateral

      H30.049   Focal chorioretinal inflammation, macular or paramacular, unspecified eye

  ● H30.1   Disseminated chorioretinal inflammation
      Disseminated chorioretinitis
      Disseminated choroiditis
      Disseminated retinitis
      Disseminated retinochoroiditis

    Excludes2   exudative retinopathy (H35.02-)

    (Ex) **For category H30.1 CC codes:** See PDX Collection 626

  ● H30.10   Unspecified disseminated chorioretinal inflammation
      Disseminated chorioretinitis NOS
      Disseminated choroiditis NOS
      Disseminated retinitis NOS
      Disseminated retinochoroiditis NOS

      H30.101   Unspecified disseminated chorioretinal inflammation, right eye

      H30.102   Unspecified disseminated chorioretinal inflammation, left eye

      H30.103   Unspecified disseminated chorioretinal inflammation, bilateral

      H30.109   Unspecified disseminated chorioretinal inflammation, unspecified eye

  ● H30.11   Disseminated chorioretinal inflammation of posterior pole

      H30.111   Disseminated chorioretinal inflammation of posterior pole, right eye

      H30.112   Disseminated chorioretinal inflammation of posterior pole, left eye

      H30.113   Disseminated chorioretinal inflammation of posterior pole, bilateral

      H30.119   Disseminated chorioretinal inflammation of posterior pole, unspecified eye

  ● H30.12   Disseminated chorioretinal inflammation, peripheral

      H30.121   Disseminated chorioretinal inflammation, peripheral right eye

      H30.122   Disseminated chorioretinal inflammation, peripheral, left eye

      H30.123   Disseminated chorioretinal inflammation, peripheral, bilateral

      H30.129   Disseminated chorioretinal inflammation, peripheral, unspecified eye

  ● H30.13   Disseminated chorioretinal inflammation, generalized

      H30.131   Disseminated chorioretinal inflammation, generalized, right eye

      H30.132   Disseminated chorioretinal inflammation, generalized, left eye

      H30.133   Disseminated chorioretinal inflammation, generalized, bilateral

      H30.139   Disseminated chorioretinal inflammation, generalized, unspecified eye

  ● H30.14   Acute posterior multifocal placoid pigment epitheliopathy

      H30.141   Acute posterior multifocal placoid pigment epitheliopathy, right eye

      H30.142   Acute posterior multifocal placoid pigment epitheliopathy, left eye

      H30.143   Acute posterior multifocal placoid pigment epitheliopathy, bilateral

      H30.149   Acute posterior multifocal placoid pigment epitheliopathy, unspecified eye

  ● H30.2   Posterior cyclitis
      Pars planitis

    H30.20   Posterior cyclitis, unspecified eye

    H30.21   Posterior cyclitis, right eye

    H30.22   Posterior cyclitis, left eye

    H30.23   Posterior cyclitis, bilateral

▶ New   ➠ Revised   ~~deleted~~ Deleted   Excludes 1   Excludes 2   Includes   Use additional   Code first   Code also   Key words

OGCR Official Guidelines   ● Unacceptable Principal Diagnosis   X Assign placeholder X   ● Use Additional Character(s)   ▶ Manifestation Code   **Coding Clinic**

● H30.8   Other chorioretinal inflammations
  ● H30.81   Harada's disease
      H30.811   Harada's disease, right eye
      H30.812   Harada's disease, left eye
      H30.813   Harada's disease, bilateral
      H30.819   Harada's disease, unspecified eye
  ● H30.89   Other chorioretinal inflammations
      (Ex) **For category H30.89 CC codes:** See PDX Collection 626
      H30.891   Other chorioretinal inflammations, right eye 🝆
      H30.892   Other chorioretinal inflammations, left eye 🝆
      H30.893   Other chorioretinal inflammations, bilateral 🝆
      H30.899   Other chorioretinal inflammations, unspecified eye 🝆
● H30.9   Unspecified chorioretinal inflammation
    Chorioretinitis NOS
    Choroiditis NOS
    Neuroretinitis NOS
    Retinitis NOS
    Retinochoroiditis NOS
    (Ex) **For category H30.9 CC codes:** See PDX Collection 626
    H30.90   Unspecified chorioretinal inflammation, unspecified eye 🝆
    H30.91   Unspecified chorioretinal inflammation, right eye 🝆
    H30.92   Unspecified chorioretinal inflammation, left eye 🝆
    H30.93   Unspecified chorioretinal inflammation, bilateral 🝆

● H31   Other disorders of choroid
  ● H31.0   Chorioretinal scars
      Excludes2   postsurgical chorioretinal scars (H59.81-)
    ● H31.00   Unspecified chorioretinal scars
      H31.001   Unspecified chorioretinal scars, right eye
      H31.002   Unspecified chorioretinal scars, left eye
      H31.003   Unspecified chorioretinal scars, bilateral
      H31.009   Unspecified chorioretinal scars, unspecified eye
    ● H31.01   Macula scars of posterior pole (postinflammatory) (post-traumatic)
      Excludes1   postprocedural chorioretinal scar (H59.81-)
      H31.011   Macula scars of posterior pole (postinflammatory) (post-traumatic), right eye
      H31.012   Macula scars of posterior pole (postinflammatory) (post-traumatic), left eye
      H31.013   Macula scars of posterior pole (postinflammatory) (post-traumatic), bilateral
      H31.019   Macula scars of posterior pole (postinflammatory) (post-traumatic), unspecified eye
    ● H31.02   Solar retinopathy
      H31.021   Solar retinopathy, right eye
      H31.022   Solar retinopathy, left eye
      H31.023   Solar retinopathy, bilateral
      H31.029   Solar retinopathy, unspecified eye

● H31.09   Other chorioretinal scars
    H31.091   Other chorioretinal scars, right eye
    H31.092   Other chorioretinal scars, left eye
    H31.093   Other chorioretinal scars, bilateral
    H31.099   Other chorioretinal scars, unspecified eye
● H31.1   Choroidal degeneration
    Excludes2   angioid streaks of macula (H35.33)
  ● H31.10   Unspecified choroidal degeneration
    Choroidal sclerosis NOS
    H31.101   Choroidal degeneration, unspecified, right eye
    H31.102   Choroidal degeneration, unspecified, left eye
    H31.103   Choroidal degeneration, unspecified, bilateral
    H31.109   Choroidal degeneration, unspecified, unspecified eye
  ● H31.11   Age-related choroidal atrophy
    H31.111   Age-related choroidal atrophy, right eye   A
    H31.112   Age-related choroidal atrophy, left eye   A
    H31.113   Age-related choroidal atrophy, bilateral   A
    H31.119   Age-related choroidal atrophy, unspecified eye   A
  ● H31.12   Diffuse secondary atrophy of choroid
    H31.121   Diffuse secondary atrophy of choroid, right eye
    H31.122   Diffuse secondary atrophy of choroid, left eye
    H31.123   Diffuse secondary atrophy of choroid, bilateral
    H31.129   Diffuse secondary atrophy of choroid, unspecified eye
● H31.2   Hereditary choroidal dystrophy
    Excludes2   hyperornithinemia (E72.4)
                  ornithinemia (E72.4)
    H31.20   Hereditary choroidal dystrophy, unspecified
    H31.21   Choroideremia
    H31.22   Choroidal dystrophy (central areolar) (generalized) (peripapillary)
    H31.23   Gyrate atrophy, choroid
    H31.29   Other hereditary choroidal dystrophy
● H31.3   Choroidal hemorrhage and rupture
  ● H31.30   Unspecified choroidal hemorrhage
    H31.301   Unspecified choroidal hemorrhage, right eye
    H31.302   Unspecified choroidal hemorrhage, left eye
    H31.303   Unspecified choroidal hemorrhage, bilateral
    H31.309   Unspecified choroidal hemorrhage, unspecified eye
  ● H31.31   Expulsive choroidal hemorrhage
    H31.311   Expulsive choroidal hemorrhage, right eye
    H31.312   Expulsive choroidal hemorrhage, left eye
    H31.313   Expulsive choroidal hemorrhage, bilateral
    H31.319   Expulsive choroidal hemorrhage, unspecified eye

CHAPTER 7 (H00-H59)

N Newborn Age: 0   **P** Pediatric Age: 0–17   **M** Maternity DX: 9–64   **A** Adult Age: 15–124   ♀ Females Only   ♂ Males Only
🝆 Complication\Comorbidity   🝆 Major C\C   (Ex) CC/MCC Exclusions   🝆 Hospital-Acquired Condition   🝆 Hierarchical Condition Category

851

● **H31.32   Choroidal rupture**
    Ⓔ **For category H31.32 CC codes:** See PDX Collection 627
    H31.321   Choroidal rupture, right eye
    H31.322   Choroidal rupture, left eye
    H31.323   Choroidal rupture, bilateral
    H31.329   Choroidal rupture, unspecified eye

● **H31.4   Choroidal detachment**
    Ⓔ **For category H31.4 CC codes:** See PDX Collection 627
  ● **H31.40   Unspecified choroidal detachment**
    H31.401   Unspecified choroidal detachment, right eye
    H31.402   Unspecified choroidal detachment, left eye
    H31.403   Unspecified choroidal detachment, bilateral
    H31.409   Unspecified choroidal detachment, unspecified eye
  ● **H31.41   Hemorrhagic choroidal detachment**
    H31.411   Hemorrhagic choroidal detachment, right eye
    H31.412   Hemorrhagic choroidal detachment, left eye
    H31.413   Hemorrhagic choroidal detachment, bilateral
    H31.419   Hemorrhagic choroidal detachment, unspecified eye
  ● **H31.42   Serous choroidal detachment**
    H31.421   Serous choroidal detachment, right eye
    H31.422   Serous choroidal detachment, left eye
    H31.423   Serous choroidal detachment, bilateral
    H31.429   Serous choroidal detachment, unspecified eye

H31.8   Other specified disorders of choroid

H31.9   Unspecified disorder of choroid

▷ **H32   *Chorioretinal disorders in diseases classified elsewhere***
    Code first underlying disease, such as:
      congenital toxoplasmosis (P37.1)
      histoplasmosis (B39.-)
      leprosy (A30.-)
    Excludes1   chorioretinitis (in):
          toxoplasmosis (acquired) (B58.01)
          tuberculosis (A18.53)

● **H33   Retinal detachments and breaks**
    Excludes1   detachment of retinal pigment epithelium (H35.72-, H35.73-)
  ● **H33.0   Retinal detachment with retinal break**
    Rhegmatogenous retinal detachment
    Excludes1   serous retinal detachment (without retinal break) (H33.2-)
    ● **H33.00   Unspecified retinal detachment with retinal break**
      H33.001   Unspecified retinal detachment with retinal break, right eye
      H33.002   Unspecified retinal detachment with retinal break, left eye
      H33.003   Unspecified retinal detachment with retinal break, bilateral
      H33.009   Unspecified retinal detachment with retinal break, unspecified eye

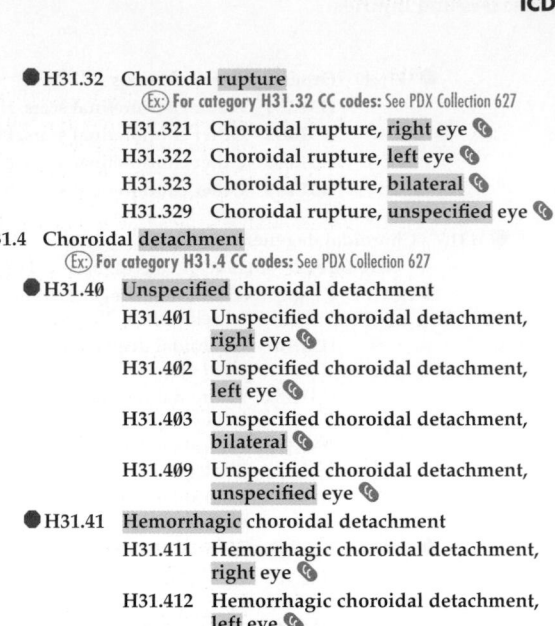
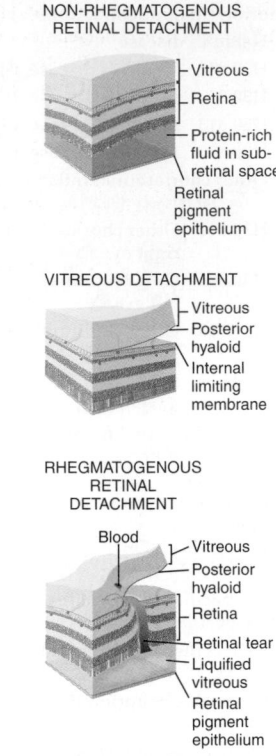

Figure 7-10   Retinal detachment. (From Kumar: Robbins and Cotran: Pathologic Basis of Disease, ed 7, Saunders, 2005)

Item 7–6   Retinal detachments and defects are conditions of the eye in which the retina separates from the underlying tissue. Initial detachment may be localized, requiring rapid treatment (medical emergency) to avoid the entire retina from detaching, which leads to vision loss and blindness.

● **H33.01   Retinal detachment with single break**
    H33.011   Retinal detachment with single break, right eye
    H33.012   Retinal detachment with single break, left eye
    H33.013   Retinal detachment with single break, bilateral
    H33.019   Retinal detachment with single break, unspecified eye
● **H33.02   Retinal detachment with multiple breaks**
    H33.021   Retinal detachment with multiple breaks, right eye
    H33.022   Retinal detachment with multiple breaks, left eye
    H33.023   Retinal detachment with multiple breaks, bilateral
    H33.029   Retinal detachment with multiple breaks, unspecified eye
● **H33.03   Retinal detachment with giant retinal tear**
    H33.031   Retinal detachment with giant retinal tear, right eye
    H33.032   Retinal detachment with giant retinal tear, left eye
    H33.033   Retinal detachment with giant retinal tear, bilateral
    H33.039   Retinal detachment with giant retinal tear, unspecified eye

▶ New   ⇒ Revised   ~~deleted~~ Deleted   Excludes 1   Excludes 2   Includes   Use additional   Code first   Code also   Key words
OGCR Official Guidelines   ● Unacceptable Principal Diagnosis   X Assign placeholder X   ● Use Additional Character(s)   ▷ Manifestation Code   **Coding Clinic**

● H33.04   Retinal detachment with retinal dialysis
    H33.041   Retinal detachment with retinal dialysis, right eye
    H33.042   Retinal detachment with retinal dialysis, left eye
    H33.043   Retinal detachment with retinal dialysis, bilateral
    H33.049   Retinal detachment with retinal dialysis, unspecified eye

● H33.05   Total retinal detachment
    H33.051   Total retinal detachment, right eye
    H33.052   Total retinal detachment, left eye
    H33.053   Total retinal detachment, bilateral
    H33.059   Total retinal detachment, unspecified eye

● H33.1   Retinoschisis and retinal cysts
    Excludes1   congenital retinoschisis (Q14.1)
                microcystoid degeneration of retina (H35.42-)

● H33.10   Unspecified retinoschisis
    H33.101   Unspecified retinoschisis, right eye
    H33.102   Unspecified retinoschisis, left eye
    H33.103   Unspecified retinoschisis, bilateral
    H33.109   Unspecified retinoschisis, unspecified eye

● H33.11   Cyst of ora serrata
    H33.111   Cyst of ora serrata, right eye
    H33.112   Cyst of ora serrata, left eye
    H33.113   Cyst of ora serrata, bilateral
    H33.119   Cyst of ora serrata, unspecified eye

● H33.12   Parasitic cyst of retina
    (Ex) **For category H33.12 CC codes:** See PDX Collection 625
    H33.121   Parasitic cyst of retina, right eye 🅒
    H33.122   Parasitic cyst of retina, left eye 🅒
    H33.123   Parasitic cyst of retina, bilateral 🅒
    H33.129   Parasitic cyst of retina, unspecified eye 🅒

● H33.19   Other retinoschisis and retinal cysts
    Pseudocyst of retina
    H33.191   Other retinoschisis and retinal cysts, right eye
    H33.192   Other retinoschisis and retinal cysts, left eye
    H33.193   Other retinoschisis and retinal cysts, bilateral
    H33.199   Other retinoschisis and retinal cysts, unspecified eye

● H33.2   Serous retinal detachment
    Retinal detachment NOS
    Retinal detachment without retinal break
    Excludes1   central serous chorioretinopathy (H35.71-)
    (Ex) **For category H33.2 CC codes:** See PDX Collection 628
    H33.20   Serous retinal detachment, unspecified eye 🅒
    H33.21   Serous retinal detachment, right eye 🅒
    H33.22   Serous retinal detachment, left eye 🅒
    H33.23   Serous retinal detachment, bilateral 🅒

● H33.3   Retinal breaks without detachment
    Excludes1   chorioretinal scars after surgery for detachment (H59.81-)
                peripheral retinal degeneration without break (H35.4-)

● H33.30   Unspecified retinal break
    H33.301   Unspecified retinal break, right eye
    H33.302   Unspecified retinal break, left eye
    H33.303   Unspecified retinal break, bilateral
    H33.309   Unspecified retinal break, unspecified eye

● H33.31   Horseshoe tear of retina without detachment
    Operculum of retina without detachment
    H33.311   Horseshoe tear of retina without detachment, right eye
    H33.312   Horseshoe tear of retina without detachment, left eye
    H33.313   Horseshoe tear of retina without detachment, bilateral
    H33.319   Horseshoe tear of retina without detachment, unspecified eye

● H33.32   Round hole of retina without detachment
    H33.321   Round hole, right eye
    H33.322   Round hole, left eye
    H33.323   Round hole, bilateral
    H33.329   Round hole, unspecified eye

● H33.33   Multiple defects of retina without detachment
    H33.331   Multiple defects of retina without detachment, right eye
    H33.332   Multiple defects of retina without detachment, left eye
    H33.333   Multiple defects of retina without detachment, bilateral
    H33.339   Multiple defects of retina without detachment, unspecified eye

● H33.4   Traction detachment of retina
    Proliferative vitreo-retinopathy with retinal detachment
    (Ex) **For category H33.4 CC codes:** See PDX Collection 628
    H33.40   Traction detachment of retina, unspecified eye 🅒
    H33.41   Traction detachment of retina, right eye 🅒
    H33.42   Traction detachment of retina, left eye 🅒
    H33.43   Traction detachment of retina, bilateral 🅒

H33.8   Other retinal detachments 🅒
    (Ex) See PDX Collection 628

● H34   Retinal vascular occlusions
    Blockage in vessel of the retina
    Excludes1   amaurosis fugax (G45.3)
    (Ex) **For category H34 CC codes:** See PDX Collection 587

● H34.0   Transient retinal artery occlusion
    H34.00   Transient retinal artery occlusion, unspecified eye 🅒
    H34.01   Transient retinal artery occlusion, right eye 🅒
    H34.02   Transient retinal artery occlusion, left eye 🅒
    H34.03   Transient retinal artery occlusion, bilateral 🅒

● H34.1   Central retinal artery occlusion
    H34.10   Central retinal artery occlusion, unspecified eye 🅒
    H34.11   Central retinal artery occlusion, right eye 🅒
    H34.12   Central retinal artery occlusion, left eye 🅒
    H34.13   Central retinal artery occlusion, bilateral 🅒

● H34.2   Other retinal artery occlusions
   ● H34.21   Partial retinal artery occlusion
    Hollenhorst's plaque
    Retinal microembolism
    H34.211   Partial retinal artery occlusion, right eye 🅒
    H34.212   Partial retinal artery occlusion, left eye 🅒
    H34.213   Partial retinal artery occlusion, bilateral 🅒
    H34.219   Partial retinal artery occlusion, unspecified eye 🅒

CHAPTER 7 (H00–H59)

N   Newborn Age: 0   P   Pediatric Age: 0–17   M   Maternity DX: 9–64   A   Adult Age: 15–124   ♀ Females Only   ♂ Males Only

🅒 Complication\Comorbidity   🅜 Major C\C   (Ex) CC/MCC Exclusions   🅗 Hospital-Acquired Condition   🅒 Hierarchical Condition Category

853

● H34.23 Retinal artery branch occlusion
    H34.231 Retinal artery branch occlusion, right eye 🔍
    H34.232 Retinal artery branch occlusion, left eye 🔍
    H34.233 Retinal artery branch occlusion, bilateral 🔍
    H34.239 Retinal artery branch occlusion, unspecified eye 🔍

● H34.8 Other retinal vascular occlusions
    Coding Clinic: 2016, Q4, P19
  ● H34.81 Central retinal vein occlusion

One of the following 7th characters is to be assigned to codes in subcategory H34.81 to designate the severity of the occlusion:

> Ø   with macular edema
> 1   with retinal neovascularization
> 2   stable
>   Old central retinal vein occlusion

    ● H34.811 Central retinal vein occlusion, right eye 🔍
    ● H34.812 Central retinal vein occlusion, left eye 🔍
    ● H34.813 Central retinal vein occlusion, bilateral 🔍
    ● H34.819 Central retinal vein occlusion, unspecified eye 🔍

  ● H34.82 Venous engorgement
    Incipient retinal vein occlusion
    Partial retinal vein occlusion
    H34.821 Venous engorgement, right eye
    H34.822 Venous engorgement, left eye
    H34.823 Venous engorgement, bilateral
    H34.829 Venous engorgement, unspecified eye

  ● H34.83 Tributary (branch) retinal vein occlusion

One of the following 7th characters is to be assigned to codes in subcategory H34.83 to designate the severity of the occlusion:

> Ø   with macular edema
> 1   with retinal neovascularization
> 2   stable
>   Old tributary (branch) retinal vein occlusion

    ● H34.831 Tributary (branch) retinal vein occlusion, right eye
    ● H34.832 Tributary (branch) retinal vein occlusion, left eye
    ● H34.833 Tributary (branch) retinal vein occlusion, bilateral
    ● H34.839 Tributary (branch) retinal vein occlusion, unspecified eye

H34.9 Unspecified retinal vascular occlusion 🔍

● H35 Other retinal disorders
  Excludes2 diabetic retinal disorders (E08.311-E08.359, E09.311-E09.359, E10.311-E10.359, E11.311-E11.359, E13.311-E13.359)

● H35.0 Background retinopathy and retinal vascular changes
  ⟾ Code also any associated hypertension (I10)
  OGCR Section I. C.9.a.5.

  Hypertensive Retinopathy
  Subcategory H35.0, Background retinopathy and retinal vascular changes, should be used with a code from category I10–I15, Hypertensive disease to include the systemic hypertension. The sequencing is based on the reason for the encounter.

H35.00 Unspecified background retinopathy
● H35.01 Changes in retinal vascular appearance
  Retinal vascular sheathing
  H35.011 Changes in retinal vascular appearance, right eye
  H35.012 Changes in retinal vascular appearance, left eye
  H35.013 Changes in retinal vascular appearance, bilateral
  H35.019 Changes in retinal vascular appearance, unspecified eye

● H35.02 Exudative retinopathy
  Coats retinopathy
  H35.021 Exudative retinopathy, right eye
  H35.022 Exudative retinopathy, left eye
  H35.023 Exudative retinopathy, bilateral
  H35.029 Exudative retinopathy, unspecified eye

● H35.03 Hypertensive retinopathy
  H35.031 Hypertensive retinopathy, right eye
  H35.032 Hypertensive retinopathy, left eye
  H35.033 Hypertensive retinopathy, bilateral
  H35.039 Hypertensive retinopathy, unspecified eye

● H35.04 Retinal micro-aneurysms, unspecified
  H35.041 Retinal micro-aneurysms, unspecified, right eye
  H35.042 Retinal micro-aneurysms, unspecified, left eye
  H35.043 Retinal micro-aneurysms, unspecified, bilateral
  H35.049 Retinal micro-aneurysms, unspecified, unspecified eye

● H35.05 Retinal neovascularization, unspecified
  H35.051 Retinal neovascularization, unspecified, right eye
  H35.052 Retinal neovascularization, unspecified, left eye
  H35.053 Retinal neovascularization, unspecified, bilateral
  H35.059 Retinal neovascularization, unspecified, unspecified eye

● H35.06 Retinal vasculitis
  Eales disease
  Retinal perivasculitis
  H35.061 Retinal vasculitis, right eye
  H35.062 Retinal vasculitis, left eye
  H35.063 Retinal vasculitis, bilateral
  H35.069 Retinal vasculitis, unspecified eye

● H35.07 Retinal telangiectasis
  H35.071 Retinal telangiectasis, right eye
  H35.072 Retinal telangiectasis, left eye
  H35.073 Retinal telangiectasis, bilateral
  H35.079 Retinal telangiectasis, unspecified eye

H35.09 Other intraretinal microvascular abnormalities
  Retinal varices

● H35.1 Retinopathy of prematurity
● H35.10 Retinopathy of prematurity, unspecified
  Retinopathy of prematurity NOS
  H35.101 Retinopathy of prematurity, unspecified, right eye
  H35.102 Retinopathy of prematurity, unspecified, left eye
  H35.103 Retinopathy of prematurity, unspecified, bilateral
  H35.109 Retinopathy of prematurity, unspecified, unspecified eye

▶ New ⟾ Revised ~~deleted~~ Deleted Excludes 1 Excludes 2 Includes Use additional Code first Code also Key words
OGCR Official Guidelines ● Unacceptable Principal Diagnosis X Assign placeholder X ● Use Additional Character(s)) Manifestation Code **Coding Clinic**

- H35.11 **Retinopathy of prematurity, stage 0**
  - H35.111 **Retinopathy of prematurity, stage 0, right eye**
  - H35.112 **Retinopathy of prematurity, stage 0, left eye**
  - H35.113 **Retinopathy of prematurity, stage 0, bilateral**
  - H35.119 **Retinopathy of prematurity, stage 0, unspecified eye**
- H35.12 **Retinopathy of prematurity, stage 1**
  - H35.121 **Retinopathy of prematurity, stage 1, right eye**
  - H35.122 **Retinopathy of prematurity, stage 1, left eye**
  - H35.123 **Retinopathy of prematurity, stage 1, bilateral**
  - H35.129 **Retinopathy of prematurity, stage 1, unspecified eye**
- H35.13 **Retinopathy of prematurity, stage 2**
  - H35.131 **Retinopathy of prematurity, stage 2, right eye**
  - H35.132 **Retinopathy of prematurity, stage 2, left eye**
  - H35.133 **Retinopathy of prematurity, stage 2, bilateral**
  - H35.139 **Retinopathy of prematurity, stage 2, unspecified eye**
- H35.14 **Retinopathy of prematurity, stage 3**
  - H35.141 **Retinopathy of prematurity, stage 3, right eye**
  - H35.142 **Retinopathy of prematurity, stage 3, left eye**
  - H35.143 **Retinopathy of prematurity, stage 3, bilateral**
  - H35.149 **Retinopathy of prematurity, stage 3, unspecified eye**
- H35.15 **Retinopathy of prematurity, stage 4**
  - H35.151 **Retinopathy of prematurity, stage 4, right eye**
  - H35.152 **Retinopathy of prematurity, stage 4, left eye**
  - H35.153 **Retinopathy of prematurity, stage 4, bilateral**
  - H35.159 **Retinopathy of prematurity, stage 4, unspecified eye**
- H35.16 **Retinopathy of prematurity, stage 5**
  - H35.161 **Retinopathy of prematurity, stage 5, right eye**
  - H35.162 **Retinopathy of prematurity, stage 5, left eye**
  - H35.163 **Retinopathy of prematurity, stage 5, bilateral**
  - H35.169 **Retinopathy of prematurity, stage 5, unspecified eye**
- H35.17 **Retrolental fibroplasia**
  - H35.171 **Retrolental fibroplasia, right eye**
  - H35.172 **Retrolental fibroplasia, left eye**
  - H35.173 **Retrolental fibroplasia, bilateral**
  - H35.179 **Retrolental fibroplasia, unspecified eye**
- H35.2 **Other non-diabetic proliferative retinopathy**
  Proliferative vitreo-retinopathy
  > **Excludes1**   proliferative vitreo-retinopathy with retinal detachment (H33.4-)
  - H35.20 **Other non-diabetic proliferative retinopathy, unspecified eye**
  - H35.21 **Other non-diabetic proliferative retinopathy, right eye**
  - H35.22 **Other non-diabetic proliferative retinopathy, left eye**
  - H35.23 **Other non-diabetic proliferative retinopathy, bilateral**
- H35.3 **Degeneration of macula and posterior pole**
  - H35.30 **Unspecified macular degeneration**   A
    Age-related macular degeneration
  - H35.31 **Nonexudative age-related macular degeneration**
    Atrophic age-related macular degeneration
    Dry age-related macular degeneration
    One of the following 7th characters is to be assigned to codes in subcategory H35.31 to designate the stage of the disease:

0	stage unspecified
1	early dry stage
2	intermediate dry stage
3	advanced atrophic without subfoveal involvement
	advanced dry stage
4	advanced atrophic with subfoveal involvement

    - H35.311 **Nonexudative age-related macular degeneration, right eye**   A
      Coding Clinic: 2016, Q4, P20-21
    - H35.312 **Nonexudative age-related macular degeneration, left eye**   A
      Coding Clinic: 2016, Q4, P20-21
    - H35.313 **Nonexudative age-related macular degeneration, bilateral**   A
      Coding Clinic: 2016, Q4, P20
    - H35.319 **Nonexudative age-related macular degeneration, unspecified eye**   A
      Coding Clinic: 2016, Q4, P20
  - H35.32 **Exudative age-related macular degeneration**
    Wet age-related macular degeneration
    One of the following 7th characters is to be assigned to codes in subcategory H35.32 to designate the stage of the disease:

0	stage unspecified
1	with active choroidal neovascularization
2	with inactive choroidal neovascularization
	with involuted or regressed neovascularization
3	with inactive scar

    Coding Clinic: 2016, Q4, P20
    - H35.321 **Exudative age-related macular degeneration, right eye** 🐾   A
    - H35.322 **Exudative age-related macular degeneration, left eye** 🐾   A
    - H35.323 **Exudative age-related macular degeneration, bilateral** 🐾   A
    - H35.329 **Exudative age-related macular degeneration, unspecified eye** 🐾   A
  - H35.33 **Angioid streaks of macula**
  - H35.34 **Macular cyst, hole, or pseudohole**
    - H35.341 **Macular cyst, hole, or pseudohole, right eye**
    - H35.342 **Macular cyst, hole, or pseudohole, left eye**
    - H35.343 **Macular cyst, hole, or pseudohole, bilateral**
    - H35.349 **Macular cyst, hole, or pseudohole, unspecified eye**

Item 7–7 Macular degeneration is typically age-related, chronic, and is evidenced by deterioration of the macula (the part of the retina that provides for central field vision), resulting in blurred vision or a blind spot in the center of visual field while not affecting peripheral vision.

CHAPTER 7 (H00-H59)

● **H35.35**   Cystoid macular degeneration
  Excludes1   cystoid macular edema following cataract surgery (H59.03-)
  H35.351   Cystoid macular degeneration, right eye
  H35.352   Cystoid macular degeneration, left eye
  H35.353   Cystoid macular degeneration, bilateral
  H35.359   Cystoid macular degeneration, unspecified eye

● **H35.36**   Drusen (degenerative) of macula
  H35.361   Drusen (degenerative) of macula, right eye
    Coding Clinic: 2016, Q4, P21
  H35.362   Drusen (degenerative) of macula, left eye
    Coding Clinic: 2016, Q4, P21
  H35.363   Drusen (degenerative) of macula, bilateral
    Coding Clinic: 2017, Q1, P51
  H35.369   Drusen (degenerative) of macula, unspecified eye

● **H35.37**   Puckering of macula
  H35.371   Puckering of macula, right eye
  H35.372   Puckering of macula, left eye
  H35.373   Puckering of macula, bilateral
  H35.379   Puckering of macula, unspecified eye

● **H35.38**   Toxic maculopathy
  Code first poisoning due to drug or toxin, if applicable (T36-T65 with fifth or sixth character 1-4 or 6)
  Use additional code for adverse effect, if applicable, to identify drug (T36-T50 with fifth or sixth character 5)
  H35.381   Toxic maculopathy, right eye
  H35.382   Toxic maculopathy, left eye
  H35.383   Toxic maculopathy, bilateral
  H35.389   Toxic maculopathy, unspecified eye

● **H35.4**   Peripheral retinal degeneration
  Excludes1   hereditary retinal degeneration (dystrophy) (H35.5-)
  peripheral retinal degeneration with retinal break (H33.3-)
  H35.40   Unspecified peripheral retinal degeneration

● **H35.41**   Lattice degeneration of retina
  Palisade degeneration of retina
  H35.411   Lattice degeneration of retina, right eye
  H35.412   Lattice degeneration of retina, left eye
  H35.413   Lattice degeneration of retina, bilateral
  H35.419   Lattice degeneration of retina, unspecified eye

● **H35.42**   Microcystoid degeneration of retina
  H35.421   Microcystoid degeneration of retina, right eye
  H35.422   Microcystoid degeneration of retina, left eye
  H35.423   Microcystoid degeneration of retina, bilateral
  H35.429   Microcystoid degeneration of retina, unspecified eye

● **H35.43**   Paving stone degeneration of retina
  H35.431   Paving stone degeneration of retina, right eye
  H35.432   Paving stone degeneration of retina, left eye

H35.433   Paving stone degeneration of retina, bilateral
H35.439   Paving stone degeneration of retina, unspecified eye

● **H35.44**   Age-related reticular degeneration of retina
  H35.441   Age-related reticular degeneration of retina, right eye   A
  H35.442   Age-related reticular degeneration of retina, left eye   A
  H35.443   Age-related reticular degeneration of retina, bilateral   A
  H35.449   Age-related reticular degeneration of retina, unspecified eye   A

● **H35.45**   Secondary pigmentary degeneration
  H35.451   Secondary pigmentary degeneration, right eye
  H35.452   Secondary pigmentary degeneration, left eye
  H35.453   Secondary pigmentary degeneration, bilateral
  H35.459   Secondary pigmentary degeneration, unspecified eye

● **H35.46**   Secondary vitreoretinal degeneration
  H35.461   Secondary vitreoretinal degeneration, right eye
  H35.462   Secondary vitreoretinal degeneration, left eye
  H35.463   Secondary vitreoretinal degeneration, bilateral
  H35.469   Secondary vitreoretinal degeneration, unspecified eye

● **H35.5**   Hereditary retinal dystrophy
  Excludes1   dystrophies primarily involving Bruch's membrane (H31.1-)
  H35.50   Unspecified hereditary retinal dystrophy
  H35.51   Vitreoretinal dystrophy
  H35.52   Pigmentary retinal dystrophy
    Albipunctate retinal dystrophy
    Retinitis pigmentosa
    Tapetoretinal dystrophy
  H35.53   Other dystrophies primarily involving the sensory retina
    Stargardt's disease
  H35.54   Dystrophies primarily involving the retinal pigment epithelium
    Vitelliform retinal dystrophy

● **H35.6**   Retinal hemorrhage
  H35.60   Retinal hemorrhage, unspecified eye
  H35.61   Retinal hemorrhage, right eye
  H35.62   Retinal hemorrhage, left eye
  H35.63   Retinal hemorrhage, bilateral

● **H35.7**   Separation of retinal layers
  Excludes1   retinal detachment (serous) (H33.2-)
  rhegmatogenous retinal detachment (H33.0-)
  (Ex) **For category H35.7 CC codes: See PDX Collection 628**
  H35.70   Unspecified separation of retinal layers ⬧
● **H35.71**   Central serous chorioretinopathy
  H35.711   Central serous chorioretinopathy, right eye
  H35.712   Central serous chorioretinopathy, left eye
  H35.713   Central serous chorioretinopathy, bilateral
  H35.719   Central serous chorioretinopathy, unspecified eye

▶ New   ⇒ Revised   ~~deleted~~ Deleted   Excludes 1   Excludes 2   Includes   Use additional   Code first   Code also   Key words
OGCR Official Guidelines   ● Unacceptable Principal Diagnosis   X Assign placeholder X   ● Use Additional Character(s)   ▶ Manifestation Code   Coding Clinic

● H35.72 **Serous** detachment of retinal pigment epithelium

    H35.721 Serous detachment of retinal pigment epithelium, **right eye** 🅒

    H35.722 Serous detachment of retinal pigment epithelium, **left eye** 🅒

    H35.723 Serous detachment of retinal pigment epithelium, **bilateral** 🅒

    H35.729 Serous detachment of retinal pigment epithelium, **unspecified eye** 🅒

● H35.73 **Hemorrhagic** detachment of retinal pigment epithelium

    H35.731 Hemorrhagic detachment of retinal pigment epithelium, **right eye** 🅒

    H35.732 Hemorrhagic detachment of retinal pigment epithelium, **left eye** 🅒

    H35.733 Hemorrhagic detachment of retinal pigment epithelium, **bilateral** 🅒

    H35.739 Hemorrhagic detachment of retinal pigment epithelium, **unspecified eye** 🅒

● H35.8 **Other** specified retinal disorders

    Excludes2 retinal hemorrhage (H35.6-)

    H35.81 Retinal **edema**
        Retinal cotton wool spots

    H35.82 Retinal **ischemia** 🅒
        (Ex:) See PDX Collection 629

    H35.89 **Other** specified retinal disorders

● H35.9 **Unspecified** retinal disorder

▶ H36 *Retinal disorders in diseases classified elsewhere*

    Code first underlying disease, such as:
        lipid storage disorders (E75.-)
        sickle-cell disorders (D57.-)

    Excludes1 arteriosclerotic retinopathy (H35.0-)
          diabetic retinopathy (E08.3-, E09.3-, E10.3-, E11.3-, E13.3-)

GLAUCOMA (H40-H42)

● H40 Glaucoma

    Intraocular pressure (IOP) that is too high results from too much aqueous humor and because of excess production or inadequate drainage, optic nerve damage and vision loss may occur.

    Excludes1 absolute glaucoma (H44.51-)
          congenital glaucoma (Q15.0)
          traumatic glaucoma due to birth injury (P15.3)

● H40.0 Glaucoma **suspect**

  ● H40.00 **Preglaucoma, unspecified**

    H40.001 Preglaucoma, unspecified, **right eye**

    H40.002 Preglaucoma, unspecified, **left eye**

    H40.003 Preglaucoma, unspecified, **bilateral**

    H40.009 Preglaucoma, unspecified, **unspecified eye**

  ● H40.01 **Open angle** with borderline findings, **low risk**
        Open angle, low risk

    H40.011 Open angle with borderline findings, low risk, **right eye**

    H40.012 Open angle with borderline findings, low risk, **left eye**

    H40.013 Open angle with borderline findings, low risk, **bilateral**

    H40.019 Open angle with borderline findings, low risk, **unspecified eye**

  ● H40.02 **Open angle** with borderline findings, **high risk**
        Open angle, high risk

    H40.021 Open angle with borderline findings, high risk, **right eye**

    H40.022 Open angle with borderline findings, high risk, **left eye**

    H40.023 Open angle with borderline findings, high risk, **bilateral**

    H40.029 Open angle with borderline findings, high risk, **unspecified eye**

● H40.03 **Anatomical narrow** angle
    Primary angle closure suspect

    H40.031 Anatomical narrow angle, **right eye**

    H40.032 Anatomical narrow angle, **left eye**

    H40.033 Anatomical narrow angle, **bilateral**

    H40.039 Anatomical narrow angle, **unspecified eye**

● H40.04 **Steroid responder**

    H40.041 Steroid responder, **right eye**

    H40.042 Steroid responder, **left eye**

    H40.043 Steroid responder, **bilateral**

    H40.049 Steroid responder, **unspecified eye**

● H40.05 Ocular **hypertension**

    H40.051 Ocular hypertension, **right eye**

    H40.052 Ocular hypertension, **left eye**

    H40.053 Ocular hypertension, **bilateral**

    H40.059 Ocular hypertension, **unspecified eye**

● H40.06 Primary angle closure **without glaucoma damage**

    H40.061 Primary angle closure without glaucoma damage, **right eye**

    H40.062 Primary angle closure without glaucoma damage, **left eye**

    H40.063 Primary angle closure without glaucoma damage, **bilateral**

    H40.069 Primary angle closure without glaucoma damage, **unspecified eye**

● H40.1 Open-angle glaucoma

  X● H40.10 **Unspecified open-angle glaucoma**

    One of the following 7th characters is to be assigned to code H40.10 to designate the stage of glaucoma

0	stage unspecified
1	mild stage
2	moderate stage
3	severe stage
4	indeterminate stage

● H40.11 **Primary open-angle glaucoma**
    Chronic simple glaucoma

    One of the following 7th characters is to be assigned to each code in subcategory H40.11 to designate the stage of glaucoma

0	stage unspecified
1	mild stage
2	moderate stage
3	severe stage
4	indeterminate stage

    Coding Clinic: 2016, Q4, P22

  ● H40.111 Primary open-angle glaucoma, **right eye**
        Coding Clinic: 2019, Q2, P31

  ● H40.112 Primary open-angle glaucoma, **left eye**

  ● H40.113 Primary open-angle glaucoma, **bilateral**

  ● H40.119 Primary open-angle glaucoma, **unspecified eye**

N Newborn Age: 0   P Pediatric Age: 0–17   M Maternity DX: 9–64   A Adult Age: 15–124   ♀ Females Only   ♂ Males Only

🅒 Complication\Comorbidity   🅒 Major C\C   (Ex:) CC/MCC Exclusions   🅒 Hospital-Acquired Condition   🅒 Hierarchical Condition Category

857

● H40.12   **Low-tension** glaucoma

One of the following 7th characters is to be assigned to each code in subcategory H40.12 to designate the stage of glaucoma

0	stage unspecified
1	mild stage
2	moderate stage
3	severe stage
4	indeterminate stage

●● H40.121   Low-tension glaucoma, **right** eye
●● H40.122   Low-tension glaucoma, **left** eye
●● H40.123   Low-tension glaucoma, **bilateral**
●● H40.129   Low-tension glaucoma, **unspecified** eye

● H40.13   **Pigmentary** glaucoma

One of the following 7th characters is to be assigned to each code in subcategory H40.13 to designate the stage of glaucoma

0	stage unspecified
1	mild stage
2	moderate stage
3	severe stage
4	indeterminate stage

●● H40.131   Pigmentary glaucoma, **right** eye
●● H40.132   Pigmentary glaucoma, **left** eye
●● H40.133   Pigmentary glaucoma, **bilateral**
●● H40.139   Pigmentary glaucoma, **unspecified** eye

● H40.14   **Capsular** glaucoma **with pseudoexfoliation** of lens

One of the following 7th characters is to be assigned to each code in subcategory H40.14 to designate the stage of glaucoma

0	stage unspecified
1	mild stage
2	moderate stage
3	severe stage
4	indeterminate stage

● H40.141   Capsular glaucoma with pseudoexfoliation of lens, **right** eye
● H40.142   Capsular glaucoma with pseudoexfoliation of lens, **left** eye
● H40.143   Capsular glaucoma with pseudoexfoliation of lens, **bilateral**
● H40.149   Capsular glaucoma with pseudoexfoliation of lens, **unspecified** eye

● H40.15   **Residual stage** of open-angle glaucoma
● H40.151   Residual stage of open-angle glaucoma, **right** eye
● H40.152   Residual stage of open-angle glaucoma, **left** eye
● H40.153   Residual stage of open-angle glaucoma, **bilateral**
● H40.159   Residual stage of open-angle glaucoma, **unspecified** eye

● H40.2   **Primary angle-closure glaucoma**

Excludes1   aqueous misdirection (H40.83-)
         malignant glaucoma (H40.83-)

X● H40.20   **Unspecified** primary angle-closure glaucoma

One of the following 7th characters is to be assigned to code H40.20 to designate the stage of glaucoma

0	stage unspecified
1	mild stage
2	moderate stage
3	severe stage
4	indeterminate stage

● H40.21   **Acute** angle-closure glaucoma

Acute angle-closure glaucoma attack
Acute angle-closure glaucoma crisis

(Ex) **For category H40.21 CC codes:** See PDX Collection 630

H40.211   Acute angle-closure glaucoma, **right** eye ✎
H40.212   Acute angle-closure glaucoma, **left** eye ✎
H40.213   Acute angle-closure glaucoma, **bilateral** ✎
H40.219   Acute angle-closure glaucoma, **unspecified** eye ✎

● H40.22   **Chronic** angle-closure glaucoma

Chronic primary angle closure glaucoma

One of the following 7th characters is to be assigned to each code in subcategory H40.22 to designate the stage of glaucoma

0	stage unspecified
1	mild stage
2	moderate stage
3	severe stage
4	indeterminate stage

● H40.221   Chronic angle-closure glaucoma, **right** eye
● H40.222   Chronic angle-closure glaucoma, **left** eye
● H40.223   Chronic angle-closure glaucoma, **bilateral**
● H40.229   Chronic angle-closure glaucoma, **unspecified** eye

● H40.23   **Intermittent** angle-closure glaucoma
H40.231   Intermittent angle-closure glaucoma, **right** eye
H40.232   Intermittent angle-closure glaucoma, **left** eye
H40.233   Intermittent angle-closure glaucoma, **bilateral**
H40.239   Intermittent angle-closure glaucoma, **unspecified** eye

● H40.24   **Residual stage** of angle-closure glaucoma
H40.241   Residual stage of angle-closure glaucoma, **right** eye
H40.242   Residual stage of angle-closure glaucoma, **left** eye
H40.243   Residual stage of angle-closure glaucoma, **bilateral**
H40.249   Residual stage of angle-closure glaucoma, **unspecified** eye

▶ New   ➡ Revised   ~~deleted~~ Deleted   Excludes 1   Excludes 2   Includes   Use additional   Code first   Code also   Key words

858   OGCR Official Guidelines   ● Unacceptable Principal Diagnosis   X Assign placeholder X   ● Use Additional Character(s)   ▶ Manifestation Code   **Coding Clinic**

● H40.3   Glaucoma secondary to eye trauma
  Code also underlying condition
  One of the following 7th characters is to be assigned to
  each code in subcategory H40.3 to designate the
  stage of glaucoma

0	stage unspecified
1	mild stage
2	moderate stage
3	severe stage
4	indeterminate stage

X● H40.30   Glaucoma secondary to eye trauma, unspecified
    eye
X● H40.31   Glaucoma secondary to eye trauma, right eye
X● H40.32   Glaucoma secondary to eye trauma, left eye
X● H40.33   Glaucoma secondary to eye trauma, bilateral

● H40.4   Glaucoma secondary to eye inflammation
  Code also underlying condition
  One of the following 7th characters is to be assigned to
  each code in subcategory H40.4 to designate the
  stage of glaucoma

0	stage unspecified
1	mild stage
2	moderate stage
3	severe stage
4	indeterminate stage

X● H40.40   Glaucoma secondary to eye inflammation,
    unspecified eye
X● H40.41   Glaucoma secondary to eye inflammation, right
    eye
X● H40.42   Glaucoma secondary to eye inflammation, left
    eye
X● H40.43   Glaucoma secondary to eye inflammation,
    bilateral

● H40.5   Glaucoma secondary to other eye disorders
  Code also underlying eye disorder
  One of the following 7th characters is to be assigned to
  each code in subcategory H40.5 to designate the
  stage of glaucoma

0	stage unspecified
1	mild stage
2	moderate stage
3	severe stage
4	indeterminate stage

X● H40.50   Glaucoma secondary to other eye disorders,
    unspecified eye
X● H40.51   Glaucoma secondary to other eye disorders,
    right eye
X● H40.52   Glaucoma secondary to other eye disorders, left
    eye
X● H40.53   Glaucoma secondary to other eye disorders,
    bilateral

● H40.6   Glaucoma secondary to drugs
  Use additional code for adverse effect, if applicable,
  to identify drug (T36-T50 with fifth or sixth
  character 5)
  One of the following 7th characters is to be assigned to
  each code in subcategory H40.6 to designate the
  stage of glaucoma

0	stage unspecified
1	mild stage
2	moderate stage
3	severe stage
4	indeterminate stage

X● H40.60   Glaucoma secondary to drugs, unspecified eye
X● H40.61   Glaucoma secondary to drugs, right eye

X● H40.62   Glaucoma secondary to drugs, left eye
X● H40.63   Glaucoma secondary to drugs, bilateral
● H40.8   Other glaucoma
 ● H40.81   Glaucoma with increased episcleral venous
    pressure
    H40.811   Glaucoma with increased episcleral
       venous pressure, right eye
    H40.812   Glaucoma with increased episcleral
       venous pressure, left eye
    H40.813   Glaucoma with increased episcleral
       venous pressure, bilateral
    H40.819   Glaucoma with increased episcleral
       venous pressure, unspecified eye
 ● H40.82   Hypersecretion glaucoma
    H40.821   Hypersecretion glaucoma, right eye
    H40.822   Hypersecretion glaucoma, left eye
    H40.823   Hypersecretion glaucoma, bilateral
    H40.829   Hypersecretion glaucoma, unspecified
       eye
 ● H40.83   Aqueous misdirection
    Malignant glaucoma
    H40.831   Aqueous misdirection, right eye
    H40.832   Aqueous misdirection, left eye
    H40.833   Aqueous misdirection, bilateral
    H40.839   Aqueous misdirection, unspecified
       eye
  H40.89   Other specified glaucoma
 H40.9   Unspecified glaucoma

▸ H42   *Glaucoma in diseases classified elsewhere*
  Code first underlying condition, such as:
   amyloidosis (E85.-)
   aniridia (Q13.1)
   glaucoma (in) diabetes mellitus (E08.39, E09.39, E10.39,
    E11.39, E13.39)
   Lowe's syndrome (E72.03)
   Reiger's anomaly (Q13.81)
   specified metabolic disorder (E70-E88)
  Excludes1 glaucoma (in) onchocerciasis (B73.02)
       glaucoma (in) syphilis (A52.71)
       glaucoma (in) tuberculous (A18.59)

DISORDERS OF VITREOUS BODY AND GLOBE (H43-H44)

● H43   Disorders of vitreous body
 ● H43.0   Vitreous prolapse
   Excludes1 vitreous syndrome following cataract
      surgery (H59.0-)
      traumatic vitreous prolapse (S05.2-)
   H43.00   Vitreous prolapse, unspecified eye
   H43.01   Vitreous prolapse, right eye
   H43.02   Vitreous prolapse, left eye
   H43.03   Vitreous prolapse, bilateral
 ● H43.1   Vitreous hemorrhage
   H43.10   Vitreous hemorrhage, unspecified eye ▨
   H43.11   Vitreous hemorrhage, right eye ▨
   H43.12   Vitreous hemorrhage, left eye ▨
   H43.13   Vitreous hemorrhage, bilateral ▨
 ● H43.2   Crystalline deposits in vitreous body
   H43.20   Crystalline deposits in vitreous body,
      unspecified eye
   H43.21   Crystalline deposits in vitreous body, right eye
   H43.22   Crystalline deposits in vitreous body, left eye
   H43.23   Crystalline deposits in vitreous body, bilateral

CHAPTER 7 (H00-H59)

N Newborn Age: 0	**P** Pediatric Age: 0–17	**M** Maternity DX: 9–64	**A** Adult Age: 15–124	♀ Females Only	♂ Males Only	
▨ Complication\Comorbidity	▨ Major C\C	(Ex) CC/MCC Exclusions	▨ Hospital-Acquired Condition	▨ Hierarchical Condition Category		

● **H43.3   Other vitreous opacities**
  ● **H43.31   Vitreous membranes and strands**
    H43.311   Vitreous membranes and strands, right eye
    H43.312   Vitreous membranes and strands, left eye
    H43.313   Vitreous membranes and strands, bilateral
    H43.319   Vitreous membranes and strands, unspecified eye
  ● **H43.39   Other vitreous opacities**
    Vitreous floaters
        Small clumps of cells that float in the vitreous of the eye, appearing as black specks or dots in the field of vision and common in the aging eye.
    H43.391   Other vitreous opacities, right eye
    H43.392   Other vitreous opacities, left eye
    H43.393   Other vitreous opacities, bilateral
    H43.399   Other vitreous opacities, unspecified eye
● **H43.8   Other disorders of vitreous body**
    Excludes1   proliferative vitreo-retinopathy with retinal detachment (H33.4)
    Excludes2   vitreous abscess (H44.02-)
  ● **H43.81   Vitreous degeneration**
    Vitreous detachment
    H43.811   Vitreous degeneration, right eye
    H43.812   Vitreous degeneration, left eye
    H43.813   Vitreous degeneration, bilateral
    H43.819   Vitreous degeneration, unspecified eye
  ● **H43.82   Vitreomacular adhesion**
    Vitreomacular traction
    H43.821   Vitreomacular adhesion, right eye   A
    H43.822   Vitreomacular adhesion, left eye   A
    H43.823   Vitreomacular adhesion, bilateral   A
    H43.829   Vitreomacular adhesion, unspecified eye   A
  H43.89   Other disorders of vitreous body
  H43.9   Unspecified disorder of vitreous body

● **H44   Disorders of globe**
    Includes   disorders affecting multiple structures of eye
  ● **H44.0   Purulent endophthalmitis**
    Use additional code to identify organism
    Excludes1   bleb associated endophthalmitis (H59.4-)
  ● **H44.00   Unspecified purulent endophthalmitis**
    (Ex) **For category H44.00 CC codes:** See PDX Collection 625
    H44.001   Unspecified purulent endophthalmitis, right eye 🛇
    H44.002   Unspecified purulent endophthalmitis, left eye 🛇
    H44.003   Unspecified purulent endophthalmitis, bilateral 🛇
    H44.009   Unspecified purulent endophthalmitis, unspecified eye 🛇
  ● **H44.01   Panophthalmitis (acute)**
    (Ex) **For category H44.01 CC codes:** See PDX Collection 625
    H44.011   Panophthalmitis (acute), right eye 🛇
    H44.012   Panophthalmitis (acute), left eye 🛇
    H44.013   Panophthalmitis (acute), bilateral 🛇
    H44.019   Panophthalmitis (acute), unspecified eye 🛇

  ● **H44.02   Vitreous abscess (chronic)**
    (Ex) **For category H44.02 CC codes:** See PDX Collection 631
    H44.021   Vitreous abscess (chronic), right eye 🛇
    H44.022   Vitreous abscess (chronic), left eye 🛇
    H44.023   Vitreous abscess (chronic), bilateral 🛇
    H44.029   Vitreous abscess (chronic), unspecified eye 🛇
  ● **H44.1   Other endophthalmitis**
    Excludes1   bleb associated endophthalmitis (H59.4-)
    Excludes2   ophthalmia nodosa (H16.2-)
  ● **H44.11   Panuveitis**
    (Ex) **For category H44.11 CC codes:** See PDX Collection 632
    H44.111   Panuveitis, right eye 🛇
    H44.112   Panuveitis, left eye 🛇
    H44.113   Panuveitis, bilateral 🛇
    H44.119   Panuveitis, unspecified eye 🛇
  ● **H44.12   Parasitic endophthalmitis, unspecified**
    (Ex) **For category H44.12 CC codes:** See PDX Collection 625
    H44.121   Parasitic endophthalmitis, unspecified, right eye 🛇
    H44.122   Parasitic endophthalmitis, unspecified, left eye 🛇
    H44.123   Parasitic endophthalmitis, unspecified, bilateral 🛇
    H44.129   Parasitic endophthalmitis, unspecified, unspecified eye 🛇
  ● **H44.13   Sympathetic uveitis**
    (Ex) **For category H44.13 CC codes:** See PDX Collection 632
    H44.131   Sympathetic uveitis, right eye 🛇
    H44.132   Sympathetic uveitis, left eye 🛇
    H44.133   Sympathetic uveitis, bilateral 🛇
    H44.139   Sympathetic uveitis, unspecified eye 🛇
  H44.19   Other endophthalmitis 🛇
    (Ex) See PDX Collection 625
  ● **H44.2   Degenerative myopia**
    Malignant myopia
    H44.20   Degenerative myopia, unspecified eye
    H44.21   Degenerative myopia, right eye
    H44.22   Degenerative myopia, left eye
    H44.23   Degenerative myopia, bilateral
  ● **H44.2A   Degenerative myopia with choroidal neovascularization**
    Use Additional code for any associated choroid disorders (H31.-)
    H44.2A1   Degenerative myopia with choroidal neovascularization, right eye
    H44.2A2   Degenerative myopia with choroidal neovascularization, left eye
    H44.2A3   Degenerative myopia with choroidal neovascularization, bilateral eye
    H44.2A9   Degenerative myopia with choroidal neovascularization, unspecified eye
  ● **H44.2B   Degenerative myopia with macular hole**
    H44.2B1   Degenerative myopia with macular hole, right eye
    H44.2B2   Degenerative myopia with macular hole, left eye
    H44.2B3   Degenerative myopia with macular hole, bilateral eye
    H44.2B9   Degenerative myopia with macular hole, unspecified eye

▶ New   ⇒ Revised   ~~deleted~~ Deleted   Excludes 1   Excludes 2   Includes   Use additional   Code first   Code also   Key words

860   OGCR Official Guidelines   ● Unacceptable Principal Diagnosis   X Assign placeholder X   ● Use Additional Character(s)   ▶ Manifestation Code   Coding Clinic

● H44.2C   Degenerative myopia with retinal detachment
     Use Additional code to identify the retinal detachment (H33.-)
     H44.2C1   Degenerative myopia with retinal detachment, right eye
     H44.2C2   Degenerative myopia with retinal detachment, left eye
     H44.2C3   Degenerative myopia with retinal detachment, bilateral eye
     H44.2C9   Degenerative myopia with retinal detachment, unspecified eye

● H44.2D   Degenerative myopia with foveoschisis
     H44.2D1   Degenerative myopia with foveoschisis, right eye
     H44.2D2   Degenerative myopia with foveoschisis, left eye
     H44.2D3   Degenerative myopia with foveoschisis, bilateral eye
     H44.2D9   Degenerative myopia with foveoschisis, unspecified eye

● H44.2E   Degenerative myopia with other maculopathy
     H44.2E1   Degenerative myopia with other maculopathy, right eye
     H44.2E2   Degenerative myopia with other maculopathy, left eye
     H44.2E3   Degenerative myopia with other maculopathy, bilateral eye
     H44.2E9   Degenerative myopia with other maculopathy, unspecified eye

● H44.3   Other and unspecified degenerative disorders of globe
     H44.30   Unspecified degenerative disorder of globe
● H44.31   Chalcosis
     H44.311   Chalcosis, right eye
     H44.312   Chalcosis, left eye
     H44.313   Chalcosis, bilateral
     H44.319   Chalcosis, unspecified eye
● H44.32   Siderosis of eye
     H44.321   Siderosis of eye, right eye
     H44.322   Siderosis of eye, left eye
     H44.323   Siderosis of eye, bilateral
     H44.329   Siderosis of eye, unspecified eye
● H44.39   Other degenerative disorders of globe
     H44.391   Other degenerative disorders of globe, right eye
     H44.392   Other degenerative disorders of globe, left eye
     H44.393   Other degenerative disorders of globe, bilateral
     H44.399   Other degenerative disorders of globe, unspecified eye

● H44.4   Hypotony of eye
     H44.40   Unspecified hypotony of eye
● H44.41   Flat anterior chamber hypotony of eye
     H44.411   Flat anterior chamber hypotony of right eye
     H44.412   Flat anterior chamber hypotony of left eye
     H44.413   Flat anterior chamber hypotony of eye, bilateral
     H44.419   Flat anterior chamber hypotony of unspecified eye
● H44.42   Hypotony of eye due to ocular fistula
     H44.421   Hypotony of right eye due to ocular fistula
     H44.422   Hypotony of left eye due to ocular fistula

     H44.423   Hypotony of eye due to ocular fistula, bilateral
     H44.429   Hypotony of unspecified eye due to ocular fistula
● H44.43   Hypotony of eye due to other ocular disorders
     H44.431   Hypotony of eye due to other ocular disorders, right eye
     H44.432   Hypotony of eye due to other ocular disorders, left eye
     H44.433   Hypotony of eye due to other ocular disorders, bilateral
     H44.439   Hypotony of eye due to other ocular disorders, unspecified eye
● H44.44   Primary hypotony of eye
     H44.441   Primary hypotony of right eye
     H44.442   Primary hypotony of left eye
     H44.443   Primary hypotony of eye, bilateral
     H44.449   Primary hypotony of unspecified eye

● H44.5   Degenerated conditions of globe
     H44.50   Unspecified degenerated conditions of globe
● H44.51   Absolute glaucoma
     H44.511   Absolute glaucoma, right eye
     H44.512   Absolute glaucoma, left eye
     H44.513   Absolute glaucoma, bilateral
     H44.519   Absolute glaucoma, unspecified eye
● H44.52   Atrophy of globe
     Phthisis bulbi
     H44.521   Atrophy of globe, right eye
     H44.522   Atrophy of globe, left eye
     H44.523   Atrophy of globe, bilateral
     H44.529   Atrophy of globe, unspecified eye
● H44.53   Leucocoria
     H44.531   Leucocoria, right eye
     H44.532   Leucocoria, left eye
     H44.533   Leucocoria, bilateral
     H44.539   Leucocoria, unspecified eye

● H44.6   Retained (old) intraocular foreign body, magnetic
     Use additional code to identify magnetic foreign body (Z18.11)
     Excludes 1   current intraocular foreign body (S05.-)
     Excludes 2   retained foreign body in eyelid (H02.81-)
             retained (old) foreign body following penetrating wound of orbit (H05.5-)
             retained (old) intraocular foreign body, nonmagnetic (H44.7-)
● H44.60   Unspecified retained (old) intraocular foreign body, magnetic
     H44.601   Unspecified retained (old) intraocular foreign body, magnetic, right eye
     H44.602   Unspecified retained (old) intraocular foreign body, magnetic, left eye
     H44.603   Unspecified retained (old) intraocular foreign body, magnetic, bilateral
     H44.609   Unspecified retained (old) intraocular foreign body, magnetic, unspecified eye
● H44.61   Retained (old) magnetic foreign body in anterior chamber
     H44.611   Retained (old) magnetic foreign body in anterior chamber, right eye
     H44.612   Retained (old) magnetic foreign body in anterior chamber, left eye
     H44.613   Retained (old) magnetic foreign body in anterior chamber, bilateral
     H44.619   Retained (old) magnetic foreign body in anterior chamber, unspecified eye

CHAPTER 7 (H00-H59)

N Newborn Age: 0   **P** Pediatric Age: 0–17   **M** Maternity DX: 9–64   **A** Adult Age: 15–124   ♀ Females Only   ♂ Males Only
Complication\Comorbidity   Major C\C   (Ex) CC/MCC Exclusions   Hospital-Acquired Condition   Hierarchical Condition Category

861

CHAPTER 7 (H00-H59)

● H44.62   Retained (old) magnetic foreign body in iris or ciliary body

     H44.621   Retained (old) magnetic foreign body in iris or ciliary body, right eye

     H44.622   Retained (old) magnetic foreign body in iris or ciliary body, left eye

     H44.623   Retained (old) magnetic foreign body in iris or ciliary body, bilateral

     H44.629   Retained (old) magnetic foreign body in iris or ciliary body, unspecified eye

● H44.63   Retained (old) magnetic foreign body in lens

     H44.631   Retained (old) magnetic foreign body in lens, right eye

     H44.632   Retained (old) magnetic foreign body in lens, left eye

     H44.633   Retained (old) magnetic foreign body in lens, bilateral

     H44.639   Retained (old) magnetic foreign body in lens, unspecified eye

● H44.64   Retained (old) magnetic foreign body in posterior wall of globe

     H44.641   Retained (old) magnetic foreign body in posterior wall of globe, right eye

     H44.642   Retained (old) magnetic foreign body in posterior wall of globe, left eye

     H44.643   Retained (old) magnetic foreign body in posterior wall of globe, bilateral

     H44.649   Retained (old) magnetic foreign body in posterior wall of globe, unspecified eye

● H44.65   Retained (old) magnetic foreign body in vitreous body

     H44.651   Retained (old) magnetic foreign body in vitreous body, right eye

     H44.652   Retained (old) magnetic foreign body in vitreous body, left eye

     H44.653   Retained (old) magnetic foreign body in vitreous body, bilateral

     H44.659   Retained (old) magnetic foreign body in vitreous body, unspecified eye

● H44.69   Retained (old) intraocular foreign body, magnetic, in other or multiple sites

     H44.691   Retained (old) intraocular foreign body, magnetic, in other or multiple sites, right eye

     H44.692   Retained (old) intraocular foreign body, magnetic, in other or multiple sites, left eye

     H44.693   Retained (old) intraocular foreign body, magnetic, in other or multiple sites, bilateral

     H44.699   Retained (old) intraocular foreign body, magnetic, in other or multiple sites, unspecified eye

● H44.7   Retained (old) intraocular foreign body, nonmagnetic

Use additional code to identify nonmagnetic foreign body (Z18.01-Z18.10, Z18.12, Z18.2-Z18.9)

Excludes1   current intraocular foreign body (S05.-)

Excludes2   retained foreign body in eyelid (H02.81-)
retained (old) foreign body following penetrating wound of orbit (H05.5-)
retained (old) intraocular foreign body, magnetic (H44.6-)

● H44.70   Unspecified retained (old) intraocular foreign body, nonmagnetic

     H44.701   Unspecified retained (old) intraocular foreign body, nonmagnetic, right eye

     H44.702   Unspecified retained (old) intraocular foreign body, nonmagnetic, left eye

     H44.703   Unspecified retained (old) intraocular foreign body, nonmagnetic, bilateral

     H44.709   Unspecified retained (old) intraocular foreign body, nonmagnetic, unspecified eye
Retained (old) intraocular foreign body NOS

● H44.71   Retained (nonmagnetic) (old) foreign body in anterior chamber

     H44.711   Retained (nonmagnetic) (old) foreign body in anterior chamber, right eye

     H44.712   Retained (nonmagnetic) (old) foreign body in anterior chamber, left eye

     H44.713   Retained (nonmagnetic) (old) foreign body in anterior chamber, bilateral

     H44.719   Retained (nonmagnetic) (old) foreign body in anterior chamber, unspecified eye

● H44.72   Retained (nonmagnetic) (old) foreign body in iris or ciliary body

     H44.721   Retained (nonmagnetic) (old) foreign body in iris or ciliary body, right eye

     H44.722   Retained (nonmagnetic) (old) foreign body in iris or ciliary body, left eye

     H44.723   Retained (nonmagnetic) (old) foreign body in iris or ciliary body, bilateral

     H44.729   Retained (nonmagnetic) (old) foreign body in iris or ciliary body, unspecified eye

● H44.73   Retained (nonmagnetic) (old) foreign body in lens

     H44.731   Retained (nonmagnetic) (old) foreign body in lens, right eye

     H44.732   Retained (nonmagnetic) (old) foreign body in lens, left eye

     H44.733   Retained (nonmagnetic) (old) foreign body in lens, bilateral

     H44.739   Retained (nonmagnetic) (old) foreign body in lens, unspecified eye

● H44.74   Retained (nonmagnetic) (old) foreign body in posterior wall of globe

     H44.741   Retained (nonmagnetic) (old) foreign body in posterior wall of globe, right eye

     H44.742   Retained (nonmagnetic) (old) foreign body in posterior wall of globe, left eye

     H44.743   Retained (nonmagnetic) (old) foreign body in posterior wall of globe, bilateral

     H44.749   Retained (nonmagnetic) (old) foreign body in posterior wall of globe, unspecified eye

● H44.75   Retained (nonmagnetic) (old) foreign body in vitreous body

     H44.751   Retained (nonmagnetic) (old) foreign body in vitreous body, right eye

     H44.752   Retained (nonmagnetic) (old) foreign body in vitreous body, left eye

     H44.753   Retained (nonmagnetic) (old) foreign body in vitreous body, bilateral

     H44.759   Retained (nonmagnetic) (old) foreign body in vitreous body, unspecified eye

▶ New   ⇒ Revised   ~~deleted~~ Deleted   Excludes 1   Excludes 2   Includes   Use additional   Code first   Code also   Key words

OGCR Official Guidelines   ● Unacceptable Principal Diagnosis   X Assign placeholder X   ● Use Additional Character(s)   ▶ Manifestation Code   **Coding Clinic**

● H44.79   Retained (old) intraocular foreign body, nonmagnetic, in other or multiple sites

    H44.791   Retained (old) intraocular foreign body, nonmagnetic, in other or multiple sites, right eye

    H44.792   Retained (old) intraocular foreign body, nonmagnetic, in other or multiple sites, left eye

    H44.793   Retained (old) intraocular foreign body, nonmagnetic, in other or multiple sites, bilateral

    H44.799   Retained (old) intraocular foreign body, nonmagnetic, in other or multiple sites, unspecified eye

● H44.8   Other disorders of globe

   ● H44.81   Hemophthalmos

     H44.811   Hemophthalmos, right eye

     H44.812   Hemophthalmos, left eye

     H44.813   Hemophthalmos, bilateral

     H44.819   Hemophthalmos, unspecified eye

   ● H44.82   Luxation of globe

     H44.821   Luxation of globe, right eye

     H44.822   Luxation of globe, left eye

     H44.823   Luxation of globe, bilateral

     H44.829   Luxation of globe, unspecified eye

   H44.89   Other disorders of globe

  H44.9   Unspecified disorder of globe

★ (See Plate 7 of the Anatomy Illustrations.)

DISORDERS OF OPTIC NERVE AND VISUAL PATHWAYS (H46-H47)

● H46   Optic neuritis

    Excludes2   ischemic optic neuropathy (H47.01-)
               neuromyelitis optica [Devic] (G36.0)

    (Ex) **For category H46 CC codes:** See PDX Collection 633

   ● H46.0   Optic papillitis

     H46.00   Optic papillitis, unspecified eye

     H46.01   Optic papillitis, right eye

     H46.02   Optic papillitis, left eye

     H46.03   Optic papillitis, bilateral

   ● H46.1   Retrobulbar neuritis

     Retrobulbar neuritis NOS

     Excludes1   syphilitic retrobulbar neuritis (A52.15)

     H46.10   Retrobulbar neuritis, unspecified eye

     H46.11   Retrobulbar neuritis, right eye

     H46.12   Retrobulbar neuritis, left eye

     H46.13   Retrobulbar neuritis, bilateral

   H46.2   Nutritional optic neuropathy

   H46.3   Toxic optic neuropathy

     Code first (T51-T65) *to identify cause*

   H46.8   Other optic neuritis

   H46.9   Unspecified optic neuritis

● H47   Other disorders of optic [2nd] nerve and visual pathways

   ● H47.0   Disorders of optic nerve, not elsewhere classified

    ● H47.01   Ischemic optic neuropathy

     H47.011   Ischemic optic neuropathy, right eye

     H47.012   Ischemic optic neuropathy, left eye

     H47.013   Ischemic optic neuropathy, bilateral

     H47.019   Ischemic optic neuropathy, unspecified eye

● H47.02   Hemorrhage in optic nerve sheath

    H47.021   Hemorrhage in optic nerve sheath, right eye

    H47.022   Hemorrhage in optic nerve sheath, left eye

    H47.023   Hemorrhage in optic nerve sheath, bilateral

    H47.029   Hemorrhage in optic nerve sheath, unspecified eye

● H47.03   Optic nerve hypoplasia

    H47.031   Optic nerve hypoplasia, right eye

    H47.032   Optic nerve hypoplasia, left eye

    H47.033   Optic nerve hypoplasia, bilateral

    H47.039   Optic nerve hypoplasia, unspecified eye

● H47.09   Other disorders of optic nerve, not elsewhere classified

    Compression of optic nerve

    H47.091   Other disorders of optic nerve, not elsewhere classified, right eye

    H47.092   Other disorders of optic nerve, not elsewhere classified, left eye

    H47.093   Other disorders of optic nerve, not elsewhere classified, bilateral

    H47.099   Other disorders of optic nerve, not elsewhere classified, unspecified eye

● H47.1   Papilledema

   H47.10   Unspecified papilledema
     (Ex) See PDX Collection 634

   H47.11   Papilledema associated with increased intracranial pressure
     (Ex) See PDX Collection 634

   H47.12   Papilledema associated with decreased ocular pressure

   H47.13   Papilledema associated with retinal disorder

● H47.14   Foster-Kennedy syndrome

    H47.141   Foster-Kennedy syndrome, right eye

    H47.142   Foster-Kennedy syndrome, left eye

    H47.143   Foster-Kennedy syndrome, bilateral

    H47.149   Foster-Kennedy syndrome, unspecified eye

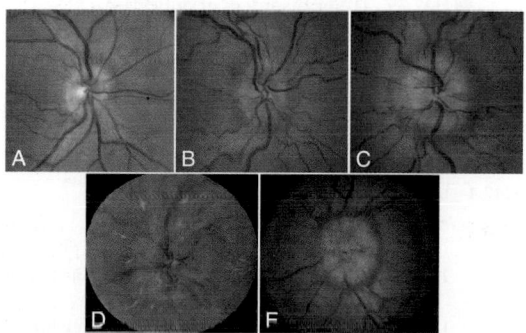

Figure 7-11   Stages of papilledema according to the Frisén grading scale. **A,** Very eary papilledema (Frisén stage 1). **B,** Early papilledema (Frisén stage 2). **C,** Moderate papilledema (Frisén stage 3). **D,** Marked papilledema (Frisén stage 4). **E,** Severe papilledema. (From Youmans JR, Winn HR: Youmans Neurological Surgery, Philadelphia, PA, Elsevier/Saunders, 2011)

Item 7-8   Papilledema is swelling of the optic disc caused by increased intracranial pressure. It is most often bilateral and occurs quickly (hours) or over weeks of time. It is a common symptom of a brain tumor. The term should not be used to describe optic disc swelling with underlying infectious, infiltrative, or inflammatory etiologies.

N Newborn Age: 0   **P** Pediatric Age: 0–17   **M** Maternity DX: 9–64   **A** Adult Age: 15–124   ♀ Females Only   ♂ Males Only

Complication\Comorbidity   Major C\C   (Ex) CC/MCC Exclusions   Hospital-Acquired Condition   Hierarchical Condition Category

863

CHAPTER 7 (H00-H59)

● **H47.2**   **Optic atrophy**
    H47.20   Unspecified optic atrophy
  ● **H47.21**   Primary optic atrophy
       H47.211   Primary optic atrophy, right eye
       H47.212   Primary optic atrophy, left eye
       H47.213   Primary optic atrophy, bilateral
       H47.219   Primary optic atrophy, unspecified eye
    H47.22   Hereditary optic atrophy
          Leber's optic atrophy
  ● **H47.23**   Glaucomatous optic atrophy
       H47.231   Glaucomatous optic atrophy, right eye
       H47.232   Glaucomatous optic atrophy, left eye
       H47.233   Glaucomatous optic atrophy, bilateral
       H47.239   Glaucomatous optic atrophy, unspecified eye
  ● **H47.29**   Other optic atrophy
          Temporal pallor of optic disc
       H47.291   Other optic atrophy, right eye
       H47.292   Other optic atrophy, left eye
       H47.293   Other optic atrophy, bilateral
       H47.299   Other optic atrophy, unspecified eye

● **H47.3**   Other disorders of optic disc
  ● **H47.31**   Coloboma of optic disc
       H47.311   Coloboma of optic disc, right eye
       H47.312   Coloboma of optic disc, left eye
       H47.313   Coloboma of optic disc, bilateral
       H47.319   Coloboma of optic disc, unspecified eye
  ● **H47.32**   Drusen of optic disc
       H47.321   Drusen of optic disc, right eye
       H47.322   Drusen of optic disc, left eye
       H47.323   Drusen of optic disc, bilateral
       H47.329   Drusen of optic disc, unspecified eye
  ● **H47.33**   Pseudopapilledema of optic disc
       H47.331   Pseudopapilledema of optic disc, right eye
       H47.332   Pseudopapilledema of optic disc, left eye
       H47.333   Pseudopapilledema of optic disc, bilateral
       H47.339   Pseudopapilledema of optic disc, unspecified eye
  ● **H47.39**   Other disorders of optic disc
       H47.391   Other disorders of optic disc, right eye
       H47.392   Other disorders of optic disc, left eye
       H47.393   Other disorders of optic disc, bilateral
       H47.399   Other disorders of optic disc, unspecified eye

● **H47.4**   Disorders of optic chiasm
      Code also underlying condition
      Ⓔ⨯ **For category H47.4 CC codes:** See PDX Collection 635
    H47.41   Disorders of optic chiasm in (due to) inflammatory disorders 🅜
    H47.42   Disorders of optic chiasm in (due to) neoplasm 🅜
    H47.43   Disorders of optic chiasm in (due to) vascular disorders 🅜
    H47.49   Disorders of optic chiasm in (due to) other disorders 🅜

● **H47.5**   Disorders of other visual pathways
      Disorders of optic tracts, geniculate nuclei and optic radiations
      Code also underlying condition
      Ⓔ⨯ **For category H47.5 CC codes:** See PDX Collection 635
  ● **H47.51**   Disorders of visual pathways in (due to) inflammatory disorders
       H47.511   Disorders of visual pathways in (due to) inflammatory disorders, right side 🅜
       H47.512   Disorders of visual pathways in (due to) inflammatory disorders, left side 🅜
       H47.519   Disorders of visual pathways in (due to) inflammatory disorders, unspecified side 🅜
  ● **H47.52**   Disorders of visual pathways in (due to) neoplasm
       H47.521   Disorders of visual pathways in (due to) neoplasm, right side 🅜
       H47.522   Disorders of visual pathways in (due to) neoplasm, left side 🅜
       H47.529   Disorders of visual pathways in (due to) neoplasm, unspecified side 🅜
  ● **H47.53**   Disorders of visual pathways in (due to) vascular disorders
       H47.531   Disorders of visual pathways in (due to) vascular disorders, right side 🅜
       H47.532   Disorders of visual pathways in (due to) vascular disorders, left side 🅜
       H47.539   Disorders of visual pathways in (due to) vascular disorders, unspecified side 🅜

● **H47.6**   Disorders of visual cortex
      Code also underlying condition
      Excludes1   injury to visual cortex S04.04-
      Ⓔ⨯ **For category H47.6 CC codes:** See PDX Collection 636
  ● **H47.61**   Cortical blindness
       H47.611   Cortical blindness, right side of brain
       H47.612   Cortical blindness, left side of brain
       H47.619   Cortical blindness, unspecified side of brain
  ● **H47.62**   Disorders of visual cortex in (due to) inflammatory disorders
       H47.621   Disorders of visual cortex in (due to) inflammatory disorders, right side of brain 🅜
       H47.622   Disorders of visual cortex in (due to) inflammatory disorders, left side of brain 🅜
       H47.629   Disorders of visual cortex in (due to) inflammatory disorders, unspecified side of brain 🅜
  ● **H47.63**   Disorders of visual cortex in (due to) neoplasm
       H47.631   Disorders of visual cortex in (due to) neoplasm, right side of brain 🅜
       H47.632   Disorders of visual cortex in (due to) neoplasm, left side of brain 🅜
       H47.639   Disorders of visual cortex in (due to) neoplasm, unspecified side of brain 🅜

▶ New   ⇒ Revised   ~~deleted~~ Deleted   Excludes 1   Excludes 2   Includes   Use additional   Code first   Code also   Key words

864   **OGCR** Official Guidelines   ● Unacceptable Principal Diagnosis   X Assign placeholder X   ● Use Additional Character(s)   🅜 Manifestation Code   **Coding Clinic**

Item 7–10 Disorders of refraction: **Hypermetropia,** or farsightedness, means focus at a distance is adequate but not on close objects. **Myopia** is near-sightedness or short-sightedness and means the focus on nearby objects is clear but distant objects appear blurred. **Astigmatism** is warping of the curvature of the cornea so light rays entering do not meet a single focal point, resulting in a distorted image. **Anisometropia** is unequal refractive power in which one eye may be myopic (near-sighted) and the other hyperopic (far-sighted). **Presbyopia** is the loss of focus on near objects, which occurs with age because the lens loses elasticity.

- ● H52.2   Astigmatism
  - ● H52.20   Unspecified astigmatism
    - H52.201   Unspecified astigmatism, right eye
    - H52.202   Unspecified astigmatism, left eye
    - H52.203   Unspecified astigmatism, bilateral
    - H52.209   Unspecified astigmatism, unspecified eye
  - ● H52.21   Irregular astigmatism
    - H52.211   Irregular astigmatism, right eye
    - H52.212   Irregular astigmatism, left eye
    - H52.213   Irregular astigmatism, bilateral
    - H52.219   Irregular astigmatism, unspecified eye
  - ● H52.22   Regular astigmatism
    - H52.221   Regular astigmatism, right eye
    - H52.222   Regular astigmatism, left eye
    - H52.223   Regular astigmatism, bilateral
    - H52.229   Regular astigmatism, unspecified eye
- ● H52.3   Anisometropia and aniseikonia
  - H52.31   Anisometropia
  - H52.32   Aniseikonia
- H52.4   Presbyopia
- ● H52.5   Disorders of accommodation
  - ● H52.51   Internal ophthalmoplegia (complete) (total)
    - H52.511   Internal ophthalmoplegia (complete) (total), right eye
    - H52.512   Internal ophthalmoplegia (complete) (total), left eye
    - H52.513   Internal ophthalmoplegia (complete) (total), bilateral
    - H52.519   Internal ophthalmoplegia (complete) (total), unspecified eye
  - ● H52.52   Paresis of accommodation
    - H52.521   Paresis of accommodation, right eye
    - H52.522   Paresis of accommodation, left eye
    - H52.523   Paresis of accommodation, bilateral
    - H52.529   Paresis of accommodation, unspecified eye
  - ● H52.53   Spasm of accommodation
    - H52.531   Spasm of accommodation, right eye
    - H52.532   Spasm of accommodation, left eye
    - H52.533   Spasm of accommodation, bilateral
    - H52.539   Spasm of accommodation, unspecified eye
- H52.6   Other disorders of refraction
- H52.7   Unspecified disorder of refraction

VISUAL DISTURBANCES AND BLINDNESS (H53-H54)

- ● H53   Visual disturbances
  - ● H53.0   Amblyopia ex anopsia
    - **Excludes1**   amblyopia due to vitamin A deficiency (E50.5)
    - ● H53.00   Unspecified amblyopia
      - H53.001   Unspecified amblyopia, right eye
      - H53.002   Unspecified amblyopia, left eye
      - H53.003   Unspecified amblyopia, bilateral
      - H53.009   Unspecified amblyopia, unspecified eye
    - ● H53.01   Deprivation amblyopia
      - H53.011   Deprivation amblyopia, right eye
      - H53.012   Deprivation amblyopia, left eye
      - H53.013   Deprivation amblyopia, bilateral
      - H53.019   Deprivation amblyopia, unspecified eye
    - ● H53.02   Refractive amblyopia
      - H53.021   Refractive amblyopia, right eye
      - H53.022   Refractive amblyopia, left eye
      - H53.023   Refractive amblyopia, bilateral
      - H53.029   Refractive amblyopia, unspecified eye
    - ● H53.03   Strabismic amblyopia
      - **Excludes1**   strabismus (H50.-)
      - H53.031   Strabismic amblyopia, right eye
      - H53.032   Strabismic amblyopia, left eye
      - H53.033   Strabismic amblyopia, bilateral
      - H53.039   Strabismic amblyopia, unspecified eye
    - ● H53.04   Amblyopia suspect
      - Coding Clinic: 2016, Q4, P22
      - H53.041   Amblyopia suspect, right eye
      - H53.042   Amblyopia suspect, left eye
      - H53.043   Amblyopia suspect, bilateral
      - H53.049   Amblyopia suspect, unspecified eye
  - ● H53.1   Subjective visual disturbances
    - **Excludes1**   subjective visual disturbances due to vitamin A deficiency (E50.5) visual hallucinations (R44.1)
    - H53.10   Unspecified subjective visual disturbances
    - H53.11   Day blindness
      - Hemeralopia
    - ● H53.12   Transient visual loss
      - Scintillating scotoma
      - **Excludes1**   amaurosis fugax (G45.3-) transient retinal artery occlusion (H34.0-)
      - (Ex) For category H53.12 CC codes: See PDX Collection 637
      - H53.121   Transient visual loss, right eye ℅
      - H53.122   Transient visual loss, left eye ℅
      - H53.123   Transient visual loss, bilateral ℅
      - H53.129   Transient visual loss, unspecified eye ℅
    - ● H53.13   Sudden visual loss
      - (Ex) For category H53.13 CC codes: See PDX Collection 637
      - H53.131   Sudden visual loss, right eye ℅
      - H53.132   Sudden visual loss, left eye ℅
      - H53.133   Sudden visual loss, bilateral ℅
      - H53.139   Sudden visual loss, unspecified eye ℅

CHAPTER 7 (H00-H59)

N Newborn Age: 0   **P** Pediatric Age: 0–17   **M** Maternity DX: 9–64   **A** Adult Age: 15–124   ♀ Females Only   ♂ Males Only

℅ Complication\Comorbidity   ℅ Major C\C   (Ex) CC/MCC Exclusions   ℅ Hospital-Acquired Condition   ℅ Hierarchical Condition Category

867

● H53.14   **Visual discomfort**
     Asthenopia
     Photophobia
     H53.141   Visual discomfort, right eye
     H53.142   Visual discomfort, left eye
     H53.143   Visual discomfort, bilateral
     H53.149   Visual discomfort, unspecified

H53.15   **Visual distortions of shape and size**
     Metamorphopsia

H53.16   **Psychophysical visual disturbances**

H53.19   **Other subjective visual disturbances**
     Visual halos

H53.2   **Diplopia**
     Double vision

● H53.3   **Other and unspecified disorders of binocular vision**

H53.30   **Unspecified disorder of binocular vision**

H53.31   **Abnormal retinal correspondence**

H53.32   **Fusion with defective stereopsis**

H53.33   **Simultaneous visual perception without fusion**

H53.34   **Suppression of binocular vision**

● H53.4   **Visual field defects**

H53.40   **Unspecified visual field defects**

● H53.41   **Scotoma involving central area**
     Central scotoma
     H53.411   Scotoma involving central area, right eye
     H53.412   Scotoma involving central area, left eye
     H53.413   Scotoma involving central area, bilateral
     H53.419   Scotoma involving central area, unspecified eye

● H53.42   **Scotoma of blind spot area**
     Enlarged blind spot
     H53.421   Scotoma of blind spot area, right eye
     H53.422   Scotoma of blind spot area, left eye
     H53.423   Scotoma of blind spot area, bilateral
     H53.429   Scotoma of blind spot area, unspecified eye

● H53.43   **Sector or arcuate defects**
     Arcuate scotoma
     Bjerrum scotoma
     H53.431   Sector or arcuate defects, right eye
     H53.432   Sector or arcuate defects, left eye
     H53.433   Sector or arcuate defects, bilateral
     H53.439   Sector or arcuate defects, unspecified eye

● H53.45   **Other localized visual field defect**
     Peripheral visual field defect
     Ring scotoma NOS
     Scotoma NOS
     H53.451   Other localized visual field defect, right eye
     H53.452   Other localized visual field defect, left eye
     H53.453   Other localized visual field defect, bilateral
     H53.459   Other localized visual field defect, unspecified eye

● H53.46   **Homonymous bilateral field defects**
     Homonymous hemianopia
     Homonymous hemianopsia
     Quadrant anopia
     Quadrant anopsia
     H53.461   Homonymous bilateral field defects, right side
     H53.462   Homonymous bilateral field defects, left side
     H53.469   Homonymous bilateral field defects, unspecified side
         Homonymous bilateral field defects NOS

H53.47   **Heteronymous bilateral field defects**
     Heteronymous hemianop(s)ia

● H53.48   **Generalized contraction of visual field**
     H53.481   Generalized contraction of visual field, right eye
     H53.482   Generalized contraction of visual field, left eye
     H53.483   Generalized contraction of visual field, bilateral
     H53.489   Generalized contraction of visual field, unspecified eye

● H53.5   **Color vision deficiencies**
     Color blindness

     Excludes2   day blindness (H53.11)

H53.50   **Unspecified color vision deficiencies**
     Color blindness NOS

H53.51   **Achromatopsia**

H53.52   **Acquired color vision deficiency**

H53.53   **Deuteranomaly**
     Deuteranopia

H53.54   **Protanomaly**
     Protanopia

H53.55   **Tritanomaly**
     Tritanopia

H53.59   **Other color vision deficiencies**

● H53.6   **Night blindness**

     Excludes1   night blindness due to vitamin A deficiency (E50.5)

H53.60   **Unspecified night blindness**

H53.61   **Abnormal dark adaptation curve**

H53.62   **Acquired night blindness**

H53.63   **Congenital night blindness**

H53.69   **Other night blindness**

● H53.7   **Vision sensitivity deficiencies**

H53.71   **Glare sensitivity**

H53.72   **Impaired contrast sensitivity**

H53.8   **Other visual disturbances**

H53.9   **Unspecified visual disturbance**

▶ New   ⇒ Revised   ~~deleted~~ Deleted   Excludes 1   Excludes 2   Includes   Use additional   Code first   Code also   Key words

868   OGCR Official Guidelines   ● Unacceptable Principal Diagnosis   X Assign placeholder X   ● Use Additional Character(s)   ▶ Manifestation Code   Coding Clinic

● **H54   Blindness and low vision**

    Note: For definition of visual impairment categories see table below.

    Code first any associated underlying cause of the blindness

    Excludes1   amaurosis fugax (G45.3)

● **H54.0   Blindness, both eyes**

    Visual impairment categories 3, 4, 5 in both eyes.

    ● **H54.0X   Blindness, both eyes, different category levels**

       H54.0X3   Blindness right eye, category 3

          H54.0X33   Blindness right eye category 3, blindness left eye category 3

          H54.0X34   Blindness right eye category 3, blindness left eye category 4

          H54.0X35   Blindness right eye category 3, blindness left eye category 5

       ● **H54.0X4   Blindness right eye, category 4**

          H54.0X43   Blindness right eye category 4, blindness left eye category 3

          H54.0X44   Blindness right eye category 4, blindness left eye category 4

          H54.0X45   Blindness right eye category 4, blindness left eye category 5

       ● **H54.0X5   Blindness right eye, category 5**

          H54.0X53   Blindness right eye category 5, blindness left eye category 3

          H54.0X54   Blindness right eye category 5, blindness left eye category 4

          H54.0X55   Blindness right eye category 5, blindness left eye category 5

● **H54.1   Blindness, one eye, low vision other eye**

    Visual impairment categories 3, 4, 5 in one eye, with categories 1 or 2 in the other eye.

    H54.10   Blindness, one eye, low vision other eye, unspecified eyes

    ● **H54.11   Blindness, right eye, low vision left eye**

       ● **H54.113   Blindness right eye category 3, low vision left eye**

          H54.1131   Blindness right eye category 3, low vision left eye category 1

          H54.1132   Blindness right eye category 3, low vision left eye category 2

       ● **H54.114   Blindness right eye category 4, low vision left eye**

          H54.1141   Blindness right eye category 4, low vision left eye category 1

          H54.1142   Blindness right eye category 4, low vision left eye category 2

● **H54.115   Blindness right eye category 5, low vision left eye**

    H54.1151   Blindness right eye category 5, low vision left eye category 1

    H54.1152   Blindness right eye category 5, low vision left eye category 2

● **H54.12   Blindness, left eye, low vision right eye**

    ● **H54.121   Low vision right eye category 1, blindness left eye**

       H54.1213   Low vision right eye category 1, blindness left eye category 3

       H54.1214   Low vision right eye category 1, blindness left eye category 4

       H54.1215   Low vision right eye category 1, blindness left eye category 5

    ● **H54.122   Low vision right eye category 2, blindness left eye**

       H54.1223   Low vision right eye category 2, blindness left eye category 3

       H54.1224   Low vision right eye category 2, blindness left eye category 4

       H54.1225   Low vision right eye category 2, blindness left eye category 5

● **H54.2   Low vision, both eyes**

    Visual impairment categories 1 or 2 in both eyes.

    ● **H54.2X   Low vision, both eyes, different category levels**

       ● **H54.2X1   Low vision, right eye, category 1**

          H54.2X11   Low vision right eye category 1, low vision left eye category 1

          H54.2X12   Low vision right eye category 1, low vision left eye category 2

       ● **H54.2X2   Low vision, right eye, category 2**

          H54.2X21   Low vision right eye category 2, low vision left eye category 1

          H54.2X22   Low vision right eye category 2, low vision left eye category 2

    H54.3   Unqualified visual loss, both eyes

       Visual impairment category 9 in both eyes.

N   Newborn Age: 0   **P**   Pediatric Age: 0–17   **M**   Maternity DX: 9–64   **A**   Adult Age: 15–124   ♀   Females Only   ♂   Males Only

🍎   Complication\Comorbidity   🍎   Major C\C   (Ex)   CC/MCC Exclusions   🍎   Hospital-Acquired Condition   🍎   Hierarchical Condition Category

869

CHAPTER 7 (H00-H59)

● **H54.4**   **Blindness, one eye**
Visual impairment categories 3, 4, 5 in one eye [normal vision in other eye]

    H54.40   Blindness, one eye, unspecified eye

●   **H54.41**   Blindness, right eye, normal vision left eye

   ●   **H54.413**   Blindness, right eye, category 3

      H54.413A   Blindness right eye category 3, normal vision left eye

   ●   **H54.414**   Blindness, right eye, category 4

      H54.414A   Blindness right eye category 4, normal vision left eye

   ●   **H54.415**   Blindness, right eye, category 5

      H54.415A   Blindness right eye category 5, normal vision left eye

●   **H54.42**   Blindness, left eye, normal vision right eye

   ●   **H54.42A**   Blindness, left eye, category 3-5

      H54.42A3   Blindness left eye category 3, normal vision right eye

      H54.42A4   Blindness left eye category 4, normal vision right eye

      H54.42A5   Blindness left eye category 5, normal vision right eye

● **H54.5**   **Low vision, one eye**
Visual impairment categories 1 or 2 in one eye [normal vision in other eye].

    H54.50   Low vision, one eye, unspecified eye

●   **H54.51**   Low vision, right eye, normal vision left eye

   ●   **H54.511**   Low vision, right eye, category 1-2

      H54.511A   Low vision right eye category 1, normal vision left eye

      H54.512A   Low vision right eye category 2, normal vision left eye

●   **H54.52**   Low vision, left eye, normal vision right eye

   ●   **H54.52A**   Low vision, left eye, category 1-2

      H54.52A1   Low vision left eye category 1, normal vision right eye

      H54.52A2   Low vision left eye category 2, normal vision right eye

● **H54.6**   **Unqualified visual loss, one eye**
Visual impairment category 9 in one eye [normal vision in other eye].

    H54.60   Unqualified visual loss, one eye, unspecified

    H54.61   Unqualified visual loss, right eye, normal vision left eye

    H54.62   Unqualified visual loss, left eye, normal vision right eye

    H54.7   **Unspecified visual loss**
Visual impairment category 9 NOS

    H54.8   **Legal blindness, as defined in USA**
Blindness NOS according to USA definition

     Excludes1   legal blindness with specification of impairment level (H54.0-H54.7)

     Note: The table below gives a classification of severity of visual impairment recommended by a WHO Study Group on the Prevention of Blindness, Geneva, 6-10 November 1972.

     The term "low vision" in category H54 comprises categories 1 and 2 of the table, the term "blindness" categories 3, 4, and 5, and the term "unqualified visual loss" category 9.

     If the extent of the visual field is taken into account, patients with a field no greater than 10 but greater than 5 around central fixation should be placed in category 3 and patients with a field no greater than 5 around central fixation should be placed in category 4, even if the central acuity is not impaired.

(Document 508 compliance requires all cells in the following table to be filled.)

Category of visual impairment	Visual acuity with best possible correction	
	Maximum less than:	**Minimum equal to or better than:**
—	6/18	6/60
3/10 (0.3)	1/10 (0.1)	—
20/70	20/200	
—	6/60	3/60
1/10 (0.1)	1/20 (0.05)	—
20/200	20/400	
—	3/60	1/60 (finger counting at one meter)
1/20 (0.05)	1/50 (0.02)	—
20/400	5/300 (20/1200)	—
—	1/60 (finger counting at one meter)	Light perception
1/50 (0.02)	—	—
5/300	—	—
—	No light perception	—
—	Undetermined or unspecified	—

OGCR   Section I.C.7.b.

Blindness

If "blindness" or "low vision" of both eyes is documented but the visual impairment category is not documented, assign code H54.3, Unqualified visual loss, both eyes. If "blindness" or "low vision" in one eye is documented but the visual impairment category is not documented, assign a code from H54.6-, Unqualified visual loss, one eye. If "blindness" or "visual loss" is documented without any information about whether one or both eyes are affected, assign code H54.7, Unspecified visual loss.

▶ New   ⇒ Revised   ~~deleted~~ Deleted   Excludes 1   Excludes 2   Includes   Use additional   Code first   Code also   Key words

OGCR Official Guidelines   ● Unacceptable Principal Diagnosis   X Assign placeholder X   ● Use Additional Character(s)   ▷ Manifestation Code   **Coding Clinic**

OTHER DISORDERS OF EYE AND ADNEXA (H55-H57)

- ● **H55 Nystagmus and other irregular eye movements**
  - ● **H55.0 Nystagmus**
    Rapid, involuntary movements of the eyes in the horizontal or vertical direction
    - H55.00 **Unspecified** nystagmus
    - H55.01 **Congenital** nystagmus
    - H55.02 **Latent** nystagmus
    - H55.03 **Visual deprivation** nystagmus
    - H55.04 **Dissociated** nystagmus
    - H55.09 **Other** forms of nystagmus
  - ● **H55.8 Other irregular eye movements**
    - H55.81 Deficient **saccadic** eye movements
    - H55.82 Deficient smooth pursuit eye movements
    - H55.89 **Other** irregular eye movements

- ● **H57 Other disorders of eye and adnexa**
  - ● **H57.0 Anomalies of pupillary function**
    - H57.00 **Unspecified** anomaly of pupillary function
    - H57.01 Argyll Robertson pupil, atypical
      > **Excludes1**   syphilitic Argyll Robertson pupil (A52.19)
    - H57.02 **Anisocoria**
    - H57.03 **Miosis**
    - H57.04 **Mydriasis**
    - ● H57.05 **Tonic pupil**
      - H57.051 Tonic pupil, **right eye**
      - H57.052 Tonic pupil, **left eye**
      - H57.053 Tonic pupil, **bilateral**
      - H57.059 Tonic pupil, **unspecified eye**
    - H57.09 **Other anomalies** of pupillary function
  - ● **H57.1 Ocular pain**
    - H57.10 Ocular pain, **unspecified eye**
    - H57.11 Ocular pain, **right eye**
    - H57.12 Ocular pain, **left eye**
    - H57.13 Ocular pain, **bilateral**
  - ● **H57.8 Other** specified disorders of eye and adnexa
    - ● H57.81 **Brow ptosis**
      - H57.811   Brow ptosis, right
        > (Ex) See PDX Collection 634
      - H57.812   Brow ptosis, left
        > (Ex) See PDX Collection 634
      - H57.813   Brow ptosis, bilateral
        > (Ex) See PDX Collection 634
      - H57.819   Brow ptosis, unspecified
        > (Ex) See PDX Collection 634
    - H57.89 Other specified disorders of eye and adnexa
  - ● **H57.9 Unspecified** disorder of eye and adnexa

INTRAOPERATIVE AND POSTPROCEDURAL COMPLICATIONS AND DISORDERS OF EYE AND ADNEXA, NOT ELSEWHERE CLASSIFIED (H59)

- ● **H59 Intraoperative and postprocedural complications and disorders of eye and adnexa, not elsewhere classified**
  > **Excludes1**   mechanical complication of intraocular lens (T85.2)
  > mechanical complication of other ocular prosthetic devices, implants and grafts (T85.3)
  > pseudophakia (Z96.1)
  > secondary cataracts (H26.4-)
  - ● **H59.0 Disorders of the eye following cataract surgery**
    > (Ex) For category H59.0 CC codes: See PDX Collection 638
    - ● H59.01 **Keratopathy** (bullous aphakic) following cataract surgery
      Vitreal corneal syndrome
      Vitreous (touch) syndrome
      - H59.011   Keratopathy (bullous aphakic) following cataract surgery, **right eye** 🦠
      - H59.012   Keratopathy (bullous aphakic) following cataract surgery, **left eye** 🦠
      - H59.013   Keratopathy (bullous aphakic) following cataract surgery, **bilateral** 🦠
      - H59.019   Keratopathy (bullous aphakic) following cataract surgery, **unspecified eye** 🦠
    - ● H59.02 **Cataract** (lens) **fragments** in eye following cataract surgery
      - H59.021   Cataract (lens) fragments in eye following cataract surgery, **right eye**
      - H59.022   Cataract (lens) fragments in eye following cataract surgery, **left eye**
      - H59.023   Cataract (lens) fragments in eye following cataract surgery, **bilateral**
      - H59.029   Cataract (lens) fragments in eye following cataract surgery, **unspecified eye**
    - ● H59.03 **Cystoid macular edema** following cataract surgery
      - H59.031   Cystoid macular edema following cataract surgery, **right eye** 🦠
      - H59.032   Cystoid macular edema following cataract surgery, **left eye** 🦠
      - H59.033   Cystoid macular edema following cataract surgery, **bilateral** 🦠
      - H59.039   Cystoid macular edema following cataract surgery, **unspecified eye** 🦠
    - ● H59.09 **Other** disorders of the eye following cataract surgery
      - H59.091   Other disorders of the **right eye** following cataract surgery 🦠
      - H59.092   Other disorders of the **left eye** following cataract surgery 🦠
      - H59.093   Other disorders of the eye following cataract surgery, **bilateral** 🦠
      - H59.099   Other disorders of **unspecified** eye following cataract surgery 🦠

CHAPTER 7 (H00-H59)

N   Newborn Age: 0   **P**   Pediatric Age: 0–17   **M**   Maternity DX: 9–64   **A**   Adult Age: 15–124   ♀   Females Only   ♂   Males Only

🦠 Complication\Comorbidity   🦠 Major C\C   (Ex) CC/MCC Exclusions   🦠 Hospital-Acquired Condition   🦠 Hierarchical Condition Category

871

● H59.1 Intraoperative hemorrhage and hematoma of eye and adnexa complicating a procedure

  Excludes1   intraoperative hemorrhage and hematoma of eye and adnexa due to accidental puncture or laceration during a procedure (H59.2-)

  Ⓔⓧ For category H59.1 CC codes: See PDX Collection 639

  ● H59.11 Intraoperative hemorrhage and hematoma of eye and adnexa complicating an ophthalmic procedure

    H59.111 Intraoperative hemorrhage and hematoma of right eye and adnexa complicating an ophthalmic procedure 🅒

    H59.112 Intraoperative hemorrhage and hematoma of left eye and adnexa complicating an ophthalmic procedure 🅒

    H59.113 Intraoperative hemorrhage and hematoma of eye and adnexa complicating an ophthalmic procedure, bilateral 🅒

    H59.119 Intraoperative hemorrhage and hematoma of unspecified eye and adnexa complicating an ophthalmic procedure 🅒

  ● H59.12 Intraoperative hemorrhage and hematoma of eye and adnexa complicating other procedure

    H59.121 Intraoperative hemorrhage and hematoma of right eye and adnexa complicating other procedure 🅒

    H59.122 Intraoperative hemorrhage and hematoma of left eye and adnexa complicating other procedure 🅒

    H59.123 Intraoperative hemorrhage and hematoma of eye and adnexa complicating other procedure, bilateral 🅒

    H59.129 Intraoperative hemorrhage and hematoma of unspecified eye and adnexa complicating other procedure 🅒

● H59.2 Accidental puncture and laceration of eye and adnexa during a procedure

  Ⓔⓧ For category H59.2 CC codes: See PDX Collection 509

  ● H59.21 Accidental puncture and laceration of eye and adnexa during an ophthalmic procedure

    H59.211 Accidental puncture and laceration of right eye and adnexa during an ophthalmic procedure 🅒

    H59.212 Accidental puncture and laceration of left eye and adnexa during an ophthalmic procedure 🅒

    H59.213 Accidental puncture and laceration of eye and adnexa during an ophthalmic procedure, bilateral 🅒

    H59.219 Accidental puncture and laceration of unspecified eye and adnexa during an ophthalmic procedure 🅒

  ● H59.22 Accidental puncture and laceration of eye and adnexa during other procedure

    H59.221 Accidental puncture and laceration of right eye and adnexa during other procedure 🅒

    H59.222 Accidental puncture and laceration of left eye and adnexa during other procedure 🅒

    H59.223 Accidental puncture and laceration of eye and adnexa during other procedure, bilateral 🅒

    H59.229 Accidental puncture and laceration of unspecified eye and adnexa during other procedure 🅒

● H59.3 Postprocedural hemorrhage, hematoma, and seroma of eye and adnexa following other procedure

  Ⓔⓧ For category H59.3 CC codes: See PDX Collection 639

  Coding Clinic: 2016, Q4, P10

  ● H59.31 Postprocedural hemorrhage of eye and adnexa following an ophthalmic procedure

    H59.311 Postprocedural hemorrhage of right eye and adnexa following an ophthalmic procedure 🅒

    H59.312 Postprocedural hemorrhage of left eye and adnexa following an ophthalmic procedure 🅒

    H59.313 Postprocedural hemorrhage of eye and adnexa following an ophthalmic procedure, bilateral 🅒

    H59.319 Postprocedural hemorrhage of unspecified eye and adnexa following an ophthalmic procedure 🅒

  ● H59.32 Postprocedural hemorrhage of eye and adnexa following other procedure

    H59.321 Postprocedural hemorrhage of right eye and adnexa following other procedure 🅒

    H59.322 Postprocedural hemorrhage of left eye and adnexa following other procedure 🅒

    H59.323 Postprocedural hemorrhage of eye and adnexa following other procedure, bilateral 🅒

    H59.329 Postprocedural hemorrhage of unspecified eye and adnexa following other procedure 🅒

  ● H59.33 Postprocedural hematoma of eye and adnexa following an ophthalmic procedure

    H59.331 Postprocedural hematoma of right eye and adnexa following an ophthalmic procedure 🅒

    H59.332 Postprocedural hematoma of left eye and adnexa following an ophthalmic procedure 🅒

    H59.333 Postprocedural hematoma of eye and adnexa following an ophthalmic procedure, bilateral 🅒

    H59.339 Postprocedural hematoma of unspecified eye and adnexa following an ophthalmic procedure 🅒

  ● H59.34 Postprocedural hematoma of eye and adnexa following other procedure

    H59.341 Postprocedural hematoma of right eye and adnexa following other procedure 🅒

    H59.342 Postprocedural hematoma of left eye and adnexa following other procedure 🅒

    H59.343 Postprocedural hematoma of eye and adnexa following other procedure, bilateral 🅒

    H59.349 Postprocedural hematoma of unspecified eye and adnexa following other procedure 🅒

▶ New   ⇛ Revised   d̶e̶l̶e̶t̶e̶d̶ Deleted   Excludes 1   Excludes 2   Includes   Use additional   Code first   Code also   Key words
OGCR Official Guidelines   ● Unacceptable Principal Diagnosis   X Assign placeholder X   ● Use Additional Character(s)   ▶ Manifestation Code   Coding Clinic

● H59.35   Postprocedural seroma of eye and adnexa following an ophthalmic procedure

     H59.351   Postprocedural seroma of right eye and adnexa following an ophthalmic procedure 🔾

     H59.352   Postprocedural seroma of left eye and adnexa following an ophthalmic procedure 🔾

     H59.353   Postprocedural seroma of eye and adnexa following an ophthalmic procedure, bilateral 🔾

     H59.359   Postprocedural seroma of unspecified eye and adnexa following an ophthalmic procedure 🔾

● H59.36   Postprocedural seroma of eye and adnexa following other procedure

     H59.361   Postprocedural seroma of right eye and adnexa following other procedure 🔾

     H59.362   Postprocedural seroma of left eye and adnexa following other procedure 🔾

     H59.363   Postprocedural seroma of eye and adnexa following other procedure, bilateral 🔾

     H59.369   Postprocedural seroma of unspecified eye and adnexa following other procedure 🔾

● H59.4   Inflammation (infection) of postprocedural bleb

     Postprocedural blebitis

     Excludes1   filtering (vitreous) bleb after glaucoma surgery status (Z98.83)

     H59.40   Inflammation (infection) of postprocedural bleb, unspecified

     H59.41   Inflammation (infection) of postprocedural bleb, stage 1

     H59.42   Inflammation (infection) of postprocedural bleb, stage 2

     H59.43   Inflammation (infection) of postprocedural bleb, stage 3

         Bleb endophthalmitis

● H59.8   Other intraoperative and postprocedural complications and disorders of eye and adnexa, not elsewhere classified

     Ⓔⓧ **For category H59.8 CC codes:** See PDX Collection 638

   ● H59.81   Chorioretinal scars after surgery for detachment

     H59.811   Chorioretinal scars after surgery for detachment, right eye 🔾

     H59.812   Chorioretinal scars after surgery for detachment, left eye 🔾

     H59.813   Chorioretinal scars after surgery for detachment, bilateral 🔾

     H59.819   Chorioretinal scars after surgery for detachment, unspecified eye 🔾

     H59.88   Other intraoperative complications of eye and adnexa, not elsewhere classified 🔾

     H59.89   Other postprocedural complications and disorders of eye and adnexa, not elsewhere classified 🔾

CHAPTER 7 (H00–H59)

N Newborn Age: 0   **P** Pediatric Age: 0–17   **M** Maternity DX: 9–64   **A** Adult Age: 15–124   ♀ Females Only   ♂ Males Only

🔾 Complication\Comorbidity   🔾 Major C\C   Ⓔⓧ CC/MCC Exclusions   🔾 Hospital-Acquired Condition   🔾 Hierarchical Condition Category

873

CHAPTER 8

DISEASES OF THE EAR AND MASTOID PROCESS (H60-H95)

OGCR Chapter-Specific Coding Guidelines

 8. Chapter 8: Diseases of the Ear and Mastoid Process (H60-H95)
  Reserved for future guideline expansion

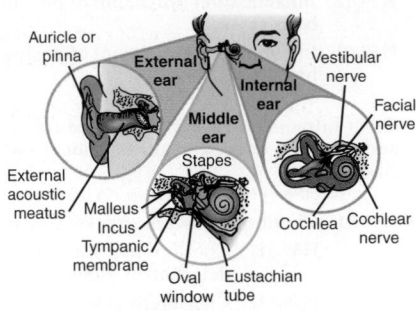

Figure 8-1 Auditory system. (From Buck CJ: Step-by-Step Medical Coding, ed 2016, St. Louis, Elsevier, 2016)

★ **(See Plate 20 of the Anatomy Illustrations.)**

CHAPTER 8

DISEASES OF THE EAR AND MASTOID PROCESS (H60-H95)

 Note: Use an external cause code following the code for the ear condition, if applicable, to identify the cause of the ear condition

 Excludes2 certain conditions originating in the perinatal period (P04-P96)
    certain infectious and parasitic diseases (A00-B99)
    complications of pregnancy, childbirth and the puerperium (O00-O9A)
    congenital malformations, deformations and chromosomal abnormalities (Q00-Q99)
    endocrine, nutritional and metabolic diseases (E00-E88)
    injury, poisoning and certain other consequences of external causes (S00-T88)
    neoplasms (C00-D49)
    symptoms, signs and abnormal clinical and laboratory findings, not elsewhere classified (R00-R94)

 This chapter contains the following blocks:

H60-H62	Diseases of external ear
H65-H75	Diseases of middle ear and mastoid
H80-H83	Diseases of inner ear
H90-H94	Other disorders of ear
H95	Intraoperative and postprocedural complications and disorders of ear and mastoid process, not elsewhere classified

DISEASES OF EXTERNAL EAR (H60-H62)

● **H60** **Otitis externa**

 ● **H60.0** **Abscess of external ear**
  Boil of external ear
  Carbuncle of auricle or external auditory canal
  Furuncle of external ear
  H60.00 Abscess of external ear, unspecified ear
  H60.01 Abscess of right external ear
  H60.02 Abscess of left external ear
  H60.03 Abscess of external ear, bilateral

● **H60.1** **Cellulitis of external ear**
 Cellulitis of auricle
 Cellulitis of external auditory canal
 H60.10 Cellulitis of external ear, unspecified ear
 H60.11 Cellulitis of right external ear
 H60.12 Cellulitis of left external ear
 H60.13 Cellulitis of external ear, bilateral

● **H60.2** **Malignant otitis externa**
  (Ex.) **For category H60.2 CC codes:** See PDX Collection 640
 H60.20 Malignant otitis externa, unspecified ear 🕸
 H60.21 Malignant otitis externa, right ear 🕸
 H60.22 Malignant otitis externa, left ear 🕸
 H60.23 Malignant otitis externa, bilateral 🕸

● **H60.3** **Other infective otitis externa**
 ● **H60.31** **Diffuse otitis externa**
  H60.311 Diffuse otitis externa, right ear
  H60.312 Diffuse otitis externa, left ear
  H60.313 Diffuse otitis externa, bilateral
  H60.319 Diffuse otitis externa, unspecified ear
 ● **H60.32** **Hemorrhagic otitis externa**
  H60.321 Hemorrhagic otitis externa, right ear
  H60.322 Hemorrhagic otitis externa, left ear
  H60.323 Hemorrhagic otitis externa, bilateral
  H60.329 Hemorrhagic otitis externa, unspecified ear
 ● **H60.33** **Swimmer's ear**
  H60.331 Swimmer's ear, right ear
  H60.332 Swimmer's ear, left ear
  H60.333 Swimmer's ear, bilateral
  H60.339 Swimmer's ear, unspecified ear
 ● **H60.39** **Other infective otitis externa**
  H60.391 Other infective otitis externa, right ear
  H60.392 Other infective otitis externa, left ear
  H60.393 Other infective otitis externa, bilateral
  H60.399 Other infective otitis externa, unspecified ear

● **H60.4** **Cholesteatoma of external ear**
 Keratosis obturans of external ear (canal)
 Excludes2 cholesteatoma of middle ear (H71.-)
    recurrent cholesteatoma of postmastoidectomy cavity (H95.0-)
 H60.40 Cholesteatoma of external ear, unspecified ear
 H60.41 Cholesteatoma of right external ear
 H60.42 Cholesteatoma of left external ear
 H60.43 Cholesteatoma of external ear, bilateral

● **H60.5** **Acute noninfective otitis externa**
 ● **H60.50** **Unspecified acute noninfective otitis externa**
  Acute otitis externa NOS
  H60.501 Unspecified acute noninfective otitis externa, right ear
  H60.502 Unspecified acute noninfective otitis externa, left ear
  H60.503 Unspecified acute noninfective otitis externa, bilateral
  H60.509 Unspecified acute noninfective otitis externa, unspecified ear
 ● **H60.51** **Acute actinic otitis externa**
  H60.511 Acute actinic otitis externa, right ear
  H60.512 Acute actinic otitis externa, left ear
  H60.513 Acute actinic otitis externa, bilateral
  H60.519 Acute actinic otitis externa, unspecified ear

● **H60.52 Acute chemical otitis externa**
- H60.521 Acute chemical otitis externa, right ear
- H60.522 Acute chemical otitis externa, left ear
- H60.523 Acute chemical otitis externa, bilateral
- H60.529 Acute chemical otitis externa, unspecified ear

● **H60.53 Acute contact otitis externa**
- H60.531 Acute contact otitis externa, right ear
- H60.532 Acute contact otitis externa, left ear
- H60.533 Acute contact otitis externa, bilateral
- H60.539 Acute contact otitis externa, unspecified ear

● **H60.54 Acute eczematoid otitis externa**
- H60.541 Acute eczematoid otitis externa, right ear
- H60.542 Acute eczematoid otitis externa, left ear
- H60.543 Acute eczematoid otitis externa, bilateral
- H60.549 Acute eczematoid otitis externa, unspecified ear

● **H60.55 Acute reactive otitis externa**
- H60.551 Acute reactive otitis externa, right ear
- H60.552 Acute reactive otitis externa, left ear
- H60.553 Acute reactive otitis externa, bilateral
- H60.559 Acute reactive otitis externa, unspecified ear

● **H60.59 Other noninfective acute otitis externa**
- H60.591 Other noninfective acute otitis externa, right ear
- H60.592 Other noninfective acute otitis externa, left ear
- H60.593 Other noninfective acute otitis externa, bilateral
- H60.599 Other noninfective acute otitis externa, unspecified ear

● **H60.6 Unspecified chronic otitis externa**
- H60.60 Unspecified chronic otitis externa, unspecified ear
- H60.61 Unspecified chronic otitis externa, right ear
- H60.62 Unspecified chronic otitis externa, left ear
- H60.63 Unspecified chronic otitis externa, bilateral

● **H60.8 Other otitis externa**
● **H60.8X Other otitis externa**
- H60.8X1 Other otitis externa, right ear
- H60.8X2 Other otitis externa, left ear
- H60.8X3 Other otitis externa, bilateral
- H60.8X9 Other otitis externa, unspecified ear

● **H60.9 Unspecified otitis externa**
- H60.90 Unspecified otitis externa, unspecified ear
- H60.91 Unspecified otitis externa, right ear
- H60.92 Unspecified otitis externa, left ear
- H60.93 Unspecified otitis externa, bilateral

● **H61 Other disorders of external ear**
● **H61.0 Chondritis and perichondritis of external ear**
Chondrodermatitis nodularis chronica helicis
Perichondritis of auricle
Perichondritis of pinna

● **H61.00 Unspecified perichondritis of external ear**
- H61.001 Unspecified perichondritis of right external ear
- H61.002 Unspecified perichondritis of left external ear
- H61.003 Unspecified perichondritis of external ear, bilateral
- H61.009 Unspecified perichondritis of external ear, unspecified ear

● **H61.01 Acute perichondritis of external ear**
- H61.011 Acute perichondritis of right external ear
- H61.012 Acute perichondritis of left external ear
- H61.013 Acute perichondritis of external ear, bilateral
- H61.019 Acute perichondritis of external ear, unspecified ear

● **H61.02 Chronic perichondritis of external ear**
- H61.021 Chronic perichondritis of right external ear
- H61.022 Chronic perichondritis of left external ear
- H61.023 Chronic perichondritis of external ear, bilateral
- H61.029 Chronic perichondritis of external ear, unspecified ear

● **H61.03 Chondritis of external ear**
Chondritis of auricle
Chondritis of pinna
- H61.031 Chondritis of right external ear
- H61.032 Chondritis of left external ear
  Coding Clinic: 2015, Q1, P18
- H61.033 Chondritis of external ear, bilateral
- H61.039 Chondritis of external ear, unspecified ear

● **H61.1 Noninfective disorders of pinna**
  Excludes2 cauliflower ear (M95.1-)
  gouty tophi of ear (M1A.-)

● **H61.10 Unspecified noninfective disorders of pinna**
Disorder of pinna NOS
- H61.101 Unspecified noninfective disorders of pinna, right ear
- H61.102 Unspecified noninfective disorders of pinna, left ear
- H61.103 Unspecified noninfective disorders of pinna, bilateral
- H61.109 Unspecified noninfective disorders of pinna, unspecified ear

● **H61.11 Acquired deformity of pinna**
Acquired deformity of auricle
  Excludes2 cauliflower ear (M95.1-)
- H61.111 Acquired deformity of pinna, right ear
- H61.112 Acquired deformity of pinna, left ear
- H61.113 Acquired deformity of pinna, bilateral
- H61.119 Acquired deformity of pinna, unspecified ear

● **H61.12 Hematoma of pinna**
Hematoma of auricle
- H61.121 Hematoma of pinna, right ear
- H61.122 Hematoma of pinna, left ear
- H61.123 Hematoma of pinna, bilateral
- H61.129 Hematoma of pinna, unspecified ear

● **H61.19 Other noninfective disorders of pinna**
- H61.191 Noninfective disorders of pinna, right ear
- H61.192 Noninfective disorders of pinna, left ear
- H61.193 Noninfective disorders of pinna, bilateral
- H61.199 Noninfective disorders of pinna, unspecified ear

N Newborn Age: 0   **P** Pediatric Age: 0–17   **M** Maternity DX: 9–64   **A** Adult Age: 15–124   ♀ Females Only   ♂ Males Only
Complication\Comorbidity   Major C\C   (Ex) CC/MCC Exclusions   Hospital-Acquired Condition   Hierarchical Condition Category
875

CHAPTER 8 (H60-H95)

H61.2 Impacted cerumen
Wax in ear
  H61.20 Impacted cerumen, unspecified ear
MCE: Questionable admission when principal dx
  H61.21 Impacted cerumen, right ear
MCE: Questionable admission when principal dx
  H61.22 Impacted cerumen, left ear
MCE: Questionable admission when principal dx
  H61.23 Impacted cerumen, bilateral
MCE: Questionable admission when principal dx

H61.3 Acquired stenosis of external ear canal
Collapse of external ear canal
Excludes1 postprocedural stenosis of external ear canal (H95.81-)
  H61.30 Acquired stenosis of external ear canal, unspecified
    H61.301 Acquired stenosis of right external ear canal, unspecified
    H61.302 Acquired stenosis of left external ear canal, unspecified
    H61.303 Acquired stenosis of external ear canal, unspecified, bilateral
    H61.309 Acquired stenosis of external ear canal, unspecified, unspecified ear
  H61.31 Acquired stenosis of external ear canal secondary to trauma
    H61.311 Acquired stenosis of right external ear canal secondary to trauma
    H61.312 Acquired stenosis of left external ear canal secondary to trauma
    H61.313 Acquired stenosis of external ear canal secondary to trauma, bilateral
    H61.319 Acquired stenosis of external ear canal secondary to trauma, unspecified ear
  H61.32 Acquired stenosis of external ear canal secondary to inflammation and infection
    H61.321 Acquired stenosis of right external ear canal secondary to inflammation and infection
    H61.322 Acquired stenosis of left external ear canal secondary to inflammation and infection
    H61.323 Acquired stenosis of external ear canal secondary to inflammation and infection, bilateral
    H61.329 Acquired stenosis of external ear canal secondary to inflammation and infection, unspecified ear
  H61.39 Other acquired stenosis of external ear canal
    H61.391 Other acquired stenosis of right external ear canal
    H61.392 Other acquired stenosis of left external ear canal
    H61.393 Other acquired stenosis of external ear canal, bilateral
    H61.399 Other acquired stenosis of external ear canal, unspecified ear

H61.8 Other specified disorders of external ear
  H61.81 Exostosis of external canal
    H61.811 Exostosis of right external canal
    H61.812 Exostosis of left external canal
    H61.813 Exostosis of external canal, bilateral
    H61.819 Exostosis of external canal, unspecified ear
  H61.89 Other specified disorders of external ear
    H61.891 Other specified disorders of right external ear
    H61.892 Other specified disorders of left external ear
    H61.893 Other specified disorders of external ear, bilateral
    H61.899 Other specified disorders of external ear, unspecified ear

H61.9 Disorder of external ear, unspecified
  H61.90 Disorder of external ear, unspecified, unspecified ear
  H61.91 Disorder of right external ear, unspecified
  H61.92 Disorder of left external ear, unspecified
  H61.93 Disorder of external ear, unspecified, bilateral

H62 Disorders of external ear in diseases classified elsewhere
  H62.4 Otitis externa in other diseases classified elsewhere
Code first underlying disease, such as:
  erysipelas (A46)
  impetigo (L01.0)
Excludes1 otitis externa (in):
  candidiasis (B37.84)
  herpes viral [herpes simplex] (B00.1)
  herpes zoster (B02.8)
    H62.40 Otitis externa in other diseases classified elsewhere, unspecified ear
    H62.41 Otitis externa in other diseases classified elsewhere, right ear
    H62.42 Otitis externa in other diseases classified elsewhere, left ear
    H62.43 Otitis externa in other diseases classified elsewhere, bilateral
  H62.8 Other disorders of external ear in diseases classified elsewhere
Code first underlying disease, such as:
  gout (M1A.-, M10.-)
    H62.8X Other disorders of external ear in diseases classified elsewhere
      H62.8X1 Other disorders of right external ear in diseases classified elsewhere
      H62.8X2 Other disorders of left external ear in diseases classified elsewhere
      H62.8X3 Other disorders of external ear in diseases classified elsewhere, bilateral
      H62.8X9 Other disorders of external ear in diseases classified elsewhere, unspecified ear

DISEASES OF MIDDLE EAR AND MASTOID (H65-H75)

★ **(See Plate 21 of the Anatomy Illustrations.)**

H65 Nonsuppurative otitis media
Bacterial or viral infection or inflammation of the middle ear; may result in fluid accumulation with pain and temporary hearing loss.
Includes nonsuppurative otitis media with myringitis
Use additional code for any associated perforated tympanic membrane (H72.-)
Use additional code to identify:
  exposure to environmental tobacco smoke (Z77.22)
  exposure to tobacco smoke in the perinatal period (P96.81)
  history of tobacco dependence (Z87.891)
  infectious agent (B95-B97)
  occupational exposure to environmental tobacco smoke (Z57.31)
  tobacco dependence (F17.-)
  tobacco use (Z72.0)
  H65.0 Acute serous otitis media
Acute and subacute secretory otitis
    H65.00 Acute serous otitis media, unspecified ear
    H65.01 Acute serous otitis media, right ear
    H65.02 Acute serous otitis media, left ear
    H65.03 Acute serous otitis media, bilateral
    H65.04 Acute serous otitis media, recurrent, right ear
    H65.05 Acute serous otitis media, recurrent, left ear
    H65.06 Acute serous otitis media, recurrent, bilateral
    H65.07 Acute serous otitis media, recurrent, unspecified ear

- ● **H65.1** **Other acute nonsuppurative otitis media**
  - **Excludes1**   otitic barotrauma (T70.Ø)
    otitis media (acute) NOS (H66.9)
  - ● **H65.11** **Acute and subacute allergic otitis media (mucoid) (sanguinous) (serous)**
    - **H65.111** Acute and subacute allergic otitis media (mucoid) (sanguinous) (serous), right ear
    - **H65.112** Acute and subacute allergic otitis media (mucoid) (sanguinous) (serous), left ear
    - **H65.113** Acute and subacute allergic otitis media (mucoid) (sanguinous) (serous), bilateral
    - **H65.114** Acute and subacute allergic otitis media (mucoid) (sanguinous) (serous), recurrent, right ear
    - **H65.115** Acute and subacute allergic otitis media (mucoid) (sanguinous) (serous), recurrent, left ear
    - **H65.116** Acute and subacute allergic otitis media (mucoid) (sanguinous) (serous), recurrent, bilateral
    - **H65.117** Acute and subacute allergic otitis media (mucoid) (sanguinous) (serous), recurrent, unspecified ear
    - **H65.119** Acute and subacute allergic otitis media (mucoid) (sanguinous) (serous), unspecified ear
  - ● **H65.19** **Other acute nonsuppurative otitis media**
    Acute and subacute mucoid otitis media
    Acute and subacute nonsuppurative otitis media NOS
    Acute and subacute sanguinous otitis media
    Acute and subacute seromucinous otitis media
    - **H65.191** Other acute nonsuppurative otitis media, right ear
    - **H65.192** Other acute nonsuppurative otitis media, left ear
    - **H65.193** Other acute nonsuppurative otitis media, bilateral
    - **H65.194** Other acute nonsuppurative otitis media, recurrent, right ear
    - **H65.195** Other acute nonsuppurative otitis media, recurrent, left ear
    - **H65.196** Other acute nonsuppurative otitis media, recurrent, bilateral
    - **H65.197** Other acute nonsuppurative otitis media recurrent, unspecified ear
    - **H65.199** Other acute nonsuppurative otitis media, unspecified ear
- ● **H65.2** **Chronic serous otitis media**
  Chronic tubotympanal catarrh
  - **H65.20** Chronic serous otitis media, unspecified ear
  - **H65.21** Chronic serous otitis media, right ear
  - **H65.22** Chronic serous otitis media, left ear
  - **H65.23** Chronic serous otitis media, bilateral
- ● **H65.3** **Chronic mucoid otitis media**
  Chronic mucinous otitis media
  Chronic secretory otitis media
  Chronic transudative otitis media
  Glue ear
  - **Excludes1**   adhesive middle ear disease (H74.1)
  - **H65.30** Chronic mucoid otitis media, unspecified ear
  - **H65.31** Chronic mucoid otitis media, right ear
  - **H65.32** Chronic mucoid otitis media, left ear
  - **H65.33** Chronic mucoid otitis media, bilateral
- ● **H65.4** **Other chronic nonsuppurative otitis media**
  - ● **H65.41** **Chronic allergic otitis media**
    - **H65.411** Chronic allergic otitis media, right ear
    - **H65.412** Chronic allergic otitis media, left ear

- **H65.413** Chronic allergic otitis media, bilateral
- **H65.419** Chronic allergic otitis media, unspecified ear
- ● **H65.49** **Other chronic nonsuppurative otitis media**
  Chronic exudative otitis media
  Chronic nonsuppurative otitis media NOS
  Chronic otitis media with effusion (nonpurulent)
  Chronic seromucinous otitis media
  - **H65.491** Other chronic nonsuppurative otitis media, right ear
  - **H65.492** Other chronic nonsuppurative otitis media, left ear
  - **H65.493** Other chronic nonsuppurative otitis media, bilateral
  - **H65.499** Other chronic nonsuppurative otitis media, unspecified ear
- ● **H65.9** **Unspecified nonsuppurative otitis media**
  Allergic otitis media NOS
  Catarrhal otitis media NOS
  Exudative otitis media NOS
  Mucoid otitis media NOS
  Otitis media with effusion (nonpurulent) NOS
  Secretory otitis media NOS
  Seromucinous otitis media NOS
  Serous otitis media NOS
  Transudative otitis media NOS
  - **H65.90** Unspecified nonsuppurative otitis media, unspecified ear
  - **H65.91** Unspecified nonsuppurative otitis media, right ear
  - **H65.92** Unspecified nonsuppurative otitis media, left ear
  - **H65.93** Unspecified nonsuppurative otitis media, bilateral
- ● **H66** **Suppurative and unspecified otitis media**
  Suppurative: Discharging pus
  - **Includes**   suppurative and unspecified otitis media with myringitis
  Use additional code to identify:
    exposure to environmental tobacco smoke (Z77.22)
    exposure to tobacco smoke in the perinatal period (P96.81)
    history of tobacco dependence (Z87.891)
    occupational exposure to environmental tobacco smoke (Z57.31)
    tobacco dependence (F17.-)
    tobacco use (Z72.Ø)
  - ● **H66.0** **Acute suppurative otitis media**
    - ● **H66.00** **Acute suppurative otitis media without spontaneous rupture of ear drum**
      - **H66.001** Acute suppurative otitis media without spontaneous rupture of ear drum, right ear
        Coding Clinic: 2016, Q1, P34
      - **H66.002** Acute suppurative otitis media without spontaneous rupture of ear drum, left ear
      - **H66.003** Acute suppurative otitis media without spontaneous rupture of ear drum, bilateral
      - **H66.004** Acute suppurative otitis media without spontaneous rupture of ear drum, recurrent, right ear
      - **H66.005** Acute suppurative otitis media without spontaneous rupture of ear drum, recurrent, left ear
      - **H66.006** Acute suppurative otitis media without spontaneous rupture of ear drum, recurrent, bilateral
      - **H66.007** Acute suppurative otitis media without spontaneous rupture of ear drum, recurrent, unspecified ear
      - **H66.009** Acute suppurative otitis media without spontaneous rupture of ear drum, unspecified ear

● H66.01   **Acute suppurative otitis media with spontaneous rupture of ear drum**

     H66.011   **Acute suppurative otitis media with spontaneous rupture of ear drum, right ear**

     H66.012   **Acute suppurative otitis media with spontaneous rupture of ear drum, left ear**

     H66.013   **Acute suppurative otitis media with spontaneous rupture of ear drum, bilateral**

     H66.014   **Acute suppurative otitis media with spontaneous rupture of ear drum, recurrent, right ear**

     H66.015   **Acute suppurative otitis media with spontaneous rupture of ear drum, recurrent, left ear**

     H66.016   **Acute suppurative otitis media with spontaneous rupture of ear drum, recurrent, bilateral**

     H66.017   **Acute suppurative otitis media with spontaneous rupture of ear drum, recurrent, unspecified ear**

     H66.019   **Acute suppurative otitis media with spontaneous rupture of ear drum, unspecified ear**

● H66.1   **Chronic tubotympanic suppurative otitis media**

     Benign chronic suppurative otitis media

     Chronic tubotympanic disease

     Use additional code for any associated perforated tympanic membrane (H72.-)

     H66.10   **Chronic tubotympanic suppurative otitis media, unspecified**

     H66.11   **Chronic tubotympanic suppurative otitis media, right ear**

     H66.12   **Chronic tubotympanic suppurative otitis media, left ear**

     H66.13   **Chronic tubotympanic suppurative otitis media, bilateral**

● H66.2   **Chronic atticoantral suppurative otitis media**

     Chronic atticoantral disease

     Use additional code for any associated perforated tympanic membrane (H72.-)

     H66.20   **Chronic atticoantral suppurative otitis media, unspecified ear**

     H66.21   **Chronic atticoantral suppurative otitis media, right ear**

     H66.22   **Chronic atticoantral suppurative otitis media, left ear**

     H66.23   **Chronic atticoantral suppurative otitis media, bilateral**

● H66.3   **Other chronic suppurative otitis media**

     Chronic suppurative otitis media NOS

     Use additional code for any associated perforated tympanic membrane (H72.-)

     Excludes1   tuberculous otitis media (A18.6)

● H66.3X   **Other chronic suppurative otitis media**

     H66.3X1   **Other chronic suppurative otitis media, right ear**

     H66.3X2   **Other chronic suppurative otitis media, left ear**

     H66.3X3   **Other chronic suppurative otitis media, bilateral**

     H66.3X9   **Other chronic suppurative otitis media, unspecified ear**

● H66.4   **Suppurative otitis media, unspecified**

     Purulent otitis media NOS

     Use additional code for any associated perforated tympanic membrane (H72.-)

     H66.40   **Suppurative otitis media, unspecified, unspecified ear**

     H66.41   **Suppurative otitis media, unspecified, right ear**

     H66.42   **Suppurative otitis media, unspecified, left ear**

     H66.43   **Suppurative otitis media, unspecified, bilateral**

● H66.9   **Otitis media, unspecified**

     Otitis media NOS

     Acute otitis media NOS

     Chronic otitis media NOS

     Use additional code for any associated perforated tympanic membrane (H72.-)

     H66.90   **Otitis media, unspecified, unspecified ear**

     H66.91   **Otitis media, unspecified, right ear**

     H66.92   **Otitis media, unspecified, left ear**

     H66.93   **Otitis media, unspecified, bilateral**

● H67   **Otitis media in diseases classified elsewhere**

     Code first underlying disease, such as:

        plasminogen deficiency (E88.02)

        viral disease NEC (B00-B34)

     Use additional code for any associated perforated tympanic membrane (H72.-)

     Excludes1   otitis media in:

        influenza (J09.X9, J10.83, J11.83)

        measles (B05.3)

        scarlet fever (A38.0)

        tuberculosis (A18.6)

     ▷ H67.1   *Otitis media in diseases classified elsewhere, right ear*

     ▷ H67.2   *Otitis media in diseases classified elsewhere, left ear*

     ▷ H67.3   *Otitis media in diseases classified elsewhere, bilateral*

     ▷ H67.9   *Otitis media in diseases classified elsewhere, unspecified ear*

● H68   **Eustachian salpingitis and obstruction**

● H68.0   **Eustachian salpingitis**

     ● H68.00   **Unspecified Eustachian salpingitis**

        H68.001   **Unspecified Eustachian salpingitis, right ear**

        H68.002   **Unspecified Eustachian salpingitis, left ear**

        H68.003   **Unspecified Eustachian salpingitis, bilateral**

        H68.009   **Unspecified Eustachian salpingitis, unspecified ear**

     ● H68.01   **Acute Eustachian salpingitis**

        H68.011   **Acute Eustachian salpingitis, right ear**

        H68.012   **Acute Eustachian salpingitis, left ear**

        H68.013   **Acute Eustachian salpingitis, bilateral**

        H68.019   **Acute Eustachian salpingitis, unspecified ear**

     ● H68.02   **Chronic Eustachian salpingitis**

        H68.021   **Chronic Eustachian salpingitis, right ear**

        H68.022   **Chronic Eustachian salpingitis, left ear**

        H68.023   **Chronic Eustachian salpingitis, bilateral**

        H68.029   **Chronic Eustachian salpingitis, unspecified ear**

▶ New   ⇒ Revised   ~~deleted~~ Deleted   Excludes 1   Excludes 2   Includes   Use additional   Code first   Code also   Key words

878   OGCR Official Guidelines   ● Unacceptable Principal Diagnosis   X Assign placeholder X   ▷ Use Additional Character(s)   ▷ Manifestation Code   Coding Clinic

- ● **H68.1 Obstruction of Eustachian tube**
  Stenosis of Eustachian tube
  Stricture of Eustachian tube
  - ● H68.10 Unspecified obstruction of Eustachian tube
    - H68.101 Unspecified obstruction of Eustachian tube, right ear
    - H68.102 Unspecified obstruction of Eustachian tube, left ear
    - H68.103 Unspecified obstruction of Eustachian tube, bilateral
    - H68.109 Unspecified obstruction of Eustachian tube, unspecified ear
  - ● H68.11 Osseous obstruction of Eustachian tube
    - H68.111 Osseous obstruction of Eustachian tube, right ear
    - H68.112 Osseous obstruction of Eustachian tube, left ear
    - H68.113 Osseous obstruction of Eustachian tube, bilateral
    - H68.119 Osseous obstruction of Eustachian tube, unspecified ear
  - ● H68.12 Intrinsic cartilagenous obstruction of Eustachian tube
    - H68.121 Intrinsic cartilagenous obstruction of Eustachian tube, right ear
    - H68.122 Intrinsic cartilagenous obstruction of Eustachian tube, left ear
    - H68.123 Intrinsic cartilagenous obstruction of Eustachian tube, bilateral
    - H68.129 Intrinsic cartilagenous obstruction of Eustachian tube, unspecified ear
  - ● H68.13 Extrinsic cartilagenous obstruction of Eustachian tube
    Compression of Eustachian tube
    - H68.131 Extrinsic cartilagenous obstruction of Eustachian tube, right ear
    - H68.132 Extrinsic cartilagenous obstruction of Eustachian tube, left ear
    - H68.133 Extrinsic cartilagenous obstruction of Eustachian tube, bilateral
    - H68.139 Extrinsic cartilagenous obstruction of Eustachian tube, unspecified ear
- ● **H69 Other and unspecified disorders of Eustachian tube**
  - ● H69.0 Patulous Eustachian tube
    - H69.00 Patulous Eustachian tube, unspecified ear
    - H69.01 Patulous Eustachian tube, right ear
    - H69.02 Patulous Eustachian tube, left ear
    - H69.03 Patulous Eustachian tube, bilateral
  - ● H69.8 Other specified disorders of Eustachian tube
    - H69.80 Other specified disorders of Eustachian tube, unspecified ear
    - H69.81 Other specified disorders of Eustachian tube, right ear
    - H69.82 Other specified disorders of Eustachian tube, left ear
    - H69.83 Other specified disorders of Eustachian tube, bilateral
  - ● H69.9 Unspecified Eustachian tube disorder
    - H69.90 Unspecified Eustachian tube disorder, unspecified ear
    - H69.91 Unspecified Eustachian tube disorder, right ear
    - H69.92 Unspecified Eustachian tube disorder, left ear
    - H69.93 Unspecified Eustachian tube disorder, bilateral

- ● **H70 Mastoiditis and related conditions**
  - ● H70.0 Acute mastoiditis
    Abscess of mastoid
    Empyema of mastoid
    (Ex) For category H70.0 CC codes: See PDX Collection 641
    - ● H70.00 Acute mastoiditis without complications
      - H70.001 Acute mastoiditis without complications, right ear
      - H70.002 Acute mastoiditis without complications, left ear
      - H70.003 Acute mastoiditis without complications, bilateral
      - H70.009 Acute mastoiditis without complications, unspecified ear
    - ● H70.01 Subperiosteal abscess of mastoid
      - H70.011 Subperiosteal abscess of mastoid, right ear
      - H70.012 Subperiosteal abscess of mastoid, left ear
      - H70.013 Subperiosteal abscess of mastoid, bilateral
      - H70.019 Subperiosteal abscess of mastoid, unspecified ear
    - ● H70.09 Acute mastoiditis with other complications
      - H70.091 Acute mastoiditis with other complications, right ear
      - H70.092 Acute mastoiditis with other complications, left ear
      - H70.093 Acute mastoiditis with other complications, bilateral
      - H70.099 Acute mastoiditis with other complications, unspecified ear
  - ● H70.1 Chronic mastoiditis
    Caries of mastoid
    Fistula of mastoid
    Excludes1 tuberculous mastoiditis (A18.03)
    - H70.10 Chronic mastoiditis, unspecified ear
    - H70.11 Chronic mastoiditis, right ear
    - H70.12 Chronic mastoiditis, left ear
    - H70.13 Chronic mastoiditis, bilateral
  - ● H70.2 Petrositis
    Inflammation of petrous bone
    - ● H70.20 Unspecified petrositis
      - H70.201 Unspecified petrositis, right ear
      - H70.202 Unspecified petrositis, left ear
      - H70.203 Unspecified petrositis, bilateral
      - H70.209 Unspecified petrositis, unspecified ear
    - ● H70.21 Acute petrositis
      - H70.211 Acute petrositis, right ear
      - H70.212 Acute petrositis, left ear
      - H70.213 Acute petrositis, bilateral
      - H70.219 Acute petrositis, unspecified ear
    - ● H70.22 Chronic petrositis
      - H70.221 Chronic petrositis, right ear
      - H70.222 Chronic petrositis, left ear
      - H70.223 Chronic petrositis, bilateral
      - H70.229 Chronic petrositis, unspecified ear

Item 8-1 Mastoiditis is an infection of the portion of the temporal bone of the skull that is behind the ear (mastoid process) caused by an untreated otitis media, leading to an infection of the surrounding structures which may include the brain.

● H70.8   Other mastoiditis and related conditions
    Excludes1   preauricular sinus and cyst (Q18.1)
        sinus, fistula, and cyst of branchial cleft
        (Q18.0)
  ● H70.81   Postauricular fistula
    H70.811   Postauricular fistula, right ear
    H70.812   Postauricular fistula, left ear
    H70.813   Postauricular fistula, bilateral
    H70.819   Postauricular fistula, unspecified ear
  ● H70.89   Other mastoiditis and related conditions
    H70.891   Other mastoiditis and related
        conditions, right ear
    H70.892   Other mastoiditis and related
        conditions, left ear
    H70.893   Other mastoiditis and related
        conditions, bilateral
    H70.899   Other mastoiditis and related
        conditions, unspecified ear

● H70.9   Unspecified mastoiditis
  H70.90   Unspecified mastoiditis, unspecified ear
  H70.91   Unspecified mastoiditis, right ear
  H70.92   Unspecified mastoiditis, left ear
  H70.93   Unspecified mastoiditis, bilateral

● H71   Cholesteatoma of middle ear
    Excludes2   cholesteatoma of external ear (H60.4-)
        recurrent cholesteatoma of postmastoidectomy
        cavity (H95.0-)
● H71.0   Cholesteatoma of attic
  H71.00   Cholesteatoma of attic, unspecified ear
  H71.01   Cholesteatoma of attic, right ear
  H71.02   Cholesteatoma of attic, left ear
  H71.03   Cholesteatoma of attic, bilateral
● H71.1   Cholesteatoma of tympanum
  H71.10   Cholesteatoma of tympanum, unspecified ear
  H71.11   Cholesteatoma of tympanum, right ear
  H71.12   Cholesteatoma of tympanum, left ear
  H71.13   Cholesteatoma of tympanum, bilateral
● H71.2   Cholesteatoma of mastoid
  H71.20   Cholesteatoma of mastoid, unspecified ear
  H71.21   Cholesteatoma of mastoid, right ear
  H71.22   Cholesteatoma of mastoid, left ear
  H71.23   Cholesteatoma of mastoid, bilateral
● H71.3   Diffuse cholesteatosis
  H71.30   Diffuse cholesteatosis, unspecified ear
  H71.31   Diffuse cholesteatosis, right ear
  H71.32   Diffuse cholesteatosis, left ear
  H71.33   Diffuse cholesteatosis, bilateral
● H71.9   Unspecified cholesteatoma
  H71.90   Unspecified cholesteatoma, unspecified ear
  H71.91   Unspecified cholesteatoma, right ear
  H71.92   Unspecified cholesteatoma, left ear
  H71.93   Unspecified cholesteatoma, bilateral

★ (See Plate 22 of the Anatomy Illustrations.)

● H72   Perforation of tympanic membrane
    Hole or rupture in ear drum
    Includes   persistent post-traumatic perforation of ear drum
        postinflammatory perforation of ear drum
    Code first any associated otitis media (H65.-, H66.1-, H66.2-,
    H66.3-, H66.4-, H66.9-, H67.-)
    Excludes1   acute suppurative otitis media with rupture of
        the tympanic membrane (H66.01-)
        traumatic rupture of ear drum (S09.2-)
● H72.0   Central perforation of tympanic membrane
  H72.00   Central perforation of tympanic membrane,
    unspecified ear
  H72.01   Central perforation of tympanic membrane,
    right ear
  H72.02   Central perforation of tympanic membrane, left
    ear
  H72.03   Central perforation of tympanic membrane,
    bilateral
● H72.1   Attic perforation of tympanic membrane
    Perforation of pars flaccida
  H72.10   Attic perforation of tympanic membrane,
    unspecified ear
  H72.11   Attic perforation of tympanic membrane, right
    ear
  H72.12   Attic perforation of tympanic membrane, left
    ear
  H72.13   Attic perforation of tympanic membrane,
    bilateral
● H72.2   Other marginal perforations of tympanic membrane
  ● H72.2X   Other marginal perforations of tympanic
    membrane
    H72.2X1   Other marginal perforations of
        tympanic membrane, right ear
    H72.2X2   Other marginal perforations of
        tympanic membrane, left ear
    H72.2X3   Other marginal perforations of
        tympanic membrane, bilateral
    H72.2X9   Other marginal perforations of
        tympanic membrane, unspecified ear
● H72.8   Other perforations of tympanic membrane
  ● H72.81   Multiple perforations of tympanic membrane
    H72.811   Multiple perforations of tympanic
        membrane, right ear
    H72.812   Multiple perforations of tympanic
        membrane, left ear
    H72.813   Multiple perforations of tympanic
        membrane, bilateral
    H72.819   Multiple perforations of tympanic
        membrane, unspecified ear
  ● H72.82   Total perforations of tympanic membrane
    H72.821   Total perforations of tympanic
        membrane, right ear
    H72.822   Total perforations of tympanic
        membrane, left ear
    H72.823   Total perforations of tympanic
        membrane, bilateral
    H72.829   Total perforations of tympanic
        membrane, unspecified ear
● H72.9   Unspecified perforation of tympanic membrane
  H72.90   Unspecified perforation of tympanic
    membrane, unspecified ear
  H72.91   Unspecified perforation of tympanic
    membrane, right ear
  H72.92   Unspecified perforation of tympanic
    membrane, left ear
  H72.93   Unspecified perforation of tympanic
    membrane, bilateral

▶ New   ⟹ Revised   ~~deleted~~ Deleted   Excludes 1   Excludes 2   Includes   Use additional   Code first   Code also   Key words
OGCR Official Guidelines   ● Unacceptable Principal Diagnosis   X Assign placeholder X   ● Use Additional Character(s)   ▶ Manifestation Code   Coding Clinic

● **H73 Other disorders of tympanic membrane**
  ● **H73.0 Acute myringitis**
      Excludes1   acute myringitis with otitis media (H65, H66)
    ● **H73.00 Unspecified acute myringitis**
          Acute tympanitis NOS
        H73.001 Acute myringitis, right ear
        H73.002 Acute myringitis, left ear
        H73.003 Acute myringitis, bilateral
        H73.009 Acute myringitis, unspecified ear
    ● **H73.01 Bullous myringitis**
        H73.011 Bullous myringitis, right ear
        H73.012 Bullous myringitis, left ear
        H73.013 Bullous myringitis, bilateral
        H73.019 Bullous myringitis, unspecified ear
    ● **H73.09 Other acute myringitis**
        H73.091 Other acute myringitis, right ear
        H73.092 Other acute myringitis, left ear
        H73.093 Other acute myringitis, bilateral
        H73.099 Other acute myringitis, unspecified ear
  ● **H73.1 Chronic myringitis**
        Chronic tympanitis
        Excludes1   chronic myringitis with otitis media (H65, H66)
      H73.10 Chronic myringitis, unspecified ear
      H73.11 Chronic myringitis, right ear
      H73.12 Chronic myringitis, left ear
      H73.13 Chronic myringitis, bilateral
  ● **H73.2 Unspecified myringitis**
      H73.20 Unspecified myringitis, unspecified ear
      H73.21 Unspecified myringitis, right ear
      H73.22 Unspecified myringitis, left ear
      H73.23 Unspecified myringitis, bilateral
  ● **H73.8 Other specified disorders of tympanic membrane**
    ● **H73.81 Atrophic flaccid tympanic membrane**
        H73.811 Atrophic flaccid tympanic membrane, right ear
        H73.812 Atrophic flaccid tympanic membrane, left ear
        H73.813 Atrophic flaccid tympanic membrane, bilateral
        H73.819 Atrophic flaccid tympanic membrane, unspecified ear
    ● **H73.82 Atrophic nonflaccid tympanic membrane**
        H73.821 Atrophic nonflaccid tympanic membrane, right ear
        H73.822 Atrophic nonflaccid tympanic membrane, left ear
        H73.823 Atrophic nonflaccid tympanic membrane, bilateral
        H73.829 Atrophic nonflaccid tympanic membrane, unspecified ear
    ● **H73.89 Other specified disorders of tympanic membrane**
        H73.891 Other specified disorders of tympanic membrane, right ear
        H73.892 Other specified disorders of tympanic membrane, left ear
        H73.893 Other specified disorders of tympanic membrane, bilateral
        H73.899 Other specified disorders of tympanic membrane, unspecified ear

● **H73.9 Unspecified disorder of tympanic membrane**
      H73.90 Unspecified disorder of tympanic membrane, unspecified ear
      H73.91 Unspecified disorder of tympanic membrane, right ear
      H73.92 Unspecified disorder of tympanic membrane, left ear
      H73.93 Unspecified disorder of tympanic membrane, bilateral
● **H74 Other disorders of middle ear mastoid**
      Excludes2   mastoiditis (H70.-)
  ● **H74.0 Tympanosclerosis**
      H74.01 Tympanosclerosis, right ear
      H74.02 Tympanosclerosis, left ear
      H74.03 Tympanosclerosis, bilateral
      H74.09 Tympanosclerosis, unspecified ear
  ● **H74.1 Adhesive middle ear disease**
        Adhesive otitis
        Excludes1   glue ear (H65.3-)
      H74.11 Adhesive right middle ear disease
      H74.12 Adhesive left middle ear disease
      H74.13 Adhesive middle ear disease, bilateral
      H74.19 Adhesive middle ear disease, unspecified ear
  ● **H74.2 Discontinuity and dislocation of ear ossicles**
      H74.20 Discontinuity and dislocation of ear ossicles, unspecified ear
      H74.21 Discontinuity and dislocation of right ear ossicles
      H74.22 Discontinuity and dislocation of left ear ossicles
      H74.23 Discontinuity and dislocation of ear ossicles, bilateral
  ● **H74.3 Other acquired abnormalities of ear ossicles**
    ● **H74.31 Ankylosis of ear ossicles**
        H74.311 Ankylosis of ear ossicles, right ear
        H74.312 Ankylosis of ear ossicles, left ear
        H74.313 Ankylosis of ear ossicles, bilateral
        H74.319 Ankylosis of ear ossicles, unspecified ear
    ● **H74.32 Partial loss of ear ossicles**
        H74.321 Partial loss of ear ossicles, right ear
        H74.322 Partial loss of ear ossicles, left ear
        H74.323 Partial loss of ear ossicles, bilateral
        H74.329 Partial loss of ear ossicles, unspecified ear
    ● **H74.39 Other acquired abnormalities of ear ossicles**
        H74.391 Other acquired abnormalities of right ear ossicles
        H74.392 Other acquired abnormalities of left ear ossicles
        H74.393 Other acquired abnormalities of ear ossicles, bilateral
        H74.399 Other acquired abnormalities of ear ossicles, unspecified ear
  ● **H74.4 Polyp of middle ear**
      H74.40 Polyp of middle ear, unspecified ear
      H74.41 Polyp of right middle ear
      H74.42 Polyp of left middle ear
      H74.43 Polyp of middle ear, bilateral

CHAPTER 8 (H60-H95)

N Newborn Age: 0   P Pediatric Age: 0–17   M Maternity DX: 9–64   A Adult Age: 15–124   ♀ Females Only   ♂ Males Only
Complication\Comorbidity   Major C\C   (Ex) CC/MCC Exclusions   Hospital-Acquired Condition   Hierarchical Condition Category

881

● H74.8 Other specified disorders of middle ear and mastoid
   ● H74.8X Other specified disorders of middle ear and mastoid
      H74.8X1 Other specified disorders of right middle ear and mastoid
      H74.8X2 Other specified disorders of left middle ear and mastoid
      H74.8X3 Other specified disorders of middle ear and mastoid, bilateral
      H74.8X9 Other specified disorders of middle ear and mastoid, unspecified ear
  ● H74.9 Unspecified disorder of middle ear and mastoid
      H74.90 Unspecified disorder of middle ear and mastoid, unspecified ear
      H74.91 Unspecified disorder of right middle ear and mastoid
      H74.92 Unspecified disorder of left middle ear and mastoid
      H74.93 Unspecified disorder of middle ear and mastoid, bilateral

● H75 Other disorders of middle ear and mastoid in diseases classified elsewhere
  Code first underlying disease
  ● H75.0 Mastoiditis in infectious and parasitic diseases classified elsewhere
    Excludes1 mastoiditis (in):
      syphilis (A52.77)
      tuberculosis (A18.03)
    ▸ H75.00 *Mastoiditis in infectious and parasitic diseases classified elsewhere, unspecified ear*
    ▸ H75.01 *Mastoiditis in infectious and parasitic diseases classified elsewhere, right ear*
    ▸ H75.02 *Mastoiditis in infectious and parasitic diseases classified elsewhere, left ear*
    ▸ H75.03 *Mastoiditis in infectious and parasitic diseases classified elsewhere, bilateral*
  ● H75.8 Other specified disorders of middle ear and mastoid in diseases classified elsewhere
    ▸ H75.80 *Other specified disorders of middle ear and mastoid in diseases classified elsewhere, unspecified ear*
    ▸ H75.81 *Other specified disorders of right middle ear and mastoid in diseases classified elsewhere*
    ▸ H75.82 *Other specified disorders of left middle ear and mastoid in diseases classified elsewhere*
    ▸ H75.83 *Other specified disorders of middle ear and mastoid in diseases classified elsewhere, bilateral*

DISEASES OF INNER EAR (H80-H83)

★ **(See Plate 23 of the Anatomy Illustrations.)**

● H80 Otosclerosis
  Inherited middle ear spongelike bone growth causing hearing loss
  Includes Otospongiosis
  ● H80.0 Otosclerosis involving oval window, nonobliterative
      H80.00 Otosclerosis involving oval window, nonobliterative, unspecified ear
      H80.01 Otosclerosis involving oval window, nonobliterative, right ear
      H80.02 Otosclerosis involving oval window, nonobliterative, left ear
      H80.03 Otosclerosis involving oval window, nonobliterative, bilateral

● H80.1 Otosclerosis involving oval window, obliterative
      H80.10 Otosclerosis involving oval window, obliterative, unspecified ear
      H80.11 Otosclerosis involving oval window, obliterative, right ear
      H80.12 Otosclerosis involving oval window, obliterative, left ear
      H80.13 Otosclerosis involving oval window, obliterative, bilateral
● H80.2 Cochlear otosclerosis
  Otosclerosis involving otic capsule
  Otosclerosis involving round window
      H80.20 Cochlear otosclerosis, unspecified ear
      H80.21 Cochlear otosclerosis, right ear
      H80.22 Cochlear otosclerosis, left ear
      H80.23 Cochlear otosclerosis, bilateral
● H80.8 Other otosclerosis
      H80.80 Other otosclerosis, unspecified ear
      H80.81 Other otosclerosis, right ear
      H80.82 Other otosclerosis, left ear
      H80.83 Other otosclerosis, bilateral
● H80.9 Unspecified otosclerosis
      H80.90 Unspecified otosclerosis, unspecified ear
      H80.91 Unspecified otosclerosis, right ear
      H80.92 Unspecified otosclerosis, left ear
      H80.93 Unspecified otosclerosis, bilateral

● H81 Disorders of vestibular function
  Excludes1 epidemic vertigo (A88.1)
    vertigo NOS (R42)
  ● H81.0 Ménière's disease
    Vestibular disorder that produces recurring symptoms including severe and intermittent hearing loss including the feeling of ear pressure or pain
    Labyrinthine hydrops
    Ménière's syndrome or vertigo
      H81.01 Ménière's disease, right ear
      H81.02 Ménière's disease, left ear
      H81.03 Ménière's disease, bilateral
      H81.09 Ménière's disease, unspecified ear
  ● H81.1 Benign paroxysmal vertigo
      H81.10 Benign paroxysmal vertigo, unspecified ear
      H81.11 Benign paroxysmal vertigo, right ear
      H81.12 Benign paroxysmal vertigo, left ear
      H81.13 Benign paroxysmal vertigo, bilateral
  ● H81.2 Vestibular neuronitis
      H81.20 Vestibular neuronitis, unspecified ear
      H81.21 Vestibular neuronitis, right ear
      H81.22 Vestibular neuronitis, left ear
      H81.23 Vestibular neuronitis, bilateral
  ● H81.3 Other peripheral vertigo
    ● H81.31 Aural vertigo
      H81.311 Aural vertigo, right ear
      H81.312 Aural vertigo, left ear
      H81.313 Aural vertigo, bilateral
      H81.319 Aural vertigo, unspecified ear
    ● H81.39 Other peripheral vertigo
      Lermoyez' syndrome
      Otogenic vertigo
      Peripheral vertigo NOS
      H81.391 Other peripheral vertigo, right ear
      H81.392 Other peripheral vertigo, left ear
      H81.393 Other peripheral vertigo, bilateral
      H81.399 Other peripheral vertigo, unspecified ear
  H81.4 Vertigo of central origin
    Central positional nystagmus

▶ New ⇒ Revised deleted Deleted Excludes 1 Excludes 2 Includes Use additional Code first Code also Key words
OGCR Official Guidelines ● Unacceptable Principal Diagnosis X Assign placeholder X ● Use Additional Character(s) ▸ Manifestation Code Coding Clinic

● **H81.8 Other disorders of vestibular function**
  ● **H81.8X** Other disorders of vestibular function
    H81.8X1 Other disorders of vestibular function, right ear
    H81.8X2 Other disorders of vestibular function, left ear
    H81.8X3 Other disorders of vestibular function, bilateral
    H81.8X9 Other disorders of vestibular function, unspecified ear

● **H81.9 Unspecified disorder of vestibular function**
    Vertiginous syndrome NOS
  H81.90 Unspecified disorder of vestibular function, unspecified ear
  H81.91 Unspecified disorder of vestibular function, right ear
  H81.92 Unspecified disorder of vestibular function, left ear
  H81.93 Unspecified disorder of vestibular function, bilateral

● **H82 Vertiginous syndromes in diseases classified elsewhere**
  Code first underlying disease
  Excludes1 epidemic vertigo (A88.1)
  ⟩ *H82.1 Vertiginous syndromes in diseases classified elsewhere, right ear*
  ⟩ *H82.2 Vertiginous syndromes in diseases classified elsewhere, left ear*
  ⟩ *H82.3 Vertiginous syndromes in diseases classified elsewhere, bilateral*
  ⟩ *H82.9 Vertiginous syndromes in diseases classified elsewhere, unspecified ear*

● **H83 Other diseases of inner ear**
  ● **H83.0 Labyrinthitis**
    Balance disorder that follows URI or head injury
    H83.01 Labyrinthitis, right ear
    H83.02 Labyrinthitis, left ear
    H83.03 Labyrinthitis, bilateral
    H83.09 Labyrinthitis, unspecified ear
  ● **H83.1 Labyrinthine fistula**
    H83.11 Labyrinthine fistula, right ear
    H83.12 Labyrinthine fistula, left ear
    H83.13 Labyrinthine fistula, bilateral
    H83.19 Labyrinthine fistula, unspecified ear
  ● **H83.2 Labyrinthine dysfunction**
    Labyrinthine hypersensitivity
    Labyrinthine hypofunction
    Labyrinthine loss of function
    ● **H83.2X** Labyrinthine dysfunction
      H83.2X1 Labyrinthine dysfunction, right ear
      H83.2X2 Labyrinthine dysfunction, left ear
      H83.2X3 Labyrinthine dysfunction, bilateral
      H83.2X9 Labyrinthine dysfunction, unspecified ear
  ● **H83.3 Noise effects on inner ear**
    Acoustic trauma of inner ear
    Noise-induced hearing loss of inner ear
    ● **H83.3X** Noise effects on inner ear
      H83.3X1 Noise effects on right inner ear
      H83.3X2 Noise effects on left inner ear
      H83.3X3 Noise effects on inner ear, bilateral
      H83.3X9 Noise effects on inner ear, unspecified ear

● **H83.8 Other specified diseases of inner ear**
  ● **H83.8X** Other specified diseases of inner ear
    H83.8X1 Other specified diseases of right inner ear
    H83.8X2 Other specified diseases of left inner ear
    H83.8X3 Other specified diseases of inner ear, bilateral
    H83.8X9 Other specified diseases of inner ear, unspecified ear

● **H83.9 Unspecified disease of inner ear**
  H83.90 Unspecified disease of inner ear, unspecified ear
  H83.91 Unspecified disease of right inner ear
  H83.92 Unspecified disease of left inner ear
  H83.93 Unspecified disease of inner ear, bilateral

OTHER DISORDERS OF EAR (H90-H94)

● **H90 Conductive and sensorineural hearing loss**
  Excludes1 deaf nonspeaking NEC (H91.3)
             deafness NOS (H91.9-)
             hearing loss NOS (H91.9-)
             noise-induced hearing loss (H83.3-)
             ototoxic hearing loss (H91.0-)
             sudden (idiopathic) hearing loss (H91.2-)
  H90.0 Conductive hearing loss, bilateral
  ● **H90.1** Conductive hearing loss, unilateral with unrestricted hearing on the contralateral side
    H90.11 Conductive hearing loss, unilateral, right ear, with unrestricted hearing on the contralateral side
    H90.12 Conductive hearing loss, unilateral, left ear, with unrestricted hearing on the contralateral side
  H90.2 Conductive hearing loss, unspecified
    Conductive deafness NOS
  H90.3 Sensorineural hearing loss, bilateral
  ● **H90.4** Sensorineural hearing loss, unilateral with unrestricted hearing on the contralateral side
    H90.41 Sensorineural hearing loss, unilateral, right ear, with unrestricted hearing on the contralateral side
    H90.42 Sensorineural hearing loss, unilateral, left ear, with unrestricted hearing on the contralateral side
  H90.5 Unspecified sensorineural hearing loss
    Central hearing loss NOS
    Congenital deafness NOS
    Neural hearing loss NOS
    Perceptive hearing loss NOS
    Sensorineural deafness NOS
    Sensory hearing loss NOS
    Excludes1 abnormal auditory perception (H93.2-)
            psychogenic deafness (F44.6)
  H90.6 Mixed conductive and sensorineural hearing loss, bilateral
    Coding Clinic: 2015, Q2, P7
  ● **H90.7** Mixed conductive and sensorineural hearing loss, unilateral with unrestricted hearing on the contralateral side
    H90.71 Mixed conductive and sensorineural hearing loss, unilateral, right ear, with unrestricted hearing on the contralateral side
    H90.72 Mixed conductive and sensorineural hearing loss, unilateral, left ear, with unrestricted hearing on the contralateral side
  H90.8 Mixed conductive and sensorineural hearing loss, unspecified

CHAPTER 8 (H60-H95)

N Newborn Age: 0   P Pediatric Age: 0–17   M Maternity DX: 9–64   A Adult Age: 15–124   ♀ Females Only   ♂ Males Only

🅒 Complication\Comorbidity   🅜 Major C\C   (Ex) CC/MCC Exclusions   🅗 Hospital-Acquired Condition   🅗 Hierarchical Condition Category

883

● **H90.A   Conductive and sensorineural hearing loss with restricted hearing on the contralateral side**
Coding Clinic: 2016, Q4, P23-24

● H90.A1 Conductive hearing loss, unilateral, with restricted hearing on the contralateral side

H90.A11 Conductive hearing loss, unilateral, right ear with restricted hearing on the contralateral side

H90.A12 Conductive hearing loss, unilateral, left ear with restricted hearing on the contralateral side
Coding Clinic: 2016, Q4, P25

● H90.A2 Sensorineural hearing loss, unilateral, with restricted hearing on the contralateral side

H90.A21 Sensorineural hearing loss, unilateral, right ear, with restricted hearing on the contralateral side

H90.A22 Sensorineural hearing loss, unilateral, left ear, with restricted hearing on the contralateral side

● H90.A3 Mixed conductive and sensorineural hearing loss, unilateral with restricted hearing on the contralateral side

H90.A31 Mixed conductive and sensorineural hearing loss, unilateral, right ear with restricted hearing on the contralateral side

H90.A32 Mixed conductive and sensorineural hearing loss, unilateral, left ear with restricted hearing on the contralateral side

● H91 Other and unspecified hearing loss
Excludes1   abnormal auditory perception (H93.2-)
hearing loss as classified in H90.-
impacted cerumen (H61.2-)
noise-induced hearing loss (H83.3-)
psychogenic deafness (F44.6)
transient ischemic deafness (H93.01-)

● H91.0 Ototoxic hearing loss
Code first poisoning due to drug or toxin, if applicable (T36-T65 with fifth or sixth character 1-4 or 6)
Use additional code for adverse effect, if applicable, to identify drug (T36-T50 with fifth or sixth character 5)

H91.01 Ototoxic hearing loss, right ear
H91.02 Ototoxic hearing loss, left ear
H91.03 Ototoxic hearing loss, bilateral
H91.09 Ototoxic hearing loss, unspecified ear

● H91.1 Presbycusis
Presbyacusia

H91.10 Presbycusis, unspecified ear
H91.11 Presbycusis, right ear
H91.12 Presbycusis, left ear
H91.13 Presbycusis, bilateral

● H91.2 Sudden idiopathic hearing loss
Sudden hearing loss NOS

H91.20 Sudden idiopathic hearing loss, unspecified ear
H91.21 Sudden idiopathic hearing loss, right ear
H91.22 Sudden idiopathic hearing loss, left ear
H91.23 Sudden idiopathic hearing loss, bilateral

H91.3 Deaf nonspeaking, not elsewhere classified

● H91.8 Other specified hearing loss

● H91.8X Other specified hearing loss
H91.8X1 Other specified hearing loss, right ear
H91.8X2 Other specified hearing loss, left ear
H91.8X3 Other specified hearing loss, bilateral
H91.8X9 Other specified hearing loss, unspecified ear

● H91.9 **Unspecified hearing loss**
Deafness NOS
High frequency deafness
Low frequency deafness

H91.90 Unspecified hearing loss, unspecified ear
H91.91 Unspecified hearing loss, right ear
H91.92 Unspecified hearing loss, left ear
H91.93 Unspecified hearing loss, bilateral

● H92 Otalgia and effusion of ear

● H92.0 Otalgia
H92.01 Otalgia, right ear
H92.02 Otalgia, left ear
H92.03 Otalgia, bilateral
H92.09 Otalgia, unspecified ear

● H92.1 Otorrhea
Excludes1   leakage of cerebrospinal fluid through ear (G96.0)

H92.10 Otorrhea, unspecified ear
H92.11 Otorrhea, right ear
H92.12 Otorrhea, left ear
H92.13 Otorrhea, bilateral

● H92.2 Otorrhagia
Excludes1   traumatic otorrhagia - code to injury

H92.20 Otorrhagia, unspecified ear
H92.21 Otorrhagia, right ear
H92.22 Otorrhagia, left ear
H92.23 Otorrhagia, bilateral

● H93 Other disorders of ear, not elsewhere classified

● H93.0 Degenerative and vascular disorders of ear
Excludes1   presbycusis (H91.1)

● H93.01 Transient ischemic deafness
H93.011 Transient ischemic deafness, right ear
H93.012 Transient ischemic deafness, left ear
H93.013 Transient ischemic deafness, bilateral
H93.019 Transient ischemic deafness, unspecified ear

● H93.09 Unspecified degenerative and vascular disorders of ear
H93.091 Unspecified degenerative and vascular disorders of right ear
H93.092 Unspecified degenerative and vascular disorders of left ear
H93.093 Unspecified degenerative and vascular disorders of ear, bilateral
H93.099 Unspecified degenerative and vascular disorders of unspecified ear

● H93.1 Tinnitus
Perception of sound (ringing, buzzing, humming, whistling tunes, or singing)

H93.11 Tinnitus, right ear
H93.12 Tinnitus, left ear
H93.13 Tinnitus, bilateral
H93.19 Tinnitus, unspecified ear

● H93.A Pulsatile tinnitus
Coding Clinic: 2016, Q4, P25

H93.A1 Pulsatile tinnitus, right ear
Coding Clinic: 2016, Q4, P26
H93.A2 Pulsatile tinnitus, left ear
H93.A3 Pulsatile tinnitus, bilateral
H93.A9 Pulsatile tinnitus, unspecified ear

▶ New   ⇒ Revised   ~~deleted~~ Deleted   Excludes 1   Excludes 2   Includes   Use additional   Code first   Code also   Key words

OGCR Official Guidelines   ● Unacceptable Principal Diagnosis   X Assign placeholder X   ● Use Additional Character(s)   ▶ Manifestation Code   Coding Clinic

● **H93.2**   **Other abnormal auditory perceptions**
     Excludes2   auditory hallucinations (R44.0)
   ● **H93.21**   **Auditory recruitment**
     H93.211   Auditory recruitment, right ear
     H93.212   Auditory recruitment, left ear
     H93.213   Auditory recruitment, bilateral
     H93.219   Auditory recruitment, unspecified ear
   ● **H93.22**   **Diplacusis**
     H93.221   Diplacusis, right ear
     H93.222   Diplacusis, left ear
     H93.223   Diplacusis, bilateral
     H93.229   Diplacusis, unspecified ear
   ● **H93.23**   **Hyperacusis**
     H93.231   Hyperacusis, right ear
     H93.232   Hyperacusis, left ear
     H93.233   Hyperacusis, bilateral
     H93.239   Hyperacusis, unspecified ear
   ● **H93.24**   **Temporary auditory threshold shift**
     H93.241   Temporary auditory threshold shift, right ear
     H93.242   Temporary auditory threshold shift, left ear
     H93.243   Temporary auditory threshold shift, bilateral
     H93.249   Temporary auditory threshold shift, unspecified ear
   H93.25   **Central auditory processing disorder**
     Congenital auditory imperception
     Word deafness
     Excludes1   mixed receptive-expressive language disorder (F80.2)
   ● **H93.29**   **Other abnormal auditory perceptions**
     H93.291   Other abnormal auditory perceptions, right ear
     H93.292   Other abnormal auditory perceptions, left ear
     H93.293   Other abnormal auditory perceptions, bilateral
     H93.299   Other abnormal auditory perceptions, unspecified ear
● **H93.3**   **Disorders of acoustic nerve**
     Disorder of 8th cranial nerve
     Excludes1   acoustic neuroma (D33.3)
             syphilitic acoustic neuritis (A52.15)
   ● **H93.3X**   **Disorders of acoustic nerve**
     H93.3X1   Disorders of right acoustic nerve
     H93.3X2   Disorders of left acoustic nerve
     H93.3X3   Disorders of bilateral acoustic nerves
     H93.3X9   Disorders of unspecified acoustic nerve
● **H93.8**   **Other specified disorders of ear**
   ● **H93.8X**   **Other specified disorders of ear**
     H93.8X1   Other specified disorders of right ear
     H93.8X2   Other specified disorders of left ear
     H93.8X3   Other specified disorders of ear, bilateral
     H93.8X9   Other specified disorders of ear, unspecified ear
● **H93.9**   **Unspecified disorder of ear**
   ● H93.90   Unspecified disorder of ear, unspecified ear
   ● H93.91   Unspecified disorder of right ear
   ● H93.92   Unspecified disorder of left ear
   ● H93.93   Unspecified disorder of ear, bilateral

● **H94**   **Other disorders of ear in diseases classified elsewhere**
   ● **H94.0**   **Acoustic neuritis in infectious and parasitic diseases classified elsewhere**
     Code first underlying disease, such as:
     parasitic disease (B65-B89)
     Excludes1   acoustic neuritis (in):
             herpes zoster (B02.29)
             syphilis (A52.15)
     ▶ *H94.00*   *Acoustic neuritis in infectious and parasitic diseases classified elsewhere, unspecified ear*
     ▶ *H94.01*   *Acoustic neuritis in infectious and parasitic diseases classified elsewhere, right ear*
     ▶ *H94.02*   *Acoustic neuritis in infectious and parasitic diseases classified elsewhere, left ear*
     ▶ *H94.03*   *Acoustic neuritis in infectious and parasitic diseases classified elsewhere, bilateral*
   ● **H94.8**   **Other specified disorders of ear in diseases classified elsewhere**
     Code first underlying disease, such as:
     congenital syphilis (A50.0)
     Excludes1   aural myiasis (B87.4)
             syphilitic labyrinthitis (A52.79)
     ▶ *H94.80*   *Other specified disorders of ear in diseases classified elsewhere, unspecified ear*
     ▶ *H94.81*   *Other specified disorders of right ear in diseases classified elsewhere*
     ▶ *H94.82*   *Other specified disorders of left ear in diseases classified elsewhere*
     ▶ *H94.83*   *Other specified disorders of ear in diseases classified elsewhere, bilateral*

INTRAOPERATIVE AND POSTPROCEDURAL COMPLICATIONS AND DISORDERS OF EAR AND MASTOID PROCESS, NOT ELSEWHERE CLASSIFIED (H95)

● **H95**   **Intraoperative and postprocedural complications and disorders of ear and mastoid process, not elsewhere classified**
     Coding Clinic: 2016, Q4, P10
   ● **H95.0**   **Recurrent cholesteatoma of postmastoidectomy cavity**
     H95.00   Recurrent cholesteatoma of postmastoidectomy cavity, unspecified ear
     H95.01   Recurrent cholesteatoma of postmastoidectomy cavity, right ear
     H95.02   Recurrent cholesteatoma of postmastoidectomy cavity, left ear
     H95.03   Recurrent cholesteatoma of postmastoidectomy cavity, bilateral ears
   ● **H95.1**   **Other disorders of ear and mastoid process following mastoidectomy**
     ● **H95.11**   **Chronic inflammation of postmastoidectomy cavity**
       H95.111   Chronic inflammation of postmastoidectomy cavity, right ear
       H95.112   Chronic inflammation of postmastoidectomy cavity, left ear
       H95.113   Chronic inflammation of postmastoidectomy cavity, bilateral ears
       H95.119   Chronic inflammation of postmastoidectomy cavity, unspecified ear
     ● **H95.12**   **Granulation of postmastoidectomy cavity**
       H95.121   Granulation of postmastoidectomy cavity, right ear
       H95.122   Granulation of postmastoidectomy cavity, left ear
       H95.123   Granulation of postmastoidectomy cavity, bilateral ears
       H95.129   Granulation of postmastoidectomy cavity, unspecified ear

CHAPTER 8 (H60-H95)

N   Newborn Age: 0   P   Pediatric Age: 0–17   M   Maternity DX: 9–64   A   Adult Age: 15–124   ♀   Females Only   ♂   Males Only

🔧   Complication\Comorbidity   🔧   Major C\C   (Ex)   CC/MCC Exclusions   🔧   Hospital-Acquired Condition   🔧   Hierarchical Condition Category

- H95.13 Mucosal cyst of postmastoidectomy cavity
  - H95.131 Mucosal cyst of postmastoidectomy cavity, right ear
  - H95.132 Mucosal cyst of postmastoidectomy cavity, left ear
  - H95.133 Mucosal cyst of postmastoidectomy cavity, bilateral ears
  - H95.139 Mucosal cyst of postmastoidectomy cavity, unspecified ear
- H95.19 Other disorders following mastoidectomy
  - H95.191 Other disorders following mastoidectomy, right ear
  - H95.192 Other disorders following mastoidectomy, left ear
  - H95.193 Other disorders following mastoidectomy, bilateral ears
  - H95.199 Other disorders following mastoidectomy, unspecified ear
- H95.2 Intraoperative hemorrhage and hematoma of ear and mastoid process complicating a procedure

  Excludes1 intraoperative hemorrhage and hematoma of ear and mastoid process due to accidental puncture or laceration during a procedure (H95.3-)

  (Ex) For category H95.2 CC codes: See PDX Collection 642
  - H95.21 Intraoperative hemorrhage and hematoma of ear and mastoid process complicating a procedure on the ear and mastoid process
  - H95.22 Intraoperative hemorrhage and hematoma of ear and mastoid process complicating other procedure
- H95.3 Accidental puncture and laceration of ear and mastoid process during a procedure

  (Ex) For category H95.3 CC codes: See PDX Collection 509
  - H95.31 Accidental puncture and laceration of the ear and mastoid process during a procedure on the ear and mastoid process
  - H95.32 Accidental puncture and laceration of the ear and mastoid process during other procedure
- H95.4 Postprocedural hemorrhage of ear and mastoid process following a procedure

  (Ex) For category H95.4 CC codes: See PDX Collection 642
  - H95.41 Postprocedural hemorrhage of ear and mastoid process following a procedure on the ear and mastoid process
  - H95.42 Postprocedural hemorrhage of ear and mastoid process following other procedure

- H95.5 Postprocedural hematoma and seroma of ear and mastoid process following a procedure

  (Ex) For category H95.5 CC codes: See PDX Collection 642
  - H95.51 Postprocedural hematoma of ear and mastoid process following a procedure on the ear and mastoid process
  - H95.52 Postprocedural hematoma of ear and mastoid process following other procedure
  - H95.53 Postprocedural seroma of ear and mastoid process following a procedure on the ear and mastoid process
  - H95.54 Postprocedural seroma of ear and mastoid process following other procedure
- H95.8 Other intraoperative and postprocedural complications and disorders of the ear and mastoid process, not elsewhere classified

  Excludes2 postprocedural complications and disorders following mastoidectomy (H95.0-, H95.1-)

  (Ex) For category H95.8 CC codes: See PDX Collection 643
  - H95.81 Postprocedural stenosis of external ear canal
    - H95.811 Postprocedural stenosis of right external ear canal
    - H95.812 Postprocedural stenosis of left external ear canal
    - H95.813 Postprocedural stenosis of external ear canal, bilateral
    - H95.819 Postprocedural stenosis of unspecified external ear canal
  - H95.88 Other intraoperative complications and disorders of the ear and mastoid process, not elsewhere classified

    Use additional code, if applicable, to further specify disorder
  - H95.89 Other postprocedural complications and disorders of the ear and mastoid process, not elsewhere classified

    Use additional code, if applicable, to further specify disorder

CHAPTER 9

DISEASES OF THE CIRCULATORY SYSTEM (I00-I99)

OGCR Chapter-Specific Coding Guidelines

9. Chapter 9: Diseases of the Circulatory System (I00-I99)

a. Hypertension

The classification presumes a causal relationship between hypertension and heart involvement and between hypertension and kidney involvement, as the two conditions are linked by the term "with" in the Alphabetic Index. These conditions should be coded as related even in the absence of provider documentation explicitly linking them, unless the documentation clearly states the conditions are unrelated.

For hypertension and conditions not specifically linked by relational terms such as "with," "associated with" or "due to" in the classification, provider documentation must link the conditions in order to code them as related.

1) Hypertension with Heart Disease

Hypertension with heart conditions classified to I50.- or I51.4-I51.7, I51.89, I51.9, are assigned to, a code from category I11, Hypertensive heart disease. Use additional code(s) from category I50, Heart failure, to identify the type(s) of heart failure in those patients with heart failure.

The same heart conditions (I50.-, I51.4-I51.7, I51.89, I51.9) with hypertension, are coded separately if the provider has documented they are unrelated to the hypertension. Sequence according to the circumstances of the admission/encounter.

2) Hypertensive Chronic Kidney Disease

Assign codes from category I12, Hypertensive chronic kidney disease, when both hypertension and a condition classifiable to category N18, Chronic kidney disease (CKD), are present. CKD should not be coded as hypertensive if the provider indicates the CKD is not related to the hypertension.

The appropriate code from category N18 should be used as a secondary code with a code from category I12 to identify the stage of chronic kidney disease.

See Section I.C.14. Chronic kidney disease.

If a patient has hypertensive chronic kidney disease and acute renal failure, an additional code for the acute renal failure is required.

3) Hypertensive Heart and Chronic Kidney Disease

Assign codes from combination category I13, Hypertensive heart and chronic kidney disease, when there is hypertension with both heart and kidney involvement. If heart failure is present, assign an additional code from category I50 to identify the type of heart failure.

The appropriate code from category N18, Chronic kidney disease, should be used as a secondary code with a code from category I13 to identify the stage of chronic kidney disease.

See Section I.C.14. Chronic kidney disease.

The codes in category I13, Hypertensive heart and chronic kidney disease, are combination codes that include hypertension, heart disease and chronic kidney disease. The Includes note at I13 specifies that the conditions included at I11 and I12 are included together in I13. If a patient has hypertension, heart disease and chronic kidney disease then a code from I13 should be used, not individual codes for hypertension, heart disease and chronic kidney disease, or codes from I11 or I12.

For patients with both acute renal failure and chronic kidney disease an additional code for acute renal failure is required.

4) Hypertensive Cerebrovascular Disease

For hypertensive cerebrovascular disease, first assign the appropriate code from categories I60-I69, followed by the appropriate hypertension code.

5) Hypertensive Retinopathy

Subcategory I135.0, Background retinopathy and retinal vascular changes, should be used with a code from category I10 – I15, Hypertensive disease to include the systemic hypertension. The sequencing is based on the reason for the encounter.

6) Hypertension, Secondary

Secondary hypertension is due to an underlying condition. Two codes are required: one to identify the underlying etiology and one from category I15 to identify the hypertension. Sequencing of codes is determined by the reason for admission/encounter.

7) Hypertension, Transient

Assign code R03.0, Elevated blood pressure reading without diagnosis of hypertension, unless patient has an established diagnosis of hypertension. Assign code O13.-, Gestational [pregnancy-induced] hypertension without significant proteinuria, or O14.-, Pre-eclampsia, for transient hypertension of pregnancy.

8) Hypertension, Controlled

This diagnostic statement usually refers to an existing state of hypertension under control by therapy. Assign the appropriate code from categories I10-I15, Hypertensive diseases.

9) Hypertension, Uncontrolled

Uncontrolled hypertension may refer to untreated hypertension or hypertension not responding to current therapeutic regimen. In either case, assign the appropriate code from categories I10-I15, Hypertensive diseases.

10) Hypertensive Crisis

Assign a code from category I16, Hypertensive crisis, for documented hypertensive urgency, hypertensive emergency or unspecified hypertensive crisis. Code also any identified hypertensive disease (I10-I15). The sequencing is based on the reason for the encounter.

11) Pulmonary Hypertension

Pulmonary hypertension is classified to category I27, Other pulmonary heart diseases. For secondary pulmonary hypertension (I27.1, I27.2-), code also any associated conditions or adverse effects of drugs or toxins. The sequencing is based on the reason for the encounter, except for adverse effects of drugs.

See Section I.C.19.e Adverse Effects, Poisoning, Underdosing and Toxic Effects.

b. Atherosclerotic Coronary Artery Disease and Angina

ICD-10-CM has combination codes for atherosclerotic heart disease with angina pectoris. The subcategories for these codes are I25.11, Atherosclerotic heart disease of native coronary artery with angina pectoris and I25.7, Atherosclerosis of coronary artery bypass graft(s) and coronary artery of transplanted heart with angina pectoris.

When using one of these combination codes it is not necessary to use an additional code for angina pectoris. A causal relationship can be assumed in a patient with both atherosclerosis and angina pectoris, unless the documentation indicates the angina is due to something other than the atherosclerosis.

If a patient with coronary artery disease is admitted due to an acute myocardial infarction (AMI), the AMI should be sequenced before the coronary artery disease.

See Section I.C.9. Acute myocardial infarction (AMI).

c. Intraoperative and Postprocedural Cerebrovascular Accident

Medical record documentation should clearly specify the cause-and-effect relationship between the medical intervention and the cerebrovascular accident in order to assign a code for intraoperative or postprocedural cerebrovascular accident.

Proper code assignment depends on whether it was an infarction or hemorrhage and whether it occurred intraoperatively or postoperatively. If it was a cerebral hemorrhage, code assignment depends on the type of procedure performed.

d. Sequelae of Cerebrovascular Disease

1) Category I69, Sequelae of Cerebrovascular disease

Category I69 is used to indicate conditions classifiable to categories I60-I67 as the causes of sequela (neurologic deficits), themselves classified elsewhere. These "late effects" include neurologic deficits that persist after initial onset of conditions classifiable to categories I60-I67. The neurologic deficits caused by cerebrovascular disease may be present from the onset or may arise at any time after the onset of the condition classifiable to categories I60-I67.

Codes from category I69, Sequelae of cerebrovascular disease, that specify hemiplegia, hemiparesis and monoplegia identify whether the dominant or nondominant side is affected. Should the affected side be documented, but not specified as dominant or nondominant, and the classification system does not indicate a default, code selection is as follows:

- For ambidextrous patients, the default should be dominant.
- If the left side is affected, the default is nondominant.
- If the right side is affected, the default is dominant.

2) Codes from category I69 with codes from I60-I67

Codes from category I69 may be assigned on a health care record with codes from I60-I67, if the patient has a current cerebrovascular disease and deficits from an old cerebrovascular disease.

3) Codes from category I69 and Personal history of transient ischemic attack (TIA) and cerebral infarction (Z86.73)

Codes from category I69 should not be assigned if the patient does not have neurologic deficits.

See Section I.C.21. 4. History (of) for use of personal history codes.

e. **Acute myocardial infarction (AMI)**

1) **Type 1 ST elevation myocardial infarction (STEMI) and non-ST elevation myocardial infarction (NSTEMI)**

The ICD-10-CM codes for acute type 1 myocardial infarction (AMI) identify the site, such as anterolateral wall or true posterior wall. Subcategories I21.0-I21.2 and code I21.3 are used for type 1 ST elevation (NSTEMI) myocardial infarction (STEMI). Code I21.4, non-ST elevation (NSTEMI) myocardial infarction, is used for type 1 non-ST elevation myocardial infarction (NSTEMI) and nontransmural MIs.

If a type 1 NSTEMI evolves to STEMI, assign the STEMI code. If a type 1 STEMI converts to NSTEMI due to thrombolytic therapy, it is still coded as STEMI.

For encounters occurring while the myocardial infarction is equal to, or less than, four weeks old, including transfers to another acute setting or a postacute setting, and the myocardial infarction meets the definition for "other diagnoses" (see Section III, Reporting Additional Diagnoses), codes from category I21 may continue to be reported. For encounters after the 4-week time frame and the patient is still receiving care related to the myocardial infarction, the appropriate aftercare code should be assigned, rather than a code from category I21. For old or healed myocardial infarctions not requiring further care, code I25.2, Old myocardial infarction, may be assigned.

2) **Acute myocardial infarction, unspecified**

Code I21.9, Acute myocardial infarction, unspecified, is the default for unspecified acute myocardial infarction or unspecified type. If only type 1 STEMI or transmural MI without the site is documented, assign code I21.3, ST elevation (STEMI) myocardial infarction of unspecified site.

3) **AMI documented as nontransmural or subendocardial but site provided**

If an AMI is documented as nontransmural or subendocardial, but the site is provided, it is still coded as a subendocardial AMI.

See Section I.C.21.3 for information on coding status post administration of tPA in a different facility within the last 24 hours.

4) **Subsequent acute myocardial infarction**

A code from category I22, Subsequent ST elevation (STEMI) and non-ST elevation (NSTEMI) myocardial infarction, is to be used when a patient who has suffered a type 1 or unspecified AMI has a new AMI within the 4-week time frame of the initial AMI. A code from category I22 must be used in conjunction with a code from category I21. The sequencing of the I22 and I21 codes depends on the circumstances of the encounter.

Do not assign code I22 for subsequent myocardial infarctions other than type 1 or unspecified. For subsequent type 2 AMI assign only code I21.A1. For subsequent type 4 or type 5 AMI, assign only code I21.A9.

If a subsequent myocardial infarction of one type occurs within 4 weeks of a myocardial infarction of a different type, assign the appropriate codes from category I21 to identify each type. Do not assign a code from I22. Codes from category I22 should only be assigned if both the initial and subsequent myocardial infarctions are type 1 or unspecified.

5) **Other Types of Myocardial Infarction**

The ICD-10-CM provides codes for different types of myocardial infarction. Type 1 myocardial infarctions are assigned to codes I21.0-I21.4 and I21.9.

Type 2 myocardial infarction, and myocardial infarction due to demand ischemia or secondary to ischemic balance, is assigned to code I21.A1, Myocardial infarction type 2 with a code for the underlying cause. Do not assign code I24.8, Other forms of acute ischemic heart disease for the demand ischemia. Sequencing of type 2 AMI or the underlying cause is dependent on the circumstances of admission. When a type 2 AMI code is described as NSTEMI or STEMI, only assign code I21.A1. Codes I21.01-I21.4 should only be assigned for type 1 AMIs.

Acute myocardial infarctions type 3, 4a, 4b, 4c, and 5 are assigned to code I21.A9, Other myocardial infarction type.

The "Code also" and "Code first" notes should be followed related to complications, and for coding of postprocedural myocardial infarctions during or following cardiac surgery.

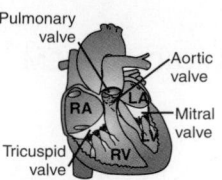

Figure 9-1 Cardiovascular valves.

Item 9–1 Rheumatic fever is the inflammation of the valve(s) of the heart, usually the mitral or aortic, which leads to valve damage. Rheumatic heart inflammations are usually **pericarditis** (sac surrounding heart), **endocarditis** (heart cavity), or **myocarditis** (heart muscle).

CHAPTER 9

DISEASES OF THE CIRCULATORY SYSTEM (I00–I99)

Excludes2   certain conditions originating in the perinatal period (P04-P96)
certain infectious and parasitic diseases (A00-B99)
complications of pregnancy, childbirth and the puerperium (O00-O9A)
congenital malformations, deformations, and chromosomal abnormalities (Q00-Q99)
endocrine, nutritional and metabolic diseases (E00-E88)
injury, poisoning and certain other consequences of external causes (S00-T88)
neoplasms (C00-D49)
symptoms, signs and abnormal clinical and laboratory findings, not elsewhere classified (R00-R94)
systemic connective tissue disorders (M30-M36)
transient cerebral ischemic attacks and related syndromes (G45.-)

This chapter contains the following blocks:

I00-I02	Acute rheumatic fever
I05-I09	Chronic rheumatic heart diseases
I10-I16	Hypertensive diseases
I20-I25	Ischemic heart diseases
I26-I28	Pulmonary heart disease and diseases of pulmonary circulation
I30-I5A	Other forms of heart disease
I60-I69	Cerebrovascular diseases
I70-I79	Diseases of arteries, arterioles and capillaries
I80-I89	Diseases of veins, lymphatic vessels and lymph nodes, not elsewhere classified
I95-I99	Other and unspecified disorders of the circulatory system

ACUTE RHEUMATIC FEVER (I00-I02)

I00   **Rheumatic fever without heart involvement**

Includes   arthritis, rheumatic, acute or subacute

Excludes1   rheumatic fever with heart involvement (I01.0-I01.9)

● **I01**   **Rheumatic fever with heart involvement**

Excludes1   chronic diseases of rheumatic origin (I05-I09) unless rheumatic fever is also present or there is evidence of reactivation or activity of the rheumatic process.

I01.0   **Acute rheumatic pericarditis** 🔖
Any condition in I00 with pericarditis
Rheumatic pericarditis (acute)

Excludes1   acute pericarditis not specified as rheumatic (I30.-)

(Ex:) See PDX Collection 188

I01.1   **Acute rheumatic endocarditis** 🔖
Any condition in I00 with endocarditis or valvulitis
Acute rheumatic valvulitis

(Ex:) See PDX Collection 644

▶ New   ⇒ Revised   ~~deleted~~ Deleted   Excludes 1   Excludes 2   Includes   Use additional   Code first   Code also   Key words

OGCR Official Guidelines   ● Unacceptable Principal Diagnosis   X Assign placeholder X   ● Use Additional Character(s)   ▶ Manifestation Code   **Coding Clinic**

Item 9-2 Rheumatic chorea, also called Sydenham's, juvenile, minor, simple, or St. Vitus' dance, is a major symptom of rheumatic fever and is characterized by ceaseless, involuntary, jerky, purposeless movements.

     I01.2   **Acute rheumatic myocarditis** 🔹
         Any condition in I00 with myocarditis
         (Ex:) See PDX Collection 186

     I01.8   **Other acute rheumatic heart disease** 🔹
         Any condition in I00 with other or multiple types of heart involvement
         Acute rheumatic pancarditis
         (Ex:) See PDX Collection 645

     I01.9   **Acute rheumatic heart disease, unspecified** 🔹
         Any condition in I00 with unspecified type of heart involvement
         Rheumatic carditis, acute
         Rheumatic heart disease, active or acute
         (Ex:) See PDX Collection 646

● **I02**   **Rheumatic chorea**
     Includes   Sydenham's chorea
     Excludes1   chorea NOS (G25.5)
           Huntington's chorea (G10)

     I02.0   **Rheumatic chorea with heart involvement** 🔹
         Chorea NOS with heart involvement
         Rheumatic chorea with heart involvement of any type classifiable under I01.-
         (Ex:) See PDX Collection 645

     I02.9   **Rheumatic chorea without heart involvement** 🔹
         Rheumatic chorea NOS
         (Ex:) See PDX Collection 646

CHRONIC RHEUMATIC HEART DISEASES (I05-I09)

● **I05**   **Rheumatic mitral valve diseases**
     Includes   conditions classifiable to both I05.0 and I05.2-I05.9, whether specified as rheumatic or not
     Excludes1   mitral valve disease specified as nonrheumatic (I34.-)
           mitral valve disease with aortic and/or tricuspid valve involvement (I08.-)

     I05.0   **Rheumatic mitral stenosis**
         Mitral (valve) obstruction (rheumatic)

     I05.1   **Rheumatic mitral insufficiency**
         Rheumatic mitral incompetence
         Rheumatic mitral regurgitation
         Excludes1   mitral insufficiency not specified as rheumatic (I34.0)

     I05.2   **Rheumatic mitral stenosis with insufficiency**
         Rheumatic mitral stenosis with incompetence or regurgitation

     I05.8   **Other rheumatic mitral valve diseases**
         Rheumatic mitral (valve) failure

     I05.9   **Rheumatic mitral valve disease, unspecified**
         Rheumatic mitral (valve) disorder (chronic) NOS

● **I06**   **Rheumatic aortic valve diseases**
     Excludes1   aortic valve disease not specified as rheumatic (I35.-)
           aortic valve disease with mitral and/or tricuspid valve involvement (I08.-)

     I06.0   **Rheumatic aortic stenosis**
         Rheumatic aortic (valve) obstruction

     I06.1   **Rheumatic aortic insufficiency**
         Rheumatic aortic incompetence
         Rheumatic aortic regurgitation

     I06.2   **Rheumatic aortic stenosis with insufficiency**
         Rheumatic aortic stenosis with incompetence or regurgitation

★ **(See Plate 33 of the Anatomy Illustrations.)**

Item 9-3 Mitral stenosis is the narrowing of the mitral valve separating the left atrium from the left ventricle. **Mitral insufficiency** is the improper closure of the mitral valve, which may lead to enlargement (hypertrophy) of the left atrium.

Item 9-4 Aortic stenosis is the narrowing of the aortic valve located between the left ventricle and the aorta. **Aortic insufficiency** is the improper closure of the aortic valve, which may lead to enlargement (hypertrophy) of the left ventricle.

     I06.8   **Other rheumatic aortic valve diseases**

     I06.9   **Rheumatic aortic valve disease, unspecified**
         Rheumatic aortic (valve) disease NOS

● **I07**   **Rheumatic tricuspid valve diseases**
     Includes   rheumatic tricuspid valve diseases specified as rheumatic or unspecified
     Excludes1   tricuspid valve disease specified as nonrheumatic (I36.-)
           tricuspid valve disease with aortic and/or mitral valve involvement (I08.-)

     I07.0   **Rheumatic tricuspid stenosis**
         Tricuspid (valve) stenosis (rheumatic)

     I07.1   **Rheumatic tricuspid insufficiency**
         Tricuspid (valve) insufficiency (rheumatic)

     I07.2   **Rheumatic tricuspid stenosis and insufficiency**

     I07.8   **Other rheumatic tricuspid valve diseases**

     I07.9   **Rheumatic tricuspid valve disease, unspecified**
         Rheumatic tricuspid valve disorder NOS

● **I08**   **Multiple valve diseases**
     Includes   multiple valve diseases specified as rheumatic or unspecified
     Excludes1   endocarditis, valve unspecified (I38)
           multiple valve disease specified a nonrheumatic (I34.-, I35.-, I36.-, I37.-, I38.-, Q22.-, Q23.-, Q24.8-)
           rheumatic valve disease NOS (I09.1)
     Coding Clinic: 2019, Q2, P5

     I08.0   **Rheumatic disorders of both mitral and aortic valves**
         Involvement of both mitral and aortic valves specified as rheumatic or unspecified
         Coding Clinic: 2019, Q2, P5

     I08.1   **Rheumatic disorders of both mitral and tricuspid valves**

     I08.2   **Rheumatic disorders of both aortic and tricuspid valves**

     I08.3   **Combined rheumatic disorders of mitral, aortic and tricuspid valves**

     I08.8   **Other rheumatic multiple valve diseases**

     I08.9   **Rheumatic multiple valve disease, unspecified**

● **I09**   **Other rheumatic heart diseases**
     I09.0   **Rheumatic myocarditis** 🔹
         Excludes1   myocarditis not specified as rheumatic (I51.4)
         (Ex:) See PDX Collection 647

     I09.1   **Rheumatic diseases of endocardium, valve unspecified**
         Rheumatic endocarditis (chronic)
         Rheumatic valvulitis (chronic)
         Excludes1   endocarditis, valve unspecified (I38)

     I09.2   **Chronic rheumatic pericarditis** 🔹
         Adherent pericardium, rheumatic
         Chronic rheumatic mediastinopericarditis
         Chronic rheumatic myopericarditis
         Excludes1   chronic pericarditis not specified as rheumatic (I31.-)
         (Ex:) See PDX Collection 188

     ● **I09.8**   **Other specified rheumatic heart diseases**
         I09.81   **Rheumatic heart failure** 🔹🔹
             Use additional code to identify type of heart failure (I50.-)
             (Ex:) See PDX Collection 648

         I09.89   **Other specified rheumatic heart diseases**
             Rheumatic disease of pulmonary valve

     I09.9   **Rheumatic heart disease, unspecified**
         Rheumatic carditis
         Excludes1   rheumatoid carditis (M05.31)

N Newborn Age: 0   **P** Pediatric Age: 0–17   **M** Maternity DX: 9–64   **A** Adult Age: 15–124   ♀ Females Only   ♂ Males Only
🔹 Complication\Comorbidity   🔹 Major C\C   (Ex:) CC/MCC Exclusions   🔹 Hospital-Acquired Condition   🔹 Hierarchical Condition Category

889

CHAPTER 9 (I00-I99)

Item 9–5 Hypertension is caused by high arterial blood pressure in the arteries. **Essential, primary,** or **idiopathic** hypertension occurs without identifiable organic cause. **Secondary** hypertension is that which has an organic cause. **Malignant** hypertension is severely elevated blood pressure. **Benign** hypertension is mildly elevated blood pressure.

HYPERTENSIVE DISEASES (I10-I16)

Use additional code to identify:
exposure to environmental tobacco smoke (Z77.22)
history of tobacco dependence (Z87.891)
occupational exposure to environmental tobacco smoke (Z57.31)
tobacco dependence (F17.-)
tobacco use (Z72.0)

Excludes1 neonatal hypertension (P29.2)
primary pulmonary hypertension (I27.0)

Excludes2 hypertensive disease complicating pregnancy, childbirth and the puerperium (O10-O11, O13-O16)

I10 **Essential (primary) hypertension**

Includes high blood pressure
hypertension (arterial) (benign) (essential) (malignant) (primary) (systemic)

Excludes1 hypertensive disease complicating pregnancy, childbirth and the puerperium (O10-O11, O13-O16)

Excludes2 essential (primary) hypertension involving vessels of brain (I60-I69)
essential (primary) hypertension involving vessels of eye (H35.0-)

MCE: Questionable admission when principal dx

● **I11** **Hypertensive heart disease**

Includes any condition in I50.- or I51.4-I51.7, I51.89, I51.9 due to hypertension

I11.0 **Hypertensive heart disease with heart failure** 🔒
Hypertensive heart failure
Use additional code to identify type of heart failure (I50.-)
Coding Clinic: 2017, Q1, P47

I11.9 **Hypertensive heart disease without heart failure**
Hypertensive heart disease NOS

OGCR Section I.C.9.a.2.

Hypertensive Chronic Kidney Disease
Assign codes from category I12, Hypertensive chronic kidney disease, when both hypertension and a condition classifiable to category N18, Chronic kidney disease (CKD), are present. **CKD should not be coded as hypertensive if the physician has specifically documented a different cause.**
The appropriate code from category N18 should be used as a secondary code with a code from category I12 to identify the stage of chronic kidney disease.
See Section I.C.14. Chronic kidney disease.
If a patient has hypertensive chronic kidney disease and acute renal failure, an additional code for the acute renal failure is required.

● **I12** **Hypertensive chronic kidney disease**

Includes any condition in N18 and N26 - due to hypertension
arteriosclerosis of kidney
arteriosclerotic nephritis (chronic) (interstitial)
hypertensive nephropathy
nephrosclerosis

Excludes1 hypertension due to kidney disease (I15.0, I15.1)
renovascular hypertension (I15.0)
secondary hypertension (I15.-)

Excludes2 acute kidney failure (N17.-)

Coding Clinic: 2018, Q4, P89; 2016, Q4, P123

I12.0 **Hypertensive chronic kidney disease with stage 5 chronic kidney disease or end stage renal disease** 🔒🔒
Use additional code to identify the stage of chronic kidney disease (N18.5, N18.6)
Ex: See PDX Collection 649
Coding Clinic: 2016, Q3, P23

I12.9 **Hypertensive chronic kidney disease with stage 1 through stage 4 chronic kidney disease, or unspecified chronic kidney disease**
Hypertensive chronic kidney disease NOS
Hypertensive renal disease NOS
Use additional code to identify the stage of chronic kidney disease (N18.1-N18.4, N18.9)
Coding Clinic: 2018, Q4, P88

OGCR Section I.c.9.a.3.

Hypertensive Heart and Chronic Kidney Disease
Assign codes from combination category I13, Hypertensive heart and chronic kidney disease, when **there is hypertension with both heart and kidney involvement.** If heart failure is present, assign an additional code from category I50 to identify the type of heart failure.
The appropriate code from category N18, Chronic kidney disease, should be used as a secondary code with a code from category I13 to identify the stage of chronic kidney disease.
See Section I.C.14. Chronic kidney disease.
The codes in category I13, Hypertensive heart and chronic kidney disease, are combination codes that include hypertension, heart disease and chronic kidney disease. The Includes note at I13 specifies that the conditions included at I11 and I12 are included together in I13. If a patient has hypertension, heart disease and chronic kidney disease then a code from I13 should be used, not individual codes for hypertension, heart disease and chronic kidney disease, or codes from I11 or I12.
For patients with both acute renal failure and chronic kidney disease an additional code for acute renal failure is required.

● **I13** **Hypertensive heart and chronic kidney disease**

Includes any condition in I11.- with any condition in I12.-
cardiorenal disease
cardiovascular renal disease

Ex: For category I13 CC codes: See PDX Collection 650
Coding Clinic: 2016, Q4, P123

I13.0 **Hypertensive heart and chronic kidney disease with heart failure and stage 1 through stage 4 chronic kidney disease, or unspecified chronic kidney disease** 🔒🔒
Use additional code to identify type of heart failure (I50.-)
Use additional code to identify stage of chronic kidney disease (N18.1-N18.4, N18.9)

● **I13.1** **Hypertensive heart and chronic kidney disease without heart failure**

I13.10 **Hypertensive heart and chronic kidney disease without heart failure, with stage 1 through stage 4 chronic kidney disease, or unspecified chronic kidney disease**
Hypertensive heart disease and hypertensive chronic kidney disease NOS
Use additional code to identify the stage of chronic kidney disease (N18.1-N18.4, N18.9)

I13.11 **Hypertensive heart and chronic kidney disease without heart failure, with stage 5 chronic kidney disease, or end stage renal disease** 🔒🔒
Use additional code to identify the stage of chronic kidney disease (N18.5, N18.6)

I13.2 **Hypertensive heart and chronic kidney disease with heart failure and with stage 5 chronic kidney disease, or end stage renal disease** 🔒🔒
Use additional code to identify type of heart failure (I50.-)
Use additional code to identify the stage of chronic kidney disease (N18.5, N18.6)

▶ New   ⇛ Revised   ~~deleted~~ Deleted   Excludes 1   Excludes 2   Includes   Use additional   Code first   Code also   Key words

OGCR Official Guidelines   ● Unacceptable Principal Diagnosis   X Assign placeholder X   ● Use Additional Character(s)   ▷ Manifestation Code   **Coding Clinic**

OGCR Section I.9.a.6.

Hypertension, Secondary
Secondary hypertension is due to an underlying condition.
Two codes are required: one to identify the underlying
etiology and one from category I15 to identify the
hypertension. Sequencing of codes is determined by the
reason for admission/encounter.

● **I15**   **Secondary hypertension**
         Code also underlying condition
         Excludes1   postprocedural hypertension (I97.3)
         Excludes2   secondary hypertension involving vessels of
                         brain (I60-I69)
                         secondary hypertension involving vessels of eye
                         (H35.0-)
    I15.0   **Renovascular** hypertension
    I15.1   **Hypertension secondary to other** renal disorders
               Coding Clinic: 2016, Q3, P23
    I15.2   **Hypertension secondary to** endocrine disorders
    I15.8   **Other** secondary hypertension
    I15.9   **Secondary hypertension,** unspecified

● **I16**   **Hypertensive crisis**
         Code also any identified hypertensive disease (I10-I15)
         Coding Clinic: 2016, Q4, P26-27, 123
    I16.0   **Hypertensive** urgency 🐾
               Ⓔ No exclusions
    I16.1   **Hypertensive** emergency
               Ⓔ See PDX Collection 3595
    I16.9   **Hypertensive crisis,** unspecified 🐾
               Ⓔ See PDX Collection 3596

ISCHEMIC HEART DISEASES (I20-I25)

~~Use additional code to identify presence of hypertension
(I10-I16)~~

▶ Code also the presence of hypertension (I10-I16)

● **I20**   **Angina pectoris**
         *Chest pain/discomfort due to lack of oxygen to the heart muscle.
         Principal symptom of myocardial infarction.*
         Use additional code to identify:
           exposure to environmental tobacco smoke (Z77.22)
           history of tobacco dependence (Z87.891)
           occupational exposure to environmental tobacco smoke
           (Z57.31)
           tobacco dependence (F17.-)
           tobacco use (Z72.0)
         Excludes1   angina pectoris with atherosclerotic heart disease
                         of native coronary arteries (I25.1-)
                         atherosclerosis of coronary artery bypass graft(s)
                         and coronary artery of transplanted heart
                         with angina pectoris (I25.7-)
                         postinfarction angina (I23.7)
    I20.0   **Unstable angina** 🐾🐾
               Accelerated angina
               Crescendo angina
               De novo effort angina
               Intermediate coronary syndrome
               Preinfarction syndrome
               Worsening effort angina
               Ⓔ See PDX Collection 651
    I20.1   **Angina pectoris with** documented spasm 🐾🐾
               Angiospastic angina
               Prinzmetal angina
               Spasm-induced angina
               Variant angina
               Ⓔ See PDX Collection 652

I20.8   **Other forms of angina pectoris** 🐾
           Angina equivalent
           Angina of effort
           Coronary slow flow syndrome
           Stable angina
           Stenocardia
           Use additional code(s) for symptoms associated with
           angina equivalent
I20.9   **Angina pectoris,** unspecified 🐾
           Angina NOS
           Anginal syndrome
           Cardiac angina
           Ischemic chest pain

● **I21**   **Acute myocardial infarction**
         Includes   cardiac infarction
                         coronary (artery) embolism
                         coronary (artery) occlusion
                         coronary (artery) rupture
                         coronary (artery) thrombosis
                         infarction of heart, myocardium, or ventricle
                         myocardial infarction specified as acute or with a
                         stated duration of 4 weeks (28 days) or less
                         from onset
         Use additional code, if applicable, to identify:
           exposure to environmental tobacco smoke (Z77.22)
           history of tobacco dependence (Z87.891)
           occupational exposure to environmental tobacco smoke
           (Z57.31)
           status post administration of tPA (rtPA) in a different facility
           within the last 24 hours prior to admission to current
           facility (Z92.82)
           tobacco dependence (F17.-)
           tobacco use (Z72.0)
         Excludes2   old myocardial infarction (I25.2)
                         postmyocardial infarction syndrome (I24.1)
                         subsequent type 1 myocardial infarction (I22.-)
         Ⓔ For category I21 CC codes: See PDX Collection 653
         Coding Clinic: 2016, Q4, P140; 2013, Q1, P25-26; 2012, Q4, P103
● **I21.0**   **ST elevation (STEMI) myocardial infarction of** anterior
             wall
             Type 1 ST elevation myocardial infarction of anterior
             wall
             Coding Clinic: 2013, Q1, P26
    I21.01   **ST elevation (STEMI) myocardial infarction
                 involving** left main coronary artery 🐾🐾
    I21.02   **ST elevation (STEMI) myocardial infarction
                 involving** left anterior descending coronary
                 artery 🐾🐾
                 ST elevation (STEMI) myocardial infarction
                 involving diagonal coronary artery
                 Coding Clinic: 2013, Q1, P26
    I21.09   **ST elevation (STEMI) myocardial infarction
                 involving** other coronary artery **of anterior
                 wall** 🐾🐾
                 Acute transmural myocardial infarction of
                 anterior wall
                 Anteroapical transmural (Q wave) infarction
                 (acute)
                 Anterolateral transmural (Q wave) infarction
                 (acute)
                 Anteroseptal transmural (Q wave) infarction
                 (acute)
                 Transmural (Q wave) infarction (acute) (of)
                 anterior (wall) NOS
                 Coding Clinic: 2012, Q4, P102, 104

N Newborn Age: 0   P Pediatric Age: 0–17   M Maternity DX: 9–64   A Adult Age: 15–124   ♀ Females Only   ♂ Males Only

🐾 Complication\Comorbidity   🐾 Major C\C   Ⓔ CC/MCC Exclusions   🐾 Hospital-Acquired Condition   🐾 Hierarchical Condition Category

CHAPTER 9 (I00-I99)

● **I21.1** **ST elevation (STEMI) myocardial infarction of inferior wall**
   Type 1 ST elevation myocardial infarction of inferior wall
   Coding Clinic: 2013, Q1, P26

  I21.11 **ST elevation (STEMI) myocardial infarction involving right coronary artery**
   Inferoposterior transmural (Q wave) infarction (acute)

  I21.19 **ST elevation (STEMI) myocardial infarction involving other coronary artery of inferior wall**
   Acute transmural myocardial infarction of inferior wall
   Inferolateral transmural (Q wave) infarction (acute)
   Transmural (Q wave) infarction (acute) (of) diaphragmatic wall
   Transmural (Q wave) infarction (acute) (of) inferior (wall) NOS

    Excludes2 ST elevation (STEMI) myocardial infarction involving left circumflex coronary artery (I21.21)
    Coding Clinic: 2012, Q4, P97

● **I21.2** **ST elevation (STEMI) myocardial infarction of other sites**
   Type 1 ST elevation myocardial infarction of other sites
   Coding Clinic: 2013, Q1, P26

  I21.21 **ST elevation (STEMI) myocardial infarction involving left circumflex coronary artery**
   ST elevation (STEMI) myocardial infarction involving oblique marginal coronary artery

  I21.29 **ST elevation (STEMI) myocardial infarction involving other sites**
   Acute transmural myocardial infarction of other sites
   Apical-lateral transmural (Q wave) infarction (acute)
   Basal-lateral transmural (Q wave) infarction (acute)
   High lateral transmural (Q wave) infarction (acute)
   Lateral (wall) NOS transmural (Q wave) infarction (acute)
   Posterior (true) transmural (Q wave) infarction (acute)
   Posterobasal transmural (Q wave) infarction (acute)
   Posterolateral transmural (Q wave) infarction (acute)
   Posteroseptal transmural (Q wave) infarction (acute)
   Septal transmural (Q wave) infarction (acute) NOS

OGCR Section I.c.9.e.2.

Acute myocardial infarction, unspecified
Code I21.9, Acute myocardial infarction, unspecified, is the default for unspecified acute myocardial infarction or unspecified type. If only type 1 STEMI or transmural MI without the site is documented, assign I21.3, ST elevation (STEMI) myocardial infarction of unspecified site.

  I21.3 **ST elevation (STEMI) myocardial infarction of unspecified site**
   Acute transmural myocardial infarction of unspecified site
   Transmural (Q wave) myocardial infarction NOS
   Type 1 ST elevation myocardial infarction of unspecified site
   Coding Clinic: 2013, Q1, P26

  I21.4 **Non-ST elevation (NSTEMI) myocardial infarction**
   Acute subendocardial myocardial infarction
   Non-Q wave myocardial infarction NOS
   Nontransmural myocardial infarction NOS
   Type 1 non-ST elevation myocardial infarction
   Coding Clinic: 2017, Q1, P44; 2015, Q2, P16; 2013, Q1, P26

I21.9 **Acute myocardial infarction, unspecified**
  Myocardial infarction (acute) NOS

● **I21.A** **Other type of myocardial infarction**
  I21.A1 **Myocardial infarction type 2**
   Myocardial infarction due to demand ischemia
   Myocardial infarction secondary to ischemic imbalance
   Code first the underlying cause, such as:
   anemia (D50.0-D64.9)
   chronic obstructive pulmonary disease (J44.-)
   paroxysmal tachycardia (I47.0-I47.9)
   shock (R57.0-R57.9)
   Coding Clinic: 2017, Q4, P13-14

  I21.A9 **Other myocardial infarction type**
   Myocardial infarction associated with revascularization procedure
   Myocardial infarction type 3
   Myocardial infarction type 4a
   Myocardial infarction type 4b
   Myocardial infarction type 4c
   Myocardial infarction type 5
   Code first, if applicable, postprocedural myocardial infarction following cardiac surgery (I97.190), or postprocedural myocardial infarction during cardiac surgery (I97.790)
   Code also complication, if known and applicable, such as:
   (acute) stent occlusion (T82.897-)
   (acute) stent stenosis (T82.857-)
   (acute) stent thrombosis (T82.865-)
   cardiac arrest due to underlying cardiac condition (I46.2)
   complication of percutaneous coronary intervention (PCI) (I97.89)
   occlusion of coronary artery bypass graft (T82.218-)
   Coding Clinic: 2019, Q2, P32-33

● **I22** **Subsequent ST elevation (STEMI) and non-ST elevation (NSTEMI) myocardial infarction**
  Includes acute myocardial infarction occurring within four weeks (28 days) of a previous acute myocardial infarction, regardless of site
   cardiac infarction
   coronary (artery) embolism
   coronary (artery) occlusion
   coronary (artery) rupture
   coronary (artery) thrombosis
   infarction of heart, myocardium, or ventricle
   recurrent myocardial infarction
   reinfarction of myocardium
   rupture of heart, myocardium, or ventricle
   subsequent type 1 myocardial infarction

  Excludes1 subsequent myocardial infarction, type 2 (I21.A1)
   subsequent myocardial infarction of other type (type 3) (type 4) (type 5) (I21.A9)

Use additional code, if applicable, to identify:
exposure to environmental tobacco smoke (Z77.22)
history of tobacco dependence (Z87.891)
occupational exposure to environmental tobacco smoke (Z57.31)
status post administration of tPA (rtPA) in a different facility within the last 24 hours prior to admission to current facility (Z92.82)
tobacco dependence (F17.-)
tobacco use (Z72.0)
Ⓔ **For category I22 CC codes:** See PDX Collection 653
Coding Clinic: 2017, Q4, P14; 2013, Q1, P25; 2012, Q4, P103

▶ New   ⮞ Revised   deleted Deleted   Excludes 1   Excludes 2   Includes   Use additional   Code first   Code also   Key words
OGCR Official Guidelines   ● Unacceptable Principal Diagnosis   X Assign placeholder X   ● Use Additional Character(s)   ▶ Manifestation Code   Coding Clinic

CHAPTER 9 (I00-I99)

I22.0   **Subsequent ST elevation (STEMI) myocardial infarction of anterior wall** 🔖🔖
> Subsequent acute transmural myocardial infarction of anterior wall
> Subsequent transmural (Q wave) infarction (acute)(of) anterior (wall) NOS
> Subsequent anteroapical transmural (Q wave) infarction (acute)
> Subsequent anterolateral transmural (Q wave) infarction (acute)
> Subsequent anteroseptal transmural (Q wave) infarction (acute)

I22.1   **Subsequent ST elevation (STEMI) myocardial infarction of inferior wall** 🔖🔖
> Subsequent acute transmural myocardial infarction of inferior wall
> Subsequent transmural (Q wave) infarction (acute)(of) diaphragmatic wall
> Subsequent transmural (Q wave) infarction (acute)(of) inferior (wall) NOS
> Subsequent inferolateral transmural (Q wave) infarction (acute)
> Subsequent inferoposterior transmural (Q wave) infarction (acute)
>
> Coding Clinic: 2012, Q4, P97, 102, 104

I22.2   **Subsequent non-ST elevation (NSTEMI) myocardial infarction** 🔖🔖
> Subsequent acute subendocardial myocardial infarction
> Subsequent non-Q wave myocardial infarction NOS
> Subsequent nontransmural myocardial infarction NOS

I22.8   **Subsequent ST elevation (STEMI) myocardial infarction of other sites** 🔖🔖
> Subsequent acute transmural myocardial infarction of other sites
> Subsequent apical-lateral transmural (Q wave) myocardial infarction (acute)
> Subsequent basal-lateral transmural (Q wave) myocardial infarction (acute)
> Subsequent high lateral transmural (Q wave) myocardial infarction (acute)
> Subsequent transmural (Q wave) myocardial infarction (acute)(of) lateral (wall) NOS
> Subsequent posterior (true) transmural (Q wave) myocardial infarction (acute)
> Subsequent posterobasal transmural (Q wave) myocardial infarction (acute)
> Subsequent posterolateral transmural (Q wave) myocardial infarction (acute)
> Subsequent posteroseptal transmural (Q wave) myocardial infarction (acute)
> Subsequent septal NOS transmural (Q wave) myocardial infarction (acute)

I22.9   **Subsequent ST elevation (STEMI) myocardial infarction of unspecified site** 🔖🔖
> Subsequent acute myocardial infarction of unspecified site
> Subsequent myocardial infarction (acute) NOS

● **I23**   **Certain current complications following ST elevation (STEMI) and non-ST elevation (NSTEMI) myocardial infarction (within the 28 day period)**
> (Ex:) For category I23 CC codes unless otherwise indicated: See PDX Collection 3500
> Coding Clinic: 2017, Q2, P11

I23.0   **Hemopericardium as current complication following acute myocardial infarction** 🔖🔖   A
> **Excludes1**   hemopericardium not specified as current complication following acute myocardial infarction (I31.2)

I23.1   **Atrial septal defect as current complication following acute myocardial infarction** 🔖🔖   A
> **Excludes1**   acquired atrial septal defect not specified as current complication following acute myocardial infarction (I51.0)

I23.2   **Ventricular septal defect as current complication following acute myocardial infarction** 🔖🔖   A
> **Excludes1**   acquired ventricular septal defect not specified as current complication following acute myocardial infarction (I51.0)

I23.3   **Rupture of cardiac wall without hemopericardium as current complication following acute myocardial infarction** 🔖🔖   A
> Coding Clinic: 2017, Q2, P11

I23.4   **Rupture of chordae tendineae as current complication following acute myocardial infarction** 🔖🔖
> **Excludes1**   rupture of chordae tendineae not specified as current complication following acute myocardial infarction (I51.1)
>
> (Ex:) See PDX Collection 655

I23.5   **Rupture of papillary muscle as current complication following acute myocardial infarction** 🔖🔖
> **Excludes1**   rupture of papillary muscle not specified as current complication following acute myocardial infarction (I51.2)
>
> (Ex:) See PDX Collection 656

I23.6   **Thrombosis of atrium, auricular appendage, and ventricle as current complications following acute myocardial infarction** 🔖🔖   A
> **Excludes1**   thrombosis of atrium, auricular appendage, and ventricle not specified as current complication following acute myocardial infarction (I51.3)

I23.7   **Postinfarction angina** 🔖🔖   A
> Coding Clinic: 2015, Q2, P16-17

I23.8   **Other current complications following acute myocardial infarction** 🔖🔖   A

● **I24**   **Other acute ischemic heart diseases**
> **Excludes1**   angina pectoris (I20.-)
>   transient myocardial ischemia in newborn (P29.4)
> ▶ **Excludes2**   non-ischemic myocardial injury (I5A)
> (Ex:) For category I24 CC codes unless otherwise indicated: See PDX Collection 657

I24.0   **Acute coronary thrombosis not resulting in myocardial infarction** 🔖🔖
> Acute coronary (artery) (vein) embolism not resulting in myocardial infarction
> Acute coronary (artery) (vein) occlusion not resulting in myocardial infarction
> Acute coronary (artery) (vein) thromboembolism not resulting in myocardial infarction
> **Excludes1**   atherosclerotic heart disease (I25.1-)
> Coding Clinic: 2013, Q1, P24

I24.1   **Dressler's syndrome** 🔖🔖
> Postmyocardial infarction syndrome
> **Excludes1**   postinfarction angina (I23.7)
> (Ex:) See PDX Collection 658

I24.8   **Other forms of acute ischemic heart disease** 🔖🔖
> **Excludes1**   myocardial infarction due to demand ischemia (I21.A1)
> Coding Clinic: 2017, Q4, P13

I24.9   **Acute ischemic heart disease, unspecified** 🔖🔖
> **Excludes1**   ischemic heart disease (chronic) NOS (I25.9)

● **I25**   **Chronic ischemic heart disease**
> ▶ **Excludes2**   non-ischemic myocardial injury (I5A)
>
> Use additional code to identify:
> chronic total occlusion of coronary artery (I25.82)
> exposure to environmental tobacco smoke (Z77.22)
> history of tobacco dependence (Z87.891)
> occupational exposure to environmental tobacco smoke (Z57.31)
> tobacco dependence (F17.-)
> tobacco use (Z72.0)

N   Newborn Age: 0   P   Pediatric Age: 0–17   M   Maternity DX: 9–64   A   Adult Age: 15–124   ♀   Females Only   ♂   Males Only

🔖 Complication\Comorbidity   🔖 Major C\C   (Ex:) CC/MCC Exclusions   🔖 Hospital-Acquired Condition   🔖 Hierarchical Condition Category

893

Item 9–6 **Classification** is based on the location of the atherosclerosis. **"Of native coronary artery"** indicates the atherosclerosis is within an original heart artery. **"Of autologous vein bypass graft"** indicates that the atherosclerosis is within a vein graft that was taken from within the patient. **"Of nonautologous biological bypass graft"** indicates the atherosclerosis is within a vessel grafted from other than the patient. **"Of artery bypass graft"** indicates the atherosclerosis is within an artery that was grafted from within the patient.

★ **(See Plates 218 and 219 on pages 74 and 75.)**

● I25.1　**Atherosclerotic heart disease of native coronary artery**
　　　　Disease in which fatty deposits form on the walls of arteries
　　　　Atherosclerotic cardiovascular disease
　　　　Coronary (artery) atheroma
　　　　Coronary (artery) atherosclerosis
　　　　Coronary (artery) disease
　　　　Coronary (artery) sclerosis

　　　　Use additional code, if applicable, to identify:
　　　　　　coronary atherosclerosis due to calcified coronary lesion (I25.84)
　　　　　　coronary atherosclerosis due to lipid rich plaque (I25.83)

　　　　Excludes2　atheroembolism (I75.-)
　　　　　　　　　　atherosclerosis of coronary artery bypass graft(s) and transplanted heart (I25.7-)

　　I25.10　**Atherosclerotic heart disease of native coronary artery without angina pectoris**　　A
　　　　　　Atherosclerotic heart disease NOS
　　　　　　Coding Clinic: 2015, Q2, P17; 2012, Q4, P92

OGCR　See Section I.9.b.

Atherosclerotic Coronary Artery Disease and Angina

ICD-10-CM has combination codes for atherosclerotic heart disease with angina pectoris. The subcategories for these codes are I25.11, Atherosclerotic heart disease of native coronary artery with angina pectoris and I25.7, Atherosclerosis of coronary artery bypass graft(s) and coronary artery of transplanted heart with angina pectoris.

When using one of these combination codes it is not necessary to use an additional code for angina pectoris. A causal relationship can be assumed in a patient with both atherosclerosis and angina pectoris, unless the documentation indicates the angina is due to something other than the atherosclerosis.

If a patient with coronary artery disease is admitted due to an acute myocardial infarction (AMI), the AMI should be sequenced before the coronary artery disease.

See Section I.C.9. Acute myocardial infarction (AMI).

　● I25.11　**Atherosclerotic heart disease of native coronary artery with angina pectoris**

　　　I25.110　**Atherosclerotic heart disease of native coronary artery with unstable angina pectoris** 🦠🦠　　A

　　　　　　Excludes1　unstable angina without atherosclerotic heart disease (I20.0)

　　　　　　CC when PDx is its own CC
　　　　　　ⒺⓍ See PDX Collection 3712

Figure 9-2　Atherosclerotic plaque.

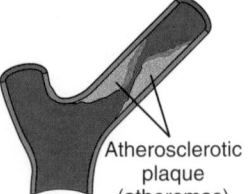

Atherosclerotic
plaque
(atheromas)

　　　I25.111　**Atherosclerotic heart disease of native coronary artery with angina pectoris with documented spasm** 🦠　　A

　　　　　　Excludes1　angina pectoris with documented spasm without atherosclerotic heart disease (I20.1)

　　　I25.118　**Atherosclerotic heart disease of native coronary artery with other forms of angina pectoris** 🦠　　A

　　　　　　Excludes1　other forms of angina pectoris without atherosclerotic heart disease (I20.8)

　　　　　　Coding Clinic: 2015, Q2, P16-17

　　　I25.119　**Atherosclerotic heart disease of native coronary artery with unspecified angina pectoris** 🦠　　A
　　　　　　Atherosclerotic heart disease with angina NOS
　　　　　　Atherosclerotic heart disease with ischemic chest pain

　　　　　　Excludes1　unspecified angina pectoris without atherosclerotic heart disease (I20.9)

　I25.2　**Old myocardial infarction**
　　　　Healed myocardial infarction
　　　　Past myocardial infarction diagnosed by ECG or other investigation, but currently presenting no symptoms

　I25.3　**Aneurysm of heart** 🦠
　　　　Mural aneurysm
　　　　Ventricular aneurysm
　　　　ⒺⓍ See PDX Collection 659

● I25.4　**Coronary artery aneurysm and dissection**

　　I25.41　**Coronary artery aneurysm**
　　　　　　Coronary arteriovenous fistula, acquired
　　　　　　Excludes1　congenital coronary (artery) aneurysm (Q24.5)

　　I25.42　**Coronary artery dissection** 🦠
　　　　　　ⒺⓍ See PDX Collection 660

　I25.5　**Ischemic cardiomyopathy**
　　　　Excludes2　coronary atherosclerosis (I25.1-, I25.7-)

　I25.6　**Silent myocardial ischemia**

● I25.7　**Atherosclerosis of coronary artery bypass graft(s) and coronary artery of transplanted heart with angina pectoris**

　　　　Use additional code, if applicable, to identify:
　　　　　　coronary atherosclerosis due to calcified coronary lesion (I25.84)
　　　　　　coronary atherosclerosis due to lipid rich plaque (I25.83)

　　　　Excludes1　atherosclerosis of bypass graft(s) of transplanted heart without angina pectoris (I25.812)
　　　　　　　　atherosclerosis of coronary artery bypass graft(s) without angina pectoris (I25.810)
　　　　　　　　atherosclerosis of native coronary artery of transplanted heart without angina pectoris (I25.811)

▶ New　➠ Revised　d̶e̶l̶e̶t̶e̶d̶ Deleted　Excludes 1　Excludes 2　Includes　Use additional　Code first　Code also　Key words
OGCR Official Guidelines　● Unacceptable Principal Diagnosis　X Assign placeholder X　● Use Additional Character(s)　▶ Manifestation Code　Coding Clinic

● **I25.70** **Atherosclerosis of coronary artery bypass graft(s), unspecified, with angina pectoris**

    I25.700 **Atherosclerosis of coronary artery bypass graft(s), unspecified, with unstable angina pectoris** 🩸🩸   A

        Excludes1   unstable angina pectoris without atherosclerosis of coronary artery bypass graft (I20.0)

        CC when PDx is its own CC

        (Ex) See PDX Collection 3714

    I25.701 **Atherosclerosis of coronary artery bypass graft(s), unspecified, with angina pectoris with documented spasm** 🩸   A

        Excludes1   angina pectoris with documented spasm without atherosclerosis of coronary artery bypass graft (I20.1)

    I25.708 **Atherosclerosis of coronary artery bypass graft(s), unspecified, with other forms of angina pectoris** 🩸   A

        Excludes1   other forms of angina pectoris without atherosclerosis of coronary artery bypass graft (I20.8)

    I25.709 **Atherosclerosis of coronary artery bypass graft(s), unspecified, with unspecified angina pectoris** 🩸   A

        Excludes1   unspecified angina pectoris without atherosclerosis of coronary artery bypass graft (I20.9)

● **I25.71** **Atherosclerosis of autologous vein coronary artery bypass graft(s) with angina pectoris**

    (Ex) **For category I25.71 CC codes unless otherwise indicated:** See PDX Collection 662

    I25.710 **Atherosclerosis of autologous vein coronary artery bypass graft(s) with unstable angina pectoris** 🩸🩸   A

        Excludes1   unstable angina without atherosclerosis of autologous vein coronary artery bypass graft(s) (I20.0)

        Excludes2   embolism or thrombus of coronary artery bypass graft(s) (T82.8-)

        CC when PDx is its own CC

        (Ex) See PDX Collection 661

    I25.711 **Atherosclerosis of autologous vein coronary artery bypass graft(s) with angina pectoris with documented spasm** 🩸🩸   A

        Excludes1   angina pectoris with documented spasm without atherosclerosis of autologous vein coronary artery bypass graft(s) (I20.1)

    I25.718 **Atherosclerosis of autologous vein coronary artery bypass graft(s) with other forms of angina pectoris** 🩸🩸   A

        Excludes1   other forms of angina pectoris without atherosclerosis of autologous vein coronary artery bypass graft(s) (I20.8)

    I25.719 **Atherosclerosis of autologous vein coronary artery bypass graft(s) with unspecified angina pectoris** 🩸🩸   A

        Excludes1   unspecified angina pectoris without atherosclerosis of autologous vein coronary artery bypass graft(s) (I20.9)

● **I25.72** **Atherosclerosis of autologous artery coronary artery bypass graft(s) with angina pectoris**

    Atherosclerosis of internal mammary artery graft with angina pectoris

    (Ex) **For category I25.72 CC codes unless otherwise indicated:** See PDX Collection 662

    I25.720 **Atherosclerosis of autologous artery coronary artery bypass graft(s) with unstable angina pectoris** 🩸🩸   A

        Excludes1   unstable angina without atherosclerosis of autologous artery coronary artery bypass graft(s) (I20.0)

        CC when PDx is its own CC

        (Ex) See PDX Collection 661

    I25.721 **Atherosclerosis of autologous artery coronary artery bypass graft(s) with angina pectoris with documented spasm** 🩸🩸   A

        Excludes1   angina pectoris with documented spasm without atherosclerosis of autologous artery coronary artery bypass graft(s) (I20.1)

    I25.728 **Atherosclerosis of autologous artery coronary artery bypass graft(s) with other forms of angina pectoris** 🩸🩸   A

        Excludes1   other forms of angina pectoris without atherosclerosis of autologous artery coronary artery bypass graft(s) (I20.8)

    I25.729 **Atherosclerosis of autologous artery coronary artery bypass graft(s) with unspecified angina pectoris** 🩸🩸   A

        Excludes1   unspecified angina pectoris without atherosclerosis of autologous artery coronary artery bypass graft(s) (I20.9)

CHAPTER 9 (I00-I99)

N Newborn Age: 0   **P** Pediatric Age: 0–17   **M** Maternity DX: 9–64   **A** Adult Age: 15–124   ♀ Females Only   ♂ Males Only

🩸 Complication\Comorbidity   🩸 Major C\C   (Ex) CC/MCC Exclusions   🩸 Hospital-Acquired Condition   🩸 Hierarchical Condition Category

895

● **I25.73** **Atherosclerosis of nonautologous biological coronary artery bypass graft(s) with angina pectoris**
> (Ex:) **For category I25.73 CC codes unless otherwise indicated:**
> See PDX Collection 662

I25.730 **Atherosclerosis of nonautologous biological coronary artery bypass graft(s) with unstable angina pectoris** 🔷🔷 A
> **Excludes1** unstable angina without atherosclerosis of nonautologous biological coronary artery bypass graft(s) (I20.0)
> CC when PDx is its own CC
> (Ex:) See PDX Collection 661

I25.731 **Atherosclerosis of nonautologous biological coronary artery bypass graft(s) with angina pectoris with documented spasm** 🔷🔷 A
> **Excludes1** angina pectoris with documented spasm without atherosclerosis of nonautologous biological coronary artery bypass graft(s) (I20.1)

I25.738 **Atherosclerosis of nonautologous biological coronary artery bypass graft(s) with other forms of angina pectoris** 🔷🔷 A
> **Excludes1** other forms of angina pectoris without atherosclerosis of nonautologous biological coronary artery bypass graft(s) (I20.8)

I25.739 **Atherosclerosis of nonautologous biological coronary artery bypass graft(s) with unspecified angina pectoris** 🔷🔷 A
> **Excludes1** unspecified angina pectoris without atherosclerosis of nonautologous biological coronary artery bypass graft(s) (I20.9)

● **I25.75** **Atherosclerosis of native coronary artery of transplanted heart with angina pectoris**
> **Excludes1** atherosclerosis of native coronary artery of transplanted heart without angina pectoris (I25.811)
> (Ex:) **For category I25.75 CC codes unless otherwise indicated:**
> See PDX Collection 664

I25.750 **Atherosclerosis of native coronary artery of transplanted heart with unstable angina** 🔷🔷
> CC when PDx is its own CC
> (Ex:) See PDX Collection 663

I25.751 **Atherosclerosis of native coronary artery of transplanted heart with angina pectoris with documented spasm** 🔷🔷

I25.758 **Atherosclerosis of native coronary artery of transplanted heart with other forms of angina pectoris** 🔷🔷

I25.759 **Atherosclerosis of native coronary artery of transplanted heart with unspecified angina pectoris** 🔷🔷

● **I25.76** **Atherosclerosis of bypass graft of coronary artery of transplanted heart with angina pectoris**
> **Excludes1** atherosclerosis of bypass graft of coronary artery of transplanted heart without angina pectoris (I25.812)

I25.760 **Atherosclerosis of bypass graft of coronary artery of transplanted heart with unstable angina** 🔷🔷 A
> CC when PDx is its own CC
> (Ex:) See PDX Collection 665

I25.761 **Atherosclerosis of bypass graft of coronary artery of transplanted heart with angina pectoris with documented spasm** 🔷🔷 A
> (Ex:) See PDX Collection 3717

I25.768 **Atherosclerosis of bypass graft of coronary artery of transplanted heart with other forms of angina pectoris** 🔷🔷 A
> (Ex:) See PDX Collection 3719

I25.769 **Atherosclerosis of bypass graft of coronary artery of transplanted heart with unspecified angina pectoris** 🔷🔷 A
> (Ex:) See PDX Collection 3721

● **I25.79** **Atherosclerosis of other coronary artery bypass graft(s) with angina pectoris** A
> (Ex:) **For category I25.79 CC codes unless otherwise indicated:**
> No exclusions

I25.790 **Atherosclerosis of other coronary artery bypass graft(s) with unstable angina pectoris** 🔷🔷
> **Excludes1** unstable angina without atherosclerosis of other coronary artery bypass graft(s) (I20.0)
> CC when PDx is its own CC
> (Ex:) See PDX Collection 3723

I25.791 **Atherosclerosis of other coronary artery bypass graft(s) with angina pectoris with documented spasm** 🔷🔷 A
> **Excludes1** angina pectoris with documented spasm without atherosclerosis of other coronary artery bypass graft(s) (I20.1)

I25.798 **Atherosclerosis of other coronary artery bypass graft(s) with other forms of angina pectoris** 🔷🔷 A
> **Excludes1** other forms of angina pectoris without atherosclerosis of other coronary artery bypass graft(s) (I20.8)
> (Ex:) See PDX Collection 3598

I25.799 **Atherosclerosis of other coronary artery bypass graft(s) with unspecified angina pectoris** 🔷🔷 A
> **Excludes1** unspecified angina pectoris without atherosclerosis of other coronary artery bypass graft(s) (I20.9)
> (Ex:) See PDX Collection 3599

● **I25.8   Other forms of chronic ischemic heart disease**
  ● **I25.81   Atherosclerosis of other coronary vessels without angina pectoris**

Use additional code, if applicable, to identify:
coronary atherosclerosis due to calcified coronary lesion (I25.84)
coronary atherosclerosis due to lipid rich plaque (I25.83)

> **Excludes2**   atherosclerotic heart disease of native coronary artery without angina pectoris (I25.10)

  I25.810   Atherosclerosis of coronary artery bypass graft(s) without angina pectoris 🔗   **A**

Atherosclerosis of coronary artery bypass graft NOS

> **Excludes1**   atherosclerosis of coronary bypass graft(s) with angina pectoris (I25.70- -I25.73-, I25.79-)

(Ex:) See PDX Collection 3226
Coding Clinic: 2016, Q4, P86

  I25.811   Atherosclerosis of native coronary artery of transplanted heart without angina pectoris 🔗

Atherosclerosis of native coronary artery of transplanted heart NOS

> **Excludes1**   atherosclerosis of native coronary artery of transplanted heart with angina pectoris (I25.75-)

(Ex:) See PDX Collection 664

  I25.812   Atherosclerosis of bypass graft of coronary artery of transplanted heart without angina pectoris 🔗   **A**

Atherosclerosis of bypass graft of transplanted heart NOS

> **Excludes1**   atherosclerosis of bypass graft of transplanted heart with angina pectoris (I25.76)

  ● **I25.82   Chronic total occlusion of coronary artery**

Complete occlusion of coronary artery
Total occlusion of coronary artery

Code first coronary atherosclerosis (I25.1-, I25.7-, I25.81-)

> **Excludes1**   acute coronary occlusion with myocardial infarction (I21.0-I21.9, I22.-)
> acute coronary occlusion without myocardial infarction (I24.0)

(Ex:) See PDX Collection 666

  ● **I25.83   Coronary atherosclerosis due to lipid rich plaque**   **A**

Code first coronary atherosclerosis (I25.1 , I25.7 , I25.81-)

  ● **I25.84   Coronary atherosclerosis due to calcified coronary lesion**

Coronary atherosclerosis due to severely calcified coronary lesion

Code first coronary atherosclerosis (I25.1-, I25.7-, I25.81-)

  I25.89   Other forms of chronic ischemic heart disease
  I25.9   Chronic ischemic heart disease, unspecified
Ischemic heart disease (chronic) NOS

PULMONARY HEART DISEASE AND DISEASES OF PULMONARY CIRCULATION (I26-I28)

● **I26   Pulmonary embolism**

> **Includes**   pulmonary (acute)(artery)(vein) infarction
> pulmonary (acute)(artery)(vein) thromboembolism
> pulmonary (acute)(artery)(vcin) thrombosis

> **Excludes2**   chronic pulmonary embolism (I27.82)
> personal history of pulmonary embolism (Z86.711)
> pulmonary embolism due to trauma (T79.0, T79.1)
> pulmonary embolism due to complications of surgical and medical care (T80.0, T81.7-, T82.8-)
> pulmonary embolism complicating abortion, ectopic or molar pregnancy (O00-O07, O08.2)
> pulmonary embolism complicating pregnancy, childbirth and the puerperium (O88.-)
> septic (non-pulmonary) arterial embolism (I76)

Coding Clinic: 2021, Q2, P10

● **I26.0   Pulmonary embolism with acute cor pulmonale**
(Ex:) For category I26.0 CC codes: See PDX Collection 667

  ● **I26.01   Septic pulmonary embolism with acute cor pulmonale** 🔗🔗

Code first underlying infection
MCC when PDx is its own MCC

  I26.02   Saddle embolus of pulmonary artery with acute cor pulmonale 🔗🔗🔗
MCC when PDx is its own MCC

  I26.09   Other pulmonary embolism with acute cor pulmonale 🔗🔗🔗
Acute cor pulmonale NOS
MCC when PDx is its own MCC

● **I26.9   Pulmonary embolism without acute cor pulmonale**
  ● **I26.90   Septic pulmonary embolism without acute cor pulmonale** 🔗🔗

Code first underlying infection
(Ex:) See PDX Collection 668

  I26.92   Saddle embolus of pulmonary artery without acute cor pulmonale 🔗🔗🔗
(Ex:) See PDX Collection 669

  I26.93   Single subsegmental pulmonary embolism without acute cor pulmonale 🔗🔗
Subsegmental pulmonary embolism NOS
(Ex:) See PDX Collection 670

  I26.94   Multiple subsegmental pulmonary emboli without acute cor pulmonale 🔗🔗
(Ex:) See PDX Collection 670
Coding Clinic: 2021, Q2, P10

  I26.99   Other pulmonary embolism without acute cor pulmonale 🔗🔗🔗
Acute pulmonary embolism NOS
Pulmonary embolism NOS
(Ex:) See PDX Collection 670
Coding Clinic: 2019, Q2, P22-23

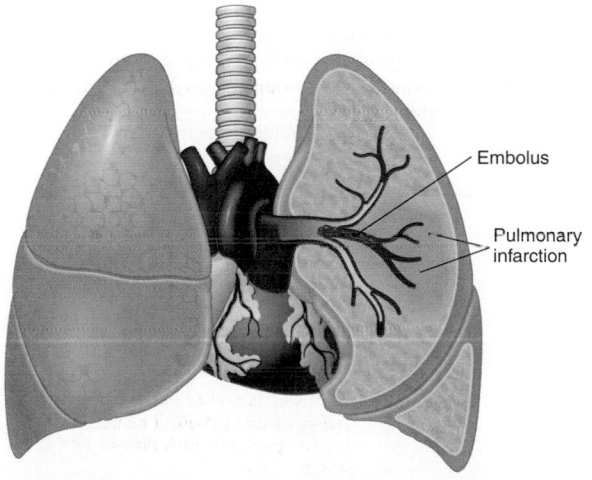

— Embolus
— Pulmonary infarction

Figure 9-3 Pulmonary embolism. (From Chabner: The Language of Medicine, ed 8, St. Louis, Saunders, 2007)

N Newborn Age: 0   **P** Pediatric Age: 0–17   **M** Maternity DX: 9–64   **A** Adult Age: 15–124   ♀ Females Only   ♂ Males Only

🔗 Complication\Comorbidity   🔗 Major C\C   (Ex:) CC/MCC Exclusions   🔗 Hospital-Acquired Condition   🔗 Hierarchical Condition Category

CHAPTER 9 (I00-I99)

897

Item 9–7 Pulmonary heart disease or **cor pulmonale** is right ventricle hypertrophy or RVH as a result of a respiratory disorder increasing back flow pressure to the right ventricle. Left untreated, cor pulmonale leads to right-heart failure and death.

● **I27 Other pulmonary heart diseases**

I27.0 Primary pulmonary hypertension 🔖🔖
  Heritable pulmonary arterial hypertension
  Idiopathic pulmonary arterial hypertension
  Primary group 1 pulmonary hypertension
  Primary pulmonary arterial hypertension

Excludes1 persistent pulmonary hypertension of newborn (P29.30)
  pulmonary hypertension NOS (I27.20)
  secondary pulmonary arterial hypertension (I27.21)
  secondary pulmonary hypertension (I27.29)

(Ex) See PDX Collection 671

I27.1 Kyphoscoliotic heart disease 🔖🔖
(Ex) See PDX Collection 533

● **I27.2 Other secondary pulmonary hypertension**
  Code also associated underlying condition

Excludes1 Eisenmenger's syndrome (I27.83)

Coding Clinic: 2016, Q2, P8

I27.20 Pulmonary hypertension, unspecified 🔖
  Pulmonary hypertension NOS

I27.21 Secondary pulmonary arterial hypertension 🔖
  (Associated) (drug-induced) (toxin-induced) pulmonary arterial hypertension NOS
  (Associated) (drug-induced) (toxin-induced) (secondary) group 1 pulmonary hypertension

Code also associated conditions if applicable, or adverse effects of drugs or toxins, such as:
  adverse effect of appetite depressants (T50.5X5)
  congenital heart disease (Q20-Q28)
  human immunodeficiency virus [HIV] disease (B20)
  polymyositis (M33.2-)
  portal hypertension (K76.6)
  rheumatoid arthritis (M05.-)
  schistosomiasis (B65.-)
  Sjögren syndrome (M35.0-)
  systemic sclerosis (M34.-)

I27.22 Pulmonary hypertension due to left heart disease 🔖
  Group 2 pulmonary hypertension
  Code also associated left heart disease, if known, such as:
    multiple valve disease (I08.-)
    rheumatic mitral valve diseases (I05.-)
    rheumatic aortic valve diseases (I06.-)

I27.23 Pulmonary hypertension due to lung diseases and hypoxia 🔖
  Group 3 pulmonary hypertension
  Code also associated lung disease, if known, such as:
    bronchiectasis (J47.-)
    cystic fibrosis with pulmonary manifestations (E84.0)
    interstitial lung disease (J84.-)
    pleural effusion (J90)
    sleep apnea (G47.3-)

I27.24 Chronic thromboembolic pulmonary hypertension 🔖
  Group 4 pulmonary hypertension
  Code also associated pulmonary embolism, if applicable (I26.-, I27.82)

I27.29 Other secondary pulmonary hypertension 🔖
  Group 5 pulmonary hypertension
  Pulmonary hypertension with unclear multifactorial mechanisms
  Pulmonary hypertension due to hematologic disorders
  Pulmonary hypertension due to metabolic disorders
  Pulmonary hypertension due to other systemic disorders
  Code also other associated disorders, if known, such as:
    chronic myeloid leukemia (C92.10-C92.22)
    essential thrombocythemia (D47.3)
    Gaucher disease (E75.22)
    hypertensive chronic kidney disease with end stage renal disease (I12.0, I13.11, I13.2)
    hyperthyroidism (E05.-)
    hypothyroidism (E00-E03)
    polycythemia vera (D45)
    sarcoidosis (D86.-)

● **I27.8 Other specified pulmonary heart diseases**

I27.81 Cor pulmonale (chronic) 🔖
  Cor pulmonale NOS

Excludes1 acute cor pulmonale (I26.0-)

I27.82 Chronic pulmonary embolism 🔖🔖
  Use additional code, if applicable, for associated long-term (current) use of anticoagulants (Z79.01)

Excludes1 personal history of pulmonary embolism (Z86.711)

(Ex) See PDX Collection 669
Coding Clinic: 2021, Q2, P10

I27.83 Eisenmenger's syndrome 🔖
  Eisenmenger's complex
  (Irreversible) Eisenmenger's disease
  Pulmonary hypertension with right to left shunt related to congenital heart disease
  Code also underlying heart defect, if known, such as:
    atrial septal defect (Q21.1)
    Eisenmenger's defect (Q21.8)
    patent ductus arteriosus (Q25.0)
    ventricular septal defect (Q21.0)

I27.89 Other specified pulmonary heart diseases 🔖

I27.9 Pulmonary heart disease, unspecified 🔖
  Chronic cardiopulmonary disease

● **I28 Other diseases of pulmonary vessels**
(Ex) For category I28 CC codes: See PDX Collection 672

I28.0 Arteriovenous fistula of pulmonary vessels 🔖🔖
Excludes1 congenital arteriovenous fistula (Q25.72)

I28.1 Aneurysm of pulmonary artery 🔖🔖
Excludes1 congenital aneurysm (Q25.79)
  congenital arteriovenous aneurysm (Q25.72)

I28.8 Other diseases of pulmonary vessels 🔖
  Pulmonary arteritis
  Pulmonary endarteritis
  Rupture of pulmonary vessels
  Stenosis of pulmonary vessels
  Stricture of pulmonary vessels

I28.9 Disease of pulmonary vessels, unspecified 🔖

● **I44**   Atrioventricular and left bundle-branch block
*Conduction problem resulting in arrhythmias/dysrhythmias due to a
luck of electrical impulses being transmitted normally through
the heart*

I44.0   Atrioventricular block, first degree

I44.1   Atrioventricular block, second degree
Atrioventricular block, type I and II
Möbitz block, type I and II
Second degree block, type I and II
Wenckebach's block

I44.2   Atrioventricular block, complete 🝔🝔
Complete heart block NOS
Third degree block
(Ex) See PDX Collection 679
Coding Clinic: 2019, Q2, P4

● I44.3   Other and unspecified atrioventricular block
Atrioventricular block NOS

I44.30   Unspecified atrioventricular block

I44.39   Other atrioventricular block

I44.4   Left anterior fascicular block
MCE: Questionable admission when principal dx

I44.5   Left posterior fascicular block
MCE: Questionable admission when principal dx

● I44.6   Other and unspecified fascicular block

I44.60   Unspecified fascicular block
Left bundle-branch hemiblock NOS
MCE: Questionable admission when principal dx

I44.69   Other fascicular block
MCE: Questionable admission when principal dx

I44.7   Left bundle-branch block, unspecified
MCE: Questionable admission when principal dx

● **I45**   Other conduction disorders

I45.0   Right fascicular block
MCE: Questionable admission when principal dx

● I45.1   Other and unspecified right bundle-branch block

I45.10   Unspecified right bundle-branch block
Right bundle-branch block NOS
MCE: Questionable admission when principal dx

I45.19   Other right bundle-branch block
MCE: Questionable admission when principal dx

I45.2   Bifascicular block 🝔
(Ex) See PDX Collection 679

I45.3   Trifascicular block 🝔
(Ex) See PDX Collection 679

I45.4   Nonspecific intraventricular block
Bundle-branch block NOS

I45.5   Other specified heart block
Sinoatrial block
Sinoauricular block
Excludes1   heart block NOS (I45.9)

I45.6   Pre-excitation syndrome
Accelerated atrioventricular conduction
Accessory atrioventricular conduction
Anomalous atrioventricular excitation
Lown-Ganong-Levine syndrome
Pre-excitation atrioventricular conduction
Wolff-Parkinson-White syndrome

● I45.8   Other specified conduction disorders

I45.81   Long QT syndrome

I45.89   Other specified conduction disorders 🝔
Atrioventricular [AV] dissociation
Interference dissociation
Isorhythmic dissociation
Nonparoxysmal AV nodal tachycardia
(Ex) See PDX Collection 679
Coding Clinic: 2013, Q2, P32

I45.9   Conduction disorder, unspecified
Heart block NOS
Stokes-Adams syndrome

● **I46**   Cardiac arrest
Excludes2   cardiogenic shock (R57.0)
(Ex) **For category I46 CC codes:** See PDX Collection 680

I46.2   Cardiac arrest due to underlying cardiac condition 🝔🝔
Code first underlying cardiac condition
MCC: If patient discharged alive

I46.8   Cardiac arrest due to other underlying condition 🝔🝔
Code first underlying condition
MCC: If patient discharged alive

I46.9   Cardiac arrest, cause unspecified 🝔🝔
MCC: If patient discharged alive

● **I47**   Paroxysmal tachycardia
Code first tachycardia complicating:
abortion or ectopic or molar pregnancy (O00-O07, O08.8)
obstetric surgery and procedures (O75.4)
Excludes1   tachycardia NOS (R00.0)
sinoauricular tachycardia NOS (R00.0)
sinus [sinusal] tachycardia NOS (R00.0)
(Ex) **For category I47 CC codes:** See PDX Collection 679

I47.0   Re-entry ventricular arrhythmia 🝔🝔

I47.1   Supraventricular tachycardia 🝔🝔
Atrial (paroxysmal) tachycardia
Atrioventricular [AV] (paroxysmal) tachycardia
Atrioventricular re-entrant (nodal) tachycardia
[AVNRT] [AVRT]
Junctional (paroxysmal) tachycardia
Nodal (paroxysmal) tachycardia

I47.2   Ventricular tachycardia 🝔🝔
Coding Clinic: 2013, Q3, P23

I47.9   Paroxysmal tachycardia, unspecified 🝔
Bouveret (-Hoffman) syndrome

● **I48**   Atrial fibrillation and flutter
*Most common abnormal heart rhythm (arrhythmia) presenting
as irregular, rapid beating (tachycardia) of the heart's upper
chamber.*
(Ex) **For category I48 CC codes:** See PDX Collection 679

I48.0   Paroxysmal atrial fibrillation 🝔

● I48.1   Persistent atrial fibrillation 🝔
Rapid contractions of the upper heart chamber
Excludes1   Permanent atrial fibrillation (I48.21)
Coding Clinic: 2019, Q2, P3-4

I48.11   Longstanding persistent atrial fibrillation 🝔

I48.19   Other persistent atrial fibrillation 🝔
Chronic persistent atrial fibrillation
Persistent atrial fibrillation, NOS

● I48.2   Chronic atrial fibrillation 🝔
Coding Clinic: 2019, Q2, P3

I48.20   Chronic atrial fibrillation, unspecified 🝔
Excludes1   Chronic persistent atrial
fibrillation (I48.19)

I48.21   Permanent atrial fibrillation 🝔

I48.3   Typical atrial flutter 🝔🝔
Type I atrial flutter

I48.4   Atypical atrial flutter 🝔🝔
Type II atrial flutter

● I48.9   Unspecified atrial fibrillation and atrial flutter

I48.91   Unspecified atrial fibrillation 🝔

I48.92   Unspecified atrial flutter 🝔🝔

N Newborn Age: 0   **P** Pediatric Age: 0–17   **M** Maternity DX: 9–64   **A** Adult Age: 15–124   ♀ Females Only   ♂ Males Only

🝔 Complication\Comorbidity   🝔 Major C\C   (Ex) CC/MCC Exclusions   🝔 Hospital-Acquired Condition   🝔 Hierarchical Condition Category

● **I49   Other cardiac arrhythmias**

    Code first cardiac arrhythmia complicating:
        abortion or ectopic or molar pregnancy (O00-O07, O08.8)
        obstetric surgery and procedures (O75.4)

    Excludes1   neonatal dysrhythmia (P29.1-)
                        sinoatrial bradycardia (R00.1)
                        sinus bradycardia (R00.1)
                        vagal bradycardia (R00.1)

    Excludes2   bradycardia NOS (R00.1)

●   **I49.0   Ventricular fibrillation and flutter**
      (Ex:) **For category I49.0 CC codes:** See PDX Collection 679

      I49.01   Ventricular fibrillation 🔹🔹
            MCC: If patient   discharged alive

      I49.02   Ventricular flutter 🔹🔹

  I49.1   Atrial premature depolarization
      Atrial premature beats

  I49.2   Junctional premature depolarization 🔹🔹
      (Ex:) See PDX Collection 679

  I49.3   Ventricular premature depolarization

●   **I49.4   Other and unspecified premature depolarization**

      I49.40   Unspecified premature depolarization
            Premature beats NOS

      I49.49   Other premature depolarization
            Ectopic beats
            Extrasystoles
            Extrasystolic arrhythmias
            Premature contractions

  I49.5   Sick sinus syndrome 🔹
      Tachycardia-bradycardia syndrome
      Coding Clinic: 2019, Q1, P33

  I49.8   Other specified cardiac arrhythmias
      Brugada syndrome
      Coronary sinus rhythm disorder
      Ectopic rhythm disorder
      Nodal rhythm disorder

  I49.9   Cardiac arrhythmia, unspecified
      Arrhythmia (cardiac) NOS

● **I50   Heart failure**

    Code first heart failure complicating abortion or ectopic or molar
        pregnancy (O00-O07, O08.8)
      heart failure due to hypertension (I11.0)
      heart failure due to hypertension with chronic kidney disease
        (I13.-)
      heart failure following surgery (I97.13-)
      obstetric surgery and procedures (O75.4)
      rheumatic heart failure (I09.81)

    ~~**Excludes1**~~   ~~neonatal cardiac failure (P29.0)~~

    Excludes2   cardiac arrest (I46.-)
                 ▶ neonatal cardiac failure (P20.0)
    Coding Clinic: 2017, Q1, P47; 2016, Q4, P122-123, Q1, P38; 2015, Q2, P15

  I50.1   Left ventricular failure, unspecified 🔹🔹
      Cardiac asthma
      Edema of lung with heart disease NOS
      Edema of lung with heart failure
      Left heart failure
      Pulmonary edema with heart disease NOS
      Pulmonary edema with heart failure

      Excludes1   edema of lung without heart disease or
                 heart failure (J81.-)
                 pulmonary edema without heart disease
                 or failure (J81.-)

      (Ex:) See PDX Collection 681

●   **I50.2   Systolic (congestive) heart failure**
      Heart failure with reduced ejection fraction [HFrEF]
      Systolic left ventricular heart failure
      Code also end stage heart failure, if applicable (I50.84)

      Excludes1   combined systolic (congestive) and
                 diastolic (congestive) heart failure
                 (I50.4-)
      (Ex:) **For category I50.2 CC codes:** See PDX Collection 682

      **I50.20   Unspecified systolic (congestive) heart
            failure** 🔹🔹

      I50.21   Acute systolic (congestive) heart failure 🔹🔹
            Presenting a short and relatively severe episode

      I50.22   Chronic systolic (congestive) heart failure 🔹🔹
            Long-lasting, presenting over time

      **I50.23   Acute on chronic systolic (congestive) heart
            failure** 🔹🔹
            *Combination code. What was a chronic condition
               now has an acute exacerbation (to make more
               severe).*
            Coding Clinic: 2013, Q2, P33

●   **I50.3   Diastolic (congestive) heart failure**
      Diastolic left ventricular heart failure
      Heart failure with normal ejection fraction
      Heart failure with preserved ejection fraction [HFpEF]
      Code also end stage heart failure, if applicable (I50.84)

      Excludes1   combined systolic (congestive) and
                 diastolic (congestive) heart failure
                 (I50.4-)
      (Ex:) **For category I50.3 CC codes:** See PDX Collection 682

      **I50.30   Unspecified diastolic (congestive) heart
            failure** 🔹🔹

      I50.31   Acute diastolic (congestive) heart failure 🔹🔹
            Coding Clinic: 2017, Q1, P46

      I50.32   Chronic diastolic (congestive) heart failure 🔹🔹

      **I50.33   Acute on chronic diastolic (congestive) heart
            failure** 🔹🔹

●   **I50.4   Combined systolic (congestive) and diastolic
      (congestive) heart failure**
      Combined systolic and diastolic left ventricular heart
        failure
      Heart failure with reduced ejection fraction and
        diastolic dysfunction
      Code also end stage heart failure, if applicable (I50.84)
      (Ex:) **For category I50.4 CC codes:** See PDX Collection 682

      **I50.40   Unspecified combined systolic (congestive) and
            diastolic (congestive) heart failure** 🔹🔹

      **I50.41   Acute combined systolic (congestive) and
            diastolic (congestive) heart failure** 🔹🔹

      **I50.42   Chronic combined systolic (congestive) and
            diastolic (congestive) heart failure** 🔹🔹

      **I50.43   Acute on chronic combined systolic
            (congestive) and diastolic (congestive) heart
            failure** 🔹🔹

●   **I50.8   Other heart failure**

  ●   **I50.81   Right heart failure**
            Right ventricular failure

      I50.810   Right heart failure, unspecified 🔹
               Right heart failure without mention
                 of left heart failure
               Right ventricular failure NOS

      I50.811   Acute right heart failure 🔹
               Acute isolated right heart failure
               Acute (isolated) right ventricular
                 failure

      I50.812   Chronic right heart failure 🔹
               Chronic isolated right heart failure
               Chronic (isolated) right ventricular
                 failure

Item 9–8 Congestive heart failure (CHF) is a condition in which the left ventricle of the heart cannot pump enough blood to the body. The blood flow from the heart slows or returns to the heart from the venous system (back flow) resulting in congestion (fluid accumulation) particularly in the abdomen. Most commonly, fluid collects in the lungs and results in shortness of breath, especially when in a reclining position.

▶ New   ⟹ Revised   ~~deleted~~ Deleted   Excludes 1   Excludes 2   Includes   Use additional   Code first   Code also   Key words

OGCR Official Guidelines   ● Unacceptable Principal Diagnosis   X Assign placeholder X   ● Use Additional Character(s)   ▸ Manifestation Code   Coding Clinic

I50.813 **Acute on chronic** right heart failure 🅑
 Acute on chronic isolated right heart failure
 Acute on chronic (isolated) right ventricular failure
 Acute decompensation of chronic (isolated) right ventricular failure
 Acute exacerbation of chronic (isolated) right ventricular failure

I50.814 **Right heart failure** due to left heart failure 🅑
 Right ventricular failure secondary to left ventricular failure
 Code also the type of left ventricular failure, if known (I50.2-I50.43)

 Excludes1 Right heart failure with but not due to left heart failure (I50.82)

I50.82 **Biventricular** heart failure 🅑
 Code also the type of left ventricular failure as systolic, diastolic, or combined, if known **(I50.2-I50.43)**

I50.83 **High output** heart failure 🅑

I50.84 **End stage** heart failure 🅑
 Stage D heart failure
 Code also the type of heart failure as systolic, diastolic, or combined, if known (I50.2-I50.43)

I50.89 **Other** heart failure 🅑

I50.9 Heart failure, **unspecified** 🅑
 Cardiac, heart or myocardial failure NOS
 Congestive heart disease
 Congestive heart failure NOS

 Excludes2 fluid overload unrelated to congestive heart failure (E87.70)

Coding Clinic: 2017, Q1, P45-46; 2015, Q2, P15; 2012, Q4, P92

●I51 Complications and ill-defined descriptions of heart disease
 Excludes1 any condition in I51.4-I51.9 due to hypertension (I11.-)
  any condition in I51.4-I51.9 due to hypertension and chronic kidney disease (I13.-)
  heart disease specified as rheumatic (I00-I09)

I51.0 **Cardiac septal defect, acquired** 🅑   A
 Acquired septal atrial defect (old)
 Acquired septal auricular defect (old)
 Acquired septal ventricular defect (old)

 Excludes1 cardiac septal defect as current complication following acute myocardial infarction (I23.1, I23.2)

 (Ex) See PDX Collection 3500

I51.1 **Rupture of chordae tendineae, not elsewhere classified** 🅑🅑

 Excludes1 rupture of chordae tendineae as current complication following acute myocardial infarction (I23.4)

 (Ex) See PDX Collection 655

I51.2 **Rupture of papillary muscle, not elsewhere classified** 🅑🅑

 Excludes1 rupture of papillary muscle as current complication following acute myocardial infarction (I23.5)

 (Ex) See PDX Collection 656

I51.3 **Intracardiac thrombosis, not elsewhere classified**
 Apical thrombosis (old)
 Atrial thrombosis (old)
 Auricular thrombosis (old)
 Mural thrombosis (old)
 Ventricular thrombosis (old)

 Excludes1 intracardiac thrombosis as current complication following acute myocardial infarction (I23.6)

Coding Clinic: 2013, Q1, P24

I51.4 **Myocarditis,** unspecified 🅑
 Chronic (interstitial) myocarditis
 Myocardial fibrosis
 Myocarditis NOS

 Excludes1 acute or subacute myocarditis (I40.-)

Coding Clinic: 2016, Q4, P122

I51.5 **Myocardial degeneration** 🅑
 Fatty degeneration of heart or myocardium
 Myocardial disease
 Senile degeneration of heart or myocardium

Coding Clinic: 2016, Q4, P122

I51.7 **Cardiomegaly**
 Cardiac dilatation
 Cardiac hypertrophy
 Ventricular dilatation

Coding Clinic: 2016, Q4, P122

●I51.8 **Other ill-defined heart diseases**

Coding Clinic: 2016, Q4, P122

I51.81 **Takotsubo syndrome** 🅑
 Reversible left ventricular dysfunction following sudden emotional stress
 Stress induced cardiomyopathy
 Takotsubo cardiomyopathy
 Transient left ventricular apical ballooning syndrome

 (Ex) See PDX Collection 683

I51.89 **Other ill-defined heart diseases**
 Carditis (acute)(chronic)
 Pancarditis (acute)(chronic)

Coding Clinic: 2019, Q2, P6

I51.9 **Heart disease,** unspecified

Coding Clinic: 2016, Q4, P122

▶I52 *Other heart disorders in diseases classified elsewhere*
 Code first underlying disease, such as:
 congenital syphilis (A50.5)
 mucopolysaccharidosis (E76.3)
 schistosomiasis (B65.0-B65.9)

 Excludes1 heart disease (in):
  gonococcal infection (A54.83)
  meningococcal infection (A39.50)
  rheumatoid arthritis (M05.31)
  syphilis (A52.06)

CEREBROVASCULAR DISEASES (I60-I69)

Use additional code to identify presence of:
alcohol abuse and dependence (F10.-)
exposure to environmental tobacco smoke (Z77.22)
history of tobacco dependence (Z87.891)
hypertension (I10-I16)
occupational exposure to environmental tobacco smoke (Z57.31)
tobacco dependence (F17.-)
tobacco use (Z72.0)

Excludes1 traumatic intracranial hemorrhage (S06.-)

Coding Clinic: 2015, Q4, P40

N Newborn Age: 0 P Pediatric Age: 0–17 M Maternity DX: 9–64 A Adult Age: 15–124 ♀ Females Only ♂ Males Only

🅑 Complication\Comorbidity 🅑 Major C\C (Ex) CC/MCC Exclusions 🅑 Hospital-Acquired Condition 🅑 Hierarchical Condition Category

903

▶**I5A**   **Non-ischemic myocardial injury (non-traumatic)**
  ▶Acute (non-ischemic) myocardial injury
  ▶Chronic (non-ischemic) myocardial injury
  ▶Unspecified (non-ischemic) myocardial injury
  ▶*Code first the underlying cause, if known and applicable, such as:*
     ▶acute kidney failure (N17.-)
     ▶acute myocarditis (I40.-)
     ▶cardiomyopathy (I42.-)
     ▶chronic kidney disease (CKD) (N18.-)
     ▶heart failure (I50.-)
     ▶hypertensive urgency (I16.0)
     ▶nonrheumatic aortic valve disorders (I35.-)
     ▶paroxysmal tachycardia (I47.-)
     ▶pulmonary embolism (I26.-)
     ▶pulmonary hypertension (I27.0, I27.2-)
     ▶sepsis (A41.-)
     ▶takotsubo syndrome (I51.81)

  ▶**Excludes1**   acute myocardial infarction (I21.-)
            injury of heart (S26.-)

  ▶**Excludes2**   other acute ischemic heart diseases (I24.-)

● **I60**   **Nontraumatic subarachnoid hemorrhage**

  Excludes1   syphilitic ruptured cerebral aneurysm (A52.05)

  Excludes2   sequelae of subarachnoid hemorrhage (I69.0-)

  (Ex) **For category I60 CC codes:** See PDX Collection 684

  ● **I60.0**   **Nontraumatic subarachnoid hemorrhage from carotid siphon and bifurcation**

    I60.00   **Nontraumatic subarachnoid hemorrhage from unspecified carotid siphon and bifurcation**

    I60.01   **Nontraumatic subarachnoid hemorrhage from right carotid siphon and bifurcation**

    I60.02   **Nontraumatic subarachnoid hemorrhage from left carotid siphon and bifurcation**

  ● **I60.1**   **Nontraumatic subarachnoid hemorrhage from middle cerebral artery**

    I60.10   **Nontraumatic subarachnoid hemorrhage from unspecified middle cerebral artery**

    I60.11   **Nontraumatic subarachnoid hemorrhage from right middle cerebral artery**

    I60.12   **Nontraumatic subarachnoid hemorrhage from left middle cerebral artery**

  I60.2   **Nontraumatic subarachnoid hemorrhage from anterior communicating artery**

  ● **I60.3**   **Nontraumatic subarachnoid hemorrhage from posterior communicating artery**

    I60.30   **Nontraumatic subarachnoid hemorrhage from unspecified posterior communicating artery**

    I60.31   **Nontraumatic subarachnoid hemorrhage from right posterior communicating artery**

    I60.32   **Nontraumatic subarachnoid hemorrhage from left posterior communicating artery**

  I60.4   **Nontraumatic subarachnoid hemorrhage from basilar artery**

  ● **I60.5**   **Nontraumatic subarachnoid hemorrhage from vertebral artery**

    I60.50   **Nontraumatic subarachnoid hemorrhage from unspecified vertebral artery**

    I60.51   **Nontraumatic subarachnoid hemorrhage from right vertebral artery**

    I60.52   **Nontraumatic subarachnoid hemorrhage from left vertebral artery**

  I60.6   **Nontraumatic subarachnoid hemorrhage from other intracranial arteries**

  I60.7   **Nontraumatic subarachnoid hemorrhage from unspecified intracranial artery**
     Ruptured (congenital) berry aneurysm
     Ruptured (congenital) cerebral aneurysm
     Subarachnoid hemorrhage (nontraumatic) from cerebral artery NOS
     Subarachnoid hemorrhage (nontraumatic) from communicating artery NOS

    Excludes1   berry aneurysm, nonruptured (I67.1)

  I60.8   **Other nontraumatic subarachnoid hemorrhage**
     Meningeal hemorrhage
     Rupture of cerebral arteriovenous malformation

  I60.9   **Nontraumatic subarachnoid hemorrhage, unspecified**

● **I61**   **Nontraumatic intracerebral hemorrhage**

  Excludes2   sequelae of intracerebral hemorrhage (I69.1-)

  (Ex) **For category I61 CC codes:** See PDX Collection 684
  Coding Clinic: 2017, Q2, P10

  I61.0   **Nontraumatic intracerebral hemorrhage in hemisphere, subcortical**
     Deep intracerebral hemorrhage (nontraumatic)
     Coding Clinic: 2016, Q4, P27

  I61.1   **Nontraumatic intracerebral hemorrhage in hemisphere, cortical**
     Cerebral lobe hemorrhage (nontraumatic)
     Superficial intracerebral hemorrhage (nontraumatic)
     Coding Clinic: 2016, Q4, P28

  I61.2   **Nontraumatic intracerebral hemorrhage in hemisphere, unspecified**

  I61.3   **Nontraumatic intracerebral hemorrhage in brain stem**

  I61.4   **Nontraumatic intracerebral hemorrhage in cerebellum**

  I61.5   **Nontraumatic intracerebral hemorrhage, intraventricular**

  I61.6   **Nontraumatic intracerebral hemorrhage, multiple localized**

  I61.8   **Other nontraumatic intracerebral hemorrhage**

  I61.9   **Nontraumatic intracerebral hemorrhage, unspecified**

● **I62**   **Other and unspecified nontraumatic intracranial hemorrhage**

  Excludes2   sequelae of intracranial hemorrhage (I69.2)

  (Ex) **For category I62 CC codes:** See PDX Collection 684

  ● **I62.0**   **Nontraumatic subdural hemorrhage**

    I62.00   **Nontraumatic subdural hemorrhage, unspecified**

    I62.01   **Nontraumatic acute subdural hemorrhage**

    I62.02   **Nontraumatic subacute subdural hemorrhage**

    I62.03   **Nontraumatic chronic subdural hemorrhage**

  I62.1   **Nontraumatic extradural hemorrhage**
     Nontraumatic epidural hemorrhage

  I62.9   **Nontraumatic intracranial hemorrhage, unspecified**

★ **(See Plate 31 of the Anatomy Illustrations.)**

● **I63**   **Cerebral infarction**

  Excludes1   neonatal cerebral infarction (P91.82-)

  Includes   occlusion and stenosis of cerebral and precerebral arteries, resulting in cerebral infarction

  Use additional code, if applicable, to identify status post administration of tPA (rtPA) in a different facility within the last 24 hours prior to admission to current facility (Z92.82)

  Use additional code, if known, to indicate National Institutes of Health Stroke Scale (NIHSS) score (R29.7-)

  Excludes2   sequelae of cerebral infarction (I69.3-)

  Coding Clinic: 2016, Q4, P28, 61, 127

  ● **I63.0**   **Cerebral infarction due to thrombosis of precerebral arteries**

    I63.00   **Cerebral infarction due to thrombosis of unspecified precerebral artery**
       (Ex) See PDX Collection 3605

▶ New   ⇛ Revised   ~~deleted~~ Deleted   Excludes 1   Excludes 2   Includes   Use additional   Code first   Code also   Key words
OGCR Official Guidelines   ● Unacceptable Principal Diagnosis   X Assign placeholder X   ● Use Additional Character(s)   ▸ Manifestation Code   Coding Clinic

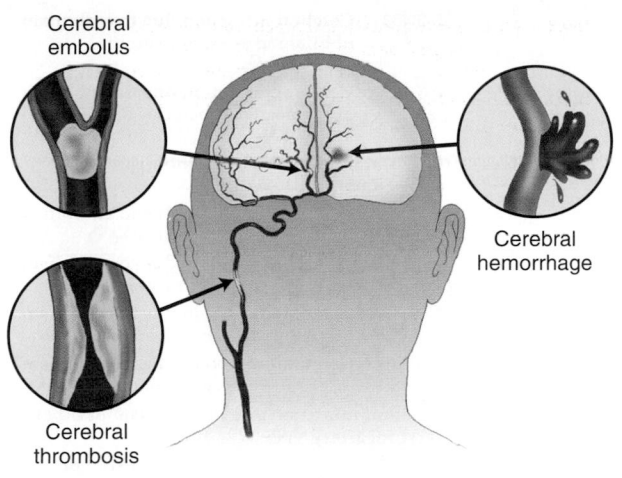

Cerebral embolus

Cerebral hemorrhage

Cerebral thrombosis

Figure 9-4 Events causing a stroke. (From Shiland: Mastering Healthcare Terminology, ed 1, St. Louis, Mosby, 2003)

● I63.01   Cerebral infarction due to thrombosis of vertebral artery
          (Ex:) For category I63.01 CC codes: See PDX Collection 3606
    I63.011   Cerebral infarction due to thrombosis of right vertebral artery 🔖🔖
    I63.012   Cerebral infarction due to thrombosis of left vertebral artery 🔖🔖
    I63.013   Cerebral infarction due to thrombosis of bilateral vertebral arteries 🔖🔖
    I63.019   Cerebral infarction due to thrombosis of unspecified vertebral artery 🔖🔖
    I63.02   Cerebral infarction due to thrombosis of basilar artery 🔖🔖
          (Ex:) See PDX Collection 3605
● I63.03   Cerebral infarction due to thrombosis of carotid artery
          (Ex:) For category I63.03 CC codes: See PDX Collection 3607
    I63.031   Cerebral infarction due to thrombosis of right carotid artery 🔖🔖
    I63.032   Cerebral infarction due to thrombosis of left carotid artery 🔖🔖
    I63.033   Cerebral infarction due to thrombosis of bilateral carotid arteries 🔖🔖
    I63.039   Cerebral infarction due to thrombosis of unspecified carotid artery 🔖🔖
    I63.09   Cerebral infarction due to thrombosis of other precerebral artery 🔖🔖
          (Ex:) See PDX Collection 3605
● I63.1   Cerebral infarction due to embolism of precerebral arteries
    I63.10   Cerebral infarction due to embolism of unspecified precerebral artery 🔖🔖
          (Ex:) See PDX Collection 3605
● I63.11   Cerebral infarction due to embolism of vertebral artery
          (Ex:) For category I63.11 CC codes: See PDX Collection 3606
    I63.111   Cerebral infarction due to embolism of right vertebral artery 🔖🔖
    I63.112   Cerebral infarction due to embolism of left vertebral artery 🔖🔖
    I63.113   Cerebral infarction due to embolism of bilateral vertebral arteries 🔖🔖
    I63.119   Cerebral infarction due to embolism of unspecified vertebral artery 🔖🔖
    I63.12   Cerebral infarction due to embolism of basilar artery 🔖🔖
          (Ex:) See PDX Collection 685

● I63.13   Cerebral infarction due to embolism of carotid artery
          (Ex:) For category I63.13 CC codes: See PDX Collection 3607
    I63.131   Cerebral infarction due to embolism of right carotid artery 🔖🔖
    I63.132   Cerebral infarction due to embolism of left carotid artery 🔖🔖
    I63.133   Cerebral infarction due to embolism of bilateral carotid arteries 🔖🔖
    I63.139   Cerebral infarction due to embolism of unspecified carotid artery 🔖🔖
    I63.19   Cerebral infarction due to embolism of other precerebral artery 🔖🔖
          (Ex:) See PDX Collection 3605
● I63.2   Cerebral infarction due to unspecified occlusion or stenosis of precerebral arteries
    I63.20   Cerebral infarction due to unspecified occlusion or stenosis of unspecified precerebral arteries 🔖🔖
          (Ex:) See PDX Collection 3605
● I63.21   Cerebral infarction due to unspecified occlusion or stenosis of vertebral artery
          (Ex:) For category I63.21 CC codes: See PDX Collection 3606
    I63.211   Cerebral infarction due to unspecified occlusion or stenosis of right vertebral artery 🔖🔖
    I63.212   Cerebral infarction due to unspecified occlusion or stenosis of left vertebral artery 🔖🔖
    I63.213   Cerebral infarction due to unspecified occlusion or stenosis of bilateral vertebral arteries 🔖🔖
    I63.219   Cerebral infarction due to unspecified occlusion or stenosis of unspecified vertebral artery 🔖🔖
    I63.22   Cerebral infarction due to unspecified occlusion or stenosis of basilar artery 🔖🔖
          (Ex:) See PDX Collection 3605
● I63.23   Cerebral infarction due to unspecified occlusion or stenosis of carotid arteries
          (Ex:) For category I63.23 CC codes: See PDX Collection 3607
    I63.231   Cerebral infarction due to unspecified occlusion or stenosis of right carotid arteries 🔖🔖
    I63.232   Cerebral infarction due to unspecified occlusion or stenosis of left carotid arteries 🔖🔖
    I63.233   Cerebral infarction due to unspecified occlusion or stenosis of bilateral carotid arteries 🔖🔖
    I63.239   Cerebral infarction due to unspecified occlusion or stenosis of unspecified carotid arteries 🔖🔖
    I63.29   Cerebral infarction due to unspecified occlusion or stenosis of other precerebral arteries 🔖🔖
          (Ex:) See PDX Collection 3605
● I63.3   Cerebral infarction due to thrombosis of cerebral arteries
          (Ex:) For category I63.3 CC codes: See PDX Collection 3608
    I63.30   Cerebral infarction due to thrombosis of unspecified cerebral artery 🔖🔖
● I63.31   Cerebral infarction due to thrombosis of middle cerebral artery
    I63.311   Cerebral infarction due to thrombosis of right middle cerebral artery 🔖🔖
    I63.312   Cerebral infarction due to thrombosis of left middle cerebral artery 🔖🔖
    I63.313   Cerebral infarction due to thrombosis of bilateral middle cerebral arteries 🔖🔖
    I63.319   Cerebral infarction due to thrombosis of unspecified middle cerebral artery 🔖🔖

N Newborn Age: Ø   **P** Pediatric Age: Ø–17   **M** Maternity DX: 9–64   **A** Adult Age: 15–124   ♀ Females Only   ♂ Males Only

🔖 Complication\Comorbidity   🔖 Major C\C   (Ex:) CC/MCC Exclusions   🔖 Hospital-Acquired Condition   🔖 Hierarchical Condition Category

CHAPTER 9 (I00-I99)

● I63.32   Cerebral infarction due to thrombosis of anterior cerebral artery
    I63.321   Cerebral infarction due to thrombosis of right anterior cerebral artery ✎ ℞
    I63.322   Cerebral infarction due to thrombosis of left anterior cerebral artery ✎ ℞
    I63.323   Cerebral infarction due to thrombosis of bilateral anterior cerebral arteries ✎ ℞
    I63.329   Cerebral infarction due to thrombosis of unspecified anterior cerebral artery ✎ ℞

● I63.33   Cerebral infarction due to thrombosis of posterior cerebral artery
    I63.331   Cerebral infarction due to thrombosis of right posterior cerebral artery ✎ ℞
    I63.332   Cerebral infarction due to thrombosis of left posterior cerebral artery ✎ ℞
    I63.333   Cerebral infarction due to thrombosis of bilateral posterior cerebral arteries ✎ ℞
    I63.339   Cerebral infarction due to thrombosis of unspecified posterior cerebral artery ✎ ℞

● I63.34   Cerebral infarction due to thrombosis of cerebellar artery
    I63.341   Cerebral infarction due to thrombosis of right cerebellar artery ✎ ℞
    I63.342   Cerebral infarction due to thrombosis of left cerebellar artery ✎ ℞
    I63.343   Cerebral infarction due to thrombosis of bilateral cerebellar arteries ✎ ℞
    I63.349   Cerebral infarction due to thrombosis of unspecified cerebellar artery ✎ ℞

   I63.39   Cerebral infarction due to thrombosis of other cerebral artery ✎ ℞

● I63.4   Cerebral infarction due to embolism of cerebral arteries
    Ⓔⓧ For category I63.4 CC codes: See PDX Collection 3608

   I63.40   Cerebral infarction due to embolism of unspecified cerebral artery ✎ ℞

● I63.41   Cerebral infarction due to embolism of middle cerebral artery
    I63.411   Cerebral infarction due to embolism of right middle cerebral artery ✎ ℞
    I63.412   Cerebral infarction due to embolism of left middle cerebral artery ✎ ℞
    I63.413   Cerebral infarction due to embolism of bilateral middle cerebral arteries ✎ ℞
    I63.419   Cerebral infarction due to embolism of unspecified middle cerebral artery ✎ ℞

● I63.42   Cerebral infarction due to embolism of anterior cerebral artery
    I63.421   Cerebral infarction due to embolism of right anterior cerebral artery ✎ ℞
    I63.422   Cerebral infarction due to embolism of left anterior cerebral artery ✎ ℞
    I63.423   Cerebral infarction due to embolism of bilateral anterior cerebral arteries ✎ ℞
    I63.429   Cerebral infarction due to embolism of unspecified anterior cerebral artery ✎ ℞

● I63.43   Cerebral infarction due to embolism of posterior cerebral artery
    I63.431   Cerebral infarction due to embolism of right posterior cerebral artery ✎ ℞
    I63.432   Cerebral infarction due to embolism of left posterior cerebral artery ✎ ℞

    I63.433   Cerebral infarction due to embolism of bilateral posterior cerebral arteries ✎ ℞
    I63.439   Cerebral infarction due to embolism of unspecified posterior cerebral artery ✎ ℞

● I63.44   Cerebral infarction due to embolism of cerebellar artery
    I63.441   Cerebral infarction due to embolism of right cerebellar artery ✎ ℞
    I63.442   Cerebral infarction due to embolism of left cerebellar artery ✎ ℞
    I63.443   Cerebral infarction due to embolism of bilateral cerebellar arteries ✎ ℞
    I63.449   Cerebral infarction due to embolism of unspecified cerebellar artery ✎ ℞

   I63.49   Cerebral infarction due to embolism of other cerebral artery ✎ ℞

● I63.5   Cerebral infarction due to unspecified occlusion or stenosis of cerebral arteries
    Ⓔⓧ For category I63.5 CC codes: See PDX Collection 3608

   I63.50   Cerebral infarction due to unspecified occlusion or stenosis of unspecified cerebral artery ✎ ℞

● I63.51   Cerebral infarction due to unspecified occlusion or stenosis of middle cerebral artery
    I63.511   Cerebral infarction due to unspecified occlusion or stenosis of right middle cerebral artery ✎ ℞
    I63.512   Cerebral infarction due to unspecified occlusion or stenosis of left middle cerebral artery ✎ ℞
    I63.513   Cerebral infarction due to unspecified occlusion or stenosis of bilateral middle cerebral arteries ✎ ℞
    I63.519   Cerebral infarction due to unspecified occlusion or stenosis of unspecified middle cerebral artery ✎ ℞

● I63.52   Cerebral infarction due to unspecified occlusion or stenosis of anterior cerebral artery
    I63.521   Cerebral infarction due to unspecified occlusion or stenosis of right anterior cerebral artery ✎ ℞
    I63.522   Cerebral infarction due to unspecified occlusion or stenosis of left anterior cerebral artery ✎ ℞
    I63.523   Cerebral infarction due to unspecified occlusion or stenosis of bilateral anterior cerebral arteries ✎ ℞
    I63.529   Cerebral infarction due to unspecified occlusion or stenosis of unspecified anterior cerebral artery ✎ ℞

● I63.53   Cerebral infarction due to unspecified occlusion or stenosis of posterior cerebral artery
    I63.531   Cerebral infarction due to unspecified occlusion or stenosis of right posterior cerebral artery ✎ ℞
    I63.532   Cerebral infarction due to unspecified occlusion or stenosis of left posterior cerebral artery ✎ ℞
        Coding Clinic: 2017, Q2, P10
    I63.533   Cerebral infarction due to unspecified occlusion or stenosis of bilateral posterior cerebral arteries ✎ ℞
    I63.539   Cerebral infarction due to unspecified occlusion or stenosis of unspecified posterior cerebral artery ✎ ℞

● I63.54   Cerebral infarction due to unspecified occlusion or stenosis of cerebellar artery
    I63.541   Cerebral infarction due to unspecified occlusion or stenosis of right cerebellar artery ✎ ℞
    I63.542   Cerebral infarction due to unspecified occlusion or stenosis of left cerebellar artery ✎ ℞

▶ New   ⇒ Revised   ~~deleted~~ Deleted   Excludes 1   Excludes 2   Includes   Use additional   Code first   Code also   Key words

OGCR Official Guidelines   ● Unacceptable Principal Diagnosis   X Assign placeholder X   ● Use Additional Character(s)   ▶ Manifestation Code   Coding Clinic

I63.543 Cerebral infarction due to unspecified occlusion or stenosis of bilateral cerebellar arteries 🏥🏥

I63.549 Cerebral infarction due to unspecified occlusion or stenosis of unspecified cerebellar artery 🏥🏥

I63.59 Cerebral infarction due to unspecified occlusion or stenosis of other cerebral artery 🏥🏥

I63.6 Cerebral infarction due to cerebral venous thrombosis, nonpyogenic 🏥🏥
Ex: See PDX Collection 3608

● I63.8 Other cerebral infarction 🏥🏥
Ex: For category I63.8 MCC codes: See PDX Collection 3608

I63.81 Other cerebral infarction due to occlusion or stenosis of small artery 🏥🏥
Lacunar infarction
Coding Clinic: 2018, Q4, P16

I63.89 Other cerebral infarction 🏥🏥
Coding Clinic: 2017, Q2, P9

I63.9 Cerebral infarction, unspecified 🏥🏥
Stroke NOS

Excludes2 transient cerebral ischemic attacks and related syndromes (G45.-)
Ex: See PDX Collection 688
Coding Clinic: 2016, Q4, P62; 2015, Q1, P26

● I65 Occlusion and stenosis of precerebral arteries, not resulting in cerebral infarction

Includes embolism of precerebral artery
narrowing of precerebral artery
obstruction (complete) (partial) of precerebral artery
thrombosis of precerebral artery

Excludes1 insufficiency, NOS, of precerebral artery (G45.-)
insufficiency of precerebral arteries causing cerebral infarction (I63.0-I63.2)

● I65.0 Occlusion and stenosis of vertebral artery

I65.01 Occlusion and stenosis of right vertebral artery

I65.02 Occlusion and stenosis of left vertebral artery

I65.03 Occlusion and stenosis of bilateral vertebral arteries

I65.09 Occlusion and stenosis of unspecified vertebral artery

I65.1 Occlusion and stenosis of basilar artery

● I65.2 Occlusion and stenosis of carotid artery

I65.21 Occlusion and stenosis of right carotid artery

I65.22 Occlusion and stenosis of left carotid artery

I65.23 Occlusion and stenosis of bilateral carotid arteries
Coding Clinic: 2021, Q1, P4

I65.29 Occlusion and stenosis of unspecified carotid artery

I65.8 Occlusion and stenosis of other precerebral arteries

I65.9 Occlusion and stenosis of unspecified precerebral artery
Occlusion and stenosis of precerebral artery NOS

● I66 Occlusion and stenosis of cerebral arteries, not resulting in cerebral infarction

Includes embolism of cerebral artery
narrowing of cerebral artery
obstruction (complete) (partial) of cerebral artery
thrombosis of cerebral artery

Excludes1 occlusion and stenosis of cerebral artery causing cerebral infarction (I63.3-I63.5)

● I66.0 Occlusion and stenosis of middle cerebral artery

I66.01 Occlusion and stenosis of right middle cerebral artery

I66.02 Occlusion and stenosis of left middle cerebral artery

I66.03 Occlusion and stenosis of bilateral middle cerebral arteries

I66.09 Occlusion and stenosis of unspecified middle cerebral artery

● I66.1 Occlusion and stenosis of anterior cerebral artery

I66.11 Occlusion and stenosis of right anterior cerebral artery

I66.12 Occlusion and stenosis of left anterior cerebral artery

I66.13 Occlusion and stenosis of bilateral anterior cerebral arteries

I66.19 Occlusion and stenosis of unspecified anterior cerebral artery

● I66.2 Occlusion and stenosis of posterior cerebral artery

I66.21 Occlusion and stenosis of right posterior cerebral artery

I66.22 Occlusion and stenosis of left posterior cerebral artery

I66.23 Occlusion and stenosis of bilateral posterior cerebral arteries

I66.29 Occlusion and stenosis of unspecified posterior cerebral artery

I66.3 Occlusion and stenosis of cerebellar arteries

I66.8 Occlusion and stenosis of other cerebral arteries
Occlusion and stenosis of perforating arteries

I66.9 Occlusion and stenosis of unspecified cerebral artery

● I67 Other cerebrovascular diseases

Excludes2 sequelae of the listed conditions (I69.8)

I67.0 Dissection of cerebral arteries, nonruptured 🏥🏥

Excludes1 ruptured cerebral arteries (I60.7)
Ex: See PDX Collection 689

I67.1 Cerebral aneurysm, nonruptured
Cerebral aneurysm NOS
Cerebral arteriovenous fistula, acquired
Internal carotid artery aneurysm, intracranial portion
Internal carotid artery aneurysm, NOS

Excludes1 congenital cerebral aneurysm, nonruptured (Q28.-)
ruptured cerebral aneurysm (I60.7)

I67.2 Cerebral atherosclerosis   A
Atheroma of cerebral and precerebral arteries

I67.3 Progressive vascular leukoencephalopathy 🏥
Binswanger's disease
Ex: See PDX Collection 133

I67.4 Hypertensive encephalopathy 🏥

Excludes2 insufficiency, NOS, of precerebral arteries (G45.2)
Ex: See PDX Collection 690

I67.5 Moyamoya disease 🏥
Ex: See PDX Collection 691

I67.6 Nonpyogenic thrombosis of intracranial venous system 🏥
Nonpyogenic thrombosis of cerebral vein
Nonpyogenic thrombosis of intracranial venous sinus

Excludes1 nonpyogenic thrombosis of intracranial venous system causing infarction (I63.6)
Ex: See PDX Collection 692

I67.7 Cerebral arteritis, not elsewhere classified 🏥
Granulomatous angiitis of the nervous system

Excludes1 allergic granulomatous angiitis (M30.1)
Ex: See PDX Collection 693

● I67.8 Other specified cerebrovascular diseases

I67.81 Acute cerebrovascular insufficiency 🏥
Acute cerebrovascular insufficiency unspecified as to location or reversibility
Ex: See PDX Collection 694

I67.82 Cerebral ischemia 🏥
Chronic cerebral ischemia
Ex: See PDX Collection 694

I67.83 Posterior reversible encephalopathy syndrome 🏥
PRES
Ex: See PDX Collection 610

N Newborn Age: 0   P Pediatric Age: 0–17   M Maternity DX: 9–64   A Adult Age: 15–124   ♀ Females Only   ♂ Males Only

🏥 Complication\Comorbidity   🏥 Major C\C   Ex: CC/MCC Exclusions   🏥 Hospital-Acquired Condition   🏥 Hierarchical Condition Category

● **I67.84**   **Cerebral vasospasm and vasoconstriction**
Ex: For category I67.84 CC codes: See PDX Collection 586

    I67.841   **Reversible cerebrovascular vasoconstriction syndrome** 🔗
        Call-Fleming syndrome
        Code first underlying condition, if applicable, such as eclampsia (O15.00-O15.9)

    I67.848   **Other cerebrovascular vasospasm and vasoconstriction** 🔗

● **I67.85**   **Hereditary cerebrovascular diseases**

    I67.850   **Cerebral autosomal dominant arteriopathy with subcortical infarcts and leukoencephalopathy** 🔗
        CADASIL

        Code also any associated diagnoses, such as:
          epilepsy (G40.-), stroke (I63.-)
          vascular dementia (F01.-)
        Ex: See PDX Collection 694

    I67.858   **Other hereditary cerebrovascular disease** 🔗
        Ex: See PDX Collection 694

    I67.89   **Other cerebrovascular disease** 🔗
        Ex: See PDX Collection 694

  I67.9   **Cerebrovascular disease, unspecified**

● **I68**   **Cerebrovascular disorders in diseases classified elsewhere**

▷ *I68.0*   *Cerebral amyloid angiopathy*
    Code first underlying amyloidosis (E85.-)

▷ *I68.2*   *Cerebral arteritis in other diseases classified elsewhere* 🔗
    Code first underlying disease
    Excludes1   cerebral arteritis (in):
        listerosis (A32.89)
        systemic lupus erythematosus (M32.19)
        syphilis (A52.04)
        tuberculosis (A18.89)
      Ex: See PDX Collection 693

▷ *I68.8*   *Other cerebrovascular disorders in diseases classified elsewhere*
    Code first underlying disease
    Excludes1   syphilitic cerebral aneurysm (A52.05)

  OGCR Section I.c.9.d.

Sequelae of Cerebrovascular Disease

1) Category I69, Sequelae of Cerebrovascular disease

Category I69 is used to indicate conditions classifiable to categories I60-I67 as the causes of sequela (neurologic deficits), themselves classified elsewhere. These "late effects" include neurologic deficits that persist after initial onset of conditions classifiable to categories I60-I67. The neurologic deficits caused by cerebrovascular disease may be present from the onset of may arise at any time after the onset of the condition classifiable to categories I60-I67.

Codes from category I69, Sequelae of cerebrovascular disease, that specify hemiplegia, hemiparesis and monoplegia identify whether the dominant or nondominant side is affected. Should the affected side be documented, but not specified as dominant or nondominant, and the classification system does not indicate a default, code selection is as follows:

For ambidextrous patients, the default should be dominant.

If the left side is affected, the default is nondominant.

If the right side is affected, the default is dominant.

2) Codes from category I69 with codes from I60-I67

Codes from category I69 may be assigned on a health care record with codes from I60-I67, if the patient has a current cerebrovascular disease and deficits from an old cerebrovascular disease.

● **I69**   **Sequelae of cerebrovascular disease**
Note: Category I69 is to be used to indicate conditions in I60-I67 as the cause of sequelae. The 'sequelae' include conditions specified as such or as residuals which may occur at any time after the onset of the causal condition.
  Excludes1   personal history of cerebral infarction without residual deficit (Z86.73)
      personal history of prolonged reversible ischemic neurologic deficit (PRIND) (Z86.73)
      personal history of reversible ischemic neurologcial deficit (RIND) (Z86.73)
      sequelae of traumatic intracranial injury (S06.-)
  Coding Clinic: 2016, Q4, P28; 2015, Q4, P40; 2012, Q4, P107

● **I69.0**   **Sequelae of nontraumatic subarachnoid hemorrhage**

  I69.00   **Unspecified sequelae of nontraumatic subarachnoid hemorrhage**

●   **I69.01**   **Cognitive deficits following nontraumatic subarachnoid hemorrhage**

    I69.010   **Attention and concentration deficit following nontraumatic subarachnoid hemorrhage**

    I69.011   **Memory deficit following nontraumatic subarachnoid hemorrhage**

    I69.012   **Visuospatial deficit and spatial neglect following nontraumatic subarachnoid hemorrhage**

    I69.013   **Psychomotor deficit following nontraumatic subarachnoid hemorrhage**

    I69.014   **Frontal lobe and executive function deficit following nontraumatic subarachnoid hemorrhage**

    I69.015   **Cognitive social or emotional deficit following nontraumatic subarachnoid hemorrhage**

    I69.018   **Other symptoms and signs involving cognitive functions following nontraumatic subarachnoid hemorrhage**

    I69.019   **Unspecified symptoms and signs involving cognitive functions following nontraumatic subarachnoid hemorrhage**

●   **I69.02**   **Speech and language deficits following nontraumatic subarachnoid hemorrhage**

    I69.020   **Aphasia following nontraumatic subarachnoid hemorrhage**

    I69.021   **Dysphasia following nontraumatic subarachnoid hemorrhage**

    I69.022   **Dysarthria following nontraumatic subarachnoid hemorrhage**

    I69.023   **Fluency disorder following nontraumatic subarachnoid hemorrhage**
        Stuttering following nontraumatic subarachnoid hemorrhage

    I69.028   **Other speech and language deficits following nontraumatic subarachnoid hemorrhage**

● I69.03 Monoplegia of upper limb following nontraumatic subarachnoid hemorrhage

    I69.031 Monoplegia of upper limb following nontraumatic subarachnoid hemorrhage affecting right dominant side 🔖

    I69.032 Monoplegia of upper limb following nontraumatic subarachnoid hemorrhage affecting left dominant side 🔖

    I69.033 Monoplegia of upper limb following nontraumatic subarachnoid hemorrhage affecting right non-dominant side 🔖

    I69.034 Monoplegia of upper limb following nontraumatic subarachnoid hemorrhage affecting left non-dominant side 🔖

    I69.039 Monoplegia of upper limb following nontraumatic subarachnoid hemorrhage affecting unspecified side 🔖

● I69.04 Monoplegia of lower limb following nontraumatic subarachnoid hemorrhage

    I69.041 Monoplegia of lower limb following nontraumatic subarachnoid hemorrhage affecting right dominant side 🔖

    I69.042 Monoplegia of lower limb following nontraumatic subarachnoid hemorrhage affecting left dominant side 🔖

    I69.043 Monoplegia of lower limb following nontraumatic subarachnoid hemorrhage affecting right non-dominant side 🔖

    I69.044 Monoplegia of lower limb following nontraumatic subarachnoid hemorrhage affecting left non-dominant side 🔖

    I69.049 Monoplegia of lower limb following nontraumatic subarachnoid hemorrhage affecting unspecified side 🔖

● I69.05 Hemiplegia and hemiparesis following nontraumatic subarachnoid hemorrhage

    I69.051 Hemiplegia and hemiparesis following nontraumatic subarachnoid hemorrhage affecting right dominant side 🔖 🔖
        (Ex:) See PDX Collection 695

    I69.052 Hemiplegia and hemiparesis following nontraumatic subarachnoid hemorrhage affecting left dominant side 🔖 🔖
        (Ex:) See PDX Collection 695

    I69.053 Hemiplegia and hemiparesis following nontraumatic subarachnoid hemorrhage affecting right non-dominant side 🔖 🔖
        (Ex:) See PDX Collection 696

    I69.054 Hemiplegia and hemiparesis following nontraumatic subarachnoid hemorrhage affecting left non-dominant side 🔖 🔖
        (Ex:) See PDX Collection 696

    I69.059 Hemiplegia and hemiparesis following nontraumatic subarachnoid hemorrhage affecting unspecified side 🔖 🔖
        (Ex:) See PDX Collection 697

● I69.06 Other paralytic syndrome following nontraumatic subarachnoid hemorrhage

    Use additional code to identify type of paralytic syndrome, such as:
    locked-in state (G83.5)
    quadriplegia (G82.5-)

    Excludes 1 hemiplegia/hemiparesis following nontraumatic subarachnoid hemorrhage (I69.05-)
        monoplegia of lower limb following nontraumatic subarachnoid hemorrhage (I69.04-)
        monoplegia of upper limb following nontraumatic subarachnoid hemorrhage (I69.03-)

    I69.061 Other paralytic syndrome following nontraumatic subarachnoid hemorrhage affecting right dominant side 🔖

    I69.062 Other paralytic syndrome following nontraumatic subarachnoid hemorrhage affecting left dominant side 🔖

    I69.063 Other paralytic syndrome following nontraumatic subarachnoid hemorrhage affecting right non-dominant side 🔖

    I69.064 Other paralytic syndrome following nontraumatic subarachnoid hemorrhage affecting left non-dominant side 🔖

    I69.065 Other paralytic syndrome following nontraumatic subarachnoid hemorrhage, bilateral 🔖

    I69.069 Other paralytic syndrome following nontraumatic subarachnoid hemorrhage affecting unspecified side 🔖

● I69.09 Other sequelae of nontraumatic subarachnoid hemorrhage

    I69.090 Apraxia following nontraumatic subarachnoid hemorrhage

    I69.091 Dysphagia following nontraumatic subarachnoid hemorrhage
        Use additional code to identify the type of dysphagia, if known (R13.1-)

    I69.092 Facial weakness following nontraumatic subarachnoid hemorrhage
        Facial droop following nontraumatic subarachnoid hemorrhage

    I69.093 Ataxia following nontraumatic subarachnoid hemorrhage

    I69.098 Other sequelae following nontraumatic subarachnoid hemorrhage
        Alterations of sensation following nontraumatic subarachnoid hemorrhage
        Disturbance of vision following nontraumatic subarachnoid hemorrhage
        Use additional code to identify the sequelae

N Newborn Age: 0   **P** Pediatric Age: 0–17   **M** Maternity DX: 9–64   **A** Adult Age: 15–124   ♀ Females Only   ♂ Males Only

🔖 Complication\Comorbidity   🔖 Major C\C   (Ex:) CC/MCC Exclusions   🔖 Hospital-Acquired Condition   🔖 Hierarchical Condition Category

909

CHAPTER 9 (I00-I99)

● I69.1   Sequelae of nontraumatic intracerebral hemorrhage

   I69.10   Unspecified sequelae of nontraumatic intracerebral hemorrhage

● I69.11   Cognitive deficits following nontraumatic intracerebral hemorrhage

     I69.110   Attention and concentration deficit following nontraumatic intracerebral hemorrhage

     I69.111   Memory deficit following nontraumatic intracerebral hemorrhage

     I69.112   Visuospatial deficit and spatial neglect following nontraumatic intracerebral hemorrhage

     I69.113   Psychomotor deficit following nontraumatic intracerebral hemorrhage

     I69.114   Frontal lobe and executive function deficit following nontraumatic intracerebral hemorrhage

     I69.115   Cognitive social or emotional deficit following nontraumatic intracerebral hemorrhage

     I69.118   Other symptoms and signs involving cognitive functions following nontraumatic intracerebral hemorrhage

     I69.119   Unspecified symptoms and signs involving cognitive functions following nontraumatic intracerebral hemorrhage

● I69.12   Speech and language deficits following nontraumatic intracerebral hemorrhage

     I69.120   Aphasia following nontraumatic intracerebral hemorrhage

     I69.121   Dysphasia following nontraumatic intracerebral hemorrhage

     I69.122   Dysarthria following nontraumatic intracerebral hemorrhage

     I69.123   Fluency disorder following nontraumatic intracerebral hemorrhage

        Stuttering following nontraumatic intracerebral hemorrhage

     I69.128   Other speech and language deficits following nontraumatic intracerebral hemorrhage

● I69.13   Monoplegia of upper limb following nontraumatic intracerebral hemorrhage

     I69.131   Monoplegia of upper limb following nontraumatic intracerebral hemorrhage affecting right dominant side 🦠

     I69.132   Monoplegia of upper limb following nontraumatic intracerebral hemorrhage affecting left dominant side 🦠

     I69.133   Monoplegia of upper limb following nontraumatic intracerebral hemorrhage affecting right non-dominant side 🦠

     I69.134   Monoplegia of upper limb following nontraumatic intracerebral hemorrhage affecting left non-dominant side 🦠

     I69.139   Monoplegia of upper limb following nontraumatic intracerebral hemorrhage affecting unspecified side 🦠

● I69.14   Monoplegia of lower limb following nontraumatic intracerebral hemorrhage

     I69.141   Monoplegia of lower limb following nontraumatic intracerebral hemorrhage affecting right dominant side 🦠

     I69.142   Monoplegia of lower limb following nontraumatic intracerebral hemorrhage affecting left dominant side 🦠

     I69.143   Monoplegia of lower limb following nontraumatic intracerebral hemorrhage affecting right non-dominant side 🦠

     I69.144   Monoplegia of lower limb following nontraumatic intracerebral hemorrhage affecting left non-dominant side 🦠

     I69.149   Monoplegia of lower limb following nontraumatic intracerebral hemorrhage affecting unspecified side 🦠

● I69.15   Hemiplegia and hemiparesis following nontraumatic intracerebral hemorrhage

     I69.151   Hemiplegia and hemiparesis following nontraumatic intracerebral hemorrhage affecting right dominant side 🦠 🦠
        (Ex:) See PDX Collection 695

     I69.152   Hemiplegia and hemiparesis following nontraumatic intracerebral hemorrhage affecting left dominant side 🦠 🦠
        (Ex:) See PDX Collection 695

     I69.153   Hemiplegia and hemiparesis following nontraumatic intracerebral hemorrhage affecting right non-dominant side 🦠 🦠
        (Ex:) See PDX Collection 696

     I69.154   Hemiplegia and hemiparesis following nontraumatic intracerebral hemorrhage affecting left non-dominant side 🦠 🦠
        (Ex:) See PDX Collection 696

     I69.159   Hemiplegia and hemiparesis following nontraumatic intracerebral hemorrhage affecting unspecified side 🦠 🦠
        (Ex:) See PDX Collection 697

● I69.16   Other paralytic syndrome following nontraumatic intracerebral hemorrhage

    Use additional code to identify type of paralytic syndrome, such as:
    locked-in state (G83.5)
    quadriplegia (G82.5-)

    Excludes1   hemiplegia/hemiparesis following nontraumatic intracerebral hemorrhage (I69.15-)
        monoplegia of lower limb following nontraumatic intracerebral hemorrhage (I69.14-)
        monoplegia of upper limb following nontraumatic intracerebral hemorrhage (I69.13-)

     I69.161   Other paralytic syndrome following nontraumatic intracerebral hemorrhage affecting right dominant side 🦠

▶ New   ⇨ Revised   ~~deleted~~ Deleted | Excludes 1 | | Excludes 2 | | Includes | | Use additional | | Code first | Code also | Key words |

OGCR Official Guidelines   ● Unacceptable Principal Diagnosis   X Assign placeholder X   ● Use Additional Character(s)   ▶ Manifestation Code   **Coding Clinic**

I69.162 Other paralytic syndrome following nontraumatic intracerebral hemorrhage affecting left dominant side 🖋

I69.163 Other paralytic syndrome following nontraumatic intracerebral hemorrhage affecting right non-dominant side 🖋

I69.164 Other paralytic syndrome following nontraumatic intracerebral hemorrhage affecting left non-dominant side 🖋

I69.165 Other paralytic syndrome following nontraumatic intracerebral hemorrhage, bilateral 🖋

I69.169 Other paralytic syndrome following nontraumatic intracerebral hemorrhage affecting unspecified side 🖋

● I69.19 Other sequelae of nontraumatic intracerebral hemorrhage

I69.190 Apraxia following nontraumatic intracerebral hemorrhage

I69.191 Dysphagia following nontraumatic intracerebral hemorrhage

    Use additional code to identify the type of dysphagia, if known (R13.1-)

I69.192 Facial weakness following nontraumatic intracerebral hemorrhage

    Facial droop following nontraumatic intracerebral hemorrhage

I69.193 Ataxia following nontraumatic intracerebral hemorrhage

I69.198 Other sequelae of nontraumatic intracerebral hemorrhage

    Alteration of sensations following nontraumatic intracerebral hemorrhage

    Disturbance of vision following nontraumatic intracerebral hemorrhage

    Use additional code to identify the sequelae

● I69.2 Sequelae of other nontraumatic intracranial hemorrhage

I69.20 Unspecified sequelae of other nontraumatic intracranial hemorrhage

● I69.21 Cognitive deficits following other nontraumatic intracranial hemorrhage

I69.210 Attention and concentration deficit following other nontraumatic intracranial hemorrhage

I69.211 Memory deficit following other nontraumatic intracranial hemorrhage

I69.212 Visuospatial deficit and spatial neglect following other nontraumatic intracranial hemorrhage

I69.213 Psychomotor deficit following other nontraumatic intracranial hemorrhage

I69.214 Frontal lobe and executive function deficit following other nontraumatic intracranial hemorrhage

I69.215 Cognitive social or emotional deficit following other nontraumatic intracranial hemorrhage

I69.218 Other symptoms and signs involving cognitive functions following other nontraumatic intracranial hemorrhage

I69.219 Unspecified symptoms and signs involving cognitive functions following other nontraumatic intracranial hemorrhage

● I69.22 Speech and language deficits following other nontraumatic intracranial hemorrhage

I69.220 Aphasia following other nontraumatic intracranial hemorrhage

I69.221 Dysphasia following other nontraumatic intracranial hemorrhage

I69.222 Dysarthria following other nontraumatic intracranial hemorrhage

I69.223 Fluency disorder following other nontraumatic intracranial hemorrhage

    Stuttering following other nontraumatic intracranial hemorrhage

I69.228 Other speech and language deficits following other nontraumatic intracranial hemorrhage

● I69.23 Monoplegia of upper limb following other nontraumatic intracranial hemorrhage

I69.231 Monoplegia of upper limb following other nontraumatic intracranial hemorrhage affecting right dominant side 🖋

I69.232 Monoplegia of upper limb following other nontraumatic intracranial hemorrhage affecting left dominant side 🖋

I69.233 Monoplegia of upper limb following other nontraumatic intracranial hemorrhage affecting right non-dominant side 🖋

I69.234 Monoplegia of upper limb following other nontraumatic intracranial hemorrhage affecting left non-dominant side 🖋

I69.239 Monoplegia of upper limb following other nontraumatic intracranial hemorrhage affecting unspecified side 🖋

● I69.24 Monoplegia of lower limb following other nontraumatic intracranial hemorrhage

I69.241 Monoplegia of lower limb following other nontraumatic intracranial hemorrhage affecting right dominant side 🖋

I69.242 Monoplegia of lower limb following other nontraumatic intracranial hemorrhage affecting left dominant side 🖋

I69.243 Monoplegia of lower limb following other nontraumatic intracranial hemorrhage affecting right non-dominant side 🖋

I69.244 Monoplegia of lower limb following other nontraumatic intracranial hemorrhage affecting left non-dominant side 🖋

I69.249 Monoplegia of lower limb following other nontraumatic intracranial hemorrhage affecting unspecified side 🖋

CHAPTER 9 (I00-I99)

N Newborn Age: 0   **P** Pediatric Age: 0–17   **M** Maternity DX: 9–64   **A** Adult Age: 15–124   ♀ Females Only   ♂ Males Only

🔧 Complication\Comorbidity   🔧 Major C\C   (Ex) CC/MCC Exclusions   🔧 Hospital-Acquired Condition   🖋 Hierarchical Condition Category

911

● **I69.25** **Hemiplegia and hemiparesis** following other nontraumatic intracranial hemorrhage

    I69.251   **Hemiplegia and hemiparesis** following other nontraumatic intracranial hemorrhage affecting **right dominant side**
          Ex: See PDX Collection 695

    I69.252   **Hemiplegia and hemiparesis** following other nontraumatic intracranial hemorrhage affecting **left dominant side**
          Ex: See PDX Collection 695

    I69.253   **Hemiplegia and hemiparesis** following other nontraumatic intracranial hemorrhage affecting **right non-dominant side**
          Ex: See PDX Collection 696

    I69.254   **Hemiplegia and hemiparesis** following other nontraumatic intracranial hemorrhage affecting **left non-dominant side**
          Ex: See PDX Collection 696

    I69.259   **Hemiplegia and hemiparesis** following other nontraumatic intracranial hemorrhage affecting **unspecified side**
          Ex: See PDX Collection 697

● **I69.26** **Other paralytic syndrome** following other nontraumatic intracranial hemorrhage

    Use additional code to identify type of paralytic syndrome, such as:
      locked-in state (G83.5)
      quadriplegia (G82.5-)

    Excludes1   hemiplegia/hemiparesis following other nontraumatic intracranial hemorrhage (I69.25-)
              monoplegia of lower limb following other nontraumatic intracranial hemorrhage (I69.24-)
              monoplegia of upper limb following other nontraumatic intracranial hemorrhage (I69.23-)

    I69.261   **Other paralytic syndrome** following other nontraumatic intracranial hemorrhage affecting **right dominant side**

    I69.262   **Other paralytic syndrome** following other nontraumatic intracranial hemorrhage affecting **left dominant side**

    I69.263   **Other paralytic syndrome** following other nontraumatic intracranial hemorrhage affecting **right non-dominant side**

    I69.264   **Other paralytic syndrome** following other nontraumatic intracranial hemorrhage affecting **left non-dominant side**

    I69.265   **Other paralytic syndrome** following other nontraumatic intracranial hemorrhage, **bilateral**

    I69.269   **Other paralytic syndrome** following other nontraumatic intracranial hemorrhage affecting **unspecified side**

● **I69.29** **Other sequelae** of other nontraumatic intracranial hemorrhage

    I69.290   **Apraxia** following other nontraumatic intracranial hemorrhage

    I69.291   **Dysphagia** following other nontraumatic intracranial hemorrhage
         Use additional code to identify the type of dysphagia, if known (R13.1-)

    I69.292   **Facial weakness** following other nontraumatic intracranial hemorrhage
         Facial droop following other nontraumatic intracranial hemorrhage

    I69.293   **Ataxia** following other nontraumatic intracranial hemorrhage

    I69.298   **Other** sequelae of other nontraumatic intracranial hemorrhage
         Alteration of sensation following other nontraumatic intracranial hemorrhage
         Disturbance of vision following other nontraumatic intracranial hemorrhage
         Use additional code to identify the sequelae

● **I69.3** **Sequelae of cerebral infarction**
    Sequelae of stroke NOS
    Coding Clinic: 2012, Q4, P92, 95

  I69.30   **Unspecified** sequelae of cerebral infarction

● **I69.31** **Cognitive deficits** following cerebral infarction

    I69.310   **Attention and concentration** deficit following cerebral infarction

    I69.311   **Memory** deficit following cerebral infarction

    I69.312   **Visuospatial** deficit and spatial neglect following cerebral infarction

    I69.313   **Psychomotor** deficit following cerebral infarction

    I69.314   **Frontal lobe and executive function** deficit following cerebral infarction

    I69.315   **Cognitive social or emotional** deficit following cerebral infarction

    I69.318   **Other** symptoms and signs involving cognitive functions following cerebral infarction

    I69.319   **Unspecified** symptoms and signs involving cognitive functions following cerebral infarction

● **I69.32** **Speech and language** deficits following cerebral infarction

    I69.320   **Aphasia** following cerebral infarction

    I69.321   **Dysphasia** following cerebral infarction
         Coding Clinic: 2012, Q4, P91

    I69.322   **Dysarthria** following cerebral infarction
         Excludes2   transient ischemic attack (TIA) (G45.9)

    I69.323   **Fluency disorder** following cerebral infarction
         Stuttering following cerebral infarction

    I69.328   **Other speech and language deficits** following cerebral infarction

● **I69.33**   **Monoplegia of upper limb** following cerebral infarction
     Coding Clinic: 2017, Q1, P47

     I69.331   Monoplegia of upper limb following cerebral infarction affecting **right dominant side** 🐾

     I69.332   Monoplegia of upper limb following cerebral infarction affecting **left dominant side** 🐾

     I69.333   Monoplegia of upper limb following cerebral infarction affecting **right non-dominant side** 🐾

     I69.334   Monoplegia of upper limb following cerebral infarction affecting **left non-dominant side** 🐾

     I69.339   Monoplegia of upper limb following cerebral infarction affecting **unspecified side** 🐾

● **I69.34**   **Monoplegia of lower limb** following cerebral infarction
     Coding Clinic: 2017, Q1, P47

     I69.341   Monoplegia of lower limb following cerebral infarction affecting **right dominant side** 🐾

     I69.342   Monoplegia of lower limb following cerebral infarction affecting **left dominant side** 🐾

     I69.343   Monoplegia of lower limb following cerebral infarction affecting **right non-dominant side** 🐾

     I69.344   Monoplegia of lower limb following cerebral infarction affecting **left non-dominant side** 🐾

     I69.349   Monoplegia of lower limb following cerebral infarction affecting **unspecified side** 🐾

● **I69.35**   **Hemiplegia and hemiparesis** following cerebral infarction

     I69.351   Hemiplegia and hemiparesis following cerebral infarction affecting **right dominant side** 🐾 🐾

         Excludes2   transient ischemic attack (TIA) (G45.9)

         (Ex:) See PDX Collection 695
         Coding Clinic: 2015, Q1, P25

     I69.352   Hemiplegia and hemiparesis following cerebral infarction affecting **left dominant side** 🐾 🐾
         (Ex:) See PDX Collection 695

     I69.353   Hemiplegia and hemiparesis following cerebral infarction affecting **right non-dominant side** 🐾 🐾
         (Ex:) See PDX Collection 696

     I69.354   Hemiplegia and hemiparesis following cerebral infarction affecting **left non-dominant side** 🐾 🐾
         (Ex:) See PDX Collection 696
         Coding Clinic: 2012, Q4, P91

     I69.359   Hemiplegia and hemiparesis following cerebral infarction affecting **unspecified side** 🐾 🐾
         (Ex:) See PDX Collection 697

● **I69.36**   **Other paralytic syndrome** following cerebral infarction

     Use additional code to identify type of paralytic syndrome, such as:
     locked-in state (G83.5)
     quadriplegia (G82.5-)

         Excludes1   hemiplegia/hemiparesis following cerebral infarction (I69.35-)
                 monoplegia of lower limb following cerebral infarction (I69.34-)
                 monoplegia of upper limb following cerebral infarction (I69.33-)

     I69.361   Other paralytic syndrome following cerebral infarction affecting **right dominant side** 🐾

     I69.362   Other paralytic syndrome following cerebral infarction affecting **left dominant side** 🐾

     I69.363   Other paralytic syndrome following cerebral infarction affecting **right non-dominant side** 🐾

     I69.364   Other paralytic syndrome following cerebral infarction affecting **left non-dominant side** 🐾

     I69.365   Other paralytic syndrome following cerebral infarction, **bilateral** 🐾

     I69.369   Other paralytic syndrome following cerebral infarction affecting **unspecified side** 🐾

● **I69.39**   **Other sequelae** of cerebral infarction

     I69.390   **Apraxia** following cerebral infarction

     I69.391   **Dysphagia** following cerebral infarction

         Use additional code to identify the type of dysphagia, if known (R13.1-)

     I69.392   **Facial weakness** following cerebral infarction
         Facial droop following cerebral infarction

     I69.393   **Ataxia** following cerebral infarction

     I69.398   **Other sequelae** of cerebral infarction
         Alteration of sensation following cerebral infarction
         Disturbance of vision following cerebral infarction
         Use additional code to identify the sequelae

● **I69.8**   **Sequelae of other cerebrovascular diseases**

     Excludes1   sequelae of traumatic intracranial injury (S06.-)

     I69.80   **Unspecified sequelae** of other cerebrovascular disease

● **I69.81**   **Cognitive deficits** following other cerebrovascular disease

     I69.810   **Attention and concentration** deficit following other cerebrovascular disease

     I69.811   **Memory** deficit following other cerebrovascular disease

     I69.812   **Visuospatial** deficit and spatial neglect following other cerebrovascular disease

CHAPTER 9 (I00-I99)

N   Newborn Age: 0   P   Pediatric Age: 0–17   M   Maternity DX: 9–64   A   Adult Age: 15–124   ♀   Females Only   ♂   Males Only

🐾 Complication\Comorbidity   🐾 Major C\C   (Ex:) CC/MCC Exclusions   🐾 Hospital-Acquired Condition   🐾 Hierarchical Condition Category

913

I69.813　Psychomotor deficit following other cerebrovascular disease

I69.814　Frontal lobe and executive function deficit following other cerebrovascular disease

I69.815　Cognitive social or emotional deficit following other cerebrovascular disease

I69.818　Other symptoms and signs involving cognitive functions following other cerebrovascular disease

I69.819　Unspecified symptoms and signs involving cognitive functions following other cerebrovascular disease

● **I69.82**　Speech and language deficits following other cerebrovascular disease

I69.820　Aphasia following other cerebrovascular disease

I69.821　Dysphasia following other cerebrovascular disease

I69.822　Dysarthria following other cerebrovascular disease

I69.823　Fluency disorder following other cerebrovascular disease
Stuttering following other cerebrovascular disease

I69.828　Other speech and language deficits following other cerebrovascular disease
Coding Clinic: 2019, Q3, P9

● **I69.83**　Monoplegia of upper limb following other cerebrovascular disease

I69.831　Monoplegia of upper limb following other cerebrovascular disease affecting right dominant side

I69.832　Monoplegia of upper limb following other cerebrovascular disease affecting left dominant side

I69.833　Monoplegia of upper limb following other cerebrovascular disease affecting right non-dominant side

I69.834　Monoplegia of upper limb following other cerebrovascular disease affecting left non-dominant side

I69.839　Monoplegia of upper limb following other cerebrovascular disease affecting unspecified side

● **I69.84**　Monoplegia of lower limb following other cerebrovascular disease

I69.841　Monoplegia of lower limb following other cerebrovascular disease affecting right dominant side

I69.842　Monoplegia of lower limb following other cerebrovascular disease affecting left dominant side

I69.843　Monoplegia of lower limb following other cerebrovascular disease affecting right non-dominant side

I69.844　Monoplegia of lower limb following other cerebrovascular disease affecting left non-dominant side

I69.849　Monoplegia of lower limb following other cerebrovascular disease affecting unspecified side

● **I69.85**　Hemiplegia and hemiparesis following other cerebrovascular disease

I69.851　Hemiplegia and hemiparesis following other cerebrovascular disease affecting right dominant side
(Ex:) See PDX Collection 695

I69.852　Hemiplegia and hemiparesis following other cerebrovascular disease affecting left dominant side
(Ex:) See PDX Collection 695

I69.853　Hemiplegia and hemiparesis following other cerebrovascular disease affecting right non-dominant side
(Ex:) See PDX Collection 696

I69.854　Hemiplegia and hemiparesis following other cerebrovascular disease affecting left non-dominant side
(Ex:) See PDX Collection 696

I69.859　Hemiplegia and hemiparesis following other cerebrovascular disease affecting unspecified side
(Ex:) See PDX Collection 697

● **I69.86**　Other paralytic syndrome following other cerebrovascular disease

Use additional code to identify type of paralytic syndrome, such as:
locked-in state (G83.5)
quadriplegia (G82.5-)

Excludes1　hemiplegia/hemiparesis following other cerebrovascular disease (I69.85-)
monoplegia of lower limb following other cerebrovascular disease (I69.84-)
monoplegia of upper limb following other cerebrovascular disease (I69.83-)

I69.861　Other paralytic syndrome following other cerebrovascular disease affecting right dominant side

I69.862　Other paralytic syndrome following other cerebrovascular disease affecting left dominant side

I69.863　Other paralytic syndrome following other cerebrovascular disease affecting right non-dominant side

I69.864　Other paralytic syndrome following other cerebrovascular disease affecting left non-dominant side

I69.865　Other paralytic syndrome following other cerebrovascular disease, bilateral

I69.869　Other paralytic syndrome following other cerebrovascular disease affecting unspecified side

▶ New　⇒ Revised　~~deleted~~ Deleted　Excludes 1　Excludes 2　Includes　Use additional　Code first　Code also　Key words
OGCR Official Guidelines　● Unacceptable Principal Diagnosis　X Assign placeholder X　● Use Additional Character(s)　▸ Manifestation Code　Coding Clinic

● **I69.89**   Other sequelae of other cerebrovascular disease

     I69.890   **Apraxia** following other cerebrovascular disease

     I69.891   **Dysphagia** following other cerebrovascular disease

         Use additional code to identify the type of dysphagia, if known (R13.1-)

     I69.892   **Facial weakness** following other cerebrovascular disease

         Facial droop following other cerebrovascular disease

     I69.893   **Ataxia** following other cerebrovascular disease

     I69.898   **Other** sequelae of other cerebrovascular disease

         Alteration of sensation following other cerebrovascular disease

         Disturbance of vision following other cerebrovascular disease

         Use additional code to identify the sequelae

● **I69.9**   Sequelae of unspecified cerebrovascular diseases

     Excludes1   sequelae of stroke (I69.3)

                 sequelae of traumatic intracranial injury (S06.-)

     I69.90   Unspecified sequelae of unspecified cerebrovascular disease

● **I69.91**   Cognitive deficits following unspecified cerebrovascular disease

     I69.910   **Attention and concentration** deficit following unspecified cerebrovascular disease

     I69.911   **Memory** deficit following unspecified cerebrovascular disease

     I69.912   **Visuospatial** deficit and spatial neglect following unspecified cerebrovascular disease

     I69.913   **Psychomotor** deficit following unspecified cerebrovascular disease

     I69.914   **Frontal lobe and executive function** deficit following unspecified cerebrovascular disease

     I69.915   **Cognitive social or emotional** deficit following unspecified cerebrovascular disease

     I69.918   **Other** symptoms and signs involving cognitive functions following unspecified cerebrovascular disease

     I69.919   **Unspecified** symptoms and signs involving cognitive functions following unspecified cerebrovascular disease

● **I69.92**   Speech and language deficits following unspecified cerebrovascular disease

     I69.920   **Aphasia** following unspecified cerebrovascular disease

     I69.921   **Dysphasia** following unspecified cerebrovascular disease

     I69.922   **Dysarthria** following unspecified cerebrovascular disease

     I69.923   **Fluency disorder** following unspecified cerebrovascular disease

         Stuttering following unspecified cerebrovascular disease

     I69.928   **Other** speech and language deficits following unspecified cerebrovascular disease

● **I69.93**   Monoplegia of upper limb following unspecified cerebrovascular disease

     I69.931   Monoplegia of upper limb following unspecified cerebrovascular disease affecting **right dominant side** 🐾

     I69.932   Monoplegia of upper limb following unspecified cerebrovascular disease affecting **left dominant side** 🐾

     I69.933   Monoplegia of upper limb following unspecified cerebrovascular disease affecting **right non-dominant side** 🐾

     I69.934   Monoplegia of upper limb following unspecified cerebrovascular disease affecting **left non-dominant side** 🐾

     I69.939   Monoplegia of upper limb following unspecified cerebrovascular disease affecting **unspecified side** 🐾

● **I69.94**   Monoplegia of lower limb following unspecified cerebrovascular disease

     I69.941   Monoplegia of lower limb following unspecified cerebrovascular disease affecting **right dominant side** 🐾

     I69.942   Monoplegia of lower limb following unspecified cerebrovascular disease affecting **left dominant side** 🐾

     I69.943   Monoplegia of lower limb following unspecified cerebrovascular disease affecting **right non-dominant side** 🐾

     I69.944   Monoplegia of lower limb following unspecified cerebrovascular disease affecting **left non-dominant side** 🐾

     I69.949   Monoplegia of lower limb following unspecified cerebrovascular disease affecting **unspecified side** 🐾

● **I69.95**   Hemiplegia and hemiparesis following unspecified cerebrovascular disease

     I69.951   Hemiplegia and hemiparesis following unspecified cerebrovascular disease affecting **right dominant side** 🐾 🐾

         (Ex:) See PDX Collection 695

     I69.952   Hemiplegia and hemiparesis following unspecified cerebrovascular disease affecting **left dominant side** 🐾 🐾

         (Ex:) See PDX Collection 695

     I69.953   Hemiplegia and hemiparesis following unspecified cerebrovascular disease affecting **right non-dominant side** 🐾 🐾

         (Ex:) See PDX Collection 696

     I69.954   Hemiplegia and hemiparesis following unspecified cerebrovascular disease affecting **left non-dominant side** 🐾 🐾

         (Ex:) See PDX Collection 696

     I69.959   Hemiplegia and hemiparesis following unspecified cerebrovascular disease affecting **unspecified side** 🐾 🐾

         (Ex:) See PDX Collection 697

CHAPTER 9 (I00-I99)

N Newborn Age: 0   **P** Pediatric Age: 0–17   **M** Maternity DX: 9–64   **A** Adult Age: 15–124   ♀ Females Only   ♂ Males Only

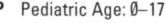 Complication\Comorbidity   🐾 Major C\C   (Ex:) CC/MCC Exclusions   Hospital-Acquired Condition   🐾 Hierarchical Condition Category

915

● **I69.96** **Other paralytic syndrome following unspecified cerebrovascular disease**

Use additional code to identify type of paralytic syndrome, such as:
locked-in state (G83.5)
quadriplegia (G82.5-)

Excludes1 hemiplegia/hemiparesis following unspecified cerebrovascular disease (I69.95-)
monoplegia of lower limb following unspecified cerebrovascular disease (I69.94-)
monoplegia of upper limb following unspecified cerebrovascular disease (I69.93-)

I69.961 Other paralytic syndrome following unspecified cerebrovascular disease affecting right dominant side 🔎

I69.962 Other paralytic syndrome following unspecified cerebrovascular disease affecting left dominant side 🔎

I69.963 Other paralytic syndrome following unspecified cerebrovascular disease affecting right non-dominant side 🔎

I69.964 Other paralytic syndrome following unspecified cerebrovascular disease affecting left non-dominant side 🔎

I69.965 Other paralytic syndrome following unspecified cerebrovascular disease, bilateral 🔎

I69.969 Other paralytic syndrome following unspecified cerebrovascular disease affecting unspecified side 🔎

● **I69.99** **Other sequelae of unspecified cerebrovascular disease**

I69.990 Apraxia following unspecified cerebrovascular disease

I69.991 Dysphagia following unspecified cerebrovascular disease

Use additional code to identify the type of dysphagia, if known (R13.1-)

I69.992 Facial weakness following unspecified cerebrovascular disease
Facial droop following unspecified cerebrovascular disease

I69.993 Ataxia following unspecified cerebrovascular disease

I69.998 Other sequelae following unspecified cerebrovascular disease
Alteration in sensation following unspecified cerebrovascular disease
Disturbance of vision following unspecified cerebrovascular disease
Use additional code to identify the sequelae

DISEASES OF ARTERIES, ARTERIOLES AND CAPILLARIES (I70-I79)

● **I70** **Atherosclerosis**

Includes arteriolosclerosis
arterial degeneration
arteriosclerosis
arteriosclerotic vascular disease
arteriovascular degeneration
atheroma
endarteritis deformans or obliterans
senile arteritis
senile endarteritis
vascular degeneration

Use additional code to identify:
exposure to environmental tobacco smoke (Z77.22)
history of tobacco dependence (Z87.891)
occupational exposure to environmental tobacco smoke (Z57.31)
tobacco dependence (F17.-)
tobacco use (Z72.0)

Excludes2 arteriosclerotic cardiovascular disease (I25.1-)
arteriosclerotic heart disease (I25.1-)
atheroembolism (I75.-)
cerebral atherosclerosis (I67.2)
coronary atherosclerosis (I25.1-)
mesenteric atherosclerosis (K55.1)
precerebral atherosclerosis (I67.2)
primary pulmonary atherosclerosis (I27.0)

I70.0 Atherosclerosis of aorta 🔎   A
I70.1 Atherosclerosis of renal artery 🔎   A
Goldblatt's kidney
Excludes2 atherosclerosis of renal arterioles (I12.-)

★ **(See Plates 500, 501, and 502 on pages 60 – 62.)**

● **I70.2** **Atherosclerosis of native arteries of the extremities**
Mönckeberg's (medial) sclerosis
Use additional code, if applicable, to identify chronic total occlusion of artery of extremity (I70.92)
Excludes2 atherosclerosis of bypass graft of extremities (I70.30-I70.79)

● **I70.20** **Unspecified atherosclerosis of native arteries of extremities**

I70.201 Unspecified atherosclerosis of native arteries of extremities, right leg 🔎   A
I70.202 Unspecified atherosclerosis of native arteries of extremities, left leg 🔎   A
I70.203 Unspecified atherosclerosis of native arteries of extremities, bilateral legs 🔎   A
I70.208 Unspecified atherosclerosis of native arteries of extremities, other extremity 🔎   A
I70.209 Unspecified atherosclerosis of native arteries of extremities, unspecified extremity 🔎   A

● **I70.21** **Atherosclerosis of native arteries of extremities with intermittent claudication**

I70.211 Atherosclerosis of native arteries of extremities with intermittent claudication, right leg 🔎   A
I70.212 Atherosclerosis of native arteries of extremities with intermittent claudication, left leg 🔎   A
I70.213 Atherosclerosis of native arteries of extremities with intermittent claudication, bilateral legs 🔎   A
I70.218 Atherosclerosis of native arteries of extremities with intermittent claudication, other extremity 🔎   A
I70.219 Atherosclerosis of native arteries of extremities with intermittent claudication, unspecified extremity 🔎   A

▶ New   ⇒ Revised   ~~deleted~~ Deleted   Excludes 1   Excludes 2   Includes   Use additional   Code first   Code also   Key words
OGCR Official Guidelines   ● Unacceptable Principal Diagnosis   X Assign placeholder X   ● Use Additional Character(s)   ▷ Manifestation Code   Coding Clinic

● **I70.22**   **Atherosclerosis of native arteries of extremities with rest pain**

> **Includes**   any condition classifiable to I70.21-
> chronic limb-threatening ischemia NOS of native arteries of extremities
> chronic limb-threatening ischemia of native arteries of extremities with rest pain
> critical limb ischemia NOS of native arteries of extremities
> critical limb ischemia of native arteries of extremities with rest pain

     I70.221   Atherosclerosis of native arteries of extremities with rest pain, right leg 🦠   A

     I70.222   Atherosclerosis of native arteries of extremities with rest pain, left leg 🦠   A

     I70.223   Atherosclerosis of native arteries of extremities with rest pain, bilateral legs 🦠   A

     I70.228   Atherosclerosis of native arteries of extremities with rest pain, other extremity 🦠   A

     I70.229   Atherosclerosis of native arteries of extremities with rest pain, unspecified extremity 🦠   A

● **I70.23**   **Atherosclerosis of native arteries of right leg with ulceration**

> **Includes**   any condition classifiable to I70.211 and I70.221
> chronic limb-threatening ischemia of native arteries of right leg with ulceration
> critical limb ischemia of native arteries of right leg with ulceration

Use additional code to identify severity of ulcer (L97.-)

     I70.231   Atherosclerosis of native arteries of right leg with ulceration of thigh 🦠   A

     I70.232   Atherosclerosis of native arteries of right leg with ulceration of calf 🦠   A

     I70.233   Atherosclerosis of native arteries of right leg with ulceration of ankle 🦠   A

     I70.234   Atherosclerosis of native arteries of right leg with ulceration of heel and midfoot 🦠   A
> Atherosclerosis of native arteries of right leg with ulceration of plantar surface of midfoot

     I70.235   Atherosclerosis of native arteries of right leg with ulceration of other part of foot 🦠   A
> Atherosclerosis of native arteries of right leg extremities with ulceration of toe

     I70.238   Atherosclerosis of native arteries of right leg with ulceration of other part of lower leg 🦠   A

     I70.239   Atherosclerosis of native arteries of right leg with ulceration of unspecified site 🦠   A

● **I70.24**   **Atherosclerosis of native arteries of left leg with ulceration**

> **Includes**   any condition classifiable to I70.212 and I70.222
> chronic limb-threatening ischemia of native arteries of left leg with ulceration
> critical limb ischemia of native arteries of left leg with ulceration

Use additional code to identify severity of ulcer (L97.-)

     I70.241   Atherosclerosis of native arteries of left leg with ulceration of thigh 🦠   A

     I70.242   Atherosclerosis of native arteries of left leg with ulceration of calf 🦠   A

     I70.243   Atherosclerosis of native arteries of left leg with ulceration of ankle 🦠   A

     I70.244   Atherosclerosis of native arteries of left leg with ulceration of heel and midfoot 🦠   A
> Atherosclerosis of native arteries of left leg with ulceration of plantar surface of midfoot

     I70.245   Atherosclerosis of native arteries of left leg with ulceration of other part of foot 🦠   A
> Atherosclerosis of native arteries of left leg extremities with ulceration of toe

     I70.248   Atherosclerosis of native arteries of left leg with ulceration of other part of lower leg 🦠   A

     I70.249   Atherosclerosis of native arteries of left leg with ulceration of unspecified site 🦠   A

  I70.25   Atherosclerosis of native arteries of other extremities with ulceration 🦠   A

> **Includes**   any condition classifiable to I70.218 and I70.228

Use additional code to identify the severity of the ulcer (L98.49-)

● **I70.26**   **Atherosclerosis of native arteries of extremities with gangrene**

> **Includes**   any condition classifiable to I70.21-, I70.22-, I70.23-, I70.24-, and I70.25-
> chronic limb-threatening ischemia of native arteries of extremities with gangrene
> critical limb ischemia of native arteries of extremities with gangrene

Use additional code to identify the severity of any ulcer (L97.-, L98.49-), if applicable

(Ex) **For category I70.26 CC codes:** See PDX Collection 519

     I70.261   Atherosclerosis of native arteries of extremities with gangrene, right leg 🦠   A

     I70.262   Atherosclerosis of native arteries of extremities with gangrene, left leg 🦠🦠   A

     I70.263   Atherosclerosis of native arteries of extremities with gangrene, bilateral legs 🦠🦠   A

     I70.268   Atherosclerosis of native arteries of extremities with gangrene, other extremity 🦠🦠   A

     I70.269   Atherosclerosis of native arteries of extremities with gangrene, unspecified extremity 🦠🦠   A

N   Newborn Age: 0   **P**   Pediatric Age: 0–17   **M**   Maternity DX: 9–64   **A**   Adult Age: 15–124   ♀ Females Only   ♂ Males Only

🦠 Complication\Comorbidity   🦠 Major C\C   (Ex) CC/MCC Exclusions   🦠 Hospital-Acquired Condition   🦠 Hierarchical Condition Category

CHAPTER 9 (I00-I99)

- **I70.29** Other atherosclerosis of native arteries of extremities
  - **I70.291** Other atherosclerosis of native arteries of extremities, right leg A
  - **I70.292** Other atherosclerosis of native arteries of extremities, left leg A
  - **I70.293** Other atherosclerosis of native arteries of extremities, bilateral legs A
  - **I70.298** Other atherosclerosis of native arteries of extremities, other extremity A
  - **I70.299** Other atherosclerosis of native arteries of extremities, unspecified extremity A
- **I70.3** Atherosclerosis of unspecified type of bypass graft(s) of the extremities

  Use additional code, if applicable, to identify chronic total occlusion of artery of extremity (I70.92)

  Excludes1 embolism or thrombus of bypass graft(s) of extremities (T82.8-)
  - **I70.30** Unspecified atherosclerosis of unspecified type of bypass graft(s) of the extremities
    - **I70.301** Unspecified atherosclerosis of unspecified type of bypass graft(s) of the extremities, right leg A
    - **I70.302** Unspecified atherosclerosis of unspecified type of bypass graft(s) of the extremities, left leg A
    - **I70.303** Unspecified atherosclerosis of unspecified type of bypass graft(s) of the extremities, bilateral legs A
    - **I70.308** Unspecified atherosclerosis of unspecified type of bypass graft(s) of the extremities, other extremity A
    - **I70.309** Unspecified atherosclerosis of unspecified type of bypass graft(s) of the extremities, unspecified extremity A
  - **I70.31** Atherosclerosis of unspecified type of bypass graft(s) of the extremities with intermittent claudication
    - **I70.311** Atherosclerosis of unspecified type of bypass graft(s) of the extremities with intermittent claudication, right leg A
    - **I70.312** Atherosclerosis of unspecified type of bypass graft(s) of the extremities with intermittent claudication, left leg A
    - **I70.313** Atherosclerosis of unspecified type of bypass graft(s) of the extremities with intermittent claudication, bilateral legs A
    - **I70.318** Atherosclerosis of unspecified type of bypass graft(s) of the extremities with intermittent claudication, other extremity A
    - **I70.319** Atherosclerosis of unspecified type of bypass graft(s) of the extremities with intermittent claudication, unspecified extremity A
- **I70.32** Atherosclerosis of unspecified type of bypass graft(s) of the extremities with rest pain

  Includes any condition classifiable to I70.31-
  chronic limb-threatening ischemia NOS of unspecified type of bypass graft(s) of the extremities
  chronic limb-threatening ischemia of unspecified type of bypass graft(s) of the extremities with rest pain, right leg
  critical limb ischemia NOS of unspecified type of bypass graft(s) of the extremities
  critical limb ischemia of unspecified type of bypass graft(s) of the extremities with rest pain
  - **I70.321** Atherosclerosis of unspecified type of bypass graft(s) of the extremities with rest pain, right leg A
  - **I70.322** Atherosclerosis of unspecified type of bypass graft(s) of the extremities with rest pain, left leg A
  - **I70.323** Atherosclerosis of unspecified type of bypass graft(s) of the extremities with rest pain, bilateral legs A
  - **I70.328** Atherosclerosis of unspecified type of bypass graft(s) of the extremities with rest pain, other extremity A
  - **I70.329** Atherosclerosis of unspecified type of bypass graft(s) of the extremities with rest pain, unspecified extremity A
- **I70.33** Atherosclerosis of unspecified type of bypass graft(s) of the right leg with ulceration

  Includes any condition classifiable to I70.311 and I70.321
  chronic limb-threatening ischemia of unspecified type of bypass graft(s) of the right leg with ulceration
  critical limb ischemia of unspecified type of bypass graft(s) of the right leg with ulceration

  Use additional code to identify severity of ulcer (L97.-)

  For category I70.33 CC codes unless otherwise indicated: See PDX Collection 698
  - **I70.331** Atherosclerosis of unspecified type of bypass graft(s) of the right leg with ulceration of thigh A
    CC when PDx is its own CC
    See PDX Collection 3300
  - **I70.332** Atherosclerosis of unspecified type of bypass graft(s) of the right leg with ulceration of calf A
    CC when PDx is its own CC
    See PDX Collection 3301
  - **I70.333** Atherosclerosis of unspecified type of bypass graft(s) of the right leg with ulceration of ankle A
    CC when PDx is its own CC
    See PDX Collection 3302

I7Ø.334　**Atherosclerosis of unspecified type of bypass graft(s) of the right leg with ulceration of heel and midfoot** 🔘🔘 A
　Atherosclerosis of unspecified type of bypass graft(s) of right leg with ulceration of plantar surface of midfoot
　CC when PDx is its own CC
　(Ex:) See PDX Collection 33Ø3

I7Ø.335　**Atherosclerosis of unspecified type of bypass graft(s) of the right leg with ulceration of other part of foot** 🔘 A
　Atherosclerosis of unspecified type of bypass graft(s) of the right leg with ulceration of toe

I7Ø.338　**Atherosclerosis of unspecified type of bypass graft(s) of the right leg with ulceration of other part of lower leg** 🔘🔘 A
　CC when PDx is its own CC
　(Ex:) See PDX Collection 33Ø4

I7Ø.339　**Atherosclerosis of unspecified type of bypass graft(s) of the right leg with ulceration of unspecified site** 🔘🔘 A
　CC when PDx is its own CC
　(Ex:) See PDX Collection 33Ø5

●I7Ø.34　**Atherosclerosis of unspecified type of bypass graft(s) of the left leg with ulceration**
　Includes　any condition classifiable to I7Ø.312 and I7Ø.322
　chronic limb-threatening ischemia of unspecified type of bypass graft(s) of the left leg with ulceration
　critical limb ischemia of unspecified type of bypass graft(s) of the left leg with ulceration
　Use additional code to identify severity of ulcer (L97.-)
　(Ex:) **For category I7Ø.34 CC codes unless otherwise indicated:** See PDX Collection 698

I7Ø.341　**Atherosclerosis of unspecified type of bypass graft(s) of the left leg with ulceration of thigh** 🔘🔘 A
　CC when PDx is its own CC
　(Ex:) See PDX Collection 33Ø6

I7Ø.342　**Atherosclerosis of unspecified type of bypass graft(s) of the left leg with ulceration of calf** 🔘🔘 A
　CC when PDx is its own CC
　(Ex:) See PDX Collection 33Ø7

I7Ø.343　**Atherosclerosis of unspecified type of bypass graft(s) of the left leg with ulceration of ankle** 🔘🔘 A
　CC when PDx is its own CC
　(Ex:) See PDX Collection 33Ø8

I7Ø.344　**Atherosclerosis of unspecified type of bypass graft(s) of the left leg with ulceration of heel and midfoot** 🔘🔘 A
　Atherosclerosis of unspecified type of bypass graft(s) of left leg with ulceration of plantar surface of midfoot
　CC when PDx is its own CC
　(Ex:) See PDX Collection 33Ø9

I7Ø.345　**Atherosclerosis of unspecified type of bypass graft(s) of the left leg with ulceration of other part of foot** 🔘 A
　Atherosclerosis of unspecified type of bypass graft(s) of the left leg with ulceration of toe

I7Ø.348　**Atherosclerosis of unspecified type of bypass graft(s) of the left leg with ulceration of other part of lower leg** 🔘🔘 A
　CC when PDx is its own CC
　(Ex:) See PDX Collection 331Ø

I7Ø.349　**Atherosclerosis of unspecified type of bypass graft(s) of the left leg with ulceration of unspecified site** 🔘🔘 A
　CC when PDx is its own CC
　(Ex:) See PDX Collection 3311

I7Ø.35　**Atherosclerosis of unspecified type of bypass graft(s) of other extremity with ulceration** 🔘 A
　Includes　any condition classifiable to I7Ø.318 and I7Ø.328
　Use additional code to identify severity of ulcer (L98.49-)

●I7Ø.36　**Atherosclerosis of unspecified type of bypass graft(s) of the extremities with gangrene**
　Includes　any condition classifiable to I7Ø.31-, I7Ø.32-, I7Ø.33-, I7Ø.34-, I7Ø.35
　chronic limb-threatening ischemia of unspecified type of bypass graft(s) of the extremities with gangrene
　critical limb ischemia of unspecified type of bypass graft(s) of the extremities with gangrene
　Use additional code to identify the severity of any ulcer (L97.-, L98.49-), if applicable

I7Ø.361　**Atherosclerosis of unspecified type of bypass graft(s) of the extremities with gangrene, right leg** 🔘🔘 A
　CC when PDx is its own CC
　(Ex:) See PDX Collection 3312

I7Ø.362　**Atherosclerosis of unspecified type of bypass graft(s) of the extremities with gangrene, left leg** 🔘🔘 A
　CC when PDx is its own CC
　(Ex:) See PDX Collection 3313

I7Ø.363　**Atherosclerosis of unspecified type of bypass graft(s) of the extremities with gangrene, bilateral legs** 🔘🔘 A
　CC when PDx is its own CC
　(Ex:) See PDX Collection 3314

I7Ø.368　**Atherosclerosis of unspecified type of bypass graft(s) of the extremities with gangrene, other extremity** 🔘🔘 A
　CC when PDx is its own CC
　(Ex:) See PDX Collection 3315

I7Ø.369　**Atherosclerosis of unspecified type of bypass graft(s) of the extremities with gangrene, unspecified extremity** 🔘🔘A
　CC when PDx is its own CC
　(Ex:) See PDX Collection 3316

●I7Ø.39　**Other atherosclerosis of unspecified type of bypass graft(s) of the extremities**

I7Ø.391　**Other atherosclerosis of unspecified type of bypass graft(s) of the extremities, right leg** 🔘 A

I7Ø.392　**Other atherosclerosis of unspecified type of bypass graft(s) of the extremities, left leg** 🔘 A

I7Ø.393　**Other atherosclerosis of unspecified type of bypass graft(s) of the extremities, bilateral legs** 🔘 A

I7Ø.398　**Other atherosclerosis of unspecified type of bypass graft(s) of the extremities, other extremity** 🔘 A

I7Ø.399　**Other atherosclerosis of unspecified type of bypass graft(s) of the extremities, unspecified extremity** 🔘 A

CHAPTER 9 (IØØ-I99)

N　Newborn Age: Ø　　P　Pediatric Age: Ø–17　　M　Maternity DX: 9–64　　A　Adult Age: 15–124　　♀ Females Only　　♂　Males Only

🔘 Complication\Comorbidity　　🔘　Major C\C　　(Ex:) CC/MCC Exclusions　　🔘　Hospital-Acquired Condition　　🔘　Hierarchical Condition Category

919

● I70.4   Atherosclerosis of autologous vein bypass graft(s) of the extremities
Use additional code, if applicable, to identify chronic total occlusion of artery of extremity (I70.92)

● I70.40   Unspecified atherosclerosis of autologous vein bypass graft(s) of the extremities

I70.401   Unspecified atherosclerosis of autologous vein bypass graft(s) of the extremities, right leg 🐾   A

I70.402   Unspecified atherosclerosis of autologous vein bypass graft(s) of the extremities, left leg 🐾   A

I70.403   Unspecified atherosclerosis of autologous vein bypass graft(s) of the extremities, bilateral legs 🐾   A

I70.408   Unspecified atherosclerosis of autologous vein bypass graft(s) of the extremities, other extremity 🐾   A

I70.409   Unspecified atherosclerosis of autologous vein bypass graft(s) of the extremities, unspecified extremity 🐾 A

● I70.41   Atherosclerosis of autologous vein bypass graft(s) of the extremities with intermittent claudication

I70.411   Atherosclerosis of autologous vein bypass graft(s) of the extremities with intermittent claudication, right leg 🐾A

I70.412   Atherosclerosis of autologous vein bypass graft(s) of the extremities with intermittent claudication, left leg 🐾   A

I70.413   Atherosclerosis of autologous vein bypass graft(s) of the extremities with intermittent claudication, bilateral legs 🐾   A

I70.418   Atherosclerosis of autologous vein bypass graft(s) of the extremities with intermittent claudication, other extremity 🐾   A

I70.419   Atherosclerosis of autologous vein bypass graft(s) of the extremities with intermittent claudication, unspecified extremity 🐾   A

● I70.42   Atherosclerosis of autologous vein bypass graft(s) of the extremities with rest pain

Includes   any condition classifiable to I70.41-
chronic limb-threatening ischemia NOS of autologous vein bypass graft(s) of the extremities
chronic limb-threatening ischemia of autologous vein bypass graft(s) of the extremities with rest pain
critical limb ischemia NOS of autologous vein bypass graft(s) of the extremities
critical limb ischemia of autologous vein bypass graft(s) of the extremities with rest pain

I70.421   Atherosclerosis of autologous vein bypass graft(s) of the extremities with rest pain, right leg 🐾   A

I70.422   Atherosclerosis of autologous vein bypass graft(s) of the extremities with rest pain, left leg 🐾   A

I70.423   Atherosclerosis of autologous vein bypass graft(s) of the extremities with rest pain, bilateral legs 🐾   A

I70.428   Atherosclerosis of autologous vein bypass graft(s) of the extremities with rest pain, other extremity 🐾   A

I70.429   Atherosclerosis of autologous vein bypass graft(s) of the extremities with rest pain, unspecified extremity 🐾   A

● I70.43   Atherosclerosis of autologous vein bypass graft(s) of the right leg with ulceration

Includes   any condition classifiable to I70.411 and I70.421
chronic limb-threatening ischemia of autologous vein bypass graft(s) of the right leg with ulceration
critical limb ischemia of autologous vein bypass graft(s) of the right leg with ulceration

Use additional code to identify severity of ulcer (L97.-)
Ⓔ⨯ For category I70.43 CC codes unless otherwise indicated: See PDX Collection 698

I70.431   Atherosclerosis of autologous vein bypass graft(s) of the right leg with ulceration of thigh 🐾🐾   A
CC when PDx is its own CC
Ⓔ⨯ See PDX Collection 3317

I70.432   Atherosclerosis of autologous vein bypass graft(s) of the right leg with ulceration of calf 🐾🐾   A
CC when PDx is its own CC
Ⓔ⨯ See PDX Collection 3318

I70.433   Atherosclerosis of autologous vein bypass graft(s) of the right leg with ulceration of ankle 🐾🐾   A
CC when PDx is its own CC
Ⓔ⨯ See PDX Collection 3319

I70.434   Atherosclerosis of autologous vein bypass graft(s) of the right leg with ulceration of heel and midfoot 🐾🐾 A
Atherosclerosis of autologous vein bypass graft(s) of right leg with ulceration of plantar surface of midfoot
CC when PDx is its own CC
Ⓔ⨯ See PDX Collection 3320

I70.435   Atherosclerosis of autologous vein bypass graft(s) of the right leg with ulceration of other part of foot 🐾   A
Atherosclerosis of autologous vein bypass graft(s) of right leg with ulceration of toe

I70.438   Atherosclerosis of autologous vein bypass graft(s) of the right leg with ulceration of other part of lower leg 🐾🐾   A
CC when PDx is its own CC
Ⓔ⨯ See PDX Collection 3321

I70.439   Atherosclerosis of autologous vein bypass graft(s) of the right leg with ulceration of unspecified site 🐾🐾   A
CC when PDx is its own CC
Ⓔ⨯ See PDX Collection 3322

▶ New   ⇒ Revised   ~~deleted~~ Deleted   Excludes 1   Excludes 2   Includes   Use additional   Code first   Code also   Key words
OGCR Official Guidelines   ● Unacceptable Principal Diagnosis   X Assign placeholder X   ● Use Additional Character(s)   ▌ Manifestation Code   Coding Clinic

● **I70.44   Atherosclerosis of autologous vein bypass graft(s) of the left leg with ulceration**

> **Includes**   any condition classifiable to I70.412 and I70.422
> chronic limb-threatening ischemia of autologous vein bypass graft(s) of the left leg with ulceration
> critical limb ischemia of autologous vein bypass graft(s) of the left leg with ulceration

Use additional code to identify severity of ulcer (L97.-)

(Ex:) **For category I70.44 CC codes unless otherwise indicated:** See PDX Collection 698

I70.441   Atherosclerosis of autologous vein bypass graft(s) of the left leg with ulceration of thigh 🦠🦠   A
> CC when PDx is its own CC
> (Ex:) See PDX Collection 3323

I70.442   Atherosclerosis of autologous vein bypass graft(s) of the left leg with ulceration of calf 🦠🦠   A
> CC when PDx is its own CC
> (Ex:) See PDX Collection 3324

I70.443   Atherosclerosis of autologous vein bypass graft(s) of the left leg with ulceration of ankle 🦠🦠   A
> CC when PDx is its own CC
> (Ex:) See PDX Collection 3325

I70.444   Atherosclerosis of autologous vein bypass graft(s) of the left leg with ulceration of heel and midfoot 🦠🦠   A
> Atherosclerosis of autologous vein bypass graft(s) of left leg with ulceration of plantar surface of midfoot
> CC when PDx is its own CC
> (Ex:) See PDX Collection 3326

I70.445   Atherosclerosis of autologous vein bypass graft(s) of the left leg with ulceration of other part of foot 🦠   A
> Atherosclerosis of autologous vein bypass graft(s) of left leg with ulceration of toe

I70.448   Atherosclerosis of autologous vein bypass graft(s) of the left leg with ulceration of other part of lower leg 🦠🦠   A
> CC when PDx is its own CC
> (Ex:) See PDX Collection 3327

I70.449   Atherosclerosis of autologous vein bypass graft(s) of the left leg with ulceration of unspecified site 🦠🦠   A
> CC when PDx is its own CC
> (Ex:) See PDX Collection 3328

I70.45   Atherosclerosis of autologous vein bypass graft(s) of other extremity with ulceration 🦠   A
> **Includes**   any condition classifiable to I70.418, I70.428, and I70.438

Use additional code to identify severity of ulcer (L98.49-)

● **I70.46   Atherosclerosis of autologous vein bypass graft(s) of the extremities with gangrene**

> **Includes**   any condition classifiable to I70.41-, I70.42-, and I70.43-, I70.44-, I70.45
> chronic limb-threatening ischemia of autologous vein bypass graft(s) of the extremities with gangrene
> critical limb ischemia of autologous vein bypass graft(s) of the extremities with gangrene

Use additional code to identify the severity of any ulcer (L97.-, L98.49-), if applicable

I70.461   Atherosclerosis of autologous vein bypass graft(s) of the extremities with gangrene, right leg 🦠   A
> CC when PDx is its own CC
> (Ex:) See PDX Collection 3329

I70.462   Atherosclerosis of autologous vein bypass graft(s) of the extremities with gangrene, left leg 🦠🦠   A
> CC when PDx is its own CC
> (Ex:) See PDX Collection 3330

I70.463   Atherosclerosis of autologous vein bypass graft(s) of the extremities with gangrene, bilateral legs 🦠🦠   A
> CC when PDx is its own CC
> (Ex:) See PDX Collection 3331

I70.468   Atherosclerosis of autologous vein bypass graft(s) of the extremities with gangrene, other extremity 🦠🦠   A
> CC when PDx is its own CC
> (Ex:) See PDX Collection 3332

I70.469   Atherosclerosis of autologous vein bypass graft(s) of the extremities with gangrene, unspecified extremity 🦠🦠 A
> CC when PDx is its own CC
> (Ex:) See PDX Collection 3333

● **I70.49   Other atherosclerosis of autologous vein bypass graft(s) of the extremities**

I70.491   Other atherosclerosis of autologous vein bypass graft(s) of the extremities, right leg 🦠   A

I70.492   Other atherosclerosis of autologous vein bypass graft(s) of the extremities, left leg 🦠   A

I70.493   Other atherosclerosis of autologous vein bypass graft(s) of the extremities, bilateral legs 🦠   A

I70.498   Other atherosclerosis of autologous vein bypass graft(s) of the extremities, other extremity 🦠   A

I70.499   Other atherosclerosis of autologous vein bypass graft(s) of the extremities, unspecified extremity 🦠   A

● **I70.5   Atherosclerosis of nonautologous biological bypass graft(s) of the extremities**

Use additional code, if applicable, to identify chronic total occlusion of artery of extremity (I70.92)

● **I70.50   Unspecified atherosclerosis of nonautologous biological bypass graft(s) of the extremities**

I70.501   Unspecified atherosclerosis of nonautologous biological bypass graft(s) of the extremities, right leg 🦠   A

I70.502   Unspecified atherosclerosis of nonautologous biological bypass graft(s) of the extremities, left leg 🦠   A

I70.503   Unspecified atherosclerosis of nonautologous biological bypass graft(s) of the extremities, bilateral legs 🦠   A

CHAPTER 9 (I00-I99)

N Newborn Age: 0   **P** Pediatric Age: 0–17   **M** Maternity DX: 9–64   **A** Adult Age: 15–124   ♀ Females Only   ♂ Males Only

🦠 Complication\Comorbidity   🦠 Major C\C   (Ex:) CC/MCC Exclusions   🦠 Hospital-Acquired Condition   🦠 Hierarchical Condition Category

921

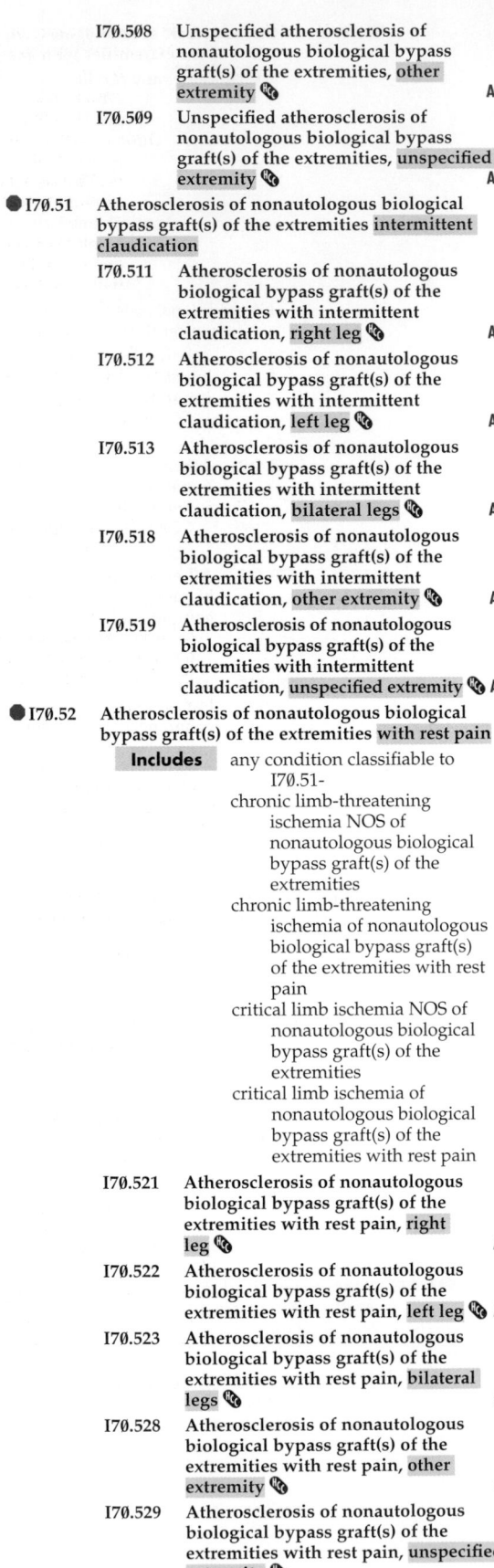

I70.508   Unspecified atherosclerosis of nonautologous biological bypass graft(s) of the extremities, other extremity   A

I70.509   Unspecified atherosclerosis of nonautologous biological bypass graft(s) of the extremities, unspecified extremity   A

● I70.51   Atherosclerosis of nonautologous biological bypass graft(s) of the extremities intermittent claudication

     I70.511   Atherosclerosis of nonautologous biological bypass graft(s) of the extremities with intermittent claudication, right leg   A

     I70.512   Atherosclerosis of nonautologous biological bypass graft(s) of the extremities with intermittent claudication, left leg   A

     I70.513   Atherosclerosis of nonautologous biological bypass graft(s) of the extremities with intermittent claudication, bilateral legs   A

     I70.518   Atherosclerosis of nonautologous biological bypass graft(s) of the extremities with intermittent claudication, other extremity   A

     I70.519   Atherosclerosis of nonautologous biological bypass graft(s) of the extremities with intermittent claudication, unspecified extremity A

● I70.52   Atherosclerosis of nonautologous biological bypass graft(s) of the extremities with rest pain

     Includes   any condition classifiable to I70.51-

             chronic limb-threatening ischemia NOS of nonautologous biological bypass graft(s) of the extremities

             chronic limb-threatening ischemia of nonautologous biological bypass graft(s) of the extremities with rest pain

             critical limb ischemia NOS of nonautologous biological bypass graft(s) of the extremities

             critical limb ischemia of nonautologous biological bypass graft(s) of the extremities with rest pain

     I70.521   Atherosclerosis of nonautologous biological bypass graft(s) of the extremities with rest pain, right leg   A

     I70.522   Atherosclerosis of nonautologous biological bypass graft(s) of the extremities with rest pain, left leg A

     I70.523   Atherosclerosis of nonautologous biological bypass graft(s) of the extremities with rest pain, bilateral legs   A

     I70.528   Atherosclerosis of nonautologous biological bypass graft(s) of the extremities with rest pain, other extremity   A

     I70.529   Atherosclerosis of nonautologous biological bypass graft(s) of the extremities with rest pain, unspecified extremity   A

● I70.53   Atherosclerosis of nonautologous biological bypass graft(s) of the right leg with ulceration

     Includes   any condition classifiable to I70.511 and I70.521

             chronic limb-threatening ischemia of nonautologous biological bypass graft(s) of the right leg with ulceration

             critical limb ischemia of nonautologous biological bypass graft(s) of the right leg with ulceration

     Use additional code to identify severity of ulcer (L97.-)

     (Ex:) **For category I70.53 CC codes unless otherwise indicated:** See PDX Collection 698

     I70.531   Atherosclerosis of nonautologous biological bypass graft(s) of the right leg with ulceration of thigh   A

           CC when PDx is its own CC

           (Ex:) See PDX Collection 3334

     I70.532   Atherosclerosis of nonautologous biological bypass graft(s) of the right leg with ulceration of calf   A

           CC when PDx is its own CC

           (Ex:) See PDX Collection 3335

     I70.533   Atherosclerosis of nonautologous biological bypass graft(s) of the right leg with ulceration of ankle   A

           CC when PDx is its own CC

           (Ex:) See PDX Collection 3336

     I70.534   Atherosclerosis of nonautologous biological bypass graft(s) of the right leg with ulceration of heel and midfoot   A

           Atherosclerosis of nonautologous biological bypass graft(s) of right leg with ulceration of plantar surface of midfoot

           CC when PDx is its own CC

           (Ex:) See PDX Collection 3337

     I70.535   Atherosclerosis of nonautologous biological bypass graft(s) of the right leg with ulceration of other part of foot   A

           Atherosclerosis of nonautologous biological bypass graft(s) of the right leg with ulceration of toe

     I70.538   Atherosclerosis of nonautologous biological bypass graft(s) of the right leg with ulceration of other part of lower leg   A

           CC when PDx is its own CC

           (Ex:) See PDX Collection 3338

     I70.539   Atherosclerosis of nonautologous biological bypass graft(s) of the right leg with ulceration of unspecified site   A

           CC when PDx is its own CC

           (Ex:) See PDX Collection 3339

▶ New   ⇒ Revised   ~~deleted~~ Deleted   Excludes 1   Excludes 2   Includes   Use additional   Code first   Code also   Key words

OGCR Official Guidelines   ● Unacceptable Principal Diagnosis   X Assign placeholder X   ● Use Additional Character(s)   ▶ Manifestation Code   **Coding Clinic**

● **I70.54** **Atherosclerosis of nonautologous biological bypass graft(s) of the left leg with ulceration**

Includes   any condition classifiable to I70.512 and I70.522

chronic limb-threatening ischemia of nonautologous biological bypass graft(s) of the left leg with ulceration

critical limb ischemia of nonautologous biological bypass graft(s) of the left leg with ulceration

Use additional code to identify severity of ulcer (L97.-)

(Ex:) **For category I70.54 CC codes unless otherwise indicated:** See PDX Collection 698

I70.541 Atherosclerosis of nonautologous biological bypass graft(s) of the left leg with ulceration of thigh 🖒🖒   A
     CC when PDx is its own CC
     (Ex:) See PDX Collection 3340

I70.542 Atherosclerosis of nonautologous biological bypass graft(s) of the left leg with ulceration of calf 🖒🖒   A
     CC when PDx is its own CC
     (Ex:) See PDX Collection 3341

I70.543 Atherosclerosis of nonautologous biological bypass graft(s) of the left leg with ulceration of ankle 🖒🖒   A
     CC when PDx is its own CC
     (Ex:) See PDX Collection 3342

I70.544 Atherosclerosis of nonautologous biological bypass graft(s) of the left leg with ulceration of heel and midfoot 🖒🖒   A
     Atherosclerosis of nonautologous biological bypass graft(s) of left leg with ulceration of plantar surface of midfoot
     CC when PDx is its own CC
     (Ex:) See PDX Collection 3343

I70.545 Atherosclerosis of nonautologous biological bypass graft(s) of the left leg with ulceration of other part of foot 🖒   A
     Atherosclerosis of nonautologous biological bypass graft(s) of the left leg with ulceration of toe

I70.548 Atherosclerosis of nonautologous biological bypass graft(s) of the left leg with ulceration of other part of lower leg 🖒🖒   A
     CC when PDx is its own CC
     (Ex:) See PDX Collection 3344

I70.549 Atherosclerosis of nonautologous biological bypass graft(s) of the left leg with ulceration of unspecified site 🖒🖒   A
     CC when PDx is its own CC
     (Ex:) See PDX Collection 3345

I70.55 **Atherosclerosis of nonautologous biological bypass graft(s) of other extremity with ulceration** 🖒   A

Includes   any condition classifiable to I70.518, I70.528, and I70.538

Use additional code to identify severity of ulcer (L98.49)

● **I70.56** **Atherosclerosis of nonautologous biological bypass graft(s) of the extremities with gangrene**

Includes   any condition classifiable to I70.51-, I70.52-, and I70.53-, I70.54-, I70.55

chronic limb-threatening ischemia of nonautologous biological bypass graft(s) of the extremities with gangrene

critical limb ischemia of nonautologous biological bypass graft(s) of the extremities with gangrene

Use additional code to identify the severity of any ulcer (L97.-, L98.49-), if applicable

I70.561 Atherosclerosis of nonautologous biological bypass graft(s) of the extremities with gangrene, right leg 🖒🖒   A
     CC when PDx is its own CC
     (Ex:) See PDX Collection 3346

I70.562 Atherosclerosis of nonautologous biological bypass graft(s) of the extremities with gangrene, left leg 🖒🖒   A
     CC when PDx is its own CC
     (Ex:) See PDX Collection 3347

I70.563 Atherosclerosis of nonautologous biological bypass graft(s) of the extremities with gangrene, bilateral legs 🖒🖒   A
     CC when PDx is its own CC
     (Ex:) See PDX Collection 3348

I70.568 Atherosclerosis of nonautologous biological bypass graft(s) of the extremities with gangrene, other extremity 🖒🖒   A
     CC when PDx is its own CC
     (Ex:) See PDX Collection 3349

I70.569 Atherosclerosis of nonautologous biological bypass graft(s) of the extremities with gangrene, unspecified extremity 🖒🖒   A
     CC when PDx is its own CC
     (Ex:) See PDX Collection 3350

● **I70.59** **Other atherosclerosis of nonautologous biological bypass graft(s) of the extremities**

I70.591 Other atherosclerosis of nonautologous biological bypass graft(s) of the extremities, right leg 🖒   A

I70.592 Other atherosclerosis of nonautologous biological bypass graft(s) of the extremities, left leg 🖒   A

I70.593 Other atherosclerosis of nonautologous biological bypass graft(s) of the extremities, bilateral legs 🖒   A

I70.598 Other atherosclerosis of nonautologous biological bypass graft(s) of the extremities, other extremity 🖒   A

I70.599 Other atherosclerosis of nonautologous biological bypass graft(s) of the extremities, unspecified extremity 🖒   A

CHAPTER 9 (I00-I99)

- **I70.6** Atherosclerosis of nonbiological bypass graft(s) of the extremities

  Use additional code, if applicable, to identify chronic total occlusion of artery of extremity (I70.92)

  - **I70.60** Unspecified atherosclerosis of nonbiological bypass graft(s) of the extremities
    - I70.601 Unspecified atherosclerosis of nonbiological bypass graft(s) of the extremities, right leg 🅰
    - I70.602 Unspecified atherosclerosis of nonbiological bypass graft(s) of the extremities, left leg 🅰
    - I70.603 Unspecified atherosclerosis of nonbiological bypass graft(s) of the extremities, bilateral legs 🅰
    - I70.608 Unspecified atherosclerosis of nonbiological bypass graft(s) of the extremities, other extremity 🅰
    - I70.609 Unspecified atherosclerosis of nonbiological bypass graft(s) of the extremities, unspecified extremity 🅰
  - **I70.61** Atherosclerosis of nonbiological bypass graft(s) of the extremities with intermittent claudication
    - I70.611 Atherosclerosis of nonbiological bypass graft(s) of the extremities with intermittent claudication, right leg 🅰
    - I70.612 Atherosclerosis of nonbiological bypass graft(s) of the extremities with intermittent claudication, left leg 🅰
    - I70.613 Atherosclerosis of nonbiological bypass graft(s) of the extremities with intermittent claudication, bilateral legs 🅰
    - I70.618 Atherosclerosis of nonbiological bypass graft(s) of the extremities with intermittent claudication, other extremity 🅰
    - I70.619 Atherosclerosis of nonbiological bypass graft(s) of the extremities with intermittent claudication, unspecified extremity 🅰
  - **I70.62** Atherosclerosis of nonbiological bypass graft(s) of the extremities with rest pain

    Includes any condition classifiable to I70.61-
    chronic limb-threatening ischemia NOS of nonbiological bypass graft(s) of the extremities
    chronic limb-threatening ischemia of nonbiological bypass graft(s) of the extremities with rest pain
    critical limb ischemia NOS of nonbiological bypass graft(s) of the extremities
    critical limb ischemia of nonbiological bypass graft(s) of the extremities with rest pain
    - I70.621 Atherosclerosis of nonbiological bypass graft(s) of the extremities with rest pain, right leg 🅰
    - I70.622 Atherosclerosis of nonbiological bypass graft(s) of the extremities with rest pain, left leg 🅰
    - I70.623 Atherosclerosis of nonbiological bypass graft(s) of the extremities with rest pain, bilateral legs 🅰
    - I70.628 Atherosclerosis of nonbiological bypass graft(s) of the extremities with rest pain, other extremity 🅰
    - I70.629 Atherosclerosis of nonbiological bypass graft(s) of the extremities with rest pain, unspecified extremity 🅰
  - **I70.63** Atherosclerosis of nonbiological bypass graft(s) of the right leg with ulceration

    Includes any condition classifiable to I70.611 and I70.621
    chronic limb-threatening ischemia of nonbiological bypass graft(s) of the right leg with ulceration
    critical limb ischemia of nonbiological bypass graft(s) of the right leg with ulceration

    Use additional code to identify severity of ulcer (L97.-)

    Ⓔ For category I70.63 CC codes unless otherwise indicated: See PDX Collection 698
    - I70.631 Atherosclerosis of nonbiological bypass graft(s) of the right leg with ulceration of thigh 🅰
      CC when PDx is its own CC
      Ⓔ See PDX Collection 3351
    - I70.632 Atherosclerosis of nonbiological bypass graft(s) of the right leg with ulceration of calf 🅰
      CC when PDx is its own CC
      Ⓔ See PDX Collection 3352
    - I70.633 Atherosclerosis of nonbiological bypass graft(s) of the right leg with ulceration of ankle 🅰
      CC when PDx is its own CC
      Ⓔ See PDX Collection 3353
    - I70.634 Atherosclerosis of nonbiological bypass graft(s) of the right leg with ulceration of heel and midfoot 🅰
      Atherosclerosis of nonbiological bypass graft(s) of right leg with ulceration of plantar surface of midfoot
      CC when PDx is its own CC
      Ⓔ See PDX Collection 3354
    - I70.635 Atherosclerosis of nonbiological bypass graft(s) of the right leg with ulceration of other part of foot 🅰
      Atherosclerosis of nonbiological bypass graft(s) of the right leg with ulceration of toe
    - I70.638 Atherosclerosis of nonbiological bypass graft(s) of the right leg with ulceration of other part of lower leg 🅰
      CC when PDx is its own CC
      Ⓔ See PDX Collection 3355
    - I70.639 Atherosclerosis of nonbiological bypass graft(s) of the right leg with ulceration of unspecified site 🅰
      CC when PDx is its own CC
      Ⓔ See PDX Collection 3356

● **I70.64**   **Atherosclerosis of nonbiological bypass graft(s) of the left leg with ulceration**

> **Includes**   any condition classifiable to I70.612 and I70.622
> chronic limb-threatening ischemia of nonbiological bypass graft(s) of the left leg with ulceration
> critical limb ischemia of nonbiological bypass graft(s) of the left leg with ulceration

Use additional code to identify severity of ulcer (L97.-)

(Ex:) **For category I70.64 CC codes unless otherwise indicated:** See PDX Collection 698

     I70.641   Atherosclerosis of nonbiological bypass graft(s) of the left leg with ulceration of thigh 🦠🦠   **A**
       CC when PDx is its own CC
       (Ex:) See PDX Collection 3357

     I70.642   Atherosclerosis of nonbiological bypass graft(s) of the left leg with ulceration of calf 🦠🦠   **A**
       CC when PDx is its own CC
       (Ex:) See PDX Collection 3358

     I70.643   Atherosclerosis of nonbiological bypass graft(s) of the left leg with ulceration of ankle 🦠🦠   **A**
       CC when PDx is its own CC
       (Ex:) See PDX Collection 3359

     I70.644   Atherosclerosis of nonbiological bypass graft(s) of the left leg with ulceration of heel and midfoot 🦠🦠 **A**
       Atherosclerosis of nonbiological bypass graft(s) of left leg with ulceration of plantar surface of midfoot
       CC when PDx is its own CC
       (Ex:) See PDX Collection 3360

     I70.645   Atherosclerosis of nonbiological bypass graft(s) of the left leg with ulceration of other part of foot 🦠   **A**
       Atherosclerosis of nonbiological bypass graft(s) of the left leg with ulceration of toe

     I70.648   Atherosclerosis of nonbiological bypass graft(s) of the left leg with ulceration of other part of lower leg 🦠🦠   **A**
       CC when PDx is its own CC
       (Ex:) See PDX Collection 3361

     I70.649   Atherosclerosis of nonbiological bypass graft(s) of the left leg with ulceration of unspecified site 🦠🦠   **A**
       CC when PDx is its own CC
       (Ex:) See PDX Collection 3362

I70.65   **Atherosclerosis of nonbiological bypass graft(s) of other extremity with ulceration** 🦠   **A**

> **Includes**   any condition classifiable to I70.618 and I70.628

Use additional code to identify severity of ulcer (L98.49-)

● **I70.66**   **Atherosclerosis of nonbiological bypass graft(s) of the extremities with gangrene**

> **Includes**   any condition classifiable to I70.61-, I70.62-, I70.63-, I70.64-, I70.65
> chronic limb-threatening ischemia of nonbiological bypass graft(s) of the extremities with gangrene
> critical limb ischemia of nonbiological bypass graft(s) of the extremities with gangrene

Use additional code to identify the severity of any ulcer (L97.-, L98.49-), if applicable

     I70.661   Atherosclerosis of nonbiological bypass graft(s) of the extremities with gangrene, right leg 🦠🦠   **A**
       CC when PDx is its own CC
       (Ex:) See PDX Collection 3363

     I70.662   Atherosclerosis of nonbiological bypass graft(s) of the extremities with gangrene, left leg 🦠🦠   **A**
       CC when PDx is its own CC
       (Ex:) See PDX Collection 3364

     I70.663   Atherosclerosis of nonbiological bypass graft(s) of the extremities with gangrene, bilateral legs 🦠🦠   **A**
       CC when PDx is its own CC
       (Ex:) See PDX Collection 3365

     I70.668   Atherosclerosis of nonbiological bypass graft(s) of the extremities with gangrene, other extremity 🦠🦠   **A**
       CC when PDx is its own CC
       (Ex:) See PDX Collection 3366

     I70.669   Atherosclerosis of nonbiological bypass graft(s) of the extremities with gangrene, unspecified extremity 🦠🦠**A**
       CC when PDx is its own CC
       (Ex:) See PDX Collection 3367

● **I70.69**   **Other atherosclerosis of nonbiological bypass graft(s) of the extremities**

     I70.691   Other atherosclerosis of nonbiological bypass graft(s) of the extremities, right leg 🦠   **A**

     I70.692   Other atherosclerosis of nonbiological bypass graft(s) of the extremities, left leg 🦠   **A**

     I70.693   Other atherosclerosis of nonbiological bypass graft(s) of the extremities, bilateral legs 🦠   **A**

     I70.698   Other atherosclerosis of nonbiological bypass graft(s) of the extremities, other extremity 🦠   **A**

     I70.699   Other atherosclerosis of nonbiological bypass graft(s) of the extremities, unspecified extremity 🦠   **A**

● **I70.7**   **Atherosclerosis of other type of bypass graft(s) of the extremities**

Use additional code, if applicable, to identify chronic total occlusion of artery of extremity (I70.92)

● **I70.70**   **Unspecified atherosclerosis of other type of bypass graft(s) of the extremities**

     I70.701   Unspecified atherosclerosis of other type of bypass graft(s) of the extremities, right leg 🦠   **A**

     I70.702   Unspecified atherosclerosis of other type of bypass graft(s) of the extremities, left leg 🦠   **A**

N Newborn Age: 0   **P** Pediatric Age: 0–17   **M** Maternity DX: 9–64   **A** Adult Age: 15–124   ♀ Females Only   ♂ Males Only

🦠 Complication\Comorbidity   🦠 Major C\C   (Ex:) CC/MCC Exclusions   🦠 Hospital-Acquired Condition   🦠 Hierarchical Condition Category

925

CHAPTER 9 (I00-I99)

I70.703　Unspecified atherosclerosis of other type of bypass graft(s) of the extremities, bilateral legs 🐾　　A

I70.708　Unspecified atherosclerosis of other type of bypass graft(s) of the extremities, other extremity 🐾　　A

I70.709　Unspecified atherosclerosis of other type of bypass graft(s) of the extremities, unspecified extremity 🐾 A

● **I70.71**　Atherosclerosis of other type of bypass graft(s) of the extremities with intermittent claudication

I70.711　Atherosclerosis of other type of bypass graft(s) of the extremities with intermittent claudication, right leg 🐾A

I70.712　Atherosclerosis of other type of bypass graft(s) of the extremities with intermittent claudication, left leg 🐾　A

I70.713　Atherosclerosis of other type of bypass graft(s) of the extremities with intermittent claudication, bilateral legs 🐾　　A

I70.718　Atherosclerosis of other type of bypass graft(s) of the extremities with intermittent claudication, other extremity 🐾　　A

I70.719　Atherosclerosis of other type of bypass graft(s) of the extremities with intermittent claudication, unspecified extremity 🐾　A

● **I70.72**　Atherosclerosis of other type of bypass graft(s) of the extremities with rest pain

> **Includes**　any condition classifiable to I70.71-
> chronic limb-threatening ischemia NOS of other type of bypass graft(s) of the extremities
> chronic limb-threatening ischemia of other type of bypass graft(s) of the extremities with rest pain
> critical limb ischemia NOS of other type of bypass graft(s) of the extremities
> critical limb ischemia of other type of bypass graft(s) of the extremities with rest pain

I70.721　Atherosclerosis of other type of bypass graft(s) of the extremities with rest pain, right leg 🐾　　A

I70.722　Atherosclerosis of other type of bypass graft(s) of the extremities with rest pain, left leg 🐾　　A

I70.723　Atherosclerosis of other type of bypass graft(s) of the extremities with rest pain, bilateral legs 🐾　　A

I70.728　Atherosclerosis of other type of bypass graft(s) of the extremities with rest pain, other extremity 🐾　　A

I70.729　Atherosclerosis of other type of bypass graft(s) of the extremities with rest pain, unspecified extremity 🐾　A

● **I70.73**　Atherosclerosis of other type of bypass graft(s) of the right leg with ulceration

> **Includes**　any condition classifiable to I70.711 and I70.721
> chronic limb-threatening ischemia of other type of bypass graft(s) of the right leg with ulceration
> critical limb ischemia of other type of bypass graft(s) of the right leg with ulceration

Use additional code to identify severity of ulcer (L97.-)

(Ex:) For category I70.73 CC codes unless otherwise indicated: See PDX Collection 698

I70.731　Atherosclerosis of other type of bypass graft(s) of the right leg with ulceration of thigh 🐾🐾　　A
　　　　CC when PDx is its own CC
　　　　(Ex:) See PDX Collection 3368

I70.732　Atherosclerosis of other type of bypass graft(s) of the right leg with ulceration of calf 🐾🐾　　A
　　　　CC when PDx is its own CC
　　　　(Ex:) See PDX Collection 3369

I70.733　Atherosclerosis of other type of bypass graft(s) of the right leg with ulceration of ankle 🐾🐾　　A
　　　　CC when PDx is its own CC
　　　　(Ex:) See PDX Collection 3370

I70.734　Atherosclerosis of other type of bypass graft(s) of the right leg with ulceration of heel and midfoot 🐾🐾 A
　　　　Atherosclerosis of other type of bypass graft(s) of right leg with ulceration of plantar surface of midfoot
　　　　CC when PDx is its own CC
　　　　(Ex:) See PDX Collection 3371

I70.735　Atherosclerosis of other type of bypass graft(s) of the right leg with ulceration of other part of foot 🐾　　A
　　　　Atherosclerosis of other type of bypass graft(s) of right leg with ulceration of toe

I70.738　Atherosclerosis of other type of bypass graft(s) of the right leg with ulceration of other part of lower leg 🐾🐾　　A
　　　　CC when PDx is its own CC
　　　　(Ex:) See PDX Collection 3372

I70.739　Atherosclerosis of other type of bypass graft(s) of the right leg with ulceration of unspecified site 🐾🐾　A
　　　　CC when PDx is its own CC
　　　　(Ex:) See PDX Collection 3373

● **I70.74**　Atherosclerosis of other type of bypass graft(s) of the left leg with ulceration

> **Includes**　any condition classifiable to I70.712 and I70.722
> chronic limb-threatening ischemia of other type of bypass graft(s) of the left leg with ulceration
> critical limb ischemia of other type of bypass graft(s) of the left leg with ulceration

Use additional code to identify severity of ulcer (L97.-)

(Ex:) For category I70.74 CC codes unless otherwise indicated: See PDX Collection 698

I70.741　Atherosclerosis of other type of bypass graft(s) of the left leg with ulceration of thigh 🐾🐾　　A
　　　　CC when PDx is its own CC
　　　　(Ex:) See PDX Collection 3374

CHAPTER 9 (I00-I99)

▶ New　⇒ Revised　~~deleted~~ Deleted　Excludes 1　Excludes 2　Includes　Use additional　Code first　Code also　Key words

OGCR Official Guidelines　● Unacceptable Principal Diagnosis　X Assign placeholder X　● Use Additional Character(s)　▶ Manifestation Code　Coding Clinic

I70.742   Atherosclerosis of other type of bypass graft(s) of the left leg with ulceration of calf 🔹🔹   A
     CC when PDx is its own CC
     (Ex) See PDX Collection 3375

I70.743   Atherosclerosis of other type of bypass graft(s) of the left leg with ulceration of ankle 🔹🔹   A
     CC when PDx is its own CC
     (Ex) See PDX Collection 3376

I70.744   Atherosclerosis of other type of bypass graft(s) of the left leg with ulceration of heel and midfoot 🔹🔹   A
     Atherosclerosis of other type of bypass graft(s) of left leg with ulceration of plantar surface of midfoot
     CC when PDx is its own CC
     (Ex) See PDX Collection 3377

I70.745   Atherosclerosis of other type of bypass graft(s) of the left leg with ulceration of other part of foot 🔹   A
     Atherosclerosis of other type of bypass graft(s) of left leg with ulceration of toe

I70.748   Atherosclerosis of other type of bypass graft(s) of the left leg with ulceration of other part of lower leg 🔹🔹   A
     CC when PDx is its own CC
     (Ex) See PDX Collection 3378

I70.749   Atherosclerosis of other type of bypass graft(s) of the left leg with ulceration of unspecified site 🔹🔹   A
     CC when PDx is its own CC
     (Ex) See PDX Collection 3379

I70.75   Atherosclerosis of other type of bypass graft(s) of other extremity with ulceration 🔹   A

     Includes   any condition classifiable to I70.718 and I70.728

     Use additional code to identify severity of ulcer (L98.49)

● I70.76   Atherosclerosis of other type of bypass graft(s) of the extremities with gangrene

     Includes   any condition classifiable to I70.71-, I70.72-, I70.73-, I70.74-, I70.75
                chronic limb-threatening ischemia of other type of bypass graft(s) of the extremities with gangrene
                critical limb ischemia of other type of bypass graft(s) of the extremities with gangrene

     Use additional code to identify the severity of any ulcer (L97.-, L98.49-), if applicable

I70.761   Atherosclerosis of other type of bypass graft(s) of the extremities with gangrene, right leg 🔹🔹   A
     CC when PDx is its own CC
     (Ex) See PDX Collection 3380

I70.762   Atherosclerosis of other type of bypass graft(s) of the extremities with gangrene, left leg 🔹🔹   A
     CC when PDx is its own CC
     (Ex) See PDX Collection 3381

I70.763   Atherosclerosis of other type of bypass graft(s) of the extremities with gangrene, bilateral legs 🔹🔹   A
     CC when PDx is its own CC
     (Ex) See PDX Collection 3382

I70.768   Atherosclerosis of other type of bypass graft(s) of the extremities with gangrene, other extremity 🔹🔹   A
     CC when PDx is its own CC
     (Ex) See PDX Collection 3383

I70.769   Atherosclerosis of other type of bypass graft(s) of the extremities with gangrene, unspecified extremity 🔹🔹 A
     CC when PDx is its own CC
     (Ex) See PDX Collection 3384

● I70.79   Other atherosclerosis of other type of bypass graft(s) of the extremities

I70.791   Other atherosclerosis of other type of bypass graft(s) of the extremities, right leg 🔹   A

I70.792   Other atherosclerosis of other type of bypass graft(s) of the extremities, left leg 🔹   A

I70.793   Other atherosclerosis of other type of bypass graft(s) of the extremities, bilateral legs 🔹   A

I70.798   Other atherosclerosis of other type of bypass graft(s) of the extremities, other extremity 🔹   A

I70.799   Other atherosclerosis of other type of bypass graft(s) of the extremities, unspecified extremity 🔹   A

I70.8   Atherosclerosis of other arteries   A

● I70.9   Other and unspecified atherosclerosis

I70.90   Unspecified atherosclerosis   A

I70.91   Generalized atherosclerosis   A

● I70.92   Chronic total occlusion of artery of the extremities 🔹🔹   A
     Complete occlusion of artery of the extremities
     Total occlusion of artery of the extremities
     Code first atherosclerosis of arteries of the extremities (I70.2-, I70.3-, I70.4-, I70.5-, I70.6-, I70.7-)
     (Ex) See PDX Collection 699

● I71   Aortic aneurysm and dissection

     Excludes1   aortic ectasia (I77.81-)
                 syphilitic aortic aneurysm (A52.01)
                 traumatic aortic aneurysm (S25.09, S35.09)
     (Ex) For category I71 CC codes: See PDX Collection 700

● I71.0   **Dissection of aorta**

I71.00   Dissection of unspecified site of aorta 🔹🔹

I71.01   Dissection of thoracic aorta 🔹🔹

I71.02   Dissection of abdominal aorta 🔹🔹

I71.03   Dissection of thoracoabdominal aorta 🔹🔹

I71.1   Thoracic aortic aneurysm, ruptured 🔹🔹

I71.2   Thoracic aortic aneurysm, without rupture 🔹

I71.3   Abdominal aortic aneurysm, ruptured 🔹🔹

I71.4   Abdominal aortic aneurysm, without rupture 🔹

I71.5   Thoracoabdominal aortic aneurysm, ruptured 🔹🔹

I71.6   Thoracoabdominal aortic aneurysm, without rupture 🔹

I71.8   Aortic aneurysm of unspecified site, ruptured 🔹🔹
     Rupture of aorta NOS

I71.9   Aortic aneurysm of unspecified site, without rupture 🔹
     Aneurysm of aorta
     Dilatation of aorta
     Hyaline necrosis of aorta

CHAPTER 9 (I00–I99)

N Newborn Age: 0   **P** Pediatric Age: 0–17   **M** Maternity DX: 9–64   **A** Adult Age: 15–124   ♀ Females Only   ♂ Males Only

🔹 Complication\Comorbidity   🔹 Major C\C   (Ex) CC/MCC Exclusions   🔹 Hospital-Acquired Condition   🔹 Hierarchical Condition Category

927

● **I72**   **Other aneurysm**

> | **Includes** | aneurysm (cirsoid) (false) (ruptured) |
> |---|---|
> | **Excludes2** | acquired aneurysm (I77.0) |

         aneurysm (of) aorta (I71.-)
         aneurysm (of) arteriovenous NOS (Q27.3-)
         carotid artery dissection (I77.71)
         cerebral (nonruptured) aneurysm (I67.1)
         coronary aneurysm (I25.4)
         coronary artery dissection (I25.42)
         dissection of artery NEC (I77.79)
         dissection of precerebral artery, congenital
            (nonruptured) (Q28.1)
         heart aneurysm (I25.3)
         iliac artery dissection (I77.72)
         precerebral artery, congential (nonruptured) (Q28.1)
         pulmonary artery aneurysm (I28.1)
         renal artery dissection (I77.73)
         retinal aneurysm (H35.0)
         ruptured cerebral aneurysm (I60.7)
         varicose aneurysm (I77.0)
         vertebral artery dissection (I77.74)

     I72.0   **Aneurysm of carotid artery** 🔍
         Aneurysm of common carotid artery
         Aneurysm of external carotid artery
         Aneurysm of internal carotid artery, extracranial
            portion

> | **Excludes1** | aneurysm of internal carotid artery, intracranial portion (I67.1) |
> |---|---|
> | | aneurysm of internal carotid artery NOS (I67.1) |

     I72.1   **Aneurysm of artery of upper extremity** 🔍
     I72.2   **Aneurysm of renal artery** 🔍
     I72.3   **Aneurysm of iliac artery** 🔍
     I72.4   **Aneurysm of artery of lower extremity** 🔍
         Coding Clinic: 2019, Q2, P22
     I72.5   **Aneurysm of other precerebral arteries** 🔍
         Aneurysm of basilar artery (trunk)

> | **Excludes2** | aneurysm of carotid artery (I72.0) |
> |---|---|
> | | aneurysm of vertebral artery (I72.6) |
> | | dissection of carotid artery (I77.71) |
> | | dissection of other precerebral arteries (I77.75) |
> | | dissection of vertebral artery (I77.74) |

         Coding Clinic: 2016, Q4, P28
     I72.6   **Aneurysm of vertebral artery** 🔍

> | **Excludes2** | dissection of vertebral artery (I77.74) |
> |---|---|

         Coding Clinic: 2016, Q4, P28
     I72.8   **Aneurysm of other specified arteries** 🔍
     I72.9   **Aneurysm of unspecified site** 🔍

● **I73**   **Other peripheral vascular diseases**

> | **Excludes2** | chilblains (T69.1) |
> |---|---|
> | | frostbite (T33-T34) |
> | | immersion hand or foot (T69.0-) |
> | | spasm of cerebral artery (G45.9) |

     Coding Clinic: 2018, Q4, P87-88

●   **I73.0**   **Raynaud's syndrome**
         Diminishing oxygen supply to fingers, toes, nose, and ears
            when exposed to temperature changes or stress
         Raynaud's disease
         Raynaud's phenomenon (secondary)

         I73.00   **Raynaud's syndrome without gangrene**
         I73.01   **Raynaud's syndrome with gangrene** 🔍🔍
            CC when PDx is its own CC
            (Ex) See PDX Collection 3385

     I73.1   **Thromboangiitis obliterans [Buerger's disease]** 🔍
         Inflammatory occlusive disease resulting in poor circulation
            to the legs, feet, and sometimes the hands due to
            progressive inflammatory narrowing and eventually
            obliteration of the small arteries

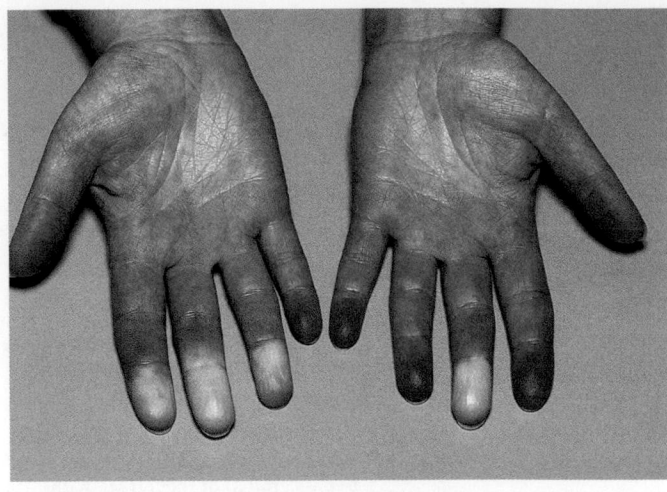

Figure 9-5   Raynaud's syndrome. (From Hallett: Comprehensive Vascular and Endovascular Surgery, ed 2, Philadelphia, Mosby Ltd., 2010)

●   **I73.8**   **Other specified peripheral vascular diseases**

> | **Excludes1** | diabetic (peripheral) angiopathy (E08-E13 with .51-.52) |
> |---|---|

         I73.81   **Erythromelalgia** 🔍
         I73.89   **Other specified peripheral vascular diseases** 🔍
            Acrocyanosis
            Erythrocyanosis
            Simple acroparesthesia [Schultze's type]
            Vasomotor acroparesthesia [Nothnagel's type]

     I73.9   **Peripheral vascular disease, unspecified** 🔍
         Intermittent claudication
         Peripheral angiopathy NOS
         Spasm of artery

> | **Excludes1** | atherosclerosis of the extremities (I70.2—I70.7-) |
> |---|---|

         Coding Clinic: 2018, Q4, P87

● **I74**   **Arterial embolism and thrombosis**

> | **Includes** | embolic infarction |
> |---|---|
> | | embolic occlusion |
> | | thrombotic infarction |
> | | thrombotic occlusion |

Code first embolism and thrombosis complicating abortion or
     ectopic or molar pregnancy (O00-O07, O08.2)
     embolism and thrombosis complicating pregnancy, childbirth
     and the puerperium (O88.-)

> | **Excludes2** | atheroembolism (I75.-) |
> |---|---|
> | | basilar embolism and thrombosis (I63.0-I63.2, I65.1) |
> | | carotid embolism and thrombosis (I63.0-I63.2, I65.2) |
> | | cerebral embolism and thrombosis (I63.3-I63.5, I66.-) |
> | | coronary embolism and thrombosis (I21-I25) |
> | | mesenteric embolism and thrombosis (K55.0-) |
> | | ophthalmic embolism and thrombosis (H34.-) |
> | | precerebral embolism and thrombosis NOS (I63.0-I63.2, I65.9) |
> | | pulmonary embolism and thrombosis (I26.-) |
> | | renal embolism and thrombosis (N28.0) |
> | | retinal embolism and thrombosis (H34.-) |
> | | septic embolism and thrombosis (I76) |
> | | vertebral embolism and thrombosis (I63.0-I63.2, I65.0) |

●   **I74.0**   **Embolism and thrombosis of abdominal aorta**
         (Ex) For category I74.0 CC codes: See PDX Collection 669

         I74.01   **Saddle embolus of abdominal aorta** 🔍🔍
         I74.09   **Other arterial embolism and thrombosis of abdominal aorta** 🔍🔍
            Aortic bifurcation syndrome
            Aortoiliac obstruction
            Leriche's syndrome

▶ New   ⇒ Revised   ~~deleted~~ Deleted   Excludes 1   Excludes 2   Includes   Use additional   Code first   Code also   Key words

OGCR Official Guidelines   ● Unacceptable Principal Diagnosis   X Assign placeholder X   ● Use Additional Character(s)   ▶ Manifestation Code   **Coding Clinic**

Item 9–9 An **embolus** is a mass of undissolved matter present in the blood that is transported by the blood current. A **thrombus** is a blood clot that occludes or shuts off a vessel. When a thrombus is dislodged, it becomes an embolus.

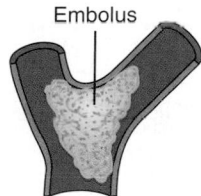

Embolus

Figure 9-6 An arterial embolus.

● **I74.1** Embolism and thrombosis of other and unspecified parts of aorta
　　Ⓔⓧ **For category I74.1 CC codes unless otherwise indicated:** See PDX Collection 669

　　I74.10 Embolism and thrombosis of unspecified parts of aorta 🏥🏥

　　I74.11 Embolism and thrombosis of thoracic aorta 🏥🏥
　　　　Ⓔⓧ See PDX Collection 701

　　I74.19 Embolism and thrombosis of other parts of aorta 🏥🏥

● **I74.2** Embolism and thrombosis of arteries of the upper extremities 🏥🏥
　　Ⓔⓧ See PDX Collection 702

● **I74.3** Embolism and thrombosis of arteries of the lower extremities 🏥🏥
　　Ⓔⓧ See PDX Collection 703

● **I74.4** Embolism and thrombosis of arteries of extremities, unspecified 🏥🏥
　　Peripheral arterial embolism NOS
　　Ⓔⓧ See PDX Collection 703

I74.5 Embolism and thrombosis of iliac artery 🏥🏥
　　Ⓔⓧ See PDX Collection 704

I74.8 Embolism and thrombosis of other arteries 🏥🏥
　　Ⓔⓧ See PDX Collection 705

I74.9 Embolism and thrombosis of unspecified artery 🏥🏥
　　Ⓔⓧ See PDX Collection 705

● **I75** Atheroembolism
　　Includes atherothrombotic microembolism
　　　　　　cholesterol embolism

● **I75.0** Atheroembolism of extremities

　● **I75.01** Atheroembolism of upper extremity
　　　Ⓔⓧ **For category I75.01 CC codes:** See PDX Collection 706

　　I75.011 Atheroembolism of right upper extremity 🏥🏥

　　I75.012 Atheroembolism of left upper extremity 🏥🏥

　　I75.013 Atheroembolism of bilateral upper extremities 🏥🏥

　　I75.019 Atheroembolism of unspecified upper extremity 🏥🏥

　● **I75.02** Atheroembolism of lower extremity
　　　Ⓔⓧ **For category I75.02 CC codes:** See PDX Collection 707

　　I75.021 Atheroembolism of right lower extremity 🏥🏥

　　I75.022 Atheroembolism of left lower extremity 🏥🏥

　　I75.023 Atheroembolism of bilateral lower extremities 🏥🏥

　　I75.029 Atheroembolism of unspecified lower extremity 🏥🏥

● **I75.8** Atheroembolism of other sites

　I75.81 Atheroembolism of kidney 🏥🏥
　　Use additional code for any associated acute kidney failure and chronic kidney disease (N17.-, N18.-)
　　Ⓔⓧ See PDX Collection 708

　I75.89 Atheroembolism of other site 🏥🏥
　　Ⓔⓧ See PDX Collection 709

● **I76** Septic arterial embolism 🏥🏥
　　Code first underlying infection, such as:
　　　infective endocarditis (I33.0)
　　　lung abscess (J85.-)
　　Use additional code to identify the site of the embolism (I74.-)
　　Excludes2 septic pulmonary embolism (I26.01, I26.90)
　　Ⓔⓧ See PDX Collection 705

● **I77** Other disorders of arteries and arterioles
　　Excludes2 collagen (vascular) diseases (M30-M36)
　　　　　　　hypersensitivity angiitis (M31.0)
　　　　　　　pulmonary artery (I28.-)

　I77.0 Arteriovenous fistula, acquired 🏥
　　Aneurysmal varix
　　Arteriovenous aneurysm, acquired
　　Excludes1 arteriovenous aneurysm NOS (Q27.3-)
　　　　　　　presence of arteriovenous shunt (fistula) for dialysis (Z99.2)
　　　　　　　traumatic - see injury of blood vessel by body region
　　Excludes2 cerebral (I67.1)
　　　　　　　coronary (I25.4)

　I77.1 Stricture of artery 🏥
　　Narrowing of artery

　I77.2 Rupture of artery 🏥🏥
　　Erosion of artery
　　Fistula of artery
　　Ulcer of artery
　　Excludes1 traumatic rupture of artery - see injury of blood vessel by body region
　　Ⓔⓧ See PDX Collection 710

　I77.3 Arterial fibromuscular dysplasia 🏥
　　Fibromuscular hyperplasia (of) carotid artery
　　Fibromuscular hyperplasia (of) renal artery

　I77.4 Celiac artery compression syndrome 🏥🏥
　　Ⓔⓧ See PDX Collection 711

　I77.5 Necrosis of artery 🏥🏥
　　Ⓔⓧ See PDX Collection 712

　I77.6 Arteritis, unspecified 🏥
　　Aortitis NOS
　　Endarteritis NOS
　　Excludes1 arteritis or endarteritis:
　　　　　　　aortic arch (M31.4)
　　　　　　　cerebral NEC (I67.7)
　　　　　　　coronary (I25.89)
　　　　　　　deformans (I70.-)
　　　　　　　giant cell (M31.5, M31.6)
　　　　　　　obliterans (I70.-)
　　　　　　　senile (I70.-)

● **I77.7** Other arterial dissection
　　Excludes2 dissection of aorta (I71.0-)
　　　　　　　dissection of coronary artery (I25.42)
　　Ⓔⓧ **For category I77.7 CC codes unless otherwise indicated:** See PDX Collection 689

　　I77.70 Dissection of unspecified artery 🏥🏥
　　　Ⓔⓧ See PDX Collection 3727
　　　Coding Clinic 2016, Q4, P28

　　I77.71 Dissection of carotid artery 🏥🏥
　　　Ⓔⓧ See PDX Collection 3386

　　I77.72 Dissection of iliac artery 🏥🏥
　　　Ⓔⓧ See PDX Collection 3729

　　I77.73 Dissection of renal artery 🏥🏥
　　　Ⓔⓧ See PDX Collection 3731

　　I77.74 Dissection of vertebral artery 🏥🏥
　　　Excludes2 aneurysm of vertebral artery (I72.6)
　　　Ⓔⓧ See PDX Collection 3732

CHAPTER 9 (I00-I99)

N Newborn Age: 0　　**P** Pediatric Age: 0–17　　**M** Maternity DX: 9–64　　**A** Adult Age: 15–124　　♀ Females Only　　♂ Males Only

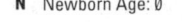 Complication\Comorbidity　　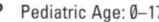 Major C\C　　Ⓔⓧ CC/MCC Exclusions　　🏥 Hospital-Acquired Condition　　Hierarchical Condition Category

CHAPTER 9 (I00-I99)

I77.75   **Dissection of other precerebral arteries** 🔹🔹
Dissection of basilar artery (trunk)
     Excludes2   aneurysm of carotid artery (I72.0)
                   aneurysm of other precerebral
                      arteries (I72.5)
                   aneurysm of vertebral artery
                      (I72.6)
                   dissection of carotid artery
                      (I77.71)
                   dissection of vertebral artery
                      (I77.74)
         (Ex:) See PDX Collection 3734
         Coding Clinic 2016, Q4, P28

I77.76   **Dissection of artery of upper extremity** 🔹🔹
         (Ex:) See PDX Collection 3736
         Coding Clinic 2016, Q4, P28

I77.77   **Dissection of artery of lower extremity** 🔹🔹
         (Ex:) See PDX Collection 3738
         Coding Clinic 2016, Q4, P28

I77.79   **Dissection of other specified artery** 🔹🔹
         Coding Clinic 2016, Q4, P28

● I77.8   **Other specified disorders of arteries and arterioles**

I77.81   **Aortic ectasia**
Ectasis aorta
     Excludes1   aortic aneurysm and dissection
                      (I71.0-)
      I77.810   **Thoracic aortic ectasia** 🔹
      I77.811   **Abdominal aortic ectasia** 🔹
      I77.812   **Thoracoabdominal aortic ectasia** 🔹
      I77.819   **Aortic ectasia, unspecified site** 🔹

I77.89   **Other specified disorders of arteries and arterioles** 🔹
         Coding Clinic 2021, Q1, P23

I77.9   **Disorder of arteries and arterioles, unspecified** 🔹
     Coding Clinic 2021, Q1, P4

● I78   **Diseases of capillaries**

I78.0   **Hereditary hemorrhagic telangiectasia** 🔹
Rendu-Osler-Weber disease

I78.1   **Nevus, non-neoplastic**
Araneus nevus   Spider nevus
Senile nevus   Stellar nevus
     Excludes1   nevus NOS (D22.-)
                      vascular NOS (Q82.5)
     Excludes2   blue nevus (D22.-)
                      flammeus nevus (Q82.5)
                      hairy nevus (D22.-)
                      melanocytic nevus (D22.-)
                      pigmented nevus (D22.-)
                      portwine nevus (Q82.5)
                      sanguineous nevus (Q82.5)
                      strawberry nevus (Q82.5)
                      verrucous nevus (Q82.5)
     Coding Clinic: 2019, Q1, P21

I78.8   **Other diseases of capillaries**

I78.9   **Disease of capillaries, unspecified**

● I79   **Disorders of arteries, arterioles and capillaries in diseases classified elsewhere**

▷ *I79.0*   *Aneurysm of aorta in diseases classified elsewhere* 🔹
     Code first underlying disease
     Excludes1   syphilitic aneurysm (A52.01)

▷ *I79.1*   *Aortitis in diseases classified elsewhere* 🔹
     Code first underlying disease
     Excludes1   syphilitic aortitis (A52.02)

▷ *I79.8*   *Other disorders of arteries, arterioles and capillaries in diseases classified elsewhere* 🔹
     Code first underlying disease, such as:
         amyloidosis (E85.-)
     Excludes1   diabetic (peripheral) angiopathy
                      (E08-E13 with .51-.52)
                      syphilitic endarteritis (A52.09)
                      tuberculous endarteritis (A18.89)

DISEASES OF VEINS, LYMPHATIC VESSELS AND LYMPH NODES, NOT ELSEWHERE CLASSIFIED (I80-I89)

● I80   **Phlebitis and thrombophlebitis**
Inflammation of a vein with infiltration of walls (phlebitis)
     Includes   endophlebitis
                  inflammation, vein
                  periphlebitis
                  suppurative phlebitis
   Code first phlebitis and thrombophlebitis complicating
     abortion, ectopic or molar pregnancy (O00-O07, O08.7)
     phlebitis and thrombophlebitis complicating pregnancy,
     childbirth and the puerperium (O22.-, O87.-)
     Excludes1   venous embolism and thrombosis of lower
                      extremities (I82.4-, I82.5-, I82.81-)

● I80.0   **Phlebitis and thrombophlebitis of superficial vessels of lower extremities**
Phlebitis and thrombophlebitis of femoropopliteal vein

     I80.00   **Phlebitis and thrombophlebitis of superficial vessels of unspecified lower extremity**
     I80.01   **Phlebitis and thrombophlebitis of superficial vessels of right lower extremity**
     I80.02   **Phlebitis and thrombophlebitis of superficial vessels of left lower extremity**
     I80.03   **Phlebitis and thrombophlebitis of superficial vessels of lower extremities, bilateral**

● I80.1   **Phlebitis and thrombophlebitis of femoral vein**
Phlebitis and thrombophlebitis of common femoral vein
Phlebitis and thrombophlebitis of deep femoral vein
     (Ex:) **For category I80.1 CC codes: See PDX Collection 713**

     I80.10   **Phlebitis and thrombophlebitis of unspecified femoral vein** 🔹🔹
     I80.11   **Phlebitis and thrombophlebitis of right femoral vein** 🔹🔹
     I80.12   **Phlebitis and thrombophlebitis of left femoral vein** 🔹🔹
     I80.13   **Phlebitis and thrombophlebitis of femoral vein, bilateral** 🔹🔹

● I80.2   **Phlebitis and thrombophlebitis of other and unspecified deep vessels of lower extremities**
     (Ex:) **For category I80.2 CC codes: See PDX Collection 713**

     ● I80.20   **Phlebitis and thrombophlebitis of unspecified deep vessels of lower extremities**
        I80.201   **Phlebitis and thrombophlebitis of unspecified deep vessels of right lower extremity** 🔹🔹
        I80.202   **Phlebitis and thrombophlebitis of unspecified deep vessels of left lower extremity** 🔹🔹
        I80.203   **Phlebitis and thrombophlebitis of unspecified deep vessels of lower extremities, bilateral** 🔹🔹
        I80.209   **Phlebitis and thrombophlebitis of unspecified deep vessels of unspecified lower extremity** 🔹🔹

     ● I80.21   **Phlebitis and thrombophlebitis of iliac vein**
Phlebitis and thrombophlebitis of common iliac vein
Phlebitis and thrombophlebitis of external iliac vein
Phlebitis and thrombophlebitis of internal iliac vein
        I80.211   **Phlebitis and thrombophlebitis of right iliac vein** 🔹🔹
        I80.212   **Phlebitis and thrombophlebitis of left iliac vein** 🔹🔹
        I80.213   **Phlebitis and thrombophlebitis of iliac vein, bilateral** 🔹🔹
        I80.219   **Phlebitis and thrombophlebitis of unspecified iliac vein** 🔹🔹

● **I80.22**   **Phlebitis and thrombophlebitis of popliteal vein**
    I80.221   Phlebitis and thrombophlebitis of right popliteal vein 🔹🔹
    I80.222   Phlebitis and thrombophlebitis of left popliteal vein 🔹🔹
    I80.223   Phlebitis and thrombophlebitis of popliteal vein, bilateral 🔹🔹
    I80.229   Phlebitis and thrombophlebitis of unspecified popliteal vein 🔹🔹

● **I80.23**   **Phlebitis and thrombophlebitis of tibial vein**
    Phlebitis and thrombophlebitis of anterior tibial vein
    Phlebitis and thrombophlebitis of posterior tibial vein
    I80.231   Phlebitis and thrombophlebitis of right tibial vein 🔹🔹
    I80.232   Phlebitis and thrombophlebitis of left tibial vein 🔹🔹
    I80.233   Phlebitis and thrombophlebitis of tibial vein, bilateral 🔹🔹
    I80.239   Phlebitis and thrombophlebitis of unspecified tibial vein 🔹🔹

● **I80.24**   **Phlebitis and thrombophlebitis of peroneal vein**
    I80.241   Phlebitis and thrombophlebitis of right peroneal vein 🔹
    I80.242   Phlebitis and thrombophlebitis of left peroneal vein 🔹
    I80.243   Phlebitis and thrombophlebitis of peroneal vein, bilateral 🔹
    I80.249   Phlebitis and thrombophlebitis of unspecified peroneal vein 🔹

● **I80.25**   **Phlebitis and thrombophlebitis of calf muscular vein**
    Phlebitis and thrombophlebitis of calf muscular vein, NOS
    Phlebitis and thrombophlebitis of gastrocnemial vein
    Phlebitis and thrombophlebitis of soleal vein
    I80.251   Phlebitis and thrombophlebitis of right calf muscular vein
    I80.252   Phlebitis and thrombophlebitis of left calf muscular vein
    I80.253   Phlebitis and thrombophlebitis of calf muscular vein, bilateral
    I80.259   Phlebitis and thrombophlebitis of unspecified calf muscular vein

● **I80.29**   **Phlebitis and thrombophlebitis of other deep vessels of lower extremities**
    I80.291   Phlebitis and thrombophlebitis of other deep vessels of right lower extremity 🔹🔹
    I80.292   Phlebitis and thrombophlebitis of other deep vessels of left lower extremity 🔹🔹
    I80.293   Phlebitis and thrombophlebitis of other deep vessels of lower extremity, bilateral 🔹🔹
    I80.299   Phlebitis and thrombophlebitis of other deep vessels of unspecified lower extremity 🔹🔹

I80.3   Phlebitis and thrombophlebitis of lower extremities, unspecified

I80.8   Phlebitis and thrombophlebitis of other sites

I80.9   Phlebitis and thrombophlebitis of unspecified site

I81   **Portal vein thrombosis** 🔹
    Portal (vein) obstruction
    Excludes2   hepatic vein thrombosis (I82.0)
               phlebitis of portal vein (K75.1)
    (Ex) See PDX Collection 714
    Coding Clinic: 2019, Q4, P68

● **I82**   **Other venous embolism and thrombosis**
    Code first venous embolism and thrombosis complicating:
    abortion, ectopic or molar pregnancy (O00-O07, O08.7)
    pregnancy, childbirth and the puerperium (O22.-, O87.-)
    Excludes2   venous embolism and thrombosis (of):
               cerebral (I63.6, I67.6)
               coronary (I21-I25)
               intracranial and intraspinal, septic or NOS (G08)
               intracranial, nonpyogenic (I67.6)
               intraspinal, nonpyogenic (G95.1)
               mesenteric (K55.0-)
               portal (I81)
               pulmonary (I26.-)

    I82.0   **Budd-Chiari syndrome** 🔹🔹
        Hepatic vein thrombosis
        (Ex) See PDX Collection 715

    I82.1   **Thrombophlebitis migrans** 🔹
        "White leg" is the other term to describe a migrating thrombus.
        (Ex) See PDX Collection 716

● **I82.2**   **Embolism and thrombosis of vena cava and other thoracic veins**
        (Ex) **For category I82.2 CC codes unless otherwise indicated:** See PDX Collection 717

    ● **I82.21**   **Embolism and thrombosis of superior vena cava**
        I82.210   **Acute** embolism and thrombosis of superior vena cava 🔹🔹
               Embolism and thrombosis of superior vena cava NOS
        I82.211   **Chronic** embolism and thrombosis of superior vena cava 🔹🔹

    ● **I82.22**   **Embolism and thrombosis of inferior vena cava**
        (Ex) **For category I82.22 CC codes:** See PDX Collection 718
        I82.220   **Acute** embolism and thrombosis of inferior vena cava 🔹🔹
               Embolism and thrombosis of inferior vena cava NOS
        I82.221   **Chronic** embolism and thrombosis of inferior vena cava 🔹🔹

    ● **I82.29**   **Embolism and thrombosis of other thoracic veins**
        Embolism and thrombosis of brachiocephalic (innominate) vein
        I82.290   **Acute** embolism and thrombosis of other thoracic veins 🔹🔹
        I82.291   **Chronic** embolism and thrombosis of other thoracic veins 🔹🔹

    I82.3   **Embolism and thrombosis of renal vein** 🔹🔹
        (Ex) See PDX Collection 719

N Newborn Age: 0   **P** Pediatric Age: 0–17   **M** Maternity DX: 9–64   **A** Adult Age: 15–124   ♀ Females Only   ♂ Males Only

🔹 Complication\Comorbidity   🔹 Major C\C   (Ex) CC/MCC Exclusions   🔹 Hospital-Acquired Condition   🔹 Hierarchical Condition Category   **931**

● **I82.4** Acute embolism and thrombosis of deep veins of lower extremity

(Ex) For category I82.4 CC codes: See PDX Collection 717

I82.40 Acute embolism and thrombosis of unspecified deep veins of lower extremity
Deep vein thrombosis NOS
DVT NOS

> **Excludes1**   acute embolism and thrombosis of unspecified deep veins of distal lower extremity (I82.4Z-)
> acute embolism and thrombosis of unspecified deep veins of proximal lower extremity (I82.4Y-)

I82.401 Acute embolism and thrombosis of unspecified deep veins of right lower extremity

I82.402 Acute embolism and thrombosis of unspecified deep veins of left lower extremity

I82.403 Acute embolism and thrombosis of unspecified deep veins of lower extremity, bilateral

I82.409 Acute embolism and thrombosis of unspecified deep veins of unspecified lower extremity

● **I82.41** Acute embolism and thrombosis of femoral vein
Acute embolism and thrombosis of common femoral vein
Acute embolism and thrombosis of deep femoral vein

I82.411 Acute embolism and thrombosis of right femoral vein

I82.412 Acute embolism and thrombosis of left femoral vein

I82.413 Acute embolism and thrombosis of femoral vein, bilateral

I82.419 Acute embolism and thrombosis of unspecified femoral vein

● **I82.42** Acute embolism and thrombosis of iliac vein
Acute embolism and thrombosis of common iliac vein
Acute embolism and thrombosis of external iliac vein
Acute embolism and thrombosis of internal iliac vein

I82.421 Acute embolism and thrombosis of right iliac vein

I82.422 Acute embolism and thrombosis of left iliac vein

I82.423 Acute embolism and thrombosis of iliac vein, bilateral

I82.429 Acute embolism and thrombosis of unspecified iliac vein

● **I82.43** Acute embolism and thrombosis of popliteal vein

I82.431 Acute embolism and thrombosis of right popliteal vein

I82.432 Acute embolism and thrombosis of left popliteal vein

I82.433 Acute embolism and thrombosis of popliteal vein, bilateral

I82.439 Acute embolism and thrombosis of unspecified popliteal vein

● **I82.44** Acute embolism and thrombosis of tibial vein
Acute embolism and thrombosis of anterior tibial vein
Acute embolism and thrombosis of posterior tibial vein

I82.441 Acute embolism and thrombosis of right tibial vein

I82.442 Acute embolism and thrombosis of left tibial vein

I82.443 Acute embolism and thrombosis of tibial vein, bilateral

I82.449 Acute embolism and thrombosis of unspecified tibial vein

● **I82.45** Acute embolism and thrombosis of peroneal vein

I82.451 Acute embolism and thrombosis of right peroneal vein

I82.452 Acute embolism and thrombosis of left peroneal vein

I82.453 Acute embolism and thrombosis of peroneal vein, bilateral

I82.459 Acute embolism and thrombosis of unspecified peroneal vein

● **I82.46** Acute embolism and thrombosis of calf muscular vein
Acute embolism and thrombosis of calf muscular vein, NOS
Acute embolism and thrombosis of gastrocnemial vein
Acute embolism and thrombosis of soleal vein

I82.461 Acute embolism and thrombosis of right calf muscular vein

I82.462 Acute embolism and thrombosis of left calf muscular vein

I82.463 Acute embolism and thrombosis of calf muscular vein, bilateral

I82.469 Acute embolism and thrombosis of unspecified calf muscular vein

● **I82.49** Acute embolism and thrombosis of other specified deep vein of lower extremity

I82.491 Acute embolism and thrombosis of other specified deep vein of right lower extremity

I82.492 Acute embolism and thrombosis of other specified deep vein of left lower extremity

I82.493 Acute embolism and thrombosis of other specified deep vein of lower extremity, bilateral

I82.499 Acute embolism and thrombosis of other specified deep vein of unspecified lower extremity

● **I82.4Y** Acute embolism and thrombosis of unspecified deep veins of proximal lower extremity
Acute embolism and thrombosis of deep vein of thigh NOS
Acute embolism and thrombosis of deep vein of upper leg NOS

I82.4Y1 Acute embolism and thrombosis of unspecified deep veins of right proximal lower extremity

I82.4Y2 Acute embolism and thrombosis of unspecified deep veins of left proximal lower extremity

I82.4Y3 Acute embolism and thrombosis of unspecified deep veins of proximal lower extremity, bilateral

I82.4Y9 Acute embolism and thrombosis of unspecified deep veins of unspecified proximal lower extremity

● **I82.4Z** Acute embolism and thrombosis of unspecified deep veins of distal lower extremity
Acute embolism and thrombosis of deep vein of calf NOS
Acute embolism and thrombosis of deep vein of lower leg NOS

I82.4Z1 Acute embolism and thrombosis of unspecified deep veins of right distal lower extremity

I82.4Z2   Acute embolism and thrombosis of unspecified deep veins of left distal lower extremity 🔹🔹🔹

I82.4Z3   Acute embolism and thrombosis of unspecified deep veins of distal lower extremity, bilateral 🔹🔹🔹

I82.4Z9   Acute embolism and thrombosis of unspecified deep veins of unspecified distal lower extremity 🔹🔹🔹

● **I82.5 Chronic embolism and thrombosis of deep veins of lower extremity**

Use additional code, if applicable, for associated long-term (current) use of anticoagulants (Z79.01)

Excludes1   personal history of venous embolism and thrombosis (Z86.718)

(Ex) **For category I82.5 CC codes:** See PDX Collection 717

● **I82.50 Chronic embolism and thrombosis of unspecified deep veins of lower extremity**

Excludes1   chronic embolism and thrombosis of unspecified deep veins of distal lower extremity (I82.5Z-)
chronic embolism and thrombosis of unspecified deep veins of proximal lower extremity (I82.5Y-)

I82.501   Chronic embolism and thrombosis of unspecified deep veins of right lower extremity 🔹🔹

I82.502   Chronic embolism and thrombosis of unspecified deep veins of left lower extremity 🔹🔹

I82.503   Chronic embolism and thrombosis of unspecified deep veins of lower extremity, bilateral 🔹🔹

I82.509   Chronic embolism and thrombosis of unspecified deep veins of unspecified lower extremity 🔹🔹

● **I82.51 Chronic embolism and thrombosis of femoral vein**

Chronic embolism and thrombosis of common femoral vein
Chronic embolism and thrombosis of deep femoral vein

I82.511   Chronic embolism and thrombosis of right femoral vein 🔹🔹

I82.512   Chronic embolism and thrombosis of left femoral vein 🔹🔹

I82.513   Chronic embolism and thrombosis of femoral vein, bilateral 🔹🔹

I82.519   Chronic embolism and thrombosis of unspecified femoral vein 🔹🔹

● **I82.52 Chronic embolism and thrombosis of iliac vein**

Chronic embolism and thrombosis of common iliac vein
Chronic embolism and thrombosis of external iliac vein
Chronic embolism and thrombosis of internal iliac vein

I82.521   Chronic embolism and thrombosis of right iliac vein 🔹🔹

I82.522   Chronic embolism and thrombosis of left iliac vein 🔹🔹

I82.523   Chronic embolism and thrombosis of iliac vein, bilateral 🔹🔹

I82.529   Chronic embolism and thrombosis of unspecified iliac vein 🔹🔹

● **I82.53 Chronic embolism and thrombosis of popliteal vein**

I82.531   Chronic embolism and thrombosis of right popliteal vein 🔹🔹

I82.532   Chronic embolism and thrombosis of left popliteal vein 🔹🔹

Item 9–10 Varicose/Varicosities (varix = singular, varices = plural): Enlarged, engorged, tortuous, twisted vascular vessels (veins, arteries, lymphatics). As such, the condition can present in various parts of the body, although the most familiar locations are the lower extremities. A common complication of varices is thrombophlebitis. Varicosities of the anus and rectum are called hemorrhoids.

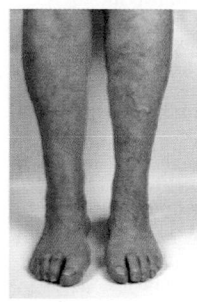

Figure 9-7   Varicose veins of the legs. (Getty Image)

I82.533   Chronic embolism and thrombosis of popliteal vein, bilateral 🔹🔹

I82.539   Chronic embolism and thrombosis of unspecified popliteal vein 🔹🔹

● **I82.54 Chronic embolism and thrombosis of tibial vein**

Chronic embolism and thrombosis of anterior tibial vein
Chronic embolism and thrombosis of posterior tibial vein

I82.541   Chronic embolism and thrombosis of right tibial vein 🔹🔹

I82.542   Chronic embolism and thrombosis of left tibial vein 🔹🔹

I82.543   Chronic embolism and thrombosis of tibial vein, bilateral 🔹🔹

I82.549   Chronic embolism and thrombosis of unspecified tibial vein 🔹🔹

● **I82.55 Chronic embolism and thrombosis of peroneal vein**

I82.551   Chronic embolism and thrombosis of right peroneal vein 🔹

I82.552   Chronic embolism and thrombosis of left peroneal vein 🔹

I82.553   Chronic embolism and thrombosis of peroneal vein, bilateral 🔹

I82.559   Chronic embolism and thrombosis of unspecified peroneal vein 🔹

● **I82.56 Chronic embolism and thrombosis of calf muscular vein**

Chronic embolism and thrombosis of calf muscular vein NOS
Chronic embolism and thrombosis of gastrocnemial vein
Chronic embolism and thrombosis of soleal vein

I82.561   Chronic embolism and thrombosis of right calf muscular vein

I82.562   Chronic embolism and thrombosis of left calf muscular vein

I82.563   Chronic embolism and thrombosis of calf muscular vein, bilateral

I82.569   Chronic embolism and thrombosis of unspecified calf muscular vein

● **I82.59 Chronic embolism and thrombosis of other specified deep vein of lower extremity**

I82.591   Chronic embolism and thrombosis of other specified deep vein of right lower extremity 🔹🔹

I82.592   Chronic embolism and thrombosis of other specified deep vein of left lower extremity 🔹🔹

CHAPTER 9 (I00-I99)

N   Newborn Age: 0   **P**   Pediatric Age: 0–17   **M**   Maternity DX: 9–64   **A**   Adult Age: 15–124   ♀ Females Only   ♂ Males Only

🔹 Complication\Comorbidity   🔹 Major C\C   (Ex) CC/MCC Exclusions   🔹 Hospital-Acquired Condition   🔹 Hierarchical Condition Category

933

I82.593 Chronic embolism and thrombosis of other specified deep vein of lower extremity, bilateral

I82.599 Chronic embolism and thrombosis of other specified deep vein of unspecified lower extremity

● I82.5Y Chronic embolism and thrombosis of unspecified deep veins of proximal lower extremity
  Chronic embolism and thrombosis of deep veins of thigh NOS
  Chronic embolism and thrombosis of deep veins of upper leg NOS

  I82.5Y1 Chronic embolism and thrombosis of unspecified deep veins of right proximal lower extremity

  I82.5Y2 Chronic embolism and thrombosis of unspecified deep veins of left proximal lower extremity

  I82.5Y3 Chronic embolism and thrombosis of unspecified deep veins of proximal lower extremity, bilateral

  I82.5Y9 Chronic embolism and thrombosis of unspecified deep veins of unspecified proximal lower extremity

● I82.5Z Chronic embolism and thrombosis of unspecified deep veins of distal lower extremity
  Chronic embolism and thrombosis of deep veins of calf NOS
  Chronic embolism and thrombosis of deep veins of lower leg NOS

  I82.5Z1 Chronic embolism and thrombosis of unspecified deep veins of right distal lower extremity

  I82.5Z2 Chronic embolism and thrombosis of unspecified deep veins of left distal lower extremity

  I82.5Z3 Chronic embolism and thrombosis of unspecified deep veins of distal lower extremity, bilateral

  I82.5Z9 Chronic embolism and thrombosis of unspecified deep veins of unspecified distal lower extremity

● I82.6 Acute embolism and thrombosis of veins of upper extremity
  Ex: For category I82.6 CC codes: See PDX Collection 717

  ● I82.60 Acute embolism and thrombosis of unspecified veins of upper extremity

    I82.601 Acute embolism and thrombosis of unspecified veins of right upper extremity

    I82.602 Acute embolism and thrombosis of unspecified veins of left upper extremity

    I82.603 Acute embolism and thrombosis of unspecified veins of upper extremity, bilateral

    I82.609 Acute embolism and thrombosis of unspecified veins of unspecified upper extremity

  ● I82.61 Acute embolism and thrombosis of superficial veins of upper extremity
    Acute embolism and thrombosis of antecubital vein
    Acute embolism and thrombosis of basilic vein
    Acute embolism and thrombosis of cephalic vein

    I82.611 Acute embolism and thrombosis of superficial veins of right upper extremity

    I82.612 Acute embolism and thrombosis of superficial veins of left upper extremity

    I82.613 Acute embolism and thrombosis of superficial veins of upper extremity, bilateral

    I82.619 Acute embolism and thrombosis of superficial veins of unspecified upper extremity

  ● I82.62 Acute embolism and thrombosis of deep veins of upper extremity
    Acute embolism and thrombosis of brachial vein
    Acute embolism and thrombosis of radial vein
    Acute embolism and thrombosis of ulnar vein

    I82.621 Acute embolism and thrombosis of deep veins of right upper extremity

    I82.622 Acute embolism and thrombosis of deep veins of left upper extremity

    I82.623 Acute embolism and thrombosis of deep veins of upper extremity, bilateral

    I82.629 Acute embolism and thrombosis of deep veins of unspecified upper extremity

● I82.7 Chronic embolism and thrombosis of veins of upper extremity
  Use additional code, if applicable, for associated long-term (current) use of anticoagulants (Z79.01)
  Excludes1 personal history of venous embolism and thrombosis (Z86.718)
  Ex: For category I82.7 CC codes: See PDX Collection 717

  ● I82.70 Chronic embolism and thrombosis of unspecified veins of upper extremity

    I82.701 Chronic embolism and thrombosis of unspecified veins of right upper extremity

    I82.702 Chronic embolism and thrombosis of unspecified veins of left upper extremity

    I82.703 Chronic embolism and thrombosis of unspecified veins of upper extremity, bilateral

    I82.709 Chronic embolism and thrombosis of unspecified veins of unspecified upper extremity

  ● I82.71 Chronic embolism and thrombosis of superficial veins of upper extremity
    Chronic embolism and thrombosis of antecubital vein
    Chronic embolism and thrombosis of basilic vein
    Chronic embolism and thrombosis of cephalic vein

    I82.711 Chronic embolism and thrombosis of superficial veins of right upper extremity

    I82.712 Chronic embolism and thrombosis of superficial veins of left upper extremity

    I82.713 Chronic embolism and thrombosis of superficial veins of upper extremity, bilateral

    I82.719 Chronic embolism and thrombosis of superficial veins of unspecified upper extremity

  ● I82.72 Chronic embolism and thrombosis of deep veins of upper extremity
    Chronic embolism and thrombosis of brachial vein
    Chronic embolism and thrombosis of radial vein
    Chronic embolism and thrombosis of ulnar vein

I82.721   Chronic embolism and thrombosis of deep veins of right upper extremity 🅒 🅡🅒

I82.722   Chronic embolism and thrombosis of deep veins of left upper extremity 🅒 🅡🅒

I82.723   Chronic embolism and thrombosis of deep veins of upper extremity, bilateral 🅒 🅡🅒

I82.729   Chronic embolism and thrombosis of deep veins of unspecified upper extremity 🅒 🅡🅒

● I82.A   Embolism and thrombosis of axillary vein

     (Ex) **For category I82.A CC codes:** See PDX Collection 717

  ● I82.A1   Acute embolism and thrombosis of axillary vein

     I82.A11   Acute embolism and thrombosis of right axillary vein 🅒 🅡🅒

     I82.A12   Acute embolism and thrombosis of left axillary vein 🅒 🅡🅒

     I82.A13   Acute embolism and thrombosis of axillary vein, bilateral 🅒 🅡🅒

     I82.A19   Acute embolism and thrombosis of unspecified axillary vein 🅒 🅡🅒

  ● I82.A2   Chronic embolism and thrombosis of axillary vein

     I82.A21   Chronic embolism and thrombosis of right axillary vein 🅒 🅡🅒

     I82.A22   Chronic embolism and thrombosis of left axillary vein 🅒 🅡🅒

     I82.A23   Chronic embolism and thrombosis of axillary vein, bilateral 🅒 🅡🅒

     I82.A29   Chronic embolism and thrombosis of unspecified axillary vein 🅒 🅡🅒

● I82.B   Embolism and thrombosis of subclavian vein

     (Ex) **For category I82.B CC codes:** See PDX Collection 717

  ● I82.B1   Acute embolism and thrombosis of subclavian vein

     I82.B11   Acute embolism and thrombosis of right subclavian vein 🅒 🅡🅒

     I82.B12   Acute embolism and thrombosis of left subclavian vein 🅒 🅡🅒

     I82.B13   Acute embolism and thrombosis of subclavian vein, bilateral 🅒 🅡🅒

     I82.B19   Acute embolism and thrombosis of unspecified subclavian vein 🅒 🅡🅒

  ● I82.B2   Chronic embolism and thrombosis of subclavian vein

     I82.B21   Chronic embolism and thrombosis of right subclavian vein 🅒 🅡🅒

     I82.B22   Chronic embolism and thrombosis of left subclavian vein 🅒 🅡🅒

     I82.B23   Chronic embolism and thrombosis of subclavian vein, bilateral 🅒 🅡🅒

     I82.B29   Chronic embolism and thrombosis of unspecified subclavian vein 🅒 🅡🅒

● I82.C   Embolism and thrombosis of internal jugular vein

     (Ex) **For category I82.C CC codes:** See PDX Collection 717

  ● I82.C1   Acute embolism and thrombosis of internal jugular vein

     I82.C11   Acute embolism and thrombosis of right internal jugular vein 🅒 🅡🅒

     I82.C12   Acute embolism and thrombosis of left internal jugular vein 🅒 🅡🅒

     I82.C13   Acute embolism and thrombosis of internal jugular vein, bilateral 🅒 🅡🅒

     I82.C19   Acute embolism and thrombosis of unspecified internal jugular vein 🅒 🅡🅒

● I82.C2   Chronic embolism and thrombosis of internal jugular vein

     I82.C21   Chronic embolism and thrombosis of right internal jugular vein 🅒 🅡🅒

     I82.C22   Chronic embolism and thrombosis of left internal jugular vein 🅒 🅡🅒

     I82.C23   Chronic embolism and thrombosis of internal jugular vein, bilateral 🅒 🅡🅒

     I82.C29   Chronic embolism and thrombosis of unspecified internal jugular vein 🅒 🅡🅒

● I82.8   Embolism and thrombosis of other specified veins

     Use additional code, if applicable, for associated long-term (current) use of anticoagulants (Z79.01)

     (Ex) **For category I82.8 CC codes:** See PDX Collection 717

  ● I82.81   Embolism and thrombosis of superficial veins of lower extremities

     Embolism and thrombosis of saphenous vein (greater) (lesser)

     I82.811   Embolism and thrombosis of superficial veins of right lower extremity 🅒

     I82.812   Embolism and thrombosis of superficial veins of left lower extremity 🅒

     I82.813   Embolism and thrombosis of superficial veins of lower extremities, bilateral 🅒

     I82.819   Embolism and thrombosis of superficial veins of unspecified lower extremity 🅒

  ● I82.89   Embolism and thrombosis of other specified veins

     I82.890   Acute embolism and thrombosis of other specified veins 🅒

     I82.891   Chronic embolism and thrombosis of other specified veins 🅒

● I82.9   Embolism and thrombosis of unspecified vein

     (Ex) **For category I82.9 CC codes:** See PDX Collection 717

     I82.90   Acute embolism and thrombosis of unspecified vein 🅒

       Embolism of vein NOS

       Thrombosis (vein) NOS

     I82.91   Chronic embolism and thrombosis of unspecified vein 🅒

● I83   Varicose veins of lower extremities

     ~~**Excludes1**   varicose veins complicating pregnancy (O22.0-)~~
       ~~varicose veins complicating the puerperium (O87.4)~~

   ▶ **Excludes2**   varicose veins complicating pregnancy (O22.0-)
       ▶varicose veins complicating the puerperium (O87.4)

● I83.0   Varicose veins of lower extremities with ulcer

     Use additional code to identify severity of ulcer (L97.-)

  ● I83.00   Varicose veins of unspecified lower extremity with ulcer

     I83.001   Varicose veins of unspecified lower extremity with ulcer of thigh 🅒   **A**

     I83.002   Varicose veins of unspecified lower extremity with ulcer of calf 🅒   **A**

     I83.003   Varicose veins of unspecified lower extremity with ulcer of ankle 🅒   **A**

     I83.004   Varicose veins of unspecified lower extremity with ulcer of heel and midfoot 🅒   **A**

       Varicose veins of unspecified lower extremity with ulcer of plantar surface of midfoot

     I83.005   Varicose veins of unspecified lower extremity with ulcer other part of foot 🅒   **A**

       Varicose veins of unspecified lower extremity with ulcer of toe

N Newborn Age: 0   **P** Pediatric Age: 0–17   **M** Maternity DX: 9–64   **A** Adult Age: 15–124   ♀ Females Only   ♂ Males Only

🅒 Complication\Comorbidity   🅜 Major C\C   (Ex) CC/MCC Exclusions   🅗 Hospital-Acquired Condition   🅡🅒 Hierarchical Condition Category

935

CHAPTER 9 (I00–I99)

I83.008   Varicose veins of unspecified lower extremity with ulcer other part of lower leg 🌟   A

I83.009   Varicose veins of unspecified lower extremity with ulcer of unspecified site 🌟   A

● I83.01   Varicose veins of right lower extremity with ulcer

I83.011   Varicose veins of right lower extremity with ulcer of thigh 🌟   A

I83.012   Varicose veins of right lower extremity with ulcer of calf 🌟   A

I83.013   Varicose veins of right lower extremity with ulcer of ankle 🌟   A

I83.014   Varicose veins of right lower extremity with ulcer of heel and midfoot 🌟   A

     Varicose veins of right lower extremity with ulcer of plantar surface of midfoot

I83.015   Varicose veins of right lower extremity with ulcer other part of foot 🌟   A

     Varicose veins of right lower extremity with ulcer of toe

I83.018   Varicose veins of right lower extremity with ulcer other part of lower leg 🌟   A

I83.019   Varicose veins of right lower extremity with ulcer of unspecified site 🌟   A

● I83.02   Varicose veins of left lower extremity with ulcer

I83.021   Varicose veins of left lower extremity with ulcer of thigh 🌟   A

I83.022   Varicose veins of left lower extremity with ulcer of calf 🌟   A

I83.023   Varicose veins of left lower extremity with ulcer of ankle 🌟   A

I83.024   Varicose veins of left lower extremity with ulcer of heel and midfoot 🌟   A

     Varicose veins of left lower extremity with ulcer of plantar surface of midfoot

I83.025   Varicose veins of left lower extremity with ulcer other part of foot 🌟   A

     Varicose veins of left lower extremity with ulcer of toe

I83.028   Varicose veins of left lower extremity with ulcer other part of lower leg 🌟   A

I83.029   Varicose veins of left lower extremity with ulcer of unspecified site 🌟   A

● I83.1   Varicose veins of lower extremities with inflammation

I83.10   Varicose veins of unspecified lower extremity with inflammation   A

I83.11   Varicose veins of right lower extremity with inflammation   A

I83.12   Varicose veins of left lower extremity with inflammation   A

● I83.2   Varicose veins of lower extremities with both ulcer and inflammation

     Use additional code to identify severity of ulcer (L97.-)

     Ex: **For category I83.2 CC codes:** See PDX Collection 720

● I83.20   Varicose veins of unspecified lower extremity with both ulcer and inflammation

I83.201   Varicose veins of unspecified lower extremity with both ulcer of thigh and inflammation 🌟🌟   A

I83.202   Varicose veins of unspecified lower extremity with both ulcer of calf and inflammation 🌟🌟   A

I83.203   Varicose veins of unspecified lower extremity with both ulcer of ankle and inflammation 🌟🌟   A

I83.204   Varicose veins of unspecified lower extremity with both ulcer of heel and midfoot and inflammation 🌟🌟   A

     Varicose veins of unspecified lower extremity with both ulcer of plantar surface of midfoot and inflammation

I83.205   Varicose veins of unspecified lower extremity with both ulcer other part of foot and inflammation 🌟🌟   A

     Varicose veins of unspecified lower extremity with both ulcer of toe and inflammation

I83.208   Varicose veins of unspecified lower extremity with both ulcer of other part of lower extremity and inflammation 🌟🌟   A

I83.209   Varicose veins of unspecified lower extremity with both ulcer of unspecified site and inflammation 🌟🌟   A

● I83.21   Varicose veins of right lower extremity with both ulcer and inflammation

I83.211   Varicose veins of right lower extremity with both ulcer of thigh and inflammation 🌟🌟   A

I83.212   Varicose veins of right lower extremity with both ulcer of calf and inflammation 🌟🌟   A

I83.213   Varicose veins of right lower extremity with both ulcer of ankle and inflammation 🌟🌟   A

I83.214   Varicose veins of right lower extremity with both ulcer of heel and midfoot and inflammation 🌟🌟   A

     Varicose veins of right lower extremity with both ulcer of plantar surface of midfoot and inflammation

I83.215   Varicose veins of right lower extremity with both ulcer other part of foot and inflammation 🌟🌟   A

     Varicose veins of right lower extremity with both ulcer of toe and inflammation

I83.218   Varicose veins of right lower extremity with both ulcer of other part of lower extremity and inflammation 🌟🌟   A

I83.219   Varicose veins of right lower extremity with both ulcer of unspecified site and inflammation 🌟🌟   A

● I83.22   Varicose veins of left lower extremity with both ulcer and inflammation

I83.221   Varicose veins of left lower extremity with both ulcer of thigh and inflammation 🌟🌟   A

I83.222   Varicose veins of left lower extremity with both ulcer of calf and inflammation 🌟🌟   A

I83.223   Varicose veins of left lower extremity with both ulcer of ankle and inflammation 🌟🌟   A

I83.224   Varicose veins of left lower extremity with both ulcer of heel and midfoot and inflammation 🌟🌟   A

     Varicose veins of left lower extremity with both ulcer of plantar surface of midfoot and inflammation

▶ New   ⇒ Revised   ~~deleted~~ Deleted   Excludes 1   Excludes 2   Includes   Use additional   Code first   Code also   Key words

OGCR Official Guidelines   ● Unacceptable Principal Diagnosis   X Assign placeholder X   🌟 Use Additional Character(s)   ▶ Manifestation Code   **Coding Clinic**

I83.225   Varicose veins of left lower extremity with both ulcer other part of foot and inflammation 🅒🅒   A
> Varicose veins of left lower extremity with both ulcer of toe and inflammation

I83.228   Varicose veins of left lower extremity with both ulcer of other part of lower extremity and inflammation 🅒🅒   A

I83.229   Varicose veins of left lower extremity with both ulcer of unspecified site and inflammation 🅒🅒   A

● **I83.8**   **Varicose veins of lower extremities with other complications**

  ● **I83.81**   Varicose veins of lower extremities with pain

I83.811   Varicose veins of right lower extremity with pain   A

I83.812   Varicose veins of left lower extremity with pain   A

I83.813   Varicose veins of bilateral lower extremities with pain   A

I83.819   Varicose veins of unspecified lower extremity with pain   A

  ● **I83.89**   Varicose veins of lower extremities with other complications
> Varicose veins of lower extremities with edema
> Varicose veins of lower extremities with swelling

I83.891   Varicose veins of right lower extremity with other complications   A

I83.892   Varicose veins of left lower extremity with other complications   A

I83.893   Varicose veins of bilateral lower extremities with other complications   A

I83.899   Varicose veins of unspecified lower extremity with other complications   A

● **I83.9**   **Asymptomatic varicose veins of lower extremities**
> Phlebectasia of lower extremities
> Varicose veins of lower extremities
> Varix of lower extremities

I83.90   Asymptomatic varicose veins of unspecified lower extremity   A
> Varicose veins NOS

I83.91   Asymptomatic varicose veins of right lower extremity   A

I83.92   Asymptomatic varicose veins of left lower extremity   A

I83.93   Asymptomatic varicose veins of bilateral lower extremities   A

● **I85**   **Esophageal varices**
> Use additional code to identify:
> alcohol abuse and dependence (F10.-)

● **I85.0**   **Esophageal varices**
> Idiopathic esophageal varices
> Primary esophageal varices

I85.00   Esophageal varices without bleeding 🅒🅒
> (Ex:) See PDX Collection 721

I85.01   Esophageal varices with bleeding 🅒🅒
> (Ex:) See PDX Collection 722

● **I85.1**   **Secondary esophageal varices**
> Esophageal varices secondary to alcoholic liver disease
> Esophageal varices secondary to cirrhosis of liver
> Esophageal varices secondary to schistosomiasis
> Esophageal varices secondary to toxic liver disease
> *Code first underlying disease*

I85.10   Secondary esophageal varices without bleeding 🅒🅒
> (Ex:) See PDX Collection 723

I85.11   Secondary esophageal varices with bleeding 🅒🅒
> (Ex:) See PDX Collection 724

● **I86**   **Varicose veins of other sites**
> **Excludes1**   varicose veins of unspecified site (I83.9-)
> **Excludes2**   retinal varices (H35.0-)

I86.0   **Sublingual varices**

I86.1   **Scrotal varices** ♂
> Varicocele

I86.2   **Pelvic varices**

I86.3   **Vulval varices** ♀
> **Excludes1**   vulval varices complicating childbirth and the puerperium (O87.8)
> vulval varices complicating pregnancy (O22.1-)

I86.4   **Gastric varices**

I86.8   **Varicose veins of other specified sites**   A
> Varicose ulcer of nasal septum

● **I87**   **Other disorders of veins**

  ● **I87.0**   **Postthrombotic syndrome**
> Chronic venous hypertension due to deep vein thrombosis
> Postphlebitic syndrome
> **Excludes1**   chronic venous hypertension without deep vein thrombosis (I87.3-)

  ● **I87.00**   Postthrombotic syndrome without complications
> Asymptomatic Postthrombotic syndrome

I87.001   Postthrombotic syndrome without complications of right lower extremity

I87.002   Postthrombotic syndrome without complications of left lower extremity

I87.003   Postthrombotic syndrome without complications of bilateral lower extremity

I87.009   Postthrombotic syndrome without complications of unspecified extremity
> Postthrombotic syndrome NOS

  ● **I87.01**   Postthrombotic syndrome with ulcer
> Use additional code to specify site and severity of ulcer (L97.-)

I87.011   Postthrombotic syndrome with ulcer of right lower extremity 🅒🅒
> (Ex:) See PDX Collection 3387

I87.012   Postthrombotic syndrome with ulcer of left lower extremity 🅒🅒
> (Ex:) See PDX Collection 3388

I87.013   Postthrombotic syndrome with ulcer of bilateral lower extremity 🅒🅒
> (Ex:) See PDX Collection 3389

I87.019   Postthrombotic syndrome with ulcer of unspecified lower extremity 🅒🅒
> (Ex:) See PDX Collection 3390

  ● **I87.02**   Postthrombotic syndrome with inflammation

I87.021   Postthrombotic syndrome with inflammation of right lower extremity

I87.022   Postthrombotic syndrome with inflammation of left lower extremity

I87.023   Postthrombotic syndrome with inflammation of bilateral lower extremity

I87.029   Postthrombotic syndrome with inflammation of unspecified lower extremity

  ● **I87.03**   Postthrombotic syndrome with ulcer and inflammation
> Use additional code to specify site and severity of ulcer (L97.-)

I87.031   Postthrombotic syndrome with ulcer and inflammation of right lower extremity 🅒🅒
> (Ex:) See PDX Collection 3391

N Newborn Age: 0   **P** Pediatric Age: 0–17   **M** Maternity DX: 9–64   **A** Adult Age: 15–124   ♀ Females Only   ♂ Males Only

🅒 Complication\Comorbidity   🅒 Major C\C   (Ex:) CC/MCC Exclusions   Hospital-Acquired Condition   Hierarchical Condition Category

937

- I87.032 Postthrombotic syndrome with ulcer and inflammation of left lower extremity
  - (Ex:) See PDX Collection 3392
- I87.033 Postthrombotic syndrome with ulcer and inflammation of bilateral lower extremity
  - (Ex:) See PDX Collection 3393
- I87.039 Postthrombotic syndrome with ulcer and inflammation of unspecified lower extremity
  - (Ex:) See PDX Collection 3394
- ● I87.09 Postthrombotic syndrome with other complications
  - I87.091 Postthrombotic syndrome with other complications of right lower extremity
  - I87.092 Postthrombotic syndrome with other complications of left lower extremity
  - I87.093 Postthrombotic syndrome with other complications of bilateral lower extremity
  - I87.099 Postthrombotic syndrome with other complications of unspecified lower extremity

I87.1 Compression of vein
Stricture of vein
Vena cava syndrome (inferior) (superior)
Excludes2 compression of pulmonary vein (I28.8)
(Ex:) See PDX Collection 726

I87.2 Venous insufficiency (chronic) (peripheral)
Stasis dermatitis
Excludes1 stasis dermatitis with varicose veins of lower extremities (I83.1-, I83.2-)

● I87.3 Chronic venous hypertension (idiopathic)
Stasis edema
Excludes1 chronic venous hypertension due to deep vein thrombosis (I87.0-)
varicose veins of lower extremities (I83.-)

- ● I87.30 Chronic venous hypertension (idiopathic) without complications
Asymptomatic chronic venous hypertension (idiopathic)
  - I87.301 Chronic venous hypertension (idiopathic) without complications of right lower extremity
  - I87.302 Chronic venous hypertension (idiopathic) without complications of left lower extremity
  - I87.303 Chronic venous hypertension (idiopathic) without complications of bilateral lower extremity
  - I87.309 Chronic venous hypertension (idiopathic) without complications of unspecified lower extremity
Chronic venous hypertension NOS
- ● I87.31 Chronic venous hypertension (idiopathic) with ulcer
Use additional code to specify site and severity of ulcer (L97.-)
  - I87.311 Chronic venous hypertension (idiopathic) with ulcer of right lower extremity
    - (Ex:) See PDX Collection 3395
  - I87.312 Chronic venous hypertension (idiopathic) with ulcer of left lower extremity
    - (Ex:) See PDX Collection 3396
  - I87.313 Chronic venous hypertension (idiopathic) with ulcer of bilateral lower extremity
    - (Ex:) See PDX Collection 3397
  - I87.319 Chronic venous hypertension (idiopathic) with ulcer of unspecified lower extremity
    - (Ex:) See PDX Collection 3398

- ● I87.32 Chronic venous hypertension (idiopathic) with inflammation
  - I87.321 Chronic venous hypertension (idiopathic) with inflammation of right lower extremity
  - I87.322 Chronic venous hypertension (idiopathic) with inflammation of left lower extremity
  - I87.323 Chronic venous hypertension (idiopathic) with inflammation of bilateral lower extremity
  - I87.329 Chronic venous hypertension (idiopathic) with inflammation of unspecified lower extremity
- ● I87.33 Chronic venous hypertension (idiopathic) with ulcer and inflammation
Use additional code to specify site and severity of ulcer (L97.-)
  - I87.331 Chronic venous hypertension (idiopathic) with ulcer and inflammation of right lower extremity
    - (Ex:) See PDX Collection 3399
  - I87.332 Chronic venous hypertension (idiopathic) with ulcer and inflammation of left lower extremity
    - (Ex:) See PDX Collection 3400
  - I87.333 Chronic venous hypertension (idiopathic) with ulcer and inflammation of bilateral lower extremity
    - (Ex:) See PDX Collection 3401
  - I87.339 Chronic venous hypertension (idiopathic) with ulcer and inflammation of unspecified lower extremity
    - (Ex:) See PDX Collection 3402
- ● I87.39 Chronic venous hypertension (idiopathic) with other complications
  - I87.391 Chronic venous hypertension (idiopathic) with other complications of right lower extremity
  - I87.392 Chronic venous hypertension (idiopathic) with other complications of left lower extremity
  - I87.393 Chronic venous hypertension (idiopathic) with other complications of bilateral lower extremity
  - I87.399 Chronic venous hypertension (idiopathic) with other complications of unspecified lower extremity

I87.8 Other specified disorders of veins
Phlebosclerosis
Venofibrosis

I87.9 Disorder of vein, unspecified

● I88 Nonspecific lymphadenitis
Excludes1 acute lymphadenitis, except mesenteric (L04.-)
enlarged lymph nodes NOS (R59.-)
human immunodeficiency virus [HIV] disease resulting in generalized lymphadenopathy (B20)

I88.0 Nonspecific mesenteric lymphadenitis
Mesenteric lymphadenitis (acute)(chronic)

I88.1 Chronic lymphadenitis, except mesenteric
Adenitis
Lymphadenitis

I88.8 Other nonspecific lymphadenitis

I88.9 Nonspecific lymphadenitis, unspecified
Lymphadenitis NOS

▶ New ⟹ Revised ~~deleted~~ Deleted | Excludes 1 | Excludes 2 | Includes | Use additional | Code first | Code also | Key words |
OGCR Official Guidelines ● Unacceptable Principal Diagnosis X Assign placeholder X ● Use Additional Character(s) ▶ Manifestation Code **Coding Clinic**

● **I89**   **Other noninfective disorders of lymphatic vessels and lymph nodes**

     Excludes1   chylocele, tunica vaginalis (nonfilarial) NOS (N50.89)
               enlarged lymph nodes NOS (R59.-)
               filarial chylocele (B74.-)
               hereditary lymphedema (Q82.0)

     I89.0   **Lymphedema, not elsewhere classified**
           Elephantiasis (nonfilarial) NOS
           Lymphangiectasis
           Obliteration, lymphatic vessel
           Praecox lymphedema
           Secondary lymphedema

         Excludes1   postmastectomy lymphedema (I97.2)

     I89.1   **Lymphangitis**
           Chronic lymphangitis
           Lymphangitis NOS
           Subacute lymphangitis

         Excludes1   acute lymphangitis (L03.-)

     I89.8   **Other specified noninfective disorders of lymphatic vessels and lymph nodes**
           Chylocele (nonfilarial)
           Chylous ascites
           Chylous cyst
           Lipomelanotic reticulosis
           Lymph node or vessel fistula
           Lymph node or vessel infarction
           Lymph node or vessel rupture

     I89.9   **Noninfective disorder of lymphatic vessels and lymph nodes, unspecified**
           Disease of lymphatic vessels NOS

OTHER AND UNSPECIFIED DISORDERS OF THE CIRCULATORY SYSTEM (I95-I99)

● **I95**   **Hypotension**
     Subnormal arterial blood pressure

     Excludes1   cardiovascular collapse (R57.9)
               maternal hypotension syndrome (O26.5-)
               nonspecific low blood pressure reading NOS (R03.1)

     I95.0   **Idiopathic hypotension**

     I95.1   **Orthostatic hypotension**
           Hypotension, postural
           Moving from a sitting or reclining position to a standing position precipitates a sudden drop in blood pressure (hypotension).

         Excludes1   neurogenic orthostatic hypotension [Shy-Drager] (G90.3)
                     orthostatic hypotension due to drugs (I95.2)

     I95.2   **Hypotension due to drugs**
           Orthostatic hypotension due to drugs
           Use additional code for adverse effect, if applicable, to identify drug (T36-T50 with fifth or sixth character 5)

     I95.3   **Hypotension of hemodialysis**
           Intra-dialytic hypotension

  ● **I95.8**   **Other hypotension**

     I95.81   **Postprocedural hypotension**

     I95.89   **Other hypotension**
           Chronic hypotension

     I95.9   **Hypotension, unspecified**

● **I96**   **Gangrene, not elsewhere classified** 🔹🔹
     Gangrenous cellulitis

     Excludes1   gangrene in atherosclerosis of native arteries of the extremities (I70.26)
               gangrene of certain specified sites - *see* Alphabetical Index
               gangrene in hernia (K40.1, K40.4, K41.1, K41.4, K42.1, K43.1-, K44.1, K45.1, K46.1)
               gangrene in other peripheral vascular diseases (I73.-)
               gas gangrene (A48.0)
               pyoderma gangrenosum (L88)

     Excludes2   gangrene in diabetes mellitus (E08-E13 with .52)

     (Ex:) See PDX Collection 519
     Coding Clinic: 2018, Q4, P87; 2017, Q3, P6; 2013, Q2, P35

● **I97**   **Intraoperative and postprocedural complications and disorders of circulatory system, not elsewhere classified**

     Excludes2   postprocedural shock (T81.1-)
     Coding Clinic: 2019, Q2, P22

     I97.0   **Postcardiotomy syndrome**

  ● **I97.1**   **Other postprocedural cardiac functional disturbances**

     Excludes2   acute pulmonary insufficiency following thoracic surgery (J95.1)
               intraoperative cardiac functional disturbances (I97.7-)
     (Ex:) For category I97.1 CC codes: See PDX Collection 728

  ● **I97.11**   **Postprocedural cardiac insufficiency**

     I97.110   **Postprocedural cardiac insufficiency following cardiac surgery** 🔹

     I97.111   **Postprocedural cardiac insufficiency following other surgery** 🔹

  ● **I97.12**   **Postprocedural cardiac arrest**

     I97.120   **Postprocedural cardiac arrest following cardiac surgery** 🔹

     I97.121   **Postprocedural cardiac arrest following other surgery** 🔹

  ● **I97.13**   **Postprocedural heart failure**
           Use additional code to identify the heart failure (I50.-)

     I97.130   **Postprocedural heart failure following cardiac surgery** 🔹

     I97.131   **Postprocedural heart failure following other surgery** 🔹

  ● **I97.19**   **Other postprocedural cardiac functional disturbances**
           Use additional code, if applicable, to further specify disorder

     I97.190   **Other postprocedural cardiac functional disturbances following cardiac surgery** 🔹
             Use Additional code, if applicable, for type 4 or type 5 myocardial infarction, to further specify disorder
             Coding Clinic: 2019, Q2, P32-33

     I97.191   **Other postprocedural cardiac functional disturbances following other surgery** 🔹

     I97.2   **Postmastectomy lymphedema syndrome**   A
           Elephantiasis due to mastectomy
           Obliteration of lymphatic vessels

     I97.3   **Postprocedural hypertension**

  ● **I97.4**   **Intraoperative hemorrhage and hematoma of a circulatory system organ or structure complicating a procedure**

     Excludes1   intraoperative hemorrhage and hematoma of a circulatory system organ or structure due to accidental puncture and laceration during a procedure (I97.5-)

     Excludes2   intraoperative cerebrovascular hemorrhage complicating a procedure (G97.3-)
     (Ex:) For category I97.4 CC codes: See PDX Collection 729

  ● **I97.41**   **Intraoperative hemorrhage and hematoma of a circulatory system organ or structure complicating a circulatory system procedure**

     I97.410   **Intraoperative hemorrhage and hematoma of a circulatory system organ or structure complicating a cardiac catheterization** 🔹

     I97.411   **Intraoperative hemorrhage and hematoma of a circulatory system organ or structure complicating a cardiac bypass** 🔹

N   Newborn Age: 0   P   Pediatric Age: 0–17   M   Maternity DX: 9–64   A   Adult Age: 15–124   ♀   Females Only   ♂   Males Only

🔹 Complication\Comorbidity   🔹 Major C\C   (Ex:) CC/MCC Exclusions   🔹 Hospital-Acquired Condition   🔹 Hierarchical Condition Category

939

I97.418   Intraoperative hemorrhage and hematoma of a circulatory system organ or structure complicating other circulatory system procedure 🔖

I97.42   Intraoperative hemorrhage and hematoma of a circulatory system organ or structure complicating other procedure 🔖
Coding Clinic: 2020, Q1, P20; 2016, Q4, P100

● I97.5   Accidental puncture and laceration of a circulatory system organ or structure during a procedure

Excludes2   accidental puncture and laceration of brain during a procedure (G97.4-)

Ⓔⓧ For category I97.5 CC codes: See PDX Collection 509

I97.51   Accidental puncture and laceration of a circulatory system organ or structure during a circulatory system procedure 🔖
Coding Clinic: 2019, Q2, P24

I97.52   Accidental puncture and laceration of a circulatory system organ or structure during other procedure 🔖

● I97.6   Postprocedural hemorrhage, hematoma and seroma of a circulatory system organ or structure following a procedure

Excludes2   postprocedural cerebrovascular hemorrhage complicating a procedure (G97.5-)

Ⓔⓧ For category I97.6 CC codes: See PDX Collection 729
Coding Clinic: 2016, Q4, P10

● I97.61   Postprocedural hemorrhage of a circulatory system organ or structure following a circulatory system procedure

I97.610   Postprocedural hemorrhage of a circulatory system organ or structure following a cardiac catheterization 🔖

I97.611   Postprocedural hemorrhage of a circulatory system organ or structure following cardiac bypass 🔖

I97.618   Postprocedural hemorrhage of a circulatory system organ or structure following other circulatory system procedure 🔖

● I97.62   Postprocedural hemorrhage, hematoma and seroma of a circulatory system organ or structure following other procedure

I97.620   Postprocedural hemorrhage of a circulatory system organ or structure following other procedure 🔖

I97.621   Postprocedural hematoma of a circulatory system organ or structure following other procedure 🔖

I97.622   Postprocedural seroma of a circulatory system organ or structure following other procedure 🔖

● I97.63   Postprocedural hematoma of a circulatory system organ or structure following a circulatory system procedure

I97.630   Postprocedural hematoma of a circulatory system organ or structure following a cardiac catheterization 🔖

I97.631   Postprocedural hematoma of a circulatory system organ or structure following cardiac bypass 🔖

I97.638   Postprocedural hematoma of a circulatory system organ or structure following other circulatory system procedure 🔖

● I97.64   Postprocedural seroma of a circulatory system organ or structure following a circulatory system procedure

I97.640   Postprocedural seroma of a circulatory system organ or structure following a cardiac catheterization 🔖

I97.641   Postprocedural seroma of a circulatory system organ or structure following cardiac bypass 🔖

I97.648   Postprocedural seroma of a circulatory system organ or structure following other circulatory system procedure 🔖

● I97.7   Intraoperative cardiac functional disturbances

Excludes2   acute pulmonary insufficiency following thoracic surgery (J95.1)
postprocedural cardiac functional disturbances (I97.1-)

Ⓔⓧ For category I97.7 CC codes: See PDX Collection 728

● I97.71   Intraoperative cardiac arrest

I97.710   Intraoperative cardiac arrest during cardiac surgery 🔖

I97.711   Intraoperative cardiac arrest during other surgery 🔖

● I97.79   Other intraoperative cardiac functional disturbances

Use additional code, if applicable, to further specify disorder

I97.790   Other intraoperative cardiac functional disturbances during cardiac surgery 🔖

I97.791   Other intraoperative cardiac functional disturbances during other surgery 🔖

● I97.8   Other intraoperative and postprocedural complications and disorders of the circulatory system, not elsewhere classified

Use additional code, if applicable, to further specify disorder

Ⓔⓧ For category I97.8 CC codes unless otherwise indicated: See PDX Collection 617

● I97.81   Intraoperative cerebrovascular infarction

I97.810   Intraoperative cerebrovascular infarction during cardiac surgery 🔖🔖

I97.811   Intraoperative cerebrovascular infarction during other surgery 🔖🔖

● I97.82   Postprocedural cerebrovascular infarction

I97.820   Postprocedural cerebrovascular infarction following cardiac surgery 🔖🔖

I97.821   Postprocedural cerebrovascular infarction following other surgery 🔖🔖

I97.88   Other intraoperative complications of the circulatory system, not elsewhere classified 🔖
Ⓔⓧ See PDX Collection 728

I97.89   Other postprocedural complications and disorders of the circulatory system, not elsewhere classified 🔖
Ⓔⓧ See PDX Collection 728
Coding Clinic: 2019, Q2, P32-33

● I99   Other and unspecified disorders of circulatory system

I99.8   Other disorder of circulatory system

I99.9   Unspecified disorder of circulatory system

CHAPTER 10

DISEASES OF THE RESPIRATORY SYSTEM (J00-J99)

OGCR Chapter-Specific Coding Guidelines

10. **Chapter 10: Diseases of the Respiratory System (J00-J99)**

    a. **Chronic Obstructive Pulmonary Disease [COPD] and Asthma**

       1) **Acute exacerbation of chronic obstructive bronchitis and asthma**

    The codes in categories J44 and J45 distinguish between uncomplicated cases and those in acute exacerbation. An acute exacerbation is a worsening or a decompensation of a chronic condition. An acute exacerbation is not equivalent to an infection superimposed on a chronic condition, though an exacerbation may be triggered by an infection.

    b. **Acute Respiratory Failure**

       1) **Acute respiratory failure as principal diagnosis**

    A code from subcategory J96.0, Acute respiratory failure, or subcategory J96.2, Acute and chronic respiratory failure, may be assigned as a principal diagnosis when it is the condition established after study to be chiefly responsible for occasioning the admission to the hospital, and the selection is supported by the Alphabetic Index and Tabular List. However, chapter-specific coding guidelines (such as obstetrics, poisoning, HIV, newborn) that provide sequencing direction take precedence.

       2) **Acute respiratory failure as secondary diagnosis**

    Respiratory failure may be listed as a secondary diagnosis if it occurs after admission, or if it is present on admission, but does not meet the definition of principal diagnosis.

       3) **Sequencing of acute respiratory failure and another acute condition**

    When a patient is admitted with respiratory failure and another acute condition (e.g., myocardial infarction, cerebrovascular accident, aspiration pneumonia), the principal diagnosis will not be the same in every situation. This applies whether the other acute condition is a respiratory or nonrespiratory condition. Selection of the principal diagnosis will be dependent on the circumstances of admission. If both the respiratory failure and the other acute condition are equally responsible for occasioning the admission to the hospital, and there are no chapter-specific sequencing rules, the guideline regarding two or more diagnoses that equally meet the definition for principal diagnosis (*Section II, C.*) may be applied in these situations.

    If the documentation is not clear as to whether acute respiratory failure and another condition are equally responsible for occasioning the admission, query the provider for clarification.

    c. **Influenza due to certain identified influenza viruses**

    Code only confirmed cases of influenza due to certain identified influenza viruses (category J09), and due to other identified influenza virus (category J10). This is an exception to the hospital inpatient guideline Section II, H. (Uncertain Diagnosis).

    In this context, "confirmation" does not require documentation of positive laboratory testing specific for avian or other novel influenza A or other identified influenza virus. However, coding should be based on the provider's diagnostic statement that the patient has avian influenza, or other novel influenza A, for category J09, or has another particular identified strain of influenza, such as H1N1 or H3N2, but not identified as novel or variant, for category J10.

    If the provider records "suspected" or "possible" or "probable" avian influenza, or novel influenza, or other identified influenza, then the appropriate influenza code from category J11, Influenza due to unidentified influenza virus, should be assigned. A code from category J09, Influenza due to certain identified influenza viruses, should not be assigned nor should a code from category J10, Influenza due to other identified influenza virus.

    d. **Ventilator associated Pneumonia**

       1) **Documentation of Ventilator associated Pneumonia**

    As with all procedural or postprocedural complications, code assignment is based on the provider's documentation of the relationship between the condition and the procedure.

    Code J95.851, Ventilator associated pneumonia, should be assigned only when the provider has documented ventilator associated pneumonia (VAP). An additional code to identify the organism (e.g., Pseudomonas aeruginosa, code B96.5) should also be assigned. Do not assign an additional code from categories J12-J18 to identify the type of pneumonia.

    Code J95.851 should not be assigned for cases where the patient has pneumonia and is on a mechanical ventilator and the provider has not specifically stated that the pneumonia is ventilator associated pneumonia. If the documentation is unclear as to whether the patient has a pneumonia that is a complication attributable to the mechanical ventilator, query the provider.

       2) **Ventilator associated Pneumonia Develops after Admission**

    A patient may be admitted with one type of pneumonia (e.g., code J13, Pneumonia due to Streptococcus pneumonia) and subsequently develop VAP. In this instance, the principal diagnosis would be the appropriate code from categories J12-J18 for the pneumonia diagnosed at the time of admission. Code J95.851, Ventilator associated pneumonia, would be assigned as an additional diagnosis when the provider has also documented the presence of ventilator associated pneumonia.

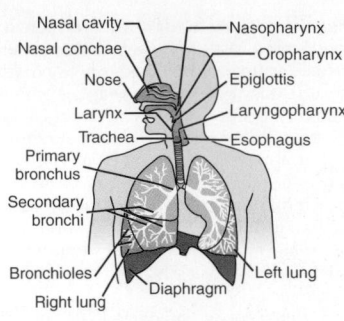

Figure 10-1   Respiratory system. (From Buck CJ: Step-by-Step Medical Coding, ed 2016, St. Louis, Elsevier, 2016)

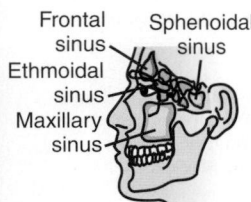

Figure 10-2   Paranasal sinuses. (From Buck CJ: Step-by-Step Medical Coding, ed 2016, St. Louis, Elsevier, 2016)

Item 10–1   Pharyngitis is painful inflammation of the pharynx (sore throat). Ninety percent of the infections are caused by a virus with the remaining being bacterial and rarely a fungus (candidiasis). Other irritants such as pollutants, chemicals, or smoke may cause similar symptoms.

CHAPTER 10

DISEASES OF THE RESPIRATORY SYSTEM (J00-J99)

Note: When a respiratory condition is described as occurring in more than one site and is not specifically indexed, it should be classified to the lower anatomic site (e.g., tracheobronchitis to bronchitis in J40).

Use additional code, where applicable, to identify:
exposure to environmental tobacco smoke (Z77.22)
exposure to tobacco smoke in the perinatal period (P96.81)
history of tobacco dependence (Z87.891)
occupational exposure to environmental tobacco smoke (Z57.31)
tobacco dependence (F17.-)
tobacco use (Z72.0)

Excludes2   certain conditions originating in the perinatal period (P04-P96)
certain infectious and parasitic diseases (A00-B99)
complications of pregnancy, childbirth and the puerperium (O00-O99A)
congenital malformations, deformations and chromosomal abnormalities (Q00-Q99)
endocrine, nutritional and metabolic diseases (E00-E88)
injury, poisoning and certain other consequences of external causes (S00-T88)
neoplasms (C00-D49)
smoke inhalation (T59.81-)
symptoms, signs and abnormal clinical and laboratory findings, not elsewhere classified (R00-R94)

This chapter contains the following blocks:

J00-J06	Acute upper respiratory infections
J09-J18	Influenza and pneumonia
J20-J22	Other acute lower respiratory infections
J30-J39	Other diseases of upper respiratory tract
J40-J47	Chronic lower respiratory diseases
J60-J70	Lung diseases due to external agents
J80-J84	Other respiratory diseases principally affecting the interstitium
J85-J86	Suppurative and necrotic conditions of the lower respiratory tract
J90-J94	Other diseases of the pleura
J95	Intraoperative and postprocedural complications and disorders of respiratory system, not elsewhere classified
J96-J99	Other diseases of the respiratory system

ACUTE UPPER RESPIRATORY INFECTIONS (J00-J06)

Excludes1   chronic obstructive pulmonary disease with acute lower respiratory infection (J44.0)

J00   **Acute nasopharyngitis [common cold]**
Acute rhinitis
Coryza (acute)
Infective nasopharyngitis NOS
Infective rhinitis
Nasal catarrh, acute
Nasopharyngitis NOS

Excludes1   acute pharyngitis (J02.-)
acute sore throat NOS (J02.9)
influenza virus with other respiratory manifestations (J09.X2, J10.1, J11.1)
pharyngitis NOS (J02.9)
rhinitis NOS (J31.0)
sore throat NOS (J02.9)

Excludes2   allergic rhinitis (J30.1-J30.9)
chronic pharyngitis (J31.2)
chronic rhinitis (J31.0)
chronic sore throat (J31.2)
nasopharyngitis, chronic (J31.1)
vasomotor rhinitis (J30.0)

★ **(See Plate 27 of the Anatomy Illustrations.)**

● **J01**   **Acute sinusitis**

Includes   acute abscess of sinus
acute empyema of sinus
acute infection of sinus
acute inflammation of sinus
acute suppuration of sinus

Use additional code (B95-B97) to identify infectious agent.

Excludes1   sinusitis NOS (J32.9)

Excludes2   chronic sinusitis (J32.0-J32.8)

● **J01.0**   **Acute maxillary sinusitis**
Acute antritis

    J01.00   **Acute maxillary sinusitis, unspecified**

    J01.01   **Acute recurrent maxillary sinusitis**

● **J01.1**   **Acute frontal sinusitis**

    J01.10   **Acute frontal sinusitis, unspecified**

    J01.11   **Acute recurrent frontal sinusitis**

● **J01.2**   **Acute ethmoidal sinusitis**

    J01.20   **Acute ethmoidal sinusitis, unspecified**

    J01.21   **Acute recurrent ethmoidal sinusitis**

● **J01.3**   **Acute sphenoidal sinusitis**

    J01.30   **Acute sphenoidal sinusitis, unspecified**

    J01.31   **Acute recurrent sphenoidal sinusitis**

● **J01.4**   **Acute pansinusitis**

    J01.40   **Acute pansinusitis, unspecified**

    J01.41   **Acute recurrent pansinusitis**

▶ New   ⇒ Revised   ~~deleted~~ Deleted   Excludes 1   Excludes 2   Includes   Use additional   Code first   Code also   Key words
OGCR Official Guidelines   ● Unacceptable Principal Diagnosis   X Assign placeholder X   ● Use Additional Character(s)   ▶ Manifestation Code   **Coding Clinic**

● **J01.8　Other acute sinusitis**

　　J01.80　　Other acute sinusitis
　　　　　　　Acute sinusitis involving more than one sinus
　　　　　　　but not pansinusitis

　　J01.81　　Other acute recurrent sinusitis
　　　　　　　Acute recurrent sinusitis involving more than
　　　　　　　one sinus but not pansinusitis

● **J01.9　Acute sinusitis, unspecified**

　　J01.90　　**Acute sinusitis, unspecified**

　　J01.91　　**Acute recurrent sinusitis, unspecified**

● **J02　Acute pharyngitis**

　　Includes　　acute sore throat
　　Excludes1　acute laryngopharyngitis (J06.0)
　　　　　　　peritonsillar abscess (J36)
　　　　　　　pharyngeal abscess (J39.1)
　　　　　　　retropharyngeal abscess (J39.0)
　　Excludes2　chronic pharyngitis (J31.2)

　J02.0　　**Streptococcal pharyngitis**
　　　　　Septic pharyngitis
　　　　　Streptococcal sore throat
　　　　　Excludes2　scarlet fever (A38.-)

　J02.8　　**Acute pharyngitis due to other specified organisms**
　　　　　Use additional code (B95-B97) to identify infectious
　　　　　　agent
　　　　　Excludes1　pharyngitis due to coxsackie virus (B08.5)
　　　　　　　　　　pharyngitis due to gonococcus (A54.5)
　　　　　　　　　　acute pharyngitis due to herpes [simplex]
　　　　　　　　　　　virus (B00.2)
　　　　　　　　　　acute pharyngitis due to infectious
　　　　　　　　　　　mononucleosis (B27.-)
　　　　　　　　　　enteroviral vesicular pharyngitis (B08.5)

　J02.9　　**Acute pharyngitis, unspecified**
　　　　　Gangrenous pharyngitis (acute)
　　　　　Infective pharyngitis (acute) NOS
　　　　　Pharyngitis (acute) NOS
　　　　　Sore throat (acute) NOS
　　　　　Suppurative pharyngitis (acute)
　　　　　Ulcerative pharyngitis (acute)
　　　　　Excludes1　influenza virus with other respiratory
　　　　　　　　　　manifestations (J09.X2, J10.1, J11.1)

● **J03　Acute tonsillitis**

　　Inflammation of pharyngeal tonsils caused by virus or bacteria
　　Excludes1　acute sore throat (J02.-)
　　　　　　　hypertrophy of tonsils (J35.1)
　　　　　　　peritonsillar abscess (J36)
　　　　　　　sore throat NOS (J02.9)
　　　　　　　streptococcal sore throat (J02.0)
　　Excludes2　chronic tonsillitis (J35.0)

　J03.0　　**Streptococcal tonsillitis**

　　J03.00　　**Acute streptococcal tonsillitis, unspecified**

　　J03.01　　**Acute recurrent streptococcal tonsillitis**

　J03.8　　**Acute tonsillitis due to other specified organisms**
　　　　　Use additional code (B95-B97) to identify infectious
　　　　　　agent.
　　　　　Excludes1　diphtheritic tonsillitis (A36.0)
　　　　　　　　　　herpesviral pharyngotonsillitis (B00.2)
　　　　　　　　　　streptococcal tonsillitis (J03.0)
　　　　　　　　　　tuberculous tonsillitis (A15.8)
　　　　　　　　　　Vincent's tonsillitis (A69.1)

　　J03.80　　**Acute tonsillitis due to other specified
　　　　　　　organisms**

　　J03.81　　**Acute recurrent tonsillitis due to other specified
　　　　　　　organisms**

Item 10-2　Laryngitis is an inflammation of the larynx (voice box) resulting in hoarse voice or the complete loss of the voice. **Tracheitis** is an inflammation of the trachea (often following a URI) commonly caused by *staphylococcus aureus* resulting in inspiratory stridor (crowing sound on inspiration) and a crouplike cough.

● **J03.9　Acute tonsillitis, unspecified**
　　　　Follicular tonsillitis (acute)
　　　　Gangrenous tonsillitis (acute)
　　　　Infective tonsillitis (acute)
　　　　Tonsillitis (acute) NOS
　　　　Ulcerative tonsillitis (acute)
　　　　Excludes1　influenza virus with other respiratory
　　　　　　　　　manifestations (J09.X2, J10.1, J11.1)

　　J03.90　　**Acute tonsillitis, unspecified**

　　J03.91　　**Acute recurrent tonsillitis, unspecified**

● **J04　Acute laryngitis and tracheitis**

　　Use additional code (B95-B97) to identify infectious agent.
　　Code also influenza, if present, such as:
　　　influenza due to identified novel influenza A virus with other
　　　　respiratory manifestations (J09.X2)
　　　influenza due to other identified influenza virus with other
　　　　respiratory manifestations (J10.1)
　　　influenza due to unidentified influenza virus with other
　　　　respiratory manifestations (J11.1)
　　Excludes1　acute obstructive laryngitis [croup] and
　　　　　　　epiglottitis (J05.-)
　　Excludes2　laryngismus (stridulus) (J38.5)

　J04.0　　**Acute laryngitis**
　　　　　Edematous laryngitis (acute)
　　　　　Laryngitis (acute) NOS
　　　　　Subglottic laryngitis (acute)
　　　　　Suppurative laryngitis (acute)
　　　　　Ulcerative laryngitis (acute)
　　　　　Excludes1　acute obstructive laryngitis (J05.0)
　　　　　Excludes2　chronic laryngitis (J37.0)

● **J04.1**　　**Acute tracheitis**
　　　　　Acute viral tracheitis
　　　　　Catarrhal tracheitis (acute)
　　　　　Tracheitis (acute) NOS
　　　　　Excludes2　chronic tracheitis (J42)

　　J04.10　　**Acute tracheitis without obstruction**

　　J04.11　　**Acute tracheitis with obstruction** 🔗
　　　　　　　(Ex) See PDX Collection 730

　J04.2　　**Acute laryngotracheitis**
　　　　　Laryngotracheitis NOS
　　　　　Tracheitis (acute) with laryngitis (acute)
　　　　　Excludes1　acute obstructive laryngotracheitis (J05.0)
　　　　　Excludes2　chronic laryngotracheitis (J37.1)

● **J04.3**　　**Supraglottitis, unspecified**

　　J04.30　　**Supraglottitis, unspecified, without obstruction**

　　J04.31　　**Supraglottitis, unspecified, with obstruction** 🔗
　　　　　　　(Ex) See PDX Collection 731

● **J05　Acute obstructive laryngitis [croup] and epiglottitis**

　　Use additional code (B95-B97) to identify infectious agent.
　➡ Code also influenza, if present, such as:
　　　influenza due to identified novel influenza A virus with other
　　　　respiratory manifestations (J09.X2)
　　　influenza due to other identified influenza virus with other
　　　　respiratory manifestations (J10.1)
　　　influenza due to unidentified influenza virus with other
　　　　respiratory manifestations (J11.1)

　J05.0　　**Acute obstructive laryngitis [croup]**
　　　　　Obstructive laryngitis (acute) NOS
　　　　　Obstructive laryngotracheitis NOS

N Newborn Age: 0　　**P** Pediatric Age: 0-17　　**M** Maternity DX: 9-64　　**A** Adult Age: 15-124　　♀ Females Only　　♂ Males Only

🔗 Complication\Comorbidity　　🔗 Major C\C　　(Ex) CC/MCC Exclusions　　🔗 Hospital-Acquired Condition　　🔗 Hierarchical Condition Category

943

● **J05.1** **Acute epiglottitis**
  Excludes2 epiglottitis, chronic (J37.0)
  J05.10 **Acute epiglottitis without obstruction** 🔖
      Epiglottitis NOS
      Ⓔ See PDX Collection 732
  J05.11 **Acute epiglottitis with obstruction** 🔖
      Ⓔ See PDX Collection 730

● **J06** **Acute upper respiratory infections of multiple and unspecified sites**
  Excludes1 acute respiratory infection NOS (J22)
      influenza virus with other respiratory manifestations (J09.X2, J10.1, J11.1)
      streptococcal pharyngitis (J02.0)
  Coding Clinic: 2020, Q1, P22

  J06.0 **Acute laryngopharyngitis**
  J06.9 **Acute upper respiratory infection, unspecified**
      Upper respiratory disease, acute
      Upper respiratory infection NOS
      Use additional code (B95-B97) to identify infectious agent, if known, such as:
      respiratory syncytial virus (RSV) (B97.4)

INFLUENZA AND PNEUMONIA (J09-J18)

Excludes2 allergic or eosinophilic pneumonia (J82)
      aspiration pneumonia NOS (J69.0)
      meconium pneumonia (P24.01)
      neonatal aspiration pneumonia (P24.-)
      pneumonia due to solids and liquids (J69.-)
      congenital pneumonia (P23.9)
      lipid pneumonia (J69.1)
      rheumatic pneumonia (I00)
      ventilator associated pneumonia (J95.851)
Coding Clinic: 2020, Q1, P22

● **J09** **Influenza due to certain identified influenza viruses**
  Excludes1 influenza A/H1N1 (J10.-)
      influenza due to other influenza viruses (J10.-)
      influenza due to unidentified influenza virus (J11.-)
      seasonal influenza due to other identified influenza virus (J10.-)
      seasonal influenza due to unidentified influenza virus (J11.-)

  ● **J09.X** **Influenza due to identified novel influenza A virus**
      Avian influenza
      Bird influenza
      Influenza A/H5N1
      Influenza of other animal origin, not bird or swine
      Swine influenza virus (viruses that normally cause infections in pigs)
      Coding Clinic: 2016, Q3, P11

  J09.X1 **Influenza due to identified novel influenza A virus with pneumonia** 🔖
      Code also , if applicable, associated:
      lung abscess (J85.1)
      other specified type of pneumonia
      Ⓔ See PDX Collection 110

  J09.X2 **Influenza due to identified novel influenza A virus with other respiratory manifestations**
      Influenza due to identified novel influenza A virus NOS
      Influenza due to identified novel influenza A virus with laryngitis
      Influenza due to identified novel influenza A virus with pharyngitis
      Influenza due to identified novel influenza A virus with upper respiratory symptoms
      Use additional code, if applicable, for associated:
      pleural effusion (J91.8)
      sinusitis (J01.-)

  J09.X3 **Influenza due to identified novel influenza A virus with gastrointestinal manifestations**
      Influenza due to identified novel influenza A virus gastroenteritis
      Excludes1 'intestinal flu' [viral gastroenteritis] (A08.-)

  J09.X9 **Influenza due to identified novel influenza A virus with other manifestations**
      Influenza due to identified novel influenza A virus with encephalopathy
      Influenza due to identified novel influenza A virus with myocarditis
      Influenza due to identified novel influenza A virus with otitis media
      Use additional code to identify manifestation

● **J10** **Influenza due to other identified influenza virus**
  Includes influenza A (non-novel)
      influenza B
      influenza C
  Excludes1 influenza due to avian influenza virus (J09.X-)
      influenza due to swine flu (J09.X-)
      influenza due to unidentified influenza virus (J11.-)

  ● **J10.0** **Influenza due to other identified influenza virus with pneumonia**
      Code also associated lung abscess, if applicable (J85.1)
  J10.00 **Influenza due to other identified influenza virus with unspecified type of pneumonia** 🔖
      Ⓔ See PDX Collection 110
  J10.01 **Influenza due to other identified influenza virus with the same other identified influenza virus pneumonia** 🔖
      Ⓔ See PDX Collection 110
  J10.08 **Influenza due to other identified influenza virus with other specified pneumonia** 🔖
      Code also other specified type of pneumonia
      Ⓔ See PDX Collection 733
      Coding Clinic: 2017, Q4, P96

  J10.1 **Influenza due to other identified influenza virus with other respiratory manifestations**
      Influenza due to other identified influenza virus NOS
      Influenza due to other identified influenza virus with laryngitis
      Influenza due to other identified influenza virus with pharyngitis
      Influenza due to other identified influenza virus with upper respiratory symptoms
      Use additional code for associated pleural effusion, if applicable (J91.8)
      Use additional code for associated sinusitis, if applicable (J01.-)
      Coding Clinic: 2016, Q3, P11

  J10.2 **Influenza due to other identified influenza virus with gastrointestinal manifestations**
      Influenza due to other identified influenza virus gastroenteritis
      Excludes1 'intestinal flu' [viral gastroenteritis] (A08.-)

  ● **J10.8** **Influenza due to other identified influenza virus with other manifestations**
  J10.81 **Influenza due to other identified influenza virus with encephalopathy**
  J10.82 **Influenza due to other identified influenza virus with myocarditis**
  J10.83 **Influenza due to other identified influenza virus with otitis media**
      Use additional code for any associated perforated tympanic membrane (H72.-)
  J10.89 **Influenza due to other identified influenza virus with other manifestations**
      Use additional codes to identify the manifestations

● **J11   Influenza due to unidentified influenza virus**
  ● **J11.0   Influenza due to unidentified influenza virus with pneumonia**

      Code also associated lung abscess, if applicable (J85.1)

      (Ex) **For category J11.0 CC codes:** See PDX Collection 110

    J11.00   Influenza due to unidentified influenza virus with unspecified type of pneumonia 🖤
          Influenza with pneumonia NOS
          Coding Clinic: 2016, Q3, P12

    J11.08   Influenza due to unidentified influenza virus with specified pneumonia 🖤
          Code also other specified type of pneumonia

  J11.1   Influenza due to unidentified influenza virus with other respiratory manifestations
        Influenza NOS
        Influenzal laryngitis NOS
        Influenzal pharyngitis NOS
        Influenza with upper respiratory symptoms NOS

      Use additional code for associated pleural effusion, if applicable (J91.8)

      Use additional code for associated sinusitis, if applicable (J01.-)

  J11.2   Influenza due to unidentified influenza virus with gastrointestinal manifestations
        Influenza gastroenteritis NOS

      Excludes 1   'intestinal flu' [viral gastroenteritis] (A08.-)

  ● **J11.8   Influenza due to unidentified influenza virus with other manifestations**

    J11.81   Influenza due to unidentified influenza virus with encephalopathy
          Influenzal encephalopathy NOS

    J11.82   Influenza due to unidentified influenza virus with myocarditis
          Influenzal myocarditis NOS

    J11.83   Influenza due to unidentified influenza virus with otitis media
          Influenzal otitis media NOS

        Use additional code for any associated perforated tympanic membrane (H72.-)

    J11.89   Influenza due to unidentified influenza virus with other manifestations
          Use additional codes to identify the manifestations

● **J12   Viral pneumonia, not elsewhere classified**
    Includes   bronchopneumonia due to viruses other than influenza viruses

    Code first associated influenza, if applicable (J09.X1, J10.0-, J11.0-)

    Code also associated abscess, if applicable (J85.1)

    Excludes 1   aspiration pneumonia due to anesthesia during labor and delivery (O74.0)
          aspiration pneumonia due to anesthesia during pregnancy (O29)
          aspiration pneumonia due to anesthesia during puerperium (O89.0)
          aspiration pneumonia due to solids and liquids (J69.-)
          aspiration pneumonia NOS (J69.0)
          congenital pneumonia (P23.0)
          congenital rubella pneumonitis (P35.0)
          interstitial pneumonia NOS (J84.9)
          lipid pneumonia (J69.1)
          neonatal aspiration pneumonia (P24.-)

    (Ex) **For category J12 CC codes unless otherwise indicated:** See PDX Collection 734
    Coding Clinic: 2021, Q1, P34

  J12.0   Adenoviral pneumonia 🖤
  J12.1   Respiratory syncytial virus pneumonia 🖤
          RSV pneumonia
  J12.2   Parainfluenza virus pneumonia 🖤
  J12.3   Human metapneumovirus pneumonia 🖤

● **J12.8   Other viral pneumonia**

    J12.81   Pneumonia due to SARS-associated coronavirus 🖤
          Severe acute respiratory syndrome NOS
          (Ex) See PDX Collection 735

  ● **J12.82   Pneumonia due to coronavirus disease 2019** 🖤🖤
          Pneumonia due to 2019 novel coronavirus (SARS-CoV-2)
          Pneumonia due to COVID-19

        Code first COVID-19 (U07.1)
          (Ex) See PDX Collection 4128
          Coding Clinic: 2021, Q1, P33-34, 42, 47, 49

    J12.89   Other viral pneumonia 🖤
          Coding Clinic: 2021, Q1, P33-34

  J12.9   Viral pneumonia, unspecified 🖤

Item 10–3   Pneumonia is an infection of the lungs, caused by a variety of microorganisms, including viruses, most commonly the Streptococcus pneumoniae (pneumococcus) bacteria, fungi, and parasites. Pneumonia occurs when the immune system is weakened, often by a URI or influenza.

J13   Pneumonia due to Streptococcus pneumoniae 🖤🖤
        Bronchopneumonia due to S. pneumoniae
      Code first associated influenza, if applicable (J09.X1, J10.0-, J11.0-)
      Code also associated abscess, if applicable (J85.1)
      Excludes 1   congenital pneumonia due to S. pneumoniae (P23.6)
              lobar pneumonia, unspecified organism (J18.1)
              pneumonia due to other streptococci (J15.3-J15.4)
        (Ex) See PDX Collection 110

J14   Pneumonia due to Hemophilus influenzae 🖤🖤
        Bronchopneumonia due to H. influenzae
      Code first associated influenza, if applicable (J09.X1, J10.0-, J11.0-)
      Code also associated abscess, if applicable (J85.1)
      Excludes 1   congenital pneumonia due to H. influenzae (P23.6)
        (Ex) See PDX Collection 110

● **J15   Bacterial pneumonia, not elsewhere classified**
    Includes   bronchopneumonia due to bacteria other than S. pneumoniae and H. influenzae
      Code first associated influenza, if applicable (J09.X1, J10.0-, J11.0-)
      Code also associated abscess, if applicable (J85.1)
      Excludes 1   chlamydial pneumonia (J16.0)
              congenital pneumonia (P23.-)
              Legionnaires' disease (A48.1)
              spirochetal pneumonia (A69.8)
        (Ex) **For category J15 CC codes:** See PDX Collection 110

  J15.0   Pneumonia due to Klebsiella pneumoniae 🖤🖤
  J15.1   Pneumonia due to Pseudomonas 🖤🖤
  ● **J15.2   Pneumonia due to staphylococcus**

    J15.20   Pneumonia due to staphylococcus, unspecified 🖤🖤

    ● **J15.21   Pneumonia due to staphylococcus aureus**

        J15.211   Pneumonia due to Methicillin susceptible Staphylococcus aureus 🖤🖤
              MSSA pneumonia
              Pneumonia due to Staphylococcus aureus NOS

        J15.212   Pneumonia due to Methicillin resistant Staphylococcus aureus 🖤🖤

      J15.29   Pneumonia due to other staphylococcus 🖤🖤

  J15.3   Pneumonia due to streptococcus, group B 🖤🖤
  J15.4   Pneumonia due to other streptococci 🖤🖤
      Excludes 1   pneumonia due to streptococcus, group B (J15.3)
              pneumonia due to Streptococcus pneumoniae (J13)

  J15.5   Pneumonia due to Escherichia coli 🖤🖤
  J15.6   Pneumonia due to other Gram-negative bacteria 🖤🖤
          Pneumonia due to other aerobic Gram-negative bacteria
          Pneumonia due to Serratia marcescens

N Newborn Age: 0   **P** Pediatric Age: 0–17   **M** Maternity DX: 9–64   **A** Adult Age: 15–124   ♀ Females Only   ♂ Males Only

🖤 Complication\Comorbidity   🖤 Major C\C   (Ex) CC/MCC Exclusions   🖤 Hospital-Acquired Condition   🖤 Hierarchical Condition Category

CHAPTER 10 (J00-J99)

J15.7   Pneumonia due to Mycoplasma pneumoniae 🔖

J15.8   Pneumonia due to other specified bacteria 🔖🔖

J15.9   Unspecified bacterial pneumonia 🔖
      Pneumonia due to gram-positive bacteria
      Coding Clinic: 2017, Q4, P96

● J16   Pneumonia due to other infectious organisms, not elsewhere classified
      Code first associated influenza, if applicable (J09.X1, J10.0-, J11.0-)
      Code also associated abscess, if applicable (J85.1)

      Excludes1 congenital pneumonia (P23.-)
                  ornithosis (A70)
                  pneumocystosis (B59)
                  pneumonia NOS (J18.9)
      Ⓔⓧ **For category J16 CC codes: See PDX Collection 110**

J16.0   Chlamydial pneumonia 🔖

J16.8   Pneumonia due to other specified infectious organisms 🔖

▷ J17   *Pneumonia in diseases classified elsewhere* 🔖
      Code first underlying disease, such as:
      Q fever (A78)
      rheumatic fever (I00)
      schistosomiasis (B65.0-B65.9)

      Excludes1 candidial pneumonia (B37.1)
                  chlamydial pneumonia (J16.0)
                  gonorrheal pneumonia (A54.84)
                  histoplasmosis pneumonia (B39.0-B39.2)
                  measles pneumonia (B05.2)
                  nocardiosis pneumonia (A43.0)
                  pneumocystosis (B59)
                  pneumonia due to Pneumocystis carinii (B59)
                  pneumonia due to Pneumocystis jiroveci (B59)
                  pneumonia in actinomycosis (A42.0)
                  pneumonia in anthrax (A22.1)
                  pneumonia in ascariasis (B77.81)
                  pneumonia in aspergillosis (B44.0-B44.1)
                  pneumonia in coccidioidomycosis (B38.0-B38.2)
                  pneumonia in cytomegalovirus disease (B25.0)
                  pneumonia in toxoplasmosis (B58.3)
                  rubella pneumonia (B06.81)
                  salmonella pneumonia (A02.22)
                  spirochetal infection NEC with pneumonia (A69.8)
                  tularemia pneumonia (A21.2)
                  typhoid fever with pneumonia (A01.03)
                  varicella pneumonia (B01.2)
                  whooping cough with pneumonia (A37 with
                      fifth-character 1)
      Ⓔⓧ See PDX Collection 110

● J18   Pneumonia, unspecified organism
      Code first associated influenza, if applicable (J09.X1, J10.0-, J11.0-)

      Excludes1 abscess of lung with pneumonia (J85.1)
                  aspiration pneumonia due to anesthesia during
                      labor and delivery (O74.0)
                  aspiration pneumonia due to anesthesia during
                      pregnancy (O29)
                  aspiration pneumonia due to anesthesia during
                      puerperium (O89.0)
                  aspiration pneumonia due to solids and liquids
                      (J69.-)
                  aspiration pneumonia NOS (J69.0)
                  congenital pneumonia (P23.0)
                  drug-induced interstitial lung disorder (J70.2-J70.4)
                  interstitial pneumonia NOS (J84.9)
                  lipid pneumonia (J69.1)
                  neonatal aspiration pneumonia (P24.-)
                  pneumonitis due to external agents (J67-J70)
                  pneumonitis due to fumes and vapors (J68.0)
                  usual interstitial pneumonia (J84.178)
      Ⓔⓧ **For category J18 CC code unless otherwise indicated: See PDX Collection 110**

J18.0   Bronchopneumonia, unspecified organism
        Excludes1 hypostatic bronchopneumonia (J18.2)
                    lipid pneumonia (J69.1)
        Excludes2 acute bronchiolitis (J21.-)
                    chronic bronchiolitis (J44.9)

J18.1   Lobar pneumonia, unspecified organism 🔖🔖
      Coding Clinic: 2016, Q3, P15

J18.2   Hypostatic pneumonia, unspecified organism 🔖
      Hypostatic bronchopneumonia
      Passive pneumonia
      Ⓔⓧ See PDX Collection 736

J18.8   Other pneumonia, unspecified organism 🔖

J18.9   Pneumonia, unspecified organism 🔖
      **Coding Clinic: Q3, P15; 2019, Q2, P28; Q1, P36; 2016, Q3, P15;
      2012, Q4, P94**

OTHER ACUTE LOWER RESPIRATORY INFECTIONS (J20-J22)

      Excludes2 chronic obstructive pulmonary disease with acute
                  lower respiratory infection (J44.0)

● J20   Acute bronchitis
      *Inflammation/irritation of the bronchial tubes lasting 2-3 weeks, most
      commonly caused by a virus*

      Includes   acute and subacute bronchitis (with) bronchospasm
                acute and subacute bronchitis (with) tracheitis
                acute and subacute bronchitis (with)
                  tracheobronchitis, acute
                acute and subacute fibrinous bronchitis
                acute and subacute membranous bronchitis
                acute and subacute purulent bronchitis
                acute and subacute septic bronchitis

      Excludes1 bronchitis NOS (J40)
                  tracheobronchitis NOS (J40)

      Excludes2 acute bronchitis with bronchiectasis (J47.0)
                  acute bronchitis with chronic obstructive asthma
                    (J44.0)
                  acute bronchitis with chronic obstructive
                    pulmonary disease (J44.0)
                  allergic bronchitis NOS (J45.909-)
                  bronchitis due to chemicals, fumes and vapors
                    (J68.0)
                  chronic bronchitis NOS (J42)
                  chronic mucopurulent bronchitis (J41.1)
                  chronic obstructive bronchitis (J44.-)
                  chronic obstructive tracheobronchitis (J44.-)
                  chronic simple bronchitis (J41.0)
                  chronic tracheobronchitis (J42)

J20.0   Acute bronchitis due to Mycoplasma pneumoniae

J20.1   Acute bronchitis due to Hemophilus influenzae

J20.2   Acute bronchitis due to streptococcus

J20.3   Acute bronchitis due to coxsackievirus

J20.4   Acute bronchitis due to parainfluenza virus

J20.5   Acute bronchitis due to respiratory syncytial virus
      Acute bronchitis due to RSV

J20.6   Acute bronchitis due to rhinovirus
      Coding Clinic: 2016, Q3, P10

J20.7   Acute bronchitis due to echovirus

J20.8   Acute bronchitis due to other specified organisms
      Coding Clinic: 2016, Q3, P11

J20.9   Acute bronchitis, unspecified
      Coding Clinic: 2019, Q1, P35; 2016, Q3, P16

● J21   Acute bronchiolitis
      *Bronchiolitis obliterans with organizing pneumonia (BOOP)
      inflammation of bronchioles and surrounding tissue in lung*

      Includes   acute bronchiolitis with bronchospasm
      Excludes2 respiratory bronchiolitis interstitial lung disease
                  (J84.115)
      Ⓔⓧ **For category J21 CC codes unless otherwise indicated: See PDX Collection 738**

J21.0   Acute bronchiolitis due to respiratory syncytial virus 🔖
      Acute bronchitis due to RSV
      Ⓔⓧ See PDX Collection 737

J21.1   Acute bronchiolitis due to human metapneumovirus 🔖

J21.8   Acute bronchiolitis due to other specified organisms 🔖

J21.9   Acute bronchiolitis, unspecified 🔖
      Bronchiolitis (acute)
      Excludes1 chronic bronchiolitis (J44.-)

J22   Unspecified acute lower respiratory infection
      Acute (lower) respiratory (tract) infection NOS
      Excludes1 upper respiratory infection (acute) (J06.9)
      Coding Clinic: 2020, Q1, P22-23

▶ New   ⟹ Revised   ~~deleted~~ Deleted   Excludes 1   Excludes 2   Includes   Use additional   Code first   Code also   Key words

OGCR Official Guidelines   ● Unacceptable Principal Diagnosis   X Assign placeholder X   ● Use Additional Character(s)   ▶ Manifestation Code   **Coding Clinic**

OTHER DISEASES OF UPPER RESPIRATORY TRACT (J30-J39)

● **J30   Vasomotor and allergic rhinitis**

  Includes   spasmodic rhinorrhea

  Excludes1   allergic rhinitis with asthma (bronchial) (J45.909)
  rhinitis NOS (J31.0)

  J30.0   **Vasomotor rhinitis**

  J30.1   **Allergic rhinitis due to pollen**
  Allergy NOS due to pollen
  Hay fever
  Pollinosis

  J30.2   **Other seasonal allergic rhinitis**

  J30.5   **Allergic rhinitis due to food**

  ● J30.8   **Other allergic rhinitis**

    J30.81   **Allergic rhinitis due to animal (cat) (dog) hair and dander**

    J30.89   **Other allergic rhinitis**
    Perennial allergic rhinitis

  J30.9   **Allergic rhinitis, unspecified**

● **J31   Chronic rhinitis, nasopharyngitis and pharyngitis**

  Use additional code to identify:
  exposure to environmental tobacco smoke (Z77.22)
  exposure to tobacco smoke in the perinatal period (P96.81)
  history of tobacco dependence (Z87.891)
  occupational exposure to environmental tobacco smoke (Z57.31)
  tobacco dependence (F17.-)
  tobacco use (Z72.0)

  J31.0   **Chronic rhinitis**
  Atrophic rhinitis (chronic)
  Granulomatous rhinitis (chronic)
  Hypertrophic rhinitis (chronic)
  Obstructive rhinitis (chronic)
  Ozena
  Purulent rhinitis (chronic)
  Rhinitis (chronic) NOS
  Ulcerative rhinitis (chronic)

    Excludes1   allergic rhinitis (J30.1-J30.9)
    vasomotor rhinitis (J30.0)

  J31.1   **Chronic nasopharyngitis**

    Excludes2   acute nasopharyngitis (J00)

  J31.2   **Chronic pharyngitis**
  Chronic sore throat
  Atrophic pharyngitis (chronic)
  Granular pharyngitis (chronic)
  Hypertrophic pharyngitis (chronic)

    Excludes2   acute pharyngitis (J02.9)

● **J32   Chronic sinusitis**

  Includes   sinus abscess
  sinus empyema
  sinus infection
  sinus suppuration

  Use additional code to identify:
  exposure to environmental tobacco smoke (Z77.22)
  exposure to tobacco smoke in the perinatal period (P96.81)
  history of tobacco dependence (Z87.891)
  infectious agent (B95-B97)
  occupational exposure to environmental tobacco smoke (Z57.31)
  tobacco dependence (F17.-)
  tobacco use (Z72.0)

  Excludes2   acute sinusitis (J01.-)

  J32.0   **Chronic maxillary sinusitis**
  Antritis (chronic)
  Maxillary sinusitis NOS

  J32.1   **Chronic frontal sinusitis**
  Frontal sinusitis NOS

Item 10–4 Nasal polyps are an abnormal growth of tissue (tumor) projecting from a mucous membrane and attached to the surface by a narrow elongated stalk (pedunculated). Nasal polyps usually originate in the ethmoid sinus but also may occur in the maxillary sinus. Symptoms are nasal block, sinusitis, anosmia, and secondary infections.

  J32.2   **Chronic ethmoidal sinusitis**
  Ethmoidal sinusitis NOS

    Excludes1   Woakes' ethmoiditis (J33.1)

  J32.3   **Chronic sphenoidal sinusitis**
  Sphenoidal sinusitis NOS

  J32.4   **Chronic pansinusitis**
  Pansinusitis NOS

  J32.8   **Other chronic sinusitis**
  Sinusitis (chronic) involving more than one sinus but not pansinusitis

  J32.9   **Chronic sinusitis, unspecified**
  Sinusitis (chronic) NOS

● **J33   Nasal polyp**

  Use additional code to identify:
  exposure to environmental tobacco smoke (Z77.22)
  exposure to tobacco smoke in the perinatal period (P96.81)
  history of tobacco dependence (Z87.891)
  occupational exposure to environmental tobacco smoke (Z57.31)
  tobacco dependence (F17.-)
  tobacco use (Z72.0)

  Excludes1   adenomatous polyps (D14.0)

  J33.0   **Polyp of nasal cavity**
  Choanal polyp
  Nasopharyngeal polyp

  J33.1   **Polypoid sinus degeneration**
  Woakes' syndrome or ethmoiditis

  J33.8   **Other polyp of sinus**
  Accessory polyp of sinus
  Ethmoidal polyp of sinus
  Maxillary polyp of sinus
  Sphenoidal polyp of sinus

  J33.9   **Nasal polyp, unspecified**

● **J34   Other and unspecified disorders of nose and nasal sinuses**

  Excludes2   varicose ulcer of nasal septum (I86.8)

  J34.0   **Abscess, furuncle and carbuncle of nose**
  Cellulitis of nose
  Necrosis of nose
  Ulceration of nose

  J34.1   **Cyst and mucocele of nose and nasal sinus**

  J34.2   **Deviated nasal septum**
  Deflection or deviation of septum (nasal) (acquired)

    Excludes1   congenital deviated nasal septum (Q67.4)

  J34.3   **Hypertrophy of nasal turbinates**

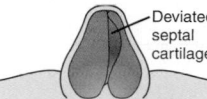
Deviated septal cartilage

Figure 10-3 Deviated nasal septum.

Item 10–5 A **deviated nasal septum** is the displacement of the septal cartilage that separates the nares. This displacement causes obstructed air flow through the nasal passages. A child can be born with this displacement (congenital), or the condition may be acquired through trauma, such as a sports injury. Symptoms include nasal block, sinusitis, and related secondary infections. Septoplasty is surgical repair of this condition.

CHAPTER 10 (J00-J99)

N Newborn Age: 0   P Pediatric Age: 0–17   M Maternity DX: 9–64   A Adult Age: 15–124   ♀ Females Only   ♂ Males Only

🅒 Complication\Comorbidity   🅒 Major C\C   (Exc) CC/MCC Exclusions   🅗 Hospital-Acquired Condition   🅗 Hierarchical Condition Category

947

● **J34.8   Other specified disorders of nose and nasal sinuses**

    J34.81   Nasal mucositis (ulcerative)

        Code also type of associated therapy, such as:
           antineoplastic and immunosuppressive
             drugs (T45.1X-)
           radiological procedure and radiotherapy
             (Y84.2)

        Excludes2 gastrointestinal mucositis
                (ulcerative) (K92.81)
                mucositis (ulcerative) of vagina
                  and vulva (N76.81)
                oral mucositis (ulcerative)
                  (K12.3-)

    **J34.89   Other specified disorders of nose and nasal
             sinuses**
        Perforation of nasal septum NOS
        Rhinolith

J34.9   Unspecified disorder of nose and nasal sinuses

● **J35   Chronic diseases of tonsils and adenoids**

    Use additional code to identify:
      exposure to environmental tobacco smoke (Z77.22)
      exposure to tobacco smoke in the perinatal period (P96.81)
      history of tobacco dependence (Z87.891)
      occupational exposure to environmental tobacco smoke
        (Z57.31)
      tobacco dependence (F17.-)
      tobacco use (Z72.0)

● **J35.0   Chronic tonsillitis and adenoiditis**

        Excludes2 acute tonsillitis (J03.-)

    J35.01   Chronic tonsillitis

    J35.02   Chronic adenoiditis

    J35.03   Chronic tonsillitis and adenoiditis

  J35.1   Hypertrophy of tonsils
      Enlargement of tonsils

      Excludes1 hypertrophy of tonsils with tonsillitis
              (J35.0-)

  J35.2   Hypertrophy of adenoids
      Enlargement of adenoids

      Excludes1 hypertrophy of adenoids with adenoiditis
              (J35.0-)

  J35.3   Hypertrophy of tonsils with hypertrophy of adenoids

      Excludes1 hypertrophy of tonsils and adenoids with
              tonsillitis and adenoiditis (J35.03)

  J35.8   Other chronic diseases of tonsils and adenoids
      Adenoid vegetations
      Amygdalolith
      Calculus, tonsil
      Cicatrix of tonsil (and adenoid)
      Tonsillar tag
      Ulcer of tonsil

  J35.9   Chronic disease of tonsils and adenoids, unspecified
      Disease (chronic) of tonsils and adenoids NOS

J36   Peritonsillar abscess 🔗

  Includes   abscess of tonsil
          peritonsillar cellulitis
          quinsy

  Use additional code (B95-B97) to identify infectious agent.

  Excludes1 acute tonsillitis (J03.-)
         chronic tonsillitis (J35.0)
         retropharyngeal abscess (J39.0)
         tonsillitis NOS (J03.9-)

  Ex: See PDX Collection 739

● **J37   Chronic laryngitis and laryngotracheitis**

    Use additional code to identify:
      exposure to environmental tobacco smoke (Z77.22)
      exposure to tobacco smoke in the perinatal period (P96.81)
      history of tobacco dependence (Z87.891)
      infectious agent (B95-B97)
      occupational exposure to environmental tobacco smoke
        (Z57.31)
      tobacco dependence (F17.-)
      tobacco use (Z72.0)

  J37.0   Chronic laryngitis
      Catarrhal laryngitis
      Hypertrophic laryngitis
      Sicca laryngitis

      Excludes2 acute laryngitis (J04.0)
             obstructive (acute) laryngitis (J05.0)

  J37.1   Chronic laryngotracheitis
      Laryngitis, chronic, with tracheitis (chronic)
      Tracheitis, chronic, with laryngitis

      Excludes1 chronic tracheitis (J42)

      Excludes2 acute laryngotracheitis (J04.2)
             acute tracheitis (J04.1)

● **J38   Diseases of vocal cords and larynx, not elsewhere classified**

    Use additional code to identify:
      exposure to environmental tobacco smoke (Z77.22)
      exposure to tobacco smoke in the perinatal period (P96.81)
      history of tobacco dependence (Z87.891)
      occupational exposure to environmental tobacco smoke
        (Z57.31)
      tobacco dependence (F17.-)
      tobacco use (Z72.0)

    Excludes1 congenital laryngeal stridor (P28.89)
         obstructive laryngitis (acute) (J05.0)
         postprocedural subglottic stenosis (J95.5)
         stridor (R06.1)
         ulcerative laryngitis (J04.0)

● **J38.0   Paralysis of vocal cords and larynx**
      Laryngoplegia
      Paralysis of glottis

    J38.00   Paralysis of vocal cords and larynx, unspecified

    J38.01   Paralysis of vocal cords and larynx, unilateral

    J38.02   Paralysis of vocal cords and larynx, bilateral

  J38.1   Polyp of vocal cord and larynx

      Excludes1 adenomatous polyps (D14.1)

  J38.2   Nodules of vocal cords
      Chorditis (fibrinous)(nodosa)(tuberosa)
      Singer's nodes
      Teacher's nodes

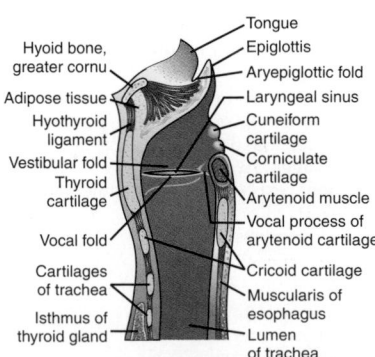

Figure 10-4 Coronal section of the larynx.

Item 10-6 The **larynx** extends from the tongue to the trachea and is divided into an upper and lower portion separated by folds. The framework of the larynx is cartilage composed of the single cricoid, thyroid, and epiglottic cartilages, and the paired arytenoid, cuneiform, and corniculate cartilages.

▶ New   ⇒ Revised   ~~deleted~~ Deleted   Excludes 1   Excludes 2   Includes   Use additional   Code first   Code also   Key words

OGCR Official Guidelines   ● Unacceptable Principal Diagnosis   X Assign placeholder X   ● Use Additional Character(s)   ▶ Manifestation Code   Coding Clinic

J38.3   **Other diseases of vocal cords**
Abscess of vocal cords
Cellulitis of vocal cords
Granuloma of vocal cords
Leukokeratosis of vocal cords
Leukoplakia of vocal cords

J38.4   **Edema of larynx**
Edema (of) glottis
Subglottic edema
Supraglottic edema

     Excludes1   acute obstructive laryngitis [croup] (J05.0)
                      edematous laryngitis (J04.0)

J38.5   **Laryngeal spasm**
Laryngismus (stridulus)

J38.6   **Stenosis of larynx**

J38.7   **Other diseases of larynx**
Abscess of larynx
Cellulitis of larynx
Disease of larynx NOS
Necrosis of larynx
Pachyderma of larynx
Perichondritis of larynx
Ulcer of larynx

● **J39**   **Other diseases of upper respiratory tract**

     Excludes1   acute respiratory infection NOS (J22)
                      acute upper respiratory infection (J06.9)
                      upper respiratory inflammation due to chemicals,
                      gases, fumes or vapors (J68.2)

J39.0   **Retropharyngeal and parapharyngeal abscess** 🅒
Peripharyngeal abscess

     Excludes1   peritonsillar abscess (J36)

     (Ex) See PDX Collection 740

J39.1   **Other abscess of pharynx** 🅒
Cellulitis of pharynx
Nasopharyngeal abscess

     (Ex) See PDX Collection 740

J39.2   **Other diseases of pharynx**
Cyst of pharynx
Edema of pharynx

     Excludes2   chronic pharyngitis (J31.2)
                      ulcerative pharyngitis (J02.9)

J39.3   **Upper respiratory tract hypersensitivity reaction, site
unspecified**

     Excludes1   hypersensitivity reaction of upper
                      respiratory tract, such as:
                      extrinsic allergic alveolitis (J67.9)
                      pneumoconiosis (J60-J67.9)

J39.8   **Other specified diseases of upper respiratory tract**

J39.9   **Disease of upper respiratory tract, unspecified**

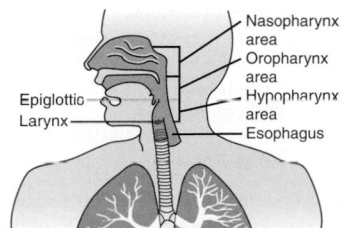

Figure 10-5   The pharynx.

Item 10-7   The **pharynx** is the passage for both food and air between
the mouth and the esophagus and is divided into three areas: nasopharynx,
oropharynx, and hypopharynx. The hypopharynx branches into the esophagus
and the voice box.

Item 10-8   **Chronic bronchitis** is usually defined as being present in
any patient who has persistent cough with sputum production for at least three
months in at least two consecutive years. **Simple chronic bronchitis** is
marked by a productive cough but no pathological airflow obstruction. **Chronic
obstructive pulmonary disease (COPD)** is a group of conditions—
bronchitis, emphysema, asthma, bronchiectasis, allergic alveolitis—marked
by dyspnea. **Catarrhal** bronchitis is an acute form of bronchitis marked by
profuse mucus and pus production (**mucopurulent** discharge). **Croupous**
bronchitis, also known as pseudomembranous, fibrinous, plastic, exudative, or
membranous, is marked by a violent cough and dyspnea.

CHRONIC LOWER RESPIRATORY DISEASES (J40-J47)

     Excludes1   bronchitis due to chemicals, gases, fumes and
                      vapors (J68.0)

     Excludes2   cystic fibrosis (E84.-)

J40   **Bronchitis, not specified as acute or chronic**
Bronchitis NOS
Catarrhal bronchitis
Bronchitis with tracheitis NOS
Tracheobronchitis NOS

Use additional code to identify:
     exposure to environmental tobacco smoke (Z77.22)
     exposure to tobacco smoke in the perinatal period (P96.81)
     history of tobacco dependence (Z87.891)
     occupational exposure to environmental tobacco smoke
       (Z57.31)
     tobacco dependence (F17.-)
     tobacco use (Z72.0)

     Excludes1   acute bronchitis (J20.-)
                      allergic bronchitis NOS (J45.909)
                      asthmatic bronchitis NOS (J45.9)
                      bronchitis due to chemicals, gases, fumes and
                      vapors (J68.0)

● **J41**   **Simple and mucopurulent chronic bronchitis**
Use additional code to identify:
     exposure to environmental tobacco smoke (Z77.22)
     exposure to tobacco smoke in the perinatal period (P96.81)
     history of tobacco dependence (Z87.891)
     occupational exposure to environmental tobacco smoke
       (Z57.31)
     tobacco dependence (F17.-)
     tobacco use (Z72.0)

     Excludes1   chronic bronchitis NOS (J42)
                      chronic obstructive bronchitis (J44.-)

J41.0   **Simple chronic bronchitis** 🅒

J41.1   **Mucopurulent chronic bronchitis** 🅒

J41.8   **Mixed simple and mucopurulent chronic bronchitis** 🅒

J42   **Unspecified chronic bronchitis** 🅒
Chronic bronchitis NOS
Chronic tracheitis
Chronic tracheobronchitis

Use additional code to identify:
     exposure to environmental tobacco smoke (Z77.22)
     exposure to tobacco smoke in the perinatal period (P96.81)
     history of tobacco dependence (Z87.891)
     occupational exposure to environmental tobacco smoke
       (Z57.31)
     tobacco dependence (F17.-)
     tobacco use (Z72.0)

     Excludes1   chronic asthmatic bronchitis (J44.-)
                      chronic bronchitis with airways obstruction (J44.-)
                      chronic emphysematous bronchitis (J44.-)
                      chronic obstructive pulmonary disease NOS
                      (J44.9)
                      simple and mucopurulent chronic bronchitis
                      (J41.-)

CHAPTER 10 (J00-J99)

N Newborn Age: 0   **P** Pediatric Age: 0–17   **M** Maternity DX: 9–64   **A** Adult Age: 15–124   ♀ Females Only   ♂ Males Only
🅒 Complication\Comorbidity   🅜 Major C\C   (Ex) CC/MCC Exclusions   🅗 Hospital-Acquired Condition   🅗 Hierarchical Condition Category

949

● J43   **Emphysema**
         Use additional code to identify:
             exposure to environmental tobacco smoke (Z77.22)
             history of tobacco dependence (Z87.891)
             occupational exposure to environmental tobacco smoke
                 (Z57.31)
             tobacco dependence (F17.-)
             tobacco use (Z72.0)

         Excludes1   compensatory emphysema (J98.3)
                          emphysema due to inhalation of chemicals, gases,
                              fumes or vapors (J68.4)
                          emphysema with chronic (obstructive) bronchitis
                              (J44.-)
                          emphysematous (obstructive) bronchitis (J44.-)
                          interstitial emphysema (J98.2)
                          mediastinal emphysema (J98.2)
                          neonatal interstitial emphysema (P25.0)
                          surgical (subcutaneous) emphysema (T81.82)

         Excludes2   traumatic subcutaneous emphysema (T79.7)

    J43.0   **Unilateral pulmonary emphysema [MacLeod's
             syndrome]** 🄬
                 Swyer-James syndrome
                 Unilateral emphysema
                 Unilateral hyperlucent lung
                 Unilateral pulmonary artery functional hypoplasia
                 Unilateral transparency of lung

    J43.1   **Panlobular emphysema** 🄬
                 Panacinar emphysema

    J43.2   **Centrilobular emphysema** 🄬

    J43.8   **Other emphysema** 🄬

    J43.9   **Emphysema, unspecified** 🄬
                 Bullous emphysema (lung)(pulmonary)
                 Emphysema (lung)(pulmonary) NOS
                 Emphysematous bleb
                 Vesicular emphysema (lung)(pulmonary)
                 Coding Clinic: 2019, Q1, P35-37; 2017, Q4, P97-98

● J44   **Other chronic obstructive pulmonary disease**
         Includes   asthma with chronic obstructive pulmonary
                         disease
                         chronic asthmatic (obstructive) bronchitis
                    ⇒ chronic bronchitis with airway obstruction
                         chronic bronchitis with emphysema
                         chronic emphysematous bronchitis
                         chronic obstructive asthma
                         chronic obstructive bronchitis
                         chronic obstructive tracheobronchitis

         Code also type of asthma, if applicable (J45.-)

         Use additional code to identify:
             exposure to environmental tobacco smoke (Z77.22)
             history of tobacco dependence (Z87.891)
             occupational exposure to environmental tobacco smoke
                 (Z57.31)
             tobacco dependence (F17.-)
             tobacco use (Z72.0)

         Excludes1   bronchiectasis (J47.-)
                          chronic bronchitis NOS (J42)
                          chronic simple and mucopurulent bronchitis
                              (J41.-)
                          chronic tracheitis (J42)
                          chronic tracheobronchitis (J42)
                          emphysema without chronic bronchitis (J43.-)
         Coding Clinic: 2019, Q1, P34-36; 2017, Q4, P97; 2017, Q1, P25; 2016, Q3, P16

    J44.0   **Chronic obstructive pulmonary disease with (acute)
             lower respiratory infection** 🄬 🄬
                 Code also to identify the infection
                 (Ex:) See PDX Collection 741
                 **Coding Clinic: 2019, Q1, P35-36; 2017, Q4, P96; 2017, Q2, P30, Q1,
                 P24-25; 2016, Q3, P15-16**

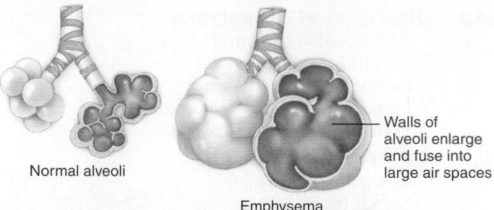

    J44.1   **Chronic obstructive pulmonary disease with (acute)
             exacerbation** 🄬 🄬
                 Decompensated COPD
                 Decompensated COPD with (acute) exacerbation
                 Excludes2   chronic obstructive pulmonary disease
                                  [COPD] with acute bronchitis (J44.0)
                                  lung diseases due to external agents
                                      (J60-J70)
                 (Ex:) See PDX Collection 741
                 **Coding Clinic: 2019, Q1, P34-35; 2017, Q4, P96; 2017, Q1, P26; 2016,
                 Q3, P15-16, Q1, P36**

    J44.9   **Chronic obstructive pulmonary disease, unspecified** 🄬
                 Chronic obstructive airway disease NOS
                 Chronic obstructive lung disease NOS
                 Excludes2   lung diseases due to external agents
                                  (J60-J70)
                 **Coding Clinic: 2019, Q1, P36; 2017, Q4, P96-97; 2017, Q1, P24-25;
                 2016, Q1, P37**

● J45   **Asthma**
             Allergic (predominantly) asthma
             Allergic bronchitis NOS
             Allergic rhinitis with asthma
             Atopic asthma
             Extrinsic allergic asthma
             Hay fever with asthma
             Idiosyncratic asthma
             Intrinsic nonallergic asthma
             Nonallergic asthma

         Use additional code to identify:
             eosinophilic asthma (J82.83)
             exposure to environmental tobacco smoke (Z77.22)
             exposure to tobacco smoke in the perinatal period (P96.81)
             history of tobacco dependence (Z87.891)
             occupational exposure to environmental tobacco smoke (Z57.31)
             tobacco dependence (F17.-)
             tobacco use (Z72.0)

         Excludes1   detergent asthma (J69.8)
                          eosinophilic asthma (J82)
                          miner's asthma (J60)
                          wheezing NOS (R06.2)
                          wood asthma (J67.8)

         Excludes2   asthma with chronic obstructive pulmonary
                              disease (J44.9)
                          chronic asthmatic (obstructive) bronchitis (J44.9)
                          chronic obstructive asthma (J44.9)
         (Ex:) For category J45 CC codes: See PDX Collection 742
         Coding Clinic: 2019, Q1, P37; 2017, Q1, P25

    ● J45.2   **Mild intermittent asthma**
        J45.20   **Mild intermittent asthma, uncomplicated**
                     Mild intermittent asthma NOS
        J45.21   **Mild intermittent asthma with (acute)
                  exacerbation** 🄬
        J45.22   **Mild intermittent asthma with status
                  asthmaticus** 🄬

Item 10–9   Asthma is a bronchial condition marked by airway obstruction,
hyper-responsiveness, and inflammation. **Extrinsic** asthma, also known as
allergic asthma, is characterized by the same symptoms that occur with exposure
to allergens and is divided into the following types: **atopic, occupational,**
and **allergic bronchopulmonary aspergillosis. Intrinsic** asthma
occurs in patients who have no history of allergy or sensitivities to allergens
and is divided into the following types: **nonreaginic** and **pharmacologic.**
Status asthmaticus is the most severe form of asthma attack and can last
for days or weeks.

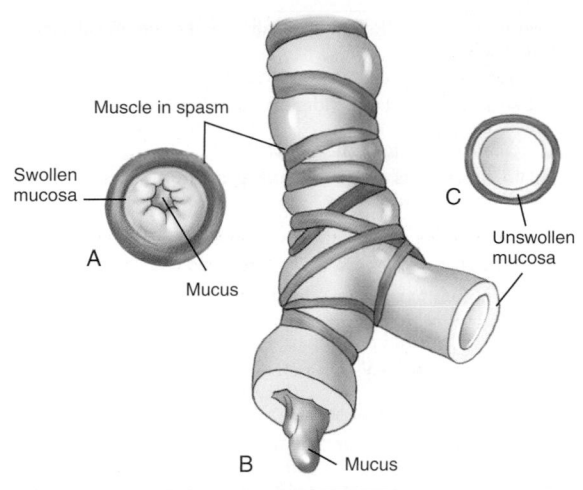

Figure 10-7   Factors causing expiratory obstruction in asthma. **A.** Cross section of a bronchiole occluded by muscle spasm, swollen mucosa, and mucus. **B.** Longitudinal section of an obstructed bronchiole. **C.** Cross section of a clear bronchiole. (From Shiland: Mastering Healthcare Terminology, ed 1, St. Louis, Mosby, 2003)

● J45.3   Mild persistent asthma
  J45.30   Mild persistent asthma, uncomplicated
            Mild persistent asthma NOS
  J45.31   Mild persistent asthma with (acute) exacerbation
            Coding Clinic: 2016, Q1, P35
  J45.32   Mild persistent asthma with status asthmaticus

● J45.4   Moderate persistent asthma
  J45.40   Moderate persistent asthma, uncomplicated
            Moderate persistent asthma NOS
  J45.41   Moderate persistent asthma with (acute) exacerbation
            Coding Clinic: 2017, Q1, P26
  J45.42   Moderate persistent asthma with status asthmaticus

● J45.5   Severe persistent asthma
  J45.50   Severe persistent asthma, uncomplicated
            Severe persistent asthma NOS
  J45.51   Severe persistent asthma with (acute) exacerbation
  J45.52   Severe persistent asthma with status asthmaticus

● J45.9   Other and unspecified asthma
  ● J45.90   Unspecified asthma
            Asthmatic bronchitis NOS
            Childhood asthma NOS
            Late onset asthma
    J45.901   Unspecified asthma with (acute) exacerbation
              Coding Clinic: 2017, Q4, P96
    J45.902   Unspecified asthma with status asthmaticus
    J45.909   Unspecified asthma, uncomplicated
              Asthma NOS
              Excludes2   lung diseases due to external agents (J60-J70)
              Coding Clinic: 2017, Q4, P96; 2017, Q1, P25
  ● J45.99   Other asthma
    J45.990   Exercise induced bronchospasm
    J45.991   Cough variant asthma
    J45.998   Other asthma

● J47   Bronchiectasis
       Includes   bronchiolectasis
       Use additional code to identify:
          exposure to environmental tobacco smoke (Z77.22)
          exposure to tobacco smoke in the perinatal period (P96.81)
          history of tobacco dependence (Z87.891)
          occupational exposure to environmental tobacco smoke (Z57.31)
          tobacco dependence (F17.-)
          tobacco use (Z72.0)
       Excludes1   congenital bronchiectasis (Q33.4)
                     tuberculous bronchiectasis (current disease) (A15.0)
       (Ex) For category J47 CC codes: See PDX Collection 743
  J47.0   Bronchiectasis with acute lower respiratory infection
           Bronchiectasis with acute bronchitis
           ~~Use additional code to identify the infection~~
           ▶ Code also to identify infection, if applicable
  J47.1   Bronchiectasis with (acute) exacerbation
           Coding Clinic: 2021, Q1, P24
  J47.9   Bronchiectasis, uncomplicated
           Bronchiectasis NOS

LUNG DISEASES DUE TO EXTERNAL AGENTS (J60-J70)

       Excludes2   asthma (J45.-)
                    malignant neoplasm of bronchus and lung (C34.-)

J60   Coalworker's pneumoconiosis   A
       Anthracosilicosis
       Anthracosis
       Black lung disease
       Coalworker's lung
       Excludes1   coalworker pneumoconiosis with tuberculosis, any type in A15 (J65)

J61   Pneumoconiosis due to asbestos and other mineral fibers   A
       Asbestosis
       Excludes1   pleural plaque with asbestosis (J92.0)
                    pneumoconiosis with tuberculosis, any type in A15 (J65)

● J62   Pneumoconiosis due to dust containing silica
       Includes   silicotic fibrosis (massive) of lung
       Excludes1   pneumoconiosis with tuberculosis, any type in A15 (J65)
  J62.0   Pneumoconiosis due to talc dust
  J62.8   Pneumoconiosis due to other dust containing silica
           Silicosis NOS

● J63   Pneumoconiosis due to other inorganic dusts
       Excludes1   pneumoconiosis with tuberculosis, any type in A15 (J65)
       Coding Clinic: 2019, Q3, P8
  J63.0   Aluminosis (of lung)
  J63.1   Bauxite fibrosis (of lung)
  J63.2   Berylliosis
  J63.3   Graphite fibrosis (of lung)
  J63.4   Siderosis
           Coding Clinic: 2019, Q3, P8

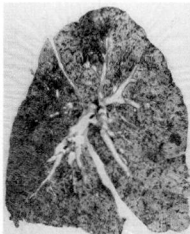

Figure 10-8   Progressive massive fibrosis superimposed on coal workers' pneumoconiosis. The large, blackened scars are located principally in the upper lobe. (From Frazier MS, Drzymkowski JW: Essentials of Human Diseases and Conditions, St. Louis, MO, Saunders, 2004)

Item 10–10   Pneumoconiosis refers to a lung condition resulting from exposure to inorganic or organic airborne particles, such as coal dust or moldy hay, as well as chemical fumes and vapors, such as insecticides. In this condition, the lungs retain the airborne particles.

N Newborn Age: 0   **P** Pediatric Age: 0–17   **M** Maternity DX: 9–64   **A** Adult Age: 15–124   ♀ Females Only   ♂ Males Only

 Complication\Comorbidity   Major C\C   (Ex) CC/MCC Exclusions   Hospital-Acquired Condition   Hierarchical Condition Category

951

J63.5   **Stannosis** 🔑

J63.6   **Pneumoconiosis due to other specified inorganic dusts** 🔑

J64   **Unspecified pneumoconiosis** 🔑

> **Excludes1**   pneumonoconiosis with tuberculosis, any type in A15 (J65)

J65   **Pneumoconiosis associated with tuberculosis** 🔑
Any condition in J60-J64 with tuberculosis, any type in A15
Silicotuberculosis

● J66   **Airway disease due to specific organic dust**

> **Excludes2**   allergic alveolitis (J67.-)
> asbestosis (J61)
> bagassosis (J67.1)
> farmer's lung (J67.0)
> hypersensitivity pneumonitis due to organic dust (J67.-)
> reactive airways dysfunction syndrome (J68.3)

J66.0   **Byssinosis** 🔑
Airway disease due to cotton dust

J66.1   **Flax-dressers' disease** 🔑

J66.2   **Cannabinosis** 🔑

J66.8   **Airway disease due to other specific organic dusts** 🔑

● J67   **Hypersensitivity pneumonitis due to organic dust**

> **Includes**   allergic alveolitis and pneumonitis due to inhaled organic dust and particles of fungal, actinomycetic or other origin

> **Excludes1**   pneumonitis due to inhalation of chemicals, gases, fumes or vapors (J68.0)

J67.0   **Farmer's lung** 🔑
Harvester's lung
Haymaker's lung
Moldy hay disease

J67.1   **Bagassosis** 🔑
Bagasse disease
Bagasse pneumonitis

J67.2   **Bird fancier's lung** 🔑
Budgerigar fancier's disease or lung
Pigeon fancier's disease or lung

J67.3   **Suberosis** 🔑
Corkhandler's disease or lung
Corkworker's disease or lung

J67.4   **Maltworker's lung** 🔑
Alveolitis due to Aspergillus clavatus

J67.5   **Mushroom-worker's lung** 🔑

J67.6   **Maple-bark-stripper's lung** 🔑
Alveolitis due to Cryptostroma corticale
Cryptostromosis

J67.7   **Air conditioner and humidifier lung** 🔑🔑
Allergic alveolitis due to fungal, thermophilic actinomycetes and other organisms growing in ventilation [air conditioning] systems
Ⓔ See PDX Collection 110

J67.8   **Hypersensitivity pneumonitis due to other organic dusts** 🔑🔑
Cheese-washer's lung
Coffee-worker's lung
Fish-meal worker's lung
Furrier's lung
Sequoiosis
Ⓔ See PDX Collection 3604

J67.9   **Hypersensitivity pneumonitis due to unspecified organic dust** 🔑🔑
Allergic alveolitis (extrinsic) NOS
Hypersensitivity pneumonitis NOS
Ⓔ See PDX Collection 3604

● J68   **Respiratory conditions due to inhalation of chemicals, gases, fumes and vapors**

> *Code first (T51-T65) to identify cause*
> Use additional code to identify associated respiratory conditions, such as:
> acute respiratory failure (J96.0-)

J68.0   **Bronchitis and pneumonitis due to chemicals, gases, fumes and vapors** 🔑🔑
Chemical bronchitis (acute)
Ⓔ See PDX Collection 3604
Coding Clinic: 2019, Q2, P31-32

J68.1   **Pulmonary edema due to chemicals, gases, fumes and vapors** 🔑🔑
Chemical pulmonary edema (acute) (chronic)

> **Excludes1**   pulmonary edema (acute) (chronic) NOS (J81.-)

Ⓔ See PDX Collection 3604

J68.2   **Upper respiratory inflammation due to chemicals, gases, fumes and vapors, not elsewhere classified** 🔑

J68.3   **Other acute and subacute respiratory conditions due to chemicals, gases, fumes and vapors** 🔑
Reactive airways dysfunction syndrome

J68.4   **Chronic respiratory conditions due to chemicals, gases, fumes and vapors** 🔑
Emphysema (diffuse) (chronic) due to inhalation of chemicals, gases, fumes and vapors
Obliterative bronchiolitis (chronic) (subacute) due to inhalation of chemicals, gases, fumes and vapors
Pulmonary fibrosis (chronic) due to inhalation of chemicals, gases, fumes and vapors

> **Excludes1**   chronic pulmonary edema due to chemicals, gases, fumes and vapors (J68.1)

J68.8   **Other respiratory conditions due to chemicals, gases, fumes and vapors** 🔑

J68.9   **Unspecified respiratory condition due to chemicals, gases, fumes and vapors** 🔑

● J69   **Pneumonitis due to solids and liquids**

> **Excludes1**   neonatal aspiration syndromes (P24.-)
> postprocedural pneumonitis (J95.4)

Ⓔ For category J69 CC codes: See PDX Collection 110

J69.0   **Pneumonitis due to inhalation of food and vomit** 🔑🔑
Aspiration pneumonia NOS
Aspiration pneumonia (due to) food (regurgitated)
Aspiration pneumonia (due to) gastric secretions
Aspiration pneumonia (due to) milk
Aspiration pneumonia (due to) vomit
Code also any associated foreign body in respiratory tract (T17.-)

> **Excludes1**   chemical pneumonitis due to anesthesia (J95.4)
> obstetric aspiration pneumonitis (O74.0)

Coding Clinic: 2021, Q1, P34; 2019, Q2, P7, 31-32; 2017, Q1, P24

J69.1   **Pneumonitis due to inhalation of oils and essences** 🔑🔑
Exogenous lipoid pneumonia
Lipid pneumonia NOS
Code first (T51-T65) to identify substance

> **Excludes1**   endogenous lipoid pneumonia (J84.89)

Ⓔ See PDX Collection 3604

J69.8   **Pneumonitis due to inhalation of other solids and liquids** 🔑🔑
Pneumonitis due to aspiration of blood
Pneumonitis due to aspiration of detergent
Code first (T51-T65) to identify substance

▶ New   ⇒ Revised   ~~deleted~~ Deleted   Excludes 1   Excludes 2   Includes   Use additional   Code first   Code also   Key words
OGCR Official Guidelines   ● Unacceptable Principal Diagnosis   X Assign placeholder X   ● Use Additional Character(s)   ▸ Manifestation Code   **Coding Clinic**

● **J70** **Respiratory conditions due to other external agents**

     J70.0 **Acute pulmonary manifestations due to radiation** 🔹🔹

         Radiation pneumonitis

         Use additional code (W88-W90, X39.0-) to identify the external cause

         Ⓔ See PDX Collection 110

     J70.1 **Chronic and other pulmonary manifestations due to radiation** 🔹🔹

         Fibrosis of lung following radiation

         Use additional code (W88-W90, X39.0-) to identify the external cause

         Ⓔ See PDX Collection 110

     J70.2 **Acute drug-induced interstitial lung disorders** 🔹

         Use additional code for adverse effect, if applicable, to identify drug (T36-T50 with fifth or sixth character 5)

         Excludes1   interstitial pneumonia NOS (J84.9)
                      lymphoid interstitial pneumonia (J84.2)

         Coding Clinic: 2019, Q2, P28

     J70.3 **Chronic drug-induced interstitial lung disorders** 🔹

         Use additional code for adverse effect, if applicable, to identify drug (T36-T50 with fifth or sixth character 5)

         Excludes1   interstitial pneumonia NOS (J84.9)
                      lymphoid interstitial pneumonia (J84.2)

     J70.4 **Drug-induced interstitial lung disorders, unspecified** 🔹

         Use additional code for adverse effect, if applicable, to identify drug (T36-T50 with fifth or sixth character 5)

         Excludes1   interstitial pneumonia NOS (J84.9)
                      lymphoid interstitial pneumonia (J84.2)

         Coding Clinic: 2019, Q2, P28

     J70.5 **Respiratory conditions due to smoke inhalation** 🔹

         Code first smoke inhalation (T59.81-)

         Excludes2   smoke inhalation due to chemicals, gases, fumes and vapors (J68.9)

     J70.8 **Respiratory conditions due to other specified external agents** 🔹

         Code first (T51-T65) to identify the external agent

     J70.9 **Respiratory conditions due to unspecified external agent** 🔹

         Code first (T51-T65) to identify the external agent

OTHER RESPIRATORY DISEASES PRINCIPALLY AFFECTING THE INTERSTITIUM (J80-J84)

J80 **Acute respiratory distress syndrome** 🔹🔹

     Acute respiratory distress syndrome in adult or child

     Adult hyaline membrane disease

     Excludes1   respiratory distress syndrome in newborn (perinatal) (P22.0)

     Ⓔ See PDX Collection 744

     Coding Clinic: 2017, Q1, P26-27

● **J81** **Pulmonary edema**

     Use additional code to identify:

         exposure to environmental tobacco smoke (Z77.22)

         history of tobacco dependence (Z87.891)

         occupational exposure to environmental tobacco smoke (Z57.31)

         tobacco dependence (F17.-)

         tobacco use (Z72.0)

     Excludes1   chemical (acute) pulmonary edema (J68.1)
                     hypostatic pneumonia (J18.2)
                     passive pneumonia (J18.2)
                     pulmonary edema due to external agents (J60-J70)
                     pulmonary edema with heart disease NOS (I50.1)
                     pulmonary edema with heart failure (I50.1)

     J81.0 **Acute pulmonary edema** 🔹🔹

         Acute edema of lung

         Ⓔ See PDX Collection 745

         Coding Clinic: 2017, Q1, P26

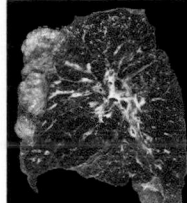

Figure 10-9   Bullous emphysema with large subpleural bullae *(upper left)*. (From Kumar: Robbins and Cotran: Pathologic Basis of Disease, ed 8, Saunders, An Imprint of Elsevier, 2009)

     J81.1 **Chronic pulmonary edema** 🔹

         Pulmonary congestion (chronic) (passive)

         Pulmonary edema NOS

         Ⓔ See PDX Collection 736

J82 **Pulmonary eosinophilia, not elsewhere classified** 🔹🔹

     Excludes2   pulmonary eosinophilia due to aspergillosis (B44.-)
                     pulmonary eosinophilia due to drugs (J70.2-J70.4)
                     pulmonary eosinophilia due to specified parasitic infection (B50-B83)
                     pulmonary eosinophilia due to systemic connective tissue disorders (M30-M36)
                     pulmonary infiltrate NOS (R91.8)

● **J82.8** **Pulmonary eosinophilia, not elsewhere classified**

     J82.81 **Chronic eosinophilic pneumonia** 🔹

         Eosinophilic pneumonia, NOS

         Ⓔ See PDX Collection 4066

     J82.82 **Acute eosinophilic pneumonia** 🔹

         Ⓔ See PDX Collection 4066

     J82.83 **Eosinophilic asthma** 🔹

         Code first asthma, by type, such as:

             mild intermittent asthma (J45.2-)

             mild persistent asthma (J45.3-)

             moderate persistent asthma (J45.4-)

             severe persistent asthma (J45.5-)

         Ⓔ See PDX Collection 4066

     J82.89 **Other pulmonary eosinophilia, not elsewhere classified** 🔹

         Allergic pneumonia

         Löffler's pneumonia

         Tropical (pulmonary) eosinophilia NOS

         Ⓔ See PDX Collection 4066

● **J84** **Other interstitial pulmonary diseases**

     Excludes1   drug-induced interstitial lung disorders (J70.2-J70.4)
                     interstitial emphysema (J98.2)

     Excludes2   lung diseases due to external agents (J60-J70)

     Ⓔ For category J84 CC codes unless otherwise indicated: See PDX Collection 747

     Coding Clinic: 2019, Q2, P28

● **J84.0** **Alveolar and parieto-alveolar conditions**

     J84.01 **Alveolar proteinosis** 🔹🔹

     J84.02 **Pulmonary alveolar microlithiasis** 🔹🔹

     ▷ **J84.03** *Idiopathic pulmonary hemosiderosis* 🔹🔹

         Essential brown induration of lung

         Code first underlying disease, such as:

             disorders of iron metabolism (E83.1-)

         Excludes1   acute idiopathic pulmonary hemorrhage in infants [AIPHI] (R04.81)

     J84.09 **Other alveolar and parieto-alveolar conditions** 🔹🔹

N   Newborn Age: 0   **P**   Pediatric Age: 0-17   **M**   Maternity DX: 9-64   **A**   Adult Age: 15-124   ♀   Females Only   ♂   Males Only

🔹 Complication\Comorbidity   🔹 Major C\C   Ⓔ CC/MCC Exclusions   🔹 Hospital-Acquired Condition   🔹 Hierarchical Condition Category

953

CHAPTER 10 (J00-J99)

● **J84.1 Other interstitial pulmonary diseases with fibrosis**
  Excludes1 pulmonary fibrosis (chronic) due to inhalation of chemicals, gases, fumes or vapors (J68.4)
  pulmonary fibrosis (chronic) following radiation (J70.1)

  J84.10 Pulmonary fibrosis, unspecified
    Capillary fibrosis of lung
    Cirrhosis of lung (chronic) NOS
    Fibrosis of lung (atrophic) (chronic) (confluent) (massive) (perialveolar) (peribronchial) NOS
    Induration of lung (chronic) NOS
    Postinflammatory pulmonary fibrosis

● **J84.11 Idiopathic interstitial pneumonia**
    Excludes1 lymphoid interstitial pneumonia (J84.2)
    pneumocystis pneumonia (B59)

    J84.111 Idiopathic interstitial pneumonia, not otherwise specified

    J84.112 Idiopathic pulmonary fibrosis
      Cryptogenic fibrosing alveolitis
      Idiopathic fibrosing alveolitis

    J84.113 Idiopathic non-specific interstitial pneumonitis
      Excludes1 non-specific interstitial pneumonia NOS, or due to known underlying cause (J84.89)

    J84.114 Acute interstitial pneumonitis
      Hamman-Rich syndrome
      Excludes1 pneumocystis pneumonia (B59)

    J84.115 Respiratory bronchiolitis interstitial lung disease

    J84.116 Cryptogenic organizing pneumonia
      Excludes1 organizing pneumonia NOS, or due to known underlying cause (J84.89)

    J84.117 Desquamative interstitial pneumonia

●▶ **J84.17 Other interstitial pulmonary diseases with fibrosis in diseases classified elsewhere**

  ▶ **J84.170 Interstitial lung disease with progressive fibrotic phenotype in diseases classified elsewhere**
    Progressive fibrotic interstitial lung disease
    Code first underlying disease, such as:
      lung diseases due to external agents (J60-J70)
      rheumatoid arthritis (M05.00-M06.9)
      sarcoidosis (D86)
      systemic connective tissue disorders (M30-M36)

  ▶ **J84.178 Other interstitial pulmonary diseases with fibrosis in diseases classified elsewhere**
    Interstitial pneumonia (nonspecific) (usual) due to collagen vascular disease
    Interstitial pneumonia (nonspecific) (usual) in diseases classified elsewhere
    Organizing pneumonia due to collagen vascular disease
    Organizing pneumonia in diseases classified elsewhere
    Code first underlying disease, such as:
      progressive systemic sclerosis (M34.0)
      rheumatoid arthritis (M05.00-M06.9)
      systemic lupus erythematosis (M32.0-M32.9)

J84.2 Lymphoid interstitial pneumonia
  Lymphoid interstitial pneumonitis

● **J84.8 Other specified interstitial pulmonary diseases**
  Excludes1 exogenous lipoid pneumonia (J69.1)
  unspecified lipoid pneumonia (J69.1)

  J84.81 Lymphangioleiomyomatosis
    Lymphangiomyomatosis

  J84.82 Adult pulmonary Langerhans cell histiocytosis   A
    Adult PLCH

  J84.83 Surfactant mutations of the lung
    (Ex:) See PDX Collection 748

● **J84.84 Other interstitial lung diseases of childhood**
    (Ex:) **For category J84.84 CC codes:** See PDX Collection 748

    J84.841 Neuroendocrine cell hyperplasia of infancy

    J84.842 Pulmonary interstitial glycogenosis

    J84.843 Alveolar capillary dysplasia with vein misalignment

    J84.848 Other interstitial lung diseases of childhood

  J84.89 Other specified interstitial pulmonary diseases
    Endogenous lipoid pneumonia
    Interstitial pneumonitis
    Non-specific interstitial pneumonitis NOS
    Organizing pneumonia NOS
    Code first, if applicable:
      poisoning due to drug or toxin (T51-T65 with fifth or sixth character to indicate intent), for toxic pneumonopathy
      underlying cause of pneumonopathy, if known
    Use additional code, for adverse effect, to identify drug (T36-T50 with fifth or sixth character 5), if drug-induced
    Excludes1 cryptogenic organizing pneumonia (J84.116)
      idiopathic non-specific interstitial pneumonitis (J84.113)
      lipoid pneumonia, exogenous or unspecified (J69.1)
      lymphoid interstitial pneumonia (J84.2)
    Coding Clinic: 2021, Q1, P48; 2019, Q2, P28

▶ New   ⇒ Revised   ~~deleted~~ Deleted   Excludes 1   Excludes 2   Includes   Use additional   Code first   Code also   Key words
OGCR Official Guidelines   ● Unacceptable Principal Diagnosis   X Assign placeholder X   ● Use Additional Character(s)   ▶ Manifestation Code   **Coding Clinic**

J84.9   Interstitial pulmonary disease, unspecified 🔹🔹
       Interstitial pneumonia NOS

SUPPURATIVE AND NECROTIC CONDITIONS OF THE LOWER RESPIRATORY TRACT (J85-J86)

● **J85**   Abscess of lung and mediastinum
       Use additional code (B95-B97) to identify infectious agent.
       (Ex) For category J85 CC codes unless otherwise indicated: See PDX Collection 749

   J85.0   Gangrene and necrosis of lung 🔹🔹

   J85.1   Abscess of lung with pneumonia 🔹🔹
         Code also the type of pneumonia

   J85.2   Abscess of lung without pneumonia 🔹🔹
         Abscess of lung NOS

   J85.3   Abscess of mediastinum 🔹🔹
         (Ex) See PDX Collection 750

● **J86**   Pyothorax
       Use additional code (B95-B97) to identify infectious agent.

       Excludes1   abscess of lung (J85.-)
                 pyothorax due to tuberculosis (A15.6)
       (Ex) For category J86 CC codes: See PDX Collection 751

   J86.0   Pyothorax with fistula 🔹🔹
         Bronchocutaneous fistula
         Bronchopleural fistula
         Hepatopleural fistula
         Mediastinal fistula
         Pleural fistula
         Thoracic fistula
         Any condition classifiable to J86.9 with fistula

   J86.9   Pyothorax without fistula 🔹🔹
         Abscess of pleura
         Abscess of thorax
         Empyema (chest) (lung) (pleura)
         Fibrinopurulent pleurisy
         Purulent pleurisy
         Pyopneumothorax
         Septic pleurisy
         Seropurulent pleurisy
         Suppurative pleurisy

OTHER DISEASES OF THE PLEURA (J90-J94)

J90   Pleural effusion, not elsewhere classified 🔹
       Encysted pleurisy
       Pleural effusion NOS
       Pleurisy with effusion (exudative) (serous)

       Excludes1   chylous (pleural) effusion (J94.0)
                 malignant pleural effusion (J91.0))
                 pleurisy NOS (R09.1)
                 tuberculous pleural effusion (A15.6)
       (Ex) See PDX Collection 752
       Coding Clinic: 2015, Q2, P16

● **J91**   Pleural effusion in conditions classified elsewhere
       Excludes2   pleural effusion in heart failure (I50.-)
                 pleural effusion in systemic lupus erythematosus
                 (M32.13)

   ▸ *J91.0*   *Malignant pleural effusion* 🔹
         Code first underlying neoplasm
         (Ex) See PDX Collection 753

   ▸ *J91.8*   *Pleural effusion in other conditions classified elsewhere* 🔹
         Code first underlying disease, such as:
           filariasis (B74.0-B74.9)
           influenza (J09.X2, J10.1, J11.1)
         (Ex) See PDX Collection 752
         Coding Clinic: 2015, Q2, P16

● **J92**   Pleural plaque
       Includes   pleural thickening

   J92.0   Pleural plaque with presence of asbestos

   J92.9   Pleural plaque without asbestos
         Pleural plaque NOS

● **J93**   Pneumothorax and air leak
       Collapsed lung

       Excludes1   congenital or perinatal pneumothorax (P25.1)
                 postprocedural air leak (J95.812)
                 postprocedural pneumothorax (J95.811)
                 traumatic pneumothorax (S27.0)
                 tuberculous (current disease) pneumothorax
                 (A15.-)
                 pyopneumothorax (J86.-)
       (Ex) For category J93 CC codes: See PDX Collection 754

   J93.0   Spontaneous tension pneumothorax 🔹
         Tension pneumothorax (most serious type) occurs when air (positive pressure) collects in the pleural space

   ● **J93.1**   Other spontaneous pneumothorax

     J93.11   Primary spontaneous pneumothorax 🔹

     ● **J93.12**   Secondary spontaneous pneumothorax 🔹
         Code first underlying condition, such as:
           catamenial pneumothorax due to
             endometriosis (N80.8)
           cystic fibrosis (E84.-)
           eosinophilic pneumonia (J82)
           lymphangioleiomyomatosis (J84.81)
           malignant neoplasm of bronchus and lung
             (C34.-)
           Marfan's syndrome (Q87.4)
           pneumonia due to Pneumocystis carinii
             (B59)
           secondary malignant neoplasm of lung
             (C78.0-)
           spontaneous rupture of the esophagus
             (K22.3)

   ● **J93.8**   Other pneumothorax and air leak

     J93.81   Chronic pneumothorax 🔹

     J93.82   Other air leak 🔹
         Persistent air leak

     J93.83   Other pneumothorax 🔹
         Acute pneumothorax
         Spontaneous pneumothorax NOS

   J93.9   Pneumothorax, unspecified 🔹
         Pneumothorax NOS

● **J94**   Other pleural conditions
       Excludes1   pleurisy NOS (R09.1)
                 traumatic hemopneumothorax (S27.2)
                 traumatic hemothorax (S27.1)
                 tuberculous pleural conditions (current disease)
                 (A15.-)
       (Ex) For category J94 CC codes unless otherwise indicated: See PDX Collection 752

   J94.0   Chylous effusion 🔹
         Chyliform effusion

   J94.1   Fibrothorax

   J94.2   Hemothorax 🔹
         Hemopneumothorax

   J94.8   Other specified pleural conditions 🔹
         Hydropneumothorax
         Hydrothorax
         (Ex) See PDX Collection 3600
         Coding Clinic: 2021, Q1, P49

   J94.9   Pleural condition, unspecified

Item 10–11   **Empyema** is a condition in which pus accumulates in a body cavity. Empyema **with fistula** occurs when the pus passes from one cavity to another organ or structure.

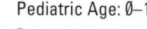 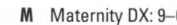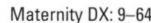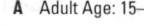

CHAPTER 10 (J00-J99)

INTRAOPERATIVE AND POSTPROCEDURAL COMPLICATIONS AND DISORDERS OF RESPIRATORY SYSTEM, NOT ELSEWHERE CLASSIFIED (J95)

● **J95** **Intraoperative and postprocedural complications and disorders of respiratory system, not elsewhere classified**

Excludes2 aspiration pneumonia (J69.-)
emphysema (subcutaneous) resulting from a procedure (T81.82)
hypostatic pneumonia (J18.2)
pulmonary manifestations due to radiation (J70.0- J70.1)

● **J95.0** **Tracheostomy complications**
(Ex) For category J95.0 CC codes: See PDX Collection 755

J95.00 **Unspecified tracheostomy complication**

J95.01 **Hemorrhage from tracheostomy stoma**

J95.02 **Infection of tracheostomy stoma**
Use additional code to identify type of infection, such as:
cellulitis of neck (L03.221)
sepsis (A40, A41.-)

J95.03 **Malfunction of tracheostomy stoma**
Mechanical complication of tracheostomy stoma
Obstruction of tracheostomy airway
Tracheal stenosis due to tracheostomy

J95.04 **Tracheo-esophageal fistula following tracheostomy**

J95.09 **Other tracheostomy complication**

J95.1 **Acute pulmonary insufficiency following thoracic surgery**
Excludes2 functional disturbances following cardiac surgery (I97.0, I97.1-)
(Ex) See PDX Collection 756

J95.2 **Acute pulmonary insufficiency following nonthoracic surgery**
Excludes2 functional disturbances following cardiac surgery (I97.0, I97.1-)
(Ex) See PDX Collection 756

J95.3 **Chronic pulmonary insufficiency following surgery**
Excludes2 functional disturbances following cardiac surgery (I97.0, I97.1-)
(Ex) See PDX Collection 756

J95.4 **Chemical pneumonitis due to anesthesia**
Mendelson's syndrome
Postprocedural aspiration pneumonia
Use additional code for adverse effect, if applicable, to identify drug (T41.- with fifth or sixth character 5)
Excludes1 aspiration pneumonitis due to anesthesia complicating labor and delivery (O74.0)
aspiration pneumonitis due to anesthesia complicating pregnancy (O29)
aspiration pneumonitis due to anesthesia complicating the puerperium (O89.01)
(Ex) See PDX Collection 757

J95.5 **Postprocedural subglottic stenosis**
(Ex) See PDX Collection 757

● **J95.6** **Intraoperative hemorrhage and hematoma of a respiratory system organ or structure complicating a procedure**
Excludes1 intraoperative hemorrhage and hematoma of a respiratory system organ or structure due to accidental puncture and laceration during procedure (J95.7-)
(Ex) For category J95.6 CC codes: See PDX Collection 758

J95.61 **Intraoperative hemorrhage and hematoma of a respiratory system organ or structure complicating a respiratory system procedure**

J95.62 **Intraoperative hemorrhage and hematoma of a respiratory system organ or structure complicating other procedure**

● **J95.7** **Accidental puncture and laceration of a respiratory system organ or structure during a procedure**
Excludes2 postprocedural pneumothorax (J95.811)
(Ex) For category J95.7 CC codes: See PDX Collection 509

J95.71 **Accidental puncture and laceration of a respiratory system organ or structure during a respiratory system procedure**

J95.72 **Accidental puncture and laceration of a respiratory system organ or structure during other procedure**

● **J95.8** **Other intraoperative and postprocedural complications and disorders of respiratory system, not elsewhere classified**
Coding Clinic: 2016, Q4, P10

● **J95.81** **Postprocedural pneumothorax and air leak**
(Ex) For category J95.81 CC codes: See PDX Collection 754

J95.811 **Postprocedural pneumothorax**
Coding Clinic: 2021, Q1, P49

J95.812 **Postprocedural air leak**

● **J95.82** **Postprocedural respiratory failure**
Excludes1 Respiratory failure in other conditions (J96.-)
(Ex) For category J95.82 CC codes: See PDX Collection 756

J95.821 **Acute postprocedural respiratory failure**
Postprocedural respiratory failure NOS

J95.822 **Acute and chronic postprocedural respiratory failure**

● **J95.83** **Postprocedural hemorrhage of a respiratory system organ or structure following a procedure**
(Ex) For category J95.83 CC codes: See PDX Collection 758

J95.830 **Postprocedural hemorrhage of a respiratory system organ or structure following a respiratory system procedure**

J95.831 **Postprocedural hemorrhage of a respiratory system organ or structure following other procedure**

J95.84 **Transfusion-related acute lung injury (TRALI)**
(Ex) See PDX Collection 757

● **J95.85** **Complication of respirator [ventilator]**

J95.850 **Mechanical complication of respirator**
Excludes1 encounter for respirator [ventilator] dependence during power failure (Z99.12)
(Ex) See PDX Collection 759

J95.851 **Ventilator associated pneumonia**
Ventilator associated pneumonitis
Use additional code to identify the organism, if known (B95.-, B96.-, B97.-)
Excludes1 ventilator lung in newborn (P27.8)
(Ex) See PDX Collection 3227
Coding Clinic: 2017, Q1, P25

J95.859 **Other complication of respirator [ventilator]**
(Ex) See PDX Collection 3228
Coding Clinic: 2021, Q1, P49

▶ New   ⇒ Revised   ~~deleted~~ Deleted   Excludes 1   Excludes 2   Includes   Use additional   Code first   Code also   Key words
OGCR Official Guidelines   ● Unacceptable Principal Diagnosis   X Assign placeholder X   ● Use Additional Character(s)   ▶ Manifestation Code   Coding Clinic

● **J95.86**   Postprocedural hematoma and seroma of a respiratory system organ or structure following a procedure
> (Ex) **For category J95.86 CC codes:** See PDX Collection 758

     J95.860   Postprocedural hematoma of a respiratory system organ or structure following a respiratory system procedure 🝙

     J95.861   Postprocedural hematoma of a respiratory system organ or structure following other procedure 🝙

     J95.862   Postprocedural seroma of a respiratory system organ or structure following a respiratory system procedure 🝙

     J95.863   Postprocedural seroma of a respiratory system organ or structure following other procedure 🝙

J95.88   Other intraoperative complications of respiratory system, not elsewhere classified 🝙
> (Ex) See PDX Collection 757

J95.89   Other postprocedural complications and disorders of respiratory system, not elsewhere classified 🝙

> Use additional code to identify disorder, such as:
> aspiration pneumonia (J69.-)
> bacterial or viral pneumonia (J12-J18)

> **Excludes2**   acute pulmonary insufficiency following thoracic surgery (J95.1)
> postprocedural subglottic stenosis (J95.5)
> (Ex) See PDX Collection 757

OTHER DISEASES OF THE RESPIRATORY SYSTEM (J96-J99)

● **J96**   Respiratory failure, not elsewhere classified

> **Excludes1**   acute respiratory distress syndrome (J80)
> cardiorespiratory failure (R09.2)
> newborn respiratory distress syndrome (P22.0)
> postprocedural respiratory failure (J95.82-)
> respiratory arrest (R09.2)
> respiratory arrest of newborn (P28.81)
> respiratory failure of newborn (P28.5)
> (Ex) **For category J96 CC codes:** See PDX Collection 744

● **J96.0**   Acute respiratory failure

     J96.00   Acute respiratory failure, unspecified whether with hypoxia or hypercapnia 🝙🝙
> Coding Clinic: 2016, Q3, P14

     J96.01   Acute respiratory failure with hypoxia 🝙🝙

     J96.02   Acute respiratory failure with hypercapnia 🝙🝙

● **J96.1**   Chronic respiratory failure

     J96.10   Chronic respiratory failure, unspecified whether with hypoxia or hypercapnia 🝙🝙
> Coding Clinic: 2021, Q1, P46; 2016, Q1, P38; 2015, Q1, P21

     J96.11   Chronic respiratory failure with hypoxia 🝙🝙

     J96.12   Chronic respiratory failure with hypercapnia 🝙🝙

● **J96.2**   Acute and chronic respiratory failure
> Acute on chronic respiratory failure

     J96.20   Acute and chronic respiratory failure, unspecified whether with hypoxia or hypercapnia 🝙🝙

     J96.21   Acute and chronic respiratory failure with hypoxia 🝙🝙

     J96.22   Acute and chronic respiratory failure with hypercapnia 🝙🝙

● **J96.9**   Respiratory failure, unspecified

     J96.90   Respiratory failure, unspecified, unspecified whether with hypoxia or hypercapnia 🝙🝙
> Coding Clinic: 2021, Q1, P44

     J96.91   Respiratory failure, unspecified with hypoxia 🝙🝙

     J96.92   Respiratory failure, unspecified with hypercapnia 🝙🝙

● **J98**   Other respiratory disorders

> Use additional code to identify:
> exposure to environmental tobacco smoke (Z77.22)
> exposure to tobacco smoke in the perinatal period (P96.81)
> history of tobacco dependence (Z87.891)
> occupational exposure to environmental tobacco smoke (Z57.31)
> tobacco dependence (F17.-)
> tobacco use (Z72.0)

> **Excludes1**   newborn apnea (P28.4)
> newborn sleep apnea (P28.3)

> **Excludes2**   apnea NOS (R06.81)
> sleep apnea (G47.3-)

● **J98.0**   Diseases of bronchus, not elsewhere classified

     J98.01   Acute bronchospasm

> **Excludes1**   acute bronchiolitis with bronchospasm (J21.-)
> acute bronchitis with bronchospasm (J20.-)
> asthma (J45.-)
> exercise induced bronchospasm (J45.990)

     J98.09   Other diseases of bronchus, not elsewhere classified
> Broncholithiasis
> Calcification of bronchus
> Stenosis of bronchus
> Tracheobronchial collapse
> Tracheobronchial dyskinesia
> Ulcer of bronchus

● **J98.1**   Pulmonary collapse

> **Excludes1**   therapeutic collapse of lung status (Z98.3)
> (Ex) **For category J98.1 CC codes:** See PDX Collection 760

     J98.11   Atelectasis 🝙

> **Excludes1**   newborn atelectasis
> tuberculous atelectasis (current disease) (A15)

     J98.19   Other pulmonary collapse 🝙

J98.2   Interstitial emphysema 🝙
> Mediastinal emphysema

> **Excludes1**   emphysema NOS (J43.9)
> emphysema in newborn (P25.0)
> surgical emphysema (subcutaneous) (T81.82)
> traumatic subcutaneous emphysema (T79.7)

J98.3   Compensatory emphysema 🝙

J98.4   Other disorders of lung
> Calcification of lung
> Cystic lung disease (acquired)
> Lung disease NOS
> Pulmolithiasis

> **Excludes1**   acute interstitial pneumonitis (J84.114)
> pulmonary insufficiency following surgery (J95.1-J95.2)

N	Newborn Age: 0	P	Pediatric Age: 0–17	M	Maternity DX: 9–64	A	Adult Age: 15–124	♀	Females Only	♂	Males Only

🝙 Complication\Comorbidity   🝙 Major C\C   (Ex) CC/MCC Exclusions   🝙 Hospital-Acquired Condition   🝙 Hierarchical Condition Category

● **J98.5**   **Diseases of mediastinum, not elsewhere classified**
       Excludes2   abscess of mediastinum (J85.3)
       Coding Clinic: 2016, Q4, P29

       J98.51   **Mediastinitis** 🔖🔖
               Code first underlying condition, if applicable, such
                   as postoperative mediastinitis (T81.-)
               (Ex:) No Exclusions

       J98.59   **Other diseases of mediastinum, not elsewhere**
               classified 🔖🔖
               Fibrosis of mediastinum
               Hernia of mediastinum
               Retraction of mediastinum
               (Ex:) No Exclusions

J98.6   **Disorders of diaphragm**
       Diaphragmatitis
       Paralysis of diaphragm
       Relaxation of diaphragm
       Excludes1   congenital malformation of diaphragm
                   NEC (Q79.1)
                   congenital diaphragmatic hernia (Q79.0)
       Excludes2   diaphragmatic hernia (K44.-)

J98.8   **Other specified respiratory disorders**

J98.9   **Respiratory disorder, unspecified**
       Respiratory disease (chronic) NOS

▷ **J99**   *Respiratory disorders in diseases classified elsewhere* 🔖
       Code first underlying disease, such as:
          amyloidosis (E85.-)
          ankylosing spondylitis (M45)
          congenital syphilis (A50.5)
          cryoglobulinemia (D89.1)
          early congenital syphilis (A50.0)
          plasminogen deficiency (E88.02)
          schistosomiasis (B65.0-B65.9)
       Excludes1   respiratory disorders in:
               amebiasis (A06.5)
               blastomycosis (B40.0-B40.2)
               candidiasis (B37.1)
               coccidioidomycosis (B38.0-B38.2)
               cystic fibrosis with pulmonary manifestations
                  (E84.0)
               dermatomyositis (M33.01, M33.11)
               histoplasmosis (B39.0-B39.2)
               late syphilis (A52.72, A52.73)
               polymyositis (M33.21)
      ⟹ Sjögren syndrome (M35.02)
               systemic lupus erythematosus (M32.13)
               systemic sclerosis (M34.81)
               Wegener's granulomatosis (M31.30-M31.31)

CHAPTER 10 (J00-J99)

▶ New   ⟹ Revised   ~~deleted~~ Deleted   Excludes 1   Excludes 2   Includes   Use additional   Code first   Code also   Key words
OGCR Official Guidelines   ● Unacceptable Principal Diagnosis   X Assign placeholder X   ● Use Additional Character(s)   ▷ Manifestation Code   Coding Clinic

CHAPTER 11

DISEASES OF THE DIGESTIVE SYSTEM (K00-K95)

OGCR Chapter-Specific Coding Guidelines

11. Chapter 11: Diseases of the Digestive System (K00-K95)
Reserved for future guideline expansion

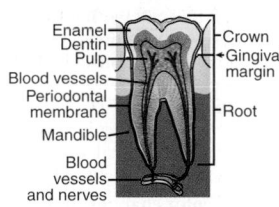

Figure 11-1 Anatomy of a tooth.

Item 11–1 **Anodontia** is the congenital absence of teeth. **Hypodontia** is partial anodontia. **Oligodontia** is the congenital absence of some teeth, whereas **supernumerary** is having more teeth than the normal number. **Mesiodens** are small extra teeth that often appear in pairs, although single small teeth are not uncommon.

CHAPTER 11

DISEASES OF THE DIGESTIVE SYSTEM (K00-K95)

> **Excludes2** certain conditions originating in the perinatal period (P04-P96)
> certain infectious and parasitic diseases (A00-B99)
> complications of pregnancy, childbirth and the puerperium (O00-O9A)
> congenital malformations, deformations and chromosomal abnormalities (Q00-Q99)
> endocrine, nutritional and metabolic diseases (E00-E88)
> injury, poisoning and certain other consequences of external causes (S00-T88)
> neoplasms (C00-D49)
> symptoms, signs and abnormal clinical and laboratory findings, not elsewhere classified (R00-R94)

This chapter contains the following blocks:

K00-K14	Diseases of oral cavity and salivary glands
K20-K31	Diseases of esophagus, stomach and duodenum
K35-K38	Diseases of appendix
K40-K46	Hernia
K50-K52	Noninfective enteritis and colitis
K55-K64	Other diseases of intestines
K65-K68	Diseases of peritoneum and retroperitoneum
K70-K77	Diseases of liver
K80-K87	Disorders of gallbladder, biliary tract and pancreas
K90-K95	Other diseases of the digestive system

DISEASES OF ORAL CAVITY AND SALIVARY GLANDS (K00-K14)

● **K00** **Disorders of tooth development and eruption**
> **Excludes2** embedded and impacted teeth (K01.-)

K00.0 **Anodontia**
Hypodontia
Oligodontia
> **Excludes1** acquired absence of teeth (K08.1-)

K00.1 **Supernumerary teeth**
Distomolar
Fourth molar
Mesiodens
Paramolar
Supplementary teeth
> **Excludes2** supernumerary roots (K00.2)

K00.2 **Abnormalities of size and form of teeth**
Concrescence of teeth
Fusion of teeth
Gemination of teeth
Dens evaginatus
Dens in dente
Dens invaginatus
Enamel pearls
Macrodontia
Microdontia
Peg-shaped [conical] teeth
Supernumerary roots
Taurodontism
Tuberculum paramolare
> **Excludes1** abnormalities of teeth due to congenital syphilis (A50.5)
> tuberculum Carabelli, which is regarded as a normal variation and should not be coded

K00.3 **Mottled teeth**
Dental fluorosis
Mottling of enamel
Nonfluoride enamel opacities
> **Excludes2** deposits [accretions] on teeth (K03.6)

K00.4 **Disturbances in tooth formation**
Aplasia and hypoplasia of cementum
Dilaceration of tooth
Enamel hypoplasia (neonatal) (postnatal) (prenatal)
Regional odontodysplasia
Turner's tooth
> **Excludes1** Hutchinson's teeth and mulberry molars in congenital syphilis (A50.5)
> **Excludes2** mottled teeth (K00.3)

K00.5 **Hereditary disturbances in tooth structure, not elsewhere classified**
Amelogenesis imperfecta
Dentinogenesis imperfecta
Odontogenesis imperfecta
Dentinal dysplasia
Shell teeth

K00.6 **Disturbances in tooth eruption**
Dentia praecox
Natal tooth
Neonatal tooth
Premature eruption of tooth
Premature shedding of primary [deciduous] tooth
Prenatal teeth
Retained [persistent] primary tooth
> **Excludes2** embedded and impacted teeth (K01.-)

K00.7 **Teething syndrome**

K00.8 **Other disorders of tooth development**
Color changes during tooth formation
Intrinsic staining of teeth NOS
> **Excludes2** posteruptive color changes (K03.7)

K00.9 **Disorder of tooth development, unspecified**
Disorder of odontogenesis NOS

● **K01** **Embedded and impacted teeth**
> **Excludes1** abnormal position of fully erupted teeth (M26.3-)

K01.0 **Embedded teeth**

K01.1 **Impacted teeth**

N Newborn Age: 0   **P** Pediatric Age: 0–17   **M** Maternity DX: 9–64   **A** Adult Age: 15–124   ♀ Females Only   ♂ Males Only
🔴 Complication\Comorbidity   🔴 Major C\C   (Ex) CC/MCC Exclusions   🔴 Hospital-Acquired Condition   🔴 Hierarchical Condition Category

959

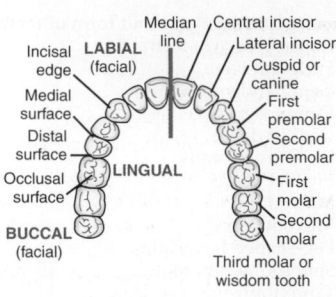

Median line
Central incisor
Lateral incisor
Cuspid or canine
First premolar
Second premolar
First molar
Second molar
Third molar or wisdom tooth
Incisal edge
LABIAL (facial)
Medial surface
Distal surface
Occlusal surface
LINGUAL
BUCCAL (facial)

Figure 11-2 The permanent teeth within the dental arch.

Item 11–2 Each dental arch (jaw) normally contains 16 teeth. Tooth decay or **dental caries** is a disease of the enamel, dentin, and cementum of the tooth and can result in a cavity.

● **K02 Dental caries**
     Includes   caries of dentine
                dental cavities
                early childhood caries
                pre-eruptive caries
                recurrent caries (dentino enamel junction) (enamel) (to the pulp)
                tooth decay

    K02.3 Arrested dental caries
          Arrested coronal and root caries
● **K02.5 Dental caries on pit and fissure surface**
          Dental caries on chewing surface of tooth
       K02.51 Dental caries on pit and fissure surface limited to enamel
            White spot lesions [initial caries] on pit and fissure surface of tooth
       K02.52 Dental caries on pit and fissure surface penetrating into dentin
            Primary dental caries, cervical origin
       K02.53 Dental caries on pit and fissure surface penetrating into pulp
● **K02.6 Dental caries on smooth surface**
       K02.61 Dental caries on smooth surface limited to enamel
            White spot lesions [initial caries] on smooth surface of tooth
       K02.62 Dental caries on smooth surface penetrating into dentin
       K02.63 Dental caries on smooth surface penetrating into pulp
    K02.7 Dental root caries
    K02.9 Dental caries, unspecified

● **K03 Other diseases of hard tissues of teeth**
     Excludes2   bruxism (F45.8)
                 dental caries (K02.-)
                 teeth-grinding NOS (F45.8)
    K03.0 Excessive attrition of teeth
          Approximal wear of teeth
          Occlusal wear of teeth
    K03.1 Abrasion of teeth
          Dentifrice abrasion of teeth
          Habitual abrasion of teeth
          Occupational abrasion of teeth
          Ritual abrasion of teeth
          Traditional abrasion of teeth
          Wedge defect NOS
    K03.2 Erosion of teeth
          Erosion of teeth due to diet
          Erosion of teeth due to drugs and medicaments
          Erosion of teeth due to persistent vomiting
          Erosion of teeth NOS
          Idiopathic erosion of teeth
          Occupational erosion of teeth

    K03.3 Pathological resorption of teeth
          Internal granuloma of pulp
          Resorption of teeth (external)
    K03.4 Hypercementosis
          Cementation hyperplasia
    K03.5 Ankylosis of teeth
    K03.6 Deposits [accretions] on teeth
          Betel deposits [accretions] on teeth
          Black deposits [accretions] on teeth
          Extrinsic staining of teeth NOS
          Green deposits [accretions] on teeth
          Materia alba deposits [accretions] on teeth
          Orange deposits [accretions] on teeth
          Staining of teeth NOS
          Subgingival dental calculus
          Supragingival dental calculus
          Tobacco deposits [accretions] on teeth
    K03.7 Posteruptive color changes of dental hard tissues
          Excludes2   deposits [accretions] on teeth (K03.6)
● **K03.8 Other specified diseases of hard tissues of teeth**
       K03.81 Cracked tooth
            Excludes1   asymptomatic craze lines in enamel - omit code
                             broken or fractured tooth due to trauma (S02.5)
       K03.89 Other specified diseases of hard tissues of teeth
    K03.9 Disease of hard tissues of teeth, unspecified

 K04 Diseases of pulp and periapical tissues
     Coding Clinic: 2016, Q4, P29
● **K04.0 Pulpitis**
          Acute pulpitis
          Chronic (hyperplastic) (ulcerative) pulpitis
          (Ex) **For category K04.0 CC codes:** See PDX Collection 761
       K04.01 Reversible pulpitis 🔗
       K04.02 Irreversible pulpitis 🔗
    K04.1 Necrosis of pulp
          Pulpal gangrene
    K04.2 Pulp degeneration
          Denticles
          Pulpal calcifications
          Pulpal stones
    K04.3 Abnormal hard tissue formation in pulp
          Secondary or irregular dentine
    K04.4 Acute apical periodontitis of pulpal origin 🔗
          Acute apical periodontitis NOS
          Excludes1   acute periodontitis (K05.2-)
          (Ex) See PDX Collection 761
    K04.5 Chronic apical periodontitis
          Apical or periapical granuloma
          Apical periodontitis NOS
          Excludes1   chronic periodontitis (K05.3-)
    K04.6 Periapical abscess with sinus
          Dental abscess with sinus
          Dentoalveolar abscess with sinus
    K04.7 Periapical abscess without sinus
          Dental abscess without sinus
          Dentoalveolar abscess without sinus
    K04.8 Radicular cyst
          Apical (periodontal) cyst
          Periapical cyst
          Residual radicular cyst
          Excludes2   lateral periodontal cyst (K09.0)
● **K04.9 Other and unspecified diseases of pulp and periapical tissues**
       K04.90 Unspecified diseases of pulp and periapical tissues
       K04.99 Other diseases of pulp and periapical tissues

▶ New   ⇒ Revised   ~~deleted~~ Deleted   Excludes 1   Excludes 2   Includes   Use additional   Code first   Code also   Key words
OGCR Official Guidelines   ● Unacceptable Principal Diagnosis   X Assign placeholder X   ● Use Additional Character(s)   ▶ Manifestation Code   **Coding Clinic**

Item 11–3 Acute gingivitis, also known as orilitis or ulitis, is the short-term, severe inflammation of the gums (gingiva) caused by bacteria. **Chronic gingivitis** is persistent inflammation of the gums. When the gingivitis moves into the periodontium it is called periodontitis, also known as paradentitis.

● **K05   Gingivitis and periodontal diseases**
     Use additional code to identify:
       alcohol abuse and dependence (F10.-)
       exposure to environmental tobacco smoke (Z77.22)
       exposure to tobacco smoke in the perinatal period (P96.81)
       history of tobacco dependence (Z87.891)
       occupational exposure to environmental tobacco smoke
         (Z57.31)
       tobacco dependence (F17.-)
       tobacco use (Z72.0)
     Coding Clinic: 2016, Q4, P29

● **K05.0 Acute gingivitis**
     Excludes1   acute necrotizing ulcerative gingivitis
               (A69.1)
              herpesviral [herpes simplex]
                 gingivostomatitis (B00.2)

     K05.00 Acute gingivitis, plaque induced
         Acute gingivitis NOS
         Plaque induced gingival disease
     K05.01 Acute gingivitis, non-plaque induced

● **K05.1 Chronic gingivitis**
     Desquamative gingivitis (chronic)
     Gingivitis (chronic) NOS
     Hyperplastic gingivitis (chronic)
     Pregnancy associated gingivitis
     Simple marginal gingivitis (chronic)
     Ulcerative gingivitis (chronic)
     Code first, if applicable, diseases of the digestive system
         complicating pregnancy (O99.61-)

     K05.10 Chronic gingivitis, plaque induced
         Chronic gingivitis NOS
         Gingivitis NOS
     K05.11 Chronic gingivitis, non-plaque induced

● **K05.2 Aggressive periodontitis**
     Acute pericoronitis
     Excludes1   acute apical periodontitis (K04.4)
              periapical abscess (K04.7)
              periapical abscess with sinus (K04.6)

     K05.20 Aggressive periodontitis, unspecified
     ● **K05.21 Aggressive periodontitis, localized**
         Periodontal abscess
         K05.211 Aggressive periodontitis, localized,
                 slight
         K05.212 Aggressive periodontitis, localized,
                 moderate
         K05.213 Aggressive periodontitis, localized,
                 severe
         K05.219 Aggressive periodontitis, localized,
                 unspecified severity
     ● **K05.22 Aggressive periodontitis, generalized**
         K05.221 Aggressive periodontitis, generalized,
                 slight
         K05.222 Aggressive periodontitis, generalized,
                 moderate
         K05.223 Aggressive periodontitis, generalized,
                 severe
         K05.229 Aggressive periodontitis, generalized,
                 unspecified severity

● **K05.3 Chronic periodontitis**
     Chronic pericoronitis
     Complex periodontitis
     Periodontitis NOS
     Simplex periodontitis
     Excludes1   chronic apical periodontitis (K04.5)

     K05.30 Chronic periodontitis, unspecified
     ● **K05.31 Chronic periodontitis, localized**
         K05.311 Chronic periodontitis, localized,
                 slight
         K05.312 Chronic periodontitis, localized,
                 moderate
         K05.313 Chronic periodontitis, localized,
                 severe
         K05.319 Chronic periodontitis, localized,
                 unspecified severity
     ● **K05.32 Chronic periodontitis, generalized**
         K05.321 Chronic periodontitis, generalized,
                 slight
         K05.322 Chronic periodontitis, generalized,
                 moderate
         K05.323 Chronic periodontitis, generalized,
                 severe
         K05.329 Chronic periodontitis, generalized,
                 unspecified severity

  K05.4 Periodontosis
     Juvenile periodontosis

  K05.5 Other periodontal diseases
     Combined periodontic-endodontic lesion
     Narrow gingival width (of periodontal soft tissue)
     Excludes2   leukoplakia of gingiva (K13.21)

  K05.6 Periodontal disease, unspecified

● **K06   Other disorders of gingiva and edentulous alveolar ridge**
     Excludes2   acute gingivitis (K05.0)
              atrophy of edentulous alveolar ridge (K08.2)
              chronic gingivitis (K05.1)
              gingivitis NOS (K05.1)
     Coding Clinic: 2016, Q4, P29

● **K06.0 Gingival recession**
     Gingival recession (postinfective) (postprocedural)
     ● **K06.01 Gingival recession, localized**
         K06.010 Localized gingival recession,
                 unspecified
                    Localized gingival recession, NOS
         K06.011 Localized gingival recession, minimal
         K06.012 Localized gingival recession,
                 moderate
         K06.013 Localized gingival recession, severe
     ● **K06.02 Gingival recession, generalized**
         K06.020 Generalized gingival recession,
                 unspecified
                    Generalized gingival recession, NOS
         K06.021 Generalized gingival recession,
                 minimal
         K06.022 Generalized gingival recession,
                 moderate
         K06.023 Generalized gingival recession,
                 severe

  K06.1 Gingival enlargement
     Gingival fibromatosis

  K06.2 Gingival and edentulous alveolar ridge lesions
     associated with trauma
     Irritative hyperplasia of edentulous ridge [denture
       hyperplasia]
     Use additional code (Chapter 20) to identify external
       cause or denture status (Z97.2)

  K06.3 Horizontal alveolar bone loss

N Newborn Age: 0   **P** Pediatric Age: 0–17   **M** Maternity DX: 9–64   **A** Adult Age: 15–124   ♀ Females Only   ♂ Males Only

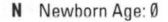 Complication\Comorbidity   Major C\C   (Ex) CC/MCC Exclusions   Hospital-Acquired Condition   Hierarchical Condition Category   **961**

K06.8 **Other specified disorders of gingiva and edentulous alveolar ridge**
Fibrous epulis
Flabby alveolar ridge
Giant cell epulis
Peripheral giant cell granuloma of gingiva
Pyogenic granuloma of gingiva
Vertical ridge deficiency
Excludes2 gingival cyst (K09.0)

K06.9 **Disorder of gingiva and edentulous alveolar ridge, unspecified**

● K08 **Other disorders of teeth and supporting structures**
Excludes2 dentofacial anomalies [including malocclusion] (M26.-)
disorders of jaw (M27.-)
Coding Clinic: 2016, Q4, P29

K08.0 **Exfoliation of teeth due to systemic causes**
Code also underlying systemic condition

● K08.1 **Complete loss of teeth**
Acquired loss of teeth, complete
Excludes1 congenital absence of teeth (K00.0)
exfoliation of teeth due to systemic causes (K08.0)
partial loss of teeth (K08.4-)

● K08.10 **Complete loss of teeth, unspecified cause**
K08.101 Complete loss of teeth, unspecified cause, class I
K08.102 Complete loss of teeth, unspecified cause, class II
K08.103 Complete loss of teeth, unspecified cause, class III
K08.104 Complete loss of teeth, unspecified cause, class IV
K08.109 Complete loss of teeth, unspecified cause, unspecified class
Edentulism NOS

● K08.11 **Complete loss of teeth due to trauma**
K08.111 Complete loss of teeth due to trauma, class I
K08.112 Complete loss of teeth due to trauma, class II
K08.113 Complete loss of teeth due to trauma, class III
K08.114 Complete loss of teeth due to trauma, class IV
K08.119 Complete loss of teeth due to trauma, unspecified class

● K08.12 **Complete loss of teeth due to periodontal diseases**
K08.121 Complete loss of teeth due to periodontal diseases, class I
K08.122 Complete loss of teeth due to periodontal diseases, class II
K08.123 Complete loss of teeth due to periodontal diseases, class III
K08.124 Complete loss of teeth due to periodontal diseases, class IV
K08.129 Complete loss of teeth due to periodontal diseases, unspecified class

● K08.13 **Complete loss of teeth due to caries**
K08.131 Complete loss of teeth due to caries, class I
K08.132 Complete loss of teeth due to caries, class II
K08.133 Complete loss of teeth due to caries, class III
K08.134 Complete loss of teeth due to caries, class IV
K08.139 Complete loss of teeth due to caries, unspecified class

● K08.19 **Complete loss of teeth due to other specified cause**
K08.191 Complete loss of teeth due to other specified cause, class I
K08.192 Complete loss of teeth due to other specified cause, class II
K08.193 Complete loss of teeth due to other specified cause, class III
K08.194 Complete loss of teeth due to other specified cause, class IV
K08.199 Complete loss of teeth due to other specified cause, unspecified class

● K08.2 **Atrophy of edentulous alveolar ridge**
K08.20 **Unspecified atrophy of edentulous alveolar ridge**
Atrophy of the mandible NOS
Atrophy of the maxilla NOS
K08.21 **Minimal atrophy of the mandible**
Minimal atrophy of the edentulous mandible
K08.22 **Moderate atrophy of the mandible**
Moderate atrophy of the edentulous mandible
K08.23 **Severe atrophy of the mandible**
Severe atrophy of the edentulous mandible
K08.24 **Minimal atrophy of maxilla**
Minimal atrophy of the edentulous maxilla
K08.25 **Moderate atrophy of the maxilla**
Moderate atrophy of the edentulous maxilla
K08.26 **Severe atrophy of the maxilla**
Severe atrophy of the edentulous maxilla

K08.3 **Retained dental root**
● K08.4 **Partial loss of teeth**
Acquired loss of teeth, partial
Excludes1 complete loss of teeth (K08.1-)
congenital absence of teeth (K00.0)
Excludes2 exfoliation of teeth due to systemic causes (K08.0)

● K08.40 **Partial loss of teeth, unspecified cause**
K08.401 Partial loss of teeth, unspecified cause, class I
K08.402 Partial loss of teeth, unspecified cause, class II
K08.403 Partial loss of teeth, unspecified cause, class III
K08.404 Partial loss of teeth, unspecified cause, class IV
K08.409 Partial loss of teeth, unspecified cause, unspecified class
Tooth extraction status NOS

● K08.41 **Partial loss of teeth due to trauma**
K08.411 Partial loss of teeth due to trauma, class I
K08.412 Partial loss of teeth due to trauma, class II
K08.413 Partial loss of teeth due to trauma, class III
K08.414 Partial loss of teeth due to trauma, class IV
K08.419 Partial loss of teeth due to trauma, unspecified class

● K08.42 **Partial loss of teeth due to periodontal diseases**
K08.421 Partial loss of teeth due to periodontal diseases, class I
K08.422 Partial loss of teeth due to periodontal diseases, class II
K08.423 Partial loss of teeth due to periodontal diseases, class III
K08.424 Partial loss of teeth due to periodontal diseases, class IV
K08.429 Partial loss of teeth due to periodontal diseases, unspecified class

▶ New   ⇒ Revised   ~~deleted~~ Deleted   Excludes 1   Excludes 2   Includes   Use additional   Code first   Code also   Key words
OGCR Official Guidelines   ● Unacceptable Principal Diagnosis   X Assign placeholder X   ● Use Additional Character(s)   ▶ Manifestation Code   **Coding Clinic**

● **K08.43**   Partial loss of teeth due to caries

    K08.431   Partial loss of teeth due to caries, class I

    K08.432   Partial loss of teeth due to caries, class II

    K08.433   Partial loss of teeth due to caries, class III

    K08.434   Partial loss of teeth due to caries, class IV

    K08.439   Partial loss of teeth due to caries, unspecified class

● **K08.49**   Partial loss of teeth due to other specified cause

    K08.491   Partial loss of teeth due to other specified cause, class I

    K08.492   Partial loss of teeth due to other specified cause, class II

    K08.493   Partial loss of teeth due to other specified cause, class III

    K08.494   Partial loss of teeth due to other specified cause, class IV

    K08.499   Partial loss of teeth due to other specified cause, unspecified class

● **K08.5**   Unsatisfactory restoration of tooth
     Defective bridge, crown, filling
     Defective dental restoration

    Excludes1   dental restoration status (Z98.811)

    Excludes2   endosseous dental implant failure (M27.6-)
                 unsatisfactory endodontic treatment (M27.5-)

    K08.50   Unsatisfactory restoration of tooth, unspecified
          Defective dental restoration NOS

    K08.51   Open restoration margins of tooth
          Dental restoration failure of marginal integrity
          Open margin on tooth restoration
          Poor gingival margin to tooth restoration

    K08.52   Unrepairable overhanging of dental restorative materials
          Overhanging of tooth restoration

●   K08.53   Fractured dental restorative material

      Excludes1   cracked tooth (K03.81)
                 traumatic fracture of tooth (S02.5)

      K08.530   Fractured dental restorative material without loss of material

      K08.531   Fractured dental restorative material with loss of material

      K08.539   Fractured dental restorative material, unspecified

    K08.54   Contour of existing restoration of tooth biologically incompatible with oral health
          Dental restoration failure of periodontal anatomical integrity
          Unacceptable contours of existing restoration of tooth
          Unacceptable morphology of existing restoration of tooth

    K08.55   Allergy to existing dental restorative material

          Use additional code to identify the specific type of allergy

    K08.56   Poor aesthetic of existing restoration of tooth
          Dental restoration aesthetically inadequate or displeasing

    K08.59   Other unsatisfactory restoration of tooth
          Other defective dental restoration

● **K08.8**   Other specified disorders of teeth and supporting structures

    K08.81   Primary occlusal trauma

    K08.82   Secondary occlusal trauma

    K08.89   Other specified disorders of teeth and supporting structures
          Enlargement of alveolar ridge NOS
          Insufficient anatomic crown height
          Insufficient clinical crown length
          Irregular alveolar process
          Toothache NOS

   K08.9   Disorder of teeth and supporting structures, unspecified

● **K09**   Cysts of oral region, not elsewhere classified

    Includes   lesions showing histological features both of aneurysmal cyst and of another fibro-osseous lesion

    Excludes2   cysts of jaw (M27.0-, M27.4-)
                 radicular cyst (K04.8)

   K09.0   Developmental odontogenic cysts
          Dentigerous cyst
          Eruption cyst
          Follicular cyst
          Gingival cyst
          Lateral periodontal cyst
          Primordial cyst

    Excludes2   keratocysts (D16.4, D16.5)
                 odontogenic keratocystic tumors (D16.4, D16.5)

   K09.1   Developmental (nonodontogenic) cysts of oral region
          Cyst (of) incisive canal
          Cyst (of) palatine of papilla
          Globulomaxillary cyst
          Median palatal cyst
          Nasoalveolar cyst
          Nasolabial cyst
          Nasopalatine duct cyst

   K09.8   Other cysts of oral region, not elsewhere classified
          Dermoid cyst
          Epidermoid cyst
          Lymphoepithelial cyst
          Epstein's pearl

   K09.9   Cyst of oral region, unspecified

★ **(See Plate 28 of the Anatomy Illustrations.)**

● **K11**   Diseases of salivary glands
      Use additional code to identify:
         alcohol abuse and dependence (F10.-)
         exposure to environmental tobacco smoke (Z77.22)
         exposure to tobacco smoke in the perinatal period (P96.81)
         history of tobacco dependence (Z87.891)
         occupational exposure to environmental tobacco smoke (Z57.31)
         tobacco dependence (F17.-)
         tobacco use (Z72.0)

   K11.0   Atrophy of salivary gland

   K11.1   Hypertrophy of salivary gland

Item 11–4 Atrophy is wasting away of a tissue or organ, whereas **hypertrophy** is overdevelopment or enlargement of a tissue or organ. **Sialoadenitis** is salivary gland inflammation. **Parotitis** is the inflammation of the parotid gland. In the epidemic form, parotitis is also known as mumps. **Sialolithiasis** is the formation of calculus within a salivary gland. **Mucocele** is a polyp composed of mucus.

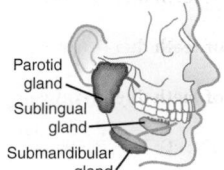

Figure 11-3   Major salivary glands.

Parotid gland
Sublingual gland
Submandibular gland

N   Newborn Age: 0   P   Pediatric Age: 0–17   M   Maternity DX: 9–64   A   Adult Age: 15–124   ♀   Females Only   ♂   Males Only

🅒 Complication\Comorbidity   🅜 Major C\C   Ⓔⓧ CC/MCC Exclusions   🅗 Hospital-Acquired Condition   🅗ⓒⓒ Hierarchical Condition Category   963

CHAPTER 11 (K00-K95)

● **K11.2 Sialoadenitis**
Parotitis
> **Excludes1** epidemic parotitis (B26.-)
> mumps (B26.-)
> uveoparotid fever [Heerfordt] (D86.89)

K11.20 Sialoadenitis, unspecified
K11.21 Acute sialoadenitis
> **Excludes1** acute recurrent sialoadenitis (K11.22)

K11.22 Acute recurrent sialoadenitis
K11.23 Chronic sialoadenitis
K11.3 Abscess of salivary gland 🔗
(Ex:) See PDX Collection 762

K11.4 Fistula of salivary gland 🔗
> **Excludes1** congenital fistula of salivary gland (Q38.4)
(Ex:) See PDX Collection 762

K11.5 Sialolithiasis
Calculus of salivary gland or duct
Stone of salivary gland or duct

K11.6 Mucocele of salivary gland
Mucous extravasation cyst of salivary gland
Mucous retention cyst of salivary gland
Ranula

K11.7 Disturbances of salivary secretion
Hypoptyalism
Ptyalism
Xerostomia
> **Excludes2** dry mouth NOS (R68.2)

K11.8 Other diseases of salivary glands
Benign lymphoepithelial lesion of salivary gland
Mikulicz' disease
Necrotizing sialometaplasia
Sialectasia
Stenosis of salivary duct
Stricture of salivary duct
> ⮕ **Excludes1** Sjögren syndrome (M35.0-)

K11.9 Disease of salivary gland, unspecified
Sialoadenopathy NOS

● **K12 Stomatitis and related lesions**
Use additional code to identify:
alcohol abuse and dependence (F10.-)
exposure to environmental tobacco smoke (Z77.22)
exposure to tobacco smoke in the perinatal period (P96.81)
history of tobacco dependence (Z87.891)
occupational exposure to environmental tobacco smoke (Z57.31)
tobacco dependence (F17.-)
tobacco use (Z72.0)
> **Excludes1** cancrum oris (A69.0)
> cheilitis (K13.0)
> gangrenous stomatitis (A69.0)
> herpesviral [herpes simplex] gingivostomatitis (B00.2)
> noma (A69.0)

K12.0 Recurrent oral aphthae
Aphthous stomatitis (major) (minor)
Bednar's aphthae
Periadenitis mucosa necrotica recurrens
Recurrent aphthous ulcer
Stomatitis herpetiformis

K12.1 Other forms of stomatitis
Stomatitis NOS
Denture stomatitis
Ulcerative stomatitis
Vesicular stomatitis
> **Excludes1** acute necrotizing ulcerative stomatitis (A69.1)
> Vincent's stomatitis (A69.1)

K12.2 Cellulitis and abscess of mouth 🔗
Cellulitis of mouth (floor)
Submandibular abscess
> **Excludes2** abscess of salivary gland (K11.3)
> abscess of tongue (K14.0)
> periapical abscess (K04.6-K04.7)
> periodontal abscess (K05.21)
> peritonsillar abscess (J36)
(Ex:) See PDX Collection 763

● **K12.3 Oral mucositis (ulcerative)**
Mucositis (oral) (oropharyneal)
> **Excludes2** gastrointestinal mucositis (ulcerative) (K92.81)
> mucositis (ulcerative) of vagina and vulva (N76.81)
> nasal mucositis (ulcerative) (J34.81)

K12.30 Oral mucositis (ulcerative), unspecified
K12.31 Oral mucositis (ulcerative) due to antineoplastic therapy
Use additional code for adverse effect, if applicable, to identify antineoplastic and immunosuppressive drugs (T45.1X5)
Use additional code for other antineoplastic therapy, such as:
radiological procedure and radiotherapy (Y84.2)

K12.32 Oral mucositis (ulcerative) due to other drugs
Use additional code for adverse effect, if applicable, to identify drug (T36-T50 with fifth or sixth character 5)

K12.33 Oral mucositis (ulcerative) due to radiation
Use additional external cause code (W88-W90, X39.0-) to identify cause

K12.39 Other oral mucositis (ulcerative)
Viral oral mucositis (ulcerative)

● **K13 Other diseases of lip and oral mucosa**
> **Includes** epithelial disturbances of tongue
Use additional code to identify:
alcohol abuse and dependence (F10.-)
exposure to environmental tobacco smoke (Z77.22)
exposure to tobacco smoke in the perinatal period (P96.81)
history of tobacco dependence (Z87.891)
occupational exposure to environmental tobacco smoke (Z57.31)
tobacco dependence (F17.-)
tobacco use (Z72.0)
> **Excludes2** certain disorders of gingiva and edentulous alveolar ridge (K05-K06)
> cysts of oral region (K09.-)
> diseases of tongue (K14.-)
> stomatitis and related lesions (K12.-)

K13.0 Diseases of lips
Abscess of lips   Exfoliative cheilitis
Angular cheilitis   Fistula of lips
Cellulitis of lips   Glandular cheilitis
Cheilitis NOS   Hypertrophy of lips
Cheilodynia   Perlèche NEC
Cheilosis
> **Excludes1** ariboflavinosis (E53.0)
> cheilitis due to radiation-related disorders (L55-L59)
> congenital fistula of lips (Q38.0)
> congenital hypertrophy of lips (Q18.6)
> Perlèche due to candidiasis (B37.83)
> Perlèche due to riboflavin deficiency (E53.0)

K13.1 Cheek and lip biting

Item 11-5 Stomatitis is the inflammation of the oral mucosa. **Mucositis** is the inflammation of the mucous membranes lining the digestive tract from the mouth to the anus. It is a common side effect of chemotherapy and of radiotherapy that involves any part of the digestive tract.

▶ New   ⮕ Revised   deleted Deleted   Excludes 1   Excludes 2   Includes   Use additional   Code first   Code also   Key words
OGCR Official Guidelines   ● Unacceptable Principal Diagnosis   X Assign placeholder X   ● Use Additional Character(s)   ▶ Manifestation Code   Coding Clinic

CHAPTER 11 (K00-K95)

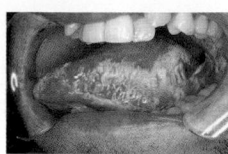

Figure 11-4 Oral leukoplakia and associated. (From Swartz MH: Textbook of Physical Diagnosis: History and Examination, Philadelphia, PA, Saunders/Elsevier, 2010)

● K13.2 **Leukoplakia and other disturbances of oral epithelium, including tongue**

> **Excludes1**   carcinoma in situ of oral epithelium (D00.0-)
> hairy leukoplakia (K13.3)

K13.21 **Leukoplakia of oral mucosa, including tongue**
Considered precancerous and evidenced by thickened white patches of epithelium on mucous membranes
Leukokeratosis of oral mucosa
Leukoplakia of gingiva, lips, tongue

> **Excludes1**   hairy leukoplakia (K13.3)
> leukokeratosis nicotina palati (K13.24)

K13.22 **Minimal keratinized residual ridge mucosa**
Minimal keratinization of alveolar ridge mucosa

K13.23 **Excessive keratinized residual ridge mucosa**
Excessive keratinization of alveolar ridge mucosa

K13.24 **Leukokeratosis nicotina palati**
Smoker's palate

K13.29 **Other disturbances of oral epithelium, including tongue**
Erythroplakia of mouth or tongue
Focal epithelial hyperplasia of mouth or tongue
Leukoedema of mouth or tongue
Other oral epithelium disturbances

K13.3 **Hairy leukoplakia**

K13.4 **Granuloma and granuloma-like lesions of oral mucosa**
Eosinophilic granuloma
Granuloma pyogenicum
Verrucous xanthoma

K13.5 **Oral submucous fibrosis**
Submucous fibrosis of tongue

K13.6 **Irritative hyperplasia of oral mucosa**

> **Excludes2**   irritative hyperplasia of edentulous ridge [denture hyperplasia] (K06.2)

● K13.7 **Other and unspecified lesions of oral mucosa**

K13.70 **Unspecified lesions of oral mucosa**

K13.79 **Other lesions of oral mucosa**
Focal oral mucinosis

★ **(See Plate 26 of the Anatomy Illustrations.)**

● K14 **Diseases of tongue**
Use additional code to identify:
alcohol abuse and dependence (F10.-)
exposure to environmental tobacco smoke (Z77.22)
history of tobacco dependence (Z87.891)
occupational exposure to environmental tobacco smoke (Z57.31)
tobacco dependence (F17.-)
tobacco use (Z72.0)

> **Excludes2**   erythroplakia (K13.29)
> focal epithelial hyperplasia (K13.29)
> leukedema of tongue (K13.29)
> leukoplakia of tongue (K13.21)
> hairy leukoplakia (K13.3)
> macroglossia (congenital) (Q38.2)
> submucous fibrosis of tongue (K13.5)

K14.0 **Glossitis**
Abscess of tongue
Ulceration (traumatic) of tongue

> **Excludes1**   atrophic glossitis (K14.4)

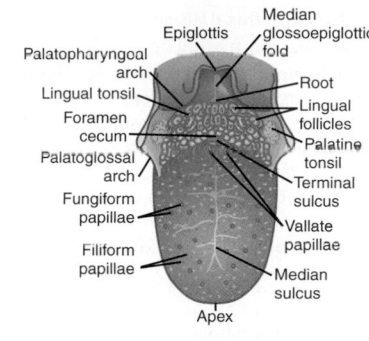

Figure 11-5   Structure of the tongue.

K14.1 **Geographic tongue**
Benign migratory glossitis
Glossitis areata exfoliativa

K14.2 **Median rhomboid glossitis**

K14.3 **Hypertrophy of tongue papillae**
Black hairy tongue
Coated tongue
Hypertrophy of foliate papillae
Lingua villosa nigra

K14.4 **Atrophy of tongue papillae**
Atrophic glossitis

K14.5 **Plicated tongue**
Fissured tongue   Scrotal tongue
Furrowed tongue

> **Excludes1**   fissured tongue, congenital (Q38.3)

K14.6 **Glossodynia**
Glossopyrosis   Painful tongue

K14.8 **Other diseases of tongue**
Atrophy of tongue   Glossocele
Crenated tongue   Glossoptosis
Enlargement of tongue   Hypertrophy of tongue

K14.9 **Disease of tongue, unspecified**
Glossopathy NOS

DISEASES OF ESOPHAGUS, STOMACH AND DUODENUM (K20-K31)

> **Excludes2**   hiatus hernia (K44.-)

● K20 **Esophagitis**
Use additional code to identify:
alcohol abuse and dependence (F10.-)

> **Excludes1**   erosion of esophagus (K22.1-)
> esophagitis with gastro-esophageal reflux disease (K21.0-)
> reflux esophagitis (K21.0-)
> ulcerative esophagitis (K22.1-)

> **Excludes2**   eosinophilic gastritis or gastroenteritis (K52.81)

K20.0 **Eosinophilic esophagitis**

● K20.8 **Other esophagitis**

K20.80 **Other esophagitis without bleeding**
Abscess of esophagus
Other esophagitis NOS

K20.81 **Other esophagitis with bleeding** 🔗
(Ex:) See PDX Collection 4079

● K20.9 **Esophagitis, unspecified**

K20.90 **Esophagitis, unspecified without bleeding**
Esophagitis NOS

K20.91 **Esophagitis, unspecified with bleeding** 🔗
(Ex:) See PDX Collection 4079

N Newborn Age: 0   **P** Pediatric Age: 0–17   **M** Maternity DX: 9–64   **A** Adult Age: 15–124   ♀ Females Only   ♂ Males Only

🔗 Complication\Comorbidity   🔗 Major C\C   (Ex:) CC/MCC Exclusions   🔗 Hospital-Acquired Condition   🔗 Hierarchical Condition Category

965

CHAPTER 11 (K00-K95)

● **K21**   Gastro-esophageal reflux disease

     Excludes1   newborn esophageal reflux (P78.83)

    ● **K21.0**   Gastro-esophageal reflux disease with esophagitis

       K21.00   Gastro-esophageal reflux disease with esophagitis, without bleeding
          Reflux esophagitis

       K21.01   Gastro-esophageal reflux disease with esophagitis, with bleeding
          Ex: See PDX Collection 4079

     K21.9   Gastro-esophageal reflux disease without esophagitis
        Esophageal reflux NOS
        Coding Clinic: 2016, Q1, P18

● **K22**   Other diseases of esophagus

     Excludes2   esophageal varices (I85.-)

     K22.0   **Achalasia of cardia**
        Achalasia NOS
        Cardiospasm

       Excludes1   congenital cardiospasm (Q39.5)

    ● **K22.1**   **Ulcer of esophagus**
        Barrett's ulcer
        Erosion of esophagus
        Fungal ulcer of esophagus
        Peptic ulcer of esophagus
        Ulcer of esophagus due to ingestion of chemicals
        Ulcer of esophagus due to ingestion of drugs and medicaments
        Ulcerative esophagitis

        Code first poisoning due to drug or toxin, if applicable (T36-T65 with fifth or sixth character 1-4 or 6)

        Use additional code for adverse effect, if applicable, to identify drug (T36-T50 with fifth or sixth character 5)

       Excludes1   Barrett's esophagus (K22.87-)

       K22.10   Ulcer of esophagus without bleeding
          Ulcer of esophagus NOS
          Ex: See PDX Collection 764

       K22.11   Ulcer of esophagus with bleeding

         Excludes2   bleeding esophageal varices (I85.01, I85.11)
         Ex: See PDX Collection 765

     K22.2   **Esophageal obstruction**
        Compression of esophagus
        Constriction of esophagus
        Stenosis of esophagus
        Stricture of esophagus

       Excludes1   congenital stenosis or stricture of esophagus (Q39.3)

     K22.3   **Perforation of esophagus**
        Rupture of esophagus

       Excludes1   traumatic perforation of (thoracic) esophagus (S27.8-)
         Ex: See PDX Collection 766

     K22.4   **Dyskinesia of esophagus**
        Difficulty in moving
        Corkscrew esophagus
        Diffuse esophageal spasm
        Spasm of esophagus

       Excludes1   cardiospasm (K22.0)

     K22.5   **Diverticulum of esophagus, acquired**
        Esophageal pouch, acquired

       Excludes1   diverticulum of esophagus (congenital) (Q39.6)

     K22.6   **Gastro-esophageal laceration-hemorrhage syndrome**
        Mallory-Weiss syndrome
        Ex: See PDX Collection 767

Item 11-6   **Esophageal reflux** is the return flow of the contents of the stomach to the esophagus and is referred to as GERD and/or "heartburn." **Gastroesophageal reflux** is the return flow of the contents of the stomach and duodenum to the esophagus. **Esophageal leukoplakia** are white areas on the mucous membrane of the esophagus for which no specific cause can be identified.

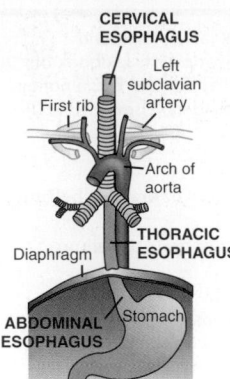

Figure 11-6   The esophagus is the muscular tube that connects the pharynx and the stomach. The 10-inch (25 cm) long esophagus is divided into three parts: **cervical, thoracic,** and **abdominal.**

Item 11-7   **Achalasia** is a condition in which the smooth muscle fibers of the esophagus do not relax. Most frequently, this condition occurs at the esophagogastric sphincter. **Cardiospasm,** also known as **megaesophagus,** is achalasia of the thoracic esophagus.

    ● **K22.7**   **Barrett's esophagus**
        Barrett's disease
        Barrett's syndrome

       Excludes1   Barrett's ulcer (K22.1)
          malignant neoplasm of esophagus (C15.-)

       K22.70   Barrett's esophagus without dysplasia
          Barrett's esophagus NOS

    ● **K22.71**   Barrett's esophagus with dysplasia

         K22.710   Barrett's esophagus with low grade dysplasia

         K22.711   Barrett's esophagus with high grade dysplasia

         K22.719   Barrett's esophagus with dysplasia, unspecified

    ● **K22.8**   **Other specified diseases of esophagus**
        ~~Hemorrhage of esophagus NOS~~

      ▶ **K22.81**   Esophageal polyp

       ▶ **Excludes1**   benign neoplasm of esophagus (D13.0)

      ▶ **K22.82**   Esophagogastric junction polyp

       ▶ **Excludes1**   benign neoplasm of stomach (D13.1)

      ▶ **K22.89**   Other specified disease of esophagus
        ▶ Hemorrhage of esophagus NOS

       Excludes2   esophageal varices (I85.-)
          Paterson-Kelly syndrome (D50.1)
       Coding Clinic: 2020, Q1, P16

     K22.9   **Disease of esophagus, unspecified**

 ▶ **K23**   *Disorders of esophagus in diseases classified elsewhere*
        Code first underlying disease, such as:
        congenital syphilis (A50.5)

       Excludes1   late syphilis (A52.79)
          megaesophagus due to Chagas' disease (B57.31)
          tuberculosis (A18.83)

● **K25**   **Gastric ulcer**

     Includes   erosion (acute) of stomach
          pylorus ulcer (peptic)
          stomach ulcer (peptic)

     Use additional code to identify:
     alcohol abuse and dependence (F10.-)

     Excludes1   acute gastritis (K29.0-)
        peptic ulcer NOS (K27.-)
       Ex: For category K25 CC codes: See PDX Collection 765

     K25.0   **Acute gastric ulcer with hemorrhage**

     K25.1   **Acute gastric ulcer with perforation**

     K25.2   **Acute gastric ulcer with both hemorrhage and perforation**

     K25.3   **Acute gastric ulcer without hemorrhage or perforation**

     K25.4   **Chronic or unspecified gastric ulcer with hemorrhage**
        Coding Clinic: 2017, Q3, P27

▶ New   ⟹ Revised   ~~deleted~~ Deleted   Excludes 1   Excludes 2   Includes   Use additional   Code first   Code also   Key words

OGCR Official Guidelines   ● Unacceptable Principal Diagnosis   X Assign placeholder X   ● Use Additional Character(s)   ▶ Manifestation Code   **Coding Clinic**

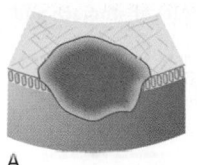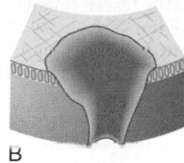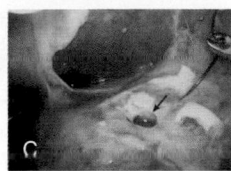

Figure 11-7 A. Ulcer. **B.** Perforated ulcer. **C.** Laparoscopic view of a perforated duodenal ulcer *(arrow)* with fibrinous exudate on the adjacent peritoneum. (**C** from Feldman: Sleisenger & Fordtran's Gastrointestinal and Liver Disease, ed 8, Saunders, An Imprint of Elsevier, 2006)

Item 11–8   Gastric ulcers are lesions of the stomach that result in the death of the tissue and a defect of the surface. **Perforated ulcers** are those in which the lesion penetrates the gastric wall, leaving a hole. **Peptic ulcers** are lesions of the stomach or the duodenum. **Peptic** refers to the gastric juice, pepsin.

K25.5   **Chronic or unspecified gastric ulcer with perforation** 🔹🔹

K25.6   **Chronic or unspecified gastric ulcer with both hemorrhage and perforation** 🔹🔹

K25.7   **Chronic gastric ulcer without hemorrhage or perforation**

K25.9   **Gastric ulcer, unspecified as acute or chronic, without hemorrhage or perforation**
          Coding Clinic: 2021, Q1, P12

● K26   **Duodenal ulcer**
          Includes   erosion (acute) of duodenum
                         duodenum ulcer (peptic)
                         postpyloric ulcer (peptic)
          Use additional code to identify:
             alcohol abuse and dependence (F10.-)
          Excludes1   peptic ulcer NOS (K27.-)
          (Ex) **For category K26 CC codes unless otherwise indicated:** See PDX Collection 768

K26.0   **Acute duodenal ulcer with hemorrhage** 🔹🔹

K26.1   **Acute duodenal ulcer with perforation** 🔹🔹

K26.2   **Acute duodenal ulcer with both hemorrhage and perforation** 🔹🔹

K26.3   **Acute duodenal ulcer without hemorrhage or perforation** 🔹
          (Ex) See PDX Collection 769

K26.4   **Chronic or unspecified duodenal ulcer with hemorrhage** 🔹
          Coding Clinic: 2016, Q1, P14

K26.5   **Chronic or unspecified duodenal ulcer with perforation** 🔹🔹

K26.6   **Chronic or unspecified duodenal ulcer with both hemorrhage and perforation** 🔹🔹

K26.7   **Chronic duodenal ulcer without hemorrhage or perforation**

K26.9   **Duodenal ulcer, unspecified as acute or chronic, without hemorrhage or perforation**

● K27   **Peptic ulcer, site unspecified**
          Includes   gastroduodenal ulcer NOS
                         peptic ulcer NOS
          Use additional code to identify:
             alcohol abuse and dependence (F10.-)
          Excludes1   peptic ulcer of newborn (P78.82)
          (Ex) **For category K27 CC codes:** See PDX Collection 768

K27.0   **Acute peptic ulcer, site unspecified, with hemorrhage** 🔹

K27.1   **Acute peptic ulcer, site unspecified, with perforation** 🔹🔹

K27.2   **Acute peptic ulcer, site unspecified, with both hemorrhage and perforation** 🔹🔹

K27.3   **Acute peptic ulcer, site unspecified, without hemorrhage or perforation** 🔹

K27.4   **Chronic or unspecified peptic ulcer, site unspecified, with hemorrhage** 🔹

K27.5   **Chronic or unspecified peptic ulcer, site unspecified, with perforation** 🔹🔹

K27.6   **Chronic or unspecified peptic ulcer, site unspecified, with both hemorrhage and perforation** 🔹🔹

K27.7   **Chronic peptic ulcer, site unspecified, without hemorrhage or perforation**

K27.9   **Peptic ulcer, site unspecified, unspecified as acute or chronic, without hemorrhage or perforation**

● K28   **Gastrojejunal ulcer**
          Includes   anastomotic ulcer (peptic) or erosion
                         gastrocolic ulcer (peptic) or erosion
                         gastrointestinal ulcer (peptic) or erosion
                         gastrojejunal ulcer (peptic) or erosion
                         jejunal ulcer (peptic) or erosion
                         marginal ulcer (peptic) or erosion
                         stomal ulcer (peptic) or erosion
          Use additional code to identify:
             alcohol abuse and dependence (F10.-)
          Excludes1   primary ulcer of small intestine (K63.3)
          (Ex) **For category K28 CC codes:** See PDX Collection 765

K28.0   **Acute gastrojejunal ulcer with hemorrhage** 🔹

K28.1   **Acute gastrojejunal ulcer with perforation** 🔹🔹

K28.2   **Acute gastrojejunal ulcer with both hemorrhage and perforation** 🔹🔹

K28.3   **Acute gastrojejunal ulcer without hemorrhage or perforation** 🔹

K28.4   **Chronic or unspecified gastrojejunal ulcer with hemorrhage** 🔹

K28.5   **Chronic or unspecified gastrojejunal ulcer with perforation** 🔹🔹

K28.6   **Chronic or unspecified gastrojejunal ulcer with both hemorrhage and perforation** 🔹🔹

K28.7   **Chronic gastrojejunal ulcer without hemorrhage or perforation**

K28.9   **Gastrojejunal ulcer, unspecified as acute or chronic, without hemorrhage or perforation**

● K29   **Gastritis and duodenitis**
          Excludes1   eosinophilic gastritis or gastroenteritis (K52.81)
                         Zollinger-Ellison syndrome (E16.4)
          (Ex) **For category K29 CC codes:** See PDX Collection 770

● K29.0   **Acute gastritis**
          Use additional code to identify:
             alcohol abuse and dependence (F10.-)
          Excludes1   erosion (acute) of stomach (K25.-)

K29.00   **Acute gastritis without bleeding**

K29.01   **Acute gastritis with bleeding** 🔹

● K29.2   **Alcoholic gastritis**
          Use additional code to identify:
             alcohol abuse and dependence (F10.-)

K29.20   **Alcoholic gastritis without bleeding**

K29.21   **Alcoholic gastritis with bleeding** 🔹

● K29.3   **Chronic superficial gastritis**

K29.30   **Chronic superficial gastritis without bleeding**

K29.31   **Chronic superficial gastritis with bleeding** 🔹

● K29.4   **Chronic atrophic gastritis**
          Gastric atrophy

K29.40   **Chronic atrophic gastritis without bleeding**

K29.41   **Chronic atrophic gastritis with bleeding** 🔹

● K29.5   **Unspecified chronic gastritis**
          Chronic antral gastritis
          Chronic fundal gastritis

K29.50   **Unspecified chronic gastritis without bleeding**

K29.51   **Unspecified chronic gastritis with bleeding** 🔹

● K29.6   **Other gastritis**
          Giant hypertrophic gastritis
          Granulomatous gastritis
          Ménétrier's disease

K29.60   **Other gastritis without bleeding**

K29.61   **Other gastritis with bleeding** 🔹

● K29.7   **Gastritis, unspecified**

K29.70   **Gastritis, unspecified, without bleeding**

K29.71   **Gastritis, unspecified, with bleeding** 🔹

N Newborn Age: 0   **P** Pediatric Age: 0–17   **M** Maternity DX: 9–64   **A** Adult Age: 15–124   ♀ Females Only   ♂ Males Only

🔹 Complication\Comorbidity   🔹 Major C\C   (Ex) CC/MCC Exclusions   🔹 Hospital-Acquired Condition   🔹 Hierarchical Condition Category

967

CHAPTER 11 (K00-K95)

Item 11–9 **Gastritis** is a severe inflammation of the stomach. **Atrophic gastritis** is a chronic inflammation of the stomach that results in destruction of the cells of the mucosa of the stomach. Duodenitis is an inflammation of the duodenum, the first section of the small intestine.

- ● **K29.8** **Duodenitis**
  - **K29.80** Duodenitis without bleeding
  - **K29.81** Duodenitis with bleeding
- ● **K29.9** **Gastroduodenitis, unspecified**
  - **K29.90** Gastroduodenitis, unspecified, without bleeding
  - **K29.91** Gastroduodenitis, unspecified, with bleeding

K30 **Functional dyspepsia**
Indigestion
> **Excludes1**   dyspepsia NOS (R10.13)
> heartburn (R12)
> nervous dyspepsia (F45.8)
> neurotic dyspepsia (F45.8)
> psychogenic dyspepsia (F45.8)

- ● **K31** **Other diseases of stomach and duodenum**
  Includes   functional disorders of stomach
  > **Excludes2**   diabetic gastroparesis (E08.43, E09.43, E10.43, E11.43, E13.43)
  > diverticulum of duodenum (K57.00-K57.13)

  - **K31.0** **Acute dilatation of stomach**
    Acute distention of stomach
    (Ex:) See PDX Collection 771
  - **K31.1** **Adult hypertrophic pyloric stenosis**   A
    Pyloric stenosis NOS
    > **Excludes1**   congenital or infantile pyloric stenosis (Q40.0)
    (Ex:) See PDX Collection 772
  - **K31.2** **Hourglass stricture and stenosis of stomach**
    > **Excludes1**   congenital hourglass stomach (Q40.2)
    > hourglass contraction of stomach (K31.89)
  - **K31.3** **Pylorospasm, not elsewhere classified**
    > **Excludes1**   congenital or infantile pylorospasm (Q40.0)
    > neurotic pylorospasm (F45.8)
    > psychogenic pylorospasm (F45.8)
  - **K31.4** **Gastric diverticulum**
    > **Excludes1**   congenital diverticulum of stomach (Q40.2)
  - **K31.5** **Obstruction of duodenum**
    Constriction of duodenum
    Duodenal ileus (chronic)
    Stenosis of duodenum
    Narrowing
    Stricture of duodenum
    Narrowing
    Volvulus of duodenum
    Twisting/knotting
    > **Excludes1**   congenital stenosis of duodenum (Q41.0)
    (Ex:) See PDX Collection 773
  - **K31.6** **Fistula of stomach and duodenum**
    Gastrocolic fistula
    Gastrojejunocolic fistula
    (Ex:) See PDX Collection 774
  - **K31.7** **Polyp of stomach and duodenum**
    > **Excludes1**   adenomatous polyp of stomach (D13.1)
    Coding Clinic: 2020, Q1, P16
  - ● **K31.8** **Other specified diseases of stomach and duodenum**
    - ● **K31.81** Angiodysplasia of stomach and duodenum
      - **K31.811** Angiodysplasia of stomach and duodenum with bleeding
        (Ex:) See PDX Collection 770
      - **K31.819** Angiodysplasia of stomach and duodenum without bleeding
        Angiodysplasia of stomach and duodenum NOS

Item 11–10 **Achlorhydria,** also known as gastric anacidity, is the absence of gastric acid.

- **K31.82** Dieulafoy lesion (hemorrhagic) of stomach and duodenum
  > **Excludes2**   Dieulafoy lesion of intestine (K63.81)
  (Ex:) See PDX Collection 775
- **K31.83** Achlorhydria
- **K31.84** Gastroparesis
  Gastroparalysis
  Code first underlying disease, if known, such as:
  anorexia nervosa (F50.0-)
  diabetes mellitus (E08.43, E09.43, E10.43, E11.43, E13.43)
  scleroderma (M34.-)
- **K31.89** Other diseases of stomach and duodenum
  Coding Clinic: 2020, Q1, P16; 2017, Q1, P28
- **K31.9** **Disease of stomach and duodenum, unspecified**
- ▶● **K31.A** **Gastric intestinal metaplasia**
  - ▶ **K31.A0** Gastric intestinal metaplasia, unspecified
    ▶ Gastric intestinal metaplasia indefinite for dysplasia
    ▶ Gastric intestinal metaplasia NOS
  - ▶● **K31.A1** Gastric intestinal metaplasia without dysplasia
    - ▶ **K31.A11** Gastric intestinal metaplasia without dysplasia, involving the antrum
    - ▶ **K31.A12** Gastric intestinal metaplasia without dysplasia, involving the body(corpus)
    - ▶ **K31.A13** Gastric intestinal metaplasia without dysplasia, involving the fundus involving the cardia
    - ▶ **K31.A14** Gastric intestinal metaplasia without dysplasia, involving the cardia
    - ▶ **K31.A15** Gastric intestinal metaplasia without dysplasia, involving multiple sites
    - ▶ **K31.A19** Gastric intestinal metaplasia without dysplasia, unspecified site
  - ▶● **K31.A2** Gastric intestinal metaplasia with dysplasia
    - ▶ **K31.A21** Gastric intestinal metaplasia with low grade dysplasia
    - ▶ **K31.A22** Gastric intestinal metaplasia with high grade dysplasia
    - ▶ **K31.A29** Gastric intestinal metaplasia with dysplasia, unspecified

DISEASES OF APPENDIX (K35-K38)

- ● **K35** **Acute appendicitis**
  (Ex:) **For category K35 CC codes: See PDX Collection 776**
  - ● **K35.2** **Acute appendicitis with generalized peritonitis**
    Appendicitis (acute) with generalized (diffuse) peritonitis following rupture or perforation of appendix
    - **K35.20** Acute appendicitis with generalized peritonitis, without abscess (Acute) appendicitis with generalized peritonitis NOS
      Coding Clinic: 2018, Q4, P18
    - **K35.21** Acute appendicitis with generalized peritonitis, with abscess
  - ● **K35.3** **Acute appendicitis with localized peritonitis**
    - **K35.30** Acute appendicitis with localized peritonitis, without perforation or gangrene
      Acute appendicitis with localized peritonitis NOS
    - **K35.31** Acute appendicitis with localized peritonitis and gangrene, without perforation
    - **K35.32** Acute appendicitis with perforation and localized peritonitis, without abscess
      (Acute) appendicitis with perforation NOS
      Perforated appendix NOS
      Ruptured appendix (with localized peritonitis) NOS
      Coding Clinic: 2020, Q1, P16; 2018, Q4, P18
    - **K35.33** Acute appendicitis with perforation and localized peritonitis, with abscess
      (Acute) appendicitis with (peritoneal) abscess NOS
      Ruptured appendix with localized peritonitis and abscess
- ● **K35.8** **Other and unspecified acute appendicitis**

▶ New   ⟶ Revised   ~~deleted~~ Deleted   Excludes 1   Excludes 2   Includes   Use additional   Code first   Code also   Key words
OGCR Official Guidelines   ● Unacceptable Principal Diagnosis   X Assign placeholder X   ● Use Additional Character(s)   ▶ Manifestation Code   **Coding Clinic**

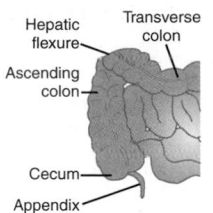

Figure 11-8 Acute appendicitis is the inflammation of the appendix, usually associated with obstruction. Most often this is a disease of adolescents and young adults.

Hepatic flexure
Transverse colon
Ascending colon
Cecum
Appendix

     K35.80   **Unspecified acute appendicitis** 🔹
           Acute appendicitis NOS
           Acute appendicitis without (localized)
             (generalized) peritonitis

 ⬤ **K35.89**   **Other acute appendicitis**
        K35.890   **Other acute appendicitis without**
                 perforation or gangrene 🔹
        K35.891   **Other acute appendicitis without**
                 perforation, with gangrene 🔹
                 (Acute) appendicitis with gangrene
                   NOS

K36   **Other appendicitis**
     Chronic appendicitis
     Recurrent appendicitis

K37   **Unspecified appendicitis**
     ⮕ **Excludes1**   unspecified appendicitis with peritonitis
                        (K35.2-, K35.3)

⬤ **K38**   **Other diseases of appendix**
     K38.0   **Hyperplasia of appendix**
     K38.1   **Appendicular concretions**
           Fecalith of appendix
           Stercolith of appendix
     K38.2   **Diverticulum of appendix**
     K38.3   **Fistula of appendix**
     K38.8   **Other specified diseases of appendix**
           Intussusception of appendix
     K38.9   **Disease of appendix, unspecified**

HERNIA (K40-K46)

     Note: Hernia with both gangrene and obstruction is classified
        to hernia with gangrene.
     Includes   acquired hernia
                    congenital [except diaphragmatic or hiatus] hernia
                    recurrent hernia

⬤ **K40**   **Inguinal hernia**
     Includes   bubonocele
                    direct inguinal hernia
                    double inguinal hernia
                    indirect inguinal hernia
                    inguinal hernia NOS
                    oblique inguinal hernia
                    scrotal hernia
     Ⓔⓧ **For category K40 CC codes:** See PDX Collection 777

 ⬤ **K40.0**   **Bilateral inguinal hernia, with obstruction, without**
          gangrene
          Inguinal hernia (bilateral) causing obstruction without
             gangrene
          Incarcerated inguinal hernia (bilateral) without gangrene
          Irreducible inguinal hernia (bilateral) without gangrene
          Strangulated inguinal hernia (bilateral) without
            gangrene
        K40.00   **Bilateral inguinal hernia, with obstruction,**
                 without gangrene, not specified as recurrent 🔹
                 Bilateral inguinal hernia, with obstruction,
                   without gangrene NOS
        K40.01   **Bilateral inguinal hernia, with obstruction,**
                 without gangrene, recurrent 🔹

 ⬤ **K40.1**   **Bilateral inguinal hernia, with gangrene**
        K40.10   **Bilateral inguinal hernia, with gangrene, not**
                 specified as recurrent 🔹
                 Bilateral inguinal hernia, with gangrene NOS
        K40.11   **Bilateral inguinal hernia, with gangrene,**
                 recurrent 🔹

Item 11-11   **Hernias** of the groin are the most common type, accounting for 80 percent of all hernias. There are two major types of inguinal hernias: indirect (oblique) affecting men only and direct. **Indirect inguinal hernias** result when the intestines emerge through the abdominal wall in an indirect fashion through the inguinal canal. **Direct inguinal hernias** penetrate through the abdominal wall in a direct fashion. **Femoral hernias** occur at the femoral ring where the femoral vessels enter the thigh and is most common in women. An abdominal wall hernia is also called a ventral or epigastric hernia and occurs in both sexes. Classification is based on location of the hernia and whether there is obstruction or gangrene.

     Ventral, epigastric, or incisional hernia occurs on the abdominal surface caused by musculature weakness or a tear at a previous surgical site and is evidenced by a bulge that changes in size, becoming larger with exertion. An **incarcerated** hernia is one in which the intestines become trapped in the hernia. A **strangulated** hernia is one in which the blood supply to the intestines is lost. **Hiatal hernia** occurs when a loop of the stomach protrudes upward through the small opening in the diaphragm through which the esophagus passes, leaving the abdominal cavity and entering the chest. It occurs in both sexes.

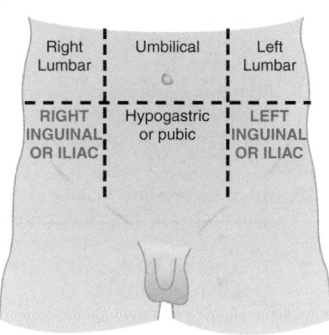

Right Lumbar   Umbilical   Left Lumbar

RIGHT INGUINAL OR ILIAC   Hypogastric or pubic   LEFT INGUINAL OR ILIAC

Figure 11-9 Inguinal hernias are those that are located in the inguinal or iliac areas of the abdomen.

 ⬤ **K40.2**   **Bilateral inguinal hernia, without obstruction or gangrene**
        K40.20   **Bilateral inguinal hernia, without obstruction**
                 or gangrene, not specified as recurrent
                 Bilateral inguinal hernia NOS
        K40.21   **Bilateral inguinal hernia, without obstruction**
                 or gangrene, recurrent

 ⬤ **K40.3**   **Unilateral inguinal hernia, with obstruction, without gangrene**
          Inguinal hernia (unilateral) causing obstruction without
            gangrene
          Incarcerated inguinal hernia (unilateral) without
            gangrene
          Irreducible inguinal hernia (unilateral) without gangrene
          Strangulated inguinal hernia (unilateral) without
            gangrene
        K40.30   **Unilateral inguinal hernia, with obstruction,**
                 without gangrene, not specified as recurrent 🔹
                 Inguinal hernia, with obstruction NOS
                 Unilateral inguinal hernia, with obstruction,
                 without gangrene NOS
        K40.31   **Unilateral inguinal hernia, with obstruction,**
                 without gangrene, recurrent 🔹

 ⬤ **K40.4**   **Unilateral inguinal hernia, with gangrene**
        K40.40   **Unilateral inguinal hernia, with gangrene, not**
                 specified as recurrent 🔹
                 Inguinal hernia with gangrene NOS
                 Unilateral inguinal hernia with gangrene NOS
        K40.41   **Unilateral inguinal hernia, with gangrene,**
                 recurrent 🔹

 ⬤ **K40.9**   **Unilateral inguinal hernia, without obstruction or gangrene**
        K40.90   **Unilateral inguinal hernia, without obstruction**
                 or gangrene, not specified as recurrent
                 Inguinal hernia NOS
                 Unilateral inguinal hernia NOS
        K40.91   **Unilateral inguinal hernia, without obstruction**
                 or gangrene, recurrent

N Newborn Age: 0   **P** Pediatric Age: 0–17   **M** Maternity DX: 9–64   **A** Adult Age: 15–124   ♀ Females Only   ♂ Males Only

🔹 Complication\Comorbidity   🔸 Major C\C   Ⓔⓧ CC/MCC Exclusions   🔹 Hospital-Acquired Condition   🔹 Hierarchical Condition Category   **969**

CHAPTER 11 (K00-K95)

● **K41**   Femoral hernia

   ● **K41.0**   **Bilateral femoral hernia, with obstruction, without gangrene**

     Femoral hernia (bilateral) causing obstruction, without gangrene

     Incarcerated femoral hernia (bilateral), without gangrene

     Irreducible femoral hernia (bilateral), without gangrene

     Strangulated femoral hernia (bilateral), without gangrene

     (Ex:) **For category K41.0 CC codes:** See PDX Collection 778

     K41.00   Bilateral femoral hernia, with obstruction, without gangrene, not specified as recurrent
        Bilateral femoral hernia, with obstruction, without gangrene NOS

     K41.01   Bilateral femoral hernia, with obstruction, without gangrene, recurrent

   ● **K41.1**   **Bilateral femoral hernia, with gangrene**

     (Ex:) **For category K41.1 CC codes:** See PDX Collection 779

     K41.10   Bilateral femoral hernia, with gangrene, not specified as recurrent
        Bilateral femoral hernia, with gangrene NOS

     K41.11   Bilateral femoral hernia, with gangrene, recurrent

   ● **K41.2**   **Bilateral femoral hernia, without obstruction or gangrene**

     K41.20   Bilateral femoral hernia, without obstruction or gangrene, not specified as recurrent
        Bilateral femoral hernia NOS

     K41.21   Bilateral femoral hernia, without obstruction or gangrene, recurrent

   ● **K41.3**   **Unilateral femoral hernia, with obstruction, without gangrene**

     Femoral hernia (unilateral) causing obstruction, without gangrene

     Incarcerated femoral hernia (unilateral), without gangrene

     Irreducible femoral hernia (unilateral), without gangrene

     Strangulated femoral hernia (unilateral), without gangrene

     (Ex:) **For category K41.3 CC codes:** See PDX Collection 778

     K41.30   Unilateral femoral hernia, with obstruction, without gangrene, not specified as recurrent
        Femoral hernia, with obstruction NOS
        Unilateral femoral hernia, with obstruction NOS

     K41.31   Unilateral femoral hernia, with obstruction, without gangrene, recurrent

   ● **K41.4**   **Unilateral femoral hernia, with gangrene**

     (Ex:) **For category K41.4 CC codes:** See PDX Collection 779

     K41.40   Unilateral femoral hernia, with gangrene, not specified as recurrent
        Femoral hernia, with gangrene NOS
        Unilateral femoral hernia, with gangrene NOS

     K41.41   Unilateral femoral hernia, with gangrene, recurrent

   ● **K41.9**   **Unilateral femoral hernia, without obstruction or gangrene**

     K41.90   Unilateral femoral hernia, without obstruction or gangrene, not specified as recurrent
        Femoral hernia NOS
        Unilateral femoral hernia NOS

     K41.91   Unilateral femoral hernia, without obstruction or gangrene, recurrent

● **K42**   Umbilical hernia

   Includes   paraumbilical hernia

   Excludes1   omphalocele (Q79.2)

   K42.0   Umbilical hernia with obstruction, without gangrene

     Umbilical hernia causing obstruction, without gangrene

     Incarcerated umbilical hernia, without gangrene

     Irreducible umbilical hernia, without gangrene

     Strangulated umbilical hernia, without gangrene

     (Ex:) See PDX Collection 780

   K42.1   Umbilical hernia with gangrene

     Gangrenous umbilical hernia

     (Ex:) See PDX Collection 781

   K42.9   Umbilical hernia without obstruction or gangrene

     Umbilical hernia NOS

● **K43**   Ventral hernia

   K43.0   Incisional hernia with obstruction, without gangrene

     Incisional hernia causing obstruction, without gangrene

     Incarcerated incisional hernia, without gangrene

     Irreducible incisional hernia, without gangrene

     Strangulated incisional hernia, without gangrene

     (Ex:) See PDX Collection 780

   K43.1   Incisional hernia with gangrene

     Gangrenous incisional hernia

     (Ex:) See PDX Collection 781

   K43.2   Incisional hernia without obstruction or gangrene

     Incisional hernia NOS

   K43.3   Parastomal hernia with obstruction, without gangrene

     Incarcerated parastomal hernia, without gangrene

     Irreducible parastomal hernia, without gangrene

     Parastomal hernia causing obstruction, without gangrene

     Strangulated parastomal hernia, without gangrene

     (Ex:) See PDX Collection 780

   K43.4   Parastomal hernia with gangrene

     Gangrenous parastomal hernia

     (Ex:) See PDX Collection 781

   K43.5   Parastomal hernia without obstruction or gangrene

     Parastomal hernia NOS

   K43.6   Other and unspecified ventral hernia with obstruction, without gangrene

     Epigastric hernia causing obstruction, without gangrene

     Hypogastric hernia causing obstruction, without gangrene

     Incarcerated epigastric hernia without gangrene

     Incarcerated hypogastric hernia without gangrene

     Incarcerated midline hernia without gangrene

     Incarcerated spigelian hernia without gangrene

     Incarcerated subxiphoid hernia without gangrene

     Irreducible epigastric hernia without gangrene

     Irreducible hypogastric hernia without gangrene

     Irreducible midline hernia without gangrene

     Irreducible spigelian hernia without gangrene

     Irreducible subxiphoid hernia without gangrene

     Midline hernia causing obstruction, without gangrene

     Spigelian hernia causing obstruction, without gangrene

     Strangulated epigastric hernia without gangrene

     Strangulated hypogastric hernia without gangrene

     Strangulated midline hernia without gangrene

     Strangulated spigelian hernia without gangrene

     Strangulated subxiphoid hernia without gangrene

     Subxiphoid hernia causing obstruction, without gangrene

     (Ex:) See PDX Collection 780

   K43.7   Other and unspecified ventral hernia with gangrene

     Any condition listed under K43.6 specified as gangrenous

     (Ex:) See PDX Collection 781

   K43.9   Ventral hernia without obstruction or gangrene

     Epigastric hernia

     Ventral hernia NOS

▶ New   ⇒ Revised   ~~deleted~~ Deleted   Excludes 1   Excludes 2   Includes   Use additional   Code first   Code also   Key words

OGCR Official Guidelines   ● Unacceptable Principal Diagnosis   X Assign placeholder X   ● Use Additional Character(s)   ⟩ Manifestation Code   Coding Clinic

● **K44** **Diaphragmatic hernia**
　　Includes　hiatus hernia (esophageal) (sliding)
　　　　　　　　paraesophageal hernia
　　Excludes1　congenital diaphragmatic hernia (Q79.0)
　　　　　　　　congenital hiatus hernia (Q40.1)
　　(Ex) **For category K44 CC codes:** See PDX Collection 782

　　K44.0 **Diaphragmatic hernia with obstruction, without gangrene** 🦠
　　　　　Diaphragmatic hernia causing obstruction
　　　　　Incarcerated diaphragmatic hernia
　　　　　Irreducible diaphragmatic hernia
　　　　　Strangulated diaphragmatic hernia

　　K44.1 **Diaphragmatic hernia with gangrene** 🦠
　　　　　Gangrenous diaphragmatic hernia

　　K44.9 **Diaphragmatic hernia without obstruction or gangrene**
　　　　　Diaphragmatic hernia NOS
　　　　　Coding Clinic: 2017, Q1, P7

● **K45** **Other abdominal hernia**
　　Includes　abdominal hernia, specified site NEC
　　　　　　　　lumbar hernia
　　　　　　　　obturator hernia
　　　　　　　　pudendal hernia
　　　　　　　　retroperitoneal hernia
　　　　　　　　sciatic hernia

　　K45.0 **Other specified abdominal hernia with obstruction, without gangrene** 🦠
　　　　　Other specified abdominal hernia causing obstruction
　　　　　Other specified incarcerated abdominal hernia
　　　　　Other specified irreducible abdominal hernia
　　　　　Other specified strangulated abdominal hernia
　　　　　(Ex) See PDX Collection 783

　　K45.1 **Other specified abdominal hernia with gangrene** 🦠
　　　　　Any condition listed under K45 specified as gangrenous
　　　　　(Ex) See PDX Collection 784

　　K45.8 **Other specified abdominal hernia without obstruction or gangrene**

● **K46** **Unspecified abdominal hernia**
　　Includes　enterocele
　　　　　　　　epiplocele
　　　　　　　　hernia NOS
　　　　　　　　interstitial hernia
　　　　　　　　intestinal hernia
　　　　　　　　intra-abdominal hernia
　　Excludes1　vaginal enterocele (N81.5)

　　K46.0 **Unspecified abdominal hernia with obstruction, without gangrene** 🦠
　　　　　Unspecified abdominal hernia causing obstruction
　　　　　Unspecified incarcerated abdominal hernia
　　　　　Unspecified irreducible abdominal hernia
　　　　　Unspecified strangulated abdominal hernia
　　　　　(Ex) See PDX Collection 783

　　K46.1 **Unspecified abdominal hernia with gangrene** 🦠
　　　　　Any condition listed under K46 specified as gangrenous
　　　　　(Ex) See PDX Collection 784

　　K46.9 **Unspecified abdominal hernia without obstruction or gangrene**
　　　　　Abdominal hernia NOS

★ **(See Plate 32 of the Anatomy Illustrations.)**

NONINFECTIVE ENTERITIS AND COLITIS (K50-K52)
　　Includes　noninfective inflammatory bowel disease
　　Excludes1　irritable bowel syndrome (K58.-)
　　　　　　　　megacolon (K59.3-)

● **K50** **Crohn's disease [regional enteritis]**
　　Includes　granulomatous enteritis
　　Use additional code to identify manifestations, such as:
　　　　pyoderma gangrenosum (L88)
　　Excludes1　ulcerative colitis (K51.-)
　　(Ex) **For category K50 CC codes unless otherwise indicated:** See PDX Collection 785

● **K50.0** **Crohn's disease of small intestine**
　　　　　Crohn's disease [regional enteritis] of duodenum
　　　　　Crohn's disease [regional enteritis] of ileum
　　　　　Crohn's disease [regional enteritis] of jejunum
　　　　　Regional ileitis
　　　　　Terminal ileitis
　　Excludes1　Crohn's disease of both small and large intestine (K50.8-)

　　K50.00 **Crohn's disease of small intestine without complications** 🦠🦠

● **K50.01** **Crohn's disease of small intestine with complications**

　　　K50.011 **Crohn's disease of small intestine with rectal bleeding** 🦠🦠

　　　K50.012 **Crohn's disease of small intestine with intestinal obstruction** 🦠🦠
　　　　　　CC when PDx is its own CC

　　　K50.013 **Crohn's disease of small intestine with fistula** 🦠🦠
　　　　　　CC when PDx is its own CC

　　　K50.014 **Crohn's disease of small intestine with abscess** 🦠🦠
　　　　　　CC when PDx is its own CC
　　　　　　Coding Clinic: 2012, Q4, P104

　　　K50.018 **Crohn's disease of small intestine with other complication** 🦠🦠

　　　K50.019 **Crohn's disease of small intestine with unspecified complications** 🦠🦠

● **K50.1** **Crohn's disease of large intestine**
　　　　　Crohn's disease [regional enteritis] of colon
　　　　　Crohn's disease [regional enteritis] of large bowel
　　　　　Crohn's disease [regional enteritis] of rectum
　　　　　Granulomatous colitis
　　　　　Regional colitis
　　Excludes1　Crohn's disease of both small and large intestine (K50.8)

　　K50.10 **Crohn's disease of large intestine without complications** 🦠🦠

● **K50.11** **Crohn's disease of large intestine with complications**

　　　K50.111 **Crohn's disease of large intestine with rectal bleeding** 🦠🦠

　　　K50.112 **Crohn's disease of large intestine with intestinal obstruction** 🦠🦠
　　　　　　CC when PDx is its own CC

　　　K50.113 **Crohn's disease of large intestine with fistula** 🦠🦠
　　　　　　CC when PDx is its own CC

　　　K50.114 **Crohn's disease of large intestine with abscess** 🦠🦠
　　　　　　CC when PDx is its own CC
　　　　　　Coding Clinic: 2012, Q4, P104

　　　K50.118 **Crohn's disease of large intestine with other complication** 🦠🦠

　　　K50.119 **Crohn's disease of large intestine with unspecified complications** 🦠🦠

Item 11-12 Crohn's disease, also known as **regional enteritis,** is a chronic inflammatory disease of the intestines. Classification is based on location in the small (duodenum, ileum, jejunum) or large (cecum, colon, rectum, anal canal) intestine.

N Newborn Age: 0　**P** Pediatric Age: 0–17　**M** Maternity DX: 9–64　**A** Adult Age: 15–124　♀ Females Only　♂ Males Only
🦠 Complication\Comorbidity　🦠 Major C\C　(Ex) CC/MCC Exclusions　Hospital-Acquired Condition　Hierarchical Condition Category

CHAPTER 11 (K00-K95)

971

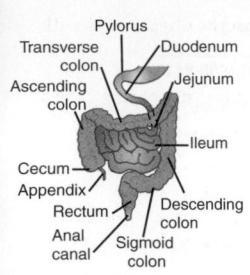

Figure 11-10   Small and large intestines.

Item 11–13   **Ulcerative colitis** attacks the colonic mucosa and forms abscesses. The disease involves the intestines. Classification is based on the location:

- Enterocolitis: large and small intestine
- Ileocolitis: ileum and colon
- Proctitis: rectum
- Proctosigmoiditis: sigmoid colon and rectum

● K50.8   Crohn's disease of both small and large intestine

    K50.80   Crohn's disease of both small and large intestine without complications

● K50.81   Crohn's disease of both small and large intestine with complications

      K50.811   Crohn's disease of both small and large intestine with rectal bleeding

      K50.812   Crohn's disease of both small and large intestine with intestinal obstruction
         CC when PDx is its own CC

      K50.813   Crohn's disease of both small and large intestine with fistula
         CC when PDx is its own CC

      K50.814   Crohn's disease of both small and large intestine with abscess
         CC when PDx is its own CC
         Coding Clinic: 2012, Q4, P104

      K50.818   Crohn's disease of both small and large intestine with other complication

      K50.819   Crohn's disease of both small and large intestine with unspecified complications

● K50.9   Crohn's disease, unspecified
      (Ex:) For category K50.9 CC codes: See PDX Collection 786

    K50.90   Crohn's disease, unspecified, without complications
      Crohn's disease NOS
      Regional enteritis NOS

● K50.91   Crohn's disease, unspecified, with complications

      K50.911   Crohn's disease, unspecified, with rectal bleeding

      K50.912   Crohn's disease, unspecified, with intestinal obstruction
         CC when PDx is its own CC

      K50.913   Crohn's disease, unspecified, with fistula
         CC when PDx is its own CC

      K50.914   Crohn's disease, unspecified, with abscess
         CC when PDx is its own CC
         Coding Clinic: 2012, Q4, P104

      K50.918   Crohn's disease, unspecified, with other complication

      K50.919   Crohn's disease, unspecified, with unspecified complications

● K51   Ulcerative colitis

    Use additional code to identify manifestations, such as: pyoderma gangrenosum (L88)

    Excludes1   Crohn's disease [regional enteritis] (K50.-)

    (Ex:) For category K51 CC codes unless otherwise indicated: See PDX Collection 785

● K51.0   Ulcerative (chronic) pancolitis
      Backwash ileitis

    K51.00   Ulcerative (chronic) pancolitis without complications
      Ulcerative (chronic) pancolitis NOS

● K51.01   Ulcerative (chronic) pancolitis with complications

      K51.011   Ulcerative (chronic) pancolitis with rectal bleeding

      K51.012   Ulcerative (chronic) pancolitis with intestinal obstruction
         CC when PDx is its own CC

      K51.013   Ulcerative (chronic) pancolitis with fistula
         CC when PDx is its own CC

      K51.014   Ulcerative (chronic) pancolitis with abscess
         CC when PDx is its own CC

      K51.018   Ulcerative (chronic) pancolitis with other complication

      K51.019   Ulcerative (chronic) pancolitis with unspecified complications

● K51.2   Ulcerative (chronic) proctitis

    K51.20   Ulcerative (chronic) proctitis without complications
      Ulcerative (chronic) proctitis NOS

● K51.21   Ulcerative (chronic) proctitis with complications

      K51.211   Ulcerative (chronic) proctitis with rectal bleeding

      K51.212   Ulcerative (chronic) proctitis with intestinal obstruction
         CC when PDx is its own CC

      K51.213   Ulcerative (chronic) proctitis with fistula
         CC when PDx is its own CC

      K51.214   Ulcerative (chronic) proctitis with abscess
         CC when PDx is its own CC

      K51.218   Ulcerative (chronic) proctitis with other complication

      K51.219   Ulcerative (chronic) proctitis with unspecified complications

● K51.3   Ulcerative (chronic) rectosigmoiditis

    K51.30   Ulcerative (chronic) rectosigmoiditis without complications
      Ulcerative (chronic) rectosigmoiditis NOS

● K51.31   Ulcerative (chronic) rectosigmoiditis with complications

      K51.311   Ulcerative (chronic) rectosigmoiditis with rectal bleeding

      K51.312   Ulcerative (chronic) rectosigmoiditis with intestinal obstruction
         CC when PDx is its own CC

      K51.313   Ulcerative (chronic) rectosigmoiditis with fistula
         CC when PDx is its own CC

      K51.314   Ulcerative (chronic) rectosigmoiditis with abscess
         CC when PDx is its own CC

      K51.318   Ulcerative (chronic) rectosigmoiditis with other complication

      K51.319   Ulcerative (chronic) rectosigmoiditis with unspecified complications

▶ New   ⇒ Revised   ~~deleted~~ Deleted   Excludes 1   Excludes 2   Includes   Use additional   Code first   Code also   Key words

972

OGCR Official Guidelines   ● Unacceptable Principal Diagnosis   X Assign placeholder X   ● Use Additional Character(s)   ▶ Manifestation Code   **Coding Clinic**

● **K51.4 Inflammatory polyps of colon**

    Excludes1   adenomatous polyp of colon (D12.6)
                 polyposis of colon (D12.6)
                 polyps of colon NOS (K63.5)

    K51.40 Inflammatory polyps of colon without complications
         Inflammatory polyps of colon NOS

●   **K51.41 Inflammatory polyps of colon with complications**

        K51.411 Inflammatory polyps of colon with rectal bleeding

        K51.412 Inflammatory polyps of colon with intestinal obstruction
              CC when PDx is its own CC

        K51.413 Inflammatory polyps of colon with fistula
              CC when PDx is its own CC

        K51.414 Inflammatory polyps of colon with abscess
              CC when PDx is its own CC

        K51.418 Inflammatory polyps of colon with other complication

        K51.419 Inflammatory polyps of colon with unspecified complications

● **K51.5 Left sided colitis**
     Left hemicolitis

    K51.50 Left sided colitis without complications
         Left sided colitis NOS

●   **K51.51 Left sided colitis with complications**

        K51.511 Left sided colitis with rectal bleeding

        K51.512 Left sided colitis with intestinal obstruction
              CC when PDx is its own CC

        K51.513 Left sided colitis with fistula
              CC when PDx is its own CC

        K51.514 Left sided colitis with abscess
              CC when PDx is its own CC

        K51.518 Left sided colitis with other complication

        K51.519 Left sided colitis with unspecified complications

● **K51.8 Other ulcerative colitis**

    K51.80 Other ulcerative colitis without complications

●   **K51.81 Other ulcerative colitis with complications**

        K51.811 Other ulcerative colitis with rectal bleeding

        K51.812 Other ulcerative colitis with intestinal obstruction
              CC when PDx is its own CC

        K51.813 Other ulcerative colitis with fistula
              CC when PDx is its own CC

        K51.814 Other ulcerative colitis with abscess
              CC when PDx is its own CC

        K51.818 Other ulcerative colitis with other complication

        K51.819 Other ulcerative colitis with unspecified complications

● **K51.9 Ulcerative colitis, unspecified**
    (Ex:) **For category K51.9 CC codes:** See PDX Collection 787

    K51.90 Ulcerative colitis, unspecified, without complications

●   **K51.91 Ulcerative colitis, unspecified, with complications**

        K51.911 Ulcerative colitis, unspecified with rectal bleeding

        K51.912 Ulcerative colitis, unspecified with intestinal obstruction
              CC when PDx is its own CC

        K51.913 Ulcerative colitis, unspecified with fistula
              CC when PDx is its own CC

        K51.914 Ulcerative colitis, unspecified with abscess
              CC when PDx is its own CC

        K51.918 Ulcerative colitis, unspecified with other complication

        K51.919 Ulcerative colitis, unspecified with unspecified complications

● **K52 Other and unspecified noninfective gastroenteritis and colitis**

    K52.0 Gastroenteritis and colitis due to radiation
        (Ex:) See PDX Collection 788

    K52.1 Toxic gastroenteritis and colitis
         Drug-induced gastroenteritis and colitis
         Code first (T51-T65) to identify toxic agent
         Use additional code for adverse effect, if applicable, to identify drug (T36-T50 with fifth or sixth character 5)
        (Ex:) See PDX Collection 789
         Coding Clinic: 2019, Q1, P17

●   **K52.2 Allergic and dietetic gastroenteritis and colitis**
         Food hypersensitivity gastroenteritis or colitis
         Use additional code to identify type of food allergy (Z91.01-, Z91.02-)

        Excludes2   allergic eosinophilic colitis (K52.82)
                      allergic eosinophilic esophagitis (K20.0)
                      allergic eosinophilic gastritis (K52.81)
                      allergic eosinophilic gastroenteritis (K52.81)
                      ~~food protein-induced proctocolitis (K52.82)~~

         Coding Clinic: 2016, Q4, P30-31

        K52.21 Food protein-induced enterocolitis syndrome
              FPIES
              Use additional code for hypovolemic shock, if present (R57.1)

        K52.22 Food protein-induced enteropathy

        K52.29 Other allergic and dietetic gastroenteritis and colitis
              ▶Allergic proctocolitis
              Food hypersensitivity gastroenteritis or colitis
              ▶Food-induced eosinophilic proctocolitis
              ▶Food protein-induced proctocolitis
              Immediate gastrointestinal hypersensitivity
              ▶Milk protein-induced proctocolitis

    K52.3 Indeterminate colitis
         Colonic inflammatory bowel disease unclassified (IBDU)
        Excludes1   unspecified colitis (K52.9)

●   **K52.8 Other specified noninfective gastroenteritis and colitis**

    K52.81 Eosinophilic gastritis or gastroenteritis
         Eosinophilic enteritis
        Excludes2   eosinophilic esophagitis (K20.0)

    K52.82 Eosinophilic colitis
         ~~Allergic proctocolitis~~
         ~~Food-induced eosinophilic proctocolitis~~
         ~~Food protein-induced proctocolitis~~
         ~~Milk protein-induced proctocolitis~~

        ▶ **Excludes2**   allergic proctocolitis (K52.29)
        ▶food-induced eosinophilic proctocolitis (K52.29)
        ▶food protein induced enterocolitis syndrome (FPIES) (K52.21)
        ▶food protein-induced proctocolitis (K52.29)
        ▶milk protein-induced proctocolitis (K52.29)

●   **K52.83 Microscopic colitis**
         Coding Clinic: 2016, Q4, P30-31

        K52.831 Collagenous colitis

        K52.832 Lymphocytic colitis

        K52.838 Other microscopic colitis

        K52.839 Microscopic colitis, unspecified

    K52.89 Other specified noninfective gastroenteritis and colitis
         Coding Clinic: 2019, Q1, P21

N Newborn Age: 0   **P** Pediatric Age: 0–17   **M** Maternity DX: 9–64   **A** Adult Age: 15–124   ♀ Females Only   ♂ Males Only

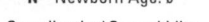 Complication\Comorbidity   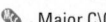 Major C\C   (Ex:) CC/MCC Exclusions   Hospital-Acquired Condition   Hierarchical Condition Category

973

CHAPTER 11 (K00-K95)

K52.9   **Noninfective gastroenteritis and colitis, unspecified**
Colitis NOS   Ileitis NOS
Enteritis NOS   Jejunitis NOS
Gastroenteritis NOS   Sigmoiditis NOS
> **Excludes1**   diarrhea NOS (R19.7)
>   functional diarrhea (K59.1)
>   infectious gastroenteritis and colitis NOS
>   (A09)
>   neonatal diarrhea (noninfective) (P78.3)
>   psychogenic diarrhea (F45.8)

OTHER DISEASES OF INTESTINES (K55-K64)

● **K55**   **Vascular disorders of intestine**
> **Excludes1**   necrotizing enterocolitis of newborn (P77.-)
> (Ex) **For category K55 CC codes unless otherwise indicated:** See PDX Collection 790

● **K55.0**   **Acute vascular disorders of intestine**
Infarction of appendices epiploicae
Mesenteric (artery) (vein) embolism
Mesenteric (artery) (vein) infarction
Mesenteric (artery) (vein) thrombosis
Coding Clinic: 2019, Q4, P68

   ● **K55.01**   **Acute (reversible) ischemia of small intestine**
     Coding Clinic: 2016, Q4, P32

     K55.011   **Focal (segmental) acute (reversible) ischemia of small intestine** 🐾🐾

     K55.012   **Diffuse acute (reversible) ischemia of small intestine** 🐾🐾

     K55.019   **Acute (reversible) ischemia of small intestine, extent unspecified** 🐾🐾

   ● **K55.02**   **Acute infarction of small intestine**
     Gangrene of small intestine
     Necrosis of small intestine
     Coding Clinic: 2016, Q4, P32

     K55.021   **Focal (segmental) acute infarction of small intestine** 🐾🐾

     K55.022   **Diffuse acute infarction of small intestine** 🐾🐾

     K55.029   **Acute infarction of small intestine, extent unspecified** 🐾🐾

   ● **K55.03**   **Acute (reversible) ischemia of large intestine**
     Acute fulminant ischemic colitis
     Subacute ischemic colitis
     Coding Clinic: 2016, Q4, P32

     K55.031   **Focal (segmental) acute (reversible) ischemia of large intestine** 🐾🐾

     K55.032   **Diffuse acute (reversible) ischemia of large intestine** 🐾🐾

     K55.039   **Acute (reversible) ischemia of large intestine, extent unspecified** 🐾🐾
       Coding Clinic: 2019, Q4, P68

   ● **K55.04**   **Acute infarction of large intestine**
     Gangrene of large intestine
     Necrosis of large intestine
     Coding Clinic: 2016, Q4, P32

     K55.041   **Focal (segmental) acute infarction of large intestine** 🐾🐾

     K55.042   **Diffuse acute infarction of large intestine** 🐾🐾

     K55.049   **Acute infarction of large intestine, extent unspecified** 🐾🐾

   ● **K55.05**   **Acute (reversible) ischemia of intestine, part unspecified**

     K55.051   **Focal (segmental) acute (reversible) ischemia of intestine, part unspecified** 🐾🐾

     K55.052   **Diffuse acute (reversible) ischemia of intestine, part unspecified** 🐾🐾

     K55.059   **Acute (reversible) ischemia of intestine, part and extent unspecified** 🐾🐾

   ● **K55.06**   **Acute infarction of intestine, part unspecified**
     Acute intestinal infarction
     Gangrene of intestine
     Necrosis of intestine

     K55.061   **Focal (segmental) acute infarction of intestine, part unspecified** 🐾🐾

     K55.062   **Diffuse acute infarction of intestine, part unspecified** 🐾🐾

     K55.069   **Acute infarction of intestine, part and extent unspecified** 🐾🐾

● **K55.1**   **Chronic vascular disorders of intestine** 🐾🐾
Chronic ischemic colitis
Chronic ischemic enteritis
Chronic ischemic enterocolitis
Ischemic stricture of intestine
Mesenteric atherosclerosis
Mesenteric vascular insufficiency
(Ex) See PDX Collection 791

● **K55.2**   **Angiodysplasia of colon**

   K55.20   **Angiodysplasia of colon without hemorrhage**

   K55.21   **Angiodysplasia of colon with hemorrhage** 🐾
     (Ex) See PDX Collection 770

● **K55.3**   **Necrotizing enterocolitis**
> **Excludes1**   necrotizing enterocolitis of newborn (P77.-)
> **Excludes2**   necrotizing enterocolitis due to
>   Clostridium difficile (A04.7-)

   K55.30   **Necrotizing enterocolitis, unspecified** 🐾🐾
     Necrotizing enterocolitis, NOS

   K55.31   **Stage 1 necrotizing enterocolitis** 🐾🐾
     Necrotizing enterocolitis without pneumatosis, without perforation
     Coding Clinic: 2016, Q4, P32

   K55.32   **Stage 2 necrotizing enterocolitis** 🐾🐾
     Necrotizing enterocolitis with pneumatosis, without perforation
     Coding Clinic: 2016, Q4, P32

   K55.33   **Stage 3 necrotizing enterocolitis** 🐾🐾
     Necrotizing enterocolitis with perforation
     Necrotizing enterocolitis with pneumatosis and perforation
     Coding Clinic: 2016, Q4, P32

K55.8   **Other vascular disorders of intestine** 🐾🐾
   (Ex) See PDX Collection 791

K55.9   **Vascular disorder of intestine, unspecified** 🐾🐾
Ischemic colitis
Ischemic enteritis
Ischemic enterocolitis
(Ex) See PDX Collection 791

● **K56**   **Paralytic ileus and intestinal obstruction without hernia**
> **Excludes1**   congenital stricture or stenosis of intestine
>   (Q41-Q42)
>   cystic fibrosis with meconium ileus (E84.11)
>   ischemic stricture of intestine (K55.1)
>   meconium ileus NOS (P76.0)
>   neonatal intestinal obstructions classifiable to P76.-
>   obstruction of duodenum (K31.5)
>   postprocedural intestinal obstruction (K91.3-)
> **Excludes2**   stenosis of anus or rectum (K62.4)
> (Ex) **For category K56 CC codes:** See PDX Collection 792

K56.0   **Paralytic ileus** 🐾🐾
Paralysis of bowel
Paralysis of colon
Paralysis of intestine
> **Excludes1**   gallstone ileus (K56.3)
>   ileus NOS (K56.7)
>   obstructive ileus NOS (K56.69-)

K56.1   **Intussusception** 🐾🐾
Intussusception or invagination of bowel
Intussusception or invagination of colon
Intussusception or invagination of intestine
Intussusception or invagination of rectum
> **Excludes2**   intussusception of appendix (K38.8)

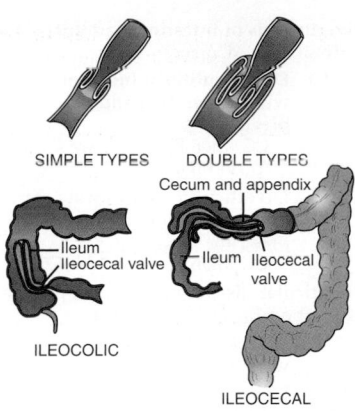

SIMPLE TYPES   DOUBLE TYPES

Cecum and appendix

Ileum
Ileocecal valve

Ileum   Ileocecal valve

ILEOCOLIC

ILEOCECAL

Figure 11-11   Types of intussusception.

Item 11–14   **Intussusception** is the prolapse (telescoping) of a part of the intestine into another adjacent part of the intestine. Intussusception may be enteric (ileoileal, jejunoileal, jejunojejunal), colic (colocolic), or intracolic (ileocecal, ileocolic).

Item 11–15   **Volvulus** is the twisting of a segment of the intestine, resulting in obstruction. Paralytic ileus is paralysis of the intestine. It need not be a complete paralysis, but it must prohibit the passage of food through the intestine and lead to intestinal blockage. It is a common aftermath of some types of surgery.

K56.2   **Volvulus** 🪙🪙
     Strangulation of colon or intestine
     Torsion of colon or intestine
     Twist of colon or intestine
     Excludes2   volvulus of duodenum (K31.5)

K56.3   **Gallstone ileus** 🪙🪙
     Obstruction of intestine by gallstone

K56.4   **Other impaction of intestine**
     K56.41   **Fecal impaction** 🪙
         Excludes1   constipation (K59.0-)
              incomplete defecation (R15.0)

     K56.49   **Other impaction of intestine** 🪙🪙

K56.5   **Intestinal adhesions [bands] with obstruction (postinfection)**
     Abdominal hernia due to adhesions with obstruction
     Peritoneal adhesions [bands] with intestinal obstruction (postinfection)

     K56.50   **Intestinal adhesions [bands], unspecified as to partial versus complete obstruction** 🪙🪙
         Intestinal adhesions with obstruction NOS

     K56.51   **Intestinal adhesions [bands], with partial obstruction** 🪙🪙
         Intestinal adhesions with incomplete obstruction

     K56.52   **Intestinal adhesions [bands] with complete obstruction** 🪙🪙

K56.6   **Other and unspecified intestinal obstruction**
     K56.60   **Unspecified intestinal obstruction**
         Coding Clinic: 2017, Q2, P12

         K56.600   **Partial intestinal obstruction, unspecified as to cause** 🪙🪙
              Incomplete intestinal obstruction, NOS

         K56.601   **Complete intestinal obstruction, unspecified as to cause** 🪙🪙

         K56.609   **Unspecified intestinal obstruction, unspecified as to partial versus complete obstruction** 🪙🪙
              Intestinal obstruction NOS

K56.69   **Other intestinal obstruction**
     Enterostenosis NOS
     Obstructive ileus NOS
     Occlusion of colon or intestine NOS
     Stenosis of colon or intestine NOS
     Stricture of colon or intestine NOS
     Excludes1   intestinal obstruction due to specified condition-code to condition
     Coding Clinic: 2017, Q2, P12

     K56.690   **Other partial intestinal obstruction** 🪙🪙
         Other incomplete intestinal obstruction

     K56.691   **Other complete intestinal obstruction** 🪙🪙

     K56.699   **Other intestinal obstruction unspecified as to partial versus complete obstruction** 🪙🪙
         Other intestinal obstruction, NEC

K56.7   **Ileus, unspecified** 🪙🪙
     Excludes1   obstructive ileus (K56.69-)
     Excludes2   intestinal obstruction with hernia (K40-K46)
     Coding Clinic: 2017, Q1, P41

K57   **Diverticular disease of intestine**
     Code also if applicable peritonitis K65.-
     Excludes1   congenital diverticulum of intestine (Q43.8)
              Meckel's diverticulum (Q43.0)
     Excludes2   diverticulum of appendix (K38.2)
     (Ex) For category K57 CC codes unless otherwise indicated: See PDX Collection 770

K57.0   **Diverticulitis of small intestine with perforation and abscess**
     Excludes1   diverticulitis of both small and large intestine with perforation and abscess (K57.4-)

     K57.00   **Diverticulitis of small intestine with perforation and abscess without bleeding** 🪙
         CC when PDx is its own CC
         (Ex) See PDX Collection 793

     K57.01   **Diverticulitis of small intestine with perforation and abscess with bleeding** 🪙🪙
         CC when PDx is its own CC

K57.1   **Diverticular disease of small intestine without perforation or abscess**
     Excludes1   diverticular disease of both small and large intestine without perforation or abscess (K57.5-)

     K57.10   **Diverticulosis of small intestine without perforation or abscess without bleeding**
         Diverticular disease of small intestine NOS

     K57.11   **Diverticulosis of small intestine without perforation or abscess with bleeding** 🪙

     K57.12   **Diverticulitis of small intestine without perforation or abscess without bleeding** 🪙
         (Ex) See PDX Collection 793

     K57.13   **Diverticulitis of small intestine without perforation or abscess with bleeding** 🪙

K57.2   **Diverticulitis of large intestine with perforation and abscess**
     Excludes1   diverticulitis of both small and large intestine with perforation and abscess (K57.4-)

     K57.20   **Diverticulitis of large intestine with perforation and abscess without bleeding** 🪙
         CC when PDx is its own CC
         (Ex) See PDX Collection 794

     K57.21   **Diverticulitis of large intestine with perforation and abscess with bleeding** 🪙
         CC when PDx is its own CC

N Newborn Age: 0   **P** Pediatric Age: 0–17   **M** Maternity DX: 9–64   **A** Adult Age: 15–124   ♀ Females Only   ♂ Males Only

🪙 Complication\Comorbidity   🪙 Major C\C   (Ex) CC/MCC Exclusions   🪙 Hospital-Acquired Condition   🪙 Hierarchical Condition Category

975

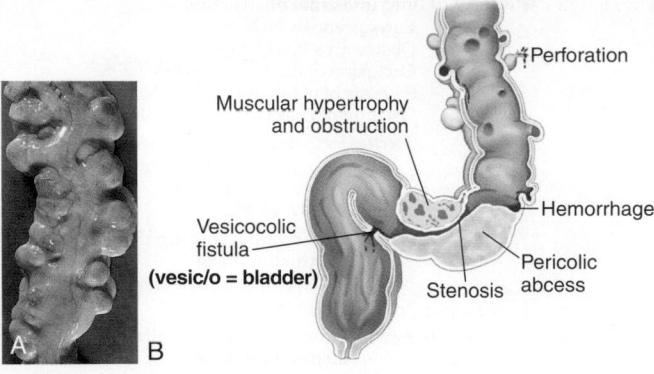

Figure 11-12 Diverticulosis. (From Shiland: Mastering Healthcare Terminology, ed 4, St. Louis, Mosby, 2012)

Item 11–16 Diverticula of the intestines are acquired herniations of the mucosa. Diverticulum (singular): Pocket or pouch that bulges outward through a weak spot (herniation) in the colon. Diverticula (plural). **Diverticulosis** is the condition of having diverticula. **Diverticulitis** is inflammation of these pouches or herniations. Classification is based on location (small intestine or colon) and whether it occurs with or without hemorrhage.

● **K57.3** Diverticular disease of large intestine without perforation or abscess

    Excludes1 diverticular disease of both small and large intestine without perforation or abscess (K57.5-)

    K57.30 Diverticulosis of large intestine without perforation or abscess without bleeding
        Diverticular disease of colon NOS

    K57.31 Diverticulosis of large intestine without perforation or abscess with bleeding 🔖

    K57.32 Diverticulitis of large intestine without perforation or abscess without bleeding 🔖
        Ⓔⓧ See PDX Collection 794

    K57.33 Diverticulitis of large intestine without perforation or abscess with bleeding 🔖

● **K57.4** Diverticulitis of both small and large intestine with perforation and abscess

    K57.40 Diverticulitis of both small and large intestine with perforation and abscess without bleeding 🔖
        CC when PDx is its own CC
        Ⓔⓧ See PDX Collection 794

    K57.41 Diverticulitis of both small and large intestine with perforation and abscess with bleeding 🔖🔖
        CC when PDx is its own CC

● **K57.5** Diverticular disease of both small and large intestine without perforation or abscess

    K57.50 Diverticulosis of both small and large intestine without perforation or abscess without bleeding
        Diverticular disease of both small and large intestine NOS

    K57.51 Diverticulosis of both small and large intestine without perforation or abscess with bleeding 🔖

    K57.52 Diverticulitis of both small and large intestine without perforation or abscess without bleeding 🔖
        CC when PDx is its own CC
        Ⓔⓧ See PDX Collection 794

    K57.53 Diverticulitis of both small and large intestine without perforation or abscess with bleeding 🔖

● **K57.8** Diverticulitis of intestine, part unspecified, with perforation and abscess

    K57.80 Diverticulitis of intestine, part unspecified, with perforation and abscess without bleeding 🔖
        CC when PDx is its own CC
        Ⓔⓧ See PDX Collection 794

    K57.81 Diverticulitis of intestine, part unspecified, with perforation and abscess with bleeding 🔖🔖
        CC when PDx is its own CC

● **K57.9** Diverticular disease of intestine, part unspecified, without perforation or abscess

    K57.90 Diverticulosis of intestine, part unspecified, without perforation or abscess without bleeding
        Diverticular disease of intestine NOS
        Coding Clinic: 2021, Q1, P12

    K57.91 Diverticulosis of intestine, part unspecified, without perforation or abscess with bleeding 🔖

    K57.92 Diverticulitis of intestine, part unspecified, without perforation or abscess without bleeding 🔖
        Ⓔⓧ See PDX Collection 794

    K57.93 Diverticulitis of intestine, part unspecified, without perforation or abscess with bleeding 🔖

● **K58** Irritable bowel syndrome

    Includes   irritable colon
                spastic colon

    K58.0 Irritable bowel syndrome with diarrhea

    K58.1 Irritable bowel syndrome with constipation
        Coding Clinic: 2016, Q4, P32

    K58.2 Mixed irritable bowel syndrome
        Coding Clinic: 2016, Q4, P32

    K58.8 Other irritable bowel syndrome
        Coding Clinic: 2016, Q4, P32

    K58.9 Irritable bowel syndrome without diarrhea
        Irritable bowel syndrome NOS

● **K59** Other functional intestinal disorders

    Excludes1 change in bowel habit NOS (R19.4)
               intestinal malabsorption (K90.-)
               psychogenic intestinal disorders (F45.8)

    Excludes2 functional disorders of stomach (K31.-)

● **K59.0** Constipation

    Excludes1 fecal impaction (K56.41)
               incomplete defecation (R15.0)

    K59.00 Constipation, unspecified
    K59.01 Slow transit constipation
    K59.02 Outlet dysfunction constipation
    K59.03 Drug induced constipation

        Use additional code for adverse effect, if applicable, to identify drug (T36-T50 with fifth or sixth character 5)
        Coding Clinic: 2016, Q4, P33

    K59.04 Chronic idiopathic constipation
        Functional constipation
        Coding Clinic: 2016, Q4, P33

    K59.09 Other constipation
        Chronic constipation

    K59.1 Functional diarrhea

    Excludes1 diarrhea NOS (R19.7)
               irritable bowel syndrome with diarrhea (K58.0)

    K59.2 Neurogenic bowel, not elsewhere classified 🔖
        Ⓔⓧ See PDX Collection 795

▶ New ⇒ Revised ~~deleted~~ Deleted Excludes 1 Excludes 2 Includes Use additional Code first Code also Key words

976   OGCR Official Guidelines ● Unacceptable Principal Diagnosis X Assign placeholder X ● Use Additional Character(s) ▶ Manifestation Code **Coding Clinic**

● **K59.3 Megacolon, not elsewhere classified**
Dilatation of colon
Code first, if applicable (T51-T65) to identify toxic agent

Excludes1 congenital megacolon (aganglionic)
(Q43.1)
megacolon (due to) (in) Chagas' disease
(B57.32)
megacolon (due to) (in) Clostridium
difficile (A04.7-)
megacolon (due to) (in) Hirschsprung's
disease (Q43.1)

(Ex) For category K59.3 CC codes: See PDX Collection 795
Coding Clinic: 2016, Q4, P33

K59.31 Toxic megacolon 🏥🅜
K59.39 Other megacolon 🏥
Megacolon NOS

K59.4 Anal spasm
Proctalgia fugax

● **K59.8 Other specified functional intestinal disorders**
K59.81 Ogilvie syndrome
Acute colonic pseudo-obstruction (ACPO)
K59.89 Other specified functional intestinal disorders
Atony of colon
Pseudo-obstruction (acute) (chronic) of
intestine

K59.9 Functional intestinal disorder, unspecified

● **K60 Fissure and fistula of anal and rectal regions**
Excludes1 fissure and fistula of anal and rectal regions with
abscess or cellulitis (K61.-)
Excludes2 anal sphincter tear (healed) (nontraumatic) (old)
(K62.81)

K60.0 Acute anal fissure
K60.1 Chronic anal fissure
K60.2 Anal fissure, unspecified
K60.3 Anal fistula
K60.4 Rectal fistula
Fistula of rectum to skin
Excludes1 rectovaginal fistula (N82.3)
vesicorectal fistula (N32.1)

K60.5 Anorectal fistula

● **K61 Abscess of anal and rectal regions**
Includes abscess of anal and rectal regions
cellulitis of anal and rectal regions
(Ex) For category K61 CC codes: See PDX Collection 796

K61.0 Anal abscess 🏥
Perianal abscess
Excludes2 intrasphincteric abscess (K61.4)
K61.1 Rectal abscess 🏥
Perirectal abscess
Excludes1 ischiorectal abscess (K61.39)
Coding Clinic: 2012, Q4, P104
K61.2 Anorectal abscess 🏥
K61.3 Ischiorectal abscess
K61.31 Horseshoe abscess 🏥
K61.39 Other ischiorectal abscess 🏥
Abscess of ischiorectal fossa
Ischiorectal abscess, NOS
K61.4 Intrasphincteric abscess 🏥
Intersphincteric abscess
K61.5 Supralevator abscess

● **K62 Other diseases of anus and rectum**
Includes anal canal
Excludes2 colostomy and enterostomy malfunction (K94.0-,
K91.4-)
fecal incontinence (R15.-)
hemorrhoids (K64.-)

K62.0 Anal polyp
Coding Clinic: 2018, Q1, P7
K62.1 Rectal polyp
Excludes1 adenomatous polyp (D12.8)
Coding Clinic: 2018, Q1, P7
K62.2 Anal prolapse
Prolapse of anal canal
K62.3 Rectal prolapse
Prolapse of rectal mucosa
K62.4 Stenosis of anus and rectum
Stricture of anus (sphincter)
Coding Clinic: 2019, Q2, P13
K62.5 Hemorrhage of anus and rectum 🏥
Excludes1 gastrointestinal bleeding NOS (K92.2)
melena (K92.1)
neonatal rectal hemorrhage (P54.2)
(Ex) See PDX Collection 770
K62.6 Ulcer of anus and rectum 🏥
Solitary ulcer of anus and rectum
Stercoral ulcer of anus and rectum
Excludes1 fissure and fistula of anus and rectum
(K60.-)
ulcerative colitis (K51.-)
(Ex) See PDX Collection 797
K62.7 Radiation proctitis
Use additional code to identify the type of radiation
(W88.-) or radiation therapy (Y84.2)
Coding Clinic: 2019, Q1, P21

● **K62.8 Other specified diseases of anus and rectum**
Excludes2 ulcerative proctitis (K51.2)
**K62.81 Anal sphincter tear (healed) (nontraumatic)
(old)**
Tear of anus, nontraumatic
Use additional code for any associated fecal
incontinence (R15.-)
Excludes2 anal fissure (K60.-)
anal sphincter tear (healed)
(old) complicating delivery
(O34.7-)
traumatic tear of anal sphincter
(S31.831)

K62.82 Dysplasia of anus
Anal intraepithelial neoplasia I and II (AIN I
and II) (histologically confirmed)
Dysplasia of anus NOS
Mild and moderate dysplasia of anus
(histologically confirmed)
Excludes1 abnormal results from anal
cytologic examination
without histologic
confirmation (R85.61-)
anal intraepithelial neoplasia III
(D01.3)
carcinoma in situ of anus (D01.3)
HGSIL of anus (R85.613)
severe dysplasia of anus (D01.3)

K62.89 Other specified diseases of anus and rectum
Proctitis NOS
Use additional code for any associated fecal
incontinence (R15.-)

K62.9 Disease of anus and rectum, unspecified

Item 11–17 A **fissure** is a groove in the surface, whereas a **fistula** is an
abnormal passage. An **abscess** is an accumulation of pus in a tissue cavity
resulting from a bacterial or parasitic infection.

CHAPTER 11 (K00-K95)

N Newborn Age: 0   P Pediatric Age: 0–17   M Maternity DX: 9–64   A Adult Age: 15–124   ♀ Females Only   ♂ Males Only
🏥 Complication\Comorbidity   🅜 Major C\C   (Ex) CC/MCC Exclusions   🏥 Hospital-Acquired Condition   🏥 Hierarchical Condition Category

977

● K63   **Other diseases of intestine**

     K63.0   **Abscess of intestine** 🔖

         Excludes1   abscess of intestine with Crohn's disease (K50.014, K50.114, K50.814, K50.914)

                   abscess of intestine with diverticular disease (K57.0, K57.2, K57.4, K57.8)

                   abscess of intestine with ulcerative colitis (K51.014, K51.214, K51.314, K51.414, K51.514, K51.814, K51.914)

         Excludes2   abscess of anal and rectal regions (K61.-)

                   abscess of appendix (K35.3-)

         (Ex:) See PDX Collection 798

     K63.1   **Perforation of intestine (nontraumatic)** 🔖🔖

         Perforation (nontraumatic) of rectum

         Excludes1   perforation (nontraumatic) of duodenum (K26.-)

                   perforation (nontraumatic) of intestine with diverticular disease (K57.0, K57.2, K57.4, K57.8)

         Excludes2   perforation (nontraumatic) of appendix (K35.2-, K35.3)

         (Ex:) See PDX Collection 799

     K63.2   **Fistula of intestine** 🔖

         Excludes1   fistula of duodenum (K31.6)

                   fistula of intestine with Crohn's disease (K50.013, K50.113, K50.813, K50.913)

                   fistula of intestine with ulcerative colitis (K51.013, K51.213, K51.313, K51.413, K51.513, K51.813, K51.913)

         Excludes2   fistula of anal and rectal regions (K60.-)

                   fistula of appendix (K38.3)

                   intestinal-genital fistula, female (N82.2-N82.4)

                   vesicointestinal fistula (N32.1)

         (Ex:) See PDX Collection 800

         Coding Clinic: 2017, Q3, P4

     K63.3   **Ulcer of intestine** 🔖

         Primary ulcer of small intestine

         Excludes1   duodenal ulcer (K26.-)

                   gastrointestinal ulcer (K28.-)

                   gastrojejunal ulcer (K28.-)

                   jejunal ulcer (K28.-)

                   peptic ulcer, site unspecified (K27.-)

                   ulcer of intestine with perforation (K63.1)

                   ulcer of anus or rectum (K62.6)

                   ulcerative colitis (K51.-)

         (Ex:) See PDX Collection 801

     K63.4   **Enteroptosis**

     K63.5   **Polyp of colon**

         Excludes1   adenomatous polyp of colon (D12.-)

                   inflammatory polyp of colon (K51.4-)

                   polyposis of colon (D12.6)

         Coding Clinic: 2019, Q1, P33; 2017, Q1, P15-16; 2015, Q2, P14

●   K63.8   **Other specified diseases of intestine**

     K63.81   **Dieulafoy lesion of intestine** 🔖

         Excludes2   Dieulafoy lesion of stomach and duodenum (K31.82)

         (Ex:) See PDX Collection 802

     K63.89   **Other specified diseases of intestine**

         Coding Clinic: 2013, Q2, P31

     K63.9   **Disease of intestine, unspecified**

● K64   **Hemorrhoids and perianal venous thrombosis**

     Includes   piles

     Excludes1   hemorrhoids complicating childbirth and the puerperium (O87.2)

                   hemorrhoids complicating pregnancy (O22.4)

     K64.0   **First degree hemorrhoids**

         Grade/stage I hemorrhoids

         Hemorrhoids (bleeding) without prolapse outside of anal canal

     K64.1   **Second degree hemorrhoids**

         Grade/stage II hemorrhoids

         Hemorrhoids (bleeding) that prolapse with straining, but retract spontaneously

     K64.2   **Third degree hemorrhoids**

         Grade/stage III hemorrhoids

         Hemorrhoids (bleeding) that prolapse with straining and require manual replacement back inside anal canal

     K64.3   **Fourth degree hemorrhoids**

         Grade/stage IV hemorrhoids

         Hemorrhoids (bleeding) with prolapsed tissue that cannot be manually replaced

     K64.4   **Residual hemorrhoidal skin tags**

         External hemorrhoids, NOS

         Skin tags of anus

     K64.5   **Perianal venous thrombosis**

         External hemorrhoids with thrombosis

         Perianal hematoma

         Thrombosed hemorrhoids NOS

     K64.8   **Other hemorrhoids**

         Internal hemorrhoids, without mention of degree

         Prolapsed hemorrhoids, degree not specified

     K64.9   **Unspecified hemorrhoids**

         Hemorrhoids (bleeding) NOS

         Hemorrhoids (bleeding) without mention of degree

DISEASES OF PERITONEUM AND RETROPERITONEUM (K65-K68)

● K65   **Peritonitis**

     Use additional code (B95-B97), to identify infectious agent, if known

     Code also if applicable diverticular disease of intestine (K57.-)

     Excludes1   acute appendicitis with generalized peritonitis (K35.2-)

                   aseptic peritonitis (T81.6)

                   benign paroxysmal peritonitis (E85.0)

                   chemical peritonitis (T81.6)

                   gonococcal peritonitis (A54.85)

                   neonatal peritonitis (P78.0-P78.1)

                   pelvic peritonitis, female (N73.3-N73.5)

                   periodic familial peritonitis (E85.0)

                   peritonitis due to talc or other foreign substance (T81.6)

                   peritonitis in chlamydia (A74.81)

                   peritonitis in diphtheria (A36.89)

                   peritonitis in syphilis (late) (A52.74)

                   peritonitis in tuberculosis (A18.31)

                   peritonitis with or following abortion or ectopic or molar pregnancy (O00-O07, O08.0)

                   peritonitis with or following appendicitis (K35.-)

                   puerperal peritonitis (O85)

                   retroperitoneal infections (K68.-)

     (Ex:) **For category K65 CC codes: See PDX Collection 803**

     K65.0   **Generalized (acute) peritonitis** 🔖🔖

         Pelvic peritonitis (acute), male

         Subphrenic peritonitis (acute)

         Suppurative peritonitis (acute)

Item 11-18   **Peritonitis** is an inflammation of the lining (peritoneum) of the abdominal cavity and surface of the intestines.

▶ New   ⇒ Revised   ~~deleted~~ Deleted   Excludes 1   Excludes 2   Includes   Use additional   Code first   Code also   Key words

OGCR Official Guidelines   ● Unacceptable Principal Diagnosis   X Assign placeholder X   ● Use Additional Character(s)   ▶ Manifestation Code   **Coding Clinic**

K65.1 Peritoneal abscess 🦠🦠
    Abdominopelvic abscess
    Abscess (of) omentum
    Abscess (of) peritoneum
    Mesenteric abscess
    Retrocecal abscess
    Subdiaphragmatic abscess
    Subhepatic abscess
    Subphrenic abscess
    Coding Clinic: 2019, Q1, P15

K65.2 Spontaneous bacterial peritonitis 🦠🦠
    Excludes1   bacterial peritonitis NOS (K65.9)

K65.3 Choleperitonitis 🦠🦠
    Peritonitis due to bile

K65.4 Sclerosing mesenteritis 🦠🦠
    Fat necrosis of peritoneum
    (Idiopathic) sclerosing mesenteric fibrosis
    Mesenteric lipodystrophy
    Mesenteric panniculitis
    Retractile mesenteritis

K65.8 Other peritonitis 🦠🦠
    Chronic proliferative peritonitis
    Peritonitis due to urine

K65.9 Peritonitis, unspecified 🦠🦠
    Bacterial peritonitis NOS
    Coding Clinic: 2013, Q2, P31

● **K66** Other disorders of peritoneum
    Excludes2   ascites (R18.-)
            peritoneal effusion (chronic) (R18.8)

K66.0 Peritoneal adhesions (postprocedural) (postinfection)
    Adhesions (of) abdominal (wall)
    Adhesions (of) diaphragm
    Adhesions (of) intestine
    Adhesions (of) male pelvis
    Adhesions (of) omentum
    Adhesions (of) stomach
    Adhesive bands
    Mesenteric adhesions
    Excludes1   female pelvic adhesions [bands] (N73.6)
            peritoneal adhesions with intestinal
            obstruction (K56.5-)

K66.1 Hemoperitoneum 🦠
    Excludes1   traumatic hemoperitoneum (S36.8-)
    (Ex:) See PDX Collection 804

K66.8 Other specified disorders of peritoneum

K66.9 Disorder of peritoneum, unspecified

▷ *K67* *Disorders of peritoneum in infectious diseases classified*
elsewhere 🦠🦠
    Code first underlying disease, such as:
    congenital syphilis (A50.0)
    helminthiasis (B65.0-B83.9)
    Excludes1   peritonitis in chlamydia (A74.81)
            peritonitis in diphtheria (A36.89)
            peritonitis in gonococcal (A54.85)
            peritonitis in syphilis (late) (A52.74)
            peritonitis in tuberculosis (A18.31)
    (Ex:) See PDX Collection 803

● **K68** Disorders of retroperitoneum
 ● **K68.1** Retroperitoneal abscess
    K68.11 Postprocedural retroperitoneal abscess 🦠🦠
        Excludes2   infection following procedure
                (T81.44)
        (Ex:) See PDX Collection 805
    K68.12 Psoas muscle abscess 🦠🦠
        (Ex:) See PDX Collection 806

K68.19 Other retroperitoneal abscess 🦠🦠
    (Ex:) See PDX Collection 803
    Coding Clinic: 2019, Q1, P15

K68.9 Other disorders of retroperitoneum 🦠
    (Ex:) See PDX Collection 803

DISEASES OF LIVER (K70-K77)

  Excludes1   jaundice NOS (R17)

  Excludes2   hemochromatosis (E83.11-)
              Reye's syndrome (G93.7)
              viral hepatitis (B15-B19)
              Wilson's disease (E83.0)

● **K70** Alcoholic liver disease
    Use additional code to identify:
    alcohol abuse and dependence (F10.-)

    K70.0 Alcoholic fatty liver   A
 ● **K70.1** Alcoholic hepatitis
    K70.10 Alcoholic hepatitis without ascites A
    K70.11 Alcoholic hepatitis with ascites   A
    K70.2 Alcoholic fibrosis and sclerosis of liver A
 ● **K70.3** Alcoholic cirrhosis of liver
    Alcoholic cirrhosis NOS
    K70.30 Alcoholic cirrhosis of liver without ascites 🦠 A
    K70.31 Alcoholic cirrhosis of liver with ascites 🦠 A
        Coding Clinic: 2018, Q1, P5
 ● **K70.4** Alcoholic hepatic failure
    Acute alcoholic hepatic failure
    Alcoholic hepatic failure NOS
    Chronic alcoholic hepatic failure
    Subacute alcoholic hepatic failure
    K70.40 Alcoholic hepatic failure without coma 🦠 A
    K70.41 Alcoholic hepatic failure with coma 🦠🦠 A
        MCC when PDx is its own MCC
        (Ex:) See PDX Collection 3276
    K70.9 Alcoholic liver disease, unspecified 🦠 A

● **K71** Toxic liver disease
  Includes   drug-induced idiosyncratic (unpredictable) liver
             disease
            drug induced toxic (predictable) liver disease
    Code first poisoning due to drug or toxin, if applicable (T36-T65 with
    fifth or sixth character 1-4 or 6)
    Use additional code for adverse effect, if applicable, to identify
    drug (T36-T50 with fifth or sixth character 5)
    Excludes2   alcoholic liver disease (K70.-)
            Budd-Chiari syndrome (I82.0)

K71.0 Toxic liver disease with cholestasis
    Cholestasis with hepatocyte injury
    'Pure' cholestasis

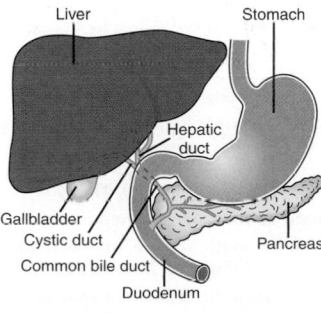

Figure 11-13 Liver and bile ducts.

Item 11-19 Retroperitoneal infections occur between the posterior parietal peritoneum and posterior abdominal wall where the kidneys, adrenal glands, ureters, duodenum, ascending colon, descending colon, pancreas, and the large vessels and nerves are located.

Item 11-20 Cirrhosis is the progressive fibrosis of the liver resulting in loss of liver function. The main causes of cirrhosis of the liver are alcohol abuse, chronic hepatitis (inflammation of the liver), biliary disease, and excessive amounts of iron. **Alcoholic cirrhosis of the liver** is also called portal, Laënnec's, or fatty nutritional cirrhosis.

N Newborn Age: 0   **P** Pediatric Age: 0–17   **M** Maternity DX: 9–64   **A** Adult Age: 15–124   ♀ Females Only   ♂ Males Only

🦠 Complication\Comorbidity   🦠 Major C\C   (Ex:) CC/MCC Exclusions   🦠 Hospital-Acquired Condition   🦠 Hierarchical Condition Category

979

CHAPTER 11 (K00-K95)

CHAPTER 11 (K00-K95)

● **K71.1** **Toxic liver disease with hepatic necrosis**
    Hepatic failure (acute) (chronic) due to drugs

    K71.10 **Toxic liver disease with hepatic necrosis, without coma**

    K71.11 **Toxic liver disease with hepatic necrosis, with coma** 🔧🔧
        MCC when PDx is its own MCC
        (Ex:) See PDX Collection 807

  K71.2 **Toxic liver disease with acute hepatitis**

  K71.3 **Toxic liver disease with chronic persistent hepatitis**

  K71.4 **Toxic liver disease with chronic lobular hepatitis**

● **K71.5** **Toxic liver disease with chronic active hepatitis**
    Toxic liver disease with lupoid hepatitis

    K71.50 **Toxic liver disease with chronic active hepatitis without ascites**

    K71.51 **Toxic liver disease with chronic active hepatitis with ascites**
        Coding Clinic: 2018, Q1, P4

  K71.6 **Toxic liver disease with hepatitis, not elsewhere classified**

  K71.7 **Toxic liver disease with fibrosis and cirrhosis of liver**

  K71.8 **Toxic liver disease with other disorders of liver**
    Toxic liver disease with focal nodular hyperplasia
    Toxic liver disease with hepatic granulomas
    Toxic liver disease with peliosis hepatis
    Toxic liver disease with veno-occlusive disease of liver

  K71.9 **Toxic liver disease, unspecified**

● **K72** **Hepatic failure, not elsewhere classified**

  Includes   fulminant hepatitis NEC, with hepatic failure
        hepatic encephalopathy NOS
        liver (cell) necrosis with hepatic failure
        malignant hepatitis NEC, with hepatic failure
        yellow liver atrophy or dystrophy

  Excludes1   alcoholic hepatic failure (K70.4)
        hepatic failure with toxic liver disease (K71.1-)
        icterus of newborn (P55-P59)
        postprocedural hepatic failure (K91.82)

  Excludes2   hepatic failure complicating abortion or ectopic or molar pregnancy (O00-O07, O08.8)
        hepatic failure complicating pregnancy, childbirth and the puerperium (O26.6-)
        viral hepatitis with hepatic coma (B15-B19)

● **K72.0** **Acute and subacute hepatic failure**
    Acute non-viral hepatitis NOS
    (Ex:) For category K72.0 CC codes: See PDX Collection 808
    Coding Clinic: 2015, Q2, P17

    K72.00 **Acute and subacute hepatic failure without coma** 🔧
        Coding Clinic: 2021, Q1, P13; 2015, Q2, P17

    K72.01 **Acute and subacute hepatic failure with coma** 🔧🔧
        MCC when PDx is its own MCC

● **K72.1** **Chronic hepatic failure**
    ▶ End stage liver disease

    K72.10 **Chronic hepatic failure without coma** 🔧🔧
        Coding Clinic: 2021, Q1, P13; 2017, Q1, P41

    K72.11 **Chronic hepatic failure with coma** 🔧🔧
        MCC when PDx is its own MCC
        (Ex:) See PDX Collection 3277
        Coding Clinic: 2020, Q1, P15

● **K72.9** **Hepatic failure, unspecified**

    K72.90 **Hepatic failure, unspecified without coma** 🔧
        Coding Clinic: 2018, Q4, P21

    K72.91 **Hepatic failure, unspecified with coma** 🔧🔧
        Hepatic coma NOS
        (Ex:) See PDX Collection 807
        Coding Clinic: 2016, Q2, P35

● **K73** **Chronic hepatitis, not elsewhere classified**

  Excludes1   alcoholic hepatitis (chronic) (K70.1-)
        drug-induced hepatitis (chronic) (K71.-)
        granulomatous hepatitis (chronic) NEC (K75.3)
        reactive, nonspecific hepatitis (chronic) (K75.2)
        viral hepatitis (chronic) (B15-B19)

  K73.0 **Chronic persistent hepatitis, not elsewhere classified** 🔧

  K73.1 **Chronic lobular hepatitis, not elsewhere classified** 🔧

  K73.2 **Chronic active hepatitis, not elsewhere classified** 🔧

  K73.8 **Other chronic hepatitis, not elsewhere classified** 🔧

  K73.9 **Chronic hepatitis, unspecified** 🔧

● **K74** **Fibrosis and cirrhosis of liver**
    Code also, if applicable, viral hepatitis (acute) (chronic) (B15-B19)

  Excludes1   alcoholic cirrhosis (of liver) (K70.3)
        alcoholic fibrosis of liver (K70.2)
        cardiac sclerosis of liver (K76.1)
        cirrhosis (of liver) with toxic liver disease (K71.7)
        congenital cirrhosis (of liver) (P78.81)
        pigmentary cirrhosis (of liver) (E83.110)

● **K74.0** **Hepatic fibrosis**
    Code first underlying liver disease, such as:
      nonalcoholic steatohepatitis (NASH) (K75.81)

  ● **K74.00** **Hepatic fibrosis, unspecified**

  ● **K74.01** **Hepatic fibrosis, early fibrosis**
        Hepatic fibrosis, stage F1 or stage F2

  ● **K74.02** **Hepatic fibrosis, advanced fibrosis**
        Hepatic fibrosis, stage F3

      Excludes1   cirrhosis of liver (K74.6-)
          hepatic fibrosis, stage F4 (K74.6-)

  K74.1 **Hepatic sclerosis**

  K74.2 **Hepatic fibrosis with hepatic sclerosis**

  K74.3 **Primary biliary cirrhosis** 🔧
    Chronic nonsuppurative destructive cholangitis
    Primary biliary cholangitis

    Excludes2   primary sclerosing cholangitis (K83.01)

  K74.4 **Secondary biliary cirrhosis** 🔧

  K74.5 **Biliary cirrhosis, unspecified** 🔧

● **K74.6** **Other and unspecified cirrhosis of liver**

    K74.60 **Unspecified cirrhosis of liver** 🔧
        Cirrhosis (of liver) NOS
        Coding Clinic: 2018, Q1, P4

    K74.69 **Other cirrhosis of liver** 🔧
        Cryptogenic cirrhosis (of liver)
        Macronodular cirrhosis (of liver)
        Micronodular cirrhosis (of liver)
        Mixed type cirrhosis (of liver)
        Portal cirrhosis (of liver)
        Postnecrotic cirrhosis (of liver)

● **K75** **Other inflammatory liver diseases**

  Excludes2   toxic liver disease (K71.-)

  K75.0 **Abscess of liver** 🔧
    Cholangitic hepatic abscess
    Hematogenic hepatic abscess
    Hepatic abscess NOS
    Lymphogenic hepatic abscess
    Pylephlebitic hepatic abscess

    Excludes1   amebic liver abscess (A06.4)
        cholangitis without liver abscess (K83.09)
        pylephlebitis without liver abscess (K75.1)

    Excludes2   acute or subacute hepatitis NOS (B17.9)
        acute or subacute non-viral hepatitis (K72.0)
        chronic hepatitis NEC (K73.8)
    (Ex:) See PDX Collection 809

  K75.1 **Phlebitis of portal vein** 🔧
    Pylephlebitis

    Excludes1   pylephlebitic liver abscess (K75.0)
    (Ex:) See PDX Collection 809

▶ New   ⇒ Revised   ~~deleted~~ Deleted   Excludes 1   Excludes 2   Includes   Use additional   Code first   Code also   Key words
OGCR Official Guidelines   ● Unacceptable Principal Diagnosis   X Assign placeholder X   ● Use Additional Character(s)   ▶ Manifestation Code   Coding Clinic

K75.2   Nonspecific reactive hepatitis
> **Excludes1**   acute or subacute hepatitis (K72.0-)
> chronic hepatitis NEC (K73.-)
> viral hepatitis (B15-B19)

K75.3   Granulomatous hepatitis, not elsewhere classified
> **Excludes1**   acute or subacute hepatitis (K72.0)
> chronic hepatitis NEC (K73.-)
> viral hepatitis (B15-B19)

K75.4   Autoimmune hepatitis 🔾
> Lupoid hepatitis NEC

● **K75.8   Other specified inflammatory liver diseases**

> **K75.81   Nonalcoholic steatohepatitis (NASH)**
>> Use additional code, if applicable, hepatic fibrosis (K74.0-)

> **K75.89   Other specified inflammatory liver diseases**

K75.9   Inflammatory liver disease, unspecified
> Hepatitis NOS
> **Excludes1**   acute or subacute hepatitis (K72.0-)
> chronic hepatitis NEC (K73.-)
> viral hepatitis (B15-B19)
> **Coding Clinic: 2015, Q2, P17**

● **K76   Other diseases of liver**
> **Excludes2**   alcoholic liver disease (K70.-)
> amyloid degeneration of liver (E85.-)
> cystic disease of liver (congenital) (Q44.6)
> hepatic vein thrombosis (I82.0)
> hepatomegaly NOS (R16.0)
> pigmentary cirrhosis (of liver) (E83.110)
> portal vein thrombosis (I81)
> toxic liver disease (K71.-)

K76.0   Fatty (change of) liver, not elsewhere classified
> Nonalcoholic fatty liver disease (NAFLD)
> **Excludes1**   nonalcoholic steatohepatitis (NASH) (K75.81)

K76.1   Chronic passive congestion of liver
> Cardiac cirrhosis
> Cardiac sclerosis

K76.2   Central hemorrhagic necrosis of liver 🔾
> **Excludes1**   liver necrosis with hepatic failure (K72.-)
> Ⓔ See PDX Collection 808

K76.3   Infarction of liver 🔾
> Ⓔ See PDX Collection 808

K76.4   Peliosis hepatis
> Hepatic angiomatosis

K76.5   Hepatic veno-occlusive disease
> **Excludes1**   Budd-Chiari syndrome (I82.0)

K76.6   Portal hypertension 🔾🔾
> Use additional code for any associated complications, such as:
> portal hypertensive gastropathy (K31.89)
> Ⓔ See PDX Collection 810
> **Coding Clinic: 2020, Q1, P15**

K76.7   Hepatorenal syndrome 🔾🔾
> **Excludes1**   hepatorenal syndrome following labor and delivery (O90.4)
> postprocedural hepatorenal syndrome (K91.83)
> Ⓔ See PDX Collection 811

● **K76.8   Other specified diseases of liver**

> ● **K76.81   Hepatopulmonary syndrome** 🔾
>> *Code first underlying liver disease, such as:*
>> alcoholic cirrhosis of liver (K70.3-)
>> cirrhosis of liver without mention of alcohol (K74.6-)

> **K76.89   Other specified diseases of liver**
>> Cyst (simple) of liver
>> Focal nodular hyperplasia of liver
>> Hepatoptosis

K76.9   Liver disease, unspecified

▶ **K77   Liver disorders in diseases classified elsewhere** 🔾
> *Code first underlying disease, such as:*
> amyloidosis (E85.-)
> congenital syphilis (A50.0, A50.5)
> congenital toxoplasmosis (P37.1)
> ▶infectious mononucleosis with liver disease (B27.0-B27.9 with .9)
> schistosomiasis (B65.0-B65.9)

> **Excludes1**   alcoholic hepatitis (K70.1-)
> alcoholic liver disease (K70.-)
> cytomegaloviral hepatitis (B25.1)
> herpesviral [herpes simplex] hepatitis (B00.81)
> ~~infectious mononucleosis with liver disease (B27.0-B27.9 with .9)~~
> mumps hepatitis (B26.81)
> sarcoidosis with liver disease (D86.89)
> secondary syphilis with liver disease (A51.45)
> syphilis (late) with liver disease (A52.74)
> toxoplasmosis (acquired) hepatitis (B58.1)
> tuberculosis with liver disease (A18.83)
> Ⓔ See PDX Collection 3229

DISORDERS OF GALLBLADDER, BILIARY TRACT AND PANCREAS (K80–K87)

● **K80   Cholelithiasis**
> *Presence or formation of gallstones*
> **Excludes1**   retained cholelithiasis following cholecystectomy (K91.86)

● **K80.0   Calculus of gallbladder with acute cholecystitis**
> Any condition listed in K80.2 with acute cholecystitis
> Use additional code if applicable for associated gangrene of gallbladder (K82.A1), or perforation of gallbladder (K82.A2)
> *Check documentation for acute/chronic gallbladder/common bile duct either with or without obstruction.*

> **K80.00   Calculus of gallbladder with acute cholecystitis without obstruction** 🔾
>> Ⓔ See PDX Collection 812
>> **Coding Clinic: 2018, Q4, P20**

> **K80.01   Calculus of gallbladder with acute cholecystitis with obstruction** 🔾
>> Ⓔ See PDX Collection 813

● **K80.1   Calculus of gallbladder with other cholecystitis**
> Use additional code if applicable for associated gangrene of gallbladder (K82.A1), or perforation of gallbladder (K82.A2)
> Ⓔ **For category K80.1 CC codes unless otherwise indicated:** See PDX Collection 813

> **K80.10   Calculus of gallbladder with chronic cholecystitis without obstruction** 🔾
>> Cholelithiasis with cholecystitis NOS

> **K80.11   Calculus of gallbladder with chronic cholecystitis with obstruction** 🔾

> **K80.12   Calculus of gallbladder with acute and chronic cholecystitis without obstruction** 🔾
>> Ⓔ See PDX Collection 812

> **K80.13   Calculus of gallbladder with acute and chronic cholecystitis with obstruction** 🔾

> **K80.18   Calculus of gallbladder with other cholecystitis without obstruction** 🔾

> **K80.19   Calculus of gallbladder with other cholecystitis with obstruction** 🔾

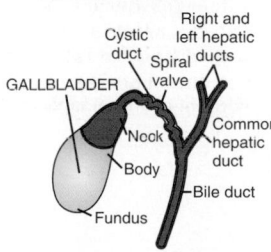

Figure 11-14   Gallbladder and bile ducts.

N Newborn Age: 0   P Pediatric Age: 0–17   M Maternity DX: 9–64   A Adult Age: 15–124   ♀ Females Only   ♂ Males Only

🔾 Complication\Comorbidity   🔾 Major C\C   Ⓔ CC/MCC Exclusions   🔾 Hospital-Acquired Condition   🔾 Hierarchical Condition Category

981

● **K80.2 Calculus of gallbladder without cholecystitis**
Cholecystolithiasis without cholecystitis
Cholelithiasis (without cholecystitis)
Colic (recurrent) of gallbladder (without cholecystitis)
Gallstone (impacted) of cystic duct (without cholecystitis)
Gallstone (impacted) of gallbladder (without cholecystitis)

K80.20 **Calculus of gallbladder without cholecystitis without obstruction**

K80.21 **Calculus of gallbladder without cholecystitis with obstruction** 🔗
(Ex:) See PDX Collection 813

● **K80.3 Calculus of bile duct with cholangitis**
Any condition listed in K80.5 with cholangitis

K80.30 **Calculus of bile duct with cholangitis, unspecified, without obstruction** 🔗
CC when PDx is its own CC
(Ex:) See PDX Collection 3744

K80.31 **Calculus of bile duct with cholangitis, unspecified, with obstruction** 🔗
CC when PDx is its own CC
(Ex:) See PDX Collection 815

K80.32 **Calculus of bile duct with acute cholangitis without obstruction** 🔗
CC when PDx is its own CC
(Ex:) See PDX Collection 3746

K80.33 **Calculus of bile duct with acute cholangitis with obstruction** 🔗
CC when PDx is its own CC
(Ex:) See PDX Collection 815

K80.34 **Calculus of bile duct with chronic cholangitis without obstruction** 🔗
CC when PDx is its own CC
(Ex:) See PDX Collection 3748

K80.35 **Calculus of bile duct with chronic cholangitis with obstruction** 🔗
CC when PDx is its own CC
(Ex:) See PDX Collection 815

K80.36 **Calculus of bile duct with acute and chronic cholangitis without obstruction** 🔗
CC when PDx is its own CC
(Ex:) See PDX Collection 3750

K80.37 **Calculus of bile duct with acute and chronic cholangitis with obstruction** 🔗
CC when PDx is its own CC
(Ex:) See PDX Collection 815

● **K80.4 Calculus of bile duct with cholecystitis**
Any condition listed in K80.5 with cholecystitis (with cholangitis)
Code also fistula of bile duct (K83.3)
Use additional code if applicable for associated gangrene of gallbladder (K82.A1), or perforation of gallbladder (K82.A2)
(Ex:) **For category K80.4 CC codes:** See PDX Collection 815

K80.40 **Calculus of bile duct with cholecystitis, unspecified, without obstruction** 🔗

K80.41 **Calculus of bile duct with cholecystitis, unspecified, with obstruction** 🔗
Coding Clinic: 2019, Q1, P18

K80.42 **Calculus of bile duct with acute cholecystitis without obstruction** 🔗

K80.43 **Calculus of bile duct with acute cholecystitis with obstruction** 🔗

K80.44 **Calculus of bile duct with chronic cholecystitis without obstruction** 🔗

K80.45 **Calculus of bile duct with chronic cholecystitis with obstruction** 🔗

K80.46 **Calculus of bile duct with acute and chronic cholecystitis without obstruction** 🔗

K80.47 **Calculus of bile duct with acute and chronic cholecystitis with obstruction** 🔗

● **K80.5 Calculus of bile duct without cholangitis or cholecystitis**
Choledocholithiasis (without cholangitis or cholecystitis)
Gallstone (impacted) of bile duct NOS (without cholangitis or cholecystitis)
Gallstone (impacted) of common duct (without cholangitis or cholecystitis)
Gallstone (impacted) of hepatic duct (without cholangitis or cholecystitis)
Hepatic cholelithiasis (without cholangitis or cholecystitis)
Hepatic colic (recurrent) (without cholangitis or cholecystitis)

K80.50 **Calculus of bile duct without cholangitis or cholecystitis without obstruction**

K80.51 **Calculus of bile duct without cholangitis or cholecystitis with obstruction** 🔗
(Ex:) See PDX Collection 815

● **K80.6 Calculus of gallbladder and bile duct with cholecystitis**
Use additional code if applicable for associated gangrene of gallbladder (K82.A1), or perforation of gallbladder (K82.A2)

K80.60 **Calculus of gallbladder and bile duct with cholecystitis, unspecified, without obstruction** 🔗
(Ex:) See PDX Collection 815

K80.61 **Calculus of gallbladder and bile duct with cholecystitis, unspecified, with obstruction** 🔗
(Ex:) See PDX Collection 815

K80.62 **Calculus of gallbladder and bile duct with acute cholecystitis without obstruction** 🔗
(Ex:) See PDX Collection 816

K80.63 **Calculus of gallbladder and bile duct with acute cholecystitis with obstruction** 🔗
(Ex:) See PDX Collection 816

K80.64 **Calculus of gallbladder and bile duct with chronic cholecystitis without obstruction** 🔗
(Ex:) See PDX Collection 815

K80.65 **Calculus of gallbladder and bile duct with chronic cholecystitis with obstruction** 🔗
(Ex:) See PDX Collection 815

K80.66 **Calculus of gallbladder and bile duct with acute and chronic cholecystitis without obstruction** 🔗
(Ex:) See PDX Collection 817

K80.67 **Calculus of gallbladder and bile duct with acute and chronic cholecystitis with obstruction** 🔗
(Ex:) See PDX Collection 817

● **K80.7 Calculus of gallbladder and bile duct without cholecystitis**

K80.70 **Calculus of gallbladder and bile duct without cholecystitis without obstruction**

K80.71 **Calculus of gallbladder and bile duct without cholecystitis with obstruction** 🔗
(Ex:) See PDX Collection 815

● **K80.8 Other cholelithiasis**

K80.80 **Other cholelithiasis without obstruction**

K80.81 **Other cholelithiasis with obstruction** 🔗
(Ex:) See PDX Collection 815

● **K81 Cholecystitis**
Chronic or acute inflammation of the gallbladder
    Use additional code if applicable for associated gangrene of gallbladder (K82.A1), or perforation of gallbladder (K82.A2)

    Excludes1   cholecystitis with cholelithiasis (K80.-)

    K81.0   Acute cholecystitis 🔗
        Abscess of gallbladder
        Angiocholecystitis
        Emphysematous (acute) cholecystitis
        Empyema of gallbladder
        Gangrene of gallbladder
        Gangrenous cholecystitis
        Suppurative cholecystitis
        (Ex:) See PDX Collection 818

    K81.1   Chronic cholecystitis

    K81.2   Acute cholecystitis with chronic cholecystitis 🔗
        (Ex:) See PDX Collection 819

    K81.9   Cholecystitis, unspecified

● **K82 Other diseases of gallbladder**

    Excludes1   nonvisualization of gallbladder (R93.2)
             postcholecystectomy syndrome (K91.5)

    (Ex:) For category K82 CC codes: See PDX Collection 820

    K82.0   Obstruction of gallbladder 🔗
        Occlusion of cystic duct or gallbladder without cholelithiasis
        Stenosis of cystic duct or gallbladder without cholelithiasis
        Stricture of cystic duct or gallbladder without cholelithiasis

        Excludes1   obstruction of gallbladder with cholelithiasis (K80.-)

    K82.1   Hydrops of gallbladder 🔗
        Mucocele of gallbladder

    K82.2   Perforation of gallbladder 🔗
        Rupture of cystic duct or gallbladder

        Excludes1   Perforation of gallbladder in cholecystitis (K82.A2)

    K82.3   Fistula of gallbladder 🔗
        Cholecystocolic fistula
        Cholecystoduodenal fistula
        Coding Clinic: 2019, Q1, P18

    K82.4   Cholesterolosis of gallbladder
        Strawberry gallbladder

        Excludes1   cholesterolosis of gallbladder with cholecystitis (K81.-)
                   cholesterolosis of gallbladder with cholelithiasis (K80.-)

    K82.8   Other specified diseases of gallbladder
        Adhesions of cystic duct or gallbladder
        Atrophy of cystic duct or gallbladder
        Cyst of cystic duct or gallbladder
        Dyskinesia of cystic duct or gallbladder
        Hypertrophy of cystic duct or gallbladder
        Nonfunctioning of cystic duct or gallbladder
        Ulcer of cystic duct or gallbladder

    K82.9   Disease of gallbladder, unspecified

    ● **K82.A   Disorders of gallbladder in diseases classified elsewhere**
        Code first the type of cholecystitis (K81.-), or cholelithiasis with cholecystitis (K80.00-K80.19, K80.40-K80.47, K80.60-K80.67)

      ▶ **K82.A1   Gangrene of gallbladder in cholecystitis** 🔗
         (Ex:) See PDX Collection 820
         Coding Clinic: 2018, Q4, P20

      ● **K82.A2   Perforation of gallbladder in cholecystitis** 🔗
         (Ex:) See PDX Collection 820
         Coding Clinic: 2018, Q4, P20

● **K83 Other diseases of biliary tract**

    Excludes1   postcholecystectomy syndrome (K91.5)
    Excludes2   conditions involving the gallbladder (K81-K82)
                 conditions involving the cystic duct (K81-K82)

    ● **K83.0   Cholangitis**

        Excludes1   cholangitic liver abscess (K75.0)
                  cholangitis with choledocholithiasis (K80.3-, K80.4-)

        Excludes2   chronic nonsuppurative destructive cholangitis (K74.3)
                  primary biliary cholangitis (K74.3)
                  primary biliary cirrhosis (K74.3)

      K83.01   Primary sclerosing cholangitis 🔗
         (Ex:) See PDX Collection 814
         Coding Clinic: 2018, Q4, P21

      K83.09   Other cholangitis 🔗
         Ascending cholangitis
         Cholangitis NOS
         Primary cholangitis
         Recurrent cholangitis
         Sclerosing cholangitis
         Secondary cholangitis
         Stenosing cholangitis
         Suppurative cholangitis
         (Ex:) See PDX Collection 814

    K83.1   Obstruction of bile duct 🔗
        Occlusion of bile duct without cholelithiasis
        Stenosis of bile duct without cholelithiasis
        Stricture of bile duct without cholelithiasis

        Excludes1   congenital obstruction of bile duct (Q44.3)
                  obstruction of bile duct with cholelithiasis (K80.-)
        (Ex:) See PDX Collection 821
        Coding Clinic: 2016, Q1, P18

    K83.2   Perforation of bile duct 🔗
        Rupture of bile duct
        (Ex:) See PDX Collection 822

    K83.3   Fistula of bile duct 🔗
        Choledochoduodenal fistula
        (Ex:) See PDX Collection 822

    K83.4   Spasm of sphincter of Oddi

    K83.5   Biliary cyst

    K83.8   Other specified diseases of biliary tract
        Adhesions of biliary tract
        Atrophy of biliary tract
        Hypertrophy of biliary tract
        Ulcer of biliary tract

    K83.9   Disease of biliary tract, unspecified

● **K85 Acute pancreatitis**
Inflammatory process in which pancreatic enzymes autodigest the gland

    Includes   acute (recurrent) pancreatitis
               subacute pancreatitis
    (Ex:) For category K85 CC codes: See PDX Collection 177
    Coding Clinic: 2016, Q4, P34

    ● **K85.0   Idiopathic acute pancreatitis**

      K85.00   Idiopathic acute pancreatitis without necrosis or infection 🔗

      K85.01   Idiopathic acute pancreatitis with uninfected necrosis 🔗

      K85.02   Idiopathic acute pancreatitis with infected necrosis 🔗

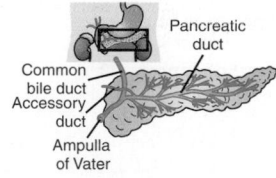

Figure 11-15 Pancreatic ductal system.

N Newborn Age: 0   **P** Pediatric Age: 0–17   **M** Maternity DX: 9–64   **A** Adult Age: 15–124   ♀ Females Only   ♂ Males Only

🔗 Complication\Comorbidity   🔗 Major C\C   (Ex:) CC/MCC Exclusions   🔗 Hospital-Acquired Condition   🔗 Hierarchical Condition Category

983

CHAPTER 11 (K00-K95)

● **K85.1** ▸ **Biliary acute pancreatitis**
  Gallstone pancreatitis

  K85.10 **Biliary acute pancreatitis without necrosis or infection** 🔖

  K85.11 **Biliary acute pancreatitis with uninfected necrosis** 🔖

  K85.12 **Biliary acute pancreatitis with infected necrosis** 🔖

● **K85.2** **Alcohol induced acute pancreatitis**

  Excludes2 alcohol induced chronic pancreatitis (K86.0)

  K85.20 **Alcohol induced acute pancreatitis without necrosis or infection** 🔖
    Coding Clinic: 2020, Q1, P9

  K85.21 **Alcohol induced acute pancreatitis with uninfected necrosis** 🔖

  K85.22 **Alcohol induced acute pancreatitis with infected necrosis** 🔖

● **K85.3** **Drug induced acute pancreatitis**
  Use additional code for adverse effect, if applicable, to identify drug (T36-T50 with fifth or sixth character 5)
  Use additional code to identify drug abuse and dependence (F11.-F17.-)

  K85.30 **Drug induced acute pancreatitis without necrosis or infection** 🔖

  K85.31 **Drug induced acute pancreatitis with uninfected necrosis** 🔖

  K85.32 **Drug induced acute pancreatitis with infected necrosis** 🔖

● **K85.8** **Other acute pancreatitis**

  K85.80 **Other acute pancreatitis without necrosis or infection** 🔖

  K85.81 **Other acute pancreatitis with uninfected necrosis** 🔖

  K85.82 **Other acute pancreatitis with infected necrosis** 🔖

● **K85.9** **Acute pancreatitis, unspecified**
  Pancreatitis NOS

  K85.90 **Acute pancreatitis without necrosis or infection, unspecified** 🔖

  K85.91 **Acute pancreatitis with uninfected necrosis, unspecified** 🔖

  K85.92 **Acute pancreatitis with infected necrosis, unspecified** 🔖

● **K86** **Other diseases of pancreas**

  Excludes2 fibrocystic disease of pancreas (E84.-)
    islet cell tumor (of pancreas) (D13.7)
    pancreatic steatorrhea (K90.3)

  K86.0 **Alcohol-induced chronic pancreatitis** 🔖 🔖
    Use additional code to identify:
      alcohol abuse and dependence (F10.-)
    Code also exocrine pancreatic insufficiency (K86.81)
    Excludes2 alcohol induced acute pancreatitis (K85.2-)
    (Ex:) See PDX Collection 823

  K86.1 **Other chronic pancreatitis** 🔖 🔖
    Chronic pancreatitis NOS
    Infectious chronic pancreatitis
    Recurrent chronic pancreatitis
    Relapsing chronic pancreatitis
    Code also exocrine pancreatic insufficiency (K86.81)
    (Ex:) See PDX Collection 823

  K86.2 **Cyst of pancreas** 🔖
    (Ex:) See PDX Collection 824

  K86.3 **Pseudocyst of pancreas** 🔖
    (Ex:) See PDX Collection 824

● **K86.8** **Other specified diseases of pancreas**
    Coding Clinic: 2016, Q4, P34

  K86.81 **Exocrine pancreatic insufficiency**

  K86.89 **Other specified diseases of pancreas**
    Aseptic pancreatic necrosis, unrelated to acute pancreatitis
    Atrophy of pancreas
    Calculus of pancreas
    Cirrhosis of pancreas
    Fibrosis of pancreas
    Pancreatic fat necrosis, unrelated to acute pancreatitis
    Pancreatic infantilism
    Pancreatic necrosis NOS, unrelated to acute pancreatitis

  K86.9 **Disease of pancreas, unspecified**

▸ *K87* *Disorders of gallbladder, biliary tract and pancreas in diseases classified elsewhere*
    Code first underlying disease
    Excludes1 cytomegaloviral pancreatitis (B25.2)
      mumps pancreatitis (B26.3)
      syphilitic gallbladder (A52.74)
      syphilitic pancreas (A52.74)
      tuberculosis of gallbladder (A18.83)
      tuberculosis of pancreas (A18.83)

OTHER DISEASES OF THE DIGESTIVE SYSTEM (K90-K95)

● **K90** **Intestinal malabsorption**
    Excludes1 intestinal malabsorption following gastrointestinal surgery (K91.2)
    (Ex:) **For category K90 cc does unless otherwise indicated:** See PDX Collection 825

  K90.0 **Celiac disease**
    Celiac disease with steatorrhea
    Celiac gluten-sensitive enteropathy
    Nontropical sprue
    Use additional code for associated disorders including:
      dermatitis herpetiformis (L13.0)
      gluten ataxia (G32.81)
    Code also exocrine pancreatic insufficiency (K86.81)

  K90.1 **Tropical sprue** 🔖
    Sprue NOS
    Tropical steatorrhea

  K90.2 **Blind loop syndrome, not elsewhere classified** 🔖
    Blind loop syndrome NOS
    Excludes1 congenital blind loop syndrome (Q43.8)
      postsurgical blind loop syndrome (K91.2)

  K90.3 **Pancreatic steatorrhea** 🔖

● **K90.4** **Other malabsorption due to intolerance**
    Excludes2 celiac gluten-sensitive enteropathy (K90.0)
      lactose intolerance (E73.-)
    Coding Clinic: 2016, Q4, P35-36

  K90.41 **Non-celiac gluten sensitivity** 🔖
    Gluten sensitivity NOS
    Non-celiac gluten sensitive enteropathy

  K90.49 **Malabsorption due to intolerance, not elsewhere classified** 🔖
    Malabsorption due to intolerance to carbohydrate
    Malabsorption due to intolerance to fat
    Malabsorption due to intolerance to protein
    Malabsorption due to intolerance to starch

● **K90.8** **Other intestinal malabsorption**

  K90.81 **Whipple's disease** 🔖
    (Ex:) See PDX Collection 826

  K90.89 **Other intestinal malabsorption** 🔖

  K90.9 **Intestinal malabsorption, unspecified** 🔖
    Coding Clinic: 2017, Q4, P108-109

▶ New   ⫸ Revised   ~~deleted~~ Deleted   Excludes 1   Excludes 2   Includes   Use additional   Code first   Code also   Key words
OGCR Official Guidelines   ● Unacceptable Principal Diagnosis   X Assign placeholder X   ● Use Additional Character(s)   ▸ Manifestation Code   **Coding Clinic**

● **K91　Intraoperative and postprocedural complications and disorders of digestive system, not elsewhere classified**

> **Excludes2**　complications of artificial opening of digestive system (K94.-)
> complications of bariatric procedures (K95.-)
> gastrojejunal ulcer (K28.-)
> postprocedural (radiation) retroperitoneal abscess (K68.11)
> radiation colitis (K52.0)
> radiation gastroenteritis (K52.0)
> radiation proctitis (K62.7)

Coding Clinic: 2016, Q4, P10

K91.0　Vomiting following gastrointestinal surgery

K91.1　Postgastric surgery syndromes
Dumping syndrome
Postgastrectomy syndrome
Postvagotomy syndrome

K91.2　Postsurgical malabsorption, not elsewhere classified 🔗
Postsurgical blind loop syndrome

> **Excludes1**　malabsorption osteomalacia in adults (M83.2)
> malabsorption osteoporosis, postsurgical (M80.8-, M81.8)

(Ex:) See PDX Collection 827

● **K91.3　Postprocedural intestinal obstruction**
(Ex:) For category K91.3 CC codes: See PDX Collection 792
Coding Clinic: 2017, Q1, P40-41

K91.30　Postprocedural intestinal obstruction, unspecified as to partial versus complete 🔗
Postprocedural intestinal obstruction NOS

K91.31　Postprocedural partial intestinal obstruction
Postprocedural incomplete intestinal obstruction

K91.32　Postprocedural complete intestinal obstruction 🔗

K91.5　Postcholecystectomy syndrome

● **K91.6　Intraoperative hemorrhage and hematoma of a digestive system organ or structure complicating a procedure**

> **Excludes1**　intraoperative hemorrhage and hematoma of a digestive system organ or structure due to accidental puncture and laceration during a procedure (K91.7-)

(Ex:) For category K91.6 CC codes: See PDX Collection 829

K91.61　Intraoperative hemorrhage and hematoma of a digestive system organ or structure complicating a digestive system procedure 🔗
Coding Clinic: 2020, Q1, P20

K91.62　Intraoperative hemorrhage and hematoma of a digestive system organ or structure complicating other procedure 🔗

● **K91.7　Accidental puncture and laceration of a digestive system organ or structure during a procedure**
(Ex:) For category K91.7 CC codes: See PDX Collection 509

K91.71　Accidental puncture and laceration of a digestive system organ or structure during a digestive system procedure 🔗
Coding Clinic: 2021, Q2, P12

K91.72　Accidental puncture and laceration of a digestive system organ or structure during other procedure 🔗
Coding Clinic: 2019, Q2, P24

● **K91.8　Other intraoperative and postprocedural complications and disorders of digestive system**
(Ex:) For category K91.8 CC codes unless otherwise indicated: See PDX Collection 828

K91.81　Other intraoperative complications of digestive system 🔗

K91.82　Postprocedural hepatic failure 🔗

K91.83　Postprocedural hepatorenal syndrome 🔗

● **K91.84　Postprocedural hemorrhage of a digestive system organ or structure following a procedure**
(Ex:) For category K91.84 CC codes: See PDX Collection 829

K91.840　Postprocedural hemorrhage of a digestive system organ or structure following a digestive system procedure 🔗
Coding Clinic: 2016, Q1, P15

K91.841　Postprocedural hemorrhage of a digestive system organ or structure following other procedure 🔗

● **K91.85　Complications of intestinal pouch**

K91.850　Pouchitis 🔗🔗
Inflammation of internal ileoanal pouch

K91.858　Other complications of intestinal pouch 🔗🔗
Coding Clinic: 2019, Q2, P13

K91.86　Retained cholelithiasis following cholecystectomy 🔗

● **K91.87　Postprocedural hematoma and seroma of a digestive system organ or structure following a procedure**
(Ex:) For category K97.87 CC codes: See PDX Collection 829

K91.870　Postprocedural hematoma of a digestive system organ or structure following a digestive system procedure 🔗

K91.871　Postprocedural hematoma of a digestive system organ or structure following other procedure 🔗

K91.872　Postprocedural seroma of a digestive system organ or structure following a digestive system procedure 🔗

K91.873　Postprocedural seroma of a digestive system organ or structure following other procedure 🔗

K91.89　Other postprocedural complications and disorders of digestive system 🔗
Use additional code, if applicable, to further specify disorder

> **Excludes2**　postprocedural retroperitoneal abscess (K68.11)

(Ex:) See PDX Collection 828
Coding Clinic: 2017, Q1, P41

● **K92　Other diseases of digestive system**

> **Excludes1**　neonatal gastrointestinal hemorrhage (P54.0-P54.3)

(Ex:) For category K92 CC codes unless otherwise indicated: See PDX Collection 770

K92.0　Hematemesis 🔗

K92.1　Melena 🔗

> **Excludes1**　occult blood in feces (R19.5)

K92.2　Gastrointestinal hemorrhage, unspecified 🔗
Gastric hemorrhage NOS
Intestinal hemorrhage NOS

> **Excludes1**　acute hemorrhagic gastritis (K29.01)
> hemorrhage of anus and rectum (K62.5)
> angiodysplasia of stomach with hemorrhage (K31.811)
> diverticular disease with hemorrhage (K57.-)
> gastritis and duodenitis with hemorrhage (K29.-)
> peptic ulcer with hemorrhage (K25-K28)

Coding Clinic: 2021, Q1, P12

CHAPTER 11 (K00-K95)

N　Newborn Age: 0　　P　Pediatric Age: 0–17　　M　Maternity DX: 9–64　　A　Adult Age: 15–124　　♀ Females Only　　♂ Males Only

🔗 Complication\Comorbidity　　🔗 Major C\C　　(Ex:) CC/MCC Exclusions　　🔗 Hospital-Acquired Condition　　🔗 Hierarchical Condition Category

985

● K92.8 ▶ **Other specified diseases of the digestive system**

K92.81 **Gastrointestinal mucositis (ulcerative)** 🔑

Code also type of associated therapy, such as:
antineoplastic and immunosuppressive
drugs (T45.1X-)
radiological procedure and radiotherapy
(Y84.2)

Excludes2 mucositis (ulcerative) of vagina
and vulva (N76.81)
nasal mucositis (ulcerative)
(J34.81)
oral mucositis (ulcerative) (K12.3-)

(Ex) See PDX Collection 765

K92.89 **Other specified diseases of the digestive system**

K92.9 **Disease of digestive system, unspecified**

● K94 **Complications of artificial openings of the digestive system**

● K94.0 **Colostomy complications**

(Ex) **For category K94.0 CC does unless otherwise indicated:** See PDX
Collection 830

K94.00 **Colostomy complication, unspecified** 🔑

K94.01 **Colostomy hemorrhage** 🔑🔑

K94.02 **Colostomy infection** 🔑🔑

Use additional code to specify type of
infection, such as:
cellulitis of abdominal wall (L03.311)
sepsis (A40.-, A41.-)

K94.03 **Colostomy malfunction** 🔑🔑

Mechanical complication of colostomy
(Ex) See PDX Collection 831

K94.09 **Other complications of colostomy** 🔑🔑

● K94.1 **Enterostomy complications**

(Ex) **For category K94.1 CC does unless otherwise indicated:** See PDX
Collection 830

K94.10 **Enterostomy complication, unspecified** 🔑

K94.11 **Enterostomy hemorrhage** 🔑🔑

K94.12 **Enterostomy infection** 🔑🔑

Use additional code to specify type of
infection, such as:
cellulitis of abdominal wall (L03.311)
sepsis (A40.-, A41.-)

K94.13 **Enterostomy malfunction** 🔑🔑

Mechanical complication of enterostomy
(Ex) See PDX Collection 831

K94.19 **Other complications of enterostomy** 🔑🔑

● K94.2 **Gastrostomy complications**

K94.20 **Gastrostomy complication, unspecified** 🔑

K94.21 **Gastrostomy hemorrhage** 🔑

K94.22 **Gastrostomy infection** 🔑🔑

Use additional code to specify type of
infection, such as:
cellulitis of abdominal wall (L03.311)
sepsis (A40.-, A41.-)
(Ex) See PDX Collection 828

K94.23 **Gastrostomy malfunction** 🔑🔑

Mechanical complication of gastrostomy
(Ex) See PDX Collection 828

K94.29 **Other complications of gastrostomy** 🔑

● K94.3 **Esophagostomy complications**

(Ex) **For category K94.3 CC codes:** See PDX Collection 828

K94.30 **Esophagostomy complications, unspecified** 🔑🔑

K94.31 **Esophagostomy hemorrhage** 🔑🔑

K94.32 **Esophagostomy infection** 🔑🔑

Use additional code to identify the infection

K94.33 **Esophagostomy malfunction** 🔑🔑

Mechanical complication of esophagostomy

K94.39 **Other complications of esophagostomy** 🔑🔑

● K95 **Complications of bariatric procedures**

(Ex) **For category K95 CC codes:** See PDX Collection 828

● K95.0 **Complications of gastric band procedure**

K95.01 **Infection due to gastric band procedure** 🔑🔑

Use additional code to specify type of infection
or organism, such as:
bacterial and viral infectious agents (B95.-,
B96.-)
cellulitis of abdominal wall (L03.311)
sepsis (A40.-, A41.-)

K95.09 **Other complications of gastric band
procedure** 🔑

Use additional code, if applicable, to further
specify complication

● K95.8 **Complications of other bariatric procedure**

Excludes1 complications of gastric band surgery
(K95.0-)

K95.81 **Infection due to other bariatric procedure** 🔑🔑

Use additional code to specify type of infection
or organism, such as:
bacterial and viral infectious agents (B95.-,
B96.-)
cellulitis of abdominal wall (L03.311)
sepsis (A40.-, A41.-)

K95.89 **Other complications of other bariatric
procedure** 🔑

Use additional code, if applicable, to further
specify complication

CHAPTER 12

DISEASES OF THE SKIN AND SUBCUTANEOUS TISSUE (L00-L99)

OGCR Chapter-Specific Coding Guidelines

12. Chapter 12: Diseases of the Skin and Subcutaneous Tissue (L00-L99)

   a. Pressure ulcer stage codes

   1) **Pressure ulcer stages**
   Codes from category L89, Pressure ulcer, identify the site of the pressure ulcer as well as the stage of the ulcer.
   The ICD-10-CM classifies pressure ulcer stages based on severity, which is designated by stages 1-4, unspecified stage and unstageable.
   Assign as many codes from category L89 as needed to identify all the pressure ulcers the patient has, if applicable.
   See Section I.B.14 for pressure ulcer stage documentation by clinicians other than patient's provider.

   2) **Unstageable pressure ulcers**
   Assignment of the code for unstageable pressure ulcer (L89.--0) should be based on the clinical documentation. These codes are used for pressure ulcers whose stage cannot be clinically determined (e.g., the ulcer is covered by eschar or has been treated with a skin or muscle graft) and pressure ulcers that are documented as deep tissue injury but not documented as due to trauma. This code should not be confused with the codes for unspecified stage (L89.--9). When there is no documentation regarding the stage of the pressure ulcer, assign the appropriate code for unspecified stage (L89.--9).

   3) **Documented pressure ulcer stage**
   Assignment of the pressure ulcer stage code should be guided by clinical documentation of the stage or documentation of the terms found in the Alphabetic Index. For clinical terms describing the stage that are not found in the Alphabetic Index, and there is no documentation of the stage, the provider should be queried.

   4) **Patients admitted with pressure ulcers documented as healed**
   No code is assigned if the documentation states that the pressure ulcer is completely healed.

   5) **Patients admitted with pressure ulcers documented as healing**
   Pressure ulcers described as healing should be assigned the appropriate pressure ulcer stage code based on the documentation in the medical record. If the documentation does not provide information about the stage of the healing pressure ulcer, assign the appropriate code for unspecified stage.
   If the documentation is unclear as to whether the patient has a current (new) pressure ulcer or if the patient is being treated for a healing pressure ulcer, query the provider.
   For ulcers that were present on admission but healed at the time of discharge, assign the code for the site and stage of the pressure ulcer at the time of admission.

   6) **Patient admitted with pressure ulcer evolving into another stage during the admission**
   If a patient is admitted to an inpatient hospital with a pressure ulcer at one stage and it progresses to a higher stage, two separate codes should be assigned: one code for the site and stage of the ulcer on admission and a second code for the same ulcer site and the highest stage reported during the stay.

   b. Non-Pressure Chronic Ulcers

   1) **Patients admitted with non-pressure ulcers documented as healed**
   No code is assigned if the documentation states that the non-pressure ulcer is completely healed.

   2) **Patients admitted with non-pressure ulcers documented as healing**
   Non-pressure ulcers described as healing should be assigned the appropriate non-pressure ulcer code based on the documentation in the medical record. If the documentation does not provide information about the severity of the healing non-pressure ulcer, assign the appropriate code for unspecified severity.
   If the documentation is unclear as to whether the patient has a current (new) non-pressure ulcer or if the patient is being treated for a healing non-pressure ulcer, query the provider.
   For ulcers that were present on admission but healed at the time of discharge, assign the code for the site and severity of the non-pressure ulcer at the time of admission.

   3) **Patient admitted with non-pressure ulcer that progresses to another severity level during the admission**
   If a patient is admitted to an inpatient hospital with a non-pressure ulcer at one severity level and it progresses to a higher severity level, two separate codes should be assigned: one code for the site and severity level of the ulcer on admission and a second code for the same ulcer site and the highest severity level reported during the stay.
   See Section I.B.14 for pressure ulcer stage documentation by clinicians other than patient's provider.

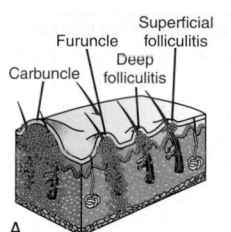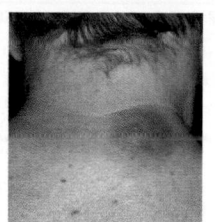

Figure 12-1 Furuncle, also known as a boil, is a staphylococcal infection. The organism enters the body through a hair follicle and so furuncles usually appear in hairy areas of the body. A cluster of furuncles is known as a carbuncle and involves infection into the deep subcutaneous fascia. These usually appear on the back and neck. (**B** from Habif TP, Binnick AN, Meyerson LB: Clinical Dermatology: A Color Guide to Diagnosis and Therapy, S.l., Mosby Elsevier, 2010)

CHAPTER 12

DISEASES OF THE SKIN AND SUBCUTANEOUS TISSUE (L00-L99)

Excludes2 certain conditions originating in the perinatal period (P04-P96)
certain infectious and parasitic diseases (A00-B99)
complications of pregnancy, childbirth and the puerperium (O00-O9A)
congenital malformations, deformations, and chromosomal abnormalities (Q00-Q99)
endocrine, nutritional and metabolic diseases (E00-E88)
lipomelanotic reticulosis (I89.8)
neoplasms (C00-D49)
symptoms, signs and abnormal clinical and laboratory findings, not elsewhere classified (R00-R94)
systemic connective tissue disorders (M30-M36)
viral warts (B07.-)

This chapter contains the following blocks:

L00-L08	Infections of the skin and subcutaneous tissue
L10-L14	Bullous disorders
L20-L30	Dermatitis and eczema
L40-L45	Papulosquamous disorders
L49-L54	Urticaria and erythema
L55-L59	Radiation-related disorders of the skin and subcutaneous tissue
L60-L75	Disorders of skin appendages
L76	Intraoperative and postprocedural complications of skin and subcutaneous tissue
L80-L99	Other disorders of the skin and subcutaneous tissue

N Newborn Age: 0   **P** Pediatric Age: 0-17   **M** Maternity DX: 9-64   **A** Adult Age: 15-124   ♀ Females Only   ♂ Males Only

🐾 Complication\Comorbidity   🐾 Major C\C   (Ex:) CC/MCC Exclusions   🐾 Hospital-Acquired Condition   🐾 Hierarchical Condition Category

987

CHAPTER 12 (L00-L99)

INFECTIONS OF THE SKIN AND SUBCUTANEOUS TISSUE (L00-L08)

Use additional code (B95-B97) to identify infectious agent.

Excludes2   hordeolum (H00.0)
infective dermatitis (L30.3)
local infections of skin classified in Chapter 1
lupus panniculitis (L93.2)
panniculitis NOS (M79.3)
panniculitis of neck and back (M54.0-)
Perlèche NOS (K13.0)
Perlèche due to candidiasis (B37.0)
Perlèche due to riboflavin deficiency (E53.0)
pyogenic granuloma (L98.0)
relapsing panniculitis [Weber-Christian] (M35.6)
viral warts (B07.-)
zoster (B02.-)

L00   **Staphylococcal scalded skin syndrome**
Ritter's disease

Use additional code to identify percentage of skin exfoliation (L49.-)

Excludes1   bullous impetigo (L01.03)
pemphigus neonatorum (L01.03)
toxic epidermal necrolysis [Lyell] (L51.2)

● **L01**   **Impetigo**
Contagious skin infection caused by a streptococcus or staphylococcus aureus, common skin infections among children

Excludes1   impetigo herpetiformis (L40.1)

● **L01.0**   **Impetigo**
Impetigo contagiosa
Impetigo vulgaris

L01.00   **Impetigo, unspecified**
Impetigo NOS

L01.01   **Non-bullous impetigo**

L01.02   **Bockhart's impetigo**
Impetigo follicularis
Perifolliculitis NOS
Superficial pustular perifolliculitis

L01.03   **Bullous impetigo**
Impetigo neonatorum
Pemphigus neonatorum
Neonate = newborn

L01.09   **Other impetigo**
Ulcerative impetigo

L01.1   **Impetiginization of other dermatoses**

● **L02**   **Cutaneous abscess, furuncle and carbuncle**
Use additional code to identify organism (B95-B96)

Excludes2   abscess of anus and rectal regions (K61.-)
abscess of female genital organs (external) (N76.4)
abscess of male genital organs (external) (N48.2, N49.-)

● **L02.0**   **Cutaneous abscess, furuncle and carbuncle of face**

Excludes2   abscess of ear, external (H60.0)
abscess of eyelid (H00.0)
abscess of head [any part, except face] (L02.8)
abscess of lacrimal gland (H04.0)
abscess of lacrimal passages (H04.3)
abscess of mouth (K12.2)
abscess of nose (J34.0)
abscess of orbit (H05.0)
submandibular abscess (K12.2)

L02.01   **Cutaneous abscess of face** 🔗
Ex: See PDX Collection 3230

L02.02   **Furuncle of face**
Boil of face
Folliculitis of face

L02.03   **Carbuncle of face**

● **L02.1**   **Cutaneous abscess, furuncle and carbuncle of neck**

L02.11   **Cutaneous abscess of neck** 🔗
Ex: See PDX Collection 832

L02.12   **Furuncle of neck**
Boil of neck
Folliculitis of neck

L02.13   **Carbuncle of neck**

● **L02.2**   **Cutaneous abscess, furuncle and carbuncle of trunk**

Excludes1   non-newborn omphalitis (L08.82)
omphalitis of newborn (P38.-)

Excludes2   abscess of breast (N61.1)
abscess of buttocks (L02.3)
abscess of female external genital organs (N76.4)
abscess of male external genital organs (N48.2, N49.-)
abscess of hip (L02.4)

● **L02.21**   **Cutaneous abscess of trunk**
Ex: For category L02.21 CC codes: See PDX Collection 833

L02.211   **Cutaneous abscess of abdominal wall** 🔗

L02.212   **Cutaneous abscess of back [any part, except buttock]** 🔗

L02.213   **Cutaneous abscess of chest wall** 🔗

L02.214   **Cutaneous abscess of groin** 🔗

L02.215   **Cutaneous abscess of perineum** 🔗

L02.216   **Cutaneous abscess of umbilicus** 🔗

L02.219   **Cutaneous abscess of trunk, unspecified** 🔗

● **L02.22**   **Furuncle of trunk**
Boil of trunk
Folliculitis of trunk

L02.221   **Furuncle of abdominal wall**

L02.222   **Furuncle of back [any part, except buttock]**

L02.223   **Furuncle of chest wall**

L02.224   **Furuncle of groin**

L02.225   **Furuncle of perineum**

L02.226   **Furuncle of umbilicus**

L02.229   **Furuncle of trunk, unspecified**

● **L02.23**   **Carbuncle of trunk**

L02.231   **Carbuncle of abdominal wall**

L02.232   **Carbuncle of back [any part, except buttock]**

L02.233   **Carbuncle of chest wall**

L02.234   **Carbuncle of groin**

L02.235   **Carbuncle of perineum**

L02.236   **Carbuncle of umbilicus**

L02.239   **Carbuncle of trunk, unspecified**

● **L02.3**   **Cutaneous abscess, furuncle and carbuncle of buttock**

Excludes1   pilonidal cyst with abscess (L05.01)

L02.31   **Cutaneous abscess of buttock** 🔗
Cutaneous abscess of gluteal region
Ex: See PDX Collection 834

L02.32   **Furuncle of buttock**
Boil of buttock
Folliculitis of buttock
Furuncle of gluteal region

L02.33   **Carbuncle of buttock**
Carbuncle of gluteal region

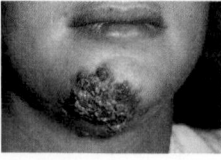

Figure 12-2 Impetigo. A thick, honey-yellow adherent crust covers the entire eroded surface. (From James WD, Elston DM, Berger TG, Andrews GC: Andrews' Diseases of the Skin: Clinical Dermatology, London, Saunders/Elsevier, 2011)

▶ New   ⇒ Revised   ~~deleted~~ Deleted   Excludes 1   Excludes 2   Includes   Use additional   Code first   Code also   Key words
OGCR Official Guidelines   ● Unacceptable Principal Diagnosis   X Assign placeholder X   ● Use Additional Character(s)   ▶ Manifestation Code   **Coding Clinic**

● **L02.4**   **Cutaneous abscess, furuncle and carbuncle of limb**
    Excludes2   Cutaneous abscess, furuncle and carbuncle of groin (L02.214, L02.224, L02.234)
      Cutaneous abscess, furuncle and carbuncle of hand (L02.5-)
      Cutaneous abscess, furuncle and carbuncle of foot (L02.6-)

   ● **L02.41**   **Cutaneous abscess of limb**
     L02.411   Cutaneous abscess of **right axilla**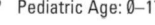
        (Ex:) See PDX Collection 835
     L02.412   Cutaneous abscess of **left axilla**
        (Ex:) See PDX Collection 835
     L02.413   Cutaneous abscess of **right upper limb**
        (Ex:) See PDX Collection 835
     L02.414   Cutaneous abscess of **left upper limb**
        (Ex:) See PDX Collection 835
     L02.415   Cutaneous abscess of **right lower limb**
        (Ex:) See PDX Collection 836
     L02.416   Cutaneous abscess of **left lower limb**
        (Ex:) See PDX Collection 836
     L02.419   Cutaneous abscess of limb, **unspecified**
        (Ex:) See PDX Collection 836

   ● **L02.42**   **Furuncle of limb**
     Boil of limb
     Folliculitis of limb
     L02.421   Furuncle of **right axilla**
     L02.422   Furuncle of **left axilla**
     L02.423   Furuncle of **right upper** limb
     L02.424   Furuncle of **left upper** limb
     L02.425   Furuncle of **right lower** limb
     L02.426   Furuncle of **left lower** limb
     L02.429   Furuncle of limb, **unspecified**

   ● **L02.43**   **Carbuncle of limb**
     L02.431   Carbuncle of **right axilla**
     L02.432   Carbuncle of **left axilla**
     L02.433   Carbuncle of **right upper** limb
     L02.434   Carbuncle of **left upper** limb
     L02.435   Carbuncle of **right lower** limb
     L02.436   Carbuncle of **left lower** limb
     L02.439   Carbuncle of limb, **unspecified**

● **L02.5**   Cutaneous abscess, furuncle and carbuncle of **hand**
   ● **L02.51**   **Cutaneous abscess of hand**
        (Ex:) **For category L02.51 CC codes:** See PDX Collection 837
     L02.511   Cutaneous abscess of **right hand**
     L02.512   Cutaneous abscess of **left hand**
     L02.519   Cutaneous abscess of **unspecified** hand

   ● **L02.52**   **Furuncle hand**
     Boil of hand
     Folliculitis of hand
     L02.521   Furuncle **right** hand
     L02.522   Furuncle **left** hand
     L02.529   Furuncle **unspecified** hand

   ● **L02.53**   **Carbuncle of hand**
     L02.531   Carbuncle of **right** hand
     L02.532   Carbuncle of **left** hand
     L02.539   Carbuncle of **unspecified** hand

● **L02.6**   Cutaneous abscess, furuncle and carbuncle of **foot**
   ● **L02.61**   **Cutaneous abscess of foot**
        (Ex:) **For category L02.61 CC codes:** See PDX Collection 838
     L02.611   Cutaneous abscess of **right foot**
     L02.612   Cutaneous abscess of **left foot**
     L02.619   Cutaneous abscess of **unspecified foot**

   ● **L02.62**   **Furuncle of foot**
     Boil of foot
     Folliculitis of foot
     L02.621   Furuncle of **right** foot
     L02.622   Furuncle of **left** foot
     L02.629   Furuncle of **unspecified** foot

   ● **L02.63**   **Carbuncle of foot**
     L02.631   Carbuncle of **right foot**
     L02.632   Carbuncle of **left foot**
     L02.639   Carbuncle of **unspecified foot**

● **L02.8**   Cutaneous abscess, furuncle and carbuncle of **other sites**
   ● **L02.81**   **Cutaneous abscess of other sites**
        (Ex:) **For category L02.81 CC codes:** See PDX Collection 839
     L02.811   Cutaneous abscess of **head** [any part, except face]
     L02.818   Cutaneous abscess of **other sites**

   ● **L02.82**   **Furuncle of other sites**
     Boil of other sites
     Folliculitis of other sites
     L02.821   Furuncle of **head** [any part, except face]
     L02.828   Furuncle of **other sites**

   ● **L02.83**   **Carbuncle of other sites**
     L02.831   Carbuncle of **head** [any part, except face]
     L02.838   Carbuncle of **other sites**

● **L02.9**   Cutaneous abscess, furuncle and carbuncle, **unspecified**
     L02.91   **Cutaneous abscess, unspecified**
        (Ex:) See PDX Collection 839
     L02.92   **Furuncle, unspecified**
        Boil NOS
        Furunculosis NOS
     L02.93   **Carbuncle, unspecified**

● **L03**   **Cellulitis and acute lymphangitis**
    Excludes2   cellulitis of anal and rectal region (K61.-)
      cellulitis of external auditory canal (H60.1)
      cellulitis of eyelid (H00.0)
      cellulitis of female external genital organs (N76.4)
      cellulitis of lacrimal apparatus (H04.3)
      cellulitis of male external genital organs (N48.2, N49.-)
      cellulitis of mouth (K12.2)
      cellulitis of nose (J34.0)
      eosinophilic cellulitis [Wells] (L98.3)
      febrile neutrophilic dermatosis [Sweet] (L98.2)
      lymphangitis (chronic) (subacute) (I89.1)

● **L03.0**   Cellulitis and acute lymphangitis of **finger and toe**
     Infection of nail
     Onychia
     Paronychia
     Perionychia
   ● **L03.01**   **Cellulitis of finger**
     Felon
     Whitlow
       Excludes1   herpetic whitlow (B00.89)
     L03.011   Cellulitis of **right** finger
     L03.012   Cellulitis of **left** finger
     L03.019   Cellulitis of **unspecified** finger

Item 12-1   **Onychia** is an inflammation of the tissue surrounding the nail with pus accumulation and loss of the nail, resulting from microscopic pathogens entering through small wounds. **Paronychia** is a nail disease also known as felon or whitlow and is a bacterial or fungal infection.

N Newborn Age: 0   **P** Pediatric Age: 0–17   **M** Maternity DX: 9–64   **A** Adult Age: 15–124   ♀ Females Only   ♂ Males Only

Complication\Comorbidity   Major C\C   (Ex:) CC/MCC Exclusions   Hospital-Acquired Condition   Hierarchical Condition Category

CHAPTER 12 (L00-L99)

- ● **L03.02** **Acute lymphangitis of finger**
      Hangnail with lymphangitis of finger
      - **L03.021** Acute lymphangitis of **right** finger
      - **L03.022** Acute lymphangitis of **left** finger
      - **L03.029** Acute lymphangitis of **unspecified** finger
- ● **L03.03** **Cellulitis of toe**
      - **L03.031** Cellulitis of **right** toe
      - **L03.032** Cellulitis of **left** toe
      - **L03.039** Cellulitis of **unspecified** toe
- ● **L03.04** **Acute lymphangitis of toe**
      Hangnail with lymphangitis of toe
      - **L03.041** Acute lymphangitis of **right** toe
      - **L03.042** Acute lymphangitis of **left** toe
      - **L03.049** Acute lymphangitis of **unspecified** toe
- ● **L03.1** Cellulitis and acute lymphangitis of **other parts of limb**
  - ● **L03.11** **Cellulitis of other parts of limb**
      Excludes2 cellulitis of fingers (L03.01-)
                    cellulitis of toes (L03.03-)
                    groin (L03.314)
      - **L03.111** Cellulitis of **right axilla** 🐾
                      (Ex:) See PDX Collection 835
      - **L03.112** Cellulitis of **left axilla** 🐾
                      (Ex:) See PDX Collection 835
      - **L03.113** Cellulitis of **right upper limb** 🐾
                      (Ex:) See PDX Collection 835
      - **L03.114** Cellulitis of **left upper limb** 🐾
                      (Ex:) See PDX Collection 835
                      Coding Clinic: 2019, Q1, P13
      - **L03.115** Cellulitis of **right lower limb** 🐾
                      (Ex:) See PDX Collection 836
      - **L03.116** Cellulitis of **left lower limb** 🐾
                      (Ex:) See PDX Collection 836
      - **L03.119** Cellulitis of **unspecified** part of limb 🐾
                      (Ex:) See PDX Collection 836
  - ● **L03.12** **Acute lymphangitis of other parts of limb**
      Excludes2 acute lymphangitis of fingers (L03.2-)
                    acute lymphangitis of toes (L03.04-)
                    acute lymphangitis of groin (L03.324)
      - **L03.121** Acute lymphangitis of **right axilla** 🐾
                      (Ex:) See PDX Collection 835
      - **L03.122** Acute lymphangitis of **left axilla** 🐾
                      (Ex:) See PDX Collection 835
      - **L03.123** Acute lymphangitis of **right upper** limb 🐾
                      (Ex:) See PDX Collection 835
      - **L03.124** Acute lymphangitis of **left upper** limb 🐾
                      (Ex:) See PDX Collection 835
      - **L03.125** Acute lymphangitis of **right lower** limb 🐾
                      (Ex:) See PDX Collection 836
      - **L03.126** Acute lymphangitis of **left lower** limb 🐾
                      (Ex:) See PDX Collection 836
      - **L03.129** Acute lymphangitis of **unspecified** part of limb 🐾
                      (Ex:) See PDX Collection 836

Item 12–2 **Cellulitis** is an acute spreading bacterial infection below the surface of the skin characterized by redness (erythema), warmth, swelling, pain, fever, chills, and enlarged lymph nodes ("swollen glands").

- ● **L03.2** Cellulitis and acute lymphangitis of **face and neck**
  - ● **L03.21** Cellulitis and acute lymphangitis of **face**
      - **L03.211** **Cellulitis of face** 🐾
                      Excludes2 abscess of orbit (H05.01-)
                                    cellulitis of ear (H60.1-)
                                    cellulitis of eyelid (H00.0-)
                                    cellulitis of head (L03.81)
                                    cellulitis of lacrimal apparatus (H04.3)
                                    cellulitis of lip (K13.0)
                                    cellulitis of mouth (K12.2)
                                    cellulitis of nose (internal) (J34.0)
                                    cellulitis of orbit (H05.01-)
                                    cellulitis of scalp (L03.81)
                      (Ex:) See PDX Collection 840
      - **L03.212** **Acute lymphangitis of face** 🐾
                      (Ex:) See PDX Collection 3231
      - **L03.213** **Periorbital cellulitis** 🐾
                      Preseptal cellulitis
                      (Ex:) See PDX Collection 840
                      Coding Clinic: 2016, Q4, P36
  - ● **L03.22** Cellulitis and acute lymphangitis of **neck**
                  (Ex:) For category L03.22 CC codes: See PDX Collection 832
      - **L03.221** **Cellulitis of neck** 🐾
      - **L03.222** **Acute lymphangitis of neck** 🐾
- ● **L03.3** Cellulitis and acute lymphangitis of **trunk**
  - ● **L03.31** **Cellulitis of trunk**
      Excludes2 cellulitis of anal and rectal regions (K61.-)
                    cellulitis of breast NOS (N61.0)
                    cellulitis of female external genital organs (N76.4)
                    cellulitis of male external genital organs (N48.2, N49.-)
                    omphalitis of newborn (P38.-)
                    puerperal cellulitis of breast (O91.2)
                  (Ex:) For category L03.31 CC codes unless otherwise indicated:
                        See PDX Collection 833
      - **L03.311** Cellulitis of **abdominal wall** 🐾
                      Excludes2 cellulitis of umbilicus (L03.316)
                                    cellulitis of groin (L03.314)
      - **L03.312** Cellulitis of **back [any part except buttock]** 🐾
      - **L03.313** Cellulitis of **chest wall** 🐾
      - **L03.314** Cellulitis of **groin** 🐾
      - **L03.315** Cellulitis of **perineum** 🐾
      - **L03.316** Cellulitis of **umbilicus** 🐾
      - **L03.317** Cellulitis of **buttock** 🐾
                      (Ex:) See PDX Collection 834
      - **L03.319** Cellulitis of trunk, **unspecified** 🐾

▶ New   ⇒ Revised   ~~deleted~~ Deleted   Excludes 1   Excludes 2   Includes   Use additional   Code first   Code also   Key words

990   OGCR Official Guidelines   ● Unacceptable Principal Diagnosis   X Assign placeholder X   ● Use Additional Character(s)   ▶ Manifestation Code   Coding Clinic

● **L03.32**   **Acute lymphangitis of trunk**
    (Ex) **For category L03.32 CC codes unless otherwise indicated:**
    See PDX Collection 833

    L03.321   Acute lymphangitis of **abdominal wall** 🐾

    L03.322   Acute lymphangitis of **back** [any part except buttock] 🐾

    L03.323   Acute lymphangitis of **chest wall** 🐾

    L03.324   Acute lymphangitis of **groin** 🐾

    L03.325   Acute lymphangitis of **perineum** 🐾

    L03.326   Acute lymphangitis of **umbilicus** 🐾

    L03.327   Acute lymphangitis of **buttock** 🐾
        (Ex) See PDX Collection 834

    L03.329   Acute lymphangitis of **trunk, unspecified** 🐾

● **L03.8**   **Cellulitis and acute lymphangitis of other sites**
    (Ex) **For category L03.8 CC codes:** See PDX Collection 839

  ● **L03.81**   **Cellulitis of other sites**

    L03.811   Cellulitis of **head** [any part, except face] 🐾
        Cellulitis of scalp

        Excludes2   cellulitis of face (L03.211)

    L03.818   Cellulitis of **other sites** 🐾

  ● **L03.89**   **Acute lymphangitis of other sites**

    L03.891   Acute lymphangitis of **head** [any part, except face] 🐾

    L03.898   Acute lymphangitis of **other sites** 🐾

● **L03.9**   **Cellulitis and acute lymphangitis, unspecified**
    (Ex) **For category L03.9 CC codes:** See PDX Collection 839

    L03.90   **Cellulitis, unspecified** 🐾

    L03.91   **Acute lymphangitis, unspecified** 🐾

        Excludes1   lymphangitis NOS (I89.1)

● **L04**   **Acute lymphadenitis**
Short-term inflammation of lymph nodes which can be regionalized to involve a given area of the lymph system or systemic involving much of the body

  Includes   abscess (acute) of lymph nodes, except mesenteric
        acute lymphadenitis, except mesenteric

  Excludes1   chronic or subacute lymphadenitis, except mesenteric (I88.1)
        enlarged lymph nodes (R59.-)
        human immunodeficiency virus [HIV] disease resulting in generalized lymphadenopathy (B20)
        lymphadenitis NOS (I88.9)
        nonspecific mesenteric lymphadenitis (I88.0)

L04.0   Acute lymphadenitis of **face, head and neck**

L04.1   Acute lymphadenitis of **trunk**

L04.2   Acute lymphadenitis of **upper limb**
    Acute lymphadenitis of axilla
    Acute lymphadenitis of shoulder

L04.3   Acute lymphadenitis of **lower limb**
    Acute lymphadenitis of hip
    Excludes2   acute lymphadenitis of groin (L04.1)

L04.8   Acute lymphadenitis of **other sites**

L04.9   Acute lymphadenitis, **unspecified**

Item 12–3   **Abscess** is a localized collection of pus in tissues or organs and is a sign of infection, resulting in swelling and inflammation.

Item 12–4   **Pilonidal cyst,** also called a coccygeal cyst, is the result of a disorder called pilonidal disease. The cyst usually contains hair and pus.

● **L05**   **Pilonidal cyst and sinus**

  ● **L05.0**   **Pilonidal cyst and sinus with abscess**
    (Ex) **For category L05.0 CC codes:** See PDX Collection 841

    L05.01   **Pilonidal cyst with abscess** 🐾
        Pilonidal abscess
        Pilonidal dimple with abscess
        Postanal dimple with abscess

        Excludes2   congenital sacral dimple (Q82.6)
            parasacral dimple (Q82.6)

    L05.02   **Pilonidal sinus with abscess** 🐾
        Coccygeal fistula with abscess
        Coccygeal sinus with abscess
        Pilonidal fistula with abscess

  ● **L05.9**   **Pilonidal cyst and sinus without abscess**

    L05.91   **Pilonidal cyst without abscess**
        Pilonidal dimple
        Postanal dimple
        Pilonidal cyst NOS

        Excludes2   congenital sacral dimple (Q82.6)
            parasacral dimple (Q82.6)

    L05.92   **Pilonidal sinus without abscess**
        Coccygeal fistula
        Coccygeal sinus without abscess
        Pilonidal fistula

● **L08**   **Other local infections of skin and subcutaneous tissue**

  L08.0   **Pyoderma**
    Dermatitis gangrenosa
    Purulent dermatitis
    Septic dermatitis
    Suppurative dermatitis
    Excludes1   pyoderma gangrenosum (L88)
        pyoderma vegetans (L08.81)

  L08.1   **Erythrasma** 🐾
    (Ex) See PDX Collection 107

  ● **L08.8**   **Other specified local infections of the skin and subcutaneous tissue**

    L08.81   **Pyoderma vegetans**
        Excludes1   pyoderma gangrenosum (L88)
            pyoderma NOS (L08.0)

    L08.82   **Omphalitis not of newborn**
        Excludes1   omphalitis of newborn (P38.-)

    L08.89   **Other specified local infections of the skin and subcutaneous tissue**

  L08.9   **Local infection of the skin and subcutaneous tissue, unspecified**

BULLOUS DISORDERS (L10-L14)

  Excludes1   benign familial pemphigus [Hailey-Hailey] (Q82.8)
        staphylococcal scalded skin syndrome (L00)
        toxic epidermal necrolysis [Lyell] (L51.2)

CHAPTER 12 (L00-L99)

N Newborn Age: 0   **P** Pediatric Age: 0–17   **M** Maternity DX: 9–64   **A** Adult Age: 15–124   ♀ Females Only   ♂ Males Only

🐾 Complication\Comorbidity   🐾 Major C\C   (Ex) CC/MCC Exclusions   🐾 Hospital-Acquired Condition   🐾 Hierarchical Condition Category

991

CHAPTER 12 (L00-L99)

● **L10** **Pemphigus**

     Excludes1   pemphigus neonatorum (L01.03)

     (Ex) **For category L10 CC codes:** See PDX Collection 842

     L10.0   Pemphigus vulgaris

     L10.1   Pemphigus vegetans

     L10.2   Pemphigus foliaceous

     L10.3   Brazilian pemphigus [fogo selvagem]

     L10.4   Pemphigus erythematosus

            Senear-Usher syndrome

     L10.5   Drug-induced pemphigus

            Use additional code for adverse effect, if applicable, to identify drug (T36-T50 with fifth or sixth character 5)

   ● **L10.8**   Other pemphigus

         L10.81   Paraneoplastic pemphigus

         L10.89   Other pemphigus

     L10.9   Pemphigus, unspecified

● **L11** **Other acantholytic disorders**

     L11.0   Acquired keratosis follicularis

         Excludes1   keratosis follicularis (congenital) [Darier-White] (Q82.8)

     L11.1   Transient acantholytic dermatosis [Grover]

     L11.8   Other specified acantholytic disorders

     L11.9   Acantholytic disorder, unspecified

● **L12** **Pemphigoid**

     Excludes1   herpes gestationis (O26.4-)

                      impetigo herpetiformis (L40.1)

     L12.0   Bullous pemphigoid

         (Ex) See PDX Collection 842

     L12.1   Cicatricial pemphigoid

            Benign mucous membrane pemphigoid

     L12.2   Chronic bullous disease of childhood   P

            Juvenile dermatitis herpetiformis

   ● **L12.3**   Acquired epidermolysis bullosa

         Excludes1   epidermolysis bullosa (congenital) (Q81.-)

         (Ex) **For category L12.3 CC codes:** See PDX Collection 843

         L12.30   Acquired epidermolysis bullosa, unspecified

         L12.31   Epidermolysis bullosa due to drug

                 Use additional code for adverse effect, if applicable, to identify drug (T36-T50 with fifth or sixth character 5)

         L12.35   Other acquired epidermolysis bullosa

     L12.8   Other pemphigoid

         (Ex) See PDX Collection 842

     L12.9   Pemphigoid, unspecified

         (Ex) See PDX Collection 842

Item 12–5 Dermatitis herpetiformis, also known as Duhring's disease, is a systemic disease characterized by small blisters (3 to 5 mm) and occasionally large bullae (> 5 mm).

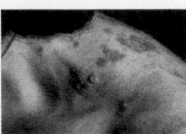

Figure 12-3   Dermatitis herpetiformis. (From Terhorst D: BASICS Dermatologie, München, Elsevier, Urban & Fischer, 2011)

● **L13** **Other bullous disorders**

     L13.0   Dermatitis herpetiformis

            Duhring's disease

            Hydroa herpetiformis

         Excludes1   juvenile dermatitis herpetiformis (L12.2)

                       senile dermatitis herpetiformis (L12.0)

     L13.1   Subcorneal pustular dermatitis

            Sneddon-Wilkinson disease

     L13.8   Other specified bullous disorders

     L13.9   Bullous disorder, unspecified

▷ **L14** *Bullous disorders in diseases classified elsewhere*

     Code first underlying disease

DERMATITIS AND ECZEMA (L20-L30)

     Note: In this block the terms dermatitis and eczema are used synonymously and interchangeably.

     Excludes2   chronic (childhood) granulomatous disease (D71)

                      dermatitis gangrenosa (L08.0)

                      dermatitis herpetiformis (L13.0)

                      dry skin dermatitis (L85.3)

                      factitial dermatitis (L98.1)

                      perioral dermatitis (L71.0)

                      radiation-related disorders of the skin and subcutaneous tissue (L55-L59)

                      stasis dermatitis (I87.2)

● **L20** **Atopic dermatitis**

     L20.0   Besnier's prurigo

   ● **L20.8**   Other atopic dermatitis

         Excludes2   circumscribed neurodermatitis (L28.0)

         L20.81   Atopic neurodermatitis

                 Diffuse neurodermatitis

         L20.82   Flexural eczema

         L20.83   Infantile (acute) (chronic) eczema   P

         L20.84   Intrinsic (allergic) eczema

         L20.89   Other atopic dermatitis

     L20.9   Atopic dermatitis, unspecified

● **L21** **Seborrheic dermatitis**

     Excludes2   infective dermatitis (L30.3)

                      seborrheic keratosis (L82.-)

     L21.0   Seborrhea capitis

            Cradle cap

            Coding Clinic: 2018, Q1, P6

     L21.1   Seborrheic infantile dermatitis   P

     L21.8   Other seborrheic dermatitis

     L21.9   Seborrheic dermatitis, unspecified

            Seborrhea NOS

Item 12–6 Seborrheic dermatitis is characterized by greasy, scaly, red patches and is associated with oily skin and scalp.

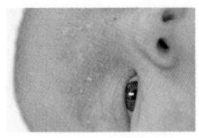

Figure 12-4   Seborrheic dermatitis. (Getty Image)

▶ New   ⮕ Revised   ~~deleted~~ Deleted   Excludes 1   Excludes 2   Includes   Use additional   Code first   Code also   Key words

OGCR Official Guidelines   ● Unacceptable Principal Diagnosis   X Assign placeholder X   ● Use Additional Character(s)   ▷ Manifestation Code   **Coding Clinic**

Item 12–7 **Atopic dermatitis,** also known as atopic eczema, infantile eczema, disseminated neuro dermatitis, flexural eczema, and *prurigo diathesique* (Besnier), is characterized by intense itching and is often hereditary.

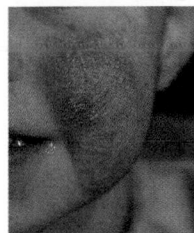

Figure 12-5 Atopic dermatitis. (From Chabner D-E: The Language of Medicine, St. Louis, MO, Saunders/Elsevier, 2007)

L22   **Diaper dermatitis**
  Diaper erythema
  Diaper rash
  Psoriasiform diaper rash

● L23   **Allergic contact dermatitis**
  Excludes1 allergy NOS (T78.4Ø)
     contact dermatitis NOS (L25.9)
     dermatitis NOS (L3Ø.9)
  Excludes2 dermatitis due to substances taken internally (L27.-)
     dermatitis of eyelid (HØ1.1-)
     diaper dermatitis (L22)
     eczema of external ear (H6Ø.5-)
     irritant contact dermatitis (L24.-)
     perioral dermatitis (L71.Ø)
     radiation-related disorders of the skin and subcutaneous tissue (L55-L59)

L23.Ø   **Allergic contact dermatitis due to metals**
  Allergic contact dermatitis due to chromium
  Allergic contact dermatitis due to nickel

L23.1   **Allergic contact dermatitis due to adhesives**

L23.2   **Allergic contact dermatitis due to cosmetics**

L23.3   **Allergic contact dermatitis due to drugs in contact with skin**
  Use additional code for adverse effect, if applicable, to identify drug (T36-T5Ø with fifth or sixth character 5)
  Excludes2 dermatitis due to ingested drugs and medicaments (L27.Ø-L27.1)

L23.4   **Allergic contact dermatitis due to dyes**

L23.5   **Allergic contact dermatitis due to other chemical products**
  Allergic contact dermatitis due to cement
  Allergic contact dermatitis due to insecticide
  Allergic contact dermatitis due to plastic
  Allergic contact dermatitis due to rubber

L23.6   **Allergic contact dermatitis due to food in contact with the skin**
  Excludes2 dermatitis due to ingested food (L27.2)

L23.7   **Allergic contact dermatitis due to plants, except food**
  Excludes2 allergy NOS due to pollen (J3Ø.1)

● L23.8   **Allergic contact dermatitis due to other agents**
  L23.81   **Allergic contact dermatitis due to animal (cat) (dog) dander**
    Allergic contact dermatitis due to animal (cat) (dog) hair
  L23.89   **Allergic contact dermatitis due to other agents**

L23.9   **Allergic contact dermatitis, unspecified cause**
  Allergic contact eczema NOS

● L24   **Irritant contact dermatitis**
  Excludes1 allergy NOS (T78.4Ø)
     contact dermatitis NOS (L25.9)
     dermatitis NOS (L3Ø.9)
  Excludes2 allergic contact dermatitis (L23.-)
     dermatitis due to substances taken internally (L27.-)
     dermatitis of eyelid (HØ1.1-)
     diaper dermatitis (L22)
     eczema of external ear (H6Ø.5-)
     perioral dermatitis (L71.Ø)
     radiation-related disorders of the skin and subcutaneous tissue (L55-L59)

L24.Ø   **Irritant contact dermatitis due to detergents**

L24.1   **Irritant contact dermatitis due to oils and greases**

L24.2   **Irritant contact dermatitis due to solvents**
  Irritant contact dermatitis due to chlorocompound
  Irritant contact dermatitis due to cyclohexane
  Irritant contact dermatitis due to ester
  Irritant contact dermatitis due to glycol
  Irritant contact dermatitis due to hydrocarbon
  Irritant contact dermatitis due to ketone

L24.3   **Irritant contact dermatitis due to cosmetics**

L24.4   **Irritant contact dermatitis due to drugs in contact with skin**
  Use additional code for adverse effect, if applicable, to identify drug (T36-T5Ø with fifth or sixth character 5)

L24.5   **Irritant contact dermatitis due to other chemical products**
  Irritant contact dermatitis due to cement
  Irritant contact dermatitis due to insecticide
  Irritant contact dermatitis due to plastic
  Irritant contact dermatitis due to rubber

L24.6   **Irritant contact dermatitis due to food in contact with skin**
  Excludes2 dermatitis due to ingested food (L27.2)

L24.7   **Irritant contact dermatitis due to plants, except food**
  Excludes2 allergy NOS to pollen (J3Ø.1)

● L24.8   **Irritant contact dermatitis due to other agents**
  L24.81   **Irritant contact dermatitis due to metals**
    Irritant contact dermatitis due to chromium
    Irritant contact dermatitis due to nickel
  L24.89   **Irritant contact dermatitis due to other agents**
    Irritant contact dermatitis due to dyes

L24.9   **Irritant contact dermatitis, unspecified cause**
  Irritant contact eczema NOS

▶● L24.A   **Irritant contact dermatitis due to friction or contact with body fluids**
  ▶**Excludes1** virritant contact dermatitis related to stoma or fistula (L24.B-)
  ▶**Excludes2** erythema intertrigo (L3Ø.4)
  ▶ L24.AØ   **Irritant contact dermatitis due to friction or contact with body fluids, unspecified**
  ▶ L24.A1   **Irritant contact dermatitis due to saliva**
  ▶ L24.A2   **Irritant contact dermatitis due to fecal, urinary or dual incontinence**
    ▶**Excludes1** diaper dermatitis (L22)
  ▶ L24.A9   **Irritant contact dermatitis due friction or contact with other specified body fluids**
    ▶ Irritant contact dermatitis related to endotracheal tube
    ▶ Wound fluids, exudate

▶● L24.B   **Irritant contact dermatitis related to stoma or fistula**
  ▶ Use additional code to identify any artificial opening status (Z93.-), if applicable, for contact dermatitis related to stoma secretions
  ▶ L24.BØ   **Irritant contact dermatitis related to unspecified stoma or fistula**
    ▶ Irritant contact dermatitis related to fistula NOS
    ▶ Irritant contact dermatitis related to stoma NOS
  ▶ L24.B1   **Irritant contact dermatitis related to digestive stoma or fistula**
    ▶ Irritant contact dermatitis related to gastrostomy
    ▶ Irritant contact dermatitis related to jejunostomy
    ▶ Irritant contact dermatitis related to saliva or spit fistula
  ▶ L24.B2   **Irritant contact dermatitis related to respiratory stoma or fistula**
    ▶ Irritant contact dermatitis related to tracheostomy
  ▶ L24.B3   **Irritant contact dermatitis related to fecal or urinary stoma or fistula**
    ▶ Irritant contact dermatitis related to colostomy
    ▶ Irritant contact dermatitis related to enterocutaneous fistula
    ▶ Irritant contact dermatitis related to ileostomy

N Newborn Age: Ø **P** Pediatric Age: Ø–17 **M** Maternity DX: 9–64 **A** Adult Age: 15–124 ♀ Females Only ♂ Males Only

🔴 Complication\Comorbidity 🔴 Major C\C (Ex) CC/MCC Exclusions 🔴 Hospital-Acquired Condition 🔴 Hierarchical Condition Category

993

CHAPTER 12 (LØØ-L99)

● **L25**   **Unspecified contact dermatitis**

     Excludes1   allergic contact dermatitis (L23.-)
                    allergy NOS (T78.40)
                    dermatitis NOS (L30.9)
                    irritant contact dermatitis (L24.-)

     Excludes2   dermatitis due to ingested substances (L27.-)
                    dermatitis of eyelid (H01.1-)
                    eczema of external ear (H60.5-)
                    perioral dermatitis (L71.0)
                    radiation-related disorders of the skin and
                       subcutaneous tissue (L55-L59)

     L25.0   Unspecified contact dermatitis due to cosmetics

     L25.1   Unspecified contact dermatitis due to drugs in contact with skin

           Use additional code for adverse effect, if applicable, to identify drug (T36-T50 with fifth or sixth character 5)

           Excludes2   dermatitis due to ingested drugs and medicaments (L27.0-L27.1)

     L25.2   Unspecified contact dermatitis due to dyes

     L25.3   Unspecified contact dermatitis due to other chemical products
           Unspecified contact dermatitis due to cement
           Unspecified contact dermatitis due to insecticide

     L25.4   Unspecified contact dermatitis due to food in contact with skin

           Excludes2   dermatitis due to ingested food (L27.2)

     L25.5   Unspecified contact dermatitis due to plants, except food
           Excludes1   nettle rash (L50.9)
           Excludes2   allergy NOS due to pollen (J30.1)

     L25.8   Unspecified contact dermatitis due to other agents

     L25.9   Unspecified contact dermatitis, unspecified cause
           Contact dermatitis (occupational) NOS
           Contact eczema (occupational) NOS

L26   **Exfoliative dermatitis**
     Hebra's pityriasis
     Excludes1   Ritter's disease (L00)

● **L27**   **Dermatitis due to substances taken internally**
     Excludes1   allergy NOS (T78.40)
     Excludes2   adverse food reaction, except dermatitis (T78.0-T78.1)
                    contact dermatitis (L23-L25)
                    drug photoallergic response (L56.1)
                    drug phototoxic response (L56.0)
                    urticaria (L50.-)

     L27.0   Generalized skin eruption due to drugs and medicaments taken internally
           Use additional code for adverse effect, if applicable, to identify drug (T36-T50 with fifth or sixth character 5)

     L27.1   Localized skin eruption due to drugs and medicaments taken internally
           Use additional code for adverse effect, if applicable, to identify drug (T36-T50 with fifth or sixth character 5)

     L27.2   Dermatitis due to ingested food
           Excludes2   dermatitis due to food in contact with skin (L23.6, L24.6, L25.4)

     L27.8   Dermatitis due to other substances taken internally

     L27.9   Dermatitis due to unspecified substance taken internally

● **L28**   **Lichen simplex chronicus and prurigo**
     L28.0   Lichen simplex chronicus
           Circumscribed neurodermatitis
           Lichen NOS

     L28.1   Prurigo nodularis

     L28.2   Other prurigo
           Prurigo NOS   Prurigo mitis
           Prurigo Hebra   Urticaria papulosa

● **L29**   **Pruritus**
     Excludes1   neurotic excoriation (L98.1)
                    psychogenic pruritus (F45.8)

     L29.0   Pruritus ani
     L29.1   Pruritus scroti ♂
     L29.2   Pruritus vulvae ♀
     L29.3   Anogenital pruritus, unspecified
     L29.8   Other pruritus
     L29.9   Pruritus, unspecified
           Itch NOS

● **L30**   **Other and unspecified dermatitis**
     Excludes2   contact dermatitis (L23-L25)
                    dry skin dermatitis (L85.3)
                    small plaque parapsoriasis (L41.3)
                    stasis dermatitis (I87.2)

     L30.0   Nummular dermatitis
     L30.1   Dyshidrosis [pompholyx]
     L30.2   Cutaneous autosensitization
           Candidid [levurid]   Eczematid
           Dermatophytid

     L30.3   Infective dermatitis
           Infectious eczematoid dermatitis

     L30.4   Erythema intertrigo

     L30.5   Pityriasis alba
           Coding Clinic: 2018, Q1, P6

     L30.8   Other specified dermatitis

     L30.9   Dermatitis, unspecified
           Eczema NOS

PAPULOSQUAMOUS DISORDERS (L40-L45)

● **L40**   **Psoriasis**
     L40.0   Psoriasis vulgaris
           Nummular psoriasis   Plaque psoriasis

     L40.1   Generalized pustular psoriasis
           Impetigo herpetiformis   Von Zumbusch's disease

     L40.2   Acrodermatitis continua
     L40.3   Pustulosis palmaris et plantaris
     L40.4   Guttate psoriasis
     ● **L40.5**   Arthropathic psoriasis
           L40.50   Arthropathic psoriasis, unspecified
           L40.51   Distal interphalangeal psoriatic arthropathy
           L40.52   Psoriatic arthritis mutilans
           L40.53   Psoriatic spondylitis
           L40.54   Psoriatic juvenile arthropathy
           L40.59   Other psoriatic arthropathy

     L40.8   Other psoriasis
           Flexural psoriasis

     L40.9   Psoriasis, unspecified

● **L41**   **Parapsoriasis**
     Excludes1   poikiloderma vasculare atrophicans (L94.5)
     L41.0   Pityriasis lichenoides et varioliformis acuta
           Mucha-Habermann disease
     L41.1   Pityriasis lichenoides chronica
     L41.3   Small plaque parapsoriasis
     L41.4   Large plaque parapsoriasis
     L41.5   Retiform parapsoriasis
     L41.8   Other parapsoriasis
     L41.9   Parapsoriasis, unspecified

     L42   Pityriasis rosea

Item 12-8 Psoriasis is a chronic, recurrent inflammatory skin disease characterized by small patches covered with thick, silvery scales. **Parapsoriasis** is a treatment-resistant erythroderma. **Pityriasis rosea** is characterized by a herald patch that is a single large lesion and that usually appears on the trunk and is followed by scattered, smaller lesions.

● **L43**   **Lichen planus**
    Excludes1   lichen planopilaris (L66.1)
    L43.0   **Hypertrophic** lichen planus
    L43.1   **Bullous** lichen planus
    L43.2   Lichenoid **drug reaction**
        Use additional code for adverse effect, if applicable, to identify drug (T36-T50 with fifth or sixth character 5)
    L43.3   **Subacute (active)** lichen planus
        Lichen planus tropicus
    L43.8   **Other** lichen planus
    L43.9   Lichen planus, **unspecified**

● **L44**   **Other papulosquamous disorders**
    L44.0   Pityriasis rubra pilaris
    L44.1   Lichen nitidus
    L44.2   Lichen striatus
    L44.3   Lichen ruber moniliformis
    L44.4   Infantile papular acrodermatitis [Gianotti-Crosti]   **P**
    L44.8   Other specified papulosquamous disorders
    L44.9   Papulosquamous disorder, **unspecified**

▹ *L45*   *Papulosquamous disorders in diseases classified elsewhere*
    Code first underlying disease

URTICARIA AND ERYTHEMA (L49-L54)

    Excludes1   Lyme disease (A69.2-)
                 rosacea (L71.-)

● **L49**   **Exfoliation due to erythematous conditions according to extent of body surface involved**
    Code first erythematous condition causing exfoliation, such as:
        Ritter's disease (L00)
        (Staphylococcal) scalded skin syndrome (L00)
        Stevens-Johnson syndrome (L51.1)
        Stevens-Johnson syndrome-toxic epidermal necrolysis overlap syndrome (L51.3)
        Toxic epidermal necrolysis (L51.2)
  ● **L49.0**   **Exfoliation due to erythematous condition involving less than 10 percent of body surface**
        Exfoliation due to erythematous condition NOS
  ● **L49.1**   **Exfoliation due to erythematous condition involving 10-19 percent of body surface**
  ● **L49.2**   **Exfoliation due to erythematous condition involving 20-29 percent of body surface**
  ● **L49.3**   **Exfoliation due to erythematous condition involving 30-39 percent of body surface**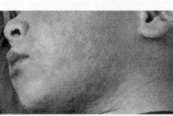
        (Ex:) See PDX Collection 844
  ● **L49.4**   **Exfoliation due to erythematous condition involving 40-49 percent of body surface**
        (Ex:) See PDX Collection 845
  ● **L49.5**   **Exfoliation due to erythematous condition involving 50-59 percent of body surface**
        (Ex:) See PDX Collection 846
  ● **L49.6**   **Exfoliation due to erythematous condition involving 60-69 percent of body surface**
        (Ex:) See PDX Collection 847
  ● **L49.7**   **Exfoliation due to erythematous condition involving 70-79 percent of body surface**
        (Ex:) See PDX Collection 848

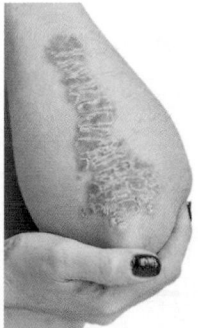

Figure 12-6   Erythematous plaques with silvery scales in a patient with psoriasis. (Getty Image)

Figure 12-7   Urticaria (hives). *(Courtesy of David Effron, MD.)* (Getty Image)

Item 12–9   **Urticaria** is a vascular reaction in which wheals surrounded by a red halo appear and cause severe itching. The causes of urticaria or hives are extensive and varied (e.g., food, heat, cold, drugs, stress, infections).

  ● **L49.8**   **Exfoliation due to erythematous condition involving 80-89 percent of body surface**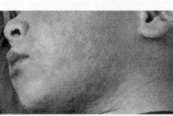
        (Ex:) See PDX Collection 849
  ● **L49.9**   **Exfoliation due to erythematous condition involving 90 or more percent of body surface**
        (Ex:) See PDX Collection 850

● **L50**   **Urticaria**
    Excludes1   allergic contact dermatitis (L23.-)
                 angioneurotic edema (T78.3)
                 giant urticaria (T78.3)
                 hereditary angio-edema (D84.1)
                 Quincke's edema (T78.3)
                 serum urticaria (T80.6-)
                 solar urticaria (L56.3)
                 urticaria neonatorum (P83.8)
                 urticaria papulosa (L28.2)
                 urticaria pigmentosa (D47.01)
    L50.0   **Allergic urticaria**
    L50.1   **Idiopathic urticaria**
    L50.2   **Urticaria due to cold and heat**
        Excludes2   familial cold urticaria (M04.2)
    L50.3   **Dermatographic urticaria**
    L50.4   **Vibratory urticaria**
    L50.5   **Cholinergic urticaria**
    L50.6   **Contact urticaria**
    L50.8   **Other urticaria**
        Chronic urticaria
        Recurrent periodic urticaria
    L50.9   Urticaria, **unspecified**

● **L51**   **Erythema multiforme**
    Use additional code for adverse effect, if applicable, to identify drug (T36-T50 with fifth or sixth character 5)
    Use additional code to identify associated manifestations, such as:
        arthropathy associated with dermatological disorders (M14.8-)
        conjunctival edema (H11.42)
        conjunctivitis (H10.22-)
        corneal scars and opacities (H17.-)
        corneal ulcer (H16.0-)
        edema of eyelid (H02.84-)
        inflammation of eyelid (H01.8)
        keratoconjunctivitis sicca (H16.22-)
        mechanical lagophthalmos (H02.22-)
        stomatitis (K12.-)
        symblepharon (H11.23-)
    Use additional code to identify percentage of skin exfoliation (L49.-)
    Excludes1   staphylococcal scalded skin syndrome (L00)
                 Ritter's disease (L00)
    (Ex:) **For category L51 CC codes:** See PDX Collection 843
    L51.0   **Nonbullous erythema multiforme**
    L51.1   **Stevens-Johnson syndrome**
    L51.2   **Toxic epidermal necrolysis [Lyell]**
    L51.3   **Stevens-Johnson syndrome-toxic epidermal necrolysis overlap syndrome**
        SJS-TEN overlap syndrome
    L51.8   **Other erythema multiforme**
    L51.9   **Erythema multiforme, unspecified**
        Erythema iris
        Erythema multiforme major NOS
        Erythema multiforme minor NOS
        Herpes iris

N Newborn Age: 0   **P** Pediatric Age: 0–17   **M** Maternity DX: 9–64   **A** Adult Age: 15–124   ♀ Females Only   ♂ Males Only

Complication\Comorbidity   Major C\C   (Ex:) CC/MCC Exclusions   Hospital-Acquired Condition   Hierarchical Condition Category   **995**

L52   **Erythema nodosum**
     Excludes1   tuberculous erythema nodosum (A18.4)

● L53   **Other erythematous conditions**
     Excludes1   erythema ab igne (L59.0)
                   erythema due to external agents in contact with
                         skin (L23-L25)
                   erythema intertrigo (L30.4)
     (Ex) **For category L53 CC codes:** See PDX Collection 851

     L53.0   **Toxic erythema** 🖐
         Code first poisoning due to drug or toxin, if applicable
             (T36-T65 with fifth or sixth character 1-4 or 6)
         Use additional code for adverse effect, if applicable,
             to identify drug (T36-T50 with fifth or sixth
             character 5)
         Excludes1   neonatal erythema toxicum (P83.1)

     L53.1   **Erythema** annulare centrifugum 🖐
     L53.2   **Erythema** marginatum 🖐
     L53.3   **Other** chronic figurate **erythema** 🖐
     L53.8   **Other** specified erythematous conditions
     L53.9   **Erythematous condition,** unspecified
            Erythema NOS
            Erythroderma NOS

▷ *L54*   *Erythema in diseases classified elsewhere*
       Code first underlying disease

RADIATION-RELATED DISORDERS OF THE SKIN AND SUBCUTANEOUS TISSUE (L55-L59)

● L55   **Sunburn**
     L55.0   **Sunburn of** first degree
     L55.1   **Sunburn of** second degree
     L55.2   **Sunburn of** third degree
     L55.9   **Sunburn,** unspecified

● L56   **Other acute skin changes due to ultraviolet radiation**
     Use additional code to identify the source of the ultraviolet
       radiation (W89, X32)

     L56.0   **Drug phototoxic response**
         Use additional code for adverse effect, if applicable,
             to identify drug (T36-T50 with fifth or sixth
             character 5)
     L56.1   **Drug photoallergic response**
         Use additional code for adverse effect, if applicable,
             to identify drug (T36-T50 with fifth or sixth
             character 5)
     L56.2   **Photocontact dermatitis [berloque dermatitis]**
     L56.3   **Solar urticaria**
     L56.4   **Polymorphous light eruption**
     L56.5   **Disseminated superficial actinic porokeratosis (DSAP)**
     L56.8   **Other specified acute skin changes due to ultraviolet
          radiation**
     L56.9   **Acute skin change due to ultraviolet radiation,**
          unspecified

● L57   **Skin changes due to chronic exposure to nonionizing radiation**
     Use additional code to identify the source of the ultraviolet
       radiation (W89), or other nonionizing radiation (W90)

     L57.0   **Actinic keratosis**
         Keratosis NOS   Solar keratosis
         Senile keratosis
     L57.1   **Actinic reticuloid**
     L57.2   **Cutis rhomboidalis nuchae**
     L57.3   **Poikiloderma of Civatte**
     L57.4   **Cutis laxa senilis**
         Elastosis senilis
     L57.5   **Actinic granuloma**

     L57.8   **Other skin changes due to chronic exposure to
          nonionizing radiation**
         Farmer's skin   Solar dermatitis
         Sailor's skin
     L57.9   **Skin changes due to chronic exposure to nonionizing
          radiation,** unspecified

● L58   **Radiodermatitis**
     Use additional code to identify the source of the radiation
       (W88, W90)
     L58.0   **Acute radiodermatitis**
     L58.1   **Chronic radiodermatitis**
     L58.9   **Radiodermatitis,** unspecified

● L59   **Other disorders of skin and subcutaneous tissue related to
      radiation**
     L59.0   **Erythema ab igne [dermatitis ab igne]**
     L59.8   **Other specified disorders of the skin and subcutaneous
          tissue related to radiation**
         Coding Clinic: 2017, Q1, P34
     L59.9   **Disorder of the skin and subcutaneous tissue related to
          radiation,** unspecified

DISORDERS OF SKIN APPENDAGES (L60-L75)

     Excludes1   congenital malformations of integument (Q84.-)

● L60   **Nail disorders**
     Excludes2   clubbing of nails (R68.3)
                   onychia and paronychia (L03.0-)

     L60.0   **Ingrowing nail**
     L60.1   **Onycholysis**
     L60.2   **Onychogryphosis**
     L60.3   **Nail dystrophy**
     L60.4   **Beau's lines**
     L60.5   **Yellow nail syndrome**
     L60.8   **Other nail disorders**
     L60.9   **Nail disorder,** unspecified

▷ *L62*   *Nail disorders in diseases classified elsewhere*
       Code first underlying disease, such as:
         pachydermoperiostosis (M89.4-)

● L63   **Alopecia areata**
     L63.0   **Alopecia (capitis)** totalis
     L63.1   **Alopecia** universalis
     L63.2   **Ophiasis**
     L63.8   **Other alopecia areata**
     L63.9   **Alopecia areata,** unspecified

Item 12–10   **Alopecia** is lack of hair and takes many forms. The most common is male pattern alopecia, also known as **androgenetic alopecia. Telogen effluvium** is early and excessive loss of hair resulting from a trauma to the hair follicle (fever, drugs, surgery, etc.).

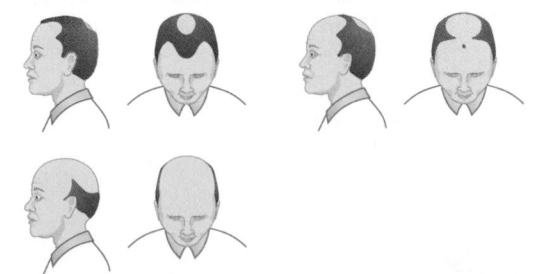

Figure 12-8   Male pattern alopecia.

▶ New   ⇒ Revised   ~~deleted~~ Deleted   Excludes 1   Excludes 2   Includes   Use additional   Code first   Code also   Key words
OGCR Official Guidelines   ● Unacceptable Principal Diagnosis   X Assign placeholder X   ● Use Additional Character(s)   ▷ Manifestation Code   Coding Clinic

● **L64   Androgenic alopecia**
　　　Includes　　male-pattern baldness
　　L64.0   Drug-induced androgenic alopecia
　　　　　Use additional code for adverse effect, if applicable,
　　　　　　to identify drug (T36-T50 with fifth or sixth
　　　　　　character 5)
　　L64.8   Other androgenic alopecia
　　L64.9   Androgenic alopecia, unspecified

● **L65   Other nonscarring hair loss**
　　　　Use additional code for adverse effect, if applicable, to identify
　　　　　drug (T36-T50 with fifth or sixth character 5)
　　　Excludes1　　trichotillomania (F63.3)
　　L65.0   Telogen effluvium
　　L65.1   Anagen effluvium
　　L65.2   Alopecia mucinosa
　　L65.8   Other specified nonscarring hair loss
　　L65.9   Nonscarring hair loss, unspecified
　　　　　Alopecia NOS

● **L66   Cicatricial alopecia [scarring hair loss]**
　　L66.0   Pseudopelade
　　L66.1   Lichen planopilaris
　　　　　Follicular lichen planus
　　L66.2   Folliculitis decalvans
　　L66.3   Perifolliculitis capitis abscedens
　　L66.4   Folliculitis ulerythematosa reticulata
　　L66.8   Other cicatricial alopecia
　　　　　Coding Clinic: 2015, Q1, P19
　　L66.9   Cicatricial alopecia, unspecified

● **L67   Hair color and hair shaft abnormalities**
　　　Excludes1　　monilethrix (Q84.1)
　　　　　　　　pili annulati (Q84.1)
　　　　　　　　telogen effluvium (L65.0)
　　L67.0   Trichorrhexis nodosa
　　L67.1   Variations in hair color
　　　　　Canities
　　　　　Greyness, hair (premature)
　　　　　Heterochromia of hair
　　　　　Poliosis circumscripta, acquired
　　　　　Poliosis NOS
　　L67.8   Other hair color and hair shaft abnormalities
　　　　　Fragilitas crinium
　　L67.9   Hair color and hair shaft abnormality, unspecified

● **L68   Hypertrichosis**
　　　Includes　　excess hair
　　　Excludes1　　congenital hypertrichosis (Q84.2)
　　　　　　　　persistent lanugo (Q84.2)
　　L68.0   Hirsutism
　　　　　Excessive growth of hair
　　L68.1   Acquired hypertrichosis lanuginosa
　　L68.2   Localized hypertrichosis
　　L68.3   Polytrichia
　　L68.8   Other hypertrichosis
　　L68.9   Hypertrichosis, unspecified

● **L70   Acne**
　　　Excludes2　　acne keloid (L73.0)
　　L70.0   Acne vulgaris
　　L70.1   Acne conglobata
　　L70.2   Acne varioliformis
　　　　　Acne necrotica miliaris

　　L70.3   Acne tropica
　　L70.4   Infantile acne   P
　　L70.5   Acné excoriée
　　　　　Acné excoriée des jeunes filles
　　　　　Picker's acne
　　L70.8   Other acne
　　L70.9   Acne, unspecified

● **L71   Rosacea**
　　　　Use additional code for adverse effect, if applicable, to identify
　　　　　drug (T36-T50 with fifth or sixth character 5)
　　L71.0   Perioral dermatitis
　　L71.1   Rhinophyma
　　L71.8   Other rosacea
　　　　　Coding Clinic: 2018, Q4, P15
　　L71.9   Rosacea, unspecified

● **L72   Follicular cysts of skin and subcutaneous tissue**
　　L72.0   Epidermal cyst
　● **L72.1   Pilar and trichodermal cyst**
　　　　L72.11   Pilar cyst
　　　　L72.12   Trichodermal cyst
　　　　　　Trichilemmal (proliferating) cyst
　　L72.3   Sebaceous cyst
　　　Excludes2　　pilar cyst (L72.11)
　　　　　　　　trichilemmal (proliferating) cyst (L72.12)
　　L72.2   Steatocystoma multiplex
　　L72.8   Other follicular cysts of the skin and subcutaneous tissue
　　L72.9   Follicular cyst of the skin and subcutaneous tissue, unspecified

● **L73   Other follicular disorders**
　　L73.0   Acne keloid
　　L73.1   Pseudofolliculitis barbae
　　L73.2   Hidradenitis suppurativa
　　L73.8   Other specified follicular disorders
　　　　　Sycosis barbae
　　L73.9   Follicular disorder, unspecified

● **L74   Eccrine sweat disorders**
　　　Excludes2　　generalized hyperhidrosis (R61)
　　L74.0   Miliaria rubra
　　L74.1   Miliaria crystallina
　　L74.2   Miliaria profunda
　　　　　Miliaria tropicalis
　　L74.3   Miliaria, unspecified
　　L74.4   Anhidrosis
　　　　　Hypohidrosis
　● **L74.5   Focal hyperhidrosis**
　　　● **L74.51   Primary focal hyperhidrosis**
　　　　　　L74.510   Primary focal hyperhidrosis, axilla
　　　　　　L74.511   Primary focal hyperhidrosis, face
　　　　　　L74.512   Primary focal hyperhidrosis, palms
　　　　　　L74.513   Primary focal hyperhidrosis, soles
　　　　　　L74.519   Primary focal hyperhidrosis, unspecified
　　　　L74.52   Secondary focal hyperhidrosis
　　　　　　Frey's syndrome
　　L74.8   Other eccrine sweat disorders
　　L74.9   Eccrine sweat disorder, unspecified
　　　　　Sweat gland disorder NOS

CHAPTER 12 (L00-L99)

N Newborn Age: 0　　**P** Pediatric Age: 0–17　　**M** Maternity DX: 9–64　　**A** Adult Age: 15–124　　♀ Females Only　　♂ Males Only

🅒 Complication\Comorbidity　　🅜 Major C\C　　Ⓔⓧ CC/MCC Exclusions　　🅗 Hospital-Acquired Condition　　🅗 Hierarchical Condition Category

997

● **L75**   **Apocrine sweat disorders**
    Excludes1   dyshidrosis (L30.1)
                 hidradenitis suppurativa (L73.2)
   L75.0   **Bromhidrosis**
   L75.1   **Chromhidrosis**
   L75.2   **Apocrine miliaria**
         Fox-Fordyce disease
   L75.8   **Other apocrine sweat disorders**
   L75.9   **Apocrine sweat disorder, unspecified**
         Intraoperative and postprocedural complications of skin and subcutaneous tissue (L76)

INTRAOPERATIVE AND POSTPROCEDURAL COMPLICATIONS OF SKIN AND SUBCUTANEOUS TISSUE (L76)

● **L76**   **Intraoperative and postprocedural complications of skin and subcutaneous tissue**
   (Ex) For category L76 CC codes unless otherwise indicated: See PDX Collection 852
   Coding Clinic: 2016, Q4, P10
   ● **L76.0**   **Intraoperative hemorrhage and hematoma of skin and subcutaneous tissue complicating a procedure**
       Excludes1   intraoperative hemorrhage and hematoma of skin and subcutaneous tissue due to accidental puncture and laceration during a procedure (L76.1-)
     L76.01   Intraoperative hemorrhage and hematoma of skin and subcutaneous tissue complicating a dermatologic procedure
     L76.02   Intraoperative hemorrhage and hematoma of skin and subcutaneous tissue complicating other procedure
   ● **L76.1**   **Accidental puncture and laceration of skin and subcutaneous tissue during a procedure**
       (Ex) For category L76.1 CC codes: See PDX Collection 509
     L76.11   Accidental puncture and laceration of skin and subcutaneous tissue during a dermatologic procedure
     L76.12   Accidental puncture and laceration of skin and subcutaneous tissue during other procedure
   ● **L76.2**   **Postprocedural hemorrhage of skin and subcutaneous tissue following a procedure**
     L76.21   Postprocedural hemorrhage of skin and subcutaneous tissue following a dermatologic procedure
     L76.22   Postprocedural hemorrhage of skin and subcutaneous tissue following other procedure
   ● **L76.3**   **Postprocedural hematoma and seroma of skin and subcutaneous tissue following a procedure**
     L76.31   Postprocedural hematoma of skin and subcutaneous tissue following a dermatologic procedure
     L76.32   Postprocedural hematoma of skin and subcutaneous tissue following other procedure
     L76.33   Postprocedural seroma of skin and subcutaneous tissue following a dermatologic procedure
     L76.34   Postprocedural seroma of skin and subcutaneous tissue following other procedure
   ● **L76.8**   **Other intraoperative and postprocedural complications of skin and subcutaneous tissue**
       Use additional code, if applicable, to further specify disorder
     L76.81   Other intraoperative complications of skin and subcutaneous tissue
     L76.82   Other postprocedural complications of skin and subcutaneous tissue
       Coding Clinic: 2017, Q3, P6

OTHER DISORDERS OF THE SKIN AND SUBCUTANEOUS TISSUE (L80-L99)

  L80   **Vitiligo**
    Excludes2   vitiligo of eyelids (H02.73-)
                 vitiligo of vulva (N90.89)
● **L81**   **Other disorders of pigmentation**
    Excludes1   birthmark NOS (Q82.5)
                 Peutz-Jeghers syndrome (Q85.8)
    Excludes2   nevus - see Alphabetical Index
   L81.0   **Postinflammatory hyperpigmentation**
   L81.1   **Chloasma**
   L81.2   **Freckles**
   L81.3   **Café au lait spots**
   L81.4   **Other melanin hyperpigmentation**
         Lentigo
   L81.5   **Leukoderma, not elsewhere classified**
   L81.6   **Other disorders of diminished melanin formation**
   L81.7   **Pigmented purpuric dermatosis**
         Angioma serpiginosum
   L81.8   **Other specified disorders of pigmentation**
         Iron pigmentation
         Tattoo pigmentation
   L81.9   **Disorder of pigmentation, unspecified**
● **L82**   **Seborrheic keratosis**
    Includes   basal cell papilloma
               dermatosis papulosa nigra
               Leser-Trélat disease
    Excludes2   seborrheic dermatitis (L21.-)
   L82.0   **Inflamed seborrheic keratosis**
   L82.1   **Other seborrheic keratosis**
         Seborrheic keratosis NOS
  L83   **Acanthosis nigricans**
         Confluent and reticulated papillomatosis
  L84   **Corns and callosities**
         Callus
         Clavus
● **L85**   **Other epidermal thickening**
    Excludes2   hypertrophic disorders of the skin (L91.-)
   L85.0   **Acquired ichthyosis**
       Excludes1   congenital ichthyosis (Q80.-)
   L85.1   **Acquired keratosis [keratoderma] palmaris et plantaris**
       Excludes1   inherited keratosis palmaris et plantaris (Q82.8)
   L85.2   **Keratosis punctata (palmaris et plantaris)**
   L85.3   **Xerosis cutis**
         Dry skin dermatitis
   L85.8   **Other specified epidermal thickening**
         Cutaneous horn
   L85.9   **Epidermal thickening, unspecified**
▷ *L86*   *Keratoderma in diseases classified elsewhere*
         Firm horny papules that have a cobblestone appearance
         Code first underlying disease, such as:
         Reiter's disease (M02.3-)
    Excludes1   gonococcal keratoderma (A54.89)
                 gonococcal keratosis (A54.89)
                 keratoderma due to vitamin A deficiency (E50.8)
                 keratosis due to vitamin A deficiency (E50.8)
                 xeroderma due to vitamin A deficiency (E50.8)

998

▶ New   ⇒ Revised   ~~deleted~~ Deleted   Excludes 1   Excludes 2   Includes   Use additional   Code first   Code also   Key words
OGCR Official Guidelines   ● Unacceptable Principal Diagnosis   X Assign placeholder X   ● Use Additional Character(s)   ▷ Manifestation Code   **Coding Clinic**

● **L87**   **Transepidermal elimination disorders**
> **Excludes1**   granuloma annulare (perforating) (L92.0)

    L87.0   **Keratosis follicularis et parafollicularis in cutem penetrans**
> Kyrle disease
> Hyperkeratosis follicularis penetrans

    L87.1   **Reactive perforating collagenosis**

    L87.2   **Elastosis perforans serpiginosa**

    L87.8   **Other transepidermal elimination disorders**

    L87.9   **Transepidermal elimination disorder, unspecified**

● **L88**   **Pyoderma gangrenosum** 🔵
> Phagedenic pyoderma
> **Excludes1**   dermatitis gangrenosa (L08.0)

   Ⓔⓧ See PDX Collection 853

OGCR   Section I.B.14.

> General Coding Guidelines
>
> Documentation for BMI, *Depth of* Non-pressure ulcers, Pressure Ulcer Stages, **Coma Scale, and** *NIH Stroke Scale*
>
> For the Body Mass Index (BMI), depth of non-pressure chronic ulcers, pressure ulcer stage, **and NIH stroke scale (NIHSS) codes,** code assignment may be based on medical record documentation from clinicians who are not the patient's provider (i.e., physician or other qualified healthcare practitioner legally accountable for establishing the patient's diagnosis), since this information is typically documented by other clinicians involved in the care of the patient (e.g., a dietitian often documents the BMI, a nurse often documents the pressure ulcer stages, **and an emergency medical technician often documents the coma scale**). However, the associated diagnosis (such as overweight, obesity, **acute stroke,** or pressure ulcer) must be documented by the patient's provider. If there is conflicting medical record documentation, either from the same clinician or different clinicians, the patient's attending provider should be queried for clarification.
>
> The BMI, **coma scale, and NHSS** codes should only be reported as secondary diagnoses.

● **L89**   **Pressure ulcer**

   Includes   bed sore   pressure area
                decubitus ulcer   pressure sore
                plaster ulcer

   Code first any associated gangrene (I96)

   Excludes2   decubitus (trophic) ulcer of cervix (uteri) (N86)
                diabetic ulcers (E08.621, E08.622, E09.621, E09.622, E10.621, E10.622, E11.621, E11.622, E13.621, E13.622)
                non-pressure chronic ulcer of skin (L97.-)
                skin infections (L00-L08)
                varicose ulcer (I83.0, I83.2)

   Ⓔⓧ **For category L89 CC codes:** See PDX Collection 854
   Coding Clinic: 2019, Q4, P11; 2018, Q2, P22; 2016, Q4, P124

● **L89.0**   **Pressure ulcer of elbow**

   ● **L89.00**   **Pressure ulcer of unspecified elbow**

       L89.000   **Pressure ulcer of unspecified elbow, unstageable** 🔵

       L89.001   **Pressure ulcer of unspecified elbow, stage 1**
> Healing pressure ulcer of unspecified elbow, stage 1
> Pressure pre-ulcer skin changes limited to persistent focal edema, unspecified elbow

       L89.002   **Pressure ulcer of unspecified elbow, stage 2**
> Healing pressure ulcer of unspecified elbow, stage 2
> Pressure ulcer with abrasion, blister, partial thickness skin loss involving epidermis and/or dermis, unspecified elbow

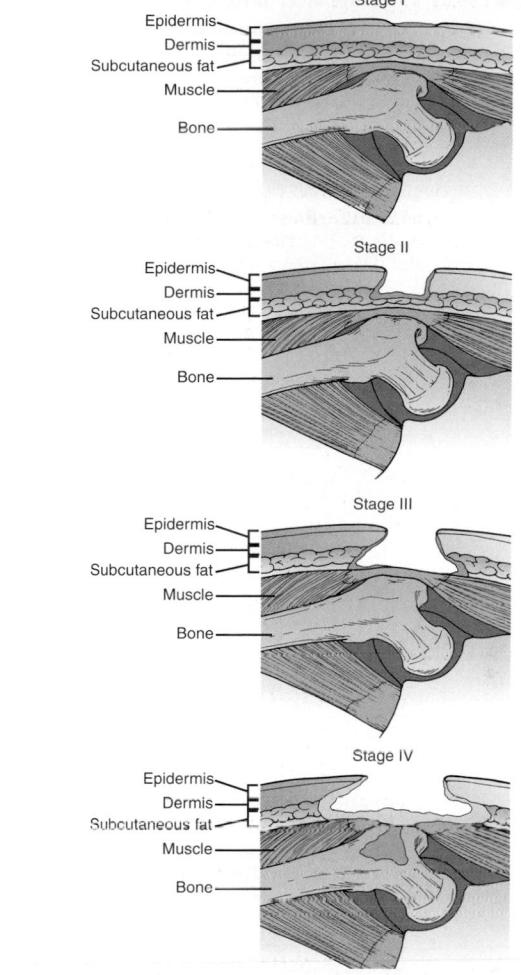

Figure 12-9   Stage I, II, III, and IV of pressure ulcers.

   L89.003   **Pressure ulcer of unspecified elbow, stage 3** 🔵 🔵🔵
> Healing pressure ulcer of unspecified elbow, stage 3
> Pressure ulcer with full thickness skin loss involving damage or necrosis of subcutaneous tissue, unspecified elbow
> MCC when PDx is its own MCC

   L89.004   **Pressure ulcer of unspecified elbow, stage 4** 🔵 🔵🔵
> Healing pressure ulcer of unspecified elbow, stage 4
> Pressure ulcer with necrosis of soft tissues through to underlying muscle, tendon, or bone, unspecified elbow
> MCC when PDx is its own MCC

   L89.006   **Pressure-induced deep tissue damage of unspecified elbow**

   L89.009   **Pressure ulcer of unspecified elbow, unspecified stage**
> Healing pressure ulcer of elbow NOS
> Healing pressure ulcer of unspecified elbow, unspecified stage

N Newborn Age: 0   **P** Pediatric Age: 0–17   **M** Maternity DX: 9–64   **A** Adult Age: 15–124   ♀ Females Only   ♂ Males Only

🔵 Complication\Comorbidity   🔵 Major C\C   Ⓔⓧ CC/MCC Exclusions   🔵 Hospital-Acquired Condition   🔵 Hierarchical Condition Category

999

CHAPTER 12 (L00-L99)

● L89.01　Pressure ulcer of right elbow
　　　L89.010　Pressure ulcer of right elbow, unstageable 🔖
　　　L89.011　Pressure ulcer of right elbow, stage 1
　　　　　　Healing pressure ulcer of right elbow, stage 1
　　　　　　Pressure pre-ulcer skin changes limited to persistent focal edema, right elbow
　　　L89.012　Pressure ulcer of right elbow, stage 2
　　　　　　Healing pressure ulcer of right elbow, stage 2
　　　　　　Pressure ulcer with abrasion, blister, partial thickness skin loss involving epidermis and/or dermis, right elbow
　　　L89.013　Pressure ulcer of right elbow, stage 3 🔖🔖🔖
　　　　　　Healing pressure ulcer of right elbow, stage 3
　　　　　　Pressure ulcer with full thickness skin loss involving damage or necrosis of subcutaneous tissue, right elbow
　　　　　　MCC when PDx is its own MCC
　　　L89.014　Pressure ulcer of right elbow, stage 4 🔖🔖🔖
　　　　　　Healing pressure ulcer of right elbow, stage 4
　　　　　　Pressure ulcer with necrosis of soft tissues through to underlying muscle, tendon, or bone, right elbow
　　　　　　MCC when PDx is its own MCC
　　　L89.016　Pressure-induced deep tissue damage of right elbow
　　　L89.019　Pressure ulcer of right elbow, unspecified stage
　　　　　　⟿ Healing pressure ulcer of right elbow NOS
　　　　　　Healing pressure ulcer of right elbow, unspecified stage

● L89.02　Pressure ulcer of left elbow
　　　L89.020　Pressure ulcer of left elbow, unstageable 🔖
　　　L89.021　Pressure ulcer of left elbow, stage 1
　　　　　　Healing pressure ulcer of left elbow, stage 1
　　　　　　Pressure pre-ulcer skin changes limited to persistent focal edema, left elbow
　　　L89.022　Pressure ulcer of left elbow, stage 2
　　　　　　Healing pressure ulcer of left elbow, stage 2
　　　　　　Pressure ulcer with abrasion, blister, partial thickness skin loss involving epidermis and/or dermis, left elbow
　　　L89.023　Pressure ulcer of left elbow, stage 3 🔖🔖🔖
　　　　　　Healing pressure ulcer of left elbow, stage 3
　　　　　　Pressure ulcer with full thickness skin loss involving damage or necrosis of subcutaneous tissue, left elbow
　　　　　　MCC when PDx is its own MCC
　　　L89.024　Pressure ulcer of left elbow, stage 4 🔖🔖🔖
　　　　　　Healing pressure ulcer of left elbow, stage 4
　　　　　　Pressure ulcer with necrosis of soft tissues through to underlying muscle, tendon, or bone, left elbow
　　　　　　MCC when PDx is its own MCC

　　　L89.026　Pressure-induced deep tissue damage of left elbow
　　　L89.029　Pressure ulcer of left elbow, unspecified stage
　　　　　　⟿ Healing pressure ulcer of left elbow NOS
　　　　　　Healing pressure ulcer of left elbow, unspecified stage

● L89.1　Pressure ulcer of back
　● L89.10　Pressure ulcer of unspecified part of back
　　　L89.100　Pressure ulcer of unspecified part of back, unstageable 🔖
　　　L89.101　Pressure ulcer of unspecified part of back, stage 1
　　　　　　Healing pressure ulcer of unspecified part of back, stage 1
　　　　　　Pressure pre-ulcer skin changes limited to persistent focal edema, unspecified part of back
　　　L89.102　Pressure ulcer of unspecified part of back, stage 2
　　　　　　Healing pressure ulcer of unspecified part of back, stage 2
　　　　　　Pressure ulcer with abrasion, blister, partial thickness skin loss involving epidermis and/or dermis, unspecified part of back
　　　L89.103　Pressure ulcer of unspecified part of back, stage 3 🔖🔖🔖
　　　　　　Healing pressure ulcer of unspecified part of back, stage 3
　　　　　　Pressure ulcer with full thickness skin loss involving damage or necrosis of subcutaneous tissue, unspecified part of back
　　　　　　MCC when PDx is its own MCC
　　　L89.104　Pressure ulcer of unspecified part of back, stage 4 🔖🔖🔖
　　　　　　Healing pressure ulcer of unspecified part of back, stage 4
　　　　　　Pressure ulcer with necrosis of soft tissues through to underlying muscle, tendon, or bone, unspecified part of back
　　　　　　MCC when PDx is its own MCC
　　　L89.106　Pressure-induced deep tissue damage of unspecified part of back
　　　L89.109　Pressure ulcer of unspecified part of back, unspecified stage
　　　　　　Healing pressure ulcer of unspecified part of back NOS
　　　　　　Healing pressure ulcer of unspecified part of back, unspecified stage

　● L89.11　Pressure ulcer of right upper back
　　　　Pressure ulcer of right shoulder blade
　　　L89.110　Pressure ulcer of right upper back, unstageable 🔖
　　　L89.111　Pressure ulcer of right upper back, stage 1
　　　　　　Healing pressure ulcer of right upper back, stage 1
　　　　　　Pressure pre-ulcer skin changes limited to persistent focal edema, right upper back
　　　L89.112　Pressure ulcer of right upper back, stage 2
　　　　　　Healing pressure ulcer of right upper back, stage 2
　　　　　　Pressure ulcer with abrasion, blister, partial thickness skin loss involving epidermis and/or dermis, right upper back

▶ New　⟿ Revised　~~deleted~~ Deleted　Excludes 1　Excludes 2　Includes　Use additional　Code first　Code also　Key words
OGCR Official Guidelines　● Unacceptable Principal Diagnosis　X Assign placeholder X　● Use Additional Character(s)　▷ Manifestation Code　Coding Clinic

L89.113   **Pressure ulcer of right upper back, stage 3** 🔘🔘🔘
     Healing pressure ulcer of right upper back, stage 3
     Pressure ulcer with full thickness skin loss involving damage or necrosis of subcutaneous tissue, right upper back
     MCC when PDx is its own MCC

L89.114   **Pressure ulcer of right upper back, stage 4** 🔘🔘🔘
     Healing pressure ulcer of right upper back, stage 4
     Pressure ulcer with necrosis of soft tissues through to underlying muscle, tendon, or bone, right upper back
     MCC when PDx is its own MCC

L89.116   **Pressure-induced deep tissue damage of right upper back**

L89.119   **Pressure ulcer of right upper back, unspecified stage**
     Healing pressure ulcer of right upper back NOS
     Healing pressure ulcer of right upper back, unspecified stage

⬤ L89.12   **Pressure ulcer of left upper back**
     Pressure ulcer of left shoulder blade

L89.120   **Pressure ulcer of left upper back, unstageable** 🔘

L89.121   **Pressure ulcer of left upper back, stage 1**
     Healing pressure ulcer of left upper back, stage 1
     Pressure pre-ulcer skin changes limited to persistent focal edema, left upper back

L89.122   **Pressure ulcer of left upper back, stage 2**
     Healing pressure ulcer of left upper back, stage 2
     Pressure ulcer with abrasion, blister, partial thickness skin loss involving epidermis and/or dermis, left upper back

L89.123   **Pressure ulcer of left upper back, stage 3** 🔘🔘🔘
     Healing pressure ulcer of left upper back, stage 3
     Pressure ulcer with full thickness skin loss involving damage or necrosis of subcutaneous tissue, left upper back
     MCC when PDx is its own MCC

L89.124   **Pressure ulcer of left upper back, stage 4** 🔘🔘🔘
     Healing pressure ulcer of left upper back, stage 4
     Pressure ulcer with necrosis of soft tissues through to underlying muscle, tendon, or bone, left upper back
     MCC when PDx is its own MCC

L89.126   **Pressure-induced deep tissue damage of left upper back**

L89.129   **Pressure ulcer of left upper back, unspecified stage**
     Healing pressure ulcer of left upper back NOS
     Healing pressure ulcer of left upper back, unspecified stage

⬤ L89.13   **Pressure ulcer of right lower back**

L89.130   **Pressure ulcer of right lower back, unstageable** 🔘

L89.131   **Pressure ulcer of right lower back, stage 1**
     Healing pressure ulcer of right lower back, stage 1
     Pressure pre-ulcer skin changes limited to persistent focal edema, right lower back

L89.132   **Pressure ulcer of right lower back, stage 2**
     Healing pressure ulcer of right lower back, stage 2
     Pressure ulcer with abrasion, blister, partial thickness skin loss involving epidermis and/or dermis, right lower back

L89.133   **Pressure ulcer of right lower back, stage 3** 🔘🔘🔘
     Healing pressure ulcer of right lower back, stage 3
     Pressure ulcer with full thickness skin loss involving damage or necrosis of subcutaneous tissue, right lower back
     MCC when PDx is its own MCC

L89.134   **Pressure ulcer of right lower back, stage 4** 🔘🔘🔘
     Healing pressure ulcer of right lower back, stage 4
     Pressure ulcer with necrosis of soft tissues through to underlying muscle, tendon, or bone, right lower back
     MCC when PDx is its own MCC

L89.136   **Pressure-induced deep tissue damage of right lower back**

L89.139   **Pressure ulcer of right lower back, unspecified stage**
     Healing pressure ulcer of right lower back NOS
     Healing pressure ulcer of right lower back, unspecified stage

⬤ L89.14   **Pressure ulcer of left lower back**

L89.140   **Pressure ulcer of left lower back, unstageable** 🔘

L89.141   **Pressure ulcer of left lower back, stage 1**
     Healing pressure ulcer of left lower back, stage 1
     Pressure pre-ulcer skin changes limited to persistent focal edema, left lower back

L89.142   **Pressure ulcer of left lower back, stage 2**
     Healing pressure ulcer of left lower back, stage 2
     Pressure ulcer with abrasion, blister, partial thickness skin loss involving epidermis and/or dermis, left lower back

L89.143   **Pressure ulcer of left lower back, stage 3** 🔘🔘🔘
     Healing pressure ulcer of left lower back, stage 3
     Pressure ulcer with full thickness skin loss involving damage or necrosis of subcutaneous tissue, left lower back
     MCC when PDx is its own MCC

CHAPTER 12 (L00-L99)

N   Newborn Age: 0   **P**   Pediatric Age: 0–17   **M**   Maternity DX: 9–64   **A**   Adult Age: 15–124   ♀   Females Only   ♂   Males Only

🔘   Complication\Comorbidity   🔘   Major C\C   (Ex)   CC/MCC Exclusions   🔘   Hospital-Acquired Condition   🔘   Hierarchical Condition Category

1001

L89.144 Pressure ulcer of left lower back, stage 4
  Healing pressure ulcer of left lower back, stage 4
  Pressure ulcer with necrosis of soft tissues through to underlying muscle, tendon, or bone, left lower back
  MCC when PDx is its own MCC

L89.146 Pressure-induced deep tissue damage of left lower back

L89.149 Pressure ulcer of left lower back, unspecified stage
  Healing pressure ulcer of left lower back NOS
  Healing pressure ulcer of left lower back, unspecified stage

● **L89.15 Pressure ulcer of sacral region**
  Pressure ulcer of coccyx
  Pressure ulcer of tailbone

L89.150 Pressure ulcer of sacral region, unstageable

L89.151 Pressure ulcer of sacral region, stage 1
  Healing pressure ulcer of sacral region, stage 1
  Pressure pre-ulcer skin changes limited to persistent focal edema, sacral region

L89.152 Pressure ulcer of sacral region, stage 2
  Healing pressure ulcer of sacral region, stage 2
  Pressure ulcer with abrasion, blister, partial thickness skin loss involving epidermis and/or dermis, sacral region

L89.153 Pressure ulcer of sacral region, stage 3
  Healing pressure ulcer of sacral region, stage 3
  Pressure ulcer with full thickness skin loss involving damage or necrosis of subcutaneous tissue, sacral region
  MCC when PDx is its own MCC

L89.154 Pressure ulcer of sacral region, stage 4
  Healing pressure ulcer of sacral region, stage 4
  Pressure ulcer with necrosis of soft tissues through to underlying muscle, tendon, or bone, sacral region
  MCC when PDx is its own MCC
  Coding Clinic: 2021, Q1, P24

L89.156 Pressure-induced deep tissue damage of sacral region

L89.159 Pressure ulcer of sacral region, unspecified stage
  Healing pressure ulcer of sacral region NOS
  Healing pressure ulcer of sacral region, unspecified stage

● **L89.2 Pressure ulcer of hip**

  ● **L89.20 Pressure ulcer of unspecified hip**

L89.200 Pressure ulcer of unspecified hip, unstageable

L89.201 Pressure ulcer of unspecified hip, stage 1
  Healing pressure ulcer of unspecified hip back, stage 1
  Pressure pre-ulcer skin changes limited to persistent focal edema, unspecified hip

L89.202 Pressure ulcer of unspecified hip, stage 2
  Healing pressure ulcer of unspecified hip, stage 2
  Pressure ulcer with abrasion, blister, partial thickness skin loss involving epidermis and/or dermis, unspecified hip

L89.203 Pressure ulcer of unspecified hip, stage 3
  Healing pressure ulcer of unspecified hip, stage 3
  Pressure ulcer with full thickness skin loss involving damage or necrosis of subcutaneous tissue, unspecified hip
  MCC when PDx is its own MCC

L89.204 Pressure ulcer of unspecified hip, stage 4
  Healing pressure ulcer of unspecified hip, stage 4
  Pressure ulcer with necrosis of soft tissues through to underlying muscle, tendon, or bone, unspecified hip
  MCC when PDx is its own MCC

L89.206 Pressure-induced deep tissue damage of unspecified hip

L89.209 Pressure ulcer of unspecified hip, unspecified stage
  Healing pressure ulcer of unspecified hip NOS
  Healing pressure ulcer of unspecified hip, unspecified stage

● **L89.21 Pressure ulcer of right hip**

L89.210 Pressure ulcer of right hip, unstageable

L89.211 Pressure ulcer of right hip, stage 1
  Healing pressure ulcer of right hip back, stage 1
  Pressure pre-ulcer skin changes limited to persistent focal edema, right hip

L89.212 Pressure ulcer of right hip, stage 2
  Healing pressure ulcer of right hip, stage 2
  Pressure ulcer with abrasion, blister, partial thickness skin loss involving epidermis and/or dermis, right hip

L89.213 Pressure ulcer of right hip, stage 3
  Healing pressure ulcer of right hip, stage 3
  Pressure ulcer with full thickness skin loss involving damage or necrosis of subcutaneous tissue, right hip
  MCC when PDx is its own MCC

L89.214 Pressure ulcer of right hip, stage 4
  Healing pressure ulcer of right hip, stage 4
  Pressure ulcer with necrosis of soft tissues through to underlying muscle, tendon, or bone, right hip
  MCC when PDx is its own MCC

L89.216 Pressure-induced deep tissue damage of right hip

L89.219 **Pressure ulcer of right hip, unspecified stage**
Healing pressure ulcer of right hip NOS
Healing pressure ulcer of right hip, unspecified stage

● L89.22 **Pressure ulcer of left hip**

L89.220 **Pressure ulcer of left hip, unstageable** 🅒

L89.221 **Pressure ulcer of left hip, stage 1**
Healing pressure ulcer of left hip back, stage 1
Pressure pre-ulcer skin changes limited to persistent focal edema, left hip

L89.222 **Pressure ulcer of left hip, stage 2**
Healing pressure ulcer of left hip, stage 2
Pressure ulcer with abrasion, blister, partial thickness skin loss involving epidermis and/or dermis, left hip

L89.223 **Pressure ulcer of left hip, stage 3** 🅒🅒🅒
Healing pressure ulcer of left hip, stage 3
Pressure ulcer with full thickness skin loss involving damage or necrosis of subcutaneous tissue, left hip
MCC when PDx is its own MCC

L89.224 **Pressure ulcer of left hip, stage 4** 🅒🅒🅒
Healing pressure ulcer of left hip, stage 4
Pressure ulcer with necrosis of soft tissues through to underlying muscle, tendon, or bone, left hip
MCC when PDx is its own MCC

L89.226 **Pressure-induced deep tissue damage of left hip**

L89.229 **Pressure ulcer of left hip, unspecified stage**
Healing pressure ulcer of left hip NOS
Healing pressure ulcer of left hip, unspecified stage

● L89.3 **Pressure ulcer of buttock**

● L89.30 **Pressure ulcer of unspecified buttock**

L89.300 **Pressure ulcer of unspecified buttock, unstageable** 🅒

L89.301 **Pressure ulcer of unspecified buttock, stage 1**
Healing pressure ulcer of unspecified buttock, stage 1
Pressure pre-ulcer skin changes limited to persistent focal edema, unspecified buttock

L89.302 **Pressure ulcer of unspecified buttock, stage 2**
Healing pressure ulcer of unspecified buttock, stage 2
Pressure ulcer with abrasion, blister, partial thickness skin loss involving epidermis and/or dermis, unspecified buttock

L89.303 **Pressure ulcer of unspecified buttock, stage 3** 🅒🅒🅒
Healing pressure ulcer of unspecified buttock, stage 3
Pressure ulcer with full thickness skin loss involving damage or necrosis of subcutaneous tissue, unspecified buttock
MCC when PDx is its own MCC

L89.304 **Pressure ulcer of unspecified buttock, stage 4** 🅒🅒
Healing pressure ulcer of unspecified buttock, stage 4
Pressure ulcer with necrosis of soft tissues through to underlying muscle, tendon, or bone, unspecified buttock
MCC when PDx is its own MCC

L89.306 **Pressure-induced deep tissue damage of unspecified buttock**

L89.309 **Pressure ulcer of unspecified buttock, unspecified stage**
Healing pressure ulcer of unspecified buttock NOS
Healing pressure ulcer of unspecified buttock, unspecified stage

● L89.31 **Pressure ulcer of right buttock**

L89.310 **Pressure ulcer of right buttock, unstageable** 🅒

L89.311 **Pressure ulcer of right buttock, stage 1**
Healing pressure ulcer of right buttock, stage 1
Pressure pre-ulcer skin changes limited to persistent focal edema, right buttock

L89.312 **Pressure ulcer of right buttock, stage 2**
Healing pressure ulcer of right buttock, stage 2
Pressure ulcer with abrasion, blister, partial thickness skin loss involving epidermis and/or dermis, right buttock

L89.313 **Pressure ulcer of right buttock, stage 3** 🅒🅒🅒
Healing pressure ulcer of right buttock, stage 3
Pressure ulcer with full thickness skin loss involving damage or necrosis of subcutaneous tissue, right buttock
MCC when PDx is its own MCC

L89.314 **Pressure ulcer of right buttock, stage 4** 🅒🅒🅒
Healing pressure ulcer of right buttock, stage 4
Pressure ulcer with necrosis of soft tissues through to underlying muscle, tendon, or bone, right buttock
MCC when PDx is its own MCC

L89.316 **Pressure-induced deep tissue damage of right buttock**

L89.319 **Pressure ulcer of right buttock, unspecified stage**
Healing pressure ulcer of right buttock NOS
Healing pressure ulcer of right buttock, unspecified stage

● L89.32 **Pressure ulcer of left buttock**

L89.320 **Pressure ulcer of left buttock, unstageable** 🅒

L89.321 **Pressure ulcer of left buttock, stage 1**
Healing pressure ulcer of left buttock, stage 1
Pressure pre-ulcer skin changes limited to persistent focal edema, left buttock

L89.322 **Pressure ulcer of left buttock, stage 2**
Healing pressure ulcer of left buttock, stage 2
Pressure ulcer with abrasion, blister, partial thickness skin loss involving epidermis and/or dermis, left buttock

N Newborn Age: 0   **P** Pediatric Age: 0–17   **M** Maternity DX: 9–64   **A** Adult Age: 15–124   ♀ Females Only   ♂ Males Only
🅒 Complication\Comorbidity   🅒 Major C\C   Ⓔ CC/MCC Exclusions   Hospital-Acquired Condition   🅒 Hierarchical Condition Category

1003

CHAPTER 12 (L00-L99)

L89.323 Pressure ulcer of left buttock, stage 3 🦠🦠🦠
    Healing pressure ulcer of left buttock, stage 3
    Pressure ulcer with full thickness skin loss involving damage or necrosis of subcutaneous tissue, left buttock
    MCC when PDx is its own MCC

L89.324 Pressure ulcer of left buttock, stage 4 🦠🦠🦠
    Healing pressure ulcer of left buttock, stage 4
    Pressure ulcer with necrosis of soft tissues through to underlying muscle, tendon, or bone, left buttock
    MCC when PDx is its own MCC

L89.326 Pressure-induced deep tissue damage of left buttock

L89.329 Pressure ulcer of left buttock, unspecified stage
    Healing pressure ulcer of left buttock NOS
    Healing pressure ulcer of left buttock, unspecified stage

● **L89.4 Pressure ulcer of contiguous site of back, buttock and hip**

L89.40 Pressure ulcer of contiguous site of back, buttock and hip, unspecified stage
    Healing pressure ulcer of contiguous site of back, buttock and hip NOS
    Healing pressure ulcer of contiguous site of back, buttock and hip, unspecified stage

L89.41 Pressure ulcer of contiguous site of back, buttock and hip, stage 1
    Healing pressure ulcer of contiguous site of back, buttock and hip, stage 1
    Pressure pre-ulcer skin changes limited to persistent focal edema, contiguous site of back, buttock and hip

L89.42 Pressure ulcer of contiguous site of back, buttock and hip, stage 2
    Healing pressure ulcer of contiguous site of back, buttock and hip, stage 2
    Pressure ulcer with abrasion, blister, partial thickness skin loss involving epidermis and/or dermis, contiguous site of back, buttock and hip

L89.43 Pressure ulcer of contiguous site of back, buttock and hip, stage 3 🦠🦠🦠
    Healing pressure ulcer of contiguous site of back, buttock and hip, stage 3
    Pressure ulcer with full thickness skin loss involving damage or necrosis of subcutaneous tissue, contiguous site of back, buttock and hip
    MCC when PDx is its own MCC

L89.44 Pressure ulcer of contiguous site of back, buttock and hip, stage 4 🦠🦠🦠
    Healing pressure ulcer of contiguous site of back, buttock and hip, stage 4
    Pressure ulcer with necrosis of soft tissues through to underlying muscle, tendon, or bone, contiguous site of back, buttock and hip
    MCC when PDx is its own MCC

L89.45 Pressure ulcer of contiguous site of back, buttock and hip, unstageable 🦠

L89.46 Pressure-induced deep tissue damage of contiguous site of back, buttock and hip

● **L89.5 Pressure ulcer of ankle**

● **L89.50 Pressure ulcer of unspecified ankle**

L89.500 Pressure ulcer of unspecified ankle, unstageable 🦠

L89.501 Pressure ulcer of unspecified ankle, stage 1
    Healing pressure ulcer of unspecified ankle, stage 1
    Pressure pre-ulcer skin changes limited to persistent focal edema, unspecified ankle

L89.502 Pressure ulcer of unspecified ankle, stage 2
    Healing pressure ulcer of unspecified ankle, stage 2
    Pressure ulcer with abrasion, blister, partial thickness skin loss involving epidermis and/or dermis, unspecified ankle

L89.503 Pressure ulcer of unspecified ankle, stage 3 🦠🦠
    Healing pressure ulcer of unspecified ankle, stage 3
    Pressure ulcer with full thickness skin loss involving damage or necrosis of subcutaneous tissue, unspecified ankle
    MCC when PDx is its own MCC

L89.504 Pressure ulcer of unspecified ankle, stage 4 🦠🦠🦠
    Healing pressure ulcer of unspecified ankle, stage 4
    Pressure ulcer with necrosis of soft tissues through to underlying muscle, tendon, or bone, unspecified ankle
    MCC when PDx is its own MCC

L89.506 Pressure-induced deep tissue damage of unspecified ankle

L89.509 Pressure ulcer of unspecified ankle, unspecified stage
    Healing pressure ulcer of unspecified ankle NOS
    Healing pressure ulcer of unspecified ankle, unspecified stage

● **L89.51 Pressure ulcer of right ankle**

L89.510 Pressure ulcer of right ankle, unstageable 🦠

L89.511 Pressure ulcer of right ankle, stage 1
    Healing pressure ulcer of right ankle, stage 1
    Pressure pre-ulcer skin changes limited to persistent focal edema, right ankle

L89.512 Pressure ulcer of right ankle, stage 2
    Healing pressure ulcer of right ankle, stage 2
    Pressure ulcer with abrasion, blister, partial thickness skin loss involving epidermis and/or dermis, right ankle

L89.513 Pressure ulcer of right ankle, stage 3 🦠🦠🦠
    Healing pressure ulcer of right ankle, stage 3
    Pressure ulcer with full thickness skin loss involving damage or necrosis of subcutaneous tissue, right ankle
    MCC when PDx is its own MCC

▶ New   ⇒ Revised   ~~deleted~~ Deleted   Excludes 1   Excludes 2   Includes   Use additional   Code first   Code also   Key words
OGCR Official Guidelines   ● Unacceptable Principal Diagnosis   X Assign placeholder X   ● Use Additional Character(s)   ▷ Manifestation Code   Coding Clinic

L89.514   **Pressure ulcer of right ankle,
           stage 4** 🏷🏷🏷
           Healing pressure ulcer of right
               ankle, stage 4
           Pressure ulcer with necrosis of soft
               tissues through to underlying
               muscle, tendon, or bone, right
               ankle
           MCC when PDx is its own MCC

L89.516   **Pressure-induced deep tissue damage
           of right ankle**

L89.519   **Pressure ulcer of right ankle,
           unspecified stage**
           Healing pressure ulcer of right ankle
               NOS
           Healing pressure ulcer of right
               ankle, unspecified stage

● L89.52   **Pressure ulcer of left ankle**

L89.520   **Pressure ulcer of left ankle,
           unstageable**

L89.521   **Pressure ulcer of left ankle, stage 1**
           Healing pressure ulcer of left ankle,
               stage 1
           Pressure pre-ulcer skin changes
               limited to persistent focal
               edema, left ankle

L89.522   **Pressure ulcer of left ankle, stage 2**
           Healing pressure ulcer of left ankle,
               stage 2
           Pressure ulcer with abrasion, blister,
               partial thickness skin loss
               involving epidermis and/or
               dermis, left ankle

L89.523   **Pressure ulcer of left ankle,
           stage 3** 🏷🏷🏷
           Healing pressure ulcer of left ankle,
               stage 3
           Pressure ulcer with full thickness
               skin loss involving damage or
               necrosis of subcutaneous tissue,
               left ankle
           MCC when PDx is its own MCC

L89.524   **Pressure ulcer of left ankle,
           stage 4** 🏷🏷🏷
           Healing pressure ulcer of left ankle,
               stage 4
           Pressure ulcer with necrosis of soft
               tissues through to underlying
               muscle, tendon, or bone, left
               ankle
           MCC when PDx is its own MCC

L89.526   **Pressure-induced deep tissue damage
           of left ankle**

L89.529   **Pressure ulcer of left ankle,
           unspecified stage**
           Healing pressure ulcer of left ankle
               NOS
           Healing pressure ulcer of left ankle,
               unspecified stage

● L89.6   **Pressure ulcer of heel**
  ● L89.60 **Pressure ulcer of unspecified heel**

L89.600   **Pressure ulcer of unspecified heel,
           unstageable** 🏷

L89.601   **Pressure ulcer of unspecified heel,
           stage 1**
           Healing pressure ulcer of
               unspecified heel, stage 1
           Pressure pre-ulcer skin changes
               limited to persistent focal
               edema, unspecified heel

L89.602   **Pressure ulcer of unspecified heel,
           stage 2**
           Healing pressure ulcer of
               unspecified heel, stage 2
           Pressure ulcer with abrasion, blister,
               partial thickness skin loss
               involving epidermis and/or
               dermis, unspecified heel

L89.603   **Pressure ulcer of unspecified heel,
           stage 3** 🏷🏷🏷
           Healing pressure ulcer of
               unspecified heel, stage 3
           Pressure ulcer with full thickness
               skin loss involving damage or
               necrosis of subcutaneous tissue,
               unspecified heel
           MCC when PDx is its own MCC

L89.604   **Pressure ulcer of unspecified heel,
           stage 4** 🏷🏷🏷
           Healing pressure ulcer of
               unspecified heel, stage 4
           Pressure ulcer with necrosis of soft
               tissues through to underlying
               muscle, tendon, or bone,
               unspecified heel
           MCC when PDx is its own MCC

L89.606   **Pressure-induced deep tissue damage
           of unspecified heel**

L89.609   **Pressure ulcer of unspecified heel,
           unspecified stage**
           Healing pressure ulcer of
               unspecified heel NOS
           Healing pressure ulcer of
               unspecified heel, unspecified
               stage

● L89.61   **Pressure ulcer of right heel**

L89.610   **Pressure ulcer of right heel,
           unstageable** 🏷

L89.611   **Pressure ulcer of right heel, stage 1**
           Healing pressure ulcer of right heel,
               stage 1
           Pressure pre-ulcer skin changes
               limited to persistent focal
               edema, right heel

L89.612   **Pressure ulcer of right heel, stage 2**
           Healing pressure ulcer of right heel,
               stage 2
           Pressure ulcer with abrasion, blister,
               partial thickness skin loss
               involving epidermis and/or
               dermis, right heel

L89.613   **Pressure ulcer of right heel,
           stage 3** 🏷🏷🏷
           Healing pressure ulcer of right heel,
               stage 3
           Pressure ulcer with full thickness
               skin loss involving damage or
               necrosis of subcutaneous tissue,
               right heel
           MCC when PDx is its own MCC

L89.614   **Pressure ulcer of right heel,
           stage 4** 🏷🏷🏷
           Healing pressure ulcer of right heel,
               stage 4
           Pressure ulcer with necrosis of soft
               tissues through to underlying
               muscle, tendon, or bone, right
               heel
           MCC when PDx is its own MCC

N Newborn Age: 0   **P** Pediatric Age: 0–17   **M** Maternity DX: 9–64   **A** Adult Age: 15–124   ♀ Females Only   ♂ Males Only
🏷 Complication\Comorbidity   🏷 Major C\C   Ⓔⓧ CC/MCC Exclusions   🏷 Hospital-Acquired Condition   🏷 Hierarchical Condition Category

1005

CHAPTER 12 (L00-L99)

L89.616 Pressure-induced deep tissue damage of right heel

L89.619 Pressure ulcer of right heel, unspecified stage
Healing pressure ulcer of right heel NOS
Healing pressure ulcer of right heel, unspecified stage

● L89.62 Pressure ulcer of left heel

L89.620 Pressure ulcer of left heel, unstageable 🔍

L89.621 Pressure ulcer of left heel, stage 1
Healing pressure ulcer of left heel, stage 1
Pressure pre-ulcer skin changes limited to persistent focal edema, left heel

L89.622 Pressure ulcer of left heel, stage 2
Healing pressure ulcer of left heel, stage 2
Pressure ulcer with abrasion, blister, partial thickness skin loss involving epidermis and/or dermis, left heel
Coding Clinic: 2016, Q4, P142

L89.623 Pressure ulcer of left heel, stage 3 🔍🔍🔍
Healing pressure ulcer of left heel, stage 3
Pressure ulcer with full thickness skin loss involving damage or necrosis of subcutaneous tissue, left heel
MCC when PDx is its own MCC
Coding Clinic: 2016, Q4, P142

L89.624 Pressure ulcer of left heel, stage 4 🔍🔍🔍
Healing pressure ulcer of left heel, stage 4
Pressure ulcer with necrosis of soft tissues through to underlying muscle, tendon, or bone, left heel
MCC when PDx is its own MCC

L89.626 Pressure-induced deep tissue damage of left heel

L89.629 Pressure ulcer of left heel, unspecified stage
Healing pressure ulcer of left heel NOS
Healing pressure ulcer of left heel, unspecified stage

● L89.8 Pressure ulcer of other site

● L89.81 Pressure ulcer of head
Pressure ulcer of face

L89.810 Pressure ulcer of head, unstageable 🔍

L89.811 Pressure ulcer of head, stage 1
Healing pressure ulcer of head, stage 1
Pressure pre-ulcer skin changes limited to persistent focal edema, head

L89.812 Pressure ulcer of head, stage 2
Healing pressure ulcer of head, stage 2
Pressure ulcer with abrasion, blister, partial thickness skin loss involving epidermis and/or dermis, head

L89.813 Pressure ulcer of head, stage 3 🔍🔍🔍
Healing pressure ulcer of head, stage 3
Pressure ulcer with full thickness skin loss involving damage or necrosis of subcutaneous tissue, head
MCC when PDx is its own MCC

L89.814 Pressure ulcer of head, stage 4 🔍🔍🔍
Healing pressure ulcer of head, stage 4
Pressure ulcer with necrosis of soft tissues through to underlying muscle, tendon, or bone, head
MCC when PDx is its own MCC

L89.816 Pressure-induced deep tissue damage of head

L89.819 Pressure ulcer of head, unspecified stage
Healing pressure ulcer of head NOS
Healing pressure ulcer of head, unspecified stage

● L89.89 Pressure ulcer of other site

L89.890 Pressure ulcer of other site, unstageable 🔍

L89.891 Pressure ulcer of other site, stage 1
Healing pressure ulcer of other site, stage 1
Pressure pre-ulcer skin changes limited to persistent focal edema, other site

L89.892 Pressure ulcer of other site, stage 2
Healing pressure ulcer of other site, stage 2
Pressure ulcer with abrasion, blister, partial thickness skin loss involving epidermis and/or dermis, other site

L89.893 Pressure ulcer of other site, stage 3 🔍🔍🔍
Healing pressure ulcer of other site, stage 3
Pressure ulcer with full thickness skin loss involving damage or necrosis of subcutaneous tissue, other site
MCC when PDx is its own MCC

L89.894 Pressure ulcer of other site, stage 4 🔍🔍🔍
Healing pressure ulcer of other site, stage 4
Pressure ulcer with necrosis of soft tissues through to underlying muscle, tendon, or bone, other site
MCC when PDx is its own MCC

L89.899 Pressure ulcer of other site, unspecified stage
Healing pressure ulcer of other site NOS
Healing pressure ulcer of other site, unspecified stage

● L89.9 Pressure ulcer of unspecified site

L89.90 Pressure ulcer of unspecified site, unspecified stage
Healing pressure ulcer of unspecified site NOS
Healing pressure ulcer of unspecified site, unspecified stage

L89.91 Pressure ulcer of unspecified site, stage 1
Healing pressure ulcer of unspecified site, stage 1
Pressure pre-ulcer skin changes limited to persistent focal edema, unspecified site

▶ New   ⇒ Revised   ~~deleted~~ Deleted   Excludes 1   Excludes 2   Includes   Use additional   Code first   Code also   Key words
OGCR Official Guidelines   ● Unacceptable Principal Diagnosis   X Assign placeholder X   ● Use Additional Character(s)   ▷ Manifestation Code   Coding Clinic

L89.92   **Pressure ulcer of unspecified site, stage 2**
Healing pressure ulcer of unspecified site, stage 2
Pressure ulcer with abrasion, blister, partial thickness skin loss involving epidermis and/or dermis, unspecified site

L89.93   **Pressure ulcer of unspecified site, stage 3** 🗫 🗫 🗫
Healing pressure ulcer of unspecified site, stage 3
Pressure ulcer with full thickness skin loss involving damage or necrosis of subcutaneous tissue, unspecified site
MCC when PDx is its own MCC

L89.94   **Pressure ulcer of unspecified site, stage 4** 🗫 🗫 🗫
Healing pressure ulcer of unspecified site, stage 4
Pressure ulcer with necrosis of soft tissues through to underlying muscle, tendon, or bone, unspecified site
MCC when PDx is its own MCC

L89.95   **Pressure ulcer of unspecified site, unstageable** 🗫

L89.96   **Pressure-induced deep tissue damage of unspecified site**

● **L90**   **Atrophic disorders of skin**

L90.0   **Lichen sclerosus et atrophicus**
> **Excludes2**   lichen sclerosus of external female genital organs (N90.4)
> lichen sclerosus of external male genital organs (N48.0)

L90.1   **Anetoderma of Schweninger-Buzzi**

L90.2   **Anetoderma of Jadassohn-Pellizzari**

L90.3   **Atrophoderma of Pasini and Pierini**

L90.4   **Acrodermatitis chronica atrophicans**

L90.5   **Scar conditions and fibrosis of skin**
Adherent scar (skin)
Cicatrix
Disfigurement of skin due to scar
Fibrosis of skin NOS
Scar NOS
> **Excludes2**   hypertrophic scar (L91.0)
> keloid scar (L91.0)
> Coding Clinic: 2016, Q2, P5; 2015, Q1, P19

L90.6   **Striae atrophicae**

L90.8   **Other atrophic disorders of skin**

L90.9   **Atrophic disorder of skin, unspecified**

● **L91**   **Hypertrophic disorders of skin**

L91.0   **Keloid scar**
Hypertrophic scar
Keloid
> **Excludes2**   acne keloid (L73.0)
> scar NOS (L90.5)

L91.8   **Other hypertrophic disorders of the skin**

L91.9   **Hypertrophic disorder of the skin, unspecified**

● **L92**   **Granulomatous disorders of skin and subcutaneous tissue**
> **Excludes2**   actinic granuloma (L57.5)

L92.0   **Granuloma annulare**
Perforating granuloma annulare

L92.1   **Necrobiosis lipoidica, not elsewhere classified**
> **Excludes1**   necrobiosis lipoidica associated with diabetes mellitus (E08-E13 with .620)

Item 12–11   **Scleroderma** means hard skin. It is a group of diseases that causes abnormal growth of connective tissues that support the skin and organs. There are two types: localized scleroderma affecting the skin and systemic scleroderma affecting blood vessels and internal organs and the skin.

L92.2   **Granuloma faciale [eosinophilic granuloma of skin]**

L92.3   **Foreign body granuloma of the skin and subcutaneous tissue**
Use additional code to identify the type of retained foreign body (Z18.-)

L92.8   **Other granulomatous disorders of the skin and subcutaneous tissue**

L92.9   **Granulomatous disorder of the skin and subcutaneous tissue, unspecified**
> **Excludes2**   umbilical granuloma (P83.81)

● **L93**   **Lupus erythematosus**
Use additional code for adverse effect, if applicable, to identify drug (T36-T50 with fifth or sixth character 5)
> **Excludes1**   lupus exedens (A18.4)
> lupus vulgaris (A18.4)
> scleroderma (M34.-)
> systemic lupus erythematosus (M32.-)

L93.0   **Discoid lupus erythematosus**
Lupus erythematosus NOS

L93.1   **Subacute cutaneous lupus erythematosus**

L93.2   **Other local lupus erythematosus**
Lupus erythematosus profundus
Lupus panniculitis

● **L94**   **Other localized connective tissue disorders**
> **Excludes1**   systemic connective tissue disorders (M30-M36)

L94.0   **Localized scleroderma [morphea]**
Circumscribed scleroderma

L94.1   **Linear scleroderma**
En coup de sabre lesion

L94.2   **Calcinosis cutis**

L94.3   **Sclerodactyly**

L94.4   **Gottron's papules**

L94.5   **Poikiloderma vasculare atrophicans**

L94.6   **Ainhum**

L94.8   **Other specified localized connective tissue disorders**

L94.9   **Localized connective tissue disorder, unspecified**

● **L95**   **Vasculitis limited to skin, not elsewhere classified**
> **Excludes1**   angioma serpiginosum (L81.7)
> Henoch(-Schönlein) purpura (D69.0)
> hypersensitivity angiitis (M31.0)
> lupus panniculitis (L93.2)
> panniculitis NOS (M79.3)
> panniculitis of neck and back (M54.0-)
> polyarteritis nodosa (M30.0)
> relapsing panniculitis (M35.6)
> rheumatoid vasculitis (M05.2)
> serum sickness (T80.6-)
> urticaria (L50.-)
> Wegener's granulomatosis (M31.3-)

L95.0   **Livedoid vasculitis**
Atrophie blanche (en plaque)

L95.1   **Erythema elevatum diutinum**

L95.8   **Other vasculitis limited to the skin**

L95.9   **Vasculitis limited to the skin, unspecified**

CHAPTER 12 (L00-L99)

N Newborn Age: 0   **P** Pediatric Age: 0–17   **M** Maternity DX: 9–64   **A** Adult Age: 15–124   ♀ Females Only   ♂ Males Only

🗫 Complication\Comorbidity   🗫 Major C\C   (Ex) CC/MCC Exclusions   🗫 Hospital-Acquired Condition   🗫 Hierarchical Condition Category   **1007**

CHAPTER 12 (L00-L99)

● **L97** Non-pressure chronic ulcer of lower limb, not elsewhere classified

Includes chronic ulcer of skin of lower limb NOS
non-healing ulcer of skin
non-infected sinus of skin
trophic ulcer NOS
tropical ulcer NOS
ulcer of skin of lower limb NOS

Code first any associated underlying condition, such as:
any associated gangrene (I96)
atherosclerosis of the lower extremities (I70.23-, I70.24-, I70.33-, I70.34-, I70.43-, I70.44-, I70.53-, I70.54-, I70.63-, I70.64-, I70.73-, I70.74-)
chronic venous hypertension (I87.31-, I87.33-)
diabetic ulcers (E08.621, E08.622, E09.621, E09.622, E10.621, E10.622, E11.621, E11.622, E13.621, E13.622)
postphlebitic syndrome (I87.01-, I87.03-)
postthrombotic syndrome (I87.01-, I87.03-)
varicose ulcer (I83.0-, I83.2-)

Excludes2 pressure ulcer (pressure area) (L89.-)
skin infections (L00-L08)
specific infections classified to A00-B99

(Ex) For category **L97** CC codes: See PDX Collection 698

● **L97.1** Non-pressure chronic ulcer of thigh
　● **L97.10** Non-pressure chronic ulcer of unspecified thigh
　　L97.101 Non-pressure chronic ulcer of unspecified thigh limited to breakdown of skin
　　L97.102 Non-pressure chronic ulcer of unspecified thigh with fat layer exposed
　　L97.103 Non-pressure chronic ulcer of unspecified thigh with necrosis of muscle
　　L97.104 Non-pressure chronic ulcer of unspecified thigh with necrosis of bone
　　L97.105 Non-pressure chronic ulcer of unspecified thigh with muscle involvement without evidence of necrosis
　　L97.106 Non-pressure chronic ulcer of unspecified thigh with bone involvement without evidence of necrosis
　　L97.108 Non-pressure chronic ulcer of unspecified thigh with other specified severity
　　L97.109 Non-pressure chronic ulcer of unspecified thigh with unspecified severity
　● **L97.11** Non-pressure chronic ulcer of right thigh
　　L97.111 Non-pressure chronic ulcer of right thigh limited to breakdown of skin
　　L97.112 Non-pressure chronic ulcer of right thigh with fat layer exposed
　　L97.113 Non-pressure chronic ulcer of right thigh with necrosis of muscle
　　L97.114 Non-pressure chronic ulcer of right thigh with necrosis of bone
　　L97.115 Non-pressure chronic ulcer of right thigh with muscle involvement without evidence of necrosis
　　L97.116 Non-pressure chronic ulcer of right thigh with bone involvement without evidence of necrosis
　　L97.118 Non-pressure chronic ulcer of right thigh with other specified severity
　　L97.119 Non-pressure chronic ulcer of right thigh with unspecified severity

● **L97.12** Non-pressure chronic ulcer of left thigh
　　L97.121 Non-pressure chronic ulcer of left thigh limited to breakdown of skin
　　L97.122 Non-pressure chronic ulcer of left thigh with fat layer exposed
　　L97.123 Non-pressure chronic ulcer of left thigh with necrosis of muscle
　　L97.124 Non-pressure chronic ulcer of left thigh with necrosis of bone
　　L97.125 Non-pressure chronic ulcer of left thigh with muscle involvement without evidence of necrosis
　　L97.126 Non-pressure chronic ulcer of left thigh with bone involvement without evidence of necrosis
　　L97.128 Non-pressure chronic ulcer of left thigh with other specified severity
　　L97.129 Non-pressure chronic ulcer of left thigh with unspecified severity

● **L97.2** Non-pressure chronic ulcer of calf
　● **L97.20** Non-pressure chronic ulcer of unspecified calf
　　L97.201 Non-pressure chronic ulcer of unspecified calf limited to breakdown of skin
　　L97.202 Non-pressure chronic ulcer of unspecified calf with fat layer exposed
　　L97.203 Non-pressure chronic ulcer of unspecified calf with necrosis of muscle
　　L97.204 Non-pressure chronic ulcer of unspecified calf with necrosis of bone
　　L97.205 Non-pressure chronic ulcer of unspecified calf with muscle involvement without evidence of necrosis
　　L97.206 Non-pressure chronic ulcer of unspecified calf with bone involvement without evidence of necrosis
　　L97.208 Non-pressure chronic ulcer of unspecified calf with other specified severity
　　L97.209 Non-pressure chronic ulcer of unspecified calf with unspecified severity
　● **L97.21** Non-pressure chronic ulcer of right calf
　　L97.211 Non-pressure chronic ulcer of right calf limited to breakdown of skin
　　L97.212 Non-pressure chronic ulcer of right calf with fat layer exposed
　　L97.213 Non-pressure chronic ulcer of right calf with necrosis of muscle
　　L97.214 Non-pressure chronic ulcer of right calf with necrosis of bone
　　L97.215 Non-pressure chronic ulcer of right calf with muscle involvement without evidence of necrosis
　　L97.216 Non-pressure chronic ulcer of right calf with bone involvement without evidence of necrosis
　　L97.218 Non-pressure chronic ulcer of right calf with other specified severity
　　L97.219 Non-pressure chronic ulcer of right calf with unspecified severity

▶ New   ⇒ Revised   ~~deleted~~ Deleted   Excludes 1   Excludes 2   Includes   Use additional   Code first   Code also   Key words
OGCR Official Guidelines   ● Unacceptable Principal Diagnosis   X Assign placeholder X   ● Use Additional Character(s)   ▶ Manifestation Code   **Coding Clinic**

● **L97.22**   Non-pressure chronic ulcer of left calf

     L97.221   Non-pressure chronic ulcer of left calf limited to breakdown of skin 🔹🔹

     L97.222   Non-pressure chronic ulcer of left calf with fat layer exposed 🔹🔹

     L97.223   Non-pressure chronic ulcer of left calf with necrosis of muscle 🔹🔹

     L97.224   Non-pressure chronic ulcer of left calf with necrosis of bone 🔹🔹

     L97.225   Non-pressure chronic ulcer of left calf with muscle involvement without evidence of necrosis 🔹🔹

     L97.226   Non-pressure chronic ulcer of left calf with bone involvement without evidence of necrosis 🔹🔹

     L97.228   Non-pressure chronic ulcer of left calf with other specified severity 🔹🔹

     L97.229   Non-pressure chronic ulcer of left calf with unspecified severity 🔹🔹

● **L97.3**   Non-pressure chronic ulcer of ankle

  ● **L97.30**   Non-pressure chronic ulcer of unspecified ankle

     L97.301   Non-pressure chronic ulcer of unspecified ankle limited to breakdown of skin 🔹🔹

     L97.302   Non-pressure chronic ulcer of unspecified ankle with fat layer exposed 🔹🔹

     L97.303   Non-pressure chronic ulcer of unspecified ankle with necrosis of muscle 🔹🔹

     L97.304   Non-pressure chronic ulcer of unspecified ankle with necrosis of bone 🔹🔹

     L97.305   Non-pressure chronic ulcer of unspecified ankle with muscle involvement without evidence of necrosis 🔹🔹

     L97.306   Non-pressure chronic ulcer of unspecified ankle with bone involvement without evidence of necrosis 🔹🔹

     L97.308   Non-pressure chronic ulcer of unspecified ankle with other specified severity 🔹🔹

     L97.309   Non-pressure chronic ulcer of unspecified ankle with unspecified severity 🔹🔹

  ● **L97.31**   Non-pressure chronic ulcer of right ankle

     L97.311   Non-pressure chronic ulcer of right ankle limited to breakdown of skin 🔹🔹

     L97.312   Non-pressure chronic ulcer of right ankle with fat layer exposed 🔹🔹

     L97.313   Non-pressure chronic ulcer of right ankle with necrosis of muscle 🔹🔹

     L97.314   Non-pressure chronic ulcer of right ankle with necrosis of bone 🔹🔹

     L97.315   Non-pressure chronic ulcer of right ankle with muscle involvement without evidence of necrosis 🔹🔹
         Coding Clinic: 2017, Q4, P17

     L97.316   Non-pressure chronic ulcer of right ankle with bone involvement without evidence of necrosis 🔹🔹

     L97.318   Non-pressure chronic ulcer of right ankle with other specified severity 🔹🔹

     L97.319   Non-pressure chronic ulcer of right ankle with unspecified severity 🔹🔹

● **L97.32**   Non-pressure chronic ulcer of left ankle

     L97.321   Non-pressure chronic ulcer of left ankle limited to breakdown of skin 🔹🔹

     L97.322   Non-pressure chronic ulcer of left ankle with fat layer exposed 🔹🔹
         Coding Clinic: 2021, Q1, P8

     L97.323   Non-pressure chronic ulcer of left ankle with necrosis of muscle 🔹🔹

     L97.324   Non-pressure chronic ulcer of left ankle with necrosis of bone 🔹🔹

     L97.325   Non-pressure chronic ulcer of left ankle with muscle involvement without evidence of necrosis 🔹🔹

     L97.326   Non-pressure chronic ulcer of left ankle with bone involvement without evidence of necrosis 🔹🔹

     L97.328   Non-pressure chronic ulcer of left ankle with other specified severity 🔹🔹

     L97.329   Non-pressure chronic ulcer of left ankle with unspecified severity 🔹🔹

● **L97.4**   Non-pressure chronic ulcer of heel and midfoot
     Non-pressure chronic ulcer of plantar surface of midfoot

  ● **L97.40**   Non-pressure chronic ulcer of unspecified heel and midfoot

     L97.401   Non-pressure chronic ulcer of unspecified heel and midfoot limited to breakdown of skin 🔹🔹

     L97.402   Non-pressure chronic ulcer of unspecified heel and midfoot with fat layer exposed 🔹🔹

     L97.403   Non-pressure chronic ulcer of unspecified heel and midfoot with necrosis of muscle 🔹🔹

     L97.404   Non-pressure chronic ulcer of unspecified heel and midfoot with necrosis of bone 🔹🔹

     L97.405   Non-pressure chronic ulcer of unspecified heel and midfoot with muscle involvement without evidence of necrosis 🔹🔹

     L97.406   Non-pressure chronic ulcer of unspecified heel and midfoot with bone involvement without evidence of necrosis 🔹🔹

     L97.408   Non-pressure chronic ulcer of unspecified heel and midfoot with other specified severity 🔹🔹

     L97.409   Non-pressure chronic ulcer of unspecified heel and midfoot with unspecified severity 🔹🔹

N Newborn Age: 0   **P** Pediatric Age: 0–17   **M** Maternity DX: 9–64   **A** Adult Age: 15–124   ♀ Females Only   ♂ Males Only

🔹 Complication\Comorbidity   🔹 Major C\C   (Ex) CC/MCC Exclusions   🔹 Hospital-Acquired Condition   🔹 Hierarchical Condition Category

1009

CHAPTER 12 (L00–L99)

● **L97.41**   Non-pressure chronic ulcer of right heel and midfoot

     L97.411   Non-pressure chronic ulcer of right heel and midfoot limited to breakdown of skin 🟢🟢

     L97.412   Non-pressure chronic ulcer of right heel and midfoot with fat layer exposed 🟢🟢

     L97.413   Non-pressure chronic ulcer of right heel and midfoot with necrosis of muscle 🟢🟢

     L97.414   Non-pressure chronic ulcer of right heel and midfoot with necrosis of bone 🟢🟢

     L97.415   Non-pressure chronic ulcer of right heel and midfoot with muscle involvement without evidence of necrosis 🟢🟢

     L97.416   Non-pressure chronic ulcer of right heel and midfoot with bone involvement without evidence of necrosis 🟢🟢

     L97.418   Non-pressure chronic ulcer of right heel and midfoot with other specified severity 🟢🟢

     L97.419   Non-pressure chronic ulcer of right heel and midfoot with unspecified severity 🟢🟢

● **L97.42**   Non-pressure chronic ulcer of left heel and midfoot

     L97.421   Non-pressure chronic ulcer of left heel and midfoot limited to breakdown of skin 🟢🟢
            Coding Clinic: 2016, Q1, P13

     L97.422   Non-pressure chronic ulcer of left heel and midfoot with fat layer exposed 🟢🟢

     L97.423   Non-pressure chronic ulcer of left heel and midfoot with necrosis of muscle 🟢🟢

     L97.424   Non-pressure chronic ulcer of left heel and midfoot with necrosis of bone 🟢🟢

     L97.425   Non-pressure chronic ulcer of left heel and midfoot with muscle involvement without evidence of necrosis 🟢🟢

     L97.426   Non-pressure chronic ulcer of left heel and midfoot with bone involvement without evidence of necrosis 🟢🟢

     L97.428   Non-pressure chronic ulcer of left heel and midfoot with other specified severity 🟢🟢

     L97.429   Non-pressure chronic ulcer of left heel and midfoot with unspecified severity 🟢🟢

● **L97.5**   Non-pressure chronic ulcer of other part of foot
     Non-pressure chronic ulcer of toe

● **L97.50**   Non-pressure chronic ulcer of other part of unspecified foot

     L97.501   Non-pressure chronic ulcer of other part of unspecified foot limited to breakdown of skin 🟢

     L97.502   Non-pressure chronic ulcer of other part of unspecified foot with fat layer exposed 🟢

     L97.503   Non-pressure chronic ulcer of other part of unspecified foot with necrosis of muscle 🟢

     L97.504   Non-pressure chronic ulcer of other part of unspecified foot with necrosis of bone 🟢

     L97.505   Non-pressure chronic ulcer of other part of unspecified foot with muscle involvement without evidence of necrosis 🟢

     L97.506   Non-pressure chronic ulcer of other part of unspecified foot with bone involvement without evidence of necrosis 🟢

     L97.508   Non-pressure chronic ulcer of other part of unspecified foot with other specified severity 🟢🟢

     L97.509   Non-pressure chronic ulcer of other part of unspecified foot with unspecified severity 🟢

● **L97.51**   Non-pressure chronic ulcer of other part of right foot

     L97.511   Non-pressure chronic ulcer of other part of right foot limited to breakdown of skin 🟢
            Coding Clinic: 2020, Q1, P12

     L97.512   Non-pressure chronic ulcer of other part of right foot with fat layer exposed 🟢

     L97.513   Non-pressure chronic ulcer of other part of right foot with necrosis of muscle 🟢

     L97.514   Non-pressure chronic ulcer of other part of right foot with necrosis of bone 🟢

     L97.515   Non-pressure chronic ulcer of other part of right foot with muscle involvement without evidence of necrosis 🟢🟢

     L97.516   Non-pressure chronic ulcer of other part of right foot with bone involvement without evidence of necrosis 🟢🟢

     L97.518   Non-pressure chronic ulcer of other part of right foot with other specified severity 🟢🟢

     L97.519   Non-pressure chronic ulcer of other part of right foot with unspecified severity 🟢

▶ New   ⟹ Revised   ~~deleted~~ Deleted   Excludes 1   Excludes 2   Includes   Use additional   Code first   Code also   Key words
OGCR Official Guidelines   ● Unacceptable Principal Diagnosis   X Assign placeholder X   ● Use Additional Character(s)   ▶ Manifestation Code   **Coding Clinic**

● **L97.52**   **Non-pressure chronic ulcer of other part of left foot**

     L97.521   Non-pressure chronic ulcer of other part of left foot limited to breakdown of skin 🦠🦠

     L97.522   Non-pressure chronic ulcer of other part of left foot with fat layer exposed 🦠

     L97.523   Non-pressure chronic ulcer of other part of left foot with necrosis of muscle 🦠

     L97.524   Non-pressure chronic ulcer of other part of left foot with necrosis of bone 🦠

     L97.525   Non-pressure chronic ulcer of other part of left foot with muscle involvement without evidence of necrosis 🦠🦠

     L97.526   Non-pressure chronic ulcer of other part of left foot with bone involvement without evidence of necrosis 🦠🦠

     L97.528   Non-pressure chronic ulcer of other part of left foot with other specified severity 🦠🦠

     L97.529   Non-pressure chronic ulcer of other part of left foot with unspecified severity 🦠

● **L97.8**   **Non-pressure chronic ulcer of other part of lower leg**

● **L97.80**   **Non-pressure chronic ulcer of other part of unspecified lower leg**

     L97.801   Non-pressure chronic ulcer of other part of unspecified lower leg limited to breakdown of skin 🦠🦠

     L97.802   Non-pressure chronic ulcer of other part of unspecified lower leg with fat layer exposed 🦠🦠

     L97.803   Non-pressure chronic ulcer of other part of unspecified lower leg with necrosis of muscle 🦠🦠

     L97.804   Non-pressure chronic ulcer of other part of unspecified lower leg with necrosis of bone 🦠🦠

     L97.805   Non-pressure chronic ulcer of other part of unspecified lower leg with muscle involvement without evidence of necrosis 🦠🦠

     L97.806   Non-pressure chronic ulcer of other part of unspecified lower leg with bone involvement without evidence of necrosis 🦠🦠

     L97.808   Non-pressure chronic ulcer of other part of unspecified lower leg with other specified severity 🦠🦠

     L97.809   Non-pressure chronic ulcer of other part of unspecified lower leg with unspecified severity 🦠🦠

● **L97.81**   **Non-pressure chronic ulcer of other part of right lower leg**

     L97.811   Non-pressure chronic ulcer of other part of right lower leg limited to breakdown of skin 🦠🦠

     L97.812   Non-pressure chronic ulcer of other part of right lower leg with fat layer exposed 🦠🦠

     L97.813   Non-pressure chronic ulcer of other part of right lower leg with necrosis of muscle 🦠🦠

     L97.814   Non-pressure chronic ulcer of other part of right lower leg with necrosis of bone 🦠🦠

     L97.815   Non-pressure chronic ulcer of other part of right lower leg with muscle involvement without evidence of necrosis 🦠🦠

     L97.816   Non-pressure chronic ulcer of other part of right lower leg with bone involvement without evidence of necrosis 🦠🦠

     L97.818   Non-pressure chronic ulcer of other part of right lower leg with other specified severity 🦠🦠

     L97.819   Non-pressure chronic ulcer of other part of right lower leg with unspecified severity 🦠🦠

● **L97.82**   **Non-pressure chronic ulcer of other part of left lower leg**

     L97.821   Non-pressure chronic ulcer of other part of left lower leg limited to breakdown of skin 🦠🦠

     L97.822   Non-pressure chronic ulcer of other part of left lower leg with fat layer exposed 🦠🦠

     L97.823   Non-pressure chronic ulcer of other part of left lower leg with necrosis of muscle 🦠🦠

     L97.824   Non-pressure chronic ulcer of other part of left lower leg with necrosis of bone 🦠🦠

     L97.825   Non-pressure chronic ulcer of other part of left lower leg with muscle involvement without evidence of necrosis 🦠🦠

     L97.826   Non-pressure chronic ulcer of other part of left lower leg with bone involvement without evidence of necrosis 🦠🦠

     L97.828   Non-pressure chronic ulcer of other part of left lower leg with other specified severity 🦠🦠

     L97.829   Non-pressure chronic ulcer of other part of left lower leg with unspecified severity 🦠🦠

CHAPTER 12 (L00-L99)

N Newborn Age: 0   **P** Pediatric Age: 0–17   **M** Maternity DX: 9–64   **A** Adult Age: 15–124   ♀ Females Only   ♂ Males Only

🦠 Complication\Comorbidity   🦠 Major C\C   Ⓔⓧ CC/MCC Exclusions   🦠 Hospital-Acquired Condition   🦠 Hierarchical Condition Category   **1011**

● **L97.9**   Non-pressure chronic ulcer of unspecified part of lower leg

   ● **L97.90**   Non-pressure chronic ulcer of unspecified part of unspecified lower leg

       L97.901   Non-pressure chronic ulcer of unspecified part of unspecified lower leg limited to breakdown of skin 🔵 🔵

       L97.902   Non-pressure chronic ulcer of unspecified part of unspecified lower leg with fat layer exposed 🔵 🔵

       L97.903   Non-pressure chronic ulcer of unspecified part of unspecified lower leg with necrosis of muscle 🔵 🔵

       L97.904   Non-pressure chronic ulcer of unspecified part of unspecified lower leg with necrosis of bone 🔵 🔵

       L97.905   Non-pressure chronic ulcer of unspecified part of unspecified lower leg with muscle involvement without evidence of necrosis 🔵 🔵

       L97.906   Non-pressure chronic ulcer of unspecified part of unspecified lower leg with bone involvement without evidence of necrosis 🔵 🔵

       L97.908   Non-pressure chronic ulcer of unspecified part of unspecified lower leg with other specified severity 🔵 🔵

       L97.909   Non-pressure chronic ulcer of unspecified part of unspecified lower leg with unspecified severity 🔵 🔵

   ● **L97.91**   Non-pressure chronic ulcer of unspecified part of right lower leg

       L97.911   Non-pressure chronic ulcer of unspecified part of right lower leg limited to breakdown of skin 🔵 🔵

       L97.912   Non-pressure chronic ulcer of unspecified part of right lower leg with fat layer exposed 🔵 🔵

       L97.913   Non-pressure chronic ulcer of unspecified part of right lower leg with necrosis of muscle 🔵 🔵

       L97.914   Non-pressure chronic ulcer of unspecified part of right lower leg with necrosis of bone 🔵 🔵

       L97.915   Non-pressure chronic ulcer of unspecified part of right lower leg with muscle involvement without evidence of necrosis 🔵 🔵

       L97.916   Non-pressure chronic ulcer of unspecified part of right lower leg with bone involvement without evidence of necrosis 🔵 🔵

       L97.918   Non-pressure chronic ulcer of unspecified part of right lower leg with other specified severity 🔵 🔵

       L97.919   Non-pressure chronic ulcer of unspecified part of right lower leg with unspecified severity 🔵 🔵

● **L97.92**   Non-pressure chronic ulcer of unspecified part of left lower leg

       L97.921   Non-pressure chronic ulcer of unspecified part of left lower leg limited to breakdown of skin 🔵 🔵

       L97.922   Non-pressure chronic ulcer of unspecified part of left lower leg with fat layer exposed 🔵 🔵

       L97.923   Non-pressure chronic ulcer of unspecified part of left lower leg with necrosis of muscle 🔵 🔵

       L97.924   Non-pressure chronic ulcer of unspecified part of left lower leg with necrosis of bone 🔵 🔵

       L97.925   Non-pressure chronic ulcer of unspecified part of left lower leg with muscle involvement without evidence of necrosis 🔵 🔵

       L97.926   Non-pressure chronic ulcer of unspecified part of left lower leg with bone involvement without evidence of necrosis 🔵 🔵

       L97.928   Non-pressure chronic ulcer of unspecified part of left lower leg with other specified severity 🔵 🔵

       L97.929   Non-pressure chronic ulcer of unspecified part of left lower leg with unspecified severity 🔵 🔵

● **L98**   Other disorders of skin and subcutaneous tissue, not elsewhere classified

    L98.0   Pyogenic granuloma

       Excludes2   pyogenic granuloma of gingiva (K06.8)
               pyogenic granuloma of maxillary alveolar ridge (K04.5)
               pyogenic granuloma of oral mucosa (K13.4)

    L98.1   Factitial dermatitis
       Neurotic excoriation

       Excludes1   Excoriation (skin-picking) disorder (F42.4)

       Coding Clinic: 2016, Q4, P15

    L98.2   Febrile neutrophilic dermatosis [Sweet]

    L98.3   Eosinophilic cellulitis [Wells] 🔵
       (Ex:) See PDX Collection 839

   ● **L98.4**   Non-pressure chronic ulcer of skin, not elsewhere classified
       Chronic ulcer of skin NOS
       Tropical ulcer NOS
       Ulcer of skin NOS

       Excludes2   pressure ulcer (pressure area) (L89.-)
               gangrene (I96) 🔵
               skin infections (L00-L08)
               specific infections classified to A00-B99
               ulcer of lower limb NEC (L97.-)
               varicose ulcer (I83.0-I83.93)

   ● **L98.41**   Non-pressure chronic ulcer of buttock

       L98.411   Non-pressure chronic ulcer of buttock limited to breakdown of skin 🔵

       L98.412   Non-pressure chronic ulcer of buttock with fat layer exposed 🔵

▶ New   ⟾ Revised   ~~deleted~~ Deleted   Excludes 1   Excludes 2   Includes   Use additional   Code first   Code also   Key words
OGCR Official Guidelines   ● Unacceptable Principal Diagnosis   X Assign placeholder X   ● Use Additional Character(s)   ▶ Manifestation Code   Coding Clinic

L98.413   Non-pressure chronic ulcer of buttock with necrosis of muscle 🔵🔵

L98.414   Non-pressure chronic ulcer of buttock with necrosis of bone 🔵

L98.415   Non-pressure chronic ulcer of buttock with muscle involvement without evidence of necrosis 🔵🔵

L98.416   Non-pressure chronic ulcer of buttock with bone involvement without evidence of necrosis 🔵🔵

L98.418   Non-pressure chronic ulcer of buttock with other specified severity 🔵🔵

L98.419   Non-pressure chronic ulcer of buttock with unspecified severity 🔵

● **L98.42**   Non-pressure chronic ulcer of back

L98.421   Non-pressure chronic ulcer of back limited to breakdown of skin 🔵

L98.422   Non-pressure chronic ulcer of back with fat layer exposed 🔵

L98.423   Non-pressure chronic ulcer of back with necrosis of muscle 🔵

L98.424   Non-pressure chronic ulcer of back with necrosis of bone 🔵

L98.425   Non-pressure chronic ulcer of back with muscle involvement without evidence of necrosis 🔵🔵

L98.426   Non-pressure chronic ulcer of back with bone involvement without evidence of necrosis 🔵🔵

L98.428   Non-pressure chronic ulcer of back with other specified severity 🔵🔵

L98.429   Non-pressure chronic ulcer of back with unspecified severity 🔵

● **L98.49**   Non-pressure chronic ulcer of skin of other sites
Non-pressure chronic ulcer of skin NOS

L98.491   Non-pressure chronic ulcer of skin of other sites limited to breakdown of skin 🔵

L98.492   Non-pressure chronic ulcer of skin of other sites with fat layer exposed 🔵

L98.493   Non-pressure chronic ulcer of skin of other sites with necrosis of muscle 🔵

L98.494   Non-pressure chronic ulcer of skin of other sites with necrosis of bone 🔵

L98.495   Non-pressure chronic ulcer of skin of other sites with muscle involvement without evidence of necrosis 🔵🔵

L98.496   Non-pressure chronic ulcer of skin of other sites with bone involvement without evidence of necrosis 🔵🔵

L98.498   Non-pressure chronic ulcer of skin of other sites with other specified severity 🔵🔵

L98.499   Non-pressure chronic ulcer of skin of other sites with unspecified severity 🔵

L98.5   **Mucinosis of the skin**
Focal mucinosis
Lichen myxedematosus
Reticular erythematous mucinosis

     Excludes 1   focal oral mucinosis (K13.79)
                   myxedema (E03.9)

L98.6   **Other infiltrative disorders of the skin and subcutaneous tissue**

     Excludes 1   hyalinosis cutis et mucosae (E78.89)

L98.7   **Excessive and redundant skin and subcutaneous tissue**
Loose or sagging skin following bariatric surgery weight loss
Loose or sagging skin following dietary weight loss
Loose or sagging skin, NOS

     Excludes 2   acquired excess or redundant skin of eyelid (H02.3-)
                   congenital excess or redundant skin of eyelid (Q10.3)
                   skin changes due to chronic exposure to nonionizing radiation (L57.-)

     Coding Clinic: 2016, Q4, P36

L98.8   **Other specified disorders of the skin and subcutaneous tissue**

     Coding Clinic: 2013, Q2, P32

L98.9   **Disorder of the skin and subcutaneous tissue, unspecified**

▷ *L99*   *Other disorders of skin and subcutaneous tissue in diseases classified elsewhere*

     Code first underlying disease, such as:
     amyloidosis (E85.-)

  ⟹ **Excludes 1**   skin disorders in diabetes (E08-E13 with .62-)
                   skin disorders in gonorrhea (A54.89)
                   skin disorders in syphilis (A51.31, A52.79)

CHAPTER 12 (L00–L99)

N Newborn Age: 0   **P** Pediatric Age: 0–17   **M** Maternity DX: 9–64   **A** Adult Age: 15–124   ♀ Females Only   ♂ Males Only

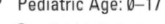 Complication\Comorbidity   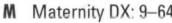 Major C\C   (Ex) CC/MCC Exclusions   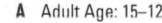 Hospital-Acquired Condition   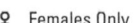 Hierarchical Condition Category   **1013**

CHAPTER 13

DISEASES OF THE MUSCULOSKELETAL SYSTEM AND CONNECTIVE TISSUE (M00-M99)

OGCR Chapter-Specific Coding Guidelines

13. Chapter 13: Diseases of the Musculoskeletal System and Connective Tissue (M00-M99)

  a. **Site and laterality**
  Most of the codes within Chapter 13 have site and laterality designations. The site represents the bone, joint or the muscle involved. For some conditions where more than one bone, joint or muscle is usually involved, such as osteoarthritis, there is a "multiple sites" code available. For categories where no multiple site code is provided and more than one bone, joint or muscle is involved, multiple codes should be used to indicate the different sites involved.

  1) **Bone versus joint**
  For certain conditions, the bone may be affected at the upper or lower end (e.g., avascular necrosis of bone, M87, Osteoporosis, M80, M81). Though the portion of the bone affected may be at the joint, the site designation will be the bone, not the joint.

  b. **Acute traumatic versus chronic or recurrent musculoskeletal conditions**
  Many musculoskeletal conditions are a result of previous injury or trauma to a site, or are recurrent conditions. Bone, joint or muscle conditions that are the result of a healed injury are usually found in Chapter 13. Recurrent bone, joint or muscle conditions are also usually found in Chapter 13. Any current, acute injury should be coded to the appropriate injury code from Chapter 19. Chronic or recurrent conditions should generally be coded with a code from Chapter 13. If it is difficult to determine from the documentation in the record which code is best to describe a condition, query the provider.

  c. **Coding of Pathologic Fractures**
  7th character A is for use as long as the patient is receiving active treatment for the fracture. While the patient may be seen by a new or different provider over the course of treatment for a pathological fracture, assignment of the 7th character is based on whether the patient is undergoing active treatment and not whether the provider is seeing the patient for the first time.

  7th character, D is to be used for encounters after the patient has completed active treatment for the fracture and is receiving routine care for the fracture during the healing or recovery phase. The other 7th characters, listed under each subcategory in the Tabular List, are to be used for subsequent encounters for treatment of problems associated with the healing, such as malunions, nonunions, and sequelae.

  Care for complications of surgical treatment for fracture repairs during the healing or recovery phase should be coded with the appropriate complication codes.

  See Section I.C.19. Coding of traumatic fractures.

  d. **Osteoporosis**
  Osteoporosis is a systemic condition, meaning that all bones of the musculoskeletal system are affected. Therefore, site is not a component of the codes under category M81, Osteoporosis without current pathological fracture. The site codes under category M80, Osteoporosis with current pathological fracture, identify the site of the fracture, not the osteoporosis.

  1) **Osteoporosis without pathological fracture**
  Category M81, Osteoporosis without current pathological fracture, is for use for patients with osteoporosis who do not currently have a pathologic fracture due to the osteoporosis, even if they have had a fracture in the past. For patients with a history of osteoporosis fractures, status code Z87.310, Personal history of (healed) osteoporosis fracture, should follow the code from M81.

  2) **Osteoporosis with current pathological fracture**
  Category M80, Osteoporosis with current pathological fracture, is for patients who have a current pathologic fracture at the time of an encounter. The codes under M80 identify the site of the fracture. A code from category M80, not a traumatic fracture code, should be used for any patient with known osteoporosis who suffers a fracture, even if the patient had a minor fall or trauma, if that fall or trauma would not usually break a normal, healthy bone.

CHAPTER 13

DISEASES OF THE MUSCULOSKELETAL SYSTEM AND CONNECTIVE TISSUE (M00-M99)

Note: Use an external cause code following the code for the musculoskeletal condition, if applicable, to identify the cause of the musculoskeletal condition

Excludes2 arthropathic psoriasis (L40.5-)
  certain conditions originating in the perinatal period (P04-P96)
  certain infectious and parasitic diseases (A00-B99)
  compartment syndrome (traumatic) (T79.A-)
  complications of pregnancy, childbirth and the puerperium (O00-O9A)
  congenital malformations, deformations, and chromosomal abnormalities (Q00-Q99)
  endocrine, nutritional and metabolic diseases (E00-E88)
  injury, poisoning and certain other consequences of external causes (S00-T88)
  neoplasms (C00-D49)
  symptoms, signs and abnormal clinical and laboratory findings, not elsewhere classified (R00-R94)

This chapter contains the following blocks:

M00-M02	Infectious arthropathies
M04	Autoinflammatory syndromes
M05-M14	Inflammatory polyarthropathies
M15-M19	Osteoarthritis
M20-M25	Other joint disorders
M26-M27	Dentofacial anomalies [including malocclusion] and other disorders of jaw
M30-M36	Systemic connective tissue disorders
M40-M43	Deforming dorsopathies
M45-M49	Spondylopathies
M50-M54	Other dorsopathies
M60-M63	Disorders of muscles
M65-M67	Disorders of synovium and tendon
M70-M79	Other soft tissue disorders
M80-M85	Disorders of bone density and structure
M86-M90	Other osteopathies
M91-M94	Chondropathies
M95	Other disorders of the musculoskeletal system and connective tissue
M96	Intraoperative and postprocedural complications and disorders of musculoskeletal system, not elsewhere classified
M97	Periprosthetic fracture around internal prosthetic joint
M99	Biomechanical lesions, not elsewhere classified

Coding Clinic: 2016, Q4, P124

ARTHROPATHIES (M00-M25)

Includes Disorders affecting predominantly peripheral (limb) joints

INFECTIOUS ARTHROPATHIES (M00-M02)

Note: This block comprises arthropathies due to microbiological agents.

Distinction is made between the following types of etiological relationship:

a) direct infection of joint, where organisms invade synovial tissue and microbial antigen is present in the joint;

b) indirect infection, which may be of two types: a reactive arthropathy, where microbial infection of the body is established but neither organisms nor antigens can be identified in the joint, and a postinfective arthropathy, where microbial antigen is present but recovery of an organism is inconstant and evidence of local multiplication is lacking.

▶ New   ⇒ Revised   deleted Deleted   Excludes 1   Excludes 2   Includes   Use additional   Code first   Code also   Key words

OGCR Official Guidelines   ● Unacceptable Principal Diagnosis   X Assign placeholder X   ● Use Additional Character(s)   ▷ Manifestation Code   Coding Clinic

● M00   **Pyogenic arthritis**
   Excludes2   infection and inflammatory reaction due to
               internal joint prosthesis (T84.5-)
● M00.0   **Staphylococcal** arthritis and polyarthritis
         Use additional code (B95.61-B95.8) to identify bacterial
         agent
      M00.00   Staphylococcal arthritis, unspecified joint 🔵🔵
               Ex: See PDX Collection 855
   ● M00.01   Staphylococcal arthritis, shoulder
               Ex: For category M00.01 CC codes: See PDX Collection 856
         M00.011   Staphylococcal arthritis, right
                   shoulder 🔵🔵
         M00.012   Staphylococcal arthritis, left
                   shoulder 🔵🔵
         M00.019   Staphylococcal arthritis, unspecified
                   shoulder 🔵🔵
   ● M00.02   Staphylococcal arthritis, elbow
               Ex: For category M00.02 CC codes: See PDX Collection 857
         M00.021   Staphylococcal arthritis, right
                   elbow 🔵🔵
         M00.022   Staphylococcal arthritis, left
                   elbow 🔵🔵
         M00.029   Staphylococcal arthritis, unspecified
                   elbow 🔵🔵
   ● M00.03   Staphylococcal arthritis, wrist
               Staphylococcal arthritis of carpal bones
               Ex: For category M00.03 CC codes: See PDX Collection 858
         M00.031   Staphylococcal arthritis, right
                   wrist 🔵🔵
         M00.032   Staphylococcal arthritis, left
                   wrist 🔵🔵
         M00.039   Staphylococcal arthritis, unspecified
                   wrist 🔵🔵
   ● M00.04   Staphylococcal arthritis, hand
               Staphylococcal arthritis of metacarpus and
               phalanges
               Ex: For category M00.04 CC codes: See PDX Collection 859
         M00.041   Staphylococcal arthritis, right
                   hand 🔵🔵
         M00.042   Staphylococcal arthritis, left
                   hand 🔵🔵
         M00.049   Staphylococcal arthritis, unspecified
                   hand 🔵🔵
   ● M00.05   Staphylococcal arthritis, hip
               Ex: For category M00.05 CC codes: See PDX Collection 860
         M00.051   Staphylococcal arthritis, right hip 🔵🔵
         M00.052   Staphylococcal arthritis, left hip 🔵🔵
         M00.059   Staphylococcal arthritis, unspecified
                   hip 🔵🔵
   ● M00.06   Staphylococcal arthritis, knee
               Ex: For category M00.06 CC codes: See PDX Collection 861
         M00.061   Staphylococcal arthritis, right
                   knee 🔵🔵
         M00.062   Staphylococcal arthritis, left
                   knee 🔵🔵
         M00.069   Staphylococcal arthritis, unspecified
                   knee 🔵🔵
   ● M00.07   Staphylococcal arthritis, ankle and foot
               Staphylococcal arthritis, tarsus, metatarsus and
               phalanges
               Ex: For category M00.07 CC codes: See PDX Collection 862
         M00.071   Staphylococcal arthritis, right ankle
                   and foot 🔵🔵
         M00.072   Staphylococcal arthritis, left ankle
                   and foot 🔵🔵
         M00.079   Staphylococcal arthritis, unspecified
                   ankle and foot 🔵🔵

      M00.08   Staphylococcal arthritis, vertebrae 🔵🔵
               Ex: See PDX Collection 855
      M00.09   Staphylococcal polyarthritis 🔵🔵
               Ex: See PDX Collection 855
● M00.1   Pneumococcal arthritis and polyarthritis
      M00.10   Pneumococcal arthritis, unspecified joint 🔵🔵
               Ex: See PDX Collection 855
   ● M00.11   Pneumococcal arthritis, shoulder
               Ex: For category M00.11 CC codes: See PDX Collection 856
         M00.111   Pneumococcal arthritis, right
                   shoulder 🔵🔵
         M00.112   Pneumococcal arthritis, left
                   shoulder 🔵🔵
         M00.119   Pneumococcal arthritis, unspecified
                   shoulder 🔵🔵
   ● M00.12   Pneumococcal arthritis, elbow
               Ex: For category M00.12 CC codes: See PDX Collection 857
         M00.121   Pneumococcal arthritis, right
                   elbow 🔵🔵
         M00.122   Pneumococcal arthritis, left
                   elbow 🔵🔵
         M00.129   Pneumococcal arthritis, unspecified
                   elbow 🔵🔵
   ● M00.13   Pneumococcal arthritis, wrist
               Pneumococcal arthritis of carpal bones
               Ex: For category M00.13 CC codes: See PDX Collection 858
         M00.131   Pneumococcal arthritis, right
                   wrist 🔵🔵
         M00.132   Pneumococcal arthritis, left wrist 🔵🔵
         M00.139   Pneumococcal arthritis, unspecified
                   wrist 🔵🔵
   ● M00.14   Pneumococcal arthritis, hand
               Pneumococcal arthritis of metacarpus and
               phalanges
               Ex: For category M00.14 CC codes: See PDX Collection 859
         M00.141   Pneumococcal arthritis, right
                   hand 🔵🔵
         M00.142   Pneumococcal arthritis, left hand 🔵🔵
         M00.149   Pneumococcal arthritis, unspecified
                   hand 🔵🔵
   ● M00.15   Pneumococcal arthritis, hip
               Ex: For category M00.15 CC codes: See PDX Collection 860
         M00.151   Pneumococcal arthritis, right hip 🔵🔵
         M00.152   Pneumococcal arthritis, left hip 🔵🔵
         M00.159   Pneumococcal arthritis, unspecified
                   hip 🔵🔵
   ● M00.16   Pneumococcal arthritis, knee
               Ex: For category M00.16 CC codes: See PDX Collection 861
         M00.161   Pneumococcal arthritis, right
                   knee 🔵🔵
         M00.162   Pneumococcal arthritis, left knee 🔵🔵
         M00.169   Pneumococcal arthritis, unspecified
                   knee 🔵🔵
   ● M00.17   Pneumococcal arthritis, ankle and foot
               Pneumococcal arthritis, tarsus, metatarsus and
               phalanges
               Ex: For category M00.17 CC codes: See PDX Collection 862
         M00.171   Pneumococcal arthritis, right ankle
                   and foot 🔵🔵
         M00.172   Pneumococcal arthritis, left ankle and
                   foot 🔵🔵
         M00.179   Pneumococcal arthritis, unspecified
                   ankle and foot 🔵🔵
      M00.18   Pneumococcal arthritis, vertebrae 🔵🔵
               Ex: See PDX Collection 855
      M00.19   Pneumococcal polyarthritis 🔵🔵
               Ex: See PDX Collection 855

CHAPTER 13 (M00-M99)

N Newborn Age: 0   **P** Pediatric Age: 0–17   **M** Maternity DX: 9–64   **A** Adult Age: 15–124   ♀ Females Only   ♂ Males Only
🔵 Complication\Comorbidity   🔵 Major C\C   Ex: CC/MCC Exclusions   🔵 Hospital-Acquired Condition   🔵 Hierarchical Condition Category

1015

● **M00.2 Other streptococcal arthritis and polyarthritis**
    Use additional code (B95.0-B95.2, B95.4-B95.5) to identify bacterial agent

    M00.20 Other streptococcal arthritis, unspecified joint 🦴🦴
        (Ex:) See PDX Collection 855

    ● **M00.21 Other streptococcal arthritis, shoulder**
        (Ex:) For category M00.21 CC codes: See PDX Collection 856
        M00.211 Other streptococcal arthritis, right shoulder 🦴🦴
        M00.212 Other streptococcal arthritis, left shoulder 🦴🦴
        M00.219 Other streptococcal arthritis, unspecified shoulder 🦴🦴

    ● **M00.22 Other streptococcal arthritis, elbow**
        (Ex:) For category M00.22 CC codes: See PDX Collection 857
        M00.221 Other streptococcal arthritis, right elbow 🦴🦴
        M00.222 Other streptococcal arthritis, left elbow 🦴🦴
        M00.229 Other streptococcal arthritis, unspecified elbow 🦴🦴

    ● **M00.23 Other streptococcal arthritis, wrist**
        Other streptococcal arthritis of carpal bones
        (Ex:) For category M00.23 CC codes: See PDX Collection 858
        M00.231 Other streptococcal arthritis, right wrist 🦴🦴
        M00.232 Other streptococcal arthritis, left wrist 🦴🦴
        M00.239 Other streptococcal arthritis, unspecified wrist 🦴🦴

    ● **M00.24 Other streptococcal arthritis, hand**
        Other streptococcal arthritis metacarpus and phalanges
        (Ex:) For category M00.24 CC codes: See PDX Collection 859
        M00.241 Other streptococcal arthritis, right hand 🦴🦴
        M00.242 Other streptococcal arthritis, left hand 🦴🦴
        M00.249 Other streptococcal arthritis, unspecified hand 🦴🦴

    ● **M00.25 Other streptococcal arthritis, hip**
        (Ex:) For category M00.25 CC codes: See PDX Collection 860
        M00.251 Other streptococcal arthritis, right hip 🦴🦴
        M00.252 Other streptococcal arthritis, left hip 🦴🦴
        M00.259 Other streptococcal arthritis, unspecified hip 🦴🦴

    ● **M00.26 Other streptococcal arthritis, knee**
        (Ex:) For category M00.26 CC codes: See PDX Collection 861
        M00.261 Other streptococcal arthritis, right knee 🦴🦴
        M00.262 Other streptococcal arthritis, left knee 🦴🦴
        M00.269 Other streptococcal arthritis, unspecified knee 🦴🦴

    ● **M00.27 Other streptococcal arthritis, ankle and foot**
        Other streptococcal arthritis, tarsus, metatarsus and phalanges
        (Ex:) For category M00.27 CC codes: See PDX Collection 862
        M00.271 Other streptococcal arthritis, right ankle and foot 🦴🦴
        M00.272 Other streptococcal arthritis, left ankle and foot 🦴🦴
        M00.279 Other streptococcal arthritis, unspecified ankle and foot 🦴🦴

    M00.28 Other streptococcal arthritis, vertebrae 🦴🦴
        (Ex:) See PDX Collection 855

    M00.29 Other streptococcal polyarthritis 🦴🦴
        (Ex:) See PDX Collection 855

● **M00.8 Arthritis and polyarthritis due to other bacteria**
    Use additional code (B96) to identify bacteria

    M00.80 Arthritis due to other bacteria, unspecified joint 🦴🦴
        (Ex:) See PDX Collection 855

    ● **M00.81 Arthritis due to other bacteria, shoulder**
        (Ex:) For category M00.81 CC codes: See PDX Collection 856
        M00.811 Arthritis due to other bacteria, right shoulder 🦴🦴
        M00.812 Arthritis due to other bacteria, left shoulder 🦴🦴
        M00.819 Arthritis due to other bacteria, unspecified shoulder 🦴🦴

    ● **M00.82 Arthritis due to other bacteria, elbow**
        (Ex:) For category M00.82 CC codes: See PDX Collection 857
        M00.821 Arthritis due to other bacteria, right elbow 🦴🦴
        M00.822 Arthritis due to other bacteria, left elbow 🦴🦴
        M00.829 Arthritis due to other bacteria, unspecified elbow 🦴🦴

    ● **M00.83 Arthritis due to other bacteria, wrist**
        Arthritis due to other bacteria, carpal bones
        (Ex:) For category M00.83 CC codes: See PDX Collection 858
        M00.831 Arthritis due to other bacteria, right wrist 🦴🦴
        M00.832 Arthritis due to other bacteria, left wrist 🦴🦴
        M00.839 Arthritis due to other bacteria, unspecified wrist 🦴🦴

    ● **M00.84 Arthritis due to other bacteria, hand**
        Arthritis due to other bacteria, metacarpus and phalanges
        (Ex:) For category M00.84 CC codes: See PDX Collection 859
        M00.841 Arthritis due to other bacteria, right hand 🦴🦴
        M00.842 Arthritis due to other bacteria, left hand 🦴🦴
        M00.849 Arthritis due to other bacteria, unspecified hand 🦴🦴

    ● **M00.85 Arthritis due to other bacteria, hip**
        (Ex:) For category M00.85 CC codes: See PDX Collection 860
        M00.851 Arthritis due to other bacteria, right hip 🦴🦴
        M00.852 Arthritis due to other bacteria, left hip 🦴🦴
        M00.859 Arthritis due to other bacteria, unspecified hip 🦴🦴

    ● **M00.86 Arthritis due to other bacteria, knee**
        (Ex:) For category M00.86 CC codes: See PDX Collection 861
        M00.861 Arthritis due to other bacteria, right knee 🦴🦴
        M00.862 Arthritis due to other bacteria, left knee 🦴🦴
           Coding Clinic: 2019, Q3, P16
        M00.869 Arthritis due to other bacteria, unspecified knee 🦴🦴

    ● **M00.87 Arthritis due to other bacteria, ankle and foot**
        Arthritis due to other bacteria, tarsus, metatarsus, and phalanges
        (Ex:) For category M00.87 CC codes: See PDX Collection 862
        M00.871 Arthritis due to other bacteria, right ankle and foot 🦴🦴
        M00.872 Arthritis due to other bacteria, left ankle and foot 🦴🦴
        M00.879 Arthritis due to other bacteria, unspecified ankle and foot 🦴🦴

    M00.88 Arthritis due to other bacteria, vertebrae 🦴🦴
        (Ex:) See PDX Collection 855

    M00.89 Polyarthritis due to other bacteria 🦴🦴
        (Ex:) See PDX Collection 855

M00.9 Pyogenic arthritis, unspecified 🦴🦴
    Infective arthritis NOS
        (Ex:) See PDX Collection 855

▶ New   ⇒ Revised   ~~deleted~~ Deleted   Excludes 1   Excludes 2   Includes   Use additional   Code first   Code also   Key words
OGCR Official Guidelines   ● Unacceptable Principal Diagnosis   X Assign placeholder X   ● Use Additional Character(s)   ▶ Manifestation Code   Coding Clinic

● **M01**   **Direct infections of joint in infectious and parasitic diseases classified elsewhere**

> *Code first underlying disease, such as:*
> leprosy [Hansen's disease] (A30.-)
> mycoses (B35-B49)
> O'nyong-nyong fever (A92.1)
> paratyphoid fever (A01.1-A01.4)
>
> **Excludes1**   arthropathy in Lyme disease (A69.23)
> gonococcal arthritis (A54.42)
> meningococcal arthritis (A39.83)
> mumps arthritis (B26.85)
> postinfective arthropathy (M02.-)
> postmeningococcal arthritis (A39.84)
> reactive arthritis (M02.3)
> rubella arthritis (B06.82)
> sarcoidosis arthritis (D86.86)
> typhoid fever arthritis (A01.04)
> tuberculosis arthritis (A18.01-A18.02)

● **M01.X**   **Direct infection of joint in infectious and parasitic diseases classified elsewhere**

> (Ex) For category M01.X CC codes unless otherwise indicated: See PDX Collection 863

> ▶ *M01.X0*   *Direct infection of unspecified joint in infectious and parasitic diseases classified elsewhere* 🔲 🔲

● *M01.X1*   **Direct infection of shoulder joint in infectious and parasitic diseases classified elsewhere**

> (Ex) For category M01.X1 CC codes: See PDX Collection 864

> ▶ *M01.X11*   *Direct infection of right shoulder in infectious and parasitic diseases classified elsewhere* 🔲 🔲

> ▶ *M01.X12*   *Direct infection of left shoulder in infectious and parasitic diseases classified elsewhere* 🔲 🔲

> ▶ *M01.X19*   *Direct infection of unspecified shoulder in infectious and parasitic diseases classified elsewhere* 🔲 🔲

● **M01.X2**   **Direct infection of elbow in infectious and parasitic diseases classified elsewhere**

> ▶ *M01.X21*   *Direct infection of right elbow in infectious and parasitic diseases classified elsewhere* 🔲 🔲

> ▶ *M01.X22*   *Direct infection of left elbow in infectious and parasitic diseases classified elsewhere* 🔲 🔲

> ▶ *M01.X29*   *Direct infection of unspecified elbow in infectious and parasitic diseases classified elsewhere* 🔲 🔲

● **M01.X3**   **Direct infection of wrist in infectious and parasitic diseases classified elsewhere**
> Direct infection of carpal bones in infectious and parasitic diseases classified elsewhere

> ▶ *M01.X31*   *Direct infection of right wrist in infectious and parasitic diseases classified elsewhere* 🔲 🔲

> ▶ *M01.X32*   *Direct infection of left wrist in infectious and parasitic diseases classified elsewhere* 🔲 🔲

> ▶ *M01.X39*   *Direct infection of unspecified wrist in infectious and parasitic diseases classified elsewhere* 🔲 🔲

● **M01.X4**   **Direct infection of hand in infectious and parasitic diseases classified elsewhere**
> Direct infection of metacarpus and phalanges in infectious and parasitic diseases classified elsewhere

> ▶ *M01.X41*   *Direct infection of right hand in infectious and parasitic diseases classified elsewhere* 🔲 🔲

> ▶ *M01.X42*   *Direct infection of left hand in infectious and parasitic diseases classified elsewhere* 🔲 🔲

> ▶ *M01.X49*   *Direct infection of unspecified hand in infectious and parasitic diseases classified elsewhere* 🔲 🔲

● **M01.X5**   **Direct infection of hip in infectious and parasitic diseases classified elsewhere**

> ▶ *M01.X51*   *Direct infection of right hip in infectious and parasitic diseases classified elsewhere* 🔲 🔲

> ▶ *M01.X52*   *Direct infection of left hip in infectious and parasitic diseases classified elsewhere* 🔲 🔲

> ▶ *M01.X59*   *Direct infection of unspecified hip in infectious and parasitic diseases classified elsewhere* 🔲 🔲

● **M01.X6**   **Direct infection of knee in infectious and parasitic diseases classified elsewhere**

> ▶ *M01.X61*   *Direct infection of right knee in infectious and parasitic diseases classified elsewhere* 🔲 🔲

> ▶ *M01.X62*   *Direct infection of left knee in infectious and parasitic diseases classified elsewhere* 🔲 🔲

> ▶ *M01.X69*   *Direct infection of unspecified knee in infectious and parasitic diseases classified elsewhere* 🔲 🔲

● **M01.X7**   **Direct infection of ankle and foot in infectious and parasitic diseases classified elsewhere**
> Direct infection of tarsus, metatarsus and phalanges in infectious and parasitic diseases classified elsewhere

> ▶ *M01.X71*   *Direct infection of right ankle and foot in infectious and parasitic diseases classified elsewhere* 🔲 🔲

> ▶ *M01.X72*   *Direct infection of left ankle and foot in infectious and parasitic diseases classified elsewhere* 🔲 🔲

> ▶ *M01.X79*   *Direct infection of unspecified ankle and foot in infectious and parasitic diseases classified elsewhere* 🔲 🔲

> ▶ *M01.X8*   *Direct infection of vertebrae in infectious and parasitic diseases classified elsewhere* 🔲 🔲

> ▶ *M01.X9*   *Direct infection of multiple joints in infectious and parasitic diseases classified elsewhere* 🔲 🔲

● **M02**   **Postinfective and reactive arthropathies**

> *Code first underlying disease, such as:*
> congenital syphilis [Clutton's joints] (A50.5)
> enteritis due to Yersinia enterocolitica (A04.6)
> infective endocarditis (I33.0)
> viral hepatitis (B15-B19)
>
> **Excludes1**   Behçet's disease (M35.2)
> direct infections of joint in infectious and parasitic diseases classified elsewhere (M01.-)
> postmeningococcal arthritis (A39.84)
> mumps arthritis (B26.85)
> rubella arthritis (B06.82)
> syphilis arthritis (late) (A52.77)
> rheumatic fever (I00)
> tabetic arthropathy [Charcôt's] (A52.16)

> (Ex) For category M02 CC codes unless otherwise indicated: See PDX Collection 4014

● **M02.0**   **Arthropathy following intestinal bypass**

>   **M02.00**   Arthropathy following intestinal bypass, unspecified site

> ● **M02.01**   Arthropathy following intestinal bypass, shoulder

>   **M02.011**   Arthropathy following intestinal bypass, right shoulder

>   **M02.012**   Arthropathy following intestinal bypass, left shoulder

>   **M02.019**   Arthropathy following intestinal bypass, unspecified shoulder

> ● **M02.02**   Arthropathy following intestinal bypass, elbow

>   **M02.021**   Arthropathy following intestinal bypass, right elbow

>   **M02.022**   Arthropathy following intestinal bypass, left elbow

>   **M02.029**   Arthropathy following intestinal bypass, unspecified elbow

N   Newborn Age: 0   **P**   Pediatric Age: 0–17   **M**   Maternity DX: 9–64   **A**   Adult Age: 15–124   ♀   Females Only

🔲 Complication\Comorbidity   🔲 Major C\C   (Ex) CC/MCC Exclusions   🔲 Hospital-Acquired Condition   🔲 Hierarchical Condition Category

1017

CHAPTER 13 (M00-M99)

- M02.03   Arthropathy following intestinal bypass, wrist
  Arthropathy following intestinal bypass, carpal bones
  - M02.031   Arthropathy following intestinal bypass, right wrist
  - M02.032   Arthropathy following intestinal bypass, left wrist
  - M02.039   Arthropathy following intestinal bypass, unspecified wrist
- M02.04   Arthropathy following intestinal bypass, hand
  Arthropathy following intestinal bypass, metacarpals and phalanges
  - M02.041   Arthropathy following intestinal bypass, right hand
  - M02.042   Arthropathy following intestinal bypass, left hand
  - M02.049   Arthropathy following intestinal bypass, unspecified hand
- M02.05   Arthropathy following intestinal bypass, hip
  - M02.051   Arthropathy following intestinal bypass, right hip
  - M02.052   Arthropathy following intestinal bypass, left hip
  - M02.059   Arthropathy following intestinal bypass, unspecified hip
- M02.06   Arthropathy following intestinal bypass, knee
  - M02.061   Arthropathy following intestinal bypass, right knee
  - M02.062   Arthropathy following intestinal bypass, left knee
  - M02.069   Arthropathy following intestinal bypass, unspecified knee
- M02.07   Arthropathy following intestinal bypass, ankle and foot
  Arthropathy following intestinal bypass, tarsus, metatarsus and phalanges
  - M02.071   Arthropathy following intestinal bypass, right ankle and foot
  - M02.072   Arthropathy following intestinal bypass, left ankle and foot
  - M02.079   Arthropathy following intestinal bypass, unspecified ankle and foot
  - M02.08   Arthropathy following intestinal bypass, vertebrae
  - M02.09   Arthropathy following intestinal bypass, multiple sites
- M02.1   Postdysenteric arthropathy
  - M02.10   Postdysenteric arthropathy, unspecified site ⚫⚫
  - M02.11   Postdysenteric arthropathy, shoulder
    - M02.111   Postdysenteric arthropathy, right shoulder ⚫⚫
    - M02.112   Postdysenteric arthropathy, left shoulder ⚫⚫
    - M02.119   Postdysenteric arthropathy, unspecified shoulder ⚫⚫
  - M02.12   Postdysenteric arthropathy, elbow
    - M02.121   Postdysenteric arthropathy, right elbow ⚫⚫
    - M02.122   Postdysenteric arthropathy, left elbow ⚫⚫
    - M02.129   Postdysenteric arthropathy, unspecified elbow ⚫⚫
  - M02.13   Postdysenteric arthropathy, wrist
    Postdysenteric arthropathy, carpal bones
    - M02.131   Postdysenteric arthropathy, right wrist ⚫⚫
    - M02.132   Postdysenteric arthropathy, left wrist ⚫⚫
    - M02.139   Postdysenteric arthropathy, unspecified wrist ⚫⚫

- M02.14   Postdysenteric arthropathy, hand
  Postdysenteric arthropathy, metacarpus and phalanges
  - M02.141   Postdysenteric arthropathy, right hand ⚫⚫
  - M02.142   Postdysenteric arthropathy, left hand ⚫⚫
  - M02.149   Postdysenteric arthropathy, unspecified hand ⚫⚫
- M02.15   Postdysenteric arthropathy, hip
  - M02.151   Postdysenteric arthropathy, right hip ⚫⚫
  - M02.152   Postdysenteric arthropathy, left hip ⚫⚫
  - M02.159   Postdysenteric arthropathy, unspecified hip ⚫⚫
- M02.16   Postdysenteric arthropathy, knee
  (Ex) **For category M02.16 CC codes:** See PDX Collection 865
  - M02.161   Postdysenteric arthropathy, right knee ⚫⚫
  - M02.162   Postdysenteric arthropathy, left knee ⚫⚫
  - M02.169   Postdysenteric arthropathy, unspecified knee ⚫⚫
- M02.17   Postdysenteric arthropathy, ankle and foot
  Postdysenteric arthropathy, tarsus, metatarsus and phalanges
  - M02.171   Postdysenteric arthropathy, right ankle and foot ⚫⚫
  - M02.172   Postdysenteric arthropathy, left ankle and foot ⚫⚫
  - M02.179   Postdysenteric arthropathy, unspecified ankle and foot ⚫⚫
  - M02.18   Postdysenteric arthropathy, vertebrae ⚫⚫
  - M02.19   Postdysenteric arthropathy, multiple sites ⚫⚫
- M02.2   Postimmunization arthropathy
  - M02.20   Postimmunization arthropathy, unspecified site
  - M02.21   Postimmunization arthropathy, shoulder
    - M02.211   Postimmunization arthropathy, right shoulder
    - M02.212   Postimmunization arthropathy, left shoulder
    - M02.219   Postimmunization arthropathy, unspecified shoulder
  - M02.22   Postimmunization arthropathy, elbow
    - M02.221   Postimmunization arthropathy, right elbow
    - M02.222   Postimmunization arthropathy, left elbow
    - M02.229   Postimmunization arthropathy, unspecified elbow
  - M02.23   Postimmunization arthropathy, wrist
    Postimmunization arthropathy, carpal bones
    - M02.231   Postimmunization arthropathy, right wrist
    - M02.232   Postimmunization arthropathy, left wrist
    - M02.239   Postimmunization arthropathy, unspecified wrist
  - M02.24   Postimmunization arthropathy, hand
    Postimmunization arthropathy, metacarpus and phalanges
    - M02.241   Postimmunization arthropathy, right hand
    - M02.242   Postimmunization arthropathy, left hand
    - M02.249   Postimmunization arthropathy, unspecified hand

▶ New   ⟹ Revised   ~~deleted~~ Deleted   Excludes 1   Excludes 2   Includes   Use additional   Code first   Code also   Key words
OGCR Official Guidelines   ⚫ Unacceptable Principal Diagnosis   X Assign placeholder X   ⚫ Use Additional Character(s)   ▶ Manifestation Code   **Coding Clinic**

● **M02.25**   Postimmunization arthropathy, hip

     M02.251   Postimmunization arthropathy, right hip

     M02.252   Postimmunization arthropathy, left hip

     M02.259   Postimmunization arthropathy, unspecified hip

● **M02.26**   Postimmunization arthropathy, knee

     M02.261   Postimmunization arthropathy, right knee

     M02.262   Postimmunization arthropathy, left knee

     M02.269   Postimmunization arthropathy, unspecified knee

● **M02.27**   Postimmunization arthropathy, ankle and foot
     Postimmunization arthropathy, tarsus, metatarsus and phalanges

     M02.271   Postimmunization arthropathy, right ankle and foot

     M02.272   Postimmunization arthropathy, left ankle and foot

     M02.279   Postimmunization arthropathy, unspecified ankle and foot

     M02.28   Postimmunization arthropathy, vertebrae

     M02.29   Postimmunization arthropathy, multiple sites

● **M02.3**   Reiter's disease
     Reactive arthritis

     M02.30   Reiter's disease, unspecified site 🦠 🦠
         CC when PDx is its own CC

● **M02.31**   Reiter's disease, shoulder

     M02.311   Reiter's disease, right shoulder 🦠 🦠
         (Ex:) See PDX Collection 3752
         CC when PDx is its own CC

     M02.312   Reiter's disease, left shoulder 🦠 🦠
         (Ex:) See PDX Collection 3754
         CC when PDx is its own CC

     M02.319   Reiter's disease, unspecified shoulder 🦠 🦠
         CC when PDx is its own CC

● **M02.32**   Reiter's disease, elbow

     M02.321   Reiter's disease, right elbow 🦠 🦠
         (Ex:) See PDX Collection 3756
         CC when PDx is its own CC

     M02.322   Reiter's disease, left elbow 🦠 🦠
         (Ex:) See PDX Collection 3758
         CC when PDx is its own CC

     M02.329   Reiter's disease, unspecified elbow 🦠 🦠
         CC when PDx is its own CC

● **M02.33**   Reiter's disease, wrist
     Reiter's disease, carpal bones

     M02.331   Reiter's disease, right wrist 🦠 🦠
         (Ex:) See PDX Collection 3760
         CC when PDx is its own CC

     M02.332   Reiter's disease, left wrist 🦠 🦠
         (Ex:) See PDX Collection 3762
         CC when PDx is its own CC

     M02.339   Reiter's disease, unspecified wrist 🦠 🦠
         CC when PDx is its own CC

● **M02.34**   Reiter's disease, hand
     Reiter's disease, metacarpus and phalanges

     M02.341   Reiter's disease, right hand 🦠 🦠
         (Ex:) See PDX Collection 3764
         CC when PDx is its own CC

     M02.342   Reiter's disease, left hand 🦠 🦠
         (Ex:) See PDX Collection 3766
         CC when PDx is its own CC

     M02.349   Reiter's disease, unspecified hand 🦠 🦠
         CC when PDx is its own CC

● **M02.35**   Reiter's disease, hip

     M02.351   Reiter's disease, right hip 🦠 🦠
         (Ex:) See PDX Collection 3768
         CC when PDx is its own CC

     M02.352   Reiter's disease, left hip 🦠 🦠
         (Ex:) See PDX Collection 3770
         CC when PDx is its own CC

     M02.359   Reiter's disease, unspecified hip 🦠 🦠
         CC when PDx is its own CC

● **M02.36**   Reiter's disease, knee

     M02.361   Reiter's disease, right knee 🦠 🦠
         (Ex:) See PDX Collection 3772
         CC when PDx is its own CC

     M02.362   Reiter's disease, left knee 🦠 🦠
         (Ex:) See PDX Collection 3774
         CC when PDx is its own CC

     M02.369   Reiter's disease, unspecified knee 🦠 🦠
         CC when PDx is its own CC

● **M02.37**   Reiter's disease, ankle and foot
     Reiter's disease, tarsus, metatarsus and phalanges

     M02.371   Reiter's disease, right ankle and foot 🦠 🦠
         (Ex:) See PDX Collection 3776
         CC when PDx is its own CC

     M02.372   Reiter's disease, left ankle and foot 🦠 🦠
         (Ex:) See PDX Collection 3778
         CC when PDx is its own CC

     M02.379   Reiter's disease, unspecified ankle and foot 🦠 🦠
         CC when PDx is its own CC

     M02.38   Reiter's disease, vertebrae 🦠 🦠
         CC when PDx is its own CC

     M02.39   Reiter's disease, multiple sites 🦠 🦠
         CC when PDx is its own CC

● **M02.8**   Other reactive arthropathies

▷ *M02.80*   *Other reactive arthropathies, unspecified site* 🦠 🦠

● **M02.81**   Other reactive arthropathies, shoulder
         (Ex:) For category M02.81 CC codes: See PDX Collection 4014

     ▷ *M02.811*   *Other reactive arthropathies, right shoulder* 🦠 🦠

     ▷ *M02.812*   *Other reactive arthropathies, left shoulder* 🦠 🦠

     ▷ *M02.819*   *Other reactive arthropathies, unspecified shoulder* 🦠 🦠

● **M02.82**   Other reactive arthropathies, elbow

     ▷ *M02.821*   *Other reactive arthropathies, right elbow* 🦠 🦠

     ▷ *M02.822*   *Other reactive arthropathies, left elbow* 🦠 🦠

     ▷ *M02.829*   *Other reactive arthropathies, unspecified elbow* 🦠 🦠

● **M02.83**   Other reactive arthropathies, wrist
     Other reactive arthropathies, carpal bones

     ▷ *M02.831*   *Other reactive arthropathies, right wrist* 🦠 🦠

     ▷ *M02.832*   *Other reactive arthropathies, left wrist* 🦠 🦠

     ▷ *M02.839*   *Other reactive arthropathies, unspecified wrist* 🦠 🦠

● **M02.84**   Other reactive arthropathies, hand
     Other reactive arthropathies, metacarpus and phalanges

     ▷ *M02.841*   *Other reactive arthropathies, right hand* 🦠 🦠

     ▷ *M02.842*   *Other reactive arthropathies, left hand* 🦠 🦠

     ▷ *M02.849*   *Other reactive arthropathies, unspecified hand* 🦠 🦠

CHAPTER 13 (M00-M99)

N Newborn Age: 0   **P** Pediatric Age: 0–17   **M** Maternity DX: 9–64   **A** Adult Age: 15–124   ♀ Females Only   ♂ Males Only

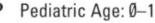 Complication\Comorbidity   🦠 Major C\C   (Ex:) CC/MCC Exclusions   🦠 Hospital-Acquired Condition   🦠 Hierarchical Condition Category

1019

● M02.85　Other reactive arthropathies, hip
- ▸ M02.851　*Other reactive arthropathies, right hip* 🔍 🔍
- ▸ M02.852　*Other reactive arthropathies, left hip* 🔍 🔍
- ▸ M02.859　*Other reactive arthropathies, unspecified hip* 🔍 🔍

● M02.86　Other reactive arthropathies, knee
- ▸ M02.861　*Other reactive arthropathies, right knee* 🔍 🔍
- ▸ M02.862　*Other reactive arthropathies, left knee* 🔍 🔍
- ▸ M02.869　*Other reactive arthropathies, unspecified knee* 🔍 🔍

● M02.87　Other reactive arthropathies, ankle and foot
　　Other reactive arthropathies, tarsus, metatarsus and phalanges
- ▸ M02.871　*Other reactive arthropathies, right ankle and foot* 🔍 🔍
- ▸ M02.872　*Other reactive arthropathies, left ankle and foot* 🔍 🔍
- ▸ M02.879　*Other reactive arthropathies, unspecified ankle and foot* 🔍 🔍
- ▸ M02.88　*Other reactive arthropathies, vertebrae* 🔍 🔍
- ▸ M02.89　*Other reactive arthropathies, multiple sites* 🔍 🔍

▸ M02.9　*Reactive arthropathy, unspecified* 🔍

AUTOINFLAMMATORY SYNDROMES (M04)

● M04　Autoinflammatory syndromes
> **Excludes2**　Crohn's disease (K50.-)
> Coding Clinic: 2016, Q4, P37

M04.1　Periodic fever syndromes 🔍
　　Familial Mediterranean fever
　　Hyperimmunoglobin D syndrome
　　Mevalonate kinase deficiency
　　Tumor necrosis factor receptor associated periodic syndrome [TRAPS]

M04.2　Cryopyrin-associated periodic syndromes 🔍
　　Chronic infantile neurological, cutaneous and articular syndrome [CINCA]
　　Familial cold autoinflammatory syndrome
　　Familial cold urticaria
　　Muckle-Wells syndrome
　　Neonatal onset multisystemic inflammatory disorder [NOMID]

M04.8　Other autoinflammatory syndromes 🔍
　　Blau syndrome
　　Deficiency of interleukin 1 receptor antagonist [DIRA]
　　Majeed syndrome
　　Periodic fever, aphthous stomatitis, pharyngitis, and adenopathy syndrome [PFAPA]
　　Pyogenic arthritis, pyoderma gangrenosum, and acne syndrome [PAPA]

M04.9　Autoinflammatory syndrome, unspecified 🔍

INFLAMMATORY POLYARTHROPATHIES (M05-M14)

● M05　Rheumatoid arthritis with rheumatoid factor
> **Excludes1**　rheumatic fever (I00)
> 　　juvenile rheumatoid arthritis (M08.-)
> 　　rheumatoid arthritis of spine (M45.-)

● M05.0　Felty's syndrome
　　Rheumatoid arthritis with splenoadenomegaly and leukopenia

M05.00　Felty's syndrome, unspecified site 🔍

Item 13-1　Rheumatoid arthritis (RA) is a chronic systemic inflammatory autoimmune disease of undetermined etiology involving primarily the synovial membranes and articular structures of multiple joints. It can also affect other organs, including the eyes, blood vessels, heart, and lungs. The disease is often progressive. In late stages, deformity, ankylosis, and other **inflammatory polyarthropathies** develop.

● M05.01　Felty's syndrome, shoulder
- M05.011　Felty's syndrome, right shoulder 🔍
- M05.012　Felty's syndrome, left shoulder 🔍
- M05.019　Felty's syndrome, unspecified shoulder 🔍

● M05.02　Felty's syndrome, elbow
- M05.021　Felty's syndrome, right elbow 🔍
- M05.022　Felty's syndrome, left elbow 🔍
- M05.029　Felty's syndrome, unspecified elbow 🔍

● M05.03　Felty's syndrome, wrist
　　Felty's syndrome, carpal bones
- M05.031　Felty's syndrome, right wrist 🔍
- M05.032　Felty's syndrome, left wrist 🔍
- M05.039　Felty's syndrome, unspecified wrist 🔍

● M05.04　Felty's syndrome, hand
　　Felty's syndrome, metacarpus and phalanges
- M05.041　Felty's syndrome, right hand 🔍
- M05.042　Felty's syndrome, left hand 🔍
- M05.049　Felty's syndrome, unspecified hand 🔍

● M05.05　Felty's syndrome, hip
- M05.051　Felty's syndrome, right hip 🔍
- M05.052　Felty's syndrome, left hip 🔍
- M05.059　Felty's syndrome, unspecified hip 🔍

● M05.06　Felty's syndrome, knee
- M05.061　Felty's syndrome, right knee 🔍
- M05.062　Felty's syndrome, left knee 🔍
- M05.069　Felty's syndrome, unspecified knee 🔍

● M05.07　Felty's syndrome, ankle and foot
　　Felty's syndrome, tarsus, metatarsus and phalanges
- M05.071　Felty's syndrome, right ankle and foot 🔍
- M05.072　Felty's syndrome, left ankle and foot 🔍
- M05.079　Felty's syndrome, unspecified ankle and foot 🔍

M05.09　Felty's syndrome, multiple sites 🔍

● M05.1　Rheumatoid lung disease with rheumatoid arthritis

M05.10　Rheumatoid lung disease with rheumatoid arthritis of unspecified site 🔍

● M05.11　Rheumatoid lung disease with rheumatoid arthritis of shoulder
- M05.111　Rheumatoid lung disease with rheumatoid arthritis of right shoulder 🔍
- M05.112　Rheumatoid lung disease with rheumatoid arthritis of left shoulder 🔍
- M05.119　Rheumatoid lung disease with rheumatoid arthritis of unspecified shoulder 🔍

● M05.12　Rheumatoid lung disease with rheumatoid arthritis of elbow
- M05.121　Rheumatoid lung disease with rheumatoid arthritis of right elbow 🔍
- M05.122　Rheumatoid lung disease with rheumatoid arthritis of left elbow 🔍
- M05.129　Rheumatoid lung disease with rheumatoid arthritis of unspecified elbow 🔍

● M05.13　Rheumatoid lung disease with rheumatoid arthritis of wrist
　　Rheumatoid lung disease with rheumatoid arthritis, carpal bones
- M05.131　Rheumatoid lung disease with rheumatoid arthritis of right wrist 🔍
- M05.132　Rheumatoid lung disease with rheumatoid arthritis of left wrist 🔍
- M05.139　Rheumatoid lung disease with rheumatoid arthritis of unspecified wrist 🔍

▶ New　⇒ Revised　~~deleted~~ Deleted　Excludes 1　Excludes 2　Includes　Use additional　Code first　Code also　Key words
OGCR Official Guidelines　● Unacceptable Principal Diagnosis　X Assign placeholder X　● Use Additional Character(s)　▸ Manifestation Code　Coding Clinic

● **M05.14**   Rheumatoid lung disease with rheumatoid arthritis of hand
    Rheumatoid lung disease with rheumatoid arthritis, metacarpus and phalanges

    M05.141   Rheumatoid lung disease with rheumatoid arthritis of right hand 🝝

    M05.142   Rheumatoid lung disease with rheumatoid arthritis of left hand 🝝

    M05.149   Rheumatoid lung disease with rheumatoid arthritis of unspecified hand 🝝

● **M05.15**   Rheumatoid lung disease with rheumatoid arthritis of hip

    M05.151   Rheumatoid lung disease with rheumatoid arthritis of right hip 🝝

    M05.152   Rheumatoid lung disease with rheumatoid arthritis of left hip 🝝

    M05.159   Rheumatoid lung disease with rheumatoid arthritis of unspecified hip 🝝

● **M05.16**   Rheumatoid lung disease with rheumatoid arthritis of knee

    M05.161   Rheumatoid lung disease with rheumatoid arthritis of right knee 🝝

    M05.162   Rheumatoid lung disease with rheumatoid arthritis of left knee 🝝

    M05.169   Rheumatoid lung disease with rheumatoid arthritis of unspecified knee 🝝

● **M05.17**   Rheumatoid lung disease with rheumatoid arthritis of ankle and foot
    Rheumatoid lung disease with rheumatoid arthritis, tarsus, metatarsus and phalanges

    M05.171   Rheumatoid lung disease with rheumatoid arthritis of right ankle and foot 🝝

    M05.172   Rheumatoid lung disease with rheumatoid arthritis of left ankle and foot 🝝

    M05.179   Rheumatoid lung disease with rheumatoid arthritis of unspecified ankle and foot 🝝

    M05.19   Rheumatoid lung disease with rheumatoid arthritis of multiple sites 🝝

● **M05.2**   Rheumatoid vasculitis with rheumatoid arthritis

    M05.20   Rheumatoid vasculitis with rheumatoid arthritis of unspecified site 🝝

● **M05.21**   Rheumatoid vasculitis with rheumatoid arthritis of shoulder

    M05.211   Rheumatoid vasculitis with rheumatoid arthritis of right shoulder 🝝

    M05.212   Rheumatoid vasculitis with rheumatoid arthritis of left shoulder 🝝

    M05.219   Rheumatoid vasculitis with rheumatoid arthritis of unspecified shoulder 🝝

● **M05.22**   Rheumatoid vasculitis with rheumatoid arthritis of elbow

    M05.221   Rheumatoid vasculitis with rheumatoid arthritis of right elbow 🝝

    M05.222   Rheumatoid vasculitis with rheumatoid arthritis of left elbow 🝝

    M05.229   Rheumatoid vasculitis with rheumatoid arthritis of unspecified elbow 🝝

● **M05.23**   Rheumatoid vasculitis with rheumatoid arthritis of wrist
    Rheumatoid vasculitis with rheumatoid arthritis, carpal bones

    M05.231   Rheumatoid vasculitis with rheumatoid arthritis of right wrist 🝝

    M05.232   Rheumatoid vasculitis with rheumatoid arthritis of left wrist 🝝

    M05.239   Rheumatoid vasculitis with rheumatoid arthritis of unspecified wrist 🝝

● **M05.24**   Rheumatoid vasculitis with rheumatoid arthritis of hand
    Rheumatoid vasculitis with rheumatoid arthritis, metacarpus and phalanges

    M05.241   Rheumatoid vasculitis with rheumatoid arthritis of right hand 🝝

    M05.242   Rheumatoid vasculitis with rheumatoid arthritis of left hand 🝝

    M05.249   Rheumatoid vasculitis with rheumatoid arthritis of unspecified hand 🝝

● **M05.25**   Rheumatoid vasculitis with rheumatoid arthritis of hip

    M05.251   Rheumatoid vasculitis with rheumatoid arthritis of right hip 🝝

    M05.252   Rheumatoid vasculitis with rheumatoid arthritis of left hip 🝝

    M05.259   Rheumatoid vasculitis with rheumatoid arthritis of unspecified hip 🝝

● **M05.26**   Rheumatoid vasculitis with rheumatoid arthritis of knee

    M05.261   Rheumatoid vasculitis with rheumatoid arthritis of right knee 🝝

    M05.262   Rheumatoid vasculitis with rheumatoid arthritis of left knee 🝝

    M05.269   Rheumatoid vasculitis with rheumatoid arthritis of unspecified knee 🝝

● **M05.27**   Rheumatoid vasculitis with rheumatoid arthritis of ankle and foot
    Rheumatoid vasculitis with rheumatoid arthritis, tarsus, metatarsus and phalanges

    M05.271   Rheumatoid vasculitis with rheumatoid arthritis of right ankle and foot 🝝

    M05.272   Rheumatoid vasculitis with rheumatoid arthritis of left ankle and foot 🝝

    M05.279   Rheumatoid vasculitis with rheumatoid arthritis of unspecified ankle and foot 🝝

    M05.29   Rheumatoid vasculitis with rheumatoid arthritis of multiple sites 🝝

● **M05.3**   Rheumatoid heart disease with rheumatoid arthritis
    Rheumatoid carditis
    Rheumatoid endocarditis
    Rheumatoid myocarditis
    Rheumatoid pericarditis

    M05.30   Rheumatoid heart disease with rheumatoid arthritis of unspecified site 🝝

● **M05.31**   Rheumatoid heart disease with rheumatoid arthritis of shoulder

    M05.311   Rheumatoid heart disease with rheumatoid arthritis of right shoulder 🝝

    M05.312   Rheumatoid heart disease with rheumatoid arthritis of left shoulder 🝝

    M05.319   Rheumatoid heart disease with rheumatoid arthritis of unspecified shoulder 🝝

CHAPTER 13 (M00–M99)

N   Newborn Age: 0   **P**   Pediatric Age: 0–17   **M**   Maternity DX: 9–64   **A**   Adult Age: 15–124   ♀   Females Only   ♂   Males Only

🝝 Complication\Comorbidity   🝝 Major C\C   (Ex) CC/MCC Exclusions   🝝 Hospital-Acquired Condition   🝝 Hierarchical Condition Category

● M05.32 Rheumatoid heart disease with rheumatoid
          arthritis of elbow
    M05.321 Rheumatoid heart disease with
             rheumatoid arthritis of right elbow 🐾
    M05.322 Rheumatoid heart disease with
             rheumatoid arthritis of left elbow 🐾
    M05.329 Rheumatoid heart disease with
             rheumatoid arthritis of unspecified
             elbow 🐾
● M05.33 Rheumatoid heart disease with rheumatoid
          arthritis of wrist
          Rheumatoid heart disease with rheumatoid
             arthritis, carpal bones
    M05.331 Rheumatoid heart disease with
             rheumatoid arthritis of right wrist 🐾
    M05.332 Rheumatoid heart disease with
             rheumatoid arthritis of left wrist 🐾
    M05.339 Rheumatoid heart disease with
             rheumatoid arthritis of unspecified
             wrist 🐾
● M05.34 Rheumatoid heart disease with rheumatoid
          arthritis of hand
          Rheumatoid heart disease with rheumatoid
             arthritis, metacarpus and phalanges
    M05.341 Rheumatoid heart disease with
             rheumatoid arthritis of right hand 🐾
    M05.342 Rheumatoid heart disease with
             rheumatoid arthritis of left hand 🐾
    M05.349 Rheumatoid heart disease with
             rheumatoid arthritis of unspecified
             hand 🐾
● M05.35 Rheumatoid heart disease with rheumatoid
          arthritis of hip
    M05.351 Rheumatoid heart disease with
             rheumatoid arthritis of right hip 🐾
    M05.352 Rheumatoid heart disease with
             rheumatoid arthritis of left hip 🐾
    M05.359 Rheumatoid heart disease with
             rheumatoid arthritis of unspecified
             hip 🐾
● M05.36 Rheumatoid heart disease with rheumatoid
          arthritis of knee
    M05.361 Rheumatoid heart disease with
             rheumatoid arthritis of right knee 🐾
    M05.362 Rheumatoid heart disease with
             rheumatoid arthritis of left knee 🐾
    M05.369 Rheumatoid heart disease with
             rheumatoid arthritis of unspecified
             knee 🐾
● M05.37 Rheumatoid heart disease with rheumatoid
          arthritis of ankle and foot
          Rheumatoid heart disease with rheumatoid
             arthritis, tarsus, metatarsus and phalanges
    M05.371 Rheumatoid heart disease with
             rheumatoid arthritis of right ankle
             and foot 🐾
    M05.372 Rheumatoid heart disease with
             rheumatoid arthritis of left ankle and
             foot 🐾
    M05.379 Rheumatoid heart disease with
             rheumatoid arthritis of unspecified
             ankle and foot 🐾
  M05.39 Rheumatoid heart disease with rheumatoid
          arthritis of multiple sites 🐾

● M05.4 Rheumatoid myopathy with rheumatoid arthritis
         Ⓔⓧ For category M05.4 CC codes: See PDX Collection 867, 3780-3822
    M05.40 Rheumatoid myopathy with rheumatoid
            arthritis of unspecified site 🐾 🐾
            CC when PDx is its own CC
● M05.41 Rheumatoid myopathy with rheumatoid
          arthritis of shoulder
    M05.411 Rheumatoid myopathy with
             rheumatoid arthritis of right
             shoulder 🐾 🐾
             CC when PDx is its own CC
    M05.412 Rheumatoid myopathy with
             rheumatoid arthritis of left
             shoulder 🐾 🐾
             CC when PDx is its own CC
    M05.419 Rheumatoid myopathy with
             rheumatoid arthritis of unspecified
             shoulder 🐾 🐾
             CC when PDx is its own CC
● M05.42 Rheumatoid myopathy with rheumatoid
          arthritis of elbow
    M05.421 Rheumatoid myopathy with
             rheumatoid arthritis of right
             elbow 🐾 🐾
             CC when PDx is its own CC
    M05.422 Rheumatoid myopathy with
             rheumatoid arthritis of left
             elbow 🐾 🐾
             CC when PDx is its own CC
    M05.429 Rheumatoid myopathy with
             rheumatoid arthritis of unspecified
             elbow 🐾 🐾
             CC when PDx is its own CC
● M05.43 Rheumatoid myopathy with rheumatoid
          arthritis of wrist
          Rheumatoid myopathy with rheumatoid
             arthritis, carpal bones
    M05.431 Rheumatoid myopathy with
             rheumatoid arthritis of right wrist 🐾 🐾
             CC when PDx is its own CC
    M05.432 Rheumatoid myopathy with
             rheumatoid arthritis of left wrist 🐾 🐾
             CC when PDx is its own CC
    M05.439 Rheumatoid myopathy with
             rheumatoid arthritis of unspecified
             wrist 🐾 🐾
             CC when PDx is its own CC
● M05.44 Rheumatoid myopathy with rheumatoid
          arthritis of hand
          Rheumatoid myopathy with rheumatoid
             arthritis, metacarpus and phalanges
    M05.441 Rheumatoid myopathy with
             rheumatoid arthritis of right
             hand 🐾 🐾
             CC when PDx is its own CC
    M05.442 Rheumatoid myopathy with
             rheumatoid arthritis of left hand 🐾 🐾
             CC when PDx is its own CC
    M05.449 Rheumatoid myopathy with
             rheumatoid arthritis of unspecified
             hand 🐾 🐾
             CC when PDx is its own CC
● M05.45 Rheumatoid myopathy with rheumatoid
          arthritis of hip
    M05.451 Rheumatoid myopathy with
             rheumatoid arthritis of right hip 🐾 🐾
             CC when PDx is its own CC
    M05.452 Rheumatoid myopathy with
             rheumatoid arthritis of left hip 🐾 🐾
             CC when PDx is its own CC
    M05.459 Rheumatoid myopathy with
             rheumatoid arthritis of unspecified
             hip 🐾 🐾
             CC when PDx is its own CC

▶ New   ⇒ Revised   ~~deleted~~ Deleted | Excludes 1 | | Excludes 2 | | Includes | Use additional   Code first   Code also | Key words |
OGCR Official Guidelines   ● Unacceptable Principal Diagnosis   X Assign placeholder X   ● Use Additional Character(s)   ▶ Manifestation Code   Coding Clinic

● **M05.46** Rheumatoid myopathy with rheumatoid arthritis of knee

     M05.461 Rheumatoid myopathy with rheumatoid arthritis of right knee 🜚 🜚
         CC when PDx is its own CC

     M05.462 Rheumatoid myopathy with rheumatoid arthritis of left knee 🜚 🜚
         CC when PDx is its own CC

     M05.469 Rheumatoid myopathy with rheumatoid arthritis of unspecified knee 🜚 🜚
         CC when PDx is its own CC

● **M05.47** Rheumatoid myopathy with rheumatoid arthritis of ankle and foot
     Rheumatoid myopathy with rheumatoid arthritis, tarsus, metatarsus and phalanges

     M05.471 Rheumatoid myopathy with rheumatoid arthritis of right ankle and foot 🜚 🜚
         CC when PDx is its own CC

     M05.472 Rheumatoid myopathy with rheumatoid arthritis of left ankle and foot 🜚 🜚
         CC when PDx is its own CC

     M05.479 Rheumatoid myopathy with rheumatoid arthritis of unspecified ankle and foot 🜚 🜚
         CC when PDx is its own CC

     M05.49 Rheumatoid myopathy with rheumatoid arthritis of multiple sites 🜚 🜚
         CC when PDx is its own CC

● **M05.5** Rheumatoid polyneuropathy with rheumatoid arthritis

     M05.50 Rheumatoid polyneuropathy with rheumatoid arthritis of unspecified site 🜚

● **M05.51** Rheumatoid polyneuropathy with rheumatoid arthritis of shoulder

     M05.511 Rheumatoid polyneuropathy with rheumatoid arthritis of right shoulder 🜚

     M05.512 Rheumatoid polyneuropathy with rheumatoid arthritis of left shoulder 🜚

     M05.519 Rheumatoid polyneuropathy with rheumatoid arthritis of unspecified shoulder 🜚

● **M05.52** Rheumatoid polyneuropathy with rheumatoid arthritis of elbow

     M05.521 Rheumatoid polyneuropathy with rheumatoid arthritis of right elbow 🜚

     M05.522 Rheumatoid polyneuropathy with rheumatoid arthritis of left elbow 🜚

     M05.529 Rheumatoid polyneuropathy with rheumatoid arthritis of unspecified elbow 🜚

● **M05.53** Rheumatoid polyneuropathy with rheumatoid arthritis of wrist
     Rheumatoid polyneuropathy with rheumatoid arthritis, carpal bones

     M05.531 Rheumatoid polyneuropathy with rheumatoid arthritis of right wrist 🜚

     M05.532 Rheumatoid polyneuropathy with rheumatoid arthritis of left wrist 🜚

     M05.539 Rheumatoid polyneuropathy with rheumatoid arthritis of unspecified wrist 🜚

● **M05.54** Rheumatoid polyneuropathy with rheumatoid arthritis of hand
     Rheumatoid polyneuropathy with rheumatoid arthritis, metacarpus and phalanges

     M05.541 Rheumatoid polyneuropathy with rheumatoid arthritis of right hand 🜚

     M05.542 Rheumatoid polyneuropathy with rheumatoid arthritis of left hand 🜚

     M05.549 Rheumatoid polyneuropathy with rheumatoid arthritis of unspecified hand 🜚

● **M05.55** Rheumatoid polyneuropathy with rheumatoid arthritis of hip

     M05.551 Rheumatoid polyneuropathy with rheumatoid arthritis of right hip 🜚

     M05.552 Rheumatoid polyneuropathy with rheumatoid arthritis of left hip 🜚

     M05.559 Rheumatoid polyneuropathy with rheumatoid arthritis of unspecified hip 🜚

● **M05.56** Rheumatoid polyneuropathy with rheumatoid arthritis of knee

     M05.561 Rheumatoid polyneuropathy with rheumatoid arthritis of right knee 🜚

     M05.562 Rheumatoid polyneuropathy with rheumatoid arthritis of left knee 🜚

     M05.569 Rheumatoid polyneuropathy with rheumatoid arthritis of unspecified knee 🜚

● **M05.57** Rheumatoid polyneuropathy with rheumatoid arthritis of ankle and foot
     Rheumatoid polyneuropathy with rheumatoid arthritis, tarsus, metatarsus and phalanges

     M05.571 Rheumatoid polyneuropathy with rheumatoid arthritis of right ankle and foot 🜚

     M05.572 Rheumatoid polyneuropathy with rheumatoid arthritis of left ankle and foot 🜚

     M05.579 Rheumatoid polyneuropathy with rheumatoid arthritis of unspecified ankle and foot 🜚

     M05.59 Rheumatoid polyneuropathy with rheumatoid arthritis of multiple sites 🜚

● **M05.6** Rheumatoid arthritis with involvement of other organs and systems

     M05.60 Rheumatoid arthritis of unspecified site with involvement of other organs and systems 🜚

● **M05.61** Rheumatoid arthritis of shoulder with involvement of other organs and systems

     M05.611 Rheumatoid arthritis of right shoulder with involvement of other organs and systems 🜚

     M05.612 Rheumatoid arthritis of left shoulder with involvement of other organs and systems 🜚

     M05.619 Rheumatoid arthritis of unspecified shoulder with involvement of other organs and systems 🜚

● **M05.62** Rheumatoid arthritis of elbow with involvement of other organs and systems

     M05.621 Rheumatoid arthritis of right elbow with involvement of other organs and systems 🜚

     M05.622 Rheumatoid arthritis of left elbow with involvement of other organs and systems 🜚

     M05.629 Rheumatoid arthritis of unspecified elbow with involvement of other organs and systems 🜚

N Newborn Age: 0   **P** Pediatric Age: 0–17   **M** Maternity DX: 9–64   **A** Adult Age: 15–124   ♀ Females Only   ♂ Males Only

🜚 Complication\Comorbidity   🜚 Major C\C   Ⓔⅹ CC/MCC Exclusions   🜚 Hospital-Acquired Condition   🜚 Hierarchical Condition Category   **1023**

● **M05.63 Rheumatoid arthritis of wrist with involvement of other organs and systems**
Rheumatoid arthritis of carpal bones with involvement of other organs and systems

     M05.631 Rheumatoid arthritis of right wrist with involvement of other organs and systems 🐾

     M05.632 Rheumatoid arthritis of left wrist with involvement of other organs and systems 🐾

     M05.639 Rheumatoid arthritis of unspecified wrist with involvement of other organs and systems 🐾

● **M05.64 Rheumatoid arthritis of hand with involvement of other organs and systems**
Rheumatoid arthritis of metacarpus and phalanges with involvement of other organs and systems

     M05.641 Rheumatoid arthritis of right hand with involvement of other organs and systems 🐾

     M05.642 Rheumatoid arthritis of left hand with involvement of other organs and systems 🐾

     M05.649 Rheumatoid arthritis of unspecified hand with involvement of other organs and systems 🐾

● **M05.65 Rheumatoid arthritis of hip with involvement of other organs and systems**

     M05.651 Rheumatoid arthritis of right hip with involvement of other organs and systems 🐾

     M05.652 Rheumatoid arthritis of left hip with involvement of other organs and systems 🐾

     M05.659 Rheumatoid arthritis of unspecified hip with involvement of other organs and systems 🐾

● **M05.66 Rheumatoid arthritis of knee with involvement of other organs and systems**

     M05.661 Rheumatoid arthritis of right knee with involvement of other organs and systems 🐾

     M05.662 Rheumatoid arthritis of left knee with involvement of other organs and systems 🐾

     M05.669 Rheumatoid arthritis of unspecified knee with involvement of other organs and systems 🐾

● **M05.67 Rheumatoid arthritis of ankle and foot with involvement of other organs and systems**
Rheumatoid arthritis of tarsus, metatarsus and phalanges with involvement of other organs and systems

     M05.671 Rheumatoid arthritis of right ankle and foot with involvement of other organs and systems 🐾

     M05.672 Rheumatoid arthritis of left ankle and foot with involvement of other organs and systems 🐾

     M05.679 Rheumatoid arthritis of unspecified ankle and foot with involvement of other organs and systems 🐾

   M05.69 Rheumatoid arthritis of multiple sites with involvement of other organs and systems 🐾

● **M05.7 Rheumatoid arthritis with rheumatoid factor without organ or systems involvement**

   M05.70 Rheumatoid arthritis with rheumatoid factor of unspecified site without organ or systems involvement 🐾

● **M05.71 Rheumatoid arthritis with rheumatoid factor of shoulder without organ or systems involvement**

     M05.711 Rheumatoid arthritis with rheumatoid factor of right shoulder without organ or systems involvement 🐾

     M05.712 Rheumatoid arthritis with rheumatoid factor of left shoulder without organ or systems involvement 🐾

     M05.719 Rheumatoid arthritis with rheumatoid factor of unspecified shoulder without organ or systems involvement 🐾

● **M05.72 Rheumatoid arthritis with rheumatoid factor of elbow without organ or systems involvement**

     M05.721 Rheumatoid arthritis with rheumatoid factor of right elbow without organ or systems involvement 🐾

     M05.722 Rheumatoid arthritis with rheumatoid factor of left elbow without organ or systems involvement 🐾

     M05.729 Rheumatoid arthritis with rheumatoid factor of unspecified elbow without organ or systems involvement 🐾

● **M05.73 Rheumatoid arthritis with rheumatoid factor of wrist without organ or systems involvement**

     M05.731 Rheumatoid arthritis with rheumatoid factor of right wrist without organ or systems involvement 🐾

     M05.732 Rheumatoid arthritis with rheumatoid factor of left wrist without organ or systems involvement 🐾

     M05.739 Rheumatoid arthritis with rheumatoid factor of unspecified wrist without organ or systems involvement 🐾

● **M05.74 Rheumatoid arthritis with rheumatoid factor of hand without organ or systems involvement**

     M05.741 Rheumatoid arthritis with rheumatoid factor of right hand without organ or systems involvement 🐾

     M05.742 Rheumatoid arthritis with rheumatoid factor of left hand without organ or systems involvement 🐾

     M05.749 Rheumatoid arthritis with rheumatoid factor of unspecified hand without organ or systems involvement 🐾

● M05.75   Rheumatoid arthritis with rheumatoid factor of hip without organ or systems involvement
     M05.751   Rheumatoid arthritis with rheumatoid factor of right hip without organ or systems involvement 🔹
     M05.752   Rheumatoid arthritis with rheumatoid factor of left hip without organ or systems involvement 🔹
     M05.759   Rheumatoid arthritis with rheumatoid factor of unspecified hip without organ or systems involvement 🔹

● M05.76   Rheumatoid arthritis with rheumatoid factor of knee without organ or systems involvement
     M05.761   Rheumatoid arthritis with rheumatoid factor of right knee without organ or systems involvement 🔹
     M05.762   Rheumatoid arthritis with rheumatoid factor of left knee without organ or systems involvement 🔹
     M05.769   Rheumatoid arthritis with rheumatoid factor of unspecified knee without organ or systems involvement 🔹

● M05.77   Rheumatoid arthritis with rheumatoid factor of ankle and foot without organ or systems involvement
     M05.771   Rheumatoid arthritis with rheumatoid factor of right ankle and foot without organ or systems involvement 🔹
     M05.772   Rheumatoid arthritis with rheumatoid factor of left ankle and foot without organ or systems involvement 🔹
     M05.779   Rheumatoid arthritis with rheumatoid factor of unspecified ankle and foot without organ or systems involvement 🔹

     M05.79   Rheumatoid arthritis with rheumatoid factor of multiple sites without organ or systems involvement 🔹

     M05.7A   Rheumatoid arthritis with rheumatoid factor of other specified site without organ or systems involvement

● M05.8   Other rheumatoid arthritis with rheumatoid factor
     M05.80   Other rheumatoid arthritis with rheumatoid factor of unspecified site 🔹

● M05.81   Other rheumatoid arthritis with rheumatoid factor of shoulder
     M05.811   Other rheumatoid arthritis with rheumatoid factor of right shoulder 🔹
     M05.812   Other rheumatoid arthritis with rheumatoid factor of left shoulder 🔹
     M05.819   Other rheumatoid arthritis with rheumatoid factor of unspecified shoulder 🔹

● M05.82   Other rheumatoid arthritis with rheumatoid factor of elbow
     M05.821   Other rheumatoid arthritis with rheumatoid factor of right elbow 🔹
     M05.822   Other rheumatoid arthritis with rheumatoid factor of left elbow 🔹
     M05.829   Other rheumatoid arthritis with rheumatoid factor of unspecified elbow 🔹

● M05.83   Other rheumatoid arthritis with rheumatoid factor of wrist
     M05.831   Other rheumatoid arthritis with rheumatoid factor of right wrist 🔹
     M05.832   Other rheumatoid arthritis with rheumatoid factor of left wrist 🔹
     M05.839   Other rheumatoid arthritis with rheumatoid factor of unspecified wrist 🔹

● M05.84   Other rheumatoid arthritis with rheumatoid factor of hand
     M05.841   Other rheumatoid arthritis with rheumatoid factor of right hand 🔹
     M05.842   Other rheumatoid arthritis with rheumatoid factor of left hand 🔹
     M05.849   Other rheumatoid arthritis with rheumatoid factor of unspecified hand 🔹

● M05.85   Other rheumatoid arthritis with rheumatoid factor of hip
     M05.851   Other rheumatoid arthritis with rheumatoid factor of right hip 🔹
     M05.852   Other rheumatoid arthritis with rheumatoid factor of left hip 🔹
     M05.859   Other rheumatoid arthritis with rheumatoid factor of unspecified hip 🔹

● M05.86   Other rheumatoid arthritis with rheumatoid factor of knee
     M05.861   Other rheumatoid arthritis with rheumatoid factor of right knee 🔹
     M05.862   Other rheumatoid arthritis with rheumatoid factor of left knee 🔹
     M05.869   Other rheumatoid arthritis with rheumatoid factor of unspecified knee 🔹

● M05.87   Other rheumatoid arthritis with rheumatoid factor of ankle and foot
     M05.871   Other rheumatoid arthritis with rheumatoid factor of right ankle and foot 🔹
     M05.872   Other rheumatoid arthritis with rheumatoid factor of left ankle and foot 🔹
     M05.879   Other rheumatoid arthritis with rheumatoid factor of unspecified ankle and foot 🔹

     M05.89   Other rheumatoid arthritis with rheumatoid factor of multiple sites 🔹

     M05.8A   Other rheumatoid arthritis with rheumatoid factor of other specified site

     M05.9   Rheumatoid arthritis with rheumatoid factor, unspecified 🔹

● M06   Other rheumatoid arthritis
   ● M06.0   Rheumatoid arthritis without rheumatoid factor
     M06.00   Rheumatoid arthritis without rheumatoid factor, unspecified site 🔹
   ● M06.01   Rheumatoid arthritis without rheumatoid factor, shoulder
     M06.011   Rheumatoid arthritis without rheumatoid factor, right shoulder 🔹
     M06.012   Rheumatoid arthritis without rheumatoid factor, left shoulder 🔹
     M06.019   Rheumatoid arthritis without rheumatoid factor, unspecified shoulder 🔹

N Newborn Age: 0   **P** Pediatric Age: 0–17   **M** Maternity DX: 9–64   **A** Adult Age: 15–124   ♀ Females Only   ♂ Males Only

🔹 Complication\Comorbidity   🔹 Major C\C   (Ex:) CC/MCC Exclusions   🔹 Hospital-Acquired Condition   🔹 Hierarchical Condition Category

1025

CHAPTER 13 (M00–M99)

● M06.02 Rheumatoid arthritis without rheumatoid factor, elbow

    M06.021 Rheumatoid arthritis without rheumatoid factor, right elbow 🏷

    M06.022 Rheumatoid arthritis without rheumatoid factor, left elbow 🏷

    M06.029 Rheumatoid arthritis without rheumatoid factor, unspecified elbow 🏷

● M06.03 Rheumatoid arthritis without rheumatoid factor, wrist

    M06.031 Rheumatoid arthritis without rheumatoid factor, right wrist 🏷

    M06.032 Rheumatoid arthritis without rheumatoid factor, left wrist 🏷

    M06.039 Rheumatoid arthritis without rheumatoid factor, unspecified wrist 🏷

● M06.04 Rheumatoid arthritis without rheumatoid factor, hand

    M06.041 Rheumatoid arthritis without rheumatoid factor, right hand 🏷

    M06.042 Rheumatoid arthritis without rheumatoid factor, left hand 🏷

    M06.049 Rheumatoid arthritis without rheumatoid factor, unspecified hand 🏷

● M06.05 Rheumatoid arthritis without rheumatoid factor, hip

    M06.051 Rheumatoid arthritis without rheumatoid factor, right hip 🏷

    M06.052 Rheumatoid arthritis without rheumatoid factor, left hip 🏷

    M06.059 Rheumatoid arthritis without rheumatoid factor, unspecified hip 🏷

● M06.06 Rheumatoid arthritis without rheumatoid factor, knee

    M06.061 Rheumatoid arthritis without rheumatoid factor, right knee 🏷

    M06.062 Rheumatoid arthritis without rheumatoid factor, left knee 🏷

    M06.069 Rheumatoid arthritis without rheumatoid factor, unspecified knee 🏷

● M06.07 Rheumatoid arthritis without rheumatoid factor, ankle and foot

    M06.071 Rheumatoid arthritis without rheumatoid factor, right ankle and foot 🏷

    M06.072 Rheumatoid arthritis without rheumatoid factor, left ankle and foot 🏷

    M06.079 Rheumatoid arthritis without rheumatoid factor, unspecified ankle and foot 🏷

M06.08 Rheumatoid arthritis without rheumatoid factor, vertebrae 🏷

M06.09 Rheumatoid arthritis without rheumatoid factor, multiple sites 🏷

M06.0A Rheumatoid arthritis without rheumatoid factor, other specified site

M06.1 Adult-onset Still's disease 🏷   A

    Excludes1   Still's disease NOS (M08.2-)

● M06.2 Rheumatoid bursitis

    M06.20 Rheumatoid bursitis, unspecified site 🏷

● M06.21 Rheumatoid bursitis, shoulder

    M06.211 Rheumatoid bursitis, right shoulder 🏷

    M06.212 Rheumatoid bursitis, left shoulder 🏷

    M06.219 Rheumatoid bursitis, unspecified shoulder 🏷

● M06.22 Rheumatoid bursitis, elbow

    M06.221 Rheumatoid bursitis, right elbow 🏷

    M06.222 Rheumatoid bursitis, left elbow 🏷

    M06.229 Rheumatoid bursitis, unspecified elbow 🏷

● M06.23 Rheumatoid bursitis, wrist

    M06.231 Rheumatoid bursitis, right wrist 🏷

    M06.232 Rheumatoid bursitis, left wrist 🏷

    M06.239 Rheumatoid bursitis, unspecified wrist 🏷

● M06.24 Rheumatoid bursitis, hand

    M06.241 Rheumatoid bursitis, right hand 🏷

    M06.242 Rheumatoid bursitis, left hand 🏷

    M06.249 Rheumatoid bursitis, unspecified hand 🏷

● M06.25 Rheumatoid bursitis, hip

    M06.251 Rheumatoid bursitis, right hip 🏷

    M06.252 Rheumatoid bursitis, left hip 🏷

    M06.259 Rheumatoid bursitis, unspecified hip 🏷

● M06.26 Rheumatoid bursitis, knee

    M06.261 Rheumatoid bursitis, right knee 🏷

    M06.262 Rheumatoid bursitis, left knee 🏷

    M06.269 Rheumatoid bursitis, unspecified knee 🏷

● M06.27 Rheumatoid bursitis, ankle and foot

    M06.271 Rheumatoid bursitis, right ankle and foot 🏷

    M06.272 Rheumatoid bursitis, left ankle and foot 🏷

    M06.279 Rheumatoid bursitis, unspecified ankle and foot 🏷

    M06.28 Rheumatoid bursitis, vertebrae 🏷

    M06.29 Rheumatoid bursitis, multiple sites 🏷

● M06.3 Rheumatoid nodule

    M06.30 Rheumatoid nodule, unspecified site 🏷

● M06.31 Rheumatoid nodule, shoulder

    M06.311 Rheumatoid nodule, right shoulder 🏷

    M06.312 Rheumatoid nodule, left shoulder 🏷

    M06.319 Rheumatoid nodule, unspecified shoulder 🏷

● M06.32 Rheumatoid nodule, elbow

    M06.321 Rheumatoid nodule, right elbow 🏷

    M06.322 Rheumatoid nodule, left elbow 🏷

    M06.329 Rheumatoid nodule, unspecified elbow 🏷

● M06.33 Rheumatoid nodule, wrist

    M06.331 Rheumatoid nodule, right wrist 🏷

    M06.332 Rheumatoid nodule, left wrist 🏷

    M06.339 Rheumatoid nodule, unspecified wrist 🏷

● M06.34   Rheumatoid nodule, hand
     M06.341   Rheumatoid nodule, right hand 🅗
     M06.342   Rheumatoid nodule, left hand 🅗
     M06.349   Rheumatoid nodule, unspecified hand 🅗

● M06.35   Rheumatoid nodule, hip
     M06.351   Rheumatoid nodule, right hip 🅗
     M06.352   Rheumatoid nodule, left hip 🅗
     M06.359   Rheumatoid nodule, unspecified hip 🅗

● M06.36   Rheumatoid nodule, knee
     M06.361   Rheumatoid nodule, right knee 🅗
     M06.362   Rheumatoid nodule, left knee 🅗
     M06.369   Rheumatoid nodule, unspecified knee 🅗

● M06.37   Rheumatoid nodule, ankle and foot
     M06.371   Rheumatoid nodule, right ankle and foot 🅗
     M06.372   Rheumatoid nodule, left ankle and foot 🅗
     M06.379   Rheumatoid nodule, unspecified ankle and foot 🅗

     M06.38   Rheumatoid nodule, vertebrae 🅗
     M06.39   Rheumatoid nodule, multiple sites 🅗

M06.4   Inflammatory polyarthropathy 🅗
     Excludes1   polyarthritis NOS (M13.0)

● M06.8   Other specified rheumatoid arthritis
     M06.80   Other specified rheumatoid arthritis, unspecified site 🅗

● M06.81   Other specified rheumatoid arthritis, shoulder
     M06.811   Other specified rheumatoid arthritis, right shoulder 🅗
     M06.812   Other specified rheumatoid arthritis, left shoulder 🅗
     M06.819   Other specified rheumatoid arthritis, unspecified shoulder 🅗

● M06.82   Other specified rheumatoid arthritis, elbow
     M06.821   Other specified rheumatoid arthritis, right elbow 🅗
     M06.822   Other specified rheumatoid arthritis, left elbow 🅗
     M06.829   Other specified rheumatoid arthritis, unspecified elbow 🅗

● M06.83   Other specified rheumatoid arthritis, wrist
     M06.831   Other specified rheumatoid arthritis, right wrist 🅗
     M06.832   Other specified rheumatoid arthritis, left wrist 🅗
     M06.839   Other specified rheumatoid arthritis, unspecified wrist 🅗

● M06.84   Other specified rheumatoid arthritis, hand
     M06.841   Other specified rheumatoid arthritis, right hand 🅗
     M06.842   Other specified rheumatoid arthritis, left hand 🅗
     M06.849   Other specified rheumatoid arthritis, unspecified hand 🅗

● M06.85   Other specified rheumatoid arthritis, hip
     M06.851   Other specified rheumatoid arthritis, right hip 🅗
     M06.852   Other specified rheumatoid arthritis, left hip 🅗
     M06.859   Other specified rheumatoid arthritis, unspecified hip 🅗

● M06.86   Other specified rheumatoid arthritis, knee
     M06.861   Other specified rheumatoid arthritis, right knee 🅗
     M06.862   Other specified rheumatoid arthritis, left knee 🅗
     M06.869   Other specified rheumatoid arthritis, unspecified knee 🅗

● M06.87   Other specified rheumatoid arthritis, ankle and foot
     M06.871   Other specified rheumatoid arthritis, right ankle and foot 🅗
     M06.872   Other specified rheumatoid arthritis, left ankle and foot 🅗
     M06.879   Other specified rheumatoid arthritis, unspecified ankle and foot 🅗

     M06.88   Other specified rheumatoid arthritis, vertebrae 🅗
     M06.89   Other specified rheumatoid arthritis, multiple sites 🅗
     M06.8A   Other specified rheumatoid arthritis, other specified site

M06.9   Rheumatoid arthritis, unspecified 🅗

● M07   Enteropathic arthropathies
     Code also associated enteropathy, such as:
       regional enteritis [Crohn's disease] (K50.-)
       ulcerative colitis (K51.-)
     Excludes1   psoriatic arthropathies (L40.5-)

● M07.6   Enteropathic arthropathies
     M07.60   Enteropathic arthropathies, unspecified site

● M07.61   Enteropathic arthropathies, shoulder
     M07.611   Enteropathic arthropathies, right shoulder
     M07.612   Enteropathic arthropathies, left shoulder
     M07.619   Enteropathic arthropathies, unspecified shoulder

● M07.62   Enteropathic arthropathies, elbow
     M07.621   Enteropathic arthropathies, right elbow
     M07.622   Enteropathic arthropathies, left elbow
     M07.629   Enteropathic arthropathies, unspecified elbow

● M07.63   Enteropathic arthropathies, wrist
     M07.631   Enteropathic arthropathies, right wrist
     M07.632   Enteropathic arthropathies, left wrist
     M07.639   Enteropathic arthropathies, unspecified wrist

● M07.64   Enteropathic arthropathies, hand
     M07.641   Enteropathic arthropathies, right hand
     M07.642   Enteropathic arthropathies, left hand
     M07.649   Enteropathic arthropathies, unspecified hand

● M07.65   Enteropathic arthropathies, hip
     M07.651   Enteropathic arthropathies, right hip
     M07.652   Enteropathic arthropathies, left hip
     M07.659   Enteropathic arthropathies, unspecified hip

● M07.66   Enteropathic arthropathies, knee
     M07.661   Enteropathic arthropathies, right knee
     M07.662   Enteropathic arthropathies, left knee
     M07.669   Enteropathic arthropathies, unspecified knee

N   Newborn Age: 0   P   Pediatric Age: 0–17   M   Maternity DX: 9–64   A   Adult Age: 15–124   ♀   Females Only   ♂   Males Only
🅒   Complication\Comorbidity   🅜   Major C\C   Ⓔ🅍   CC/MCC Exclusions   🅗   Hospital-Acquired Condition   🅗   Hierarchical Condition Category

1027

● M07.67   Enteropathic arthropathies, ankle and foot
  M07.671 Enteropathic arthropathies, right ankle and foot
  M07.672 Enteropathic arthropathies, left ankle and foot
  M07.679 Enteropathic arthropathies, unspecified ankle and foot
 M07.68 Enteropathic arthropathies, vertebrae
 M07.69 Enteropathic arthropathies, multiple sites

● M08 Juvenile arthritis
 Code also any associated underlying condition, such as:
  regional enteritis [Crohn's disease] (K50.-)
  ulcerative colitis (K51.-)

 Excludes1 arthropathy in Whipple's disease (M14.8)
     Felty's syndrome (M05.0)
     juvenile dermatomyositis (M33.0-)
     psoriatic juvenile arthropathy (L40.54)

● M08.0 Unspecified juvenile rheumatoid arthritis
 Juvenile rheumatoid arthritis with or without rheumatoid factor
 M08.00 Unspecified juvenile rheumatoid arthritis of unspecified site 🐾
 ● M08.01 Unspecified juvenile rheumatoid arthritis, shoulder
  M08.011 Unspecified juvenile rheumatoid arthritis, right shoulder 🐾
  M08.012 Unspecified juvenile rheumatoid arthritis, left shoulder 🐾
  M08.019 Unspecified juvenile rheumatoid arthritis, unspecified shoulder 🐾
 ● M08.02 Unspecified juvenile rheumatoid arthritis of elbow
  M08.021 Unspecified juvenile rheumatoid arthritis, right elbow 🐾
  M08.022 Unspecified juvenile rheumatoid arthritis, left elbow 🐾
  M08.029 Unspecified juvenile rheumatoid arthritis, unspecified elbow 🐾
 ● M08.03 Unspecified juvenile rheumatoid arthritis, wrist
  M08.031 Unspecified juvenile rheumatoid arthritis, right wrist 🐾
  M08.032 Unspecified juvenile rheumatoid arthritis, left wrist 🐾
  M08.039 Unspecified juvenile rheumatoid arthritis, unspecified wrist 🐾
 ● M08.04 Unspecified juvenile rheumatoid arthritis, hand
  M08.041 Unspecified juvenile rheumatoid arthritis, right hand 🐾
  M08.042 Unspecified juvenile rheumatoid arthritis, left hand 🐾
  M08.049 Unspecified juvenile rheumatoid arthritis, unspecified hand 🐾
 ● M08.05 Unspecified juvenile rheumatoid arthritis, hip
  M08.051 Unspecified juvenile rheumatoid arthritis, right hip 🐾
  M08.052 Unspecified juvenile rheumatoid arthritis, left hip 🐾
  M08.059 Unspecified juvenile rheumatoid arthritis, unspecified hip 🐾
 ● M08.06 Unspecified juvenile rheumatoid arthritis, knee
  M08.061 Unspecified juvenile rheumatoid arthritis, right knee 🐾
  M08.062 Unspecified juvenile rheumatoid arthritis, left knee 🐾
  M08.069 Unspecified juvenile rheumatoid arthritis, unspecified knee 🐾

 ● M08.07 Unspecified juvenile rheumatoid arthritis, ankle and foot
  M08.071 Unspecified juvenile rheumatoid arthritis, right ankle and foot 🐾
  M08.072 Unspecified juvenile rheumatoid arthritis, left ankle and foot 🐾
  M08.079 Unspecified juvenile rheumatoid arthritis, unspecified ankle and foot 🐾
 M08.08 Unspecified juvenile rheumatoid arthritis, vertebrae 🐾
 M08.09 Unspecified juvenile rheumatoid arthritis, multiple sites 🐾
 M08.0A Unspecified juvenile rheumatoid arthritis, other specified site

M08.1 Juvenile ankylosing spondylitis 🐾
 Excludes1 ankylosing spondylitis in adults (M45.0-)

● M08.2 Juvenile rheumatoid arthritis with systemic onset
 Still's disease NOS
 Excludes1 adult-onset Still's disease (M06.1-)
 M08.20 Juvenile rheumatoid arthritis with systemic onset, unspecified site 🐾
 ● M08.21 Juvenile rheumatoid arthritis with systemic onset, shoulder
  M08.211 Juvenile rheumatoid arthritis with systemic onset, right shoulder 🐾
  M08.212 Juvenile rheumatoid arthritis with systemic onset, left shoulder 🐾
  M08.219 Juvenile rheumatoid arthritis with systemic onset, unspecified shoulder 🐾
 ● M08.22 Juvenile rheumatoid arthritis with systemic onset, elbow
  M08.221 Juvenile rheumatoid arthritis with systemic onset, right elbow 🐾
  M08.222 Juvenile rheumatoid arthritis with systemic onset, left elbow 🐾
  M08.229 Juvenile rheumatoid arthritis with systemic onset, unspecified elbow 🐾
 ● M08.23 Juvenile rheumatoid arthritis with systemic onset, wrist
  M08.231 Juvenile rheumatoid arthritis with systemic onset, right wrist 🐾
  M08.232 Juvenile rheumatoid arthritis with systemic onset, left wrist 🐾
  M08.239 Juvenile rheumatoid arthritis with systemic onset, unspecified wrist 🐾
 ● M08.24 Juvenile rheumatoid arthritis with systemic onset, hand
  M08.241 Juvenile rheumatoid arthritis with systemic onset, right hand 🐾
  M08.242 Juvenile rheumatoid arthritis with systemic onset, left hand 🐾
  M08.249 Juvenile rheumatoid arthritis with systemic onset, unspecified hand 🐾
 ● M08.25 Juvenile rheumatoid arthritis with systemic onset, hip
  M08.251 Juvenile rheumatoid arthritis with systemic onset, right hip 🐾
  M08.252 Juvenile rheumatoid arthritis with systemic onset, left hip 🐾
  M08.259 Juvenile rheumatoid arthritis with systemic onset, unspecified hip 🐾

▶ New ⇢ Revised ~~deleted~~ Deleted Excludes 1 Excludes 2 Includes Use additional Code first Code also Key words
OGCR Official Guidelines ● Unacceptable Principal Diagnosis X Assign placeholder X ● Use Additional Character(s) ▷ Manifestation Code Coding Clinic

● M08.26   Juvenile rheumatoid arthritis with systemic onset, knee

     M08.261   Juvenile rheumatoid arthritis with systemic onset, right knee 🐾

     M08.262   Juvenile rheumatoid arthritis with systemic onset, left knee 🐾

     M08.269   Juvenile rheumatoid arthritis with systemic onset, unspecified knee 🐾

● M08.27   Juvenile rheumatoid arthritis with systemic onset, ankle and foot

     M08.271   Juvenile rheumatoid arthritis with systemic onset, right ankle and foot 🐾

     M08.272   Juvenile rheumatoid arthritis with systemic onset, left ankle and foot 🐾

     M08.279   Juvenile rheumatoid arthritis with systemic onset, unspecified ankle and foot 🐾

   M08.28   Juvenile rheumatoid arthritis with systemic onset, vertebrae 🐾

   M08.29   Juvenile rheumatoid arthritis with systemic onset, multiple sites 🐾

   M08.2A   Juvenile rheumatoid arthritis with systemic onset, other specified site

M08.3   Juvenile rheumatoid polyarthritis (seronegative)

● M08.4   Pauciarticular juvenile rheumatoid arthritis

   M08.40   Pauciarticular juvenile rheumatoid arthritis, unspecified site 🐾

● M08.41   Pauciarticular juvenile rheumatoid arthritis, shoulder

     M08.411   Pauciarticular juvenile rheumatoid arthritis, right shoulder 🐾

     M08.412   Pauciarticular juvenile rheumatoid arthritis, left shoulder 🐾

     M08.419   Pauciarticular juvenile rheumatoid arthritis, unspecified shoulder 🐾

● M08.42   Pauciarticular juvenile rheumatoid arthritis, elbow

     M08.421   Pauciarticular juvenile rheumatoid arthritis, right elbow 🐾

     M08.422   Pauciarticular juvenile rheumatoid arthritis, left elbow 🐾

     M08.429   Pauciarticular juvenile rheumatoid arthritis, unspecified elbow 🐾

● M08.43   Pauciarticular juvenile rheumatoid arthritis, wrist

     M08.431   Pauciarticular juvenile rheumatoid arthritis, right wrist 🐾

     M08.432   Pauciarticular juvenile rheumatoid arthritis, left wrist 🐾

     M08.439   Pauciarticular juvenile rheumatoid arthritis, unspecified wrist 🐾

● M08.44   Pauciarticular juvenile rheumatoid arthritis, hand

     M08.441   Pauciarticular juvenile rheumatoid arthritis, right hand 🐾

     M08.442   Pauciarticular juvenile rheumatoid arthritis, left hand 🐾

     M08.449   Pauciarticular juvenile rheumatoid arthritis, unspecified hand 🐾

● M08.45   Pauciarticular juvenile rheumatoid arthritis, hip

     M08.451   Pauciarticular juvenile rheumatoid arthritis, right hip 🐾

     M08.452   Pauciarticular juvenile rheumatoid arthritis, left hip 🐾

     M08.459   Pauciarticular juvenile rheumatoid arthritis, unspecified hip 🐾

● M08.46   Pauciarticular juvenile rheumatoid arthritis, knee

     M08.461   Pauciarticular juvenile rheumatoid arthritis, right knee 🐾

     M08.462   Pauciarticular juvenile rheumatoid arthritis, left knee 🐾

     M08.469   Pauciarticular juvenile rheumatoid arthritis, unspecified knee 🐾

● M08.47   Pauciarticular juvenile rheumatoid arthritis, ankle and foot

     M08.471   Pauciarticular juvenile rheumatoid arthritis, right ankle and foot 🐾

     M08.472   Pauciarticular juvenile rheumatoid arthritis, left ankle and foot 🐾

     M08.479   Pauciarticular juvenile rheumatoid arthritis, unspecified ankle and foot 🐾

   M08.48   Pauciarticular juvenile rheumatoid arthritis, vertebrae 🐾

   M08.4A   Pauciarticular juvenile rheumatoid arthritis, other specified site

● M08.8   Other juvenile arthritis

   M08.80   Other juvenile arthritis, unspecified site 🐾

● M08.81   Other juvenile arthritis, shoulder

     M08.811   Other juvenile arthritis, right shoulder 🐾

     M08.812   Other juvenile arthritis, left shoulder 🐾

     M08.819   Other juvenile arthritis, unspecified shoulder 🐾

● M08.82   Other juvenile arthritis, elbow

     M08.821   Other juvenile arthritis, right elbow 🐾

     M08.822   Other juvenile arthritis, left elbow 🐾

     M08.829   Other juvenile arthritis, unspecified elbow 🐾

● M08.83   Other juvenile arthritis, wrist

     M08.831   Other juvenile arthritis, right wrist 🐾

     M08.832   Other juvenile arthritis, left wrist 🐾

     M08.839   Other juvenile arthritis, unspecified wrist 🐾

● M08.84   Other juvenile arthritis, hand

     M08.841   Other juvenile arthritis, right hand 🐾

     M08.842   Other juvenile arthritis, left hand 🐾

     M08.849   Other juvenile arthritis, unspecified hand 🐾

● M08.85   Other juvenile arthritis, hip

     M08.851   Other juvenile arthritis, right hip 🐾

     M08.852   Other juvenile arthritis, left hip 🐾

     M08.859   Other juvenile arthritis, unspecified hip 🐾

● M08.86   Other juvenile arthritis, knee

     M08.861   Other juvenile arthritis, right knee 🐾

     M08.862   Other juvenile arthritis, left knee 🐾

     M08.869   Other juvenile arthritis, unspecified knee 🐾

● M08.87   Other juvenile arthritis, ankle and foot

     M08.871   Other juvenile arthritis, right ankle and foot 🐾

     M08.872   Other juvenile arthritis, left ankle and foot 🐾

     M08.879   Other juvenile arthritis, unspecified ankle and foot 🐾

   M08.88   Other juvenile arthritis, other specified site 🐾
       Other juvenile arthritis, vertebrae

   M08.89   Other juvenile arthritis, multiple sites 🐾

N   Newborn Age: 0   **P**   Pediatric Age: 0–17   **M**   Maternity DX: 9–64   **A**   Adult Age: 15–124   ♀ Females Only   ♂ Males Only

🐾 Complication\Comorbidity   🐾 Major C\C   (Ex) CC/MCC Exclusions   🐾 Hospital-Acquired Condition   🐾 Hierarchical Condition Category

1029

CHAPTER 13 (M00-M99)

● M08.9 Juvenile arthritis, unspecified
     Excludes1   juvenile rheumatoid arthritis, unspecified (M08.0-)

   M08.90 Juvenile arthritis, unspecified, unspecified site 🐾

● M08.91 Juvenile arthritis, unspecified, shoulder
     M08.911 Juvenile arthritis, unspecified, right shoulder 🐾
     M08.912 Juvenile arthritis, unspecified, left shoulder 🐾
     M08.919 Juvenile arthritis, unspecified, unspecified shoulder 🐾

● M08.92 Juvenile arthritis, unspecified, elbow
     M08.921 Juvenile arthritis, unspecified, right elbow 🐾
     M08.922 Juvenile arthritis, unspecified, left elbow 🐾
     M08.929 Juvenile arthritis, unspecified, unspecified elbow 🐾

● M08.93 Juvenile arthritis, unspecified, wrist
     M08.931 Juvenile arthritis, unspecified, right wrist 🐾
     M08.932 Juvenile arthritis, unspecified, left wrist 🐾
     M08.939 Juvenile arthritis, unspecified, unspecified wrist 🐾

● M08.94 Juvenile arthritis, unspecified, hand
     M08.941 Juvenile arthritis, unspecified, right hand 🐾
     M08.942 Juvenile arthritis, unspecified, left hand 🐾
     M08.949 Juvenile arthritis, unspecified, unspecified hand 🐾

● M08.95 Juvenile arthritis, unspecified, hip
     M08.951 Juvenile arthritis, unspecified, right hip 🐾
     M08.952 Juvenile arthritis, unspecified, left hip 🐾
     M08.959 Juvenile arthritis, unspecified, unspecified hip 🐾

● M08.96 Juvenile arthritis, unspecified, knee
     M08.961 Juvenile arthritis, unspecified, right knee 🐾
     M08.962 Juvenile arthritis, unspecified, left knee 🐾
     M08.969 Juvenile arthritis, unspecified, unspecified knee 🐾

● M08.97 Juvenile arthritis, unspecified, ankle and foot
     M08.971 Juvenile arthritis, unspecified, right ankle and foot 🐾
     M08.972 Juvenile arthritis, unspecified, left ankle and foot 🐾
     M08.979 Juvenile arthritis, unspecified, unspecified ankle and foot 🐾

   M08.98 Juvenile arthritis, unspecified, vertebrae 🐾
   M08.99 Juvenile arthritis, unspecified, multiple sites 🐾
   M08.9A Juvenile arthritis, unspecified, other specified site

● M1A Chronic gout
    Use additional code to identify:
     Autonomic neuropathy in diseases classified elsewhere (G99.0)
     Calculus of urinary tract in diseases classified elsewhere (N22)
     Cardiomyopathy in diseases classified elsewhere (I43)
     Disorders of external ear in diseases classified elsewhere (H61.1-, H62.8-)
     Disorders of iris and ciliary body in diseases classified elsewhere (H22)
     Glomerular disorders in diseases classified elsewhere (N08)

    Excludes1   gout NOS (M10.-)

    Excludes2   acute gout (M10.-)

    The appropriate 7th character is to be added to each code from category M1A

0	without tophus (tophi)
1	with tophus (tophi)

● M1A.0 Idiopathic chronic gout
    Chronic gouty bursitis
    Primary chronic gout

  X ● M1A.00 Idiopathic chronic gout, unspecified site
    ● M1A.01 Idiopathic chronic gout, shoulder
      ● M1A.011 Idiopathic chronic gout, right shoulder
      ● M1A.012 Idiopathic chronic gout, left shoulder
      ● M1A.019 Idiopathic chronic gout, unspecified shoulder

    ● M1A.02 Idiopathic chronic gout, elbow
      ● M1A.021 Idiopathic chronic gout, right elbow
      ● M1A.022 Idiopathic chronic gout, left elbow
      ● M1A.029 Idiopathic chronic gout, unspecified elbow

    ● M1A.03 Idiopathic chronic gout, wrist
      ● M1A.031 Idiopathic chronic gout, right wrist
      ● M1A.032 Idiopathic chronic gout, left wrist
      ● M1A.039 Idiopathic chronic gout, unspecified wrist

    ● M1A.04 Idiopathic chronic gout, hand
      ● M1A.041 Idiopathic chronic gout, right hand
      ● M1A.042 Idiopathic chronic gout, left hand
      ● M1A.049 Idiopathic chronic gout, unspecified hand

    ● M1A.05 Idiopathic chronic gout, hip
      ● M1A.051 Idiopathic chronic gout, right hip
      ● M1A.052 Idiopathic chronic gout, left hip
      ● M1A.059 Idiopathic chronic gout, unspecified hip

    ● M1A.06 Idiopathic chronic gout, knee
      ● M1A.061 Idiopathic chronic gout, right knee
      ● M1A.062 Idiopathic chronic gout, left knee
      ● M1A.069 Idiopathic chronic gout, unspecified knee

    ● M1A.07 Idiopathic chronic gout, ankle and foot
      ● M1A.071 Idiopathic chronic gout, right ankle and foot
      ● M1A.072 Idiopathic chronic gout, left ankle and foot
      ● M1A.079 Idiopathic chronic gout, unspecified ankle and foot

  X ● M1A.08 Idiopathic chronic gout, vertebrae
  X ● M1A.09 Idiopathic chronic gout, multiple sites

▶ New   ⇒ Revised   ~~deleted~~ Deleted   Excludes 1   Excludes 2   Includes   Use additional   Code first   Code also   Key words
OGCR Official Guidelines   ● Unacceptable Principal Diagnosis   X Assign placeholder X   ● Use Additional Character(s)   ▶ Manifestation Code   **Coding Clinic**

● M1A.1 Lead-induced chronic gout

> *Code first toxic effects of lead and its compounds (T56.0-)*

X● M1A.10 Lead-induced chronic gout, unspecified site

● M1A.11 Lead-induced chronic gout, shoulder
- ● M1A.111 Lead-induced chronic gout, right shoulder
- ● M1A.112 Lead-induced chronic gout, left shoulder
- ● M1A.119 Lead-induced chronic gout, unspecified shoulder

● M1A.12 Lead-induced chronic gout, elbow
- ● M1A.121 Lead-induced chronic gout, right elbow
- ● M1A.122 Lead-induced chronic gout, left elbow
- ● M1A.129 Lead-induced chronic gout, unspecified elbow

● M1A.13 Lead-induced chronic gout, wrist
- ● M1A.131 Lead-induced chronic gout, right wrist
- ● M1A.132 Lead-induced chronic gout, left wrist
- ● M1A.139 Lead-induced chronic gout, unspecified wrist

● M1A.14 Lead-induced chronic gout, hand
- ● M1A.141 Lead-induced chronic gout, right hand
- ● M1A.142 Lead-induced chronic gout, left hand
- ● M1A.149 Lead-induced chronic gout, unspecified hand

● M1A.15 Lead-induced chronic gout, hip
- ● M1A.151 Lead-induced chronic gout, right hip
- ● M1A.152 Lead-induced chronic gout, left hip
- ● M1A.159 Lead-induced chronic gout, unspecified hip

● M1A.16 Lead-induced chronic gout, knee
- ● M1A.161 Lead-induced chronic gout, right knee
- ● M1A.162 Lead-induced chronic gout, left knee
- ● M1A.169 Lead-induced chronic gout, unspecified knee

● M1A.17 Lead-induced chronic gout, ankle and foot
- ● M1A.171 Lead-induced chronic gout, right ankle and foot
- ● M1A.172 Lead-induced chronic gout, left ankle and foot
- ● M1A.179 Lead-induced chronic gout, unspecified ankle and foot

X● M1A.18 Lead-induced chronic gout, vertebrae

X● M1A.19 Lead-induced chronic gout, multiple sites

● M1A.2 Drug-induced chronic gout

> *Use additional code for adverse effect, if applicable, to identify drug (T36-T50 with fifth or sixth character 5)*

X● M1A.20 Drug-induced chronic gout, unspecified site

● M1A.21 Drug-induced chronic gout, shoulder
- ● M1A.211 Drug-induced chronic gout, right shoulder
- ● M1A.212 Drug-induced chronic gout, left shoulder
- ● M1A.219 Drug-induced chronic gout, unspecified shoulder

● M1A.22 Drug-induced chronic gout, elbow
- ● M1A.221 Drug-induced chronic gout, right elbow
- ● M1A.222 Drug-induced chronic gout, left elbow
- ● M1A.229 Drug-induced chronic gout, unspecified elbow

● M1A.23 Drug-induced chronic gout, wrist
- ● M1A.231 Drug-induced chronic gout, right wrist
- ● M1A.232 Drug-induced chronic gout, left wrist
- ● M1A.239 Drug-induced chronic gout, unspecified wrist

● M1A.24 Drug-induced chronic gout, hand
- ● M1A.241 Drug-induced chronic gout, right hand
- ● M1A.242 Drug-induced chronic gout, left hand
- ● M1A.249 Drug-induced chronic gout, unspecified hand

● M1A.25 Drug-induced chronic gout, hip
- ● M1A.251 Drug-induced chronic gout, right hip
- ● M1A.252 Drug-induced chronic gout, left hip
- ● M1A.259 Drug-induced chronic gout, unspecified hip

● M1A.26 Drug-induced chronic gout, knee
- ● M1A.261 Drug-induced chronic gout, right knee
- ● M1A.262 Drug-induced chronic gout, left knee
- ● M1A.269 Drug-induced chronic gout, unspecified knee

● M1A.27 Drug-induced chronic gout, ankle and foot
- ● M1A.271 Drug-induced chronic gout, right ankle and foot
- ● M1A.272 Drug-induced chronic gout, left ankle and foot
- ● M1A.279 Drug-induced chronic gout, unspecified ankle and foot

X● M1A.28 Drug-induced chronic gout, vertebrae

X● M1A.29 Drug-induced chronic gout, multiple sites

● M1A.3 Chronic gout due to renal impairment

> *Code first associated renal disease*

X● M1A.30 Chronic gout due to renal impairment, unspecified site

● M1A.31 Chronic gout due to renal impairment, shoulder
- ● M1A.311 Chronic gout due to renal impairment, right shoulder
- ● M1A.312 Chronic gout due to renal impairment, left shoulder
- ● M1A.319 Chronic gout due to renal impairment, unspecified shoulder

● M1A.32 Chronic gout due to renal impairment, elbow
- ● M1A.321 Chronic gout due to renal impairment, right elbow
- ● M1A.322 Chronic gout due to renal impairment, left elbow
- ● M1A.329 Chronic gout due to renal impairment, unspecified elbow

● M1A.33 Chronic gout due to renal impairment, wrist
- ● M1A.331 Chronic gout due to renal impairment, right wrist
- ● M1A.332 Chronic gout due to renal impairment, left wrist
- ● M1A.339 Chronic gout due to renal impairment, unspecified wrist

● M1A.34 Chronic gout due to renal impairment, hand
- ● M1A.341 Chronic gout due to renal impairment, right hand
- ● M1A.342 Chronic gout due to renal impairment, left hand
- ● M1A.349 Chronic gout due to renal impairment, unspecified hand

CHAPTER 13 (M00-M99)

N Newborn Age: 0   P Pediatric Age: 0–17   M Maternity DX: 9–64   A Adult Age: 15–124   ♀ Females Only   ♂ Males Only

Complication\Comorbidity   Major C\C   (Ex) CC/MCC Exclusions   Hospital-Acquired Condition   Hierarchical Condition Category   1031

CHAPTER 13 (M00-M99)

● M1A.35 Chronic gout due to renal impairment, hip
- ● M1A.351 Chronic gout due to renal impairment, right hip
- ● M1A.352 Chronic gout due to renal impairment, left hip
- ● M1A.359 Chronic gout due to renal impairment, unspecified hip

● M1A.36 Chronic gout due to renal impairment, knee
- ● M1A.361 Chronic gout due to renal impairment, right knee
- ● M1A.362 Chronic gout due to renal impairment, left knee
- ● M1A.369 Chronic gout due to renal impairment, unspecified knee

● M1A.37 Chronic gout due to renal impairment, ankle and foot
- ● M1A.371 Chronic gout due to renal impairment, right ankle and foot
- ● M1A.372 Chronic gout due to renal impairment, left ankle and foot
- ● M1A.379 Chronic gout due to renal impairment, unspecified ankle and foot

X● M1A.38 Chronic gout due to renal impairment, vertebrae

X● M1A.39 Chronic gout due to renal impairment, multiple sites

● M1A.4 Other secondary chronic gout
Code first associated condition

X● M1A.40 Other secondary chronic gout, unspecified site

● M1A.41 Other secondary chronic gout, shoulder
- ● M1A.411 Other secondary chronic gout, right shoulder
- ● M1A.412 Other secondary chronic gout, left shoulder
- ● M1A.419 Other secondary chronic gout, unspecified shoulder

● M1A.42 Other secondary chronic gout, elbow
- ● M1A.421 Other secondary chronic gout, right elbow
- ● M1A.422 Other secondary chronic gout, left elbow
- ● M1A.429 Other secondary chronic gout, unspecified elbow

● M1A.43 Other secondary chronic gout, wrist
- ● M1A.431 Other secondary chronic gout, right wrist
- ● M1A.432 Other secondary chronic gout, left wrist
- ● M1A.439 Other secondary chronic gout, unspecified wrist

● M1A.44 Other secondary chronic gout, hand
- ● M1A.441 Other secondary chronic gout, right hand
- ● M1A.442 Other secondary chronic gout, left hand
- ● M1A.449 Other secondary chronic gout, unspecified hand

● M1A.45 Other secondary chronic gout, hip
- ● M1A.451 Other secondary chronic gout, right hip
- ● M1A.452 Other secondary chronic gout, left hip
- ● M1A.459 Other secondary chronic gout, unspecified hip

● M1A.46 Other secondary chronic gout, knee
- ● M1A.461 Other secondary chronic gout, right knee
- ● M1A.462 Other secondary chronic gout, left knee
- ● M1A.469 Other secondary chronic gout, unspecified knee

● M1A.47 Other secondary chronic gout, ankle and foot
- ● M1A.471 Other secondary chronic gout, right ankle and foot
- ● M1A.472 Other secondary chronic gout, left ankle and foot
- ● M1A.479 Other secondary chronic gout, unspecified ankle and foot

X● M1A.48 Other secondary chronic gout, vertebrae

X● M1A.49 Other secondary chronic gout, multiple sites

X● M1A.9 Chronic gout, unspecified

● M10 Gout
Accumulation of uric acid that results in swollen, red, hot, painful, stiff joints
Acute gout
Gout attack
Gout flare
Podagra
Use additional code to identify:
   Autonomic neuropathy in diseases classified elsewhere (G99.0)
   Calculus of urinary tract in diseases classified elsewhere (N22)
   Cardiomyopathy in diseases classified elsewhere (I43)
   Disorders of external ear in diseases classified elsewhere (H61.1-, H62.8-)
   Disorders of iris and ciliary body in diseases classified elsewhere (H22)
   Glomerular disorders in diseases classified elsewhere (N08)

Excludes2   chronic gout (M1A.-)

● M10.0 Idiopathic gout
Gouty bursitis
Primary gout

M10.00 Idiopathic gout, unspecified site

● M10.01 Idiopathic gout, shoulder
- M10.011 Idiopathic gout, right shoulder
- M10.012 Idiopathic gout, left shoulder
- M10.019 Idiopathic gout, unspecified shoulder

● M10.02 Idiopathic gout, elbow
- M10.021 Idiopathic gout, right elbow
- M10.022 Idiopathic gout, left elbow
- M10.029 Idiopathic gout, unspecified elbow

● M10.03 Idiopathic gout, wrist
- M10.031 Idiopathic gout, right wrist
- M10.032 Idiopathic gout, left wrist
- M10.039 Idiopathic gout, unspecified wrist

● M10.04 Idiopathic gout, hand
- M10.041 Idiopathic gout, right hand
- M10.042 Idiopathic gout, left hand
- M10.049 Idiopathic gout, unspecified hand

● M10.05 Idiopathic gout, hip
- M10.051 Idiopathic gout, right hip
- M10.052 Idiopathic gout, left hip
- M10.059 Idiopathic gout, unspecified hip

● M10.06 Idiopathic gout, knee
- M10.061 Idiopathic gout, right knee
- M10.062 Idiopathic gout, left knee
- M10.069 Idiopathic gout, unspecified knee

● M10.07 Idiopathic gout, ankle and foot
   M10.071 Idiopathic gout, right ankle and foot
   M10.072 Idiopathic gout, left ankle and foot
   M10.079 Idiopathic gout, unspecified ankle and foot
  M10.08 Idiopathic gout, vertebrae
  M10.09 Idiopathic gout, multiple sites
● M10.1 Lead-induced gout
    Code first toxic effects of lead and its compounds (T56.0-)
  M10.10 Lead-induced gout, unspecified site
● M10.11 Lead-induced gout, shoulder
   M10.111 Lead-induced gout, right shoulder
   M10.112 Lead-induced gout, left shoulder
   M10.119 Lead-induced gout, unspecified shoulder
● M10.12 Lead-induced gout, elbow
   M10.121 Lead-induced gout, right elbow
   M10.122 Lead-induced gout, left elbow
   M10.129 Lead-induced gout, unspecified elbow
● M10.13 Lead-induced gout, wrist
   M10.131 Lead-induced gout, right wrist
   M10.132 Lead-induced gout, left wrist
   M10.139 Lead-induced gout, unspecified wrist
● M10.14 Lead-induced gout, hand
   M10.141 Lead-induced gout, right hand
   M10.142 Lead-induced gout, left hand
   M10.149 Lead-induced gout, unspecified hand
● M10.15 Lead-induced gout, hip
   M10.151 Lead-induced gout, right hip
   M10.152 Lead-induced gout, left hip
   M10.159 Lead-induced gout, unspecified hip
● M10.16 Lead-induced gout, knee
   M10.161 Lead-induced gout, right knee
   M10.162 Lead-induced gout, left knee
   M10.169 Lead-induced gout, unspecified knee
● M10.17 Lead-induced gout, ankle and foot
   M10.171 Lead-induced gout, right ankle and foot
   M10.172 Lead-induced gout, left ankle and foot
   M10.179 Lead-induced gout, unspecified ankle and foot
  M10.18 Lead-induced gout, vertebrae
  M10.19 Lead-induced gout, multiple sites
● M10.2 Drug-induced gout
    Use additional code for adverse effect, if applicable, to identify drug (T36-T50 with fifth or sixth character 5)
  M10.20 Drug-induced gout, unspecified site
● M10.21 Drug-induced gout, shoulder
   M10.211 Drug-induced gout, right shoulder
   M10.212 Drug-induced gout, left shoulder
   M10.219 Drug-induced gout, unspecified shoulder
● M10.22 Drug-induced gout, elbow
   M10.221 Drug-induced gout, right elbow
   M10.222 Drug-induced gout, left elbow
   M10.229 Drug-induced gout, unspecified elbow
● M10.23 Drug-induced gout, wrist
   M10.231 Drug-induced gout, right wrist
   M10.232 Drug-induced gout, left wrist
   M10.239 Drug-induced gout, unspecified wrist

● M10.24 Drug-induced gout, hand
   M10.241 Drug-induced gout, right hand
   M10.242 Drug-induced gout, left hand
   M10.249 Drug-induced gout, unspecified hand
● M10.25 Drug-induced gout, hip
   M10.251 Drug-induced gout, right hip
   M10.252 Drug-induced gout, left hip
   M10.259 Drug-induced gout, unspecified hip
● M10.26 Drug-induced gout, knee
   M10.261 Drug-induced gout, right knee
   M10.262 Drug-induced gout, left knee
   M10.269 Drug-induced gout, unspecified knee
● M10.27 Drug-induced gout, ankle and foot
   M10.271 Drug-induced gout, right ankle and foot
   M10.272 Drug-induced gout, left ankle and foot
   M10.279 Drug-induced gout, unspecified ankle and foot
  M10.28 Drug-induced gout, vertebrae
  M10.29 Drug-induced gout, multiple sites
● M10.3 Gout due to renal impairment
    Code also associated renal disease
  M10.30 Gout due to renal impairment, unspecified site
● M10.31 Gout due to renal impairment, shoulder
   M10.311 Gout due to renal impairment, right shoulder
   M10.312 Gout due to renal impairment, left shoulder
   M10.319 Gout due to renal impairment, unspecified shoulder
● M10.32 Gout due to renal impairment, elbow
   M10.321 Gout due to renal impairment, right elbow
   M10.322 Gout due to renal impairment, left elbow
   M10.329 Gout due to renal impairment, unspecified elbow
● M10.33 Gout due to renal impairment, wrist
   M10.331 Gout due to renal impairment, right wrist
   M10.332 Gout due to renal impairment, left wrist
   M10.339 Gout due to renal impairment, unspecified wrist
● M10.34 Gout due to renal impairment, hand
   M10.341 Gout due to renal impairment, right hand
   M10.342 Gout due to renal impairment, left hand
   M10.349 Gout due to renal impairment, unspecified hand
● M10.35 Gout due to renal impairment, hip
   M10.351 Gout due to renal impairment, right hip
   M10.352 Gout due to renal impairment, left hip
   M10.359 Gout due to renal impairment, unspecified hip
● M10.36 Gout due to renal impairment, knee
   M10.361 Gout due to renal impairment, right knee
   M10.362 Gout due to renal impairment, left knee
   M10.369 Gout due to renal impairment, unspecified knee

CHAPTER 13 (M00-M99)

N Newborn Age: 0   **P** Pediatric Age: 0–17   **M** Maternity DX: 9–64   **A** Adult Age: 15–124   ♀ Females Only   ♂ Males Only

Complication\Comorbidity   Major C\C   (Ex) CC/MCC Exclusions   Hospital-Acquired Condition   Hierarchical Condition Category

1033

● M10.37   Gout due to renal impairment, ankle and foot
    M10.371   Gout due to renal impairment, right ankle and foot
    M10.372   Gout due to renal impairment, left ankle and foot
    M10.379   Gout due to renal impairment, unspecified ankle and foot
  M10.38   Gout due to renal impairment, vertebrae
  M10.39   Gout due to renal impairment, multiple sites

● M10.4   Other secondary gout
    Code first associated condition
  M10.40   Other secondary gout, unspecified site
● M10.41   Other secondary gout, shoulder
    M10.411   Other secondary gout, right shoulder
    M10.412   Other secondary gout, left shoulder
    M10.419   Other secondary gout, unspecified shoulder
● M10.42   Other secondary gout, elbow
    M10.421   Other secondary gout, right elbow
    M10.422   Other secondary gout, left elbow
    M10.429   Other secondary gout, unspecified elbow
● M10.43   Other secondary gout, wrist
    M10.431   Other secondary gout, right wrist
    M10.432   Other secondary gout, left wrist
    M10.439   Other secondary gout, unspecified wrist
● M10.44   Other secondary gout, hand
    M10.441   Other secondary gout, right hand
    M10.442   Other secondary gout, left hand
    M10.449   Other secondary gout, unspecified hand
● M10.45   Other secondary gout, hip
    M10.451   Other secondary gout, right hip
    M10.452   Other secondary gout, left hip
    M10.459   Other secondary gout, unspecified hip
● M10.46   Other secondary gout, knee
    M10.461   Other secondary gout, right knee
    M10.462   Other secondary gout, left knee
    M10.469   Other secondary gout, unspecified knee
● M10.47   Other secondary gout, ankle and foot
    M10.471   Other secondary gout, right ankle and foot
    M10.472   Other secondary gout, left ankle and foot
    M10.479   Other secondary gout, unspecified ankle and foot
  M10.48   Other secondary gout, vertebrae
  M10.49   Other secondary gout, multiple sites

M10.9   Gout, unspecified
    Gout NOS

● M11   Other crystal arthropathies
● M11.0   Hydroxyapatite deposition disease
  M11.00   Hydroxyapatite deposition disease, unspecified site
● M11.01   Hydroxyapatite deposition disease, shoulder
    M11.011   Hydroxyapatite deposition disease, right shoulder
    M11.012   Hydroxyapatite deposition disease, left shoulder
    M11.019   Hydroxyapatite deposition disease, unspecified shoulder

● M11.02   Hydroxyapatite deposition disease, elbow
    M11.021   Hydroxyapatite deposition disease, right elbow
    M11.022   Hydroxyapatite deposition disease, left elbow
    M11.029   Hydroxyapatite deposition disease, unspecified elbow
● M11.03   Hydroxyapatite deposition disease, wrist
    M11.031   Hydroxyapatite deposition disease, right wrist
    M11.032   Hydroxyapatite deposition disease, left wrist
    M11.039   Hydroxyapatite deposition disease, unspecified wrist
● M11.04   Hydroxyapatite deposition disease, hand
    M11.041   Hydroxyapatite deposition disease, right hand
    M11.042   Hydroxyapatite deposition disease, left hand
    M11.049   Hydroxyapatite deposition disease, unspecified hand
● M11.05   Hydroxyapatite deposition disease, hip
    M11.051   Hydroxyapatite deposition disease, right hip
    M11.052   Hydroxyapatite deposition disease, left hip
    M11.059   Hydroxyapatite deposition disease, unspecified hip
● M11.06   Hydroxyapatite deposition disease, knee
    M11.061   Hydroxyapatite deposition disease, right knee
    M11.062   Hydroxyapatite deposition disease, left knee
    M11.069   Hydroxyapatite deposition disease, unspecified knee
● M11.07   Hydroxyapatite deposition disease, ankle and foot
    M11.071   Hydroxyapatite deposition disease, right ankle and foot
    M11.072   Hydroxyapatite deposition disease, left ankle and foot
    M11.079   Hydroxyapatite deposition disease, unspecified ankle and foot
  M11.08   Hydroxyapatite deposition disease, vertebrae
  M11.09   Hydroxyapatite deposition disease, multiple sites

● M11.1   Familial chondrocalcinosis
  M11.10   Familial chondrocalcinosis, unspecified site
● M11.11   Familial chondrocalcinosis, shoulder
    M11.111   Familial chondrocalcinosis, right shoulder
    M11.112   Familial chondrocalcinosis, left shoulder
    M11.119   Familial chondrocalcinosis, unspecified shoulder
● M11.12   Familial chondrocalcinosis, elbow
    M11.121   Familial chondrocalcinosis, right elbow
    M11.122   Familial chondrocalcinosis, left elbow
    M11.129   Familial chondrocalcinosis, unspecified elbow
● M11.13   Familial chondrocalcinosis, wrist
    M11.131   Familial chondrocalcinosis, right wrist
    M11.132   Familial chondrocalcinosis, left wrist
    M11.139   Familial chondrocalcinosis, unspecified wrist

▶ New   ⇒ Revised   ~~deleted~~ Deleted   Excludes 1   Excludes 2   Includes   Use additional   Code first   Code also   Key words
OGCR Official Guidelines   ● Unacceptable Principal Diagnosis   X Assign placeholder X   ● Use Additional Character(s)   ▷ Manifestation Code   **Coding Clinic**

● M11.14   Familial chondrocalcinosis, hand
    M11.141   Familial chondrocalcinosis, right hand
    M11.142   Familial chondrocalcinosis, left hand
    M11.149   Familial chondrocalcinosis, unspecified hand
● M11.15   Familial chondrocalcinosis, hip
    M11.151   Familial chondrocalcinosis, right hip
    M11.152   Familial chondrocalcinosis, left hip
    M11.159   Familial chondrocalcinosis, unspecified hip
● M11.16   Familial chondrocalcinosis, knee
    M11.161   Familial chondrocalcinosis, right knee
    M11.162   Familial chondrocalcinosis, left knee
    M11.169   Familial chondrocalcinosis, unspecified knee
● M11.17   Familial chondrocalcinosis, ankle and foot
    M11.171   Familial chondrocalcinosis, right ankle and foot
    M11.172   Familial chondrocalcinosis, left ankle and foot
    M11.179   Familial chondrocalcinosis, unspecified ankle and foot
    M11.18   Familial chondrocalcinosis, vertebrae
    M11.19   Familial chondrocalcinosis, multiple sites
● M11.2   Other chondrocalcinosis
    Chondrocalcinosis NOS
    M11.20   Other chondrocalcinosis, unspecified site
● M11.21   Other chondrocalcinosis, shoulder
    M11.211   Other chondrocalcinosis, right shoulder
    M11.212   Other chondrocalcinosis, left shoulder
    M11.219   Other chondrocalcinosis, unspecified shoulder
● M11.22   Other chondrocalcinosis, elbow
    M11.221   Other chondrocalcinosis, right elbow
    M11.222   Other chondrocalcinosis, left elbow
    M11.229   Other chondrocalcinosis, unspecified elbow
● M11.23   Other chondrocalcinosis, wrist
    M11.231   Other chondrocalcinosis, right wrist
    M11.232   Other chondrocalcinosis, left wrist
    M11.239   Other chondrocalcinosis, unspecified wrist
● M11.24   Other chondrocalcinosis, hand
    M11.241   Other chondrocalcinosis, right hand
    M11.242   Other chondrocalcinosis, left hand
    M11.249   Other chondrocalcinosis, unspecified hand
● M11.25   Other chondrocalcinosis, hip
    M11.251   Other chondrocalcinosis, right hip
    M11.252   Other chondrocalcinosis, left hip
    M11.259   Other chondrocalcinosis, unspecified hip
● M11.26   Other chondrocalcinosis, knee
    M11.261   Other chondrocalcinosis, right knee
    M11.262   Other chondrocalcinosis, left knee
    M11.269   Other chondrocalcinosis, unspecified knee

● M11.27   Other chondrocalcinosis, ankle and foot
    M11.271   Other chondrocalcinosis, right ankle and foot
    M11.272   Other chondrocalcinosis, left ankle and foot
    M11.279   Other chondrocalcinosis, unspecified ankle and foot
    M11.28   Other chondrocalcinosis, vertebrae
    M11.29   Other chondrocalcinosis, multiple sites
● M11.8   Other specified crystal arthropathies
    M11.80   Other specified crystal arthropathies, unspecified site
● M11.81   Other specified crystal arthropathies, shoulder
    M11.811   Other specified crystal arthropathies, right shoulder
    M11.812   Other specified crystal arthropathies, left shoulder
    M11.819   Other specified crystal arthropathies, unspecified shoulder
● M11.82   Other specified crystal arthropathies, elbow
    M11.821   Other specified crystal arthropathies, right elbow
    M11.822   Other specified crystal arthropathies, left elbow
    M11.829   Other specified crystal arthropathies, unspecified elbow
● M11.83   Other specified crystal arthropathies, wrist
    M11.831   Other specified crystal arthropathies, right wrist
    M11.832   Other specified crystal arthropathies, left wrist
    M11.839   Other specified crystal arthropathies, unspecified wrist
● M11.84   Other specified crystal arthropathies, hand
    M11.841   Other specified crystal arthropathies, right hand
    M11.842   Other specified crystal arthropathies, left hand
    M11.849   Other specified crystal arthropathies, unspecified hand
● M11.85   Other specified crystal arthropathies, hip
    M11.851   Other specified crystal arthropathies, right hip
    M11.852   Other specified crystal arthropathies, left hip
    M11.859   Other specified crystal arthropathies, unspecified hip
● M11.86   Other specified crystal arthropathies, knee
    M11.861   Other specified crystal arthropathies, right knee
    M11.862   Other specified crystal arthropathies, left knee
    M11.869   Other specified crystal arthropathies, unspecified knee
● M11.87   Other specified crystal arthropathies, ankle and foot
    M11.871   Other specified crystal arthropathies, right ankle and foot
    M11.872   Other specified crystal arthropathies, left ankle and foot
    M11.879   Other specified crystal arthropathies, unspecified ankle and foot
    M11.88   Other specified crystal arthropathies, vertebrae
    M11.89   Other specified crystal arthropathies, multiple sites
    M11.9   Crystal arthropathy, unspecified

CHAPTER 13 (M00–M99)

● **M12 Other and unspecified arthropathy**
    Excludes1   arthrosis (M15-M19)
                cricoarytenoid arthropathy (J38.7)
   ● **M12.0 Chronic postrheumatic arthropathy [Jaccoud]**
      M12.00   Chronic postrheumatic arthropathy [Jaccoud], unspecified site 🔖
     ● M12.01   Chronic postrheumatic arthropathy [Jaccoud], shoulder
         M12.011   Chronic postrheumatic arthropathy [Jaccoud], right shoulder 🔖
         M12.012   Chronic postrheumatic arthropathy [Jaccoud], left shoulder 🔖
         M12.019   Chronic postrheumatic arthropathy [Jaccoud], unspecified shoulder 🔖
     ● M12.02   Chronic postrheumatic arthropathy [Jaccoud], elbow
         M12.021   Chronic postrheumatic arthropathy [Jaccoud], right elbow 🔖
         M12.022   Chronic postrheumatic arthropathy [Jaccoud], left elbow 🔖
         M12.029   Chronic postrheumatic arthropathy [Jaccoud], unspecified elbow 🔖
     ● M12.03   Chronic postrheumatic arthropathy [Jaccoud], wrist
         M12.031   Chronic postrheumatic arthropathy [Jaccoud], right wrist 🔖
         M12.032   Chronic postrheumatic arthropathy [Jaccoud], left wrist 🔖
         M12.039   Chronic postrheumatic arthropathy [Jaccoud], unspecified wrist 🔖
     ● M12.04   Chronic postrheumatic arthropathy [Jaccoud], hand
         M12.041   Chronic postrheumatic arthropathy [Jaccoud], right hand 🔖
         M12.042   Chronic postrheumatic arthropathy [Jaccoud], left hand 🔖
         M12.049   Chronic postrheumatic arthropathy [Jaccoud], unspecified hand 🔖
     ● M12.05   Chronic postrheumatic arthropathy [Jaccoud], hip
         M12.051   Chronic postrheumatic arthropathy [Jaccoud], right hip 🔖
         M12.052   Chronic postrheumatic arthropathy [Jaccoud], left hip 🔖
         M12.059   Chronic postrheumatic arthropathy [Jaccoud], unspecified hip 🔖
     ● M12.06   Chronic postrheumatic arthropathy [Jaccoud], knee
         M12.061   Chronic postrheumatic arthropathy [Jaccoud], right knee 🔖
         M12.062   Chronic postrheumatic arthropathy [Jaccoud], left knee 🔖
         M12.069   Chronic postrheumatic arthropathy [Jaccoud], unspecified knee 🔖
     ● M12.07   Chronic postrheumatic arthropathy [Jaccoud], ankle and foot
         M12.071   Chronic postrheumatic arthropathy [Jaccoud], right ankle and foot 🔖
         M12.072   Chronic postrheumatic arthropathy [Jaccoud], left ankle and foot 🔖
         M12.079   Chronic postrheumatic arthropathy [Jaccoud], unspecified ankle and foot 🔖
      M12.08   Chronic postrheumatic arthropathy [Jaccoud], other specified site 🔖
         Chronic postrheumatic arthropathy [Jaccoud], vertebrae
      M12.09   Chronic postrheumatic arthropathy [Jaccoud], multiple sites 🔖

   ● **M12.1 Kaschin-Beck disease**
        Osteochondroarthrosis deformans endemica
      M12.10   Kaschin-Beck disease, unspecified site
     ● M12.11   Kaschin-Beck disease, shoulder
         M12.111   Kaschin-Beck disease, right shoulder
         M12.112   Kaschin-Beck disease, left shoulder
         M12.119   Kaschin-Beck disease, unspecified shoulder
     ● M12.12   Kaschin-Beck disease, elbow
         M12.121   Kaschin-Beck disease, right elbow
         M12.122   Kaschin-Beck disease, left elbow
         M12.129   Kaschin-Beck disease, unspecified elbow
     ● M12.13   Kaschin-Beck disease, wrist
         M12.131   Kaschin-Beck disease, right wrist
         M12.132   Kaschin-Beck disease, left wrist
         M12.139   Kaschin-Beck disease, unspecified wrist
     ● M12.14   Kaschin-Beck disease, hand
         M12.141   Kaschin-Beck disease, right hand
         M12.142   Kaschin-Beck disease, left hand
         M12.149   Kaschin-Beck disease, unspecified hand
     ● M12.15   Kaschin-Beck disease, hip
         M12.151   Kaschin-Beck disease, right hip
         M12.152   Kaschin-Beck disease, left hip
         M12.159   Kaschin-Beck disease, unspecified hip
     ● M12.16   Kaschin-Beck disease, knee
         M12.161   Kaschin-Beck disease, right knee
         M12.162   Kaschin-Beck disease, left knee
         M12.169   Kaschin-Beck disease, unspecified knee
     ● M12.17   Kaschin-Beck disease, ankle and foot
         M12.171   Kaschin-Beck disease, right ankle and foot
         M12.172   Kaschin-Beck disease, left ankle and foot
         M12.179   Kaschin-Beck disease, unspecified ankle and foot
      M12.18   Kaschin-Beck disease, vertebrae
      M12.19   Kaschin-Beck disease, multiple sites
   ● **M12.2 Villonodular synovitis (pigmented)**
      M12.20   Villonodular synovitis (pigmented), unspecified site
     ● M12.21   Villonodular synovitis (pigmented), shoulder
         M12.211   Villonodular synovitis (pigmented), right shoulder
         M12.212   Villonodular synovitis (pigmented), left shoulder
         M12.219   Villonodular synovitis (pigmented), unspecified shoulder
     ● M12.22   Villonodular synovitis (pigmented), elbow
         M12.221   Villonodular synovitis (pigmented), right elbow
         M12.222   Villonodular synovitis (pigmented), left elbow
         M12.229   Villonodular synovitis (pigmented), unspecified elbow
     ● M12.23   Villonodular synovitis (pigmented), wrist
         M12.231   Villonodular synovitis (pigmented), right wrist
         M12.232   Villonodular synovitis (pigmented), left wrist
         M12.239   Villonodular synovitis (pigmented), unspecified wrist

● M12.24 Villonodular synovitis (pigmented), hand
   M12.241 Villonodular synovitis (pigmented), right hand
   M12.242 Villonodular synovitis (pigmented), left hand
   M12.249 Villonodular synovitis (pigmented), unspecified hand
● M12.25 Villonodular synovitis (pigmented), hip
   M12.251 Villonodular synovitis (pigmented), right hip
   M12.252 Villonodular synovitis (pigmented), left hip
   M12.259 Villonodular synovitis (pigmented), unspecified hip
● M12.26 Villonodular synovitis (pigmented), knee
   M12.261 Villonodular synovitis (pigmented), right knee
   M12.262 Villonodular synovitis (pigmented), left knee
   M12.269 Villonodular synovitis (pigmented), unspecified knee
● M12.27 Villonodular synovitis (pigmented), ankle and foot
   M12.271 Villonodular synovitis (pigmented), right ankle and foot
   M12.272 Villonodular synovitis (pigmented), left ankle and foot
   M12.279 Villonodular synovitis (pigmented), unspecified ankle and foot
  M12.28 Villonodular synovitis (pigmented), other specified site
    Villonodular synovitis (pigmented), vertebrae
  M12.29 Villonodular synovitis (pigmented), multiple sites
● M12.3 Palindromic rheumatism
  M12.30 Palindromic rheumatism, unspecified site
● M12.31 Palindromic rheumatism, shoulder
   M12.311 Palindromic rheumatism, right shoulder
   M12.312 Palindromic rheumatism, left shoulder
   M12.319 Palindromic rheumatism, unspecified shoulder
● M12.32 Palindromic rheumatism, elbow
   M12.321 Palindromic rheumatism, right elbow
   M12.322 Palindromic rheumatism, left elbow
   M12.329 Palindromic rheumatism, unspecified elbow
● M12.33 Palindromic rheumatism, wrist
   M12.331 Palindromic rheumatism, right wrist
   M12.332 Palindromic rheumatism, left wrist
   M12.339 Palindromic rheumatism, unspecified wrist
● M12.34 Palindromic rheumatism, hand
   M12.341 Palindromic rheumatism, right hand
   M12.342 Palindromic rheumatism, left hand
   M12.349 Palindromic rheumatism, unspecified hand
● M12.35 Palindromic rheumatism, hip
   M12.351 Palindromic rheumatism, right hip
   M12.352 Palindromic rheumatism, left hip
   M12.359 Palindromic rheumatism, unspecified hip

● M12.36 Palindromic rheumatism, knee
   M12.361 Palindromic rheumatism, right knee
   M12.362 Palindromic rheumatism, left knee
   M12.369 Palindromic rheumatism, unspecified knee
● M12.37 Palindromic rheumatism, ankle and foot
   M12.371 Palindromic rheumatism, right ankle and foot
   M12.372 Palindromic rheumatism, left ankle and foot
   M12.379 Palindromic rheumatism, unspecified ankle and foot
  M12.38 Palindromic rheumatism, other specified site
    Palindromic rheumatism, vertebrae
  M12.39 Palindromic rheumatism, multiple sites
● M12.4 Intermittent hydrarthrosis
  M12.40 Intermittent hydrarthrosis, unspecified site
● M12.41 Intermittent hydrarthrosis, shoulder
   M12.411 Intermittent hydrarthrosis, right shoulder
   M12.412 Intermittent hydrarthrosis, left shoulder
   M12.419 Intermittent hydrarthrosis, unspecified shoulder
● M12.42 Intermittent hydrarthrosis, elbow
   M12.421 Intermittent hydrarthrosis, right elbow
   M12.422 Intermittent hydrarthrosis, left elbow
   M12.429 Intermittent hydrarthrosis, unspecified elbow
● M12.43 Intermittent hydrarthrosis, wrist
   M12.431 Intermittent hydrarthrosis, right wrist
   M12.432 Intermittent hydrarthrosis, left wrist
   M12.439 Intermittent hydrarthrosis, unspecified wrist
● M12.44 Intermittent hydrarthrosis, hand
   M12.441 Intermittent hydrarthrosis, right hand
   M12.442 Intermittent hydrarthrosis, left hand
   M12.449 Intermittent hydrarthrosis, unspecified hand
● M12.45 Intermittent hydrarthrosis, hip
   M12.451 Intermittent hydrarthrosis, right hip
   M12.452 Intermittent hydrarthrosis, left hip
   M12.459 Intermittent hydrarthrosis, unspecified hip
● M12.46 Intermittent hydrarthrosis, knee
   M12.461 Intermittent hydrarthrosis, right knee
   M12.462 Intermittent hydrarthrosis, left knee
   M12.469 Intermittent hydrarthrosis, unspecified knee
● M12.47 Intermittent hydrarthrosis, ankle and foot
   M12.471 Intermittent hydrarthrosis, right ankle and foot
   M12.472 Intermittent hydrarthrosis, left ankle and foot
   M12.479 Intermittent hydrarthrosis, unspecified ankle and foot
  M12.48 Intermittent hydrarthrosis, other site
  M12.49 Intermittent hydrarthrosis, multiple sites

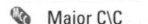
CHAPTER 13 (M00-M99)

● **M12.5** **Traumatic arthropathy**
    Excludes1 current injury–see Alphabetic Index
                  post-traumatic osteoarthritis of first
                     carpometacarpal joint (M18.2-M18.3)
                  post-traumatic osteoarthritis of hip
                     (M16.4-M16.5)
                  post-traumatic osteoarthritis of knee
                     (M17.2-M17.3)
                  post-traumatic osteoarthritis NOS
                     (M19.1-)
                  post-traumatic osteoarthritis of other
                     single joints (M19.1-)
    M12.50 Traumatic arthropathy, unspecified site
●   **M12.51** Traumatic arthropathy, shoulder
        M12.511 Traumatic arthropathy, right shoulder
        M12.512 Traumatic arthropathy, left shoulder
        M12.519 Traumatic arthropathy, unspecified
                 shoulder
●   **M12.52** Traumatic arthropathy, elbow
        M12.521 Traumatic arthropathy, right elbow
        M12.522 Traumatic arthropathy, left elbow
        M12.529 Traumatic arthropathy, unspecified
                 elbow
●   **M12.53** Traumatic arthropathy, wrist
        M12.531 Traumatic arthropathy, right wrist
        M12.532 Traumatic arthropathy, left wrist
        M12.539 Traumatic arthropathy, unspecified
                 wrist
●   **M12.54** Traumatic arthropathy, hand
        M12.541 Traumatic arthropathy, right hand
        M12.542 Traumatic arthropathy, left hand
        M12.549 Traumatic arthropathy, unspecified
                 hand
●   **M12.55** Traumatic arthropathy, hip
        M12.551 Traumatic arthropathy, right hip
        M12.552 Traumatic arthropathy, left hip
                 Coding Clinic: 2015, Q1, P17
        M12.559 Traumatic arthropathy, unspecified
                 hip
●   **M12.56** Traumatic arthropathy, knee
        M12.561 Traumatic arthropathy, right knee
        M12.562 Traumatic arthropathy, left knee
        M12.569 Traumatic arthropathy, unspecified
                 knee
●   **M12.57** Traumatic arthropathy, ankle and foot
        M12.571 Traumatic arthropathy, right ankle
                 and foot
        M12.572 Traumatic arthropathy, left ankle and
                 foot
        M12.579 Traumatic arthropathy, unspecified
                 ankle and foot
    M12.58 Traumatic arthropathy, other specified site
            Traumatic arthropathy, vertebrae
    M12.59 Traumatic arthropathy, multiple sites
● **M12.8** Other specific arthropathies, not elsewhere classified
        Transient arthropathy
    M12.80 Other specific arthropathies, not elsewhere
           classified, unspecified site
●   **M12.81** Other specific arthropathies, not elsewhere
           classified, shoulder
        M12.811 Other specific arthropathies, not
                 elsewhere classified, right shoulder
        M12.812 Other specific arthropathies, not
                 elsewhere classified, left shoulder
        M12.819 Other specific arthropathies, not
                 elsewhere classified, unspecified
                 shoulder

●   **M12.82** Other specific arthropathies, not elsewhere
           classified, elbow
        M12.821 Other specific arthropathies, not
                 elsewhere classified, right elbow
        M12.822 Other specific arthropathies, not
                 elsewhere classified, left elbow
        M12.829 Other specific arthropathies, not
                 elsewhere classified, unspecified
                 elbow
●   **M12.83** Other specific arthropathies, not elsewhere
           classified, wrist
        M12.831 Other specific arthropathies, not
                 elsewhere classified, right wrist
        M12.832 Other specific arthropathies, not
                 elsewhere classified, left wrist
        M12.839 Other specific arthropathies, not
                 elsewhere classified, unspecified wrist
●   **M12.84** Other specific arthropathies, not elsewhere
           classified, hand
        M12.841 Other specific arthropathies, not
                 elsewhere classified, right hand
        M12.842 Other specific arthropathies, not
                 elsewhere classified, left hand
        M12.849 Other specific arthropathies, not
                 elsewhere classified, unspecified hand
●   **M12.85** Other specific arthropathies, not elsewhere
           classified, hip
        M12.851 Other specific arthropathies, not
                 elsewhere classified, right hip
        M12.852 Other specific arthropathies, not
                 elsewhere classified, left hip
        M12.859 Other specific arthropathies, not
                 elsewhere classified, unspecified hip
●   **M12.86** Other specific arthropathies, not elsewhere
           classified, knee
        M12.861 Other specific arthropathies, not
                 elsewhere classified, right knee
        M12.862 Other specific arthropathies, not
                 elsewhere classified, left knee
        M12.869 Other specific arthropathies, not
                 elsewhere classified, unspecified knee
●   **M12.87** Other specific arthropathies, not elsewhere
           classified, ankle and foot
        M12.871 Other specific arthropathies, not
                 elsewhere classified, right ankle and
                 foot
        M12.872 Other specific arthropathies, not
                 elsewhere classified, left ankle and
                 foot
        M12.879 Other specific arthropathies, not
                 elsewhere classified, unspecified
                 ankle and foot
    M12.88 Other specific arthropathies, not elsewhere
           classified, other specified site
             Other specific arthropathies, not elsewhere
               classified, vertebrae
    M12.89 Other specific arthropathies, not elsewhere
           classified, multiple sites
M12.9 Arthropathy, unspecified

▶ New   ⇛ Revised   ~~deleted~~ Deleted   Excludes 1   Excludes 2   Includes   Use additional   Code first   Code also   Key words
OGCR Official Guidelines   ● Unacceptable Principal Diagnosis   X Assign placeholder X   ● Use Additional Character(s)   ▶ Manifestation Code   **Coding Clinic**

● **M13 Other arthritis**

    Excludes1   arthrosis (M15-M19)

            osteoarthritis (M15-M19)

     M13.0   Polyarthritis, unspecified

● M13.1   Monoarthritis, not elsewhere classified

       M13.10   Monoarthritis, not elsewhere classified, unspecified site

     ● M13.11   Monoarthritis, not elsewhere classified, shoulder

         M13.111   Monoarthritis, not elsewhere classified, right shoulder

         M13.112   Monoarthritis, not elsewhere classified, left shoulder

         M13.119   Monoarthritis, not elsewhere classified, unspecified shoulder

     ● M13.12   Monoarthritis, not elsewhere classified, elbow

         M13.121   Monoarthritis, not elsewhere classified, right elbow

         M13.122   Monoarthritis, not elsewhere classified, left elbow

         M13.129   Monoarthritis, not elsewhere classified, unspecified elbow

     ● M13.13   Monoarthritis, not elsewhere classified, wrist

         M13.131   Monoarthritis, not elsewhere classified, right wrist

         M13.132   Monoarthritis, not elsewhere classified, left wrist

         M13.139   Monoarthritis, not elsewhere classified, unspecified wrist

     ● M13.14   Monoarthritis, not elsewhere classified, hand

         M13.141   Monoarthritis, not elsewhere classified, right hand

         M13.142   Monoarthritis, not elsewhere classified, left hand

         M13.149   Monoarthritis, not elsewhere classified, unspecified hand

     ● M13.15   Monoarthritis, not elsewhere classified, hip

         M13.151   Monoarthritis, not elsewhere classified, right hip

         M13.152   Monoarthritis, not elsewhere classified, left hip

         M13.159   Monoarthritis, not elsewhere classified, unspecified hip

     ● M13.16   Monoarthritis, not elsewhere classified, knee

         M13.161   Monoarthritis, not elsewhere classified, right knee

         M13.162   Monoarthritis, not elsewhere classified, left knee

         M13.169   Monoarthritis, not elsewhere classified, unspecified knee

     ● M13.17   Monoarthritis, not elsewhere classified, ankle and foot

         M13.171   Monoarthritis, not elsewhere classified, right ankle and foot

         M13.172   Monoarthritis, not elsewhere classified, left ankle and foot

         M13.179   Monoarthritis, not elsewhere classified, unspecified ankle and foot

● M13.8   Other specified arthritis

     Allergic arthritis

    Excludes1   osteoarthritis (M15-M19)

       M13.80   Other specified arthritis, unspecified site

     ● M13.81   Other specified arthritis, shoulder

         M13.811   Other specified arthritis, right shoulder

         M13.812   Other specified arthritis, left shoulder

         M13.819   Other specified arthritis, unspecified shoulder

     ● M13.82   Other specified arthritis, elbow

         M13.821   Other specified arthritis, right elbow

         M13.822   Other specified arthritis, left elbow

         M13.829   Other specified arthritis, unspecified elbow

     ● M13.83   Other specified arthritis, wrist

         M13.831   Other specified arthritis, right wrist

         M13.832   Other specified arthritis, left wrist

         M13.839   Other specified arthritis, unspecified wrist

     ● M13.84   Other specified arthritis, hand

         M13.841   Other specified arthritis, right hand

         M13.842   Other specified arthritis, left hand

         M13.849   Other specified arthritis, unspecified hand

     ● M13.85   Other specified arthritis, hip

         M13.851   Other specified arthritis, right hip

         M13.852   Other specified arthritis, left hip

         M13.859   Other specified arthritis, unspecified hip

     ● M13.86   Other specified arthritis, knee

         M13.861   Other specified arthritis, right knee

         M13.862   Other specified arthritis, left knee

         M13.869   Other specified arthritis, unspecified knee

     ● M13.87   Other specified arthritis, ankle and foot

         M13.871   Other specified arthritis, right ankle and foot

         M13.872   Other specified arthritis, left ankle and foot

         M13.879   Other specified arthritis, unspecified ankle and foot

       M13.88   Other specified arthritis, other site

       M13.89   Other specified arthritis, multiple sites

● M14   Arthropathies in other diseases classified elsewhere

    Excludes1   arthropathy in:

         diabetes mellitus (E08 E13 with .61-)

         hematological disorders (M36.2-M36.3)

         hypersensitivity reactions (M36.4)

         neoplastic disease (M36.1)

         neurosyphillis (A52.16)

         sarcoidosis (D86.86)

       enteropathic arthropathies (M07.0-)

       juvenile psoriatic arthropathy (L40.54)

       lipoid dermatoarthritis (E78.81)

● M14.6   Charcôt's joint

     Neuropathic arthropathy

    Excludes1   Charcôt's joint in diabetes mellitus (E08-E13 with .610)

         Charcôt's joint in tabes dorsalis (A52.16)

       M14.60   Charcôt's joint, unspecified site

     ● M14.61   Charcôt's joint, shoulder

         M14.611   Charcôt's joint, right shoulder

         M14.612   Charcôt's joint, left shoulder

         M14.619   Charcôt's joint, unspecified shoulder

     ● M14.62   Charcôt's joint, elbow

         M14.621   Charcôt's joint, right elbow

         M14.622   Charcôt's joint, left elbow

         M14.629   Charcôt's joint, unspecified elbow

     ● M14.63   Charcôt's joint, wrist

         M14.631   Charcôt's joint, right wrist

         M14.632   Charcôt's joint, left wrist

         M14.639   Charcôt's joint, unspecified wrist

CHAPTER 13 (M00-M99)

N Newborn Age: 0   P Pediatric Age: 0–17   M Maternity DX: 9–64   A Adult Age: 15–124   ♀ Females Only   ♂ Males Only

Complication\Comorbidity   Major C\C   (Ex) CC/MCC Exclusions   Hospital-Acquired Condition   Hierarchical Condition Category   1039

● M14.64 Charcôt's joint, hand
 M14.641 Charcôt's joint, right hand
 M14.642 Charcôt's joint, left hand
 M14.649 Charcôt's joint, unspecified hand
● M14.65 Charcôt's joint, hip
 M14.651 Charcôt's joint, right hip
 M14.652 Charcôt's joint, left hip
 M14.659 Charcôt's joint, unspecified hip
● M14.66 Charcôt's joint, knee
 M14.661 Charcôt's joint, right knee
 M14.662 Charcôt's joint, left knee
 M14.669 Charcôt's joint, unspecified knee
● M14.67 Charcôt's joint, ankle and foot
 M14.671 Charcôt's joint, right ankle and foot
 M14.672 Charcôt's joint, left ankle and foot
 M14.679 Charcôt's joint, unspecified ankle and foot
M14.68 Charcôt's joint, vertebrae
M14.69 Charcôt's joint, multiple sites

● M14.8 Arthropathies in other specified diseases classified elsewhere
Code first underlying disease, such as:
 amyloidosis (E85.-)
 erythema multiforme (L51.-)
 erythema nodosum (L52)
 hemochromatosis (E83.11-)
 hyperparathyroidism (E21.-)
 hypothyroidism (E00-E03)
 sickle-cell disorders (D57.-)
 thyrotoxicosis [hyperthyroidism] (E05.-)
 Whipple's disease (K90.81)

▸ *M14.80 Arthropathies in other specified diseases classified elsewhere, unspecified site*
● M14.81 Arthropathies in other specified diseases classified elsewhere, shoulder
 ▸ *M14.811 ...right shoulder*
 ▸ *M14.812 ...left shoulder*
 ▸ *M14.819 ...unspecified shoulder*
● M14.82 Arthropathies in other specified diseases classified elsewhere, elbow
 ▸ *M14.821 ...right elbow*
 ▸ *M14.822 ...left elbow*
 ▸ *M14.829 ...unspecified elbow*
● M14.83 Arthropathies in other specified diseases classified elsewhere, wrist
 ▸ *M14.831 ...right wrist*
 ▸ *M14.832 ...left wrist*
 ▸ *M14.839 ...unspecified wrist*

● M14.84 Arthropathies in other specified diseases classified elsewhere, hand
 ▸ *M14.841 ...right hand*
 ▸ *M14.842 ...left hand*
 ▸ *M14.849 ...unspecified hand*
● M14.85 ...hip
 ▸ *M14.851 ...right hip*
 ▸ *M14.852 ...left hip*
 ▸ *M14.859 ...unspecified hip*
● M14.86 ...knee
 ▸ *M14.861 ...right knee*
 ▸ *M14.862 ...left knee*
 ▸ *M14.869 ...unspecified knee*
● M14.87 ...ankle and foot
 ▸ *M14.871 ...right ankle and foot*
 ▸ *M14.872 ...left ankle and foot*
 ▸ *M14.879 ...unspecified ankle and foot*
▸ *M14.88 ...vertebrae*
▸ *M14.89 ...multiple sites*

OSTEOARTHRITIS (M15-M19)

Osteoarthritis is the most common degenerative joint disease and form of arthritis that breaks down the cartilage causing pain, swelling, and reduced motion in the joints.

Excludes2 osteoarthritis of spine (M47.-)

● M15 Polyosteoarthritis
Includes arthritis of multiple sites
Excludes1 bilateral involvement of single joint (M16-M19)
M15.0 Primary generalized (osteo)arthritis
M15.1 Heberden's nodes (with arthropathy)
 Interphalangeal distal osteoarthritis
M15.2 Bouchard's nodes (with arthropathy)
 Juxtaphalangeal distal osteoarthritis
M15.3 Secondary multiple arthritis
 Post-traumatic polyosteoarthritis
M15.4 Erosive (osteo)arthritis
M15.8 Other polyosteoarthritis
M15.9 Polyosteoarthritis, unspecified
 Generalized osteoarthritis NOS

● **M16   Osteoarthritis of hip**

    M16.0   Bilateral primary osteoarthritis of hip
        Coding Clinic: 2018, Q2, P15; 2016, Q4, P146

   ● **M16.1   Unilateral primary osteoarthritis of hip**
        Primary osteoarthritis of hip NOS

       M16.10   Unilateral primary osteoarthritis, unspecified hip

       M16.11   Unilateral primary osteoarthritis, right hip

       M16.12   Unilateral primary osteoarthritis, left hip

    M16.2   Bilateral osteoarthritis resulting from hip dysplasia

   ● **M16.3   Unilateral osteoarthritis resulting from hip dysplasia**
        Dysplastic osteoarthritis of hip NOS

       M16.30   Unilateral osteoarthritis resulting from hip dysplasia, unspecified hip

       M16.31   Unilateral osteoarthritis resulting from hip dysplasia, right hip

       M16.32   Unilateral osteoarthritis resulting from hip dysplasia, left hip

    M16.4   Bilateral post-traumatic osteoarthritis of hip

   ● **M16.5   Unilateral post-traumatic osteoarthritis of hip**
        Post-traumatic osteoarthritis of hip NOS

       M16.50   Unilateral post-traumatic osteoarthritis, unspecified hip

       M16.51   Unilateral post-traumatic osteoarthritis, right hip

       M16.52   Unilateral post-traumatic osteoarthritis, left hip

    M16.6   Other bilateral secondary osteoarthritis of hip

    M16.7   Other unilateral secondary osteoarthritis of hip
        Secondary osteoarthritis of hip NOS

    M16.9   Osteoarthritis of hip, unspecified

● **M17   Osteoarthritis of knee**

    M17.0   Bilateral primary osteoarthritis of knee

   ● **M17.1   Unilateral primary osteoarthritis of knee**
        Primary osteoarthritis of knee NOS

       M17.10   Unilateral primary osteoarthritis, unspecified knee
          Coding Clinic: 2016, Q4, P147

       M17.11   Unilateral primary osteoarthritis, right knee

       M17.12   Unilateral primary osteoarthritis, left knee
          Coding Clinic: 2016, Q4, P146

    M17.2   Bilateral post-traumatic osteoarthritis of knee

   ● **M17.3   Unilateral post-traumatic osteoarthritis of knee**
        Post-traumatic osteoarthritis of knee NOS

       M17.30   Unilateral post-traumatic osteoarthritis, unspecified knee

       M17.31   Unilateral post-traumatic osteoarthritis, right knee

       M17.32   Unilateral post-traumatic osteoarthritis, left knee

    M17.4   Other bilateral secondary osteoarthritis of knee

    M17.5   Other unilateral secondary osteoarthritis of knee
        Secondary osteoarthritis of knee NOS

    M17.9   Osteoarthritis of knee, unspecified
        Coding Clinic: 2016, Q4, P146

● **M18   Osteoarthritis of first carpometacarpal joint**

    M18.0   Bilateral primary osteoarthritis of first carpometacarpal joints

   ● **M18.1   Unilateral primary osteoarthritis of first carpometacarpal joint**
        Primary osteoarthritis of first carpometacarpal joint NOS

       M18.10   Unilateral primary osteoarthritis of first carpometacarpal joint, unspecified hand

       M18.11   Unilateral primary osteoarthritis of first carpometacarpal joint, right hand

       M18.12   Unilateral primary osteoarthritis of first carpometacarpal joint, left hand

    M18.2   Bilateral post-traumatic osteoarthritis of first carpometacarpal joints

   ● **M18.3   Unilateral post-traumatic osteoarthritis of first carpometacarpal joint**
        Post-traumatic osteoarthritis of first carpometacarpal joint NOS

       M18.30   Unilateral post-traumatic osteoarthritis of first carpometacarpal joint, unspecified hand

       M18.31   Unilateral post-traumatic osteoarthritis of first carpometacarpal joint, right hand

       M18.32   Unilateral post-traumatic osteoarthritis of first carpometacarpal joint, left hand

    M18.4   Other bilateral secondary osteoarthritis of first carpometacarpal joints

   ● **M18.5   Other unilateral secondary osteoarthritis of first carpometacarpal joint**
        Secondary osteoarthritis of first carpometacarpal joint NOS

       M18.50   Other unilateral secondary osteoarthritis of first carpometacarpal joint, unspecified hand

       M18.51   Other unilateral secondary osteoarthritis of first carpometacarpal joint, right hand

       M18.52   Other unilateral secondary osteoarthritis of first carpometacarpal joint, left hand

    M18.9   Osteoarthritis of first carpometacarpal joint, unspecified

● **M19   Other and unspecified osteoarthritis**

    Excludes1   polyarthritis (M15.-)

    Excludes2   arthrosis of spine (M47.-)
             hallux rigidus (M20.2)
             osteoarthritis of spine (M47.-)

   ● **M19.0   Primary osteoarthritis of other joints**

     ● **M19.01   Primary osteoarthritis, shoulder**

         M19.011   Primary osteoarthritis, right shoulder
            Coding Clinic: 2016, Q4, P145

         M19.012   Primary osteoarthritis, left shoulder

         M19.019   Primary osteoarthritis, unspecified shoulder

     ● **M19.02   Primary osteoarthritis, elbow**

         M19.021   Primary osteoarthritis, right elbow

         M19.022   Primary osteoarthritis, left elbow

         M19.029   Primary osteoarthritis, unspecified elbow

     ● **M19.03   Primary osteoarthritis, wrist**

         M19.031   Primary osteoarthritis, right wrist

         M19.032   Primary osteoarthritis, left wrist

         M19.039   Primary osteoarthritis, unspecified wrist

     ● **M19.04   Primary osteoarthritis, hand**

        Excludes2   primary osteoarthritis of first carpometacarpal joint (M18.0-, M18.1-)

         M19.041   Primary osteoarthritis, right hand

         M19.042   Primary osteoarthritis, left hand

         M19.049   Primary osteoarthritis, unspecified hand

     ● **M19.07   Primary osteoarthritis ankle and foot**

         M19.071   Primary osteoarthritis, right ankle and foot

         M19.072   Primary osteoarthritis, left ankle and foot

         M19.079   Primary osteoarthritis, unspecified ankle and foot

       M19.09   Primary osteoarthritis, other specified site

N   Newborn Age: 0   **P**   Pediatric Age: 0–17   **M**   Maternity DX: 9–64   **A**   Adult Age: 15–124   ♀   Females Only   ♂   Males Only

🅒 Complication\Comorbidity   🅜 Major C\C   Ⓔ🄰 CC/MCC Exclusions   🅗 Hospital-Acquired Condition   🅗🅒 Hierarchical Condition Category

1041

● **M19.1** Post-traumatic osteoarthritis of other joints
  ● **M19.11** Post-traumatic osteoarthritis, shoulder
     M19.111 Post-traumatic osteoarthritis, right shoulder
     M19.112 Post-traumatic osteoarthritis, left shoulder
     M19.119 Post-traumatic osteoarthritis, unspecified shoulder
  ● **M19.12** Post-traumatic osteoarthritis, elbow
     M19.121 Post-traumatic osteoarthritis, right elbow
     M19.122 Post-traumatic osteoarthritis, left elbow
     M19.129 Post-traumatic osteoarthritis, unspecified elbow
  ● **M19.13** Post-traumatic osteoarthritis, wrist
     M19.131 Post-traumatic osteoarthritis, right wrist
     M19.132 Post-traumatic osteoarthritis, left wrist
     M19.139 Post-traumatic osteoarthritis, unspecified wrist
  ● **M19.14** Post-traumatic osteoarthritis, hand
     Excludes2   post-traumatic osteoarthritis of first carpometacarpal joint (M18.2-, M18.3-)
     M19.141 Post-traumatic osteoarthritis, right hand
     M19.142 Post-traumatic osteoarthritis, left hand
     M19.149 Post-traumatic osteoarthritis, unspecified hand
  ● **M19.17** Post-traumatic osteoarthritis, ankle and foot
     M19.171 Post-traumatic osteoarthritis, right ankle and foot
     M19.172 Post-traumatic osteoarthritis, left ankle and foot
     M19.179 Post-traumatic osteoarthritis, unspecified ankle and foot
     M19.19 Post-traumatic osteoarthritis, other specified site
● **M19.2** Secondary osteoarthritis of other joints
  ● **M19.21** Secondary osteoarthritis, shoulder
     M19.211 Secondary osteoarthritis, right shoulder
     M19.212 Secondary osteoarthritis, left shoulder
     M19.219 Secondary osteoarthritis, unspecified shoulder
  ● **M19.22** Secondary osteoarthritis, elbow
     M19.221 Secondary osteoarthritis, right elbow
     M19.222 Secondary osteoarthritis, left elbow
     M19.229 Secondary osteoarthritis, unspecified elbow
  ● **M19.23** Secondary osteoarthritis, wrist
     M19.231 Secondary osteoarthritis, right wrist
     M19.232 Secondary osteoarthritis, left wrist
     M19.239 Secondary osteoarthritis, unspecified wrist
  ● **M19.24** Secondary osteoarthritis, hand
     M19.241 Secondary osteoarthritis, right hand
     M19.242 Secondary osteoarthritis, left hand
     M19.249 Secondary osteoarthritis, unspecified hand
  ● **M19.27** Secondary osteoarthritis, ankle and foot
     M19.271 Secondary osteoarthritis, right ankle and foot
     M19.272 Secondary osteoarthritis, left ankle and foot
     M19.279 Secondary osteoarthritis, unspecified ankle and foot
     M19.29 Secondary osteoarthritis, other specified site

● **M19.9** Osteoarthritis, unspecified site
   M19.90 Unspecified osteoarthritis, unspecified site
     Arthrosis NOS
     Arthritis NOS
     Osteoarthritis NOS
     Coding Clinic: 2016, Q4, P147
   M19.91 Primary osteoarthritis, unspecified site
     Primary osteoarthritis NOS
   M19.92 Post-traumatic osteoarthritis, unspecified site
     Post-traumatic osteoarthritis NOS
   M19.93 Secondary osteoarthritis, unspecified site
     Secondary osteoarthritis NOS

OTHER JOINT DISORDERS (M20-M25)

Excludes2   joints of the spine (M40-M54)

● **M20** Acquired deformities of fingers and toes
   Excludes1   acquired absence of fingers and toes (Z89.-)
     congenital absence of fingers and toes (Q71.3-, Q72.3-)
     congenital deformities and malformations of fingers and toes (Q66.-, Q68-Q70, Q74.-)
  ● **M20.0** Deformity of finger(s)
     Excludes1   clubbing of fingers (R68.3)
      palmar fascial fibromatosis [Dupuytren] (M72.0)
      trigger finger (M65.3)
   ● **M20.00** Unspecified deformity of finger(s)
     M20.001 Unspecified deformity of right finger(s)
     M20.002 Unspecified deformity of left finger(s)
     M20.009 Unspecified deformity of unspecified finger(s)
   ● **M20.01** Mallet finger
     M20.011 Mallet finger of right finger(s)
     M20.012 Mallet finger of left finger(s)
     M20.019 Mallet finger of unspecified finger(s)
   ● **M20.02** Boutonnière deformity
     M20.021 Boutonnière deformity of right finger(s)
     M20.022 Boutonnière deformity of left finger(s)
     M20.029 Boutonnière deformity of unspecified finger(s)
   ● **M20.03** Swan-neck deformity
     M20.031 Swan-neck deformity of right finger(s)
     M20.032 Swan-neck deformity of left finger(s)
     M20.039 Swan-neck deformity of unspecified finger(s)
   ● **M20.09** Other deformity of finger(s)
     M20.091 Other deformity of right finger(s)
     M20.092 Other deformity of left finger(s)
     M20.099 Other deformity of finger(s), unspecified finger(s)
  ● **M20.1** Hallux valgus (acquired)
     Excludes2   bunion (M21.6-)
     Coding Clinic: 2016, Q4, P38
     M20.10 Hallux valgus (acquired), unspecified foot
     M20.11 Hallux valgus (acquired), right foot
     M20.12 Hallux valgus (acquired), left foot
  ● **M20.2** Hallux rigidus
     M20.20 Hallux rigidus, unspecified foot
     M20.21 Hallux rigidus, right foot
     M20.22 Hallux rigidus, left foot

▶ New   ⇒ Revised   ~~deleted~~ Deleted   Excludes 1   Excludes 2   Includes   Use additional   Code first   Code also   Key words
OGCR Official Guidelines   ● Unacceptable Principal Diagnosis   X Assign placeholder X   ● Use Additional Character(s)   ▷ Manifestation Code   **Coding Clinic**

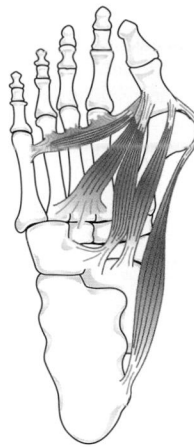

Figure 13-1   Hallux valgus.

Item 13–2 Hallux valgus is a sometimes painful structural deformity caused by an inflammation of the bursal sac at the base of the metatarsophalangeal joint (big toe). **Hallus varus** is a deviation of the great toe to the inner side of the foot or away from the next toe.

● M20.3   Hallux varus (acquired)

     M20.30   Hallux varus (acquired), unspecified foot

     M20.31   Hallux varus (acquired), right foot

     M20.32   Hallux varus (acquired), left foot

● M20.4   Other hammer toe(s) (acquired)

     M20.40   Other hammer toe(s) (acquired), unspecified foot

     M20.41   Other hammer toe(s) (acquired), right foot

     M20.42   Other hammer toe(s) (acquired), left foot

● M20.5   Other deformities of toe(s) (acquired)

    ● M20.5X   Other deformities of toe(s) (acquired)

       M20.5X1   Other deformities of toe(s) (acquired), right foot

       M20.5X2   Other deformities of toe(s) (acquired), left foot

       M20.5X9   Other deformities of toe(s) (acquired), unspecified foot

● M20.6   Acquired deformities of toe(s), unspecified

     M20.60   Acquired deformities of toe(s), unspecified, unspecified foot

     M20.61   Acquired deformities of toe(s), unspecified, right foot

     M20.62   Acquired deformities of toe(s), unspecified, left foot

● M21   Other acquired deformities of limbs

    Excludes1   acquired absence of limb (Z89.-)
              congenital absence of limbs (Q71-Q73)
              congenital deformities and malformations of limbs (Q65-Q66, Q68-Q74)

    Excludes2   acquired deformities of fingers or toes (M20.-)
              coxa plana (M91.2)

   ● M21.0   Valgus deformity, not elsewhere classified

      Excludes1   metatarsus valgus (Q66.6)
                 talipes calcaneovalgus (Q66.4-)

     M21.00   Valgus deformity, not elsewhere classified, unspecified site

    ● M21.02   Valgus deformity, not elsewhere classified, elbow
         Cubitus valgus

       M21.021   Valgus deformity, not elsewhere classified, right elbow

       M21.022   Valgus deformity, not elsewhere classified, left elbow

       M21.029   Valgus deformity, not elsewhere classified, unspecified elbow

Item 13–3 Cubitus valgus is a deformity of the elbow resulting in an increased carrying angle in which the arm extends at the side and the palm faces forward, which results in the forearm and hand extended at greater than 15 degrees.

Item 13–4 Cubitus varus is a deformity of the elbow resulting in the arm extended at the side and the palm facing forward so that the forearm and hand are held at less than 5 degrees, decreasing the carrying angle.

   ● M21.05   Valgus deformity, not elsewhere classified, hip

       M21.051   Valgus deformity, not elsewhere classified, right hip

       M21.052   Valgus deformity, not elsewhere classified, left hip

       M21.059   Valgus deformity, not elsewhere classified, unspecified hip

   ● M21.06   Valgus deformity, not elsewhere classified, knee
         Genu valgum
         Knock knee

       M21.061   Valgus deformity, not elsewhere classified, right knee

       M21.062   Valgus deformity, not elsewhere classified, left knee

       M21.069   Valgus deformity, not elsewhere classified, unspecified knee

   ● M21.07   Valgus deformity, not elsewhere classified, ankle

       M21.071   Valgus deformity, not elsewhere classified, right ankle

       M21.072   Valgus deformity, not elsewhere classified, left ankle

       M21.079   Valgus deformity, not elsewhere classified, unspecified ankle

● M21.1   Varus deformity, not elsewhere classified

    Excludes1   metatarsus varus (Q66.22-)
                tibia vara (M92.51-)

     M21.10   Varus deformity, not elsewhere classified, unspecified site

   ● M21.12   Varus deformity, not elsewhere classified, elbow
         Cubitus varus, elbow

       M21.121   Varus deformity, not elsewhere classified, right elbow

       M21.122   Varus deformity, not elsewhere classified, left elbow

       M21.129   Varus deformity, not elsewhere classified, unspecified elbow

   ● M21.15   Varus deformity, not elsewhere classified, hip

       M21.151   Varus deformity, not elsewhere classified, right hip

       M21.152   Varus deformity, not elsewhere classified, left hip

       M21.159   Varus deformity, not elsewhere classified, unspecified

   ● M21.16   Varus deformity, not elsewhere classified, knee
         Bow leg
         Genu varum

       M21.161   Varus deformity, not elsewhere classified, right knee

       M21.162   Varus deformity, not elsewhere classified, left knee

       M21.169   Varus deformity, not elsewhere classified, unspecified knee

   ● M21.17   Varus deformity, not elsewhere classified, ankle

       M21.171   Varus deformity, not elsewhere classified, right ankle

       M21.172   Varus deformity, not elsewhere classified, left ankle

       M21.179   Varus deformity, not elsewhere classified, unspecified ankle

N Newborn Age: 0   **P** Pediatric Age: 0–17   **M** Maternity DX: 9–64   **A** Adult Age: 15–124   ♀ Females Only   ♂ Males Only

🔵 Complication\Comorbidity   🔵 Major C\C   (Ex:) CC/MCC Exclusions   🔵 Hospital-Acquired Condition   🔵 Hierarchical Condition Category

1043

● M21.2 Flexion deformity
   M21.20 Flexion deformity, unspecified site
  ● M21.21 Flexion deformity, shoulder
     M21.211 Flexion deformity, right shoulder
     M21.212 Flexion deformity, left shoulder
     M21.219 Flexion deformity, unspecified shoulder
  ● M21.22 Flexion deformity, elbow
     M21.221 Flexion deformity, right elbow
     M21.222 Flexion deformity, left elbow
     M21.229 Flexion deformity, unspecified elbow
  ● M21.23 Flexion deformity, wrist
     M21.231 Flexion deformity, right wrist
     M21.232 Flexion deformity, left wrist
     M21.239 Flexion deformity, unspecified wrist
  ● M21.24 Flexion deformity, finger joints
     M21.241 Flexion deformity, right finger joints
     M21.242 Flexion deformity, left finger joints
     M21.249 Flexion deformity, unspecified finger joints
  ● M21.25 Flexion deformity, hip
     M21.251 Flexion deformity, right hip
     M21.252 Flexion deformity, left hip
     M21.259 Flexion deformity, unspecified hip
  ● M21.26 Flexion deformity, knee
     M21.261 Flexion deformity, right knee
     M21.262 Flexion deformity, left knee
     M21.269 Flexion deformity, unspecified knee
  ● M21.27 Flexion deformity, ankle and toes
     M21.271 Flexion deformity, right ankle and toes
     M21.272 Flexion deformity, left ankle and toes
     M21.279 Flexion deformity, unspecified ankle and toes
● M21.3 Wrist or foot drop (acquired)
  ● M21.33 Wrist drop (acquired)
     M21.331 Wrist drop, right wrist
     M21.332 Wrist drop, left wrist
     M21.339 Wrist drop, unspecified wrist
  ● M21.37 Foot drop (acquired)
     M21.371 Foot drop, right foot
     M21.372 Foot drop, left foot
     M21.379 Foot drop, unspecified foot
● M21.4 Flat foot [pes planus] (acquired)
    Excludes1 congenital pes planus (Q66.5-)
   M21.40 Flat foot [pes planus] (acquired), unspecified foot
   M21.41 Flat foot [pes planus] (acquired), right foot
   M21.42 Flat foot [pes planus] (acquired), left foot
● M21.5 Acquired clawhand, clubhand, clawfoot and clubfoot
    Excludes1 clubfoot, not specified as acquired (Q66.89)
  ● M21.51 Acquired clawhand
     M21.511 Acquired clawhand, right hand
     M21.512 Acquired clawhand, left hand
     M21.519 Acquired clawhand, unspecified hand
  ● M21.52 Acquired clubhand
     M21.521 Acquired clubhand, right hand
     M21.522 Acquired clubhand, left hand
     M21.529 Acquired clubhand, unspecified hand

● M21.53 Acquired clawfoot
     M21.531 Acquired clawfoot, right foot
     M21.532 Acquired clawfoot, left foot
     M21.539 Acquired clawfoot, unspecified foot
● M21.54 Acquired clubfoot
     M21.541 Acquired clubfoot, right foot
     M21.542 Acquired clubfoot, left foot
     M21.549 Acquired clubfoot, unspecified foot
● M21.6 Other acquired deformities of foot
    Excludes2 deformities of toe (acquired) (M20.1-M20.6-)
  ● M21.61 Bunion
     Coding Clinic: 2016, Q4, P38
     M21.611 Bunion of right foot
     M21.612 Bunion of left foot
     M21.619 Bunion of unspecified foot
  ● M21.62 Bunionette
     Coding Clinic: 2016, Q4, P38
     M21.621 Bunionette of right foot
     M21.622 Bunionette of left foot
     M21.629 Bunionette of unspecified foot
  ● M21.6X Other acquired deformities of foot
     M21.6X1 Other acquired deformities of right foot
     M21.6X2 Other acquired deformities of left foot
     M21.6X9 Other acquired deformities of unspecified foot
● M21.7 Unequal limb length (acquired)
   Note: The site used should correspond to the shorter limb.
   M21.70 Unequal limb length (acquired), unspecified site
  ● M21.72 Unequal limb length (acquired), humerus
     M21.721 Unequal limb length (acquired), right humerus
     M21.722 Unequal limb length (acquired), left humerus
     M21.729 Unequal limb length (acquired), unspecified humerus
  ● M21.73 Unequal limb length (acquired), ulna and radius
     M21.731 Unequal limb length (acquired), right ulna
     M21.732 Unequal limb length (acquired), left ulna
     M21.733 Unequal limb length (acquired), right radius
     M21.734 Unequal limb length (acquired), left radius
     M21.739 Unequal limb length (acquired), unspecified ulna and radius
  ● M21.75 Unequal limb length (acquired), femur
     M21.751 Unequal limb length (acquired), right femur
     M21.752 Unequal limb length (acquired), left femur
     M21.759 Unequal limb length (acquired), unspecified femur

● **M21.76** Unequal limb length (acquired), tibia and fibula

     M21.761 Unequal limb length (acquired), right tibia

     M21.762 Unequal limb length (acquired), left tibia

     M21.763 Unequal limb length (acquired), right fibula

     M21.764 Unequal limb length (acquired), left fibula

     M21.769 Unequal limb length (acquired), unspecified tibia and fibula

● **M21.8** Other specified acquired deformities of limbs

     Excludes2   coxa plana (M91.2)

     M21.80 Other specified acquired deformities of unspecified limb

●   M21.82 Other specified acquired deformities of upper arm

     M21.821 Other specified acquired deformities of right upper arm

     M21.822 Other specified acquired deformities of left upper arm

     M21.829 Other specified acquired deformities of unspecified upper arm

●   M21.83 Other specified acquired deformities of forearm

     M21.831 Other specified acquired deformities of right forearm

     M21.832 Other specified acquired deformities of left forearm

     M21.839 Other specified acquired deformities of unspecified forearm

●   M21.85 Other specified acquired deformities of thigh

     M21.851 Other specified acquired deformities of right thigh

     M21.852 Other specified acquired deformities of left thigh

     M21.859 Other specified acquired deformities of unspecified thigh

●   M21.86 Other specified acquired deformities of lower leg

     M21.861 Other specified acquired deformities of right lower leg

     M21.862 Other specified acquired deformities of left lower leg

     M21.869 Other specified acquired deformities of unspecified lower leg

● **M21.9** Unspecified acquired deformity of limb and hand

     M21.90 Unspecified acquired deformity of unspecified limb

●   M21.92 Unspecified acquired deformity of upper arm

     M21.921 Unspecified acquired deformity of right upper arm

     M21.922 Unspecified acquired deformity of left upper arm

     M21.929 Unspecified acquired deformity of unspecified upper arm

●   M21.93 Unspecified acquired deformity of forearm

     M21.931 Unspecified acquired deformity of right forearm

     M21.932 Unspecified acquired deformity of left forearm

     M21.939 Unspecified acquired deformity of unspecified forearm

●   M21.94 Unspecified acquired deformity of hand

     M21.941 Unspecified acquired deformity of hand, right hand

     M21.942 Unspecified acquired deformity of hand, left hand

     M21.949 Unspecified acquired deformity of hand, unspecified hand

●   M21.95 Unspecified acquired deformity of thigh

     M21.951 Unspecified acquired deformity of right thigh

     M21.952 Unspecified acquired deformity of left thigh

     M21.959 Unspecified acquired deformity of unspecified thigh

●   M21.96 Unspecified acquired deformity of lower leg

     M21.961 Unspecified acquired deformity of right lower leg

     M21.962 Unspecified acquired deformity of left lower leg

     M21.969 Unspecified acquired deformity of unspecified lower leg

● **M22** Disorder of patella

     Excludes2   traumatic dislocation of patella (S83.0-)

●   **M22.0** Recurrent dislocation of patella

     M22.00 Recurrent dislocation of patella, unspecified knee

     M22.01 Recurrent dislocation of patella, right knee

     M22.02 Recurrent dislocation of patella, left knee

●   **M22.1** Recurrent subluxation of patella

     Incomplete dislocation of patella

     M22.10 Recurrent subluxation of patella, unspecified knee

     M22.11 Recurrent subluxation of patella, right knee

     M22.12 Recurrent subluxation of patella, left knee

●   **M22.2** Patellofemoral disorders

●   M22.2X Patellofemoral disorders

     M22.2X1 Patellofemoral disorders, right knee

     M22.2X2 Patellofemoral disorders, left knee

     M22.2X9 Patellofemoral disorders, unspecified knee

●   **M22.3** Other derangements of patella

●   M22.3X Other derangements of patella

     M22.3X1 Other derangements of patella, right knee

     M22.3X2 Other derangements of patella, left knee

     M22.3X9 Other derangements of patella, unspecified knee

●   **M22.4** Chondromalacia patellae

     M22.40 Chondromalacia patellae, unspecified knee

     M22.41 Chondromalacia patellae, right knee

     M22.42 Chondromalacia patellae, left knee

●   **M22.8** Other disorders of patella

●   M22.8X Other disorders of patella

     M22.8X1 Other disorders of patella, right knee

     M22.8X2 Other disorders of patella, left knee

     M22.8X9 Other disorders of patella, unspecified knee

●   **M22.9** Unspecified disorder of patella

     M22.90 Unspecified disorder of patella, unspecified knee

     M22.91 Unspecified disorder of patella, right knee

     M22.92 Unspecified disorder of patella, left knee

CHAPTER 13 (M00-M99)

N Newborn Age: 0   **P** Pediatric Age: 0–17   **M** Maternity DX: 9–64   **A** Adult Age: 15–124   ♀ Females Only   ♂ Males Only

Complication\Comorbidity   Major C\C   (Ex) CC/MCC Exclusions   Hospital-Acquired Condition   Hierarchical Condition Category

1045

● **M23**   **Internal derangement of knee**

     Excludes1   ankylosis (M24.66)
                 deformity of knee (M21.-)
                 osteochondritis dissecans (M93.2)

     Excludes2   current injury - see injury of knee and lower leg
                 (S80-S89)
                 recurrent dislocation or subluxation of joints
                 (M24.4)
                 recurrent dislocation or subluxation of patella
                 (M22.0-M22.1)

     Coding Clinic: 2019, Q2, P26

● **M23.0**   **Cystic meniscus**

   ● **M23.00**   Cystic meniscus, unspecified meniscus
          Cystic meniscus, unspecified lateral meniscus
          Cystic meniscus, unspecified medial meniscus

     M23.000   Cystic meniscus, unspecified lateral meniscus, right knee
     M23.001   Cystic meniscus, unspecified lateral meniscus, left knee
     M23.002   Cystic meniscus, unspecified lateral meniscus, unspecified knee
     M23.003   Cystic meniscus, unspecified medial meniscus, right knee
     M23.004   Cystic meniscus, unspecified medial meniscus, left knee
     M23.005   Cystic meniscus, unspecified medial meniscus, unspecified knee
     M23.006   Cystic meniscus, unspecified meniscus, right knee
     M23.007   Cystic meniscus, unspecified meniscus, left knee
     M23.009   Cystic meniscus, unspecified meniscus, unspecified knee

   ● **M23.01**   Cystic meniscus, anterior horn of medial meniscus
     M23.011   Cystic meniscus, anterior horn of medial meniscus, right knee
     M23.012   Cystic meniscus, anterior horn of medial meniscus, left knee
     M23.019   Cystic meniscus, anterior horn of medial meniscus, unspecified knee

   ● **M23.02**   Cystic meniscus, posterior horn of medial meniscus
     M23.021   Cystic meniscus, posterior horn of medial meniscus, right knee
     M23.022   Cystic meniscus, posterior horn of medial meniscus, left knee
     M23.029   Cystic meniscus, posterior horn of medial meniscus, unspecified knee

   ● **M23.03**   Cystic meniscus, other medial meniscus
     M23.031   Cystic meniscus, other medial meniscus, right knee
     M23.032   Cystic meniscus, other medial meniscus, left knee
     M23.039   Cystic meniscus, other medial meniscus, unspecified knee

   ● **M23.04**   Cystic meniscus, anterior horn of lateral meniscus
     M23.041   Cystic meniscus, anterior horn of lateral meniscus, right knee
     M23.042   Cystic meniscus, anterior horn of lateral meniscus, left knee
     M23.049   Cystic meniscus, anterior horn of lateral meniscus, unspecified knee

   ● **M23.05**   Cystic meniscus, posterior horn of lateral meniscus
     M23.051   Cystic meniscus, posterior horn of lateral meniscus, right knee
     M23.052   Cystic meniscus, posterior horn of lateral meniscus, left knee
     M23.059   Cystic meniscus, posterior horn of lateral meniscus, unspecified knee

   ● **M23.06**   Cystic meniscus, other lateral meniscus
     M23.061   Cystic meniscus, other lateral meniscus, right knee
     M23.062   Cystic meniscus, other lateral meniscus, left knee
     M23.069   Cystic meniscus, other lateral meniscus, unspecified knee

★ **(See Plate 34 of the Anatomy Illustrations.)**

   ● **M23.2**   Derangement of meniscus due to old tear or injury
        Old bucket-handle tear

   ● **M23.20**   Derangement of unspecified meniscus due to old tear or injury
        Derangement of unspecified lateral meniscus due to old tear or injury
        Derangement of unspecified medial meniscus due to old tear or injury

     M23.200   Derangement of unspecified lateral meniscus due to old tear or injury, right knee
     M23.201   Derangement of unspecified lateral meniscus due to old tear or injury, left knee
     M23.202   Derangement of unspecified lateral meniscus due to old tear or injury, unspecified knee
     M23.203   Derangement of unspecified medial meniscus due to old tear or injury, right knee
     M23.204   Derangement of unspecified medial meniscus due to old tear or injury, left knee
     M23.205   Derangement of unspecified medial meniscus due to old tear or injury, unspecified knee
     M23.206   Derangement of unspecified meniscus due to old tear or injury, right knee
     M23.207   Derangement of unspecified meniscus due to old tear or injury, left knee
     M23.209   Derangement of unspecified meniscus due to old tear or injury, unspecified knee

   ● **M23.21**   Derangement of anterior horn of medial meniscus due to old tear or injury
     M23.211   Derangement of anterior horn of medial meniscus due to old tear or injury, right knee
     M23.212   Derangement of anterior horn of medial meniscus due to old tear or injury, left knee
     M23.219   Derangement of anterior horn of medial meniscus due to old tear or injury, unspecified knee

   ● **M23.22**   Derangement of posterior horn of medial meniscus due to old tear or injury
     M23.221   Derangement of posterior horn of medial meniscus due to old tear or injury, right knee
     M23.222   Derangement of posterior horn of medial meniscus due to old tear or injury, left knee
     M23.229   Derangement of posterior horn of medial meniscus due to old tear or injury, unspecified knee

▶ New   ⇒ Revised   ~~deleted~~ Deleted   Excludes 1   Excludes 2   Includes   Use additional   Code first   Code also   Key words

OGCR Official Guidelines   ● Unacceptable Principal Diagnosis   X Assign placeholder X   ● Use Additional Character(s)   ▶ Manifestation Code   Coding Clinic

● **M23.23** Derangement of other medial meniscus due to old tear or injury

    M23.231 Derangement of other medial meniscus due to old tear or injury, right knee

    M23.232 Derangement of other medial meniscus due to old tear or injury, left knee

    M23.239 Derangement of other medial meniscus due to old tear or injury, unspecified knee

● **M23.24** Derangement of anterior horn of lateral meniscus due to old tear or injury

    M23.241 Derangement of anterior horn of lateral meniscus due to old tear or injury, right knee

    M23.242 Derangement of anterior horn of lateral meniscus due to old tear or injury, left knee

    M23.249 Derangement of anterior horn of lateral meniscus due to old tear or injury, unspecified knee

● **M23.25** Derangement of posterior horn of lateral meniscus due to old tear or injury

    M23.251 Derangement of posterior horn of lateral meniscus due to old tear or injury, right knee

    M23.252 Derangement of posterior horn of lateral meniscus due to old tear or injury, left knee

    M23.259 Derangement of posterior horn of lateral meniscus due to old tear or injury, unspecified knee

● **M23.26** Derangement of other lateral meniscus due to old tear or injury

    M23.261 Derangement of other lateral meniscus due to old tear or injury, right knee

    M23.262 Derangement of other lateral meniscus due to old tear or injury, left knee

    M23.269 Derangement of other lateral meniscus due to old tear or injury, unspecified knee

● **M23.3** Other meniscus derangements
Degenerate meniscus
Detached meniscus
Retained meniscus

● **M23.30** Other meniscus derangements, unspecified meniscus
Other meniscus derangements, unspecified lateral meniscus
Other meniscus derangements, unspecified medial meniscus

    M23.300 Other meniscus derangements, unspecified lateral meniscus, right knee

    M23.301 Other meniscus derangements, unspecified lateral meniscus, left knee

    M23.302 Other meniscus derangements, unspecified lateral meniscus, unspecified knee

    M23.303 Other meniscus derangements, unspecified medial meniscus, right knee

    M23.304 Other meniscus derangements, unspecified medial meniscus, left knee

    M23.305 Other meniscus derangements, unspecified medial meniscus, unspecified knee

    M23.306 Other meniscus derangements, unspecified meniscus, right knee

    M23.307 Other meniscus derangements, unspecified meniscus, left knee

    M23.309 Other meniscus derangements, unspecified meniscus, unspecified knee

● **M23.31** Other meniscus derangements, anterior horn of medial meniscus

    M23.311 Other meniscus derangements, anterior horn of medial meniscus, right knee

    M23.312 Other meniscus derangements, anterior horn of medial meniscus, left knee

    M23.319 Other meniscus derangements, anterior horn of medial meniscus, unspecified knee

● **M23.32** Other meniscus derangements, posterior horn of medial meniscus

    M23.321 Other meniscus derangements, posterior horn of medial meniscus, right knee

    M23.322 Other meniscus derangements, posterior horn of medial meniscus, left knee

    M23.329 Other meniscus derangements, posterior horn of medial meniscus, unspecified knee

● **M23.33** Other meniscus derangements, other medial meniscus

    M23.331 Other meniscus derangements, other medial meniscus, right knee

    M23.332 Other meniscus derangements, other medial meniscus, left knee

    M23.339 Other meniscus derangements, other medial meniscus, unspecified knee

● **M23.34** Other meniscus derangements, anterior horn of lateral meniscus

    M23.341 Other meniscus derangements, anterior horn of lateral meniscus, right knee

    M23.342 Other meniscus derangements, anterior horn of lateral meniscus, left knee

    M23.349 Other meniscus derangements, anterior horn of lateral meniscus, unspecified knee

● **M23.35** Other meniscus derangements, posterior horn of lateral meniscus

    M23.351 Other meniscus derangements, posterior horn of lateral meniscus, right knee

    M23.352 Other meniscus derangements, posterior horn of lateral meniscus, left knee

    M23.359 Other meniscus derangements, posterior horn of lateral meniscus, unspecified knee

● **M23.36** Other meniscus derangements, other lateral meniscus

    M23.361 Other meniscus derangements, other lateral meniscus, right knee

    M23.362 Other meniscus derangements, other lateral meniscus, left knee

    M23.369 Other meniscus derangements, other lateral meniscus, unspecified knee

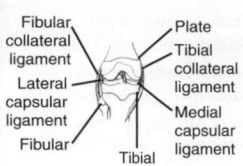

Fibular collateral ligament
Lateral capsular ligament
Fibular
Tibial
Plate
Tibial collateral ligament
Medial capsular ligament

Figure 13-2 Collateral and cruciate ligament of knee. (From DeLee: DeLee and Drez's Orthopaedic Sports Medicine, ed 3, Saunders, 2009)

● **M23.4　Loose body in knee**
　　M23.40　Loose body in knee, unspecified knee
　　M23.41　Loose body in knee, right knee
　　M23.42　Loose body in knee, left knee
● **M23.5　Chronic instability of knee**
　　M23.50　Chronic instability of knee, unspecified knee
　　M23.51　Chronic instability of knee, right knee
　　M23.52　Chronic instability of knee, left knee
● **M23.6　Other spontaneous disruption of ligament(s) of knee**
　● M23.60　Other spontaneous disruption of unspecified ligament of knee
　　　M23.601　Other spontaneous disruption of unspecified ligament of right knee
　　　M23.602　Other spontaneous disruption of unspecified ligament of left knee
　　　M23.609　Other spontaneous disruption of unspecified ligament of unspecified knee
　● M23.61　Other spontaneous disruption of anterior cruciate ligament of knee
　　　M23.611　Other spontaneous disruption of anterior cruciate ligament of right knee
　　　M23.612　Other spontaneous disruption of anterior cruciate ligament of left knee
　　　M23.619　Other spontaneous disruption of anterior cruciate ligament of unspecified knee
　● M23.62　Other spontaneous disruption of posterior cruciate ligament of knee
　　　M23.621　Other spontaneous disruption of posterior cruciate ligament of right knee
　　　M23.622　Other spontaneous disruption of posterior cruciate ligament of left knee
　　　M23.629　Other spontaneous disruption of posterior cruciate ligament of unspecified knee
　● M23.63　Other spontaneous disruption of medial collateral ligament of knee
　　　M23.631　Other spontaneous disruption of medial collateral ligament of right knee
　　　M23.632　Other spontaneous disruption of medial collateral ligament of left knee
　　　M23.639　Other spontaneous disruption of medial collateral ligament of unspecified knee
　● M23.64　Other spontaneous disruption of lateral collateral ligament of knee
　　　M23.641　Other spontaneous disruption of lateral collateral ligament of right knee
　　　M23.642　Other spontaneous disruption of lateral collateral ligament of left knee
　　　M23.649　Other spontaneous disruption of lateral collateral ligament of unspecified knee

● M23.67　Other spontaneous disruption of capsular ligament of knee
　　M23.671　Other spontaneous disruption of capsular ligament of right knee
　　M23.672　Other spontaneous disruption of capsular ligament of left knee
　　M23.679　Other spontaneous disruption of capsular ligament of unspecified knee
● **M23.8　Other internal derangements of knee**
　　Laxity of ligament of knee
　　Snapping knee
　● M23.8X　Other internal derangements of knee
　　　M23.8X1　Other internal derangements of right knee
　　　M23.8X2　Other internal derangements of left knee
　　　M23.8X9　Other internal derangements of unspecified knee
● **M23.9　Unspecified internal derangement of knee**
　　M23.90　Unspecified internal derangement of unspecified knee
　　M23.91　Unspecified internal derangement of right knee
　　M23.92　Unspecified internal derangement of left knee

● **M24　Other specific joint derangements**
　　Excludes1　current injury - see injury of joint by body region
　　Excludes2　ganglion (M67.4)
　　　　　　　snapping knee (M23.8-)
　　　　　　　temporomandibular joint disorders (M26.6-)
● **M24.0　Loose body in joint**
　　Excludes2　loose body in knee (M23.4)
　　M24.00　Loose body in unspecified joint
　● M24.01　Loose body in shoulder
　　　M24.011　Loose body in right shoulder
　　　M24.012　Loose body in left shoulder
　　　M24.019　Loose body in unspecified shoulder
　● M24.02　Loose body in elbow
　　　M24.021　Loose body in right elbow
　　　M24.022　Loose body in left elbow
　　　M24.029　Loose body in unspecified elbow
　● M24.03　Loose body in wrist
　　　M24.031　Loose body in right wrist
　　　M24.032　Loose body in left wrist
　　　M24.039　Loose body in unspecified wrist
　● M24.04　Loose body in finger joints
　　　M24.041　Loose body in right finger joint(s)
　　　M24.042　Loose body in left finger joint(s)
　　　M24.049　Loose body in unspecified finger joint(s)
　● M24.05　Loose body in hip
　　　M24.051　Loose body in right hip
　　　M24.052　Loose body in left hip
　　　M24.059　Loose body in unspecified hip
　● M24.07　Loose body in ankle and toe joints
　　　M24.071　Loose body in right ankle
　　　M24.072　Loose body in left ankle
　　　M24.073　Loose body in unspecified ankle
　　　M24.074　Loose body in right toe joint(s)
　　　M24.075　Loose body in left toe joint(s)
　　　M24.076　Loose body in unspecified toe joints
　　M24.08　Loose body, other site

▶ New　⇒ Revised　deleted Deleted　Excludes 1　Excludes 2　Includes　Use additional　Code first　Code also　Key words
OGCR Official Guidelines　● Unacceptable Principal Diagnosis　X Assign placeholder X　● Use Additional Character(s)　▶ Manifestation Code　Coding Clinic

● **M24.1** Other articular cartilage disorders

     Excludes2   chondrocalcinosis (M11.1, M11.2-)
                        internal derangement of knee (M23.-)
                        metastatic calcification (E83.5)
                        ochronosis (E70.2)

     M24.10   Other articular cartilage disorders, unspecified site

● M24.11   Other articular cartilage disorders, shoulder

     M24.111   Other articular cartilage disorders, right shoulder

     M24.112   Other articular cartilage disorders, left shoulder

     M24.119   Other articular cartilage disorders, unspecified shoulder

● M24.12   Other articular cartilage disorders, elbow

     M24.121   Other articular cartilage disorders, right elbow

     M24.122   Other articular cartilage disorders, left elbow

     M24.129   Other articular cartilage disorders, unspecified elbow

● M24.13   Other articular cartilage disorders, wrist

     M24.131   Other articular cartilage disorders, right wrist

     M24.132   Other articular cartilage disorders, left wrist

     M24.139   Other articular cartilage disorders, unspecified wrist

● M24.14   Other articular cartilage disorders, hand

     M24.141   Other articular cartilage disorders, right hand

     M24.142   Other articular cartilage disorders, left hand

     M24.149   Other articular cartilage disorders, unspecified hand

● M24.15   Other articular cartilage disorders, hip

     M24.151   Other articular cartilage disorders, right hip

     M24.152   Other articular cartilage disorders, left hip

     M24.159   Other articular cartilage disorders, unspecified hip

● M24.17   Other articular cartilage disorders, ankle and foot

     M24.171   Other articular cartilage disorders, right ankle

     M24.172   Other articular cartilage disorders, left ankle

     M24.173   Other articular cartilage disorders, unspecified ankle

     M24.174   Other articular cartilage disorders, right foot

     M24.175   Other articular cartilage disorders, left foot

     M24.176   Other articular cartilage disorders, unspecified foot

     M24.19   Other articular cartilage disorders, other specified site

● M24.2   Disorder of ligament

     Instability secondary to old ligament injury
     Ligamentous laxity NOS

     Excludes1   familial ligamentous laxity (M35.7)

     Excludes2   internal derangement of knee (M23.5-M23.8X9)

     M24.20   Disorder of ligament, unspecified site

● M24.21   Disorder of ligament, shoulder

     M24.211   Disorder of ligament, right shoulder

     M24.212   Disorder of ligament, left shoulder

     M24.219   Disorder of ligament, unspecified shoulder

● M24.22   Disorder of ligament, elbow

     M24.221   Disorder of ligament, right elbow

     M24.222   Disorder of ligament, left elbow

     M24.229   Disorder of ligament, unspecified elbow

● M24.23   Disorder of ligament, wrist

     M24.231   Disorder of ligament, right wrist

     M24.232   Disorder of ligament, left wrist

     M24.239   Disorder of ligament, unspecified wrist

● M24.24   Disorder of ligament, hand

     M24.241   Disorder of ligament, right hand

     M24.242   Disorder of ligament, left hand

     M24.249   Disorder of ligament, unspecified hand

● M24.25   Disorder of ligament, hip

     M24.251   Disorder of ligament, right hip

     M24.252   Disorder of ligament, left hip

     M24.259   Disorder of ligament, unspecified hip

● M24.27   Disorder of ligament, ankle and foot

     M24.271   Disorder of ligament, right ankle

     M24.272   Disorder of ligament, left ankle

     M24.273   Disorder of ligament, unspecified ankle

     M24.274   Disorder of ligament, right foot

     M24.275   Disorder of ligament, left foot

     M24.276   Disorder of ligament, unspecified foot

     M24.28   Disorder of ligament, vertebrae

     M24.29   Disorder of ligament, other specified site

● M24.3   Pathological dislocation of joint, not elsewhere classified

     Excludes1   congenital dislocation or displacement of joint - see congenital malformations and deformations of the musculoskeletal system (Q65-Q79)
                      current injury - see injury of joints and ligaments by body region
                      recurrent dislocation of joint (M24.4-)

     M24.30   Pathological dislocation of unspecified joint, not elsewhere classified

● M24.31   Pathological dislocation of shoulder, not elsewhere classified

     M24.311   Pathological dislocation of right shoulder, not elsewhere classified

     M24.312   Pathological dislocation of left shoulder, not elsewhere classified

     M24.319   Pathological dislocation of unspecified shoulder, not elsewhere classified

● M24.32   Pathological dislocation of elbow, not elsewhere classified

     M24.321   Pathological dislocation of right elbow, not elsewhere classified

     M24.322   Pathological dislocation of left elbow, not elsewhere classified

     M24.329   Pathological dislocation of unspecified elbow, not elsewhere classified

● M24.33   Pathological dislocation of wrist, not elsewhere classified

     M24.331   Pathological dislocation of right wrist, not elsewhere classified

     M24.332   Pathological dislocation of left wrist, not elsewhere classified

     M24.339   Pathological dislocation of unspecified wrist, not elsewhere classified

CHAPTER 13 (M00-M99)

N   Newborn Age: 0   P   Pediatric Age: 0–17   M   Maternity DX: 9–64   A   Adult Age: 15–124   ♀   Females Only   ♂   Males Only

🅒 Complication\Comorbidity   🅒 Major C\C   (Ex) CC/MCC Exclusions   🅒 Hospital-Acquired Condition   🅒 Hierarchical Condition Category

1049

CHAPTER 13 (M00-M99)

● M24.34   Pathological dislocation of hand, not elsewhere classified
     M24.341   Pathological dislocation of right hand, not elsewhere classified
     M24.342   Pathological dislocation of left hand, not elsewhere classified
     M24.349   Pathological dislocation of unspecified hand, not elsewhere classified

● M24.35   Pathological dislocation of hip, not elsewhere classified
     M24.351   Pathological dislocation of right hip, not elsewhere classified
     M24.352   Pathological dislocation of left hip, not elsewhere classified
     M24.359   Pathological dislocation of unspecified hip, not elsewhere classified

● M24.36   Pathological dislocation of knee, not elsewhere classified
     M24.361   Pathological dislocation of right knee, not elsewhere classified
     M24.362   Pathological dislocation of left knee, not elsewhere classified
     M24.369   Pathological dislocation of unspecified knee, not elsewhere classified

● M24.37   Pathological dislocation of ankle and foot, not elsewhere classified
     M24.371   Pathological dislocation of right ankle, not elsewhere classified
     M24.372   Pathological dislocation of left ankle, not elsewhere classified
     M24.373   Pathological dislocation of unspecified ankle, not elsewhere classified
     M24.374   Pathological dislocation of right foot, not elsewhere classified
     M24.375   Pathological dislocation of left foot, not elsewhere classified
     M24.376   Pathological dislocation of unspecified foot, not elsewhere classified

   M24.39   Pathological dislocation of other specified joint, not elsewhere classified

● M24.4   Recurrent dislocation of joint
     Recurrent subluxation of joint
     Excludes2   recurrent dislocation of patella (M22.0-M22.1)
               recurrent vertebral dislocation (M43.3-, M43.4, M43.5-)

   M24.40   Recurrent dislocation, unspecified joint

● M24.41   Recurrent dislocation, shoulder
     M24.411   Recurrent dislocation, right shoulder
     M24.412   Recurrent dislocation, left shoulder
     M24.419   Recurrent dislocation, unspecified shoulder

● M24.42   Recurrent dislocation, elbow
     M24.421   Recurrent dislocation, right elbow
     M24.422   Recurrent dislocation, left elbow
     M24.429   Recurrent dislocation, unspecified elbow

● M24.43   Recurrent dislocation, wrist
     M24.431   Recurrent dislocation, right wrist
     M24.432   Recurrent dislocation, left wrist
     M24.439   Recurrent dislocation, unspecified wrist

● M24.44   Recurrent dislocation, hand and finger(s)
     M24.441   Recurrent dislocation, right hand
     M24.442   Recurrent dislocation, left hand
     M24.443   Recurrent dislocation, unspecified hand
     M24.444   Recurrent dislocation, right finger
     M24.445   Recurrent dislocation, left finger
     M24.446   Recurrent dislocation, unspecified finger

● M24.45   Recurrent dislocation, hip
     M24.451   Recurrent dislocation, right hip
     M24.452   Recurrent dislocation, left hip
     M24.459   Recurrent dislocation, unspecified hip

● M24.46   Recurrent dislocation, knee
     M24.461   Recurrent dislocation, right knee
     M24.462   Recurrent dislocation, left knee
     M24.469   Recurrent dislocation, unspecified knee

● M24.47   Recurrent dislocation, ankle, foot and toes
     M24.471   Recurrent dislocation, right ankle
     M24.472   Recurrent dislocation, left ankle
     M24.473   Recurrent dislocation, unspecified ankle
     M24.474   Recurrent dislocation, right foot
     M24.475   Recurrent dislocation, left foot
     M24.476   Recurrent dislocation, unspecified foot
     M24.477   Recurrent dislocation, right toe(s)
     M24.478   Recurrent dislocation, left toe(s)
     M24.479   Recurrent dislocation, unspecified toe(s)

   M24.49   Recurrent dislocation, other specified joint

● M24.5   Contracture of joint
     Excludes1   contracture of muscle without contracture of joint (M62.4-)
               contracture of tendon (sheath) without contracture of joint (M62.4-)
               Dupuytren's contracture (M72.0)
     Excludes2   acquired deformities of limbs (M20-M21)

   M24.50   Contracture, unspecified joint

● M24.51   Contracture, shoulder
     M24.511   Contracture, right shoulder
     M24.512   Contracture, left shoulder
     M24.519   Contracture, unspecified shoulder

● M24.52   Contracture, elbow
     M24.521   Contracture, right elbow
     M24.522   Contracture, left elbow
     M24.529   Contracture, unspecified elbow

● M24.53   Contracture, wrist
     M24.531   Contracture, right wrist
     M24.532   Contracture, left wrist
     M24.539   Contracture, unspecified wrist

● M24.54   Contracture, hand
     M24.541   Contracture, right hand
     M24.542   Contracture, left hand
     M24.549   Contracture, unspecified hand

● M24.55   Contracture, hip
     M24.551   Contracture, right hip
          Coding Clinic: 2016, Q2, P6
     M24.552   Contracture, left hip
          Coding Clinic: 2016, Q2, P6
     M24.559   Contracture, unspecified hip

▶ New   ⇒ Revised   ~~deleted~~ Deleted   Excludes 1   Excludes 2   Includes   Use additional   Code first   Code also   Key words
OGCR Official Guidelines   ● Unacceptable Principal Diagnosis   X Assign placeholder X   ● Use Additional Character(s)   ▶ Manifestation Code   **Coding Clinic**

Item 13–5 Ankylosis or arthrokleisis is a consolidation of a joint due to disease, injury, or surgical procedure. Spondylosis is the degeneration of the vertebral processes and formation of osteophytes and commonly occurs with age. **Spondylitis** or ankylosing spondylitis is a type of arthritis that affects the spine or backbone, causing back pain and stiffness.

● M24.56   Contracture, knee

     M24.561   Contracture, right knee
             Coding Clinic: 2016, Q2, P6

     M24.562   Contracture, left knee
             Coding Clinic: 2016, Q2, P6

     M24.569   Contracture, unspecified knee

● M24.57   Contracture, ankle and foot

     M24.571   Contracture, right ankle

     M24.572   Contracture, left ankle

     M24.573   Contracture, unspecified ankle

     M24.574   Contracture, right foot

     M24.575   Contracture, left foot

     M24.576   Contracture, unspecified foot

   M24.59   Contracture, other specified joint

● M24.6   Ankylosis of joint

     Excludes1   stiffness of joint without ankylosis (M25.6-)

     Excludes2   spine (M43.2-)

   M24.60   Ankylosis, unspecified joint

● M24.61   Ankylosis, shoulder

     M24.611   Ankylosis, right shoulder

     M24.612   Ankylosis, left shoulder

     M24.619   Ankylosis, unspecified shoulder

● M24.62   Ankylosis, elbow

     M24.621   Ankylosis, right elbow

     M24.622   Ankylosis, left elbow

     M24.629   Ankylosis, unspecified elbow

● M24.63   Ankylosis, wrist

     M24.631   Ankylosis, right wrist

     M24.632   Ankylosis, left wrist

     M24.639   Ankylosis, unspecified wrist

● M24.64   Ankylosis, hand

     M24.641   Ankylosis, right hand

     M24.642   Ankylosis, left hand

     M24.649   Ankylosis, unspecified hand

● M24.65   Ankylosis, hip

     M24.651   Ankylosis, right hip

     M24.652   Ankylosis, left hip

     M24.659   Ankylosis, unspecified hip

● M24.66   Ankylosis, knee

     M24.661   Ankylosis, right knee

     M24.662   Ankylosis, left knee

     M24.669   Ankylosis, unspecified knee

● M24.67   Ankylosis, ankle and foot

     M24.671   Ankylosis, right ankle

     M24.672   Ankylosis, left ankle

     M24.673   Ankylosis, unspecified ankle

     M24.674   Ankylosis, right foot

     M24.675   Ankylosis, left foot

     M24.676   Ankylosis, unspecified foot

   M24.69   Ankylosis, other specified joint

  M24.7   Protrusio acetabuli

● M24.8   Other specific joint derangements, not elsewhere classified

     Excludes2   iliotibial band syndrome (M76.3)

   M24.80   Other specific joint derangements of unspecified joint, not elsewhere classified

● M24.81   Other specific joint derangements of shoulder, not elsewhere classified

     M24.811   Other specific joint derangements of right shoulder, not elsewhere classified

     M24.812   Other specific joint derangements of left shoulder, not elsewhere classified

     M24.819   Other specific joint derangements of unspecified shoulder, not elsewhere classified

● M24.82   Other specific joint derangements of elbow, not elsewhere classified

     M24.821   Other specific joint derangements of right elbow, not elsewhere classified

     M24.822   Other specific joint derangements of left elbow, not elsewhere classified

     M24.829   Other specific joint derangements of unspecified elbow, not elsewhere classified

● M24.83   Other specific joint derangements of wrist, not elsewhere classified

     M24.831   Other specific joint derangements of right wrist, not elsewhere classified

     M24.832   Other specific joint derangements of left wrist, not elsewhere classified

     M24.839   Other specific joint derangements of unspecified wrist, not elsewhere classified

● M24.84   Other specific joint derangements of hand, not elsewhere classified

     M24.841   Other specific joint derangements of right hand, not elsewhere classified

     M24.842   Other specific joint derangements of left hand, not elsewhere classified

     M24.849   Other specific joint derangements of unspecified hand, not elsewhere classified

● M24.85   Other specific joint derangements of hip, not elsewhere classified
        Irritable hip

     M24.851   Other specific joint derangements of right hip, not elsewhere classified

     M24.852   Other specific joint derangements of left hip, not elsewhere classified

     M24.859   Other specific joint derangements of unspecified hip, not elsewhere classified

● M24.87   Other specific joint derangements of ankle and foot, not elsewhere classified

     M24.871   Other specific joint derangements of right ankle, not elsewhere classified

     M24.872   Other specific joint derangements of left ankle, not elsewhere classified

     M24.873   Other specific joint derangements of unspecified ankle, not elsewhere classified

     M24.874   Other specific joint derangements of right foot, not elsewhere classified

     M24.875   Other specific joint derangements left foot, not elsewhere classified

     M24.876   Other specific joint derangements of unspecified foot, not elsewhere classified

   M24.89   Other specific joint derangement of other specified joint, not elsewhere classified

  M24.9   Joint derangement, unspecified

CHAPTER 13 (M00-M99)

N Newborn Age: 0   **P** Pediatric Age: 0–17   **M** Maternity DX: 9–64   **A** Adult Age: 15–124   ♀ Females Only   ♂ Males Only

 Complication\Comorbidity   Major C\C   (Ex) CC/MCC Exclusions   Hospital-Acquired Condition   Hierarchical Condition Category   **1051**

● M25   **Other joint disorder, not elsewhere classified**

     Excludes2   abnormality of gait and mobility (R26.-)
                      acquired deformities of limb (M20-M21)
                      calcification of bursa (M71.4-)
                      calcification of shoulder (joint) (M75.3)
                      calcification of tendon (M65.2-)
                      difficulty in walking (R26.2)
                      temporomandibular joint disorder (M26.6-)

● M25.0   **Hemarthrosis**

     Excludes1   current injury - see injury of joint by body region
                      hemophilic arthropathy (M36.2)

     M25.00   Hemarthrosis, unspecified joint   ⬯
         Ⓔⓧ See PDX Collection 868

     ● M25.01   Hemarthrosis, shoulder
         Ⓔⓧ For category M25.01 CC codes: See PDX Collection 869
         M25.011   Hemarthrosis, right shoulder ⬯
         M25.012   Hemarthrosis, left shoulder ⬯
         M25.019   Hemarthrosis, unspecified shoulder ⬯

     ● M25.02   Hemarthrosis, elbow
         Ⓔⓧ For category M25.02 CC codes: See PDX Collection 870
         M25.021   Hemarthrosis, right elbow ⬯
         M25.022   Hemarthrosis, left elbow ⬯
         M25.029   Hemarthrosis, unspecified elbow ⬯

     ● M25.03   Hemarthrosis, wrist
         Ⓔⓧ For category M25.03 CC codes: See PDX Collection 871
         M25.031   Hemarthrosis, right wrist ⬯
         M25.032   Hemarthrosis, left wrist ⬯
         M25.039   Hemarthrosis, unspecified wrist ⬯

     ● M25.04   Hemarthrosis, hand
         Ⓔⓧ For category M25.04 CC codes: See PDX Collection 872
         M25.041   Hemarthrosis, right hand ⬯
         M25.042   Hemarthrosis, left hand ⬯
         M25.049   Hemarthrosis, unspecified hand ⬯

     ● M25.05   Hemarthrosis, hip
         Ⓔⓧ For category M25.05 CC codes: See PDX Collection 868
         M25.051   Hemarthrosis, right hip ⬯
         M25.052   Hemarthrosis, left hip ⬯
         M25.059   Hemarthrosis, unspecified hip ⬯

     ● M25.06   Hemarthrosis, knee
         Ⓔⓧ For category M25.06 CC codes: See PDX Collection 873
         M25.061   Hemarthrosis, right knee ⬯
         M25.062   Hemarthrosis, left knee ⬯
         M25.069   Hemarthrosis, unspecified knee ⬯

     ● M25.07   Hemarthrosis, ankle and foot
         Ⓔⓧ For category M25.07 CC codes: See PDX Collection 873
         M25.071   Hemarthrosis, right ankle ⬯
         M25.072   Hemarthrosis, left ankle ⬯
         M25.073   Hemarthrosis, unspecified ankle ⬯
         M25.074   Hemarthrosis, right foot ⬯
         M25.075   Hemarthrosis, left foot ⬯
         M25.076   Hemarthrosis, unspecified foot ⬯

     M25.08   Hemarthrosis, other specified site ⬯
         Hemarthrosis, vertebrae
         Ⓔⓧ See PDX Collection 868

● M25.1   **Fistula of joint**

     M25.10   Fistula, unspecified joint

     ● M25.11   Fistula, shoulder
         M25.111   Fistula, right shoulder
         M25.112   Fistula, left shoulder
         M25.119   Fistula, unspecified shoulder

     ● M25.12   Fistula, elbow
         M25.121   Fistula, right elbow
         M25.122   Fistula, left elbow
         M25.129   Fistula, unspecified elbow

     ● M25.13   Fistula, wrist
         M25.131   Fistula, right wrist
         M25.132   Fistula, left wrist
         M25.139   Fistula, unspecified wrist

     ● M25.14   Fistula, hand
         M25.141   Fistula, right hand
         M25.142   Fistula, left hand
         M25.149   Fistula, unspecified hand

     ● M25.15   Fistula, hip
         M25.151   Fistula, right hip
         M25.152   Fistula, left hip
         M25.159   Fistula, unspecified hip

     ● M25.16   Fistula, knee
         M25.161   Fistula, right knee
         M25.162   Fistula, left knee
         M25.169   Fistula, unspecified knee

     ● M25.17   Fistula, ankle and foot
         M25.171   Fistula, right ankle
         M25.172   Fistula, left ankle
         M25.173   Fistula, unspecified ankle
         M25.174   Fistula, right foot
         M25.175   Fistula, left foot
         M25.176   Fistula, unspecified foot

     M25.18   Fistula, other specified site
         Fistula, vertebrae

● M25.2   **Flail joint**

     M25.20   Flail joint, unspecified joint

     ● M25.21   Flail joint, shoulder
         M25.211   Flail joint, right shoulder
         M25.212   Flail joint, left shoulder
         M25.219   Flail joint, unspecified shoulder

     ● M25.22   Flail joint, elbow
         M25.221   Flail joint, right elbow
         M25.222   Flail joint, left elbow
         M25.229   Flail joint, unspecified elbow

     ● M25.23   Flail joint, wrist
         M25.231   Flail joint, right wrist
         M25.232   Flail joint, left wrist
         M25.239   Flail joint, unspecified wrist

     ● M25.24   Flail joint, hand
         M25.241   Flail joint, right hand
         M25.242   Flail joint, left hand
         M25.249   Flail joint, unspecified hand

     ● M25.25   Flail joint, hip
         M25.251   Flail joint, right hip
         M25.252   Flail joint, left hip
         M25.259   Flail joint, unspecified hip

     ● M25.26   Flail joint, knee
         M25.261   Flail joint, right knee
         M25.262   Flail joint, left knee
         M25.269   Flail joint, unspecified knee

     ● M25.27   Flail joint, ankle and foot
         M25.271   Flail joint, right ankle and foot
         M25.272   Flail joint, left ankle and foot
         M25.279   Flail joint, unspecified ankle and foot

     M25.28   Flail joint, other site

▶ New   ⬤ Revised   ~~deleted~~ Deleted   Excludes 1   Excludes 2   Includes   Use additional   Code first   Code also   Key words

OGCR Official Guidelines   ● Unacceptable Principal Diagnosis   X Assign placeholder X   ● Use Additional Character(s)   ▶ Manifestation Code   Coding Clinic

● **M25.3 Other instability of joint**
> **Excludes1**   instability of joint secondary to old ligament injury (M24.2-)
> instability of joint secondary to removal of joint prosthesis (M96.8-)
>
> **Excludes2**   spinal instabilities (M53.2-)

M25.30   Other instability, unspecified joint
● M25.31   Other instability, shoulder
    M25.311   Other instability, right shoulder
    M25.312   Other instability, left shoulder
    M25.319   Other instability, unspecified shoulder
● M25.32   Other instability, elbow
    M25.321   Other instability, right elbow
    M25.322   Other instability, left elbow
    M25.329   Other instability, unspecified elbow
● M25.33   Other instability, wrist
    M25.331   Other instability, right wrist
    M25.332   Other instability, left wrist
    M25.339   Other instability, unspecified wrist
● M25.34   Other instability, hand
    M25.341   Other instability, right hand
    M25.342   Other instability, left hand
    M25.349   Other instability, unspecified hand
● M25.35   Other instability, hip
    M25.351   Other instability, right hip
    M25.352   Other instability, left hip
    M25.359   Other instability, unspecified hip
● M25.36   Other instability, knee
    M25.361   Other instability, right knee
    M25.362   Other instability, left knee
    M25.369   Other instability, unspecified knee
● M25.37   Other instability, ankle and foot
    M25.371   Other instability, right ankle
    M25.372   Other instability, left ankle
    M25.373   Other instability, unspecified ankle
    M25.374   Other instability, right foot
    M25.375   Other instability, left foot
    M25.376   Other instability, unspecified foot
M25.39   Other instability of joint
● **M25.4 Effusion of joint**
> **Excludes1**   hydrarthrosis in yaws (A66.6)
> intermittent hydrarthrosis (M12.4-)
> other infective (teno)synovitis (M65.1-)

M25.40   Effusion, unspecified joint
● M25.41   Effusion, shoulder
    M25.411   Effusion, right shoulder
    M25.412   Effusion, left shoulder
    M25.419   Effusion, unspecified shoulder
● M25.42   Effusion, elbow
    M25.421   Effusion, right elbow
    M25.422   Effusion, left elbow
    M25.429   Effusion, unspecified elbow
● M25.43   Effusion, wrist
    M25.431   Effusion, right wrist
    M25.432   Effusion, left wrist
    M25.439   Effusion, unspecified wrist
● M25.44   Effusion, hand
    M25.441   Effusion, right hand
    M25.442   Effusion, left hand
    M25.449   Effusion, unspecified hand

● M25.45   Effusion, hip
    M25.451   Effusion, right hip
    M25.452   Effusion, left hip
    M25.459   Effusion, unspecified hip
● M25.46   Effusion, knee
    M25.461   Effusion, right knee
    M25.462   Effusion, left knee
    M25.469   Effusion, unspecified knee
● M25.47   Effusion, ankle and foot
    M25.471   Effusion, right ankle
    M25.472   Effusion, left ankle
    M25.473   Effusion, unspecified ankle
    M25.474   Effusion, right foot
    M25.475   Effusion, left foot
    M25.476   Effusion, unspecified foot
M25.48   Effusion, other site
● **M25.5 Pain in joint**
> **Excludes2**   pain in hand (M79.64-)
> pain in fingers (M79.64-)
> pain in foot (M79.67-)
> pain in limb (M79.6-)
> pain in toes (M79.67-)

M25.50   Pain in unspecified joint
● M25.51   Pain in shoulder
    M25.511   Pain in right shoulder
    M25.512   Pain in left shoulder
    M25.519   Pain in unspecified shoulder
● M25.52   Pain in elbow
    M25.521   Pain in right elbow
    M25.522   Pain in left elbow
    M25.529   Pain in unspecified elbow
● M25.53   Pain in wrist
    M25.531   Pain in right wrist
    M25.532   Pain in left wrist
    M25.539   Pain in unspecified wrist
● M25.54   Pain in joints of hand
    Coding Clinic: 2016, Q4, P38
    M25.541   Pain in joints of right hand
    M25.542   Pain in joints of left hand
    M25.549   Pain in joints of unspecified hand
      Pain in joints of hand NOS
● M25.55   Pain in hip
    M25.551   Pain in right hip
    M25.552   Pain in left hip
    M25.559   Pain in unspecified hip
● M25.56   Pain in knee
    M25.561   Pain in right knee
    M25.562   Pain in left knee
    M25.569   Pain in unspecified knee
● M25.57   Pain in ankle and joints of foot
    M25.571   Pain in right ankle and joints of right foot
    M25.572   Pain in left ankle and joints of left foot
    M25.579   Pain in unspecified ankle and joints of unspecified foot
M25.59   Pain in other specified joint

CHAPTER 13 (M00-M99)

CHAPTER 13 (M00-M99)

● M25.6   Stiffness of joint, not elsewhere classified
      Excludes1   ankylosis of joint (M24.6-)
                     contracture of joint (M24.5-)

   M25.60   Stiffness of unspecified joint, not elsewhere classified

● M25.61   Stiffness of shoulder, not elsewhere classified
      M25.611   Stiffness of right shoulder, not elsewhere classified
      M25.612   Stiffness of left shoulder, not elsewhere classified
      M25.619   Stiffness of unspecified shoulder, not elsewhere classified

● M25.62   Stiffness of elbow, not elsewhere classified
      M25.621   Stiffness of right elbow, not elsewhere classified
      M25.622   Stiffness of left elbow, not elsewhere classified
      M25.629   Stiffness of unspecified elbow, not elsewhere classified

● M25.63   Stiffness of wrist, not elsewhere classified
      M25.631   Stiffness of right wrist, not elsewhere classified
      M25.632   Stiffness of left wrist, not elsewhere classified
      M25.639   Stiffness of unspecified wrist, not elsewhere classified

● M25.64   Stiffness of hand, not elsewhere classified
      M25.641   Stiffness of right hand, not elsewhere classified
      M25.642   Stiffness of left hand, not elsewhere classified
      M25.649   Stiffness of unspecified hand, not elsewhere classified

● M25.65   Stiffness of hip, not elsewhere classified
      M25.651   Stiffness of right hip, not elsewhere classified
      M25.652   Stiffness of left hip, not elsewhere classified
      M25.659   Stiffness of unspecified hip, not elsewhere classified

● M25.66   Stiffness of knee, not elsewhere classified
      M25.661   Stiffness of right knee, not elsewhere classified
      M25.662   Stiffness of left knee, not elsewhere classified
      M25.669   Stiffness of unspecified knee, not elsewhere classified

● M25.67   Stiffness of ankle and foot, not elsewhere classified
      M25.671   Stiffness of right ankle, not elsewhere classified
      M25.672   Stiffness of left ankle, not elsewhere classified
      M25.673   Stiffness of unspecified ankle, not elsewhere classified
      M25.674   Stiffness of right foot, not elsewhere classified
      M25.675   Stiffness of left foot, not elsewhere classified
      M25.676   Stiffness of unspecified foot, not elsewhere classified

   M25.69   Stiffness of other specified joint, not elsewhere classified

● M25.7   Osteophyte
   M25.70   Osteophyte, unspecified joint

● M25.71   Osteophyte, shoulder
      M25.711   Osteophyte, right shoulder
      M25.712   Osteophyte, left shoulder
      M25.719   Osteophyte, unspecified shoulder

● M25.72   Osteophyte, elbow
      M25.721   Osteophyte, right elbow
      M25.722   Osteophyte, left elbow
      M25.729   Osteophyte, unspecified elbow

● M25.73   Osteophyte, wrist
      M25.731   Osteophyte, right wrist
      M25.732   Osteophyte, left wrist
      M25.739   Osteophyte, unspecified wrist

● M25.74   Osteophyte, hand
      M25.741   Osteophyte, right hand
      M25.742   Osteophyte, left hand
      M25.749   Osteophyte, unspecified hand

● M25.75   Osteophyte, hip
      M25.751   Osteophyte, right hip
      M25.752   Osteophyte, left hip
      M25.759   Osteophyte, unspecified hip

● M25.76   Osteophyte, knee
      M25.761   Osteophyte, right knee
      M25.762   Osteophyte, left knee
      M25.769   Osteophyte, unspecified knee

● M25.77   Osteophyte, ankle and foot
      M25.771   Osteophyte, right ankle
      M25.772   Osteophyte, left ankle
      M25.773   Osteophyte, unspecified ankle
      M25.774   Osteophyte, right foot
      M25.775   Osteophyte, left foot
      M25.776   Osteophyte, unspecified foot

   M25.78   Osteophyte, vertebrae

● M25.8   Other specified joint disorders
   M25.80   Other specified joint disorders, unspecified joint

● M25.81   Other specified joint disorders, shoulder
      M25.811   Other specified joint disorders, right shoulder
      M25.812   Other specified joint disorders, left shoulder
      M25.819   Other specified joint disorders, unspecified shoulder

● M25.82   Other specified joint disorders, elbow
      M25.821   Other specified joint disorders, right elbow
      M25.822   Other specified joint disorders, left elbow
      M25.829   Other specified joint disorders, unspecified elbow

● M25.83   Other specified joint disorders, wrist
      M25.831   Other specified joint disorders, right wrist
      M25.832   Other specified joint disorders, left wrist
      M25.839   Other specified joint disorders, unspecified wrist

● M25.84   Other specified joint disorders, hand

     M25.841   Other specified joint disorders, right hand

     M25.842   Other specified joint disorders, left hand

     M25.849   Other specified joint disorders, unspecified hand

● M25.85   Other specified joint disorders, hip

     M25.851   Other specified joint disorders, right hip

     M25.852   Other specified joint disorders, left hip

     M25.859   Other specified joint disorders, unspecified hip

● M25.86   Other specified joint disorders, knee

     M25.861   Other specified joint disorders, right knee

     M25.862   Other specified joint disorders, left knee

     M25.869   Other specified joint disorders, unspecified knee

● M25.87   Other specified joint disorders, ankle and foot

     M25.871   Other specified joint disorders, right ankle and foot

     M25.872   Other specified joint disorders, left ankle and foot

     M25.879   Other specified joint disorders, unspecified ankle and foot

M25.9   Joint disorder, unspecified

DENTOFACIAL ANOMALIES [INCLUDING MALOCCLUSION] AND OTHER DISORDERS OF JAW (M26–M27)

     Excludes1   hemifacial atrophy or hypertrophy (Q67.4)
                    unilateral condylar hyperplasia or hypoplasia (M27.8)

● M26   Dentofacial anomalies [including malocclusion]

   ● M26.0   Major anomalies of jaw size

     Excludes1   acromegaly (E22.0)
                   Robin's syndrome (Q87.0)

     M26.00   Unspecified anomaly of jaw size

     M26.01   Maxillary hyperplasia

     M26.02   Maxillary hypoplasia

     M26.03   Mandibular hyperplasia

     M26.04   Mandibular hypoplasia

     M26.05   Macrogenia

     M26.06   Microgenia

     M26.07   Excessive tuberosity of jaw
              Entire maxillary tuberosity

     M26.09   Other specified anomalies of jaw size

   ● M26.1   Anomalies of jaw-cranial base relationship

     M26.10   Unspecified anomaly of jaw-cranial base relationship

     M26.11   Maxillary asymmetry

     M26.12   Other jaw asymmetry

     M26.19   Other specified anomalies of jaw-cranial base relationship
              Coding Clinic: 2020, Q1, P21

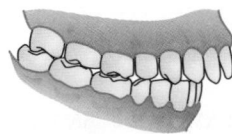

Figure 13-3   Dentofacial malocclusion.

● M26.2   Anomalies of dental arch relationship

     M26.20   Unspecified anomaly of dental arch relationship

   ● M26.21   Malocclusion, Angle's class

     M26.211   Malocclusion, Angle's class I
              Neutro-occlusion

     M26.212   Malocclusion, Angle's class II
              Disto-occlusion Division I
              Disto-occlusion Division II

     M26.213   Malocclusion, Angle's class III
              Mesio-occlusion

     M26.219   Malocclusion, Angle's class, unspecified

   ● M26.22   Open occlusal relationship

     M26.220   Open anterior occlusal relationship
              Anterior open bite

     M26.221   Open posterior occlusal relationship
              Posterior open bite

     M26.23   Excessive horizontal overlap
              Excessive horizontal overjet

     M26.24   Reverse articulation
              Crossbite (anterior) (posterior)

     M26.25   Anomalies of interarch distance

     M26.29   Other anomalies of dental arch relationship
              Midline deviation of dental arch
              Overbite (excessive) deep
              Overbite (excessive) horizontal
              Overbite (excessive) vertical
              Posterior lingual occlusion of mandibular teeth

● M26.3   Anomalies of tooth position of fully erupted tooth or teeth

     Excludes2   embedded and impacted teeth (K01.-)

     M26.30   Unspecified anomaly of tooth position of fully erupted tooth or teeth
              Abnormal spacing of fully erupted tooth or teeth NOS
              Displacement of fully erupted tooth or teeth NOS
              Transposition of fully erupted tooth or teeth NOS

     M26.31   Crowding of fully erupted teeth

     M26.32   Excessive spacing of fully erupted teeth
              Diastema of fully erupted tooth or teeth NOS

     M26.33   Horizontal displacement of fully erupted tooth or teeth
              Tipped tooth or teeth
              Tipping of fully erupted tooth

     M26.34   Vertical displacement of fully erupted tooth or teeth
              Extruded tooth
              Infraeruption of tooth or teeth
              Supraeruption of tooth or teeth

     M26.35   Rotation of fully erupted tooth or teeth

     M26.36   Insufficient interocclusal distance of fully erupted teeth (ridge)
              Lack of adequate intermaxillary vertical dimension of fully erupted teeth

     M26.37   Excessive interocclusal distance of fully erupted teeth
              Excessive intermaxillary vertical dimension of fully erupted teeth
              Loss of occlusal vertical dimension of fully erupted teeth

     M26.39   Other anomalies of tooth position of fully erupted tooth or teeth

M26.4   Malocclusion, unspecified

Item 13–6 Hyperplasia is a condition of overdevelopment, whereas **hypoplasia** is a condition of underdevelopment. **Macrogenia** is overdevelopment of the chin, whereas **microgenia** is underdevelopment of the chin.

CHAPTER 13 (M00-M99)

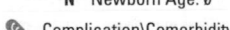

N Newborn Age: 0   **P** Pediatric Age: 0–17   **M** Maternity DX: 9–64   **A** Adult Age: 15–124   ♀ Females Only   ♂ Males Only

🔹 Complication\Comorbidity   🔹 Major C\C   (Ex) CC/MCC Exclusions   🔹 Hospital-Acquired Condition   🔹 Hierarchical Condition Category

1055

CHAPTER 13 (M00-M99)

● M26.5 **Dentofacial functional abnormalities**
> **Excludes1**   bruxism (F45.8)
> > teeth-grinding NOS (F45.8)

M26.50 **Dentofacial functional abnormalities, unspecified**

M26.51 **Abnormal jaw closure**

M26.52 **Limited mandibular range of motion**

M26.53 **Deviation in opening and closing of the mandible**

M26.54 **Insufficient anterior guidance**
> Insufficient anterior occlusal guidance

M26.55 **Centric occlusion maximum intercuspation discrepancy**
> > **Excludes1**   centric occlusion NOS (M26.59)

M26.56 **Non-working side interference**
> Balancing side interference

M26.57 **Lack of posterior occlusal support**

M26.59 **Other dentofacial functional abnormalities**
> Centric occlusion (of teeth) NOS
> Malocclusion due to abnormal swallowing
> Malocclusion due to mouth breathing
> Malocclusion due to tongue, lip or finger habits

● M26.6 **Temporomandibular joint disorders**
> **Excludes2**   current temporomandibular joint
> > dislocation (S03.0)
> > current temporomandibular joint sprain
> > (S03.4)

> Coding Clinic: 2016, Q4, P38-39

● M26.60 **Temporomandibular joint disorder, unspecified**

M26.601 **Right temporomandibular joint disorder, unspecified**

M26.602 **Left temporomandibular joint disorder, unspecified**

M26.603 **Bilateral temporomandibular joint disorder, unspecified**

M26.609 **Unspecified temporomandibular joint disorder, unspecified side**
> Temporomandibular joint disorder NOS

● M26.61 **Adhesions and ankylosis of temporomandibular joint**

M26.611 **Adhesions and ankylosis of right temporomandibular joint**

M26.612 **Adhesions and ankylosis of left temporomandibular joint**

M26.613 **Adhesions and ankylosis of bilateral temporomandibular joint**

M26.619 **Adhesions and ankylosis of temporomandibular joint, unspecified side**

● M26.62 **Arthralgia of temporomandibular joint**

M26.621 **Arthralgia of right temporomandibular joint**

M26.622 **Arthralgia of left temporomandibular joint**

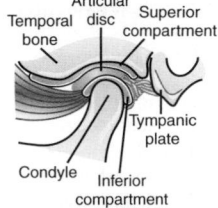

Temporal bone / Articular disc / Superior compartment / Tympanic plate / Condyle / Inferior compartment

Figure 13-4 Temporomandibular joint.

Item 13–7 Dysfunction of the temporomandibular joint is termed **temporomandibular joint (TMJ) syndrome** and is characterized by pain and tenderness/spasm of the muscles of mastication, joint noise, and in the later stages, limited mandibular movement.

M26.623 **Arthralgia of bilateral temporomandibular joint**

M26.629 **Arthralgia of temporomandibular joint, unspecified side**

● M26.63 **Articular disc disorder of temporomandibular joint**

M26.631 **Articular disc disorder of right temporomandibular joint**

M26.632 **Articular disc disorder of left temporomandibular joint**

M26.633 **Articular disc disorder of bilateral temporomandibular joint**

M26.639 **Articular disc disorder of temporomandibular joint, unspecified side**

● M26.64 **Arthritis of temporomandibular joint**

M26.641 **Arthritis of right temporomandibular joint**

M26.642 **Arthritis of left temporomandibular joint**

M26.643 **Arthritis of bilateral temporomandibular joint**

M26.649 **Arthritis of unspecified temporomandibular joint**

● M26.65 **Arthropathy of temporomandibular joint**

M26.651 **Arthropathy of right temporomandibular joint**

M26.652 **Arthropathy of left temporomandibular joint**

M26.653 **Arthropathy of bilateral temporomandibular joint**

M26.659 **Arthropathy of unspecified temporomandibular joint**

M26.69 **Other specified disorders of temporomandibular joint**

● M26.7 **Dental alveolar anomalies**

M26.70 **Unspecified alveolar anomaly**

M26.71 **Alveolar maxillary hyperplasia**

M26.72 **Alveolar mandibular hyperplasia**

M26.73 **Alveolar maxillary hypoplasia**

M26.74 **Alveolar mandibular hypoplasia**

M26.79 **Other specified alveolar anomalies**

● M26.8 **Other dentofacial anomalies**

M26.81 **Anterior soft tissue impingement**
> Anterior soft tissue impingement on teeth

M26.82 **Posterior soft tissue impingement**
> Posterior soft tissue impingement on teeth

M26.89 **Other dentofacial anomalies**

M26.9 **Dentofacial anomaly, unspecified**

● M27 **Other diseases of jaws**

M27.0 **Developmental disorders of jaws**
> Latent bone cyst of jaw
> Stafne's cyst
> Torus mandibularis
> Torus palatinus

M27.1 **Giant cell granuloma, central**
> Giant cell granuloma NOS
> > **Excludes1**   peripheral giant cell granuloma (K06.8)

M27.2 **Inflammatory conditions of jaws**
> Osteitis of jaw(s)
> Osteomyelitis (neonatal) jaw(s)
> Osteoradionecrosis jaw(s)
> Periostitis jaw(s)
> Sequestrum of jaw bone
> Use additional code (W88-W90, X39.0) to identify radiation, if radiation-induced
> > **Excludes2**   osteonecrosis of jaw due to drug (M87.180)

M27.3 **Alveolitis of jaws**
> Alveolar osteitis
> Dry socket

▶ Now ⇶ Revised ~~deleted~~ Deleted Excludes 1 Excludes 2 Includes Use additional Code first Code also Key words
OGCR Official Guidelines ● Unacceptable Principal Diagnosis X Assign placeholder X ● Use Additional Character(s) ▶ Manifestation Code **Coding Clinic**

- **M27.4 Other and unspecified cysts of jaw**
  - **Excludes1**   cysts of oral region (K09.-)
    - latent bone cyst of jaw (M27.0)
    - Stafne's cyst (M27.0)
  - **M27.40 Unspecified cyst of jaw**
    - Cyst of jaw NOS
  - **M27.49 Other cysts of jaw**
    - Aneurysmal cyst of jaw
    - Hemorrhagic cyst of jaw
    - Traumatic cyst of jaw
- **M27.5 Periradicular pathology associated with previous endodontic treatment**
  - **M27.51 Perforation of root canal space due to endodontic treatment**
  - **M27.52 Endodontic overfill**
  - **M27.53 Endodontic underfill**
  - **M27.59 Other periradicular pathology associated with previous endodontic treatment**
- **M27.6 Endosseous dental implant failure**
  - **M27.61 Osseointegration failure of dental implant**
    - Hemorrhagic complications of dental implant placement
    - Iatrogenic osseointegration failure of dental implant
    - Osseointegration failure of dental implant due to complications of systemic disease
    - Osseointegration failure of dental implant due to poor bone quality
    - Pre-integration failure of dental implant NOS
    - Pre-osseointegration failure of dental implant
  - **M27.62 Post-osseointegration biological failure of dental implant**
    - Failure of dental implant due to lack of attached gingiva
    - Failure of dental implant due to occlusal trauma (caused by poor prosthetic design)
    - Failure of dental implant due to parafunctional habits
    - Failure of dental implant due to periodontal infection (peri implantitis)
    - Failure of dental implant due to poor oral hygiene
    - Iatrogenic post-osseointegration failure of dental implant
    - Post-osseointegration failure of dental implant due to complications of systemic disease
  - **M27.63 Post-osseointegration mechanical failure of dental implant**
    - Failure of dental prosthesis causing loss of dental implant
    - Fracture of dental implant
    - **Excludes2**   cracked tooth (K03.81)
      - fractured dental restorative material with loss of material (K08.531)
      - fractured dental restorative material without loss of material (K08.530)
      - fractured tooth (S02.5)
  - **M27.69 Other endosseous dental implant failure**
    - Dental implant failure NOS
- **M27.8 Other specified diseases of jaws**
  - Cherubism
  - Exostosis
  - Fibrous dysplasia
  - Unilateral condylar hyperplasia
  - Unilateral condylar hypoplasia
  - **Excludes1**   jaw pain (R68.84)
- **M27.9 Disease of jaws, unspecified**

SYSTEMIC CONNECTIVE TISSUE DISORDERS (M30-M36)

- **Includes**   autoimmune disease NOS
  - collagen (vascular) disease NOS
  - systemic autoimmune disease
  - systemic collagen (vascular) disease
- **Excludes1**   autoimmune disease, single organ or single cell-type - code to relevant condition category
- **M30 Polyarteritis nodosa and related conditions**
  - **Excludes1**   microscopic polyarteritis (M31.7)
  - (Ex) For category M30 CC codes unless otherwise indicated: See PDX Collection 874
  - **M30.0 Polyarteritis nodosa**
  - **M30.1 Polyarteritis with lung involvement [Churg-Strauss]**
    - Allergic granulomatous angiitis
    - Eosinophilic granulomatosis with polyangiitis [EGPA]
    - Coding Clinic: 2021, Q1, P23
  - **M30.2 Juvenile polyarteritis**
  - **M30.3 Mucocutaneous lymph node syndrome [Kawasaki]**
    - (Ex) See PDX Collection 875
  - **M30.8 Other conditions related to polyarteritis nodosa**
    - Polyangiitis overlap syndrome
- **M31 Other necrotizing vasculopathies**
  - (Ex) For category M31 CC codes unless otherwise indicated: See PDX Collection 874
  - **M31.0 Hypersensitivity angiitis**
    - Goodpasture's syndrome
  - **M31.1 Thrombotic microangiopathy**
    - Thrombotic thrombocytopenic purpura
    - **M31.10 Thrombotic microangiopathy, unspecified**
    - **M31.11 Hematopoietic stem cell transplantation-associated thrombotic microangiopathy [HSCT-TMA]**
      - Transplant-associated thrombotic microangiopathy [TA-TMA]
      - *Code first* if applicable:
        - complications of bone marrow transplant (T86.0-)
        - complications of stem cell transplant (T86.5)
      - Use Additional code to identify specific organ dysfunction, such as:
        - acute kidney failure (N17.-)
        - acute respiratory distress syndrome (J80)
        - capillary leak syndrome (I78.8)
        - diffuse alveolar hemorrhage (R04.89)
        - encephalopathy (metabolic) (septic) (G93.41)
        - fluid overload, unspecified (E87.70)
        - graft versus host disease (D89.81-)
        - hemolytic uremic syndrome (D59.3)
        - hepatic failure (K72.-)
        - hepatic veno-occlusive disease (K76.5)
        - idiopathic interstitial pneumonia (J84.11-)
        - sinusoidal obstruction syndrome (K76.5)
    - **M31.19 Other thrombotic microangiopathy**
      - Thrombotic thrombocytopenic purpura
  - **M31.2 Lethal midline granuloma**
  - **M31.3 Wegener's granulomatosis**
    - Granulomatosis with polyangiitis
    - Necrotizing respiratory granulomatosis
    - Coding Clinic: 2021, Q1, P23
    - **M31.30 Wegener's granulomatosis without renal involvement**
      - Wegener's granulomatosis NOS
      - Coding Clinic: 2021, Q2, P10
    - **M31.31 Wegener's granulomatosis with renal involvement**
  - **M31.4 Aortic arch syndrome [Takayasu]**
  - **M31.5 Giant cell arteritis with polymyalgia rheumatica**
  - **M31.6 Other giant cell arteritis**

CHAPTER 13 (M00-M99)

N Newborn Age: 0   **P** Pediatric Age: 0–17   **M** Maternity DX: 9–64   **A** Adult Age: 15–124   ♀ Females Only   ♂ Males Only

Complication\Comorbidity   Major C\C   (Ex) CC/MCC Exclusions   Hospital-Acquired Condition   Hierarchical Condition Category

1057

M31.7 **Microscopic polyangiitis** 🔹🔹
Microscopic polyarteritis
> **Excludes1** polyarteritis nodosa (M30.0)
> *Coding Clinic: 2021, Q1, P23*

M31.8 **Other specified necrotizing vasculopathies** 🔹🔹
Hypocomplementemic vasculitis
Septic vasculitis
(Ex:) See PDX Collection 712

M31.9 **Necrotizing vasculopathy, unspecified** 🔹🔹
(Ex:) See PDX Collection 712

● **M32** **Systemic lupus erythematosus (SLE)**
Autoimmune inflammatory connective tissue disease of unknown cause that occurs most often in women
> **Excludes1** lupus erythematosus (discoid) (NOS) (L93.0)

M32.0 **Drug-induced systemic lupus erythematosus** 🔹
> Use additional code for adverse effect, if applicable, to identify drug (T36-T50 with fifth or sixth character 5)

● **M32.1** **Systemic lupus erythematosus with organ or system involvement**

M32.10 **Systemic lupus erythematosus, organ or system involvement unspecified** 🔹

M32.11 **Endocarditis in systemic lupus erythematosus** 🔹🔹
Libman-Sacks disease
CC when PDx is its own CC
(Ex:) See PDX Collection 3825

M32.12 **Pericarditis in systemic lupus erythematosus** 🔹🔹
Lupus pericarditis
CC when PDx is its own CC
(Ex:) See PDX Collection 3827

M32.13 **Lung involvement in systemic lupus erythematosus** 🔹
Pleural effusion due to systemic lupus erythematosus

M32.14 **Glomerular disease in systemic lupus erythematosus** 🔹
Lupus renal disease NOS

M32.15 **Tubulo-interstitial nephropathy in systemic lupus erythematosus** 🔹

M32.19 **Other organ or system involvement in systemic lupus erythematosus** 🔹

M32.8 **Other forms of systemic lupus erythematosus** 🔹

M32.9 **Systemic lupus erythematosus, unspecified** 🔹
SLE NOS
Systemic lupus erythematosus NOS
Systemic lupus erythematosus without organ involvement

● **M33** **Dermatopolymyositis**
(Ex:) **For category M33 CC codes unless otherwise indicated:** See PDX Collection 876

● **M33.0** **Juvenile dermatomyositis**

M33.00 **Juvenile dermatomyositis, organ involvement unspecified** 🔹🔹

M33.01 **Juvenile dermatomyositis with respiratory involvement** 🔹🔹

M33.02 **Juvenile dermatomyositis with myopathy** 🔹🔹
CC when PDx is its own CC
(Ex:) See PDX Collection 877

M33.03 **Juvenile dermatomyositis without myopathy** 🔹🔹

M33.09 **Juvenile dermatomyositis with other organ involvement** 🔹🔹

● **M33.1** **Other dermatomyositis**
Adult dermatomyositis

M33.10 **Other dermatomyositis, organ involvement unspecified** 🔹🔹

M33.11 **Other dermatomyositis with respiratory involvement** 🔹🔹

M33.12 **Other dermatomyositis with myopathy** 🔹🔹
CC when PDx is its own CC
(Ex:) See PDX Collection 877

M33.13 **Other dermatomyositis without myopathy** 🔹🔹
Dermatomyositis NOS

M33.19 **Other dermatomyositis with other organ involvement** 🔹🔹

● **M33.2** **Polymyositis**

M33.20 **Polymyositis, organ involvement unspecified** 🔹🔹
(Ex:) See PDX Collection 878

M33.21 **Polymyositis with respiratory involvement** 🔹🔹
(Ex:) See PDX Collection 878

M33.22 **Polymyositis with myopathy** 🔹🔹
CC when PDx is its own CC
(Ex:) See PDX Collection 879

M33.29 **Polymyositis with other organ involvement** 🔹🔹
(Ex:) See PDX Collection 878

● **M33.9** **Dermatopolymyositis, unspecified**

M33.90 **Dermatopolymyositis, unspecified, organ involvement unspecified** 🔹🔹

M33.91 **Dermatopolymyositis, unspecified with respiratory involvement** 🔹🔹

M33.92 **Dermatopolymyositis, unspecified with myopathy** 🔹🔹
CC when PDx is its own CC
(Ex:) See PDX Collection 877

M33.93 **Dermatopolymyositis, unspecified without myopathy** 🔹🔹

M33.99 **Dermatopolymyositis, unspecified with other organ involvement** 🔹🔹

● **M34** **Systemic sclerosis [scleroderma]**
> **Excludes1** circumscribed scleroderma (L94.0)
> neonatal scleroderma (P83.88)

M34.0 **Progressive systemic sclerosis** 🔹

M34.1 **CR(E)ST syndrome** 🔹
Combination of calcinosis, Raynaud's phenomenon, esophageal dysfunction, sclerodactyly, telangiectasia

M34.2 **Systemic sclerosis induced by drug and chemical** 🔹
Code first poisoning due to drug or toxin, if applicable (T36-T65 with fifth or sixth character 1-4 or 6)
> Use additional code for adverse effect, if applicable, to identify drug (T36-T50 with fifth or sixth character 5)

● **M34.8** **Other forms of systemic sclerosis** 🔹

M34.81 **Systemic sclerosis with lung involvement** 🔹🔹
▶ Code also if applicable:
▶ other interstitial pulmonary diseases (J84.89)
▶ secondary pulmonary arterial hypertension (I27.21)
CC when PDx is its own CC
(Ex:) See PDX Collection 3232

M34.82 **Systemic sclerosis with myopathy** 🔹🔹
CC when PDx is its own CC
(Ex:) See PDX Collection 3403

M34.83 **Systemic sclerosis with polyneuropathy** 🔹

M34.89 **Other systemic sclerosis** 🔹
(Ex:) **For category M35.8 CC codes unless otherwise indicated:** See PDX Collection 4125

M34.9 **Systemic sclerosis, unspecified** 🔹

● **M35** **Other systemic involvement of connective tissue**
> **Excludes1** reactive perforating collagenosis (L87.1)

⇒● **M35.0** **Sjögren syndrome**
▶ Sicca syndrome
▶ Use Additional code to identify associated manifestations
> **Excludes1** dry mouth, unspecified (R68.2)

M35.00 **Sjögren syndrome, unspecified** 🔹

M35.01 **Sjögren syndrome with keratoconjunctivitis** 🔹

M35.02 **Sjögren syndrome with lung involvement** 🔹

M35.03 **Sjögren syndrome with myopathy** 🔹🔹
CC when PDx is its own CC
(Ex:) See PDX Collection 3404

▶ New   ⇒ Revised   ~~deleted~~ Deleted   Excludes 1   Excludes 2   Includes   Use additional   Code first   Code also   Key words

OGCR Official Guidelines   ● Unacceptable Principal Diagnosis   X Assign placeholder X   ● Use Additional Character(s)   ▶ Manifestation Code   Coding Clinic

Item 13–8   **Polymyalgia rheumatica** is a syndrome characterized by aching and morning stiffness and is related to aging and hereditary predisposition.

   M35.04   Sjögren syndrome with tubulo-interstitial nephropathy 🅒🅒
       Renal tubular acidosis in sicca syndrome

▶ **M35.05**   Sjögren syndrome with inflammatory arthritis

▶ **M35.06**   Sjögren syndrome with peripheral nervous system involvement

▶ **M35.07**   Sjögren syndrome with central nervous system involvement

▶ **M35.08**   Sjögren syndrome with gastrointestinal involvement

   M35.09   Sjögren syndrome with other organ involvement 🅒🅒

▶ **M35.0A**   Sjögren syndrome with glomerular disease

▶ **M35.0B**   Sjögren syndrome with vasculitis

▶ **M35.0C**   Sjögren syndrome with dental involvement

M35.1   Other overlap syndromes 🅒🅒
       Mixed connective tissue disease

     Excludes1   polyangiitis overlap syndrome (M30.8)

     Ⓔⓧ See PDX Collection 880

M35.2   Behçet's disease 🅒🅒
     Ⓔⓧ See PDX Collection 863

M35.3   Polymyalgia rheumatica 🅒🅒

     Excludes1   polymyalgia rheumatica with giant cell arteritis (M31.5)

M35.4   Diffuse (eosinophilic) fasciitis

M35.5   Multifocal fibrosclerosis 🅒🅒
     Ⓔⓧ See PDX Collection 880

M35.6   Relapsing panniculitis [Weber-Christian]

     Excludes1   lupus panniculitis (L93.2)
                panniculitis NOS (M79.3-)

M35.7   Hypermobility syndrome
       Familial ligamentous laxity

     Excludes1   Ehlers-Danlos syndromes (Q79.6-)
                ligamentous laxity, NOS (M24.2-)

     Excludes2   Ehlers-Danlos syndromes (Q79.6-)

● **M35.8**   Other specified systemic involvement of connective tissue 🅒🅒
     Ⓔⓧ For category M35.8 CC codes unless otherwise indicated: See PDX Collection 4125
     Coding Clinic: 2021, Q1, P36

   M35.81   Multisystem inflammatory syndrome 🅒
       MIS-A
       MIS-C
       Multisystem inflammatory syndrome in adults
       Multisystem inflammatory syndrome in children
       Pediatric inflammatory multisystem syndrome
       PIMS

       Code first, if applicable, COVID-19 (U07.1)

       Code also any associated complications such as:
         acute hepatic failure (K72.0-)
         acute kidney failure (N17.-)
         acute myocarditis (I40.-)
         acute respiratory distress syndrome (J80)
         cardiac arrhythmia (I47-I49.-)
         pneumonia due to COVID-19 (J12.82)
         severe sepsis (R65.2-)
         viral cardiomyopathy (B33.24)
         viral pericarditis (B33.23)

       Use additional code, if applicable, for:
         exposure to COVID-19 or SARS-C
         personal history of COVID-19 (Z86.16)
         sequelae of COVID-19 (B94.8)
       ▶ post COVID-19 condition (U09.9)
       Coding Clinic: 2021, Q1, P36, 42

   M35.89   Other specified systemic involvement of connective tissue 🅒

M35.9   Systemic involvement of connective tissue, unspecified 🅒
       Autoimmune disease (systemic) NOS
       Collagen (vascular) disease NOS

● **M36**   Systemic disorders of connective tissue in diseases classified elsewhere

     Excludes2   arthropathies in diseases classified elsewhere (M14.-)

▶ *M36.0*   *Dermato(poly)myositis in neoplastic disease* 🅒🅒
       Code first underlying neoplasm (C00-D49)
     Ⓔⓧ See PDX Collection 876

▶ *M36.1*   *Arthropathy in neoplastic disease*
       Code first underlying neoplasm, such as:
         leukemia (C91-C95)
         malignant histiocytosis (C96.A)
         multiple myeloma (C90.0)

▶ *M36.2*   *Hemophilic arthropathy*
       Hemarthrosis in hemophilic arthropathy
       Code first underlying disease, such as:
         factor VIII deficiency (D66)
         with vascular defect (D68.0)
         factor IX deficiency (D67)
         hemophilia (classical) (D66)
         hemophilia B (D67)
         hemophilia C (D68.1)

▶ *M36.3*   *Arthropathy in other blood disorders*

▶ *M36.4*   *Arthropathy in hypersensitivity reactions classified elsewhere*
       Code first underlying disease, such as:
         Henoch (-Schönlein) purpura (D69.0)
         serum sickness (T80.6-)

▶ *M36.8*   *Systemic disorders of connective tissue in other diseases classified elsewhere* 🅒
       Code first underlying disease, such as:
         alkaptonuria (E70.2)
         hypogammaglobulinemia (D80.-)
         ochronosis (E70.2)

DORSOPATHIES (M40-M54)

DEFORMING DORSOPATHIES (M40-M43)

● **M40**   Kyphosis and lordosis

     Excludes1   congenital kyphosis and lordosis (Q76.4)
                kyphoscoliosis (M41.-)
                postprocedural kyphosis and lordosis (M96.-)

▶ *Code first underlying disease*

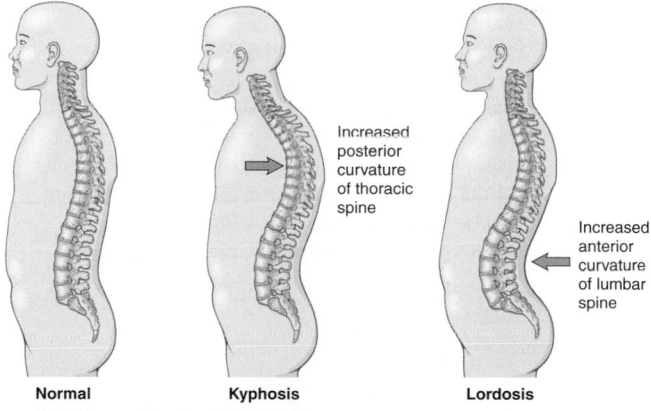

Normal   Kyphosis   Lordosis

Figure 13-5   Kyphosis, Lordosis, Scoliosis. (From Chabner: The Language of Medicine, ed 8, St. Louis, Saunders, 2007)

Item 13–9   **Kyphosis** is an abnormal curvature of the spine. **Senile kyphosis** is a result of disc degeneration causing ossification (turning to bone). **Adolescent** or **juvenile** kyphosis is also known as **Scheuermann's disease,** a condition in which the discs of the lower thoracic spine herniate, causing the disc space to narrow and the spine to tilt forward. This condition is attributed to poor posture. **Lordosis or swayback** is an abnormal curvature of the spine resulting in an inward curve of the lumbar spine just above the buttocks. **Scoliosis** causes a sideways curve to the spine. The curves are S- or C-shaped, and it is most commonly acquired in late childhood and early teen years, when growth is fast.

N Newborn Age: 0   **P** Pediatric Age: 0–17   **M** Maternity DX: 9–64   **A** Adult Age: 15–124   ♀ Females Only   ♂ Males Only

🅒 Complication\Comorbidity   🅒 Major C\C   Ⓔⓧ CC/MCC Exclusions   🅒 Hospital-Acquired Condition   🅒 Hierarchical Condition Category

1059

CHAPTER 13 (M00-M99)

CHAPTER 13 (M00-M99)

● M40.0 **Postural kyphosis**
  Excludes1 osteochondrosis of spine (M42.-)
  M40.00 Postural kyphosis, site unspecified
  M40.03 Postural kyphosis, cervicothoracic region
  M40.04 Postural kyphosis, thoracic region
  M40.05 Postural kyphosis, thoracolumbar region
● M40.1 **Other secondary kyphosis**
  M40.10 Other secondary kyphosis, site unspecified
  M40.12 Other secondary kyphosis, cervical region
  M40.13 Other secondary kyphosis, cervicothoracic region
  M40.14 Other secondary kyphosis, thoracic region
  M40.15 Other secondary kyphosis, thoracolumbar region
● M40.2 Other and unspecified kyphosis
  ● M40.20 **Unspecified kyphosis**
    M40.202 Unspecified kyphosis, cervical region
    M40.203 Unspecified kyphosis, cervicothoracic region
    M40.204 Unspecified kyphosis, thoracic region
    M40.205 Unspecified kyphosis, thoracolumbar region
    M40.209 Unspecified kyphosis, site unspecified
  ● M40.29 **Other kyphosis**
    M40.292 Other kyphosis, cervical region
    M40.293 Other kyphosis, cervicothoracic region
    M40.294 Other kyphosis, thoracic region
    M40.295 Other kyphosis, thoracolumbar region
    M40.299 Other kyphosis, site unspecified
● M40.3 **Flatback** syndrome
  M40.30 Flatback syndrome, site unspecified
  M40.35 Flatback syndrome, thoracolumbar region
  M40.36 Flatback syndrome, lumbar region
  M40.37 Flatback syndrome, lumbosacral region
● M40.4 **Postural lordosis**
    Abnormal increase in the normal curvature of the lumbar spine (sway back)
    Acquired lordosis
  M40.40 Postural lordosis, site unspecified
  M40.45 Postural lordosis, thoracolumbar region
  M40.46 Postural lordosis, lumbar region
  M40.47 Postural lordosis, lumbosacral region
● M40.5 **Lordosis, unspecified**
  M40.50 Lordosis, unspecified, site unspecified
  M40.55 Lordosis, unspecified, thoracolumbar region
  M40.56 Lordosis, unspecified, lumbar region
  M40.57 Lordosis, unspecified, lumbosacral region
● M41 Scoliosis
  Includes kyphoscoliosis
  Excludes1 congenital scoliosis NOS (Q67.5)
    congenital scoliosis due to bony malformation (Q76.3)
    postural congenital scoliosis (Q67.5)
    kyphoscoliotic heart disease (I27.1)
    postprocedural scoliosis (M96.-)
  ▶ **Excludes2** postprocedural scoliosis (M96.-)
● M41.0 **Infantile idiopathic scoliosis**
  M41.00 Infantile idiopathic scoliosis, site unspecified
  M41.02 Infantile idiopathic scoliosis, cervical region
  M41.03 Infantile idiopathic scoliosis, cervicothoracic region
  M41.04 Infantile idiopathic scoliosis, thoracic region
  M41.05 Infantile idiopathic scoliosis, thoracolumbar region
  M41.06 Infantile idiopathic scoliosis, lumbar region

M41.07 Infantile idiopathic scoliosis, lumbosacral region
M41.08 Infantile idiopathic scoliosis, sacral and sacrococcygeal region
● M41.1 Juvenile and adolescent idiopathic scoliosis
  ● M41.11 Juvenile idiopathic scoliosis
    M41.112 Juvenile idiopathic scoliosis, cervical region
    M41.113 Juvenile idiopathic scoliosis, cervicothoracic region
    M41.114 Juvenile idiopathic scoliosis, thoracic region
    M41.115 Juvenile idiopathic scoliosis, thoracolumbar region
    M41.116 Juvenile idiopathic scoliosis, lumbar region
    M41.117 Juvenile idiopathic scoliosis, lumbosacral region
    M41.119 Juvenile idiopathic scoliosis, site unspecified
  ● M41.12 Adolescent scoliosis
    M41.122 Adolescent idiopathic scoliosis, cervical region
    M41.123 Adolescent idiopathic scoliosis, cervicothoracic region
    M41.124 Adolescent idiopathic scoliosis, thoracic region
    M41.125 Adolescent idiopathic scoliosis, thoracolumbar region
    M41.126 Adolescent idiopathic scoliosis, lumbar region
    M41.127 Adolescent idiopathic scoliosis, lumbosacral region
    M41.129 Adolescent idiopathic scoliosis, site unspecified
● M41.2 **Other idiopathic** scoliosis
  M41.20 Other idiopathic scoliosis, site unspecified
  M41.22 Other idiopathic scoliosis, cervical region
  M41.23 Other idiopathic scoliosis, cervicothoracic region
  M41.24 Other idiopathic scoliosis, thoracic region
  M41.25 Other idiopathic scoliosis, thoracolumbar region
  M41.26 Other idiopathic scoliosis, lumbar region
  M41.27 Other idiopathic scoliosis, lumbosacral region
● M41.3 **Thoracogenic** scoliosis
  M41.30 Thoracogenic scoliosis, site unspecified
  M41.34 Thoracogenic scoliosis, thoracic region
  M41.35 Thoracogenic scoliosis, thoracolumbar region
● M41.4 **Neuromuscular** scoliosis
    Scoliosis secondary to cerebral palsy, Friedreich's ataxia, poliomyelitis and other neuromuscular disorders
    Code also underlying condition
  M41.40 Neuromuscular scoliosis, site unspecified
  M41.41 **Neuromuscular scoliosis, occipito-atlanto-axial region**
  M41.42 Neuromuscular scoliosis, cervical region
  M41.43 Neuromuscular scoliosis, cervicothoracic region
  M41.44 Neuromuscular scoliosis, thoracic region
  M41.45 Neuromuscular scoliosis, thoracolumbar region
  M41.46 Neuromuscular scoliosis, lumbar region
  M41.47 Neuromuscular scoliosis, lumbosacral region
● M41.5 **Other secondary scoliosis**
    Coding Clinic: 2019, Q1, P19
    ▶ *Code first underlying disease*
  M41.50 Other secondary scoliosis, site unspecified
  M41.52 Other secondary scoliosis, cervical region
  M41.53 Other secondary scoliosis, cervicothoracic region

▶ New ⇒ Revised ~~deleted~~ Deleted `Excludes 1` `Excludes 2` `Includes` Use additional Code first Code also `Key words`
OGCR Official Guidelines ● Unacceptable Principal Diagnosis X Assign placeholder X ● Use Additional Character(s) ▶ Manifestation Code **Coding Clinic**

M41.54   Other secondary scoliosis, thoracic region
M41.55   Other secondary scoliosis, thoracolumbar region
M41.56   Other secondary scoliosis, lumbar region
M41.57   Other secondary scoliosis, lumbosacral region
● M41.8   **Other forms of scoliosis**
M41.80   Other forms of scoliosis, site unspecified
M41.82   Other forms of scoliosis, cervical region
M41.83   Other forms of scoliosis, cervicothoracic region
M41.84   Other forms of scoliosis, thoracic region
M41.85   Other forms of scoliosis, thoracolumbar region
M41.86   Other forms of scoliosis, lumbar region
M41.87   Other forms of scoliosis, lumbosacral region
M41.9   Scoliosis, unspecified
● **M42**   **Spinal osteochondrosis**
● M42.0   **Juvenile osteochondrosis of spine**
Calvé's disease
Scheuermann's disease

Excludes1   postural kyphosis (M40.0)

M42.00   Juvenile osteochondrosis of spine, site unspecified
M42.01   Juvenile osteochondrosis of spine, occipito-atlanto-axial region
M42.02   Juvenile osteochondrosis of spine, cervical region
M42.03   Juvenile osteochondrosis of spine, cervicothoracic region
M42.04   Juvenile osteochondrosis of spine, thoracic region
M42.05   Juvenile osteochondrosis of spine, thoracolumbar region
M42.06   Juvenile osteochondrosis of spine, lumbar region
M42.07   Juvenile osteochondrosis of spine, lumbosacral region
M42.08   Juvenile osteochondrosis of spine, sacral and sacrococcygeal region
M42.09   Juvenile osteochondrosis of spine, multiple sites in spine
● M42.1   **Adult osteochondrosis of spine**
M42.10   Adult osteochondrosis of spine, site unspecified   A
M42.11   Adult osteochondrosis of spine, occipitoatlanto-axial region   A
M42.12   Adult osteochondrosis of spine, cervical region   A
M42.13   Adult osteochondrosis of spine, cervicothoracic region   A
M42.14   Adult osteochondrosis of spine, thoracic region   A
M42.15   Adult osteochondrosis of spine, thoracolumbar region   A
M42.16   Adult osteochondrosis of spine, lumbar region   A
M42.17   Adult osteochondrosis of spine, lumbosacral region   A
M42.18   Adult osteochondrosis of spine, sacral and sacrococcygeal region   A
M42.19   Adult osteochondrosis of spine, multiple sites in spine   A
M42.9   Spinal osteochondrosis, unspecified
● **M43**   **Other deforming dorsopathies**

Excludes1   congenital spondylolysis and spondylolisthesis (Q76.2)
hemivertebra (Q76.3-Q76.4)
Klippel-Feil syndrome (Q76.1)
lumbarization and sacralization (Q76.4)
platyspondylisis (Q76.4)
spina bifida occulta (Q76.0)
spinal curvature in osteoporosis (M80.-)
spinal curvature in Paget's disease of bone [osteitis deformans] (M88.-)

Item 13–10   **Spondylolisthesis** is a condition caused by the slipping forward of one disc over another.

● M43.0   **Spondylolysis**

Excludes1   congenital spondylolysis (Q76.2)
spondylolisthesis (M43.1)

M43.00   Spondylolysis, site unspecified
M43.01   Spondylolysis, occipito-atlanto-axial region
M43.02   Spondylolysis, cervical region
M43.03   Spondylolysis, cervicothoracic region
M43.04   Spondylolysis, thoracic region
M43.05   Spondylolysis, thoracolumbar region
M43.06   Spondylolysis, lumbar region
M43.07   Spondylolysis, lumbosacral region
M43.08   Spondylolysis, sacral and sacrococcygeal region
M43.09   Spondylolysis, multiple sites in spine
● M43.1   **Spondylolisthesis**

Excludes1   acute traumatic of lumbosacral region (S33.1)
acute traumatic of sites other than lumbosacral - code to Fracture, vertebra, by region
congenital spondylolisthesis (Q76.2)

M43.10   Spondylolisthesis, site unspecified
M43.11   Spondylolisthesis, occipito-atlanto-axial region
M43.12   Spondylolisthesis, cervical region
M43.13   Spondylolisthesis, cervicothoracic region
M43.14   Spondylolisthesis, thoracic region
M43.15   Spondylolisthesis, thoracolumbar region
M43.16   Spondylolisthesis, lumbar region
M43.17   Spondylolisthesis, lumbosacral region
M43.18   Spondylolisthesis, sacral and sacrococcygeal region
M43.19   Spondylolisthesis, multiple sites in spine
● M43.2   **Fusion of spine**
Ankylosis of spinal joint

Excludes1   ankylosing spondylitis (M45.0-)
congenital fusion of spine (Q76.4)

Excludes2   arthrodesis status (Z98.1)
pseudoarthrosis after fusion or arthrodesis (M96.0)

M43.20   Fusion of spine, site unspecified
M43.21   Fusion of spine, occipito-atlanto-axial region
M43.22   Fusion of spine, cervical region
M43.23   Fusion of spine, cervicothoracic region
M43.24   Fusion of spine, thoracic region
M43.25   Fusion of spine, thoracolumbar region
M43.26   Fusion of spine, lumbar region
M43.27   Fusion of spine, lumbosacral region
M43.28   Fusion of spine, sacral and sacrococcygeal region
M43.3   Recurrent atlantoaxial dislocation with myelopathy
M43.4   Other recurrent atlantoaxial dislocation
● M43.5   **Other recurrent vertebral dislocation**

Excludes1   biomechanical lesions NEC (M99.-)

● M43.5X   **Other recurrent vertebral dislocation**
M43.5X2   Other recurrent vertebral dislocation, cervical region
M43.5X3   Other recurrent vertebral dislocation, cervicothoracic region
M43.5X4   Other recurrent vertebral dislocation, thoracic region
M43.5X5   Other recurrent vertebral dislocation, thoracolumbar region
M43.5X6   Other recurrent vertebral dislocation, lumbar region
M43.5X7   Other recurrent vertebral dislocation, lumbosacral region
M43.5X8   Other recurrent vertebral dislocation, sacral and sacrococcygeal region
M43.5X9   Other recurrent vertebral dislocation, site unspecified

CHAPTER 13 (M00-M99)

N Newborn Age: 0   **P** Pediatric Age: 0–17   **M** Maternity DX: 9–64   **A** Adult Age: 15–124   ♀ Females Only   ♂ Males Only

Complication\Comorbidity   Major C\C   (Ex) CC/MCC Exclusions   Hospital-Acquired Condition   Hierarchical Condition Category

M43.6 Torticollis

Excludes1   congenital (sternomastoid) torticollis (Q68.0)
current injury - see Injury, of spine, by body region ocular torticollis (R29.891)
psychogenic torticollis (F45.8)
spasmodic torticollis (G24.3)
torticollis due to birth injury (P15.2)

M43.8 Other specified deforming dorsopathies

Excludes2   kyphosis and lordosis (M40.-)
scoliosis (M41.-)

M43.8X Other specified deforming dorsopathies

M43.8X1 Other specified deforming dorsopathies, occipito-atlanto-axial region

M43.8X2 Other specified deforming dorsopathies, cervical region

M43.8X3 Other specified deforming dorsopathies, cervicothoracic region

M43.8X4 Other specified deforming dorsopathies, thoracic region

M43.8X5 Other specified deforming dorsopathies, thoracolumbar region

M43.8X6 Other specified deforming dorsopathies, lumbar region

M43.8X7 Other specified deforming dorsopathies, lumbosacral region

M43.8X8 Other specified deforming dorsopathies, sacral and sacrococcygeal region

M43.8X9 Other specified deforming dorsopathies, site unspecified

M43.9 Deforming dorsopathy, unspecified
Curvature of spine NOS

SPONDYLOPATHIES (M45-M49)

M45 Ankylosing spondylitis
Rheumatoid arthritis of spine

Excludes1   arthropathy in Reiter's disease (M02.3-)
juvenile (ankylosing) spondylitis (M08.1)

Excludes2   Behçet's disease (M35.2)

M45.0 Ankylosing spondylitis of multiple sites in spine

M45.1 Ankylosing spondylitis of occipito-atlanto-axial region

M45.2 Ankylosing spondylitis of cervical region

M45.3 Ankylosing spondylitis of cervicothoracic region

M45.4 Ankylosing spondylitis of thoracic region

M45.5 Ankylosing spondylitis of thoracolumbar region

M45.6 Ankylosing spondylitis lumbar region

M45.7 Ankylosing spondylitis of lumbosacral region

M45.8 Ankylosing spondylitis sacral and sacrococcygeal region

M45.9 Ankylosing spondylitis of unspecified sites in spine

M45.A Non-radiographic axial spondyloarthritis

M45.A0 Non-radiographic axial spondyloarthritis of unspecified sites in spine

M45.A1 Non-radiographic axial spondyloarthritis of occipito-atlanto-axial region

M45.A2 Non-radiographic axial spondyloarthritis of cervical region

M45.A3 Non-radiographic axial spondyloarthritis of cervicothoracic region

M45.A4 Non-radiographic axial spondyloarthritis of thoracic region

M45.A5 Non-radiographic axial spondyloarthritis of thoracolumbar region

M45.A6 Non-radiographic axial spondyloarthritis of lumbar region

M45.A7 Non-radiographic axial spondyloarthritis of lumbosacral region

M45.A8 Non-radiographic axial spondyloarthritis of sacral and sacrococcygeal region

M45.AB Non-radiographic axial spondyloarthritis of multiple sites in spine

M46 Other inflammatory spondylopathies

M46.0 Spinal enthesopathy
Disorder of ligamentous or muscular attachments of spine

M46.00 Spinal enthesopathy, site unspecified

M46.01 Spinal enthesopathy, occipito-atlanto-axial region

M46.02 Spinal enthesopathy, cervical region

M46.03 Spinal enthesopathy, cervicothoracic region

M46.04 Spinal enthesopathy, thoracic region

M46.05 Spinal enthesopathy, thoracolumbar region

M46.06 Spinal enthesopathy, lumbar region

M46.07 Spinal enthesopathy, lumbosacral region

M46.08 Spinal enthesopathy, sacral and sacrococcygeal region

M46.09 Spinal enthesopathy, multiple sites in spine

M46.1 Sacroiliitis, not elsewhere classified

M46.2 Osteomyelitis of vertebra
(Ex) For category M46.2 CC codes: See PDX Collection 881

M46.20 Osteomyelitis of vertebra, site unspecified

M46.21 Osteomyelitis of vertebra, occipito-atlanto-axial region

M46.22 Osteomyelitis of vertebra, cervical region

M46.23 Osteomyelitis of vertebra, cervicothoracic region

M46.24 Osteomyelitis of vertebra, thoracic region

M46.25 Osteomyelitis of vertebra, thoracolumbar region

M46.26 Osteomyelitis of vertebra, lumbar region

M46.27 Osteomyelitis of vertebra, lumbosacral region

M46.28 Osteomyelitis of vertebra, sacral and sacrococcygeal region

M46.3 Infection of intervertebral disc (pyogenic)
Use additional code (B95-B97) to identify infectious agent
(Ex) For category M46.3 CC codes: See PDX Collection 882

M46.30 Infection of intervertebral disc (pyogenic), site unspecified

M46.31 Infection of intervertebral disc (pyogenic), occipito-atlanto-axial region

M46.32 Infection of intervertebral disc (pyogenic), cervical region

M46.33 Infection of intervertebral disc (pyogenic), cervicothoracic region

M46.34 Infection of intervertebral disc (pyogenic), thoracic region

M46.35 Infection of intervertebral disc (pyogenic), thoracolumbar region

M46.36 Infection of intervertebral disc (pyogenic), lumbar region

M46.37 Infection of intervertebral disc (pyogenic), lumbosacral region

M46.38 Infection of intervertebral disc (pyogenic), sacral and sacrococcygeal region

M46.39 Infection of intervertebral disc (pyogenic), multiple sites in spine

M46.4 Discitis, unspecified

M46.40 Discitis, unspecified, site unspecified

M46.41 Discitis, unspecified, occipito-atlanto-axial region

M46.42 Discitis, unspecified, cervical region

M46.43 Discitis, unspecified, cervicothoracic region

M46.44 Discitis, unspecified, thoracic region

M46.45 Discitis, unspecified, thoracolumbar region

M46.46 Discitis, unspecified, lumbar region

M46.47 Discitis, unspecified, lumbosacral region

M46.48 Discitis, unspecified, sacral and sacrococcygeal region

M46.49 Discitis, unspecified, multiple sites in spine

- M46.5   Other infective spondylopathies
  - M46.50   Other infective spondylopathies, site unspecified 🦠
  - M46.51   Other infective spondylopathies, occipitoatlanto-axial region 🦠
  - M46.52   Other infective spondylopathies, cervical region 🦠
  - M46.53   Other infective spondylopathies, cervicothoracic region 🦠
  - M46.54   Other infective spondylopathies, thoracic region 🦠
  - M46.55   Other infective spondylopathies, thoracolumbar region 🦠
  - M46.56   Other infective spondylopathies, lumbar region 🦠
  - M46.57   Other infective spondylopathies, lumbosacral region 🦠
  - M46.58   Other infective spondylopathies, sacral and sacrococcygeal region 🦠
  - M46.59   Other infective spondylopathies, multiple sites in spine 🦠
- M46.8   Other specified inflammatory spondylopathies
  - M46.80   Other specified inflammatory spondylopathies, site unspecified 🦠
  - M46.81   Other specified inflammatory spondylopathies, occipito-atlanto-axial region 🦠
  - M46.82   Other specified inflammatory spondylopathies, cervical region 🦠
  - M46.83   Other specified inflammatory spondylopathies, cervicothoracic region 🦠
  - M46.84   Other specified inflammatory spondylopathies, thoracic region 🦠
  - M46.85   Other specified inflammatory spondylopathies, thoracolumbar region 🦠
  - M46.86   Other specified inflammatory spondylopathies, lumbar region 🦠
  - M46.87   Other specified inflammatory spondylopathies, lumbosacral region 🦠
  - M46.88   Other specified inflammatory spondylopathies, sacral and sacrococcygeal region 🦠
  - M46.89   Other specified inflammatory spondylopathies, multiple sites in spine 🦠
- M46.9   Unspecified inflammatory spondylopathy
  - M46.90   Unspecified inflammatory spondylopathy, site unspecified 🦠
  - M46.91   Unspecified inflammatory spondylopathy, occipito-atlanto-axial region 🦠
  - M46.92   Unspecified inflammatory spondylopathy, cervical region 🦠
    Coding Clinic: 2019, Q3, P10
  - M46.93   Unspecified inflammatory spondylopathy, cervicothoracic region 🦠
  - M46.94   Unspecified inflammatory spondylopathy, thoracic region 🦠
  - M46.95   Unspecified inflammatory spondylopathy, thoracolumbar region 🦠
  - M46.96   Unspecified inflammatory spondylopathy, lumbar region 🦠
  - M46.97   Unspecified inflammatory spondylopathy, lumbosacral region 🦠
  - M46.98   Unspecified inflammatory spondylopathy, sacral and sacrococcygeal region 🦠
  - M46.99   Unspecified inflammatory spondylopathy, multiple sites in spine 🦠
- M47   Spondylosis
  - **Includes**   arthrosis or osteoarthritis of spine
    degeneration of facet joints
  - M47.0   Anterior spinal and vertebral artery compression syndromes
    (Ex:) **For category M47.0 CC codes: See PDX Collection 883**
    Coding Clinic: 2019, Q3, P10

- M47.01   Anterior spinal artery compression syndromes
  - M47.011   Anterior spinal artery compression syndromes, occipito-atlanto-axial region 🦠
  - M47.012   Anterior spinal artery compression syndromes, cervical region 🦠
  - M47.013   Anterior spinal artery compression syndromes, cervicothoracic region 🦠
  - M47.014   Anterior spinal artery compression syndromes, thoracic region 🦠
  - M47.015   Anterior spinal artery compression syndromes, thoracolumbar region 🦠
  - M47.016   Anterior spinal artery compression syndromes, lumbar region 🦠
  - M47.019   Anterior spinal artery compression syndromes, site unspecified 🦠
- M47.02   Vertebral artery compression syndromes
  - M47.021   Vertebral artery compression syndromes, occipito-atlanto-axial region 🦠
  - M47.022   Vertebral artery compression syndromes, cervical region 🦠
  - M47.029   Vertebral artery compression syndromes, site unspecified 🦠
- M47.1   Other spondylosis with myelopathy
  Spondylogenic compression of spinal cord
  Excludes1   vertebral subluxation (M43.3-M43.5X9)
  - M47.10   Other spondylosis with myelopathy, site unspecified 🦠
    (Ex:) See PDX Collection 884
  - M47.11   Other spondylosis with myelopathy, occipito-atlanto-axial region 🦠
    (Ex:) See PDX Collection 883
  - M47.12   Other spondylosis with myelopathy, cervical region 🦠
    (Ex:) See PDX Collection 883
    Coding Clinic: 2020, Q1, P17
  - M47.13   Other spondylosis with myelopathy, cervicothoracic region 🦠
    (Ex:) See PDX Collection 883
  - M47.14   Other spondylosis with myelopathy, thoracic region 🦠
    (Ex:) See PDX Collection 885
  - M47.15   Other spondylosis with myelopathy, thoracolumbar region 🦠
    (Ex:) See PDX Collection 885
  - M47.16   Other spondylosis with myelopathy, lumbar region 🦠
    (Ex:) See PDX Collection 886
- M47.2   Other spondylosis with radiculopathy
  - M47.20   Other spondylosis with radiculopathy, site unspecified
  - M47.21   Other spondylosis with radiculopathy, occipito-atlanto-axial region
  - M47.22   Other spondylosis with radiculopathy, cervical region
    Coding Clinic: 2020, Q1, P17
  - M47.23   Other spondylosis with radiculopathy, cervicothoracic region
  - M47.24   Other spondylosis with radiculopathy, thoracic region
  - M47.25   Other spondylosis with radiculopathy, thoracolumbar region
  - M47.26   Other spondylosis with radiculopathy, lumbar region
  - M47.27   Other spondylosis with radiculopathy, lumbosacral region
  - M47.28   Other spondylosis with radiculopathy, sacral and sacrococcygeal region

N Newborn Age: 0   **P** Pediatric Age: 0–17   **M** Maternity DX: 9–64   **A** Adult Age: 15–124   ♀ Females Only   ♂ Males Only

🦠 Complication\Comorbidity   🦠 Major C\C   (Ex:) CC/MCC Exclusions   🦠 Hospital-Acquired Condition   🦠 Hierarchical Condition Category

1063

CHAPTER 13 (M00-M99)

CHAPTER 13 (M00-M99)

● M47.8   Other spondylosis
  ● M47.81   Spondylosis without myelopathy or radiculopathy
    M47.811   Spondylosis without myelopathy or radiculopathy, occipito-atlanto-axial region
    M47.812   Spondylosis without myelopathy or radiculopathy, cervical region
          Coding Clinic: 2019, Q3, P10-11; 2018, Q2, P15
    M47.813   Spondylosis without myelopathy or radiculopathy, cervicothoracic region
    M47.814   Spondylosis without myelopathy or radiculopathy, thoracic region
    M47.815   Spondylosis without myelopathy or radiculopathy, thoracolumbar region
    M47.816   Spondylosis without myelopathy or radiculopathy, lumbar region
    M47.817   Spondylosis without myelopathy or radiculopathy, lumbosacral region
    M47.818   Spondylosis without myelopathy or radiculopathy, sacral and sacrococcygeal region
    M47.819   Spondylosis without myelopathy or radiculopathy, site unspecified
  ● M47.89   Other spondylosis
    M47.891   Other spondylosis, occipito-atlanto-axial region
    M47.892   Other spondylosis, cervical region
    M47.893   Other spondylosis, cervicothoracic region
    M47.894   Other spondylosis, thoracic region
    M47.895   Other spondylosis, thoracolumbar region
    M47.896   Other spondylosis, lumbar region
    M47.897   Other spondylosis, lumbosacral region
    M47.898   Other spondylosis, sacral and sacrococcygeal region
    M47.899   Other spondylosis, site unspecified
  M47.9   Spondylosis, unspecified

● M48   Other spondylopathies
  ● M48.0   Spinal stenosis
       Caudal stenosis
    M48.00   Spinal stenosis, site unspecified
    M48.01   Spinal stenosis, occipito-atlanto-axial region
    M48.02   Spinal stenosis, cervical region
          Coding Clinic: 2020, Q1, P17
    M48.03   Spinal stenosis, cervicothoracic region
    M48.04   Spinal stenosis, thoracic region
    M48.05   Spinal stenosis, thoracolumbar region
    ● M48.06   Spinal stenosis, lumbar region
          Coding Clinic: 2017, Q3, P24
      M48.061   Spinal stenosis, lumbar region without neurogenic claudication
           Spinal stenosis, lumbar region NOS
      M48.062   Spinal stenosis, lumbar region with neurogenic claudication
           Coding Clinic: 2017, Q4, P19
    M48.07   Spinal stenosis, lumbosacral region
    M48.08   Spinal stenosis, sacral and sacrococcygeal region
  ● M48.1   Ankylosing hyperostosis [Forestier]
       Diffuse idiopathic skeletal hyperostosis [DISH]
    M48.10   Ankylosing hyperostosis [Forestier], site unspecified
    M48.11   Ankylosing hyperostosis [Forestier], occipito-atlanto-axial region
    M48.12   Ankylosing hyperostosis [Forestier], cervical region
    M48.13   Ankylosing hyperostosis [Forestier], cervicothoracic region

M48.14   Ankylosing hyperostosis [Forestier], thoracic region
M48.15   Ankylosing hyperostosis [Forestier], thoracolumbar region
M48.16   Ankylosing hyperostosis [Forestier], lumbar region
M48.17   Ankylosing hyperostosis [Forestier], lumbosacral region
M48.18   Ankylosing hyperostosis [Forestier], sacral and sacrococcygeal region
M48.19   Ankylosing hyperostosis [Forestier], multiple sites in spine
● M48.2   Kissing spine
  M48.20   Kissing spine, site unspecified
  M48.21   Kissing spine, occipito-atlanto-axial region
  M48.22   Kissing spine, cervical region
  M48.23   Kissing spine, cervicothoracic region
  M48.24   Kissing spine, thoracic region
  M48.25   Kissing spine, thoracolumbar region
  M48.26   Kissing spine, lumbar region
  M48.27   Kissing spine, lumbosacral region
● M48.3   Traumatic spondylopathy
  Ex: **For category M48.3 CC codes:** See PDX Collection 887
  M48.30   Traumatic spondylopathy, site unspecified
  M48.31   Traumatic spondylopathy, occipito-atlanto-axial region
  M48.32   Traumatic spondylopathy, cervical region
  M48.33   Traumatic spondylopathy, cervicothoracic region
  M48.34   Traumatic spondylopathy, thoracic region
  M48.35   Traumatic spondylopathy, thoracolumbar region
  M48.36   Traumatic spondylopathy, lumbar region
  M48.37   Traumatic spondylopathy, lumbosacral region
  M48.38   Traumatic spondylopathy, sacral and sacrococcygeal region
● M48.4   Fatigue fracture of vertebra
  Stress fracture of vertebra
  Excludes1   pathological fracture NOS (M84.4-)
      pathological fracture of vertebra due to neoplasm (M84.58)
      pathological fracture of vertebra due to other diagnosis (M84.68)
      pathological fracture of vertebra due to osteoporosis (M80.-)
      traumatic fracture of vertebrae (S12.0-S12.3-, S22.0-, S32.0-)
  The appropriate 7th character is to be added to each code from subcategory M48.4:

A	initial encounter for fracture
D	subsequent encounter for fracture with routine healing
G	subsequent encounter for fracture with delayed healing
S	sequela of fracture

X ● M48.40   Fatigue fracture of vertebra, site unspecified
X ● M48.41   Fatigue fracture of vertebra, occipitoatlanto-axial region
X ● M48.42   Fatigue fracture of vertebra, cervical region
X ● M48.43   Fatigue fracture of vertebra, cervicothoracic region
X ● M48.44   Fatigue fracture of vertebra, thoracic region
X ● M48.45   Fatigue fracture of vertebra, thoracolumbar region
X ● M48.46   Fatigue fracture of vertebra, lumbar region
X ● M48.47   Fatigue fracture of vertebra, lumbosacral region
X ● M48.48   Fatigue fracture of vertebra, sacral and sacrococcygeal region

▶ New   ⇒ Revised   ~~deleted~~ Deleted   Excludes 1   Excludes 2   Includes   Use additional   Code first   Code also   Key words
OGCR Official Guidelines   ● Unacceptable Principal Diagnosis   X Assign placeholder X   ▶ Use Additional Character(s)   ▶ Manifestation Code   **Coding Clinic**

● **M48.5   Collapsed vertebra, not elsewhere classified**
     Collapsed vertebra NOS
     Compression fracture of vertebra NOS
     Wedging of vertebra NOS

     Excludes1   current injury - see Injury of spine, by
                 body region
                 fatigue fracture of vertebra (M48.4)
                 pathological fracture of vertebra due to
                 neoplasm (M84.58)
                 pathological fracture of vertebra due to
                 other diagnosis (M84.68)
                 pathological fracture of vertebra due to
                 osteoporosis (M80.-)
                 pathological fracture NOS (M84.4-)
                 stress fracture of vertebra (M48.4-)
                 traumatic fracture of vertebra (S12.-, S22.-,
                 S32.-)

     The appropriate 7th character is to be added to each
     code from subcategory M48.5:

> | | |
> |---|---|
> | A | initial encounter for fracture |
> | D | subsequent encounter for fracture with routine healing |
> | G | subsequent encounter for fracture with delayed healing |
> | S | sequela of fracture |

     (Ex) For category **M48.5** CC codes: See PDX Collection 888

X ● **M48.50   Collapsed vertebra, not elsewhere classified,**
        site unspecified A 🦠, A 🦠

X ● **M48.51   Collapsed vertebra, not elsewhere classified,**
        occipito-atlanto-axial region A 🦠, A 🦠

X ● **M48.52   Collapsed vertebra, not elsewhere classified,**
        cervical region A 🦠, A 🦠

X ● **M48.53   Collapsed vertebra, not elsewhere classified,**
        cervicothoracic region A 🦠, A 🦠

X ● **M48.54   Collapsed vertebra, not elsewhere classified,**
        thoracic region A 🦠, A 🦠

X ● **M48.55   Collapsed vertebra, not elsewhere classified,**
        thoracolumbar region A 🦠, A 🦠

X ● **M48.56   Collapsed vertebra, not elsewhere classified,**
        lumbar region A 🦠, A 🦠

X ● **M48.57   Collapsed vertebra, not elsewhere classified,**
        lumbosacral region A 🦠, A 🦠

X ● **M48.58   Collapsed vertebra, not elsewhere classified,**
        sacral and sacrococcygeal region A 🦠, A 🦠

● **M48.8   Other specified spondylopathies**
     Ossification of posterior longitudinal ligament

     ● **M48.8X   Other specified spondylopathies**

         M48.8X1   Other specified spondylopathies,
                 occipito-atlanto-axial region 🦠

         M48.8X2   Other specified spondylopathies,
                 cervical region 🦠

         M48.8X3   Other specified spondylopathies,
                 cervicothoracic region 🦠

         M48.8X4   Other specified spondylopathies,
                 thoracic region 🦠

         M48.8X5   Other specified spondylopathies,
                 thoracolumbar region 🦠

         M48.8X6   Other specified spondylopathies,
                 lumbar region 🦠

         M48.8X7   Other specified spondylopathies,
                 lumbosacral region 🦠

         M48.8X8   Other specified spondylopathies,
                 sacral and sacrococcygeal region 🦠

         M48.8X9   Other specified spondylopathies, site
                 unspecified 🦠

     M48.9   Spondylopathy, unspecified

● **M49   Spondylopathies in diseases classified elsewhere**

     Includes   curvature of spine in diseases classified elsewhere
                deformity of spine in diseases classified elsewhere
                kyphosis in diseases classified elsewhere
                scoliosis in diseases classified elsewhere
                spondylopathy in diseases classified elsewhere

     Code first underlying disease, such as:
     brucellosis (A23.-)
     Charcot-Marie-Tooth disease (G60.0)
     enterobacterial infections (A01-A04)
     osteitis fibrosa cystica (E21.0)

     Excludes1   curvature of spine in tuberculosis [Pott's] (A18.01)
                enteropathic arthropathies (M07.-)
                gonococcal spondylitis (A54.41)
                neuropathic [tabes dorsalis] spondylitis (A52.11)
                neuropathic spondylopathy in syringomyelia
                (G95.0)
                neuropathic spondylopathy in tabes dorsalis
                (A52.11)
                nonsyphilitic neuropathic spondylopathy NEC
                (G98.0)
                spondylitis in syphilis (acquired) (A52.77)
                tuberculous spondylitis (A18.01)
                typhoid fever spondylitis (A01.05)

     ● **M49.8   Spondylopathy in diseases classified elsewhere**

        ▶ *M49.80   Spondylopathy in diseases classified elsewhere,*
                site unspecified 🦠

        ▶ *M49.81   Spondylopathy in diseases classified elsewhere,*
                occipito-atlanto-axial region 🦠

        ▶ *M49.82   Spondylopathy in diseases classified elsewhere,*
                cervical region 🦠

        ▶ *M49.83   Spondylopathy in diseases classified elsewhere,*
                cervicothoracic region 🦠

        ▶ *M49.84   Spondylopathy in diseases classified elsewhere,*
                thoracic region 🦠

        ▶ *M49.85   Spondylopathy in diseases classified elsewhere,*
                thoracolumbar region 🦠

        ▶ *M49.86   Spondylopathy in diseases classified elsewhere,*
                lumbar region 🦠

        ▶ *M49.87   Spondylopathy in diseases classified elsewhere,*
                lumbosacral region 🦠

        ▶ *M49.88   Spondylopathy in diseases classified elsewhere,*
                sacral and sacrococcygeal region 🦠

        ▶ *M49.89   Spondylopathy in diseases classified elsewhere,*
                multiple sites in spine 🦠

OTHER DORSOPATHIES (M50-M54)

     Excludes1   current injury - see injury of spine by body region
                discitis NOS (M46.4-)

● **M50   Cervical disc disorders**

     Note: Code to the most superior level of disorder.

     Includes   cervicothoracic disc disorders with cervicalgia
                cervicothoracic disc disorders
     Coding Clinic: 2016, Q1, P17

     ● **M50.0   Cervical disc disorder with myelopathy**
        (Ex) For category **M50.0** CC codes: See PDX Collection 889

         M50.00   Cervical disc disorder with myelopathy,
                 unspecified cervical region 🦠

         M50.01   Cervical disc disorder with myelopathy, high
                 cervical region 🦠
                 C2-C3 disc disorder with myelopathy
                 C3-C4 disc disorder with myelopathy
                 Coding Clinic: 2016, Q1, P17

        ● **M50.02   Cervical disc disorder with myelopathy,**
                 mid-cervical region
                 Coding Clinic: 2016, Q4, P39-40

                 M50.020   Cervical disc disorder with
                       myelopathy, mid-cervical region,
                       unspecified level 🦠

                 M50.021   Cervical disc disorder at C4-C5 level
                       with myelopathy 🦠
                       C4-C5 disc disorder with
                       myelopathy

N   Newborn Age: 0   **P**   Pediatric Age: 0–17   **M**   Maternity DX: 9–64   **A**   Adult Age: 15–124   ♀   Females Only   ♂   Males Only

🦠   Complication\Comorbidity   🦠   Major C\C   (Ex)   CC/MCC Exclusions   🦠   Hospital-Acquired Condition   🦠   Hierarchical Condition Category

1065

M50.022   Cervical disc disorder at C5-C6 level
with myelopathy 🖱
C5-C6 disc disorder with myelopathy

M50.023   Cervical disc disorder at C6-C7 level
with myelopathy 🖱
C6-C7 disc disorder with myelopathy

M50.03   Cervical disc disorder with myelopathy,
cervicothoracic region 🖱
C7-T1 disc disorder with myelopathy

● M50.1   Cervical disc disorder with radiculopathy

    Excludes2   brachial radiculitis NOS (M54.13)

M50.10   Cervical disc disorder with radiculopathy,
unspecified cervical region

M50.11   Cervical disc disorder with radiculopathy, high
cervical region
C2-C3 disc disorder with radiculopathy
C3 radiculopathy due to disc disorder
C3-C4 disc disorder with radiculopathy
C4 radiculopathy due to disc disorder

● M50.12   Cervical disc disorder with radiculopathy,
mid-cervical region
Coding Clinic: 2016, Q4, P39-40

M50.120   Mid-cervical disc disorder,
unspecified level

M50.121   Cervical disc disorder at C4-C5 level
with radiculopathy
C4-C5 disc disorder with
radiculopathy
C5 radiculopathy due to disc
disorder

M50.122   Cervical disc disorder at C5-C6 level
with radiculopathy
C5-C6 disc disorder with
radiculopathy
C6 radiculopathy due to disc
disorder

M50.123   Cervical disc disorder at C6-C7 level
with radiculopathy
C6-C7 disc disorder with
radiculopathy
C7 radiculopathy due to disc
disorder

M50.13   Cervical disc disorder with radiculopathy,
cervicothoracic region
C7-T1 disc disorder with radiculopathy
C8 radiculopathy due to disc disorder

● M50.2   Other cervical disc displacement
Coding Clinic: 2016, Q4, P40

M50.20   Other cervical disc displacement, unspecified
cervical region

M50.21   Other cervical disc displacement, high cervical
region
Other C2-C3 cervical disc displacement
Other C3-C4 cervical disc displacement

● M50.22   Other cervical disc displacement, mid-cervical
region

M50.220   Other cervical disc displacement,
mid-cervical region, unspecified
level

M50.221   Other cervical disc displacement at
C4-C5 level
Other C4-C5 cervical disc
displacement

M50.222   Other cervical disc displacement at
C5-C6 level
Other C5-C6 cervical disc
displacement

M50.223   Other cervical disc displacement at
C6-C7 level
Other C6-C7 cervical disc
displacement

M50.23   Other cervical disc displacement,
cervicothoracic region
Other C7-T1 cervical disc displacement

● M50.3   Other cervical disc degeneration
Coding Clinic: 2016, Q4, P40

M50.30   Other cervical disc degeneration, unspecified
cervical region

M50.31   Other cervical disc degeneration, high cervical
region
Other C2-C3 cervical disc degeneration
Other C3-C4 cervical disc degeneration

● M50.32   Other cervical disc degeneration, mid-cervical
region

M50.320   Other cervical disc degeneration,
mid-cervical region, unspecified
level

M50.321   Other cervical disc degeneration at
C4-C5 level
Other C4-C5 cervical disc
degeneration

M50.322   Other cervical disc degeneration at
C5-C6 level
Other C5-C6 cervical disc
degeneration

M50.323   Other cervical disc degeneration at
C6-C7 level
Other C6-C7 cervical disc
degeneration

M50.33   Other cervical disc degeneration,
cervicothoracic region
Other C7-T1 cervical disc degeneration

● M50.8   Other cervical disc disorders
Coding Clinic: 2016, Q4, P40

M50.80   Other cervical disc disorders, unspecified
cervical region

M50.81   Other cervical disc disorders, high cervical
region
Other C2-C3 cervical disc disorders
Other C3-C4 cervical disc disorders

● M50.82   Other cervical disc disorders, mid-cervical
region

M50.820   Other cervical disc disorders,
mid-cervical region, unspecified
level

M50.821   Other cervical disc disorders at C4-C5
level
Other C4-C5 cervical disc
disorders

M50.822   Other cervical disc disorders at C5-C6
level
Other C5-C6 cervical disc
disorders

M50.823   Other cervical disc disorders at C6-C7
level
Other C6-C7 cervical disc
disorders

M50.83   Other cervical disc disorders, cervicothoracic
region
Other C7-T1 cervical disc disorders

● M50.9   Cervical disc disorder, unspecified
     Coding Clinic: 2016, Q4, P40

   M50.90   Cervical disc disorder, unspecified, unspecified cervical region

   M50.91   Cervical disc disorder, unspecified, high cervical region
       C2-C3 cervical disc disorder, unspecified
       C3-C4 cervical disc disorder, unspecified

  ● M50.92   Cervical disc disorder, unspecified, mid-cervical region

     M50.920   Unspecified cervical disc disorder, mid-cervical region, unspecified level

     M50.921   Unspecified cervical disc disorder at C4-C5 level
         Unspecified C4-C5 cervical disc disorder

     M50.922   Unspecified cervical disc disorder at C5-C6 level
         Unspecified C5-C6 cervical disc disorder

     M50.923   Unspecified cervical disc disorder at C6-C7 level
         Unspecified C6-C7 cervical disc disorder

   M50.93   Cervical disc disorder, unspecified, cervicothoracic region
       C7-T1 cervical disc disorder, unspecified

● M51   Thoracic, thoracolumbar, and lumbosacral intervertebral disc disorders

    Excludes2   cervical and cervicothoracic disc disorders (M50.-)
           sacral and sacrococcygeal disorders (M53.3)

  ● M51.0   Thoracic, thoracolumbar and lumbosacral intervertebral disc disorders with myelopathy
     (Ex) For category M51.0 CC codes unless otherwise indicated: See PDX Collection 890

   M51.04   Intervertebral disc disorders with myelopathy, thoracic region 🆚

   M51.05   Intervertebral disc disorders with myelopathy, thoracolumbar region 🆚

   M51.06   Intervertebral disc disorders with myelopathy, lumbar region 🆚
     (Ex) See PDX Collection 891

  ● M51.1   Thoracic, thoracolumbar and lumbosacral intervertebral disc disorders with radiculopathy
     Sciatica due to intervertebral disc disorder

    Excludes1   lumbar radiculitis NOS (M54.16)
           sciatica NOS (M54.3)

   M51.14   Intervertebral disc disorders with radiculopathy, thoracic region

   M51.15   Intervertebral disc disorders with radiculopathy, thoracolumbar region

   M51.16   Intervertebral disc disorders with radiculopathy, lumbar region

   M51.17   Intervertebral disc disorders with radiculopathy, lumbosacral region

  ● M51.2   Other thoracic, thoracolumbar and lumbosacral intervertebral disc displacement
     Lumbago due to displacement of intervertebral disc

   M51.24   Other intervertebral disc displacement, thoracic region

   M51.25   Other intervertebral disc displacement, thoracolumbar region

   M51.26   Other intervertebral disc displacement, lumbar region

   M51.27   Other intervertebral disc displacement, lumbosacral region

● M51.3   Other thoracic, thoracolumbar and lumbosacral intervertebral disc degeneration
     Coding Clinic: 2013, Q3, P22

   M51.34   Other intervertebral disc degeneration, thoracic region

   M51.35   Other intervertebral disc degeneration, thoracolumbar region

   M51.36   Other intervertebral disc degeneration, lumbar region
       Coding Clinic: 2018, Q2, P15

   M51.37   Other intervertebral disc degeneration, lumbosacral region

● M51.4   Schmorl's nodes

   M51.44   Schmorl's nodes, thoracic region

   M51.45   Schmorl's nodes, thoracolumbar region

   M51.46   Schmorl's nodes, lumbar region

   M51.47   Schmorl's nodes, lumbosacral region

● M51.8   Other thoracic, thoracolumbar and lumbosacral intervertebral disc disorders

   M51.84   Other intervertebral disc disorders, thoracic region

   M51.85   Other intervertebral disc disorders, thoracolumbar region

   M51.86   Other intervertebral disc disorders, lumbar region

   M51.87   Other intervertebral disc disorders, lumbosacral region

  M51.9   Unspecified thoracic, thoracolumbar and lumbosacral intervertebral disc disorder

● M53   Other and unspecified dorsopathies, not elsewhere classified

  M53.0   Cervicocranial syndrome
     Posterior cervical sympathetic syndrome

  M53.1   Cervicobrachial syndrome

    Excludes2   cervical disc disorder (M50.-)
           thoracic outlet syndrome (G54.0)

● M53.2   Spinal instabilities

  ● M53.2X   Spinal instabilities

     M53.2X1   Spinal instabilities, occipito-atlanto-axial region

     M53.2X2   Spinal instabilities, cervical region

     M53.2X3   Spinal instabilities, cervicothoracic region

     M53.2X4   Spinal instabilities, thoracic region

     M53.2X5   Spinal instabilities, thoracolumbar region

     M53.2X6   Spinal instabilities, lumbar region

     M53.2X7   Spinal instabilities, lumbosacral region

     M53.2X8   Spinal instabilities, sacral and sacrococcygeal region

     M53.2X9   Spinal instabilities, site unspecified

  M53.3   Sacrococcygeal disorders, not elsewhere classified
     Coccygodynia

● M53.8   Other specified dorsopathies

   M53.80   Other specified dorsopathies, site unspecified

   M53.81   Other specified dorsopathies, occipito-atlanto-axial region

   M53.82   Other specified dorsopathies, cervical region

   M53.83   Other specified dorsopathies, cervicothoracic region

   M53.84   Other specified dorsopathies, thoracic region

   M53.85   Other specified dorsopathies, thoracolumbar region

   M53.86   Other specified dorsopathies, lumbar region

   M53.87   Other specified dorsopathies, lumbosacral region

   M53.88   Other specified dorsopathies, sacral and sacrococcygeal region

  M53.9   Dorsopathy, unspecified

CHAPTER 13 (M00-M99)

N   Newborn Age: 0   **P**   Pediatric Age: 0–17   **M**   Maternity DX: 9–64   **A**   Adult Age: 15–124   ♀   Females Only   ♂   Males Only

🆚   Complication\Comorbidity   🆚   Major C\C   (Ex)   CC/MCC Exclusions   🆚   Hospital-Acquired Condition   🆚   Hierarchical Condition Category

● M54   Dorsalgia
     Excludes1   psychogenic dorsalgia (F45.41)
 ● M54.0   Panniculitis affecting regions of neck and back
       Excludes1   lupus panniculitis (L93.2)
                panniculitis NOS (M79.3)
                relapsing [Weber-Christian] panniculitis
                   (M35.6)
     M54.00   Panniculitis affecting regions of neck and back, site unspecified
     M54.01   Panniculitis affecting regions of neck and back, occipito-atlanto-axial region
     M54.02   Panniculitis affecting regions of neck and back, cervical region
     M54.03   Panniculitis affecting regions of neck and back, cervicothoracic region
     M54.04   Panniculitis affecting regions of neck and back, thoracic region
     M54.05   Panniculitis affecting regions of neck and back, thoracolumbar region
     M54.06   Panniculitis affecting regions of neck and back, lumbar region
     M54.07   Panniculitis affecting regions of neck and back, lumbosacral region
     M54.08   Panniculitis affecting regions of neck and back, sacral and sacrococcygeal region
     M54.09   Panniculitis affecting regions, neck and back, multiple sites in spine

 ● M54.1   Radiculopathy
      Brachial neuritis or radiculitis NOS
      Lumbar neuritis or radiculitis NOS
      Lumbosacral neuritis or radiculitis NOS
      Thoracic neuritis or radiculitis NOS
      Radiculitis NOS
       Excludes1   neuralgia and neuritis NOS (M79.2)
               radiculopathy with cervical disc disorder
                 (M50.1)
               radiculopathy with lumbar and other
                 intervertebral disc disorder (M51.1-)
               radiculopathy with spondylosis (M47.2-)
     M54.10   Radiculopathy, site unspecified
     M54.11   Radiculopathy, occipito-atlanto-axial region
     M54.12   Radiculopathy, cervical region
     M54.13   Radiculopathy, cervicothoracic region
     M54.14   Radiculopathy, thoracic region
     M54.15   Radiculopathy, thoracolumbar region
     M54.16   Radiculopathy, lumbar region
     M54.17   Radiculopathy, lumbosacral region
     M54.18   Radiculopathy, sacral and sacrococcygeal region

   M54.2   Cervicalgia
       Excludes1   cervicalgia due to intervertebral cervical disc disorder (M50.-)

 ● M54.3   Sciatica
       Excludes1   lesion of sciatic nerve (G57.0)
               sciatica due to intervertebral disc disorder
                 (M51.1-)
               sciatica with lumbago (M54.4-)
     M54.30   Sciatica, unspecified side
     M54.31   Sciatica, right side
     M54.32   Sciatica, left side

 ● M54.4   Lumbago with sciatica
       Excludes1   lumbago with sciatica due to
               intervertebral disc disorder (M51.1-)
     M54.40   Lumbago with sciatica, unspecified side
     M54.41   Lumbago with sciatica, right side
     M54.42   Lumbago with sciatica, left side
         Coding Clinic: 2016, Q2, P7

● M54.5   Low back pain
      ~~Loin pain~~
      ~~Lumbago NOS~~
       Excludes1   low back strain (S39.012)
              lumbago due to intervertebral disc
                displacement (M51.2-)
              lumbago with sciatica (M54.4-)
  ▶ M54.50   Low back pain, unspecified
       ▶Loin pain
       ▶Lumbago NOS
  ▶ M54.51   Vertebrogenic low back pain
       ▶Low back vertebral endplate pain
  ▶ M54.59   Other low back pain
   M54.6   Pain in thoracic spine
       Excludes1   pain in thoracic spine due to
               intervertebral disc disorder (M51.)

● M54.8   Other dorsalgia
       Excludes1   dorsalgia in thoracic region (M54.6)
             ⇨low back pain (M54.5-)
     M54.81   Occipital neuralgia
     M54.89   Other dorsalgia
   M54.9   Dorsalgia, unspecified
      Backache NOS
      Back pain NOS

SOFT TISSUE DISORDERS (M60-M79)

DISORDERS OF MUSCLES (M60-M63)

   Excludes1   dermatopolymyositis (M33.-)
            muscular dystrophies and myopathies (G71-G72)
            myopathy in amyloidosis (E85.-)
            myopathy in polyarteritis nodosa (M30.0)
            myopathy in rheumatoid arthritis (M05.32)
            myopathy in scleroderma (M34.-)
            myopathy in Sjögren's syndrome (M35.03)
            myopathy in systemic lupus erythematosus
              (M32.-)

● M60   Myositis
     Excludes2   inclusion body myositis [IBM] (G72.41)
 ● M60.0   Infective myositis
      Tropical pyomyositis
      Use additional code (B95-B97) to identify infectious agent
      Ex: **For category M60.0 CC codes:** See PDX Collection 806
  ● M60.00   Infective myositis, unspecified site
     M60.000   Infective myositis, unspecified right arm 🔧
         Infective myositis, right upper limb NOS
     M60.001   Infective myositis, unspecified left arm 🔧
         Infective myositis, left upper limb NOS
     M60.002   Infective myositis, unspecified arm 🔧
         Infective myositis, upper limb NOS
     M60.003   Infective myositis, unspecified right leg 🔧
         Infective myositis, right lower limb NOS
     M60.004   Infective myositis, unspecified left leg 🔧
         Infective myositis, left lower limb NOS
     M60.005   Infective myositis, unspecified leg 🔧
         Infective myositis, lower limb NOS
     M60.009   Infective myositis, unspecified site 🔧
  ● M60.01   Infective myositis, shoulder
     M60.011   Infective myositis, right shoulder 🔧
     M60.012   Infective myositis, left shoulder 🔧
     M60.019   Infective myositis, unspecified shoulder 🔧

▶ New   ⇨ Revised   ~~deleted~~ Deleted   Excludes 1   Excludes 2   Includes   Use additional   Code first   Code also   Key words
OGCR Official Guidelines   ● Unacceptable Principal Diagnosis   X Assign placeholder X   ● Use Additional Character(s)   ▶ Manifestation Code   Coding Clinic

● M60.02 Infective myositis, upper arm
    M60.021 Infective myositis, right upper arm 🦠
    M60.022 Infective myositis, left upper arm 🦠
    M60.029 Infective myositis, unspecified upper arm 🦠
● M60.03 Infective myositis, forearm
    M60.031 Infective myositis, right forearm 🦠
    M60.032 Infective myositis, left forearm 🦠
    M60.039 Infective myositis, unspecified forearm 🦠
● M60.04 Infective myositis, hand and fingers
    M60.041 Infective myositis, right hand 🦠
    M60.042 Infective myositis, left hand 🦠
    M60.043 Infective myositis, unspecified hand 🦠
    M60.044 Infective myositis, right finger(s) 🦠
    M60.045 Infective myositis, left finger(s) 🦠
    M60.046 Infective myositis, unspecified finger(s) 🦠
● M60.05 Infective myositis, thigh
    M60.051 Infective myositis, right thigh 🦠
    M60.052 Infective myositis, left thigh 🦠
    M60.059 Infective myositis, unspecified thigh 🦠
● M60.06 Infective myositis, lower leg
    M60.061 Infective myositis, right lower leg 🦠
    M60.062 Infective myositis, left lower leg 🦠
    M60.069 Infective myositis, unspecified lower leg 🦠
● M60.07 Infective myositis, ankle, foot and toes
    M60.070 Infective myositis, right ankle 🦠
    M60.071 Infective myositis, left ankle 🦠
    M60.072 Infective myositis, unspecified ankle 🦠
    M60.073 Infective myositis, right foot 🦠
    M60.074 Infective myositis, left foot 🦠
    M60.075 Infective myositis, unspecified foot 🦠
    M60.076 Infective myositis, right toe(s) 🦠
    M60.077 Infective myositis, left toe(s) 🦠
    M60.078 Infective myositis, unspecified toe(s) 🦠
    M60.08 Infective myositis, other site 🦠
    M60.09 Infective myositis, multiple sites 🦠
● M60.1 Interstitial myositis
    M60.10 Interstitial myositis of unspecified site
● M60.11 Interstitial myositis, shoulder
    M60.111 Interstitial myositis, right shoulder
    M60.112 Interstitial myositis, left shoulder
    M60.119 Interstitial myositis, unspecified shoulder
● M60.12 Interstitial myositis, upper arm
    M60.121 Interstitial myositis, right upper arm
    M60.122 Interstitial myositis, left upper arm
    M60.129 Interstitial myositis, unspecified upper arm
● M60.13 Interstitial myositis, forearm
    M60.131 Interstitial myositis, right forearm
    M60.132 Interstitial myositis, left forearm
    M60.139 Interstitial myositis, unspecified forearm

● M60.14 Interstitial myositis, hand
    M60.141 Interstitial myositis, right hand
    M60.142 Interstitial myositis, left hand
    M60.149 Interstitial myositis, unspecified hand
● M60.15 Interstitial myositis, thigh
    M60.151 Interstitial myositis, right thigh
    M60.152 Interstitial myositis, left thigh
    M60.159 Interstitial myositis, unspecified thigh
● M60.16 Interstitial myositis, lower leg
    M60.161 Interstitial myositis, right lower leg
    M60.162 Interstitial myositis, left lower leg
    M60.169 Interstitial myositis, unspecified lower leg
● M60.17 Interstitial myositis, ankle and foot
    M60.171 Interstitial myositis, right ankle and foot
    M60.172 Interstitial myositis, left ankle and foot
    M60.179 Interstitial myositis, unspecified ankle and foot
    M60.18 Interstitial myositis, other site
    M60.19 Interstitial myositis, multiple sites
● M60.2 Foreign body granuloma of soft tissue, not elsewhere classified

    Use additional code to identify the type of retained foreign body (Z18.-)

    Excludes1 foreign body granuloma of skin and subcutaneous tissue (L92.3)

    M60.20 Foreign body granuloma of soft tissue, not elsewhere classified, unspecified site
● M60.21 Foreign body granuloma of soft tissue, not elsewhere classified, shoulder
    M60.211 Foreign body granuloma of soft tissue, not elsewhere classified, right shoulder
    M60.212 Foreign body granuloma of soft tissue, not elsewhere classified, left shoulder
    M60.219 Foreign body granuloma of soft tissue, not elsewhere classified, unspecified shoulder
● M60.22 Foreign body granuloma of soft tissue, not elsewhere classified, upper arm
    M60.221 Foreign body granuloma of soft tissue, not elsewhere classified, right upper arm
    M60.222 Foreign body granuloma of soft tissue, not elsewhere classified, left upper arm
    M60.229 Foreign body granuloma of soft tissue, not elsewhere classified, unspecified upper arm
● M60.23 Foreign body granuloma of soft tissue, not elsewhere classified, forearm
    M60.231 Foreign body granuloma of soft tissue, not elsewhere classified, right forearm
    M60.232 Foreign body granuloma of soft tissue, not elsewhere classified, left forearm
    M60.239 Foreign body granuloma of soft tissue, not elsewhere classified, unspecified forearm

N Newborn Age: 0   **P** Pediatric Age: 0–17   **M** Maternity DX: 9–64   **A** Adult Age: 15–124   ♀ Females Only   ♂ Males Only

🦠 Complication\Comorbidity   🦠 Major C\C   (Ex) CC/MCC Exclusions   🦠 Hospital-Acquired Condition   🦠 Hierarchical Condition Category

1069

CHAPTER 13 (M00-M99)

CHAPTER 13 (M00-M99)

● M60.24   Foreign body granuloma of soft tissue, not elsewhere classified, hand
- M60.241   Foreign body granuloma of soft tissue, not elsewhere classified, right hand
- M60.242   Foreign body granuloma of soft tissue, not elsewhere classified, left hand
- M60.249   Foreign body granuloma of soft tissue, not elsewhere classified, unspecified hand

● M60.25   Foreign body granuloma of soft tissue, not elsewhere classified, thigh
- M60.251   Foreign body granuloma of soft tissue, not elsewhere classified, right thigh
- M60.252   Foreign body granuloma of soft tissue, not elsewhere classified, left thigh
- M60.259   Foreign body granuloma of soft tissue, not elsewhere classified, unspecified thigh

● M60.26   Foreign body granuloma of soft tissue, not elsewhere classified, lower leg
- M60.261   Foreign body granuloma of soft tissue, not elsewhere classified, right lower leg
- M60.262   Foreign body granuloma of soft tissue, not elsewhere classified, left lower leg
- M60.269   Foreign body granuloma of soft tissue, not elsewhere classified, unspecified lower leg

● M60.27   Foreign body granuloma of soft tissue, not elsewhere classified, ankle and foot
- M60.271   Foreign body granuloma of soft tissue, not elsewhere classified, right ankle and foot
- M60.272   Foreign body granuloma of soft tissue, not elsewhere classified, left ankle and foot
- M60.279   Foreign body granuloma of soft tissue, not elsewhere classified, unspecified ankle and foot

M60.28   Foreign body granuloma of soft tissue, not elsewhere classified, other site

● M60.8   Other myositis
M60.80   Other myositis, unspecified site

● M60.81   Other myositis shoulder
- M60.811   Other myositis, right shoulder
- M60.812   Other myositis, left shoulder
- M60.819   Other myositis, unspecified shoulder

● M60.82   Other myositis, upper arm
- M60.821   Other myositis, right upper arm
- M60.822   Other myositis, left upper arm
- M60.829   Other myositis, unspecified upper arm

● M60.83   Other myositis, forearm
- M60.831   Other myositis, right forearm
- M60.832   Other myositis, left forearm
- M60.839   Other myositis, unspecified forearm

● M60.84   Other myositis, hand
- M60.841   Other myositis, right hand
- M60.842   Other myositis, left hand
- M60.849   Other myositis, unspecified hand

● M60.85   Other myositis, thigh
- M60.851   Other myositis, right thigh
- M60.852   Other myositis, left thigh
- M60.859   Other myositis, unspecified thigh

● M60.86   Other myositis, lower leg
- M60.861   Other myositis, right lower leg
- M60.862   Other myositis, left lower leg
- M60.869   Other myositis, unspecified lower leg

● M60.87   Other myositis, ankle and foot
- M60.871   Other myositis, right ankle and foot
- M60.872   Other myositis, left ankle and foot
- M60.879   Other myositis, unspecified ankle and foot

M60.88   Other myositis, other site

M60.89   Other myositis, multiple sites

M60.9   Myositis, unspecified

● M61   Calcification and ossification of muscle

  ● M61.0   Myositis ossificans traumatica
M61.00   Myositis ossificans traumatica, unspecified site

● M61.01   Myositis ossificans traumatica, shoulder
- M61.011   Myositis ossificans traumatica, right shoulder
- M61.012   Myositis ossificans traumatica, left shoulder
- M61.019   Myositis ossificans traumatica, unspecified shoulder

● M61.02   Myositis ossificans traumatica, upper arm
- M61.021   Myositis ossificans traumatica, right upper arm
- M61.022   Myositis ossificans traumatica, left upper arm
- M61.029   Myositis ossificans traumatica, unspecified upper arm

● M61.03   Myositis ossificans traumatica, forearm
- M61.031   Myositis ossificans traumatica, right forearm
- M61.032   Myositis ossificans traumatica, left forearm
- M61.039   Myositis ossificans traumatica, unspecified forearm

● M61.04   Myositis ossificans traumatica, hand
- M61.041   Myositis ossificans traumatica, right hand
- M61.042   Myositis ossificans traumatica, left hand
- M61.049   Myositis ossificans traumatica, unspecified hand

● M61.05   Myositis ossificans traumatica, thigh
- M61.051   Myositis ossificans traumatica, right thigh
- M61.052   Myositis ossificans traumatica, left thigh
- M61.059   Myositis ossificans traumatica, unspecified thigh

● M61.06   Myositis ossificans traumatica, lower leg
- M61.061   Myositis ossificans traumatica, right lower leg
- M61.062   Myositis ossificans traumatica, left lower leg
- M61.069   Myositis ossificans traumatica, unspecified lower leg

● M61.07   Myositis ossificans traumatica, ankle and foot
- M61.071   Myositis ossificans traumatica, right ankle and foot
- M61.072   Myositis ossificans traumatica, left ankle and foot
- M61.079   Myositis ossificans traumatica, unspecified ankle and foot

M61.08   Myositis ossificans traumatica, other site

M61.09   Myositis ossificans traumatica, multiple sites

▶ New   ⇒ Revised   ~~deleted~~ Deleted   Excludes 1   Excludes 2   Includes   Use additional   Code first   Code also   Key words
OGCR Official Guidelines   ● Unacceptable Principal Diagnosis   X Assign placeholder X   ● Use Additional Character(s)   ▌ Manifestation Code   **Coding Clinic**

● M61.1   Myositis ossificans progressiva
     Fibrodysplasia ossificans progressiva
    M61.10   Myositis ossificans progressiva, unspecified site
● M61.11   Myositis ossificans progressiva, shoulder
     M61.111   Myositis ossificans progressiva, right shoulder
     M61.112   Myositis ossificans progressiva, left shoulder
     M61.119   Myositis ossificans progressiva, unspecified shoulder
● M61.12   Myositis ossificans progressiva, upper arm
     M61.121   Myositis ossificans progressiva, right upper arm
     M61.122   Myositis ossificans progressiva, left upper arm
     M61.129   Myositis ossificans progressiva, unspecified arm
● M61.13   Myositis ossificans progressiva, forearm
     M61.131   Myositis ossificans progressiva, right forearm
     M61.132   Myositis ossificans progressiva, left forearm
     M61.139   Myositis ossificans progressiva, unspecified forearm
● M61.14   Myositis ossificans progressiva, hand and finger(s)
     M61.141   Myositis ossificans progressiva, right hand
     M61.142   Myositis ossificans progressiva, left hand
     M61.143   Myositis ossificans progressiva, unspecified hand
     M61.144   Myositis ossificans progressiva, right finger(s)
     M61.145   Myositis ossificans progressiva, left finger(s)
     M61.146   Myositis ossificans progressiva, unspecified finger(s)
● M61.15   Myositis ossificans progressiva, thigh
     M61.151   Myositis ossificans progressiva, right thigh
     M61.152   Myositis ossificans progressiva, left thigh
     M61.159   Myositis ossificans progressiva, unspecified thigh
● M61.16   Myositis ossificans progressiva, lower leg
     M61.161   Myositis ossificans progressiva, right lower leg
     M61.162   Myositis ossificans progressiva, left lower leg
     M61.169   Myositis ossificans progressiva, unspecified lower leg
● M61.17   Myositis ossificans progressiva, ankle, foot and toe(s)
     M61.171   Myositis ossificans progressiva, right ankle
     M61.172   Myositis ossificans progressiva, left ankle
     M61.173   Myositis ossificans progressiva, unspecified ankle
     M61.174   Myositis ossificans progressiva, right foot
     M61.175   Myositis ossificans progressiva, left foot

     M61.176   Myositis ossificans progressiva, unspecified foot
     M61.177   Myositis ossificans progressiva, right toe(s)
     M61.178   Myositis ossificans progressiva, left toe(s)
     M61.179   Myositis ossificans progressiva, unspecified toe(s)
    M61.18   Myositis ossificans progressiva, other site
    M61.19   Myositis ossificans progressiva, multiple sites
● M61.2   Paralytic calcification and ossification of muscle
     Myositis ossificans associated with quadriplegia or paraplegia
    M61.20   Paralytic calcification and ossification of muscle, unspecified site
● M61.21   Paralytic calcification and ossification of muscle, shoulder
     M61.211   Paralytic calcification and ossification of muscle, right shoulder
     M61.212   Paralytic calcification and ossification of muscle, left shoulder
     M61.219   Paralytic calcification and ossification of muscle, unspecified shoulder
● M61.22   Paralytic calcification and ossification of muscle, upper arm
     M61.221   Paralytic calcification and ossification of muscle, right upper arm
     M61.222   Paralytic calcification and ossification of muscle, left upper arm
     M61.229   Paralytic calcification and ossification of muscle, unspecified upper arm
● M61.23   Paralytic calcification and ossification of muscle, forearm
     M61.231   Paralytic calcification and ossification of muscle, right forearm
     M61.232   Paralytic calcification and ossification of muscle, left forearm
     M61.239   Paralytic calcification and ossification of muscle, unspecified forearm
● M61.24   Paralytic calcification and ossification of muscle, hand
     M61.241   Paralytic calcification and ossification of muscle, right hand
     M61.242   Paralytic calcification and ossification of muscle, left hand
     M61.249   Paralytic calcification and ossification of muscle, unspecified hand
● M61.25   Paralytic calcification and ossification of muscle, thigh
     M61.251   Paralytic calcification and ossification of muscle, right thigh
     M61.252   Paralytic calcification and ossification of muscle, left thigh
     M61.259   Paralytic calcification and ossification of muscle, unspecified thigh
● M61.26   Paralytic calcification and ossification of muscle, lower leg
     M61.261   Paralytic calcification and ossification of muscle, right lower leg
     M61.262   Paralytic calcification and ossification of muscle, left lower leg
     M61.269   Paralytic calcification and ossification of muscle, unspecified lower leg

CHAPTER 13 (M00-M99)

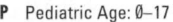

N   Newborn Age: 0   **P**   Pediatric Age: 0–17   **M**   Maternity DX: 9–64   **A**   Adult Age: 15–124   ♀   Females Only   ♂   Males Only

🄯   Complication\Comorbidity   🄯   Major C\C   (Ex)   CC/MCC Exclusions   🄯   Hospital-Acquired Condition   🄯   Hierarchical Condition Category

1071

● M61.27 Paralytic calcification and ossification of muscle, ankle and foot

  M61.271 Paralytic calcification and ossification of muscle, right ankle and foot

  M61.272 Paralytic calcification and ossification of muscle, left ankle and foot

  M61.279 Paralytic calcification and ossification of muscle, unspecified ankle and foot

M61.28 Paralytic calcification and ossification of muscle, other site

M61.29 Paralytic calcification and ossification of muscle, multiple sites

● M61.3 Calcification and ossification of muscles associated with burns
  Myositis ossificans associated with burns

M61.30 Calcification and ossification of muscles associated with burns, unspecified site

● M61.31 Calcification and ossification of muscles associated with burns, shoulder

  M61.311 Calcification and ossification of muscles associated with burns, right shoulder

  M61.312 Calcification and ossification of muscles associated with burns, left shoulder

  M61.319 Calcification and ossification of muscles associated with burns, unspecified shoulder

● M61.32 Calcification and ossification of muscles associated with burns, upper arm

  M61.321 Calcification and ossification of muscles associated with burns, right upper arm

  M61.322 Calcification and ossification of muscles associated with burns, left upper arm

  M61.329 Calcification and ossification of muscles associated with burns, unspecified upper arm

● M61.33 Calcification and ossification of muscles associated with burns, forearm

  M61.331 Calcification and ossification of muscles associated with burns, right forearm

  M61.332 Calcification and ossification of muscles associated with burns, left forearm

  M61.339 Calcification and ossification of muscles associated with burns, unspecified forearm

● M61.34 Calcification and ossification of muscles associated with burns, hand

  M61.341 Calcification and ossification of muscles associated with burns, right hand

  M61.342 Calcification and ossification of muscles associated with burns, left hand

  M61.349 Calcification and ossification of muscles associated with burns, unspecified hand

● M61.35 Calcification and ossification of muscles associated with burns, thigh

  M61.351 Calcification and ossification of muscles associated with burns, right thigh

  M61.352 Calcification and ossification of muscles associated with burns, left thigh

  M61.359 Calcification and ossification of muscles associated with burns, unspecified thigh

● M61.36 Calcification and ossification of muscles associated with burns, lower leg

  M61.361 Calcification and ossification of muscles associated with burns, right lower leg

  M61.362 Calcification and ossification of muscles associated with burns, left lower leg

  M61.369 Calcification and ossification of muscles associated with burns, unspecified lower leg

● M61.37 Calcification and ossification of muscles associated with burns, ankle and foot

  M61.371 Calcification and ossification of muscles associated with burns, right ankle and foot

  M61.372 Calcification and ossification of muscles associated with burns, left ankle and foot

  M61.379 Calcification and ossification of muscles associated with burns, unspecified ankle and foot

M61.38 Calcification and ossification of muscles associated with burns, other site

M61.39 Calcification and ossification of muscles associated with burns, multiple sites

● M61.4 Other calcification of muscle

  Excludes1   calcific tendinitis NOS (M65.2-)
              calcific tendinitis of shoulder (M75.3)

M61.40 Other calcification of muscle, unspecified site

● M61.41 Other calcification of muscle, shoulder

  M61.411 Other calcification of muscle, right shoulder

  M61.412 Other calcification of muscle, left shoulder

  M61.419 Other calcification of muscle, unspecified shoulder

● M61.42 Other calcification of muscle, upper arm

  M61.421 Other calcification of muscle, right upper arm

  M61.422 Other calcification of muscle, left upper arm

  M61.429 Other calcification of muscle, unspecified upper arm

● M61.43 Other calcification of muscle, forearm

  M61.431 Other calcification of muscle, right forearm

  M61.432 Other calcification of muscle, left forearm

  M61.439 Other calcification of muscle, unspecified forearm

● M61.44 Other calcification of muscle, hand

  M61.441 Other calcification of muscle, right hand

  M61.442 Other calcification of muscle, left hand

  M61.449 Other calcification of muscle, unspecified hand

● M61.45 Other calcification of muscle, thigh

  M61.451 Other calcification of muscle, right thigh

  M61.452 Other calcification of muscle, left thigh

  M61.459 Other calcification of muscle, unspecified thigh

● M61.46   Other calcification of muscle, lower leg

     M61.461   Other calcification of muscle, right lower leg

     M61.462   Other calcification of muscle, left lower leg

     M61.469   Other calcification of muscle, unspecified lower leg

● M61.47   Other calcification of muscle, ankle and foot

     M61.471   Other calcification of muscle, right ankle and foot

     M61.472   Other calcification of muscle, left ankle and foot

     M61.479   Other calcification of muscle, unspecified ankle and foot

   M61.48   Other calcification of muscle, other site

   M61.49   Other calcification of muscle, multiple sites

● M61.5   Other ossification of muscle

   M61.50   Other ossification of muscle, unspecified site

● M61.51   Other ossification of muscle, shoulder

     M61.511   Other ossification of muscle, right shoulder

     M61.512   Other ossification of muscle, left shoulder

     M61.519   Other ossification of muscle, unspecified shoulder

● M61.52   Other ossification of muscle, upper arm

     M61.521   Other ossification of muscle, right upper arm

     M61.522   Other ossification of muscle, left upper arm

     M61.529   Other ossification of muscle, unspecified upper arm

● M61.53   Other ossification of muscle, forearm

     M61.531   Other ossification of muscle, right forearm

     M61.532   Other ossification of muscle, left forearm

     M61.539   Other ossification of muscle, unspecified forearm

● M61.54   Other ossification of muscle, hand

     M61.541   Other ossification of muscle, right hand

     M61.542   Other ossification of muscle, left hand

     M61.549   Other ossification of muscle, unspecified hand

● M61.55   Other ossification of muscle, thigh

     M61.551   Other ossification of muscle, right thigh

     M61.552   Other ossification of muscle, left thigh

     M61.559   Other ossification of muscle, unspecified thigh

● M61.56   Other ossification of muscle, lower leg

     M61.561   Other ossification of muscle, right lower leg

     M61.562   Other ossification of muscle, left lower leg

     M61.569   Other ossification of muscle, unspecified lower leg

● M61.57   Other ossification of muscle, ankle and foot

     M61.571   Other ossification of muscle, right ankle and foot

     M61.572   Other ossification of muscle, left ankle and foot

     M61.579   Other ossification of muscle, unspecified ankle and foot

   M61.58   Other ossification of muscle, other site

   M61.59   Other ossification of muscle, multiple sites

  M61.9   Calcification and ossification of muscle, unspecified

● M62   Other disorders of muscle

   Excludes1   alcoholic myopathy (G72.1)
        cramp and spasm (R25.2)
        drug-induced myopathy (G72.0)
        myalgia (M79.1-)
        stiff-man syndrome (G25.82)

   Excludes2   nontraumatic hematoma of muscle (M79.81)

● M62.0   **Separation of muscle (nontraumatic)**
     Diastasis of muscle

     Excludes1   diastasis recti complicating pregnancy, labor and delivery (O71.8)
          traumatic separation of muscle - see strain of muscle by body region

   M62.00   Separation of muscle (nontraumatic), unspecified site

● M62.01   Separation of muscle (nontraumatic), shoulder

     M62.011   Separation of muscle (nontraumatic), right shoulder

     M62.012   Separation of muscle (nontraumatic), left shoulder

     M62.019   Separation of muscle (nontraumatic), unspecified shoulder

● M62.02   Separation of muscle (nontraumatic), upper arm

     M62.021   Separation of muscle (nontraumatic), right upper arm

     M62.022   Separation of muscle (nontraumatic), left upper arm

     M62.029   Separation of muscle (nontraumatic), unspecified upper arm

● M62.03   Separation of muscle (nontraumatic), forearm

     M62.031   Separation of muscle (nontraumatic), right forearm

     M62.032   Separation of muscle (nontraumatic), left forearm

     M62.039   Separation of muscle (nontraumatic), unspecified forearm

● M62.04   Separation of muscle (nontraumatic), hand

     M62.041   Separation of muscle (nontraumatic), right hand

     M62.042   Separation of muscle (nontraumatic), left hand

     M62.049   Separation of muscle (nontraumatic), unspecified hand

● M62.05   Separation of muscle (nontraumatic), thigh

     M62.051   Separation of muscle (nontraumatic), right thigh

     M62.052   Separation of muscle (nontraumatic), left thigh

     M62.059   Separation of muscle (nontraumatic), unspecified thigh

● M62.06   Separation of muscle (nontraumatic), lower leg

     M62.061   Separation of muscle (nontraumatic), right lower leg

     M62.062   Separation of muscle (nontraumatic), left lower leg

     M62.069   Separation of muscle (nontraumatic), unspecified lower leg

● M62.07   Separation of muscle (nontraumatic), ankle and foot

     M62.071   Separation of muscle (nontraumatic), right ankle and foot

     M62.072   Separation of muscle (nontraumatic), left ankle and foot

     M62.079   Separation of muscle (nontraumatic), unspecified ankle and foot

   M62.08   Separation of muscle (nontraumatic), other site

N Newborn Age: 0   **P** Pediatric Age: 0–17   **M** Maternity DX: 9–64   **A** Adult Age: 15–124   ♀ Females Only   ♂ Males Only

◔ Complication\Comorbidity   ◔ Major C\C   (Ex) CC/MCC Exclusions   ◔ Hospital-Acquired Condition   ◔ Hierarchical Condition Category

1073

● M62.1   **Other rupture of muscle (nontraumatic)**
-     **Excludes1**   traumatic rupture of muscle - see strain of muscle by body region
-     **Excludes2**   rupture of tendon (M66.-)

M62.10   Other rupture of muscle (nontraumatic), **unspecified** site

● M62.11   Other rupture of muscle (nontraumatic), **shoulder**
- M62.111   Other rupture of muscle (nontraumatic), **right** shoulder
- M62.112   Other rupture of muscle (nontraumatic), **left** shoulder
- M62.119   Other rupture of muscle (nontraumatic), **unspecified** shoulder

● M62.12   Other rupture of muscle (nontraumatic), **upper arm**
- M62.121   Other rupture of muscle (nontraumatic), **right** upper arm
- M62.122   Other rupture of muscle (nontraumatic), **left** upper arm
- M62.129   Other rupture of muscle (nontraumatic), **unspecified** upper arm

● M62.13   Other rupture of muscle (nontraumatic), **forearm**
- M62.131   Other rupture of muscle (nontraumatic), **right** forearm
- M62.132   Other rupture of muscle (nontraumatic), **left** forearm
- M62.139   Other rupture of muscle (nontraumatic), **unspecified** forearm

● M62.14   Other rupture of muscle (nontraumatic), **hand**
- M62.141   Other rupture of muscle (nontraumatic), **right** hand
- M62.142   Other rupture of muscle (nontraumatic), **left** hand
- M62.149   Other rupture of muscle (nontraumatic), **unspecified** hand

● M62.15   Other rupture of muscle (nontraumatic), **thigh**
- M62.151   Other rupture of muscle (nontraumatic), **right** thigh
- M62.152   Other rupture of muscle (nontraumatic), **left** thigh
- M62.159   Other rupture of muscle (nontraumatic), **unspecified** thigh

● M62.16   Other rupture of muscle (nontraumatic), **lower leg**
- M62.161   Other rupture of muscle (nontraumatic), **right** lower leg
- M62.162   Other rupture of muscle (nontraumatic), **left** lower leg
- M62.169   Other rupture of muscle (nontraumatic), **unspecified** lower leg

● M62.17   Other rupture of muscle (nontraumatic), **ankle and foot**
- M62.171   Other rupture of muscle (nontraumatic), **right** ankle and foot
- M62.172   Other rupture of muscle (nontraumatic), **left** ankle and foot
- M62.179   Other rupture of muscle (nontraumatic), **unspecified** ankle and foot

M62.18   Other rupture of muscle (nontraumatic), **other** site

● M62.2   **Nontraumatic ischemic infarction of muscle**
-     **Excludes1**   compartment syndrome (traumatic) (T79.A-)
  - nontraumatic compartment syndrome (M79.A-)
  - traumatic ischemia of muscle (T79.6)
  - rhabdomyolysis (M62.82)
  - Volkmann's ischemic contracture (T79.6)

M62.20   Nontraumatic ischemic infarction of muscle, **unspecified** site

● M62.21   Nontraumatic ischemic infarction of muscle, **shoulder**
- M62.211   Nontraumatic ischemic infarction of muscle, **right** shoulder
- M62.212   Nontraumatic ischemic infarction of muscle, **left** shoulder
- M62.219   Nontraumatic ischemic infarction of muscle, **unspecified** shoulder

● M62.22   Nontraumatic ischemic infarction of muscle, **upper arm**
- M62.221   Nontraumatic ischemic infarction of muscle, **right** upper arm
- M62.222   Nontraumatic ischemic infarction of muscle, **left** upper arm
- M62.229   Nontraumatic ischemic infarction of muscle, **unspecified** upper arm

● M62.23   Nontraumatic ischemic infarction of muscle, **forearm**
- M62.231   Nontraumatic ischemic infarction of muscle, **right** forearm
- M62.232   Nontraumatic ischemic infarction of muscle, **left** forearm
- M62.239   Nontraumatic ischemic infarction of muscle, **unspecified** forearm

● M62.24   Nontraumatic ischemic infarction of muscle, **hand**
- M62.241   Nontraumatic ischemic infarction of muscle, **right** hand
- M62.242   Nontraumatic ischemic infarction of muscle, **left** hand
- M62.249   Nontraumatic ischemic infarction of muscle, **unspecified** hand

● M62.25   Nontraumatic ischemic infarction of muscle, **thigh**
- M62.251   Nontraumatic ischemic infarction of muscle, **right** thigh
- M62.252   Nontraumatic ischemic infarction of muscle, **left** thigh
- M62.259   Nontraumatic ischemic infarction of muscle, **unspecified** thigh

● M62.26   Nontraumatic ischemic infarction of muscle, **lower leg**
- M62.261   Nontraumatic ischemic infarction of muscle, **right** lower leg
- M62.262   Nontraumatic ischemic infarction of muscle, **left** lower leg
- M62.269   Nontraumatic ischemic infarction of muscle, **unspecified** lower leg

● M62.27   Nontraumatic ischemic infarction of muscle, **ankle and foot**
- M62.271   Nontraumatic ischemic infarction of muscle, **right** ankle and foot
- M62.272   Nontraumatic ischemic infarction of muscle, **left** ankle and foot
- M62.279   Nontraumatic ischemic infarction of muscle, **unspecified** ankle and foot

M62.28   Nontraumatic ischemic infarction of muscle, **other site**

▶ New   ⇒ Revised   ~~deleted~~ Deleted   Excludes 1   Excludes 2   Includes   Use additional   Code first   Code also   Key words

OGCR Official Guidelines   ● Unacceptable Principal Diagnosis   X Assign placeholder X   ● Use Additional Character(s)   ▶ Manifestation Code   **Coding Clinic**

M62.3 **Immobility syndrome (paraplegic)**

M62.4 **Contracture of muscle**
Contracture of tendon (sheath)
> **Excludes1**   contracture of joint (M24.5-)

  M62.40 Contracture of muscle, unspecified site

● M62.41 Contracture of muscle, shoulder
   M62.411 Contracture of muscle, right shoulder
   M62.412 Contracture of muscle, left shoulder
   M62.419 Contracture of muscle, unspecified shoulder

● M62.42 Contracture of muscle, upper arm
   M62.421 Contracture of muscle, right upper arm
   M62.422 Contracture of muscle, left upper arm
   M62.429 Contracture of muscle, unspecified upper arm

● M62.43 Contracture of muscle, forearm
   M62.431 Contracture of muscle, right forearm
   M62.432 Contracture of muscle, left forearm
   M62.439 Contracture of muscle, unspecified forearm

● M62.44 Contracture of muscle, hand
   M62.441 Contracture of muscle, right hand
   M62.442 Contracture of muscle, left hand
   M62.449 Contracture of muscle, unspecified hand

● M62.45 Contracture of muscle, thigh
   M62.451 Contracture of muscle, right thigh
   M62.452 Contracture of muscle, left thigh
   M62.459 Contracture of muscle, unspecified thigh

● M62.46 Contracture of muscle, lower leg
   M62.461 Contracture of muscle, right lower leg
   M62.462 Contracture of muscle, left lower leg
   M62.469 Contracture of muscle, unspecified lower leg

● M62.47 Contracture of muscle, ankle and foot
   M62.471 Contracture of muscle, right ankle and foot
   M62.472 Contracture of muscle, left ankle and foot
   M62.479 Contracture of muscle, unspecified ankle and foot

  M62.48 Contracture of muscle, other site

  M62.49 Contracture of muscle, multiple sites

● M62.5 **Muscle wasting and atrophy, not elsewhere classified**
Disuse atrophy NEC
> **Excludes1**   neuralgic amyotrophy (G54.5)
> progressive muscular atrophy (G12.21)
> sarcopenia (M62.84)
>
> **Excludes2**   pelvic muscle wasting (N81.84)

  M62.50 Muscle wasting and atrophy, not elsewhere classified, unspecified site

● M62.51 Muscle wasting and atrophy, not elsewhere classified, shoulder
   M62.511 Muscle wasting and atrophy, not elsewhere classified, right shoulder
   M62.512 Muscle wasting and atrophy, not elsewhere classified, left shoulder
   M62.519 Muscle wasting and atrophy, not elsewhere classified, unspecified shoulder

● M62.52 Muscle wasting and atrophy, not elsewhere classified, upper arm
   M62.521 Muscle wasting and atrophy, not elsewhere classified, right upper arm
   M62.522 Muscle wasting and atrophy, not elsewhere classified, left upper arm
   M62.529 Muscle wasting and atrophy, not elsewhere classified, unspecified upper arm

● M62.53 Muscle wasting and atrophy, not elsewhere classified, forearm
   M62.531 Muscle wasting and atrophy, not elsewhere classified, right forearm
   M62.532 Muscle wasting and atrophy, not elsewhere classified, left forearm
   M62.539 Muscle wasting and atrophy, not elsewhere classified, unspecified forearm

● M62.54 Muscle wasting and atrophy, not elsewhere classified, hand
   M62.541 Muscle wasting and atrophy, not elsewhere classified, right hand
   M62.542 Muscle wasting and atrophy, not elsewhere classified, left hand
   M62.549 Muscle wasting and atrophy, not elsewhere classified, unspecified hand

● M62.55 Muscle wasting and atrophy, not elsewhere classified, thigh
   M62.551 Muscle wasting and atrophy, not elsewhere classified, right thigh
   M62.552 Muscle wasting and atrophy, not elsewhere classified, left thigh
   M62.559 Muscle wasting and atrophy, not elsewhere classified, unspecified thigh

● M62.56 Muscle wasting and atrophy, not elsewhere classified, lower leg
   M62.561 Muscle wasting and atrophy, not elsewhere classified, right lower leg
   M62.562 Muscle wasting and atrophy, not elsewhere classified, left lower leg
   M62.569 Muscle wasting and atrophy, not elsewhere classified, unspecified lower leg

● M62.57 Muscle wasting and atrophy, not elsewhere classified, ankle and foot
   M62.571 Muscle wasting and atrophy, not elsewhere classified, right ankle and foot
   M62.572 Muscle wasting and atrophy, not elsewhere classified, left ankle and foot
   M62.579 Muscle wasting and atrophy, not elsewhere classified, unspecified ankle and foot

  M62.58 Muscle wasting and atrophy, not elsewhere classified, other site

  M62.59 Muscle wasting and atrophy, not elsewhere classified, multiple sites

● **M62.8   Other specified disorders of muscle**
   Excludes2 nontraumatic hematoma of muscle (M79.81)

  M62.81   Muscle weakness (generalized)
      Excludes1 muscle weakness in sarcopenia (M62.84)

  M62.82   Rhabdomyolysis 🔖
      Excludes1 traumatic rhabdomyolysis (T79.6)
      Ex: See PDX Collection 892
      Coding Clinic: 2019, Q2, P12

  ● **M62.83   Muscle spasm**
     M62.830   Muscle spasm of back
     M62.831   Muscle spasm of calf
         Charley-horse
     M62.838   Other muscle spasm

  M62.84   Sarcopenia
     Age-related sarcopenia
     Code first underlying disease, if applicable, such as:
       disorders of myoneural junction and muscle disease in diseases classified elsewhere (G73.-)
       other and unspecified myopathies (G72.-)
       primary disorders of muscles (G71.-)
     Coding Clinic: 2016, Q4, P41

  M62.89   Other specified disorders of muscle
     Muscle (sheath) hernia

M62.9   Disorder of muscle, unspecified

● **M63   Disorders of muscle in diseases classified elsewhere**
   Code first underlying disease, such as:
    leprosy (A30.-)
    neoplasm (C49.-, C79.89, D21.-, D48.1)
    schistosomiasis (B65.-)
    trichinellosis (B75)
   Excludes1 myopathy in cysticercosis (B69.81)
       myopathy in endocrine diseases (G73.7)
       myopathy in metabolic diseases (G73.7)
       myopathy in sarcoidosis (D86.87)
       myopathy in secondary syphilis (A51.49)
       myopathy in syphilis (late) (A52.78)
       myopathy in toxoplasmosis (B58.82)
       myopathy in tuberculosis (A18.09)

  ● **M63.8   Disorders of muscle in diseases classified elsewhere**
    ▷ *M63.80   Disorders of muscle in diseases classified elsewhere, unspecified site*

    ● **M63.81   Disorders of muscle in diseases classified elsewhere, shoulder**
      ▷ *M63.811   Disorders of muscle in diseases classified elsewhere, right shoulder*
      ▷ *M63.812   Disorders of muscle in diseases classified elsewhere, left shoulder*
      ▷ *M63.819   Disorders of muscle in diseases classified elsewhere, unspecified shoulder*

    ● **M63.82   Disorders of muscle in diseases classified elsewhere, upper arm**
      ▷ *M63.821   Disorders of muscle in diseases classified elsewhere, right upper arm*
      ▷ *M63.822   Disorders of muscle in diseases classified elsewhere, left upper arm*
      ▷ *M63.829   Disorders of muscle in diseases classified elsewhere, unspecified upper arm*

● **M63.83   Disorders of muscle in diseases classified elsewhere, forearm**
   ▷ *M63.831   Disorders of muscle in diseases classified elsewhere, right forearm*
   ▷ *M63.832   Disorders of muscle in diseases classified elsewhere, left forearm*
   ▷ *M63.839   Disorders of muscle in diseases classified elsewhere, unspecified forearm*

● **M63.84   Disorders of muscle in diseases classified elsewhere, hand**
   ▷ *M63.841   Disorders of muscle in diseases classified elsewhere, right hand*
   ▷ *M63.842   Disorders of muscle in diseases classified elsewhere, left hand*
   ▷ *M63.849   Disorders of muscle in diseases classified elsewhere, unspecified hand*

● **M63.85   Disorders of muscle in diseases classified elsewhere, thigh**
   ▷ *M63.851   Disorders of muscle in diseases classified elsewhere, right thigh*
   ▷ *M63.852   Disorders of muscle in diseases classified elsewhere, left thigh*
   ▷ *M63.859   Disorders of muscle in diseases classified elsewhere, unspecified thigh*

● **M63.86   Disorders of muscle in diseases classified elsewhere, lower leg**
   ▷ *M63.861   Disorders of muscle in diseases classified elsewhere, right lower leg*
   ▷ *M63.862   Disorders of muscle in diseases classified elsewhere, left lower leg*
   ▷ *M63.869   Disorders of muscle in diseases classified elsewhere, unspecified lower leg*

● **M63.87   Disorders of muscle in diseases classified elsewhere, ankle and foot**
   ▷ *M63.871   Disorders of muscle in diseases classified elsewhere, right ankle and foot*
   ▷ *M63.872   Disorders of muscle in diseases classified elsewhere, left ankle and foot*
   ▷ *M63.879   Disorders of muscle in diseases classified elsewhere, unspecified ankle and foot*

  ▷ *M63.88   Disorders of muscle in diseases classified elsewhere, other site*
  ▷ *M63.89   Disorders of muscle in diseases classified elsewhere, multiple sites*

DISORDERS OF SYNOVIUM AND TENDON (M65-M67)

● **M65   Synovitis and tenosynovitis**
   Excludes1 chronic crepitant synovitis of hand and wrist (M70.0-)
       current injury - see injury of ligament or tendon by body region
       soft tissue disorders related to use, overuse and pressure (M70.-)

● **M65.0   Abscess of tendon sheath**
   Use additional code (B95-B96) to identify bacterial agent
  M65.00   Abscess of tendon sheath, unspecified site
  ● **M65.01   Abscess of tendon sheath, shoulder**
     M65.011   Abscess of tendon sheath, right shoulder
     M65.012   Abscess of tendon sheath, left shoulder
     M65.019   Abscess of tendon sheath, unspecified shoulder

Item 13–11 **Synovitis** is an inflammation of a synovial membrane resulting in pain on motion and is characterized by fluctuating swelling due to effusion in a synovial sac. **Tenosynovitis** is an inflammation of a tendon sheath and occurs most commonly in the wrists, hands, and feet. Bursitis is inflammation of a bursa (fluid-filled sac) caused by repetitive use, trauma, infection, or systemic inflammatory disease. Bursae act as protectors and facilitate movement between bones and overlapping muscles (deep bursae) or between bones and tendons/skin (superficial bursae).

● **M65.02** Abscess of tendon sheath, upper arm
　　　M65.021 Abscess of tendon sheath, right upper arm
　　　M65.022 Abscess of tendon sheath, left upper arm
　　　M65.029 Abscess of tendon sheath, unspecified upper arm
● **M65.03** Abscess of tendon sheath, forearm
　　　M65.031 Abscess of tendon sheath, right forearm
　　　M65.032 Abscess of tendon sheath, left forearm
　　　M65.039 Abscess of tendon sheath, unspecified forearm
● **M65.04** Abscess of tendon sheath, hand
　　　M65.041 Abscess of tendon sheath, right hand
　　　M65.042 Abscess of tendon sheath, left hand
　　　M65.049 Abscess of tendon sheath, unspecified hand
● **M65.05** Abscess of tendon sheath, thigh
　　　M65.051 Abscess of tendon sheath, right thigh
　　　M65.052 Abscess of tendon sheath, left thigh
　　　M65.059 Abscess of tendon sheath, unspecified thigh
● **M65.06** Abscess of tendon sheath, lower leg
　　　M65.061 Abscess of tendon sheath, right lower leg
　　　M65.062 Abscess of tendon sheath, left lower leg
　　　M65.069 Abscess of tendon sheath, unspecified lower leg
● **M65.07** Abscess of tendon sheath, ankle and foot
　　　M65.071 Abscess of tendon sheath, right ankle and foot
　　　M65.072 Abscess of tendon sheath, left ankle and foot
　　　M65.079 Abscess of tendon sheath, unspecified ankle and foot
　　　M65.08 Abscess of tendon sheath, other site
● **M65.1** Other infective (teno)synovitis
　　　M65.10 Other infective (teno)synovitis, unspecified site
● **M65.11** Other infective (teno)synovitis, shoulder
　　　M65.111 Other infective (teno)synovitis, right shoulder
　　　M65.112 Other infective (teno)synovitis, left shoulder
　　　M65.119 Other infective (teno)synovitis, unspecified shoulder
● **M65.12** Other infective (teno)synovitis, elbow
　　　M65.121 Other infective (teno)synovitis, right elbow
　　　M65.122 Other infective (teno)synovitis, left elbow
　　　M65.129 Other infective (teno)synovitis, unspecified elbow

● **M65.13** Other infective (teno)synovitis, wrist
　　　M65.131 Other infective (teno)synovitis, right wrist
　　　M65.132 Other infective (teno)synovitis, left wrist
　　　M65.139 Other infective (teno)synovitis, unspecified wrist
● **M65.14** Other infective (teno)synovitis, hand
　　　M65.141 Other infective (teno)synovitis, right hand
　　　M65.142 Other infective (teno)synovitis, left hand
　　　M65.149 Other infective (teno)synovitis, unspecified hand
● **M65.15** Other infective (teno)synovitis, hip
　　　M65.151 Other infective (teno)synovitis, right hip
　　　M65.152 Other infective (teno)synovitis, left hip
　　　M65.159 Other infective (teno)synovitis, unspecified hip
● **M65.16** Other infective (teno)synovitis, knee
　　　M65.161 Other infective (teno)synovitis, right knee
　　　M65.162 Other infective (teno)synovitis, left knee
　　　M65.169 Other infective (teno)synovitis, unspecified knee
● **M65.17** Other infective (teno)synovitis, ankle and foot
　　　M65.171 Other infective (teno)synovitis, right ankle and foot
　　　M65.172 Other infective (teno)synovitis, left ankle and foot
　　　M65.179 Other infective (teno)synovitis, unspecified ankle and foot
　　　M65.18 Other infective (teno)synovitis, other site
　　　M65.19 Other infective (teno)synovitis, multiple sites
● **M65.2** Calcific tendinitis
　　　Excludes1　tendinitis as classified in M75 M77 calcified tendinitis of shoulder (M75.3)
　　　M65.20 Calcific tendinitis, unspecified site
● **M65.22** Calcific tendinitis, upper arm
　　　M65.221 Calcific tendinitis, right upper arm
　　　M65.222 Calcific tendinitis, left upper arm
　　　M65.229 Calcific tendinitis, unspecified upper arm
● **M65.23** Calcific tendinitis, forearm
　　　M65.231 Calcific tendinitis, right forearm
　　　M65.232 Calcific tendinitis, left forearm
　　　M65.239 Calcific tendinitis, unspecified forearm
● **M65.24** Calcific tendinitis, hand
　　　M65.241 Calcific tendinitis, right hand
　　　M65.242 Calcific tendinitis, left hand
　　　M65.249 Calcific tendinitis, unspecified hand
● **M65.25** Calcific tendinitis, thigh
　　　M65.251 Calcific tendinitis, right thigh
　　　M65.252 Calcific tendinitis, left thigh
　　　M65.259 Calcific tendinitis, unspecified thigh
● **M65.26** Calcific tendinitis, lower leg
　　　M65.261 Calcific tendinitis, right lower leg
　　　M65.262 Calcific tendinitis, left lower leg
　　　M65.269 Calcific tendinitis, unspecified lower leg

CHAPTER 13 (M00–M99)

N　Newborn Age: 0　　P　Pediatric Age: 0–17　　M　Maternity DX: 9–64　　A　Adult Age: 15–124　　♀　Females Only　　♂　Males Only
🅒 Complication\Comorbidity　　🅜 Major C\C　　🅔🅧 CC/MCC Exclusions　　🅗 Hospital-Acquired Condition　　🅗 Hierarchical Condition Category

1077

● M65.27 Calcific tendinitis, ankle and foot
    M65.271 Calcific tendinitis, right ankle and foot
    M65.272 Calcific tendinitis, left ankle and foot
    M65.279 Calcific tendinitis, unspecified ankle and foot
  M65.28 Calcific tendinitis, other site
  M65.29 Calcific tendinitis, multiple sites
● M65.3 Trigger finger
    Nodular tendinous disease
  M65.30 Trigger finger, unspecified finger
● M65.31 Trigger thumb
    M65.311 Trigger thumb, right thumb
    M65.312 Trigger thumb, left thumb
    M65.319 Trigger thumb, unspecified thumb
● M65.32 Trigger finger, index finger
    M65.321 Trigger finger, right index finger
    M65.322 Trigger finger, left index finger
    M65.329 Trigger finger, unspecified index finger
● M65.33 Trigger finger, middle finger
    M65.331 Trigger finger, right middle finger
    M65.332 Trigger finger, left middle finger
    M65.339 Trigger finger, unspecified middle finger
● M65.34 Trigger finger, ring finger
    M65.341 Trigger finger, right ring finger
    M65.342 Trigger finger, left ring finger
    M65.349 Trigger finger, unspecified ring finger
● M65.35 Trigger finger, little finger
    M65.351 Trigger finger, right little finger
    M65.352 Trigger finger, left little finger
    M65.359 Trigger finger, unspecified little finger
  M65.4 Radial styloid tenosynovitis [de Quervain]
● M65.8 Other synovitis and tenosynovitis
  M65.80 Other synovitis and tenosynovitis, unspecified site
● M65.81 Other synovitis and tenosynovitis, shoulder
    M65.811 Other synovitis and tenosynovitis, right shoulder
    M65.812 Other synovitis and tenosynovitis, left shoulder
    M65.819 Other synovitis and tenosynovitis, unspecified shoulder
● M65.82 Other synovitis and tenosynovitis, upper arm
    M65.821 Other synovitis and tenosynovitis, right upper arm
    M65.822 Other synovitis and tenosynovitis, left upper arm
    M65.829 Other synovitis and tenosynovitis, unspecified upper arm
● M65.83 Other synovitis and tenosynovitis, forearm
    M65.831 Other synovitis and tenosynovitis, right forearm
    M65.832 Other synovitis and tenosynovitis, left forearm
    M65.839 Other synovitis and tenosynovitis, unspecified forearm
● M65.84 Other synovitis and tenosynovitis, hand
    M65.841 Other synovitis and tenosynovitis, right hand
    M65.842 Other synovitis and tenosynovitis, left hand
    M65.849 Other synovitis and tenosynovitis, unspecified hand

● M65.85 Other synovitis and tenosynovitis, thigh
    M65.851 Other synovitis and tenosynovitis, right thigh
    M65.852 Other synovitis and tenosynovitis, left thigh
    M65.859 Other synovitis and tenosynovitis, unspecified thigh
● M65.86 Other synovitis and tenosynovitis, lower leg
    M65.861 Other synovitis and tenosynovitis, right lower leg
    M65.862 Other synovitis and tenosynovitis, left lower leg
    M65.869 Other synovitis and tenosynovitis, unspecified lower leg
● M65.87 Other synovitis and tenosynovitis, ankle and foot
    M65.871 Other synovitis and tenosynovitis, right ankle and foot
    M65.872 Other synovitis and tenosynovitis, left ankle and foot
    M65.879 Other synovitis and tenosynovitis, unspecified ankle and foot
  M65.88 Other synovitis and tenosynovitis, other site
  M65.89 Other synovitis and tenosynovitis, multiple sites
  M65.9 Synovitis and tenosynovitis, unspecified

● M66 Spontaneous rupture of synovium and tendon
  Includes rupture that occurs when a normal force is applied to tissues that are inferred to have less than normal strength
  Excludes2 rotator cuff syndrome (M75.1-)
    rupture where an abnormal force is applied to normal tissue - see injury of tendon by body region
  M66.0 Rupture of popliteal cyst
● M66.1 Rupture of synovium
    Rupture of synovial cyst
    Excludes2 rupture of popliteal cyst (M66.0)
  M66.10 Rupture of synovium, unspecified joint
● M66.11 Rupture of synovium, shoulder
    M66.111 Rupture of synovium, right shoulder
    M66.112 Rupture of synovium, left shoulder
    M66.119 Rupture of synovium, unspecified shoulder
● M66.12 Rupture of synovium, elbow
    M66.121 Rupture of synovium, right elbow
    M66.122 Rupture of synovium, left elbow
    M66.129 Rupture of synovium, unspecified elbow
● M66.13 Rupture of synovium, wrist
    M66.131 Rupture of synovium, right wrist
    M66.132 Rupture of synovium, left wrist
    M66.139 Rupture of synovium, unspecified wrist
● M66.14 Rupture of synovium, hand and fingers
    M66.141 Rupture of synovium, right hand
    M66.142 Rupture of synovium, left hand
    M66.143 Rupture of synovium, unspecified hand
    M66.144 Rupture of synovium, right finger(s)
    M66.145 Rupture of synovium, left finger(s)
    M66.146 Rupture of synovium, unspecified finger(s)

● M66.15　Rupture of synovium, hip
　　　　M66.151　Rupture of synovium, right hip
　　　　M66.152　Rupture of synovium, left hip
　　　　M66.159　Rupture of synovium, unspecified hip
● M66.17　Rupture of synovium, ankle, foot and toes
　　　　M66.171　Rupture of synovium, right ankle
　　　　M66.172　Rupture of synovium, left ankle
　　　　M66.173　Rupture of synovium, unspecified ankle
　　　　M66.174　Rupture of synovium, right foot
　　　　M66.175　Rupture of synovium, left foot
　　　　M66.176　Rupture of synovium, unspecified foot
　　　　M66.177　Rupture of synovium, right toe(s)
　　　　M66.178　Rupture of synovium, left toe(s)
　　　　M66.179　Rupture of synovium, unspecified toe(s)
　　　　M66.18　Rupture of synovium, other site
● M66.2　Spontaneous rupture of extensor tendons
　　　　M66.20　Spontaneous rupture of extensor tendons, unspecified site
● M66.21　Spontaneous rupture of extensor tendons, shoulder
　　　　M66.211　Spontaneous rupture of extensor tendons, right shoulder
　　　　M66.212　Spontaneous rupture of extensor tendons, left shoulder
　　　　M66.219　Spontaneous rupture of extensor tendons, unspecified shoulder
● M66.22　Spontaneous rupture of extensor tendons, upper arm
　　　　M66.221　Spontaneous rupture of extensor tendons, right upper arm
　　　　M66.222　Spontaneous rupture of extensor tendons, left upper arm
　　　　M66.229　Spontaneous rupture of extensor tendons, unspecified upper arm
● M66.23　Spontaneous rupture of extensor tendons, forearm
　　　　M66.231　Spontaneous rupture of extensor tendons, right forearm
　　　　M66.232　Spontaneous rupture of extensor tendons, left forearm
　　　　M66.239　Spontaneous rupture of extensor tendons, unspecified forearm
● M66.24　Spontaneous rupture of extensor tendons, hand
　　　　M66.241　Spontaneous rupture of extensor tendons, right hand
　　　　M66.242　Spontaneous rupture of extensor tendons, left hand
　　　　M66.249　Spontaneous rupture of extensor tendons, unspecified hand
● M66.25　Spontaneous rupture of extensor tendons, thigh
　　　　M66.251　Spontaneous rupture of extensor tendons, right thigh
　　　　M66.252　Spontaneous rupture of extensor tendons, left thigh
　　　　M66.259　Spontaneous rupture of extensor tendons, unspecified thigh
● M66.26　Spontaneous rupture of extensor tendons, lower leg
　　　　M66.261　Spontaneous rupture of extensor tendons, right lower leg
　　　　M66.262　Spontaneous rupture of extensor tendons, left lower leg
　　　　M66.269　Spontaneous rupture of extensor tendons, unspecified lower leg

● M66.27　Spontaneous rupture of extensor tendons, ankle and foot
　　　　M66.271　Spontaneous rupture of extensor tendons, right ankle and foot
　　　　M66.272　Spontaneous rupture of extensor tendons, left ankle and foot
　　　　M66.279　Spontaneous rupture of extensor tendons, unspecified ankle and foot
　　　　M66.28　Spontaneous rupture of extensor tendons, other site
　　　　M66.29　Spontaneous rupture of extensor tendons, multiple sites
● M66.3　Spontaneous rupture of flexor tendons
　　　　M66.30　Spontaneous rupture of flexor tendons, unspecified site
● M66.31　Spontaneous rupture of flexor tendons, shoulder
　　　　M66.311　Spontaneous rupture of flexor tendons, right shoulder
　　　　M66.312　Spontaneous rupture of flexor tendons, left shoulder
　　　　M66.319　Spontaneous rupture of flexor tendons, unspecified shoulder
● M66.32　Spontaneous rupture of flexor tendons, upper arm
　　　　M66.321　Spontaneous rupture of flexor tendons, right upper arm
　　　　M66.322　Spontaneous rupture of flexor tendons, left upper arm
　　　　M66.329　Spontaneous rupture of flexor tendons, unspecified upper arm
● M66.33　Spontaneous rupture of flexor tendons, forearm
　　　　M66.331　Spontaneous rupture of flexor tendons, right forearm
　　　　M66.332　Spontaneous rupture of flexor tendons, left forearm
　　　　M66.339　Spontaneous rupture of flexor tendons, unspecified forearm
● M66.34　Spontaneous rupture of flexor tendons, hand
　　　　M66.341　Spontaneous rupture of flexor tendons, right hand
　　　　M66.342　Spontaneous rupture of flexor tendons, left hand
　　　　M66.349　Spontaneous rupture of flexor tendons, unspecified hand
● M66.35　Spontaneous rupture of flexor tendons, thigh
　　　　M66.351　Spontaneous rupture of flexor tendons, right thigh
　　　　M66.352　Spontaneous rupture of flexor tendons, left thigh
　　　　M66.359　Spontaneous rupture of flexor tendons, unspecified thigh
● M66.36　Spontaneous rupture of flexor tendons, lower leg
　　　　M66.361　Spontaneous rupture of flexor tendons, right lower leg
　　　　M66.362　Spontaneous rupture of flexor tendons, left lower leg
　　　　M66.369　Spontaneous rupture of flexor tendons, unspecified lower leg
● M66.37　Spontaneous rupture of flexor tendons, ankle and foot
　　　　M66.371　Spontaneous rupture of flexor tendons, right ankle and foot
　　　　M66.372　Spontaneous rupture of flexor tendons, left ankle and foot
　　　　M66.379　Spontaneous rupture of flexor tendons, unspecified ankle and foot

CHAPTER 13 (M00-M99)

N　Newborn Age: 0　　P　Pediatric Age: 0–17　　M　Maternity DX: 9–64　　A　Adult Age: 15–124　　♀　Females Only　　♂　Males Only
　Complication\Comorbidity　　　Major C\C　　(Ex)　CC/MCC Exclusions　　　Hospital-Acquired Condition　　　Hierarchical Condition Category

1079

M66.38 Spontaneous rupture of flexor tendons, other site

M66.39 Spontaneous rupture of flexor tendons, multiple sites

● **M66.8** Spontaneous rupture of other tendons

M66.80 Spontaneous rupture of other tendons, unspecified site

● **M66.81** Spontaneous rupture of other tendons, shoulder

　　M66.811 Spontaneous rupture of other tendons, right shoulder

　　M66.812 Spontaneous rupture of other tendons, left shoulder

　　M66.819 Spontaneous rupture of other tendons, unspecified shoulder

● **M66.82** Spontaneous rupture of other tendons, upper arm

　　M66.821 Spontaneous rupture of other tendons, right upper arm

　　M66.822 Spontaneous rupture of other tendons, left upper arm

　　M66.829 Spontaneous rupture of other tendons, unspecified upper arm

● **M66.83** Spontaneous rupture of other tendons, forearm

　　M66.831 Spontaneous rupture of other tendons, right forearm

　　M66.832 Spontaneous rupture of other tendons, left forearm

　　M66.839 Spontaneous rupture of other tendons, unspecified forearm

● **M66.84** Spontaneous rupture of other tendons, hand

　　M66.841 Spontaneous rupture of other tendons, right hand

　　M66.842 Spontaneous rupture of other tendons, left hand

　　M66.849 Spontaneous rupture of other tendons, unspecified hand

● **M66.85** Spontaneous rupture of other tendons, thigh

　　M66.851 Spontaneous rupture of other tendons, right thigh

　　M66.852 Spontaneous rupture of other tendons, left thigh

　　M66.859 Spontaneous rupture of other tendons, unspecified thigh

● **M66.86** Spontaneous rupture of other tendons, lower leg

　　M66.861 Spontaneous rupture of other tendons, right lower leg

　　M66.862 Spontaneous rupture of other tendons, left lower leg

　　M66.869 Spontaneous rupture of other tendons, unspecified lower leg

● **M66.87** Spontaneous rupture of other tendons, ankle and foot

　　M66.871 Spontaneous rupture of other tendons, right ankle and foot

　　M66.872 Spontaneous rupture of other tendons, left ankle and foot

　　M66.879 Spontaneous rupture of other tendons, unspecified ankle and foot

M66.88 Spontaneous rupture of other tendons, other sites

M66.89 Spontaneous rupture of other tendons, multiple sites

M66.9 Spontaneous rupture of unspecified tendon

　　Rupture at musculotendinous junction, nontraumatic

● **M67** Other disorders of synovium and tendon

　Excludes1　palmar fascial fibromatosis [Dupuytren] (M72.0)
　　　　　　tendinitis NOS (M77.9-)
　　　　　　xanthomatosis localized to tendons (E78.2)

● **M67.0** Short Achilles tendon (acquired)

M67.00 Short Achilles tendon (acquired), unspecified ankle

M67.01 Short Achilles tendon (acquired), right ankle

M67.02 Short Achilles tendon (acquired), left ankle

● **M67.2** Synovial hypertrophy, not elsewhere classified

　Excludes1　villonodular synovitis (pigmented) (M12.2-)

M67.20 Synovial hypertrophy, not elsewhere classified, unspecified site

● **M67.21** Synovial hypertrophy, not elsewhere classified, shoulder

　　M67.211 Synovial hypertrophy, not elsewhere classified, right shoulder

　　M67.212 Synovial hypertrophy, not elsewhere classified, left shoulder

　　M67.219 Synovial hypertrophy, not elsewhere classified, unspecified shoulder

● **M67.22** Synovial hypertrophy, not elsewhere classified, upper arm

　　M67.221 Synovial hypertrophy, not elsewhere classified, right upper arm

　　M67.222 Synovial hypertrophy, not elsewhere classified, left upper arm

　　M67.229 Synovial hypertrophy, not elsewhere classified, unspecified upper arm

● **M67.23** Synovial hypertrophy, not elsewhere classified, forearm

　　M67.231 Synovial hypertrophy, not elsewhere classified, right forearm

　　M67.232 Synovial hypertrophy, not elsewhere classified, left forearm

　　M67.239 Synovial hypertrophy, not elsewhere classified, unspecified forearm

● **M67.24** Synovial hypertrophy, not elsewhere classified, hand

　　M67.241 Synovial hypertrophy, not elsewhere classified, right hand

　　M67.242 Synovial hypertrophy, not elsewhere classified, left hand

　　M67.249 Synovial hypertrophy, not elsewhere classified, unspecified hand

● **M67.25** Synovial hypertrophy, not elsewhere classified, thigh

　　M67.251 Synovial hypertrophy, not elsewhere classified, right thigh

　　M67.252 Synovial hypertrophy, not elsewhere classified, left thigh

　　M67.259 Synovial hypertrophy, not elsewhere classified, unspecified thigh

● **M67.26** Synovial hypertrophy, not elsewhere classified, lower leg

　　M67.261 Synovial hypertrophy, not elsewhere classified, right lower leg

　　M67.262 Synovial hypertrophy, not elsewhere classified, left lower leg

　　M67.269 Synovial hypertrophy, not elsewhere classified, unspecified lower leg

CHAPTER 13 (M00-M99)

● M67.27   Synovial hypertrophy, not elsewhere classified, ankle and foot
    M67.271   Synovial hypertrophy, not elsewhere classified, right ankle and foot
    M67.272   Synovial hypertrophy, not elsewhere classified, left ankle and foot
    M67.279   Synovial hypertrophy, not elsewhere classified, unspecified ankle and foot
  M67.28   Synovial hypertrophy, not elsewhere classified, other site
  M67.29   Synovial hypertrophy, not elsewhere classified, multiple sites

● M67.3   Transient synovitis
    Toxic synovitis
    Excludes1   palindromic rheumatism (M12.3-)
  M67.30   Transient synovitis, unspecified site
● M67.31   Transient synovitis, shoulder
    M67.311   Transient synovitis, right shoulder
    M67.312   Transient synovitis, left shoulder
    M67.319   Transient synovitis, unspecified shoulder
● M67.32   Transient synovitis, elbow
    M67.321   Transient synovitis, right elbow
    M67.322   Transient synovitis, left elbow
    M67.329   Transient synovitis, unspecified elbow
● M67.33   Transient synovitis, wrist
    M67.331   Transient synovitis, right wrist
    M67.332   Transient synovitis, left wrist
    M67.339   Transient synovitis, unspecified wrist
● M67.34   Transient synovitis, hand
    M67.341   Transient synovitis, right hand
    M67.342   Transient synovitis, left hand
    M67.349   Transient synovitis, unspecified hand
● M67.35   Transient synovitis, hip
    M67.351   Transient synovitis, right hip
    M67.352   Transient synovitis, left hip
    M67.359   Transient synovitis, unspecified hip
● M67.36   Transient synovitis, knee
    M67.361   Transient synovitis, right knee
    M67.362   Transient synovitis, left knee
    M67.369   Transient synovitis, unspecified knee
● M67.37   Transient synovitis, ankle and foot
    M67.371   Transient synovitis, right ankle and foot
    M67.372   Transient synovitis, left ankle and foot
    M67.379   Transient synovitis, unspecified ankle and foot
  M67.38   Transient synovitis, other site
  M67.39   Transient synovitis, multiple sites

● M67.4   Ganglion
    Ganglion of joint or tendon (sheath)
    Excludes1   ganglion in yaws (A66.6)
    Excludes2   cyst of bursa (M71.2-M71.3)
               cyst of synovium (M71.2-M71.3)
  M67.40   Ganglion, unspecified site
● M67.41   Ganglion, shoulder
    M67.411   Ganglion, right shoulder
    M67.412   Ganglion, left shoulder
    M67.419   Ganglion, unspecified shoulder

● M67.42   Ganglion, elbow
    M67.421   Ganglion, right elbow
    M67.422   Ganglion, left elbow
    M67.429   Ganglion, unspecified elbow
● M67.43   Ganglion, wrist
    M67.431   Ganglion, right wrist
    M67.432   Ganglion, left wrist
    M67.439   Ganglion, unspecified wrist
● M67.44   Ganglion, hand
    M67.441   Ganglion, right hand
    M67.442   Ganglion, left hand
    M67.449   Ganglion, unspecified hand
● M67.45   Ganglion, hip
    M67.451   Ganglion, right hip
    M67.452   Ganglion, left hip
    M67.459   Ganglion, unspecified hip
● M67.46   Ganglion, knee
    M67.461   Ganglion, right knee
    M67.462   Ganglion, left knee
    M67.469   Ganglion, unspecified knee
● M67.47   Ganglion, ankle and foot
    M67.471   Ganglion, right ankle and foot
    M67.472   Ganglion, left ankle and foot
    M67.479   Ganglion, unspecified ankle and foot
  M67.48   Ganglion, other site
  M67.49   Ganglion, multiple sites

● M67.5   Plica syndrome
    Plica knee
    M67.50   Plica syndrome, unspecified knee
    M67.51   Plica syndrome, right knee
    M67.52   Plica syndrome, left knee

● M67.8   Other specified disorders of synovium and tendon
    M67.80   Other specified disorders of synovium and tendon, unspecified site
● M67.81   Other specified disorders of synovium and tendon, shoulder
    M67.811   Other specified disorders of synovium, right shoulder
    M67.812   Other specified disorders of synovium, left shoulder
    M67.813   Other specified disorders of tendon, right shoulder
    M67.814   Other specified disorders of tendon, left shoulder
    M67.819   Other specified disorders of synovium and tendon, unspecified shoulder
● M67.82   Other specified disorders of synovium and tendon, elbow
    M67.821   Other specified disorders of synovium, right elbow
    M67.822   Other specified disorders of synovium, left elbow
    M67.823   Other specified disorders of tendon, right elbow
    M67.824   Other specified disorders of tendon, left elbow
    M67.829   Other specified disorders of synovium and tendon, unspecified elbow

CHAPTER 13 (M00-M99)

N Newborn Age: 0   P Pediatric Age: 0–17   M Maternity DX: 9–64   A Adult Age: 15–124   ♀ Females Only   ♂ Males Only

mplication\Comorbidity   Major C\C   (Ex) CC/MCC Exclusions   Hospital-Acquired Condition   Hierarchical Condition Category   1081

CHAPTER 13 (M00-M99)

● M67.83   Other specified disorders of synovium and
           tendon, wrist
   M67.831   Other specified disorders of
             synovium, right wrist
   M67.832   Other specified disorders of
             synovium, left wrist
   M67.833   Other specified disorders of tendon,
             right wrist
   M67.834   Other specified disorders of tendon,
             left wrist
   M67.839   Other specified disorders of
             synovium and tendon, unspecified
             wrist
● M67.84   Other specified disorders of synovium and
           tendon, hand
   M67.841   Other specified disorders of
             synovium, right hand
   M67.842   Other specified disorders of
             synovium, left hand
   M67.843   Other specified disorders of tendon,
             right hand
   M67.844   Other specified disorders of tendon,
             left hand
   M67.849   Other specified disorders of
             synovium and tendon, unspecified
             hand
● M67.85   Other specified disorders of synovium and
           tendon, hip
   M67.851   Other specified disorders of
             synovium, right hip
   M67.852   Other specified disorders of
             synovium, left hip
   M67.853   Other specified disorders of tendon,
             right hip
   M67.854   Other specified disorders of tendon,
             left hip
   M67.859   Other specified disorders of
             synovium and tendon, unspecified
             hip
● M67.86   Other specified disorders of synovium and
           tendon, knee
   M67.861   Other specified disorders of
             synovium, right knee
   M67.862   Other specified disorders of
             synovium, left knee
   M67.863   Other specified disorders of tendon,
             right knee
   M67.864   Other specified disorders of tendon,
             left knee
   M67.869   Other specified disorders of
             synovium and tendon, unspecified
             knee
● M67.87   Other specified disorders of synovium and
           tendon, ankle and foot
   M67.871   Other specified disorders of
             synovium, right ankle and foot
   M67.872   Other specified disorders of
             synovium, left ankle and foot
   M67.873   Other specified disorders of tendon,
             right ankle and foot
   M67.874   Other specified disorders of tendon,
             left ankle and foot
   M67.879   Other specified disorders of
             synovium and tendon, unspecified
             ankle and foot
   M67.88   Other specified disorders of synovium and
            tendon, other site
   M67.89   Other specified disorders of synovium and
            tendon, multiple sites

● M67.9   Unspecified disorder of synovium and tendon
   M67.90   Unspecified disorder of synovium and tendon,
            unspecified site
● M67.91   Unspecified disorder of synovium and tendon,
           shoulder
   M67.911   Unspecified disorder of synovium
             and tendon, right shoulder
   M67.912   Unspecified disorder of synovium
             and tendon, left shoulder
   M67.919   Unspecified disorder of synovium
             and tendon, unspecified shoulder
● M67.92   Unspecified disorder of synovium and tendon,
           upper arm
   M67.921   Unspecified disorder of synovium
             and tendon, right upper arm
   M67.922   Unspecified disorder of synovium
             and tendon, left upper arm
   M67.929   Unspecified disorder of synovium
             and tendon, unspecified upper arm
● M67.93   Unspecified disorder of synovium and tendon,
           forearm
   M67.931   Unspecified disorder of synovium
             and tendon, right forearm
   M67.932   Unspecified disorder of synovium
             and tendon, left forearm
   M67.939   Unspecified disorder of synovium
             and tendon, unspecified forearm
● M67.94   Unspecified disorder of synovium and tendon,
           hand
   M67.941   Unspecified disorder of synovium
             and tendon, right hand
   M67.942   Unspecified disorder of synovium
             and tendon, left hand
   M67.949   Unspecified disorder of synovium
             and tendon, unspecified hand
● M67.95   Unspecified disorder of synovium and tendon,
           thigh
   M67.951   Unspecified disorder of synovium
             and tendon, right thigh
   M67.952   Unspecified disorder of synovium
             and tendon, left thigh
   M67.959   Unspecified disorder of synovium
             and tendon, unspecified thigh
● M67.96   Unspecified disorder of synovium and tendon,
           lower leg
   M67.961   Unspecified disorder of synovium
             and tendon, right lower leg
   M67.962   Unspecified disorder of synovium
             and tendon, left lower leg
   M67.969   Unspecified disorder of synovium
             and tendon, unspecified lower leg
● M67.97   Unspecified disorder of synovium and tendon,
           ankle and foot
   M67.971   Unspecified disorder of synovium
             and tendon, right ankle and foot
   M67.972   Unspecified disorder of synovium
             and tendon, left ankle and foot
   M67.979   Unspecified disorder of synovium
             and tendon, unspecified ankle and
             foot
   M67.98   Unspecified disorder of synovium and tendon,
            other site
   M67.99   Unspecified disorder of synovium and tendon,
            multiple sites

▶ New   ⇒ Revised   deleted Deleted   Excludes 1   Excludes 2   Includes   Use additional   Code first   Code also   Key
OGCR Official Guidelines   ● Unacceptable Principal Diagnosis   X Assign placeholder X   ● Use Additional Character(s)   ▶ Manifestation Code   C

● M72 Fibroblastic disorders
    Excludes2   retroperitoneal fibromatosis (D48.3)
    M72.0 Palmar fascial fibromatosis [Dupuytren]   A
    M72.1 Knuckle pads
    M72.2 Plantar fascial fibromatosis
           Plantar fasciitis
    M72.4 Pseudosarcomatous fibromatosis
           Nodular fasciitis
    M72.6 Necrotizing fasciitis 🔖 🔖
           Use additional code (B95.-, B96.-) to identify causative
               organism
           Ⓔⓧ See PDX Collection 806
    M72.8 Other fibroblastic disorders
           Abscess of fascia
           Fasciitis NEC
           Other infective fasciitis
           Use additional code to (B95.-, B96.-) identify causative
               organism
           Excludes1   diffuse (eosinophilic) fasciitis (M35.4)
                            necrotizing fasciitis (M72.6)
                            nodular fasciitis (M72.4)
                            perirenal fasciitis NOS (N13.5)
                            perirenal fasciitis with infection (N13.6)
                            plantar fasciitis (M72.2)
    M72.9 Fibroblastic disorder, unspecified
           Fasciitis NOS
           Fibromatosis NOS

● M75 Shoulder lesions
    Excludes2   shoulder-hand syndrome (M89.0-)
    ● M75.0 Adhesive capsulitis of shoulder
             Frozen shoulder
             Periarthritis of shoulder
             M75.00 Adhesive capsulitis of unspecified shoulder
             M75.01 Adhesive capsulitis of right shoulder
             M75.02 Adhesive capsulitis of left shoulder
                     Coding Clinic: 2015, Q2, P23
    ● M75.1 Rotator cuff tear or rupture, not specified as traumatic
             Rotator cuff syndrome
             Supraspinatus syndrome
             Supraspinatus tear or rupture, not specified as
                 traumatic
             Excludes1   tear of rotator cuff, traumatic (S46.01-)
             Gradual onset due to repetitive stress to rotator cuff
             ● M75.10 Unspecified rotator cuff tear or rupture, not
                       specified as traumatic
                       M75.100 Unspecified rotator cuff tear or
                                rupture of unspecified shoulder, not
                                specified as traumatic
                       M75.101 Unspecified rotator cuff tear or
                                rupture of right shoulder, not
                                specified as traumatic
                       M75.102 Unspecified rotator cuff tear or
                                rupture of left shoulder, not specified
                                as traumatic
             ● M75.11 Incomplete rotator cuff tear or rupture not
                       specified as traumatic
                       M75.110 Incomplete rotator cuff tear or rupture
                                of unspecified shoulder, not specified
                                as traumatic
                       M75.111 Incomplete rotator cuff tear or rupture
                                of right shoulder, not specified as
                                traumatic
                       M75.112 Incomplete rotator cuff tear or rupture
                                of left shoulder, not specified as
                                traumatic

● M75.12 Complete rotator cuff tear or rupture not
          specified as traumatic
          M75.120 Complete rotator cuff tear or rupture
                   of unspecified shoulder, not specified
                   as traumatic
          M75.121 Complete rotator cuff tear or rupture
                   of right shoulder, not specified as
                   traumatic
          M75.122 Complete rotator cuff tear or rupture
                   of left shoulder, not specified as
                   traumatic
● M75.2 Bicipital tendinitis
         M75.20 Bicipital tendinitis, unspecified shoulder
         M75.21 Bicipital tendinitis, right shoulder
         M75.22 Bicipital tendinitis, left shoulder
● M75.3 Calcific tendinitis of shoulder
         Calcified bursa of shoulder
         M75.30 Calcific tendinitis of unspecified shoulder
         M75.31 Calcific tendinitis of right shoulder
         M75.32 Calcific tendinitis of left shoulder
● M75.4 Impingement syndrome of shoulder
         M75.40 Impingement syndrome of unspecified
                 shoulder
         M75.41 Impingement syndrome of right shoulder
         M75.42 Impingement syndrome of left shoulder
● M75.5 Bursitis of shoulder
         M75.50 Bursitis of unspecified shoulder
         M75.51 Bursitis of right shoulder
         M75.52 Bursitis of left shoulder
● M75.8 Other shoulder lesions
         M75.80 Other shoulder lesions, unspecified shoulder
         M75.81 Other shoulder lesions, right shoulder
         M75.82 Other shoulder lesions, left shoulder
● M75.9 Shoulder lesion, unspecified
         M75.90 Shoulder lesion, unspecified, unspecified
                 shoulder
         M75.91 Shoulder lesion, unspecified, right shoulder
         M75.92 Shoulder lesion, unspecified, left shoulder

● M76 Enthesopathies, lower limb, excluding foot
    Excludes2   bursitis due to use, overuse and pressure (M70.-)
                    enthesopathies of ankle and foot (M77.5-)
    ● M76.0 Gluteal tendinitis
             M76.00 Gluteal tendinitis, unspecified hip
             M76.01 Gluteal tendinitis, right hip
             M76.02 Gluteal tendinitis, left hip
    ● M76.1 Psoas tendinitis
             M76.10 Psoas tendinitis, unspecified hip
             M76.11 Psoas tendinitis, right hip
             M76.12 Psoas tendinitis, left hip
    ● M76.2 Iliac crest spur
             M76.20 Iliac crest spur, unspecified hip
             M76.21 Iliac crest spur, right hip
             M76.22 Iliac crest spur, left hip
    ● M76.3 Iliotibial band syndrome
             M76.30 Iliotibial band syndrome, unspecified leg
             M76.31 Iliotibial band syndrome, right leg
             M76.32 Iliotibial band syndrome, left leg
    ● M76.4 Tibial collateral bursitis [Pellegrini-Stieda]
             M76.40 Tibial collateral bursitis [Pellegrini-Stieda],
                     unspecified leg
             M76.41 Tibial collateral bursitis [Pellegrini-Stieda],
                     right leg
             M76.42 Tibial collateral bursitis [Pellegrini-Stieda], left
                     leg

CHAPTER 13 (M00-M99)

N Newborn Age: 0   **P** Pediatric Age: 0–17   **M** Maternity DX: 9–64   **A** Adult Age: 15–124   ♀ Females Only   ♂ Males Only
🔖 Complication\Comorbidity   🔖 Major C\C   Ⓔⓧ CC/MCC Exclusions   🔖 Hospital-Acquired Condition   🔖 Hierarchical Condition Category

1087

CHAPTER 13 (M00-M99)

● **M76.5 Patellar** tendinitis
    M76.50 Patellar tendinitis, unspecified knee
    M76.51 Patellar tendinitis, right knee
    M76.52 Patellar tendinitis, left knee
● **M76.6 Achilles** tendinitis
    Achilles bursitis
    M76.60 Achilles tendinitis, unspecified leg
    M76.61 Achilles tendinitis, right leg
    M76.62 Achilles tendinitis, left leg
● **M76.7 Peroneal** tendinitis
    M76.70 Peroneal tendinitis, unspecified leg
    M76.71 Peroneal tendinitis, right leg
    M76.72 Peroneal tendinitis, left leg
● **M76.8 Other** specified enthesopathies of lower limb, excluding foot
  ● **M76.81 Anterior** tibial syndrome
      M76.811 Anterior tibial syndrome, right leg
      M76.812 Anterior tibial syndrome, left leg
      M76.819 Anterior tibial syndrome, unspecified leg
  ● **M76.82 Posterior** tibial tendinitis
      M76.821 Posterior tibial tendinitis, right leg
      M76.822 Posterior tibial tendinitis, left leg
      M76.829 Posterior tibial tendinitis, unspecified leg
  ● **M76.89 Other** specified enthesopathies of lower limb, excluding foot
      M76.891 Other specified enthesopathies of right lower limb, excluding foot
      M76.892 Other specified enthesopathies of left lower limb, excluding foot
      M76.899 Other specified enthesopathies of unspecified lower limb, excluding foot
    M76.9 Unspecified enthesopathy, lower limb, excluding foot

● **M77 Other enthesopathies**
    Excludes1 bursitis NOS (M71.9-)
    Excludes2 bursitis due to use, overuse and pressure (M70.-)
               osteophyte (M25.7)
               spinal enthesopathy (M46.0-)
  ● **M77.0 Medial** epicondylitis
      M77.00 Medial epicondylitis, unspecified elbow
      M77.01 Medial epicondylitis, right elbow
      M77.02 Medial epicondylitis, left elbow
  ● **M77.1 Lateral** epicondylitis
      Tennis elbow
      M77.10 Lateral epicondylitis, unspecified elbow
      M77.11 Lateral epicondylitis, right elbow
      M77.12 Lateral epicondylitis, left elbow
  ● **M77.2 Periarthritis** of wrist
      M77.20 Periarthritis, unspecified wrist
      M77.21 Periarthritis, right wrist
      M77.22 Periarthritis, left wrist
  ● **M77.3 Calcaneal** spur
      M77.30 Calcaneal spur, unspecified foot
      M77.31 Calcaneal spur, right foot
      M77.32 Calcaneal spur, left foot
  ● **M77.4 Metatarsalgia**
      Excludes1 Morton's metatarsalgia (G57.6)
      M77.40 Metatarsalgia, unspecified foot
      M77.41 Metatarsalgia, right foot
      M77.42 Metatarsalgia, left foot

● **M77.5 Other** enthesopathy of foot and ankle
    M77.50 Other enthesopathy of unspecified foot and ankle
    M77.51 Other enthesopathy of right foot and ankle
    M77.52 Other enthesopathy of left foot and ankle
    M77.8 Other enthesopathies, not elsewhere classified
    M77.9 Enthesopathy, unspecified
      Bone spur NOS
      Capsulitis NOS
      Periarthritis NOS
      Tendinitis NOS

● **M79 Other and unspecified soft tissue disorders, not elsewhere classified**
    Excludes1 psychogenic rheumatism (F45.8)
               soft tissue pain, psychogenic (F45.41)
    M79.0 Rheumatism, unspecified
      Excludes1 fibromyalgia (M79.7)
               palindromic rheumatism (M12.3-)
  ● **M79.1 Myalgia**
      Myofascial pain syndrome
      M79.10 Myalgia, unspecified site
      M79.11 Myalgia of mastication muscle
      M79.12 Myalgia of auxiliary muscles, head and neck
      M79.18 Myalgia, other site
        Excludes1 fibromyalgia (M79.7)
                myositis (M60.-)
    M79.2 Neuralgia and neuritis, unspecified
      Excludes1 brachial radiculitis NOS (M54.1)
               lumbosacral radiculitis NOS (M54.1)
               mononeuropathies (G56-G58)
               radiculitis NOS (M54.1)
               sciatica (M54.3-M54.4)
    M79.3 Panniculitis, unspecified
      Excludes1 lupus panniculitis (L93.2)
               neck and back panniculitis (M54.0-)
               relapsing [Weber-Christian] panniculitis (M35.6)
    M79.4 Hypertrophy of (infrapatellar) fat pad
    M79.5 Residual foreign body in soft tissue
      Excludes1 foreign body granuloma of skin and subcutaneous tissue (L92.3)
               foreign body granuloma of soft tissue (M60.2-)
  ● **M79.6 Pain in limb, hand, foot, fingers and toes**
      Excludes2 pain in joint (M25.5-)
    ● **M79.60 Pain in limb, unspecified**
        M79.601 Pain in right arm
          Pain in right upper limb NOS
        M79.602 Pain in left arm
          Pain in left upper limb NOS
        M79.603 Pain in arm, unspecified
          Pain in upper limb NOS
        M79.604 Pain in right leg
          Pain in right lower limb NOS
        M79.605 Pain in left leg
          Pain in left lower limb NOS
        M79.606 Pain in leg, unspecified
          Pain in lower limb NOS
        M79.609 Pain in unspecified limb
          Pain in limb NOS
    ● **M79.62 Pain in upper arm**
        Pain in axillary region
        M79.621 Pain in right upper arm
        M79.622 Pain in left upper arm
        M79.629 Pain in unspecified upper arm
    ● **M79.63 Pain in forearm**
        M79.631 Pain in right forearm
        M79.632 Pain in left forearm
        M79.639 Pain in unspecified forearm

● M79.64 Pain in hand and fingers
    M79.641 Pain in right hand
    M79.642 Pain in left hand
    M79.643 Pain in unspecified hand
    M79.644 Pain in right finger(s)
    M79.645 Pain in left finger(s)
    M79.646 Pain in unspecified finger(s)

● M79.65 Pain in thigh
    M79.651 Pain in right thigh
    M79.652 Pain in left thigh
    M79.659 Pain in unspecified thigh

● M79.66 Pain in lower leg
    M79.661 Pain in right lower leg
    M79.662 Pain in left lower leg
    M79.669 Pain in unspecified lower leg

● M79.67 Pain in foot and toes
    M79.671 Pain in right foot
    M79.672 Pain in left foot
    M79.673 Pain in unspecified foot
    M79.674 Pain in right toe(s)
    M79.675 Pain in left toe(s)
    M79.676 Pain in unspecified toe(s)

M79.7 Fibromyalgia
    Fibromyositis
    Fibrositis
    Myofibrositis

● M79.A Nontraumatic compartment syndrome
    Code first, if applicable, associated postprocedural complication
    Excludes1 compartment syndrome NOS (T79.A-)
               fibromyalgia (M79.7) nontraumatic
                  ischemic infarction of muscle (M62.2-)
               traumatic compartment syndrome (T79.A-)

  ● M79.A1 Nontraumatic compartment syndrome of upper extremity
      Nontraumatic compartment syndrome of shoulder, arm, forearm, wrist, hand, and fingers
      M79.A11 Nontraumatic compartment syndrome of right upper extremity 🅗
          (Ex:) See PDX Collection 3278
      M79.A12 Nontraumatic compartment syndrome of left upper extremity 🅗
          (Ex:) See PDX Collection 3279
      M79.A19 Nontraumatic compartment syndrome of unspecified upper extremity 🅗
          (Ex:) See PDX Collection 3280

  ● M79.A2 Nontraumatic compartment syndrome of lower extremity
      Nontraumatic compartment syndrome of hip, buttock, thigh, leg, foot, and toes
      (Ex:) **For category M79.A2 CC codes:** See PDX Collection 984, 3829, 3831
      M79.A21 Nontraumatic compartment syndrome of right lower extremity 🅗
      M79.A22 Nontraumatic compartment syndrome of left lower extremity 🅗
      M79.A29 Nontraumatic compartment syndrome of unspecified lower extremity 🅗

  M79.A3 Nontraumatic compartment syndrome of abdomen 🅗
      (Ex:) See PDX Collection 895

  M79.A9 Nontraumatic compartment syndrome of other sites 🅗
      (Ex:) See PDX Collection 3281

● M79.8 Other specified soft tissue disorders
  M79.81 Nontraumatic hematoma of soft tissue
    Nontraumatic hematoma of muscle
    Nontraumatic seroma of muscle and soft tissue
  M79.89 Other specified soft tissue disorders
    Polyalgia

M79.9 Soft tissue disorder, unspecified

OGCR See Section I.C., Chapter 13.d.

Osteoporosis

Osteoporosis is a systemic condition, meaning that all bones of the musculoskeletal system are affected. Therefore, site is not a component of the codes under category M81, Osteoporosis without current pathological fracture. The site codes under category M80, Osteoporosis with current pathological fracture, identify the site of the fracture, not the osteoporosis.

1) Osteoporosis without pathological fracture

Category M81, Osteoporosis without current pathological fracture, is for use for patients with osteoporosis who do not currently have a pathologic fracture due to the osteoporosis, even if they have had a fracture in the past. For patients with a history of osteoporosis fractures, status code Z87.310, Personal history of (healed) osteoporosis fracture, should follow the code from M81.

2) Osteoporosis with current pathological fracture

Category M80, Osteoporosis with current pathological fracture, is for patients who have a current pathologic fracture at the time of an encounter. The codes under M80 identify the site of the fracture. A code from category M80, not a traumatic fracture code, should be used for any patient with known osteoporosis who suffers a fracture, even if the patient had a minor fall or trauma, if that fall or trauma would not usually break a normal, healthy bone.

OSTEOPATHIES AND CHONDROPATHIES (M80-M94)

DISORDERS OF BONE DENSITY AND STRUCTURE (M80-M85)

M80 Osteoporosis with current pathological fracture
    Excessive skeletal fragility (porous bone) resulting in bone fractures
    Includes osteoporosis with current fragility fracture
    Use additional code to identify major osseous defect, if applicable (M89.7-)
    Excludes1 collapsed vertebra NOS (M48.5)
               pathological fracture NOS (M84.4)
               wedging of vertebra NOS (M48.5)
    Excludes2 personal history of (healed) osteoporosis fracture (Z87.310)
    Coding Clinic: 2018, Q2, P12

The appropriate 7th character is to be added to each code from category M80:

A	initial encounter for fracture *All encounters involving diagnosis and treatment*
D	subsequent encounter for fracture with routine healing
G	subsequent encounter for fracture with delayed healing *Encounters for attention to casting or fixation devices, medication, and follow-up visits during the healing phase*
K	subsequent encounter for fracture with nonunion *Total failure of fracture healing*
P	subsequent encounter for fracture with malunion *Fracture ends do not heal together correctly.*
S	sequela

    (Ex:) **For category M80[A] CC codes:** See PDX Collection 888
             For category M80[K,P] CC codes: See PDX Collection 561

● M80.0 Age-related osteoporosis with current pathological fracture
    Involutional osteoporosis with current pathological fracture
    Osteoporosis NOS with current pathological fracture
    Postmenopausal osteoporosis with current pathological fracture
    Senile osteoporosis with current pathological fracture

  X● M80.00 Age-related osteoporosis with current pathological fracture, unspecified site
      A, K, P 🅗   A

N Newborn Age: 0   **P** Pediatric Age: 0–17   **M** Maternity DX: 9–64   **A** Adult Age: 15–124   ♀ Females Only   ♂ Males Only

🅗 Complication\Comorbidity   🅗 Major C\C   (Ex:) CC/MCC Exclusions   🅗 Hospital-Acquired Condition   🅗 Hierarchical Condition Category

1089

CHAPTER 13 (M00-M99)

● M80.01   Age-related osteoporosis with current pathological fracture, shoulder

    ● M80.011   Age-related osteoporosis with current pathological fracture, right shoulder A, K, P 🔍   A

    ● M80.012   Age-related osteoporosis with current pathological fracture, left shoulder A, K, P 🔍   A

    ● M80.019   Age-related osteoporosis with current pathological fracture, unspecified shoulder A, K, P 🔍   A

● M80.02   Age-related osteoporosis with current pathological fracture, humerus

    ● M80.021   Age-related osteoporosis with current pathological fracture, right humerus A, K, P 🔍   A

    ● M80.022   Age-related osteoporosis with current pathological fracture, left humerus A, K, P 🔍   A

    ● M80.029   Age-related osteoporosis with current pathological fracture, unspecified humerus A, K, P 🔍   A

● M80.03   Age-related osteoporosis with current pathological fracture, forearm
    Age-related osteoporosis with current pathological fracture of wrist

    ● M80.031   Age-related osteoporosis with current pathological fracture, right forearm A, K, P 🔍   A

    ● M80.032   Age-related osteoporosis with current pathological fracture, left forearm A, K, P 🔍   A

    ● M80.039   Age-related osteoporosis with current pathological fracture, unspecified forearm A, K, P 🔍   A

● M80.04   Age-related osteoporosis with current pathological fracture, hand

    ● M80.041   Age-related osteoporosis with current pathological fracture, right hand A, K, P 🔍   A

    ● M80.042   Age-related osteoporosis with current pathological fracture, left hand A, K, P 🔍   A

    ● M80.049   Age-related osteoporosis with current pathological fracture, unspecified hand A, K, P 🔍   A

● M80.05   Age-related osteoporosis with current pathological fracture, femur
    Age-related osteoporosis with current pathological fracture of hip

    ● M80.051   Age-related osteoporosis with current pathological fracture, right femur A, K, P 🔍, A 🔍   A

    ● M80.052   Age-related osteoporosis with current pathological fracture, left femur A, K, P 🔍, A 🔍   A
        Coding Clinic: 2018, Q2, P12

    ● M80.059   Age-related osteoporosis with current pathological fracture, unspecified femur A, K, P 🔍, A 🔍   A

● M80.06   Age-related osteoporosis with current pathological fracture, lower leg

    ● M80.061   Age-related osteoporosis with current pathological fracture, right lower leg A, K, P 🔍   A

    ● M80.062   Age-related osteoporosis with current pathological fracture, left lower leg A, K, P 🔍   A

    ● M80.069   Age-related osteoporosis with current pathological fracture, unspecified lower leg A, K, P 🔍   A

● M80.07   Age-related osteoporosis with current pathological fracture, ankle and foot

    ● M80.071   Age-related osteoporosis with current pathological fracture, right ankle and foot A, K, P 🔍   A

    ● M80.072   Age-related osteoporosis with current pathological fracture, left ankle and foot A, K, P 🔍   A

    ● M80.079   Age-related osteoporosis with current pathological fracture, unspecified ankle and foot A, K, P 🔍   A

X ● M80.08   Age-related osteoporosis with current pathological fracture, vertebra(e) A, K, P 🔍, A 🔍   A

M80.0A   Age-related osteoporosis with current pathological fracture, other site A, D, G, K, P, S 🔍   A

● M80.8   Other osteoporosis with current pathological fracture
    Drug-induced osteoporosis with current pathological fracture
    Idiopathic osteoporosis with current pathological fracture
    Osteoporosis of disuse with current pathological fracture
    Postoophorectomy osteoporosis with current pathological fracture
    Postsurgical malabsorption osteoporosis with current pathological fracture
    Post-traumatic osteoporosis with current pathological fracture
    Use additional code for adverse effect, if applicable, to identify drug (T36-T50 with fifth or sixth character 5)

X ● M80.80   Other osteoporosis with current pathological fracture, unspecified site A, K, P 🔍   A

● M80.81   Other osteoporosis with pathological fracture, shoulder

    ● M80.811   Other osteoporosis with current pathological fracture, right shoulder A, K, P 🔍

    ● M80.812   Other osteoporosis with current pathological fracture, left shoulder A, K, P 🔍

    ● M80.819   Other osteoporosis with current pathological fracture, unspecified shoulder A, K, P 🔍

● M80.82   Other osteoporosis with current pathological fracture, humerus

    ● M80.821   Other osteoporosis with current pathological fracture, right humerus A, K, P 🔍

    ● M80.822   Other osteoporosis with current pathological fracture, left humerus A, K, P 🔍

    ● M80.829   Other osteoporosis with current pathological fracture, unspecified humerus A, K, P 🔍

● M80.83   Other osteoporosis with current pathological fracture, forearm
    Other osteoporosis with current pathological fracture of wrist

    ● M80.831   Other osteoporosis with current pathological fracture, right forearm A, K, P 🔍

    ● M80.832   Other osteoporosis with current pathological fracture, left forearm A, K, P 🔍

    ● M80.839   Other osteoporosis with current pathological fracture, unspecified forearm A, K, P 🔍

M80.8A   Other osteoporosis with current pathological fracture, other site A, K, P 🔍
    Ⓔˣ **For category M80.8A[A,K,P] CC codes:** See PDX Collection 4046, 4084, 4086

▶ New   ⇒ Revised   ~~deleted~~ Deleted   Excludes 1   Excludes 2   Includes   Use additional   Code first   Code also   Key words
OGCR Official Guidelines   ● Unacceptable Principal Diagnosis   X Assign placeholder X   ● Use Additional Character(s)   ▶ Manifestation Code   **Coding Clinic**

● **M80.84 Other osteoporosis with current pathological fracture, hand**
  ● **M80.841 Other osteoporosis with current pathological fracture, right hand** A, K, P 🔵
  ● **M80.842 Other osteoporosis with current pathological fracture, left hand** A, K, P 🔵
  ● **M80.849 Other osteoporosis with current pathological fracture, unspecified hand** A, K, P 🔵

● **M80.85 Other osteoporosis with current pathological fracture, femur**
    Other osteoporosis with current pathological fracture of hip
  ● **M80.851 Other osteoporosis with current pathological fracture, right femur** A, K, P 🔵, A 🔵
  ● **M80.852 Other osteoporosis with current pathological fracture, left femur** A, K, P 🔵, A 🔵
  ● **M80.859 Other osteoporosis with current pathological fracture, unspecified femur** A, K, P 🔵, A 🔵

● **M80.86 Other osteoporosis with current pathological fracture, lower leg**
  ● **M80.861 Other osteoporosis with current pathological fracture, right lower leg** A, K, P 🔵
  ● **M80.862 Other osteoporosis with current pathological fracture, left lower leg** A, K, P 🔵
  ● **M80.869 Other osteoporosis with current pathological fracture, unspecified lower leg** A, K, P 🔵

● **M80.87 Other osteoporosis with current pathological fracture, ankle and foot**
  ● **M80.871 Other osteoporosis with current pathological fracture, right ankle and foot** A, K, P 🔵
  ● **M80.872 Other osteoporosis with current pathological fracture, left ankle and foot** A, K, P 🔵
  ● **M80.879 Other osteoporosis with current pathological fracture, unspecified ankle and foot** A, K, P 🔵

X ● **M80.88 Other osteoporosis with current pathological fracture, vertebra(e)** A, K, P 🔵, A 🔵

● **M81 Osteoporosis without current pathological fracture**
    Use additional code to identify:
      major osseous defect, if applicable (M89.7-)
      personal history of (healed) osteoporosis fracture, if applicable (Z87.310)

    | **Excludes1** | osteoporosis with current pathological fracture (M80.-) |
    | | Sudeck's atrophy (M89.0) |

  M81.0 Age-related osteoporosis without current pathological fracture   A
    Involutional osteoporosis without current pathological fracture
    Osteoporosis NOS
    Postmenopausal osteoporosis without current pathological fracture
    Senile osteoporosis without current pathological fracture

  M81.6 Localized osteoporosis [Lequesne]
    | **Excludes1** | Sudeck's atrophy (M89.0) |

M81.8 Other osteoporosis without current pathological fracture
    Drug-induced osteoporosis without current pathological fracture
    Idiopathic osteoporosis without current pathological fracture
    Osteoporosis of disuse without current pathological fracture
    Postoophorectomy osteoporosis without current pathological fracture
    Postsurgical malabsorption osteoporosis without current pathological fracture
    Post-traumatic osteoporosis without current pathological fracture
    Use additional code for adverse effect, if applicable, to identify drug (T36-T50 with fifth or sixth character 5)

● **M83 Adult osteomalacia**
    | **Excludes1** | infantile and juvenile osteomalacia (E55.0) |
    | | renal osteodystrophy (N25.0) |
    | | rickets (active) (E55.0) |
    | | rickets (active) sequelae (E64.3) |
    | | vitamin D-resistant osteomalacia (E83.3) |
    | | vitamin D-resistant rickets (active) (E83.3) |

  M83.0 Puerperal osteomalacia ♀   M
  M83.1 Senile osteomalacia   A
  M83.2 Adult osteomalacia due to malabsorption   A
    Postsurgical malabsorption osteomalacia in adults
  M83.3 Adult osteomalacia due to malnutrition   A
  M83.4 Aluminum bone disease
  M83.5 Other drug-induced osteomalacia in adults   A
    Use additional code for adverse effect, if applicable, to identify drug (T36-T50 with fifth or sixth character 5)
  M83.8 Other adult osteomalacia   A
  M83.9 Adult osteomalacia, unspecified   A

● **M84 Disorder of continuity of bone**
    | **Excludes2** | traumatic fracture of bone-see fracture, by site |

  ● **M84.3 Stress fracture**
    Fatigue fracture
    March fracture
    Stress fracture NOS
    Stress reaction
    Use additional external cause code(s) to identify the cause of the stress fracture

    | **Excludes1** | pathological fracture NOS (M84.4.-) |
    | | pathological fracture due to osteoporosis (M80.-) |
    | | traumatic fracture (S12.-, S22.-, S32.-, S42.-, S52.-, S62.-, S72.-, S82.-, S92.-) |

    | **Excludes2** | personal history of (healed) stress (fatigue) fracture (Z87.312) |
    | | stress fracture of vertebra (M48.4-) |

    The appropriate 7th character is to be added to each code from subcategory M84.3:

A	initial encounter for fracture
D	subsequent encounter for fracture with routine healing
G	subsequent encounter for fracture with delayed healing
K	subsequent encounter for fracture with nonunion
P	subsequent encounter for fracture with malunion
S	sequela

    (Ex:) **For category M84[A] CC codes:** See PDX Collection 888
    For category M84[K,P] CC codes: See PDX Collection 561

  X ● **M84.30 Stress fracture, unspecified site** K, P 🔵
  ● **M84.31 Stress fracture, shoulder**
    ● **M84.311 Stress fracture, right shoulder** K, P 🔵
    ● **M84.312 Stress fracture, left shoulder** K, P 🔵
    ● **M84.319 Stress fracture, unspecified shoulder** K, P 🔵

N Newborn Age: 0   **P** Pediatric Age: 0–17   **M** Maternity DX: 9–64   **A** Adult Age: 15–124   ♀ Females Only   ♂ Males Only

🔵 Complication\Comorbidity   🔵 Major C\C   (Ex:) CC/MCC Exclusions   🔵 Hospital-Acquired Condition   🔵 Hierarchical Condition Category

1091

● M84.32   Stress fracture, humerus
- ● M84.321   Stress fracture, right humerus K, P
- ● M84.322   Stress fracture, left humerus K, P
- ● M84.329   Stress fracture, unspecified humerus K, P

● M84.33   Stress fracture, ulna and radius
- ● M84.331   Stress fracture, right ulna K, P
- ● M84.332   Stress fracture, left ulna K, P
- ● M84.333   Stress fracture, right radius K, P
- ● M84.334   Stress fracture, left radius K, P
- ● M84.339   Stress fracture, unspecified ulna and radius K, P

● M84.34   Stress fracture, hand and fingers
- ● M84.341   Stress fracture, right hand K, P
- ● M84.342   Stress fracture, left hand K, P
- ● M84.343   Stress fracture, unspecified hand K, P
- ● M84.344   Stress fracture, right finger(s) K, P
- ● M84.345   Stress fracture, left finger(s) K, P
- ● M84.346   Stress fracture, unspecified finger(s) K, P

● M84.35   Stress fracture, pelvis and femur
    Stress fracture, hip
- ● M84.350   Stress fracture, pelvis K, P
- ● M84.351   Stress fracture, right femur K, P
- ● M84.352   Stress fracture, left femur K, P
- ● M84.353   Stress fracture, unspecified femur K, P
- ● M84.359   Stress fracture, hip, unspecified K, P

● M84.36   Stress fracture, tibia and fibula
- ● M84.361   Stress fracture, right tibia K, P
- ● M84.362   Stress fracture, left tibia K, P
- ● M84.363   Stress fracture, right fibula K, P
- ● M84.364   Stress fracture, left fibula K, P
- ● M84.369   Stress fracture, unspecified tibia and fibula K, P

● M84.37   Stress fracture, ankle, foot and toes
- ● M84.371   Stress fracture, right ankle K, P
- ● M84.372   Stress fracture, left ankle K, P
- ● M84.373   Stress fracture, unspecified ankle K, P
- ● M84.374   Stress fracture, right foot K, P
- ● M84.375   Stress fracture, left foot K, P
- ● M84.376   Stress fracture, unspecified foot K, P
- ● M84.377   Stress fracture, right toe(s) K, P
- ● M84.378   Stress fracture, left toe(s) K, P
- ● M84.379   Stress fracture, unspecified toe(s) K, P

X ● M84.38   Stress fracture, other site K, P
     Excludes2   stress fracture of vertebra (M48.4-)

● M84.4   Pathological fracture, not elsewhere classified
    Chronic fracture
    Pathological fracture NOS
    Excludes1   collapsed vertebra NEC (M48.5)
             pathological fracture in neoplastic disease (M84.5-)
             pathological fracture in osteoporosis (M80.-)
             pathological fracture in other disease (M84.6-)
             stress fracture (M84.3-)
             traumatic fracture (S12.-, S22.-, S32.-, S42.-, S52.-, S62.-, S72.-, S82.-, S92.-)
    Excludes2   personal history of (healed) pathological fracture (Z87.311)

The appropriate 7th character is to be added to each code from subcategory M84.4:

> A   initial encounter for fracture
> D   subsequent encounter for fracture with routine healing
> G   subsequent encounter for fracture with delayed healing
> K   subsequent encounter for fracture with nonunion
> P   subsequent encounter for fracture with malunion
> S   sequela

(Ex:) **For category M80[A] CC codes:** See PDX Collection 888
     For category M80[K,P] CC codes: See PDX Collection 561

X ● M84.40   Pathological fracture, unspecified site A, K, P

● M84.41   Pathological fracture, shoulder
- ● M84.411   Pathological fracture, right shoulder A, K, P
- ● M84.412   Pathological fracture, left shoulder A, K, P
- ● M84.419   Pathological fracture, unspecified shoulder A, K, P

● M84.42   Pathological fracture, humerus
- ● M84.421   Pathological fracture, right humerus A, K, P
- ● M84.422   Pathological fracture, left humerus A, K, P
- ● M84.429   Pathological fracture, unspecified humerus A, K, P

● M84.43   Pathological fracture, ulna and radius
- ● M84.431   Pathological fracture, right ulna A, K, P
- ● M84.432   Pathological fracture, left ulna A, K, P
- ● M84.433   Pathological fracture, right radius A, K, P
- ● M84.434   Pathological fracture, left radius A, K, P
- ● M84.439   Pathological fracture, unspecified ulna and radius A, K, P

● M84.44   Pathological fracture, hand and fingers
    ● M84.441   Pathological fracture, right hand
           A, K, P
    ● M84.442   Pathological fracture, left hand
           A, K, P
    ● M84.443   Pathological fracture, unspecified
           hand A, K, P
    ● M84.444   Pathological fracture, right finger(s)
           A, K, P
    ● M84.445   Pathological fracture, left finger(s)
           A, K, P
    ● M84.446   Pathological fracture, unspecified
           finger(s) A, K, P
● M84.45   Pathological fracture, femur and pelvis
    ● M84.451   Pathological fracture, right femur
           A, K, P, A
    ● M84.452   Pathological fracture, left femur
           A, K, P, A
    ● M84.453   Pathological fracture, unspecified
           femur A, K, P, A
    ● M84.454   Pathological fracture, pelvis
           A, K, P, A
           Coding Clinic: 2016, Q4, P43
    ● M84.459   Pathological fracture, hip, unspecified
           A, K, P, A
● M84.46   Pathological fracture, tibia and fibula
    ● M84.461   Pathological fracture, right tibia
           A, K, P
    ● M84.462   Pathological fracture, left tibia
           A, K, P
    ● M84.463   Pathological fracture, right fibula
           A, K, P
    ● M84.464   Pathological fracture, left fibula
           A, K, P
    ● M84.469   Pathological fracture, unspecified
           tibia and fibula A, K, P
● M84.47   Pathological fracture, ankle, foot and toes
    ● M84.471   Pathological fracture, right ankle
           A, K, P
    ● M84.472   Pathological fracture, left ankle
           A, K, P
    ● M84.473   Pathological fracture, unspecified
           ankle A, K, P
    ● M84.474   Pathological fracture, right foot
           A, K, P
    ● M84.475   Pathological fracture, left foot
           A, K, P
    ● M84.476   Pathological fracture, unspecified foot
           A, K, P
    ● M84.477   Pathological fracture, right toe(s)
           A, K, P
    ● M84.478   Pathological fracture, left toe(s)
           A, K, P
    ● M84.479   Pathological fracture, unspecified
           toe(s) A, K, P
X ● M84.48   Pathological fracture, other site A, K, P

OGCR Section I.C. 13.C.

Coding of Pathologic Fractures

7th character A is for use as long as the patient is receiving active treatment for the fracture. While the patient may be seen by a new or different provider over the course of treatment for a pathological fracture, assignment of the 7th character is based on whether the patient is undergoing active treatment and not whether the provider is seeing the patient for the first time.

7th character, D is to be used for encounters after the patient has completed active treatment for the fracture and is receiving routine care for the fracture during the healing or recovery phase. The other 7th characters, listed under each subcategory in the Tabular List, are to be used for subsequent encounters for treatment of problems associated with the healing, such as malunions, nonunions, and sequelae.

Care for complications of surgical treatment for fracture repairs during the healing or recovery phase should be coded with the appropriate complication codes.

See Section I.C.19. Coding of traumatic fractures.

● M84.5   Pathological fracture in neoplastic disease
    Code also underlying neoplasm
    The appropriate 7th character is to be added to each code from subcategory M84.5:

A	initial encounter for fracture
D	subsequent encounter for fracture with routine healing
G	subsequent encounter for fracture with delayed healing
K	subsequent encounter for fracture with nonunion
P	subsequent encounter for fracture with malunion
S	sequela

(Ex) **For category M80[A] CC codes:** See PDX Collection 888
     For category M80[K,P] CC codes: See PDX Collection 561

X ● M84.50   Pathological fracture in neoplastic disease, unspecified site A, K, P
   ● M84.51   Pathological fracture in neoplastic disease, shoulder
     ● M84.511   Pathological fracture in neoplastic disease, right shoulder A, K, P
     ● M84.512   Pathological fracture in neoplastic disease, left shoulder A, K, P
     ● M84.519   Pathological fracture in neoplastic disease, unspecified shoulder A, K, P
   ● M84.52   Pathological fracture in neoplastic disease, humerus
     ● M84.521   Pathological fracture in neoplastic disease, right humerus A, K, P
     ● M84.522   Pathological fracture in neoplastic disease, left humerus A, K, P
     ● M84.529   Pathological fracture in neoplastic disease, unspecified humerus A, K, P

CHAPTER 13 (M00-M99)

N   Newborn Age: 0   **P**   Pediatric Age: 0–17   **M**   Maternity DX: 9–64   **A**   Adult Age: 15–124   ♀   Females Only   ♂   Males Only

Complication\Comorbidity   Major C\C   (Ex)   CC/MCC Exclusions   Hospital-Acquired Condition   Hierarchical Condition Category

1093

● M84.53 Pathological fracture in neoplastic disease, ulna and radius
  ● M84.531 Pathological fracture in neoplastic disease, right ulna A, K, P 🏷
  ● M84.532 Pathological fracture in neoplastic disease, left ulna A, K, P 🏷
  ● M84.533 Pathological fracture in neoplastic disease, right radius A, K, P 🏷
  ● M84.534 Pathological fracture in neoplastic disease, left radius A, K, P 🏷
  ● M84.539 Pathological fracture in neoplastic disease, unspecified ulna and radius A, K, P 🏷

● M84.54 Pathological fracture in neoplastic disease, hand
  ● M84.541 Pathological fracture in neoplastic disease, right hand A, K, P 🏷
  ● M84.542 Pathological fracture in neoplastic disease, left hand A, K, P 🏷
  ● M84.549 Pathological fracture in neoplastic disease, unspecified hand A, K, P 🏷

● M84.55 Pathological fracture in neoplastic disease, pelvis and femur
  ● M84.550 Pathological fracture in neoplastic disease, pelvis A, K, P 🏷
  ● M84.551 Pathological fracture in neoplastic disease, right femur A, K, P 🏷, A 🏷
  ● M84.552 Pathological fracture in neoplastic disease, left femur A, K, P 🏷, A 🏷
  ● M84.553 Pathological fracture in neoplastic disease, unspecified femur A, K, P 🏷, A 🏷
  ● M84.559 Pathological fracture in neoplastic disease, hip, unspecified A, K, P 🏷, A 🏷

● M84.56 Pathological fracture in neoplastic disease, tibia and fibula
  ● M84.561 Pathological fracture in neoplastic disease, right tibia A, K, P 🏷
  ● M84.562 Pathological fracture in neoplastic disease, left tibia A, K, P 🏷
  ● M84.563 Pathological fracture in neoplastic disease, right fibula A, K, P 🏷
  ● M84.564 Pathological fracture in neoplastic disease, left fibula A, K, P 🏷
  ● M84.569 Pathological fracture in neoplastic disease, unspecified tibia and fibula A, K, P 🏷

● M84.57 Pathological fracture in neoplastic disease, ankle and foot
  ● M84.571 Pathological fracture in neoplastic disease, right ankle A, K, P 🏷
  ● M84.572 Pathological fracture in neoplastic disease, left ankle A, K, P 🏷
  ● M84.573 Pathological fracture in neoplastic disease, unspecified ankle A, K, P 🏷
  ● M84.574 Pathological fracture in neoplastic disease, right foot A, K, P 🏷
  ● M84.575 Pathological fracture in neoplastic disease, left foot A, K, P 🏷
  ● M84.576 Pathological fracture in neoplastic disease, unspecified foot A, K, P 🏷

X ● M84.58 Pathological fracture in neoplastic disease, other specified site A, K, P 🏷
  Pathological fracture in neoplastic disease, vertebrae

● M84.6 Pathological fracture in other disease
  Code also underlying condition
  Excludes1   pathological fracture in osteoporosis (M80.-)
  The appropriate 7th character is to be added to each code from subcategory M84.6:

A	initial encounter for fracture
D	subsequent encounter for fracture with routine healing
G	subsequent encounter for fracture with delayed healing
K	subsequent encounter for fracture with nonunion
P	subsequent encounter for fracture with malunion
S	sequela

  (Ex:) **For category M80[A] CC codes:** See PDX Collection 888
  For category M80[K,P] CC codes: See PDX Collection 561

  X ● M84.60 Pathological fracture in other disease, unspecified site A, K, P 🏷
  ● M84.61 Pathological fracture in other disease, shoulder
    ● M84.611 Pathological fracture in other disease, right shoulder A, K, P 🏷
    ● M84.612 Pathological fracture in other disease, left shoulder A, K, P 🏷
    ● M84.619 Pathological fracture in other disease, unspecified shoulder A, K, P 🏷
  ● M84.62 Pathological fracture in other disease, humerus
    ● M84.621 Pathological fracture in other disease, right humerus A, K, P 🏷
    ● M84.622 Pathological fracture in other disease, left humerus A, K, P 🏷
    ● M84.629 Pathological fracture in other disease, unspecified humerus A, K, P 🏷
  ● M84.63 Pathological fracture in other disease, ulna and radius
    ● M84.631 Pathological fracture in other disease, right ulna A, K, P 🏷
    ● M84.632 Pathological fracture in other disease, left ulna A, K, P 🏷
    ● M84.633 Pathological fracture in other disease, right radius A, K, P 🏷
    ● M84.634 Pathological fracture in other disease, left radius A, K, P 🏷
    ● M84.639 Pathological fracture in other disease, unspecified ulna and radius A, K, P 🏷
  ● M84.64 Pathological fracture in other disease, hand
    ● M84.641 Pathological fracture in other disease, right hand A, K, P 🏷
    ● M84.642 Pathological fracture in other disease, left hand A, K, P 🏷
    ● M84.649 Pathological fracture in other disease, unspecified hand A, K, P 🏷
  ● M84.65 Pathological fracture in other disease, pelvis and femur
    ● M84.650 Pathological fracture in other disease, pelvis A, K, P 🏷
    ● M84.651 Pathological fracture in other disease, right femur A, K, P 🏷, A 🏷
    ● M84.652 Pathological fracture in other disease, left femur A, K, P 🏷, A 🏷
    ● M84.653 Pathological fracture in other disease, unspecified femur A, K, P 🏷, A 🏷
    ● M84.659 Pathological fracture in other disease, hip, unspecified A, K, P 🏷, A 🏷

▶ New   ⇒ Revised   ~~deleted~~ Deleted   Excludes 1   Excludes 2   Includes   Use additional   Code first   Code also   Key words
OGCR Official Guidelines   ● Unacceptable Principal Diagnosis   X Assign placeholder X   ● Use Additional Character(s)   ▶ Manifestation Code   Coding Clinic

● M84.66   Pathological fracture in other disease, tibia and fibula
   ● M84.661   Pathological fracture in other disease, right tibia A, K, P 🅒
   ● M84.662   Pathological fracture in other disease, left tibia A, K, P 🅒
   ● M84.663   Pathological fracture in other disease, right fibula A, K, P 🅒
   ● M84.664   Pathological fracture in other disease, left fibula A, K, P 🅒
   ● M84.669   Pathological fracture in other disease, unspecified tibia and fibula A, K, P 🅒

● M84.67   Pathological fracture in other disease, ankle and foot
   ● M84.671   Pathological fracture in other disease, right ankle A, K, P 🅒
   ● M84.672   Pathological fracture in other disease, left ankle A, K, P 🅒
   ● M84.673   Pathological fracture in other disease, unspecified ankle A, K, P 🅒
   ● M84.674   Pathological fracture in other disease, right foot A, K, P 🅒
   ● M84.675   Pathological fracture in other disease, left foot A, K, P 🅒
   ● M84.676   Pathological fracture in other disease, unspecified foot A, K, P 🅒

X ● M84.68   Pathological fracture in other disease, other site A, K, P 🅒

● M84.7   Nontraumatic fracture, not elsewhere classified
   ● M84.75   Atypical femoral fracture

The appropriate 7th character is to be added to each code from M84.75:

A	initial encounter for fracture
D	subsequent encounter for fracture with routine healing
G	subsequent encounter for fracture with delayed healing
K	subsequent encounter for fracture with nonunion
P	subsequent encounter for fracture with malunion
S	sequela

(Ex) For category M80[A] CC codes: See PDX Collection 888
For category M80[K,P] CC codes: See PDX Collection 561
Coding Clinic: 2016, Q4, P41

   ● M84.750   Atypical femoral fracture, unspecified A, K, P 🅒
   ● M84.751   Incomplete atypical femoral fracture, right leg A, K, P 🅒
   ● M84.752   Incomplete atypical femoral fracture, left leg A, K, P 🅒
   ● M84.753   Incomplete atypical femoral fracture, unspecified leg A, K, P 🅒
   ● M84.754   Complete transverse atypical femoral fracture, right leg A, K, P 🅒, A 🅜🅒🅒
   ● M84.755   Complete transverse atypical femoral fracture, left leg A, K, P 🅒, A 🅜🅒🅒
   ● M84.756   Complete transverse atypical femoral fracture, unspecified leg A, K, P 🅒, A 🅜🅒🅒
   ● M84.757   Complete oblique atypical femoral fracture, right leg A, K, P 🅒, A 🅜🅒🅒
   ● M84.758   Complete oblique atypical femoral fracture, left leg A, K, P 🅒, A 🅜🅒🅒
   ● M84.759   Complete oblique atypical femoral fracture, unspecified leg A, K, P 🅒, A 🅜🅒🅒

● M84.8   Other disorders of continuity of bone
   M84.80   Other disorders of continuity of bone, unspecified site
   ● M84.81   Other disorders of continuity of bone, shoulder
     M84.811   Other disorders of continuity of bone, right shoulder
     M84.812   Other disorders of continuity of bone, left shoulder
     M84.819   Other disorders of continuity of bone, unspecified shoulder
   ● M84.82   Other disorders of continuity of bone, humerus
     M84.821   Other disorders of continuity of bone, right humerus
     M84.822   Other disorders of continuity of bone, left humerus
     M84.829   Other disorders of continuity of bone, unspecified humerus
   ● M84.83   Other disorders of continuity of bone, ulna and radius
     M84.831   Other disorders of continuity of bone, right ulna
     M84.832   Other disorders of continuity of bone, left ulna
     M84.833   Other disorders of continuity of bone, right radius
     M84.834   Other disorders of continuity of bone, left radius
     M84.839   Other disorders of continuity of bone, unspecified ulna and radius
   ● M84.84   Other disorders of continuity of bone, hand
     M84.841   Other disorders of continuity of bone, right hand
     M84.842   Other disorders of continuity of bone, left hand
     M84.849   Other disorders of continuity of bone, unspecified hand
   ● M84.85   Other disorders of continuity of bone, pelvic region and thigh
     M84.851   Other disorders of continuity of bone, right pelvic region and thigh
     M84.852   Other disorders of continuity of bone, left pelvic region and thigh
     M84.859   Other disorders of continuity of bone, unspecified pelvic region and thigh
   ● M84.86   Other disorders of continuity of bone, tibia and fibula
     M84.861   Other disorders of continuity of bone, right tibia
     M84.862   Other disorders of continuity of bone, left tibia
     M84.863   Other disorders of continuity of bone, right fibula
     M84.864   Other disorders of continuity of bone, left fibula
     M84.869   Other disorders of continuity of bone, unspecified tibia and fibula
   ● M84.87   Other disorders of continuity of bone, ankle and foot
     M84.871   Other disorders of continuity of bone, right ankle and foot
     M84.872   Other disorders of continuity of bone, left ankle and foot
     M84.879   Other disorders of continuity of bone, unspecified ankle and foot
   M84.88   Other disorders of continuity of bone, other site
   M84.9   Disorder of continuity of bone, unspecified

CHAPTER 13 (M00-M99)

N   Newborn Age: 0   P   Pediatric Age: 0–17   M   Maternity DX: 9–64   A   Adult Age: 15–124   ♀ Females Only   ♂ Males Only

🅒 Complication\Comorbidity   🅜🅒 Major C\C   (Ex) CC/MCC Exclusions   🅗 Hospital-Acquired Condition   🅒 Hierarchical Condition Category

1095

● **M85 Other disorders of bone density and structure**

    Excludes1 osteogenesis imperfecta (Q78.0)
        osteopetrosis (Q78.2)
        osteopoikilosis (Q78.8)
        polyostotic fibrous dysplasia (Q78.1)

● **M85.0 Fibrous dysplasia (monostotic)**

    Excludes2 fibrous dysplasia of jaw (M27.8)

    M85.00 Fibrous dysplasia (monostotic), unspecified site

●   M85.01 Fibrous dysplasia (monostotic), shoulder

      M85.011 Fibrous dysplasia (monostotic), right shoulder
      M85.012 Fibrous dysplasia (monostotic), left shoulder
      M85.019 Fibrous dysplasia (monostotic), unspecified shoulder

●   M85.02 Fibrous dysplasia (monostotic), upper arm

      M85.021 Fibrous dysplasia (monostotic), right upper arm
      M85.022 Fibrous dysplasia (monostotic), left upper arm
      M85.029 Fibrous dysplasia (monostotic), unspecified upper arm

●   M85.03 Fibrous dysplasia (monostotic), forearm

      M85.031 Fibrous dysplasia (monostotic), right forearm
      M85.032 Fibrous dysplasia (monostotic), left forearm
      M85.039 Fibrous dysplasia (monostotic), unspecified forearm

●   M85.04 Fibrous dysplasia (monostotic), hand

      M85.041 Fibrous dysplasia (monostotic), right hand
      M85.042 Fibrous dysplasia (monostotic), left hand
      M85.049 Fibrous dysplasia (monostotic), unspecified hand

●   M85.05 Fibrous dysplasia (monostotic), thigh

      M85.051 Fibrous dysplasia (monostotic), right thigh
      M85.052 Fibrous dysplasia (monostotic), left thigh
      M85.059 Fibrous dysplasia (monostotic), unspecified thigh

●   M85.06 Fibrous dysplasia (monostotic), lower leg

      M85.061 Fibrous dysplasia (monostotic), right lower leg
      M85.062 Fibrous dysplasia (monostotic), left lower leg
      M85.069 Fibrous dysplasia (monostotic), unspecified lower leg

●   M85.07 Fibrous dysplasia (monostotic), ankle and foot

      M85.071 Fibrous dysplasia (monostotic), right ankle and foot
      M85.072 Fibrous dysplasia (monostotic), left ankle and foot
      M85.079 Fibrous dysplasia (monostotic), unspecified ankle and foot

    M85.08 Fibrous dysplasia (monostotic), other site

    M85.09 Fibrous dysplasia (monostotic), multiple sites

● **M85.1 Skeletal fluorosis**

    M85.10 Skeletal fluorosis, unspecified site

●   M85.11 Skeletal fluorosis, shoulder

      M85.111 Skeletal fluorosis, right shoulder
      M85.112 Skeletal fluorosis, left shoulder
      M85.119 Skeletal fluorosis, unspecified shoulder

●   M85.12 Skeletal fluorosis, upper arm

      M85.121 Skeletal fluorosis, right upper arm
      M85.122 Skeletal fluorosis, left upper arm
      M85.129 Skeletal fluorosis, unspecified upper arm

●   M85.13 Skeletal fluorosis, forearm

      M85.131 Skeletal fluorosis, right forearm
      M85.132 Skeletal fluorosis, left forearm
      M85.139 Skeletal fluorosis, unspecified forearm

●   M85.14 Skeletal fluorosis, hand

      M85.141 Skeletal fluorosis, right hand
      M85.142 Skeletal fluorosis, left hand
      M85.149 Skeletal fluorosis, unspecified hand

●   M85.15 Skeletal fluorosis, thigh

      M85.151 Skeletal fluorosis, right thigh
      M85.152 Skeletal fluorosis, left thigh
      M85.159 Skeletal fluorosis, unspecified thigh

●   M85.16 Skeletal fluorosis, lower leg

      M85.161 Skeletal fluorosis, right lower leg
      M85.162 Skeletal fluorosis, left lower leg
      M85.169 Skeletal fluorosis, unspecified lower leg

●   M85.17 Skeletal fluorosis, ankle and foot

      M85.171 Skeletal fluorosis, right ankle and foot
      M85.172 Skeletal fluorosis, left ankle and foot
      M85.179 Skeletal fluorosis, unspecified ankle and foot

    M85.18 Skeletal fluorosis, other site

    M85.19 Skeletal fluorosis, multiple sites

M85.2 Hyperostosis of skull

● **M85.3 Osteitis condensans**

    M85.30 Osteitis condensans, unspecified site

●   M85.31 Osteitis condensans, shoulder

      M85.311 Osteitis condensans, right shoulder
      M85.312 Osteitis condensans, left shoulder
      M85.319 Osteitis condensans, unspecified shoulder

●   M85.32 Osteitis condensans, upper arm

      M85.321 Osteitis condensans, right upper arm
      M85.322 Osteitis condensans, left upper arm
      M85.329 Osteitis condensans, unspecified upper arm

●   M85.33 Osteitis condensans, forearm

      M85.331 Osteitis condensans, right forearm
      M85.332 Osteitis condensans, left forearm
      M85.339 Osteitis condensans, unspecified forearm

●   M85.34 Osteitis condensans, hand

      M85.341 Osteitis condensans, right hand
      M85.342 Osteitis condensans, left hand
      M85.349 Osteitis condensans, unspecified hand

● M85.35   Osteitis condensans, thigh
    M85.351   Osteitis condensans, right thigh
    M85.352   Osteitis condensans, left thigh
    M85.359   Osteitis condensans, unspecified thigh
● M85.36   Osteitis condensans, lower leg
    M85.361   Osteitis condensans, right lower leg
    M85.362   Osteitis condensans, left lower leg
    M85.369   Osteitis condensans, unspecified lower leg
● M85.37   Osteitis condensans, ankle and foot
    M85.371   Osteitis condensans, right ankle and foot
    M85.372   Osteitis condensans, left ankle and foot
    M85.379   Osteitis condensans, unspecified ankle and foot
   M85.38   Osteitis condensans, other site
   M85.39   Osteitis condensans, multiple sites
● M85.4   Solitary bone cyst
    Excludes2   solitary cyst of jaw (M27.4)
   M85.40   Solitary bone cyst, unspecified site
● M85.41   Solitary bone cyst, shoulder
    M85.411   Solitary bone cyst, right shoulder
    M85.412   Solitary bone cyst, left shoulder
    M85.419   Solitary bone cyst, unspecified shoulder
● M85.42   Solitary bone cyst, humerus
    M85.421   Solitary bone cyst, right humerus
    M85.422   Solitary bone cyst, left humerus
    M85.429   Solitary bone cyst, unspecified humerus
● M85.43   Solitary bone cyst, ulna and radius
    M85.431   Solitary bone cyst, right ulna and radius
    M85.432   Solitary bone cyst, left ulna and radius
    M85.439   Solitary bone cyst, unspecified ulna and radius
● M85.44   Solitary bone cyst, hand
    M85.441   Solitary bone cyst, right hand
    M85.442   Solitary bone cyst, left hand
    M85.449   Solitary bone cyst, unspecified hand
● M85.45   Solitary bone cyst, pelvis
    M85.451   Solitary bone cyst, right pelvis
    M85.452   Solitary bone cyst, left pelvis
    M85.459   Solitary bone cyst, unspecified pelvis
● M85.46   Solitary bone cyst, tibia and fibula
    M85.461   Solitary bone cyst, right tibia and fibula
    M85.462   Solitary bone cyst, left tibia and fibula
    M85.469   Solitary bone cyst, unspecified tibia and fibula
● M85.47   Solitary bone cyst, ankle and foot
    M85.471   Solitary bone cyst, right ankle and foot
    M85.472   Solitary bone cyst, left ankle and foot
    M85.479   Solitary bone cyst, unspecified ankle and foot
   M85.48   Solitary bone cyst, other site

● M85.5   Aneurysmal bone cyst
    Excludes2   aneurysmal cyst of jaw (M27.4)
   M85.50   Aneurysmal bone cyst, unspecified site
● M85.51   Aneurysmal bone cyst, shoulder
    M85.511   Aneurysmal bone cyst, right shoulder
    M85.512   Aneurysmal bone cyst, left shoulder
    M85.519   Aneurysmal bone cyst, unspecified shoulder
● M85.52   Aneurysmal bone cyst, upper arm
    M85.521   Aneurysmal bone cyst, right upper arm
    M85.522   Aneurysmal bone cyst, left upper arm
    M85.529   Aneurysmal bone cyst, unspecified upper arm
● M85.53   Aneurysmal bone cyst, forearm
    M85.531   Aneurysmal bone cyst, right forearm
    M85.532   Aneurysmal bone cyst, left forearm
    M85.539   Aneurysmal bone cyst, unspecified forearm
● M85.54   Aneurysmal bone cyst, hand
    M85.541   Aneurysmal bone cyst, right hand
    M85.542   Aneurysmal bone cyst, left hand
    M85.549   Aneurysmal bone cyst, unspecified hand
● M85.55   Aneurysmal bone cyst, thigh
    M85.551   Aneurysmal bone cyst, right thigh
    M85.552   Aneurysmal bone cyst, left thigh
    M85.559   Aneurysmal bone cyst, unspecified thigh
● M85.56   Aneurysmal bone cyst, lower leg
    M85.561   Aneurysmal bone cyst, right lower leg
    M85.562   Aneurysmal bone cyst, left lower leg
    M85.569   Aneurysmal bone cyst, unspecified lower leg
● M85.57   Aneurysmal bone cyst, ankle and foot
    M85.571   Aneurysmal bone cyst, right ankle and foot
    M85.572   Aneurysmal bone cyst, left ankle and foot
    M85.579   Aneurysmal bone cyst, unspecified ankle and foot
   M85.58   Aneurysmal bone cyst, other site
   M85.59   Aneurysmal bone cyst, multiple sites
● M85.6   Other cyst of bone
    Excludes1   cyst of jaw NEC (M27.4)
            osteitis fibrosa cystica generalisata [von Recklinghausen's disease of bone] (E21.0)
   M85.60   Other cyst of bone, unspecified site
● M85.61   Other cyst of bone, shoulder
    M85.611   Other cyst of bone, right shoulder
    M85.612   Other cyst of bone, left shoulder
    M85.619   Other cyst of bone, unspecified shoulder
● M85.62   Other cyst of bone, upper arm
    M85.621   Other cyst of bone, right upper arm
    M85.622   Other cyst of bone, left upper arm
    M85.629   Other cyst of bone, unspecified upper arm
● M85.63   Other cyst of bone, forearm
    M85.631   Other cyst of bone, right forearm
    M85.632   Other cyst of bone, left forearm
    M85.639   Other cyst of bone, unspecified forearm

CHAPTER 13 (M00–M99)

N Newborn Age: 0   **P** Pediatric Age: 0–17   **M** Maternity DX: 9–64   **A** Adult Age: 15–124   ♀ Females Only   ♂ Males Only

Complication\Comorbidity   Major C\C   (Ex:) CC/MCC Exclusions   Hospital-Acquired Condition   Hierarchical Condition Category

1097

● M85.64   Other cyst of bone, hand
    M85.641   Other cyst of bone, right hand
    M85.642   Other cyst of bone, left hand
    M85.649   Other cyst of bone, unspecified hand

● M85.65   Other cyst of bone, thigh
    M85.651   Other cyst of bone, right thigh
    M85.652   Other cyst of bone, left thigh
    M85.659   Other cyst of bone, unspecified thigh

● M85.66   Other cyst of bone, lower leg
    M85.661   Other cyst of bone, right lower leg
    M85.662   Other cyst of bone, left lower leg
    M85.669   Other cyst of bone, unspecified lower leg

● M85.67   Other cyst of bone, ankle and foot
    M85.671   Other cyst of bone, right ankle and foot
    M85.672   Other cyst of bone, left ankle and foot
    M85.679   Other cyst of bone, unspecified ankle and foot

   M85.68   Other cyst of bone, other site
   M85.69   Other cyst of bone, multiple sites

● M85.8   **Other specified disorders of bone density and structure**
    Hyperostosis of bones, except skull
    Osteosclerosis, acquired

    Excludes1   diffuse idiopathic skeletal hyperostosis [DISH] (M48.1)
              osteosclerosis congenita (Q77.4)
              osteosclerosis fragilitas (generalista) (Q78.2)
              osteosclerosis myelofibrosis (D75.81)

   M85.80   Other specified disorders of bone density and structure, unspecified site

● M85.81   Other specified disorders of bone density and structure, shoulder
    M85.811   Other specified disorders of bone density and structure, right shoulder
    M85.812   Other specified disorders of bone density and structure, left shoulder
    M85.819   Other specified disorders of bone density and structure, unspecified shoulder

● M85.82   Other specified disorders of bone density and structure, upper arm
    M85.821   Other specified disorders of bone density and structure, right upper arm
    M85.822   Other specified disorders of bone density and structure, left upper arm
    M85.829   Other specified disorders of bone density and structure, unspecified upper arm

● M85.83   Other specified disorders of bone density and structure, forearm
    M85.831   Other specified disorders of bone density and structure, right forearm
    M85.832   Other specified disorders of bone density and structure, left forearm
    M85.839   Other specified disorders of bone density and structure, unspecified forearm

● M85.84   Other specified disorders of bone density and structure, hand
    M85.841   Other specified disorders of bone density and structure, right hand
    M85.842   Other specified disorders of bone density and structure, left hand
    M85.849   Other specified disorders of bone density and structure, unspecified hand

● M85.85   Other specified disorders of bone density and structure, thigh
    M85.851   Other specified disorders of bone density and structure, right thigh
    M85.852   Other specified disorders of bone density and structure, left thigh
    M85.859   Other specified disorders of bone density and structure, unspecified thigh

● M85.86   Other specified disorders of bone density and structure, lower leg
    M85.861   Other specified disorders of bone density and structure, right lower leg
    M85.862   Other specified disorders of bone density and structure, left lower leg
    M85.869   Other specified disorders of bone density and structure, unspecified lower leg

● M85.87   Other specified disorders of bone density and structure, ankle and foot
    M85.871   Other specified disorders of bone density and structure, right ankle and foot
    M85.872   Other specified disorders of bone density and structure, left ankle and foot
    M85.879   Other specified disorders of bone density and structure, unspecified ankle and foot

   M85.88   Other specified disorders of bone density and structure, other site
   M85.89   Other specified disorders of bone density and structure, multiple sites

   M85.9   Disorder of bone density and structure, unspecified

OTHER OSTEOPATHIES (M86-M90)

Excludes1   postprocedural osteopathies (M96.-)

● M86   **Osteomyelitis**
    Use additional code (B95-B97) to identify infectious agent
    Use additional code to identify major osseous defect, if applicable (M89.7-)

    Excludes1   osteomyelitis due to:
              echinococcus (B67.2)
              gonococcus (A54.43)
              salmonella (A02.24)

    Excludes2   ostemyelitis of:
              orbit (H05.0-)
              petrous bone (H70.2-)
              vertebra (M46.2-)

● M86.0   Acute hematogenous osteomyelitis
    M86.00   Acute hematogenous osteomyelitis, unspecified site 🔵🔵
       Ex: See PDX Collection 898

    ● M86.01   Acute hematogenous osteomyelitis, shoulder
       Ex: For category M86.01 CC codes: See PDX Collection 3833, 3835, 3837

       M86.011   Acute hematogenous osteomyelitis, right shoulder 🔵🔵
       M86.012   Acute hematogenous osteomyelitis, left shoulder 🔵🔵
       M86.019   Acute hematogenous osteomyelitis, unspecified shoulder 🔵🔵

    ● M86.02   Acute hematogenous osteomyelitis, humerus
       Ex: For category M86.02 CC codes: See PDX Collection 3839, 3841, 3843

       M86.021   Acute hematogenous osteomyelitis, right humerus 🔵🔵
       M86.022   Acute hematogenous osteomyelitis, left humerus 🔵🔵
       M86.029   Acute hematogenous osteomyelitis, unspecified humerus 🔵🔵

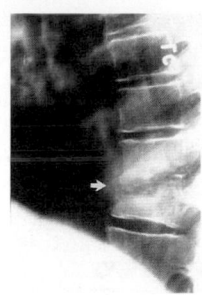

Figure 13-6 Osteomyelitis of the spine. A lateral view of the lower thoracic spine demonstrates destruction of the disk space *(arrow)* as well as destruction of the adjoining vertebral bodies. (From Mettler: Essentials of Radiology, ed 2, Saunders, An Imprint of Elsevier, 2005)

Item 13-12 Osteomyelitis is an inflammation of the bone. **Acute osteomyelitis** is a rapidly destructive, pus-producing infection capable of causing severe bone destruction. **Chronic osteomyelitis** can remain long after the initial acute episode has passed and may lead to a recurrence of the acute phase. **Brodie's abscess** is an encapsulated focal abscess that must be surgically drained. **Periostitis** is an inflammation of the periosteum, a dense membrane composed of fibrous connective tissue that closely wraps all bone, except those with articulating surfaces in joints, which are covered by synovial membranes.

● M86.03 Acute hematogenous osteomyelitis, radius and ulna
  (Ex) For category M86.03 CC codes: See PDX Collection 3845, 3847, 3849

  M86.031 Acute hematogenous osteomyelitis, right radius and ulna
  M86.032 Acute hematogenous osteomyelitis, left radius and ulna
  M86.039 Acute hematogenous osteomyelitis, unspecified radius and ulna

● M86.04 Acute hematogenous osteomyelitis, hand
  (Ex) For category M86.04 CC codes: See PDX Collection 3851, 3853, 3855

  M86.041 Acute hematogenous osteomyelitis, right hand
  M86.042 Acute hematogenous osteomyelitis, left hand
  M86.049 Acute hematogenous osteomyelitis, unspecified hand

● M86.05 Acute hematogenous osteomyelitis, femur
  (Ex) For category M86.05 CC codes: See PDX Collection 3857, 3859, 3861

  M86.051 Acute hematogenous osteomyelitis, right femur
  M86.052 Acute hematogenous osteomyelitis, left femur
  M86.059 Acute hematogenous osteomyelitis, unspecified femur

● M86.06 Acute hematogenous osteomyelitis, tibia and fibula
  (Ex) For category M86.06 CC codes: See PDX Collection 3863, 3865, 3867

  M86.061 Acute hematogenous osteomyelitis, right tibia and fibula
  M86.062 Acute hematogenous osteomyelitis, left tibia and fibula
  M86.069 Acute hematogenous osteomyelitis, unspecified tibia and fibula

● M86.07 Acute hematogenous osteomyelitis, ankle and foot
  (Ex) For category M86.07 CC codes: See PDX Collection 3869, 3871, 3873

  M86.071 Acute hematogenous osteomyelitis, right ankle and foot
  M86.072 Acute hematogenous osteomyelitis, left ankle and foot
  M86.079 Acute hematogenous osteomyelitis, unspecified ankle and foot

M86.08 Acute hematogenous osteomyelitis, other sites
  (Ex) See PDX Collection 882
M86.09 Acute hematogenous osteomyelitis, multiple sites
  (Ex) See PDX Collection 898
● M86.1 Other acute osteomyelitis
  M86.10 Other acute osteomyelitis, unspecified site
    (Ex) See PDX Collection 898
● M86.11 Other acute osteomyelitis, shoulder
    (Ex) For category M86.11 CC codes: See PDX Collection 3875, 3877, 3879
  M86.111 Other acute osteomyelitis, right shoulder
  M86.112 Other acute osteomyelitis, left shoulder
  M86.119 Other acute osteomyelitis, unspecified shoulder
● M86.12 Other acute osteomyelitis, humerus
    (Ex) For category M86.12 CC codes: See PDX Collection 3881, 3883, 3885
  M86.121 Other acute osteomyelitis, right humerus
  M86.122 Other acute osteomyelitis, left humerus
  M86.129 Other acute osteomyelitis, unspecified humerus
● M86.13 Other acute osteomyelitis, radius and ulna
    (Ex) For category M86.13 CC codes: See PDX Collection 3887, 3889, 3891
  M86.131 Other acute osteomyelitis, right radius and ulna
  M86.132 Other acute osteomyelitis, left radius and ulna
  M86.139 Other acute osteomyelitis, unspecified radius and ulna
● M86.14 Other acute osteomyelitis, hand
    (Ex) For category M86.14 CC codes: See PDX Collection 3893, 3895, 3897
  M86.141 Other acute osteomyelitis, right hand
  M86.142 Other acute osteomyelitis, left hand
  M86.149 Other acute osteomyelitis, unspecified hand
● M86.15 Other acute osteomyelitis, femur
    (Ex) For category M86.15 CC codes: See PDX Collection 3899, 3901, 3903
  M86.151 Other acute osteomyelitis, right femur
  M86.152 Other acute osteomyelitis, left femur
  M86.159 Other acute osteomyelitis, unspecified femur
● M86.16 Other acute osteomyelitis, tibia and fibula
    (Ex) For category M86.16 CC codes: See PDX Collection 3905, 3907, 3909
  M86.161 Other acute osteomyelitis, right tibia and fibula
  M86.162 Other acute osteomyelitis, left tibia and fibula
  M86.169 Other acute osteomyelitis, unspecified tibia and fibula
● M86.17 Other acute osteomyelitis, ankle and foot
    (Ex) For category M86.17 CC codes: See PDX Collection 3911, 3913, 3915
  M86.171 Other acute osteomyelitis, right ankle and foot
    Coding Clinic: 2020, Q1, P12
  M86.172 Other acute osteomyelitis, left ankle and foot
  M86.179 Other acute osteomyelitis, unspecified ankle and foot

CHAPTER 13 (M00-M99)

N Newborn Age: 0   P Pediatric Age: 0–17   M Maternity DX: 9–64   A Adult Age: 15–124   ♀ Females Only   ♂ Males Only
Complication\Comorbidity   Major C\C   (Ex) CC/MCC Exclusions   Hospital-Acquired Condition   Hierarchical Condition Category

M86.18   Other acute osteomyelitis, other site
(Ex:) See PDX Collection 882

M86.19   Other acute osteomyelitis, multiple sites
(Ex:) See PDX Collection 898

● M86.2   Subacute osteomyelitis

M86.20   Subacute osteomyelitis, unspecified site
(Ex:) See PDX Collection 898

● M86.21   Subacute osteomyelitis, shoulder
(Ex:) For category M86.21 CC codes: See PDX Collection 899

    M86.211   Subacute osteomyelitis, right shoulder
(Ex:) See PDX Collection 3917

    M86.212   Subacute osteomyelitis, left shoulder
(Ex:) See PDX Collection 3919

    M86.219   Subacute osteomyelitis, unspecified shoulder

● M86.22   Subacute osteomyelitis, humerus
(Ex:) For category M86.22 CC codes: See PDX Collection 900

    M86.221   Subacute osteomyelitis, right humerus
(Ex:) See PDX Collection 3921

    M86.222   Subacute osteomyelitis, left humerus
(Ex:) See PDX Collection 3923

    M86.229   Subacute osteomyelitis, unspecified humerus

● M86.23   Subacute osteomyelitis, radius and ulna
(Ex:) For category M86.23 CC codes: See PDX Collection 901

    M86.231   Subacute osteomyelitis, right radius and ulna
(Ex:) See PDX Collection 3925

    M86.232   Subacute osteomyelitis, left radius and ulna
(Ex:) See PDX Collection 3927

    M86.239   Subacute osteomyelitis, unspecified radius and ulna

● M86.24   Subacute osteomyelitis, hand
(Ex:) For category M86.24 CC codes: See PDX Collection 902

    M86.241   Subacute osteomyelitis, right hand
(Ex:) See PDX Collection 3929

    M86.242   Subacute osteomyelitis, left hand
(Ex:) See PDX Collection 3931

    M86.249   Subacute osteomyelitis, unspecified hand

● M86.25   Subacute osteomyelitis, femur
(Ex:) For category M86.25 CC codes: See PDX Collection 903

    M86.251   Subacute osteomyelitis, right femur
(Ex:) See PDX Collection 3933

    M86.252   Subacute osteomyelitis, left femur
(Ex:) See PDX Collection 3935

    M86.259   Subacute osteomyelitis, unspecified femur

● M86.26   Subacute osteomyelitis, tibia and fibula
(Ex:) For category M86.26 CC codes: See PDX Collection 904

    M86.261   Subacute osteomyelitis, right tibia and fibula
(Ex:) See PDX Collection 3937

    M86.262   Subacute osteomyelitis, left tibia and fibula
(Ex:) See PDX Collection 3939

    M86.269   Subacute osteomyelitis, unspecified tibia and fibula

● M86.27   Subacute osteomyelitis, ankle and foot
(Ex:) For category M86.27 CC codes: See PDX Collection 905

    M86.271   Subacute osteomyelitis, right ankle and foot
(Ex:) See PDX Collection 3941

    M86.272   Subacute osteomyelitis, left ankle and foot
(Ex:) See PDX Collection 3943

    M86.279   Subacute osteomyelitis, unspecified ankle and foot

M86.28   Subacute osteomyelitis, other site
(Ex:) See PDX Collection 882

M86.29   Subacute osteomyelitis, multiple sites
(Ex:) See PDX Collection 898

● M86.3   Chronic multifocal osteomyelitis
(Ex:) For category M86.3 CC codes unless otherwise indicated: See PDX Collection 881

M86.30   Chronic multifocal osteomyelitis, unspecified site
(Ex:) See PDX Collection 906

● M86.31   Chronic multifocal osteomyelitis, shoulder

    M86.311   Chronic multifocal osteomyelitis, right shoulder

    M86.312   Chronic multifocal osteomyelitis, left shoulder

    M86.319   Chronic multifocal osteomyelitis, unspecified shoulder

● M86.32   Chronic multifocal osteomyelitis, humerus

    M86.321   Chronic multifocal osteomyelitis, right humerus

    M86.322   Chronic multifocal osteomyelitis, left humerus

    M86.329   Chronic multifocal osteomyelitis, unspecified humerus

● M86.33   Chronic multifocal osteomyelitis, radius and ulna

    M86.331   Chronic multifocal osteomyelitis, right radius and ulna

    M86.332   Chronic multifocal osteomyelitis, left radius and ulna

    M86.339   Chronic multifocal osteomyelitis, unspecified radius and ulna

● M86.34   Chronic multifocal osteomyelitis, hand

    M86.341   Chronic multifocal osteomyelitis, right hand

    M86.342   Chronic multifocal osteomyelitis, left hand

    M86.349   Chronic multifocal osteomyelitis, unspecified hand

● M86.35   Chronic multifocal osteomyelitis, femur

    M86.351   Chronic multifocal osteomyelitis, right femur

    M86.352   Chronic multifocal osteomyelitis, left femur

    M86.359   Chronic multifocal osteomyelitis, unspecified femur

● M86.36   Chronic multifocal osteomyelitis, tibia and fibula

    M86.361   Chronic multifocal osteomyelitis, right tibia and fibula

    M86.362   Chronic multifocal osteomyelitis, left tibia and fibula

    M86.369   Chronic multifocal osteomyelitis, unspecified tibia and fibula

● M86.37   Chronic multifocal osteomyelitis, ankle and foot

    M86.371   Chronic multifocal osteomyelitis, right ankle and foot

    M86.372   Chronic multifocal osteomyelitis, left ankle and foot

    M86.379   Chronic multifocal osteomyelitis, unspecified ankle and foot

▶ New   ⟹ Revised   ~~deleted~~ Deleted   Excludes 1   Excludes 2   Includes   Use additional   Code first   Code also   Key words

OGCR Official Guidelines   ● Unacceptable Principal Diagnosis   X Assign placeholder X   ● Use Additional Character(s)   ▷ Manifestation Code   **Coding Clinic**

M86.38   Chronic multifocal osteomyelitis, other site 🝢 🝢

M86.39   Chronic multifocal osteomyelitis, multiple sites 🝢 🝢

● M86.4   Chronic osteomyelitis with draining sinus

    (Ex) For category M86.4 CC codes unless otherwise indicated: See PDX Collection 881

M86.40   Chronic osteomyelitis with draining sinus, unspecified site 🝢 🝢

    (Ex) See PDX Collection 906

● M86.41   Chronic osteomyelitis with draining sinus, shoulder

    M86.411   Chronic osteomyelitis with draining sinus, right shoulder 🝢 🝢

    M86.412   Chronic osteomyelitis with draining sinus, left shoulder 🝢 🝢

    M86.419   Chronic osteomyelitis with draining sinus, unspecified shoulder 🝢 🝢

● M86.42   Chronic osteomyelitis with draining sinus, humerus

    M86.421   Chronic osteomyelitis with draining sinus, right humerus 🝢 🝢

    M86.422   Chronic osteomyelitis with draining sinus, left humerus 🝢 🝢

    M86.429   Chronic osteomyelitis with draining sinus, unspecified humerus 🝢 🝢

● M86.43   Chronic osteomyelitis with draining sinus, radius and ulna

    M86.431   Chronic osteomyelitis with draining sinus, right radius and ulna 🝢 🝢

    M86.432   Chronic osteomyelitis with draining sinus, left radius and ulna 🝢 🝢

    M86.439   Chronic osteomyelitis with draining sinus, unspecified radius and ulna 🝢 🝢

● M86.44   Chronic osteomyelitis with draining sinus, hand

    M86.441   Chronic osteomyelitis with draining sinus, right hand 🝢 🝢

    M86.442   Chronic osteomyelitis with draining sinus, left hand 🝢 🝢

    M86.449   Chronic osteomyelitis with draining sinus, unspecified hand 🝢 🝢

● M86.45   Chronic osteomyelitis with draining sinus, femur

    M86.451   Chronic osteomyelitis with draining sinus, right femur 🝢 🝢

    M86.452   Chronic osteomyelitis with draining sinus, left femur 🝢 🝢

    M86.459   Chronic osteomyelitis with draining sinus, unspecified femur 🝢 🝢

● M86.46   Chronic osteomyelitis with draining sinus, tibia and fibula

    M86.461   Chronic osteomyelitis with draining sinus, right tibia and fibula 🝢 🝢

    M86.462   Chronic osteomyelitis with draining sinus, left tibia and fibula 🝢 🝢

    M86.469   Chronic osteomyelitis with draining sinus, unspecified tibia and fibula 🝢 🝢

● M86.47   Chronic osteomyelitis with draining sinus, ankle and foot

    M86.471   Chronic osteomyelitis with draining sinus, right ankle and foot 🝢 🝢

    M86.472   Chronic osteomyelitis with draining sinus, left ankle and foot 🝢 🝢

    M86.479   Chronic osteomyelitis with draining sinus, unspecified ankle and foot 🝢 🝢

M86.48   Chronic osteomyelitis with draining sinus, other site 🝢 🝢

M86.49   Chronic osteomyelitis with draining sinus, multiple sites 🝢 🝢

● M86.5   Other chronic hematogenous osteomyelitis

    (Ex) For category M86.5 CC codes unless otherwise indicated: See PDX Collection 881

M86.50   Other chronic hematogenous osteomyelitis, unspecified site 🝢 🝢

    (Ex) See PDX Collection 906

● M86.51   Other chronic hematogenous osteomyelitis, shoulder

    M86.511   Other chronic hematogenous osteomyelitis, right shoulder 🝢 🝢

    M86.512   Other chronic hematogenous osteomyelitis, left shoulder 🝢 🝢

    M86.519   Other chronic hematogenous osteomyelitis, unspecified shoulder 🝢 🝢

● M86.52   Other chronic hematogenous osteomyelitis, humerus

    M86.521   Other chronic hematogenous osteomyelitis, right humerus 🝢 🝢

    M86.522   Other chronic hematogenous osteomyelitis, left humerus 🝢 🝢

    M86.529   Other chronic hematogenous osteomyelitis, unspecified humerus 🝢 🝢

● M86.53   Other chronic hematogenous osteomyelitis, radius and ulna

    M86.531   Other chronic hematogenous osteomyelitis, right radius and ulna 🝢 🝢

    M86.532   Other chronic hematogenous osteomyelitis, left radius and ulna 🝢 🝢

    M86.539   Other chronic hematogenous osteomyelitis, unspecified radius and ulna 🝢 🝢

● M86.54   Other chronic hematogenous osteomyelitis, hand

    M86.541   Other chronic hematogenous osteomyelitis, right hand 🝢 🝢

    M86.542   Other chronic hematogenous osteomyelitis, left hand 🝢 🝢

    M86.549   Other chronic hematogenous osteomyelitis, unspecified hand 🝢 🝢

● M86.55   Other chronic hematogenous osteomyelitis, femur

    M86.551   Other chronic hematogenous osteomyelitis, right femur 🝢 🝢

    M86.552   Other chronic hematogenous osteomyelitis, left femur 🝢 🝢

    M86.559   Other chronic hematogenous osteomyelitis, unspecified femur 🝢 🝢

● M86.56   Other chronic hematogenous osteomyelitis, tibia and fibula

    M86.561   Other chronic hematogenous osteomyelitis, right tibia and fibula 🝢 🝢

    M86.562   Other chronic hematogenous osteomyelitis, left tibia and fibula 🝢 🝢

    M86.569   Other chronic hematogenous osteomyelitis, unspecified tibia and fibula 🝢 🝢

● M86.57   Other chronic hematogenous osteomyelitis, ankle and foot

    M86.571   Other chronic hematogenous osteomyelitis, right ankle and foot 🝢 🝢

    M86.572   Other chronic hematogenous osteomyelitis, left ankle and foot 🝢 🝢

    M86.579   Other chronic hematogenous osteomyelitis, unspecified ankle and foot 🝢 🝢

CHAPTER 13 (M00-M99)

N   Newborn Age: 0   **P**   Pediatric Age: 0–17   **M**   Maternity DX: 9–64   **A**   Adult Age: 15–124   ♀   Females Only   ♂   Males Only

🝢   Complication\Comorbidity   🝢   Major C\C   (Ex)   CC/MCC Exclusions   🝢   Hospital-Acquired Condition   🝢   Hierarchical Condition Category

M86.58 Other chronic hematogenous osteomyelitis, other site

M86.59 Other chronic hematogenous osteomyelitis, multiple sites

M86.6 Other chronic osteomyelitis
(Ex:) For category M86.6 CC codes unless otherwise indicated: See PDX Collection 881

M86.60 Other chronic osteomyelitis, unspecified site
(Ex:) See PDX Collection 906

M86.61 Other chronic osteomyelitis, shoulder

M86.611 Other chronic osteomyelitis, right shoulder

M86.612 Other chronic osteomyelitis, left shoulder

M86.619 Other chronic osteomyelitis, unspecified shoulder

M86.62 Other chronic osteomyelitis, humerus

M86.621 Other chronic osteomyelitis, right humerus

M86.622 Other chronic osteomyelitis, left humerus

M86.629 Other chronic osteomyelitis, unspecified humerus

M86.63 Other chronic osteomyelitis, radius and ulna

M86.631 Other chronic osteomyelitis, right radius and ulna

M86.632 Other chronic osteomyelitis, left radius and ulna

M86.639 Other chronic osteomyelitis, unspecified radius and ulna

M86.64 Other chronic osteomyelitis, hand

M86.641 Other chronic osteomyelitis, right hand

M86.642 Other chronic osteomyelitis, left hand

M86.649 Other chronic osteomyelitis, unspecified hand

M86.65 Other chronic osteomyelitis, thigh

M86.651 Other chronic osteomyelitis, right thigh

M86.652 Other chronic osteomyelitis, left thigh

M86.659 Other chronic osteomyelitis, unspecified thigh

M86.66 Other chronic osteomyelitis, tibia and fibula

M86.661 Other chronic osteomyelitis, right tibia and fibula

M86.662 Other chronic osteomyelitis, left tibia and fibula

M86.669 Other chronic osteomyelitis, unspecified tibia and fibula

M86.67 Other chronic osteomyelitis, ankle and foot

M86.671 Other chronic osteomyelitis, right ankle and foot
Coding Clinic: 2016, Q1, P13

M86.672 Other chronic osteomyelitis, left ankle and foot

M86.679 Other chronic osteomyelitis, unspecified ankle and foot

M86.68 Other chronic osteomyelitis, other site

M86.69 Other chronic osteomyelitis, multiple sites

M86.8 Other osteomyelitis
Brodie's abscess
(Ex:) For category M86.8 CC codes unless otherwise indicated: See PDX Collection 881

M86.8X Other osteomyelitis

M86.8X0 Other osteomyelitis, multiple sites

M86.8X1 Other osteomyelitis, shoulder

M86.8X2 Other osteomyelitis, upper arm

M86.8X3 Other osteomyelitis, forearm

M86.8X4 Other osteomyelitis, hand

M86.8X5 Other osteomyelitis, thigh

M86.8X6 Other osteomyelitis, lower leg

M86.8X7 Other osteomyelitis, ankle and foot

M86.8X8 Other osteomyelitis, other site

M86.8X9 Other osteomyelitis, unspecified sites
(Ex:) See PDX Collection 906

M86.9 Osteomyelitis, unspecified
Infection of bone NOS
Periostitis without osteomyelitis
(Ex:) See PDX Collection 906

M87 Osteonecrosis
Includes avascular necrosis of bone
Use additional code to identify major osseous defect, if applicable (M89.7-)
Excludes1 juvenile osteonecrosis (M91-M92)
osteochondropathies (M90-M93)
(Ex:) For category M87 CC codes unless otherwise indicated: See PDX Collection 907

M87.0 Idiopathic aseptic necrosis of bone

M87.00 Idiopathic aseptic necrosis of unspecified bone

M87.01 Idiopathic aseptic necrosis of shoulder
Idiopathic aseptic necrosis of clavicle and scapula
(Ex:) For category M87.01 CC codes: See PDX Collection 908

M87.011 Idiopathic aseptic necrosis of right shoulder

M87.012 Idiopathic aseptic necrosis of left shoulder

M87.019 Idiopathic aseptic necrosis of unspecified shoulder

M87.02 Idiopathic aseptic necrosis of humerus
(Ex:) For category M87.02 CC codes: See PDX Collection 908

M87.021 Idiopathic aseptic necrosis of right humerus

M87.022 Idiopathic aseptic necrosis of left humerus

M87.029 Idiopathic aseptic necrosis of unspecified humerus

M87.03 Idiopathic aseptic necrosis of radius, ulna and carpus

M87.031 Idiopathic aseptic necrosis of right radius

M87.032 Idiopathic aseptic necrosis of left radius

M87.033 Idiopathic aseptic necrosis of unspecified radius

M87.034 Idiopathic aseptic necrosis of right ulna

M87.035 Idiopathic aseptic necrosis of left ulna

M87.036 Idiopathic aseptic necrosis of unspecified ulna

M87.037 Idiopathic aseptic necrosis of right carpus

M87.038 Idiopathic aseptic necrosis of left carpus

M87.039 Idiopathic aseptic necrosis of unspecified carpus

● M87.04   **Idiopathic aseptic necrosis of hand and fingers**
Idiopathic aseptic necrosis of metacarpals and phalanges of hands

    M87.041   Idiopathic aseptic necrosis of right hand 🔹 🔹

    M87.042   Idiopathic aseptic necrosis of left hand 🔹 🔹

    M87.043   Idiopathic aseptic necrosis of unspecified hand 🔹 🔹

    M87.044   Idiopathic aseptic necrosis of right finger(s) 🔹 🔹

    M87.045   Idiopathic aseptic necrosis of left finger(s) 🔹 🔹

    M87.046   Idiopathic aseptic necrosis of unspecified finger(s) 🔹 🔹

● M87.05   **Idiopathic aseptic necrosis of pelvis and femur**

    M87.050   Idiopathic aseptic necrosis of pelvis 🔹 🔹

    M87.051   Idiopathic aseptic necrosis of right femur 🔹 🔹
       (Ex:) See PDX Collection 909

    M87.052   Idiopathic aseptic necrosis of left femur 🔹 🔹
       (Ex:) See PDX Collection 909

    M87.059   Idiopathic aseptic necrosis of unspecified femur 🔹 🔹
       Idiopathic aseptic necrosis of hip NOS
       (Ex:) See PDX Collection 909

● M87.06   **Idiopathic aseptic necrosis of tibia and fibula**

    M87.061   Idiopathic aseptic necrosis of right tibia 🔹 🔹

    M87.062   Idiopathic aseptic necrosis of left tibia 🔹 🔹

    M87.063   Idiopathic aseptic necrosis of unspecified tibia 🔹 🔹

    M87.064   Idiopathic aseptic necrosis of right fibula 🔹 🔹

    M87.065   Idiopathic aseptic necrosis of left fibula 🔹 🔹

    M87.066   Idiopathic aseptic necrosis of unspecified fibula 🔹 🔹

● M87.07   **Idiopathic aseptic necrosis of ankle, foot and toes**
       Idiopathic aseptic necrosis of metatarsus, tarsus, and phalanges of toes

    M87.071   Idiopathic aseptic necrosis of right ankle 🔹 🔹

    M87.072   Idiopathic aseptic necrosis of left ankle 🔹 🔹

    M87.073   Idiopathic aseptic necrosis of unspecified ankle 🔹 🔹

    M87.074   Idiopathic aseptic necrosis of right foot 🔹 🔹
       (Ex:) See PDX Collection 910

    M87.075   Idiopathic aseptic necrosis of left foot 🔹 🔹
       (Ex:) See PDX Collection 910

    M87.076   Idiopathic aseptic necrosis of unspecified foot 🔹 🔹
       (Ex:) See PDX Collection 910

    M87.077   Idiopathic aseptic necrosis of right toe(s) 🔹 🔹

    M87.078   Idiopathic aseptic necrosis of left toe(s) 🔹 🔹

    M87.079   Idiopathic aseptic necrosis of unspecified toe(s) 🔹 🔹

   M87.08   Idiopathic aseptic necrosis of bone, other site 🔹 🔹

   M87.09   Idiopathic aseptic necrosis of bone, multiple sites 🔹 🔹

● M87.1   **Osteonecrosis due to drugs**
       Use additional code for adverse effect, if applicable, to identify drug (T36-T50 with fifth or sixth character 5)
       (Ex:) For category M87 CC codes unless otherwise indicated: See PDX Collection 907

   M87.10   Osteonecrosis due to drugs, unspecified bone 🔹 🔹

● M87.11   Osteonecrosis due to drugs, shoulder

    M87.111   Osteonecrosis due to drugs, right shoulder 🔹 🔹

    M87.112   Osteonecrosis due to drugs, left shoulder 🔹 🔹

    M87.119   Osteonecrosis due to drugs, unspecified shoulder 🔹 🔹

● M87.12   Osteonecrosis due to drugs, humerus
       (Ex:) For category M87.12 CC codes: See PDX Collection 908

    M87.121   Osteonecrosis due to drugs, right humerus 🔹 🔹

    M87.122   Osteonecrosis due to drugs, left humerus 🔹 🔹

    M87.129   Osteonecrosis due to drugs, unspecified humerus 🔹 🔹

● M87.13   Osteonecrosis due to drugs of radius, ulna and carpus

    M87.131   Osteonecrosis due to drugs of right radius 🔹 🔹

    M87.132   Osteonecrosis due to drugs of left radius 🔹 🔹

    M87.133   Osteonecrosis due to drugs of unspecified radius 🔹 🔹

    M87.134   Osteonecrosis due to drugs of right ulna 🔹 🔹

    M87.135   Osteonecrosis due to drugs of left ulna 🔹 🔹

    M87.136   Osteonecrosis due to drugs of unspecified ulna 🔹 🔹

    M87.137   Osteonecrosis due to drugs of right carpus 🔹 🔹

    M87.138   Osteonecrosis due to drugs of left carpus 🔹 🔹

    M87.139   Osteonecrosis due to drugs of unspecified carpus 🔹 🔹

● M87.14   Osteonecrosis due to drugs, hand and fingers

    M87.141   Osteonecrosis due to drugs, right hand 🔹 🔹

    M87.142   Osteonecrosis due to drugs, left hand 🔹 🔹

    M87.143   Osteonecrosis due to drugs, unspecified hand 🔹 🔹

    M87.144   Osteonecrosis due to drugs, right finger(s) 🔹 🔹

    M87.145   Osteonecrosis due to drugs, left finger(s) 🔹 🔹

    M87.146   Osteonecrosis due to drugs, unspecified finger(s) 🔹 🔹

● M87.15   Osteonecrosis due to drugs, pelvis and femur
       (Ex:) For category M87.15 CC codes: See PDX Collection 909

    M87.150   Osteonecrosis due to drugs, pelvis 🔹 🔹

    M87.151   Osteonecrosis due to drugs, right femur 🔹 🔹

    M87.152   Osteonecrosis due to drugs, left femur 🔹 🔹

    M87.159   Osteonecrosis due to drugs, unspecified femur 🔹 🔹

N   Newborn Age: 0   **P**   Pediatric Age: 0–17   **M**   Maternity DX: 9–64   **A**   Adult Age: 15–124   ♀   Females Only   ♂   Males Only

🔹 Complication\Comorbidity   🔹 Major C\C   (Ex:) CC/MCC Exclusions   🔹 Hospital-Acquired Condition   🔹 Hierarchical Condition Category

● **M87.16** Osteonecrosis due to drugs, tibia and fibula

    M87.161 Osteonecrosis due to drugs, right tibia 🪙 🔴

    M87.162 Osteonecrosis due to drugs, left tibia 🪙 🔴

    M87.163 Osteonecrosis due to drugs, unspecified tibia 🪙 🔴

    M87.164 Osteonecrosis due to drugs, right fibula 🪙 🔴

    M87.165 Osteonecrosis due to drugs, left fibula 🪙 🔴

    M87.166 Osteonecrosis due to drugs, unspecified fibula 🪙 🔴

● **M87.17** Osteonecrosis due to drugs, ankle, foot and toes

    M87.171 Osteonecrosis due to drugs, right ankle 🪙 🔴

    M87.172 Osteonecrosis due to drugs, left ankle 🪙 🔴

    M87.173 Osteonecrosis due to drugs, unspecified ankle 🪙 🔴

    M87.174 Osteonecrosis due to drugs, right foot 🪙 🔴
        (Ex:) See PDX Collection 910

    M87.175 Osteonecrosis due to drugs, left foot 🪙 🔴
        (Ex:) See PDX Collection 910

    M87.176 Osteonecrosis due to drugs, unspecified foot 🪙 🔴
        (Ex:) See PDX Collection 910

    M87.177 Osteonecrosis due to drugs, right toe(s) 🪙 🔴

    M87.178 Osteonecrosis due to drugs, left toe(s) 🪙 🔴

    M87.179 Osteonecrosis due to drugs, unspecified toe(s) 🪙 🔴

● **M87.18** Osteonecrosis due to drugs, other site

    M87.180 Osteonecrosis due to drugs, jaw 🪙 🔴

    M87.188 Osteonecrosis due to drugs, other site 🪙 🔴

  M87.19 Osteonecrosis due to drugs, multiple sites 🪙 🔴

● **M87.2** Osteonecrosis due to previous trauma
    (Ex:) **For category M87 CC codes unless otherwise indicated:** See PDX Collection 907

  M87.20 Osteonecrosis due to previous trauma, unspecified bone 🪙 🔴

● **M87.21** Osteonecrosis due to previous trauma, shoulder

    M87.211 Osteonecrosis due to previous trauma, right shoulder 🪙 🔴

    M87.212 Osteonecrosis due to previous trauma, left shoulder 🪙 🔴

    M87.219 Osteonecrosis due to previous trauma, unspecified shoulder 🪙 🔴

● **M87.22** Osteonecrosis due to previous trauma, humerus
    (Ex:) **For category M87.22 CC codes:** See PDX Collection 908

    M87.221 Osteonecrosis due to previous trauma, right humerus 🪙 🔴

    M87.222 Osteonecrosis due to previous trauma, left humerus 🪙 🔴

    M87.229 Osteonecrosis due to previous trauma, unspecified humerus 🪙 🔴

● **M87.23** Osteonecrosis due to previous trauma of radius, ulna and carpus

    M87.231 Osteonecrosis due to previous trauma of right radius 🪙 🔴

    M87.232 Osteonecrosis due to previous trauma of left radius 🪙 🔴

    M87.233 Osteonecrosis due to previous trauma of unspecified radius 🪙 🔴

    M87.234 Osteonecrosis due to previous trauma of right ulna 🪙 🔴

    M87.235 Osteonecrosis due to previous trauma of left ulna 🪙 🔴

    M87.236 Osteonecrosis due to previous trauma of unspecified ulna 🪙 🔴

    M87.237 Osteonecrosis due to previous trauma of right carpus 🪙 🔴

    M87.238 Osteonecrosis due to previous trauma of left carpus 🪙 🔴

    M87.239 Osteonecrosis due to previous trauma of unspecified carpus 🪙 🔴

● **M87.24** Osteonecrosis due to previous trauma, hand and fingers

    M87.241 Osteonecrosis due to previous trauma, right hand 🪙 🔴

    M87.242 Osteonecrosis due to previous trauma, left hand 🪙 🔴

    M87.243 Osteonecrosis due to previous trauma, unspecified hand 🪙 🔴

    M87.244 Osteonecrosis due to previous trauma, right finger(s) 🪙 🔴

    M87.245 Osteonecrosis due to previous trauma, left finger(s) 🪙 🔴

    M87.246 Osteonecrosis due to previous trauma, unspecified finger(s) 🪙 🔴

● **M87.25** Osteonecrosis due to previous trauma, pelvis and femur

    M87.250 Osteonecrosis due to previous trauma, pelvis 🪙 🔴

    M87.251 Osteonecrosis due to previous trauma, right femur 🪙 🔴
        (Ex:) See PDX Collection 909

    M87.252 Osteonecrosis due to previous trauma, left femur 🪙 🔴
        (Ex:) See PDX Collection 909

    M87.256 Osteonecrosis due to previous trauma, unspecified femur 🪙 🔴
        (Ex:) See PDX Collection 909

● **M87.26** Osteonecrosis due to previous trauma, tibia and fibula

    M87.261 Osteonecrosis due to previous trauma, right tibia 🪙 🔴

    M87.262 Osteonecrosis due to previous trauma, left tibia 🪙 🔴

    M87.263 Osteonecrosis due to previous trauma, unspecified tibia 🪙 🔴

    M87.264 Osteonecrosis due to previous trauma, right fibula 🪙 🔴

    M87.265 Osteonecrosis due to previous trauma, left fibula 🪙 🔴

    M87.266 Osteonecrosis due to previous trauma, unspecified fibula 🪙 🔴

▶ New   ⇒ Revised   ~~deleted~~ Deleted   Excludes 1   Excludes 2   Includes   Use additional   Code first   Code also   Key words

OGCR Official Guidelines   ● Unacceptable Principal Diagnosis   X Assign placeholder X   ● Use Additional Character(s)   ▶ Manifestation Code   Coding Clinic

● M87.27 Osteonecrosis due to previous trauma, ankle, foot and toes

    M87.271 Osteonecrosis due to previous trauma, right ankle 🅲 🅷

    M87.272 Osteonecrosis due to previous trauma, left ankle 🅲 🅷

    M87.273 Osteonecrosis due to previous trauma, unspecified ankle 🅲 🅷

    M87.274 Osteonecrosis due to previous trauma, right foot 🅲 🅷
        (Ex:) See PDX Collection 910

    M87.275 Osteonecrosis due to previous trauma, left foot 🅲 🅷
        (Ex:) See PDX Collection 910

    M87.276 Osteonecrosis due to previous trauma, unspecified foot 🅲 🅷
        (Ex:) See PDX Collection 910

    M87.277 Osteonecrosis due to previous trauma, right toe(s) 🅲 🅷

    M87.278 Osteonecrosis due to previous trauma, left toe(s) 🅲 🅷

    M87.279 Osteonecrosis due to previous trauma, unspecified toe(s) 🅲 🅷

  M87.28 Osteonecrosis due to previous trauma, other site 🅲 🅷

  M87.29 Osteonecrosis due to previous trauma, multiple sites 🅲 🅷

● M87.3 Other secondary osteonecrosis
    (Ex:) For category M87 CC codes unless otherwise indicated: See PDX Collection 907

  M87.30 Other secondary osteonecrosis, unspecified bone 🅲 🅷

● M87.31 Other secondary osteonecrosis, shoulder

    M87.311 Other secondary osteonecrosis, right shoulder 🅲 🅷

    M87.312 Other secondary osteonecrosis, left shoulder 🅲 🅷

    M87.319 Other secondary osteonecrosis, unspecified shoulder 🅲 🅷

● M87.32 Other secondary osteonecrosis, humerus
    (Ex:) For category M87.32 CC codes: See PDX Collection 908

    M87.321 Other secondary osteonecrosis, right humerus 🅲 🅷

    M87.322 Other secondary osteonecrosis, left humerus 🅲 🅷

    M87.329 Other secondary osteonecrosis, unspecified humerus 🅲 🅷

● M87.33 Other secondary osteonecrosis of radius, ulna and carpus

    M87.331 Other secondary osteonecrosis of right radius 🅲 🅷

    M87.332 Other secondary osteonecrosis of left radius 🅲 🅷

    M87.333 Other secondary osteonecrosis of unspecified radius 🅲 🅷

    M87.334 Other secondary osteonecrosis of right ulna 🅲 🅷

    M87.335 Other secondary osteonecrosis of left ulna 🅲 🅷

    M87.336 Other secondary osteonecrosis of unspecified ulna 🅲 🅷

    M87.337 Other secondary osteonecrosis of right carpus 🅲 🅷

    M87.338 Other secondary osteonecrosis of left carpus 🅲 🅷

    M87.339 Other secondary osteonecrosis of unspecified carpus 🅲 🅷

● M87.34 Other secondary osteonecrosis, hand and fingers

    M87.341 Other secondary osteonecrosis, right hand 🅲 🅷

    M87.342 Other secondary osteonecrosis, left hand 🅲 🅷

    M87.343 Other secondary osteonecrosis, unspecified hand 🅲 🅷

    M87.344 Other secondary osteonecrosis, right finger(s) 🅲 🅷

    M87.345 Other secondary osteonecrosis, left finger(s) 🅲 🅷

    M87.346 Other secondary osteonecrosis, unspecified finger(s) 🅲 🅷

● M87.35 Other secondary osteonecrosis, pelvis and femur
    (Ex:) For category M87.35 CC codes: See PDX Collection 909

    M87.350 Other secondary osteonecrosis, pelvis 🅲 🅷

    M87.351 Other secondary osteonecrosis, right femur 🅲 🅷

    M87.352 Other secondary osteonecrosis, left femur 🅲 🅷

    M87.353 Other secondary osteonecrosis, unspecified femur 🅲 🅷

● M87.36 Other secondary osteonecrosis, tibia and fibula

    M87.361 Other secondary osteonecrosis, right tibia 🅲 🅷

    M87.362 Other secondary osteonecrosis, left tibia 🅲 🅷

    M87.363 Other secondary osteonecrosis, unspecified tibia 🅲 🅷

    M87.364 Other secondary osteonecrosis, right fibula 🅲 🅷

    M87.365 Other secondary osteonecrosis, left fibula 🅲 🅷

    M87.366 Other secondary osteonecrosis, unspecified fibula 🅲 🅷

● M87.37 Other secondary osteonecrosis, ankle and foot

    M87.371 Other secondary osteonecrosis, right ankle 🅲 🅷

    M87.372 Other secondary osteonecrosis, left ankle 🅲 🅷

    M87.373 Other secondary osteonecrosis, unspecified ankle 🅲 🅷

    M87.374 Other secondary osteonecrosis, right foot 🅲 🅷
        (Ex:) See PDX Collection 910

    M87.375 Other secondary osteonecrosis, left foot 🅲 🅷
        (Ex:) See PDX Collection 910

    M87.376 Other secondary osteonecrosis, unspecified foot 🅲 🅷
        (Ex:) See PDX Collection 910

    M87.377 Other secondary osteonecrosis, right toe(s) 🅲 🅷

    M87.378 Other secondary osteonecrosis, left toe(s) 🅲 🅷

    M87.379 Other secondary osteonecrosis, unspecified toe(s) 🅲 🅷

  M87.38 Other secondary osteonecrosis, other site 🅲 🅷

  M87.39 Other secondary osteonecrosis, multiple sites 🅲 🅷

N Newborn Age: 0   **P** Pediatric Age: 0–17   **M** Maternity DX: 9–64   **A** Adult Age: 15–124   ♀ Females Only   ♂ Males Only

🅲 Complication\Comorbidity   🅷 Major C\C   (Ex:) CC/MCC Exclusions   Hospital-Acquired Condition   Hierarchical Condition Category

1105

● M87.8 **Other osteonecrosis**
 (Ex:) **For category M87 CC codes unless otherwise indicated:** See PDX
        Collection 907

 M87.80 Other osteonecrosis, unspecified bone 🪙 🪙

● M87.81 Other osteonecrosis, shoulder

 M87.811 Other osteonecrosis, right
          shoulder 🪙 🪙

 M87.812 Other osteonecrosis, left
          shoulder 🪙 🪙

 M87.819 Other osteonecrosis, unspecified
          shoulder 🪙 🪙

● M87.82 Other osteonecrosis, humerus
 (Ex:) **For category M87.82 CC codes:** See PDX Collection 908

 M87.821 Other osteonecrosis, right
          humerus 🪙 🪙

 M87.822 Other osteonecrosis, left
          humerus 🪙 🪙

 M87.829 Other osteonecrosis, unspecified
          humerus 🪙 🪙

● M87.83 Other osteonecrosis of radius, ulna and carpus

 M87.831 Other osteonecrosis of right
          radius 🪙 🪙

 M87.832 Other osteonecrosis of left
          radius 🪙 🪙

 M87.833 Other osteonecrosis of unspecified
          radius 🪙 🪙

 M87.834 Other osteonecrosis of right ulna 🪙 🪙

 M87.835 Other osteonecrosis of left ulna 🪙 🪙

 M87.836 Other osteonecrosis of unspecified
          ulna 🪙 🪙

 M87.837 Other osteonecrosis of right
          carpus 🪙 🪙

 M87.838 Other osteonecrosis of left
          carpus 🪙 🪙

 M87.839 Other osteonecrosis of unspecified
          carpus 🪙 🪙

● M87.84 Other osteonecrosis, hand and fingers

 M87.841 Other osteonecrosis, right hand 🪙 🪙

 M87.842 Other osteonecrosis, left hand 🪙 🪙

 M87.843 Other osteonecrosis, unspecified
          hand 🪙 🪙

 M87.844 Other osteonecrosis, right
          finger(s) 🪙 🪙

 M87.845 Other osteonecrosis, left finger(s) 🪙 🪙

 M87.849 Other osteonecrosis, unspecified
          finger(s) 🪙 🪙

● M87.85 Other osteonecrosis, pelvis and femur
 (Ex:) **For category M87.85 CC codes:** See PDX Collection 909

 M87.850 Other osteonecrosis, pelvis 🪙 🪙

 M87.851 Other osteonecrosis, right femur 🪙 🪙

 M87.852 Other osteonecrosis, left femur 🪙 🪙

 M87.859 Other osteonecrosis, unspecified
          femur 🪙 🪙

● M87.86 Other osteonecrosis, tibia and fibula

 M87.861 Other osteonecrosis, right tibia 🪙 🪙

 M87.862 Other osteonecrosis, left tibia 🪙 🪙

 M87.863 Other osteonecrosis, unspecified
          tibia 🪙 🪙

 M87.864 Other osteonecrosis, right fibula 🪙 🪙

 M87.865 Other osteonecrosis, left fibula 🪙 🪙

 M87.869 Other osteonecrosis, unspecified
          fibula 🪙 🪙

● M87.87 Other osteonecrosis, ankle, foot and toes

 M87.871 Other osteonecrosis, right ankle 🪙 🪙

 M87.872 Other osteonecrosis, left ankle 🪙 🪙

 M87.873 Other osteonecrosis, unspecified
          ankle 🪙 🪙

 M87.874 Other osteonecrosis, right foot 🪙 🪙
 (Ex:) See PDX Collection 910

 M87.875 Other osteonecrosis, left foot 🪙 🪙
 (Ex:) See PDX Collection 910

 M87.876 Other osteonecrosis, unspecified
          foot 🪙 🪙
 (Ex:) See PDX Collection 910

 M87.877 Other osteonecrosis, right toe(s) 🪙 🪙

 M87.878 Other osteonecrosis, left toe(s) 🪙 🪙

 M87.879 Other osteonecrosis, unspecified
          toe(s) 🪙 🪙

 M87.88 Other osteonecrosis, other site 🪙 🪙

 M87.89 Other osteonecrosis, multiple sites 🪙 🪙

● M87.9 Osteonecrosis, unspecified 🪙 🪙
         Necrosis of bone NOS
 (Ex:) **For category M87 CC codes unless otherwise indicated:** See PDX
        Collection 907

● M88 **Osteitis deformans [Paget's disease of bone]**
       Chronic disorder that results in enlarged and deformed bones. The
       excessive breakdown and formation of bone tissue causes bones
       to weaken and results in bone pain, arthritis, deformities, and
       fractures.

 Excludes1 osteitis deformans in neoplastic disease (M90.6)

 M88.0 Osteitis deformans of skull

 M88.1 Osteitis deformans of vertebrae

● M88.8 Osteitis deformans of other bones

● M88.81 Osteitis deformans of shoulder

 M88.811 Osteitis deformans of right shoulder

 M88.812 Osteitis deformans of left shoulder

 M88.819 Osteitis deformans of unspecified
          shoulder

● M88.82 Osteitis deformans of upper arm

 M88.821 Osteitis deformans of right upper arm

 M88.822 Osteitis deformans of left upper arm

 M88.829 Osteitis deformans of unspecified
          upper arm

● M88.83 Osteitis deformans of forearm

 M88.831 Osteitis deformans of right forearm

 M88.832 Osteitis deformans of left forearm

 M88.839 Osteitis deformans of unspecified
          forearm

● M88.84 Osteitis deformans of hand

 M88.841 Osteitis deformans of right hand

 M88.842 Osteitis deformans of left hand

 M88.849 Osteitis deformans of unspecified
          hand

● M88.85 Osteitis deformans of thigh

 M88.851 Osteitis deformans of right thigh

 M88.852 Osteitis deformans of left thigh

 M88.859 Osteitis deformans of unspecified
          thigh

● M88.86 Osteitis deformans of lower leg

 M88.861 Osteitis deformans of right lower leg

 M88.862 Osteitis deformans of left lower leg

 M88.869 Osteitis deformans of unspecified
          lower leg

● M88.87 Osteitis deformans of ankle and foot

 M88.871 Osteitis deformans of right ankle and
          foot

 M88.872 Osteitis deformans of left ankle and
          foot

 M88.879 Osteitis deformans of unspecified
          ankle and foot

 M88.88 Osteitis deformans of other bones

 Excludes2 osteitis deformans of skull
              (M88.0)
              osteitis deformans of vertebrae
              (M88.1)

 M88.89 Osteitis deformans of multiple sites

 M88.9 Osteitis deformans of unspecified bone

▶ New   ⇒ Revised   ~~deleted~~ Deleted   Excludes 1   Excludes 2   Includes   Use additional   Code first   Code also   Key words

OGCR Official Guidelines   ● Unacceptable Principal Diagnosis   X Assign placeholder X   ● Use Additional Character(s)   ▶ Manifestation Code   **Coding Clinic**

● **M89** Other disorders of bone
  ● **M89.0** Algoneurodystrophy
      Shoulder-hand syndrome
      Sudeck's atrophy
      Excludes 1   causalgia, lower limb (G57.7-)
                causalgia, upper limb (G56.4-)
                complex regional pain syndrome II, lower
                    limb (G57.7-)
                complex regional pain syndrome II,
                    upper limb (G56.4-)
                reflex sympathetic dystrophy (G90.5-)
      M89.00 Algoneurodystrophy, unspecified site
    ● M89.01 Algoneurodystrophy, shoulder
        M89.011 Algoneurodystrophy, right shoulder
        M89.012 Algoneurodystrophy, left shoulder
        M89.019 Algoneurodystrophy, unspecified
                 shoulder
    ● M89.02 Algoneurodystrophy, upper arm
        M89.021 Algoneurodystrophy, right upper arm
        M89.022 Algoneurodystrophy, left upper arm
        M89.029 Algoneurodystrophy, unspecified
                 upper arm
    ● M89.03 Algoneurodystrophy, forearm
        M89.031 Algoneurodystrophy, right forearm
        M89.032 Algoneurodystrophy, left forearm
        M89.039 Algoneurodystrophy, unspecified
                 forearm
    ● M89.04 Algoneurodystrophy, hand
        M89.041 Algoneurodystrophy, right hand
        M89.042 Algoneurodystrophy, left hand
        M89.049 Algoneurodystrophy, unspecified
                 hand
    ● M89.05 Algoneurodystrophy, thigh
        M89.051 Algoneurodystrophy, right thigh
        M89.052 Algoneurodystrophy, left thigh
        M89.059 Algoneurodystrophy, unspecified
                 thigh
    ● M89.06 Algoneurodystrophy, lower leg
        M89.061 Algoneurodystrophy, right lower leg
        M89.062 Algoneurodystrophy, left lower leg
        M89.069 Algoneurodystrophy, unspecified
                 lower leg
    ● M89.07 Algoneurodystrophy, ankle and foot
        M89.071 Algoneurodystrophy, right ankle and
                 foot
        M89.072 Algoneurodystrophy, left ankle and
                 foot
        M89.079 Algoneurodystrophy, unspecified
                 ankle and foot
      M89.08 Algoneurodystrophy, other site
      M89.09 Algoneurodystrophy, multiple sites
  ● **M89.1** Physeal arrest
      Arrest of growth plate
      Epiphyseal arrest
      Growth plate arrest
    ● M89.12 Physeal arrest, humerus
        M89.121 Complete physeal arrest, right
                 proximal humerus
        M89.122 Complete physeal arrest, left proximal
                 humerus
        M89.123 Partial physeal arrest, right proximal
                 humerus
        M89.124 Partial physeal arrest, left proximal
                 humerus
        M89.125 Complete physeal arrest, right distal
                 humerus

        M89.126 Complete physeal arrest, left distal
                 humerus
        M89.127 Partial physeal arrest, right distal
                 humerus
        M89.128 Partial physeal arrest, left distal
                 humerus
        M89.129 Physeal arrest, humerus, unspecified
    ● M89.13 Physeal arrest, forearm
        M89.131 Complete physeal arrest, right distal
                 radius
        M89.132 Complete physeal arrest, left distal
                 radius
        M89.133 Partial physeal arrest, right distal
                 radius
        M89.134 Partial physeal arrest, left distal
                 radius
        M89.138 Other physeal arrest of forearm
        M89.139 Physeal arrest, forearm, unspecified
    ● M89.15 Physeal arrest, femur
        M89.151 Complete physeal arrest, right
                 proximal femur
        M89.152 Complete physeal arrest, left proximal
                 femur
        M89.153 Partial physeal arrest, right proximal
                 femur
        M89.154 Partial physeal arrest, left proximal
                 femur
        M89.155 Complete physeal arrest, right distal
                 femur
        M89.156 Complete physeal arrest, left distal
                 femur
        M89.157 Partial physeal arrest, right distal
                 femur
        M89.158 Partial physeal arrest, left distal femur
        M89.159 Physeal arrest, femur, unspecified
    ● M89.16 Physeal arrest, lower leg
        M89.160 Complete physeal arrest, right
                 proximal tibia
        M89.161 Complete physeal arrest, left proximal
                 tibia
        M89.162 Partial physeal arrest, right proximal
                 tibia
        M89.163 Partial physeal arrest, left proximal
                 tibia
        M89.164 Complete physeal arrest, right distal
                 tibia
        M89.165 Complete physeal arrest, left distal
                 tibia
        M89.166 Partial physeal arrest, right distal
                 tibia
        M89.167 Partial physeal arrest, left distal tibia
        M89.168 Other physeal arrest of lower leg
        M89.169 Physeal arrest, lower leg, unspecified
      M89.18 Physeal arrest, other site
  ● **M89.2** Other disorders of bone development and growth
      M89.20 Other disorders of bone development and
               growth, unspecified site
    ● M89.21 Other disorders of bone development and
               growth, shoulder
        M89.211 Other disorders of bone development
                 and growth, right shoulder
        M89.212 Other disorders of bone development
                 and growth, left shoulder
        M89.219 Other disorders of bone development
                 and growth, unspecified shoulder

CHAPTER 13 (M00-M99)

● M89.22 Other disorders of bone development and growth, humerus
  M89.221 Other disorders of bone development and growth, right humerus
  M89.222 Other disorders of bone development and growth, left humerus
  M89.229 Other disorders of bone development and growth, unspecified humerus
● M89.23 Other disorders of bone development and growth, ulna and radius
  M89.231 Other disorders of bone development and growth, right ulna
  M89.232 Other disorders of bone development and growth, left ulna
  M89.233 Other disorders of bone development and growth, right radius
  M89.234 Other disorders of bone development and growth, left radius
  M89.239 Other disorders of bone development and growth, unspecified ulna and radius
● M89.24 Other disorders of bone development and growth, hand
  M89.241 Other disorders of bone development and growth, right hand
  M89.242 Other disorders of bone development and growth, left hand
  M89.249 Other disorders of bone development and growth, unspecified hand
● M89.25 Other disorders of bone development and growth, femur
  M89.251 Other disorders of bone development and growth, right femur
  M89.252 Other disorders of bone development and growth, left femur
  M89.259 Other disorders of bone development and growth, unspecified femur
● M89.26 Other disorders of bone development and growth, tibia and fibula
  M89.261 Other disorders of bone development and growth, right tibia
  M89.262 Other disorders of bone development and growth, left tibia
  M89.263 Other disorders of bone development and growth, right fibula
  M89.264 Other disorders of bone development and growth, left fibula
  M89.269 Other disorders of bone development and growth, unspecified lower leg
● M89.27 Other disorders of bone development and growth, ankle and foot
  M89.271 Other disorders of bone development and growth, right ankle and foot
  M89.272 Other disorders of bone development and growth, left ankle and foot
  M89.279 Other disorders of bone development and growth, unspecified ankle and foot
  M89.28 Other disorders of bone development and growth, other site
  M89.29 Other disorders of bone development and growth, multiple sites
● M89.3 Hypertrophy of bone
  M89.30 Hypertrophy of bone, unspecified site
● M89.31 Hypertrophy of bone, shoulder
  M89.311 Hypertrophy of bone, right shoulder
  M89.312 Hypertrophy of bone, left shoulder
  M89.319 Hypertrophy of bone, unspecified shoulder

● M89.32 Hypertrophy of bone, humerus
  M89.321 Hypertrophy of bone, right humerus
  M89.322 Hypertrophy of bone, left humerus
  M89.329 Hypertrophy of bone, unspecified humerus
● M89.33 Hypertrophy of bone, ulna and radius
  M89.331 Hypertrophy of bone, right ulna
  M89.332 Hypertrophy of bone, left ulna
  M89.333 Hypertrophy of bone, right radius
  M89.334 Hypertrophy of bone, left radius
  M89.339 Hypertrophy of bone, unspecified ulna and radius
● M89.34 Hypertrophy of bone, hand
  M89.341 Hypertrophy of bone, right hand
  M89.342 Hypertrophy of bone, left hand
  M89.349 Hypertrophy of bone, unspecified hand
● M89.35 Hypertrophy of bone, femur
  M89.351 Hypertrophy of bone, right femur
  M89.352 Hypertrophy of bone, left femur
  M89.359 Hypertrophy of bone, unspecified femur
● M89.36 Hypertrophy of bone, tibia and fibula
  M89.361 Hypertrophy of bone, right tibia
  M89.362 Hypertrophy of bone, left tibia
  M89.363 Hypertrophy of bone, right fibula
  M89.364 Hypertrophy of bone, left fibula
  M89.369 Hypertrophy of bone, unspecified tibia and fibula
● M89.37 Hypertrophy of bone, ankle and foot
  M89.371 Hypertrophy of bone, right ankle and foot
  M89.372 Hypertrophy of bone, left ankle and foot
  M89.379 Hypertrophy of bone, unspecified ankle and foot
  M89.38 Hypertrophy of bone, other site
  M89.39 Hypertrophy of bone, multiple sites
● M89.4 Other hypertrophic osteoarthropathy
    Marie-Bamberger disease
    Pachydermoperiostosis
  M89.40 Other hypertrophic osteoarthropathy, unspecified site
● M89.41 Other hypertrophic osteoarthropathy, shoulder
  M89.411 Other hypertrophic osteoarthropathy, right shoulder
  M89.412 Other hypertrophic osteoarthropathy, left shoulder
  M89.419 Other hypertrophic osteoarthropathy, unspecified shoulder
● M89.42 Other hypertrophic osteoarthropathy, upper arm
  M89.421 Other hypertrophic osteoarthropathy, right upper arm
  M89.422 Other hypertrophic osteoarthropathy, left upper arm
  M89.429 Other hypertrophic osteoarthropathy, unspecified upper arm
● M89.43 Other hypertrophic osteoarthropathy, forearm
  M89.431 Other hypertrophic osteoarthropathy, right forearm
  M89.432 Other hypertrophic osteoarthropathy, left forearm
  M89.439 Other hypertrophic osteoarthropathy, unspecified forearm

● M89.44　Other hypertrophic osteoarthropathy, hand
　　　M89.441　Other hypertrophic osteoarthropathy, right hand
　　　M89.442　Other hypertrophic osteoarthropathy, left hand
　　　M89.449　Other hypertrophic osteoarthropathy, unspecified hand
● M89.45　Other hypertrophic osteoarthropathy, thigh
　　　M89.451　Other hypertrophic osteoarthropathy, right thigh
　　　M89.452　Other hypertrophic osteoarthropathy, left thigh
　　　M89.459　Other hypertrophic osteoarthropathy, unspecified thigh
● M89.46　Other hypertrophic osteoarthropathy, lower leg
　　　M89.461　Other hypertrophic osteoarthropathy, right lower leg
　　　M89.462　Other hypertrophic osteoarthropathy, left lower leg
　　　M89.469　Other hypertrophic osteoarthropathy, unspecified lower leg
● M89.47　Other hypertrophic osteoarthropathy, ankle and foot
　　　M89.471　Other hypertrophic osteoarthropathy, right ankle and foot
　　　M89.472　Other hypertrophic osteoarthropathy, left ankle and foot
　　　M89.479　Other hypertrophic osteoarthropathy, unspecified ankle and foot
　　M89.48　Other hypertrophic osteoarthropathy, other site
　　M89.49　Other hypertrophic osteoarthropathy, multiple sites
● M89.5　Osteolysis
　　　Use additional code to identify major osseous defect, if applicable (M89.7-)
　　　Excludes2　periprosthetic osteolysis of internal prosthetic joint (T84.05-)
　　M89.50　Osteolysis, unspecified site
● M89.51　Osteolysis, shoulder
　　　M89.511　Osteolysis, right shoulder
　　　M89.512　Osteolysis, left shoulder
　　　M89.519　Osteolysis, unspecified shoulder
● M89.52　Osteolysis, upper arm
　　　M89.521　Osteolysis, right upper arm
　　　M89.522　Osteolysis, left upper arm
　　　M89.529　Osteolysis, unspecified upper arm
● M89.53　Osteolysis, forearm
　　　M89.531　Osteolysis, right forearm
　　　M89.532　Osteolysis, left forearm
　　　M89.539　Osteolysis, unspecified forearm
● M89.54　Osteolysis, hand
　　　M89.541　Osteolysis, right hand
　　　M89.542　Osteolysis, left hand
　　　M89.549　Osteolysis, unspecified hand
● M89.55　Osteolysis, thigh
　　　M89.551　Osteolysis, right thigh
　　　M89.552　Osteolysis, left thigh
　　　M89.559　Osteolysis, unspecified thigh
● M89.56　Osteolysis, lower leg
　　　M89.561　Osteolysis, right lower leg
　　　M89.562　Osteolysis, left lower leg
　　　M89.569　Osteolysis, unspecified lower leg

● M89.57　Osteolysis, ankle and foot
　　　M89.571　Osteolysis, right ankle and foot
　　　M89.572　Osteolysis, left ankle and foot
　　　M89.579　Osteolysis, unspecified ankle and foot
　　M89.58　Osteolysis, other site
　　M89.59　Osteolysis, multiple sites
● M89.6　Osteopathy after poliomyelitis
　　　Use additional code (B91) to identify previous poliomyelitis
　　　Excludes1　postpolio syndrome (G14)
　　M89.60　Osteopathy after poliomyelitis, unspecified site 🦠
● M89.61　Osteopathy after poliomyelitis, shoulder
　　　M89.611　Osteopathy after poliomyelitis, right shoulder 🦠
　　　M89.612　Osteopathy after poliomyelitis, left shoulder 🦠
　　　M89.619　Osteopathy after poliomyelitis, unspecified shoulder 🦠
● M89.62　Osteopathy after poliomyelitis, upper arm
　　　M89.621　Osteopathy after poliomyelitis, right upper arm 🦠
　　　M89.622　Osteopathy after poliomyelitis, left upper arm 🦠
　　　M89.629　Osteopathy after poliomyelitis, unspecified upper arm 🦠
● M89.63　Osteopathy after poliomyelitis, forearm
　　　M89.631　Osteopathy after poliomyelitis, right forearm 🦠
　　　M89.632　Osteopathy after poliomyelitis, left forearm 🦠
　　　M89.639　Osteopathy after poliomyelitis, unspecified forearm 🦠
● M89.64　Osteopathy after poliomyelitis, hand
　　　M89.641　Osteopathy after poliomyelitis, right hand 🦠
　　　M89.642　Osteopathy after poliomyelitis, left hand 🦠
　　　M89.649　Osteopathy after poliomyelitis, unspecified hand 🦠
● M89.65　Osteopathy after poliomyelitis, thigh
　　　M89.651　Osteopathy after poliomyelitis, right thigh 🦠
　　　M89.652　Osteopathy after poliomyelitis, left thigh 🦠
　　　M89.659　Osteopathy after poliomyelitis, unspecified thigh 🦠
● M89.66　Osteopathy after poliomyelitis, lower leg
　　　M89.661　Osteopathy after poliomyelitis, right lower leg 🦠
　　　M89.662　Osteopathy after poliomyelitis, left lower leg 🦠
　　　M89.669　Osteopathy after poliomyelitis, unspecified lower leg 🦠
● M89.67　Osteopathy after poliomyelitis, ankle and foot
　　　M89.671　Osteopathy after poliomyelitis, right ankle and foot 🦠
　　　M89.672　Osteopathy after poliomyelitis, left ankle and foot 🦠
　　　M89.679　Osteopathy after poliomyelitis, unspecified ankle and foot 🦠
　　M89.68　Osteopathy after poliomyelitis, other site 🦠
　　M89.69　Osteopathy after poliomyelitis, multiple sites 🦠

CHAPTER 13 (M00-M99)

● **M89.7 Major osseous defect**
  Code first underlying disease, if known, such as:
    aseptic necrosis of bone (M87.-)
    malignant neoplasm of bone (C40.-)
    osteolysis (M89.5)
    osteomyelitis (M86.-)
    osteonecrosis (M87.-)
    osteoporosis (M80.-, M81.-)
    periprosthetic osteolysis (T84.05-)

  M89.70 Major osseous defect, unspecified site

  ● M89.71 Major osseous defect, shoulder region
        Major osseous defect clavicle or scapula
      M89.711 Major osseous defect, right shoulder region
      M89.712 Major osseous defect, left shoulder region
      M89.719 Major osseous defect, unspecified shoulder region

  ● M89.72 Major osseous defect, humerus
      M89.721 Major osseous defect, right humerus
      M89.722 Major osseous defect, left humerus
      M89.729 Major osseous defect, unspecified humerus

  ● M89.73 Major osseous defect, forearm
        Major osseous defect of radius and ulna
      M89.731 Major osseous defect, right forearm
      M89.732 Major osseous defect, left forearm
      M89.739 Major osseous defect, unspecified forearm

  ● M89.74 Major osseous defect, hand
        Major osseous defect of carpus, fingers, metacarpus
      M89.741 Major osseous defect, right hand
      M89.742 Major osseous defect, left hand
      M89.749 Major osseous defect, unspecified hand

  ● M89.75 Major osseous defect, pelvic region and thigh
        Major osseous defect of femur and pelvis
      M89.751 Major osseous defect, right pelvic region and thigh
      M89.752 Major osseous defect, left pelvic region and thigh
      M89.759 Major osseous defect, unspecified pelvic region and thigh

  ● M89.76 Major osseous defect, lower leg
        Major osseous defect of fibula and tibia
      M89.761 Major osseous defect, right lower leg
      M89.762 Major osseous defect, left lower leg
      M89.769 Major osseous defect, unspecified lower leg

  ● M89.77 Major osseous defect, ankle and foot
        Major osseous defect of metatarsus, tarsus, toes
      M89.771 Major osseous defect, right ankle and foot
      M89.772 Major osseous defect, left ankle and foot
      M89.779 Major osseous defect, unspecified ankle and foot

  M89.78 Major osseous defect, other site
  M89.79 Major osseous defect, multiple sites

● **M89.8 Other specified disorders of bone**
    Infantile cortical hyperostoses
    Post-traumatic subperiosteal ossification

  ● M89.8X Other specified disorders of bone
      M89.8X0 Other specified disorders of bone, multiple sites
      M89.8X1 Other specified disorders of bone, shoulder
      M89.8X2 Other specified disorders of bone, upper arm
      M89.8X3 Other specified disorders of bone, forearm
            Coding Clinic: 2019, Q3, P10
      M89.8X4 Other specified disorders of bone, hand
      M89.8X5 Other specified disorders of bone, thigh
      M89.8X6 Other specified disorders of bone, lower leg
      M89.8X7 Other specified disorders of bone, ankle and foot
      M89.8X8 Other specified disorders of bone, other site
      M89.8X9 Other specified disorders of bone, unspecified site

  M89.9 Disorder of bone, unspecified

● **M90 Osteopathies in diseases classified elsewhere**
    Excludes1 osteochondritis, osteomyelitis, and osteopathy (in):
        cryptococcosis (B45.3)
        diabetes mellitus (E08-E13 with .69-)
        gonococcal (A54.43)
        neurogenic syphilis (A52.11)
        renal osteodystrophy (N25.0)
        salmonellosis (A02.24)
        secondary syphilis (A51.46)
        syphilis (late) (A52.77)

● **M90.5 Osteonecrosis in diseases classified elsewhere**
    Code first underlying disease, such as:
      caisson disease (T70.3)
      hemoglobinopathy (D50-D64)
    (Ex) **For category M90.5 CC codes unless otherwise indicated:** See PDX Collection 907

  ▌ *M90.50 Osteonecrosis in diseases classified elsewhere, unspecified site* 🔖 🔖
        CC when PDx is its own CC

  ● M90.51 Osteonecrosis in diseases classified elsewhere, shoulder
        (Ex) **For category M90.51 CC codes:** See PDX Collection 908
      ▌ *M90.511 Osteonecrosis in diseases classified elsewhere, right shoulder* 🔖 🔖
            CC when PDx is its own CC
      ▌ *M90.512 Osteonecrosis in diseases classified elsewhere, left shoulder* 🔖 🔖
            CC when PDx is its own CC
      ▌ *M90.519 Osteonecrosis in diseases classified elsewhere, unspecified shoulder* 🔖 🔖
            CC when PDx is its own CC

  ● M90.52 Osteonecrosis in diseases classified elsewhere, upper arm
      ▌ *M90.521 Osteonecrosis in diseases classified elsewhere, right upper arm* 🔖 🔖
            CC when PDx is its own CC
      ▌ *M90.522 Osteonecrosis in diseases classified elsewhere, left upper arm* 🔖 🔖
            CC when PDx is its own CC
      ▌ *M90.529 Osteonecrosis in diseases classified elsewhere, unspecified upper arm* 🔖 🔖
            CC when PDx is its own CC

▶ New   ⇒ Revised   ~~deleted~~ Deleted | Excludes 1 | | Excludes 2 | | Includes | | Use additional | | Code first | | Code also | | Key words |
OGCR Official Guidelines   ● Unacceptable Principal Diagnosis   X Assign placeholder X   ● Use Additional Character(s)   ▌ Manifestation Code   **Coding Clinic**

● **M90.53** Osteonecrosis in diseases classified elsewhere, forearm

   ▶ *M90.531*   *Osteonecrosis in diseases classified elsewhere, right forearm* 🦠 🦠
        CC when PDx is its own CC

   ▶ *M90.532*   *Osteonecrosis in diseases classified elsewhere, left forearm* 🦠 🦠
        CC when PDx is its own CC

   ▶ *M90.539*   *Osteonecrosis in diseases classified elsewhere, unspecified forearm* 🦠 🦠
        CC when PDx is its own CC

● **M90.54** Osteonecrosis in diseases classified elsewhere, hand

   ▶ *M90.541*   *Osteonecrosis in diseases classified elsewhere, right hand* 🦠 🦠
        CC when PDx is its own CC

   ▶ *M90.542*   *Osteonecrosis in diseases classified elsewhere, left hand* 🦠 🦠
        CC when PDx is its own CC

   ▶ *M90.549*   *Osteonecrosis in diseases classified elsewhere, unspecified hand* 🦠 🦠
        CC when PDx is its own CC

● **M90.55** Osteonecrosis in diseases classified elsewhere, thigh
        (Ex) **For category M90.55 CC codes:** See PDX Collection 909

   ▶ *M90.551*   *Osteonecrosis in diseases classified elsewhere, right thigh* 🦠 🦠
        CC when PDx is its own CC

   ▶ *M90.552*   *Osteonecrosis in diseases classified elsewhere, left thigh* 🦠 🦠
        CC when PDx is its own CC

   ▶ *M90.559*   *Osteonecrosis in diseases classified elsewhere, unspecified thigh* 🦠 🦠
        CC when PDx is its own CC

● **M90.56** Osteonecrosis in diseases classified elsewhere, lower leg

   ▶ *M90.561*   *Osteonecrosis in diseases classified elsewhere, right lower leg* 🦠 🦠
        CC when PDx is its own CC

   ▶ *M90.562*   *Osteonecrosis in diseases classified elsewhere, left lower leg* 🦠 🦠
        CC when PDx is its own CC

   ▶ *M90.569*   *Osteonecrosis in diseases classified elsewhere, unspecified lower leg* 🦠 🦠
        CC when PDx is its own CC

● **M90.57** Osteonecrosis in diseases classified elsewhere, ankle and foot

   ▶ *M90.571*   *Osteonecrosis in diseases classified elsewhere, right ankle and foot* 🦠 🦠
        CC when PDx is its own CC

   ▶ *M90.572*   *Osteonecrosis in diseases classified elsewhere, left ankle and foot* 🦠 🦠
        CC when PDx is its own CC

   ▶ *M90.579*   *Osteonecrosis in diseases classified elsewhere, unspecified ankle and foot* 🦠 🦠
        CC when PDx is its own CC

   ▶ *M90.58*   *Osteonecrosis in diseases classified elsewhere, other site* 🦠 🦠
        CC when PDx is its own CC

   ▶ *M90.59*   *Osteonecrosis in diseases classified elsewhere, multiple sites* 🦠 🦠
        CC when PDx is its own CC

● **M90.6** Osteitis deformans in neoplastic diseases
       Osteitis deformans in malignant neoplasm of bone
       Code first the neoplasm (C40.-, C41.-)
       Excludes1   osteitis deformans [Paget's disease of bone] (M88.-)

   ▶ *M90.60*   *Osteitis deformans in neoplastic diseases, unspecified site*

● **M90.61** Osteitis deformans in neoplastic diseases, shoulder

   ▶ *M90.611*   *Osteitis deformans in neoplastic diseases, right shoulder*

   ▶ *M90.612*   *Osteitis deformans in neoplastic diseases, left shoulder*

   ▶ *M90.619*   *Osteitis deformans in neoplastic diseases, unspecified shoulder*

● **M90.62** Osteitis deformans in neoplastic diseases, upper arm

   ▶ *M90.621*   *Osteitis deformans in neoplastic diseases, right upper arm*

   ▶ *M90.622*   *Osteitis deformans in neoplastic diseases, left upper arm*

   ▶ *M90.629*   *Osteitis deformans in neoplastic diseases, unspecified upper arm*

● **M90.63** Osteitis deformans in neoplastic diseases, forearm

   ▶ *M90.631*   *Osteitis deformans in neoplastic diseases, right forearm*

   ▶ *M90.632*   *Osteitis deformans in neoplastic diseases, left forearm*

   ▶ *M90.639*   *Osteitis deformans in neoplastic diseases, unspecified forearm*

● **M90.64** Osteitis deformans in neoplastic diseases, hand

   ▶ *M90.641*   *Osteitis deformans in neoplastic diseases, right hand*

   ▶ *M90.642*   *Osteitis deformans in neoplastic diseases, left hand*

   ▶ *M90.649*   *Osteitis deformans in neoplastic diseases, unspecified hand*

● **M90.65** Osteitis deformans in neoplastic diseases, thigh

   ▶ *M90.651*   *Osteitis deformans in neoplastic diseases, right thigh*

   ▶ *M90.652*   *Osteitis deformans in neoplastic diseases, left thigh*

   ▶ *M90.659*   *Osteitis deformans in neoplastic diseases, unspecified thigh*

● **M90.66** Osteitis deformans in neoplastic diseases, lower leg

   ▶ *M90.661*   *Osteitis deformans in neoplastic diseases, right lower leg*

   ▶ *M90.662*   *Osteitis deformans in neoplastic diseases, left lower leg*

   ▶ *M90.669*   *Osteitis deformans in neoplastic diseases, unspecified lower leg*

● **M90.67** Osteitis deformans in neoplastic diseases, ankle and foot

   ▶ *M90.671*   *Osteitis deformans in neoplastic diseases, right ankle and foot*

   ▶ *M90.672*   *Osteitis deformans in neoplastic diseases, left ankle and foot*

   ▶ *M90.679*   *Osteitis deformans in neoplastic diseases, unspecified ankle and foot*

   ▶ *M90.68*   *Osteitis deformans in neoplastic diseases, other site*

   ▶ *M90.69*   *Osteitis deformans in neoplastic diseases, multiple sites*

CHAPTER 13 (M00-M99)

● M90.8   **Osteopathy in diseases classified elsewhere**
     Code first underlying disease, such as:
       rickets (E55.0)
       vitamin-D-resistant rickets (E83.3)
   ▶ *M90.80*   *Osteopathy in diseases classified elsewhere, unspecified site*
   ● M90.81   **Osteopathy in diseases classified elsewhere, shoulder**
     ▶ *M90.811*   *Osteopathy in diseases classified elsewhere, right shoulder*
     ▶ *M90.812*   *Osteopathy in diseases classified elsewhere, left shoulder*
     ▶ *M90.819*   *Osteopathy in diseases classified elsewhere, unspecified shoulder*
   ● M90.82   **Osteopathy in diseases classified elsewhere, upper arm**
     ▶ *M90.821*   *Osteopathy in diseases classified elsewhere, right upper arm*
     ▶ *M90.822*   *Osteopathy in diseases classified elsewhere, left upper arm*
     ▶ *M90.829*   *Osteopathy in diseases classified elsewhere, unspecified upper arm*
   ● M90.83   **Osteopathy in diseases classified elsewhere, forearm**
     ▶ *M90.831*   *Osteopathy in diseases classified elsewhere, right forearm*
     ▶ *M90.832*   *Osteopathy in diseases classified elsewhere, left forearm*
     ▶ *M90.839*   *Osteopathy in diseases classified elsewhere, unspecified forearm*
   ● M90.84   **Osteopathy in diseases classified elsewhere, hand**
     ▶ *M90.841*   *Osteopathy in diseases classified elsewhere, right hand*
     ▶ *M90.842*   *Osteopathy in diseases classified elsewhere, left hand*
     ▶ *M90.849*   *Osteopathy in diseases classified elsewhere, unspecified hand*
   ● M90.85   **Osteopathy in diseases classified elsewhere, thigh**
     ▶ *M90.851*   *Osteopathy in diseases classified elsewhere, right thigh*
     ▶ *M90.852*   *Osteopathy in diseases classified elsewhere, left thigh*
     ▶ *M90.859*   *Osteopathy in diseases classified elsewhere, unspecified thigh*
   ● M90.86   **Osteopathy in diseases classified elsewhere, lower leg**
     ▶ *M90.861*   *Osteopathy in diseases classified elsewhere, right lower leg*
     ▶ *M90.862*   *Osteopathy in diseases classified elsewhere, left lower leg*
     ▶ *M90.869*   *Osteopathy in diseases classified elsewhere, unspecified lower leg*
   ● M90.87   **Osteopathy in diseases classified elsewhere, ankle and foot**
     ▶ *M90.871*   *Osteopathy in diseases classified elsewhere, right ankle and foot*
     ▶ *M90.872*   *Osteopathy in diseases classified elsewhere, left ankle and foot*
     ▶ *M90.879*   *Osteopathy in diseases classified elsewhere, unspecified ankle and foot*
   ▶ *M90.88*   *Osteopathy in diseases classified elsewhere, other site*
   ▶ *M90.89*   *Osteopathy in diseases classified elsewhere, multiple sites*

CHONDROPATHIES (M91-M94)

   Excludes1   postprocedural chondropathies (M96.-)

● M91   **Juvenile osteochondrosis of hip and pelvis**
   Excludes1   slipped upper femoral epiphysis (nontraumatic) (M93.0)
   M91.0   **Juvenile osteochondrosis of pelvis**
     Osteochondrosis (juvenile) of acetabulum
     Osteochondrosis (juvenile) of iliac crest [Buchanan]
     Osteochondrosis (juvenile) of ischiopubic synchondrosis [van Neck]
     Osteochondrosis (juvenile) of symphysis pubis [Pierson]
   ● M91.1   **Juvenile osteochondrosis of head of femur [Legg-Calvé-Perthes]**
     M91.10   Juvenile osteochondrosis of head of femur [Legg-Calvé-Perthes], unspecified leg
     M91.11   Juvenile osteochondrosis of head of femur [Legg-Calvé-Perthes], right leg
     M91.12   Juvenile osteochondrosis of head of femur [Legg-Calvé-Perthes], left leg
   ● M91.2   **Coxa plana**
     Hip deformity due to previous juvenile osteochondrosis
     M91.20   Coxa plana, unspecified hip
     M91.21   Coxa plana, right hip
     M91.22   Coxa plana, left hip
   ● M91.3   **Pseudocoxalgia**
     M91.30   Pseudocoxalgia, unspecified hip
     M91.31   Pseudocoxalgia, right hip
     M91.32   Pseudocoxalgia, left hip
   ● M91.4   **Coxa magna**
     M91.40   Coxa magna, unspecified hip
     M91.41   Coxa magna, right hip
     M91.42   Coxa magna, left hip
   ● M91.8   **Other juvenile osteochondrosis of hip and pelvis**
     Juvenile osteochondrosis after reduction of congenital dislocation of hip
     M91.80   Other juvenile osteochondrosis of hip and pelvis, unspecified leg
     M91.81   Other juvenile osteochondrosis of hip and pelvis, right leg
     M91.82   Other juvenile osteochondrosis of hip and pelvis, left leg
   ● M91.9   **Juvenile osteochondrosis of hip and pelvis, unspecified**
     M91.90   Juvenile osteochondrosis of hip and pelvis, unspecified, unspecified leg
     M91.91   Juvenile osteochondrosis of hip and pelvis, unspecified, right leg
     M91.92   Juvenile osteochondrosis of hip and pelvis, unspecified, left leg

● M92   **Other juvenile osteochondrosis**
   ● M92.0   **Juvenile osteochondrosis of humerus**
     Osteochondrosis (juvenile) of capitulum of humerus [Panner]
     Osteochondrosis (juvenile) of head of humerus [Haas]
     M92.00   Juvenile osteochondrosis of humerus, unspecified arm
     M92.01   Juvenile osteochondrosis of humerus, right arm
     M92.02   Juvenile osteochondrosis of humerus, left arm
   ● M92.1   **Juvenile osteochondrosis of radius and ulna**
     Osteochondrosis (juvenile) of lower ulna [Burns]
     Osteochondrosis (juvenile) of radial head [Brailsford]
     M92.10   Juvenile osteochondrosis of radius and ulna, unspecified arm
     M92.11   Juvenile osteochondrosis of radius and ulna, right arm
     M92.12   Juvenile osteochondrosis of radius and ulna, left arm

● M92.2   Juvenile osteochondrosis, hand
   ● M92.20   Unspecified juvenile osteochondrosis, hand
     M92.201   Unspecified juvenile osteochondrosis, right hand
     M92.202   Unspecified juvenile osteochondrosis, left hand
     M92.209   Unspecified juvenile osteochondrosis, unspecified hand
   ● M92.21   Osteochondrosis (juvenile) of carpal lunate [Kienböck]
     M92.211   Osteochondrosis (juvenile) of carpal lunate [Kienböck], right hand
     M92.212   Osteochondrosis (juvenile) of carpal lunate [Kienböck], left hand
     M92.219   Osteochondrosis (juvenile) of carpal lunate [Kienböck], unspecified hand
   ● M92.22   Osteochondrosis (juvenile) of metacarpal heads [Mauclaire]
     M92.221   Osteochondrosis (juvenile) of metacarpal heads [Mauclaire], right hand
     M92.222   Osteochondrosis (juvenile) of metacarpal heads [Mauclaire], left hand
     M92.229   Osteochondrosis (juvenile) of metacarpal heads [Mauclaire], unspecified hand
   ● M92.29   Other juvenile osteochondrosis, hand
     M92.291   Other juvenile osteochondrosis, right hand
     M92.292   Other juvenile osteochondrosis, left hand
     M92.299   Other juvenile osteochondrosis, unspecified hand
● M92.3   Other juvenile osteochondrosis, upper limb
     M92.30   Other juvenile osteochondrosis, unspecified upper limb
     M92.31   Other juvenile osteochondrosis, right upper limb
     M92.32   Other juvenile osteochondrosis, left upper limb
● M92.4   Juvenile osteochondrosis of patella
     Osteochondrosis (juvenile) of primary patellar center [Köhler]
     Osteochondrosis (juvenile) of secondary patellar center [Sinding Larsen]
     M92.40   Juvenile osteochondrosis of patella, unspecified knee
     M92.41   Juvenile osteochondrosis of patella, right knee
     M92.42   Juvenile osteochondrosis of patella, left knee
● M92.5   Juvenile osteochondrosis of tibia and fibula
   ● M92.50   Unspecified juvenile osteochondrosis of tibia and fibula
     M92.501   Unspecified juvenile osteochondrosis, right leg
     M92.502   Unspecified juvenile osteochondrosis, left leg
     M92.503   Unspecified juvenile osteochondrosis, bilateral leg
     M92.509   Unspecified juvenile osteochondrosis, unspecified leg
   ● M92.51   Juvenile osteochondrosis of proximal tibia
     Blount disease
     Tibia vara
     M92.511   Juvenile osteochondrosis of proximal tibia, right leg
     M92.512   Juvenile osteochondrosis of proximal tibia, left leg

     M92.513   Juvenile osteochondrosis of proximal tibia, bilateral
     M92.519   Juvenile osteochondrosis of proximal tibia, unspecified leg
   ● M92.52   Juvenile osteochondrosis of tibia tubercle
     Osgood-Schlatter disease
     M92.521   Juvenile osteochondrosis of tibia tubercle, right leg
     M92.522   Juvenile osteochondrosis of tibia tubercle, left leg
     M92.523   Juvenile osteochondrosis of tibia tubercle, bilateral
     M92.529   Juvenile osteochondrosis of tibia tubercle, unspecified leg
     M92.59   Other juvenile osteochondrosis of tibia and fibula
     M92.591   Other juvenile osteochondrosis of tibia and fibula, right leg
     M92.592   Other juvenile osteochondrosis of tibia and fibula, left leg
     M92.593   Other juvenile osteochondrosis of tibia and fibula, bilateral
     M92.599   Other juvenile osteochondrosis of tibia and fibula, unspecified leg
● M92.6   Juvenile osteochondrosis of tarsus
     Osteochondrosis (juvenile) of calcaneum [Sever]
     Osteochondrosis (juvenile) of os tibiale externum [Haglund]
     Osteochondrosis (juvenile) of talus [Diaz]
     Osteochondrosis (juvenile) of tarsal navicular [Köhler]
     M92.60   Juvenile osteochondrosis of tarsus, unspecified ankle
     M92.61   Juvenile osteochondrosis of tarsus, right ankle
     M92.62   Juvenile osteochondrosis of tarsus, left ankle
● M92.7   Juvenile osteochondrosis of metatarsus
     Osteochondrosis (juvenile) of fifth metatarsus [Iselin]
     Osteochondrosis (juvenile) of second metatarsus [Freiberg]
     M92.70   Juvenile osteochondrosis of metatarsus, unspecified foot
     M92.71   Juvenile osteochondrosis of metatarsus, right foot
     M92.72   Juvenile osteochondrosis of metatarsus, left foot
   M92.8   Other specified juvenile osteochondrosis
     Calcaneal apophysitis
   M92.9   Juvenile osteochondrosis, unspecified
     Juvenile apophysitis NOS
     Juvenile epiphysitis NOS
     Juvenile osteochondritis NOS
     Juvenile osteochondrosis NOS
● M93   Other osteochondropathies
   Excludes2   osteochondrosis of spine (M42.-)
● M93.0   Slipped upper femoral epiphysis (nontraumatic)
     Use additional code for associated chondrolysis (M94.3)
   ● M93.00   Unspecified slipped upper femoral epiphysis (nontraumatic)
     M93.001   Unspecified slipped upper femoral epiphysis (nontraumatic), right hip
     M93.002   Unspecified slipped upper femoral epiphysis (nontraumatic), left hip
     M93.003   Unspecified slipped upper femoral epiphysis (nontraumatic), unspecified hip
   ● M93.01   Acute slipped upper femoral epiphysis (nontraumatic)
     M93.011   Acute slipped upper femoral epiphysis (nontraumatic), right hip
     M93.012   Acute slipped upper femoral epiphysis (nontraumatic), left hip
     M93.013   Acute slipped upper femoral epiphysis (nontraumatic), unspecified hip

CHAPTER 13 (M00-M99)

N   Newborn Age: 0   **P**   Pediatric Age: 0–17   **M**   Maternity DX: 9–64   **A**   Adult Age: 15–124   ♀   Females Only   ♂   Males Only

🏥 Complication\Comorbidity   🏥 Major C\C   (Ex) CC/MCC Exclusions   🏥 Hospital-Acquired Condition   🏥 Hierarchical Condition Category

1113

● M93.02   Chronic slipped upper femoral epiphysis (nontraumatic)

    M93.021   Chronic slipped upper femoral epiphysis (nontraumatic), right hip

    M93.022   Chronic slipped upper femoral epiphysis (nontraumatic), left hip

    M93.023   Chronic slipped upper femoral epiphysis (nontraumatic), unspecified hip

● M93.03   Acute on chronic slipped upper femoral epiphysis (nontraumatic)

    M93.031   Acute on chronic slipped upper femoral epiphysis (nontraumatic), right hip

    M93.032   Acute on chronic slipped upper femoral epiphysis (nontraumatic), left hip

    M93.033   Acute on chronic slipped upper femoral epiphysis (nontraumatic), unspecified hip

M93.1   Kienböck's disease of adults   A
    Adult osteochondrosis of carpal lunates

● M93.2   Osteochondritis dissecans

  M93.20   Osteochondritis dissecans of unspecified site

● M93.21   Osteochondritis dissecans of shoulder

    M93.211   Osteochondritis dissecans, right shoulder

    M93.212   Osteochondritis dissecans, left shoulder

    M93.219   Osteochondritis dissecans, unspecified shoulder

● M93.22   Osteochondritis dissecans of elbow

    M93.221   Osteochondritis dissecans, right elbow

    M93.222   Osteochondritis dissecans, left elbow

    M93.229   Osteochondritis dissecans, unspecified elbow

● M93.23   Osteochondritis dissecans of wrist

    M93.231   Osteochondritis dissecans, right wrist

    M93.232   Osteochondritis dissecans, left wrist

    M93.239   Osteochondritis dissecans, unspecified wrist

● M93.24   Osteochondritis dissecans of joints of hand

    M93.241   Osteochondritis dissecans, joints of right hand

    M93.242   Osteochondritis dissecans, joints of left hand

    M93.249   Osteochondritis dissecans, joints of unspecified hand

● M93.25   Osteochondritis dissecans of hip

    M93.251   Osteochondritis dissecans, right hip

    M93.252   Osteochondritis dissecans, left hip

    M93.259   Osteochondritis dissecans, unspecified hip

● M93.26   Osteochondritis dissecans knee

    M93.261   Osteochondritis dissecans, right knee

    M93.262   Osteochondritis dissecans, left knee

    M93.269   Osteochondritis dissecans, unspecified knee

● M93.27   Osteochondritis dissecans of ankle and joints of foot

    M93.271   Osteochondritis dissecans, right ankle and joints of right foot

    M93.272   Osteochondritis dissecans, left ankle and joints of left foot

    M93.279   Osteochondritis dissecans, unspecified ankle and joints of foot

  M93.28   Osteochondritis dissecans other site

  M93.29   Osteochondritis dissecans multiple sites

● M93.8   Other specified osteochondropathies

  M93.80   Other specified osteochondropathies of unspecified site

● M93.81   Other specified osteochondropathies of shoulder

    M93.811   Other specified osteochondropathies, right shoulder

    M93.812   Other specified osteochondropathies, left shoulder

    M93.819   Other specified osteochondropathies, unspecified shoulder

● M93.82   Other specified osteochondropathies of upper arm

    M93.821   Other specified osteochondropathies, right upper arm

    M93.822   Other specified osteochondropathies, left upper arm

    M93.829   Other specified osteochondropathies, unspecified upper arm

● M93.83   Other specified osteochondropathies of forearm

    M93.831   Other specified osteochondropathies, right forearm

    M93.832   Other specified osteochondropathies, left forearm

    M93.839   Other specified osteochondropathies, unspecified forearm

● M93.84   Other specified osteochondropathies of hand

    M93.841   Other specified osteochondropathies, right hand

    M93.842   Other specified osteochondropathies, left hand

    M93.849   Other specified osteochondropathies, unspecified hand

● M93.85   Other specified osteochondropathies of thigh

    M93.851   Other specified osteochondropathies, right thigh

    M93.852   Other specified osteochondropathies, left thigh

    M93.859   Other specified osteochondropathies, unspecified thigh

● M93.86   Other specified osteochondropathies lower leg

    M93.861   Other specified osteochondropathies, right lower leg

    M93.862   Other specified osteochondropathies, left lower leg

    M93.869   Other specified osteochondropathies, unspecified lower leg

● M93.87   Other specified osteochondropathies of ankle and foot

    M93.871   Other specified osteochondropathies, right ankle and foot

    M93.872   Other specified osteochondropathies, left ankle and foot

    M93.879   Other specified osteochondropathies, unspecified ankle and foot

  M93.88   Other specified osteochondropathies other

  M93.89   Other specified osteochondropathies multiple sites

M93.9   Osteochondropathy, unspecified
    Apophysitis NOS
    Epiphysitis NOS
    Osteochondritis NOS
    Osteochondrosis NOS

  M93.90   Osteochondropathy, unspecified of unspecified site

● M93.91   Osteochondropathy, unspecified of shoulder

    M93.911   Osteochondropathy, unspecified, right shoulder

    M93.912   Osteochondropathy, unspecified, left shoulder

    M93.919   Osteochondropathy, unspecified, unspecified shoulder

▶ New   ⇒ Revised   ~~deleted~~ Deleted   Excludes 1   Excludes 2   Includes   Use additional   Code first   Code also   Key words
OGCR Official Guidelines   ● Unacceptable Principal Diagnosis   X Assign placeholder X   ● Use Additional Character(s)   ▶ Manifestation Code   Coding Clinic

● M93.92   Osteochondropathy, unspecified of upper arm
    M93.921   Osteochondropathy, unspecified, right upper arm
    M93.922   Osteochondropathy, unspecified, left upper arm
    M93.929   Osteochondropathy, unspecified, unspecified upper arm

● M93.93   Osteochondropathy, unspecified of forearm
    M93.931   Osteochondropathy, unspecified, right forearm
    M93.932   Osteochondropathy, unspecified, left forearm
    M93.939   Osteochondropathy, unspecified, unspecified forearm

● M93.94   Osteochondropathy, unspecified of hand
    M93.941   Osteochondropathy, unspecified, right hand
    M93.942   Osteochondropathy, unspecified, left hand
    M93.949   Osteochondropathy, unspecified, unspecified hand

● M93.95   Osteochondropathy, unspecified of thigh
    M93.951   Osteochondropathy, unspecified, right thigh
    M93.952   Osteochondropathy, unspecified, left thigh
    M93.959   Osteochondropathy, unspecified, unspecified thigh

● M93.96   Osteochondropathy, unspecified lower leg
    M93.961   Osteochondropathy, unspecified, right lower leg
    M93.962   Osteochondropathy, unspecified, left lower leg
    M93.969   Osteochondropathy, unspecified, unspecified lower leg

● M93.97   Osteochondropathy, unspecified of ankle and foot
    M93.971   Osteochondropathy, unspecified, right ankle and foot
    M93.972   Osteochondropathy, unspecified, left ankle and foot
    M93.979   Osteochondropathy, unspecified, unspecified ankle and foot

    M93.98   Osteochondropathy, unspecified other
    M93.99   Osteochondropathy, unspecified multiple sites

● M94   Other disorders of cartilage
    M94.0   Chondrocostal junction syndrome [Tietze]
       Costochondritis

    M94.1   Relapsing polychondritis

● M94.2   Chondromalacia
       Excludes1   chondromalacia patellae (M22.4)
    M94.20   Chondromalacia, unspecified site
● M94.21   Chondromalacia, shoulder
    M94.211   Chondromalacia, right shoulder
    M94.212   Chondromalacia, left shoulder
    M94.219   Chondromalacia, unspecified shoulder
● M94.22   Chondromalacia, elbow
    M94.221   Chondromalacia, right elbow
    M94.222   Chondromalacia, left elbow
    M94.229   Chondromalacia, unspecified elbow
● M94.23   Chondromalacia, wrist
    M94.231   Chondromalacia, right wrist
    M94.232   Chondromalacia, left wrist
    M94.239   Chondromalacia, unspecified wrist
● M94.24   Chondromalacia, joints of hand
    M94.241   Chondromalacia, joints of right hand
    M94.242   Chondromalacia, joints of left hand
    M94.249   Chondromalacia, joints of unspecified hand

● M94.25   Chondromalacia, hip
    M94.251   Chondromalacia, right hip
    M94.252   Chondromalacia, left hip
    M94.259   Chondromalacia, unspecified hip
● M94.26   Chondromalacia, knee
    M94.261   Chondromalacia, right knee
    M94.262   Chondromalacia, left knee
    M94.269   Chondromalacia, unspecified knee
● M94.27   Chondromalacia, ankle and joints of foot
    M94.271   Chondromalacia, right ankle and joints of right foot
    M94.272   Chondromalacia, left ankle and joints of left foot
    M94.279   Chondromalacia, unspecified ankle and joints of foot

    M94.28   Chondromalacia, other site
    M94.29   Chondromalacia, multiple sites

● M94.3   Chondrolysis
    Code first any associated slipped upper femoral epiphysis (nontraumatic) (M93.0-)
● M94.35   Chondrolysis, hip
    M94.351   Chondrolysis, right hip
    M94.352   Chondrolysis, left hip
    M94.359   Chondrolysis, unspecified hip

● M94.8   Other specified disorders of cartilage
● M94.8X   Other specified disorders of cartilage
    M94.8X0   Other specified disorders of cartilage, multiple sites
    M94.8X1   Other specified disorders of cartilage, shoulder
    M94.8X2   Other specified disorders of cartilage, upper arm
    M94.8X3   Other specified disorders of cartilage, forearm
    M94.8X4   Other specified disorders of cartilage, hand
    M94.8X5   Other specified disorders of cartilage, thigh
    M94.8X6   Other specified disorders of cartilage, lower leg
    M94.8X7   Other specified disorders of cartilage, ankle and foot
    M94.8X8   Other specified disorders of cartilage, other site
    M94.8X9   Other specified disorders of cartilage, unspecified sites

    M94.9   Disorder of cartilage, unspecified

OTHER DISORDERS OF THE MUSCULOSKELETAL SYSTEM AND CONNECTIVE TISSUE (M95)

● M95   Other acquired deformities of musculoskeletal system and connective tissue
       Excludes2   acquired absence of limbs and organs (Z89-Z90)
                acquired deformities of limbs (M20-M21)
                congenital malformations and deformations of the musculoskeletal system (Q65-Q79)
                deforming dorsopathies (M40-M43)
                dentofacial anomalies [including malocclusion] (M26.-)
                postprocedural musculoskeletal disorders (M96.-)
    M95.0   Acquired deformity of nose
       Excludes2   deviated nasal septum (J34.2)
● M95.1   Cauliflower ear
       Excludes2   other acquired deformities of ear (H61.1)
    M95.10   Cauliflower ear, unspecified ear
    M95.11   Cauliflower ear, right ear
    M95.12   Cauliflower ear, left ear

CHAPTER 13 (M00-M99)

N Newborn Age: 0   **P** Pediatric Age: 0–17   **M** Maternity DX: 9–64   **A** Adult Age: 15–124   ♀ Females Only   ♂ Males Only

🅺 Complication\Comorbidity   🅺 Major C\C   (Ex) CC/MCC Exclusions   🅺 Hospital-Acquired Condition   🅺 Hierarchical Condition Category

1115

M95.2 Other acquired deformity of head

M95.3 Acquired deformity of neck

M95.4 Acquired deformity of chest and rib

M95.5 Acquired deformity of pelvis

> **Excludes1**   maternal care for known or suspected disproportion (O33.-)

M95.8 Other specified acquired deformities of musculoskeletal system

M95.9 Acquired deformity of musculoskeletal system, unspecified

---

INTRAOPERATIVE AND POSTPROCEDURAL COMPLICATIONS AND DISORDERS OF MUSCULOSKELETAL SYSTEM, NOT ELSEWHERE CLASSIFIED (M96)

● **M96** Intraoperative and postprocedural complications and disorders of musculoskeletal system, not elsewhere classified

> **Excludes2**   arthropathy following intestinal bypass (M02.0-)
> complications of internal orthopedic prosthetic devices, implants and grafts (T84.-)
> disorders associated with osteoporosis (M80)
> periprosthetic fracture around internal prosthetic joint (M97.-)
> presence of functional implants and other devices (Z96-Z97)

M96.0 Pseudarthrosis after fusion or arthrodesis 🔍

> (Ex:) See PDX Collection 3233

M96.1 Postlaminectomy syndrome, not elsewhere classified

M96.2 Postradiation kyphosis

M96.3 Postlaminectomy kyphosis

M96.4 Postsurgical lordosis

M96.5 Postradiation scoliosis

● **M96.6** Fracture of bone following insertion of orthopedic implant, joint prosthesis, or bone plate

> Intraoperative fracture of bone during insertion of orthopedic implant, joint prosthesis, or bone plate
>
> **Excludes2**   complication of internal orthopedic devices, implants or grafts (T84.-)
>
> (Ex:) For category M96.6 CC codes: See PDX Collection 911

    ● **M96.62** Fracture of humerus following insertion of orthopedic implant, joint prosthesis, or bone plate

        M96.621 Fracture of humerus following insertion of orthopedic implant, joint prosthesis, or bone plate, right arm 🔍🔍

        M96.622 Fracture of humerus following insertion of orthopedic implant, joint prosthesis, or bone plate, left arm 🔍🔍

        M96.629 Fracture of humerus following insertion of orthopedic implant, joint prosthesis, or bone plate, unspecified arm 🔍🔍

    ● **M96.63** Fracture of radius or ulna following insertion of orthopedic implant, joint prosthesis, or bone plate

        M96.631 Fracture of radius or ulna following insertion of orthopedic implant, joint prosthesis, or bone plate, right arm 🔍🔍

        M96.632 Fracture of radius or ulna following insertion of orthopedic implant, joint prosthesis, or bone plate, left arm 🔍🔍

        M96.639 Fracture of radius or ulna following insertion of orthopedic implant, joint prosthesis, or bone plate, unspecified arm 🔍🔍

    M96.65 Fracture of pelvis following insertion of orthopedic implant, joint prosthesis, or bone plate 🔍🔍

● **M96.66** Fracture of femur following insertion of orthopedic implant, joint prosthesis, or bone plate

    M96.661 Fracture of femur following insertion of orthopedic implant, joint prosthesis, or bone plate, right leg 🔍🔍

    M96.662 Fracture of femur following insertion of orthopedic implant, joint prosthesis, or bone plate, left leg 🔍🔍

    M96.669 Fracture of femur following insertion of orthopedic implant, joint prosthesis, or bone plate, unspecified leg 🔍🔍

● **M96.67** Fracture of tibia or fibula following insertion of orthopedic implant, joint prosthesis, or bone plate

    M96.671 Fracture of tibia or fibula following insertion of orthopedic implant, joint prosthesis, or bone plate, right leg 🔍🔍

    M96.672 Fracture of tibia or fibula following insertion of orthopedic implant, joint prosthesis, or bone plate, left leg 🔍🔍

    M96.679 Fracture of tibia or fibula following insertion of orthopedic implant, joint prosthesis, or bone plate, unspecified leg 🔍🔍

    M96.69 Fracture of other bone following insertion of orthopedic implant, joint prosthesis, or bone plate 🔍🔍

● **M96.8** Other intraoperative and postprocedural complications and disorders of musculoskeletal system, not elsewhere classified

> Coding Clinic: 2016, Q4, P10

● **M96.81** Intraoperative hemorrhage and hematoma of a musculoskeletal structure complicating a procedure

> **Excludes1**   intraoperative hemorrhage and hematoma of a musculoskeletal structure due to accidental puncture and laceration during a procedure (M96.82-)
>
> (Ex:) For category M96.81 CC codes: See PDX Collection 912

    M96.810 Intraoperative hemorrhage and hematoma of a musculoskeletal structure complicating a musculoskeletal system procedure 🔍

    M96.811 Intraoperative hemorrhage and hematoma of a musculoskeletal structure complicating other procedure 🔍

● **M96.82** Accidental puncture and laceration of a musculoskeletal structure during a procedure

> (Ex:) For category M96.82 CC codes: See PDX Collection 509

    M96.820 Accidental puncture and laceration of a musculoskeletal structure during a musculoskeletal system procedure 🔍

    M96.821 Accidental puncture and laceration of a musculoskeletal structure during other procedure 🔍

● **M96.83** Postprocedural hemorrhage of a musculoskeletal structure following a procedure

> (Ex:) For category M96.83 CC codes: See PDX Collection 912

    M96.830 Postprocedural hemorrhage of a musculoskeletal structure following a musculoskeletal system procedure 🔍

    M96.831 Postprocedural hemorrhage of a musculoskeletal structure following other procedure 🔍

▶ New   ⇒ Revised   ~~deleted~~ Deleted   Excludes 1   Excludes 2   Includes   Use additional   Code first   Code also   Key words

OGCR Official Guidelines   ● Unacceptable Principal Diagnosis   X Assign placeholder X   ● Use Additional Character(s)   ▶ Manifestation Code   **Coding Clinic**

● M96.84 **Postprocedural hematoma and seroma** of a musculoskeletal structure following a procedure
     (Ex:) For category M96.84 CC codes: See PDX Collection 912

     M96.840 **Postprocedural hematoma** of a musculoskeletal structure following a **musculoskeletal system procedure** 🔹

     M96.841 **Postprocedural hematoma** of a musculoskeletal structure following **other procedure** 🔹
         Coding Clinic: 2016, Q4, P10

     M96.842 **Postprocedural seroma** of a musculoskeletal structure following a **musculoskeletal system procedure** 🔹

     M96.843 **Postprocedural seroma** of a musculoskeletal structure following **other procedure** 🔹

M96.89 **Other intraoperative and postprocedural complications and disorders of the musculoskeletal system** 🔹
     Instability of joint secondary to removal of joint prosthesis
     Use additional code, if applicable, to further specify disorder
     (Ex:) See PDX Collection 643
     Coding Clinic: 2021, Q1, P5

PERIPROSTHETIC FRACTURE AROUND INTERNAL PROSTHETIC JOINT (M97)

● M97 **Periprosthetic fracture around internal prosthetic joint**
     Excludes2   fracture of bone following insertion of orthopedic implant, joint prosthesis or bone plate (M96.6-)
         breakage (fracture) of prosthetic joint (T84.01-)
     Coding Clinic: 2016, Q4, P42

The appropriate 7th character is to be added to each code from category M97:

A	initial encounter
D	subsequent encounter
S	sequela

     (Ex:) For category M97 CC codes: See PDX Collection 911

● M97.0 **Periprosthetic fracture around internal prosthetic hip joint**
   X ● M97.01 **Periprosthetic fracture around internal prosthetic right hip joint** A 🔹🔹
       Coding Clinic: 2016, Q4, P43

   X ● M97.02 **Periprosthetic fracture around internal prosthetic left hip joint** A 🔹🔹

● M97.1 **Periprosthetic fracture around internal prosthetic knee joint**
   X ● M97.11 **Periprosthetic fracture around internal prosthetic right knee joint** A 🔹

   X ● M97.12 **Periprosthetic fracture around internal prosthetic left knee joint** A 🔹

● M97.2 **Periprosthetic fracture around internal prosthetic ankle joint**
   X ● M97.21 **Periprosthetic fracture around internal prosthetic right ankle joint** A 🔹

   X ● M97.22 **Periprosthetic fracture around internal prosthetic left ankle joint** A 🔹

● M97.3 **Periprosthetic fracture around internal prosthetic shoulder joint**
   X ● M97.31 **Periprosthetic fracture around internal prosthetic right shoulder joint** A 🔹

   X ● M97.32 **Periprosthetic fracture around internal prosthetic left shoulder joint** A 🔹

● M97.4 **Periprosthetic fracture around internal prosthetic elbow joint**
   X ● M97.41 **Periprosthetic fracture around internal prosthetic right elbow joint** A 🔹

   X ● M97.42 **Periprosthetic fracture around internal prosthetic left elbow joint** A 🔹

X ● M97.8 **Periprosthetic fracture around other internal prosthetic joint** A 🔹
     Periprosthetic fracture around internal prosthetic finger joint
     Periprosthetic fracture around internal prosthetic spinal joint
     Periprosthetic fracture around internal prosthetic toe joint
     Periprosthetic fracture around internal prosthetic wrist joint
     Use additional code to identify the joint (Z96.6-)

X ● M97.9 **Periprosthetic fracture around unspecified internal prosthetic joint** A 🔹

BIOMECHANICAL LESIONS, NOT ELSEWHERE CLASSIFIED (M99)

● M99 **Biomechanical lesions, not elsewhere classified**
     Note: This category should not be used if the condition can be classified elsewhere.

● M99.0 **Segmental and somatic dysfunction**
     M99.00 **Segmental and somatic dysfunction of head region**

     M99.01 **Segmental and somatic dysfunction of cervical region**

     M99.02 **Segmental and somatic dysfunction of thoracic region**

     M99.03 **Segmental and somatic dysfunction of lumbar region**

     M99.04 **Segmental and somatic dysfunction of sacral region**

     M99.05 **Segmental and somatic dysfunction of pelvic region**

     M99.06 **Segmental and somatic dysfunction of lower extremity**

     M99.07 **Segmental and somatic dysfunction of upper extremity**

     M99.08 **Segmental and somatic dysfunction of rib cage**

     M99.09 **Segmental and somatic dysfunction of abdomen and other regions**

● M99.1 **Subluxation complex (vertebral)**
     M99.10 **Subluxation complex (vertebral) of head region** 🔹🔹
        (Ex:) See PDX Collection 913

     M99.11 **Subluxation complex (vertebral) of cervical region** 🔹🔹
        (Ex:) See PDX Collection 913

     M99.12 **Subluxation complex (vertebral) of thoracic region**

     M99.13 **Subluxation complex (vertebral) of lumbar region**

     M99.14 **Subluxation complex (vertebral) of sacral region**

     M99.15 **Subluxation complex (vertebral) of pelvic region**

     M99.16 **Subluxation complex (vertebral) of lower extremity**

     M99.17 **Subluxation complex (vertebral) of upper extremity**

     M99.18 **Subluxation complex (vertebral) of rib cage** 🔹🔹
        (Ex:) See PDX Collection 914

     M99.19 **Subluxation complex (vertebral) of abdomen and other regions**

N   Newborn Age: 0   **P**   Pediatric Age: 0–17   **M**   Maternity DX: 9–64   **A**   Adult Age: 15–124   ♀   Females Only   ♂   Males Only
🔹   Complication\Comorbidity   🔹   Major C\C   (Ex:)   CC/MCC Exclusions   🔹   Hospital-Acquired Condition   🔹   Hierarchical Condition Category

1117

● **M99.2　Subluxation stenosis of neural canal**

M99.2Ø　Subluxation stenosis of neural canal of head region

M99.21　Subluxation stenosis of neural canal of cervical region

M99.22　Subluxation stenosis of neural canal of thoracic region

M99.23　Subluxation stenosis of neural canal of lumbar region

M99.24　Subluxation stenosis of neural canal of sacral region

M99.25　Subluxation stenosis of neural canal of pelvic region

M99.26　Subluxation stenosis of neural canal of lower extremity

M99.27　Subluxation stenosis of neural canal of upper extremity

M99.28　Subluxation stenosis of neural canal of rib cage

M99.29　Subluxation stenosis of neural canal of abdomen and other regions

● **M99.3　Osseous stenosis of neural canal**

M99.3Ø　Osseous stenosis of neural canal of head region

M99.31　Osseous stenosis of neural canal of cervical region

M99.32　Osseous stenosis of neural canal of thoracic region

M99.33　Osseous stenosis of neural canal of lumbar region

M99.34　Osseous stenosis of neural canal of sacral region

M99.35　Osseous stenosis of neural canal of pelvic region

M99.36　Osseous stenosis of neural canal of lower extremity

M99.37　Osseous stenosis of neural canal of upper extremity

M99.38　Osseous stenosis of neural canal of rib cage

M99.39　Osseous stenosis of neural canal of abdomen and other regions

● **M99.4　Connective tissue stenosis of neural canal**

M99.4Ø　Connective tissue stenosis of neural canal of head region

M99.41　Connective tissue stenosis of neural canal of cervical region

M99.42　Connective tissue stenosis of neural canal of thoracic region

M99.43　Connective tissue stenosis of neural canal of lumbar region

M99.44　Connective tissue stenosis of neural canal of sacral region

M99.45　Connective tissue stenosis of neural canal of pelvic region

M99.46　Connective tissue stenosis of neural canal of lower extremity

M99.47　Connective tissue stenosis of neural canal of upper extremity

M99.48　Connective tissue stenosis of neural canal of rib cage

M99.49　Connective tissue stenosis of neural canal of abdomen and other regions

● **M99.5　Intervertebral disc stenosis of neural canal**

M99.5Ø　Intervertebral disc stenosis of neural canal of head region

M99.51　Intervertebral disc stenosis of neural canal of cervical region

M99.52　Intervertebral disc stenosis of neural canal of thoracic region

M99.53　Intervertebral disc stenosis of neural canal of lumbar region

M99.54　Intervertebral disc stenosis of neural canal of sacral region

M99.55　Intervertebral disc stenosis of neural canal of pelvic region

M99.56　Intervertebral disc stenosis of neural canal of lower extremity

M99.57　Intervertebral disc stenosis of neural canal of upper extremity

M99.58　Intervertebral disc stenosis of neural canal of rib cage

M99.59　Intervertebral disc stenosis of neural canal of abdomen and other regions

● **M99.6　Osseous and subluxation stenosis of intervertebral foramina**

M99.6Ø　Osseous and subluxation stenosis of intervertebral foramina of head region

M99.61　Osseous and subluxation stenosis of intervertebral foramina of cervical region

M99.62　Osseous and subluxation stenosis of intervertebral foramina of thoracic region

M99.63　Osseous and subluxation stenosis of intervertebral foramina of lumbar region

M99.64　Osseous and subluxation stenosis of intervertebral foramina of sacral region

M99.65　Osseous and subluxation stenosis of intervertebral foramina of pelvic region

M99.66　Osseous and subluxation stenosis of intervertebral foramina of lower extremity

M99.67　Osseous and subluxation stenosis of intervertebral foramina of upper extremity

M99.68　Osseous and subluxation stenosis of intervertebral foramina of rib cage

M99.69　Osseous and subluxation stenosis of intervertebral foramina of abdomen and other regions

● **M99.7　Connective tissue and disc stenosis of intervertebral foramina**

M99.7Ø　Connective tissue and disc stenosis of intervertebral foramina of head region

M99.71　Connective tissue and disc stenosis of intervertebral foramina of cervical region

M99.72　Connective tissue and disc stenosis of intervertebral foramina of thoracic region

M99.73　Connective tissue and disc stenosis of intervertebral foramina of lumbar region

M99.74　Connective tissue and disc stenosis of intervertebral foramina of sacral region

M99.75　Connective tissue and disc stenosis of intervertebral foramina of pelvic region

M99.76　Connective tissue and disc stenosis of intervertebral foramina of lower extremity

M99.77　Connective tissue and disc stenosis of intervertebral foramina of upper extremity

M99.78　Connective tissue and disc stenosis of intervertebral foramina of rib cage

M99.79　Connective tissue and disc stenosis of intervertebral foramina of abdomen and other regions

● **M99.8　Other biomechanical lesions**

M99.8Ø　Other biomechanical lesions of head region

M99.81　Other biomechanical lesions of cervical region

M99.82　Other biomechanical lesions of thoracic region

M99.83　Other biomechanical lesions of lumbar region

M99.84　Other biomechanical lesions of sacral region

M99.85　Other biomechanical lesions of pelvic region

M99.86　Other biomechanical lesions of lower extremity

M99.87　Other biomechanical lesions of upper extremity

M99.88　Other biomechanical lesions of rib cage

M99.89　Other biomechanical lesions of abdomen and other regions

M99.9　Biomechanical lesion, unspecified

▶ New　⇒ Revised　deleted Deleted　Excludes 1　Excludes 2　Includes　Use additional　Code first　Code also　Key words

1118　OGCR Official Guidelines　● Unacceptable Principal Diagnosis　X Assign placeholder X　● Use Additional Character(s)　▶ Manifestation Code　Coding Clinic

CHAPTER 14

DISEASES OF THE GENITOURINARY SYSTEM (N00-N99)

OGCR Chapter-Specific Coding Guidelines

14. Chapter 14: Diseases of Genitourinary System (N00-N99)

   a. **Chronic kidney disease**

     1) Stages of chronic kidney disease (CKD)
The ICD-10-CM classifies CKD based on severity. The severity of CKD is designated by stages 1-5. Stage 2, code N18.2, equates to mild CKD; stage 3, code N18.3, equates to moderate CKD; and stage 4, code N18.4, equates to severe CKD. Code N18.6, End stage renal disease (ESRD), is assigned when the provider has documented end-stage-renal disease (ESRD).

     If both a stage of CKD and ESRD are documented, assign code N18.6 only.

     2) Chronic kidney disease and kidney transplant status
Patients who have undergone kidney transplant may still have some form of chronic kidney disease CKD because the kidney transplant may not fully restore kidney function. Therefore, the presence of CKD alone does not constitute a transplant complication. Assign the appropriate N18 code for the patient's stage of CKD and code Z94.0, Kidney transplant status. If a transplant complication such as failure or rejection or other transplant complication is documented, see Section I.C.19.g for information on coding complications of a kidney transplant. If the documentation is unclear as to whether the patient has a complication of the transplant, query the provider.

     3) Chronic kidney disease with other conditions
Patients with CKD may also suffer from other serious conditions, most commonly diabetes mellitus and hypertension. The sequencing of the CKD code in relationship to codes for other contributing conditions is based on the conventions in the Tabular List.

       See I.C.9. Hypertensive chronic kidney disease.
       See I.C.19. Chronic kidney disease and kidney transplant complications.

Item 14–1 Nephritis (inflammation) or **nephropathy** (disease) **with lesion of proliferative glomerulonephritis** results from a streptococcal infection.

Nephritis (inflammation) or **nephropathy** (disease) **with lesion of membranous glomerulonephritis** is characterized by deposits along the epithelial side of the basement membrane.

Nephritis (inflammation) or **nephropathy** (disease) **with lesion of membranoproliferative glomerulonephritis** is characterized by alterations in the basement membranes of the kidney and the glomerular cells.

Nephritis (inflammation) or **nephropathy** (disease) **with lesion of rapidly progressive glomerulonephritis** is characterized by rapid and progressive decline in renal function.

Nephritis (inflammation) or **nephropathy** (disease) **with lesion of renal cortical necrosis** is characterized by death of the cortical tissues.

Nephritis (inflammation) or **nephropathy** (disease) **with lesion of renal medullary necrosis** is characterized by death of the tissues that collect urine.

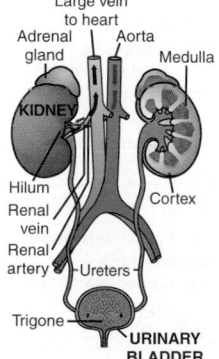

Figure 14-1   Kidneys within the urinary system.

Item 14–2 Glomerulonephritis is nephritis accompanied by inflammation of the glomeruli of the kidney, resulting in the degeneration of the glomeruli and the nephrons.

   Acute glomerulonephritis primarily affects children and young adults and is usually a result of a streptococcal infection.

   Proliferative glomerulonephritis is the acute form of the disease resulting from a streptococcal infection.

   Rapidly progressive glomerulonephritis, also known as **crescentic** or **malignant glomerulonephritis**, is the acute form of the disease, which leads quickly to rapid and progressive decline in renal function.

CHAPTER 14

DISEASES OF THE GENITOURINARY SYSTEM (N00-N99)

   Excludes2   certain conditions originating in the perinatal period (P04-P96)

              certain infectious and parasitic diseases (A00-B99)

              complications of pregnancy, childbirth and the puerperium (O00-O9A)

              congenital malformations, deformations and chromosomal abnormalities (Q00-Q99)

              endocrine, nutritional and metabolic diseases (E00-E88)

              injury, poisoning and certain other consequences of external causes (S00-T88)

              neoplasms (C00-D49)

              symptoms, signs and abnormal clinical and laboratory findings, not elsewhere classified (R00-R94)

   This chapter contains the following blocks:

N00-N08	Glomerular diseases
N10-N16	Renal tubulo-interstitial diseases
N17-N19	Acute kidney failure and chronic kidney disease
N20-N23	Urolithiasis
N25-N29	Other disorders of kidney and ureter
N30-N39	Other diseases of the urinary system
N40-N53	Diseases of male genital organs
N60-N65	Disorders of breast
N70-N77	Inflammatory diseases of female pelvic organs
N80-N98	Noninflammatory disorders of female genital tract
N99	Intraoperative and postprocedural complications and disorders of genitourinary system, not elsewhere classified

GLOMERULAR DISEASES (N00-N08)

   Code also any associated kidney failure (N17-N19)

   Excludes1   hypertensive chronic kidney disease (I12.-)

● **N00** **Acute nephritic syndrome**

   Includes   acute glomerular disease
                acute glomerulonephritis
                acute nephritis

   Excludes1   acute tubulo-interstitial nephritis (N10)
                nephritic syndrome NOS (N05.-)

   (Ex) **For category N00 CC codes unless otherwise indicated:** See PDX Collection 915

   N00.0 **Acute nephritic syndrome with minor glomerular abnormality**
        Acute nephritic syndrome with minimal change lesion

   N00.1 **Acute nephritic syndrome with focal and segmental glomerular lesions**
        Acute nephritic syndrome with focal and segmental hyalinosis
        Acute nephritic syndrome with focal and segmental sclerosis
        Acute nephritic syndrome with focal glomerulonephritis

   N00.2 **Acute nephritic syndrome with diffuse membranous glomerulonephritis**

   N00.3 **Acute nephritic syndrome with diffuse mesangial proliferative glomerulonephritis**

   N00.4 **Acute nephritic syndrome with diffuse endocapillary proliferative glomerulonephritis**

N Newborn Age: 0	**P** Pediatric Age: 0–17	**M** Maternity DX: 9–64	**A** Adult Age: 15–124	♀ Females Only	♂ Males Only

🔹 Complication\Comorbidity   🔹 Major C\C   (Ex) CC/MCC Exclusions   🔹 Hospital-Acquired Condition   🔹 Hierarchical Condition Category   **1119**

CHAPTER 14 (N00–N99)

N00.5   **Acute nephritic syndrome with** diffuse mesangiocapillary glomerulonephritis 🔖
     Acute nephritic syndrome with membranoproliferative glomerulonephritis, types 1 and 3, or NOS

     Excludes1   Acute nephritic syndrome with C3 glomerulonephritis (N00.A)
                Acute nephritic syndrome with C3 glomerulopathy (N00.A)

N00.6   **Acute nephritic syndrome with** dense deposit disease 🔖
     Acute nephritic syndrome with C3 glomerulopathy with dense deposit disease
     Acute nephritic syndrome with membranoproliferative glomerulonephritis, type 2

N00.7   **Acute nephritic syndrome with** diffuse crescentic glomerulonephritis 🔖
     Acute nephritic syndrome with extracapillary glomerulonephritis

N00.8   **Acute nephritic syndrome with** other morphologic changes 🔖
     Acute nephritic syndrome with proliferative glomerulonephritis NOS
     (Ex:) See PDX Collection 916

N00.9   **Acute nephritic syndrome with** unspecified morphologic changes 🔖

N00.A   **Acute nephritic syndrome with C3 glomerulonephritis** 🔖
     Acute nephritic syndrome with C3 glomerulopathy, NOS

     Excludes1   Acute nephritic syndrome (with C3 glomerulopathy) with dense deposit disease(N00.6)
     (Ex:) See PDX Collection 4069

● **N01**   **Rapidly progressive nephritic syndrome**
     Includes   rapidly progressive glomerular disease
                 rapidly progressive glomerulonephritis
                 rapidly progressive nephritis

     Excludes1   nephritic syndrome NOS (N05.-)
     (Ex:) **For category N01 CC codes:** See PDX Collection 915

N01.0   **Rapidly progressive nephritic syndrome with** minor glomerular abnormality 🔖
     Rapidly progressive nephritic syndrome with minimal change lesion

N01.1   **Rapidly progressive nephritic syndrome with** focal and segmental glomerular lesions 🔖
     Rapidly progressive nephritic syndrome with focal and segmental hyalinosis
     Rapidly progressive nephritic syndrome with focal and segmental sclerosis
     Rapidly progressive nephritic syndrome with focal glomerulonephritis

N01.2   **Rapidly progressive nephritic syndrome with** diffuse membranous glomerulonephritis 🔖

N01.3   **Rapidly progressive nephritic syndrome with** diffuse mesangial proliferative glomerulonephritis 🔖

N01.4   **Rapidly progressive nephritic syndrome with** diffuse endocapillary proliferative glomerulonephritis 🔖

N01.5   **Rapidly progressive nephritic syndrome with** diffuse mesangiocapillary glomerulonephritis 🔖
     Rapidly progressive nephritic syndrome with membranoproliferative glomerulonephritis, types 1 and 3, or NOS

     Excludes1   Rapidly progressive nephritic syndrome with C3 glomerulonephritis (N01.A)
                Rapidly progressive nephritic syndrome with C3 glomerulopathy (N01.A)

N01.6   **Rapidly progressive nephritic syndrome with** dense deposit disease 🔖
     Rapidly progressive nephritic syndrome with C3 glomerulopathy with dense deposit disease
     Rapidly progressive nephritic syndrome with membranoproliferative glomerulonephritis, type 2

N01.7   **Rapidly progressive nephritic syndrome with** diffuse crescentic glomerulonephritis 🔖
     Rapidly progressive nephritic syndrome with extracapillary glomerulonephritis

N01.8   **Rapidly progressive nephritic syndrome with** other morphologic changes 🔖
     Rapidly progressive nephritic syndrome with proliferative glomerulonephritis NOS

N01.9   **Rapidly progressive nephritic syndrome with** unspecified morphologic changes 🔖

N01.A   **Rapidly progressive nephritic syndrome with C3 glomerulonephritis** 🔖
     Rapidly progressive nephritic syndrome with C3 glomerulopathy, NOS

     Excludes1   Rapidly progressive nephritic syndrome (with C3 glomerulopathy) with dense deposit disease (N01.6)
     (Ex:) See PDX Collection 4070

● **N02**   **Recurrent and persistent hematuria**
     Excludes1   acute cystitis with hematuria (N30.01)
                hematuria NOS (R31.9)
                hematuria not associated with specified morphologic lesions (R31.-)
     (Ex:) **For category N02 CC codes unless otherwise indicated:** See PDX Collection 917

N02.0   **Recurrent and persistent hematuria with** minor glomerular abnormality 🔖
     Recurrent and persistent hematuria with minimal change lesion

N02.1   **Recurrent and persistent hematuria with** focal and segmental glomerular lesions 🔖
     Recurrent and persistent hematuria with focal and segmental hyalinosis
     Recurrent and persistent hematuria with focal and segmental sclerosis
     Recurrent and persistent hematuria with focal glomerulonephritis

N02.2   **Recurrent and persistent hematuria with** diffuse membranous glomerulonephritis 🔖

N02.3   **Recurrent and persistent hematuria with** diffuse mesangial proliferative glomerulonephritis 🔖

N02.4   **Recurrent and persistent hematuria with** diffuse endocapillary proliferative glomerulonephritis 🔖

N02.5   **Recurrent and persistent hematuria with** diffuse mesangiocapillary glomerulonephritis 🔖
     Recurrent and persistent hematuria with membranoproliferative glomerulonephritis, types 1 and 3, or NOS

     Excludes1   Recurrent and persistent hematuria with C3 glomerulonephritis (N02.A)
                Recurrent and persistent hematuria with C3 glomerulopathy (N02.A)

N02.6   **Recurrent and persistent hematuria with** dense deposit disease 🔖
     Recurrent and persistent hematuria with C3 glomerulopathy with dense deposit disease
     Recurrent and persistent hematuria with membranoproliferative glomerulonephritis, type 2

N02.7   **Recurrent and persistent hematuria with** diffuse crescentic glomerulonephritis 🔖
     Recurrent and persistent hematuria with extracapillary glomerulonephritis

N02.8   **Recurrent and persistent hematuria with** other morphologic changes 🔖
     Recurrent and persistent hematuria with proliferative glomerulonephritis NOS
     (Ex:) See PDX Collection 915

N02.9   **Recurrent and persistent hematuria with** unspecified morphologic changes 🔖
     (Ex:) See PDX Collection 915
     Coding Clinic: 2017, Q2, P5

N02.A   **Recurrent and persistent hematuria with C3 glomerulonephritis** 🔖
     Recurrent and persistent hematuria with C3 glomerulopathy

     Excludes1   Recurrent and persistent hematuria (with C3 glomerulopathy) with dense deposit disease (N02.6)
     (Ex:) See PDX Collection 4070

▶ New   ⇒ Revised   ~~deleted~~ Deleted   Excludes 1   Excludes 2   Includes   Use additional   Code first   Code also   Key words

OGCR Official Guidelines   ● Unacceptable Principal Diagnosis   X Assign placeholder X   ● Use Additional Character(s)   ▶ Manifestation Code   **Coding Clinic**

Item 14–3 Chronic glomerulonephritis (GN) persists over a period of years, with remissions and exacerbation.

Chronic GN with lesion of proliferative glomerulonephritis results from a streptococcal infection.

Chronic GN with lesion of membranous glomerulonephritis, also known as membranous nephropathy, is characterized by deposits along the epithelial side of the basement membrane.

Chronic GN with lesion of membrano-proliferative glomerulonephritis (MPGN) is a group of disorders characterized by alterations in the basement membranes of the kidney and the glomerular cells.

Chronic GN with lesion of rapidly progressive glomerulonephritis is characterized by necrosis, endothelial proliferation, and mesangial proliferation. The condition is marked by rapid and progressive decline in renal function.

● **N03   Chronic nephritic syndrome**

Includes   chronic glomerular disease
chronic glomerulonephritis
chronic nephritis

Excludes1   chronic tubulo-interstitial nephritis (N11.-)
diffuse sclerosing glomerulonephritis (N05.8-)
nephritic syndrome NOS (N05.-)

(Ex:) **For category N03 CC codes:** See PDX Collection 918

N03.0   Chronic nephritic syndrome with minor glomerular abnormality 🔹
Chronic nephritic syndrome with minimal change lesion

N03.1   Chronic nephritic syndrome with focal and segmental glomerular lesions 🔹
Chronic nephritic syndrome with focal and segmental hyalinosis
Chronic nephritic syndrome with focal and segmental sclerosis
Chronic nephritic syndrome with focal glomerulonephritis

N03.2   Chronic nephritic syndrome with diffuse membranous glomerulonephritis 🔹

N03.3   Chronic nephritic syndrome with diffuse mesangial proliferative glomerulonephritis 🔹

N03.4   Chronic nephritic syndrome with diffuse endocapillary proliferative glomerulonephritis 🔹

N03.5   Chronic nephritic syndrome with diffuse mesangiocapillary glomerulonephritis 🔹
Chronic nephritic syndrome with membranoproliferative glomerulonephritis, types 1 and 3, or NOS

Excludes1   Chronic nephritic syndrome with C3 glomerulonephritis (N03.A)
Chronic nephritic syndrome with C3 glomerulopathy (N03.A)

N03.6   Chronic nephritic syndrome with dense deposit disease 🔹
Chronic nephritic syndrome with C3 glomerulopathy with dense deposit disease
Chronic nephritic syndrome with membranoproliferative glomerulonephritis, type 2

N03.7   Chronic nephritic syndrome with diffuse crescentic glomerulonephritis 🔹
Chronic nephritic syndrome with extracapillary glomerulonephritis

N03.8   Chronic nephritic syndrome with other morphologic changes 🔹
Chronic nephritic syndrome with proliferative glomerulonephritis NOS

N03.9   Chronic nephritic syndrome with unspecified morphologic changes 🔹

N03.A   Chronic nephritic syndrome with C3 glomerulonephritis 🔹
Chronic nephritic syndrome with C3 glomerulopathy

Excludes1   Chronic nephritic syndrome (with C3 glomerulopathy) with dense deposit disease(N03.6)

(Ex:) See PDX Collection 4070

● **N04   Nephrotic syndrome**

Includes   congenital nephrotic syndrome
lipoid nephrosis

(Ex:) **For category N04 CC codes unless otherwise indicated:** See PDX Collection 917

N04.0   Nephrotic syndrome with minor glomerular abnormality 🔹
Nephrotic syndrome with minimal change lesion

N04.1   Nephrotic syndrome with focal and segmental glomerular lesions 🔹
Nephrotic syndrome with focal and segmental hyalinosis
Nephrotic syndrome with focal and segmental sclerosis
Nephrotic syndrome with focal glomerulonephritis

N04.2   Nephrotic syndrome with diffuse membranous glomerulonephritis 🔹

N04.3   Nephrotic syndrome with diffuse mesangial proliferative glomerulonephritis 🔹

N04.4   Nephrotic syndrome with diffuse endocapillary proliferative glomerulonephritis 🔹

N04.5   Nephrotic syndrome with diffuse mesangiocapillary glomerulonephritis 🔹
Nephrotic syndrome with membranoproliferative glomerulonephritis, types 1 and 3, or NOS

Excludes1   Nephrotic syndrome with C3 glomerulonephritis (N04.A)
Nephrotic syndrome with C3 glomerulopathy (N04.A)

N04.6   Nephrotic syndrome with dense deposit disease 🔹
Nephrotic syndrome with C3 glomerulopathy with dense deposit disease
Nephrotic syndrome with membranoproliferative glomerulonephritis, type 2

N04.7   Nephrotic syndrome with diffuse crescentic glomerulonephritis 🔹
Nephrotic syndrome with extracapillary glomerulonephritis
(Ex:) See PDX Collection 915

N04.8   Nephrotic syndrome with other morphologic changes 🔹
Nephrotic syndrome with proliferative glomerulonephritis NOS
(Ex:) See PDX Collection 915

N04.9   Nephrotic syndrome with unspecified morphologic changes 🔹
(Ex:) See PDX Collection 915

N04.A   Nephrotic syndrome with C3 glomerulonephritis 🔹
Nephrotic syndrome with C3 glomerulopathy

Excludes1   Nephrotic syndrome (with C3 glomerulopathy) with dense deposit disease (N04.6)

(Ex:) See PDX Collection 4070

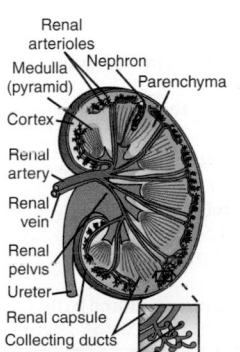

Renal arterioles
Medulla (pyramid)   Nephron
Parenchyma
Cortex
Renal artery
Renal vein
Renal pelvis
Ureter
Renal capsule
Collecting ducts
Glomeruli (microscopic)

Figure 14-2   Kidney cross section.

Item 14–4 Nephrotic syndrome (NS) is marked by massive proteinuria (protein in the urine) and water retention. Patients with NS are particularly vulnerable to staphylococcal and pneumococcal infections. NS with lesion of proliferative glomerulonephritis results from a streptococcal infection. NS with lesion of membranous glomerulonephritis results in thickening of the capillary walls. NS with lesion of minimal change glomerulonephritis is usually a benign disorder that occurs mostly in children and requires electron microscopy (biopsy) to verify changes in the glomeruli.

CHAPTER 14 (N00-N99)

N Newborn Age: 0   **P** Pediatric Age: 0–17   **M** Maternity DX: 9–64   **A** Adult Age: 15–124   ♀ Females Only   ♂ Males Only

🔹 Complication\Comorbidity   🔹 Major C\C   (Ex:) CC/MCC Exclusions   🔹 Hospital-Acquired Condition   🔹 Hierarchical Condition Category

1121

● **N05** **Unspecified nephritic syndrome**

    Includes   glomerular disease NOS
                     glomerulonephritis NOS
                     nephritis NOS
                     nephropathy NOS and renal disease NOS with
                           morphological lesion specified in .0-.8

    Excludes1   nephropathy NOS with no stated morphological
                          lesion (N28.9)
                        renal disease NOS with no stated morphological
                          lesion (N28.9)
                        tubulo-interstitial nephritis NOS (N12)

  N05.0 **Unspecified nephritic syndrome with minor glomerular abnormality**
       Unspecified nephritic syndrome with minimal change lesion

  N05.1 **Unspecified nephritic syndrome with focal and segmental glomerular lesions**
       Unspecified nephritic syndrome with focal and segmental hyalinosis
       Unspecified nephritic syndrome with focal and segmental sclerosis
       Unspecified nephritic syndrome with focal glomerulonephritis

  N05.2 **Unspecified nephritic syndrome with diffuse membranous glomerulonephritis** 🔎
       (Ex:) See PDX Collection 918

  N05.3 **Unspecified nephritic syndrome with diffuse mesangial proliferative glomerulonephritis** 🔎
       (Ex:) See PDX Collection 918

  N05.4 **Unspecified nephritic syndrome with diffuse endocapillary proliferative glomerulonephritis** 🔎
       (Ex:) See PDX Collection 918

  N05.5 **Unspecified nephritic syndrome with diffuse mesangiocapillary glomerulonephritis** 🔎
       Unspecified nephritic syndrome with membranoproliferative glomerulonephritis, types 1 and 3, or NOS

      Excludes1   Unspecified nephritic syndrome with C3 glomerulonephritis (N05.A)
                         Unspecified nephritic syndrome with C3 glomerulopathy (N05.A)
       (Ex:) See PDX Collection 918

  N05.6 **Unspecified nephritic syndrome with dense deposit disease**
       Unspecified nephritic syndrome with C3 glomerulopathy with dense deposit disease
       Unspecified nephritic syndrome with membranoproliferative glomerulonephritis, type 2

  N05.7 **Unspecified nephritic syndrome with diffuse crescentic glomerulonephritis**
       Unspecified nephritic syndrome with extracapillary glomerulonephritis

  N05.8 **Unspecified nephritic syndrome with other morphologic changes**
       Unspecified nephritic syndrome with proliferative glomerulonephritis NOS

  N05.9 **Unspecified nephritic syndrome with unspecified morphologic changes**

  N05.A **Unspecified nephritic syndrome with C3 glomerulonephritis** 🔎
       Unspecified nephritic syndrome with C3 glomerulopathy

      Excludes1   Unspecified nephritic syndrome (with C3 glomerulopathy) with dense deposit disease(N05.6)
       (Ex:) See PDX Collection 4070

● **N06** **Isolated proteinuria with specified morphological lesion**

    Excludes1   proteinuria not associated with specific morphologic lesions (R80.0)

  N06.0 **Isolated proteinuria with minor glomerular abnormality**
       Isolated proteinuria with minimal change lesion

  N06.1 **Isolated proteinuria with focal and segmental glomerular lesions**
       Isolated proteinuria with focal and segmental hyalinosis
       Isolated proteinuria with focal and segmental sclerosis
       Isolated proteinuria with focal glomerulonephritis

  N06.2 **Isolated proteinuria with diffuse membranous glomerulonephritis** 🔎
       (Ex:) See PDX Collection 918

  N06.3 **Isolated proteinuria with diffuse mesangial proliferative glomerulonephritis** 🔎
       (Ex:) See PDX Collection 918

  N06.4 **Isolated proteinuria with diffuse endocapillary proliferative glomerulonephritis** 🔎
       (Ex:) See PDX Collection 918

  N06.5 **Isolated proteinuria with diffuse mesangiocapillary glomerulonephritis** 🔎
       Isolated proteinuria with membranoproliferative glomerulonephritis, types 1 and 3, or NOS

      Excludes1   Isolated proteinuria with C3 glomerulonephritis (N06.A)
                         Isolated proteinuria with C3 glomerulopathy (N06.A)
       (Ex:) See PDX Collection 918

  N06.6 **Isolated proteinuria with dense deposit disease**
       Isolated proteinuria with C3 glomerulopathy with dense deposit disease
       Isolated proteinuria with membranoproliferative glomerulonephritis, type 2

  N06.7 **Isolated proteinuria with diffuse crescentic glomerulonephritis**
       Isolated proteinuria with extracapillary glomerulonephritis

  N06.8 **Isolated proteinuria with other morphologic lesion**
       Isolated proteinuria with proliferative glomerulonephritis NOS

  N06.9 **Isolated proteinuria with unspecified morphologic lesion**

  N06.A **Isolated proteinuria with C3 glomerulonephritis** 🔎
       Isolated proteinuria with C3 glomerulopathy

      Excludes1   Isolated proteinuria (with C3 glomerulopathy) with dense deposit disease (N06.6)
       (Ex:) See PDX Collection 4070

● **N07** **Hereditary nephropathy, not elsewhere classified**

    Excludes2   Alport's syndrome (Q87.81-)
                        hereditary amyloid nephropathy (E85.-)
                        nail patella syndrome (Q87.2)
                        non-neuropathic heredofamilial amyloidosis (E85.-)

  N07.0 **Hereditary nephropathy, not elsewhere classified with minor glomerular abnormality**
       Hereditary nephropathy, not elsewhere classified with minimal change lesion

  N07.1 **Hereditary nephropathy, not elsewhere classified with focal and segmental glomerular lesions**
       Hereditary nephropathy, not elsewhere classified with focal and segmental hyalinosis
       Hereditary nephropathy, not elsewhere classified with focal and segmental sclerosis
       Hereditary nephropathy, not elsewhere classified with focal glomerulonephritis

  N07.2 **Hereditary nephropathy, not elsewhere classified with diffuse membranous glomerulonephritis** 🔎
       (Ex:) See PDX Collection 918

▶ New   ⇒ Revised   ~~deleted~~ Deleted   Excludes 1   Excludes 2   Includes   Use additional   Code first   Code also   Key words
OGCR Official Guidelines   ● Unacceptable Principal Diagnosis   X Assign placeholder X   ● Use Additional Character(s)   ▷ Manifestation Code   **Coding Clinic**

N07.3 **Hereditary nephropathy, not elsewhere classified with diffuse mesangial proliferative glomerulonephritis**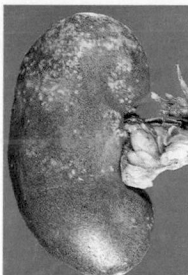
    (Ex) See PDX Collection 918

N07.4 **Hereditary nephropathy, not elsewhere classified with diffuse endocapillary proliferative glomerulonephritis**
    (Ex) See PDX Collection 918

N07.5 **Hereditary nephropathy, not elsewhere classified with diffuse mesangiocapillary glomerulonephritis**
    Hereditary nephropathy, not elsewhere classified with membranoproliferative glomerulonephritis, types 1 and 3, or NOS

    Excludes1   Hereditary nephropathy, not elsewhere classified with C3 glomerulonephritis (N07.A)
                Hereditary nephropathy, not elsewhere classified with C3 glomerulopathy (N07.A)
    (Ex) See PDX Collection 918

N07.6 **Hereditary nephropathy, not elsewhere classified with dense deposit disease**
    Hereditary nephropathy, not elsewhere classified with C3 glomerulopathy with dense deposit disease
    Hereditary nephropathy, not elsewhere classified with membranoproliferative glomerulonephritis, type 2

N07.7 **Hereditary nephropathy, not elsewhere classified with diffuse crescentic glomerulonephritis**
    Hereditary nephropathy, not elsewhere classified with extracapillary glomerulonephritis

N07.8 **Hereditary nephropathy, not elsewhere classified with other morphologic lesions**
    Hereditary nephropathy, not elsewhere classified with proliferative glomerulonephritis NOS

N07.9 **Hereditary nephropathy, not elsewhere classified with unspecified morphologic lesions**

N07.A **Hereditary nephropathy, not elsewhere classified with C3 glomerulonephritis**
    Hereditary nephropathy, not elsewhere classified with C3 glomerulopathy

    Excludes1   Hereditary nephropathy, not elsewhere classified (with C3 glomerulopathy) with dense deposit disease (N07.6)
    (Ex) See PDX Collection 4070

N08 *Glomerular disorders in diseases classified elsewhere*
    Glomerulonephritis
    Nephritis
    Nephropathy

    Code first underlying disease, such as:
      amyloidosis (E85.-)
      congenital syphilis (A50.5)
      cryoglobulinemia (D89.1)
      disseminated intravascular coagulation (D65)
      gout (M1A.-, M10.-)
      microscopic polyangiitis (M31.7)
      multiple myeloma (C90.0-)
      sepsis (A40.0-A41.9)
      sickle-cell disease (D57.0-D57.8)

    Excludes1   glomerulonephritis, nephritis and nephropathy (in):
                antiglomerular basement membrane disease (M31.0)
                diabetes (E08-E13 with .21)
                gonococcal (A54.21)
                Goodpasture's syndrome (M31.0)
                hemolytic-uremic syndrome (D59.3)
                lupus (M32.14)
                mumps (B26.83)
                syphilis (A52.75)
                systemic lupus erythematosus (M32.14)
                Wegener's granulomatosis (M31.31)
            pyelonephritis in diseases classified elsewhere (N16)
            renal tubulo-interstitial disorders classified elsewhere (N16)

Figure 14-3 Acute pyelonephritis. Cortical surface exhibits grayish white areas of inflammation and abscess formation. (From Frazier MS, Drzymkowski JW: Essentials of Human Diseases and Conditions, St. Louis, Saunders/Elsevier, 2009)

Item 14-5 Pyelonephritis is an infection of the kidneys and ureters and may be chronic or acute in one or both kidneys.

RENAL TUBULO-INTERSTITIAL DISEASES (N10-N16)

Includes   pyelonephritis

Excludes1   pyeloureteritis cystica (N28.85)

N10 **Acute pyelonephritis**
    Acute infectious interstitial nephritis
    Acute pyelitis
    Acute tubulo-interstitial nephritis
    Hemoglobin nephrosis
    Myoglobin nephrosis
    Use additional code (B95-B97), to identify infectious agent
    (Ex) See PDX Collection 2919
    Coding Clinic: 2019, Q3, P13-14

● **N11** **Chronic tubulo-interstitial nephritis**
    Includes   chronic infectious interstitial nephritis
                    chronic pyelitis
                    chronic pyelonephritis
    Use additional code (B95-B97), to identify infectious agent

  N11.0 **Nonobstructive reflux-associated chronic pyelonephritis**
    Pyelonephritis (chronic) associated with (vesicoureteral) reflux

    Excludes1   vesicoureteral reflux NOS (N13.70)

  N11.1 **Chronic obstructive pyelonephritis**
    Pyelonephritis (chronic) associated with anomaly of pelviureteric junction
    Pyelonephritis (chronic) associated with anomaly of pyeloureteric junction
    Pyelonephritis (chronic) associated with crossing of vessel
    Pyelonephritis (chronic) associated with kinking of ureter
    Pyelonephritis (chronic) associated with obstruction of ureter
    Pyelonephritis (chronic) associated with stricture of pelviureteric junction
    Pyelonephritis (chronic) associated with stricture of ureter

    Excludes1   calculous pyelonephritis (N20.9)
                   obstructive uropathy (N13.-)
    CC when PDx is its own CC
    (Ex) See PDX Collection 920

  N11.8 **Other chronic tubulo-interstitial nephritis**
    Nonobstructive chronic pyelonephritis NOS
    (Ex) See PDX Collection 921

  N11.9 **Chronic tubulo-interstitial nephritis, unspecified**
    Chronic interstitial nephritis NOS
    Chronic pyelitis NOS
    Chronic pyelonephritis NOS
    (Ex) See PDX Collection 4047

N12 **Tubulo-interstitial nephritis, not specified as acute or chronic**
    Interstitial nephritis NOS
    Pyelitis NOS
    Pyelonephritis NOS

    Excludes1   calculous pyelonephritis (N20.9)
    (Ex) See PDX Collection 4047

CHAPTER 14 (N00-N99)

N   Newborn Age: 0   **P**   Pediatric Age: 0-17   **M**   Maternity DX: 9-64   **A**   Adult Age: 15-124   ♀   Females Only   ♂   Males Only

Complication\Comorbidity   Major C\C   (Ex) CC/MCC Exclusions   Hospital-Acquired Condition   Hierarchical Condition Category

1123

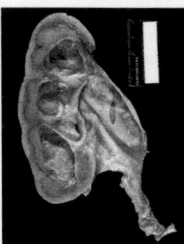

Figure 14-4 Hydronephrosis of the kidney, with marked dilatation of pelvis and calyces and thinning of renal parenchyma. (From Kumar: Robbins and Cotran: Pathologic Basis of Disease, ed 8, Saunders, An Imprint of Elsevier, 2009)

CHAPTER 14 (N00-N99)

● **N13 Obstructive and reflux uropathy**

     Excludes2   calculus of kidney and ureter without hydronephrosis (N20.-)
                 congenital obstructive defects of renal pelvis and ureter (Q62.0-Q62.3)
                 hydronephrosis with ureteropelvic junction obstruction (Q62.11)
                 obstructive pyelonephritis (N11.1)

     (Ex:) **For category N13 CC codes unless otherwise indicated:** See PDX Collection 4015

N13.0 Hydronephrosis with ureteropelvic junction obstruction 🔧
     Hydronephrosis due to acquired occlusion of ureteropelvic junction
         Excludes2   Hydronephrosis with ureteropelvic junction obstruction due to calculus (N13.2)
     CC when PDx is its own CC
     Coding Clinic: 2016, Q4, P43

N13.1 Hydronephrosis with ureteral stricture, not elsewhere classified 🔧
         Excludes1   hydronephrosis with ureteral stricture with infection (N13.6)
     CC when PDx is its own CC

N13.2 Hydronephrosis with renal and ureteral calculous obstruction 🔧
         Excludes1   hydronephrosis with renal and ureteral calculous obstruction with infection (N13.6)
     CC when PDx is its own CC

● **N13.3 Other and unspecified hydronephrosis**
         Excludes1   hydronephrosis with infection (N13.6)
     N13.30 Unspecified hydronephrosis 🔧
     N13.39 Other hydronephrosis 🔧

N13.4 Hydroureter 🔧
         Excludes1   congenital hydroureter (Q62.3-)
                 hydroureter with infection (N13.6)
                 vesicoureteral-reflux with hydroureter (N13.73-)
     (Ex:) See PDX Collection 923

N13.5 Crossing vessel and stricture of ureter without hydronephrosis
     Kinking and stricture of ureter without hydronephrosis
         Excludes1   crossing vessel and stricture of ureter without hydronephrosis with infection (N13.6)
     Coding Clinic: 2016, Q4, P43

N13.6 Pyonephrosis 🔧 🔧
     Conditions in N13.0-N13.5 with infection
     Obstructive uropathy with infection
     Use additional code (B95-B97), to identify infectious agent
     Coding Clinic: 2018, Q2, P21

● **N13.7 Vesicoureteral-reflux**
     Excludes1   reflux-associated pyelonephritis (N11.0)

     N13.70 Vesicoureteral-reflux, unspecified
         Occurs when urine flows from bladder back into ureters
         Vesicoureteral-reflux NOS

     N13.71 Vesicoureteral-reflux without reflux nephropathy

     ● **N13.72 Vesicoureteral-reflux with reflux nephropathy without hydroureter**
         N13.721 Vesicoureteral-reflux with reflux nephropathy without hydroureter, unilateral
         N13.722 Vesicoureteral-reflux with reflux nephropathy without hydroureter, bilateral
         N13.729 Vesicoureteral-reflux with reflux nephropathy without hydroureter, unspecified

     ● **N13.73 Vesicoureteral-reflux with reflux nephropathy with hydroureter**
         N13.731 Vesicoureteral-reflux with reflux nephropathy with hydroureter, unilateral
         N13.732 Vesicoureteral-reflux with reflux nephropathy with hydroureter, bilateral
         N13.739 Vesicoureteral-reflux with reflux nephropathy with hydroureter, unspecified

N13.8 Other obstructive and reflux uropathy 🔧
     Urinary tract obstruction due to specified cause
     Code first, if applicable, any causal condition first, such as: enlarged prostate (N40.1)
     (Ex:) See PDX Collection 920

N13.9 Obstructive and reflux uropathy, unspecified
     Urinary tract obstruction NOS

● **N14 Drug- and heavy-metal-induced tubulo-interstitial and tubular conditions**
     Code first poisoning due to drug or toxin, if applicable (T36-T65 with fifth or sixth character 1-4 or 6)
     Use additional code for adverse effect, if applicable, to identify drug (T36-T50 with fifth or sixth character 5)

N14.0 Analgesic nephropathy
N14.1 Nephropathy induced by other drugs, medicaments and biological substances
N14.2 Nephropathy induced by unspecified drug, medicament or biological substance
N14.3 Nephropathy induced by heavy metals
N14.4 Toxic nephropathy, not elsewhere classified

● **N15 Other renal tubulo-interstitial diseases**
N15.0 Balkan nephropathy
     Balkan endemic nephropathy
N15.1 Renal and perinephric abscess 🔧 🔧
     (Ex:) See PDX Collection 919

N15.8 Other specified renal tubulo-interstitial diseases
N15.9 Renal tubulo-interstitial disease, unspecified
     Infection of kidney NOS
         Excludes1   urinary tract infection NOS (N39.0)

▶ New   ⟹ Revised   ~~deleted~~ Deleted   Excludes 1   Excludes 2   Includes   Use additional   Code first   Code also   Key words

1124   OGCR Official Guidelines   ● Unacceptable Principal Diagnosis   X Assign placeholder X   ● Use Additional Character(s)   ▶ Manifestation Code   Coding Clinic

▶ **N16** *Renal tubulo-interstitial disorders in diseases classified elsewhere*

    Pyelonephritis

    Tubulo-interstitial nephritis

    Code first underlying disease, such as:

        brucellosis (A23.0-A23.9)

        cryoglobulinemia (D89.1)

        glycogen storage disease (E74.0)

        leukemia (C91-C95)

        lymphoma (C81.0-C85.9, C96.0-C96.9)

        multiple myeloma (C90.0-)

        sepsis (A40.0-A41.9)

        Wilson's disease (E83.0)

      Excludes1   diphtheritic pyelonephritis and tubulo-interstitial nephritis (A36.84)

              pyelonephritis and tubulo-interstitial nephritis in candidiasis (B37.49)

              pyelonephritis and tubulo-interstitial nephritis in cystinosis (E72.04)

              pyelonephritis and tubulo-interstitial nephritis in salmonella infection (A02.25)

              pyelonephritis and tubulo-interstitial nephritis in sarcoidosis (D86.84)

            ➡ pyelonephritis and tubulo-interstitial nephritis in Sjögren syndrome (M35.04)

              pyelonephritis and tubulo-interstitial nephritis in systemic lupus erythematosus (M32.15)

              pyelonephritis and tubulo-interstitial nephritis in toxoplasmosis (B58.83)

              renal tubular degeneration in diabetes (E08-E13 with .29)

              syphilitic pyelonephritis and tubulo-interstitial nephritis (A52.75)

ACUTE KIDNEY FAILURE AND CHRONIC KIDNEY DISEASE (N17-N19)

    Excludes2   congenital renal failure (P96.0)

           drug- and heavy-metal-induced tubulo-interstitial and tubular conditions (N14.-)

           extrarenal uremia (R39.2)

           hemolytic-uremic syndrome (D59.3)

           hepatorenal syndrome (K76.7)

           postpartum hepatorenal syndrome (O90.4)

           posttraumatic renal failure (T79.5)

           prerenal uremia (R39.2)

           renal failure complicating abortion or ectopic or molar pregnancy (O00-O07, O08.4)

           renal failure following labor and delivery (O90.4)

           renal failure postprocedural (N99.0)

● **N17** **Acute kidney failure**

    Code also associated underlying condition

      Excludes1   posttraumatic renal failure (T79.5)

      (Ex:) **For category N17 CC codes unless otherwise indicated:** See PDX Collection 284

    N17.0 **Acute kidney failure with tubular necrosis** 🔹🔹

        Acute tubular necrosis

        Renal tubular necrosis

        Tubular necrosis NOS

    N17.1 **Acute kidney failure with acute cortical necrosis** 🔹🔹

        Acute cortical necrosis

        Cortical necrosis NOS

        Renal cortical necrosis

    N17.2 **Acute kidney failure with medullary necrosis** 🔹🔹

        Medullary [papillary] necrosis NOS

        Acute medullary [papillary] necrosis

        Renal medullary [papillary] necrosis

    N17.8 **Other acute kidney failure** 🔹🔹

      (Ex:) See PDX Collection 250

    N17.9 **Acute kidney failure, unspecified** 🔹🔹

        Acute kidney injury (nontraumatic)

      Excludes2   traumatic kidney injury (S37.0-)

      Coding Clinic: 2019, Q2, P7,25

Item 14–6 Decreased blood flow is the usual cause of **acute renal failure** that offers a good prognosis for recovery.

    Chronic renal failure is usually the result of long-standing kidney disease and is a very serious condition that generally results in death.

● **N18** **Chronic kidney disease (CKD)**

    Code first any associated:

      diabetic chronic kidney disease (E08.22, E09.22, E10.22, E11.22, E13.22)

      hypertensive chronic kidney disease (I12.-, I13.-)

    Use additional code to identify kidney transplant status, if applicable, (Z94.0)

    Coding Clinic: 2018, Q4, P89; 2016, Q4, P123

    N18.1 **Chronic kidney disease, stage 1**

    N18.2 **Chronic kidney disease, stage 2 (mild)**

  ● **N18.3** **Chronic kidney disease, stage 3 (moderate)**

      N18.30 **Chronic kidney disease, stage 3 unspecified**

      N18.31 **Chronic kidney disease, stage 3a**

      N18.32 **Chronic kidney disease, stage 3b**

    N18.4 **Chronic kidney disease, stage 4 (severe)** 🔹🔹

      (Ex:) See PDX Collection 282

      Coding Clinic: 2013, Q1, P24

    N18.5 **Chronic kidney disease, stage 5** 🔹🔹

      Excludes1   chronic kidney disease, stage 5 requiring chronic dialysis (N18.6)

      (Ex:) See PDX Collection 282

    N18.6 **End stage renal disease** 🔹🔹

        Chronic kidney disease requiring chronic dialysis

        Use additional code to identify dialysis status (Z99.2)

      (Ex:) See PDX Collection 283

      Coding Clinic: 2016, Q3, P23, Q1, P13

    N18.9 **Chronic kidney disease, unspecified**

        Chronic renal disease

        Chronic renal failure NOS

        Chronic renal insufficiency

        Chronic uremia NOS

        Diffuse sclerosing glomerulonephritis NOS

      Coding Clinic: 2018, Q4, P88

N19 **Unspecified kidney failure**

    Uremia NOS

      Excludes1   acute kidney failure (N17.-)

            chronic kidney disease (N18.)

            chronic uremia (N18.9)

            extrarenal uremia (R39.2)

            prerenal uremia (R39.2)

            renal insufficiency (acute) (N28.9)

            uremia of newborn (P96.0)

UROLITHIASIS (N20-N23)

● **N20** **Calculus of kidney and ureter**

    Calculous pyelonephritis

      Excludes1   nephrocalcinosis (E83.5)

            that with hydronephrosis (N13.2)

    Coding Clinic: 2019, Q3, P14

    N20.0 **Calculus of kidney**

        Nephrolithiasis NOS   Staghorn calculus

        Renal calculus   Stone in kidney

        Renal stone

      Coding Clinic: 2019, Q3, P13; 2017, Q1, P5

    N20.1 **Calculus of ureter** 🔹

        Calculus of the ureteropelvic junction

        Ureteric stone

      (Ex:) See PDX Collection 928

      Coding Clinic: 2016, Q3, P24

    N20.2 **Calculus of kidney with calculus of ureter** 🔹

      (Ex:) See PDX Collection 928

    N20.9 **Urinary calculus, unspecified**

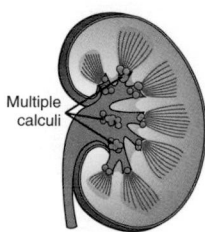

Figure 14-5   Multiple urinary calculi.

Multiple calculi

N Newborn Age: 0   P Pediatric Age: 0–17   M Maternity DX: 9–64   A Adult Age: 15–124   ♀ Females Only   ♂ Males Only

🔹 Complication\Comorbidity   🔹 Major C\C   (Ex:) CC/MCC Exclusions   🔹 Hospital-Acquired Condition   🔹 Hierarchical Condition Category

● **N21**   **Calculus of lower urinary tract**
>   **Includes**   calculus of lower urinary tract with cystitis and urethritis

    N21.0   **Calculus in bladder**
       Calculus in diverticulum of bladder
       Urinary bladder stone
>   **Excludes2**   staghorn calculus (N20.0)
>   Coding Clinic: 2015, Q2, P9

    N21.1   **Calculus in urethra**
>   **Excludes2**   calculus of prostate (N42.0)

    N21.8   **Other lower urinary tract calculus**

    N21.9   **Calculus of lower urinary tract, unspecified**
>   **Excludes1**   calculus of urinary tract NOS (N20.9)

▷ **N22**   *Calculus of urinary tract in diseases classified elsewhere*
>   *Code first underlying disease, such as:*
>   gout (M1A.-, M10.-)
>   schistosomiasis (B65.0-B65.9)

N23   **Unspecified renal colic**

OTHER DISORDERS OF KIDNEY AND URETER (N25-N29)
>   **Excludes2**   disorders of kidney and ureter with urolithiasis (N20-N23)

● **N25**   **Disorders resulting from impaired renal tubular function**

    N25.0   **Renal osteodystrophy**
       Azotemic osteodystrophy
       Phosphate-losing tubular disorders
       Renal rickets
       Renal short stature
>   **Excludes2**   metabolic disorders classifiable to E70-E88

    N25.1   **Nephrogenic diabetes insipidus** 🔒 🔒
>   **Excludes1**   diabetes insipidus NOS (E23.2)
>   (Ex) See PDX Collection 929

●   **N25.8**   **Other disorders resulting from impaired renal tubular function**

       N25.81   **Secondary hyperparathyroidism of renal origin** 🔒 🔒
>   **Excludes1**   secondary hyperparathyroidism, non-renal (E21.1)
>   **Excludes2**   metabolic disorders classifiable to E70-E88
>   (Ex) See PDX Collection 930

       N25.89   **Other disorders resulting from impaired renal tubular function**
          Hypokalemic nephropathy
          Lightwood-Albright syndrome
          Renal tubular acidosis NOS

    N25.9   **Disorder resulting from impaired renal tubular function, unspecified**

● **N26**   **Unspecified contracted kidney**
>   **Excludes1**   contracted kidney due to hypertension (I12.-)
>   diffuse sclerosing glomerulonephritis (N05.8-)
>   hypertensive nephrosclerosis (arteriolar) (arteriosclerotic) (I12.-)
>   small kidney of unknown cause (N27.-)

    N26.1   **Atrophy of kidney (terminal)**

    N26.2   **Page kidney**

    N26.9   **Renal sclerosis, unspecified**

● **N27**   **Small kidney of unknown cause**
>   **Includes**   oligonephronia

    N27.0   **Small kidney, unilateral**

    N27.1   **Small kidney, bilateral**

    N27.9   **Small kidney, unspecified**

● **N28**   **Other disorders of kidney and ureter, not elsewhere classified**

    N28.0   **Ischemia and infarction of kidney** 🔒 🔒
       Renal artery embolism
       Renal artery obstruction
       Renal artery occlusion
       Renal artery thrombosis
       Renal infarct
>   **Excludes1**   atherosclerosis of renal artery (extrarenal part) (I70.1)
>   congenital stenosis of renal artery (Q27.1)
>   Goldblatt's kidney (I70.1)
>   (Ex) See PDX Collection 931

    N28.1   **Cyst of kidney, acquired**
       Cyst (multiple) (solitary) of kidney, (acquired)
>   **Excludes1**   cystic kidney disease (congenital) (Q61.-)

● **N28.8**   **Other specified disorders of kidney and ureter**
>   **Excludes1**   hydroureter (N13.4)
>   ureteric stricture with hydronephrosis (N13.1)
>   ureteric stricture without hydronephrosis (N13.5)

       N28.81   **Hypertrophy of kidney**

       N28.82   **Megaloureter**

       N28.83   **Nephroptosis**

       N28.84   **Pyelitis cystica** 🔒 🔒
>   (Ex) See PDX Collection 4015

       N28.85   **Pyeloureteritis cystica** 🔒 🔒
>   (Ex) See PDX Collection 4015

       N28.86   **Ureteritis cystica** 🔒 🔒
>   (Ex) See PDX Collection 4015

       N28.89   **Other specified disorders of kidney and ureter**

    N28.9   **Disorder of kidney and ureter, unspecified**
       Nephropathy NOS
       Renal disease (acute) NOS
       Renal insufficiency (acute)
>   **Excludes1**   chronic renal insufficiency (N18.9)
>   unspecified nephritic syndrome (N05.-)
>   Coding Clinic: 2016, Q1, P13

▷ **N29**   *Other disorders of kidney and ureter in diseases classified elsewhere*
>   *Code first underlying disease, such as:*
>   amyloidosis (E85.-)
>   nephrocalcinosis (E83.5)
>   schistosomiasis (B65.0-B65.9)
>   **Excludes1**   disorders of kidney and ureter in:
>   cystinosis (E72.0)
>   gonorrhea (A54.21)
>   syphilis (A52.75)
>   tuberculosis (A18.11)

OTHER DISEASES OF THE URINARY SYSTEM (N30-N39)
>   ~~**Excludes1**   urinary infection (complicating):~~
>   ~~abortion or ectopic or molar pregnancy (O00-O07, O08.8)~~
>   ~~pregnancy, childbirth and the puerperium (O23.-, O75.3, O86.2-)~~

>   ▶ **Excludes2**   urinary infection (complicating):
>   ▶ abortion or ectopic or molar pregnancy (O00-O07, O08.8)
>   ▶ pregnancy, childbirth and the puerperium (O23.-, O75.3, O86.2-)

● **N30**   **Cystitis**
>   *Infection of bladder and irritation in lower urinary tract*
>   Use additional code to identify infectious agent (B95-B97)
>   **Excludes1**   prostatocystitis (N41.3)

● **N30.0**   **Acute cystitis**
>   **Excludes1**   irradiation cystitis (N30.4-)
>   trigonitis (N30.3-)
>   (Ex) For category N30.0 CC codes: See PDX Collection 2932

       N30.00   **Acute cystitis without hematuria** 🔒 🔒

       N30.01   **Acute cystitis with hematuria** 🔒 🔒

● **N30.1 Interstitial cystitis (chronic)**
    Ongoing infection of kidney glomeruli and tubules
    N30.10 Interstitial cystitis (chronic) without hematuria
    N30.11 Interstitial cystitis (chronic) with hematuria

● **N30.2 Other chronic cystitis**
    N30.20 Other chronic cystitis without hematuria
    N30.21 Other chronic cystitis with hematuria

● **N30.3 Trigonitis**
    Inflammation of triangular area of bladder (where the ureters
    and urethra come together)
    Urethrotrigonitis
    N30.30 Trigonitis without hematuria
    N30.31 Trigonitis with hematuria

● **N30.4 Irradiation cystitis**
    (Ex) **For category N30.4 CC codes: See PDX Collection 932**
    N30.40 Irradiation cystitis without hematuria 🅒
    N30.41 Irradiation cystitis with hematuria 🅒

● **N30.8 Other cystitis**
    Abscess of bladder
    N30.80 Other cystitis without hematuria
    N30.81 Other cystitis with hematuria

● **N30.9 Cystitis, unspecified**
    N30.90 Cystitis, unspecified without hematuria
    N30.91 Cystitis, unspecified with hematuria

● **N31 Neuromuscular dysfunction of bladder, not elsewhere classified**
    Use additional code to identify any associated urinary
    incontinence (N39.3-N39.4-)
    Excludes1 cord bladder NOS (G95.89)
        neurogenic bladder due to cauda equina
            syndrome (G83.4)
        neuromuscular dysfunction due to spinal cord
            lesion (G95.89)

    N31.0 Uninhibited neuropathic bladder, not elsewhere classified
    N31.1 Reflex neuropathic bladder, not elsewhere classified
    N31.2 Flaccid neuropathic bladder, not elsewhere classified
        Atonic (motor) (sensory) neuropathic bladder
        Diminished tone of bladder muscle
        Autonomous neuropathic bladder
        Nonreflex neuropathic bladder
    N31.8 Other neuromuscular dysfunction of bladder
    N31.9 Neuromuscular dysfunction of bladder, unspecified
        Neurogenic bladder dysfunction NOS

● **N32 Other disorders of bladder**
    Excludes2 calculus of bladder (N21.0)
        cystocele (N81.1-)
        hernia or prolapse of bladder, female (N81.1-)

    N32.0 Bladder-neck obstruction
        Bladder-neck stenosis (acquired)
        Excludes1 congenital bladder-neck obstruction
            (Q64.3-)

    N32.1 Vesicointestinal fistula 🅒
        Vesicorectal fistula
        (Ex) See PDX Collection 933

    N32.2 Vesical fistula, not elsewhere classified 🅒
        Excludes1 fistula between bladder and female
            genital tract (N82.0-N82.1)
        (Ex) See PDX Collection 933

    N32.3 Diverticulum of bladder
        Formation of sac from a herniation of wall of bladder
        Excludes1 congenital diverticulum of bladder (Q64.6)
            diverticulitis of bladder (N30.8-)

● **N32.8 Other specified disorders of bladder**
    N32.81 Overactive bladder
        Detrusor muscle hyperactivity
        Excludes1 frequent urination due to
            specified bladder condition-
            code to condition

    N32.89 Other specified disorders of bladder
        Bladder hemorrhage
        Bladder hypertrophy
        Calcified bladder
        Contracted bladder

    N32.9 Bladder disorder, unspecified

▷ **N33 Bladder disorders in diseases classified elsewhere**
    Code first underlying disease, such as:
      schistosomiasis (B65.0-B65.9)
    Excludes1 bladder disorder in syphilis (A52.76)
        bladder disorder in tuberculosis (A18.12)
        candidal cystitis (B37.41)
        chlamydial cystitis(A56.01)
        cystitis in gonorrhea (A54.01)
        cystitis in neurogenic bladder (N31.-)
        diphtheritic cystitis (A36.85)
        syphilitic cystitis (A52.76)
        trichomonal cystitis (A59.03)

● **N34 Urethritis and urethral syndrome**
    Use additional code (B95-B97), to identify infectious agent
    Excludes2 Reiter's disease (M02.3-)
        urethritis in diseases with a predominantly sexual
            mode of transmission (A50-A64)
        urethrotrigonitis (N30.3-)

    N34.0 Urethral abscess 🅒 🅒
        Abscess (of) Cowper's gland
        Abscess (of) Littré's gland
        Abscess (of) urethral (gland)
        Periurethral abscess
        Excludes1 urethral caruncle (N36.2)
        (Ex) See PDX Collection 934

    N34.1 Nonspecific urethritis
        Nongonococcal urethritis
        Nonvenereal urethritis

    N34.2 Other urethritis
        Inflammation of urethra
        Meatitis, urethral
        Postmenopausal urethritis
        Ulcer of urethra (meatus)
        Urethritis NOS

    N34.3 Urethral syndrome, unspecified

● **N35 Urethral stricture**
    Narrowing of lumen of urethra caused by scarring due to infection or
    injury
    Excludes1 congenital urethral stricture (Q64.3-)
        postprocedural urethral stricture (N99.1-)

● **N35.0 Post-traumatic urethral stricture**
    Urethral stricture due to injury
    Excludes1 postprocedural urethral stricture (N99.1-)
    ● **N35.01 Post-traumatic urethral stricture, male**
        N35.010 Post-traumatic urethral stricture,
            male, meatal ♂
        N35.011 Post-traumatic bulbous urethral
            stricture ♂
        N35.012 Post-traumatic membranous urethral
            stricture ♂
        N35.013 Post-traumatic anterior urethral
            stricture ♂
        N35.014 Post-traumatic urethral stricture,
            male, unspecified ♂
        N35.016 Post-traumatic urethral stricture,
            male, overlapping sites ♂
            (Ex) See PDX Collection 934

    ● **N35.02 Post-traumatic urethral stricture, female**
        N35.021 Urethral stricture due to childbirth ♀
        N35.028 Other post-traumatic urethral
            stricture, female ♀

N Newborn Age: 0   **P** Pediatric Age: 0-17   **M** Maternity DX: 9-64   **A** Adult Age: 15-124   ♀ Females Only   ♂ Males Only

🅒 Complication\Comorbidity   🅒 Major C\C   (Ex) CC/MCC Exclusions   🅗 Hospital-Acquired Condition   🅗 Hierarchical Condition Category

1127

CHAPTER 14 (N00-N99)

● N35.1   Postinfective urethral stricture, not elsewhere classified
    Excludes1   urethral stricture associated with
                schistosomiasis (B65.-, N29)
            gonococcal urethral stricture (A54.01)
            syphilitic urethral stricture (A52.76)

    ● N35.11   Postinfective urethral stricture, not elsewhere
            classified, male
        N35.111   Postinfective urethral stricture, not
                elsewhere classified, male, meatal ♂
        N35.112   Postinfective bulbous urethral stricture,
                not elsewhere classified, male ♂
        N35.113   Postinfective membranous urethral
                stricture, not elsewhere classified,
                male ♂
        N35.114   Postinfective anterior urethral
                stricture, not elsewhere classified,
                male ♂
        N35.116   Postinfective urethral stricture,
                not elsewhere classified, male,
                overlapping sites ♂
        N35.119   Postinfective urethral stricture,
                not elsewhere classified, male,
                unspecified ♂
    N35.12   Postinfective urethral stricture, not elsewhere
            classified, female ♀

● N35.8   Other urethral stricture
    Excludes1   postprocedural urethral stricture (N99.1-)
    ● N35.81   Other urethral stricture, male
        N35.811   Other urethral stricture, male,
                meatal ♂
                (Ex:) See PDX Collection 934
        N35.812   Other urethral bulbous stricture,
                male ♂
                (Ex:) See PDX Collection 934
        N35.813   Other membranous urethral stricture,
                male ♂
                (Ex:) See PDX Collection 934
        N35.814   Other anterior urethral stricture,
                male ♂
                (Ex:) See PDX Collection 934
        N35.816   Other urethral stricture, male,
                overlapping sites ♂
                (Ex:) See PDX Collection 934
        N35.819   Other urethral stricture, male,
                unspecified site ♂
                (Ex:) See PDX Collection 934
    N35.82   Other urethral stricture, female ♀

● N35.9   Urethral stricture, unspecified
    ● N35.91   Urethral stricture, unspecified, male
        N35.911   Unspecified urethral stricture, male,
                meatal ♂
                (Ex:) See PDX Collection 934
        N35.912   Unspecified bulbous urethral
                stricture, male ♂
                (Ex:) See PDX Collection 934
        N35.913   Unspecified membranous urethral
                stricture, male ♂
                (Ex:) See PDX Collection 934
        N35.914   Unspecified anterior urethral
                stricture, male ♂
                (Ex:) See PDX Collection 934
        N35.916   Unspecified urethral stricture, male,
                overlapping sites ♂
                (Ex:) See PDX Collection 934
        N35.919   Unspecified urethral stricture, male,
                unspecified site ♂
                Pinhole meatus NOS
                Urethral stricture NOS
                (Ex:) See PDX Collection 934
    N35.92   Unspecified urethral stricture, female ♀

● N36   Other disorders of urethra
    N36.0   Urethral fistula 🅶
            Urethroperineal fistula
            Urethrorectal fistula
            Urinary fistula NOS
        Excludes1   urethroscrotal fistula (N50.89)
                urethrovaginal fistula (N82.1)
                urethrovesicovaginal fistula (N82.1)
        (Ex:) See PDX Collection 935
    N36.1   Urethral diverticulum
    N36.2   Urethral caruncle
    ● N36.4   Urethral functional and muscular disorders
            Use additional code to identify associated urinary stress
                incontinence (N39.3)
        N36.41   Hypermobility of urethra
        N36.42   Intrinsic sphincter deficiency (ISD)
        N36.43   Combined hypermobility of urethra and
                intrinsic sphincter deficiency
        N36.44   Muscular disorders of urethra
                Bladder sphincter dyssynergy
    N36.5   Urethral false passage
    N36.8   Other specified disorders of urethra
        Excludes1   congenital urethrocele (Q64.7)
                female urethrocele (N81.0)
    N36.9   Urethral disorder, unspecified

▷ N37   *Urethral disorders in diseases classified elsewhere*
        Code first underlying disease
        Excludes1   urethritis (in):
                candidal infection (B37.41)
                chlamydial (A56.01)
                gonorrhea (A54.01)
                syphilis (A52.76)
                trichomonal infection (A59.03)
                tuberculosis (A18.13)

● N39   Other disorders of urinary system
    Excludes2   hematuria NOS (R31.-)
            recurrent or persistent hematuria (N02.-)
            recurrent or persistent hematuria with specified
                morphological lesion (N02.-)
            proteinuria NOS (R80.-)
    N39.0   Urinary tract infection, site not specified 🅶 🅶
            Use additional code (B95-B97), to identify infectious
                agent
        Excludes1   candidiasis of urinary tract (B37.4-)
                neonatal urinary tract infection (P39.3)
                pyuria (R82.81)
                urinary tract infection of specified site,
                    such as:
                    cystitis (N30.-)
                    urethritis (N34.-)
        (Ex:) See PDX Collection 936
        Coding Clinic: 2018, Q2, P22; Q1, P16; 2012, Q4, P94
    N39.3   Stress incontinence (female) (male)
            Code also any associated overactive bladder (N32.81)
        Excludes1   mixed incontinence (N39.46)
    ● N39.4   Other specified urinary incontinence
            Code also any associated overactive bladder (N32.81)
        Excludes1   enuresis NOS (R32)
                functional urinary incontinence (R39.81)
                urinary incontinence associated with
                    cognitive impairment (R39.81)
                urinary incontinence NOS (R32)
                urinary incontinence of nonorganic origin
                    (F98.0)
        N39.41   Urge incontinence
            Excludes1   mixed incontinence (N39.46)
        N39.42   Incontinence without sensory awareness
                Insensible (urinary) incontinence
        N39.43   Post-void dribbling

▶ New   ⇒ Revised   ~~deleted~~ Deleted   Excludes 1   Excludes 2   Includes   Use additional   Code first   Code also   Key words
OGCR Official Guidelines   ● Unacceptable Principal Diagnosis   X Assign placeholder X   ● Use Additional Character(s)   ▷ Manifestation Code   Coding Clinic

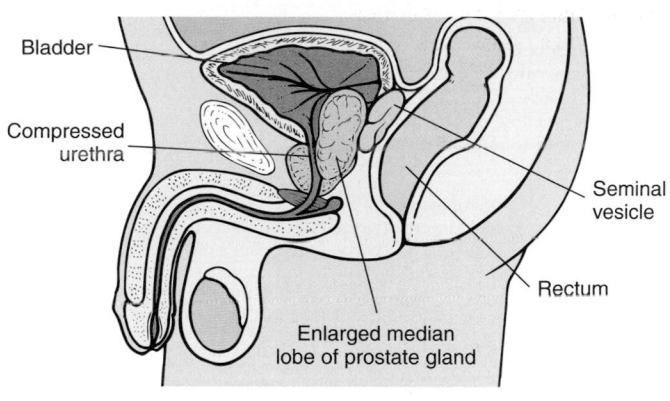

Figure 14-6   Benign prostatic hyperplasia. (From Shiland: Mastering Healthcare Terminology, ed 3, St. Louis, Mosby, 2010)

N39.44   **Nocturnal enuresis**
> **Excludes2**   nocturnal polyuria (R35.81)

N39.45   **Continuous leakage**

N39.46   **Mixed incontinence**
     Urge and stress incontinence

● **N39.49**   **Other specified urinary incontinence**

     N39.490   **Overflow incontinence**

     N39.491   **Coital incontinence**
         Coding Clinic: 2016, Q4, P44

     N39.492   **Postural (urinary) incontinence**
         Coding Clinic: 2016, Q4, P44

     N39.498   **Other specified urinary incontinence**
         Reflex incontinence
         Total incontinence

N39.8   **Other** specified disorders of urinary system

N39.9   **Disorder of urinary system, unspecified**

DISEASES OF MALE GENITAL ORGANS (N40-N53)

★ **(See Plate 5 of the Anatomy Illustrations.)**

● **N40**   **Benign prostatic hyperplasia**

     Includes   adenofibromatous hypertrophy of prostate
         benign hypertrophy of the prostate
         Enlargement of prostate gland usually occurring
           with age and causing obstructed urine flow
         benign prostatic hypertrophy
         BPH
         enlarged prostate
         nodular prostate
         polyp of prostate

     Excludes1   benign neoplasms of prostate (adenoma, benign)
         (fibroadenoma) (fibroma) (myoma) (D29.1)
         malignant neoplasm of prostate (C61)

N40.0   **Benign prostatic hyperplasia without lower urinary tract symptoms** ♂   **A**
     Enlarged prostate without LUTS
     Enlarged prostate NOS

N40.1   **Benign prostatic hyperplasia with lower urinary tract symptoms** ♂   **A**
     Enlarged prostate with LUTS
     Use additional code for associated symptoms, when
         specified:
         incomplete bladder emptying (R39.14)
         nocturia (R35.1)
         straining on urination (R39.16)
         urinary frequency (R35.0)
         urinary hesitancy (R39.11)
         urinary incontinence (N39.4-)
         urinary obstruction (N13.8)
         urinary retention (R33.8)
         urinary urgency (R39.15)
         weak urinary stream (R39.12)
     Coding Clinic: 2018, Q4, P55

N40.2   **Nodular prostate without lower urinary tract symptoms** ♂   **A**
     Nodular prostate without LUTS

N40.3   **Nodular prostate with lower urinary tract symptoms** ♂   **A**
     Use additional code for associated symptoms, when
         specified:
     incomplete bladder emptying (R39.14)
     nocturia (R35.1)
     straining on urination (R39.16)
     urinary frequency (R35.0)
     urinary hesitancy (R39.11)
     urinary incontinence (N39.4-)
     urinary obstruction (N13.8)
     urinary retention (R33.8)
     urinary urgency (R39.15)
     weak urinary stream (R39.12)

● **N41**   **Inflammatory diseases of prostate**
     Use additional code (B95-B97), to identify infectious agent

N41.0   **Acute prostatitis** ♂ 🦠   **A**
     (Ex:) See PDX Collection 937

N41.1   **Chronic prostatitis** ♂   **A**

N41.2   **Abscess of prostate** ♂ 🦠   **A**
     (Ex:) See PDX Collection 937

N41.3   **Prostatocystitis** ♂   **A**

N41.4   **Granulomatous prostatitis** ♂   **A**

N41.8   **Other inflammatory diseases of prostate** ♂   **A**

N41.9   **Inflammatory disease of prostate, unspecified** ♂   **A**
     Prostatitis NOS

● **N42**   **Other and unspecified disorders of prostate**

N42.0   **Calculus of prostate** ♂   **A**
     Prostatic stone

N42.1   **Congestion and hemorrhage of prostate** ♂   **A**

     Excludes1   enlarged prostate (N40.-)
         hematuria (R31.-)
         hyperplasia of prostate (N40.-)
         inflammatory diseases of prostate (N41.-)

● **N42.3**   **Dysplasia of prostate**
     Coding Clinic: 2016, Q4, P44

     N42.30   **Unspecified dysplasia of prostate** ♂

     N42.31   **Prostatic intraepithelial neoplasia** ♂
         PIN
         Prostatic intraepithelial neoplasia I (PIN I)
         Prostatic intraepithelial neoplasia II (PIN II)

         Excludes1   prostatic intraepithelial neoplasia
           III (PIN III) (D07.5)

     N42.32   **Atypical small acinar proliferation of prostate** ♂

     N42.39   **Other dysplasia of prostate** ♂

● **N42.8**   **Other specified disorders of prostate**

     N42.81   **Prostatodynia syndrome** ♂   **A**
         Painful prostate syndrome

     N42.82   **Prostatosis syndrome** ♂   **A**

     N42.83   **Cyst of prostate** ♂   **A**

     N42.89   **Other specified disorders of prostate** ♂   **A**

N42.9   **Disorder of prostate, unspecified** ♂   **A**

● **N43**   **Hydrocele and spermatocele**

     Includes   hydrocele of spermatic cord, testis or tunica
         vaginalis

     Excludes1   congenital hydrocele (P83.5)

N43.0   **Encysted hydrocele** ♂

N43.1   **Infected hydrocele** ♂ 🦠
     Use additional code (B95-B97), to identify infectious
         agent
     (Ex:) See PDX Collection 938

N43.2   **Other hydrocele** ♂

Item 14-7   **Hydrocele** is a sac of fluid accumulating in the testes membrane.

N   Newborn Age: 0   **P**   Pediatric Age: 0–17   **M**   Maternity DX: 9–64   **A**   Adult Age: 15–124   ♀ Females Only   ♂ Males Only
🦠 Complication\Comorbidity   🦠 Major C\C   (Ex:) CC/MCC Exclusions   🦠 Hospital-Acquired Condition   🦠 Hierarchical Condition Category

CHAPTER 14 (N00-N99)

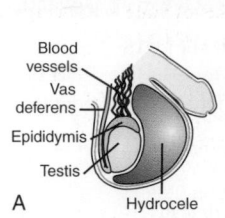
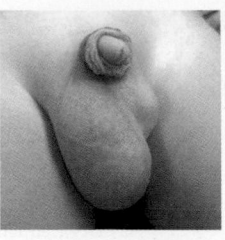

Figure 14-7 A. Hydrocele. **B.** Newborn with large right hydrocele. (**B** from Nelson WE, Kliegman R: Nelson Textbook of Pediatrics, Philadelphia, Saunders Elsevier, 2011)

N43.3   Hydrocele, unspecified ♂
● N43.4   Spermatocele of epididymis
          Spermatic cyst
          N43.40   Spermatocele of epididymis, unspecified ♂
          N43.41   Spermatocele of epididymis, single ♂
          N43.42   Spermatocele of epididymis, multiple ♂
● N44 Noninflammatory disorders of testis
   ● N44.0   Torsion of testis
             (Ex:) **For category N44.0 CC codes:** See PDX Collection 939
             N44.00   Torsion of testis, unspecified ♂ 🦠
             N44.01   Extravaginal torsion of spermatic cord ♂ 🦠
             N44.02   Intravaginal torsion of spermatic cord ♂ 🦠
                      Torsion of spermatic cord NOS
             N44.03   Torsion of appendix testis ♂ 🦠
             N44.04   Torsion of appendix epididymis ♂ 🦠
      N44.1   Cyst of tunica albuginea testis ♂
      N44.2   Benign cyst of testis ♂
      N44.8   Other noninflammatory disorders of the testis ♂
● N45 Orchitis and epididymitis
       Orchitis is inflammation of one or both of the testes as a result of mumps or other infection, trauma, or metastasis. Epididymitis is inflammation of the tubular structure that connects the testicle with the vas deferens.
       Use additional code (B95-B97), to identify infectious agent
      N45.1   Epididymitis ♂
      N45.2   Orchitis ♂
      N45.3   Epididymo-orchitis ♂
      N45.4   Abscess of epididymis or testis ♂ 🦠
              (Ex:) See PDX Collection 940
● N46 Male infertility
       Excludes1   vasectomy status (Z98.52)
   ● N46.0   Azoospermia
             Absolute male infertility
             Male infertility due to germinal (cell) aplasia
             Male infertility due to spermatogenic arrest (complete)
             N46.01   Organic azoospermia ♂   A
                      Azoospermia NOS
          ● N46.02   Azoospermia due to extratesticular causes
                     Code also associated cause
                     N46.021   Azoospermia due to drug therapy ♂   A
                     N46.022   Azoospermia due to infection ♂   A
                     N46.023   Azoospermia due to obstruction of
                               efferent ducts ♂   A
                     N46.024   Azoospermia due to radiation ♂   A
                     N46.025   Azoospermia due to systemic
                               disease ♂   A
                     N46.029   Azoospermia due to other
                               extratesticular causes ♂   A

Item 14-8 Male infertility is the inability of the female sex partner to conceive after one year of unprotected intercourse.
    Azoospermia is no sperm ejaculated and **oligospermia** is few sperm ejaculated—both resulting in infertility. Extratesticular causes such as injury, infections, radiation, and chemotherapy may also cause male infertility.

   ● N46.1   Oligospermia
             Male infertility due to germinal cell desquamation
             Male infertility due to hypospermatogenesis
             Male infertility due to incomplete spermatogenic arrest
             N46.11   Organic oligospermia ♂   A
                      Oligospermia NOS
          ● N46.12   Oligospermia due to extratesticular causes
                     Code also associated cause
                     N46.121   Oligospermia due to drug therapy ♂ A
                     N46.122   Oligospermia due to infection ♂   A
                     N46.123   Oligospermia due to obstruction of
                               efferent ducts ♂   A
                     N46.124   Oligospermia due to radiation ♂   A
                     N46.125   Oligospermia due to systemic
                               disease ♂   A
                     N46.129   Oligospermia due to other
                               extratesticular causes ♂
      N46.8   Other male infertility ♂   A
      N46.9   Male infertility, unspecified ♂   A
● N47 Disorders of prepuce
      N47.0   Adherent prepuce, newborn ♂   N
      N47.1   Phimosis ♂
      N47.2   Paraphimosis ♂
      N47.3   Deficient foreskin ♂
      N47.4   Benign cyst of prepuce ♂
      N47.5   Adhesions of prepuce and glans penis ♂
      N47.6   Balanoposthitis ♂
              Use additional code (B95-B97), to identify infectious
              agent
              Excludes1   balanitis (N48.1)
      N47.7   Other inflammatory diseases of prepuce ♂
              Use additional code (B95-B97), to identify infectious
              agent
      N47.8   Other disorders of prepuce ♂
● N48 Other disorders of penis
      N48.0   Leukoplakia of penis ♂
              Balanitis xerotica obliterans
              Kraurosis of penis
              Lichen sclerosus of external male genital organs
              Excludes1   carcinoma in situ of penis (D07.4)
      N48.1   Balanitis ♂
              Use additional code (B95-B97), to identify infectious
              agent
              Excludes1   amebic balanitis (A06.8)
                              balanitis xerotica obliterans (N48.0)
                              candidal balanitis (B37.42)
                              gonococcal balanitis (A54.23)
                              herpesviral [herpes simplex] balanitis
                                (A60.01)
   ● N48.2   Other inflammatory disorders of penis
             Use additional code (B95-B97), to identify infectious
             agent
             Excludes1   balanitis (N48.1)
                             balanitis xerotica obliterans (N48.0)
                             balanoposthitis (N47.6)
             N48.21   Abscess of corpus cavernosum and penis ♂
             N48.22   Cellulitis of corpus cavernosum and penis ♂
             N48.29   Other inflammatory disorders of penis ♂

▶ New   ⇒ Revised   ~~deleted~~ Deleted   Excludes 1   Excludes 2   Includes   Use additional   Code first   Code also   Key words

1130   OGCR Official Guidelines   ● Unacceptable Principal Diagnosis   X Assign placeholder X   ● Use Additional Character(s)   ▶ Manifestation Code   **Coding Clinic**

● N48.3   **Priapism**
    Painful erection
    Code first underlying cause
    Ⓔ **For category N48.3 CC codes:** See PDX Collection 941
    N48.30   **Priapism, unspecified** ♂ 🅖
    N48.31   **Priapism due to trauma** ♂ 🅖
    ▸ N48.32   *Priapism due to disease classified elsewhere* ♂ 🅖
    N48.33   **Priapism, drug-induced** ♂ 🅖
    N48.39   **Other priapism** ♂ 🅖

N48.5   **Ulcer of penis** ♂

N48.6   **Induratio penis plastica** ♂
    Peyronie's disease
    Plastic induration of penis

● N48.8   **Other specified disorders of penis**
    N48.81   **Thrombosis of superficial vein of penis** ♂
    N48.82   **Acquired torsion of penis** ♂
       Acquired torsion of penis NOS
       Excludes1   congenital torsion of penis
           (Q55.63)
    N48.83   **Acquired buried penis** ♂
       Excludes1   congenital hidden penis (Q55.64)
    N48.89   **Other specified disorders of penis** ♂

N48.9   **Disorder of penis, unspecified** ♂

● N49   **Inflammatory disorders of male genital organs, not elsewhere classified**
    Use additional code (B95-B97), to identify infectious agent
    Excludes1   inflammation of penis (N48.1, N48.2-)
           orchitis and epididymitis (N45.-)

N49.0   **Inflammatory disorders of seminal vesicle** ♂
    Vesiculitis NOS

N49.1   **Inflammatory disorders of spermatic cord, tunica vaginalis and vas deferens** ♂
    Vasitis

N49.2   **Inflammatory disorders of scrotum** ♂

N49.3   **Fournier gangrene** ♂

N49.8   **Inflammatory disorders of other specified male genital organs** ♂
    Inflammation of multiple sites in male genital organs

N49.9   **Inflammatory disorder of unspecified male genital organ** ♂
    Abscess of unspecified male genital organ
    Boil of unspecified male genital organ
    Carbuncle of unspecified male genital organ
    Cellulitis of unspecified male genital organ

Item 14–9 Seminal vesiculitis is an inflammation of the seminal vesicle. **Spermatocele** is a benign cystic accumulation of sperm arising from the head of the epididymis. **Torsion of the testis** is a medical emergency occurring most commonly in boys 7 to 12 years of age and results from a congenital abnormality of the covering of the testis allowing the testis to twist within its sac and cutting off the blood supply to the testis.

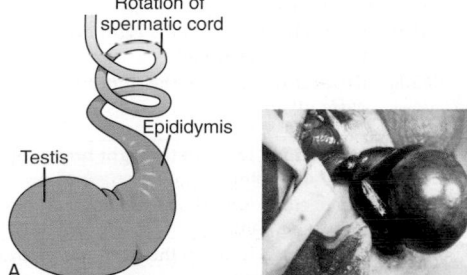

Rotation of spermatic cord

Epididymis

Testis

A   B

Figure 14-8 A. Torsion of testis. **B.** Torsion of the testis. (**B** from Kliegman R, Nelson WE: Nelson Textbook of Pediatrics, Philadelphia, Saunders, 2007)

● N50   **Other and unspecified disorders of male genital organs**
    Excludes2   torsion of testis (N44.0-)

N50.0   **Atrophy of testis** ♂

N50.1   **Vascular disorders of male genital organs** ♂
    Hematocele, NOS, of male genital organs
    Hemorrhage of male genital organs
    Thrombosis of male genital organs

N50.3   **Cyst of epididymis** ♂

● N50.8   **Other specified disorders of male genital organs**
    Coding Clinic: 2016, Q4, P45
    ● N50.81   **Testicular pain**
       N50.811   **Right testicular pain** ♂
       N50.812   **Left testicular pain** ♂
       N50.819   **Testicular pain, unspecified** ♂
    N50.82   **Scrotal pain** ♂
    N50.89   **Other specified disorders of the male genital organs** ♂
       Atrophy of scrotum, seminal vesicle, spermatic cord, tunica vaginalis and vas deferens
       Chylocele, tunica vaginalis (nonfilarial) NOS
       Edema of scrotum, seminal vesicle, spermatic cord, tunica vaginalis and vas deferens
       Hypertrophy of scrotum, seminal vesicle, spermatic cord, tunica vaginalis and vas deferens
       Stricture of spermatic cord, tunica vaginalis, and vas deferens
       Ulcer of scrotum, seminal vesicle, spermatic cord, testis, tunica vaginalis and vas deferens
       Urethroscrotal fistula

N50.9   **Disorder of male genital organs, unspecified** ♂

▸ N51   *Disorders of male genital organs in diseases classified elsewhere* ♂
    Code first underlying disease, such as:
    filariasis (B74.0-B74.9)
    Excludes1   amebic balanitis (A06.8)
           candidal balanitis (B37.42)
           gonococcal balanitis (A54.23)
           gonococcal prostatitis (A54.22)
           herpesviral [herpes simplex] balanitis (A60.01)
           trichomonal prostatitis (A59.02)
           tuberculous prostatitis (A18.14)

● N52   **Male erectile dysfunction**
    Excludes1   psychogenic impotence (F52.21)
    ● N52.0   **Vasculogenic erectile dysfunction**
       N52.01   **Erectile dysfunction due to arterial insufficiency** ♂   A
       N52.02   **Corporo-venous occlusive erectile dysfunction** ♂   A
       N52.03   **Combined arterial insufficiency and corporo-venous occlusive erectile dysfunction** ♂   A
    ▸ N52.1   *Erectile dysfunction due to diseases classified elsewhere* ♂   A
       Code first underlying disease
    N52.2   **Drug-induced erectile dysfunction** ♂   A
    ● N52.3   **Postprocedural erectile dysfunction**
       N52.31   **Erectile dysfunction following radical prostatectomy** ♂   A
       N52.32   **Erectile dysfunction following radical cystectomy** ♂   A
       N52.33   **Erectile dysfunction following urethral surgery** ♂   A
       N52.34   **Erectile dysfunction following simple prostatectomy** ♂   A
       N52.35   **Erectile dysfunction following radiation therapy** ♂   A
       Coding Clinic: 2016, Q4, P45

N Newborn Age: 0   **P** Pediatric Age: 0–17   **M** Maternity DX: 9–64   **A** Adult Age: 15–124   ♀ Females Only   ♂ Males Only

🅒 Complication\Comorbidity   🅜 Major C\C   Ⓔ CC/MCC Exclusions   🅗 Hospital-Acquired Condition   🅖 Hierarchical Condition Category

N52.36   Erectile dysfunction following interstitial seed therapy ♂   A
     Coding Clinic: 2016, Q4, P45

N52.37   Erectile dysfunction following prostate ablative therapy ♂   A
     Erectile dysfunction following cryotherapy
     Erectile dysfunction following other prostate ablative therapies
     Erectile dysfunction following ultrasound ablative therapies
     Coding Clinic: 2016, Q4, P45

N52.39   Other and unspecified postprocedural erectile dysfunction ♂   A

N52.8   Other male erectile dysfunction ♂   A

N52.9   Male erectile dysfunction, unspecified ♂   A
     Impotence NOS

● N53   Other male sexual dysfunction
     Excludes1   psychogenic sexual dysfunction (F52.-)

● N53.1   Ejaculatory dysfunction
     Excludes1   premature ejaculation (F52.4)

N53.11   Retarded ejaculation ♂

N53.12   Painful ejaculation ♂

N53.13   Anejaculatory orgasm ♂

N53.14   Retrograde ejaculation ♂

N53.19   Other ejaculatory dysfunction ♂
     Ejaculatory dysfunction NOS

N53.8   Other male sexual dysfunction ♂

N53.9   Unspecified male sexual dysfunction ♂

DISORDERS OF BREAST (N60-N65)

Excludes1   disorders of breast associated with childbirth (O91-O92)

● N60   Benign mammary dysplasia
     Benign lumpiness of breast
     Includes   fibrocystic mastopathy

● N60.0   Solitary cyst of breast
     Cyst of breast

N60.01   Solitary cyst of right breast

N60.02   Solitary cyst of left breast

N60.09   Solitary cyst of unspecified breast

● N60.1   Diffuse cystic mastopathy
     Cystic breast
     Fibrocystic disease of breast
     Excludes1   diffuse cystic mastopathy with epithelial proliferation (N60.3-)

N60.11   Diffuse cystic mastopathy of right breast   A

N60.12   Diffuse cystic mastopathy of left breast   A

N60.19   Diffuse cystic mastopathy of unspecified breast   A

● N60.2   Fibroadenosis of breast
     Adenofibrosis of breast
     Excludes2   fibroadenoma of breast (D24.-)

N60.21   Fibroadenosis of right breast

N60.22   Fibroadenosis of left breast

N60.29   Fibroadenosis of unspecified breast

● N60.3   Fibrosclerosis of breast
     Cystic mastopathy with epithelial proliferation

N60.31   Fibrosclerosis of right breast

N60.32   Fibrosclerosis of left breast

N60.39   Fibrosclerosis of unspecified breast

● N60.4   Mammary duct ectasia

N60.41   Mammary duct ectasia of right breast

N60.42   Mammary duct ectasia of left breast

N60.49   Mammary duct ectasia of unspecified breast

● N60.8   Other benign mammary dysplasias

N60.81   Other benign mammary dysplasias of right breast

N60.82   Other benign mammary dysplasias of left breast

N60.89   Other benign mammary dysplasias of unspecified breast

● N60.9   Unspecified benign mammary dysplasia

N60.91   Unspecified benign mammary dysplasia of right breast

N60.92   Unspecified benign mammary dysplasia of left breast

N60.99   Unspecified benign mammary dysplasia of unspecified breast

● N61   Inflammatory disorders of breast
     Excludes1   inflammatory carcinoma of breast (C50.9)
       inflammatory disorder of breast associated with childbirth (O91.-)
       neonatal infective mastitis (P39.0)
       thrombophlebitis of breast [Mondor's disease] (I80.8)

N61.0   Mastitis without abscess
     Infective mastitis (acute) (nonpuerperal) (subacute)
     Mastitis (acute) (nonpuerperal) (subacute) NOS
     Cellulitis (acute) (nonpuerperal) (subacute) of breast NOS
     Cellulitis (acute) (nonpuerperal) (subacute) of nipple NOS

N61.1   Abscess of the breast and nipple
     Abscess (acute) (chronic) (nonpuerperal) of areola
     Abscess (acute) (chronic) (nonpuerperal) of breast
     Carbuncle of breast
     Mastitis with abscess

● N61.2   Granulomatous mastitis

N61.20   Granulomatous mastitis, unspecified breast

N61.21   Granulomatous mastitis, right breast

N61.22   Granulomatous mastitis, left breast

N61.23   Granulomatous mastitis, bilateral breast

N62   Hypertrophy of breast
     Gynecomastia
     Hypertrophy of breast NOS
     Massive pubertal hypertrophy of breast
     Excludes1   breast engorgement of newborn (P83.4)
       disproportion of reconstructed breast (N65.1)

● N63   Unspecified lump in breast
     Nodule(s) NOS in breast

N63.0   Unspecified lump in unspecified breast

● N63.1   Unspecified lump in the right breast

N63.10   Unspecified lump in the right breast, unspecified quadrant

N63.11   Unspecified lump in the right breast, upper outer quadrant
     Coding Clinic: 2017, Q4, P19

N63.12   Unspecified lump in the right breast, upper inner quadrant

N63.13   Unspecified lump in the right breast, lower outer quadrant

N63.14   Unspecified lump in the right breast, lower inner quadrant

N63.15   Unspecified lump in the right breast, overlapping quadrants

Figure 14-9   Breast.

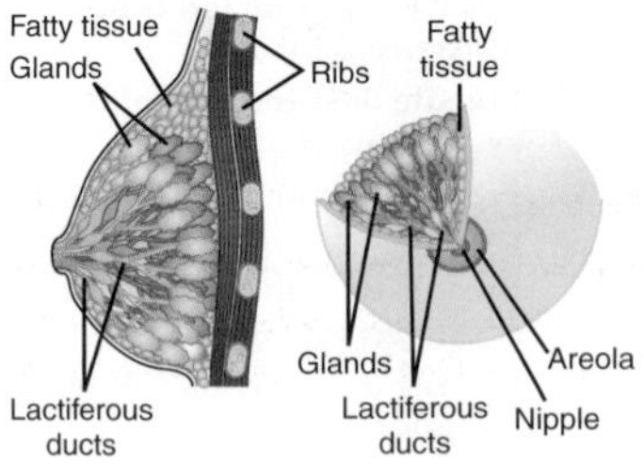

Fatty tissue / Glands / Ribs / Fatty tissue / Glands / Lactiferous ducts / Lactiferous ducts / Areola / Nipple

▶ New   ⇒ Revised   ~~deleted~~ Deleted   Excludes 1   Excludes 2   Includes   Use additional   Code first   Code also   Key words
OGCR Official Guidelines   ● Unacceptable Principal Diagnosis   X Assign placeholder X   ● Use Additional Character(s)   ▷ Manifestation Code   Coding Clinic

● **N63.2**   Unspecified lump in the left breast

     N63.20   Unspecified lump in the left breast, unspecified quadrant

     N63.21   Unspecified lump in the left breast, upper outer quadrant

     N63.22   Unspecified lump in the left breast, upper inner quadrant

     N63.23   Unspecified lump in the left breast, lower outer quadrant

     N63.24   Unspecified lump in the left breast, lower inner quadrant

     N63.25   Unspecified lump in the left breast, overlapping quadrants

● **N63.3**   Unspecified lump in axillary tail

     N63.31   Unspecified lump in axillary tail of the right breast

     N63.32   Unspecified lump in axillary tail of the left breast

● **N63.4**   Unspecified lump in breast, subareolar

     N63.41   Unspecified lump in right breast, subareolar

     N63.42   Unspecified lump in left breast, subareolar

● **N64**   Other disorders of breast

     Excludes2   mechanical complication of breast prosthesis and implant (T85.4-)

     N64.0   Fissure and fistula of nipple

●   N64.1   Fat necrosis of breast

         Fat necrosis (segmental) of breast

         Code first breast necrosis due to breast graft (T85.898)

     N64.2   Atrophy of breast

     N64.3   Galactorrhea not associated with childbirth

         Excessive or spontaneous flow of milk

     N64.4   Mastodynia

●   N64.5   Other signs and symptoms in breast

         Excludes2   abnormal findings on diagnostic imaging of breast (R92.-)

     N64.51   Induration of breast

     N64.52   Nipple discharge

         Excludes1   abnormal findings in nipple discharge (R89.-)

     N64.53   Retraction of nipple

     N64.59   Other signs and symptoms in breast

●   N64.8   Other specified disorders of breast

     N64.81   Ptosis of breast   A

         Excludes1   ptosis of native breast in relation to reconstructed breast (N65.1)

     N64.82   Hypoplasia of breast   A

         Micromastia

         Excludes1   congenital absence of breast (Q83.0)

             hypoplasia of native breast in relation to reconstructed breast (N65.1)

     N64.89   Other specified disorders of breast

         Galactocele

         Subinvolution of breast (postlactational)

         Coding Clinic: 2019, Q1, P32; 2018, Q1, P4

     N64.9   Disorder of breast, unspecified

         Coding Clinic: 2018, Q1, P4

● **N65**   Deformity and disproportion of reconstructed breast

     N65.0   Deformity of reconstructed breast   A

         Contour irregularity in reconstructed breast

         Excess tissue in reconstructed breast

         Misshapen reconstructed breast

     N65.1   Disproportion of reconstructed breast   A

         Breast asymmetry between native breast and reconstructed breast

         Disproportion between native breast and reconstructed breast

---

INFLAMMATORY DISEASES OF FEMALE PELVIC ORGANS (N70-N77)

     Excludes1   inflammatory diseases of female pelvic organs complicating:

         abortion or ectopic or molar pregnancy (O00-O07, O08.0)

         pregnancy, childbirth and the puerperium (O23.-, O75.3, O85, O86.-)

★ **(See Plate 35 of the Anatomy Illustrations.)**

● **N70**   Salpingitis and oophoritis

     Oophoritis = inflammation of ovary

     Salpingitis = inflammation of fallopian tube

     Includes   abscess (of) fallopian tube

         abscess (of) ovary

         pyosalpinx

         salpingo-oophoritis

         tubo-ovarian abscess

         tubo-ovarian inflammatory disease

     Use additional code (B95-B97), to identify infectious agent

     Excludes1   gonococcal infection (A54.24)

         tuberculous infection (A18.17)

●   N70.0   Acute salpingitis and oophoritis

     (Ex:) **For category N70.0 CC codes: See PDX Collection 942**

     N70.01   Acute salpingitis ♀ %

     N70.02   Acute oophoritis ♀ %

     N70.03   Acute salpingitis and oophoritis ♀ %

●   N70.1   Chronic salpingitis and oophoritis

     Hydrosalpinx

     N70.11   Chronic salpingitis ♀

     N70.12   Chronic oophoritis ♀

     N70.13   Chronic salpingitis and oophoritis ♀

●   N70.9   Salpingitis and oophoritis, unspecified

     N70.91   Salpingitis, unspecified ♀

     N70.92   Oophoritis, unspecified ♀

     N70.93   Salpingitis and oophoritis, unspecified ♀

● **N71**   Inflammatory disease of uterus, except cervix

     Includes   endo (myo) metritis

         metritis

         myometritis

         pyometra

         uterine abscess

     Use additional code (B95-B97), to identify infectious agent

     Excludes1   hyperplastic endometritis (N85.0-)

         infection of uterus following delivery (O85, O86.-)

     N71.0   Acute inflammatory disease of uterus ♀ %

         (Ex:) **See PDX Collection 943**

     N71.1   Chronic inflammatory disease of uterus ♀

     N71.9   Inflammatory disease of uterus, unspecified ♀

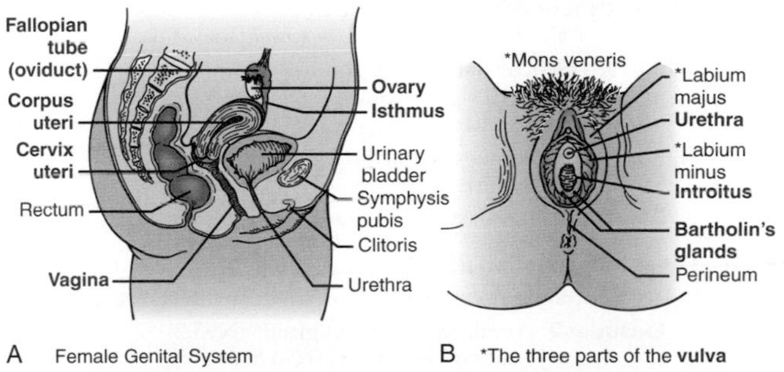

Figure 14-10   A. Female genital system. **B.** External female genital system. (From Buck CJ: Step-by-Step Medical Coding, ed 2016, St. Louis, Elsevier, 2016)

Item 14–10 Salpingitis is an infection of one or both fallopian tubes. **Oophoritis** is an infection of one or both ovaries.

N   Newborn Age: 0   P   Pediatric Age: 0–17   M   Maternity DX: 9–64   A   Adult Age: 15–124   ♀   Females Only   ♂   Males Only

%   Complication\Comorbidity   %   Major C\C   (Ex:)   CC/MCC Exclusions   %   Hospital-Acquired Condition   %   Hierarchical Condition Category

1133

CHAPTER 14 (N00-N99)

N72   Inflammatory disease of cervix uteri ♀
  Includes   cervicitis (with or without erosion or ectropion)
          endocervicitis (with or without erosion or
            ectropion)
          exocervicitis (with or without erosion or ectropion)
      Use additional code (B95-B97), to identify infectious agent
  Excludes1   erosion and ectropion of cervix without cervicitis
          (N86)

● **N73   Other female pelvic inflammatory diseases**
      Use additional code (B95-B97), to identify infectious agent
  N73.0   Acute parametritis and pelvic cellulitis ♀ ⚕
          Abscess of broad ligament
          Abscess of parametrium
          Pelvic cellulitis, female
          (Ex:) See PDX Collection 942
  N73.1   Chronic parametritis and pelvic cellulitis ♀
          Any condition in N73.0 specified as chronic
      Excludes1   tuberculous parametritis and pelvic
              cellulitis (A18.17)
  N73.2   Unspecified parametritis and pelvic cellulitis ♀
          Any condition in N73.0 unspecified whether acute or
            chronic
  N73.3   Female acute pelvic peritonitis ♀ ⚕
          (Ex:) See PDX Collection 942
  N73.4   Female chronic pelvic peritonitis ♀ ⚕
      Excludes1   tuberculous pelvic (female) peritonitis
              (A18.17)
          (Ex:) See PDX Collection 942
  N73.5   Female pelvic peritonitis, unspecified ♀
  N73.6   Female pelvic peritoneal adhesions (postinfective) ♀
      Excludes2   postprocedural pelvic peritoneal
              adhesions (N99.4)
  N73.8   Other specified female pelvic inflammatory diseases ♀
  N73.9   Female pelvic inflammatory disease, unspecified ♀
          Female pelvic infection or inflammation NOS

▌ **N74   Female pelvic inflammatory disorders in diseases classified
      elsewhere ♀**
      Code first underlying disease
      Excludes1   chlamydial cervicitis (A56.02)
              chlamydial pelvic inflammatory disease (A56.11)
              gonococcal cervicitis (A54.03)
              gonococcal pelvic inflammatory disease (A54.24)
              herpesviral [herpes simplex] cervicitis (A60.03)
              herpesviral [herpes simplex] pelvic inflammatory
                disease (A60.09)
              syphilitic cervicitis (A52.76)
              syphilitic pelvic inflammatory disease (A52.76)
              trichomonal cervicitis (A59.09)
              tuberculous cervicitis (A18.16)
              tuberculous pelvic inflammatory disease (A18.17)

● **N75   Diseases of Bartholin's gland**
  N75.0   Cyst of Bartholin's gland ♀
          Cysts filled with liquid or semisolid material
  N75.1   Abscess of Bartholin's gland ♀ ⚕
          Localized collection of pus
          (Ex:) See PDX Collection 944
  N75.8   Other diseases of Bartholin's gland ♀
          Bartholinitis
  N75.9   Disease of Bartholin's gland, unspecified ♀

● **N76   Other inflammation of vagina and vulva**
      Use additional code (B95-B97), to identify infectious agent
  Excludes2   senile (atrophic) vaginitis (N95.2)
          vulvar vestibulitis (N94.810)
  N76.0   Acute vaginitis ♀
          Acute vulvovaginitis
          Vaginitis NOS
          Vulvovaginitis NOS
  N76.1   Subacute and chronic vaginitis ♀
          Chronic vulvovaginitis
          Subacute vulvovaginitis

  N76.2   Acute vulvitis ♀
          Vulvitis NOS
  N76.3   Subacute and chronic vulvitis ♀
  N76.4   Abscess of vulva ♀ ⚕
          Furuncle of vulva
          (Ex:) See PDX Collection 944
  N76.5   Ulceration of vagina ♀
  N76.6   Ulceration of vulva ♀
● **N76.8   Other specified inflammation of vagina and vulva**
      N76.81   Mucositis (ulcerative) of vagina and vulva ♀ ⚕
              Code also type of associated therapy, such as:
                antineoplastic and immunosuppressive
                  drugs (T45.1X-)
                radiological procedure and radiotherapy
                  (Y84.2)
          Excludes2   gastrointestinal mucositis
                  (ulcerative) (K92.81)
                  nasal mucositis (ulcerative)
                    (J34.81)
                  oral mucositis (ulcerative) (K12.3-)
              (Ex:) See PDX Collection 945
      **N76.89   Other specified inflammation of vagina and
              vulva ♀**

● **N77   Vulvovaginal ulceration and inflammation in diseases classified
      elsewhere**
  ▌ **N77.0   Ulceration of vulva in diseases classified elsewhere ♀**
          Code first underlying disease, such as:
            Behçet's disease (M35.2)
      Excludes1   ulceration of vulva in gonococcal
              infection (A54.02)
              ulceration of vulva in herpesviral [herpes
                simplex] infection (A60.04)
              ulceration of vulva in syphilis (A51.0)
              ulceration of vulva in tuberculosis (A18.18)
  ▌ **N77.1   Vaginitis, vulvitis and vulvovaginitis in diseases
          classified elsewhere ♀**
          Code first underlying disease, such as:
            pinworm (B80)
      Excludes1   candidial vulvovaginitis (B37.3)
              chlamydial vulvovaginitis (A56.02)
              gonococcal vulvovaginitis (A54.02)
              herpesviral [herpes simplex]
                vulvovaginitis (A60.04)
              trichomonal vulvovaginitis (A59.01)
              tuberculous vulvovaginitis (A18.18)
              vulvovaginitis in early syphilis (A51.0)
              vulvovaginitis in late syphilis (A52.76)

NONINFLAMMATORY DISORDERS OF FEMALE GENITAL TRACT (N80-N98)

● **N80   Endometriosis**
  N80.0   Endometriosis of uterus ♀
          Adenomyosis
      Excludes1   stromal endometriosis (D39.0)
  N80.1   Endometriosis of ovary ♀
  N80.2   Endometriosis of fallopian tube ♀
  N80.3   Endometriosis of pelvic peritoneum ♀
  N80.4   Endometriosis of rectovaginal septum and vagina ♀
  N80.5   Endometriosis of intestine ♀
  N80.6   Endometriosis in cutaneous scar ♀
  N80.8   Other endometriosis ♀
          Endometriosis of thorax
  N80.9   Endometriosis, unspecified ♀

Item 14-11 Endometriosis is a condition for which no clear cause has
been identified. Endometrial tissue is expelled from the uterus into the abdominal
cavity and can implant onto a variety of organs. Classification is based on the
site of implant of the endometrial tissue.

▶ New   ⮕ Revised   ~~deleted~~ Deleted   Excludes 1   Excludes 2   Includes   Use additional   Code first   Code also   Key words

OGCR Official Guidelines   ● Unacceptable Principal Diagnosis   X Assign placeholder X   ● Use Additional Character(s)   ▌ Manifestation Code   Coding Clinic

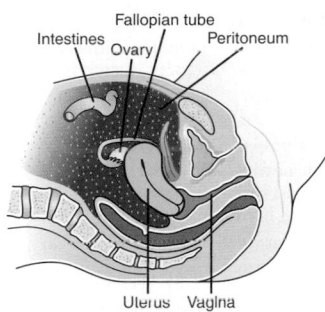

Figure 14-11   Sites of potential endometrial implants.

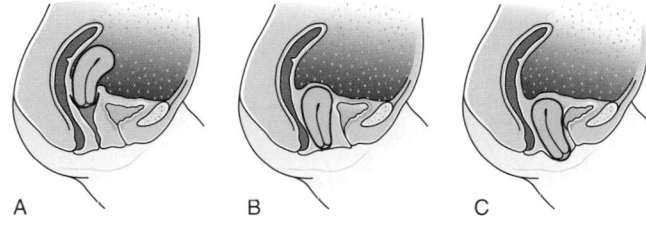

Figure 14-12   Three stages of uterine prolapse. **A.** Uterus is prolapsed. **B.** Vagina and uterus are prolapsed (incomplete uterovaginal prolapse). **C.** Vagina and uterus are completely prolapsed and are exposed through the external genitalia (complete uterovaginal prolapse).

●N81   **Female genital prolapse**

> **Excludes1**   genital prolapse complicating pregnancy, labor or delivery (O34.5-)
> prolapse and hernia of ovary and fallopian tube (N83.4-)
> prolapse of vaginal vault after hysterectomy (N99.3)

N81.0   **Urethrocele** ♀

> **Excludes1**   urethrocele with cystocele (N81.1-)
> urethrocele with prolapse of uterus (N81.2-N81.4)

●N81.1   **Cystocele**
> Cystocele with urethrocele
> Cystourethrocele
> **Excludes1**   cystocele with prolapse of uterus (N81.2-N81.4)

    N81.10   **Cystocele, unspecified** ♀
> Prolapse of (anterior) vaginal wall NOS

    N81.11   **Cystocele, midline** ♀

    N81.12   **Cystocele, lateral** ♀
> Paravaginal cystocele

N81.2   **Incomplete uterovaginal prolapse** ♀
> First degree uterine prolapse
> Prolapse of cervix NOS
> Second degree uterine prolapse
> **Excludes1**   cervical stump prolapse (N81.85)

N81.3   **Complete uterovaginal prolapse** ♀
> Procidentia (uteri) NOS
> Third degree uterine prolapse

N81.4   **Uterovaginal prolapse, unspecified** ♀
> Prolapse of uterus NOS

N81.5   **Vaginal enterocele** ♀
> **Excludes1**   enterocele with prolapse of uterus (N81.2-N81.4)

N81.6   **Rectocele** ♀
> Prolapse of posterior vaginal wall
> Use additional code for any associated fecal incontinence, if applicable (R15.-)
> **Excludes2**   perineocele (N81.81)
> rectal prolapse (K62.3)
> rectocele with prolapse of uterus (N81.2-N81.4)

●N81.8   **Other female genital prolapse**

    N81.81   **Perineocele** ♀

    N81.82   **Incompetence or weakening of pubocervical tissue** ♀

    N81.83   **Incompetence or weakening of rectovaginal tissue** ♀

    N81.84   **Pelvic muscle wasting** ♀
> Disuse atrophy of pelvic muscles and anal sphincter

    N81.85   **Cervical stump prolapse** ♀

    N81.89   **Other female genital prolapse** ♀
> Deficient perineum
> Old laceration of muscles of pelvic floor

N81.9   **Female genital prolapse, unspecified** ♀

●N82   **Fistulae involving female genital tract**
> **Excludes1**   vesicointestinal fistulae (N32.1)
> (Ex) For category N82 CC codes: See PDX Collection 946

N82.0   **Vesicovaginal fistula** ♀ 🅒

N82.1   **Other female urinary-genital tract fistulae** ♀ 🅒
> Cervicovesical fistula
> Ureterovaginal fistula
> Urethrovaginal fistula
> Uteroureteric fistula
> Uterovesical fistula
> **Coding Clinic: 2017, Q3, P4**

N82.2   **Fistula of vagina to small intestine** ♀ 🅒

N82.3   **Fistula of vagina to large intestine** ♀ 🅒
> Rectovaginal fistula

N82.4   **Other female intestinal-genital tract fistulae** ♀ 🅒
> Intestinouterine fistula

N82.5   **Female genital tract-skin fistulae** ♀ 🅒
> Uterus to abdominal wall fistula
> Vaginoperineal fistula

N82.8   **Other female genital tract fistulae** ♀ 🅒

N82.9   **Female genital tract fistula, unspecified** ♀ 🅒

●N83   **Noninflammatory disorders of ovary, fallopian tube and broad ligament**
> **Excludes2**   hydrosalpinx (N70.1-)

●N83.0   **Follicular cyst of ovary**
> Cyst of graafian follicle
> Hemorrhagic follicular cyst (of ovary)
> **Coding Clinic: 2016, Q4, P46**

    N83.00   **Follicular cyst of ovary, unspecified side** ♀

    N83.01   **Follicular cyst of right ovary** ♀

    N83.02   **Follicular cyst of left ovary** ♀

●N83.1   **Corpus luteum cyst**
> Hemorrhagic corpus luteum cyst
> **Coding Clinic: 2016, Q4, P46**

    N83.10   **Corpus luteum cyst of ovary, unspecified side** ♀

    N83.11   **Corpus luteum cyst of right ovary** ♀

    N83.12   **Corpus luteum cyst of left ovary** ♀

●N83.2   **Other and unspecified ovarian cysts**
> **Excludes1**   developmental ovarian cyst (Q50.1)
> neoplastic ovarian cyst (D27.-)
> polycystic ovarian syndrome (E28.2)
> Stein-Leventhal syndrome (E28.2)
> **Coding Clinic: 2016, Q4, P46**

    ●N83.20   **Unspecified ovarian cysts**

       N83.201   **Unspecified ovarian cyst, right side** ♀

       N83.202   **Unspecified ovarian cyst, left side** ♀

       N83.209   **Unspecified ovarian cyst, unspecified side** ♀
> Ovarian cyst, NOS

N Newborn Age: 0   **P** Pediatric Age: 0–17   **M** Maternity DX: 9–64   **A** Adult Age: 15–124   ♀ Females Only   ♂ Males Only

🅒 Complication\Comorbidity   🅒 Major C\C   (Ex) CC/MCC Exclusions   Hospital-Acquired Condition   🅒 Hierarchical Condition Category

CHAPTER 14 (N00-N99)

1135

● **N83.29**   **Other ovarian cysts**
     Retention cyst of ovary
     Simple cyst of ovary
     N83.291   Other ovarian cyst, right side ♀
     N83.292   Other ovarian cyst, left side ♀
     N83.299   Other ovarian cyst, unspecified side ♀

● **N83.3**   **Acquired atrophy of ovary and fallopian tube**
     Coding Clinic: 2016, Q4, P46
   ● **N83.31**   **Acquired atrophy of ovary**
     N83.311   Acquired atrophy of right ovary ♀
     N83.312   Acquired atrophy of left ovary ♀
     N83.319   Acquired atrophy of ovary, unspecified side ♀
         Acquired atrophy of ovary, NOS
   ● **N83.32**   **Acquired atrophy of fallopian tube**
     N83.321   Acquired atrophy of right fallopian tube ♀
     N83.322   Acquired atrophy of left fallopian tube ♀
     N83.329   Acquired atrophy of fallopian tube, unspecified side ♀
         Acquired atrophy of fallopian tube, NOS
   ● **N83.33**   **Acquired atrophy of ovary and fallopian tube**
     N83.331   Acquired atrophy of right ovary and fallopian tube ♀
     N83.332   Acquired atrophy of left ovary and fallopian tube ♀
     N83.339   Acquired atrophy of ovary and fallopian tube, unspecified side ♀
         Acquired atrophy of ovary and fallopian tube, NOS

● **N83.4**   **Prolapse and hernia of ovary and fallopian tube**
     Coding Clinic: 2016, Q4, P46
     N83.40   Prolapse and hernia of ovary and fallopian tube, unspecified side ♀
         Prolapse and hernia of ovary and fallopian tube, NOS
     N83.41   Prolapse and hernia of right ovary and fallopian tube ♀
     N83.42   Prolapse and hernia of left ovary and fallopian tube ♀

● **N83.5**   **Torsion of ovary, ovarian pedicle and fallopian tube**
     Torsion of accessory tube
     Ⓔⓧ For category N83.5 CC codes: See PDX Collection 947
     Coding Clinic: 2016, Q4, P46
   ● **N83.51**   **Torsion of ovary and ovarian pedicle**
     N83.511   Torsion of right ovary and ovarian pedicle ♀ 🗢
     N83.512   Torsion of left ovary and ovarian pedicle ♀ 🗢
     N83.519   Torsion of ovary and ovarian pedicle, unspecified side ♀ 🗢
         Torsion of ovary and ovarian pedicle, NOS
   ● **N83.52**   **Torsion of fallopian tube**
     Torsion of hydatid of Morgagni
     N83.521   Torsion of right fallopian tube ♀ 🗢
     N83.522   Torsion of left fallopian tube ♀ 🗢
     N83.529   Torsion of fallopian tube, unspecified side ♀ 🗢
         Torsion of fallopian tube, NOS
     N83.53   Torsion of ovary, ovarian pedicle and fallopian tube ♀ 🗢

● **N83.6**   **Hematosalpinx** ♀
     Excludes1   hematosalpinx (with) (in):
         hematocolpos (N89.7)
         hematometra (N85.7)
         tubal pregnancy (O00.1-)
   N83.7   **Hematoma of broad ligament** ♀
   N83.8   **Other noninflammatory disorders of ovary, fallopian tube and broad ligament** ♀
     Broad ligament laceration syndrome [Allen-Masters]
   N83.9   **Noninflammatory disorder of ovary, fallopian tube and broad ligament, unspecified** ♀

● **N84**   **Polyp of female genital tract**
     Excludes1   adenomatous polyp (D28.-)
               placental polyp (O90.89)
   N84.0   **Polyp of corpus uteri** ♀
     Polyp of endometrium
     Polyp of uterus NOS
     Excludes1   polypoid endometrial hyperplasia (N85.0-)
   N84.1   **Polyp of cervix uteri** ♀
     Mucous polyp of cervix
   N84.2   **Polyp of vagina** ♀
   N84.3   **Polyp of vulva** ♀
     Polyp of labia
   N84.8   **Polyp of other parts of female genital tract** ♀
   N84.9   **Polyp of female genital tract, unspecified** ♀

● **N85**   **Other noninflammatory disorders of uterus, except cervix**
     Excludes1   endometriosis (N80.-)
               inflammatory diseases of uterus (N71.-)
               noninflammatory disorders of cervix, except malposition (N86-N88)
               polyp of corpus uteri (N84.0)
               uterine prolapse (N81.-)
   ● **N85.0**   **Endometrial hyperplasia**
     N85.00   Endometrial hyperplasia, unspecified ♀
         Hyperplasia (adenomatous) (cystic) (glandular) of endometrium
         Hyperplastic endometritis
     N85.01   Benign endometrial hyperplasia ♀
         Endometrial hyperplasia (complex) (simple) without atypia
     N85.02   Endometrial intraepithelial neoplasia [EIN] ♀
         Endometrial hyperplasia with atypia
         Excludes1   malignant neoplasm of endometrium (with endometrial intraepithelial neoplasia [EIN]) (C54.1)
   N85.2   **Hypertrophy of uterus** ♀
     Bulky or enlarged uterus
     Excludes1   puerperal hypertrophy of uterus (O90.89)
   N85.3   **Subinvolution of uterus** ♀
     Excludes1   puerperal subinvolution of uterus (O90.89)
   N85.4   **Malposition of uterus** ♀
     Anteversion of uterus
     Retroflexion of uterus
     Retroversion of uterus
     Excludes1   malposition of uterus complicating pregnancy, labor or delivery (O34.5-, O65.5)
   N85.5   **Inversion of uterus** ♀
     Excludes1   current obstetric trauma (O71.2)
               postpartum inversion of uterus (O71.2)
   N85.6   **Intrauterine synechiae** ♀
   N85.7   **Hematometra** ♀
     Hematosalpinx with hematometra
     Excludes1   hematometra with hematocolpos (N89.7)

▶ New   ⇒ Revised   ~~deleted~~ Deleted   Excludes 1   Excludes 2   Includes   Use additional   Code first   Code also   Key words
OGCR Official Guidelines   ● Unacceptable Principal Diagnosis   X Assign placeholder X   ● Use Additional Character(s)   ▷ Manifestation Code   Coding Clinic

N85.8   Other specified noninflammatory disorders of uterus ♀
> Atrophy of uterus, acquired
> Fibrosis of uterus NOS

N85.9   Noninflammatory disorder of uterus, unspecified ♀
> Disorder of uterus NOS

N86   Erosion and ectropion of cervix uteri ♀
> Decubitus (trophic) ulcer of cervix
> Eversion of cervix
> **Excludes1**   erosion and ectropion of cervix with cervicitis (N72)

● **N87   Dysplasia of cervix uteri**
> **Excludes1**   abnormal results from cervical cytologic examination without histologic confirmation (R87.61-)
> > carcinoma in situ of cervix uteri (D06.-)
> > cervical intraepithelial neoplasia III [CIN III] (D06.-)
> > HGSIL of cervix (R87.613)
> > severe dysplasia of cervix uteri (D06.-)

N87.0   Mild cervical dysplasia ♀
> Cervical intraepithelial neoplasia I [CIN I]

N87.1   Moderate cervical dysplasia ♀
> Cervical intraepithelial neoplasia II [CIN II]

N87.9   Dysplasia of cervix uteri, unspecified ♀
> Anaplasia of cervix
> Cervical atypism
> Cervical dysplasia NOS

● **N88   Other noninflammatory disorders of cervix uteri**
> **Excludes2**   inflammatory disease of cervix (N72)
> > polyp of cervix (N84.1)

N88.0   Leukoplakia of cervix uteri ♀

N88.1   Old laceration of cervix uteri ♀
> Adhesions of cervix
> **Excludes1**   current obstetric trauma (O71.3)

N88.2   Stricture and stenosis of cervix uteri ♀
> **Excludes1**   stricture and stenosis of cervix uteri complicating labor (O65.5)

N88.3   Incompetence of cervix uteri ♀
> Investigation and management of (suspected) cervical incompetence in a nonpregnant woman
> **Excludes1**   cervical incompetence complicating pregnancy (O34.3-)

N88.4   Hypertrophic elongation of cervix uteri ♀

N88.8   Other specified noninflammatory disorders of cervix uteri ♀
> **Excludes1**   current obstetric trauma (O71.3)

N88.9   Noninflammatory disorder of cervix uteri, unspecified ♀

● **N89   Other noninflammatory disorders of vagina**
> **Excludes1**   abnormal results from vaginal cytologic examination without histologic confirmation (R87.62-)
> > carcinoma in situ of vagina (D07.2)
> > HGSIL of vagina (R87.623)
> > inflammation of vagina (N76.-)
> > senile (atrophic) vaginitis (N95.2)
> > severe dysplasia of vagina (D07.2)
> > trichomonal leukorrhea (A59.00)
> > vaginal intraepithelial neoplasia [VAIN], grade III (D07.2)

N89.0   Mild vaginal dysplasia ♀
> Vaginal intraepithelial neoplasia [VAIN], grade I

N89.1   Moderate vaginal dysplasia ♀
> Vaginal intraepithelial neoplasia [VAIN], grade II

N89.3   Dysplasia of vagina, unspecified ♀

N89.4   Leukoplakia of vagina ♀

N89.5   Stricture and atresia of vagina ♀
> Vaginal adhesions   Vaginal stenosis
> **Excludes1**   congenital atresia or stricture (Q52.4)
> > postprocedural adhesions of vagina (N99.2)

N89.6   Tight hymenal ring ♀
> Rigid hymen   Tight introitus
> **Excludes1**   imperforate hymen (Q52.3)

N89.7   Hematocolpos ♀
> Hematocolpos with hematometra or hematosalpinx
> Coding Clinic: 2016, Q4, P59

N89.8   Other specified noninflammatory disorders of vagina ♀
> Leukorrhea NOS
> Old vaginal laceration
> Pessary ulcer of vagina
> **Excludes1**   current obstetric trauma (O70.-, O71.4, O71.7-O71.8)
> > old laceration involving muscles of pelvic floor (N81.8)

N89.9   Noninflammatory disorder of vagina, unspecified ♀

● **N90   Other noninflammatory disorders of vulva and perineum**
> **Excludes1**   anogenital (venereal) warts (A63.0)
> > carcinoma in situ of vulva (D07.1)
> > condyloma acuminatum (A63.0)
> > current obstetric trauma (O70.-, O71.7-O71.8)
> > inflammation of vulva (N76.-)
> > severe dysplasia of vulva (D07.1)
> > vulvar intraepithelial neoplasm III [VIN III] (D07.1)

N90.0   Mild vulvar dysplasia ♀
> Vulvar intraepithelial neoplasia [VIN], grade I

N90.1   Moderate vulvar dysplasia ♀
> Vulvar intraepithelial neoplasia [VIN], grade II

N90.3   Dysplasia of vulva, unspecified ♀

N90.4   Leukoplakia of vulva ♀
> Dystrophy of vulva
> Kraurosis of vulva
> Lichen sclerosus of external female genital organs

N90.5   Atrophy of vulva ♀
> Stenosis of vulva

● **N90.6   Hypertrophy of vulva**
> Coding Clinic: 2016, Q4, P46

> **N90.60   Unspecified hypertrophy of vulva ♀**
> > Unspecified hypertrophy of labia

> **N90.61   Childhood asymmetric labium majus enlargement ♀**
> > CALME

> **N90.69   Other specified hypertrophy of vulva ♀**
> > Other specified hypertrophy of labia

N90.7   Vulvar cyst ♀

● **N90.8   Other specified noninflammatory disorders of vulva and perineum**

> ● **N90.81   Female genital mutilation status**
> > Female genital cutting status

> > **N90.810   Female genital mutilation status, unspecified ♀**
> > > Female genital cutting status, unspecified
> > > Female genital mutilation status NOS

> > **N90.811   Female genital mutilation Type I status ♀**
> > > Clitorectomy status
> > > Female genital cutting Type I status

> > **N90.812   Female genital mutilation Type II status ♀**
> > > Clitorectomy with excision of labia minora status
> > > Female genital cutting Type II status

N Newborn Age: 0   **P** Pediatric Age: 0–17   **M** Maternity DX: 9–64   **A** Adult Age: 15–124   ♀ Females Only   ♂ Males Only

🔲 Complication\Comorbidity   🔲 Major C\C   (Ex) CC/MCC Exclusions   🔲 Hospital-Acquired Condition   🔲 Hierarchical Condition Category

1137

N90.813 **Female genital mutilation** Type III **status** ♀
  Female genital cutting Type III status
  Infibulation status

N90.818 **Other female genital mutilation status** ♀
  Female genital cutting Type IV status
  Female genital mutilation Type IV status
  Other female genital cutting status

N90.89 **Other specified noninflammatory disorders of vulva and perineum** ♀
  Adhesions of vulva
  Hypertrophy of clitoris

N90.9 **Noninflammatory disorder of vulva and perineum, unspecified** ♀

● N91 **Absent, scanty and rare menstruation**

> **Excludes1**   ovarian dysfunction (E28.-)

N91.0 **Primary amenorrhea** ♀

N91.1 **Secondary amenorrhea** ♀

N91.2 **Amenorrhea, unspecified** ♀

N91.3 **Primary oligomenorrhea** ♀

N91.4 **Secondary oligomenorrhea** ♀

N91.5 **Oligomenorrhea, unspecified** ♀
  Hypomenorrhea NOS

● N92 **Excessive, frequent and irregular menstruation**

> **Excludes1**   postmenopausal bleeding (N95.0)
> precocious puberty (menstruation) (E30.1)

N92.0 **Excessive and frequent menstruation with regular cycle** ♀
  Heavy periods NOS   Polymenorrhea
  Menorrhagia NOS

N92.1 **Excessive and frequent menstruation with irregular cycle** ♀
  Irregular intermenstrual bleeding
  Irregular, shortened intervals between menstrual bleeding
  Menometrorrhagia
  Metrorrhagia

N92.2 **Excessive menstruation at puberty** ♀   P
  Excessive bleeding associated with onset of menstrual periods
  Pubertal menorrhagia
  Puberty bleeding

N92.3 **Ovulation bleeding** ♀
  Regular intermenstrual bleeding

N92.4 **Excessive bleeding in the premenopausal period** ♀
  Climacteric menorrhagia or metrorrhagia
  Menopausal menorrhagia or metrorrhagia
  Perimenopausal bleeding
  Perimenopausal menorrhagia or metrorrhagia
  Preclimacteric menorrhagia or metrorrhagia
  Premenopausal menorrhagia or metrorrhagia

N92.5 **Other specified irregular menstruation** ♀

N92.6 **Irregular menstruation, unspecified** ♀
  Irregular bleeding NOS
  Irregular periods NOS

> **Excludes1**   irregular menstruation with:
> lengthened intervals or scanty bleeding (N91.3-N91.5)
> shortened intervals or excessive bleeding (N92.1)

● N93 **Other abnormal uterine and vaginal bleeding**

> **Excludes1**   neonatal vaginal hemorrhage (P54.6)
> precocious puberty (menstruation) (E30.1)
> pseudomenses (P54.6)

N93.0 **Postcoital and contact bleeding** ♀

N93.1 **Pre-pubertal vaginal bleeding** ♀
  Coding Clinic: 2016, Q4, P47

N93.8 **Other specified abnormal uterine and vaginal bleeding** ♀
  Dysfunctional or functional uterine or vaginal bleeding NOS

N93.9 **Abnormal uterine and vaginal bleeding, unspecified** ♀

● N94 **Pain and other conditions associated with female genital organs and menstrual cycle**

N94.0 **Mittelschmerz** ♀
  Ovulation pain

● N94.1 **Dyspareunia**
  Painful intercourse/coitus

> **Excludes1**   psychogenic dyspareunia (F52.6)
> Coding Clinic: 2016, Q4, P47

N94.10 **Unspecified dyspareunia** ♀

N94.11 **Superficial (introital) dyspareunia** ♀

N94.12 **Deep dyspareunia** ♀

N94.19 **Other specified dyspareunia** ♀

N94.2 **Vaginismus** ♀
  Vagina tightness

> **Excludes1**   psychogenic vaginismus (F52.5)

N94.3 **Premenstrual tension syndrome** ♀
  AKA: PMS
  Code also associated menstrual migraine (G43.82-, G43.83-)

> **Excludes1**   Premenstrual dysphoric disorder (F32.81)
> Coding Clinic: 2016, Q4, P14

N94.4 **Primary dysmenorrhea** ♀
  Lifelong painful menstruation

N94.5 **Secondary dysmenorrhea** ♀
  Later onset of painful menstruation

N94.6 **Dysmenorrhea, unspecified** ♀

> **Excludes1**   psychogenic dysmenorrhea (F45.8)

● N94.8 **Other specified conditions associated with female genital organs and menstrual cycle**

● N94.81 **Vulvodynia**

N94.810 **Vulvar vestibulitis** ♀

N94.818 **Other vulvodynia** ♀

N94.819 **Vulvodynia, unspecified** ♀
  Vulvodynia NOS

N94.89 **Other specified conditions associated with female genital organs and menstrual cycle** ♀

N94.9 **Unspecified condition associated with female genital organs and menstrual cycle** ♀

● N95 **Menopausal and other perimenopausal disorders**
  Menopausal and other perimenopausal disorders due to naturally occurring (age-related) menopause and perimenopause

> **Excludes1**   excessive bleeding in the premenopausal period (N92.4)
> menopausal and perimenopausal disorders due to artificial or premature menopause (E89.4-, E28.31-)
> premature menopause (E28.31-)

> **Excludes2**   postmenopausal osteoporosis (M81.0-)
> postmenopausal osteoporosis with current pathological fracture (M80.0-)
> postmenopausal urethritis (N34.2)

N95.0 **Postmenopausal bleeding** ♀

N95.1 **Menopausal and female climacteric states** ♀
  Symptoms such as flushing, sleeplessness, headache, lack of concentration, associated with natural (age-related) menopause
  Use additional code for associated symptoms

> **Excludes1**   asymptomatic menopausal state (Z78.0)
> symptoms associated with artificial menopause (E89.41)
> symptoms associated with premature menopause (E28.310)

N95.2   Postmenopausal atrophic vaginitis ♀
     Senile (atrophic) vaginitis

N95.8   Other specified menopausal and perimenopausal disorders ♀

N95.9   Unspecified menopausal and perimenopausal disorder ♀

N96   Recurrent pregnancy loss ♀
     Investigation or care in a nonpregnant woman with history of recurrent pregnancy loss
     Excludes1   recurrent pregnancy loss with current pregnancy (O26.2-)

● **N97   Female infertility**
     Includes   inability to achieve a pregnancy
         sterility, female NOS
     ~~Excludes1~~   ~~female infertility associated with:~~
         ~~hypopituitarism (E23.0)~~
         ~~Stein-Leventhal syndrome (E28.2)~~
     ▶ **Excludes2**   female infertility associated with:
         hypopituitarism (E23.0)
         Stein-Leventhal syndrome (E28.2)
         incompetence of cervix uteri (N88.3)

N97.0   Female infertility associated with anovulation ♀

N97.1   Female infertility of tubal origin ♀
     Female infertility associated with congenital anomaly of tube
     Female infertility due to tubal block
     Female infertility due to tubal occlusion
     Female infertility due to tubal stenosis

N97.2   Female infertility of uterine origin ♀
     Female infertility associated with congenital anomaly of uterus
     Female infertility due to nonimplantation of ovum

N97.8   Female infertility of other origin ♀

N97.9   Female infertility, unspecified ♀

● **N98   Complications associated with artificial fertilization**
     (Ex:) For category N98 CC codes unless otherwise indicated: See PDX Collection 643

N98.0   Infection associated with artificial insemination ♀ 🦠
     (Ex:) See PDX Collection 948

N98.1   Hyperstimulation of ovaries ♀ 🦠
     Hyperstimulation of ovaries NOS
     Hyperstimulation of ovaries associated with induced ovulation

N98.2   Complications of attempted introduction of fertilized ovum following in vitro fertilization ♀ 🦠

N98.3   Complications of attempted introduction of embryo in embryo transfer ♀ 🦠

N98.8   Other complications associated with artificial fertilization ♀ 🦠

N98.9   Complication associated with artificial fertilization, unspecified ♀ 🦠

INTRAOPERATIVE AND POSTPROCEDURAL COMPLICATIONS AND DISORDERS OF GENITOURINARY SYSTEM, NOT ELSEWHERE CLASSIFIED (N99)

● **N99   Intraoperative and postprocedural complications and disorders of genitourinary system, not elsewhere classified**
     Excludes2   irradiation cystitis (N30.4-)
         postoophorectomy osteoporosis with current pathological fracture (M80.8-)
         postoophorectomy osteoporosis without current pathological fracture (M81.8)

N99.0   Postprocedural (acute) (chronic) kidney failure
     Use additional code to type of kidney disease

● N99.1   Postprocedural urethral stricture
     Postcatheterization urethral stricture

     ● N99.11   Postprocedural urethral stricture, male

         N99.110   Postprocedural urethral stricture, male, meatal ♂

         N99.111   Postprocedural bulbous urethral stricture, male ♂

         N99.112   Postprocedural membranous urethral stricture, male ♂

         N99.113   Postprocedural anterior bulbous urethral stricture, male ♂
            Coding Clinic: 2016, Q4, P48

         N99.114   Postprocedural urethral stricture, male, unspecified ♂

         N99.115   Postprocedural fossa navicularis urethral stricture ♂
            Coding Clinic: 2016, Q4, P47

         N99.116   Postprocedural urethral stricture, male, overlapping sites ♂
            (Ex:) See PDX Collection 935

     N99.12   Postprocedural urethral stricture, female ♀

N99.2   Postprocedural adhesions of vagina ♀

N99.3   Prolapse of vaginal vault after hysterectomy ♀

N99.4   Postprocedural pelvic peritoneal adhesions
     Excludes2   pelvic peritoneal adhesions NOS (N73.6)
         postinfective pelvic peritoneal adhesions (N73.6)

● N99.5   Complications of stoma of urinary tract
     Excludes2   mechanical complication of urinary catheter (T83.0-)

     ● N99.51   Complication of cystostomy

         N99.510   Cystostomy hemorrhage 🦠 🦠
            (Ex:) See PDX Collection 949

         N99.511   Cystostomy infection 🦠 🦠
            (Ex:) See PDX Collection 950

         N99.512   Cystostomy malfunction 🦠 🦠
            (Ex:) See PDX Collection 951

         N99.518   Other cystostomy complication 🦠 🦠
            (Ex:) See PDX Collection 949

     ● N99.52   Complication of incontinent external stoma of urinary tract

         N99.520   Hemorrhage of incontinent external stoma of urinary tract 🦠

         N99.521   Infection of incontinent external stoma of urinary tract 🦠
            Coding Clinic: 2016, Q4, P48

         N99.522   Malfunction of incontinent external stoma of urinary tract 🦠

         N99.523   Herniation of incontinent stoma of urinary tract 🦠
            Coding Clinic: 2016, Q4, P48

         N99.524   Stenosis of incontinent stoma of urinary tract 🦠
            Coding Clinic: 2016, Q4, P48

         N99.528   Other complication of incontinent external stoma of urinary tract 🦠

     ● N99.53   Complication of continent stoma of urinary tract

         N99.530   Hemorrhage of continent stoma of urinary tract 🦠

         N99.531   Infection of continent stoma of urinary tract 🦠

         N99.532   Malfunction of continent stoma of urinary tract 🦠

         N99.533   Herniation of continent stoma of urinary tract 🦠
            Coding Clinic: 2016, Q4, P48

         N99.534   Stenosis of continent stoma of urinary tract 🦠
            Coding Clinic: 2016, Q4, P48

         N99.538   Other complication of continent stoma of urinary tract 🦠

N   Newborn Age: 0   **P**   Pediatric Age: 0–17   **M**   Maternity DX: 9–64   **A**   Adult Age: 15–124   ♀   Females Only   ♂   Males Only

🦠   Complication\Comorbidity   🦠   Major C\C   (Ex:)   CC/MCC Exclusions   🦠   Hospital-Acquired Condition   🦠   Hierarchical Condition Category

1139

CHAPTER 14 (N00-N99)

● N99.6   **Intraoperative hemorrhage and hematoma** of a **genitourinary system organ or structure complicating a procedure**

      Excludes1   intraoperative hemorrhage and hematoma of a genitourinary system organ or structure due to accidental puncture or laceration during a procedure (N99.7-)

       (Ex:) **For category N99.6 CC codes:** See PDX Collection 952

   N99.61   Intraoperative hemorrhage and hematoma of a genitourinary system organ or structure complicating a **genitourinary system procedure** 🔖

   N99.62   Intraoperative hemorrhage and hematoma of a genitourinary system organ or structure complicating **other procedure** 🔖

● N99.7   **Accidental puncture and laceration** of a genitourinary system organ or structure during a procedure

       (Ex:) **For category N99.7 CC codes:** See PDX Collection 509

   N99.71   Accidental puncture and laceration of a genitourinary system organ or structure during a **genitourinary system procedure** 🔖

   N99.72   Accidental puncture and laceration of a genitourinary system organ or structure during **other procedure** 🔖

● N99.8   **Other intraoperative and postprocedural** complications and disorders of genitourinary system

       Coding Clinic: 2016, Q4, P10

   N99.81   **Other** intraoperative complications of genitourinary system

●   N99.82   **Postprocedural hemorrhage** of a genitourinary system organ or structure following a procedure

       (Ex:) **For category N99.82 CC codes:** See PDX Collection 952

     N99.820   Postprocedural hemorrhage of a genitourinary system organ or structure following a **genitourinary system procedure** 🔖

     N99.821   Postprocedural hemorrhage of a genitourinary system organ or structure following **other procedure** 🔖

N99.83   Residual ovary syndrome ♀

● N99.84   **Postprocedural hematoma and seroma** of a genitourinary system organ or structure following a procedure

       (Ex:) **For category N99.84 CC codes:** See PDX Collection 952

     N99.840   Postprocedural **hematoma** of a genitourinary system organ or structure following a **genitourinary system procedure** 🔖

     N99.841   Postprocedural **hematoma** of a genitourinary system organ or structure following **other procedure** 🔖

     N99.842   Postprocedural **seroma** of a genitourinary system organ or structure following a **genitourinary system procedure** 🔖

     N99.843   Postprocedural **seroma** of a genitourinary system organ or structure following **other procedure** 🔖

N99.85   Post endometrial ablation syndrome

       Coding Clinic: 2019, Q4, P12

N99.89   **Other** postprocedural complications and disorders of genitourinary system

CHAPTER 15

PREGNANCY, CHILDBIRTH, AND THE PUERPERIUM (O00-O9A)

OGCR Chapter-Specific Coding Guidelines

15. **Chapter 15: Pregnancy, Childbirth, and the Puerperium (O00-O9A)**

a. **General Rules for Obstetric Cases**

1) **Codes from Chapter 15 and sequencing priority**
Obstetric cases require codes from Chapter 15, codes in the range O00-O9A, Pregnancy, Childbirth, and the Puerperium. Chapter 15 codes have sequencing priority over codes from other chapters. Additional codes from other chapters may be used in conjunction with Chapter 15 codes to further specify conditions. Should the provider document that the pregnancy is incidental to the encounter, then code Z33.1, Pregnant state, incidental, should be used in place of any Chapter 15 codes. It is the provider's responsibility to state that the condition being treated is not affecting the pregnancy.

2) **Chapter 15 codes used only on the maternal record**
Chapter 15 codes are to be used only on the maternal record, never on the record of the newborn.

3) **Final character for trimester**
The majority of codes in Chapter 15 have a final character indicating the trimester of pregnancy. The timeframes for the trimesters are indicated at the beginning of the chapter. If trimester is not a component of a code it is because the condition always occurs in a specific trimester, or the concept of trimester of pregnancy is not applicable. Certain codes have characters for only certain trimesters because the condition does not occur in all trimesters, but it may occur in more than just one.

Assignment of the final character for trimester should be based on the provider's documentation of the trimester (or number of weeks) for the current admission/encounter. This applies to the assignment of trimester for pre-existing conditions as well as those that develop during or are due to the pregnancy. The provider's documentation of the number of weeks may be used to assign the appropriate code identifying the trimester.

Whenever delivery occurs during the current admission, and there is an "in childbirth" option for the obstetric complication being coded, the "in childbirth" code should be assigned.

4) **Selection of trimester for inpatient admissions that encompass more than one trimester**
In instances when a patient is admitted to a hospital for complications of pregnancy during one trimester and remains in the hospital into a subsequent trimester, the trimester character for the antepartum complication code should be assigned on the basis of the trimester when the complication developed, not the trimester of the discharge. If the condition developed prior to the current admission/encounter or represents a pre-existing condition, the trimester character for the trimester at the time of the admission/encounter should be assigned.

5) **Unspecified trimester**
Each category that includes codes for trimester has a code for "unspecified trimester." The "unspecified trimester" code should rarely be used, such as when the documentation in the record is insufficient to determine the trimester and it is not possible to obtain clarification.

6) **7th character for Fetus Identification**
Where applicable, a 7th character is to be assigned for certain categories (O31, O32, O33.3 - O33.6, O35, O36, O40, O41, O60.1, O60.2, O64, and O69) to identify the fetus for which the complication code applies.

Assign 7th character "0":
- For single gestations
- When the documentation in the record is insufficient to determine the fetus affected and it is not possible to obtain clarification.
- When it is not possible to clinically determine which fetus is affected.

b. **Selection of OB Principal or First-listed Diagnosis**

1) **Routine outpatient prenatal visits**
For routine outpatient prenatal visits when no complications are present, a code from category Z34, Encounter for supervision of normal pregnancy, should be used as the first-listed diagnosis. These codes should not be used in conjunction with Chapter 15 codes.

2) **Supervision of High-Risk Pregnancy**
Codes from category O09, Supervision of high-risk pregnancy, are intended for use only during the prenatal period. For complications during the labor or delivery episode as a result of a high-risk pregnancy, assign the applicable complication codes from Chapter 15. If there are no complications during the labor or delivery episode, assign code O80, Encounter for full-term uncomplicated delivery.

For routine prenatal outpatient visits for patients with high-risk pregnancies, a code from category O09, Supervision of high-risk pregnancy, should be used as the first-listed diagnosis. Secondary Chapter 15 codes may be used in conjunction with these codes if appropriate.

3) **Episodes when no delivery occurs**
In episodes when no delivery occurs, the principal diagnosis should correspond to the principal complication of the pregnancy which necessitated the encounter. Should more than one complication exist, all of which are treated or monitored, any of the complications codes may be sequenced first.

4) **When a delivery occurs**
When an obstetric patient is admitted and delivers during that admission, the condition that prompted the admission should be sequenced as the principal diagnosis. If multiple conditions prompted the admission, sequence the one most related to the delivery as the principal diagnosis. A code for any complication of the delivery should be assigned as an additional diagnosis. In cases of cesarean delivery, if the patient was admitted with a condition that resulted in the performance of a cesarean procedure, that condition should be selected as the principal diagnosis. If the reason for the admission was unrelated to the condition resulting in the cesarean delivery, the condition related to the reason for the admission should be selected as the principal diagnosis.

5) **Outcome of delivery**
A code from category Z37, Outcome of delivery, should be included on every maternal record when a delivery has occurred. These codes are not to be used on subsequent records or on the newborn record.

c. **Pre-existing conditions versus conditions due to the pregnancy**
Certain categories in Chapter 15 distinguish between conditions of the mother that existed prior to pregnancy (pre-existing) and those that are a direct result of pregnancy. When assigning codes from Chapter 15, it is important to assess if a condition was pre-existing prior to pregnancy or developed during or due to the pregnancy in order to assign the correct code.

Categories that do not distinguish between pre-existing and pregnancy-related conditions may be used for either. It is acceptable to use codes specifically for the puerperium with codes complicating pregnancy and childbirth if a condition arises postpartum during the delivery encounter.

d. **Pre-existing hypertension in pregnancy**
Category O10, Pre-existing hypertension complicating pregnancy, childbirth and the puerperium, includes codes for hypertensive heart and hypertensive chronic kidney disease. When assigning one of the O10 codes that includes hypertensive heart disease or hypertensive chronic kidney disease, it is necessary to add a secondary code from the appropriate hypertension category to specify the type of heart failure or chronic kidney disease.
See Section I.C.9. Hypertension.

e. **Fetal Conditions Affecting the Management of the Mother**

1) **Codes from categories O35 and O36**
Codes from categories O35, Maternal care for known or suspected fetal abnormality and damage, and O36, Maternal care for other fetal problems, are assigned only when the fetal condition is actually responsible for modifying the management of the mother, i.e., by requiring diagnostic studies, additional observation, special care, or termination of pregnancy. The fact that the fetal condition exists does not justify assigning a code from this series to the mother's record.

2) **In utero surgery**
In cases when surgery is performed on the fetus, a diagnosis code from category O35, Maternal care for known or suspected fetal abnormality and damage, should be assigned identifying the fetal condition. Assign the appropriate procedure code for the procedure performed.

No code from Chapter 16, the perinatal codes, should be used on the mother's record to identify fetal conditions. Surgery performed in utero on a fetus is still to be coded as an obstetric encounter.

f. **HIV Infection in Pregnancy, Childbirth, and the Puerperium**
During pregnancy, childbirth or the puerperium, a patient admitted because of an HIV-related illness should receive a principal diagnosis from subcategory O98.7-, Human immunodeficiency [HIV] disease complicating pregnancy, childbirth and the puerperium, followed by the code(s) for the HIV-related illness(es).

Patients with asymptomatic HIV infection status admitted during pregnancy, childbirth, or the puerperium should receive codes of O98.7- and Z21, Asymptomatic human immunodeficiency virus [HIV] infection status.

g. **Diabetes mellitus in pregnancy**
Diabetes mellitus is a significant complicating factor in pregnancy. Pregnant women who are diabetic should be assigned a code from category O24, Diabetes mellitus in pregnancy, childbirth, and the puerperium, first, followed by the appropriate diabetes code(s) (E08-E13) from Chapter 4.

h. Long-term use of insulin and oral hypoglycemics
See Section I.C.4.a.3 for information on the long-term use of insulin and oral hypoglycemic.

i. Gestational (pregnancy induced) diabetes
Gestational (pregnancy induced) diabetes can occur during the second and third trimester of pregnancy in women who were not diabetic prior to pregnancy. Gestational diabetes can cause complications in the pregnancy similar to those of pre-existing diabetes mellitus. It also puts the woman at greater risk of developing diabetes after the pregnancy. Codes for gestational diabetes are in subcategory O24.4, Gestational diabetes mellitus. No other code from category O24, Diabetes mellitus in pregnancy, childbirth, and the puerperium, should be used with a code from O24.4.

The codes under subcategory O24.4 include diet controlled, insulin controlled, and controlled by oral hypoglycemic drugs. If a patient with gestational diabetes is treated with both diet and insulin, only the code for insulin-controlled is required. If a patient with gestational diabetes is treated with both diet and oral hypoglycemic medications, only the code for "controlled by oral hypoglycemic drugs" is required. Code Z79.4, Long-term (current) use of insulin or code Z79.84, Long-term (current) use of oral hypoglycemic drugs, should not be assigned with codes from subcategory O24.4.

An abnormal glucose tolerance in pregnancy is assigned a code from subcategory O99.81, Abnormal glucose complicating pregnancy, childbirth, and the puerperium.

j. Sepsis and septic shock complicating abortion, pregnancy, childbirth and the puerperium
When assigning a Chapter 15 code for sepsis complicating abortion, pregnancy, childbirth, and the puerperium, a code for the specific type of infection should be assigned as an additional diagnosis. If severe sepsis is present, a code from subcategory R65.2, Severe sepsis, and code(s) for associated organ dysfunction(s) should also be assigned as additional diagnoses.

k. Puerperal sepsis
Code O85, Puerperal sepsis, should be assigned with a secondary code to identify the causal organism (e.g., for a bacterial infection, assign a code from category B95-B96, Bacterial infections in conditions classified elsewhere). A code from category A40, Streptococcal sepsis, or A41, Other sepsis, should not be used for puerperal sepsis. If applicable, use additional codes to identify severe sepsis (R65.2-) and any associated acute organ dysfunction.

l. Alcohol, tobacco and drug use during pregnancy, childbirth and the puerperium

1) Alcohol use during pregnancy, childbirth and the puerperium
Codes under subcategory O99.31, Alcohol use complicating pregnancy, childbirth, and the puerperium, should be assigned for any pregnancy case when a mother uses alcohol during the pregnancy or postpartum. A secondary code from category F10, Alcohol-related disorders, should also be assigned to identify manifestations of the alcohol use.

2) Tobacco use during pregnancy, childbirth, and the puerperium
Codes under subcategory O99.33, Smoking (tobacco) complicating pregnancy, childbirth, and the puerperium, should be assigned for any pregnancy case when a mother uses any type of tobacco product during the pregnancy or postpartum. A secondary code from category F17, Nicotine dependence, should also be assigned to identify the type of nicotine dependence.

3) Drug use during pregnancy, childbirth and the puerperium
Codes under subcategory O99.32, Drug use complicating pregnancy, childbirth, and the puerperium, should be assigned for any pregnancy case when a mother uses drugs during the pregnancy or postpartum. This can involve illegal drugs, or inappropriate use or abuse of prescription drugs. Secondary code(s) from categories F11-F16 and F18F19 should also be assigned to identify manifestations of the drug use.

m. Poisoning, toxic effects, adverse effects and underdosing in a pregnant patient
A code from subcategory O9A.2, Injury, poisoning and certain other consequences of external causes complicating pregnancy, childbirth, and the puerperium, should be sequenced first, followed by the appropriate injury, poisoning, toxic effect, adverse effect or underdosing code, and then the additional code(s) that specifies the condition caused by the poisoning, toxic effect, adverse effect or underdosing.
See Section I.C.19. Adverse effects, poisoning, underdosing and toxic effects.

n. Normal Delivery, Code O80

1) Encounter for full-term uncomplicated delivery
Code O80 should be assigned when a woman is admitted for a full-term normal delivery and delivers a single, healthy infant without any complications antepartum, during the delivery, or postpartum during the delivery episode. Code O80 is always a principal diagnosis. It is not to be used if any other code from Chapter 15 is needed to describe a current complication of the antenatal, delivery, or perinatal period. Additional codes from other chapters may be used with code O80 if they are not related to or are in any way complicating the pregnancy.

2) Uncomplicated delivery with resolved antepartum complication
Code O80 may be used if the patient had a complication at some point during the pregnancy, but the complication is not present at the time of the admission for delivery.

3) Outcome of delivery for O80
Z37.0, Single live birth, is the only outcome of delivery code appropriate for use with O80.

o. The Peripartum and Postpartum Periods

1) Peripartum and Postpartum periods
The postpartum period begins immediately after delivery and continues for six weeks following delivery. The peripartum period is defined as the last month of pregnancy to five months postpartum.

2) Peripartum and postpartum complication
A postpartum complication is any complication occurring within the six-week period.

3) Pregnancy-related complications after 6 week period
Chapter 15 codes may also be used to describe pregnancy-related complications after the peripartum or postpartum period if the provider documents that a condition is pregnancy related.

4) Admission for routine postpartum care following delivery outside hospital
When the mother delivers outside the hospital prior to admission and is admitted for routine postpartum care and no complications are noted, code Z39.0, Encounter for care and examination of mother immediately after delivery, should be assigned as the principal diagnosis.

5) Pregnancy associated cardiomyopathy
Pregnancy associated cardiomyopathy, code O90.3, is unique in that it may be diagnosed in the third trimester of pregnancy but may continue to progress months after delivery. For this reason, it is referred to as peripartum cardiomyopathy. Code O90.3 is only for use when the cardiomyopathy develops as a result of pregnancy in a woman who did not have pre-existing heart disease.

p. Code O94, Sequelae of complication of pregnancy, childbirth, and the puerperium

1) Code O94
Code O94, Sequelae of complication of pregnancy, childbirth, and the puerperium, is for use in those cases when an initial complication of a pregnancy develops a sequelae requiring care or treatment at a future date.

2) After the initial postpartum period
This code may be used at any time after the initial postpartum period.

3) Sequencing of Code O94
This code, like all sequela codes, is to be sequenced following the code describing the sequelae of the complication.

q. Termination of Pregnancy and Spontaneous abortions

1) Abortion with Liveborn Fetus
When an attempted termination of pregnancy results in a liveborn fetus assign code Z33.2, Encounter for elective termination of pregnancy and a code from category Z37, Outcome of Delivery.

2) Retained Products of Conception following an abortion
Subsequent encounters for retained products of conception following a spontaneous abortion or elective termination of pregnancy, without complications are assigned O03.4, Incomplete spontaneous, abortion without complication, or codes O07.4, Failed attempted termination of pregnancy without complication. This advice is appropriate even when the patient was discharged previously with a discharge diagnosis of complete abortion. If the patient has a specific complication associated with the spontaneous abortion or elective termination of pregnancy in addition to retained products of conception, assign the appropriate complication in category O03 or O07 instead of code O03.4 or O07.4

3) Complications leading to abortion
Codes from Chapter 15 may be used as additional codes to identify any documented complications of the pregnancy in conjunction with codes in categories in O04, O07 and O08.

r. Abuse in a pregnant patient
For suspected or confirmed cases of abuse of a pregnant patient, a code(s) from subcategories O9A.3, Physical abuse complicating pregnancy, childbirth, and the puerperium, O9A.4, Sexual abuse complicating pregnancy, childbirth, and the puerperium, and O9A.5, Psychological abuse complicating pregnancy, childbirth, and the puerperium, should be sequenced first, followed by the appropriate codes (if applicable) to identify any associated current injury due to physical abuse, sexual abuse, and the perpetrator of abuse.
See Section I.C.19. Adult and child abuse, neglect and other maltreatment.

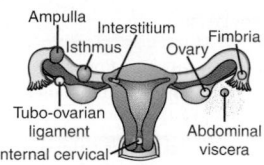

Figure 15-1 Implantation sites of ectopic pregnancy.

Item 15-1 Ectopic pregnancy most often occurs in the fallopian tube. Pregnancy outside the uterus may end in a lifethreatening rupture.

★ **(See Plate 4 of the Anatomy Illustrations.)**

CHAPTER 15

PREGNANCY, CHILDBIRTH, AND THE PUERPERIUM (O00-O9A)

Note: CODES FROM THIS CHAPTER ARE FOR USE ONLY ON MATERNAL RECORDS, NEVER ON NEWBORN RECORDS

Codes from this chapter are for use for conditions related to or aggravated by the pregnancy, childbirth, or by the puerperium (maternal causes or obstetric causes)

Trimesters are counted from the first day of the last menstrual period. They are defined as follows:

1st trimester - less than 14 weeks 0 days

2nd trimester - 14 weeks 0 days to less than 28 weeks 0 days

3rd trimester - 28 weeks 0 days until delivery

Use additional code from category Z3A, Weeks of gestation, to identify the specific week of the pregnancy, if known.

Excludes1 supervision of normal pregnancy (Z34.-)

Excludes2 mental and behavioral disorders associated with the puerperium (F53.-)
obstetrical tetanus (A34)
postpartum necrosis of pituitary gland (E23.0)
puerperal osteomalacia (M83.0)

This chapter contains the following blocks:

O00-O08	Pregnancy with abortive outcome
O09	Supervision of high risk pregnancy
O10-O16	Edema, proteinuria and hypertensive disorders in pregnancy, childbirth and the puerperium
O20-O29	Other maternal disorders predominantly related to pregnancy
O30-O48	Maternal care related to the fetus and amniotic cavity and possible delivery problems
O60-O77	Complications of labor and delivery
O80, O82	Encounter for delivery
O85-O92	Complications predominantly related to the puerperium
O94-O9A	Other obstetric conditions, not elsewhere classified

PREGNANCY WITH ABORTIVE OUTCOME (O00-O08)

Excludes1 continuing pregnancy in multiple gestation after abortion of one fetus or more (O31.1-, O31.3-)
Coding Clinic: 2016, Q4, P130

● **O00 Ectopic pregnancy**

Includes ruptured ectopic pregnancy

Use additional code from category O08 to identify any associated complication

(Ex) For category O00 CC codes: See PDX Collection 953

● **O00.0 Abdominal pregnancy**

Excludes1 maternal care for viable fetus in abdominal pregnancy (O36.7-)
Coding Clinic: 2016, Q4, P49

    O00.00 Abdominal pregnancy without intrauterine pregnancy ♀ 🔵   **M**
        Abdominal pregnancy NOS

    O00.01 Abdominal pregnancy with intrauterine pregnancy ♀ 🔵   **M**

● **O00.1 Tubal pregnancy**
    Fallopian pregnancy
    Rupture of (fallopian) tube due to pregnancy
    Tubal abortion
    Coding Clinic: 2016, Q4, P49

  ● **O00.10 Tubal pregnancy without intrauterine pregnancy**
        Tubal pregnancy NOS

        O00.101 Right tubal pregnancy without intrauterine pregnancy ♀ 🔵   **M**

        O00.102 Left tubal pregnancy without intrauterine pregnancy ♀ 🔵   **M**

        O00.109 Unspecified tubal pregnancy without intrauterine pregnancy ♀ 🔵   **M**

  ● **O00.11 Tubal pregnancy with intrauterine pregnancy**

        O00.111 Right tubal pregnancy with intrauterine pregnancy ♀ 🔵   **M**

        O00.112 Left tubal pregnancy with intrauterine pregnancy ♀ 🔵   **M**

        O00.119 Unspecified tubal pregnancy with intrauterine pregnancy ♀ 🔵   **M**

● **O00.2 Ovarian pregnancy**
    Coding Clinic: 2016, Q4, P49

  ● **O00.20 Ovarian pregnancy without intrauterine pregnancy**
        Ovarian pregnancy NOS

        O00.201 Right ovarian pregnancy without intrauterine pregnancy ♀ 🔵   **M**

        O00.202 Left ovarian pregnancy without intrauterine pregnancy ♀ 🔵   **M**

        O00.209 Unspecified ovarian pregnancy without intrauterine pregnancy ♀ 🔵 **M**

  ● **O00.21 Ovarian pregnancy with intrauterine pregnancy**

        O00.211 Right ovarian pregnancy with intrauterine pregnancy ♀ 🔵   **M**

        O00.212 Left ovarian pregnancy with intrauterine pregnancy ♀ 🔵   **M**

        O00.219 Unspecified ovarian pregnancy with intrauterine pregnancy ♀ 🔵   **M**

● **O00.8 Other ectopic pregnancy**
    Cervical pregnancy
    Cornual pregnancy
    Intraligamentous pregnancy
    Mural pregnancy
    Coding Clinic: 2016, Q4, P49

    O00.80 Other ectopic pregnancy without intrauterine pregnancy ♀ 🔵   **M**
        Other ectopic pregnancy NOS

    O00.81 Other ectopic pregnancy with intrauterine pregnancy ♀ 🔵   **M**

N Newborn Age: 0   **P** Pediatric Age: 0–17   **M** Maternity DX: 9–64   **A** Adult Age: 15-124   ♀ Females Only   ♂ Males Only

🔵 Complication\Comorbidity   🔵 Major C\C   (Ex) CC/MCC Exclusions   🔵 Hospital-Acquired Condition   🔵 Hierarchical Condition Category

● O00.9 **Ectopic pregnancy, unspecified**
Coding Clinic: 2016, Q4, P49

    O00.90 **Unspecified ectopic pregnancy without intrauterine pregnancy** ♀ 🖉   M
        Ectopic pregnancy NOS

    O00.91 **Unspecified ectopic pregnancy with intrauterine pregnancy** ♀ 🖉   M

● O01 **Hydatidiform mole**
    Use additional code from category O08 to identify any associated complication

    Excludes1 chorioadenoma (destruens) (D39.2)
           malignant hydatidiform mole (D39.2)

  O01.0 **Classical hydatidiform mole** ♀   M
    Complete hydatidiform mole

  O01.1 **Incomplete and partial hydatidiform mole** ♀   M

  O01.9 **Hydatidiform mole, unspecified** ♀   M
    Trophoblastic disease NOS
    Vesicular mole NOS

● O02 **Other abnormal products of conception**
    Use additional code from category O08 to identify any associated complication

    Excludes1 papyraceous fetus (O31.0-)

  O02.0 **Blighted ovum and nonhydatidiform mole** ♀   M
    Carneous mole   Molar pregnancy NEC
    Fleshy mole   Pathological ovum
    Intrauterine mole NOS

  O02.1 **Missed abortion** ♀   M
    Early fetal death, before completion of 20 weeks of gestation, with retention of dead fetus

    Excludes1 failed induced abortion (O07.-)
           fetal death (intrauterine) (late) (O36.4)
           missed abortion with blighted ovum (O02.0)
           missed abortion with hydatidiform mole (O01.-)
           missed abortion with nonhydatidiform (O02.0)
           missed abortion with other abnormal products of conception (O02.8-)
           missed delivery (O36.4)
           stillbirth (P95)

    Coding Clinic: 2019, Q3, P12

● O02.8 **Other specified abnormal products of conception**
    Excludes1 abnormal products of conception with blighted ovum (O02.0)
           abnormal products of conception with hydatidiform mole (O01.-)
           abnormal products of conception with nonhydatidiform mole (O02.0)

  O02.81 **Inappropriate change in quantitative human chorionic gonadotropin (hCG) in early pregnancy** ♀   M
    Biochemical pregnancy
    Chemical pregnancy
    Inappropriate level of quantitative human chorionic gonadotropin (hCG) for gestational age in early pregnancy

  O02.89 **Other abnormal products of conception** ♀   M

  O02.9 **Abnormal product of conception, unspecified** ♀   M

● O03 **Spontaneous abortion**
    (Ex) For category O03 CC codes: See PDX Collection 954

    Note: Incomplete abortion includes retained products of conception following spontaneous abortion.

    Includes miscarriage

  O03.0 **Genital tract and pelvic infection following incomplete spontaneous abortion** ♀ 🖉   M
    Endometritis following incomplete spontaneous abortion
    Oophoritis following incomplete spontaneous abortion
    Parametritis following incomplete spontaneous abortion
    Pelvic peritonitis following incomplete spontaneous abortion
    Salpingitis following incomplete spontaneous abortion
    Salpingo-oophoritis following incomplete spontaneous abortion

    Excludes1 sepsis following incomplete spontaneous abortion (O03.37)
           urinary tract infection following incomplete spontaneous abortion (O03.38)

  O03.1 **Delayed or excessive hemorrhage following incomplete spontaneous abortion** ♀   M
    Afibrinogenemia following incomplete spontaneous abortion
    Defibrination syndrome following incomplete spontaneous abortion
    Hemolysis following incomplete spontaneous abortion
    Intravascular coagulation following incomplete spontaneous abortion

  O03.2 **Embolism following incomplete spontaneous abortion** ♀ 🖉   M
    Air embolism following incomplete spontaneous abortion
    Amniotic fluid embolism following incomplete spontaneous abortion
    Blood-clot embolism following incomplete spontaneous abortion
    Embolism NOS following incomplete spontaneous abortion
    Fat embolism following incomplete spontaneous abortion
    Pulmonary embolism following incomplete spontaneous abortion
    Pyemic embolism following incomplete spontaneous abortion
    Septic or septicopyemic embolism following incomplete spontaneous abortion
    Soap embolism following incomplete spontaneous abortion

● O03.3 **Other and unspecified complications following incomplete spontaneous abortion**

  O03.30 **Unspecified complication following incomplete spontaneous abortion** ♀ 🖉   M

  O03.31 **Shock following incomplete spontaneous abortion** ♀ 🖉   M
    Circulatory collapse following incomplete spontaneous abortion
    Shock (postprocedural) following incomplete spontaneous abortion

    Excludes1 shock due to infection following incomplete spontaneous abortion (O03.37)

  O03.32 **Renal failure following incomplete spontaneous abortion** ♀ 🖉   M
    Kidney failure (acute) following incomplete spontaneous abortion
    Oliguria following incomplete spontaneous abortion
    Renal shutdown following incomplete spontaneous abortion
    Renal tubular necrosis following incomplete spontaneous abortion
    Uremia following incomplete spontaneous abortion

Item 15–2 A **hydatidiform** mole is an overproduction of placental tissue. The tumor secretes a hormone, chorionic gonadotropic hormone (CGH), that indicates a positive pregnancy test. There is no viable fetus. More than 80% of hydatidiform moles are noncancerous.

▶ New ⇒ Revised ~~deleted~~ Deleted Excludes 1 Excludes 2 Includes Use additional Code first Code also Key words
OGCR Official Guidelines ● Unacceptable Principal Diagnosis X Assign placeholder X ● Use Additional Character(s) ▶ Manifestation Code Coding Clinic

O03.33 **Metabolic disorder** following incomplete spontaneous abortion ♀ 🅒 **M**

O03.34 **Damage to pelvic organs** following incomplete spontaneous abortion ♀ 🅒 **M**

Laceration, perforation, tear or chemical damage of bladder following incomplete spontaneous abortion

Laceration, perforation, tear or chemical damage of bowel following incomplete spontaneous abortion

Laceration, perforation, tear or chemical damage of broad ligament following incomplete spontaneous abortion

Laceration, perforation, tear or chemical damage of cervix following incomplete spontaneous abortion

Laceration, perforation, tear or chemical damage of periurethral tissue following incomplete spontaneous abortion

Laceration, perforation, tear or chemical damage of uterus following incomplete spontaneous abortion

Laceration, perforation, tear or chemical damage of vagina following incomplete spontaneous abortion

O03.35 **Other venous complications** following incomplete spontaneous abortion ♀ 🅒 **M**

O03.36 **Cardiac arrest** following incomplete spontaneous abortion ♀ 🅒 **M**

O03.37 **Sepsis** following incomplete spontaneous abortion ♀ 🅒 **M**

Use additional code to identify infectious agent (B95-B97)

Use additional code to identify severe sepsis, if applicable (R65.2-)

Excludes1 septic or septicopyemic embolism following incomplete spontaneous abortion (O03.2)

O03.38 **Urinary tract infection** following incomplete spontaneous abortion ♀ 🅒 **M**

Cystitis following incomplete spontaneous abortion

O03.39 **Incomplete spontaneous abortion with other complications** ♀ 🅒 **M**

O03.4 **Incomplete spontaneous abortion without complication** ♀ **M**

O03.5 **Genital tract and pelvic infection** following complete or unspecified spontaneous abortion ♀ 🅒 **M**

Endometritis following complete or unspecified spontaneous abortion

Oophoritis following complete or unspecified spontaneous abortion

Parametritis following complete or unspecified spontaneous abortion

Pelvic peritonitis following complete or unspecified spontaneous abortion

Salpingitis following complete or unspecified spontaneous abortion

Salpingo-oophoritis following complete or unspecified spontaneous abortion

Excludes1 sepsis following complete or unspecified spontaneous abortion (O03.87)
urinary tract infection following complete or unspecified spontaneous abortion (O03.88)

O03.6 **Delayed or excessive hemorrhage** following complete or unspecified spontaneous abortion ♀ **M**

Afibrinogenemia following complete or unspecified spontaneous abortion

Defibrination syndrome following complete or unspecified spontaneous abortion

Hemolysis following complete or unspecified spontaneous abortion

Intravascular coagulation following complete or unspecified spontaneous abortion

O03.7 **Embolism** following **complete** or **unspecified** spontaneous abortion ♀ 🅒 **M**

Air embolism following complete or unspecified spontaneous abortion

Amniotic fluid embolism following complete or unspecified spontaneous abortion

Blood-clot embolism following complete or unspecified spontaneous abortion

Embolism NOS following complete or unspecified spontaneous abortion

Fat embolism following complete or unspecified spontaneous abortion

Pulmonary embolism following complete or unspecified spontaneous abortion

Pyemic embolism following complete or unspecified spontaneous abortion

Septic or septicopyemic embolism following complete or unspecified spontaneous abortion

Soap embolism following complete or unspecified spontaneous abortion

● O03.8 **Other and unspecified complications following complete or unspecified** spontaneous abortion

O03.80 **Unspecified complication** following complete or unspecified spontaneous abortion ♀ 🅒 **M**

O03.81 **Shock** following complete or **unspecified** spontaneous abortion ♀ 🅒 **M**

Circulatory collapse following complete or unspecified spontaneous abortion

Shock (postprocedural) following complete or unspecified spontaneous abortion

Excludes1 shock due to infection following complete or unspecified spontaneous abortion (O03.87)

O03.82 **Renal failure** following **complete** or **unspecified** spontaneous abortion ♀ 🅒 **M**

Kidney failure (acute) following complete or unspecified spontaneous abortion

Oliguria following complete or unspecified spontaneous abortion

Renal shutdown following complete or unspecified spontaneous abortion

Renal tubular necrosis following complete or unspecified spontaneous abortion

Uremia following complete or unspecified spontaneous abortion

O03.83 **Metabolic disorder** following **complete or unspecified** spontaneous abortion ♀ 🅒 **M**

O03.84 **Damage to pelvic organs** following **complete or unspecified** spontaneous abortion ♀ 🅒 **M**

Laceration, perforation, tear or chemical damage of bladder following complete or unspecified spontaneous abortion

Laceration, perforation, tear or chemical damage of bowel following complete or unspecified spontaneous abortion

Laceration, perforation, tear or chemical damage of broad ligament following complete or unspecified spontaneous abortion

Laceration, perforation, tear or chemical damage of cervix following complete or unspecified spontaneous abortion

Laceration, perforation, tear or chemical damage of periurethral tissue following complete or unspecified spontaneous abortion

Laceration, perforation, tear or chemical damage of uterus following complete or unspecified spontaneous abortion

Laceration, perforation, tear or chemical damage of vagina following complete or unspecified spontaneous abortion

N Newborn Age: 0   **P** Pediatric Age: 0–17   **M** Maternity DX: 9–64   **A** Adult Age: 15–124   ♀ Females Only   ♂ Males Only

🅒 Complication\Comorbidity   🅒 Major C\C   (Ex:) CC/MCC Exclusions   🅒 Hospital-Acquired Condition   🅒 Hierarchical Condition Category

O03.85   Other venous complications following complete or unspecified spontaneous abortion ♀ 🔖   M

O03.86   Cardiac arrest following complete or unspecified spontaneous abortion ♀ 🔖   M

O03.87   Sepsis following complete or unspecified spontaneous abortion ♀ 🔖   M

> Use additional code to identify infectious agent (B95-B97)
>
> Use additional code to identify severe sepsis, if applicable (R65.2-)
>
> **Excludes1**   septic or septicopyemic embolism following complete or unspecified spontaneous abortion (O03.7)

O03.88   Urinary tract infection following complete or unspecified spontaneous abortion ♀ 🔖   M

> Cystitis following complete or unspecified spontaneous abortion

O03.89   Complete or unspecified spontaneous abortion with other complications ♀ 🔖   M

O03.9   Complete or unspecified spontaneous abortion without complication ♀   M

> Miscarriage NOS
>
> Spontaneous abortion NOS

● **O04**   **Complications following (induced) termination of pregnancy**

> **Includes**   complications following (induced) termination of pregnancy
>
> **Excludes1**   encounter for elective termination of pregnancy, uncomplicated (Z33.2)
>
>   failed attempted termination of pregnancy (O07.-)
>
> (Ex:) **For category O04 CC codes unless otherwise indicated:** See PDX Collection 954

O04.5   Genital tract and pelvic infection following (induced) termination of pregnancy ♀   M

> Endometritis following (induced) termination of pregnancy
>
> Oophoritis following (induced) termination of pregnancy
>
> Parametritis following (induced) termination of pregnancy
>
> Pelvic peritonitis following (induced) termination of pregnancy
>
> Salpingitis following (induced) termination of pregnancy
>
> Salpingo-oophoritis following (induced) termination of pregnancy
>
> **Excludes1**   sepsis following (induced) termination of pregnancy (O04.87)
>
>   urinary tract infection following (induced) termination of pregnancy (O04.88)

O04.6   Delayed or excessive hemorrhage following (induced) termination of pregnancy ♀   M

> Afibrinogenemia following (induced) termination of pregnancy
>
> Defibrination syndrome following (induced) termination of pregnancy
>
> Hemolysis following (induced) termination of pregnancy
>
> Intravascular coagulation following (induced) termination of pregnancy
>
> **Coding Clinic: 2019, Q3, P12**

O04.7   Embolism following (induced) termination of pregnancy ♀ 🔖   M

> Air embolism following (induced) termination of pregnancy
>
> Amniotic fluid embolism following (induced) termination of pregnancy
>
> Blood-clot embolism following (induced) termination of pregnancy
>
> Embolism NOS following (induced) termination of pregnancy
>
> Fat embolism following (induced) termination of pregnancy
>
> Pulmonary embolism following (induced) termination of pregnancy
>
> Pyemic embolism following (induced) termination of pregnancy
>
> Septic or septicopyemic embolism following (induced) termination of pregnancy
>
> Soap embolism following (induced) termination of pregnancy

● **O04.8**   (Induced) termination of pregnancy with other and unspecified complications

O04.80   (Induced) termination of pregnancy with unspecified complications ♀ 🔖   M

O04.81   Shock following (induced) termination of pregnancy ♀ 🔖   M

> Circulatory collapse following (induced) termination of pregnancy
>
> Shock (postprocedural) following (induced) termination of pregnancy
>
> **Excludes1**   shock due to infection following (induced) termination of pregnancy (O04.87)

O04.82   Renal failure following (induced) termination of pregnancy ♀   M

> Kidney failure (acute) following (induced) termination of pregnancy
>
> Oliguria following (induced) termination of pregnancy
>
> Renal shutdown following (induced) termination of pregnancy
>
> Renal tubular necrosis following (induced) termination of pregnancy
>
> Uremia following (induced) termination of pregnancy

O04.83   Metabolic disorder following (induced) termination of pregnancy ♀ 🔖   M

O04.84   Damage to pelvic organs following (induced) termination of pregnancy ♀ 🔖   M

> Laceration, perforation, tear or chemical damage of bladder following (induced) termination of pregnancy
>
> Laceration, perforation, tear or chemical damage of bowel following (induced) termination of pregnancy
>
> Laceration, perforation, tear or chemical damage of broad ligament following (induced) termination of pregnancy
>
> Laceration, perforation, tear or chemical damage of cervix following (induced) termination of pregnancy
>
> Laceration, perforation, tear or chemical damage of periurethral tissue following (induced) termination of pregnancy
>
> Laceration, perforation, tear or chemical damage of uterus following (induced) termination of pregnancy
>
> Laceration, perforation, tear or chemical damage of vagina following (induced) termination of pregnancy

O04.85   Other venous complications following (induced) termination of pregnancy ♀ 🔖   M

O04.86   Cardiac arrest following (induced) termination of pregnancy ♀ 🔖   M

▶ New   ⮕ Revised   ~~deleted~~ Deleted   Excludes 1   Excludes 2   Includes   Use additional   Code first   Code also   Key words

OGCR Official Guidelines   ● Unacceptable Principal Diagnosis   X Assign placeholder X   ● Use Additional Character(s)   ▷ Manifestation Code   Coding Clinic

O04.87   **Sepsis following (induced) termination of pregnancy** ♀ 🐾   **M**

     Use additional code to identify infectious agent (B95-B97)

     Use additional code to identify severe sepsis, if applicable (R65.2-)

     Excludes1   septic or septicopyemic embolism following (induced) termination of pregnancy (O04.7)

     (Ex:) See PDX Collection 954

O04.88   **Urinary tract infection following (induced) termination of pregnancy** ♀ 🐾   **M**

     Cystitis following (induced) termination of pregnancy

O04.89   **(Induced) termination of pregnancy with other complications** ♀ 🐾   **M**

● O07   **Failed attempted termination of pregnancy**

     Includes   failure of attempted induction of termination of pregnancy
                incomplete elective abortion

     Excludes1   incomplete spontaneous abortion (O03.0-)

O07.0   **Genital tract and pelvic infection following failed attempted termination of pregnancy** ♀ 🐾   **M**

     Endometritis following failed attempted termination of pregnancy

     Oophoritis following failed attempted termination of pregnancy

     Parametritis following failed attempted termination of pregnancy

     Pelvic peritonitis following failed attempted termination of pregnancy

     Salpingitis following failed attempted termination of pregnancy

     Salpingo-oophoritis following failed attempted termination of pregnancy

     Excludes1   sepsis following failed attempted termination of pregnancy (O07.37)
                  urinary tract infection following failed attempted termination of pregnancy (O07.38)

     (Ex:) See PDX Collection 956

O07.1   **Delayed or excessive hemorrhage following failed attempted termination of pregnancy** ♀ 🐾   **M**

     Afibrinogenemia following failed attempted termination of pregnancy

     Defibrination syndrome following failed attempted termination of pregnancy

     Hemolysis following failed attempted termination of pregnancy

     Intravascular coagulation following failed attempted termination of pregnancy

     (Ex:) See PDX Collection 957

O07.2   **Embolism following failed attempted termination of pregnancy** ♀ 🐾   **M**

     Air embolism following failed attempted termination of pregnancy

     Amniotic fluid embolism following failed attempted termination of pregnancy

     Blood-clot embolism following failed attempted termination of pregnancy

     Embolism NOS following failed attempted termination of pregnancy

     Fat embolism following failed attempted termination of pregnancy

     Pulmonary embolism following failed attempted termination of pregnancy

     Pyemic embolism following failed attempted termination of pregnancy

     Septic or septicopyemic embolism following failed attempted termination of pregnancy

     Soap embolism following failed attempted termination of pregnancy

     (Ex:) See PDX Collection 958

● O07.3   **Failed attempted termination of pregnancy with other and unspecified complications**

O07.30   **Failed attempted termination of pregnancy with unspecified complications** ♀ 🐾   **M**
     (Ex:) See PDX Collection 954

O07.31   **Shock following failed attempted termination of pregnancy** ♀ 🐾   **M**

     Circulatory collapse following failed attempted termination of pregnancy

     Shock (postprocedural) following failed attempted termination of pregnancy

     Excludes1   shock due to infection following failed attempted termination of pregnancy (O07.37)

     (Ex:) See PDX Collection 959

O07.32   **Renal failure following failed attempted termination of pregnancy** ♀ 🐾   **M**

     Kidney failure (acute) following failed attempted termination of pregnancy

     Oliguria following failed attempted termination of pregnancy

     Renal shutdown following failed attempted termination of pregnancy

     Renal tubular necrosis following failed attempted termination of pregnancy

     Uremia following failed attempted termination of pregnancy

     (Ex:) See PDX Collection 960

O07.33   **Metabolic disorder following failed attempted termination of pregnancy** ♀ 🐾   **M**
     (Ex:) See PDX Collection 954

O07.34   **Damage to pelvic organs following failed attempted termination of pregnancy** ♀ 🐾   **M**

     Laceration, perforation, tear or chemical damage of bladder following failed attempted termination of pregnancy

     Laceration, perforation, tear or chemical damage of bowel following failed attempted termination of pregnancy

     Laceration, perforation, tear or chemical damage of broad ligament following failed attempted termination of pregnancy

     Laceration, perforation, tear or chemical damage of cervix following failed attempted termination of pregnancy

     Laceration, perforation, tear or chemical damage of periurethral tissue following failed attempted termination of pregnancy

     Laceration, perforation, tear or chemical damage of uterus following failed attempted termination of pregnancy

     Laceration, perforation, tear or chemical damage of vagina following failed attempted termination of pregnancy

     (Ex:) See PDX Collection 961

O07.35   **Other venous complications following failed attempted termination of pregnancy** ♀ 🐾   **M**
     (Ex:) See PDX Collection 954

O07.36   **Cardiac arrest following failed attempted termination of pregnancy** ♀ 🐾   **M**
     (Ex:) See PDX Collection 954

O07.37   **Sepsis following failed attempted termination of pregnancy** ♀ 🐾   **M**

     Use additional code (B95-B97), to identify infectious agent

     Use additional code (R65.2-) to identify severe sepsis, if applicable

     Excludes1   septic or septicopyemic embolism following failed attempted termination of pregnancy (O07.2)

     (Ex:) See PDX Collection 956

CHAPTER 15 (O00-O9A)

N   Newborn Age: 0   **P**   Pediatric Age: 0–17   **M**   Maternity DX: 9–64   **A**   Adult Age: 15–124   ♀   Females Only   ♂   Males Only

🐾   Complication\Comorbidity   🐾   Major C\C   (Ex:)   CC/MCC Exclusions   🐾   Hospital-Acquired Condition   🐾   Hierarchical Condition Category

1147

O07.38   **Urinary tract infection** following failed attempted termination of pregnancy ♀ 🔒   M

Cystitis following failed attempted termination of pregnancy ♀ 🔒

(Ex:) See PDX Collection 954

O07.39   **Failed attempted termination of pregnancy with other complications** ♀ 🔒   M

(Ex:) See PDX Collection 954

O07.4   **Failed attempted termination of pregnancy without complication** ♀   M

● **O08**   **Complications following ectopic and molar pregnancy**

This category is for use with categories O00-O02 to identify any associated complications.

(Ex:) **For category O08 CC codes unless otherwise indicated:** See PDX Collection 963

O08.0   **Genital tract and pelvic infection** following ectopic and molar pregnancy ♀ 🔒   M

Endometritis following ectopic and molar pregnancy

Oophoritis following ectopic and molar pregnancy

Parametritis following ectopic and molar pregnancy

Pelvic peritonitis following ectopic and molar pregnancy

Salpingitis following ectopic and molar pregnancy

Salpingo-oophoritis following ectopic and molar pregnancy

Excludes1   sepsis following ectopic and molar pregnancy (O08.82)

urinary tract infection (O08.83)

(Ex:) See PDX Collection 85

O08.1   **Delayed or excessive hemorrhage** following ectopic and molar pregnancy ♀ 🔒   M

Afibrinogenemia following ectopic and molar pregnancy

Defibrination syndrome following ectopic and molar pregnancy

Hemolysis following ectopic and molar pregnancy

Intravascular coagulation following ectopic and molar pregnancy

Excludes1   delayed or excessive hemorrhage due to incomplete abortion (O03.1)

(Ex:) See PDX Collection 962

O08.2   **Embolism following ectopic and molar pregnancy** ♀ 🔒 M

Air embolism following ectopic and molar pregnancy

Amniotic fluid embolism following ectopic and molar pregnancy

Blood-clot embolism following ectopic and molar pregnancy

Embolism NOS following ectopic and molar pregnancy

Fat embolism following ectopic and molar pregnancy

Pulmonary embolism following ectopic and molar pregnancy

Pyemic embolism following ectopic and molar pregnancy

Septic or septicopyemic embolism following ectopic and molar pregnancy

Soap embolism following ectopic and molar pregnancy

O08.3   **Shock following ectopic and molar pregnancy** ♀ 🔒   M

Circulatory collapse following ectopic and molar pregnancy

Shock (postprocedural) following ectopic and molar pregnancy

Excludes1   shock due to infection following ectopic and molar pregnancy (O08.82)

O08.4   **Renal failure** following ectopic and molar pregnancy ♀ 🔒   M

Kidney failure (acute) following ectopic and molar pregnancy

Oliguria following ectopic and molar pregnancy

Renal shutdown following ectopic and molar pregnancy

Renal tubular necrosis following ectopic and molar pregnancy

Uremia following ectopic and molar pregnancy

O08.5   **Metabolic disorders** following an ectopic and molar pregnancy ♀ 🔒   M

O08.6   **Damage to pelvic organs and tissues** following an ectopic and molar pregnancy ♀ 🔒   M

Laceration, perforation, tear or chemical damage of bladder following an ectopic and molar pregnancy

Laceration, perforation, tear or chemical damage of bowel following an ectopic and molar pregnancy

Laceration, perforation, tear or chemical damage of broad ligament following an ectopic and molar pregnancy

Laceration, perforation, tear or chemical damage of cervix following an ectopic and molar pregnancy

Laceration, perforation, tear or chemical damage of periurethral tissue following an ectopic and molar pregnancy

Laceration, perforation, tear or chemical damage of uterus following an ectopic and molar pregnancy

Laceration, perforation, tear or chemical damage of vagina following an ectopic and molar pregnancy

O08.7   **Other venous** complications following an ectopic and molar pregnancy ♀ 🔒   M

● **O08.8**   **Other complications** following an ectopic and molar pregnancy

O08.81   **Cardiac arrest** following an ectopic and molar pregnancy ♀ 🔒   M

O08.82   **Sepsis** following ectopic and molar pregnancy ♀ 🔒   M

Use additional code (B95-B97), to identify infectious agent

Use additional code (R65.2-) to identify severe sepsis, if applicable

Excludes1   septic or septicopyemic embolism following ectopic and molar pregnancy (O08.2)

(Ex:) See PDX Collection 85

O08.83   **Urinary tract infection** following an ectopic and molar pregnancy ♀ 🔒   M

Cystitis following an ectopic and molar pregnancy

O08.89   **Other** complications following an ectopic and molar pregnancy ♀ 🔒   M

O08.9   **Unspecified** complication following an ectopic and molar pregnancy ♀ 🔒   M

SUPERVISION OF HIGH RISK PREGNANCY (O09)

● **O09**   **Supervision of high risk pregnancy**

Coding Clinic: 2016, Q4, P125, 150

● **O09.0**   **Supervision of pregnancy with history of infertility**

● **O09.00**   Supervision of pregnancy with history of infertility, **unspecified trimester** ♀   M

● **O09.01**   Supervision of pregnancy with history of infertility, **first trimester** ♀   M

● **O09.02**   Supervision of pregnancy with history of infertility, **second trimester** ♀   M

● **O09.03**   Supervision of pregnancy with history of infertility, **third trimester** ♀   M

● **O09.1**   **Supervision of pregnancy with history of ectopic pregnancy**

Coding Clinic: 2016, Q4, P49-50

● **O09.10**   Supervision of pregnancy with history of ectopic pregnancy, **unspecified trimester** ♀   M

● **O09.11**   Supervision of pregnancy with history of ectopic pregnancy, **first trimester** ♀   M

● **O09.12**   Supervision of pregnancy with history of ectopic pregnancy, **second trimester** ♀   M

● **O09.13**   Supervision of pregnancy with history of ectopic pregnancy, **third trimester** ♀   M

▶ New   ⇒ Revised   ~~deleted~~ Deleted   Excludes 1   Excludes 2   Includes   Use additional   Code first   Code also   Key words

OGCR Official Guidelines   ● Unacceptable Principal Diagnosis   X Assign placeholder X   ● Use Additional Character(s)   ⫸ Manifestation Code   Coding Clinic

- ● **O09.A** Supervision of pregnancy with history of molar pregnancy
  Coding Clinic: 2016, Q4, P50
  - ● **O09.A0** Supervision of pregnancy with history of molar pregnancy, unspecified trimester ♀   M
  - ● **O09.A1** Supervision of pregnancy with history of molar pregnancy, first trimester ♀   M
  - ● **O09.A2** Supervision of pregnancy with history of molar pregnancy, second trimester ♀   M
  - ● **O09.A3** Supervision of pregnancy with history of molar pregnancy, third trimester ♀   M
- ● **O09.2** Supervision of pregnancy with other poor reproductive or obstetric history
  Excludes2   pregnancy care for patient with history of recurrent pregnancy loss (O26.2‐)
  - ● **O09.21** Supervision of pregnancy with history of pre-term labor
    - ● **O09.211** Supervision of pregnancy with history of pre-term labor, first trimester ♀   M
    - ● **O09.212** Supervision of pregnancy with history of pre-term labor, second trimester ♀ M
    - ● **O09.213** Supervision of pregnancy with history of pre-term labor, third trimester ♀   M
    - ● **O09.219** Supervision of pregnancy with history of pre-term labor, unspecified trimester ♀   M
  - ● **O09.29** Supervision of pregnancy with other poor reproductive or obstetric history
    Supervision of pregnancy with history of neonatal death
    Supervision of pregnancy with history of stillbirth
    - ● **O09.291** Supervision of pregnancy with other poor reproductive or obstetric history, first trimester ♀   M
    - ● **O09.292** Supervision of pregnancy with other poor reproductive or obstetric history, second trimester ♀   M
    - ● **O09.293** Supervision of pregnancy with other poor reproductive or obstetric history, third trimester ♀   M
    - ● **O09.299** Supervision of pregnancy with other poor reproductive or obstetric history, unspecified trimester ♀   M
- ● **O09.3** Supervision of pregnancy with insufficient antenatal care
  Supervision of concealed pregnancy
  Supervision of hidden pregnancy
  - ● **O09.30** Supervision of pregnancy with insufficient antenatal care, unspecified trimester ♀   M
  - ● **O09.31** Supervision of pregnancy with insufficient antenatal care, first trimester ♀   M
  - ● **O09.32** Supervision of pregnancy with insufficient antenatal care, second trimester ♀   M
  - ● **O09.33** Supervision of pregnancy with insufficient antenatal care, third trimester ♀   M
- ● **O09.4** Supervision of pregnancy with grand multiparity
  - ● **O09.40** Supervision of pregnancy with grand multiparity, unspecified trimester ♀   M
  - ● **O09.41** Supervision of pregnancy with grand multiparity, first trimester ♀   M
  - ● **O09.42** Supervision of pregnancy with grand multiparity, second trimester ♀   M
  - ● **O09.43** Supervision of pregnancy with grand multiparity, third trimester ♀   M

- ● **O09.5** Supervision of elderly primigravida and multigravida
  Pregnancy for a female 35 years and older at expected date of delivery
  - ● **O09.51** Supervision of elderly primigravida
    - ● **O09.511** Supervision of elderly primigravida, first trimester ♀   M
    - ● **O09.512** Supervision of elderly primigravida, second trimester ♀   M
    - ● **O09.513** Supervision of elderly primigravida, third trimester ♀   M
    - ● **O09.519** Supervision of elderly primigravida, unspecified trimester ♀   M
  - ● **O09.52** Supervision of elderly multigravida
    - ● **O09.521** Supervision of elderly multigravida, first trimester ♀   M
    - ● **O09.522** Supervision of elderly multigravida, second trimester ♀   M
    - ● **O09.523** Supervision of elderly multigravida, third trimester ♀   M
      Coding Clinic: 2016, Q4, P150
    - ● **O09.529** Supervision of elderly multigravida, unspecified trimester ♀   M
- ● **O09.6** Supervision of young primigravida and multigravida
  Supervision of pregnancy for a female less than 16 years old at expected date of delivery
  - ● **O09.61** Supervision of young primigravida
    - ● **O09.611** Supervision of young primigravida, first trimester ♀   M
    - ● **O09.612** Supervision of young primigravida, second trimester ♀   M
    - ● **O09.613** Supervision of young primigravida, third trimester ♀   M
    - ● **O09.619** Supervision of young primigravida, unspecified trimester ♀   M
  - ● **O09.62** Supervision of young multigravida
    - ● **O09.621** Supervision of young multigravida, first trimester ♀   M
    - ● **O09.622** Supervision of young multigravida, second trimester ♀   M
    - ● **O09.623** Supervision of young multigravida, third trimester ♀   M
    - ● **O09.629** Supervision of young multigravida, unspecified trimester ♀   M
- ● **O09.7** Supervision of high risk pregnancy due to social problems
  - ● **O09.70** Supervision of high risk pregnancy due to social problems, unspecified trimester ♀   M
  - ● **O09.71** Supervision of high risk pregnancy due to social problems, first trimester ♀   M
  - ● **O09.72** Supervision of high risk pregnancy due to social problems, second trimester ♀   M
  - ● **O09.73** Supervision of high risk pregnancy due to social problems, third trimester ♀   M
- ● **O09.8** Supervision of other high risk pregnancies
  - ● **O09.81** Supervision of pregnancy resulting from assisted reproductive technology
    Supervision of pregnancy resulting from in-vitro fertilization
    Excludes2   gestational carrier status (Z33.3)
    - ● **O09.811** Supervision of pregnancy resulting from assisted reproductive technology, first trimester ♀   M
    - ● **O09.812** Supervision of pregnancy resulting from assisted reproductive technology, second trimester ♀   M

CHAPTER 15 (O00-O9A)

N Newborn Age: 0   **P** Pediatric Age: 0–17   **M** Maternity DX: 9–64   **A** Adult Age: 15–124   ♀ Females Only   ♂ Males Only

Complication\Comorbidity   Major C\C   (Ex) CC/MCC Exclusions   Hospital-Acquired Condition   Hierarchical Condition Category   1149

● O09.813   Supervision of pregnancy resulting from assisted reproductive technology, third trimester ♀   M

● O09.819   Supervision of pregnancy resulting from assisted reproductive technology, unspecified trimester ♀   M

● O09.82   Supervision of pregnancy with history of in utero procedure during previous pregnancy

  ● O09.821   Supervision of pregnancy with history of in utero procedure during previous pregnancy, first trimester ♀   M

  ● O09.822   Supervision of pregnancy with history of in utero procedure during previous pregnancy, second trimester ♀   M

  ● O09.823   Supervision of pregnancy with history of in utero procedure during previous pregnancy, third trimester ♀   M

  ● O09.829   Supervision of pregnancy with history of in utero procedure during previous pregnancy, unspecified trimester ♀   M

      Excludes1   supervision of pregnancy affected by in utero procedure during current pregnancy (O35.7)

● O09.89   Supervision of other high risk pregnancies

  ● O09.891   Supervision of other high risk pregnancies, first trimester ♀   M

  ● O09.892   Supervision of other high risk pregnancies, second trimester ♀   M

  ● O09.893   Supervision of other high risk pregnancies, third trimester ♀   M

  ● O09.899   Supervision of other high risk pregnancies, unspecified trimester ♀   M

● O09.9   Supervision of high risk pregnancy, unspecified

  ● O09.90   Supervision of high risk pregnancy, unspecified, unspecified trimester ♀   M

  ● O09.91   Supervision of high risk pregnancy, unspecified, first trimester ♀   M

  ● O09.92   Supervision of high risk pregnancy, unspecified, second trimester ♀   M

  ● O09.93   Supervision of high risk pregnancy, unspecified, third trimester ♀   M

EDEMA, PROTEINURIA AND HYPERTENSIVE DISORDERS IN PREGNANCY, CHILDBIRTH AND THE PUERPERIUM (O10-O16)

● O10   Pre-existing hypertension complicating pregnancy, childbirth and the puerperium

   Includes   pre-existing hypertension with pre-existing proteinuria complicating pregnancy, childbirth and the puerperium

   Excludes2   pre-existing hypertension with superimposed pre-eclampsia complicating pregnancy, childbirth and the puerperium (O11.-)

   (Ex) **For category O10 CC codes:** See PDX Collection 4042-4043

   Coding Clinic: 2016, Q4, P50

● O10.0   Pre-existing essential hypertension complicating pregnancy, childbirth and the puerperium

   Any condition in I10 specified as a reason for obstetric care during pregnancy, childbirth or the puerperium

  ● O10.01   Pre-existing essential hypertension complicating pregnancy

     O10.011   Pre-existing essential hypertension complicating pregnancy, first trimester ♀ 🔗   M

     O10.012   Pre-existing essential hypertension complicating pregnancy, second trimester ♀ 🔗   M

     O10.013   Pre-existing essential hypertension complicating pregnancy, third trimester ♀ 🔗   M

     O10.019   Pre-existing essential hypertension complicating pregnancy, unspecified trimester ♀   M

   O10.02   Pre-existing essential hypertension complicating childbirth ♀ 🔗   M

     (Ex) See PDX Collection 4059

   O10.03   Pre-existing essential hypertension complicating the puerperium ♀   M

● O10.1   Pre-existing hypertensive heart disease complicating pregnancy, childbirth and the puerperium

   Any condition in I11 specified as a reason for obstetric care during pregnancy, childbirth or the puerperium

   Use additional code from I11 to identify the type of hypertensive heart disease

  ● O10.11   Pre-existing hypertensive heart disease complicating pregnancy

     O10.111   Pre-existing hypertensive heart disease complicating pregnancy, first trimester ♀   M

     O10.112   Pre-existing hypertensive heart disease complicating pregnancy, second trimester ♀   M

     O10.113   Pre-existing hypertensive heart disease complicating pregnancy, third trimester ♀   M

     O10.119   Pre-existing hypertensive heart disease complicating pregnancy, unspecified trimester ♀   M

   O10.12   Pre-existing hypertensive heart disease complicating childbirth ♀   M

   O10.13   Pre-existing hypertensive heart disease complicating the puerperium ♀   M

● O10.2   Pre-existing hypertensive chronic kidney disease complicating pregnancy, childbirth and the puerperium

   Any condition in I12 specified as a reason for obstetric care during pregnancy, childbirth or the puerperium

   Use additional code from I12 to identify the type of hypertensive chronic kidney disease

  ● O10.21   Pre-existing hypertensive chronic kidney disease complicating pregnancy

     O10.211   Pre-existing hypertensive chronic kidney disease complicating pregnancy, first trimester ♀   M

     O10.212   Pre-existing hypertensive chronic kidney disease complicating pregnancy, second trimester ♀   M

     O10.213   Pre-existing hypertensive chronic kidney disease complicating pregnancy, third trimester ♀   M

     O10.219   Pre-existing hypertensive chronic kidney disease complicating pregnancy, unspecified trimester ♀   M

   O10.22   Pre-existing hypertensive chronic kidney disease complicating childbirth ♀   M

   O10.23   Pre-existing hypertensive chronic kidney disease complicating the puerperium ♀   M

▶ New   ⟹ Revised   ~~deleted~~ Deleted   Excludes 1   Excludes 2   Includes   Use additional   Code first   Code also   Key words

1150   OGCR Official Guidelines   ● Unacceptable Principal Diagnosis   X Assign placeholder X   ● Use Additional Character(s)   ▶ Manifestation Code   Coding Clinic

● **O10.3** **Pre-existing hypertensive heart and chronic kidney disease** complicating pregnancy, childbirth and the puerperium

    Any condition in I13 specified as a reason for obstetric care during pregnancy, childbirth or the puerperium

    Use additional code from I13 to identify the type of hypertensive heart and chronic kidney disease

  ● **O10.31** Pre-existing hypertensive heart and chronic kidney disease complicating pregnancy

    O10.311   Pre-existing hypertensive heart and chronic kidney disease complicating pregnancy, first trimester ♀   M

    O10.312   Pre-existing hypertensive heart and chronic kidney disease complicating pregnancy, second trimester ♀   M

    O10.313   Pre-existing hypertensive heart and chronic kidney disease complicating pregnancy, third trimester ♀   M

    O10.319   Pre-existing hypertensive heart and chronic kidney disease complicating pregnancy, unspecified trimester ♀   M

   O10.32   Pre-existing hypertensive heart and chronic kidney disease complicating childbirth ♀   M

   O10.33   Pre-existing hypertensive heart and chronic kidney disease complicating the puerperium ♀   M

● **O10.4** Pre-existing secondary hypertension complicating pregnancy, childbirth and the puerperium

    Any condition in I15 specified as a reason for obstetric care during pregnancy, childbirth or the puerperium

    Use additional code from I15 to identify the type of secondary hypertension

  ● **O10.41** Pre-existing secondary hypertension complicating pregnancy

    O10.411   Pre-existing secondary hypertension complicating pregnancy, first trimester ♀ 🏷   M

    O10.412   Pre-existing secondary hypertension complicating pregnancy, second trimester ♀ 🏷   M

    O10.413   Pre-existing secondary hypertension complicating pregnancy, third trimester ♀ 🏷   M

    O10.419   Pre-existing secondary hypertension complicating pregnancy, unspecified trimester ♀   M

   O10.42   Pre-existing secondary hypertension complicating childbirth ♀ 🏷   M

      (Ex:) See PDX Collection 4059

   O10.43   Pre-existing secondary hypertension complicating the puerperium ♀ 🏷   M

      (Ex:) See PDX Collection 4063

● **O10.9** Unspecified pre-existing hypertension complicating pregnancy, childbirth and the puerperium

  ● **O10.91** Unspecified pre-existing hypertension complicating pregnancy

    O10.911   Unspecified pre-existing hypertension complicating pregnancy, first trimester ♀ 🏷   M

    O10.912   Unspecified pre-existing hypertension complicating pregnancy, second trimester ♀ 🏷   M

    O10.913   Unspecified pre-existing hypertension complicating pregnancy, third trimester ♀ 🏷   M

    O10.919   Unspecified pre-existing hypertension complicating pregnancy, unspecified trimester ♀   M

   O10.92   Unspecified pre-existing hypertension complicating childbirth ♀ 🏷   M

   O10.93   Unspecified pre-existing hypertension complicating the puerperium ♀   M

● **O11** Pre-existing hypertension with pre-eclampsia

    Includes   conditions in O10 complicated by pre-eclampsia pre-eclampsia superimposed pre-existing hypertension

    Use additional code from O10 to identify the type of hypertension

    (Ex:) For category O11 CC codes: See PDX Collection 964, 4042-4043

    Coding Clinic: 2016, Q4, P50

  O11.1   Pre-existing hypertension with pre-eclampsia, first trimester ♀ 🏷   M

  O11.2   Pre-existing hypertension with pre-eclampsia, second trimester ♀ 🏷   M

  O11.3   Pre-existing hypertension with pre-eclampsia, third trimester ♀ 🏷   M

  O11.4   Pre-existing hypertension with pre-eclampsia, complicating childbirth ♀   M

  O11.5   Pre-existing hypertension with pre-eclampsia, complicating the puerperium ♀   M

  O11.9   Pre-existing hypertension with pre-eclampsia, unspecified trimester ♀   M

● **O12** Gestational [pregnancy-induced] edema and proteinuria without hypertension

    (Ex:) For category O12 CC codes: See PDX Collection 965

    Coding Clinic: 2016, Q4, P50

  ● **O12.0** Gestational edema

    O12.00   Gestational edema, unspecified trimester ♀   M

    O12.01   Gestational edema, first trimester ♀   M

    O12.02   Gestational edema, second trimester ♀   M

    O12.03   Gestational edema, third trimester ♀   M

    O12.04   Gestational edema, complicating childbirth ♀   M

    O12.05   Gestational edema, complicating the puerperium ♀   M

  ● **O12.1** Gestational proteinuria

    O12.10   Gestational proteinuria, unspecified trimester ♀   M

    O12.11   Gestational proteinuria, first trimester ♀ 🏷   M

    O12.12   Gestational proteinuria, second trimester ♀ 🏷 M

    O12.13   Gestational proteinuria, third trimester ♀ 🏷   M

    O12.14   Gestational proteinuria, complicating childbirth ♀   M

    O12.15   Gestational proteinuria, complicating the puerperium ♀   M

  ● **O12.2** Gestational edema with proteinuria

    O12.20   Gestational edema with proteinuria, unspecified trimester ♀   M

    O12.21   Gestational edema with proteinuria, first trimester ♀ 🏷   M

       CC when PDx is its own CC

    O12.22   Gestational edema with proteinuria, second trimester ♀ 🏷   M

       CC when PDx is its own CC

    O12.23   Gestational edema with proteinuria, third trimester ♀ 🏷   M

       CC when PDx is its own CC

    O12.24   Gestational edema with proteinuria, complicating childbirth ♀   M

    O12.25   Gestational edema with proteinuria, complicating the puerperium ♀   M

N Newborn Age: 0   **P** Pediatric Age: 0–17   **M** Maternity DX: 9–64   **A** Adult Age: 15–124   ♀ Females Only   ♂ Males Only

🏷 Complication\Comorbidity   🏷 Major C\C   (Ex:) CC/MCC Exclusions   🏷 Hospital-Acquired Condition   🏷 Hierarchical Condition Category

1151

● **O13   Gestational [pregnancy-induced] hypertension without significant proteinuria**

Includes   gestational hypertension NOS
transient hypertension of pregnancy ♀

Coding Clinic: 2016, Q4, P50

O13.1   Gestational [pregnancy-induced] hypertension without significant proteinuria, first trimester ♀   M

O13.2   Gestational [pregnancy-induced] hypertension without significant proteinuria, second trimester ♀   M

O13.3   Gestational [pregnancy-induced] hypertension without significant proteinuria, third trimester ♀   M

O13.4   Gestational [pregnancy-induced] hypertension without significant proteinuria, complicating childbirth ♀   M

O13.5   Gestational [pregnancy-induced] hypertension without significant proteinuria, complicating the puerperium ♀   M

O13.9   Gestational [pregnancy-induced] hypertension without significant proteinuria, unspecified trimester ♀   M

● **O14   Pre-eclampsia**

Excludes1   pre-existing hypertension with pre-eclampsia (O11)

(Ex) **For category O14 CC codes:** See PDX Collection 964, 4042-4043
Coding Clinic: 2016, Q4, P50

● O14.0   Mild to moderate pre-eclampsia

O14.00   Mild to moderate pre-eclampsia, unspecified trimester ♀   M

O14.02   Mild to moderate pre-eclampsia, second trimester ♀   M

O14.03   Mild to moderate pre-eclampsia, third trimester ♀   M

O14.04   Mild to moderate pre-eclampsia, complicating childbirth ♀
       Coding Clinic: 2019, Q2, P8   M

O14.05   Mild to moderate pre-eclampsia, complicating the puerperium ♀   M

● O14.1   Severe pre-eclampsia

Excludes1   HELLP syndrome (O14.2-)

H=hemolysis, EL=elevated liver enzymes, LP=low platelet count
Coding Clinic: 2019, Q3, P12

O14.10   Severe pre-eclampsia, unspecified trimester ♀   M

O14.12   Severe pre-eclampsia, second trimester ♀   M

O14.13   Severe pre-eclampsia, third trimester ♀   M

O14.14   Severe pre-eclampsia complicating childbirth ♀   M

O14.15   Severe pre-eclampsia, complicating the puerperium ♀   M

● O14.2   HELLP syndrome

Severe pre-eclampsia with hemolysis, elevated liver enzymes and low platelet count (HELLP)

O14.20   HELLP syndrome (HELLP), unspecified trimester ♀   M

O14.22   HELLP syndrome (HELLP), second trimester ♀   M

O14.23   HELLP syndrome (HELLP), third trimester ♀   M

O14.24   HELLP syndrome, complicating childbirth ♀   M

O14.25   HELLP syndrome, complicating the puerperium ♀   M

● O14.9   Unspecified pre-eclampsia

O14.90   Unspecified pre-eclampsia, unspecified trimester ♀   M

O14.92   Unspecified pre-eclampsia, second trimester ♀   M

O14.93   Unspecified pre-eclampsia, third trimester ♀   M

O14.94   Unspecified pre-eclampsia, complicating childbirth ♀   M

O14.95   Unspecified pre-eclampsia, complicating the puerperium ♀   M

● **O15   Eclampsia**

Includes   convulsions following conditions in O10-O14 and O16

(Ex) **For category O15 CC codes:** See PDX Collection 964

● O15.0   Eclampsia complicating pregnancy
Coding Clinic: 2016, Q4, P50

O15.00   Eclampsia complicating pregnancy, unspecified trimester ♀   M

O15.02   Eclampsia complicating pregnancy, second trimester ♀   M
       (Ex) See PDX Collection 4042

O15.03   Eclampsia complicating pregnancy, third trimester ♀   M
       (Ex) See PDX Collection 4043

O15.1   Eclampsia complicating labor ♀   M
       (Ex) See PDX Collection 4059

O15.2   Eclampsia complicating the puerperium ♀   M
       (Ex) See PDX Collection 4063

O15.9   Eclampsia, unspecified as to time period ♀   M
Eclampsia NOS

● **O16   Unspecified maternal hypertension**

(Ex) **For category O16 CC codes:** See PDX Collection 964, 4402-4403
Coding Clinic: 2016, Q4, P50

O16.1   Unspecified maternal hypertension, first trimester ♀   M

O16.2   Unspecified maternal hypertension, second trimester ♀   M

O16.3   Unspecified maternal hypertension, third trimester ♀   M

O16.4   Unspecified maternal hypertension, complicating childbirth ♀   M

O16.5   Unspecified maternal hypertension, complicating the puerperium ♀   M

O16.9   Unspecified maternal hypertension, unspecified trimester ♀   M

OTHER MATERNAL DISORDERS PREDOMINANTLY RELATED TO PREGNANCY (O20-O29)

Excludes2   maternal care related to the fetus and amniotic cavity and possible delivery problems (O30-O48)
maternal diseases classifiable elsewhere but complicating pregnancy, labor and delivery, and the puerperium (O98-O99)

● **O20   Hemorrhage in early pregnancy**

Includes   hemorrhage before completion of 20 weeks gestation

Excludes1   pregnancy with abortive outcome (O00-O08)

(Ex) **For category O20 CC codes:** See PDX Collection 966, 4011

O20.0   Threatened abortion ♀   M
Hemorrhage specified as due to threatened abortion

O20.8   Other hemorrhage in early pregnancy ♀   M

O20.9   Hemorrhage in early pregnancy, unspecified ♀   M

● **O21   Excessive vomiting in pregnancy**

O21.0   Mild hyperemesis gravidarum ♀   M
Hyperemesis gravidarum, mild or unspecified, starting before the end of the 20th week of gestation

O21.1   Hyperemesis gravidarum with metabolic disturbance ♀
Hyperemesis gravidarum, starting before the end of the 20th week of gestation, with metabolic disturbance such as carbohydrate depletion
Hyperemesis gravidarum, starting before the end of the 20th week of gestation, with metabolic disturbance such as dehydration
Hyperemesis gravidarum, starting before the end of the 20th week of gestation, with metabolic disturbance such as electrolyte imbalance

O21.2   Late vomiting of pregnancy ♀   M
Excessive vomiting starting after 20 completed weeks of gestation

---

▶ New   ⇒ Revised   ~~deleted~~ Deleted   Excludes 1   Excludes 2   Includes   Use additional   Code first   Code also   Key words

OGCR Official Guidelines   ● Unacceptable Principal Diagnosis   X Assign placeholder X   ● Use Additional Character(s)   ▶ Manifestation Code   Coding Clinic

O21.8   Other vomiting complicating pregnancy ♀   **M**
Vomiting due to diseases classified elsewhere,
complicating pregnancy
Use additional code, to identify cause

O21.9   Vomiting of pregnancy, unspecified ♀   **M**

● **O22**   Venous complications and hemorrhoids in pregnancy

Excludes1   venous complications of:
abortion NOS (O03.9)
ectopic or molar pregnancy (O08.7)
failed attempted abortion (O07.35)
induced abortion (O04.85)
spontaneous abortion (O03.89)

Excludes2   obstetric pulmonary embolism (O88.-)
venous complications and hemorrhoids of
childbirth and the puerperium (O87.-)

Ex: For category O22 CC codes: See PDX Collection 967, 4012

● **O22.0**   Varicose veins of lower extremity in pregnancy
Varicose veins NOS in pregnancy

O22.00   Varicose veins of lower extremity in pregnancy,
unspecified trimester ♀   **M**

O22.01   Varicose veins of lower extremity in pregnancy,
first trimester ♀   **M**

O22.02   Varicose veins of lower extremity in pregnancy,
second trimester ♀   **M**

O22.03   Varicose veins of lower extremity in pregnancy,
third trimester ♀   **M**

● **O22.1**   Genital varices in pregnancy
Perineal varices in pregnancy
Vaginal varices in pregnancy
Vulval varices in pregnancy

O22.10   Genital varices in pregnancy, unspecified
trimester ♀   **M**

O22.11   Genital varices in pregnancy, first trimester ♀ **M**

O22.12   Genital varices in pregnancy, second
trimester ♀   **M**

O22.13   Genital varices in pregnancy, third trimester ♀ **M**

● **O22.2**   Superficial thrombophlebitis in pregnancy
Phlebitis in pregnancy NOS
Thrombophlebitis of legs in pregnancy
Thrombosis in pregnancy NOS
Use additional code to identify the superficial
thrombophlebitis (I80.0-)

O22.20   Superficial thrombophlebitis in pregnancy,
unspecified trimester ♀ 🦠   **M**

O22.21   Superficial thrombophlebitis in pregnancy, first
trimester ♀ 🦠   **M**

O22.22   Superficial thrombophlebitis in pregnancy,
second trimester ♀ 🦠   **M**

O22.23   Superficial thrombophlebitis in pregnancy,
third trimester ♀ 🦠   **M**

● **O22.3**   Deep phlebothrombosis in pregnancy
Deep vein thrombosis, antepartum
➡ Use additional code to identify the deep vein
thrombosis (I82.4-, I82.5-, I82.62-, I82.72-)
Use additional code, if applicable, for associated long-
term (current) use of anticoagulants (Z79.01)

O22.30   Deep phlebothrombosis in pregnancy,
unspecified trimester ♀ 🦠   **M**

O22.31   Deep phlebothrombosis in pregnancy,
first trimester ♀ 🦠   **M**

O22.32   Deep phlebothrombosis in pregnancy, second
trimester ♀ 🦠   **M**

O22.33   Deep phlebothrombosis in pregnancy, third
trimester ♀ 🦠   **M**

● **O22.4**   Hemorrhoids in pregnancy

O22.40   Hemorrhoids in pregnancy, unspecified
trimester ♀ 🦠   **M**

O22.41   Hemorrhoids in pregnancy, first trimester ♀ 🦠 **M**

O22.42   Hemorrhoids in pregnancy, second
trimester ♀ 🦠   **M**

O22.43   Hemorrhoids in pregnancy, third
trimester ♀ 🦠   **M**

● **O22.5**   Cerebral venous thrombosis in pregnancy
Cerebrovenous sinus thrombosis in pregnancy

O22.50   Cerebral venous thrombosis in pregnancy,
unspecified trimester ♀ 🦠   **M**

O22.51   Cerebral venous thrombosis in pregnancy, first
trimester ♀ 🦠   **M**

O22.52   Cerebral venous thrombosis in pregnancy,
second trimester ♀ 🦠   **M**

O22.53   Cerebral venous thrombosis in pregnancy, third
trimester ♀ 🦠   **M**

● **O22.8**   Other venous complications in pregnancy

● **O22.8X**   Other venous complications in pregnancy

O22.8X1   Other venous complications in
pregnancy, first trimester ♀ 🦠   **M**

O22.8X2   Other venous complications in
pregnancy, second trimester ♀ 🦠   **M**

O22.8X3   Other venous complications in
pregnancy, third trimester ♀ 🦠   **M**

O22.8X9   Other venous complications in
pregnancy, unspecified
trimester ♀ 🦠   **M**

● **O22.9**   Venous complication in pregnancy, unspecified
Gestational phlebitis NOS
Gestational phlebopathy NOS
Gestational thrombosis NOS

O22.90   Venous complication in pregnancy, unspecified,
unspecified trimester ♀ 🦠   **M**

O22.91   Venous complication in pregnancy, unspecified,
first trimester ♀   **M**

O22.92   Venous complication in pregnancy, unspecified,
second trimester ♀   **M**

O22.93   Venous complication in pregnancy, unspecified,
third trimester ♀   **M**

● **O23**   Infections of genitourinary tract in pregnancy
Use additional code to identify organism (B95.-, B96.-)

Excludes2   gonococcal infections complicating pregnancy,
childbirth and the puerperium (O98.2)
infections with a predominantly sexual mode of
transmission NOS complicating pregnancy,
childbirth and the puerperium (O98.3)
syphilis complicating pregnancy, childbirth and
the puerperium (O98.1)
tuberculosis of genitourinary system
complicating pregnancy, childbirth and the
puerperium (O98.0)
venereal disease NOS complicating pregnancy,
childbirth and the puerperium (O98.3)

Ex: For category O23 CC codes: See PDX Collection 968, 4052-4053

● **O23.0**   Infections of kidney in pregnancy
Pyelonephritis in pregnancy

O23.00   Infections of kidney in pregnancy, unspecified
trimester ♀   **M**

O23.01   Infections of kidney in pregnancy, first
trimester ♀ 🦠   **M**

O23.02   Infections of kidney in pregnancy, second
trimester ♀ 🦠   **M**

O23.03   Infections of kidney in pregnancy, third
trimester ♀ 🦠   **M**

● **O23.1**   Infections of bladder in pregnancy

O23.10   Infections of bladder in pregnancy, unspecified
trimester ♀   **M**

O23.11   Infections of bladder in pregnancy, first
trimester ♀ 🦠   **M**

O23.12   Infections of bladder in pregnancy, second
trimester ♀ 🦠   **M**

O23.13   Infections of bladder in pregnancy, third
trimester ♀ 🦠   **M**

N Newborn Age: 0   **P** Pediatric Age: 0–17   **M** Maternity DX: 9–64   **A** Adult Age: 15–124   ♀ Females Only   ♂ Males Only

🦠 Complication\Comorbidity   🦠 Major C\C   Ex: CC/MCC Exclusions   🦠 Hospital-Acquired Condition   🦠 Hierarchical Condition Category

1153

O23.2   **Infections of urethra in pregnancy**
- O23.20   Infections of urethra in pregnancy, unspecified trimester ♀ **M**
- O23.21   Infections of urethra in pregnancy, first trimester ♀ 🔒 **M**
- O23.22   Infections of urethra in pregnancy, second trimester ♀ 🔒 **M**
- O23.23   Infections of urethra in pregnancy, third trimester ♀ 🔒 **M**

O23.3   **Infections of other parts of urinary tract in pregnancy**
- O23.30   Infections of other parts of urinary tract in pregnancy, unspecified trimester ♀ **M**
- O23.31   Infections of other parts of urinary tract in pregnancy, first trimester ♀ 🔒 **M**
- O23.32   Infections of other parts of urinary tract in pregnancy, second trimester ♀ 🔒 **M**
- O23.33   Infections of other parts of urinary tract in pregnancy, third trimester ♀ 🔒 **M**

O23.4   **Unspecified infection of urinary tract in pregnancy**
- O23.40   Unspecified infection of urinary tract in pregnancy, unspecified trimester ♀ **M**
- O23.41   Unspecified infection of urinary tract in pregnancy, first trimester ♀ 🔒 **M**
- O23.42   Unspecified infection of urinary tract in pregnancy, second trimester ♀ 🔒 **M**
- O23.43   Unspecified infection of urinary tract in pregnancy, third trimester ♀ 🔒 **M**

O23.5   **Infections of the genital tract in pregnancy**
- O23.51   Infection of cervix in pregnancy
  - O23.511   Infections of cervix in pregnancy, first trimester ♀ 🔒 **M**
  - O23.512   Infections of cervix in pregnancy, second trimester ♀ 🔒 **M**
  - O23.513   Infections of cervix in pregnancy, third trimester ♀ 🔒 **M**
  - O23.519   Infections of cervix in pregnancy, unspecified trimester ♀ **M**
- O23.52   Salpingo-oophoritis in pregnancy
  Oophoritis = inflammation of ovary
  Salpingitis = inflammation of fallopian tube
  Oophoritis in pregnancy
  Salpingitis in pregnancy
  - O23.521   Salpingo-oophoritis in pregnancy, first trimester ♀ 🔒 **M**
  - O23.522   Salpingo-oophoritis in pregnancy, second trimester ♀ 🔒 **M**
  - O23.523   Salpingo-oophoritis in pregnancy, third trimester ♀ 🔒 **M**
  - O23.529   Salpingo-oophoritis in pregnancy, unspecified trimester ♀ **M**
- O23.59   Infection of other part of genital tract in pregnancy
  - O23.591   Infection of other part of genital tract in pregnancy, first trimester ♀ 🔒 **M**
  - O23.592   Infection of other part of genital tract in pregnancy, second trimester ♀ 🔒 **M**
  - O23.593   Infection of other part of genital tract in pregnancy, third trimester ♀ 🔒 **M**
  - O23.599   Infection of other part of genital tract in pregnancy, unspecified trimester ♀ **M**

O23.9   **Unspecified genitourinary tract infection in pregnancy**
  Genitourinary tract infection in pregnancy NOS
- O23.90   Unspecified genitourinary tract infection in pregnancy, unspecified trimester ♀ **M**
- O23.91   Unspecified genitourinary tract infection in pregnancy, first trimester ♀ 🔒 **M**
- O23.92   Unspecified genitourinary tract infection in pregnancy, second trimester ♀ 🔒 **M**
- O23.93   Unspecified genitourinary tract infection in pregnancy, third trimester ♀ 🔒 **M**

OGCR Section I.C.15.g.

Diabetes mellitus in pregnancy
Diabetes mellitus is a significant complicating factor in pregnancy. Pregnant women who are diabetic should be assigned a code from category O24, Diabetes mellitus in pregnancy, childbirth, and the puerperium, first, followed by the appropriate diabetes code(s) (E08-E13) from Chapter 4.

O24   **Diabetes mellitus in pregnancy, childbirth, and the puerperium**
  Ex: For category O24 CC codes: See PDX Collection 969, 3999-4003

O24.0   **Pre-existing type 1 diabetes mellitus, in pregnancy, childbirth and the puerperium**
  Juvenile onset diabetes mellitus, in pregnancy, childbirth and the puerperium
  Ketosis-prone diabetes mellitus in pregnancy, childbirth and the puerperium
  Use additional code from category E10 to further identify any manifestations
- O24.01   Pre-existing type 1 diabetes mellitus, in pregnancy
  - O24.011   Pre-existing type 1 diabetes mellitus, in pregnancy, first trimester ♀ 🔒 **M**
  - O24.012   Pre-existing type 1 diabetes mellitus, in pregnancy, second trimester ♀ 🔒 **M**
  - O24.013   Pre-existing type 1 diabetes mellitus, in pregnancy, third trimester ♀ 🔒 **M**
  - O24.019   Pre-existing type 1 diabetes mellitus, in pregnancy, unspecified trimester ♀ **M**
- O24.02   Pre-existing type 1 diabetes mellitus, in childbirth ♀ 🔒 **M**
- O24.03   Pre-existing type 1 diabetes mellitus, in the puerperium ♀ 🔒 **M**

O24.1   **Pre-existing type 2 diabetes mellitus, in pregnancy, childbirth and the puerperium**
  Insulin-resistant diabetes mellitus in pregnancy, childbirth and the puerperium
  Use additional code (for):
    from category E11 to further identify any manifestations
    long-term (current) use of insulin (Z79.4)
- O24.11   Pre-existing type 2 diabetes mellitus, in pregnancy
  - O24.111   Pre-existing type 2 diabetes mellitus, in pregnancy, first trimester ♀ 🔒 **M**
  - O24.112   Pre-existing type 2 diabetes mellitus, in pregnancy, second trimester ♀ 🔒 **M**
  - O24.113   Pre-existing type 2 diabetes mellitus, in pregnancy, third trimester ♀ 🔒 **M**
  - O24.119   Pre-existing type 2 diabetes mellitus, in pregnancy, unspecified trimester ♀ **M**
- O24.12   Pre-existing type 2 diabetes mellitus, in childbirth ♀ 🔒 **M**
- O24.13   Pre-existing type 2 diabetes mellitus, in the puerperium ♀ 🔒 **M**

▶ New ⇒ Revised ~~deleted~~ Deleted Excludes 1 Excludes 2 Includes Use additional Code first Code also Key words
OGCR Official Guidelines ● Unacceptable Principal Diagnosis X Assign placeholder X ● Use Additional Character(s) ▷ Manifestation Code Coding Clinic

● O24.3   **Unspecified pre-existing diabetes mellitus in pregnancy, childbirth and the puerperium**

     Use additional code (for):
         from category E11 to further identify any manifestation
         long-term (current) use of insulin (Z79.4)

   ● O24.31   **Unspecified pre-existing diabetes mellitus in pregnancy**

       O24.311   Unspecified pre-existing diabetes mellitus in pregnancy, **first trimester** ♀ 🦠   M

       O24.312   Unspecified pre-existing diabetes mellitus in pregnancy, **second trimester** ♀ 🦠   M

       O24.313   Unspecified pre-existing diabetes mellitus in pregnancy, **third trimester** ♀   M

       O24.319   Unspecified pre-existing diabetes mellitus in pregnancy, **unspecified trimester** ♀   M

     O24.32   Unspecified pre-existing diabetes mellitus in **childbirth** ♀ 🦠   M

     O24.33   Unspecified pre-existing diabetes mellitus in **the puerperium** ♀ 🦠   M

● O24.4   **Gestational diabetes mellitus**
     Diabetes mellitus arising in pregnancy
     Gestational diabetes mellitus NOS
     Coding Clinic: 2016, Q4, P50, 126

   ● O24.41   Gestational diabetes mellitus in **pregnancy**

       O24.410   Gestational diabetes mellitus in pregnancy, **diet controlled** ♀   M

       O24.414   Gestational diabetes mellitus in pregnancy, **insulin controlled** ♀   M

       O24.415   Gestational diabetes mellitus in pregnancy, **controlled by oral hypoglycemic drugs** ♀   M
           Gestational diabetes mellitus in pregnancy, controlled by oral antidiabetic drugs
           Coding Clinic: 2016, Q4, P50

       O24.419   Gestational diabetes mellitus in pregnancy, **unspecified control** ♀   M
           Coding Clinic: 2015, Q4, P34

   ● O24.42   Gestational diabetes mellitus in **childbirth**

       O24.420   Gestational diabetes mellitus in childbirth, **diet controlled** ♀   M

       O24.424   Gestational diabetes mellitus in childbirth, **insulin controlled** ♀   M

       O24.425   Gestational diabetes mellitus in childbirth, **controlled by oral hypoglycemic drugs** ♀   M
           Gestational diabetes mellitus in childbirth, controlled by oral antidiabetic drugs
           Coding Clinic: 2016, Q4, P50

       O24.429   Gestational diabetes mellitus in childbirth, **unspecified control** ♀   M

OGCR Section I.C.15.i.

Gestational (pregnancy induced) diabetes

Gestational (pregnancy induced) diabetes can occur during the second and third trimester of pregnancy in women who were not diabetic prior to pregnancy. Gestational diabetes can cause complications in the pregnancy similar to those of pre-existing diabetes mellitus. It also puts the woman at greater risk of developing diabetes after the pregnancy. Codes for gestational diabetes are in subcategory O24.4, Gestational diabetes mellitus. No other code from category O24, Diabetes mellitus in pregnancy, childbirth, and the puerperium, should be used with a code from O24.4

The codes under subcategory O24.4 include diet controlled, insulin controlled, **and controlled by oral hypoglycemic drugs.** If a patient with gestational diabetes is treated with both diet and insulin, only the code for insulin-controlled is required. **If a patient with gestational diabetes is treated with both diet and oral hypoglycemic medications, only the code for "controlled by oral hypoglycemic drugs" is required.** Code Z79.4, Long-term (current) use of insulin or code Z79.84, Long-term (current) use of oral hypoglycemic drugs, should not be assigned with codes from subcategory O24.4.

An abnormal glucose tolerance in pregnancy is assigned a code from subcategory O99.81, Abnormal glucose complicating pregnancy, childbirth, and the puerperium.

   ● O24.43   Gestational diabetes mellitus in the **puerperium**

       O24.430   Gestational diabetes mellitus in the puerperium, **diet controlled** ♀   M

       O24.434   Gestational diabetes mellitus in the puerperium, **insulin controlled** ♀   M

       O24.435   Gestational diabetes mellitus in puerperium, **controlled by oral hypoglycemic drugs** ♀   M
           Gestational diabetes mellitus in puerperium, controlled by oral antidiabetic drugs
           Coding Clinic: 2016, Q4, P50

       O24.439   Gestational diabetes mellitus in the puerperium, **unspecified control** ♀   M

● O24.8   **Other pre-existing diabetes mellitus in pregnancy, childbirth, and the puerperium**

     Use additional code (for):
         from categories E08, E09 and E13 to further identify any manifestation
         long-term (current) use of insulin (Z79.4)

   ● O24.81   Other pre-existing diabetes mellitus in pregnancy

       O24.811   Other pre-existing diabetes mellitus in pregnancy, **first trimester** ♀ 🦠 M

       O24.812   Other pre-existing diabetes mellitus in pregnancy, **second trimester** ♀ 🦠 M

       O24.813   Other pre-existing diabetes mellitus in pregnancy, **third trimester** ♀ 🦠 M

       O24.819   Other pre-existing diabetes mellitus in pregnancy, **unspecified trimester** ♀ 🦠   M

     O24.82   Other pre-existing diabetes mellitus in **childbirth** ♀ 🦠   M

     O24.83   Other pre-existing diabetes mellitus in the **puerperium** ♀ 🦠   M

N   Newborn Age: 0   **P**   Pediatric Age: 0–17   **M**   Maternity DX: 9–64   **A**   Adult Age: 15–124   ♀   Females Only   ♂   Males Only

🦠   Complication\Comorbidity   🦠   Major C\C   (Ex)   CC/MCC Exclusions   🦠   Hospital-Acquired Condition   🦠   Hierarchical Condition Category

CHAPTER 15 (O00-O9A)

- **O24.9** **Unspecified** diabetes mellitus in pregnancy, childbirth and the puerperium
  Use additional code for long-term (current) use of insulin (Z79.4)
  Unknown whether patient was diabetic before pregnancy occurred
  - **O24.91** **Unspecified** diabetes mellitus in **pregnancy**
    - O24.911 Unspecified diabetes mellitus in pregnancy, **first trimester** ♀ 🅒   M
    - O24.912 Unspecified diabetes mellitus in pregnancy, **second trimester** ♀ 🅒   M
    - O24.913 Unspecified diabetes mellitus in pregnancy, **third trimester** ♀ 🅒   M
    - O24.919 Unspecified diabetes mellitus in pregnancy, **unspecified trimester** ♀ 🅒   M
  - O24.92 **Unspecified** diabetes mellitus in **childbirth** ♀   M
  - O24.93 **Unspecified** diabetes mellitus in the **puerperium** ♀ 🅒   M

- **O25** **Malnutrition** in pregnancy, childbirth and the puerperium
  - **O25.1** Malnutrition in **pregnancy**
    - O25.10 Malnutrition in pregnancy, **unspecified trimester** ♀   M
    - O25.11 Malnutrition in pregnancy, **first trimester** ♀   M
    - O25.12 Malnutrition in pregnancy, **second trimester** ♀ M
    - O25.13 Malnutrition in pregnancy, **third trimester** ♀   M
  - O25.2 Malnutrition in **childbirth** ♀   M
  - O25.3 Malnutrition in the **puerperium** ♀   M

- **O26** Maternal care for other conditions predominantly related to pregnancy
  - **O26.0** **Excessive weight gain** in pregnancy
    Excludes2 gestational edema (O12.0, O12.2)
    - O26.00 Excessive weight gain in pregnancy, **unspecified trimester** ♀   M
    - O26.01 Excessive weight gain in pregnancy, **first trimester** ♀   M
    - O26.02 Excessive weight gain in pregnancy, **second trimester** ♀   M
    - O26.03 Excessive weight gain in pregnancy, **third trimester** ♀   M
  - **O26.1** **Low weight gain** in pregnancy
    - O26.10 Low weight gain in pregnancy, **unspecified trimester** ♀   M
    - O26.11 Low weight gain in pregnancy, **first trimester** ♀   M
    - O26.12 Low weight gain in pregnancy, **second trimester** ♀   M
    - O26.13 Low weight gain in pregnancy, **third trimester** ♀   M
  - **O26.2** Pregnancy care for patient with **recurrent pregnancy loss**
    - O26.20 Pregnancy care for patient with recurrent pregnancy loss, **unspecified trimester** ♀   M
    - O26.21 Pregnancy care for patient with recurrent pregnancy loss, **first trimester** ♀   M
    - O26.22 Pregnancy care for patient with recurrent pregnancy loss, **second trimester** ♀   M
    - O26.23 Pregnancy care for patient with recurrent pregnancy loss, **third trimester** ♀   M

- **O26.3** Retained intrauterine contraceptive device in pregnancy
  - O26.30 Retained intrauterine contraceptive device in pregnancy, **unspecified trimester** ♀   M
  - O26.31 Retained intrauterine contraceptive device in pregnancy, **first trimester** ♀   M
  - O26.32 Retained intrauterine contraceptive device in pregnancy, **second trimester** ♀   M
  - O26.33 Retained intrauterine contraceptive device in pregnancy, **third trimester** ♀   M
- **O26.4** Herpes gestationis
  - O26.40 Herpes gestationis, **unspecified trimester** ♀   M
  - O26.41 Herpes gestationis, **first trimester** ♀   M
  - O26.42 Herpes gestationis, **second trimester** ♀   M
  - O26.43 Herpes gestationis, **third trimester** ♀   M
- **O26.5** Maternal hypotension syndrome
  Supine hypotensive syndrome
  - O26.50 Maternal hypotension syndrome, **unspecified trimester** ♀   M
  - O26.51 Maternal hypotension syndrome, **first trimester** ♀   M
  - O26.52 Maternal hypotension syndrome, **second trimester** ♀   M
  - O26.53 Maternal hypotension syndrome, **third trimester** ♀   M
- **O26.6** Liver and biliary tract disorders in pregnancy, childbirth and the puerperium
  Use additional code to identify the specific disorder
  Excludes2 hepatorenal syndrome following labor and delivery (O90.4)
  - **O26.61** Liver and biliary tract disorders in **pregnancy**
    (Ex:) For category O26.61 CC codes: See PDX Collection 972
    - O26.611 Liver and biliary tract disorders in pregnancy, **first trimester** ♀ 🅒   M
      (Ex:) See PDX Collection 4054
    - O26.612 Liver and biliary tract disorders in pregnancy, **second trimester** ♀ 🅒   M
      (Ex:) See PDX Collection 4054
    - O26.613 Liver and biliary tract disorders in pregnancy, **third trimester** ♀ 🅒   M
    - O26.619 Liver and biliary tract disorders in pregnancy, **unspecified trimester** ♀   M
  - O26.62 Liver and biliary tract disorders in **childbirth** ♀ 🅒   M
    (Ex:) See PDX Collection 4008
  - O26.63 Liver and biliary tract disorders in the **puerperium** ♀   M
- **O26.7** Subluxation of symphysis (pubis) in pregnancy, childbirth and the puerperium
  Excludes1 traumatic separation of symphysis (pubis) during childbirth (O71.6)
  - **O26.71** Subluxation of symphysis (pubis) in **pregnancy**
    - O26.711 Subluxation of symphysis (pubis) in pregnancy, **first trimester** ♀   M
    - O26.712 Subluxation of symphysis (pubis) in pregnancy, **second trimester** ♀   M
    - O26.713 Subluxation of symphysis (pubis) in pregnancy, **third trimester** ♀   M
    - O26.719 Subluxation of symphysis (pubis) in pregnancy, **unspecified trimester** ♀ M
  - O26.72 Subluxation of symphysis (pubis) in **childbirth** ♀   M
  - O26.73 Subluxation of symphysis (pubis) in the **puerperium** ♀   M

● **O26.8**   Other specified pregnancy related conditions
  ● **O26.81**   Pregnancy related exhaustion and fatigue
     O26.811   Pregnancy related exhaustion and fatigue, first trimester ♀   **M**
     O26.812   Pregnancy related exhaustion and fatigue, second trimester ♀   **M**
     O26.813   Pregnancy related exhaustion and fatigue, third trimester ♀   **M**
     O26.819   Pregnancy related exhaustion and fatigue, unspecified trimester ♀   **M**
  ● **O26.82**   Pregnancy related peripheral neuritis
     O26.821   Pregnancy related peripheral neuritis, first trimester ♀   **M**
     O26.822   Pregnancy related peripheral neuritis, second trimester ♀   **M**
     O26.823   Pregnancy related peripheral neuritis, third trimester ♀   **M**
     O26.829   Pregnancy related peripheral neuritis, unspecified trimester ♀   **M**
  ● **O26.83**   Pregnancy related renal disease
     Use additional code to identify the specific disorder
     (Ex:) **For category O26.83 CC codes:** See PDX Collection 965
     O26.831   Pregnancy related renal disease, first trimester ♀ 🔹   **M**
     O26.832   Pregnancy related renal disease, second trimester ♀ 🔹   **M**
     O26.833   Pregnancy related renal disease, third trimester ♀ 🔹   **M**
     O26.839   Pregnancy related renal disease, unspecified trimester ♀   **M**
  ● **O26.84**   Uterine size-date discrepancy complicating pregnancy
     Excludes1   encounter for suspected problem with fetal growth ruled out (Z03.74)
     O26.841   Uterine size-date discrepancy, first trimester ♀   **M**
     O26.842   Uterine size-date discrepancy, second trimester ♀   **M**
     O26.843   Uterine size-date discrepancy, third trimester ♀   **M**
     O26.849   Uterine size-date discrepancy, unspecified trimester ♀   **M**
  ● **O26.85**   Spotting complicating pregnancy
     O26.851   Spotting complicating pregnancy, first trimester ♀   **M**
     O26.852   Spotting complicating pregnancy, second trimester ♀   **M**
     O26.853   Spotting complicating pregnancy, third trimester ♀   **M**
     O26.859   Spotting complicating pregnancy, unspecified trimester ♀   **M**
     O26.86   Pruritic urticarial papules and plaques of pregnancy (PUPPP) ♀   **M**
     Polymorphic eruption of pregnancy
  ● **O26.87**   Cervical shortening
     Excludes1   encounter for suspected cervical shortening ruled out (Z03.75)
     (Ex:) **For category O26.87 CC codes:** See PDX Collection 973
     O26.872   Cervical shortening, second trimester ♀ 🔹   **M**
     O26.873   Cervical shortening, third trimester ♀ 🔹   **M**
     O26.879   Cervical shortening, unspecified trimester ♀ 🔹   **M**

  ● **O26.89**   Other specified pregnancy related conditions
     O26.891   Other specified pregnancy related conditions, first trimester ♀   **M**
     O26.892   Other specified pregnancy related conditions, second trimester ♀   **M**
     O26.893   Other specified pregnancy related conditions, third trimester ♀   **M**
       Coding Clinic: 2015, Q3, P40
     O26.899   Other specified pregnancy related conditions, unspecified trimester ♀   **M**
● **O26.9**   Pregnancy related conditions, unspecified
     O26.90   Pregnancy related conditions, unspecified, unspecified trimester ♀   **M**
     O26.91   Pregnancy related conditions, unspecified, first trimester ♀   **M**
     O26.92   Pregnancy related conditions, unspecified, second trimester ♀   **M**
     O26.93   Pregnancy related conditions, unspecified, third trimester ♀   **M**

● **O28**   Abnormal findings on antenatal screening of mother
     Excludes1   diagnostic findings classified elsewhere - see Alphabetical Index
   O28.0   Abnormal hematological finding on antenatal screening of mother ♀   **M**
   O28.1   Abnormal biochemical finding on antenatal screening of mother ♀   **M**
   O28.2   Abnormal cytological finding on antenatal screening of mother ♀   **M**
   O28.3   Abnormal ultrasonic finding on antenatal screening of mother ♀   **M**
       Coding Clinic: 2016, Q4, P5
   O28.4   Abnormal radiological finding on antenatal screening of mother ♀   **M**
   O28.5   Abnormal chromosomal and genetic finding on antenatal screening of mother ♀   **M**
   O28.8   Other abnormal findings on antenatal screening of mother ♀   **M**
   O28.9   Unspecified abnormal findings on antenatal screening of mother ♀   **M**

● **O29**   Complications of anesthesia during pregnancy
     Includes   maternal complications arising from the administration of a general, regional or local anesthetic, analgesic or other sedation during pregnancy
     Use additional code, if necessary, to identify the complication
     Excludes2   complications of anesthesia during labor and delivery (O74.-)
       complications of anesthesia during the puerperium (O89.-)
  ● **O29.0**   Pulmonary complications of anesthesia during pregnancy
    ● **O29.01**   Aspiration pneumonitis due to anesthesia during pregnancy
       Inhalation of stomach contents or secretions NOS due to anesthesia during pregnancy
       Mendelson's syndrome due to anesthesia during pregnancy
       O29.011   Aspiration pneumonitis due to anesthesia during pregnancy, first trimester ♀   **M**
       O29.012   Aspiration pneumonitis due to anesthesia during pregnancy, second trimester ♀   **M**
       O29.013   Aspiration pneumonitis due to anesthesia during pregnancy, third trimester ♀   **M**
       O29.019   Aspiration pneumonitis due to anesthesia during pregnancy, unspecified trimester ♀   **M**

N   Newborn Age: 0   **P**   Pediatric Age: 0–17   **M**   Maternity DX: 9–64   **A**   Adult Age: 15–124   ♀   Females Only   ♂   Males Only

🔹 Complication\Comorbidity   🔹 Major C\C   (Ex:) CC/MCC Exclusions   🔹 Hospital-Acquired Condition   🔹 Hierarchical Condition Category   **1157**

● O29.02   Pressure collapse of lung due to anesthesia during pregnancy

     O29.021   Pressure collapse of lung due to anesthesia during pregnancy, first trimester ♀   M

     O29.022   Pressure collapse of lung due to anesthesia during pregnancy, second trimester ♀   M

     O29.023   Pressure collapse of lung due to anesthesia during pregnancy, third trimester ♀   M

     O29.029   Pressure collapse of lung due to anesthesia during pregnancy, unspecified trimester ♀   M

● O29.09   Other pulmonary complications of anesthesia during pregnancy

     O29.091   Other pulmonary complications of anesthesia during pregnancy, first trimester ♀   M

     O29.092   Other pulmonary complications of anesthesia during pregnancy, second trimester ♀   M

     O29.093   Other pulmonary complications of anesthesia during pregnancy, third trimester ♀   M

     O29.099   Other pulmonary complications of anesthesia during pregnancy, unspecified trimester ♀   M

● O29.1   Cardiac complications of anesthesia during pregnancy

  ● O29.11   Cardiac arrest due to anesthesia during pregnancy

     O29.111   Cardiac arrest due to anesthesia during pregnancy, first trimester ♀   M

     O29.112   Cardiac arrest due to anesthesia during pregnancy, second trimester ♀   M

     O29.113   Cardiac arrest due to anesthesia during pregnancy, third trimester ♀   M

     O29.119   Cardiac arrest due to anesthesia during pregnancy, unspecified trimester ♀   M

  ● O29.12   Cardiac failure due to anesthesia during pregnancy

     O29.121   Cardiac failure due to anesthesia during pregnancy, first trimester ♀   M

     O29.122   Cardiac failure due to anesthesia during pregnancy, second trimester ♀   M

     O29.123   Cardiac failure due to anesthesia during pregnancy, third trimester ♀   M

     O29.129   Cardiac failure due to anesthesia during pregnancy, unspecified trimester ♀   M

  ● O29.19   Other cardiac complications of anesthesia during pregnancy

     O29.191   Other cardiac complications of anesthesia during pregnancy, first trimester ♀   M

     O29.192   Other cardiac complications of anesthesia during pregnancy, second trimester ♀   M

     O29.193   Other cardiac complications of anesthesia during pregnancy, third trimester ♀   M

     O29.199   Other cardiac complications of anesthesia during pregnancy, unspecified trimester ♀   M

● O29.2   Central nervous system complications of anesthesia during pregnancy

  ● O29.21   Cerebral anoxia due to anesthesia during pregnancy

     O29.211   Cerebral anoxia due to anesthesia during pregnancy, first trimester ♀   M

     O29.212   Cerebral anoxia due to anesthesia during pregnancy, second trimester ♀   M

     O29.213   Cerebral anoxia due to anesthesia during pregnancy, third trimester ♀   M

     O29.219   Cerebral anoxia due to anesthesia during pregnancy, unspecified trimester ♀   M

  ● O29.29   Other central nervous system complications of anesthesia during pregnancy

     O29.291   Other central nervous system complications of anesthesia during pregnancy, first trimester ♀   M

     O29.292   Other central nervous system complications of anesthesia during pregnancy, second trimester ♀   M

     O29.293   Other central nervous system complications of anesthesia during pregnancy, third trimester ♀   M

     O29.299   Other central nervous system complications of anesthesia during pregnancy, unspecified trimester ♀   M

● O29.3   Toxic reaction to local anesthesia during pregnancy

  ● O29.3X   Toxic reaction to local anesthesia during pregnancy

     O29.3X1   Toxic reaction to local anesthesia during pregnancy, first trimester ♀   M

     O29.3X2   Toxic reaction to local anesthesia during pregnancy, second trimester ♀   M

     O29.3X3   Toxic reaction to local anesthesia during pregnancy, third trimester ♀   M

     O29.3X9   Toxic reaction to local anesthesia during pregnancy, unspecified trimester ♀   M

● O29.4   Spinal and epidural anesthesia induced headache during pregnancy

     O29.40   Spinal and epidural anesthesia induced headache during pregnancy, unspecified trimester ♀   M

     O29.41   Spinal and epidural anesthesia induced headache during pregnancy, first trimester ♀   M

     O29.42   Spinal and epidural anesthesia induced headache during pregnancy, second trimester ♀   M

     O29.43   Spinal and epidural anesthesia induced headache during pregnancy, third trimester ♀   M

● O29.5   Other complications of spinal and epidural anesthesia during pregnancy

  ● O29.5X   Other complications of spinal and epidural anesthesia during pregnancy

     O29.5X1   Other complications of spinal and epidural anesthesia during pregnancy, first trimester ♀   M

     O29.5X2   Other complications of spinal and epidural anesthesia during pregnancy, second trimester ♀   M

     O29.5X3   Other complications of spinal and epidural anesthesia during pregnancy, third trimester ♀   M

     O29.5X9   Other complications of spinal and epidural anesthesia during pregnancy, unspecified trimester ♀   M

▶ New   ⇒ Revised   ~~deleted~~ Deleted   Excludes 1   Excludes 2   Includes   Use additional   Code first   Code also   Key words

OGCR Official Guidelines   ● Unacceptable Principal Diagnosis   X Assign placeholder X   ● Use Additional Character(s)   ▷ Manifestation Code   **Coding Clinic**

● O29.6 Failed or difficult intubation for anesthesia during pregnancy

O29.60 Failed or difficult intubation for anesthesia during pregnancy, unspecified trimester ♀ M

O29.61 Failed or difficult intubation for anesthesia during pregnancy, first trimester ♀ M

O29.62 Failed or difficult intubation for anesthesia during pregnancy, second trimester ♀ M

O29.63 Failed or difficult intubation for anesthesia during pregnancy, third trimester ♀ M

● O29.8 Other complications of anesthesia during pregnancy

● O29.8X Other complications of anesthesia during pregnancy

O29.8X1 Other complications of anesthesia during pregnancy, first trimester ♀ M

O29.8X2 Other complications of anesthesia during pregnancy, second trimester ♀ M

O29.8X3 Other complications of anesthesia during pregnancy, third trimester ♀ M

O29.8X9 Other complications of anesthesia during pregnancy, unspecified trimester ♀ M

● O29.9 Unspecified complication of anesthesia during pregnancy

O29.90 Unspecified complication of anesthesia during pregnancy, unspecified trimester ♀ M

O29.91 Unspecified complication of anesthesia during pregnancy, first trimester ♀ M

O29.92 Unspecified complication of anesthesia during pregnancy, second trimester ♀ M

O29.93 Unspecified complication of anesthesia during pregnancy, third trimester ♀ M

MATERNAL CARE RELATED TO THE FETUS AND AMNIOTIC CAVITY AND POSSIBLE DELIVERY PROBLEMS (O30-O48)

● O30 Multiple gestation

Code also any complications specific to multiple gestation
Coding Clinic: 2016, Q4, P51

● O30.0 Twin pregnancy

● O30.00 Twin pregnancy, unspecified number of placenta and unspecified number of amniotic sacs

O30.001 Twin pregnancy, unspecified number of placenta and unspecified number of amniotic sacs, first trimester ♀ M

O30.002 Twin pregnancy, unspecified number of placenta and unspecified number of amniotic sacs, second trimester ♀ M

O30.003 Twin pregnancy, unspecified number of placenta and unspecified number of amniotic sacs, third trimester ♀ M

O30.009 Twin pregnancy, unspecified number of placenta and unspecified number of amniotic sacs, unspecified trimester ♀ M

● O30.01 Twin pregnancy, monochorionic/monoamniotic
Twin pregnancy, one placenta, one amniotic sac

Excludes1 conjoined twins (O30.02-)

O30.011 Twin pregnancy, monochorionic/monoamniotic, first trimester ♀ M

O30.012 Twin pregnancy, monochorionic/monoamniotic, second trimester ♀ M

O30.013 Twin pregnancy, monochorionic/monoamniotic, third trimester ♀ M

O30.019 Twin pregnancy, monochorionic/monoamniotic, unspecified trimester ♀ M

● O30.02 Conjoined twin pregnancy

O30.021 Conjoined twin pregnancy, first trimester ♀ M

O30.022 Conjoined twin pregnancy, second trimester ♀ M

O30.023 Conjoined twin pregnancy, third trimester ♀ M

O30.029 Conjoined twin pregnancy, unspecified trimester ♀ M

● O30.03 Twin pregnancy, monochorionic/diamniotic
Twin pregnancy, one placenta, two amniotic sacs

O30.031 Twin pregnancy, monochorionic/diamniotic, first trimester ♀ M

O30.032 Twin pregnancy, monochorionic/diamniotic, second trimester ♀ M

O30.033 Twin pregnancy, monochorionic/diamniotic, third trimester ♀ M

O30.039 Twin pregnancy, monochorionic/diamniotic, unspecified trimester ♀ M

● O30.04 Twin pregnancy, dichorionic/diamniotic
Twin pregnancy, two placentae, two amniotic sacs

O30.041 Twin pregnancy, dichorionic/diamniotic, first trimester ♀ M

O30.042 Twin pregnancy, dichorionic/diamniotic, second trimester ♀ M

O30.043 Twin pregnancy, dichorionic/diamniotic, third trimester ♀ M

O30.049 Twin pregnancy, dichorionic/diamniotic, unspecified trimester ♀ M

● O30.09 Twin pregnancy, unable to determine number of placenta and number of amniotic sacs

O30.091 Twin pregnancy, unable to determine number of placenta and number of amniotic sacs, first trimester ♀ M

O30.092 Twin pregnancy, unable to determine number of placenta and number of amniotic sacs, second trimester ♀ M

O30.093 Twin pregnancy, unable to determine number of placenta and number of amniotic sacs, third trimester ♀ M

O30.099 Twin pregnancy, unable to determine number of placenta and number of amniotic sacs, unspecified trimester ♀ M

● O30.1 Triplet pregnancy
Ex: For category O30.1 CC codes: See PDX Collection 976

● O30.10 Triplet pregnancy, unspecified number of placenta and unspecified number of amniotic sacs

O30.101 Triplet pregnancy, unspecified number of placenta and unspecified number of amniotic sacs, first trimester ♀ 🦠 M

O30.102 Triplet pregnancy, unspecified number of placenta and unspecified number of amniotic sacs, second trimester ♀ 🦠 M

O30.103 Triplet pregnancy, unspecified number of placenta and unspecified number of amniotic sacs, third trimester ♀ 🦠 M
Coding Clinic: 2016, Q2, P8

O30.109 Triplet pregnancy, unspecified number of placenta and unspecified number of amniotic sacs, unspecified trimester ♀ M

N Newborn Age: 0   P Pediatric Age: 0–17   M Maternity DX: 9–64   A Adult Age: 15–124   ♀ Females Only   ♂ Males Only

🦠 Complication\Comorbidity   🦠 Major C\C   Ex: CC/MCC Exclusions   🦠 Hospital-Acquired Condition   🦠 Hierarchical Condition Category

1159

CHAPTER 15 (O00-O9A)

● **O30.11 Triplet pregnancy with two or more monochorionic fetuses**

     O30.111   Triplet pregnancy with two or more monochorionic fetuses, first trimester ♀ 🐾   M

     O30.112   Triplet pregnancy with two or more monochorionic fetuses, second trimester ♀ 🐾   M

     O30.113   Triplet pregnancy with two or more monochorionic fetuses, third trimester ♀ 🐾   M

     O30.119   Triplet pregnancy with two or more monochorionic fetuses, unspecified trimester ♀   M

● **O30.12 Triplet pregnancy with two or more monoamniotic fetuses**

     O30.121   Triplet pregnancy with two or more monoamniotic fetuses, first trimester ♀ 🐾   M

     O30.122   Triplet pregnancy with two or more monoamniotic fetuses, second trimester ♀ 🐾   M

     O30.123   Triplet pregnancy with two or more monoamniotic fetuses, third trimester ♀ 🐾   M

     O30.129   Triplet pregnancy with two or more monoamniotic fetuses, unspecified trimester ♀   M

● **O30.13 Triplet pregnancy, trichorionic/triamniotic**

     O30.131   Triplet pregnancy, trichorionic/triamniotic, first trimester ♀ 🐾   M

     O30.132   Triplet pregnancy, trichorionic/triamniotic, second trimester ♀ 🐾   M

     O30.133   Triplet pregnancy, trichorionic/triamniotic, third trimester ♀ 🐾   M

     O30.139   Triplet pregnancy, trichorionic/triamniotic, unspecified trimester ♀   M

● **O30.19 Triplet pregnancy, unable to determine number of placenta and number of amniotic sacs**

     O30.191   Triplet pregnancy, unable to determine number of placenta and number of amniotic sacs, first trimester ♀ 🐾   M

     O30.192   Triplet pregnancy, unable to determine number of placenta and number of amniotic sacs, second trimester ♀ 🐾   M

     O30.193   Triplet pregnancy, unable to determine number of placenta and number of amniotic sacs, third trimester ♀ 🐾   M

     O30.199   Triplet pregnancy, unable to determine number of placenta and number of amniotic sacs, unspecified trimester ♀   M

● **O30.2 Quadruplet pregnancy**

     Ⓔⓧ **For category O30.2 CC codes:** See PDX Collection 976

● **O30.20 Quadruplet pregnancy, unspecified number of placenta and unspecified number of amniotic sacs**

     O30.201   Quadruplet pregnancy, unspecified number of placenta and unspecified number of amniotic sacs, first trimester ♀   M

     O30.202   Quadruplet pregnancy, unspecified number of placenta and unspecified number of amniotic sacs, second trimester ♀   M

     O30.203   Quadruplet pregnancy, unspecified number of placenta and unspecified number of amniotic sacs, third trimester ♀   M

     O30.209   Quadruplet pregnancy, unspecified number of placenta and unspecified number of amniotic sacs, unspecified trimester ♀   M

● **O30.21 Quadruplet pregnancy with two or more monochorionic fetuses**

     O30.211   Quadruplet pregnancy with two or more monochorionic fetuses, first trimester ♀ 🐾   M

     O30.212   Quadruplet pregnancy with two or more monochorionic fetuses, second trimester ♀ 🐾   M

     O30.213   Quadruplet pregnancy with two or more monochorionic fetuses, third trimester ♀ 🐾   M

     O30.219   Quadruplet pregnancy with two or more monochorionic fetuses, unspecified trimester ♀   M

● **O30.22 Quadruplet pregnancy with two or more monoamniotic fetuses**

     O30.221   Quadruplet pregnancy with two or more monoamniotic fetuses, first trimester ♀ 🐾   M

     O30.222   Quadruplet pregnancy with two or more monoamniotic fetuses, second trimester ♀ 🐾   M

     O30.223   Quadruplet pregnancy with two or more monoamniotic fetuses, third trimester ♀ 🐾   M

     O30.229   Quadruplet pregnancy with two or more monoamniotic fetuses, unspecified trimester ♀   M

● **O30.23 Quadruplet pregnancy, quadrachorionic/quadra-amniotic**

     O30.231   Quadruplet pregnancy, quadrachorionic/quadra-amniotic, first trimester ♀ 🐾   M

     O30.232   Quadruplet pregnancy, quadrachorionic/quadra-amniotic, second trimester ♀ 🐾   M

     O30.233   Quadruplet pregnancy, quadrachorionic/quadra-amniotic, third trimester ♀ 🐾   M

     O30.239   Quadruplet pregnancy, quadrachorionic/quadra-amniotic, unspecifiedtrimester ♀ 🐾   M

● **O30.29 Quadruplet pregnancy, unable to determine number of placenta and number of amniotic sacs**

     O30.291   Quadruplet pregnancy, unable to determine number of placenta and number of amniotic sacs, first trimester ♀ 🐾   M

     O30.292   Quadruplet pregnancy, unable to determine number of placenta and number of amniotic sacs, second trimester ♀ 🐾   M

     O30.293   Quadruplet pregnancy, unable to determine number of placenta and number of amniotic sacs, third trimester ♀ 🐾   M

     O30.299   Quadruplet pregnancy, unable to determine number of placenta and number of amniotic sacs, unspecified trimester ♀   M

● **O30.8 Other specified multiple gestation**

     Multiple gestation pregnancy greater then quadruplets

     Ⓔⓧ **For category O30.8 CC codes:** See PDX Collection 976

● **O30.80 Other specified multiple gestation, unspecified number of placenta and unspecified number of amniotic sacs**

▶ New   ⇒ Revised   ~~deleted~~ Deleted   Excludes 1   Excludes 2   Includes   Use additional   Code first   Code also   Key words

OGCR Official Guidelines   ● Unacceptable Principal Diagnosis   X Assign placeholder X   ● Use Additional Character(s)   ▶ Manifestation Code   **Coding Clinic**

O30.801   Other specified multiple gestation, unspecified number of placenta and unspecified number of amniotic sacs, first trimester ♀ 🦠   M

O30.802   Other specified multiple gestation, unspecified number of placenta and unspecified number of amniotic sacs, second trimester ♀ 🦠   M

O30.803   Other specified multiple gestation, unspecified number of placenta and unspecified number of amniotic sacs, third trimester ♀ 🦠   M

O30.809   Other specified multiple gestation, unspecified number of placenta and unspecified number of amniotic sacs, unspecified trimester ♀   M

● **O30.81** Other specified multiple gestation with two or more monochorionic fetuses

O30.811   Other specified multiple gestation with two or more monochorionic fetuses, first trimester ♀ 🦠   M

O30.812   Other specified multiple gestation with two or more monochorionic fetuses, second trimester ♀ 🦠   M

O30.813   Other specified multiple gestation with two or more monochorionic fetuses, third trimester ♀ 🦠   M

O30.819   Other specified multiple gestation with two or more monochorionic fetuses, unspecified trimester ♀   M

● **O30.82** Other specified multiple gestation with two or more monoamniotic fetuses

O30.821   Other specified multiple gestation with two or more monoamniotic fetuses, first trimester ♀ 🦠   M

O30.822   Other specified multiple gestation with two or more monoamniotic fetuses, second trimester ♀ 🦠   M

O30.823   Other specified multiple gestation with two or more monoamniotic fetuses, third trimester ♀ 🦠   M

O30.829   Other specified multiple gestation with two or more monoamniotic fetuses, unspecified trimester ♀   M

● **O30.83** Other specified multiple gestation, number of chorions and amnions are both equal to the number of fetuses
    Pentachorionic, penta-amniotic pregnancy (quintuplets)
    Hexachorionic, hexa-amniotic pregnancy (sextuplets)
    Heptachorionic, hepta-amniotic pregnancy (septuplets)

O30.831   Other specified multiple gestation, number of chorions and amnions are both equal to the number of fetuses, first trimester ♀ 🦠   M

O30.832   Other specified multiple gestation, number of chorions and amnions are both equal to the number of fetuses, second trimester ♀ 🦠   M

O30.833   Other specified multiple gestation, number of chorions and amnions are both equal to the number of fetuses, third trimester ♀ 🦠   M

O30.839   Other specified multiple gestation, number of chorions and amnions are both equal to the number of fetuses, unspecified trimester ♀ 🦠   M

● **O30.89**   Other specified multiple gestation, unable to determine number of placenta and number of amniotic sacs

O30.891   Other specified multiple gestation, unable to determine number of placenta and number of amniotic sacs, first trimester ♀ 🦠   M

O30.892   Other specified multiple gestation, unable to determine number of placenta and number of amniotic sacs, second trimester ♀ 🦠   M

O30.893   Other specified multiple gestation, unable to determine number of placenta and number of amniotic sacs, third trimester ♀ 🦠   M

O30.899   Other specified multiple gestation, unable to determine number of placenta and number of amniotic sacs, unspecified trimester ♀   M

● **O30.9** Multiple gestation, unspecified
    Multiple pregnancy NOS

O30.90   Multiple gestation, unspecified, unspecified trimester ♀   M

O30.91   Multiple gestation, unspecified, first trimester ♀   M

O30.92   Multiple gestation, unspecified, second trimester ♀   M

O30.93   Multiple gestation, unspecified, third trimester ♀   M

● **O31**   Complications specific to multiple gestation

    Excludes2   delayed delivery of second twin, triplet, etc. (O63.2)
                malpresentation of one fetus or more (O32.9)
                placental transfusion syndromes (O43.0-)

    Coding Clinic: 2012, Q4, P107

    One of the following 7th characters is to be assigned to each code under category O31. 7th character Ø is for single gestations and multiple gestations where the fetus is unspecified. 7th characters 1 through 9 are for cases of multiple gestations to identify the fetus for which the code applies. The appropriate code from category O30, Multiple gestation, must also be assigned when assigning a code from category O31 that has a 7th character of 1 through 9.

Ø	not applicable or unspecified
1	fetus 1
2	fetus 2
3	fetus 3
4	fetus 4
5	fetus 5
9	other fetus

● **O31.0**   Papyraceous fetus
    Fetus compressus

X ● **O31.00**   Papyraceous fetus, unspecified trimester ♀   M

X ● **O31.01**   Papyraceous fetus, first trimester ♀   M

X ● **O31.02**   Papyraceous fetus, second trimester ♀   M

X ● **O31.03**   Papyraceous fetus, third trimester ♀   M

● **O31.1**   Continuing pregnancy after spontaneous abortion of one fetus or more

X ● **O31.10**   Continuing pregnancy after spontaneous abortion of one fetus or more, unspecified trimester ♀   M

X ● **O31.11**   Continuing pregnancy after spontaneous abortion of one fetus or more, first trimester ♀ M

X ● **O31.12**   Continuing pregnancy after spontaneous abortion of one fetus or more, second trimester ♀   M

X ● **O31.13**   Continuing pregnancy after spontaneous abortion of one fetus or more, third trimester ♀   M

CHAPTER 15 (O00–O9A)

N   Newborn Age: Ø   **P**   Pediatric Age: Ø–17   **M**   Maternity DX: 9–64   **A**   Adult Age: 15–124   ♀   Females Only   ♂   Males Only

🦠 Complication\Comorbidity   🦠 Major C\C   (Ex.) CC/MCC Exclusions   🦠 Hospital-Acquired Condition   🦠 Hierarchical Condition Category

1161

● O31.2   Continuing pregnancy after intrauterine death of one fetus or more

X● O31.20   Continuing pregnancy after intrauterine death of one fetus or more, unspecified trimester ♀   M

X● O31.21   Continuing pregnancy after intrauterine death of one fetus or more, first trimester ♀   M

X● O31.22   Continuing pregnancy after intrauterine death of one fetus or more, second trimester ♀   M

X● O31.23   Continuing pregnancy after intrauterine death of one fetus or more, third trimester ♀   M

● O31.3   Continuing pregnancy after elective fetal reduction of one fetus or more

Continuing pregnancy after selective termination of one fetus or more

X● O31.30   Continuing pregnancy after elective fetal reduction of one fetus or more, unspecified trimester ♀   M

X● O31.31   Continuing pregnancy after elective fetal reduction of one fetus or more, first trimester ♀   M

X● O31.32   Continuing pregnancy after elective fetal reduction of one fetus or more, second trimester ♀   M

X● O31.33   Continuing pregnancy after elective fetal reduction of one fetus or more, third trimester ♀   M

● O31.8   Other complications specific to multiple gestation

Ex: For category O31.8 CC codes: See PDX Collection 976

● O31.8X   Other complications specific to multiple gestation

● O31.8X1   Other complications specific to multiple gestation, first trimester ♀   M

● O31.8X2   Other complications specific to multiple gestation, second trimester ♀   M

● O31.8X3   Other complications specific to multiple gestation, third trimester ♀   M

● O31.8X9   Other complications specific to multiple gestation, unspecified trimester ♀   M

● O32   Maternal care for malpresentation of fetus

Includes   the listed conditions as a reason for observation, hospitalization or other obstetric care of the mother, or for cesarean delivery before onset of labor

Excludes1   malpresentation of fetus with obstructed labor (O64.-)

Coding Clinic: 2012, Q4, P107

One of the following 7th characters is to be assigned to each code under category O32. 7th character Ø is for single gestations and multiple gestations where the fetus is unspecified. 7th characters 1 through 9 are for cases of multiple gestations to identify the fetus for which the code applies. The appropriate code from category O30, Multiple gestation, must also be assigned when assigning a code from category O32 that has a 7th character of 1 through 9.

Ø	not applicable or unspecified
1	fetus 1
2	fetus 2
3	fetus 3
4	fetus 4
5	fetus 5
9	other fetus

X● O32.0   Maternal care for unstable lie ♀   M

X● O32.1   Maternal care for breech presentation ♀   M

Maternal care for buttocks presentation
Maternal care for complete breech
Maternal care for frank breech

Excludes1   footling presentation (O32.8)
incomplete breech (O32.8)

X● O32.2   Maternal care for transverse and oblique lie ♀   M

Maternal care for oblique presentation
Maternal care for transverse presentation

X● O32.3   Maternal care for face, brow and chin presentation ♀   M

X● O32.4   Maternal care for high head at term ♀   M

Maternal care for failure of head to enter pelvic brim

X● O32.6   Maternal care for compound presentation ♀   M

X● O32.8   Maternal care for other malpresentation of fetus ♀   M

Maternal care for footling presentation
Maternal care for incomplete breech

X● O32.9   Maternal care for malpresentation of fetus, unspecified ♀   M

● O33   Maternal care for disproportion

Includes   the listed conditions as a reason for observation, hospitalization or other obstetric care of the mother, or for cesarean delivery before onset of labor

Excludes1   disproportion with obstructed labor (O65-O66)

O33.0   Maternal care for disproportion due to deformity of maternal pelvic bones ♀ 🔖   M

Maternal care for disproportion due to pelvic deformity causing disproportion NOS

Ex: See PDX Collection 977

O33.1   Maternal care for disproportion due to generally contracted pelvis ♀   M

Maternal care for disproportion due to contracted pelvis NOS causing disproportion

O33.2   Maternal care for disproportion due to inlet contraction of pelvis ♀   M

Maternal care for disproportion due to inlet contraction (pelvis) causing disproportion

X● O33.3   Maternal care for disproportion due to outlet contraction of pelvis ♀   M

Maternal care for disproportion due to mid-cavity contraction (pelvis)
Maternal care for disproportion due to outlet contraction (pelvis)

One of the following 7th characters is to be assigned to code O33.3. 7th character Ø is for single gestations and multiple gestations where the fetus is unspecified. 7th characters 1 through 9 are for cases of multiple gestations to identify the fetus for which the code applies. The appropriate code from category O30, Multiple gestation, must also be assigned when assigning code O33.3 with a 7th character of 1 through 9.

Ø	not applicable or unspecified
1	fetus 1
2	fetus 2
3	fetus 3
4	fetus 4
5	fetus 5
9	other fetus

X● O33.4   Maternal care for disproportion of mixed maternal and fetal origin ♀   M

One of the following 7th characters is to be assigned to code O33.4. 7th character Ø is for single gestations and multiple gestations where the fetus is unspecified. 7th characters 1 through 9 are for cases of multiple gestations to identify the fetus for which the code applies. The appropriate code from category O30, Multiple gestation, must also be assigned when assigning code O33.4 with a 7th character of 1 through 9.

Ø	not applicable or unspecified
1	fetus 1
2	fetus 2
3	fetus 3
4	fetus 4
5	fetus 5
9	other fetus

▶ New   ⇒ Revised   ~~deleted~~ Deleted   Excludes 1   Excludes 2   Includes   Use additional   Code first   Code also   Key words

OGCR Official Guidelines   ● Unacceptable Principal Diagnosis   X Assign placeholder X   ● Use Additional Character(s)   ▷ Manifestation Code   **Coding Clinic**

X ● **O33.5 Maternal care for disproportion due to unusually large fetus** ♀   M

> Maternal care for disproportion due to disproportion of fetal origin with normally formed fetus
> Maternal care for disproportion due to fetal disproportion NOS
>
> One of the following 7th characters is to be assigned to code O33.5. 7th character Ø is for single gestations and multiple gestations where the fetus is unspecified. 7th characters 1 through 9 are for cases of multiple gestations to identify the fetus for which the code applies. The appropriate code from category O3Ø, Multiple gestation, must also be assigned when assigning code O33.5 with a 7th character of 1 through 9.

> | Ø | not applicable or unspecified |
> |---|---|
> | 1 | fetus 1 |
> | 2 | fetus 2 |
> | 3 | fetus 3 |
> | 4 | fetus 4 |
> | 5 | fetus 5 |
> | 9 | other fetus |

X ● **O33.6 Maternal care for disproportion due to hydrocephalic fetus** ♀   M

> One of the following 7th characters is to be assigned to code O33.6. 7th character Ø is for single gestations and multiple gestations where the fetus is unspecified. 7th characters 1 through 9 are for cases of multiple gestations to identify the fetus for which the code applies. The appropriate code from category O3Ø, Multiple gestation, must also be assigned when assigning code O33.6 with a 7th character of 1 through 9.

> | Ø | not applicable or unspecified |
> |---|---|
> | 1 | fetus 1 |
> | 2 | fetus 2 |
> | 3 | fetus 3 |
> | 4 | fetus 4 |
> | 5 | fetus 5 |
> | 9 | other fetus |

X ● **O33.7 Maternal care for disproportion due to other fetal deformities** ♀   M

> Maternal care for disproportion due to fetal ascites
> Maternal care for disproportion due to fetal hydrops
> Maternal care for disproportion due to fetal meningomyelocele
> Maternal care for disproportion due to fetal sacral teratoma
> Maternal care for disproportion due to fetal tumor
>
> **Excludes1**   obstructed labor due to other fetal deformities (O66.3)
>
> Coding Clinic: 2016, Q4, P51
>
> One of the following 7th characters is to be assigned to code O33.7. 7th character Ø is for single gestations and multiple gestations where the fetus is unspecified. 7th characters 1 through 9 are for cases of multiple gestations to identify the fetus for which the code applies. The appropriate code from category O3Ø, Multiple gestation, must also be assigned when assigning code O33.7 with a 7th character of 1 through 9.

> | Ø | not applicable or unspecified |
> |---|---|
> | 1 | fetus 1 |
> | 2 | fetus 2 |
> | 3 | fetus 3 |
> | 4 | fetus 4 |
> | 5 | fetus 5 |
> | 9 | other fetus |

O33.8 Maternal care for disproportion of other origin ♀   M

O33.9 Maternal care for disproportion, unspecified ♀   M

> Maternal care for disproportion due to cephalopelvic disproportion NOS
> Maternal care for disproportion due to fetopelvic disproportion NOS

● **O34 Maternal care for abnormality of pelvic organs**

> **Includes**   the listed conditions as a reason for hospitalization or other obstetric care of the mother, or for cesarean delivery before onset of labor
>
> *Code first any associated obstructed labor (O65.5)*
> Use additional code for specific condition

● **O34.0 Maternal care for congenital malformation of uterus**

> Maternal care for double uterus
> Maternal care for uterus bicornis

> **O34.00 Maternal care for unspecified congenital malformation of uterus, unspecified trimester** ♀   M
>
> **O34.01 Maternal care for unspecified congenital malformation of uterus, first trimester** ♀   M
>
> **O34.02 Maternal care for unspecified congenital malformation of uterus, second trimester** ♀   M
>
> **O34.03 Maternal care for unspecified congenital malformation of uterus, third trimester** ♀   M

● **O34.1 Maternal care for benign tumor of corpus uteri**

> **Excludes2**   maternal care for benign tumor of cervix (O34.4-)
> maternal care for malignant neoplasm of uterus (O9A.1-)

> **O34.10 Maternal care for benign tumor of corpus uteri, unspecified trimester** ♀   M
>
> **O34.11 Maternal care for benign tumor of corpus uteri, first trimester** ♀   M
>
> **O34.12 Maternal care for benign tumor of corpus uteri, second trimester** ♀   M
>
> **O34.13 Maternal care for benign tumor of corpus uteri, third trimester** ♀   M

● **O34.2 Maternal care due to uterine scar from previous surgery**

> Coding Clinic: 2016, Q4, P76

> ● **O34.21 Maternal care for scar from previous cesarean delivery**
>
> > Coding Clinic: 2016, Q4, P51
>
> > **O34.211 Maternal care for low transverse scar from previous cesarean delivery** ♀   M
> >
> > **O34.212 Maternal care for vertical scar from previous cesarean delivery** ♀   M
> > > Maternal care for classical scar from previous cesarean delivery
> >
> > **O34.218 Maternal care for other type scar from previous cesarean delivery** ♀   M
> > > Mid-transverse T incision
> >
> > **O34.219 Maternal care for unspecified type scar from previous cesarean delivery** ♀   M
>
> **O34.22 Maternal care for cesarean scar defect (isthmocele)** ♀   M
>
> **O34.29 Maternal care due to uterine scar from other previous surgery** ♀   M
> > Maternal care due to uterine scar from other transmural uterine incision

● **O34.3 Maternal care for cervical incompetence**

> Maternal care for cerclage with or without cervical incompetence
> Maternal care for Shirodkar suture with or without cervical incompetence
> (Ex) **For category O34.3 CC codes:** See PDX Collection 973

> **O34.30 Maternal care for cervical incompetence, unspecified trimester** ♀   M
>
> **O34.31 Maternal care for cervical incompetence, first trimester** ♀ 🗞   M
>
> **O34.32 Maternal care for cervical incompetence, second trimester** ♀ 🗞   M
>
> **O34.33 Maternal care for cervical incompetence, third trimester** ♀ 🗞   M

N Newborn Age: Ø   **P** Pediatric Age: Ø–17   **M** Maternity DX: 9–64   **A** Adult Age: 15–124   ♀ Females Only   ♂ Males Only

🗞 Complication\Comorbidity   🗞 Major C\C   (Ex) CC/MCC Exclusions   🗞 Hospital-Acquired Condition   🗞 Hierarchical Condition Category

1163

● O34.4   Maternal care for other abnormalities of cervix
    O34.40   Maternal care for other abnormalities of cervix, unspecified trimester ♀   M
    O34.41   Maternal care for other abnormalities of cervix, first trimester ♀   M
    O34.42   Maternal care for other abnormalities of cervix, second trimester ♀   M
    O34.43   Maternal care for other abnormalities of cervix, third trimester ♀   M

● O34.5   Maternal care for other abnormalities of gravid uterus
  ● O34.51   Maternal care for incarceration of gravid uterus
    O34.511   Maternal care for incarceration of gravid uterus, first trimester ♀   M
    O34.512   Maternal care for incarceration of gravid uterus, second trimester ♀   M
    O34.513   Maternal care for incarceration of gravid uterus, third trimester ♀   M
    O34.519   Maternal care for incarceration of gravid uterus, unspecified trimester ♀   M

  ● O34.52   Maternal care for prolapse of gravid uterus
    O34.521   Maternal care for prolapse of gravid uterus, first trimester ♀   M
    O34.522   Maternal care for prolapse of gravid uterus, second trimester ♀   M
    O34.523   Maternal care for prolapse of gravid uterus, third trimester ♀   M
    O34.529   Maternal care for prolapse of gravid uterus, unspecified trimester ♀   M

  ● O34.53   Maternal care for retroversion of gravid uterus
    O34.531   Maternal care for retroversion of gravid uterus, first trimester ♀   M
    O34.532   Maternal care for retroversion of gravid uterus, second trimester ♀   M
    O34.533   Maternal care for retroversion of gravid uterus, third trimester ♀   M
    O34.539   Maternal care for retroversion of gravid uterus, unspecified trimester ♀   M

  ● O34.59   Maternal care for other abnormalities of gravid uterus
    O34.591   Maternal care for other abnormalities of gravid uterus, first trimester ♀   M
    O34.592   Maternal care for other abnormalities of gravid uterus, second trimester ♀   M
    O34.593   Maternal care for other abnormalities of gravid uterus, third trimester ♀   M
    O34.599   Maternal care for other abnormalities of gravid uterus, unspecified trimester ♀   M

● O34.6   Maternal care for abnormality of vagina
    Excludes2   maternal care for vaginal varices in pregnancy (O22.1-)
    O34.60   Maternal care for abnormality of vagina, unspecified trimester ♀   M
    O34.61   Maternal care for abnormality of vagina, first trimester ♀   M
    O34.62   Maternal care for abnormality of vagina, second trimester ♀   M
    O34.63   Maternal care for abnormality of vagina, third trimester ♀   M

● O34.7   Maternal care for abnormality of vulva and perineum
    Excludes2   maternal care for perineal and vulval varices in pregnancy (O22.1-)
    O34.70   Maternal care for abnormality of vulva and perineum, unspecified trimester ♀   M
    O34.71   Maternal care for abnormality of vulva and perineum, first trimester ♀   M
    O34.72   Maternal care for abnormality of vulva and perineum, second trimester ♀   M
    O34.73   Maternal care for abnormality of vulva and perineum, third trimester ♀   M

● O34.8   Maternal care for other abnormalities of pelvic organs
    O34.80   Maternal care for other abnormalities of pelvic organs, unspecified trimester ♀   M
    O34.81   Maternal care for other abnormalities of pelvic organs, first trimester ♀   M
    O34.82   Maternal care for other abnormalities of pelvic organs, second trimester ♀   M
    O34.83   Maternal care for other abnormalities of pelvic organs, third trimester ♀   M

● O34.9   Maternal care for abnormality of pelvic organ, unspecified
    O34.90   Maternal care for abnormality of pelvic organ, unspecified, unspecified trimester ♀   M
    O34.91   Maternal care for abnormality of pelvic organ, unspecified, first trimester ♀   M
    O34.92   Maternal care for abnormality of pelvic organ, unspecified, second trimester ♀   M
    O34.93   Maternal care for abnormality of pelvic organ, unspecified, third trimester ♀   M

● O35   Maternal care for known or suspected fetal abnormality and damage
    Includes   the listed conditions in the fetus as a reason for hospitalization or other obstetric care to the mother, or for termination of pregnancy
    Code also any associated maternal condition
    Excludes1   encounter for suspected maternal and fetal conditions ruled out (Z03.7-)
    One of the following 7th characters is to be assigned to each code under category O35. 7th character Ø is for single gestations and multiple gestations where the fetus is unspecified. 7th characters 1 through 9 are for cases of multiple gestations to identify the fetus for which the code applies. The appropriate code from category O30, Multiple gestation, must also be assigned when assigning a code from category O35 that has a 7th character of 1 through 9.

Ø	not applicable or unspecified
1	fetus 1
2	fetus 2
3	fetus 3
4	fetus 4
5	fetus 5
9	other fetus

X ● O35.0   Maternal care for (suspected) central nervous system malformation in fetus ♀   M
    Maternal care for fetal anencephaly
    Maternal care for fetal hydrocephalus
    Maternal care for fetal spina bifida
    Excludes2   chromosomal abnormality in fetus (O35.1)
X ● O35.1   Maternal care for (suspected) chromosomal abnormality in fetus ♀   M

▶ New   ⟹ Revised   deleted Deleted   Excludes 1   Excludes 2   Includes   Use additional   Code first   Code also   Key words
OGCR Official Guidelines   ● Unacceptable Principal Diagnosis   X Assign placeholder X   ● Use Additional Character(s)   ▷ Manifestation Code   Coding Clinic

CHAPTER 15 (O00-O9A)

X ● **O35.2** **Maternal care for (suspected) hereditary disease in fetus** ♀   M

      Excludes2   chromosomal abnormality in fetus (O35.1)

X ● **O35.3** **Maternal care for (suspected) damage to fetus from viral disease in mother** ♀   M

      Maternal care for damage to fetus from maternal cytomegalovirus infection

      Maternal care for damage to fetus from maternal rubella

      Coding Clinic: 2016, Q4, P6

X ● **O35.4** **Maternal care for (suspected) damage to fetus from alcohol** ♀   M

X ● **O35.5** **Maternal care for (suspected) damage to fetus by drugs** ♀   M

      Maternal care for damage to fetus from drug addiction

X ● **O35.6** **Maternal care for (suspected) damage to fetus by radiation** ♀   M

X ● **O35.7** **Maternal care for (suspected) damage to fetus by other medical procedures** ♀   M

      Maternal care for damage to fetus by amniocentesis

      Maternal care for damage to fetus by biopsy procedures

      Maternal care for damage to fetus by hematological investigation

      Maternal care for damage to fetus by intrauterine contraceptive device

      Maternal care for damage to fetus by intrauterine surgery

X ● **O35.8** **Maternal care for other (suspected) fetal abnormality and damage** ♀   M

      Maternal care for damage to fetus from maternal listeriosis

      Maternal care for damage to fetus from maternal toxoplasmosis

X ● **O35.9** **Maternal care for (suspected) fetal abnormality and damage, unspecified** ♀   M

● **O36** **Maternal care for other fetal problems**

    Includes   the listed conditions in the fetus as a reason for hospitalization or other obstetric care of the mother, or for termination of pregnancy

    Excludes1   encounter for suspected maternal and fetal conditions ruled out (Z03.7-)

        placental transfusion syndromes (O43.0-)

    Excludes2   labor and delivery complicated by fetal stress (O77.-)

One of the following 7th characters is to be assigned to each code under category O36. 7th character 0 is for single gestations and multiple gestations where the fetus is unspecified. 7th characters 1 through 9 are for cases of multiple gestations to identify the fetus for which the code applies. The appropriate code from category O30, Multiple gestation, must also be assigned when assigning a code from category O36 that has a 7th character of 1 through 9.

0	not applicable or unspecified
1	fetus 1
2	fetus 2
3	fetus 3
4	fetus 4
5	fetus 5
9	other fetus

Coding Clinic: 2015, Q3, P40

● **O36.0** **Maternal care for rhesus isoimmunization**

    Maternal care for Rh incompatibility (with hydrops fetalis)

    (Ex) **For category O36.0 CC codes:** See PDX Collection 978

  ● **O36.01** **Maternal care for anti-D [Rh] antibodies**

    ● **O36.011** Maternal care for anti-D [Rh] antibodies, first trimester ♀ 🝆   M

    ● **O36.012** Maternal care for anti-D [Rh] antibodies, second trimester ♀ 🝆   M

    ● **O36.013** Maternal care for anti-D [Rh] antibodies, third trimester ♀ 🝆   M

    ● **O36.019** Maternal care for anti-D [Rh] antibodies, unspecified trimester ♀   M

  ● **O36.09** **Maternal care for other rhesus isoimmunization**

    ● **O36.091** Maternal care for other rhesus isoimmunization, first trimester ♀ 🝆   M

    ● **O36.092** Maternal care for other rhesus isoimmunization, second trimester ♀ 🝆   M

    ● **O36.093** Maternal care for other rhesus isoimmunization, third trimester ♀ 🝆   M

        Coding Clinic: 2015, Q3, P40

    ● **O36.099** Maternal care for other rhesus isoimmunization, unspecified trimester ♀   M

● **O36.1** **Maternal care for other isoimmunization**

    Maternal care for ABO isoimmunization

  ● **O36.11** **Maternal care for Anti-A sensitization**

    Maternal care for isoimmunization NOS (with hydrops fetalis)

    ● **O36.111** Maternal care for Anti-A sensitization, first trimester ♀   M

    ● **O36.112** Maternal care for Anti-A sensitization, second trimester ♀   M

    ● **O36.113** Maternal care for Anti-A sensitization, third trimester ♀   M

    ● **O36.119** Maternal care for Anti-A sensitization, unspecified trimester ♀   M

OGCR Section I.C.15.e.1.

Fetal Conditions Affecting the Management of the Mother

1) Code from categories O35 and O36

Codes from categories O35, Maternal care for known or suspected fetal abnormality and damage, and O36, Maternal care for other fetal problems, are assigned only when the fetal condition is actually responsible for modifying the management of the mother, i.e., by requiring diagnostic studies, additional observation, special care, or termination of pregnancy. The fact that the fetal condition exists does not justify assigning a code from this series to the mother's record.

2) In utero surgery

In cases when surgery is performed on the fetus, a diagnosis code from category O35, Maternal care for known or suspected fetal abnormality and damage, should be assigned identifying the fetal condition. Assign the appropriate procedure code for the procedure performed.

No code from Chapter 16, the perinatal codes, should be used on the mother's record to identify fetal conditions. Surgery performed in utero on a fetus is still to be coded as an obstetric encounter.

N Newborn Age: 0   **P** Pediatric Age: 0–17   **M** Maternity DX: 9–64   **A** Adult Age: 15–124   ♀ Females Only   ♂ Males Only

🝆 Complication\Comorbidity   🝆 Major C\C   (Ex) CC/MCC Exclusions   🝆 Hospital-Acquired Condition   🝆 Hierarchical Condition Category

● **O36.19 Maternal care for other isoimmunization**
Maternal care for Anti-B sensitization
   ● **O36.191 Maternal care for other isoimmunization, first trimester** ♀ M
   ● **O36.192 Maternal care for other isoimmunization, second trimester** ♀ M
   ● **O36.193 Maternal care for other isoimmunization, third trimester** ♀ M
   ● **O36.199 Maternal care for other isoimmunization, unspecified trimester** ♀ M

● **O36.2 Maternal care for hydrops fetalis**
Maternal care for hydrops fetalis NOS
Maternal care for hydrops fetalis not associated with isoimmunization
   Excludes1 hydrops fetalis associated with ABO isoimmunization (O36.1-)
           hydrops fetalis associated with rhesus isoimmunization (O36.0-)
   ● **O36.20 Maternal care for hydrops fetalis, unspecified trimester** ♀ M
   ● **O36.21 Maternal care for hydrops fetalis, first trimester** ♀ M
   ● **O36.22 Maternal care for hydrops fetalis, second trimester** ♀ M
   ● **O36.23 Maternal care for hydrops fetalis, third trimester** ♀ M

● **O36.4 Maternal care for intrauterine death** ♀ 🔒 M
Maternal care for intrauterine fetal death NOS
Maternal care for intrauterine fetal death after completion of 20 weeks of gestation
Maternal care for late fetal death
Maternal care for missed delivery
   Excludes1 missed abortion (O02.1)
           stillbirth (P95)
   Ex See PDX Collection 979

● **O36.5 Maternal care for known or suspected poor fetal growth**
  ● **O36.51 Maternal care for known or suspected placental insufficiency**
   ● **O36.511 Maternal care for known or suspected placental insufficiency, first trimester** ♀ M
   ● **O36.512 Maternal care for known or suspected placental insufficiency, second trimester** ♀ M
   ● **O36.513 Maternal care for known or suspected placental insufficiency, third trimester** ♀ M
   ● **O36.519 Maternal care for known or suspected placental insufficiency, unspecified trimester** ♀ M
  ● **O36.59 Maternal care for other known or suspected poor fetal growth**
Maternal care for known or suspected light-for-dates NOS
Maternal care for known or suspected small-for-dates NOS
   ● **O36.591 Maternal care for other known or suspected poor fetal growth, first trimester** ♀ M
   ● **O36.592 Maternal care for other known or suspected poor fetal growth, second trimester** ♀ M
   ● **O36.593 Maternal care for other known or suspected poor fetal growth, third trimester** ♀ M
   ● **O36.599 Maternal care for other known or suspected poor fetal growth, unspecified trimester** ♀ M

● **O36.6 Maternal care for excessive fetal growth**
Maternal care for known or suspected large-for-dates
  X● **O36.60 Maternal care for excessive fetal growth, unspecified trimester** ♀ M
  X● **O36.61 Maternal care for excessive fetal growth, first trimester** ♀ M
  X● **O36.62 Maternal care for excessive fetal growth, second trimester** ♀ M
  X● **O36.63 Maternal care for excessive fetal growth, third trimester** ♀ M

● **O36.7 Maternal care for viable fetus in abdominal pregnancy**
  X● **O36.70 Maternal care for viable fetus in abdominal pregnancy, unspecified trimester** ♀ M
  X● **O36.71 Maternal care for viable fetus in abdominal pregnancy, first trimester** ♀ M
  X● **O36.72 Maternal care for viable fetus in abdominal pregnancy, second trimester** ♀ M
  X● **O36.73 Maternal care for viable fetus in abdominal pregnancy, third trimester** ♀ M

● **O36.8 Maternal care for other specified fetal problems**
  ●X● **O36.80 Pregnancy with inconclusive fetal viability** ♀ M
Encounter to determine fetal viability of pregnancy
Coding Clinic: 2019, Q2, P29
  ● **O36.81 Decreased fetal movements**
   ● **O36.812 Decreased fetal movements, second trimester** ♀ M
   ● **O36.813 Decreased fetal movements, third trimester** ♀ M
   ● **O36.819 Decreased fetal movements, unspecified trimester** ♀ M
  ● **O36.82 Fetal anemia and thrombocytopenia**
   ● **O36.821 Fetal anemia and thrombocytopenia, first trimester** ♀ M
   ● **O36.822 Fetal anemia and thrombocytopenia, second trimester** ♀ M
   ● **O36.823 Fetal anemia and thrombocytopenia, third trimester** ♀ M
   ● **O36.829 Fetal anemia and thrombocytopenia, unspecified trimester** ♀ M
  ● **O36.83 Maternal care for abnormalities of the fetal heart rate or rhythm**
Maternal care for depressed fetal heart rate tones
Maternal care for fetal bradycardia
Maternal care for fetal heart rate abnormal variability
Maternal care for fetal heart rate decelerations
Maternal care for fetal heart rate irregularity
Maternal care for fetal tachycardia
Maternal care for non-reassuring fetal heart rate or rhythm
   ● **O36.831 Maternal care for abnormalities of the fetal heart rate or rhythm, first trimester** ♀ M
   ● **O36.832 Maternal care for abnormalities of the fetal heart rate or rhythm, second trimester** ♀ M
   ● **O36.833 Maternal care for abnormalities of the fetal heart rate or rhythm, third trimester** ♀ M
   ● **O36.839 Maternal care for abnormalities of the fetal heart rate or rhythm, unspecified trimester** ♀ M
  ● **O36.89 Maternal care for other specified fetal problems**
   ● **O36.891 Maternal care for other specified fetal problems, first trimester** ♀ M
   ● **O36.892 Maternal care for other specified fetal problems, second trimester** ♀ M
   ● **O36.893 Maternal care for other specified fetal problems, third trimester** ♀ M
   ● **O36.899 Maternal care for other specified fetal problems, unspecified trimester** ♀ M

● O36.9   Maternal care for fetal problem, unspecified

   X ● O36.90   Maternal care for fetal problem, unspecified, unspecified trimester ♀   M

   X ● O36.91   Maternal care for fetal problem, unspecified, first trimester ♀   M

   X ● O36.92   Maternal care for fetal problem, unspecified, second trimester ♀   M

   X ● O36.93   Maternal care for fetal problem, unspecified, third trimester ♀   M

● O40   Polyhydramnios

   Overabundance of amniotic fluid

   | **Includes** | hydramnios |
   | **Excludes1** | encounter for suspected maternal and fetal conditions ruled out (Z03.7-) |

   One of the following 7th characters is to be assigned to each code under category O40. 7th character Ø is for single gestations and multiple gestations where the fetus is unspecified. 7th characters 1 through 9 are for cases of multiple gestations to identify the fetus for which the code applies. The appropriate code from category O30, Multiple gestation, must also be assigned when assigning a code from category O40 that has a 7th character of 1 through 9.

Ø	not applicable or unspecified
1	fetus 1
2	fetus 2
3	fetus 3
4	fetus 4
5	fetus 5
9	other fetus

   X ● O40.1   Polyhydramnios, first trimester ♀   M

   X ● O40.2   Polyhydramnios, second trimester ♀   M

   X ● O40.3   Polyhydramnios, third trimester ♀   M

   X ● O40.9   Polyhydramnios, unspecified trimester ♀   M

● O41   Other disorders of amniotic fluid and membranes

   | **Excludes1** | encounter for suspected maternal and fetal conditions ruled out (Z03.7-) |

   One of the following 7th characters is to be assigned to each code under category O41. 7th character Ø is for single gestations and multiple gestations where the fetus is unspecified. 7th characters 1 through 9 are for cases of multiple gestations to identify the fetus for which the code applies. The appropriate code from category O30, Multiple gestation, must also be assigned when assigning a code from category O41 that has a 7th character of 1 through 9.

Ø	not applicable or unspecified
1	fetus 1
2	fetus 2
3	fetus 3
4	fetus 4
5	fetus 5
9	other fetus

   ● O41.0   Oligohydramnios

     Scant volume of amniotic fluid

     Oligohydramnios without rupture of membranes

     (Ex) **For category O41.0 CC codes:** See PDX Collection 982

   X ● O41.00   Oligohydramnios, unspecified trimester ♀   M

   X ● O41.01   Oligohydramnios, first trimester ♀ 🦠   M

   X ● O41.02   Oligohydramnios, second trimester ♀ 🦠   M

   X ● O41.03   Oligohydramnios, third trimester ♀ 🦠   M

● O41.1   Infection of amniotic sac and membranes

   (Ex) **For category O41.1 CC codes:** See PDX Collection 983

   ● O41.10   Infection of amniotic sac and membranes, unspecified

     ● O41.101   Infection of amniotic sac and membranes, unspecified, first trimester ♀ 🦠   M

     ● O41.102   Infection of amniotic sac and membranes, unspecified, second trimester ♀ 🦠   M

     ● O41.103   Infection of amniotic sac and membranes, unspecified, third trimester ♀ 🦠   M

     ● O41.109   Infection of amniotic sac and membranes, unspecified, unspecified trimester ♀   M

   ● O41.12   Chorioamnionitis

     Coding Clinic: 2019, Q2, P34-35

     ● O41.121   Chorioamnionitis, first trimester ♀ 🦠   M

     ● O41.122   Chorioamnionitis, second trimester ♀ 🦠   M

     ● O41.123   Chorioamnionitis, third trimester ♀ 🦠   M

     ● O41.129   Chorioamnionitis, unspecified trimester ♀   M

   ● O41.14   Placentitis

     ● O41.141   Placentitis, first trimester ♀ 🦠   M

     ● O41.142   Placentitis, second trimester ♀ 🦠   M

     ● O41.143   Placentitis, third trimester ♀ 🦠   M

     ● O41.149   Placentitis, unspecified trimester ♀   M

● O41.8   Other specified disorders of amniotic fluid and membranes

   ● O41.8X   Other specified disorders of amniotic fluid and membranes

     ● O41.8X1   Other specified disorders of amniotic fluid and membranes, first trimester ♀   M

     ● O41.8X2   Other specified disorders of amniotic fluid and membranes, second trimester ♀   M

     ● O41.8X3   Other specified disorders of amniotic fluid and membranes, third trimester ♀   M

     ● O41.8X9   Other specified disorders of amniotic fluid and membranes, unspecified trimester ♀   M

● O41.9   Disorder of amniotic fluid and membranes, unspecified

   X ● O41.90   Disorder of amniotic fluid and membranes, unspecified, unspecified trimester ♀   M

   X ● O41.91   Disorder of amniotic fluid and membranes, unspecified, first trimester ♀   M

   X ● O41.92   Disorder of amniotic fluid and membranes, unspecified, second trimester ♀   M

   X ● O41.93   Disorder of amniotic fluid and membranes, unspecified, third trimester ♀   M

N Newborn Age: Ø   **P** Pediatric Age: Ø–17   **M** Maternity DX: 9–64   **A** Adult Age: 15–124   ♀ Females Only   ♂ Males Only

🦠 Complication\Comorbidity   🦠 Major C\C   (Ex) CC/MCC Exclusions   Hospital-Acquired Condition   Hierarchical Condition Category

● **O42   Premature rupture of membranes**

   ● **O42.0   Premature rupture of membranes, onset of labor within 24 hours of rupture**

     O42.00   Premature rupture of membranes, onset of labor within 24 hours of rupture, unspecified weeks of gestation ♀   **M**

     ● **O42.01   Preterm premature rupture of membranes, onset of labor within 24 hours of rupture**
        Premature rupture of membranes before 37 completed weeks of gestation

        O42.011   Preterm premature rupture of membranes, onset of labor within 24 hours of rupture, first trimester ♀   **M**

        O42.012   Preterm premature rupture of membranes, onset of labor within 24 hours of rupture, second trimester ♀ **M**

        O42.013   Preterm premature rupture of membranes, onset of labor within 24 hours of rupture, third trimester ♀   **M**

        O42.019   Preterm premature rupture of membranes, onset of labor within 24 hours of rupture, unspecified trimester ♀   **M**

     O42.02   Full-term premature rupture of membranes, onset of labor within 24 hours of rupture ♀   **M**
        Premature rupture of membranes at or after 37 completed weeks of gestation, onset of labor within 24 hours of rupture

   ● **O42.1   Premature rupture of membranes, onset of labor more than 24 hours following rupture**

     O42.10   Premature rupture of membranes, onset of labor more than 24 hours following rupture, unspecified weeks of gestation ♀   **M**

     ● **O42.11   Preterm premature rupture of membranes, onset of labor more than 24 hours following rupture**
        Premature rupture of membranes before 37 completed weeks of gestation

        O42.111   Preterm premature rupture of membranes, onset of labor more than 24 hours following rupture, first trimester ♀   **M**

        O42.112   Preterm premature rupture of membranes, onset of labor more than 24 hours following rupture, second trimester ♀   **M**

        O42.113   Preterm premature rupture of membranes, onset of labor more than 24 hours following rupture, third trimester ♀   **M**

        O42.119   Preterm premature rupture of membranes, onset of labor more than 24 hours following rupture, unspecified trimester ♀   **M**

     O42.12   Full-term premature rupture of membranes, onset of labor more than 24 hours following rupture ♀   **M**
        Premature rupture of membranes at or after 37 completed weeks of gestation, onset of labor more than 24 hours following rupture

   ● **O42.9   Premature rupture of membranes, unspecified as to length of time between rupture and onset of labor**

     O42.90   Premature rupture of membranes, unspecified as to length of time between rupture and onset of labor, unspecified weeks of gestation ♀   **M**

     ● **O42.91   Preterm premature rupture of membranes, unspecified as to length of time between rupture and onset of labor**
        Premature rupture of membranes before 37 completed weeks of gestation

        O42.911   Preterm premature rupture of membranes, unspecified as to length of time between rupture and onset of labor, first trimester ♀   **M**

        O42.912   Preterm premature rupture of membranes, unspecified as to length of time between rupture and onset of labor, second trimester ♀   **M**

        O42.913   Preterm premature rupture of membranes, unspecified as to length of time between rupture and onset of labor, third trimester ♀

        O42.919   Preterm premature rupture of membranes, unspecified as to length of time between rupture and onset of labor, unspecified trimester ♀   **M**

     O42.92   Full-term premature rupture of membranes, unspecified as to length of time between rupture and onset of labor ♀   **M**
        Premature rupture of membranes at or after 37 completed weeks of gestation, unspecified as to length of time between rupture and onset of labor

● **O43   Placental disorders**

   Excludes2   maternal care for poor fetal growth due to placental insufficiency (O36.5-)
                placenta previa (O44.-)
                placental polyp (O90.89)
                placentitis (O41.14-)
                premature separation of placenta [abruptio placentae] (O45.-)

   ● **O43.0   Placental transfusion syndromes**

     ● **O43.01   Fetomaternal placental transfusion syndrome**
        Maternofetal placental transfusion syndrome

        O43.011   Fetomaternal placental transfusion syndrome, first trimester ♀   **M**

        O43.012   Fetomaternal placental transfusion syndrome, second trimester ♀   **M**

        O43.013   Fetomaternal placental transfusion syndrome, third trimester ♀   **M**

        O43.019   Fetomaternal placental transfusion syndrome, unspecified trimester ♀   **M**

     ● **O43.02   Fetus-to-fetus placental transfusion syndrome**

        O43.021   Fetus-to-fetus placental transfusion syndrome, first trimester ♀   **M**

        O43.022   Fetus-to-fetus placental transfusion syndrome, second trimester ♀   **M**

        O43.023   Fetus-to-fetus placental transfusion syndrome, third trimester ♀   **M**

        O43.029   Fetus-to-fetus placental transfusion syndrome, unspecified trimester ♀   **M**

● O43.1   Malformation of placenta
   ● O43.10   Malformation of placenta, unspecified
         Abnormal placenta NOS
       O43.101   Malformation of placenta, unspecified, first trimester ♀   M
       O43.102   Malformation of placenta, unspecified, second trimester ♀   M
       O43.103   Malformation of placenta, unspecified, third trimester ♀   M
       O43.109   Malformation of placenta, unspecified, unspecified trimester ♀   M
   ● O43.11   Circumvallate placenta
       O43.111   Circumvallate placenta, first trimester ♀   M
       O43.112   Circumvallate placenta, second trimester ♀   M
       O43.113   Circumvallate placenta, third trimester ♀   M
       O43.119   Circumvallate placenta, unspecified trimester ♀   M
   ● O43.12   Velamentous insertion of umbilical cord
       O43.121   Velamentous insertion of umbilical cord, first trimester ♀   M
       O43.122   Velamentous insertion of umbilical cord, second trimester ♀   M
       O43.123   Velamentous insertion of umbilical cord, third trimester ♀   M
       O43.129   Velamentous insertion of umbilical cord, unspecified trimester ♀   M
   ● O43.19   Other malformation of placenta
       O43.191   Other malformation of placenta, first trimester ♀   M
       O43.192   Other malformation of placenta, second trimester ♀   M
       O43.193   Other malformation of placenta, third trimester ♀   M
       O43.199   Other malformation of placenta, unspecified trimester ♀   M

● O43.2   Morbidly adherent placenta
     Code also associated third stage postpartum hemorrhage, if applicable (O72.0)
     Excludes1   retained placenta (O73.-)
   ● O43.21   Placenta accreta
       O43.211   Placenta accreta, first trimester ♀   M
       O43.212   Placenta accreta, second trimester ♀   M
       O43.213   Placenta accreta, third trimester ♀   M
       O43.219   Placenta accreta, unspecified trimester ♀   M
   ● O43.22   Placenta increta
       O43.221   Placenta increta, first trimester ♀   M
       O43.222   Placenta increta, second trimester ♀   M
       O43.223   Placenta increta, third trimester ♀   M
       O43.229   Placenta increta, unspecified trimester ♀   M
   ● O43.23   Placenta percreta
       O43.231   Placenta percreta, first trimester ♀   M
       O43.232   Placenta percreta, second trimester ♀ M
       O43.233   Placenta percreta, third trimester ♀   M
       O43.239   Placenta percreta, unspecified trimester ♀   M

● O43.8   Other placental disorders
   ● O43.81   Placental infarction
       O43.811   Placental infarction, first trimester ♀ M
       O43.812   Placental infarction, second trimester ♀   M
       O43.813   Placental infarction, third trimester ♀   M
       O43.819   Placental infarction, unspecified trimester ♀   M
   ● O43.89   Other placental disorders
         Placental dysfunction
       O43.891   Other placental disorders, first trimester ♀   M
       O43.892   Other placental disorders, second trimester ♀   M
       O43.893   Other placental disorders, third trimester ♀   M
       O43.899   Other placental disorders, unspecified trimester ♀   M

● O43.9   Unspecified placental disorder
       O43.90   Unspecified placental disorder, unspecified trimester ♀   M
       O43.91   Unspecified placental disorder, first trimester ♀   M
       O43.92   Unspecified placental disorder, second trimester ♀   M
       O43.93   Unspecified placental disorder, third trimester ♀   M

● O44   Placenta previa
     (Ex) **For category O44 CC codes:** See PDX Collection 966, 4010-4011
     Coding Clinic: 2016, Q4, P52
  ● O44.0   Complete placenta previa NOS or without hemorrhage
         Placenta previa NOS
       O44.00   Complete placenta previa NOS or without hemorrhage, unspecified trimester ♀   M
       O44.01   Complete placenta previa NOS or without hemorrhage, first trimester ♀ ◔   M
       O44.02   Complete placenta previa NOS or without hemorrhage, second trimester ♀ ◔   M
       O44.03   Complete placenta previa NOS or without hemorrhage, third trimester ♀ ◔   M
  ● O44.1   Complete placenta previa with hemorrhage
     Excludes1   labor and delivery complicated by hemorrhage from vasa previa (O69.4)
       O44.10   Complete placenta previa with hemorrhage, unspecified trimester ♀   M
       O44.11   Complete placenta previa with hemorrhage, first trimester ♀ ◔   M
       O44.12   Complete placenta previa with hemorrhage, second trimester ♀ ◔   M
       O44.13   Complete placenta previa with hemorrhage, third trimester ♀ ◔   M

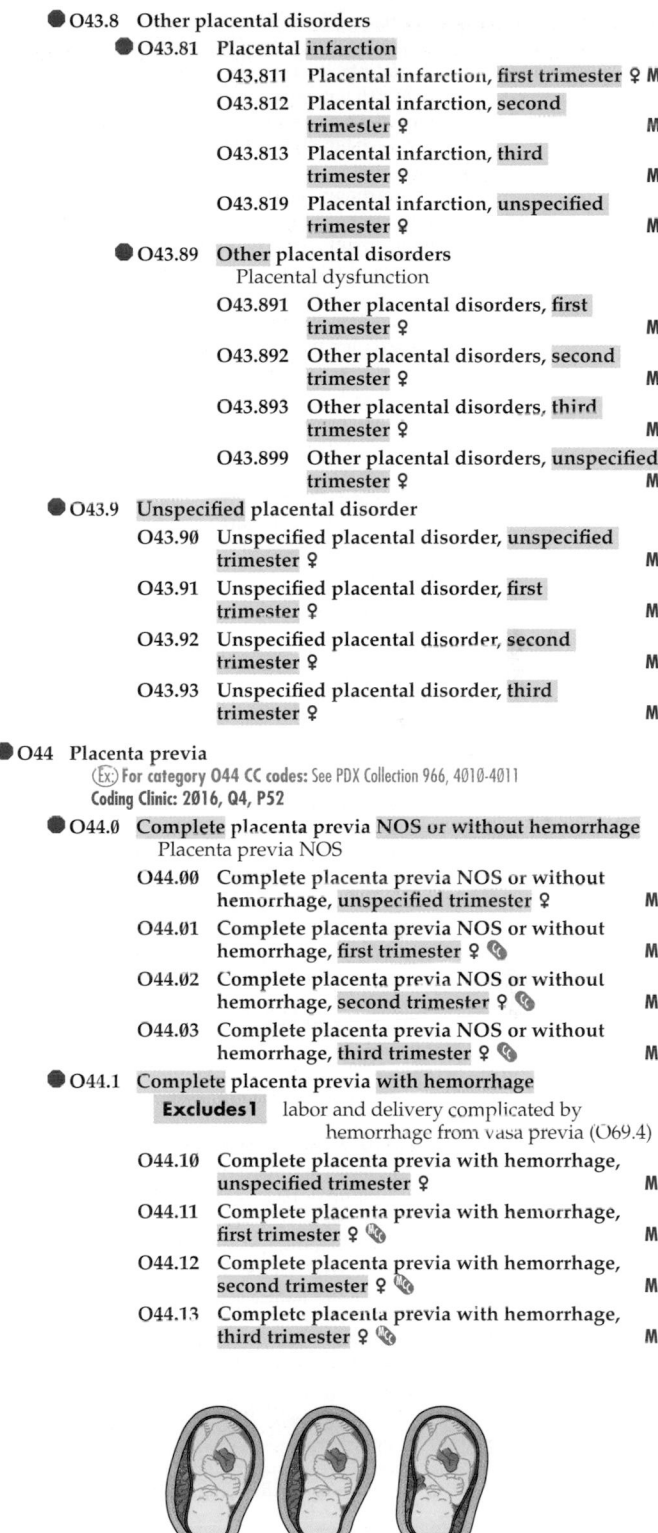

A   B   C

Figure 15-2   **A.** Marginal placenta previa. **B.** Partial placenta previa. **C.** Total placenta previa.

Item 15–3   Placenta previa is a condition in which the opening of the cervix is obstructed by the displaced placenta. The three types, marginal, partial, and total, are varying degrees of placenta displacement. Placenta abruption is the premature breaking away of the placenta from the site of the uterine implant before the delivery of the fetus.

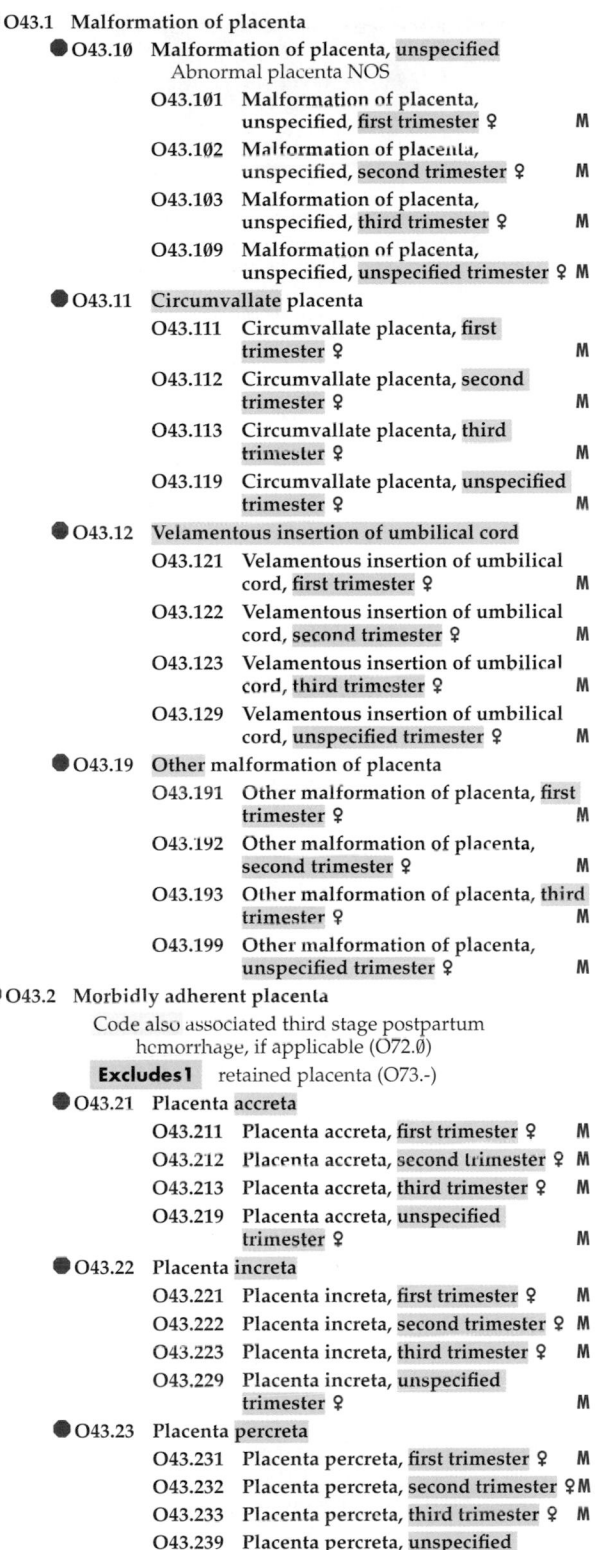

N Newborn Age: 0   **P** Pediatric Age: 0–17   **M** Maternity DX: 9–64   **A** Adult Age: 15–124   ♀ Females Only   ♂ Males Only

◔ Complication\Comorbidity   ◔ Major C\C   (Ex) CC/MCC Exclusions   ◔ Hospital-Acquired Condition   ◔ Hierarchical Condition Category   **1169**

● **O44.2** **Partial placenta previa without hemorrhage**
Marginal placenta previa, NOS or without hemorrhage

       O44.20   Partial placenta previa NOS or without hemorrhage, unspecified trimester ♀   M

       O44.21   Partial placenta previa NOS or without hemorrhage, first trimester ♀ 🔍   M

       O44.22   Partial placenta previa NOS or without hemorrhage, second trimester ♀   M

       O44.23   Partial placenta previa NOS or without hemorrhage, third trimester ♀ 🔍   M

● **O44.3** **Partial placenta previa with hemorrhage**
Marginal placenta previa with hemorrhage

       O44.30   Partial placenta previa with hemorrhage, unspecified trimester ♀   M

       O44.31   Partial placenta previa with hemorrhage, first trimester ♀ 🔍   M

       O44.32   Partial placenta previa with hemorrhage, second trimester ♀ 🔍   M

       O44.33   Partial placenta previa with hemorrhage, third trimester ♀ 🔍   M

● **O44.4** **Low lying placenta NOS or without hemorrhage**
Low implantation of placenta NOS or without hemorrhage

       O44.40   Low lying placenta NOS or without hemorrhage, unspecified trimester ♀   M

       O44.41   Low lying placenta NOS or without hemorrhage, first trimester ♀ 🔍   M

       O44.42   Low lying placenta NOS or without hemorrhage, second trimester ♀   M

       O44.43   Low lying placenta NOS or without hemorrhage, third trimester ♀ 🔍   M

● **O44.5** **Low lying placenta with hemorrhage**
Low implantation of placenta with hemorrhage

       O44.50   Low lying placenta with hemorrhage, unspecified trimester ♀   M

       O44.51   Low lying placenta with hemorrhage, first trimester ♀ 🔍   M

       O44.52   Low lying placenta with hemorrhage, second trimester ♀ 🔍   M

       O44.53   Low lying placenta with hemorrhage, third trimester ♀ 🔍   M

● **O45** **Premature separation of placenta [abruptio placentae]**

  ● **O45.0** **Premature separation of placenta with coagulation defect**
       (Ex) **For category O45.0 CC codes:** See PDX Collection 985, 4005-4006

    ● **O45.00** **Premature separation of placenta with coagulation defect, unspecified**

       O45.001   Premature separation of placenta with coagulation defect, unspecified, first trimester ♀ 🔍   M

       O45.002   Premature separation of placenta with coagulation defect, unspecified, second trimester ♀ 🔍   M

       O45.003   Premature separation of placenta with coagulation defect, unspecified, third trimester ♀ 🔍   M

       O45.009   Premature separation of placenta with coagulation defect, unspecified, unspecified trimester ♀   M

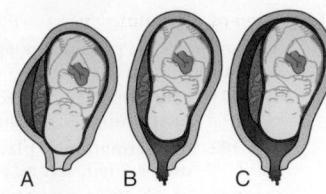

Figure 15-3   Abruptio placentae is classified according to the grade of separation of the placenta from the uterine wall. **A.** Mild separation in which hemorrhage is internal. **B.** Moderate separation in which there is external hemorrhage. **C.** Severe separation in which there is external hemorrhage and extreme separation.

  ● **O45.01** **Premature separation of placenta with afibrinogenemia**
Premature separation of placenta with hypofibrinogenemia

       O45.011   Premature separation of placenta with afibrinogenemia, first trimester ♀ 🔍 M

       O45.012   Premature separation of placenta with afibrinogenemia, second trimester ♀ 🔍   M

       O45.013   Premature separation of placenta with afibrinogenemia, third trimester ♀ 🔍   M

       O45.019   Premature separation of placenta with afibrinogenemia, unspecified trimester ♀   M

  ● **O45.02** **Premature separation of placenta with disseminated intravascular coagulation**

       O45.021   Premature separation of placenta with disseminated intravascular coagulation, first trimester ♀ 🔍   M

       O45.022   Premature separation of placenta with disseminated intravascular coagulation, second trimester ♀ 🔍 M

       O45.023   Premature separation of placenta with disseminated intravascular coagulation, third trimester ♀ 🔍   M

       O45.029   Premature separation of placenta with disseminated intravascular coagulation, unspecified trimester ♀ M

  ● **O45.09** **Premature separation of placenta with other coagulation defect**

       O45.091   Premature separation of placenta with other coagulation defect, first trimester ♀ 🔍   M

       O45.092   Premature separation of placenta with other coagulation defect, second trimester ♀ 🔍   M

       O45.093   Premature separation of placenta with other coagulation defect, third trimester ♀ 🔍   M

       O45.099   Premature separation of placenta with other coagulation defect, unspecified trimester ♀   M

  ● **O45.8** **Other premature separation of placenta**
       (Ex) **For category O45.8 CC codes:** See PDX Collection 986, 4061-4062

    ● **O45.8X** **Other premature separation of placenta**

       O45.8X1   Other premature separation of placenta, first trimester ♀ 🔍   M

       O45.8X2   Other premature separation of placenta, second trimester ♀ 🔍   M

       O45.8X3   Other premature separation of placenta, third trimester ♀ 🔍   M

       O45.8X9   Other premature separation of placenta, unspecified trimester ♀   M

CHAPTER 15 (O00-O9A)

▶ New   ⇒ Revised   ~~deleted~~ Deleted   Excludes 1   Excludes 2   Includes   Use additional   Code first   Code also   Key words

OGCR Official Guidelines   ● Unacceptable Principal Diagnosis   X Assign placeholder X   ● Use Additional Character(s)   ▶ Manifestation Code   **Coding Clinic**

● **O45.9 Premature separation of placenta, unspecified**
Abruptio placentae NOS
(Ex) **For category O45.9 CC codes:** See PDX Collection 986, 4061-4062

     O45.90   Premature separation of placenta, unspecified, unspecified trimester ♀   M

     O45.91   Premature separation of placenta, unspecified, first trimester ♀ 🐾   M

     O45.92   Premature separation of placenta, unspecified, second trimester ♀ 🐾   M

     O45.93   Premature separation of placenta, unspecified, third trimester ♀ 🐾   M

● **O46 Antepartum hemorrhage, not elsewhere classified**
Excludes1   hemorrhage in early pregnancy (O20.-)
intrapartum hemorrhage NEC (O67.-)
placenta previa (O44.-)
premature separation of placenta [abruptio placentae] (O45.-)

● **O46.0 Antepartum hemorrhage with coagulation defect**
(Ex) **For category O46.0 CC codes:** See PDX Collection 985, 4005-4006

●   O46.00   Antepartum hemorrhage with coagulation defect, unspecified

     O46.001   Antepartum hemorrhage with coagulation defect, unspecified, first trimester ♀ 🐾   M

     O46.002   Antepartum hemorrhage with coagulation defect, unspecified, second trimester ♀ 🐾   M

     O46.003   Antepartum hemorrhage with coagulation defect, unspecified, third trimester ♀ 🐾   M

     O46.009   Antepartum hemorrhage with coagulation defect, unspecified, unspecified trimester ♀   M

●   O46.01   Antepartum hemorrhage with afibrinogenemia
Antepartum hemorrhage with hypofibrinogenemia

     O46.011   Antepartum hemorrhage with afibrinogenemia, first trimester ♀ 🐾 M

     O46.012   Antepartum hemorrhage with afibrinogenemia, second trimester ♀ 🐾   M

     O46.013   Antepartum hemorrhage with afibrinogenemia, third trimester ♀ 🐾   M

     O46.019   Antepartum hemorrhage with afibrinogenemia, unspecified trimester ♀   M

●   O46.02   Antepartum hemorrhage with disseminated intravascular coagulation

     O46.021   Antepartum hemorrhage with disseminated intravascular coagulation, first trimester ♀ 🐾   M

     O46.022   Antepartum hemorrhage with disseminated intravascular coagulation, second trimester ♀ 🐾   M

     O46.023   Antepartum hemorrhage with disseminated intravascular coagulation, third trimester ♀ 🐾   M

     O46.029   Antepartum hemorrhage with disseminated intravascular coagulation, unspecified trimester ♀ M

●   O46.09   Antepartum hemorrhage with other coagulation defect

     O46.091   Antepartum hemorrhage with other coagulation defect, first trimester ♀ 🐾   M

     O46.092   Antepartum hemorrhage with other coagulation defect, second trimester ♀ 🐾   M

     O46.093   Antepartum hemorrhage with other coagulation defect, third trimester ♀ 🐾   M

     O46.099   Antepartum hemorrhage with other coagulation defect, unspecified trimester ♀   M

● **O46.8 Other antepartum hemorrhage**
●   O46.8x   Other antepartum hemorrhage

     O46.8x1   Other antepartum hemorrhage, first trimester ♀   M

     O46.8x2   Other antepartum hemorrhage, second trimester ♀   M

     O46.8x3   Other antepartum hemorrhage, third trimester ♀   M

     O46.8x9   Other antepartum hemorrhage, unspecified trimester ♀   M

● **O46.9 Antepartum hemorrhage, unspecified**

     O46.90   Antepartum hemorrhage, unspecified, unspecified trimester ♀   M

     O46.91   Antepartum hemorrhage, unspecified, first trimester ♀   M

     O46.92   Antepartum hemorrhage, unspecified, second trimester ♀   M

     O46.93   Antepartum hemorrhage, unspecified, third trimester ♀   M

● **O47 False labor**
Includes   Braxton Hicks contractions
threatened labor
Excludes1   preterm labor (O60.-)
(Ex) **For category O47 CC codes:** See PDX Collection 987, 4050-4051

● **O47.0 False labor before 37 completed weeks of gestation**

     O47.00   False labor before 37 completed weeks of gestation, unspecified trimester ♀   M

     O47.02   False labor before 37 completed weeks of gestation, second trimester ♀ 🐾   M

     O47.03   False labor before 37 completed weeks of gestation, third trimester ♀ 🐾   M

O47.1   False labor at or after 37 completed weeks of gestation ♀ 🐾   M
Coding Clinic: 2021, Q1, P10

O47.9   False labor, unspecified ♀   M

● **O48 Late pregnancy**
O48.0   Post-term pregnancy ♀   M
Pregnancy over 40 completed weeks to 42 completed weeks gestation

O48.1   Prolonged pregnancy ♀   M
Pregnancy which has advanced beyond 42 completed weeks gestation

CHAPTER 15 (O00-O9A)

CHAPTER 15 (O00-O9A)

COMPLICATIONS OF LABOR AND DELIVERY (O60-O77)

● **O60**   **Preterm labor**

     Includes   onset (spontaneous) of labor before 37 completed weeks of gestation

     Excludes1   false labor (O47.0-)
                      threatened labor NOS (O47.0-)

     (Ex:) **For category O60 CC codes:** See PDX Collection 4033

● **O60.0**   **Preterm labor without delivery**

     O60.00   **Preterm labor without delivery, unspecified trimester** ♀   **M**

     O60.02   **Preterm labor without delivery, second trimester** ♀ 🔖   **M**
             (Ex:) See PDX Collection 4050

     O60.03   **Preterm labor without delivery, third trimester** ♀ 🔖   **M**
             (Ex:) See PDX Collection 4051

● **O60.1**   **Preterm labor with preterm delivery**

One of the following 7th characters is to be assigned to each code under subcategory O60.1. 7th character 0 is for single gestations and multiple gestations where the fetus is unspecified. 7th characters 1 through 9 are for cases of multiple gestations to identify the fetus for which the code applies. The appropriate code from category O30, Multiple gestation, must also be assigned when assigning a code from subcategory O60.1 that has a 7th character of 1 through 9.

0	not applicable or unspecified
1	fetus 1
2	fetus 2
3	fetus 3
4	fetus 4
5	fetus 5
9	other fetus

Coding Clinic: 2016, Q2, P11

X ● **O60.10**   **Preterm labor with preterm delivery, unspecified trimester** ♀ 🔖   **M**
             Preterm labor with delivery NOS

X ● **O60.12**   **Preterm labor second trimester with preterm delivery second trimester** ♀ 🔖   **M**

X ● **O60.13**   **Preterm labor second trimester with preterm delivery third trimester** ♀ 🔖   **M**

X ● **O60.14**   **Preterm labor third trimester with preterm delivery third trimester** ♀ 🔖   **M**
            Coding Clinic: 2016, Q2, P10

● **O60.2**   **Term delivery with preterm labor**

One of the following 7th characters is to be assigned to each code under subcategory O60.2. 7th character 0 is for single gestations and multiple gestations where the fetus is unspecified. 7th characters 1 through 9 are for cases of multiple gestations to identify the fetus for which the code applies. The appropriate code from category O30, Multiple gestation, must also be assigned when assigning a code from subcategory O60.2 that has a 7th character of 1 through 9.

0	not applicable or unspecified
1	fetus 1
2	fetus 2
3	fetus 3
4	fetus 4
5	fetus 5
9	other fetus

X ● **O60.20**   **Term delivery with preterm labor, unspecified trimester** ♀ 🔖   **M**

X ● **O60.22**   **Term delivery with preterm labor, second trimester** ♀ 🔖   **M**

X ● **O60.23**   **Term delivery with preterm labor, third trimester** ♀ 🔖   **M**

● **O61**   **Failed induction of labor**

     O61.0   **Failed medical induction of labor** ♀   **M**
            Failed induction (of labor) by oxytocin
            Failed induction (of labor) by prostaglandins

     O61.1   **Failed instrumental induction of labor** ♀   **M**
            Failed mechanical induction (of labor)
            Failed surgical induction (of labor)

     O61.8   **Other failed induction of labor** ♀   **M**

     O61.9   **Failed induction of labor, unspecified** ♀   **M**

● **O62**   **Abnormalities of forces of labor**

     O62.0   **Primary inadequate contractions** ♀   **M**
            Failure of cervical dilatation
            Primary hypotonic uterine dysfunction
            Uterine inertia during latent phase of labor

     O62.1   **Secondary uterine inertia** ♀   **M**
            Arrested active phase of labor
            Secondary hypotonic uterine dysfunction

     O62.2   **Other uterine inertia** ♀   **M**
            Atony of uterus without hemorrhage
            Atony of uterus NOS
            Desultory labor
            Hypotonic uterine dysfunction NOS
            Irregular labor
            Poor contractions
            Slow slope active phase of labor
            Uterine inertia NOS

        Excludes1   atony of uterus with hemorrhage (postpartum) (O72.1)
                       postpartum atony of uterus without hemorrhage (O75.89)

     O62.3   **Precipitate labor** ♀   **M**

     O62.4   **Hypertonic, incoordinate, and prolonged uterine contractions** ♀   **M**
            Cervical spasm
            Contraction ring dystocia
            Dyscoordinate labor
            Hour-glass contraction of uterus
            Hypertonic uterine dysfunction
            Incoordinate uterine action
            Tetanic contractions
            Uterine dystocia NOS
            Uterine spasm

        Excludes1   dystocia (fetal) (maternal) NOS (O66.9)

     O62.8   **Other abnormalities of forces of labor** ♀   **M**

     O62.9   **Abnormality of forces of labor, unspecified** ♀   **M**

● **O63**   **Long labor**

     O63.0   **Prolonged first stage (of labor)** ♀   **M**

     O63.1   **Prolonged second stage (of labor)** ♀   **M**

     O63.2   **Delayed delivery of second twin, triplet, etc.** ♀   **M**

     O63.9   **Long labor, unspecified** ♀ 🔖   **M**
            Prolonged labor NOS
            (Ex:) See PDX Collection 988

▶ New   ⇒ Revised   ~~deleted~~ Deleted   Excludes 1   Excludes 2   Includes   Use additional   Code first   Code also   Key words

OGCR Official Guidelines   ● Unacceptable Principal Diagnosis   X Assign placeholder X   ● Use Additional Character(s)   ▶ Manifestation Code   Coding Clinic

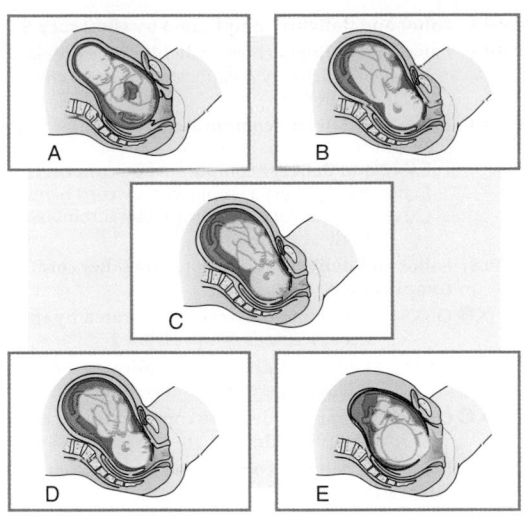

Figure 15-4 Five types of malposition and malpresentation of the fetus:
A. Breech. **B.** Vertex. **C.** Face. **D.** Brow. **E.** Shoulder.

● O64　Obstructed labor due to malposition and malpresentation of fetus

One of the following 7th characters is to be assigned to each code under category O64. 7th character Ø is for single gestations and multiple gestations where the fetus is unspecified. 7th characters 1 through 9 are for cases of multiple gestations to identify the fetus for which the code applies. The appropriate code from category O30, Multiple gestation, must also be assigned when assigning a code from category O64 that has a 7th character of 1 through 9.

Ø	not applicable or unspecified
1	fetus 1
2	fetus 2
3	fetus 3
4	fetus 4
5	fetus 5
9	other fetus

X ● O64.0　Obstructed labor due to incomplete rotation of fetal head ♀　　　M
　　　Deep transverse arrest
　　　Obstructed labor due to persistent occipitoiliac (position)
　　　Obstructed labor due to persistent occipitoposterior (position)
　　　Obstructed labor due to persistent occipitosacral (position)
　　　Obstructed labor due to persistent occipitotransverse (position)

X ● O64.1　Obstructed labor due to breech presentation ♀　　　M
　　　Obstructed labor due to buttocks presentation
　　　Obstructed labor due to complete breech presentation
　　　Obstructed labor due to frank breech presentation

X ● O64.2　Obstructed labor due to face presentation ♀　　　M
　　　Obstructed labor due to chin presentation

X ● O64.3　Obstructed labor due to brow presentation ♀　　　M

X ● O64.4　Obstructed labor due to shoulder presentation ♀　　　M
　　　Prolapsed arm
　　　Excludes1　impacted shoulders (O66.0)
　　　　　　　　shoulder dystocia (O66.0)

X ● O64.5　Obstructed labor due to compound presentation ♀　　　M

X ● O64.8　Obstructed labor due to other malposition and malpresentation ♀　　　M
　　　Obstructed labor due to footling presentation
　　　Obstructed labor due to incomplete breech presentation

X ● O64.9　Obstructed labor due to malposition and malpresentation, unspecified ♀　　　M

● O65　Obstructed labor due to maternal pelvic abnormality
　O65.0　Obstructed labor due to deformed pelvis ♀　　　M
　O65.1　Obstructed labor due to generally contracted pelvis ♀　　　M
　O65.2　Obstructed labor due to pelvic inlet contraction ♀　　　M
　O65.3　Obstructed labor due to pelvic outlet and mid-cavity contraction ♀　　　M
　O65.4　Obstructed labor due to fetopelvic disproportion, unspecified ♀　　　M
　　　Excludes1　dystocia due to abnormality of fetus (O66.2-O66.3)
　O65.5　Obstructed labor due to abnormality of maternal pelvic organs ♀　　　M
　　　Obstructed labor due to conditions listed in O34.-
　　　Use additional code to identify abnormality of pelvic organs O34.-
　O65.8　Obstructed labor due to other maternal pelvic abnormalities ♀　　　M
　O65.9　Obstructed labor due to maternal pelvic abnormality, unspecified ♀　　　M

● O66　Other obstructed labor
　O66.0　Obstructed labor due to shoulder dystocia ♀　　　M
　　　Impacted shoulders
　O66.1　Obstructed labor due to locked twins ♀　　　M
　O66.2　Obstructed labor due to unusually large fetus ♀　　　M
　O66.3　Obstructed labor due to other abnormalities of fetus ♀　M
　　　Dystocia due to fetal ascites
　　　Dystocia due to fetal hydrops
　　　Dystocia due to fetal meningomyelocele
　　　Dystocia due to fetal sacral teratoma
　　　Dystocia due to fetal tumor
　　　Dystocia due to hydrocephalic fetus
　　　Use additional code to identify cause of obstruction
　● O66.4　Failed trial of labor
　　O66.40　Failed trial of labor, unspecified ♀　　　M
　　O66.41　Failed attempted vaginal birth after previous cesarean delivery ♀　　　M
　　　　Code first rupture of uterus, if applicable (O71.0-, O71.1)
　O66.5　Attempted application of vacuum extractor and forceps ♀　　　M
　　　Attempted application of vacuum or forceps, with subsequent delivery by forceps or cesarean delivery
　O66.6　Obstructed labor due to other multiple fetuses ♀　　　M
　O66.8　Other specified obstructed labor ♀　　　M
　　　Use additional code to identify cause of obstruction
　O66.9　Obstructed labor, unspecified ♀　　　M
　　　Dystocia NOS
　　　Fetal dystocia NOS
　　　Maternal dystocia NOS

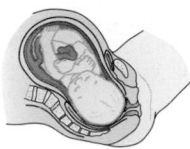

Figure 15-5 Hydrocephalic fetus causing disproportion.

N Newborn Age: Ø　**P** Pediatric Age: Ø–17　**M** Maternity DX: 9–64　**A** Adult Age: 15–124　♀ Females Only　♂ Males Only

🅒 Complication\Comorbidity　🅜 Major C\C　Ⓔ CC/MCC Exclusions　🅗 Hospital-Acquired Condition　🅗 Hierarchical Condition Category

1173

CHAPTER 15 (OØØ-O9A)

● **O67 Labor and delivery complicated by intrapartum hemorrhage, not elsewhere classified**

> **Excludes1** antepartum hemorrhage NEC (O46.-)
> placenta previa (O44.-)
> premature separation of placenta [abruptio placentae] (O45.-)
>
> **Excludes2** postpartum hemorrhage (O72.-)

   O67.0 Intrapartum hemorrhage with coagulation defect ♀ 🔖 M
> Intrapartum hemorrhage (excessive) associated with afibrinogenemia
> Intrapartum hemorrhage (excessive) associated with disseminated intravascular coagulation
> Intrapartum hemorrhage (excessive) associated with hyperfibrinolysis
> Intrapartum hemorrhage (excessive) associated with hypofibrinogenemia
> (Ex:) See PDX Collection 4005

   O67.8 Other intrapartum hemorrhage ♀ M
> Excessive intrapartum hemorrhage

   O67.9 Intrapartum hemorrhage, unspecified ♀ M

● **O68 Labor and delivery complicated by abnormality of fetal acid-base balance** ♀ 🔖 M
> Fetal acidemia complicating labor and delivery
> Fetal acidosis complicating labor and delivery
> Fetal alkalosis complicating labor and delivery
> Fetal metabolic acidemia complicating labor and delivery

> **Excludes1** fetal stress NOS (O77.9)
> labor and delivery complicated by electrocardiographic evidence of fetal stress (O77.8)
> labor and delivery complicated by ultrasonic evidence of fetal stress (O77.8)
>
> **Excludes2** abnormality in fetal heart rate or rhythm (O76)
> labor and delivery complicated by meconium in amniotic fluid (O77.0)
>
> (Ex:) See PDX Collection 989

● **O69 Labor and delivery complicated by umbilical cord complications**

> One of the following 7th characters is to be assigned to each code under category O69. 7th character 0 is for single gestations and multiple gestations where the fetus is unspecified. 7th characters 1 through 9 are for cases of multiple gestations to identify the fetus for which the code applies. The appropriate code from category O30, Multiple gestation, must also be assigned when assigning a code from category O69 that has a 7th character of 1 through 9.

0	not applicable or unspecified
1	fetus 1
2	fetus 2
3	fetus 3
4	fetus 4
5	fetus 5
9	other fetus

X● **O69.0 Labor and delivery complicated by prolapse of cord** ♀ M

X● **O69.1 Labor and delivery complicated by cord around neck, with compression** ♀ M
> **Excludes1** labor and delivery complicated by cord around neck, without compression (O69.81)

X● **O69.2 Labor and delivery complicated by other cord entanglement, with compression** ♀ M
> Labor and delivery complicated by compression of cord NOS
> Labor and delivery complicated by entanglement of cords of twins in monoamniotic sac
> Labor and delivery complicated by knot in cord
> **Excludes1** labor and delivery complicated by other cord entanglement, without compression (O69.82)

X● **O69.3 Labor and delivery complicated by short cord** ♀ M
X● **O69.4 Labor and delivery complicated by vasa previa** ♀ M
> Labor and delivery complicated by hemorrhage from vasa previa

X● **O69.5 Labor and delivery complicated by vascular lesion of cord** ♀ M
> Labor and delivery complicated by cord bruising
> Labor and delivery complicated by cord hematoma
> Labor and delivery complicated by thrombosis of umbilical vessels

● **O69.8 Labor and delivery complicated by other cord complications**
   X● **O69.81 Labor and delivery complicated by cord around neck, without compression** ♀ M
   X● **O69.82 Labor and delivery complicated by other cord entanglement, without compression** ♀ M
   X● **O69.89 Labor and delivery complicated by other cord complications** ♀ M

X● **O69.9 Labor and delivery complicated by cord complication, unspecified** ♀ M

● **O70 Perineal laceration during delivery**
> **Includes** episiotomy extended by laceration
> **Excludes1** obstetric high vaginal laceration alone (O71.4)

   O70.0 First degree perineal laceration during delivery ♀ M
> Perineal laceration, rupture or tear involving fourchette during delivery
> Perineal laceration, rupture or tear involving labia during delivery
> Perineal laceration, rupture or tear involving skin during delivery
> Perineal laceration, rupture or tear involving vagina during delivery
> Perineal laceration, rupture or tear involving vulva during delivery
> Slight perineal laceration, rupture or tear during delivery

   O70.1 Second degree perineal laceration during delivery ♀ M
> Perineal laceration, rupture or tear during delivery as in O70.0, also involving pelvic floor
> Perineal laceration, rupture or tear during delivery as in O70.0, also involving perineal muscles
> Perineal laceration, rupture or tear during delivery as in O70.0, also involving vaginal muscles
> **Excludes1** perineal laceration involving anal sphincter (O70.2)
> **Coding Clinic: 2016, CODING CIQ4, P53, Q2, P34**

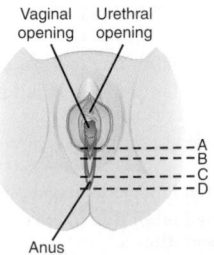

Figure 15-6 Perineal lacerations: **A.** First-degree is laceration of superficial tissues. **B.** Second-degree is limited to the pelvic floor and may involve the perineal or vaginal muscles. **C.** Third-degree involves the anal sphincter. **D.** Fourth-degree involves anal or rectal mucosa.

● **O70.2**   **Third degree perineal laceration during delivery**
Perineal laceration, rupture or tear during delivery as in O70.1, also involving anal sphincter
Perineal laceration, rupture or tear during delivery as in O70.1, also involving rectovaginal septum
Perineal laceration, rupture or tear during delivery as in O70.1, also involving sphincter NOS

> **Excludes1**   anal sphincter tear during delivery without third degree perineal laceration (O70.4)
> perineal laceration involving anal or rectal mucosa (O70.3)

(Ex:) **For category O70.2 CC codes:** See PDX Collection 992

    O70.20   **Third degree perineal laceration during delivery, unspecified** ♀ 🦠   **M**

    O70.21   **Third degree perineal laceration during delivery, IIIa** ♀ 🦠   **M**
Third degree perineal laceration during delivery with less than 50% of external anal sphincter (EAS) thickness torn

    O70.22   **Third degree perineal laceration during delivery, IIIb** ♀ 🦠   **M**
Third degree perineal laceration during delivery with more than 50% external anal sphincter (EAS) thickness torn

    O70.23   **Third degree perineal laceration during delivery, IIIc** ♀ 🦠   **M**
Third degree perineal laceration during delivery with both external anal sphincter (EAS) and internal anal sphincter (IAS) torn

O70.3   **Fourth degree perineal laceration during delivery** ♀ 🦠 **M**
Perineal laceration, rupture or tear during delivery as in O70.2, also involving anal mucosa
Perineal laceration, rupture or tear during delivery as in O70.2, also involving rectal mucosa

(Ex:) See PDX Collection 991

O70.4   **Anal sphincter tear complicating delivery, not associated with third degree laceration** ♀ 🦠   **M**

> **Excludes1**   anal sphincter tear with third degree perineal laceration (O70.2)

(Ex:) See PDX Collection 992

O70.9   **Perineal laceration during delivery, unspecified** ♀   **M**

● **O71**   **Other obstetric trauma**

> **Includes**   obstetric damage from instruments

 ● **O71.0**   **Rupture of uterus (spontaneous) before onset of labor**

> **Excludes1**   disruption of (current) cesarean delivery wound (O90.0)
> laceration of uterus, NEC (O71.81)

(Ex:) **For category O71.0 CC codes:** See PDX Collection 993

    O71.00   **Rupture of uterus before onset of labor, unspecified trimester** ♀   **M**

    O71.02   **Rupture of uterus before onset of labor, second trimester** ♀ 🦠   **M**

    O71.03   **Rupture of uterus before onset of labor, third trimester** ♀ 🦠   **M**

O71.1   **Rupture of uterus during labor** ♀ 🦠   **M**
Rupture of uterus not stated as occurring before onset of labor

> **Excludes1**   disruption of cesarean delivery wound (O90.0)
> laceration of uterus, NEC (O71.81)

(Ex:) See PDX Collection 993

O71.2   **Postpartum inversion of uterus** ♀ 🦠   **M**
(Ex:) See PDX Collection 994

O71.3   **Obstetric laceration of cervix** ♀ 🦠   **M**
Annular detachment of cervix
(Ex:) See PDX Collection 995

O71.4   **Obstetric high vaginal laceration alone** ♀ 🦠   **M**
Laceration of vaginal wall without perineal laceration

> **Excludes1**   obstetric high vaginal laceration with perineal laceration (O70.-)

(Ex:) See PDX Collection 996

O71.5   **Other obstetric injury to pelvic organs** ♀ 🦠   **M**
Obstetric injury to bladder
Obstetric injury to urethra

> **Excludes2**   obstetric periurethral trauma (O71.82)

(Ex:) See PDX Collection 993

O71.6   **Obstetric damage to pelvic joints and ligaments** ♀ 🦠 **M**
Obstetric avulsion of inner symphyseal cartilage
Obstetric damage to coccyx
Obstetric traumatic separation of symphysis (pubis)
(Ex:) See PDX Collection 997

O71.7   **Obstetric hematoma of pelvis** ♀ 🦠   **M**
Obstetric hematoma of perineum
Obstetric hematoma of vagina
Obstetric hematoma of vulva
(Ex:) See PDX Collection 998

● **O71.8**   **Other specified obstetric trauma**

    O71.81   **Laceration of uterus, not elsewhere classified** ♀   **M**

    O71.82   **Other specified trauma to perineum and vulva** ♀   **M**
Obstetric periurethral trauma

    O71.89   **Other specified obstetric trauma** ♀   **M**

O71.9   **Obstetric trauma, unspecified** ♀   **M**

● **O72**   **Postpartum hemorrhage**

> **Includes**   hemorrhage after delivery of fetus or infant

O72.0   **Third-stage hemorrhage** ♀ 🦠   **M**
Hemorrhage associated with retained, trapped or adherent placenta
Retained placenta NOS
Code also type of adherent placenta (O43.2-)
(Ex:) See PDX Collection 999

O72.1   **Other immediate postpartum hemorrhage** ♀ 🦠   **M**
Hemorrhage following delivery of placenta
Postpartum hemorrhage (atonic) NOS
Uterine atony with hemorrhage

> **Excludes1**   uterine atony NOS (O62.2)
> uterine atony without hemorrhage (O62.2)
> postpartum atony of uterus without hemorrhage (O75.89)

(Ex:) See PDX Collection 1000

O72.2   **Delayed and secondary postpartum hemorrhage** ♀ 🦠   **M**
Hemorrhage associated with retained portions of placenta or membranes after the first 24 hours following delivery of placenta
Retained products of conception NOS, following delivery
(Ex:) See PDX Collection 1001

O72.3   **Postpartum coagulation defects** ♀   **M**
Postpartum afibrinogenemia
Postpartum fibrinolysis

● **O73**   **Retained placenta and membranes, without hemorrhage**

> **Excludes1**   placenta accreta (O43.21-)
> placenta increta (O43.22-)
> placenta percreta (O43.23-)

O73.0   **Retained placenta without hemorrhage** ♀   **M**
Adherent placenta, without hemorrhage
Trapped placenta without hemorrhage

O73.1   **Retained portions of placenta and membranes, without hemorrhage** ♀   **M**
Retained products of conception following delivery, without hemorrhage

---

N   Newborn Age: 0   **P**   Pediatric Age: 0–17   **M**   Maternity DX: 9–64   **A**   Adult Age: 15–124   ♀   Females Only   ♂   Males Only

🦠 Complication\Comorbidity   🦠 Major C\C   (Ex:) CC/MCC Exclusions   🦠 Hospital-Acquired Condition   🦠 Hierarchical Condition Category

● **O74**   **Complications of anesthesia during labor and delivery**

    Includes   maternal complications arising from the administration of a general, regional or local anesthetic, analgesic or other sedation during labor and delivery

    Use additional code, if applicable, to identify specific complication

    O74.0   **Aspiration pneumonitis** due to anesthesia during labor and delivery ♀   M

        Inhalation of stomach contents or secretions NOS due to anesthesia during labor and delivery

        Mendelson's syndrome due to anesthesia during labor and delivery

    O74.1   **Other pulmonary complications** of anesthesia during labor and delivery ♀   M

    O74.2   **Cardiac complications** of anesthesia during labor and delivery ♀   M

    O74.3   **Central nervous system** complications of anesthesia during labor and delivery ♀   M

    O74.4   **Toxic reaction** to local anesthesia during labor and delivery ♀   M

    O74.5   **Spinal and epidural anesthesia-induced headache** during labor and delivery ♀   M

    O74.6   **Other complications of spinal and epidural** anesthesia during labor and delivery ♀   M

    O74.7   **Failed or difficult intubation** for anesthesia during labor and delivery ♀   M

    O74.8   **Other complications** of anesthesia during labor and delivery ♀   M

    O74.9   **Complication of anesthesia during labor and delivery, unspecified** ♀   M

● **O75**   **Other complications of labor and delivery, not elsewhere classified**

    Excludes2   puerperal (postpartum) infection (O86.-)

                 puerperal (postpartum) sepsis (O85)

    O75.0   **Maternal distress** during labor and delivery ♀   M

    O75.1   **Shock during or following labor and delivery** ♀ 🦠   M

        Obstetric shock following labor and delivery

        Ⓔⓧ See PDX Collection 1002

    O75.2   **Pyrexia during labor, not elsewhere classified** ♀ 🦠   M

        Ⓔⓧ See PDX Collection 1003

    O75.3   **Other infection during labor** ♀ 🦠   M

        Sepsis during labor

        Use additional code (B95-B97), to identify infectious agent

        Ⓔⓧ See PDX Collection 1004

    O75.4   **Other complications of obstetric surgery and procedures** ♀   M

        Cardiac arrest following obstetric surgery or procedures

        Cardiac failure following obstetric surgery or procedures

        Cerebral anoxia following obstetric surgery or procedures

        Pulmonary edema following obstetric surgery or procedures

        Use additional code to identify specific complication

        Excludes2   complications of anesthesia during labor and delivery (O74.-)

                 disruption of obstetrical (surgical) wound (O90.0-O90.1)

                 hematoma of obstetrical (surgical) wound (O90.2)

                 infection of obstetrical (surgical) wound (O86.0-)

    O75.5   **Delayed delivery after artificial rupture of membranes** ♀   M

● **O75.8**   **Other specified complications of labor and delivery**

    O75.81   **Maternal exhaustion complicating labor and delivery** ♀   M

    O75.82   **Onset (spontaneous) of labor after 37 completed weeks of gestation but before 39 completed weeks gestation, with delivery by (planned) cesarean section** ♀   M

        Delivery by (planned) cesarean section occurring after 37 completed weeks of gestation but before 39 completed weeks gestation due to (spontaneous) onset of labor

        Code first to specify reason for planned cesarean section such as:

           cephalopelvic disproportion (normally formed fetus) (O33.9)

           previous cesarean delivery (O34.21)

    O75.89   **Other specified complications of labor and delivery** ♀   M

    O75.9   **Complication of labor and delivery, unspecified** ♀   M

  O76   **Abnormality in fetal heart rate and rhythm complicating labor and delivery** ♀   M

    Depressed fetal heart rate tones complicating labor and delivery

    Fetal bradycardia complicating labor and delivery

    Fetal heart rate decelerations complicating labor and delivery

    Fetal heart rate irregularity complicating labor and delivery

    Fetal heart rate abnormal variability complicating labor and delivery

    Fetal tachycardia complicating labor and delivery

    Non-reassuring fetal heart rate or rhythm complicating labor and delivery

    Excludes1   fetal stress NOS (O77.9)

                 labor and delivery complicated by electrocardiographic evidence of fetal stress (O77.8)

                 labor and delivery complicated by ultrasonic evidence of fetal stress (O77.8)

    Excludes2   fetal metabolic acidemia (O68)

                 other fetal stress (O77.0-O77.1)

● **O77**   **Other fetal stress complicating labor and delivery**

    O77.0   **Labor and delivery complicated by meconium in amniotic fluid** ♀   M

    O77.1   **Fetal stress in labor or delivery due to drug administration** ♀   M

    O77.8   **Labor and delivery complicated by other evidence of fetal stress** ♀   M

        Labor and delivery complicated by electrocardiographic evidence of fetal stress

        Labor and delivery complicated by ultrasonic evidence of fetal stress

        Excludes1   abnormality of fetal acid-base balance (O68)

                 abnormality in fetal heart rate or rhythm (O76)

                 fetal metabolic acidemia (O68)

    O77.9   **Labor and delivery complicated by fetal stress, unspecified** ♀   M

        Excludes1   abnormality of fetal acid-base balance (O68)

                 abnormality in fetal heart rate or rhythm (O76)

                 fetal metabolic acidemia (O68)

▶ New   ⇒ Revised   ~~deleted~~ Deleted   Excludes 1   Excludes 2   Includes   Use additional   Code first   Code also   Key words

OGCR Official Guidelines   ● Unacceptable Principal Diagnosis   X Assign placeholder X   ● Use Additional Character(s)   ▶ Manifestation Code   **Coding Clinic**

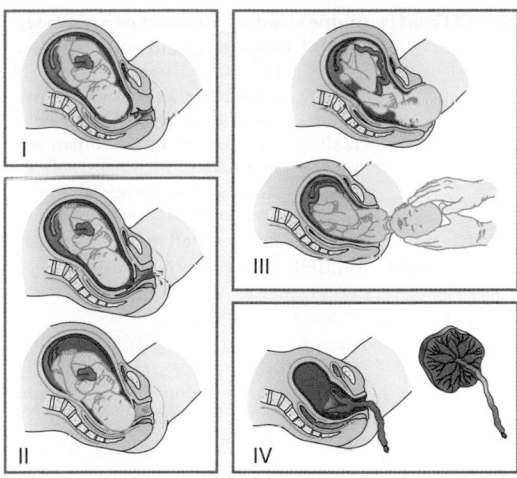

Figure 15-7 The four stages of normal delivery: **I.** Lightening, which occurs 2 to 4 weeks before birth, at which time the fetus turns with head toward the vagina. **II.** Regular contractions begin, the amniotic sac ruptures, and dilation is complete. **III.** Delivery of the head and rotation. **IV.** Expulsion of placenta.

OGCR Section I.C., Chapter 15.n.

Normal Delivery, Code O80

1) Encounter for full-term uncomplicated delivery

Code O80 should be assigned when a woman is admitted for a full-term normal delivery and delivers a single, healthy infant without any complications antepartum, during the delivery, or postpartum during the delivery episode. Code O80 is always a principal diagnosis. It is not to be used if any other code from Chapter 15 is needed to describe a current complication of the antenatal, delivery, or perinatal period. Additional codes from other chapters may be used with code O80 if they are not related to or are in any way complicating the pregnancy.

2) Uncomplicated delivery with resolved antepartum complication

Code O80 may be used if the patient had a complication at some point during the pregnancy, but the complication is not present at the time of the admission for delivery.

3) Outcome of delivery for O80

Z37.0, Single live brith, is the only outcome of delivery code appropriate for use with O80.

ENCOUNTER FOR DELIVERY (O80-O82)

O80 **Encounter for full-term uncomplicated delivery** ♀   **M**
   Delivery requiring minimal or no assistance, with or without episiotomy, without fetal manipulation [e.g., rotation version] or instrumentation [forceps] of a spontaneous, cephalic, vaginal, full-term, single, live-born infant. This code is for use as a single diagnosis code and is not to be used with any other code from Chapter 15.
   Use additional code to indicate outcome of delivery (Z37.0)
   Coding Clinic: 2016, Q4, P124, 150

O82 **Encounter for cesarean delivery without indication** ♀   **M**
   Use additional code to indicate outcome of delivery (Z37.0)

COMPLICATIONS PREDOMINANTLY RELATED TO THE PUERPERIUM (O85-O92)

   Excludes2 mental and behavioral disorders associated with the puerperium (F53.-)
      obstetrical tetanus (A34)
      puerperal osteomalacia (M83.0)

O85 **Puerperal sepsis** ♀ 🐾   **M**
   Postpartum sepsis
   Puerperal peritonitis
   Puerperal pyemia
   Use additional code (B95-B97), to identify infectious agent
   Use additional code (R65.2-) to identify severe sepsis, if applicable
   Excludes1 fever of unknown origin following delivery (O86.4)
      genital tract infection following delivery (O86.1-)
      obstetric pyemic and septic embolism (O88.3-)
      puerperal septic thrombophlebitis (O86.81)
      urinary tract infection following delivery (O86.2-)
   Excludes2 sepsis during labor (O75.3)
   Ⓔⓧ See PDX Collection 4039
   Coding Clinic: 2018, Q4, P23

● O86 **Other puerperal infections**
   Use additional code (B95-B97), to identify infectious agent
   Excludes2 infection during labor (O75.3)
      obstetrical tetanus (A34)
   Ⓔⓧ **For category O86 CC codes unless otherwise indicated:** See PDX Collection 4036

● O86.0 **Infection of obstetric surgical wound**
   Infected cesarean delivery wound following delivery
   Infected perineal repair following delivery
   Excludes1 complications of procedures, not elsewhere classified (T81.44)
      postprocedural fever NOS (R50.82)
      postprocedural retroperitoneal abscess (K68.11)

   O86.00 **Infection of obstetric surgical wound, unspecified**   **M**

   O86.01 **Infection of obstetric surgical wound, superficial incisional site** ♀   **M**
      Subcutaneous abscess following an obstetrical procedure
      Stitch abscess following an obstetrical procedure

   O86.02 **Infection of obstetric surgical wound, deep incisional site** ♀   **M**
      Intramuscular abscess following an obstetrical procedure
      Sub-fascial abscess following an obstetrical procedure
      Coding Clinic: 2018, Q4, P23

   O86.03 **Infection of obstetric surgical wound, organ and space site** ♀   **M**
      Intraabdominal abscess following an obstetrical procedure
      Subphrenic abscess following an obstetrical procedure

   O86.04 **Sepsis following an obstetrical procedure** ♀ 🐾   **M**
      Use additional code to identify the sepsis
      Ⓔⓧ See PDX Collection 4040

   O86.09 **Infection of obstetric surgical wound, other surgical site** ♀   **M**

● O86.1 **Other infection of genital tract following delivery**
   O86.11 **Cervicitis following delivery** ♀ 🐾   **M**
   O86.12 **Endometritis following delivery** ♀ 🐾   **M**
      Ⓔⓧ See PDX Collection 4039
   O86.13 **Vaginitis following delivery** ♀ 🐾   **M**
   O86.19 **Other infection of genital tract following delivery** ♀ 🐾   **M**

N Newborn Age: 0   **P** Pediatric Age: 0–17   **M** Maternity DX: 9–64   **A** Adult Age: 15–124   ♀ Females Only   ♂ Males Only
🐾 Complication\Comorbidity   🐾 Major C\C   Ⓔⓧ CC/MCC Exclusions   🐾 Hospital-Acquired Condition   🐾 Hierarchical Condition Category

1177

● O86.2   Urinary tract infection following delivery

     O86.20   Urinary tract infection following delivery, unspecified ♀ 🦠   M
           Puerperal urinary tract infection NOS

     O86.21   Infection of kidney following delivery ♀ 🦠   M

     O86.22   Infection of bladder following delivery ♀ 🦠   M
           Infection of urethra following delivery

     O86.29   Other urinary tract infection following delivery ♀ 🦠   M

● O86.4   Pyrexia of unknown origin following delivery ♀ 🦠   M
      Puerperal infection NOS following delivery
      Puerperal pyrexia NOS following delivery

     Excludes2   pyrexia during labor (O75.2)

     (Ex:) See PDX Collection 1006

● O86.8   Other specified puerperal infections
     (Ex:) For category O86.8 CC codes: See PDX Collection 4039

     O86.81   Puerperal septic thrombophlebitis ♀ 🦠   M

     O86.89   Other specified puerperal infections ♀ 🦠   M

● O87   Venous complications and hemorrhoids in the puerperium

     Includes   venous complications in labor, delivery and the puerperium

     Excludes2   obstetric embolism (O88.-)
                 puerperal septic thrombophlebitis (O86.81)
                 venous complications in pregnancy (O22.-)

     (Ex:) For category O87 CC codes: See PDX Collection 4041

     O87.0   Superficial thrombophlebitis in the puerperium ♀ 🦠   M
         Puerperal phlebitis NOS
         Puerperal thrombosis NOS

     O87.1   Deep phlebothrombosis in the puerperium ♀ 🦠   M
         Deep vein thrombosis, postpartum
         Pelvic thrombophlebitis, postpartum

      ⟹ Use additional code to identify the deep vein thrombosis (I82.4-, I82.5-, I82.62-, I82.72-)

       Use additional code, if applicable, for associated long-term (current) use of anticoagulants (Z79.01)

     O87.2   Hemorrhoids in the puerperium ♀ 🦠   M

     O87.3   Cerebral venous thrombosis in the puerperium ♀ 🦠   M
         Cerebrovenous sinus thrombosis in the puerperium

     O87.4   Varicose veins of lower extremity in the puerperium ♀ M

     O87.8   Other venous complications in the puerperium ♀ 🦠   M
         Genital varices in the puerperium

     O87.9   Venous complication in the puerperium, unspecified ♀ M
         Puerperal phlebopathy NOS

O88   Obstetric embolism

     Excludes1   embolism complicating abortion NOS (O03.2)
                 embolism complicating ectopic or molar pregnancy (O08.2)
                 embolism complicating failed attempted abortion (O07.2)
                 embolism complicating induced abortion (O04.7)
                 embolism complicating spontaneous abortion (O03.2, O03.7)

     (Ex:) For category O88 CC codes: See PDX Collection 4020-4021, 4030-4031

● O88.0   Obstetric air embolism

     ● O88.01   Obstetric air embolism in pregnancy

         O88.011   Air embolism in pregnancy, first trimester ♀ 🦠   M

         O88.012   Air embolism in pregnancy, second trimester ♀ 🦠   M

         O88.013   Air embolism in pregnancy, third trimester ♀ 🦠   M

         O88.019   Air embolism in pregnancy, unspecified trimester ♀   M

     O88.02   Air embolism in childbirth ♀ 🦠   M

     O88.03   Air embolism in the puerperium ♀ 🦠   M

● O88.1   Amniotic fluid embolism
      Anaphylactoid syndrome in pregnancy

     ● O88.11   Amniotic fluid embolism in pregnancy

         O88.111   Amniotic fluid embolism in pregnancy, first trimester ♀ 🦠   M

         O88.112   Amniotic fluid embolism in pregnancy, second trimester ♀ 🦠   M

         O88.113   Amniotic fluid embolism in pregnancy, third trimester ♀ 🦠   M

         O88.119   Amniotic fluid embolism in pregnancy, unspecified trimester ♀   M

     O88.12   Amniotic fluid embolism in childbirth ♀ 🦠   M

     O88.13   Amniotic fluid embolism in the puerperium ♀ 🦠   M

● O88.2   Obstetric thromboembolism

     ● O88.21   Thromboembolism in pregnancy
         Obstetric (pulmonary) embolism NOS

         O88.211   Thromboembolism in pregnancy, first trimester ♀ 🦠   M

         O88.212   Thromboembolism in pregnancy, second trimester ♀ 🦠   M

         O88.213   Thromboembolism in pregnancy, third trimester ♀ 🦠   M

         O88.219   Thromboembolism in pregnancy, unspecified trimester ♀   M

     O88.22   Thromboembolism in childbirth ♀ 🦠   M

     O88.23   Thromboembolism in the puerperium ♀ 🦠   M
         Puerperal (pulmonary) embolism NOS

● O88.3   Obstetric pyemic and septic embolism

     ● O88.31   Pyemic and septic embolism in pregnancy

         O88.311   Pyemic and septic embolism in pregnancy, first trimester ♀ 🦠   M

         O88.312   Pyemic and septic embolism in pregnancy, second trimester ♀ 🦠   M

         O88.313   Pyemic and septic embolism in pregnancy, third trimester ♀ 🦠   M

         O88.319   Pyemic and septic embolism in pregnancy, unspecified trimester ♀   M

     O88.32   Pyemic and septic embolism in childbirth ♀ 🦠   M

     O88.33   Pyemic and septic embolism in the puerperium ♀ 🦠   M

● O88.8   Other obstetric embolism
      Obstetric fat embolism

     ● O88.81   Other embolism in pregnancy

         O88.811   Other embolism in pregnancy, first trimester ♀ 🦠   M

         O88.812   Other embolism in pregnancy, second trimester ♀ 🦠   M

         O88.813   Other embolism in pregnancy, third trimester ♀ 🦠   M

         O88.819   Other embolism in pregnancy, unspecified trimester ♀   M

     O88.82   Other embolism in childbirth ♀ 🦠   M

     O88.83   Other embolism in the puerperium ♀ 🦠   M

● O89   Complications of anesthesia during the puerperium

     Includes   maternal complications arising from the administration of a general, regional or local anesthetic, analgesic or other sedation during the puerperium

     Use additional code, if applicable, to identify specific complication

     ● O89.0   Pulmonary complications of anesthesia during the puerperium

         O89.01   Aspiration pneumonitis due to anesthesia during the puerperium ♀   M
           Inhalation of stomach contents or secretions NOS due to anesthesia during the puerperium
           Mendelson's syndrome due to anesthesia during the puerperium

         O89.09   Other pulmonary complications of anesthesia during the puerperium ♀   M

O89.1   Cardiac complications of anesthesia during the puerperium ♀   **M**

O89.2   Central nervous system complications of anesthesia during the puerperium ♀   **M**

O89.3   Toxic reaction to local anesthesia during the puerperium ♀   **M**

O89.4   Spinal and epidural anesthesia-induced headache during the puerperium ♀   **M**

O89.5   Other complications of spinal and epidural anesthesia during the puerperium ♀   **M**

O89.6   Failed or difficult intubation for anesthesia during the puerperium ♀   **M**

O89.8   Other complications of anesthesia during the puerperium ♀   **M**

O89.9   Complication of anesthesia during the puerperium, unspecified ♀   **M**

● O90   Complications of the puerperium, not elsewhere classified

O90.0   Disruption of cesarean delivery wound ♀   **M**
    Dehiscence of cesarean delivery wound

> **Excludes1**   rupture of uterus (spontaneous) before onset of labor (O71.0-)
> rupture of uterus during labor (O71.1)

O90.1   Disruption of perineal obstetric wound ♀   **M**
    Disruption of wound of episiotomy
    Disruption of wound of perineal laceration
    Secondary perineal tear

O90.2   Hematoma of obstetric wound ♀   **M**

O90.3   Peripartum cardiomyopathy ♀ 🅗   **M**
    Conditions in I42.- arising during pregnancy and the puerperium

> **Excludes1**   pre-existing heart disease complicating pregnancy and the puerperium (O99.4-)

    (Ex:) See PDX Collection 1008

O90.4   Postpartum acute kidney failure ♀ 🅗   **M**
    Hepatorenal syndrome following labor and delivery
    (Ex:) See PDX Collection 1009

O90.5   Postpartum thyroiditis ♀   **M**

O90.6   Postpartum mood disturbance ♀   **M**
    Postpartum blues   Postpartum sadness
    Postpartum dysphoria

> **Excludes1**   postpartum depression (F53.0)
> puerperal psychosis (F53.1)

● O90.8   Other complications of the puerperium, not elsewhere classified

O90.81   Anemia of the puerperium ♀   **M**
    Postpartum anemia NOS

> **Excludes1**   pre-existing anemia complicating the puerperium (O99.03)

O90.89   Other complications of the puerperium, not elsewhere classified ♀   **M**
    Placental polyp

O90.9   Complication of the puerperium, unspecified ♀   **M**

● O91   Infections of breast associated with pregnancy, the puerperium and lactation

Use additional code to identify infection

● O91.0   Infection of nipple associated with pregnancy, the puerperium and lactation

● O91.01   Infection of nipple associated with pregnancy
    Gestational abscess of nipple

O91.011   Infection of nipple associated with pregnancy, first trimester ♀   **M**

O91.012   Infection of nipple associated with pregnancy, second trimester ♀   **M**

O91.013   Infection of nipple associated with pregnancy, third trimester ♀   **M**

O91.019   Infection of nipple associated with pregnancy, unspecified trimester ♀   **M**

O91.02   Infection of nipple associated with the puerperium ♀   **M**
    Puerperal abscess of nipple

O91.03   Infection of nipple associated with lactation ♀ **M**
    Abscess of nipple associated with lactation

● O91.1   Abscess of breast associated with pregnancy, the puerperium and lactation

● O91.11   Abscess of breast associated with pregnancy
    Gestational mammary abscess
    Gestational purulent mastitis
    Gestational subareolar abscess

O91.111   Abscess of breast associated with pregnancy, first trimester ♀   **M**

O91.112   Abscess of breast associated with pregnancy, second trimester ♀   **M**

O91.113   Abscess of breast associated with pregnancy, third trimester ♀   **M**

O91.119   Abscess of breast associated with pregnancy, unspecified trimester ♀   **M**

O91.12   Abscess of breast associated with the puerperium ♀   **M**
    Puerperal mammary abscess
    Puerperal purulent mastitis
    Puerperal subareolar abscess

O91.13   Abscess of breast associated with lactation ♀   **M**
    Mammary abscess associated with lactation
    Purulent mastitis associated with lactation
    Subareolar abscess associated with lactation

● O91.2   Nonpurulent mastitis associated with pregnancy, the puerperium and lactation

● O91.21   Nonpurulent mastitis associated with pregnancy
    Gestational interstitial mastitis
    Gestational lymphangitis of breast
    Gestational mastitis NOS
    Gestational parenchymatous mastitis

O91.211   Nonpurulent mastitis associated with pregnancy, first trimester ♀   **M**

O91.212   Nonpurulent mastitis associated with pregnancy, second trimester ♀   **M**

O91.213   Nonpurulent mastitis associated with pregnancy, third trimester ♀   **M**

O91.219   Nonpurulent mastitis associated with pregnancy, unspecified trimester ♀   **M**

O91.22   Nonpurulent mastitis associated with the puerperium ♀   **M**
    Puerperal interstitial mastitis
    Puerperal lymphangitis of breast
    Puerperal mastitis NOS
    Puerperal parenchymatous mastitis

O91.23   Nonpurulent mastitis associated with lactation ♀   **M**
    Interstitial mastitis associated with lactation
    Lymphangitis of breast associated with lactation
    Mastitis NOS associated with lactation
    Parenchymatous mastitis associated with lactation

● O92   Other disorders of breast and disorders of lactation associated with pregnancy and the puerperium

● O92.0   Retracted nipple associated with pregnancy, the puerperium, and lactation

● O92.01   Retracted nipple associated with pregnancy

O92.011   Retracted nipple associated with pregnancy, first trimester ♀   **M**

O92.012   Retracted nipple associated with pregnancy, second trimester ♀   **M**

O92.013   Retracted nipple associated with pregnancy, third trimester ♀   **M**

O92.019   Retracted nipple associated with pregnancy, unspecified trimester ♀   **M**

O92.02   Retracted nipple associated with the puerperium ♀   **M**

O92.03   Retracted nipple associated with lactation ♀   **M**

N Newborn Age: 0   **P** Pediatric Age: 0–17   **M** Maternity DX: 9–64   **A** Adult Age: 15–124   ♀ Females Only   ♂ Males Only

🅗 Complication\Comorbidity   Major C\C   (Ex:) CC/MCC Exclusions   Hospital-Acquired Condition   Hierarchical Condition Category

1179

● **O92.1 Cracked nipple** associated with pregnancy, the puerperium, and lactation
    Fissure of nipple, gestational or puerperal

  ● **O92.11** Cracked nipple associated with **pregnancy**
      O92.111 Cracked nipple associated with pregnancy, **first trimester** ♀   M
      O92.112 Cracked nipple associated with pregnancy, **second trimester** ♀   M
      O92.113 Cracked nipple associated with pregnancy, **third trimester** ♀   M
      O92.119 Cracked nipple associated with pregnancy, **unspecified trimester** ♀   M
  O92.12 Cracked nipple associated with the **puerperium** ♀   M
  O92.13 Cracked nipple associated with **lactation** ♀   M

● **O92.2** Other and unspecified disorders of breast associated with pregnancy and the puerperium
  O92.20 **Unspecified** disorder of breast associated with pregnancy and the puerperium ♀   M
  O92.29 **Other** disorders of breast associated with pregnancy and the puerperium ♀   M

O92.3 Agalactia ♀   M
  Primary agalactia
    Excludes1 elective agalactia (O92.5)
                secondary agalactia (O92.5)
                therapeutic agalactia (O92.5)

O92.4 Hypogalactia ♀   M
O92.5 Suppressed lactation ♀   M
  Elective agalactia   Therapeutic agalactia
  Secondary agalactia
    Excludes1 primary agalactia (O92.3)

O92.6 Galactorrhea ♀   M
● **O92.7** Other and unspecified disorders of lactation
  O92.70 **Unspecified** disorders of lactation ♀   M
  O92.79 Other disorders of lactation ♀   M
         Puerperal galactocele

OTHER OBSTETRIC CONDITIONS, NOT ELSEWHERE CLASSIFIED (O94-O9A)

● **O94** Sequelae of complication of pregnancy, childbirth, and the puerperium ♀   M
  Note: This category is to be used to indicate conditions in O00-O77.-, O85-O94 and O98-O9A.- as the cause of late effects. The "sequelae" include conditions specified as such, or as late effects, which may occur at any time after the puerperium.
  Code first condition resulting from (sequela) of complication of pregnancy, childbirth, and the puerperium

O98 Maternal infectious and parasitic diseases classifiable elsewhere but complicating pregnancy, childbirth and the puerperium
  Includes the listed conditions when complicating the pregnant state, when aggravated by the pregnancy, or as a reason for obstetric care
  Use additional code (Chapter 1), to identify specific infectious or parasitic disease
  Excludes2 herpes gestationis (O26.4-)
         infectious carrier state (O99.82-, O99.83-)
         obstetrical tetanus (A34)
         puerperal infection (O86.-)
         puerperal sepsis (O85)
         when the reason for maternal care is that the disease is known or suspected to have affected the fetus (O35-O36)

● **O98.0** Tuberculosis complicating pregnancy, childbirth and the puerperium
  Conditions in A15-A19
  (Ex) **For category O98.0 CC codes:** See PDX Collection 1011, 4034-4035, 4065
  ● **O98.01** Tuberculosis complicating **pregnancy**
    O98.011 Tuberculosis complicating pregnancy, **first trimester** ♀ 🔖   M
    O98.012 Tuberculosis complicating pregnancy, **second trimester** ♀ 🔖   M

    O98.013 Tuberculosis complicating pregnancy, **third trimester** ♀ 🔖   M
    O98.019 Tuberculosis complicating pregnancy, **unspecified trimester** ♀   M
  O98.02 Tuberculosis complicating **childbirth** ♀ 🔖   M
  O98.03 Tuberculosis complicating the **puerperium** ♀ 🔖   M

● **O98.1** **Syphilis** complicating pregnancy, childbirth and the puerperium
  Conditions in A50-A53
  (Ex) **For category O98.1 CC codes:** See PDX Collection 1012
  ● **O98.11** Syphilis complicating **pregnancy**
    O98.111 Syphilis complicating pregnancy, **first** trimester ♀ 🔖   M
    O98.112 Syphilis complicating pregnancy, **second trimester** ♀ 🔖   M
    O98.113 Syphilis complicating pregnancy, **third trimester** ♀ 🔖   M
    O98.119 Syphilis complicating pregnancy, **unspecified trimester** ♀   M
  O98.12 Syphilis complicating **childbirth** ♀ 🔖   M
  O98.13 Syphilis complicating the **puerperium** ♀ 🔖   M

● **O98.2** **Gonorrhea** complicating pregnancy, childbirth and the puerperium
  Conditions in A54.-
  (Ex) **For category O98.2 CC codes:** See PDX Collection 4017
  ● **O98.21** Gonorrhea complicating **pregnancy**
    O98.211 Gonorrhea complicating pregnancy, **first trimester** ♀ 🔖   M
    O98.212 Gonorrhea complicating pregnancy, **second trimester** ♀ 🔖   M
    O98.213 Gonorrhea complicating pregnancy, **third trimester** ♀ 🔖   M
    O98.219 Gonorrhea complicating pregnancy, **unspecified trimester** ♀   M
  O98.22 Gonorrhea complicating **childbirth** ♀ 🔖   M
  O98.23 Gonorrhea complicating the **puerperium** ♀ 🔖 M

● **O98.3** **Other infections with a predominantly sexual mode of transmission** complicating pregnancy, childbirth and the puerperium
  Conditions in A55-A64
  (Ex) **For category O98.3 CC codes:** See PDX Collection 4017
  ● **O98.31** Other infections with a predominantly sexual mode of transmission complicating **pregnancy**
    O98.311 Other infections with a predominantly sexual mode of transmission complicating pregnancy, **first trimester** ♀ 🔖   M
    O98.312 Other infections with a predominantly sexual mode of transmission complicating pregnancy, **second trimester** ♀ 🔖   M
    O98.313 Other infections with a predominantly sexual mode of transmission complicating pregnancy, **third trimester** ♀ 🔖   M
    O98.319 Other infections with a predominantly sexual mode of transmission complicating pregnancy, **unspecified trimester** ♀   M
  O98.32 Other infections with a predominantly sexual mode of transmission complicating **childbirth** ♀ 🔖   M
    Coding Clinic: 2020, Q1, P20
  O98.33 Other infections with a predominantly sexual mode of transmission complicating the **puerperium** ♀ 🔖   M

▶ New   ⇛ Revised   ~~deleted~~ Deleted   Excludes 1   Excludes 2   Includes   Use additional   Code first   Code also   Key words

OGCR Official Guidelines   ● Unacceptable Principal Diagnosis   X Assign placeholder X   ● Use Additional Character(s)   ▶ Manifestation Code   **Coding Clinic**

● O98.4 Viral hepatitis complicating pregnancy, childbirth and the puerperium
   Conditions in B15-B19
   (Ex) For category O98.4 CC codes: See PDX Collection 1013

   ● O98.41 Viral hepatitis complicating pregnancy
       O98.411 Viral hepatitis complicating pregnancy, first trimester ♀ (C)   M
       O98.412 Viral hepatitis complicating pregnancy, second trimester ♀ (C)   M
       O98.413 Viral hepatitis complicating pregnancy, third trimester ♀ (C)   M
       O98.419 Viral hepatitis complicating pregnancy, unspecified trimester ♀   M
   O98.42 Viral hepatitis complicating childbirth ♀ (C)   M
   O98.43 Viral hepatitis complicating the puerperium ♀ (C)   M

● O98.5 Other viral diseases complicating pregnancy, childbirth and the puerperium
   Conditions in A80-B09, B25-B34, R87.81-, R87.82-
   Excludes:1 human immunodeficiency virus [HIV] disease complicating pregnancy, childbirth and the puerperium (O98.7-)
   (Ex) For category O98.5 CC codes: See PDX Collection 1013

   ● O98.51 Other viral diseases complicating pregnancy
       O98.511 Other viral diseases complicating pregnancy, first trimester ♀ (C)   M
       O98.512 Other viral diseases complicating pregnancy, second trimester ♀ (C)   M
                Coding Clinic: 2016, Q4, P5-6
       O98.513 Other viral diseases complicating pregnancy, third trimester ♀ (C)   M
                Coding Clinic: 2016, Q4, P6
       O98.519 Other viral diseases complicating pregnancy, unspecified trimester ♀   M
   O98.52 Other viral diseases complicating childbirth ♀ (C)   M
   O98.53 Other viral diseases complicating the puerperium ♀ (C)   M

● O98.6 Protozoal diseases complicating pregnancy, childbirth and the puerperium
   Conditions in B50-B64

   ● O98.61 Protozoal diseases complicating pregnancy
       (Ex) For category O98.61 CC codes: See PDX Collection 1014, 4002, 4067
       O98.611 Protozoal diseases complicating pregnancy, first trimester ♀ (C)   M
       O98.612 Protozoal diseases complicating pregnancy, second trimester ♀ (C)   M
       O98.613 Protozoal diseases complicating pregnancy, third trimester ♀ (C)   M
       O98.619 Protozoal diseases complicating pregnancy, unspecified trimester ♀   M
   O98.62 Protozoal diseases complicating childbirth ♀ (C)   M
       (Ex) See PDX Collection 1015
   O98.63 Protozoal diseases complicating the puerperium ♀ (C)   M
       (Ex) See PDX Collection 1015

● O98.7 Human immunodeficiency virus [HIV] disease complicating pregnancy, childbirth and the puerperium
   Use additional code to identify the type of HIV disease:
       Acquired immune deficiency syndrome (AIDS) (B20)
       Asymptomatic HIV status (Z21)
       HIV positive NOS (Z21)
       Symptomatic HIV disease (B20)
   OGCR Section I.C.15.f.

   HIV Infection in Pregnancy, Childbirth and the Puerperium
   During pregnancy, childbirth or the puerperium, a patient admitted because of an HIV-related illness should receive a principal diagnosis from subcategory O98.7-. Human immunodeficiency [HIV] disease complicating pregnancy, childbirth and the puerperium, followed by the code(s) for the HIV-related illness(es).

   Patients with asymptomatic HIV infection status admitted during pregnancy, childbirth, or the puerperium should receive codes of O98.7- and Z21, Asymptomatic human immunodeficiency virus [HIV] infection status.

   (Ex) For category O98.7 CC codes: See PDX Collection 1013

   ● O98.71 Human immunodeficiency virus [HIV] disease complicating pregnancy
       O98.711 Human immunodeficiency virus [HIV] disease complicating pregnancy, first trimester ♀ (C)   M
       O98.712 Human immunodeficiency virus [HIV] disease complicating pregnancy, second trimester ♀ (C)   M
       O98.713 Human immunodeficiency virus [HIV] disease complicating pregnancy, third trimester ♀ (C)   M
       O98.719 Human immunodeficiency virus [HIV] disease complicating pregnancy, unspecified trimester ♀   M
   O98.72 Human immunodeficiency virus [HIV] disease complicating childbirth ♀ (C)   M
   O98.73 Human immunodeficiency virus [HIV] disease complicating the puerperium ♀ (C)   M

● O98.8 Other maternal infectious and parasitic diseases complicating pregnancy, childbirth and the puerperium
   (Ex) For category O98.8 CC codes: See PDX Collection 1013

   ● O98.81 Other maternal infectious and parasitic diseases complicating pregnancy
       O98.811 Other maternal infectious and parasitic diseases complicating pregnancy, first trimester ♀ (C)   M
       O98.812 Other maternal infectious and parasitic diseases complicating pregnancy, second trimester ♀ (C)   M
       O98.813 Other maternal infectious and parasitic diseases complicating pregnancy, third trimester ♀ (C)   M
       O98.819 Other maternal infectious and parasitic diseases complicating pregnancy, unspecified trimester ♀   M
   O98.82 Other maternal infectious and parasitic diseases complicating childbirth ♀ (C)   M
       Coding Clinic: 2020, Q1, P10
   O98.83 Other maternal infectious and parasitic diseases complicating the puerperium ♀ (C)   M

● **O98.9** Unspecified maternal infectious and parasitic disease complicating pregnancy, childbirth and the puerperium
Ex: For category O98.9 CC codes: See PDX Collection 1013

● **O98.91** Unspecified maternal infectious and parasitic disease complicating pregnancy

O98.911 Unspecified maternal infectious and parasitic disease complicating pregnancy, first trimester ♀   M

O98.912 Unspecified maternal infectious and parasitic disease complicating pregnancy, second trimester ♀   M

O98.913 Unspecified maternal infectious and parasitic disease complicating pregnancy, third trimester ♀   M

O98.919 Unspecified maternal infectious and parasitic disease complicating pregnancy, unspecified trimester ♀   M

O98.92 Unspecified maternal infectious and parasitic disease complicating childbirth ♀   M

O98.93 Unspecified maternal infectious and parasitic disease complicating the puerperium ♀   M

● **O99** Other maternal diseases classifiable elsewhere but complicating pregnancy, childbirth and the puerperium

Includes: conditions which complicate the pregnant state, are aggravated by the pregnancy or are a main reason for obstetric care

Use additional code to identify specific condition

Excludes2 when the reason for maternal care is that the condition is known or suspected to have affected the fetus (O35-O36)

Coding Clinic: 2018, Q4, P8-9

● **O99.0** Anemia complicating pregnancy, childbirth and the puerperium
Conditions in D50-D64

Excludes1 anemia arising in the puerperium (O90.81)
postpartum anemia NOS (O90.81)

● **O99.01** Anemia complicating pregnancy

O99.011 Anemia complicating pregnancy, first trimester ♀   M

O99.012 Anemia complicating pregnancy, second trimester ♀   M

O99.013 Anemia complicating pregnancy, third trimester ♀   M

O99.019 Anemia complicating pregnancy, unspecified trimester ♀   M

O99.02 Anemia complicating childbirth ♀   M

O99.03 Anemia complicating the puerperium ♀   M

Excludes1 postpartum anemia not pre-existing prior to delivery (O90.81)

● **O99.1** Other diseases of the blood and blood-forming organs and certain disorders involving the immune mechanism complicating pregnancy, childbirth and the puerperium
Conditions in D65-D89

Excludes1 hemorrhage with coagulation defects (O45.-, O46.0-, O67.0, O72.3)

● **O99.11** Other diseases of the blood and blood-forming organs and certain disorders involving the immune mechanism complicating pregnancy

O99.111 Other diseases of the blood and blood-forming organs and certain disorders involving the immune mechanism complicating pregnancy, first trimester ♀   M
Ex: See PDX Collection 3945

O99.112 Other diseases of the blood and blood-forming organs and certain disorders involving the immune mechanism complicating pregnancy, second trimester ♀   M
Ex: See PDX Collection 3947

O99.113 Other diseases of the blood and blood-forming organs and certain disorders involving the immune mechanism complicating pregnancy, third trimester ♀   M
Ex: See PDX Collection 3949

O99.119 Other diseases of the blood and blood-forming organs and certain disorders involving the immune mechanism complicating pregnancy, unspecified trimester ♀   M
Ex: See PDX Collection 1017

O99.12 Other diseases of the blood and blood-forming organs and certain disorders involving the immune mechanism complicating childbirth ♀   M
Ex: See PDX Collection 3952

O99.13 Other diseases of the blood and blood-forming organs and certain disorders involving the immune mechanism complicating the puerperium ♀   M
Ex: See PDX Collection 3954

● **O99.2** Endocrine, nutritional and metabolic diseases complicating pregnancy, childbirth and the puerperium
Conditions in E00-E89

Excludes2 diabetes mellitus (O24.-)
malnutrition (O25.-)
postpartum thyroiditis (O90.5)

● **O99.21** Obesity complicating pregnancy, childbirth, and the puerperium
Use additional code to identify the type of obesity (E66.-)

O99.210 Obesity complicating pregnancy, unspecified trimester ♀   M

O99.211 Obesity complicating pregnancy, first trimester ♀   M

O99.212 Obesity complicating pregnancy, second trimester ♀   M

O99.213 Obesity complicating pregnancy, third trimester ♀   M

O99.214 Obesity complicating childbirth ♀ M
Coding Clinic: 2021, Q2, P10-11; 2018, Q4, P80

O99.215 Obesity complicating the puerperium ♀   M

● **O99.28** Other endocrine, nutritional and metabolic diseases complicating pregnancy, childbirth and the puerperium

O99.280 Endocrine, nutritional and metabolic diseases complicating pregnancy, unspecified trimester ♀   M

O99.281 Endocrine, nutritional and metabolic diseases complicating pregnancy, first trimester ♀   M

O99.282 Endocrine, nutritional and metabolic diseases complicating pregnancy, second trimester ♀   M

O99.283 Endocrine, nutritional and metabolic diseases complicating pregnancy, third trimester ♀   M

O99.284 Endocrine, nutritional and metabolic diseases complicating childbirth ♀   M

O99.285 Endocrine, nutritional and metabolic diseases complicating the puerperium ♀   M
Coding Clinic: 2021, Q1, P9

● **O99.3   Mental disorders and diseases of the nervous system complicating pregnancy, childbirth and the puerperium**

  ● **O99.31   Alcohol use complicating pregnancy, childbirth, and the puerperium**

    Use additional code(s) from F10 to identify manifestations of the alcohol use

    O99.310   Alcohol use complicating pregnancy, unspecified trimester ♀   M

    O99.311   Alcohol use complicating pregnancy, first trimester ♀   M

    O99.312   Alcohol use complicating pregnancy, second trimester ♀   M

    O99.313   Alcohol use complicating pregnancy, third trimester ♀   M

    O99.314   Alcohol use complicating childbirth ♀   M

    O99.315   Alcohol use complicating the puerperium ♀   M

  ● **O99.32   Drug use complicating pregnancy, childbirth, and the puerperium**

    Use additional code(s) from F11-F16 and F18-F19 to identify manifestations of the drug use

    (Ex:) **For category O99.32 CC codes unless otherwise indicated:** See PDX Collection 4023

    O99.320   Drug use complicating pregnancy, unspecified trimester ♀   M
      (Ex:) See PDX Collection 1018

    O99.321   Drug use complicating pregnancy, first trimester ♀ 🅗   M

    O99.322   Drug use complicating pregnancy, second trimester ♀ 🅗   M

    O99.323   Drug use complicating pregnancy, third trimester ♀ 🅗   M
      (Ex:) See PDX Collection 4024

    O99.324   Drug use complicating childbirth ♀ 🅗   M
      (Ex:) See PDX Collection 4025

    O99.325   Drug use complicating the puerperium ♀ 🅗   M
      (Ex:) See PDX Collection 4026

  ● **O99.33   Tobacco use disorder complicating pregnancy, childbirth, and the puerperium**

    Smoking complicating pregnancy, childbirth, and the puerperium

    Use additional code from category F17 to identify type of tobacco nicotine dependence

    O99.330   Smoking (tobacco) complicating pregnancy, unspecified trimester ♀   M

    O99.331   Smoking (tobacco) complicating pregnancy, first trimester ♀   M

    O99.332   Smoking (tobacco) complicating pregnancy, second trimester ♀   M

    O99.333   Smoking (tobacco) complicating pregnancy, third trimester ♀   M

    O99.334   Smoking (tobacco) complicating childbirth ♀   M

    O99.335   Smoking (tobacco) complicating the puerperium ♀   M

  ● **O99.34   Other mental disorders complicating pregnancy, childbirth, and the puerperium**

    Conditions in F01-F09, F20-F52 and F54-F99

    Excludes2   postpartum mood disturbance (O90.6)
                  postnatal psychosis (F53.1)
                  puerperal psychosis (F53.1)

    Coding Clinic: 2018, Q4, P9

    O99.340   Other mental disorders complicating pregnancy, unspecified trimester ♀   M

    O99.341   Other mental disorders complicating pregnancy, first trimester ♀   M

    O99.342   Other mental disorders complicating pregnancy, second trimester ♀   M

    O99.343   Other mental disorders complicating pregnancy, third trimester ♀   M

    O99.344   Other mental disorders complicating childbirth ♀   M

    O99.345   Other mental disorders complicating the puerperium ♀   M

    Coding Clinic: 2018, Q4, P8-9

  ● **O99.35   Diseases of the nervous system complicating pregnancy, childbirth, and the puerperium**

    Conditions in G00-G99

    Excludes2   pregnancy related peripheral neuritis (O26.8-)

    O99.350   Diseases of the nervous system complicating pregnancy, unspecified trimester ♀   M

    O99.351   Diseases of the nervous system complicating pregnancy, first trimester ♀   M

    O99.352   Diseases of the nervous system complicating pregnancy, second trimester ♀   M

    O99.353   Diseases of the nervous system complicating pregnancy, third trimester ♀   M

    O99.354   Diseases of the nervous system complicating childbirth ♀ 🅗   M
      (Ex:) See PDX Collection 3956

    O99.355   Diseases of the nervous system complicating the puerperium ♀ 🅗   M
      (Ex:) See PDX Collection 1016

● **O99.4   Diseases of the circulatory system complicating pregnancy, childbirth and the puerperium**

    Conditions in I00-I99

    Excludes1   peripartum cardiomyopathy (O90.3)
    Excludes2   hypertensive disorders (O10-O16)
                  obstetric embolism (O88.-)
                  venous complications and cerebrovenous sinus thrombosis in labor, childbirth and the puerperium (O87.-)
                  venous complications and cerebrovenous sinus thrombosis in pregnancy (O22.-)

    (Ex:) **For category O99.4 CC codes unless otherwise indicated:** See PDX Collection 1019

  ● **O99.41   Diseases of the circulatory system complicating pregnancy**

    Coding Clinic: 2016, Q2, P8

    O99.411   Diseases of the circulatory system complicating pregnancy, first trimester ♀ 🅗   M
      (Ex:) See PDX Collection 4060

    O99.412   Diseases of the circulatory system complicating pregnancy, second trimester ♀ 🅗   M
      (Ex:) See PDX Collection 4060

    O99.413   Diseases of the circulatory system complicating pregnancy, third trimester ♀ 🅗   M

    O99.419   Diseases of the circulatory system complicating pregnancy, unspecified trimester ♀   M

    O99.42   Diseases of the circulatory system complicating childbirth ♀ 🅗   M
      (Ex:) See PDX Collection 4037

    O99.43   Diseases of the circulatory system complicating the puerperium ♀ 🅗   M
      (Ex:) See PDX Collection 4038

N Newborn Age: 0   **P** Pediatric Age: 0–17   **M** Maternity DX: 9–64   **A** Adult Age: 15–124   ♀ Females Only   ♂ Males Only

🅒 Complication\Comorbidity   🅜 Major C\C   (Ex:) CC/MCC Exclusions   🅗 Hospital-Acquired Condition   🅗 Hierarchical Condition Category

1183

CHAPTER 15 (O00-O9A)

● **O99.5** **Diseases of the respiratory system** complicating pregnancy, childbirth and the puerperium
Conditions in J00-J99

  ● **O99.51** Diseases of the respiratory system complicating **pregnancy**

     O99.511 Diseases of the respiratory system complicating pregnancy, **first trimester** ♀   M

     O99.512 Diseases of the respiratory system complicating pregnancy, **second trimester** ♀   M

     O99.513 Diseases of the respiratory system complicating pregnancy, **third trimester** ♀   M

     O99.519 Diseases of the respiratory system complicating pregnancy, **unspecified trimester** ♀   M

   O99.52 Diseases of the respiratory system complicating **childbirth** ♀   M

   O99.53 Diseases of the respiratory system complicating the **puerperium** ♀   M

● **O99.6** **Diseases of the digestive system** complicating pregnancy, childbirth and the puerperium
Conditions in K00-K93

   Excludes2   hemorrhoids in pregnancy (O22.4-)
                  liver and biliary tract disorders in pregnancy, childbirth and the puerperium (O26.6-)

  ● **O99.61** Diseases of the digestive system complicating **pregnancy**

     O99.611 Diseases of the digestive system complicating pregnancy, **first trimester** ♀   M

     O99.612 Diseases of the digestive system complicating pregnancy, **second trimester** ♀   M

     O99.613 Diseases of the digestive system complicating pregnancy, **third trimester** ♀   M

     O99.619 Diseases of the digestive system complicating pregnancy, **unspecified trimester** ♀   M

   O99.62 Diseases of the digestive system complicating **childbirth** ♀   M

   O99.63 Diseases of the digestive system complicating the **puerperium** ♀   M

● **O99.7** **Diseases of the skin and subcutaneous tissue** complicating pregnancy, childbirth and the puerperium
Conditions in L00-L99

   Excludes2   herpes gestationis (O26.4)
                  pruritic urticarial papules and plaques of pregnancy (PUPPP) (O26.86)

  ● **O99.71** Diseases of the skin and subcutaneous tissue complicating **pregnancy**

     O99.711 Diseases of the skin and subcutaneous tissue complicating pregnancy, **first trimester** ♀   M

     O99.712 Diseases of the skin and subcutaneous tissue complicating pregnancy, **second trimester** ♀   M

     O99.713 Diseases of the skin and subcutaneous tissue complicating pregnancy, **third trimester** ♀   M

     O99.719 Diseases of the skin and subcutaneous tissue complicating pregnancy, **unspecified trimester** ♀   M

   O99.72 Diseases of the skin and subcutaneous tissue complicating **childbirth** ♀   M

   O99.73 Diseases of the skin and subcutaneous tissue complicating the **puerperium** ♀   M

● **O99.8** **Other specified diseases and conditions** complicating pregnancy, childbirth and the puerperium
Conditions in D00-D48, H00-H95, M00-N99, and Q00-Q99

   Use additional code to identify condition

   Excludes2   genitourinary infections in pregnancy (O23.-)
                  infection of genitourinary tract following delivery (O86.1-O86.4)
                  malignant neoplasm complicating pregnancy, childbirth and the puerperium (O9A.1-)
                  maternal care for known or suspected abnormality of maternal pelvic organs (O34.-)
                  postpartum acute kidney failure (O90.4)
                  traumatic injuries in pregnancy (O9A.2-)

  ● **O99.81** **Abnormal glucose** complicating pregnancy, childbirth and the puerperium

     Excludes1   gestational diabetes (O24.4-)

     O99.810 Abnormal glucose complicating **pregnancy** ♀   M

     O99.814 Abnormal glucose complicating **childbirth** ♀   M

     O99.815 Abnormal glucose complicating the **puerperium** ♀   M

  ● **O99.82** **Streptococcus B carrier state** complicating pregnancy, childbirth and the puerperium

     Excludes1   Carrier of streptococcus group B (GBS) in a nonpregnant woman (Z22.330)

    ● O99.820 Streptococcus B carrier state complicating **pregnancy** ♀   M

     O99.824 Streptococcus B carrier state complicating **childbirth** ♀   M
                Coding Clinic: 2019, Q2, P9

    ● O99.825 Streptococcus B carrier state complicating the **puerperium** ♀   M

  ● **O99.83** **Other infection carrier state** complicating pregnancy, childbirth and the puerperium

     Use additional code to identify the carrier state (Z22.-)

     (Ex) **For category O99.83 CC codes:** See PDX Collection 1013

     O99.830 Other infection carrier state complicating **pregnancy** ♀ 🔗   M

     O99.834 Other infection carrier state complicating **childbirth** ♀ 🔗   M

     O99.835 Other infection carrier state complicating the **puerperium** ♀ 🔗   M

  ● **O99.84** **Bariatric surgery status** complicating pregnancy, childbirth and the puerperium
     Gastric banding status complicating pregnancy, childbirth and the puerperium
     Gastric bypass status for obesity complicating pregnancy, childbirth and the puerperium
     Obesity surgery status complicating pregnancy, childbirth and the puerperium

     O99.840 Bariatric surgery status complicating pregnancy, **unspecified trimester** ♀ M

     O99.841 Bariatric surgery status complicating pregnancy, **first trimester** ♀   M

     O99.842 Bariatric surgery status complicating pregnancy, **second trimester** ♀   M

     O99.843 Bariatric surgery status complicating pregnancy, **third trimester** ♀   M

     O99.844 Bariatric surgery status complicating **childbirth** ♀   M

     O99.845 Bariatric surgery status complicating the **puerperium** ♀   M

▶ New   ⇒ Revised   ~~deleted~~ Deleted   Excludes 1   Excludes 2   Includes   Use additional   Code first   Code also   Key words
OGCR Official Guidelines   ● Unacceptable Principal Diagnosis   X Assign placeholder X   ● Use Additional Character(s)   ▶ Manifestation Code   **Coding Clinic**

● O99.89 Other specified diseases and conditions complicating pregnancy, childbirth and the puerperium ♀   M

O99.891 Other specified diseases and conditions complicating pregnancy ♀   M

O99.892 Other specified diseases and conditions complicating childbirth ♀   M

O99.893 Other specified diseases and conditions complicating puerperium ♀   M

OGCR Section I.C.2.l.3.

Malignant neoplasm in a pregnant patient

When a pregnant woman has a malignant neoplasm, a code from subcategory O9A.1-, Malignant neoplasm complicating pregnancy, childbirth, and the puerperium, should be sequenced first, followed by the appropriate code from Chapter 2 to indicate the type of neoplasm.

● O9A Maternal malignant neoplasms, traumatic injuries and abuse classifiable elsewhere but complicating pregnancy, childbirth and the puerperium

● O9A.1 Malignant neoplasm complicating pregnancy, childbirth and the puerperium

Conditions in C00-C96

Use additional code to identify neoplasm

Excludes2 maternal care for benign tumor of corpus uteri (O34.1-)
maternal care for benign tumor of cervix (O34.4-)

● O9A.11 Malignant neoplasm complicating pregnancy

O9A.111 Malignant neoplasm complicating pregnancy, first trimester ♀   M

O9A.112 Malignant neoplasm complicating pregnancy, second trimester ♀   M

O9A.113 Malignant neoplasm complicating pregnancy, third trimester ♀   M

O9A.119 Malignant neoplasm complicating pregnancy, unspecified trimester ♀   M

O9A.12 Malignant neoplasm complicating childbirth ♀   M

O9A.13 Malignant neoplasm complicating the puerperium ♀   M
Coding Clinic: 2015, Q3, P19

● O9A.2 Injury, poisoning and certain other consequences of external causes complicating pregnancy, childbirth and the puerperium

Conditions in S00-T88, except T74 and T76

Use additional code(s) to identify the injury or poisoning

Excludes2 physical, sexual and psychological abuse complicating pregnancy, childbirth and the puerperium (O9A.3-, O9A.4-, O9A.5-)

● O9A.21 Injury, poisoning and certain other consequences of external causes complicating pregnancy

O9A.211 Injury, poisoning and certain other consequences of external causes complicating pregnancy, first trimester ♀   M

O9A.212 Injury, poisoning and certain other consequences of external causes complicating pregnancy, second trimester ♀   M

O9A.213 Injury, poisoning and certain other consequences of external causes complicating pregnancy, third trimester ♀   M

O9A.219 Injury, poisoning and certain other consequences of external causes complicating pregnancy, unspecified trimester ♀   M

O9A.22 Injury, poisoning and certain other consequences of external causes complicating childbirth ♀   M

O9A.23 Injury, poisoning and certain other consequences of external causes complicating the puerperium ♀   M

● O9A.3 Physical abuse complicating pregnancy, childbirth and the puerperium

Conditions in T74.11 or T76.11

Use additional code (if applicable):
to identify any associated current injury due to physical abuse
to identify the perpetrator of abuse (Y07.-)

Excludes2 sexual abuse complicating pregnancy, childbirth and the puerperium (O9A.4)

● O9A.31 Physical abuse complicating pregnancy

O9A.311 Physical abuse complicating pregnancy, first trimester ♀   M

O9A.312 Physical abuse complicating pregnancy, second trimester ♀   M

O9A.313 Physical abuse complicating pregnancy, third trimester ♀   M

O9A.319 Physical abuse complicating pregnancy, unspecified trimester ♀   M

O9A.32 Physical abuse complicating childbirth ♀   M

O9A.33 Physical abuse complicating the puerperium ♀   M

● O9A.4 Sexual abuse complicating pregnancy, childbirth and the puerperium

Conditions in T74.21 or T76.21

Use additional code (if applicable):
to identify any associated current injury due to sexual abuse
to identify the perpetrator of abuse (Y07.-)

● O9A.41 Sexual abuse complicating pregnancy

O9A.411 Sexual abuse complicating pregnancy, first trimester ♀   M

O9A.412 Sexual abuse complicating pregnancy, second trimester ♀   M

O9A.413 Sexual abuse complicating pregnancy, third trimester ♀   M

O9A.419 Sexual abuse complicating pregnancy, unspecified trimester ♀   M

O9A.42 Sexual abuse complicating childbirth ♀   M

O9A.43 Sexual abuse complicating the puerperium ♀   M

● O9A.5 Psychological abuse complicating pregnancy, childbirth and the puerperium

Conditions in T74.31 or T76.31

Use additional code to identify the perpetrator of abuse (Y07.-)

● O9A.51 Psychological abuse complicating pregnancy

O9A.511 Psychological abuse complicating pregnancy, first trimester ♀   M

O9A.512 Psychological abuse complicating pregnancy, second trimester ♀   M

O9A.513 Psychological abuse complicating pregnancy, third trimester ♀   M

O9A.519 Psychological abuse complicating pregnancy, unspecified trimester ♀   M

O9A.52 Psychological abuse complicating childbirth ♀ M

O9A.53 Psychological abuse complicating the puerperium ♀   M

CHAPTER 15 (O00-O9A)

N Newborn Age: 0   P Pediatric Age: 0–17   M Maternity DX: 9–64   A Adult Age: 15–124   ♀ Females Only   ♂ Males Only

Complication\Comorbidity   Major C\C   (Ex) CC/MCC Exclusions   Hospital-Acquired Condition   Hierarchical Condition Category

CHAPTER 16

CERTAIN CONDITIONS ORIGINATING IN THE PERINATAL PERIOD (P00-P96)

OGCR Chapter-Specific Coding Guidelines

16. **Chapter 16: Certain Conditions Originating in the Perinatal Period (P00-P96)**

For coding and reporting purposes the perinatal period is defined as before birth through the 28th day following birth. The following guidelines are provided for reporting purposes

a. General Perinatal Rules

1) **Use of Chapter 16 Codes**

Codes in this chapter are <u>never</u> for use on the maternal record. Codes from Chapter 15, the obstetric chapter, are never permitted on the newborn record. Chapter 16 codes may be used throughout the life of the patient if the condition is still present.

2) **Principal Diagnosis for Birth Record**

When coding the birth episode in a newborn record, assign a code from category Z38, Liveborn infants according to place of birth and type of delivery, as the principal diagnosis. A code from category Z38 is assigned only once, to a newborn at the time of birth. If a newborn is transferred to another institution, a code from category Z38 should not be used at the receiving hospital.

A code from category Z38 is used only on the newborn record, not on the mother's record.

3) **Use of Codes from other Chapters with Codes from Chapter 16**

Codes from other chapters may be used with codes from chapter 16 if the codes from the other chapters provide more specific detail. Codes for signs and symptoms may be assigned when a definitive diagnosis has not been established. If the reason for the encounter is a perinatal condition, the code from Chapter 16 should be sequenced first.

4) **Use of Chapter 16 Codes after the Perinatal Period**

Should a condition originate in the perinatal period, and continue throughout the life of the patient, the perinatal code should continue to be used regardless of the patient's age.

5) **Birth process or community acquired conditions**

If a newborn has a condition that may be either due to the birth process or community acquired and the documentation does not indicate which it is, the default is due to the birth process and the code from Chapter 16 should be used. If the condition is community-acquired, a code from Chapter 16 should not be assigned.

6) **Code all clinically significant conditions**

All clinically significant conditions noted on routine newborn examination should be coded. A condition is clinically significant if it requires:

- clinical evaluation; or
- therapeutic treatment; or
- diagnostic procedures; or
- extended length of hospital stay; or
- increased nursing care and/or monitoring; or
- has implications for future health care needs

Note: The perinatal guidelines listed above are the same as the general coding guidelines for "additional diagnoses", except for the final point regarding implications for future health care needs. Codes should be assigned for conditions that have been specified by the provider as having implications for future health care needs.

b. Observation and Evaluation of Newborns for Suspected Conditions Not Found

1) **Use of Z05 codes**

Assign a code from category Z05, Observation and evaluation of newborns and infants for suspected conditions ruled out, to identify those instances when a healthy newborn is evaluated for a suspected condition that is determined after study not to be present. Do not use a code from category Z05 when the patient has identified signs or symptoms of a suspected problem; in such cases code the sign or symptom.

2) **Z05 on Other than the Birth Record**

A code from category Z05 may also be assigned as a principal or first-listed code for readmissions or encounters when the code from category Z38 code no longer applies. Codes from category Z05 are for use only for healthy newborns and infants for which no condition after study is found to be present.

3) **Z05 on a birth record**

A code from category Z05 is to be used as a secondary code after the code from category Z38, Liveborn infants according to place of birth and type of delivery.

c. Coding Additional Perinatal Diagnoses

1) **Assigning codes for conditions that require treatment**

Assign codes for conditions that require treatment or further investigation, prolong the length of stay, or require resource utilization.

2) **Codes for conditions specified as having implications for future health care needs**

Assign codes for conditions that have been specified by the provider as having implications for future health care needs.

Note: This guideline should not be used for adult patients.

d. Prematurity and Fetal Growth Retardation

Providers utilize different criteria in determining prematurity. A code for prematurity should not be assigned unless it is documented. Assignment of codes in categories P05, Disorders of newborn related to slow fetal growth and fetal malnutrition, and P07, Disorders of newborn related to short gestation and low birth weight, not elsewhere classified, should be based on the recorded birth weight and estimated gestational age.

When both birth weight and gestational age are available, two codes from category P07 should be assigned, with the code for birth weight sequenced before the code for gestational age.

e. Low birth weight and immaturity status

Codes from category P07, Disorders of newborn related to short gestation and low birth weight, not elsewhere classified, are for use for a child or adult who was premature or had a low birth weight as a newborn and this is affecting the patient's current health status.

See Section I.C.21. Factors influencing health status and contact with health services, Status.

f. Bacterial Sepsis of Newborn

Category P36, Bacterial sepsis of newborn, includes congenital sepsis. If a perinate is documented as having sepsis without documentation of congenital or community acquired, the default is congenital and a code from category P36 should be assigned. If the P36 code includes the causal organism, an additional code from category B95, Streptococcus, Staphylococcus, and Enterococcus as the cause of diseases classified elsewhere, or B96, Other bacterial agents as the cause of diseases classified elsewhere, should not be assigned. If the P36 code does not include the causal organism, assign an additional code from category B96. If applicable, use additional codes to identify severe sepsis (R65.2-) and any associated acute organ dysfunction.

g. Stillbirth

Code P95, Stillbirth, is only for use in institutions that maintain separate records for stillbirths. No other code should be used with P95. Code P95 should not be used on the mother's record.

CHAPTER 16

CERTAIN CONDITIONS ORIGINATING IN THE PERINATAL PERIOD (P00-P96)

Note: Codes from this chapter are for use on newborn records only, never on maternal records.

Includes	conditions that have their origin in the fetal or perinatal period (before birth through the first 28 days after birth) even if morbidity occurs later

Excludes2	congenital malformations, deformations and chromosomal abnormalities (Q00-Q99)
	endocrine, nutritional and metabolic diseases (E00-E88)
	injury, poisoning and certain other consequences of external causes (S00-T88)
	neoplasms (C00-D49)
	tetanus neonatorum (A33)

This chapter contains the following blocks:

P00-P04	Newborn affected by maternal factors and by complications of pregnancy, labor, and delivery
P05-P08	Disorders of newborns related to length of gestation and fetal growth
P09	Abnormal findings on neonatal screening
P10-P15	Birth trauma
P19-P29	Respiratory and cardiovascular disorders specific to the perinatal period
P35-P39	Infections specific to the perinatal period
P50-P61	Hemorrhagic and hematological disorders of newborn
P70-P74	Transitory endocrine and metabolic disorders specific to newborn
P76-P78	Digestive system disorders of newborn
P80-P83	Conditions involving the integument and temperature regulation of newborn
P84	Other problems with newborn
P90-P96	Other disorders originating in the perinatal period

NEWBORN AFFECTED BY MATERNAL FACTORS AND BY COMPLICATIONS OF PREGNANCY, LABOR, AND DELIVERY (P00-P04)

Note: These codes are for use when the listed maternal conditions are specified as the cause of confirmed morbidity or potential morbidity which have their origin in the perinatal period (before birth through the first 28 days after birth).

● **P00**   Newborn affected by maternal conditions that may be unrelated to present pregnancy

Code first any current condition in newborn

Excludes2	encounter for observation of newborn for suspected diseases and conditions ruled out (Z05.-)
	newborn affected by maternal complications of pregnancy (P01.-)
	newborn affected by maternal endocrine and metabolic disorders (P70–P74)
	newborn affected by noxious substances transmitted via placenta or breast milk (P04.-)

Coding Clinic: 2016, Q4, P54

P00.0   Newborn affected by maternal hypertensive disorders
Newborn affected by maternal conditions classifiable to O10-O11, O13-O16

P00.1   Newborn affected by maternal renal and urinary tract diseases
Newborn affected by maternal conditions classifiable to N00-N39

P00.2   Newborn affected by maternal infectious and parasitic diseases
Newborn affected by maternal infectious disease classifiable to A00-B99, J09 and J10

Excludes1	maternal genital tract or other localized infections (P00.8)

Excludes2	infections specific to the perinatal period (P35-P39)
	▶newborn affected by (positive) maternal group B streptococcus (GBS) colonization (P00.82)

Coding Clinic: 2019, Q2, P10; 2015, Q3, P21

P00.3   Newborn affected by other maternal circulatory and respiratory diseases
Newborn affected by maternal conditions classifiable to I00-I99, J00-J99, Q20-Q34 and not included in P00.0, P00.2

P00.4   Newborn affected by maternal nutritional disorders
Newborn affected by maternal disorders classifiable to E40-E64
Maternal malnutrition NOS

P00.5   Newborn affected by maternal injury
Newborn affected by maternal conditions classifiable to O9A.2-

P00.6   Newborn affected by surgical procedure on mother
Newborn affected by amniocentesis

Excludes1	Cesarean delivery for present delivery (P03.4)
	damage to placenta from amniocentesis, cesarean delivery or surgical induction (P02.1)
	previous surgery to uterus or pelvic organs (P03.89)

Excludes2	newborn affected by complication of (fetal) intrauterine procedure (P96.5)

P00.7   Newborn affected by other medical procedures on mother, not elsewhere classified
Newborn affected by radiation to mother

Excludes1	damage to placenta from amniocentesis, cesarean delivery or surgical induction (P02.1)
	newborn affected by other complications of labor and delivery (P03.-)

● **P00.8**   Newborn affected by other maternal conditions

P00.81   Newborn affected by periodontal disease in mother

▶**P00.82**   Newborn affected by (positive) maternal group B streptococcus (GBS) colonization
▶Contact with positive maternal group B streptococcus

P00.89   Newborn affected by other maternal conditions
Newborn affected by conditions classifiable to T80-T88
Newborn affected by maternal genital tract or other localized infections
Newborn affected by maternal systemic lupus erythematosus
Use additional code to identify infectious agent, if known

▶ **Excludes2**	newborn affected by positive maternal group B streptococcus (GBS) colonization (P00.82)

Coding Clinic: 2019, Q2, P9

P00.9   Newborn affected by unspecified maternal condition

● **P01**   Newborn affected by maternal complications of pregnancy
Code first any current condition in newborn

Excludes2	encounter for observation of newborn for suspected diseases and conditions ruled out (Z05.-)

Coding Clinic: 2016, Q4, P54

P01.0   Newborn affected by incompetent cervix

P01.1   Newborn affected by premature rupture of membranes

N Newborn Age: 0   **P** Pediatric Age: 0–17   **M** Maternity DX: 9–64   **A** Adult Age: 15–124   ♀ Females Only   ♂ Males Only

🔾 Complication\Comorbidity   🔾 Major C\C   (Ex) CC/MCC Exclusions   🔾 Hospital-Acquired Condition   🔾 Hierarchical Condition Category

1187

CHAPTER 16 (P00-P96)

CHAPTER 16 (P00-P96)

P01.2 Newborn affected by oligohydramnios
> **Excludes1**   oligohydramnios due to premature rupture of membranes (P01.1)

P01.3 Newborn affected by polyhydramnios
Excess of amniotic fluid, usually > 2000 mL
Newborn affected by hydramnios

P01.4 Newborn affected by ectopic pregnancy
Newborn affected by abdominal pregnancy

P01.5 Newborn affected by multiple pregnancy
Newborn affected by triplet (pregnancy)
Newborn affected by twin (pregnancy)

P01.6 Newborn affected by maternal death

P01.7 Newborn affected by malpresentation before labor
Newborn affected by breech presentation before labor
Newborn affected by external version before labor
Newborn affected by face presentation before labor
Newborn affected by transverse lie before labor
Newborn affected by unstable lie before labor

P01.8 Newborn affected by other maternal complications of pregnancy

P01.9 Newborn affected by maternal complication of pregnancy, unspecified

● **P02 Newborn affected by complications of placenta, cord and membranes**
> *Code first any current condition in newborn*
> **Excludes2**   encounter for observation of newborn for suspected diseases and conditions ruled out (Z05.-)

Coding Clinic: 2016, Q4, P54

P02.0 Newborn affected by placenta previa

P02.1 Newborn affected by other forms of placental separation and hemorrhage
Newborn affected by abruptio placenta
Newborn affected by accidental hemorrhage
Newborn affected by antepartum hemorrhage
Newborn affected by damage to placenta from amniocentesis, cesarean delivery or surgical induction
Newborn affected by maternal blood loss
Newborn affected by premature separation of placenta

● **P02.2 Newborn affected by other and unspecified morphological and functional abnormalities of placenta**

  P02.20 Newborn affected by unspecified morphological and functional abnormalities of placenta

  P02.29 Newborn affected by other morphological and functional abnormalities of placenta
Newborn affected by placental dysfunction
Newborn affected by placental infarction
Newborn affected by placental insufficiency

P02.3 Newborn affected by placental transfusion syndromes
Newborn affected by placental and cord abnormalities resulting in twin-to-twin or other transplacental transfusion

P02.4 Newborn affected by prolapsed cord

P02.5 Newborn affected by other compression of umbilical cord
Newborn affected by umbilical cord (tightly) around neck
Newborn affected by entanglement of umbilical cord
Newborn affected by knot in umbilical cord

● **P02.6 Newborn affected by other and unspecified conditions of umbilical cord**

  P02.60 Newborn affected by unspecified conditions of umbilical cord

  P02.69 Newborn affected by other conditions of umbilical cord
Newborn affected by short umbilical cord
Newborn affected by vasa previa
> **Excludes1**   newborn affected by single umbilical artery (Q27.0)

● **P02.7 Newborn affected by chorioamnionitis**
Inflammation of chorion and amnion

  P02.70 Newborn affected by fetal inflammatory response syndrome ⚕
Newborn affected by FIRS

  P02.78 Newborn affected by other conditions from chorioamnionitis
Newborn affected by amnionitis
Newborn affected by membranitis
Newborn affected by placentitis

P02.8 Newborn affected by other abnormalities of membranes

P02.9 Newborn affected by abnormality of membranes, unspecified

● **P03 Newborn affected by other complications of labor and delivery**
> *Code first any current condition in newborn*
> **Excludes2**   encounter for observation of newborn for suspected diseases and conditions ruled out (Z05.-)

Coding Clinic: 2016, Q4, P54

P03.0 Newborn affected by breech delivery and extraction

P03.1 Newborn affected by other malpresentation, malposition and disproportion during labor and delivery
Newborn affected by contracted pelvis
Newborn affected by conditions classifiable to O64-O66
Newborn affected by persistent occipitoposterior
Newborn affected by transverse lie

P03.2 Newborn affected by forceps delivery

P03.3 Newborn affected by delivery by vacuum extractor [ventouse]

P03.4 Newborn affected by Cesarean delivery

P03.5 Newborn affected by precipitate delivery
Newborn affected by rapid second stage

P03.6 Newborn affected by abnormal uterine contractions
Newborn affected by conditions classifiable to O62.-, except O62.3
Newborn affected by hypertonic labor
Newborn affected by uterine inertia

● **P03.8 Newborn affected by other specified complications of labor and delivery**

  ● **P03.81 Newborn affected by abnormality in fetal (intrauterine) heart rate or rhythm**
> **Excludes1**   neonatal cardiac dysrhythmia (P29.1-)

    P03.810 Newborn affected by abnormality in fetal (intrauterine) heart rate or rhythm before the onset of labor

    P03.811 Newborn affected by abnormality in fetal (intrauterine) heart rate or rhythm during labor

    P03.819 Newborn affected by abnormality in fetal (intrauterine) heart rate or rhythm, unspecified as to time of onset

  P03.82 Meconium passage during delivery
> **Excludes1**   meconium aspiration (P24.00, P24.01)
> meconium staining (P96.83)

  P03.89 Newborn affected by other specified complications of labor and delivery
Newborn affected by abnormality of maternal soft tissues
Newborn affected by conditions classifiable to O60-O75 and by procedures used in labor and delivery not included in P02.- and P03.0-P03.6
Newborn affected by induction of labor

P03.9 Newborn affected by complication of labor and delivery, unspecified

▶ New   ⇒ Revised   ~~deleted~~ Deleted   Excludes 1   Excludes 2   Includes   Use additional   Code first   Code also   Key words
OGCR Official Guidelines   ● Unacceptable Principal Diagnosis   X Assign placeholder X   ● Use Additional Character(s)   ▸ Manifestation Code   Coding Clinic

● **P04**   **Newborn affected by** noxious substances transmitted via placenta or breast milk

Code first any current condition in newborn, if applicable

Includes   nonteratogenic effects of substances transmitted via placenta

Excludes2   congenital malformations (Q00-Q99)

encounter for observation of newborn for suspected diseases and conditions ruled out (Z05.-)

neonatal jaundice from excessive hemolysis due to drugs or toxins transmitted from mother (P58.4)

newborn in contact with and (suspected) exposures hazardous to health not transmitted via placenta or breast milk (Z77.-)

Coding Clinic: 2016, Q4, P54

P04.0   **Newborn affected by maternal** anesthesia and analgesia **in pregnancy, labor and delivery**

Newborn affected by reactions and intoxications from maternal opiates and tranquilizers administered for procedures during pregnancy or labor and delivery

Excludes2   newborn affected by other maternal medication (P04.1-)

● **P04.1**   **Newborn affected by** other maternal medication

Code first withdrawal symptoms from maternal use of drugs of addiction, if applicable (P96.1)

Excludes1   dysmorphism due to warfarin (Q86.2)

fetal hydantoin syndrome (Q86.1)

Excludes2   maternal anesthesia and analgesia in pregnancy, labor and delivery (P04.0)

maternal use of drugs of addiction (P04.4-)

   P04.11   Newborn affected by maternal antineoplastic chemotherapy

   P04.12   Newborn affected by maternal cytotoxic drugs

   P04.13   Newborn affected by maternal use of anticonvulsants

   P04.14   Newborn affected by maternal use of opiates

   P04.15   Newborn affected by maternal use of antidepressants

   P04.16   Newborn affected by maternal use of amphetamines

   P04.17   Newborn affected by maternal use of sedative-hypnotics

   P04.1A   Newborn affected by maternal use of anxiolytics

   P04.18   Newborn affected by other maternal medication

   P04.19   Newborn affected by maternal use of unspecified medication

     Coding Clinic: 2016, Q4, P55

P04.2   **Newborn affected by maternal** use of tobacco

Newborn affected by exposure in utero to tobacco smoke

Excludes2   newborn exposure to environmental tobacco smoke (P96.81)

P04.3   **Newborn affected by maternal** use of alcohol

Excludes1   fetal alcohol syndrome (Q86.0)

● **P04.4**   **Newborn affected by maternal use of** drugs of addiction

   P04.40   Newborn affected by maternal use of unspecified drugs of addiction

   P04.41   Newborn affected by maternal use of cocaine

   P04.42   Newborn affected by maternal use of hallucinogens

     Excludes2   newborn affected by other maternal medication (P04.1-)

   P04.49   Newborn affected by maternal use of other drugs of addiction

     Excludes2   newborn affected by maternal anesthesia and analgesia (P04.0)

withdrawal symptoms from maternal use of drugs of addiction (P96.1)

P04.5   **Newborn affected by maternal use of** nutritional chemical substances

P04.6   **Newborn affected by maternal** exposure to environmental chemical substances

● **P04.8**   **Newborn affected by** other maternal noxious substances

   P04.81   Newborn affected by maternal use of cannabis

   P04.89   Newborn affected by other maternal noxious substances

P04.9   **Newborn affected by maternal noxious substance, unspecified**

OGCR   Section I.C.16.d.

Prematurity and Fetal Growth Retardation

Providers utilize different criteria in determining prematurity. A code for prematurity should not be assigned unless it is documented. Assignment of codes in categories P05, Disorders of newborn related to slow fetal growth and fetal malnutrition, and P07, Disorders of newborn related to short gestation and low birth weight, not elsewhere classified, should be based on the recorded birth weight and estimated gestational age.

When both birth weight and gestational age are available, two codes from category P07 should be assigned, with the code for birth weight sequenced before the code for gestational age.

DISORDERS OF NEWBORN RELATED TO LENGTH OF GESTATION AND FETAL GROWTH (P05-P08)

● **P05**   **Disorders of newborn related to slow fetal growth and fetal malnutrition**

Coding Clinic: 2016, Q4, P56

● **P05.0**   **Newborn** light for gestational age

Newborn light-for-dates

Weight below but length above 10th percentile for gestational age

   P05.00   Newborn light for gestational age, unspecified weight

   P05.01   Newborn light for gestational age, less than 500 grams

   P05.02   Newborn light for gestational age, 500-749 grams

   P05.03   Newborn light for gestational age, 750-999 grams

   P05.04   Newborn light for gestational age, 1000-1249 grams

   P05.05   Newborn light for gestational age, 1250-1499 grams

   P05.06   Newborn light for gestational age, 1500-1749 grams

   P05.07   Newborn light for gestational age, 1750-1999 grams

   P05.08   Newborn light for gestational age, 2000-2499 grams

   P05.09   Newborn light for gestational age, 2500 grams and over

Newborn light for gestational age, other

Coding Clinic: 2016, Q4, P55

N   Newborn Age: 0   **P**   Pediatric Age: 0–17   **M**   Maternity DX: 9–64   **A**   Adult Age: 15–124   ♀   Females Only   ♂   Males Only

🔹 Complication\Comorbidity   🔹 Major C\C   (Ex) CC/MCC Exclusions   🔹 Hospital-Acquired Condition   🔹 Hierarchical Condition Category   **1189**

CHAPTER 16 (P00-P96)

● **P05.1** **Newborn small for gestational age**
Newborn small-and-light-for-dates
Newborn small-for-dates
Weight and length below 10th percentile for gestational age

     P05.10 **Newborn small for gestational age, unspecified weight**

     P05.11 **Newborn small for gestational age, less than 500 grams**

     P05.12 **Newborn small for gestational age, 500-749 grams**

     P05.13 **Newborn small for gestational age, 750-999 grams**

     P05.14 **Newborn small for gestational age, 1000-1249 grams**

     P05.15 **Newborn small for gestational age, 1250-1499 grams**

     P05.16 **Newborn small for gestational age, 1500-1749 grams**

     P05.17 **Newborn small for gestational age, 1750-1999 grams**

     P05.18 **Newborn small for gestational age, 2000-2499 grams**

     P05.19 **Newborn small for gestational age, other**
Newborn small for gestational age, 2500 grams and over
Coding Clinic: 2016, Q4, P55

   P05.2 **Newborn affected by fetal (intrauterine) malnutrition not light or small for gestational age**
Infant, not light or small for gestational age, showing signs of fetal malnutrition, such as dry, peeling skin and loss of subcutaneous tissue

     Excludes1   newborn affected by fetal malnutrition with light for gestational age (P05.0-)
newborn affected by fetal malnutrition with small for gestational age (P05.1-)

   P05.9 **Newborn affected by slow intrauterine growth, unspecified**
Newborn affected by fetal growth retardation NOS

● **P07** **Disorders of newborn related to short gestation and low birth weight, not elsewhere classified**
Note: When both birth weight and gestational age of the newborn are available, both should be coded with birth weight sequenced before gestational age.

     Includes   the listed conditions, without further specification, as the cause of morbidity or additional care, in newborn

● **P07.0** **Extremely low birth weight newborn**
Newborn birth weight 999 g. or less

     Excludes1   low birth weight due to slow fetal growth and fetal malnutrition (P05.-)

     P07.00 **Extremely low birth weight newborn, unspecified weight**

     P07.01 **Extremely low birth weight newborn, less than 500 grams**

     P07.02 **Extremely low birth weight newborn, 500-749 grams**

     P07.03 **Extremely low birth weight newborn, 750-999 grams**

● **P07.1** **Other low birth weight newborn**
Newborn birth weight 1000-2499 g.

     Excludes1   low birth weight due to slow fetal growth and fetal malnutrition (P05.-)

     P07.10 **Other low birth weight newborn, unspecified weight**

     P07.14 **Other low birth weight newborn, 1000-1249 grams**

     P07.15 **Other low birth weight newborn, 1250-1499 grams**

     P07.16 **Other low birth weight newborn, 1500-1749 grams**

     P07.17 **Other low birth weight newborn, 1750-1999 grams**

     P07.18 **Other low birth weight newborn, 2000-2499 grams**

● **P07.2** **Extreme immaturity of newborn**
Less than 28 completed weeks (less than 196 completed days) of gestation

     P07.20 **Extreme immaturity of newborn, unspecified weeks of gestation**
Gestational age less than 28 completed weeks NOS

     P07.21 **Extreme immaturity of newborn, gestational age less than 23 completed weeks**
Extreme immaturity of newborn, gestational age less than 23 weeks, 0 days

     P07.22 **Extreme immaturity of newborn, gestational age 23 completed weeks**
Extreme immaturity of newborn, gestational age 23 weeks, 0 days through 23 weeks, 6 days

     P07.23 **Extreme immaturity of newborn, gestational age 24 completed weeks**
Extreme immaturity of newborn, gestational age 24 weeks, 0 days through 24 weeks, 6 days

     P07.24 **Extreme immaturity of newborn, gestational age 25 completed weeks**
Extreme immaturity of newborn, gestational age 25 weeks, 0 days through 25 weeks, 6 days

     P07.25 **Extreme immaturity of newborn, gestational age 26 completed weeks**
Extreme immaturity of newborn, gestational age 26 weeks, 0 days through 26 weeks, 6 days

     P07.26 **Extreme immaturity of newborn, gestational age 27 completed weeks**
Extreme immaturity of newborn, gestational age 27 weeks, 0 days through 27 weeks, 6 days

● **P07.3** **Preterm [premature] newborn [other]**
28 completed weeks or more but less than 37 completed weeks (196 completed days but less than 259 completed days) of gestation
Prematurity NOS

     P07.30 **Preterm newborn, unspecified weeks of gestation**

     P07.31 **Preterm newborn, gestational age 28 completed weeks**
Preterm newborn, gestational age 28 weeks, 0 days through 28 weeks, 6 days

     P07.32 **Preterm newborn, gestational age 29 completed weeks**
Preterm newborn, gestational age 29 weeks, 0 days through 29 weeks, 6 days

     P07.33 **Preterm newborn, gestational age 30 completed weeks**
Preterm newborn, gestational age 30 weeks, 0 days through 30 weeks, 6 days

     P07.34 **Preterm newborn, gestational age 31 completed weeks**
Preterm newborn, gestational age 31 weeks, 0 days through 31 weeks, 6 days

     P07.35 **Preterm newborn, gestational age 32 completed weeks**
Preterm newborn, gestational age 32 weeks, 0 days through 32 weeks, 6 days

     P07.36 **Preterm newborn, gestational age 33 completed weeks**
Preterm newborn, gestational age 33 weeks, 0 days through 33 weeks, 6 days

▶ New   ⇒ Revised   ~~deleted~~ Deleted   Excludes 1   Excludes 2   Includes   Use additional   Code first   Code also   Key words
OGCR Official Guidelines   ● Unacceptable Principal Diagnosis   X Assign placeholder X   ● Use Additional Character(s)   ▶ Manifestation Code   Coding Clinic

P07.37 **Preterm newborn, gestational age 34 completed weeks**
Preterm newborn, gestational age 34 weeks, 0 days through 34 weeks, 6 days
Coding Clinic: 2017, Q2, P7

P07.38 **Preterm newborn, gestational age 35 completed weeks**
Preterm newborn, gestational age 35 weeks, 0 days through 35 weeks, 6 days

P07.39 **Preterm newborn, gestational age 36 completed weeks**
Preterm newborn, gestational age 36 weeks, 0 days through 36 weeks, 6 days
Coding Clinic: 2017, Q3, P26

● P08 **Disorders of newborn related to long gestation and high birth weight**
Note: When both birth weight and gestational age of the newborn are available, priority of assignment should be given to birth weight.
Includes the listed conditions, without further specification, as causes of morbidity or additional care, in newborn

P08.0 **Exceptionally large newborn baby**
Usually implies a birth weight of 4500 g. or more
Excludes1 syndrome of infant of diabetic mother (P70.1)
syndrome of infant of mother with gestational diabetes (P70.0)

P08.1 **Other heavy for gestational age newborn**
Other newborn heavy- or large-for-dates regardless of period of gestation
Usually implies a birth weight of 4000 g. to 4499 g.
Excludes1 newborn with a birth weight of 4500 or more (P08.0)
syndrome of infant of diabetic mother (P70.1)
syndrome of infant of mother with gestational diabetes (P70.0)

● P08.2 **Late newborn, not heavy for gestational age**
P08.21 **Post-term newborn**
Newborn with gestation period over 40 completed weeks to 42 completed weeks

P08.22 **Prolonged gestation of newborn**
Newborn with gestation period over 42 completed weeks (294 days or more), not heavy- or large-for-dates
Postmaturity NOS

ABNORMAL FINDINGS ON NEONATAL SCREENING (P09)

● P09 **Abnormal findings on neonatal screening**
Use additional code to identify signs, symptoms and conditions associated with the screening
▶Includes: Abnormal findings on state mandated newborn screens
▶Failed newborn screening
Excludes2 nonspecific serologic evidence of human immunodeficiency virus [HIV] (R75)

▶P09.1 **Abnormal findings on neonatal screening for inborn errors of metabolism**

▶P09.2 **Abnormal findings on neonatal screening for congenital endocrine disease**
▶Abnormal findings on neonatal screening for congenital adrenal hyperplasia
▶Abnormal findings on neonatal screening for hypothyroidism screen

▶P09.3 **Abnormal findings on neonatal screening for congenital hematologic disorders**
▶Abnormal findings for hemoglobinothies screen
▶Abnormal findings on red cell membrane defects screen
▶Abnormal findings on sickle cell screen

▶P09.4 **Abnormal findings on neonatal screening for cystic fibrosis**

▶P09.5 **Abnormal findings on neonatal screening for critical congenital heart disease**
▶Neonatal congenital heart disease screening failure

▶P09.6 **Abnormal findings on neonatal screening for neonatal hearing loss**
▶**Excludes2** encounter for hearing examination following failed hearing screening (Z01.110)

▶P09.8 **Other abnormal findings on neonatal screening**

▶P09.9 **Abnormal findings on neonatal screening, unspecified**

BIRTH TRAUMA (P10-P15)

● P10 **Intracranial laceration and hemorrhage due to birth injury**
Excludes1 intracranial hemorrhage of newborn NOS (P52.9)
intracranial hemorrhage of newborn due to anoxia or hypoxia (P52.-)
nontraumatic intracranial hemorrhage of newborn (P52.-)
(Ex) **For category P10 CC codes unless otherwise indicated:** See PDX Collection 1020

P10.0 **Subdural hemorrhage due to birth injury** 🅗
Subdural hematoma (localized) due to birth injury
Excludes1 subdural hemorrhage accompanying tentorial tear (P10.4)

P10.1 **Cerebral hemorrhage due to birth injury** 🅗

P10.2 **Intraventricular hemorrhage due to birth injury** 🅒
(Ex) See PDX Collection 1021

P10.3 **Subarachnoid hemorrhage due to birth injury** 🅗
(Ex) See PDX Collection 1022

P10.4 **Tentorial tear due to birth injury** 🅗
Pertaining to tentorium of cerebellum (extension of dura mater that separates cerebellum from inferior portion of occipital lobes)

P10.8 **Other intracranial lacerations and hemorrhages due to birth injury** 🅗

P10.9 **Unspecified intracranial laceration and hemorrhage due to birth injury** 🅗

● P11 **Other birth injuries to central nervous system**
P11.0 **Cerebral edema due to birth injury** 🅗
(Ex) See PDX Collection 1020

P11.1 **Other specified brain damage due to birth injury**

P11.2 **Unspecified brain damage due to birth injury** 🅗
(Ex) See PDX Collection 1020

P11.3 **Birth injury to facial nerve**
Facial palsy due to birth injury

P11.4 **Birth injury to other cranial nerves**

P11.5 **Birth injury to spine and spinal cord**
Fracture of spine due to birth injury

P11.9 **Birth injury to central nervous system, unspecified** 🅗
(Ex) See PDX Collection 1020

● P12 **Birth injury to scalp**
P12.0 **Cephalhematoma due to birth injury**

P12.1 **Chignon (from vacuum extraction) due to birth injury**

P12.2 **Epicranial subaponeurotic hemorrhage due to birth injury** 🅒
Subgaleal hemorrhage
(Ex) See PDX Collection 1023

P12.3 **Bruising of scalp due to birth injury**

P12.4 **Injury of scalp of newborn due to monitoring equipment**
Sampling incision of scalp of newborn
Scalp clip (electrode) injury of newborn

● P12.8 **Other birth injuries to scalp**
P12.81 **Caput succedaneum**
P12.89 **Other birth injuries to scalp**

P12.9 **Birth injury to scalp, unspecified**

● P13 **Birth injury to skeleton**

N Newborn Age: 0   **P** Pediatric Age: 0–17   **M** Maternity DX: 9–64   **A** Adult Age: 15–124   ♀ Females Only   ♂ Males Only

🅒 Complication\Comorbidity   🅗 Major C\C   (Ex) CC/MCC Exclusions   🅗 Hospital-Acquired Condition   🅗 Hierarchical Condition Category

CHAPTER 16 (P00-P96)

Excludes2   birth injury to spine (P11.5)

P13.0   **Fracture of skull due to birth injury**

P13.1   **Other birth injuries to skull**

     Excludes1   cephalhematoma (P12.0)

P13.2   **Birth injury to femur**

P13.3   **Birth injury to other long bones**

P13.4   **Fracture of clavicle due to birth injury**

P13.8   **Birth injuries to other parts of skeleton**

P13.9   **Birth injury to skeleton, unspecified**

● P14   **Birth injury to peripheral nervous system**

P14.0   **Erb's paralysis due to birth injury**

P14.1   **Klumpke's paralysis due to birth injury**

P14.2   **Phrenic nerve paralysis due to birth injury**

P14.3   **Other brachial plexus birth injuries**

P14.8   **Birth injuries to other parts of peripheral nervous system**

P14.9   **Birth injury to peripheral nervous system, unspecified**

● P15   **Other birth injuries**

P15.0   **Birth injury to liver**

     Rupture of liver due to birth injury

P15.1   **Birth injury to spleen**

     Rupture of spleen due to birth injury

Item 16–1   The **peripheral nervous system** consists of 31 pairs of spinal nerves, 12 pairs of cranial nerves, and the autonomic nerves, which are divided into the parasympathetic and sympathetic nerves. The cranial nerves are: olfactory (I), optic (II), oculomotor (III), trochlear (IV), trigeminal (V), abducens (VI), facial (VII), vestibulocochlear (VIII), glossopharyngeal (IX), vagus (X), accessory (XI), and hypoglossal (XII).

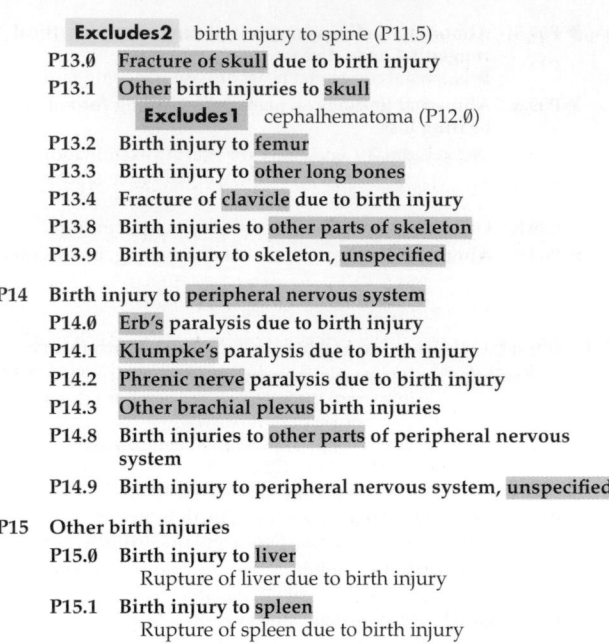
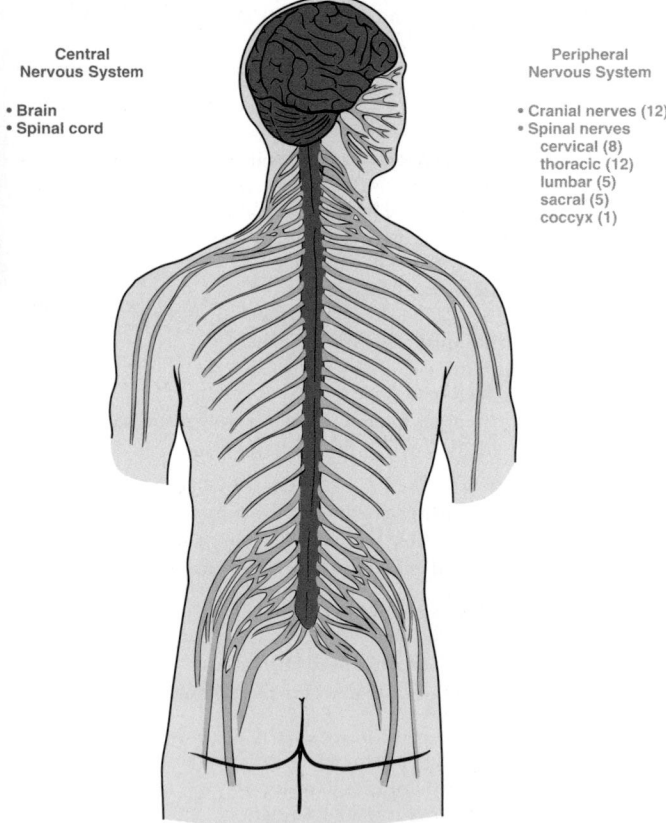

Central Nervous System

• Brain
• Spinal cord

Peripheral Nervous System

• Cranial nerves (12)
• Spinal nerves
   cervical (8)
   thoracic (12)
   lumbar (5)
   sacral (5)
   coccyx (1)

Figure 16-1   The central nervous system consists of the brain and spinal cord. The peripheral nervous system consists of nerves that lie outside the skull and spinal cord. (From Stoy: Mosby's EMT-Basic Textbook, ed 2, St. Louis, Mosby, 2007)

P15.2   **Sternomastoid injury due to birth injury**

P15.3   **Birth injury to eye**

     Subconjunctival hemorrhage due to birth injury

     Traumatic glaucoma due to birth injury

P15.4   **Birth injury to face**

     Facial congestion due to birth injury

P15.5   **Birth injury to external genitalia**

P15.6   **Subcutaneous fat necrosis due to birth injury**

P15.8   **Other specified birth injuries**

P15.9   **Birth injury, unspecified**

RESPIRATORY AND CARDIOVASCULAR DISORDERS SPECIFIC TO THE PERINATAL PERIOD (P19-P29)

● P19   **Metabolic acidemia in newborn**

     Includes   metabolic acidemia in newborn

P19.0   **Metabolic acidemia in newborn first noted before onset of labor**

P19.1   **Metabolic acidemia in newborn first noted during labor**

P19.2   **Metabolic acidemia noted at birth**

P19.9   **Metabolic acidemia, unspecified**

● P22   **Respiratory distress of newborn**

     Coding Clinic: 2019, Q2, P29

P22.0   **Respiratory distress syndrome of newborn** 🔖

     Cardiorespiratory distress syndrome of newborn

     Hyaline membrane disease

     Idiopathic respiratory distress syndrome [IRDS or RDS] of newborn

     Pulmonary hypoperfusion syndrome

     Respiratory distress syndrome, type I

     Excludes2   respiratory arrest of newborn (P28.81)

         respiratory failure of newborn NOS (P28.5)

     (Ex) See PDX Collection 748

     Coding Clinic: 2019, Q2, P29

P22.1   **Transient tachypnea of newborn**

     Idiopathic tachypnea of newborn

     Respiratory distress syndrome, type II

     Wet lung syndrome

P22.8   **Other respiratory distress of newborn**

     Excludes1   respiratory arrest of newborn (P28.81)

         respiratory failure of newborn NOS (P28.5)

P22.9   **Respiratory distress of newborn, unspecified**

     Excludes1   respiratory arrest of newborn (P28.81)

         respiratory failure of newborn NOS (P28.5)

● P23   **Congenital pneumonia**

     Includes   infective pneumonia acquired in utero or during birth

     Excludes1   neonatal pneumonia resulting from aspiration (P24.-)

     (Ex) **For category P23 CC codes:** See PDX Collection 748

P23.0   **Congenital pneumonia due to viral agent** 🔖

     Use additional code (B97) to identify organism

     Excludes1   congenital rubella pneumonitis (P35.0)

P23.1   **Congenital pneumonia due to Chlamydia** 🔖

P23.2   **Congenital pneumonia due to staphylococcus** 🔖

P23.3   **Congenital pneumonia due to streptococcus, group B** 🔖

P23.4   **Congenital pneumonia due to Escherichia coli** 🔖

P23.5   **Congenital pneumonia due to Pseudomonas** 🔖

P23.6   **Congenital pneumonia due to other bacterial agents** 🔖

     Congenital pneumonia due to Hemophilus influenzae

     Congenital pneumonia due to Klebsiella pneumoniae

     Congenital pneumonia due to Mycoplasma

     Congenital pneumonia due to Streptococcus, except group B

     Use additional code (B95-B96) to identify organism

P23.8   **Congenital pneumonia due to other organisms** 🔖

P23.9   **Congenital pneumonia, unspecified** 🔖

▶ New   ⇒ Revised   ~~deleted~~ Deleted   Excludes 1   Excludes 2   Includes   Use additional   Code first   Code also   Key words

OGCR Official Guidelines   ● Unacceptable Principal Diagnosis   X Assign placeholder X   ● Use Additional Character(s)   🔖 Manifestation Code   Coding Clinic

● **P24**   **Neonatal aspiration**
     Includes   aspiration in utero and during delivery

● **P24.0**   **Meconium aspiration**
     Excludes1   meconium passage (without aspiration)
           during delivery (P03.82)
           meconium staining (P96.83)

     P24.00   **Meconium aspiration without respiratory symptoms**
         Meconium aspiration NOS

     P24.01   **Meconium aspiration with respiratory symptoms** 🦠
         Meconium aspiration pneumonia
         Meconium aspiration pneumonitis
         Meconium aspiration syndrome NOS

         Use additional code to identify any secondary
         pulmonary hypertension, if applicable
         (I27.2-)
         (Ex:) See PDX Collection 748

● **P24.1**   **Neonatal aspiration of (clear) amniotic fluid and mucus**
     Neonatal aspiration of liquor (amnii)

     P24.10   **Neonatal aspiration of (clear) amniotic fluid and mucus without respiratory symptoms**
         Neonatal aspiration of amniotic fluid and mucus NOS

     P24.11   **Neonatal aspiration of (clear) amniotic fluid and mucus with respiratory symptoms** 🦠
         Neonatal aspiration of amniotic fluid and mucus with pneumonia
         Neonatal aspiration of amniotic fluid and mucus with pneumonitis

         Use additional code to identify any secondary
         pulmonary hypertension, if applicable
         (I27.2-)
         (Ex:) See PDX Collection 748

● **P24.2**   **Neonatal aspiration of blood**

     P24.20   **Neonatal aspiration of blood without respiratory symptoms**
         Neonatal aspiration of blood NOS

     P24.21   **Neonatal aspiration of blood with respiratory symptoms** 🦠
         Neonatal aspiration of blood with pneumonia
         Neonatal aspiration of blood with pneumonitis

         Use additional code to identify any secondary
         pulmonary hypertension, if applicable
         (I27.2-)
         (Ex:) See PDX Collection 748

● **P24.3**   **Neonatal aspiration of milk and regurgitated food**
     Neonatal aspiration of stomach contents

     P24.30   **Neonatal aspiration of milk and regurgitated food without respiratory symptoms**
         Neonatal aspiration of milk and regurgitated food NOS

     P24.31   **Neonatal aspiration of milk and regurgitated food with respiratory symptoms** 🦠
         Neonatal aspiration of milk and regurgitated food with pneumonia
         Neonatal aspiration of milk and regurgitated food with pneumonitis

         Use additional code to identify any secondary
         pulmonary hypertension, if applicable
         (I27.2-)
         (Ex:) See PDX Collection 748

● **P24.8**   **Other neonatal aspiration**

     P24.80   **Other neonatal aspiration without respiratory symptoms**
         Neonatal aspiration NEC

     P24.81   **Other neonatal aspiration with respiratory symptoms** 🦠
         Neonatal aspiration pneumonia NEC
         Neonatal aspiration with pneumonitis NEC
         Neonatal aspiration with pneumonia NOS
         Neonatal aspiration with pneumonitis NOS

         Use additional code to identify any secondary
         pulmonary hypertension, if applicable
         (I27.2-)
         (Ex:) See PDX Collection 748

     P24.9   **Neonatal aspiration, unspecified**

● **P25**   **Interstitial emphysema and related conditions originating in the perinatal period**
     (Ex:) For category P25 CC codes: See PDX Collection 748

     P25.0   **Interstitial emphysema originating in the perinatal period** 🦠

     P25.1   **Pneumothorax originating in the perinatal period** 🦠

     P25.2   **Pneumomediastinum originating in the perinatal period** 🦠

     P25.3   **Pneumopericardium originating in the perinatal period** 🦠

     P25.8   **Other conditions related to interstitial emphysema originating in the perinatal period** 🦠

● **P26**   **Pulmonary hemorrhage originating in the perinatal period**
     Excludes1   acute idiopathic hemorrhage in infants over 28 days old (R04.81)
     (Ex:) For category P26 CC codes: See PDX Collection 748

     P26.0   **Tracheobronchial hemorrhage originating in the perinatal period** 🦠

     P26.1   **Massive pulmonary hemorrhage originating in the perinatal period** 🦠

     P26.8   **Other pulmonary hemorrhages originating in the perinatal period** 🦠

     P26.9   **Unspecified pulmonary hemorrhage originating in the perinatal period** 🦠

● **P27**   **Chronic respiratory disease originating in the perinatal period**
     Excludes2   respiratory distress of newborn (P22.0-P22.9)
     (Ex:) For category P27 CC codes: See PDX Collection 748

     P27.0   **Wilson-Mikity syndrome** 🦠
         Pulmonary dysmaturity

     P27.1   **Bronchopulmonary dysplasia originating in the perinatal period** 🦠

     P27.8   **Other chronic respiratory diseases originating in the perinatal period** 🦠
         Congenital pulmonary fibrosis
         Ventilator lung in newborn

     P27.9   **Unspecified chronic respiratory disease originating in the perinatal period** 🦠

● **P28**   **Other respiratory conditions originating in the perinatal period**
     Excludes1   congenital malformations of the respiratory system (Q30-Q34)

     P28.0   **Primary atelectasis of newborn** 🦠
         Failure of lungs to expand properly at birth
         Primary failure to expand terminal respiratory units
         Pulmonary hypoplasia associated with short gestation
         Pulmonary immaturity NOS
         (Ex:) See PDX Collection 748

● **P28.1**   **Other and unspecified atelectasis of newborn**
     (Ex:) For category P28.1 CC codes: See PDX Collection 748

     P28.10   **Unspecified atelectasis of newborn** 🦠
         Atelectasis of newborn NOS

     P28.11   **Resorption atelectasis without respiratory distress syndrome** 🦠
         Excludes1   resorption atelectasis with respiratory distress syndrome (P22.0)

     P28.19   **Other atelectasis of newborn** 🦠
         Partial atelectasis of newborn
         Secondary atelectasis of newborn

     P28.2   **Cyanotic attacks of newborn** 🦠
         Excludes1   apnea of newborn (P28.3-P28.4)
         (Ex:) See PDX Collection 1024

     P28.3   **Primary sleep apnea of newborn** 🦠
         Central sleep apnea of newborn
         Obstructive sleep apnea of newborn
         Sleep apnea of newborn NOS
         (Ex:) See PDX Collection 1025

     P28.4   **Other apnea of newborn** 🦠
         Apnea of prematurity
         Obstructive apnea of newborn
         Excludes1   obstructive sleep apnea of newborn (P28.3)
         (Ex:) See PDX Collection 1026

N Newborn Age: 0   **P** Pediatric Age: 0–17   **M** Maternity DX: 9–64   **A** Adult Age: 15–124   ♀ Females Only   ♂ Males Only

🦠 Complication\Comorbidity   🦠 Major C\C   (Ex:) CC/MCC Exclusions   🦠 Hospital-Acquired Condition   🦠 Hierarchical Condition Category

1193

CHAPTER 16 (P00-P96)

P28.5 **Respiratory failure of newborn** 🔊
  Excludes1 respiratory arrest of newborn (P28.81)
  respiratory distress of newborn (P22.0-)
  Ⓔ See PDX Collection 748
  Coding Clinic: 2019, Q2, P29

● **P28.8** **Other specified respiratory conditions of newborn**
  P28.81 **Respiratory arrest of newborn** 🔊
    Ⓔ See PDX Collection 1027
    Coding Clinic: 2017, Q2, P6

  P28.89 **Other specified respiratory conditions of newborn**
    Congenital laryngeal stridor
    Sniffles in newborn
    Snuffles in newborn
    Excludes1 early congenital syphilitic
    rhinitis (A50.05)

P28.9 **Respiratory condition of newborn, unspecified**
    Respiratory depression in newborn

● **P29** **Cardiovascular disorders originating in the perinatal period**
  ~~**Excludes1** congenital malformations of the circulatory system (Q20-Q28)~~
  ▶ **Excludes2** congenital malformations of the circulatory
    system (Q20-Q28)

  P29.0 **Neonatal cardiac failure**
● **P29.1** **Neonatal cardiac dysrhythmia**
    P29.11 **Neonatal tachycardia**
    P29.12 **Neonatal bradycardia**
  P29.2 **Neonatal hypertension**
● **P29.3** **Persistent fetal circulation**
    P29.30 **Pulmonary hypertension of newborn** 🔊
      Persistent pulmonary hypertension of newborn
      Ⓔ See PDX Collection 3959
    P29.38 **Other persistent fetal circulation** 🔊
      Delayed closure of ductus arteriosus
      Ⓔ See PDX Collection 1028
  P29.4 **Transient myocardial ischemia in newborn**
● **P29.8** **Other cardiovascular disorders originating in the perinatal period**
    P29.81 **Cardiac arrest of newborn** 🔊
      Ⓔ See PDX Collection 1029
    P29.89 **Other cardiovascular disorders originating in the perinatal period**
  P29.9 **Cardiovascular disorder originating in the perinatal period, unspecified**

INFECTIONS SPECIFIC TO THE PERINATAL PERIOD (P35-P39)
  Infections acquired in utero, during birth via the umbilicus, or
    during the first 28 days after birth
  Excludes2 asymptomatic human immunodeficiency virus
    [HIV] infection status (Z21)
    congenital gonococcal infection (A54.-)
    congenital pneumonia (P23.-)
    congenital syphilis (A50.-)
    human immunodeficiency virus [HIV] disease (B20)
    infant botulism (A48.51)
    infectious diseases not specific to the perinatal
      period (A00-B99, J09, J10.-)
    intestinal infectious disease (A00 A09)
    laboratory evidence of human immunodeficiency
      virus [HIV] (R75)
    tetanus neonatorum (A33)

● **P35** **Congenital viral diseases**
  Includes infections acquired in utero or during birth
  Ⓔ For category P35 CC codes unless otherwise indicated: See PDX Collection 4049
  P35.0 **Congenital rubella syndrome** 🔊
    Congenital rubella pneumonitis
    Ⓔ See PDX Collection 1030
  P35.1 **Congenital cytomegalovirus infection** 🔊
    *Viruses transmitted by multiple routes that cause mild/
      subclinical infection*
    Ⓔ See PDX Collection 1030
  P35.2 **Congenital herpesviral [herpes simplex] infection** 🔊

P35.3 **Congenital viral hepatitis** 🔊
P35.4 **Congenital Zika virus disease** 🔊
    Use additional code to identify manifestations of
      congenital Zika virus disease
    Coding Clinic: 2018, Q4, P26
P35.8 **Other congenital viral diseases** 🔊
    Congenital varicella [chickenpox]
    Coding Clinic: 2016, Q4, P7
P35.9 **Congenital viral disease, unspecified** 🔊

● **P36** **Bacterial sepsis of newborn**
  Includes congenital sepsis
  Use additional code(s), if applicable, to identify severe sepsis
    (R65.2-) and associated acute organ dysfunction(s)
  Ⓔ For category P36 CC codes: See PDX Collection 1031
  P36.0 **Sepsis of newborn due to streptococcus, group B** 🔊🔊
● **P36.1** **Sepsis of newborn due to other and unspecified streptococci**
    P36.10 **Sepsis of newborn due to unspecified streptococci** 🔊🔊
    P36.19 **Sepsis of newborn due to other streptococci** 🔊🔊
  P36.2 **Sepsis of newborn due to Staphylococcus aureus** 🔊🔊
● **P36.3** **Sepsis of newborn due to other and unspecified staphylococci**
    P36.30 **Sepsis of newborn due to unspecified staphylococci** 🔊🔊
    P36.39 **Sepsis of newborn due to other staphylococci** 🔊🔊
  P36.4 **Sepsis of newborn due to Escherichia coli** 🔊🔊
  P36.5 **Sepsis of newborn due to anaerobes** 🔊🔊
  P36.8 **Other bacterial sepsis of newborn** 🔊🔊
    Use additional code from category B96 to identify
      organism
  P36.9 **Bacterial sepsis of newborn, unspecified** 🔊🔊

● **P37** **Other congenital infectious and parasitic diseases**
  Excludes2 congenital syphilis (A50.-)
    infectious neonatal diarrhea (A00-A09)
    necrotizing enterocolitis in newborn (P77.-)
    noninfectious neonatal diarrhea (P78.3)
    ophthalmia neonatorum due to gonococcus
      (A54.31)
    tetanus neonatorum (A33)
  Ⓔ For category P37 CC codes: See PDX Collection 562
  P37.0 **Congenital tuberculosis** 🔊
    Ⓔ See PDX Collection 4049
  P37.1 **Congenital toxoplasmosis** 🔊
    Parasitic infection, often causing mild flu-like illness
    Hydrocephalus due to congenital toxoplasmosis
  P37.2 **Neonatal (disseminated) listeriosis** 🔊
    *Acquired transplacentally or during/after parturition in
      which symptoms are those of sepsis*
  P37.3 **Congenital falciparum malaria** 🔊
  P37.4 **Other congenital malaria** 🔊
  P37.5 **Neonatal candidiasis**
  P37.8 **Other specified congenital infectious and parasitic diseases** 🔊
  P37.9 **Congenital infectious or parasitic disease, unspecified** 🔊

● **P38** **Omphalitis of newborn**
  Inflammation of umbilicus
  Excludes1 omphalitis not of newborn (L08.82)
    tetanus omphalitis (A33)
    umbilical hemorrhage of newborn (P51.-)
  P38.1 **Omphalitis with mild hemorrhage** 🔊
    Ⓔ See PDX Collection 3961
  P38.9 **Omphalitis without hemorrhage** 🔊
    Omphalitis of newborn NOS
    Ⓔ See PDX Collection 3963

▶ New ⇒ Revised ~~deleted~~ Deleted Excludes 1 Excludes 2 Includes Use additional Code first Code also Key words
OGCR Official Guidelines ● Unacceptable Principal Diagnosis X Assign placeholder X ● Use Additional Character(s) ▶ Manifestation Code Coding Clinic

● **P39**　**Other infections specific to the perinatal period**
　　　Use additional code to identify organism or specific infection
　　　(Ex:) **For category P39 CC codes unless otherwise indicated:** See PDX Collection 1033

　　P39.0　**Neonatal infective mastitis** 🦠
　　　　　Excludes1　breast engorgement of newborn (P83.4)
　　　　　　　　　　　noninfective mastitis of newborn (P83.4)
　　　　　(Ex:) See PDX Collection 1032

　　P39.1　**Neonatal conjunctivitis and dacryocystitis**
　　　　　Neonatal chlamydial conjunctivitis
　　　　　Ophthalmia neonatorum NOS
　　　　　　Neonate – newborn
　　　　　Excludes1　gonococcal conjunctivitis (A54.31)

　　P39.2　**Intra-amniotic infection affecting newborn, not elsewhere classified** 🦠

　　P39.3　**Neonatal urinary tract infection** 🦠
　　　　　(Ex:) See PDX Collection 1034

　　P39.4　**Neonatal skin infection** 🦠
　　　　　Neonatal pyoderma
　　　　　Excludes1　pemphigus neonatorum (L00)
　　　　　　　　　　　staphylococcal scalded skin syndrome (L00)

　　P39.8　**Other specified infections specific to the perinatal period** 🦠

　　P39.9　**Infection specific to the perinatal period, unspecified** 🦠

HEMORRHAGIC AND HEMATOLOGICAL DISORDERS OF NEWBORN (P50-P61)

　　Excludes1　congenital stenosis and stricture of bile ducts (Q44.3)
　　　　　　　Crigler-Najjar syndrome (E80.5)
　　　　　　　Dubin-Johnson syndrome (E80.6)
　　　　　　　Gilbert syndrome (E80.4)
　　　　　　　hereditary hemolytic anemias (D55-D58)

● **P50**　**Newborn affected by intrauterine (fetal) blood loss**
　　　　　Excludes1　congenital anemia from intrauterine (fetal) blood loss (P61.3)

　　P50.0　**Newborn affected by intrauterine (fetal) blood loss from vasa previa**

　　P50.1　**Newborn affected by intrauterine (fetal) blood loss from ruptured cord**

　　P50.2　**Newborn affected by intrauterine (fetal) blood loss from placenta**

　　P50.3　**Newborn affected by hemorrhage into co-twin**

　　P50.4　**Newborn affected by hemorrhage into maternal circulation**

　　P50.5　**Newborn affected by intrauterine (fetal) blood loss from cut end of co-twin's cord**

　　P50.8　**Newborn affected by other intrauterine (fetal) blood loss**

　　P50.9　**Newborn affected by intrauterine (fetal) blood loss, unspecified**
　　　　　Newborn affected by fetal hemorrhage NOS

● **P51**　**Umbilical hemorrhage of newborn**
　　　　　Excludes1　omphalitis with mild hemorrhage (P38.1)
　　　　　　　　　　　umbilical hemorrhage from cut end of co-twins cord (P50.5)

　　P51.0　**Massive umbilical hemorrhage of newborn**

　　P51.8　**Other umbilical hemorrhages of newborn**
　　　　　Slipped umbilical ligature NOS

　　P51.9　**Umbilical hemorrhage of newborn, unspecified**

● **P52**　**Intracranial nontraumatic hemorrhage of newborn**
　　　　　Includes　intracranial hemorrhage due to anoxia or hypoxia
　　　　　Excludes1　intracranial hemorrhage due to birth injury (P10.-)
　　　　　　　　　　　intracranial hemorrhage due to other injury (S06.-)

　　P52.0　**Intraventricular (nontraumatic) hemorrhage, grade 1, of newborn** 🦠
　　　　　Subependymal hemorrhage (without intraventricular extension)
　　　　　Bleeding into germinal matrix
　　　　　(Ex:) See PDX Collection 1021

　　P52.1　**Intraventricular (nontraumatic) hemorrhage, grade 2, of newborn** 🦠
　　　　　Subependymal hemorrhage with intraventricular extension
　　　　　Bleeding into ventricle
　　　　　(Ex:) See PDX Collection 1021

● **P52.2**　**Intraventricular (nontraumatic) hemorrhage, grade 3 and grade 4, of newborn**

　　P52.21　**Intraventricular (nontraumatic) hemorrhage, grade 3, of newborn** 🦠
　　　　　Subependymal hemorrhage with intraventricular extension with enlargement of ventricle
　　　　　(Ex:) See PDX Collection 1021

　　P52.22　**Intraventricular (nontraumatic) hemorrhage, grade 4, of newborn** 🦠
　　　　　Bleeding into cerebral cortex
　　　　　Subependymal hemorrhage with intracerebral extension
　　　　　(Ex:) See PDX Collection 1021

　　P52.3　**Unspecified intraventricular (nontraumatic) hemorrhage of newborn** 🦠
　　　　　(Ex:) See PDX Collection 1021

　　P52.4　**Intracerebral (nontraumatic) hemorrhage of newborn** 🦠
　　　　　(Ex:) See PDX Collection 1020

　　P52.5　**Subarachnoid (nontraumatic) hemorrhage of newborn** 🦠
　　　　　(Ex:) See PDX Collection 1022

　　P52.6　**Cerebellar (nontraumatic) and posterior fossa hemorrhage of newborn** 🦠
　　　　　(Ex:) See PDX Collection 1020

　　P52.8　**Other intracranial (nontraumatic) hemorrhages of newborn** 🦠
　　　　　(Ex:) See PDX Collection 1020

　　P52.9　**Intracranial (nontraumatic) hemorrhage of newborn, unspecified** 🦠
　　　　　(Ex:) See PDX Collection 1020

○ **P53**　**Hemorrhagic disease of newborn** 🦠
　　　　　Vitamin K deficiency of newborn
　　　　　(Ex:) See PDX Collection 1035

● **P54**　**Other neonatal hemorrhages**
　　　　　Excludes1　newborn affected by (intrauterine) blood loss (P50.-)
　　　　　　　　　　　pulmonary hemorrhage originating in the perinatal period (P26.-)

　　P54.0　**Neonatal hematemesis**
　　　　　Vomiting of blood
　　　　　Excludes1　neonatal hematemesis due to swallowed maternal blood (P78.2)

　　P54.1　**Neonatal melena** 🦠
　　　　　Dark-colored feces stained with blood pigments
　　　　　Excludes1　neonatal melena due to swallowed maternal blood (P78.2)
　　　　　(Ex:) See PDX Collection 1036

　　P54.2　**Neonatal rectal hemorrhage** 🦠
　　　　　(Ex:) See PDX Collection 1036

　　P54.3　**Other neonatal gastrointestinal hemorrhage** 🦠
　　　　　(Ex:) See PDX Collection 1036

　　P54.4　**Neonatal adrenal hemorrhage** 🦠
　　　　　(Ex:) See PDX Collection 1036

　　P54.5　**Neonatal cutaneous hemorrhage**
　　　　　Neonatal bruising
　　　　　Neonatal ecchymoses
　　　　　Neonatal petechiae
　　　　　Neonatal superficial hematomata
　　　　　Excludes2　bruising of scalp due to birth injury (P12.3)
　　　　　　　　　　　cephalhematoma due to birth injury (P12.0)

　　P54.6　**Neonatal vaginal hemorrhage** ♀
　　　　　Neonatal pseudomenses

　　P54.8　**Other specified neonatal hemorrhages**

　　P54.9　**Neonatal hemorrhage, unspecified**

N Newborn Age: 0　　**P** Pediatric Age: 0 17　　**M** Maternity DX: 9–64　　**A** Adult Age: 15–124　　♀ Females Only　　♂ Males Only

🦠 Complication\Comorbidity　　🦠 Major C\C　　(Ex:) CC/MCC Exclusions　　🦠 Hospital-Acquired Condition　　🦠 Hierarchical Condition Category

1195

CHAPTER 16 (P00-P96)

● **P55 Hemolytic disease of newborn**
AKA erythroblastosis fetalis and is due to Rh isoimmunization, result of Rh blood factor incompatibilities between mother (Rh negative) and fetus (Rh positive)

P55.0 Rh isoimmunization of newborn

P55.1 ABO isoimmunization of newborn
Coding Clinic: 2015, Q3, P20

P55.8 Other hemolytic diseases of newborn

P55.9 Hemolytic disease of newborn, unspecified

● **P56 Hydrops fetalis due to hemolytic disease**
Caused by maternal sensitization to fetal blood group antigen

Excludes1 hydrops fetalis NOS (P83.2)

(Ex:) For category P56 CC codes: See PDX Collection 1037

P56.0 Hydrops fetalis due to isoimmunization

● P56.9 Hydrops fetalis due to other and unspecified hemolytic disease

P56.90 Hydrops fetalis due to unspecified hemolytic disease

P56.99 Hydrops fetalis due to other hemolytic disease

● **P57 Kernicterus**
High levels of bilirubin in blood, with severe neural symptoms

(Ex:) For category P57 CC codes unless otherwise indicated: See PDX Collection 1038

P57.0 Kernicterus due to isoimmunization
(Ex:) See PDX Collection 1037

P57.8 Other specified kernicterus
Excludes1 Crigler-Najjar syndrome (E80.5)

P57.9 Kernicterus, unspecified

● **P58 Neonatal jaundice due to other excessive hemolysis**
Excludes1 jaundice due to isoimmunization (P55-P57)

P58.0 Neonatal jaundice due to bruising

P58.1 Neonatal jaundice due to bleeding

P58.2 Neonatal jaundice due to infection

P58.3 Neonatal jaundice due to polycythemia

● P58.4 Neonatal jaundice due to drugs or toxins transmitted from mother or given to newborn
Code first poisoning due to drug or toxin, if applicable (T36-T65 with fifth or sixth character 1-4 or 6)
Use additional code for adverse effect, if applicable, to identify drug (T36-T50 with fifth or sixth character 5)

● P58.41 Neonatal jaundice due to drugs or toxins transmitted from mother

● P58.42 Neonatal jaundice due to drugs or toxins given to newborn

P58.5 Neonatal jaundice due to swallowed maternal blood

P58.8 Neonatal jaundice due to other specified excessive hemolysis

P58.9 Neonatal jaundice due to excessive hemolysis, unspecified

● **P59 Neonatal jaundice from other and unspecified causes**
Excludes1 jaundice due to inborn errors of metabolism (E70-E88)
kernicterus (P57.-)

P59.0 Neonatal jaundice associated with preterm delivery
Hyperbilirubinemia of prematurity
Jaundice due to delayed conjugation associated with preterm delivery

P59.1 Inspissated bile syndrome
(Ex:) See PDX Collection 1038

● P59.2 Neonatal jaundice from other and unspecified hepatocellular damage
Excludes1 congenital viral hepatitis (P35.3)
(Ex:) For category P59.2 CC codes unless otherwise indicated: See PDX Collection 1038

P59.20 Neonatal jaundice from unspecified hepatocellular damage

P59.29 Neonatal jaundice from other hepatocellular damage
Neonatal giant cell hepatitis
Neonatal (idiopathic) hepatitis

P59.3 Neonatal jaundice from breast milk inhibitor

P59.8 Neonatal jaundice from other specified causes

P59.9 Neonatal jaundice, unspecified
Neonatal physiological jaundice (intense)(prolonged) NOS
Coding Clinic: 2015, Q3, P20

P60 Disseminated intravascular coagulation of newborn
Defibrination syndrome of newborn
(Ex:) See PDX Collection 1035

● **P61 Other perinatal hematological disorders**
Excludes1 transient hypogammaglobulinemia of infancy (D80.7)

P61.0 Transient neonatal thrombocytopenia
Lack of sufficient numbers of circulating thrombocytes (platelets)
Neonatal thrombocytopenia due to exchange transfusion
Neonatal thrombocytopenia due to idiopathic maternal thrombocytopenia
Neonatal thrombocytopenia due to isoimmunization
(Ex:) See PDX Collection 1035

P61.1 Polycythemia neonatorum
Neonate = newborn

P61.2 Anemia of prematurity
(Ex:) See PDX Collection 1039

P61.3 Congenital anemia from fetal blood loss
(Ex:) See PDX Collection 1039

P61.4 Other congenital anemias, not elsewhere classified
Congenital anemia NOS
(Ex:) See PDX Collection 1039

P61.5 Transient neonatal neutropenia
Low levels of granulocytic neutrophilic white blood cells
Excludes1 congenital neutropenia (nontransient) (D70.0)
(Ex:) See PDX Collection 1040

P61.6 Other transient neonatal disorders of coagulation
(Ex:) See PDX Collection 1035

P61.8 Other specified perinatal hematological disorders

P61.9 Perinatal hematological disorder, unspecified

TRANSITORY ENDOCRINE AND METABOLIC DISORDERS SPECIFIC TO NEWBORN (P70-P74)

Includes transitory endocrine and metabolic disturbances caused by the infant's response to maternal endocrine and metabolic factors, or its adjustment to extrauterine environment

● **P70 Transitory disorders of carbohydrate metabolism specific to newborn**

P70.0 Syndrome of infant of mother with gestational diabetes
Newborn (with hypoglycemia) affected by maternal gestational diabetes
Excludes1 newborn (with hypoglycemia) affected by maternal (pre-existing) diabetes mellitus (P70.1)
syndrome of infant of a diabetic mother (P70.1)

P70.1 Syndrome of infant of a diabetic mother
Newborn (with hypoglycemia) affected by maternal (pre-existing) diabetes mellitus
Excludes1 newborn (with hypoglycemia) affected by maternal gestational diabetes (P70.0)
syndrome of infant of mother with gestational diabetes (P70.0)

P70.2 Neonatal diabetes mellitus
(Ex:) See PDX Collection 1041

P70.3 Iatrogenic neonatal hypoglycemia

P70.4 Other neonatal hypoglycemia
Transitory neonatal hypoglycemia

P70.8 Other transitory disorders of carbohydrate metabolism of newborn
(Ex:) See PDX Collection 3458

P70.9 Transitory disorder of carbohydrate metabolism of newborn, unspecified

▶ New　⮕ Revised　deleted Deleted　Excludes 1　Excludes 2　Includes　Use additional　Code first　Code also　Key words
OGCR Official Guidelines　● Unacceptable Principal Diagnosis　X Assign placeholder X　● Use Additional Character(s)　▶ Manifestation Code　Coding Clinic

● **P71** Transitory neonatal disorders of calcium and magnesium metabolism
    Ⓔₓ **For category P71 CC codes:** See PDX Collection 1041

    P71.0 Cow's milk hypocalcemia in newborn ◔

    P71.1 Other neonatal hypocalcemia ◔
        Excludes1 neonatal hypoparathyroidism (P71.4)

    P71.2 Neonatal hypomagnesemia ◔

    P71.3 Neonatal tetany without calcium or magnesium deficiency ◔
        Neonatal tetany NOS

    P71.4 Transitory neonatal hypoparathyroidism ◔

    P71.8 Other transitory neonatal disorders of calcium and magnesium metabolism ◔
        Coding Clinic: 2016, Q4, P55

    P71.9 Transitory neonatal disorder of calcium and magnesium metabolism, unspecified ◔

● **P72** Other transitory neonatal endocrine disorders
    Excludes1 congenital hypothyroidism with or without goiter (E03.0-E03.1)
             dyshormogenetic goiter (E07.1)
             Pendred's syndrome (E07.1)
    Ⓔₓ **For category P72 CC codes unless otherwise noted:** See PDX Collection 1042

    P72.0 Neonatal goiter, not elsewhere classified ◔
        Transitory congenital goiter with normal functioning
        Ⓔₓ See PDX Collection 3459

    P72.1 Transitory neonatal hyperthyroidism ◔
        Neonatal thyrotoxicosis
        Ⓔₓ See PDX Collection 1041

    P72.2 Other transitory neonatal disorders of thyroid function, not elsewhere classified ◔
        Ⓔₓ See PDX Collection 3460
        Transitory neonatal hypothyroidism

    P72.8 Other specified transitory neonatal endocrine disorders ◔
        Ⓔₓ See PDX Collection 3461

    P72.9 Transitory neonatal endocrine disorder, unspecified

● **P74** Other transitory neonatal electrolyte and metabolic disturbances
    P74.0 Late metabolic acidosis of newborn ◔
        Excludes1 (fetal) metabolic acidosis of newborn (P19)
        Ⓔₓ See PDX Collection 1041

    P74.1 Dehydration of newborn

  ● P74.2 Disturbances of sodium balance of newborn
        Coding Clinic: 2018, Q2, P6

        P74.21 Hypernatremia of newborn
        P74.22 Hyponatremia of newborn

  ● P74.3 Disturbances of potassium balance of newborn
        P74.31 Hyperkalemia of newborn
        P74.32 Hypokalemia of newborn

  ● P74.4 Other transitory electrolyte disturbances of newborn
        P74.41 Alkalosis of newborn ◔
            Hyperbicarbonatemia
            Ⓔₓ See PDX Collection 1042

      ● P74.42 Disturbances of chlorine balance of newborn
            P74.421 Hyperchloremia of newborn
                 Hyperchloremic metabolic acidosis
                 Excludes2 late metabolic acidosis of the newborn (P74.0)
            P74.422 Hypochloremia of newborn

        P74.49 Other transitory electrolyte disturbance of newborn

    P74.5 Transitory tyrosinemia of newborn ◔
        Ⓔₓ See PDX Collection 3462

    P74.6 Transitory hyperammonemia of newborn ◔
        Ⓔₓ See PDX Collection 3463

    P74.8 Other transitory metabolic disturbances of newborn ◔
        Amino-acid metabolic disorders described as transitory
        Ⓔₓ See PDX Collection 3464

    P74.9 Transitory metabolic disturbance of newborn, unspecified

DIGESTIVE SYSTEM DISORDERS OF NEWBORN (P76-P78)

● **P76** Other intestinal obstruction of newborn
    P76.0 Meconium plug syndrome
        Fetal stool obstruction in large intestine, present at birth; may be symptom of organic disease.
        Meconium ileus NOS
        Excludes1 meconium ileus in cystic fibrosis (E84.11)

    P76.1 Transitory ileus of newborn ◔
        Temporary obstruction of ileus (small intestine)
        Excludes1 Hirschsprung's disease (Q43.1)
        Ⓔₓ See PDX Collection 1043

    P76.2 Intestinal obstruction due to inspissated milk
        Being thickened, dried, or made less fluid

    P76.8 Other specified intestinal obstruction of newborn
        Excludes1 intestinal obstruction classifiable to K56.-

    P76.9 Intestinal obstruction of newborn, unspecified

● **P77** Necrotizing enterocolitis of newborn
    Ⓔₓ **For category P77 CC codes:** See PDX Collection 1044

    P77.1 Stage 1 necrotizing enterocolitis in newborn ◔
        Necrotizing enterocolitis without pneumatosis, without perforation

    P77.2 Stage 2 necrotizing enterocolitis in newborn ◔
        Necrotizing enterocolitis with pneumatosis, without perforation

    P77.3 Stage 3 necrotizing enterocolitis in newborn ◔
        Necrotizing enterocolitis with perforation
        Necrotizing enterocolitis with pneumatosis and perforation

    P77.9 Necrotizing enterocolitis in newborn, unspecified ◔
        Necrotizing enterocolitis in newborn, NOS

● **P78** Other perinatal digestive system disorders
    Excludes1 cystic fibrosis (E84.0-E84.9)
             neonatal gastrointestinal hemorrhages (P54.0-P54.3)

    P78.0 Perinatal intestinal perforation ◔
        Meconium peritonitis
        Ⓔₓ See PDX Collection 1044

    P78.1 Other neonatal peritonitis
        Neonatal peritonitis NOS

    P78.2 Neonatal hematemesis and melena due to swallowed maternal blood

    P78.3 Noninfective neonatal diarrhea
        Neonatal diarrhea NOS

  ● P78.8 Other specified perinatal digestive system disorders
        P78.81 Congenital cirrhosis (of liver)
        P78.82 Peptic ulcer of newborn
        P78.83 Newborn esophageal reflux
            Neonatal esophageal reflux
        P78.84 Gestational alloimmune liver disease
            GALD
            Neonatal hemochromatosis
            Excludes1 hemochromatosis (E83.11-)
        P78.89 Other specified perinatal digestive system disorders

    P78.9 Perinatal digestive system disorder, unspecified

N Newborn Age: 0 **P** Pediatric Age: 0–17 **M** Maternity DX: 9–64 **A** Adult Age: 15–124 ♀ Females Only ♂ Males Only

◔ Complication\Comorbidity ◕ Major C\C Ⓔₓ CC/MCC Exclusions ◔ Hospital-Acquired Condition ● Hierarchical Condition Category

CHAPTER 16 (P00-P96)

1197

CONDITIONS INVOLVING THE INTEGUMENT AND TEMPERATURE REGULATION OF NEWBORN (P80-P83)

● **P80   Hypothermia of newborn**

   P80.0   Cold injury syndrome
            Severe and usually chronic hypothermia associated
               with a pink flushed appearance, edema and
               neurological and biochemical abnormalities.
            Excludes1   mild hypothermia of newborn (P80.8)

   P80.8   Other hypothermia of newborn
            Mild hypothermia of newborn

   P80.9   Hypothermia of newborn, unspecified

● **P81   Other disturbances of temperature regulation of newborn**

   P81.0   Environmental hyperthermia of newborn

   **P81.8   Other specified disturbances of temperature regulation
            of newborn**

   **P81.9   Disturbance of temperature regulation of newborn,
            unspecified**
            Fever of newborn NOS

● **P83   Other conditions of integument specific to newborn**
            Excludes1   congenital malformations of skin and integument
                        (Q80-Q84)
                        hydrops fetalis due to hemolytic disease (P56.-)
                        neonatal skin infection (P39.4)
                        staphylococcal scalded skin syndrome (L00)
            Excludes2   cradle cap (L21.0)
                        diaper [napkin] dermatitis (L22)

   P83.0   Sclerema neonatorum 🅲
            Neonate = newborn
            (Ex:) See PDX Collection 1045

   P83.1   Neonatal erythema toxicum
            *Benign, generalized, transient pustules that become firm
               vesicles*

   P83.2   Hydrops fetalis not due to hemolytic disease 🅲
            *Severe, life-threatening problem of severe edema (swelling)
               as a result of too much fluid leaving blood and entering
               tissue*
            Hydrops fetalis NOS
            (Ex:) See PDX Collection 1046

● **P83.3   Other and unspecified edema specific to newborn**
            (Ex:) **For category P83.3 CC codes:** See PDX Collection 1047

      P83.30   Unspecified edema specific to newborn 🅲
      P83.39   Other edema specific to newborn 🅲

   P83.4   Breast engorgement of newborn
            Noninfective mastitis of newborn

   P83.5   Congenital hydrocele ♂

   P83.6   Umbilical polyp of newborn

● **P83.8   Other specified conditions of integument specific to
            newborn**

      P83.81   Umbilical granuloma
               Excludes2   Granulomatous disorder of the
                           skin and subcutaneous
                           tissue, unspecified (L92.9)

      **P83.88   Other specified conditions of integument
               specific to newborn**
               Bronze baby syndrome
               Neonatal scleroderma
               Urticaria neonatorum

   **P83.9   Condition of the integument specific to newborn,
            unspecified**

OTHER PROBLEMS WITH NEWBORN (P84)

P84   Other problems with newborn
      Acidemia of newborn
      Acidosis of newborn
      Anoxia of newborn NOS
      Asphyxia of newborn NOS
      Hypercapnia of newborn
      Hypoxemia of newborn
      Hypoxia of newborn NOS
      Mixed metabolic and respiratory acidosis of newborn
      Excludes1   intracranial hemorrhage due to anoxia or hypoxia
                  (P52.-)
                  hypoxic ischemic encephalopathy [HIE] (P91.6-)
                  late metabolic acidosis of newborn (P74.0)

OTHER DISORDERS ORIGINATING IN THE PERINATAL PERIOD (P90-P96)

P90   Convulsions of newborn 🅲
      Excludes1   benign myoclonic epilepsy in infancy (G40.3-)
                  benign neonatal convulsions (familial) (G40.3-)
      (Ex:) See PDX Collection 1048

● **P91   Other disturbances of cerebral status of newborn**

   P91.0   Neonatal cerebral ischemia 🅲
            Excludes1   Neonatal cerebral infarction (P91.82-)
            (Ex:) See PDX Collection 1049

   P91.1   Acquired periventricular cysts of newborn 🅲
            (Ex:) See PDX Collection 1049

   P91.2   Neonatal cerebral leukomalacia 🅲
            *Degeneration of white matter adjacent to cerebral ventricles
               following cerebral hypoxia or brain ischemia in neonates*
            Periventricular leukomalacia
            (Ex:) See PDX Collection 1022

   P91.3   Neonatal cerebral irritability 🅲
            (Ex:) See PDX Collection 1049

   P91.4   Neonatal cerebral depression 🅲
            (Ex:) See PDX Collection 1049

   P91.5   Neonatal coma 🅲
            (Ex:) See PDX Collection 1049

● **P91.6   Hypoxic ischemic encephalopathy [HIE]**
            Excludes1   Neonatal cerebral depression (P91.4)
                        Neonatal cerebral irritability (P91.3)
                        Neonatal coma (P91.5)
            (Ex:) **For category P91.6 CC codes:** See PDX Collection 1050

      **P91.60   Hypoxic ischemic encephalopathy [HIE],
               unspecified** 🅲
      **P91.61   Mild hypoxic ischemic encephalopathy
               [HIE]** 🅲
      **P91.62   Moderate hypoxic ischemic encephalopathy
               [HIE]** 🅲
      **P91.63   Severe hypoxic ischemic encephalopathy
               [HIE]** 🅲

● **P91.8   Other specified disturbances of cerebral status of
            newborn**

   ● **P91.81   Neonatal encephalopathy**

      ▶ *P91.811   Neonatal encephalopathy in diseases
                  classified elsewhere*
                  *Code first underlying condition, if known,
                     such as:*
                  congenital cirrhosis (of liver) (P78.81)
                  intracranial nontraumatic
                     hemorrhage of newborn (P52.-)
                  kernicterus (P57.-)

      P91.819   Neonatal encephalopathy, unspecified

▶ New   ➡ Revised   ~~deleted~~ Deleted   Excludes 1   Excludes 2   Includes   Use additional   Code first   Code also   Key words

OGCR Official Guidelines   ● Unacceptable Principal Diagnosis   X Assign placeholder X   ● Use Additional Character(s)   ▶ Manifestation Code   Coding Clinic

● **P91.82**   **Neonatal cerebral infarction**
Neonatal stroke
Perinatal arterial ischemic stroke
Perinatal cerebral infarction
Excludes1   cerebral infarction (I63.-)
Excludes2   intracranial hemorrhage of
newborn (P52.-)
(Ex) For category P91.82 MCC codes: See PDX Collection 4083

P91.821   **Neonatal cerebral infarction, right side of brain** 🔖

P91.822   **Neonatal cerebral infarction, left side of brain** 🔖

P91.823   **Neonatal cerebral infarction, bilateral** 🔖

P91.829   **Neonatal cerebral infarction, unspecified side** 🔖

P91.88   **Other specified disturbances of cerebral status of newborn**

P91.9   **Disturbance of cerebral status of newborn, unspecified**

● **P92**   **Feeding problems of newborn**
~~**Excludes1**   eating disorders (F50.-)~~
~~feeding problems in child over 28 days old (R63.3)~~
▶ **Excludes2**   feeding problems in child over 28 days old (R63.3)
Coding Clinic: 2017, Q1, P28; 2016, Q3, P19

● **P92.0**   **Vomiting of newborn**
Excludes1   vomiting of child over 28 days old (R11.-)

P92.01   **Bilious vomiting of newborn** 🔖
Excludes1   bilious vomiting in child over 28 days old (R11.14)
(Ex) See PDX Collection 1051

P92.09   **Other vomiting of newborn**
Excludes1   regurgitation of food in newborn (P92.1)

P92.1   **Regurgitation and rumination of newborn**

P92.2   **Slow feeding of newborn**

P92.3   **Underfeeding of newborn**

P92.4   **Overfeeding of newborn**

P92.5   **Neonatal difficulty in feeding at breast**
Coding Clinic: 2017, Q1, P28; 2016, Q3, P19

P92.6   **Failure to thrive in newborn**
Excludes1   failure to thrive in child over 28 days old (R62.51)

P92.8   **Other feeding problems of newborn**

P92.9   **Feeding problem of newborn, unspecified**

● **P93**   **Reactions and intoxications due to drugs administered to newborn**
Includes   reactions and intoxications due to drugs administered to fetus affecting newborn
Excludes1   jaundice due to drugs or toxins transmitted from mother or given to newborn (P58.4-)
reactions and intoxications from maternal opiates, tranquilizers and other medication (P04.0-P04.1, P04.4-)
withdrawal symptoms from maternal use of drugs of addiction (P96.1)
withdrawal symptoms from therapeutic use of drugs in newborn (P96.2)
(Ex) For category P93 CC codes: See PDX Collection 1052

P93.0   **Grey baby syndrome** 🔖
Grey syndrome from chloramphenicol administration in newborn

P93.8   **Other reactions and intoxications due to drugs administered to newborn** 🔖
Use additional code for adverse effect, if applicable, to identify drug (T36-T50 with fifth or sixth character 5)

● **P94**   **Disorders of muscle tone of newborn**

P94.0   **Transient neonatal myasthenia gravis** 🔖
Excludes1   myasthenia gravis (G70.0)
(Ex) See PDX Collection 1041

P94.1   **Congenital hypertonia**

P94.2   **Congenital hypotonia**
Floppy baby syndrome, unspecified

P94.8   **Other disorders of muscle tone of newborn**

P94.9   **Disorder of muscle tone of newborn, unspecified**

OGCR Section I.C.16.g.

Stillbirth

Code P95, Stillbirth, is only for use for institutions that maintain separate records for stillbirths. No other code should be used with P95. Code P95 should not be used on the mother's record.

P95   **Stillbirth**
Deadborn fetus NOS
Fetal death of unspecified cause
Stillbirth NOS
Excludes1   maternal care for intrauterine death (O36.4)
missed abortion (O02.1)
outcome of delivery, stillbirth (Z37.1, Z37.3, Z37.4, Z37.7)

● **P96**   **Other conditions originating in the perinatal period**

P96.0   **Congenital renal failure**
Uremia of newborn

P96.1   **Neonatal withdrawal symptoms from maternal use of drugs of addiction** 🔖
Drug withdrawal syndrome in infant of dependent mother
Neonatal abstinence syndrome
Excludes1   reactions and intoxications from maternal opiates and tranquilizers administered during labor and delivery (P04.0)
(Ex) See PDX Collection 1052

P96.2   **Withdrawal symptoms from therapeutic use of drugs in newborn** 🔖
(Ex) See PDX Collection 1052

P96.3   **Wide cranial sutures of newborn**
Neonatal craniotabes

P96.5   **Complication to newborn due to (fetal) intrauterine procedure**
Excludes2   newborn affected by amniocentesis (P00.6)

● **P96.8**   **Other specified conditions originating in the perinatal period**

P96.81   **Exposure to (parental) (environmental) tobacco smoke in the perinatal period**
Excludes2   newborn affected by in utero exposure to tobacco (P04.2)
exposure to environmental tobacco smoke after the perinatal period (Z77.22)

P96.82   **Delayed separation of umbilical cord**

P96.83   **Meconium staining**
Excludes1   meconium aspiration (P24.00, P24.01)
meconium passage during delivery (P03.82)

P96.89   **Other specified conditions originating in the perinatal period**
Use additional code to specify condition

P96.9   **Condition originating in the perinatal period, unspecified**
Congenital debility NOS

CHAPTER 16 (P00-P96)

N   Newborn Age: 0   **P**   Pediatric Age: 0–17   **M**   Maternity DX: 9–64   **A**   Adult Age: 15–124   ♀   Females Only   ♂   Males Only
🔖 Complication\Comorbidity   🔖 Major C\C   (Ex) CC/MCC Exclusions   🔖 Hospital-Acquired Condition   🔖 Hierarchical Condition Category

1199

CHAPTER 17 (Q00-Q99)

CHAPTER 17

CONGENITAL MALFORMATIONS, DEFORMATIONS, AND CHROMOSOMAL ABNORMALITIES (Q00-Q99)

OGCR Chapter-Specific Coding Guidelines

17. Chapter 17: Congenital malformations, deformations, and chromosomal abnormalities (Q00-Q99)

Assign an appropriate code(s) from categories Q00-Q99, Congenital malformations, deformations, and chromosomal abnormalities when a malformation/deformation or chromosomal abnormality is documented. A malformation/deformation/ or chromosomal abnormality may be the principal/first-listed diagnosis on a record or a secondary diagnosis.

When a malformation/deformation/or chromosomal abnormality does not have a unique code assignment, assign additional code(s) for any manifestations that may be present.

When the code assignment specifically identifies the malformation/deformation/or chromosomal abnormality, manifestations that are an inherent component of the anomaly should not be coded separately. Additional codes should be assigned for manifestations that are not an inherent component.

Codes from Chapter 17 may be used throughout the life of the patient. If a congenital malformation or deformity has been corrected, a personal history code should be used to identify the history of the malformation or deformity. Although present at birth, malformation/deformation/or chromosomal abnormality may not be identified until later in life. Whenever the condition is diagnosed by the physician, it is appropriate to assign a code from codes Q00-Q99.

For the birth admission, the appropriate code from category Z38, Liveborn infants, according to place of birth and type of delivery, should be sequenced as the principal diagnosis, followed by any congenital anomaly codes, Q00-Q99.

CHAPTER 17

CONGENITAL MALFORMATIONS, DEFORMATIONS, AND CHROMOSOMAL ABNORMALITIES (Q00-Q99)

Note: Codes from this chapter are not for use on maternal records

Excludes2 inborn errors of metabolism (E70-E88)

This chapter contains the following blocks:

Q00-Q07	Congenital malformations of the nervous system
Q10-Q18	Congenital malformations of eye, ear, face and neck
Q20-Q28	Congenital malformations of the circulatory system
Q30-Q34	Congenital malformations of the respiratory system
Q35-Q37	Cleft lip and cleft palate
Q38-Q45	Other congenital malformations of the digestive system
Q50-Q56	Congenital malformations of genital organs
Q60-Q64	Congenital malformations of the urinary system
Q65-Q79	Congenital malformations and deformations of the musculoskeletal system
Q80-Q89	Other congenital malformations
Q90-Q99	Chromosomal abnormalities, not elsewhere classified

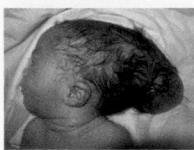

Figure 17-1 An infant with a large occipital encephalocele. The large skin-covered encephalocele is visible. (From Swaiman KF, Ashwal S, Ferriero DM: Pediatric Neurology: Principles and Practice, Philadelphia, Saunders, 2012)

CONGENITAL MALFORMATIONS OF THE NERVOUS SYSTEM (Q00–Q07)

● **Q00 Anencephaly and similar malformations**
Ex: For category Q00 CC codes: See PDX Collection 1053

Q00.0 Anencephaly
Absence of skull with cerebral hemispheres missing or reduced to small masses attached to base of cranium
Acephaly
Acrania
Amyelencephaly
Hemianencephaly
Hemicephaly

Q00.1 Craniorachischisis
Developmental anomaly consisting of fissure of cranium and vertebral column

Q00.2 Iniencephaly
Developmental anomaly characterized by enlargement of foramen magnum and absence of laminae and spinous processes of cervical, dorsal

● **Q01 Encephalocele**
Sac-like protrusions of brain and membranes visible through an opening in skull

Includes   Arnold-Chiari syndrome, type III
encephalocystocele
encephalomyelocele
hydroencephalocele
hydromeningocele, cranial
meningocele, cerebral
meningoencephalocele

Excludes1   Meckel-Gruber syndrome (Q61.9)

Ex: For category Q01 CC codes: See PDX Collection 1054

Q01.0 Frontal encephalocele
Q01.1 Nasofrontal encephalocele
Q01.2 Occipital encephalocele
Q01.8 Encephalocele of other sites
Q01.9 Encephalocele, unspecified

Q02 Microcephaly
Head size measures significantly below normal based on standardized charts

Includes   hydromicrocephaly
micrencephalon

Code first, if applicable, congenital Zika virus disease

Excludes1   Meckel-Gruber syndrome (Q61.9)

Coding Clinic: 2018, Q4, P26; 2016, Q4, P7

● **Q03 Congenital hydrocephalus**
Accumulation of cerebrospinal fluid in ventricles resulting in swelling and enlargement

Includes   hydrocephalus in newborn
Excludes1   Arnold-Chiari syndrome, type II (Q07.0-)
acquired hydrocephalus (G91.-)
hydrocephalus due to congenital toxoplasmosis (P37.1)
hydrocephalus with spina bifida (Q05.0-Q05.4)

Q03.0 Malformations of aqueduct of Sylvius
Anomaly of aqueduct of Sylvius
Obstruction of aqueduct of Sylvius, congenital
Stenosis of aqueduct of Sylvius

Q03.1 Atresia of foramina of Magendie and Luschka
Dandy-Walker syndrome

Q03.8 Other congenital hydrocephalus
Q03.9 Congenital hydrocephalus, unspecified

▶ New   ⇒ Revised   ~~deleted~~ Deleted   Excludes 1   Excludes 2   Includes   Use additional   Code first   Code also   Key words

OGCR Official Guidelines   ● Unacceptable Principal Diagnosis   X Assign placeholder X   ● Use Additional Character(s)   ▶ Manifestation Code   Coding Clinic

● **Q04   Other congenital malformations of brain**

Excludes1   cyclopia (Q87.0)
macrocephaly (Q75.3)

(Ex:) For category Q04 CC codes Q04.0-Q04.3: See PDX Collection 1054
For category Q04 CC codes Q04.4-Q04.8: See PDX Collection 1055

Q04.0   Congenital malformations of corpus callosum 🔵 🔵
Agenesis of corpus callosum

Q04.1   Arhinencephaly 🔵 🔵
Congenital absence of olfactory bulbs, tract, or nerves

Q04.2   Holoprosencephaly 🔵 🔵
Failure of cleavage of forebrain (prosencephalon) resulting in incomplete or absent cortical separation and deficits in midline facial development

Q04.3   Other reduction deformities of brain 🔵 🔵
Absence of part of brain
Agenesis of part of brain
Cerebral cortex are not fully formed, brain surface is smooth
Agyria
Aplasia of part of brain
Hydranencephaly
Hypoplasia of part of brain
Lissencephaly
Congenital malformation or absence of convolutions of cerebral cortex
Microgyria
Malformation of brain characterized by excessive number of small convolutions (gyri) on surface
Pachygyria
Reduction in number of sulci of cerebrum

Excludes1   congenital malformations of corpus callosum (Q04.0)

Q04.4   Septo-optic dysplasia of brain 🔵 🔵

Q04.5   Megalencephaly 🔵 🔵
Abnormally large brain

Q04.6   Congenital cerebral cysts 🔵 🔵
Porencephaly   Schizencephaly

Excludes1   acquired porencephalic cyst (G93.0)

Q04.8   Other specified congenital malformations of brain 🔵 🔵
Arnold-Chiari syndrome, type IV
Macrogyria

Q04.9   Congenital malformation of brain, unspecified 🔵
Congenital anomaly NOS of brain
Congenital deformity NOS of brain
Congenital disease or lesion NOS of brain
Multiple anomalies NOS of brain, congenital

● **Q05   Spina bifida**
Developmental anomaly characterized by defective closure of vertebral arch, through which spinal cord and meninges may protrude

Includes   hydromeningocele (spinal)
meningocele (spinal)
meningomyelocele
myelocele
myelomeningocele
rachischisis
spina bifida (aperta)(cystica)
syringomyelocele

Use additional code for any associated paraplegia (paraparesis) (G82.2-)

Excludes1   Arnold-Chiari syndrome, type II (Q07.0-)
spina bifida occulta (Q76.0)

(Ex:) **For category Q05 CC codes unless otherwise indicated:** See PDX Collection 1056

Q05.0   Cervical spina bifida with hydrocephalus 🔵 🔵
(Ex:) See PDX Collection 3501

Q05.1   Thoracic spina bifida with hydrocephalus 🔵 🔵
Dorsal spina bifida with hydrocephalus
Thoracolumbar spina bifida with hydrocephalus
(Ex:) See PDX Collection 3501

Q05.2   Lumbar spina bifida with hydrocephalus 🔵 🔵
Lumbosacral spina bifida with hydrocephalus
(Ex:) See PDX Collection 3501

Q05.3   Sacral spina bifida with hydrocephalus 🔵 🔵
(Ex:) See PDX Collection 3501

Q05.4   Unspecified spina bifida with hydrocephalus 🔵 🔵
(Ex:) See PDX Collection 3501

Q05.5   Cervical spina bifida without hydrocephalus 🔵

Q05.6   Thoracic spina bifida without hydrocephalus 🔵
Dorsal spina bifida NOS
Thoracolumbar spina bifida NOS

Q05.7   Lumbar spina bifida without hydrocephalus 🔵
Lumbosacral spina bifida NOS

Q05.8   Sacral spina bifida without hydrocephalus 🔵

Q05.9   Spina bifida, unspecified 🔵

● **Q06   Other congenital malformations of spinal cord**

Q06.0   Amyelia 🔵
Congenital absence of spinal cord

Q06.1   Hypoplasia and dysplasia of spinal cord 🔵
Underdevelopment of spinal cord
Atelomyelia
Congenitally incomplete development of spinal cord
Myelatelia
Myelodysplasia of spinal cord
Defective development of spinal cord, especially lower segments

Q06.2   Diastematomyelia 🔵
Congenital anomaly, associated with spina bifida, in which spinal cord is split into halves and surrounded by dural sac

Q06.3   Other congenital cauda equina malformations 🔵

Q06.4   Hydromyelia 🔵
Dilation of central canal of spinal cord with increased fluid accumulation
Hydrorachis

Q06.8   Other specified congenital malformations of spinal cord 🔵

Q06.9   Congenital malformation of spinal cord, unspecified 🔵
Congenital anomaly NOS of spinal cord
Congenital deformity NOS of spinal cord
Congenital disease or lesion NOS of spinal cord

● **Q07   Other congenital malformations of nervous system**

Excludes2   congenital central alveolar hypoventilation syndrome (G47.35)
familial dysautonomia [Riley-Day] (G90.1)
neurofibromatosis (nonmalignant) (Q85.0-)

● **Q07.0   Arnold-Chiari syndrome**
Herniation of cerebellar tonsils and vermis through foramen magnum into spinal canal
Arnold-Chiari syndrome, type II

Excludes1   Arnold-Chiari syndrome, type III (Q01.-)
Arnold-Chiari syndrome, type IV (Q04.8)

Q07.00   Arnold-Chiari syndrome without spina bifida or hydrocephalus 🔵

Q07.01   Arnold-Chiari syndrome with spina bifida 🔵

Q07.02   Arnold-Chiari syndrome with hydrocephalus 🔵 🔵
(Ex:) See PDX Collection 3501

Q07.03   Arnold-Chiari syndrome with spina bifida and hydrocephalus 🔵 🔵
(Ex:) See PDX Collection 3501

Q07.8   Other specified congenital malformations of nervous system 🔵
Agenesis of nerve
Displacement of brachial plexus
Jaw-winking syndrome
Marcus Gunn's syndrome

Q07.9   Congenital malformation of nervous system, unspecified 🔵
Congenital anomaly NOS of nervous system
Congenital deformity NOS of nervous system
Congenital disease or lesion NOS of nervous system

N Newborn Age: 0   **P** Pediatric Age: 0–17   **M** Maternity DX: 9–64   **A** Adult Age: 15–124   ♀ Females Only   ♂ Males Only

🔵 Complication\Comorbidity   🔵 Major C\C   (Ex:) CC/MCC Exclusions   🔵 Hospital-Acquired Condition   🔵 Hierarchical Condition Category

1201

CONGENITAL MALFORMATIONS OF EYE, EAR, FACE AND NECK (Q10-Q18)

> **Excludes2**   cleft lip and cleft palate (Q35-Q37)
> congenital malformation of cervical spine (Q05.0,
> Q05.5, Q67.5, Q76.0-Q76.4)
> congenital malformation of larynx (Q31.-)
> congenital malformation of lip NEC (Q38.0)
> congenital malformation of nose (Q30.-)
> congenital malformation of parathyroid gland
> (Q89.2)
> congenital malformation of thyroid gland (Q89.2)

● **Q10   Congenital malformations of eyelid, lacrimal apparatus and orbit**

> **Excludes1**   cryptophthalmos NOS (Q11.2)
> cryptophthalmos syndrome (Q87.0)

Q10.0   Congenital ptosis
> *Prolapse or drooping of upper eyelid from paralysis of third*
> *nerve or from sympathetic innervations*

Q10.1   Congenital ectropion
> *Outward turning of eyelid*

Q10.2   Congenital entropion
> *Inward turning of eyelid*

Q10.3   Other congenital malformations of eyelid
> Ablepharon
> Blepharophimosis, congenital
> Coloboma of eyelid
> Congenital absence or agenesis of cilia
> Congenital absence or agenesis of eyelid
> Congenital accessory eyelid
> Congenital accessory eye muscle
> Congenital malformation of eyelid NOS

Q10.4   Absence and agenesis of lacrimal apparatus
> Congenital absence of punctum lacrimale

Q10.5   Congenital stenosis and stricture of lacrimal duct

Q10.6   Other congenital malformations of lacrimal apparatus
> Congenital malformation of lacrimal apparatus NOS

Q10.7   Congenital malformation of orbit

● **Q11   Anophthalmos, microphthalmos and macrophthalmos**
> *Absence of eye and optic pit*

Q11.0   Cystic eyeball

Q11.1   Other anophthalmos
> Anophthalmos NOS
> Agenesis of eye
> > *Absence of eye*
> Aplasia of eye

Q11.2   Microphthalmos
> *Partial absence of eye and optic pit*
> Cryptophthalmos NOS
> Dysplasia of eye
> Hypoplasia of eye
> Rudimentary eye
> > **Excludes1**   cryptophthalmos syndrome (Q87.0)

Q11.3   Macrophthalmos
> *Congenital enlargement of eyes*
> > **Excludes1**   macrophthalmos in congenital glaucoma
> > (Q15.0)

● **Q12   Congenital lens malformations**

Q12.0   Congenital cataract

Q12.1   Congenital displaced lens

Q12.2   Coloboma of lens

Q12.3   Congenital aphakia

Q12.4   Spherophakia
> *Smaller, more spherical optic lens than normal*

Q12.8   Other congenital lens malformations
> Microphakia

Q12.9   Congenital lens malformation, unspecified

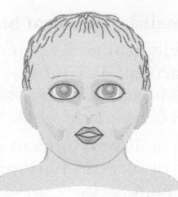

Figure 17-2   Bilateral congenital **hydrophthalmia,** in which the eyes are very large in comparison to the other facial features due to glaucoma.

● **Q13   Congenital malformations of anterior segment of eye**

Q13.0   Coloboma of iris
> Coloboma NOS

Q13.1   Absence of iris
> Aniridia
> Use additional code for associated glaucoma (H42)

Q13.2   Other congenital malformations of iris
> Anisocoria, congenital
> Atresia of pupil
> Congenital malformation of iris NOS
> Corectopia

Q13.3   Congenital corneal opacity

Q13.4   Other congenital corneal malformations
> Congenital malformation of cornea NOS
> Microcornea
> Peter's anomaly

Q13.5   Blue sclera
> *Condition of unusual blueness of sclera; not harmful*

● **Q13.8   Other congenital malformations of anterior segment of eye**

Q13.81   Rieger's anomaly
> Use additional code for associated glaucoma
> (H42)

Q13.89   Other congenital malformations of anterior segment of eye

Q13.9   Congenital malformation of anterior segment of eye, unspecified

● **Q14   Congenital malformations of posterior segment of eye**

> **Excludes2**   optic nerve hypoplasia (H47.03-)

Q14.0   Congenital malformation of vitreous humor
> Congenital vitreous opacity

Q14.1   Congenital malformation of retina
> Congenital retinal aneurysm

Q14.2   Congenital malformation of optic disc
> Coloboma of optic disc

Q14.3   Congenital malformation of choroid

Q14.8   Other congenital malformations of posterior segment of eye
> Coloboma of the fundus

Q14.9   Congenital malformation of posterior segment of eye, unspecified

● **Q15   Other congenital malformations of eye**

> **Excludes1**   congenital nystagmus (H55.01)
> ocular albinism (E70.31-)
> optic nerve hypoplasia (H47.03-)
> retinitis pigmentosa (H35.52)

Q15.0   Congenital glaucoma
> Axenfeld's anomaly
> Buphthalmos
> > *Congenital syndrome characterized by enlargement of the*
> > *eye with symptoms of glaucoma.*
> Glaucoma of childhood
> Glaucoma of newborn
> Hydrophthalmos
> Keratoglobus, congenital, with glaucoma
> Macrocornea with glaucoma
> Macrophthalmos in congenital glaucoma
> Megalocornea with glaucoma

CHAPTER 17 (Q00-Q99)

Q15.8 **Other specified congenital malformations of eye**

Q15.9 **Congenital malformation of eye, unspecified**
   Congenital anomaly of eye
   Congenital deformity of eye

● Q16 **Congenital malformations of ear causing impairment of hearing**
   Excludes1   congenital deafness (H90.-)

Q16.0 **Congenital absence of (ear) auricle**

Q16.1 **Congenital absence, atresia and stricture of auditory canal (external)**
   Congenital atresia or stricture of osseous meatus

Q16.2 **Absence of eustachian tube**

Q16.3 **Congenital malformation of ear ossicles**
   Congenital fusion of ear ossicles

Q16.4 **Other congenital malformations of middle ear**
   Congenital malformation of middle ear NOS

Q16.5 **Congenital malformation of inner ear**
   Congenital anomaly of membranous labyrinth
   Congenital anomaly of organ of Corti

Q16.9 **Congenital malformation of ear causing impairment of hearing, unspecified**
   Congenital absence of ear NOS

● Q17 **Other congenital malformations of ear**
   Excludes1   congenital malformations of ear with impairment
                        of hearing (Q16.0-Q16.9)
                        preauricular sinus (Q18.1)

Q17.0 **Accessory auricle**
   Accessory tragus
   Polyotia
   Preauricular appendage or tag
   Supernumerary ear
   Supernumerary lobule

Q17.1 **Macrotia**
   Enlarged ears

Q17.2 **Microtia**
   An abnormally small or underdeveloped external ear

Q17.3 **Other misshapen ear**
   Pointed ear

Q17.4 **Misplaced ear**
   Low-set ears
   Excludes1   cervical auricle (Q18.2)

Q17.5 **Prominent ear**
   Bat ear

Q17.8 **Other specified congenital malformations of ear**
   Congenital absence of lobe of ear

Q17.9 **Congenital malformation of ear, unspecified**
   Congenital anomaly of ear NOS

● Q18 **Other congenital malformations of face and neck**
   Excludes1   cleft lip and cleft palate (Q35-Q37)
                        conditions classified to Q67.0-Q67.4
                        congenital malformations of skull and face bones
                           (Q75.-)
                        cyclopia (Q87.0)
                        dentofacial anomalies [including malocclusion]
                           (M26.-)
                        malformation syndromes affecting facial
                           appearance (Q87.0)
                        persistent thyroglossal duct (Q89.2)

Q18.0 **Sinus, fistula and cyst of branchial cleft**
   Branchial vestige
      *Branchial remnants (cysts, fistula, skin tags) that are
         developmental anomalies*

Q18.1 **Preauricular sinus and cyst**
   Fistula of auricle, congenital
   Cervicoaural fistula
      *Abnormal passage in neck originating from first branchial
         cleft*

Q18.2 **Other branchial cleft malformations**
   Branchial cleft malformation NOS
   Cervical auricle
   Otocephaly

Q18.3 **Webbing of neck**
   Pterygium colli
      Thick fold of skin on side of neck

Q18.4 **Macrostomia**
   *Results from failure of union of maxillary and mandibular
      processes, results in abnormally large mouth*

Q18.5 **Microstomia**

Q18.6 **Macrocheilia**
   Excessive size of lips
   Hypertrophy of lip, congenital

Q18.7 **Microcheilia**
   Abnormal smallness of lips

Q18.8 **Other specified congenital malformations of face and neck**
   Medial cyst of face and neck
   Medial fistula of face and neck
   Medial sinus of face and neck

Q18.9 **Congenital malformation of face and neck, unspecified**
   Congenital anomaly NOS of face and neck

CONGENITAL MALFORMATIONS OF THE CIRCULATORY SYSTEM (Q20-Q28)

● Q20 **Congenital malformations of cardiac chambers and connections**
   Excludes1   dextrocardia with situs inversus (Q89.3)
                        mirror-image atrial arrangement with situs
                           inversus (Q89.3)
   (Ex:) **For category Q20 CC codes unless otherwise indicated:** See PDX Collection 1057

Q20.0 **Common arterial trunk** 🔵
   Persistent truncus arteriosus
   Excludes1   aortic septal defect (Q21.4)
   (Ex:) See PDX Collection 3502

Q20.1 **Double outlet right ventricle** 🔵
   Taussig-Bing syndrome
   (Ex:) See PDX Collection 3502

Q20.2 **Double outlet left ventricle** 🔵
   (Ex:) See PDX Collection 3502

Q20.3 **Discordant ventriculoarterial connection** 🔵
   Dextrotransposition of aorta
   Transposition of great vessels (complete)
   (Ex:) See PDX Collection 3502

Q20.4 **Double inlet ventricle** 🔵
   Common ventricle
   Cor triloculare biatriatum
   Single ventricle
   (Ex:) See PDX Collection 3502

Q20.5 **Discordant atrioventricular connection** 🔵
   Corrected transposition
   Levotransposition
   Ventricular inversion
   (Ex:) See PDX Collection 3502

Q20.6 **Isomerism of atrial appendages**
   Isomerism of atrial appendages with asplenia or
      polysplenia

Q20.8 **Other congenital malformations of cardiac chambers and connections**
   Cor binoculare

Q20.9 **Congenital malformation of cardiac chambers and connections, unspecified**

● Q21 **Congenital malformations of cardiac septa**
   Excludes1   acquired cardiac septal defect (I51.0)

Q21.0 **Ventricular septal defect** 🔵
   Roger's disease
   (Ex:) See PDX Collection 1057

Q21.1 **Atrial septal defect** 🔵
   Coronary sinus defect
   Patent or persistent foramen ovale
   Patent or persistent ostium secundum defect (type II)
   Patent or persistent sinus venosus defect
   (Ex:) See PDX Collection 1058

Q21.2 **Atrioventricular septal defect** 🔊
   Common atrioventricular canal
   Endocardial cushion defect
   Ostium primum atrial septal defect (type I)
   (Ex:) See PDX Collection 1057

Q21.3 **Tetralogy of Fallot** 🔊
   Ventricular septal defect with pulmonary stenosis or
      atresia, dextroposition of aorta and hypertrophy of
      right ventricle.
   (Ex:) See PDX Collection 3502

Q21.4 **Aortopulmonary septal defect**
   Aortic septal defect
   Aortopulmonary window

Q21.8 **Other congenital malformations of cardiac septa**
   Eisenmenger's defect
   Pentalogy of Fallot
   ➥ Code also, if applicable:
      Eisenmenger's complex (I27.83)
      Eisenmenger's syndrome (I27.83)

Q21.9 **Congenital malformation of cardiac septum, unspecified**
   Septal (heart) defect NOS

● Q22 **Congenital malformations of pulmonary and tricuspid valves**
   Q22.0 **Pulmonary valve atresia** 🔊
      (Ex:) See PDX Collection 3502

   Q22.1 **Congenital pulmonary valve stenosis** 🔊
      (Ex:) See PDX Collection 1059

   Q22.2 **Congenital pulmonary valve insufficiency** 🔊
      Congenital pulmonary valve regurgitation
      (Ex:) See PDX Collection 1060

   Q22.3 **Other congenital malformations of pulmonary valve** 🔊
      Congenital malformation of pulmonary valve NOS
      Supernumerary cusps of pulmonary valve
      (Ex:) See PDX Collection 1060

   Q22.4 **Congenital tricuspid stenosis** 🔊
      Congenital tricuspid atresia
      (Ex:) See PDX Collection 3504

   Q22.5 **Ebstein's anomaly** 🔊
      Malformation of tricuspid valve
      (Ex:) See PDX Collection 3504

   Q22.6 **Hypoplastic right heart syndrome** 🔊
      (Ex:) See PDX Collection 3504

   Q22.8 **Other congenital malformations of tricuspid valve** 🔊
      (Ex:) See PDX Collection 3504

   Q22.9 **Congenital malformation of tricuspid valve, unspecified** 🔊
      (Ex:) See PDX Collection 3504

● Q23 **Congenital malformations of aortic and mitral valves**
   (Ex:) **For category Q23 CC codes unless otherwise indicated:** See PDX Collection 1061
   Q23.0 **Congenital stenosis of aortic valve** 🔊
      Congenital aortic atresia
      Congenital aortic stenosis NOS
      Excludes1 congenital stenosis of aortic valve in
         hypoplastic left heart syndrome
         (Q23.4)
         congenital subaortic stenosis (Q24.4)
         supravalvular aortic stenosis (congenital)
         (Q25.3)

   Q23.1 **Congenital insufficiency of aortic valve** 🔊
      Bicuspid aortic valve
      Congenital aortic insufficiency

   Q23.2 **Congenital mitral stenosis** 🔊
      Congenital mitral atresia

   Q23.3 **Congenital mitral insufficiency** 🔊

   Q23.4 **Hypoplastic left heart syndrome** 🔊
      (Ex:) See PDX Collection 3504

   Q23.8 **Other congenital malformations of aortic and mitral valves**

   Q23.9 **Congenital malformation of aortic and mitral valves, unspecified**

● Q24 **Other congenital malformations of heart**
   Excludes1 endocardial fibroelastosis (I42.4)
   Q24.0 **Dextrocardia** 🔊
      Heart is located in right hemithorax
      Excludes1 dextrocardia with situs inversus (Q89.3)
         isomerism of atrial appendages (with
            asplenia or polysplenia) (Q20.6)
         mirror-image atrial arrangement with
            situs inversus (Q89.3)
      (Ex:) See PDX Collection 1062

   Q24.1 **Levocardia** 🔊
      Normal position of heart but related structures on wrong side
      (Ex:) See PDX Collection 1062

   Q24.2 **Cor triatriatum** 🔊
      Congenital heart defect; left atrium is subdivided
      (Ex:) See PDX Collection 3505

   Q24.3 **Pulmonary infundibular stenosis** 🔊
      Subvalvular pulmonic stenosis
      (Ex:) See PDX Collection 3505

   Q24.4 **Congenital subaortic stenosis** 🔊
      (Ex:) See PDX Collection 3505

   Q24.5 **Malformation of coronary vessels** 🔊
      Congenital coronary (artery) aneurysm
      (Ex:) See PDX Collection 1064

   Q24.6 **Congenital heart block** 🔊
      (Ex:) See PDX Collection 3406

   Q24.8 **Other specified congenital malformations of heart**
      Congenital diverticulum of left ventricle
      Congenital malformation of myocardium
      Congenital malformation of pericardium
      Malposition of heart
      Uhl's disease

   Q24.9 **Congenital malformation of heart, unspecified**
      Congenital anomaly of heart
      Congenital disease of heart

● Q25 **Congenital malformations of great arteries**
   Q25.0 **Patent ductus arteriosus** 🔊
      *Fetal blood vessel connecting left pulmonary artery directly
         to descending aorta*
      Patent ductus Botallo
      Persistent ductus arteriosus
      (Ex:) See PDX Collection 1066

   Q25.1 **Coarctation of aorta** 🔊
      Coarctation of aorta (preductal) (postductal)
      Stenosis of aorta
      (Ex:) See PDX Collection 1067
      Coding Clinic: 2016, Q4, P56-57

● Q25.2 **Atresia of aorta**
      (Ex:) **For category Q25.2 CC codes:** See PDX Collection 3507
      Coding Clinic: 2016, Q4, P56

   Q25.21 **Interruption of aortic arch** 🔊
      Atresia of aortic arch

   Q25.29 **Other atresia of aorta** 🔊
      Atresia of aorta

   Q25.3 **Supravalvular aortic stenosis** 🔊
      Excludes1 congenital aortic stenosis NOS (Q23.0)
         congenital stenosis of aortic valve (Q23.0)
      (Ex:) See PDX Collection 3507

● Q25.4 **Other congenital malformations of aorta**
      Excludes1 hypoplasia of aorta in hypoplastic left
         heart syndrome (Q23.4)
      (Ex:) **For category Q25.4 CC codes:** See PDX Collection 1069
      Coding Clinic: 2016, Q4, P57

   Q25.40 **Congenital malformation of aorta unspecified** 🔊

   Q25.41 **Absence and aplasia of aorta** 🔊

   Q25.42 **Hypoplasia of aorta** 🔊

▶ New   ➥ Revised   ~~deleted~~ Deleted   Excludes 1   Excludes 2   Includes   Use additional   Code first   Code also   Key words
OGCR Official Guidelines   ● Unacceptable Principal Diagnosis   X Assign placeholder X   ● Use Additional Character(s)   ▶ Manifestation Code   Coding Clinic

Q25.43 **Congenital aneurysm of aorta** 🅗
    Congenital aneurysm of aortic root
    Congenital aneurysm of aortic sinus

Q25.44 **Congenital dilation of aorta** 🅗

Q25.45 **Double aortic arch** 🅗
    Vascular ring of aorta

Q25.46 **Tortuous aortic arch** 🅗
    Persistent convolutions of aortic arch

Q25.47 **Right aortic arch** 🅗
    Persistent right aortic arch

Q25.48 **Anomalous origin of subclavian artery** 🅗

Q25.49 **Other congenital malformations of aorta** 🅗
    Aortic arch
    Bovine arch

Q25.5 **Atresia of pulmonary artery** 🅗
    (Ex:) See PDX Collection 1070

Q25.6 **Stenosis of pulmonary artery** 🅗
    Supravalvular pulmonary stenosis
    (Ex:) See PDX Collection 1070

● Q25.7 **Other congenital malformations of pulmonary artery**
    (Ex:) **For category Q25.7 CC codes:** See PDX Collection 1070

Q25.71 **Coarctation of pulmonary artery** 🅗

Q25.72 **Congenital pulmonary arteriovenous malformation** 🅗
    Congenital pulmonary arteriovenous aneurysm

Q25.79 **Other congenital malformations of pulmonary artery** 🅗
    Aberrant pulmonary artery
    Agenesis of pulmonary artery
    Congenital aneurysm of pulmonary artery
    Congenital anomaly of pulmonary artery
    Hypoplasia of pulmonary artery

Q25.8 **Other congenital malformations of other great arteries** 🅗
    (Ex:) See PDX Collection 1069

Q25.9 **Congenital malformation of great arteries, unspecified** 🅗
    (Ex:) See PDX Collection 1069

● Q26 **Congenital malformations of great veins**

Q26.0 **Congenital stenosis of vena cava** 🅗
    Congenital stenosis of vena cava (inferior)(superior)
    (Ex:) See PDX Collection 1071

Q26.1 **Persistent left superior vena cava** 🅗
    (Ex:) See PDX Collection 1071

Q26.2 **Total anomalous pulmonary venous connection** 🅗
    Total anomalous pulmonary venous return [TAPVR], subdiaphragmatic
    Total anomalous pulmonary venous return [TAPVR], supradiaphragmatic
    (Ex:) See PDX Collection 1072

Q26.3 **Partial anomalous pulmonary venous connection** 🅗
    Partial anomalous pulmonary venous return
    (Ex:) See PDX Collection 1073

Q26.4 **Anomalous pulmonary venous connection, unspecified** 🅗
    (Ex:) See PDX Collection 1073

Q26.5 **Anomalous portal venous connection**

Q26.6 **Portal vein-hepatic artery fistula**

Q26.8 **Other congenital malformations of great veins** 🅗
    Absence of vena cava (inferior) (superior)
    Azygos continuation of inferior vena cava
    Persistent left posterior cardinal vein
    Scimitar syndrome
    (Ex:) See PDX Collection 1071

Q26.9 **Congenital malformation of great vein, unspecified** 🅗
    Congenital anomaly of vena cava (inferior) (superior) NOS
    (Ex:) See PDX Collection 1074

● Q27 **Other congenital malformations of peripheral vascular system**
    Excludes2 anomalies of cerebral and precerebral vessels (Q28.0-Q28.3)
        anomalies of coronary vessels (Q24.5)
        anomalies of pulmonary artery (Q25.5-Q25.7)
        congenital retinal aneurysm (Q14.1)
        hemangioma and lymphangioma (D18.-)

Q27.0 **Congenital absence and hypoplasia of umbilical artery**
    Single umbilical artery

Q27.1 **Congenital renal artery stenosis**

Q27.2 **Other congenital malformations of renal artery**
    Congenital malformation of renal artery NOS
    Multiple renal arteries

● Q27.3 **Arteriovenous malformation (peripheral)**
    Arteriovenous aneurysm
    Excludes1 acquired arteriovenous aneurysm (I77.0)
    Excludes2 arteriovenous malformation of cerebral vessels (Q28.2)
        arteriovenous malformation of precerebral vessels (Q28.0)

Q27.30 **Arteriovenous malformation, site unspecified** 🅗
    (Ex:) See PDX Collection 1075

Q27.31 **Arteriovenous malformation of vessel of upper limb**

Q27.32 **Arteriovenous malformation of vessel of lower limb**

Q27.33 **Arteriovenous malformation of digestive system vessel**

Q27.34 **Arteriovenous malformation of renal vessel**

Q27.39 **Arteriovenous malformation, other site**

Q27.4 **Congenital phlebectasia** 🅗
    (Ex:) See PDX Collection 1075

Q27.8 **Other specified congenital malformations of peripheral vascular system**
    Absence of peripheral vascular system
    Atresia of peripheral vascular system
    Congenital aneurysm (peripheral)
    Congenital stricture, artery
    Congenital varix
    Excludes1 arteriovenous malformation (Q27.3-)

Q27.9 **Congenital malformation of peripheral vascular system, unspecified**
    Anomaly of artery or vein NOS

● Q28 **Other congenital malformations of circulatory system**
    Excludes1 congenital aneurysm NOS (Q27.8)
        congenital coronary aneurysm (Q24.5)
        ruptured cerebral arteriovenous malformation (I60.8)
        ruptured malformation of precerebral vessels (I72.0)
    Excludes2 congenital peripheral aneurysm (Q27.8)
        congenital pulmonary aneurysm (Q25.79)
        congenital retinal aneurysm (Q14.1)

Q28.0 **Arteriovenous malformation of precerebral vessels** 🅗
    Congenital arteriovenous precerebral aneurysm (nonruptured)
    (Ex:) See PDX Collection 1075

Q28.1 **Other malformations of precerebral vessels** 🅗
    Congenital malformation of precerebral vessels NOS
    Congenital precerebral aneurysm (nonruptured)
    (Ex:) See PDX Collection 1075

Q28.2 **Arteriovenous malformation of cerebral vessels** 🅗
    Arteriovenous malformation of brain NOS
    Congenital arteriovenous cerebral aneurysm (nonruptured)
    (Ex:) See PDX Collection 1076

Q28.3 **Other malformations of cerebral vessels** 🅗
    Congenital cerebral aneurysm (nonruptured)
    Congenital malformation of cerebral vessels NOS
    Developmental venous anomaly
    (Ex:) See PDX Collection 1076

CHAPTER 17 (Q00-Q99)

N Newborn Age: 0   **P** Pediatric Age: 0–17   **M** Maternity DX: 9–64   **A** Adult Age: 15–124   ♀ Females Only   ♂ Males Only

🅗 Complication\Comorbidity   🅗 Major C\C   (Ex:) CC/MCC Exclusions   🅗 Hospital-Acquired Condition   🅗 Hierarchical Condition Category

1205

CHAPTER 17 (Q00-Q99)

Q28.8   Other specified congenital malformations of circulatory system 🔍
     Congenital aneurysm, specified site NEC
     Spinal vessel anomaly
     (Ex:) See PDX Collection 1075

Q28.9   Congenital malformation of circulatory system, unspecified 🔍
     (Ex:) See PDX Collection 1077

CONGENITAL MALFORMATIONS OF THE RESPIRATORY SYSTEM (Q30-Q34)

● **Q30**   Congenital malformations of nose
     Excludes1   congenital deviation of nasal septum (Q67.4)

Q30.0   Choanal atresia
     Atresia of nares (anterior) (posterior)
     Congenital stenosis of nares (anterior) (posterior)

Q30.1   Agenesis and underdevelopment of nose
     Congenital absent of nose

Q30.2   Fissured, notched and cleft nose

Q30.3   Congenital perforated nasal septum

Q30.8   Other congenital malformations of nose
     Accessory nose
     Congenital anomaly of nasal sinus wall

Q30.9   Congenital malformation of nose, unspecified

● **Q31**   Congenital malformations of larynx
     Excludes1   congenital laryngeal stridor NOS (P28.89)
     (Ex:) For category Q31 CC codes: See PDX Collection 1078

Q31.0   Web of larynx
     Glottic web of larynx
     Subglottic web of larynx
     Web of larynx NOS

Q31.1   Congenital subglottic stenosis 🔍

Q31.2   Laryngeal hypoplasia 🔍

Q31.3   Laryngocele 🔍

Q31.5   Congenital laryngomalacia 🔍

Q31.8   Other congenital malformations of larynx 🔍
     Absence of larynx
     Agenesis of larynx
     Atresia of larynx
     Congenital cleft thyroid cartilage
     Congenital fissure of epiglottis
     Congenital stenosis of larynx NEC
     Posterior cleft of cricoid cartilage

Q31.9   Congenital malformation of larynx, unspecified 🔍

● **Q32**   Congenital malformations of trachea and bronchus
     Excludes1   congenital bronchiectasis (Q33.4)
     (Ex:) For category Q32 CC codes: See PDX Collection 1078

Q32.0   Congenital tracheomalacia 🔍

Q32.1   Other congenital malformations of trachea 🔍
     Atresia of trachea
     Congenital anomaly of tracheal cartilage
     Congenital dilatation of trachea
     Congenital malformation of trachea
     Congenital stenosis of trachea
     Congenital tracheocele

Q32.2   Congenital bronchomalacia 🔍

Q32.3   Congenital stenosis of bronchus 🔍

Q32.4   Other congenital malformations of bronchus 🔍
     Absence of bronchus
     Agenesis of bronchus
     Atresia of bronchus
     Congenital diverticulum of bronchus
     Congenital malformation of bronchus NOS

● **Q33**   Congenital malformations of lung

Q33.0   Congenital cystic lung 🔍
     Congenital cystic lung disease
     Congenital honeycomb lung
     Congenital polycystic lung disease
     Excludes1   cystic fibrosis (E84.0)
                  cystic lung disease, acquired or unspecified (J98.4)
     (Ex:) See PDX Collection 1079

Q33.1   Accessory lobe of lung
     Azygos lobe (fissured), lung

Q33.2   Sequestration of lung 🔍
     (Ex:) See PDX Collection 1079

Q33.3   Agenesis of lung 🔍
     Congenital absence of lung (lobe)
     (Ex:) See PDX Collection 1079

Q33.4   Congenital bronchiectasis 🔍
     (Ex:) See PDX Collection 1080

Q33.5   Ectopic tissue in lung

Q33.6   Congenital hypoplasia and dysplasia of lung 🔍
     Excludes1   pulmonary hypoplasia associated with short gestation (P28.0)
     (Ex:) See PDX Collection 1079

Q33.8   Other congenital malformations of lung

Q33.9   Congenital malformation of lung, unspecified

● **Q34**   Other congenital malformations of respiratory system
     Excludes2   congenital central alveolar hypoventilation syndrome (G47.35)

Q34.0   Anomaly of pleura

Q34.1   Congenital cyst of mediastinum

Q34.8   Other specified congenital malformations of respiratory system
     Atresia of nasopharynx

Q34.9   Congenital malformation of respiratory system, unspecified
     Congenital absence of respiratory system
     Congenital anomaly of respiratory system NOS

CLEFT LIP AND CLEFT PALATE (Q35-Q37)

Use additional code to identify associated malformation of the nose (Q30.2)

~~**Excludes1**~~ ~~Robin's syndrome (Q87.0)~~

Excludes2   Robin's syndrome (Q87.0)

● **Q35**   Cleft palate
     Includes   fissure of palate
                palatoschisis
     Excludes1   cleft palate with cleft lip (Q37.-)

Q35.1   Cleft hard palate

Q35.3   Cleft soft palate

Q35.5   Cleft hard palate with cleft soft palate

Q35.7   Cleft uvula

Q35.9   Cleft palate, unspecified
     Cleft palate NOS

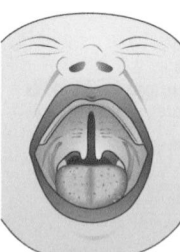

Figure 17-3   Cleft palate.

▶ New   ⇒ Revised   ~~deleted~~ Deleted   Excludes 1   Excludes 2   Includes   Use additional   Code first   Code also   Key words
OGCR Official Guidelines   ● Unacceptable Principal Diagnosis   X Assign placeholder X   ● Use Additional Character(s)   ⟩ Manifestation Code   Coding Clinic

● **Q36**   Cleft lip
> **Includes**   cheiloschisis
> congenital fissure of lip
> harelip
> labium leporinum
> **Excludes1**   cleft lip with cleft palate (Q37.-)

     Q36.0   Cleft lip, bilateral
     Q36.1   Cleft lip, median
     Q36.9   Cleft lip, unilateral
           Cleft lip NOS

● **Q37**   Cleft palate with cleft lip
> **Includes**   cheilopalatoschisis

     Q37.0   Cleft hard palate with bilateral cleft lip
     Q37.1   Cleft hard palate with unilateral cleft lip
           Cleft hard palate with cleft lip NOS
     Q37.2   Cleft soft palate with bilateral cleft lip
     Q37.3   Cleft soft palate with unilateral cleft lip
           Cleft soft palate with cleft lip NOS
     Q37.4   Cleft hard and soft palate with bilateral cleft lip
     Q37.5   Cleft hard and soft palate with unilateral cleft lip
           Cleft hard and soft palate with cleft lip NOS
     Q37.8   Unspecified cleft palate with bilateral cleft lip
     Q37.9   Unspecified cleft palate with unilateral cleft lip
           Cleft palate with cleft lip NOS

OTHER CONGENITAL MALFORMATIONS OF THE DIGESTIVE SYSTEM (Q38-Q45)

● **Q38**   Other congenital malformations of tongue, mouth and pharynx
> **Excludes1**   dentofacial anomalies (M26.-)
> macrostomia (Q18.4)
> microstomia (Q18.5)

     Q38.0   Congenital malformations of lips, not elsewhere classified
           Congenital fistula of lip
           Congenital malformation of lip NOS
           Van der Woude's syndrome
> **Excludes1**   cleft lip (Q36.-)
> cleft lip with cleft palate (Q37.-)
> macrocheilia (Q18.6)
> microcheilia (Q18.7)

     Q38.1   Ankyloglossia
           Restricted movement of tongue resulting in speech difficulty
           Tongue tie
     Q38.2   Macroglossia
           Excessive size of tongue
           Congenital hypertrophy of tongue
     Q38.3   Other congenital malformations of tongue
           Aglossia
           Bifid tongue
           Congenital adhesion of tongue
           Congenital fissure of tongue
           Congenital malformation of tongue NOS
           Double tongue
           Hypoglossia
           Hypoplasia of tongue
           Microglossia
     Q38.4   Congenital malformations of salivary glands and ducts
           Atresia of salivary glands and ducts
           Congenital absence of salivary glands and ducts
           Congenital accessory salivary glands and ducts
           Congenital fistula of salivary gland
     Q38.5   Congenital malformations of palate, not elsewhere classified
           Congenital absence of uvula
           Congenital malformation of palate NOS
           Congenital high arched palate
> **Excludes1**   cleft palate (Q35.-)
> cleft palate with cleft lip (Q37.-)

     Q38.6   Other congenital malformations of mouth
           Congenital malformation of mouth NOS
     Q38.7   Congenital pharyngeal pouch
           Congenital diverticulum of pharynx
> **Excludes1**   pharyngeal pouch syndrome (D82.1)

     Q38.8   Other congenital malformations of pharynx
           Congenital malformation of pharynx NOS
           Imperforate pharynx

● **Q39**   Congenital malformations of esophagus
> (Ex:) For category Q39 CC codes Q39.0-Q39.4: See PDX Collection 1081
> For category Q39 CC codes Q39.5-Q39.9: See PDX Collection 1082

     Q39.0   Atresia of esophagus without fistula
           Atresia of esophagus NOS
     Q39.1   Atresia of esophagus with tracheo-esophageal fistula
           Atresia of esophagus with broncho-esophageal fistula
     Q39.2   Congenital tracheo-esophageal fistula without atresia
           Congenital tracheo-esophageal fistula NOS
     Q39.3   Congenital stenosis and stricture of esophagus
     Q39.4   Esophageal web
     Q39.5   Congenital dilatation of esophagus
           Congenital cardiospasm
     Q39.6   Congenital diverticulum of esophagus
           Congenital esophageal pouch
     Q39.8   Other congenital malformations of esophagus
           Congenital absence of esophagus
           Congenital displacement of esophagus
           Congenital duplication of esophagus
     Q39.9   Congenital malformation of esophagus, unspecified

● **Q40**   Other congenital malformations of upper alimentary tract
     Q40.0   Congenital hypertrophic pyloric stenosis
           Congenital or infantile constriction
           Congenital or infantile hypertrophy
           Congenital or infantile spasm
           Congenital or infantile stenosis
           Congenital or infantile stricture
     Q40.1   Congenital hiatus hernia
           Congenital displacement of cardia through esophageal hiatus
> **Excludes1**   congenital diaphragmatic hernia (Q79.0)

     Q40.2   Other specified congenital malformations of stomach
           Congenital displacement of stomach
           Congenital diverticulum of stomach
           Congenital hourglass stomach
           Congenital duplication of stomach
           Megalogastria
           Microgastria
     Q40.3   Congenital malformation of stomach, unspecified
     Q40.8   Other specified congenital malformations of upper alimentary tract
     Q40.9   Congenital malformation of upper alimentary tract, unspecified
           Congenital anomaly of upper alimentary tract
           Congenital deformity of upper alimentary tract

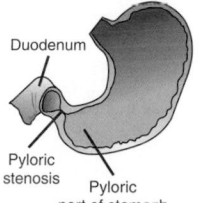

Figure 17-4   Pyloric stenosis.

Duodenum
Pyloric stenosis
Pyloric part of stomach

CHAPTER 17 (Q00-Q99)

N   Newborn Age: 0   P   Pediatric Age: 0-17   M   Maternity DX: 9-64   A   Adult Age: 15-124   ♀ Females Only   ♂ Males Only

Complication\Comorbidity   Major C\C   (Ex:) CC/MCC Exclusions   Hospital-Acquired Condition   Hierarchical Condition Category   1207

Q41   Congenital absence, atresia and stenosis of small intestine

> **Includes**   congenital obstruction, occlusion or stricture of small intestine or intestine NOS
>
> **Excludes1**   cystic fibrosis with intestinal manifestation (E84.11)
> meconium ileus NOS (without cystic fibrosis) (P76.0)
>
> Ex: For category Q41 CC codes: See PDX Collection 1083

Q41.0   Congenital absence, atresia and stenosis of duodenum

Q41.1   Congenital absence, atresia and stenosis of jejunum
> Apple peel syndrome
> Imperforate jejunum

Q41.2   Congenital absence, atresia and stenosis of ileum

Q41.8   Congenital absence, atresia and stenosis of other specified parts of small intestine

Q41.9   Congenital absence, atresia and stenosis of small intestine, part unspecified
> Congenital absence, atresia and stenosis of intestine NOS

Q42   Congenital absence, atresia and stenosis of large intestine

> **Includes**   congenital obstruction, occlusion and stricture of large intestine
>
> Ex: For category Q42 CC codes: See PDX Collection 1084

Q42.0   Congenital absence, atresia and stenosis of rectum with fistula

Q42.1   Congenital absence, atresia and stenosis of rectum without fistula
> Imperforate rectum

Q42.2   Congenital absence, atresia and stenosis of anus with fistula

Q42.3   Congenital absence, atresia and stenosis of anus without fistula
> Imperforate anus

Q42.8   Congenital absence, atresia and stenosis of other parts of large intestine

Q42.9   Congenital absence, atresia and stenosis of large intestine, part unspecified

Q43   Other congenital malformations of intestine

> Ex: For category Q43 CC codes unless otherwise indicated: See PDX Collection 1087

Q43.0   Meckel's diverticulum (displaced) (hypertrophic)
> *Congenital abnormality in which a pouch remains on the lower end of the small intestine*
> Persistent omphalomesenteric duct
> Persistent vitelline duct

Q43.1   Hirschsprung's disease
> *Developmental disorder of enteric nervous system characterized by absence of ganglion cells in distal colon resulting in functional obstruction*
> Aganglionosis
> Congenital (aganglionic) megacolon
> Ex: See PDX Collection 1085

Q43.2   Other congenital functional disorders of colon
> Congenital dilatation of colon
> Ex: See PDX Collection 1085

Q43.3   Congenital malformations of intestinal fixation
> Congenital omental, anomalous adhesions [bands]
> Congenital peritoneal adhesions [bands]
> Incomplete rotation of cecum and colon
> Insufficient rotation of cecum and colon
> Jackson's membrane
> Malrotation of colon
> Rotation failure of cecum and colon
> Universal mesentery
> Ex: See PDX Collection 1086

Q43.4   Duplication of intestine

Q43.5   Ectopic anus
> *Anal opening in abnormal location*

Q43.6   Congenital fistula of rectum and anus

> **Excludes1**   congenital fistula of anus with absence, atresia and stenosis (Q42.2)
> congenital fistula of rectum with absence, atresia and stenosis (Q42.0)
> congenital rectovaginal fistula (Q52.2)
> congenital urethrorectal fistula (Q64.73)
> pilonidal fistula or sinus (L05.-)

Q43.7   Persistent cloaca
> *Malformation in which rectum, vagina, and urinary tract form one channel; AKA congenital cloaca*
> Cloaca NOS

Q43.8   Other specified congenital malformations of intestine
> Congenital blind loop syndrome
> Congenital diverticulitis, colon
> Congenital diverticulum, intestine
> Dolichocolon
> Megaloappendix
> Megaloduodenum
> Microcolon
> Transposition of appendix
> Transposition of colon
> Transposition of intestine

Q43.9   Congenital malformation of intestine, unspecified

Q44   Congenital malformations of gallbladder, bile ducts and liver

> Ex: For category Q44 CC codes unless otherwise indicated: See PDX Collection 1088

Q44.0   Agenesis, aplasia and hypoplasia of gallbladder
> Congenital absence of gallbladder

Q44.1   Other congenital malformations of gallbladder
> Congenital malformation of gallbladder NOS
> Intrahepatic gallbladder

Q44.2   Atresia of bile ducts
> Ex: See PDX Collection 1089

Q44.3   Congenital stenosis and stricture of bile ducts
> Ex: See PDX Collection 1089

Q44.4   Choledochal cyst

Q44.5   Other congenital malformations of bile ducts
> Accessory hepatic duct
> Biliary duct duplication
> Congenital malformation of bile duct NOS
> Cystic duct duplication

Q44.6   Cystic disease of liver
> Fibrocystic disease of liver
> Ex: See PDX Collection 1090

Q44.7   Other congenital malformations of liver
> Accessory liver
> Alagille's syndrome
> Congenital absence of liver
> Congenital hepatomegaly
> Congenital malformation of liver NOS

Q45   Other congenital malformations of digestive system

> **Excludes2**   congenital diaphragmatic hernia (Q79.0)
> congenital hiatus hernia (Q40.1)
>
> Ex: For category Q45 CC codes: See PDX Collection 1091

Q45.0   Agenesis, aplasia and hypoplasia of pancreas
> Congenital absence of pancreas

Q45.1   Annular pancreas

Q45.2   Congenital pancreatic cyst

Q45.3   Other congenital malformations of pancreas and pancreatic duct
> Accessory pancreas
> Congenital malformation of pancreas or pancreatic duct NOS
>
> **Excludes1**   congenital diabetes mellitus (E10.-)
> cystic fibrosis (E84.0-E84.9)
> fibrocystic disease of pancreas (E84.-)
> neonatal diabetes mellitus (P70.2)

▶ New   ⇒ Revised   ~~deleted~~ Deleted   Excludes 1   Excludes 2   Includes   Use additional   Code first   Code also   Key words

OGCR Official Guidelines   ● Unacceptable Principal Diagnosis   X Assign placeholder X   ● Use Additional Character(s)   ▷ Manifestation Code   Coding Clinic

Q45.8   **Other specified congenital malformations of digestive system**
- Absence (complete) (partial) of alimentary tract NOS
- Duplication of digestive system
- Malposition, congenital of digestive system

Q45.9   **Congenital malformation of digestive system, unspecified**
- Congenital anomaly of digestive system
- Congenital deformity of digestive system

CONGENITAL MALFORMATIONS OF GENITAL ORGANS (Q50–Q56)

Excludes1   androgen insensitivity syndrome (E34.5-)
syndromes associated with anomalies in the number and form of chromosomes (Q90–Q99)

● Q50   Congenital malformations of ovaries, fallopian tubes and broad ligaments

  ● Q50.0   Congenital absence of ovary
     Excludes1   Turner's syndrome (Q96.-)
     Q50.01   Congenital absence of ovary, unilateral ♀
     Q50.02   Congenital absence of ovary, bilateral ♀

   Q50.1   Developmental ovarian cyst ♀

   Q50.2   Congenital torsion of ovary ♀

  ● Q50.3   Other congenital malformations of ovary
     Q50.31   Accessory ovary ♀
     Q50.32   Ovarian streak ♀
       Inadequate ovaries with absent follicular and hormonal function
       46, XX with streak gonads
     Q50.39   Other congenital malformation of ovary ♀
       Congenital malformation of ovary NOS

   Q50.4   Embryonic cyst of fallopian tube ♀
     Fimbrial cyst

   Q50.5   Embryonic cyst of broad ligament ♀
     Epoophoron cyst
     Parovarian cyst

   Q50.6   Other congenital malformations of fallopian tube and broad ligament ♀
     Absence of fallopian tube and broad ligament
     Accessory fallopian tube and broad ligament
     Atresia of fallopian tube and broad ligament
     Congenital malformation of fallopian tube or broad ligament NOS

● Q51   Congenital malformations of uterus and cervix

   Q51.0   Agenesis and aplasia of uterus ♀
     Congenital absence of uterus

  ● Q51.1   Doubling of uterus with doubling of cervix and vagina
     Q51.10   Doubling of uterus with doubling of cervix and vagina without obstruction ♀
       Doubling of uterus with doubling of cervix and vagina NOS
     Q51.11   Doubling of uterus with doubling of cervix and vagina with obstruction ♀

  ● Q51.2   Other doubling of uterus
     Doubling of uterus NOS
     Septate uterus
     ~~Q51.20   Other doubling of uterus, unspecified~~
       ~~Septate uterus, unspecified~~
     Q51.21   Complete doubling of uterus ♀
       Complete septate uterus
     Q51.22   Partial doubling of uterus ♀
       Partial septate uterus
     Q51.28   Other and unspecified doubling of uterus ♀
       Septate uterus NOS

   Q51.3   Bicornate uterus ♀
     Bicornate uterus, complete or partial
     Birth defect in which uterus has two separate "horns" that form top of uterus

Q51.4   Unicornate uterus ♀
- Unicornate uterus with or without a separate uterine horn
- Uterus with only one functioning horn
- *Uterus with half being undeveloped*

Q51.5   Agenesis and aplasia of cervix ♀
- Congenital absence of cervix

Q51.6   Embryonic cyst of cervix ♀

Q51.7   Congenital fistulae between uterus and digestive and urinary tracts ♀

● Q51.8   Other congenital malformations of uterus and cervix
  ● Q51.81   Other congenital malformations of uterus
     Q51.810   Arcuate uterus ♀
       Arcuatus uterus
     Q51.811   Hypoplasia of uterus ♀
     Q51.818   Other congenital malformations of uterus ♀
       Müllerian anomaly of uterus NEC
  ● Q51.82   Other congenital malformations of cervix
     Q51.820   Cervical duplication ♀
     Q51.821   Hypoplasia of cervix ♀
     Q51.828   Other congenital malformations of cervix ♀

Q51.9   Congenital malformation of uterus and cervix, unspecified ♀

● Q52   Other congenital malformations of female genitalia

   Q52.0   Congenital absence of vagina ♀
     Vaginal agenesis, total or partial

  ● Q52.1   Doubling of vagina
     Excludes1   doubling of vagina with doubling of uterus and cervix (Q51.1-)
     Q52.10   Doubling of vagina, unspecified ♀
       Septate vagina NOS
     Q52.11   Transverse vaginal septum ♀
  ● Q52.12   Longitudinal vaginal septum
     Coding Clinic: 2016, Q4, P58
     Q52.120   Longitudinal vaginal septum, nonobstructing ♀
     Q52.121   Longitudinal vaginal septum, obstructing, right side ♀
     Q52.122   Longitudinal vaginal septum, obstructing, left side ♀
     Q52.123   Longitudinal vaginal septum, microperforate, right side ♀
     Q52.124   Longitudinal vaginal septum, microperforate, left side ♀
       Coding Clinic: 2016, Q4, P59
     Q52.129   Other and unspecified longitudinal vaginal septum ♀

   Q52.2   Congenital rectovaginal fistula ♀
     Excludes1   cloaca (Q43.7)

   Q52.3   Imperforate hymen ♀
     Membrane (hymen) completely closes vaginal orifice

   Q52.4   Other congenital malformations of vagina ♀
     Canal of Nuck cyst, congenital
     Congenital malformation of vagina NOS
     Embryonic vaginal cyst
     Gartner's duct cyst

   Q52.5   Fusion of labia ♀

   Q52.6   Congenital malformation of clitoris ♀

  ● Q52.7   Other and unspecified congenital malformations of vulva
     Q52.70   Unspecified congenital malformations of vulva ♀
       Congenital malformation of vulva NOS
     Q52.71   Congenital absence of vulva ♀
     Q52.79   Other congenital malformations of vulva ♀
       Congenital cyst of vulva

N   Newborn Age: 0   **P**   Podiatric Age: 0–17   **M**   Maternity DX: 9–64   **A**   Adult Age: 15–124   ♀   Females Only   ♂   Males Only

Complication\Comorbidity   Major C\C   (Ex)   CC/MCC Exclusions   Hospital-Acquired Condition   Hierarchical Condition Category   **1209**

Item 17-1   Testes form in the abdomen of the male and only descend into the scrotum during normal embryonic development. "Ectopic" testes are out of their normal place or "retained" (left behind) in the abdomen. Crypto (hidden) orchism (testicle) is a major risk factor for testicular cancer.

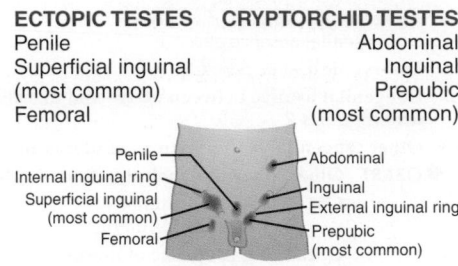

ECTOPIC TESTES	CRYPTORCHID TESTES
Penile	Abdominal
Superficial inguinal	Inguinal
(most common)	Prepubic
Femoral	(most common)

Figure 17-5   Undescended testes and the positions of the testes in various types of cryptorchidism or abnormal paths of descent.

Q52.8   Other specified congenital malformations of female genitalia ♀

Q52.9   Congenital malformation of female genitalia, unspecified ♀

● Q53   Undescended and ectopic testicle

  ● Q53.0   Ectopic testis

     Q53.00   Ectopic testis, unspecified ♂

     Q53.01   Ectopic testis, unilateral ♂

     Q53.02   Ectopic testes, bilateral ♂

  ● Q53.1   Undescended testicle, unilateral

     Q53.10   Unspecified undescended testicle, unilateral ♂

    ● Q53.11   Abdominal testis, unilateral

       Q53.111   Unilateral intraabdominal testis ♂

       Q53.112   Unilateral inguinal testis ♂

     Q53.12   Ectopic perineal testis, unilateral ♂

     Q53.13   Unilateral high scrotal testis ♂

  ● Q53.2   Undescended testicle, bilateral

     Q53.20   Undescended testicle, unspecified, bilateral ♂

    ● Q53.21   Abdominal testis, bilateral

       Q53.211   Bilateral intraabdominal testes ♂

       Q53.212   Bilateral inguinal testes ♂

     Q53.22   Ectopic perineal testis, bilateral ♂

     Q53.23   Bilateral high scrotal testes ♂

   Q53.9   Undescended testicle, unspecified ♂

     Cryptorchism NOS

● Q54   Hypospadias

   Birth defect of male; urethra opens in abnormal location on shaft

   Excludes1   epispadias (Q64.0)

   Q54.0   Hypospadias, balanic ♂

     Hypospadias, coronal

     Hypospadias, glandular

   Q54.1   Hypospadias, penile ♂

   Q54.2   Hypospadias, penoscrotal ♂

   Q54.3   Hypospadias, perineal ♂

   Q54.4   Congenital chordee ♂

     Chordee without hypospadias

   Q54.8   Other hypospadias ♂

     Hypospadias with intersex state

   Q54.9   Hypospadias, unspecified ♂

● Q55   Other congenital malformations of male genital organs

   Excludes1   congenital hydrocele (P83.5)

     hypospadias (Q54.-)

   Q55.0   Absence and aplasia of testis ♂

     Monorchism

   Q55.1   Hypoplasia of testis and scrotum ♂

     Fusion of testes

● Q55.2   Other and unspecified congenital malformations of testis and scrotum

   Q55.20   Unspecified congenital malformations of testis and scrotum ♂

     Congenital malformation of testis or scrotum NOS

   Q55.21   Polyorchism ♂

     Developmental anomaly characterized by presence of more than two testes

   Q55.22   Retractile testis ♂

   Q55.23   Scrotal transposition ♂

   Q55.29   Other congenital malformations of testis and scrotum ♂

Q55.3   Atresia of vas deferens ♂

   Code first any associated cystic fibrosis (E84.-)

Q55.4   Other congenital malformations of vas deferens, epididymis, seminal vesicles and prostate ♂

   Absence or aplasia of prostate

   Absence or aplasia of spermatic cord

   Congenital malformation of vas deferens, epididymis, seminal vesicles or prostate NOS

Q55.5   Congenital absence and aplasia of penis ♂

● Q55.6   Other congenital malformations of penis

   Q55.61   Curvature of penis (lateral) ♂

   Q55.62   Hypoplasia of penis ♂

     Underdevelopment penis

     Micropenis

   Q55.63   Congenital torsion of penis ♂

     Excludes1   acquired torsion of penis (N48.82)

   Q55.64   Hidden penis ♂

     Buried penis

     Concealed penis

     Excludes1   acquired buried penis (N48.83)

   Q55.69   Other congenital malformation of penis ♂

     Congenital malformation of penis NOS

Q55.7   Congenital vasocutaneous fistula ♂

   Abnormal opening between vas deferens and skin

Q55.8   Other specified congenital malformations of male genital organs ♂

Q55.9   Congenital malformation of male genital organ, unspecified ♂

   Congenital anomaly of male genital organ

   Congenital deformity of male genital organ

● Q56   Indeterminate sex and pseudohermaphroditism

   Internal reproductive organs are opposite external physical characteristics.

   Excludes1   46,XX true hermaphrodite (Q99.1)

     androgen insensitivity syndrome (E34.5-)

     chimera 46,XX/46,XY true hermaphrodite (Q99.0)

     female pseudohermaphroditism with adrenocortical disorder (E25.-)

     pseudohermaphroditism with specified chromosomal anomaly (Q96-Q99)

     pure gonadal dysgenesis (Q99.1)

   Q56.0   Hermaphroditism, not elsewhere classified

     Ovotestis

   Q56.1   Male pseudohermaphroditism, not elsewhere classified ♂

     46, XY with streak gonads

     Male pseudohermaphroditism NOS

   Q56.2   Female pseudohermaphroditism, not elsewhere classified ♀

     Female pseudohermaphroditism NOS

   Q56.3   Pseudohermaphroditism, unspecified

   Q56.4   Indeterminate sex, unspecified

     Ambiguous genitalia

▶ New   ⇒ Revised   ~~deleted~~ Deleted   Excludes 1   Excludes 2   Includes   Use additional   Code first   Code also   Key words

1210   OGCR Official Guidelines   ● Unacceptable Principal Diagnosis   X Assign placeholder X   ● Use Additional Character(s)   ▶ Manifestation Code   **Coding Clinic**

CONGENITAL MALFORMATIONS OF THE URINARY SYSTEM (Q60-Q64)

● **Q60**   **Renal agenesis and other reduction defects of kidney**

     Includes   congenital absence of kidney
                      congenital atrophy of kidney
                      infantile atrophy of kidney
    (Ex) **For category Q60 CC codes:** See PDX Collection 1092

    Q60.0   Renal agenesis, unilateral 🔹
    Q60.1   Renal agenesis, bilateral 🔹
    Q60.2   Renal agenesis, unspecified 🔹
    Q60.3   Renal hypoplasia, unilateral 🔹
    Q60.4   Renal hypoplasia, bilateral 🔹
    Q60.5   Renal hypoplasia, unspecified 🔹
    Q60.6   Potter's syndrome 🔹

● **Q61**   **Cystic kidney disease**

    Cysts that develop in failing kidney due to end-stage renal disease

     Excludes1   acquired cyst of kidney (N28.1)
                       Potter's syndrome (Q60.6)

   ● Q61.0   Congenital renal cyst

       Q61.00   Congenital renal cyst, unspecified 🔹
           Cyst of kidney NOS (congenital)
           (Ex) See PDX Collection 1093

       Q61.01   Congenital single renal cyst 🔹
           (Ex) See PDX Collection 1094

       Q61.02   Congenital multiple renal cysts 🔹
           (Ex) See PDX Collection 1095

   ● Q61.1   Polycystic kidney, infantile type
      Polycystic kidney, autosomal recessive
      (Ex) **For category Q61.1 CC codes:** See PDX Collection 1096

       Q61.11   Cystic dilatation of collecting ducts 🔹
       Q61.19   Other polycystic kidney, infantile type 🔹

    Q61.2   Polycystic kidney, adult type 🔹
      Polycystic kidney, autosomal dominant
      (Ex) See PDX Collection 1096

    Q61.3   Polycystic kidney, unspecified 🔹
      (Ex) See PDX Collection 1096
      Coding Clinic: 2016, Q3, P23

    Q61.4   Renal dysplasia 🔹
      Multicystic dysplastic kidney
      Multicystic kidney (development)
      Multicystic kidney disease
      Multicystic renal dysplasia

      Excludes1   polycystic kidney disease (Q61.11-Q61.3)
      (Ex) See PDX Collection 1097

    Q61.5   Medullary cystic kidney 🔹
      ⟱ Nephronophthisis
      Sponge kidney NOS
      (Ex) See PDX Collection 1095

    Q61.8   Other cystic kidney diseases 🔹
      Fibrocystic kidney
      Fibrocystic renal degeneration or disease
      (Ex) See PDX Collection 1095

    Q61.9   Cystic kidney disease, unspecified 🔹
      Meckel-Gruber syndrome
      (Ex) See PDX Collection 1093

● **Q62**   **Congenital obstructive defects of renal pelvis and congenital malformations of ureter**

    Q62.0   Congenital hydronephrosis 🔹
      (Ex) See PDX Collection 1098

   ● Q62.1   Congenital occlusion of ureter
      Atresia and stenosis of ureter
      (Ex) **For category Q62.1 CC codes:** See PDX Collection 1098

       Q62.10   Congenital occlusion of ureter, unspecified 🔹
       Q62.11   Congenital occlusion of ureteropelvic junction 🔹
       Q62.12   Congenital occlusion of ureterovesical orifice 🔹

    Q62.2   Congenital megaureter 🔹
      Congenital dilatation of ureter
      (Ex) See PDX Collection 1098

   ● Q62.3   Other obstructive defects of renal pelvis and ureter
      (Ex) **For category Q62.3 CC codes:** See PDX Collection 1098

       Q62.31   Congenital ureterocele, orthotopic 🔹
           (Ex) See PDX Collection 3966

       Q62.32   Cecoureterocele 🔹
           Ectopic ureterocele
           (Ex) See PDX Collection 3968

       Q62.39   Other obstructive defects of renal pelvis and ureter 🔹
           Ureteropelvic junction obstruction NOS

    Q62.4   Agenesis of ureter
      Congenital absence ureter

    Q62.5   Duplication of ureter
      Accessory ureter
      Double ureter

   ● Q62.6   Malposition of ureter
       Q62.60   Malposition of ureter, unspecified
       Q62.61   Deviation of ureter
       Q62.62   Displacement of ureter
       Q62.63   Anomalous implantation of ureter
           Ectopia of ureter
           Ectopic ureter
       Q62.69   Other malposition of ureter

    Q62.7   Congenital vesico-uretero-renal reflux

    Q62.8   Other congenital malformations of ureter
      Anomaly of ureter NOS

● **Q63**   **Other congenital malformations of kidney**

     Excludes1   congenital nephrotic syndrome (N04.-)

    Q63.0   Accessory kidney
    Q63.1   Lobulated, fused and horseshoe kidney
    Q63.2   Ectopic kidney
      Congenital displaced kidney
      Malrotation of kidney
    Q63.3   Hyperplastic and giant kidney
      Compensatory hypertrophy of kidney
    Q63.8   Other specified congenital malformations of kidney
      Congenital renal calculi
    Q63.9   Congenital malformation of kidney, unspecified

● **Q64**   **Other congenital malformations of urinary system**

    Q64.0   Epispadias
      Urethral opening somewhere on dorsum of penis

      Excludes1   hypospadias (Q54.-)

   ● Q64.1   Exstrophy of urinary bladder
      Bladder is exposed, inside out, and protrudes through abdominal wall
      (Ex) **For category Q64.1 CC codes:** See PDX Collection 1099

       Q64.10   Exstrophy of urinary bladder, unspecified 🔹
           Ectopia vesicae
       Q64.11   Supravesical fissure of urinary bladder 🔹
       Q64.12   Cloacal exstrophy of urinary bladder 🔹
       Q64.19   Other exstrophy of urinary bladder 🔹
           Extroversion of bladder

    Q64.2   Congenital posterior urethral valves 🔹
      (Ex) See PDX Collection 1100

   ● Q64.3   Other atresia and stenosis of urethra and bladder neck
      (Ex) **For category Q64.3 CC codes:** See PDX Collection 1100

       Q64.31   Congenital bladder neck obstruction 🔹
           Congenital obstruction of vesicourethral orifice
       Q64.32   Congenital stricture of urethra 🔹
       Q64.33   Congenital stricture of urinary meatus 🔹
       Q64.39   Other atresia and stenosis of urethra and bladder neck 🔹
           Atresia and stenosis of urethra and bladder neck NOS

    Q64.4   Malformation of urachus
      Cyst of urachus
      Patent urachus
      Prolapse of urachus

    Q64.5   Congenital absence of bladder and urethra
    Q64.6   Congenital diverticulum of bladder

N Newborn Age: 0   **P** Pediatric Age: 0–17   **M** Maternity DX: 9–64   **A** Adult Age: 15–124   ♀ Females Only   ♂ Males Only

🔹 Complication\Comorbidity   🔹 Major C\C   (Ex) CC/MCC Exclusions   🔹 Hospital-Acquired Condition   🔹 Hierarchical Condition Category

CHAPTER 17 (Q00-Q99)

- **Q64.7 Other and unspecified congenital malformations of bladder and urethra**
  Excludes1   congenital prolapse of bladder (mucosa) (Q79.4)
  - Q64.70 **Unspecified congenital malformation of bladder and urethra**
    Malformation of bladder or urethra NOS
  - Q64.71 **Congenital prolapse of urethra**
  - Q64.72 **Congenital prolapse of urinary meatus**
  - Q64.73 **Congenital urethrorectal fistula**
  - Q64.74 **Double urethra**
  - Q64.75 **Double urinary meatus**
  - Q64.79 **Other congenital malformations of bladder and urethra**
- **Q64.8 Other specified congenital malformations of urinary system**
- **Q64.9 Congenital malformation of urinary system, unspecified**
  Congenital anomaly NOS of urinary system
  Congenital deformity NOS of urinary system

CONGENITAL MALFORMATIONS AND DEFORMATIONS OF THE MUSCULOSKELETAL SYSTEM (Q65-Q79)

- **Q65 Congenital deformities of hip**
  Excludes1   clicking hip (R29.4)
  - **Q65.0 Congenital dislocation of hip, unilateral**
    - Q65.00 **Congenital dislocation of unspecified hip, unilateral**
    - Q65.01 **Congenital dislocation of right hip, unilateral**
    - Q65.02 **Congenital dislocation of left hip, unilateral**
  - Q65.1 **Congenital dislocation of hip, bilateral**
  - Q65.2 **Congenital dislocation of hip, unspecified**
  - **Q65.3 Congenital partial dislocation of hip, unilateral**
    - Q65.30 **Congenital partial dislocation of unspecified hip, unilateral**
    - Q65.31 **Congenital partial dislocation of right hip, unilateral**
    - Q65.32 **Congenital partial dislocation of left hip, unilateral**
  - Q65.4 **Congenital partial dislocation of hip, bilateral**
  - Q65.5 **Congenital partial dislocation of hip, unspecified**
  - Q65.6 **Congenital unstable hip**
    Congenital dislocatable hip
  - **Q65.8 Other congenital deformities of hip**
    - Q65.81 **Congenital coxa valga**
    - Q65.82 **Congenital coxa vara**
    - Q65.89 **Other specified congenital deformities of hip**
      Anteversion of femoral neck
      Congenital acetabular dysplasia
  - Q65.9 **Congenital deformity of hip, unspecified**
- **Q66 Congenital deformities of feet**
  Excludes1   reduction defects of feet (Q72.-)
  valgus deformities (acquired) (M21.0-)
  varus deformities (acquired) (M21.1-)
  - **Q66.0 Congenital talipes equinovarus**
    Heel is turned inward from midline and foot is plantar flexed; AKA clubfoot
    - Q66.00 **Congenital talipes equinovarus, unspecified foot**
    - Q66.01 **Congenital talipes equinovarus, right foot**
    - Q66.02 **Congenital talipes equinovarus, left foot**
  - **Q66.1 Congenital talipes calcaneovarus**
    Deformity of foot in which heel is turned toward midline of body and anterior of foot is elevated
    - Q66.10 **Congenital talipes calcaneovarus, unspecified foot**
    - Q66.11 **Congenital talipes calcaneovarus, right foot**
    - Q66.12 **Congenital talipes calcaneovarus, left foot**

Item 17-2   **Equinus foot** is a term referring to the hoof of a horse. The deformity is usually congenital or spastic. **Talipes equinovarus** is referred to as clubfoot. The foot tends to be smaller than normal, with the heel pointing downward and the forefoot turning inward. The heel cord (Achilles tendon) is tight, causing the heel to be drawn up toward the leg.

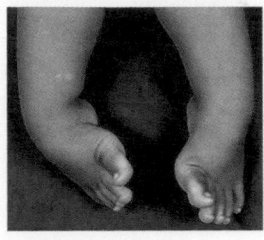

Figure 17-6   Supination and cavus deformity of forefoot. (From Kliegman R, Nelson WE: Nelson Textbook of Pediatrics, Philadelphia, Saunders, 2007)

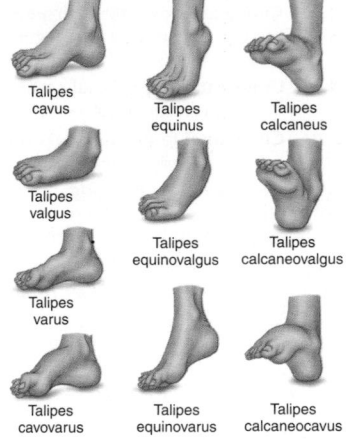

Figure 17-7   Talipes. (From Dorland: Dorland's Illustrated Medical Dictionary, ed 31, Saunders, 2007, p 1893)

- **Q66.2 Congenital metatarsus (primus) varus**
  Angulation of first metatarsal bone toward midline of body
  Coding Clinic: 2016, Q4, P59
  - **Q66.21 Congenital metatarsus primus varus**
    - Q66.211 **Congenital metatarsus primus varus, right foot**
    - Q66.212 **Congenital metatarsus primus varus, left foot**
    - Q66.219 **Congenital metatarsus primus varus, unspecified foot**
  - **Q66.22 Congenital metatarsus adductus**
    Congenital metatarsus varus
    - Q66.221 **Congenital metatarsus adductus, right foot**
    - Q66.222 **Congenital metatarsus adductus, left foot**
    - Q66.229 **Congenital metatarsus adductus, unspecified foot**
- **Q66.3 Other congenital varus deformities of feet**
  Hallux varus, congenital
  - Q66.30 **Other congenital varus deformities of feet, unspecified foot**
  - Q66.31 **Other congenital varus deformities of feet, right foot**
  - Q66.32 **Other congenital varus deformities of feet, left foot**

▶ New   ⇒ Revised   ~~deleted~~ Deleted   Excludes 1   Excludes 2   Includes   Use additional   Code first   Code also   Key words
OGCR Official Guidelines   ● Unacceptable Principal Diagnosis   X Assign placeholder X   ● Use Additional Character(s)   ▷ Manifestation Code   **Coding Clinic**

● Q66.4   Congenital talipes calcaneovalgus

     Q66.40   Congenital talipes calcaneovalgus, unspecified foot

     Q66.41   Congenital talipes calcaneovalgus, right foot

     Q66.42   Congenital talipes calcaneovalgus, left foot

● Q66.5   Congenital pes planus

     Congenital flat foot

     Congenital rigid flat foot

     Congenital spastic (everted) flat foot

     Excludes1   pes planus, acquired (M21.4)

     Q66.50   Congenital pes planus, unspecified foot

     Q66.51   Congenital pes planus, right foot

     Q66.52   Congenital pes planus, left foot

● Q66.6   Other congenital valgus deformities of feet

     Inward angulation

     Congenital metatarsus valgus

● Q66.7   Congenital pes cavus

     Q66.70   Congenital pes cavus, unspecified foot

     Q66.71   Congenital pes cavus, right foot

     Q66.72   Congenital pes cavus, left foot

● Q66.8   Other congenital deformities of feet

     Q66.80   Congenital vertical talus deformity, unspecified foot

     Q66.81   Congenital vertical talus deformity, right foot

     Q66.82   Congenital vertical talus deformity, left foot

     Q66.89   Other specified congenital deformities of feet

        Congenital asymmetric talipes

        Congenital clubfoot NOS

        Congenital talipes NOS

        Congenital tarsal coalition

        Hammer toe, congenital

● Q66.9   Congenital deformity of feet, unspecified

     Q66.90   Congenital deformity of feet, unspecified, unspecified foot

     Q66.91   Congenital deformity of feet, unspecified, right foot

     Q66.92   Congenital deformity of feet, unspecified, left foot

● Q67   Congenital musculoskeletal deformities of head, face, spine and chest

     Excludes1   congenital malformation syndromes classified to Q87.-

          Potter's syndrome (Q60.6)

    Q67.0   Congenital facial asymmetry

    Q67.1   Congenital compression facies

    Q67.2   Dolichocephaly

       Long head dimension

    Q67.3   Plagiocephaly

       Asymmetric shape of head resulting from irregular closure of cranial sutures

    Q67.4   Other congenital deformities of skull, face and jaw

       Congenital depressions in skull

       Congenital hemifacial atrophy or hypertrophy

       Deviation of nasal septum, congenital

       Squashed or bent nose, congenital

       Excludes1   dentofacial anomalies [including malocclusion] (M26.-)

           syphilitic saddle nose (A50.5)

    Q67.5   Congenital deformity of spine 🔗

       Congenital postural scoliosis

       Congenital scoliosis NOS

       Excludes1   infantile idiopathic scoliosis (M41.0)

           scoliosis due to congenital bony malformation (Q76.3)

       (Ex:) See PDX Collection 1101

    Q67.6   Pectus excavatum

       Congenital funnel chest

       Funnel-shaped chest depression

    Q67.7   Pectus carinatum

       Congenital pigeon chest

    Q67.8   Other congenital deformities of chest 🔗

       Congenital deformity of chest wall NOS

       (Ex:) See PDX Collection 1102

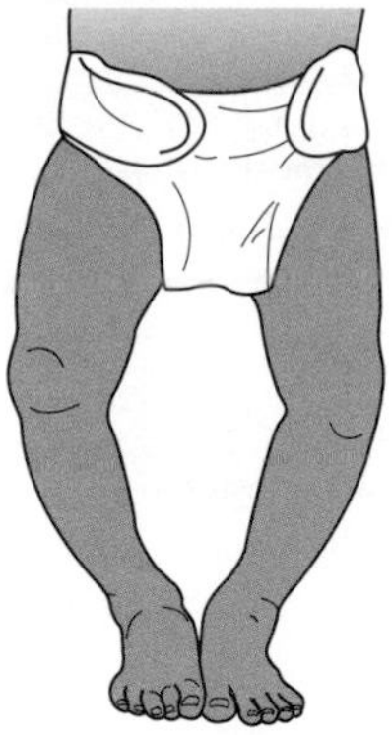

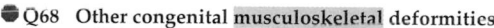

Figure 17-8   Mild to moderate inbowing of the lower leg. (From Lissauer T, Clayden G: Illustrated Textbook of Paediatrics, Edinburgh, Mosby, 2011)

◐ Q68   Other congenital musculoskeletal deformities

     Excludes1   reduction defects of limb(s) (Q71-Q73)

     Excludes2   congenital myotonic chondrodystrophy (G71.13)

    Q68.0   Congenital deformity of sternocleidomastoid muscle

       Congenital contracture of sternocleidomastoid (muscle)

       Congenital (sternomastoid) torticollis

       Sternomastoid tumor (congenital)

    Q68.1   Congenital deformity of finger(s) and hand 🔗

       Congenital clubfinger

       Spade-like hand (congenital)

       (Ex:) See PDX Collection 1102

    Q68.2   Congenital deformity of knee

       Congenital dislocation of knee

       Congenital genu recurvatum

       Hyperextension of knee resulting from hypermobility

    Q68.3   Congenital bowing of femur

       Excludes1   anteversion of femur (neck) (Q65.89)

    Q68.4   Congenital bowing of tibia and fibula

    Q68.5   Congenital bowing of long bones of leg, unspecified

    Q68.6   Discoid meniscus

    Q68.8   Other specified congenital musculoskeletal deformities

       Congenital deformity of clavicle

       Congenital deformity of elbow

       Congenital deformity of forearm

       Congenital deformity of scapula

       Congenital deformity of wrist

       Congenital dislocation of elbow

       Congenital dislocation of shoulder

       Congenital dislocation of wrist

● Q69   Polydactyly

     AKA hyperdactyly, consists of supernumerary fingers or toes

    Q69.0   Accessory finger(s)

    Q69.1   Accessory thumb(s)

    Q69.2   Accessory toe(s)

       Accessory hallux

    Q69.9   Polydactyly, unspecified

       Supernumerary digit(s) NOS

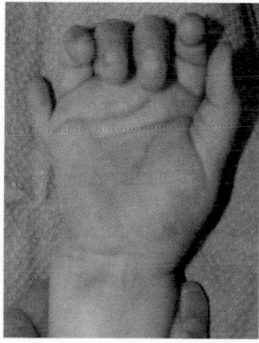

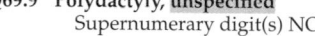

Figure 17-9   Thumb and index finger. (From Chung K: Hand and Upper Extremity Reconstruction, 1e, Saunders, 2008)

CHAPTER 17 (Q00-Q99)

N Newborn Age: 0   **P** Pediatric Age: 0–17   **M** Maternity DX: 9–64   **A** Adult Age: 15–124   ♀ Females Only   ♂ Males Only

🔗 Complication\Comorbidity   🔗 Major C\C   (Ex:) CC/MCC Exclusions   🔗 Hospital-Acquired Condition   🔗 Hierarchical Condition Category

● **Q70　Syndactyly**
　　　Webbing between distal phalanges of adjacent digits
　● **Q70.0　Fused fingers**
　　　　Complex syndactyly of fingers with synostosis
　　　Q70.00　Fused fingers, unspecified hand
　　　Q70.01　Fused fingers, right hand
　　　Q70.02　Fused fingers, left hand
　　　Q70.03　Fused fingers, bilateral
　● **Q70.1　Webbed fingers**
　　　　Simple syndactyly of fingers without synostosis
　　　Q70.10　Webbed fingers, unspecified hand
　　　Q70.11　Webbed fingers, right hand
　　　Q70.12　Webbed fingers, left hand
　　　Q70.13　Webbed fingers, bilateral
　● **Q70.2　Fused toes**
　　　　Complex syndactyly of toes with synostosis
　　　Q70.20　Fused toes, unspecified foot
　　　Q70.21　Fused toes, right foot
　　　Q70.22　Fused toes, left foot
　　　Q70.23　Fused toes, bilateral
　● **Q70.3　Webbed toes**
　　　　Simple syndactyly of toes without synostosis
　　　Q70.30　Webbed toes, unspecified foot
　　　Q70.31　Webbed toes, right foot
　　　Q70.32　Webbed toes, left foot
　　　Q70.33　Webbed toes, bilateral
　　Q70.4　Polysyndactyly, unspecified
　　　　　Excludes1　specified syndactyly of hand and
　　　　　　　　　feet - code to specified conditions
　　　　　　　　　(Q70.0- -Q70.3-)
　　　　　Extra and webbed digits
　　Q70.9　Syndactyly, unspecified
　　　　Symphalangy NOS

● **Q71　Reduction defects of upper limb**
　● **Q71.0　Congenital complete absence of upper limb**
　　　Q71.00　Congenital complete absence of unspecified
　　　　　　　upper limb
　　　Q71.01　Congenital complete absence of right upper limb
　　　Q71.02　Congenital complete absence of left upper limb
　　　Q71.03　Congenital complete absence of upper limb,
　　　　　　　bilateral
　● **Q71.1　Congenital absence of upper arm and forearm with hand
　　　present**
　　　Q71.10　Congenital absence of unspecified upper arm
　　　　　　　and forearm with hand present
　　　Q71.11　Congenital absence of right upper arm and
　　　　　　　forearm with hand present
　　　Q71.12　Congenital absence of left upper arm and
　　　　　　　forearm with hand present
　　　Q71.13　Congenital absence of upper arm and forearm
　　　　　　　with hand present, bilateral
　● **Q71.2　Congenital absence of both forearm and hand**
　　　Q71.20　Congenital absence of both forearm and hand,
　　　　　　　unspecified upper limb
　　　Q71.21　Congenital absence of both forearm and hand,
　　　　　　　right upper limb
　　　Q71.22　Congenital absence of both forearm and hand,
　　　　　　　left upper limb
　　　Q71.23　Congenital absence of both forearm and hand,
　　　　　　　bilateral
　● **Q71.3　Congenital absence of hand and finger**
　　　Q71.30　Congenital absence of unspecified hand and
　　　　　　　finger
　　　Q71.31　Congenital absence of right hand and finger
　　　Q71.32　Congenital absence of left hand and finger
　　　Q71.33　Congenital absence of hand and finger, bilateral

● **Q71.4　Longitudinal reduction defect of radius**
　　　Clubhand (congenital)
　　　Radial clubhand
　　　Q71.40　Longitudinal reduction defect of unspecified
　　　　　　　radius
　　　Q71.41　Longitudinal reduction defect of right radius
　　　Q71.42　Longitudinal reduction defect of left radius
　　　Q71.43　Longitudinal reduction defect of radius,
　　　　　　　bilateral
　● **Q71.5　Longitudinal reduction defect of ulna**
　　　Q71.50　Longitudinal reduction defect of unspecified ulna
　　　Q71.51　Longitudinal reduction defect of right ulna
　　　Q71.52　Longitudinal reduction defect of left ulna
　　　Q71.53　Longitudinal reduction defect of ulna, bilateral
　● **Q71.6　Lobster-claw hand**
　　　Q71.60　Lobster-claw hand, unspecified hand
　　　Q71.61　Lobster-claw right hand
　　　Q71.62　Lobster-claw left hand
　　　Q71.63　Lobster-claw hand, bilateral
　● **Q71.8　Other reduction defects of upper limb**
　　● **Q71.81　Congenital shortening of upper limb**
　　　　　Q71.811　Congenital shortening of right upper
　　　　　　　　　limb
　　　　　Q71.812　Congenital shortening of left upper
　　　　　　　　　limb
　　　　　Q71.813　Congenital shortening of upper limb,
　　　　　　　　　bilateral
　　　　　Q71.819　Congenital shortening of unspecified
　　　　　　　　　upper limb
　　● **Q71.89　Other reduction defects of upper limb**
　　　　　Q71.891　Other reduction defects of right upper
　　　　　　　　　limb
　　　　　Q71.892　Other reduction defects of left upper
　　　　　　　　　limb
　　　　　Q71.893　Other reduction defects of upper
　　　　　　　　　limb, bilateral
　　　　　Q71.899　Other reduction defects of
　　　　　　　　　unspecified upper limb
　● **Q71.9　Unspecified reduction defect of upper limb**
　　　Q71.90　Unspecified reduction defect of unspecified
　　　　　　　upper limb
　　　Q71.91　Unspecified reduction defect of right upper
　　　　　　　limb
　　　Q71.92　Unspecified reduction defect of left upper limb
　　　Q71.93　Unspecified reduction defect of upper limb,
　　　　　　　bilateral

● **Q72　Reduction defects of lower limb**
　● **Q72.0　Congenital complete absence of lower limb**
　　　Q72.00　Congenital complete absence of unspecified
　　　　　　　lower limb
　　　Q72.01　Congenital complete absence of right lower
　　　　　　　limb
　　　Q72.02　Congenital complete absence of left lower limb
　　　Q72.03　Congenital complete absence of lower limb,
　　　　　　　bilateral
　● **Q72.1　Congenital absence of thigh and lower leg with foot
　　　present**
　　　Q72.10　Congenital absence of unspecified thigh and
　　　　　　　lower leg with foot present
　　　Q72.11　Congenital absence of right thigh and lower leg
　　　　　　　with foot present
　　　Q72.12　Congenital absence of left thigh and lower leg
　　　　　　　with foot present
　　　Q72.13　Congenital absence of thigh and lower leg with
　　　　　　　foot present, bilateral

▶ New　⏵ Revised　~~deleted~~ Deleted　Excludes 1　Excludes 2　Includes　Use additional　Code first　Code also　Key words
OGCR Official Guidelines　● Unacceptable Principal Diagnosis　X Assign placeholder X　● Use Additional Character(s)　▶ Manifestation Code　Coding Clinic

● **Q72.2 Congenital absence of both lower leg and foot**

Q72.20   Congenital absence of both lower leg and foot, unspecified lower limb

Q72.21   Congenital absence of both lower leg and foot, right lower limb

Q72.22   Congenital absence of both left lower leg and foot, left lower limb

Q72.23   Congenital absence of both lower leg and foot, bilateral

● **Q72.3 Congenital absence of foot and toe(s)**

Q72.30   Congenital absence of unspecified foot and toe(s)

Q72.31   Congenital absence of right foot and toe(s)

Q72.32   Congenital absence of left foot and toe(s)

Q72.33   Congenital absence of foot and toe(s), bilateral

● **Q72.4 Longitudinal reduction defect of femur**

Proximal femoral focal deficiency

Q72.40   Longitudinal reduction defect of unspecified femur

Q72.41   Longitudinal reduction defect of right femur

Q72.42   Longitudinal reduction defect of left femur

Q72.43   Longitudinal reduction defect of femur, bilateral

● **Q72.5 Longitudinal reduction defect of tibia**

Q72.50   Longitudinal reduction defect of unspecified tibia

Q72.51   Longitudinal reduction defect of right tibia

Q72.52   Longitudinal reduction defect of left tibia

Q72.53   Longitudinal reduction defect of tibia, bilateral

● **Q72.6 Longitudinal reduction defect of fibula**

Q72.60   Longitudinal reduction defect of unspecified fibula

Q72.61   Longitudinal reduction defect of right fibula

Q72.62   Longitudinal reduction defect of left fibula

Q72.63   Longitudinal reduction defect of fibula, bilateral

● **Q72.7 Split foot**

Q72.70   Split foot, unspecified lower limb

Q72.71   Split foot, right lower limb

Q72.72   Split foot, left lower limb

Q72.73   Split foot, bilateral

● **Q72.8 Other reduction defects of lower limb**

● Q72.81   Congenital shortening of lower limb

Q72.811   Congenital shortening of right lower limb

Q72.812   Congenital shortening of left lower limb

Q72.813   Congenital shortening of lower limb, bilateral

Q72.819   Congenital shortening of unspecified lower limb

● Q72.89   Other reduction defects of lower limb

Q72.891   Other reduction defects of right lower limb

Q72.892   Other reduction defects of left lower limb

Q72.893   Other reduction defects of lower limb, bilateral

Q72.899   Other reduction defects of unspecified lower limb

● **Q72.9 Unspecified reduction defect of lower limb**

Q72.90   Unspecified reduction defect of unspecified lower limb

Q72.91   Unspecified reduction defect of right lower limb

Q72.92   Unspecified reduction defect of left lower limb

Q72.93   Unspecified reduction defect of lower limb, bilateral

● **Q73 Reduction defects of unspecified limb**

Q73.0   **Congenital absence of unspecified limb(s)**

Amelia NOS

Q73.1   **Phocomelia, unspecified limb(s)**

Phocomelia NOS

Absence/shortening of long bones primarily as a result of thalidomide

Q73.8   **Other reduction defects of unspecified limb(s)**

Longitudinal reduction deformity of unspecified limb(s)

Ectromelia of limb NOS

Gross hypoplasia or aplasia of one or more long bones of limb(s)

Hemimelia of limb NOS

Absence of one-half of long bone

Reduction defect of limb NOS

● **Q74 Other congenital malformations of limb(s)**

Excludes1   polydactyly (Q69.-)

reduction defect of limb (Q71-Q73)

syndactyly (Q70.-)

Q74.0   **Other congenital malformations of upper limb(s), including shoulder girdle**

Accessory carpal bones

Cleidocranial dysostosis

Congenital pseudarthrosis of clavicle

Macrodactylia (fingers)

Madelung's deformity

Radioulnar synostosis

Sprengel's deformity

Triphalangeal thumb

Q74.1   **Congenital malformation of knee**

Congenital absence of patella

Congenital dislocation of patella

Congenital genu valgum

Congenital genu varum

Rudimentary patella

Excludes1   congenital dislocation of knee (Q68.2)

congenital genu recurvatum (Q68.2)

nail patella syndrome (Q87.2)

Q74.2   **Other congenital malformations of lower limb(s), including pelvic girdle**

Congenital fusion of sacroiliac joint

Congenital malformation of ankle joint

Congenital malformation of sacroiliac joint

Excludes1   anteversion of femur (neck) (Q65.89)

Q74.3   **Arthrogryposis multiplex congenita** 🅗

Q74.8   **Other specified congenital malformations of limb(s)**

Q74.9   **Unspecified congenital malformation of limb(s)**

Congenital anomaly of limb(s) NOS

● **Q75 Other congenital malformations of skull and face bones**

Excludes1   congenital malformation of face NOS (Q18.-)

congenital malformation syndromes classified to Q87.-

dentofacial anomalies [including malocclusion] (M26.-)

musculoskeletal deformities of head and face (Q67.0-Q67.4)

skull defects associated with congenital anomalies of brain such as:

anencephaly (Q00.0)

encephalocele (Q01.-)

hydrocephalus (Q03.-)

microcephaly (Q02)

Q75.0   **Craniosynostosis**

Premature closure of sutures of skull

Acrocephaly

Imperfect fusion of skull

Oxycephaly

Trigonocephaly

Q75.1   **Craniofacial dysostosis**

Congenital deformity of head

Crouzon's disease

Q75.2   **Hypertelorism**

Q75.3   **Macrocephaly**

Unusually large size of head; AKA megalocephaly

N Newborn Age: 0   **P** Pediatric Age: 0–17   **M** Maternity DX: 9–64   **A** Adult Age: 15–124   ♀ Females Only   ♂ Males Only

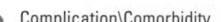 Complication\Comorbidity   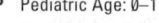 Major C\C   (Ex) CC/MCC Exclusions   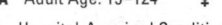 Hospital-Acquired Condition   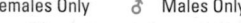 Hierarchical Condition Category

1215

CHAPTER 17 (Q00–Q99)

Item 17–3 Anencephalus is a congenital deformity of the cranial vault. **Craniosynostosis,** also known as craniostenosis and stenocephaly, signifies any form of congenital deformity of the skull that results from the premature closing of the sutures of the skull. **Iniencephaly** is a deformity in which the head and neck are flexed backward to a great extent and the head is very large in comparison to the shortened body.

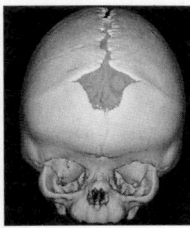

Figure 17-10 Generalized craniosynostosis without symptoms or signs of increased intracranial pressure. (From Goetz C: Textbook of Clinical Neurology, St. Louis, MO, Elsevier, 2007)

Q75.4 Mandibulofacial dysostosis
    Franceschetti syndrome
    Treacher Collins syndrome

Q75.5 Oculomandibular dysostosis
    Ossification of occular and mandibular bones

Q75.8 Other specified congenital malformations of skull and face bones
    Absence of skull bone, congenital
    Congenital deformity of forehead
    Platybasia

Q75.9 Congenital malformation of skull and face bones, unspecified
    Congenital anomaly of face bones NOS
    Congenital anomaly of skull NOS

● **Q76 Congenital malformations of spine and bony thorax**
    Excludes1 congenital musculoskeletal deformities of spine and chest (Q67.5-Q67.8)

Q76.0 Spina bifida occulta
    Excludes1 meningocele (spinal) (Q05.-)
              spina bifida (aperta) (cystica) (Q05.-)

Q76.1 Klippel-Feil syndrome
    Cervical fusion syndrome

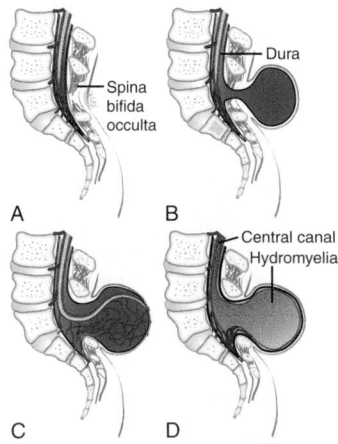

Figure 17-11 A. Spina bifida occulta. **B.** Meningocele. **C.** Myelomeningocele. **D.** Myelocystocele (syringomyelocele) or hydromyelia.

Item 17–4 Spina bifida is a midline spinal defect in which one or more vertebrae fail to fuse, leaving an opening in the vertebral canal. When the defect is not visible, it is called spina bifida occulta, and when it is visible, it is called spina bifida cystica.

Q76.2 Congenital spondylolisthesis
    Congenital spondylolysis
    Excludes1 spondylolisthesis (acquired) (M43.1-)
              spondylolysis (acquired) (M43.0-)

Q76.3 Congenital scoliosis due to congenital bony malformation 🔖
    Hemivertebra fusion or failure of segmentation with scoliosis
    (Ex) See PDX Collection 1101

● **Q76.4 Other congenital malformations of spine, not associated with scoliosis**
    ● **Q76.41 Congenital kyphosis**
        Abnormal increase in convexity curvature of thoracic spinal column; AKA humpback
        Q76.411 Congenital kyphosis, occipito-atlanto-axial region
        Q76.412 Congenital kyphosis, cervical region
        Q76.413 Congenital kyphosis, cervicothoracic region
        Q76.414 Congenital kyphosis, thoracic region
        Q76.415 Congenital kyphosis, thoracolumbar region
        Q76.419 Congenital kyphosis, unspecified region

    ● **Q76.42 Congenital lordosis**
        An abnormal increase in curvature of lumbar spine (sway back)
        (Ex) **For category Q76.42 CC codes:** See PDX Collection 1101
        Q76.425 Congenital lordosis, thoracolumbar region 🔖
        Q76.426 Congenital lordosis, lumbar region 🔖
        Q76.427 Congenital lordosis, lumbosacral region 🔖
        Q76.428 Congenital lordosis, sacral and sacrococcygeal region 🔖
        Q76.429 Congenital lordosis, unspecified region 🔖

    Q76.49 Other congenital malformations of spine, not associated with scoliosis
        Congenital absence of vertebra NOS
        Congenital fusion of spine NOS
        Congenital malformation of lumbosacral (joint) (region) NOS
        Congenital malformation of spine NOS
        Hemivertebra NOS
        Malformation of spine NOS
        Platyspondylisis NOS
        Supernumerary vertebra NOS

Q76.5 Cervical rib
    Supernumerary rib in cervical region

Q76.6 Other congenital malformations of ribs 🔖
    Accessory rib
    Congenital absence of rib
    Congenital fusion of ribs
    Congenital malformation of ribs NOS
    Excludes1 short rib syndrome (Q77.2)
    (Ex) See PDX Collection 1103

Q76.7 Congenital malformation of sternum 🔖
    Congenital absence of sternum
    Sternum bifidum
    (Ex) See PDX Collection 1103

Q76.8 Other congenital malformations of bony thorax 🔖
    (Ex) See PDX Collection 1103

Q76.9 Congenital malformation of bony thorax, unspecified 🔖
    (Ex) See PDX Collection 1103

▶ New   ⇒ Revised   ~~deleted~~ Deleted   Excludes 1   Excludes 2   Includes   Use additional   Code first   Code also   Key words

1216   OGCR Official Guidelines   ● Unacceptable Principal Diagnosis   X Assign placeholder X   ● Use Additional Character(s)   ▶ Manifestation Code   **Coding Clinic**

● Q77　Osteochondrodysplasia with defects of growth of tubular bones and spine

> **Excludes1**　mucopolysaccharidosis (E76.0-E76.3)
>
> **Excludes2**　congenital myotonic chondrodystrophy (G71.13)

Q77.0　**Achondrogenesis**
Hypochondrogenesis

Q77.1　**Thanatophoric short stature**

Q77.2　**Short rib syndrome** 🐾
Asphyxiating thoracic dysplasia [Jeune]
🔘 See PDX Collection 1103

Q77.3　**Chondrodysplasia punctata**
Benign cartilaginous neoplasms

> **Excludes1**　rhizomelic chondrodysplasia punctata (E71.43)

Q77.4　**Achondroplasia**
Disturbance of epiphyseal chondroblastic growth and maturation, results in dwarfism
Hypochondroplasia
Osteosclerosis congenita

Q77.5　**Diastrophic dysplasia**

Q77.6　**Chondroectodermal dysplasia**
Defective development of skin, hair, teeth, with polydactyly and defect of cardiac septum
Ellis-van Creveld syndrome

Q77.7　**Spondyloepiphyseal dysplasia**

Q77.8　**Other osteochondrodysplasia with defects of growth of tubular bones and spine**

Q77.9　**Osteochondrodysplasia with defects of growth of tubular bones and spine, unspecified**

● Q78　Other osteochondrodysplasias
Disorder of development of bone and cartilage; common cause of dwarfism

> **Excludes2**　congenital myotonic chondrodystrophy (G71.13)

Q78.0　**Osteogenesis imperfecta** 🐾
Fragilitas ossium
Osteopsathyrosis
🔘 See PDX Collection 1104

Q78.1　**Polyostotic fibrous dysplasia**
Albright(-McCune)(-Sternberg) syndrome

Q78.2　**Osteopetrosis** 🐾
Abnormally dense bone; AKA marble bones disease, ivory bones
Albers-Schönberg syndrome
Osteosclerosis NOS
🔘 See PDX Collection 1104

Q78.3　**Progressive diaphyseal dysplasia**
Camurati-Engelmann syndrome

Q78.4　**Enchondromatosis**
Thinning of overlying cortex of bone and distorted length
Maffucci's syndrome
Ollier's disease

Q78.5　**Metaphyseal dysplasia**
Disturbance in enchondral bone growth, causing ends of shafts to remain larger than normal in circumference
Pyle's syndrome

Q78.6　**Multiple congenital exostoses**
Diaphyseal aclasis

Q78.8　**Other specified osteochondrodysplasias**
Osteopoikilosis

Q78.9　**Osteochondrodysplasia, unspecified**
Chondrodystrophy NOS
AKA skeletal dysplasia (dwarfism) caused by genetic mutations affecting hyaline cartilage capping long bones and vertebrae
Osteodystrophy NOS

● Q79　Congenital malformations of musculoskeletal system, not elsewhere classified

> **Excludes2**　congenital (sternomastoid) torticollis (Q68.0)

Q79.0　**Congenital diaphragmatic hernia** 🐾

> **Excludes1**　congenital hiatus hernia (Q40.1)

🔘 See PDX Collection 1105

Q79.1　**Other congenital malformations of diaphragm** 🐾
Absence of diaphragm
Congenital malformation of diaphragm NOS
Eventration of diaphragm
🔘 See PDX Collection 1105

Q79.2　**Exomphalos** 🐾
Abdominal hernia in which part of intestine protrudes at umbilicus; AKA exomphalos and exumbilication
Omphalocele

> **Excludes1**　umbilical hernia (K42.-)

🔘 See PDX Collection 1106

Q79.3　**Gastroschisis** 🐾
Congenital fissure of anterior abdominal wall often with protrusion of small/large intestine
🔘 See PDX Collection 1106

Q79.4　**Prune belly syndrome** 🐾
Congenital prolapse of bladder mucosa
Eagle-Barrett syndrome
🔘 See PDX Collection 1106

● Q79.5　**Other congenital malformations of abdominal wall**

> **Excludes1**　umbilical hernia (K42.-)

🔘 For category Q79.5 CC codes: See PDX Collection 1106

Q79.51　**Congenital hernia of bladder** 🐾

Q79.59　**Other congenital malformations of abdominal wall** 🐾

● Q79.6　**Ehlers-Danlos syndromes**
🔘 See PDX Collection 3467
Group of inherited disorders of connective tissue; AKA cutis hyperelastica

Q79.60　**Ehlers-Danlos syndrome, unspecified** 🐾

Q79.61　**Classical Ehlers-Danlos syndrome** 🐾
Classical EDS (cEDS)

Q79.62　**Hypermobile Ehlers-Danlos syndrome** 🐾
Hypermobile EDS (hEDS)

Q79.63　**Vascular Ehlers-Danlos syndrome** 🐾
Vascular EDS (vEDS)

Q79.69　**Other Ehlers-Danlos syndromes** 🐾

Q79.8　**Other congenital malformations of musculoskeletal system**
Absence of muscle
Absence of tendon
Accessory muscle
Amyotrophia congenita
Congenital constricting bands
Congenital shortening of tendon
Poland syndrome

Q79.9　**Congenital malformation of musculoskeletal system, unspecified**
Congenital anomaly of musculoskeletal system NOS
Congenital deformity of musculoskeletal system NOS

N Newborn Age: 0　　**P** Pediatric Age: 0–17　　**M** Maternity DX: 9–64　　**A** Adult Age: 15–124　　♀ Females Only　　♂ Males Only

🐾 Complication\Comorbidity　　🐾 Major C\C　　🔘 CC/MCC Exclusions　　🐾 Hospital-Acquired Condition　　🐾 Hierarchical Condition Category

1217

OTHER CONGENITAL MALFORMATIONS (Q80-Q89)

● **Q80   Congenital ichthyosis**
Characterized by increased keratinization, resulting in noninflammatory scaling of skin

> **Excludes1**   Refsum's disease (G60.1)

Q80.0   Ichthyosis vulgaris

Q80.1   X-linked ichthyosis

Q80.2   Lamellar ichthyosis
Collodion baby

Q80.3   Congenital bullous ichthyosiform erythroderma

Q80.4   Harlequin fetus

Q80.8   Other congenital ichthyosis

Q80.9   Congenital ichthyosis, unspecified

● **Q81   Epidermolysis bullosa**
Loosening of epidermis

Q81.0   Epidermolysis bullosa simplex

> **Excludes1**   Cockayne's syndrome (Q87.19)

Q81.1   Epidermolysis bullosa letalis
Herlitz' syndrome

Q81.2   Epidermolysis bullosa dystrophica

Q81.8   Other epidermolysis bullosa

Q81.9   Epidermolysis bullosa, unspecified

● **Q82   Other congenital malformations of skin**

> **Excludes1**   acrodermatitis enteropathica (E83.2)
> congenital erythropoietic porphyria (E80.0)
> pilonidal cyst or sinus (L05.-)
> Sturge-Weber (-Dimitri) syndrome (Q85.8)

Q82.0   Hereditary lymphedema
Characterized by swelling of subcutaneous tissue caused by obstruction of lymphatic vessels and resulting edema of lymph fluid

Q82.1   Xeroderma pigmentosum
Extreme sensitivity to ultraviolet rays that most commonly affects the eyes and skin, but may also involve the nervous system

Q82.2   Congenital cutaneous mastocytosis
Characterized by infiltrates of mast cells in tissues/organs
Congenital diffuse cutaneous mastocytosis
Congenital maculopapular cutaneous mastocytosis
Congenital urticaria pigmentosa

> **Excludes1**   cutaneous mastocytosis NOS (D47.01)
> diffuse cutaneous mastocytosis (with onset after newborn period) (D47.01)
> malignant mastocytosis (C96.2-)
> systemic mastocytosis (D47.02)
> urticaria pigmentosa (non-congenital) (with onset after newborn period) (D47.01)

Q82.3   Incontinentia pigmenti
Characterized by hypopigmented cutaneous in adults and early childhood

Q82.4   Ectodermal dysplasia (anhidrotic)
Absence/deficiency of tissues/structures, including teeth, hair, nails, and certain glands

> **Excludes1**   Ellis-van Creveld syndrome (Q77.6)

Q82.5   Congenital non-neoplastic nevus
Birthmark NOS
Flammeus Nevus
Portwine Nevus
Sanguineous Nevus
Strawberry Nevus
Vascular Nevus NOS
Verrucous Nevus

> **Excludes2**   Café au lait spots (L81.3)
> lentigo (L81.4)
> nevus NOS (D22.-)
> araneus nevus (I78.1)
> melanocytic nevus (D22.-)
> pigmented nevus (D22.-)
> spider nevus (I78.1)
> stellar nevus (I78.1)

Q82.6   Congenital sacral dimple
Parasacral dimple

> **Excludes2**   pilonidal cyst with abscess (L05.01)
> pilonidal cyst without abscess (L05.91)

Coding Clinic: 2016, Q4, P60

Q82.8   Other specified congenital malformations of skin
Abnormal palmar creases
Accessory skin tags
Benign familial pemphigus [Hailey-Hailey]
Congenital poikiloderma
Cutis laxa (hyperelastica)
Dermatoglyphic anomalies
Inherited keratosis palmaris et plantaris
Keratosis follicularis [Darier-White]

> **Excludes1**   Ehlers-Danlos syndromes (Q79.6-)

Coding Clinic: 2016, Q1, P17

Q82.9   Congenital malformation of skin, unspecified

● **Q83   Congenital malformations of breast**

> **Excludes2**   absence of pectoral muscle (Q79.8)
> hypoplasia of breast (N64.82)
> micromastia (N64.82)

Q83.0   Congenital absence of breast with absent nipple

Q83.1   Accessory breast
Supernumerary breast

Q83.2   Absent nipple

Q83.3   Accessory nipple
Supernumerary nipple

Q83.8   Other congenital malformations of breast

Q83.9   Congenital malformation of breast, unspecified

● **Q84   Other congenital malformations of integument**

Q84.0   Congenital alopecia
Congenital atrichosis

Q84.1   Congenital morphological disturbances of hair, not elsewhere classified
Beaded hair
Monilethrix
Pili annulati

> **Excludes1**   Menkes' kinky hair syndrome (E83.0)

Q84.2   Other congenital malformations of hair
Congenital hypertrichosis
Congenital malformation of hair NOS
Persistent lanugo

Q84.3   Anonychia
Absence of nail

> **Excludes1**   nail patella syndrome (Q87.2)

Q84.4   Congenital leukonychia
Opaque, whitish discoloration of nails; AKA leukopathia unguium

Q84.5   Enlarged and hypertrophic nails
Congenital onychauxis
Pachyonychia

Q84.6   Other congenital malformations of nails
Congenital clubnail
Congenital koilonychia
Congenital malformation of nail NOS

Q84.8   Other specified congenital malformations of integument
Aplasia cutis congenita

Q84.9   Congenital malformation of integument, unspecified
Congenital anomaly of integument NOS
Congenital deformity of integument NOS

▶ New   ⇒ Revised   ~~deleted~~ Deleted   Excludes 1   Excludes 2   Includes   Use additional   Code first   Code also   Key words
OGCR Official Guidelines   ● Unacceptable Principal Diagnosis   X Assign placeholder X   ● Use Additional Character(s)   ▷ Manifestation Code   **Coding Clinic**

● **Q85 Phakomatoses, not elsewhere classified**
  Excludes1 ataxia telangiectasia [Louis-Bar] (G11.3)
       familial dysautonomia [Riley-Day] (G90.1)

 ● **Q85.0 Neurofibromatosis (nonmalignant)**
   Developmental changes in nervous system and other
   structures, with formation of neurofibromas
  Q85.00 Neurofibromatosis, unspecified 🔹
  Q85.01 Neurofibromatosis, type 1 🔹
    Von Recklinghausen disease
  Q85.02 Neurofibromatosis, type 2 🔹
    Acoustic neurofibromatosis
  Q85.03 Schwannomatosis 🔹
  Q85.09 Other neurofibromatosis 🔹

 Q85.1 Tuberous sclerosis 🔹🔹
   Bourneville's disease
   Epiloia
   (Ex:) See PDX Collection 1108

 Q85.8 Other phakomatoses, not elsewhere classified 🔹🔹
   Peutz-Jeghers Syndrome
   Sturge-Weber(-Dimitri) syndrome
   von Hippel-Lindau syndrome
  Excludes1 Meckel-Gruber syndrome (Q61.9)
   (Ex:) See PDX Collection 1109

 Q85.9 Phakomatosis, unspecified 🔹🔹
   Hamartosis NOS
   (Ex:) See PDX Collection 1109

● **Q86 Congenital malformation syndromes due to known exogenous causes, not elsewhere classified**
  Excludes2 iodine-deficiency-related hypothyroidism
      (E00-E02)
     nonteratogenic effects of substances transmitted
     via placenta or breast milk (P04.-)

 Q86.0 Fetal alcohol syndrome (dysmorphic)

 Q86.1 Fetal hydantoin syndrome
   Meadow's syndrome

 Q86.2 Dysmorphism due to warfarin

 Q86.8 Other congenital malformation syndromes due to known exogenous causes

● **Q87 Other specified congenital malformation syndromes affecting multiple systems**
  Use additional code(s) to identify all associated manifestations

 Q87.0 Congenital malformation syndromes predominantly affecting facial appearance
   Acrocephalopolysyndactyly
   Acrocephalosyndactyly [Apert]
   Cryptophthalmos syndrome
   Cyclopia
   Goldenhar syndrome
   Moebius syndrome
   Oro-facial-digital syndrome
   Robin syndrome
   Whistling face

● **Q87.1 Congenital malformation syndromes predominantly associated with short stature**
   (Ex:) See PDX Collection 2979

 Q87.11 Prader-Willi syndrome 🔹

 Q87.19 Other congenital malformation syndromes predominantly associated with short stature 🔹
   Aarskog syndrome
   Cockayne syndrome
   De Lange syndrome
   Dubowitz syndrome
   Noonan syndrome
   Robinow-Silverman-Smith syndrome
   Russell-Silver syndrome
   Seckel syndrome
  Excludes1 Ellis-van Creveld syndrome (Q77.6)
      Smith-Lemli-Opitz syndrome (E78.72)
   (Ex:) See PDX Collection 1110

 Q87.2 Congenital malformation syndromes predominantly involving limbs 🔹
   Holt-Oram syndrome
   Klippel-Trenaunay-Weber syndrome
   Nail patella syndrome
   Rubinstein-Taybi syndrome
   Sirenomelia syndrome
   Thrombocytopenia with absent radius [TAR] syndrome
   VATER syndrome

 Q87.3 Congenital malformation syndromes involving early overgrowth 🔹
   Beckwith-Wiedemann syndrome
   Sotos' syndrome
   Weaver syndrome
   (Ex:) See PDX Collection 540

● **Q87.4 Marfan's syndrome**
   (Ex:) For category Q87.4 CC codes: See PDX Collection 3508

 Q87.40 Marfan's syndrome, unspecified 🔹

 ● **Q87.41 Marfan's syndrome with cardiovascular manifestations**
  Q87.410 Marfan's syndrome with aortic dilation 🔹
  Q87.418 Marfan's syndrome with other cardiovascular manifestations 🔹

 Q87.42 Marfan's syndrome with ocular manifestations 🔹

 Q87.43 Marfan's syndrome with skeletal manifestation 🔹

 Q87.5 Other congenital malformation syndromes with other skeletal changes 🔹
   (Ex:) See PDX Collection 3499

● **Q87.8 Other specified congenital malformation syndromes, not elsewhere classified**
  Excludes1 Zellweger syndrome (E71.510)
   (Ex:) For category Q87.8 CC codes: See PDX Collection 540

 Q87.81 Alport syndrome 🔹
   Progressive sensorineural hearing loss, progressive
   pyelonephritis or glomerulonephritis, and
   ocular defects
   Use additional code to identify stage of chronic kidney disease (N18.1-N18.6)

 Q87.82 Arterial tortuosity syndrome 🔹
  Coding Clinic: 2016, Q4, P60-61

 Q87.89 Other specified congenital malformation syndromes, not elsewhere classified 🔹
   Laurence-Moon (-Bardet)-Biedl syndrome

CHAPTER 17 (Q00-Q99)

N Newborn Age: 0 **P** Pediatric Age: 0–17 **M** Maternity DX: 9–64 **A** Adult Age: 15–124 ♀ Females Only ♂ Males Only

🔹 Complication\Comorbidity 🔹 Major C\C (Ex:) CC/MCC Exclusions 🔹 Hospital-Acquired Condition 🔹 Hierarchical Condition Category

1219

CHAPTER 17 (Q00–Q99)

● Q89 **Other congenital malformations, not elsewhere classified**

   ● Q89.0 **Congenital absence and malformations of spleen**
      Excludes1 isomerism of atrial appendages (with asplenia or polysplenia) (Q20.6)
      (Ex:) **For category Q87.8 CC codes:** See PDX Collection 1111

      Q89.01 **Asplenia (congenital)** 🐾

      Q89.09 **Congenital malformations of spleen** 🐾
          Congenital splenomegaly

   Q89.1 **Congenital malformations of adrenal gland**
      Excludes1 adrenogenital disorders (E25.-)
               congenital adrenal hyperplasia (E25.0)

   Q89.2 **Congenital malformations of other endocrine glands**
      Congenital malformation of parathyroid or thyroid gland
      Persistent thyroglossal duct
      Thyroglossal cyst
      Excludes1 congenital goiter (E03.0)
               congenital hypothyroidism (E03.1)

   Q89.3 **Situs inversus** 🐾
      Lateral transposition of viscera of thorax and abdomen
      Dextrocardia with situs inversus
      Mirror-image atrial arrangement with situs inversus
      Situs inversus or transversus abdominalis
      Situs inversus or transversus thoracis
      Transposition of abdominal viscera
      Transposition of thoracic viscera
      Excludes1 dextrocardia NOS (Q24.0)
      (Ex:) See PDX Collection 1112

   Q89.4 **Conjoined twins** 🐾
      Craniopagus
      Dicephaly
      Pygopagus
      Thoracopagus
      (Ex:) See PDX Collection 1113

   Q89.7 **Multiple congenital malformations, not elsewhere classified** 🐾
      Multiple congenital anomalies NOS
      Multiple congenital deformities NOS
      Excludes1 congenital malformation syndromes affecting multiple systems (Q87.-)
      (Ex:) See PDX Collection 1112

   Q89.8 **Other specified congenital malformations** 🐾
      Use additional code(s) to identify all associated manifestations
      (Ex:) See PDX Collection 540

   Q89.9 **Congenital malformation, unspecified**
      Congenital anomaly NOS
      Congenital deformity NOS

CHROMOSOMAL ABNORMALITIES, NOT ELSEWHERE CLASSIFIED (Q90–Q99)

   Excludes2 mitochondrial metabolic disorders (E88.4-)

● Q90 **Down syndrome**
   Use additional code(s) to identify any associated physical conditions and degree of intellectual disabilities (F70-F79)

   Q90.0 **Trisomy 21, nonmosaicism (meiotic nondisjunction)**
      Trisomy 21, nondisjunction, accounts for 95% of Downs syndrome cases

   Q90.1 **Trisomy 21, mosaicism (mitotic nondisjunction)**

   Q90.2 **Trisomy 21, translocation**

   Q90.9 **Down syndrome, unspecified**
      Trisomy 21 NOS

● Q91 **Trisomy 18 and Trisomy 13**
   (Ex:) **For category Q91 CC codes:** See PDX Collection 1114

   Q91.0 **Trisomy 18, nonmosaicism (meiotic nondisjunction)** 🐾
   Q91.1 **Trisomy 18, mosaicism (mitotic nondisjunction)** 🐾
   Q91.2 **Trisomy 18, translocation** 🐾
   Q91.3 **Trisomy 18, unspecified** 🐾
   Q91.4 **Trisomy 13, nonmosaicism (meiotic nondisjunction)** 🐾
   Q91.5 **Trisomy 13, mosaicism (mitotic nondisjunction)** 🐾
   Q91.6 **Trisomy 13, translocation** 🐾
   Q91.7 **Trisomy 13, unspecified** 🐾

● Q92 **Other trisomies and partial trisomies of the autosomes, not elsewhere classified**
   Includes unbalanced translocations and insertions
   Excludes1 trisomies of chromosomes 13, 18, 21 (Q90-Q91)

   Q92.0 **Whole chromosome trisomy, nonmosaicism (meiotic nondisjunction)**

   Q92.1 **Whole chromosome trisomy, mosaicism (mitotic nondisjunction)**

   Q92.2 **Partial trisomy**
      Less than whole arm duplicated
      Whole arm or more duplicated
      Excludes1 partial trisomy due to unbalanced translocation (Q92.5)

   Q92.5 **Duplications with other complex rearrangements**
      Partial trisomy due to unbalanced translocations
      Code also any associated deletions due to unbalanced translocations, inversions and insertions (Q93.7)

   ● Q92.6 **Marker chromosomes**
      Trisomies due to dicentrics
      Trisomies due to extra rings
      Trisomies due to isochromosomes
      Individual with marker heterochromatin
      Q92.61 **Marker chromosomes in normal individual**
      Q92.62 **Marker chromosomes in abnormal individual**

   Q92.7 **Triploidy and polyploidy**

   Q92.8 **Other specified trisomies and partial trisomies of autosomes**
      Duplications identified by fluorescence in situ hybridization (FISH)
      Duplications identified by in situ hybridization (ISH)
      Duplications seen only at prometaphase

   Q92.9 **Trisomy and partial trisomy of autosomes, unspecified**

● Q93 **Monosomies and deletions from the autosomes, not elsewhere classified**
   (Ex:) **For category Q93 CC codes unless otherwise indicated:** See PDX Collection 1115

   Q93.0 **Whole chromosome monosomy, nonmosaicism (meiotic nondisjunction)**

   Q93.1 **Whole chromosome monosomy, mosaicism (mitotic nondisjunction)**

   Q93.2 **Chromosome replaced with ring, dicentric or isochromosome**

   Q93.3 **Deletion of short arm of chromosome 4** 🐾
      Wolff-Hirschorn syndrome
      (Ex:) See PDX Collection 3970

   Q93.4 **Deletion of short arm of chromosome 5** 🐾
      Cri-du-chat syndrome
      (Ex:) See PDX Collection 1116

   ● Q93.5 **Other deletions of part of a chromosome**
      Q93.51 **Angelman syndrome** 🐾
          (Ex:) See PDX Collection 1114
      Q93.59 **Other deletions of part of a chromosome** 🐾
          (Ex:) See PDX Collection 1114

   Q93.7 **Deletions with other complex rearrangements** 🐾
      Deletions due to unbalanced translocations, inversions and insertions
      Code also any associated duplications due to unbalanced translocations, inversions and insertions (Q92.5)
      (Ex:) See PDX Collection 3972

▶ New   ⇒ Revised   ~~deleted~~ Deleted   Excludes 1   Excludes 2   Includes   Use additional   Code first   Code also   Key words

OGCR Official Guidelines   ● Unacceptable Principal Diagnosis   X Assign placeholder X   ● Use Additional Character(s)   ▶ Manifestation Code   **Coding Clinic**

● **Q93.8 Other deletions from the autosomes**

    Q93.81 Velo-cardio-facial syndrome 🅖
        Deletion 22q11.2
        (Ex) See PDX Collection 1117
        Coding Clinic: 2019, Q3, P14

    Q93.82 Williams syndrome 🅖
        (Ex) See PDX Collection 1114

    Q93.88 Other microdeletions Miller-Dieker syndrome 🅖
        Smith-Magenis syndrome
        (Ex) See PDX Collection 1118

    Q93.89 Other deletions from the autosomes 🅖
        Deletions identified by fluorescence in situ hybridization (FISH)
        Deletions identified by in situ hybridization (ISH)
        Deletions seen only at prometaphase
        (Ex) See PDX Collection 3974

Q93.9 Deletion from autosomes, unspecified 🅖

● **Q95 Balanced rearrangements and structural markers, not elsewhere classified**

    Includes   Robertsonian and balanced reciprocal translocations and insertions

Q95.0 Balanced translocation and insertion in normal individual

Q95.1 Chromosome inversion in normal individual

Q95.2 Balanced autosomal rearrangement in abnormal individual

Q95.3 Balanced sex/autosomal rearrangement in abnormal individual

Q95.5 Individual with autosomal fragile site

Q95.8 Other balanced rearrangements and structural markers

Q95.9 Balanced rearrangement and structural marker, unspecified

● **Q96 Turner's syndrome**
Caused by missing or incomplete X chromosome affecting growth and sexual development

    Excludes1   Noonan syndrome (Q87.19)

Q96.0 Karyotype 45, X ♀

Q96.1 Karyotype 46, X iso (Xq) ♀
    Karyotype 46, isochromosome Xq

Q96.2 Karyotype 46, X with abnormal sex chromosome, except iso (Xq) ♀
    Karyotype 46, X with abnormal sex chromosome, except isochromosome Xq

Q96.3 Mosaicism, 45, X/46, XX or XY ♀

Q96.4 Mosaicism, 45, X/other cell line(s) with abnormal sex chromosome ♀

Q96.8 Other variants of Turner's syndrome ♀

Q96.9 Turner's syndrome, unspecified ♀

● **Q97 Other sex chromosome abnormalities, female phenotype, not elsewhere classified**

    Excludes1   Turner's syndrome (Q96.-)

Q97.0 Karyotype 47, XXX ♀

Q97.1 Female with more than three X chromosomes ♀

Q97.2 Mosaicism, lines with various numbers of X chromosomes ♀

Q97.3 Female with 46, XY karyotype ♀

Q97.8 Other specified sex chromosome abnormalities, female phenotype ♀

Q97.9 Sex chromosome abnormality, female phenotype, unspecified ♀

● **Q98 Other sex chromosome abnormalities, male phenotype, not elsewhere classified**

Q98.0 Klinefelter syndrome karyotype 47, XXY ♂

Q98.1 Klinefelter syndrome, male with more than two X chromosomes ♂

Q98.3 Other male with 46, XX karyotype ♂

Q98.4 Klinefelter syndrome, unspecified ♂

Q98.5 Karyotype 47, XYY

Q98.6 Male with structurally abnormal sex chromosome ♂

Q98.7 Male with sex chromosome mosaicism ♂

Q98.8 Other specified sex chromosome abnormalities, male phenotype ♂

Q98.9 Sex chromosome abnormality, male phenotype, unspecified ♂

● **Q99 Other chromosome abnormalities, not elsewhere classified**

Q99.0 Chimera 46, XX/46, XY
    Chimera 46, XX/46, XY true hermaphrodite

Q99.1 46, XX true hermaphrodite
    46, XX with streak gonads
    46, XY with streak gonads
    Pure gonadal dysgenesis

Q99.2 Fragile X chromosome
    Fragile X syndrome

Q99.8 Other specified chromosome abnormalities

Q99.9 Chromosomal abnormality, unspecified

CHAPTER 17 (Q00-Q99)

N Newborn Age: 0   **P** Pediatric Age: 0–17   **M** Maternity DX: 9–64   **A** Adult Age: 15–124   ♀ Females Only   ♂ Males Only

🅖 Complication\Comorbidity   🅖 Major C\C   (Ex) CC/MCC Exclusions   🅖 Hospital-Acquired Condition   🅖 Hierarchical Condition Category

1221

CHAPTER 18

SYMPTOMS, SIGNS, AND ABNORMAL CLINICAL AND LABORATORY FINDINGS, NOT ELSEWHERE CLASSIFIED (R00-R99)

OGCR Chapter-Specific Coding Guidelines

18. **Chapter 18: Symptoms, signs, and abnormal clinical and laboratory findings, not elsewhere classified (R00-R99)**

Chapter 18 includes symptoms, signs, abnormal results of clinical or other investigative procedures, and ill-defined conditions regarding which no diagnosis classifiable elsewhere is recorded. Signs and symptoms that point to a specific diagnosis have been assigned to a category in other chapters of the classification.

a. Use of symptom codes

Codes that describe symptoms and signs are acceptable for reporting purposes when a related definitive diagnosis has not been established (confirmed) by the provider.

b. Use of a symptom code with a definitive diagnosis code

Codes for signs and symptoms may be reported in addition to a related definitive diagnosis when the sign or symptom is not routinely associated with that diagnosis, such as the various signs and symptoms associated with complex syndromes. The definitive diagnosis code should be sequenced before the symptom code.

Signs or symptoms that are associated routinely with a disease process should not be assigned as additional codes, unless otherwise instructed by the classification.

c. Combination codes that include symptoms

ICD-10-CM contains a number of combination codes that identify both the definitive diagnosis and common symptoms of that diagnosis. When using one of these combination codes, an additional code should not be assigned for the symptom.

d. Repeated falls

Code R29.6, Repeated falls, is for use for encounters when a patient has recently fallen and the reason for the fall is being investigated.

Code Z91.81, History of falling, is for use when a patient has fallen in the past and is at risk for future falls. When appropriate, both codes R29.6 and Z91.81 may be assigned together.

e. Coma scale

The coma scale codes (R40.2-) can be used in conjunction with traumatic brain injury codes, acute cerebrovascular disease or sequelae of cerebrovascular disease codes. These codes are primarily for use by trauma registries, but they may be used in any setting where this information is collected. The coma scale may also be used to assess the status of the central nervous system for other non-trauma conditions, such as monitoring patients in the intensive care unit regardless of medical condition. The coma scale codes should be sequenced after the diagnosis code(s).

These codes, one from each subcategory, are needed to complete the scale. The 7th character indicates when the scale was recorded. The 7th character should match for all three codes.

At a minimum, report the initial score documented on presentation at your facility. This may be a score from the emergency medicine technician (EMT) or in the emergency department. If desired, a facility may choose to capture multiple coma scale scores.

Assign code R40.24, Glasgow coma scale, total score, when only the total score is documented in the medical record and not the individual score(s).

Do not report codes for individual or total Glasgow coma scale scores for a patient with a medically induced coma or a sedated patient.

See Section I.B.14 for coma scale documentation by clinicians other than patient's provider.

f. Functional quadriplegia

GUIDELINE HAS BEEN DELETED EFFECTIVE OCTOBER 1, 2017

g. SIRS due to Non-Infectious Process

The systemic inflammatory response syndrome (SIRS) can develop as a result of certain non-infectious disease processes, such as trauma, malignant neoplasm, or pancreatitis. When SIRS is documented with a noninfectious condition, and no subsequent infection is documented, the code for the underlying condition, such as an injury, should be assigned, followed by code R65.10, Systemic inflammatory response syndrome (SIRS) of non-infectious origin without acute organ dysfunction, or code R65.11, Systemic inflammatory response syndrome (SIRS) of non-infectious origin with acute organ dysfunction. If an associated acute organ dysfunction is documented, the appropriate code(s) for the specific type of organ dysfunction(s) should be assigned in addition to code R65.11. If acute organ dysfunction is documented, but it cannot be determined if the acute organ dysfunction is associated with SIRS or due to another condition (e.g., directly due to the trauma), the provider should be queried.

h. Death NOS

Code R99, Ill-defined and unknown cause of mortality, is only for use in the very limited circumstance when a patient who has already died is brought into an emergency department or other healthcare facility and is pronounced dead upon arrival. It does not represent the discharge disposition of death.

i. NIHSS Stroke Scale

The NIH stroke scale (NIHSS) codes (R29.7- -) can be used in conjunction with acute stroke codes (I63) to identify the patient's neurological status and the severity of the stroke. The stroke scale codes should be sequenced after the acute stroke diagnosis code(s).

At a minimum, report the initial score documented. If desired, a facility may choose to capture multiple stroke scale scores.

See Section I.B.14 for NIHSS stroke scale documentation by clinicians other than patient's provider.

CHAPTER 18

SYMPTOMS, SIGNS, AND ABNORMAL CLINICAL AND LABORATORY FINDINGS, NOT ELSEWHERE CLASSIFIED (R00-R99)

Note: This chapter includes symptoms, signs, abnormal results of clinical or other investigative procedures, and ill-defined conditions regarding which no diagnosis classifiable elsewhere is recorded.

Signs and symptoms that point rather definitely to a given diagnosis have been assigned to a category in other chapters of the classification. In general, categories in this chapter include the less well-defined conditions and symptoms that, without the necessary study of the case to establish a final diagnosis, point perhaps equally to two or more diseases or to two or more systems of the body. Practically all categories in the chapter could be designated "not otherwise specified", "unknown etiology" or "transient". The Alphabetical Index should be consulted to determine which symptoms and signs are to be allocated here and which to other chapters. The residual subcategories, numbered .8, are generally provided for other relevant symptoms that cannot be allocated elsewhere in the classification.

The conditions and signs or symptoms included in categories R00-R94 consist of:

(a) cases for which no more specific diagnosis can be made even after all the facts bearing on the case have been investigated;

(b) signs or symptoms existing at the time of initial encounter that proved to be transient and whose causes could not be determined;

(c) provisional diagnosis in a patient who failed to return for further investigation or care;

(d) cases referred elsewhere for investigation or treatment before the diagnosis was made;

(e) cases in which a more precise diagnosis was not available for any other reason;

(f) certain symptoms, for which supplementary information is provided, that represent important problems in medical care in their own right.

Excludes2   abnormal findings on antenatal screening of mother (O28.-)

certain conditions originating in the perinatal period (P04-P96)

signs and symptoms classified in the body system chapters

signs and symptoms of breast (N63, N64.5)

This chapter contains the following blocks:

R00-R09	Symptoms and signs involving the circulatory and respiratory systems
R10-R19	Symptoms and signs involving the digestive system and abdomen
R20-R23	Symptoms and signs involving the skin and subcutaneous tissue
R25-R29	Symptoms and signs involving the nervous and musculoskeletal systems
R30-R39	Symptoms and signs involving the genitourinary system
R40-R46	Symptoms and signs involving cognition, perception, emotional state and behavior
R47-R49	Symptoms and signs involving speech and voice
R50-R69	General symptoms and signs
R70-R79	Abnormal findings on examination of blood, without diagnosis
R80-R82	Abnormal findings on examination of urine, without diagnosis
R83-R89	Abnormal findings on examination of other body fluids, substances and tissues, without diagnosis
R90-R94	Abnormal findings on diagnostic imaging and in function studies, without diagnosis
R97	Abnormal tumor markers
R99	Ill-defined and unknown cause of mortality

SYMPTOMS AND SIGNS INVOLVING THE CIRCULATORY AND RESPIRATORY SYSTEMS (R00-R09)

● **R00**   **Abnormalities of heart beat**

    Excludes1   abnormalities originating in the perinatal period (P29.1-)

    Excludes2   specified arrhythmias (I47-I49)

   R00.0   **Tachycardia, unspecified**

     Rapid heart rate >100 beats

     Rapid heart beat

     Sinoauricular tachycardia NOS

     Sinus [sinusal] tachycardia NOS

     Excludes1   neonatal tachycardia (P29.11)

                paroxysmal tachycardia (I47.-)

   R00.1   **Bradycardia, unspecified**

     Slow heart rate, <60

     Sinoatrial bradycardia

     Sinus bradycardia

     Slow heart beat

     Vagal bradycardia

     Use additional code for adverse effect, if applicable, to identify drug (T36-T50 with fifth or sixth character 5)

     Excludes1   neonatal bradycardia (P29.12)

   R00.2   **Palpitations**

     Awareness of heart beat

   R00.8   **Other abnormalities of heart beat**

   R00.9   **Unspecified abnormalities of heart beat**

N Newborn Age: 0   **P** Pediatric Age: 0–17   **M** Maternity DX: 9–64   **A** Adult Age: 15–124   ♀ Females Only   ♂ Males Only

Complication\Comorbidity   Major C\C   (Ex:) CC/MCC Exclusions   Hospital-Acquired Condition   Hierarchical Condition Category   **1223**

CHAPTER 18 (R00-R99)

● **R01**   **Cardiac murmurs and other cardiac sounds**

     Excludes1   cardiac murmurs and sounds originating in the perinatal period (P29.8)

     R01.0   **Benign and innocent cardiac murmurs**
         Functional cardiac murmur

     R01.1   **Cardiac murmur, unspecified**
         Cardiac bruit NOS
         Heart murmur NOS
         Systolic murmur NOS

     R01.2   **Other cardiac sounds**
         Cardiac dullness, increased or decreased
         Precordial friction

OGCR Section I.C.9.a.7.

> Hypertension, Transient
>
> Assign code R03.0, Elevated blood pressure reading without diagnosis of hypertension, unless patient has an established diagnosis of hypertension. Assign code O13.-, Gestational [pregnancy-induced] hypertension with significant proteinuria, or O14.-, Pre-eclampsia, for transient hypertension of pregnancy.

● **R03**   **Abnormal blood-pressure reading, without diagnosis**

     R03.0   **Elevated blood-pressure reading, without diagnosis of hypertension**
         Note: This category is to be used to record an episode of elevated blood pressure in a patient in whom no formal diagnosis of hypertension has been made, or as an isolated incidental finding.
         MCE: Questionable admission when principal dx

     R03.1   **Nonspecific low blood-pressure reading**
         Excludes1   hypotension (I95.-)
                   maternal hypotension syndrome (O26.5-)
                   neurogenic orthostatic hypotension (G90.3)

● **R04**   **Hemorrhage from respiratory passages**
     (Ex:) **For category R04 CC codes: See PDX Collection 1119**

     R04.0   **Epistaxis**
         Hemorrhage from nose
         Nosebleed
         Coding Clinic: 2018, Q4, P38

     R04.1   **Hemorrhage from throat**
         Excludes2   hemoptysis (R04.2)

     R04.2   **Hemoptysis** 🦠
         Blood-stained sputum
         Cough with hemorrhage

    ● **R04.8**   **Hemorrhage from other sites in respiratory passages**

         R04.81   **Acute idiopathic pulmonary hemorrhage in infants** 🦠   **P**
                  AIPHI
                  Acute idiopathic hemorrhage in infants over 28 days old
                  Excludes1   perinatal pulmonary hemorrhage (P26.-)
                                von Willebrand's disease (D68.0)

         R04.89   **Hemorrhage from other sites in respiratory passages** 🦠
                  Pulmonary hemorrhage NOS

     R04.9   **Hemorrhage from respiratory passages, unspecified** 🦠

● **R05**   **Cough**
     Excludes1   ~~cough with hemorrhage (R04.2)~~
                ▶paroxysmal cough due to Bordetella pertussis (A37.0-)
                smoker's cough (J41.0)
     ▶**Excludes2**   cough with hemorrhage (R04.2))

    ▶ **R05.1**   **Acute cough**
    ▶ **R05.2**   **Subacute cough**
    ▶ **R05.3**   **Chronic cough**
         ▶Persistent cough
         ▶Refractory cough
         ▶Unexplained cough

    ▶ **R05.4**   **Cough syncope**
         ▶*Code first syncope and collapse (R55)*
    ▶ **R05.8**   **Other specified cough**
    ▶ **R05.9**   **Cough, unspecified**

● **R06**   **Abnormalities of breathing**
     Excludes1   acute respiratory distress syndrome (J80)
                  respiratory arrest (R09.2)
                  respiratory arrest of newborn (P28.81)
                  respiratory distress syndrome of newborn (P22.-)
                  respiratory failure (J96.-)
                  respiratory failure of newborn (P28.5)

    ● **R06.0**   **Dyspnea**
         Excludes1   tachypnea NOS (R06.82)
                  transient tachypnea of newborn (P22.1)

         R06.00   **Dyspnea, unspecified**
              Coding Clinic: 2017, Q1, P26-27
         R06.01   **Orthopnea**
         R06.02   **Shortness of breath**
         R06.03   **Acute respiratory distress**
         R06.09   **Other forms of dyspnea**

     R06.1   **Stridor**
         Harsh, high-pitched breath sound
         Excludes1   congenital laryngeal stridor (P28.89)
                  laryngismus (stridulus) (J38.5)

     R06.2   **Wheezing**
         Excludes1   Asthma (J45.-)
         Coding Clinic: 2016, Q2, P34

     R06.3   **Periodic breathing** 🦠
         Cheyne-Stokes breathing
         An abnormal pattern of breathing with gradually increasing and decreasing tidal volume with some periods of apnea
         (Ex:) See PDX Collection 1120

     R06.4   **Hyperventilation**
         Excludes1   psychogenic hyperventilation (F45.8)

     R06.5   **Mouth breathing**
         Excludes2   dry mouth NOS (R68.2)

     R06.6   **Hiccough**
         Excludes1   psychogenic hiccough (F45.8)

     R06.7   **Sneezing**

    ● **R06.8**   **Other abnormalities of breathing**

         R06.81   **Apnea, not elsewhere classified**
              Apnea NOS
              Excludes1   apnea (of) newborn (P28.4)
                         sleep apnea (G47.3-)
                         sleep apnea of newborn (primary) (P28.3)

         R06.82   **Tachypnea, not elsewhere classified**
              Tachypnea NOS
              Excludes1   transitory tachypnea of newborn (P22.1)

         R06.83   **Snoring**
         R06.89   **Other abnormalities of breathing**
              Breath-holding (spells)
              Sighing

     R06.9   **Unspecified abnormalities of breathing**

● **R07**   **Pain in throat and chest**
     Excludes1   epidemic myalgia (B33.0)
     Excludes2   jaw pain R68.84
                  pain in breast (N64.4)

     R07.0   **Pain in throat**
         Excludes1   chronic sore throat (J31.2)
                  sore throat (acute) NOS (J02.9)
         Excludes2   dysphagia (R13.1-)
                  pain in neck (M54.2)

     R07.1   **Chest pain on breathing**
         Painful respiration

     R07.2   **Precordial pain**

▶ New   ⇒ Revised   ~~deleted~~ Deleted   Excludes 1   Excludes 2   Includes   Use additional   Code first   Code also   Key words

OGCR Official Guidelines   ● Unacceptable Principal Diagnosis   X Assign placeholder X   ● Use Additional Character(s)   ▌ Manifestation Code   **Coding Clinic**

- R07.8   **Other chest pain**
  - R07.81   **Pleurodynia**
    - Pleurodynia NOS
    - **Excludes1**   epidemic pleurodynia (B33.0)
  - R07.82   **Intercostal pain**
  - R07.89   **Other chest pain**
    - Anterior chest-wall pain NOS
    - Coding Clinic: 2021, Q1, P42
  - R07.9   **Chest pain, unspecified**
- R09   **Other symptoms and signs involving the circulatory and respiratory system**
  - **Excludes1**   acute respiratory distress syndrome (J80)
    - respiratory arrest of newborn (P28.81)
    - respiratory distress syndrome of newborn (P22.0)
    - respiratory failure (J96.-)
    - respiratory failure of newborn (P28.5)
  - R09.0   **Asphyxia and hypoxemia**
    - **Excludes1**   asphyxia due to carbon monoxide (T58.-)
      - asphyxia due to foreign body in respiratory tract (T17.-)
      - birth (intrauterine) asphyxia (P84)
      - hyperventilation (R06.4)
      - traumatic asphyxia (T71.-)
    - **Excludes2**   hypercapnia (R06.89)
    - R09.01   **Asphyxia** 🖇
      - (Ex:) See PDX Collection 1121
    - R09.02   **Hypoxemia**
      - Coding Clinic: 2019, Q3, P15
  - R09.1   **Pleurisy**
    - *Occurs when double membrane (pleura) lining chest cavity and lung surface becomes inflamed, causing sharp pain on inspiration/expiration*
    - **Excludes1**   pleurisy with effusion (J90)
  - R09.2   **Respiratory arrest** 🖇🖇
    - Cardiorespiratory failure
    - **Excludes1**   cardiac arrest (I46.-)
      - respiratory arrest of newborn (P28.81)
      - respiratory distress of newborn (P22.0)
      - respiratory failure (J96.-)
      - respiratory failure of newborn (P28.5)
      - respiratory insufficiency (R06.89)
      - respiratory insufficiency of newborn (P28.5)
    - MCC: Only if patient discharged alive
    - (Ex:) See PDX Collection 1121
  - R09.3   **Abnormal sputum**
    - Abnormal amount of sputum
    - Abnormal color of sputum
    - Abnormal odor of sputum
    - Excessive sputum
    - **Excludes1**   blood-stained sputum (R04.2)
  - R09.8   **Other specified symptoms and signs involving the circulatory and respiratory systems**
    - R09.81   **Nasal congestion**
    - R09.82   **Postnasal drip**
    - R09.89   **Other specified symptoms and signs involving the circulatory and respiratory systems**
      - Bruit (arterial)
      - Abnormal chest percussion
      - Feeling of foreign body in throat
      - Friction sounds in chest
      - Chest tympany
      - Choking sensation
      - Rales
        - *Wet rattling, clicking, crackling sounds on auscultation*
      - Weak pulse
      - **Excludes2**   foreign body in throat (T17.2-)
        - wheezing (R06.2)
      - Coding Clinic: 2021, Q1, P42

SYMPTOMS AND SIGNS INVOLVING THE DIGESTIVE SYSTEM AND ABDOMEN (R10-R19)

Excludes2   congenital or infantile pylorospasm (Q40.0)
- gastrointestinal hemorrhage (K92.0-K92.2)
- intestinal obstruction (K56.-)
- newborn gastrointestinal hemorrhage (P54.0-P54.3)
- newborn intestinal obstruction (P76.-)
- pylorospasm (K31.3)
- signs and symptoms involving the urinary system (R30-R39)
- symptoms referable to female genital organs (N94.-)
- symptoms referable to male genital organs (N48-N50)

- R10   **Abdominal and pelvic pain**
  - **Excludes1**   renal colic (N23)
  - **Excludes2**   dorsalgia (M54.-)
    - flatulence and related conditions (R14.-)
  - R10.0   **Acute abdomen**
    - Severe abdominal pain (generalized) (with abdominal rigidity)
    - **Excludes1**   abdominal rigidity NOS (R19.3)
      - generalized abdominal pain NOS (R10.84)
      - localized abdominal pain (R10.1-R10.3-)
  - R10.1   **Pain localized to upper abdomen**
    - R10.10   **Upper abdominal pain, unspecified**
    - R10.11   **Right upper quadrant pain**
    - R10.12   **Left upper quadrant pain**
    - R10.13   **Epigastric pain**
      - Dyspepsia
      - **Excludes1**   functional dyspepsia (K30)
  - R10.2   **Pelvic and perineal pain**
    - **Excludes1**   vulvodynia (N94.81)
  - R10.3   **Pain localized to other parts of lower abdomen**
    - R10.30   **Lower abdominal pain, unspecified**
    - R10.31   **Right lower quadrant pain**
    - R10.32   **Left lower quadrant pain**
    - R10.33   **Periumbilical pain**
  - R10.8   **Other abdominal pain**
    - R10.81   **Abdominal tenderness**
      - Abdominal tenderness NOS
      - R10.811   **Right upper quadrant abdominal tenderness**
      - R10.812   **Left upper quadrant abdominal tenderness**
      - R10.813   **Right lower quadrant abdominal tenderness**
      - R10.814   **Left lower quadrant abdominal tenderness**
      - R10.815   **Periumbilic abdominal tenderness**
      - R10.816   **Epigastric abdominal tenderness**
      - R10.817   **Generalized abdominal tenderness**
      - R10.819   **Abdominal tenderness, unspecified site**
    - R10.82   **Rebound abdominal tenderness**
      - R10.821   **Right upper quadrant rebound abdominal tenderness**
      - R10.822   **Left upper quadrant rebound abdominal tenderness**
      - R10.823   **Right lower quadrant rebound abdominal tenderness**
      - R10.824   **Left lower quadrant rebound abdominal tenderness**
      - R10.825   **Periumbilic rebound abdominal tenderness**
      - R10.826   **Epigastric rebound abdominal tenderness**

CHAPTER 18 (R00-R99)

N Newborn Age: 0   **P** Pediatric Age: 0–17   **M** Maternity DX: 9–64   **A** Adult Age: 15–124   ♀ Females Only   ♂ Males Only

🖇 Complication\Comorbidity   🖇 Major C\C   (Ex:) CC/MCC Exclusions   🖇 Hospital-Acquired Condition   🖇 Hierarchical Condition Category

1225

R10.827   Generalized rebound abdominal tenderness

R10.829   Rebound abdominal tenderness, unspecified site

R10.83   Colic   P
Colic NOS
Infantile colic
Excludes1   colic in adult and child over 12 months old (R10.84)

R10.84   Generalized abdominal pain
Excludes1   generalized abdominal pain associated with acute abdomen (R10.0)

R10.9   Unspecified abdominal pain

● R11   Nausea and vomiting
Excludes1   cyclical vomiting associated with migraine (G43.A-)
excessive vomiting in pregnancy (O21.-)
hematemesis (K92.0)
neonatal hematemesis (P54.0)
newborn vomiting (P92.0-)
psychogenic vomiting (F50.89)
vomiting associated with bulimia nervosa (F50.2)
vomiting following gastrointestinal surgery (K91.0)
Coding Clinic: 2017, Q1, P27

● R11.0   Nausea
Nausea NOS
Nausea without vomiting

● R11.1   Vomiting

R11.10   Vomiting, unspecified
Vomiting NOS

R11.11   Vomiting without nausea

R11.12   Projectile vomiting

R11.13   Vomiting of fecal matter

R11.14   Bilious vomiting
Bilious emesis

R11.15   Cyclical vomiting syndrome unrelated to migraine
Cyclic vomiting syndrome NOS
Persistent vomiting
Excludes1   cyclical vomiting in migraine (G43.A-)
Excludes2   bulimia nervosa (F50.2)
diabetes mellitus due to underlying condition (E08.-)

R11.2   Nausea with vomiting, unspecified
Persistent nausea with vomiting NOS
Coding Clinic: 2020, Q1, P8

R12   Heartburn
Excludes1   dyspepsia NOS (R10.13)
functional dyspepsia (K30)

● R13   Aphagia and dysphagia

R13.0   Aphagia
Inability to swallow
Excludes1   psychogenic aphagia (F50.9)

● R13.1   Dysphagia
Difficulty swallowing
Code first, if applicable, dysphagia following cerebrovascular disease (I69. with final characters -91)
Excludes1   psychogenic dysphagia (F45.8)

R13.10   Dysphagia, unspecified
Difficulty in swallowing NOS

R13.11   Dysphagia, oral phase

R13.12   Dysphagia, oropharyngeal phase

R13.13   Dysphagia, pharyngeal phase

R13.14   Dysphagia, pharyngoesophageal phase

R13.19   Other dysphagia
Cervical dysphagia
Neurogenic dysphagia

● R14   Flatulence and related conditions
Excludes1   psychogenic aerophagy (F45.8)

R14.0   Abdominal distension (gaseous)
Bloating
Tympanites (abdominal) (intestinal)

R14.1   Gas pain

R14.2   Eructation
Belching air from stomach through mouth

R14.3   Flatulence

● R15   Fecal incontinence
Includes   encopresis NOS
Excludes1   fecal incontinence of nonorganic origin (F98.1)

R15.0   Incomplete defecation
Excludes1   constipation (K59.0-)
fecal impaction (K56.41)

R15.1   Fecal smearing
Fecal soiling

R15.2   Fecal urgency

R15.9   Full incontinence of feces
Fecal incontinence NOS

● R16   Hepatomegaly and splenomegaly, not elsewhere classified
Enlargement of liver or spleen

R16.0   Hepatomegaly, not elsewhere classified
Hepatomegaly NOS

R16.1   Splenomegaly, not elsewhere classified
Splenomegaly NOS

R16.2   Hepatomegaly with splenomegaly, not elsewhere classified
Hepatosplenomegaly NOS

R17   Unspecified jaundice ⊗
Excludes1   neonatal jaundice (P55, P57-P59)
(Ex:) See PDX Collection 1122

● R18   Ascites
Includes   fluid in peritoneal cavity
Excludes1   ascites in alcoholic cirrhosis (K70.31)
ascites in alcoholic hepatitis (K70.11)
ascites in toxic liver disease with chronic active hepatitis (K71.51)
(Ex:) For category R18 CC codes: See PDX Collection 1123

● R18.0   Malignant ascites ⊗
Code first malignancy, such as:
malignant neoplasm of ovary (C56.-)
secondary malignant neoplasm of retroperitoneum and peritoneum (C78.6)

R18.8   Other ascites ⊗
Ascites NOS
Peritoneal effusion (chronic)
Coding Clinic: 2018, Q1, P4

● R19   Other symptoms and signs involving the digestive system and abdomen
Excludes1   acute abdomen (R10.0)

● R19.0   Intra-abdominal and pelvic swelling, mass and lump
Excludes1   abdominal distension (gaseous) (R14.-)
ascites (R18.-)

R19.00   Intra-abdominal and pelvic swelling, mass and lump, unspecified site

R19.01   Right upper quadrant abdominal swelling, mass and lump

R19.02   Left upper quadrant abdominal swelling, mass and lump

R19.03   Right lower quadrant abdominal swelling, mass and lump

R19.04   Left lower quadrant abdominal swelling, mass and lump

▶ New   ⇒ Revised   ~~deleted~~ Deleted   Excludes 1   Excludes 2   Includes   Use additional   Code first   Code also   Key words

OGCR Official Guidelines   ● Unacceptable Principal Diagnosis   X Assign placeholder X   ● Use Additional Character(s)   ▌ Manifestation Code   Coding Clinic

       R19.05 **Periumbilic swelling, mass or lump**
            Diffuse or generalized umbilical swelling or mass

       R19.06 **Epigastric swelling, mass or lump**

       R19.07 **Generalized intra-abdominal and pelvic swelling, mass and lump**
            Diffuse or generalized intra-abdominal swelling or mass NOS
            Diffuse or generalized pelvic swelling or mass NOS

       R19.09 **Other intra-abdominal and pelvic swelling, mass and lump**

● R19.1 **Abnormal bowel sounds**

       R19.11 **Absent bowel sounds**

       R19.12 **Hyperactive bowel sounds**

       R19.15 **Other abnormal bowel sounds**
            Abnormal bowel sounds NOS

R19.2 **Visible peristalsis**
     Hyperperistalsis

● R19.3 **Abdominal rigidity**
     Excludes1 abdominal rigidity with severe abdominal pain (R10.0)

       R19.30 **Abdominal rigidity, unspecified site**

       R19.31 **Right upper quadrant abdominal rigidity**

       R19.32 **Left upper quadrant abdominal rigidity**

       R19.33 **Right lower quadrant abdominal rigidity**

       R19.34 **Left lower quadrant abdominal rigidity**

       R19.35 **Periumbilic abdominal rigidity**

       R19.36 **Epigastric abdominal rigidity**

       R19.37 **Generalized abdominal rigidity**

R19.4 **Change in bowel habit**
     Excludes1 constipation (K59.0-)
               functional diarrhea (K59.1)

R19.5 **Other fecal abnormalities**
     Abnormal stool color
     Bulky stools
     Mucus in stools
     Occult blood in feces
     Occult blood in stools
     Excludes1 melena (K92.1)
               neonatal melena (P54.1)
     Coding Clinic: 2021, Q1, P10; 2019, Q1, P32

R19.6 **Halitosis**

R19.7 **Diarrhea, unspecified**
     Diarrhea NOS
     Excludes1 functional diarrhea (K59.1)
               neonatal diarrhea (P78.3)
               psychogenic diarrhea (F45.8)

R19.8 **Other specified symptoms and signs involving the digestive system and abdomen**

SYMPTOMS AND SIGNS INVOLVING THE SKIN AND SUBCUTANEOUS TISSUE (R20-R23)

     Excludes2 symptoms relating to breast (N64.4-N64.5)

● R20 **Disturbances of skin sensation**
     Excludes1 dissociative anesthesia and sensory loss (F44.6)
               psychogenic disturbances (F45.8)

R20.0 **Anesthesia of skin**
     Loss of sensation

R20.1 **Hypoesthesia of skin**
     Unpleasant abnormal sensation

R20.2 **Paresthesia of skin**
     Abnormal touch sensation, including burning, prickling, often in absence of external stimulus
     Formication   Tingling skin
     Pins and needles
     Excludes1 acroparesthesia (I73.8)

R20.3 **Hyperesthesia**

R20.8 **Other disturbances of skin sensation**

R20.9 **Unspecified disturbances of skin sensation**

R21 **Rash and other nonspecific skin eruption**
     Includes rash NOS
     Excludes1 specified type of rash- code to condition
               vesicular eruption (R23.8)

● R22 **Localized swelling, mass and lump of skin and subcutaneous tissue**
     Includes subcutaneous nodules (localized) (superficial)
     Excludes1 abnormal findings on diagnostic imaging (R90-R93)
               edema (R60.-)
               enlarged lymph nodes (R59.-)
               localized adiposity (E65)
               swelling of joint (M25.4-)

R22.0 **Localized swelling, mass and lump, head**

R22.1 **Localized swelling, mass and lump, neck**

R22.2 **Localized swelling, mass and lump, trunk**
     Excludes1 intra-abdominal or pelvic mass and lump (R19.0-)
               intra-abdominal or pelvic swelling (R19.0-)
     Excludes2 breast mass and lump (N63)

● R22.3 **Localized swelling, mass and lump, upper limb**
       R22.30 **Localized swelling, mass and lump, unspecified upper limb**
       R22.31 **Localized swelling, mass and lump, right upper limb**
       R22.32 **Localized swelling, mass and lump, left upper limb**
       R22.33 **Localized swelling, mass and lump, upper limb, bilateral**

● R22.4 **Localized swelling, mass and lump, lower limb**
       R22.40 **Localized swelling, mass and lump, unspecified lower limb**
       R22.41 **Localized swelling, mass and lump, right lower limb**
       R22.42 **Localized swelling, mass and lump, left lower limb**
       R22.43 **Localized swelling, mass and lump, lower limb, bilateral**

R22.9 **Localized swelling, mass and lump, unspecified**

● R23 **Other skin changes**

R23.0 **Cyanosis**
     Excludes1 acrocyanosis (I73.8)
               cyanotic attacks of newborn (P28.2)

R23.1 **Pallor**
     Clammy skin

R23.2 **Flushing**
     Excessive blushing
     Code first, if applicable, menopausal and female climacteric states (N95.1)

R23.3 **Spontaneous ecchymoses**
     Small hemorrhagic spot of skin; AKA black and blue spot
     Petechiae
     Excludes1 ecchymoses of newborn (P54.5)
               purpura (D69.-)

R23.4 **Changes in skin texture**
     Desquamation of skin   Scaling of skin
     Induration of skin
     Excludes1 epidermal thickening NOS (L85.9)

R23.8 **Other skin changes**

R23.9 **Unspecified skin changes**

N Newborn Age: 0   **P** Pediatric Age: 0–17   **M** Maternity DX: 9–64   **A** Adult Age: 15–124   ♀ Females Only   ♂ Males Only

  Complication\Comorbidity   Major C\C   (Ex) CC/MCC Exclusions   Hospital-Acquired Condition   Hierarchical Condition Category

1227

SYMPTOMS AND SIGNS INVOLVING THE NERVOUS AND MUSCULOSKELETAL SYSTEMS (R25-R29)

● R25   **Abnormal involuntary movements**
> **Excludes1**   specific movement disorders (G20-G26)
> stereotyped movement disorders (F98.4)
> tic disorders (F95.-)

R25.0   **Abnormal head movements**

R25.1   **Tremor, unspecified**
> **Excludes1**   chorea NOS (G25.5)
> essential tremor (G25.0)
> hysterical tremor (F44.4)
> intention tremor (G25.2)

R25.2   **Cramp and spasm**
> **Excludes2**   carpopedal spasm (R29.0)
> charley-horse (M62.831)
> infantile spasms (G40.4-)
> muscle spasm of back (M62.830)
> muscle spasm of calf (M62.831)

R25.3   **Fasciculation**
> Twitching NOS

R25.8   **Other abnormal involuntary movements**

R25.9   **Unspecified abnormal involuntary movements**

● R26   **Abnormalities of gait and mobility**
> **Excludes1**   ataxia NOS (R27.0)
> hereditary ataxia (G11.-)
> locomotor (syphilitic) ataxia (A52.11)
> immobility syndrome (paraplegic) (M62.3)

R26.0   **Ataxic gait**
> Staggering gait

R26.1   **Paralytic gait**
> Spastic gait

R26.2   **Difficulty in walking, not elsewhere classified**
> **Excludes1**   falling (R29.6)
> unsteadiness on feet (R26.81)
> Coding Clinic: 2016, Q2, P7

● R26.8   **Other abnormalities of gait and mobility**

   R26.81   **Unsteadiness on feet**

   R26.89   **Other abnormalities of gait and mobility**

R26.9   **Unspecified abnormalities of gait and mobility**

● R27   **Other lack of coordination**
> **Excludes1**   ataxic gait (R26.0)
> hereditary ataxia (G11.-)
> vertigo NOS (R42)

R27.0   **Ataxia, unspecified**
> **Excludes1**   ataxia following cerebrovascular disease (I69. with final characters -93)

R27.8   **Other lack of coordination**

R27.9   **Unspecified lack of coordination**

● R29   **Other symptoms and signs involving the nervous and musculoskeletal systems**

R29.0   **Tetany** 🔧
> *Hyperexcitability of nerves and muscles characterized by spasm, twitching, and cramps*
> Carpopedal spasm
> **Excludes1**   hysterical tetany (F44.5)
> neonatal tetany (P71.3)
> parathyroid tetany (E20.9)
> post-thyroidectomy tetany (E89.2)
> (Ex:) See PDX Collection 1124

R29.1   **Meningismus** 🔧
> (Ex:) See PDX Collection 1125

R29.2   **Abnormal reflex**
> **Excludes2**   abnormal pupillary reflex (H57.0)
> hyperactive gag reflex (J39.2)
> vasovagal reaction or syncope (R55)

R29.3   **Abnormal posture**

R29.4   **Clicking hip**
> **Excludes1**   congenital deformities of hip (Q65.-)

R29.5   **Transient paralysis** 🔧
> *Code first any associated spinal cord injury (S14.0, S14.1-, S24.0, S24.1-, S34.0-, S34.1-)*
> **Excludes1**   transient ischemic attack (G45.9)
> (Ex:) See PDX Collection 1126

R29.6   **Repeated falls**
> Falling
> Tendency to fall
> **Excludes2**   at risk for falling (Z91.81)
> history of falling (Z91.81)

> **OGCR** Section I.C.18.d.
> Repeated falls
> Code R29.6, Repeated falls, is for use for encounters when a patient has recently fallen and the reason for the fall is being investigated.
> Code Z91.81, History of falling, is for use when a patient has fallen in the past and is at risk for future falls. When appropriate, both codes R29.6 and Z91.81 may be assigned together.

> Coding Clinic: 2016, Q2, P7

● R29.7   **National Institutes of Health Stroke Scale (NIHSS) score**
> *Code first the type of cerebral infarction (I63.-)*
> Coding Clinic: 2016, Q4, P61, 127

● R29.70   **NIHSS score 0-9**
- ● R29.700   **NIHSS score 0**
- ● R29.701   **NIHSS score 1**
- ● R29.702   **NIHSS score 2**
- ● R29.703   **NIHSS score 3**
- ● R29.704   **NIHSS score 4**
- ● R29.705   **NIHSS score 5**
- ● R29.706   **NIHSS score 6**
- ● R29.707   **NIHSS score 7**
- ● R29.708   **NIHSS score 8**
- ● R29.709   **NIHSS score 9**

● R29.71   **NIHSS score 10-19**
- ● R29.710   **NIHSS score 10**
- ● R29.711   **NIHSS score 11**
- ● R29.712   **NIHSS score 12**
- ● R29.713   **NIHSS score 13**
- ● R29.714   **NIHSS score 14**
- ● R29.715   **NIHSS score 15**
- ● R29.716   **NIHSS score 16**
- ● R29.717   **NIHSS score 17**
- ● R29.718   **NIHSS score 18**
- ● R29.719   **NIHSS score 19**

● R29.72   **NIHSS score 20-29**
- ● R29.720   **NIHSS score 20**
- ● R29.721   **NIHSS score 21**
- ● R29.722   **NIHSS score 22**
- ● R29.723   **NIHSS score 23**
- ● R29.724   **NIHSS score 24**
- ● R29.725   **NIHSS score 25**
- ● R29.726   **NIHSS score 26**
- ● R29.727   **NIHSS score 27**
- ● R29.728   **NIHSS score 28**
- ● R29.729   **NIHSS score 29**

> **OGCR** Section I.C.18.i.
> NIHSS Stroke Scale
> The NIH stroke scale (NIHSS) codes (R29.7- -) can be used in conjunction with acute stroke codes (I63) to identify the patient's neurological status and the severity of the stroke. The stroke scale codes should be sequenced after the acute stroke diagnosis code(s).
> At a minimum, report the initial score documented. If desired, a facility may choose to capture multiple stroke scale scores.

▶ New   ⟹ Revised   ~~deleted~~ Deleted   Excludes 1   Excludes 2   Includes   Use additional   Code first   Code also   Key words

OGCR Official Guidelines   ● Unacceptable Principal Diagnosis   X Assign placeholder X   ● Use Additional Character(s)   ▶ Manifestation Code   **Coding Clinic**

● R29.73   NIHSS score 30-39
     ● R29.730   NIHSS score 30
         Coding Clinic: 2016, Q4, P62
     ● R29.731   NIHSS score 31
     ● R29.732   NIHSS score 32
     ● R29.733   NIHSS score 33
     ● R29.734   NIHSS score 34
     ● R29.735   NIHSS score 35
     ● R29.736   NIHSS score 36
     ● R29.737   NIHSS score 37
     ● R29.738   NIHSS score 38
     ● R29.739   NIHSS score 39
● R29.74   NIHSS score 40-42
     ● R29.740   NIHSS score 40
     ● R29.741   NIHSS score 41
     ● R29.742   NIHSS score 42

● R29.8   Other symptoms and signs involving the nervous and musculoskeletal systems
   ● R29.81   Other symptoms and signs involving the nervous system
     R29.810   Facial weakness
         Facial droop
         Excludes1   Bell's palsy (G51.0) facial weakness following cerebrovascular disease (I69. with final characters -92)
     R29.818   Other symptoms and signs involving the nervous system
   ● R29.89   Other symptoms and signs involving the musculoskeletal system
         Excludes2   pain in limb (M79.6-)
     R29.890   Loss of height
         Excludes1   osteoporosis (M80-M81)
     R29.891   Ocular torticollis
         Excludes1   congenital (sterno-mastoid) torticollis Q68.0 psychogenic torticollis (F45.8) spasmodic torticollis (G24.3) torticollis due to birth injury (P15.8) torticollis NOS M43.6
     R29.898   Other symptoms and signs involving the musculoskeletal system
● R29.9   Unspecified symptoms and signs involving the nervous and musculoskeletal systems
     R29.90   Unspecified symptoms and signs involving the nervous system
     R29.91   Unspecified symptoms and signs involving the musculoskeletal system

---

SYMPTOMS AND SIGNS INVOLVING THE GENITOURINARY SYSTEM (R30-R39)

● R30   Pain associated with micturition
     Excludes1   psychogenic pain associated with micturition (F45.8)
   R30.0   Dysuria
       Painful urination
       Strangury
   R30.1   Vesical tenesmus
       Straining to urinate, with sensation of a full bladder even when empty
   R30.9   Painful micturition, unspecified
       Painful urination NOS

● R31   Hematuria
     Excludes1   hematuria included with underlying conditions, such as: acute cystitis with hematuria (N30.01) recurrent and persistent hematuria in glomerular diseases (N02.-)
   R31.0   Gross hematuria
       Coding Clinic: 2017, Q1, P17
   R31.1   Benign essential microscopic hematuria
   ● R31.2   Other microscopic hematuria
       Coding Clinic: 2016, Q4, P62
     R31.21   Asymptomatic microscopic hematuria
         AMH
     R31.29   Other microscopic hematuria
   R31.9   Hematuria, unspecified
       Coding Clinic: 2017, Q1, P6

R32   Unspecified urinary incontinence
     Enuresis NOS
     Excludes1   functional urinary incontinence (R39.81) nonorganic enuresis (F98.0) stress incontinence and other specified urinary incontinence (N39.3-N39.4-) urinary incontinence associated with cognitive impairment (R39.81)

● R33   Retention of urine
     Excludes1   psychogenic retention of urine (F45.8)
   R33.0   Drug induced retention of urine
       Use additional code for adverse effect, if applicable, to identify drug (T36-T50 with fifth or sixth character 5)
   R33.8   Other retention of urine
       Code first, if applicable, any causal condition, such as: enlarged prostate (N40.1)
       Coding Clinic: 2018, Q4, P55
   R33.9   Retention of urine, unspecified

R34   Anuria and oliguria
     Excludes1   anuria and oliguria complicating abortion or ectopic or molar pregnancy (O00-O07, O08.4) anuria and oliguria complicating pregnancy (O26.83-) anuria and oliguria complicating the puerperium (O90.4)

● R35   Polyuria
     Passage of excessive volume of urine
     Code first, if applicable, any causal condition, such as: enlarged prostate (N40.1)
     Excludes1   psychogenic polyuria (F45.8)
   R35.0   Frequency of micturition
       Discharge or passage of urine; AKA uresis
   R35.1   Nocturia
       Urinary frequency at night
   ● R35.8   Other polyuria
       ~~Polyuria NOS~~
     ▶ R35.81   Nocturnal polyuria
       ▶ **Excludes2**   nocturnal enuresis (N39.44)
     ▶ R35.89   Other polyuria
       ▶ Polyuria NOS

● R36   Urethral discharge
   R36.0   Urethral discharge without blood
   R36.1   Hematospermia ♂
       Presence of blood in semen
   R36.9   Urethral discharge, unspecified
       Penile discharge NOS
       Urethrorrhea

R37   Sexual dysfunction, unspecified

N   Newborn Age: 0   P   Pediatric Age: 0–17   M   Maternity DX: 9–64   A   Adult Age: 15–124   ♀   Females Only   ♂   Males Only

🍏 Complication\Comorbidity   🍏 Major C\C   (Ex) CC/MCC Exclusions   🍏 Hospital-Acquired Condition   🍏 Hierarchical Condition Category

1229

CHAPTER 18 (R00-R99)

● R39   **Other and unspecified symptoms and signs involving the genitourinary system**

     R39.0   **Extravasation of urine** 🅒
         Leakage, discharge
         (Ex:) See PDX Collection 1127

    ● **R39.1**   **Other difficulties with micturition**
         Code first, if applicable, any causal condition, such as:
           enlarged prostate (N40.1)

         R39.11   **Hesitancy of micturition**

         R39.12   **Poor urinary stream**
           Weak urinary steam

         R39.13   **Splitting of urinary stream**

         R39.14   **Feeling of incomplete bladder emptying**

         R39.15   **Urgency of urination**
           Excludes1   urge incontinence (N39.41, N39.46)

         R39.16   **Straining to void**

   ● **R39.19**   **Other difficulties with micturition**
           Coding Clinic: 2016, Q4, P63

           R39.191   **Need to immediately re-void**

           R39.192   **Position dependent micturition**

           R39.198   **Other difficulties with micturition**

     R39.2   **Extrarenal uremia**
         Prerenal uremia
         Excludes1   uremia NOS (N19)

    ● **R39.8**   **Other symptoms and signs involving the genitourinary system**

         R39.81   **Functional urinary incontinence**
           Urinary incontinence due to cognitive impairment, or severe physical disability or immobility
           Excludes1   stress incontinence and other specified urinary incontinence (N39.3-N39.4-)
                     urinary incontinence NOS (R32)

         R39.82   **Chronic bladder pain**
           Coding Clinic: 2016, Q4, P64

         R39.83   **Unilateral non-palpable testicle** ♂

         R39.84   **Bilateral non-palpable testicles** ♂

         R39.89   **Other symptoms and signs involving the genitourinary system**
           Coding Clinic: 2016, Q4, P64

     R39.9   **Unspecified symptoms and signs involving the genitourinary system**

SYMPTOMS AND SIGNS INVOLVING COGNITION, PERCEPTION, EMOTIONAL STATE AND BEHAVIOR (R40-R46)

Excludes2   symptoms and signs constituting part of a pattern of mental disorder (F01-F99)
Coding Clinic: 2015, Q4, P40

● R40   **Somnolence, stupor and coma**
     Excludes1   neonatal coma (P91.5)
                somnolence, stupor and coma in diabetes (E08-E13)
                somnolence, stupor and coma in hepatic failure (K72.-)
                somnolence, stupor and coma in hypoglycemia (nondiabetic) (E15)

     R40.0   **Somnolence**
         Drowsiness
         Excludes1   coma (R40.2-)

     R40.1   **Stupor**
         Lowered level of consciousness
         Catatonic stupor
         Semicoma
         Excludes1   catatonic schizophrenia (F20.2)
                     coma (R40.2-)
                     depressive stupor (F31-F33)
                     dissociative stupor (F44.2)
                     manic stupor (F30.2)

OGCR Section I.C.18.e.

Coma scale

The coma scale codes (R40.2-) can be used in conjunction with traumatic brain injury codes, acute cerebrovascular disease or sequelae of cerebrovascular disease codes. These codes are primarily for use by trauma registries, but they may be used in any setting where this information is collected. The coma scale may also be used to assess the status of the central nervous system for other non-trauma conditions, such as monitoring patients in the intensive care unit regardless of medical condition. The coma scale codes should be sequenced after the diagnosis code(s).

These codes, one from each subcategory, are needed to complete the scale. The 7th character indicates when the scale was recorded. The 7th character should match for all three codes.

At a minimum, report the initial score documented on presentation at your facility. This may be a score from the emergency medicine technician (EMT) or in the emergency department. If desired, a facility may choose to capture multiple coma scale scores.

Assign code R40.24, Glasgow coma scale, total score, when only the total score is documented in the medical record and not the individual score(s).

● **R40.2**   **Coma**
     Code first any associated:
         fracture of skull (S02.-)
         intracranial injury (S06.-)
     Note: One code from each subcategory R40.21-R40-23 is required to complete the coma scale
     (Ex:) **For category R40.2 CC codes:** See PDX Collection 515
     Coding Clinic: 2016, Q4, P127

    ● **R40.20**   **Unspecified coma** 🅒🅒
         Coma NOS
         Unconsciousness NOS

    ● **R40.21**   **Coma scale, eyes open**
         The following appropriate 7th character is to be added to subcategory R40.21-:

0	unspecified time
1	in the field [EMT or ambulance]
2	at arrival to emergency department
3	at hospital admission
4	24 hours or more after hospital admission

         Coding Clinic: 2017, Q4, P25; 2015, Q2, P18

   ●● **R40.211**   **Coma scale, eyes open, never** 🅒🅒
           Coma scale eye opening score of 1

   ●● **R40.212**   **Coma scale, eyes open, to pain** 🅒🅒
           Coma scale eye opening score of 2

   ●● **R40.213**   **Coma scale, eyes open, to sound**
           Coma scale eye opening score of 3

   ●● **R40.214**   **Coma scale, eyes open, spontaneous**
           Coma scale eye opening score of 4

    ● **R40.22**   **Coma scale, best verbal response**
         The following appropriate 7th character is to be added to subcategory R40.22-:

0	unspecified time
1	in the field [EMT or ambulance]
2	at arrival to emergency department
3	at hospital admission
4	24 hours or more after hospital admission

         Coding Clinic: 2017, Q4, P25; 2015, Q2, P18

   ●● **R40.221**   **Coma scale, best verbal response, none** 🅒🅒
           Coma scale verbal score of 1

   ●● **R40.222**   **Coma scale, best verbal response, incomprehensible words** 🅒🅒
           Coma scale verbal score of 2
           Incomprehensible sounds (2-5 years of age)
           Moans/grunts to pain; restless (<2 years old)

▶ New   ⬛ Revised   ~~deleted~~ Deleted   Excludes 1   Excludes 2   Includes   Use additional   Code first   Code also   Key words

OGCR Official Guidelines   ● Unacceptable Principal Diagnosis   X Assign placeholder X   ● Use Additional Character(s)   ▶ Manifestation Code   Coding Clinic

1230

Glasgow Coma Scale

Eye Opening Response	
• Spontaneous--open with blinking at baseline	4 points
• To verbal stimuli, command, speech	3 points
• To pain only (not applied to face)	2 points
• No response	1 point
Verbal Response	
• Oriented	5 points
• Confused conversation, but able to answer questions	4 points
• Inappropriate words	3 points
• Incomprehensible speech	2 points
• No response	1 point
Motor Response	
• Obeys commands for movement	6 points
• Purposeful movement to painful stimulus	5 points
• Withdraws in response to pain	4 points
• Flexion in response to pain (decorticate posturing)	3 points
• Extension response in response to pain (decerebrate posturing)	2 points
• No response	1 point
Categorization:	
Coma: No eye opening, no ability to follow commands, no word verbalizations (3-8)	
Head Injury Classification:	
Severe Head Injury--GCS score of 8 or less	
Moderate Head Injury--GCS score of 9 to 12	
Mild head injury--GCS score of 13 to 15	
(Adapted from: Advanced Trauma Life Support: Course for Physicians, American College of Surgeons, 1993). http://www.bt.cdc.gov/masscasulatires/gscale.asp	

Figure 18-1

● ● R40.223   **Coma scale, best verbal response, inappropriate words**
      Coma scale verbal score of 3
      Inappropriate crying or screaming (< 2 years of age)
      Screaming (2-5 years of age)

● ● R40.224   **Coma scale, best verbal response, confused conversation**
      Coma scale verbal score of 4
      Inappropriate words (2-5 years of age)
      Irritable cries (< 2 years of age)

● ● R40.225   **Coma scale, best verbal response, oriented**
      Coma scale verbal score of 5
      Cooing or babbling or crying appropriately (< 2 years of age)
      Uses appropriate words (2- 5 years of age)

● R40.23   **Coma scale, best motor response**
      The following appropriate 7th character is to be added to subcategory R40.23-:

0	unspecified time
1	in the field [EMT or ambulance]
2	at arrival to emergency department
3	at hospital admission
4	24 hours or more after hospital admission

      Coding Clinic: 2017, Q4, P25; 2015, Q2, P18

● ● R40.231   **Coma scale, best motor response, none**
      Coma scale motor score of 1

● ● R40.232   **Coma scale, best motor response, extension**
      Abnormal extensor posturing to pain or noxious stimuli (< 2 years of age)
      Coma scale motor score of 2
      Extensor posturing to pain or noxious stimuli (2-5 years of age)

● ● R40.233   **Coma scale, best motor response, abnormal flexion**
      Coma scale motor score of 3
      Abnormal flexure posturing to pain or noxious stimuli (2-5 years of age)
      Flexion/decorticate posturing (< 2 years of age)

● ● R40.234   **Coma scale, best motor response, flexion withdrawal**
      Coma scale motor score of 4
      Withdraws from pain or noxious stimuli (2-5 years of age)

● ● R40.235   **Coma scale, best motor response, localizes pain**
      Coma scale motor score of 5
      Localizes pain (2-5 years of age)
      Withdraws to touch (< 2 years of age)

● ● R40.236   **Coma scale, best motor response, obeys commands**
      Coma scale motor score of 6
      Normal or spontaneous movement (< 2 years of age)
      Obeys commands (2-5 years of age)

● R40.24   **Glasgow coma scale, total score**
      Note: Assign a code from subcategory R40.24, when only the total coma score is documented
      The following appropriate 7th character is to be added to subcategory R40.24-:

0	unspecified time
1	in the field [EMT or ambulance]
2	at arrival to emergency department
3	at hospital admission
4	24 hours or more after hospital admission

      Coding Clinic: 2016, Q4, P64; 2015, Q2, P18

● ● R40.241   Glasgow coma scale score 13-15
● ● R40.242   Glasgow coma scale score 9-12
● ● R40.243   Glasgow coma scale score 3-8
● ● R40.244   Other coma, without documented Glasgow coma scale score, or with partial score reported

R40.3   **Persistent vegetative state**
      (Ex) See PDX Collection 515

R40.4   **Transient alteration of awareness**

● R41   **Other symptoms and signs involving cognitive functions and awareness**
      Excludes1   dissociative [conversion] disorders (F44.-)
               mild cognitive impairment, so stated (G31.84)

R41.0   **Disorientation, unspecified**
      Confusion NOS   Delirium NOS
      Coding Clinic: 2019, Q2, P34; 2016, Q4, P71

R41.1   **Anterograde amnesia**

R41.2   **Retrograde amnesia**

N Newborn Age: 0   **P** Pediatric Age: 0–17   **M** Maternity DX: 9–64   **A** Adult Age: 15–124   ♀ Females Only   ♂ Males Only

Complication\Comorbidity   Major C\C   (Ex) CC/MCC Exclusions   Hospital-Acquired Condition   Hierarchical Condition Category

1231

CHAPTER 18 (R00-R99)

R41.3 **Other amnesia**
Amnesia NOS
Memory loss NOS

> **Excludes1** amnestic disorder due to known
> physiologic condition (F04)
> amnestic syndrome due to psychoactive
> substance use (F10-F19 with 5th
> character .6)
> mild memory disturbance due to known
> physiological condition (F06.8)
> transient global amnesia (G45.4)

R41.4 **Neurologic neglect syndrome** 🔗
Asomatognosia   Left-sided neglect
Hemi-akinesia   Sensory neglect
Hemi-inattention   Visuospatial neglect
Hemispatial neglect

> **Excludes1** visuospatial deficit (R41.842)

Ⓔⓧ See PDX Collection 1128

● **R41.8** **Other symptoms and signs involving cognitive functions and awareness**

R41.81 **Age-related cognitive decline**   A
Senility NOS

R41.82 **Altered mental status, unspecified**
Change in mental status NOS

> **Excludes1** altered level of consciousness
> (R40.-)
> altered mental status due to
> known condition - code to
> condition
> delirium NOS (R41.0)

Coding Clinic: 2012, Q4, P98

● **R41.83** **Borderline intellectual functioning**
IQ level 71 to 84

> **Excludes1** intellectual disabilities (F70-F79)

● **R41.84** **Other specified cognitive deficit**

> **Excludes1** cognitive deficits as sequelae
> of cerebrovascular disease
> (I69.01-, I69.11-, I69.21-,
> I69.31-, I69.81-, I69.91-)

R41.840 **Attention and concentration deficit**

> **Excludes1** attention-deficit
> hyperactivity
> disorders (F90.-)

R41.841 **Cognitive communication deficit**

R41.842 **Visuospatial deficit**

R41.843 **Psychomotor deficit**

R41.844 **Frontal lobe and executive function deficit**

R41.89 **Other symptoms and signs involving cognitive functions and awareness**
Anosognosia

R41.9 **Unspecified symptoms and signs involving cognitive functions and awareness**
Unspecified neurocognitive disorder

R42 **Dizziness and giddiness**
Light-headedness
Vertigo NOS

> **Excludes1** vertiginous syndromes (H81.-)
> vertigo from infrasound (T75.23)

Coding Clinic: 2015, Q4, P40

● **R43** **Disturbances of smell and taste**

R43.0 **Anosmia**
Absence of sense of smell; AKA anosphresia and olfactory anesthesia

R43.1 **Parosmia**

R43.2 **Parageusia**
Perversion of sense of taste or bad taste in mouth; AKA dysgeusia

R43.8 **Other disturbances of smell and taste**
Mixed disturbance of smell and taste

R43.9 **Unspecified disturbances of smell and taste**

● **R44** **Other symptoms and signs involving general sensations and perceptions**

> **Excludes1** alcoholic hallucinations (F10.151, F10.251,
> F10.951)
> hallucinations in drug psychosis (F11-F19 with
> fifth to sixth characters 51)
> hallucinations in mood disorders with psychotic
> symptoms (F30.2, F31.5, F32.3, F33.3)
> hallucinations in schizophrenia, schizotypal and
> delusional disorders (F20-F29)
>
> **Excludes2** disturbances of skin sensation (R20.-)

R44.0 **Auditory hallucinations** 🔗
Ⓔⓧ See PDX Collection 1129

R44.1 **Visual hallucinations**

R44.2 **Other hallucinations** 🔗
Ⓔⓧ See PDX Collection 1129

R44.3 **Hallucinations, unspecified** 🔗
Ⓔⓧ See PDX Collection 1129

R44.8 **Other symptoms and signs involving general sensations and perceptions**

R44.9 **Unspecified symptoms and signs involving general sensations and perceptions**

● **R45** **Symptoms and signs involving emotional state**

R45.0 **Nervousness**
Nervous tension

R45.1 **Restlessness and agitation**

R45.2 **Unhappiness**

R45.3 **Demoralization and apathy**

> **Excludes1** anhedonia (R45.84)

R45.4 **Irritability and anger**

R45.5 **Hostility**

R45.6 **Violent behavior**

R45.7 **State of emotional shock and stress, unspecified**

● **R45.8** **Other symptoms and signs involving emotional state**

R45.81 **Low self-esteem**

R45.82 **Worries**

R45.83 **Excessive crying of child, adolescent or adult**

> **Excludes1** excessive crying of infant (baby)
> R68.11

R45.84 **Anhedonia**
Total loss of feeling of pleasure in pleasurable acts

● **R45.85** **Homicidal and suicidal ideations**

> **Excludes1** suicide attempt (T14.91)

● **R45.850** **Homicidal ideations**

R45.851 **Suicidal ideations** 🔗
Ⓔⓧ See PDX Collection 1130

R45.86 **Emotional lability**

R45.87 **Impulsiveness**

▶ **R45.88** **Nonsuicidal self-harm**
▶Nonsuicidal self-injury
▶Nonsuicidal self-mutilation
▶Self-inflicted injury without suicidal intent
▶Code also injury, if known

R45.89 **Other symptoms and signs involving emotional state**

● **R46** **Symptoms and signs involving appearance and behavior**

> **Excludes1** appearance and behavior in schizophrenia,
> schizotypal and delusional disorders
> (F20-F29)
> mental and behavioral disorders (F01-F99)

R46.0 **Very low level of personal hygiene**

R46.1 **Bizarre personal appearance**

R46.2 **Strange and inexplicable behavior**

R46.3 **Overactivity**

R46.4 **Slowness and poor responsiveness**

> **Excludes1** stupor (R40.1)

R46.5 **Suspiciousness and marked evasiveness**

R46.6 **Undue concern and preoccupation with stressful events**

R46.7   **Verbosity and circumstantial detail obscuring reason for contact**

● **R46.8**   **Other symptoms and signs involving appearance and behavior**

    ● **R46.81**   **Obsessive-compulsive behavior**

       Excludes1   obsessive-compulsive disorder (F42.-)

    ● **R46.89**   **Other symptoms and signs involving appearance and behavior**

SYMPTOMS AND SIGNS INVOLVING SPEECH AND VOICE (R47-R49)

● **R47**   **Speech disturbances, not elsewhere classified**

    Excludes1   autism (F84.0)
                cluttering (F80.81)
                specific developmental disorders of speech and language (F80.-)
                stuttering (F80.81)

● **R47.0**   **Dysphasia and aphasia**

    R47.01   **Aphasia** 🅒🅒

       Excludes1   aphasia following cerebrovascular disease (I69. with final characters -20)
               progressive isolated aphasia (G31.01)

       (Ex:) See PDX Collection 1131

    R47.02   **Dysphasia**
       Impairment in comprehension of speech, caused by left-sided brain damage

       Excludes1   dysphasia following cerebrovascular disease (I69. with final characters -21)

R47.1   **Dysarthria and anarthria**
    Motor speech disorder

    Excludes1   dysarthria following cerebrovascular disease (I69. with final characters -22)

● **R47.8**   **Other speech disturbances**

    Excludes1   dysarthria following cerebrovascular disease (I69. with final characters -28)

    R47.81   **Slurred speech**

    ▸ **R47.82**   *Fluency disorder in conditions classified elsewhere*
       Stuttering in conditions classified elsewhere

       Code first underlying disease or condition, such as:
       Parkinson's disease (G20)

       Excludes1   adult onset fluency disorder (F98.5)
               childhood onset fluency disorder (F80.81)
               fluency disorder (stuttering) following cerebrovascular disease (I69. with final characters -23)

    R47.89   **Other speech disturbances**

R47.9   **Unspecified speech disturbances**

● **R48**   **Dyslexia and other symbolic dysfunctions, not elsewhere classified**

    Excludes1   specific developmental disorders of scholastic skills (F81.-)

R48.0   **Dyslexia and alexia**

R48.1   **Agnosia**
    Loss of ability to recognize objects, persons, sounds, shapes, or smells
    Astereognosia (astereognosis)
    Autotopagnosia

    Excludes1   visual object agnosia (R48.3)

R48.2   **Apraxia**
    Loss of ability to execute or carry out learned purposeful movements

    Excludes1   apraxia following cerebrovascular disease (I69. with final characters -90)

R48.3   **Visual agnosia**
    Prosopagnosia
    Simultanagnosia (asimultagnosia)

R48.8   **Other symbolic dysfunctions**
    Acalculia
    Difficulty performing simple mathematical tasks resulting from neurological injury
    Agraphia
    Coding Clinic: 2017, Q1, P27

R48.9   **Unspecified symbolic dysfunctions**

● **R49**   **Voice and resonance disorders**

    Excludes1   psychogenic voice and resonance disorders (F44.4)

R49.0   **Dysphonia**
    Hoarseness

R49.1   **Aphonia**
    Loss of voice

● **R49.2**   **Hypernasality and hyponasality**

    R49.21   **Hypernasality**

    R49.22   **Hyponasality**

R49.8   **Other voice and resonance disorders**

R49.9   **Unspecified voice and resonance disorder**
    Change in voice NOS
    Resonance disorder NOS

GENERAL SYMPTOMS AND SIGNS (R50-R69)

● **R50**   **Fever of other and unknown origin**

    Excludes1   chills without fever (R68.83)
               febrile convulsions (R56.0-)
               fever of unknown origin during labor (O75.2)
               fever of unknown origin in newborn (P81.9)
               hypothermia due to illness (R68.0)
               malignant hyperthermia due to anesthesia (T88.3)
               puerperal pyrexia NOS (O86.4)

R50.2   **Drug induced fever**
    Use additional code for adverse effect, if applicable, to identify drug (T36-T50 with fifth or sixth character 5)

    Excludes1   postvaccination (postimmunization) fever (R50.83)

● **R50.8**   **Other specified fever**

    ▸ **R50.81**   *Fever presenting with conditions classified elsewhere*

       Code first underlying condition when associated fever is present, such as with:
       leukemia (C91-C95)
       neutropenia (D70.-)
       sickle-cell disease (D57.-)
       Coding Clinic: 2019, Q2, P25

    R50.82   **Postprocedural fever**

       Excludes1   postprocedural infection (T81.44)
               posttransfusion fever (R50.84)
               postvaccination (postimmunization) fever (R50.83)

    R50.83   **Postvaccination fever**
       Postimmunization fever

    R50.84   **Febrile nonhemolytic transfusion reaction**
       FNHTR
       Posttransfusion fever

● **R50.9**   **Fever, unspecified**
    Fever NOS
    Fever of unknown origin [FUO]
    Fever with chills
    Fever with rigors
    Hyperpyrexia NOS
    Persistent fever
    Pyrexia NOS

N Newborn Age: 0   **P** Pediatric Age: 0–17   **M** Maternity DX: 9–64   **A** Adult Age: 15–124   ♀ Females Only   ♂ Males Only

🅒🅒 Complication\Comorbidity   🅒🅒 Major C\C   (Ex:) CC/MCC Exclusions   🅗 Hospital-Acquired Condition   🅒 Hierarchical Condition Category

1233

CHAPTER 18 (R00-R99)

● **R51   Headache**
    Excludes2   atypical face pain (G50.1)
                   migraine and other headache syndromes
                       (G43-G44)
                   trigeminal neuralgia (G50.0)

     R51.0   Headache with orthostatic component, not elsewhere classified
         Headache with positional component, not elsewhere classified

     R51.9 Headache, unspecified
         Facial pain NOS

   R52   **Pain, unspecified**
       Acute pain NOS
       Generalized pain NOS
      Excludes1   acute and chronic pain, not elsewhere classified (G89.-)
                   localized pain, unspecified type - code to pain by site, such as:
                       abdomen pain (R10.-)
                       back pain (M54.9)
                       breast pain (N64.4)
                       chest pain (R07.1-R07.9)
                       ear pain (H92.0-)
                       eye pain (H57.1)
                       headache (R51.9)
                       joint pain (M25.5-)
                       limb pain (M79.6-)
           ➡ lumbar region pain (M54.5-)
                       pelvic and perineal pain (R10.2)
                       shoulder pain (M25.51-)
                       spine pain (M54.-)
                       throat pain (R07.0)
                       tongue pain (K14.6)
                       tooth pain (K08.8)
                       renal colic (N23)
                   pain disorders exclusively related to psychological factors (F45.41)

● **R53   Malaise and fatigue**
     R53.0   Neoplastic (malignant) related fatigue
         Code first associated neoplasm

     R53.1   Weakness
         Asthenia NOS
       Excludes1   age-related weakness (R54)
                    muscle weakness (generalized) (M62.81)
                    sarcopenia (M62.84)
                    senile asthenia (R54)
       Coding Clinic: 2017, Q1, P7

     R53.2   Functional quadriplegia 🔖 🔖
         Complete immobility due to severe physical disability or frailty
       Excludes1   frailty NOS (R54)
                    hysterical paralysis (F44.4)
                    immobility syndrome (M62.3)
                    neurologic quadriplegia (G82.5-)
                    quadriplegia (G82.50)
         (Ex:) See PDX Collection 595
         Coding Clinic: 2016, Q2, P6

● **R53.8   Other malaise and fatigue**
       Excludes1   combat exhaustion and fatigue (F43.0)
                    congenital debility (P96.9)
                    exhaustion and fatigue due to excessive exertion (T73.3)
                    exhaustion and fatigue due to exposure (T73.2)
                    exhaustion and fatigue due to heat (T67.-)
                    exhaustion and fatigue due to pregnancy (O26.8-)
                    exhaustion and fatigue due to recurrent depressive episode (F33)
                    exhaustion and fatigue due to senile debility (R54)

     R53.81   Other malaise
         Chronic debility
         Debility NOS
         General physical deterioration
         Malaise NOS
         Nervous debility
         Excludes1   age-related physical debility (R54)
         Coding Clinic: 2021, Q1, P43

     R53.82   Chronic fatigue, unspecified
         Chronic fatigue syndrome NOS
         Excludes1   postviral fatigue syndrome (G93.3)

     R53.83   Other fatigue
         Fatigue NOS   Lethargy
         Lack of energy   Tiredness
         Excludes2   exhaustion and fatigue due to depressive episode (F32.-)
         Coding Clinic: 2017, Q1, P7

   R54   **Age-related physical debility**   A
       Frailty   Senile asthenia
       Old age   Senile debility
       Senescence
      Excludes1   age-related cognitive decline (R41.81)
                   sarcopenia (M62.84)
                   senile psychosis (F03)
                   senility NOS (R41.81)

   R55   **Syncope and collapse**
       Blackout
       Fainting
       Vasovagal attack
      Excludes1   cardiogenic shock (R57.0)
                   carotid sinus syncope (G90.01)
                   heat syncope (T67.1)
                   neurocirculatory asthenia (F45.8)
                   neurogenic orthostatic hypotension (G90.3)
                   orthostatic hypotension (I95.1)
                   postprocedural shock (T81.1-)
                   psychogenic syncope (F48.8)
                   shock NOS (R57.9)
                   shock complicating or following abortion or ectopic or molar pregnancy (O00-O07, O08.3)
                   shock complicating or following labor and delivery (O75.1)
                   Stokes-Adams attack (I45.9)
                   unconsciousness NOS (R40.2-)

● **R56   Convulsions, not elsewhere classified**
      Excludes1   dissociative convulsions and seizures (F44.5)
                   epileptic convulsions and seizures (G40.-)
                   newborn convulsions and seizures (P90)

● **R56.0   Febrile convulsions**
         (Ex:) **For category R56.0 CC codes:** See PDX Collection 1132

     R56.00   Simple febrile convulsions 🔖 🔖
         Febrile convulsion NOS
         Febrile seizure NOS

     R56.01   Complex febrile convulsions 🔖 🔖
         Atypical febrile seizure
         Complex febrile seizure
         Complicated febrile seizure
         Excludes1   status epilepticus (G40.901)

▶ New   ➡ Revised   ~~deleted~~ Deleted   Excludes 1   Excludes 2   Includes   Use additional   Code first   Code also   Key words

OGCR Official Guidelines   ● Unacceptable Principal Diagnosis   X Assign placeholder X   ● Use Additional Character(s)   ▶ Manifestation Code   Coding Clinic

R56.1   **Post traumatic seizures** 🔹🔹

     Excludes1   post traumatic epilepsy (G40.-)

     (Ex:) See PDX Collection 582

R56.9   **Unspecified convulsions** 🔹

     Convulsion disorder   Recurrent convulsions
     Fit NOS   Seizure(s) (convulsive) NOS

     Coding Clinic: 2021, Q1, P3; 2019, Q4, P18

● R57   **Shock, not elsewhere classified**

     Excludes1   anaphylactic shock NOS (T78.2)
                 anaphylactic reaction or shock due to adverse food reaction (T78.0-)
                 anaphylactic shock due to adverse effect of correct drug or medicament properly administered (T88.6)
                 anaphylactic shock due to serum (T80.5-)
                 anesthetic shock (T88.3)
                 electric shock (T75.4)
                 obstetric shock (O75.1)
                 postprocedural shock (T81.1-)
                 psychic shock (F43.0)
                 shock complicating or following ectopic or molar pregnancy (O00-O07, O08.3)
                ▶shock due to anesthesia (T88.2)
                 shock due to lightning (T75.01)
                 traumatic shock (T79.4)
                 toxic shock syndrome (A48.3)

     (Ex:) **For category R57 CC codes: See PDX Collection 1133**

R57.0   **Cardiogenic shock** 🔹🔹

     Excludes2   septic shock (R65.21)

     MCC: Only if patient discharged alive

R57.1   **Hypovolemic shock** 🔹🔹
     Decreased blood volume (loss)
     MCC: Only if patient discharged alive
     Coding Clinic: 2019, Q2, P7-8

R57.8   **Other shock** 🔹🔹
     MCC: Only if patient discharged alive

R57.9   **Shock, unspecified** 🔹🔹
     Failure of peripheral circulation NOS
     Resulting in significant blood pressure drop

R58   **Hemorrhage, not elsewhere classified**
     Hemorrhage NOS

     Excludes1   hemorrhage included with underlying conditions, such as:
                 acute duodenal ulcer with hemorrhage (K26.0)
                 acute gastritis with bleeding (K29.01)
                 ulcerative enterocolitis with rectal bleeding (K51.01)

● R59   **Enlarged lymph nodes**

     Includes   swollen glands

     Excludes1   lymphadenitis NOS (I88.9)
                 acute lymphadenitis (L04.-)
                 chronic lymphadenitis (I88.1)
                 mesenteric (acute) (chronic) lymphadenitis (I88.0)

R59.0   **Localized** enlarged lymph nodes

R59.1   **Generalized** enlarged lymph nodes
     Lymphadenopathy NOS

R59.9   **Enlarged lymph nodes, unspecified**

● R60   **Edema, not elsewhere classified**

     Excludes1   angioneurotic edema (T78.3)
                 ascites (R18.-)
                 cerebral edema (G93.6)
                 cerebral edema due to birth injury (P11.0)
                 edema of larynx (J38.4)
                 edema of nasopharynx (J39.2)
                 edema of pharynx (J39.2)
                 gestational edema (O12.0-)
                 hereditary edema (Q82.0)
                 hydrops fetalis NOS (P83.2)
                 hydrothorax (J94.8)
                 hydrops fetalis NOS (P83.2)
                 newborn edema (P83.3)
                 pulmonary edema (J81.-)

R60.0   **Localized edema**

R60.1   **Generalized edema**

     Excludes2   nutritional edema (E40-E46)

R60.9   **Edema, unspecified**
     Fluid retention NOS

R61   **Generalized hyperhidrosis**
     Excessive sweating
     Night sweats
     Secondary hyperhidrosis

     Code first, if applicable, menopausal and female climacteric states (N95.1)

     Excludes1   focal (primary) (secondary) hyperhidrosis (L74.5-)
                 Frey's syndrome (L74.52)
                 localized (primary) (secondary) hyperhidrosis (L74.5-)

● R62   **Lack of expected normal physiological development in childhood and adults**

     Excludes1   delayed puberty (E30.0)
                 gonadal dysgenesis (Q99.1)
                 hypopituitarism (E23.0)

R62.0   **Delayed milestone in childhood**   **P**
     Delayed attainment of expected physiological developmental stage
     Late talker
     Late walker

● R62.5   **Other and unspecified lack of expected normal physiological development in childhood**

     Excludes1   HIV disease resulting in failure to thrive (B20)
                 physical retardation due to malnutrition (E45)

R62.50   **Unspecified** lack of expected normal physiological development in childhood
     Infantilism NOS

R62.51   **Failure to thrive (child)**   **P**
     Failure to gain weight

     Excludes1   failure to thrive in child under 28 days old (P92.6)

     Coding Clinic: 2018, Q4, P82

R62.52   **Short stature (child)**
     Lack of growth   Short stature NOS
     Physical retardation

     Excludes1   short stature due to endocrine disorder (E34.3)

R62.59   **Other lack of expected normal physiological development in childhood**

R62.7   **Adult failure to thrive**   **A**

CHAPTER 18 (R00-R99)

N Newborn Age: 0   **P** Pediatric Age: 0–17   **M** Maternity DX: 9–64   **A** Adult Age: 15–124   ♀ Females Only   ♂ Males Only

🔹 Complication\Comorbidity   🔹 Major C\C   (Ex:) CC/MCC Exclusions   🔹 Hospital-Acquired Condition   🔹 Hierarchical Condition Category

1235

● R63   Symptoms and signs concerning food and fluid intake
         Excludes1   bulimia NOS (F50.2)
    R63.0   Anorexia
             Loss of appetite
             Excludes1   anorexia nervosa (F50.0-)
                          loss of appetite of nonorganic origin
                               (F50.89)
    R63.1   Polydipsia
             Excessive thirst
    R63.2   Polyphagia
             Excessive eating   Hyperalimentation NOS
● R63.3   Feeding difficulties
           Feeding problem (elderly) (infant) NOS
           Picky eater
           Excludes1   eating disorders (F50.-)
                        feeding problems of newborn (P92.-)
                        infant feeding disorder of nonorganic
                             origin (F98.2-)

           ▶ Excludes2   eating disorders (F50.-)
                          ▶feeding problems of newborn (P92.-)
                          ▶infant feeding disorder of nonorganic
                               origin (F98.2-)
    ▶ R63.30   Feeding difficulties, unspecified
    ▶ R63.31   Pediatric feeding disorder, acute
                ▶Pediatric feeding dysfunction, acute
                ▶Code also, if applicable, associated conditions
                     such as:
                ▶aspiration pneumonia (J69.0)
                ▶dysphagia (R13.1-)
                ▶gastro-esophageal reflux disease (K21.-)
                ▶malnutrition (E40-E46)
    ▶ R63.32   Pediatric feeding disorder, chronic
                ▶Pediatric feeding dysfunction, chronic
                ▶Code also, if applicable, associated conditions
                     such as:
                ▶aspiration pneumonia (J69.0)
                ▶dysphagia (R13.1-)
                ▶gastro-esophageal reflux disease (K21.-)
                ▶malnutrition (E40-E46)
    ▶ R63.39   Other feeding difficulties
                ▶Feeding problem (elderly) (infant) NOS
                ▶Picky eater
                Coding Clinic: 2017, Q1, P27; 2016, Q3, P19
    R63.4   Abnormal weight loss
    R63.5   Abnormal weight gain
             Excludes1   excessive weight gain in pregnancy (O26.0-)
                          obesity (E66.-)
    R63.6   Underweight
             Use additional code to identify body mass index (BMI),
                  if known (Z68.-)
             Excludes1   abnormal weight loss (R63.4)
                          anorexia nervosa (F50.0-)
                          malnutrition (E40-E46)
    R63.8   Other symptoms and signs concerning food and fluid
             intake

R64   Cachexia 🏷️ 🏷️
         Wasting syndrome
         Code first underlying condition, if known
         Excludes1   abnormal weight loss (R63.4)
                      nutritional marasmus (E41)
         (Ex:) See PDX Collection 1134
         Coding Clinic: 2017, Q3, P25
● R65   Symptoms and signs specifically associated with systemic
         inflammation and infection
         (Ex:) For category R65 CC codes unless otherwise indicated: See PDX Collection 71
    ● R65.1   Systemic inflammatory response syndrome (SIRS) of
               non-infectious origin
               Code first underlying condition, such as:
                  heatstroke (T67.0-)
                  injury and trauma (S00-T88)
               Excludes1   sepsis - code to infection
                            severe sepsis (R65.2)
               Coding Clinic: 2019, Q2, P38

    ● R65.10   Systemic inflammatory response syndrome
                (SIRS) of non-infectious origin without acute
                organ dysfunction 🏷️ 🏷️
                Systemic inflammatory response syndrome
                     (SIRS) NOS
                Coding Clinic: 2019, Q2, P25, 38
    ● R65.11   Systemic inflammatory response syndrome
                (SIRS) of non-infectious origin with acute
                organ dysfunction 🏷️ 🏷️
                Use additional code to identify specific acute
                     organ dysfunction, such as:
                acute kidney failure (N17.-)
                acute respiratory failure (J96.0-)
                critical illness myopathy (G72.81)
                critical illness polyneuropathy (G62.81)
                disseminated intravascular coagulopathy
                     [DIC] (D65)
                encephalopathy (metabolic) (septic) (G93.41)
                hepatic failure (K72.0-)

OGCR Section I.C.18.g.

SIRS due to Non-Infectious Process
The systemic inflammatory response syndrome (SIRS) can develop as
a result of certain non-infectious disease processes, such as trauma,
malignant neoplasm, or pancreatitis. When SIRS is documented
with a noninfectious condition, and no subsequent infection is
documented, the code for the underlying condition, such as an injury,
should be assigned, followed by code R65.10. Systemic inflammatory
response syndrome (SIRS) of non-infectious origin without
acute organ dysfunction, or code R65.11, Systemic inflammatory
response syndrome (SIRS) of non-infectious origin with acute organ
dysfunction. If an associated acute organ dysfunction is documented,
the appropriate code(s) for the specific type of organ dysfunction(s)
should be assigned in addition to code R65.11. If acute organ
dysfunction is documented, but it cannot be determined if the acute
organ dysfunction is associated with SIRS or due to another condition
(e.g., directly due to the trauma), the provider should be queried.

    ● R65.2   Severe sepsis
               Infection with associated acute organ dysfunction
               Sepsis with acute organ dysfunction
               Sepsis with multiple organ dysfunction
               Systemic inflammatory response syndrome due to
                    infectious process with acute organ dysfunction
               Code first underlying infection, such as:
                  infection following a procedure (T81.44)
                  infections following infusion, transfusion and
                       therapeutic injection (T80.2-)
                  puerperal sepsis (O85)
                  sepsis following complete or unspecified
                       spontaneous abortion (O03.87)
                  sepsis following ectopic and molar pregnancy
                       (O08.82)
                  sepsis following incomplete spontaneous abortion
                       (O03.37)
                  sepsis following (induced) termination of pregnancy
                       (O04.87)
                  sepsis NOS (A41.9)
               Use additional code to identify specific acute organ
                    dysfunction, such as:
                  acute kidney failure (N17.-)
                  acute respiratory failure (J96.0-)
                  critical illness myopathy (G72.81)
                  critical illness polyneuropathy (G62.81)
                  disseminated intravascular coagulopathy [DIC] (D65)
                  encephalopathy (metabolic) (septic) (G93.41)
                  hepatic failure (K72.0-)
               Coding Clinic: 2017, Q4, P99; 2016, Q3, P8
    ● R65.20   Severe sepsis without septic shock 🏷️ 🏷️
                Severe sepsis NOS
                Coding Clinic: 2019, Q1, P14; 2018, Q4, P90; 2016, Q3, P14
    ● R65.21   Severe sepsis with septic shock 🏷️ 🏷️
                MCC when PDx is its own MCC
                (Ex:) See PDX Collection 1133

▶ New   ⇒ Revised   deleted Deleted   Excludes 1   Excludes 2   Includes   Use additional   Code first   Code also   Key words

OGCR Official Guidelines   ● Unacceptable Principal Diagnosis   X Assign placeholder X   ● Use Additional Character(s)   ▶ Manifestation Code   Coding Clinic

CHAPTER 18 (R00-R99)

● **R68**   **Other general symptoms and signs**

    R68.0   **Hypothermia, not associated with low environmental temperature**

        Excludes1   hypothermia NOS (accidental) (T68)
                hypothermia due to anesthesia (T88.51)
                hypothermia due to low environmental temperature (T68)
                newborn hypothermia (P80.-)

   ● **R68.1**   **Nonspecific symptoms peculiar to infancy**

        Excludes1   colic, infantile (R10.83)
                neonatal cerebral irritability (P91.3)
                teething syndrome (K00.7)

      R68.11   **Excessive crying of infant (baby)**   **P**

          Excludes1   excessive crying of child, adolescent, or adult (R45.83)

      R68.12   **Fussy infant (baby)**   **P**
          Irritable infant

      R68.13   **Apparent life threatening event in infant (ALTE)**   **P**
          Apparent life threatening event in newborn
          Brief resolved unexplained event (BRUE)
          Code first confirmed diagnosis, if known
          Use additional code(s) for associated signs and symptoms if no confirmed diagnosis established, or if signs and symptoms are not associated routinely with confirmed diagnosis, or provide additional information for cause of ALTE

      R68.19   **Other nonspecific symptoms peculiar to infancy**   **P**

    R68.2   **Dry mouth, unspecified**

        Excludes1   dry mouth due to dehydration (E86.0)
        ➠ dry mouth due to Sjögren syndrome (M35.0-)
                salivary gland hyposecretion (K11.7)

    R68.3   **Clubbing of fingers**
        Clubbing of nails

        Excludes1   congenital clubfinger (Q68.1)

   ● **R68.8**   **Other general symptoms and signs**

      R68.81   **Early satiety**

      R68.82   **Decreased libido**   **A**
          Decreased sexual desire

      R68.83   **Chills (without fever)**
          Chills NOS

          Excludes1   chills with fever (R50.9)

      R68.84   **Jaw pain**
          Mandibular pain
          Maxilla pain

          Excludes1   temporomandibular joint arthralgia (M26.62-)

      R68.89   **Other general symptoms and signs**

R69   **Illness, unspecified**
    Unknown and unspecified cases of morbidity

ABNORMAL FINDINGS ON EXAMINATION OF BLOOD, WITHOUT DIAGNOSIS (R70-R79)

        Excludes2   abnormal findings on antenatal screening of mother (O28.-)
                abnormalities of lipids (E78.-)
                abnormalities of platelets and thrombocytes (D69.-)
                abnormalities of white blood cells classified elsewhere (D70-D72)
                coagulation hemorrhagic disorders (D65-D68)
                diagnostic abnormal findings classified elsewhere —*see* Alphabetical Index
                hemorrhagic and hematological disorders of newborn (P50-P61)

● **R70**   **Elevated erythrocyte sedimentation rate and abnormality of plasma viscosity**

    R70.0   **Elevated erythrocyte sedimentation rate**

    R70.1   **Abnormal plasma viscosity**

● **R71**   **Abnormality of red blood cells**

        Excludes1   anemias (D50-D64)
                anemia of premature infant (P61.2)
                benign (familial) polycythemia (D75.0)
                congenital anemias (P61.2-P61.4)
                newborn anemia due to isoimmunization (P55.-)
                polycythemia neonatorum (P61.1)
                polycythemia NOS (D75.1)
                polycythemia vera (D45)
                secondary polycythemia (D75.1)

    R71.0   **Precipitous drop in hematocrit** 🦠
        Drop (precipitous) in hemoglobin
        Drop in hematocrit
        Blood volume that has decreased red blood cells
        (Ex) See PDX Collection 3453

    R71.8   **Other abnormality of red blood cells**
        Abnormal red-cell morphology NOS
        Abnormal red-cell volume NOS
        Anisocytosis
        Red blood cells of unequal size
        Poikilocytosis
        Red blood cells of abnormal shape

● **R73**   **Elevated blood glucose level**

        Excludes1   diabetes mellitus (E08-E13)
                diabetes mellitus in pregnancy, childbirth and the puerperium (O24.-)
                neonatal disorders (P70.0-P70.2)
                postsurgical hypoinsulinemia (E89.1)

   ● **R73.0**   **Abnormal glucose**

        Excludes1   abnormal glucose in pregnancy (O99.81-)
                diabetes mellitus (E08-E13)
                dysmetabolic syndrome X (E88.81)
                gestational diabetes (O24.4-)
                glycosuria (R81)
                hypoglycemia (E16.2)

      R73.01   **Impaired fasting glucose**
          Elevated fasting glucose

      R73.02   **Impaired glucose tolerance (oral)**
          Elevated glucose tolerance

      R73.03   **Prediabetes**
          Latent diabetes
          Coding Clinic: 2016, Q4, P65

      R73.09   **Other abnormal glucose**
          Abnormal glucose NOS
          Abnormal non-fasting glucose tolerance
          Coding Clinic: 2016, Q4, P65

    R73.9   **Hyperglycemia, unspecified**

● **R74**   **Abnormal serum enzyme levels**

   ● **R74.0**   **Nonspecific elevation of levels of transaminase and lactic acid dehydrogenase [LDH]**

      R74.01   **Elevation of levels of liver transaminase levels**
          Elevation of levels of alanine transaminase (ALT)
          Elevation of levels of aspartate transaminase (AST)

      R74.02   **Elevation of levels of lactic acid dehydrogenase [LDH]**

    R74.8   **Abnormal levels of other serum enzymes**
        Abnormal level of acid phosphatase
        Abnormal level of alkaline phosphatase
        Abnormal level of amylase
        Abnormal level of lipase [triacylglycerol lipase]
        Coding Clinic: 2019, Q2, P6

    R74.9   **Abnormal serum enzyme level, unspecified**

R75   **Inconclusive laboratory evidence of human immunodeficiency virus [HIV]**
    Nonconclusive HIV-test finding in infants

        Excludes1   asymptomatic human immunodeficiency virus [HIV] infection status (Z21)
                human immunodeficiency virus [HIV] disease (B20)

CHAPTER 18 (R00-R99)

N Newborn Age: 0   **P** Pediatric Age: 0–17   **M** Maternity DX: 9–64   **A** Adult Age: 15–124   ♀ Females Only   ♂ Males Only

🦠 Complication\Comorbidity   🦠 Major C\C   (Ex) CC/MCC Exclusions   🦠 Hospital-Acquired Condition   🦠 Hierarchical Condition Category

1237

CHAPTER 18 (R00-R99)

● **R76   Other abnormal immunological findings in serum**

    R76.0   Raised antibody titer

       Excludes1   isoimmunization in pregnancy (O36.0-O36.1)

                     isoimmunization affecting newborn (P55.-)

            Coding Clinic: 2021, Q1, P7

●   **R76.1   Nonspecific reaction to test for tuberculosis**

       R76.11   Nonspecific reaction to tuberculin skin test without active tuberculosis

           Abnormal result of Mantoux test

           PPD positive

           Tuberculin (skin test) positive

           Tuberculin (skin test) reactor

           Excludes1   nonspecific reaction to cell mediated immunity measurement of gamma interferon antigen response without active tuberculosis (R76.12)

       R76.12   Nonspecific reaction to cell mediated immunity measurement of gamma interferon antigen response without active tuberculosis

           Nonspecific reaction to QuantiFERON-TB test (QFT) without active tuberculosis

           Excludes1   nonspecific reaction to tuberculin skin test without active tuberculosis (R76.11)

                     positive tuberculin skin test (R76.11)

    R76.8   Other specified abnormal immunological findings in serum

       Raised level of immunoglobulins NOS

       Coding Clinic: 2021, Q1, P7

    R76.9   Abnormal immunological finding in serum, unspecified

● **R77   Other abnormalities of plasma proteins**

    Excludes1   disorders of plasma-protein metabolism (E88.0-)

    R77.0   Abnormality of albumin

    R77.1   Abnormality of globulin

       Hyperglobulinemia NOS

    R77.2   Abnormality of alphafetoprotein

    R77.8   Other specified abnormalities of plasma proteins

       Coding Clinic: 2019, Q2, P6

    R77.9   Abnormality of plasma protein, unspecified

       Coding Clinic: 2019, Q2, P6

● **R78   Findings of drugs and other substances, not normally found in blood**

    Use additional code to identify any retained foreign body, if applicable (Z18.-)

    Excludes1   mental or behavioral disorders due to psychoactive substance use (F10-F19)

    R78.0   Finding of alcohol in blood

       Use additional external cause code (Y90.-), for detail regarding alcohol level.

    R78.1   Finding of opiate drug in blood

    R78.2   Finding of cocaine in blood

    R78.3   Finding of hallucinogen in blood

    R78.4   Finding of other drugs of addictive potential in blood

    R78.5   Finding of other psychotropic drug in blood

    R78.6   Finding of steroid agent in blood

●   **R78.7   Finding of abnormal level of heavy metals in blood**

       R78.71   Abnormal lead level in blood

           Excludes1   lead poisoning (T56.0-)

       R78.79   Finding of abnormal level of heavy metals in blood

●   **R78.8   Finding of other specified substances, not normally found in blood**

       R78.81   Bacteremia 🔗

           Blood poisoning/bacteremia

           Excludes1   sepsis-code to specified infection

           Ex: See PDX Collection 1136

       R78.89   Finding of other specified substances, not normally found in blood

           Finding of abnormal level of lithium in blood

    R78.9   Finding of unspecified substance, not normally found in blood

● **R79   Other abnormal findings of blood chemistry**

    Use additional code to identify any retained foreign body, if applicable (Z18.-)

    Excludes1   asymptomatic hyperuricemia (E79.0)

                     hyperglycemia NOS (R73.9)

                     hypoglycemia NOS (E16.2)

                     neonatal hypoglycemia (P70.3-P70.4)

                     specific findings indicating disorder of amino-acid metabolism (E70-E72)

                     specific findings indicating disorder of carbohydrate metabolism (E73-E74)

                     specific findings indicating disorder of lipid metabolism (E75.-)

    R79.0   Abnormal level of blood mineral

       Abnormal blood level of cobalt

       Abnormal blood level of copper

       Abnormal blood level of iron

       Abnormal blood level of magnesium

       Abnormal blood level of mineral NEC

       Abnormal blood level of zinc

       Excludes1   abnormal level of lithium (R78.89)

                  disorders of mineral metabolism (E83.-)

                  neonatal hypomagnesemia (P71.2)

                  nutritional mineral deficiency (E58-E61)

    R79.1   Abnormal coagulation profile

       Abnormal or prolonged bleeding time

       Abnormal or prolonged coagulation time

       Abnormal or prolonged partial thromboplastin time [PTT]

       Abnormal or prolonged prothrombin time [PT]

       Excludes1   coagulation defects (D68.-)

       Excludes2   abnormality of fluid, electrolyte or acid-base balance (E86-E87)

●   **R79.8   Other specified abnormal findings of blood chemistry**

       R79.81   Abnormal blood-gas level

       R79.82   Elevated C-reactive protein (CRP)

▶   **R79.83   Abnormal findings of blood amino-acid level**

       ▶Homocysteinemia

           Excludes1   disorders of amino-acid metabolism (E70-E72)

       R79.89   Other specified abnormal findings of blood chemistry

           Coding Clinic: 2019, Q2, P6

    R79.9   Abnormal finding of blood chemistry, unspecified

ABNORMAL FINDINGS ON EXAMINATION OF URINE, WITHOUT DIAGNOSIS (R80-R82)

    Excludes1   abnormal findings on antenatal screening of mother (O28.-)

                  diagnostic abnormal findings classified elsewhere - see Alphabetical Index

                  specific findings indicating disorder of amino-acid metabolism (E70-E72)

                  specific findings indicating disorder of carbohydrate metabolism (E73-E74)

▶ New   ⇒ Revised   ~~deleted~~ Deleted   Excludes 1   Excludes 2   Includes   Use additional   Code first   Code also   Key words

1238   OGCR Official Guidelines   ● Unacceptable Principal Diagnosis   X Assign placeholder X   ● Use Additional Character(s)   ▶ Manifestation Code   Coding Clinic

● R80   Proteinuria
        Excludes1   gestational proteinuria (O12.1-)
        R80.0   **Isolated proteinuria**
                Idiopathic proteinuria
                Excludes1   isolated proteinuria with specific
                                morphological lesion (N06.-)
        R80.1   **Persistent proteinuria, unspecified**
        R80.2   **Orthostatic proteinuria, unspecified**
                Postural proteinuria
        R80.3   **Bence Jones proteinuria**
        R80.8   **Other proteinuria**
        R80.9   **Proteinuria, unspecified**
                Albuminuria NOS

R81   Glycosuria
        Excludes1   renal glycosuria (E74.818)

● R82   Other and unspecified abnormal findings in urine
        Includes   chromoabnormalities in urine
                Use additional code to identify any retained foreign body, if
                applicable (Z18.-)
        Excludes2   hematuria (R31.-)
        R82.0   **Chyluria** 🐾
                White milky urine
                Excludes1   filarial chyluria (B74.-)
                Ⓔ See PDX Collection 1137
        R82.1   **Myoglobinuria** 🐾
                Presence of myoglobin (iron containing protein) in urine
                Ⓔ See PDX Collection 1138
        R82.2   **Biliuria**
                Presence of bile pigments/salts in urine
        R82.3   **Hemoglobinuria**
                Presence of hemoglobin in urine
                Excludes1   hemoglobinuria due to hemolysis from
                                external causes NEC (D59.6)
                                hemoglobinuria due to paroxysmal
                                nocturnal [Marchiafava-Micheli]
                                (D59.5)
        R82.4   **Acetonuria**
                Ketonuria
        R82.5   **Elevated urine levels of drugs, medicaments and
                biological substances**
                Elevated urine levels of catecholamines
                Elevated urine levels of indoleacetic acid
                Elevated urine levels of 17-ketosteroids
                Elevated urine levels of steroids
        R82.6   **Abnormal urine levels of substances chiefly
                nonmedicinal as to source**
                Abnormal urine level of heavy metals
● R82.7   Abnormal findings on microbiological examination of
        urine
                Excludes1   colonization status (Z22.-)
                Coding Clinic: 2016, Q4, P65
        R82.71   **Bacteriuria**
        R82.79   **Other abnormal findings on microbiological
                examination of urine**
                Positive culture findings of urine
● R82.8   Abnormal findings on cytological and histological
        examination of urine
        R82.81   **Pyuria**
                Sterile pyuria
                Coding Clinic: 2019, Q4, P16
        R82.89   **Other abnormal findings on cytological and
                histological examination of urine**
● R82.9   Other and unspecified abnormal findings in urine
        R82.90   **Unspecified abnormal findings in urine**
        R82.91   **Other chromoabnormalities of urine**
                Chromoconversion (dipstick)
                Idiopathic dipstick converts positive for blood
                        with no cellular forms in sediment
                Excludes1   hemoglobinuria (R82.3)
                                myoglobinuria (R82.1)

● R82.99   Other abnormal findings in urine
        R82.991   **Hypocitraturia** 🐾
                Ⓔ See PDX Collection 1137
        R82.992   **Hyperoxaluria** 🐾
                Excludes1   Primary hyperoxaluria
                                (E72.53)
                Ⓔ See PDX Collection 1137
        R82.993   **Hyperuricosuria** 🐾
                Ⓔ See PDX Collection 1137
        R82.994   **Hypercalciuria** 🐾
                Idiopathic hypercalciuria
                Ⓔ See PDX Collection 1137
        R82.998   **Other abnormal findings in urine** 🐾
                Cells and casts in urine
                Crystalluria
                Melanuria
                Ⓔ See PDX Collection 1137

**ABNORMAL FINDINGS ON EXAMINATION OF OTHER BODY FLUIDS,
SUBSTANCES AND TISSUES, WITHOUT DIAGNOSIS (R83-R89)**

        Excludes1   abnormal findings on antenatal screening of
                        mother (O28.-)
                        diagnostic abnormal findings classified elsewhere
                        - see Alphabetical Index
        Excludes2   abnormal findings on examination of blood,
                        without diagnosis (R70-R79)
                        abnormal findings on examination of urine,
                        without diagnosis (R80-R82)
                        abnormal tumor markers (R97.-)

● R83   Abnormal findings in cerebrospinal fluid
        R83.0   Abnormal level of enzymes in cerebrospinal fluid
        R83.1   Abnormal level of hormones in cerebrospinal fluid
        R83.2   Abnormal level of other drugs, medicaments and
                biological substances in cerebrospinal fluid
        R83.3   Abnormal level of substances chiefly nonmedicinal as to
                source in cerebrospinal fluid
        R83.4   Abnormal immunological findings in cerebrospinal
                fluid
        R83.5   Abnormal microbiological findings in cerebrospinal
                fluid
                Positive culture findings in cerebrospinal fluid
                Excludes1   colonization status (Z22.-)
        R83.6   Abnormal cytological findings in cerebrospinal fluid
        R83.8   Other abnormal findings in cerebrospinal fluid
                Abnormal chromosomal findings in cerebrospinal fluid
        R83.9   Unspecified abnormal finding in cerebrospinal fluid

● R84   Abnormal findings in specimens from respiratory organs and
        thorax
        Includes   abnormal findings in bronchial washings
                        abnormal findings in nasal secretions
                        abnormal findings in pleural fluid
                        abnormal findings in sputum
                        abnormal findings in throat scrapings
        Excludes1   blood-stained sputum (R04.2)
        R84.0   Abnormal level of enzymes in specimens from
                respiratory organs and thorax
        R84.1   Abnormal level of hormones in specimens from
                respiratory organs and thorax
        R84.2   Abnormal level of other drugs, medicaments and
                biological substances in specimens from respiratory
                organs and thorax
        R84.3   Abnormal level of substances chiefly nonmedicinal as to
                source in specimens from respiratory organs and thorax
        R84.4   Abnormal immunological findings in specimens from
                respiratory organs and thorax
        R84.5   Abnormal microbiological findings in specimens from
                respiratory organs and thorax
                Positive culture findings in specimens from respiratory
                        organs and thorax
                Excludes1   colonization status (Z22.-)

N   Newborn Age: 0   P   Pediatric Age: 0-17   M   Maternity DX: 9-64   A   Adult Age: 15-124   ♀   Females Only   ♂   Males Only
🐾   Complication\Comorbidity   🐾   Major C\C   Ⓔ   CC/MCC Exclusions   🐾   Hospital-Acquired Condition   🐾   Hierarchical Condition Category

R84.6   Abnormal cytological findings in specimens from respiratory organs and thorax

R84.7   Abnormal histological findings in specimens from respiratory organs and thorax

R84.8   Other abnormal findings in specimens from respiratory organs and thorax

> Abnormal chromosomal findings in specimens from respiratory organs and thorax

R84.9   Unspecified abnormal finding in specimens from respiratory organs and thorax

●**R85**   Abnormal findings in specimens from digestive organs and abdominal cavity

> **Includes**   abnormal findings in peritoneal fluid
> abnormal findings in saliva

> **Excludes1**   cloudy peritoneal dialysis effluent (R88.0)
> fecal abnormalities (R19.5)

R85.0   Abnormal level of enzymes in specimens from digestive organs and abdominal cavity

R85.1   Abnormal level of hormones in specimens from digestive organs and abdominal cavity

R85.2   Abnormal level of other drugs, medicaments and biological substances in specimens from digestive organs and abdominal cavity

R85.3   Abnormal level of substances chiefly nonmedicinal as to source in specimens from digestive organs and abdominal cavity

R85.4   Abnormal immunological findings in specimens from digestive organs and abdominal cavity

R85.5   Abnormal microbiological findings in specimens from digestive organs and abdominal cavity

> Positive culture findings in specimens from digestive organs and abdominal cavity

> **Excludes1**   colonization status (Z22.-)

●**R85.6**   Abnormal cytological findings in specimens from digestive organs and abdominal cavity

     ●**R85.61**   Abnormal cytologic smear of anus

> **Excludes1**   abnormal cytological findings in specimens from other digestive organs and abdominal cavity (R85.69)
> carcinoma in situ of anus (histologically confirmed) (D01.3)
> anal intraepithelial neoplasia I [AIN I] (K62.82)
> anal intraepithelial neoplasia II [AIN II] (K62.82)
> anal intraepithelial neoplasia III [AIN III] (D01.3)
> dysplasia (mild) (moderate) of anus (histologically confirmed) (K62.82)
> severe dysplasia of anus (histologically confirmed) (D01.3)

> **Excludes2**   anal high risk human papillomavirus (HPV) DNA test positive (R85.81)
> anal low risk human papillomavirus (HPV) DNA test positive (R85.82)

         R85.610   Atypical squamous cells of undetermined significance on cytologic smear of anus (ASC-US)

         R85.611   Atypical squamous cells cannot exclude high grade squamous intraepithelial lesion on cytologic smear of anus (ASC-H)

         R85.612   Low grade squamous intraepithelial lesion on cytologic smear of anus (LGSIL)

         R85.613   High grade squamous intraepithelial lesion on cytologic smear of anus (HGSIL)

         R85.614   Cytologic evidence of malignancy on smear of anus

         R85.615   Unsatisfactory cytologic smear of anus

> Inadequate sample of cytologic smear of anus

         R85.616   Satisfactory anal smear but lacking transformation zone

         R85.618   Other abnormal cytological findings on specimens from anus

         R85.619   Unspecified abnormal cytological findings in specimens from anus

> Abnormal anal cytology NOS
> Atypical glandular cells of anus NOS

     R85.69   Abnormal cytological findings in specimens from other digestive organs and abdominal cavity

R85.7   Abnormal histological findings in specimens from digestive organs and abdominal cavity

●**R85.8**   Other abnormal findings in specimens from digestive organs and abdominal cavity

     R85.81   Anal high risk human papillomavirus (HPV) DNA test positive

> **Excludes1**   anogenital warts due to human papillomavirus (HPV) (A63.0)
> condyloma acuminatum (A63.0)

     R85.82   Anal low risk human papillomavirus (HPV) DNA test positive

> Use additional code for associated human papillomavirus (B97.7)

     R85.89   Other abnormal findings in specimens from digestive organs and abdominal cavity

> Abnormal chromosomal findings in specimens from digestive organs and abdominal cavity

R85.9   Unspecified abnormal finding in specimens from digestive organs and abdominal cavity

●**R86**   Abnormal findings in specimens from male genital organs

> **Includes**   abnormal findings in prostatic secretions
> abnormal findings in semen, seminal fluid
> abnormal spermatozoa

> **Excludes1**   azoospermia (N46.0-)
> oligospermia (N46.1-)

R86.0   Abnormal level of enzymes in specimens from male genital organs ♂

R86.1   Abnormal level of hormones in specimens from male genital organs ♂

R86.2   Abnormal level of other drugs, medicaments and biological substances in specimens from male genital organs ♂

R86.3   Abnormal level of substances chiefly nonmedicinal as to source in specimens from male genital organs ♂

R86.4   Abnormal immunological findings in specimens from male genital organs ♂

R86.5   Abnormal microbiological findings in specimens from male genital organs ♂

> Positive culture findings in specimens from male genital organs

> **Excludes1**   colonization status (Z22.-)

R86.6   Abnormal cytological findings in specimens from male genital organs ♂

R86.7   Abnormal histological findings in specimens from male genital organs ♂

R86.8   Other abnormal findings in specimens from male genital organs ♂

> Abnormal chromosomal findings in specimens from male genital organs

R86.9   Unspecified abnormal finding in specimens from male genital organs ♂

▶ New   ⇒ Revised   ~~deleted~~ Deleted   Excludes 1   Excludes 2   Includes   Use additional   Code first   Code also   Key words

OGCR Official Guidelines   ● Unacceptable Principal Diagnosis   X Assign placeholder X   ● Use Additional Character(s)   ▶ Manifestation Code   **Coding Clinic**

● R87 Abnormal findings in specimens from female genital organs

    Includes   abnormal findings in secretion and smears from cervix uteri

            abnormal findings in secretion and smears from vagina

            abnormal findings in secretion and smears from vulva

R87.0   Abnormal level of enzymes in specimens from female genital organs ♀

R87.1   Abnormal level of hormones in specimens from female genital organs ♀

R87.2   Abnormal level of other drugs, medicaments and biological substances in specimens from female genital organs ♀

R87.3   Abnormal level of substances chiefly nonmedicinal as to source in specimens from female genital organs ♀

R87.4   Abnormal immunological findings in specimens from female genital organs ♀

R87.5   Abnormal microbiological findings in specimens from female genital organs ♀

    Positive culture findings in specimens from female genital organs

    Excludes1   colonization status (Z22.-)

● R87.6 Abnormal cytological findings in specimens from female genital organs

  ● R87.61 Abnormal cytological findings in specimens from cervix uteri

      Excludes1   abnormal cytological findings in specimens from other female genital organs (R87.69)

                abnormal cytological findings in specimens from vagina (R87.62-)

                carcinoma in situ of cervix uteri (histologically confirmed) (D06.-)

                cervical intraepithelial neoplasia I [CIN I] (N87.0)

                cervical intraepithelial neoplasia II [CIN II] (N87.1)

                cervical intraepithelial neoplasia III [CIN III] (D06.-)

                dysplasia (mild) (moderate) of cervix uteri (histologically confirmed) (N87.-)

                severe dysplasia of cervix uteri (histologically confirmed) (D06.-)

      Excludes2   cervical high risk human papillomavirus (HPV) DNA test positive (R87.810)

                cervical low risk human papillomavirus (HPV) DNA test positive (R87.820)

      R87.610   Atypical squamous cells of undetermined significance on cytologic smear of cervix (ASC-US) ♀

      R87.611   Atypical squamous cells cannot exclude high grade squamous intraepithelial lesion on cytologic smear of cervix (ASC-H) ♀

      R87.612   Low grade squamous intraepithelial lesion on cytologic smear of cervix (LGSIL) ♀

      R87.613   High grade squamous intraepithelial lesion on cytologic smear of cervix (HGSIL) ♀

      R87.614   Cytologic evidence of malignancy on smear of cervix ♀

      R87.615   Unsatisfactory cytologic smear of cervix ♀

          Inadequate sample of cytologic smear of cervix

R87.616   Satisfactory cervical smear but lacking transformation zone ♀

R87.618   Other abnormal cytological findings on specimens from cervix uteri ♀

R87.619   Unspecified abnormal cytological findings in specimens from cervix uteri ♀

    Abnormal cervical cytology NOS

    Abnormal Papanicolaou smear of cervix NOS

    Abnormal thin preparation smear of cervix NOS

    Atypical endocervical cells of cervix NOS

    Atypical endometrial cells of cervix NOS

    Atypical glandular cells of cervix NOS

● R87.62 Abnormal cytological findings in specimens from vagina

    Use additional code to identify acquired absence of uterus and cervix, if applicable (Z90.71-)

    Excludes1   abnormal cytological findings in specimens from cervix uteri (R87.61-)

              abnormal cytological findings in specimens from other female genital organs (R87.69)

              carcinoma in situ of vagina (histologically confirmed) (D07.2)

              vaginal intraepithelial neoplasia I [VAIN I] (N89.0)

              vaginal intraepithelial neoplasia II [VAIN II] (N89.1)

              vaginal intraepithelial neoplasia III [VAIN III] (D07.2)

              dysplasia (mild) (moderate) of vagina (histologically confirmed) (N89.-)

              severe dysplasia of vagina (histologically confirmed) (D07.2)

    Excludes2   vaginal high risk human papillomavirus (HPV) DNA test positive (R87.811)

              vaginal low risk human papillomavirus (HPV) DNA test positive (R87.821)

R87.620   Atypical squamous cells of undetermined significance on cytologic smear of vagina (ASC-US) ♀

R87.621   Atypical squamous cells cannot exclude high grade squamous intraepithelial lesion on cytologic smear of vagina (ASC-H) ♀

R87.622   Low grade squamous intraepithelial lesion on cytologic smear of vagina (LGSIL) ♀

R87.623   High grade squamous intraepithelial lesion on cytologic smear of vagina (HGSIL) ♀

R87.624   Cytologic evidence of malignancy on smear of vagina ♀

R87.625   Unsatisfactory cytologic smear of vagina ♀

    Inadequate sample of cytologic smear of vagina

R87.628   Other abnormal cytological findings on specimens from vagina ♀

N Newborn Age: 0   **P** Pediatric Age: 0–17   **M** Maternity DX: 9–64   **A** Adult Age: 15–124   ♀ Females Only   ♂ Males Only

℞ Complication\Comorbidity   ℞ Major C\C   (Ex) CC/MCC Exclusions   ℞ Hospital-Acquired Condition   ℞ Hierarchical Condition Category

1241

CHAPTER 18 (R00-R99)

R87.629   Unspecified abnormal cytological findings in specimens from vagina ♀
Abnormal Papanicolaou smear of vagina NOS
Abnormal thin preparation smear of vagina NOS
Abnormal vaginal cytology NOS
Atypical endocervical cells of vagina NOS
Atypical endometrial cells of vagina NOS
Atypical glandular cells of vagina NOS

R87.69   Abnormal cytological findings in specimens from other female genital organs ♀
Abnormal cytological findings in specimens from female genital organs NOS

     Excludes1   dysplasia of vulva (histologically confirmed) (N90.0-N90.3)

R87.7   Abnormal histological findings in specimens from female genital organs ♀

     Excludes1   carcinoma in situ (histologically confirmed) of female genital organs (D06-D07.3)
cervical intraepithelial neoplasia I [CIN I] (N87.0)
cervical intraepithelial neoplasia II [CIN II] (N87.1)
cervical intraepithelial neoplasia III [CIN III] (D06.-)
dysplasia (mild) (moderate) of cervix uteri (histologically confirmed) (N87.-)
dysplasia (mild) (moderate) of vagina (histologically confirmed) (N89.-)
vaginal intraepithelial neoplasia I [VAIN I] (N89.0)
vaginal intraepithelial neoplasia II [VAIN II] (N89.1)
vaginal intraepithelial neoplasia III [VAIN III] (D07.2)
severe dysplasia of cervix uteri (histologically confirmed) (D06.-)
severe dysplasia of vagina (histologically confirmed) (D07.2)

● R87.8   Other abnormal findings in specimens from female genital organs

   ● R87.81   High risk human papillomavirus (HPV) DNA test positive from female genital organs

       Excludes1   anogenital warts due to human papillomavirus (HPV) (A63.0)
condyloma acuminatum (A63.0)

     R87.810   Cervical high risk human papillomavirus (HPV) DNA test positive ♀

     R87.811   Vaginal high risk human papillomavirus (HPV) DNA test positive ♀

   ● R87.82   Low risk human papillomavirus (HPV) DNA test positive from female genital organs
Use additional code for associated human papillomavirus (B97.7)

     R87.820   Cervical low risk human papillomavirus (HPV) DNA test positive ♀

     R87.821   Vaginal low risk human papillomavirus (HPV) DNA test positive ♀

   R87.89   Other abnormal findings in specimens from female genital organs ♀
Abnormal chromosomal findings in specimens from female genital organs

R87.9   Unspecified abnormal finding in specimens from female genital organs ♀

● R88   Abnormal findings in other body fluids and substances
R88.0   Cloudy (hemodialysis) (peritoneal) dialysis effluent
R88.8   Abnormal findings in other body fluids and substances

● R89   Abnormal findings in specimens from other organs, systems and tissues

     Includes   abnormal findings in nipple discharge
abnormal findings in synovial fluid
abnormal findings in wound secretions

R89.0   Abnormal level of enzymes in specimens from other organs, systems and tissues

R89.1   Abnormal level of hormones in specimens from other organs, systems and tissues

R89.2   Abnormal level of other drugs, medicaments and biological substances in specimens from other organs, systems and tissues

R89.3   Abnormal level of substances chiefly nonmedicinal as to source in specimens from other organs, systems and tissues

R89.4   Abnormal immunological findings in specimens from other organs, systems and tissues

R89.5   Abnormal microbiological findings in specimens from other organs, systems and tissues
Positive culture findings in specimens from other organs, systems and tissues

     Excludes1   colonization status (Z22.-)

R89.6   Abnormal cytological findings in specimens from other organs, systems and tissues

R89.7   Abnormal histological findings in specimens from other organs, systems and tissues

R89.8   Other abnormal findings in specimens from other organs, systems and tissues
Abnormal chromosomal findings in specimens from other organs, systems and tissues

R89.9   Unspecified abnormal finding in specimens from other organs, systems and tissues

---

ABNORMAL FINDINGS ON DIAGNOSTIC IMAGING AND IN FUNCTION STUDIES, WITHOUT DIAGNOSIS (R90-R94)

     Includes   nonspecific abnormal findings on diagnostic imaging by computerized axial tomography [CAT scan]
nonspecific abnormal findings on diagnostic imaging by magnetic resonance imaging [MRI][NMR]
nonspecific abnormal findings on diagnostic imaging by positron emission tomography [PET scan]
nonspecific abnormal findings on diagnostic imaging by thermography
nonspecific abnormal findings on diagnostic imaging by ultrasound [echogram]
nonspecific abnormal findings on diagnostic imaging by X-ray examination

     Excludes1   abnormal findings on antenatal screening of mother (O28.-)
diagnostic abnormal findings classified elsewhere - see Alphabetical Index

● R90   Abnormal findings on diagnostic imaging of central nervous system

R90.0   Intracranial space-occupying lesion found on diagnostic imaging of central nervous system

   ● R90.8   Other abnormal findings on diagnostic imaging of central nervous system

     R90.81   Abnormal echoencephalogram

     R90.82   White matter disease, unspecified

     R90.89   Other abnormal findings on diagnostic imaging of central nervous system
Other cerebrovascular abnormality found on diagnostic imaging of central nervous system

● **R91 Abnormal findings on diagnostic imaging of lung**

    R91.1 Solitary pulmonary nodule
        Coin lesion lung
        Solitary pulmonary nodule, subsegmental branch of the bronchial tree

    R91.8 Other nonspecific abnormal finding of lung field
        Lung mass NOS found on diagnostic imaging of lung
        Pulmonary infiltrate NOS
        Shadow, lung

● **R92 Abnormal and inconclusive findings on diagnostic imaging of breast**

    R92.0 Mammographic microcalcification found on diagnostic imaging of breast
        Excludes2   mammographic calcification (calculus) found on diagnostic imaging of breast (R92.1)

    R92.1 Mammographic calcification found on diagnostic imaging of breast
        Mammographic calculus found on diagnostic imaging of breast

    R92.2 Inconclusive mammogram
        Dense breasts NOS
        Inconclusive mammogram NEC
        Inconclusive mammography due to dense breasts
        Inconclusive mammography NEC
        Coding Clinic: 2015, Q1, P24

    R92.8 Other abnormal and inconclusive findings on diagnostic imaging of breast

● **R93 Abnormal findings on diagnostic imaging of other body structures**

    R93.0 Abnormal findings on diagnostic imaging of skull and head, not elsewhere classified
        Excludes1   intracranial space-occupying lesion found on diagnostic imaging (R90.0)

    R93.1 Abnormal findings on diagnostic imaging of heart and coronary circulation
        Abnormal echocardiogram NOS
        Abnormal heart shadow

    R93.2 Abnormal findings on diagnostic imaging of liver and biliary tract
        Nonvisualization of gallbladder

    R93.3 Abnormal findings on diagnostic imaging of other parts of digestive tract

    ● **R93.4 Abnormal findings on diagnostic imaging of urinary organs**
        Excludes2   hypertrophy of kidney (N28.81)
        Coding Clinic: 2016, Q4, P66

        R93.41 Abnormal radiologic findings on diagnostic imaging of renal pelvis, ureter, or bladder
            Filling defect of bladder found on diagnostic imaging
            Filling defect of renal pelvis found on diagnostic imaging
            Filling defect of ureter found on diagnostic imaging

        ● **R93.42 Abnormal radiologic findings on diagnostic imaging of kidney**
            R93.421 Abnormal radiologic findings on diagnostic imaging of right kidney
            R93.422 Abnormal radiologic findings on diagnostic imaging of left kidney
            R93.429 Abnormal radiologic findings on diagnostic imaging of unspecified kidney

        R93.49 Abnormal radiologic findings on diagnostic imaging of other urinary organs

    R93.5 Abnormal findings on diagnostic imaging of other abdominal regions, including retroperitoneum

    R93.6 Abnormal findings on diagnostic imaging of limbs
        Excludes2   abnormal finding in skin and subcutaneous tissue (R93.8-)
        Coding Clinic: 2020, Q1, P14

    R93.7 Abnormal findings on diagnostic imaging of other parts of musculoskeletal system
        Excludes2   abnormal findings on diagnostic imaging of skull (R93.0)

    ● **R93.8 Abnormal findings on diagnostic imaging of other specified body structures**

        ● **R93.81 Abnormal radiologic findings on diagnostic imaging of testis**
            R93.811 Abnormal radiologic findings on diagnostic imaging of right testicle ♂
            R93.812 Abnormal radiologic findings on diagnostic imaging of left testicle ♂
            R93.813 Abnormal radiologic findings on diagnostic imaging of testicles, bilateral ♂
            R93.819 Abnormal radiologic findings on diagnostic imaging of unspecified testicle ♂

        R93.89 Abnormal findings on diagnostic imaging of other specified body structures
            Abnormal finding by radioisotope localization of placenta
            Abnormal radiological finding in skin and subcutaneous tissue
            Mediastinal shift

    R93.9 Diagnostic imaging inconclusive due to excess body fat of patient

● **R94 Abnormal results of function studies**
        Includes   abnormal results of radionuclide [radioisotope] uptake studies
            abnormal results of scintigraphy

    ● **R94.0 Abnormal results of function studies of central nervous system**
        R94.01 Abnormal electroencephalogram [EEG]
        R94.02 Abnormal brain scan
        R94.09 Abnormal results of other function studies of central nervous system

    ● **R94.1 Abnormal results of function studies of peripheral nervous system and special senses**

        ● **R94.11 Abnormal results of function studies of eye**
            R94.110 Abnormal electro-oculogram [EOG]
            R94.111 Abnormal electroretinogram [ERG]
                Abnormal retinal function study
            R94.112 Abnormal visually evoked potential [VEP]
            R94.113 Abnormal oculomotor study
            R94.118 Abnormal results of other function studies of eye

        ● **R94.12 Abnormal results of function studies of ear and other special senses**
            R94.120 Abnormal auditory function study
                Coding Clinic: 2016, Q3, P17
            R94.121 Abnormal vestibular function study
            R94.128 Abnormal results of other function studies of ear and other special senses

CHAPTER 18 (R00-R99)

N Newborn Age: 0   **P** Pediatric Age: 0–17   **M** Maternity DX: 9–64   **A** Adult Age: 15–124   ♀ Females Only   ♂ Males Only

🅒 Complication\Comorbidity   🅜 Major C\C   Ⓔⓧ CC/MCC Exclusions   🅗 Hospital-Acquired Condition   🅗 Hierarchical Condition Category   **1243**

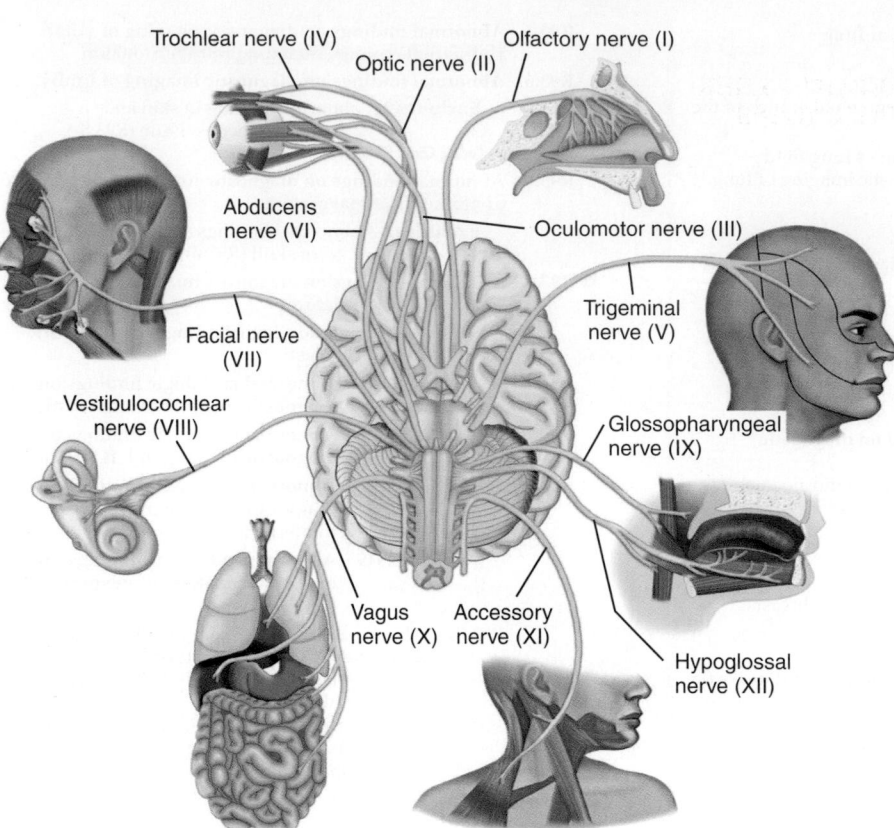

Figure 18-2 Cranial nerves. (From Patton and Thibodeau: Anatomy and physiology, ed 7, St. Louis, Mosby, 2009)

Trochlear nerve (IV)
Optic nerve (II)
Olfactory nerve (I)
Abducens nerve (VI)
Oculomotor nerve (III)
Facial nerve (VII)
Trigeminal nerve (V)
Vestibulocochlear nerve (VIII)
Glossopharyngeal nerve (IX)
Vagus nerve (X)
Accessory nerve (XI)
Hypoglossal nerve (XII)

Item 18–1 The **peripheral nervous system** consists of 31 pairs of spinal nerves, 12 pairs of cranial nerves, and the autonomic nerves, which are divided into the parasympathetic and sympathetic nerves. The cranial nerves are: olfactory (I), optic (II), oculomotor (III), trochlear (IV), trigeminal (V), abducens (VI), facial (VII), vestibulocochlear (VIII), glossopharyngeal (IX), vagus (X), accessory (XI), and hypoglossal (XII).

● **R94.13   Abnormal results of function studies of peripheral nervous system**

    R94.130   Abnormal response to nerve stimulation, unspecified

    R94.131   Abnormal electromyogram [EMG]
       Excludes1   electromyogram of eye (R94.113)

    R94.138   Abnormal results of other function studies of peripheral nervous system

R94.2   Abnormal results of pulmonary function studies
  Reduced ventilatory capacity
  Reduced vital capacity

● **R94.3   Abnormal results of cardiovascular function studies**

    R94.30   Abnormal result of cardiovascular function study, unspecified

    R94.31   Abnormal electrocardiogram [ECG] [EKG]
       Excludes1   long QT syndrome (I45.81)

    R94.39   Abnormal result of other cardiovascular function study
      Abnormal electrophysiological intracardiac studies
      Abnormal phonocardiogram
      Abnormal vectorcardiogram

R94.4   Abnormal results of kidney function studies
  Abnormal renal function test

R94.5   Abnormal results of liver function studies

R94.6   Abnormal results of thyroid function studies

R94.7   Abnormal results of other endocrine function studies
    Excludes2   abnormal glucose (R73.0-)

R94.8   Abnormal results of function studies of other organs and systems
  Abnormal basal metabolic rate [BMR]
  Abnormal bladder function test
  Abnormal splenic function test

ABNORMAL TUMOR MARKERS (R97)

● **R97   Abnormal tumor markers**
  Elevated tumor associated antigens [TAA]
  Elevated tumor specific antigens [TSA]

R97.0   Elevated carcinoembryonic antigen [CEA]

R97.1   Elevated cancer antigen 125 [CA 125]

● **R97.2   Elevated prostate specific antigen [PSA]**
  Coding Clinic: 2016, Q4, P66

    R97.20   Elevated prostate specific antigen [PSA] ♂   A
      MCE: Questionable admission when principal dx

    R97.21   Rising PSA following treatment for malignant neoplasm of prostate ♂   A
      MCE: Questionable admission when principal dx

R97.8   Other abnormal tumor markers

ILL-DEFINED AND UNKNOWN CAUSE OF MORTALITY (R99)

R99   Ill-defined and unknown cause of mortality
  Death (unexplained) NOS
  Unspecified cause of mortality
  OGCR Section I.C.18.h.

  Death NOS
  Code R99, Ill-defined and unknown cause of mortality, is only for use in the very limited circumstance when a patient who has already died is brought into the emergency department or other healthcare facility and is pronounced dead upon arrival. It does not represent the discharge disposition of death.

▶ New   ⇒ Revised   ~~deleted~~ Deleted   Excludes 1   Excludes 2   Includes   Use additional   Code first   Code also   Key words
OGCR Official Guidelines   ● Unacceptable Principal Diagnosis   X Assign placeholder X   ● Use Additional Character(s)   ▷ Manifestation Code   **Coding Clinic**

CHAPTER 19

INJURY, POISONING AND CERTAIN OTHER CONSEQUENCES OF EXTERNAL CAUSES (S00-T88)

OGCR Chapter-Specific Coding Guidelines

19. Chapter 19: Injury, poisoning, and certain other consequences of external causes (S00-T88)

a. Application of 7th Characters in Chapter 19

Most categories in Chapter 19 have a 7th character requirement for each applicable code. Most categories in this chapter have three 7th character values (with the exception of fractures): A, initial encounter, D, subsequent encounter and S, sequela. Categories for traumatic fractures have additional 7th character values. While the patient may be seen by a new or different provider over the course of treatment for an injury, assignment of the 7th character is based on whether the patient is undergoing active treatment and not whether the provider is seeing the patient for the first time.

For complication codes, active treatment refers to treatment for the condition described by the code, even though it may be related to an earlier precipitating problem. For example, code T84.50XA, Infection and inflammatory reaction due to unspecified internal joint prosthesis, initial encounter, is used when active treatment is provided for the infection, even though the condition relates to the prosthetic device, implant or graft that was placed at a previous encounter.

7th character "A", initial encounter is used for each encounter where the patient is receiving active treatment for the condition.

7th character "D" subsequent encounter is used for encounters after the patient has completed active treatment of the condition and is receiving routine care for the condition during the healing or recovery phase.

The aftercare Z codes should not be used for aftercare for conditions such as injuries or poisonings, where 7th characters are provided to identify subsequent care. For example, for aftercare of an injury, assign the acute injury code with the 7th character "D" (subsequent encounter).

7th character "S", sequela, is for use for complications or conditions that arise as a direct result of a condition, such as scar formation after a burn. The scars are sequelae of the burn. When using 7th character "S", it is necessary to use both the injury code that precipitated the sequela and the code for the sequela itself. The "S" is added only to the injury code, not the sequela code. The 7th character "S" identifies the injury responsible for the sequela. The specific type of sequela (e.g. scar) is sequenced first, followed by the injury code.

See Section I.B.10. Sequelae, (Late Effects).

b. Coding of Injuries

When coding injuries, assign separate codes for each injury unless a combination code is provided, in which case the combination code is assigned. Codes from category T07, Unspecified multiple injuries should not be assigned in the inpatient setting unless information for a more specific code is not available. Traumatic injury codes (S00-T14.9) are not to be used for normal, healing surgical wounds or to identify complications of surgical wounds.

The code for the most serious injury, as determined by the provider and the focus of treatment, is sequenced first.

1) Superficial injuries

Superficial injuries such as abrasions or contusions are not coded when associated with more severe injuries of the same site.

2) Primary injury with damage to nerves/blood vessels

When a primary injury results in minor damage to peripheral nerves or blood vessels, the primary injury is sequenced first with additional code(s) for injuries to nerves and spinal cord (such as category S04), and/or injury to blood vessels (such as category S15). When the primary injury is to the blood vessels or nerves, that injury should be sequenced first.

c. Coding of Traumatic Fractures

The principles of multiple coding of injuries should be followed in coding fractures. Fractures of specified sites are coded individually by site in accordance with both the provisions within categories S02, S12, S22, S32, S42, S49, S52, S59, S62, S72, S79, S82, S89, S92 and the level of detail furnished by medical record content.

A fracture not indicated as open or closed should be coded to closed. A fracture not indicated whether displaced or not displaced should be coded to displaced.

More specific guidelines are as follows:

1) Initial vs. Subsequent Encounter for Fractures

Traumatic fractures are coded using the appropriate 7th character for initial encounter (A, B, C) for each encounter where the patient is receiving active treatment for the fracture. The appropriate 7th character for initial encounter should also be assigned for a patient who delayed seeking treatment for the fracture or nonunion.

Fractures are coded using the appropriate 7th character for subsequent care for encounters after the patient has completed active treatment of the fracture and is receiving routine care for the fracture during the healing or recovery phase.

Care for complications of surgical treatment for fracture repairs during the healing or recovery phase should be coded with the appropriate complication codes.

Care of complications of fractures, such as malunion and nonunion, should be reported with the appropriate 7th character for subsequent care with nonunion (K, M, N,) or subsequent care with malunion (P, Q, R).

Malunion/nonunion: The appropriate 7th character for initial encounter should also be assigned for a patient who delayed seeking treatment for the fracture or nonunion.

The open fracture designations in the assignment of the 7th character for fractures of the forearm, femur and lower leg, including ankle are based on the Gustilo open fracture classification. When the Gustilo classification type is not specified for an open fracture, the 7th character for open fracture type I or II should be assigned (B, E, H, M, Q).

A code from category M80, not a traumatic fracture code, should be used for any patient with known osteoporosis who suffers a fracture, even if the patient had a minor fall or trauma, if that fall or trauma would not usually break a normal, healthy bone.

See Section I.C.13. Osteoporosis.

The aftercare Z codes should not be used for aftercare for traumatic fractures. For aftercare of a traumatic fracture, assign the acute fracture code with the appropriate 7th character.

2) Multiple fractures sequencing

Multiple fractures are sequenced in accordance with the severity of the fracture.

d. Coding of Burns and Corrosions

The ICD-10-CM makes a distinction between burns and corrosions. The burn codes are for thermal burns, except sunburns, that come from a heat source, such as a fire or hot appliance. The burn codes are also for burns resulting from electricity and radiation. Corrosions are burns due to chemicals. The guidelines are the same for burns and corrosions.

Current burns (T20-T25) are classified by depth, extent and by agent (X code). Burns are classified by depth as first degree (erythema), second degree (blistering), and third degree (full-thickness involvement). Burns of the eye and internal organs (T26-T28) are classified by site, but not by degree.

1) Sequencing of burn and related condition codes

Sequence first the code that reflects the highest degree of burn when more than one burn is present.

  a. When the reason for the admission or encounter is for treatment of external multiple burns, sequence first the code that reflects the burn of the highest degree.

  b. When a patient has both internal and external burns, the circumstances of admission govern the selection of the principal diagnosis or first-listed diagnosis.

  c. When a patient is admitted for burn injuries and other related conditions such as smoke inhalation and/or respiratory failure, the circumstances of admission govern the selection of the principal or first-listed diagnosis.

2) Burns of the same *anatomic* site

Classify burns of the same anatomic site and on the same side but of different degrees to the subcategory identifying the highest degree recorded in the diagnosis (e.g., for second- and third-degree burns of right thigh, assign only code T24.311-).

3) Non-healing burns

Non-healing burns are coded as acute burns.

Necrosis of burned skin should be coded as a non-healed burn.

4) Infected Burn

For any documented infected burn site, use an additional code for the infection.

5) Assign separate codes for each burn site

When coding burns, assign separate codes for each burn site. Category T30, Burn and corrosion, body region unspecified is extremely vague and should rarely be used.

Codes for burns of "multiple sites" should only be assigned when the medical record documentation does not specify the individual sites.

6) Burns and Corrosions Classified According to Extent of Body Surface Involved

Assign codes from category T31, Burns classified according to extent of body surface involved, or T32, Corrosions classified according to extent of body surface involved, when the site of the burn is not specified or when there is a need for additional data. It is advisable to use category T31 as additional coding when needed to provide data for evaluating burn mortality, such as that needed by burn units. It is also advisable to use category T31 as an additional code for reporting purposes when there is mention of a third-degree burn involving 20 percent or more of the body surface.

Categories T31 and T32 are based on the classic "rule of nines" in estimating body surface involved: head and neck are assigned nine percent, each arm nine percent, each leg 18 percent, the anterior trunk 18 percent, posterior trunk 18 percent, and genitalia one percent. Providers may change these percentage assignments where necessary to accommodate infants and children who have proportionately larger heads than adults, and patients who have large buttocks, thighs, or abdomen that involve burns.

7) Encounters for treatment of sequela of burns

Encounters for the treatment of the late effects of burns or corrosions (i.e., scars or joint contractures) should be coded with a burn or corrosion code with the 7th character "S" for sequela.

8) Sequelae with a late effect code and current burn

When appropriate, both a code for a current burn or corrosion with 7th character "A" or "D" and a burn or corrosion code with 7th character "S" may be assigned on the same record (when both a current burn and sequelae of an old burn exist). Burns and corrosions do not heal at the same rate and a current healing wound may still exist with sequela of a healed burn or corrosion.

See Section I.B.10. Sequela, (Late Effects).

9) Use of an external cause code with burns and corrosions

An external cause code should be used with burns and corrosions to identify the source and intent of the burn, as well as the place where it occurred.

e. Adverse Effects, Poisoning , Underdosing and Toxic Effects

Codes in categories T36-T65 are combination codes that include the substance that was taken as well as the intent. No additional external cause code is required for poisonings, toxic effects, adverse effects and underdosing codes.

1) Do not code directly from the Table of Drugs

Do not code directly from the Table of Drugs and Chemicals. Always refer back to the Tabular List.

2) Use as many codes as necessary to describe

Use as many codes as necessary to describe completely all drugs, medicinal or biological substances.

3) If the same code would describe the causative agent

If the same code would describe the causative agent for more than one adverse reaction, poisoning, toxic effect or underdosing, assign the code only once.

4) If two or more drugs, medicinal or biological substances

If two or more drugs, medicinal or biological substances are reported, code each individually unless a combination code is listed in the Table of Drugs and Chemicals.

5) The occurrence of drug toxicity is classified in ICD-10-CM as follows:

(a) Adverse Effect

When coding an adverse effect of a drug that has been correctly prescribed and properly administered, assign the appropriate code for the nature of the adverse effect followed by the appropriate code for the adverse effect of the drug (T36-T50). The code for the drug should have a 5th or 6th character "5" (for example T36.0X5-) Examples of the nature of an adverse effect are tachycardia, delirium, gastrointestinal hemorrhaging, vomiting, hypokalemia, hepatitis, renal failure, or respiratory failure.

(b) Poisoning

When coding a poisoning or reaction to the improper use of a medication (e.g., overdose, wrong substance given or taken in error, wrong route of administration), first assign the appropriate code from categories T36-T50. The poisoning codes have an associated intent as their 5th or 6th character (accidental, intentional self-harm, assault and undetermined). If the intent of the poisoning is unknown or unspecified, code the intent as accidental intent. The undetermined intent is only for use if the documentation in the record specifies that the intent cannot be determined. Use additional code(s) for all manifestations of poisonings.

If there is also a diagnosis of abuse or dependence of the substance, the abuse or dependence is assigned as an additional code.

Examples of poisoning include:

(i) Error was made in drug prescription
Errors made in drug prescription or in the administration of the drug by provider, nurse, patient, or other person.

(ii) Overdose of a drug intentionally taken If an overdose of a drug was intentionally taken or administered and resulted in drug toxicity, it would be coded as a poisoning.

(iii) Nonprescribed drug taken with correctly prescribed and properly administered drug. If a nonprescribed drug or medicinal agent was taken in combination with a correctly prescribed and properly administered drug, any drug toxicity or other reaction resulting from the interaction of the two drugs would be classified as a poisoning.

(iv) Interaction of drug(s) and alcohol. When a reaction results from the interaction of a drug(s) and alcohol, this would be classified as poisoning.

See Section I.C.4. if poisoning is the result of insulin pump malfunctions.

(c) Underdosing

Underdosing refers to taking less of a medication than is prescribed by a provider or a manufacturer's instruction. Discontinuing the use of a prescribed medication on the patient's own initiative (not directed by the patient's provider) is also classified as an underdosing. For underdosing, assign the code from categories T36-T50 (fifth or sixth character "6").

Codes for underdosing should never be assigned as principal or first-listed codes. If a patient has a relapse or exacerbation of the medical condition for which the drug is prescribed because of the reduction in dose, then the medical condition itself should be coded.

Noncompliance (Z91.12-, Z91.13- and Z91.14-) or complication of care (Y63.6-Y63.9) codes are to be used with an underdosing code to indicate intent, if known.

(d) Toxic Effects

When a harmful substance is ingested or comes in contact with a person, this is classified as a toxic effect. The toxic effect codes are in categories T51-T65.

Toxic effect codes have an associated intent: accidental, intentional self-harm, assault and undetermined.

f. Adult and child abuse, neglect and other maltreatment

Sequence first the appropriate code from categories T74 (Adult and child abuse, neglect and other maltreatment, confirmed) or T76 (Adult and child abuse, neglect and other maltreatment, suspected) for abuse, neglect and other maltreatment, followed by any accompanying mental health or injury code(s).

If the documentation in the medical record states abuse or neglect it is coded as confirmed (T74.-). It is coded as suspected if it is documented as suspected (T76.-).

For cases of confirmed abuse or neglect an external cause code from the assault section (X92-Y09) should be added to identify the cause of any physical injuries. A perpetrator code (Y07) should be added when the perpetrator of the abuse is known. For suspected cases of abuse or neglect, do not report external cause or perpetrator code.

If a suspected case of abuse, neglect or mistreatment is ruled out during an encounter code Z04.71, Encounter for examination and observation following alleged physical adult abuse, ruled out, or code Z04.72, Encounter for examination and observation following alleged child physical abuse, ruled out, should be used, not a code from T76.

If a suspected case of alleged rape or sexual abuse is ruled out during an encounter code Z04.41, Encounter for examination and observation following alleged adult rape or code Z04.42, Encounter for examination and observation following alleged child rape, should be used, not a code from T76.

If a suspected case of forced sexual exploitation or forced labor exploitation is ruled out during an encounter, code Z04.81, Encounter for examination and observation of victim following forced sexual exploitation, or code Z04.82, Encounter for examination and observation of victim following forced labor exploitation, should be used, not a code from T76.

See Section I.C.15. Abuse in a pregnant patient.

g. Complications of care

1) General guidelines for complications of care

(a) Documentation of complications of care

See Section I.B.16. for information on documentation of complications of care.

2) Pain due to medical devices

Pain associated with devices, implants or grafts left in a surgical site (for example painful hip prosthesis) is assigned to the appropriate code(s) found in Chapter 19, Injury, poisoning, and

certain other consequences of external causes. Specific codes for pain due to medical devices are found in the T code section of the ICD-10-CM. Use additional code(s) from category G89 to identify acute or chronic pain due to presence of the device, implant or graft (G89.18 or G89.28).

3) Transplant complications

(a) Transplant complications other than kidney

Codes under category T86, Complications of transplanted organs and tissues, are for use for both complications and rejection of transplanted organs. A transplant complication code is only assigned if the complication affects the function of the transplanted organ. Two codes are required to fully describe a transplant complication: the appropriate code from category T86 and a secondary code that identifies the complication.

Pre-existing conditions or conditions that develop after the transplant are not coded as complications unless they affect the function of the transplanted organs.

See I.C.21. for transplant organ removal status.

See I.C.2. for malignant neoplasm associated with transplanted organ.

(b) Kidney transplant complications

Patients who have undergone kidney transplant may still have some form of chronic kidney disease (CKD) because the kidney transplant may not fully restore kidney function. Code T86.1- should be assigned for documented complications of a kidney transplant, such as transplant failure or rejection or other transplant complication. Code T86.1- should not be assigned for post kidney transplant patients who have chronic kidney (CKD) unless a transplant complication such as transplant failure or rejection is documented. If the documentation is unclear as to whether the patient has a complication of the transplant, query the provider.

Conditions that affect the function of the transplanted kidney, other than CKD, should be assigned a code from subcategory T86.1, Complications of transplanted organ, Kidney, and a secondary code that identifies the complication.

For patients with CKD following a kidney transplant, but who do not have a complication such as failure or rejection, *see Section I.C.14. Chronic kidney disease and kidney transplant status.*

4) Complication codes that include the external cause

As with certain other T codes, some of the complications of care codes have the external cause included in the code. The code includes the nature of the complication as well as the type of procedure that caused the complication. No external cause code indicating the type of procedure is necessary for these codes.

5) Complications of care codes within the body system chapters

Intraoperative and postprocedural complication codes are found within the body system chapters with codes specific to the organs and structures of that body system. These codes should be sequenced first, followed by a code(s) for the specific complication, if applicable.

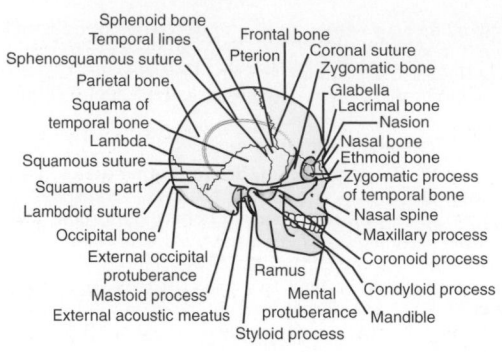

Figure 19-1 Lateral view of skull.

Figure 19-2 Frontal view of skull.

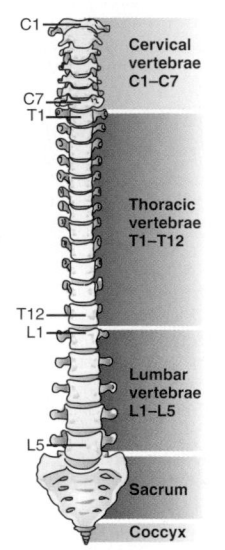

Figure 19-3 Anterior view of vertebral column.

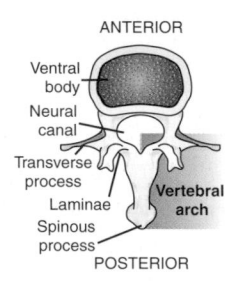

Figure 19-4 Vertebra viewed from above.

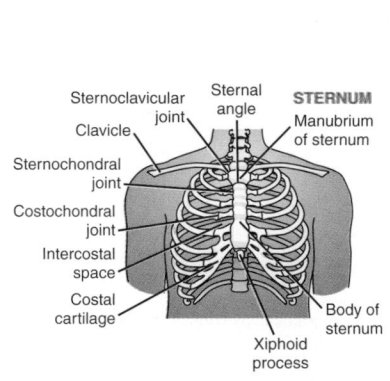

Figure 19-5 Anterior view of rib cage.

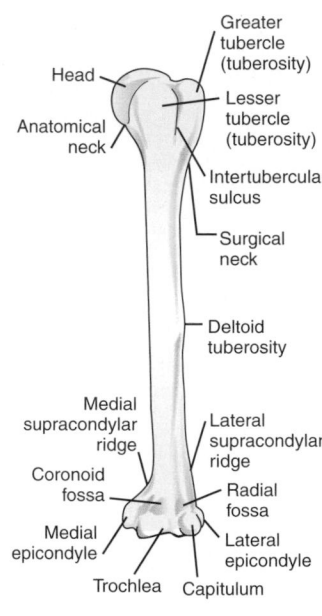

Figure 19-6 Anterior aspect of left humerus.

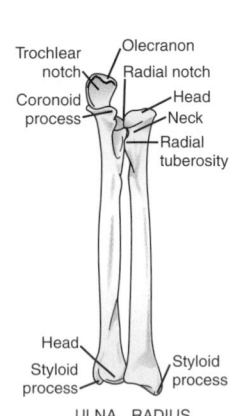

Figure 19-7 Anterior aspect of left radius and ulna.

Figure 19-8 Right hand and wrist: **A.** Dorsal surface. **B.** Palmar surface.

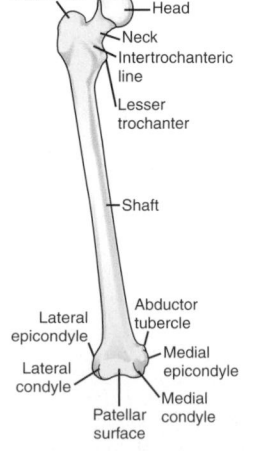

Figure 19-9 Anterior aspect of right femur.

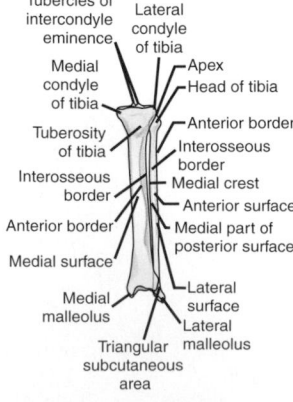

Figure 19-10 Anterior aspect of left tibia and fibula.

▶ New   ⫸ Revised   ~~deleted~~ Deleted   Excludes 1   Excludes 2   Includes   Use additional   Code first   Code also   Key words

OGCR Official Guidelines   ● Unacceptable Principal Diagnosis   **X** Assign placeholder X   ● Use Additional Character(s)   ▶ Manifestation Code   **Coding Clinic**

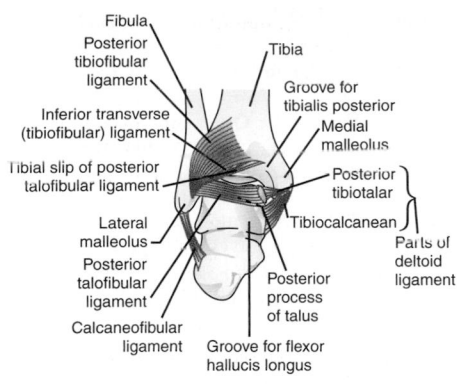

Figure 19-11 Posterior aspect of the left ankle joint.

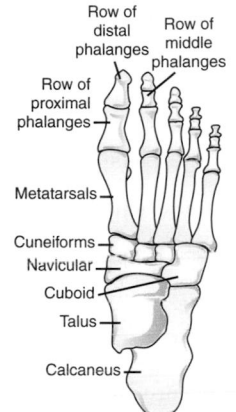

Figure 19-12 Right foot viewed from above.

CHAPTER 19

INJURY, POISONING AND CERTAIN OTHER CONSEQUENCES OF EXTERNAL CAUSES (S00-T88)

Note: Use secondary code(s) from Chapter 20, External causes of morbidity, to indicate cause of injury. Codes within the T section that include the external cause do not require an additional external cause code.

Use additional code to identify any retained foreign body, if applicable (Z18.-)

Excludes1 birth trauma (P10-P15)
             obstetric trauma (O70-O71)

Note: The chapter uses the S-section for coding different types of injuries related to single body regions and the T-section to cover injuries to unspecified body regions as well as poisoning and certain other consequences of external causes.

This chapter contains the following blocks:

S00-S09	Injuries to the head
S10-S19	Injuries to the neck
S20-S29	Injuries to the thorax
S30-S39	Injuries to the abdomen, lower back, lumbar spine, pelvis and external genitals
S40-S49	Injuries to the shoulder and upper arm
S50-S59	Injuries to the elbow and forearm
S60-S69	Injuries to the wrist, hand, and fingers
S70-S79	Injuries to the hip and thigh
S80-S89	Injuries to the knee and lower leg
S90-S99	Injuries to the ankle and foot

T07	Injuries involving multiple body regions	
T14	Injury of unspecified body region	
T15-T19	Effects of foreign body entering through natural orifice	
T20-T25	Burns and corrosions of external body surface, specified by site	
T26-T28	Burns and corrosions confined to eye and internal organs	
T30-T32	Burns and corrosions of multiple and unspecified body regions	
T33-T34	Frostbite	
T36-T50	Poisoning by, adverse effect of and underdosing of drugs, medicaments and biological substances	
T51-T65	Toxic effects of substances chiefly nonmedicinal as to source	
T66-T78	Other and unspecified effects of external causes	
T79	Certain early complications of trauma	
T80-T88	Complications of surgical and medical care, not elsewhere classified	

INJURIES TO THE HEAD (S00-S09)

Includes injuries of ear
               injuries of eye
               injuries of face [any part]
               injuries of gum
               injuries of jaw
               injuries of oral cavity
               injuries of palate
               injuries of periocular area
               injuries of scalp
               injuries of temporomandibular joint area
               injuries of tongue
               injuries of tooth

Code also for any associated infection

Excludes2 burns and corrosions (T20-T32)
             effects of foreign body in ear (T16)
             effects of foreign body in larynx (T17.3)
             effects of foreign body in mouth NOS (T18.0)
             effects of foreign body in nose (T17.0-T17.1)
             effects of foreign body in pharynx (T17.2)
             effects of foreign body on external eye (T15.-)
             frostbite (T33-T34)
             insect bite or sting, venomous (T63.4)

● **S00** **Superficial injury of head**

    Excludes1 diffuse cerebral contusion (S06.2-)
                 focal cerebral contusion (S06.3)
                 injury of eye and orbit (S05.-)
                 open wound of head (S01.-)

The appropriate 7th character is to be added to each code from category S00

A	initial encounter
	All encounters involving diagnosis and treatment
D	subsequent encounter
	Encounters during the healing phase
S	sequela

● **S00.0** **Superficial injury of scalp**
  X● **S00.00** **Unspecified** superficial injury of scalp
  X● **S00.01** **Abrasion** of scalp
  X● **S00.02** **Blister (nonthermal)** of scalp
  X● **S00.03** **Contusion** of scalp
            Bruise of scalp
            Hematoma of scalp
  X● **S00.04** **External constriction** of part of scalp
  X● **S00.05** **Superficial foreign body** of scalp
            Splinter in the scalp
  X● **S00.06** **Insect bite (nonvenomous)** of scalp
  X● **S00.07** **Other** superficial bite of scalp
        Excludes1 open bite of scalp (S01.05)

N Newborn Age: 0   **P** Pediatric Age: 0–17   **M** Maternity DX: 9–64   **A** Adult Age: 15–124   ♀ Females Only   ♂ Males Only

🅒 Complication\Comorbidity   🅜 Major C\C   (Ex) CC/MCC Exclusions   🅗 Hospital-Acquired Condition   🅗 Hierarchical Condition Category

CHAPTER 19 (S00-T88)

● **S00.1**   Contusion of eyelid and periocular area
         Black eye
         Excludes2   contusion of eyeball and orbital tissues (S05.1-)

X ● **S00.10**   Contusion of unspecified eyelid and periocular area
X ● **S00.11**   Contusion of right eyelid and periocular area
X ● **S00.12**   Contusion of left eyelid and periocular area

● **S00.2**   Other and unspecified superficial injuries of eyelid and periocular area
         Excludes2   superficial injury of conjunctiva and cornea (S05.0-)

● **S00.20**   Unspecified superficial injury of eyelid and periocular area
     ● **S00.201**   Unspecified superficial injury of right eyelid and periocular area
     ● **S00.202**   Unspecified superficial injury of left eyelid and periocular area
     ● **S00.209**   Unspecified superficial injury of unspecified eyelid and periocular area

● **S00.21**   Abrasion of eyelid and periocular area
     ● **S00.211**   Abrasion of right eyelid and periocular area
     ● **S00.212**   Abrasion of left eyelid and periocular area
     ● **S00.219**   Abrasion of unspecified eyelid and periocular area

● **S00.22**   Blister (nonthermal) of eyelid and periocular area
     ● **S00.221**   Blister (nonthermal) of right eyelid and periocular area
     ● **S00.222**   Blister (nonthermal) of left eyelid and periocular area
     ● **S00.229**   Blister (nonthermal) of unspecified eyelid and periocular area

● **S00.24**   External constriction of eyelid and periocular area
     ● **S00.241**   External constriction of right eyelid and periocular area
     ● **S00.242**   External constriction of left eyelid and periocular area
     ● **S00.249**   External constriction of unspecified eyelid and periocular area

● **S00.25**   Superficial foreign body of eyelid and periocular area
         Splinter of eyelid and periocular area
         Excludes2   retained foreign body in eyelid (H02.81-)
     ● **S00.251**   Superficial foreign body of right eyelid and periocular area
     ● **S00.252**   Superficial foreign body of left eyelid and periocular area
     ● **S00.259**   Superficial foreign body of unspecified eyelid and periocular area

● **S00.26**   Insect bite (nonvenomous) of eyelid and periocular area
     ● **S00.261**   Insect bite (nonvenomous) of right eyelid and periocular area
     ● **S00.262**   Insect bite (nonvenomous) of left eyelid and periocular area
     ● **S00.269**   Insect bite (nonvenomous) of unspecified eyelid and periocular area

● **S00.27**   Other superficial bite of eyelid and periocular area
         Excludes1   open bite of eyelid and periocular area (S01.15)
     ● **S00.271**   Other superficial bite of right eyelid and periocular area
     ● **S00.272**   Other superficial bite of left eyelid and periocular area
     ● **S00.279**   Other superficial bite of unspecified eyelid and periocular area

● **S00.3**   Superficial injury of nose
X ● **S00.30**   Unspecified superficial injury of nose
X ● **S00.31**   Abrasion of nose
X ● **S00.32**   Blister (nonthermal) of nose
X ● **S00.33**   Contusion of nose
         Bruise of nose
         Hematoma of nose
X ● **S00.34**   External constriction of nose
X ● **S00.35**   Superficial foreign body of nose
         Splinter in the nose
X ● **S00.36**   Insect bite (nonvenomous) of nose
X ● **S00.37**   Other superficial bite of nose
         Excludes1   open bite of nose (S01.25)

● **S00.4**   Superficial injury of ear
● **S00.40**   Unspecified superficial injury of ear
     ● **S00.401**   Unspecified superficial injury of right ear
     ● **S00.402**   Unspecified superficial injury of left ear
     ● **S00.409**   Unspecified superficial injury of unspecified ear

● **S00.41**   Abrasion of ear
     ● **S00.411**   Abrasion of right ear
     ● **S00.412**   Abrasion of left ear
     ● **S00.419**   Abrasion of unspecified ear

● **S00.42**   Blister (nonthermal) of ear
     ● **S00.421**   Blister (nonthermal) of right ear
     ● **S00.422**   Blister (nonthermal) of left ear
     ● **S00.429**   Blister (nonthermal) of unspecified ear

● **S00.43**   Contusion of ear
         Bruise of ear
         Hematoma of ear
     ● **S00.431**   Contusion of right ear
     ● **S00.432**   Contusion of left ear
     ● **S00.439**   Contusion of unspecified ear

● **S00.44**   External constriction of ear
     ● **S00.441**   External constriction of right ear
     ● **S00.442**   External constriction of left ear
     ● **S00.449**   External constriction of unspecified ear

● **S00.45**   Superficial foreign body of ear
         Splinter in the ear
     ● **S00.451**   Superficial foreign body of right ear
     ● **S00.452**   Superficial foreign body of left ear
     ● **S00.459**   Superficial foreign body of unspecified ear

● **S00.46**   Insect bite (nonvenomous) of ear
     ● **S00.461**   Insect bite (nonvenomous) of right ear
     ● **S00.462**   Insect bite (nonvenomous) of left ear
     ● **S00.469**   Insect bite (nonvenomous) of unspecified ear

▶ New   ⇒ Revised   ~~deleted~~ Deleted   Excludes 1   Excludes 2   Includes   Use additional   Code first   Code also   Key words

OGCR Official Guidelines   ● Unacceptable Principal Diagnosis   X Assign placeholder X   ● Use Additional Character(s)   ▶ Manifestation Code   **Coding Clinic**

● **S00.47**   Other superficial bite of ear
       Excludes1   open bite of ear (S01.35)
    ● **S00.471**   Other superficial bite of right ear
    ● **S00.472**   Other superficial bite of left ear
    ● **S00.479**   Other superficial bite of unspecified ear

● **S00.5**   Superficial injury of lip and oral cavity
   ● **S00.50**   Unspecified superficial injury of lip and oral cavity
    ● **S00.501**   Unspecified superficial injury of lip
    ● **S00.502**   Unspecified superficial injury of oral cavity
   ● **S00.51**   Abrasion of lip and oral cavity
    ● **S00.511**   Abrasion of lip
    ● **S00.512**   Abrasion of oral cavity
   ● **S00.52**   Blister (nonthermal) of lip and oral cavity
    ● **S00.521**   Blister (nonthermal) of lip
    ● **S00.522**   Blister (nonthermal) of oral cavity
   ● **S00.53**   Contusion of lip and oral cavity
    ● **S00.531**   Contusion of lip
       Bruise of lip
       Hematoma of lip
    ● **S00.532**   Contusion of oral cavity
       Bruise of oral cavity
       Hematoma of oral cavity
   ● **S00.54**   External constriction of lip and oral cavity
    ● **S00.541**   External constriction of lip
    ● **S00.542**   External constriction of oral cavity
   ● **S00.55**   Superficial foreign body of lip and oral cavity
    ● **S00.551**   Superficial foreign body of lip
       Splinter of lip and oral cavity
    ● **S00.552**   Superficial foreign body of oral cavity
       Splinter of lip and oral cavity
   ● **S00.56**   Insect bite (nonvenomous) of lip and oral cavity
    ● **S00.561**   Insect bite (nonvenomous) of lip
    ● **S00.562**   Insect bite (nonvenomous) of oral cavity
   ● **S00.57**   Other superficial bite of lip and oral cavity
    ● **S00.571**   Other superficial bite of lip
       Excludes1   open bite of lip (S01.551)
    ● **S00.572**   Other superficial bite of oral cavity
       Excludes1   open bite of oral cavity (S01.552)

● **S00.8**   Superficial injury of other parts of head
    Superficial injuries of face [any part]
  X ● **S00.80**   Unspecified superficial injury of other part of head
  X ● **S00.81**   Abrasion of other part of head
  X ● **S00.82**   Blister (nonthermal) of other part of head
  X ● **S00.83**   Contusion of other part of head
       Bruise of other part of head
       Hematoma of other part of head
  X ● **S00.84**   External constriction of other part of head
  X ● **S00.85**   Superficial foreign body of other part of head
       Splinter in other part of head
  X ● **S00.86**   Insect bite (nonvenomous) of other part of head
  X ● **S00.87**   Other superficial bite of other part of head
       Excludes1   open bite of other part of head (S01.85)

● **S00.9**   Superficial injury of unspecified part of head
  X ● **S00.90**   Unspecified superficial injury of unspecified part of head
  X ● **S00.91**   Abrasion of unspecified part of head
  X ● **S00.92**   Blister (nonthermal) of unspecified part of head
  X ● **S00.93**   Contusion of unspecified part of head
       Bruise of head
       Hematoma of head

X ● **S00.94**   External constriction of unspecified part of head
X ● **S00.95**   Superficial foreign body of unspecified part of head
       Splinter of head
X ● **S00.96**   Insect bite (nonvenomous) of unspecified part of head
X ● **S00.97**   Other superficial bite of unspecified part of head
       Excludes1   open bite of head (S01.95)

● **S01**   Open wound of head
    Code also any associated:
      injury of cranial nerve (S04.-)
      injury of muscle and tendon of head (S09.1-)
      intracranial injury (S06.-)
      wound infection
    Excludes1   open skull fracture (S02.- with 7th character B)
    Excludes2   injury of eye and orbit (S05.-)
                traumatic amputation of part of head (S08.-)
    The appropriate 7th character is to be added to each code from category S01

A	initial encounter
D	subsequent encounter
S	sequela

● **S01.0**   Open wound of scalp
    ➡ **Excludes1**   avulsion of scalp (S08.0-)
  X ● **S01.00**   Unspecified open wound of scalp
  X ● **S01.01**   Laceration without foreign body of scalp
  X ● **S01.02**   Laceration with foreign body of scalp
       Coding Clinic: 2015, Q1, P5-7
  X ● **S01.03**   Puncture wound without foreign body of scalp
  X ● **S01.04**   Puncture wound with foreign body of scalp
  X ● **S01.05**   Open bite of scalp
       Bite of scalp NOS
       Excludes1   superficial bite of scalp (S00.06, S00.07-)

● **S01.1**   Open wound of eyelid and periocular area
    Open wound of eyelid and periocular area with or without involvement of lacrimal passages
   ● **S01.10**   Unspecified open wound of eyelid and periocular area
       (Ex) For category S01.10 CC codes: See PDX Collection 1139
    ● **S01.101**   Unspecified open wound of right eyelid and periocular area A
    ● **S01.102**   Unspecified open wound of left eyelid and periocular area A
    ● **S01.109**   Unspecified open wound of unspecified eyelid and periocular area A
   ● **S01.11**   Laceration without foreign body of eyelid and periocular area
    ● **S01.111**   Laceration without foreign body of right eyelid and periocular area
    ● **S01.112**   Laceration without foreign body of left eyelid and periocular area
    ● **S01.119**   Laceration without foreign body of unspecified eyelid and periocular area
   ● **S01.12**   Laceration with foreign body of eyelid and periocular area
    ● **S01.121**   Laceration with foreign body of right eyelid and periocular area
    ● **S01.122**   Laceration with foreign body of left eyelid and periocular area
    ● **S01.129**   Laceration with foreign body of unspecified eyelid and periocular area

N Newborn Age: 0   **P** Pediatric Age: 0–17   **M** Maternity DX: 9–64   **A** Adult Age: 15–124   ♀ Females Only   ♂ Males Only
🌢 Complication\Comorbidity   🌢 Major C\C   (Ex) CC/MCC Exclusions   🌢 Hospital-Acquired Condition   🌢 Hierarchical Condition Category

1251

- S01.13 **Puncture wound without foreign body** of eyelid and periocular area
  - S01.131 Puncture wound without foreign body of **right** eyelid and periocular area
  - S01.132 Puncture wound without foreign body of **left** eyelid and periocular area
  - S01.139 Puncture wound without foreign body of **unspecified** eyelid and periocular area
- S01.14 **Puncture wound with foreign body** of eyelid and periocular area
  - S01.141 Puncture wound with foreign body of **right** eyelid and periocular area
  - S01.142 Puncture wound with foreign body of **left** eyelid and periocular area
  - S01.149 Puncture wound with foreign body of **unspecified** eyelid and periocular area
- S01.15 **Open bite of eyelid and periocular area**
  Bite of eyelid and periocular area NOS
  Excludes1 superficial bite of eyelid and periocular area (S00.26, S00.27)
  - S01.151 Open bite of **right** eyelid and periocular area
  - S01.152 Open bite of **left** eyelid and periocular area
  - S01.159 Open bite of **unspecified** eyelid and periocular area
- S01.2 Open wound of **nose**
  - X● S01.20 **Unspecified** open wound of nose
  - X● S01.21 **Laceration without foreign body** of nose
    Coding Clinic: 2015, Q1, P5-6
  - X● S01.22 **Laceration with foreign body** of nose
  - X● S01.23 **Puncture wound without foreign body** of nose
  - X● S01.24 **Puncture wound with foreign body** of nose
  - X● S01.25 **Open bite of nose**
    Bite of nose NOS
    Excludes1 superficial bite of nose (S00.36, S00.37)
- S01.3 Open wound of **ear**
  - S01.30 **Unspecified** open wound of ear
    - S01.301 Unspecified open wound of **right** ear
    - S01.302 Unspecified open wound of **left** ear
    - S01.309 Unspecified open wound of **unspecified** ear
  - S01.31 **Laceration without foreign body** of ear
    - S01.311 Laceration without foreign body of **right** ear
    - S01.312 Laceration without foreign body of **left** ear
    - S01.319 Laceration without foreign body of **unspecified** ear
  - S01.32 **Laceration with foreign body** of ear
    - S01.321 Laceration with foreign body of **right** ear
    - S01.322 Laceration with foreign body of **left** ear
    - S01.329 Laceration with foreign body of **unspecified** ear

- S01.33 **Puncture wound without foreign body** of ear
  - S01.331 Puncture wound without foreign body of **right** ear
  - S01.332 Puncture wound without foreign body of **left** ear
  - S01.339 Puncture wound without foreign body of **unspecified** ear
- S01.34 **Puncture wound with foreign body** of ear
  - S01.341 Puncture wound with foreign body of **right** ear
  - S01.342 Puncture wound with foreign body of **left** ear
  - S01.349 Puncture wound with foreign body of **unspecified** ear
- S01.35 **Open bite of ear**
  Bite of ear NOS
  Excludes1 superficial bite of ear (S00.46, S00.47)
  - S01.351 Open bite of **right** ear
  - S01.352 Open bite of **left** ear
  - S01.359 Open bite of **unspecified** ear
- S01.4 Open wound of **cheek and temporomandibular area**
  - S01.40 **Unspecified** open wound of cheek and temporomandibular area
    - S01.401 Unspecified open wound of **right** cheek and temporomandibular area
    - S01.402 Unspecified open wound of **left** cheek and temporomandibular area
    - S01.409 Unspecified open wound of **unspecified** cheek and temporomandibular area
  - S01.41 **Laceration without foreign body** of cheek and temporomandibular area
    - S01.411 Laceration without foreign body of **right** cheek and temporomandibular area
      Coding Clinic: 2015, Q1, P5-7
    - S01.412 Laceration without foreign body of **left** cheek and temporomandibular area
    - S01.419 Laceration without foreign body of **unspecified** cheek and temporomandibular area
  - S01.42 **Laceration with foreign body** of cheek and temporomandibular area
    - S01.421 Laceration with foreign body of **right** cheek and temporomandibular area
    - S01.422 Laceration with foreign body of **left** cheek and temporomandibular area
    - S01.429 Laceration with foreign body of **unspecified** cheek and temporomandibular area
  - S01.43 **Puncture wound without foreign body** of cheek and temporomandibular area
    - S01.431 Puncture wound without foreign body of **right** cheek and temporomandibular area
    - S01.432 Puncture wound without foreign body of **left** cheek and temporomandibular area
    - S01.439 Puncture wound without foreign body of **unspecified** cheek and temporomandibular area

CHAPTER 19 (S00-T88)

● S01.44 Puncture wound with foreign body of cheek and temporomandibular area
    ● S01.441 Puncture wound with foreign body of right cheek and temporomandibular area
    ● S01.442 Puncture wound with foreign body of left cheek and temporomandibular area
    ● S01.449 Puncture wound with foreign body of unspecified cheek and temporomandibular area
● S01.45 Open bite of cheek and temporomandibular area
    Bite of cheek and temporomandibular area NOS
    Excludes2 superficial bite of cheek and temporomandibular area (S00.86, S00.87)
    ● S01.451 Open bite of right cheek and temporomandibular area
    ● S01.452 Open bite of left cheek and temporomandibular area
    ● S01.459 Open bite of unspecified cheek and temporomandibular area

● S01.5 Open wound of lip and oral cavity
    Excludes2 tooth dislocation (S03.2)
                tooth fracture (S02.5)
  ● S01.50 Unspecified open wound of lip and oral cavity
    ● S01.501 Unspecified open wound of lip
    ● S01.502 Unspecified open wound of oral cavity
  ● S01.51 Laceration of lip and oral cavity without foreign body
    ● S01.511 Laceration without foreign body of lip
    ● S01.512 Laceration without foreign body of oral cavity
  ● S01.52 Laceration of lip and oral cavity with foreign body
    ● S01.521 Laceration with foreign body of lip
    ● S01.522 Laceration with foreign body of oral cavity
  ● S01.53 Puncture wound of lip and oral cavity without foreign body
    ● S01.531 Puncture wound without foreign body of lip
    ● S01.532 Puncture wound without foreign body of oral cavity
  ● S01.54 Puncture wound of lip and oral cavity with foreign body
    ● S01.541 Puncture wound with foreign body of lip
    ● S01.542 Puncture wound with foreign body of oral cavity
  ● S01.55 Open bite of lip and oral cavity
    ● S01.551 Open bite of lip
        Bite of lip NOS
        Excludes1 superficial bite of lip (S00.571)
    ● S01.552 Open bite of oral cavity
        Bite of oral cavity NOS
        Excludes1 superficial bite of oral cavity (S00.572)

● S01.8 Open wound of other parts of head
  X● S01.80 Unspecified open wound of other part of head
  X● S01.81 Laceration without foreign body of other part of head
  X● S01.82 Laceration with foreign body of other part of head
  X● S01.83 Puncture wound without foreign body of other part of head
  X● S01.84 Puncture wound with foreign body of other part of head
  X● S01.85 Open bite of other part of head
    Bite of other part of head NOS
    Excludes1 superficial bite of other part of head (S00.87)

● S01.9 Open wound of unspecified part of head
  X● S01.90 Unspecified open wound of unspecified part of head
  X● S01.91 Laceration without foreign body of unspecified part of head
  X● S01.92 Laceration with foreign body of unspecified part of head
  X● S01.93 Puncture wound without foreign body of unspecified part of head
  X● S01.94 Puncture wound with foreign body of unspecified part of head
  X● S01.95 Open bite of unspecified part of head
    Bite of head NOS
    Excludes1 superficial bite of head NOS (S00.97)

● S02 Fracture of skull and facial bones
  Note: A fracture not indicated as open or closed should be coded to closed
    The appropriate 7th character is to be added to each code from category S02

A	initial encounter for closed fracture
B	initial encounter for open fracture
D	subsequent encounter for fracture with routine healing
G	subsequent encounter for fracture with delayed healing
K	subsequent encounter for fracture with nonunion
S	sequela

  Code also any associated intracranial injury (S06.-)
  X● S02.0 Fracture of vault of skull A, K 🐾, B 🐾, A, B 🐾, **A, B, S** 🐾
    Fracture of frontal bone
    Fracture of parietal bone
    (Ex) **For category S02.0 CC codes S02.0[A,B]: See PDX Collection 1140** For S02.0[K]: See PDX Collection 897
  ● S02.1 Fracture of base of skull
    Excludes2 lateral orbital wall (S02.84-)
            medial orbital wall (S02.83-)
            orbital floor (S02.3-)
    (Ex) **For category S02.1 CC codes: For S02.1[A,B] CC codes: See PDX Collection 1140** For S02.1[K] CC codes: See PDX Collection 897
    Coding Clinic: 2016, Q4, P66
    ● S02.10 Unspecified fracture of base of skull
      ● S02.101 Fracture of base of skull, right side A, K 🐾, B 🐾, A, B 🐾, **A, B, S** 🐾
      ● S02.102 Fracture of base of skull, left side A, K 🐾, B 🐾, A, B 🐾, **A, B, S** 🐾
      ● S02.109 Fracture of base of skull, unspecified side A, K 🐾, B 🐾, A, B 🐾, **A, B, S** 🐾

N Newborn Age: 0   **P** Pediatric Age: 0–17   **M** Maternity DX: 9–64   **A** Adult Age: 15–124   ♀ Females Only   ♂ Males Only

🐾 Complication\Comorbidity   🐾 Major C\C   (Ex) CC/MCC Exclusions   🐾 Hospital-Acquired Condition   🐾 Hierarchical Condition Category

1253

● **S02.11**   Fracture of occiput

     ● **S02.110**   Type I occipital condyle fracture, unspecified side A, K 🔧, B 🔧, A, B 🔧, A, B, S 🔧

     ● **S02.111**   Type II occipital condyle fracture, unspecified side A, K 🔧, B 🔧, A, B 🔧, A, B, S 🔧

     ● **S02.112**   Type III occipital condyle fracture, unspecified side A, K 🔧, B 🔧, A, B 🔧, A, B, S 🔧

     ● **S02.113**   Unspecified occipital condyle fracture A, K 🔧, B 🔧, A, B 🔧, A, B, S 🔧

     ● **S02.118**   Other fracture of occiput, unspecified side A, K 🔧, B 🔧, A, B 🔧, A, B, S 🔧

     ● **S02.119**   Unspecified fracture of occiput A, K 🔧, B 🔧, A, B 🔧, A, B, S 🔧

     ● **S02.11A**   Type I occipital condyle fracture, right side A, K 🔧, B 🔧, A, B 🔧, A, B, S 🔧

     ● **S02.11B**   Type I occipital condyle fracture, left side A, K 🔧, B 🔧, A, B 🔧, A, B, S 🔧

     ● **S02.11C**   Type II occipital condyle fracture, right side A, K 🔧, B 🔧, A, B 🔧, A, B, S 🔧

     ● **S02.11D**   Type II occipital condyle fracture, left side A, K 🔧, B 🔧, A, B 🔧, A, B, S 🔧

     ● **S02.11E**   Type III occipital condyle fracture, right side A, K 🔧, B 🔧, A, B 🔧, A, B, S 🔧

     ● **S02.11F**   Type III occipital condyle fracture, left side A, K 🔧, B 🔧, A, B 🔧, A, B, S 🔧

     ● **S02.11G**   Other fracture of occiput, right side A, K 🔧, B 🔧, A, B 🔧, A, B, S 🔧

     ● **S02.11H**   Other fracture of occiput, left side A, K 🔧, B 🔧, A, B 🔧, A, B, S 🔧

S02.12   Fracture of orbital roof

     (Ex) **For category S02.12[A,B]: See PDX Collection 1140**
     For category S02.12[K]: See PDX Collection 897

     S02.121   Fracture of orbital roof, right side A, K 🔧, B 🔧, A, B 🔧

     S02.122   Fracture of orbital roof, left side A, K 🔧, B 🔧, A, B 🔧

     S02.129   Fracture of orbital roof, unspecified side A, K 🔧, B 🔧, A, B 🔧

X ● **S02.19**   Other fracture of base of skull A, K 🔧, B 🔧, A, B 🔧, A, B, S 🔧

     Fracture of anterior fossa of base of skull
     Fracture of ethmoid sinus
     Fracture of frontal sinus
     Fracture of middle fossa of base of skull
     Fracture of posterior fossa of base of skull
     Fracture of sphenoid
     Fracture of temporal bone

X ● **S02.2**   Fracture of nasal bones B, K 🔧, B 🔧

     (Ex) **For category S02.2 CC codes S02.2[B]: See PDX Collection 1141**
     For S02.2[K]: See PDX Collection 897

● **S02.3**   Fracture of orbital floor

     Fracture of inferior orbital wall

     Excludes1   orbit NOS (S02.85)

     Excludes2   lateral orbital wall (S02.84-)
                       medial orbital wall (S02.83-)
                       orbital roof (S02.1-)

     (Ex) **For category S02.3 CC codes S02.3[A,B]: See PDX Collection 1142**
     For S02.3[K]: See PDX Collection 897

     Coding Clinic: 2016, Q4, P66

X ● **S02.30**   Fracture of orbital floor, unspecified side A, B, K 🔧, A, B 🔧, A, B, S 🔧

X ● **S02.31**   Fracture of orbital floor, right side A, B, K 🔧, A, B 🔧, A, B, S 🔧

X ● **S02.32**   Fracture of orbital floor, left side A, B, K 🔧, A, B 🔧, A, B, S 🔧

● **S02.4**   Fracture of malar, maxillary and zygoma bones

     Fracture of superior maxilla
     Fracture of upper jaw (bone)
     Fracture of zygomatic process of temporal bone

     (Ex) **For category S02.4 CC codes S02.4[A,B] unless otherwise indicated: See PDX Collection 1143 For S02.4[K]: See PDX Collection 897**

     Coding Clinic: 2016, Q4, P66

     ● **S02.40**   Fracture of malar, maxillary and zygoma bones, unspecified

         ● **S02.400**   Malar fracture unspecified side A, B, K 🔧, A, B 🔧, A, B, S 🔧

         ● **S02.401**   Maxillary fracture, unspecified side A, B, K 🔧, A, B 🔧, A, B, S 🔧

         ● **S02.402**   Zygomatic fracture, unspecified side A, B, K 🔧, A, B 🔧, A, B, S 🔧

         ● **S02.40A**   Malar fracture, right side A, B, K 🔧, A, B 🔧, A, B, S 🔧

         ● **S02.40B**   Malar fracture, left side A, B, K 🔧, A, B 🔧, A, B, S 🔧

         ● **S02.40C**   Maxillary fracture, right side A, B, K 🔧, A, B 🔧, A, B, S 🔧

         ● **S02.40D**   Maxillary fracture, left side A, B, K 🔧, A, B 🔧, A, B, S 🔧

         ● **S02.40E**   Zygomatic fracture, right side A, B, K 🔧, A, B 🔧, A, B, S 🔧

         ● **S02.40F**   Zygomatic fracture, left side A, B, K 🔧, A, B 🔧, A, B, S 🔧

     ● **S02.41**   LeFort fracture

         ● **S02.411**   LeFort I fracture A, B, K 🔧, A, B 🔧, A, B, S 🔧

         ● **S02.412**   LeFort II fracture A, B, K 🔧, A, B 🔧, A, B, S 🔧

         ● **S02.413**   LeFort III fracture A, B, K 🔧, A, B 🔧, A, B, S 🔧

X ● **S02.42**   Fracture of alveolus of maxilla A, B, K 🔧, A, B 🔧, A, B, S 🔧

     (Ex) **For S02.42[A,B]: See PDX Collection 1142 For S02.42[K]: See PDX Collection 897**

X ● **S02.5**   Fracture of tooth (traumatic) Broken tooth K 🔧

     Excludes1   cracked tooth (nontraumatic) (K03.81)

     (Ex) See PDX Collection 897

● **S02.6**   Fracture of mandible

     Fracture of lower jaw (bone)

     (Ex) **For category S02.6 CC codes S02.6[A,B]: See PDX Collection 1143**
     For S02.6[K]: See PDX Collection 897

     Coding Clinic: 2016, Q4, P66

     ● **S02.60**   Fracture of mandible of unspecified site

         ● **S02.600**   Fracture of unspecified part of body of mandible, unspecified side A, B, K 🔧, A, B 🔧, A, B, S 🔧

         ● **S02.601**   Fracture of unspecified part of body of right mandible A, B, K 🔧, A, B 🔧, A, B, S 🔧

         ● **S02.602**   Fracture of unspecified part of body of left mandible A, B, K 🔧, A, B 🔧, A, B, S 🔧

         ● **S02.609**   Fracture of mandible, unspecified A, B, K 🔧, A, B 🔧, A, B, S 🔧

     ● **S02.61**   Fracture of condylar process of mandible

         ● **S02.610**   Fracture of condylar process of mandible, unspecified side A, B, K 🔧, A, B 🔧, A, B, S 🔧

         ● **S02.611**   Fracture of condylar process of right mandible A, B, K 🔧, A, B 🔧, A, B, S 🔧

             Coding Clinic: 2021, Q1, P6

         ● **S02.612**   Fracture of condylar process of left mandible A, B, K 🔧, A, B 🔧, A, B, S 🔧

▶ New   ⇒ Revised   ~~deleted~~ Deleted   Excludes 1   Excludes 2   Includes   Use additional   Code first   Code also   Key words

OGCR Official Guidelines   ● Unacceptable Principal Diagnosis   X Assign placeholder X   ● Use Additional Character(s)   ▶ Manifestation Code   **Coding Clinic**

● S02.62   Fracture of subcondylar process of mandible
   ● S02.620   Fracture of subcondylar process of mandible, unspecified side A, B, K 🐾, A, B 🐾, A, B, S 🐾
   ● S02.621   Fracture of subcondylar process of right mandible A, B, K 🐾, A, B 🐾, A, B, S 🐾
   ● S02.622   Fracture of subcondylar process of left mandible A, B, K 🐾, A, B 🐾, A, B, S 🐾

● S02.63   Fracture of coronoid process of mandible
   ● S02.630   Fracture of coronoid process of mandible, unspecified side A, B, K 🐾, A, B 🐾, A, B, S 🐾
   ● S02.631   Fracture of coronoid process of right mandible A, B, K 🐾, A, B 🐾, A, B, S 🐾
   ● S02.632   Fracture of coronoid process of left mandible A, B, K 🐾, A, B 🐾, A, B, S 🐾

● S02.64   Fracture of ramus of mandible
   ● S02.640   Fracture of ramus of mandible, unspecified side A, B, K 🐾, A, B 🐾, A, B, S 🐾
   ● S02.641   Fracture of ramus of right mandible A, B, K 🐾, A, B 🐾, A, B, S 🐾
   ● S02.642   Fracture of ramus of left mandible A, B, K 🐾, A, B 🐾, A, B, S 🐾

● S02.65   Fracture of angle of mandible
   ● S02.650   Fracture of angle of mandible, unspecified side A, B, K 🐾, A, B 🐾, A, B, S 🐾
   ● S02.651   Fracture of angle of right mandible A, B, K 🐾, A, B 🐾, A, B, S 🐾
   ● S02.652   Fracture of angle of left mandible A, B, K 🐾, A, B 🐾, A, B, S 🐾

X ● S02.66   Fracture of symphysis of mandible A, B, K 🐾, A, B 🐾, A, B, S 🐾
     Coding Clinic: 2021, Q1, P6

● S02.67   Fracture of alveolus of mandible
   ● S02.670   Fracture of alveolus of mandible, unspecified side A, B, K 🐾, A, B 🐾, A, B, S 🐾
   ● S02.671   Fracture of alveolus of right mandible A, B, K 🐾, A, B 🐾, A, B, S 🐾
   ● S02.672   Fracture of alveolus of left mandible A, B, K 🐾, A, B 🐾, A, B, S 🐾

X ● S02.69   Fracture of mandible of other specified site A, B, K 🐾, A, B 🐾, A, B, S 🐾

● S02.8   Fractures of other specified skull and facial bones
   Fracture of palate
   Excludes2   lateral orbital wall (S02.84-)
           medial orbital wall (S02.83-)
   (Ex:) For category S02.8 CC codes S02.8[A,B]: See PDX Collection 1142
     For S02.8[K]: See PDX Collection 897
   Coding Clinic: 2016, Q4, P66
X ● S02.80   Fracture of other specified skull and facial bones, unspecified side A, B, K 🐾, A, B 🐾, A, B, S 🐾
X ● S02.81   Fracture of other specified skull and facial bones, right side A, B, K 🐾, A, B 🐾, A, B, S 🐾
X ● S02.82   Fracture of other specified skull and facial bones, left side A, B, K 🐾, A, B 🐾, A, B, S 🐾

● S02.83   Fracture of medial orbital wall
   Excludes2   orbital floor (S02.3-)
           orbital roof (S02.12-)
   (Ex:) For category S02.83[A,B]: See PDX Collection 1142
     For S02.83[K]: See PDX Collection 897
   S02.831   Fracture of medial orbital wall, right side A, B, K 🐾, A, B 🐾
   S02.832   Fracture of medial orbital wall, left side A, B, K 🐾, A, B 🐾
   S02.839   Fracture of medial orbital wall, unspecified side A, B, K 🐾, A, B 🐾

● S02.84   Fracture of lateral orbital wall
   Excludes2   orbital floor (S02.3-)
           orbital roof (S02.12-)
   (Ex:) For category S02.84[A,B]: See PDX Collection 1142
     For category S02.84[K]: See PDX Collection 897
   S02.841   Fracture of lateral orbital wall, right side A, B, K 🐾, A, B 🐾
   S02.842   Fracture of lateral orbital wall, left side A, B, K 🐾, A, B 🐾
   S02.849   Fracture of lateral orbital wall, unspecified side A, B, K 🐾, A, B 🐾

● S02.85   Fracture of orbit, unspecified A, B, K 🐾, A, B 🐾
   Fracture of orbit NOS
   Fracture of orbit wall NOS
   Excludes1   lateral orbital wall (S02.84-)
           medial orbital wall (S02.83-)
           orbital floor (S02.3-)
           orbital roof (S02.12-)
   (Ex:) For category S02.85[A,B]: See PDX Collection 1142
     For category S02.85[K]: See PDX Collection 897

● S02.9   Fracture of unspecified skull and facial bones
X ● S02.91   Unspecified fracture of skull A, K 🐾, B 🐾, A, B 🐾, A, B, S 🐾
   (Ex:) For category S02.91 CC codes S02.91[A,B]: See PDX Collection 1140 For S02.91[K]: See PDX Collection 897
X ● S02.92   Unspecified fracture of facial bones A, B, K 🐾, A, B 🐾, A, B, S 🐾
   (Ex:) For category S02.92 CC codes S02.92[A,B]: See PDX Collection 1142 For S02.92[K]: See PDX Collection 897

● S03   Dislocation and sprain of joints and ligaments of head
   Includes   avulsion of joint (capsule) or ligament of head
     laceration of cartilage, joint (capsule) or ligament of head
     sprain of cartilage, joint (capsule) or ligament of head
     traumatic hemarthrosis of joint or ligament of head
     traumatic rupture of joint or ligament of head
     traumatic subluxation of joint or ligament of head
     traumatic tear of joint or ligament of head
   Code also any associated open wound
   Excludes2   Strain of muscle or tendon of head (S09.1)
   The appropriate 7th character is to be added to each code from category S03

     | A | initial encounter |
     | D | subsequent encounter |
     | S | sequela |

● S03.0   Dislocation of jaw
   Dislocation of jaw (cartilage) (meniscus)
   Dislocation of mandible
   Dislocation of temporomandibular (joint)
   Coding Clinic: 2016, Q4, P67
   X ● S03.00   Dislocation of jaw, unspecified side
   X ● S03.01   Dislocation of jaw, right side
   X ● S03.02   Dislocation of jaw, left side
   X ● S03.03   Dislocation of jaw, bilateral side
X ● S03.1   Dislocation of septal cartilage of nose
X ● S03.2   Dislocation of tooth

N Newborn Age: 0   **P** Pediatric Age: 0–17   **M** Maternity DX: 9–64   **A** Adult Age: 15–124   ♀ Females Only   ♂ Males Only

🐾 Complication\Comorbidity   🐾 Major C\C   (Ex:) CC/MCC Exclusions   🐾 Hospital-Acquired Condition   🐾 Hierarchical Condition Category

1255

CHAPTER 19 (S00-T88)

● S03.4   Sprain of jaw
            Sprain of temporomandibular (joint) (ligament)
            Coding Clinic: 2016, Q4, P67
    X● S03.40   Sprain of jaw, unspecified side
    X● S03.41   Sprain of jaw, right side
    X● S03.42   Sprain of jaw, left side
    X● S03.43   Sprain of jaw, bilateral side
X● S03.8   Sprain of joints and ligaments of other parts of head
X● S03.9   Sprain of joints and ligaments of unspecified parts of
            head

● S04   Injury of cranial nerve
            The selection of side should be based on the side of the body
                being affected
            Code first any associated intracranial injury (S06.-)
            Code also any associated:
                open wound of head (S01.-)
                skull fracture (S02.-)
            The appropriate 7th character is to be added to each code from
                category S04

            | A | initial encounter |
            | D | subsequent encounter |
            | S | sequela |

    ● S04.0   Injury of optic nerve and pathways
                Use additional code to identify any visual field defect
                    or blindness (H53.4-, H54.-)
                (Ex) **For category S04.0 CC codes:** See PDX Collection 1144
        ● S04.01   Injury of optic nerve
                    Injury of 2nd cranial nerve
            ● S04.011   Injury of optic nerve, right eye A 🝙
            ● S04.012   Injury of optic nerve, left eye A 🝙
            ● S04.019   Injury of optic nerve, unspecified eye
                        A 🝙
                        Injury of optic nerve NOS
        X● S04.02   Injury of optic chiasm A 🝙

● S04.03   Injury of optic tract and pathways
            Injury of optic radiation
    ● S04.031   Injury of optic tract and pathways,
                right side A 🝙
    ● S04.032   Injury of optic tract and pathways,
                left side A 🝙
    ● S04.039   Injury of optic tract and pathways,
                unspecified side A 🝙
                Injury of optic tract and pathways
                    NOS
● S04.04   Injury of visual cortex
    ● S04.041   Injury of visual cortex, right side A 🝙
    ● S04.042   Injury of visual cortex, left side A 🝙
    ● S04.049   Injury of visual cortex, unspecified
                side A 🝙
                Injury of visual cortex NOS
● S04.1   Injury of oculomotor nerve
            Injury of 3rd cranial nerve
            (Ex) **For category S04.1 CC codes:** See PDX Collection 1145
    X● S04.10   Injury of oculomotor nerve, unspecified side
                A 🝙
    X● S04.11   Injury of oculomotor nerve, right side A 🝙
    X● S04.12   Injury of oculomotor nerve, left side A 🝙
● S04.2   Injury of trochlear nerve
            Injury of 4th cranial nerve
            (Ex) **For category S04.2 CC codes:** See PDX Collection 1146
    X● S04.20   Injury of trochlear nerve, unspecified side A 🝙
    X● S04.21   Injury of trochlear nerve, right side A 🝙
    X● S04.22   Injury of trochlear nerve, left side A 🝙
● S04.3   Injury of trigeminal nerve
            Injury of 5th cranial nerve
            (Ex) **For category S04.3 CC codes:** See PDX Collection 1147
    X● S04.30   Injury of trigeminal nerve, unspecified side A 🝙
    X● S04.31   Injury of trigeminal nerve, right side A 🝙
    X● S04.32   Injury of trigeminal nerve, left side A 🝙

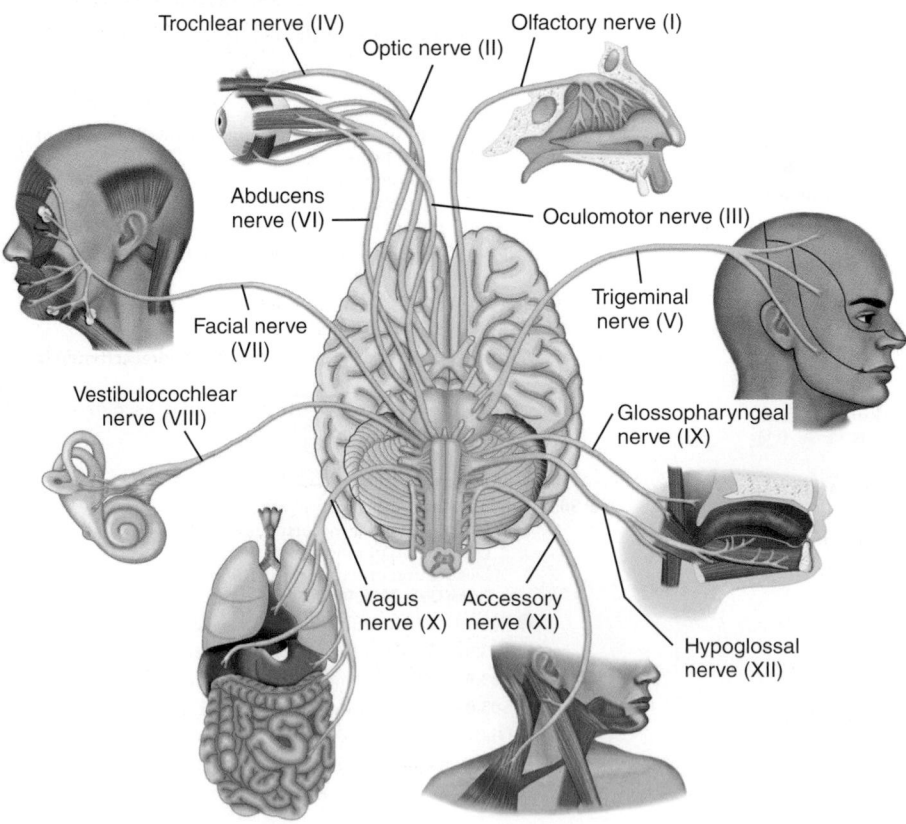

Figure 19-13 Cranial nerves. (From Patton
and Thibodeau: Anatomy and physiology, ed 7,
St. Louis, Mosby, 2009)

Trochlear nerve (IV)
Optic nerve (II)
Olfactory nerve (I)
Abducens nerve (VI)
Oculomotor nerve (III)
Facial nerve (VII)
Trigeminal nerve (V)
Vestibulocochlear nerve (VIII)
Glossopharyngeal nerve (IX)
Vagus nerve (X)
Accessory nerve (XI)
Hypoglossal nerve (XII)

▶ New   ⇒ Revised   ~~deleted~~ Deleted   Excludes 1   Excludes 2   Includes   Use additional   Code first   Code also   Key words

1256   OGCR Official Guidelines   ● Unacceptable Principal Diagnosis   X Assign placeholder X   ● Use Additional Character(s)   ▶ Manifestation Code   Coding Clinic

● **S04.4** Injury of abducent nerve
Injury of 6th cranial nerve
Ⓔ For category S04.4 CC codes: See PDX Collection 1148

X ● **S04.40** Injury of abducent nerve, unspecified side A Ⓗ
X ● **S04.41** Injury of abducent nerve, right side A Ⓗ
X ● **S04.42** Injury of abducent nerve, left side A Ⓗ

● **S04.5** Injury of facial nerve
Injury of 7th cranial nerve
Ⓔ For category S04.5 CC codes: See PDX Collection 1149

X ● **S04.50** Injury of facial nerve, unspecified side A Ⓗ
X ● **S04.51** Injury of facial nerve, right side A Ⓗ
X ● **S04.52** Injury of facial nerve, left side A Ⓗ

● **S04.6** Injury of acoustic nerve
Injury of auditory nerve
Injury of 8th cranial nerve
Ⓔ For category S04.6 CC codes: See PDX Collection 1150

X ● **S04.60** Injury of acoustic nerve, unspecified side A Ⓗ
X ● **S04.61** Injury of acoustic nerve, right side A Ⓗ
X ● **S04.62** Injury of acoustic nerve, left side A Ⓗ

● **S04.7** Injury of accessory nerve
Injury of 11th cranial nerve
Ⓔ For category S04.7 CC codes: See PDX Collection 1151

X ● **S04.70** Injury of accessory nerve, unspecified side A Ⓗ
X ● **S04.71** Injury of accessory nerve, right side A Ⓗ
X ● **S04.72** Injury of accessory nerve, left side A Ⓗ

● **S04.8** Injury of other cranial nerves
Ⓔ For category S04.8 CC codes: See PDX Collection 1152

● **S04.81** Injury of olfactory [1st] nerve
● **S04.811** Injury of olfactory [1st] nerve, right side A Ⓗ
● **S04.812** Injury of olfactory [1st] nerve, left side A Ⓗ
● **S04.819** Injury of olfactory [1st] nerve, unspecified side A Ⓗ

● **S04.89** Injury of other cranial nerves
Injury of vagus [10th] nerve
● **S04.891** Injury of other cranial nerves, right side A Ⓗ
● **S04.892** Injury of other cranial nerves, left side A Ⓗ
● **S04.899** Injury of other cranial nerves, unspecified side A Ⓗ

X ● **S04.9** Injury of unspecified cranial nerve A Ⓗ
Ⓔ See PDX Collection 1152

● **S05** Injury of eye and orbit
Includes open wound of eye and orbit
Excludes2 2nd cranial [optic] nerve injury (S04.0-)
3rd cranial [oculomotor] nerve injury (S04.1-)
open wound of eyelid and periocular area (S01.1-)
orbital bone fracture (S02.1-, S02.3-, S02.8-)
superficial injury of eyelid (S00.1-S00.2)

The appropriate 7th character is to be added to each code from category S05

A   initial encounter
D   subsequent encounter
S   sequela

● **S05.0** Injury of conjunctiva and corneal abrasion without foreign body
Excludes1 foreign body in conjunctival sac (T15.1)
foreign body in cornea (T15.0)
Ⓔ For category S05 CC codes unless otherwise indicated: See PDX Collection 1139

X ● **S05.00** Injury of conjunctiva and corneal abrasion without foreign body, unspecified eye
X ● **S05.01** Injury of conjunctiva and corneal abrasion without foreign body, right eye
X ● **S05.02** Injury of conjunctiva and corneal abrasion without foreign body, left eye

● **S05.1** Contusion of eyeball and orbital tissues
Traumatic hyphema
Excludes2 black eye NOS (S00.1)
contusion of eyelid and periocular area (S00.1)

X ● **S05.10** Contusion of eyeball and orbital tissues, unspecified eye
X ● **S05.11** Contusion of eyeball and orbital tissues, right eye
X ● **S05.12** Contusion of eyeball and orbital tissues, left eye

● **S05.2** Ocular laceration and rupture with prolapse or loss of intraocular tissue
X ● **S05.20** Ocular laceration and rupture with prolapse or loss of intraocular tissue, unspecified eye A Ⓗ
X ● **S05.21** Ocular laceration and rupture with prolapse or loss of intraocular tissue, right eye A Ⓗ
X ● **S05.22** Ocular laceration and rupture with prolapse or loss of intraocular tissue, left eye A Ⓗ

● **S05.3** Ocular laceration without prolapse or loss of intraocular tissue
Laceration of eye NOS
X ● **S05.30** Ocular laceration without prolapse or loss of intraocular tissue, unspecified eye A Ⓗ
X ● **S05.31** Ocular laceration without prolapse or loss of intraocular tissue, right eye A Ⓗ
X ● **S05.32** Ocular laceration without prolapse or loss of intraocular tissue, left eye A Ⓗ

● **S05.4** Penetrating wound of orbit with or without foreign body
Excludes2 retained (old) foreign body following penetrating wound in orbit (H05.5-)
X ● **S05.40** Penetrating wound of orbit with or without foreign body, unspecified eye A Ⓗ
X ● **S05.41** Penetrating wound of orbit with or without foreign body, right eye A Ⓗ
X ● **S05.42** Penetrating wound of orbit with or without foreign body, left eye A Ⓗ

● **S05.5** Penetrating wound with foreign body of eyeball
Excludes2 retained (old) intraocular foreign body (H44.6-, H44.7)
Ⓔ For category S05.5 CC codes: See PDX Collection 1153
X ● **S05.50** Penetrating wound with foreign body of unspecified eyeball A Ⓗ
X ● **S05.51** Penetrating wound with foreign body of right eyeball A Ⓗ
X ● **S05.52** Penetrating wound with foreign body of left eyeball A Ⓗ

● **S05.6** Penetrating wound without foreign body of eyeball
Ocular penetration NOS
X ● **S05.60** Penetrating wound without foreign body of unspecified eyeball
X ● **S05.61** Penetrating wound without foreign body of right eyeball
X ● **S05.62** Penetrating wound without foreign body of left eyeball

● **S05.7** Avulsion of eye
Traumatic enucleation
X ● **S05.70** Avulsion of unspecified eye A Ⓗ
X ● **S05.71** Avulsion of right eye A Ⓗ
X ● **S05.72** Avulsion of left eye A Ⓗ

● **S05.8** Other injuries of eye and orbit
Lacrimal duct injury
● **S05.8X** Other injuries of eye and orbit
● **S05.8X1** Other injuries of right eye and orbit A Ⓗ
● **S05.8X2** Other injuries of left eye and orbit A Ⓗ
● **S05.8X9** Other injuries of unspecified eye and orbit A Ⓗ

CHAPTER 19 (S00-T88)

N Newborn Age: 0   **P** Pediatric Age: 0–17   **M** Maternity DX: 9–64   **A** Adult Age: 15–124   ♀ Females Only   ♂ Males Only

Ⓒ Complication\Comorbidity   Ⓜ Major C\C   Ⓔ CC/MCC Exclusions   Ⓗ Hospital-Acquired Condition   Ⓗ Hierarchical Condition Category   **1257**

CHAPTER 19 (S00-T88)

- **S05.9**   Unspecified injury of eye and orbit
  Injury of eye NOS
  - X● **S05.90**   Unspecified injury of unspecified eye and orbit
  - X● **S05.91**   Unspecified injury of right eye and orbit A 🐾
  - X● **S05.92**   Unspecified injury of left eye and orbit A 🐾

- ● **S06**   Intracranial injury
  Includes   traumatic brain injury
  Code also any associated:
     open wound of head (S01.-)
     skull fracture (S02.-)
  Excludes1   head injury NOS (S09.90)
  The appropriate 7th character is to be added to each code from category S06

  > A   initial encounter
  > D   subsequent encounter
  > S   sequela

  Note: 7th characters D and S do not apply to codes in category S06 with 6th character 7 - death due to brain injury prior to regaining consciousness, or 8 - death due to other cause prior to regaining consciousness.
  (Ex:) For category S06 CC codes unless otherwise indicated: See PDX Collection 1154
  Coding Clinic: 2015, Q4, P40

  - ● **S06.0**   Concussion
    Commotio cerebri
    Excludes1   concussion with other intracranial injuries classified in subcategories S06.1- to S06.6- , S06.81- and S06.82- code to specified intracranial injury
    Coding Clinic: 2016, Q4, P67
    - ● **S06.0X**   Concussion
      - ● **S06.0X0**   Concussion without loss of consciousness S 🐾
      - ● **S06.0X1**   Concussion with loss of consciousness of 30 minutes or less A 🐾, A 🐾, S 🐾
      - ● **S06.0X9**   Concussion with loss of consciousness of unspecified duration A 🐾, A 🐾, S 🐾
        Concussion NOS
        Coding Clinic: 2016, Q4, P68

  - ● **S06.1**   Traumatic cerebral edema
    Diffuse traumatic cerebral edema
    Focal traumatic cerebral edema
    Coding Clinic: 2016, Q4, P67
    - ● **S06.1X**   Traumatic cerebral edema
      - ● **S06.1X0**   Traumatic cerebral edema without loss of consciousness A 🐾, A, S 🐾
        MCC when PDx is its own MCC
        (Ex:) See PDX Collection 3977
        Coding Clinic: 2015, Q1, P12
      - ● **S06.1X1**   Traumatic cerebral edema with loss of consciousness of 30 minutes or less A 🐾, A 🐾, A, S 🐾
        MCC when PDx is its own MCC
        (Ex:) See PDX Collection 1155
      - ● **S06.1X2**   Traumatic cerebral edema with loss of consciousness of 31 minutes to 59 minutes A 🐾, A 🐾, A, S 🐾
        MCC when PDx is its own MCC
        (Ex:) See PDX Collection 1155
      - ● **S06.1X3**   Traumatic cerebral edema with loss of consciousness of 1 hour to 5 hours 59 minutes A 🐾, A 🐾, A, S 🐾
        MCC when PDx is its own MCC
        (Ex:) See PDX Collection 1155
      - ● **S06.1X4**   Traumatic cerebral edema with loss of consciousness of 6 hours to 24 hours A 🐾, A 🐾, A, S 🐾
        MCC when PDx is its own MCC
        (Ex:) See PDX Collection 1155

  - ● **S06.1X5**   Traumatic cerebral edema with loss of consciousness greater than 24 hours with return to pre-existing conscious level A 🐾, A 🐾, A, S 🐾
    MCC when PDx is its own MCC
    (Ex:) See PDX Collection 1155
  - ● **S06.1X6**   Traumatic cerebral edema with loss of consciousness greater than 24 hours without return to pre-existing conscious level with patient surviving A 🐾, A 🐾, A, S 🐾
    MCC when PDx is its own MCC
  - ● **S06.1X7**   Traumatic cerebral edema with loss of consciousness of any duration with death due to brain injury prior to regaining consciousness A 🐾, A 🐾
    MCC when PDx is its own MCC
  - ● **S06.1X8**   Traumatic cerebral edema with loss of consciousness of any duration with death due to other cause prior to regaining consciousness A 🐾, A 🐾
    MCC when PDx is its own MCC
  - ● **S06.1X9**   Traumatic cerebral edema with loss of consciousness of unspecified duration A 🐾, A 🐾, A, S 🐾
    Traumatic cerebral edema NOS
    MCC when PDx is its own MCC
    (Ex:) See PDX Collection 1155

  - ● **S06.2**   Diffuse traumatic brain injury
    Diffuse axonal brain injury
    Excludes1   traumatic diffuse cerebral edema (S06.1X-)
    ▶ Use Additional code, if applicable, for traumatic brain compression or herniation (S06.A-)
    - ● **S06.2X**   Diffuse traumatic brain injury
      - ● **S06.2X0**   Diffuse traumatic brain injury without loss of consciousness A, S 🐾
      - ● **S06.2X1**   Diffuse traumatic brain injury with loss of consciousness of 30 minutes or less A 🐾, A 🐾, A, S 🐾
      - ● **S06.2X2**   Diffuse traumatic brain injury with loss of consciousness of 31 minutes to 59 minutes A 🐾, A 🐾, A, S 🐾
      - ● **S06.2X3**   Diffuse traumatic brain injury with loss of consciousness of 1 hour to 5 hours 59 minutes A 🐾, A 🐾, A, S 🐾
      - ● **S06.2X4**   Diffuse traumatic brain injury with loss of consciousness of 6 hours to 24 hours A 🐾, A 🐾, A, S 🐾
      - ● **S06.2X5**   Diffuse traumatic brain injury with loss of consciousness greater than 24 hours with return to pre-existing conscious levels A 🐾, A 🐾, A, S 🐾
      - ● **S06.2X6**   Diffuse traumatic brain injury with loss of consciousness greater than 24 hours without return to pre-existing conscious level with patient surviving A 🐾, A 🐾, A, S 🐾
      - ● **S06.2X7**   Diffuse traumatic brain injury with loss of consciousness of any duration with death due to brain injury prior to regaining consciousness A 🐾, A 🐾
      - ● **S06.2X8**   Diffuse traumatic brain injury with loss of consciousness of any duration with death due to other cause prior to regaining consciousness A 🐾, A 🐾
      - ● **S06.2X9**   Diffuse traumatic brain injury with loss of consciousness of unspecified duration A 🐾, A 🐾, A, S 🐾
        Diffuse traumatic brain injury NOS

▶ New   ⇒ Revised   ~~deleted~~ Deleted   Excludes 1   Excludes 2   Includes   Use additional   Code first   Code also   Key words
OGCR Official Guidelines   ● Unacceptable Principal Diagnosis   X Assign placeholder X   ● Use Additional Character(s)   ▶ Manifestation Code   Coding Clinic

● **S06.3** **Focal traumatic brain injury**

　　Excludes1　any condition classifiable to S06.4–S06.6

　　Excludes2　focal cerebral edema (S06.1)

　　▶ Use Additional code, if applicable, for traumatic brain compression or herniation (S06.A-)

● **S06.30** Unspecified focal traumatic brain injury

　● **S06.300** Unspecified focal traumatic brain injury without loss of consciousness A, S 🔸

　● **S06.301** Unspecified focal traumatic brain injury with loss of consciousness of 30 minutes or less A 🔸, A 🔸, A, S 🔸

　● **S06.302** Unspecified focal traumatic brain injury with loss of consciousness of 31 minutes to 59 minutes A 🔸, A 🔸, A, S 🔸

　● **S06.303** Unspecified focal traumatic brain injury with loss of consciousness of 1 hour to 5 hours 59 minutes A 🔸, A 🔸, A, S 🔸

　● **S06.304** Unspecified focal traumatic brain injury with loss of consciousness of 6 hours to 24 hours A 🔸, A 🔸, A, S 🔸

　● **S06.305** Unspecified focal traumatic brain injury with loss of consciousness greater than 24 hours with return to pre-existing conscious level A 🔸, A 🔸, A, S 🔸

　● **S06.306** Unspecified focal traumatic brain injury with loss of consciousness greater than 24 hours without return to pre-existing conscious level with patient surviving A 🔸, A 🔸, A, S 🔸

　● **S06.307** Unspecified focal traumatic brain injury with loss of consciousness of any duration with death due to brain injury prior to regaining consciousness A 🔸, A 🔸

　● **S06.308** Unspecified focal traumatic brain injury with loss of consciousness of any duration with death due to other cause prior to regaining consciousness A 🔸, A 🔸

　● **S06.309** Unspecified focal traumatic brain injury with loss of consciousness of unspecified duration A 🔸, A 🔸, A, S 🔸

　　　Unspecified focal traumatic brain injury NOS

● **S06.31** Contusion and laceration of right cerebrum

　● **S06.310** Contusion and laceration of right cerebrum without loss of consciousness A 🔸, A 🔸, A, S 🔸

　● **S06.311** Contusion and laceration of right cerebrum with loss of consciousness of 30 minutes or less A 🔸, A 🔸, A, S 🔸

　● **S06.312** Contusion and laceration of right cerebrum with loss of consciousness of 31 minutes to 59 minutes A 🔸, A 🔸, A, S 🔸

　● **S06.313** Contusion and laceration of right cerebrum with loss of consciousness of 1 hour to 5 hours 59 minutes A 🔸, A 🔸, A, S 🔸

　● **S06.314** Contusion and laceration of right cerebrum with loss of consciousness of 6 hours to 24 hours A 🔸, A 🔸, A, S 🔸

● **S06.315** Contusion and laceration of right cerebrum with loss of consciousness greater than 24 hours with return to pre-existing conscious level A 🔸, A 🔸, A, S 🔸

● **S06.316** Contusion and laceration of right cerebrum with loss of consciousness greater than 24 hours without return to pre-existing conscious level with patient surviving A 🔸, A 🔸, A, S 🔸

● **S06.317** Contusion and laceration of right cerebrum with loss of consciousness of any duration with death due to brain injury prior to regaining consciousness A 🔸, A 🔸

● **S06.318** Contusion and laceration of right cerebrum with loss of consciousness of any duration with death due to other cause prior to regaining consciousness A 🔸, A 🔸

● **S06.319** Contusion and laceration of right cerebrum with loss of consciousness of unspecified duration A 🔸, A 🔸, A, S 🔸

　　　Contusion and laceration of right cerebrum NOS

● **S06.32** Contusion and laceration of left cerebrum

● **S06.320** Contusion and laceration of left cerebrum without loss of consciousness A 🔸, A 🔸, A, S 🔸

● **S06.321** Contusion and laceration of left cerebrum with loss of consciousness of 30 minutes or less A 🔸, A 🔸, A, S 🔸

● **S06.322** Contusion and laceration of left cerebrum with loss of consciousness of 31 minutes to 59 minutes A 🔸, A 🔸, A, S 🔸

● **S06.323** Contusion and laceration of left cerebrum with loss of consciousness of 1 hour to 5 hours 59 minutes A 🔸, A 🔸, A, S 🔸

● **S06.324** Contusion and laceration of left cerebrum with loss of consciousness of 6 hours to 24 hours A 🔸, A 🔸, A, S 🔸

● **S06.325** Contusion and laceration of left cerebrum with loss of consciousness greater than 24 hours with return to pre-existing conscious level A 🔸, A 🔸, A, S 🔸

● **S06.326** Contusion and laceration of left cerebrum with loss of consciousness greater than 24 hours without return to pre-existing conscious level with patient surviving A 🔸, A 🔸, A, S 🔸

● **S06.327** Contusion and laceration of left cerebrum with loss of consciousness of any duration with death due to brain injury prior to regaining consciousness A 🔸, A 🔸

● **S06.328** Contusion and laceration of left cerebrum with loss of consciousness of any duration with death due to other cause prior to regaining consciousness A 🔸, A 🔸

● **S06.329** Contusion and laceration of left cerebrum with loss of consciousness of unspecified duration A 🔸, A 🔸, A, S 🔸

　　　Contusion and laceration of left cerebrum NOS

N Newborn Age: 0　　**P** Pediatric Age: 0–17　　**M** Maternity DX: 9–64　　**A** Adult Age: 15–124　　♀ Females Only　　♂ Males Only

🔸 Complication\Comorbidity　　🔸 Major C\C　　(Ex) CC/MCC Exclusions　　🔸 Hospital-Acquired Condition　　🔸 Hierarchical Condition Category

1259

- S06.33 **Contusion and laceration of cerebrum, unspecified**
  - S06.330 Contusion and laceration of cerebrum, unspecified, without loss of consciousness A 🐾, A 🐾, A, S 🐾
  - S06.331 Contusion and laceration of cerebrum, unspecified, with loss of consciousness of **30 minutes or less** A 🐾, A 🐾, A, S 🐾
  - S06.332 Contusion and laceration of cerebrum, unspecified, with loss of consciousness of **31 minutes to 59 minutes** A 🐾, A 🐾, A, S 🐾
  - S06.333 Contusion and laceration of cerebrum, unspecified, with loss of consciousness of **1 hour to 5 hours 59 minutes** A 🐾, A 🐾, A, S 🐾
  - S06.334 Contusion and laceration of cerebrum, unspecified, with loss of consciousness of **6 hours to 24 hours** A 🐾, A 🐾, A, S 🐾
  - S06.335 Contusion and laceration of cerebrum, unspecified, with loss of consciousness **greater than 24 hours** with **return to pre-existing conscious level** A 🐾, A 🐾, A, S 🐾
  - S06.336 Contusion and laceration of cerebrum, unspecified, with loss of consciousness **greater than 24 hours without return to pre-existing conscious level with patient surviving** A 🐾, A 🐾, A, S 🐾
  - S06.337 Contusion and laceration of cerebrum, unspecified, with loss of consciousness of **any duration with death due to brain injury** prior to regaining consciousness A 🐾, A 🐾
  - S06.338 Contusion and laceration of cerebrum, unspecified, with loss of consciousness of **any duration with death due to other cause** prior to regaining consciousness A 🐾, A 🐾
  - S06.339 Contusion and laceration of cerebrum, unspecified, with loss of consciousness of **unspecified duration** A 🐾, A 🐾, A, S 🐾
    Contusion and laceration of cerebrum NOS
- S06.34 **Traumatic hemorrhage of right cerebrum**
  Traumatic intracerebral hemorrhage and hematoma of right cerebrum
  - S06.340 Traumatic hemorrhage of right cerebrum **without loss of consciousness** A 🐾, A 🐾, A, S 🐾
    Coding Clinic: 2015, Q1, P12
  - S06.341 Traumatic hemorrhage of right cerebrum with loss of consciousness of **30 minutes or less** A 🐾, A 🐾, A, S 🐾
  - S06.342 Traumatic hemorrhage of right cerebrum with loss of consciousness of **31 minutes to 59 minutes** A 🐾, A 🐾, A, S 🐾
  - S06.343 Traumatic hemorrhage of right cerebrum with loss of consciousness of **1 hours to 5 hours 59 minutes** A 🐾, A 🐾, A, S 🐾
  - S06.344 Traumatic hemorrhage of right cerebrum with loss of consciousness of **6 hours to 24 hours** A 🐾, A 🐾, A, S 🐾

- S06.345 Traumatic hemorrhage of right cerebrum with loss of consciousness **greater than 24 hours with return to pre-existing conscious level** A 🐾, A 🐾, A, S 🐾
- S06.346 Traumatic hemorrhage of right cerebrum with loss of consciousness **greater than 24 hours without return to pre-existing conscious level with patient surviving** A 🐾, A 🐾, A, S 🐾
- S06.347 Traumatic hemorrhage of right cerebrum with loss of consciousness of **any duration with death due to brain injury** prior to regaining consciousness A 🐾, A 🐾
- S06.348 Traumatic hemorrhage of right cerebrum with loss of consciousness of **any duration with death due to other cause** prior to regaining consciousness A 🐾, A 🐾
- S06.349 Traumatic hemorrhage of right cerebrum with loss of consciousness of **unspecified duration** A 🐾, A 🐾, A, S 🐾
  Traumatic hemorrhage of right cerebrum NOS
- S06.35 **Traumatic hemorrhage of left cerebrum**
  Traumatic intracerebral hemorrhage and hematoma of left cerebrum
  - S06.350 Traumatic hemorrhage of left cerebrum **without loss of consciousness** A 🐾, A 🐾, A, S 🐾
  - S06.351 Traumatic hemorrhage of left cerebrum with loss of consciousness of **30 minutes or less** A 🐾, A 🐾, A, S 🐾
  - S06.352 Traumatic hemorrhage of left cerebrum with loss of consciousness of **31 minutes to 59 minutes** A 🐾, A 🐾, A, S 🐾
  - S06.353 Traumatic hemorrhage of left cerebrum with loss of consciousness of **1 hours to 5 hours 59 minutes** A 🐾, A 🐾, A, S 🐾
  - S06.354 Traumatic hemorrhage of left cerebrum with loss of consciousness of **6 hours to 24 hours** A 🐾, A 🐾, A, S 🐾
  - S06.355 Traumatic hemorrhage of left cerebrum with loss of consciousness **greater than 24 hours with return to pre-existing conscious level** A 🐾, A 🐾, A, S 🐾
  - S06.356 Traumatic hemorrhage of left cerebrum with loss of consciousness **greater than 24 hours without return to pre-existing conscious level with patient surviving** A 🐾, A 🐾, A, S 🐾
  - S06.357 Traumatic hemorrhage of left cerebrum with loss of consciousness of **any duration with death due to brain injury** prior to regaining consciousness A 🐾, A 🐾
  - S06.358 Traumatic hemorrhage of left cerebrum with loss of consciousness of **any duration with death due to other cause** prior to regaining consciousness A 🐾, A 🐾
  - S06.359 Traumatic hemorrhage of left cerebrum with loss of consciousness of **unspecified duration** A 🐾, A 🐾, A, S 🐾
    Traumatic hemorrhage of left cerebrum NOS

▶ New   ➡ Revised   ~~deleted~~ Deleted   Excludes 1   Excludes 2   Includes   Use additional   Code first   Code also   Key words
OGCR Official Guidelines   ● Unacceptable Principal Diagnosis   X Assign placeholder X   ● Use Additional Character(s)   ▷ Manifestation Code   Coding Clinic

● S06.36   **Traumatic hemorrhage of cerebrum, unspecified**
            Traumatic intracerebral hemorrhage and
            hematoma, unspecified
  ● S06.360   Traumatic hemorrhage of cerebrum,
               unspecified, without loss of
               consciousness A 🔴, A 🔴, A, S 🔴
  ● S06.361   Traumatic hemorrhage of cerebrum,
               unspecified, with loss of
               consciousness of 30 minutes or less
               A 🔴, A 🔴, A, S 🔴
  ● S06.362   Traumatic hemorrhage of cerebrum,
               unspecified, with loss of
               consciousness of 31 minutes to
               59 minutes A 🔴, A 🔴, A, S 🔴
  ● S06.363   Traumatic hemorrhage of cerebrum,
               unspecified, with loss of
               consciousness of 1 hours to 5 hours
               59 minutes A 🔴, A 🔴, A, S 🔴
  ● S06.364   Traumatic hemorrhage of cerebrum,
               unspecified, with loss of
               consciousness of 6 hours to 24 hours
               A 🔴, A 🔴, A, S 🔴
  ● S06.365   Traumatic hemorrhage of cerebrum,
               unspecified, with loss of
               consciousness greater than 24 hours
               with return to pre-existing conscious
               level A 🔴, A 🔴, A, S 🔴
  ● S06.366   Traumatic hemorrhage of cerebrum,
               unspecified, with loss of
               consciousness greater than 24 hours
               without return to pre-existing
               conscious level with patient surviving
               A 🔴, A 🔴, A, S 🔴
  ● S06.367   Traumatic hemorrhage of cerebrum,
               unspecified, with loss of
               consciousness of any duration with
               death due to brain injury prior to
               regaining consciousness A 🔴, A 🔴
  ● S06.368   Traumatic hemorrhage of cerebrum,
               unspecified, with loss of
               consciousness of any duration with
               death due to other cause prior to
               regaining consciousness A 🔴, A 🔴
  ● S06.369   Traumatic hemorrhage of cerebrum,
               unspecified, with loss of
               consciousness of unspecified duration
               A 🔴, A 🔴, A, S 🔴
               Traumatic hemorrhage of cerebrum
                   NOS
               (Ex:) See PDX Collection 3601

● S06.37   **Contusion, laceration, and hemorrhage of
            cerebellum**
  ● S06.370   Contusion, laceration, and hemorrhage
               of cerebellum without loss of
               consciousness A 🔴, A 🔴, A, S 🔴
               (Ex:) No exclusions
  ● S06.371   Contusion, laceration, and
               hemorrhage of cerebellum with loss
               of consciousness of 30 minutes or less
               A 🔴, A 🔴, A, S 🔴
  ● S06.372   Contusion, laceration, and
               hemorrhage of cerebellum with loss
               of consciousness of 31 minutes to
               59 minutes A 🔴, A 🔴, A, S 🔴
  ● S06.373   Contusion, laceration, and
               hemorrhage of cerebellum with loss
               of consciousness of 1 hour to 5 hours
               59 minutes A 🔴, A 🔴, A, S 🔴

  ● S06.374   Contusion, laceration, and
               hemorrhage of cerebellum with loss
               of consciousness of 6 hours to
               24 hours A 🔴, A 🔴, A, S 🔴
  ● S06.375   Contusion, laceration, and
               hemorrhage of cerebellum with loss
               of consciousness greater than 24
               hours with return to pre-existing
               conscious level A 🔴, A 🔴, A, S 🔴
  ● S06.376   Contusion, laceration, and
               hemorrhage of cerebellum with loss
               of consciousness greater than 24
               hours without return to pre-existing
               conscious level with patient surviving
               A 🔴, A 🔴, A, S 🔴
  ● S06.377   Contusion, laceration, and
               hemorrhage of cerebellum with loss
               of consciousness of any duration with
               death due to brain injury prior to
               regaining consciousness A 🔴, A 🔴
  ● S06.378   Contusion, laceration, and
               hemorrhage of cerebellum with loss
               of consciousness of any duration with
               death due to other cause prior to
               regaining consciousness A 🔴, A 🔴
  ● S06.379   Contusion, laceration, and
               hemorrhage of cerebellum with loss
               of consciousness of unspecified
               duration A 🔴, A 🔴, A, S 🔴
               Contusion, laceration, and
                   hemorrhage of cerebellum NOS

● S06.38   **Contusion, laceration, and hemorrhage of
            brainstem**
  ● S06.380   Contusion, laceration, and
               hemorrhage of brainstem without loss
               of consciousness A 🔴, A 🔴, A, S 🔴
               (Ex:) See PDX Collection 3602
  ● S06.381   Contusion, laceration, and
               hemorrhage of brainstem with loss of
               consciousness of 30 minutes or less
               A 🔴, A 🔴, A, S 🔴
  ● S06.382   Contusion, laceration, and
               hemorrhage of brainstem with loss of
               consciousness of 31 minutes to
               59 minutes A 🔴, A 🔴, A, S 🔴
  ● S06.383   Contusion, laceration, and
               hemorrhage of brainstem with loss of
               consciousness of 1 hour to 5 hours
               59 minutes A 🔴, A 🔴, A, S 🔴
  ● S06.384   Contusion, laceration, and
               hemorrhage of brainstem with loss of
               consciousness of 6 hours to 24 hours
               A 🔴, A 🔴, A, S 🔴
  ● S06.385   Contusion, laceration, and
               hemorrhage of brainstem with loss of
               consciousness greater than 24 hours
               with return to pre-existing conscious
               level A 🔴, A 🔴, A, S 🔴
  ● S06.386   Contusion, laceration, and
               hemorrhage of brainstem with loss of
               consciousness greater than 24 hours
               without return to pre-existing
               conscious level with patient surviving
               A 🔴, A 🔴, A, S 🔴
  ● S06.387   Contusion, laceration, and
               hemorrhage of brainstem with loss of
               consciousness of any duration with
               death due to brain injury prior to
               regaining consciousness A 🔴, A 🔴

CHAPTER 19 (S00-T88)

N Newborn Age: 0   **P** Pediatric Age: 0–17   **M** Maternity DX: 9–64   **A** Adult Age: 15–124   ♀ Females Only   ♂ Males Only

🔴 Complication\Comorbidity   🔴 Major C\C   (Ex:) CC/MCC Exclusions   🔴 Hospital-Acquired Condition   🔴 Hierarchical Condition Category

1261

● S06.388   Contusion, laceration, and hemorrhage of brainstem with loss of consciousness of any duration with death due to other cause prior to regaining consciousness A 🔟, A 🔟

● S06.389   Contusion, laceration, and hemorrhage of brainstem with loss of consciousness of unspecified duration A 🔟, A 🔟, A, S 🔟

       Contusion, laceration, and hemorrhage of brainstem NOS

● S06.4   Epidural hemorrhage
       Situated outside dura mater
       Extradural hemorrhage NOS
       Intracranial hemorrhage due to trauma
       Extradural hemorrhage (traumatic)

   ● S06.4X   Epidural hemorrhage

     ● S06.4X0   Epidural hemorrhage without loss of consciousness A 🔟, A 🔟, A, S 🔟

     ● S06.4X1   Epidural hemorrhage with loss of consciousness of 30 minutes or less A 🔟, A 🔟, A, S 🔟

     ● S06.4X2   Epidural hemorrhage with loss of consciousness of 31 minutes to 59 minutes A 🔟, A 🔟, A, S 🔟

     ● S06.4X3   Epidural hemorrhage with loss of consciousness of 1 hour to 5 hours 59 minutes A 🔟, A 🔟, A, S 🔟

     ● S06.4X4   Epidural hemorrhage with loss of consciousness of 6 hours to 24 hours A 🔟, A 🔟, A, S 🔟

     ● S06.4X5   Epidural hemorrhage with loss of consciousness greater than 24 hours with return to pre-existing conscious level A 🔟, A 🔟, A, S 🔟

     ● S06.4X6   Epidural hemorrhage with loss of consciousness greater than 24 hours without return to pre-existing conscious level with patient surviving A 🔟, A 🔟, A, S 🔟

     ● S06.4X7   Epidural hemorrhage with loss of consciousness of any duration with death due to brain injury prior to regaining consciousness A 🔟, A 🔟

     ● S06.4X8   Epidural hemorrhage with loss of consciousness of any duration with death due to other causes prior to regaining consciousness A 🔟, A 🔟

     ● S06.4X9   Epidural hemorrhage with loss of consciousness of unspecified duration A 🔟, A 🔟, A, S 🔟
       Epidural hemorrhage NOS

● S06.5   Traumatic subdural hemorrhage
   ▶ Use Additional code, if applicable, for traumatic brain compression or herniation (S06.A-)

   ● S06.5X   Traumatic subdural hemorrhage

     ● S06.5X0   Traumatic subdural hemorrhage without loss of consciousness A 🔟, A 🔟, A, S 🔟
       Coding Clinic: 2021, Q1, P4; 2018, Q2, P13; 2015, Q3, P37

     ● S06.5X1   Traumatic subdural hemorrhage with loss of consciousness of 30 minutes or less A 🔟, A 🔟, A, S 🔟

     ● S06.5X2   Traumatic subdural hemorrhage with loss of consciousness of 31 minutes to 59 minutes A 🔟, A 🔟, A, S 🔟

     ● S06.5X3   Traumatic subdural hemorrhage with loss of consciousness of 1 hour to 5 hours 59 minutes A 🔟, A 🔟, A, S 🔟

     ● S06.5X4   Traumatic subdural hemorrhage with loss of consciousness of 6 hours to 24 hours A 🔟, A 🔟, A, S 🔟

● S06.5X5   Traumatic subdural hemorrhage with loss of consciousness greater than 24 hours with return to pre-existing conscious level A 🔟, A 🔟, A, S 🔟

● S06.5X6   Traumatic subdural hemorrhage with loss of consciousness greater than 24 hours without return to pre-existing conscious level with patient surviving A 🔟, A 🔟, A, S 🔟
       Coding Clinic: 2021, Q2, P5

● S06.5X7   Traumatic subdural hemorrhage with loss of consciousness of any duration with death due to brain injury before regaining consciousness A 🔟, A 🔟

● S06.5X8   Traumatic subdural hemorrhage with loss of consciousness of any duration with death due to other cause before regaining consciousness A 🔟, A 🔟

● S06.5X9   Traumatic subdural hemorrhage with loss of consciousness of unspecified duration A 🔟, A 🔟, A, S 🔟
       Traumatic subdural hemorrhage NOS

● S06.6   Traumatic subarachnoid hemorrhage
       Between arachnoid and pia mater
   ▶ Use Additional code, if applicable, for traumatic brain compression or herniation (S06.A-)
       Coding Clinic: 2016, Q4, P67

   ● S06.6X   Traumatic subarachnoid hemorrhage

     ● S06.6X0   Traumatic subarachnoid hemorrhage without loss of consciousness A 🔟, A 🔟, A, S 🔟
       Coding Clinic: 2015, Q3, P37

     ● S06.6X1   Traumatic subarachnoid hemorrhage with loss of consciousness of 30 minutes or less A 🔟, A 🔟, A, S 🔟

     ● S06.6X2   Traumatic subarachnoid hemorrhage with loss of consciousness of 31 minutes to 59 minutes A 🔟, A 🔟, A, S 🔟

     ● S06.6X3   Traumatic subarachnoid hemorrhage with loss of consciousness of 1 hour to 5 hours 59 minutes A 🔟, A 🔟, A, S 🔟

     ● S06.6X4   Traumatic subarachnoid hemorrhage with loss of consciousness of 6 hours to 24 hours A 🔟, A 🔟, A, S 🔟

     ● S06.6X5   Traumatic subarachnoid hemorrhage with loss of consciousness greater than 24 hours with return to pre-existing conscious level A 🔟, A 🔟, A, S 🔟

     ● S06.6X6   Traumatic subarachnoid hemorrhage with loss of consciousness greater than 24 hours without return to pre-existing conscious level with patient surviving A 🔟, A 🔟, A, S 🔟
       Coding Clinic: 2021, Q2, P5

     ● S06.6X7   Traumatic subarachnoid hemorrhage with loss of consciousness of any duration with death due to brain injury prior to regaining consciousness A 🔟, A 🔟

     ● S06.6X8   Traumatic subarachnoid hemorrhage with loss of consciousness of any duration with death due to other cause prior to regaining consciousness A 🔟, A 🔟

     ● S06.6X9   Traumatic subarachnoid hemorrhage with loss of consciousness of unspecified duration A 🔟, A 🔟, A, S 🔟
       Traumatic subarachnoid hemorrhage NOS

▶ New   ➡ Revised   ~~deleted~~ Deleted   Excludes 1   Excludes 2   Includes   Use additional   Code first   Code also   Key words

OGCR Official Guidelines   ● Unacceptable Principal Diagnosis   X Assign placeholder X   ● Use Additional Character(s)   ▶ Manifestation Code   **Coding Clinic**

● **S06.8**   Other specified intracranial injuries

  ● **S06.81**   Injury of right internal carotid artery, intracranial portion, not elsewhere classified
         Coding Clinic: 2016, Q4, P67

    ● **S06.810**   Injury of right internal carotid artery, intracranial portion, not elsewhere classified without loss of consciousness A, S

    ● **S06.811**   Injury of right internal carotid artery, intracranial portion, not elsewhere classified with loss of consciousness of 30 minutes or less A, A, A, S

    ● **S06.812**   Injury of right internal carotid artery, intracranial portion, not elsewhere classified with loss of consciousness of 31 minutes to 59 minutes A, A, A, S

    ● **S06.813**   Injury of right internal carotid artery, intracranial portion, not elsewhere classified with loss of consciousness of 1 hour to 5 hours 59 minutes A, A, A, S

    ● **S06.814**   Injury of right internal carotid artery, intracranial portion, not elsewhere classified with loss of consciousness of 6 hours to 24 hours A, A, A, S

    ● **S06.815**   Injury of right internal carotid artery, intracranial portion, not elsewhere classified with loss of consciousness greater than 24 hours with return to pre-existing conscious level A, A, A, S

    ● **S06.816**   Injury of right internal carotid artery, intracranial portion, not elsewhere classified with loss of consciousness greater than 24 hours without return to pre-existing conscious level with patient surviving A, A, A, S

    ● **S06.817**   Injury of right internal carotid artery, intracranial portion, not elsewhere classified with loss of consciousness of any duration with death due to brain injury prior to regaining consciousness A, A

    ● **S06.818**   Injury of right internal carotid artery, intracranial portion, not elsewhere classified with loss of consciousness of any duration with death due to other cause prior to regaining consciousness A, A

    ● **S06.819**   Injury of right internal carotid artery, intracranial portion, not elsewhere classified with loss of consciousness of unspecified duration A, A, A, S

         Injury of right internal carotid artery, intracranial portion, not elsewhere classified NOS

  ● **S06.82**   Injury of left internal carotid artery, intracranial portion, not elsewhere classified
         Coding Clinic: 2016, Q4, P67

    ● **S06.820**   Injury of left internal carotid artery, intracranial portion, not elsewhere classified without loss of consciousness A, S

    ● **S06.821**   Injury of left internal carotid artery, intracranial portion, not elsewhere classified with loss of consciousness of 30 minutes or less A, A, A, S

    ● **S06.822**   Injury of left internal carotid artery, intracranial portion, not elsewhere classified with loss of consciousness of 31 minutes to 59 minutes A, A, A, S

    ● **S06.823**   Injury of left internal carotid artery, intracranial portion, not elsewhere classified with loss of consciousness of 1 hour to 5 hours 59 minutes A, A, A, S

    ● **S06.824**   Injury of left internal carotid artery, intracranial portion, not elsewhere classified with loss of consciousness of 6 hours to 24 hours A, A, A, S

    ● **S06.825**   Injury of left internal carotid artery, intracranial portion, not elsewhere classified with loss of consciousness greater than 24 hours with return to pre-existing conscious level A, A v

    ● **S06.826**   Injury of left internal carotid artery, intracranial portion, not elsewhere classified with loss of consciousness greater than 24 hours without return to pre-existing conscious level with patient surviving A, A, A, S

    ● **S06.827**   Injury of left internal carotid artery, intracranial portion, not elsewhere classified with loss of consciousness of any duration with death due to brain injury prior to regaining consciousness A, A

    ● **S06.828**   Injury of left internal carotid artery, intracranial portion, not elsewhere classified with loss of consciousness of any duration with death due to other cause prior to regaining consciousness A, A

    ● **S06.829**   Injury of left internal carotid artery, intracranial portion, not elsewhere classified with loss of consciousness of unspecified duration A, A, A, S

         Injury of left internal carotid artery, intracranial portion, not elsewhere classified NOS

CHAPTER 19 (S00-T88)

N Newborn Age: 0   **P** Pediatric Age: 0–17   **M** Maternity DX: 9–64   **A** Adult Age: 15–124   ♀ Females Only   ♂ Males Only

Complication\Comorbidity   Major C\C   (Ex) CC/MCC Exclusions   Hospital-Acquired Condition   Hierarchical Condition Category   **1263**

● **S06.89**   **Other specified intracranial injury**
     Excludes1   concussion (S06.0X-)

  ● **S06.890**   Other specified intracranial injury without loss of consciousness A 🔍, S 🔍

  ● **S06.891**   Other specified intracranial injury with loss of consciousness of 30 minutes or less A 🔍, A 🔍, A, S 🔍

  ● **S06.892**   Other specified intracranial injury with loss of consciousness of 31 minutes to 59 minutes A 🔍, A 🔍, A, S 🔍

  ● **S06.893**   Other specified intracranial injury with loss of consciousness of 1 hour to 5 hours 59 minutes A 🔍, A 🔍, A, S 🔍

  ● **S06.894**   Other specified intracranial injury with loss of consciousness of 6 hours to 24 hours A 🔍, A 🔍, A, S 🔍

  ● **S06.895**   Other specified intracranial injury with loss of consciousness greater than 24 hours with return to pre-existing conscious level A 🔍, A 🔍, A, S 🔍

  ● **S06.896**   Other specified intracranial injury with loss of consciousness greater than 24 hours without return to pre-existing conscious level with patient surviving A 🔍, A 🔍, A, S 🔍

  ● **S06.897**   Other specified intracranial injury with loss of consciousness of any duration with death due to brain injury prior to regaining consciousness A 🔍, A 🔍

  ● **S06.898**   Other specified intracranial injury with loss of consciousness of any duration with death due to other cause prior to regaining consciousness A 🔍, A 🔍

  ● **S06.899**   Other specified intracranial injury with loss of consciousness of unspecified duration A 🔍, A 🔍, A, S 🔍

● **S06.9**   **Unspecified intracranial injury**
     Brain injury NOS
     Head injury NOS with loss of consciousness
     Traumatic brain injury NOS
     Excludes1   conditions classifiable to S06.0- to S06.8- code to specified intracranial injury head injury NOS (S09.90)

● **S06.9X**   **Unspecified intracranial injury**

  ● **S06.9X0**   Unspecified intracranial injury without loss of consciousness A, S 🔍

  ● **S06.9X1**   Unspecified intracranial injury with loss of consciousness of 30 minutes or less A 🔍, A 🔍, A, S 🔍

  ● **S06.9X2**   Unspecified intracranial injury with loss of consciousness of 31 minutes to 59 minutes A 🔍, A 🔍, A, S 🔍

  ● **S06.9X3**   Unspecified intracranial injury with loss of consciousness of 1 hour to 5 hours 59 minutes A 🔍, A 🔍, A, S 🔍

  ● **S06.9X4**   Unspecified intracranial injury with loss of consciousness of 6 hours to 24 hours A 🔍, A 🔍, A, S 🔍

  ● **S06.9X5**   Unspecified intracranial injury with loss of consciousness greater than 24 hours with return to pre-existing conscious level A 🔍, A 🔍, A, S 🔍

  ● **S06.9X6**   Unspecified intracranial injury with loss of consciousness greater than 24 hours without return to pre-existing conscious level with patient surviving A 🔍, A 🔍, A, S 🔍

  ● **S06.9X7**   Unspecified intracranial injury with loss of consciousness of any duration with death due to brain injury prior to regaining consciousness A 🔍, A 🔍

  ● **S06.9X8**   Unspecified intracranial injury with loss of consciousness of any duration with death due to other cause prior to regaining consciousness A 🔍, A 🔍

  ● **S06.9X9**   Unspecified intracranial injury with loss of consciousness of unspecified duration A 🔍, A 🔍, A, S 🔍

▶ ● **S06.A**   **Traumatic brain compression and herniation**
     ▶ Traumatic cerebral compression
     ▶ *Code first the underlying traumatic brain injury, such as:*
         ▶ diffuse traumatic brain injury (S06.2-)
         ▶ focal traumatic brain injury (S06.3-)
         ▶ traumatic subdural hemorrhage (S06.5-)
         ▶ traumatic subarachnoid hemorrhage (S06.6-)

  ▶ **S06.A0**   **Traumatic brain compression without herniation**
     ▶ Traumatic brain compression NOS
     ▶ Traumatic cerebral compression NOS

  ▶ **S06.A1**   **Traumatic brain compression with herniation**
     ▶ Traumatic brain herniation
     ▶ Traumatic brainstem compression with herniation
     ▶ Traumatic cerebellar compression with herniation
     ▶ Traumatic cerebral compression with herniation

● **S07**   **Crushing injury of head**
     Use additional code for all associated injuries, such as:
        intracranial injuries (S06.-)
        skull fractures (S02.-)
     The appropriate 7th character is to be added to each code from category S07

A	initial encounter
D	subsequent encounter
S	sequela

     Ex: For category S07 CC codes: See PDX Collection 1156

X ● **S07.0**   Crushing injury of face A 🔍, A 🔍

X ● **S07.1**   Crushing injury of skull A 🔍, A 🔍

X ● **S07.8**   Crushing injury of other parts of head A 🔍, A 🔍

X ● **S07.9**   Crushing injury of head, part unspecified A 🔍, A 🔍

● **S08**   **Avulsion and traumatic amputation of part of head**
     An amputation not identified as partial or complete should be coded to complete
     The appropriate 7th character is to be added to each code from category S08

A	initial encounter
D	subsequent encounter
S	sequela

X ● **S08.0**   Avulsion of scalp

● **S08.1**   **Traumatic amputation of ear**

  ● **S08.11**   Complete traumatic amputation of ear
    ● **S08.111**   Complete traumatic amputation of right ear
    ● **S08.112**   Complete traumatic amputation of left ear
    ● **S08.119**   Complete traumatic amputation of unspecified ear

  ● **S08.12**   Partial traumatic amputation of ear
    ● **S08.121**   Partial traumatic amputation of right ear
    ● **S08.122**   Partial traumatic amputation of left ear
    ● **S08.129**   Partial traumatic amputation of unspecified ear

- ● **S08.8**   **Traumatic amputation of other parts of head**
  - ● **S08.81**   **Traumatic amputation of nose**
    - ● **S08.811**   **Complete** traumatic amputation of nose
    - ● **S08.812**   **Partial** traumatic amputation of nose
  - X● **S08.89**   **Traumatic amputation of other parts of head**
- ● **S09**   **Other and unspecified injuries of head**

  The appropriate 7th character is to be added to each code from category S09

A	initial encounter
D	subsequent encounter
S	sequela

  - X● **S09.0**   **Injury of blood vessels of head, not elsewhere classified** A

    Excludes1   injury of cerebral blood vessels (S06.-)
 injury of precerebral blood vessels (S15.-)

    (Ex:) See PDX Collection 1157

  - ● **S09.1**   **Injury of muscle and tendon of head**

    Code also any associated open wound (S01.-)

    Excludes2   sprain to joints and ligament of head (S03.9)

    - X● **S09.10**   **Unspecified** injury of muscle and tendon of head

      Injury of muscle and tendon of head NOS

    - X● **S09.11**   **Strain** of muscle and tendon of head
    - X● **S09.12**   **Laceration** of muscle and tendon of head
    - X● **S09.19**   **Other specified** injury of muscle and tendon of head

  - ● **S09.2**   **Traumatic rupture of ear drum**

    Excludes1   traumatic rupture of ear drum due to blast injury (S09.31-)

    (Ex:) For category S09.2 CC codes: See PDX Collection 1158

    - X● **S09.20**   **Traumatic rupture of unspecified ear drum** A
    - X● **S09.21**   **Traumatic rupture of right ear drum** A
    - X● **S09.22**   **Traumatic rupture of left ear drum** A

  - ● **S09.3**   **Other specified and unspecified injury of middle and inner ear**

    Excludes1   injury to ear NOS (S09.91-)

    Excludes2   injury to external ear (S00.4-, S01.3-, S08.1-)

    (Ex:) For category S09.3 CC codes: See PDX Collection 1158

    - ● **S09.30**   **Unspecified injury of middle and inner ear**
      - ● **S09.301**   Unspecified injury of **right** middle and inner ear A
      - ● **S09.302**   Unspecified injury of **left** middle and inner ear A
      - ● **S09.309**   Unspecified injury of **unspecified** middle and inner ear A
    - ● **S09.31**   **Primary blast injury of ear**

      Blast injury of ear NOS

      - ● **S09.311**   Primary blast injury of **right** ear A
      - ● **S09.312**   Primary blast injury of **left** ear A
      - ● **S09.313**   Primary blast injury of ear, **bilateral** A
      - ● **S09.319**   Primary blast injury of **unspecified** ear A
    - ● **S09.39**   **Other specified injury of middle and inner ear**

      Secondary blast injury to ear

      - ● **S09.391**   Other specified injury of **right** middle and inner ear A
      - ● **S09.392**   Other specified injury of **left** middle and inner ear A
      - ● **S09.399**   Other specified injury of **unspecified** middle and inner ear A

  - X● **S09.8**   **Other specified injuries of head**

- ● **S09.9**   **Unspecified injury of face and head**
  - X● **S09.90**   **Unspecified injury of head**

    Head injury NOS

    Excludes1   brain injury NOS (S06.9-)
 head injury NOS with loss of consciousness (S06.9-)
 intracranial injury NOS (S06.9-)

  - X● **S09.91**   **Unspecified injury of ear**

    Injury of ear NOS

  - X● **S09.92**   **Unspecified injury of nose**

    Injury of nose NOS

  - X● **S09.93**   **Unspecified injury of face**

    Injury of face NOS

INJURIES TO THE NECK (S10-S19)

Includes	injuries of nape injuries of supraclavicular region injuries of throat
Excludes2	burns and corrosions (T20-T32) effects of foreign body in esophagus (T18.1) effects of foreign body in larynx (T17.3) effects of foreign body in pharynx (T17.2) effects of foreign body in trachea (T17.4) frostbite (T33-T34) insect bite or sting, venomous (T63.4)

- ● **S10**   **Superficial injury of neck**

  The appropriate 7th character is to be added to each code from category S10

A	initial encounter
D	subsequent encounter
S	sequela

  - X● **S10.0**   **Contusion of throat**

    Contusion of cervical esophagus
 Contusion of larynx
 Contusion of pharynx
 Contusion of trachea

  - ● **S10.1**   **Other and unspecified superficial injuries of throat**
    - X● **S10.10**   **Unspecified** superficial injuries of throat
    - X● **S10.11**   **Abrasion** of throat
    - X● **S10.12**   **Blister (nonthermal)** of throat
    - X● **S10.14**   **External constriction** of part of throat
    - X● **S10.15**   **Superficial foreign body** of throat

      Splinter in the throat

    - X● **S10.16**   **Insect bite (nonvenomous)** of throat
    - X● **S10.17**   **Other superficial bite** of throat

      Excludes1   open bite of throat (S11.85)

  - ● **S10.8**   **Superficial injury of other specified parts of neck**
    - X● **S10.80**   **Unspecified** superficial injury of other specified part of neck
    - X● **S10.81**   **Abrasion** of other specified part of neck
    - X● **S10.82**   **Blister (nonthermal)** of other specified part of neck
    - X● **S10.83**   **Contusion** of other specified part of neck
    - X● **S10.84**   **External constriction** of other specified part of neck
    - X● **S10.85**   **Superficial foreign body** of other specified part of neck

      Splinter in other part of neck

    - X● **S10.86**   **Insect bite** of other specified part of neck
    - X● **S10.87**   **Other superficial bite** of other specified part of neck

      Excludes1   open bite of other specified parts of neck (S11.85)

N Newborn Age: 0   **P** Pediatric Age: 0–17   **M** Maternity DX: 9–64   **A** Adult Age: 15–124   ♀ Females Only   ♂ Males Only

Complication\Comorbidity   Major C\C   (Ex:) CC/MCC Exclusions   Hospital-Acquired Condition   Hierarchical Condition Category

1265

CHAPTER 19 (S00-T88)

CHAPTER 19 (S00-T88)

● S10.9 Superficial injury of unspecified part of neck
  X● S10.90 **Unspecified superficial injury of unspecified part of neck**
  X● S10.91 **Abrasion** of unspecified part of neck
  X● S10.92 **Blister** (nonthermal) of unspecified part of neck
  X● S10.93 **Contusion** of unspecified part of neck
  X● S10.94 **External constriction** of unspecified part of neck
  X● S10.95 **Superficial foreign body** of unspecified part of neck
  X● S10.96 **Insect bite** of unspecified part of neck
  X● S10.97 **Other superficial bite** of unspecified part of neck

● S11 Open wound of neck
  Code also any associated:
    spinal cord injury (S14.0, S14.1-)
    wound infection
  Excludes2 open fracture of vertebra (S12.- with 7th character B)
  The appropriate 7th character is to be added to each code from category S11

> A   initial encounter
> D   subsequent encounter
> S   sequela

● S11.0 Open wound of larynx and trachea
  (Ex:) For category S11.0 CC codes: See PDX Collection 1159
  ● S11.01 Open wound of larynx
    Excludes2 open wound of vocal cord (S11.03)
    ● S11.011 **Laceration without foreign body of larynx** A
    ● S11.012 **Laceration with foreign body of larynx** A
    ● S11.013 **Puncture wound without foreign body of larynx** A
    ● S11.014 **Puncture wound with foreign body of larynx** A
    ● S11.015 **Open bite** of larynx A
      Bite of larynx NOS
    ● S11.019 **Unspecified** open wound of larynx A
  ● S11.02 Open wound of trachea
    Open wound of cervical trachea
    Open wound of trachea NOS
    Excludes2 open wound of thoracic trachea (S27.5-)
    ● S11.021 **Laceration without foreign body of trachea** A
    ● S11.022 **Laceration with foreign body of trachea** A
    ● S11.023 **Puncture wound without foreign body of trachea** A
    ● S11.024 **Puncture wound with foreign body of trachea** A
    ● S11.025 **Open bite** of trachea A
      Bite of trachea NOS
    ● S11.029 **Unspecified** open wound of trachea A

● S11.03 Open wound of vocal cord
  ● S11.031 **Laceration without foreign body of vocal cord** A
  ● S11.032 **Laceration with foreign body of vocal cord** A
  ● S11.033 **Puncture wound without foreign body of vocal cord** A
  ● S11.034 **Puncture wound with foreign body of vocal cord** A
  ● S11.035 **Open bite** of vocal cord A
    Bite of vocal cord NOS
  ● S11.039 **Unspecified** open wound of vocal cord A

● S11.1 Open wound of thyroid gland
  (Ex:) For category S11.1 CC codes unless otherwise indicated: See PDX Collection 1160
  X● S11.10 **Unspecified** open wound of thyroid gland A
  X● S11.11 **Laceration without foreign body of thyroid gland** A
  X● S11.12 **Laceration with foreign body of thyroid gland** A
    (Ex:) See PDX Collection 1161
  X● S11.13 **Puncture wound without foreign body of thyroid gland** A
  X● S11.14 **Puncture wound with foreign body of thyroid gland** A
    (Ex:) See PDX Collection 1161
  X● S11.15 **Open bite** of thyroid gland A
    Bite of thyroid gland NOS

● S11.2 Open wound of pharynx and cervical esophagus
  Excludes1 open wound of esophagus NOS (S27.8-)
  (Ex:) For category S11.2 CC codes unless otherwise indicated: See PDX Collection 1162
  X● S11.20 **Unspecified** open wound of pharynx and cervical esophagus A
  X● S11.21 **Laceration without foreign body of pharynx and cervical esophagus** A
  X● S11.22 **Laceration with foreign body of pharynx and cervical esophagus** A
    (Ex:) See PDX Collection 1163
  X● S11.23 **Puncture wound without foreign body of pharynx and cervical esophagus** A
  X● S11.24 **Puncture wound with foreign body of pharynx and cervical esophagus** A
    (Ex:) See PDX Collection 1163
  X● S11.25 **Open bite** of pharynx and cervical esophagus A
    Bite of pharynx and cervical esophagus NOS

● S11.8 Open wound of other specified parts of neck
  X● S11.80 **Unspecified** open specified wound of other part of neck
  X● S11.81 **Laceration without foreign body of other specified part of neck**
  X● S11.82 **Laceration with foreign body of other specified part of neck**
  X● S11.83 **Puncture wound without foreign body of other specified part of neck**
  X● S11.84 **Puncture wound with foreign body of other specified part of neck**
  X● S11.85 **Open bite** of other specified part of neck
    Bite of other part of neck NOS
    Excludes1 superficial bite of other specified part of neck (S10.87)
  X● S11.89 **Other** open wound of other part of neck

● **S11.9**   Open wound of unspecified part of neck

   X ● **S11.90**   Unspecified open wound of unspecified part of neck

   X ● **S11.91**   Laceration without foreign body of unspecified part of neck

   X ● **S11.92**   Laceration with foreign body of unspecified part of neck

   X ● **S11.93**   Puncture wound without foreign body of unspecified part of neck

   X ● **S11.94**   Puncture wound with foreign body of unspecified part of neck

   X ● **S11.95**   Open bite of unspecified part of neck
       Bite of neck NOS
       Excludes1   superficial bite of neck (S10.97)

● **S12**   Fracture of cervical vertebra and other parts of neck

   Note: A fracture not indicated as displaced or nondisplaced should be coded to displaced

   A fracture not indicated as open or closed should be coded to closed

   Includes   fracture of cervical neural arch
         fracture of cervical spine
         fracture of cervical spinous process
         fracture of cervical transverse process
         fracture of cervical vertebral arch
         fracture of neck

   Code first any associated cervical spinal cord injury (S14.0, S14.1-)

   The appropriate 7th character is to be added to all codes from subcategories S12.0-S12.6

A	initial encounter for closed fracture
B	initial encounter for open fracture
D	subsequent encounter for fracture with routine healing
G	subsequent encounter for fracture with delayed healing
K	subsequent encounter for fracture with nonunion
S	sequela

   (Ex:) For category S12 CC codes S12[A,B]: See PDX Collection 1164
       For S12[K]: See PDX Collection 897 **unless otherwise indicated**

● **S12.0**   Fracture of first cervical vertebra
     Atlas

   ● **S12.00**   Unspecified fracture of first cervical vertebra

     ● **S12.000**   Unspecified displaced fracture of first cervical vertebra A, K, B, A, B, A, B

     ● **S12.001**   Unspecified nondisplaced fracture of first cervical vertebra A, K, B, A, B, A, B

   X ● **S12.01**   Stable burst fracture of first cervical vertebra A, K, B, A, B, A, B

   X ● **S12.02**   Unstable burst fracture of first cervical vertebra A, K, B, A, B, A, B

   ● **S12.03**   Posterior arch fracture of first cervical vertebra

     ● **S12.030**   Displaced posterior arch fracture of first cervical vertebra A, K, B, A, B, A, B

     ● **S12.031**   Nondisplaced posterior arch fracture of first cervical vertebra A, K, B, A, B, A, B

   ● **S12.04**   Lateral mass fracture of first cervical vertebra

     ● **S12.040**   Displaced lateral mass fracture of first cervical vertebra A, K, B, A, B, A, B

     ● **S12.041**   Nondisplaced lateral mass fracture of first cervical vertebra A, K, B, A, B, A, B

● **S12.09**   Other fracture of first cervical vertebra

   ● **S12.090**   Other displaced fracture of first cervical vertebra A, K, B, A, B, A, B

   ● **S12.091**   Other nondisplaced fracture of first cervical vertebra A, K, B, A, B, A, B

● **S12.1**   Fracture of second cervical vertebra
     Axis

   ● **S12.10**   Unspecified fracture of second cervical vertebra

     ● **S12.100**   Unspecified displaced fracture of second cervical vertebra A, K, B, A, B, A, B

     ● **S12.101**   Unspecified nondisplaced fracture of second cervical vertebra A, K, B, A, B, A, B

   ● **S12.11**   Type II dens fracture

     ● **S12.110**   Anterior displaced Type II dens fracture A, K, B, A, B, A, B

     ● **S12.111**   Posterior displaced Type II dens fracture A, K, B, A, B, A, B

     ● **S12.112**   Nondisplaced Type II dens fracture A, K, B, A, B, A, B

   ● **S12.12**   Other dens fracture

     ● **S12.120**   Other displaced dens fracture A, K, B, A, B, A, B

     ● **S12.121**   Other nondisplaced dens fracture A, K, B, A, B, A, B

   ● **S12.13**   Unspecified traumatic spondylolisthesis of second cervical vertebra

     ● **S12.130**   Unspecified traumatic displaced spondylolisthesis of second cervical vertebra A, K, B, A, B, A, B

     ● **S12.131**   Unspecified traumatic nondisplaced spondylolisthesis of second cervical vertebra A, K, B, A, B, A, B

   X ● **S12.14**   Type III traumatic spondylolisthesis of second cervical vertebra A, K, B, A, B, A, B

   ● **S12.15**   Other traumatic spondylolisthesis of second cervical vertebra

     ● **S12.150**   Other traumatic displaced spondylolisthesis of second cervical vertebra A, K, B, A, B, A, B

     ● **S12.151**   Other traumatic nondisplaced spondylolisthesis of second cervical vertebra A, K, B, A, B, A, B

   ● **S12.19**   Other fracture of second cervical vertebra

     ● **S12.190**   Other displaced fracture of second cervical vertebra A, K, B, A, B, A, B

     ● **S12.191**   Other nondisplaced fracture of second cervical vertebra A, K, B, A, B, A, B

● **S12.2**   Fracture of third cervical vertebra

   ● **S12.20**   Unspecified fracture of third cervical vertebra

     ● **S12.200**   Unspecified displaced fracture of third cervical vertebra A, K, B, A, B, A, B

     ● **S12.201**   Unspecified nondisplaced fracture of third cervical vertebra A, K, B, A, B, A, B

N Newborn Age: 0   **P** Pediatric Age: 0–17   **M** Maternity DX: 9–64   **A** Adult Age: 15–124   ♀ Females Only   ♂ Males Only

🔹 Complication\Comorbidity   🔹 Major C\C   (Ex:) CC/MCC Exclusions   🔹 Hospital-Acquired Condition   🔹 Hierarchical Condition Category

1267

CHAPTER 19 (S00-T88)

CHAPTER 19 (S00-T88)

● S12.23   Unspecified traumatic spondylolisthesis of third cervical vertebra

  ● S12.230   Unspecified traumatic displaced spondylolisthesis of third cervical vertebra A, K 🪙, B 🪙, A, B 🪙, **A, B** 🪙

  ● S12.231   Unspecified traumatic nondisplaced spondylolisthesis of third cervical vertebra A, K 🪙, B 🪙, A, B 🪙, **A, B** 🪙

X ● S12.24   Type III traumatic spondylolisthesis of third cervical vertebra A, K 🪙, B 🪙, A, B 🪙, **A, B** 🪙

● S12.25   Other traumatic spondylolisthesis of third cervical vertebra

  ● S12.250   Other traumatic displaced spondylolisthesis of third cervical vertebra A, K 🪙, B 🪙, A, B 🪙, **A, B** 🪙

  ● S12.251   Other traumatic nondisplaced spondylolisthesis of third cervical vertebra A, K 🪙, B 🪙, A, B 🪙, **A, B** 🪙

● S12.29   Other fracture of third cervical vertebra

  ● S12.290   Other displaced fracture of third cervical vertebra A, K 🪙, B 🪙, A, B 🪙, **A, B** 🪙

  ● S12.291   Other nondisplaced fracture of third cervical vertebra A, K 🪙, B 🪙, A, B 🪙, **A, B** 🪙

● S12.3   Fracture of fourth cervical vertebra

  ● S12.30   Unspecified fracture of fourth cervical vertebra

    ● S12.300   Unspecified displaced fracture of fourth cervical vertebra A, K 🪙, B 🪙, A, B 🪙, **A, B** 🪙

    ● S12.301   Unspecified nondisplaced fracture of fourth cervical vertebra A, K 🪙, B 🪙, A, B 🪙, **A, B** 🪙

  ● S12.33   Unspecified traumatic spondylolisthesis of fourth cervical vertebra

    ● S12.330   Unspecified traumatic displaced spondylolisthesis of fourth cervical vertebra A, K 🪙, B 🪙, A, B 🪙, **A, B** 🪙

    ● S12.331   Unspecified traumatic nondisplaced spondylolisthesis of fourth cervical vertebra A, K 🪙, B 🪙, A, B 🪙, **A, B** 🪙

X ● S12.34   Type III traumatic spondylolisthesis of fourth cervical vertebra A, K 🪙, B 🪙, A, B 🪙, **A, B** 🪙

  ● S12.35   Other traumatic spondylolisthesis of fourth cervical vertebra

    ● S12.350   Other traumatic displaced spondylolisthesis of fourth cervical vertebra A, K 🪙, B 🪙, A, B 🪙, **A, B** 🪙

    ● S12.351   Other traumatic nondisplaced spondylolisthesis of fourth cervical vertebra A, K 🪙, B 🪙, A, B 🪙, **A, B** 🪙

  ● S12.39   Other fracture of fourth cervical vertebra

    ● S12.390   Other displaced fracture of fourth cervical vertebra A, K 🪙, B 🪙, A, B 🪙, **A, B** 🪙

    ● S12.391   Other nondisplaced fracture of fourth cervical vertebra A, K 🪙, B 🪙, A, B 🪙, **A, B** 🪙

● S12.4   Fracture of fifth cervical vertebra

  ● S12.40   Unspecified fracture of fifth cervical vertebra

    ● S12.400   Unspecified displaced fracture of fifth cervical vertebra A, K 🪙, B 🪙, A, B 🪙, **A, B** 🪙

    ● S12.401   Unspecified nondisplaced fracture of fifth cervical vertebra A, K 🪙, B 🪙, A, B 🪙, **A, B** 🪙

● S12.43   Unspecified traumatic spondylolisthesis of fifth cervical vertebra

  ● S12.430   Unspecified traumatic displaced spondylolisthesis of fifth cervical vertebra A, K 🪙, B 🪙, A, B 🪙, **A, B** 🪙

  ● S12.431   Unspecified traumatic nondisplaced spondylolisthesis of fifth cervical vertebra A, K 🪙, B 🪙, A, B 🪙, **A, B** 🪙

X ● S12.44   Type III traumatic spondylolisthesis of fifth cervical vertebra A, K 🪙, B 🪙, A, B 🪙, **A, B** 🪙

● S12.45   Other traumatic spondylolisthesis of fifth cervical vertebra

  ● S12.450   Other traumatic displaced spondylolisthesis of fifth cervical vertebra A, K 🪙, B 🪙, A, B 🪙, **A, B** 🪙

  ● S12.451   Other traumatic nondisplaced spondylolisthesis of fifth cervical vertebra A, K 🪙, B 🪙, A, B 🪙, **A, B** 🪙

● S12.49   Other fracture of fifth cervical vertebra

  ● S12.490   Other displaced fracture of fifth cervical vertebra A, K 🪙, B 🪙, A, B 🪙, **A, B** 🪙

  ● S12.491   Other nondisplaced fracture of fifth cervical vertebra A, K 🪙, B 🪙, A, B 🪙, **A, B** 🪙

● S12.5   Fracture of sixth cervical vertebra

  ● S12.50   Unspecified fracture of sixth cervical vertebra

    ● S12.500   Unspecified displaced fracture of sixth cervical vertebra A, K 🪙, B 🪙, A, B 🪙, **A, B** 🪙

    ● S12.501   Unspecified nondisplaced fracture of sixth cervical vertebra A, K 🪙, B 🪙, A, B 🪙, **A, B** 🪙

  ● S12.53   Unspecified traumatic spondylolisthesis of sixth cervical vertebra

    ● S12.530   Unspecified traumatic displaced spondylolisthesis of sixth cervical vertebra A, K 🪙, B 🪙, A, B 🪙, **A, B** 🪙

    ● S12.531   Unspecified traumatic nondisplaced spondylolisthesis of sixth cervical vertebra A, K 🪙, B 🪙, A, B 🪙, **A, B** 🪙

X ● S12.54   Type III traumatic spondylolisthesis of sixth cervical vertebra A, K 🪙, B 🪙, A, B 🪙, **A, B** 🪙

  ● S12.55   Other traumatic spondylolisthesis of sixth cervical vertebra

    ● S12.550   Other traumatic displaced spondylolisthesis of sixth cervical vertebra A, K 🪙, B 🪙, A, B 🪙, **A, B** 🪙

    ● S12.551   Other traumatic nondisplaced spondylolisthesis of sixth cervical vertebra A, K 🪙, B 🪙, A, B 🪙, **A, B** 🪙

  ● S12.59   Other fracture of sixth cervical vertebra

    ● S12.590   Other displaced fracture of sixth cervical vertebra A, K 🪙, B 🪙, A, B 🪙, **A, B** 🪙

    ● S12.591   Other nondisplaced fracture of sixth cervical vertebra A, K 🪙, B 🪙, A, B 🪙, **A, B** 🪙

● S12.6   Fracture of seventh cervical vertebra

  S12.60   Unspecified fracture of seventh cervical vertebra

    ● S12.600   Unspecified displaced fracture of seventh cervical vertebra A, K 🪙, B 🪙, A, B 🪙, **A, B** 🪙

    ● S12.601   Unspecified nondisplaced fracture of seventh cervical vertebra A, K 🪙, B 🪙, A, B 🪙, **A, B** 🪙

▶ New   ⟹ Revised   ~~deleted~~ Deleted   Excludes 1   Excludes 2   Includes   Use additional   Code first   Code also   Key words

OGCR Official Guidelines   ● Unacceptable Principal Diagnosis   X Assign placeholder X   ● Use Additional Character(s)   ▷ Manifestation Code   **Coding Clinic**

● **S12.63** Unspecified traumatic spondylolisthesis of seventh cervical vertebra
　　● **S12.630** Unspecified traumatic displaced spondylolisthesis of seventh cervical vertebra A, K 🅒, B 🅜, A, B 🅜, **A, B** 🅗🅒
　　● **S12.631** Unspecified traumatic nondisplaced spondylolisthesis of seventh cervical vertebra A, K 🅒, B 🅜, A, B 🅜, **A, B** 🅗🅒
X ● **S12.64** Type III traumatic spondylolisthesis of seventh cervical vertebra A, K 🅒, B 🅜, A, B 🅜, **A, B** 🅗🅒
● **S12.65** Other traumatic spondylolisthesis of seventh cervical vertebra
　　● **S12.650** Other traumatic displaced spondylolisthesis of seventh cervical vertebra A, K 🅒, B 🅜, A, B 🅜, **A, B** 🅗🅒
　　● **S12.651** Other traumatic nondisplaced spondylolisthesis of seventh cervical vertebra A, K 🅒, B 🅜, A, B 🅜, **A, B** 🅗🅒
● **S12.69** Other fracture of seventh cervical vertebra
　　● **S12.690** Other displaced fracture of seventh cervical vertebra A, K 🅒, B 🅜, A, B 🅜, **A, B** 🅗🅒
　　● **S12.691** Other nondisplaced fracture of seventh cervical vertebra A, K 🅒, B 🅜, A, B 🅜, **A, B** 🅗🅒

X ● **S12.8** Fracture of other parts of neck A 🅒, A 🅜, **A** 🅗🅒
　　Hyoid bone　　　　Thyroid cartilage
　　Larynx　　　　　 Trachea

　　The appropriate 7th character is to be added to code S12.8

A	initial encounter
D	subsequent encounter
S	sequela

(Ex:) See PDX Collection 1165

X ● **S12.9** Fracture of neck, unspecified A 🅒, A 🅜, **A** 🅗🅒
　　Fracture of neck NOS
　　Fracture of cervical spine NOS
　　Fracture of cervical vertebra NOS

　　The appropriate 7th character is to be added to code S12.9

A	initial encounter
D	subsequent encounter
S	sequela

● **S13** Dislocation and sprain of joints and ligaments at neck level
　　Includes avulsion of joint or ligament at neck level
　　　　laceration of cartilage, joint or ligament at neck level
　　　　sprain of cartilage, joint or ligament at neck level
　　　　traumatic hemarthrosis of joint or ligament at neck level
　　　　traumatic rupture of joint or ligament at neck level
　　　　traumatic subluxation of joint or ligament at neck level
　　　　traumatic tear of joint or ligament at neck level
　　Code also any associated open wound
　　Excludes2 strain of muscle or tendon at neck level (S16.1)
　　The appropriate 7th character is to be added to each code from category S13

A	initial encounter
D	subsequent encounter
S	sequela

(Ex:) **For category S13 CC codes:** See PDX Collection 913

X ● **S13.0** Traumatic rupture of cervical intervertebral disc A 🅒, A 🅜
　　　　Excludes1 rupture or displacement (nontraumatic) of cervical intervertebral disc NOS (M50.-)

● **S13.1** Subluxation and dislocation of cervical vertebrae
　　Code also any associated:
　　　open wound of neck (S11.-)
　　　spinal cord injury (S14.1-)
　　Excludes2 fracture of cervical vertebrae (S12.0-S12.3-)
● **S13.10** Subluxation and dislocation of unspecified cervical vertebrae
　　● **S13.100** Subluxation of unspecified cervical vertebrae A 🅒, A 🅜
　　● **S13.101** Dislocation of unspecified cervical vertebrae A 🅒, A 🅜
● **S13.11** Subluxation and dislocation of C0/C1 cervical vertebrae
　　Subluxation and dislocation of atlantooccipital joint
　　Subluxation and dislocation of atloidooccipital joint
　　Subluxation and dislocation of occipitoatloid joint
　　● **S13.110** Subluxation of C0/C1 cervical vertebrae A 🅒, A 🅜
　　● **S13.111** Dislocation of C0/C1 cervical vertebrae A 🅒, A 🅜
● **S13.12** Subluxation and dislocation of C1/C2 cervical vertebrae
　　Subluxation and dislocation of atlantoaxial joint
　　● **S13.120** Subluxation of C1/C2 cervical vertebrae A 🅒, A 🅜
　　● **S13.121** Dislocation of C1/C2 cervical vertebrae A 🅒, A 🅜
● **S13.13** Subluxation and dislocation of C2/C3 cervical vertebrae
　　● **S13.130** Subluxation of C2/C3 cervical vertebrae A 🅒, A 🅜
　　● **S13.131** Dislocation of C2/C3 cervical vertebrae A 🅒, A 🅜
● **S13.14** Subluxation and dislocation of C3/C4 cervical vertebrae
　　● **S13.140** Subluxation of C3/C4 cervical vertebrae A 🅒, A 🅜
　　● **S13.141** Dislocation of C3/C4 cervical vertebrae A 🅒, A 🅜
● **S13.15** Subluxation and dislocation of C4/C5 cervical vertebrae
　　● **S13.150** Subluxation of C4/C5 cervical vertebrae A 🅒, A 🅜
　　● **S13.151** Dislocation of C4/C5 cervical vertebrae A 🅒, A 🅜
● **S13.16** Subluxation and dislocation of C5/C6 cervical vertebrae
　　● **S13.160** Subluxation of C5/C6 cervical vertebrae A 🅒, A 🅜
　　● **S13.161** Dislocation of C5/C6 cervical vertebrae A 🅒, A 🅜
● **S13.17** Subluxation and dislocation of C6/C7 cervical vertebrae
　　● **S13.170** Subluxation of C6/C7 cervical vertebrae A 🅒, A 🅜
　　● **S13.171** Dislocation of C6/C7 cervical vertebrae A 🅒, A 🅜

● **S13.18**   **Subluxation and dislocation of C7/T1 cervical vertebrae**
     ● **S13.180**   **Subluxation of C7/T1 cervical vertebrae** A 🔖, A 🔖
     ● **S13.181**   **Dislocation of C7/T1 cervical vertebrae** A 🔖, A 🔖

● **S13.2**   **Dislocation of other and unspecified parts of neck**
   X ● **S13.20**   **Dislocation of unspecified parts of neck** A 🔖, A 🔖
   X ● **S13.29**   **Dislocation of other parts of neck** A 🔖, A 🔖

X ● **S13.4**   **Sprain of ligaments of cervical spine**
     Sprain of anterior longitudinal (ligament), cervical
     Sprain of atlanto-axial (joints)
     Sprain of atlanto-occipital (joints)
     Whiplash injury of cervical spine

X ● **S13.5**   **Sprain of thyroid region**
     Sprain of cricoarytenoid (joint) (ligament)
     Sprain of cricothyroid (joint) (ligament)
     Sprain of thyroid cartilage

X ● **S13.8**   **Sprain of joints and ligaments of other parts of neck**

X ● **S13.9**   **Sprain of joints and ligaments of unspecified parts of neck**

● **S14**   **Injury of nerves and spinal cord at neck level**
     Note: Code to highest level of cervical cord injury
     Code also any associated:
       fracture of cervical vertebra (S12.0--S12.6.-)
       open wound of neck (S11.-)
       transient paralysis (R29.5)
     The appropriate 7th character is to be added to each code from category S14

> A   initial encounter
> D   subsequent encounter
> S   sequela

     (Ex:) **For category S14 CC codes:** See PDX Collection 1166

X ● **S14.0**   **Concussion and edema of cervical spinal cord** A 🔖, A, D, S 🔖

● **S14.1**   **Other and unspecified injuries of cervical spinal cord**
   ● **S14.10**   **Unspecified injury of cervical spinal cord**
     ● **S14.101**   **Unspecified injury at C1 level of cervical spinal cord** A 🔖, A 🔖, A, D, S 🔖
     ● **S14.102**   **Unspecified injury at C2 level of cervical spinal cord** A 🔖, A 🔖, A, D, S 🔖
     ● **S14.103**   **Unspecified injury at C3 level of cervical spinal cord** A 🔖, A 🔖, A, D, S 🔖
     ● **S14.104**   **Unspecified injury at C4 level of cervical spinal cord** A 🔖, A 🔖, A, D, S 🔖
     ● **S14.105**   **Unspecified injury at C5 level of cervical spinal cord** A 🔖, A 🔖, A, D, S 🔖
     ● **S14.106**   **Unspecified injury at C6 level of cervical spinal cord** A 🔖, A 🔖, A, D, S 🔖

● **S14.107**   **Unspecified injury at C7 level of cervical spinal cord** A 🔖, A 🔖, A, D, S 🔖
● **S14.108**   **Unspecified injury at C8 level of cervical spinal cord** A 🔖, A, D, S 🔖
● **S14.109**   **Unspecified injury at unspecified level of cervical spinal cord** A, D, S 🔖
     Injury of cervical spinal cord NOS

● **S14.11**   **Complete lesion of cervical spinal cord**
   ● **S14.111**   **Complete lesion at C1 level of cervical spinal cord** A 🔖, A 🔖, A, D, S 🔖
   ● **S14.112**   **Complete lesion at C2 level of cervical spinal cord** A 🔖, A 🔖, A, D, S 🔖
   ● **S14.113**   **Complete lesion at C3 level of cervical spinal cord** A 🔖, A 🔖, A, D, S 🔖
   ● **S14.114**   **Complete lesion at C4 level of cervical spinal cord** A 🔖, A 🔖, A, D, S 🔖
   ● **S14.115**   **Complete lesion at C5 level of cervical spinal cord** A 🔖, A 🔖, A, D, S 🔖
   ● **S14.116**   **Complete lesion at C6 level of cervical spinal cord** A 🔖, A 🔖, A, D, S 🔖
   ● **S14.117**   **Complete lesion at C7 level of cervical spinal cord** A 🔖, A 🔖, A, D, S 🔖
   ● **S14.118**   **Complete lesion at C8 level of cervical spinal cord** A 🔖, A, D, S 🔖
   ● **S14.119**   **Complete lesion at unspecified level of cervical spinal cord** A, D, S 🔖

● **S14.12**   **Central cord syndrome of cervical spinal cord**
   ● **S14.121**   **Central cord syndrome at C1 level of cervical spinal cord** A 🔖, A 🔖, A, D, S 🔖
   ● **S14.122**   **Central cord syndrome at C2 level of cervical spinal cord** A 🔖, A 🔖, A, D, S 🔖
   ● **S14.123**   **Central cord syndrome at C3 level of cervical spinal cord** A 🔖, A 🔖, A, D, S 🔖
   ● **S14.124**   **Central cord syndrome at C4 level of cervical spinal cord** A 🔖, A 🔖, A, D, S 🔖
   ● **S14.125**   **Central cord syndrome at C5 level of cervical spinal cord** A 🔖, A 🔖, A, D, S 🔖
   ● **S14.126**   **Central cord syndrome at C6 level of cervical spinal cord** A 🔖, A 🔖, A, D, S 🔖
   ● **S14.127**   **Central cord syndrome at C7 level of cervical spinal cord** A 🔖, A 🔖, A, D, S 🔖
   ● **S14.128**   **Central cord syndrome at C8 level of cervical spinal cord** A 🔖, A, D, S 🔖
   ● **S14.129**   **Central cord syndrome at unspecified level of cervical spinal cord** A, D, S 🔖

► New   ⇒ Revised   ~~deleted~~ Deleted   Excludes 1   Excludes 2   Includes   Use additional   Code first   Code also   Key words
OGCR Official Guidelines   ● Unacceptable Principal Diagnosis   X Assign placeholder X   ● Use Additional Character(s)   ▷ Manifestation Code   **Coding Clinic**

- **S14.13** Anterior cord syndrome of cervical spinal cord
  - **S14.131** Anterior cord syndrome at C1 level of cervical spinal cord A 🐾, A 🐾, A, D, S 🐾
  - **S14.132** Anterior cord syndrome at C2 level of cervical spinal cord A 🐾, A 🐾, A, D, S 🐾
  - **S14.133** Anterior cord syndrome at C3 level of cervical spinal cord A 🐾, A 🐾, A, D, S 🐾
  - **S14.134** Anterior cord syndrome at C4 level of cervical spinal cord A 🐾, A 🐾, A, D, S 🐾
  - **S14.135** Anterior cord syndrome at C5 level of cervical spinal cord A 🐾, A 🐾, A, D, S 🐾
  - **S14.136** Anterior cord syndrome at C6 level of cervical spinal cord A 🐾, A 🐾, A, D, S 🐾
  - **S14.137** Anterior cord syndrome at C7 level of cervical spinal cord A 🐾, A 🐾, A, D, S 🐾
  - **S14.138** Anterior cord syndrome at C8 level of cervical spinal cord A 🐾, A, D, S 🐾
  - **S14.139** Anterior cord syndrome at unspecified level of cervical spinal cord, A, D, S 🐾
- **S14.14** Brown-Séquard syndrome of cervical spinal cord
  - **S14.141** Brown-Séquard syndrome at C1 level of cervical spinal cord A 🐾, A, D, S 🐾
  - **S14.142** Brown-Séquard syndrome at C2 level of cervical spinal cord A 🐾, A, D, S 🐾
  - **S14.143** Brown-Séquard syndrome at C3 level of cervical spinal cord A 🐾, A, D, S 🐾
  - **S14.144** Brown-Séquard syndrome at C4 level of cervical spinal cord A 🐾, A, D, S 🐾
  - **S14.145** Brown-Séquard syndrome at C5 level of cervical spinal cord A 🐾, A, D, S 🐾
  - **S14.146** Brown-Séquard syndrome at C6 level of cervical spinal cord A 🐾, A, D, S 🐾
  - **S14.147** Brown-Séquard syndrome at C7 level of cervical spinal cord A 🐾, A, D, S 🐾
  - **S14.148** Brown-Séquard syndrome at C8 level of cervical spinal cord A 🐾, A, D, S 🐾
  - **S14.149** Brown-Séquard syndrome at unspecified level of cervical spinal cord A, D, S 🐾
- **S14.15** Other incomplete lesions of cervical spinal cord
  Incomplete lesion of cervical spinal cord NOS
  Posterior cord syndrome of cervical spinal cord
  - **S14.151** Other incomplete lesion at C1 level of cervical spinal cord A 🐾, A 🐾, A, D, S 🐾
  - **S14.152** Other incomplete lesion at C2 level of cervical spinal cord A 🐾, A 🐾, A, D, S 🐾
  - **S14.153** Other incomplete lesion at C3 level of cervical spinal cord A 🐾, A 🐾, A, D, S 🐾
  - **S14.154** Other incomplete lesion at C4 level of cervical spinal cord A 🐾, A 🐾, A, D, S 🐾
  - **S14.155** Other incomplete lesion at C5 level of cervical spinal cord A 🐾, A 🐾, A, D, S 🐾
  - **S14.156** Other incomplete lesion at C6 level of cervical spinal cord A 🐾, A 🐾, A, D, S 🐾
  - **S14.157** Other incomplete lesion at C7 level of cervical spinal cord A 🐾, A 🐾, A, D, S 🐾
  - **S14.158** Other incomplete lesion at C8 level of cervical spinal cord A 🐾, A, D, S 🐾
  - **S14.159** Other incomplete lesion at unspecified level of cervical spinal cord A, D, S 🐾
- X● **S14.2** Injury of nerve root of cervical spine
- X● **S14.3** Injury of brachial plexus
- X● **S14.4** Injury of peripheral nerves of neck
- X● **S14.5** Injury of cervical sympathetic nerves
- X● **S14.8** Injury of other specified nerves of neck
- X● **S14.9** Injury of unspecified nerves of neck

- **S15** Injury of blood vessels at neck level
  Code also any associated open wound (S11.-)
  The appropriate 7th character is to be added to each code from category S15

A	initial encounter
D	subsequent encounter
S	sequela

  - **S15.0** Injury of carotid artery of neck
    Injury of carotid artery (common) (external) (internal, extracranial portion)
    Injury of carotid artery NOS
    Excludes1   injury of internal carotid artery, intracranial portion (S06.8)
    (Ex:) **For category S15.0 CC codes unless otherwise indicated:** See PDX Collection 1167
    - **S15.00** Unspecified injury of carotid artery
      - **S15.001** Unspecified injury of right carotid artery A 🐾
        (Ex:) See PDX Collection 3405
      - **S15.002** Unspecified injury of left carotid artery A 🐾
        (Ex:) See PDX Collection 3406
      - **S15.009** Unspecified injury of unspecified carotid artery A 🐾
    - **S15.01** Minor laceration of carotid artery
      Incomplete transection of carotid artery
      Laceration of carotid artery NOS
      Superficial laceration of carotid artery
      - **S15.011** Minor laceration of right carotid artery A 🐾
        (Ex:) See PDX Collection 3407
      - **S15.012** Minor laceration of left carotid artery A 🐾
        (Ex:) See PDX Collection 3408
      - **S15.019** Minor laceration of unspecified carotid artery A 🐾
        (Ex:) See PDX Collection 3409
    - **S15.02** Major laceration of carotid artery
      Complete transection of carotid artery
      Traumatic rupture of carotid artery
      - **S15.021** Major laceration of right carotid artery A 🐾
        (Ex:) See PDX Collection 3410
      - **S15.022** Major laceration of left carotid artery A 🐾
        (Ex:) See PDX Collection 3411
      - **S15.029** Major laceration of unspecified carotid artery A 🐾
    - **S15.09** Other specified injury of carotid artery
      - **S15.091** Other specified injury of right carotid artery A 🐾
        (Ex:) See PDX Collection 3412
      - **S15.092** Other specified injury of left carotid artery A 🐾
        (Ex:) See PDX Collection 3413
      - **S15.099** Other specified injury of unspecified carotid artery A 🐾

N Newborn Age: 0	**P** Pediatric Age: 0–17	**M** Maternity DX: 9–64	**A** Adult Age: 15–124	♀ Females Only	♂ Males Only
🐾 Complication\Comorbidity	🐾 Major C\C	(Ex:) CC/MCC Exclusions	🐾 Hospital-Acquired Condition	🐾 Hierarchical Condition Category	

● **S15.1   Injury of vertebral artery**
Ex: For category S15.1 CC codes: See PDX Collection 1157

● **S15.10   Unspecified injury of vertebral artery**

● **S15.101   Unspecified injury of right vertebral artery** A 🔍

● **S15.102   Unspecified injury of left vertebral artery** A 🔍

● **S15.109   Unspecified injury of unspecified vertebral artery** A 🔍

● **S15.11   Minor laceration of vertebral artery**
Incomplete transection of vertebral artery
Laceration of vertebral artery NOS
Superficial laceration of vertebral artery

● **S15.111   Minor laceration of right vertebral artery** A 🔍

● **S15.112   Minor laceration of left vertebral artery** A 🔍

● **S15.119   Minor laceration of unspecified vertebral artery** A 🔍

● **S15.12   Major laceration of vertebral artery**
Complete transection of vertebral artery
Traumatic rupture of vertebral artery

● **S15.121   Major laceration of right vertebral artery** A 🔍

● **S15.122   Major laceration of left vertebral artery** A 🔍

● **S15.129   Major laceration of unspecified vertebral artery** A 🔍

● **S15.19   Other specified injury of vertebral artery**

● **S15.191   Other specified injury of right vertebral artery** A 🔍

● **S15.192   Other specified injury of left vertebral artery** A 🔍

● **S15.199   Other specified injury of unspecified vertebral artery** A 🔍

● **S15.2   Injury of external jugular vein**

● **S15.20   Unspecified injury of external jugular vein**

● **S15.201   Unspecified injury of right external jugular vein** A 🔍
Ex: See PDX Collection 3414

● **S15.202   Unspecified injury of left external jugular vein** A 🔍
Ex: See PDX Collection 3415

● **S15.209   Unspecified injury of unspecified external jugular vein** A 🔍
Ex: See PDX Collection 3416

● **S15.21   Minor laceration of external jugular vein**
Incomplete transection of external jugular vein
Laceration of external jugular vein NOS
Superficial laceration of external jugular vein

● **S15.211   Minor laceration of right external jugular vein** A 🔍
Ex: See PDX Collection 3417

● **S15.212   Minor laceration of left external jugular vein** A 🔍
Ex: See PDX Collection 3418

● **S15.219   Minor laceration of unspecified external jugular vein** A 🔍
Ex: See PDX Collection 3419

● **S15.22   Major laceration of external jugular vein**
Complete transection of external jugular vein
Traumatic rupture of external jugular vein

● **S15.221   Major laceration of right external jugular vein** A 🔍
Ex: See PDX Collection 3420

● **S15.222   Major laceration of left external jugular vein** A 🔍
Ex: See PDX Collection 3421

● **S15.229   Major laceration of unspecified external jugular vein** A 🔍
Ex: See PDX Collection 3422

● **S15.29   Other specified injury of external jugular vein**

● **S15.291   Other specified injury of right external jugular vein** A 🔍
Ex: See PDX Collection 3423

● **S15.292   Other specified injury of left external jugular vein** A 🔍
Ex: See PDX Collection 3424

● **S15.299   Other specified injury of unspecified external jugular vein** A 🔍
Ex: See PDX Collection 3425

● **S15.3   Injury of internal jugular vein**

● **S15.30   Unspecified injury of internal jugular vein**

● **S15.301   Unspecified injury of right internal jugular vein** A 🔍
Ex: See PDX Collection 3426

● **S15.302   Unspecified injury of left internal jugular vein** A 🔍
Ex: See PDX Collection 3427

● **S15.309   Unspecified injury of unspecified internal jugular vein** A 🔍
Ex: See PDX Collection 3428

● **S15.31   Minor laceration of internal jugular vein**
Incomplete transection of internal jugular vein
Laceration of internal jugular vein NOS
Superficial laceration of internal jugular vein

● **S15.311   Minor laceration of right internal jugular vein** A 🔍
Ex: See PDX Collection 3429

● **S15.312   Minor laceration of left internal jugular vein** A 🔍
Ex: See PDX Collection 3430

● **S15.319   Minor laceration of unspecified internal jugular vein** A 🔍
Ex: See PDX Collection 3431

● **S15.32   Major laceration of internal jugular vein**
Complete transection of internal jugular vein
Traumatic rupture of internal jugular vein

● **S15.321   Major laceration of right internal jugular vein** A 🔍
Ex: See PDX Collection 3432

● **S15.322   Major laceration of left internal jugular vein** A 🔍
Ex: See PDX Collection 3433

● **S15.329   Major laceration of unspecified internal jugular vein** A 🔍
Ex: See PDX Collection 3434

● **S15.39   Other specified injury of internal jugular vein**

● **S15.391   Other specified injury of right internal jugular vein** A 🔍
Ex: See PDX Collection 3435

● **S15.392   Other specified injury of left internal jugular vein** A 🔍
Ex: See PDX Collection 3436

● **S15.399   Other specified injury of unspecified internal jugular vein** A 🔍
Ex: See PDX Collection 3437

X ● **S15.8   Injury of other specified blood vessels at neck level** A 🔍
Ex: See PDX Collection 1157

X ● **S15.9   Injury of unspecified blood vessel at neck level** A 🔍
Ex: See PDX Collection 1157

● **S16   Injury of muscle, fascia and tendon at neck level**
Code also any associated open wound (S11.-)

Excludes2   sprain of joint or ligament at neck level (S13.9)

The appropriate 7th character is to be added to each code from category S16

A	initial encounter
D	subsequent encounter
S	sequela

X ● **S16.1   Strain of muscle, fascia and tendon at neck level**
X ● **S16.2   Laceration of muscle, fascia and tendon at neck level**

▶ New   ➡ Revised   ~~deleted~~ Deleted   Excludes 1   Excludes 2   Includes   Use additional   Code first   Code also   Key words

OGCR Official Guidelines   ● Unacceptable Principal Diagnosis   X Assign placeholder X   ● Use Additional Character(s)   ▶ Manifestation Code   Coding Clinic

X ● **S16.8**   Other specified injury of muscle, fascia and tendon at neck level
X ● **S16.9**   Unspecified injury of muscle, fascia and tendon at neck level

● **S17**   Crushing injury of neck
> Use additional code for all associated injuries, such as:
>> injury of blood vessels (S15.-)
>> open wound of neck (S11.-)
>> spinal cord injury (S14.0, S14.1-)
>> vertebral fracture (S12.0--S12.3-)
>
> The appropriate 7th character is to be added to each code from category S17

> | | |
> |---|---|
> | A | initial encounter |
> | D | subsequent encounter |
> | S | sequela |

> (Ex) **For category S17 CC codes:** See PDX Collection 123

X ● **S17.0**   Crushing injury of larynx and trachea A 🪙, A 🪙
X ● **S17.8**   Crushing injury of other specified parts of neck A 🪙, A 🪙
X ● **S17.9**   Crushing injury of neck, part unspecified A 🪙, A 🪙

● **S19**   Other and unspecified injuries of neck
> The appropriate 7th character is to be added to each code from category S19

> | | |
> |---|---|
> | A | initial encounter |
> | D | subsequent encounter |
> | S | sequela |

● **S19.8**   Other specified injuries of neck
  X ● **S19.80**   Other specified injuries of unspecified part of neck
  X ● **S19.81**   Other specified injuries of larynx
  X ● **S19.82**   Other specified injuries of cervical trachea
    > **Excludes2**   other specified injury of thoracic trachea (S27.5-)
  X ● **S19.83**   Other specified injuries of vocal cord
  X ● **S19.84**   Other specified injuries of thyroid gland
  X ● **S19.85**   Other specified injuries of pharynx and cervical esophagus
  X ● **S19.89**   Other specified injuries of other specified part of neck
X ● **S19.9**   Unspecified injury of neck

INJURIES TO THE THORAX (S20-S29)

Includes   injuries of breast
injuries of chest (wall)
injuries of interscapular area

Excludes2   burns and corrosions (T20-T32)
effects of foreign body in bronchus (T17.5)
effects of foreign body in esophagus (T18.1)
effects of foreign body in lung (T17.8)
effects of foreign body in trachea (T17.4)
frostbite (T33-T34)
injuries of axilla
injuries of clavicle
injuries of scapular region
injuries of shoulder
insect bite or sting, venomous (T63.4)

● **S20**   Superficial injury of thorax
> The appropriate 7th character is to be added to each code from category S20

> | | |
> |---|---|
> | A | initial encounter |
> | D | subsequent encounter |
> | S | sequela |

● **S20.0**   Contusion of breast
  X ● **S20.00**   Contusion of breast, unspecified breast
  X ● **S20.01**   Contusion of right breast
  X ● **S20.02**   Contusion of left breast

● **S20.1**   Other and unspecified superficial injuries of breast
  ● **S20.10**   Unspecified superficial injuries of breast
    ● **S20.101**   Unspecified superficial injuries of breast, right breast
    ● **S20.102**   Unspecified superficial injuries of breast, left breast
    ● **S20.109**   Unspecified superficial injuries of breast, unspecified breast
  ● **S20.11**   Abrasion of breast
    ● **S20.111**   Abrasion of breast, right breast
    ● **S20.112**   Abrasion of breast, left breast
    ● **S20.119**   Abrasion of breast, unspecified breast
  ● **S20.12**   Blister (nonthermal) of breast
    ● **S20.121**   Blister (nonthermal) of breast, right breast
    ● **S20.122**   Blister (nonthermal) of breast, left breast
    ● **S20.129**   Blister (nonthermal) of breast, unspecified breast
  ● **S20.14**   External constriction of part of breast
    ● **S20.141**   External constriction of part of breast, right breast
    ● **S20.142**   External constriction of part of breast, left breast
    ● **S20.149**   External constriction of part of breast, unspecified breast
  ● **S20.15**   Superficial foreign body of breast
    > Splinter in the breast
    ● **S20.151**   Superficial foreign body of breast, right breast
    ● **S20.152**   Superficial foreign body of breast, left breast
    ● **S20.159**   Superficial foreign body of breast, unspecified breast
  ● **S20.16**   Insect bite (nonvenomous) of breast
    ● **S20.161**   Insect bite (nonvenomous) of breast, right breast
    ● **S20.162**   Insect bite (nonvenomous) of breast, left breast
    ● **S20.169**   Insect bite (nonvenomous) of breast, unspecified breast
  ● **S20.17**   Other superficial bite of breast
    > **Excludes1**   open bite of breast (S21.05-)
    ● **S20.171**   Other superficial bite of breast, right breast
    ● **S20.172**   Other superficial bite of breast, left breast
    ● **S20.179**   Other superficial bite of breast, unspecified breast
● **S20.2**   Contusion of thorax
  X ● **S20.20**   Contusion of thorax, unspecified
  ● **S20.21**   Contusion of front wall of thorax
    ● **S20.211**   Contusion of right front wall of thorax
    ● **S20.212**   Contusion of left front wall of thorax
    S20.213   Contusion of bilateral front wall of thorax
    S20.214   Contusion of middle front wall of thorax
    ● **S20.219**   Contusion of unspecified front wall of thorax
  ● **S20.22**   Contusion of back wall of thorax
    ● **S20.221**   Contusion of right back wall of thorax
    ● **S20.222**   Contusion of left back wall of thorax
    S20.223   Contusion of bilateral back wall of thorax
    S20.224   Contusion of middle back wall of thorax
    ● **S20.229**   Contusion of unspecified back wall of thorax

N Newborn Age: 0   **P** Pediatric Age: 0–17   **M** Maternity DX: 9–64   **A** Adult Age: 15–124   ♀ Females Only   ♂ Males Only

🪙 Complication\Comorbidity   🪙 Major C\C   (Ex) CC/MCC Exclusions   🪙 Hospital-Acquired Condition   🪙 Hierarchical Condition Category

1273

● **S20.3**   Other and unspecified superficial injuries of front wall of thorax

  ● **S20.30**   Unspecified superficial injuries of front wall of thorax

    ● **S20.301**   Unspecified superficial injuries of right front wall of thorax

    ● **S20.302**   Unspecified superficial injuries of left front wall of thorax

    S20.303   Unspecified superficial injuries of bilateral front wall of thorax

    S20.304   Unspecified superficial injuries of middle front wall of thorax

    ● **S20.309**   Unspecified superficial injuries of unspecified front wall of thorax

  ● **S20.31**   Abrasion of front wall of thorax

    ● **S20.311**   Abrasion of right front wall of thorax

    ● **S20.312**   Abrasion of left front wall of thorax

    S20.313   Abrasion of bilateral front wall of thorax

    S20.314   Abrasion of middle front wall of thorax

    ● **S20.319**   Abrasion of unspecified front wall of thorax

  ● **S20.32**   Blister (nonthermal) of front wall of thorax

    ● **S20.321**   Blister (nonthermal) of right front wall of thorax

    ● **S20.322**   Blister (nonthermal) of left front wall of thorax

    S20.323   Blister (nonthermal) of bilateral front wall of thorax

    S20.324   Blister (nonthermal) of middle front wall of thorax

    ● **S20.329**   Blister (nonthermal) of unspecified front wall of thorax

  ● **S20.34**   External constriction of front wall of thorax

    ● **S20.341**   External constriction of right front wall of thorax

    ● **S20.342**   External constriction of left front wall of thorax

    S20.343   External constriction of bilateral front wall of thorax

    S20.344   External constriction of middle front wall of thorax

    ● **S20.349**   External constriction of unspecified front wall of thorax

  ● **S20.35**   Superficial foreign body of front wall of thorax

    Splinter in front wall of thorax

    ● **S20.351**   Superficial foreign body of right front wall of thorax

    ● **S20.352**   Superficial foreign body of left front wall of thorax

    S20.353   Superficial foreign body of bilateral front wall of thorax

    S20.354   Superficial foreign body of middle front wall of thorax

    ● **S20.359**   Superficial foreign body of unspecified front wall of thorax

  ● **S20.36**   Insect bite (nonvenomous) of front wall of thorax

    ● **S20.361**   Insect bite (nonvenomous) of right front wall of thorax

    ● **S20.362**   Insect bite (nonvenomous) of left front wall of thorax

    S20.363   Insect bite (nonvenomous) of bilateral front wall of thorax

    S20.364   Insect bite (nonvenomous) of middle front wall of thorax

    ● **S20.369**   Insect bite (nonvenomous) of unspecified front wall of thorax

  ● **S20.37**   Other superficial bite of front wall of thorax

    Excludes1   open bite of front wall of thorax (S21.14)

    ● **S20.371**   Other superficial bite of right front wall of thorax

    ● **S20.372**   Other superficial bite of left front wall of thorax

    S20.373   Other superficial bite of bilateral front wall of thorax

    S20.374   Other superficial bite of middle front wall of thorax

    ● **S20.379**   Other superficial bite of unspecified front wall of thorax

● **S20.4**   Other and unspecified superficial injuries of back wall of thorax

  ● **S20.40**   Unspecified superficial injuries of back wall of thorax

    ● **S20.401**   Unspecified superficial injuries of right back wall of thorax

    ● **S20.402**   Unspecified superficial injuries of left back wall of thorax

    ● **S20.409**   Unspecified superficial injuries of unspecified back wall of thorax

  ● **S20.41**   Abrasion of back wall of thorax

    ● **S20.411**   Abrasion of right back wall of thorax

    ● **S20.412**   Abrasion of left back wall of thorax

    ● **S20.419**   Abrasion of unspecified back wall of thorax

  ● **S20.42**   Blister (nonthermal) of back wall of thorax

    ● **S20.421**   Blister (nonthermal) of right back wall of thorax

    ● **S20.422**   Blister (nonthermal) of left back wall of thorax

    ● **S20.429**   Blister (nonthermal) of unspecified back wall of thorax

  ● **S20.44**   External constriction of back wall of thorax

    ● **S20.441**   External constriction of right back wall of thorax

    ● **S20.442**   External constriction of left back wall of thorax

    ● **S20.449**   External constriction of unspecified back wall of thorax

  ● **S20.45**   Superficial foreign body of back wall of thorax

    Splinter of back wall of thorax

    ● **S20.451**   Superficial foreign body of right back wall of thorax

    ● **S20.452**   Superficial foreign body of left back wall of thorax

    ● **S20.459**   Superficial foreign body of unspecified back wall of thorax

  ● **S20.46**   Insect bite (nonvenomous) of back wall of thorax

    ● **S20.461**   Insect bite (nonvenomous) of right back wall of thorax

    ● **S20.462**   Insect bite (nonvenomous) of left back wall of thorax

    ● **S20.469**   Insect bite (nonvenomous) of unspecified back wall of thorax

  ● **S20.47**   Other superficial bite of back wall of thorax

    Excludes1   open bite of back wall of thorax (S21.24)

    ● **S20.471**   Other superficial bite of right back wall of thorax

    ● **S20.472**   Other superficial bite of left back wall of thorax

    ● **S20.479**   Other superficial bite of unspecified back wall of thorax

▶ New   ⇒ Revised   ~~deleted~~ Deleted   Excludes 1   Excludes 2   Includes   Use additional   Code first   Code also   Key words

OGCR Official Guidelines   ● Unacceptable Principal Diagnosis   X Assign placeholder X   ● Use Additional Character(s)   ▶ Manifestation Code   **Coding Clinic**

● **S20.9**   **Superficial injury of unspecified parts of thorax**
> **Excludes1**   contusion of thorax NOS (S20.20)

X● **S20.90**   **Unspecified superficial injury of unspecified parts of thorax**
> Superficial injury of thoracic wall NOS

X● **S20.91**   **Abrasion of unspecified parts of thorax**

X● **S20.92**   **Blister (nonthermal) of unspecified parts of thorax**

X● **S20.94**   **External constriction of unspecified parts of thorax**

X● **S20.95**   **Superficial foreign body of unspecified parts of thorax**
> Splinter in thorax NOS

X● **S20.96**   **Insect bite (nonvenomous) of unspecified parts of thorax**

X● **S20.97**   **Other superficial bite of unspecified parts of thorax**
> **Excludes1**   open bite of thorax NOS (S21.95)

● **S21**   **Open wound of thorax**
> Code also any associated injury such as:
> injury of heart (S26.-)
> injury of intrathoracic organs (S27.-)
> rib fracture (S22.3-, S22.4-)
> spinal cord injury (S24.0-, S24.1-)
> traumatic hemothorax (S27.1)
> traumatic hemopneumothorax (S27.3)
> traumatic pneumothorax (S27.0)
> wound infection
>
> **Excludes1**   traumatic amputation (partial) of thorax (S28.1)
>
> The appropriate 7th character is to be added to each code from category S21

A	initial encounter
D	subsequent encounter
S	sequela

● **S21.0**   **Open wound of breast**

   ● **S21.00**   **Unspecified open wound of breast**

     ● **S21.001**   Unspecified open wound of right breast

     ● **S21.002**   Unspecified open wound of left breast

     ● **S21.009**   Unspecified open wound of unspecified breast

   ● **S21.01**   **Laceration without foreign body of breast**

     ● **S21.011**   Laceration without foreign body of right breast

     ● **S21.012**   Laceration without foreign body of left breast

     ● **S21.019**   Laceration without foreign body of unspecified breast

   ● **S21.02**   **Laceration with foreign body of breast**

     ● **S21.021**   Laceration with foreign body of right breast

     ● **S21.022**   Laceration with foreign body of left breast

     ● **S21.029**   Laceration with foreign body of unspecified breast

● **S21.03**   **Puncture wound without foreign body of breast**

   ● **S21.031**   Puncture wound without foreign body of right breast

   ● **S21.032**   Puncture wound without foreign body of left breast

   ● **S21.039**   Puncture wound without foreign body of unspecified breast

● **S21.04**   **Puncture wound with foreign body of breast**

   ● **S21.041**   Puncture wound with foreign body of right breast

   ● **S21.042**   Puncture wound with foreign body of left breast

   ● **S21.049**   Puncture wound with foreign body of unspecified breast

● **S21.05**   **Open bite of breast**
> Bite of breast NOS
> **Excludes1**   superficial bite of breast (S20.17)

   ● **S21.051**   Open bite of right breast

   ● **S21.052**   Open bite of left breast

   ● **S21.059**   Open bite of unspecified breast

● **S21.1**   **Open wound of front wall of thorax without penetration into thoracic cavity**
> Open wound of chest without penetration into thoracic cavity
> (Ex) **For category S21.1 CC codes:** See PDX Collection 1168

   ● **S21.10**   **Unspecified open wound of front wall of thorax without penetration into thoracic cavity**

     ● **S21.101**   Unspecified open wound of right front wall of thorax without penetration into thoracic cavity A 🐾

     ● **S21.102**   Unspecified open wound of left front wall of thorax without penetration into thoracic cavity A 🐾

     ● **S21.109**   Unspecified open wound of unspecified front wall of thorax without penetration into thoracic cavity A 🐾

   ● **S21.11**   **Laceration without foreign body of front wall of thorax without penetration into thoracic cavity**

     ● **S21.111**   Laceration without foreign body of right front wall of thorax without penetration into thoracic cavity A 🐾

     ● **S21.112**   Laceration without foreign body of left front wall of thorax without penetration into thoracic cavity A 🐾

     ● **S21.119**   Laceration without foreign body of unspecified front wall of thorax without penetration into thoracic cavity A 🐾

   ● **S21.12**   **Laceration with foreign body of front wall of thorax without penetration into thoracic cavity**

     ● **S21.121**   Laceration with foreign body of right front wall of thorax without penetration into thoracic cavity A 🐾

     ● **S21.122**   Laceration with foreign body of left front wall of thorax without penetration into thoracic cavity A 🐾

     ● **S21.129**   Laceration with foreign body of unspecified front wall of thorax without penetration into thoracic cavity A 🐾

Item 19-1 Pneumothorax is a collection of gas (positive air pressure) in the pleural space, resulting in the lung collapsing. A **tension pneumothorax** is life-threatening and is a result of air in the pleural space causing a displacement in the mediastinal structures and cardiopulmonary function compromise. A **traumatic pneumothorax** results from blunt or penetrating injury that disrupts the parietal/visceral pleura. **Hemothorax** is blood or bloody fluid in the pleural cavity as a result of traumatic blood vessel rupture or inflammation of the lungs from pneumonia.

CHAPTER 19 (S00-T88)

N Newborn Age: 0	**P** Pediatric Age: 0–17	**M** Maternity DX: 9–64	**A** Adult Age: 15–124	♀ Females Only	♂ Males Only	
🐾 Complication\Comorbidity	🐾 Major C\C	(Ex) CC/MCC Exclusions	🐾 Hospital-Acquired Condition	🐾 Hierarchical Condition Category		

● **S21.13** Puncture wound without foreign body of front wall of thorax without penetration into thoracic cavity

● **S21.131** Puncture wound without foreign body of right front wall of thorax without penetration into thoracic cavity A 🔍

● **S21.132** Puncture wound without foreign body of left front wall of thorax without penetration into thoracic cavity A 🔍

● **S21.139** Puncture wound without foreign body of unspecified front wall of thorax without penetration into thoracic cavity A 🔍

● **S21.14** Puncture wound with foreign body of front wall of thorax without penetration into thoracic cavity

● **S21.141** Puncture wound with foreign body of right front wall of thorax without penetration into thoracic cavity A 🔍

● **S21.142** Puncture wound with foreign body of left front wall of thorax without penetration into thoracic cavity A 🔍

● **S21.149** Puncture wound with foreign body of unspecified front wall of thorax without penetration into thoracic cavity A 🔍

● **S21.15** Open bite of front wall of thorax without penetration into thoracic cavity
Bite of front wall of thorax NOS

Excludes1 superficial bite of front wall of thorax (S20.37)

● **S21.151** Open bite of right front wall of thorax without penetration into thoracic cavity A 🔍

● **S21.152** Open bite of left front wall of thorax without penetration into thoracic cavity A 🔍

● **S21.159** Open bite of unspecified front wall of thorax without penetration into thoracic cavity A 🔍

● **S21.2** Open wound of back wall of thorax without penetration into thoracic cavity

● **S21.20** Unspecified open wound of back wall of thorax without penetration into thoracic cavity

● **S21.201** Unspecified open wound of right back wall of thorax without penetration into thoracic cavity

● **S21.202** Unspecified open wound of left back wall of thorax without penetration into thoracic cavity

● **S21.209** Unspecified open wound of unspecified back wall of thorax without penetration into thoracic cavity

● **S21.21** Laceration without foreign body of back wall of thorax without penetration into thoracic cavity

● **S21.211** Laceration without foreign body of right back wall of thorax without penetration into thoracic cavity

● **S21.212** Laceration without foreign body of left back wall of thorax without penetration into thoracic cavity

● **S21.219** Laceration without foreign body of unspecified back wall of thorax without penetration into thoracic cavity

● **S21.22** Laceration with foreign body of back wall of thorax without penetration into thoracic cavity

● **S21.221** Laceration with foreign body of right back wall of thorax without penetration into thoracic cavity

● **S21.222** Laceration with foreign body of left back wall of thorax without penetration into thoracic cavity

● **S21.229** Laceration with foreign body of unspecified back wall of thorax without penetration into thoracic cavity

● **S21.23** Puncture wound without foreign body of back wall of thorax without penetration into thoracic cavity

● **S21.231** Puncture wound without foreign body of right back wall of thorax without penetration into thoracic cavity

● **S21.232** Puncture wound without foreign body of left back wall of thorax without penetration into thoracic cavity

● **S21.239** Puncture wound without foreign body of unspecified back wall of thorax without penetration into thoracic cavity

● **S21.24** Puncture wound with foreign body of back wall of thorax without penetration into thoracic cavity

● **S21.241** Puncture wound with foreign body of right back wall of thorax without penetration into thoracic cavity

● **S21.242** Puncture wound with foreign body of left back wall of thorax without penetration into thoracic cavity

● **S21.249** Puncture wound with foreign body of unspecified back wall of thorax without penetration into thoracic cavity

● **S21.25** Open bite of back wall of thorax without penetration into thoracic cavity
Bite of back wall of thorax NOS

Excludes1 superficial bite of back wall of thorax (S20.47)

● **S21.251** Open bite of right back wall of thorax without penetration into thoracic cavity

● **S21.252** Open bite of left back wall of thorax without penetration into thoracic cavity

● **S21.259** Open bite of unspecified back wall of thorax without penetration into thoracic cavity

● **S21.3** Open wound of front wall of thorax with penetration into thoracic cavity
Open wound of chest with penetration into thoracic cavity

(Ex:) **For category S21.3 CC codes unless otherwise indicated:** See PDX Collection 1169

● **S21.30** Unspecified open wound of front wall of thorax with penetration into thoracic cavity

● **S21.301** Unspecified open wound of right front wall of thorax with penetration into thoracic cavity A 🔍

● **S21.302** Unspecified open wound of left front wall of thorax with penetration into thoracic cavity A 🔍

● **S21.309** Unspecified open wound of unspecified front wall of thorax with penetration into thoracic cavity A 🔍
(Ex:) See PDX Collection 1170

▶ New ⇒ Revised ~~deleted~~ Deleted | Excludes 1 | Excludes 2 | Includes | Use additional | Code first | Code also | Key words |
OGCR Official Guidelines ● Unacceptable Principal Diagnosis X Assign placeholder X ● Use Additional Character(s) ▶ Manifestation Code **Coding Clinic**

● S21.31 Laceration without foreign body of front wall of thorax with penetration into thoracic cavity
- ● S21.311 Laceration without foreign body of right front wall of thorax with penetration into thoracic cavity A 🦠
- ● S21.312 Laceration without foreign body of left front wall of thorax with penetration into thoracic cavity A 🦠
- ● S21.319 Laceration without foreign body of unspecified front wall of thorax with penetration into thoracic cavity A 🦠

● S21.32 Laceration with foreign body of front wall of thorax with penetration into thoracic cavity
- ● S21.321 Laceration with foreign body of right front wall of thorax with penetration into thoracic cavity A 🦠
- ● S21.322 Laceration with foreign body of left front wall of thorax with penetration into thoracic cavity A 🦠
- ● S21.329 Laceration with foreign body of unspecified front wall of thorax with penetration into thoracic cavity A 🦠

● S21.33 Puncture wound without foreign body of front wall of thorax with penetration into thoracic cavity
- ● S21.331 Puncture wound without foreign body of right front wall of thorax with penetration into thoracic cavity A 🦠
- ● S21.332 Puncture wound without foreign body of left front wall of thorax with penetration into thoracic cavity A 🦠
- ● S21.339 Puncture wound without foreign body of unspecified front wall of thorax with penetration into thoracic cavity A 🦠

● S21.34 Puncture wound with foreign body of front wall of thorax with penetration into thoracic cavity
- ● S21.341 Puncture wound with foreign body of right front wall of thorax with penetration into thoracic cavity A 🦠
- ● S21.342 Puncture wound with foreign body of left front wall of thorax with penetration into thoracic cavity A 🦠
- ● S21.349 Puncture wound with foreign body of unspecified front wall of thorax with penetration into thoracic cavity A 🦠

● S21.35 Open bite of front wall of thorax with penetration into thoracic cavity

> **Excludes1**   superficial bite of front wall of thorax (S20.37)

- ● S21.351 Open bite of right front wall of thorax with penetration into thoracic cavity A 🦠
- ● S21.352 Open bite of left front wall of thorax with penetration into thoracic cavity A 🦠
- ● S21.359 Open bite of unspecified front wall of thorax with penetration into thoracic cavity A 🦠

● S21.4 Open wound of back wall of thorax with penetration into thoracic cavity
> (Ex) **For category S21.4 CC codes:** See PDX Collection 1169

● S21.40 Unspecified open wound of back wall of thorax with penetration into thoracic cavity
- ● S21.401 Unspecified open wound of right back wall of thorax with penetration into thoracic cavity A 🦠
- ● S21.402 Unspecified open wound of left back wall of thorax with penetration into thoracic cavity A 🦠
- ● S21.409 Unspecified open wound of unspecified back wall of thorax with penetration into thoracic cavity A 🦠

● S21.41 Laceration without foreign body of back wall of thorax with penetration into thoracic cavity
- ● S21.411 Laceration without foreign body of right back wall of thorax with penetration into thoracic cavity A 🦠
- ● S21.412 Laceration without foreign body of left back wall of thorax with penetration into thoracic cavity A 🦠
- ● S21.419 Laceration without foreign body of unspecified back wall of thorax with penetration into thoracic cavity A 🦠

● S21.42 Laceration with foreign body of back wall of thorax with penetration into thoracic cavity
- ● S21.421 Laceration with foreign body of right back wall of thorax with penetration into thoracic cavity A 🦠
- ● S21.422 Laceration with foreign body of left back wall of thorax with penetration into thoracic cavity A 🦠
- ● S21.429 Laceration with foreign body of unspecified back wall of thorax with penetration into thoracic cavity A 🦠

● S21.43 Puncture wound without foreign body of back wall of thorax with penetration into thoracic cavity
- ● S21.431 Puncture wound without foreign body of right back wall of thorax with penetration into thoracic cavity A 🦠
- ● S21.432 Puncture wound without foreign body of left back wall of thorax with penetration into thoracic cavity A 🦠
- ● S21.439 Puncture wound without foreign body of unspecified back wall of thorax with penetration into thoracic cavity A 🦠

● S21.44 Puncture wound with foreign body of back wall of thorax with penetration into thoracic cavity
- ● S21.441 Puncture wound with foreign body of right back wall of thorax with penetration into thoracic cavity A 🦠
- ● S21.442 Puncture wound with foreign body of left back wall of thorax with penetration into thoracic cavity A 🦠
- ● S21.449 Puncture wound with foreign body of unspecified back wall of thorax with penetration into thoracic cavity A 🦠

● S21.45 Open bite of back wall of thorax with penetration into thoracic cavity
Bite of back wall of thorax NOS

> **Excludes1**   superficial bite of back wall of thorax (S20.47)

- ● S21.451 Open bite of right back wall of thorax with penetration into thoracic cavity A 🦠
- ● S21.452 Open bite of left back wall of thorax with penetration into thoracic cavity A 🦠
- ● S21.459 Open bite of unspecified back wall of thorax with penetration into thoracic cavity A 🦠

● S21.9 Open wound of unspecified part of thorax
Open wound of thoracic wall NOS
> (Ex) **For category S21.9 CC codes:** See PDX Collection 1168

- X ● S21.90 Unspecified open wound of unspecified part of thorax A 🦠
- X ● S21.91 Laceration without foreign body of unspecified part of thorax A 🦠
- X ● S21.92 Laceration with foreign body of unspecified part of thorax A 🦠
- X ● S21.93 Puncture wound without foreign body of unspecified part of thorax A 🦠

N Newborn Age: 0   **P** Pediatric Age: 0–17   **M** Maternity DX: 9–64   **A** Adult Age: 15–124   ♀ Females Only   ♂ Males Only

🦠 Complication\Comorbidity   🦠 Major C\C   (Ex) CC/MCC Exclusions   🦠 Hospital-Acquired Condition   🦠 Hierarchical Condition Category

1277

X ● S21.94   **Puncture wound with foreign body** of
unspecified part of thorax A 🐾

X ● S21.95   **Open bite** of unspecified part of thorax A 🐾
Excludes1   superficial bite of thorax (S20.97)

● S22   **Fracture of rib(s), sternum and thoracic spine**
Note: A fracture not indicated as displaced or nondisplaced
should be coded to displaced

A fracture not indicated as open or closed should be coded to
closed

Includes   fracture of thoracic neural arch
fracture of thoracic spinous process
fracture of thoracic transverse process
fracture of thoracic vertebra
fracture of thoracic vertebral arch

Code first any associated:
injury of intrathoracic organ (S27.-)
spinal cord injury (S24.0-, S24.1-)

Excludes1   transection of thorax (S28.1)

Excludes2   fracture of clavicle (S42.0-)
fracture of scapula (S42.1-)

The appropriate 7th character is to be added to each code from
category S22

A	initial encounter for closed fracture
B	initial encounter for open fracture
D	subsequent encounter for fracture with routine healing
G	subsequent encounter for fracture with delayed healing
K	subsequent encounter for fracture with nonunion
S	sequela

● S22.0   **Fracture of thoracic vertebra**
(Ex) **For category S22.0 CC codes S22.0[A,B]:** See PDX Collection 1171
For S22.0[K]: See PDX Collection 897

● S22.00   **Fracture of unspecified thoracic vertebra**
● S22.000   **Wedge compression** fracture of
unspecified thoracic vertebra A, K 🐾,
B 🐾, A, B 🐾, **A, B** 🐾

● S22.001   **Stable burst** fracture of unspecified
thoracic vertebra A, K 🐾, B 🐾,
A, B 🐾, **A, B** 🐾

● S22.002   **Unstable burst** fracture of unspecified
thoracic vertebra A, K 🐾, B 🐾,
A, B 🐾, **A, B** 🐾

● S22.008   **Other** fracture of unspecified thoracic
vertebra A, K 🐾, B 🐾, A, B 🐾, **A, B** 🐾

● S22.009   **Unspecified** fracture of unspecified
thoracic vertebra A, K 🐾, B 🐾,
A, B 🐾, **A, B** 🐾

● S22.01   **Fracture of first thoracic vertebra**
● S22.010   **Wedge compression** fracture of first
thoracic vertebra A, K 🐾, B 🐾,
A, B 🐾, **A, B** 🐾

● S22.011   **Stable burst** fracture of first thoracic
vertebra A, K 🐾, B 🐾, A, B 🐾, **A, B** 🐾

● S22.012   **Unstable burst** fracture of first
thoracic vertebra A, K 🐾, B 🐾,
A, B 🐾, **A, B** 🐾

● S22.018   **Other** fracture of first thoracic vertebra
A, K 🐾, B 🐾, A, B 🐾, **A, B** 🐾

● S22.019   **Unspecified** fracture of first thoracic
vertebra A, K 🐾, B 🐾, A, B 🐾, **A, B** 🐾

● S22.02   **Fracture of second thoracic vertebra**
● S22.020   **Wedge compression** fracture of
second thoracic vertebra A, K 🐾, B 🐾,
A, B 🐾, **A, B** 🐾

● S22.021   **Stable burst** fracture of second
thoracic vertebra A, K 🐾, B 🐾,
A, B 🐾, **A, B** 🐾

● S22.022   **Unstable burst** fracture of second
thoracic vertebra A, K 🐾, B 🐾,
A, B 🐾, **A, B** 🐾

● S22.028   **Other** fracture of second thoracic
vertebra A, K 🐾, B 🐾, A, B 🐾, **A, B** 🐾

● S22.029   **Unspecified** fracture of second
thoracic vertebra A, K 🐾, B 🐾,
A, B 🐾, **A, B** 🐾

● S22.03   **Fracture of third thoracic vertebra**
● S22.030   **Wedge compression** fracture of third
thoracic vertebra A, K 🐾, B 🐾,
A, B 🐾, **A, B** 🐾

● S22.031   **Stable burst** fracture of third thoracic
vertebra A, K 🐾, B 🐾, A, B 🐾, **A, B** 🐾

● S22.032   **Unstable burst** fracture of third
thoracic vertebra A, K 🐾, B 🐾,
A, B 🐾, **A, B** 🐾

● S22.038   **Other** fracture of third thoracic
vertebra A, K 🐾, B 🐾, A, B 🐾, **A, B** 🐾

● S22.039   **Unspecified** fracture of third thoracic
vertebra A, K 🐾, B 🐾, A, B 🐾, **A, B** 🐾

● S22.04   **Fracture of fourth thoracic vertebra**
● S22.040   **Wedge compression** fracture of fourth
thoracic vertebra A, K 🐾, B 🐾,
A, B 🐾, **A, B** 🐾

● S22.041   **Stable burst** fracture of fourth
thoracic vertebra A, K 🐾, B 🐾,
A, B 🐾, **A, B** 🐾

● S22.042   **Unstable burst** fracture of fourth
thoracic vertebra A, K 🐾, B 🐾,
A, B 🐾, **A, B** 🐾

● S22.048   **Other** fracture of fourth thoracic
vertebra A, K 🐾, B 🐾, A, B 🐾, **A, B** 🐾

● S22.049   **Unspecified** fracture of fourth thoracic
vertebra A, K 🐾, B 🐾, A, B 🐾, **A, B** 🐾

● S22.05   **Fracture of T5-T6 vertebra**
● S22.050   **Wedge compression** fracture of
T5-T6 vertebra A, K 🐾, B 🐾,
A, B 🐾, **A, B** 🐾

● S22.051   **Stable burst** fracture of T5-T6
vertebra A, K 🐾, B 🐾, A, B 🐾, **A, B** 🐾

● S22.052   **Unstable burst** fracture of
T5-T6 vertebra A, K 🐾, B 🐾,
A, B 🐾, **A, B** 🐾

● S22.058   **Other** fracture of T5-T6 vertebra
A, K 🐾, B 🐾, A, B 🐾, **A, B** 🐾

● S22.059   **Unspecified** fracture of T5-T6 vertebra
A, K 🐾, B 🐾, A, B 🐾, **A, B** 🐾

● S22.06   **Fracture of T7-T8 vertebra**
● S22.060   **Wedge compression** fracture of
T7-T8 vertebra A, K 🐾, B 🐾,
A, B 🐾, **A, B** 🐾

● S22.061   **Stable burst** fracture of T7-T8
vertebra A, K 🐾, B 🐾, A, B 🐾, **A, B** 🐾

● S22.062   **Unstable burst** fracture of
T7-T8 vertebra A, K 🐾, B 🐾,
A, B 🐾, **A, B** 🐾

● S22.068   **Other** fracture of T7-T8 thoracic
vertebra A, K 🐾, B 🐾, A, B 🐾, **A, B** 🐾

● S22.069   **Unspecified** fracture of T7-T8 vertebra
A, K 🐾, B 🐾, A, B 🐾, **A, B** 🐾

▶ New   ➡ Revised   ~~deleted~~ Deleted   Excludes 1   Excludes 2   Includes   Use additional   Code first   Code also   Key words

OGCR Official Guidelines   ● Unacceptable Principal Diagnosis   X Assign placeholder X   ● Use Additional Character(s)   ▶ Manifestation Code   Coding Clinic

● S22.07   Fracture of T9-T10 vertebra
   ● S22.070   Wedge compression fracture of T9-T10 vertebra A, K 🔹, B 🔹, A, B 🔹, **A, B** 🔹
   ● S22.071   Stable burst fracture of T9-T10 vertebra A, K 🔹, B 🔹, A, B 🔹, **A, B** 🔹
   ● S22.072   Unstable burst fracture of T9-T10 vertebra A, K 🔹, B 🔹, A, B 🔹, **A, B** 🔹
   ● S22.078   Other fracture of T9-T10 vertebra A, K 🔹, B 🔹, A, B 🔹, **A, B** 🔹
   ● S22.079   Unspecified fracture of T9-T10 vertebra A, K 🔹, B 🔹, A, B 🔹, **A, B** 🔹

● S22.08   Fracture of T11-T12 vertebra
   ● S22.080   Wedge compression fracture of T11-T12 vertebra A, K 🔹, B 🔹, A, B 🔹, **A, B** 🔹
   ● S22.081   Stable burst fracture of T11-T12 vertebra A, K 🔹, B 🔹, A, B 🔹, **A, B** 🔹
   ● S22.082   Unstable burst fracture of T11-T12 vertebra A, K 🔹, B 🔹, A, B 🔹, **A, B** 🔹
   ● S22.088   Other fracture of T11-T12 vertebra A, K 🔹, B 🔹, A, B 🔹, **A, B** 🔹
   ● S22.089   Unspecified fracture of T11-T12 vertebra A, K 🔹, B 🔹, A, B 🔹, **A, B** 🔹

● S22.2   Fracture of sternum
   (Ex) **For category S22.2 CC codes S22.2[A,B]: See PDX Collection 1172**
   For S22.2[K]: See PDX Collection 897
  X ● S22.20   Unspecified fracture of sternum A, K 🔹, B 🔹, A, B 🔹
  X ● S22.21   Fracture of manubrium A, K 🔹, B 🔹, A, B 🔹
  X ● S22.22   Fracture of body of sternum A, K 🔹, B 🔹, A, B 🔹
  X ● S22.23   Sternal manubrial dissociation A, K 🔹, B 🔹, A, B 🔹
  X ● S22.24   Fracture of xiphoid process A, K 🔹, B 🔹, A, B 🔹

● S22.3   Fracture of one rib
   (Ex) **For category S22.3 CC codes S22.3[A]: See PDX Collection 1173**
   For S22.3[B]: See PDX Collection 1174 For S22.3[K]: See PDX Collection 897
  X ● S22.31   Fracture of one rib, right side A, K 🔹, B 🔹, A, B 🔹
  X ● S22.32   Fracture of one rib, left side A, K 🔹, B 🔹, A, B 🔹
  X ● S22.39   Fracture of one rib, unspecified side A, K 🔹, B 🔹, A, B 🔹

● S22.4   Multiple fractures of ribs
   Fractures of two or more ribs
   Excludes1   flail chest (S22.5-)
   (Ex) **For category S22.4 CC codes S22.4[A,B]: See PDX Collection 1174**
   For S22.49[B]: See PDX Collection 3234 For S22.4[K]: See PDX Collection 897
  X ● S22.41   Multiple fractures of ribs, right side A, K 🔹, B 🔹, A, B 🔹
  X ● S22.42   Multiple fractures of ribs, left side A, K 🔹, B 🔹, A, B 🔹
  X ● S22.43   Multiple fractures of ribs, bilateral A, K 🔹, B 🔹, A, B 🔹
  X ● S22.49   Multiple fractures of ribs, unspecified side A, K 🔹, B 🔹, A, B 🔹

  X ● S22.5   Flail chest K 🔹, A, B 🔹, A, B 🔹
   Unstable chest due to sternum and/or rib fracture
   (Ex) **For category S22.5 CC codes S22.5[A,B]: See PDX Collection 1175**
   For S22.5[K]: See PDX Collection 897

  X ● S22.9   Fracture of bony thorax, part unspecified A, K 🔹, B 🔹, A, B 🔹
   (Ex) **For category S22.9 CC codes S22.9[A,B]: See PDX Collection 1176**
   For S22.9[K]: See PDX Collection 897

● S23   Dislocation and sprain of joints and ligaments of thorax
   Includes   avulsion of joint or ligament of thorax
     laceration of cartilage, joint or ligament of thorax
     sprain of cartilage, joint or ligament of thorax
     traumatic hemarthrosis of joint or ligament of thorax
     traumatic rupture of joint or ligament of thorax
     traumatic subluxation of joint or ligament of thorax
     traumatic tear of joint or ligament of thorax
   ➡ Code also any associated: open wound
   Excludes2   dislocation, sprain of sternoclavicular joint (S43.2, S43.6)
     strain of muscle or tendon of thorax (S29.01-)
   The appropriate 7th character is to be added to each code from category S23

A	initial encounter
D	subsequent encounter
S	sequela

  X ● S23.0   Traumatic rupture of thoracic intervertebral disc
   Excludes1   rupture or displacement (nontraumatic) of thoracic intervertebral disc NOS (M51.- with fifth character 4)

● S23.1   Subluxation and dislocation of thoracic vertebra
   Code also any associated
     open wound of thorax (S21.)
     spinal cord injury (S24.0-, S24.1-)
   Excludes2   fracture of thoracic vertebrae (S22.0-)
  ● S23.10   Subluxation and dislocation of unspecified thoracic vertebra
   ● S23.100   Subluxation of unspecified thoracic vertebra
   ● S23.101   Dislocation of unspecified thoracic vertebra
  ● S23.11   Subluxation and dislocation of T1/T2 thoracic vertebra
   ● S23.110   Subluxation of T1/T2 thoracic vertebra
   ● S23.111   Dislocation of T1/T2 thoracic vertebra
  ● S23.12   Subluxation and dislocation of T2/T3-T3/T4 thoracic vertebra
   ● S23.120   Subluxation of T2/T3 thoracic vertebra
   ● S23.121   Dislocation of T2/T3 thoracic vertebra
   ● S23.122   Subluxation of T3/T4 thoracic vertebra
   ● S23.123   Dislocation of T3/T4 thoracic vertebra
  ● S23.13   Subluxation and dislocation of T4/T5-T5/T6 thoracic vertebra
   ● S23.130   Subluxation of T4/T5 thoracic vertebra
   ● S23.131   Dislocation of T4/T5 thoracic vertebra
   ● S23.132   Subluxation of T5/T6 thoracic vertebra
   ● S23.133   Dislocation of T5/T6 thoracic vertebra
  ● S23.14   Subluxation and dislocation of T6/T7-T7/T8 thoracic vertebra
   ● S23.140   Subluxation of T6/T7 thoracic vertebra
   ● S23.141   Dislocation of T6/T7 thoracic vertebra
   ● S23.142   Subluxation of T7/T8 thoracic vertebra
   ● S23.143   Dislocation of T7/T8 thoracic vertebra

● **S23.15**   Subluxation and dislocation of T8/T9-T9/T10 thoracic vertebra
- ● **S23.150**   Subluxation of T8/T9 thoracic vertebra
- ● **S23.151**   Dislocation of T8/T9 thoracic vertebra
- ● **S23.152**   Subluxation of T9/T10 thoracic vertebra
- ● **S23.153**   Dislocation of T9/T10 thoracic vertebra

● **S23.16**   Subluxation and dislocation of T10/T11-T11/T12 thoracic vertebra
- ● **S23.160**   Subluxation of T10/T11 thoracic vertebra
- ● **S23.161**   Dislocation of T10/T11 thoracic vertebra
- ● **S23.162**   Subluxation of T11/T12 thoracic vertebra
- ● **S23.163**   Dislocation of T11/T12 thoracic vertebra

● **S23.17**   Subluxation and dislocation of T12/L1 thoracic vertebra
- ● **S23.170**   Subluxation of T12/L1 thoracic vertebra
- ● **S23.171**   Dislocation of T12/L1 thoracic vertebra

● **S23.2**   Dislocation of other and unspecified parts of thorax
- X● **S23.20**   Dislocation of unspecified part of thorax
- X● **S23.29**   Dislocation of other parts of thorax

X● **S23.3**   Sprain of ligaments of thoracic spine

● **S23.4**   Sprain of ribs and sternum
- X● **S23.41**   Sprain of ribs
- ● **S23.42**   Sprain of sternum
  - ● **S23.420**   Sprain of sternoclavicular (joint) (ligament)
  - ● **S23.421**   Sprain of chondrosternal joint
  - ● **S23.428**   Other sprain of sternum
  - ● **S23.429**   Unspecified sprain of sternum

X● **S23.8**   Sprain of other specified parts of thorax

X● **S23.9**   Sprain of unspecified parts of thorax

● **S24**   **Injury of nerves and spinal cord at thorax level**

> **Note:** Code to highest level of thoracic spinal cord injury.
>
> Injuries to the spinal cord (S24.0 and S24.1) refer to the cord level and not bone level injury, and can affect nerve roots at and below the level given.
>
> Code also any associated:
> fracture of thoracic vertebra (S22.0-)
> open wound of thorax (S21.-)
> transient paralysis (R29.5)

Excludes2   injury of brachial plexus (S14.3)

The appropriate 7th character is to be added to each code from category S24

A	initial encounter
D	subsequent encounter
S	sequela

(Ex:) **For category S24 CC codes:** See PDX Collection 1177

X● **S24.0**   Concussion and edema of thoracic spinal cord A 🔒, A, D, S 🔒

● **S24.1**   Other and unspecified injuries of thoracic spinal cord
- ● **S24.10**   Unspecified injury of thoracic spinal cord
  - ● **S24.101**   Unspecified injury at T1 level of thoracic spinal cord A 🔒, A 🔒, A, D, S 🔒
  - ● **S24.102**   Unspecified injury at T2-T6 level of thoracic spinal cord A 🔒, A 🔒, A, D, S 🔒
  - ● **S24.103**   Unspecified injury at T7-T10 level of thoracic spinal cord A 🔒, A 🔒, A, D, S 🔒
  - ● **S24.104**   Unspecified injury at T11-T12 level of thoracic spinal cord A 🔒, A 🔒, A, D, S 🔒
  - ● **S24.109**   Unspecified injury at unspecified level of thoracic spinal cord A, D, S 🔒
    Injury of thoracic spinal cord NOS

- ● **S24.11**   Complete lesion of thoracic spinal cord
  - ● **S24.111**   Complete lesion at T1 level of thoracic spinal cord A 🔒, A 🔒, A, D, S 🔒
  - ● **S24.112**   Complete lesion at T2-T6 level of thoracic spinal cord A 🔒, A 🔒, A, D, S 🔒
  - ● **S24.113**   Complete lesion at T7-T10 level of thoracic spinal cord A 🔒, A 🔒, A, D, S 🔒
  - ● **S24.114**   Complete lesion at T11-T12 level of thoracic spinal cord A 🔒, A 🔒, A, D, S 🔒
  - ● **S24.119**   Complete lesion at unspecified level of thoracic spinal cord A, D, S 🔒

- ● **S24.13**   Anterior cord syndrome of thoracic spinal cord
  - ● **S24.131**   Anterior cord syndrome at T1 level of thoracic spinal cord A 🔒, A 🔒, A, D, S 🔒
  - ● **S24.132**   Anterior cord syndrome at T2-T6 level of thoracic spinal cord A 🔒, A 🔒, A, D, S 🔒
  - ● **S24.133**   Anterior cord syndrome at T7-T10 level of thoracic spinal cord A 🔒, A 🔒, A, D, S 🔒
  - ● **S24.134**   Anterior cord syndrome at T11-T12 level of thoracic spinal cord A 🔒, A 🔒, A, D, S 🔒
  - ● **S24.139**   Anterior cord syndrome at unspecified level of thoracic spinal cord A, D, S 🔒

- ● **S24.14**   Brown-Séquard syndrome of thoracic spinal cord
  - ● **S24.141**   Brown-Séquard syndrome at T1 level of thoracic spinal cord A 🔒, A, D, S 🔒
  - ● **S24.142**   Brown-Séquard syndrome at T2-T6 level of thoracic spinal cord A 🔒, A, D, S 🔒
  - ● **S24.143**   Brown-Séquard syndrome at T7-T10 level of thoracic spinal cord A 🔒, A, D, S 🔒
  - ● **S24.144**   Brown-Séquard syndrome at T11-T12 level of thoracic spinal cord A 🔒, A, D, S 🔒
  - ● **S24.149**   Brown-Séquard syndrome at unspecified level of thoracic spinal cord A, D, S 🔒

- ● **S24.15**   Other incomplete lesions of thoracic spinal cord
    Incomplete lesion of thoracic spinal cord NOS
    Posterior cord syndrome of thoracic spinal cord
  - ● **S24.151**   Other incomplete lesion at T1 level of thoracic spinal cord A 🔒, A 🔒, A, D, S 🔒
  - ● **S24.152**   Other incomplete lesion at T2-T6 level of thoracic spinal cord A 🔒, A 🔒, A, D, S 🔒
  - ● **S24.153**   Other incomplete lesion at T7-T10 level of thoracic spinal cord A 🔒, A 🔒, A, D, S 🔒
  - ● **S24.154**   Other incomplete lesion at T11-T12 level of thoracic spinal cord A 🔒, A 🔒, A, D, S 🔒
  - ● **S24.159**   Other incomplete lesion at unspecified level of thoracic spinal cord A, D, S 🔒

▶ New   ⇒ Revised   ~~deleted~~ Deleted   Excludes 1   Excludes 2   Includes   Use additional   Code first   Code also   Key words

OGCR Official Guidelines   ● Unacceptable Principal Diagnosis   X Assign placeholder X   ● Use Additional Character(s)   ▶ Manifestation Code   **Coding Clinic**

X● **S24.2**   **Injury of nerve root of thoracic spine**

X● **S24.3**   **Injury of peripheral nerves of thorax**

X● **S24.4**   **Injury of thoracic sympathetic nervous system**
     Injury of cardiac plexus
     Injury of esophageal plexus
     Injury of pulmonary plexus
     Injury of stellate ganglion
     Injury of thoracic sympathetic ganglion

X● **S24.8**   **Injury of other specified nerves of thorax**

X● **S24.9**   **Injury of unspecified nerve of thorax**

● **S25**   **Injury of blood vessels of thorax**
     The appropriate 7th character is to be added to each code from category S25

A	initial encounter
D	subsequent encounter
S	sequela

     Code also any associated open wound (S21.-)

● **S25.0**   **Injury of thoracic aorta**
     Injury of aorta NOS
     (Ex:) **For category S25.0 CC codes:** See PDX Collection 1178

X● **S25.00**   **Unspecified** injury of thoracic aorta A 🐾

X● **S25.01**   **Minor laceration** of thoracic aorta A 🐾
     Incomplete transection of thoracic aorta
     Laceration of thoracic aorta NOS
     Superficial laceration of thoracic aorta

X● **S25.02**   **Major laceration** of thoracic aorta A 🐾
     Complete transection of thoracic aorta
     Traumatic rupture of thoracic aorta

X● **S25.09**   **Other** specified injury of thoracic aorta A 🐾

● **S25.1**   **Injury of innominate or subclavian artery**
     (Ex:) **For category S25.1 CC codes:** See PDX Collection 1179

● **S25.10**   **Unspecified** injury of innominate or subclavian artery

   ● **S25.101**   Unspecified injury of **right** innominate or subclavian artery A 🐾

   ● **S25.102**   Unspecified injury of **left** innominate or subclavian artery A 🐾

   ● **S25.109**   Unspecified injury of **unspecified** innominate or subclavian artery A 🐾

● **S25.11**   **Minor laceration** of innominate or subclavian artery
     Incomplete transection of innominate or subclavian artery
     Laceration of innominate or subclavian artery NOS
     Superficial laceration of innominate or subclavian artery

   ● **S25.111**   Minor laceration of **right** innominate or subclavian artery A 🐾

   ● **S25.112**   Minor laceration of **left** innominate or subclavian artery A 🐾

   ● **S25.119**   Minor laceration of **unspecified** innominate or subclavian artery A 🐾

● **S25.12**   **Major laceration** of innominate or subclavian artery
     Complete transection of innominate or subclavian artery
     Traumatic rupture of innominate or subclavian artery

   ● **S25.121**   Major laceration of **right** innominate or subclavian artery A 🐾

   ● **S25.122**   Major laceration of **left** innominate or subclavian artery A 🐾

   ● **S25.129**   Major laceration of **unspecified** innominate or subclavian artery A 🐾

● **S25.19**   **Other** specified injury of innominate or subclavian artery

   ● **S25.191**   Other specified injury of **right** innominate or subclavian artery A 🐾

   ● **S25.192**   Other specified injury of **left** innominate or subclavian artery A 🐾

   ● **S25.199**   Other specified injury of **unspecified** innominate or subclavian artery A 🐾

● **S25.2**   **Injury of superior vena cava**
     Injury of vena cava NOS
     (Ex:) **For category S25.2 CC codes:** See PDX Collection 1180

X● **S25.20**   **Unspecified** injury of superior vena cava A 🐾

X● **S25.21**   **Minor laceration** of superior vena cava A 🐾
     Incomplete transection of superior vena cava
     Laceration of superior vena cava NOS
     Superficial laceration of superior vena cava

X● **S25.22**   **Major laceration** of superior vena cava A 🐾
     Complete transection of superior vena cava
     Traumatic rupture of superior vena cava

X● **S25.29**   **Other** specified injury of superior vena cava A 🐾

● **S25.3**   **Injury of innominate or subclavian vein**
     (Ex:) **For category S25.3 CC codes:** See PDX Collection 1181

● **S25.30**   **Unspecified** injury of innominate or subclavian vein

   ● **S25.301**   Unspecified injury of **right** innominate or subclavian vein A 🐾

   ● **S25.302**   Unspecified injury of **left** innominate or subclavian vein A 🐾

   ● **S25.309**   Unspecified injury of **unspecified** innominate or subclavian vein A 🐾

● **S25.31**   **Minor laceration** of innominate or subclavian vein
     Incomplete transection of innominate or subclavian vein
     Laceration of innominate or subclavian vein NOS
     Superficial laceration of innominate or subclavian vein

   ● **S25.311**   Minor laceration of **right** innominate or subclavian vein A 🐾

   ● **S25.312**   Minor laceration of **left** innominate or subclavian vein A 🐾

   ● **S25.319**   Minor laceration of **unspecified** innominate or subclavian vein A 🐾

● **S25.32**   **Major laceration** of innominate or subclavian vein
     Complete transection of innominate or subclavian vein
     Traumatic rupture of innominate or subclavian vein

   ● **S25.321**   Major laceration of **right** innominate or subclavian vein A 🐾

   ● **S25.322**   Major laceration of **left** innominate or subclavian vein A 🐾

   ● **S25.329**   Major laceration of **unspecified** innominate or subclavian vein A 🐾

● **S25.39**   **Other** specified injury of innominate or subclavian vein

   ● **S25.391**   Other specified injury of **right** innominate or subclavian vein A 🐾

   ● **S25.392**   Other specified injury of **left** innominate or subclavian vein A 🐾

   ● **S25.399**   Other specified injury of **unspecified** innominate or subclavian vein A 🐾

CHAPTER 19 (S00-T88)

N   Newborn Age: 0   **P**   Pediatric Age: 0–17   **M**   Maternity DX: 9–64   **A**   Adult Age: 15–124   ♀   Females Only   ♂   Males Only

🐾   Complication\Comorbidity   🐾   Major C\C   (Ex:)   CC/MCC Exclusions   🐾   Hospital-Acquired Condition   🐾   Hierarchical Condition Category

● **S25.4   Injury of pulmonary blood vessels**
> Ⓔ **For category S25.4 CC codes unless otherwise indicated:** See PDX Collection 1182

    ● **S25.40   Unspecified injury of pulmonary blood vessels**

        ● S25.401   Unspecified injury of right pulmonary blood vessels A 🔖

        ● S25.402   Unspecified injury of left pulmonary blood vessels A 🔖

        ● S25.409   Unspecified injury of unspecified pulmonary blood vessels A 🔖

    ● **S25.41   Minor laceration of pulmonary blood vessels**
> Incomplete transection of pulmonary blood vessels
> Laceration of pulmonary blood vessels NOS
> Superficial laceration of pulmonary blood vessels

        ● S25.411   Minor laceration of right pulmonary blood vessels A 🔖

        ● S25.412   Minor laceration of left pulmonary blood vessels A 🔖

        ● S25.419   Minor laceration of unspecified pulmonary blood vessels A 🔖

    ● **S25.42   Major laceration of pulmonary blood vessels**
> Complete transection of pulmonary blood vessels
> Traumatic rupture of pulmonary blood vessels

        ● S25.421   Major laceration of right pulmonary blood vessels A 🔖
> Ⓔ See PDX Collection 1183

        ● S25.422   Major laceration of left pulmonary blood vessels A 🔖

        ● S25.429   Major laceration of unspecified pulmonary blood vessels A 🔖

    ● **S25.49   Other specified injury of pulmonary blood vessels**

        ● S25.491   Other specified injury of right pulmonary blood vessels A 🔖

        ● S25.492   Other specified injury of left pulmonary blood vessels A 🔖

        ● S25.499   Other specified injury of unspecified pulmonary blood vessels A 🔖

● **S25.5   Injury of intercostal blood vessels**
> Ⓔ **For category S25.5 CC codes:** See PDX Collection 1184

    ● **S25.50   Unspecified injury of intercostal blood vessels**

        ● S25.501   Unspecified injury of intercostal blood vessels, right side A 🔖

        ● S25.502   Unspecified injury of intercostal blood vessels, left side A 🔖

        ● S25.509   Unspecified injury of intercostal blood vessels, unspecified side A 🔖

    ● **S25.51   Laceration of intercostal blood vessels**

        ● S25.511   Laceration of intercostal blood vessels, right side A 🔖

        ● S25.512   Laceration of intercostal blood vessels, left side A 🔖

        ● S25.519   Laceration of intercostal blood vessels, unspecified side A 🔖

    ● **S25.59   Other specified injury of intercostal blood vessels**

        ● S25.591   Other specified injury of intercostal blood vessels, right side A 🔖

        ● S25.592   Other specified injury of intercostal blood vessels, left side A 🔖

        ● S25.599   Other specified injury of intercostal blood vessels, unspecified side A 🔖

● **S25.8   Injury of other blood vessels of thorax**
> Injury of azygos vein
> Injury of mammary artery or vein
> Ⓔ **For category S25.8 CC codes:** See PDX Collection 1185

    ● **S25.80   Unspecified injury of other blood vessels of thorax**

        ● S25.801   Unspecified injury of other blood vessels of thorax, right side A 🔖

        ● S25.802   Unspecified injury of other blood vessels of thorax, left side A 🔖

        ● S25.809   Unspecified injury of other blood vessels of thorax, unspecified side A 🔖

    ● **S25.81   Laceration of other blood vessels of thorax**

        ● S25.811   Laceration of other blood vessels of thorax, right side A 🔖

        ● S25.812   Laceration of other blood vessels of thorax, left side A 🔖

        ● S25.819   Laceration of other blood vessels of thorax, unspecified side A 🔖

    ● **S25.89   Other specified injury of other blood vessels of thorax**

        ● S25.891   Other specified injury of other blood vessels of thorax, right side A 🔖

        ● S25.892   Other specified injury of other blood vessels of thorax, left side A 🔖

        ● S25.899   Other specified injury of other blood vessels of thorax, unspecified side A 🔖

● **S25.9   Injury of unspecified blood vessel of thorax**
> Ⓔ **For category S25.9 CC codes:** See PDX Collection 1185

    X ● **S25.90   Unspecified injury of unspecified blood vessel of thorax A 🔖**

    X ● **S25.91   Laceration of unspecified blood vessel of thorax A 🔖**

    X ● **S25.99   Other specified injury of unspecified blood vessel of thorax A 🔖**

● **S26   Injury of heart**
> The appropriate 7th character is to be added to each code from category S26

> | A | initial encounter |
> |---|---|
> | D | subsequent encounter |
> | S | sequela |

> Code also any associated:
> open wound of thorax (S21.-)
> traumatic hemopneumothorax (S27.2)
> traumatic hemothorax (S27.1)
> traumatic pneumothorax (S27.0)
> Ⓔ **For category S26 CC codes unless otherwise indicated:** See PDX Collection 1187

● **S26.0   Injury of heart with hemopericardium**
> *Hemopericardium: effusion of blood within pericardium*

    X ● **S26.00   Unspecified injury of heart with hemopericardium A 🔖**
> Ⓔ See PDX Collection 1186

    X ● **S26.01   Contusion of heart with hemopericardium A 🔖**

    ● **S26.02   Laceration of heart with hemopericardium**

        ● S26.020   Mild laceration of heart with hemopericardium A 🔖
> Laceration of heart without penetration of heart chamber

        ● S26.021   Moderate laceration of heart with hemopericardium A 🔖
> Laceration of heart with penetration of heart chamber

        ● S26.022   Major laceration of heart with hemopericardium A 🔖
> Laceration of heart with penetration of multiple heart chambers

    X ● **S26.09   Other injury of heart with hemopericardium A 🔖**
> Ⓔ See PDX Collection 1186

● **S26.1   Injury of heart without hemopericardium**
　　　　Hemopericardium: effusion of blood within pericardium
　X● S26.10   **Unspecified** injury of heart without hemopericardium A ⬡
　　　　　　Ⓔⓧ See PDX Collection 1186
　X● S26.11   **Contusion** of heart without hemopericardium A ⬡
　X● S26.12   **Laceration** of heart without hemopericardium A ⬡
　X● S26.19   **Other** injury of heart without hemopericardium A ⬡
　　　　　　Ⓔⓧ See PDX Collection 1186
● **S26.9   Injury of heart, unspecified with or without hemopericardium**
　　　　Hemopericardium: effusion of blood within pericardium
　X● S26.90   **Unspecified** injury of heart, unspecified with or without hemopericardium A ⬡
　　　　　　Ⓔⓧ See PDX Collection 1186
　X● S26.91   **Contusion** of heart, unspecified with or without hemopericardium A ⬡
　X● S26.92   **Laceration** of heart, unspecified with or without hemopericardium A ⬡
　　　　Laceration of heart NOS
　X● S26.99   **Other** injury of heart, unspecified with or without hemopericardium A ⬡
　　　　　　Ⓔⓧ See PDX Collection 1186

● **S27   Injury of other and unspecified intrathoracic organs**
　　　　Code also any associated open wound of thorax (S21.-)
　　　　Excludes2　injury of cervical esophagus (S10-S19)
　　　　　　　　　injury of trachea (cervical) (S10-S19)
　　　　The appropriate 7th character is to be added to each code from category S27

A	initial encounter
D	subsequent encounter
S	sequela

　X● S27.0   **Traumatic pneumothorax** A ⬡
　　　　Excludes1　spontaneous pneumothorax (J93.-)
　　　　　　Ⓔⓧ See PDX Collection 1180
　X● S27.1   **Traumatic hemothorax** A ⬡
　　　　　　Ⓔⓧ See PDX Collection 1188
　X● S27.2   **Traumatic hemopneumothorax** A ⬡
　　　　　　Ⓔⓧ See PDX Collection 1188
● S27.3   **Other and unspecified injuries of lung**
　　　　Ⓔⓧ **For category S27.3 CC codes unless otherwise indicated:** See PDX Collection 1189
　● S27.30   **Unspecified** injury of lung
　　　● S27.301   **Unspecified** injury of lung, **unilateral** A ⬡
　　　● S27.302   **Unspecified** injury of lung, **bilateral** A ⬡
　　　● S27.309   **Unspecified** injury of lung, **unspecified** A ⬡
　● S27.31   **Primary blast** injury of lung
　　　　Blast injury of lung NOS
　　　● S27.311   **Primary blast** injury of lung, **unilateral** A ⬡
　　　● S27.312   **Primary blast** injury of lung, **bilateral** A ⬡
　　　● S27.319   **Primary blast** injury of lung, **unspecified** A ⬡

● S27.32   **Contusion of lung**
　　　● S27.321   Contusion of lung, **unilateral** A ⬡
　　　● S27.322   Contusion of lung, **bilateral** A ⬡
　　　● S27.329   Contusion of lung, **unspecified** A ⬡
● S27.33   **Laceration of lung**
　　　　Ⓔⓧ **For category S27.33 CC codes:** See PDX Collection 1190
　　　● S27.331   Laceration of lung, **unilateral** A ⬡
　　　● S27.332   Laceration of lung, **bilateral** A ⬡
　　　● S27.339   Laceration of lung, **unspecified** A ⬡
● S27.39   **Other injuries of lung**
　　　　Secondary blast injury of lung
　　　● S27.391   Other injuries of lung, **unilateral** A ⬡
　　　● S27.392   Other injuries of lung, **bilateral** A ⬡
　　　● S27.399   Other injuries of lung, **unspecified** A ⬡
● **S27.4   Injury of bronchus**
　　　　Ⓔⓧ **For category S27.4 CC codes:** See PDX Collection 1191
　● S27.40   **Unspecified** injury of bronchus
　　　● S27.401   Unspecified injury of bronchus, **unilateral** A ⬡
　　　● S27.402   Unspecified injury of bronchus, **bilateral** A ⬡
　　　● S27.409   Unspecified injury of bronchus, **unspecified** A ⬡
　● S27.41   **Primary blast injury of bronchus**
　　　　Blast injury of bronchus NOS
　　　● S27.411   **Primary blast** injury of bronchus, **unilateral** A ⬡
　　　● S27.412   **Primary blast** injury of bronchus, **bilateral** A ⬡
　　　● S27.419   **Primary blast** injury of bronchus, **unspecified** A ⬡
　● S27.42   **Contusion of bronchus**
　　　● S27.421   Contusion of bronchus, **unilateral** A ⬡
　　　● S27.422   Contusion of bronchus, **bilateral** A ⬡
　　　● S27.429   Contusion of bronchus, **unspecified** A ⬡
　● S27.43   **Laceration of bronchus**
　　　● S27.431   Laceration of bronchus, **unilateral** A ⬡
　　　● S27.432   Laceration of bronchus, **bilateral** A ⬡
　　　● S27.439   Laceration of bronchus, **unspecified** A ⬡
　● S27.49   **Other injury of bronchus**
　　　　Secondary blast injury of bronchus
　　　● S27.491   Other injury of bronchus, **unilateral** A ⬡
　　　● S27.492   Other injury of bronchus, **bilateral** A ⬡
　　　● S27.499   Other injury of bronchus, **unspecified** A ⬡

CHAPTER 19 (S00-T88)

Item 19–2 Pneumothorax is a collection of gas (positive air pressure) in the pleural space resulting in the lung collapsing. A **tension pneumothorax** is life-threatening and is a result of air in the pleural space causing a displacement in the mediastinal structures and cardiopulmonary function compromise. A **traumatic pneumothorax** results from blunt or penetrating injury that disrupts the parietal/visceral pleura. **Hemothorax** is blood or bloody fluid in the pleural cavity as a result of traumatic blood vessel rupture or inflammation of the lungs from pneumonia.

N Newborn Age: 0	**P** Pediatric Age: 0–17	**M** Maternity DX: 9–64	**A** Adult Age: 15–124	♀ Females Only	♂ Males Only

⬡ Complication\Comorbidity　　⬡ Major C\C　　Ⓔⓧ CC/MCC Exclusions　　⬡ Hospital-Acquired Condition　　⬡ Hierarchical Condition Category

● **S27.5**   Injury of thoracic trachea
    (Ex:) For category S27.5 CC codes: See PDX Collection 1169
  X ● **S27.50**   Unspecified injury of thoracic trachea A 🐾
  X ● **S27.51**   Primary blast injury of thoracic trachea A 🐾
           Blast injury of thoracic trachea NOS
  X ● **S27.52**   Contusion of thoracic trachea A 🐾
  X ● **S27.53**   Laceration of thoracic trachea A 🐾
  X ● **S27.59**   Other injury of thoracic trachea A 🐾
           Secondary blast injury of thoracic trachea

● **S27.6**   Injury of pleura
    (Ex:) For category S27.6 CC codes: See PDX Collection 1169
  X ● **S27.60**   Unspecified injury of pleura A 🐾
  X ● **S27.63**   Laceration of pleura A 🐾
  X ● **S27.69**   Other injury of pleura A 🐾

● **S27.8**   Injury of other specified intrathoracic organs
  ● **S27.80**   Injury of diaphragm
      (Ex:) For category S27.80 CC codes: See PDX Collection 1192
   ● **S27.802**   Contusion of diaphragm A 🐾
   ● **S27.803**   Laceration of diaphragm A 🐾
   ● **S27.808**   Other injury of diaphragm A 🐾
   ● **S27.809**   Unspecified injury of diaphragm A 🐾
  ● **S27.81**   Injury of esophagus (thoracic part)
      (Ex:) For category S27.81 CC codes: See PDX Collection 1193
   ● **S27.812**   Contusion of esophagus (thoracic part) A 🐾
   ● **S27.813**   Laceration of esophagus (thoracic part) A 🐾
   ● **S27.818**   Other injury of esophagus (thoracic part) A 🐾
   ● **S27.819**   Unspecified injury of esophagus (thoracic part) A 🐾
  ● **S27.89**   Injury of other specified intrathoracic organs
       Injury of lymphatic thoracic duct
       Injury of thymus gland
      (Ex:) For category S27.89 CC codes: See PDX Collection 1169
   ● **S27.892**   Contusion of other specified intrathoracic organs A 🐾
   ● **S27.893**   Laceration of other specified intrathoracic organs A 🐾
   ● **S27.898**   Other injury of other specified intrathoracic organs A 🐾
   ● **S27.899**   Unspecified injury of other specified intrathoracic organs A 🐾
  X ● **S27.9**   Injury of unspecified intrathoracic organ A 🐾
    (Ex:) See PDX Collection 1194

● **S28**   Crushing injury of thorax, and traumatic amputation of part of thorax
    The appropriate 7th character is to be added to each code from category S28

A	initial encounter
D	subsequent encounter
S	sequela

  X ● **S28.0**   Crushed chest
       Use additional code for all associated injuries
       Excludes1   flail chest (S22.5)
  X ● **S28.1**   Traumatic amputation (partial) of part of thorax, except breast A 🐾
      (Ex:) For category S28.1 CC codes: See PDX Collection 1168

● **S28.2**   Traumatic amputation of breast
  ● **S28.21**   Complete traumatic amputation of breast
       Traumatic amputation of breast NOS
   ● **S28.211**   Complete traumatic amputation of right breast
   ● **S28.212**   Complete traumatic amputation of left breast
   ● **S28.219**   Complete traumatic amputation of unspecified breast
  ● **S28.22**   Partial traumatic amputation of breast
   ● **S28.221**   Partial traumatic amputation of right breast
   ● **S28.222**   Partial traumatic amputation of left breast
   ● **S28.229**   Partial traumatic amputation of unspecified breast

● **S29**   Other and unspecified injuries of thorax
    Code also any associated open wound (S21.-)
    The appropriate 7th character is to be added to each code from category S29

A	initial encounter
D	subsequent encounter
S	sequela

  ● **S29.0**   Injury of muscle and tendon at thorax level
   ● **S29.00**   Unspecified injury of muscle and tendon of thorax
    ● **S29.001**   Unspecified injury of muscle and tendon of front wall of thorax
    ● **S29.002**   Unspecified injury of muscle and tendon of back wall of thorax
    ● **S29.009**   Unspecified injury of muscle and tendon of unspecified wall of thorax
   ● **S29.01**   Strain of muscle and tendon of thorax
    ● **S29.011**   Strain of muscle and tendon of front wall of thorax
    ● **S29.012**   Strain of muscle and tendon of back wall of thorax
    ● **S29.019**   Strain of muscle and tendon of unspecified wall of thorax
   ● **S29.02**   Laceration of muscle and tendon of thorax
      (Ex:) For category S29.02 CC codes: See PDX Collection 1168
    ● **S29.021**   Laceration of muscle and tendon of front wall of thorax A 🐾
    ● **S29.022**   Laceration of muscle and tendon of back wall of thorax
    ● **S29.029**   Laceration of muscle and tendon of unspecified wall of thorax A 🐾
   ● **S29.09**   Other injury of muscle and tendon of thorax
    ● **S29.091**   Other injury of muscle and tendon of front wall of thorax
    ● **S29.092**   Other injury of muscle and tendon of back wall of thorax
    ● **S29.099**   Other injury of muscle and tendon of unspecified wall of thorax
  X ● **S29.8**   Other specified injuries of thorax
  X ● **S29.9**   Unspecified injury of thorax

▶ New   ⇒ Revised   ~~deleted~~ Deleted   Excludes 1   Excludes 2   Includes   Use additional   Code first   Code also   Key words
OGCR Official Guidelines   ● Unacceptable Principal Diagnosis   X Assign placeholder X   ● Use Additional Character(s)   ▶ Manifestation Code   Coding Clinic

INJURIES TO THE ABDOMEN, LOWER BACK, LUMBAR SPINE
PELVIS AND EXTERNAL GENITALS (S30-S39)

Includes	injuries to the abdominal wall
	injuries to the anus
	injuries to the buttock
	injuries to the external genitalia
	injuries to the flank
	injuries to the groin

Excludes2	burns and corrosions (T20-T32)
	effects of foreign body in anus and rectum (T18.5)
	effects of foreign body in genitourinary tract (T19.-)
	effects of foreign body in stomach, small intestine and colon (T18.2-T18.4)
	frostbite (T33-T34)
	insect bite or sting, venomous (T63.4)

● **S30** **Superficial injury of abdomen, lower back, pelvis and external genitals**

Excludes2	superficial injury of hip (S70.-)

The appropriate 7th character is to be added to each code from category S30

A	initial encounter
D	subsequent encounter
S	sequela

X● **S30.0** **Contusion of lower back and pelvis**
Contusion of buttock

X● **S30.1** **Contusion of abdominal wall**
Contusion of flank
Contusion of groin

● **S30.2** **Contusion of external genital organs**
  ● **S30.20** Contusion of unspecified external genital organ
    ● **S30.201** Contusion of unspecified external genital organ, male ♂
    ● **S30.202** Contusion of unspecified external genital organ, female ♀
  X● **S30.21** Contusion of penis ♂
  X● **S30.22** Contusion of scrotum and testes ♂
  X● **S30.23** Contusion of vagina and vulva ♀

X● **S30.3** **Contusion of anus**

● **S30.8** **Other superficial injuries of abdomen, lower back, pelvis and external genitals**
  ● **S30.81** Abrasion of abdomen, lower back, pelvis and external genitals
    ● **S30.810** Abrasion of lower back and pelvis
    ● **S30.811** Abrasion of abdominal wall
    ● **S30.812** Abrasion of penis ♂
    ● **S30.813** Abrasion of scrotum and testes ♂
    ● **S30.814** Abrasion of vagina and vulva ♀
    ● **S30.815** Abrasion of unspecified external genital organs, male ♂
    ● **S30.816** Abrasion of unspecified external genital organs, female ♀
    ● **S30.817** Abrasion of anus
  ● **S30.82** Blister (nonthermal) of abdomen, lower back, pelvis and external genitals
    ● **S30.820** Blister (nonthermal) of lower back and pelvis
    ● **S30.821** Blister (nonthermal) of abdominal wall
    ● **S30.822** Blister (nonthermal) of penis ♂
    ● **S30.823** Blister (nonthermal) of scrotum and testes ♂

    ● **S30.824** Blister (nonthermal) of vagina and vulva ♀
    ● **S30.825** Blister (nonthermal) of unspecified external genital organs, male ♂
    ● **S30.826** Blister (nonthermal) of unspecified external genital organs, female ♀
    ● **S30.827** Blister (nonthermal) of anus
● **S30.84** External constriction of abdomen, lower back, pelvis and external genitals
    ● **S30.840** External constriction of lower back and pelvis
    ● **S30.841** External constriction of abdominal wall
    ● **S30.842** External constriction of penis ♂
        Hair tourniquet syndrome of penis
        Use additional cause code to identify the constricting item (W49.0-)
    ● **S30.843** External constriction of scrotum and testes ♂
    ● **S30.844** External constriction of vagina and vulva ♀
    ● **S30.845** External constriction of unspecified external genital organs, male ♂
    ● **S30.846** External constriction of unspecified external genital organs, female ♀
● **S30.85** Superficial foreign body of abdomen, lower back, pelvis and external genitals
        Splinter in the abdomen, lower back, pelvis and external genitals
    ● **S30.850** Superficial foreign body of lower back and pelvis
    ● **S30.851** Superficial foreign body of abdominal wall
    ● **S30.852** Superficial foreign body of penis ♂
    ● **S30.853** Superficial foreign body of scrotum and testes ♂
    ● **S30.854** Superficial foreign body of vagina and vulva ♀
    ● **S30.855** Superficial foreign body of unspecified external genital organs, male ♂
    ● **S30.856** Superficial foreign body of unspecified external genital organs, female ♀
    ● **S30.857** Superficial foreign body of anus
● **S30.86** Insect bite (nonvenomous) of abdomen, lower back, pelvis and external genitals
    ● **S30.860** Insect bite (nonvenomous) of lower back and pelvis
    ● **S30.861** Insect bite (nonvenomous) of abdominal wall
    ● **S30.862** Insect bite (nonvenomous) of penis ♂
    ● **S30.863** Insect bite (nonvenomous) of scrotum and testes ♂
    ● **S30.864** Insect bite (nonvenomous) of vagina and vulva ♀
    ● **S30.865** Insect bite (nonvenomous) of unspecified external genital organs, male ♂
    ● **S30.866** Insect bite (nonvenomous) of unspecified external genital organs, female ♀
    ● **S30.867** Insect bite (nonvenomous) of anus

CHAPTER 19 (S00-T88)

N Newborn Age: 0   **P** Pediatric Age: 0–17   **M** Maternity DX: 9–64   **A** Adult Age: 15–124   ♀ Females Only   ♂ Males Only

🔴 Complication\Comorbidity   🔴 Major C\C   (Ex) CC/MCC Exclusions   🔴 Hospital-Acquired Condition   🔴 Hierarchical Condition Category

1285

● S30.87   **Other superficial bite of abdomen, lower back, pelvis and external genitals**
    Excludes1   open bite of abdomen, lower back, pelvis and external genitals (S31.05, S31.15, S31.25, S31.35, S31.45, S31.55)
    ● S30.870   **Other superficial bite of lower back and pelvis**
    ● S30.871   **Other superficial bite of abdominal wall**
    ● S30.872   **Other superficial bite of penis♂**
    ● S30.873   **Other superficial bite of scrotum and testes♂**
    ● S30.874   **Other superficial bite of vagina and vulva♀**
    ● S30.875   **Other superficial bite of unspecified external genital organs, male♂**
    ● S30.876   **Other superficial bite of unspecified external genital organs, female♀**
    ● S30.877   **Other superficial bite of anus**
● S30.9   **Unspecified superficial injury of abdomen, lower back, pelvis and external genitals**
    X ● S30.91   **Unspecified superficial injury of lower back and pelvis**
    X ● S30.92   **Unspecified superficial injury of abdominal wall**
    X ● S30.93   **Unspecified superficial injury of penis♂**
    X ● S30.94   **Unspecified superficial injury of scrotum and testes♂**
    X ● S30.95   **Unspecified superficial injury of vagina and vulva♀**
    X ● S30.96   **Unspecified superficial injury of unspecified external genital organs, male ♂**
    X ● S30.97   **Unspecified superficial injury of unspecified external genital organs, female ♀**
    X ● S30.98   **Unspecified superficial injury of anus**

● S31   **Open wound of abdomen, lower back, pelvis and external genitals**
    Code also any associated:
        spinal cord injury (S24.0, S24.1-, S34.0-, S34.1-)
        wound infection
    Excludes1   traumatic amputation of part of abdomen, lower back and pelvis (S38.2-, S38.3)
    Excludes2   open wound of hip (S71.00-S71.02)
        open fracture of pelvis (S32.1--S32.9 with 7th character B)
    The appropriate 7th character is to be added to each code from category S31

A	initial encounter
D	subsequent encounter
S	sequela

    ● S31.0   **Open wound of lower back and pelvis**
        (Ex) *For category S31.0 CC codes:* See PDX Collection 1195
        ● S31.00   **Unspecified open wound of lower back and pelvis**
            ● S31.000   **Unspecified open wound of lower back and pelvis without penetration into retroperitoneum**
                Unspecified open wound of lower back and pelvis NOS
            ● S31.001   **Unspecified open wound of lower back and pelvis with penetration into retroperitoneum** A 🔌

● S31.01   **Laceration without foreign body of lower back and pelvis**
    ● S31.010   **Laceration without foreign body of lower back and pelvis without penetration into retroperitoneum**
        Laceration without foreign body of lower back and pelvis NOS
    ● S31.011   **Laceration without foreign body of lower back and pelvis with penetration into retroperitoneum** A 🔌
● S31.02   **Laceration with foreign body of lower back and pelvis**
    ● S31.020   **Laceration with foreign body of lower back and pelvis without penetration into retroperitoneum**
        Laceration with foreign body of lower back and pelvis NOS
    ● S31.021   **Laceration with foreign body of lower back and pelvis with penetration into retroperitoneum** A 🔌
● S31.03   **Puncture wound without foreign body of lower back and pelvis**
    ● S31.030   **Puncture wound without foreign body of lower back and pelvis without penetration into retroperitoneum**
        Puncture wound without foreign body of lower back and pelvis NOS
    ● S31.031   **Puncture wound without foreign body of lower back and pelvis with penetration into retroperitoneum** A 🔌
● S31.04   **Puncture wound with foreign body of lower back and pelvis**
    ● S31.040   **Puncture wound with foreign body of lower back and pelvis without penetration into retroperitoneum**
        Puncture wound with foreign body of lower back and pelvis NOS
    ● S31.041   **Puncture wound with foreign body of lower back and pelvis with penetration into retroperitoneum** A 🔌
● S31.05   **Open bite of lower back and pelvis**
    Bite of lower back and pelvis NOS
    Excludes1   superficial bite of lower back and pelvis (S30.860, S30.870)
    ● S31.050   **Open bite of lower back and pelvis without penetration into retroperitoneum**
        Open bite of lower back and pelvis NOS
    ● S31.051   **Open bite of lower back and pelvis with penetration into retroperitoneum** A 🔌
● S31.1   **Open wound of abdominal wall without penetration into peritoneal cavity**
    Open wound of abdominal wall NOS
    Excludes2   open wound of abdominal wall with penetration into peritoneal cavity (S31.6-)
    ● S31.10   **Unspecified open wound of abdominal wall without penetration into peritoneal cavity**
        ● S31.100   **Unspecified open wound of abdominal wall, right upper quadrant without penetration into peritoneal cavity**
        ● S31.101   **Unspecified open wound of abdominal wall, left upper quadrant without penetration into peritoneal cavity**

● S31.102   Unspecified open wound of abdominal wall, epigastric region without penetration into peritoneal cavity

● S31.103   Unspecified open wound of abdominal wall, right lower quadrant without penetration into peritoneal cavity

● S31.104   Unspecified open wound of abdominal wall, left lower quadrant without penetration into peritoneal cavity

● S31.105   Unspecified open wound of abdominal wall, periumbilic region without penetration into peritoneal cavity

● S31.109   Unspecified open wound of abdominal wall, unspecified quadrant without penetration into peritoneal cavity

     Unspecified open wound of abdominal wall NOS

● S31.11   Laceration without foreign body of abdominal wall without penetration into peritoneal cavity

● S31.110   Laceration without foreign body of abdominal wall, right upper quadrant without penetration into peritoneal cavity

● S31.111   Laceration without foreign body of abdominal wall, left upper quadrant without penetration into peritoneal cavity

● S31.112   Laceration without foreign body of abdominal wall, epigastric region without penetration into peritoneal cavity

● S31.113   Laceration without foreign body of abdominal wall, right lower quadrant without penetration into peritoneal cavity

● S31.114   Laceration without foreign body of abdominal wall, left lower quadrant without penetration into peritoneal cavity

● S31.115   Laceration without foreign body of abdominal wall, periumbilic region without penetration into peritoneal cavity

● S31.119   Laceration without foreign body of abdominal wall, unspecified quadrant without penetration into peritoneal cavity

● S31.12   Laceration with foreign body of abdominal wall without penetration into peritoneal cavity

● S31.120   Laceration of abdominal wall with foreign body, right upper quadrant without penetration into peritoneal cavity

● S31.121   Laceration of abdominal wall with foreign body, left upper quadrant without penetration into peritoneal cavity

● S31.122   Laceration of abdominal wall with foreign body, epigastric region without penetration into peritoneal cavity

● S31.123   Laceration of abdominal wall with foreign body, right lower quadrant without penetration into peritoneal cavity

● S31.124   Laceration of abdominal wall with foreign body, left lower quadrant without penetration into peritoneal cavity

● S31.125   Laceration of abdominal wall with foreign body, periumbilic region without penetration into peritoneal cavity

● S31.129   Laceration of abdominal wall with foreign body, unspecified quadrant without penetration into peritoneal cavity

● S31.13   Puncture wound of abdominal wall without foreign body without penetration into peritoneal cavity

● S31.130   Puncture wound of abdominal wall without foreign body, right upper quadrant without penetration into peritoneal cavity

● S31.131   Puncture wound of abdominal wall without foreign body, left upper quadrant without penetration into peritoneal cavity

● S31.132   Puncture wound of abdominal wall without foreign body, epigastric region without penetration into peritoneal cavity

● S31.133   Puncture wound of abdominal wall without foreign body, right lower quadrant without penetration into peritoneal cavity

● S31.134   Puncture wound of abdominal wall without foreign body, left lower quadrant without penetration into peritoneal cavity

● S31.135   Puncture wound of abdominal wall without foreign body, periumbilic region without penetration into peritoneal cavity

● S31.139   Puncture wound of abdominal wall without foreign body, unspecified quadrant without penetration into peritoneal cavity

● S31.14   Puncture wound of abdominal wall with foreign body without penetration into peritoneal cavity

● S31.140   Puncture wound of abdominal wall with foreign body, right upper quadrant without penetration into peritoneal cavity

● S31.141   Puncture wound of abdominal wall with foreign body, left upper quadrant without penetration into peritoneal cavity

● S31.142   Puncture wound of abdominal wall with foreign body, epigastric region without penetration into peritoneal cavity

● S31.143   Puncture wound of abdominal wall with foreign body, right lower quadrant without penetration into peritoneal cavity

● S31.144   Puncture wound of abdominal wall with foreign body, left lower quadrant without penetration into peritoneal cavity

● S31.145   Puncture wound of abdominal wall with foreign body, periumbilic region without penetration into peritoneal cavity

● S31.149   Puncture wound of abdominal wall with foreign body, unspecified quadrant without penetration into peritoneal cavity

N   Newborn Age: 0   **P**   Pediatric Age: 0–17   **M**   Maternity DX: 9–64   **A**   Adult Age: 15–124   ♀   Females Only   ♂   Males Only

🅒   Complication\Comorbidity   🅒   Major C\C   (Ex:)   CC/MCC Exclusions   🅒   Hospital-Acquired Condition   🅒   Hierarchical Condition Category

1287

● **S31.15** Open bite of abdominal wall without penetration into peritoneal cavity
Bite of abdominal wall NOS

Excludes1 superficial bite of abdominal wall (S30.871)

● **S31.150** Open bite of abdominal wall, right upper quadrant without penetration into peritoneal cavity

● **S31.151** Open bite of abdominal wall, left upper quadrant without penetration into peritoneal cavity

● **S31.152** Open bite of abdominal wall, epigastric region without penetration into peritoneal cavity

● **S31.153** Open bite of abdominal wall, right lower quadrant without penetration into peritoneal cavity

● **S31.154** Open bite of abdominal wall, left lower quadrant without penetration into peritoneal cavity

● **S31.155** Open bite of abdominal wall, periumbilic region without penetration into peritoneal cavity

● **S31.159** Open bite of abdominal wall, unspecified quadrant without penetration into peritoneal cavity

● **S31.2** Open wound of penis
X● **S31.20** Unspecified open wound of penis ♂
X● **S31.21** Laceration without foreign body of penis ♂
X● **S31.22** Laceration with foreign body of penis ♂
X● **S31.23** Puncture wound without foreign body of penis ♂
X● **S31.24** Puncture wound with foreign body of penis ♂
X● **S31.25** Open bite of penis ♂
Bite of penis NOS

Excludes1 superficial bite of penis (S30.862, S30.872)

● **S31.3** Open wound of scrotum and testes
X● **S31.30** Unspecified open wound of scrotum and testes ♂
X● **S31.31** Laceration without foreign body of scrotum and testes ♂
X● **S31.32** Laceration with foreign body of scrotum and testes ♂
X● **S31.33** Puncture wound without foreign body of scrotum and testes ♂
X● **S31.34** Puncture wound with foreign body of scrotum and testes ♂
X● **S31.35** Open bite of scrotum and testes ♂
Bite of scrotum and testes NOS

Excludes1 superficial bite of scrotum and testes (S30.863, S30.873)

● **S31.4** Open wound of vagina and vulva

Excludes1 injury to vagina and vulva during delivery (O70.-, O71.4)

X● **S31.40** Unspecified open wound of vagina and vulva ♀
X● **S31.41** Laceration without foreign body of vagina and vulva ♀
X● **S31.42** Laceration with foreign body of vagina and vulva ♀
X● **S31.43** Puncture wound without foreign body of vagina and vulva ♀
X● **S31.44** Puncture wound with foreign body of vagina and vulva ♀
X● **S31.45** Open bite of vagina and vulva ♀
Bite of vagina and vulva NOS

Excludes1 superficial bite of vagina and vulva (S30.864, S30.874)

● **S31.5** Open wound of unspecified external genital organs

Excludes1 traumatic amputation of external genital organs (S38.21, S38.22)

● **S31.50** Unspecified open wound of unspecified external genital organs
● **S31.501** Unspecified open wound of unspecified external genital organs, male ♂
● **S31.502** Unspecified open wound of unspecified external genital organs, female ♀

● **S31.51** Laceration without foreign body of unspecified external genital organs
● **S31.511** Laceration without foreign body of unspecified external genital organs, male ♂
● **S31.512** Laceration without foreign body of unspecified external genital organs, female ♀

● **S31.52** Laceration with foreign body of unspecified external genital organs
● **S31.521** Laceration with foreign body of unspecified external genital organs, male ♂
● **S31.522** Laceration with foreign body of unspecified external genital organs, female ♀

● **S31.53** Puncture wound without foreign body of unspecified external genital organs
● **S31.531** Puncture wound without foreign body of unspecified external genital organs, male ♂
● **S31.532** Puncture wound without foreign body of unspecified external genital organs, female ♀

● **S31.54** Puncture wound with foreign body of unspecified external genital organs
● **S31.541** Puncture wound with foreign body of unspecified external genital organs, male ♂
● **S31.542** Puncture wound with foreign body of unspecified external genital organs, female ♀

● **S31.55** Open bite of unspecified external genital organs
Bite of unspecified external genital organs NOS

Excludes1 superficial bite of unspecified external genital organs (S30.865, S30.866, S30.875, S30.876)

● **S31.551** Open bite of unspecified external genital organs, male ♂
● **S31.552** Open bite of unspecified external genital organs, female ♀

● **S31.6** Open wound of abdominal wall with penetration into peritoneal cavity
(Ex) **For category S31.6 CC codes:** See PDX Collection 1195

● **S31.60** Unspecified open wound of abdominal wall with penetration into peritoneal cavity
● **S31.600** Unspecified open wound of abdominal wall, right upper quadrant with penetration into peritoneal cavity A
● **S31.601** Unspecified open wound of abdominal wall, left upper quadrant with penetration into peritoneal cavity A
● **S31.602** Unspecified open wound of abdominal wall, epigastric region with penetration into peritoneal cavity A

▶ New   ⇒ Revised   ~~deleted~~ Deleted   Excludes 1   Excludes 2   Includes   Use additional   Code first   Code also   Key words
OGCR Official Guidelines   ● Unacceptable Principal Diagnosis   X Assign placeholder X   ● Use Additional Character(s)   ▶ Manifestation Code   Coding Clinic

● S31.603 Unspecified open wound of abdominal wall, **right lower** quadrant with penetration into peritoneal cavity A 🏮

● S31.604 Unspecified open wound of abdominal wall, **left lower** quadrant with penetration into peritoneal cavity A 🏮

● S31.605 Unspecified open wound of abdominal wall, **periumbilic region** with penetration into peritoneal cavity A 🏮

● S31.609 Unspecified open wound of abdominal wall, **unspecified** quadrant with penetration into peritoneal cavity A 🏮

● S31.61 Laceration without foreign body of abdominal wall with penetration into peritoneal cavity

● S31.610 Laceration without foreign body of abdominal wall, **right upper** quadrant with penetration into peritoneal cavity A 🏮

● S31.611 Laceration without foreign body of abdominal wall, **left upper** quadrant with penetration into peritoneal cavity A 🏮

● S31.612 Laceration without foreign body of abdominal wall, **epigastric region** with penetration into peritoneal cavity A 🏮

● S31.613 Laceration without foreign body of abdominal wall, **right lower** quadrant with penetration into peritoneal cavity A 🏮,
  Coding Clinic: 2015, Q4, P37

● S31.614 Laceration without foreign body of abdominal wall, **left lower** quadrant with penetration into peritoneal cavity A 🏮

● S31.615 Laceration without foreign body of abdominal wall, **periumbilic region** with penetration into peritoneal cavity A 🏮

● S31.619 Laceration without foreign body of abdominal wall, **unspecified** quadrant with penetration into peritoneal cavity A 🏮

● S31.62 Laceration with foreign body of abdominal wall with penetration into peritoneal cavity

● S31.620 Laceration with foreign body of abdominal wall, **right upper** quadrant with penetration into peritoneal cavity A 🏮

● S31.621 Laceration with foreign body of abdominal wall, **left upper** quadrant with penetration into peritoneal cavity A 🏮

● S31.622 Laceration with foreign body of abdominal wall, **epigastric region** with penetration into peritoneal cavity A 🏮

● S31.623 Laceration with foreign body of abdominal wall, **right lower** quadrant with penetration into peritoneal cavity A 🏮

● S31.624 Laceration with foreign body of abdominal wall, **left lower** quadrant with penetration into peritoneal cavity A 🏮

● S31.625 Laceration with foreign body of abdominal wall, **periumbilic region** with penetration into peritoneal cavity A 🏮

● S31.629 Laceration with foreign body of abdominal wall, **unspecified** quadrant with penetration into peritoneal cavity A 🏮

● S31.63 Puncture wound without foreign body of abdominal wall with penetration into peritoneal cavity

● S31.630 Puncture wound without foreign body of abdominal wall, **right upper** quadrant with penetration into peritoneal cavity A 🏮

● S31.631 Puncture wound without foreign body of abdominal wall, **left upper** quadrant with penetration into peritoneal cavity A 🏮

● S31.632 Puncture wound without foreign body of abdominal wall, **epigastric region** with penetration into peritoneal cavity A 🏮

● S31.633 Puncture wound without foreign body of abdominal wall, **right lower** quadrant with penetration into peritoneal cavity A 🏮

● S31.634 Puncture wound without foreign body of abdominal wall, **left lower** quadrant with penetration into peritoneal cavity A 🏮

● S31.635 Puncture wound without foreign body of abdominal wall, **periumbilic region** with penetration into peritoneal cavity A 🏮

● S31.639 Puncture wound without foreign body of abdominal wall, **unspecified** quadrant with penetration into peritoneal cavity A 🏮

● S31.64 Puncture wound with foreign body of abdominal wall with penetration into peritoneal cavity

● S31.640 Puncture wound with foreign body of abdominal wall, **right upper** quadrant with penetration into peritoneal cavity A 🏮

● S31.641 Puncture wound with foreign body of abdominal wall, **left upper** quadrant with penetration into peritoneal cavity A 🏮

● S31.642 Puncture wound with foreign body of abdominal wall, **epigastric region** with penetration into peritoneal cavity A 🏮

● S31.643 Puncture wound with foreign body of abdominal wall, **right lower** quadrant with penetration into peritoneal cavity A 🏮

● S31.644 Puncture wound with foreign body of abdominal wall, **left lower** quadrant with penetration into peritoneal cavity A 🏮

● S31.645 Puncture wound with foreign body of abdominal wall, **periumbilic region** with penetration into peritoneal cavity A 🏮

● S31.649 Puncture wound with foreign body of abdominal wall, **unspecified** quadrant with penetration into peritoneal cavity A 🏮

CHAPTER 19 (S00-T88)

● S31.65   **Open bite of abdominal wall with penetration into peritoneal cavity**
> **Excludes1**   superficial bite of abdominal wall (S30.861, S30.871)

  ● S31.650   **Open bite of abdominal wall, right upper quadrant with penetration into peritoneal cavity** A 🔣

  ● S31.651   **Open bite of abdominal wall, left upper quadrant with penetration into peritoneal cavity** A 🔣

  ● S31.652   **Open bite of abdominal wall, epigastric region with penetration into peritoneal cavity** A 🔣

  ● S31.653   **Open bite of abdominal wall, right lower quadrant with penetration into peritoneal cavity** A 🔣

  ● S31.654   **Open bite of abdominal wall, left lower quadrant with penetration into peritoneal cavity** A 🔣

  ● S31.655   **Open bite of abdominal wall, periumbilic region with penetration into peritoneal cavity** A 🔣

  ● S31.659   **Open bite of abdominal wall, unspecified quadrant with penetration into peritoneal cavity** A 🔣

● S31.8   **Open wound of other parts of abdomen, lower back and pelvis**

  ● S31.80   **Open wound of unspecified buttock**

    ● S31.801   **Laceration without foreign body of unspecified buttock**

    ● S31.802   **Laceration with foreign body of unspecified buttock**

    ● S31.803   **Puncture wound without foreign body of unspecified buttock**

    ● S31.804   **Puncture wound with foreign body of unspecified buttock**

    ● S31.805   **Open bite of unspecified buttock**
> Bite of buttock NOS
> **Excludes1**   superficial bite of buttock (S30.870)

    ● S31.809   **Unspecified open wound of unspecified buttock**

  ● S31.81   **Open wound of right buttock**

    ● S31.811   **Laceration without foreign body of right buttock**

    ● S31.812   **Laceration with foreign body of right buttock**

    ● S31.813   **Puncture wound without foreign body of right buttock**

    ● S31.814   **Puncture wound with foreign body of right buttock**

    ● S31.815   **Open bite of right buttock**
> Bite of right buttock NOS
> **Excludes1**   superficial bite of buttock (S30.870)

    ● S31.819   **Unspecified open wound of right buttock**

  ● S31.82   **Open wound of left buttock**

    ● S31.821   **Laceration without foreign body of left buttock**

    ● S31.822   **Laceration with foreign body of left buttock**

    ● S31.823   **Puncture wound without foreign body of left buttock**

    ● S31.824   **Puncture wound with foreign body of left buttock**

    ● S31.825   **Open bite of left buttock**
> Bite of left buttock NOS
> **Excludes1**   superficial bite of buttock (S30.870)

    ● S31.829   **Unspecified open wound of left buttock**

● S31.83   **Open wound of anus**

  ● S31.831   **Laceration without foreign body of anus**

  ● S31.832   **Laceration with foreign body of anus**

  ● S31.833   **Puncture wound without foreign body of anus**

  ● S31.834   **Puncture wound with foreign body of anus**

  ● S31.835   **Open bite of anus**
> Bite of anus NOS
> **Excludes1**   superficial bite of anus (S30.877)

  ● S31.839   **Unspecified open wound of anus**

● S32   **Fracture of lumbar spine and pelvis**

Note: A fracture not indicated as displaced or nondisplaced should be coded to displaced

A fracture not indicated as opened or closed should be coded to closed

> **Includes**   fracture of lumbosacral neural arch
> fracture of lumbosacral spinous process
> fracture of lumbosacral transverse process
> fracture of lumbosacral vertebra
> fracture of lumbosacral vertebral arch

Code first any associated spinal cord and spinal nerve injury (S34.-)

> **Excludes1**   transection of abdomen (S38.3)
> **Excludes2**   fracture of hip NOS (S72.0-)

The appropriate 7th character is to be added to each code from category S32

A	initial encounter for closed fracture
B	initial encounter for open fracture
D	subsequent encounter for fracture with routine healing
G	subsequent encounter for fracture with delayed healing
K	subsequent encounter for fracture with nonunion
S	sequela

● S32.0   **Fracture of lumbar vertebra**
> Fracture of lumbar spine NOS
> (Ex) **For category S32.0 CC codes S32.0[A,B]:** See PDX Collection 1196
> **For S32.0[K]:** See PDX Collection 897

  ● S32.00   **Fracture of unspecified lumbar vertebra**

    ● S32.000   **Wedge compression fracture of unspecified lumbar vertebra** A, K 🔣, B 🔣, A, B 🔣, A, B 🔣

    ● S32.001   **Stable burst fracture of unspecified lumbar vertebra** A, K 🔣, B 🔣, A, B 🔣, A, B 🔣

    ● S32.002   **Unstable burst fracture of unspecified lumbar vertebra** A, K 🔣, B 🔣, A, B 🔣, A, B 🔣

    ● S32.008   **Other fracture of unspecified lumbar vertebra** A, K 🔣, B 🔣, A, B 🔣, A, B 🔣

    ● S32.009   **Unspecified fracture of unspecified lumbar vertebra** A, K 🔣, B 🔣, A, B 🔣, A, B 🔣

  ● S32.01   **Fracture of first lumbar vertebra**

    ● S32.010   **Wedge compression fracture of first lumbar vertebra** A, K 🔣, B 🔣, A, B 🔣, A, B 🔣

    ● S32.011   **Stable burst fracture of first lumbar vertebra** A, K 🔣, B 🔣, A, B 🔣, A, B 🔣

    ● S32.012   **Unstable burst fracture of first lumbar vertebra** A, K 🔣, B 🔣, A, B 🔣, A, B 🔣

    ● S32.018   **Other fracture of first lumbar vertebra** A, K 🔣, B 🔣, A, B 🔣, A, B 🔣

    ● S32.019   **Unspecified fracture of first lumbar vertebra** A, K 🔣, B 🔣, A, B 🔣, A, B 🔣

● S32.02   Fracture of second lumbar vertebra
   ● S32.020   **Wedge compression** fracture of second lumbar vertebra A, K, B, A, B, **A, B**
   ● S32.021   **Stable burst** fracture of second lumbar vertebra A, K, B, A, B, **A, B**
   ● S32.022   **Unstable burst** fracture of second lumbar vertebra A, K, B, A, B, **A, B**
   ● S32.028   **Other** fracture of second lumbar vertebra A, K, B, A, B, **A, B**
   ● S32.029   **Unspecified** fracture of second lumbar vertebra A, K, B, A, B, **A, B**

● S32.03   Fracture of third lumbar vertebra
   ● S32.030   **Wedge compression** fracture of third lumbar vertebra A, K, B, A, B, **A, B**
   ● S32.031   **Stable burst** fracture of third lumbar vertebra A, K, B, A, B, **A, B**
   ● S32.032   **Unstable burst** fracture of third lumbar vertebra A, K, B, A, B, **A, B**
   ● S32.038   **Other** fracture of third lumbar vertebra A, K, B, A, B, **A, B**
   ● S32.039   **Unspecified** fracture of third lumbar vertebra A, K, B, A, B, **A, B**

● S32.04   Fracture of fourth lumbar vertebra
   ● S32.040   **Wedge compression** fracture of fourth lumbar vertebra A, K, B, A, B, **A, B**
   ● S32.041   **Stable burst** fracture of fourth lumbar vertebra A, K, B, A, B, **A, B**
   ● S32.042   **Unstable burst** fracture of fourth lumbar vertebra A, K, B, A, B, **A, B**
   ● S32.048   **Other** fracture of fourth lumbar vertebra A, K, B, A, B, **A, B**
   ● S32.049   **Unspecified** fracture of fourth lumbar vertebra A, K, B, A, B, **A, B**

● S32.05   Fracture of fifth lumbar vertebra
   ● S32.050   **Wedge compression** fracture of fifth lumbar vertebra A, K, B, A, B, **A, B**
   ● S32.051   **Stable burst** fracture of fifth lumbar vertebra A, K, B, A, B, **A, B**
   ● S32.052   **Unstable burst** fracture of fifth lumbar vertebra A, K, B, A, B, **A, B**
   ● S32.058   **Other** fracture of fifth lumbar vertebra A, K, B, A, B, **A, B**
   ● S32.059   **Unspecified** fracture of fifth lumbar vertebra A, K, B, A, B, **A, B**

● S32.1   Fracture of **sacrum**
For vertical fractures, code to most medial fracture extension
Use two codes if both a vertical and transverse fracture are present
Code also any associated fracture of pelvic ring (S32.8-)
(Ex) **For category S32.1 CC codes S32.1[A,B]:** See PDX Collection 1197
For S32.1[K]: See PDX Collection 897
X ● S32.10   **Unspecified** fracture of sacrum A, K, B, A, B, **A, B**
   ● S32.11   **Zone I** fracture of sacrum
Vertical sacral ala fracture of sacrum
    ● S32.110   **Nondisplaced** Zone I fracture of sacrum A, K, B, A, B, **A, B**
    ● S32.111   **Minimally displaced** Zone I fracture of sacrum A, K, B, A, B, **A, B**

    ● S32.112   **Severely displaced** Zone I fracture of sacrum A, K, B, A, B, **A, B**
    ● S32.119   **Unspecified** Zone I fracture of sacrum A, K, B, A, B, **A, B**
   ● S32.12   **Zone II** fracture of sacrum
Vertical foraminal region fracture of sacrum
    ● S32.120   **Nondisplaced** Zone II fracture of sacrum A, K, B, A, B, **A, B**
    ● S32.121   **Minimally displaced** Zone II fracture of sacrum A, K, B, A, B, **A, B**
    ● S32.122   **Severely displaced** Zone II fracture of sacrum A, K, B, A, B, **A, B**
    ● S32.129   **Unspecified** Zone II fracture of sacrum A, K, B, A, B, **A, B**
   ● S32.13   **Zone III** fracture of sacrum
Vertical fracture into spinal canal region of sacrum
    ● S32.130   **Nondisplaced** Zone III fracture of sacrum A, K, B, A, B, **A, B**
    ● S32.131   **Minimally displaced** Zone III fracture of sacrum A, K, B, A, B, **A, B**
    ● S32.132   **Severely displaced** Zone III fracture of sacrum A, K, B, A, B, **A, B**
    ● S32.139   **Unspecified** Zone III fracture of sacrum A, K, B, A, B, **A, B**
X ● S32.14   **Type 1** fracture of sacrum A, K, B, A, B, **A, B**
Transverse flexion fracture of sacrum without displacement
X ● S32.15   **Type 2** fracture of sacrum A, K, B, A, B, **A, B**
Transverse flexion fracture of sacrum with posterior displacement
X ● S32.16   **Type 3** fracture of sacrum A, K, B, A, B, **A, B**
Transverse extension fracture of sacrum with anterior displacement
X ● S32.17   **Type 4** fracture of sacrum A, K, B, A, B, **A, B**
Transverse segmental comminution of upper sacrum
X ● S32.19   **Other** fracture of sacrum A, K, B, A, B, **A, B**
X ● S32.2   Fracture of **coccyx** A, K, B, A, B, **A, B**
(Ex) **For category S32.2 CC codes S32.2[A,B]:** See PDX Collection 1197
For S32.2[K]: See PDX Collection 897
● S32.3   Fracture of **ilium**
   Excludes1   fracture of ilium with associated disruption of pelvic ring (S32.8-)
(Ex) **For category S32.3 CC codes S32.3[A]:** See PDX Collection 1176
For S32.3[B]: See PDX Collection 1198 **For S32.3[K]:** See PDX Collection 897
   ● S32.30   **Unspecified** fracture of ilium
    ● S32.301   **Unspecified** fracture of **right** ilium A, K, B, A, B, **A, B**
    ● S32.302   **Unspecified** fracture of **left** ilium A, K, B, A, B, **A, B**
    ● S32.309   **Unspecified** fracture of **unspecified** ilium A, K, B, A, B, **A, B**
   ● S32.31   **Avulsion** fracture of ilium
    ● S32.311   **Displaced avulsion** fracture of **right** ilium A, K, B, A, B, **A, B**
    ● S32.312   **Displaced avulsion** fracture of **left** ilium A, K, B, A, B, **A, B**
    ● S32.313   **Displaced avulsion** fracture of **unspecified** ilium A, K, B, A, B, **A, B**

N Newborn Age: 0   **P** Pediatric Age: 0–17   **M** Maternity DX: 9–64   **A** Adult Age: 15–124   ♀ Females Only   ♂ Males Only

Complication\Comorbidity   Major C\C   (Ex) CC/MCC Exclusions   Hospital-Acquired Condition   Hierarchical Condition Category

CHAPTER 19 (S00-T88)

1291

● S32.314   Nondisplaced avulsion fracture of right ilium A, K 🔹, B 🔹, A, B 🔹, A, B 🔹

● S32.315   Nondisplaced avulsion fracture of left ilium A, K 🔹, B 🔹, A, B 🔹, A, B 🔹

● S32.316   Nondisplaced avulsion fracture of unspecified ilium A, K 🔹, B 🔹, A, B 🔹, A, B 🔹

● S32.39   Other fracture of ilium

● S32.391   Other fracture of right ilium A, K 🔹, B 🔹, A, B 🔹, A, B 🔹

● S32.392   Other fracture of left ilium A, K 🔹, B 🔹, A, B 🔹, A, B 🔹

● S32.399   Other fracture of unspecified ilium A, K 🔹, B 🔹, A, B 🔹, A, B 🔹

● S32.4   Fracture of acetabulum

Code also any associated fracture of pelvic ring (S32.8-)

(Ex:) For category S32.4 CC codes S32.4[A]: See PDX Collection 1199
For S32.4[B]: See PDX Collection 1200 For S32.4[K]: See PDX Collection 897

● S32.40   Unspecified fracture of acetabulum

● S32.401   Unspecified fracture of right acetabulum K 🔹, A, B 🔹, A, B 🔹, A, B 🔹

● S32.402   Unspecified fracture of left acetabulum K 🔹, A, B 🔹, A, B 🔹, A, B 🔹

● S32.409   Unspecified fracture of unspecified acetabulum K 🔹, A, B 🔹, A, B 🔹, A, B 🔹

● S32.41   Fracture of anterior wall of acetabulum

● S32.411   Displaced fracture of anterior wall of right acetabulum K 🔹, A, B 🔹, A, B 🔹, A, B 🔹

● S32.412   Displaced fracture of anterior wall of left acetabulum K 🔹, A, B 🔹, A, B 🔹, A, B 🔹

● S32.413   Displaced fracture of anterior wall of unspecified acetabulum K 🔹, A, B 🔹, A, B 🔹, A, B 🔹

● S32.414   Nondisplaced fracture of anterior wall of right acetabulum K 🔹, A, B 🔹, A, B 🔹, A, B 🔹

● S32.415   Nondisplaced fracture of anterior wall of left acetabulum K 🔹, A, B 🔹, A, B 🔹, A, B 🔹

● S32.416   Nondisplaced fracture of anterior wall of unspecified acetabulum K 🔹, A, B 🔹, A, B 🔹, A, B 🔹

● S32.42   Fracture of posterior wall of acetabulum

● S32.421   Displaced fracture of posterior wall of right acetabulum K 🔹, A, B 🔹, A, B 🔹, A, B 🔹

● S32.422   Displaced fracture of posterior wall of left acetabulum K 🔹, A, B 🔹, A, B 🔹, A, B 🔹

● S32.423   Displaced fracture of posterior wall of unspecified acetabulum K 🔹, A, B 🔹, A, B 🔹, A, B 🔹

● S32.424   Nondisplaced fracture of posterior wall of right acetabulum K 🔹, A, B 🔹, A, B 🔹, A, B 🔹

● S32.425   Nondisplaced fracture of posterior wall of left acetabulum K 🔹, A, B 🔹, A, B 🔹, A, B 🔹

● S32.426   Nondisplaced fracture of posterior wall of unspecified acetabulum K 🔹, A, B 🔹, A, B 🔹, A, B 🔹

● S32.43   Fracture of anterior column [iliopubic] of acetabulum

● S32.431   Displaced fracture of anterior column [iliopubic] of right acetabulum K 🔹, A, B 🔹, A, B 🔹, A, B 🔹

● S32.432   Displaced fracture of anterior column [iliopubic] of left acetabulum K 🔹, A, B 🔹, A, B 🔹, A, B 🔹

● S32.433   Displaced fracture of anterior column [iliopubic] of unspecified acetabulum K 🔹, A, B 🔹, A, B 🔹, A, B 🔹

● S32.434   Nondisplaced fracture of anterior column [iliopubic] of right acetabulum K 🔹, A, B 🔹, A, B 🔹, A, B 🔹

● S32.435   Nondisplaced fracture of anterior column [iliopubic] of left acetabulum K 🔹, A, B 🔹, A, B 🔹, A, B 🔹

● S32.436   Nondisplaced fracture of anterior column [iliopubic] of unspecified acetabulum K 🔹, A, B 🔹, A, B 🔹, A, B 🔹

● S32.44   Fracture of posterior column [ilioischial] of acetabulum

● S32.441   Displaced fracture of posterior column [ilioischial] of right acetabulum K 🔹, A, B 🔹, A, B 🔹, A, B 🔹

● S32.442   Displaced fracture of posterior column [ilioischial] of left acetabulum K 🔹, A, B 🔹, A, B 🔹, A, B 🔹

● S32.443   Displaced fracture of posterior column [ilioischial] of unspecified acetabulum K 🔹, A, B 🔹, A, B 🔹, A, B 🔹

● S32.444   Nondisplaced fracture of posterior column [ilioischial] of right acetabulum K 🔹, A, B 🔹, A, B 🔹, A, B 🔹

● S32.445   Nondisplaced fracture of posterior column [ilioischial] of left acetabulum K 🔹, A, B 🔹, A, B 🔹, A, B 🔹

● S32.446   Nondisplaced fracture of posterior column [ilioischial] of unspecified acetabulum K 🔹, A, B 🔹, A, B 🔹, A, B 🔹

● S32.45   Transverse fracture of acetabulum

● S32.451   Displaced transverse fracture of right acetabulum K 🔹, A, B 🔹, A, B 🔹, A, B 🔹

● S32.452   Displaced transverse fracture of left acetabulum K 🔹, A, B 🔹, A, B 🔹, A, B 🔹

● S32.453   Displaced transverse fracture of unspecified acetabulum K 🔹, A, B 🔹, A, B 🔹, A, B 🔹

● S32.454   Nondisplaced transverse fracture of right acetabulum K 🔹, A, B 🔹, A, B 🔹, A, B 🔹

● S32.455   Nondisplaced transverse fracture of left acetabulum K 🔹, A, B 🔹, A, B 🔹, A, B 🔹

● S32.456   Nondisplaced transverse fracture of unspecified acetabulum K 🔹, A, B 🔹, A, B 🔹, A, B 🔹

● S32.46   Associated transverse-posterior fracture of acetabulum

● S32.461   Displaced associated transverse-posterior fracture of right acetabulum K 🔹, A, B 🔹, A, B 🔹, A, B 🔹

● S32.462   Displaced associated transverse-posterior fracture of left acetabulum K 🔹, A, B 🔹, A, B 🔹, A, B 🔹

- S32.463 Displaced associated transverse-posterior fracture of unspecified acetabulum K ⦿, A, B ⦿, A, B ⦿, **A, B** ⦿
  - S32.464 Nondisplaced associated transverse-posterior fracture of right acetabulum K ⦿, A, B ⦿, A, B ⦿, **A, B** ⦿
  - S32.465 Nondisplaced associated transverse-posterior fracture of left acetabulum K ⦿, A, B ⦿, A, B ⦿, **A, B** ⦿
  - S32.466 Nondisplaced associated transverse-posterior fracture of unspecified acetabulum K ⦿, A, B ⦿, A, B ⦿, **A, B** ⦿
- S32.47 Fracture of medial wall of acetabulum
  - S32.471 Displaced fracture of medial wall of right acetabulum K ⦿, A, B ⦿, A, B ⦿, **A, B** ⦿
  - S32.472 Displaced fracture of medial wall of left acetabulum K ⦿, A, B ⦿, A, B ⦿, **A, B** ⦿
  - S32.473 Displaced fracture of medial wall of unspecified acetabulum K ⦿, A, B ⦿, A, B ⦿, **A, B** ⦿
  - S32.474 Nondisplaced fracture of medial wall of right acetabulum K ⦿, A, B ⦿, A, B ⦿, **A, B** ⦿
  - S32.475 Nondisplaced fracture of medial wall of left acetabulum K ⦿, A, B ⦿, A, B ⦿, **A, B** ⦿
  - S32.476 Nondisplaced fracture of medial wall of unspecified acetabulum K ⦿, A, B ⦿, A, B ⦿, **A, B** ⦿
- S32.48 Dome fracture of acetabulum
  - S32.481 Displaced dome fracture of right acetabulum K ⦿, A, B ⦿, A, B ⦿, **A, B** ⦿
  - S32.482 Displaced dome fracture of left acetabulum K ⦿, A, B ⦿, A, B ⦿, **A, B** ⦿
  - S32.483 Displaced dome fracture of unspecified acetabulum K ⦿, A, B ⦿, A, B ⦿, **A, B** ⦿
  - S32.484 Nondisplaced dome fracture of right acetabulum K ⦿, A, B ⦿, A, B ⦿, **A, B** ⦿
  - S32.485 Nondisplaced dome fracture of left acetabulum K ⦿, A, B ⦿, A, B ⦿, **A, B** ⦿
  - S32.486 Nondisplaced dome fracture of unspecified acetabulum K ⦿, A, B ⦿, A, B ⦿, **A, B** ⦿
- S32.49 Other fracture of acetabulum
  - S32.491 Other fracture of right acetabulum K ⦿, A, B ⦿, A, B ⦿, **A, B** ⦿
  - S32.492 Other fracture of left acetabulum K ⦿, A, B ⦿, A, B ⦿, **A, B** ⦿
  - S32.499 Other fracture of unspecified acetabulum K ⦿, A, B ⦿, A, B ⦿, **A, B** ⦿
- S32.5 Fracture of pubis
  - **Excludes1** fracture of pubis with associated disruption of pelvic ring (S32.8-)
  - (Ex) **For category S32.5 CC codes S32.5[A,B]:** See PDX Collection 1201 **For S32.5[K]:** See PDX Collection 897
  - S32.50 Unspecified fracture of pubis
    - S32.501 Unspecified fracture of right pubis A, K ⦿, B ⦿, A, B ⦿, **A, B** ⦿
    - S32.502 Unspecified fracture of left pubis A, K ⦿, B ⦿, A, B ⦿, **A, B** ⦿
    - S32.509 Unspecified fracture of unspecified pubis A, K ⦿, B ⦿, A, B ⦿, **A, B** ⦿

- S32.51 Fracture of superior rim of pubis
  - S32.511 Fracture of superior rim of right pubis A, K ⦿, B ⦿, A, B ⦿, **A, B** ⦿
  - S32.512 Fracture of superior rim of left pubis A, K ⦿, B ⦿, A, B ⦿, **A, B** ⦿
  - S32.519 Fracture of superior rim of unspecified pubis A, K ⦿, B ⦿, A, B ⦿, **A, B** ⦿
- S32.59 Other specified fracture of pubis
  - S32.591 Other specified fracture of right pubis A, K ⦿, B ⦿, A, B ⦿, **A, B** ⦿
  - S32.592 Other specified fracture of left pubis A, K ⦿, B ⦿, A, B ⦿, **A, B** ⦿
  - S32.599 Other specified fracture of unspecified pubis A, K ⦿, B ⦿, **A, B** ⦿
- S32.6 Fracture of ischium
  - **Excludes1** fracture of ischium with associated disruption of pelvic ring (S32.8-)
  - (Ex) **For category S32.6 CC codes S32.6[A]:** See PDX Collection 1202 **For S32.6[B]:** See PDX Collection 1203 **For S32.5[K]:** See PDX Collection 897
  - S32.60 Unspecified fracture of ischium
    - S32.601 Unspecified fracture of right ischium A, K ⦿, B ⦿, A, B ⦿, **A, B** ⦿
    - S32.602 Unspecified fracture of left ischium A, K ⦿, B ⦿, A, B ⦿, **A, B** ⦿
    - S32.609 Unspecified fracture of unspecified ischium A, K ⦿, B ⦿, A, B ⦿, **A, B** ⦿
  - S32.61 Avulsion fracture of ischium
    - S32.611 Displaced avulsion fracture of right ischium A, K ⦿, B ⦿, A, B ⦿, **A, B** ⦿
    - S32.612 Displaced avulsion fracture of left ischium A, K ⦿, B ⦿, A, B ⦿, **A, B** ⦿
    - S32.613 Displaced avulsion fracture of unspecified ischium A, K ⦿, B ⦿, **A, B** ⦿
    - S32.614 Nondisplaced avulsion fracture of right ischium A, K ⦿, B ⦿, A, B ⦿, **A, B** ⦿
    - S32.615 Nondisplaced avulsion fracture of left ischium A, K ⦿, B ⦿, A, B ⦿, **A, B** ⦿
    - S32.616 Nondisplaced avulsion fracture of unspecified ischium A, K ⦿, B ⦿, **A, B** ⦿
  - S32.69 Other specified fracture of ischium
    - S32.691 Other specified fracture of right ischium A, K ⦿, B ⦿, A, B ⦿, **A, B** ⦿
    - S32.692 Other specified fracture of left ischium A, K ⦿, B ⦿, A, B ⦿, **A, B** ⦿
    - S32.699 Other specified fracture of unspecified ischium A, K ⦿, B ⦿, **A, B** ⦿
- S32.8 Fracture of other parts of pelvis
  - Code also any associated:
    - fracture of acetabulum (S32.4-)
    - sacral fracture (S32.1-)
- S32.81 Multiple fractures of pelvis with disruption of pelvic ring
  - Multiple pelvic fractures with disruption of pelvic circle
  - (Ex) **For category S32.81 CC codes S32.81[A,B]:** See PDX Collection 1204 **For S32.81[K]:** See PDX Collection 897
  - S32.810 Multiple fractures of pelvis with stable disruption of pelvic ring A, K ⦿, B ⦿, A, B ⦿, **A, B** ⦿
  - S32.811 Multiple fractures of pelvis with unstable disruption of pelvic ring A, K ⦿, B ⦿, A, B ⦿, **A, B** ⦿

N Newborn Age: 0   P   Pediatric Age: 0–17   M   Maternity DX: 9–64   A Adult Age: 15–124   ♀ Females Only   ♂ Males Only

⦿ Complication\Comorbidity   ⦿ Major C\C   (Ex) CC/MCC Exclusions   ⦿ Hospital-Acquired Condition   ⦿ Hierarchical Condition Category

1293

CHAPTER 19 (S00–T88)

X ● S32.82 **Multiple fractures of pelvis without disruption of pelvic ring** A, K 🔒, B 🔒, A, B 🔒, **A, B** 🔒
  Multiple pelvic fractures without disruption of pelvic circle
    (Ex) **For category S32.82 CC codes S32.82[A,B]:** See PDX Collection 1205, 3979 **For S32.81[K]:** See PDX Collection 897

X ● S32.89 **Fracture of other parts of pelvis** A, K 🔒, B 🔒, A, B 🔒, **A, B** 🔒
    (Ex) **For category S32.89 CC codes S32.89[A,B]:** See PDX Collection 1206 **For S32.89[K]:** See PDX Collection 897

X ● S32.9 **Fracture of unspecified parts of lumbosacral spine and pelvis** A, K 🔒, B 🔒, A, B 🔒, **A, B** 🔒
  Fracture of lumbosacral spine NOS
  Fracture of pelvis NOS
    (Ex) **For category S32.9 CC codes S32.9[A,B]:** See PDX Collection 1204 **For S32.9[K]:** See PDX Collection 897
    Coding Clinic: 2012, Q4, P93

● S33 Dislocation and sprain of joints and ligaments of lumbar spine and pelvis
  Includes avulsion of joint or ligament of lumbar spine and pelvis
    laceration of cartilage, joint or ligament of lumbar spine and pelvis
    sprain of cartilage, joint or ligament of lumbar spine and pelvis
    traumatic hemarthrosis of joint or ligament of lumbar spine and pelvis
    traumatic rupture of joint or ligament of lumbar spine and pelvis
    traumatic subluxation of joint or ligament of lumbar spine and pelvis
    traumatic tear of joint or ligament of lumbar spine and pelvis
  Code also any associated open wound
  Excludes1 nontraumatic rupture or displacement of lumbar intervertebral disc NOS (M51.-)
    obstetric damage to pelvic joints and ligaments (O71.6)
  Excludes2 dislocation and sprain of joints and ligaments of hip (S73.-)
    strain of muscle of lower back and pelvis (S39.01-)
  The appropriate 7th character is to be added to each code from category S33

A	initial encounter
D	subsequent encounter
S	sequela

X ● S33.0 **Traumatic rupture of lumbar intervertebral disc**
    Excludes1 rupture or displacement (nontraumatic) of lumbar intervertebral disc NOS (M51.- with fifth character 6)

● S33.1 **Subluxation and dislocation of lumbar vertebra**
  Code also any associated:
    open wound of abdomen, lower back and pelvis (S31)
    spinal cord injury (S24.0, S24.1-, S34.0-, S34.1-)
    Excludes2 fracture of lumbar vertebrae (S32.0-)
  ● S33.10 **Subluxation and dislocation of unspecified lumbar vertebra**
    ● S33.100 **Subluxation of unspecified lumbar vertebra**
    ● S33.101 **Dislocation of unspecified lumbar vertebra**
  ● S33.11 **Subluxation and dislocation of L1/L2 lumbar vertebra**
    ● S33.110 **Subluxation of L1/L2 lumbar vertebra**
    ● S33.111 **Dislocation of L1/L2 lumbar vertebra**

● S33.12 **Subluxation and dislocation of L2/L3 lumbar vertebra**
  ● S33.120 **Subluxation of L2/L3 lumbar vertebra**
  ● S33.121 **Dislocation of L2/L3 lumbar vertebra**
● S33.13 **Subluxation and dislocation of L3/L4 lumbar vertebra**
  ● S33.130 **Subluxation of L3/L4 lumbar vertebra**
  ● S33.131 **Dislocation of L3/L4 lumbar vertebra**
● S33.14 **Subluxation and dislocation of L4/L5 lumbar vertebra**
  ● S33.140 **Subluxation of L4/L5 lumbar vertebra**
  ● S33.141 **Dislocation of L4/L5 lumbar vertebra**
X ● S33.2 Dislocation of **sacroiliac and sacrococcygeal joint**
● S33.3 Dislocation of other and unspecified parts of lumbar spine and pelvis
  X ● S33.30 **Dislocation of unspecified parts of lumbar spine and pelvis**
  X ● S33.39 **Dislocation of other parts of lumbar spine and pelvis**
X ● S33.4 Traumatic rupture of **symphysis pubis**
X ● S33.5 Sprain of ligaments of **lumbar spine**
X ● S33.6 Sprain of **sacroiliac joint**
X ● S33.8 Sprain of **other parts** of lumbar spine and pelvis
X ● S33.9 Sprain of **unspecified** parts of lumbar spine and pelvis

● S34 Injury of lumbar and sacral spinal cord and nerves at abdomen, lower back and pelvis level
  Note: Code to highest level of lumbar cord injury
    Injuries to the spinal cord (S34.0 and S34.1) refer to the cord level and not bone level injury, and can affect nerve roots at and below the level given.
  The appropriate 7th character is to be added to each code from category S34

A	initial encounter
D	subsequent encounter
S	sequela

  Code also any associated:
    fracture of vertebra (S22.0-, S32.0-)
    open wound of abdomen, lower back and pelvis (S31.-)
    transient paralysis (R29.5)
    (Ex) **For category S34 CC codes unless otherwise indicated:** See PDX Collection 1207
  ● S34.0 **Concussion and edema of lumbar and sacral spinal cord**
    X ● S34.01 **Concussion and edema of lumbar spinal cord** A 🔒, **A, D, S** 🔒
    X ● S34.02 **Concussion and edema of sacral spinal cord** A 🔒, **A, D, S** 🔒
      Concussion and edema of conus medullaris
      (Ex) See PDX Collection 1208
  ● S34.1 Other and unspecified injury of lumbar and sacral spinal cord
    ● S34.10 **Unspecified injury to lumbar spinal cord**
      ● S34.101 **Unspecified injury to L₁ level of lumbar spinal cord** A 🔒, A 🔒, **A, D, S** 🔒
        Unspecified injury to lumbar spinal cord level 1
      ● S34.102 **Unspecified injury to L₂ level of lumbar spinal cord** A 🔒, A 🔒, **A, D, S** 🔒
        Unspecified injury to lumbar spinal cord level 2
      ● S34.103 **Unspecified injury to L₃ level of lumbar spinal cord** A 🔒, A 🔒, **A, D, S** 🔒
        Unspecified injury to lumbar spinal cord level 3

▶ New   ⇒ Revised   ~~deleted~~ Deleted   Excludes 1   Excludes 2   Includes   Use additional   Code first   Code also   Key words
OGCR Official Guidelines   ● Unacceptable Principal Diagnosis   X Assign placeholder X   ● Use Additional Character(s)   ▶ Manifestation Code   **Coding Clinic**

● S34.104   Unspecified injury to L₄ level of
            lumbar spinal cord A 🔴, A 🔴,
            A, D, S 🔴
               Unspecified injury to lumbar spinal
               cord level 4

● S34.105   Unspecified injury to L₅ level of
            lumbar spinal cord A 🔴, A 🔴,
            A, D, S 🔴
               Unspecified injury to lumbar spinal
               cord level 5

● S34.109   Unspecified injury to unspecified
            level of lumbar spinal cord A 🔴, A 🔴,
            A, D, S 🔴

● S34.11   Complete lesion of lumbar spinal cord

● S34.111   Complete lesion of L₁ level of lumbar
            spinal cord A 🔴, A 🔴, A, D, S 🔴
               Complete lesion of lumbar spinal
               cord level 1

● S34.112   Complete lesion of L₂ level of lumbar
            spinal cord A 🔴, A 🔴, A, D, S 🔴
               Complete lesion of lumbar spinal
               cord level 2

● S34.113   Complete lesion of L₃ level of lumbar
            spinal cord A 🔴, A 🔴, A, D, S 🔴
               Complete lesion of lumbar spinal
               cord level 3

● S34.114   Complete lesion of L₄ level of lumbar
            spinal cord A 🔴, A 🔴, A, D, S 🔴
               Complete lesion of lumbar spinal
               cord level 4

● S34.115   Complete lesion of L₅ level of lumbar
            spinal cord A 🔴, A 🔴, A, D, S 🔴
               Complete lesion of lumbar spinal
               cord level 5

● S34.119   Complete lesion of unspecified level
            of lumbar spinal cord A 🔴, A 🔴,
            A, D, S 🔴

● S34.12   Incomplete lesion of lumbar spinal cord

● S34.121   Incomplete lesion of L₁ level of
            lumbar spinal cord A 🔴, A 🔴,
            A, D, S 🔴
               Incomplete lesion of lumbar spinal
               cord level 1

● S34.122   Incomplete lesion of L₂ level of
            lumbar spinal cord A 🔴, A 🔴,
            A, D, S 🔴
               Incomplete lesion of lumbar spinal
               cord level 2

● S34.123   Incomplete lesion of L₃ level of
            lumbar spinal cord A 🔴, A 🔴,
            A, D, S 🔴
               Incomplete lesion of lumbar spinal
               cord level 3

● S34.124   Incomplete lesion of L₄ level of
            lumbar spinal cord A 🔴, A 🔴,
            A, D, S 🔴
               Incomplete lesion of lumbar spinal
               cord level 4

● S34.125   Incomplete lesion of L₅ level of
            lumbar spinal cord A 🔴, A 🔴,
            A, D, S 🔴
               Incomplete lesion of lumbar spinal
               cord level 5

● S34.129   Incomplete lesion of unspecified level
            of lumbar spinal cord A 🔴, A 🔴,
            A, D, S 🔴

● S34.13   Other and unspecified injury to sacral spinal
            cord
               Other injury to conus medullaris
               (Ex) For category S34.13 CC codes: See PDX Collection 1208

● S34.131   Complete lesion of sacral spinal cord
            A 🔴, A 🔴, A, D, S 🔴
               Complete lesion of conus medullaris

● S34.132   Incomplete lesion of sacral spinal
            cord A 🔴, A 🔴, A, D, S 🔴
               Incomplete lesion of conus
               medullaris

● S34.139   Unspecified injury to sacral spinal
            cord A 🔴, A 🔴, A, D, S 🔴
               Unspecified injury of conus
               medullaris

● S34.2   Injury of nerve root of lumbar and sacral spine

X● S34.21   Injury of nerve root of lumbar spine

X● S34.22   Injury of nerve root of sacral spine

X● S34.3   Injury of cauda equina A 🔴, A 🔴, A, D, S 🔴
            (Ex) See PDX Collection 1208

X● S34.4   Injury of lumbosacral plexus

X● S34.5   Injury of lumbar, sacral and pelvic sympathetic nerves
               Injury of celiac ganglion or plexus
               Injury of hypogastric plexus
               Injury of mesenteric plexus (inferior) (superior)
               Injury of splanchnic nerve

X● S34.6   Injury of peripheral nerve(s) at abdomen, lower back
            and pelvis level

X● S34.8   Injury of other nerves at abdomen, lower back and
            pelvis level

X● S34.9   Injury of unspecified nerves at abdomen, lower back
            and pelvis level

● S35   Injury of blood vessels at abdomen, lower back and pelvis level
         The appropriate 7th character is to be added to each code from
         category S35

         | A | initial encounter |
         | D | subsequent encounter |
         | S | sequela |

         Code also any associated open wound (S31.-)

● S35.0   Injury of abdominal aorta
            Excludes1   injury of aorta NOS (S25.0)
            (Ex) For category S35.0 CC codes: See PDX Collection 1209

X● S35.00   Unspecified injury of abdominal aorta A 🔴

X● S35.01   Minor laceration of abdominal aorta A 🔴
               Incomplete transection of abdominal aorta
               Laceration of abdominal aorta NOS
               Superficial laceration of abdominal aorta

X● S35.02   Major laceration of abdominal aorta A 🔴
               Complete transection of abdominal aorta
               Traumatic rupture of abdominal aorta

X● S35.09   Other injury of abdominal aorta A 🔴

● S35.1   Injury of inferior vena cava
               Injury of hepatic vein
            Excludes1   injury of vena cava NOS (S25.2)
            (Ex) For category S35.1 CC codes: See PDX Collection 1210

X● S35.10   Unspecified injury of inferior vena cava A 🔴

X● S35.11   Minor laceration of inferior vena cava A 🔴
               Incomplete transection of inferior vena cava
               Laceration of inferior vena cava NOS
               Superficial laceration of inferior vena cava

X● S35.12   Major laceration of inferior vena cava A 🔴
               Complete transection of inferior vena cava
               Traumatic rupture of inferior vena cava

X● S35.19   Other injury of inferior vena cava A 🔴

N Newborn Age: 0   P Pediatric Age: 0–17   M Maternity DX: 9–64   A Adult Age: 15–124   ♀ Females Only   ♂ Males Only

🔴 Complication\Comorbidity   🔴 Major C\C   (Ex) CC/MCC Exclusions   🔴 Hospital-Acquired Condition   🔴 Hierarchical Condition Category

1295

● **S35.2 Injury of celiac or mesenteric artery and branches**
  ● **S35.21 Injury of celiac artery**
    (Ex:) **For category S35.21 CC codes:** See PDX Collection 1211
    ● **S35.211 Minor laceration of celiac artery A** 🔒
        Incomplete transection of celiac artery
        Laceration of celiac artery NOS
        Superficial laceration of celiac artery
    ● **S35.212 Major laceration of celiac artery A** 🔒
        Complete transection of celiac artery
        Traumatic rupture of celiac artery
    ● **S35.218 Other injury of celiac artery A** 🔒
    ● **S35.219 Unspecified injury of celiac artery A** 🔒
  ● **S35.22 Injury of superior mesenteric artery**
    (Ex:) **For category S35.22 CC codes:** See PDX Collection 1212
    ● **S35.221 Minor laceration of superior mesenteric artery A** 🔒
        Incomplete transection of superior mesenteric artery
        Laceration of superior mesenteric artery NOS
        Superficial laceration of superior mesenteric artery
    ● **S35.222 Major laceration of superior mesenteric artery A** 🔒
        Complete transection of superior mesenteric artery
        Traumatic rupture of superior mesenteric artery
    ● **S35.228 Other injury of superior mesenteric artery A** 🔒
    ● **S35.229 Unspecified injury of superior mesenteric artery A** 🔒
  ● **S35.23 Injury of inferior mesenteric artery**
    (Ex:) **For category S35.23 CC codes:** See PDX Collection 1213
    ● **S35.231 Minor laceration of inferior mesenteric artery A** 🔒
        Incomplete transection of inferior mesenteric artery
        Laceration of inferior mesenteric artery NOS
        Superficial laceration of inferior mesenteric artery
    ● **S35.232 Major laceration of inferior mesenteric artery A** 🔒
        Complete transection of inferior mesenteric artery
        Traumatic rupture of inferior mesenteric artery
    ● **S35.238 Other injury of inferior mesenteric artery A** 🔒
    ● **S35.239 Unspecified injury of inferior mesenteric artery A** 🔒
  ● **S35.29 Injury of branches of celiac and mesenteric artery**
    Injury of gastric artery
    Injury of gastroduodenal artery
    Injury of hepatic artery
    Injury of splenic artery
    (Ex:) **For category S35.29 CC codes unless otherwise indicated:** See PDX Collection 1215
    ● **S35.291 Minor laceration of branches of celiac and mesenteric artery A** 🔒
        Incomplete transection of branches of celiac and mesenteric artery
        Laceration of branches of celiac and mesenteric artery NOS
        Superficial laceration of branches of celiac and mesenteric artery
        (Ex:) See PDX Collection 1214

    ● **S35.292 Major laceration of branches of celiac and mesenteric artery A** 🔒
        Complete transection of branches of celiac and mesenteric artery
        Traumatic rupture of branches of celiac and mesenteric artery
    ● **S35.298 Other injury of branches of celiac and mesenteric artery A** 🔒
    ● **S35.299 Unspecified injury of branches of celiac and mesenteric artery A** 🔒
        (Ex:) See PDX Collection 1216
● **S35.3 Injury of portal or splenic vein and branches**
  ● **S35.31 Injury of portal vein**
    (Ex:) **For category S35.31 CC codes:** See PDX Collection 1217
    ● **S35.311 Laceration of portal vein A** 🔒
    ● **S35.318 Other specified injury of portal vein A** 🔒
    ● **S35.319 Unspecified injury of portal vein A** 🔒
  ● **S35.32 Injury of splenic vein**
    (Ex:) **For category S35.32 CC codes:** See PDX Collection 1218
    ● **S35.321 Laceration of splenic vein A** 🔒
    ● **S35.328 Other specified injury of splenic vein A** 🔒
    ● **S35.329 Unspecified injury of splenic vein A** 🔒
  ● **S35.33 Injury of superior mesenteric vein**
    (Ex:) **For category S35.33 CC codes:** See PDX Collection 1219
    ● **S35.331 Laceration of superior mesenteric vein A** 🔒
    ● **S35.338 Other specified injury of superior mesenteric vein A** 🔒
    ● **S35.339 Unspecified injury of superior mesenteric vein A** 🔒
  ● **S35.34 Injury of inferior mesenteric vein**
    (Ex:) **For category S35.34 CC codes:** See PDX Collection 1220
    ● **S35.341 Laceration of inferior mesenteric vein A** 🔒
    ● **S35.348 Other specified injury of inferior mesenteric vein A** 🔒
    ● **S35.349 Unspecified injury of inferior mesenteric vein A** 🔒
● **S35.4 Injury of renal blood vessels**
  ● **S35.40 Unspecified injury of renal blood vessel**
    (Ex:) **For category S35.40 CC codes S35.401-S35.403:** See PDX Collection 1221
    For category S35.40 CC codes S35.404-S35.406: See PDX Collection 1222
    ● **S35.401 Unspecified injury of right renal artery A** 🔒
    ● **S35.402 Unspecified injury of left renal artery A** 🔒
    ● **S35.403 Unspecified injury of unspecified renal artery A** 🔒
    ● **S35.404 Unspecified injury of right renal vein A** 🔒
    ● **S35.405 Unspecified injury of left renal vein A** 🔒
    ● **S35.406 Unspecified injury of unspecified renal vein A** 🔒
  ● **S35.41 Laceration of renal blood vessel**
    (Ex:) **For category S35.41 CC codes S35.411-S35.413:** See PDX Collection 1221
    For category S35.41 CC codes S35.414-S35.416: See PDX Collection 1222
    ● **S35.411 Laceration of right renal artery A** 🔒
    ● **S35.412 Laceration of left renal artery A** 🔒
    ● **S35.413 Laceration of unspecified renal artery A** 🔒
    ● **S35.414 Laceration of right renal vein A** 🔒
    ● **S35.415 Laceration of left renal vein A** 🔒
    ● **S35.416 Laceration of unspecified renal vein A** 🔒

▶ New   ⇒ Revised   ~~deleted~~ Deleted   Excludes 1   Excludes 2   Includes   Use additional   Code first   Code also   Key words
OGCR Official Guidelines   ● Unacceptable Principal Diagnosis   X Assign placeholder X   ● Use Additional Character(s)   ▶ Manifestation Code   **Coding Clinic**

● **S35.49**   **Other specified injury of renal blood vessel**
   (Ex) **For category S35.49 CC codes S35.491-S35.493:**
     See PDX Collection 1221
   For category S35.49 CC codes S35.494-S35.496:
     See PDX Collection 1222

   ● **S35.491**   **Other specified injury of right renal artery** A 🦠

   ● **S35.492**   **Other specified injury of left renal artery** A 🦠

   ● **S35.493**   **Other specified injury of unspecified renal artery** A 🦠

   ● **S35.494**   **Other specified injury of right renal vein** A 🦠

   ● **S35.495**   **Other specified injury of left renal vein** A 🦠

   ● **S35.496**   **Other specified injury of unspecified renal vein** A 🦠

● **S35.5**   **Injury of iliac blood vessels**

   X● **S35.50**   **Injury of unspecified iliac blood vessel(s)** A 🦠
     (Ex) See PDX Collection 1223

  ● **S35.51**   **Injury of iliac artery or vein**
     Injury of hypogastric artery or vein
     (Ex) **For category S35.51 CC codes S35.511-S35.513:**
       See PDX Collection 1224
     For category S35.51 CC codes S35.514-S35.516:
       See PDX Collection 1225

   ● **S35.511**   **Injury of right iliac artery** A 🦠
   ● **S35.512**   **Injury of left iliac artery** A 🦠
   ● **S35.513**   **Injury of unspecified iliac artery** A 🦠
   ● **S35.514**   **Injury of right iliac vein** A 🦠
   ● **S35.515**   **Injury of left iliac vein** A 🦠
   ● **S35.516**   **Injury of unspecified iliac vein** A 🦠

  ● **S35.53**   **Injury of uterine artery or vein**
     (Ex) **For category S35.53 CC codes S35.531-S35.533:**
       See PDX Collection 1226
     For category S35.53 CC codes S35.534-S35.536:
       See PDX Collection 1227

   ● **S35.531**   **Injury of right uterine artery** ♀ A 🦠
   ● **S35.532**   **Injury of left uterine artery** ♀ A 🦠
   ● **S35.533**   **Injury of unspecified uterine artery** ♀ A 🦠
   ● **S35.534**   **Injury of right uterine vein** ♀ A 🦠
   ● **S35.535**   **Injury of left uterine vein** ♀ A 🦠
   ● **S35.536**   **Injury of unspecified uterine vein** ♀ A 🦠

   X● **S35.59**   **Injury of other iliac blood vessels** A 🦠
     (Ex) See PDX Collection 1223

● **S35.8**   **Injury of other blood vessels at abdomen, lower back and pelvis level**
   Injury of ovarian artery or vein
   (Ex) **For category S35.8 CC codes: See PDX Collection 1228**

  ● **S35.8X**   **Injury of other blood vessels at abdomen, lower back and pelvis level**

   ● **S35.8X1**   **Laceration of other blood vessels at abdomen, lower back and pelvis level** A 🦠

   ● **S35.8X8**   **Other specified injury of other blood vessels at abdomen, lower back and pelvis level** A 🦠

   ● **S35.8X9**   **Unspecified injury of other blood vessels at abdomen, lower back and pelvis level** A 🦠

● **S35.9**   **Injury of unspecified blood vessel at abdomen, lower back and pelvis level**
   (Ex) **For category S35.9 CC codes: See PDX Collection 1229**

   X● **S35.90**   **Unspecified injury of unspecified blood vessel at abdomen, lower back and pelvis level** A 🦠

   X● **S35.91**   **Laceration of unspecified blood vessel at abdomen, lower back and pelvis level** A 🦠

   X● **S35.99**   **Other specified injury of unspecified blood vessel at abdomen, lower back and pelvis level** A 🦠

● **S36**   **Injury of intra-abdominal organs**
   The appropriate 7th character is to be added to each code from category S36

A	initial encounter
D	subsequent encounter
S	sequela

   Code also any associated open wound (S31.-)

● **S36.0**   **Injury of spleen**
   (Ex) **For category S36.0 CC codes: See PDX Collection 1230**

   X● **S36.00**   **Unspecified injury of spleen** A 🦠

  ● **S36.02**   **Contusion of spleen**

   ● **S36.020**   **Minor contusion of spleen** A 🦠
     Contusion of spleen less than 2 cm

   ● **S36.021**   **Major contusion of spleen** A 🦠
     Contusion of spleen greater than 2 cm

   ● **S36.029**   **Unspecified contusion of spleen** A 🦠
     Coding Clinic: 2015, Q2, P36, Q1, P11

  ● **S36.03**   **Laceration of spleen**

   ● **S36.030**   **Superficial (capsular) laceration of spleen** A 🦠
     Laceration of spleen less than 1 cm
     Minor laceration of spleen

   ● **S36.031**   **Moderate laceration of spleen** A 🦠
     Laceration of spleen 1 to 3 cm
     Coding Clinic: 2015, Q2, P36, Q1, P11

   ● **S36.032**   **Major laceration of spleen** A 🦠
     Avulsion of spleen
     Laceration of spleen greater than 3 cm
     Massive laceration of spleen
     Multiple moderate lacerations of spleen
     Stellate laceration of spleen

   ● **S36.039**   **Unspecified laceration of spleen** A 🦠

   X● **S36.09**   **Other injury of spleen** A 🦠

● **S36.1**   **Injury of liver and gallbladder and bile duct**

  ● **S36.11**   **Injury of liver**
     (Ex) **For category S36.11 CC codes: See PDX Collection 1231**

   ● **S36.112**   **Contusion of liver** A 🦠
   ● **S36.113**   **Laceration of liver, unspecified degree** A 🦠

   ● **S36.114**   **Minor laceration of liver** A 🦠
     Laceration involving capsule only, or, without significant involvement of hepatic parenchyma [i.e., less than 1 cm deep]

   ● **S36.115**   **Moderate laceration of liver** A 🦠
     Laceration involving parenchyma but without major disruption of parenchyma [i.e., less than 10 cm long and less than 3 cm deep]

   ● **S36.116**   **Major laceration of liver** A 🦠
     Laceration with significant disruption of hepatic parenchyma [i.e., greater than 10 cm long and 3 cm deep]
     Multiple moderate lacerations, with or without hematoma
     Stellate laceration of liver

   ● **S36.118**   **Other injury of liver** A 🦠
   ● **S36.119**   **Unspecified injury of liver** A 🦠
     Coding Clinic: 2015, Q2, P17

N   Newborn Age: 0   **P**   Pediatric Age: 0 17   **M**   Maternity DX: 9–64   **A**   Adult Age: 15–124   ♀   Females Only   ♂   Males Only

🦠 Complication\Comorbidity   🦠 Major C\C   (Ex) CC/MCC Exclusions   🦠 Hospital-Acquired Condition   🦠 Hierarchical Condition Category

1297

● **S36.12**   Injury of gallbladder
     Ex: **For category S36.12 CC codes:** See PDX Collection 1232

     ● **S36.122**   Contusion of gallbladder A 🅒

     ● **S36.123**   Laceration of gallbladder A 🅒

     ● **S36.128**   Other injury of gallbladder A 🅒

     ● **S36.129**   Unspecified injury of gallbladder A 🅒

X ● **S36.13**   Injury of bile duct A 🅒
     Ex: See PDX Collection 1232

● **S36.2**   Injury of pancreas
     Ex: **For category S36.2 CC codes:** See PDX Collection 1233

   ● **S36.20**   Unspecified injury of pancreas

     ● **S36.200**   Unspecified injury of head of pancreas A 🅒

     ● **S36.201**   Unspecified injury of body of pancreas A 🅒

     ● **S36.202**   Unspecified injury of tail of pancreas A 🅒

     ● **S36.209**   Unspecified injury of unspecified part of pancreas A 🅒

   ● **S36.22**   Contusion of pancreas

     ● **S36.220**   Contusion of head of pancreas A 🅒

     ● **S36.221**   Contusion of body of pancreas A 🅒

     ● **S36.222**   Contusion of tail of pancreas A 🅒

     ● **S36.229**   Contusion of unspecified part of pancreas A 🅒

   ● **S36.23**   Laceration of pancreas, unspecified degree

     ● **S36.230**   Laceration of head of pancreas, unspecified degree A 🅒

     ● **S36.231**   Laceration of body of pancreas, unspecified degree A 🅒

     ● **S36.232**   Laceration of tail of pancreas, unspecified degree A 🅒

     ● **S36.239**   Laceration of unspecified part of pancreas, unspecified degree A 🅒

   ● **S36.24**   Minor laceration of pancreas

     ● **S36.240**   Minor laceration of head of pancreas A 🅒

     ● **S36.241**   Minor laceration of body of pancreas A 🅒

     ● **S36.242**   Minor laceration of tail of pancreas A 🅒

     ● **S36.249**   Minor laceration of unspecified part of pancreas A 🅒

   ● **S36.25**   Moderate laceration of pancreas

     ● **S36.250**   Moderate laceration of head of pancreas A 🅒

     ● **S36.251**   Moderate laceration of body of pancreas A 🅒

     ● **S36.252**   Moderate laceration of tail of pancreas A 🅒

     ● **S36.259**   Moderate laceration of unspecified part of pancreas A 🅒

   ● **S36.26**   Major laceration of pancreas

     ● **S36.260**   Major laceration of head of pancreas A 🅒

     ● **S36.261**   Major laceration of body of pancreas A 🅒

     ● **S36.262**   Major laceration of tail of pancreas A 🅒

     ● **S36.269**   Major laceration of unspecified part of pancreas A 🅒

   ● **S36.29**   Other injury of pancreas

     ● **S36.290**   Other injury of head of pancreas A 🅒

     ● **S36.291**   Other injury of body of pancreas A 🅒

     ● **S36.292**   Other injury of tail of pancreas A 🅒

     ● **S36.299**   Other injury of unspecified part of pancreas A 🅒

● **S36.3**   Injury of stomach
     Ex: **For category S36.3 CC codes:** See PDX Collection 1234

X ● **S36.30**   Unspecified injury of stomach A 🅒

X ● **S36.32**   Contusion of stomach A 🅒

X ● **S36.33**   Laceration of stomach A 🅒

X ● **S36.39**   Other injury of stomach A 🅒

● **S36.4**   Injury of small intestine
     Ex: **For category S36.4 CC codes:** See PDX Collection 1235

   ● **S36.40**   Unspecified injury of small intestine

     ● **S36.400**   Unspecified injury of duodenum A 🅒

     ● **S36.408**   Unspecified injury of other part of small intestine A 🅒

     ● **S36.409**   Unspecified injury of unspecified part of small intestine A 🅒

   ● **S36.41**   Primary blast injury of small intestine
     Blast injury of small intestine NOS

     ● **S36.410**   Primary blast injury of duodenum A 🅒

     ● **S36.418**   Primary blast injury of other part of small intestine A 🅒

     ● **S36.419**   Primary blast injury of unspecified part of small intestine A 🅒

   ● **S36.42**   Contusion of small intestine

     ● **S36.420**   Contusion of duodenum A 🅒

     ● **S36.428**   Contusion of other part of small intestine A 🅒

     ● **S36.429**   Contusion of unspecified part of small intestine A 🅒

   ● **S36.43**   Laceration of small intestine

     ● **S36.430**   Laceration of duodenum A 🅒

     ● **S36.438**   Laceration of other part of small intestine A 🅒

     ● **S36.439**   Laceration of unspecified part of small intestine A 🅒

   ● **S36.49**   Other injury of small intestine

     ● **S36.490**   Other injury of duodenum A 🅒

     ● **S36.498**   Other injury of other part of small intestine A 🅒

     ● **S36.499**   Other injury of unspecified part of small intestine A 🅒

● **S36.5**   Injury of colon

     Excludes2   injury of rectum (S36.6-)
     Ex: **For category S36.5 CC codes:** See PDX Collection 1236

   ● **S36.50**   Unspecified injury of colon

     ● **S36.500**   Unspecified injury of ascending [right] colon A 🅒

     ● **S36.501**   Unspecified injury of transverse colon A 🅒

     ● **S36.502**   Unspecified injury of descending [left] colon A 🅒

     ● **S36.503**   Unspecified injury of sigmoid colon A 🅒

     ● **S36.508**   Unspecified injury of other part of colon A 🅒

     ● **S36.509**   Unspecified injury of unspecified part of colon A 🅒

● **S36.51**   Primary blast injury of colon
             Blast injury of colon NOS

     ● **S36.510**   Primary blast injury of ascending [right] colon A 🦠

     ● **S36.511**   Primary blast injury of transverse colon A 🦠

     ● **S36.512**   Primary blast injury of descending [left] colon A 🦠

     ● **S36.513**   Primary blast injury of sigmoid colon A 🦠

     ● **S36.518**   Primary blast injury of other part of colon A 🦠

     ● **S36.519**   Primary blast injury of unspecified part of colon A 🦠

● **S36.52**   Contusion of colon

     ● **S36.520**   Contusion of ascending [right] colon A 🦠

     ● **S36.521**   Contusion of transverse colon A 🦠

     ● **S36.522**   Contusion of descending [left] colon A 🦠

     ● **S36.523**   Contusion of sigmoid colon A 🦠

     ● **S36.528**   Contusion of other part of colon A 🦠

     ● **S36.529**   Contusion of unspecified part of colon A 🦠

● **S36.53**   Laceration of colon

     ● **S36.530**   Laceration of ascending [right] colon A 🦠

     ● **S36.531**   Laceration of transverse colon A 🦠

     ● **S36.532**   Laceration of descending [left] colon A 🦠

     ● **S36.533**   Laceration of sigmoid colon A 🦠

     ● **S36.538**   Laceration of other part of colon A 🦠

     S36.539   Laceration of unspecified part of colon A 🦠

● **S36.59**   Other injury of colon
             Secondary blast injury of colon

     ● **S36.590**   Other injury of ascending [right] colon A 🦠

     ● **S36.591**   Other injury of transverse colon A 🦠

     ● **S36.592**   Other injury of descending [left] colon A 🦠

     ● **S36.593**   Other injury of sigmoid colon A 🦠

     ● **S36.598**   Other injury of other part of colon A 🦠

     ● **S36.599**   Other injury of unspecified part of colon A 🦠

● **S36.6**   Injury of rectum
     (Ex) **For category S36.6 CC codes:** See PDX Collection 1236

X ● **S36.60**   Unspecified injury of rectum A 🦠

X ● **S36.61**   Primary blast injury of rectum A 🦠
             Blast injury of rectum NOS

X ● **S36.62**   Contusion of rectum A 🦠

X ● **S36.63**   Laceration of rectum A 🦠

X ● **S36.69**   Other injury of rectum A 🦠
             Secondary blast injury of rectum

● **S36.8**   Injury of other intra-abdominal organs
     (Ex) **For category S36.8 CC codes:** See PDX Collection 1195

X ● **S36.81**   Injury of peritoneum A 🦠

● **S36.89**   Injury of other intra-abdominal organs
             Injury of retroperitoneum

     ● **S36.892**   Contusion of other intra-abdominal organs A 🦠

     ● **S36.893**   Laceration of other intra-abdominal organs A 🦠

     ● **S36.898**   Other injury of other intra-abdominal organs A 🦠

     S36.899   Unspecified injury of other intra-abdominal organs A 🦠

● **S36.9**   Injury of unspecified intra-abdominal organ
     (Ex) **For category S36.9 CC codes:** See PDX Collection 1195

X ● **S36.90**   Unspecified injury of unspecified intra-abdominal organ A 🦠

X ● **S36.92**   Contusion of unspecified intra-abdominal organ A 🦠

X ● **S36.93**   Laceration of unspecified intra-abdominal organ A 🦠

X ● **S36.99**   Other injury of unspecified intra-abdominal organ A 🦠

● **S37**   Injury of urinary and pelvic organs
     Code also any associated open wound (S31.-)

     Excludes1   obstetric trauma to pelvic organs (O71.-)

     Excludes2   injury of peritoneum (S36.81)
                       injury of retroperitoneum (S36.89-)

     The appropriate 7th character is to be added to each code from category S37

A	initial encounter
D	subsequent encounter
S	sequela

● **S37.0**   Injury of kidney

     Excludes2   acute kidney injury (nontraumatic) (N17.9)

     (Ex) **For category S37.0 CC codes:** See PDX Collection 1237

     ● **S37.00**   Unspecified injury of kidney

         ● **S37.001**   Unspecified injury of right kidney A 🦠

         ● **S37.002**   Unspecified injury of left kidney A 🦠

         ● **S37.009**   Unspecified injury of unspecified kidney A 🦠

     ● **S37.01**   Minor contusion of kidney
               Contusion of kidney less than 2 cm
               Contusion of kidney NOS

         ● **S37.011**   Minor contusion of right kidney A 🦠

         ● **S37.012**   Minor contusion of left kidney A 🦠

         ● **S37.019**   Minor contusion of unspecified kidney A 🦠

     ● **S37.02**   Major contusion of kidney
               Contusion of kidney greater than 2 cm

         ● **S37.021**   Major contusion of right kidney A 🦠

         ● **S37.022**   Major contusion of left kidney A 🦠

         ● **S37.029**   Major contusion of unspecified kidney A 🦠

     ● **S37.03**   Laceration of kidney, unspecified degree

         ● **S37.031**   Laceration of right kidney, unspecified degree A 🦠

         ● **S37.032**   Laceration of left kidney, unspecified degree A 🦠

         ● **S37.039**   Laceration of unspecified kidney, unspecified degree A 🦠

     ● **S37.04**   Minor laceration of kidney
               Laceration of kidney less than 1 cm

         ● **S37.041**   Minor laceration of right kidney A 🦠

         ● **S37.042**   Minor laceration of left kidney A 🦠

         ● **S37.049**   Minor laceration of unspecified kidney A 🦠

     ● **S37.05**   Moderate laceration of kidney
               Laceration of kidney 1 to 3 cm

         ● **S37.051**   Moderate laceration of right kidney A 🦠

         ● **S37.052**   Moderate laceration of left kidney A 🦠

         ● **S37.059**   Moderate laceration of unspecified kidney A 🦠

N Newborn Age: 0   **P** Pediatric Age: 0–17   **M** Maternity DX: 9–64   **A** Adult Age: 15–124   ♀ Females Only   ♂ Males Only

🦠 Complication\Comorbidity   🦠 Major C\C   (Ex) CC/MCC Exclusions   🦠 Hospital-Acquired Condition   🦠 Hierarchical Condition Category

1299

CHAPTER 19 (S00-T88)

- **S37.06** **Major laceration of kidney**
  - Avulsion of kidney
  - Laceration of kidney greater than 3 cm
  - Massive laceration of kidney
  - Multiple moderate lacerations of kidney
  - Stellate laceration of kidney
    - **S37.061** Major laceration of **right** kidney A
    - **S37.062** Major laceration of **left** kidney A
    - **S37.069** Major laceration of **unspecified** kidney A
- **S37.09** **Other** injury of kidney
  - **S37.091** Other injury of **right** kidney A
  - **S37.092** Other injury of **left** kidney A
  - **S37.099** Other injury of **unspecified** kidney A

S37.1   Injury of **ureter**
Ex) For category S37.1 CC codes: See PDX Collection 1238
- X **S37.10** **Unspecified** injury of ureter A
- X **S37.12** **Contusion** of ureter A
- X **S37.13** **Laceration** of ureter A
- X **S37.19** **Other** injury of ureter A

S37.2   Injury of **bladder**
Ex) For category S37.2 CC codes: See PDX Collection 1239
- X **S37.20** **Unspecified** injury of bladder A
- X **S37.22** **Contusion** of bladder A
- X **S37.23** **Laceration** of bladder A
- X **S37.29** **Other** injury of bladder A

S37.3   Injury of **urethra**
Ex) For category S37.3 CC codes: See PDX Collection 1239
- X **S37.30** **Unspecified** injury of urethra A
- X **S37.32** **Contusion** of urethra A
- X **S37.33** **Laceration** of urethra A
- X **S37.39** **Other** injury of urethra A

S37.4   Injury of **ovary**
- **S37.40** **Unspecified** injury of ovary
  - **S37.401** Unspecified injury of ovary, **unilateral** ♀
  - **S37.402** Unspecified injury of ovary, **bilateral** ♀
  - **S37.409** Unspecified injury of ovary, **unspecified** ♀
- **S37.42** **Contusion** of ovary
  - **S37.421** Contusion of ovary, **unilateral** ♀
  - **S37.422** Contusion of ovary, **bilateral** ♀
  - **S37.429** Contusion of ovary, **unspecified** ♀
- **S37.43** **Laceration** of ovary
  - **S37.431** Laceration of ovary, **unilateral** ♀
  - **S37.432** Laceration of ovary, **bilateral** ♀
  - **S37.439** Laceration of ovary, **unspecified** ♀
- **S37.49** **Other** injury of ovary
  - **S37.491** Other injury of ovary, **unilateral** ♀
  - **S37.492** Other injury of ovary, **bilateral** ♀
  - **S37.499** Other injury of ovary, **unspecified** ♀

S37.5   Injury of **fallopian tube**
- **S37.50** **Unspecified** injury of fallopian tube
  - **S37.501** Unspecified injury of fallopian tube, **unilateral** ♀
  - **S37.502** Unspecified injury of fallopian tube, **bilateral** ♀
  - **S37.509** Unspecified injury of fallopian tube, **unspecified** ♀

- **S37.51** **Primary blast injury of fallopian tube**
  - Blast injury of fallopian tube NOS
    - **S37.511** **Primary blast injury of fallopian tube, unilateral** ♀
    - **S37.512** **Primary blast injury of fallopian tube, bilateral** ♀
    - **S37.519** **Primary blast injury of fallopian tube, unspecified** ♀
- **S37.52** **Contusion of fallopian tube**
  - **S37.521** **Contusion of fallopian tube, unilateral** ♀
  - **S37.522** **Contusion of fallopian tube, bilateral** ♀
  - **S37.529** **Contusion of fallopian tube, unspecified** ♀
- **S37.53** **Laceration** of fallopian tube
  - **S37.531** **Laceration of fallopian tube, unilateral** ♀
  - **S37.532** **Laceration of fallopian tube, bilateral** ♀
  - **S37.539** **Laceration of fallopian tube, unspecified** ♀
- **S37.59** **Other** injury of fallopian tube
  - Secondary blast injury of fallopian tube
    - **S37.591** **Other injury of fallopian tube, unilateral** ♀
    - **S37.592** **Other injury of fallopian tube, bilateral** ♀
    - **S37.599** **Other injury of fallopian tube, unspecified** ♀

S37.6   Injury of **uterus**
Excludes1   injury to gravid uterus (O9A.2-)
             injury to uterus during delivery (O71.-)
Ex) For category S37.6 CC codes: See PDX Collection 1240
- X **S37.60** **Unspecified** injury of uterus ♀ A
- X **S37.62** **Contusion** of uterus ♀ A
- X **S37.63** **Laceration** of uterus ♀ A
- X **S37.69** **Other** injury of uterus ♀ A

S37.8   Injury of **other urinary and pelvic organs**
- **S37.81** Injury of **adrenal gland**
  Ex) For category S37.81 CC codes: See PDX Collection 1241
  - **S37.812** **Contusion** of adrenal gland A
  - **S37.813** **Laceration** of adrenal gland A
  - **S37.818** **Other** injury of adrenal gland A
  - **S37.819** **Unspecified** injury of adrenal gland A
- **S37.82** Injury of **prostate**
  - **S37.822** **Contusion** of prostate ♂
  - **S37.823** **Laceration** of prostate ♂
  - **S37.828** **Other** injury of prostate ♂
  - **S37.829** **Unspecified** injury of prostate ♂
- **S37.89** Injury of **other** urinary and pelvic organ
  Ex) For category S37.89 CC codes: See PDX Collection 1242
  - **S37.892** **Contusion** of other urinary and pelvic organ A
  - **S37.893** **Laceration** of other urinary and pelvic organ A
  - **S37.898** **Other** injury of other urinary and pelvic organ A
  - **S37.899** **Unspecified** injury of other urinary and pelvic organ A

▶ New   ⇒ Revised   ~~deleted~~ Deleted   Excludes 1   Excludes 2   Includes   Use additional   Code first   Code also   Key words
OGCR Official Guidelines   ● Unacceptable Principal Diagnosis   X Assign placeholder X   ● Use Additional Character(s)   ▸ Manifestation Code   **Coding Clinic**

● S37.9　Injury of unspecified urinary and pelvic organ
　　　(Ex.) For category S37.9 CC codes: See PDX Collection 1242

X● S37.90　Unspecified injury of unspecified urinary and pelvic organ A 🄲

X● S37.92　Contusion of unspecified urinary and pelvic organ A 🄲

X● S37.93　Laceration of unspecified urinary and pelvic organ A 🄲

X● S37.99　Other injury of unspecified urinary and pelvic organ A 🄲

● S38　Crushing injury and traumatic amputation of abdomen, lower back, pelvis and external genitals
　　An amputation not identified as partial or complete should be coded to complete
　　The appropriate 7th character is to be added to each code from category S38

A	initial encounter
D	subsequent encounter
S	sequela

● S38.0　Crushing injury of external genital organs
　　　Use additional code for any associated injuries

● S38.00　Crushing injury of unspecified external genital organs

● S38.001　Crushing injury of unspecified external genital organs, male ♂

● S38.002　Crushing injury of unspecified external genital organs, female ♀

X● S38.01　Crushing injury of penis ♂

X● S38.02　Crushing injury of scrotum and testis ♂

X● S38.03　Crushing injury of vulva ♀

X● S38.1　Crushing injury of abdomen, lower back, and pelvis
　　　Use additional code for all associated injuries, such as:
　　　fracture of thoracic or lumbar spine and pelvis (S22.0-, S32.-)
　　　injury to intra-abdominal organs (S36.-)
　　　injury to urinary and pelvic organs (S37.-)
　　　open wound of abdominal wall (S31.-)
　　　spinal cord injury (S04.0, S34.1-)
　　　Excludes2　crushing injury of external genital organs (S38.0-)

● S38.2　Traumatic amputation of external genital organs

● S38.21　Traumatic amputation of female external genital organs
　　　Traumatic amputation of clitoris
　　　Traumatic amputation of labium (majus) (minus)
　　　Traumatic amputation of vulva

● S38.211　Complete traumatic amputation of female external genital organs ♀

● S38.212　Partial traumatic amputation of female external genital organs ♀

● S38.22　Traumatic amputation of penis

● S38.221　Complete traumatic amputation of penis ♂

● S38.222　Partial traumatic amputation of penis ♂

● S38.23　Traumatic amputation of scrotum and testis

● S38.231　Complete traumatic amputation of scrotum and testis ♂

● S38.232　Partial traumatic amputation of scrotum and testis ♂

X● S38.3　Transection (partial) of abdomen

● S39　Other and unspecified injuries of abdomen, lower back, pelvis and external genitals
　　Code also any associated open wound (S31.-)
　　Excludes2　sprain of joints and ligaments of lumbar spine and pelvis (S33.-)
　　The appropriate 7th character is to be added to each code from category S39

A	initial encounter
D	subsequent encounter
S	sequela

● S39.0　Injury of muscle, fascia and tendon of abdomen, lower back and pelvis

● S39.00　Unspecified injury of muscle, fascia and tendon of abdomen, lower back and pelvis

● S39.001　Unspecified injury of muscle, fascia and tendon of abdomen

● S39.002　Unspecified injury of muscle, fascia and tendon of lower back

● S39.003　Unspecified injury of muscle, fascia and tendon of pelvis

● S39.01　Strain of muscle, fascia and tendon of abdomen, lower back and pelvis

● S39.011　Strain of muscle, fascia and tendon of abdomen

● S39.012　Strain of muscle, fascia and tendon of lower back
　　　Coding Clinic: 2016, Q4, P74

● S39.013　Strain of muscle, fascia and tendon of pelvis

● S39.02　Laceration of muscle, fascia and tendon of abdomen, lower back and pelvis

● S39.021　Laceration of muscle, fascia and tendon of abdomen

● S39.022　Laceration of muscle, fascia and tendon of lower back

● S39.023　Laceration of muscle, fascia and tendon of pelvis

● S39.09　Other injury of muscle, fascia and tendon of abdomen, lower back and pelvis

● S39.091　Other injury of muscle, fascia and tendon of abdomen

● S39.092　Other injury of muscle, fascia and tendon of lower back

● S39.093　Other injury of muscle, fascia and tendon of pelvis

● S39.8　Other specified injuries of abdomen, lower back, pelvis and external genitals

X● S39.81　Other specified injuries of abdomen

X● S39.82　Other specified injuries of lower back

X● S39.83　Other specified injuries of pelvis

● S39.84　Other specified injuries of external genitals

● S39.840　Fracture of corpus cavernosum penis ♂

● S39.848　Other specified injuries of external genitals

● S39.9　Unspecified injury of abdomen, lower back, pelvis and external genitals

X● S39.91　Unspecified injury of abdomen

X● S39.92　Unspecified injury of lower back

X● S39.93　Unspecified injury of pelvis

X● S39.94　Unspecified injury of external genitals

N Newborn Age: 0　　**P** Pediatric Age: 0–17　　**M** Maternity DX: 9–64　　**A** Adult Age: 15–124　　♀ Females Only　　♂ Males Only

🄲 Complication\Comorbidity　　🄼 Major C\C　　(Ex.) CC/MCC Exclusions　　🄷🄰🄲 Hospital-Acquired Condition　　🄷🄲🄲 Hierarchical Condition Category

1301

CHAPTER 19 (S00-T88)

INJURIES TO THE SHOULDER AND UPPER ARM (S40-S49)

Includes	injuries of axilla injuries of scapular region
Excludes2	burns and corrosions (T20-T32)
	frostbite (T33-T34)
	injuries of elbow (S50-S59)
	insect bite or sting, venomous (T63.4)

- **S40**   Superficial injury of shoulder and upper arm

  The appropriate 7th character is to be added to each code from category S40

  > A   initial encounter
  > D   subsequent encounter
  > S   sequela

  - **S40.0**   Contusion of shoulder and upper arm
    - **S40.01**   Contusion of shoulder
      - **S40.011**   Contusion of right shoulder
      - **S40.012**   Contusion of left shoulder
      - **S40.019**   Contusion of unspecified shoulder
    - **S40.02**   Contusion of upper arm
      - **S40.021**   Contusion of right upper arm
      - **S40.022**   Contusion of left upper arm
      - **S40.029**   Contusion of unspecified upper arm
  - **S40.2**   Other superficial injuries of shoulder
    - **S40.21**   Abrasion of shoulder
      - **S40.211**   Abrasion of right shoulder
      - **S40.212**   Abrasion of left shoulder
      - **S40.219**   Abrasion of unspecified shoulder
    - **S40.22**   Blister (nonthermal) of shoulder
      - **S40.221**   Blister (nonthermal) of right shoulder
      - **S40.222**   Blister (nonthermal) of left shoulder
      - **S40.229**   Blister (nonthermal) of unspecified shoulder
    - **S40.24**   External constriction of shoulder
      - **S40.241**   External constriction of right shoulder
      - **S40.242**   External constriction of left shoulder
      - **S40.249**   External constriction of unspecified shoulder
    - **S40.25**   Superficial foreign body of shoulder
      Splinter in the shoulder
      - **S40.251**   Superficial foreign body of right shoulder
      - **S40.252**   Superficial foreign body of left shoulder
      - **S40.259**   Superficial foreign body of unspecified shoulder
    - **S40.26**   Insect bite (nonvenomous) of shoulder
      - **S40.261**   Insect bite (nonvenomous) of right shoulder
      - **S40.262**   Insect bite (nonvenomous) of left shoulder
      - **S40.269**   Insect bite (nonvenomous) of unspecified shoulder
    - **S40.27**   Other superficial bite of shoulder
      > **Excludes1**   open bite of shoulder (S41.05)
      - **S40.271**   Other superficial bite of right shoulder
      - **S40.272**   Other superficial bite of left shoulder
      - **S40.279**   Other superficial bite of unspecified shoulder

- **S40.8**   Other superficial injuries of upper arm
  - **S40.81**   Abrasion of upper arm
    - **S40.811**   Abrasion of right upper arm
    - **S40.812**   Abrasion of left upper arm
    - **S40.819**   Abrasion of unspecified upper arm
  - **S40.82**   Blister (nonthermal) of upper arm
    - **S40.821**   Blister (nonthermal) of right upper arm
    - **S40.822**   Blister (nonthermal) of left upper arm
    - **S40.829**   Blister (nonthermal) of unspecified upper arm
  - **S40.84**   External constriction of upper arm
    - **S40.841**   External constriction of right upper arm
    - **S40.842**   External constriction of left upper arm
    - **S40.849**   External constriction of unspecified upper arm
  - **S40.85**   Superficial foreign body of upper arm
    Splinter in the upper arm
    - **S40.851**   Superficial foreign body of right upper arm
    - **S40.852**   Superficial foreign body of left upper arm
    - **S40.859**   Superficial foreign body of unspecified upper arm
  - **S40.86**   Insect bite (nonvenomous) of upper arm
    - **S40.861**   Insect bite (nonvenomous) of right upper arm
    - **S40.862**   Insect bite (nonvenomous) of left upper arm
    - **S40.869**   Insect bite (nonvenomous) of unspecified upper arm
  - **S40.87**   Other superficial bite of upper arm
    > **Excludes1**   open bite of upper arm (S41.14)
    > **Excludes2**   other superficial bite of shoulder (S40.27-)
    - **S40.871**   Other superficial bite of right upper arm
    - **S40.872**   Other superficial bite of left upper arm
    - **S40.879**   Other superficial bite of unspecified upper arm
- **S40.9**   Unspecified superficial injury of shoulder and upper arm
  - **S40.91**   Unspecified superficial injury of shoulder
    - **S40.911**   Unspecified superficial injury of right shoulder
    - **S40.912**   Unspecified superficial injury of left shoulder
    - **S40.919**   Unspecified superficial injury of unspecified shoulder
  - **S40.92**   Unspecified superficial injury of upper arm
    - **S40.921**   Unspecified superficial injury of right upper arm
    - **S40.922**   Unspecified superficial injury of left upper arm
    - **S40.929**   Unspecified superficial injury of unspecified upper arm

▶ New   ⇒ Revised   ~~deleted~~ Deleted   Excludes 1   Excludes 2   Includes   Use additional   Code first   Code also   Key words
OGCR Official Guidelines   ● Unacceptable Principal Diagnosis   X Assign placeholder X   ● Use Additional Character(s)   ▶ Manifestation Code   **Coding Clinic**

● **S41 Open wound of shoulder and upper arm**

Code also any associated wound infection

Excludes1 traumatic amputation of shoulder and upper arm (S48.-)

Excludes2 open fracture of shoulder and upper arm (S42.- with 7th character B or C)

The appropriate 7th character is to be added to each code from category S41

> A   initial encounter
> D   subsequent encounter
> S   sequela

● **S41.0 Open wound of shoulder**
   ● **S41.00 Unspecified open wound of shoulder**
      ● S41.001 Unspecified open wound of **right** shoulder
      ● S41.002 Unspecified open wound of **left** shoulder
      ● S41.009 Unspecified open wound of **unspecified** shoulder
   ● **S41.01 Laceration without foreign body of shoulder**
      ● S41.011 Laceration without foreign body of **right** shoulder
      ● S41.012 Laceration without foreign body of **left** shoulder
      ● S41.019 Laceration without foreign body of **unspecified** shoulder
   ● **S41.02 Laceration with foreign body of shoulder**
      ● S41.021 Laceration with foreign body of **right** shoulder
      ● S41.022 Laceration with foreign body of **left** shoulder
      ● S41.029 Laceration with foreign body of **unspecified** shoulder
   ● **S41.03 Puncture wound without foreign body of shoulder**
      ● S41.031 Puncture wound without foreign body of **right** shoulder
      ● S41.032 Puncture wound without foreign body of **left** shoulder
      ● S41.039 Puncture wound without foreign body of **unspecified** shoulder
   ● **S41.04 Puncture wound with foreign body of shoulder**
      ● S41.041 Puncture wound with foreign body of **right** shoulder
      ● S41.042 Puncture wound with foreign body of **left** shoulder
      ● S41.049 Puncture wound with foreign body of **unspecified** shoulder
   ● **S41.05 Open bite of shoulder**
      Bite of shoulder NOS

      Excludes1 superficial bite of shoulder (S40.27)

      ● S41.051 Open bite of **right** shoulder
      ● S41.052 Open bite of **left** shoulder
      ● S41.059 Open bite of **unspecified** shoulder
● **S41.1 Open wound of upper arm**
   ● **S41.10 Unspecified open wound of upper arm**
      ● S41.101 Unspecified open wound of **right** upper arm
      ● S41.102 Unspecified open wound of **left** upper arm
      ● S41.109 Unspecified open wound of **unspecified** upper arm

● **S41.11 Laceration without foreign body of upper arm**
   ● S41.111 Laceration without foreign body of **right** upper arm
   ● S41.112 Laceration without foreign body of **left** upper arm
   ● S41.119 Laceration without foreign body of **unspecified** upper arm
● **S41.12 Laceration with foreign body of upper arm**
   ● S41.121 Laceration with foreign body of **right** upper arm
   ● S41.122 Laceration with foreign body of **left** upper arm
   ● S41.129 Laceration with foreign body of **unspecified** upper arm
● **S41.13 Puncture wound without foreign body of upper arm**
   ● S41.131 Puncture wound without foreign body of **right** upper arm
   ● S41.132 Puncture wound without foreign body of **left** upper arm
   ● S41.139 Puncture wound without foreign body of **unspecified** upper arm
● **S41.14 Puncture wound with foreign body of upper arm**
   ● S41.141 Puncture wound with foreign body of **right** upper arm
   ● S41.142 Puncture wound with foreign body of **left** upper arm
   ● S41.149 Puncture wound with foreign body of **unspecified** upper arm
● **S41.15 Open bite of upper arm**
   Bite of upper arm NOS

      Excludes1 superficial bite of upper arm (S40.87)

   ● S41.151 Open bite of **right** upper arm
   ● S41.152 Open bite of **left** upper arm
   ● S41.159 Open bite of **unspecified** upper arm

● **S42 Fracture of shoulder and upper arm**

Note: A fracture not indicated as displaced or nondisplaced should be coded to displaced

A fracture not indicated as open or closed should be coded to closed

Excludes1 traumatic amputation of shoulder and upper arm (S48.-)

The appropriate 7th character is to be added to all codes from category S42

> A   initial encounter for closed fracture
> B   initial encounter for open fracture
> D   subsequent encounter for fracture with routine healing
> G   subsequent encounter for fracture with delayed healing
> K   subsequent encounter for fracture with nonunion
> P   subsequent encounter for fracture with malunion
> S   sequela

● **S42.0 Fracture of clavicle**
   (Ex) **For S42.0[B]:** See PDX Collection 1243 **For S42.0[K,P]:** See PDX Collection 897
   ● **S42.00 Fracture of unspecified part of clavicle**
      ● S42.001 Fracture of unspecified part of **right** clavicle B, K, P 🞇, B 🞇
      ● S42.002 Fracture of unspecified part of **left** clavicle B, K, P 🞇, B 🞇
      ● S42.009 Fracture of unspecified part of **unspecified** clavicle B, K, P 🞇, B 🞇
      Coding Clinic: 2012, Q4, P3

N Newborn Age: 0   P Pediatric Age: 0–17   M Maternity DX: 9–64   A Adult Age: 15–124   ♀ Females Only   ♂ Males Only
🞇 Complication\Comorbidity   🞇 Major C\C   (Ex) CC/MCC Exclusions   🞇 Hospital-Acquired Condition   🞇 Hierarchical Condition Category

1303

● S42.01   Fracture of sternal end of clavicle

  ● S42.011   Anterior displaced fracture of sternal end of right clavicle B, K, P 🔍, B 🔍

  ● S42.012   Anterior displaced fracture of sternal end of left clavicle B, K, P 🔍, B 🔍

  ● S42.013   Anterior displaced fracture of sternal end of unspecified clavicle B, K, P 🔍, B 🔍

     Displaced fracture of sternal end of clavicle NOS

  ● S42.014   Posterior displaced fracture of sternal end of right clavicle B, K, P 🔍, B 🔍

  ● S42.015   Posterior displaced fracture of sternal end of left clavicle B, K, P 🔍, B 🔍

  ● S42.016   Posterior displaced fracture of sternal end of unspecified clavicle B, K, P 🔍, B 🔍

  ● S42.017   Nondisplaced fracture of sternal end of right clavicle B, K, P 🔍, B 🔍

  ● S42.018   Nondisplaced fracture of sternal end of left clavicle B, K, P 🔍, B 🔍

  ● S42.019   Nondisplaced fracture of sternal end of unspecified clavicle B, K, P 🔍, B 🔍

● S42.02   Fracture of shaft of clavicle

  ● S42.021   Displaced fracture of shaft of right clavicle B, K, P 🔍, B 🔍

  ● S42.022   Displaced fracture of shaft of left clavicle B, K, P 🔍, B 🔍

  ● S42.023   Displaced fracture of shaft of unspecified clavicle B, K, P 🔍, B 🔍

  ● S42.024   Nondisplaced fracture of shaft of right clavicle B, K, P 🔍, B 🔍

  ● S42.025   Nondisplaced fracture of shaft of left clavicle B, K, P 🔍, B 🔍

  ● S42.026   Nondisplaced fracture of shaft of unspecified clavicle B, K, P 🔍, B 🔍

● S42.03   Fracture of lateral end of clavicle

     Fracture of acromial end of clavicle

  ● S42.031   Displaced fracture of lateral end of right clavicle B, K, P 🔍, B 🔍

  ● S42.032   Displaced fracture of lateral end of left clavicle B, K, P 🔍, B 🔍

  ● S42.033   Displaced fracture of lateral end of unspecified clavicle B, K, P 🔍, B 🔍

  ● S42.034   Nondisplaced fracture of lateral end of right clavicle B, K, P 🔍, B 🔍

  ● S42.035   Nondisplaced fracture of lateral end of left clavicle B, K, P 🔍, B 🔍

  ● S42.036   Nondisplaced fracture of lateral end of unspecified clavicle B, K, P 🔍, B 🔍

● S42.1   Fracture of scapula

  Ⓔⓧ **For S42.1[B]:** See PDX Collection 1244 **For S42.1[K,P]:** See PDX Collection 897

  ● S42.10   Fracture of unspecified part of scapula

    ● S42.101   Fracture of unspecified part of scapula, right shoulder B, K, P 🔍, B 🔍

    ● S42.102   Fracture of unspecified part of scapula, left shoulder B, K, P 🔍, B 🔍

    ● S42.109   Fracture of unspecified part of scapula, unspecified shoulder B, K, P 🔍, B 🔍

● S42.11   Fracture of body of scapula

  ● S42.111   Displaced fracture of body of scapula, right shoulder B, K, P 🔍, B 🔍

  ● S42.112   Displaced fracture of body of scapula, left shoulder B, K, P 🔍, B 🔍

  ● S42.113   Displaced fracture of body of scapula, unspecified shoulder B, K, P 🔍, B 🔍

  ● S42.114   Nondisplaced fracture of body of scapula, right shoulder B, K, P 🔍, B 🔍

  ● S42.115   Nondisplaced fracture of body of scapula, left shoulder B, K, P 🔍, B 🔍

  ● S42.116   Nondisplaced fracture of body of scapula, unspecified shoulder B, K, P 🔍, B 🔍

● S42.12   Fracture of acromial process

  ● S42.121   Displaced fracture of acromial process, right shoulder B, K, P 🔍, B 🔍

  ● S42.122   Displaced fracture of acromial process, left shoulder B, K, P 🔍, B 🔍

  ● S42.123   Displaced fracture of acromial process, unspecified shoulder B, K, P 🔍, B 🔍

  ● S42.124   Nondisplaced fracture of acromial process, right shoulder B, K, P 🔍, B 🔍

  ● S42.125   Nondisplaced fracture of acromial process, left shoulder B, K, P 🔍, B 🔍

  ● S42.126   Nondisplaced fracture, of acromial process, unspecified shoulder B, K, P 🔍, B 🔍

● S42.13   Fracture of coracoid process

  ● S42.131   Displaced fracture of coracoid process, right shoulder B, K, P 🔍, B 🔍

  ● S42.132   Displaced fracture of coracoid process, left shoulder B, K, P 🔍, B 🔍

  ● S42.133   Displaced fracture of coracoid process, unspecified shoulder B, K, P 🔍, B 🔍

  ● S42.134   Nondisplaced fracture of coracoid process, right shoulder B, K, P 🔍, B 🔍

  ● S42.135   Nondisplaced fracture of coracoid process, left shoulder B, K, P 🔍, B 🔍

  ● S42.136   Nondisplaced fracture of coracoid process, unspecified shoulder B, K, P 🔍, B 🔍

● S42.14   Fracture of glenoid cavity of scapula

  ● S42.141   Displaced fracture of glenoid cavity of scapula, right shoulder B, K, P 🔍, B 🔍

  ● S42.142   Displaced fracture of glenoid cavity of scapula, left shoulder B, K, P 🔍, B 🔍

  ● S42.143   Displaced fracture of glenoid cavity of scapula, unspecified shoulder B, K, P 🔍, B 🔍

  ● S42.144   Nondisplaced fracture of glenoid cavity of scapula, right shoulder B, K, P 🔍, B 🔍

  ● S42.145   Nondisplaced fracture of glenoid cavity of scapula, left shoulder B, K, P 🔍, B 🔍

  ● S42.146   Nondisplaced fracture of glenoid cavity of scapula, unspecified shoulder B, K, P 🔍, B 🔍

● S42.15   Fracture of neck of scapula
    ● S42.151   Displaced fracture of neck of scapula, right shoulder B, K, P 🅒, B 🅜
    ● S42.152   Displaced fracture of neck of scapula, left shoulder B, K, P 🅒, B 🅜
    ● S42.153   Displaced fracture of neck of scapula, unspecified shoulder B, K, P 🅒, B 🅜
    ● S42.154   Nondisplaced fracture of neck of scapula, right shoulder B, K, P 🅒, B 🅜
    ● S42.155   Nondisplaced fracture of neck of scapula, left shoulder B, K, P 🅒, B 🅜
    ● S42.156   Nondisplaced fracture of neck of scapula, unspecified shoulder B, K, P 🅒, B 🅜

● S42.19   Fracture of other part of scapula
    ● S42.191   Fracture of other part of scapula, right shoulder B, K, P 🅒, B 🅜
    ● S42.192   Fracture of other part of scapula, left shoulder B, K, P 🅒, B 🅜
    ● S42.199   Fracture of other part of scapula, unspecified shoulder B, K, P 🅒, B 🅜

● S42.2   Fracture of upper end of humerus
    Fracture of proximal end of humerus
    Excludes2   fracture of shaft of humerus (S42.3-)
        physeal fracture of upper end of humerus (S49.0-)

● S42.20   Unspecified fracture of upper end of humerus
    ● S42.201   Unspecified fracture of upper end of right humerus A, K, P 🅒, B 🅜, A, B 🅗
       (Ex:) For S42.201[A]: See PDX Collection 1245
         For S42.201[B]: See PDX Collection 1246
         For S42.201[K,P]: See PDX Collection 897
    ● S42.202   Unspecified fracture of upper end of left humerus A, K, P 🅒, B 🅜, A, B 🅗
       (Ex:) For category S42.202 CC codes
         S42.202[A]: See PDX Collection 1247
         For S42.202[B]: See PDX Collection 1246
         For S42.202[K,P]: See PDX Collection 897
    ● S42.209   Unspecified fracture of upper end of unspecified humerus A, K, P 🅒, B 🅜, A, B 🅗
       (Ex:) For S42.209[A]: See PDX Collection 1248
         For S42.202[B]: See PDX Collection 1246
         For S42.202[K,P]: See PDX Collection 897

● S42.21   Unspecified fracture of surgical neck of humerus
    Fracture of neck of humerus NOS
    ● S42.211   Unspecified displaced fracture of surgical neck of right humerus A, K, P 🅒, B 🅜, A, B 🅗
       (Ex:) For S42.211[A]: See PDX Collection 1245
         For S42.211[B]: See PDX Collection 1246
         For S42.211[K,P]: See PDX Collection 897
    ● S42.212   Unspecified displaced fracture of surgical neck of left humerus A, K, P 🅒, B 🅜, A, B 🅗
       (Ex:) For S42.212[A]: See PDX Collection 1247
         For S42.212[B]: See PDX Collection 1246
         For S42.212[K,P]: See PDX Collection 897

● S42.213   Unspecified displaced fracture of surgical neck of unspecified humerus A, K, P 🅒, B 🅜, A, B 🅗
       (Ex:) For S42.213[A]: See PDX Collection 1248
         For S42.213[B]: See PDX Collection 1246
         For S42.213[K,P]: See PDX Collection 897

● S42.214   Unspecified nondisplaced fracture of surgical neck of right humerus A, K, P 🅒, B 🅜, A, B 🅗
       (Ex:) For S42.214[A]: See PDX Collection 1245
         For S42.214[B]: See PDX Collection 1246
         For S42.214[K,P]: See PDX Collection 897

● S42.215   Unspecified nondisplaced fracture of surgical neck of left humerus A, K, P 🅒, B 🅜, A, B 🅗
       (Ex:) For S42.215[A]: See PDX Collection 1246
         For S42.215[B]: See PDX Collection 1246
         For S42.215[K,P]: See PDX Collection 897

● S42.216   Unspecified nondisplaced fracture of surgical neck of unspecified humerus A, K, P 🅒, B 🅜, A, B 🅗
       (Ex:) For S42.216[A]: See PDX Collection 1248
         For S42.216[B]: See PDX Collection 1246
         For S42.216[K,P]: See PDX Collection 897

● S42.22   2-part fracture of surgical neck of humerus
    ● S42.221   2-part displaced fracture of surgical neck of right humerus A, K, P 🅒, B 🅜, A, B 🅗
       (Ex:) For S42.221[A]: See PDX Collection 1245
         For S42.221[B]: See PDX Collection 1246
         For S42.221[K,P]: See PDX Collection 897
    ● S42.222   2-part displaced fracture of surgical neck of left humerus A, K, P 🅒, B 🅜, A, B 🅗
       (Ex:) For S42.222[A]: See PDX Collection 1247
         For S42.222[B]: See PDX Collection 1246
         For S42.222[K,P]: See PDX Collection 897
    ● S42.223   2-part displaced fracture of surgical neck of unspecified humerus A, K, P 🅒, B 🅜, A, B 🅗
       (Ex:) For S42.223[A]: See PDX Collection 1248
         For S42.223[B]: See PDX Collection 1246
         For S42.223[K,P]: See PDX Collection 897
    ● S42.224   2-part nondisplaced fracture of surgical neck of right humerus A, K, P 🅒, B 🅜, A, B 🅗
       (Ex:) For S42.224[A]: See PDX Collection 1245
         For S42.224[B]: See PDX Collection 1246
         For S42.224[K,P]: See PDX Collection 897
    ● S42.225   2-part nondisplaced fracture of surgical neck of left humerus A, K, P 🅒, B 🅜, A, B 🅗
       (Ex:) For S42.225[A]: See PDX Collection 1247
         For S42.225[B]: See PDX Collection 1246
         For S42.225[K,P]: See PDX Collection 897
    ● S42.226   2-part nondisplaced fracture of surgical neck of unspecified humerus A, K, P 🅒, B 🅜, A, B 🅗
       (Ex:) For S42.226[A]: See PDX Collection 1248
         For S42.226[B]: See PDX Collection 1246
         For S42.226[K,P]: See PDX Collection 897

CHAPTER 19 (S00-T88)

N   Newborn Age: 0   P   Pediatric Age: 0–17   M   Maternity DX: 9–64   A   Adult Age: 15–124   ♀   Females Only   ♂   Males Only

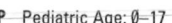 Complication\Comorbidity   🅜 Major C\C   (Ex:) CC/MCC Exclusions   🅗 Hospital-Acquired Condition   🅗🅒🅒 Hierarchical Condition Category

1305

● S42.23 **3-part fracture of surgical neck of humerus**
   ● S42.231 **3-part fracture of surgical neck of right humerus** A, K, P 🌑, B 🌑, A, B 🌑
         (Ex) **For S42.231[A]:** See PDX Collection 1245
              For S42.231[B]: See PDX Collection 1246
              For S42.231[K,P]: See PDX Collection 897
   ● S42.232 **3-part fracture of surgical neck of left humerus** A, K, P 🌑, B 🌑, A, B 🌑
         (Ex) **For S42.232[A]:** See PDX Collection 1247
              For S42.232[B]: See PDX Collection 1246
              For S42.232[K,P]: See PDX Collection 897
   ● S42.239 **3-part fracture of surgical neck of unspecified humerus** A, K, P 🌑, B 🌑, A, B 🌑
         (Ex) **For S42.239[A]:** See PDX Collection 1248
              For S42.239[B]: See PDX Collection 1246
              For S42.239[K,P]: See PDX Collection 897

● S42.24 **4-part fracture of surgical neck of humerus**
   ● S42.241 **4-part fracture of surgical neck of right humerus** A, K, P 🌑, B 🌑, A, B 🌑
         (Ex) **For S42.241[A]:** See PDX Collection 1245
              For S42.241[B]: See PDX Collection 1246
              For S42.241[K,P]: See PDX Collection 897
   ● S42.242 **4-part fracture of surgical neck of left humerus** A, K, P 🌑, B 🌑, A, B 🌑
         (Ex) **For S42.242[A]:** See PDX Collection 1247
              For S42.242[B]: See PDX Collection 1246
              For S42.242[K,P]: See PDX Collection 897
   ● S42.249 **4-part fracture of surgical neck of unspecified humerus** A, K, P 🌑, B 🌑, A, B 🌑
         (Ex) **For S42.249[A]:** See PDX Collection 1248
              For S42.249[B]: See PDX Collection 1246
              For S42.249[K,P]: See PDX Collection 897

● S42.25 **Fracture of greater tuberosity of humerus**
   ● S42.251 **Displaced fracture of greater tuberosity of right humerus** A, K, P 🌑, B 🌑, A, B 🌑
         (Ex) **For S42.251[A]:** See PDX Collection 1245
              For S42.251[B]: See PDX Collection 1246
              For S42.251[K,P]: See PDX Collection 897
   ● S42.252 **Displaced fracture of greater tuberosity of left humerus** A, K, P 🌑, B 🌑, A, B 🌑
         (Ex) **For S42.252[A]:** See PDX Collection 1247
              For S42.252[B]: See PDX Collection 1246
              For S42.252[K,P]: See PDX Collection 897
   ● S42.253 **Displaced fracture of greater tuberosity of unspecified humerus** A, K, P 🌑, B 🌑, A, B 🌑
         (Ex) **For S42.253[A]:** See PDX Collection 1248
              For S42.253[B]: See PDX Collection 1246
              For S42.253[K,P]: See PDX Collection 897
   ● S42.254 **Nondisplaced fracture of greater tuberosity of right humerus** A, K, P 🌑, B 🌑, A, B 🌑
         (Ex) **For S42.254[A]:** See PDX Collection 1245
              For S42.254[B]: See PDX Collection 1246
              For S42.254[K,P]: See PDX Collection 897
   ● S42.255 **Nondisplaced fracture of greater tuberosity of left humerus** A, K, P 🌑, B 🌑, A, B 🌑
         (Ex) **For S42.255[A]:** See PDX Collection 1247
              For S42.255[B]: See PDX Collection 1246
              For S42.255[K,P]: See PDX Collection 897
   ● S42.256 **Nondisplaced fracture of greater tuberosity of unspecified humerus** A, K, P 🌑, B 🌑, A, B 🌑
         (Ex) **For S42.256[A]:** See PDX Collection 1248
              For S42.256[B]: See PDX Collection 1246
              For S42.256[K,P]: See PDX Collection 897

● S42.26 **Fracture of lesser tuberosity of humerus**
   ● S42.261 **Displaced fracture of lesser tuberosity of right humerus** A, K, P 🌑, B 🌑, A, B 🌑
         (Ex) **For S42.261[A]:** See PDX Collection 1245
              For S42.261[B]: See PDX Collection 1246
              For S42.261[K,P]: See PDX Collection 897
   ● S42.262 **Displaced fracture of lesser tuberosity of left humerus** A, K, P 🌑, B 🌑, A, B 🌑
         (Ex) **For S42.262[A]:** See PDX Collection 1247
              For S42.262[B]: See PDX Collection 1246
              For S42.262[K,P]: See PDX Collection 897
   ● S42.263 **Displaced fracture of lesser tuberosity of unspecified humerus** A, K, P 🌑, B 🌑, A, B 🌑
         (Ex) **For S42.263[A]:** See PDX Collection 1248
              For S42.263[B]: See PDX Collection 1246
              For S42.263[K,P]: See PDX Collection 897
   ● S42.264 **Nondisplaced fracture of lesser tuberosity of right humerus** A, K, P 🌑, B 🌑, A, B 🌑
         (Ex) **For S42.264[A]:** See PDX Collection 1245
              For S42.264[B]: See PDX Collection 1246
              For S42.264[K,P]: See PDX Collection 897
   ● S42.265 **Nondisplaced fracture of lesser tuberosity of left humerus** A, K, P 🌑, B 🌑, A, B 🌑
         (Ex) **For S42.265[A]:** See PDX Collection 1247
              For S42.265[B]: See PDX Collection 1246
              For S42.265[K,P]: See PDX Collection 897
   ● S42.266 **Nondisplaced fracture of lesser tuberosity of unspecified humerus** A, K, P 🌑, B 🌑, A, B 🌑
         (Ex) **For S42.266[A]:** See PDX Collection 1248
              For S42.266[B]: See PDX Collection 1246
              For S42.266[K,P]: See PDX Collection 897

● S42.27 **Torus fracture of upper end of humerus**

The appropriate 7th character is to be added to all codes in subcategory S42.27

A	initial encounter for closed fracture
D	subsequent encounter for fracture with routine healing
G	subsequent encounter for fracture with delayed healing
K	subsequent encounter for fracture with nonunion
P	subsequent encounter for fracture with malunion
S	sequela

   ● S42.271 **Torus fracture of upper end of right humerus** A, K, P 🌑, A 🌑
         (Ex) **For S42.271[A]:** See PDX Collection 1245
              For S42.271[K,P]: See PDX Collection 897
   ● S42.272 **Torus fracture of upper end of left humerus** A, K, P 🌑, A 🌑
         (Ex) **For S42.272[A]:** See PDX Collection 1247
              For S42.272[K,P]: See PDX Collection 897
   ● S42.279 **Torus fracture of upper end of unspecified humerus** A, K, P 🌑, A 🌑
         (Ex) **For S42.279[A]:** See PDX Collection 1248
              For S42.279[K,P]: See PDX Collection 897

● **S42.29**   Other fracture of upper end of humerus
     Fracture of anatomical neck of humerus
     Fracture of articular head of humerus

   ● **S42.291**   Other displaced fracture of upper end of right humerus A, K, P 🔵, B 🔴, A, B 🔴
       Ⓔ **For S42.291[A]:** See PDX Collection 1245
       For S42.291[B]: See PDX Collection 1246
       For S42.291[K,P]: See PDX Collection 897

   ● **S42.292**   Other displaced fracture of upper end of left humerus A, K, P 🔵, B 🔴, A, B 🔴
       Ⓔ **For S42.292[A]:** See PDX Collection 1247
       For S42.292[B]: See PDX Collection 1246
       For S42.292[K,P]: See PDX Collection 897

   ● **S42.293**   Other displaced fracture of upper end of unspecified humerus A, K, P 🔵, B 🔴, A, B 🔴
       Ⓔ **For S42.293[A]:** See PDX Collection 1248
       For S42.293[B]: See PDX Collection 1246
       For S42.293[K,P]: See PDX Collection 897

   ● **S42.294**   Other nondisplaced fracture of upper end of right humerus A, K, P 🔵, B 🔴, A, B 🔴
       Ⓔ **For S42.294[A]:** See PDX Collection 1245
       For S42.294[B]: See PDX Collection 1246
       For S42.294[K,P]: See PDX Collection 897

   ● **S42.295**   Other nondisplaced fracture of upper end of left humerus A, K, P 🔵, B 🔴, A, B 🔴
       Ⓔ **For S42.295[A]:** See PDX Collection 1247
       For S42.295[B]: See PDX Collection 1246
       For S42.295[K,P]: See PDX Collection 897
       Coding Clinic: 2019, Q1, P19

   ● **S42.296**   Other nondisplaced fracture of upper end of unspecified humerus A, K, P 🔵, B 🔴, A, B 🔴
       Ⓔ **For S42.296[A]:** See PDX Collection 1248
       For S42.296[B]: See PDX Collection 1246
       For S42.296[K,P]: See PDX Collection 897

● **S42.3**   Fracture of shaft of humerus
     Fracture of humerus NOS
     Fracture of upper arm NOS
     Excludes2   physeal fractures of upper end of humerus (S49.0-)
                 physeal fractures of lower end of humerus (S49.1-)

   ● **S42.30**   Unspecified fracture of shaft of humerus

     ● **S42.301**   Unspecified fracture of shaft of humerus, right arm A, K, P 🔵, B 🔴, A, B 🔴
         Ⓔ **For S42.301[A]:** See PDX Collection 1245
         For S42.301[B]: See PDX Collection 1246
         For S42.301[K,P]: See PDX Collection 897

     ● **S42.302**   Unspecified fracture of shaft of humerus, left arm A, K, P 🔵, B 🔴, A, B 🔴
         Ⓔ **For S42.302[A]:** See PDX Collection 1247
         For S42.302[B]: See PDX Collection 1246
         For S42.302[K,P]: See PDX Collection 897

     ● **S42.309**   Unspecified fracture of shaft of humerus, unspecified arm A, K, P 🔵, B 🔴, A, B 🔴
         Ⓔ **For S42.309[A]:** See PDX Collection 1248
         For S42.309[B]: See PDX Collection 1246
         For S42.309[K,P]: See PDX Collection 897

● **S42.31**   Greenstick fracture of shaft of humerus
     The appropriate 7th character is to be added to all codes in subcategory S42.31

A	initial encounter for closed fracture
D	subsequent encounter for fracture with routine healing
G	subsequent encounter for fracture with delayed healing
K	subsequent encounter for fracture with nonunion
P	subsequent encounter for fracture with malunion
S	sequela

   ● **S42.311**   Greenstick fracture of shaft of humerus, right arm A, K, P 🔵, A 🔴
       Ⓔ **For S42.311[A]:** See PDX Collection 1249
       For S42.311[K,P]: See PDX Collection 897

   ● **S42.312**   Greenstick fracture of shaft of humerus, left arm A, K, P 🔵, A 🔴
       Ⓔ **For S42.312[A]:** See PDX Collection 1250
       For S42.312[K,P]: See PDX Collection 897

   ● **S42.319**   Greenstick fracture of shaft of humerus, unspecified arm A, K, P 🔵, A 🔴
       Ⓔ **For S42.319[A]:** See PDX Collection 1251
       For S42.319[K,P]: See PDX Collection 897

● **S42.32**   Transverse fracture of shaft of humerus

   ● **S42.321**   Displaced transverse fracture of shaft of humerus, right arm A, K, P 🔵, B 🔴, A, B 🔴
       Ⓔ **For S42.321[A]:** See PDX Collection 1250
       For S42.321[B]: See PDX Collection 1246
       For S42.321[K,P]: See PDX Collection 897

   ● **S42.322**   Displaced transverse fracture of shaft of humerus, left arm A, K, P 🔵, B 🔴, A, B 🔴
       Ⓔ **For S42.322[A]:** See PDX Collection 1250
       For S42.322[B]: See PDX Collection 1246
       For S42.322[K,P]: See PDX Collection 897

   ● **S42.323**   Displaced transverse fracture of shaft of humerus, unspecified arm A, K, P 🔵, B 🔴, A, B 🔴
       Ⓔ **For S42.323[A]:** See PDX Collection 1251
       For S42.323[B]: See PDX Collection 1246
       For S42.313[K,P]: See PDX Collection 897

   ● **S42.324**   Nondisplaced transverse fracture of shaft of humerus, right arm A, K, P 🔵, B 🔴, A, B 🔴
       Ⓔ **For S42.324[A]:** See PDX Collection 1249
       For S42.324[B]: See PDX Collection 1246
       For S42.324[K,P]: See PDX Collection 897

   ● **S42.325**   Nondisplaced transverse fracture of shaft of humerus, left arm A, K, P 🔵, B 🔴, A, B 🔴
       Ⓔ **For S42.325[A]:** See PDX Collection 1250
       For S42.325[B]: See PDX Collection 1246
       For S42.325[K,P]: See PDX Collection 897

   ● **S42.326**   Nondisplaced transverse fracture of shaft of humerus, unspecified arm A, K, P 🔵, B 🔴, A, B 🔴
       Ⓔ **For S42.326[A]:** See PDX Collection 1251
       For S42.326[B]: See PDX Collection 1246
       For S42.316[K,P]: See PDX Collection 897

CHAPTER 19 (S00-T88)

N   Newborn Age: 0   P   Pediatric Age: 0–17   M   Maternity DX: 9–64   A   Adult Age: 15–124   ♀   Females Only   ♂   Males Only

🔵 Complication\Comorbidity   🔴 Major C\C   Ⓔ CC/MCC Exclusions   🔴 Hospital-Acquired Condition   🔴 Hierarchical Condition Category

1307

- **S42.33**   Oblique fracture of shaft of humerus
  - **S42.331**   Displaced oblique fracture of shaft of humerus, right arm A, K, P, B, A, B
    - (Ex:) For S42.331[A]: See PDX Collection 1249
    - For S42.331[B]: See PDX Collection 1246
    - For S42.331[K,P]: See PDX Collection 897
  - **S42.332**   Displaced oblique fracture of shaft of humerus, left arm A, K, P, B, A, B
    - (Ex:) For S42.332[A]: See PDX Collection 1250
    - For S42.332[B]: See PDX Collection 1246
    - For S42.332[K,P]: See PDX Collection 897
  - **S42.333**   Displaced oblique fracture of shaft of humerus, unspecified arm A, K, P, B, A, B
    - (Ex:) For S42.333[A]: See PDX Collection 1251
    - For S42.333[B]: See PDX Collection 1246
    - For S42.333[K,P]: See PDX Collection 897
  - **S42.334**   Nondisplaced oblique fracture of shaft of humerus, right arm A, K, P, B, A, B
    - (Ex:) For S42.334[A]: See PDX Collection 1249
    - For S42.334[B]: See PDX Collection 1246
    - For S42.334[K,P]: See PDX Collection 897
  - **S42.335**   Nondisplaced oblique fracture of shaft of humerus, left arm A, K, P, B, A, B
    - (Ex:) For S42.335[A]: See PDX Collection 1250
    - For S42.335[B]: See PDX Collection 1246
    - For S42.335[K,P]: See PDX Collection 897
  - **S42.336**   Nondisplaced oblique fracture of shaft of humerus, unspecified arm A, K, P, B, A, B
    - (Ex:) For S42.336[A]: See PDX Collection 1251
    - For S42.336[B]: See PDX Collection 1246
    - For S42.336[K,P]: See PDX Collection 897
- **S42.34**   Spiral fracture of shaft of humerus
  - **S42.341**   Displaced spiral fracture of shaft of humerus, right arm A, K, P, B, A, B
    - (Ex:) For S42.341[A]: See PDX Collection 1249
    - For S42.341[B]: See PDX Collection 1246
    - For S42.341[K,P]: See PDX Collection 897
  - **S42.342**   Displaced spiral fracture of shaft of humerus, left arm A, K, P, B, A, B
    - (Ex:) For S42.342[A]: See PDX Collection 1250
    - For S42.342[B]: See PDX Collection 1246
    - For S42.342[K,P]: See PDX Collection 897
  - **S42.343**   Displaced spiral fracture of shaft of humerus, unspecified arm A, K, P, B, A, B
    - (Ex:) For S42.343[A]: See PDX Collection 1251
    - For S42.343[B]: See PDX Collection 1246
    - For S42.343[K,P]: See PDX Collection 897
  - **S42.344**   Nondisplaced spiral fracture of shaft of humerus, right arm A, K, P, B, A, B
    - (Ex:) For S42.344[A]: See PDX Collection 1249
    - For S42.344[B]: See PDX Collection 1246
    - For S42.344[K,P]: See PDX Collection 897
  - **S42.345**   Nondisplaced spiral fracture of shaft of humerus, left arm A, K, P, B, A, B
    - (Ex:) For S42.345[A]: See PDX Collection 1250
    - For S42.345[B]: See PDX Collection 1246
    - For S42.345[K,P]: See PDX Collection 897
  - **S42.346**   Nondisplaced spiral fracture of shaft of humerus, unspecified arm A, K, P, B, A, B
    - (Ex:) For S42.346[A]: See PDX Collection 1251
    - For S42.346[B]: See PDX Collection 1246
    - For S42.346[K,P]: See PDX Collection 897

- **S42.35**   Comminuted fracture of shaft of humerus
  - **S42.351**   Displaced comminuted fracture of shaft of humerus, right arm A, K, P, B, A, B
    - (Ex:) For S42.351[A]: See PDX Collection 1249
    - For S42.351[B]: See PDX Collection 1246
    - For S42.351[K,P]: See PDX Collection 897
  - **S42.352**   Displaced comminuted fracture of shaft of humerus, left arm A, K, P, B, A, B
    - (Ex:) For S42.352[A]: See PDX Collection 1250
    - For S42.352[B]: See PDX Collection 1246
    - For S42.352[K,P]: See PDX Collection 897
  - **S42.353**   Displaced comminuted fracture of shaft of humerus, unspecified arm A, K, P, B, A, B
    - (Ex:) For S42.353[A]: See PDX Collection 1251
    - For S42.353[B]: See PDX Collection 1246
    - For S42.353[K,P]: See PDX Collection 897
  - **S42.354**   Nondisplaced comminuted fracture of shaft of humerus, right arm A, K, P, B, A, B
    - (Ex:) For S42.354[A]: See PDX Collection 1249
    - For S42.354[B]: See PDX Collection 1246
    - For S42.354[K,P]: See PDX Collection 897
  - **S42.355**   Nondisplaced comminuted fracture of shaft of humerus, left arm A, K, P, B, A, B
    - (Ex:) For S42.355[A]: See PDX Collection 1250
    - For S42.355[B]: See PDX Collection 1246
    - For S42.355[K,P]: See PDX Collection 897
  - **S42.356**   Nondisplaced comminuted fracture of shaft of humerus, unspecified arm A, K, P, B, A, B
    - (Ex:) For S42.356[A]: See PDX Collection 1251
    - For S42.356[B]: See PDX Collection 1246
    - For S42.356[K,P]: See PDX Collection 897
- **S42.36**   Segmental fracture of shaft of humerus
  - **S42.361**   Displaced segmental fracture of shaft of humerus, right arm A, K, P, B, A, B
    - (Ex:) For S42.361[A]: See PDX Collection 1249
    - For S42.361[B]: See PDX Collection 1246
    - For S42.361[K,P]: See PDX Collection 897
  - **S42.362**   Displaced segmental fracture of shaft of humerus, left arm A, K, P, B, A, B
    - (Ex:) For S42.362[A]: See PDX Collection 1250
    - For S42.362[B]: See PDX Collection 1246
    - For S42.362[K,P]: See PDX Collection 897
  - **S42.363**   Displaced segmental fracture of shaft of humerus, unspecified arm A, K, P, B, A, B
    - (Ex:) For S42.363[A]: See PDX Collection 1251
    - For S42.363[B]: See PDX Collection 1246
    - For S42.363[K,P]: See PDX Collection 897
  - **S42.364**   Nondisplaced segmental fracture of shaft of humerus, right arm A, K, P, B, A, B
    - (Ex:) For S42.364[A]: See PDX Collection 1249
    - For S42.364[B]: See PDX Collection 1246
    - For S42.364[K,P]: See PDX Collection 897
  - **S42.365**   Nondisplaced segmental fracture of shaft of humerus, left arm A, K, P, B, A, B
    - (Ex:) For S42.365[A]: See PDX Collection 1250
    - For S42.365[B]: See PDX Collection 1246
    - For S42.365[K,P]: See PDX Collection 897
  - **S42.366**   Nondisplaced segmental fracture of shaft of humerus, unspecified arm A, K, P, B, A, B
    - (Ex:) For S42.366[A]: See PDX Collection 1251
    - For S42.366[B]: See PDX Collection 1246
    - For S42.366[K,P]: See PDX Collection 897

▶ New   ⇒ Revised   ~~deleted~~ Deleted   Excludes 1   Excludes 2   Includes   Use additional   Code first   Code also   Key words

OGCR Official Guidelines   ● Unacceptable Principal Diagnosis   X Assign placeholder X   ● Use Additional Character(s)   ▶ Manifestation Code   **Coding Clinic**

● **S42.39** Other fracture of shaft of humerus
  ● S42.391 Other fracture of shaft of right humerus A, K, P 🔾, B 🔾, A, B 🔾
    (Ex:) **For S42.391[A]:** See PDX Collection 1249
         For S42.391[B]: See PDX Collection 1246
         For S42.391[K,P]: See PDX Collection 897
  ● S42.392 Other fracture of shaft of left humerus A, K, P 🔾, B 🔾, A, B 🔾
    (Ex:) **For S42.392[A]:** See PDX Collection 1250
         For S42.392[B]: See PDX Collection 1246
         For S42.392[K,P]: See PDX Collection 897
  ● S42.399 Other fracture of shaft of unspecified humerus A, K, P 🔾, B 🔾, A, B 🔾
    (Ex:) **For S42.399[A]:** See PDX Collection 1251
         For S42.399[B]: See PDX Collection 1246
         For S42.399[K,P]: See PDX Collection 897

● **S42.4** Fracture of lower end of humerus
  Fracture of distal end of humerus

  Excludes2   fracture of shaft of humerus (S42.3-)
                  physeal fracture of lower end of humerus
                  (S49.1-)

● **S42.40** Unspecified fracture of lower end of humerus
  Fracture of elbow NOS
  ● S42.401 Unspecified fracture of lower end of right humerus A, K, P 🔾, B 🔾, A, B 🔾
    (Ex:) **For S42.401[A]:** See PDX Collection 1245
         For S42.401[B]: See PDX Collection 1246
         For S42.401[K,P]: See PDX Collection 897
  ● S42.402 Unspecified fracture of lower end of left humerus A, K, P 🔾, B 🔾, A, B 🔾
    (Ex:) **For S42.402[A]:** See PDX Collection 1247
         For S42.402[B]: See PDX Collection 1246
         For S42.402[K,P]: See PDX Collection 897
  ● S42.409 Unspecified fracture of lower end of unspecified humerus A, K, P 🔾, B 🔾, A, B 🔾
    (Ex:) **For S42.409[A]:** See PDX Collection 1248
         For S42.409[B]: See PDX Collection 1246
         For S42.409[K,P]: See PDX Collection 897

● **S42.41** Simple supracondylar fracture without intercondylar fracture of humerus
  ● S42.411 Displaced simple supracondylar fracture without intercondylar fracture of right humerus A, K, P 🔾, B 🔾, A, B 🔾
    (Ex:) **For S42.411[A]:** See PDX Collection 1245
         For S42.411[B]: See PDX Collection 1246
         For S42.411[K,P]: See PDX Collection 897
  ● S42.412 Displaced simple supracondylar fracture without intercondylar fracture of left humerus A, K, P 🔾, B 🔾, A, B 🔾
    (Ex:) **For S42.412[A]:** See PDX Collection 1247
         For S42.412[B]: See PDX Collection 1246
         For S42.412[K,P]: See PDX Collection 897
  ● S42.413 Displaced simple supracondylar fracture without intercondylar fracture of unspecified humerus A, K, P 🔾, B 🔾, A, B 🔾
    (Ex:) **For S42.413[A]:** See PDX Collection 1248
         For S42.413[B]: See PDX Collection 1246
         For S42.413[K,P]: See PDX Collection 897

● S42.414 Nondisplaced simple supracondylar fracture without intercondylar fracture of right humerus A, K, P 🔾, B 🔾, A, B 🔾
    (Ex:) **For S42.414[A]:** See PDX Collection 1245
         For S42.414[B]: See PDX Collection 1246
         For S42.414[K,P]: See PDX Collection 897
● S42.415 Nondisplaced simple supracondylar fracture without intercondylar fracture of left humerus A, K, P 🔾, B 🔾, A, B 🔾
    (Ex:) **For S42.415[A]:** See PDX Collection 1247
         For S42.415[B]: See PDX Collection 1246
         For S42.415[K,P]: See PDX Collection 897
● S42.416 Nondisplaced simple supracondylar fracture without intercondylar fracture of unspecified humerus A, K, P 🔾, B 🔾, A, B 🔾
    (Ex:) **For S42.416[A]:** See PDX Collection 1248
         For S42.416[B]: See PDX Collection 1246
         For S42.416[K,P]: See PDX Collection 897

● **S42.42** Comminuted supracondylar fracture without intercondylar fracture of humerus
  ● S42.421 Displaced comminuted supracondylar fracture without intercondylar fracture of right humerus A, K, P 🔾, B 🔾, A, B 🔾
    (Ex:) **For S42.421[A]:** See PDX Collection 1245
         For S42.421[B]: See PDX Collection 1246
         For S42.421[K,P]: See PDX Collection 897
  ● S42.422 Displaced comminuted supracondylar fracture without intercondylar fracture of left humerus A, K, P 🔾, B 🔾, A, B 🔾
    (Ex:) **For S42.422[A]:** See PDX Collection 1247
         For S42.422[B]: See PDX Collection 1246
         For S42.422[K,P]: See PDX Collection 897
  ● S42.423 Displaced comminuted supracondylar fracture without intercondylar fracture of unspecified humerus A, K, P 🔾, B 🔾, A, B 🔾
    (Ex:) **For S42.423[A]:** See PDX Collection 1248
         For S42.423[B]: See PDX Collection 1246
         For S42.423[K,P]: See PDX Collection 897
  ● S42.424 Nondisplaced comminuted supracondylar fracture without intercondylar fracture of right humerus A, K, P 🔾, B 🔾, A, B 🔾
    (Ex:) **For S42.424[A]:** See PDX Collection 1245
         For S42.424[B]: See PDX Collection 1246
         For S42.424[K,P]: See PDX Collection 897
  ● S42.425 Nondisplaced comminuted supracondylar fracture without intercondylar fracture of left humerus A, K, P 🔾, B 🔾, A, B 🔾
    (Ex:) **For S42.425[A]:** See PDX Collection 1247
         For S42.425[B]: See PDX Collection 1246
         For S42.425[K,P]: See PDX Collection 897
  ● S42.426 Nondisplaced comminuted supracondylar fracture without intercondylar fracture of unspecified humerus A, K, P 🔾, B 🔾, A, B 🔾
    (Ex:) **For S42.426[A]:** See PDX Collection 1248
         For S42.426[B]: See PDX Collection 1246
         For S42.426[K,P]: See PDX Collection 897

CHAPTER 19 (S00-T88)

N Newborn Age: 0   P Pediatric Age: 0–17   M Maternity DX: 9–64   A Adult Age: 15–124   ♀ Females Only   ♂ Males Only

🔾 Complication\Comorbidity   🔾 Major C\C   (Ex:) CC/MCC Exclusions   🔾 Hospital-Acquired Condition   🔾 Hierarchical Condition Category

1309

CHAPTER 19 (S00-T88)

● **S42.43** Fracture (avulsion) of lateral epicondyle of humerus
- ● **S42.431** Displaced fracture (avulsion) of lateral epicondyle of right humerus A, K, P 🪙, B 🪙, A, B 🪙
  - Ex: For S42.431[A]: See PDX Collection 1245
    For S42.431[B]: See PDX Collection 1246
    For S42.431[K,P]: See PDX Collection 897
- ● **S42.432** Displaced fracture (avulsion) of lateral epicondyle of left humerus A, K, P 🪙, B 🪙, A, B 🪙
  - Ex: For S42.432[A]: See PDX Collection 1247
    For S42.432[B]: See PDX Collection 1246
    For S42.432[K,P]: See PDX Collection 897
- ● **S42.433** Displaced fracture (avulsion) of lateral epicondyle of unspecified humerus A, K, P 🪙, B 🪙, A, B 🪙
  - Ex: For S42.433[A]: See PDX Collection 1248
    For S42.433[B]: See PDX Collection 1246
    For S42.433[K,P]: See PDX Collection 897
- ● **S42.434** Nondisplaced fracture (avulsion) of lateral epicondyle of right humerus A, K, P 🪙, B 🪙, A, B 🪙
  - Ex: For S42.434[A]: See PDX Collection 1245
    For S42.434[B]: See PDX Collection 1246
    For S42.434[K,P]: See PDX Collection 897
- ● **S42.435** Nondisplaced fracture (avulsion) of lateral epicondyle of left humerus A, K, P 🪙, B 🪙, A, B 🪙
  - Ex: For S42.435[A]: See PDX Collection 1247
    For S42.435[B]: See PDX Collection 1246
    For S42.435[K,P]: See PDX Collection 897
- ● **S42.436** Nondisplaced fracture (avulsion) of lateral epicondyle of unspecified humerus A, K, P 🪙, B 🪙, A, B 🪙
  - Ex: For S42.436[A]: See PDX Collection 1248
    For S42.436[B]: See PDX Collection 1246
    For S42.436[K,P]: See PDX Collection 897

● **S42.44** Fracture (avulsion) of medial epicondyle of humerus
- ● **S42.441** Displaced fracture (avulsion) of medial epicondyle of right humerus A, K, P 🪙, B 🪙, A, B 🪙
  - Ex: For S42.441[A]: See PDX Collection 1245
    For S42.441[B]: See PDX Collection 1246
    For S42.441[K,P]: See PDX Collection 897
- ● **S42.442** Displaced fracture (avulsion) of medial epicondyle of left humerus A, K, P 🪙, B 🪙, A, B 🪙
  - Ex: For S42.442[A]: See PDX Collection 1247
    For S42.442[B]: See PDX Collection 1246
    For S42.442[K,P]: See PDX Collection 897
- ● **S42.443** Displaced fracture (avulsion) of medial epicondyle of unspecified humerus A, K, P 🪙, B 🪙, A, B 🪙
  - Ex: For S42.443[A]: See PDX Collection 1248
    For S42.443[B]: See PDX Collection 1246
    For S42.443[K,P]: See PDX Collection 897
- ● **S42.444** Nondisplaced fracture (avulsion) of medial epicondyle of right humerus A, K, P 🪙, B 🪙, A, B 🪙
  - Ex: For S42.444[A]: See PDX Collection 1245
    For S42.444[B]: See PDX Collection 1246
    For S42.444[K,P]: See PDX Collection 897

- ● **S42.445** Nondisplaced fracture (avulsion) of medial epicondyle of left humerus A, K, P 🪙, B 🪙, A, B 🪙
  - Ex: For S42.445[A]: See PDX Collection 1247
    For S42.445[B]: See PDX Collection 1246
    For S42.445[K,P]: See PDX Collection 897
- ● **S42.446** Nondisplaced fracture (avulsion) of medial epicondyle of unspecified humerus A, K, P 🪙, B 🪙, A, B 🪙
  - Ex: For S42.446[A]: See PDX Collection 1248
    For S42.446[B]: See PDX Collection 1246
    For S42.446[K,P]: See PDX Collection 897
- ● **S42.447** Incarcerated fracture (avulsion) of medial epicondyle of right humerus A, K, P 🪙, B 🪙, A, B 🪙
  - Ex: For S42.447[A]: See PDX Collection 1245
    For S42.447[B]: See PDX Collection 1246
    For S42.447[K,P]: See PDX Collection 897
- ● **S42.448** Incarcerated fracture (avulsion) of medial epicondyle of left humerus A, K, P 🪙, B 🪙, A, B 🪙
  - Ex: For S42.448[A]: See PDX Collection 1247
    For S42.448[B]: See PDX Collection 1246
    For S42.448[K,P]: See PDX Collection 897
- ● **S42.449** Incarcerated fracture (avulsion) of medial epicondyle of unspecified humerus A, K, P 🪙, B 🪙, A, B 🪙
  - Ex: For S42.449[A]: See PDX Collection 1248
    For S42.449[B]: See PDX Collection 1246
    For S42.449[K,P]: See PDX Collection 897

● **S42.45** Fracture of lateral condyle of humerus
Fracture of capitellum of humerus
- ● **S42.451** Displaced fracture of lateral condyle of right humerus A, K, P 🪙, B 🪙, A, B 🪙
  - Ex: For S42.451[A]: See PDX Collection 1245
    For S42.451[B]: See PDX Collection 1246
    For S42.451[K,P]: See PDX Collection 897
- ● **S42.452** Displaced fracture of lateral condyle of left humerus A, K, P 🪙, B 🪙, A, B 🪙
  - Ex: For S42.452[A]: See PDX Collection 1247
    For S42.452[B]: See PDX Collection 1246
    For S42.452[K,P]: See PDX Collection 897
- ● **S42.453** Displaced fracture of lateral condyle of unspecified humerus A, K, P 🪙, B 🪙, A, B 🪙
  - Ex: For S42.453[A]: See PDX Collection 1248
    For S42.453[B]: See PDX Collection 1246
    For S42.453[K,P]: See PDX Collection 897
- ● **S42.454** Nondisplaced fracture of lateral condyle of right humerus A, K, P 🪙, B 🪙, A, B 🪙
  - Ex: For S42.454[A]: See PDX Collection 1245
    For S42.454[B]: See PDX Collection 1246
    For S42.454[K,P]: See PDX Collection 897
- ● **S42.455** Nondisplaced fracture of lateral condyle of left humerus A, K, P 🪙, B 🪙, A, B 🪙
  - Ex: For S42.455[A]: See PDX Collection 1247
    For S42.455[B]: See PDX Collection 1246
    For S42.455[K,P]: See PDX Collection 897
- ● **S42.456** Nondisplaced fracture of lateral condyle of unspecified humerus A, K, P 🪙, B 🪙, A, B 🪙
  - Ex: For S42.456[A]: See PDX Collection 1248
    For S42.456[B]: See PDX Collection 1246
    For S42.456[K,P]: See PDX Collection 897

▶ New ⇒ Revised ~~deleted~~ Deleted Excludes 1 Excludes 2 Includes Use additional Code first Code also Key words
OGCR Official Guidelines ● Unacceptable Principal Diagnosis X Assign placeholder X ● Use Additional Character(s) ▷ Manifestation Code **Coding Clinic**

● **S42.46**   Fracture of medial condyle of humerus
     Trochlea fracture of humerus

   ● **S42.461**   **Displaced fracture of medial condyle of right humerus** A, K, P 🅒, B 🅒, A, B 🅒
       Ⓔ For S42.461[A]: See PDX Collection 1245
         For S42.461[B]: See PDX Collection 1246
         For S42.461[K,P]: See PDX Collection 897

   ● **S42.462**   **Displaced fracture of medial condyle of left humerus** A, K, P 🅒, B 🅒, A, B 🅒
       Ⓔ For S42.462[A]: See PDX Collection 1247
         For S42.462[B]: See PDX Collection 1246
         For S42.462[K,P]: See PDX Collection 897

   ● **S42.463**   **Displaced fracture of medial condyle of unspecified humerus** A, K, P 🅒, B 🅒, A, B 🅒
       Ⓔ For S42.463[A]: See PDX Collection 1248
         For S42.463[B]: See PDX Collection 1246
         For S42.463[K,P]: See PDX Collection 897

   ● **S42.464**   **Nondisplaced fracture of medial condyle of right humerus** A, K, P 🅒, B 🅒, A, B 🅒
       Ⓔ For S42.464[A]: See PDX Collection 1245
         For S42.464[B]: See PDX Collection 1246
         For S42.464[K,P]: See PDX Collection 897

   ● **S42.465**   **Nondisplaced fracture of medial condyle of left humerus** A, K, P 🅒, B 🅒, A, B 🅒
       Ⓔ For S42.465[A]: See PDX Collection 1247
         For S42.465[B]: See PDX Collection 1246
         For S42.465[K,P]: See PDX Collection 897

   ● **S42.466**   **Nondisplaced fracture of medial condyle of unspecified humerus** A, K, P 🅒, B 🅒, A, B 🅒
       Ⓔ For S42.466[A]: See PDX Collection 1248
         For S42.466[B]: See PDX Collection 1246
         For S42.466[K,P]: See PDX Collection 897

● **S42.47**   Transcondylar fracture of humerus

   ● **S42.471**   **Displaced transcondylar fracture of right humerus** A, K, P 🅒, B 🅒, A, B 🅒
       Ⓔ For S42.471[A]: See PDX Collection 1245
         For S42.471[B]: See PDX Collection 1246
         For S42.471[K,P]: See PDX Collection 897

   ● **S42.472**   **Displaced transcondylar fracture of left humerus** A, K, P 🅒, B 🅒, A, B 🅒
       Ⓔ For S42.472[A]: See PDX Collection 1247
         For S42.472[B]: See PDX Collection 1246
         For S42.472[K,P]: See PDX Collection 897

   ● **S42.473**   **Displaced transcondylar fracture of unspecified humerus** A, K, P 🅒, B 🅒, A, B 🅒
       Ⓔ For S42.473[A]: See PDX Collection 1248
         For S42.473[B]: See PDX Collection 1246
         For S42.473[K,P]: See PDX Collection 897

   ● **S42.474**   **Nondisplaced transcondylar fracture of right humerus** A, K, P 🅒, B 🅒, A, B 🅒
       Ⓔ For S42.474[A]: See PDX Collection 1245
         For S42.474[B]: See PDX Collection 1246
         For S42.474[K,P]: See PDX Collection 897

   ● **S42.475**   **Nondisplaced transcondylar fracture of left humerus** A, K, P 🅒, B 🅒, A, B 🅒
       Ⓔ For S42.475[A]: See PDX Collection 1247
         For S42.475[B]: See PDX Collection 1246
         For S42.475[K,P]: See PDX Collection 897

   ● **S42.476**   **Nondisplaced transcondylar fracture of unspecified humerus** A, K, P 🅒, B 🅒, A, B 🅒
       Ⓔ For S42.476[A]: See PDX Collection 1248
         For S42.476[B]: See PDX Collection 1246
         For S42.476[K,P]: See PDX Collection 897

● **S42.48**   Torus fracture of lower end of humerus
     The appropriate 7th character is to be added to all codes in subcategory S42.48

> A   initial encounter for closed fracture
> D   subsequent encounter for fracture with routine healing
> G   subsequent encounter for fracture with delayed healing
> K   subsequent encounter for fracture with nonunion
> P   subsequent encounter for fracture with malunion
> S   sequela

   ● **S42.481**   **Torus fracture of lower end of right humerus** A, K, P 🅒, A 🅒
       Ⓔ For S42.481[A]: See PDX Collection 1245
         For S42.481[K,P]: See PDX Collection 897

   ● **S42.482**   **Torus fracture of lower end of left humerus** A, K, P 🅒, A 🅒
       Ⓔ For S42.482[A]: See PDX Collection 1247
         For S42.482[K,P]: See PDX Collection 897

   ● **S42.489**   **Torus fracture of lower end of unspecified humerus** A, K, P 🅒, A 🅒
       Ⓔ For S42.489[A]: See PDX Collection 1248
         For S42.489[K,P]: See PDX Collection 897

● **S42.49**   Other fracture of lower end of humerus

   ● **S42.491**   **Other displaced fracture of lower end of right humerus** A, K, P 🅒, B 🅒, A, B 🅒
       Ⓔ For S42.491[A]: See PDX Collection 1245
         For S42.491[B]: See PDX Collection 1246
         For S42.491[K,P]: See PDX Collection 897

   ● **S42.492**   **Other displaced fracture of lower end of left humerus** A, K, P 🅒, B 🅒, A, B 🅒
       Ⓔ For S42.492[A]: See PDX Collection 1247
         For S42.492[B]: See PDX Collection 1246
         For S42.492[K,P]: See PDX Collection 897

   ● **S42.493**   **Other displaced fracture of lower end of unspecified humerus** A, K, P 🅒, B 🅒, A, B 🅒
       Ⓔ For S42.493[A]: See PDX Collection 1248
         For S42.493[B]: See PDX Collection 1246
         For S42.493[K,P]: See PDX Collection 897

   ● **S42.494**   **Other nondisplaced fracture of lower end of right humerus** A, K, P 🅒, B 🅒, A, B 🅒
       Ⓔ For S42.494[A]: See PDX Collection 1245
         For S42.494[B]: See PDX Collection 1246
         For S42.494[K,P]: See PDX Collection 897

   ● **S42.495**   **Other nondisplaced fracture of lower end of left humerus** A, K, P 🅒, B 🅒, A, B 🅒
       Ⓔ For S42.495[A]: See PDX Collection 1247
         For S42.495[B]: See PDX Collection 1246
         For S42.495[K,P]: See PDX Collection 897

   ● **S42.496**   **Other nondisplaced fracture of lower end of unspecified humerus** A, K, P 🅒, B 🅒, A, B 🅒
       Ⓔ For S42.496[A]: See PDX Collection 1248
         For S42.496[B]: See PDX Collection 1246
         For S42.496[K,P]: See PDX Collection 897

● **S42.9**   Fracture of shoulder girdle, part unspecified
     Fracture of shoulder NOS
     Ⓔ For category S42.9 CC codes S42.9[A]: See PDX Collection 1248
     For S42.9[B]: See PDX Collection 1246 For S42.9[K,P]: See PDX Collection 897

   X● **S42.90**   **Fracture of unspecified shoulder girdle, part unspecified** A, K, P 🅒, B 🅒, A, B 🅒

   X● **S42.91**   **Fracture of right shoulder girdle, part unspecified** A, K, P 🅒, B 🅒, A, B 🅒

   X● **S42.92**   **Fracture of left shoulder girdle, part unspecified** A, K, P 🅒, B 🅒, A, B 🅒

CHAPTER 19 (S00-T88)

● **S43   Dislocation and sprain of joints and ligaments of shoulder girdle**

> **Includes**   avulsion of joint or ligament of shoulder girdle
> laceration of cartilage, joint or ligament of shoulder girdle
> sprain of cartilage, joint or ligament of shoulder girdle
> traumatic hemarthrosis of joint or ligament of shoulder girdle
> traumatic rupture of joint or ligament of shoulder girdle
> traumatic subluxation of joint or ligament of shoulder girdle
> traumatic tear of joint or ligament of shoulder girdle

Code also any associated open wound

> **Excludes2**   strain of muscle, fascia and tendon of shoulder and upper arm (S46.-)

The appropriate 7th character is to be added to each code from category S43

A	initial encounter
D	subsequent encounter
S	sequela

● **S43.0   Subluxation and dislocation of shoulder joint**
> Dislocation of glenohumeral joint
> Subluxation of glenohumeral joint

   ● **S43.00   Unspecified subluxation and dislocation of shoulder joint**
> Dislocation of humerus NOS
> Subluxation of humerus NOS

     ● S43.001   Unspecified subluxation of right shoulder joint
     ● S43.002   Unspecified subluxation of left shoulder joint
     ● S43.003   Unspecified subluxation of unspecified shoulder joint
     ● S43.004   Unspecified dislocation of right shoulder joint
     ● S43.005   Unspecified dislocation of left shoulder joint
     ● S43.006   Unspecified dislocation of unspecified shoulder joint

   ● **S43.01   Anterior subluxation and dislocation of humerus**
     ● S43.011   Anterior subluxation of right humerus
     ● S43.012   Anterior subluxation of left humerus
     ● S43.013   Anterior subluxation of unspecified humerus
     ● S43.014   Anterior dislocation of right humerus
     ● S43.015   Anterior dislocation of left humerus
     ● S43.016   Anterior dislocation of unspecified humerus

   ● **S43.02   Posterior subluxation and dislocation of humerus**
     ● S43.021   Posterior subluxation of right humerus
     ● S43.022   Posterior subluxation of left humerus
     ● S43.023   Posterior subluxation of unspecified humerus
     ● S43.024   Posterior dislocation of right humerus
     ● S43.025   Posterior dislocation of left humerus
     ● S43.026   Posterior dislocation of unspecified humerus

   ● **S43.03   Inferior subluxation and dislocation of humerus**
     ● S43.031   Inferior subluxation of right humerus
     ● S43.032   Inferior subluxation of left humerus
     ● S43.033   Inferior subluxation of unspecified humerus
     ● S43.034   Inferior dislocation of right humerus
     ● S43.035   Inferior dislocation of left humerus
     ● S43.036   Inferior dislocation of unspecified humerus

   ● **S43.08   Other subluxation and dislocation of shoulder joint**
     ● S43.081   Other subluxation of right shoulder joint
     ● S43.082   Other subluxation of left shoulder joint
     ● S43.083   Other subluxation of unspecified shoulder joint
     ● S43.084   Other dislocation of right shoulder joint
     ● S43.085   Other dislocation of left shoulder joint
     ● S43.086   Other dislocation of unspecified shoulder joint

● **S43.1   Subluxation and dislocation of acromioclavicular joint**

   ● **S43.10   Unspecified dislocation of acromioclavicular joint**
     ● S43.101   Unspecified dislocation of right acromioclavicular joint
     ● S43.102   Unspecified dislocation of left acromioclavicular joint
     ● S43.109   Unspecified dislocation of unspecified acromioclavicular joint

   ● **S43.11   Subluxation of acromioclavicular joint**
     ● S43.111   Subluxation of right acromioclavicular joint
     ● S43.112   Subluxation of left acromioclavicular joint
     ● S43.119   Subluxation of unspecified acromioclavicular joint

   ● **S43.12   Dislocation of acromioclavicular joint, 100%-200% displacement**
     ● S43.121   Dislocation of right acromioclavicular joint, 100%-200% displacement
     ● S43.122   Dislocation of left acromioclavicular joint, 100%-200% displacement
     ● S43.129   Dislocation of unspecified acromioclavicular joint, 100%-200% displacement

   ● **S43.13   Dislocation of acromioclavicular joint, greater than 200% displacement**
     ● S43.131   Dislocation of right acromioclavicular joint, greater than 200% displacement
     ● S43.132   Dislocation of left acromioclavicular joint, greater than 200% displacement
     ● S43.139   Dislocation of unspecified acromioclavicular joint, greater than 200% displacement

   ● **S43.14   Inferior dislocation of acromioclavicular joint**
     ● S43.141   Inferior dislocation of right acromioclavicular joint
     ● S43.142   Inferior dislocation of left acromioclavicular joint
     ● S43.149   Inferior dislocation of unspecified acromioclavicular joint

▶ New   ⇒ Revised   ~~deleted~~ Deleted   Excludes 1   Excludes 2   Includes   Use additional   Code first   Code also   Key words
OGCR Official Guidelines   ● Unacceptable Principal Diagnosis   X Assign placeholder X   ● Use Additional Character(s)   ▶ Manifestation Code   **Coding Clinic**

● S43.15   Posterior dislocation of acromioclavicular joint
  ● S43.151   Posterior dislocation of right acromioclavicular joint
  ● S43.152   Posterior dislocation of left acromioclavicular joint
  ● S43.159   Posterior dislocation of unspecified acromioclavicular joint
● S43.2   Subluxation and dislocation of sternoclavicular joint
  ● S43.20   Unspecified subluxation and dislocation of sternoclavicular joint
    ● S43.201   Unspecified subluxation of right sternoclavicular joint A 🅒, A 🅗
       (Ex:) See PDX Collection 1252
    ● S43.202   Unspecified subluxation of left sternoclavicular joint A 🅒, A 🅗
       (Ex:) See PDX Collection 1253
    ● S43.203   Unspecified subluxation of unspecified sternoclavicular joint A 🅒, A 🅗
       (Ex:) See PDX Collection 914
    ● S43.204   Unspecified dislocation of right sternoclavicular joint A 🅒, A 🅗
       (Ex:) See PDX Collection 1252
    ● S43.205   Unspecified dislocation of left sternoclavicular joint A 🅒, A 🅗
       (Ex:) See PDX Collection 1253
    ● S43.206   Unspecified dislocation of unspecified sternoclavicular joint A 🅒, A 🅗
       (Ex:) See PDX Collection 914
  ● S43.21   Anterior subluxation and dislocation of sternoclavicular joint
    ● S43.211   Anterior subluxation of right sternoclavicular joint A 🅒, A 🅗
       (Ex:) See PDX Collection 1252
    ● S43.212   Anterior subluxation of left sternoclavicular joint A 🅒, A 🅗
       (Ex:) See PDX Collection 1253
    ● S43.213   Anterior subluxation of unspecified sternoclavicular joint A 🅒, A 🅗
       (Ex:) See PDX Collection 914
    ● S43.214   Anterior dislocation of right sternoclavicular joint A 🅒, A 🅗
       (Ex:) See PDX Collection 1252
    ● S43.215   Anterior dislocation of left sternoclavicular joint A 🅒, A 🅗
       (Ex:) See PDX Collection 1253
    ● S43.216   Anterior dislocation of unspecified sternoclavicular joint A 🅒, A 🅗
       (Ex:) See PDX Collection 914
  ● S43.22   Posterior subluxation and dislocation of sternoclavicular joint
    ● S43.221   Posterior subluxation of right sternoclavicular joint A 🅒, A 🅗
       (Ex:) See PDX Collection 1252
    ● S43.222   Posterior subluxation of left sternoclavicular joint A 🅒, A 🅗
       (Ex:) See PDX Collection 1253
    ● S43.223   Posterior subluxation of unspecified sternoclavicular joint A 🅒, A 🅗
       (Ex:) See PDX Collection 914
    ● S43.224   Posterior dislocation of right sternoclavicular joint A 🅒, A 🅗
       (Ex:) See PDX Collection 1252
    ● S43.225   Posterior dislocation of left sternoclavicular joint A 🅒, A 🅗
       (Ex:) See PDX Collection 1253
    ● S43.226   Posterior dislocation of unspecified sternoclavicular joint A 🅒, A 🅗
       (Ex:) See PDX Collection 914

● S43.3   Subluxation and dislocation of other and unspecified parts of shoulder girdle
  ● S43.30   Subluxation and dislocation of unspecified parts of shoulder girdle
     Dislocation of shoulder girdle NOS
     Subluxation of shoulder girdle NOS
    ● S43.301   Subluxation of unspecified parts of right shoulder girdle
    ● S43.302   Subluxation of unspecified parts of left shoulder girdle
    ● S43.303   Subluxation of unspecified parts of unspecified shoulder girdle
    ● S43.304   Dislocation of unspecified parts of right shoulder girdle
    ● S43.305   Dislocation of unspecified parts of left shoulder girdle
    ● S43.306   Dislocation of unspecified parts of unspecified shoulder girdle
  ● S43.31   Subluxation and dislocation of scapula
    ● S43.311   Subluxation of right scapula
    ● S43.312   Subluxation of left scapula
    ● S43.313   Subluxation of unspecified scapula
    ● S43.314   Dislocation of right scapula
    ● S43.315   Dislocation of left scapula
    ● S43.316   Dislocation of unspecified scapula
  ● S43.39   Subluxation and dislocation of other parts of shoulder girdle
    ● S43.391   Subluxation of other parts of right shoulder girdle
    ● S43.392   Subluxation of other parts of left shoulder girdle
    ● S43.393   Subluxation of other parts of unspecified shoulder girdle
    ● S43.394   Dislocation of other parts of right shoulder girdle
    ● S43.395   Dislocation of other parts of left shoulder girdle
    ● S43.396   Dislocation of other parts of unspecified shoulder girdle
● S43.4   Sprain of shoulder joint
  ● S43.40   Unspecified sprain of shoulder joint
    ● S43.401   Unspecified sprain of right shoulder joint
    ● S43.402   Unspecified sprain of left shoulder joint
    ● S43.409   Unspecified sprain of unspecified shoulder joint
  ● S43.41   Sprain of coracohumeral (ligament)
    ● S43.411   Sprain of right coracohumeral (ligament)
    ● S43.412   Sprain of left coracohumeral (ligament)
    ● S43.419   Sprain of unspecified coracohumeral (ligament)
  ● S43.42   Sprain of rotator cuff capsule
     Encounters during the healing phase

     Excludes1   rotator cuff syndrome (complete) (incomplete), not specified as traumatic (M75.1-)

     Excludes2   injury of tendon of rotator cuff (S46.0-)
    ● S43.421   Sprain of right rotator cuff capsule
    ● S43.422   Sprain of left rotator cuff capsule
    ● S43.429   Sprain of unspecified rotator cuff capsule

CHAPTER 19 (S00-T88)

N Newborn Age: 0   **P** Pediatric Age: 0–17   **M** Maternity DX: 9–64   **A** Adult Age: 15–124   ♀ Females Only   ♂ Males Only

🅒 Complication\Comorbidity   🅜 Major C\C   (Ex:) CC/MCC Exclusions   🅗 Hospital-Acquired Condition   🅗 Hierarchical Condition Category

1313

CHAPTER 19 (S00-T88)

● **S43.43**   **Superior glenoid labrum lesion**
       SLAP lesion
       Coding Clinic: 2019, Q2, P27

     ● **S43.431**   Superior glenoid labrum lesion of right shoulder

     ● **S43.432**   Superior glenoid labrum lesion of left shoulder

     ● **S43.439**   Superior glenoid labrum lesion of unspecified shoulder

● **S43.49**   Other sprain of shoulder joint

     ● **S43.491**   Other sprain of right shoulder joint

     ● **S43.492**   Other sprain of left shoulder joint

     ● **S43.499**   Other sprain of unspecified shoulder joint

● **S43.5**   Sprain of acromioclavicular joint
       Sprain of acromioclavicular ligament

   X ● **S43.50**   Sprain of unspecified acromioclavicular joint

   X ● **S43.51**   Sprain of right acromioclavicular joint

   X ● **S43.52**   Sprain of left acromioclavicular joint

● **S43.6**   Sprain of sternoclavicular joint

   X ● **S43.60**   Sprain of unspecified sternoclavicular joint

   X ● **S43.61**   Sprain of right sternoclavicular joint

   X ● **S43.62**   Sprain of left sternoclavicular joint

● **S43.8**   Sprain of other specified parts of shoulder girdle

   X ● **S43.80**   Sprain of other specified parts of unspecified shoulder girdle

   X ● **S43.81**   Sprain of other specified parts of right shoulder girdle

   X ● **S43.82**   Sprain of other specified parts of left shoulder girdle

● **S43.9**   Sprain of unspecified parts of shoulder girdle

   X ● **S43.90**   Sprain of unspecified parts of unspecified shoulder girdle
         Sprain of shoulder girdle NOS

   X ● **S43.91**   Sprain of unspecified parts of right shoulder girdle

   X ● **S43.92**   Sprain of unspecified parts of left shoulder girdle

● **S44**   **Injury of nerves at shoulder and upper arm level**
       Code also any associated open wound (S41.-)

     Excludes2   injury of brachial plexus (S14.3-)

     The appropriate 7th character is to be added to each code from category S44

A	initial encounter
D	subsequent encounter
S	sequela

● **S44.0**   **Injury of ulnar nerve at upper arm level**
     Excludes1   ulnar nerve NOS (S54.0)

   X ● **S44.00**   Injury of ulnar nerve at upper arm level, unspecified arm

   X ● **S44.01**   Injury of ulnar nerve at upper arm level, right arm

   X ● **S44.02**   Injury of ulnar nerve at upper arm level, left arm

● **S44.1**   **Injury of median nerve at upper arm level**
     Excludes1   median nerve NOS (S54.1)

   X ● **S44.10**   Injury of median nerve at upper arm level, unspecified arm

   X ● **S44.11**   Injury of median nerve at upper arm level, right arm

   X ● **S44.12**   Injury of median nerve at upper arm level, left arm

● **S44.2**   **Injury of radial nerve at upper arm level**
     Excludes1   radial nerve NOS (S54.2)

   X ● **S44.20**   Injury of radial nerve at upper arm level, unspecified arm

   X ● **S44.21**   Injury of radial nerve at upper arm level, right arm

   X ● **S44.22**   Injury of radial nerve at upper arm level, left arm

● **S44.3**   **Injury of axillary nerve**

   X ● **S44.30**   Injury of axillary nerve, unspecified arm

   X ● **S44.31**   Injury of axillary nerve, right arm

   X ● **S44.32**   Injury of axillary nerve, left arm

● **S44.4**   **Injury of musculocutaneous nerve**

   X ● **S44.40**   Injury of musculocutaneous nerve, unspecified arm

   X ● **S44.41**   Injury of musculocutaneous nerve, right arm

   X ● **S44.42**   Injury of musculocutaneous nerve, left arm

● **S44.5**   **Injury of cutaneous sensory nerve at shoulder and upper arm level**

   X ● **S44.50**   Injury of cutaneous sensory nerve at shoulder and upper arm level, unspecified arm

   X ● **S44.51**   Injury of cutaneous sensory nerve at shoulder and upper arm level, right arm

   X ● **S44.52**   Injury of cutaneous sensory nerve at shoulder and upper arm level, left arm

● **S44.8**   **Injury of other nerves at shoulder and upper arm level**

   ● **S44.8X**   Injury of other nerves at shoulder and upper arm level

     ● **S44.8X1**   Injury of other nerves at shoulder and upper arm level, right arm

     ● **S44.8X2**   Injury of other nerves at shoulder and upper arm level, left arm

     ● **S44.8X9**   Injury of other nerves at shoulder and upper arm level, unspecified arm

● **S44.9**   **Injury of unspecified nerve at shoulder and upper arm level**

   X ● **S44.90**   Injury of unspecified nerve at shoulder and upper arm level, unspecified arm

   X ● **S44.91**   Injury of unspecified nerve at shoulder and upper arm level, right arm

   X ● **S44.92**   Injury of unspecified nerve at shoulder and upper arm level, left arm

● **S45**   **Injury of blood vessels at shoulder and upper arm level**
       Code also any associated open wound (S41.-)

     Excludes2   injury of subclavian artery (S25.1)
                 injury of subclavian vein (S25.3)

     The appropriate 7th character is to be added to each code from category S45

A	initial encounter
D	subsequent encounter
S	sequela

● **S45.0**   **Injury of axillary artery**

   ● **S45.00**   **Unspecified injury of axillary artery**

     ● **S45.001**   Unspecified injury of axillary artery, right side A
           (Ex) See PDX Collection 1254

     ● **S45.002**   Unspecified injury of axillary artery, left side A
           (Ex) See PDX Collection 1255

     ● **S45.009**   Unspecified injury of axillary artery, unspecified side A
           (Ex) See PDX Collection 1256

▶ New   ⇒ Revised   ~~deleted~~ Deleted   Excludes 1   Excludes 2   Includes   Use additional   Code first   Code also   Key words

OGCR Official Guidelines   ● Unacceptable Principal Diagnosis   X Assign placeholder X   ● Use Additional Character(s)   ▶ Manifestation Code   Coding Clinic

- S45.01   Laceration of axillary artery
  - S45.011   Laceration of axillary artery, right side A
    - Ex: See PDX Collection 1254
  - S45.012   Laceration of axillary artery, left side A
    - Ex: See PDX Collection 1255
  - S45.019   Laceration of axillary artery, unspecified side A
    - Ex: See PDX Collection 1256
- S45.09   Other specified injury of axillary artery
  - S45.091   Other specified injury of axillary artery, right side A
    - Ex: See PDX Collection 1254
  - S45.092   Other specified injury of axillary artery, left side A
    - Ex: See PDX Collection 1255
  - S45.099   Other specified injury of axillary artery, unspecified side A
    - Ex: See PDX Collection 1256
- S45.1   Injury of brachial artery
  - S45.10   Unspecified injury of brachial artery
    - S45.101   Unspecified injury of brachial artery, right side A
      - Ex: See PDX Collection 1257
    - S45.102   Unspecified injury of brachial artery, left side A
      - Ex: See PDX Collection 1258
    - S45.109   Unspecified injury of brachial artery, unspecified side A
      - Ex: See PDX Collection 1259
  - S45.11   Laceration of brachial artery
    - S45.111   Laceration of brachial artery, right side A
      - Ex: See PDX Collection 1257
    - S45.112   Laceration of brachial artery, left side A
      - Ex: See PDX Collection 1258
    - S45.119   Laceration of brachial artery, unspecified side A
      - Ex: See PDX Collection 1259
  - S45.19   Other specified injury of brachial artery
    - S45.191   Other specified injury of brachial artery, right side A
      - Ex: See PDX Collection 1257
    - S45.192   Other specified injury of brachial artery, left side A
      - Ex: See PDX Collection 1258
    - S45.199   Other specified injury of brachial artery, unspecified side A
      - Ex: See PDX Collection 1259
- S45.2   Injury of axillary or brachial vein
  - S45.20   Unspecified injury of axillary or brachial vein
    - S45.201   Unspecified injury of axillary or brachial vein, right side A
      - Ex: See PDX Collection 1257
    - S45.202   Unspecified injury of axillary or brachial vein, left side A
      - Ex: See PDX Collection 1258
    - S45.209   Unspecified injury of axillary or brachial vein, unspecified side A
      - Ex: See PDX Collection 1259
  - S45.21   Laceration of axillary or brachial vein
    - S45.211   Laceration of axillary or brachial vein, right side A
      - Ex: See PDX Collection 1257
    - S45.212   Laceration of axillary or brachial vein, left side A
      - Ex: See PDX Collection 1258
    - S45.219   Laceration of axillary or brachial vein, unspecified side A
      - Ex: See PDX Collection 1259

- S45.29   Other specified injury of axillary or brachial vein
  - S45.291   Other specified injury of axillary or brachial vein, right side A
    - Ex: See PDX Collection 1257
  - S45.292   Other specified injury of axillary or brachial vein, left side A
    - Ex: See PDX Collection 1258
  - S45.299   Other specified injury of axillary or brachial vein, unspecified side A
    - Ex: See PDX Collection 1259
- S45.3   Injury of superficial vein at shoulder and upper arm level
  - S45.30   Unspecified injury of superficial vein at shoulder and upper arm level
    - S45.301   Unspecified injury of superficial vein at shoulder and upper arm level, right arm A
      - Ex: See PDX Collection 1260
    - S45.302   Unspecified injury of superficial vein at shoulder and upper arm level, left arm A
      - Ex: See PDX Collection 1261
    - S45.309   Unspecified injury of superficial vein at shoulder and upper arm level, unspecified arm A
      - Ex: See PDX Collection 1262
  - S45.31   Laceration of superficial vein at shoulder and upper arm level
    - S45.311   Laceration of superficial vein at shoulder and upper arm level, right arm A
      - Ex: See PDX Collection 1260
    - S45.312   Laceration of superficial vein at shoulder and upper arm level, left arm A
      - Ex: See PDX Collection 1261
    - S45.319   Laceration of superficial vein at shoulder and upper arm level, unspecified arm A
      - Ex: See PDX Collection 1262
  - S45.39   Other specified injury of superficial vein at shoulder and upper arm level
    - S45.391   Other specified injury of superficial vein at shoulder and upper arm level, right arm A
      - Ex: See PDX Collection 1260
    - S45.392   Other specified injury of superficial vein at shoulder and upper arm level, left arm A
      - Ex: See PDX Collection 1261
    - S45.399   Other specified injury of superficial vein at shoulder and upper arm level, unspecified arm A
      - Ex: See PDX Collection 1262
- S45.8   Injury of other specified blood vessels at shoulder and upper arm level
  - S45.80   Unspecified injury of other specified blood vessels at shoulder and upper arm level
    - S45.801   Unspecified injury of other specified blood vessels at shoulder and upper arm level, right arm A
      - Ex: See PDX Collection 1260
    - S45.802   Unspecified injury of other specified blood vessels at shoulder and upper arm level, left arm A
      - Ex: See PDX Collection 1261
    - S45.809   Unspecified injury of other specified blood vessels at shoulder and upper arm level, unspecified arm A
      - Ex: See PDX Collection 1262

N Newborn Age: 0   **P** Pediatric Age: 0–17   **M** Maternity DX: 9–64   **A** Adult Age: 15–124   ♀ Females Only   ♂ Males Only

Complication\Comorbidity   Major C\C   Ex: CC/MCC Exclusions   Hospital-Acquired Condition   Hierarchical Condition Category

1315

CHAPTER 19 (S00-T88)

● **S45.81** Laceration of other specified blood vessels at shoulder and upper arm level

  ● **S45.811** Laceration of other specified blood vessels at shoulder and upper arm level, right arm A 🔒
     Ex:) See PDX Collection 1260

  ● **S45.812** Laceration of other specified blood vessels at shoulder and upper arm level, left arm A 🔒
     Ex:) See PDX Collection 1261

  ● **S45.819** Laceration of other specified blood vessels at shoulder and upper arm level, unspecified arm A 🔒
     Ex:) See PDX Collection 1262

● **S45.89** Other specified injury of other specified blood vessels at shoulder and upper arm level

  ● **S45.891** Other specified injury of other specified blood vessels at shoulder and upper arm level, right arm A 🔒
     Ex:) See PDX Collection 1260

  ● **S45.892** Other specified injury of other specified blood vessels at shoulder and upper arm level, left arm A 🔒
     Ex:) See PDX Collection 1261

  ● **S45.899** Other specified injury of other specified blood vessels at shoulder and upper arm level, unspecified arm A 🔒
     Ex:) See PDX Collection 1262

● **S45.9** Injury of unspecified blood vessel at shoulder and upper arm level

  ● **S45.90** Unspecified injury of unspecified blood vessel at shoulder and upper arm level

    ● **S45.901** Unspecified injury of unspecified blood vessel at shoulder and upper arm level, right arm A 🔒
      Ex:) See PDX Collection 1260

    ● **S45.902** Unspecified injury of unspecified blood vessel at shoulder and upper arm level, left arm A 🔒
      Ex:) See PDX Collection 1261

    ● **S45.909** Unspecified injury of unspecified blood vessel at shoulder and upper arm level, unspecified arm A 🔒
      Ex:) See PDX Collection 1262

  ● **S45.91** Laceration of unspecified blood vessel at shoulder and upper arm level

    ● **S45.911** Laceration of unspecified blood vessel at shoulder and upper arm level, right arm A 🔒
      Ex:) See PDX Collection 1260

    ● **S45.912** Laceration of unspecified blood vessel at shoulder and upper arm level, left arm A 🔒
      Ex:) See PDX Collection 1261

    ● **S45.919** Laceration of unspecified blood vessel at shoulder and upper arm level, unspecified arm A 🔒
      Ex:) See PDX Collection 1262

  ● **S45.99** Other specified injury of unspecified blood vessel at shoulder and upper arm level

    ● **S45.991** Other specified injury of unspecified blood vessel at shoulder and upper arm level, right arm A 🔒
      Ex:) See PDX Collection 1260

    ● **S45.992** Other specified injury of unspecified blood vessel at shoulder and upper arm level, left arm A 🔒
      Ex:) See PDX Collection 1261

    ● **S45.999** Other specified injury of unspecified blood vessel at shoulder and upper arm level, unspecified arm A 🔒
      Ex:) See PDX Collection 1262

● **S46** Injury of muscle, fascia and tendon at shoulder and upper arm level

  Code also any associated open wound (S41.-)

  Excludes2 injury of muscle, fascia and tendon at elbow (S56.-)
      sprain of joints and ligaments of shoulder girdle (S43.9)

  The appropriate 7th character is to be added to each code from category S46

A	initial encounter
D	subsequent encounter
S	sequela

● **S46.0** Injury of muscle(s) and tendon(s) of the rotator cuff of shoulder

  ● **S46.00** Unspecified injury of muscle(s) and tendon(s) of the rotator cuff of shoulder

    ● **S46.001** Unspecified injury of muscle(s) and tendon(s) of the rotator cuff of right shoulder

    ● **S46.002** Unspecified injury of muscle(s) and tendon(s) of the rotator cuff of left shoulder

    ● **S46.009** Unspecified injury of muscle(s) and tendon(s) of the rotator cuff of unspecified shoulder

  ● **S46.01** Strain of muscle(s) and tendon(s) of the rotator cuff of shoulder
    Acute onset due to trauma to rotator cuff muscle/tendon

    ● **S46.011** Strain of muscle(s) and tendon(s) of the rotator cuff of right shoulder

    ● **S46.012** Strain of muscle(s) and tendon(s) of the rotator cuff of left shoulder

    ● **S46.019** Strain of muscle(s) and tendon(s) of the rotator cuff of unspecified shoulder

  ● **S46.02** Laceration of muscle(s) and tendon(s) of the rotator cuff of shoulder

    ● **S46.021** Laceration of muscle(s) and tendon(s) of the rotator cuff of right shoulder A 🔒
      Ex:) See PDX Collection 1263

    ● **S46.022** Laceration of muscle(s) and tendon(s) of the rotator cuff of left shoulder A 🔒
      Ex:) See PDX Collection 1264

    ● **S46.029** Laceration of muscle(s) and tendon(s) of the rotator cuff of unspecified shoulder A 🔒
      Ex:) See PDX Collection 1265

  ● **S46.09** Other injury of muscle(s) and tendon(s) of the rotator cuff of shoulder

    ● **S46.091** Other injury of muscle(s) and tendon(s) of the rotator cuff of right shoulder

    ● **S46.092** Other injury of muscle(s) and tendon(s) of the rotator cuff of left shoulder

    ● **S46.099** Other injury of muscle(s) and tendon(s) of the rotator cuff of unspecified shoulder

● **S46.1**   Injury of muscle, fascia and tendon of long head of biceps

  ● **S46.10**   Unspecified injury of muscle, fascia and tendon of long head of biceps

    ● **S46.101**   Unspecified injury of muscle, fascia and tendon of long head of biceps, right arm

    ● **S46.102**   Unspecified injury of muscle, fascia and tendon of long head of biceps, left arm

    ● **S46.109**   Unspecified injury of muscle, fascia and tendon of long head of biceps, unspecified arm

  ● **S46.11**   Strain of muscle, fascia and tendon of long head of biceps
      Coding Clinic: 2019, Q2, P27

    ● **S46.111**   Strain of muscle, fascia and tendon of long head of biceps, right arm

    ● **S46.112**   Strain of muscle, fascia and tendon of long head of biceps, left arm

    ● **S46.119**   Strain of muscle, fascia and tendon of long head of biceps, unspecified arm

  ● **S46.12**   Laceration of muscle, fascia and tendon of long head of biceps

    ● **S46.121**   Laceration of muscle, fascia and tendon of long head of biceps, right arm A 🦠
       (Ex:) See PDX Collection 1263

    ● **S46.122**   Laceration of muscle, fascia and tendon of long head of biceps, left arm A 🦠
       (Ex:) See PDX Collection 1264

    ● **S46.129**   Laceration of muscle, fascia and tendon of long head of biceps, unspecified arm A 🦠
       (Ex:) See PDX Collection 1265

  ● **S46.19**   Other injury of muscle, fascia and tendon of long head of biceps

    ● **S46.191**   Other injury of muscle, fascia and tendon of long head of biceps, right arm

    ● **S46.192**   Other injury of muscle, fascia and tendon of long head of biceps, left arm

    ● **S46.199**   Other injury of muscle, fascia and tendon of long head of biceps, unspecified arm

● **S46.2**   Injury of muscle, fascia and tendon of other parts of biceps

  ● **S46.20**   Unspecified injury of muscle, fascia and tendon of other parts of biceps

    ● **S46.201**   Unspecified injury of muscle, fascia and tendon of other parts of biceps, right arm

    ● **S46.202**   Unspecified injury of muscle, fascia and tendon of other parts of biceps, left arm

    ● **S46.209**   Unspecified injury of muscle, fascia and tendon of other parts of biceps, unspecified arm

  ● **S46.21**   Strain of muscle, fascia and tendon of other parts of biceps

    ● **S46.211**   Strain of muscle, fascia and tendon of other parts of biceps, right arm

    ● **S46.212**   Strain of muscle, fascia and tendon of other parts of biceps, left arm

    ● **S46.219**   Strain of muscle, fascia and tendon of other parts of biceps, unspecified arm

● **S46.22**   Laceration of muscle, fascia and tendon of other parts of biceps

    ● **S46.221**   Laceration of muscle, fascia and tendon of other parts of biceps, right arm A 🦠
       (Ex:) See PDX Collection 1263

    ● **S46.222**   Laceration of muscle, fascia and tendon of other parts of biceps, left arm A 🦠
       (Ex:) See PDX Collection 1264

    ● **S46.229**   Laceration of muscle, fascia and tendon of other parts of biceps, unspecified arm A 🦠
       (Ex:) See PDX Collection 1265

  ● **S46.29**   Other injury of muscle, fascia and tendon of other parts of biceps

    ● **S46.291**   Other injury of muscle, fascia and tendon of other parts of biceps, right arm

    ● **S46.292**   Other injury of muscle, fascia and tendon of other parts of biceps, left arm

    ● **S46.299**   Other injury of muscle, fascia and tendon of other parts of biceps, unspecified arm

● **S46.3**   Injury of muscle, fascia and tendon of triceps

  ● **S46.30**   Unspecified injury of muscle, fascia and tendon of triceps

    ● **S46.301**   Unspecified injury of muscle, fascia and tendon of triceps, right arm

    ● **S46.302**   Unspecified injury of muscle, fascia and tendon of triceps, left arm

    ● **S46.309**   Unspecified injury of muscle, fascia and tendon of triceps, unspecified arm

  ● **S46.31**   Strain of muscle, fascia and tendon of triceps

    ● **S46.311**   Strain of muscle, fascia and tendon of triceps, right arm

    ● **S46.312**   Strain of muscle, fascia and tendon of triceps, left arm

    ● **S46.319**   Strain of muscle, fascia and tendon of triceps, unspecified arm

  ● **S46.32**   Laceration of muscle, fascia and tendon of triceps

    ● **S46.321**   Laceration of muscle, fascia and tendon of triceps, right arm A 🦠
       (Ex:) See PDX Collection 1263

    ● **S46.322**   Laceration of muscle, fascia and tendon of triceps, left arm A 🦠
       (Ex:) See PDX Collection 1264

    ● **S46.329**   Laceration of muscle, fascia and tendon of triceps, unspecified arm A 🦠
       (Ex:) See PDX Collection 1265

  ● **S46.39**   Other injury of muscle, fascia and tendon of triceps

    ● **S46.391**   Other injury of muscle, fascia and tendon of triceps, right arm

    ● **S46.392**   Other injury of muscle, fascia and tendon of triceps, left arm

    ● **S46.399**   Other injury of muscle, fascia and tendon of triceps, unspecified arm

● **S46.8**   Injury of other muscles, fascia and tendons at shoulder and upper arm level

  ● **S46.80**   Unspecified injury of other muscles, fascia and tendons at shoulder and upper arm level

    ● **S46.801**   Unspecified injury of other muscles, fascia and tendons at shoulder and upper arm level, right arm

    ● **S46.802**   Unspecified injury of other muscles, fascia and tendons at shoulder and upper arm level, left arm

    ● **S46.809**   Unspecified injury of other muscles, fascia and tendons at shoulder and upper arm level, unspecified arm

CHAPTER 19 (S00-T88)

N Newborn Age: 0   **P** Pediatric Age: 0–17   **M** Maternity DX: 9–64   **A** Adult Age. 15–124   ♀ Females Only   ♂ Males Only

🦠 Complication\Comorbidity   🦠 Major C\C   (Ex:) CC/MCC Exclusions   🦠 Hospital-Acquired Condition   🦠 Hierarchical Condition Category

1317

● **S46.81** Strain of other muscles, fascia and tendons at shoulder and upper arm level

   ● **S46.811** Strain of other muscles, fascia and tendons at shoulder and upper arm level, right arm

   ● **S46.812** Strain of other muscles, fascia and tendons at shoulder and upper arm level, left arm

   ● **S46.819** Strain of other muscles, fascia and tendons at shoulder and upper arm level, unspecified arm

● **S46.82** Laceration of other muscles, fascia and tendons at shoulder and upper arm level

   ● **S46.821** Laceration of other muscles, fascia and tendons at shoulder and upper arm level, right arm A 🪙
      (Ex:) See PDX Collection 1263

   ● **S46.822** Laceration of other muscles, fascia and tendons at shoulder and upper arm level, left arm A 🪙
      (Ex:) See PDX Collection 1264

   ● **S46.829** Laceration of other muscles, fascia and tendons at shoulder and upper arm level, unspecified arm A 🪙
      (Ex:) See PDX Collection 1265

● **S46.89** Other injury of other muscles, fascia and tendons at shoulder and upper arm level

   ● **S46.891** Other injury of other muscles, fascia and tendons at shoulder and upper arm level, right arm

   ● **S46.892** Other injury of other muscles, fascia and tendons at shoulder and upper arm level, left arm

   ● **S46.899** Other injury of other muscles, fascia and tendons at shoulder and upper arm level, unspecified arm

● **S46.9** Injury of unspecified muscle, fascia and tendon at shoulder and upper arm level

  ● **S46.90** Unspecified injury of unspecified muscle, fascia and tendon at shoulder and upper arm level

   ● **S46.901** Unspecified injury of unspecified muscle, fascia and tendon at shoulder and upper arm level, right arm

   ● **S46.902** Unspecified injury of unspecified muscle, fascia and tendon at shoulder and upper arm level, left arm

   ● **S46.909** Unspecified injury of unspecified muscle, fascia and tendon at shoulder and upper arm level, unspecified arm

  ● **S46.91** Strain of unspecified muscle, fascia and tendon at shoulder and upper arm level

   ● **S46.911** Strain of unspecified muscle, fascia and tendon at shoulder and upper arm level, right arm

   ● **S46.912** Strain of unspecified muscle, fascia and tendon at shoulder and upper arm level, left arm

   ● **S46.919** Strain of unspecified muscle, fascia and tendon at shoulder and upper arm level, unspecified arm

● **S46.92** Laceration of unspecified muscle, fascia and tendon at shoulder and upper arm level

   ● **S46.921** Laceration of unspecified muscle, fascia and tendon at shoulder and upper arm level, right arm A 🪙
      (Ex:) See PDX Collection 1263

   ● **S46.922** Laceration of unspecified muscle, fascia and tendon at shoulder and upper arm level, left arm A 🪙
      (Ex:) See PDX Collection 1264

   ● **S46.929** Laceration of unspecified muscle, fascia and tendon at shoulder and upper arm level, unspecified arm A 🪙
      (Ex:) See PDX Collection 1265

  ● **S46.99** Other injury of unspecified muscle, fascia and tendon at shoulder and upper arm level

   ● **S46.991** Other injury of unspecified muscle, fascia and tendon at shoulder and upper arm level, right arm

   ● **S46.992** Other injury of unspecified muscle, fascia and tendon at shoulder and upper arm level, left arm

   ● **S46.999** Other injury of unspecified muscle, fascia and tendon at shoulder and upper arm level, unspecified arm

● **S47** Crushing injury of shoulder and upper arm

  Use additional code for all associated injuries

  Excludes2 crushing injury of elbow (S57.0-)

  The appropriate 7th character is to be added to each code from category S47

A	initial encounter
D	subsequent encounter
S	sequela

X ● **S47.1** Crushing injury of right shoulder and upper arm

X ● **S47.2** Crushing injury of left shoulder and upper arm

X ● **S47.9** Crushing injury of shoulder and upper arm, unspecified arm

● **S48** Traumatic amputation of shoulder and upper arm

  An amputation not identified as partial or complete should be coded to complete

  Excludes1 traumatic amputation at elbow level (S58.0)

  The appropriate 7th character is to be added to each code from category S48

A	initial encounter
D	subsequent encounter
S	sequela

● **S48.0** Traumatic amputation at shoulder joint

  ● **S48.01** Complete traumatic amputation at shoulder joint

   ● **S48.011** Complete traumatic amputation at right shoulder joint A 🪙, A, S 🪙
      (Ex:) See PDX Collection 1266

   ● **S48.012** Complete traumatic amputation at left shoulder joint A 🪙, A, S 🪙
      (Ex:) See PDX Collection 1267

   ● **S48.019** Complete traumatic amputation at unspecified shoulder joint A 🪙, A, S 🪙
      (Ex:) See PDX Collection 1268

▶ New   ⇥ Revised   ~~deleted~~ Deleted   Excludes 1   Excludes 2   Includes   Use additional   Code first   Code also   Key words

OGCR Official Guidelines   ● Unacceptable Principal Diagnosis   X Assign placeholder X   ● Use Additional Character(s)   ▸ Manifestation Code   Coding Clinic

● **S48.02**   Partial traumatic amputation at shoulder joint

   ● **S48.021**   Partial traumatic amputation at right shoulder joint A 🅒, A, S 🅜🅒
     (Ex) See PDX Collection 1266

   ● **S48.022**   Partial traumatic amputation at left shoulder joint A 🅒, A, S 🅜🅒
     (Ex) See PDX Collection 1267

   ● **S48.029**   Partial traumatic amputation at unspecified shoulder joint A 🅒, A, S 🅜🅒
     (Ex) See PDX Collection 1268

● **S48.1**   Traumatic amputation at level between shoulder and elbow

   ● **S48.11**   Complete traumatic amputation at level between shoulder and elbow

     ● **S48.111**   Complete traumatic amputation at level between right shoulder and elbow A 🅒, A, S 🅜🅒
       (Ex) See PDX Collection 1266

     ● **S48.112**   Complete traumatic amputation at level between left shoulder and elbow A 🅒, A, S 🅜🅒
       (Ex) See PDX Collection 1267

     ● **S48.119**   Complete traumatic amputation at level between unspecified shoulder and elbow A 🅒, A, S 🅜🅒
       (Ex) See PDX Collection 1268

   ● **S48.12**   Partial traumatic amputation at level between shoulder and elbow

     ● **S48.121**   Partial traumatic amputation at level between right shoulder and elbow A 🅒, A, S 🅜🅒
       (Ex) See PDX Collection 1266

     ● **S48.122**   Partial traumatic amputation at level between left shoulder and elbow A 🅒, A, S 🅜🅒
       (Ex) See PDX Collection 1267

     ● **S48.129**   Partial traumatic amputation at level between unspecified shoulder and elbow A 🅒, A, S 🅜🅒
       (Ex) See PDX Collection 1268

● **S48.9**   Traumatic amputation of shoulder and upper arm, level unspecified

   ● **S48.91**   Complete traumatic amputation of shoulder and upper arm, level unspecified

     ● **S48.911**   Complete traumatic amputation of right shoulder and upper arm, level unspecified A 🅒, A, S 🅜🅒
       (Ex) See PDX Collection 1266

     ● **S48.912**   Complete traumatic amputation of left shoulder and upper arm, level unspecified A 🅒, A, S 🅜🅒
       (Ex) See PDX Collection 1267

     ● **S48.919**   Complete traumatic amputation of unspecified shoulder and upper arm, level unspecified A 🅒, A, S 🅜🅒
       (Ex) See PDX Collection 1268

   ● **S48.92**   Partial traumatic amputation of shoulder and upper arm, level unspecified

     ● **S48.921**   Partial traumatic amputation of right shoulder and upper arm, level unspecified A 🅒, A, S 🅜🅒
       (Ex) See PDX Collection 1266

     ● **S48.922**   Partial traumatic amputation of left shoulder and upper arm, level unspecified A 🅒, A, S 🅜🅒
       (Ex) See PDX Collection 1267

     ● **S48.929**   Partial traumatic amputation of unspecified shoulder and upper arm, level unspecified A 🅒, A, S 🅜🅒
       (Ex) See PDX Collection 1268

Item 19–3   **SALTER-HARRIS TYPE 1:** epiphysis is completely separated from end of bone, or metaphysic growth plate remains attached to epiphysis

SALTER-HARRIS TYPE 2: epiphysis and growth plate are partially separated from metaphysis, which is cracked—most common type

SALTER-HARRIS TYPE 3: fracture occurring through epiphysis and separates part of epiphysis and growth plate from metaphysis fracture, usually at distal end of tibia

SALTER-HARRIS TYPE 4: fracture runs through epiphysis, across growth plate, into metaphysic, surgery is required to restore joint surface to normal and align growth plate

● **S49**   Other and unspecified injuries of shoulder and upper arm

   The appropriate 7th character is to be added to each code from subcategories S49.0 and S49.1

A	initial encounter for closed fracture
D	subsequent encounter for fracture with routine healing
G	subsequent encounter for fracture with delayed healing
K	subsequent encounter for fracture with nonunion
P	subsequent encounter for fracture with malunion
S	sequela

● **S49.0**   Physeal fracture of upper end of humerus

   ● **S49.00**   Unspecified physeal fracture of upper end of humerus

     ● **S49.001**   Unspecified physeal fracture of upper end of humerus, right arm A, K, P 🅒, A 🅜🅒
       (Ex) For S49.001[A]: See PDX Collection 1245
       For S49.001[K,P]: See PDX Collection 897

     ● **S49.002**   Unspecified physeal fracture of upper end of humerus, left arm A, K, P 🅒, A 🅜🅒
       (Ex) For S49.002[A]: See PDX Collection 1247
       For S49.002[K,P]: See PDX Collection 897

     ● **S49.009**   Unspecified physeal fracture of upper end of humerus, unspecified arm A, K, P 🅒, A 🅜🅒
       (Ex) For S49.009[A]: See PDX Collection 1248
       For S49.009[K,P]: See PDX Collection 897

   ● **S49.01**   Salter-Harris Type I physeal fracture of upper end of humerus

     ● **S49.011**   Salter-Harris Type I physeal fracture of upper end of humerus, right arm A, K, P 🅒, A 🅜🅒
       (Ex) For S49.011[A]: See PDX Collection 1245
       For S49.011[K,P]: See PDX Collection 897

     ● **S49.012**   Salter-Harris Type I physeal fracture of upper end of humerus, left arm A, K, P 🅒, A 🅜🅒
       (Ex) For S49.012[A]: See PDX Collection 1247
       For S49.012[K,P]: See PDX Collection 897

     ● **S49.019**   Salter-Harris Type I physeal fracture of upper end of humerus, unspecified arm A, K, P 🅒, A 🅜🅒
       (Ex) For S49.019[A]: See PDX Collection 1248
       For S49.019[K,P]: See PDX Collection 897

   ● **S49.02**   Salter-Harris Type II physeal fracture of upper end of humerus

     ● **S49.021**   Salter-Harris Type II physeal fracture of upper end of humerus, right arm A, K, P 🅒, A 🅜🅒
       (Ex) For S49.021[A]: See PDX Collection 1245
       For S49.021[K,P]: See PDX Collection 897

     ● **S49.022**   Salter-Harris Type II physeal fracture of upper end of humerus, left arm A, K, P 🅒, A 🅜🅒
       (Ex) For S49.022[A]: See PDX Collection 1247
       For S49.022[K,P]: See PDX Collection 897

     ● **S49.029**   Salter-Harris Type II physeal fracture of upper end of humerus, unspecified arm A, K, P 🅒, A 🅜🅒
       (Ex) For S49.029[A]: See PDX Collection 1248
       For S49.029[K,P]: See PDX Collection 897

CHAPTER 19 (S00-T88)

N   Newborn Age: 0   P   Pediatric Age: 0–17   M   Maternity DX: 9–64   A   Adult Age: 15–124   ♀   Females Only   ♂   Males Only

🅒 Complication\Comorbidity   🅜🅒 Major C\C   (Ex) CC/MCC Exclusions   🅗 Hospital-Acquired Condition   🅗 Hierarchical Condition Category

1319

- ● S49.03 **Salter-Harris Type III** physeal fracture of upper end of humerus
  - ● S49.031 Salter-Harris Type III physeal fracture of upper end of humerus, **right arm** A, K, P 🔵, A 🔵
    - (Ex:) **For S49.031[A]:** See PDX Collection 1245
      For S49.031[K,P]: See PDX Collection 897
  - ● S49.032 Salter-Harris Type III physeal fracture of upper end of humerus, **left arm** A, K, P 🔵, A 🔵
    - (Ex:) **For S49.032[A]:** See PDX Collection 1247
      For S49.032[K,P]: See PDX Collection 897
  - ● S49.039 Salter-Harris Type III physeal fracture of upper end of humerus, **unspecified arm** A, K, P 🔵, A 🔵
    - (Ex:) **For S49.039[A]:** See PDX Collection 1248
      For S49.039[K,P]: See PDX Collection 897
- ● S49.04 **Salter-Harris Type IV** physeal fracture of upper end of humerus
  - ● S49.041 Salter-Harris Type IV physeal fracture of upper end of humerus, **right arm** A, K, P 🔵, A 🔵
    - (Ex:) **For S49.041[A]:** See PDX Collection 1245
      For S49.041[K,P]: See PDX Collection 897
  - ● S49.042 Salter-Harris Type IV physeal fracture of upper end of humerus, **left arm** A, K, P 🔵, A 🔵
    - (Ex:) **For S49.042[A]:** See PDX Collection 1247
      For S49.042[K,P]: See PDX Collection 897
  - ● S49.049 Salter-Harris Type IV physeal fracture of upper end of humerus, **unspecified arm** A, K, P 🔵, A 🔵
    - (Ex:) **For S49.049[A]:** See PDX Collection 1248
      For S49.049[K,P]: See PDX Collection 897
- ● S49.09 **Other** physeal fracture of upper end of humerus
  - ● S49.091 Other physeal fracture of upper end of humerus, **right arm** A, K, P 🔵, A 🔵
    - (Ex:) **For S49.091[A]:** See PDX Collection 1245
      For S49.091[K,P]: See PDX Collection 897
  - ● S49.092 Other physeal fracture of upper end of humerus, **left arm** A, K, P 🔵, A 🔵
    - (Ex:) **For S49.092[A]:** See PDX Collection 1247
      For S49.092[K,P]: See PDX Collection 897
  - ● S49.099 Other physeal fracture of upper end of humerus, **unspecified arm** A, K, P 🔵, A 🔵
    - (Ex:) **For S49.099[A]:** See PDX Collection 1248
      For S49.099[K,P]: See PDX Collection 897
- ● S49.1 **Physeal** fracture of **lower end of humerus**
  - ● S49.10 **Unspecified** physeal fracture of lower end of humerus
    - ● S49.101 Unspecified physeal fracture of lower end of humerus, **right arm** A, K, P 🔵, A 🔵
      - (Ex:) **For S49.101[A]:** See PDX Collection 1245
        For S49.101[K,P]: See PDX Collection 897
    - ● S49.102 Unspecified physeal fracture of lower end of humerus, **left arm** A, K, P 🔵, A 🔵
      - (Ex:) **For S49.102[A]:** See PDX Collection 1247
        For S49.102[K,P]: See PDX Collection 897
    - ● S49.109 Unspecified physeal fracture of lower end of humerus, **unspecified arm** A, K, P 🔵, A 🔵
      - (Ex:) **For S49.109[A]:** See PDX Collection 1248
        For S49.109[K,P]: See PDX Collection 897

- ● S49.11 **Salter-Harris Type I** physeal fracture of lower end of humerus
  - ● S49.111 Salter-Harris Type I physeal fracture of lower end of humerus, **right arm** A, K, P 🔵, A 🔵
    - (Ex:) **For S49.111[A]:** See PDX Collection 1245
      For S49.111[K,P]: See PDX Collection 897
  - ● S49.112 Salter-Harris Type I physeal fracture of lower end of humerus, **left arm** A, K, P 🔵, A 🔵
    - (Ex:) **For S49.112[A]:** See PDX Collection 1247
      For S49.112[K,P]: See PDX Collection 897
  - ● S49.119 Salter-Harris Type I physeal fracture of lower end of humerus, **unspecified arm** A, K, P 🔵, A 🔵
    - (Ex:) **For S49.119[A]:** See PDX Collection 1248
      For S49.119[K,P]: See PDX Collection 897
- ● S49.12 **Salter-Harris Type II** physeal fracture of lower end of humerus
  - ● S49.121 Salter-Harris Type II physeal fracture of lower end of humerus, **right arm** A, K, P 🔵, A 🔵
    - (Ex:) **For S49.121[A]:** See PDX Collection 1245
      For S49.121[K,P]: See PDX Collection 897
  - ● S49.122 Salter-Harris Type II physeal fracture of lower end of humerus, **left arm** A, K, P 🔵, A 🔵
    - (Ex:) **For S49.122[A]:** See PDX Collection 1247
      For S49.122[K,P]: See PDX Collection 897
  - ● S49.129 Salter-Harris Type II physeal fracture of lower end of humerus, **unspecified arm** A, K, P 🔵, A 🔵
    - (Ex:) **For S49.129[A]:** See PDX Collection 1248
      For S49.129[K,P]: See PDX Collection 897
- ● S49.13 **Salter-Harris Type III** physeal fracture of lower end of humerus
  - ● S49.131 Salter-Harris Type III physeal fracture of lower end of humerus, **right arm** A, K, P 🔵, A 🔵
    - (Ex:) **For S49.131[A]:** See PDX Collection 1245
      For S49.131[K,P]: See PDX Collection 897
  - ● S49.132 Salter-Harris Type III physeal fracture of lower end of humerus, **left arm** A, K, P 🔵, A 🔵
    - (Ex:) **For S49.132[A]:** See PDX Collection 1247
      For S49.132[K,P]: See PDX Collection 897
  - ● S49.139 Salter-Harris Type III physeal fracture of lower end of humerus, **unspecified arm** A, K, P 🔵, A 🔵
    - (Ex:) **For S49.139[A]:** See PDX Collection 1248
      For S49.139[K,P]: See PDX Collection 897
- ● S49.14 **Salter-Harris Type IV** physeal fracture of lower end of humerus
  - ● S49.141 Salter-Harris Type IV physeal fracture of lower end of humerus, **right arm** A, K, P 🔵, A 🔵
    - (Ex:) **For S49.141[A]:** See PDX Collection 1245
      For S49.141[K,P]: See PDX Collection 897
  - ● S49.142 Salter-Harris Type IV physeal fracture of lower end of humerus, **left arm** A, K, P 🔵, A 🔵
    - (Ex:) **For S49.142[A]:** See PDX Collection 1247
      For S49.142[K,P]: See PDX Collection 897
  - ● S49.149 Salter-Harris Type IV physeal fracture of lower end of humerus, **unspecified arm** A, K, P 🔵, A 🔵
    - (Ex:) **For S49.149[A]:** See PDX Collection 1248
      For S49.149[K,P]: See PDX Collection 897

▶ New   ⇒ Revised   ~~deleted~~ Deleted   Excludes 1   Excludes 2   Includes   Use additional   Code first   Code also   Key words

OGCR Official Guidelines   ● Unacceptable Principal Diagnosis   X Assign placeholder X   ● Use Additional Character(s)   ▶ Manifestation Code   **Coding Clinic**

● S49.19   Other physeal fracture of lower end of humerus
     ● S49.191   Other physeal fracture of lower end of humerus, right arm A, K, P 🅒, A 🅗
           Ⓔⓧ For S49.191[A]: See PDX Collection 1245
               For S49.191[K,P]: See PDX Collection 897
     ● S49.192   Other physeal fracture of lower end of humerus, left arm A, K, P 🅒, A 🅗
           Ⓔⓧ For S49.192[A]: See PDX Collection 1247
               For S49.192[K,P]: See PDX Collection 897
     ● S49.199   Other physeal fracture of lower end of humerus, unspecified arm A, K, P 🅒, A 🅗
           Ⓔⓧ For S49.199[A]: See PDX Collection 1248
               For S49.199[K,P]: See PDX Collection 897

● S49.8   Other specified injuries of shoulder and upper arm

     The appropriate 7th character is to be added to each code in subcategory S49.8

A	initial encounter
D	subsequent encounter
S	sequela

X ● S49.80   Other specified injuries of shoulder and upper arm, unspecified arm
X ● S49.81   Other specified injuries of right shoulder and upper arm
X ● S49.82   Other specified injuries of left shoulder and upper arm

● S49.9   Unspecified injury of shoulder and upper arm

     The appropriate 7th character is to be added to each code in subcategory S49.9

A	initial encounter
D	subsequent encounter
S	sequela

X ● S49.90   Unspecified injury of shoulder and upper arm, unspecified arm
X ● S49.91   Unspecified injury of right shoulder and upper arm
X ● S49.92   Unspecified injury of left shoulder and upper arm

---

INJURIES TO THE ELBOW AND FOREARM (S50-S59)

Excludes2   burns and corrosions (T20-T32)
           frostbite (T33-T34)
           injuries of wrist and hand (S60-S69)
           insect bite or sting, venomous (T63.4)

● S50   Superficial injury of elbow and forearm

     Excludes2   superficial injury of wrist and hand (S60.-)

     The appropriate 7th character is to be added to each code from category S50

A	initial encounter
D	subsequent encounter
S	sequela

● S50.0   Contusion of elbow
   X ● S50.00   Contusion of unspecified elbow
   X ● S50.01   Contusion of right elbow
   X ● S50.02   Contusion of left elbow
● S50.1   Contusion of forearm
   X ● S50.10   Contusion of unspecified forearm
   X ● S50.11   Contusion of right forearm
   X ● S50.12   Contusion of left forearm

● S50.3   Other superficial injuries of elbow
   ● S50.31   Abrasion of elbow
     ● S50.311   Abrasion of right elbow
     ● S50.312   Abrasion of left elbow
     ● S50.319   Abrasion of unspecified elbow
   ● S50.32   Blister (nonthermal) of elbow
     ● S50.321   Blister (nonthermal) of right elbow
     ● S50.322   Blister (nonthermal) of left elbow
     ● S50.329   Blister (nonthermal) of unspecified elbow
   ● S50.34   External constriction of elbow
     ● S50.341   External constriction of right elbow
     ● S50.342   External constriction of left elbow
     ● S50.349   External constriction of unspecified elbow
   ● S50.35   Superficial foreign body of elbow
       Splinter in the elbow
     ● S50.351   Superficial foreign body of right elbow
     ● S50.352   Superficial foreign body of left elbow
     ● S50.359   Superficial foreign body of unspecified elbow
   ● S50.36   Insect bite (nonvenomous) of elbow
     ● S50.361   Insect bite (nonvenomous) of right elbow
     ● S50.362   Insect bite (nonvenomous) of left elbow
     ● S50.369   Insect bite (nonvenomous) of unspecified elbow
   ● S50.37   Other superficial bite of elbow
       Excludes1   open bite of elbow (S51.04)
     ● S50.371   Other superficial bite of right elbow
     ● S50.372   Other superficial bite of left elbow
     ● S50.379   Other superficial bite of unspecified elbow
● S50.8   Other superficial injuries of forearm
   ● S50.81   Abrasion of forearm
     ● S50.811   Abrasion of right forearm
     ● S50.812   Abrasion of left forearm
     ● S50.819   Abrasion of unspecified forearm
   ● S50.82   Blister (nonthermal) of forearm
     ● S50.821   Blister (nonthermal) of right forearm
     ● S50.822   Blister (nonthermal) of left forearm
     ● S50.829   Blister (nonthermal) of unspecified forearm
   ● S50.84   External constriction of forearm
     ● S50.841   External constriction of right forearm
     ● S50.842   External constriction of left forearm
     ● S50.849   External constriction of unspecified forearm
   ● S50.85   Superficial foreign body of forearm
       Splinter in the forearm
     ● S50.851   Superficial foreign body of right forearm
     ● S50.852   Superficial foreign body of left forearm
     ● S50.859   Superficial foreign body of unspecified forearm

---

N Newborn Age: 0   **P** Pediatric Age: 0–17   **M** Maternity DX: 9–64   **A** Adult Age: 15–124   ♀ Females Only   ♂ Males Only

🅒 Complication\Comorbidity   🅜 Major C\C   Ⓔⓧ CC/MCC Exclusions   🅗 Hospital-Acquired Condition   🅗 Hierarchical Condition Category

1321

● S50.86   Insect bite (nonvenomous) of forearm
   ● S50.861   Insect bite (nonvenomous) of right forearm
   ● S50.862   Insect bite (nonvenomous) of left forearm
   ● S50.869   Insect bite (nonvenomous) of unspecified forearm
● S50.87   Other superficial bite of forearm
   Excludes1   open bite of forearm (S51.84)
   ● S50.871   Other superficial bite of right forearm
   ● S50.872   Other superficial bite of left forearm
   ● S50.879   Other superficial bite of unspecified forearm
● S50.9   Unspecified superficial injury of elbow and forearm
   ● S50.90   Unspecified superficial injury of elbow
     ● S50.901   Unspecified superficial injury of right elbow
     ● S50.902   Unspecified superficial injury of left elbow
     ● S50.909   Unspecified superficial injury of unspecified elbow
   ● S50.91   Unspecified superficial injury of forearm
     ● S50.911   Unspecified superficial injury of right forearm
     ● S50.912   Unspecified superficial injury of left forearm
     ● S50.919   Unspecified superficial injury of unspecified forearm

● S51   Open wound of elbow and forearm
   Code also any associated wound infection
   Excludes1   open fracture of elbow and forearm (S52.- with open fracture 7th character)
      traumatic amputation of elbow and forearm (S58.-)
   Excludes2   open wound of wrist and hand (S61.-)
   The appropriate 7th character is to be added to each code from category S51

A	initial encounter
D	subsequent encounter
S	sequela

   ● S51.0   Open wound of elbow
     ● S51.00   Unspecified open wound of elbow
       ● S51.001   Unspecified open wound of right elbow
         Coding Clinic: 2012, Q4, P108
       ● S51.002   Unspecified open wound of left elbow
       ● S51.009   Unspecified open wound of unspecified elbow
         Open wound of elbow NOS
     ● S51.01   Laceration without foreign body of elbow
       ● S51.011   Laceration without foreign body of right elbow
       ● S51.012   Laceration without foreign body of left elbow
       ● S51.019   Laceration without foreign body of unspecified elbow
     ● S51.02   Laceration with foreign body of elbow
       ● S51.021   Laceration with foreign body of right elbow
       ● S51.022   Laceration with foreign body of left elbow
       ● S51.029   Laceration with foreign body of unspecified elbow

● S51.03   Puncture wound without foreign body of elbow
   ● S51.031   Puncture wound without foreign body of right elbow
   ● S51.032   Puncture wound without foreign body of left elbow
   ● S51.039   Puncture wound without foreign body of unspecified elbow
● S51.04   Puncture wound with foreign body of elbow
   ● S51.041   Puncture wound with foreign body of right elbow
   ● S51.042   Puncture wound with foreign body of left elbow
   ● S51.049   Puncture wound with foreign body of unspecified elbow
● S51.05   Open bite of elbow
   Bite of elbow NOS
   Excludes1   superficial bite of elbow (S50.36, S50.37)
   ● S51.051   Open bite, right elbow
   ● S51.052   Open bite, left elbow
   ● S51.059   Open bite, unspecified elbow
● S51.8   Open wound of forearm
   Excludes2   open wound of elbow (S51.0-)
   ● S51.80   Unspecified open wound of forearm
     ● S51.801   Unspecified open wound of right forearm
     ● S51.802   Unspecified open wound of left forearm
     ● S51.809   Unspecified open wound of unspecified forearm
       Open wound of forearm NOS
   ● S51.81   Laceration without foreign body of forearm
     ● S51.811   Laceration without foreign body of right forearm
     ● S51.812   Laceration without foreign body of left forearm
     ● S51.819   Laceration without foreign body of unspecified forearm
   ● S51.82   Laceration with foreign body of forearm
     ● S51.821   Laceration with foreign body of right forearm
     ● S51.822   Laceration with foreign body of left forearm
     ● S51.829   Laceration with foreign body of unspecified forearm
   ● S51.83   Puncture wound without foreign body of forearm
     ● S51.831   Puncture wound without foreign body of right forearm
     ● S51.832   Puncture wound without foreign body of left forearm
     ● S51.839   Puncture wound without foreign body of unspecified forearm
   ● S51.84   Puncture wound with foreign body of forearm
     ● S51.841   Puncture wound with foreign body of right forearm
     ● S51.842   Puncture wound with foreign body of left forearm
     ● S51.849   Puncture wound with foreign body of unspecified forearm
   ● S51.85   Open bite of forearm
     Bite of forearm NOS
     Excludes1   superficial bite of forearm (S50.86, S50.87)
     ● S51.851   Open bite of right forearm
     ● S51.852   Open bite of left forearm
     ● S51.859   Open bite of unspecified forearm

▶ Now   ⇒ Revised   ~~deleted~~ Deleted   Excludes 1   Excludes 2   Includes   Use additional   Code first   Code also   Key words
OGCR Official Guidelines   ● Unacceptable Principal Diagnosis   X Assign placeholder X   ● Use Additional Character(s)   ▶ Manifestation Code   Coding Clinic

● **S52   Fracture of forearm**

> **Note:** A fracture not identified as displaced or nondisplaced should be coded to displaced
>
> A fracture not designated as open or closed should be coded to closed
>
> The open fracture designations are based on the Gustilo open fracture classification

> **Excludes1**   traumatic amputation of forearm (S58.-)

> **Excludes2**   fracture at wrist and hand level (S62.-)

The appropriate 7th character is to be added to all codes from category S52

A	initial encounter for closed fracture
B	initial encounter for open fracture type I or II initial encounter for open fracture NOS
C	initial encounter for open fracture type IIIA, IIIB, or IIIC
D	subsequent encounter for closed fracture with routine healing
E	subsequent encounter for open fracture type I or II with routine healing
F	subsequent encounter for open fracture type IIIA, IIIB, or IIIC with routine healing
G	subsequent encounter for closed fracture with delayed healing
H	subsequent encounter for open fracture type I or II with delayed healing
J	subsequent encounter for open fracture type IIIA, IIIB, or IIIC with delayed healing
K	subsequent encounter for closed fracture with nonunion
M	subsequent encounter for open fracture type I or II with nonunion
N	subsequent encounter for open fracture type IIIA, IIIB, or IIIC with nonunion
P	subsequent encounter for closed fracture with malunion
Q	subsequent encounter for open fracture type I or II with malunion
R	subsequent encounter for open fracture type IIIA, IIIB, or IIIC with malunion
S	sequela

Coding Clinic: 2016, Q1, P33

● **S52.0   Fracture of upper end of ulna**
> Fracture of proximal end of ulna

> **Excludes2**   fracture of elbow NOS (S42.40-)
>   fractures of shaft of ulna (S52.2-)

● **S52.00   Unspecified fracture of upper end of ulna**
> (Ex) For category S52.00 CC codes S52.00[B,C]:
> See PDX Collection 1269 For S52.00[K,M,N,P,Q,R]:
> See PDX Collection 897

● **S52.001   Unspecified fracture of upper end of right ulna** K, M, N, P, Q, R 🄲, B, C 🄼, B, C 🄷

● **S52.002   Unspecified fracture of upper end of left ulna** K, M, N, P, Q, R 🄲, B, C 🄼, B, C 🄷

● **S52.009   Unspecified fracture of upper end of unspecified ulna** K, M, N, P, Q, R 🄲, B, C 🄼, B, C 🄷

● **S52.01   Torus fracture of upper end of ulna**
> The appropriate 7th character is to be added to all codes in subcategory S52.01

A	initial encounter for closed fracture
D	subsequent encounter for fracture with routine healing
G	subsequent encounter for fracture with delayed healing
K	subsequent encounter for fracture with nonunion
P	subsequent encounter for fracture with malunion
S	sequela

● **S52.011   Torus fracture of upper end of right ulna** A, K, P 🄲, A 🄷
> (Ex) For code S52.011[A]: See PDX Collection 1270
> For S52.011[K,P]: See PDX Collection 897

● **S52.012   Torus fracture of upper end of left ulna** A, K, P 🄲, A 🄷
> (Ex) For code S52.012[A]: See PDX Collection 1271
> For S52.012[K,P]: See PDX Collection 897

● **S52.019   Torus fracture of upper end of unspecified ulna** A, K, P 🄲, A 🄷
> (Ex) For code S52.019[A]: See PDX Collection 1272
> For S52.019[K,P]: See PDX Collection 897

● **S52.02   Fracture of olecranon process without intraarticular extension of ulna**
> (Ex) For category S52.02 CC codes S52.02[B,C]: See PDX
> Collection 1273 For S52.02[K,M,N,P,Q,R]: See PDX
> Collection 897

● **S52.021   Displaced fracture of olecranon process without intraarticular extension of right ulna** K, M, N, P, Q, R 🄲, B, C 🄼, B, C 🄷

● **S52.022   Displaced fracture of olecranon process without intraarticular extension of left ulna** K, M, N, P, Q, R 🄲, B, C 🄼, B, C 🄷

● **S52.023   Displaced fracture of olecranon process without intraarticular extension of unspecified ulna** K, M, N, P, Q, R 🄲, B, C 🄼, B, C 🄷

● **S52.024   Nondisplaced fracture of olecranon process without intraarticular extension of right ulna** K, M, N, P, Q, R 🄲, B, C 🄼, B, C 🄷

● **S52.025   Nondisplaced fracture of olecranon process without intraarticular extension of left ulna** K, M, N, P, Q, R 🄲, B, C 🄼, B, C 🄷

● **S52.026   Nondisplaced fracture of olecranon process without intraarticular extension of unspecified ulna** K, M, N, P, Q, R 🄲, B, C 🄼, B, C 🄷

CHAPTER 19 (S00-T88)

N Newborn Age: 0   P Pediatric Age: 0–17   M Maternity DX: 9–64   A Adult Age: 15–124   ♀ Females Only   ♂ Males Only

🄲 Complication\Comorbidity   🄼 Major C\C   (Ex) CC/MCC Exclusions   🄷 Hospital-Acquired Condition   🄷 Hierarchical Condition Category

1323

● **S52.03** Fracture of olecranon process with intraarticular extension of ulna

(Ex:) **For category S52.03 CC codes S52.03[B,C]:** See PDX Collection 1273 **For S52.03[K,M,N,P,Q,R]:** See PDX Collection 897

  ● **S52.031** Displaced fracture of olecranon process with intraarticular extension of right ulna K, M, N, P, Q, R 🪙, B, C 🪙, B, C 🪙

  ● **S52.032** Displaced fracture of olecranon process with intraarticular extension of left ulna K, M, N, P, Q, R 🪙, B, C 🪙, B, C 🪙

  ● **S52.033** Displaced fracture of olecranon process with intraarticular extension of unspecified ulna K, M, N, P, Q, R 🪙, B, C 🪙, B, C 🪙

  ● **S52.034** Nondisplaced fracture of olecranon process with intraarticular extension of right ulna K, M, N, P, Q, R 🪙, B, C 🪙, B, C 🪙

  ● **S52.035** Nondisplaced fracture of olecranon process with intraarticular extension of left ulna K, M, N, P, Q, R 🪙, B, C 🪙, B, C 🪙

  ● **S52.036** Nondisplaced fracture of olecranon process with intraarticular extension of unspecified ulna K, M, N, P, Q, R 🪙, B, C 🪙, B, C 🪙

● **S52.04** Fracture of coronoid process of ulna

(Ex:) **For category S52.04 CC codes S52.04[B,C]:** See PDX Collection 1269 **For S52.04[K,M,N,P,Q,R]:** See PDX Collection 897

  ● **S52.041** Displaced fracture of coronoid process of right ulna K, M, N, P, Q, R 🪙, B, C 🪙, B, C 🪙

  ● **S52.042** Displaced fracture of coronoid process of left ulna K, M, N, P, Q, R 🪙, B, C 🪙, B, C 🪙

  ● **S52.043** Displaced fracture of coronoid process of unspecified ulna K, M, N, P, Q, R 🪙, B, C 🪙, B, C 🪙

  ● **S52.044** Nondisplaced fracture of coronoid process of right ulna K, M, N, P, Q, R 🪙, B, C 🪙, B, C 🪙

  ● **S52.045** Nondisplaced fracture of coronoid process of left ulna K, M, N, P, Q, R 🪙, B, C 🪙, B, C 🪙

  ● **S52.046** Nondisplaced fracture of coronoid process of unspecified ulna K, M, N, P, Q, R 🪙, B, C 🪙, B, C 🪙

● **S52.09** Other fracture of upper end of ulna

(Ex:) **For category S52.09 CC codes S52.09[B,C]:** See PDX Collection 1269 **For S52.09[K,M,N,P,Q,R]:** See PDX Collection 897

  ● **S52.091** Other fracture of upper end of right ulna K, M, N, P, Q, R 🪙, B, C 🪙, B, C 🪙

  ● **S52.092** Other fracture of upper end of left ulna K, M, N, P, Q, R 🪙, B, C 🪙, B, C 🪙

  ● **S52.099** Other fracture of upper end of unspecified ulna K, M, N, P, Q, R 🪙, B, C 🪙, B, C 🪙

● **S52.1** Fracture of upper end of radius

Fracture of proximal end of radius

Excludes2 physeal fractures of upper end of radius (S59.2-)

          fracture of shaft of radius (S52.3-)

● **S52.10** Unspecified fracture of upper end of radius

(Ex:) **For category S52.10 CC codes S52.10[B,C]:** See PDX Collection 1269 **For S52.10[K,M,N,P,Q,R]:** See PDX Collection 897

  ● **S52.101** Unspecified fracture of upper end of right radius K, M, N, P, Q, R 🪙, B, C 🪙, B, C 🪙

  ● **S52.102** Unspecified fracture of upper end of left radius K, M, N, P, Q, R 🪙, B, C 🪙, B, C 🪙

  ● **S52.109** Unspecified fracture of upper end of unspecified radius K, M, N, P, Q, R 🪙, B, C 🪙, B, C 🪙

● **S52.11** Torus fracture of upper end of radius

The appropriate 7th character is to be added to all codes in subcategory S52.11

A	initial encounter for closed fracture
D	subsequent encounter for fracture with routine healing
G	subsequent encounter for fracture with delayed healing
K	subsequent encounter for fracture with nonunion
P	subsequent encounter for fracture with malunion
S	sequela

  ● **S52.111** Torus fracture of upper end of right radius A, K, P 🪙, A 🪙

(Ex:) **For code S52.111[A]:** See PDX Collection 1270 **For S52.111[K,P]:** See PDX Collection 897

  ● **S52.112** Torus fracture of upper end of left radius A, K, P 🪙, A 🪙

(Ex:) **For code S52.112[A]:** See PDX Collection 1271 **For S52.112[K,P]:** See PDX Collection 897

  ● **S52.119** Torus fracture of upper end of unspecified radius A, K, P 🪙, A 🪙

(Ex:) **For code S52.119[A]:** See PDX Collection 1272 **For S52.119[K,P]:** See PDX Collection 897

● **S52.12** Fracture of head of radius

(Ex:) **For category S52.12 CC codes S52.12[B,C]:** See PDX Collection 1269 **For S52.12[K,M,N,P,Q,R]:** See PDX Collection 897

  ● **S52.121** Displaced fracture of head of right radius K, M, N, P, Q, R 🪙, B, C 🪙, B, C 🪙

  ● **S52.122** Displaced fracture of head of left radius K, M, N, P, Q, R 🪙, B, C 🪙, B, C 🪙

  ● **S52.123** Displaced fracture of head of unspecified radius K, M, N, P, Q, R 🪙, B, C 🪙, B, C 🪙

  ● **S52.124** Nondisplaced fracture of head of right radius K, M, N, P, Q, R 🪙, B, C 🪙, B, C 🪙

  ● **S52.125** Nondisplaced fracture of head of left radius K, M, N, P, Q, R 🪙, B, C 🪙, B, C 🪙

  ● **S52.126** Nondisplaced fracture of head of unspecified radius K, M, N, P, Q, R 🪙, B, C 🪙, B, C 🪙

▶ New   ⇒ Revised   ~~deleted~~ Deleted   Excludes 1   Excludes 2   Includes   Use additional   Code first   Code also   Key words

OGCR Official Guidelines   ● Unacceptable Principal Diagnosis   X Assign placeholder X   ● Use Additional Character(s)   ▌ Manifestation Code   **Coding Clinic**

● **S52.13**   Fracture of neck of radius
    (Ex) **For category S52.13 CC codes S52.13[B,C]:** See PDX
    Collection 1269 **For S52.13[K,M,N,P,Q,R]:** See PDX
    Collection 897

    ● **S52.131**   Displaced fracture of neck of right radius K, M, N, P, Q, R 🪙, B, C 🪙, B, C 🪙

    ● **S52.132**   Displaced fracture of neck of left radius K, M, N, P, Q, R 🪙, B, C 🪙, B, C 🪙

    ● **S52.133**   Displaced fracture of neck of unspecified radius K, M, N, P, Q, R 🪙, B, C 🪙, B, C 🪙

    ● **S52.134**   Nondisplaced fracture of neck of right radius K, M, N, P, Q R 🪙, B, C 🪙, B, C 🪙

    ● **S52.135**   Nondisplaced fracture of neck of left radius K, M, N, P, Q, R 🪙, B, C 🪙, B, C 🪙

    ● **S52.136**   Nondisplaced fracture of neck of unspecified radius K, M, N, P, Q, R 🪙, B, C 🪙, B, C 🪙

● **S52.18**   Other fracture of upper end of radius
    (Ex) **For category S52.18 CC codes S52.18[B,C]:** See PDX
    Collection 1269 **For S52.18[K,M,N,P,Q,R]:** See PDX
    Collection 897

    ● **S52.181**   Other fracture of upper end of right radius K, M, N, P, Q, R 🪙, B, C 🪙, B, C 🪙

    ● **S52.182**   Other fracture of upper end of left radius K, M, N, P, Q, R 🪙, B, C 🪙, B, C 🪙

    ● **S52.189**   Other fracture of upper end of unspecified radius K, M, N, P, Q, R 🪙, B, C 🪙, B, C 🪙

● **S52.2**   Fracture of shaft of ulna

    ● **S52.20**   Unspecified fracture of shaft of ulna
      Fracture of ulna NOS

    ● **S52.201**   Unspecified fracture of shaft of right ulna A, K, M, N, P, Q, R 🪙, B, C 🪙, A, B, C 🪙
      (Ex) **For code S52.201[A]:** See PDX Collection 1270
      For S52.201[B,C]: See PDX Collection 1269
      For S52.201[K,M,N,P,Q,R]: See PDX
      Collection 897

    ● **S52.202**   Unspecified fracture of shaft of left ulna A, K, M, N, P, Q, R 🪙, B, C 🪙, A, B, C 🪙
      (Ex) **For code S52.202[A]:** See PDX Collection 1271
      For code S52.202[B,C]: See PDX
      Collection 1269 **For S52.202[K,M,N,P,Q,R]:**
      See PDX Collection 897

    ● **S52.209**   Unspecified fracture of shaft of unspecified ulna
      A, K, M, N, P, Q, R 🪙, B, C 🪙, A, B, C 🪙
      (Ex) **For code S52.209[A]:** See PDX Collection 1272
      For code S52.209[B,C]: See PDX
      Collection 1269 **For S52.209[K,M,N,P,Q,R]:**
      See PDX Collection 897

● **S52.21**   Greenstick fracture of shaft of ulna
    The appropriate 7th character is to be added to
    all codes in subcategory S52.21

A	initial encounter for closed fracture
D	subsequent encounter for fracture with routine healing
G	subsequent encounter for fracture with delayed healing
K	subsequent encounter for fracture with nonunion
P	subsequent encounter for fracture with malunion
S	sequela

    ● **S52.211**   Greenstick fracture of shaft of right ulna A, K, P 🪙, A 🪙
      (Ex) **For code S52.211[A]:** See PDX Collection 1270
      For S52.211[K,P]: See PDX Collection 897

    ● **S52.212**   Greenstick fracture of shaft of left ulna A, K, P 🪙, A 🪙
      (Ex) **For code S52.212[A]:** See PDX Collection 1271
      For S52.202[K,P]: See PDX Collection 897

    ● **S52.219**   Greenstick fracture of shaft of unspecified ulna A, K, P 🪙, A 🪙
      (Ex) **For code S52.219[A]:** See PDX Collection 1272
      For S52.219[K,P]: See PDX Collection 897

● **S52.22**   Transverse fracture of shaft of ulna

    ● **S52.221**   Displaced transverse fracture of shaft of right ulna A, K, M, N, P, Q, R 🪙, B, C 🪙, A, B, C 🪙
      (Ex) **For code S52.221[A]:** See PDX Collection 1270
      For S52.221[B,C]: See PDX Collection 1269
      For S52.221[K,M,N,P,Q,R]: See PDX
      Collection 897

    ● **S52.222**   Displaced transverse fracture of shaft of left ulna A, K, M, N, P, Q, R 🪙, B, C 🪙, A, B, C 🪙
      (Ex) **For code S52.222[A]:** See PDX Collection 1271
      For code S52.222[B,C]: See PDX
      Collection 1269 **For S52.222[K,M,N,P,Q,R]:**
      See PDX Collection 897

    ● **S52.223**   Displaced transverse fracture of shaft of unspecified ulna
      A, K, M, N, P, Q, R 🪙, B, C 🪙, A, B, C 🪙
      (Ex) **For code S52.223[A]:** See PDX Collection 1272
      For S52.223[B,C]: See PDX
      Collection 1269 **For S52.223[K,M,N,P,Q,R]:**
      See PDX Collection 897

    ● **S52.224**   Nondisplaced transverse fracture of shaft of right ulna
      A, K, M, N, P, Q, R 🪙, B, C 🪙, A, B, C 🪙
      (Ex) **For code S52.224[A]:** See PDX Collection 1270
      For S52.224[B,C]: See PDX Collection 1269
      For S52.224[K,M,N,P,Q,R]: See PDX
      Collection 897

    ● **S52.225**   Nondisplaced transverse fracture of shaft of left ulna
      A, K, M, N, P, Q, R 🪙, B, C 🪙, A, B, C 🪙
      (Ex) **For code S52.225[A]:** See PDX Collection 1271
      For code S52.225[B,C]: See PDX
      Collection 1269 **For S52.225[K,M,N,P,Q,R]:**
      See PDX Collection 897

    ● **S52.226**   Nondisplaced transverse fracture of shaft of unspecified ulna
      A, K, M, N, P, Q, R 🪙, B, C 🪙, A, B, C 🪙
      (Ex) **For code S52.226[A]:** See PDX Collection 1272
      For code S52.226[B,C]: See PDX
      Collection 1269 **For S52.226[K,M,N,P,Q,R]:**
      See PDX Collection 897

CHAPTER 19 (S00-T88)

N Newborn Age: 0   **P** Pediatric Age: 0–17   **M** Maternity DX: 9–64   **A** Adult Age: 15–124   ♀ Females Only   ♂ Males Only

🪙 Complication\Comorbidity   🪙 Major C\C   (Ex) CC/MCC Exclusions   🪙 Hospital-Acquired Condition   🪙 Hierarchical Condition Category

1325

● **S52.23** Oblique fracture of shaft of ulna

  ● **S52.231** Displaced oblique fracture of shaft of right ulna A, K, M, N, P, Q, R 🪙, B, C 🪙, A, B, C 🪙

  (Ex) **For code S52.231[A]:** See PDX Collection 1270
  For S52.231[B,C]: See PDX Collection 1269
  For S52.231[K,M,N,P,Q,R]: See PDX Collection 897

  ● **S52.232** Displaced oblique fracture of shaft of left ulna A, K, M, N, P, Q, R 🪙, B, C 🪙, A, B, C 🪙

  (Ex) **For code S52.232[A]:** See PDX Collection 1271
  For code S52.232[B,C]: See PDX Collection 1269 **For S52.232[K,M,N,P,Q,R]:** See PDX Collection 897

  ● **S52.233** Displaced oblique fracture of shaft of unspecified ulna A, K, M, N, P, Q, R 🪙, B, C 🪙, A, B, C 🪙

  (Ex) **For code S52.233[A]:** See PDX Collection 1272
  For code S52.233[B,C]: See PDX Collection 1269 **For S52.233[K,M,N,P,Q,R]:** See PDX Collection 897

  ● **S52.234** Nondisplaced oblique fracture of shaft of right ulna A, K, M, N, P, Q, R 🪙, B, C 🪙, A, B, C 🪙

  (Ex) **For code S52.234[A]:** See PDX Collection 1270
  For S52.234[B,C]: See PDX Collection 1269
  For S52.234[K,M,N,P,Q,R]: See PDX Collection 897

  ● **S52.235** Nondisplaced oblique fracture of shaft of left ulna A, K, M, N, P, Q, R 🪙, B, C 🪙, A, B, C 🪙

  (Ex) **For code S52.235[A]:** See PDX Collection 1271
  For code S52.235[B,C]: See PDX Collection 1269 **For S52.235[K,M,N,P,Q,R]:** See PDX Collection 897

  ● **S52.236** Nondisplaced oblique fracture of shaft of unspecified ulna A, K, M, N, P, Q, R 🪙, B, C 🪙, A, B, C 🪙

  (Ex) **For code S52.236[A]:** See PDX Collection 1272
  For code S52.236[B,C]: See PDX Collection 1269 **For S52.236[K,M,N,P,Q,R]:** See PDX Collection 897

● **S52.24** Spiral fracture of shaft of ulna

  ● **S52.241** Displaced spiral fracture of shaft of ulna, right arm A, K, M, N, P, Q, R 🪙, B, C 🪙, A, B, C 🪙

  (Ex) **For code S52.241[A]:** See PDX Collection 1270
  For S52.241[B,C]: See PDX Collection 1269
  For S52.241[K,M,N,P,Q,R]: See PDX Collection 897

  ● **S52.242** Displaced spiral fracture of shaft of ulna, left arm A, K, M, N, P, Q, R 🪙, B, C 🪙, A, B, C 🪙

  (Ex) **For code S52.242[A]:** See PDX Collection 1271
  For code S52.242[B,C]: See PDX Collection 1269 **For S52.242[K,M,N,P,Q,R]:** See PDX Collection 897

  ● **S52.243** Displaced spiral fracture of shaft of ulna, unspecified arm A, K, M, N, P, Q, R 🪙, B, C 🪙, A, B, C 🪙

  (Ex) **For code S52.243[A]:** See PDX Collection 1272
  For code S52.243[B,C]: See PDX Collection 1269 **For S52.243[K,M,N,P,Q,R]:** See PDX Collection 897

● **S52.244** Nondisplaced spiral fracture of shaft of ulna, right arm A, K, M, N, P, Q, R 🪙, B, C 🪙, A, B, C 🪙

  (Ex) **For code S52.244[A]:** See PDX Collection 1270
  For S52.244[B,C]: See PDX Collection 1269
  For S52.244[K,M,N,P,Q,R]: See PDX Collection 897

● **S52.245** Nondisplaced spiral fracture of shaft of ulna, left arm A, K, M, N, P, Q, R 🪙, B, C 🪙, A, B, C 🪙

  (Ex) **For code S52.245[A]:** See PDX Collection 1271
  For S52.245[B,C]: See PDX Collection 1269 **For S52.245[K,M,N,P,Q,R]:** See PDX Collection 897

● **S52.246** Nondisplaced spiral fracture of shaft of ulna, unspecified arm A, K, M, N, P, Q, R 🪙, B, C 🪙, A, B, C 🪙

  (Ex) **For code S52.246[A]:** See PDX Collection 1272
  For S52.246[B,C]: See PDX Collection 1269 **For S52.246[K,M,N,P,Q,R]:** See PDX Collection 897

● **S52.25** Comminuted fracture of shaft of ulna

  ● **S52.251** Displaced comminuted fracture of shaft of ulna, right arm A, K, M, N, P, Q, R 🪙, B, C 🪙, A, B, C 🪙

  (Ex) **For code S52.251[A]:** See PDX Collection 1270
  For S52.251[B,C]: See PDX Collection 1269
  For S52.251[K,M,N,P,Q,R]: See PDX Collection 897

  ● **S52.252** Displaced comminuted fracture of shaft of ulna, left arm A, K, M, N, P, Q, R 🪙, B, C 🪙, A, B, C 🪙

  (Ex) **For code S52.252[A]:** See PDX Collection 1271
  For S52.252[B,C]: See PDX Collection 1269 **For S52.252[K,M,N,P,Q,R]:** See PDX Collection 897

  ● **S52.253** Displaced comminuted fracture of shaft of ulna, unspecified arm A, K, M, N, P, Q, R 🪙, B, C 🪙, A, B, C 🪙

  (Ex) **For code S52.253[A]:** See PDX Collection 1272
  For S52.253[B,C]: See PDX Collection 1269 **For S52.253[K,M,N,P,Q,R]:** See PDX Collection 897

  ● **S52.254** Nondisplaced comminuted fracture of shaft of ulna, right arm A, K, M, N, P, Q, R 🪙, B, C 🪙, A, B, C 🪙

  (Ex) **For code S52.254[A]:** See PDX Collection 1270
  For S52.254[B,C]: See PDX Collection 1269
  For S52.254[K,M,N,P,Q,R]: See PDX Collection 897

  ● **S52.255** Nondisplaced comminuted fracture of shaft of ulna, left arm A, K, M, N, P, Q, R 🪙, B, C 🪙, A, B, C 🪙

  (Ex) **For code S52.255[A]:** See PDX Collection 1271
  For code S52.255[B,C]: See PDX Collection 1269 **For S52.255[K,M,N,P,Q,R]:** See PDX Collection 897

  ● **S52.256** Nondisplaced comminuted fracture of shaft of ulna, unspecified arm A, K, M, N, P, Q, R 🪙, B, C 🪙, A, B, C 🪙

  (Ex) **For code S52.256[A]:** See PDX Collection 1272
  For S52.256[B,C]: See PDX Collection 1269 **For S52.256[K,M,N,P,Q,R]:** See PDX Collection 897

▶ New   ⇒ Revised   ~~deleted~~ Deleted   Excludes 1   Excludes 2   Includes   Use additional   Code first   Code also   Key words

OGCR Official Guidelines   ● Unacceptable Principal Diagnosis   X Assign placeholder X   ● Use Additional Character(s)   ▶ Manifestation Code   **Coding Clinic**

● **S52.26**   **Segmental fracture of shaft of ulna**

　　● **S52.261**   **Displaced segmental fracture of shaft of ulna, right arm**
　　　　A, K, M, N, P, Q, R 🦠, B, C 🦠,
　　　　A, B, C 🦠
　　　　　(Ex:) **For code S52.261[A]:** See PDX Collection 1270
　　　　　　　For S52.261[B,C]: See PDX Collection 1269
　　　　　　　For S52.261[K,M,N,P,Q,R]: See PDX
　　　　　　　Collection 897

　　● **S52.262**   **Displaced segmental fracture of shaft of ulna, left arm** A, K, M, N, P, Q, R 🦠,
　　　　B, C 🦠, A, B, C 🦠
　　　　　(Ex:) **For code S52.262[A]:** See PDX Collection 1271
　　　　　　　For code S52.262[B,C]: See PDX
　　　　　　　Collection 1269 **For S52.262[K,M,N,P,Q,R]:**
　　　　　　　See PDX Collection 897

　　● **S52.263**   **Displaced segmental fracture of shaft of ulna, unspecified arm**
　　　　A, K, M, N, P, Q, R 🦠, B, C 🦠,
　　　　A, B, C 🦠
　　　　　(Ex:) **For code S52.263[A]:** See PDX Collection 1272
　　　　　　　For code S52.263[B,C]: See PDX
　　　　　　　Collection 1269 **For S52.263[K,M,N,P,Q,R]:**
　　　　　　　See PDX Collection 897

　　● **S52.264**   **Nondisplaced segmental fracture of shaft of ulna, right arm**
　　　　A, K, M, N, P, Q, R 🦠, B, C 🦠,
　　　　A, B, C 🦠
　　　　　(Ex:) **For code S52.264[A]:** See PDX Collection 1270
　　　　　　　For S52.264[B,C]: See PDX Collection 1269
　　　　　　　For S52.264[K,M,N,P,Q,R]: See PDX
　　　　　　　Collection 897

　　● **S52.265**   **Nondisplaced segmental fracture of shaft of ulna, left arm**
　　　　A, K, M, N, P, Q, R 🦠, B, C 🦠,
　　　　A, B, C 🦠
　　　　　(Ex:) **For code S52.265[A]:** See PDX Collection 1271
　　　　　　　For code S52.265[B,C]: See PDX
　　　　　　　Collection 1269 **For S52.265[K,M,N,P,Q,R]:**
　　　　　　　See PDX Collection 897

　　● **S52.266**   **Nondisplaced segmental fracture of shaft of ulna, unspecified arm**
　　　　A, K, M, N, P, Q, R 🦠, B, C 🦠,
　　　　A, B, C 🦠
　　　　　(Ex:) **For code S52.266[A]:** See PDX Collection 1272
　　　　　　　For code S52.266[B,C]: See PDX
　　　　　　　Collection 1269 **For S52.266[K,M,N,P,Q,R]:**
　　　　　　　See PDX Collection 897

● **S52.27**   **Monteggia's fracture of ulna**
　　Fracture of upper shaft of ulna with dislocation
　　of radial head
　　(Ex:) **For category S52.27 CC codes S52.27[B,C]:** See PDX
　　　Collection 1269 **For S52.27[K,M,N,P,Q,R]:** See PDX
　　　Collection 897

　　● **S52.271**   **Monteggia's fracture of right ulna**
　　　　K, M, N, P, Q, R 🦠, B, C 🦠, B, C 🦠

　　● **S52.272**   **Monteggia's fracture of left ulna**
　　　　K, M, N, P, Q, R 🦠, B, C 🦠, B, C 🦠

　　● **S52.279**   **Monteggia's fracture of unspecified ulna** K, M, N, P, Q, R 🦠, B, C 🦠,
　　　　B, C 🦠

● **S52.28**   **Bent bone of ulna**

　　● **S52.281**   **Bent bone of right ulna**
　　　　A, K, M, N, P, Q, R 🦠, B, C 🦠,
　　　　A, B, C 🦠
　　　　　(Ex:) **For code S52.281[A]:** See PDX Collection 1270
　　　　　　　For S52.281[B,C]: See PDX Collection 1269
　　　　　　　For S52.281[K,M,N,P,Q,R]: See PDX
　　　　　　　Collection 897

　　● **S52.282**   **Bent bone of left ulna**
　　　　A, K, M, N, P, Q, R 🦠, B, C 🦠,
　　　　A, B, C 🦠
　　　　　(Ex:) **For code S52.282[A]:** See PDX Collection 1271
　　　　　　　For code S52.282[B,C]: See PDX
　　　　　　　Collection 1269 **For S52.282[K,M,N,P,Q,R]:**
　　　　　　　See PDX Collection 897

　　● **S52.283**   **Bent bone of unspecified ulna**
　　　　A, K, M, N, P, Q, R 🦠, B, C 🦠,
　　　　A, B, C 🦠
　　　　　(Ex:) **For code S52.283[A]:** See PDX Collection 1272
　　　　　　　For code S52.283[B,C]: See PDX
　　　　　　　Collection 1269 **For S52.283[K,M,N,P,Q,R]:**
　　　　　　　See PDX Collection 897

● **S52.29**   **Other fracture of shaft of ulna**

　　● **S52.291**   **Other fracture of shaft of right ulna**
　　　　A, K, M, N, P, Q, R 🦠, B, C 🦠,
　　　　A, B, C 🦠
　　　　　(Ex:) **For code S52.291[A]:** See PDX Collection 1270
　　　　　　　For S52.291[B,C]: See PDX Collection 1269
　　　　　　　For S52.291[K,M,N,P,Q,R]: See PDX
　　　　　　　Collection 897

　　● **S52.292**   **Other fracture of shaft of left ulna**
　　　　A, K, M, N, P, Q, R 🦠, B, C 🦠,
　　　　A, B, C 🦠
　　　　　(Ex:) **For code S52.292[A]:** See PDX Collection 1271
　　　　　　　For code S52.292[B,C]: See PDX
　　　　　　　Collection 1269 **For S52.292[K,M,N,P,Q,R]:**
　　　　　　　See PDX Collection 897

　　● **S52.299**   **Other fracture of shaft of unspecified ulna** A, K, M, N, P, Q, R 🦠, B, C 🦠,
　　　　A, B, C 🦠
　　　　　(Ex:) **For code S52.299[A]:** See PDX Collection 1272
　　　　　　　For code S52.299[B,C]: See PDX
　　　　　　　Collection 1269 **For S52.299[K,M,N,P,Q,R]:**
　　　　　　　See PDX Collection 897

● **S52.3**   **Fracture of shaft of radius**

　● **S52.30**   **Unspecified fracture of shaft of radius**

　　● **S52.301**   **Unspecified fracture of shaft of right radius** A, K, M, N, P, Q, R 🦠, B, C 🦠,
　　　　A, B, C 🦠
　　　　　(Ex:) **For code S52.301[A]:** See PDX Collection 1270
　　　　　　　For S52.301[B,C]: See PDX Collection 1269
　　　　　　　For S52.301[K,M,N,P,Q,R]: See PDX
　　　　　　　Collection 897

　　● **S52.302**   **Unspecified fracture of shaft of left radius** A, K, M, N, P, Q, R 🦠, B, C 🦠,
　　　　A, B, C 🦠
　　　　　(Ex:) **For code S52.302[A]:** See PDX Collection 1271
　　　　　　　For code S52.302[B,C]: See PDX
　　　　　　　Collection 1269 **For S52.302[K,M,N,P,Q,R]:**
　　　　　　　See PDX Collection 897

　　● **S52.309**   **Unspecified fracture of shaft of unspecified radius**
　　　　A, K, M, N, P, Q, R 🦠, B, C 🦠,
　　　　A, B, C 🦠
　　　　　(Ex:) **For code S52.309[A]:** See PDX Collection 1272
　　　　　　　For code S52.309[B,C]: See PDX
　　　　　　　Collection 1269 **For S52.309[K,M,N,P,Q,R]:**
　　　　　　　See PDX Collection 897

N Newborn Age: 0   **P** Pediatric Age: 0–17   **M** Maternity DX: 9–64   **A** Adult Age: 15–124   ♀ Females Only   ♂ Males Only

🦠 Complication\Comorbidity   🦠 Major C\C   (Ex:) CC/MCC Exclusions   🦠 Hospital-Acquired Condition   🦠 Hierarchical Condition Category

1327

CHAPTER 19 (S00-T88)

● **S52.31**   Greenstick fracture of shaft of radius

The appropriate 7th character is to be added to all codes in subcategory S52.31

> A   initial encounter for closed fracture
> D   subsequent encounter for fracture with routine healing
> G   subsequent encounter for fracture with delayed healing
> K   subsequent encounter for fracture with nonunion
> P   subsequent encounter for fracture with malunion
> S   sequela

● **S52.311**   **Greenstick fracture of shaft of radius, right arm** A, K, P 🖢, A 🖢
> (Ex:) **For code S52.311[A]:** See PDX Collection 1270
> **For S52.311[K,P]:** See PDX Collection 897

● **S52.312**   **Greenstick fracture of shaft of radius, left arm** A, K, P 🖢, A 🖢
> (Ex:) **For code S52.312[A]:** See PDX Collection 1271
> **For S52.312[K,P]:** See PDX Collection 897

● **S52.319**   **Greenstick fracture of shaft of radius, unspecified arm** A, K, P 🖢, A 🖢
> (Ex:) **For code S52.319[A]:** See PDX Collection 1272
> **For S52.319[K,P]:** See PDX Collection 897

● **S52.32**   Transverse fracture of shaft of radius

● **S52.321**   **Displaced transverse fracture of shaft of right radius** A, K, M, N, P, Q, R 🖢, B, C 🖢, A, B, C 🖢
> (Ex:) **For code S52.321[A]:** See PDX Collection 1270
> **For S52.321[B,C]:** See PDX Collection 1269
> **For S52.321[K,M,N,P,Q,R]:** See PDX Collection 897

● **S52.322**   **Displaced transverse fracture of shaft of left radius** A, K, M, N, P, Q, R 🖢, B, C 🖢, A, B, C 🖢
> (Ex:) **For code S52.322[A]:** See PDX Collection 1271
> **For code S52.322[B,C]:** See PDX Collection 1269 **For S52.322[K,M,N,P,Q,R]:** See PDX Collection 897

● **S52.323**   **Displaced transverse fracture of shaft of unspecified radius** A, K, M, N, P, Q, R 🖢, B, C 🖢, A, B, C 🖢
> (Ex:) **For code S52.323[A]:** See PDX Collection 1272
> **For S52.323[B,C]:** See PDX Collection 1269 **For S52.323[K,M,N,P,Q,R]:** See PDX Collection 897

● **S52.324**   **Nondisplaced transverse fracture of shaft of right radius** A, K, M, N, P, Q, R 🖢, B, C 🖢, A, B, C 🖢
> (Ex:) **For code S52.324[A]:** See PDX Collection 1270
> **For S52.324[B,C]:** See PDX Collection 1269
> **For S52.324[K,M,N,P,Q,R]:** See PDX Collection 897

● **S52.325**   **Nondisplaced transverse fracture of shaft of left radius** A, K, M, N, P, Q, R 🖢, B, C 🖢, A, B, C 🖢
> (Ex:) **For code S52.325[A]:** See PDX Collection 1271
> **For code S52.325[B,C]:** See PDX Collection 1269 **For S52.325[K,M,N,P,Q,R]:** See PDX Collection 897

● **S52.326**   **Nondisplaced transverse fracture of shaft of unspecified radius** A, K, M, N, P, Q, R 🖢, B, C 🖢, A, B, C 🖢
> (Ex:) **For code S52.326[A]:** See PDX Collection 1272
> **For S52.326[B,C]:** See PDX Collection 1269 **For S52.326[K,M,N,P,Q,R]:** See PDX Collection 897

● **S52.33**   Oblique fracture of shaft of radius

● **S52.331**   **Displaced oblique fracture of shaft of right radius** A, K, M, N, P, Q, R 🖢, B, C 🖢, A, B, C 🖢
> (Ex:) **For code S52.331[A]:** See PDX Collection 1270
> **For S52.331[B,C]:** See PDX Collection 1269
> **For S52.331[K,M,N,P,Q,R]:** See PDX Collection 897

● **S52.332**   **Displaced oblique fracture of shaft of left radius** A, K, M, N, P, Q, R 🖢, B, C 🖢, A, B, C 🖢
> (Ex:) **For code S52.332[A]:** See PDX Collection 1271
> **For code S52.332[B,C]:** See PDX Collection 1269 **For S52.332[K,M,N,P,Q,R]:** See PDX Collection 897

● **S52.333**   **Displaced oblique fracture of shaft of unspecified radius** A, K, M, N, P, Q, R 🖢, B, C 🖢, A, B, C 🖢
> (Ex:) **For code S52.333[A]:** See PDX Collection 1272
> **For S52.333[B,C]:** See PDX Collection 1269 **For S52.333[K,M,N,P,Q,R]:** See PDX Collection 897

● **S52.334**   **Nondisplaced oblique fracture of shaft of right radius** A, K, M, N, P, Q, R 🖢, B, C 🖢, A, B, C 🖢
> (Ex:) **For code S52.334[A]:** See PDX Collection 1270
> **For S52.334[B,C]:** See PDX Collection 1269
> **For S52.334[K,M,N,P,Q,R]:** See PDX Collection 897

● **S52.335**   **Nondisplaced oblique fracture of shaft of left radius** A, K, M, N, P, Q, R 🖢, B, C 🖢, A, B, C 🖢
> (Ex:) **For code S52.335[A]:** See PDX Collection 1271
> **For code S52.335[B,C]:** See PDX Collection 1269 **For S52.335[K,M,N,P,Q,R]:** See PDX Collection 897

● **S52.336**   **Nondisplaced oblique fracture of shaft of unspecified radius** A, K, M, N, P, Q, R 🖢, B, C 🖢, A, B, C 🖢
> (Ex:) **For code S52.336[A]:** See PDX Collection 1272
> **For code S52.336[B,C]:** See PDX Collection 1269 **For S52.336[K,M,N,P,Q,R]:** See PDX Collection 897

● **S52.34**   Spiral fracture of shaft of radius

● **S52.341**   **Displaced spiral fracture of shaft of radius, right arm** A, K, M, N, P, Q, R 🖢, B, C 🖢, A, B, C 🖢
> (Ex:) **For code S52.341[A]:** See PDX Collection 1270
> **For S52.341[B,C]:** See PDX Collection 1269
> **For S52.341[K,M,N,P,Q,R]:** See PDX Collection 897

● **S52.342**   **Displaced spiral fracture of shaft of radius, left arm** A, K, M, N, P, Q, R 🖢, B, C 🖢, A, B, C 🖢
> (Ex:) **For code S52.342[A]:** See PDX Collection 1271
> **For S52.342[B,C]:** See PDX Collection 1269 **For S52.342[K,M,N,P,Q,R]:** See PDX Collection 897

● **S52.343**   **Displaced spiral fracture of shaft of radius, unspecified arm** A, K, M, N, P, Q, R 🖢, B, C 🖢, A, B, C 🖢
> (Ex:) **For code S52.343[A]:** See PDX Collection 1272
> **For code S52.343[B,C]:** See PDX Collection 1269 **For S52.343[K,M,N,P,Q,R]:** See PDX Collection 897

▶ New   ⇒ Revised   ~~deleted~~ Deleted   Excludes 1   Excludes 2   Includes   Use additional   Code first   Code also   Key words
OGCR Official Guidelines   ● Unacceptable Principal Diagnosis   X Assign placeholder X   ● Use Additional Character(s)   ▶ Manifestation Code   **Coding Clinic**

● S52.344   Nondisplaced spiral fracture of shaft of radius, right arm
A, K, M, N, P, Q, R 🝙, B, C 🝙,
A, B, C 🝙
> (Ex) **For code S52.344[A]:** See PDX Collection 1270
> **For S52.344[B,C]:** See PDX Collection 1269
> **For S52.344[K,M,N,P,Q,R]:** See PDX Collection 897

● S52.345   Nondisplaced spiral fracture of shaft of radius, left arm
A, K, M, N, P, Q, R 🝙, B, C 🝙,
A, B, C 🝙
> (Ex) **For code S52.345[A]:** See PDX Collection 1271
> **For code S52.345[B,C]:** See PDX Collection 1269 **For S52.345[K,M,N,P,Q,R]:** See PDX Collection 897

● S52.346   Nondisplaced spiral fracture of shaft of radius, unspecified arm
A, K, M, N, P, Q, R 🝙, B, C 🝙,
A, B, C 🝙
> (Ex) **For code S52.346[A]:** See PDX Collection 1272
> **For code S52.346[B,C]:** See PDX Collection 1269 **For S52.346[K,M,N,P,Q,R]:** See PDX Collection 897

● S52.35   Comminuted fracture of shaft of radius

● S52.351   Displaced comminuted fracture of shaft of radius, right arm
A, K, M, N, P, Q, R 🝙, B, C 🝙,
A, B, C 🝙
> (Ex) **For code S52.351[A]:** See PDX Collection 1270
> **For S52.351[B,C]:** See PDX Collection 1269
> **For S52.351[K,M,N,P,Q,R]:** See PDX Collection 897

● S52.352   Displaced comminuted fracture of shaft of radius, left arm
A, K, M, N, P, Q, R 🝙, B, C 🝙,
A, B, C 🝙
> (Ex) **For code S52.352[A]:** See PDX Collection 1271
> **For code S52.352[B,C]:** See PDX Collection 1269 **For S52.352[K,M,N,P,Q,R]:** See PDX Collection 897

● S52.353   Displaced comminuted fracture of shaft of radius, unspecified arm
A, K, M, N, P, Q, R 🝙, B, C 🝙,
A, B, C 🝙
> (Ex) **For code S52.353[A]:** See PDX Collection 1272
> **For code S52.353[B,C]:** See PDX Collection 1269 **For S52.353[K,M,N,P,Q,R]:** See PDX Collection 897

● S52.354   Nondisplaced comminuted fracture of shaft of radius, right arm
A, K, M, N, P, Q, R 🝙, B, C 🝙,
A, B, C 🝙
> (Ex) **For code S52.354[A]:** See PDX Collection 1270
> **For S52.354[B,C]:** See PDX Collection 1269
> **For S52.354[K,M,N,P,Q,R]:** See PDX Collection 897

● S52.355   Nondisplaced comminuted fracture of shaft of radius, left arm
A, K, M, N, P, Q, R 🝙, B, C 🝙,
A, B, C 🝙
> (Ex) **For code S52.355[A]:** See PDX Collection 1271
> **For code S52.355[B,C]:** See PDX Collection 1269 **For S52.355[K,M,N,P,Q,R]:** See PDX Collection 897

● S52.356   Nondisplaced comminuted fracture of shaft of radius, unspecified arm
A, K, M, N, P, Q, R 🝙, B, C 🝙,
A, B, C 🝙
> (Ex) **For code S52.356[A]:** See PDX Collection 1272
> **For code S52.356[B,C]:** See PDX Collection 1269 **For S52.356[K,M,N,P,Q,R]:** See PDX Collection 897

● S52.36   Segmental fracture of shaft of radius

● S52.361   Displaced segmental fracture of shaft of radius, right arm
A, K, M, N, P, Q, R 🝙, B, C 🝙,
A, B, C 🝙
> (Ex) **For code S52.361[A]:** See PDX Collection 1270
> **For S52.361[B,C]:** See PDX Collection 1269
> **For S52.361[K,M,N,P,Q,R]:** See PDX Collection 897

● S52.362   Displaced segmental fracture of shaft of radius, left arm
A, K, M, N, P, Q, R 🝙, B, C 🝙,
A, B, C 🝙
> (Ex) **For code S52.362[A]:** See PDX Collection 1271
> **For code S52.362[B,C]:** See PDX Collection 1269 **For S52.362[K,M,N,P,Q,R]:** See PDX Collection 897

● S52.363   Displaced segmental fracture of shaft of radius, unspecified arm
A, K, M, N, P, Q, R 🝙, B, C 🝙,
A, B, C 🝙
> (Ex) **For code S52.363[A]:** See PDX Collection 1272
> **For code S52.363[B,C]:** See PDX Collection 1269 **For S52.363[K,M,N,P,Q,R]:** See PDX Collection 897

● S52.364   Nondisplaced segmental fracture of shaft of radius, right arm
A, K, M, N, P, Q, R 🝙, B, C 🝙,
A, B, C 🝙
> (Ex) **For code S52.364[A]:** See PDX Collection 1270
> **For S52.364[B,C]:** See PDX Collection 1269
> **For S52.364[K,M,N,P,Q,R]:** See PDX Collection 897

● S52.365   Nondisplaced segmental fracture of shaft of radius, left arm
A, K, M, N, P, Q, R 🝙, B, C 🝙,
A, B, C 🝙
> (Ex) **For code S52.365[A]:** See PDX Collection 1271
> **For code S52.365[B,C]:** See PDX Collection 1269 **For S52.365[K,M,N,P,Q,R]:** See PDX Collection 897

● S52.366   Nondisplaced segmental fracture of shaft of radius, unspecified arm
A, K, M, N, P, Q, R 🝙, B, C 🝙,
A, B, C 🝙
> (Ex) **For code S52.366[A]:** See PDX Collection 1272
> **For code S52.366[B,C]:** See PDX Collection 1269 **For S52.366[K,M,N,P,Q,R]:** See PDX Collection 897

● S52.37   Galeazzi's fracture
Fracture of lower shaft of radius with radioulnar joint dislocation

● S52.371   Galeazzi's fracture of right radius
A, K, M, N, P, Q, R 🝙, B, C 🝙,
A, B, C 🝙
> (Ex) **For code S52.371[A]:** See PDX Collection 1270
> **For S52.371[B,C]:** See PDX Collection 1269
> **For S52.371[K,M,N,P,Q,R]:** See PDX Collection 897

● S52.372   Galeazzi's fracture of left radius
A, K, M, N, P, Q, R 🝙, B, C 🝙,
A, B, C 🝙
> (Ex) **For code S52.372[A]:** See PDX Collection 1271
> **For code S52.372[B,C]:** See PDX Collection 1269 **For S52.372[K,M,N,P,Q,R]:** See PDX Collection 897

● S52.379   Galeazzi's fracture of unspecified radius A, K, M, N, P, Q, R 🝙, B, C 🝙,
A, B, C 🝙
> (Ex) **For code S52.379[A]:** See PDX Collection 1272
> **For code S52.379[B,C]:** See PDX Collection 1269 **For S52.379[K,M,N,P,Q,R]:** See PDX Collection 897

CHAPTER 19 (S00–T88)

N Newborn Age: 0   **P** Pediatric Age: 0–17   **M** Maternity DX: 9–64   **A** Adult Age: 15–124   ♀ Females Only   ♂ Males Only

🝙 Complication\Comorbidity   🝙 Major C\C   (Ex) CC/MCC Exclusions   🝙 Hospital-Acquired Condition   🝙 Hierarchical Condition Category

1329

CHAPTER 19 (S00-T88)

● S52.38   Bent bone of radius
- ● S52.381   Bent bone of right radius
A, K, M, N, P, Q, R 🔾, B, C 🔾,
A, B, C 🔾
   (Ex:) **For code S52.381[A]:** See PDX Collection 1270
For S52.381[B,C]: See PDX Collection 1269
For S52.381[K,M,N,P,Q,R]: See PDX
Collection 897
- ● S52.382   Bent bone of left radius
A, K, M, N, P, Q, R 🔾, B, C 🔾,
A, B, C 🔾
   (Ex:) **For code S52.382[A]:** See PDX Collection 1271
For S52.382[B,C]: See PDX
Collection 1269 **For S52.382[K,M,N,P,Q,R]:**
See PDX Collection 897
- ● S52.389   Bent bone of unspecified radius
A, K, M, N, P, Q, R 🔾, B, C 🔾,
A, B, C 🔾
   (Ex:) **For code S52.389[A]:** See PDX Collection 1272
For S52.389[B,C]: See PDX
Collection 1269 **For S52.389[K,M,N,P,Q,R]:**
See PDX Collection 897

● S52.39   Other fracture of shaft of radius
- ● S52.391   Other fracture of shaft of radius, right
arm A, K, M, N, P, Q, R 🔾, B, C 🔾,
A, B, C 🔾
   (Ex:) **For code S52.391[A]:** See PDX Collection 1270
For S52.391[B,C]: See PDX Collection 1269
For S52.391[K,M,N,P,Q,R]: See PDX
Collection 897
- ● S52.392   Other fracture of shaft of radius, left
arm A, K, M, N, P, Q, R 🔾, B, C 🔾,
A, B, C 🔾
   (Ex:) **For code S52.392[A]:** See PDX Collection 1271
For S52.392[B,C]: See PDX
Collection 1269 **For S52.392[K,M,N,P,Q,R]:**
See PDX Collection 897
- ● S52.399   Other fracture of shaft of radius,
unspecified arm A, K, M, N, P, Q, R 🔾,
B, C 🔾, A, B, C 🔾
   (Ex:) **For code S52.399[A]:** See PDX Collection 1272
For S52.399[B,C]: See PDX
Collection 1269 **For S52.399[K,M,N,P,Q,R]:**
See PDX Collection 897

● S52.5   Fracture of lower end of radius
Fracture of distal end of radius
   Excludes2   physeal fractures of lower end of radius
(S59.2-)

● S52.50   Unspecified fracture of the lower end of radius
- ● S52.501   Unspecified fracture of the lower end
of right radius A, K, M, N, P, Q, R 🔾,
B, C 🔾, A, B, C 🔾
   (Ex:) **For code S52.501[A]:** See PDX Collection 1270
For S52.501[B,C]: See PDX Collection 1269
For S52.501[K,M,N,P,Q,R]: See PDX
Collection 897
- ● S52.502   Unspecified fracture of the lower end
of left radius A, K, M, N, P, Q, R 🔾,
B, C 🔾, A, B, C 🔾
   (Ex:) **For code S52.502[A]:** See PDX Collection 1271
For S52.502[B,C]: See PDX
Collection 1269 **For S52.502[K,M,N,P,Q,R]:**
See PDX Collection 897
- ● S52.509   Unspecified fracture of the lower end
of unspecified radius
A, K, M, N, P, Q, R 🔾, B, C 🔾,
A, B, C 🔾
   (Ex:) **For code S52.509[A]:** See PDX Collection 1272
For code S52.509[B,C]: See PDX
Collection 1269 **For S52.509[K,M,N,P,Q,R]:**
See PDX Collection 897

● S52.51   Fracture of radial styloid process
- ● S52.511   Displaced fracture of right radial
styloid process A, K, M, N, P, Q, R 🔾,
B, C 🔾, A, B, C 🔾
   (Ex:) **For code S52.511[A]:** See PDX Collection 1270
For S52.511[B,C]: See PDX Collection 1269
For S52.511[K,M,N,P,Q,R]: See PDX
Collection 897
- ● S52.512   Displaced fracture of left radial
styloid process A, K, M, N, P, Q, R 🔾,
B, C 🔾, A, B, C 🔾
   (Ex:) **For code S52.512[A]:** See PDX Collection 1271
For S52.512[B,C]: See PDX
Collection 1269 **For S52.512[K,M,N,P,Q,R]:**
See PDX Collection 897
- ● S52.513   Displaced fracture of unspecified
radial styloid process
A, K, M, N, P, Q, R 🔾, B, C 🔾,
A, B, C 🔾
   (Ex:) **For code S52.513[A]:** See PDX Collection 1272
For S52.513[B,C]: See PDX
Collection 1269 **For S52.513[K,M,N,P,Q,R]:**
See PDX Collection 897
- ● S52.514   Nondisplaced fracture of right radial
styloid process A, K, M, N, P, Q, R 🔾,
B, C 🔾, A, B, C 🔾
   (Ex:) **For code S52.514[A]:** See PDX Collection 1270
For S52.514[B,C]: See PDX Collection 1269
For S52.514[K,M,N,P,Q,R]: See PDX
Collection 897
- ● S52.515   Nondisplaced fracture of left radial
styloid process A, K, M, N, P, Q, R 🔾,
B, C 🔾, A, B, C 🔾
   (Ex:) **For code S52.515[A]:** See PDX Collection 1271
For S52.515[B,C]: See PDX
Collection 1269 **For S52.515[K,M,N,P,Q,R]:**
See PDX Collection 897
- ● S52.516   Nondisplaced fracture of unspecified
radial styloid process
A, K, M, N, P, Q, R 🔾, B, C 🔾,
A, B, C 🔾
   (Ex:) **For code S52.516[A]:** See PDX Collection 1272
For S52.516[B,C]: See PDX
Collection 1269 **For S52.516[K,M,N,P,Q,R]:**
See PDX Collection 897

● S52.52   Torus fracture of lower end of radius
The appropriate 7th character is to be added to
all codes in subcategory S52.52

A	initial encounter for closed fracture
D	subsequent encounter for fracture with routine healing
G	subsequent encounter for fracture with delayed healing
K	subsequent encounter for fracture with nonunion
P	subsequent encounter for fracture with malunion
S	sequela

- ● S52.521   Torus fracture of lower end of right
radius A, K, P 🔾, A 🔾
   (Ex:) **For code S52.521[A]:** See PDX Collection 1270
For S52.521[K,P]: See PDX Collection 897
- ● S52.522   Torus fracture of lower end of left
radius A, K, P 🔾, A 🔾
   (Ex:) **For code S52.522[A]:** See PDX Collection 1271
For S52.522[K,P]: See PDX Collection 897
- ● S52.529   Torus fracture of lower end of
unspecified radius A, K, P 🔾, A 🔾
   (Ex:) **For code S52.529[A]:** See PDX Collection 1272
For S52.529[K,P]: See PDX Collection 897

▶ New   ⇒ Revised   ~~deleted~~ Deleted   Excludes 1   Excludes 2   Includes   Use additional   Code first   Code also   Key words
OGCR Official Guidelines   ● Unacceptable Principal Diagnosis   X Assign placeholder X   🔾 Use Additional Character(s)   ▶ Manifestation Code   **Coding Clinic**

● **S52.53**   Colles' fracture
  ● **S52.531**   Colles' fracture of right radius
     A, K, M, N, P, Q, R 🅒, B, C 🅒🅒,
     A, B, C 🅒🅒
     Ⓔⓧ **For code S52.531[A]:** See PDX Collection 1270
     For S52.531[B,C]: See PDX Collection 1269
     For S52.531[K,M,N,P,Q,R]: See PDX Collection 897

  ● **S52.532**   Colles' fracture of left radius
     A, K, M, N, P, Q, R 🅒, B, C 🅒🅒,
     A, B, C 🅒🅒
     Ⓔⓧ **For code S52.532[A]:** See PDX Collection 1271
     For S52.532[B,C]: See PDX Collection 1269 **For S52.532[K,M,N,P,Q,R]:** See PDX Collection 897
     Coding Clinic: 2016, Q2, P5

  ● **S52.539**   Colles' fracture of unspecified radius
     A, K, M, N, P, Q, R 🅒, B, C 🅒🅒,
     A, B, C 🅒🅒
     Ⓔⓧ **For code S52.539[A]:** See PDX Collection 1272
     For S52.539[B,C]: See PDX Collection 1269 **For S52.539[K,M,N,P,Q,R]:** See PDX Collection 897

● **S52.54**   Smith's fracture
  ● **S52.541**   Smith's fracture of right radius
     A, K, M, N, P, Q, R 🅒, B, C 🅒🅒,
     A, B, C 🅒🅒
     Ⓔⓧ **For code S52.541[A]:** See PDX Collection 1270
     For S52.541[B,C]: See PDX Collection 1269
     For S52.541[K,M,N,P,Q,R]: See PDX Collection 897

  ● **S52.542**   Smith's fracture of left radius
     A, K, M, N, P, Q, R 🅒, B, C 🅒🅒,
     A, B, C 🅒🅒
     Ⓔⓧ **For code S52.542[A]:** See PDX Collection 1271
     For code S52.542[B,C]: See PDX Collection 1269 **For S52.542[K,M,N,P,Q,R]:** See PDX Collection 897

  ● **S52.549**   Smith's fracture of unspecified radius
     A, K, M, N, P, Q, R 🅒, B, C 🅒🅒,
     A, B, C 🅒🅒
     Ⓔⓧ **For code S52.549[A]:** See PDX Collection 1272
     For S52.549[B,C]: See PDX Collection 1269 **For S52.549[K,M,N,P,Q,R]:** See PDX Collection 897

● **S52.55**   Other extraarticular fracture of lower end of radius
  ● **S52.551**   Other extraarticular fracture of lower end of right radius
     A, K, M, N, P, Q, R 🅒, B, C 🅒🅒,
     A, B, C 🅒🅒
     Ⓔⓧ **For code S52.551[A]:** See PDX Collection 1270
     For S52.551[B,C]: See PDX Collection 1269
     For S52.551[K,M,N,P,Q,R]: See PDX Collection 897

  ● **S52.552**   Other extraarticular fracture of lower end of left radius
     A, K, M, N, P, Q, R 🅒, B, C 🅒🅒,
     A, B, C 🅒🅒
     Ⓔⓧ **For code S52.552[A]:** See PDX Collection 1271
     For code S52.552[B,C]: See PDX Collection 1269 **For S52.552[K,M,N,P,Q,R]:** See PDX Collection 897

  ● **S52.559**   Other extraarticular fracture of lower end of unspecified radius
     A, K, M, N, P, Q, R 🅒, B, C 🅒🅒,
     A, B, C 🅒🅒
     Ⓔⓧ **For code S52.559[A]:** See PDX Collection 1272
     For S52.559[B,C]: See PDX Collection 1269 **For S52.559[K,M,N,P,Q,R]:** See PDX Collection 897

● **S52.56**   Barton's fracture
  ● **S52.561**   Barton's fracture of right radius
     A, K, M, N, P, Q, R 🅒, B, C 🅒🅒,
     A, B, C 🅒🅒
     Ⓔⓧ **For code S52.561[A]:** See PDX Collection 1270
     For S52.561[B,C]: See PDX Collection 1269
     For S52.561[K,M,N,P,Q,R]: See PDX Collection 897

  ● **S52.562**   Barton's fracture of left radius
     A, K, M, N, P, Q, R 🅒, B, C 🅒🅒,
     A, B, C 🅒🅒
     Ⓔⓧ **For code S52.562[A]:** See PDX Collection 1271
     For S52.562[B,C]: See PDX Collection 1269 **For S52.562[K,M,N,P,Q,R]:** See PDX Collection 897

  ● **S52.569**   Barton's fracture of unspecified radius
     A, K, M, N, P, Q, R 🅒, B, C 🅒🅒,
     A, B, C 🅒🅒
     Ⓔⓧ **For code S52.569[A]:** See PDX Collection 1272
     For S52.569[B,C]: See PDX Collection 1269 **For S52.569[K,M,N,P,Q,R]:** See PDX Collection 897

● **S52.57**   Other intraarticular fracture of lower end of radius
  ● **S52.571**   Other intraarticular fracture of lower end of right radius
     A, K, M, N, P, Q, R 🅒, B, C 🅒🅒,
     A, B, C 🅒🅒
     Ⓔⓧ **For code S52.571[A]:** See PDX Collection 1270
     For S52.571[B,C]: See PDX Collection 1269
     For S52.571[K,M,N,P,Q,R]: See PDX Collection 897

  ● **S52.572**   Other intraarticular fracture of lower end of left radius
     A, K, M, N, P, Q, R 🅒, B, C 🅒🅒,
     A, B, C 🅒🅒
     Ⓔⓧ **For code S52.572[A]:** See PDX Collection 1271
     For S52.572[B,C]: See PDX Collection 1269 **For S52.572[K,M,N,P,Q,R]:** See PDX Collection 897

  ● **S52.579**   Other intraarticular fracture of lower end of unspecified radius
     A, K, M, N, P, Q, R 🅒, B, C 🅒🅒,
     A, B, C 🅒🅒
     Ⓔⓧ **For code S52.579[A]:** See PDX Collection 1272
     For S52.579[B,C]: See PDX Collection 1269 **For S52.579[K,M,N,P,Q,R]:** See PDX Collection 897

● **S52.59**   Other fractures of lower end of radius
  ● **S52.591**   Other fractures of lower end of right radius A, K, M, N, P, Q, R 🅒, B, C 🅒🅒,
     A, B, C 🅒🅒
     Ⓔⓧ **For code S52.591[A]:** See PDX Collection 1270
     For S52.591[B,C]: See PDX Collection 1269
     For S52.591[K,M,N,P,Q,R]: See PDX Collection 897
     Coding Clinic: 2019, Q3, P10

  ● **S52.592**   Other fractures of lower end of left radius A, K, M, N, P, Q, R 🅒, B, C 🅒🅒,
     A, B, C 🅒🅒
     Ⓔⓧ **For code S52.592[A]:** See PDX Collection 1271
     For S52.592[B,C]: See PDX Collection 1269 **For S52.592[K,M,N,P,Q,R]:** See PDX Collection 897

  ● **S52.599**   Other fractures of lower end of unspecified radius
     A, K, M, N, P, Q, R 🅒, B, C 🅒🅒,
     A, B, C 🅒🅒
     Ⓔⓧ **For code S52.599[A]:** See PDX Collection 1272
     For S52.599[B,C]: See PDX Collection 1269 **For S52.599[K,M,N,P,Q,R]:** See PDX Collection 897

N Newborn Age: 0   **P** Pediatric Age: 0–17   **M** Maternity DX: 9–64   **A** Adult Age: 15–124   ♀ Females Only   ♂ Males Only

🅒 Complication\Comorbidity   🅒🅒 Major C\C   Ⓔⓧ CC/MCC Exclusions   🅗 Hospital-Acquired Condition   🅒 Hierarchical Condition Category

1331

CHAPTER 19 (S00–T88)

- S52.6 Fracture of lower end of ulna
  - S52.60 Unspecified fracture of lower end of ulna
    - S52.601 Unspecified fracture of lower end of right ulna A, K, M, N, P, Q, R 🔵, B, C 🔵, A, B, C 🔵
      - (Ex:) For code S52.601[A]: See PDX Collection 1270
        For S52.601[B,C]: See PDX Collection 1269
        For S52.601[K,M,N,P,Q,R]: See PDX Collection 897
    - S52.602 Unspecified fracture of lower end of left ulna A, K, M, N, P, Q, R 🔵, B, C 🔵, A, B, C 🔵
      - (Ex:) For code S52.602[A]: See PDX Collection 1271
        For code S52.602[B,C]: See PDX Collection 1269 For S52.602[K,M,N,P,Q,R]: See PDX Collection 897
    - S52.609 Unspecified fracture of lower end of unspecified ulna
      A, K, M, N, P, Q, R 🔵, B, C 🔵, A, B, C 🔵
      - (Ex:) For code S52.609[A]: See PDX Collection 1272
        For code S52.609[B,C]: See PDX Collection 1269 For S52.609[K,M,N,P,Q,R]: See PDX Collection 897
  - S52.61 Fracture of ulna styloid process
    - S52.611 Displaced fracture of right ulna styloid process A, K, M, N, P, Q, R 🔵, B, C 🔵, A, B, C 🔵
      - (Ex:) For code S52.611[A]: See PDX Collection 1270
        For S52.611[B,C]: See PDX Collection 1269
        For S52.611[K,M,N,P,Q,R]: See PDX Collection 897
    - S52.612 Displaced fracture of left ulna styloid process A, K, M, N, P, Q, R 🔵, B, C 🔵, A, B, C 🔵
      - (Ex:) For code S52.612[A]: See PDX Collection 1271
        For code S52.612[B,C]: See PDX Collection 1269 For S52.612[K,M,N,P,Q,R]: See PDX Collection 897
    - S52.613 Displaced fracture of unspecified ulna styloid process A, K, M, N, P, Q, R 🔵, B, C 🔵, A, B, C 🔵
      - (Ex:) For code S52.613[A]: See PDX Collection 1272
        For code S52.613[B,C]: See PDX Collection 1269 For S52.613[K,M,N,P,Q,R]: See PDX Collection 897
    - S52.614 Nondisplaced fracture of right ulna styloid process A, K, M, N, P, Q, R 🔵, B, C 🔵, A, B, C 🔵
      - (Ex:) For code S52.614[A]: See PDX Collection 1270
        For S52.614[B,C]: See PDX Collection 1269
        For S52.614[K,M,N,P,Q,R]: See PDX Collection 897
    - S52.615 Nondisplaced fracture of left ulna styloid process A, K, M, N, P, Q, R 🔵, B, C 🔵, A, B, C 🔵
      - (Ex:) For code S52.615[A]: See PDX Collection 1271
        For code S52.615[B,C]: See PDX Collection 1269 For S52.615[K,M,N,P,Q,R]: See PDX Collection 897
    - S52.616 Nondisplaced fracture of unspecified ulna styloid process
      A, K, M, N, P, Q, R 🔵, B, C 🔵, A, B, C 🔵
      - (Ex:) For code S52.616[A]: See PDX Collection 1272
        For code S52.616[B,C]: See PDX Collection 1269 For S52.616[K,M,N,P,Q,R]: See PDX Collection 897

- S52.62 Torus fracture of lower end of ulna

  The appropriate 7th character is to be added to all codes in subcategory S52.62

A	initial encounter for closed fracture
D	subsequent encounter for fracture with routine healing
G	subsequent encounter for fracture with delayed healing
K	subsequent encounter for fracture with nonunion
P	subsequent encounter for fracture with malunion
S	sequela

  - S52.621 Torus fracture of lower end of right ulna A, K, P 🔵, A 🔵
    - (Ex:) For code S52.621[A]: See PDX Collection 1270
      For S52.621[K,P]: See PDX Collection 897
  - S52.622 Torus fracture of lower end of left ulna A, K, P 🔵, A 🔵
    - (Ex:) For code S52.622[A]: See PDX Collection 1271
      For S52.622[K,P]: See PDX Collection 897
  - S52.629 Torus fracture of lower end of unspecified ulna A, K, P 🔵, A 🔵
    - (Ex:) For code S52.629[A]: See PDX Collection 1272
      For S52.629[K,P]: See PDX Collection 897
- S52.69 Other fracture of lower end of ulna
  - S52.691 Other fracture of lower end of right ulna A, K, M, N, P, Q, R 🔵, B, C 🔵, A, B, C 🔵
    - (Ex:) For code S52.691[A]: See PDX Collection 1270
      For S52.691[B,C]: See PDX Collection 1269
      For S52.691[K,M,N,P,Q,R]: See PDX Collection 897
    - **Coding Clinic: 2019, Q3, P10**
  - S52.692 Other fracture of lower end of left ulna A, K, M, N, P, Q, R 🔵, B, C 🔵, A, B, C 🔵
    - (Ex:) For code S52.692[A]: See PDX Collection 1271
      For code S52.692[B,C]: See PDX Collection 1269 For S52.692[K,M,N,P,Q,R]: See PDX Collection 897
  - S52.699 Other fracture of lower end of unspecified ulna
    A, K, M, N, P, Q, R 🔵, B, C 🔵, A, B, C 🔵
    - (Ex:) For code S52.699[A]: See PDX Collection 1272
      For code S52.699[B,C]: See PDX Collection 1269 For S52.699[K,M,N,P,Q,R]: See PDX Collection 897

- S52.9 Unspecified fracture of forearm
  - (Ex:) For category S52.9 CC codes S52.9[A]: See PDX Collection 1272
    For code S52.9[B,C]: See PDX Collection 1269 For S52.9[K,M,N,P,Q,R]: See PDX Collection 897
  - X● S52.90 Unspecified fracture of unspecified forearm A, K, M, N, P, Q, R 🔵, B, C 🔵, A, B, C 🔵
  - X● S52.91 Unspecified fracture of right forearm A, K, M, N, P, Q, R 🔵, B, C 🔵, A, B, C 🔵
  - X● S52.92 Unspecified fracture of left forearm A, K, M, N, P, Q, R 🔵, B, C 🔵, A, B, C 🔵

CHAPTER 19 (S00-T88)

▶ New ⇒ Revised ~~deleted~~ Deleted Excludes 1 Excludes 2 Includes Use additional Code first Code also Key words

OGCR Official Guidelines ● Unacceptable Principal Diagnosis X Assign placeholder X ● Use Additional Character(s) ▶ Manifestation Code **Coding Clinic**

● **S53** Dislocation and sprain of joints and ligaments of elbow

> **Includes** avulsion of joint or ligament of elbow
> laceration of cartilage, joint or ligament of elbow
> sprain of cartilage, joint or ligament of elbow
> traumatic hemarthrosis of joint or ligament of elbow
> traumatic rupture of joint or ligament of elbow
> traumatic subluxation of joint or ligament of elbow
> traumatic tear of joint or ligament of elbow

Code also any associated open wound

> **Excludes2** strain of muscle, fascia and tendon at forearm level (S56.-)

The appropriate 7th character is to be added to each code from category S53

A	initial encounter
D	subsequent encounter
S	sequela

● **S53.0** Subluxation and dislocation of radial head
> Dislocation of radiohumeral joint
> Subluxation of radiohumeral joint
> **Excludes1** Monteggia's fracture-dislocation (S52.27-)

● **S53.00** Unspecified subluxation and dislocation of radial head
- ● **S53.001** Unspecified subluxation of right radial head
- ● **S53.002** Unspecified subluxation of left radial head
- ● **S53.003** Unspecified subluxation of unspecified radial head
- ● **S53.004** Unspecified dislocation of right radial head
- ● **S53.005** Unspecified dislocation of left radial head
- ● **S53.006** Unspecified dislocation of unspecified radial head

● **S53.01** Anterior subluxation and dislocation of radial head
> Anteriomedial subluxation and dislocation of radial head
- ● **S53.011** Anterior subluxation of right radial head
- ● **S53.012** Anterior subluxation of left radial head
- ● **S53.013** Anterior subluxation of unspecified radial head
- ● **S53.014** Anterior dislocation of right radial head
- ● **S53.015** Anterior dislocation of left radial head
- ● **S53.016** Anterior dislocation of unspecified radial head

● **S53.02** Posterior subluxation and dislocation of radial head
> Posteriolateral subluxation and dislocation of radial head
- ● **S53.021** Posterior subluxation of right radial head
- ● **S53.022** Posterior subluxation of left radial head
- ● **S53.023** Posterior subluxation of unspecified radial head
- ● **S53.024** Posterior dislocation of right radial head
- ● **S53.025** Posterior dislocation of left radial head
- ● **S53.026** Posterior dislocation of unspecified radial head

● **S53.03** Nursemaid's elbow
- ● **S53.031** Nursemaid's elbow, right elbow
  Coding Clinic: 2015, Q1, P7-8
- ● **S53.032** Nursemaid's elbow, left elbow
- ● **S53.033** Nursemaid's elbow, unspecified elbow

● **S53.09** Other subluxation and dislocation of radial head
- ● **S53.091** Other subluxation of right radial head
- ● **S53.092** Other subluxation of left radial head
- ● **S53.093** Other subluxation of unspecified radial head
- ● **S53.094** Other dislocation of right radial head
- ● **S53.095** Other dislocation of left radial head
- ● **S53.096** Other dislocation of unspecified radial head

● **S53.1** Subluxation and dislocation of ulnohumeral joint
> Subluxation and dislocation of elbow NOS
> **Excludes1** dislocation of radial head alone (S53.0-)

● **S53.10** Unspecified subluxation and dislocation of ulnohumeral joint
- ● **S53.101** Unspecified subluxation of right ulnohumeral joint
- ● **S53.102** Unspecified subluxation of left ulnohumeral joint
- ● **S53.103** Unspecified subluxation of unspecified ulnohumeral joint
- ● **S53.104** Unspecified dislocation of right ulnohumeral joint
- ● **S53.105** Unspecified dislocation of left ulnohumeral joint
- ● **S53.106** Unspecified dislocation of unspecified ulnohumeral joint

● **S53.11** Anterior subluxation and dislocation of ulnohumeral joint
- ● **S53.111** Anterior subluxation of right ulnohumeral joint
- ● **S53.112** Anterior subluxation of left ulnohumeral joint
- ● **S53.113** Anterior subluxation of unspecified ulnohumeral joint
- ● **S53.114** Anterior dislocation of right ulnohumeral joint
  Coding Clinic: 2012, Q4, P108
- ● **S53.115** Anterior dislocation of left ulnohumeral joint
- ● **S53.116** Anterior dislocation of unspecified ulnohumeral joint

● **S53.12** Posterior subluxation and dislocation of ulnohumeral joint
- ● **S53.121** Posterior subluxation of right ulnohumeral joint
- ● **S53.122** Posterior subluxation of left ulnohumeral joint
- ● **S53.123** Posterior subluxation of unspecified ulnohumeral joint
- ● **S53.124** Posterior dislocation of right ulnohumeral joint
- ● **S53.125** Posterior dislocation of left ulnohumeral joint
- ● **S53.126** Posterior dislocation of unspecified ulnohumeral joint

CHAPTER 19 (S00-T88)

N Newborn Age: 0   **P** Pediatric Age: 0-17   **M** Maternity DX: 9-64   **A** Adult Age: 15-124   ♀ Females Only   ♂ Males Only

Complication\Comorbidity   Major C\C   (Ex) CC/MCC Exclusions   Hospital-Acquired Condition   Hierarchical Condition Category

1333

● S53.13   Medial subluxation and dislocation of
            ulnohumeral joint
    ● S53.131   Medial subluxation of right
                 ulnohumeral joint
    ● S53.132   Medial subluxation of left
                 ulnohumeral joint
    ● S53.133   Medial subluxation of unspecified
                 ulnohumeral joint
    ● S53.134   Medial dislocation of right
                 ulnohumeral joint
    ● S53.135   Medial dislocation of left
                 ulnohumeral joint
    ● S53.136   Medial dislocation of unspecified
                 ulnohumeral joint
● S53.14   Lateral subluxation and dislocation of
            ulnohumeral joint
    ● S53.141   Lateral subluxation of right
                 ulnohumeral joint
    ● S53.142   Lateral subluxation of left
                 ulnohumeral joint
    ● S53.143   Lateral subluxation of unspecified
                 ulnohumeral joint
    ● S53.144   Lateral dislocation of right
                 ulnohumeral joint
    ● S53.145   Lateral dislocation of left
                 ulnohumeral joint
    ● S53.146   Lateral dislocation of unspecified
                 ulnohumeral joint
● S53.19   Other subluxation and dislocation of
            ulnohumeral joint
    ● S53.191   Other subluxation of right
                 ulnohumeral joint
    ● S53.192   Other subluxation of left
                 ulnohumeral joint
    ● S53.193   Other subluxation of unspecified
                 ulnohumeral joint
    ● S53.194   Other dislocation of right
                 ulnohumeral joint
    ● S53.195   Other dislocation of left ulnohumeral
                 joint
    ● S53.196   Other dislocation of unspecified
                 ulnohumeral joint
● S53.2   Traumatic rupture of radial collateral ligament
    Excludes1   sprain of radial collateral ligament NOS
                     (S53.43-)
    X ● S53.20   Traumatic rupture of unspecified radial
                  collateral ligament
    X ● S53.21   Traumatic rupture of right radial collateral
                  ligament
    X ● S53.22   Traumatic rupture of left radial collateral
                  ligament
● S53.3   Traumatic rupture of ulnar collateral ligament
    Excludes1   sprain of ulnar collateral ligament
                     (S53.44-)
    X ● S53.30   Traumatic rupture of unspecified ulnar
                  collateral ligament
    X ● S53.31   Traumatic rupture of right ulnar collateral
                  ligament
    X ● S53.32   Traumatic rupture of left ulnar collateral
                  ligament

● S53.4   Sprain of elbow
    Excludes2   traumatic rupture of radial collateral
                     ligament (S53.2-)
                     traumatic rupture of ulnar collateral
                     ligament (S53.3-)
    ● S53.40   Unspecified sprain of elbow
        ● S53.401   Unspecified sprain of right elbow
        ● S53.402   Unspecified sprain of left elbow
        ● S53.409   Unspecified sprain of unspecified
                     elbow
                     Sprain of elbow NOS
    ● S53.41   Radiohumeral (joint) sprain
        ● S53.411   Radiohumeral (joint) sprain of right
                     elbow
        ● S53.412   Radiohumeral (joint) sprain of left
                     elbow
        ● S53.419   Radiohumeral (joint) sprain of
                     unspecified elbow
    ● S53.42   Ulnohumeral (joint) sprain
        ● S53.421   Ulnohumeral (joint) sprain of right
                     elbow
        ● S53.422   Ulnohumeral (joint) sprain of left
                     elbow
        ● S53.429   Ulnohumeral (joint) sprain of
                     unspecified elbow
    ● S53.43   Radial collateral ligament sprain
        ● S53.431   Radial collateral ligament sprain of
                     right elbow
        ● S53.432   Radial collateral ligament sprain of
                     left elbow
        ● S53.439   Radial collateral ligament sprain of
                     unspecified elbow
    ● S53.44   Ulnar collateral ligament sprain
        ● S53.441   Ulnar collateral ligament sprain of
                     right elbow
        ● S53.442   Ulnar collateral ligament sprain of
                     left elbow
        ● S53.449   Ulnar collateral ligament sprain of
                     unspecified elbow
    ● S53.49   Other sprain of elbow
        ● S53.491   Other sprain of right elbow
        ● S53.492   Other sprain of left elbow
        ● S53.499   Other sprain of unspecified elbow

● S54   Injury of nerves at forearm level
         Code also any associated open wound (S51.-)
         Excludes2   injury of nerves at wrist and hand level (S64.-)
         The appropriate 7th character is to be added to each code from
         category S54

         | A | initial encounter |
         | D | subsequent encounter |
         | S | sequela |

    ● S54.0   Injury of ulnar nerve at forearm level
               Injury of ulnar nerve NOS
        X ● S54.00   Injury of ulnar nerve at forearm level,
                      unspecified arm
        X ● S54.01   Injury of ulnar nerve at forearm level, right arm
        X ● S54.02   Injury of ulnar nerve at forearm level, left arm
    ● S54.1   Injury of median nerve at forearm level
               Injury of median nerve NOS
        X ● S54.10   Injury of median nerve at forearm level,
                      unspecified arm
        X ● S54.11   Injury of median nerve at forearm level, right
                      arm
        X ● S54.12   Injury of median nerve at forearm level, left
                      arm

▶ New   ⯈ Revised   deleted Deleted   Excludes 1   Excludes 2   Includes   Use additional   Code first   Code also   Key words

OGCR Official Guidelines   ● Unacceptable Principal Diagnosis   X Assign placeholder X   ● Use Additional Character(s)   ▷ Manifestation Code   **Coding Clinic**

● S54.2   Injury of radial nerve at forearm level
     Injury of radial nerve NOS
   X ● S54.20   Injury of radial nerve at forearm level, unspecified arm
   X ● S54.21   Injury of radial nerve at forearm level, right arm
   X ● S54.22   Injury of radial nerve at forearm level, left arm

● S54.3   Injury of cutaneous sensory nerve at forearm level
   X ● S54.30   Injury of cutaneous sensory nerve at forearm level, unspecified arm
   X ● S54.31   Injury of cutaneous sensory nerve at forearm level, right arm
   X ● S54.32   Injury of cutaneous sensory nerve at forearm level, left arm

● S54.8   Injury of other nerves at forearm level
   ● S54.8X   Injury of other nerves at forearm level
     ● S54.8X1   Injury of other nerves at forearm level, right arm
     ● S54.8X2   Injury of other nerves at forearm level, left arm
     ● S54.8X9   Injury of other nerves at forearm level, unspecified arm

● S54.9   Injury of unspecified nerve at forearm level
   X ● S54.90   Injury of unspecified nerve at forearm level, unspecified arm
   X ● S54.91   Injury of unspecified nerve at forearm level, right arm
   X ● S54.92   Injury of unspecified nerve at forearm level, left arm

● S55   Injury of blood vessels at forearm level
     Code also any associated open wound (S51.-)
     Excludes2   injury of blood vessels at wrist and hand level (S65.-)
             injury of brachial vessels (S45.1-S45.2)
     The appropriate 7th character is to be added to each code from category S55

A	initial encounter
D	subsequent encounter
S	sequela

● S55.0   Injury of ulnar artery at forearm level
   ● S55.00   Unspecified injury of ulnar artery at forearm level
     ● S55.001   Unspecified injury of ulnar artery at forearm level, right arm A 🌑
       (Ex:) See PDX Collection 1274
     ● S55.002   Unspecified injury of ulnar artery at forearm level, left arm A 🌑
       (Ex:) See PDX Collection 1275
     ● S55.009   Unspecified injury of ulnar artery at forearm level, unspecified arm A 🌑
       (Ex:) See PDX Collection 1276
   ● S55.01   Laceration of ulnar artery at forearm level
     ● S55.011   Laceration of ulnar artery at forearm level, right arm A 🌑
       (Ex:) See PDX Collection 1274
     ● S55.012   Laceration of ulnar artery at forearm level, left arm A 🌑
       (Ex:) See PDX Collection 1275
     ● S55.019   Laceration of ulnar artery at forearm level, unspecified arm A 🌑
       (Ex:) See PDX Collection 1276

● S55.09   Other specified injury of ulnar artery at forearm level
   ● S55.091   Other specified injury of ulnar artery at forearm level, right arm A 🌑
     (Ex:) See PDX Collection 1274
   ● S55.092   Other specified injury of ulnar artery at forearm level, left arm A 🌑
     (Ex:) See PDX Collection 1275
   ● S55.099   Other specified injury of ulnar artery at forearm level, unspecified arm A 🌑
     (Ex:) See PDX Collection 1276

● S55.1   Injury of radial artery at forearm level
   ● S55.10   Unspecified injury of radial artery at forearm level
     ● S55.101   Unspecified injury of radial artery at forearm level, right arm A 🌑
       (Ex:) See PDX Collection 1277
     ● S55.102   Unspecified injury of radial artery at forearm level, left arm A 🌑
       (Ex:) See PDX Collection 1278
     ● S55.109   Unspecified injury of radial artery at forearm level, unspecified arm A 🌑
       (Ex:) See PDX Collection 1279
   ● S55.11   Laceration of radial artery at forearm level
     ● S55.111   Laceration of radial artery at forearm level, right arm A 🌑
       (Ex:) See PDX Collection 1277
     ● S55.112   Laceration of radial artery at forearm level, left arm A 🌑
       (Ex:) See PDX Collection 1278
     ● S55.119   Laceration of radial artery at forearm level, unspecified arm A 🌑
       (Ex:) See PDX Collection 1279
   ● S55.19   Other specified injury of radial artery at forearm level
     ● S55.191   Other specified injury of radial artery at forearm level, right arm A 🌑
       (Ex:) See PDX Collection 1277
     ● S55.192   Other specified injury of radial artery at forearm level, left arm A 🌑
       (Ex:) See PDX Collection 1278
     ● S55.199   Other specified injury of radial artery at forearm level, unspecified arm A 🌑
       (Ex:) See PDX Collection 1279

● S55.2   Injury of vein at forearm level
   ● S55.20   Unspecified injury of vein at forearm level
     ● S55.201   Unspecified injury of vein at forearm level, right arm A 🌑
       (Ex:) See PDX Collection 1260
     ● S55.202   Unspecified injury of vein at forearm level, left arm A 🌑
       (Ex:) See PDX Collection 1261
     ● S55.209   Unspecified injury of vein at forearm level, unspecified arm A 🌑
       (Ex:) See PDX Collection 1262
   ● S55.21   Laceration of vein at forearm level
     ● S55.211   Laceration of vein at forearm level, right arm A 🌑
       (Ex:) See PDX Collection 1260
     ● S55.212   Laceration of vein at forearm level, left arm A 🌑
       (Ex:) See PDX Collection 1261
     ● S55.219   Laceration of vein at forearm level, unspecified arm A 🌑
       (Ex:) See PDX Collection 1262

CHAPTER 19 (S00-T88)

N Newborn Age: 0   **P** Pediatric Age: 0–17   **M** Maternity DX: 9–64   **A** Adult Age: 15–124   ♀ Females Only   ♂ Males Only

🌑 Complication\Comorbidity   🌑 Major C\C   (Ex:) CC/MCC Exclusions   🌑 Hospital-Acquired Condition   🌑 Hierarchical Condition Category   1335

● **S55.29**   Other specified injury of vein at forearm level
    ● **S55.291**   Other specified injury of vein at forearm level, right arm A 🔗
       (Ex:) See PDX Collection 1260
    ● **S55.292**   Other specified injury of vein at forearm level, left arm A 🔗
       (Ex:) See PDX Collection 1261
    ● **S55.299**   Other specified injury of vein at forearm level, unspecified arm A 🔗
       (Ex:) See PDX Collection 1262

● **S55.8**   Injury of other blood vessels at forearm level
   ● **S55.80**   Unspecified injury of other blood vessels at forearm level
    ● **S55.801**   Unspecified injury of other blood vessels at forearm level, right arm A 🔗
       (Ex:) See PDX Collection 1260
    ● **S55.802**   Unspecified injury of other blood vessels at forearm level, left arm A 🔗
       (Ex:) See PDX Collection 1261
    ● **S55.809**   Unspecified injury of other blood vessels at forearm level, unspecified arm A 🔗
       (Ex:) See PDX Collection 1262
   ● **S55.81**   Laceration of other blood vessels at forearm level
    ● **S55.811**   Laceration of other blood vessels at forearm level, right arm A 🔗
       (Ex:) See PDX Collection 1260
    ● **S55.812**   Laceration of other blood vessels at forearm level, left arm A 🔗
       (Ex:) See PDX Collection 1261
    ● **S55.819**   Laceration of other blood vessels at forearm level, unspecified arm A 🔗
       (Ex:) See PDX Collection 1262
   ● **S55.89**   Other specified injury of other blood vessels at forearm level
    ● **S55.891**   Other specified injury of other blood vessels at forearm level, right arm A 🔗
       (Ex:) See PDX Collection 1260
    ● **S55.892**   Other specified injury of other blood vessels at forearm level, left arm A 🔗
       (Ex:) See PDX Collection 1261
    ● **S55.899**   Other specified injury of other blood vessels at forearm level, unspecified arm A 🔗
       (Ex:) See PDX Collection 1262

● **S55.9**   Injury of unspecified blood vessel at forearm level
   ● **S55.90**   Unspecified injury of unspecified blood vessel at forearm level
    ● **S55.901**   Unspecified injury of unspecified blood vessel at forearm level, right arm A 🔗
       (Ex:) See PDX Collection 1260
    ● **S55.902**   Unspecified injury of unspecified blood vessel at forearm level, left arm A 🔗
       (Ex:) See PDX Collection 1261
    ● **S55.909**   Unspecified injury of unspecified blood vessel at forearm level, unspecified arm A 🔗
       (Ex:) See PDX Collection 1262

   ● **S55.91**   Laceration of unspecified blood vessel at forearm level
    ● **S55.911**   Laceration of unspecified blood vessel at forearm level, right arm A 🔗
       (Ex:) See PDX Collection 1260
    ● **S55.912**   Laceration of unspecified blood vessel at forearm level, left arm A 🔗
       (Ex:) See PDX Collection 1261
    ● **S55.919**   Laceration of unspecified blood vessel at forearm level, unspecified arm A 🔗
       (Ex:) See PDX Collection 1262
   ● **S55.99**   Other specified injury of unspecified blood vessel at forearm level
    ● **S55.991**   Other specified injury of unspecified blood vessel at forearm level, right arm A 🔗
       (Ex:) See PDX Collection 1260
    ● **S55.992**   Other specified injury of unspecified blood vessel at forearm level, left arm A 🔗
       (Ex:) See PDX Collection 1261
    ● **S55.999**   Other specified injury of unspecified blood vessel at forearm level, unspecified arm A 🔗
       (Ex:) See PDX Collection 1262

● **S56**   **Injury of muscle, fascia and tendon at forearm level**
   Code also any associated open wound (S51.-)
   Excludes2   injury of muscle, fascia and tendon at or below wrist (S66.-)
           sprain of joints and ligaments of elbow (S53.4-)
   The appropriate 7th character is to be added to each code from category S56

A	initial encounter
D	subsequent encounter
S	sequela

● **S56.0**   Injury of flexor muscle, fascia and tendon of thumb at forearm level
   ● **S56.00**   Unspecified injury of flexor muscle, fascia and tendon of thumb at forearm level
    ● **S56.001**   Unspecified injury of flexor muscle, fascia and tendon of right thumb at forearm level
    ● **S56.002**   Unspecified injury of flexor muscle, fascia and tendon of left thumb at forearm level
    ● **S56.009**   Unspecified injury of flexor muscle, fascia and tendon of unspecified thumb at forearm level
   ● **S56.01**   Strain of flexor muscle, fascia and tendon of thumb at forearm level
    ● **S56.011**   Strain of flexor muscle, fascia and tendon of right thumb at forearm level
    ● **S56.012**   Strain of flexor muscle, fascia and tendon of left thumb at forearm level
    ● **S56.019**   Strain of flexor muscle, fascia and tendon of unspecified thumb at forearm level

- **S56.02**   Laceration of flexor muscle, fascia and tendon of thumb at forearm level
  - **S56.021**   Laceration of flexor muscle, fascia and tendon of right thumb at forearm level A 🔖
    - (Ex:) See PDX Collection 1280
  - **S56.022**   Laceration of flexor muscle, fascia and of left thumb at forearm level A 🔖
    - (Ex:) See PDX Collection 1281
  - **S56.029**   Laceration of flexor muscle, fascia and tendon of unspecified thumb at forearm level A 🔖
    - (Ex:) See PDX Collection 1282
- **S56.09**   Other injury of flexor muscle, fascia and tendon of thumb at forearm level
  - **S56.091**   Other injury of flexor muscle, fascia and tendon of right thumb at forearm level
  - **S56.092**   Other injury of flexor muscle, fascia and tendon of left thumb at forearm level
  - **S56.099**   Other injury of flexor muscle, fascia and tendon of unspecified thumb at forearm level
- **S56.1**   Injury of flexor muscle, fascia and tendon of other and unspecified finger at forearm level
  - **S56.10**   Unspecified injury of flexor muscle, fascia and tendon of other and unspecified finger at forearm level
    - **S56.101**   Unspecified injury of flexor muscle, fascia and tendon of right index finger at forearm level
    - **S56.102**   Unspecified injury of flexor muscle, fascia and tendon of left index finger at forearm level
    - **S56.103**   Unspecified injury of flexor muscle, fascia and tendon of right middle finger at forearm level
    - **S56.104**   Unspecified injury of flexor muscle, fascia and tendon of left middle finger at forearm level
    - **S56.105**   Unspecified injury of flexor muscle, fascia and tendon of right ring finger at forearm level
    - **S56.106**   Unspecified injury of flexor muscle, fascia and tendon of left ring finger at forearm level
    - **S56.107**   Unspecified injury of flexor muscle, fascia and tendon of right little finger at forearm level
    - **S56.108**   Unspecified injury of flexor muscle, fascia and tendon of left little finger at forearm level
    - **S56.109**   Unspecified injury of flexor muscle, fascia and tendon of unspecified finger at forearm level
  - **S56.11**   Strain of flexor muscle, fascia and tendon of other and unspecified finger at forearm level
    - **S56.111**   Strain of flexor muscle, fascia and tendon of right index finger at forearm level
    - **S56.112**   Strain of flexor muscle, fascia and tendon of left index finger at forearm level
    - **S56.113**   Strain of flexor muscle, fascia and tendon of right middle finger at forearm level
    - **S56.114**   Strain of flexor muscle, fascia and tendon of left middle finger at forearm level
    - **S56.115**   Strain of flexor muscle, fascia and tendon of right ring finger at forearm level
    - **S56.116**   Strain of flexor muscle, fascia and tendon of left ring finger at forearm level
    - **S56.117**   Strain of flexor muscle, fascia and tendon of right little finger at forearm level
    - **S56.118**   Strain of flexor muscle, fascia and tendon of left little finger at forearm level
    - **S56.119**   Strain of flexor muscle, fascia and tendon of finger of unspecified finger at forearm level
  - **S56.12**   Laceration of flexor muscle, fascia and tendon of other and unspecified finger at forearm level
    - **S56.121**   Laceration of flexor muscle, fascia and tendon of right index finger at forearm level A 🔖
      - (Ex:) See PDX Collection 1280
    - **S56.122**   Laceration of flexor muscle, fascia and tendon of left index finger at forearm level A 🔖
      - (Ex:) See PDX Collection 1281
    - **S56.123**   Laceration of flexor muscle, fascia and tendon of right middle finger at forearm level A 🔖
      - (Ex:) See PDX Collection 1280
    - **S56.124**   Laceration of flexor muscle, fascia and tendon of left middle finger at forearm level A 🔖
      - (Ex:) See PDX Collection 1281
    - **S56.125**   Laceration of flexor muscle, fascia and tendon of right ring finger at forearm level A 🔖
      - (Ex:) See PDX Collection 1280
    - **S56.126**   Laceration of flexor muscle, fascia and tendon of left ring finger at forearm level A 🔖
      - (Ex:) See PDX Collection 1281
    - **S56.127**   Laceration of flexor muscle, fascia and tendon of right little finger at forearm level A 🔖
      - (Ex:) See PDX Collection 1280
    - **S56.128**   Laceration of flexor muscle, fascia and tendon of left little finger at forearm level A 🔖
      - (Ex:) See PDX Collection 1281
    - **S56.129**   Laceration of flexor muscle, fascia and tendon of unspecified finger at forearm level A 🔖
      - (Ex:) See PDX Collection 1282
  - **S56.19**   Other injury of flexor muscle, fascia and tendon of other and unspecified finger at forearm level
    - **S56.191**   Other injury of flexor muscle, fascia and tendon of right index finger at forearm level
    - **S56.192**   Other injury of flexor muscle, fascia and tendon of left index finger at forearm level
    - **S56.193**   Other injury of flexor muscle, fascia and tendon of right middle finger at forearm level
    - **S56.194**   Other injury of flexor muscle, fascia and tendon of left middle finger at forearm level
    - **S56.195**   Other injury of flexor muscle, fascia and tendon of right ring finger at forearm level

CHAPTER 19 (S00-T88)

N   Newborn Age: 0   **P**   Pediatric Age: 0–17   **M**   Maternity DX: 9–64   **A**   Adult Age: 15–124   ♀   Females Only   ♂   Males Only

🔖 Complication\Comorbidity   🔖 Major C\C   (Ex:) CC/MCC Exclusions   🔖 Hospital-Acquired Condition   🔖 Hierarchical Condition Category

1337
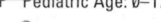

● S56.196   Other injury of flexor muscle, fascia and tendon of left ring finger at forearm level

● S56.197   Other injury of flexor muscle, fascia and tendon of right little finger at forearm level

● S56.198   Other injury of flexor muscle, fascia and tendon of left little finger at forearm level

● S56.199   Other injury of flexor muscle, fascia and tendon of unspecified finger at forearm level

● S56.2   Injury of other flexor muscle, fascia and tendon at forearm level

● S56.20   Unspecified injury of other flexor muscle, fascia and tendon at forearm level

● S56.201   Unspecified injury of other flexor muscle, fascia and tendon at forearm level, right arm

● S56.202   Unspecified injury of other flexor muscle, fascia and tendon at forearm level, left arm

● S56.209   Unspecified injury of other flexor muscle, fascia and tendon at forearm level, unspecified arm

● S56.21   Strain of other flexor muscle, fascia and tendon at forearm level

● S56.211   Strain of other flexor muscle, fascia and tendon at forearm level, right arm

● S56.212   Strain of other flexor muscle, fascia and tendon at forearm level, left arm

● S56.219   Strain of other flexor muscle, fascia and tendon at forearm level, unspecified arm

● S56.22   Laceration of other flexor muscle, fascia and tendon at forearm level

● S56.221   Laceration of other flexor muscle, fascia and tendon at forearm level, right arm A ⬡
    (Ex:) See PDX Collection 1280

● S56.222   Laceration of other flexor muscle, fascia and tendon at forearm level, left arm A ⬡
    (Ex:) See PDX Collection 1281

● S56.229   Laceration of other flexor muscle, fascia and tendon at forearm level, unspecified arm A ⬡
    (Ex:) See PDX Collection 1282

● S56.29   Other injury of other flexor muscle, fascia and tendon at forearm level

● S56.291   Other injury of other flexor muscle, fascia and tendon at forearm level, right arm

● S56.292   Other injury of other flexor muscle, fascia and tendon at forearm level, left arm

● S56.299   Other injury of other flexor muscle, fascia and tendon at forearm level, unspecified arm

● S56.3   Injury of extensor or abductor muscles, fascia and tendons of thumb at forearm level

● S56.30   Unspecified injury of extensor or abductor muscles, fascia and tendons of thumb at forearm level

● S56.301   Unspecified injury of extensor or abductor muscles, fascia and tendons of right thumb at forearm level

● S56.302   Unspecified injury of extensor or abductor muscles, fascia and tendons of left thumb at forearm level

● S56.309   Unspecified injury of extensor or abductor muscles, fascia and tendons of unspecified thumb at forearm level

● S56.31   Strain of extensor or abductor muscles, fascia and tendons of thumb at forearm level

● S56.311   Strain of extensor or abductor muscles, fascia and tendons of right thumb at forearm level

● S56.312   Strain of extensor or abductor muscles, fascia and tendons of left thumb at forearm level

● S56.319   Strain of extensor or abductor muscles, fascia and tendons of unspecified thumb at forearm level

● S56.32   Laceration of extensor or abductor muscles, fascia and tendons of thumb at forearm level

● S56.321   Laceration of extensor or abductor muscles, fascia and tendons of right thumb at forearm level A ⬡
    (Ex:) See PDX Collection 1280

● S56.322   Laceration of extensor or abductor muscles, fascia and tendons of left thumb at forearm level A ⬡
    (Ex:) See PDX Collection 1281

● S56.329   Laceration of extensor or abductor muscles, fascia and tendons of unspecified thumb at forearm level A ⬡
    (Ex:) See PDX Collection 1282

● S56.39   Other injury of extensor or abductor muscles, fascia and tendons of thumb at forearm level

● S56.391   Other injury of extensor or abductor muscles, fascia and tendons of right thumb at forearm level

● S56.392   Other injury of extensor or abductor muscles, fascia and tendons of left thumb at forearm level

● S56.399   Other injury of extensor or abductor muscles, fascia and tendons of unspecified thumb at forearm level

● S56.4   Injury of extensor muscle, fascia and tendon of other and unspecified finger at forearm level

● S56.40   Unspecified injury of extensor muscle, fascia and tendon of other and unspecified finger at forearm level

● S56.401   Unspecified injury of extensor muscle, fascia and tendon of right index finger at forearm level

● S56.402   Unspecified injury of extensor muscle, fascia and tendon of left index finger at forearm level

● S56.403   Unspecified injury of extensor muscle, fascia and tendon of right middle finger at forearm level

● S56.404   Unspecified injury of extensor muscle, fascia and tendon of left middle finger at forearm level

● S56.405   Unspecified injury of extensor muscle, fascia and tendon of right ring finger at forearm level

● S56.406   Unspecified injury of extensor muscle, fascia and tendon of left ring finger at forearm level

● S56.407   Unspecified injury of extensor muscle, fascia and tendon of right little finger at forearm level

● S56.408   Unspecified injury of extensor muscle, fascia and tendon of left little finger at forearm level

● S56.409   Unspecified injury of extensor muscle, fascia and tendon of unspecified finger at forearm level

● S56.41   Strain of extensor muscle, fascia and tendon of other and unspecified finger at forearm level

    ● S56.411   Strain of extensor muscle, fascia and tendon of right index finger at forearm level

    ● S56.412   Strain of extensor muscle, fascia and tendon of left index finger at forearm level

    ● S56.413   Strain of extensor muscle, fascia and tendon of right middle finger at forearm level

    ● S56.414   Strain of extensor muscle, fascia and tendon of left middle finger at forearm level

    ● S56.415   Strain of extensor muscle, fascia and tendon of right ring finger at forearm level

    ● S56.416   Strain of extensor muscle, fascia and tendon of left ring finger at forearm level

    ● S56.417   Strain of extensor muscle, fascia and tendon of right little finger at forearm level

    ● S56.418   Strain of extensor muscle, fascia and tendon of left little finger at forearm level

    ● S56.419   Strain of extensor muscle, fascia and tendon of finger, unspecified finger at forearm level

● S56.42   Laceration of extensor muscle, fascia and tendon of other and unspecified finger at forearm level

    ● S56.421   Laceration of extensor muscle, fascia and tendon of right index finger at forearm level A 🦠
        (Ex:) See PDX Collection 1280

    ● S56.422   Laceration of extensor muscle, fascia and tendon of left index finger at forearm level A 🦠
        (Ex:) See PDX Collection 1281

    ● S56.423   Laceration of extensor muscle, fascia and tendon of right middle finger at forearm level A 🦠
        (Ex:) See PDX Collection 1280

    ● S56.424   Laceration of extensor muscle, fascia and tendon of left middle finger at forearm level A 🦠
        (Ex:) See PDX Collection 1281

    ● S56.425   Laceration of extensor muscle, fascia and tendon of right ring finger at forearm level A 🦠
        (Ex:) See PDX Collection 1280

    ● S56.426   Laceration of extensor muscle, fascia and tendon of left ring finger at forearm level A 🦠
        (Ex:) See PDX Collection 1281

    ● S56.427   Laceration of extensor muscle, fascia and tendon of right little finger at forearm level A 🦠
        (Ex:) See PDX Collection 1280

    ● S56.428   Laceration of extensor muscle, fascia and tendon of left little finger at forearm level A 🦠
        (Ex:) See PDX Collection 1281

    ● S56.429   Laceration of extensor muscle, fascia and tendon of unspecified finger at forearm level A 🦠
        (Ex:) See PDX Collection 1282

● S56.49   Other injury of extensor muscle, fascia and tendon of other and unspecified finger at forearm level

    ● S56.491   Other injury of extensor muscle, fascia and tendon of right index finger at forearm level

    ● S56.492   Other injury of extensor muscle, fascia and tendon of left index finger at forearm level

    ● S56.493   Other injury of extensor muscle, fascia and tendon of right middle finger at forearm level

    ● S56.494   Other injury of extensor muscle, fascia and tendon of left middle finger at forearm level

    ● S56.495   Other injury of extensor muscle, fascia and tendon of right ring finger at forearm level

    ● S56.496   Other injury of extensor muscle, fascia and tendon of left ring finger at forearm level

    ● S56.497   Other injury of extensor muscle, fascia and tendon of right little finger at forearm level

    ● S56.498   Other injury of extensor muscle, fascia and tendon of left little finger at forearm level

    ● S56.499   Other injury of extensor muscle, fascia and tendon of unspecified finger at forearm level

● S56.5   Injury of other extensor muscle, fascia and tendon at forearm level

    ● S56.50   Unspecified injury of other extensor muscle, fascia and tendon at forearm level

      ● S56.501   Unspecified injury of other extensor muscle, fascia and tendon at forearm level, right arm

      ● S56.502   Unspecified injury of other extensor muscle, fascia and tendon at forearm level, left arm

      ● S56.509   Unspecified injury of other extensor muscle, fascia and tendon at forearm level, unspecified arm

    ● S56.51   Strain of other extensor muscle, fascia and tendon at forearm level

      ● S56.511   Strain of other extensor muscle, fascia and tendon at forearm level, right arm

      ● S56.512   Strain of other extensor muscle, fascia and tendon at forearm level, left arm

      ● S56.519   Strain of other extensor muscle, fascia and tendon at forearm level, unspecified arm

    ● S56.52   Laceration of other extensor muscle, fascia and tendon at forearm level

      ● S56.521   Laceration of other extensor muscle, fascia and tendon at forearm level, right arm A 🦠
          (Ex:) See PDX Collection 1280

      ● S56.522   Laceration of other extensor muscle, fascia and tendon at forearm level, left arm A 🦠
          (Ex:) See PDX Collection 1281

      ● S56.529   Laceration of other extensor muscle, fascia and tendon at forearm level, unspecified arm A 🦠
          (Ex:) See PDX Collection 1282

N   Newborn Age: 0   **P**   Pediatric Age: 0–17   **M**   Maternity DX: 9–64   **A**   Adult Age: 15–124   ♀   Females Only   ♂   Males Only

🦠   Complication\Comorbidity   🦠   Major C\C   (Ex:)   CC/MCC Exclusions   🦠   Hospital-Acquired Condition   🦠   Hierarchical Condition Category

1339

- S56.59 **Other** injury of other extensor muscle, fascia and tendon at forearm level
    - S56.591 Other injury of other extensor muscle, fascia and tendon at forearm level, **right** arm
    - S56.592 Other injury of other extensor muscle, fascia and tendon at forearm level, **left** arm
    - S56.599 Other injury of other extensor muscle, fascia and tendon at forearm level, **unspecified** arm
- S56.8 Injury of **other** muscles, fascia and tendons at forearm level
    - S56.80 **Unspecified** injury of other muscles, fascia and tendons at forearm level
        - S56.801 Unspecified injury of other muscles, fascia and tendons at forearm level, **right** arm
        - S56.802 Unspecified injury of other muscles, fascia and tendons at forearm level, **left** arm
        - S56.809 Unspecified injury of other muscles, fascia and tendons at forearm level, **unspecified** arm
    - S56.81 **Strain** of other muscles, fascia and tendons at forearm level
        - S56.811 Strain of other muscles, fascia and tendons at forearm level, **right** arm
        - S56.812 Strain of other muscles, fascia and tendons at forearm level, **left** arm
        - S56.819 Strain of other muscles, fascia and tendons at forearm level, **unspecified** arm
    - S56.82 **Laceration** of other muscles, fascia and tendons at forearm level
        - S56.821 Laceration of other muscles, fascia and tendons at forearm level, **right** arm A
            - (Ex:) See PDX Collection 1280
        - S56.822 Laceration of other muscles, fascia and tendons at forearm level, **left** arm A
            - (Ex:) See PDX Collection 1281
        - S56.829 Laceration of other muscles, fascia and tendons at forearm level, **unspecified** arm A
            - (Ex:) See PDX Collection 1282
    - S56.89 **Other** injury of other muscles, fascia and tendons at forearm level
        - S56.891 Other injury of other muscles, fascia and tendons at forearm level, **right** arm
        - S56.892 Other injury of other muscles, fascia and tendons at forearm level, **left** arm
        - S56.899 Other injury of other muscles, fascia and tendons at forearm level, **unspecified** arm
- S56.9 Injury of **unspecified** muscles, fascia and tendons at forearm level
    - S56.90 **Unspecified** injury of unspecified muscles, fascia and tendons at forearm level
        - S56.901 Unspecified injury of unspecified muscles, fascia and tendons at forearm level, **right** arm
        - S56.902 Unspecified injury of unspecified muscles, fascia and tendons at forearm level, **left** arm
        - S56.909 Unspecified injury of unspecified muscles, fascia and tendons at forearm level, **unspecified** arm

- S56.91 **Strain** of unspecified muscles, fascia and **tendons** at forearm level
    - S56.911 Strain of unspecified muscles, fascia and tendons at forearm level, **right** arm
    - S56.912 Strain of unspecified muscles, fascia and tendons at forearm level, **left** arm
    - S56.919 Strain of unspecified muscles, fascia and tendons at forearm level, **unspecified** arm
- S56.92 **Laceration** of unspecified muscles, fascia and tendons at forearm level
    - S56.921 Laceration of unspecified muscles, fascia and tendons at forearm level, **right** arm A
        - (Ex:) See PDX Collection 1280
    - S56.922 Laceration of unspecified muscles, fascia and tendons at forearm level, **left** arm A
        - (Ex:) See PDX Collection 1281
    - S56.929 Laceration of unspecified muscles, fascia and tendons at forearm level, **unspecified** arm A
        - (Ex:) See PDX Collection 1282
- S56.99 **Other** injury of unspecified muscles, fascia and tendons at forearm level
    - S56.991 Other injury of unspecified muscles, fascia and tendons at forearm level, **right** arm
    - S56.992 Other injury of unspecified muscles, fascia and tendons at forearm level, **left** arm
    - S56.999 Other injury of unspecified muscles, fascia and tendons at forearm level, **unspecified** arm

- S57 **Crushing injury of elbow and forearm**
    Use additional code(s) for all associated injuries
    Excludes2 crushing injury of wrist and hand (S67.-)
    The appropriate 7th character is to be added to each code from category S57

A	initial encounter
D	subsequent encounter
S	sequela

    - S57.0 Crushing injury of **elbow**
        - X S57.00 Crushing injury of **unspecified** elbow
        - X S57.01 Crushing injury of **right** elbow
        - X S57.02 Crushing injury of **left** elbow
    - S57.8 Crushing injury of **forearm**
        - X S57.80 Crushing injury of **unspecified** forearm
        - X S57.81 Crushing injury of **right** forearm
        - X S57.82 Crushing injury of **left** forearm

▶ New ⇒ Revised deleted Deleted Excludes 1 Excludes 2 Includes Use additional Code first Code also Key words
OGCR Official Guidelines ● Unacceptable Principal Diagnosis X Assign placeholder X ● Use Additional Character(s) ▷ Manifestation Code Coding Clinic

● **S58 Traumatic amputation of elbow and forearm**

An amputation not identified as partial or complete should be coded to complete

Excludes1 traumatic amputation of wrist and hand (S68.-)

The appropriate 7th character is to be added to each code from category S58

> A   initial encounter
> D   subsequent encounter
> S   sequela

● **S58.0 Traumatic amputation at elbow level**

  ● **S58.01 Complete traumatic amputation at elbow level**

    ● S58.011   Complete traumatic amputation at elbow level, right arm A 🐷, A, S 🐷🐷
        (Ex:) See PDX Collection 1266

    ● S58.012   Complete traumatic amputation at elbow level, left arm A 🐷, A, S 🐷🐷
        (Ex:) See PDX Collection 1267

    ● S58.019   Complete traumatic amputation at elbow level, unspecified arm A 🐷, A, S 🐷🐷
        (Ex:) See PDX Collection 1268

  ● **S58.02 Partial traumatic amputation at elbow level**

    ● S58.021   Partial traumatic amputation at elbow level, right arm A 🐷, A, S 🐷🐷
        (Ex:) See PDX Collection 1266

    ● S58.022   Partial traumatic amputation at elbow level, left arm A 🐷, A, S 🐷🐷
        (Ex:) See PDX Collection 1267

    ● S58.029   Partial traumatic amputation at elbow level, unspecified arm A 🐷, A, S 🐷🐷
        (Ex:) See PDX Collection 1268

● **S58.1 Traumatic amputation at level between elbow and wrist**

  ● **S58.11 Complete traumatic amputation at level between elbow and wrist**

    ● S58.111   Complete traumatic amputation at level between elbow and wrist, right arm A 🐷, A, S 🐷🐷
        (Ex:) See PDX Collection 1266

    ● S58.112   Complete traumatic amputation at level between elbow and wrist, left arm A 🐷, A, S 🐷🐷
        (Ex:) See PDX Collection 1267

    ● S58.119   Complete traumatic amputation at level between elbow and wrist, unspecified arm A 🐷, A, S 🐷🐷
        (Ex:) See PDX Collection 1268

  ● **S58.12 Partial traumatic amputation at level between elbow and wrist**

    ● S58.121   Partial traumatic amputation at level between elbow and wrist, right arm A 🐷, A, S 🐷🐷
        (Ex:) See PDX Collection 1266

    ● S58.122   Partial traumatic amputation at level between elbow and wrist, left arm A 🐷, A, S 🐷🐷
        (Ex:) See PDX Collection 1267

    ● S58.129   Partial traumatic amputation at level between elbow and wrist, unspecified arm A 🐷, A, S 🐷🐷
        (Ex:) See PDX Collection 1268

● **S58.9 Traumatic amputation of forearm, level unspecified**

Excludes1 traumatic amputation of wrist (S68.-)

  ● **S58.91 Complete traumatic amputation of forearm, level unspecified**

    ● S58.911   Complete traumatic amputation of right forearm, level unspecified A 🐷, A, S 🐷🐷
        (Ex:) See PDX Collection 1266

    ● S58.912   Complete traumatic amputation of left forearm, level unspecified A 🐷, A, S 🐷🐷
        (Ex:) See PDX Collection 1267

    ● S58.919   Complete traumatic amputation of unspecified forearm, level unspecified A 🐷, A, S 🐷🐷
        (Ex:) See PDX Collection 1268

  ● **S58.92 Partial traumatic amputation of forearm, level unspecified**

    ● S58.921   Partial traumatic amputation of right forearm, level unspecified A 🐷, A, S 🐷🐷
        (Ex:) See PDX Collection 1266

    ● S58.922   Partial traumatic amputation of left forearm, level unspecified A 🐷, A, S 🐷🐷
        (Ex:) See PDX Collection 1267

    ● S58.929   Partial traumatic amputation of unspecified forearm, level unspecified A 🐷, A, S 🐷🐷
        (Ex:) See PDX Collection 1268

● **S59 Other and unspecified injuries of elbow and forearm**

Excludes2 other and unspecified injuries of wrist and hand (S69.-)

The appropriate 7th character is to be added to each code from subcategories S59.0, S59.1, and S59.2

> A   initial encounter for closed fracture
> D   subsequent encounter for fracture with routine healing
> G   subsequent encounter for fracture with delayed healing
> K   subsequent encounter for fracture with nonunion
> P   subsequent encounter for fracture with malunion
> S   sequela

● **S59.0 Physeal fracture of lower end of ulna**

  ● **S59.00 Unspecified physeal fracture of lower end of ulna**

    ● S59.001   Unspecified physeal fracture of lower end of ulna, right arm A, K, P 🐷, A 🐷
        (Ex:) **For code S59.001[A]:** See PDX Collection 1270
        For S59.001[K,P]: See PDX Collection 897

    ● S59.002   Unspecified physeal fracture of lower end of ulna, left arm A, K, P 🐷, A 🐷
        (Ex:) **For code S59.002[A]:** See PDX Collection 1271
        For S59.002[K,P]: See PDX Collection 897

    ● S59.009   Unspecified physeal fracture of lower end of ulna, unspecified arm A, K, P 🐷, A 🐷
        (Ex:) **For code S59.009[A]:** See PDX Collection 1272
        For S59.009[K,P]: See PDX Collection 897

  ● **S59.01 Salter-Harris Type I physeal fracture of lower end of ulna**

    ● S59.011   Salter-Harris Type I physeal fracture of lower end of ulna, right arm A, K, P 🐷, A 🐷
        (Ex:) **For code S59.011[A]:** See PDX Collection 1270
        For S59.011[K,P]: See PDX Collection 897

    ● S59.012   Salter-Harris Type I physeal fracture of lower end of ulna, left arm A, K, P 🐷, A 🐷
        (Ex:) **For code S59.012[A]:** See PDX Collection 1271
        For S59.012[K,P]: See PDX Collection 897

    ● S59.019   Salter-Harris Type I physeal fracture of lower end of ulna, unspecified arm A, K, P 🐷, A 🐷
        (Ex:) **For code S59.019[A]:** See PDX Collection 1272
        For S59.019[K,P]: See PDX Collection 897

CHAPTER 19 (S00-T88)

N   Newborn Age: 0   P   Pediatric Age: 0–17   M   Maternity DX: 9–64   A   Adult Age: 15–124   ♀   Females Only   ♂   Males Only

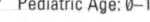 Complication\Comorbidity   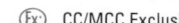 Major C\C   (Ex:) CC/MCC Exclusions   Hospital-Acquired Condition   🐷 Hierarchical Condition Category

1341

Item 19–4   **SALTER-HARRIS TYPE 1:** epiphysis is completely separated from end of bone, or metaphysic growth plate remains attached to epiphysis

    SALTER-HARRIS TYPE 2: epiphysis and growth plate are partially separated from metaphysis, which is cracked—most common type

    SALTER-HARRIS TYPE 3: fracture occurring through epiphysis and separates part of epiphysis and growth plate from metaphysis fracture, usually at distal end of tibia

    SALTER-HARRIS TYPE 4: fracture runs through epiphysis, across growth plate, into metaphysic, surgery is required to restore joint surface to normal and align growth plate

● S59.02   Salter-Harris Type II physeal fracture of lower end of ulna

    ● S59.021   Salter-Harris Type II physeal fracture of lower end of ulna, right arm A, K, P ◌, A ◌
      (Ex:) For code S59.021[A]: See PDX Collection 1270
        For S59.021[K,P]: See PDX Collection 897

    ● S59.022   Salter-Harris Type II physeal fracture of lower end of ulna, left arm A, K, P ◌, A ◌
      (Ex:) For code S59.022[A]: See PDX Collection 1271
        For S59.022[K,P]: See PDX Collection 897

    ● S59.029   Salter-Harris Type II physeal fracture of lower end of ulna, unspecified arm A, K, P ◌, A ◌
      (Ex:) For code S59.029[A]: See PDX Collection 1272
        For S59.029[K,P]: See PDX Collection 897

● S59.03   Salter-Harris Type III physeal fracture of lower end of ulna

    ● S59.031   Salter-Harris Type III physeal fracture of lower end of ulna, right arm A, K, P ◌, A ◌
      (Ex:) For code S59.031[A]: See PDX Collection 1270
        For S59.031[K,P]: See PDX Collection 897

    ● S59.032   Salter-Harris Type III physeal fracture of lower end of ulna, left arm A, K, P ◌, A ◌
      (Ex:) For code S59.032[A]: See PDX Collection 1271
        For S59.032[K,P]: See PDX Collection 897

    ● S59.039   Salter-Harris Type III physeal fracture of lower end of ulna, unspecified arm A, K, P ◌, A ◌
      (Ex:) For code S59.039[A]: See PDX Collection 1272
        For S59.039[K,P]: See PDX Collection 897

● S59.04   Salter-Harris Type IV physeal fracture of lower end of ulna

    ● S59.041   Salter-Harris Type IV physeal fracture of lower end of ulna, right arm A, K, P ◌, A ◌
      (Ex:) For code S59.041[A]: See PDX Collection 1270
        For S59.041[K,P]: See PDX Collection 897

    ● S59.042   Salter-Harris Type IV physeal fracture of lower end of ulna, left arm A, K, P ◌, A ◌
      (Ex:) For code S59.042[A]: See PDX Collection 1271
        For S59.042[K,P]: See PDX Collection 897

    ● S59.049   Salter-Harris Type IV physeal fracture of lower end of ulna, unspecified arm A, K, P ◌, A ◌
      (Ex:) For code S59.049[A]: See PDX Collection 1272
        For S59.049[K,P]: See PDX Collection 897

● S59.09   Other physeal fracture of lower end of ulna

    ● S59.091   Other physeal fracture of lower end of ulna, right arm A, K, P ◌, A ◌
      (Ex:) For code S59.091[A]: See PDX Collection 1270
        For S59.091[K,P]: See PDX Collection 897

    ● S59.092   Other physeal fracture of lower end of ulna, left arm A, K, P ◌, A ◌
      (Ex:) For code S59.092[A]: See PDX Collection 1271
        For S59.092[K,P]: See PDX Collection 897

    ● S59.099   Other physeal fracture of lower end of ulna, unspecified arm A, K, P ◌, A ◌
      (Ex:) For code S59.099[A]: See PDX Collection 1272
        For S59.099[K,P]: See PDX Collection 897

● S59.1   Physeal fracture of upper end of radius
    (Ex:) For category S59.1 CC codes: See PDX Collection 897

    ● S59.10   Unspecified physeal fracture of upper end of radius

      ● S59.101   Unspecified physeal fracture of upper end of radius, right arm K, P ◌

      ● S59.102   Unspecified physeal fracture of upper end of radius, left arm K, P ◌

      ● S59.109   Unspecified physeal fracture of upper end of radius, unspecified arm K, P ◌

    ● S59.11   Salter-Harris Type I physeal fracture of upper end of radius

      ● S59.111   Salter-Harris Type I physeal fracture of upper end of radius, right arm K, P ◌

      ● S59.112   Salter-Harris Type I physeal fracture of upper end of radius, left arm K, P ◌

      ● S59.119   Salter-Harris Type I physeal fracture of upper end of radius, unspecified arm K, P ◌

    ● S59.12   Salter-Harris Type II physeal fracture of upper end of radius

      ● S59.121   Salter-Harris Type II physeal fracture of upper end of radius, right arm K, P ◌

      ● S59.122   Salter-Harris Type II physeal fracture of upper end of radius, left arm K, P ◌

      ● S59.129   Salter-Harris Type II physeal fracture of upper end of radius, unspecified arm K, P ◌

    ● S59.13   Salter-Harris Type III physeal fracture of upper end of radius

      ● S59.131   Salter-Harris Type III physeal fracture of upper end of radius, right arm K, P ◌

      ● S59.132   Salter-Harris Type III physeal fracture of upper end of radius, left arm K, P ◌

      ● S59.139   Salter-Harris Type III physeal fracture of upper end of radius, unspecified arm K, P ◌

    ● S59.14   Salter-Harris Type IV physeal fracture of upper end of radius

      ● S59.141   Salter-Harris Type IV physeal fracture of upper end of radius, right arm K, P ◌

      ● S59.142   Salter-Harris Type IV physeal fracture of upper end of radius, left arm K, P ◌

      ● S59.149   Salter-Harris Type IV physeal fracture of upper end of radius, unspecified arm K, P ◌

▶ New   ⇒ Revised   deleted Deleted   Excludes 1   Excludes 2   Includes   Use additional   Code first   Code also   Key words

OGCR Official Guidelines   ● Unacceptable Principal Diagnosis   X Assign placeholder X   ◌ Use Additional Character(s)   ▷ Manifestation Code   **Coding Clinic**

● S59.19   Other physeal fracture of upper end of radius
   ● S59.191   Other physeal fracture of upper end of radius, right arm K, P 🪙
   ● S59.192   Other physeal fracture of upper end of radius, left arm K, P 🪙
   ● S59.199   Other physeal fracture of upper end of radius, unspecified arm K, P 🪙
● S59.2   Physeal fracture of lower end of radius
  ● S59.20   Unspecified physeal fracture of lower end of radius
   ● S59.201   Unspecified physeal fracture of lower end of radius, right arm A, K, P 🪙, A 🪙
     (Ex:) For code S59.201[A]: See PDX Collection 1270
     For S59.201[K,P]: See PDX Collection 897
   ● S59.202   Unspecified physeal fracture of lower end of radius, left arm A, K, P 🪙, A 🪙
     (Ex:) For code S59.202[A]: See PDX Collection 1271
     For S59.202[K,P]: See PDX Collection 897
   ● S59.209   Unspecified physeal fracture of lower end of radius, unspecified arm A, K, P 🪙, A 🪙
     (Ex:) For code S59.209[A]: See PDX Collection 1272
     For S59.209[K,P]: See PDX Collection 897
  ● S59.21   Salter-Harris Type I physeal fracture of lower end of radius
   ● S59.211   Salter-Harris Type I physeal fracture of lower end of radius, right arm A, K, P 🪙, A 🪙
     (Ex:) For code S59.211[A]: See PDX Collection 1270
     For S59.211[K,P]: See PDX Collection 897
   ● S59.212   Salter-Harris Type I physeal fracture of lower end of radius, left arm A, K, P 🪙, A 🪙
     (Ex:) For code S59.212[A]: See PDX Collection 1271
     For S59.212[K,P]: See PDX Collection 897
   ● S59.219   Salter-Harris Type I physeal fracture of lower end of radius, unspecified arm A, K, P 🪙, A 🪙
     (Ex:) For code S59.219[A]: See PDX Collection 1272
     For S59.219[K,P]: See PDX Collection 897
  ● S59.22   Salter-Harris Type II physeal fracture of lower end of radius
   ● S59.221   Salter-Harris Type II physeal fracture of lower end of radius, right arm A, K, P 🪙, A 🪙
     (Ex:) For code S59.221[A]: See PDX Collection 1270
     For S59.221[K,P]: See PDX Collection 897
   ● S59.222   Salter-Harris Type II physeal fracture of lower end of radius, left arm A, K, P 🪙, A 🪙
     (Ex:) For code S59.222[A]: See PDX Collection 1271
     For S59.222[K,P]: See PDX Collection 897
   ● S59.229   Salter-Harris Type II physeal fracture of lower end of radius, unspecified arm A, K, P 🪙, A 🪙
     (Ex:) For code S59.229[A]: See PDX Collection 1272
     For S59.229[K,P]: See PDX Collection 897
  ● S59.23   Salter-Harris Type III physeal fracture of lower end of radius
   ● S59.231   Salter-Harris Type III physeal fracture of lower end of radius, right arm A, K, P 🪙, A 🪙
     (Ex:) For code S59.231[A]: See PDX Collection 1270
     For S59.231[K,P]: See PDX Collection 897
   ● S59.232   Salter-Harris Type III physeal fracture of lower end of radius, left arm A, K, P 🪙, A 🪙
     (Ex:) For code S59.232[A]: See PDX Collection 1271
     For S59.232[K,P]: See PDX Collection 897
   ● S59.239   Salter-Harris Type III physeal fracture of lower end of radius, unspecified arm A, K, P 🪙, A 🪙
     (Ex:) For code S59.239[A]: See PDX Collection 1272
     For S59.239[K,P]: See PDX Collection 897

● S59.24   Salter-Harris Type IV physeal fracture of lower end of radius
   ● S59.241   Salter-Harris Type IV physeal fracture of lower end of radius, right arm A, K, P 🪙, A 🪙
     (Ex:) For code S59.241[A]: See PDX Collection 1270
     For S59.241[K,P]: See PDX Collection 897
   ● S59.242   Salter-Harris Type IV physeal fracture of lower end of radius, left arm A, K, P 🪙, A 🪙
     (Ex:) For code S59.242[A]: See PDX Collection 1271
     For S59.242[K,P]: See PDX Collection 897
   ● S59.249   Salter-Harris Type IV physeal fracture of lower end of radius, unspecified arm A, K, P 🪙, A 🪙
     (Ex:) For code S59.249[A]: See PDX Collection 1272
     For S59.249[K,P]: See PDX Collection 897
● S59.29   Other physeal fracture of lower end of radius
   ● S59.291   Other physeal fracture of lower end of radius, right arm A, K, P 🪙, A 🪙
     (Ex:) For code S59.291[A]: See PDX Collection 1270
     For S59.291[K,P]: See PDX Collection 897
   ● S59.292   Other physeal fracture of lower end of radius, left arm A, K, P 🪙, A 🪙
     (Ex:) For code S59.292[A]: See PDX Collection 1271
     For S59.292[K,P]: See PDX Collection 897
   ● S59.299   Other physeal fracture of lower end of radius, unspecified arm A, K, P 🪙, A 🪙
     (Ex:) For code S59.299[A]: See PDX Collection 1272
     For S59.299[K,P]: See PDX Collection 897

● S59.8   Other specified injuries of elbow and forearm
  The appropriate 7th character is to be added to each code in subcategory S59.8

    A   initial encounter
    D   subsequent encounter
    S   sequela

  ● S59.80   Other specified injuries of elbow
   ● S59.801   Other specified injuries of right elbow
   ● S59.802   Other specified injuries of left elbow
   ● S59.809   Other specified injuries of unspecified elbow
  ● S59.81   Other specified injuries of forearm
   ● S59.811   Other specified injuries right forearm
   ● S59.812   Other specified injuries left forearm
   ● S59.819   Other specified injuries unspecified forearm
● S59.9   Unspecified injury of elbow and forearm
  The appropriate 7th character is to be added to each code in subcategory S59.9

    A   initial encounter
    D   subsequent encounter
    S   sequela

  ● S59.90   Unspecified injury of elbow
   ● S59.901   Unspecified injury of right elbow
   ● S59.902   Unspecified injury of left elbow
   ● S59.909   Unspecified injury of unspecified elbow
  ● S59.91   Unspecified injury of forearm
   ● S59.911   Unspecified injury of right forearm
   ● S59.912   Unspecified injury of left forearm
   ● S59.919   Unspecified injury of unspecified forearm

CHAPTER 19 (S00-T88)

N   Newborn Age: 0   P   Pediatric Age: 0–17   M   Maternity DX: 9–64   A   Adult Age: 15–124   ♀   Females Only   ♂   Males Only

🪙 Complication\Comorbidity   🪙 Major C\C   (Ex:) CC/MCC Exclusions   🪙 Hospital-Acquired Condition   🪙 Hierarchical Condition Category

1343

INJURIES TO THE WRIST, HAND AND FINGERS (S60-S69)

Excludes2 burns and corrosions (T20-T32)
     frostbite (T33-T34)
     insect bite or sting, venomous (T63.4)

● S60 **Superficial injury of wrist, hand and fingers**
   The appropriate 7th character is to be added to each code from
   category S60

    A initial encounter
    D subsequent encounter
    S sequela

 ● S60.0 **Contusion of finger without damage to nail**
    Excludes1 contusion involving nail (matrix) (S60.1)
 X ● S60.00 Contusion of unspecified finger without
     damage to nail
      Contusion of finger(s) NOS
  ● S60.01 Contusion of thumb without damage to nail
   ● S60.011 Contusion of right thumb without
      damage to nail
   ● S60.012 Contusion of left thumb without
      damage to nail
   ● S60.019 Contusion of unspecified thumb
      without damage to nail
  ● S60.02 Contusion of index finger without damage to
    nail
   ● S60.021 Contusion of right index finger
      without damage to nail
   ● S60.022 Contusion of left index finger without
      damage to nail
   ● S60.029 Contusion of unspecified index finger
      without damage to nail
  ● S60.03 Contusion of middle finger without damage to
    nail
   ● S60.031 Contusion of right middle finger
      without damage to nail
   ● S60.032 Contusion of left middle finger
      without damage to nail
   ● S60.039 Contusion of unspecified middle
      finger without damage to nail
  ● S60.04 Contusion of ring finger without damage to nail
   ● S60.041 Contusion of right ring finger without
      damage to nail
   ● S60.042 Contusion of left ring finger without
      damage to nail
   ● S60.049 Contusion of unspecified ring finger
      without damage to nail
  ● S60.05 Contusion of little finger without damage to
    nail
   ● S60.051 Contusion of right little finger
      without damage to nail
   ● S60.052 Contusion of left little finger without
      damage to nail
   ● S60.059 Contusion of unspecified little finger
      without damage to nail
 ● S60.1 **Contusion of finger with damage to nail**
 X ● S60.10 Contusion of unspecified finger with damage to
    nail
  ● S60.11 Contusion of thumb with damage to nail
   ● S60.111 Contusion of right thumb with
      damage to nail
   ● S60.112 Contusion of left thumb with damage
      to nail
   ● S60.119 Contusion of unspecified thumb with
      damage to nail

  ● S60.12 Contusion of index finger with damage to nail
   ● S60.121 Contusion of right index finger with
      damage to nail
   ● S60.122 Contusion of left index finger with
      damage to nail
   ● S60.129 Contusion of unspecified index finger
      with damage to nail
  ● S60.13 Contusion of middle finger with damage to nail
   ● S60.131 Contusion of right middle finger with
      damage to nail
   ● S60.132 Contusion of left middle finger with
      damage to nail
   ● S60.139 Contusion of unspecified middle
      finger with damage to nail
  ● S60.14 Contusion of ring finger with damage to nail
   ● S60.141 Contusion of right ring finger with
      damage to nail
   ● S60.142 Contusion of left ring finger with
      damage to nail
   ● S60.149 Contusion of unspecified ring finger
      with damage to nail
  ● S60.15 Contusion of little finger with damage to nail
   ● S60.151 Contusion of right little finger with
      damage to nail
   ● S60.152 Contusion of left little finger with
      damage to nail
   ● S60.159 Contusion of unspecified little finger
      with damage to nail
 ● S60.2 **Contusion of wrist and hand**
    Excludes2 contusion of fingers (S60.0-, S60.1-)
  ● S60.21 Contusion of wrist
   ● S60.211 Contusion of right wrist
   ● S60.212 Contusion of left wrist
   ● S60.219 Contusion of unspecified wrist
  ● S60.22 Contusion of hand
   ● S60.221 Contusion of right hand
   ● S60.222 Contusion of left hand
   ● S60.229 Contusion of unspecified hand
 ● S60.3 **Other superficial injuries of thumb**
  ● S60.31 **Abrasion of thumb**
   ● S60.311 Abrasion of right thumb
   ● S60.312 Abrasion of left thumb
   ● S60.319 Abrasion of unspecified thumb
  ● S60.32 **Blister (nonthermal) of thumb**
   ● S60.321 Blister (nonthermal) of right thumb
   ● S60.322 Blister (nonthermal) of left thumb
   ● S60.329 Blister (nonthermal) of unspecified
      thumb
  ● S60.34 **External constriction of thumb**
    Hair tourniquet syndrome of thumb
    Use additional cause code to identify the
     constricting item (W49.0-)
   ● S60.341 External constriction of right thumb
   ● S60.342 External constriction of left thumb
   ● S60.349 External constriction of unspecified
      thumb
  ● S60.35 **Superficial foreign body of thumb**
    Splinter in the thumb
   ● S60.351 Superficial foreign body of right
      thumb
   ● S60.352 Superficial foreign body of left thumb
   ● S60.359 Superficial foreign body of
      unspecified thumb

▶ New ⇒ Revised ~~deleted~~ Deleted Excludes 1 Excludes 2 Includes Use additional Code first Code also Key words
OGCR Official Guidelines ● Unacceptable Principal Diagnosis X Assign placeholder X ● Use Additional Character(s) ▶ Manifestation Code Coding Clinic

- S60.36   Insect bite (nonvenomous) of thumb
  - S60.361   Insect bite (nonvenomous) of right thumb
  - S60.362   Insect bite (nonvenomous) of left thumb
  - S60.369   Insect bite (nonvenomous) of unspecified thumb
- S60.37   Other superficial bite of thumb
  - **Excludes1**   open bite of thumb (S61.05-, S61.15-)
  - S60.371   Other superficial bite of right thumb
  - S60.372   Other superficial bite of left thumb
  - S60.379   Other superficial bite of unspecified thumb
- S60.39   Other superficial injuries of thumb
  - S60.391   Other superficial injuries of right thumb
  - S60.392   Other superficial injuries of left thumb
  - S60.399   Other superficial injuries of unspecified thumb
- S60.4   Other superficial injuries of other fingers
  - S60.41   Abrasion of fingers
    - S60.410   Abrasion of right index finger
    - S60.411   Abrasion of left index finger
    - S60.412   Abrasion of right middle finger
    - S60.413   Abrasion of left middle finger
    - S60.414   Abrasion of right ring finger
    - S60.415   Abrasion of left ring finger
    - S60.416   Abrasion of right little finger
    - S60.417   Abrasion of left little finger
    - S60.418   Abrasion of other finger
      Abrasion of specified finger with unspecified laterality
    - S60.419   Abrasion of unspecified finger
  - S60.42   Blister (nonthermal) of fingers
    - S60.420   Blister (nonthermal) of right index finger
    - S60.421   Blister (nonthermal) of left index finger
    - S60.422   Blister (nonthermal) of right middle finger
    - S60.423   Blister (nonthermal) of left middle finger
    - S60.424   Blister (nonthermal) of right ring finger
    - S60.425   Blister (nonthermal) of left ring finger
    - S60.426   Blister (nonthermal) of right little finger
    - S60.427   Blister (nonthermal) of left little finger
    - S60.428   Blister (nonthermal) of other finger
      Blister (nonthermal) of specified finger with unspecified laterality
    - S60.429   Blister (nonthermal) of unspecified finger
  - S60.44   External constriction of fingers
    Hair tourniquet syndrome of finger
    Use additional cause code to identify the constricting item (W49.0-)
    - S60.440   External constriction of right index finger
    - S60.441   External constriction of left index finger
    - S60.442   External constriction of right middle finger
    - S60.443   External constriction of left middle finger
    - S60.444   External constriction of right ring finger
    - S60.445   External constriction of left ring finger
    - S60.446   External constriction of right little finger
    - S60.447   External constriction of left little finger
    - S60.448   External constriction of other finger
      External constriction of specified finger with unspecified laterality
    - S60.449   External constriction of unspecified finger
  - S60.45   Superficial foreign body of fingers
    Splinter in the finger(s)
    - S60.450   Superficial foreign body of right index finger
    - S60.451   Superficial foreign body of left index finger
    - S60.452   Superficial foreign body of right middle finger
    - S60.453   Superficial foreign body of left middle finger
    - S60.454   Superficial foreign body of right ring finger
    - S60.455   Superficial foreign body of left ring finger
    - S60.456   Superficial foreign body of right little finger
    - S60.457   Superficial foreign body of left little finger
    - S60.458   Superficial foreign body of other finger
      Superficial foreign body of specified finger with unspecified laterality
    - S60.459   Superficial foreign body of unspecified finger
  - S60.46   Insect bite (nonvenomous) of fingers
    - S60.460   Insect bite (nonvenomous) of right index finger
    - S60.461   Insect bite (nonvenomous) of left index finger
    - S60.462   Insect bite (nonvenomous) of right middle finger
    - S60.463   Insect bite (nonvenomous) of left middle finger
    - S60.464   Insect bite (nonvenomous) of right ring finger
    - S60.465   Insect bite (nonvenomous) of left ring finger
    - S60.466   Insect bite (nonvenomous) of right little finger
    - S60.467   Insect bite (nonvenomous) of left little finger
    - S60.468   Insect bite (nonvenomous) of other finger
      Insect bite (nonvenomous) of specified finger with unspecified laterality
    - S60.469   Insect bite (nonvenomous) of unspecified finger

N Newborn Age: 0   **P** Pediatric Age: 0–17   **M** Maternity DX: 9–64   **A** Adult Age: 15–124   ♀ Females Only   ♂ Males Only

Complication\Comorbidity   Major C\C   (Ex) CC/MCC Exclusions   Hospital-Acquired Condition   Hierarchical Condition Category

1345

CHAPTER 19 (S00-T88)

● **S60.47**   Other superficial bite of fingers
       Excludes1   open bite of fingers (S61.25-, S61.35-)
    ● **S60.470**   Other superficial bite of right index finger
    ● **S60.471**   Other superficial bite of left index finger
    ● **S60.472**   Other superficial bite of right middle finger
    ● **S60.473**   Other superficial bite of left middle finger
    ● **S60.474**   Other superficial bite of right ring finger
    ● **S60.475**   Other superficial bite of left ring finger
    ● **S60.476**   Other superficial bite of right little finger
    ● **S60.477**   Other superficial bite of left little finger
    ● **S60.478**   Other superficial bite of other finger
        Other superficial bite of specified finger with unspecified laterality
    ● **S60.479**   Other superficial bite of unspecified finger

● **S60.5**   Other superficial injuries of hand
       Excludes2   superficial injuries of fingers (S60.3-, S60.4-)
  ● **S60.51**   Abrasion of hand
    ● **S60.511**   Abrasion of right hand
    ● **S60.512**   Abrasion of left hand
    ● **S60.519**   Abrasion of unspecified hand
  ● **S60.52**   Blister (nonthermal) of hand
    ● **S60.521**   Blister (nonthermal) of right hand
    ● **S60.522**   Blister (nonthermal) of left hand
    ● **S60.529**   Blister (nonthermal) of unspecified hand
  ● **S60.54**   External constriction of hand
    ● **S60.541**   External constriction of right hand
    ● **S60.542**   External constriction of left hand
    ● **S60.549**   External constriction of unspecified hand
  ● **S60.55**   Superficial foreign body of hand
       Splinter in the hand
    ● **S60.551**   Superficial foreign body of right hand
    ● **S60.552**   Superficial foreign body of left hand
    ● **S60.559**   Superficial foreign body of unspecified hand
  ● **S60.56**   Insect bite (nonvenomous) of hand
    ● **S60.561**   Insect bite (nonvenomous) of right hand
    ● **S60.562**   Insect bite (nonvenomous) of left hand
    ● **S60.569**   Insect bite (nonvenomous) of unspecified hand
  ● **S60.57**   Other superficial bite of hand
       Excludes1   open bite of hand (S61.45-)
    ● **S60.571**   Other superficial bite of hand of right hand
    ● **S60.572**   Other superficial bite of hand of left hand
    ● **S60.579**   Other superficial bite of hand of unspecified hand

● **S60.8**   Other superficial injuries of wrist
  ● **S60.81**   Abrasion of wrist
    ● **S60.811**   Abrasion of right wrist
    ● **S60.812**   Abrasion of left wrist
    ● **S60.819**   Abrasion of unspecified wrist
  ● **S60.82**   Blister (nonthermal) of wrist
    ● **S60.821**   Blister (nonthermal) of right wrist
    ● **S60.822**   Blister (nonthermal) of left wrist
    ● **S60.829**   Blister (nonthermal) of unspecified wrist
  ● **S60.84**   External constriction of wrist
    ● **S60.841**   External constriction of right wrist
    ● **S60.842**   External constriction of left wrist
    ● **S60.849**   External constriction of unspecified wrist
  ● **S60.85**   Superficial foreign body of wrist
       Splinter in the wrist
    ● **S60.851**   Superficial foreign body of right wrist
    ● **S60.852**   Superficial foreign body of left wrist
    ● **S60.859**   Superficial foreign body of unspecified wrist
  ● **S60.86**   Insect bite (nonvenomous) of wrist
    ● **S60.861**   Insect bite (nonvenomous) of right wrist
    ● **S60.862**   Insect bite (nonvenomous) of left wrist
    ● **S60.869**   Insect bite (nonvenomous) of unspecified wrist
  ● **S60.87**   Other superficial bite of wrist
       Excludes1   open bite of wrist (S61.55)
    ● **S60.871**   Other superficial bite of right wrist
    ● **S60.872**   Other superficial bite of left wrist
    ● **S60.879**   Other superficial bite of unspecified wrist

● **S60.9**   Unspecified superficial injury of wrist, hand and fingers
  ● **S60.91**   Unspecified superficial injury of wrist
    ● **S60.911**   Unspecified superficial injury of right wrist
    ● **S60.912**   Unspecified superficial injury of left wrist
    ● **S60.919**   Unspecified superficial injury of unspecified wrist
  ● **S60.92**   Unspecified superficial injury of hand
    ● **S60.921**   Unspecified superficial injury of right hand
    ● **S60.922**   Unspecified superficial injury of left hand
    ● **S60.929**   Unspecified superficial injury of unspecified hand
  ● **S60.93**   Unspecified superficial injury of thumb
    ● **S60.931**   Unspecified superficial injury of right thumb
    ● **S60.932**   Unspecified superficial injury of left thumb
    ● **S60.939**   Unspecified superficial injury of unspecified thumb

▶ New   ⇒ Revised   ~~deleted~~ Deleted   Excludes 1   Excludes 2   Includes   Use additional   Code first   Code also   Key words
OGCR Official Guidelines   ● Unacceptable Principal Diagnosis   X Assign placeholder X   ● Use Additional Character(s)   ▶ Manifestation Code   Coding Clinic

- **S60.94** Unspecified superficial injury of other fingers
  - **S60.940** Unspecified superficial injury of right index finger
  - **S60.941** Unspecified superficial injury of left index finger
  - **S60.942** Unspecified superficial injury of right middle finger
  - **S60.943** Unspecified superficial injury of left middle finger
  - **S60.944** Unspecified superficial injury of right ring finger
  - **S60.945** Unspecified superficial injury of left ring finger
  - **S60.946** Unspecified superficial injury of right little finger
  - **S60.947** Unspecified superficial injury of left little finger
  - **S60.948** Unspecified superficial injury of other finger
    > Unspecified superficial injury of specified finger with unspecified laterality
  - **S60.949** Unspecified superficial injury of unspecified finger

- **S61** **Open wound of wrist, hand and fingers**
  > Code also any associated wound infection
  > **Excludes1**   open fracture of wrist, hand and finger (S62.- with 7th character B)
  > traumatic amputation of wrist and hand (S68.-)
  >
  > The appropriate 7th character is to be added to each code from category S61
  >
  > | | |
  > |---|---|
  > | A | initial encounter |
  > | D | subsequent encounter |
  > | S | sequela |

  - **S61.0** Open wound of thumb without damage to nail
    > **Excludes1**   open wound of thumb with damage to nail (S61.1-)
    - **S61.00** Unspecified open wound of thumb without damage to nail
      - **S61.001** Unspecified open wound of right thumb without damage to nail
      - **S61.002** Unspecified open wound of left thumb without damage to nail
      - **S61.009** Unspecified open wound of unspecified thumb without damage to nail
    - **S61.01** Laceration without foreign body of thumb without damage to nail
      - **S61.011** Laceration without foreign body of right thumb without damage to nail
      - **S61.012** Laceration without foreign body of left thumb without damage to nail
      - **S61.019** Laceration without foreign body of unspecified thumb without damage to nail
    - **S61.02** Laceration with foreign body of thumb without damage to nail
      - **S61.021** Laceration with foreign body of right thumb without damage to nail
      - **S61.022** Laceration with foreign body of left thumb without damage to nail
      - **S61.029** Laceration with foreign body of unspecified thumb without damage to nail

  - **S61.03** Puncture wound without foreign body of thumb without damage to nail
    - **S61.031** Puncture wound without foreign body of right thumb without damage to nail
    - **S61.032** Puncture wound without foreign body of left thumb without damage to nail
    - **S61.039** Puncture wound without foreign body of unspecified thumb without damage to nail
  - **S61.04** Puncture wound with foreign body of thumb without damage to nail
    - **S61.041** Puncture wound with foreign body of right thumb without damage to nail
    - **S61.042** Puncture wound with foreign body of left thumb without damage to nail
    - **S61.049** Puncture wound with foreign body of unspecified thumb without damage to nail
  - **S61.05** Open bite of thumb without damage to nail
    > Bite of thumb NOS
    > **Excludes1**   superficial bite of thumb (S60.36-, S60.37-)
    - **S61.051** Open bite of right thumb without damage to nail
    - **S61.052** Open bite of left thumb without damage to nail
    - **S61.059** Open bite of unspecified thumb without damage to nail

  - **S61.1** Open wound of thumb with damage to nail
    - **S61.10** Unspecified open wound of thumb with damage to nail
      - **S61.101** Unspecified open wound of right thumb with damage to nail
      - **S61.102** Unspecified open wound of left thumb with damage to nail
      - **S61.109** Unspecified open wound of unspecified thumb with damage to nail
    - **S61.11** Laceration without foreign body of thumb with damage to nail
      - **S61.111** Laceration without foreign body of right thumb with damage to nail
      - **S61.112** Laceration without foreign body of left thumb with damage to nail
      - **S61.119** Laceration without foreign body of unspecified thumb with damage to nail
    - **S61.12** Laceration with foreign body of thumb with damage to nail
      - **S61.121** Laceration with foreign body of right thumb with damage to nail
      - **S61.122** Laceration with foreign body of left thumb with damage to nail
      - **S61.129** Laceration with foreign body of unspecified thumb with damage to nail
    - **S61.13** Puncture wound without foreign body of thumb with damage to nail
      - **S61.131** Puncture wound without foreign body of right thumb with damage to nail
      - **S61.132** Puncture wound without foreign body of left thumb with damage to nail
      - **S61.139** Puncture wound without foreign body of unspecified thumb with damage to nail

N Newborn Age: 0   **P** Pediatric Age: 0–17   **M** Maternity DX: 9–64   **A** Adult Age: 15–124   ♀ Females Only   ♂ Males Only

🏷 Complication\Comorbidity   🏷 Major C\C   (Ex) CC/MCC Exclusions   🏷 Hospital-Acquired Condition   🏷 Hierarchical Condition Category

1347

● **S61.14**   **Puncture wound with foreign body** of thumb with damage to nail

     ● **S61.141**   Puncture wound with foreign body of **right** thumb with damage to nail

     ● **S61.142**   Puncture wound with foreign body of **left** thumb with damage to nail

     ● **S61.149**   Puncture wound with foreign body of **unspecified** thumb with damage to nail

● **S61.15**   Open bite of **thumb** with damage to nail

     Bite of thumb with damage to nail NOS

     Excludes1   superficial bite of thumb (S60.36-, S60.37-)

     ● **S61.151**   Open bite of **right** thumb with damage to nail

     ● **S61.152**   Open bite of **left** thumb with damage to nail

     ● **S61.159**   Open bite of **unspecified** thumb with damage to nail

● **S61.2**   Open wound of **other finger without damage to nail**

     Excludes1   open wound of finger involving nail (matrix) (S61.3-)

     Excludes2   open wound of thumb without damage to nail (S61.0-)

     ● **S61.20**   **Unspecified** open wound of other finger without damage to nail

         ● **S61.200**   Unspecified open wound of **right index** finger without damage to nail

         ● **S61.201**   Unspecified open wound of **left index** finger without damage to nail

         ● **S61.202**   Unspecified open wound of **right middle** finger without damage to nail

         ● **S61.203**   Unspecified open wound of **left middle** finger without damage to nail

         ● **S61.204**   Unspecified open wound of **right ring** finger without damage to nail

         ● **S61.205**   Unspecified open wound of **left ring** finger without damage to nail

         ● **S61.206**   Unspecified open wound of **right little** finger without damage to nail

         ● **S61.207**   Unspecified open wound of **left little** finger without damage to nail

         ● **S61.208**   Unspecified open wound of **other** finger without damage to nail

            Unspecified open wound of specified finger with unspecified laterality without damage to nail

         ● **S61.209**   Unspecified open wound of **unspecified** finger without damage to nail

     ● **S61.21**   **Laceration without foreign body** of finger without damage to nail

         ● **S61.210**   Laceration without foreign body of **right index** finger without damage to nail

         ● **S61.211**   Laceration without foreign body of **left index** finger without damage to nail

         ● **S61.212**   Laceration without foreign body of **right middle** finger without damage to nail

         ● **S61.213**   Laceration without foreign body of **left middle** finger without damage to nail

         ● **S61.214**   Laceration without foreign body of **right ring** finger without damage to nail

         ● **S61.215**   Laceration without foreign body of **left ring** finger without damage to nail

         ● **S61.216**   Laceration without foreign body of **right little** finger without damage to nail

         ● **S61.217**   Laceration without foreign body of **left little** finger without damage to nail

         ● **S61.218**   Laceration without foreign body of **other** finger without damage to nail

            Laceration without foreign body of specified finger with unspecified laterality without damage to nail

         ● **S61.219**   Laceration without foreign body of **unspecified** finger without damage to nail

     ● **S61.22**   Laceration **with foreign body** of finger without damage to nail

         ● **S61.220**   Laceration with foreign body of **right index** finger without damage to nail

         ● **S61.221**   Laceration with foreign body of **left index** finger without damage to nail

         ● **S61.222**   Laceration with foreign body of **right middle** finger without damage to nail

         ● **S61.223**   Laceration with foreign body of **left middle** finger without damage to nail

         ● **S61.224**   Laceration with foreign body of **right ring** finger without damage to nail

         ● **S61.225**   Laceration with foreign body of **left ring** finger without damage to nail

         ● **S61.226**   Laceration with foreign body of **right little** finger without damage to nail

         ● **S61.227**   Laceration with foreign body of **left little** finger without damage to nail

         ● **S61.228**   Laceration with foreign body of **other** finger without damage to nail

            Laceration with foreign body of specified finger with unspecified laterality without damage to nail

         ● **S61.229**   Laceration with foreign body of **unspecified** finger without damage to nail

     ● **S61.23**   Puncture wound **without foreign body** of finger without damage to nail

         ● **S61.230**   Puncture wound without foreign body of **right index** finger without damage to nail

         ● **S61.231**   Puncture wound without foreign body of **left index** finger without damage to nail

         ● **S61.232**   Puncture wound without foreign body of **right middle** finger without damage to nail

         ● **S61.233**   Puncture wound without foreign body of **left middle** finger without damage to nail

         ● **S61.234**   Puncture wound without foreign body of **right ring** finger without damage to nail

         ● **S61.235**   Puncture wound without foreign body of **left ring** finger without damage to nail

         ● **S61.236**   Puncture wound without foreign body of **right little** finger without damage to nail

         ● **S61.237**   Puncture wound without foreign body of **left little** finger without damage to nail

         ● **S61.238**   Puncture wound without foreign body of **other** finger without damage to nail

            Puncture wound without foreign body of specified finger with unspecified laterality without damage to nail

         ● **S61.239**   Puncture wound without foreign body of **unspecified** finger without damage to nail

▶ New   ⮞ Revised   ~~deleted~~ Deleted   Excludes 1   Excludes 2   Includes   Use additional   Code first   Code also   Key words

OGCR Official Guidelines   ● Unacceptable Principal Diagnosis   X Assign placeholder X   ● Use Additional Character(s)   ▶ Manifestation Code   Coding Clinic

● **S61.24**   Puncture wound with foreign body of finger without damage to nail

   ● S61.240   Puncture wound with foreign body of right index finger without damage to nail

   ● S61.241   Puncture wound with foreign body of left index finger without damage to nail

   ● S61.242   Puncture wound with foreign body of right middle finger without damage to nail

   ● S61.243   Puncture wound with foreign body of left middle finger without damage to nail

   ● S61.244   Puncture wound with foreign body of right ring finger without damage to nail

   ● S61.245   Puncture wound with foreign body of left ring finger without damage to nail

   ● S61.246   Puncture wound with foreign body of right little finger without damage to nail

   ● S61.247   Puncture wound with foreign body of left little finger without damage to nail

   ● S61.248   Puncture wound with foreign body of other finger without damage to nail
      Puncture wound with foreign body of specified finger with unspecified laterality without damage to nail

   ● S61.249   Puncture wound with foreign body of unspecified finger without damage to nail

● **S61.25**   Open bite of finger without damage to nail
     Bite of finger without damage to nail NOS

    Excludes1   superficial bite of finger (S60.46-, S60.47-)

   ● S61.250   Open bite of right index finger without damage to nail

   ● S61.251   Open bite of left index finger without damage to nail

   ● S61.252   Open bite of right middle finger without damage to nail

   ● S61.253   Open bite of left middle finger without damage to nail

   ● S61.254   Open bite of right ring finger without damage to nail

   ● S61.255   Open bite of left ring finger without damage to nail

   ● S61.256   Open bite of right little finger without damage to nail

   ● S61.257   Open bite of left little finger without damage to nail

   ● S61.258   Open bite of other finger without damage to nail
      Open bite of specified finger with unspecified laterality without damage to nail

   ● S61.259   Open bite of unspecified finger without damage to nail

● **S61.3**   Open wound of other finger with damage to nail

  ● **S61.30**   Unspecified open wound of finger with damage to nail

   ● S61.300   Unspecified open wound of right index finger with damage to nail

   ● S61.301   Unspecified open wound of left index finger with damage to nail

   ● S61.302   Unspecified open wound of right middle finger with damage to nail

   ● S61.303   Unspecified open wound of left middle finger with damage to nail

   ● S61.304   Unspecified open wound of right ring finger with damage to nail

   ● S61.305   Unspecified open wound of left ring finger with damage to nail

   ● S61.306   Unspecified open wound of right little finger with damage to nail

   ● S61.307   Unspecified open wound of left little finger with damage to nail

   ● S61.308   Unspecified open wound of other finger with damage to nail
      Unspecified open wound of specified finger with unspecified laterality with damage to nail

   ● S61.309   Unspecified open wound of unspecified finger with damage to nail

  ● **S61.31**   Laceration without foreign body of finger with damage to nail

   ● S61.310   Laceration without foreign body of right index finger with damage to nail

   ● S61.311   Laceration without foreign body of left index finger with damage to nail

   ● S61.312   Laceration without foreign body of right middle finger with damage to nail

   ● S61.313   Laceration without foreign body of left middle finger with damage to nail

   ● S61.314   Laceration without foreign body of right ring finger with damage to nail

   ● S61.315   Laceration without foreign body of left ring finger with damage to nail

   ● S61.316   Laceration without foreign body of right little finger with damage to nail

   ● S61.317   Laceration without foreign body of left little finger with damage to nail

   ● S61.318   Laceration without foreign body of other finger with damage to nail
      Laceration without foreign body of specified finger with unspecified laterality with damage to nail

   ● S61.319   Laceration without foreign body of unspecified finger with damage to nail

  ● **S61.32**   Laceration with foreign body of finger with damage to nail

   ● S61.320   Laceration with foreign body of right index finger with damage to nail

   ● S61.321   Laceration with foreign body of left index finger with damage to nail

   ● S61.322   Laceration with foreign body of right middle finger with damage to nail

N Newborn Age: 0   **P** Pediatric Age: 0–17   **M** Maternity DX: 9–64   **A** Adult Age: 15–124   ♀ Females Only   ♂ Males Only

🅒 Complication\Comorbidity   🅒 Major C\C   (Ex) CC/MCC Exclusions   🅒 Hospital-Acquired Condition   🅒 Hierarchical Condition Category

1349

● S61.323   Laceration with foreign body of left middle finger with damage to nail

● S61.324   Laceration with foreign body of right ring finger with damage to nail

● S61.325   Laceration with foreign body of left ring finger with damage to nail

● S61.326   Laceration with foreign body of right little finger with damage to nail

● S61.327   Laceration with foreign body of left little finger with damage to nail

● S61.328   Laceration with foreign body of other finger with damage to nail
             Laceration with foreign body of specified finger with unspecified laterality with damage to nail

● S61.329   Laceration with foreign body of unspecified finger with damage to nail

● S61.33   Puncture wound without foreign body of finger with damage to nail

● S61.330   Puncture wound without foreign body of right index finger with damage to nail

● S61.331   Puncture wound without foreign body of left index finger with damage to nail

● S61.332   Puncture wound without foreign body of right middle finger with damage to nail

● S61.333   Puncture wound without foreign body of left middle finger with damage to nail

● S61.334   Puncture wound without foreign body of right ring finger with damage to nail

● S61.335   Puncture wound without foreign body of left ring finger with damage to nail

● S61.336   Puncture wound without foreign body of right little finger with damage to nail

● S61.337   Puncture wound without foreign body of left little finger with damage to nail

● S61.338   Puncture wound without foreign body of other finger with damage to nail
             Puncture wound without foreign body of specified finger with unspecified laterality with damage to nail

● S61.339   Puncture wound without foreign body of unspecified finger with damage to nail

● S61.34   Puncture wound with foreign body of finger with damage to nail

● S61.340   Puncture wound with foreign body of right index finger with damage to nail

● S61.341   Puncture wound with foreign body of left index finger with damage to nail

● S61.342   Puncture wound with foreign body of right middle finger with damage to nail

● S61.343   Puncture wound with foreign body of left middle finger with damage to nail

● S61.344   Puncture wound with foreign body of right ring finger with damage to nail

● S61.345   Puncture wound with foreign body of left ring finger with damage to nail

● S61.346   Puncture wound with foreign body of right little finger with damage to nail

● S61.347   Puncture wound with foreign body of left little finger with damage to nail

● S61.348   Puncture wound with foreign body of other finger with damage to nail
             Puncture wound with foreign body of specified finger with unspecified laterality with damage to nail

● S61.349   Puncture wound with foreign body of unspecified finger with damage to nail

● S61.35   Open bite of finger with damage to nail
            Bite of finger with damage to nail NOS

            Excludes1   superficial bite of finger (S60.46-, S60.47-)

● S61.350   Open bite of right index finger with damage to nail

● S61.351   Open bite of left index finger with damage to nail

● S61.352   Open bite of right middle finger with damage to nail

● S61.353   Open bite of left middle finger with damage to nail

● S61.354   Open bite of right ring finger with damage to nail

● S61.355   Open bite of left ring finger with damage to nail

● S61.356   Open bite of right little finger with damage to nail

● S61.357   Open bite of left little finger with damage to nail

● S61.358   Open bite of other finger with damage to nail
             Open bite of specified finger with unspecified laterality with damage to nail

● S61.359   Open bite of unspecified finger with damage to nail

● S61.4   Open wound of hand

● S61.40   Unspecified open wound of hand

● S61.401   Unspecified open wound of right hand

● S61.402   Unspecified open wound of left hand

● S61.409   Unspecified open wound of unspecified hand

● S61.41   Laceration without foreign body of hand

● S61.411   Laceration without foreign body of right hand

● S61.412   Laceration without foreign body of left hand

● S61.419   Laceration without foreign body of unspecified hand

● S61.42   Laceration with foreign body of hand

● S61.421   Laceration with foreign body of right hand

● S61.422   Laceration with foreign body of left hand

● S61.429   Laceration with foreign body of unspecified hand

▶ New   ⟹ Revised   ~~deleted~~ Deleted   Excludes 1   Excludes 2   Includes   Use additional   Code first   Code also   Key words
OGCR Official Guidelines   ● Unacceptable Principal Diagnosis   X Assign placeholder X   ● Use Additional Character(s)   ▶ Manifestation Code   **Coding Clinic**

● **S61.43**   Puncture wound without foreign body of hand
   ● **S61.431**   Puncture wound without foreign body of right hand
   ● **S61.432**   Puncture wound without foreign body of left hand
   ● **S61.439**   Puncture wound without foreign body of unspecified hand
● **S61.44**   Puncture wound with foreign body of hand
   ● **S61.441**   Puncture wound with foreign body of right hand
   ● **S61.442**   Puncture wound with foreign body of left hand
   ● **S61.449**   Puncture wound with foreign body of unspecified hand
● **S61.45**   Open bite of hand
      Bite of hand NOS
       Excludes1   superficial bite of hand (S60.56-, S60.57-)
   ● **S61.451**   Open bite of right hand
   ● **S61.452**   Open bite of left hand
   ● **S61.459**   Open bite of unspecified hand
● **S61.5**   Open wound of wrist
● **S61.50**   Unspecified open wound of wrist
   ● **S61.501**   Unspecified open wound of right wrist
   ● **S61.502**   Unspecified open wound of left wrist
   ● **S61.509**   Unspecified open wound of unspecified wrist
● **S61.51**   Laceration without foreign body of wrist
   ● **S61.511**   Laceration without foreign body of right wrist
   ● **S61.512**   Laceration without foreign body of left wrist
   ● **S61.519**   Laceration without foreign body of unspecified wrist
● **S61.52**   Laceration with foreign body of wrist
   ● **S61.521**   Laceration with foreign body of right wrist
   ● **S61.522**   Laceration with foreign body of left wrist
   ● **S61.529**   Laceration with foreign body of unspecified wrist
● **S61.53**   Puncture wound without foreign body of wrist
   ● **S61.531**   Puncture wound without foreign body of right wrist
   ● **S61.532**   Puncture wound without foreign body of left wrist
   ● **S61.539**   Puncture wound without foreign body of unspecified wrist
● **S61.54**   Puncture wound with foreign body of wrist
   ● **S61.541**   Puncture wound with foreign body of right wrist
   ● **S61.542**   Puncture wound with foreign body of left wrist
   ● **S61.549**   Puncture wound with foreign body of unspecified wrist
● **S61.55**   Open bite of wrist
      Bite of wrist NOS
       Excludes1   superficial bite of wrist (S60.86-, S60.87-)
   ● **S61.551**   Open bite of right wrist
   ● **S61.552**   Open bite of left wrist
   ● **S61.559**   Open bite of unspecified wrist

● **S62**   Fracture at wrist and hand level
    Note: A fracture not indicated as displaced or nondisplaced should be coded to displaced
       A fracture not indicated as open or closed should be coded to closed
    Excludes1   traumatic amputation of wrist and hand (S68.-)
    Excludes2   fracture of distal parts of ulna and radius (S52.-)
    The appropriate 7th character is to be added to each code from category S62

> A   initial encounter for closed fracture
> B   initial encounter for open fracture
> D   subsequent encounter for fracture with routine healing
> G   subsequent encounter for fracture with delayed healing
> K   subsequent encounter for fracture with nonunion
> P   subsequent encounter for fracture with malunion
> S   sequela

● **S62.0**   Fracture of navicular [scaphoid] bone of wrist
    (Ex) **For category S62.0 CC codes S62.0[B]:** See PDX Collection 1283
      For S62.0[K,P]: See PDX Collection 897
  ● **S62.00**   Unspecified fracture of navicular [scaphoid] bone of wrist
   ● **S62.001**   Unspecified fracture of navicular [scaphoid] bone of right wrist
      B, K, P 🅒, B 🅜
   ● **S62.002**   Unspecified fracture of navicular [scaphoid] bone of left wrist
      B, K, P 🅒, B 🅜
       Coding Clinic: 2012, Q4, P106
   ● **S62.009**   Unspecified fracture of navicular [scaphoid] bone of unspecified wrist
      B, K, P 🅒, B 🅜
  ● **S62.01**   Fracture of distal pole of navicular [scaphoid] bone of wrist
      Fracture of volar tuberosity of navicular [scaphoid] bone of wrist
   ● **S62.011**   Displaced fracture of distal pole of navicular [scaphoid] bone of right wrist B, K, P 🅒, B 🅜
   ● **S62.012**   Displaced fracture of distal pole of navicular [scaphoid] bone of left wrist B, K, P 🅒, B 🅜
   ● **S62.013**   Displaced fracture of distal pole of navicular [scaphoid] bone of unspecified wrist B, K, P 🅒, B 🅜
   ● **S62.014**   Nondisplaced fracture of distal pole of navicular [scaphoid] bone of right wrist B, K, P 🅒, B 🅜
   ● **S62.015**   Nondisplaced fracture of distal pole of navicular [scaphoid] bone of left wrist B, K, P 🅒, B 🅜
   ● **S62.016**   Nondisplaced fracture of distal pole of navicular [scaphoid] bone of unspecified wrist B, K, P 🅒, B 🅜
  ● **S62.02**   Fracture of middle third of navicular [scaphoid] bone of wrist
   ● **S62.021**   Displaced fracture of middle third of navicular [scaphoid] bone of right wrist B, K, P 🅒, B 🅜
   ● **S62.022**   Displaced fracture of middle third of navicular [scaphoid] bone of left wrist B, K, P 🅒, B 🅜
   ● **S62.023**   Displaced fracture of middle third of navicular [scaphoid] bone of unspecified wrist B, K, P 🅒, B 🅜
   ● **S62.024**   Nondisplaced fracture of middle third of navicular [scaphoid] bone of right wrist B, K, P 🅒, B 🅜
   ● **S62.025**   Nondisplaced fracture of middle third of navicular [scaphoid] bone of left wrist B, K, P 🅒, B 🅜
   ● **S62.026**   Nondisplaced fracture of middle third of navicular [scaphoid] bone of unspecified wrist B, K, P 🅒, B 🅜

N   Newborn Age: 0   P   Pediatric Age: 0–17   M   Maternity DX: 9–64   A   Adult Age: 15–124   ♀   Females Only   ♂   Males Only

🅒   Complication\Comorbidity   🅜   Major C\C   (Ex)   CC/MCC Exclusions   Hospital-Acquired Condition   Hierarchical Condition Category

1351

- S62.03 Fracture of proximal third of navicular [scaphoid] bone of wrist
  - S62.031 Displaced fracture of proximal third of navicular [scaphoid] bone of right wrist B, K, P 🪙, B 🪙
  - S62.032 Displaced fracture of proximal third of navicular [scaphoid] bone of left wrist B, K, P 🪙, B 🪙
  - S62.033 Displaced fracture of proximal third of navicular [scaphoid] bone of unspecified wrist B, K, P 🪙, B 🪙
  - S62.034 Nondisplaced fracture of proximal third of navicular [scaphoid] bone of right wrist B, K, P 🪙, B 🪙
  - S62.035 Nondisplaced fracture of proximal third of navicular [scaphoid] bone of left wrist B, K, P 🪙, B 🪙
  - S62.036 Nondisplaced fracture of proximal third of navicular [scaphoid] bone of unspecified wrist B, K, P 🪙, B 🪙
- S62.1 Fracture of other and unspecified carpal bone(s)
  - Excludes2 fracture of scaphoid of wrist (S62.0-)
  - (Ex:) For category S62.1 CC codes S62.1[B]: See PDX Collection 1283
    For S62.0[K,P]: See PDX Collection 897
  - S62.10 Fracture of unspecified carpal bone
    Fracture of wrist NOS
    - S62.101 Fracture of unspecified carpal bone, right wrist B, K, P 🪙, B 🪙
    - S62.102 Fracture of unspecified carpal bone, left wrist B, K, P 🪙, B 🪙
      Coding Clinic: 2012, Q4, P95
    - S62.109 Fracture of unspecified carpal bone, unspecified wrist B, K, P 🪙, B 🪙
  - S62.11 Fracture of triquetrum [cuneiform] bone of wrist
    - S62.111 Displaced fracture of triquetrum [cuneiform] bone, right wrist B, K, P 🪙, B 🪙
    - S62.112 Displaced fracture of triquetrum [cuneiform] bone, left wrist B, K, P 🪙, B 🪙
    - S62.113 Displaced fracture of triquetrum [cuneiform] bone, unspecified wrist B, K, P 🪙, B 🪙
    - S62.114 Nondisplaced fracture of triquetrum [cuneiform] bone, right wrist B, K, P 🪙, B 🪙
    - S62.115 Nondisplaced fracture of triquetrum [cuneiform] bone, left wrist B, K, P 🪙, B 🪙
    - S62.116 Nondisplaced fracture of triquetrum [cuneiform] bone, unspecified wrist B, K, P 🪙, B 🪙
  - S62.12 Fracture of lunate [semilunar]
    - S62.121 Displaced fracture of lunate [semilunar], right wrist B, K, P 🪙, B 🪙
    - S62.122 Displaced fracture of lunate [semilunar], left wrist B, K, P 🪙, B 🪙
    - S62.123 Displaced fracture of lunate [semilunar], unspecified wrist B, K, P 🪙, B 🪙
    - S62.124 Nondisplaced fracture of lunate [semilunar], right wrist B, K, P 🪙, B 🪙
    - S62.125 Nondisplaced fracture of lunate [semilunar], left wrist B, K, P 🪙, B 🪙
    - S62.126 Nondisplaced fracture of lunate [semilunar], unspecified wrist B, K, P 🪙, B 🪙

- S62.13 Fracture of capitate [os magnum] bone
  - S62.131 Displaced fracture of capitate [os magnum] bone, right wrist B, K, P 🪙, B 🪙
  - S62.132 Displaced fracture of capitate [os magnum] bone, left wrist B, K, P 🪙, B 🪙
  - S62.133 Displaced fracture of capitate [os magnum] bone, unspecified wrist B, K, P 🪙, B 🪙
  - S62.134 Nondisplaced fracture of capitate [os magnum] bone, right wrist B, K, P 🪙, B 🪙
  - S62.135 Nondisplaced fracture of capitate [os magnum] bone, left wrist B, K, P 🪙, B 🪙
  - S62.136 Nondisplaced fracture of capitate [os magnum] bone, unspecified wrist B, K, P 🪙, B 🪙
- S62.14 Fracture of body of hamate [unciform] bone
  Fracture of hamate [unciform] bone NOS
  - S62.141 Displaced fracture of body of hamate [unciform] bone, right wrist B, K, P 🪙, B 🪙
  - S62.142 Displaced fracture of body of hamate [unciform] bone, left wrist B, K, P 🪙, B 🪙
  - S62.143 Displaced fracture of body of hamate [unciform] bone, unspecified wrist B, K, P 🪙, B 🪙
  - S62.144 Nondisplaced fracture of body of hamate [unciform] bone, right wrist B, K, P 🪙, B 🪙
  - S62.145 Nondisplaced fracture of body of hamate [unciform] bone, left wrist B, K, P 🪙, B 🪙
  - S62.146 Nondisplaced fracture of body of hamate [unciform] bone, unspecified wrist B, K, P 🪙, B 🪙
- S62.15 Fracture of hook process of hamate [unciform] bone
  Fracture of unciform process of hamate [unciform] bone
  - S62.151 Displaced fracture of hook process of hamate [unciform] bone, right wrist B, K, P 🪙, B 🪙
  - S62.152 Displaced fracture of hook process of hamate [unciform] bone, left wrist B, K, P 🪙, B 🪙
  - S62.153 Displaced fracture of hook process of hamate [unciform] bone, unspecified wrist B, K, P 🪙, B 🪙
  - S62.154 Nondisplaced fracture of hook process of hamate [unciform] bone, right wrist B, K, P 🪙, B 🪙
  - S62.155 Nondisplaced fracture of hook process of hamate [unciform] bone, left wrist B, K, P 🪙, B 🪙
  - S62.156 Nondisplaced fracture of hook process of hamate [unciform] bone, unspecified wrist B, K, P 🪙, B 🪙
- S62.16 Fracture of pisiform
  - S62.161 Displaced fracture of pisiform, right wrist B, K, P 🪙, B 🪙
  - S62.162 Displaced fracture of pisiform, left wrist B, K, P 🪙, B 🪙
  - S62.163 Displaced fracture of pisiform, unspecified wrist B, K, P 🪙, B 🪙
  - S62.164 Nondisplaced fracture of pisiform, right wrist B, K, P 🪙, B 🪙
  - S62.165 Nondisplaced fracture of pisiform, left wrist B, K, P 🪙, B 🪙
  - S62.166 Nondisplaced fracture of pisiform, unspecified wrist B, K, P 🪙, B 🪙

● **S62.17**   Fracture of trapezium [larger multangular]

  ● **S62.171**   Displaced fracture of trapezium [larger multangular], **right** wrist B, K, P 🅒, B 🅜

  ● **S62.172**   Displaced fracture of trapezium [larger multangular], **left** wrist B, K, P 🅒, B 🅜

  ● **S62.173**   Displaced fracture of trapezium [larger multangular], **unspecified** wrist B, K, P 🅒, B 🅜

  ● **S62.174**   Nondisplaced fracture of trapezium [larger multangular], **right** wrist B, K, P 🅒, B 🅜

  ● **S62.175**   Nondisplaced fracture of trapezium [larger multangular], **left** wrist B, K, P 🅒, B 🅜

  ● **S62.176**   Nondisplaced fracture of trapezium [larger multangular], **unspecified** wrist B, K, P 🅒, B 🅜

● **S62.18**   Fracture of trapezoid [smaller multangular]

  ● **S62.181**   Displaced fracture of trapezoid [smaller multangular], **right** wrist B, K, P 🅒, B 🅜

  ● **S62.182**   Displaced fracture of trapezoid [smaller multangular], **left** wrist B, K, P 🅒, B 🅜

  ● **S62.183**   Displaced fracture of trapezoid [smaller multangular], **unspecified** wrist B, K, P 🅒, B 🅜

  ● **S62.184**   Nondisplaced fracture of trapezoid [smaller multangular], **right** wrist B, K, P 🅒, B 🅜

  ● **S62.185**   Nondisplaced fracture of trapezoid [smaller multangular], **left** wrist B, K, P 🅒, B 🅜

  ● **S62.186**   Nondisplaced fracture of trapezoid [smaller multangular], **unspecified** wrist B, K, P 🅒, B 🅜

● **S62.2**   Fracture of first metacarpal bone

  (Ex.) For category S62.2 CC codes S62.2[B]: See PDX Collection 1284
     For S62.2[K,P]: See PDX Collection 897

  ● **S62.20**   Unspecified fracture of first metacarpal bone

    ● **S62.201**   Unspecified fracture of first metacarpal bone, **right** hand B, K, P 🅒, B 🅜

    ● **S62.202**   Unspecified fracture of first metacarpal bone, **left** hand B, K, P 🅒, B 🅜

    ● **S62.209**   Unspecified fracture of first metacarpal bone, **unspecified** hand B, K, P 🅒, B 🅜

  ● **S62.21**   Bennett's fracture

    ● **S62.211**   Bennett's fracture, **right** hand B, K, P 🅒, B 🅜

    ● **S62.212**   Bennett's fracture, **left** hand B, K, P 🅒, B 🅜

    ● **S62.213**   Bennett's fracture, **unspecified** hand B, K, P 🅒, B 🅜

  ● **S62.22**   Rolando's fracture

    ● **S62.221**   Displaced Rolando's fracture, **right** hand B, K, P 🅒, B 🅜

    ● **S62.222**   Displaced Rolando's fracture, **left** hand B, K, P 🅒, B 🅜

    ● **S62.223**   Displaced Rolando's fracture, **unspecified** hand B, K, P 🅒, B 🅜

    ● **S62.224**   Nondisplaced Rolando's fracture, **right** hand B, K, P 🅒, B 🅜

    ● **S62.225**   Nondisplaced Rolando's fracture, **left** hand B, K, P 🅒, B 🅜

    ● **S62.226**   Nondisplaced Rolando's fracture, **unspecified** hand B, K, P 🅒, B 🅜

● **S62.23**   Other fracture of base of first metacarpal bone

  ● **S62.231**   Other displaced fracture of base of first metacarpal bone, **right** hand B, K, P 🅒, B 🅜

  ● **S62.232**   Other displaced fracture of base of first metacarpal bone, **left** hand B, K, P 🅒, B 🅜

  ● **S62.233**   Other displaced fracture of base of first metacarpal bone, **unspecified** hand B, K, P 🅒, B 🅜

  ● **S62.234**   Other nondisplaced fracture of base of first metacarpal bone, **right** hand B, K, P 🅒, B 🅜

  ● **S62.235**   Other nondisplaced fracture of base of first metacarpal bone, **left** hand B, K, P 🅒, B 🅜

  ● **S62.236**   Other nondisplaced fracture of base of first metacarpal bone, **unspecified** hand B, K, P 🅒, B 🅜

● **S62.24**   Fracture of shaft of first metacarpal bone

  ● **S62.241**   Displaced fracture of shaft of first metacarpal bone, **right** hand B, K, P 🅒, B 🅜

  ● **S62.242**   Displaced fracture of shaft of first metacarpal bone, **left** hand B, K, P 🅒, B 🅜

  ● **S62.243**   Displaced fracture of shaft of first metacarpal bone, **unspecified** hand B, K, P 🅒, B 🅜

  ● **S62.244**   Nondisplaced fracture of shaft of first metacarpal bone, **right** hand B, K, P 🅒, B 🅜

  ● **S62.245**   Nondisplaced fracture of shaft of first metacarpal bone, **left** hand B, K, P 🅒, B 🅜

  ● **S62.246**   Nondisplaced fracture of shaft of first metacarpal bone, **unspecified** hand B, K, P 🅒, B 🅜

● **S62.25**   Fracture of neck of first metacarpal bone

  ● **S62.251**   Displaced fracture of neck of first metacarpal bone, **right** hand B, K, P 🅒, B 🅜

  ● **S62.252**   Displaced fracture of neck of first metacarpal bone, **left** hand B, K, P 🅒, B 🅜

  ● **S62.253**   Displaced fracture of neck of first metacarpal bone, **unspecified** hand B, K, P 🅒, B 🅜

  ● **S62.254**   Nondisplaced fracture of neck of first metacarpal bone, **right** hand B, K, P 🅒, B 🅜

  ● **S62.255**   Nondisplaced fracture of neck of first metacarpal bone, **left** hand B, K, P 🅒, B 🅜

  ● **S62.256**   Nondisplaced fracture of neck of first metacarpal bone, **unspecified** hand B, K, P 🅒, B 🅜

● **S62.29**   Other fracture of first metacarpal bone

  ● **S62.291**   Other fracture of first metacarpal bone, **right** hand B, K, P 🅒, B 🅜

  ● **S62.292**   Other fracture of first metacarpal bone, **left** hand B, K, P 🅒, B 🅜

  ● **S62.299**   Other fracture of first metacarpal bone, **unspecified** hand B, K, P 🅒, B 🅜

N Newborn Age: 0   **P** Pediatric Age: 0–17   **M** Maternity DX: 9–64   **A** Adult Age: 15–124   ♀ Females Only   ♂ Males Only

🅒 Complication\Comorbidity   🅜 Major C\C   (Ex) CC/MCC Exclusions   🅗 Hospital-Acquired Condition   🅗 Hierarchical Condition Category

1353

CHAPTER 19 (S00-T88)

● **S62.3 Fracture of other and unspecified metacarpal bone**
    Excludes2   fracture of first metacarpal bone (S62.2-)
    (Ex:) **For category S62.3 CC codes S62.3[B]:** See PDX Collection 1284
      For S62.3[K,P]: See PDX Collection 897

● **S62.30 Unspecified fracture of other metacarpal bone**

● **S62.300 Unspecified fracture of second metacarpal bone, right hand** B, K, P (c), B (ec)

● **S62.301 Unspecified fracture of second metacarpal bone, left hand** B, K, P (c), B (ec)

● **S62.302 Unspecified fracture of third metacarpal bone, right hand** B, K, P (c), B (ec)

● **S62.303 Unspecified fracture of third metacarpal bone, left hand** B, K, P (c), B (ec)

● **S62.304 Unspecified fracture of fourth metacarpal bone, right hand** B, K, P (c), B (ec)

● **S62.305 Unspecified fracture of fourth metacarpal bone, left hand** B, K, P (c), B (ec)

● **S62.306 Unspecified fracture of fifth metacarpal bone, right hand** B, K, P (c), B (ec)

● **S62.307 Unspecified fracture of fifth metacarpal bone, left hand** B, K, P (c), B (ec)

● **S62.308 Unspecified fracture of other metacarpal bone** B, K, P (c), B (ec)
    Unspecified fracture of specified metacarpal bone with unspecified laterality

● **S62.309 Unspecified fracture of unspecified metacarpal bone** B, K, P (c), B (ec)

● **S62.31 Displaced fracture of base of other metacarpal bone**

● **S62.310 Displaced fracture of base of second metacarpal bone, right hand** B, K, P (c), B (ec)

● **S62.311 Displaced fracture of base of second metacarpal bone, left hand** B, K, P (c), B (ec)

● **S62.312 Displaced fracture of base of third metacarpal bone, right hand** B, K, P (c), B (ec)

● **S62.313 Displaced fracture of base of third metacarpal bone, left hand** B, K, P (c), B (ec)

● **S62.314 Displaced fracture of base of fourth metacarpal bone, right hand** B, K, P (c), B (ec)

● **S62.315 Displaced fracture of base of fourth metacarpal bone, left hand** B, K, P (c), B (ec)

● **S62.316 Displaced fracture of base of fifth metacarpal bone, right hand** B, K, P (c), B (ec)

● **S62.317 Displaced fracture of base of fifth metacarpal bone, left hand** B, K, P (c), B (ec)

● **S62.318 Displaced fracture of base of other metacarpal bone** B, K, P (c), B (ec)
    Displaced fracture of base of specified metacarpal bone with unspecified laterality

● **S62.319 Displaced fracture of base of unspecified metacarpal bone** B, K, P (c), B (ec)

● **S62.32 Displaced fracture of shaft of other metacarpal bone**

● **S62.320 Displaced fracture of shaft of second metacarpal bone, right hand** B, K, P (c), B (ec)

● **S62.321 Displaced fracture of shaft of second metacarpal bone, left hand** B, K, P (c), B (ec)

● **S62.322 Displaced fracture of shaft of third metacarpal bone, right hand** B, K, P (c), B (ec)

● **S62.323 Displaced fracture of shaft of third metacarpal bone, left hand** B, K, P (c), B (ec)

● **S62.324 Displaced fracture of shaft of fourth metacarpal bone, right hand** B, K, P (c), B (ec)

● **S62.325 Displaced fracture of shaft of fourth metacarpal bone, left hand** B, K, P (c), B (ec)

● **S62.326 Displaced fracture of shaft of fifth metacarpal bone, right hand** B, K, P (c), B (ec)

● **S62.327 Displaced fracture of shaft of fifth metacarpal bone, left hand** B, K, P (c), B (ec)

● **S62.328 Displaced fracture of shaft of other metacarpal bone** B, K, P (c), B (ec)
    Displaced fracture of shaft of specified metacarpal bone with unspecified laterality

● **S62.329 Displaced fracture of shaft of unspecified metacarpal bone** B, K, P (c), B (ec)

● **S62.33 Displaced fracture of neck of other metacarpal bone**

● **S62.330 Displaced fracture of neck of second metacarpal bone, right hand** B, K, P (c), B (ec)

● **S62.331 Displaced fracture of neck of second metacarpal bone, left hand** B, K, P (c), B (ec)

● **S62.332 Displaced fracture of neck of third metacarpal bone, right hand** B, K, P (c), B (ec)

● **S62.333 Displaced fracture of neck of third metacarpal bone, left hand** B, K, P (c), B (ec)

● **S62.334 Displaced fracture of neck of fourth metacarpal bone, right hand** B, K, P (c), B (ec)

● **S62.335 Displaced fracture of neck of fourth metacarpal bone, left hand** B, K, P (c), B (ec)

● **S62.336 Displaced fracture of neck of fifth metacarpal bone, right hand** B, K, P (c), B (ec)

● **S62.337 Displaced fracture of neck of fifth metacarpal bone, left hand** B, K, P (c), B (ec)

● **S62.338 Displaced fracture of neck of other metacarpal bone** B, K, P (c), B (ec)
    Displaced fracture of neck of specified metacarpal bone with unspecified laterality

● **S62.339 Displaced fracture of neck of unspecified metacarpal bone** B, K, P (c), B (ec)

▶ New   ⇒ Revised   ~~deleted~~ Deleted   Excludes 1   Excludes 2   Includes   Use additional   Code first   Code also   Key words
OGCR Official Guidelines   ● Unacceptable Principal Diagnosis   X Assign placeholder X   ● Use Additional Character(s)   ▌Manifestation Code   **Coding Clinic**

● **S62.34**   Nondisplaced fracture of base of other metacarpal bone
   ● **S62.340**   Nondisplaced fracture of base of second metacarpal bone, right hand B, K, P 🔾, B 🔾
   ● **S62.341**   Nondisplaced fracture of base of second metacarpal bone, left hand B, K, P 🔾, B 🔾
   ● **S62.342**   Nondisplaced fracture of base of third metacarpal bone, right hand B, K, P 🔾, B 🔾
   ● **S62.343**   Nondisplaced fracture of base of third metacarpal bone, left hand B, K, P 🔾, B 🔾
   ● **S62.344**   Nondisplaced fracture of base of fourth metacarpal bone, right hand B, K, P 🔾, B 🔾
   ● **S62.345**   Nondisplaced fracture of base of fourth metacarpal bone, left hand B, K, P 🔾, B 🔾
   ● **S62.346**   Nondisplaced fracture of base of fifth metacarpal bone, right hand B, K, P 🔾, B 🔾
   ● **S62.347**   Nondisplaced fracture of base of fifth metacarpal bone, left hand B, K, P 🔾, B 🔾
   ● **S62.348**   Nondisplaced fracture of base of other metacarpal bone B, K, P 🔾, B 🔾
       Nondisplaced fracture of base of specified metacarpal bone with unspecified laterality
   ● **S62.349**   Nondisplaced fracture of base of unspecified metacarpal bone B, K, P 🔾, B 🔾
● **S62.35**   Nondisplaced fracture of shaft of other metacarpal bone
   ● **S62.350**   Nondisplaced fracture of shaft of second metacarpal bone, right hand B, K, P 🔾, B 🔾
   ● **S62.351**   Nondisplaced fracture of shaft of second metacarpal bone, left hand B, K, P 🔾, B 🔾
   ● **S62.352**   Nondisplaced fracture of shaft of third metacarpal bone, right hand B, K, P 🔾, B 🔾
   ● **S62.353**   Nondisplaced fracture of shaft of third metacarpal bone, left hand B, K, P 🔾, B 🔾
   ● **S62.354**   Nondisplaced fracture of shaft of fourth metacarpal bone, right hand B, K, P 🔾, B 🔾
   ● **S62.355**   Nondisplaced fracture of shaft of fourth metacarpal bone, left hand B, K, P 🔾, B 🔾
   ● **S62.356**   Nondisplaced fracture of shaft of fifth metacarpal bone, right hand B, K, P 🔾, B 🔾
   ● **S62.357**   Nondisplaced fracture of shaft of fifth metacarpal bone, left hand B, K, P 🔾, B 🔾
   ● **S62.358**   Nondisplaced fracture of shaft of other metacarpal bone B, K, P 🔾, B 🔾
       Nondisplaced fracture of shaft of specified metacarpal bone with unspecified laterality
   ● **S62.359**   Nondisplaced fracture of shaft of unspecified metacarpal bone B, K, P 🔾, B 🔾

● **S62.36**   Nondisplaced fracture of neck of other metacarpal bone
   ● **S62.360**   Nondisplaced fracture of neck of second metacarpal bone, right hand B, K, P 🔾, B 🔾
   ● **S62.361**   Nondisplaced fracture of neck of second metacarpal bone, left hand B, K, P 🔾, B 🔾
   ● **S62.362**   Nondisplaced fracture of neck of third metacarpal bone, right hand B, K, P 🔾, B 🔾
   ● **S62.363**   Nondisplaced fracture of neck of third metacarpal bone, left hand B, K, P 🔾, B 🔾
   ● **S62.364**   Nondisplaced fracture of neck of fourth metacarpal bone, right hand B, K, P 🔾, B 🔾
   ● **S62.365**   Nondisplaced fracture of neck of fourth metacarpal bone, left hand B, K, P 🔾, B 🔾
   ● **S62.366**   Nondisplaced fracture of neck of fifth metacarpal bone, right hand B, K, P 🔾, B 🔾
   ● **S62.367**   Nondisplaced fracture of neck of fifth metacarpal bone, left hand B, K, P 🔾, B 🔾
   ● **S62.368**   Nondisplaced fracture of neck of other metacarpal bone B, K, P 🔾, B 🔾
       Nondisplaced fracture of neck of specified metacarpal bone with unspecified laterality
   ● **S62.369**   Nondisplaced fracture of neck of unspecified metacarpal bone B, K, P 🔾, B 🔾
● **S62.39**   Other fracture of other metacarpal bone
   ● **S62.390**   Other fracture of second metacarpal bone, right hand B, K, P 🔾, B 🔾
   ● **S62.391**   Other fracture of second metacarpal bone, left hand B, K, P 🔾, B 🔾
   ● **S62.392**   Other fracture of third metacarpal bone, right hand B, K, P 🔾, B 🔾
   ● **S62.393**   Other fracture of third metacarpal bone, left hand B, K, P 🔾, B 🔾
   ● **S62.394**   Other fracture of fourth metacarpal bone, right hand B, K, P 🔾, B 🔾
   ● **S62.395**   Other fracture of fourth metacarpal bone, left hand B, K, P 🔾, B 🔾
   ● **S62.396**   Other fracture of fifth metacarpal bone, right hand B, K, P 🔾, B 🔾
   ● **S62.397**   Other fracture of fifth metacarpal bone, left hand B, K, P 🔾, B 🔾
   ● **S62.398**   Other fracture of other metacarpal bone B, K, P 🔾, B 🔾
       Other fracture of specified metacarpal bone with unspecified laterality
   ● **S62.399**   Other fracture of unspecified metacarpal bone B, K, P 🔾, B 🔾
● **S62.5**   Fracture of thumb
     (Ex) For category S62.5 CC codes S62.5[B]: See PDX Collection 1785
     For S62.5[K,P]: See PDX Collection 897
 ● **S62.50**   Fracture of unspecified phalanx of thumb
   ● **S62.501**   Fracture of unspecified phalanx of right thumb B, K, P 🔾, B 🔾
   ● **S62.502**   Fracture of unspecified phalanx of left thumb B, K, P 🔾, B 🔾
   ● **S62.509**   Fracture of unspecified phalanx of unspecified thumb B, K, P 🔾, B 🔾

● **S62.51**   Fracture of proximal phalanx of thumb
- ● **S62.511**   Displaced fracture of proximal phalanx of right thumb B, K, P 🔴, B 🔴
- ● **S62.512**   Displaced fracture of proximal phalanx of left thumb B, K, P 🔴, B 🔴
- ● **S62.513**   Displaced fracture of proximal phalanx of unspecified thumb B, K, P 🔴, B 🔴
- ● **S62.514**   Nondisplaced fracture of proximal phalanx of right thumb B, K, P 🔴, B 🔴
- ● **S62.515**   Nondisplaced fracture of proximal phalanx of left thumb B, K, P 🔴, B 🔴
- ● **S62.516**   Nondisplaced fracture of proximal phalanx of unspecified thumb B, K, P 🔴, B 🔴

● **S62.52**   Fracture of distal phalanx of thumb
- ● **S62.521**   Displaced fracture of distal phalanx of right thumb B, K, P 🔴, B 🔴
- ● **S62.522**   Displaced fracture of distal phalanx of left thumb B, K, P 🔴, B 🔴
- ● **S62.523**   Displaced fracture of distal phalanx of unspecified thumb B, K, P 🔴, B 🔴
- ● **S62.524**   Nondisplaced fracture of distal phalanx of right thumb B, K, P 🔴, B 🔴
- ● **S62.525**   Nondisplaced fracture of distal phalanx of left thumb B, K, P 🔴, B 🔴
- ● **S62.526**   Nondisplaced fracture of distal phalanx of unspecified thumb B, K, P 🔴, B 🔴

● **S62.6**   Fracture of other and unspecified finger(s)

     Excludes2   fracture of thumb (S62.5-)

     Ex: **For category S62.6 CC codes S62.6[B]:** See PDX Collection 1285
     For S62.5[K,P]: See PDX Collection 897

● **S62.60**   Fracture of unspecified phalanx of finger
- ● **S62.600**   Fracture of unspecified phalanx of right index finger B, K, P 🔴, B 🔴
- ● **S62.601**   Fracture of unspecified phalanx of left index finger B, K, P 🔴, B 🔴
- ● **S62.602**   Fracture of unspecified phalanx of right middle finger B, K, P 🔴, B 🔴
- ● **S62.603**   Fracture of unspecified phalanx of left middle finger B, K, P 🔴, B 🔴
- ● **S62.604**   Fracture of unspecified phalanx of right ring finger B, K, P 🔴, B 🔴
- ● **S62.605**   Fracture of unspecified phalanx of left ring finger B, K, P 🔴, B 🔴
- ● **S62.606**   Fracture of unspecified phalanx of right little finger B, K, P 🔴, B 🔴
- ● **S62.607**   Fracture of unspecified phalanx of left little finger B, K, P 🔴, B 🔴
- ● **S62.608**   Fracture of unspecified phalanx of other finger B, K, P 🔴, B 🔴
  Fracture of unspecified phalanx of specified finger with unspecified laterality
- ● **S62.609**   Fracture of unspecified phalanx of unspecified finger B, K, P 🔴, B 🔴

● **S62.61**   Displaced fracture of proximal phalanx of finger
- ● **S62.610**   Displaced fracture of proximal phalanx of right index finger B, K, P 🔴, B 🔴
- ● **S62.611**   Displaced fracture of proximal phalanx of left index finger B, K, P 🔴, B 🔴
- ● **S62.612**   Displaced fracture of proximal phalanx of right middle finger B, K, P 🔴, B 🔴

- ● **S62.613**   Displaced fracture of proximal phalanx of left middle finger B, K, P 🔴, B 🔴
- ● **S62.614**   Displaced fracture of proximal phalanx of right ring finger B, K, P 🔴, B 🔴
- ● **S62.615**   Displaced fracture of proximal phalanx of left ring finger B, K, P 🔴, B 🔴
- ● **S62.616**   Displaced fracture of proximal phalanx of right little finger B, K, P 🔴, B 🔴
- ● **S62.617**   Displaced fracture of proximal phalanx of left little finger B, K, P 🔴, B 🔴
- ● **S62.618**   Displaced fracture of proximal phalanx of other finger B, K, P 🔴, B 🔴
  Displaced fracture of proximal phalanx of specified finger with unspecified laterality
- ● **S62.619**   Displaced fracture of proximal phalanx of unspecified finger B, K, P 🔴, B 🔴

● **S62.62**   Displaced fracture of middle phalanx of finger
- ● **S62.620**   Displaced fracture of middle phalanx of right index finger B, K, P 🔴, B 🔴
- ● **S62.621**   Displaced fracture of middle phalanx of left index finger B, K, P 🔴, B 🔴
- ● **S62.622**   Displaced fracture of middle phalanx of right middle finger B, K, P 🔴, B 🔴
- ● **S62.623**   Displaced fracture of middle phalanx of left middle finger B, K, P 🔴, B 🔴
- ● **S62.624**   Displaced fracture of middle phalanx of right ring finger B, K, P 🔴, B 🔴
- ● **S62.625**   Displaced fracture of middle phalanx of left ring finger B, K, P 🔴, B 🔴
- ● **S62.626**   Displaced fracture of middle phalanx of right little finger B, K, P 🔴, B 🔴
- ● **S62.627**   Displaced fracture of middle phalanx of left little finger B, K, P 🔴, B 🔴
- ● **S62.628**   Displaced fracture of middle phalanx of other finger B, K, P 🔴, B 🔴
  Displaced fracture of middle phalanx of specified finger with unspecified laterality
- ● **S62.629**   Displaced fracture of middle phalanx of unspecified finger B, K, P 🔴, B 🔴

● **S62.63**   Displaced fracture of distal phalanx of finger
- ● **S62.630**   Displaced fracture of distal phalanx of right index finger B, K, P 🔴, B 🔴
- ● **S62.631**   Displaced fracture of distal phalanx of left index finger B, K, P 🔴, B 🔴
- ● **S62.632**   Displaced fracture of distal phalanx of right middle finger B, K, P 🔴, B 🔴
- ● **S62.633**   Displaced fracture of distal phalanx of left middle finger B, K, P 🔴, B 🔴
- ● **S62.634**   Displaced fracture of distal phalanx of right ring finger B, K, P 🔴, B 🔴
- ● **S62.635**   Displaced fracture of distal phalanx of left ring finger B, K, P 🔴, B 🔴
- ● **S62.636**   Displaced fracture of distal phalanx of right little finger B, K, P 🔴, B 🔴
- ● **S62.637**   Displaced fracture of distal phalanx of left little finger B, K, P 🔴, B 🔴
- ● **S62.638**   Displaced fracture of distal phalanx of other finger B, K, P 🔴, B 🔴
  Displaced fracture of distal phalanx of specified finger with unspecified laterality
- ● **S62.639**   Displaced fracture of distal phalanx of unspecified finger B, K, P 🔴, B 🔴

▶ New   ⇒ Revised   deleted Deleted   Excludes 1   Excludes 2   Includes   Use additional   Code first   Code also   Key words

OGCR Official Guidelines   ● Unacceptable Principal Diagnosis   X Assign placeholder X   ● Use Additional Character(s)   ▶ Manifestation Code   **Coding Clinic**

● **S62.64**   Nondisplaced fracture of proximal phalanx of finger

   ● **S62.640**   Nondisplaced fracture of proximal phalanx of right index finger B, K, P ⓒ, B ⓜ

   ● **S62.641**   Nondisplaced fracture of proximal phalanx of left index finger B, K, P ⓒ, B ⓜ

   ● **S62.642**   Nondisplaced fracture of proximal phalanx of right middle finger B, K, P ⓒ, B ⓜ

   ● **S62.643**   Nondisplaced fracture of proximal phalanx of left middle finger B, K, P ⓒ, B ⓜ

   ● **S62.644**   Nondisplaced fracture of proximal phalanx of right ring finger B, K, P ⓒ, B ⓜ

   ● **S62.645**   Nondisplaced fracture of proximal phalanx of left ring finger B, K, P ⓒ, B ⓜ

   ● **S62.646**   Nondisplaced fracture of proximal phalanx of right little finger B, K, P ⓒ, B ⓜ

   ● **S62.647**   Nondisplaced fracture of proximal phalanx of left little finger B, K, P ⓒ, B ⓜ

   ● **S62.648**   Nondisplaced fracture of proximal phalanx of other finger B, K, P ⓒ, B ⓜ
       Nondisplaced fracture of proximal phalanx of specified finger with unspecified laterality

   ● **S62.649**   Nondisplaced fracture of proximal phalanx of unspecified finger B, K, P ⓒ, B ⓜ

● **S62.65**   Nondisplaced fracture of middle phalanx of finger

   ● **S62.650**   Nondisplaced fracture of middle phalanx of right index finger B, K, P ⓒ, B ⓜ

   ● **S62.651**   Nondisplaced fracture of middle phalanx of left index finger B, K, P ⓒ, B ⓜ

   ● **S62.652**   Nondisplaced fracture of middle phalanx of right middle finger B, K, P ⓒ, B ⓜ

   ● **S62.653**   Nondisplaced fracture of middle phalanx of left middle finger B, K, P ⓒ, B ⓜ

   ● **S62.654**   Nondisplaced fracture of middle phalanx of right ring finger B, K, P ⓒ, B ⓜ

   ● **S62.655**   Nondisplaced fracture of middle phalanx of left ring finger B, K, P ⓒ, B ⓜ

   ● **S62.656**   Nondisplaced fracture of middle phalanx of right little finger B, K, P ⓒ, B ⓜ

   ● **S62.657**   Nondisplaced fracture of middle phalanx of left little finger B, K, P ⓒ, B ⓜ

   ● **S62.658**   Nondisplaced fracture of middle phalanx of other finger B, K, P ⓒ, B ⓜ
       Nondisplaced fracture of middle phalanx of specified finger with unspecified laterality

   ● **S62.659**   Nondisplaced fracture of middle phalanx of unspecified finger B, K, P ⓒ, B ⓜ

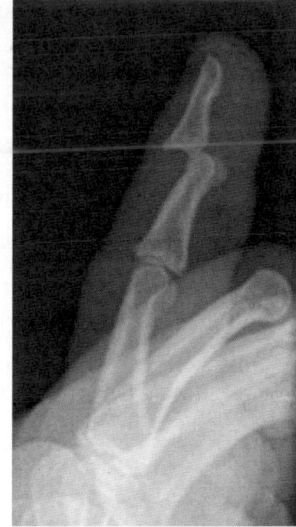

Figure 19-14   Dorsal dislocation of the distal phalanx of the index finger. (From Hardy M, Snaith B: Musculoskeletal Trauma: A Guide to Assessment and Diagnosis, 1e, Elsevier, 2011)

● **S62.66**   Nondisplaced fracture of distal phalanx of finger

   ● **S62.660**   Nondisplaced fracture of distal phalanx of right index finger B, K, P ⓒ, B ⓜ

   ● **S62.661**   Nondisplaced fracture of distal phalanx of left index finger B, K, P ⓒ, B ⓜ

   ● **S62.662**   Nondisplaced fracture of distal phalanx of right middle finger B, K, P ⓒ, B ⓜ

   ● **S62.663**   Nondisplaced fracture of distal phalanx of left middle finger B, K, P ⓒ, B ⓜ

   ● **S62.664**   Nondisplaced fracture of distal phalanx of right ring finger B, K, P ⓒ, B ⓜ

   ● **S62.665**   Nondisplaced fracture of distal phalanx of left ring finger B, K, P ⓒ, B ⓜ

   ● **S62.666**   Nondisplaced fracture of distal phalanx of right little finger B, K, P ⓒ, B ⓜ

   ● **S62.667**   Nondisplaced fracture of distal phalanx of left little finger B, K, P ⓒ, B ⓜ

   ● **S62.668**   Nondisplaced fracture of distal phalanx of other finger B, K, P ⓒ, B ⓜ
       Nondisplaced fracture of distal phalanx of specified finger with unspecified laterality

   ● **S62.669**   Nondisplaced fracture of distal phalanx of unspecified finger B, K, P ⓒ, B ⓜ

● **S62.9**   Unspecified fracture of wrist and hand

  X● **S62.90**   Unspecified fracture of unspecified wrist and hand B, K, P ⓒ, B ⓜ
       (Ex) **For S62.90[B]:** See PDX Collection 1286 **For S62.90[K,P]:** See PDX Collection 897

  X● **S62.91**   Unspecified fracture of right wrist and hand B, K, P ⓒ, B ⓜ
       (Ex) **For S62.91[B]:** See PDX Collection 1287 **For S62.91[K,P]:** See PDX Collection 897

  X● **S62.92**   Unspecified fracture of left wrist and hand B, K, P ⓒ, B ⓜ
       (Ex) **For S62.92[B]:** See PDX Collection 1287 **For S62.92[K,P]:** See PDX Collection 897

CHAPTER 19 (S00–T88)

CHAPTER 19 (S00–T88)

● **S63 Dislocation and sprain of joints and ligaments at wrist and hand level**

> **Includes** avulsion of joint or ligament at wrist and hand level
>
> laceration of cartilage, joint or ligament at wrist and hand level
>
> sprain of cartilage, joint or ligament at wrist and hand level
>
> traumatic hemarthrosis of joint or ligament at wrist and hand level
>
> traumatic rupture of joint or ligament at wrist and hand level
>
> traumatic subluxation of joint or ligament at wrist and hand level
>
> traumatic tear of joint or ligament at wrist and hand level

Code also any associated open wound

> **Excludes2** strain of muscle, fascia and tendon of wrist and hand (S66.-)

The appropriate 7th character is to be added to each code from category S63

> A   initial encounter
> D   subsequent encounter
> S   sequela

● **S63.0 Subluxation and dislocation of wrist and hand joints**

● **S63.00 Unspecified subluxation and dislocation of wrist and hand**
> Dislocation of carpal bone NOS
> Dislocation of distal end of radius NOS
> Subluxation of carpal bone NOS
> Subluxation of distal end of radius NOS

● S63.001 Unspecified subluxation of right wrist and hand

● S63.002 Unspecified subluxation of left wrist and hand

● S63.003 Unspecified subluxation of unspecified wrist and hand

● S63.004 Unspecified dislocation of right wrist and hand

● S63.005 Unspecified dislocation of left wrist and hand

● S63.006 Unspecified dislocation of unspecified wrist and hand

● **S63.01 Subluxation and dislocation of distal radioulnar joint**

● S63.011 Subluxation of distal radioulnar joint of right wrist

● S63.012 Subluxation of distal radioulnar joint of left wrist

● S63.013 Subluxation of distal radioulnar joint of unspecified wrist

● S63.014 Dislocation of distal radioulnar joint of right wrist

● S63.015 Dislocation of distal radioulnar joint of left wrist

● S63.016 Dislocation of distal radioulnar joint of unspecified wrist

● **S63.02 Subluxation and dislocation of radiocarpal joint**

● S63.021 Subluxation of radiocarpal joint of right wrist

● S63.022 Subluxation of radiocarpal joint of left wrist

● S63.023 Subluxation of radiocarpal joint of unspecified wrist

● S63.024 Dislocation of radiocarpal joint of right wrist

● S63.025 Dislocation of radiocarpal joint of left wrist

● S63.026 Dislocation of radiocarpal joint of unspecified wrist

● **S63.03 Subluxation and dislocation of midcarpal joint**

● S63.031 Subluxation of midcarpal joint of right wrist

● S63.032 Subluxation of midcarpal joint of left wrist

● S63.033 Subluxation of midcarpal joint of unspecified wrist

● S63.034 Dislocation of midcarpal joint of right wrist

● S63.035 Dislocation of midcarpal joint of left wrist

● S63.036 Dislocation of midcarpal joint of unspecified wrist

● **S63.04 Subluxation and dislocation of carpometacarpal joint of thumb**

> **Excludes2** interphalangeal subluxation and dislocation of thumb (S63.1-)

● S63.041 Subluxation of carpometacarpal joint of right thumb

● S63.042 Subluxation of carpometacarpal joint of left thumb

● S63.043 Subluxation of carpometacarpal joint of unspecified thumb

● S63.044 Dislocation of carpometacarpal joint of right thumb

● S63.045 Dislocation of carpometacarpal joint of left thumb

● S63.046 Dislocation of carpometacarpal joint of unspecified thumb

● **S63.05 Subluxation and dislocation of other carpometacarpal joint**

> **Excludes2** subluxation and dislocation of carpometacarpal joint of thumb (S63.04-)

● S63.051 Subluxation of other carpometacarpal joint of right hand

● S63.052 Subluxation of other carpometacarpal joint of left hand

● S63.053 Subluxation of other carpometacarpal joint of unspecified hand

● S63.054 Dislocation of other carpometacarpal joint of right hand

● S63.055 Dislocation of other carpometacarpal joint of left hand

● S63.056 Dislocation of other carpometacarpal joint of unspecified hand

● **S63.06 Subluxation and dislocation of metacarpal (bone), proximal end**

● S63.061 Subluxation of metacarpal (bone), proximal end of right hand

● S63.062 Subluxation of metacarpal (bone), proximal end of left hand

● S63.063 Subluxation of metacarpal (bone), proximal end of unspecified hand

● S63.064 Dislocation of metacarpal (bone), proximal end of right hand

● S63.065 Dislocation of metacarpal (bone), proximal end of left hand

● S63.066 Dislocation of metacarpal (bone), proximal end of unspecified hand

▶ New   ⇒ Revised   ~~deleted~~ Deleted   Excludes 1   Excludes 2   Includes   Use additional   Code first   Code also   Key words
OGCR Official Guidelines   ● Unacceptable Principal Diagnosis   X Assign placeholder X   ● Use Additional Character(s)   ▶ Manifestation Code   Coding Clinic

● S63.07 Subluxation and dislocation of distal end of ulna
  ● S63.071 Subluxation of distal end of right ulna
  ● S63.072 Subluxation of distal end of left ulna
  ● S63.073 Subluxation of distal end of unspecified ulna
  ● S63.074 Dislocation of distal end of right ulna
  ● S63.075 Dislocation of distal end of left ulna
  ● S63.076 Dislocation of distal end of unspecified ulna
● S63.09 Other subluxation and dislocation of wrist and hand
  ● S63.091 Other subluxation of right wrist and hand
  ● S63.092 Other subluxation of left wrist and hand
  ● S63.093 Other subluxation of unspecified wrist and hand
  ● S63.094 Other dislocation of right wrist and hand
  ● S63.095 Other dislocation of left wrist and hand
  ● S63.096 Other dislocation of unspecified wrist and hand
● S63.1 Subluxation and dislocation of thumb
  ● S63.10 Unspecified subluxation and dislocation of thumb
    ● S63.101 Unspecified subluxation of right thumb
    ● S63.102 Unspecified subluxation of left thumb
    ● S63.103 Unspecified subluxation of unspecified thumb
    ● S63.104 Unspecified dislocation of right thumb
    ● S63.105 Unspecified dislocation of left thumb
    ● S63.106 Unspecified dislocation of unspecified thumb
  ● S63.11 Subluxation and dislocation of metacarpophalangeal joint of thumb
    ● S63.111 Subluxation of metacarpophalangeal joint of right thumb
    ● S63.112 Subluxation of metacarpophalangeal joint of left thumb
    ● S63.113 Subluxation of metacarpophalangeal joint of unspecified thumb
    ● S63.114 Dislocation of metacarpophalangeal joint of right thumb
    ● S63.115 Dislocation of metacarpophalangeal joint of left thumb
    ● S63.116 Dislocation of metacarpophalangeal joint of unspecified thumb
  ● S63.12 Subluxation and dislocation of interphalangeal joint of thumb
    ● S63.121 Subluxation of interphalangeal joint of right thumb
    ● S63.122 Subluxation of interphalangeal joint of left thumb
    ● S63.123 Subluxation of interphalangeal joint of unspecified thumb
    ● S63.124 Dislocation of interphalangeal joint of right thumb
    ● S63.125 Dislocation of interphalangeal joint of left thumb
    ● S63.126 Dislocation of interphalangeal joint of unspecified thumb

● S63.2 Subluxation and dislocation of other finger(s)
  Excludes2 subluxation and dislocation of thumb (S63.1-)
  ● S63.20 Unspecified subluxation of other finger
    ● S63.200 Unspecified subluxation of right index finger
    ● S63.201 Unspecified subluxation of left index finger
    ● S63.202 Unspecified subluxation of right middle finger
    ● S63.203 Unspecified subluxation of left middle finger
    ● S63.204 Unspecified subluxation of right ring finger
    ● S63.205 Unspecified subluxation of left ring finger
    ● S63.206 Unspecified subluxation of right little finger
    ● S63.207 Unspecified subluxation of left little finger
    ● S63.208 Unspecified subluxation of other finger
      Unspecified subluxation of specified finger with unspecified laterality
    ● S63.209 Unspecified subluxation of unspecified finger
  ● S63.21 Subluxation of metacarpophalangeal joint of finger
    ● S63.210 Subluxation of metacarpophalangeal joint of right index finger
    ● S63.211 Subluxation of metacarpophalangeal joint of left index finger
    ● S63.212 Subluxation of metacarpophalangeal joint of right middle finger
    ● S63.213 Subluxation of metacarpophalangeal joint of left middle finger
    ● S63.214 Subluxation of metacarpophalangeal joint of right ring finger
    ● S63.215 Subluxation of metacarpophalangeal joint of left ring finger
    ● S63.216 Subluxation of metacarpophalangeal joint of right little finger
    ● S63.217 Subluxation of metacarpophalangeal joint of left little finger
    ● S63.218 Subluxation of metacarpophalangeal joint of other finger
      Subluxation of metacarpophalangeal joint of specified finger with unspecified laterality
    ● S63.219 Subluxation of metacarpophalangeal joint of unspecified finger

N Newborn Age: 0   P Pediatric Age: 0–17   M Maternity DX: 9–64   A Adult Age: 15–124   ♀ Females Only   ♂ Males Only

🅒 Complication\Comorbidity   🅜 Major C\C   Ⓔⓧ CC/MCC Exclusions   🅗 Hospital-Acquired Condition   🅗 Hierarchical Condition Category

1359

● S63.22   Subluxation of unspecified interphalangeal joint of finger
- ● S63.220   Subluxation of unspecified interphalangeal joint of right index finger
- ● S63.221   Subluxation of unspecified interphalangeal joint of left index finger
- ● S63.222   Subluxation of unspecified interphalangeal joint of right middle finger
- ● S63.223   Subluxation of unspecified interphalangeal joint of left middle finger
- ● S63.224   Subluxation of unspecified interphalangeal joint of right ring finger
- ● S63.225   Subluxation of unspecified interphalangeal joint of left ring finger
- ● S63.226   Subluxation of unspecified interphalangeal joint of right little finger
- ● S63.227   Subluxation of unspecified interphalangeal joint of left little finger
- ● S63.228   Subluxation of unspecified interphalangeal joint of other finger
  Subluxation of unspecified interphalangeal joint of specified finger with unspecified laterality
- ● S63.229   Subluxation of unspecified interphalangeal joint of unspecified finger

● S63.23   Subluxation of proximal interphalangeal joint of finger
- ● S63.230   Subluxation of proximal interphalangeal joint of right index finger
- ● S63.231   Subluxation of proximal interphalangeal joint of left index finger
- ● S63.232   Subluxation of proximal interphalangeal joint of right middle finger
- ● S63.233   Subluxation of proximal interphalangeal joint of left middle finger
- ● S63.234   Subluxation of proximal interphalangeal joint of right ring finger
- ● S63.235   Subluxation of proximal interphalangeal joint of left ring finger
- ● S63.236   Subluxation of proximal interphalangeal joint of right little finger
- ● S63.237   Subluxation of proximal interphalangeal joint of left little finger

- ● S63.238   Subluxation of proximal interphalangeal joint of other finger
  Subluxation of proximal interphalangeal joint of specified finger with unspecified laterality
- ● S63.239   Subluxation of proximal interphalangeal joint of unspecified finger

● S63.24   Subluxation of distal interphalangeal joint of finger
- ● S63.240   Subluxation of distal interphalangeal joint of right index finger
- ● S63.241   Subluxation of distal interphalangeal joint of left index finger
- ● S63.242   Subluxation of distal interphalangeal joint of right middle finger
- ● S63.243   Subluxation of distal interphalangeal joint of left middle finger
- ● S63.244   Subluxation of distal interphalangeal joint of right ring finger
- ● S63.245   Subluxation of distal interphalangeal joint of left ring finger
- ● S63.246   Subluxation of distal interphalangeal joint of right little finger
- ● S63.247   Subluxation of distal interphalangeal joint of left little finger
- ● S63.248   Subluxation of distal interphalangeal joint of other finger
  Subluxation of distal interphalangeal joint of specified finger with unspecified laterality
- ● S63.249   Subluxation of distal interphalangeal joint of unspecified finger

● S63.25   Unspecified dislocation of other finger
- ● S63.250   Unspecified dislocation of right index finger
- ● S63.251   Unspecified dislocation of left index finger
- ● S63.252   Unspecified dislocation of right middle finger
- ● S63.253   Unspecified dislocation of left middle finger
- ● S63.254   Unspecified dislocation of right ring finger
- ● S63.255   Unspecified dislocation of left ring finger
- ● S63.256   Unspecified dislocation of right little finger
- ● S63.257   Unspecified dislocation of left little finger
- ● S63.258   Unspecified dislocation of other finger
  Unspecified dislocation of specified finger with unspecified laterality
- ● S63.259   Unspecified dislocation of unspecified finger
  Unspecified dislocation of unspecified finger with unspecified laterality

● S63.26 Dislocation of metacarpophalangeal joint of finger
  ● S63.260 Dislocation of metacarpophalangeal joint of right index finger
  ● S63.261 Dislocation of metacarpophalangeal joint of left index finger
  ● S63.262 Dislocation of metacarpophalangeal joint of right middle finger
  ● S63.263 Dislocation of metacarpophalangeal joint of left middle finger
  ● S63.264 Dislocation of metacarpophalangeal joint of right ring finger
  ● S63.265 Dislocation of metacarpophalangeal joint of left ring finger
  ● S63.266 Dislocation of metacarpophalangeal joint of right little finger
  ● S63.267 Dislocation of metacarpophalangeal joint of left little finger
  ● S63.268 Dislocation of metacarpophalangeal joint of other finger
    Dislocation of metacarpophalangeal joint of specified finger with unspecified laterality
  ● S63.269 Dislocation of metacarpophalangeal joint of unspecified finger
● S63.27 Dislocation of unspecified interphalangeal joint of finger
  ● S63.270 Dislocation of unspecified interphalangeal joint of right index finger
  ● S63.271 Dislocation of unspecified interphalangeal joint of left index finger
  ● S63.272 Dislocation of unspecified interphalangeal joint of right middle finger
  ● S63.273 Dislocation of unspecified interphalangeal joint of left middle finger
  ● S63.274 Dislocation of unspecified interphalangeal joint of right ring finger
  ● S63.275 Dislocation of unspecified interphalangeal joint of left ring finger
  ● S63.276 Dislocation of unspecified interphalangeal joint of right little finger
  ● S63.277 Dislocation of unspecified interphalangeal joint of left little finger
  ● S63.278 Dislocation of unspecified interphalangeal joint of other finger
    Dislocation of unspecified interphalangeal joint of specified finger with unspecified laterality
  ● S63.279 Dislocation of unspecified interphalangeal joint of unspecified finger
    Dislocation of unspecified interphalangeal joint of unspecified finger without specified laterality

● S63.28 Dislocation of proximal interphalangeal joint of finger
  ● S63.280 Dislocation of proximal interphalangeal joint of right index finger
  ● S63.281 Dislocation of proximal interphalangeal joint of left index finger
  ● S63.282 Dislocation of proximal interphalangeal joint of right middle finger
  ● S63.283 Dislocation of proximal interphalangeal joint of left middle finger
  ● S63.284 Dislocation of proximal interphalangeal joint of right ring finger
  ● S63.285 Dislocation of proximal interphalangeal joint of left ring finger
  ● S63.286 Dislocation of proximal interphalangeal joint of right little finger
  ● S63.287 Dislocation of proximal interphalangeal joint of left little finger
  ● S63.288 Dislocation of proximal interphalangeal joint of other finger
    Dislocation of proximal interphalangeal joint of specified finger with unspecified laterality
  ● S63.289 Dislocation of proximal interphalangeal joint of unspecified finger
● S63.29 Dislocation of distal interphalangeal joint of finger
  ● S63.290 Dislocation of distal interphalangeal joint of right index finger
  ● S63.291 Dislocation of distal interphalangeal joint of left index finger
  ● S63.292 Dislocation of distal interphalangeal joint of right middle finger
  ● S63.293 Dislocation of distal interphalangeal joint of left middle finger
  ● S63.294 Dislocation of distal interphalangeal joint of right ring finger
  ● S63.295 Dislocation of distal interphalangeal joint of left ring finger
  ● S63.296 Dislocation of distal interphalangeal joint of right little finger
  ● S63.297 Dislocation of distal interphalangeal joint of left little finger
  ● S63.298 Dislocation of distal interphalangeal joint of other finger
    Dislocation of distal interphalangeal joint of specified finger with unspecified laterality
  ● S63.299 Dislocation of distal interphalangeal joint of unspecified finger
● S63.3 Traumatic rupture of ligament of wrist
  ● S63.30 Traumatic rupture of unspecified ligament of wrist
  ● S63.301 Traumatic rupture of unspecified ligament of right wrist
  ● S63.302 Traumatic rupture of unspecified ligament of left wrist
  ● S63.309 Traumatic rupture of unspecified ligament of unspecified wrist

● **S63.31** Traumatic rupture of collateral ligament of wrist
- ● **S63.311** Traumatic rupture of collateral ligament of right wrist
- ● **S63.312** Traumatic rupture of collateral ligament of left wrist
- ● **S63.319** Traumatic rupture of collateral ligament of unspecified wrist

● **S63.32** Traumatic rupture of radiocarpal ligament
- ● **S63.321** Traumatic rupture of right radiocarpal ligament
- ● **S63.322** Traumatic rupture of left radiocarpal ligament
- ● **S63.329** Traumatic rupture of unspecified radiocarpal ligament

● **S63.33** Traumatic rupture of ulnocarpal (palmar) ligament
- ● **S63.331** Traumatic rupture of right ulnocarpal (palmar) ligament
- ● **S63.332** Traumatic rupture of left ulnocarpal (palmar) ligament
- ● **S63.339** Traumatic rupture of unspecified ulnocarpal (palmar) ligament

● **S63.39** Traumatic rupture of other ligament of wrist
- ● **S63.391** Traumatic rupture of other ligament of right wrist
- ● **S63.392** Traumatic rupture of other ligament of left wrist
- ● **S63.399** Traumatic rupture of other ligament of unspecified wrist

● **S63.4** Traumatic rupture of ligament of finger at metacarpophalangeal and interphalangeal joint(s)
- ● **S63.40** Traumatic rupture of unspecified ligament of finger at metacarpophalangeal and interphalangeal joint
  - ● **S63.400** Traumatic rupture of unspecified ligament of right index finger at metacarpophalangeal and interphalangeal joint
  - ● **S63.401** Traumatic rupture of unspecified ligament of left index finger at metacarpophalangeal and interphalangeal joint
  - ● **S63.402** Traumatic rupture of unspecified ligament of right middle finger at metacarpophalangeal and interphalangeal joint
  - ● **S63.403** Traumatic rupture of unspecified ligament of left middle finger at metacarpophalangeal and interphalangeal joint
  - ● **S63.404** Traumatic rupture of unspecified ligament of right ring finger at metacarpophalangeal and interphalangeal joint
  - ● **S63.405** Traumatic rupture of unspecified ligament of left ring finger at metacarpophalangeal and interphalangeal joint
  - ● **S63.406** Traumatic rupture of unspecified ligament of right little finger at metacarpophalangeal and interphalangeal joint

● **S63.407** Traumatic rupture of unspecified ligament of left little finger at metacarpophalangeal and interphalangeal joint
● **S63.408** Traumatic rupture of unspecified ligament of other finger at metacarpophalangeal and interphalangeal joint

Traumatic rupture of unspecified ligament of specified finger with unspecified laterality at metacarpophalangeal and interphalangeal joint
● **S63.409** Traumatic rupture of unspecified ligament of unspecified finger at metacarpophalangeal and interphalangeal joint

● **S63.41** Traumatic rupture of collateral ligament of finger at metacarpophalangeal and interphalangeal joint
- ● **S63.410** Traumatic rupture of collateral ligament of right index finger at metacarpophalangeal and interphalangeal joint
- ● **S63.411** Traumatic rupture of collateral ligament of left index finger at metacarpophalangeal and interphalangeal joint
- ● **S63.412** Traumatic rupture of collateral ligament of right middle finger at metacarpophalangeal and interphalangeal joint
- ● **S63.413** Traumatic rupture of collateral ligament of left middle finger at metacarpophalangeal and interphalangeal joint
- ● **S63.414** Traumatic rupture of collateral ligament of right ring finger at metacarpophalangeal and interphalangeal joint
- ● **S63.415** Traumatic rupture of collateral ligament of left ring finger at metacarpophalangeal and interphalangeal joint
- ● **S63.416** Traumatic rupture of collateral ligament of right little finger at metacarpophalangeal and interphalangeal joint
- ● **S63.417** Traumatic rupture of collateral ligament of left little finger at metacarpophalangeal and interphalangeal joint
- ● **S63.418** Traumatic rupture of collateral ligament of other finger at metacarpophalangeal and interphalangeal joint

Traumatic rupture of collateral ligament of specified finger with unspecified laterality at metacarpophalangeal and interphalangeal joint
- ● **S63.419** Traumatic rupture of collateral ligament of unspecified finger at metacarpophalangeal and interphalangeal joint

▶ New   ⇒ Revised   ~~deleted~~ Deleted   Excludes 1   Excludes 2   Includes   Use additional   Code first   Code also   Key words
OGCR Official Guidelines   ● Unacceptable Principal Diagnosis   X Assign placeholder X   ● Use Additional Character(s)   ▶ Manifestation Code   **Coding Clinic**

● **S63.42**   Traumatic rupture of palmar ligament of finger at metacarpophalangeal and interphalangeal joint

  ● **S63.420**   Traumatic rupture of palmar ligament of right index finger at metacarpophalangeal and interphalangeal joint

  ● **S63.421**   Traumatic rupture of palmar ligament of left index finger at metacarpophalangeal and interphalangeal joint

  ● **S63.422**   Traumatic rupture of palmar ligament of right middle finger at metacarpophalangeal and interphalangeal joint

  ● **S63.423**   Traumatic rupture of palmar ligament of left middle finger at metacarpophalangeal and interphalangeal joint

  ● **S63.424**   Traumatic rupture of palmar ligament of right ring finger at metacarpophalangeal and interphalangeal joint

  ● **S63.425**   Traumatic rupture of palmar ligament of left ring finger at metacarpophalangeal and interphalangeal joint

  ● **S63.426**   Traumatic rupture of palmar ligament of right little finger at metacarpophalangeal and interphalangeal joint

  ● **S63.427**   Traumatic rupture of palmar ligament of left little finger at metacarpophalangeal and interphalangeal joint

  ● **S63.428**   Traumatic rupture of palmar ligament of other finger at metacarpophalangeal and interphalangeal joint

    Traumatic rupture of palmar ligament of specified finger with unspecified laterality at metacarpophalangeal and interphalangeal joint

  ● **S63.429**   Traumatic rupture of palmar ligament of unspecified finger at metacarpophalangeal and interphalangeal joint

● **S63.43**   Traumatic rupture of volar plate of finger at metacarpophalangeal and interphalangeal joint

  ● **S63.430**   Traumatic rupture of volar plate of right index finger at metacarpophalangeal and interphalangeal joint

  ● **S63.431**   Traumatic rupture of volar plate of left index finger at metacarpophalangeal and interphalangeal joint

  ● **S63.432**   Traumatic rupture of volar plate of right middle finger at metacarpophalangeal and interphalangeal joint

  ● **S63.433**   Traumatic rupture of volar plate of left middle finger at metacarpophalangeal and interphalangeal joint

  ● **S63.434**   Traumatic rupture of volar plate of right ring finger at metacarpophalangeal and interphalangeal joint

  ● **S63.435**   Traumatic rupture of volar plate of left ring finger at metacarpophalangeal and interphalangeal joint

  ● **S63.436**   Traumatic rupture of volar plate of right little finger at metacarpophalangeal and interphalangeal joint

  ● **S63.437**   Traumatic rupture of volar plate of left little finger at metacarpophalangeal and interphalangeal joint

  ● **S63.438**   Traumatic rupture of volar plate of other finger at metacarpophalangeal and interphalangeal joint

    Traumatic rupture of volar plate of specified finger with unspecified laterality at metacarpophalangeal and interphalangeal joint

  ● **S63.439**   Traumatic rupture of volar plate of unspecified finger at metacarpophalangeal and interphalangeal joint

● **S63.49**   Traumatic rupture of other ligament of finger at metacarpophalangeal and interphalangeal joint

  ● **S63.490**   Traumatic rupture of other ligament of right index finger at metacarpophalangeal and interphalangeal joint

  ● **S63.491**   Traumatic rupture of other ligament of left index finger at metacarpophalangeal and interphalangeal joint

  ● **S63.492**   Traumatic rupture of other ligament of right middle finger at metacarpophalangeal and interphalangeal joint

  ● **S63.493**   Traumatic rupture of other ligament of left middle finger at metacarpophalangeal and interphalangeal joint

  ● **S63.494**   Traumatic rupture of other ligament of right ring finger at metacarpophalangeal and interphalangeal joint

  ● **S63.495**   Traumatic rupture of other ligament of left ring finger at metacarpophalangeal and interphalangeal joint

  ● **S63.496**   Traumatic rupture of other ligament of right little finger at metacarpophalangeal and interphalangeal joint

  ● **S63.497**   Traumatic rupture of other ligament of left little finger at metacarpophalangeal and interphalangeal joint

  ● **S63.498**   Traumatic rupture of other ligament of other finger at metacarpophalangeal and interphalangeal joint

    Traumatic rupture of ligament of specified finger with unspecified laterality at metacarpophalangeal and interphalangeal joint

  ● **S63.499**   Traumatic rupture of other ligament of unspecified finger at metacarpophalangeal and interphalangeal joint

● **S63.5**   Other and unspecified sprain of wrist

  ● **S63.50**   Unspecified sprain of wrist

    ● **S63.501**   Unspecified sprain of right wrist

    ● **S63.502**   Unspecified sprain of left wrist

    ● **S63.509**   Unspecified sprain of unspecified wrist

N Newborn Age: 0   **P** Pediatric Age: 0–17   **M** Maternity DX: 9–64   **A** Adult Age: 15–124   ♀ Females Only   ♂ Males Only

🏷 Complication\Comorbidity   🏷 Major C\C   (Ex) CC/MCC Exclusions   🏷 Hospital-Acquired Condition   🏷 Hierarchical Condition Category

1363

● S63.51   Sprain of carpal (joint)
- ● S63.511   Sprain of carpal joint of right wrist
- ● S63.512   Sprain of carpal joint of left wrist
- ● S63.519   Sprain of carpal joint of unspecified wrist

● S63.52   Sprain of radiocarpal joint
> **Excludes1**   traumatic rupture of radiocarpal ligament (S63.32-)
- ● S63.521   Sprain of radiocarpal joint of right wrist
- ● S63.522   Sprain of radiocarpal joint of left wrist
- ● S63.529   Sprain of radiocarpal joint of unspecified wrist

● S63.59   Other specified sprain of wrist
- ● S63.591   Other specified sprain of right wrist
- ● S63.592   Other specified sprain of left wrist
- ● S63.599   Other specified sprain of unspecified wrist

● S63.6   Other and unspecified sprain of finger(s)
> **Excludes1**   traumatic rupture of ligament of finger at metacarpophalangeal and interphalangeal joint(s) (S63.4-)

● S63.60   Unspecified sprain of thumb
- ● S63.601   Unspecified sprain of right thumb
- ● S63.602   Unspecified sprain of left thumb
- ● S63.609   Unspecified sprain of unspecified thumb

● S63.61   Unspecified sprain of other and unspecified finger(s)
- ● S63.610   Unspecified sprain of right index finger
- ● S63.611   Unspecified sprain of left index finger
- ● S63.612   Unspecified sprain of right middle finger
- ● S63.613   Unspecified sprain of left middle finger
- ● S63.614   Unspecified sprain of right ring finger
- ● S63.615   Unspecified sprain of left ring finger
- ● S63.616   Unspecified sprain of right little finger
- ● S63.617   Unspecified sprain of left little finger
- ● S63.618   Unspecified sprain of other finger
  - Unspecified sprain of specified finger with unspecified laterality
- ● S63.619   Unspecified sprain of unspecified finger

● S63.62   Sprain of interphalangeal joint of thumb
- ● S63.621   Sprain of interphalangeal joint of right thumb
- ● S63.622   Sprain of interphalangeal joint of left thumb
- ● S63.629   Sprain of interphalangeal joint of unspecified thumb

● S63.63   Sprain of interphalangeal joint of other and unspecified finger(s)
- ● S63.630   Sprain of interphalangeal joint of right index finger
- ● S63.631   Sprain of interphalangeal joint of left index finger
- ● S63.632   Sprain of interphalangeal joint of right middle finger
- ● S63.633   Sprain of interphalangeal joint of left middle finger
- ● S63.634   Sprain of interphalangeal joint of right ring finger
- ● S63.635   Sprain of interphalangeal joint of left ring finger
- ● S63.636   Sprain of interphalangeal joint of right little finger
- ● S63.637   Sprain of interphalangeal joint of left little finger
- ● S63.638   Sprain of interphalangeal joint of other finger
- ● S63.639   Sprain of interphalangeal joint of unspecified finger

● S63.64   Sprain of metacarpophalangeal joint of thumb
- ● S63.641   Sprain of metacarpophalangeal joint of right thumb
- ● S63.642   Sprain of metacarpophalangeal joint of left thumb
- ● S63.649   Sprain of metacarpophalangeal joint of unspecified thumb

● S63.65   Sprain of metacarpophalangeal joint of other and unspecified finger(s)
- ● S63.650   Sprain of metacarpophalangeal joint of right index finger
- ● S63.651   Sprain of metacarpophalangeal joint of left index finger
- ● S63.652   Sprain of metacarpophalangeal joint of right middle finger
- ● S63.653   Sprain of metacarpophalangeal joint of left middle finger
- ● S63.654   Sprain of metacarpophalangeal joint of right ring finger
- ● S63.655   Sprain of metacarpophalangeal joint of left ring finger
- ● S63.656   Sprain of metacarpophalangeal joint of right little finger
- ● S63.657   Sprain of metacarpophalangeal joint of left little finger
- ● S63.658   Sprain of metacarpophalangeal joint of other finger
  - Sprain of metacarpophalangeal joint of specified finger with unspecified laterality
- ● S63.659   Sprain of metacarpophalangeal joint of unspecified finger

● S63.68   Other sprain of thumb
- ● S63.681   Other sprain of right thumb
- ● S63.682   Other sprain of left thumb
- ● S63.689   Other sprain of unspecified thumb

● S63.69   Other sprain of other and unspecified finger(s)
- ● S63.690   Other sprain of right index finger
- ● S63.691   Other sprain of left index finger
- ● S63.692   Other sprain of right middle finger
- ● S63.693   Other sprain of left middle finger
- ● S63.694   Other sprain of right ring finger
- ● S63.695   Other sprain of left ring finger
- ● S63.696   Other sprain of right little finger
- ● S63.697   Other sprain of left little finger
- ● S63.698   Other sprain of other finger
  - Other sprain of specified finger with unspecified laterality
- ● S63.699   Other sprain of unspecified finger

● S63.8   Sprain of other part of wrist and hand
● S63.8X   Sprain of other part of wrist and hand
- ● S63.8X1   Sprain of other part of right wrist and hand
- ● S63.8X2   Sprain of other part of left wrist and hand
- ● S63.8X9   Sprain of other part of unspecified wrist and hand

▶ New   ⇒ Revised   ~~deleted~~ Deleted   Excludes 1   Excludes 2   Includes   Use additional   Code first   Code also   Key words
OGCR Official Guidelines   ● Unacceptable Principal Diagnosis   X Assign placeholder X   ● Use Additional Character(s)   ▶ Manifestation Code   **Coding Clinic**

- S63.9   Sprain of unspecified part of wrist and hand
  - X ● S63.90   Sprain of unspecified part of unspecified wrist and hand
  - X ● S63.91   Sprain of unspecified part of right wrist and hand
  - X ● S63.92   Sprain of unspecified part of left wrist and hand

- S64   **Injury of nerves at wrist and hand level**

  The appropriate 7th character is to be added to each code from category S64

A	initial encounter
D	subsequent encounter
S	sequela

  Code also any associated open wound (S61.-)

- S64.0   Injury of ulnar nerve at wrist and hand level
  - X ● S64.00   Injury of ulnar nerve at wrist and hand level of unspecified arm
  - X ● S64.01   Injury of ulnar nerve at wrist and hand level of right arm
  - X ● S64.02   Injury of ulnar nerve at wrist and hand level of left arm
- S64.1   Injury of median nerve at wrist and hand level
  - X ● S64.10   Injury of median nerve at wrist and hand level of unspecified arm
  - X ● S64.11   Injury of median nerve at wrist and hand level of right arm
  - X ● S64.12   Injury of median nerve at wrist and hand level of left arm
- S64.2   Injury of radial nerve at wrist and hand level
  - X ● S64.20   Injury of radial nerve at wrist and hand level of unspecified arm
  - X ● S64.21   Injury of radial nerve at wrist and hand level of right arm
  - X ● S64.22   Injury of radial nerve at wrist and hand level of left arm
- S64.3   Injury of digital nerve of thumb
  - X ● S64.30   Injury of digital nerve of unspecified thumb
  - X ● S64.31   Injury of digital nerve of right thumb
  - X ● S64.32   Injury of digital nerve of left thumb
- S64.4   Injury of digital nerve of other and unspecified finger
  - X ● S64.40   Injury of digital nerve of unspecified finger
  - ● S64.49   Injury of digital nerve of other finger
    - ● S64.490   Injury of digital nerve of right index finger
    - ● S64.491   Injury of digital nerve of left index finger
    - ● S64.492   Injury of digital nerve of right middle finger
    - ● S64.493   Injury of digital nerve of left middle finger
    - ● S64.494   Injury of digital nerve of right ring finger
    - ● S64.495   Injury of digital nerve of left ring finger
    - ● S64.496   Injury of digital nerve of right little finger
    - ● S64.497   Injury of digital nerve of left little finger
    - ● S64.498   Injury of digital nerve of other finger
      Injury of digital nerve of specified finger with unspecified laterality

- S64.8   Injury of other nerves at wrist and hand level
  - ● S64.8X   Injury of other nerves at wrist and hand level
    - ● S64.8X1   Injury of other nerves at wrist and hand level of right arm
    - ● S64.8X2   Injury of other nerves at wrist and hand level of left arm
    - ● S64.8X9   Injury of other nerves at wrist and hand level of unspecified arm
- S64.9   Injury of unspecified nerve at wrist and hand level
  - X ● S64.90   Injury of unspecified nerve at wrist and hand level of unspecified arm
  - X ● S64.91   Injury of unspecified nerve at wrist and hand level of right arm
  - X ● S64.92   Injury of unspecified nerve at wrist and hand level of left arm

- S65   **Injury of blood vessels at wrist and hand level**

  The appropriate 7th character is to be added to each code from category S65

A	initial encounter
D	subsequent encounter
S	sequela

  Code also any associated open wound (S61.-)

- S65.0   Injury of ulnar artery at wrist and hand level
  - ● S65.00   Unspecified injury of ulnar artery at wrist and hand level
    - ● S65.001   Unspecified injury of ulnar artery at wrist and hand level of right arm A 🅢
      (Ex:) See PDX Collection 1274
    - ● S65.002   Unspecified injury of ulnar artery at wrist and hand level of left arm A 🅢
      (Ex:) See PDX Collection 1275
    - ● S65.009   Unspecified injury of ulnar artery at wrist and hand level of unspecified arm A 🅢
      (Ex:) See PDX Collection 1276
  - ● S65.01   Laceration of ulnar artery at wrist and hand level
    - ● S65.011   Laceration of ulnar artery at wrist and hand level of right arm A 🅢
      (Ex:) See PDX Collection 1274
    - ● S65.012   Laceration of ulnar artery at wrist and hand level of left arm A 🅢
      (Ex:) See PDX Collection 1275
    - ● S65.019   Laceration of ulnar artery at wrist and hand level of unspecified arm A 🅢
      (Ex:) See PDX Collection 1276
  - ● S65.09   Other specified injury of ulnar artery at wrist and hand level
    - ● S65.091   Other specified injury of ulnar artery at wrist and hand level of right arm A 🅢
      (Ex:) See PDX Collection 1274
    - ● S65.092   Other specified injury of ulnar artery at wrist and hand level of left arm A 🅢
      (Ex:) See PDX Collection 1275
    - ● S65.099   Other specified injury of ulnar artery at wrist and hand level of unspecified arm A 🅢
      (Ex:) See PDX Collection 1276

CHAPTER 19 (S00-T88)

N Newborn Age: 0   **P** Pediatric Age: 0–17   **M** Maternity DX: 9–64   **A** Adult Age: 15–124   ♀ Females Only   ♂ Males Only

🅒 Complication\Comorbidity   🅜 Major C\C   (Ex:) CC/MCC Exclusions   🅗 Hospital-Acquired Condition   🅗 Hierarchical Condition Category

1365

● S65.1   Injury of radial artery at wrist and hand level
   ● S65.10   Unspecified injury of radial artery at wrist and hand level
     ● S65.101   Unspecified injury of radial artery at wrist and hand level of right arm A 🅒
       Ⓔ See PDX Collection 1277
     ● S65.102   Unspecified injury of radial artery at wrist and hand level of left arm A 🅒
       Ⓔ See PDX Collection 1278
     ● S65.109   Unspecified injury of radial artery at wrist and hand level of unspecified arm A 🅒
       Ⓔ See PDX Collection 1279
   ● S65.11   Laceration of radial artery at wrist and hand level
     ● S65.111   Laceration of radial artery at wrist and hand level of right arm A 🅒
       Ⓔ See PDX Collection 1277
     ● S65.112   Laceration of radial artery at wrist and hand level of left arm A 🅒
       Ⓔ See PDX Collection 1278
     ● S65.119   Laceration of radial artery at wrist and hand level of unspecified arm A 🅒
       Ⓔ See PDX Collection 1279
   ● S65.19   Other specified injury of radial artery at wrist and hand level
     ● S65.191   Other specified injury of radial artery at wrist and hand level of right arm A 🅒
       Ⓔ See PDX Collection 1277
     ● S65.192   Other specified injury of radial artery at wrist and hand level of left arm A 🅒
       Ⓔ See PDX Collection 1278
     ● S65.199   Other specified injury of radial artery at wrist and hand level of unspecified arm A 🅒
       Ⓔ See PDX Collection 1279

● S65.2   Injury of superficial palmar arch
   ● S65.20   Unspecified injury of superficial palmar arch
     ● S65.201   Unspecified injury of superficial palmar arch of right hand A 🅒
       Ⓔ See PDX Collection 1288
     ● S65.202   Unspecified injury of superficial palmar arch of left hand A 🅒
       Ⓔ See PDX Collection 1289
     ● S65.209   Unspecified injury of superficial palmar arch of unspecified hand A 🅒
       Ⓔ See PDX Collection 1290
   ● S65.21   Laceration of superficial palmar arch
     ● S65.211   Laceration of superficial palmar arch of right hand A 🅒
       Ⓔ See PDX Collection 1288
     ● S65.212   Laceration of superficial palmar arch of left hand A 🅒
       Ⓔ See PDX Collection 1289
     ● S65.219   Laceration of superficial palmar arch of unspecified hand A 🅒
       Ⓔ See PDX Collection 1290
   ● S65.29   Other specified injury of superficial palmar arch
     ● S65.291   Other specified injury of superficial palmar arch of right hand A 🅒
       Ⓔ See PDX Collection 1288
     ● S65.292   Other specified injury of superficial palmar arch of left hand A 🅒
       Ⓔ See PDX Collection 1289
     ● S65.299   Other specified injury of superficial palmar arch of unspecified hand A 🅒
       Ⓔ See PDX Collection 1290

● S65.3   Injury of deep palmar arch
   ● S65.30   Unspecified injury of deep palmar arch
     ● S65.301   Unspecified injury of deep palmar arch of right hand A 🅒
       Ⓔ See PDX Collection 1288
     ● S65.302   Unspecified injury of deep palmar arch of left hand A 🅒
       Ⓔ See PDX Collection 1289
     ● S65.309   Unspecified injury of deep palmar arch of unspecified hand A 🅒
       Ⓔ See PDX Collection 1290
   ● S65.31   Laceration of deep palmar arch
     ● S65.311   Laceration of deep palmar arch of right hand A 🅒
       Ⓔ See PDX Collection 1288
     ● S65.312   Laceration of deep palmar arch of left hand A 🅒
       Ⓔ See PDX Collection 1289
     ● S65.319   Laceration of deep palmar arch of unspecified hand A 🅒
       Ⓔ See PDX Collection 1290
   ● S65.39   Other specified injury of deep palmar arch
     ● S65.391   Other specified injury of deep palmar arch of right hand A 🅒
       Ⓔ See PDX Collection 1288
     ● S65.392   Other specified injury of deep palmar arch of left hand A 🅒
       Ⓔ See PDX Collection 1289
     ● S65.399   Other specified injury of deep palmar arch of unspecified hand A 🅒
       Ⓔ See PDX Collection 1290

● S65.4   Injury of blood vessel of thumb
   ● S65.40   Unspecified injury of blood vessel of thumb
     ● S65.401   Unspecified injury of blood vessel of right thumb A 🅒
       Ⓔ See PDX Collection 1291
     ● S65.402   Unspecified injury of blood vessel of left thumb A 🅒
       Ⓔ See PDX Collection 1292
     ● S65.409   Unspecified injury of blood vessel of unspecified thumb A 🅒
       Ⓔ See PDX Collection 1293
   ● S65.41   Laceration of blood vessel of thumb
     ● S65.411   Laceration of blood vessel of right thumb A 🅒
       Ⓔ See PDX Collection 1291
     ● S65.412   Laceration of blood vessel of left thumb A 🅒
       Ⓔ See PDX Collection 1292
     ● S65.419   Laceration of blood vessel of unspecified thumb A 🅒
       Ⓔ See PDX Collection 1293
   ● S65.49   Other specified injury of blood vessel of thumb
     ● S65.491   Other specified injury of blood vessel of right thumb A 🅒
       Ⓔ See PDX Collection 1291
     ● S65.492   Other specified injury of blood vessel of left thumb A 🅒
       Ⓔ See PDX Collection 1292
     ● S65.499   Other specified injury of blood vessel of unspecified thumb A 🅒
       Ⓔ See PDX Collection 1293

● S65.5   **Injury of blood vessel of other and unspecified finger**
   ● S65.50   Unspecified injury of blood vessel of other and unspecified finger
      ● S65.500   Unspecified injury of blood vessel of right index finger A 🦪
         (Ex:) See PDX Collection 1291
      ● S65.501   Unspecified injury of blood vessel of left index finger A 🦪
         (Ex:) See PDX Collection 1292
      ● S65.502   Unspecified injury of blood vessel of right middle finger A 🦪
         (Ex:) See PDX Collection 1291
      ● S65.503   Unspecified injury of blood vessel of left middle finger A 🦪
         (Ex:) See PDX Collection 1292
      ● S65.504   Unspecified injury of blood vessel of right ring finger A 🦪
         (Ex:) See PDX Collection 1291
      ● S65.505   Unspecified injury of blood vessel of left ring finger A 🦪
         (Ex:) See PDX Collection 1292
      ● S65.506   Unspecified injury of blood vessel of right little finger A 🦪
         (Ex:) See PDX Collection 1291
      ● S65.507   Unspecified injury of blood vessel of left little finger A 🦪
         (Ex:) See PDX Collection 1292
      ● S65.508   Unspecified injury of blood vessel of other finger A 🦪
         Unspecified injury of blood vessel of specified finger with unspecified laterality
         (Ex:) See PDX Collection 1293
      ● S65.509   Unspecified injury of blood vessel of unspecified finger A 🦪
         (Ex:) See PDX Collection 1293
   ● S65.51   Laceration of blood vessel of other and unspecified finger
      ● S65.510   Laceration of blood vessel of right index finger A 🦪
         (Ex:) See PDX Collection 1291
      ● S65.511   Laceration of blood vessel of left index finger A 🦪
         (Ex:) See PDX Collection 1292
      ● S65.512   Laceration of blood vessel of right middle finger A 🦪
         (Ex:) See PDX Collection 1291
      ● S65.513   Laceration of blood vessel of left middle finger A 🦪
         (Ex:) See PDX Collection 1292
      ● S65.514   Laceration of blood vessel of right ring finger A 🦪
         (Ex:) See PDX Collection 1291
      ● S65.515   Laceration of blood vessel of left ring finger A 🦪
         (Ex:) See PDX Collection 1292
      ● S65.516   Laceration of blood vessel of right little finger A 🦪
         (Ex:) See PDX Collection 1291
      ● S65.517   Laceration of blood vessel of left little finger A 🦪
         (Ex:) See PDX Collection 1292
      ● S65.518   Laceration of blood vessel of other finger A 🦪
         Laceration of blood vessel of specified finger with unspecified laterality
         (Ex:) See PDX Collection 1293
      ● S65.519   Laceration of blood vessel of unspecified finger A 🦪
         (Ex:) See PDX Collection 1293

   ● S65.59   Other specified injury of blood vessel of other and unspecified finger
      ● S65.590   Other specified injury of blood vessel of right index finger A 🦪
         (Ex:) See PDX Collection 1291
      ● S65.591   Other specified injury of blood vessel of left index finger A 🦪
         (Ex:) See PDX Collection 1292
      ● S65.592   Other specified injury of blood vessel of right middle finger A 🦪
         (Ex:) See PDX Collection 1291
      ● S65.593   Other specified injury of blood vessel of left middle finger A 🦪
         (Ex:) See PDX Collection 1292
      ● S65.594   Other specified injury of blood vessel of right ring finger A 🦪
         (Ex:) See PDX Collection 1291
      ● S65.595   Other specified injury of blood vessel of left ring finger A 🦪
         (Ex:) See PDX Collection 1292
      ● S65.596   Other specified injury of blood vessel of right little finger A 🦪
         (Ex:) See PDX Collection 1291
      ● S65.597   Other specified injury of blood vessel of left little finger A 🦪
         (Ex:) See PDX Collection 1292
      ● S65.598   Other specified injury of blood vessel of other finger A 🦪
         Other specified injury of blood vessel of specified finger with unspecified laterality
         (Ex:) See PDX Collection 1293
      ● S65.599   Other specified injury of blood vessel of unspecified finger A 🦪
         (Ex:) See PDX Collection 1293
● S65.8   **Injury of other blood vessels at wrist and hand level**
   ● S65.80   Unspecified injury of other blood vessels at wrist and hand level
      ● S65.801   Unspecified injury of other blood vessels at wrist and hand level of right arm A 🦪
         (Ex:) See PDX Collection 1260
      ● S65.802   Unspecified injury of other blood vessels at wrist and hand level of left arm A 🦪
         (Ex:) See PDX Collection 1261
      ● S65.809   Unspecified injury of other blood vessels at wrist and hand level of unspecified arm A 🦪
         (Ex:) See PDX Collection 1262
   ● S65.81   Laceration of other blood vessels at wrist and hand level
      ● S65.811   Laceration of other blood vessels at wrist and hand level of right arm A 🦪
         (Ex:) See PDX Collection 1260
      ● S65.812   Laceration of other blood vessels at wrist and hand level of left arm A 🦪
         (Ex:) See PDX Collection 1261
      ● S65.819   Laceration of other blood vessels at wrist and hand level of unspecified arm A 🦪
         (Ex:) See PDX Collection 1262

CHAPTER 19 (S00-T88)

N Newborn Age: 0   P Pediatric Age: 0–17   M Maternity DX: 9–64   A Adult Age: 15–124   ♀ Females Only   ♂ Males Only

🦪 Complication\Comorbidity   🦪 Major C\C   (Ex:) CC/MCC Exclusions   🦪 Hospital-Acquired Condition   🦪 Hierarchical Condition Category

1367

- S65.89 Other specified injury of other blood vessels at wrist and hand level
  - S65.891 Other specified injury of other blood vessels at wrist and hand level of right arm A 🔊
    (Ex:) See PDX Collection 1260
  - S65.892 Other specified injury of other blood vessels at wrist and hand level of left arm A 🔊
    (Ex:) See PDX Collection 1261
  - S65.899 Other specified injury of other blood vessels at wrist and hand level of unspecified arm A 🔊
    (Ex:) See PDX Collection 1262
- S65.9 Injury of unspecified blood vessel at wrist and hand level
  - S65.90 Unspecified injury of unspecified blood vessel at wrist and hand level
    - S65.901 Unspecified injury of unspecified blood vessel at wrist and hand level of right arm A 🔊
      (Ex:) See PDX Collection 1260
    - S65.902 Unspecified injury of unspecified blood vessel at wrist and hand level of left arm A 🔊
      (Ex:) See PDX Collection 1261
    - S65.909 Unspecified injury of unspecified blood vessel at wrist and hand level of unspecified arm A 🔊
      (Ex:) See PDX Collection 1262
  - S65.91 Laceration of unspecified blood vessel at wrist and hand level
    - S65.911 Laceration of unspecified blood vessel at wrist and hand level of right arm A 🔊
      (Ex:) See PDX Collection 1260
    - S65.912 Laceration of unspecified blood vessel at wrist and hand level of left arm A 🔊
      (Ex:) See PDX Collection 1261
    - S65.919 Laceration of unspecified blood vessel at wrist and hand level of unspecified arm A 🔊
      (Ex:) See PDX Collection 1262
  - S65.99 Other specified injury of unspecified blood vessel at wrist and hand level
    - S65.991 Other specified injury of unspecified blood vessel at wrist and hand of right arm A 🔊
      (Ex:) See PDX Collection 1260
    - S65.992 Other specified injury of unspecified blood vessel at wrist and hand of left arm A 🔊
      (Ex:) See PDX Collection 1261
    - S65.999 Other specified injury of unspecified blood vessel at wrist and hand of unspecified arm A 🔊
      (Ex:) See PDX Collection 1262

- S66 Injury of muscle, fascia and tendon at wrist and hand level
  Code also any associated open wound (S61.-)

  Excludes2 sprain of joints and ligaments of wrist and hand (S63.-)

  The appropriate 7th character is to be added to each code from category S66

A	initial encounter
D	subsequent encounter
S	sequela

  - S66.0 Injury of long flexor muscle, fascia and tendon of thumb at wrist and hand level
    - S66.00 Unspecified injury of long flexor muscle, fascia and tendon of thumb at wrist and hand level
      - S66.001 Unspecified injury of long flexor muscle, fascia and tendon of right thumb at wrist and hand level
      - S66.002 Unspecified injury of long flexor muscle, fascia and tendon of left thumb at wrist and hand level
      - S66.009 Unspecified injury of long flexor muscle, fascia and tendon of unspecified thumb at wrist and hand level
    - S66.01 Strain of long flexor muscle, fascia and tendon of thumb at wrist and hand level
      - S66.011 Strain of long flexor muscle, fascia and tendon of right thumb at wrist and hand level
      - S66.012 Strain of long flexor muscle, fascia and tendon of left thumb at wrist and hand level
      - S66.019 Strain of long flexor muscle, fascia and tendon of unspecified thumb at wrist and hand level
    - S66.02 Laceration of long flexor muscle, fascia and tendon of thumb at wrist and hand level
      - S66.021 Laceration of long flexor muscle, fascia and tendon of right thumb at wrist and hand level A 🔊
        (Ex:) See PDX Collection 1294
      - S66.022 Laceration of long flexor muscle, fascia and tendon of left thumb at wrist and hand level A 🔊
        (Ex:) See PDX Collection 1295
      - S66.029 Laceration of long flexor muscle, fascia and tendon of unspecified thumb at wrist and hand level A 🔊
        (Ex:) See PDX Collection 1296
    - S66.09 Other specified injury of long flexor muscle, fascia and tendon of thumb at wrist and hand level
      - S66.091 Other specified injury of long flexor muscle, fascia and tendon of right thumb at wrist and hand level
      - S66.092 Other specified injury of long flexor muscle, fascia and tendon of left thumb at wrist and hand level
      - S66.099 Other specified injury of long flexor muscle, fascia and tendon of unspecified thumb at wrist and hand level

▶ New ⟡ Revised deleted Deleted | Excludes 1 | Excludes 2 | Includes | Use additional | Code first | Code also | Key words
OGCR Official Guidelines ● Unacceptable Principal Diagnosis X Assign placeholder X ● Use Additional Character(s) ▶ Manifestation Code **Coding Clinic**

● S66.1   Injury of flexor muscle, fascia and tendon of other and unspecified finger at wrist and hand level

     Excludes2   injury of long flexor muscle, fascia and tendon of thumb at wrist and hand level (S66.0-)

● S66.10   Unspecified injury of flexor muscle, fascia and tendon of other and unspecified finger at wrist and hand level

     ● S66.100   Unspecified injury of flexor muscle, fascia and tendon of right index finger at wrist and hand level

     ● S66.101   Unspecified injury of flexor muscle, fascia and tendon of left index finger at wrist and hand level

     ● S66.102   Unspecified injury of flexor muscle, fascia and tendon of right middle finger at wrist and hand level

     ● S66.103   Unspecified injury of flexor muscle, fascia and tendon of left middle finger at wrist and hand level

     ● S66.104   Unspecified injury of flexor muscle, fascia and tendon of right ring finger at wrist and hand level

     ● S66.105   Unspecified injury of flexor muscle, fascia and tendon of left ring finger at wrist and hand level

     ● S66.106   Unspecified injury of flexor muscle, fascia and tendon of right little finger at wrist and hand level

     ● S66.107   Unspecified injury of flexor muscle, fascia and tendon of left little finger at wrist and hand level

     ● S66.108   Unspecified injury of flexor muscle, fascia and tendon of other finger at wrist and hand level

         Unspecified injury of flexor muscle, fascia and tendon of specified finger with unspecified laterality at wrist and hand level

     ● S66.109   Unspecified injury of flexor muscle, fascia and tendon of unspecified finger at wrist and hand level

● S66.11   Strain of flexor muscle, fascia and tendon of other and unspecified finger at wrist and hand level

     ● S66.110   Strain of flexor muscle, fascia and tendon of right index finger at wrist and hand level

     ● S66.111   Strain of flexor muscle, fascia and tendon of left index finger at wrist and hand level

     ● S66.112   Strain of flexor muscle, fascia and tendon of right middle finger at wrist and hand level

     ● S66.113   Strain of flexor muscle, fascia and tendon of left middle finger at wrist and hand level

     ● S66.114   Strain of flexor muscle, fascia and tendon of right ring finger at wrist and hand level

     ● S66.115   Strain of flexor muscle, fascia and tendon of left ring finger at wrist and hand level

● S66.116   Strain of flexor muscle, fascia and tendon of right little finger at wrist and hand level

● S66.117   Strain of flexor muscle, fascia and tendon of left little finger at wrist and hand level

● S66.118   Strain of flexor muscle, fascia and tendon of other finger at wrist and hand level

     Strain of flexor muscle, fascia and tendon of specified finger with unspecified laterality at wrist and hand level

● S66.119   Strain of flexor muscle, fascia and tendon of unspecified finger at wrist and hand level

● S66.12   Laceration of flexor muscle, fascia and tendon of other and unspecified finger at wrist and hand level

     ● S66.120   Laceration of flexor muscle, fascia and tendon of right index finger at wrist and hand level A 🗇
         (Ex:) See PDX Collection 1294

     ● S66.121   Laceration of flexor muscle, fascia and tendon of left index finger at wrist and hand level A 🗇
         (Ex:) See PDX Collection 1295

     ● S66.122   Laceration of flexor muscle, fascia and tendon of right middle finger at wrist and hand level A 🗇
         (Ex:) See PDX Collection 1294

     ● S66.123   Laceration of flexor muscle, fascia and tendon of left middle finger at wrist and hand level A 🗇
         (Ex:) See PDX Collection 1295

     ● S66.124   Laceration of flexor muscle, fascia and tendon of right ring finger at wrist and hand level A 🗇
         (Ex:) See PDX Collection 1294

     ● S66.125   Laceration of flexor muscle, fascia and tendon of left ring finger at wrist and hand level A 🗇
         (Ex:) See PDX Collection 1295

     ● S66.126   Laceration of flexor muscle, fascia and tendon of right little finger at wrist and hand level A 🗇
         (Ex:) See PDX Collection 1294

     ● S66.127   Laceration of flexor muscle, fascia and tendon of left little finger at wrist and hand level A 🗇
         (Ex:) See PDX Collection 1795

     ● S66.128   Laceration of flexor muscle, fascia and tendon of other finger at wrist and hand level A 🗇

         Laceration of flexor muscle, fascia and tendon of specified finger with unspecified laterality at wrist and hand level
         (Ex:) See PDX Collection 1296

     ● S66.129   Laceration of flexor muscle, fascia and tendon of unspecified finger at wrist and hand level A 🗇
         (Ex:) See PDX Collection 1296

N   Newborn Age: 0   **P**   Pediatric Age: 0–17   **M**   Maternity DX: 9–64   **A**   Adult Age: 15–124   ♀   Females Only   ♂   Males Only

🗇   Complication\Comorbidity   🗇   Major C\C   (Ex:)   CC/MCC Exclusions   🗇   Hospital-Acquired Condition   🗇   Hierarchical Condition Category

● **S66.19**   Other injury of flexor muscle, fascia and tendon of other and unspecified finger at wrist and hand level

  ● **S66.190**   Other injury of flexor muscle, fascia and tendon of right index finger at wrist and hand level

  ● **S66.191**   Other injury of flexor muscle, fascia and tendon of left index finger at wrist and hand level

  ● **S66.192**   Other injury of flexor muscle, fascia and tendon of right middle finger at wrist and hand level

  ● **S66.193**   Other injury of flexor muscle, fascia and tendon of left middle finger at wrist and hand level

  ● **S66.194**   Other injury of flexor muscle, fascia and tendon of right ring finger at wrist and hand level

  ● **S66.195**   Other injury of flexor muscle, fascia and tendon of left ring finger at wrist and hand level

  ● **S66.196**   Other injury of flexor muscle, fascia and tendon of right little finger at wrist and hand level

  ● **S66.197**   Other injury of flexor muscle, fascia and tendon of left little finger at wrist and hand level

  ● **S66.198**   Other injury of flexor muscle, fascia and tendon of other finger at wrist and hand level

       Other injury of flexor muscle, fascia and tendon of specified finger with unspecified laterality at wrist and hand level

  ● **S66.199**   Other injury of flexor muscle, fascia and tendon of unspecified finger at wrist and hand level

● **S66.2**   Injury of extensor muscle, fascia and tendon of thumb at wrist and hand level

 ● **S66.20**   Unspecified injury of extensor muscle, fascia and tendon of thumb at wrist and hand level

  ● **S66.201**   Unspecified injury of extensor muscle, fascia and tendon of right thumb at wrist and hand level

  ● **S66.202**   Unspecified injury of extensor muscle, fascia and tendon of left thumb at wrist and hand level

  ● **S66.209**   Unspecified injury of extensor muscle, fascia and tendon of unspecified thumb at wrist and hand level

 ● **S66.21**   Strain of extensor muscle, fascia and tendon of thumb at wrist and hand level

  ● **S66.211**   Strain of extensor muscle, fascia and tendon of right thumb at wrist and hand level

  ● **S66.212**   Strain of extensor muscle, fascia and tendon of left thumb at wrist and hand level

  ● **S66.219**   Strain of extensor muscle, fascia and tendon of unspecified thumb at wrist and hand level

 ● **S66.22**   Laceration of extensor muscle, fascia and tendon of thumb at wrist and hand level

  ● **S66.221**   Laceration of extensor muscle, fascia and tendon of right thumb at wrist and hand level A 🔗
      (Ex:) See PDX Collection 1294

  ● **S66.222**   Laceration of extensor muscle, fascia and tendon of left thumb at wrist and hand level A 🔗
      (Ex:) See PDX Collection 1295

  ● **S66.229**   Laceration of extensor muscle, fascia and tendon of unspecified thumb at wrist and hand level A 🔗
      (Ex:) See PDX Collection 1296

 ● **S66.29**   Other specified injury of extensor muscle, fascia and tendon of thumb at wrist and hand level

  ● **S66.291**   Other specified injury of extensor muscle, fascia and tendon of right thumb at wrist and hand level

  ● **S66.292**   Other specified injury of extensor muscle, fascia and tendon of left thumb at wrist and hand level

  ● **S66.299**   Other specified injury of extensor muscle, fascia and tendon of unspecified thumb at wrist and hand level

● **S66.3**   Injury of extensor muscle, fascia and tendon of other and unspecified finger at wrist and hand level

    Excludes2   injury of extensor muscle, fascia and tendon of thumb at wrist and hand level (S66.2-)

 ● **S66.30**   Unspecified injury of extensor muscle, fascia and tendon of other and unspecified finger at wrist and hand level

  ● **S66.300**   Unspecified injury of extensor muscle, fascia and tendon of right index finger at wrist and hand level

  ● **S66.301**   Unspecified injury of extensor muscle, fascia and tendon of left index finger at wrist and hand level

  ● **S66.302**   Unspecified injury of extensor muscle, fascia and tendon of right middle finger at wrist and hand level

  ● **S66.303**   Unspecified injury of extensor muscle, fascia and tendon of left middle finger at wrist and hand level

  ● **S66.304**   Unspecified injury of extensor muscle, fascia and tendon of right ring finger at wrist and hand level

  ● **S66.305**   Unspecified injury of extensor muscle, fascia and tendon of left ring finger at wrist and hand level

  ● **S66.306**   Unspecified injury of extensor muscle, fascia and tendon of right little finger at wrist and hand level

  ● **S66.307**   Unspecified injury of extensor muscle, fascia and tendon of left little finger at wrist and hand level

  ● **S66.308**   Unspecified injury of extensor muscle, fascia and tendon of other finger at wrist and hand level

       Unspecified injury of extensor muscle, fascia and tendon of specified finger with unspecified laterality at wrist and hand level

  ● **S66.309**   Unspecified injury of extensor muscle, fascia and tendon of unspecified finger at wrist and hand level

▶ New   ⇒ Revised   ~~deleted~~ Deleted   Excludes 1   Excludes 2   Includes   Use additional   Code first   Code also   Key words

OGCR Official Guidelines   ● Unacceptable Principal Diagnosis   X Assign placeholder X   ● Use Additional Character(s)   ▶ Manifestation Code   **Coding Clinic**

● **S66.31**   Strain of extensor muscle, fascia and tendon of other and unspecified finger at wrist and hand level

    ● **S66.310**   Strain of extensor muscle, fascia and tendon of right index finger at wrist and hand level

    ● **S66.311**   Strain of extensor muscle, fascia and tendon of left index finger at wrist and hand level

    ● **S66.312**   Strain of extensor muscle, fascia and tendon of right middle finger at wrist and hand level

    ● **S66.313**   Strain of extensor muscle, fascia and tendon of left middle finger at wrist and hand level

    ● **S66.314**   Strain of extensor muscle, fascia and tendon of right ring finger at wrist and hand level

    ● **S66.315**   Strain of extensor muscle, fascia and tendon of left ring finger at wrist and hand level

    ● **S66.316**   Strain of extensor muscle, fascia and tendon of right little finger at wrist and hand level

    ● **S66.317**   Strain of extensor muscle, fascia and tendon of left little finger at wrist and hand level

    ● **S66.318**   Strain of extensor muscle, fascia and tendon of other finger at wrist and hand level

        Strain of extensor muscle, fascia and tendon of specified finger with unspecified laterality at wrist and hand level

    ● **S66.319**   Strain of extensor muscle, fascia and tendon of unspecified finger at wrist and hand level

● **S66.32**   Laceration of extensor muscle, fascia and tendon of other and unspecified finger at wrist and hand level

    ● **S66.320**   Laceration of extensor muscle, fascia and tendon of right index finger at wrist and hand level A 🐾
       (Ex) See PDX Collection 1294

    ● **S66.321**   Laceration of extensor muscle, fascia and tendon of left index finger at wrist and hand level A 🐾
       (Ex) See PDX Collection 1295

    ● **S66.322**   Laceration of extensor muscle, fascia and tendon of right middle finger at wrist and hand level A 🐾
       (Ex) See PDX Collection 1294

    ● **S66.323**   Laceration of extensor muscle, fascia and tendon of left middle finger at wrist and hand level A 🐾
       (Ex) See PDX Collection 1295

    ● **S66.324**   Laceration of extensor muscle, fascia and tendon of right ring finger at wrist and hand level A 🐾
       (Ex) See PDX Collection 1294

    ● **S66.325**   Laceration of extensor muscle, fascia and tendon of left ring finger at wrist and hand level A 🐾
       (Ex) See PDX Collection 1295

    ● **S66.326**   Laceration of extensor muscle, fascia and tendon of right little finger at wrist and hand level A 🐾
       (Ex) See PDX Collection 1294

    ● **S66.327**   Laceration of extensor muscle, fascia and tendon of left little finger at wrist and hand level A 🐾
       (Ex) See PDX Collection 1295

    ● **S66.328**   Laceration of extensor muscle, fascia and tendon of other finger at wrist and hand level A 🐾

        Laceration of extensor muscle, fascia and tendon of specified finger with unspecified laterality at wrist and hand level
       (Ex) See PDX Collection 1296

    ● **S66.329**   Laceration of extensor muscle, fascia and tendon of unspecified finger at wrist and hand level A 🐾
       (Ex) See PDX Collection 1296

● **S66.39**   Other injury of extensor muscle, fascia and tendon of other and unspecified finger at wrist and hand level

    ● **S66.390**   Other injury of extensor muscle, fascia and tendon of right index finger at wrist and hand level

    ● **S66.391**   Other injury of extensor muscle, fascia and tendon of left index finger at wrist and hand level

    ● **S66.392**   Other injury of extensor muscle, fascia and tendon of right middle finger at wrist and hand level

    ● **S66.393**   Other injury of extensor muscle, fascia and tendon of left middle finger at wrist and hand level

    ● **S66.394**   Other injury of extensor muscle, fascia and tendon of right ring finger at wrist and hand level

    ● **S66.395**   Other injury of extensor muscle, fascia and tendon of left ring finger at wrist and hand level

    ● **S66.396**   Other injury of extensor muscle, fascia and tendon of right little finger at wrist and hand level

    ● **S66.397**   Other injury of extensor muscle, fascia and tendon of left little finger at wrist and hand level

    ● **S66.398**   Other injury of extensor muscle, fascia and tendon of other finger at wrist and hand level

        Other injury of extensor muscle, fascia and tendon of specified finger with unspecified laterality at wrist and hand level

    ● **S66.399**   Other injury of extensor muscle, fascia and tendon of unspecified finger at wrist and hand level

● **S66.4**   Injury of intrinsic muscle, fascia and tendon of thumb at wrist and hand level

   ● **S66.40**   Unspecified injury of intrinsic muscle, fascia and tendon of thumb at wrist and hand level

    ● **S66.401**   Unspecified injury of intrinsic muscle, fascia and tendon of right thumb at wrist and hand level

    ● **S66.402**   Unspecified injury of intrinsic muscle, fascia and tendon of left thumb at wrist and hand level

    ● **S66.409**   Unspecified injury of intrinsic muscle, fascia and tendon of unspecified thumb at wrist and hand level

   ● **S66.41**   Strain of intrinsic muscle, fascia and tendon of thumb at wrist and hand level

    ● **S66.411**   Strain of intrinsic muscle, fascia and tendon of right thumb at wrist and hand level

    ● **S66.412**   Strain of intrinsic muscle, fascia and tendon of left thumb at wrist and hand level

    ● **S66.419**   Strain of intrinsic muscle, fascia and tendon of unspecified thumb at wrist and hand level

---

N Newborn Age: 0   **P** Pediatric Age: 0–17   **M** Maternity DX: 9–64   **A** Adult Age: 15–124   ♀ Females Only   ♂ Males Only

🐾 Complication\Comorbidity   🐾 Major C\C   (Ex) CC/MCC Exclusions   🐾 Hospital-Acquired Condition   🐾 Hierarchical Condition Category

1371

CHAPTER 19 (S00-T88)

● S66.42   Laceration of intrinsic muscle, fascia and tendon of thumb at wrist and hand level

  ● S66.421   Laceration of intrinsic muscle, fascia and tendon of right thumb at wrist and hand level A 🗇
    (Ex:) See PDX Collection 1294

  ● S66.422   Laceration of intrinsic muscle, fascia and tendon of left thumb at wrist and hand level A 🗇
    (Ex:) See PDX Collection 1295

  ● S66.429   Laceration of intrinsic muscle, fascia and tendon of unspecified thumb at wrist and hand level A 🗇
    (Ex:) See PDX Collection 1296

● S66.49   Other specified injury of intrinsic muscle, fascia and tendon of thumb at wrist and hand level

  ● S66.491   Other specified injury of intrinsic muscle, fascia and tendon of right thumb at wrist and hand level

  ● S66.492   Other specified injury of intrinsic muscle, fascia and tendon of left thumb at wrist and hand level

  ● S66.499   Other specified injury of intrinsic muscle, fascia and tendon of unspecified thumb at wrist and hand level

● S66.5   Injury of intrinsic muscle, fascia and tendon of other and unspecified finger at wrist and hand level

  Excludes2   injury of intrinsic muscle, fascia and tendon of thumb at wrist and hand level (S66.4-)

● S66.50   Unspecified injury of intrinsic muscle, fascia and tendon of other and unspecified finger at wrist and hand level

  ● S66.500   Unspecified injury of intrinsic muscle, fascia and tendon of right index finger at wrist and hand level

  ● S66.501   Unspecified injury of intrinsic muscle, fascia and tendon of left index finger at wrist and hand level

  ● S66.502   Unspecified injury of intrinsic muscle, fascia and tendon of right middle finger at wrist and hand level

  ● S66.503   Unspecified injury of intrinsic muscle, fascia and tendon of left middle finger at wrist and hand level

  ● S66.504   Unspecified injury of intrinsic muscle, fascia and tendon of right ring finger at wrist and hand level

  ● S66.505   Unspecified injury of intrinsic muscle, fascia and tendon of left ring finger at wrist and hand level

  ● S66.506   Unspecified injury of intrinsic muscle, fascia and tendon of right little finger at wrist and hand level

  ● S66.507   Unspecified injury of intrinsic muscle, fascia and tendon of left little finger at wrist and hand level

  ● S66.508   Unspecified injury of intrinsic muscle, fascia and tendon of other finger at wrist and hand level
    Unspecified injury of intrinsic muscle, fascia and tendon of specified finger with unspecified laterality at wrist and hand level

  ● S66.509   Unspecified injury of intrinsic muscle, fascia and tendon of unspecified finger at wrist and hand level

● S66.51   Strain of intrinsic muscle, fascia and tendon of other and unspecified finger at wrist and hand level

  ● S66.510   Strain of intrinsic muscle, fascia and tendon of right index finger at wrist and hand level

  ● S66.511   Strain of intrinsic muscle, fascia and tendon of left index finger at wrist and hand level

  ● S66.512   Strain of intrinsic muscle, fascia and tendon of right middle finger at wrist and hand level

  ● S66.513   Strain of intrinsic muscle, fascia and tendon of left middle finger at wrist and hand level

  ● S66.514   Strain of intrinsic muscle, fascia and tendon of right ring finger at wrist and hand level

  ● S66.515   Strain of intrinsic muscle, fascia and tendon of left ring finger at wrist and hand level

  ● S66.516   Strain of intrinsic muscle, fascia and tendon of right little finger at wrist and hand level

  ● S66.517   Strain of intrinsic muscle, fascia and tendon of left little finger at wrist and hand level

  ● S66.518   Strain of intrinsic muscle, fascia and tendon of other finger at wrist and hand level
    Strain of intrinsic muscle, fascia and tendon of specified finger with unspecified laterality at wrist and hand level

  ● S66.519   Strain of intrinsic muscle, fascia and tendon of unspecified finger at wrist and hand level

● S66.52   Laceration of intrinsic muscle, fascia and tendon of other and unspecified finger at wrist and hand level

  ● S66.520   Laceration of intrinsic muscle, fascia and tendon of right index finger at wrist and hand level A 🗇
    (Ex:) See PDX Collection 1294

  ● S66.521   Laceration of intrinsic muscle, fascia and tendon of left index finger at wrist and hand level A 🗇
    (Ex:) See PDX Collection 1295

  ● S66.522   Laceration of intrinsic muscle, fascia and tendon of right middle finger at wrist and hand level A 🗇
    (Ex:) See PDX Collection 1294

  ● S66.523   Laceration of intrinsic muscle, fascia and tendon of left middle finger at wrist and hand level A 🗇
    (Ex:) See PDX Collection 1295

  ● S66.524   Laceration of intrinsic muscle, fascia and tendon of right ring finger at wrist and hand level A 🗇
    (Ex:) See PDX Collection 1294

  ● S66.525   Laceration of intrinsic muscle, fascia and tendon of left ring finger at wrist and hand level A 🗇
    (Ex:) See PDX Collection 1295

  ● S66.526   Laceration of intrinsic muscle, fascia and tendon of right little finger at wrist and hand level A 🗇
    (Ex:) See PDX Collection 1294

  ● S66.527   Laceration of intrinsic muscle, fascia and tendon of left little finger at wrist and hand level A 🗇
    (Ex:) See PDX Collection 1295

● S66.528   Laceration of intrinsic muscle, fascia and tendon of other finger at wrist and hand level A ⦿
> Laceration of intrinsic muscle, fascia and tendon of specified finger with unspecified laterality at wrist and hand level
> (Ex:) See PDX Collection 1296

● S66.529   Laceration of intrinsic muscle, fascia and tendon of unspecified finger at wrist and hand level A ⦿
> (Ex:) See PDX Collection 1296

● S66.59   Other injury of intrinsic muscle, fascia and tendon of other and unspecified finger at wrist and hand level

● S66.590   Other injury of intrinsic muscle, fascia and tendon of right index finger at wrist and hand level

● S66.591   Other injury of intrinsic muscle, fascia and tendon of left index finger at wrist and hand level

● S66.592   Other injury of intrinsic muscle, fascia and tendon of right middle finger at wrist and hand level

● S66.593   Other injury of intrinsic muscle, fascia and tendon of left middle finger at wrist and hand level

● S66.594   Other injury of intrinsic muscle, fascia and tendon of right ring finger at wrist and hand level

● S66.595   Other injury of intrinsic muscle, fascia and tendon of left ring finger at wrist and hand level

● S66.596   Other injury of intrinsic muscle, fascia and tendon of right little finger at wrist and hand level

● S66.597   Other injury of intrinsic muscle, fascia and tendon of left little finger at wrist and hand level

● S66.598   Other injury of intrinsic muscle, fascia and tendon of other finger at wrist and hand level
> Other injury of intrinsic muscle, fascia and tendon of specified finger with unspecified laterality at wrist and hand level

● S66.599   Other injury of intrinsic muscle, fascia and tendon of unspecified finger at wrist and hand level

● S66.8   Injury of other specified muscles, fascia and tendons at wrist and hand level

● S66.80   Unspecified injury of other specified muscles, fascia and tendons at wrist and hand level

● S66.801   Unspecified injury of other specified muscles, fascia and tendons at wrist and hand level, right hand

● S66.802   Unspecified injury of other specified muscles, fascia and tendons at wrist and hand level, left hand

● S66.809   Unspecified injury of other specified muscles, fascia and tendons at wrist and hand level, unspecified hand

● S66.81   Strain of other specified muscles, fascia and tendons at wrist and hand level

● S66.811   Strain of other specified muscles, fascia and tendons at wrist and hand level, right hand

● S66.812   Strain of other specified muscles, fascia and tendons at wrist and hand level, left hand

● S66.819   Strain of other specified muscles, fascia and tendons at wrist and hand level, unspecified hand

● S66.82   Laceration of other specified muscles, fascia and tendons at wrist and hand level

● S66.821   Laceration of other specified muscles, fascia and tendons at wrist and hand level, right hand A ⦿
> (Ex:) See PDX Collection 1294

● S66.822   Laceration of other specified muscles, fascia and tendons at wrist and hand level, left hand A ⦿
> (Ex:) See PDX Collection 1295

● S66.829   Laceration of other specified muscles, fascia and tendons at wrist and hand level, unspecified hand A ⦿
> (Ex:) See PDX Collection 1296

● S66.89   Other injury of other specified muscles, fascia and tendons at wrist and hand level

● S66.891   Other injury of other specified muscles, fascia and tendons at wrist and hand level, right hand

● S66.892   Other injury of other specified muscles, fascia and tendons at wrist and hand level, left hand

● S66.899   Other injury of other specified muscles, fascia and tendons at wrist and hand level, unspecified hand

● S66.9   Injury of unspecified muscle, fascia and tendon at wrist and hand level

● S66.90   Unspecified injury of unspecified muscle, fascia and tendon at wrist and hand level

● S66.901   Unspecified injury of unspecified muscle, fascia and tendon at wrist and hand level, right hand

● S66.902   Unspecified injury of unspecified muscle, fascia and tendon at wrist and hand level, left hand

● S66.909   Unspecified injury of unspecified muscle, fascia and tendon at wrist and hand level, unspecified hand

● S66.91   Strain of unspecified muscle, fascia and tendon at wrist and hand level

● S66.911   Strain of unspecified muscle, fascia and tendon at wrist and hand level, right hand

● S66.912   Strain of unspecified muscle, fascia and tendon at wrist and hand level, left hand

● S66.919   Strain of unspecified muscle, fascia and tendon at wrist and hand level, unspecified hand

N Newborn Age: 0   P Pediatric Age: 0–17   M Maternity DX: 9–64   A Adult Age: 15–124   ♀ Females Only   ♂ Males Only

⦿ Complication\Comorbidity   ⦿ Major C\C   (Ex:) CC/MCC Exclusions   ⦿ Hospital-Acquired Condition   ⦿ Hierarchical Condition Category   1373

CHAPTER 19 (S00–T88)

● S66.92   Laceration of unspecified muscle, fascia and tendon at wrist and hand level

   ● S66.921   Laceration of unspecified muscle, fascia and tendon at wrist and hand level, right hand A 🔗
     (Ex:) See PDX Collection 1294

   ● S66.922   Laceration of unspecified muscle, fascia and tendon at wrist and hand level, left hand A 🔗
     (Ex:) See PDX Collection 1295

   ● S66.929   Laceration of unspecified muscle, fascia and tendon at wrist and hand level, unspecified hand A 🔗
     (Ex:) See PDX Collection 1296

● S66.99   Other injury of unspecified muscle, fascia and tendon at wrist and hand level

   ● S66.991   Other injury of unspecified muscle, fascia and tendon at wrist and hand level, right hand

   ● S66.992   Other injury of unspecified muscle, fascia and tendon at wrist and hand level, left hand

   ● S66.999   Other injury of unspecified muscle, fascia and tendon at wrist and hand level, unspecified hand

● S67   Crushing injury of wrist, hand and fingers

Use additional code for all associated injuries, such as:
fracture of wrist and hand (S62.-)
open wound of wrist and hand (S61.-)

The appropriate 7th character is to be added to each code from category S67

A	initial encounter
D	subsequent encounter
S	sequela

● S67.0   Crushing injury of thumb
   X ● S67.00   Crushing injury of unspecified thumb
   X ● S67.01   Crushing injury of right thumb
   X ● S67.02   Crushing injury of left thumb

● S67.1   Crushing injury of other and unspecified finger(s)
   Excludes2   crushing injury of thumb (S67.0-)
   X ● S67.10   Crushing injury of unspecified finger(s)
   ● S67.19   Crushing injury of other finger(s)
     ● S67.190   Crushing injury of right index finger
     ● S67.191   Crushing injury of left index finger
     ● S67.192   Crushing injury of right middle finger
     ● S67.193   Crushing injury of left middle finger
     ● S67.194   Crushing injury of right ring finger
     ● S67.195   Crushing injury of left ring finger
     ● S67.196   Crushing injury of right little finger
     ● S67.197   Crushing injury of left little finger
     ● S67.198   Crushing injury of other finger
       Crushing injury of specified finger with unspecified laterality

● S67.2   Crushing injury of hand
   Excludes2   crushing injury of fingers (S67.1-)
               crushing injury of thumb (S67.0-)
   X ● S67.20   Crushing injury of unspecified hand
   X ● S67.21   Crushing injury of right hand
   X ● S67.22   Crushing injury of left hand

● S67.3   Crushing injury of wrist
   X ● S67.30   Crushing injury of unspecified wrist
   X ● S67.31   Crushing injury of right wrist
   X ● S67.32   Crushing injury of left wrist

● S67.4   Crushing injury of wrist and hand
   Excludes1   crushing injury of hand alone (S67.2-)
               crushing injury of wrist alone (S67.3-)
   Excludes2   crushing injury of fingers (S67.1-)
               crushing injury of thumb (S67.0-)
   X ● S67.40   Crushing injury of unspecified wrist and hand
   X ● S67.41   Crushing injury of right wrist and hand
   X ● S67.42   Crushing injury of left wrist and hand

● S67.9   Crushing injury of unspecified part(s) of wrist, hand and fingers
   X ● S67.90   Crushing injury of unspecified part(s) of unspecified wrist, hand and fingers
   X ● S67.91   Crushing injury of unspecified part(s) of right wrist, hand and fingers
   X ● S67.92   Crushing injury of unspecified part(s) of left wrist, hand and fingers

● S68   Traumatic amputation of wrist, hand and fingers

An amputation not identified as partial or complete should be coded to complete

The appropriate 7th character is to be added to each code from category S68

A	initial encounter
D	subsequent encounter
S	sequela

● S68.0   Traumatic metacarpophalangeal amputation of thumb
   Traumatic amputation of thumb NOS
   ● S68.01   Complete traumatic metacarpophalangeal amputation of thumb
     ● S68.011   Complete traumatic metacarpophalangeal amputation of right thumb S 🔗
     ● S68.012   Complete traumatic metacarpophalangeal amputation of left thumb S 🔗
     ● S68.019   Complete traumatic metacarpophalangeal amputation of unspecified thumb S 🔗
   ● S68.02   Partial traumatic metacarpophalangeal amputation of thumb
     ● S68.021   Partial traumatic metacarpophalangeal amputation of right thumb S 🔗
     ● S68.022   Partial traumatic metacarpophalangeal amputation of left thumb S 🔗
     ● S68.029   Partial traumatic metacarpophalangeal amputation of unspecified thumb S 🔗

● S68.1   Traumatic metacarpophalangeal amputation of other and unspecified finger
   Traumatic amputation of finger NOS
   Excludes2   traumatic metacarpophalangeal amputation of thumb (S68.0-)
   ● S68.11   Complete traumatic metacarpophalangeal amputation of other and unspecified finger
     ● S68.110   Complete traumatic metacarpophalangeal amputation of right index finger S 🔗
     ● S68.111   Complete traumatic metacarpophalangeal amputation of left index finger S 🔗
     ● S68.112   Complete traumatic metacarpophalangeal amputation of right middle finger S 🔗
     ● S68.113   Complete traumatic metacarpophalangeal amputation of left middle finger S 🔗

● S68.114   Complete traumatic metacarpophalangeal amputation of right ring finger S 🦴

● S68.115   Complete traumatic metacarpophalangeal amputation of left ring finger S 🦴

● S68.116   Complete traumatic metacarpophalangeal amputation of right little finger S 🦴

● S68.117   Complete traumatic metacarpophalangeal amputation of left little finger S 🦴

● S68.118   Complete traumatic metacarpophalangeal amputation of other finger S 🦴

     Complete traumatic metacarpophalangeal amputation of specified finger with unspecified laterality

● S68.119   Complete traumatic metacarpophalangeal amputation of unspecified finger S 🦴

● S68.12   Partial traumatic metacarpophalangeal amputation of other and unspecified finger

● S68.120   Partial traumatic metacarpophalangeal amputation of right index finger S 🦴

● S68.121   Partial traumatic metacarpophalangeal amputation of left index finger S 🦴

● S68.122   Partial traumatic metacarpophalangeal amputation of right middle finger S 🦴

● S68.123   Partial traumatic metacarpophalangeal amputation of left middle finger S 🦴

● S68.124   Partial traumatic metacarpophalangeal amputation of right ring finger S 🦴

● S68.125   Partial traumatic metacarpophalangeal amputation of left ring finger S 🦴

● S68.126   Partial traumatic metacarpophalangeal amputation of right little finger S 🦴

● S68.127   Partial traumatic metacarpophalangeal amputation of left little finger S 🦴

● S68.128   Partial traumatic metacarpophalangeal amputation of other finger S 🦴

     Partial traumatic metacarpophalangeal amputation of specified finger with unspecified laterality

● S68.129   Partial traumatic metacarpophalangeal amputation of unspecified finger S 🦴

● S68.4   **Traumatic amputation of hand at wrist level**

Traumatic amputation of hand NOS

Traumatic amputation of wrist

● S68.41   Complete traumatic amputation of hand at wrist level

● S68.411   Complete traumatic amputation of right hand at wrist level A 🦴, A, S 🦴

     (Ex:) See PDX Collection 1266

● S68.412   Complete traumatic amputation of left hand at wrist level A 🦴, A, S 🦴

     (Ex:) See PDX Collection 1267

● S68.419   Complete traumatic amputation of unspecified hand at wrist level A 🦴, A, S 🦴

     (Ex:) See PDX Collection 1268

● S68.42   Partial traumatic amputation of hand at wrist level

● S68.421   Partial traumatic amputation of right hand at wrist level A 🦴, A, S 🦴

     (Ex:) See PDX Collection 1266

● S68.422   Partial traumatic amputation of left hand at wrist level A 🦴, A, S 🦴

     (Ex:) See PDX Collection 1267

● S68.429   Partial traumatic amputation of unspecified hand at wrist level A 🦴, A, S 🦴

     (Ex:) See PDX Collection 1268

● S68.5   **Traumatic transphalangeal amputation of thumb**

Traumatic interphalangeal joint amputation of thumb

● S68.51   Complete traumatic transphalangeal amputation of thumb

● S68.511   Complete traumatic transphalangeal amputation of right thumb S 🦴

● S68.512   Complete traumatic transphalangeal amputation of left thumb S 🦴

● S68.519   Complete traumatic transphalangeal amputation of unspecified thumb S 🦴

● S68.52   Partial traumatic transphalangeal amputation of thumb

● S68.521   Partial traumatic transphalangeal amputation of right thumb S 🦴

● S68.522   Partial traumatic transphalangeal amputation of left thumb S 🦴

● S68.529   Partial traumatic transphalangeal amputation of unspecified thumb S 🦴

● S68.6   **Traumatic transphalangeal amputation of other and unspecified finger**

● S68.61   Complete traumatic transphalangeal amputation of other and unspecified finger(s)

● S68.610   Complete traumatic transphalangeal amputation of right index finger S 🦴

● S68.611   Complete traumatic transphalangeal amputation of left index finger S 🦴

● S68.612   Complete traumatic transphalangeal amputation of right middle finger S 🦴

● S68.613   Complete traumatic transphalangeal amputation of left middle finger S 🦴

● S68.614   Complete traumatic transphalangeal amputation of right ring finger S 🦴

● S68.615   Complete traumatic transphalangeal amputation of left ring finger S 🦴

● S68.616   Complete traumatic transphalangeal amputation of right little finger S 🦴

● S68.617   Complete traumatic transphalangeal amputation of left little finger S 🦴

● S68.618   Complete traumatic transphalangeal amputation of other finger S 🦴

     Complete traumatic transphalangeal amputation of specified finger with unspecified laterality

● S68.619   Complete traumatic transphalangeal amputation of unspecified finger S 🦴

● S68.62   Partial traumatic transphalangeal amputation of other and unspecified finger

● S68.620   Partial traumatic transphalangeal amputation of right index finger S 🦴

● S68.621   Partial traumatic transphalangeal amputation of left index finger S 🦴

● S68.622   Partial traumatic transphalangeal amputation of right middle finger S 🦴

● S68.623   Partial traumatic transphalangeal amputation of left middle finger S 🦴

N Newborn Age: 0   **P** Pediatric Age: 0–17   **M** Maternity DX: 9–64   **A** Adult Age: 15–124   ♀ Females Only   ♂ Males Only

🦴 Complication\Comorbidity   🦴 Major C\C   (Ex:) CC/MCC Exclusions   🦴 Hospital-Acquired Condition   🦴 Hierarchical Condition Category

● S68.624   Partial traumatic transphalangeal amputation of **right ring finger** S 🔖

● S68.625   Partial traumatic transphalangeal amputation of **left ring finger** S 🔖

● S68.626   Partial traumatic transphalangeal amputation of **right little finger** S 🔖

● S68.627   Partial traumatic transphalangeal amputation of **left little finger** S 🔖

● S68.628   Partial traumatic transphalangeal amputation of **other finger** S 🔖

Partial traumatic transphalangeal amputation of specified finger with unspecified laterality

● S68.629   Partial traumatic transphalangeal amputation of **unspecified finger** S 🔖

● S68.7   Traumatic **transmetacarpal amputation** of **hand**

● S68.71   **Complete** traumatic transmetacarpal amputation of hand

● S68.711   Complete traumatic transmetacarpal amputation of **right hand** A 🔖, A, S 🔖
(Ex:) See PDX Collection 1266

● S68.712   Complete traumatic transmetacarpal amputation of **left hand** A 🔖, A, S 🔖
(Ex:) See PDX Collection 1267

● S68.719   Complete traumatic transmetacarpal amputation of **unspecified hand** A 🔖, A, S 🔖
(Ex:) See PDX Collection 1268

● S68.72   **Partial** traumatic transmetacarpal amputation of hand

● S68.721   Partial traumatic transmetacarpal amputation of **right hand** A 🔖, A, S 🔖
(Ex:) See PDX Collection 1266

● S68.722   Partial traumatic transmetacarpal amputation of **left hand** A 🔖, A, S 🔖
(Ex:) See PDX Collection 1267

● S68.729   Partial traumatic transmetacarpal amputation of **unspecified hand** A 🔖, A, S 🔖
(Ex:) See PDX Collection 1268

● S69   Other and unspecified injuries of wrist, hand and finger(s)

The appropriate 7th character is to be added to each code from category S69

A	initial encounter
D	subsequent encounter
S	sequela

● S69.8   **Other** specified injuries of wrist, hand and finger(s)

X● S69.80   Other specified injuries of **unspecified** wrist, hand and finger(s)

X● S69.81   Other specified injuries of **right** wrist, hand and finger(s)

X● S69.82   Other specified injuries of **left** wrist, hand and finger(s)

● S69.9   **Unspecified** injury of wrist, hand and finger(s)

X● S69.90   Unspecified injury of **unspecified** wrist, hand and finger(s)

X● S69.91   Unspecified injury of **right** wrist, hand and finger(s)

X● S69.92   Unspecified injury of **left** wrist, hand and finger(s)

INJURIES TO THE HIP AND THIGH (S70-S79)

Excludes2   burns and corrosions (T20-T32)
frostbite (T33-T34)
snake bite (T63.0-)
venomous insect bite or sting (T63.4-)

● S70   Superficial injury of hip and thigh

The appropriate 7th character is to be added to each code from category S70

A	initial encounter
D	subsequent encounter
S	sequela

● S70.0   Contusion of **hip**

X● S70.00   Contusion of **unspecified** hip

X● S70.01   Contusion of **right** hip

X● S70.02   Contusion of **left** hip

● S70.1   Contusion of **thigh**

X● S70.10   Contusion of **unspecified** thigh

X● S70.11   Contusion of **right** thigh

X● S70.12   Contusion of **left** thigh

● S70.2   Other superficial injuries of **hip**

● S70.21   **Abrasion** of hip

● S70.211   Abrasion, **right** hip

● S70.212   Abrasion, **left** hip

● S70.219   Abrasion, **unspecified** hip

● S70.22   **Blister** (nonthermal) of hip

● S70.221   Blister (nonthermal), **right** hip

● S70.222   Blister (nonthermal), **left** hip

● S70.229   Blister (nonthermal), **unspecified** hip

● S70.24   **External constriction** of hip

● S70.241   External constriction, **right** hip

● S70.242   External constriction, **left** hip

● S70.249   External constriction, **unspecified** hip

● S70.25   **Superficial foreign** body of hip

Splinter in the hip

● S70.251   Superficial foreign body, **right** hip

● S70.252   Superficial foreign body, **left** hip

● S70.259   Superficial foreign body, **unspecified** hip

● S70.26   **Insect bite** (nonvenomous) of hip

● S70.261   Insect bite (nonvenomous), **right** hip

● S70.262   Insect bite (nonvenomous), **left** hip

● S70.269   Insect bite (nonvenomous), **unspecified** hip

● S70.27   **Other superficial bite** of hip

Excludes1   open bite of hip (S71.05-)

● S70.271   Other superficial bite of hip, **right** hip

● S70.272   Other superficial bite of hip, **left** hip

● S70.279   Other superficial bite of hip, **unspecified** hip

● S70.3   Other superficial injuries of **thigh**

● S70.31   **Abrasion** of thigh

● S70.311   Abrasion, **right** thigh

● S70.312   Abrasion, **left** thigh

● S70.319   Abrasion, **unspecified** thigh

● S70.32   **Blister** (nonthermal) of thigh

● S70.321   Blister (nonthermal), **right** thigh

● S70.322   Blister (nonthermal), **left** thigh

● S70.329   Blister (nonthermal), **unspecified** thigh

▶ New   ⇒ Revised   ~~deleted~~ Deleted   Excludes 1   Excludes 2   Includes   Use additional   Code first   Code also   Key words

OGCR Official Guidelines   ● Unacceptable Principal Diagnosis   X Assign placeholder X   ● Use Additional Character(s)   ▶ Manifestation Code   Coding Clinic

● S70.34   External constriction of thigh
   ● S70.341   External constriction, right thigh
   ● S70.342   External constriction, left thigh
   ● S70.349   External constriction, unspecified thigh
● S70.35   Superficial foreign body of thigh
      Splinter in the thigh
   ● S70.351   Superficial foreign body, right thigh
   ● S70.352   Superficial foreign body, left thigh
   ● S70.359   Superficial foreign body, unspecified thigh
● S70.36   Insect bite (nonvenomous) of thigh
   ● S70.361   Insect bite (nonvenomous), right thigh
   ● S70.362   Insect bite (nonvenomous), left thigh
   ● S70.369   Insect bite (nonvenomous), unspecified thigh
● S70.37   Other superficial bite of thigh
     Excludes1   open bite of thigh (S71.15)
   ● S70.371   Other superficial bite of right thigh
   ● S70.372   Other superficial bite of left thigh
   ● S70.379   Other superficial bite of unspecified thigh
● S70.9   Unspecified superficial injury of hip and thigh
  ● S70.91   Unspecified superficial injury of hip
   ● S70.911   Unspecified superficial injury of right hip
   ● S70.912   Unspecified superficial injury of left hip
   ● S70.919   Unspecified superficial injury of unspecified hip
  ● S70.92   Unspecified superficial injury of thigh
   ● S70.921   Unspecified superficial injury of right thigh
   ● S70.922   Unspecified superficial injury of left thigh
   ● S70.929   Unspecified superficial injury of unspecified thigh

● S71   Open wound of hip and thigh
    Code also any associated wound infection
    Excludes1   open fracture of hip and thigh (S72.-)
                traumatic amputation of hip and thigh (S78.-)
    Excludes2   bite of venomous animal (T63.-)
                open wound of ankle, foot and toes (S91.-)
                open wound of knee and lower leg (S81.-)
    The appropriate 7th character is to be added to each code from category S71

A	initial encounter
D	subsequent encounter
S	sequela

● S71.0   Open wound of hip
  ● S71.00   Unspecified open wound of hip
   ● S71.001   Unspecified open wound, right hip
   ● S71.002   Unspecified open wound, left hip
   ● S71.009   Unspecified open wound, unspecified hip
  ● S71.01   Laceration without foreign body of hip
   ● S71.011   Laceration without foreign body, right hip
   ● S71.012   Laceration without foreign body, left hip
   ● S71.019   Laceration without foreign body, unspecified hip

● S71.02   Laceration with foreign body of hip
   ● S71.021   Laceration with foreign body, right hip
   ● S71.022   Laceration with foreign body, left hip
   ● S71.029   Laceration with foreign body, unspecified hip
● S71.03   Puncture wound without foreign body of hip
   ● S71.031   Puncture wound without foreign body, right hip
   ● S71.032   Puncture wound without foreign body, left hip
   ● S71.039   Puncture wound without foreign body, unspecified hip
● S71.04   Puncture wound with foreign body of hip
   ● S71.041   Puncture wound with foreign body, right hip
   ● S71.042   Puncture wound with foreign body, left hip
   ● S71.049   Puncture wound with foreign body, unspecified hip
● S71.05   Open bite of hip
      Bite of hip NOS
     Excludes1   superficial bite of hip (S70.26, S70.27)
   ● S71.051   Open bite, right hip
   ● S71.052   Open bite, left hip
   ● S71.059   Open bite, unspecified hip
● S71.1   Open wound of thigh
  ● S71.10   Unspecified open wound of thigh
   ● S71.101   Unspecified open wound, right thigh
   ● S71.102   Unspecified open wound, left thigh
   ● S71.109   Unspecified open wound, unspecified thigh
  ● S71.11   Laceration without foreign body of thigh
   ● S71.111   Laceration without foreign body, right thigh
   ● S71.112   Laceration without foreign body, left thigh
   ● S71.119   Laceration without foreign body, unspecified thigh
  ● S71.12   Laceration with foreign body of thigh
   ● S71.121   Laceration with foreign body, right thigh
   ● S71.122   Laceration with foreign body, left thigh
   ● S71.129   Laceration with foreign body, unspecified thigh
  ● S71.13   Puncture wound without foreign body of thigh
   ● S71.131   Puncture wound without foreign body, right thigh
   ● S71.132   Puncture wound without foreign body, left thigh
   ● S71.139   Puncture wound without foreign body, unspecified thigh
  ● S71.14   Puncture wound with foreign body of thigh
   ● S71.141   Puncture wound with foreign body, right thigh
   ● S71.142   Puncture wound with foreign body, left thigh
   ● S71.149   Puncture wound with foreign body, unspecified thigh
● S71.15   Open bite of thigh
      Bite of thigh NOS
     Excludes1   superficial bite of thigh (S70.37-)
   ● S71.151   Open bite, right thigh
   ● S71.152   Open bite, left thigh
   ● S71.159   Open bite, unspecified thigh

CHAPTER 19 (S00-T88)

N Newborn Age: 0	**P** Pediatric Age: 0–17	**M** Maternity DX: 9–64	**A** Adult Age: 15–124	♀ Females Only	♂ Males Only

🦠 Complication\Comorbidity   🦠 Major C\C   (Ex) CC/MCC Exclusions   🦠 Hospital-Acquired Condition   🦠 Hierarchical Condition Category

1377

● S72 Fracture of femur

> **Note:** A fracture not indicated as displaced or nondisplaced should be coded to displaced
>
> A fracture not indicated as open or closed should be coded to closed
>
> The open fracture designations are based on the Gustilo open fracture classification

> **Excludes1** traumatic amputation of hip and thigh (S78.-)
>
> **Excludes2** fracture of lower leg and ankle (S82.-)
>
> fracture of foot (S92.-)
>
> periprosthetic fracture of prosthetic implant of hip (M97.0-)

The appropriate 7th character is to be added to all codes from category S72

A	initial encounter for closed fracture
B	initial encounter for open fracture type I or II
	initial encounter for open fracture NOS
C	initial encounter for open fracture type IIIA, IIIB, or IIIC
D	subsequent encounter for closed fracture with routine healing
E	subsequent encounter for open fracture type I or II with routine healing
F	subsequent encounter for open fracture type IIIA, IIIB, or IIIC with routine healing
G	subsequent encounter for closed fracture with delayed healing
H	subsequent encounter for open fracture type I or II with delayed healing
J	subsequent encounter for open fracture type IIIA, IIIB, or IIIC with delayed healing
K	subsequent encounter for closed fracture with nonunion
M	subsequent encounter for open fracture type I or II with nonunion
N	subsequent encounter for open fracture type IIIA, IIIB, or IIIC with nonunion
P	subsequent encounter for closed fracture with malunion
Q	subsequent encounter for open fracture type I or II with malunion
R	subsequent encounter for open fracture type IIIA, IIIB, or IIIC with malunion
S	sequela

● S72.0 Fracture of head and neck of femur

> **Excludes2** physeal fracture of upper end of femur (S79.0-)

● S72.00 Fracture of unspecified part of neck of femur
> Fracture of hip NOS
> Fracture of neck of femur NOS

● S72.001 Fracture of unspecified part of neck of right femur K, M, N, P, Q, R 🔁, A, B, C 🔁, A, B, C 🔁, **A, B, C** 🔁
> (Ex) **For S72.001[A]:** See PDX Collection 1297
> **For S72.001[B,C]:** See PDX Collection 1298
> **For S72.001[K,M,N,P,Q,R]:** See PDX Collection 897

● S72.002 Fracture of unspecified part of neck of left femur K, M, N, P, Q, R 🔁, A, B, C 🔁, A, B, C 🔁, **A, B, C** 🔁
> (Ex) **For S72.002[A]:** See PDX Collection 1299
> **For S72.002[B,C]:** See PDX Collection 1298
> **For S72.002[K,M,N,P,Q,R]:** See PDX Collection 897
>
> **Coding Clinic: 2015, Q4, P37, Q1, P17**

● S72.009 Fracture of unspecified part of neck of unspecified femur K, M, N, P, Q, R 🔁, A, B, C 🔁, A, B, C 🔁, **A, B, C** 🔁
> (Ex) **For S72.009[A,B,C]:** See PDX Collection 1298
> **For S72.009[K,M,N,P,Q,R]:** See PDX Collection 897

● S72.01 Unspecified intracapsular fracture of femur
> Subcapital fracture of femur

● S72.011 Unspecified intracapsular fracture of right femur K, M, N, P, Q, R 🔁, A, B, C 🔁, A, B, C 🔁, **A, B, C** 🔁
> (Ex) **For S72.011[A]:** See PDX Collection 1297
> **For S72.011[B,C]:** See PDX Collection 1298
> **For S72.011[K,M,N,P,Q,R]:** See PDX Collection 897

● S72.012 Unspecified intracapsular fracture of left femur K, M, N, P, Q, R 🔁, A, B, C 🔁, A, B, C 🔁, **A, B, C** 🔁
> (Ex) **For S72.012[A]:** See PDX Collection 1299
> **For S72.012[B,C]:** See PDX Collection 1298
> **For S72.012[K,M,N,P,Q,R]:** See PDX Collection 897

● S72.019 Unspecified intracapsular fracture of unspecified femur K, M, N, P, Q, R 🔁, A, B, C 🔁, A, B, C 🔁, **A, B, C** 🔁
> (Ex) **For S72.019[A,B,C]:** See PDX Collection 1298
> **For S72.019[K,M,N,P,Q,R]:** See PDX Collection 897

● S72.02 Fracture of epiphysis (separation) (upper) of femur
> Transepiphyseal fracture of femur
> *Fracture and separation across growth plate*

> **Excludes1** capital femoral epiphyseal fracture (pediatric) of femur (S79.01-)
>
> Salter-Harris Type I physeal fracture of upper end of femur (S79.01-)

● S72.021 Displaced fracture of epiphysis (separation) (upper) of right femur K, M, N, P, Q, R 🔁, A, B, C 🔁, A, B, C 🔁, **A, B, C** 🔁
> (Ex) **For S72.021[A]:** See PDX Collection 1297
> **For S72.021[B,C]:** See PDX Collection 1298
> **For S72.021[K,M,N,P,Q,R]:** See PDX Collection 897

● S72.022 Displaced fracture of epiphysis (separation) (upper) of left femur K, M, N, P, Q, R 🔁, A, B, C 🔁, A, B, C 🔁, **A, B, C** 🔁
> (Ex) **For S72.022[A]:** See PDX Collection 1299
> **For S72.022[B,C]:** See PDX Collection 1298
> **For S72.022[K,M,N,P,Q,R]:** See PDX Collection 897

● S72.023 Displaced fracture of epiphysis (separation) (upper) of unspecified femur K, M, N, P, Q, R 🔁, A, B, C 🔁, A, B, C 🔁, **A, B, C** 🔁
> (Ex) **For S72.023[A,B,C]:** See PDX Collection 1298
> **For S72.023[K,M,N,P,Q,R]:** See PDX Collection 897

● S72.024 Nondisplaced fracture of epiphysis (separation) (upper) of right femur K, M, N, P, Q, R 🔁, A, B, C 🔁, A, B, C 🔁, **A, B, C** 🔁
> (Ex) **For S72.024[A]:** See PDX Collection 1297
> **For S72.024[B,C]:** See PDX Collection 1298
> **For S72.024[K,M,N,P,Q,R]:** See PDX Collection 897

● S72.025 Nondisplaced fracture of epiphysis (separation) (upper) of left femur K, M, N, P, Q, R 🔁, A, B, C 🔁, A, B, C 🔁, **A, B, C** 🔁
> (Ex) **For S72.025[A]:** See PDX Collection 1299
> **For S72.025[B,C]:** See PDX Collection 1298
> **For S72.025[K,M,N,P,Q,R]:** See PDX Collection 897

● S72.026 Nondisplaced fracture of epiphysis (separation) (upper) of unspecified femur K, M, N, P, Q, R 🔁, A, B, C 🔁, A, B, C 🔁, **A, B, C** 🔁
> (Ex) **For S72.026[A,B,C]:** See PDX Collection 1298
> **For S72.026[K,M,N,P,Q,R]:** See PDX Collection 897

● **S72.03**   Midcervical fracture of femur
     Transcervical fracture of femur NOS

   ● **S72.031**   Displaced midcervical fracture of right femur K, M, N, P, Q, R 🪙, A, B, C 🪙, A, B, C 🪙, **A, B, C** 🪙
         ⒺⓍ For S72.031[A]: See PDX Collection 1297
           For S72.031[B,C]: See PDX Collection 1298
           For S72.031[K,M,N,P,Q,R]: See PDX Collection 897

   ● **S72.032**   Displaced midcervical fracture of left femur K, M, N, P, Q, R 🪙, A, B, C 🪙, A, B, C 🪙, **A, B, C** 🪙
         ⒺⓍ For S72.032[A]: See PDX Collection 1299
           For S72.032[B,C]: See PDX Collection 1298
           For S72.032[K,M,N,P,Q,R]: See PDX Collection 897

   ● **S72.033**   Displaced midcervical fracture of unspecified femur K, M, N, P, Q, R 🪙, A, B, C 🪙, A, B, C 🪙, **A, B, C** 🪙
         ⒺⓍ For S72.033[A,B,C]: See PDX Collection 1298
           For S72.033[K,M,N,P,Q,R]: See PDX Collection 897

   ● **S72.034**   Nondisplaced midcervical fracture of right femur K, M, N, P, Q, R 🪙, A, B, C 🪙, A, B, C 🪙, **A, B, C** 🪙
         ⒺⓍ For S72.034[A]: See PDX Collection 1297
           For S72.034[B,C]: See PDX Collection 1298
           For S72.034[K,M,N,P,Q,R]: See PDX Collection 897

   ● **S72.035**   Nondisplaced midcervical fracture of left femur K, M, N, P, Q, R 🪙, A, B, C 🪙, A, B, C 🪙, **A, B, C** 🪙
         ⒺⓍ For S72.035[A]: See PDX Collection 1299
           For S72.035[B,C]: See PDX Collection 1298
           For S72.035[K,M,N,P,Q,R]: See PDX Collection 897

   ● **S72.036**   Nondisplaced midcervical fracture of unspecified femur K, M, N, P, Q, R 🪙, A, B, C 🪙, A, B, C 🪙, **A, B, C** 🪙
         ⒺⓍ For S72.036[A,B,C]: See PDX Collection 1298
           For S72.036[K,M,N,P,Q,R]: See PDX Collection 897

● **S72.04**   Fracture of base of neck of femur
     Cervicotrochanteric fracture of femur

   ● **S72.041**   Displaced fracture of base of neck of right femur K, M, N, P, Q, R 🪙, A, B, C 🪙, A, B, C 🪙, **A, B, C** 🪙
         ⒺⓍ For S72.041[A]: See PDX Collection 1297
           For S72.041[B,C]: See PDX Collection 1298
           For S72.041[K,M,N,P,Q,R]: See PDX Collection 897

   ● **S72.042**   Displaced fracture of base of neck of left femur K, M, N, P, Q, R 🪙, A, B, C 🪙, A, B, C 🪙, **A, B, C** 🪙
         ⒺⓍ For S72.042[A]: See PDX Collection 1299
           For S72.042[B,C]: See PDX Collection 1298
           For S72.042[K,M,N,P,Q,R]: See PDX Collection 897

   ● **S72.043**   Displaced fracture of base of neck of unspecified femur K, M, N, P, Q, R 🪙, A, B, C 🪙, A, B, C 🪙, **A, B, C** 🪙
         ⒺⓍ For S72.043[A,B,C]: See PDX Collection 1298
           For S72.043[K,M,N,P,Q,R]: See PDX Collection 897

   ● **S72.044**   Nondisplaced fracture of base of neck of right femur K, M, N, P, Q, R 🪙, A, B, C 🪙, A, B, C 🪙, **A, B, C** 🪙
         ⒺⓍ For S72.044[A]: See PDX Collection 1297
           For S72.044[B,C]: See PDX Collection 1298
           For S72.044[K,M,N,P,Q,R]: See PDX Collection 897

   ● **S72.045**   Nondisplaced fracture of base of neck of left femur K, M, N, P, Q, R 🪙, A, B, C 🪙, A, B, C 🪙, **A, B, C** 🪙
         ⒺⓍ For S72.045[A]: See PDX Collection 1299
           For S72.045[B,C]: See PDX Collection 1298
           For S72.045[K,M,N,P,Q,R]: See PDX Collection 897

   ● **S72.046**   Nondisplaced fracture of base of neck of unspecified femur K, M, N, P, Q, R 🪙, A, B, C 🪙, A, B, C 🪙, **A, B, C** 🪙
         ⒺⓍ For S72.046[A,B,C]: See PDX Collection 1298
           For S72.046[K,M,N,P,Q,R]: See PDX Collection 897

● **S72.05**   Unspecified fracture of head of femur
     Fracture of head of femur NOS

   ● **S72.051**   Unspecified fracture of head of right femur K, M, N, P, Q, R 🪙, A, B, C 🪙, A, B, C 🪙, **A, B, C** 🪙
         ⒺⓍ For S72.051[A]: See PDX Collection 1297
           For S72.051[B,C]: See PDX Collection 1298
           For S72.051[K,M,N,P,Q,R]: See PDX Collection 897

   ● **S72.052**   Unspecified fracture of head of left femur K, M, N, P, Q, R 🪙, A, B, C 🪙, A, B, C 🪙, **A, B, C** 🪙
         ⒺⓍ For S72.052[A]: See PDX Collection 1299
           For S72.052[B,C]: See PDX Collection 1298
           For S72.052[K,M,N,P,Q,R]: See PDX Collection 897

   ● **S72.059**   Unspecified fracture of head of unspecified femur K, M, N, P, Q, R 🪙, A, B, C 🪙, A, B, C 🪙, **A, B, C** 🪙
         ⒺⓍ For S72.059[A,B,C]: See PDX Collection 1298
           For S72.059[K,M,N,P,Q,R]: See PDX Collection 897

● **S72.06**   Articular fracture of head of femur

   ● **S72.061**   Displaced articular fracture of head of right femur K, M, N, P, Q, R 🪙, A, B, C 🪙, A, B, C 🪙, **A, B, C** 🪙
         ⒺⓍ For S72.061[A]: See PDX Collection 1297
           For S72.061[B,C]: See PDX Collection 1298
           For S72.061[K,M,N,P,Q,R]: See PDX Collection 897

   ● **S72.062**   Displaced articular fracture of head of left femur K, M, N, P, Q, R 🪙, A, B, C 🪙, A, B, C 🪙, **A, B, C** 🪙
         ⒺⓍ For S72.062[A]: See PDX Collection 1299
           For S72.062[B,C]: See PDX Collection 1298
           For S72.062[K,M,N,P,Q,R]: See PDX Collection 897

   ● **S72.063**   Displaced articular fracture of head of unspecified femur K, M, N, P, Q, R 🪙, A, B, C 🪙, A, B, C 🪙, **A, B, C** 🪙
         ⒺⓍ For S72.063[A,B,C]: See PDX Collection 1298
           For S72.063[K,M,N,P,Q,R]: See PDX Collection 897

   ● **S72.064**   Nondisplaced articular fracture of head of right femur K, M, N, P, Q, R 🪙, A, B, C 🪙, A, B, C 🪙, **A, B, C** 🪙
         ⒺⓍ For S72.064[A]: See PDX Collection 1297
           For S72.064[B,C]: See PDX Collection 1298
           For S72.064[K,M,N,P,Q,R]: See PDX Collection 897

   ● **S72.065**   Nondisplaced articular fracture of head of left femur K, M, N, P, Q, R 🪙, A, B, C 🪙, A, B, C 🪙, **A, B, C** 🪙
         ⒺⓍ For S72.065[A]: See PDX Collection 1299
           For S72.065[B,C]: See PDX Collection 1298
           For S72.065[K,M,N,P,Q,R]: See PDX Collection 897

CHAPTER 19 (S00-T88)

N   Newborn Age: 0   P   Pediatric Age: 0–17   M   Maternity DX: 9–64   A   Adult Age: 15–124   ♀   Females Only   ♂   Males Only
🪙   Complication\Comorbidity   🪙   Major C\C   ⒺⓍ   CC/MCC Exclusions   🪙   Hospital-Acquired Condition   🪙   Hierarchical Condition Category

1379

● S72.066   **Nondisplaced** articular fracture of head of **unspecified** femur K, M, N, P, Q, R ⦿, A, B, C ⦿, A, B, C ⦿, A, B, C ⦿

    Ⓔ **For S72.066[A,B,C]:** See PDX Collection 1298
    For S72.066[K,M,N,P,Q,R]: See PDX Collection 897

● S72.09   Other fracture of head and neck of femur

  ● S72.091   Other fracture of head and neck of **right** femur K, M, N, P, Q, R ⦿, A, B, C ⦿, A, B, C ⦿, A, B, C ⦿

    Ⓔ **For S72.091[A]:** See PDX Collection 1297
    For S72.091[B,C]: See PDX Collection 1298
    For S72.091[K,M,N,P,Q,R]: See PDX Collection 897

  ● S72.092   Other fracture of head and neck of **left** femur K, M, N, P, Q, R ⦿, A, B, C ⦿, A, B, C ⦿, A, B, C ⦿

    Ⓔ **For S72.092[A]:** See PDX Collection 1299
    For S72.092[B,C]: See PDX Collection 1298
    For S72.092[K,M,N,P,Q,R]: See PDX Collection 897

  ● S72.099   Other fracture of head and neck of **unspecified** femur K, M, N, P, Q, R ⦿, A, B, C ⦿, A, B, C ⦿, A, B, C ⦿

    Ⓔ **For S72.099[A,B,C]:** See PDX Collection 1298
    For S72.099[K,M,N,P,Q,R]: See PDX Collection 897

● S72.1   **Pertrochanteric fracture**
  Fracture extending close to, but not into, joint

  ● S72.10   Unspecified trochanteric fracture of femur
    Fracture of trochanter NOS

    ● S72.101   **Unspecified trochanteric** fracture of **right** femur K, M, N, P, Q, R ⦿, A, B, C ⦿, A, B, C ⦿, A, B, C ⦿

      Ⓔ **For S72.101[A]:** See PDX Collection 1297
      For S72.101[B,C]: See PDX Collection 1298
      For S72.101[K,M,N,P,Q,R]: See PDX Collection 897

    ● S72.102   **Unspecified trochanteric** fracture of **left** femur K, M, N, P, Q, R ⦿, A, B, C ⦿, A, B, C ⦿, A, B, C ⦿

      Ⓔ **For S72.102[A]:** See PDX Collection 1299
      For S72.102[B,C]: See PDX Collection 1298
      For S72.102[K,M,N,P,Q,R]: See PDX Collection 897

    ● S72.109   **Unspecified trochanteric** fracture of **unspecified** femur K, M, N, P, Q, R ⦿, A, B, C ⦿, A, B, C ⦿, A, B, C ⦿

      Ⓔ **For S72.109[A,B,C]:** See PDX Collection 1298
      For S72.109[K,M,N,P,Q,R]: See PDX Collection 897

  ● S72.11   Fracture of **greater trochanter** of femur

    ● S72.111   **Displaced** fracture of greater trochanter of **right** femur K, M, N, P, Q, R ⦿, A, B, C ⦿, A, B, C ⦿, A, B, C ⦿

      Ⓔ **For S72.111[A]:** See PDX Collection 1297
      For S72.111[B,C]: See PDX Collection 1298
      For S72.111[K,M,N,P,Q,R]: See PDX Collection 897

    ● S72.112   **Displaced** fracture of greater trochanter of **left** femur K, M, N, P, Q, R ⦿, A, B, C ⦿, A, B, C ⦿, A, B, C ⦿

      Ⓔ **For S72.112[A]:** See PDX Collection 1299
      For S72.112[B,C]: See PDX Collection 1298
      For S72.112[K,M,N,P,Q,R]: See PDX Collection 897

● S72.113   **Displaced** fracture of greater trochanter of **unspecified** femur K, M, N, P, Q, R ⦿, A, B, C ⦿, A, B, C ⦿, A, B, C ⦿

    Ⓔ **For S72.113[A,B,C]:** See PDX Collection 1298
    For S72.113[K,M,N,P,Q,R]: See PDX Collection 897

● S72.114   **Nondisplaced** fracture of greater trochanter of **right** femur K, M, N, P, Q, R ⦿, A, B, C ⦿, A, B, C ⦿, A, B, C ⦿

    Ⓔ **For S72.114[A]:** See PDX Collection 1297
    For S72.114[B,C]: See PDX Collection 1298
    For S72.114[K,M,N,P,Q,R]: See PDX Collection 897

● S72.115   **Nondisplaced** fracture of greater trochanter of **left** femur K, M, N, P, Q, R ⦿, A, B, C ⦿, A, B, C ⦿, A, B, C ⦿

    Ⓔ **For S72.115[A]:** See PDX Collection 1299
    For S72.115[B,C]: See PDX Collection 1298
    For S72.115[K,M,N,P,Q,R]: See PDX Collection 897

● S72.116   **Nondisplaced** fracture of greater trochanter of **unspecified** femur K, M, N, P, Q, R ⦿, A, B, C ⦿, A, B, C ⦿, A, B, C ⦿

    Ⓔ **For S72.116[A,B,C]:** See PDX Collection 1298
    For S72.116[K,M,N,P,Q,R]: See PDX Collection 897

● S72.12   Fracture of **lesser trochanter** of femur

  ● S72.121   **Displaced** fracture of lesser trochanter of **right** femur K, M, N, P, Q, R ⦿, A, B, C ⦿, A, B, C ⦿, A, B, C ⦿

    Ⓔ **For S72.121[A]:** See PDX Collection 1297
    For S72.121[B,C]: See PDX Collection 1298
    For S72.121[K,M,N,P,Q,R]: See PDX Collection 897

  ● S72.122   **Displaced** fracture of lesser trochanter of **left** femur K, M, N, P, Q, R ⦿, A, B, C ⦿, A, B, C ⦿, A, B, C ⦿

    Ⓔ **For S72.122[A]:** See PDX Collection 1299
    For S72.122[B,C]: See PDX Collection 1298
    For S72.122[K,M,N,P,Q,R]: See PDX Collection 897

  ● S72.123   **Displaced** fracture of lesser trochanter of **unspecified** femur K, M, N, P, Q, R ⦿, A, B, C ⦿, A, B, C ⦿, A, B, C ⦿

    Ⓔ **For S72.123[A,B,C]:** See PDX Collection 1298
    For S72.123[K,M,N,P,Q,R]: See PDX Collection 897

  ● S72.124   **Nondisplaced** fracture of lesser trochanter of **right** femur K, M, N, P, Q, R ⦿, A, B, C ⦿, A, B, C ⦿, A, B, C ⦿

    Ⓔ **For S72.124[A]:** See PDX Collection 1297
    For S72.124[B,C]: See PDX Collection 1298
    For S72.124[K,M,N,P,Q,R]: See PDX Collection 897

  ● S72.125   **Nondisplaced** fracture of lesser trochanter of **left** femur K, M, N, P, Q, R ⦿, A, B, C ⦿, A, B, C ⦿, A, B, C ⦿

    Ⓔ **For S72.125[A]:** See PDX Collection 1299
    For S72.125[B,C]: See PDX Collection 1298
    For S72.125[K,M,N,P,Q,R]: See PDX Collection 897

  ● S72.126   **Nondisplaced** fracture of lesser trochanter of **unspecified** femur K, M, N, P, Q, R ⦿, A, B, C ⦿, A, B, C ⦿, A, B, C ⦿

    Ⓔ **For S72.126[A,B,C]:** See PDX Collection 1298
    For S72.126[K,M,N,P,Q,R]: See PDX Collection 897

▶ New   ⇒ Revised   ~~deleted~~ Deleted   Excludes 1   Excludes 2   Includes   Use additional   Code first   Code also   Key words

1380   OGCR Official Guidelines   ● Unacceptable Principal Diagnosis   X Assign placeholder X   ● Use Additional Character(s)   ▶ Manifestation Code   Coding Clinic

● **S72.13**   **Apophyseal** fracture of femur
Pertaining to articulations between articular facets of adjacent vertebrae

    Excludes1   chronic (nontraumatic) slipped upper femoral epiphysis (M93.0-)

   ● **S72.131**   **Displaced** apophyseal fracture of **right** femur K, M, N, P, Q, R 🜲, A, B, C 🜲, A, B, C 🜲, **A, B, C** 🜲
     (Ex:) For S72.131[A]: See PDX Collection 1297
       For S72.131[B,C]: See PDX Collection 1298
       For S72.131[K,M,N,P,Q,R]: See PDX Collection 897

   ● **S72.132**   **Displaced** apophyseal fracture of **left** femur K, M, N, P, Q, R 🜲, A, B, C 🜲, A, B, C 🜲, **A, B, C** 🜲
     (Ex:) For S72.132[A]: See PDX Collection 1299
       For S72.132[B,C]: See PDX Collection 1298
       For S72.132[K,M,N,P,Q,R]: See PDX Collection 897

   ● **S72.133**   **Displaced** apophyseal fracture of **unspecified** femur K, M, N, P, Q, R 🜲, A, B, C 🜲, A, B, C 🜲, **A, B, C** 🜲
     (Ex:) For S72.133[A,B,C]: See PDX Collection 1298
       For S72.133[K,M,N,P,Q,R]: See PDX Collection 897

   ● **S72.134**   **Nondisplaced** apophyseal fracture of **right** femur K, M, N, P, Q, R 🜲, A, B, C 🜲, A, B, C 🜲, **A, B, C** 🜲
     (Ex:) For S72.134[A]: See PDX Collection 1297
       For S72.134[B,C]: See PDX Collection 1298
       For S72.134[K,M,N,P,Q,R]: See PDX Collection 897

   ● **S72.135**   **Nondisplaced** apophyseal fracture of **left** femur K, M, N, P, Q, R 🜲, A, B, C 🜲, A, B, C 🜲, **A, B, C** 🜲
     (Ex:) For S72.135[A]: See PDX Collection 1299
       For S72.135[B,C]: See PDX Collection 1298
       For S72.135[K,M,N,P,Q,R]: See PDX Collection 897

   ● **S72.136**   **Nondisplaced** apophyseal fracture of **unspecified** femur K, M, N, P, Q, R 🜲, A, B, C 🜲, A, B, C 🜲, **A, B, C** 🜲
     (Ex:) For S72.136[A,B,C]: See PDX Collection 1298
       For S72.136[K,M,N,P,Q,R]: See PDX Collection 897

● **S72.14**   **Intertrochanteric** fracture of femur

   ● **S72.141**   **Displaced** intertrochanteric fracture of **right** femur K, M, N, P, Q, R 🜲, A, B, C 🜲, A, B, C 🜲, **A, B, C** 🜲
     (Ex:) For S72.141[A]: See PDX Collection 1297
       For S72.141[B,C]: See PDX Collection 1298
       For S72.141[K,M,N,P,Q,R]: See PDX Collection 897
     Coding Clinic: 2016, Q3, P17

   ● **S72.142**   **Displaced** intertrochanteric fracture of **left** femur K, M, N, P, Q, R 🜲, A, B, C 🜲, A, B, C 🜲, **A, B, C** 🜲
     (Ex:) For S72.142[A]: See PDX Collection 1299
       For S72.142[B,C]: See PDX Collection 1298
       For S72.142[K,M,N,P,Q,R]: See PDX Collection 897

   ● **S72.143**   **Displaced** intertrochanteric fracture of **unspecified** femur K, M, N, P, Q, R 🜲, A, B, C 🜲, A, B, C 🜲, **A, B, C** 🜲
     (Ex:) For S72.143[A,B,C]: See PDX Collection 1298
       For S72.143[K,M,N,P,Q,R]: See PDX Collection 897

   ● **S72.144**   **Nondisplaced** intertrochanteric fracture of **right** femur K, M, N, P, Q, R 🜲, A, B, C 🜲, A, B, C 🜲, **A, B, C** 🜲
     (Ex:) For S72.144[A]: See PDX Collection 1297
       For S72.144[B,C]: See PDX Collection 1298
       For S72.144[K,M,N,P,Q,R]: See PDX Collection 897

   ● **S72.145**   **Nondisplaced** intertrochanteric fracture of **left** femur K, M, N, P, Q, R 🜲, A, B, C 🜲, A, B, C 🜲, **A, B, C** 🜲
     (Ex:) For S72.145[A]: See PDX Collection 1299
       For S72.145[B,C]: See PDX Collection 1298
       For S72.145[K,M,N,P,Q,R]: See PDX Collection 897

   ● **S72.146**   **Nondisplaced** intertrochanteric fracture of **unspecified** femur K, M, N, P, Q, R 🜲, A, B, C 🜲, A, B, C 🜲, **A, B, C** 🜲
     (Ex:) For S72.146[A,B,C]: See PDX Collection 1298
       For S72.146[K,M,N,P,Q,R]: See PDX Collection 897

● **S72.2**   **Subtrochanteric** fracture of femur
Subtrochanteric: inferior to trochanter
   (Ex:) For category S72.2 CC codes S72.2[A,B,C]: See PDX Collection 1298
     For S72.2[K,M,N,P,Q,R]: See PDX Collection 897

   X ● **S72.21**   **Displaced** subtrochanteric fracture of **right** femur K, M, N, P, Q, R 🜲, A, B, C 🜲, A, B, C 🜲, **A, B, C** 🜲

   X ● **S72.22**   **Displaced** subtrochanteric fracture of **left** femur K, M, N, P, Q, R 🜲, A, B, C 🜲, A, B, C 🜲, **A, B, C** 🜲

   X ● **S72.23**   **Displaced** subtrochanteric fracture of **unspecified** femur K, M, N, P, Q, R 🜲, A, B, C 🜲, A, B, C 🜲, **A, B, C** 🜲

   X ● **S72.24**   **Nondisplaced** subtrochanteric fracture of **right** femur K, M, N, P, Q, R 🜲, A, B, C 🜲, A, B, C 🜲, **A, B, C** 🜲

   X ● **S72.25**   **Nondisplaced** subtrochanteric fracture of **left** femur K, M, N, P, Q, R 🜲, A, B, C 🜲, A, B, C 🜲, **A, B, C** 🜲

   X ● **S72.26**   **Nondisplaced** subtrochanteric fracture of **unspecified** femur K, M, N, P, Q, R 🜲, A, B, C 🜲, A, B, C 🜲, **A, B, C** 🜲

● **S72.3**   Fracture of **shaft** of femur

   ● **S72.30**   **Unspecified** fracture of shaft of femur

     ● **S72.301**   **Unspecified** fracture of shaft of **right** femur K, M, N, P, Q, R 🜲, A, B, C 🜲, A, B, C 🜲, **A, B, C** 🜲
       (Ex:) For S72.301[A]: See PDX Collection 1297
         For S72.301[B,C]: See PDX Collection 1298
         For S72.301[K,M,N,P,Q,R]: See PDX Collection 897
       Coding Clinic: 2018, Q2, P12

     ● **S72.302**   **Unspecified** fracture of shaft of **left** femur K, M, N, P, Q, R 🜲, A, B, C 🜲, A, B, C 🜲, **A, B, C** 🜲
       (Ex:) For S72.302[A]: See PDX Collection 1299
         For S72.302[B,C]: See PDX Collection 1298
         For S72.302[K,M,N,P,Q,R]: See PDX Collection 897

     ● **S72.309**   **Unspecified** fracture of shaft of **unspecified** femur K, M, N, P, Q, R 🜲, A, B, C 🜲, A, B, C 🜲, **A, B, C** 🜲
       (Ex:) For S72.309[A,B,C]: See PDX Collection 1298
         For S72.309[K,M,N,P,Q,R]: See PDX Collection 897

   ● **S72.32**   **Transverse** fracture of shaft of femur

     ● **S72.321**   **Displaced** transverse fracture of shaft of **right** femur K, M, N, P, Q, R 🜲, A, B, C 🜲, A, B, C 🜲, **A, B, C** 🜲
       (Ex:) For S72.321[A]: See PDX Collection 1297
         For S72.321[B,C]: See PDX Collection 1298
         For S72.321[K,M,N,P,Q,R]: See PDX Collection 897

     ● **S72.322**   **Displaced** transverse fracture of shaft of **left** femur K, M, N, P, Q, R 🜲, A, B, C 🜲, A, B, C 🜲, **A, B, C** 🜲
       (Ex:) For S72.322[A]: See PDX Collection 1299
         For S72.322[B,C]: See PDX Collection 1298
         For S72.322[K,M,N,P,Q,R]: See PDX Collection 897

N   Newborn Age: 0   **P**   Pediatric Age: 0–17   **M**   Maternity DX: 9–64   **A**   Adult Age: 15–124   ♀   Females Only   ♂   Males Only
🜲   Complication\Comorbidity   🜲   Major C\C   (Ex:)   CC/MCC Exclusions   🜲   Hospital-Acquired Condition   🜲   Hierarchical Condition Category

● S72.323   **Displaced transverse fracture of shaft of unspecified femur** K, M, N, P, Q, R 🩹, A, B, C 🩹, A, B, C 🩹, A, B, C 🩹
   (Ex:) **For S72.323[A,B,C]:** See PDX Collection 1298
   For S72.323[K,M,N,P,Q,R]: See PDX Collection 897

● S72.324   **Nondisplaced transverse fracture of shaft of right femur** K, M, N, P, Q, R 🩹, A, B, C 🩹, A, B, C 🩹, A, B, C 🩹
   (Ex:) **For S72.324[A]:** See PDX Collection 1297
   For S72.324[B,C]: See PDX Collection 1298
   For S72.324[K,M,N,P,Q,R]: See PDX Collection 897

● S72.325   **Nondisplaced transverse fracture of shaft of left femur** K, M, N, P, Q, R 🩹, A, B, C 🩹, A, B, C 🩹, A, B, C 🩹
   (Ex:) **For S72.325[A]:** See PDX Collection 1299
   For S72.325[B,C]: See PDX Collection 1298
   For S72.325[K,M,N,P,Q,R]: See PDX Collection 897

● S72.326   **Nondisplaced transverse fracture of shaft of unspecified femur** K, M, N, P, Q, R 🩹, A, B, C 🩹, A, B, C 🩹, A, B, C 🩹
   (Ex:) **For S72.326[A,B,C]:** See PDX Collection 1298
   For S72.326[K,M,N,P,Q,R]: See PDX Collection 897

● S72.33   **Oblique fracture of shaft of femur**

● S72.331   **Displaced oblique fracture of shaft of right femur** K, M, N, P, Q, R 🩹, A, B, C 🩹, A, B, C 🩹, A, B, C 🩹
   (Ex:) **For S72.331[A]:** See PDX Collection 1297
   For S72.331[B,C]: See PDX Collection 1298
   For S72.331[K,M,N,P,Q,R]: See PDX Collection 897

● S72.332   **Displaced oblique fracture of shaft of left femur** K, M, N, P, Q, R 🩹, A, B, C 🩹, A, B, C 🩹, A, B, C 🩹
   (Ex:) **For S72.332[A]:** See PDX Collection 1299
   For S72.332[B,C]: See PDX Collection 1298
   For S72.332[K,M,N,P,Q,R]: See PDX Collection 897

● S72.333   **Displaced oblique fracture of shaft of unspecified femur** K, M, N, P, Q, R 🩹, A, B, C 🩹, A, B, C 🩹, A, B, C 🩹
   (Ex:) **For S72.333[A,B,C]:** See PDX Collection 1298
   For S72.333[K,M,N,P,Q,R]: See PDX Collection 897

● S72.334   **Nondisplaced oblique fracture of shaft of right femur** K, M, N, P, Q, R 🩹, A, B, C 🩹, A, B, C 🩹, A, B, C 🩹
   (Ex:) **For S72.334[A]:** See PDX Collection 1297
   For S72.334[B,C]: See PDX Collection 1298
   For S72.334[K,M,N,P,Q,R]: See PDX Collection 897

● S72.335   **Nondisplaced oblique fracture of shaft of left femur** K, M, N, P, Q, R 🩹, A, B, C 🩹, A, B, C 🩹, A, B, C 🩹
   (Ex:) **For S72.335[A]:** See PDX Collection 1299
   For S72.335[B,C]: See PDX Collection 1298
   For S72.335[K,M,N,P,Q,R]: See PDX Collection 897

● S72.336   **Nondisplaced oblique fracture of shaft of unspecified femur** K, M, N, P, Q, R 🩹, A, B, C 🩹, A, B, C 🩹, A, B, C 🩹
   (Ex:) **For S72.336[A,B,C]:** See PDX Collection 1298
   For S72.336[K,M,N,P,Q,R]: See PDX Collection 897

● S72.34   **Spiral fracture of shaft of femur**

● S72.341   **Displaced spiral fracture of shaft of right femur** K, M, N, P, Q, R 🩹, A, B, C 🩹, A, B, C 🩹, A, B, C 🩹
   (Ex:) **For S72.341[A]:** See PDX Collection 1297
   For S72.341[B,C]: See PDX Collection 1298
   For S72.341[K,M,N,P,Q,R]: See PDX Collection 897

● S72.342   **Displaced spiral fracture of shaft of left femur** K, M, N, P, Q, R 🩹, A, B, C 🩹, A, B, C 🩹, A, B, C 🩹
   (Ex:) **For S72.342[A]:** See PDX Collection 1299
   For S72.342[B,C]: See PDX Collection 1298
   For S72.342[K,M,N,P,Q,R]: See PDX Collection 897

● S72.343   **Displaced spiral fracture of shaft of unspecified femur** K, M, N, P, Q, R 🩹, A, B, C 🩹, A, B, C 🩹, A, B, C 🩹
   (Ex:) **For S72.343[A,B,C]:** See PDX Collection 1298
   For S72.343[K,M,N,P,Q,R]: See PDX Collection 897

● S72.344   **Nondisplaced spiral fracture of shaft of right femur** K, M, N, P, Q, R 🩹, A, B, C 🩹, A, B, C 🩹, A, B, C 🩹
   (Ex:) **For S72.344[A]:** See PDX Collection 1297
   For S72.344[B,C]: See PDX Collection 1298
   For S72.344[K,M,N,P,Q,R]: See PDX Collection 897

● S72.345   **Nondisplaced spiral fracture of shaft of left femur** K, M, N, P, Q, R 🩹, A, B, C 🩹, A, B, C 🩹, A, B, C 🩹
   (Ex:) **For S72.345[A]:** See PDX Collection 1299
   For S72.345[B,C]: See PDX Collection 1298
   For S72.345[K,M,N,P,Q,R]: See PDX Collection 897

● S72.346   **Nondisplaced spiral fracture of shaft of unspecified femur** K, M, N, P, Q, R 🩹, A, B, C 🩹, A, B, C 🩹, A, B, C 🩹
   (Ex:) **For S72.346[A,B,C]:** See PDX Collection 1298
   For S72.346[K,M,N,P,Q,R]: See PDX Collection 897

● S72.35   **Comminuted fracture of shaft of femur**

● S72.351   **Displaced comminuted fracture of shaft of right femur** K, M, N, P, Q, R 🩹, A, B, C 🩹, A, B, C 🩹, A, B, C 🩹
   (Ex:) **For S72.351[A]:** See PDX Collection 1297
   For S72.351[B,C]: See PDX Collection 1298
   For S72.351[K,M,N,P,Q,R]: See PDX Collection 897

● S72.352   **Displaced comminuted fracture of shaft of left femur** K, M, N, P, Q, R 🩹, A, B, C 🩹, A, B, C 🩹, A, B, C 🩹
   (Ex:) **For S72.352[A]:** See PDX Collection 1299
   For S72.352[B,C]: See PDX Collection 1298
   For S72.352[K,M,N,P,Q,R]: See PDX Collection 897

● S72.353   **Displaced comminuted fracture of shaft of unspecified femur** K, M, N, P, Q, R 🩹, A, B, C 🩹, A, B, C 🩹, A, B, C 🩹
   (Ex:) **For S72.353[A,B,C]:** See PDX Collection 1298
   For S72.353[K,M,N,P,Q,R]: See PDX Collection 897

● S72.354   **Nondisplaced comminuted fracture of shaft of right femur** K, M, N, P, Q, R 🩹, A, B, C 🩹, A, B, C 🩹, A, B, C 🩹
   (Ex:) **For S72.354[A]:** See PDX Collection 1297
   For S72.354[B,C]: See PDX Collection 1298
   For S72.354[K,M,N,P,Q,R]: See PDX Collection 897

▶ New   ➡ Revised   ~~deleted~~ Deleted   Excludes 1   Excludes 2   Includes   Use additional   Code first   Code also   Key words
OGCR Official Guidelines   ● Unacceptable Principal Diagnosis   X Assign placeholder X   ● Use Additional Character(s)   ▶ Manifestation Code   **Coding Clinic**

● S72.355   Nondisplaced comminuted fracture of shaft of left femur K, M, N, P, Q, R 🅒, A, B, C, A, B, C 🅜, A, B, C 🅗
> Ⓔⓧ **For S72.355[A]:** See PDX Collection 1299
> **For S72.355[B,C]:** See PDX Collection 1298
> **For S72.355[K,M,N,P,Q,R]:** See PDX Collection 897

● S72.356   Nondisplaced comminuted fracture of shaft of unspecified femur K, M, N, P, Q, R 🅒, A, B, C, A, B, C 🅜, A, B, C 🅗
> Ⓔⓧ **For S72.356[A,B,C]:** See PDX Collection 1298
> **For S72.356[K,M,N,P,Q,R]:** See PDX Collection 897

● S72.36   Segmental fracture of shaft of femur

● S72.361   Displaced segmental fracture of shaft of right femur K, M, N, P, Q, R 🅒, A, B, C 🅜, A, B, C 🅜, A, B, C 🅗
> Ⓔⓧ **For S72.361[A]:** See PDX Collection 1297
> **For S72.361[B,C]:** See PDX Collection 1298
> **For S72.361[K,M,N,P,Q,R]:** See PDX Collection 897

● S72.362   Displaced segmental fracture of shaft of left femur K, M, N, P, Q, R 🅒, A, B, C 🅜, A, B, C 🅜, A, B, C 🅗
> Ⓔⓧ **For S72.362[A]:** See PDX Collection 1299
> **For S72.362[B,C]:** See PDX Collection 1298
> **For S72.362[K,M,N,P,Q,R]:** See PDX Collection 897

● S72.363   Displaced segmental fracture of shaft of unspecified femur K, M, N, P, Q, R 🅒, A, B, C 🅜, A, B, C 🅜, A, B, C 🅗
> Ⓔⓧ **For S72.363[A,B,C]:** See PDX Collection 1298
> **For S72.363[K,M,N,P,Q,R]:** See PDX Collection 897

● S72.364   Nondisplaced segmental fracture of shaft of right femur K, M, N, P, Q, R 🅒, A, B, C 🅜, A, B, C 🅜, A, B, C 🅗
> Ⓔⓧ **For S72.364[A]:** See PDX Collection 1297
> **For S72.364[B,C]:** See PDX Collection 1298
> **For S72.364[K,M,N,P,Q,R]:** See PDX Collection 897

● S72.365   Nondisplaced segmental fracture of shaft of left femur K, M, N, P, Q, R 🅒, A, B, C 🅜, A, B, C 🅜, A, B, C 🅗
> Ⓔⓧ **For S72.365[A]:** See PDX Collection 1299
> **For S72.365[B,C]:** See PDX Collection 1298
> **For S72.365[K,M,N,P,Q,R]:** See PDX Collection 897

● S72.366   Nondisplaced segmental fracture of shaft of unspecified femur K, M, N, P, Q, R 🅒, A, B, C 🅜, A, B, C 🅜, A, B, C 🅗
> Ⓔⓧ **For S72.366[A,B,C]:** See PDX Collection 1298
> **For S72.366[K,M,N,P,Q,R]:** See PDX Collection 897

● S72.39   Other fracture of shaft of femur

● S72.391   Other fracture of shaft of right femur K, M, N, P, Q, R 🅒, A, B, C, A, B, C 🅜, A, B, C 🅗
> Ⓔⓧ **For S72.391[A]:** See PDX Collection 1297
> **For S72.391[B,C]:** See PDX Collection 1298
> **For S72.391[K,M,N,P,Q,R]:** See PDX Collection 897

● S72.392   Other fracture of shaft of left femur K, M, N, P, Q, R 🅒, A, B, C, A, B, C 🅜, A, B, C 🅗
> Ⓔⓧ **For S72.392[A]:** See PDX Collection 1299
> **For S72.392[B,C]:** See PDX Collection 1298
> **For S72.392[K,M,N,P,Q,R]:** See PDX Collection 897

● S72.399   Other fracture of shaft of unspecified femur K, M, N, P, Q, R 🅒, A, B, C, A, B, C 🅜, A, B, C 🅗
> Ⓔⓧ **For S72.399[A,B,C]:** See PDX Collection 1298
> **For S72.399[K,M,N,P,Q,R]:** See PDX Collection 897

● S72.4   Fracture of lower end of femur
> Fracture of distal end of femur
> **Excludes2**   fracture of shaft of femur (S72.3-)
> physeal fracture of lower end of femur (S79.1-)

● S72.40   Unspecified fracture of lower end of femur

● S72.401   Unspecified fracture of lower end of right femur A, K, M, N, P, Q, R 🅒, B, C 🅜, A, B, C 🅜, A, B, C 🅗
> Ⓔⓧ **For S72.401[A]:** See PDX Collection 1300
> **For S72.401[B,C]:** See PDX Collection 1301
> **For S72.401[K,M,N,P,Q,R]:** See PDX Collection 897

> **Coding Clinic: 2016, Q4, P43**

● S72.402   Unspecified fracture of lower end of left femur A, K, M, N, P, Q, R 🅒, B, C 🅜, A, B, C 🅜, A, B, C 🅗
> Ⓔⓧ **For S72.402[A]:** See PDX Collection 1302
> **For S72.402[B,C]:** See PDX Collection 1301
> **For S72.401[K,M,N,P,Q,R]:** See PDX Collection 897

● S72.409   Unspecified fracture of lower end of unspecified femur A, K, M, N, P, Q, R 🅒, B, C 🅜, A, B, C 🅜, A, B, C 🅗
> Ⓔⓧ **For S72.409[A,B,C]:** See PDX Collection 1301
> **For S72.401[K,M,N,P,Q,R]:** See PDX Collection 897

● S72.41   Unspecified condyle fracture of lower end of femur
> Condyle fracture of femur NOS

● S72.411   Displaced unspecified condyle fracture of lower end of right femur A, K, M, N, P, Q, R 🅒, B, C 🅜, A, B, C 🅜, A, B, C 🅗
> Ⓔⓧ **For S72.411[A]:** See PDX Collection 1300
> **For S72.411[B,C]:** See PDX Collection 1301
> **For S72.411[K,M,N,P,Q,R]:** See PDX Collection 897

● S72.412   Displaced unspecified condyle fracture of lower end of left femur A, K, M, N, P, Q, R 🅒, B, C 🅜, A, B, C 🅜, A, B, C 🅗
> Ⓔⓧ **For S72.412[A]:** See PDX Collection 1302
> **For S72.412[B,C]:** See PDX Collection 1301
> **For S72.411[K,M,N,P,Q,R]:** See PDX Collection 897

● S72.413   Displaced unspecified condyle fracture of lower end of unspecified femur A, K, M, N, P, Q, R 🅒, B, C 🅜, A, B, C 🅜, A, B, C 🅗
> Ⓔⓧ **For S72.413[A,B,C]:** See PDX Collection 1301
> **For S72.413[K,M,N,P,Q,R]:** See PDX Collection 897

● S72.414   Nondisplaced unspecified condyle fracture of lower end of right femur A, K, M, N, P, Q, R 🅒, B, C 🅜, A, B, C 🅜, A, B, C 🅗
> Ⓔⓧ **For S72.414[A]:** See PDX Collection 1300
> **For S72.414[B,C]:** See PDX Collection 1301
> **For S72.414[K,M,N,P,Q,R]:** See PDX Collection 897

● S72.415   Nondisplaced unspecified condyle fracture of lower end of left femur A, K, M, N, P, Q, R 🅒, B, C 🅜, A, B, C 🅜, A, B, C 🅗
> Ⓔⓧ **For S72.415[A]:** See PDX Collection 1302
> **For S72.415[B,C]:** See PDX Collection 1301
> **For S72.415[K,M,N,P,Q,R]:** See PDX Collection 897

● S72.416   Nondisplaced unspecified condyle fracture of lower end of unspecified femur A, K, M, N, P, Q, R 🅒, B, C 🅜, A, B, C 🅜, A, B, C 🅗
> Ⓔⓧ **For S72.416[A,B,C]:** See PDX Collection 1301
> **For S72.416[K,M,N,P,Q,R]:** See PDX Collection 897

N Newborn Age: 0   **P** Pediatric Age: 0–17   **M** Maternity DX: 9–64   **A** Adult Age: 15–124   ♀ Females Only   ♂ Males Only

🅒 Complication\Comorbidity   🅜 Major C\C   Ⓔⓧ CC/MCC Exclusions   🅗 Hospital-Acquired Condition   Hierarchical Condition Category

1383

CHAPTER 19 (S00-T88)

● S72.42 Fracture of lateral condyle of femur
   ● S72.421 Displaced fracture of lateral condyle
             of right femur A, K, M, N, P, Q, R ©,
             B, C ©, A, B, C ©, **A, B, C** ©©
               Ⓔⓧ **For S72.421[A]:** See PDX Collection 1300
                    For S72.421[B,C]: See PDX Collection 1301
                    For S72.421[K,M,N,P,Q,R]: See PDX
                    Collection 897

   ● S72.422 Displaced fracture of lateral condyle
             of left femur A, K, M, N, P, Q, R ©,
             B, C ©, A, B, C ©, **A, B, C** ©©
               Ⓔⓧ **For S72.422[A]:** See PDX Collection 1302
                    For S72.422[B,C]: See PDX Collection 1301
                    For S72.422[K,M,N,P,Q,R]: See PDX
                    Collection 897

   ● S72.423 Displaced fracture of lateral condyle
             of unspecified femur
             A, K, M, N, P, Q, R ©, B, C ©,
             A, B, C ©, **A, B, C** ©©
               Ⓔⓧ **For S72.423[A,B,C]:** See PDX Collection 1301
                    For S72.423[K,M,N,P,Q,R]: See PDX
                    Collection 897

   ● S72.424 Nondisplaced fracture of lateral
             condyle of right femur
             A, K, M, N, P, Q, R ©, B, C ©,
             A, B, C ©, **A, B, C** ©©
               Ⓔⓧ **For S72.424[A]:** See PDX Collection 1300
                    For S72.424[B,C]: See PDX Collection 1301
                    For S72.424[K,M,N,P,Q,R]: See PDX
                    Collection 897

   ● S72.425 Nondisplaced fracture of lateral
             condyle of left femur
             A, K, M, N, P, Q, R ©, B, C ©,
             A, B, C ©, **A, B, C** ©©
               Ⓔⓧ **For S72.425[A]:** See PDX Collection 1302
                    For S72.425[B,C]: See PDX Collection 1301
                    For S72.425[K,M,N,P,Q,R]: See PDX
                    Collection 897

   ● S72.426 Nondisplaced fracture of lateral
             condyle of unspecified femur
             A, K, M, N, P, Q, R ©, B, C ©,
             A, B, C ©, **A, B, C** ©©
               Ⓔⓧ **For S72.426[A,B,C]:** See PDX Collection 1301
                    For S72.426[K,M,N,P,Q,R]: See PDX
                    Collection 897

● S72.43 Fracture of medial condyle of femur
   ● S72.431 Displaced fracture of medial condyle
             of right femur A, K, M, N, P, Q, R ©,
             B, C ©, A, B, C ©, **A, B, C** ©©
               Ⓔⓧ **For S72.431[A]:** See PDX Collection 1300
                    For S72.431[B,C]: See PDX Collection 1301
                    For S72.431[K,M,N,P,Q,R]: See PDX
                    Collection 897

   ● S72.432 Displaced fracture of medial condyle
             of left femur A, K, M, N, P, Q, R ©,
             B, C ©, A, B, C ©, **A, B, C** ©©
               Ⓔⓧ **For S72.432[A]:** See PDX Collection 1302
                    For S72.432[B,C]: See PDX Collection 1301
                    For S72.432[K,M,N,P,Q,R]: See PDX
                    Collection 897

   ● S72.433 Displaced fracture of medial condyle
             of unspecified femur
             A, K, M, N, P, Q, R ©, B, C ©,
             A, B, C ©, **A, B, C** ©©
               Ⓔⓧ **For S72.433[A,B,C]:** See PDX Collection 1301
                    For S72.433[K,M,N,P,Q,R]: See PDX
                    Collection 897

   ● S72.434 Nondisplaced fracture of medial
             condyle of right femur
             A, K, M, N, P, Q, R ©, B, C ©,
             A, B, C ©, **A, B, C** ©©
               Ⓔⓧ **For S72.434[A]:** See PDX Collection 1300
                    For S72.434[B,C]: See PDX Collection 1301
                    For S72.434[K,M,N,P,Q,R]: See PDX
                    Collection 897

   ● S72.435 Nondisplaced fracture of medial
             condyle of left femur
             A, K, M, N, P, Q, R ©, B, C ©,
             A, B, C ©, **A, B, C** ©©
               Ⓔⓧ **For S72.435[A]:** See PDX Collection 1302
                    For S72.435[B,C]: See PDX Collection 1301
                    For S72.435[K,M,N,P,Q,R]: See PDX
                    Collection 897

   ● S72.436 Nondisplaced fracture of medial
             condyle of unspecified femur
             A, K, M, N, P, Q, R ©, B, C ©,
             A, B, C ©, **A, B, C** ©©
               Ⓔⓧ **For S72.436[A,B,C]:** See PDX Collection 1301
                    For S72.436[K,M,N,P,Q,R]: See PDX
                    Collection 897

● S72.44 Fracture of lower epiphysis (separation) of
        femur
       Excludes1 Salter-Harris Type I physeal
                   fracture of lower end of
                   femur (S79.11-)

   ● S72.441 Displaced fracture of lower epiphysis
             (separation) of right femur
             A, K, M, N, P, Q, R ©, B, C ©,
             A, B, C ©, **A, B, C** ©©
               Ⓔⓧ **For S72.441[A]:** See PDX Collection 1300
                    For S72.441[B,C]: See PDX Collection 1301
                    For S72.441[K,M,N,P,Q,R]: See PDX
                    Collection 897

   ● S72.442 Displaced fracture of lower epiphysis
             (separation) of left femur
             A, K, M, N, P, Q, R ©, B, C ©,
             A, B, C ©, **A, B, C** ©©
               Ⓔⓧ **For S72.442[A]:** See PDX Collection 1302
                    For S72.442[B,C]: See PDX Collection 1301
                    For S72.442[K,M,N,P,Q,R]: See PDX
                    Collection 897

   ● S72.443 Displaced fracture of lower epiphysis
             (separation) of unspecified femur
             A, K, M, N, P, Q, R ©, B, C ©,
             A, B, C ©, **A, B, C** ©©
               Ⓔⓧ **For S72.443[A,B,C]:** See PDX Collection 1301
                    For S72.443[K,M,N,P,Q,R]: See PDX
                    Collection 897

   ● S72.444 Nondisplaced fracture of lower
             epiphysis (separation) of right femur
             A, K, M, N, P, Q, R ©, B, C ©,
             A, B, C ©, **A, B, C** ©©
               Ⓔⓧ **For S72.444[A]:** See PDX Collection 1300
                    For S72.444[B,C]: See PDX Collection 1301
                    For S72.444[K,M,N,P,Q,R]: See PDX
                    Collection 897

   ● S72.445 Nondisplaced fracture of lower
             epiphysis (separation) of left femur
             A, K, M, N, P, Q, R ©, B, C ©,
             A, B, C ©, **A, B, C** ©©
               Ⓔⓧ **For S72.445[A]:** See PDX Collection 1302
                    For S72.445[B,C]: See PDX Collection 1301
                    For S72.445[K,M,N,P,Q,R]: See PDX
                    Collection 897

   ● S72.446 Nondisplaced fracture of lower
             epiphysis (separation) of unspecified
             femur A, K, M, N, P, Q, R ©, B, C ©,
             A, B, C ©, **A, B, C** ©©
               Ⓔⓧ **For S72.446[A,B,C]:** See PDX Collection 1301
                    For S72.446[K,M,N,P,Q,R]: See PDX
                    Collection 897

▶ New ⟹ Revised ~~deleted~~ Deleted Excludes 1 Excludes 2 Includes Use additional Code first Code also Key words
OGCR Official Guidelines ● Unacceptable Principal Diagnosis X Assign placeholder X ● Use Additional Character(s) ❱ Manifestation Code Coding Clinic

● **S72.45** Supracondylar fracture without intracondylar extension of lower end of femur

   Supracondylar fracture of lower end of femur NOS

   Excludes1   supracondylar fracture with intracondylar extension of lower end of femur (S72.46-)

● **S72.451** Displaced supracondylar fracture without intracondylar extension of lower end of right femur

   A, K, M, N, P, Q, R 🪙, B, C 🪙, A, B, C 🪙, A, B, C 🪙

   (Ex) For S72.451[A]: See PDX Collection 1300
   For S72.451[B,C]: See PDX Collection 1301
   For S72.451[K,M,N,P,Q,R]: See PDX Collection 897

● **S72.452** Displaced supracondylar fracture without intracondylar extension of lower end of left femur

   A, K, M, N, P, Q, R 🪙, B, C 🪙, A, B, C 🪙, A, B, C 🪙

   (Ex) For S72.452[A]: See PDX Collection 1302
   For S72.452[B,C]: See PDX Collection 1301
   For S72.452[K,M,N,P,Q,R]: See PDX Collection 897

● **S72.453** Displaced supracondylar fracture without intracondylar extension of lower end of unspecified femur

   A, K, M, N, P, Q, R 🪙, B, C 🪙, A, B, C 🪙, A, B, C 🪙

   (Ex) For S72.453[A,B,C]: See PDX Collection 1301
   For S72.453[K,M,N,P,Q,R]: See PDX Collection 897

● **S72.454** Nondisplaced supracondylar fracture without intracondylar extension of lower end of right femur

   A, K, M, N, P, Q, R 🪙, B, C 🪙, A, B, C 🪙, A, B, C 🪙

   (Ex) For S72.454[A]: See PDX Collection 1300
   For S72.454[B,C]: See PDX Collection 1301
   For S72.454[K,M,N,P,Q,R]: See PDX Collection 897

● **S72.455** Nondisplaced supracondylar fracture without intracondylar extension of lower end of left femur

   A, K, M, N, P, Q, R 🪙, B, C 🪙, A, B, C 🪙, A, B, C 🪙

   (Ex) For S72.455[A]: See PDX Collection 1302
   For S72.455[B,C]: See PDX Collection 1301
   For S72.455[K,M,N,P,Q,R]: See PDX Collection 897

● **S72.456** Nondisplaced supracondylar fracture without intracondylar extension of lower end of unspecified femur

   A, K, M, N, P, Q, R 🪙, B, C 🪙, A, B, C 🪙, A, B, C 🪙

   (Ex) For S72.456[A,B,C]: See PDX Collection 1301
   For S72.456[K,M,N,P,Q,R]: See PDX Collection 897

● **S72.46** Supracondylar fracture with intracondylar extension of lower end of femur

   Excludes1   supracondylar fracture without intracondylar extension of lower end of femur (S72.45-)

● **S72.461** Displaced supracondylar fracture with intracondylar extension of lower end of right femur

   A, K, M, N, P, Q, R 🪙, B, C 🪙, A, B, C 🪙, A, B, C 🪙

   (Ex) For S72.461[A]: See PDX Collection 1300
   For S72.461[B,C]: See PDX Collection 1301
   For S72.461[K,M,N,P,Q,R]: See PDX Collection 897

● **S72.462** Displaced supracondylar fracture with intracondylar extension of lower end of left femur

   A, K, M, N, P, Q, R 🪙, B, C 🪙, A, B, C 🪙, A, B, C 🪙

   (Ex) For S72.462[A]: See PDX Collection 1302
   For S72.462[B,C]: See PDX Collection 1301
   For S72.462[K,M,N,P,Q,R]: See PDX Collection 897

● **S72.463** Displaced supracondylar fracture with intracondylar extension of lower end of unspecified femur

   A, K, M, N, P, Q, R 🪙, B, C 🪙, A, B, C 🪙, A, B, C 🪙

   (Ex) For S72.463[A,B,C]: See PDX Collection 1301
   For S72.463[K,M,N,P,Q,R]: See PDX Collection 897

● **S72.464** Nondisplaced supracondylar fracture with intracondylar extension of lower end of right femur

   A, K, M, N, P, Q, R 🪙, B, C 🪙, A, B, C 🪙, A, B, C 🪙

   (Ex) For S72.464[A]: See PDX Collection 1300
   For S72.464[B,C]: See PDX Collection 1301
   For S72.464[K,M,N,P,Q,R]: See PDX Collection 897

● **S72.465** Nondisplaced supracondylar fracture with intracondylar extension of lower end of left femur

   A, K, M, N, P, Q, R 🪙, B, C 🪙, A, B, C 🪙, A, B, C 🪙

   (Ex) For S72.465[A]: See PDX Collection 1302
   For S72.465[B,C]: See PDX Collection 1301
   For S72.465[K,M,N,P,Q,R]: See PDX Collection 897

● **S72.466** Nondisplaced supracondylar fracture with intracondylar extension of lower end of unspecified femur

   A, K, M, N, P, Q, R 🪙, B, C 🪙, A, B, C 🪙, A, B, C 🪙

   (Ex) For S72.466[A,B,C]: See PDX Collection 1301
   For S72.466[K,M,N,P,Q,R]: See PDX Collection 897

N Newborn Age: 0   **P** Pediatric Age: 0–17   **M** Maternity DX: 9–64   **A** Adult Age: 15–124   ♀ Females Only   ♂ Males Only

🪙 Complication\Comorbidity   🪙 Major C\C   (Ex) CC/MCC Exclusions   🪙 Hospital-Acquired Condition   🪙 Hierarchical Condition Category

1385

● S72.47   Torus fracture of lower end of femur
           The appropriate 7th character is to be added to
           all codes in subcategory S72.47

A	initial encounter for closed fracture
D	subsequent encounter for fracture with routine healing
G	subsequent encounter for fracture with delayed healing
K	subsequent encounter for fracture with nonunion
P	subsequent encounter for fracture with malunion
S	sequela

    ● S72.471   Torus fracture of lower end of right
               femur A, K, P 🦻, A 🦻, A 🦻
               Ⓔⓧ For S72.471[A]: See PDX Collection 1300
                  For S72.471[K,P]: See PDX Collection 897

    ● S72.472   Torus fracture of lower end of left
               femur A, K, P 🦻, A 🦻, A 🦻
               Ⓔⓧ For S72.472[A]: See PDX Collection 1302
                  For S72.472[K,P]: See PDX Collection 897

    ● S72.479   Torus fracture of lower end of
               unspecified femur A, K, P 🦻, A 🦻,
               A 🦻
               Ⓔⓧ For S72.479[A]: See PDX Collection 1301
                  For S72.479[K,P]: See PDX Collection 897

● S72.49   Other fracture of lower end of femur

    ● S72.491   Other fracture of lower end of right
               femur A, K, M, N, P, Q, R 🦻, B, C 🦻,
               A, B, C 🦻, A, B, C 🦻
               Ⓔⓧ For S72.491[A]: See PDX Collection 1300
                  For S72.491[B,C]: See PDX Collection 1303
                  For S72.491[K,M,N,P,Q,R]: See PDX
                  Collection 897

    ● S72.492   Other fracture of lower end of left
               femur A, K, M, N, P, Q, R 🦻, B, C 🦻,
               A, B, C 🦻, A, B, C 🦻
               Ⓔⓧ For S72.492[A]: See PDX Collection 1302
                  For S72.492[B,C]: See PDX Collection 1303
                  For S72.492[K,M,N,P,Q,R]: See PDX
                  Collection 897

    ● S72.499   Other fracture of lower end of
               unspecified femur
               A, K, M, N, P, Q, R 🦻, B, C 🦻,
               A, B, C 🦻, A, B, C 🦻
               Ⓔⓧ For S72.499[A]: See PDX Collection 1301
                  For S72.499[B,C]: See PDX Collection 1303
                  For S72.499[K,M,N,P,Q,R]: See PDX
                  Collection 897

● S72.8   Other fracture of femur
          Ⓔⓧ For category S72.8 CC codes S72.8[A,B,C]: See PDX Collection 1298
             For S72.8[K,M,N,P,Q,R]: See PDX Collection 897

    ● S72.8X   Other fracture of femur

        ● S72.8X1   Other fracture of right femur K, M, N,
                   P, Q, R 🦻, A, B, C 🦻, A, B, C 🦻,
                   A, B, C 🦻

        ● S72.8X2   Other fracture of left femur K, M, N,
                   P, Q, R 🦻, A, B, C 🦻, A, B, C 🦻,
                   A, B, C 🦻

        ● S72.8X9   Other fracture of unspecified femur
                   K, M, N, P, Q, R 🦻, A, B, C 🦻,
                   A, B, C 🦻, A, B, C 🦻

● S72.9   Unspecified fracture of femur
          Fracture of thigh NOS
          Fracture of upper leg NOS
          Excludes1   fracture of hip NOS (S72.00-, S72.01-)
          Ⓔⓧ For category S72.9 CC codes S72.9[A,B,C]: See PDX Collection 1298
             For S72.9[K,M,N,P,Q,R]: See PDX Collection 897

    X ● S72.90   Unspecified fracture of unspecified femur
               K, M, N, P, Q, R 🦻, A, B, C 🦻, A, B, C 🦻,
               A, B, C 🦻
               Coding Clinic: 2012, Q4, P94

X ● S72.91   Unspecified fracture of right femur K, M, N,
            P, Q, R 🦻, A, B, C 🦻, A, B, C 🦻, A, B, C 🦻
X ● S72.92   Unspecified fracture of left femur K, M, N,
            P, Q, R 🦻, A, B, C 🦻, A, B, C 🦻, A, B, C 🦻

● S73   Dislocation and sprain of joint and ligaments of hip
        Includes   avulsion of joint or ligament of hip
                       laceration of cartilage, joint or ligament of hip
                       sprain of cartilage, joint or ligament of hip
                       traumatic hemarthrosis of joint or ligament of hip
                       traumatic rupture of joint or ligament of hip
                       traumatic subluxation of joint or ligament of hip
                       traumatic tear of joint or ligament of hip
        Code also any associated open wound
        Excludes2   strain of muscle, fascia and tendon of hip and
                       thigh (S76.-)
        The appropriate 7th character is to be added to each code from
        category S73

A	initial encounter
D	subsequent encounter
S	sequela

    ● S73.0   Subluxation and dislocation of hip
              Out of position
              Excludes2   dislocation and subluxation of hip
                             prosthesis (T84.020, T84.021)

        ● S73.00   Unspecified subluxation and dislocation of hip
                   Dislocation of hip NOS
                   Subluxation of hip NOS

            ● S73.001   Unspecified subluxation of right hip
                       A 🦻, A 🦻, A 🦻
                       Ⓔⓧ See PDX Collection 1304

            ● S73.002   Unspecified subluxation of left hip
                       A 🦻, A 🦻, A 🦻
                       Ⓔⓧ See PDX Collection 1305

            ● S73.003   Unspecified subluxation of
                       unspecified hip A 🦻, A 🦻, A 🦻
                       Ⓔⓧ See PDX Collection 1306

            ● S73.004   Unspecified dislocation of right hip
                       A 🦻, A 🦻, A 🦻
                       Ⓔⓧ See PDX Collection 1304

            ● S73.005   Unspecified dislocation of left hip
                       A 🦻, A 🦻, A 🦻
                       Ⓔⓧ See PDX Collection 1305

            ● S73.006   Unspecified dislocation of unspecified
                       hip A 🦻, A 🦻, A 🦻
                       Ⓔⓧ See PDX Collection 1306

        ● S73.01   Posterior subluxation and dislocation of hip

            ● S73.011   Posterior subluxation of right hip
                       A 🦻, A 🦻, A 🦻
                       Ⓔⓧ See PDX Collection 1307

            ● S73.012   Posterior subluxation of left hip A 🦻,
                       A 🦻, A 🦻
                       Ⓔⓧ See PDX Collection 1308

            ● S73.013   Posterior subluxation of unspecified
                       hip A 🦻, A 🦻, A 🦻
                       Ⓔⓧ See PDX Collection 1309

            ● S73.014   Posterior dislocation of right hip A 🦻,
                       A 🦻, A 🦻
                       Ⓔⓧ See PDX Collection 1307

            ● S73.015   Posterior dislocation of left hip A 🦻,
                       A 🦻, A 🦻
                       Ⓔⓧ See PDX Collection 1308

            ● S73.016   Posterior dislocation of unspecified
                       hip A 🦻, A 🦻, A 🦻
                       Ⓔⓧ See PDX Collection 1309

▶ New   ⇒ Revised   ~~deleted~~ Deleted   Excludes 1   Excludes 2   Includes   Use additional   Code first   Code also   Key words
OGCR Official Guidelines   ● Unacceptable Principal Diagnosis   X Assign placeholder X   ● Use Additional Character(s)   ▌ Manifestation Code   Coding Clinic

- ● **S73.02**   Obturator subluxation and dislocation of hip
  - ● **S73.021**   Obturator subluxation of right hip A 🪙, A 🪙, A 🪙
    - Ex: See PDX Collection 1310
  - ● **S73.022**   Obturator subluxation of left hip A 🪙, A 🪙, A 🪙
    - Ex: See PDX Collection 1311
  - ● **S73.023**   Obturator subluxation of unspecified hip A 🪙, A 🪙, A 🪙
    - Ex: See PDX Collection 1312
  - ● **S73.024**   Obturator dislocation of right hip A 🪙, A 🪙, A 🪙
    - Ex: See PDX Collection 1310
  - ● **S73.025**   Obturator dislocation of left hip A 🪙, A 🪙, A 🪙
    - Ex: See PDX Collection 1311
  - ● **S73.026**   Obturator dislocation of unspecified hip A 🪙, A 🪙, A 🪙
    - Ex: See PDX Collection 1312
- ● **S73.03**   Other anterior subluxation and dislocation of hip
  - ● **S73.031**   Other anterior subluxation of right hip A 🪙, A 🪙, A 🪙
    - Ex: See PDX Collection 1313
  - ● **S73.032**   Other anterior subluxation of left hip A 🪙, A 🪙, A 🪙
    - Ex: See PDX Collection 1314
  - ● **S73.033**   Other anterior subluxation of unspecified hip A 🪙, A 🪙, A 🪙
    - Ex: See PDX Collection 1315
  - ● **S73.034**   Other anterior dislocation of right hip A 🪙, A 🪙, A 🪙
    - Ex: See PDX Collection 1313
  - ● **S73.035**   Other anterior dislocation of left hip A 🪙, A 🪙, A 🪙
    - Ex: See PDX Collection 1314
  - ● **S73.036**   Other anterior dislocation of unspecified hip A 🪙, A 🪙, A 🪙
    - Ex: See PDX Collection 1315
- ● **S73.04**   Central subluxation and dislocation of hip
  - ● **S73.041**   Central subluxation of right hip A 🪙, A 🪙, A 🪙
    - Ex: See PDX Collection 1304
  - ● **S73.042**   Central subluxation of left hip A 🪙, A 🪙, A 🪙
    - Ex: See PDX Collection 1305
  - ● **S73.043**   Central subluxation of unspecified hip A 🪙, A 🪙, A 🪙
    - Ex: See PDX Collection 1306
  - ● **S73.044**   Central dislocation of right hip A 🪙, A 🪙, A 🪙
    - Ex: See PDX Collection 1304
  - ● **S73.045**   Central dislocation of left hip A 🪙, A 🪙, A 🪙
    - Ex: See PDX Collection 1305
  - ● **S73.046**   Central dislocation of unspecified hip A 🪙, A 🪙, A 🪙
    - Ex: See PDX Collection 1306
- ● **S73.1**   Sprain of hip
  - ● **S73.10**   Unspecified sprain of hip
    - ● **S73.101**   Unspecified sprain of right hip
    - ● **S73.102**   Unspecified sprain of left hip
    - ● **S73.109**   Unspecified sprain of unspecified hip

- ● **S73.11**   Iliofemoral ligament sprain of hip
  - ● **S73.111**   Iliofemoral ligament sprain of right hip
  - ● **S73.112**   Iliofemoral ligament sprain of left hip
  - ● **S73.119**   Iliofemoral ligament sprain of unspecified hip
- ● **S73.12**   Ischiocapsular (ligament) sprain of hip
  - ● **S73.121**   Ischiocapsular ligament sprain of right hip
  - ● **S73.122**   Ischiocapsular ligament sprain of left hip
  - ● **S73.129**   Ischiocapsular ligament sprain of unspecified hip
- ● **S73.19**   Other sprain of hip
  - ● **S73.191**   Other sprain of right hip
  - ● **S73.192**   Other sprain of left hip
  - ● **S73.199**   Other sprain of unspecified hip
- ● **S74**   Injury of nerves at hip and thigh level

  Code also any associated open wound (S71.-)

  Excludes2   injury of nerves at ankle and foot level (S94.-)
  injury of nerves at lower leg level (S84.-)

  The appropriate 7th character is to be added to each code from category S74

A	initial encounter
D	subsequent encounter
S	sequela

  - ● **S74.0**   Injury of sciatic nerve at hip and thigh level
    - X● **S74.00**   Injury of sciatic nerve at hip and thigh level, unspecified leg
    - X● **S74.01**   Injury of sciatic nerve at hip and thigh level, right leg
    - X● **S74.02**   Injury of sciatic nerve at hip and thigh level, left leg
  - ● **S74.1**   Injury of femoral nerve at hip and thigh level
    - X● **S74.10**   Injury of femoral nerve at hip and thigh level, unspecified leg
    - X● **S74.11**   Injury of femoral nerve at hip and thigh level, right leg
    - X● **S74.12**   Injury of femoral nerve at hip and thigh level, left leg
  - ● **S74.2**   Injury of cutaneous sensory nerve at hip and thigh level
    - X● **S74.20**   Injury of cutaneous sensory nerve at hip and thigh level, unspecified leg
    - X● **S74.21**   Injury of cutaneous sensory nerve at hip and high level, right leg
    - X● **S74.22**   Injury of cutaneous sensory nerve at hip and thigh level, left leg
  - ● **S74.8**   Injury of other nerves at hip and thigh level
    - ● **S74.8X**   Injury of other nerves at hip and thigh level
      - ● **S74.8X1**   Injury of other nerves at hip and thigh level, right leg
      - ● **S74.8X2**   Injury of other nerves at hip and thigh level, left leg
      - ● **S74.8X9**   Injury of other nerves at hip and thigh level, unspecified leg
  - ● **S74.9**   Injury of unspecified nerve at hip and thigh level
    - X● **S74.90**   Injury of unspecified nerve at hip and thigh level, unspecified leg
    - X● **S74.91**   Injury of unspecified nerve at hip and thigh level, right leg
    - X● **S74.92**   Injury of unspecified nerve at hip and thigh level, left leg

N Newborn Age: 0   **P** Pediatric Age: 0–17   **M** Maternity DX: 9–64   **A** Adult Age: 15–124   ♀ Females Only   ♂ Males Only
🪙 Complication\Comorbidity   🪙 Major C\C   Ex: CC/MCC Exclusions   🪙 Hospital-Acquired Condition   🪙 Hierarchical Condition Category

● **S75**   **Injury of blood vessels at hip and thigh level**

Code also any associated open wound (S71.-)

Excludes2   injury of blood vessels at lower leg level (S85.-)
injury of popliteal artery (S85.0)

The appropriate 7th character is to be added to each code from category S75

> A   initial encounter
> D   subsequent encounter
> S   sequela

● **S75.0**   **Injury of femoral artery**

   ● **S75.00**   **Unspecified injury of femoral artery**

     ● **S75.001**   **Unspecified injury of femoral artery, right leg** A 🔖
        (Ex:) See PDX Collection 1316

     ● **S75.002**   **Unspecified injury of femoral artery, left leg** A 🔖
        (Ex:) See PDX Collection 1317

     ● **S75.009**   **Unspecified injury of femoral artery, unspecified leg** A 🔖
        (Ex:) See PDX Collection 1318

   ● **S75.01**   **Minor laceration of femoral artery**
     Incomplete transection of femoral artery
     Laceration of femoral artery NOS
     Superficial laceration of femoral artery

     ● **S75.011**   **Minor laceration of femoral artery, right leg** A 🔖
        (Ex:) See PDX Collection 1316

     ● **S75.012**   **Minor laceration of femoral artery, left leg** A 🔖
        (Ex:) See PDX Collection 1317

     ● **S75.019**   **Minor laceration of femoral artery, unspecified leg** A 🔖
        (Ex:) See PDX Collection 1318

   ● **S75.02**   **Major laceration of femoral artery**
     Complete transection of femoral artery
     Traumatic rupture of femoral artery

     ● **S75.021**   **Major laceration of femoral artery, right leg** A 🔖
        (Ex:) See PDX Collection 1316

     ● **S75.022**   **Major laceration of femoral artery, left leg** A 🔖
        (Ex:) See PDX Collection 1317

     ● **S75.029**   **Major laceration of femoral artery, unspecified leg** A 🔖
        (Ex:) See PDX Collection 1318

   ● **S75.09**   **Other specified injury of femoral artery**

     ● **S75.091**   **Other specified injury of femoral artery, right leg** A 🔖
        (Ex:) See PDX Collection 1316

     ● **S75.092**   **Other specified injury of femoral artery, left leg** A 🔖
        (Ex:) See PDX Collection 1317

     ● **S75.099**   **Other specified injury of femoral artery, unspecified leg** A 🔖
        (Ex:) See PDX Collection 1318

● **S75.1**   **Injury of femoral vein at hip and thigh level**

   ● **S75.10**   **Unspecified injury of femoral vein at hip and thigh level**

     ● **S75.101**   **Unspecified injury of femoral vein at hip and thigh level, right leg** A 🔖
        (Ex:) See PDX Collection 1319

     ● **S75.102**   **Unspecified injury of femoral vein at hip and thigh level, left leg** A 🔖
        (Ex:) See PDX Collection 1320

     ● **S75.109**   **Unspecified injury of femoral vein at hip and thigh level, unspecified leg** A 🔖
        (Ex:) See PDX Collection 1321

   ● **S75.11**   **Minor laceration of femoral vein at hip and thigh level**
     Incomplete transection of femoral vein at hip and thigh level
     Laceration of femoral vein at hip and thigh level NOS
     Superficial laceration of femoral vein at hip and thigh level

     ● **S75.111**   **Minor laceration of femoral vein at hip and thigh level, right leg** A 🔖
        (Ex:) See PDX Collection 1319

     ● **S75.112**   **Minor laceration of femoral vein at hip and thigh level, left leg** A 🔖
        (Ex:) See PDX Collection 1320

     ● **S75.119**   **Minor laceration of femoral vein at hip and thigh level, unspecified leg** A 🔖
        (Ex:) See PDX Collection 1321

   ● **S75.12**   **Major laceration of femoral vein at hip and thigh level**
     Complete transection of femoral vein at hip and thigh level
     Traumatic rupture of femoral vein at hip and thigh level

     ● **S75.121**   **Major laceration of femoral vein at hip and thigh level, right leg** A 🔖
        (Ex:) See PDX Collection 1319

     ● **S75.122**   **Major laceration of femoral vein at hip and thigh level, left leg** A 🔖
        (Ex:) See PDX Collection 1320

     ● **S75.129**   **Major laceration of femoral vein at hip and thigh level, unspecified leg** A 🔖
        (Ex:) See PDX Collection 1321

   ● **S75.19**   **Other specified injury of femoral vein at hip and thigh level**

     ● **S75.191**   **Other specified injury of femoral vein at hip and thigh level, right leg** A 🔖
        (Ex:) See PDX Collection 1319

     ● **S75.192**   **Other specified injury of femoral vein at hip and thigh level, left leg** A 🔖
        (Ex:) See PDX Collection 1320

     ● **S75.199**   **Other specified injury of femoral vein at hip and thigh level, unspecified leg** A 🔖
        (Ex:) See PDX Collection 1321

● **S75.2**   **Injury of greater saphenous vein at hip and thigh level**

Excludes1   greater saphenous vein NOS (S85.3)

   ● **S75.20**   **Unspecified injury of greater saphenous vein at hip and thigh level**

     ● **S75.201**   **Unspecified injury of greater saphenous vein at hip and thigh level, right leg** A 🔖
        (Ex:) See PDX Collection 1322

     ● **S75.202**   **Unspecified injury of greater saphenous vein at hip and thigh level, left leg** A 🔖
        (Ex:) See PDX Collection 1323

     ● **S75.209**   **Unspecified injury of greater saphenous vein at hip and thigh level, unspecified leg** A 🔖
        (Ex:) See PDX Collection 1324

▶ New   ⇒ Revised   ~~deleted~~ Deleted   Excludes 1   Excludes 2   Includes   Use additional   Code first   Code also   Key words
OGCR Official Guidelines   ● Unacceptable Principal Diagnosis   X Assign placeholder X   ● Use Additional Character(s)   ▌ Manifestation Code   **Coding Clinic**

● **S75.21**   Minor laceration of greater saphenous vein at hip and thigh level
    Incomplete transection of greater saphenous vein at hip and thigh level
    Laceration of greater saphenous vein at hip and thigh level NOS
    Superficial laceration of greater saphenous vein at hip and thigh level

   ● **S75.211**   Minor laceration of greater saphenous vein at hip and thigh level, right leg A 🍂
      (Ex:) See PDX Collection 1322

   ● **S75.212**   Minor laceration of greater saphenous vein at hip and thigh level, left leg A 🍂
      (Ex:) See PDX Collection 1323

   ● **S75.219**   Minor laceration of greater saphenous vein at hip and thigh level, unspecified leg A 🍂
      (Ex:) See PDX Collection 1324

● **S75.22**   Major laceration of greater saphenous vein at hip and thigh level
    Complete transection of greater saphenous vein at hip and thigh level
    Traumatic rupture of greater saphenous vein at hip and thigh level

   ● **S75.221**   Major laceration of greater saphenous vein at hip and thigh level, right leg A 🍂
      (Ex:) See PDX Collection 1322

   ● **S75.222**   Major laceration of greater saphenous vein at hip and thigh level, left leg A 🍂
      (Ex:) See PDX Collection 1323

   ● **S75.229**   Major laceration of greater saphenous vein at hip and thigh level, unspecified leg A 🍂
      (Ex:) See PDX Collection 1324

● **S75.29**   Other specified injury of greater saphenous vein at hip and thigh level

   ● **S75.291**   Other specified injury of greater saphenous vein at hip and thigh level, right leg A 🍂
      (Ex:) See PDX Collection 1322

   ● **S75.292**   Other specified injury of greater saphenous vein at hip and thigh level, left leg A 🍂
      (Ex:) See PDX Collection 1323

   ● **S75.299**   Other specified injury of greater saphenous vein at hip and thigh level, unspecified leg A 🍂
      (Ex:) See PDX Collection 1324

● **S75.8**   Injury of other blood vessels at hip and thigh level

  ● **S75.80**   Unspecified injury of other blood vessels at hip and thigh level

   ● **S75.801**   Unspecified injury of other blood vessels at hip and thigh level, right leg A 🍂
      (Ex:) See PDX Collection 1325

   ● **S75.802**   Unspecified injury of other blood vessels at hip and thigh level, left leg A 🍂
      (Ex:) See PDX Collection 1326

   ● **S75.809**   Unspecified injury of other blood vessels at hip and thigh level, unspecified leg A 🍂
      (Ex:) See PDX Collection 1327

● **S75.81**   Laceration of other blood vessels at hip and thigh level

   ● **S75.811**   Laceration of other blood vessels at hip and thigh level, right leg A 🍂
      (Ex:) See PDX Collection 1325

   ● **S75.812**   Laceration of other blood vessels at hip and thigh level, left leg A 🍂
      (Ex:) See PDX Collection 1326

   ● **S75.819**   Laceration of other blood vessels at hip and thigh level, unspecified leg A 🍂
      (Ex:) See PDX Collection 1327

● **S75.89**   Other specified injury of other blood vessels at hip and thigh level

   ● **S75.891**   Other specified injury of other blood vessels at hip and thigh level, right leg A 🍂
      (Ex:) See PDX Collection 1325

   ● **S75.892**   Other specified injury of other blood vessels at hip and thigh level, left leg A 🍂
      (Ex:) See PDX Collection 1326

   ● **S75.899**   Other specified injury of other blood vessels at hip and thigh level, unspecified leg A 🍂
      (Ex:) See PDX Collection 1327

● **S75.9**   Injury of unspecified blood vessel at hip and thigh level

  ● **S75.90**   Unspecified injury of unspecified blood vessel at hip and thigh level

   ● **S75.901**   Unspecified injury of unspecified blood vessel at hip and thigh level, right leg A 🍂
      (Ex:) See PDX Collection 1325

   ● **S75.902**   Unspecified injury of unspecified blood vessel at hip and thigh level, left leg A 🍂
      (Ex:) See PDX Collection 1326

   ● **S75.909**   Unspecified injury of unspecified blood vessel at hip and thigh level, unspecified leg A 🍂
      (Ex:) See PDX Collection 1327

  ● **S75.91**   Laceration of unspecified blood vessel at hip and thigh level

   ● **S75.911**   Laceration of unspecified blood vessel at hip and thigh level, right leg A 🍂
      (Ex:) See PDX Collection 1325

   ● **S75.912**   Laceration of unspecified blood vessel at hip and thigh level, left leg A 🍂
      (Ex:) See PDX Collection 1326

   ● **S75.919**   Laceration of unspecified blood vessel at hip and thigh level, unspecified leg A 🍂
      (Ex:) See PDX Collection 1327

  ● **S75.99**   Other specified injury of unspecified blood vessel at hip and thigh level

   ● **S75.991**   Other specified injury of unspecified blood vessel at hip and thigh level, right leg A 🍂
      (Ex:) See PDX Collection 1325

   ● **S75.992**   Other specified injury of unspecified blood vessel at hip and thigh level, left leg A 🍂
      (Ex:) See PDX Collection 1326

   ● **S75.999**   Other specified injury of unspecified blood vessel at hip and thigh level, unspecified leg A 🍂
      (Ex:) See PDX Collection 1327

N   Newborn Age: 0   P   Pediatric Age: 0–17   M   Maternity DX: 9–64   A   Adult Age: 15–124   ♀   Females Only   ♂   Males Only

🍂 Complication\Comorbidity   🍂 Major C\C   (Ex:) CC/MCC Exclusions   🍂 Hospital-Acquired Condition   🍂 Hierarchical Condition Category

1389

● **S76   Injury of muscle, fascia and tendon at hip and thigh level**

Code also any associated open wound (S71.-)

Excludes2   injury of muscle, fascia and tendon at lower leg level (S86)

sprain of joint and ligament of hip (S73.1)

The appropriate 7th character is to be added to each code from category S76

A	initial encounter
D	subsequent encounter
S	sequela

● **S76.0   Injury of muscle, fascia and tendon of hip**

● **S76.00   Unspecified injury of muscle, fascia and tendon of hip**

● S76.001   Unspecified injury of muscle, fascia and tendon of right hip

● S76.002   Unspecified injury of muscle, fascia and tendon of left hip

● S76.009   Unspecified injury of muscle, fascia and tendon of unspecified hip

● **S76.01   Strain of muscle, fascia and tendon of hip**

● S76.011   Strain of muscle, fascia and tendon of right hip

● S76.012   Strain of muscle, fascia and tendon of left hip

● S76.019   Strain of muscle, fascia and tendon of unspecified hip

● **S76.02   Laceration of muscle, fascia and tendon of hip**

● S76.021   Laceration of muscle, fascia and tendon of right hip A 🕲
Ex: See PDX Collection 1328

● S76.022   Laceration of muscle, fascia and tendon of left hip A 🕲
Ex: See PDX Collection 1329

● S76.029   Laceration of muscle, fascia and tendon of unspecified hip A 🕲
Ex: See PDX Collection 1330

● **S76.09   Other specified injury of muscle, fascia and tendon of hip**

● S76.091   Other specified injury of muscle, fascia and tendon of right hip

● S76.092   Other specified injury of muscle, fascia and tendon of left hip

● S76.099   Other specified injury of muscle, fascia and tendon of unspecified hip

● **S76.1   Injury of quadriceps muscle, fascia and tendon**
Injury of patellar ligament (tendon)

● **S76.10   Unspecified injury of quadriceps muscle, fascia and tendon**

● S76.101   Unspecified injury of right quadriceps muscle, fascia and tendon

● S76.102   Unspecified injury of left quadriceps muscle, fascia and tendon

● S76.109   Unspecified injury of unspecified quadriceps muscle, fascia and tendon

● **S76.11   Strain of quadriceps muscle, fascia and tendon**

● S76.111   Strain of right quadriceps muscle, fascia and tendon

● S76.112   Strain of left quadriceps muscle, fascia and tendon

● S76.119   Strain of unspecified quadriceps muscle, fascia and tendon

● **S76.12   Laceration of quadriceps muscle, fascia and tendon**

● S76.121   Laceration of right quadriceps muscle, fascia and tendon A 🕲
Ex: See PDX Collection 1328

● S76.122   Laceration of left quadriceps muscle, fascia and tendon A 🕲
Ex: See PDX Collection 1329

● S76.129   Laceration of unspecified quadriceps muscle, fascia and tendon A 🕲
Ex: See PDX Collection 1330

● **S76.19   Other specified injury of quadriceps muscle, fascia and tendon**

● S76.191   Other specified injury of right quadriceps muscle, fascia and tendon

● S76.192   Other specified injury of left quadriceps muscle, fascia and tendon

● S76.199   Other specified injury of unspecified quadriceps muscle, fascia and tendon

● **S76.2   Injury of adductor muscle, fascia and tendon of thigh**

● **S76.20   Unspecified injury of adductor muscle, fascia and tendon of thigh**

● S76.201   Unspecified injury of adductor muscle, fascia and tendon of right thigh

● S76.202   Unspecified injury of adductor muscle, fascia and tendon of left thigh

● S76.209   Unspecified injury of adductor muscle, fascia and tendon of unspecified thigh

● **S76.21   Strain of adductor muscle, fascia and tendon of thigh**

● S76.211   Strain of adductor muscle, fascia and tendon of right thigh

● S76.212   Strain of adductor muscle, fascia and tendon of left thigh

● S76.219   Strain of adductor muscle, fascia and tendon of unspecified thigh

● **S76.22   Laceration of adductor muscle, fascia and tendon of thigh**

● S76.221   Laceration of adductor muscle, fascia and tendon of right thigh A 🕲
Ex: See PDX Collection 1328

● S76.222   Laceration of adductor muscle, fascia and tendon of left thigh A 🕲
Ex: See PDX Collection 1329

● S76.229   Laceration of adductor muscle, fascia and tendon of unspecified thigh A 🕲
Ex: See PDX Collection 1330

● **S76.29   Other injury of adductor muscle, fascia and tendon of thigh**

● S76.291   Other injury of adductor muscle, fascia and tendon of right thigh

● S76.292   Other injury of adductor muscle, fascia and tendon of left thigh

● S76.299   Other injury of adductor muscle, fascia and tendon of unspecified thigh

▶ New   ⠿ Revised   ~~deleted~~ Deleted   Excludes 1   Excludes 2   Includes   Use additional   Code first   Code also   Key words

OGCR Official Guidelines   ● Unacceptable Principal Diagnosis   X Assign placeholder X   ● Use Additional Character(s)   ▶ Manifestation Code   Coding Clinic

● S76.3   Injury of muscle, fascia and tendon of the posterior muscle group at thigh level

    ● S76.30   Unspecified injury of muscle, fascia and tendon of the posterior muscle group at thigh level

      ● S76.301   Unspecified injury of muscle, fascia and tendon of the posterior muscle group at thigh level, right thigh

      ● S76.302   Unspecified injury of muscle, fascia and tendon of the posterior muscle group at thigh level, left thigh

      ● S76.309   Unspecified injury of muscle, fascia and tendon of the posterior muscle group at thigh level, unspecified thigh

    ● S76.31   Strain of muscle, fascia and tendon of the posterior muscle group at thigh level

      ● S76.311   Strain of muscle, fascia and tendon of the posterior muscle group at thigh level, right thigh

      ● S76.312   Strain of muscle, fascia and tendon of the posterior muscle group at thigh level, left thigh

      ● S76.319   Strain of muscle, fascia and tendon of the posterior muscle group at thigh level, unspecified thigh

    ● S76.32   Laceration of muscle, fascia and tendon of the posterior muscle group at thigh level

      ● S76.321   Laceration of muscle, fascia and tendon of the posterior muscle group at thigh level, right thigh A 🅒
         (Ex:) See PDX Collection 1328

      ● S76.322   Laceration of muscle, fascia and tendon of the posterior muscle group at thigh level, left thigh A 🅒
         (Ex:) See PDX Collection 1329

      ● S76.329   Laceration of muscle, fascia and tendon of the posterior muscle group at thigh level, unspecified thigh A 🅒
         (Ex:) See PDX Collection 1330

    ● S76.39   Other specified injury of muscle, fascia and tendon of the posterior muscle group at thigh level

      ● S76.391   Other specified injury of muscle, fascia and tendon of the posterior muscle group at thigh level, right thigh

      ● S76.392   Other specified injury of muscle, fascia and tendon of the posterior muscle group at thigh level, left thigh

      ● S76.399   Other specified injury of muscle, fascia and tendon of the posterior muscle group at thigh level, unspecified thigh

● S76.8   Injury of other specified muscles, fascia and tendons at thigh level

    ● S76.80   Unspecified injury of other specified muscles, fascia and tendons at thigh level

      ● S76.801   Unspecified injury of other specified muscles, fascia and tendons at thigh level, right thigh

      ● S76.802   Unspecified injury of other specified muscles, fascia and tendons at thigh level, left thigh

      ● S76.809   Unspecified injury of other specified muscles, fascia and tendons at thigh level, unspecified thigh

● S76.81   Strain of other specified specified muscles, fascia and tendons at thigh level

      ● S76.811   Strain of other specified muscles, fascia and tendons at thigh level, right thigh

      ● S76.812   Strain of other specified muscles, fascia and tendons at thigh level, left thigh

      ● S76.819   Strain of other specified muscles, fascia and tendons at thigh level, unspecified thigh

● S76.82   Laceration of other specified muscles, fascia and tendons at thigh level

      ● S76.821   Laceration of other specified muscles, fascia and tendons at thigh level, right thigh A 🅒
         (Ex:) See PDX Collection 1328

      ● S76.822   Laceration of other specified muscles, fascia and tendons at thigh level, left thigh A 🅒
         (Ex:) See PDX Collection 1329

      ● S76.829   Laceration of other specified muscles, fascia and tendons at thigh level, unspecified thigh A 🅒
         (Ex:) See PDX Collection 1330

● S76.89   Other injury of other specified muscles, fascia and tendons at thigh level

      ● S76.891   Other injury of other specified muscles, fascia and tendons at thigh level, right thigh

      ● S76.892   Other injury of other specified muscles, fascia and tendons at thigh level, left thigh

      ● S76.899   Other injury of other specified muscles, fascia and tendons at thigh level, unspecified thigh

● S76.9   Injury of unspecified muscles, fascia and tendons at thigh level

    ● S76.90   Unspecified injury of unspecified muscles, fascia and tendons at thigh level

      ● S76.901   Unspecified injury of unspecified muscles, fascia and tendons at thigh level, right thigh

      ● S76.902   Unspecified injury of unspecified muscles, fascia and tendons at thigh level, left thigh

      ● S76.909   Unspecified injury of unspecified muscles, fascia and tendons at thigh level, unspecified thigh

    ● S76.91   Strain of unspecified muscles, fascia and tendons at thigh level

      ● S76.911   Strain of unspecified muscles, fascia and tendons at thigh level, right thigh

      ● S76.912   Strain of unspecified muscles, fascia and tendons at thigh level, left thigh

      ● S76.919   Strain of unspecified muscles fascia and tendons at thigh level, unspecified thigh

    ● S76.92   Laceration of unspecified muscles, fascia and tendons at thigh level

      ● S76.921   Laceration of unspecified muscles, fascia and tendons at thigh level, right thigh A 🅒
         (Ex:) See PDX Collection 1328

      ● S76.922   Laceration of unspecified muscles, fascia and tendons at thigh level, left thigh A 🅒
         (Ex:) See PDX Collection 1329

      ● S76.929   Laceration of unspecified muscles, fascia and tendons at thigh level, unspecified thigh A 🅒
         (Ex:) See PDX Collection 1330

N Newborn Age: 0   **P** Pediatric Age: 0–17   **M** Maternity DX: 9–64   **A** Adult Age: 15–124   ♀ Females Only   ♂ Males Only

🅒 Complication\Comorbidity   🅒 Major C\C   (Ex:) CC/MCC Exclusions   🅒 Hospital-Acquired Condition   🅒 Hierarchical Condition Category

● S76.99   Other specified injury of unspecified muscles, fascia and tendons at thigh level

     ● S76.991   Other specified injury of unspecified muscles, fascia and tendons at thigh level, right thigh

     ● S76.992   Other specified injury of unspecified muscles, fascia and tendons at thigh level, left thigh

     ● S76.999   Other specified injury of unspecified muscles, fascia and tendons at thigh level, unspecified thigh

● **S77**   Crushing injury of hip and thigh

     Use additional code(s) for all associated injuries

     Excludes2   crushing injury of ankle and foot (S97.-)
                     crushing injury of lower leg (S87.-)

     The appropriate 7th character is to be added to each code from category S77

A	initial encounter
D	subsequent encounter
S	sequela

     ● **S77.0**   Crushing injury of hip

         (Ex:) For category S77.0 CC codes: See PDX Collection 1331

     X ● S77.00   Crushing injury of unspecified hip A 🜂, A 🜂

     X ● S77.01   Crushing injury of right hip A 🜂, A 🜂

     X ● S77.02   Crushing injury of left hip A 🜂, A 🜂

     ● **S77.1**   Crushing injury of thigh

         (Ex:) For category S77.1 CC codes: See PDX Collection 1332

     X ● S77.10   Crushing injury of unspecified thigh A 🜂, A 🜂

     X ● S77.11   Crushing injury of right thigh A 🜂, A 🜂

     X ● S77.12   Crushing injury of left thigh A 🜂, A 🜂

     ● **S77.2**   Crushing injury of hip with thigh

     X ● S77.20   Crushing injury of unspecified hip with thigh

     X ● S77.21   Crushing injury of right hip with thigh

     X ● S77.22   Crushing injury of left hip with thigh

● **S78**   Traumatic amputation of hip and thigh

     An amputation not identified as partial or complete should be coded to complete

     Excludes1   traumatic amputation of knee (S88.0-)

     The appropriate 7th character is to be added to each code from category S78

A	initial encounter
D	subsequent encounter
S	sequela

     ● **S78.0**   Traumatic amputation at hip joint

       ● S78.01   Complete traumatic amputation at hip joint

         ● S78.011   Complete traumatic amputation at right hip joint A 🜂, A, D, S 🜂
             (Ex:) See PDX Collection 1333

         ● S78.012   Complete traumatic amputation at left hip joint A 🜂, A, D, S 🜂
             (Ex:) See PDX Collection 1334

         ● S78.019   Complete traumatic amputation at unspecified hip joint A 🜂, A, D, S 🜂
             (Ex:) See PDX Collection 1335

       ● S78.02   Partial traumatic amputation at hip joint

         ● S78.021   Partial traumatic amputation at right hip joint A 🜂, A, D, S 🜂
             (Ex:) See PDX Collection 1333

         ● S78.022   Partial traumatic amputation at left hip joint A 🜂, A, D, S 🜂
             (Ex:) See PDX Collection 1334

         ● S78.029   Partial traumatic amputation at unspecified hip joint A 🜂, A, D, S 🜂
             (Ex:) See PDX Collection 1335

● S78.1   Traumatic amputation at level between hip and knee

     Excludes1   traumatic amputation of knee (S88.0-)

     ● S78.11   Complete traumatic amputation at level between hip and knee

       ● S78.111   Complete traumatic amputation at level between right hip and knee A 🜂, A, D, S 🜂
           (Ex:) See PDX Collection 1333

       ● S78.112   Complete traumatic amputation at level between left hip and knee A 🜂, A, D, S 🜂
           (Ex:) See PDX Collection 1334

       ● S78.119   Complete traumatic amputation at level between unspecified hip and knee A 🜂, A, D, S 🜂
           (Ex:) See PDX Collection 1335

     ● S78.12   Partial traumatic amputation at level between hip and knee

       ● S78.121   Partial traumatic amputation at level between right hip and knee A 🜂, A, D, S 🜂
           (Ex:) See PDX Collection 1333

       ● S78.122   Partial traumatic amputation at level between left hip and knee A 🜂, A, D, S 🜂
           (Ex:) See PDX Collection 1334

       ● S78.129   Partial traumatic amputation at level between unspecified hip and knee A 🜂, A, D, S 🜂
           (Ex:) See PDX Collection 1335

● S78.9   Traumatic amputation of hip and thigh, level unspecified

     ● S78.91   Complete traumatic amputation of hip and thigh, level unspecified

       ● S78.911   Complete traumatic amputation of right hip and thigh, level unspecified A 🜂, A, D, S 🜂
           (Ex:) See PDX Collection 1333

       ● S78.912   Complete traumatic amputation of left hip and thigh, level unspecified A 🜂, A, D, S 🜂
           (Ex:) See PDX Collection 1334

       ● S78.919   Complete traumatic amputation of unspecified hip and thigh, level unspecified A 🜂, A, D, S 🜂
           (Ex:) See PDX Collection 1335

     ● S78.92   Partial traumatic amputation of hip and thigh, level unspecified

       ● S78.921   Partial traumatic amputation of right hip and thigh, level unspecified A 🜂, A, D, S 🜂
           (Ex:) See PDX Collection 1333

       ● S78.922   Partial traumatic amputation of left hip and thigh, level unspecified A 🜂, A, D, S 🜂
           (Ex:) See PDX Collection 1334

       ● S78.929   Partial traumatic amputation of unspecified hip and thigh, level unspecified A 🜂, A, D, S 🜂
           (Ex:) See PDX Collection 1335

▶ New   ⇒ Revised   ~~deleted~~ Deleted   Excludes 1   Excludes 2   Includes   Use additional   Code first   Code also   Key words

OGCR Official Guidelines   ● Unacceptable Principal Diagnosis   X Assign placeholder X   ● Use Additional Character(s)   ▷ Manifestation Code   **Coding Clinic**

● **S79   Other and unspecified injuries of hip and thigh**

Note: A fracture not indicated as open or closed should be coded to closed

The appropriate 7th character is to be added to each code from subcategories S79.0 and S79.1

> A   initial encounter for closed fracture
> D   subsequent encounter for fracture with routine healing
> G   subsequent encounter for fracture with delayed healing
> K   subsequent encounter for fracture with nonunion
> P   subsequent encounter for fracture with malunion
> S   sequela

● **S79.0   Physeal fracture of upper end of femur**

Excludes1   apophyseal fracture of upper end of femur (S72.13-)
nontraumatic slipped upper femoral epiphysis (M93.0-)

● **S79.00   Unspecified physeal fracture of upper end of femur**

● **S79.001   Unspecified physeal fracture of upper end of right femur** K, P 🔹, A 🔹, A 🔹, A 🔹

(Ex:) **For S79.001[A]:** See PDX Collection 1297
For S79.001[K,P]: See PDX Collection 897

● **S79.002   Unspecified physeal fracture of upper end of left femur** K, P 🔹, A 🔹, A 🔹, A 🔹

(Ex:) **For S79.002[A]:** See PDX Collection 1299
For S79.002[K,P]: See PDX Collection 897

● **S79.009   Unspecified physeal fracture of upper end of unspecified femur** K, P 🔹, A 🔹, A 🔹, A 🔹

(Ex:) **For S79.009[A]:** See PDX Collection 1298
For S79.009[K,P]: See PDX Collection 897

● **S79.01   Salter-Harris Type I physeal fracture of upper end of femur**

Acute on chronic slipped capital femoral epiphysis (traumatic)
Acute slipped capital femoral epiphysis (traumatic)
Capital femoral epiphyseal fracture

Excludes1   chronic slipped upper femoral epiphysis (nontraumatic) (M93.02-)

● **S79.011   Salter-Harris Type I physeal fracture of upper end of right femur** K, P 🔹, A 🔹, A 🔹, A 🔹

(Ex:) **For S79.011[A]:** See PDX Collection 1297
For S79.011[K,P]: See PDX Collection 897

● **S79.012   Salter-Harris Type I physeal fracture of upper end of left femur** K, P 🔹, A 🔹, A 🔹, A 🔹

(Ex:) **For S79.012[A]:** See PDX Collection 1299
For S79.012[K,P]: See PDX Collection 897

● **S79.019   Salter-Harris Type I physeal fracture of upper end of unspecified femur** K, P 🔹, A 🔹, A 🔹, A 🔹

(Ex:) **For S79.019[A]:** See PDX Collection 1298
For S79.019[K,P]: See PDX Collection 897

● **S79.09   Other physeal fracture of upper end of femur**

● **S79.091   Other physeal fracture of upper end of right femur** K, P 🔹, A 🔹, A 🔹, A 🔹

(Ex:) **For S79.091[A]:** See PDX Collection 1297
For S79.091[K,P]: See PDX Collection 897

● **S79.092   Other physeal fracture of upper end of left femur** K, P 🔹, A 🔹, A 🔹, A 🔹

(Ex:) **For S79.092[A]:** See PDX Collection 1299
For S79.092[K,P]: See PDX Collection 897

● **S79.099   Other physeal fracture of upper end of unspecified femur** K, P 🔹, A 🔹, A 🔹, A 🔹

(Ex:) **For S79.099[A]:** See PDX Collection 1298
For S79.099[K,P]: See PDX Collection 897

● **S79.1   Physeal fracture of lower end of femur**

● **S79.10   Unspecified physeal fracture of lower end of femur**

● **S79.101   Unspecified physeal fracture of lower end of right femur** A, K, P 🔹, A 🔹, A 🔹

(Ex:) **For S79.101[A]:** See PDX Collection 1300
For S79.101[K,P]: See PDX Collection 897

● **S79.102   Unspecified physeal fracture of lower end of left femur** A, K, P 🔹, A 🔹, A 🔹

(Ex:) **For S79.102[A]:** See PDX Collection 1302
For S72.102[K,P]: See PDX Collection 897

● **S79.109   Unspecified physeal fracture of lower end of unspecified femur** A, K, P 🔹, A 🔹, A 🔹

(Ex:) **For S79.109[A]:** See PDX Collection 1301
For S79.109[K,P]: See PDX Collection 897

● **S79.11   Salter-Harris Type I physeal fracture of lower end of femur**

● **S79.111   Salter-Harris Type I physeal fracture of lower end of right femur** A, K, P 🔹, A 🔹, A 🔹

(Ex:) **For S79.111[A]:** See PDX Collection 1300
For S79.111[K,P]: See PDX Collection 897

● **S79.112   Salter-Harris Type I physeal fracture of lower end of left femur** A, K, P 🔹, A 🔹, A 🔹

(Ex:) **For S79.112[A]:** See PDX Collection 1302
For S72.112[K,P]: See PDX Collection 897

● **S79.119   Salter-Harris Type I physeal fracture of lower end of unspecified femur** A, K, P 🔹, A 🔹, A 🔹

(Ex:) **For S79.119[A]:** See PDX Collection 1301
For S79.119[K,P]: See PDX Collection 897

● **S79.12   Salter-Harris Type II physeal fracture of lower end of femur**

● **S79.121   Salter-Harris Type II physeal fracture of lower end of right femur** A, K, P 🔹, A 🔹, A 🔹

(Ex:) **For S79.121[A]:** See PDX Collection 1300
For S79.121[K,P]: See PDX Collection 897

● **S79.122   Salter-Harris Type II physeal fracture of lower end of left femur** A, K, P 🔹, A 🔹, A 🔹

(Ex:) **For S79.122[A]:** See PDX Collection 1302
For S72.122[K,P]: See PDX Collection 897

● **S79.129   Salter-Harris Type II physeal fracture of lower end of unspecified femur** A, K, P 🔹, A 🔹, A 🔹

(Ex:) **For S79.129[A]:** See PDX Collection 1301
For S79.129[K,P]: See PDX Collection 897

Item 19–5   SALTER-HARRIS TYPE 1: epiphysis is completely separated from end of bone, or metaphysic growth plate remains attached to epiphysis

SALTER-HARRIS TYPE 2: epiphysis and growth plate are partially separated from metaphysis, which is cracked—most common type

SALTER-HARRIS TYPE 3: fracture occurring through epiphysis and separates part of epiphysis and growth plate from metaphysis fracture, usually at distal end of tibia

SALTER-HARRIS TYPE 4: fracture runs through epiphysis, across growth plate, into metaphysic; surgery is required to restore joint surface to normal and align growth plate

CHAPTER 19 (S00-T88)

N Newborn Age: 0   P Pediatric Age: 0–17   M Maternity DX: 9–64   A Adult Age: 15–124   ♀ Females Only   ♂ Males Only

🔹 Complication\Comorbidity   🔹 Major C\C   (Ex:) CC/MCC Exclusions   🔹 Hospital-Acquired Condition   🔹 Hierarchical Condition Category

● S79.13   Salter-Harris Type III physeal fracture of lower
           end of femur
    ● S79.131   Salter-Harris Type III physeal fracture
               of lower end of right femur A, K, P 🅒,
               A 🅒, A 🅒
               (Ex:) For S79.131[A]: See PDX Collection 1300
                     For S79.131[K,P]: See PDX Collection 897
    ● S79.132   Salter-Harris Type III physeal fracture
               of lower end of left femur A, K, P 🅒,
               A 🅒, A 🅒
               (Ex:) For S79.132[A]: See PDX Collection 1302
                     For S72.132[K,P]: See PDX Collection 897
    ● S79.139   Salter-Harris Type III physeal fracture
               of lower end of unspecified femur
               A, K, P 🅒, A 🅒, A 🅒
               (Ex:) For S79.139[A]: See PDX Collection 1301
                     For S79.139[K,P]: See PDX Collection 897
● S79.14   Salter-Harris Type IV physeal fracture of lower
           end of femur
    ● S79.141   Salter-Harris Type IV physeal fracture
               of lower end of right femur A, K, P 🅒,
               A 🅒, A 🅒
               (Ex:) For S79.141[A]: See PDX Collection 1300
                     For S79.141[K,P]: See PDX Collection 897
    ● S79.142   Salter-Harris Type IV physeal fracture
               of lower end of left femur A, K, P 🅒,
               A 🅒, A 🅒
               (Ex:) For S79.142[A]: See PDX Collection 1302
                     For S72.142[K,P]: See PDX Collection 897
    ● S79.149   Salter-Harris Type IV physeal fracture
               of lower end of unspecified femur
               A, K, P 🅒, A 🅒, A 🅒
               (Ex:) For S79.149[A]: See PDX Collection 1301
                     For S79.149[K,P]: See PDX Collection 897
● S79.19   Other physeal fracture of lower end of femur
    ● S79.191   Other physeal fracture of lower end
               of right femur A, K, P 🅒, A 🅒, A 🅒
               (Ex:) For S79.191[A]: See PDX Collection 1300
                     For S79.191[K,P]: See PDX Collection 897
    ● S79.192   Other physeal fracture of lower end
               of left femur A, K, P 🅒, A 🅒, A 🅒
               (Ex:) For S79.192[A]: See PDX Collection 1302
                     For S72.192[K,P]: See PDX Collection 897
    ● S79.199   Other physeal fracture of lower end
               of unspecified femur A, K, P 🅒, A 🅒,
               A 🅒
               (Ex:) For S79.199[A]: See PDX Collection 1301
                     For S79.199[K,P]: See PDX Collection 897

● S79.8   Other specified injuries of hip and thigh
          The appropriate 7th character is to be added to each
          code in subcategory S79.8

          | A | initial encounter |
          | D | subsequent encounter |
          | S | sequela |

    ● S79.81   Other specified injuries of hip
        ● S79.811   Other specified injuries of right hip
        ● S79.812   Other specified injuries of left hip
        ● S79.819   Other specified injuries of
                    unspecified hip
    ● S79.82   Other specified injuries of thigh
        ● S79.821   Other specified injuries of right thigh
        ● S79.822   Other specified injuries of left thigh
        ● S79.829   Other specified injuries of
                    unspecified thigh

● S79.9   Unspecified injury of hip and thigh
          The appropriate 7th character is to be added to each
          code in subcategory S79.9

          | A | initial encounter |
          | D | subsequent encounter |
          | S | sequela |

    ● S79.91   Unspecified injury of hip
        ● S79.911   Unspecified injury of right hip
        ● S79.912   Unspecified injury of left hip
        ● S79.919   Unspecified injury of unspecified hip
    ● S79.92   Unspecified injury of thigh
        ● S79.921   Unspecified injury of right thigh
        ● S79.922   Unspecified injury of left thigh
        ● S79.929   Unspecified injury of unspecified
                    thigh

INJURIES TO THE KNEE AND LOWER LEG (S80-S89)

Excludes2   burns and corrosions (T20-T32)
               frostbite (T33-T34)
               injuries of ankle and foot, except fracture of ankle
                  and malleolus (S90-S99)
               insect bite or sting, venomous (T63.4)

● S80   Superficial injury of knee and lower leg
        Excludes2   superficial injury of ankle and foot (S90.-)
        The appropriate 7th character is to be added to each code from
        category S80

        | A | initial encounter |
        | D | subsequent encounter |
        | S | sequela |

    ● S80.0   Contusion of knee
        X ● S80.00   Contusion of unspecified knee
        X ● S80.01   Contusion of right knee
        X ● S80.02   Contusion of left knee
    ● S80.1   Contusion of lower leg
        X ● S80.10   Contusion of unspecified lower leg
        X ● S80.11   Contusion of right lower leg
        X ● S80.12   Contusion of left lower leg
    ● S80.2   Other superficial injuries of knee
        ● S80.21   Abrasion of knee
            ● S80.211   Abrasion, right knee
            ● S80.212   Abrasion, left knee
            ● S80.219   Abrasion, unspecified knee
        ● S80.22   Blister (nonthermal) of knee
            ● S80.221   Blister (nonthermal), right knee
            ● S80.222   Blister (nonthermal), left knee
            ● S80.229   Blister (nonthermal), unspecified
                        knee
        ● S80.24   External constriction of knee
            ● S80.241   External constriction, right knee
            ● S80.242   External constriction, left knee
            ● S80.249   External constriction, unspecified
                        knee
        ● S80.25   Superficial foreign body of knee
                   Splinter in the knee
            ● S80.251   Superficial foreign body, right knee
            ● S80.252   Superficial foreign body, left knee
            ● S80.259   Superficial foreign body, unspecified
                        knee

▶ New   ⇒ Revised   ~~deleted~~ Deleted   Excludes 1   Excludes 2   Includes   Use additional   Code first   Code also   Key words
OGCR Official Guidelines   ● Unacceptable Principal Diagnosis   X Assign placeholder X   ● Use Additional Character(s)   ▌ Manifestation Code   Coding Clinic

● S80.26   Insect bite (nonvenomous) of knee
  ● S80.261   Insect bite (nonvenomous), right knee
  ● S80.262   Insect bite (nonvenomous), left knee
  ● S80.269   Insect bite (nonvenomous), unspecified knee
● S80.27   Other superficial bite of knee
    Excludes1   open bite of knee (S81.05-)
  ● S80.271   Other superficial bite of right knee
  ● S80.272   Other superficial bite of left knee
  ● S80.279   Other superficial bite of unspecified knee

● S80.8   Other superficial injuries of lower leg
  ● S80.81   Abrasion of lower leg
    ● S80.811   Abrasion, right lower leg
    ● S80.812   Abrasion, left lower leg
    ● S80.819   Abrasion, unspecified lower leg
  ● S80.82   Blister (nonthermal) of lower leg
    ● S80.821   Blister (nonthermal), right lower leg
    ● S80.822   Blister (nonthermal), left lower leg
    ● S80.829   Blister (nonthermal), unspecified lower leg
  ● S80.84   External constriction of lower leg
    ● S80.841   External constriction, right lower leg
    ● S80.842   External constriction, left lower leg
    ● S80.849   External constriction, unspecified lower leg
  ● S80.85   Superficial foreign body of lower leg
    Splinter in the lower leg
    ● S80.851   Superficial foreign body, right lower leg
    ● S80.852   Superficial foreign body, left lower leg
    ● S80.859   Superficial foreign body, unspecified lower leg
  ● S80.86   Insect bite (nonvenomous) of lower leg
    ● S80.861   Insect bite (nonvenomous), right lower leg
    ● S80.862   Insect bite (nonvenomous), left lower leg
    ● S80.869   Insect bite (nonvenomous), unspecified lower leg
  ● S80.87   Other superficial bite of lower leg
    Excludes1   open bite of lower leg (S81.85-)
    ● S80.871   Other superficial bite, right lower leg
    ● S80.872   Other superficial bite, left lower leg
    ● S80.879   Other superficial bite, unspecified lower leg

● S80.9   Unspecified superficial injury of knee and lower leg
  ● S80.91   Unspecified superficial injury of knee
    ● S80.911   Unspecified superficial injury of right knee
    ● S80.912   Unspecified superficial injury of left knee
    ● S80.919   Unspecified superficial injury of unspecified knee

  ● S80.92   Unspecified superficial injury of lower leg
    ● S80.921   Unspecified superficial injury of right lower leg
    ● S80.922   Unspecified superficial injury of left lower leg
    ● S80.929   Unspecified superficial injury of unspecified lower leg

● S81   Open wound of knee and lower leg
  Code also any associated wound infection
  Excludes1   open fracture of knee and lower leg (S82.-)
           traumatic amputation of lower leg (S88.-)
  Excludes2   open wound of ankle and foot (S91.-)
  The appropriate 7th character is to be added to each code from category S81

A	initial encounter
D	subsequent encounter
S	sequela

● S81.0   Open wound of knee
  ● S81.00   Unspecified open wound of knee
    ● S81.001   Unspecified open wound, right knee
    ● S81.002   Unspecified open wound, left knee
    ● S81.009   Unspecified open wound, unspecified knee
  ● S81.01   Laceration without foreign body of knee
    ● S81.011   Laceration without foreign body, right knee
    ● S81.012   Laceration without foreign body, left knee
    ● S81.019   Laceration without foreign body, unspecified knee
  ● S81.02   Laceration with foreign body of knee
    ● S81.021   Laceration with foreign body, right knee
    ● S81.022   Laceration with foreign body, left knee
    ● S81.029   Laceration with foreign body, unspecified knee
  ● S81.03   Puncture wound without foreign body of knee
    ● S81.031   Puncture wound without foreign body, right knee
    ● S81.032   Puncture wound without foreign body, left knee
    ● S81.039   Puncture wound without foreign body, unspecified knee
  ● S81.04   Puncture wound with foreign body of knee
    ● S81.041   Puncture wound with foreign body, right knee
    ● S81.042   Puncture wound with foreign body, left knee
    ● S81.049   Puncture wound with foreign body, unspecified knee

CHAPTER 19 (S00-T88)

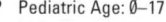

● S81.05   **Open bite of knee**
           Bite of knee NOS
           Excludes1   superficial bite of knee (S80.27-)

   ● S81.051   Open bite, **right** knee
   ● S81.052   Open bite, **left** knee
   ● S81.059   Open bite, **unspecified** knee

● S81.8   Open wound of lower leg
  ● S81.80   **Unspecified** open wound of lower leg
   ● S81.801   Unspecified open wound, **right** lower leg
   ● S81.802   Unspecified open wound, **left** lower leg
   ● S81.809   Unspecified open wound, **unspecified** lower leg

  ● S81.81   Laceration without foreign body of lower leg
   ● S81.811   Laceration without foreign body, **right** lower leg
   ● S81.812   Laceration without foreign body, **left** lower leg
   ● S81.819   Laceration without foreign body, **unspecified** lower leg

  ● S81.82   Laceration with foreign body of lower leg
   ● S81.821   Laceration with foreign body, **right** lower leg
   ● S81.822   Laceration with foreign body, **left** lower leg
   ● S81.829   Laceration with foreign body, **unspecified** lower leg

  ● S81.83   Puncture wound without foreign body of lower leg
   ● S81.831   Puncture wound without foreign body, **right** lower leg
   ● S81.832   Puncture wound without foreign body, **left** lower leg
   ● S81.839   Puncture wound without foreign body, **unspecified** lower leg

  ● S81.84   Puncture wound with foreign body of lower leg
   ● S81.841   Puncture wound with foreign body, **right** lower leg
    Coding Clinic: 2016, Q3, P46
   ● S81.842   Puncture wound with foreign body, **left** lower leg
   ● S81.849   Puncture wound with foreign body, **unspecified** lower leg

  ● S81.85   **Open bite of lower leg**
   Bite of lower leg NOS
   Excludes1   superficial bite of lower leg (S80.86-, S80.87-)

   ● S81.851   Open bite, **right** lower leg
   ● S81.852   Open bite, **left** lower leg
   ● S81.859   Open bite, **unspecified** lower leg

● S82   **Fracture of lower leg, including ankle**
  Note: A fracture not indicated as displaced or nondisplaced should be coded to displaced

  A fracture not indicated as open or closed should be coded to closed

  The open fracture designations are based on the Gustilo open fracture classification

  Includes   fracture of malleolus
  Excludes1   traumatic amputation of lower leg (S88.-)
  Excludes2   fracture of foot, except ankle (S92.-)
  ⟹ periprosthetic fracture around internal of prosthetic implant of knee joint (M97.1-)

The appropriate 7th character is to be added to all codes from category S82

A	initial encounter for closed fracture
B	initial encounter for open fracture type I or II initial encounter for open fracture NOS
C	initial encounter for open fracture type IIIA, IIIB, or IIIC
D	subsequent encounter for closed fracture with routine healing
E	subsequent encounter for open fracture type I or II with routine healing
F	subsequent encounter for open fracture type IIIA, IIIB, or IIIC with routine healing
G	subsequent encounter for closed fracture with delayed healing
H	subsequent encounter for open fracture type I or II with delayed healing
J	subsequent encounter for open fracture type IIIA, IIIB, or IIIC with delayed healing
K	subsequent encounter for closed fracture with nonunion
M	subsequent encounter for open fracture type I or II with nonunion
N	subsequent encounter for open fracture type IIIA, IIIB, or IIIC with nonunion
P	subsequent encounter for closed fracture with malunion
Q	subsequent encounter for open fracture type I or II with malunion
R	subsequent encounter for open fracture type IIIA, IIIB, or IIIC with malunion
S	sequela

● S82.0   **Fracture of patella**
  Knee cap
  ● S82.00   **Unspecified** fracture of patella
   ● S82.001   Unspecified fracture of **right** patella
    A, B, C,K,M, N, P, Q, R 🔄, A, B, C 🔄
    Ⓔ **For S82.001[A]:** See PDX Collection 1336
    For S82.001[B,C]: See PDX Collection 1337
    For S82.001[K,M,N,P,Q,R]: See PDX Collection 897

   ● S82.002   Unspecified fracture of **left** patella
    A, B, C,K,M, N, P, Q, R 🔄, A, B, C 🔄
    Ⓔ **For S82.002[A]:** See PDX Collection 1338
    For S82.002[B,C]: See PDX Collection 1337
    For S82.002[K,M,N,P,Q,R]: See PDX Collection 897

   ● S82.009   Unspecified fracture of **unspecified** patella A, B, C,K,M, N, P, Q, R 🔄, A, B, C 🔄
    Ⓔ **For S82.009[A]:** See PDX Collection 1339
    For S82.009[B,C]: See PDX Collection 1337
    For S82.009[K,M,N,P,Q,R]: See PDX Collection 897

▶ New   ⟹ Revised   ~~deleted~~ Deleted   **Excludes 1**   **Excludes 2**   **Includes**   **Use additional**   **Code first**   **Code also**   **Key words**
OGCR Official Guidelines   ● Unacceptable Principal Diagnosis   **X** Assign placeholder X   ● Use Additional Character(s)   ▶ Manifestation Code   **Coding Clinic**

● **S82.01**   Osteochondral fracture of patella
   ● **S82.011**   Displaced osteochondral fracture of right patella A, B, C,K,M, N, P, Q, R 🝊, A, B, C 🝊
     (Ex:) **For S82.011[A]:** See PDX Collection 1336
         For S82.011[B,C]: See PDX Collection 1337
         For S82.011[K,M,N,P,Q,R]: See PDX Collection 897

   ● **S82.012**   Displaced osteochondral fracture of left patella A, B, C,K,M, N, P, Q, R 🝊, A, B, C 🝊
     (Ex:) **For S82.012[A]:** See PDX Collection 1338
         For S82.012[B,C]: See PDX Collection 1337
         For S82.012[K,M,N,P,Q,R]: See PDX Collection 897

   ● **S82.013**   Displaced osteochondral fracture of unspecified patella A, B, C,K,M, N, P, Q, R 🝊, A, B, C 🝊
     (Ex:) **For S82.013[A]:** See PDX Collection 1339
         For S82.013[B,C]: See PDX Collection 1337
         For S82.013[K,M,N,P,Q,R]: See PDX Collection 897

   ● **S82.014**   Nondisplaced osteochondral fracture of right patella A, B, C,K,M, N, P, Q, R 🝊, A, B, C 🝊
     (Ex:) **For S82.014[A]:** See PDX Collection 1336
         For S82.014[B,C]: See PDX Collection 1337
         For S82.014[K,M,N,P,Q,R]: See PDX Collection 897

   ● **S82.015**   Nondisplaced osteochondral fracture of left patella A, B, C,K,M, N, P, Q, R 🝊, A, B, C 🝊
     (Ex:) **For S82.015[A]:** See PDX Collection 1338
         For S82.015[B,C]: See PDX Collection 1337
         For S82.015[K,M,N,P,Q,R]: See PDX Collection 897

   ● **S82.016**   Nondisplaced osteochondral fracture of unspecified patella A, B, C,K,M, N, P, Q, R 🝊, A, B, C 🝊
     (Ex:) **For S82.016[A]:** See PDX Collection 1339
         For S82.016[B,C]: See PDX Collection 1337
         For S82.016[K,M,N,P,Q,R]: See PDX Collection 897

● **S82.02**   Longitudinal fracture of patella
   ● **S82.021**   Displaced longitudinal fracture of right patella A, B, C,K,M, N, P, Q, R 🝊, A, B, C 🝊
     (Ex:) **For S82.021[A]:** See PDX Collection 1336
         For S82.021[B,C]: See PDX Collection 1337
         For S82.021[K,M,N,P,Q,R]: See PDX Collection 897

   ● **S82.022**   Displaced longitudinal fracture of left patella A, B, C,K,M, N, P, Q, R 🝊, A, B, C 🝊
     (Ex:) **For S82.022[A]:** See PDX Collection 1338
         For S82.022[B,C]: See PDX Collection 1337
         For S82.022[K,M,N,P,Q,R]: See PDX Collection 897

   ● **S82.023**   Displaced longitudinal fracture of unspecified patella A, B, C,K,M, N, P, Q, R 🝊, A, B, C 🝊
     (Ex:) **For S82.023[A]:** See PDX Collection 1339
         For S82.023[B,C]: See PDX Collection 1337
         For S82.023[K,M,N,P,Q,R]: See PDX Collection 897

   ● **S82.024**   Nondisplaced longitudinal fracture of right patella A, B, C,K,M, N, P, Q, R 🝊, A, B, C 🝊
     (Ex:) **For S82.024[A]:** See PDX Collection 1336
         For S82.024[B,C]: See PDX Collection 1337
         For S82.024[K,M,N,P,Q,R]: See PDX Collection 897

   ● **S82.025**   Nondisplaced longitudinal fracture of left patella A, B, C,K,M, N, P, Q, R 🝊, A, B, C 🝊
     (Ex:) **For S82.025[A]:** See PDX Collection 1338
         For S82.025[B,C]: See PDX Collection 1337
         For S82.025[K,M,N,P,Q,R]: See PDX Collection 897

   ● **S82.026**   Nondisplaced longitudinal fracture of unspecified patella A, B, C,K,M, N, P, Q, R 🝊, A, B, C 🝊
     (Ex:) **For S82.026[A]:** See PDX Collection 1339
         For S82.026[B,C]: See PDX Collection 1337
         For S82.026[K,M,N,P,Q,R]: See PDX Collection 897

● **S82.03**   Transverse fracture of patella
   ● **S82.031**   Displaced transverse fracture of right patella A, B, C,K,M, N, P, Q, R 🝊, A, B, C 🝊
     (Ex:) **For S82.031[A]:** See PDX Collection 1336
         For S82.031[B,C]: See PDX Collection 1337
         For S82.031[K,M,N,P,Q,R]: See PDX Collection 897

   ● **S82.032**   Displaced transverse fracture of left patella A, B, C,K,M, N, P, Q, R 🝊, A, B, C 🝊
     (Ex:) **For S82.032[A]:** See PDX Collection 1338
         For S82.032[B,C]: See PDX Collection 1337
         For S82.032[K,M,N,P,Q,R]: See PDX Collection 897

   ● **S82.033**   Displaced transverse fracture of unspecified patella A, B, C,K,M, N, P, Q, R 🝊, A, B, C 🝊
     (Ex:) **For S82.033[A]:** See PDX Collection 1339
         For S82.033[B,C]: See PDX Collection 1337
         For S82.033[K,M,N,P,Q,R]: See PDX Collection 897

   ● **S82.034**   Nondisplaced transverse fracture of right patella A, B, C,K,M, N, P, Q, R 🝊, A, B, C 🝊
     (Ex:) **For S82.034[A]:** See PDX Collection 1336
         For S82.034[B,C]: See PDX Collection 1337
         For S82.034[K,M,N,P,Q,R]: See PDX Collection 897

   ● **S82.035**   Nondisplaced transverse fracture of left patella A, B, C,K,M, N, P, Q, R 🝊, A, B, C 🝊
     (Ex:) **For S82.035[A]:** See PDX Collection 1338
         For S82.035[B,C]: See PDX Collection 1337
         For S82.035[K,M,N,P,Q,R]: See PDX Collection 897

   ● **S82.036**   Nondisplaced transverse fracture of unspecified patella A, B, C,K,M, N, P, Q, R 🝊, A, B, C 🝊
     (Ex:) **For S82.036[A]:** See PDX Collection 1339
         For S82.036[B,C]: See PDX Collection 1337
         For S82.036[K,M,N,P,Q,R]: See PDX Collection 897

N Newborn Age: 0   **P** Pediatric Age: 0–17   **M** Maternity DX: 9–64   **A** Adult Age: 15–124   ♀ Females Only   ♂ Males Only
🝊 Complication\Comorbidity   🝊 Major C\C   (Ex:) CC/MCC Exclusions   🝊 Hospital-Acquired Condition   🝊 Hierarchical Condition Category

CHAPTER 19 (S00–T88)

1397

● **S82.04**   Comminuted fracture of patella

   ● **S82.041**   Displaced comminuted fracture of right patella A, B, C,K,M, N, P, Q, R 🔍, A, B, C 🔍

     Ex: **For S82.041[A]:** See PDX Collection 1336
     For S82.041[B,C]: See PDX Collection 1337
     For S82.041[K,M,N,P,Q,R]: See PDX Collection 897

   ● **S82.042**   Displaced comminuted fracture of left patella A, B, C,K,M, N, P, Q, R 🔍, A, B, C 🔍

     Ex: **For S82.042[A]:** See PDX Collection 1338
     For S82.042[B,C]: See PDX Collection 1337
     For S82.042[K,M,N,P,Q,R]: See PDX Collection 897

   ● **S82.043**   Displaced comminuted fracture of unspecified patella A, B, C,K,M, N, P, Q, R 🔍, A, B, C 🔍

     Ex: **For S82.043[A]:** See PDX Collection 1339
     For S82.043[B,C]: See PDX Collection 1337
     For S82.043[K,M,N,P,Q,R]: See PDX Collection 897

   ● **S82.044**   Nondisplaced comminuted fracture of right patella A, B, C,K,M, N, P, Q, R 🔍, A, B, C 🔍

     Ex: **For S82.044[A]:** See PDX Collection 1336
     For S82.044[B,C]: See PDX Collection 1337
     For S82.044[K,M,N,P,Q,R]: See PDX Collection 897

   ● **S82.045**   Nondisplaced comminuted fracture of left patella A, B, C,K,M, N, P, Q, R 🔍, A, B, C 🔍

     Ex: **For S82.045[A]:** See PDX Collection 1338
     For S82.045[B,C]: See PDX Collection 1337
     For S82.045[K,M,N,P,Q,R]: See PDX Collection 897

   ● **S82.046**   Nondisplaced comminuted fracture of unspecified patella A, B, C,K,M, N, P, Q, R 🔍, A, B, C 🔍

     Ex: **For S82.046[A]:** See PDX Collection 1339
     For S82.046[B,C]: See PDX Collection 1337
     For S82.046[K,M,N,P,Q,R]: See PDX Collection 897

● **S82.09**   Other fracture of patella

   ● **S82.091**   Other fracture of right patella A, B, C,K,M, N, P, Q, R 🔍, A, B, C 🔍

     Ex: **For S82.091[A]:** See PDX Collection 1336
     For S82.091[B,C]: See PDX Collection 1337
     For S82.091[K,M,N,P,Q,R]: See PDX Collection 897

   ● **S82.092**   Other fracture of left patella A, B, C,K,M, N, P, Q, R 🔍, A, B, C 🔍

     Ex: **For S82.092[A]:** See PDX Collection 1338
     For S82.092[B,C]: See PDX Collection 1337
     For S82.092[K,M,N,P,Q,R]: See PDX Collection 897

   ● **S82.099**   Other fracture of unspecified patella A, B, C,K,M, N, P, Q, R 🔍, A, B, C 🔍

     Ex: **For S82.099[A]:** See PDX Collection 1339
     For S82.099[B,C]: See PDX Collection 1337
     For S82.099[K,M,N,P,Q,R]: See PDX Collection 897

● **S82.1**   Fracture of upper end of tibia
   Fracture of proximal end of tibia
   Excludes2   fracture of shaft of tibia (S82.2-)
     physeal fracture of upper end of tibia (S89.0-)

● **S82.10**   Unspecified fracture of upper end of tibia

   ● **S82.101**   Unspecified fracture of upper end of right tibia A, K, M, N, P, Q, R 🔍, B, C 🔍, A, B, C 🔍

     Ex: **For S82.101[A]:** See PDX Collection 1340
     For S82.101[B,C]: See PDX Collection 1341
     For S82.101[K,M,N,P,Q,R]: See PDX Collection 897

   ● **S82.102**   Unspecified fracture of upper end of left tibia A, K, M, N, P, Q, R 🔍, B, C 🔍, A, B, C 🔍

     Ex: **For S82.102[A]:** See PDX Collection 1342
     For S82.102[B,C]: See PDX Collection 1341
     For S82.102[K,M,N,P,Q,R]: See PDX Collection 897

   ● **S82.109**   Unspecified fracture of upper end of unspecified tibia A, K, M, N, P, Q, R 🔍, B, C 🔍, A, B, C 🔍

     Ex: **For S82.109[A,B,C]:** See PDX Collection 1341
     For S82.109[K,M,N,P,Q,R]: See PDX Collection 897

● **S82.11**   Fracture of tibial spine

   ● **S82.111**   Displaced fracture of right tibial spine A, K, M, N, P, Q, R 🔍, B, C 🔍, A, B, C 🔍

     Ex: **For S82.111[A]:** See PDX Collection 1340
     For S82.111[B,C]: See PDX Collection 1341
     For S82.111[K,M,N,P,Q,R]: See PDX Collection 897

   ● **S82.112**   Displaced fracture of left tibial spine A, K, M, N, P, Q, R 🔍, B, C 🔍, A, B, C 🔍

     Ex: **For S82.112[A]:** See PDX Collection 1342
     For S82.112[B,C]: See PDX Collection 1341
     For S82.112[K,M,N,P,Q,R]: See PDX Collection 897

   ● **S82.113**   Displaced fracture of unspecified tibial spine A, K, M, N, P, Q, R 🔍, B, C 🔍, A, B, C 🔍

     Ex: **For S82.113 [A,B,C]:** See PDX Collection 1341
     For S82.113[K,M,N,P,Q,R]: See PDX Collection 897

   ● **S82.114**   Nondisplaced fracture of right tibial spine A, K, M, N, P, Q, R 🔍, B, C 🔍, A, B, C 🔍

     Ex: **For S82.114[A]:** See PDX Collection 1340
     For S82.114[B,C]: See PDX Collection 1341
     For S82.114[K,M,N,P,Q,R]: See PDX Collection 897

   ● **S82.115**   Nondisplaced fracture of left tibial spine A, K, M, N, P, Q, R 🔍, B, C 🔍, A, B, C 🔍

     Ex: **For S82.115[A]:** See PDX Collection 1342
     For S82.115[B,C]: See PDX Collection 1341
     For S82.115[K,M,N,P,Q,R]: See PDX Collection 897

   ● **S82.116**   Nondisplaced fracture of unspecified tibial spine A, K, M, N, P, Q, R 🔍, B, C 🔍, A, B, C 🔍

     Ex: **For S82.116[A,B,C]:** See PDX Collection 1341
     For S82.116[K,M,N,P,Q,R]: See PDX Collection 897

▶ New   ⇒ Revised   deleted Deleted   Excludes 1   Excludes 2   Includes   Use additional   Code first   Code also   Key words
OGCR Official Guidelines   ● Unacceptable Principal Diagnosis   X Assign placeholder X   ● Use Additional Character(s)   ▌ Manifestation Code   Coding Clinic

● **S82.12**   Fracture of lateral condyle of tibia
 ● **S82.121**   **Displaced fracture of lateral condyle of right tibia** A, K, M, N, P, Q, R ☣, B, C ☣, A, B, C ☣
  (Ex) **For S82.121[A]:** See PDX Collection 1340
   For S82.121[B,C]: See PDX Collection 1341
   For S82.121[K,M,N,P,Q,R]: See PDX Collection 897
 ● **S82.122**   **Displaced fracture of lateral condyle of left tibia** A, K, M, N, P, Q, R ☣, B, C ☣, A, B, C ☣
  (Ex) **For S82.122[A]:** See PDX Collection 1342
   For S82.122[B,C]: See PDX Collection 1341
   For S82.122[K,M,N,P,Q,R]: See PDX Collection 897
 ● **S82.123**   **Displaced fracture of lateral condyle of unspecified tibia** A, K, M, N, P, Q, R ☣, B, C ☣, A, B, C ☣
  (Ex) **For S82.123[A,B,C]:** See PDX Collection 1341
   For S82.123[K,M,N,P,Q,R]: See PDX Collection 897
 ● **S82.124**   **Nondisplaced fracture of lateral condyle of right tibia** A, K, M, N, P, Q, R ☣, B, C ☣, A, B, C ☣
  (Ex) **For S82.124[A]:** See PDX Collection 1340
   For S82.124[B,C]: See PDX Collection 1341
   For S82.124[K,M,N,P,Q,R]: See PDX Collection 897
 ● **S82.125**   **Nondisplaced fracture of lateral condyle of left tibia** A, K, M, N, P, Q, R ☣, B, C ☣, A, B, C ☣
  (Ex) **For S82.125[A]:** See PDX Collection 1342
   For S82.125[B,C]: See PDX Collection 1341
   For S82.125[K,M,N,P,Q,R]: See PDX Collection 897
 ● **S82.126**   **Nondisplaced fracture of lateral condyle of unspecified tibia** A, K, M, N, P, Q, R ☣, B, C ☣, A, B, C ☣
  (Ex) **For S82.126[A,B,C]:** See PDX Collection 1341
   For S82.126[K,M,N,P,Q,R]: See PDX Collection 897

● **S82.13**   Fracture of medial condyle of tibia
 ● **S82.131**   **Displaced fracture of medial condyle of right tibia** A, K, M, N, P, Q, R ☣, B, C ☣, A, B, C ☣
  (Ex) **For S82.131[A]:** See PDX Collection 1340
   For S82.131[B,C]: See PDX Collection 1341
   For S82.131[K,M,N,P,Q,R]: See PDX Collection 897
 ● **S82.132**   **Displaced fracture of medial condyle of left tibia** A, K, M, N, P, Q, R ☣, B, C ☣, A, B, C ☣
  (Ex) **For S82.132[A]:** See PDX Collection 1342
   For S82.132[B,C]: See PDX Collection 1341
   For S82.132[K,M,N,P,Q,R]: See PDX Collection 897
 ● **S82.133**   **Displaced fracture of medial condyle of unspecified tibia** A, K, M, N, P, Q, R ☣, B, C ☣, A, B, C ☣
  (Ex) **For S82.133[A,B,C]:** See PDX Collection 1341
   For S82.133[K,M,N,P,Q,R]: See PDX Collection 897
 ● **S82.134**   **Nondisplaced fracture of medial condyle of right tibia** A, K, M, N, P, Q, R ☣, B, C ☣, A, B, C ☣
  (Ex) **For S82.134[A]:** See PDX Collection 1340
   For S82.134[B,C]: See PDX Collection 1341
   For S82.134[K,M,N,P,Q,R]: See PDX Collection 897

 ● **S82.135**   **Nondisplaced fracture of medial condyle of left tibia** A, K, M, N, P, Q, R ☣, B, C ☣, A, B, C ☣
  (Ex) **For S82.135[A]:** See PDX Collection 1342
   For S82.135[B,C]: See PDX Collection 1341
   For S82.135[K,M,N,P,Q,R]: See PDX Collection 897
 ● **S82.136**   **Nondisplaced fracture of medial condyle of unspecified tibia** A, K, M, N, P, Q, R ☣, B, C ☣, A, B, C ☣
  (Ex) **For S82.136[A,B,C]:** See PDX Collection 1341
   For S82.136[K,M,N,P,Q,R]: See PDX Collection 897

● **S82.14**   Bicondylar fracture of tibia
    Fracture of tibial plateau NOS
 ● **S82.141**   **Displaced bicondylar fracture of right tibia** A, K, M, N, P, Q, R ☣, B, C ☣, A, B, C ☣
  (Ex) **For S82.141[A]:** See PDX Collection 1340
   For S82.141[B,C]: See PDX Collection 1341
   For S82.141[K,M,N,P,Q,R]: See PDX Collection 897
 ● **S82.142**   **Displaced bicondylar fracture of left tibia** A, K, M, N, P, Q, R ☣, B, C ☣, A, B, C ☣
  (Ex) **For S82.142[A]:** See PDX Collection 1342
   For S82.142[B,C]: See PDX Collection 1341
   For S82.142[K,M,N,P,Q,R]: See PDX Collection 897
 ● **S82.143**   **Displaced bicondylar fracture of unspecified tibia** A, K, M, N, P, Q, R ☣, B, C ☣, A, B, C ☣
  (Ex) **For S82.143[A,B,C]:** See PDX Collection 1341
   For S82.143[K,M,N,P,Q,R]: See PDX Collection 897
 ● **S82.144**   **Nondisplaced bicondylar fracture of right tibia** A, K, M, N, P, Q, R ☣, B, C ☣, A, B, C ☣
  (Ex) **For S82.144[A]:** See PDX Collection 1340
   For S82.144[B,C]: See PDX Collection 1341
   For S82.144[K,M,N,P,Q,R]: See PDX Collection 897
 ● **S82.145**   **Nondisplaced bicondylar fracture of left tibia** A, K, M, N, P, Q, R ☣, B, C ☣, A, B, C ☣
  (Ex) **For S82.145[A]:** See PDX Collection 1342
   For S82.145[B,C]: See PDX Collection 1341
   For S82.145[K,M,N,P,Q,R]: See PDX Collection 897
 ● **S82.146**   **Nondisplaced bicondylar fracture of unspecified tibia** A, K, M, N, P, Q, R ☣, B, C ☣, A, B, C ☣
  (Ex) **For S82.146[A,B,C]:** See PDX Collection 1341
   For S82.146[K,M,N,P,Q,R]: See PDX Collection 897

● **S82.15**   Fracture of tibial tuberosity
 ● **S82.151**   **Displaced fracture of right tibial tuberosity** A, K, M, N, P, Q, R ☣, B, C ☣, A, B, C ☣
  (Ex) **For S82.151[A]:** See PDX Collection 1340
   For S82.151[B,C]: See PDX Collection 1341
   For S82.151[K,M,N,P,Q,R]: See PDX Collection 897
 ● **S82.152**   **Displaced fracture of left tibial tuberosity** A, K, M, N, P, Q, R ☣, B, C ☣, A, B, C ☣
  (Ex) **For S82.152[A]:** See PDX Collection 1342
   For S82.152[B,C]: See PDX Collection 1341
   For S82.152[K,M,N,P,Q,R]: See PDX Collection 897

CHAPTER 19 (S00-T88)

N Newborn Age: 0   **P** Pediatric Age: 0–17   **M** Maternity DX: 9–64   **A** Adult Age: 15–124   ♀ Females Only   ♂ Males Only
☣ Complication\Comorbidity   ☣ Major C\C   (Ex) CC/MCC Exclusions   ☣ Hospital-Acquired Condition   ☣ Hierarchical Condition Category

1399

● S82.153   **Displaced** fracture of **unspecified** tibial tuberosity A, K, M, N, P, Q, R 🔗, B, C 🔗, A, B, C 🔗
    Ex: **For S82.153[A,B,C]:** See PDX Collection 1341
       For S82.153[K,M,P,Q,R]: See PDX Collection 897

● S82.154   **Nondisplaced** fracture of **right** tibial tuberosity A, K, M, N, P, Q, R 🔗, B, C 🔗, A, B, C 🔗
    Ex: **For S82.154[A]:** See PDX Collection 1340
       For S82.154[B,C]: See PDX Collection 1341
       For S82.154[K,M,N,P,Q,R]: See PDX Collection 897

● S82.155   **Nondisplaced** fracture of **left** tibial tuberosity A, K, M, N, P, Q, R 🔗, B, C 🔗, A, B, C 🔗
    Ex: **For S82.155[A]:** See PDX Collection 1342
       For S82.155[B,C]: See PDX Collection 1341
       For S82.155[K,M,N,P,Q,R]: See PDX Collection 897

● S82.156   **Nondisplaced** fracture of **unspecified** tibial tuberosity A, K, M, N, P, Q, R 🔗, B, C 🔗, A, B, C 🔗
    Ex: **For S82.156[A,B,C]:** See PDX Collection 1341
       For S82.156[K,M,N,P,Q,R]: See PDX Collection 897

● S82.16   **Torus** fracture of **upper end of tibia**

The appropriate 7th character is to be added to all codes in subcategory S82.16

A	initial encounter for closed fracture
D	subsequent encounter for fracture with routine healing
G	subsequent encounter for fracture with delayed healing
K	subsequent encounter for fracture with nonunion
P	subsequent encounter for fracture with malunion
S	sequela

● S82.161   Torus fracture of upper end of **right** tibia A, K, P 🔗, A 🔗
    Ex: **For S82.161[A]:** See PDX Collection 1343
       For S82.161[K,P]: See PDX Collection 897

● S82.162   Torus fracture of upper end of **left** tibia A, K, P 🔗, A 🔗
    Ex: **For S82.162[A]:** See PDX Collection 1344
       For S82.162[K,P]: See PDX Collection 897

● S82.169   Torus fracture of upper end of **unspecified** tibia A, K, P 🔗, A 🔗
    Ex: **For S82.169[A]:** See PDX Collection 1345
       For S82.169[K,P]: See PDX Collection 897

● S82.19   **Other** fracture of upper end of tibia

● S82.191   Other fracture of upper end of **right** tibia A, K, M, N, P, Q, R 🔗, B, C 🔗, A, B, C 🔗
    Ex: **For S82.191[A]:** See PDX Collection 1340
       For S82.191[B,C]: See PDX Collection 1341
       For S82.191[K,M,N,P,Q,R]: See PDX Collection 897

● S82.192   Other fracture of upper end of **left** tibia A, K, M, N, P, Q, R 🔗, B, C 🔗, A, B, C 🔗
    Ex: **For S82.192[A]:** See PDX Collection 1342
       For S82.192[B,C]: See PDX Collection 1341
       For S82.192[K,M,N,P,Q,R]: See PDX Collection 897

● S82.199   Other fracture of upper end of **unspecified** tibia A, K, M, N, P, Q, R 🔗, B, C 🔗, A, B, C 🔗
    Ex: **For S82.199[A,B,C]:** See PDX Collection 1341
       For S82.199[K,M,N,P,Q,R]: See PDX Collection 897

● S82.2   Fracture of **shaft** of tibia

● S82.20   **Unspecified** fracture of shaft of tibia
    Fracture of tibia NOS

● S82.201   Unspecified fracture of shaft of **right** tibia A, K, M, N, P, Q, R 🔗, B, C 🔗, A, B, C 🔗
    Ex: **For S82.201[A]:** See PDX Collection 1346
       For S82.201[B,C]: See PDX Collection 1341
       For S82.201[K,M,N,P,Q,R]: See PDX Collection 897

● S82.202   Unspecified fracture of shaft of **left** tibia A, K, M, N, P, Q, R 🔗, B, C 🔗, A, B, C 🔗
    Ex: **For S82.202[A]:** See PDX Collection 1342
       For S82.202[B,C]: See PDX Collection 1341
       For S82.202[K,M,N,P,Q,R]: See PDX Collection 897

● S82.209   Unspecified fracture of shaft of **unspecified** tibia A, K, M, N, P, Q, R 🔗, B, C 🔗, A, B, C 🔗
    Ex: **For S82.209[A,B,C]:** See PDX Collection 1341
       For S82.209[K,M,N,P,Q,R]: See PDX Collection 897

● S82.22   **Transverse** fracture of shaft of tibia

● S82.221   **Displaced transverse** fracture of shaft of **right** tibia A, K, M, N, P, Q, R 🔗, B, C 🔗, A, B, C 🔗
    Ex: **For S82.221[A]:** See PDX Collection 1340
       For S82.221[B,C]: See PDX Collection 1341
       For S82.221[K,M,N,P,Q,R]: See PDX Collection 897

● S82.222   **Displaced transverse** fracture of shaft of **left** tibia A, K, M, N, P, Q, R 🔗, B, C 🔗, A, B, C 🔗
    Ex: **For S82.222[A]:** See PDX Collection 1342
       For S82.222[B,C]: See PDX Collection 1341
       For S82.222[K,M,N,P,Q,R]: See PDX Collection 897

● S82.223   **Displaced transverse** fracture of shaft of **unspecified** tibia A, K, M, N, P, Q, R 🔗, B, C 🔗, A, B, C 🔗
    Ex: **For S82.223[A,B,C]:** See PDX Collection 1341
       For S82.223[K,M,N,P,Q,R]: See PDX Collection 897

● S82.224   **Nondisplaced transverse** fracture of shaft of **right** tibia A, K, M, N, P, Q, R 🔗, B, C 🔗, A, B, C 🔗
    Ex: **For S82.224[A]:** See PDX Collection 1340
       For S82.224[B,C]: See PDX Collection 1341
       For S82.224[K,M,N,P,Q,R]: See PDX Collection 897

● S82.225   **Nondisplaced transverse** fracture of shaft of **left** tibia A, K, M, N, P, Q, R 🔗, B, C 🔗, A, B, C 🔗
    Ex: **For S82.225[A]:** See PDX Collection 1342
       For S82.225[B,C]: See PDX Collection 1341
       For S82.225[K,M,N,P,Q,R]: See PDX Collection 897

● S82.226   **Nondisplaced transverse** fracture of shaft of **unspecified** tibia A, K, M, N, P, Q, R 🔗, B, C 🔗, A, B, C 🔗
    Ex: **For S82.226[A,B,C]:** See PDX Collection 1341
       For S82.226[K,M,N,P,Q,R]: See PDX Collection 897

▶ New   ⇒ Revised   ~~deleted~~ Deleted   Excludes 1   Excludes 2   Includes   Use additional   Code first   Code also   Key words
OGCR Official Guidelines   ● Unacceptable Principal Diagnosis   X Assign placeholder X   ● Use Additional Character(s)   ▶ Manifestation Code   **Coding Clinic**

● **S82.23**   Oblique fracture of shaft of tibia

  ● **S82.231**   Displaced oblique fracture of shaft of right tibia A, K, M, N, P, Q, R 🝆, B, C 🝆, A, B, C 🝆
     (Ex:) **For S82.231[A]:** See PDX Collection 1340
        For S82.231[B,C]: See PDX Collection 1341
        For S82.231[K,M,N,P,Q,R]: See PDX Collection 897

  ● **S82.232**   Displaced oblique fracture of shaft of left tibia A, K, M, N, P, Q, R 🝆, B, C 🝆, A, B, C 🝆
     (Ex:) **For S82.232[A]:** See PDX Collection 1342
        For S82.232[B,C]: See PDX Collection 1341
        For S82.232[K,M,N,P,Q,R]: See PDX Collection 897

  ● **S82.233**   Displaced oblique fracture of shaft of unspecified tibia A, K, M, N, P, Q, R 🝆, B, C 🝆, A, B, C 🝆
     (Ex:) **For S82.233[A,B,C]:** See PDX Collection 1341
        For S82.233[K,M,N,P,Q,R]: See PDX Collection 897

  ● **S82.234**   Nondisplaced oblique fracture of shaft of right tibia A, K, M, N, P, Q, R 🝆, B, C 🝆, A, B, C 🝆
     (Ex:) **For S82.234[A]:** See PDX Collection 1340
        For S82.234[B,C]: See PDX Collection 1341
        For S82.234[K,M,N,P,Q,R]: See PDX Collection 897
     Coding Clinic: 2015, Q1, P9-10

  ● **S82.235**   Nondisplaced oblique fracture of shaft of left tibia A, K, M, N, P, Q, R 🝆, B, C 🝆, A, B, C 🝆
     (Ex:) **For S82.235[A]:** See PDX Collection 1342
        For S82.235[B,C]: See PDX Collection 1341
        For S82.235[K,M,N,P,Q,R]: See PDX Collection 897

  ● **S82.236**   Nondisplaced oblique fracture of shaft of unspecified tibia A, K, M, N, P, Q, R 🝆, B, C 🝆, A, B, C 🝆
     (Ex:) **For S82.236[A,B,C]:** See PDX Collection 1341
        For S82.236[K,M,N,P,Q,R]: See PDX Collection 897

● **S82.24**   Spiral fracture of shaft of tibia
     Toddler fracture

  ● **S82.241**   Displaced spiral fracture of shaft of right tibia A, K, M, N, P, Q, R 🝆, B, C 🝆, A, B, C 🝆
     (Ex:) **For S82.241[A]:** See PDX Collection 1340
        For S82.241[B,C]: See PDX Collection 1341
        For S82.241[K,M,N,P,Q,R]: See PDX Collection 897

  ● **S82.242**   Displaced spiral fracture of shaft of left tibia A, K, M, N, P, Q, R 🝆, B, C 🝆, A, B, C 🝆
     (Ex:) **For S82.242[A]:** See PDX Collection 1342
        For S82.242[B,C]: See PDX Collection 1341
        For S82.242[K,M,N,P,Q,R]: See PDX Collection 897

  ● **S82.243**   Displaced spiral fracture of shaft of unspecified tibia A, K, M, N, P, Q, R 🝆, B, C 🝆, A, B, C 🝆
     (Ex:) **For S82.243[A,B,C]:** See PDX Collection 1341
        For S82.243[K,M,N,P,Q,R]: See PDX Collection 897

  ● **S82.244**   Nondisplaced spiral fracture of shaft of right tibia A, K, M, N, P, Q, R 🝆, B, C 🝆, A, B, C 🝆
     (Ex:) **For S82.244[A]:** See PDX Collection 1340
        For S82.244[B,C]: See PDX Collection 1341
        For S82.244[K,M,N,P,Q,R]: See PDX Collection 897

  ● **S82.245**   Nondisplaced spiral fracture of shaft of left tibia A, K, M, N, P, Q, R 🝆, B, C 🝆, A, B, C 🝆
     (Ex:) **For S82.245[A]:** See PDX Collection 1342
        For S82.245[B,C]: See PDX Collection 1341
        For S82.245[K,M,N,P,Q,R]: See PDX Collection 897

  ● **S82.246**   Nondisplaced spiral fracture of shaft of unspecified tibia A, K, M, N, P, Q, R 🝆, B, C 🝆, A, B, C 🝆
     (Ex:) **For S82.246[A,B,C]:** See PDX Collection 1341
        For S82.246[K,M,N,P,Q,R]: See PDX Collection 897

● **S82.25**   Comminuted fracture of shaft of tibia

  ● **S82.251**   Displaced comminuted fracture of shaft of right tibia A, K, M, N, P, Q, R 🝆, B, C 🝆, A, B, C 🝆
     (Ex:) **For S82.251[A]:** See PDX Collection 1340
        For S82.251[B,C]: See PDX Collection 1341
        For S82.251[K,M,N,P,Q,R]: See PDX Collection 897
     Coding Clinic: 2015, Q2, P6

  ● **S82.252**   Displaced comminuted fracture of shaft of left tibia A, K, M, N, P, Q, R 🝆, B, C 🝆, A, B, C 🝆
     (Ex:) **For S82.252[A]:** See PDX Collection 1342
        For S82.252[B,C]: See PDX Collection 1341
        For S82.252[K,M,N,P,Q,R]: See PDX Collection 897

  ● **S82.253**   Displaced comminuted fracture of shaft of unspecified tibia A, K, M, N, P, Q, R 🝆, B, C 🝆, A, B, C 🝆
     (Ex:) **For S82.253[A,B,C]:** See PDX Collection 1341
        For S82.253[K,M,N,P,Q,R]: See PDX Collection 897

  ● **S82.254**   Nondisplaced comminuted fracture of shaft of right tibia A, K, M, N, P, Q, R 🝆, B, C 🝆, A, B, C 🝆
     (Ex:) **For S82.254[A]:** See PDX Collection 1340
        For S82.254[B,C]: See PDX Collection 1341
        For S82.254[K,M,N,P,Q,R]: See PDX Collection 897

  ● **S82.255**   Nondisplaced comminuted fracture of shaft of left tibia A, K, M, N, P, Q, R 🝆, B, C 🝆, A, B, C 🝆
     (Ex:) **For S82.255[A]:** See PDX Collection 1342
        For S82.255[B,C]: See PDX Collection 1341
        For S82.255[K,M,N,P,Q,R]: See PDX Collection 897

  ● **S82.256**   Nondisplaced comminuted fracture of shaft of unspecified tibia A, K, M, N, P, Q, R 🝆, B, C 🝆, A, B, C 🝆
     (Ex:) **For S82.256[A,B,C]:** See PDX Collection 1341
        For S82.256[K,M,N,P,Q,R]: See PDX Collection 897

● **S82.26**   Segmental fracture of shaft of tibia

  ● **S82.261**   Displaced segmental fracture of shaft of right tibia A, K, M, N, P, Q, R 🝆, B, C 🝆, A, B, C 🝆
     (Ex:) **For S82.261[A]:** See PDX Collection 1340
        For S82.261[B,C]: See PDX Collection 1341
        For S82.261[K,M,N,P,Q,R]: See PDX Collection 897

  ● **S82.262**   Displaced segmental fracture of shaft of left tibia A, K, M, N, P, Q, R 🝆, B, C 🝆, A, B, C 🝆
     (Ex:) **For S82.262[A]:** See PDX Collection 1342
        For S82.262[B,C]: See PDX Collection 1341
        For S82.262[K,M,N,P,Q,R]: See PDX Collection 897

N Newborn Age: 0   **P** Pediatric Age: 0–17   **M** Maternity DX: 9–64   **A** Adult Age: 15–124   ♀ Females Only   ♂ Males Only

🝆 Complication\Comorbidity   🝆 Major C\C   (Ex:) CC/MCC Exclusions   🝆 Hospital-Acquired Condition   🝆 Hierarchical Condition Category

CHAPTER 19 (S00-T88)

CHAPTER 19 (S00-T88)

● S82.263 **Displaced segmental fracture of shaft of unspecified tibia** A, K, M, N, P, Q, R 🔵, B, C 🔵, A, B, C 🔵
    Ⓔₓ For S82.263[A,B,C]: See PDX Collection 1341
      For S82.263[K,M,N,P,Q,R]: See PDX Collection 897

● S82.264 **Nondisplaced segmental fracture of shaft of right tibia** A, K, M, N, P, Q, R 🔵, B, C 🔵, A, B, C 🔵
    Ⓔₓ For S82.264[A]: See PDX Collection 1340
      For S82.264[B,C]: See PDX Collection 1341
      For S82.264[K,M,N,P,Q,R]: See PDX Collection 897

● S82.265 **Nondisplaced segmental fracture of shaft of left tibia** A, K, M, N, P, Q, R 🔵, B, C 🔵, A, B, C 🔵
    Ⓔₓ For S82.265[A]: See PDX Collection 1342
      For S82.265[B,C]: See PDX Collection 1341
      For S82.265[K,M,N,P,Q,R]: See PDX Collection 897

● S82.266 **Nondisplaced segmental fracture of shaft of unspecified tibia** A, K, M, N, P, Q, R 🔵, B, C 🔵, A, B, C 🔵
    Ⓔₓ For S82.266[A,B,C]: See PDX Collection 1341
      For S82.266[K,M,N,P,Q,R]: See PDX Collection 897

● S82.29 **Other fracture of shaft of tibia**

● S82.291 **Other fracture of shaft of right tibia** A, K, M, N, P, Q, R 🔵, B, C 🔵, A, B, C 🔵
    Ⓔₓ For S82.291[A]: See PDX Collection 1340
      For S82.291[B,C]: See PDX Collection 1341
      For S82.291[K,M,N,P,Q,R]: See PDX Collection 897

● S82.292 **Other fracture of shaft of left tibia** A, K, M, N, P, Q, R 🔵, B, C 🔵, A, B, C 🔵
    Ⓔₓ For S82.292[A]: See PDX Collection 1342
      For S82.292[B,C]: See PDX Collection 1341
      For S82.292[K,M,N,P,Q,R]: See PDX Collection 897

● S82.299 **Other fracture of shaft of unspecified tibia** A, K, M, N, P, Q, R 🔵, B, C 🔵, A, B, C 🔵
    Ⓔₓ For S82.299[A,B,C]: See PDX Collection 1341
      For S82.299[K,M,N,P,Q,R]: See PDX Collection 897

● S82.3 **Fracture of lower end of tibia**

   Excludes1   bimalleolar fracture of lower leg (S82.84-)
              fracture of medial malleolus alone (S82.5-)
              Maisonneuve's fracture (S82.86-)
              pilon fracture of distal tibia (S82.87-)
              trimalleolar fractures of lower leg (S82.85-)

● S82.30 **Unspecified fracture of lower end of tibia**
    Ⓔₓ For category S82.30 CC codes S82.30[B,C]: See PDX Collection 1347 For S82.30[K,M,N,P,Q,R]: See PDX Collection 897

● S82.301 **Unspecified fracture of lower end of right tibia** B, C, K, M, N, P, Q, R 🔵, B, C 🔵

● S82.302 **Unspecified fracture of lower end of left tibia** B, C, K, M, N, P, Q, R 🔵, B, C 🔵

● S82.309 **Unspecified fracture of lower end of unspecified tibia** B, C, K, M, N, P, Q, R 🔵, B, C 🔵

● S82.31 **Torus fracture of lower end of tibia**

The appropriate 7th character is to be added to all codes in subcategory S82.31

A	initial encounter for closed fracture
D	subsequent encounter for fracture with routine healing
G	subsequent encounter for fracture with delayed healing
K	subsequent encounter for fracture with nonunion
P	subsequent encounter for fracture with malunion
S	sequela

● S82.311 **Torus fracture of lower end of right tibia** A, K, P 🔵, A 🔵
    Ⓔₓ For S82.311[A]: See PDX Collection 1343
      For S82.311[K,P]: See PDX Collection 897

● S82.312 **Torus fracture of lower end of left tibia** A, K, P 🔵, A 🔵
    Ⓔₓ For S82.312[A]: See PDX Collection 1344
      For S82.312[K,P]: See PDX Collection 897

● S82.319 **Torus fracture of lower end of unspecified tibia** A, K, P 🔵, A 🔵
    Ⓔₓ For S82.319[A]: See PDX Collection 1345
      S82.319[K,P]: See PDX Collection 897

● S82.39 **Other fracture of lower end of tibia**
    Ⓔₓ For category S82.39 CC codes S82.39[B,C]: See PDX Collection 1347 For S82.39[K,M,N,P,Q,R]: See PDX Collection 897

● S82.391 **Other fracture of lower end of right tibia** B, C, K, M, N, P, Q, R 🔵, B, C 🔵

● S82.392 **Other fracture of lower end of left tibia** B, C, K, M, N, P, Q, R 🔵, B, C 🔵
    Coding Clinic: 2015, Q1, P25

● S82.399 **Other fracture of lower end of unspecified tibia** B, C, K, M, N, P, Q, R 🔵, B, C 🔵

● S82.4 **Fracture of shaft of fibula**

   Excludes2   fracture of lateral malleolus alone (S82.6-)
    Ⓔₓ For category S82.4 CC codes S82.4[B,C]: See PDX Collection 1341
      For S82.4[K,M,N,P,Q,R]: See PDX Collection 897

● S82.40 **Unspecified fracture of shaft of fibula**

● S82.401 **Unspecified fracture of shaft of right fibula** K, M, N, P, Q, R 🔵, B, C 🔵, B, C 🔵

● S82.402 **Unspecified fracture of shaft of left fibula** K, M, N, P, Q, R 🔵, B, C 🔵, B, C 🔵

● S82.409 **Unspecified fracture of shaft of unspecified fibula** K, M, N, P, Q, R 🔵, B, C 🔵, B, C 🔵

● S82.42 **Transverse fracture of shaft of fibula**

● S82.421 **Displaced transverse fracture of shaft of right fibula** K, M, N, P, Q, R 🔵, B, C 🔵, B, C 🔵

● S82.422 **Displaced transverse fracture of shaft of left fibula** K, M, N, P, Q, R 🔵, B, C 🔵, B, C 🔵

● S82.423 **Displaced transverse fracture of shaft of unspecified fibula** K, M, N, P, Q, R 🔵, B, C 🔵, B, C 🔵

● S82.424 **Nondisplaced transverse fracture of shaft of right fibula** K, M, N, P, Q, R 🔵, B, C 🔵, B, C 🔵

● S82.425 **Nondisplaced transverse fracture of shaft of left fibula** K, M, N, P, Q, R 🔵, B, C 🔵, B, C 🔵

● S82.426 **Nondisplaced transverse fracture of shaft of unspecified fibula** K, M, N, P, Q, R 🔵, B, C 🔵, B, C 🔵

▶ New   ⇛ Revised   ~~deleted~~ Doleted   Excludes 1   Excludes 2   Includes   Use additional   Code first   Code also   Key words
OGCR Official Guidelines   ● Unacceptable Principal Diagnosis   X Assign placeholder X   ● Use Additional Character(s)   ▶ Manifestation Code   Coding Clinic

● **S82.43**   Oblique fracture of shaft of fibula
    ● **S82.431**   Displaced oblique fracture of shaft of right fibula K, M, N, P, Q, R 🦠, B, C 🦠, B, C 🦠
    ● **S82.432**   Displaced oblique fracture of shaft of left fibula K, M, N, P, Q, R 🦠, B, C 🦠, B, C 🦠
    ● **S82.433**   Displaced oblique fracture of shaft of unspecified fibula K, M, N, P, Q, R 🦠, B, C 🦠, B, C 🦠
    ● **S82.434**   Nondisplaced oblique fracture of shaft of right fibula K, M, N, P, Q, R 🦠, B, C 🦠, B, C 🦠
    ● **S82.435**   Nondisplaced oblique fracture of shaft of left fibula K, M, N, P, Q, R 🦠, B, C 🦠, B, C 🦠
    ● **S82.436**   Nondisplaced oblique fracture of shaft of unspecified fibula K, M, N, P, Q, R 🦠, B, C 🦠, B, C 🦠

● **S82.44**   Spiral fracture of shaft of fibula
    ● **S82.441**   Displaced spiral fracture of shaft of right fibula K, M, N, P, Q, R 🦠, B, C 🦠, B, C 🦠
    ● **S82.442**   Displaced spiral fracture of shaft of left fibula K, M, N, P, Q, R 🦠, B, C 🦠, B, C 🦠
    ● **S82.443**   Displaced spiral fracture of shaft of unspecified fibula K, M, N, P, Q, R 🦠, B, C 🦠, B, C 🦠
    ● **S82.444**   Nondisplaced spiral fracture of shaft of right fibula K, M, N, P, Q, R 🦠, B, C 🦠, B, C 🦠
    ● **S82.445**   Nondisplaced spiral fracture of shaft of left fibula K, M, N, P, Q, R 🦠, B, C 🦠, B, C 🦠
    ● **S82.446**   Nondisplaced spiral fracture of shaft of unspecified fibula K, M, N, P, Q, R 🦠, B, C 🦠, B, C 🦠

● **S82.45**   Comminuted fracture of shaft of fibula
    ● **S82.451**   Displaced comminuted fracture of shaft of right fibula K, M, N, P, Q, R 🦠, B, C 🦠, B, C 🦠
    ● **S82.452**   Displaced comminuted fracture of shaft of left fibula K, M, N, P, Q, R 🦠, B, C 🦠, B, C 🦠
    ● **S82.453**   Displaced comminuted fracture of shaft of unspecified fibula K, M, N, P, Q, R 🦠, B, C 🦠, B, C 🦠
    ● **S82.454**   Nondisplaced comminuted fracture of shaft of right fibula K, M, N, P, Q, R 🦠, B, C 🦠, B, C 🦠
    ● **S82.455**   Nondisplaced comminuted fracture of shaft of left fibula K, M, N, P, Q, R 🦠, B, C 🦠, B, C 🦠
    ● **S82.456**   Nondisplaced comminuted fracture of shaft of unspecified fibula K, M, N, P, Q, R 🦠, B, C 🦠, B, C 🦠

● **S82.46**   Segmental fracture of shaft of fibula
    ● **S82.461**   Displaced segmental fracture of shaft of right fibula K, M, N, P, Q, R 🦠, B, C 🦠, B, C 🦠
    ● **S82.462**   Displaced segmental fracture of shaft of left fibula K, M, N, P, Q, R 🦠, B, C 🦠, B, C 🦠
    ● **S82.463**   Displaced segmental fracture of shaft of unspecified fibula K, M, N, P, Q, R 🦠, B, C 🦠, B, C 🦠
    ● **S82.464**   Nondisplaced segmental fracture of shaft of right fibula K, M, N, P, Q, R 🦠, B, C 🦠, B, C 🦠
    ● **S82.465**   Nondisplaced segmental fracture of shaft of left fibula K, M, N, P, Q, R 🦠, B, C 🦠, B, C 🦠
    ● **S82.466**   Nondisplaced segmental fracture of shaft of unspecified fibula K, M, N, P, Q, R 🦠, B, C 🦠, B, C 🦠

● **S82.49**   Other fracture of shaft of fibula
    ● **S82.491**   Other fracture of shaft of right fibula K, M, N, P, Q, R 🦠, B, C 🦠, B, C 🦠
    ● **S82.492**   Other fracture of shaft of left fibula K, M, N, P, Q, R 🦠, B, C 🦠, B, C 🦠
    ● **S82.499**   Other fracture of shaft of unspecified fibula K, M, N, P, Q, R 🦠, B, C 🦠, B, C 🦠

● **S82.5**   Fracture of medial malleolus
    Excludes1   pilon fracture of distal tibia (S82.87-)
           Salter-Harris type III of lower end of tibia (S89.13-)
           Salter-Harris type IV of lower end of tibia (S89.14-)
    (Ex) For category S82.5 CC codes S82.5[B,C]: See PDX Collection 1347
        For S82.5[K,M,N,P,Q,R]: See PDX Collection 897
    X ● **S82.51**   Displaced fracture of medial malleolus of right tibia B, C, K, M, N, P, Q, R 🦠, B, C 🦠
    X ● **S82.52**   Displaced fracture of medial malleolus of left tibia B, C, K, M, N, P, Q, R 🦠, B, C 🦠
    X ● **S82.53**   Displaced fracture of medial malleolus of unspecified tibia B, C, K, M, N, P, Q, R 🦠, B, C 🦠
    X ● **S82.54**   Nondisplaced fracture of medial malleolus of right tibia B, C, K, M, N, P, Q, R 🦠, B, C 🦠
    X ● **S82.55**   Nondisplaced fracture of medial malleolus of left tibia B, C, K, M, N, P, Q, R 🦠, B, C 🦠
    X ● **S82.56**   Nondisplaced fracture of medial malleolus of unspecified tibia B, C, K, M, N, P, Q, R 🦠, B, C 🦠

● **S82.6**   Fracture of lateral malleolus
    Excludes1   pilon fracture of distal tibia (S82.87-)
    (Ex) For category S82.6 CC codes S82.6[B,C]: See PDX Collection 1347
        For S82.6[K,M,N,P,Q,R]: See PDX Collection 897
    X ● **S82.61**   Displaced fracture of lateral malleolus of right fibula B, C, K, M, N, P, Q, R 🦠, B, C 🦠
    X ● **S82.62**   Displaced fracture of lateral malleolus of left fibula B, C, K, M, N, P, Q, R 🦠, B, C 🦠
    X ● **S82.63**   Displaced fracture of lateral malleolus of unspecified fibula B, C, K, M, N, P, Q, R 🦠, B, C 🦠
    X ● **S82.64**   Nondisplaced fracture of lateral malleolus of right fibula B, C, K, M, N, P, Q, R 🦠, B, C 🦠
    X ● **S82.65**   Nondisplaced fracture of lateral malleolus of left fibula B, C, K, M, N, P, Q, R 🦠, B, C 🦠
    X ● **S82.66**   Nondisplaced fracture of lateral malleolus of unspecified fibula B, C, K, M, N, P, Q, R 🦠, B, C 🦠

N Newborn Age: 0   **P** Pediatric Age: 0–17   **M** Maternity DX: 9–64   **A** Adult Age: 15–124   ♀ Females Only   ♂ Males Only
🦠 Complication\Comorbidity   🦠 Major C\C   (Ex) CC/MCC Exclusions   🦠 Hospital-Acquired Condition   🦠 Hierarchical Condition Category

1403

CHAPTER 19 (S00-T88)

● **S82.8   Other fractures of lower leg**
   ● **S82.81   Torus fracture of upper end of fibula**

The appropriate 7th character is to be added to all codes in subcategory S82.81

A	initial encounter for closed fracture
D	subsequent encounter for fracture with routine healing
G	subsequent encounter for fracture with delayed healing
K	subsequent encounter for fracture with nonunion
P	subsequent encounter for fracture with malunion
S	sequela

(Ex) **For category S82.81 CC codes:** See PDX Collection 897

   ● **S82.811   Torus fracture of upper end of right fibula** K, P 🐷

   ● **S82.812   Torus fracture of upper end of left fibula** K, P 🐷

   ● **S82.819   Torus fracture of upper end of unspecified fibula** K, P 🐷

   ● **S82.82   Torus fracture of lower end of fibula**

The appropriate 7th character is to be added to all codes in subcategory S82.82

A	initial encounter for closed fracture
D	subsequent encounter for fracture with routine healing
G	subsequent encounter for fracture with delayed healing
K	subsequent encounter for fracture with nonunion
P	subsequent encounter for fracture with malunion
S	sequela

(Ex) **For category S82.82 CC codes:** See PDX Collection 897

   ● **S82.821   Torus fracture of lower end of right fibula** K, P 🐷

   ● **S82.822   Torus fracture of lower end of left fibula** K, P 🐷

   ● **S82.829   Torus fracture of lower end of unspecified fibula** K, P 🐷

   ● **S82.83   Other fracture of upper and lower end of fibula**
      (Ex) **For category S82.83 CC codes S82.83[B,C]:** See PDX Collection 1341 **For S82.83[K,M,N,P,Q,R]:** See PDX Collection 897

   ● **S82.831   Other fracture of upper and lower end of right fibula** K, M, N, P, Q, R 🐷, B, C 🐷, B, C 🐷

   ● **S82.832   Other fracture of upper and lower end of left fibula** K, M, N, P, Q, R 🐷, B, C 🐷, B, C 🐷
      Coding Clinic: 2015, Q1, P9-10

   ● **S82.839   Other fracture of upper and lower end of unspecified fibula** K, M, N, P, Q, R 🐷, B, C 🐷, B, C 🐷

   ● **S82.84   Bimalleolar fracture of lower leg**
      (Ex) **For category S82.84 CC codes S82.84[B,C]:** See PDX Collection 1347 **For S82.84[K,M,N,P,Q,R]:** See PDX Collection 897

   ● **S82.841   Displaced bimalleolar fracture of right lower leg** B, C, K, M, N, P, Q, R 🐷, B, C 🐷

   ● **S82.842   Displaced bimalleolar fracture of left lower leg** B, C, K, M, N, P, Q, R 🐷, B, C 🐷

   ● **S82.843   Displaced bimalleolar fracture of unspecified lower leg** B, C, K, M, N, P, Q, R 🐷, B, C 🐷

   ● **S82.844   Nondisplaced bimalleolar fracture of right lower leg** B, C, K, M, N, P, Q, R 🐷, B, C 🐷

   ● **S82.845   Nondisplaced bimalleolar fracture of left lower leg** B, C, K, M, N, P, Q, R 🐷, B, C 🐷

   ● **S82.846   Nondisplaced bimalleolar fracture of unspecified lower leg** B, C, K, M, N, P, Q, R 🐷, B, C 🐷

   ● **S82.85   Trimalleolar fracture of lower leg**
      (Ex) **For category S82.85 CC codes S82.85[B,C]:** See PDX Collection 1347 **For S82.85[K,M,N,P,Q,R]:** See PDX Collection 897

   ● **S82.851   Displaced trimalleolar fracture of right lower leg** B, C, K, M, N, P, Q, R 🐷, B, C 🐷

   ● **S82.852   Displaced trimalleolar fracture of left lower leg** B, C, K, M, N, P, Q, R 🐷, B, C 🐷

   ● **S82.853   Displaced trimalleolar fracture of unspecified lower leg** B, C, K, M, N, P, Q, R 🐷, B, C 🐷

   ● **S82.854   Nondisplaced trimalleolar fracture of right lower leg** B, C, K, M, N, P, Q, R 🐷, B, C 🐷

   ● **S82.855   Nondisplaced trimalleolar fracture of left lower leg** B, C, K, M, N, P, Q, R 🐷, B, C 🐷

   ● **S82.856   Nondisplaced trimalleolar fracture of unspecified lower leg** B, C, K, M, N, P, Q, R 🐷, B, C 🐷

   ● **S82.86   Maisonneuve's fracture**
      (Ex) **For category S82.86 CC codes S82.86[B,C]:** See PDX Collection 1341 **For S82.86[K,M,N,P,Q,R]:** See PDX Collection 897

   ● **S82.861   Displaced Maisonneuve's fracture of right leg** K, M, N, P, Q, R 🐷, B, C 🐷, B, C 🐷

   ● **S82.862   Displaced Maisonneuve's fracture of left leg** K, M, N, P, Q, R 🐷, B, C 🐷, B, C 🐷

   ● **S82.863   Displaced Maisonneuve's fracture of unspecified leg** K, M, N, P, Q, R 🐷, B, C 🐷, B, C 🐷

   ● **S82.864   Nondisplaced Maisonneuve's fracture of right leg** K, M, N, P, Q, R 🐷, B, C 🐷, B, C 🐷

   ● **S82.865   Nondisplaced Maisonneuve's fracture of left leg** K, M, N, P, Q, R 🐷, B, C 🐷, B, C 🐷

   ● **S82.866   Nondisplaced Maisonneuve's fracture of unspecified leg** K, M, N, P, Q, R 🐷, B, C 🐷, B, C 🐷

   ● **S82.87   Pilon fracture of tibia**
      (Ex) **For category S82.87 CC codes S82.87[B,C]:** See PDX Collection 1347 **For S82.87[K,M,N,P,Q,R]:** See PDX Collection 897

   ● **S82.871   Displaced pilon fracture of right tibia** B, C, K, M, N, P, Q, R 🐷, B, C 🐷

   ● **S82.872   Displaced pilon fracture of left tibia** B, C, K, M, N, P, Q, R 🐷, B, C 🐷

   ● **S82.873   Displaced pilon fracture of unspecified tibia** B, C, K, M, N, P, Q, R 🐷, B, C 🐷

   ● **S82.874   Nondisplaced pilon fracture of right tibia** B, C, K, M, N, P, Q, R 🐷, B, C 🐷

   ● **S82.875   Nondisplaced pilon fracture of left tibia** B, C, K, M, N, P, Q, R 🐷, B, C 🐷

   ● **S82.876   Nondisplaced pilon fracture of unspecified tibia** B, C, K, M, N, P, Q, R 🐷, B, C 🐷

▶ New   ⫸ Revised   ~~deleted~~ Deleted   Excludes 1   Excludes 2   Includes   Use additional   Code first   Code also   Key words
OGCR Official Guidelines   ● Unacceptable Principal Diagnosis   X Assign placeholder X   ● Use Additional Character(s)   ▶ Manifestation Code   **Coding Clinic**

● S82.89   Other fractures of lower leg
      Fracture of ankle NOS
      (Ex) **For category S82.89 CC codes S82.89[B,C]:** See PDX
      Collection 1347 **For S82.89[K,M,N,P,Q,R]:** See PDX
      Collection 897

     ● S82.891   Other fracture of right lower leg
           B, C, K, M, N, P, Q, R 🔵 B, C 🔵

     ● S82.892   Other fracture of left lower leg
           B, C, K, M, N, P, Q, R 🔵 B, C 🔵

     ● S82.899   Other fracture of unspecified lower
           leg B, C, K, M, N, P, Q, R 🔵 B, C 🔵

● S82.9   Unspecified fracture of lower leg
      (Ex) **For category S82.9 CC codes S82.9[B,C]:** See PDX Collection 1348
      For S82.9[K,M,N,P,Q,R]: See PDX Collection 897

   X ● S82.90   Unspecified fracture of unspecified lower leg
           A, K, M, N, P, Q, R 🔵 B, C 🔵

   X ● S82.91   Unspecified fracture of right lower leg A, K, M,
           N, P, Q, R 🔵 B, C 🔵

   X ● S82.92   Unspecified fracture of left lower leg A, K, M,
           N, P, Q, R 🔵 B, C 🔵

● S83   Dislocation and sprain of joints and ligaments of knee

    Includes   avulsion of joint or ligament of knee
          laceration of cartilage, joint or ligament of knee
          sprain of cartilage, joint or ligament of knee
          traumatic hemarthrosis of joint or ligament of
             knee
          traumatic rupture of joint or ligament of knee
          traumatic subluxation of joint or ligament of knee
          traumatic tear of joint or ligament of knee

     Code also any associated open wound

    Excludes2   derangement of patella (M22.0-M22.3)
          injury of patellar ligament (tendon) (S76.1-)
          internal derangement of knee (M23.-)
          old dislocation of knee (M24.36)
          pathological dislocation of knee (M24.36)
          recurrent dislocation of knee (M22.0)
          strain of muscle, fascia and tendon of lower leg
             (S86.-)

     Coding Clinic: 2019, Q2, P26

     The appropriate 7th character is to be added to each code from
       category S83

       | | |
       | A | initial encounter |
       | D | subsequent encounter |
       | S | sequela |

● S83.0   Subluxation and dislocation of patella

     ● S83.00   Unspecified subluxation and dislocation of
           patella

       ● S83.001   Unspecified subluxation of right
             patella

       ● S83.002   Unspecified subluxation of left
             patella

       ● S83.003   Unspecified subluxation of
             unspecified patella

       ● S83.004   Unspecified dislocation of right
             patella

       ● S83.005   Unspecified dislocation of left patella

       ● S83.006   Unspecified dislocation of unspecified
             patella

     ● S83.01   Lateral subluxation and dislocation of patella

       ● S83.011   Lateral subluxation of right patella

       ● S83.012   Lateral subluxation of left patella

       ● S83.013   Lateral subluxation of unspecified
             patella

       ● S83.014   Lateral dislocation of right patella

       ● S83.015   Lateral dislocation of left patella

       ● S83.016   Lateral dislocation of unspecified
             patella

● S83.09   Other subluxation and dislocation of patella

     ● S83.091   Other subluxation of right patella

     ● S83.092   Other subluxation of left patella

     ● S83.093   Other subluxation of unspecified
           patella

     ● S83.094   Other dislocation of right patella

     ● S83.095   Other dislocation of left patella

     ● S83.096   Other dislocation of unspecified
           patella

● S83.1   Subluxation and dislocation of knee

     Excludes2   instability of knee prosthesis (T84.022,
           T84.023)

     ● S83.10   Unspecified subluxation and dislocation of
           knee

       ● S83.101   Unspecified subluxation of right knee

       ● S83.102   Unspecified subluxation of left knee

       ● S83.103   Unspecified subluxation of
             unspecified knee

       ● S83.104   Unspecified dislocation of right knee

       ● S83.105   Unspecified dislocation of left knee

       ● S83.106   Unspecified dislocation of unspecified
             knee

     ● S83.11   Anterior subluxation and dislocation of
           proximal end of tibia
           Posterior subluxation and dislocation of distal
           end of femur

       ● S83.111   Anterior subluxation of proximal end
             of tibia, right knee

       ● S83.112   Anterior subluxation of proximal end
             of tibia, left knee

       ● S83.113   Anterior subluxation of proximal end
             of tibia, unspecified knee

       ● S83.114   Anterior dislocation of proximal end
             of tibia, right knee

       ● S83.115   Anterior dislocation of proximal end
             of tibia, left knee

       ● S83.116   Anterior dislocation of proximal end
             of tibia, unspecified knee

     ● S83.12   Posterior subluxation and dislocation of
           proximal end of tibia
           Anterior dislocation of distal end of femur

       ● S83.121   Posterior subluxation of proximal end
             of tibia, right knee

       ● S83.122   Posterior subluxation of proximal end
             of tibia, left knee

       ● S83.123   Posterior subluxation of proximal end
             of tibia, unspecified knee

       ● S83.124   Posterior dislocation of proximal end
             of tibia, right knee

       ● S83.125   Posterior dislocation of proximal end
             of tibia, left knee

       ● S83.126   Posterior dislocation of proximal end
             of tibia, unspecified knee

     ● S83.13   Medial subluxation and dislocation of proximal
           end of tibia

       ● S83.131   Medial subluxation of proximal end
             of tibia, right knee

       ● S83.132   Medial subluxation of proximal end
             of tibia, left knee

       ● S83.133   Medial subluxation of proximal end
             of tibia, unspecified knee

       ● S83.134   Medial dislocation of proximal end of
             tibia, right knee

       ● S83.135   Medial dislocation of proximal end of
             tibia, left knee

       ● S83.136   Medial dislocation of proximal end of
             tibia, unspecified knee

N Newborn Age: 0   **P** Pediatric Age: 0–17   **M** Maternity DX: 9–64   **A** Adult Age: 15–124   ♀ Females Only   ♂ Males Only

🔵 Complication\Comorbidity   🔵 Major C\C   (Ex) CC/MCC Exclusions   🔵 Hospital-Acquired Condition   🔵 Hierarchical Condition Category

1405

● **S83.14**   Lateral subluxation and dislocation of proximal end of tibia
- ● S83.141   Lateral subluxation of proximal end of tibia, right knee
- ● S83.142   Lateral subluxation of proximal end of tibia, left knee
- ● S83.143   Lateral subluxation of proximal end of tibia, unspecified knee
- ● S83.144   Lateral dislocation of proximal end of tibia, right knee
- ● S83.145   Lateral dislocation of proximal end of tibia, left knee
- ● S83.146   Lateral dislocation of proximal end of tibia, unspecified knee

● **S83.19**   Other subluxation and dislocation of knee
- ● S83.191   Other subluxation of right knee
- ● S83.192   Other subluxation of left knee
- ● S83.193   Other subluxation of unspecified knee
- ● S83.194   Other dislocation of right knee
- ● S83.195   Other dislocation of left knee
- ● S83.196   Other dislocation of unspecified knee

● **S83.2**   Tear of meniscus, current injury

> **Excludes1**   old bucket-handle tear (M23.2)

● **S83.20**   Tear of unspecified meniscus, current injury
> Tear of meniscus of knee NOS
- ● S83.200   Bucket-handle tear of unspecified meniscus, current injury, right knee
- ● S83.201   Bucket-handle tear of unspecified meniscus, current injury, left knee
- ● S83.202   Bucket-handle tear of unspecified meniscus, current injury, unspecified knee
- ● S83.203   Other tear of unspecified meniscus, current injury, right knee
- ● S83.204   Other tear of unspecified meniscus, current injury, left knee
- ● S83.205   Other tear of unspecified meniscus, current injury, unspecified knee
- ● S83.206   Unspecified tear of unspecified meniscus, current injury, right knee
- ● S83.207   Unspecified tear of unspecified meniscus, current injury, left knee
- ● S83.209   Unspecified tear of unspecified meniscus, current injury, unspecified knee

● **S83.21**   Bucket-handle tear of medial meniscus, current injury
- ● S83.211   Bucket-handle tear of medial meniscus, current injury, right knee
- ● S83.212   Bucket-handle tear of medial meniscus, current injury, left knee
- ● S83.219   Bucket-handle tear of medial meniscus, current injury, unspecified knee

● **S83.22**   Peripheral tear of medial meniscus, current injury
- ● S83.221   Peripheral tear of medial meniscus, current injury, right knee
- ● S83.222   Peripheral tear of medial meniscus, current injury, left knee
- ● S83.229   Peripheral tear of medial meniscus, current injury, unspecified knee

● **S83.23**   Complex tear of medial meniscus, current injury
- ● S83.231   Complex tear of medial meniscus, current injury, right knee
- ● S83.232   Complex tear of medial meniscus, current injury, left knee
> Coding Clinic: 2019, Q2, P26
- ● S83.239   Complex tear of medial meniscus, current injury, unspecified knee

● **S83.24**   Other tear of medial meniscus, current injury
- ● S83.241   Other tear of medial meniscus, current injury, right knee
- ● S83.242   Other tear of medial meniscus, current injury, left knee
- ● S83.249   Other tear of medial meniscus, current injury, unspecified knee

● **S83.25**   Bucket-handle tear of lateral meniscus, current injury
- ● S83.251   Bucket-handle tear of lateral meniscus, current injury, right knee
- ● S83.252   Bucket-handle tear of lateral meniscus, current injury, left knee
- ● S83.259   Bucket-handle tear of lateral meniscus, current injury, unspecified knee

● **S83.26**   Peripheral tear of lateral meniscus, current injury
- ● S83.261   Peripheral tear of lateral meniscus, current injury, right knee
- ● S83.262   Peripheral tear of lateral meniscus, current injury, left knee
- ● S83.269   Peripheral tear of lateral meniscus, current injury, unspecified knee

● **S83.27**   Complex tear of lateral meniscus, current injury
- ● S83.271   Complex tear of lateral meniscus, current injury, right knee
- ● S83.272   Complex tear of lateral meniscus, current injury, left knee
- ● S83.279   Complex tear of lateral meniscus, current injury, unspecified knee

● **S83.28**   Other tear of lateral meniscus, current injury
- ● S83.281   Other tear of lateral meniscus, current injury, right knee
- ● S83.282   Other tear of lateral meniscus, current injury, left knee
- ● S83.289   Other tear of lateral meniscus, current injury, unspecified knee

● **S83.3**   Tear of articular cartilage of knee, current
- X ● S83.30   Tear of articular cartilage of unspecified knee, current
- X ● S83.31   Tear of articular cartilage of right knee, current
- X ● S83.32   Tear of articular cartilage of left knee, current

● **S83.4**   Sprain of collateral ligament of knee
- ● S83.40   Sprain of unspecified collateral ligament of knee
  - ● S83.401   Sprain of unspecified collateral ligament of right knee
  - ● S83.402   Sprain of unspecified collateral ligament of left knee
  - ● S83.409   Sprain of unspecified collateral ligament of unspecified knee
- ● S83.41   Sprain of medial collateral ligament of knee
  > Sprain of tibial collateral ligament
  - ● S83.411   Sprain of medial collateral ligament of right knee
  - ● S83.412   Sprain of medial collateral ligament of left knee
  - ● S83.419   Sprain of medial collateral ligament of unspecified knee

● **S83.42**   Sprain of lateral collateral ligament of knee
Sprain of fibular collateral ligament

     ● **S83.421**   Sprain of lateral collateral ligament of right knee

     ● **S83.422**   Sprain of lateral collateral ligament of left knee

     ● **S83.429**   Sprain of lateral collateral ligament of unspecified knee

● **S83.5**   Sprain of cruciate ligament of knee

   ● **S83.50**   Sprain of unspecified cruciate ligament of knee

     ● **S83.501**   Sprain of unspecified cruciate ligament of right knee

     ● **S83.502**   Sprain of unspecified cruciate ligament of left knee

     ● **S83.509**   Sprain of unspecified cruciate ligament of unspecified knee

   ● **S83.51**   Sprain of anterior cruciate ligament of knee

     ● **S83.511**   Sprain of anterior cruciate ligament of right knee
         Coding Clinic: 2016, Q2, P4

     ● **S83.512**   Sprain of anterior cruciate ligament of left knee

     ● **S83.519**   Sprain of anterior cruciate ligament of unspecified knee

   ● **S83.52**   Sprain of posterior cruciate ligament of knee

     ● **S83.521**   Sprain of posterior cruciate ligament of right knee

     ● **S83.522**   Sprain of posterior cruciate ligament of left knee

     ● **S83.529**   Sprain of posterior cruciate ligament of unspecified knee

● **S83.6**   Sprain of the superior tibiofibular joint and ligament

   X● **S83.60**   Sprain of the superior tibiofibular joint and ligament, unspecified knee

   X● **S83.61**   Sprain of the superior tibiofibular joint and ligament, right knee

   X● **S83.62**   Sprain of the superior tibiofibular joint and ligament, left knee

● **S83.8**   Sprain of other specified parts of knee

   ● **S83.8X**   Sprain of other specified parts of knee

     ● **S83.8X1**   Sprain of other specified parts of right knee

     ● **S83.8X2**   Sprain of other specified parts of left knee

     ● **S83.8X9**   Sprain of other specified parts of unspecified knee

● **S83.9**   Sprain of unspecified site of knee

   X● **S83.90**   Sprain of unspecified site of unspecified knee

   X● **S83.91**   Sprain of unspecified site of right knee

   X● **S83.92**   Sprain of unspecified site of left knee

● **S84**   Injury of nerves at lower leg level

Code also any associated open wound (S81.-)

Excludes2   injury of nerves at ankle and foot level (S94.-)

The appropriate 7th character is to be added to each code from category S84

A	initial encounter
D	subsequent encounter
S	sequela

● **S84.0**   Injury of tibial nerve at lower leg level

   X● **S84.00**   Injury of tibial nerve at lower leg level, unspecified leg

   X● **S84.01**   Injury of tibial nerve at lower leg level, right leg

   X● **S84.02**   Injury of tibial nerve at lower leg level, left leg

● **S84.1**   Injury of peroneal nerve at lower leg level

   X● **S84.10**   Injury of peroneal nerve at lower leg level, unspecified leg

   X● **S84.11**   Injury of peroneal nerve at lower leg level, right leg

   X● **S84.12**   Injury of peroneal nerve at lower leg level, left leg

● **S84.2**   Injury of cutaneous sensory nerve at lower leg level

   X● **S84.20**   Injury of cutaneous sensory nerve at lower leg level, unspecified leg

   X● **S84.21**   Injury of cutaneous sensory nerve at lower leg level, right leg

   X● **S84.22**   Injury of cutaneous sensory nerve at lower leg level, left leg

● **S84.8**   Injury of other nerves at lower leg level

   ● **S84.80**   Injury of other nerves at lower leg level

     ● **S84.801**   Injury of other nerves at lower leg level, right leg

     ● **S84.802**   Injury of other nerves at lower leg level, left leg

     ● **S84.809**   Injury of other nerves at lower leg level, unspecified leg

● **S84.9**   Injury of unspecified nerve at lower leg level

   X● **S84.90**   Injury of unspecified nerve at lower leg level, unspecified leg

   X● **S84.91**   Injury of unspecified nerve at lower leg level, right leg

   X● **S84.92**   Injury of unspecified nerve at lower leg level, left leg

● **S85**   Injury of blood vessels at lower leg level

Code also any associated open wound (S81.-)

Excludes2   injury of blood vessels at ankle and foot level (S95.-)

The appropriate 7th character is to be added to each code from category S85

A	initial encounter
D	subsequent encounter
S	sequela

● **S85.0**   Injury of popliteal artery

   ● **S85.00**   Unspecified injury of popliteal artery

     ● **S85.001**   Unspecified injury of popliteal artery, right leg A 🦠
         (Ex) See PDX Collection 1349

     ● **S85.002**   Unspecified injury of popliteal artery, left leg A 🦠
         (Ex) See PDX Collection 1350

     ● **S85.009**   Unspecified injury of popliteal artery, unspecified leg A 🦠
         (Ex) See PDX Collection 1351

   ● **S85.01**   Laceration of popliteal artery

     ● **S85.011**   Laceration of popliteal artery, right leg A 🦠
         (Ex) See PDX Collection 1349

     ● **S85.012**   Laceration of popliteal artery, left leg A 🦠
         (Ex) See PDX Collection 1350

     ● **S85.019**   Laceration of popliteal artery, unspecified leg A 🦠
         (Ex) See PDX Collection 1351

CHAPTER 19 (S00-T88)

N Newborn Age: 0   **P** Pediatric Age: 0–17   **M** Maternity DX: 9–64   **A** Adult Age: 15–124   ♀ Females Only   ♂ Males Only

🦠 Complication\Comorbidity   🦠 Major C\C   (Ex) CC/MCC Exclusions   🦠 Hospital-Acquired Condition   🦠 Hierarchical Condition Category

1407

CHAPTER 19 (S00-T88)

● S85.09   Other specified injury of popliteal artery
   ● S85.091   Other specified injury of popliteal artery, right leg A 🔒
       (Ex:) See PDX Collection 1349
   ● S85.092   Other specified injury of popliteal artery, left leg A 🔒
       (Ex:) See PDX Collection 1350
   ● S85.099   Other specified injury of popliteal artery, unspecified leg A 🔒
       (Ex:) See PDX Collection 1351

● S85.1   Injury of tibial artery
  ● S85.10   Unspecified injury of unspecified tibial artery
      Injury of tibial artery NOS
   ● S85.101   Unspecified injury of unspecified tibial artery, right leg A 🔒
       (Ex:) See PDX Collection 1352
   ● S85.102   Unspecified injury of unspecified tibial artery, left leg A 🔒
       (Ex:) See PDX Collection 1353
   ● S85.109   Unspecified injury of unspecified tibial artery, unspecified leg A 🔒
       (Ex:) See PDX Collection 1354
  ● S85.11   Laceration of unspecified tibial artery
   ● S85.111   Laceration of unspecified tibial artery, right leg A 🔒
       (Ex:) See PDX Collection 1352
   ● S85.112   Laceration of unspecified tibial artery, left leg A 🔒
       (Ex:) See PDX Collection 1353
   ● S85.119   Laceration of unspecified tibial artery, unspecified leg A 🔒
       (Ex:) See PDX Collection 1354
  ● S85.12   Other specified injury of unspecified tibial artery
   ● S85.121   Other specified injury of unspecified tibial artery, right leg A 🔒
       (Ex:) See PDX Collection 1352
   ● S85.122   Other specified injury of unspecified tibial artery, left leg A 🔒
       (Ex:) See PDX Collection 1353
   ● S85.129   Other specified injury of unspecified tibial artery, unspecified leg A 🔒
       (Ex:) See PDX Collection 1354
  ● S85.13   Unspecified injury of anterior tibial artery
   ● S85.131   Unspecified injury of anterior tibial artery, right leg A 🔒
       (Ex:) See PDX Collection 1355
   ● S85.132   Unspecified injury of anterior tibial artery, left leg A 🔒
       (Ex:) See PDX Collection 1356
   ● S85.139   Unspecified injury of anterior tibial artery, unspecified leg A 🔒
       (Ex:) See PDX Collection 1357
  ● S85.14   Laceration of anterior tibial artery
   ● S85.141   Laceration of anterior tibial artery, right leg A 🔒
       (Ex:) See PDX Collection 1355
   ● S85.142   Laceration of anterior tibial artery, left leg A 🔒
       (Ex:) See PDX Collection 1356
   ● S85.149   Laceration of anterior tibial artery, unspecified leg A 🔒
       (Ex:) See PDX Collection 1357

● S85.15   Other specified injury of anterior tibial artery
   ● S85.151   Other specified injury of anterior tibial artery, right leg A 🔒
       (Ex:) See PDX Collection 1355
   ● S85.152   Other specified injury of anterior tibial artery, left leg A 🔒
       (Ex:) See PDX Collection 1356
   ● S85.159   Other specified injury of anterior tibial artery, unspecified leg A 🔒
       (Ex:) See PDX Collection 1357
● S85.16   Unspecified injury of posterior tibial artery
   ● S85.161   Unspecified injury of posterior tibial artery, right leg A 🔒
       (Ex:) See PDX Collection 1358
   ● S85.162   Unspecified injury of posterior tibial artery, left leg A 🔒
       (Ex:) See PDX Collection 1359
   ● S85.169   Unspecified injury of posterior tibial artery, unspecified leg A 🔒
       (Ex:) See PDX Collection 1360
● S85.17   Laceration of posterior tibial artery
   ● S85.171   Laceration of posterior tibial artery, right leg A 🔒
       (Ex:) See PDX Collection 1358
   ● S85.172   Laceration of posterior tibial artery, left leg A 🔒
       (Ex:) See PDX Collection 1359
   ● S85.179   Laceration of posterior tibial artery, unspecified leg A 🔒
       (Ex:) See PDX Collection 1360
● S85.18   Other specified injury of posterior tibial artery
   ● S85.181   Other specified injury of posterior tibial artery, right leg A 🔒
       (Ex:) See PDX Collection 1358
   ● S85.182   Other specified injury of posterior tibial artery, left leg A 🔒
       (Ex:) See PDX Collection 1359
   ● S85.189   Other specified injury of posterior tibial artery, unspecified leg A 🔒
       (Ex:) See PDX Collection 1360
● S85.2   Injury of peroneal artery
  ● S85.20   Unspecified injury of peroneal artery
   ● S85.201   Unspecified injury of peroneal artery, right leg A 🔒
       (Ex:) See PDX Collection 1325
   ● S85.202   Unspecified injury of peroneal artery, left leg A 🔒
       (Ex:) See PDX Collection 1326
   ● S85.209   Unspecified injury of peroneal artery, unspecified leg A 🔒
       (Ex:) See PDX Collection 1327
  ● S85.21   Laceration of peroneal artery
   ● S85.211   Laceration of peroneal artery, right leg A 🔒
       (Ex:) See PDX Collection 1325
   ● S85.212   Laceration of peroneal artery, left leg A 🔒
       (Ex:) See PDX Collection 1326
   ● S85.219   Laceration of peroneal artery, unspecified leg A 🔒
       (Ex:) See PDX Collection 1327

▶ New   ⇒ Revised   ~~Deleted~~ Deleted   Excludes 1   Excludes 2   Includes   Use additional   Code first   Code also   Key words
OGCR Official Guidelines   ● Unacceptable Principal Diagnosis   X Assign placeholder X   ● Use Additional Character(s)   ▶ Manifestation Code   Coding Clinic

- S85.29   Other specified injury of peroneal artery
  - S85.291   Other specified injury of peroneal artery, right leg A 🔹
    (Ex:) See PDX Collection 1325
  - S85.292   Other specified injury of peroneal artery, left leg A 🔹
    (Ex:) See PDX Collection 1326
  - S85.299   Other specified injury of peroneal artery, unspecified leg A 🔹
    (Ex:) See PDX Collection 1327
- S85.3   Injury of greater saphenous vein at lower leg level
  Injury of greater saphenous vein NOS
  Injury of saphenous vein NOS
  - S85.30   Unspecified injury of greater saphenous vein at lower leg level
    - S85.301   Unspecified injury of greater saphenous vein at lower leg level, right leg A 🔹
      (Ex:) See PDX Collection 1322
    - S85.302   Unspecified injury of greater saphenous vein at lower leg level, left leg A 🔹
      (Ex:) See PDX Collection 1323
    - S85.309   Unspecified injury of greater saphenous vein at lower leg level, unspecified leg A 🔹
      (Ex:) See PDX Collection 1324
  - S85.31   Laceration of greater saphenous vein at lower leg level
    - S85.311   Laceration of greater saphenous vein at lower leg level, right leg A 🔹
      (Ex:) See PDX Collection 1322
    - S85.312   Laceration of greater saphenous vein at lower leg level, left leg A 🔹
      (Ex:) See PDX Collection 1323
    - S85.319   Laceration of greater saphenous vein at lower leg level, unspecified leg A 🔹
      (Ex:) See PDX Collection 1324
  - S85.39   Other specified injury of greater saphenous vein at lower leg level
    - S85.391   Other specified injury of greater saphenous vein at lower leg level, right leg A 🔹
      (Ex:) See PDX Collection 1322
    - S85.392   Other specified injury of greater saphenous vein at lower leg level, left leg A 🔹
      (Ex:) See PDX Collection 1323
    - S85.399   Other specified injury of greater saphenous vein at lower leg level, unspecified leg A 🔹
      (Ex:) See PDX Collection 1324
- S85.4   Injury of lesser saphenous vein at lower leg level
  - S85.40   Unspecified injury of lesser saphenous vein at lower leg level
    - S85.401   Unspecified injury of lesser saphenous vein at lower leg level, right leg A 🔹
      (Ex:) See PDX Collection 1322
    - S85.402   Unspecified injury of lesser saphenous vein at lower leg level, left leg A 🔹
      (Ex:) See PDX Collection 1323
    - S85.409   Unspecified injury of lesser saphenous vein at lower leg level, unspecified leg A 🔹
      (Ex:) See PDX Collection 1324

- S85.41   Laceration of lesser saphenous vein at lower leg level
  - S85.411   Laceration of lesser saphenous vein at lower leg level, right leg A 🔹
    (Ex:) See PDX Collection 1322
  - S85.412   Laceration of lesser saphenous vein at lower leg level, left leg A 🔹
    (Ex:) See PDX Collection 1323
  - S85.419   Laceration of lesser saphenous vein at lower leg level, unspecified leg A 🔹
    (Ex:) See PDX Collection 1324
- S85.49   Other specified injury of lesser saphenous vein at lower leg level
  - S85.491   Other specified injury of lesser saphenous vein at lower leg level, right leg A 🔹
    (Ex:) See PDX Collection 1322
  - S85.492   Other specified injury of lesser saphenous vein at lower leg level, left leg A 🔹
    (Ex:) See PDX Collection 1323
  - S85.499   Other specified injury of lesser saphenous vein at lower leg level, unspecified leg A 🔹
    (Ex:) See PDX Collection 1324
- S85.5   Injury of popliteal vein
  - S85.50   Unspecified injury of popliteal vein
    - S85.501   Unspecified injury of popliteal vein, right leg A 🔹
      (Ex:) See PDX Collection 1361
    - S85.502   Unspecified injury of popliteal vein, left leg A 🔹
      (Ex:) See PDX Collection 1362
    - S85.509   Unspecified injury of popliteal vein, unspecified leg A 🔹
      (Ex:) See PDX Collection 1363
  - S85.51   Laceration of popliteal vein
    - S85.511   Laceration of popliteal vein, right leg A 🔹
      (Ex:) See PDX Collection 1361
    - S85.512   Laceration of popliteal vein, left leg A 🔹
      (Ex:) See PDX Collection 1362
    - S85.519   Laceration of popliteal vein, unspecified leg A 🔹
      (Ex:) See PDX Collection 1363
  - S85.59   Other specified injury of popliteal vein
    - S85.591   Other specified injury of popliteal vein, right leg A 🔹
      (Ex:) See PDX Collection 1361
    - S85.592   Other specified injury of popliteal vein, left leg A 🔹
      (Ex:) See PDX Collection 1362
    - S85.599   Other specified injury of popliteal vein, unspecified leg A 🔹
      (Ex:) See PDX Collection 1363
- S85.8   Injury of other blood vessels at lower leg level
  - S85.80   Unspecified injury of other blood vessels at lower leg level
    - S85.801   Unspecified injury of other blood vessels at lower leg level, right leg A 🔹
      (Ex:) See PDX Collection 1325
    - S85.802   Unspecified injury of other blood vessels at lower leg level, left leg A 🔹
      (Ex:) See PDX Collection 1326
    - S85.809   Unspecified injury of other blood vessels at lower leg level, unspecified leg A 🔹
      (Ex:) See PDX Collection 1327

N   Newborn Age: 0   **P**   Pediatric Age: 0–17   **M**   Maternity DX: 9–64   **A**   Adult Age: 15–124   ♀   Females Only   ♂   Males Only

🔹   Complication\Comorbidity   🔹   Major C\C   (Ex:)   CC/MCC Exclusions   🔹   Hospital-Acquired Condition   🔹   Hierarchical Condition Category

● **S85.81** **Laceration** of other blood vessels at lower leg level

  ● **S85.811** Laceration of other blood vessels at lower leg level, **right leg** A 🔗
    (Ex:) See PDX Collection 1325

  ● **S85.812** Laceration of other blood vessels at lower leg level, **left leg** A 🔗
    (Ex:) See PDX Collection 1326

  ● **S85.819** Laceration of other blood vessels at lower leg level, **unspecified leg** A 🔗
    (Ex:) See PDX Collection 1327

● **S85.89** **Other** specified injury of other blood vessels at lower leg level

  ● **S85.891** Other specified injury of other blood vessels at lower leg level, **right leg** A 🔗
    (Ex:) See PDX Collection 1325

  ● **S85.892** Other specified injury of other blood vessels at lower leg level, **left leg** A 🔗
    (Ex:) See PDX Collection 1326

  ● **S85.899** Other specified injury of other blood vessels at lower leg level, **unspecified leg** A 🔗
    (Ex:) See PDX Collection 1327

● **S85.9** Injury of **unspecified blood vessel** at lower leg level

  ● **S85.90** **Unspecified** injury of unspecified blood vessel at lower leg level

    ● **S85.901** Unspecified injury of unspecified blood vessel at lower leg level, **right leg** A 🔗
      (Ex:) See PDX Collection 1325

    ● **S85.902** Unspecified injury of unspecified blood vessel at lower leg level, **left leg** A 🔗
      (Ex:) See PDX Collection 1326

    ● **S85.909** Unspecified injury of unspecified blood vessel at lower leg level, **unspecified leg** A 🔗
      (Ex:) See PDX Collection 1327

  ● **S85.91** **Laceration** of unspecified blood vessel at lower leg level

    ● **S85.911** Laceration of unspecified blood vessel at lower leg level, **right leg** A 🔗
      (Ex:) See PDX Collection 1325

    ● **S85.912** Laceration of unspecified blood vessel at lower leg level, **left leg** A 🔗
      (Ex:) See PDX Collection 1326

    ● **S85.919** Laceration of unspecified blood vessel at lower leg level, **unspecified leg** A 🔗
      (Ex:) See PDX Collection 1327

  ● **S85.99** **Other** specified injury of unspecified blood vessel at lower leg level

    ● **S85.991** Other specified injury of unspecified blood vessel at lower leg level, **right leg** A 🔗
      (Ex:) See PDX Collection 1325

    ● **S85.992** Other specified injury of unspecified blood vessel at lower leg level, **left leg** A 🔗
      (Ex:) See PDX Collection 1326

    ● **S85.999** Other specified injury of unspecified blood vessel at lower leg level, **unspecified leg** A 🔗
      (Ex:) See PDX Collection 1327

● **S86** Injury of muscle, fascia and tendon at lower leg level

Code also any associated open wound (S81.-)

> **Excludes2** injury of muscle, fascia and tendon at ankle (S96.-)
> injury of patellar ligament (tendon) (S76.1-)
> sprain of joints and ligaments of knee (S83.-)

The appropriate 7th character is to be added to each code from category S86

A	initial encounter
D	subsequent encounter
S	sequela

● **S86.0** Injury of **Achilles tendon**

  ● **S86.00** **Unspecified** injury of Achilles tendon

    ● **S86.001** Unspecified injury of **right** Achilles tendon

    ● **S86.002** Unspecified injury of **left** Achilles tendon

    ● **S86.009** Unspecified injury of **unspecified** Achilles tendon

  ● **S86.01** **Strain** of Achilles tendon

    ● **S86.011** Strain of **right** Achilles tendon

    ● **S86.012** Strain of **left** Achilles tendon

    ● **S86.019** Strain of **unspecified** Achilles tendon

  ● **S86.02** **Laceration** of Achilles tendon

    ● **S86.021** Laceration of **right** Achilles tendon A 🔗
      (Ex:) See PDX Collection 1364

    ● **S86.022** Laceration of **left** Achilles tendon A 🔗
      (Ex:) See PDX Collection 1365

    ● **S86.029** Laceration of **unspecified** Achilles tendon A 🔗
      (Ex:) See PDX Collection 1366

  ● **S86.09** **Other** specified injury of Achilles tendon

    ● **S86.091** Other specified injury of **right** Achilles tendon

    ● **S86.092** Other specified injury of **left** Achilles tendon

    ● **S86.099** Other specified injury of **unspecified** Achilles tendon

● **S86.1** Injury of other muscle(s) and tendon(s) of **posterior muscle group** at lower leg level

  ● **S86.10** **Unspecified** injury of other muscle(s) and tendon(s) of posterior muscle group at lower leg level

    ● **S86.101** Unspecified injury of other muscle(s) and tendon(s) of posterior muscle group at lower leg level, **right leg**

    ● **S86.102** Unspecified injury of other muscle(s) and tendon(s) of posterior muscle group at lower leg level, **left leg**

    ● **S86.109** Unspecified injury of other muscle(s) and tendon(s) of posterior muscle group at lower leg level, **unspecified leg**

  ● **S86.11** **Strain** of other muscle(s) and tendon(s) of posterior muscle group at lower leg level

    ● **S86.111** Strain of other muscle(s) and tendon(s) of posterior muscle group at lower leg level, **right leg**

    ● **S86.112** Strain of other muscle(s) and tendon(s) of posterior muscle group at lower leg level, **left leg**

    ● **S86.119** Strain of other muscle(s) and tendon(s) of posterior muscle group at lower leg level, **unspecified leg**

● S86.12   Laceration of other muscle(s) and tendon(s) of posterior muscle group at lower leg level
   ● S86.121   Laceration of other muscle(s) and tendon(s) of posterior muscle group at lower leg level, right leg A 🅒
      Ⓔⓧ See PDX Collection 1364
   ● S86.122   Laceration of other muscle(s) and tendon(s) of posterior muscle group at lower leg level, left leg A 🅒
      Ⓔⓧ See PDX Collection 1365
   ● S86.129   Laceration of other muscle(s) and tendon(s) of posterior muscle group at lower leg level, unspecified leg A 🅒
      Ⓔⓧ See PDX Collection 1366

● S86.19   Other injury of other muscle(s) and tendon(s) of posterior muscle group at lower leg level
   ● S86.191   Other injury of other muscle(s) and tendon(s) of posterior muscle group at lower leg level, right leg
   ● S86.192   Other injury of other muscle(s) and tendon(s) of posterior muscle group at lower leg level, left leg
   ● S86.199   Other injury of other muscle(s) and tendon(s) of posterior muscle group at lower leg level, unspecified leg

● S86.2   Injury of muscle(s) and tendon(s) of anterior muscle group at lower leg level
 ● S86.20   Unspecified injury of muscle(s) and tendon(s) of anterior muscle group at lower leg level
   ● S86.201   Unspecified injury of muscle(s) and tendon(s) of anterior muscle group at lower leg level, right leg
   ● S86.202   Unspecified injury of muscle(s) and tendon(s) of anterior muscle group at lower leg level, left leg
   ● S86.209   Unspecified injury of muscle(s) and tendon(s) of anterior muscle group at lower leg level, unspecified leg

 ● S86.21   Strain of muscle(s) and tendon(s) of anterior muscle group at lower leg level
   ● S86.211   Strain of muscle(s) and tendon(s) of anterior muscle group at lower leg level, right leg
   ● S86.212   Strain of muscle(s) and tendon(s) of anterior muscle group at lower leg level, left leg
   ● S86.219   Strain of muscle(s) and tendon(s) of anterior muscle group at lower leg level, unspecified leg

 ● S86.22   Laceration of muscle(s) and tendon(s) of anterior muscle group at lower leg level
   ● S86.221   Laceration of muscle(s) and tendon(s) of anterior muscle group at lower leg level, right leg A 🅒
      Ⓔⓧ See PDX Collection 1364
   ● S86.222   Laceration of muscle(s) and tendon(s) of anterior muscle group at lower leg level, left leg A 🅒
      Ⓔⓧ See PDX Collection 1365
   ● S86.229   Laceration of muscle(s) and tendon(s) of anterior muscle group at lower leg level, unspecified leg A 🅒
      Ⓔⓧ See PDX Collection 1366

● S86.29   Other injury of muscle(s) and tendon(s) of anterior muscle group at lower leg level
   ● S86.291   Other injury of muscle(s) and tendon(s) of anterior muscle group at lower leg level, right leg
   ● S86.292   Other injury of muscle(s) and tendon(s) of anterior muscle group at lower leg level, left leg
   ● S86.299   Other injury of muscle(s) and tendon(s) of anterior muscle group at lower leg level, unspecified leg

● S86.3   Injury of muscle(s) and tendon(s) of peroneal muscle group at lower leg level
 ● S86.30   Unspecified injury of muscle(s) and tendon(s) of peroneal muscle group at lower leg level
   ● S86.301   Unspecified injury of muscle(s) and tendon(s) of peroneal muscle group at lower leg level, right leg
   ● S86.302   Unspecified injury of muscle(s) and tendon(s) of peroneal muscle group at lower leg level, left leg
   ● S86.309   Unspecified injury of muscle(s) and tendon(s) of peroneal muscle group at lower leg level, unspecified leg

 ● S86.31   Strain of muscle(s) and tendon(s) of peroneal muscle group at lower leg level
   ● S86.311   Strain of muscle(s) and tendon(s) of peroneal muscle group at lower leg level, right leg
   ● S86.312   Strain of muscle(s) and tendon(s) of peroneal muscle group at lower leg level, left leg
   ● S86.319   Strain of muscle(s) and tendon(s) of peroneal muscle group at lower leg level, unspecified leg

 ● S86.32   Laceration of muscle(s) and tendon(s) of peroneal muscle group at lower leg level
   ● S86.321   Laceration of muscle(s) and tendon(s) of peroneal muscle group at lower leg level, right leg A 🅒
      Ⓔⓧ See PDX Collection 1364
   ● S86.322   Laceration of muscle(s) and tendon(s) of peroneal muscle group at lower leg level, left leg A 🅒
      Ⓔⓧ See PDX Collection 1365
   ● S86.329   Laceration of muscle(s) and tendon(s) of peroneal muscle group at lower leg level, unspecified leg A 🅒
      Ⓔⓧ See PDX Collection 1366

 ● S86.39   Other injury of muscle(s) and tendon(s) of peroneal muscle group at lower leg level
   ● S86.391   Other injury of muscle(s) and tendon(s) of peroneal muscle group at lower leg level, right leg
   ● S86.392   Other injury of muscle(s) and tendon(s) of peroneal muscle group at lower leg level, left leg
   ● S86.399   Other injury of muscle(s) and tendon(s) of peroneal muscle group at lower leg level, unspecified leg

● S86.8   Injury of other muscles and tendons at lower leg level
  ● S86.80   Unspecified injury of other muscles and tendons at lower leg level
    ● S86.801   Unspecified injury of other muscle(s) and tendon(s) at lower leg level, right leg
    ● S86.802   Unspecified injury of other muscle(s) and tendon(s) at lower leg level, left leg
    ● S86.809   Unspecified injury of other muscle(s) and tendon(s) at lower leg level, unspecified leg
  ● S86.81   Strain of other muscles and tendons at lower leg level
    ● S86.811   Strain of other muscle(s) and tendon(s) at lower leg level, right leg
    ● S86.812   Strain of other muscle(s) and tendon(s) at lower leg level, left leg
    ● S86.819   Strain of other muscle(s) and tendon(s) at lower leg level, unspecified leg
  ● S86.82   Laceration of other muscles and tendons at lower leg level
    ● S86.821   Laceration of other muscle(s) and tendon(s) at lower leg level, right leg A 🔧
        (Ex:) See PDX Collection 1364
    ● S86.822   Laceration of other muscle(s) and tendon(s) at lower leg level, left leg A 🔧
        (Ex:) See PDX Collection 1365
    ● S86.829   Laceration of other muscle(s) and tendon(s) at lower leg level, unspecified leg A 🔧
        (Ex:) See PDX Collection 1366
  ● S86.89   Other injury of other muscles and tendons at lower leg level
    ● S86.891   Other injury of other muscle(s) and tendon(s) at lower leg level, right leg
    ● S86.892   Other injury of other muscle(s) and tendon(s) at lower leg level, left leg
    ● S86.899   Other injury of other muscle(s) and tendon(s) at lower leg level, unspecified leg
● S86.9   Injury of unspecified muscle and tendon at lower leg level
  ● S86.90   Unspecified injury of unspecified muscle and tendon at lower leg level
    ● S86.901   Unspecified injury of unspecified muscle(s) and tendon(s) at lower leg level, right leg
    ● S86.902   Unspecified injury of unspecified muscle(s) and tendon(s) at lower leg level, left leg
    ● S86.909   Unspecified injury of unspecified muscle(s) and tendon(s) at lower leg level, unspecified leg
  ● S86.91   Strain of unspecified muscle and tendon at lower leg level
    ● S86.911   Strain of unspecified muscle(s) and tendon(s) at lower leg level, right leg
    ● S86.912   Strain of unspecified muscle(s) and tendon(s) at lower leg level, left leg
    ● S86.919   Strain of unspecified muscle(s) and tendon(s) at lower leg level, unspecified leg

● S86.92   Laceration of unspecified muscle and tendon at lower leg level
    ● S86.921   Laceration of unspecified muscle(s) and tendon(s) at lower leg level, right leg A 🔧
        (Ex:) See PDX Collection 1364
    ● S86.922   Laceration of unspecified muscle(s) and tendon(s) at lower leg level, left leg A 🔧
        (Ex:) See PDX Collection 1365
    ● S86.929   Laceration of unspecified muscle(s) and tendon(s) at lower leg level, unspecified leg A 🔧
        (Ex:) See PDX Collection 1366
  ● S86.99   Other injury of unspecified muscle and tendon at lower leg level
    ● S86.991   Other injury of unspecified muscle(s) and tendon(s) at lower leg level, right leg
    ● S86.992   Other injury of unspecified muscle(s) and tendon(s) at lower leg level, left leg
    ● S86.999   Other injury of unspecified muscle(s) and tendon(s) at lower leg level, unspecified leg

● S87   Crushing injury of lower leg
  Use additional code(s) for all associated injuries
  Excludes2   crushing injury of ankle and foot (S97.-)
  The appropriate 7th character is to be added to each code from category S87

A	initial encounter
D	subsequent encounter
S	sequela

  ● S87.0   Crushing injury of knee
  X ● S87.00   Crushing injury of unspecified knee
  X ● S87.01   Crushing injury of right knee
  X ● S87.02   Crushing injury of left knee
  ● S87.8   Crushing injury of lower leg
  X ● S87.80   Crushing injury of unspecified lower leg
  X ● S87.81   Crushing injury of right lower leg
  X ● S87.82   Crushing injury of left lower leg

● S88   Traumatic amputation of lower leg
  An amputation not identified as partial or complete should be coded to complete
  Excludes1   traumatic amputation of ankle and foot (S98.-)
  The appropriate 7th character is to be added to each code from category S88

A	initial encounter
D	subsequent encounter
S	sequela

  ● S88.0   Traumatic amputation at knee level
    ● S88.01   Complete traumatic amputation at knee level
      ● S88.011   Complete traumatic amputation at knee level, right lower leg A 🔧, A, D, S 🔧
        (Ex:) See PDX Collection 1333
      ● S88.012   Complete traumatic amputation at knee level, left lower leg A 🔧, A, D, S 🔧
        (Ex:) See PDX Collection 1334
      ● S88.019   Complete traumatic amputation at knee level, unspecified lower leg A 🔧, A, D, S 🔧
        (Ex:) See PDX Collection 1335

▶ New   ⇒ Revised   deleted Deleted   Excludes 1   Excludes 2   Includes   Use additional   Code first   Code also   Key words
OGCR Official Guidelines   ● Unacceptable Principal Diagnosis   X Assign placeholder X   ● Use Additional Character(s)   ▷ Manifestation Code   Coding Clinic

● **S88.02**   Partial traumatic amputation at knee level

   ● **S88.021**   Partial traumatic amputation at knee level, right lower leg A 🎗, A, D, S 🎗
      (Ex:) See PDX Collection 1333

   ● **S88.022**   Partial traumatic amputation at knee level, left lower leg A 🎗, A, D, S 🎗
      (Ex:) See PDX Collection 1334

   ● **S88.029**   Partial traumatic amputation at knee level, unspecified lower leg A 🎗, A, D, S 🎗
      (Ex:) See PDX Collection 1335

● **S88.1**   Traumatic amputation at level between knee and ankle

  ● **S88.11**   Complete traumatic amputation at level between knee and ankle

   ● **S88.111**   Complete traumatic amputation at level between knee and ankle, right lower leg A 🎗, A, D, S 🎗
      (Ex:) See PDX Collection 1333

   ● **S88.112**   Complete traumatic amputation at level between knee and ankle, left lower leg A 🎗, A, D, S 🎗
      (Ex:) See PDX Collection 1334

   ● **S88.119**   Complete traumatic amputation at level between knee and ankle, unspecified lower leg A 🎗, A, D, S 🎗
      (Ex:) See PDX Collection 1335

  ● **S88.12**   Partial traumatic amputation at level between knee and ankle

   ● **S88.121**   Partial traumatic amputation at level between knee and ankle, right lower leg A 🎗, A, D, S 🎗
      (Ex:) See PDX Collection 1333

   ● **S88.122**   Partial traumatic amputation at level between knee and ankle, left lower leg A 🎗, A, D, S 🎗
      (Ex:) See PDX Collection 1334

   ● **S88.129**   Partial traumatic amputation at level between knee and ankle, unspecified lower leg A 🎗, A, D, S 🎗
      (Ex:) See PDX Collection 1335

● **S88.9**   Traumatic amputation of lower leg, level unspecified

  ● **S88.91**   Complete traumatic amputation of lower leg, level unspecified

   ● **S88.911**   Complete traumatic amputation of right lower leg, level unspecified A 🎗, A, D, S 🎗
      (Ex:) See PDX Collection 1333

   ● **S88.912**   Complete traumatic amputation of left lower leg, level unspecified A 🎗, A, D, S 🎗
      (Ex:) See PDX Collection 1334

   ● **S88.919**   Complete traumatic amputation of unspecified lower leg, level unspecified A 🎗, A, D, S 🎗
      (Ex:) See PDX Collection 1335

  ● **S88.92**   Partial traumatic amputation of lower leg, level unspecified

   ● **S88.921**   Partial traumatic amputation of right lower leg, level unspecified A 🎗, A, D, S 🎗
      (Ex:) See PDX Collection 1333

   ● **S88.922**   Partial traumatic amputation of left lower leg, level unspecified A 🎗, A, D, S 🎗
      (Ex:) See PDX Collection 1334

   ● **S88.929**   Partial traumatic amputation of unspecified lower leg, level unspecified A 🎗, A, D, S 🎗
      (Ex:) See PDX Collection 1335

● **S89**   Other and unspecified injuries of lower leg

  Note: A fracture not indicated as open or closed should be coded to closed

  Excludes2   other and unspecified injuries of ankle and foot (S99.-)

  The appropriate 7th character is to be added to each code from subcategories S89.0, S89.1, S89.2, and S89.3

A	initial encounter for closed fracture
D	subsequent encounter for fracture with routine healing
G	subsequent encounter for fracture with delayed healing
K	subsequent encounter for fracture with nonunion
P	subsequent encounter for fracture with malunion
S	sequela

● **S89.0**   Physeal fracture of upper end of tibia

  ● **S89.00**   Unspecified physeal fracture of upper end of tibia

   ● **S89.001**   Unspecified physeal fracture of upper end of right tibia A, K, P 🎗, A 🎗
      (Ex:) For S89.001[A]: See PDX Collection 1340
      For S89.001[K,P]: See PDX Collection 897

   ● **S89.002**   Unspecified physeal fracture of upper end of left tibia A, K, P 🎗, A 🎗
      (Ex:) For S89.002[A]: See PDX Collection 1342
      For S89.002[K,P]: See PDX Collection 897

   ● **S89.009**   Unspecified physeal fracture of upper end of unspecified tibia A, K, P 🎗, A 🎗
      (Ex:) For S89.009[A]: See PDX Collection 1341
      For S89.009[K,P]: See PDX Collection 897

  ● **S89.01**   Salter-Harris Type I physeal fracture of upper end of tibia

   ● **S89.011**   Salter-Harris Type I physeal fracture of upper end of right tibia A, K, P 🎗, A 🎗
      (Ex:) For S89.011[A]: See PDX Collection 1340
      For S89.011[K,P]: See PDX Collection 897

   ● **S89.012**   Salter-Harris Type I physeal fracture of upper end of left tibia A, K, P 🎗, A 🎗
      (Ex:) For S89.012[A]: See PDX Collection 1342
      For S89.012[K,P]: See PDX Collection 897

   ● **S89.019**   Salter-Harris Type I physeal fracture of upper end of unspecified tibia A, K, P 🎗, A 🎗
      (Ex:) For S89.019[A]: See PDX Collection 1341
      For S89.019[K,P]: See PDX Collection 897

  ● **S89.02**   Salter-Harris Type II physeal fracture of upper end of tibia

   ● **S89.021**   Salter-Harris Type II physeal fracture of upper end of right tibia A, K, P 🎗, A 🎗
      (Ex:) For S89.021[A]: See PDX Collection 1340
      For S89.021[K,P]: See PDX Collection 897

   ● **S89.022**   Salter-Harris Type II physeal fracture of upper end of left tibia A, K, P 🎗, A 🎗
      (Ex:) For S89.022[A]: See PDX Collection 1342
      For S89.022[K,P]: See PDX Collection 897

   ● **S89.029**   Salter-Harris Type II physeal fracture of upper end of unspecified tibia A, K, P 🎗, A 🎗
      (Ex:) For S89.029[A]: See PDX Collection 1341
      For S89.029[K,P]: See PDX Collection 897

CHAPTER 19 (S00-T88)

N Newborn Age: 0   **P** Pediatric Age: 0–17   **M** Maternity DX: 9–64   **A** Adult Age: 15–124   ♀ Females Only   ♂ Males Only

🎗 Complication\Comorbidity   🎗 Major C\C   (Ex:) CC/MCC Exclusions   🎗 Hospital-Acquired Condition   🎗 Hierarchical Condition Category

1413

- S89.03   Salter-Harris Type III physeal fracture of upper end of tibia
  - S89.031   Salter-Harris Type III physeal fracture of upper end of right tibia A, K, P 🔵, A ⚕
    - (Ex:) **For S89.031[A]:** See PDX Collection 1340
    - **For S89.031[K,P]:** See PDX Collection 897
  - S89.032   Salter-Harris Type III physeal fracture of upper end of left tibia A, K, P 🔵, A ⚕
    - (Ex:) **For S89.032[A]:** See PDX Collection 1342
    - **For S89.032[K,P]:** See PDX Collection 897
  - S89.039   Salter-Harris Type III physeal fracture of upper end of unspecified tibia A, K, P 🔵, A ⚕
    - (Ex:) **For S89.039[A]:** See PDX Collection 1341
    - **For S89.039[K,P]:** See PDX Collection 897
- S89.04   Salter-Harris Type IV physeal fracture of upper end of tibia
  - S89.041   Salter-Harris Type IV physeal fracture of upper end of right tibia A, K, P 🔵, A ⚕
    - (Ex:) **For S89.041[A]:** See PDX Collection 1340
    - **For S89.041[K,P]:** See PDX Collection 897
  - S89.042   Salter-Harris Type IV physeal fracture of upper end of left tibia A, K, P 🔵, A ⚕
    - (Ex:) **For S89.042[A]:** See PDX Collection 1342
    - **For S89.042[K,P]:** See PDX Collection 897
  - S89.049   Salter-Harris Type IV physeal fracture of upper end of unspecified tibia A, K, P 🔵, A ⚕
    - (Ex:) **For S89.049[A]:** See PDX Collection 1341
    - **For S89.049[K,P]:** See PDX Collection 897
- S89.09   Other physeal fracture of upper end of tibia
  - S89.091   Other physeal fracture of upper end of right tibia A, K, P 🔵, A ⚕
    - (Ex:) **For S89.091[A]:** See PDX Collection 1340
    - **For S89.091[K,P]:** See PDX Collection 897
  - S89.092   Other physeal fracture of upper end of left tibia A, K, P 🔵, A ⚕
    - (Ex:) **For S89.092[A]:** See PDX Collection 1342
    - **For S89.092[K,P]:** See PDX Collection 897
  - S89.099   Other physeal fracture of upper end of unspecified tibia A, K, P 🔵, A ⚕
    - (Ex:) **For S89.099[A]:** See PDX Collection 1341
    - **For S89.099[K,P]:** See PDX Collection 897
- S89.1   Physeal fracture of lower end of tibia
  - (Ex:) **For category S89.1 CC codes:** See PDX Collection 897
  - S89.10   Unspecified physeal fracture of lower end of tibia
    - S89.101   Unspecified physeal fracture of lower end of right tibia K, P ⚕
    - S89.102   Unspecified physeal fracture of lower end of left tibia K, P ⚕
    - S89.109   Unspecified physeal fracture of lower end of unspecified tibia K, P ⚕
  - S89.11   Salter-Harris Type I physeal fracture of lower end of tibia
    - S89.111   Salter-Harris Type I physeal fracture of lower end of right tibia K, P ⚕
    - S89.112   Salter-Harris Type I physeal fracture of lower end of left tibia K, P ⚕
    - S89.119   Salter-Harris Type I physeal fracture of lower end of unspecified tibia K, P ⚕

- S89.12   Salter-Harris Type II physeal fracture of lower end of tibia
  - S89.121   Salter-Harris Type II physeal fracture of lower end of right tibia K, P ⚕
  - S89.122   Salter-Harris Type II physeal fracture of lower end of left tibia K, P ⚕
  - S89.129   Salter-Harris Type II physeal fracture of lower end of unspecified tibia K, P ⚕
- S89.13   Salter-Harris Type III physeal fracture of lower end of tibia
  - **Excludes1**   fracture of medial malleolus (adult) (S82.5-)
  - S89.131   Salter-Harris Type III physeal fracture of lower end of right tibia K, P ⚕
  - S89.132   Salter-Harris Type III physeal fracture of lower end of left tibia K, P ⚕
  - S89.139   Salter-Harris Type III physeal fracture of lower end of unspecified tibia K, P ⚕
- S89.14   Salter-Harris Type IV physeal fracture of lower end of tibia
  - **Excludes1**   fracture of medial malleolus (adult) (S82.5-)
  - S89.141   Salter-Harris Type IV physeal fracture of lower end of right tibia K, P ⚕
  - S89.142   Salter-Harris Type IV physeal fracture of lower end of left tibia K, P ⚕
  - S89.149   Salter-Harris Type IV physeal fracture of lower end of unspecified tibia K, P ⚕
- S89.19   Other physeal fracture of lower end of tibia
  - S89.191   Other physeal fracture of lower end of right tibia K, P ⚕
  - S89.192   Other physeal fracture of lower end of left tibia K, P ⚕
  - S89.199   Other physeal fracture of lower end of unspecified tibia K, P ⚕
- S89.2   Physeal fracture of upper end of fibula
  - (Ex:) **For category S89.2 CC codes:** See PDX Collection 897
  - S89.20   Unspecified physeal fracture of upper end of fibula
    - S89.201   Unspecified physeal fracture of upper end of right fibula K, P ⚕
    - S89.202   Unspecified physeal fracture of upper end of left fibula K, P ⚕
    - S89.209   Unspecified physeal fracture of upper end of unspecified fibula K, P ⚕
  - S89.21   Salter-Harris Type I physeal fracture of upper end of fibula
    - S89.211   Salter-Harris Type I physeal fracture of upper end of right fibula K, P ⚕
    - S89.212   Salter-Harris Type I physeal fracture of upper end of left fibula K, P ⚕
    - S89.219   Salter-Harris Type I physeal fracture of upper end of unspecified fibula K, P ⚕
  - S89.22   Salter-Harris Type II physeal fracture of upper end of fibula
    - S89.221   Salter-Harris Type II physeal fracture of upper end of right fibula K, P ⚕
    - S89.222   Salter-Harris Type II physeal fracture of upper end of left fibula K, P ⚕
    - S89.229   Salter-Harris Type II physeal fracture of upper end of unspecified fibula K, P ⚕

▶ New   ⇒ Revised   ~~deleted~~ Deleted   Excludes 1   Excludes 2   Includes   Use additional   Code first   Code also   Key words

OGCR Official Guidelines   ● Unacceptable Principal Diagnosis   X Assign placeholder X   ● Use Additional Character(s)   ▌ Manifestation Code   **Coding Clinic**

● S89.29   Other physeal fracture of upper end of fibula
     ● S89.291   Other physeal fracture of upper end of right fibula K, P 🦠
     ● S89.292   Other physeal fracture of upper end of left fibula K, P 🦠
     ● S89.299   Other physeal fracture of upper end of unspecified fibula K, P 🦠

● S89.3   Physeal fracture of lower end of fibula
    (Ex) For category S89.3 CC codes: See PDX Collection 897
    ● S89.30   Unspecified physeal fracture of lower end of fibula
     ● S89.301   Unspecified physeal fracture of lower end of right fibula K, P 🦠
     ● S89.302   Unspecified physeal fracture of lower end of left fibula K, P 🦠
     ● S89.309   Unspecified physeal fracture of lower end of unspecified fibula K, P 🦠
    ● S89.31   Salter-Harris Type I physeal fracture of lower end of fibula
     ● S89.311   Salter-Harris Type I physeal fracture of lower end of right fibula K, P 🦠
     ● S89.312   Salter-Harris Type I physeal fracture of lower end of left fibula K, P 🦠
     ● S89.319   Salter-Harris Type I physeal fracture of lower end of unspecified fibula K, P 🦠
    ● S89.32   Salter-Harris Type II physeal fracture of lower end of fibula
     ● S89.321   Salter-Harris Type II physeal fracture of lower end of right fibula K, P 🦠
     ● S89.322   Salter-Harris Type II physeal fracture of lower end of left fibula K, P 🦠
     ● S89.329   Salter-Harris Type II physeal fracture of lower end of unspecified fibula K, P 🦠
    ● S89.39   Other physeal fracture of lower end of fibula
     ● S89.391   Other physeal fracture of lower end of right fibula K, P 🦠
     ● S89.392   Other physeal fracture of lower end of left fibula K, P 🦠
     ● S89.399   Other physeal fracture of lower end of unspecified fibula K, P 🦠

● S89.8   Other specified injuries of lower leg
    The appropriate 7th character is to be added to each code in subcategory S89.8

A	initial encounter
D	subsequent encounter
S	sequela

    X ● S89.80   Other specified injuries of unspecified lower leg
    X ● S89.81   Other specified injuries of right lower leg
    X ● S89.82   Other specified injuries of left lower leg

● S89.9   Unspecified injury of lower leg
    The appropriate 7th character is to be added to each code in subcategory S89.9

A	initial encounter
D	subsequent encounter
S	sequela

    X ● S89.90   Unspecified injury of unspecified lower leg
    X ● S89.91   Unspecified injury of right lower leg
    X ● S89.92   Unspecified injury of left lower leg

INJURIES TO THE ANKLE AND FOOT (S90-S99)

Excludes2   burns and corrosions (T20-T32)
            fracture of ankle and malleolus (S82.-)
            frostbite (T33-T34)
            insect bite or sting, venomous (T63.4)

● S90   Superficial injury of ankle, foot and toes
    The appropriate 7th character is to be added to each code from category S90

A	initial encounter
D	subsequent encounter
S	sequela

    ● S90.0   Contusion of ankle
    X ● S90.00   Contusion of unspecified ankle
    X ● S90.01   Contusion of right ankle
    X ● S90.02   Contusion of left ankle
    ● S90.1   Contusion of toe without damage to nail
     ● S90.11   Contusion of great toe without damage to nail
      ● S90.111   Contusion of right great toe without damage to nail
      ● S90.112   Contusion of left great toe without damage to nail
      ● S90.119   Contusion of unspecified great toe without damage to nail
     ● S90.12   Contusion of lesser toe without damage to nail
      ● S90.121   Contusion of right lesser toe(s) without damage to nail
      ● S90.122   Contusion of left lesser toe(s) without damage to nail
      ● S90.129   Contusion of unspecified lesser toe(s) without damage to nail
          Contusion of toe NOS
    ● S90.2   Contusion of toe with damage to nail
     ● S90.21   Contusion of great toe with damage to nail
      ● S90.211   Contusion of right great toe with damage to nail
      ● S90.212   Contusion of left great toe with damage to nail
      ● S90.219   Contusion of unspecified great toe with damage to nail
     ● S90.22   Contusion of lesser toe with damage to nail
      ● S90.221   Contusion of right lesser toe(s) with damage to nail
      ● S90.222   Contusion of left lesser toe(s) with damage to nail
      ● S90.229   Contusion of unspecified lesser toe(s) with damage to nail
    ● S90.3   Contusion of foot
     Excludes2   contusion of toes (S90.1-, S90.2-)
    X ● S90.30   Contusion of unspecified foot
          Contusion of foot NOS
    X ● S90.31   Contusion of right foot
    X ● S90.32   Contusion of left foot
    ● S90.4   Other superficial injuries of toe
     ● S90.41   Abrasion of toe
      ● S90.411   Abrasion, right great toe
      ● S90.412   Abrasion, left great toe
      ● S90.413   Abrasion, unspecified great toe
      ● S90.414   Abrasion, right lesser toe(s)
      ● S90.415   Abrasion, left lesser toe(s)
      ● S90.416   Abrasion, unspecified lesser toe(s)

CHAPTER 19 (S00-T88)

N   Newborn Age: 0   P   Pediatric Age: 0–17   M   Maternity DX: 9–64   A   Adult Age: 15–124   ♀   Females Only   ♂   Males Only

🦠   Complication\Comorbidity   🦠   Major C\C   (Ex)   CC/MCC Exclusions   🦠   Hospital-Acquired Condition   🦠   Hierarchical Condition Category

1415

● **S90.42**   Blister (nonthermal) of toe
- ● **S90.421**   Blister (nonthermal), right great toe
- ● **S90.422**   Blister (nonthermal), left great toe
- ● **S90.423**   Blister (nonthermal), unspecified great toe
- ● **S90.424**   Blister (nonthermal), right lesser toe(s)
- ● **S90.425**   Blister (nonthermal), left lesser toe(s)
- ● **S90.426**   Blister (nonthermal), unspecified lesser toe(s)

● **S90.44**   External constriction of toe
    Hair tourniquet syndrome of toe
- ● **S90.441**   External constriction, right great toe
- ● **S90.442**   External constriction, left great toe
- ● **S90.443**   External constriction, unspecified great toe
- ● **S90.444**   External constriction, right lesser toe(s)
- ● **S90.445**   External constriction, left lesser toe(s)
- ● **S90.446**   External constriction, unspecified lesser toe(s)

● **S90.45**   Superficial foreign body of toe
    Splinter in the toe
- ● **S90.451**   Superficial foreign body, right great toe
- ● **S90.452**   Superficial foreign body, left great toe
- ● **S90.453**   Superficial foreign body, unspecified great toe
- ● **S90.454**   Superficial foreign body, right lesser toe(s)
- ● **S90.455**   Superficial foreign body, left lesser toe(s)
- ● **S90.456**   Superficial foreign body, unspecified lesser toe(s)

● **S90.46**   Insect bite (nonvenomous) of toe
- ● **S90.461**   Insect bite (nonvenomous), right great toe
- ● **S90.462**   Insect bite (nonvenomous), left great toe
- ● **S90.463**   Insect bite (nonvenomous), unspecified great toe
- ● **S90.464**   Insect bite (nonvenomous), right lesser toe(s)
- ● **S90.465**   Insect bite (nonvenomous), left lesser toe(s)
- ● **S90.466**   Insect bite (nonvenomous), unspecified lesser toe(s)

● **S90.47**   Other superficial bite of toe
    Excludes1   open bite of toe (S91.15-, S91.25-)
- ● **S90.471**   Other superficial bite of right great toe
- ● **S90.472**   Other superficial bite of left great toe
- ● **S90.473**   Other superficial bite of unspecified great toe
- ● **S90.474**   Other superficial bite of right lesser toe(s)
- ● **S90.475**   Other superficial bite of left lesser toe(s)
- ● **S90.476**   Other superficial bite of unspecified lesser toe(s)

● **S90.5**   Other superficial injuries of ankle
● **S90.51**   Abrasion of ankle
- ● **S90.511**   Abrasion, right ankle
- ● **S90.512**   Abrasion, left ankle
- ● **S90.519**   Abrasion, unspecified ankle

● **S90.52**   Blister (nonthermal) of ankle
- ● **S90.521**   Blister (nonthermal), right ankle
- ● **S90.522**   Blister (nonthermal), left ankle
- ● **S90.529**   Blister (nonthermal), unspecified ankle

● **S90.54**   External constriction of ankle
- ● **S90.541**   External constriction, right ankle
- ● **S90.542**   External constriction, left ankle
- ● **S90.549**   External constriction, unspecified ankle

● **S90.55**   Superficial foreign body of ankle
    Splinter in the ankle
- ● **S90.551**   Superficial foreign body, right ankle
- ● **S90.552**   Superficial foreign body, left ankle
- ● **S90.559**   Superficial foreign body, unspecified ankle

● **S90.56**   Insect bite (nonvenomous) of ankle
- ● **S90.561**   Insect bite (nonvenomous), right ankle
- ● **S90.562**   Insect bite (nonvenomous), left ankle
- ● **S90.569**   Insect bite (nonvenomous), unspecified ankle

● **S90.57**   Other superficial bite of ankle
    Excludes1   open bite of ankle (S91.05-)
- ● **S90.571**   Other superficial bite of ankle, right ankle
- ● **S90.572**   Other superficial bite of ankle, left ankle
- ● **S90.579**   Other superficial bite of ankle, unspecified ankle

● **S90.8**   Other superficial injuries of foot
● **S90.81**   Abrasion of foot
- ● **S90.811**   Abrasion, right foot
- ● **S90.812**   Abrasion, left foot
- ● **S90.819**   Abrasion, unspecified foot

● **S90.82**   Blister (nonthermal) of foot
- ● **S90.821**   Blister (nonthermal), right foot
- ● **S90.822**   Blister (nonthermal), left foot
- ● **S90.829**   Blister (nonthermal), unspecified foot

● **S90.84**   External constriction of foot
- ● **S90.841**   External constriction, right foot
- ● **S90.842**   External constriction, left foot
- ● **S90.849**   External constriction, unspecified foot

● **S90.85**   Superficial foreign body of foot
    Splinter in the foot
- ● **S90.851**   Superficial foreign body, right foot
- ● **S90.852**   Superficial foreign body, left foot
- ● **S90.859**   Superficial foreign body, unspecified foot

● **S90.86**   Insect bite (nonvenomous) of foot
- ● **S90.861**   Insect bite (nonvenomous), right foot
- ● **S90.862**   Insect bite (nonvenomous), left foot
- ● **S90.869**   Insect bite (nonvenomous), unspecified foot

● **S90.87**   Other superficial bite of foot
    Excludes1   open bite of foot (S91.35-)
- ● **S90.871**   Other superficial bite of right foot
- ● **S90.872**   Other superficial bite of left foot
- ● **S90.879**   Other superficial bite of unspecified foot

▶ New   ⇒ Revised   ~~deleted~~ Deleted   Excludes 1   Excludes 2   Includes   Use additional   Code first   Code also   Key words
OGCR Official Guidelines   ● Unacceptable Principal Diagnosis   X Assign placeholder X   ● Use Additional Character(s)   ▸ Manifestation Code   **Coding Clinic**

● **S90.9**   Unspecified superficial injury of ankle, foot and toe
   ● **S90.91**   Unspecified superficial injury of ankle
      ● **S90.911**   Unspecified superficial injury of right ankle
      ● **S90.912**   Unspecified superficial injury of left ankle
      ● **S90.919**   Unspecified superficial injury of unspecified ankle
   ● **S90.92**   Unspecified superficial injury of foot
      ● **S90.921**   Unspecified superficial injury of right foot
      ● **S90.922**   Unspecified superficial injury of left foot
      ● **S90.929**   Unspecified superficial injury of unspecified foot
   ● **S90.93**   Unspecified superficial injury of toes
      ● **S90.931**   Unspecified superficial injury of right great toe
      ● **S90.932**   Unspecified superficial injury of left great toe
      ● **S90.933**   Unspecified superficial injury of unspecified great toe
      ● **S90.934**   Unspecified superficial injury of right lesser toe(s)
      ● **S90.935**   Unspecified superficial injury of left lesser toe(s)
      ● **S90.936**   Unspecified superficial injury of unspecified lesser toe(s)

● **S91**   Open wound of ankle, foot and toes
   Code also any associated wound infection
   Excludes1   open fracture of ankle, foot and toes (S92.-with 7th character B)
                 traumatic amputation of ankle and foot (S98.-)
   The appropriate 7th character is to be added to each code from category S91

A	initial encounter
D	subsequent encounter
S	sequela

   ⊜ **S91.0**   Open wound of ankle
     ● **S91.00**   Unspecified open wound of ankle
        ● **S91.001**   Unspecified open wound, right ankle
        ● **S91.002**   Unspecified open wound, left ankle
        ● **S91.009**   Unspecified open wound, unspecified ankle
     ● **S91.01**   Laceration without foreign body of ankle
        ● **S91.011**   Laceration without foreign body, right ankle
        ● **S91.012**   Laceration without foreign body, left ankle
            Coding Clinic: 2021, Q1, P8
        ● **S91.019**   Laceration without foreign body, unspecified ankle
     ● **S91.02**   Laceration with foreign body of ankle
        ● **S91.021**   Laceration with foreign body, right ankle
        ● **S91.022**   Laceration with foreign body, left ankle
        ● **S91.029**   Laceration with foreign body, unspecified ankle
     ● **S91.03**   Puncture wound without foreign body of ankle
        ● **S91.031**   Puncture wound without foreign body, right ankle
        ● **S91.032**   Puncture wound without foreign body, left ankle
        ● **S91.039**   Puncture wound without foreign body, unspecified ankle

     ● **S91.04**   Puncture wound with foreign body of ankle
        ● **S91.041**   Puncture wound with foreign body, right ankle
        ● **S91.042**   Puncture wound with foreign body, left ankle
        ● **S91.049**   Puncture wound with foreign body, unspecified ankle
     ● **S91.05**   Open bite of ankle
        Excludes1   superficial bite of ankle (S90.56-, S90.57-)
        ● **S91.051**   Open bite, right ankle
        ● **S91.052**   Open bite, left ankle
        ● **S91.059**   Open bite, unspecified ankle
  ● **S91.1**   Open wound of toe without damage to nail
    ● **S91.10**   Unspecified open wound of toe without damage to nail
      ● **S91.101**   Unspecified open wound of right great toe without damage to nail
      ● **S91.102**   Unspecified open wound of left great toe without damage to nail
      ● **S91.103**   Unspecified open wound of unspecified great toe without damage to nail
      ● **S91.104**   Unspecified open wound of right lesser toe(s) without damage to nail
      ● **S91.105**   Unspecified open wound of left lesser toe(s) without damage to nail
      ● **S91.106**   Unspecified open wound of unspecified lesser toe(s) without damage to nail
      ● **S91.109**   Unspecified open wound of unspecified toe(s) without damage to nail
    ● **S91.11**   Laceration without foreign body of toe without damage to nail
      ● **S91.111**   Laceration without foreign body of right great toe without damage to nail
      ● **S91.112**   Laceration without foreign body of left great toe without damage to nail
      ● **S91.113**   Laceration without foreign body of unspecified great toe without damage to nail
      ● **S91.114**   Laceration without foreign body of right lesser toe(s) without damage to nail
      ● **S91.115**   Laceration without foreign body of left lesser toe(s) without damage to nail
      ● **S91.116**   Laceration without foreign body of unspecified lesser toe(s) without damage to nail
      ● **S91.119**   Laceration without foreign body of unspecified toe without damage to nail
    ● **S91.12**   Laceration with foreign body of toe without damage to nail
      ● **S91.121**   Laceration with foreign body of right great toe without damage to nail
      ● **S91.122**   Laceration with foreign body of left great toe without damage to nail
      ● **S91.123**   Laceration with foreign body of unspecified great toe without damage to nail
      ● **S91.124**   Laceration with foreign body of right lesser toe(s) without damage to nail

N Newborn Age: 0   **P** Pediatric Age: 0–17   **M** Maternity DX: 9–64   **A** Adult Age: 15–124   ♀ Females Only   ♂ Males Only
🅒 Complication\Comorbidity   🅒 Major C\C   (Ex) CC/MCC Exclusions   🅒 Hospital-Acquired Condition   🅒 Hierarchical Condition Category
1417

CHAPTER 19 (S00-T88)

- S91.125 Laceration with foreign body of left lesser toe(s) without damage to nail
- S91.126 Laceration with foreign body of unspecified lesser toe(s) without damage to nail
- S91.129 Laceration with foreign body of unspecified toe(s) without damage to nail

- S91.13 Puncture wound without foreign body of toe without damage to nail
  - S91.131 Puncture wound without foreign body of right great toe without damage to nail
  - S91.132 Puncture wound without foreign body of left great toe without damage to nail
  - S91.133 Puncture wound without foreign body of unspecified great toe without damage to nail
  - S91.134 Puncture wound without foreign body of right lesser toe(s) without damage to nail
  - S91.135 Puncture wound without foreign body of left lesser toe(s) without damage to nail
  - S91.136 Puncture wound without foreign body of unspecified lesser toe(s) without damage to nail
  - S91.139 Puncture wound without foreign body of unspecified toe(s) without damage to nail

- S91.14 Puncture wound with foreign body of toe without damage to nail
  - S91.141 Puncture wound with foreign body of right great toe without damage to nail
  - S91.142 Puncture wound with foreign body of left great toe without damage to nail
  - S91.143 Puncture wound with foreign body of unspecified great toe without damage to nail
  - S91.144 Puncture wound with foreign body of right lesser toe(s) without damage to nail
  - S91.145 Puncture wound with foreign body of left lesser toe(s) without damage to nail
  - S91.146 Puncture wound with foreign body of unspecified lesser toe(s) without damage to nail
  - S91.149 Puncture wound with foreign body of unspecified toe(s) without damage to nail

- S91.15 Open bite of toe without damage to nail
    Bite of toe NOS
    Excludes1   superficial bite of toe (S90.46-, S90.47-)
  - S91.151 Open bite of right great toe without damage to nail
  - S91.152 Open bite of left great toe without damage to nail
  - S91.153 Open bite of unspecified great toe without damage to nail
  - S91.154 Open bite of right lesser toe(s) without damage to nail

- S91.155 Open bite of left lesser toe(s) without damage to nail
- S91.156 Open bite of unspecified lesser toe(s) without damage to nail
- S91.159 Open bite of unspecified toe(s) without damage to nail

- S91.2 Open wound of toe with damage to nail
  - S91.20 Unspecified open wound of toe with damage to nail
    - S91.201 Unspecified open wound of right great toe with damage to nail
    - S91.202 Unspecified open wound of left great toe with damage to nail
    - S91.203 Unspecified open wound of unspecified great toe with damage to nail
    - S91.204 Unspecified open wound of right lesser toe(s) with damage to nail
    - S91.205 Unspecified open wound of left lesser toe(s) with damage to nail
    - S91.206 Unspecified open wound of unspecified lesser toe(s) with damage to nail
    - S91.209 Unspecified open wound of unspecified toe(s) with damage to nail
  - S91.21 Laceration without foreign body of toe with damage to nail
    - S91.211 Laceration without foreign body of right great toe with damage to nail
    - S91.212 Laceration without foreign body of left great toe with damage to nail
    - S91.213 Laceration without foreign body of unspecified great toe with damage to nail
    - S91.214 Laceration without foreign body of right lesser toe(s) with damage to nail
    - S91.215 Laceration without foreign body of left lesser toe(s) with damage to nail
    - S91.216 Laceration without foreign body of unspecified lesser toe(s) with damage to nail
    - S91.219 Laceration without foreign body of unspecified toe(s) with damage to nail
  - S91.22 Laceration with foreign body of toe with damage to nail
    - S91.221 Laceration with foreign body of right great toe with damage to nail
    - S91.222 Laceration with foreign body of left great toe with damage to nail
    - S91.223 Laceration with foreign body of unspecified great toe with damage to nail
    - S91.224 Laceration with foreign body of right lesser toe(s) with damage to nail
    - S91.225 Laceration with foreign body of left lesser toe(s) with damage to nail
    - S91.226 Laceration with foreign body of unspecified lesser toe(s) with damage to nail
    - S91.229 Laceration with foreign body of unspecified toe(s) with damage to nail

● S91.23　Puncture wound without foreign body of toe with damage to nail

　● S91.231　Puncture wound without foreign body of right great toe with damage to nail

　● S91.232　Puncture wound without foreign body of left great toe with damage to nail

　● S91.233　Puncture wound without foreign body of unspecified great toe with damage to nail

　● S91.234　Puncture wound without foreign body of right lesser toe(s) with damage to nail

　● S91.235　Puncture wound without foreign body of left lesser toe(s) with damage to nail

　● S91.236　Puncture wound without foreign body of unspecified lesser toe(s) with damage to nail

　● S91.239　Puncture wound without foreign body of unspecified toe(s) with damage to nail

● S91.24　Puncture wound with foreign body of toe with damage to nail

　● S91.241　Puncture wound with foreign body of right great toe with damage to nail

　● S91.242　Puncture wound with foreign body of left great toe with damage to nail

　● S91.243　Puncture wound with foreign body of unspecified great toe with damage to nail

　● S91.244　Puncture wound with foreign body of right lesser toe(s) with damage to nail

　● S91.245　Puncture wound with foreign body of left lesser toe(s) with damage to nail

　● S91.246　Puncture wound with foreign body of unspecified lesser toe(s) with damage to nail

　● S91.249　Puncture wound with foreign body of unspecified toe(s) with damage to nail

● S91.25　Open bite of toe with damage to nail
　　　　　Bite of toe with damage to nail NOS

　　Excludes1　superficial bite of toe (S90.46-, S90.47-)

　● S91.251　Open bite of right great toe with damage to nail

　● S91.252　Open bite of left great toe with damage to nail

　● S91.253　Open bite of unspecified great toe with damage to nail

　● S91.254　Open bite of right lesser toe(s) with damage to nail

　● S91.255　Open bite of left lesser toe(s) with damage to nail

　● S91.256　Open bite of unspecified lesser toe(s) with damage to nail

　● S91.259　Open bite of unspecified toe(s) with damage to nail

● S91.3　Open wound of foot

　● S91.30　Unspecified open wound of foot

　　● S91.301　Unspecified open wound, right foot

　　● S91.302　Unspecified open wound, left foot

　　● S91.309　Unspecified open wound, unspecified foot

● S91.31　Laceration without foreign body of foot

　● S91.311　Laceration without foreign body, right foot

　● S91.312　Laceration without foreign body, left foot

　● S91.319　Laceration without foreign body, unspecified foot

● S91.32　Laceration with foreign body of foot

　● S91.321　Laceration with foreign body, right foot

　● S91.322　Laceration with foreign body, left foot

　● S91.329　Laceration with foreign body, unspecified foot

● S91.33　Puncture wound without foreign body of foot

　● S91.331　Puncture wound without foreign body, right foot

　● S91.332　Puncture wound without foreign body, left foot

　● S91.339　Puncture wound without foreign body, unspecified foot

● S91.34　Puncture wound with foreign body of foot

　● S91.341　Puncture wound with foreign body, right foot

　● S91.342　Puncture wound with foreign body, left foot

　● S91.349　Puncture wound with foreign body, unspecified foot

● S91.35　Open bite of foot

　　Excludes1　superficial bite of foot (S90.86-, S90.87-)

　● S91.351　Open bite, right foot

　● S91.352　Open bite, left foot

　● S91.359　Open bite, unspecified foot

● S92　Fracture of foot and toe, except ankle

　Note:　A fracture not indicated as displaced or nondisplaced should be coded to displaced

　　A fracture not indicated as open or closed should be coded to closed

　~~**Excludes1**　traumatic amputation of ankle and foot (S98.-)~~

　Excludes2　fracture of ankle (S82.-)
　　　　　　fracture of malleolus (S82.-)
　　　　▶traumatic amputation of ankle and foot (S98.-)

　The appropriate 7th character is to be added to each code from category S92

A	initial encounter for closed fracture
B	initial encounter for open fracture
D	subsequent encounter for fracture with routine healing
G	subsequent encounter for fracture with delayed healing
K	subsequent encounter for fracture with nonunion
P	subsequent encounter for fracture with malunion
S	sequela

● S92.0　Fracture of calcaneus
　　　Heel bone　　　　　　　Os calcis

　　Excludes2　Physeal fracture of calcaneus (S99.0-)

　　(Ex) **For category S92.0 CC codes S92.0[B]:** See PDX Collection 1367
　　　For S92.0[K,P]: See PDX Collection 897

　● S92.00　Unspecified fracture of calcaneus

　　● S92.001　Unspecified fracture of right calcaneus B, K, P 🐾, B 🐾

　　● S92.002　Unspecified fracture of left calcaneus B, K, P 🐾, B 🐾

　　● S92.009　Unspecified fracture of unspecified calcaneus B, K, P 🐾, B 🐾

N Newborn Age: 0　　**P** Pediatric Age: 0–17　　**M** Maternity DX: 9–64　　**A** Adult Age: 15–124　　♀ Females Only　　♂ Males Only

🐾 Complication\Comorbidity　　🐾 Major C\C　　(Ex) CC/MCC Exclusions　　🐾 Hospital-Acquired Condition　　🐾 Hierarchical Condition Category

1419

● **S92.01** Fracture of body of calcaneus
  ● S92.011 Displaced fracture of body of right calcaneus B, K, P 🔹, B 🔹
  ● S92.012 Displaced fracture of body of left calcaneus B, K, P 🔹, B 🔹
  ● S92.013 Displaced fracture of body of unspecified calcaneus B, K, P 🔹, B 🔹
  ● S92.014 Nondisplaced fracture of body of right calcaneus B, K, P 🔹, B 🔹
  ● S92.015 Nondisplaced fracture of body of left calcaneus B, K, P 🔹, B 🔹
  ● S92.016 Nondisplaced fracture of body of unspecified calcaneus B, K, P 🔹, B 🔹

● **S92.02** Fracture of anterior process of calcaneus
  ● S92.021 Displaced fracture of anterior process of right calcaneus B, K, P 🔹, B 🔹
  ● S92.022 Displaced fracture of anterior process of left calcaneus B, K, P 🔹, B 🔹
  ● S92.023 Displaced fracture of anterior process of unspecified calcaneus B, K, P 🔹, B 🔹
  ● S92.024 Nondisplaced fracture of anterior process of right calcaneus B, K, P 🔹, B 🔹
  ● S92.025 Nondisplaced fracture of anterior process of left calcaneus B, K, P 🔹, B 🔹
  ● S92.026 Nondisplaced fracture of anterior process of unspecified calcaneus B, K, P 🔹, B 🔹

● **S92.03** Avulsion fracture of tuberosity of calcaneus
  ● S92.031 Displaced avulsion fracture of tuberosity of right calcaneus B, K, P 🔹, B 🔹
  ● S92.032 Displaced avulsion fracture of tuberosity of left calcaneus B, K, P 🔹, B 🔹
  ● S92.033 Displaced avulsion fracture of tuberosity of unspecified calcaneus B, K, P 🔹, B 🔹
  ● S92.034 Nondisplaced avulsion fracture of tuberosity of right calcaneus B, K, P 🔹, B 🔹
  ● S92.035 Nondisplaced avulsion fracture of tuberosity of left calcaneus B, K, P 🔹, B 🔹
  ● S92.036 Nondisplaced avulsion fracture of tuberosity of unspecified calcaneus B, K, P 🔹, B 🔹

● **S92.04** Other fracture of tuberosity of calcaneus
  ● S92.041 Displaced other fracture of tuberosity of right calcaneus B, K, P 🔹, B 🔹
  ● S92.042 Displaced other fracture of tuberosity of left calcaneus B, K, P 🔹, B 🔹
  ● S92.043 Displaced other fracture of tuberosity of unspecified calcaneus B, K, P 🔹, B 🔹
  ● S92.044 Nondisplaced other fracture of tuberosity of right calcaneus B, K, P 🔹, B 🔹
  ● S92.045 Nondisplaced other fracture of tuberosity of left calcaneus B, K, P 🔹, B 🔹
  ● S92.046 Nondisplaced other fracture of tuberosity of unspecified calcaneus B, K, P 🔹, B 🔹

● **S92.05** Other extraarticular fracture of calcaneus
  ● S92.051 Displaced other extraarticular fracture of right calcaneus B, K, P 🔹, B 🔹
  ● S92.052 Displaced other extraarticular fracture of left calcaneus B, K, P 🔹, B 🔹
  ● S92.053 Displaced other extraarticular fracture of unspecified calcaneus B, K, P 🔹, B 🔹
  ● S92.054 Nondisplaced other extraarticular fracture of right calcaneus B, K, P 🔹, B 🔹
  ● S92.055 Nondisplaced other extraarticular fracture of left calcaneus B, K, P 🔹, B 🔹
  ● S92.056 Nondisplaced other extraarticular fracture of unspecified calcaneus B, K, P 🔹, B 🔹

● **S92.06** Intraarticular fracture of calcaneus
  ● S92.061 Displaced intraarticular fracture of right calcaneus B, K, P 🔹, B 🔹
  ● S92.062 Displaced intraarticular fracture of left calcaneus B, K, P 🔹, B 🔹
  ● S92.063 Displaced intraarticular fracture of unspecified calcaneus B, K, P 🔹, B 🔹
  ● S92.064 Nondisplaced intraarticular fracture of right calcaneus B, K, P 🔹, B 🔹
  ● S92.065 Nondisplaced intraarticular fracture of left calcaneus B, K, P 🔹, B 🔹
  ● S92.066 Nondisplaced intraarticular fracture of unspecified calcaneus B, K, P 🔹, B 🔹

● **S92.1** Fracture of talus
  Astragalus
  Ⓔⓧ For category S92.1 CC codes S92.1[B]: See PDX Collection 1368
  For S92.1[K,P]: See PDX Collection 897
  ● **S92.10** Unspecified fracture of talus
    ● S92.101 Unspecified fracture of right talus B, K, P 🔹, B 🔹
    ● S92.102 Unspecified fracture of left talus B, K, P 🔹, B 🔹
    ● S92.109 Unspecified fracture of unspecified talus B, K, P 🔹, B 🔹
  ● **S92.11** Fracture of neck of talus
    ● S92.111 Displaced fracture of neck of right talus B, K, P 🔹, B 🔹
    ● S92.112 Displaced fracture of neck of left talus B, K, P 🔹, B 🔹
    ● S92.113 Displaced fracture of neck of unspecified talus B, K, P 🔹, B 🔹
    ● S92.114 Nondisplaced fracture of neck of right talus B, K, P 🔹, B 🔹
    ● S92.115 Nondisplaced fracture of neck of left talus B, K, P 🔹, B 🔹
    ● S92.116 Nondisplaced fracture of neck of unspecified talus B, K, P 🔹, B 🔹
  ● **S92.12** Fracture of body of talus
    ● S92.121 Displaced fracture of body of right talus B, K, P 🔹, B 🔹
    ● S92.122 Displaced fracture of body of left talus B, K, P 🔹, B 🔹
    ● S92.123 Displaced fracture of body of unspecified talus B, K, P 🔹, B 🔹
    ● S92.124 Nondisplaced fracture of body of right talus B, K, P 🔹, B 🔹
    ● S92.125 Nondisplaced fracture of body of left talus B, K, P 🔹, B 🔹
    ● S92.126 Nondisplaced fracture of body of unspecified talus B, K, P 🔹, B 🔹

▶ New ⇒ Revised ~~deleted~~ Deleted Excludes 1 Excludes 2 Includes Use additional Code first Code also Key words
OGCR Official Guidelines ● Unacceptable Principal Diagnosis X Assign placeholder X ● Use Additional Character(s) ▶ Manifestation Code Coding Clinic

● S92.13   Fracture of posterior process of talus
    ● S92.131   Displaced fracture of posterior process of right talus B, K, P 🅒, B 🅜
    ● S92.132   Displaced fracture of posterior process of left talus B, K, P 🅒, B 🅜
    ● S92.133   Displaced fracture of posterior process of unspecified talus B, K, P 🅒, B 🅜
    ● S92.134   Nondisplaced fracture of posterior process of right talus B, K, P 🅒, B 🅜
    ● S92.135   Nondisplaced fracture of posterior process of left talus B, K, P 🅒, B 🅜
    ● S92.136   Nondisplaced fracture of posterior process of unspecified talus B, K, P 🅒, B 🅜

● S92.14   Dome fracture of talus
    Excludes1   osteochondritis dissecans (M93.2)
    ● S92.141   Displaced dome fracture of right talus B, K, P 🅒, B 🅜
    ● S92.142   Displaced dome fracture of left talus B, K, P 🅒, B 🅜
    ● S92.143   Displaced dome fracture of unspecified talus B, K, P 🅒, B 🅜
    ● S92.144   Nondisplaced dome fracture of right talus B, K, P 🅒, B 🅜
    ● S92.145   Nondisplaced dome fracture of left talus B, K, P 🅒, B 🅜
    ● S92.146   Nondisplaced dome fracture of unspecified talus B, K, P 🅒, B 🅜

● S92.15   Avulsion fracture (chip fracture) of talus
    ● S92.151   Displaced avulsion fracture (chip fracture) of right talus B, K, P 🅒, B 🅜
    ● S92.152   Displaced avulsion fracture (chip fracture) of left talus B, K, P 🅒, B 🅜
    ● S92.153   Displaced avulsion fracture (chip fracture) of unspecified talus B, K, P 🅒, B 🅜
    ● S92.154   Nondisplaced avulsion fracture (chip fracture) of right talus B, K, P 🅒, B 🅜
    ● S92.155   Nondisplaced avulsion fracture (chip fracture) of left talus B, K, P 🅒, B 🅜
    ● S92.156   Nondisplaced avulsion fracture (chip fracture) of unspecified talus B, K, P 🅒, B 🅜

● S92.19   Other fracture of talus
    ● S92.191   Other fracture of right talus B, K, P 🅒, B 🅜
    ● S92.192   Other fracture of left talus B, K, P 🅒, B 🅜
    ● S92.199   Other fracture of unspecified talus B, K, P 🅒, B 🅜

● S92.2   Fracture of other and unspecified tarsal bone(s)
    (Ex) **For category S92.2 CC codes S92.2[B]:** See PDX Collection 1368
    For S92.2[K,P]: See PDX Collection 897 **unless otherwise indicated**

● S92.20   Fracture of unspecified tarsal bone(s)
    (Ex) **For category S92.20 CC codes S92.20[B]:** See PDX Collection 1369 **For S92.20[K,P]:** See PDX Collection 897
    ● S92.201   Fracture of unspecified tarsal bone(s) of right foot B, K, P 🅒, B 🅜
    ● S92.202   Fracture of unspecified tarsal bone(s) of left foot B, K, P 🅒, B 🅜
    ● S92.209   Fracture of unspecified tarsal bone(s) of unspecified foot B, K, P 🅒, B 🅜

● S92.21   Fracture of cuboid bone
    ● S92.211   Displaced fracture of cuboid bone of right foot B, K, P 🅒, B 🅜
    ● S92.212   Displaced fracture of cuboid bone of left foot B, K, P 🅒, B 🅜
    ● S92.213   Displaced fracture of cuboid bone of unspecified foot B, K, P 🅒, B 🅜
    ● S92.214   Nondisplaced fracture of cuboid bone of right foot B, K, P 🅒, B 🅜
    ● S92.215   Nondisplaced fracture of cuboid bone of left foot B, K, P 🅒, B 🅜
    ● S92.216   Nondisplaced fracture of cuboid bone of unspecified foot B, K, P 🅒, B 🅜

● S92.22   Fracture of lateral cuneiform
    ● S92.221   Displaced fracture of lateral cuneiform of right foot B, K, P 🅒, B 🅜
    ● S92.222   Displaced fracture of lateral cuneiform of left foot B, K, P 🅒, B 🅜
    ● S92.223   Displaced fracture of lateral cuneiform of unspecified foot B, K, P 🅒, B 🅜
    ● S92.224   Nondisplaced fracture of lateral cuneiform of right foot B, K, P 🅒, B 🅜
    ● S92.225   Nondisplaced fracture of lateral cuneiform of left foot B, K, P 🅒, B 🅜
    ● S92.226   Nondisplaced fracture of lateral cuneiform of unspecified foot B, K, P 🅒, B 🅜

● S92.23   Fracture of intermediate cuneiform
    ● S92.231   Displaced fracture of intermediate cuneiform of right foot B, K, P 🅒, B 🅜
    ● S92.232   Displaced fracture of intermediate cuneiform of left foot B, K, P 🅒, B 🅜
    ● S92.233   Displaced fracture of intermediate cuneiform of unspecified foot B, K, P 🅒, B 🅜
    ● S92.234   Nondisplaced fracture of intermediate cuneiform of right foot B, K, P 🅒, B 🅜
    ● S92.235   Nondisplaced fracture of intermediate cuneiform of left foot B, K, P 🅒, B 🅜
    ● S92.236   Nondisplaced fracture of intermediate cuneiform of unspecified foot B, K, P 🅒, B 🅜

● S92.24   Fracture of medial cuneiform
    ● S92.241   Displaced fracture of medial cuneiform of right foot B, K, P 🅒, B 🅜
    ● S92.242   Displaced fracture of medial cuneiform of left foot B, K, P 🅒, B 🅜
    ● S92.243   Displaced fracture of medial cuneiform of unspecified foot B, K, P 🅒, B 🅜
    ● S92.244   Nondisplaced fracture of medial cuneiform of right foot B, K, P 🅒, B 🅜
    ● S92.245   Nondisplaced fracture of medial cuneiform of left foot B, K, P 🅒, B 🅜
    ● S92.246   Nondisplaced fracture of medial cuneiform of unspecified foot B, K, P 🅒, B 🅜

N Newborn Age: 0   **P** Pediatric Age: 0–17   **M** Maternity DX: 9–64   **A** Adult Age: 15–124   ♀ Females Only   ♂ Males Only

🅒 Complication\Comorbidity   🅜 Major C\C   (Ex) CC/MCC Exclusions   🅗 Hospital-Acquired Condition   🅗 Hierarchical Condition Category

1421

CHAPTER 19 (S00-T88)

CHAPTER 19 (S00-T88)

● S92.25   Fracture of navicular [scaphoid] of foot
- ● S92.251   Displaced fracture of navicular [scaphoid] of right foot B, K, P 🝙, B 🝙
- ● S92.252   Displaced fracture of navicular [scaphoid] of left foot B, K, P 🝙, B 🝙
- ● S92.253   Displaced fracture of navicular [scaphoid] of unspecified foot B, K, P 🝙, B 🝙
- ● S92.254   Nondisplaced fracture of navicular [scaphoid] of right foot B, K, P 🝙, B 🝙
- ● S92.255   Nondisplaced fracture of navicular [scaphoid] of left foot B, K, P 🝙, B 🝙
- ● S92.256   Nondisplaced fracture of navicular [scaphoid] of unspecified foot B, K, P 🝙, B 🝙

● S92.3   Fracture of metatarsal bone(s)

> **Excludes2**   Physeal fracture of metatarsal (S99.1-)

> (Ex) **For category S92.3 CC codes S92.3[B]:** See PDX Collection 1368
> **For S92.3[K,P]:** See PDX Collection 897

- ● S92.30   Fracture of unspecified metatarsal bone(s)
  - ● S92.301   Fracture of unspecified metatarsal bone(s), right foot B, K, P 🝙, B 🝙
  - ● S92.302   Fracture of unspecified metatarsal bone(s), left foot B, K, P 🝙, B 🝙
  - ● S92.309   Fracture of unspecified metatarsal bone(s), unspecified foot B, K, P 🝙, B 🝙

- ● S92.31   Fracture of first metatarsal bone
  - ● S92.311   Displaced fracture of first metatarsal bone, right foot B, K, P 🝙, B 🝙
  - ● S92.312   Displaced fracture of first metatarsal bone, left foot B, K, P 🝙, B 🝙
  - ● S92.313   Displaced fracture of first metatarsal bone, unspecified foot B, K, P 🝙, B 🝙
  - ● S92.314   Nondisplaced fracture of first metatarsal bone, right foot B, K, P 🝙, B 🝙
  - ● S92.315   Nondisplaced fracture of first metatarsal bone, left foot B, K, P 🝙, B 🝙
  - ● S92.316   Nondisplaced fracture of first metatarsal bone, unspecified foot B, K, P 🝙, B 🝙

- ● S92.32   Fracture of second metatarsal bone
  - ● S92.321   Displaced fracture of second metatarsal bone, right foot B, K, P 🝙, B 🝙
  - ● S92.322   Displaced fracture of second metatarsal bone, left foot B, K, P 🝙, B 🝙
  - ● S92.323   Displaced fracture of second metatarsal bone, unspecified foot B, K, P 🝙, B 🝙
  - ● S92.324   Nondisplaced fracture of second metatarsal bone, right foot B, K, P 🝙, B 🝙
  - ● S92.325   Nondisplaced fracture of second metatarsal bone, left foot B, K, P 🝙, B 🝙
  - ● S92.326   Nondisplaced fracture of second metatarsal bone, unspecified foot B, K, P 🝙, B 🝙

● S92.33   Fracture of third metatarsal bone
> Coding Clinic: 2018, Q1, P3
- ● S92.331   Displaced fracture of third metatarsal bone, right foot B, K, P 🝙, B 🝙
- ● S92.332   Displaced fracture of third metatarsal bone, left foot B, K, P 🝙, B 🝙
- ● S92.333   Displaced fracture of third metatarsal bone, unspecified foot B, K, P 🝙, B 🝙
- ● S92.334   Nondisplaced fracture of third metatarsal bone, right foot B, K, P 🝙, B 🝙
- ● S92.335   Nondisplaced fracture of third metatarsal bone, left foot B, K, P 🝙, B 🝙
- ● S92.336   Nondisplaced fracture of third metatarsal bone, unspecified foot B, K, P 🝙, B 🝙

● S92.34   Fracture of fourth metatarsal bone
- ● S92.341   Displaced fracture of fourth metatarsal bone, right foot B, K, P 🝙, B 🝙
- ● S92.342   Displaced fracture of fourth metatarsal bone, left foot B, K, P 🝙, B 🝙
- ● S92.343   Displaced fracture of fourth metatarsal bone, unspecified foot B, K, P 🝙, B 🝙
- ● S92.344   Nondisplaced fracture of fourth metatarsal bone, right foot B, K, P 🝙, B 🝙
- ● S92.345   Nondisplaced fracture of fourth metatarsal bone, left foot B, K, P 🝙, B 🝙
- ● S92.346   Nondisplaced fracture of fourth metatarsal bone, unspecified foot B, K, P 🝙, B 🝙

● S92.35   Fracture of fifth metatarsal bone
- ● S92.351   Displaced fracture of fifth metatarsal bone, right foot B, K, P 🝙, B 🝙
- ● S92.352   Displaced fracture of fifth metatarsal bone, left foot B, K, P 🝙, B 🝙
- ● S92.353   Displaced fracture of fifth metatarsal bone, unspecified foot B, K, P 🝙, B 🝙
- ● S92.354   Nondisplaced fracture of fifth metatarsal bone, right foot B, K, P 🝙, B 🝙
- ● S92.355   Nondisplaced fracture of fifth metatarsal bone, left foot B, K, P 🝙, B 🝙
- ● S92.356   Nondisplaced fracture of fifth metatarsal bone, unspecified foot B, K, P 🝙, B 🝙

● S92.4   Fracture of great toe

> **Excludes2**   Physeal fracture of phalanx of toe (S99.2-)

> (Ex) **For category S92.4 CC codes:** See PDX Collection 897

- ● S92.40   Unspecified fracture of great toe
  - ● S92.401   Displaced unspecified fracture of right great toe K, P 🝙
  - ● S92.402   Displaced unspecified fracture of left great toe K, P 🝙
  - ● S92.403   Displaced unspecified fracture of unspecified great toe K, P 🝙
  - ● S92.404   Nondisplaced unspecified fracture of right great toe K, P 🝙
  - ● S92.405   Nondisplaced unspecified fracture of left great toe K, P 🝙
  - ● S92.406   Nondisplaced unspecified fracture of unspecified great toe K, P 🝙

▶ New   ⫸ Revised   ~~deleted~~ Deleted   Excludes 1   Excludes 2   Includes   Use additional   Code first   Code also   Key words

OGCR Official Guidelines   ● Unacceptable Principal Diagnosis   X Assign placeholder X   🝙 Use Additional Character(s)   〗 Manifestation Code   **Coding Clinic**

● S92.41   Fracture of proximal phalanx of great toe
- ● S92.411   Displaced fracture of proximal phalanx of right great toe K, P ●
- ● S92.412   Displaced fracture of proximal phalanx of left great toe K, P ●
- ● S92.413   Displaced fracture of proximal phalanx of unspecified great toe K, P ●
- ● S92.414   Nondisplaced fracture of proximal phalanx of right great toe K, P ●
- ● S92.415   Nondisplaced fracture of proximal phalanx of left great toe K, P ●
- ● S92.416   Nondisplaced fracture of proximal phalanx of unspecified great toe K, P ●

● S92.42   Fracture of distal phalanx of great toe
- ● S92.421   Displaced fracture of distal phalanx of right great toe K, P ●
- ● S92.422   Displaced fracture of distal phalanx of left great toe K, P ●
- ● S92.423   Displaced fracture of distal phalanx of unspecified great toe K, P ●
- ● S92.424   Nondisplaced fracture of distal phalanx of right great toe K, P ●
- ● S92.425   Nondisplaced fracture of distal phalanx of left great toe K, P ●
- ● S92.426   Nondisplaced fracture of distal phalanx of unspecified great toe K, P ●

● S92.49   Other fracture of great toe
- ● S92.491   Other fracture of right great toe K, P ●
- ● S92.492   Other fracture of left great toe K, P ●
- ● S92.499   Other fracture of unspecified great toe K, P ●

● S92.5   Fracture of lesser toe(s)

> **Excludes2**   Physeal fracture of phalanx of toe (S99.2-)
>
> (Ex:) For category S92.5 CC codes: See PDX Collection 897

● S92.50   Unspecified fracture of lesser toe(s)
- ● S92.501   Displaced unspecified fracture of right lesser toe(s) K, P ●
- ● S92.502   Displaced unspecified fracture of left lesser toe(s) K, P ●
- ● S92.503   Displaced unspecified fracture of unspecified lesser toe(s) K, P ●
- ● S92.504   Nondisplaced unspecified fracture of right lesser toe(s) K, P ●
- ● S92.505   Nondisplaced unspecified fracture of left lesser toe(s) K, P ●
- ● S92.506   Nondisplaced unspecified fracture of unspecified lesser toe(s) K, P ●

● S92.51   Fracture of proximal phalanx of lesser toe(s)
- ● S92.511   Displaced fracture of proximal phalanx of right lesser toe(s) K, P ●
- ● S92.512   Displaced fracture of proximal phalanx of left lesser toe(s) K, P ●
- ● S92.513   Displaced fracture of proximal phalanx of unspecified lesser toe(s) K, P ●
- ● S92.514   Nondisplaced fracture of proximal phalanx of right lesser toe(s) K, P ●
- ● S92.515   Nondisplaced fracture of proximal phalanx of left lesser toe(s) K, P ●
- ● S92.516   Nondisplaced fracture of proximal phalanx of unspecified lesser toe(s) K, P ●

● S92.52   Fracture of middle phalanx of lesser toe(s)
- ● S92.521   Displaced fracture of middle phalanx of right lesser toe(s) K, P ●
- ● S92.522   Displaced fracture of middle phalanx of left lesser toe(s) K, P ●
- ● S92.523   Displaced fracture of middle phalanx of unspecified lesser toe(s) K, P ●
- ● S92.524   Nondisplaced fracture of middle phalanx of right lesser toe(s) K, P ●
- ● S92.525   Nondisplaced fracture of middle phalanx of left lesser toe(s) K, P ●
- ● S92.526   Nondisplaced fracture of middle phalanx of unspecified lesser toe(s) K, P ●

● S92.53   Fracture of distal phalanx of lesser toe(s)
- ● S92.531   Displaced fracture of distal phalanx of right lesser toe(s) K, P ●
- ● S92.532   Displaced fracture of distal phalanx of left lesser toe(s) K, P ●
- ● S92.533   Displaced fracture of distal phalanx of unspecified lesser toe(s) K, P ●
- ● S92.534   Nondisplaced fracture of distal phalanx of right lesser toe(s) K, P ●
- ● S92.535   Nondisplaced fracture of distal phalanx of left lesser toe(s) K, P ●
- ● S92.536   Nondisplaced fracture of distal phalanx of unspecified lesser toe(s) K, P ●

● S92.59   Other fracture of lesser toe(s)
- ● S92.591   Other fracture of right lesser toe(s) K, P ●
- ● S92.592   Other fracture of left lesser toe(s) K, P ●
- ● S92.599   Other fracture of unspecified lesser toe(s) K, P ●

● S92.8   Other fracture of foot, except ankle

> (Ex:) For category S92.8 CC codes S92.8[B]: See PDX Collection 1369
> For S92.90[K,P]: See PDX Collection 897

● S92.81   Other fracture of foot
Sesamoid fracture of foot
Coding Clinic: 2016, Q4, P68
- ● S92.811   Other fracture of right foot B, K, P ●, B ●
- ● S92.812   Other fracture of left foot B, K, P ●, B ●
- ● S92.819   Other fracture of unspecified foot B, K, P ●, B ●

● S92.9   Unspecified fracture of foot and toe

● S92.90   Unspecified fracture of foot

> (Ex:) For category S92.90 CC codes S92.90[B]: See PDX Collection 1369 For S92.90[K,P]: See PDX Collection 897

- ● S92.901   Unspecified fracture of right foot B, K, P ●, B ●
- ● S92.902   Unspecified fracture of left foot B, K, P ●, B ●
- ● S92.909   Unspecified fracture of unspecified foot B, K, P ●, B ●

● S92.91   Unspecified fracture of toe

> (Ex:) For category S92.91 CC codes: See PDX Collection 897

- ● S92.911   Unspecified fracture of right toe(s) K, P ●
- ● S92.912   Unspecified fracture of left toe(s) K, P ●
- ● S92.919   Unspecified fracture of unspecified toe(s) K, P ●

N Newborn Age: 0   **P** Pediatric Age: 0–17   **M** Maternity DX: 9–64   **A** Adult Age: 15–124   ♀ Females Only   ♂ Males Only

● Complication\Comorbidity   ● Major C\C   (Ex:) CC/MCC Exclusions   ● Hospital-Acquired Condition   ● Hierarchical Condition Category

1423

● **S93   Dislocation and sprain of joints and ligaments at ankle, foot and toe level**

Includes   avulsion of joint or ligament of ankle, foot and toe

laceration of cartilage, joint or ligament of ankle, foot and toe

sprain of cartilage, joint or ligament of ankle, foot and toe

traumatic hemarthrosis of joint or ligament of ankle, foot and toe

traumatic rupture of joint or ligament of ankle, foot and toe

traumatic subluxation of joint or ligament of ankle, foot and toe

traumatic tear of joint or ligament of ankle, foot and toe

Code also any associated open wound

Excludes2   strain of muscle and tendon of ankle and foot (S96.-)

The appropriate 7th character is to be added to each code from category S93

A	initial encounter
D	subsequent encounter
S	sequela

● **S93.0   Subluxation and dislocation of ankle joint**

Subluxation and dislocation of astragalus

Subluxation and dislocation of fibula, lower end

Subluxation and dislocation of talus

Subluxation and dislocation of tibia, lower end

X● S93.01   Subluxation of right ankle joint

X● S93.02   Subluxation of left ankle joint

X● S93.03   Subluxation of unspecified ankle joint

X● S93.04   Dislocation of right ankle joint

X● S93.05   Dislocation of left ankle joint

X● S93.06   Dislocation of unspecified ankle joint

● **S93.1   Subluxation and dislocation of toe**

● **S93.10   Unspecified subluxation and dislocation of toe**

Dislocation of toe NOS

Subluxation of toe NOS

● S93.101   Unspecified subluxation of right toe(s)

● S93.102   Unspecified subluxation of left toe(s)

● S93.103   Unspecified subluxation of unspecified toe(s)

● S93.104   Unspecified dislocation of right toe(s)

● S93.105   Unspecified dislocation of left toe(s)

● S93.106   Unspecified dislocation of unspecified toe(s)

● **S93.11   Dislocation of interphalangeal joint**

● S93.111   Dislocation of interphalangeal joint of right great toe

● S93.112   Dislocation of interphalangeal joint of left great toe

● S93.113   Dislocation of interphalangeal joint of unspecified great toe

● S93.114   Dislocation of interphalangeal joint of right lesser toe(s)

● S93.115   Dislocation of interphalangeal joint of left lesser toe(s)

● S93.116   Dislocation of interphalangeal joint of unspecified lesser toe(s)

● S93.119   Dislocation of interphalangeal joint of unspecified toe(s)

● **S93.12   Dislocation of metatarsophalangeal joint**

● S93.121   Dislocation of metatarsophalangeal joint of right great toe

● S93.122   Dislocation of metatarsophalangeal joint of left great toe

● S93.123   Dislocation of metatarsophalangeal joint of unspecified great toe

● S93.124   Dislocation of metatarsophalangeal joint of right lesser toe(s)

● S93.125   Dislocation of metatarsophalangeal joint of left lesser toe(s)

● S93.126   Dislocation of metatarsophalangeal joint of unspecified lesser toe(s)

● S93.129   Dislocation of metatarsophalangeal joint of unspecified toe(s)

● **S93.13   Subluxation of interphalangeal joint**

● S93.131   Subluxation of interphalangeal joint of right great toe

● S93.132   Subluxation of interphalangeal joint of left great toe

● S93.133   Subluxation of interphalangeal joint of unspecified great toe

● S93.134   Subluxation of interphalangeal joint of right lesser toe(s)

● S93.135   Subluxation of interphalangeal joint of left lesser toe(s)

● S93.136   Subluxation of interphalangeal joint of unspecified lesser toe(s)

● S93.139   Subluxation of interphalangeal joint of unspecified toe(s)

● **S93.14   Subluxation of metatarsophalangeal joint**

● S93.141   Subluxation of metatarsophalangeal joint of right great toe

● S93.142   Subluxation of metatarsophalangeal joint of left great toe

● S93.143   Subluxation of metatarsophalangeal joint of unspecified great toe

● S93.144   Subluxation of metatarsophalangeal joint of right lesser toe(s)

● S93.145   Subluxation of metatarsophalangeal joint of left lesser toe(s)

● S93.146   Subluxation of metatarsophalangeal joint of unspecified lesser toe(s)

● S93.149   Subluxation of metatarsophalangeal joint of unspecified toe(s)

● **S93.3   Subluxation and dislocation of foot**

Excludes2   dislocation of toe (S93.1-)

● **S93.30   Unspecified subluxation and dislocation of foot**

Dislocation of foot NOS

Subluxation of foot NOS

● S93.301   Unspecified subluxation of right foot

● S93.302   Unspecified subluxation of left foot

● S93.303   Unspecified subluxation of unspecified foot

● S93.304   Unspecified dislocation of right foot

● S93.305   Unspecified dislocation of left foot

● S93.306   Unspecified dislocation of unspecified foot

● **S93.31   Subluxation and dislocation of tarsal joint**

● S93.311   Subluxation of tarsal joint of right foot

● S93.312   Subluxation of tarsal joint of left foot

● S93.313   Subluxation of tarsal joint of unspecified foot

● S93.314   Dislocation of tarsal joint of right foot

● S93.315   Dislocation of tarsal joint of left foot

● S93.316   Dislocation of tarsal joint of unspecified foot

▶ New   ⇒ Revised   deleted Deleted   Excludes 1   Excludes 2   Includes   Use additional   Code first   Code also   Key words

OGCR Official Guidelines   ● Unacceptable Principal Diagnosis   X Assign placeholder X   ● Use Additional Character(s)   ▷ Manifestation Code   **Coding Clinic**

● **S93.32**   Subluxation and dislocation of tarsometatarsal joint
  ● **S93.321**   Subluxation of tarsometatarsal joint of right foot
  ● **S93.322**   Subluxation of tarsometatarsal joint of left foot
  ● **S93.323**   Subluxation of tarsometatarsal joint of unspecified foot
  ● **S93.324**   Dislocation of tarsometatarsal joint of right foot
  ● **S93.325**   Dislocation of tarsometatarsal joint of left foot
  ● **S93.326**   Dislocation of tarsometatarsal joint of unspecified foot
● **S93.33**   Other subluxation and dislocation of foot
  ● **S93.331**   Other subluxation of right foot
  ● **S93.332**   Other subluxation of left foot
  ● **S93.333**   Other subluxation of unspecified foot
  ● **S93.334**   Other dislocation of right foot
  ● **S93.335**   Other dislocation of left foot
  ● **S93.336**   Other dislocation of unspecified foot
● **S93.4**   Sprain of ankle
  Injury to ligaments when one or more is stretched/torn
  Excludes2   injury of Achilles tendon (S86.0-)
  ● **S93.40**   Sprain of unspecified ligament of ankle
    Sprain of ankle NOS
    Sprained ankle NOS
    ● **S93.401**   Sprain of unspecified ligament of right ankle
    ● **S93.402**   Sprain of unspecified ligament of left ankle
    ● **S93.409**   Sprain of unspecified ligament of unspecified ankle
  ● **S93.41**   Sprain of calcaneofibular ligament
    ● **S93.411**   Sprain of calcaneofibular ligament of right ankle
    ● **S93.412**   Sprain of calcaneofibular ligament of left ankle
    ● **S93.419**   Sprain of calcaneofibular ligament of unspecified ankle
  ● **S93.42**   Sprain of deltoid ligament
    ● **S93.421**   Sprain of deltoid ligament of right ankle
    ● **S93.422**   Sprain of deltoid ligament of left ankle
    ● **S93.429**   Sprain of deltoid ligament of unspecified ankle
  ● **S93.43**   Sprain of tibiofibular ligament
    ● **S93.431**   Sprain of tibiofibular ligament of right ankle
    ● **S93.432**   Sprain of tibiofibular ligament of left ankle
    ● **S93.439**   Sprain of tibiofibular ligament of unspecified ankle
  ● **S93.49**   Sprain of other ligament of ankle
    Sprain of internal collateral ligament
    Sprain of talofibular ligament
    ● **S93.491**   Sprain of other ligament of right ankle
    ● **S93.492**   Sprain of other ligament of left ankle
    ● **S93.499**   Sprain of other ligament of unspecified ankle

● **S93.5**   Sprain of toe
  ● **S93.50**   Unspecified sprain of toe
    ● **S93.501**   Unspecified sprain of right great toe
    ● **S93.502**   Unspecified sprain of left great toe
    ● **S93.503**   Unspecified sprain of unspecified great toe
    ● **S93.504**   Unspecified sprain of right lesser toe(s)
    ● **S93.505**   Unspecified sprain of left lesser toe(s)
    ● **S93.506**   Unspecified sprain of unspecified lesser toe(s)
    ● **S93.509**   Unspecified sprain of unspecified toe(s)
  ● **S93.51**   Sprain of interphalangeal joint of toe
    ● **S93.511**   Sprain of interphalangeal joint of right great toe
    ● **S93.512**   Sprain of interphalangeal joint of left great toe
    ● **S93.513**   Sprain of interphalangeal joint of unspecified great toe
    ● **S93.514**   Sprain of interphalangeal joint of right lesser toe(s)
    ● **S93.515**   Sprain of interphalangeal joint of left lesser toe(s)
    ● **S93.516**   Sprain of interphalangeal joint of unspecified lesser toe(s)
    ● **S93.519**   Sprain of interphalangeal joint of unspecified toe(s)
  ● **S93.52**   Sprain of metatarsophalangeal joint of toe
    ● **S93.521**   Sprain of metatarsophalangeal joint of right great toe
    ● **S93.522**   Sprain of metatarsophalangeal joint of left great toe
    ● **S93.523**   Sprain of metatarsophalangeal joint of unspecified great toe
    ● **S93.524**   Sprain of metatarsophalangeal joint of right lesser toe(s)
    ● **S93.525**   Sprain of metatarsophalangeal joint of left lesser toe(s)
    ● **S93.526**   Sprain of metatarsophalangeal joint of unspecified lesser toe(s)
    ● **S93.529**   Sprain of metatarsophalangeal joint of unspecified toe(s)
● **S93.6**   Sprain of foot
  Excludes2   sprain of metatarsophalangeal joint of toe (S93.52-)
    sprain of toe (S93.5-)
  ● **S93.60**   Unspecified sprain of foot
    ● **S93.601**   Unspecified sprain of right foot
    ● **S93.602**   Unspecified sprain of left foot
    ● **S93.609**   Unspecified sprain of unspecified foot
  ● **S93.61**   Sprain of tarsal ligament of foot
    ● **S93.611**   Sprain of tarsal ligament of right foot
    ● **S93.612**   Sprain of tarsal ligament of left foot
    ● **S93.619**   Sprain of tarsal ligament of unspecified foot
  ● **S93.62**   Sprain of tarsometatarsal ligament of foot
    ● **S93.621**   Sprain of tarsometatarsal ligament of right foot
    ● **S93.622**   Sprain of tarsometatarsal ligament of left foot
    ● **S93.629**   Sprain of tarsometatarsal ligament of unspecified foot
  ● **S93.69**   Other sprain of foot
    ● **S93.691**   Other sprain of right foot
    ● **S93.692**   Other sprain of left foot
    ● **S93.699**   Other sprain of unspecified foot

CHAPTER 19 (S00-T88)

N Newborn Age: 0   **P** Pediatric Age: 0–17   **M** Maternity DX: 9–64   **A** Adult Age: 15–124   ♀ Females Only   ♂ Males Only
● Complication\Comorbidity   ● Major C\C   ⒺⓍ CC/MCC Exclusions   ● Hospital-Acquired Condition   ● Hierarchical Condition Category

1425

CHAPTER 19 (S00-T88)

● **S94**   **Injury of nerves at ankle and foot level**

The appropriate 7th character is to be added to each code from category S94

A	initial encounter
D	subsequent encounter
S	sequela

Code also any associated open wound (S91.-)

● **S94.0**   Injury of lateral plantar nerve

   X● **S94.00**   Injury of lateral plantar nerve, unspecified leg

   X● **S94.01**   Injury of lateral plantar nerve, right leg

   X● **S94.02**   Injury of lateral plantar nerve, left leg

● **S94.1**   Injury of medial plantar nerve

   X● **S94.10**   Injury of medial plantar nerve, unspecified leg

   X● **S94.11**   Injury of medial plantar nerve, right leg

   X● **S94.12**   Injury of medial plantar nerve, left leg

● **S94.2**   Injury of deep peroneal nerve at ankle and foot level

    Injury of terminal, lateral branch of deep peroneal nerve

   X● **S94.20**   Injury of deep peroneal nerve at ankle and foot level, unspecified leg

   X● **S94.21**   Injury of deep peroneal nerve at ankle and foot level, right leg

   X● **S94.22**   Injury of deep peroneal nerve at ankle and foot level, left leg

● **S94.3**   Injury of cutaneous sensory nerve at ankle and foot level

   X● **S94.30**   Injury of cutaneous sensory nerve at ankle and foot level, unspecified leg

   X● **S94.31**   Injury of cutaneous sensory nerve at ankle and foot level, right leg

   X● **S94.32**   Injury of cutaneous sensory nerve at ankle and foot level, left leg

● **S94.8**   Injury of other nerves at ankle and foot level

   ● **S94.8X**   Injury of other nerves at ankle and foot level

     ● **S94.8X1**   Injury of other nerves at ankle and foot level, right leg

     ● **S94.8X2**   Injury of other nerves at ankle and foot level, left leg

     ● **S94.8X9**   Injury of other nerves at ankle and foot level, unspecified leg

● **S94.9**   Injury of unspecified nerve at ankle and foot level

   X● **S94.90**   Injury of unspecified nerve at ankle and foot level, unspecified leg

   X● **S94.91**   Injury of unspecified nerve at ankle and foot level, right leg

   X● **S94.92**   Injury of unspecified nerve at ankle and foot level, left leg

● **S95**   **Injury of blood vessels at ankle and foot level**

Code also any associated open wound (S91.-)

   Excludes2   injury of posterior tibial artery and vein (S85.1-, S85.8-)

The appropriate 7th character is to be added to each code from category S95

A	initial encounter
D	subsequent encounter
S	sequela

● **S95.0**   Injury of dorsal artery of foot

   ● **S95.00**   Unspecified injury of dorsal artery of foot

     ● **S95.001**   Unspecified injury of dorsal artery of right foot A 🔕

       (Ex:) See PDX Collection 1325

     ● **S95.002**   Unspecified injury of dorsal artery of left foot A 🔕

       (Ex:) See PDX Collection 1326

     ● **S95.009**   Unspecified injury of dorsal artery of unspecified foot A 🔕

       (Ex:) See PDX Collection 1327

● **S95.01**   Laceration of dorsal artery of foot

   ● **S95.011**   Laceration of dorsal artery of right foot A 🔕

     (Ex:) See PDX Collection 1325

   ● **S95.012**   Laceration of dorsal artery of left foot A 🔕

     (Ex:) See PDX Collection 1326

   ● **S95.019**   Laceration of dorsal artery of unspecified foot A 🔕

     (Ex:) See PDX Collection 1327

● **S95.09**   Other specified injury of dorsal artery of foot

   ● **S95.091**   Other specified injury of dorsal artery of right foot A 🔕

     (Ex:) See PDX Collection 1325

   ● **S95.092**   Other specified injury of dorsal artery of left foot A 🔕

     (Ex:) See PDX Collection 1326

   ● **S95.099**   Other specified injury of dorsal artery of unspecified foot A 🔕

     (Ex:) See PDX Collection 1327

● **S95.1**   Injury of plantar artery of foot

   ● **S95.10**   Unspecified injury of plantar artery of foot

     ● **S95.101**   Unspecified injury of plantar artery of right foot A 🔕

       (Ex:) See PDX Collection 1370

     ● **S95.102**   Unspecified injury of plantar artery of left foot A 🔕

       (Ex:) See PDX Collection 1371

     ● **S95.109**   Unspecified injury of plantar artery of unspecified foot A 🔕

       (Ex:) See PDX Collection 1372

   ● **S95.11**   Laceration of plantar artery of foot

     ● **S95.111**   Laceration of plantar artery of right foot A 🔕

       (Ex:) See PDX Collection 1370

     ● **S95.112**   Laceration of plantar artery of left foot A 🔕

       (Ex:) See PDX Collection 1371

     ● **S95.119**   Laceration of plantar artery of unspecified foot A 🔕

       (Ex:) See PDX Collection 1372

   ● **S95.19**   Other specified injury of plantar artery of foot

     ● **S95.191**   Other specified injury of plantar artery of right foot A 🔕

       (Ex:) See PDX Collection 1370

     ● **S95.192**   Other specified injury of plantar artery of left foot A 🔕

       (Ex:) See PDX Collection 1371

     ● **S95.199**   Other specified injury of plantar artery of unspecified foot A 🔕

       (Ex:) See PDX Collection 1372

● **S95.2**   Injury of dorsal vein of foot

   ● **S95.20**   Unspecified injury of dorsal vein of foot

     ● **S95.201**   Unspecified injury of dorsal vein of right foot A 🔕

       (Ex:) See PDX Collection 1325

     ● **S95.202**   Unspecified injury of dorsal vein of left foot A 🔕

       (Ex:) See PDX Collection 1326

     ● **S95.209**   Unspecified injury of dorsal vein of unspecified foot A 🔕

       (Ex:) See PDX Collection 1327

   ● **S95.21**   Laceration of dorsal vein of foot

     ● **S95.211**   Laceration of dorsal vein of right foot A 🔕

       (Ex:) See PDX Collection 1325

     ● **S95.212**   Laceration of dorsal vein of left foot A 🔕

       (Ex:) See PDX Collection 1326

     ● **S95.219**   Laceration of dorsal vein of unspecified foot A 🔕

       (Ex:) See PDX Collection 1327

▶ New   ⇒ Revised   deleted Deleted   Excludes 1   Excludes 2   Includes   Use additional   Code first   Code also   Key words

OGCR Official Guidelines   ● Unacceptable Principal Diagnosis   X Assign placeholder X   ● Use Additional Character(s)   ▶ Manifestation Code   **Coding Clinic**

- **S95.29**   Other specified injury of dorsal vein of foot
  - **S95.291**   Other specified injury of dorsal vein of right foot A 🝋
    - (Ex:) See PDX Collection 1325
  - **S95.292**   Other specified injury of dorsal vein of left foot A 🝋
    - (Ex:) See PDX Collection 1326
  - **S95.299**   Other specified injury of dorsal vein of unspecified foot A 🝋
    - (Ex:) See PDX Collection 1327
- **S95.8**   Injury of other blood vessels at ankle and foot level
  - **S95.80**   Unspecified injury of other blood vessels at ankle and foot level
    - **S95.801**   Unspecified injury of other blood vessels at ankle and foot level, right leg A 🝋
      - (Ex:) See PDX Collection 1325
    - **S95.802**   Unspecified injury of other blood vessels at ankle and foot level, left leg A 🝋
      - (Ex:) See PDX Collection 1326
    - **S95.809**   Unspecified injury of other blood vessels at ankle and foot level, unspecified leg A 🝋
      - (Ex:) See PDX Collection 1327
  - **S95.81**   Laceration of other blood vessels at ankle and foot level
    - **S95.811**   Laceration of other blood vessels at ankle and foot level, right leg A 🝋
      - (Ex:) See PDX Collection 1325
    - **S95.812**   Laceration of other blood vessels at ankle and foot level, left leg A 🝋
      - (Ex:) See PDX Collection 1326
    - **S95.819**   Laceration of other blood vessels at ankle and foot level, unspecified leg A 🝋
      - (Ex:) See PDX Collection 1327
  - **S95.89**   Other specified injury of other blood vessels at ankle and foot level
    - **S95.891**   Other specified injury of other blood vessels at ankle and foot level, right leg A 🝋
      - (Ex:) See PDX Collection 1325
    - **S95.892**   Other specified injury of other blood vessels at ankle and foot level, left leg A 🝋
      - (Ex:) See PDX Collection 1326
    - **S95.899**   Other specified injury of other blood vessels at ankle and foot level, unspecified leg A 🝋
      - (Ex:) See PDX Collection 1327
- **S95.9**   Injury of unspecified blood vessel at ankle and foot level
  - **S95.90**   Unspecified injury of unspecified blood vessel at ankle and foot level
    - **S95.901**   Unspecified injury of unspecified blood vessel at ankle and foot level, right leg A 🝋
      - (Ex:) See PDX Collection 1325
    - **S95.902**   Unspecified injury of unspecified blood vessel at ankle and foot level, left leg A 🝋
      - (Ex:) See PDX Collection 1326
    - **S95.909**   Unspecified injury of unspecified blood vessel at ankle and foot level, unspecified leg A 🝋
      - (Ex:) See PDX Collection 1327

- **S95.91**   Laceration of unspecified blood vessel at ankle and foot level
  - **S95.911**   Laceration of unspecified blood vessel at ankle and foot level, right leg A 🝋
    - (Ex:) See PDX Collection 1325
  - **S95.912**   Laceration of unspecified blood vessel at ankle and foot level, left leg A 🝋
    - (Ex:) See PDX Collection 1326
  - **S95.919**   Laceration of unspecified blood vessel at ankle and foot level, unspecified leg A 🝋
    - (Ex:) See PDX Collection 1327
- **S95.99**   Other specified injury of unspecified blood vessel at ankle and foot level
  - **S95.991**   Other specified injury of unspecified blood vessel at ankle and foot level, right leg A 🝋
    - (Ex:) See PDX Collection 1325
  - **S95.992**   Other specified injury of unspecified blood vessel at ankle and foot level, left leg A 🝋
    - (Ex:) See PDX Collection 1326
  - **S95.999**   Other specified injury of unspecified blood vessel at ankle and foot level, unspecified leg A 🝋
    - (Ex:) See PDX Collection 1327

- **S96**   **Injury of muscle and tendon at ankle and foot level**
  - Code also any associated open wound (S91.-)
  - **Excludes2**   injury of Achilles tendon (S86.0-)
    - sprain of joints and ligaments of ankle and foot (S93.-)
  - The appropriate 7th character is to be added to each code from category S96

A	initial encounter
D	subsequent encounter
S	sequela

  - **S96.0**   Injury of muscle and tendon of long flexor muscle of toe at ankle and foot level
    - **S96.00**   Unspecified injury of muscle and tendon of long flexor muscle of toe at ankle and foot level
      - **S96.001**   Unspecified injury of muscle and tendon of long flexor muscle of toe at ankle and foot level, right foot
      - **S96.002**   Unspecified injury of muscle and tendon of long flexor muscle of toe at ankle and foot level, left foot
      - **S96.009**   Unspecified injury of muscle and tendon of long flexor muscle of toe at ankle and foot level, unspecified foot
    - **S96.01**   Strain of muscle and tendon of long flexor muscle of toe at ankle and foot level
      - **S96.011**   Strain of muscle and tendon of long flexor muscle of toe at ankle and foot level, right foot
      - **S96.012**   Strain of muscle and tendon of long flexor muscle of toe at ankle and foot level, left foot
      - **S96.019**   Strain of muscle and tendon of long flexor muscle of toe at ankle and foot level, unspecified foot

N Newborn Age: 0   **P** Pediatric Age: 0–17   **M** Maternity DX: 9–64   **A** Adult Age: 15–124   ♀ Females Only   ♂ Males Only

🝋 Complication\Comorbidity   🝋 Major C\C   (Ex:) CC/MCC Exclusions   Hospital-Acquired Condition   🝋 Hierarchical Condition Category

1427

- **S96.02** Laceration of muscle and tendon of long flexor muscle of toe at ankle and foot level
  - **S96.021** Laceration of muscle and tendon of long flexor muscle of toe at ankle and foot level, right foot A 🔵
    - (Ex:) See PDX Collection 1364
  - **S96.022** Laceration of muscle and tendon of long flexor muscle of toe at ankle and foot level, left foot A 🔵
    - (Ex:) See PDX Collection 1365
  - **S96.029** Laceration of muscle and tendon of long flexor muscle of toe at ankle and foot level, unspecified foot A 🔵
    - (Ex:) See PDX Collection 1366
- **S96.09** Other injury of muscle and tendon of long flexor muscle of toe at ankle and foot level
  - **S96.091** Other injury of muscle and tendon of long flexor muscle of toe at ankle and foot level, right foot
  - **S96.092** Other injury of muscle and tendon of long flexor muscle of toe at ankle and foot level, left foot
  - **S96.099** Other injury of muscle and tendon of long flexor muscle of toe at ankle and foot level, unspecified foot
- **S96.1** Injury of muscle and tendon of long extensor muscle of toe at ankle and foot level
  - **S96.10** Unspecified injury of muscle and tendon of long extensor muscle of toe at ankle and foot level
    - **S96.101** Unspecified injury of muscle and tendon of long extensor muscle of toe at ankle and foot level, right foot
    - **S96.102** Unspecified injury of muscle and tendon of long extensor muscle of toe at ankle and foot level, left foot
    - **S96.109** Unspecified injury of muscle and tendon of long extensor muscle of toe at ankle and foot level, unspecified foot
  - **S96.11** Strain of muscle and tendon of long extensor muscle of toe at ankle and foot level
    - **S96.111** Strain of muscle and tendon of long extensor muscle of toe at ankle and foot level, right foot
    - **S96.112** Strain of muscle and tendon of long extensor muscle of toe at ankle and foot level, left foot
    - **S96.119** Strain of muscle and tendon of long extensor muscle of toe at ankle and foot level, unspecified foot
  - **S96.12** Laceration of muscle and tendon of long extensor muscle of toe at ankle and foot level
    - **S96.121** Laceration of muscle and tendon of long extensor muscle of toe at ankle and foot level, right foot A 🔵
      - (Ex:) See PDX Collection 1364
    - **S96.122** Laceration of muscle and tendon of long extensor muscle of toe at ankle and foot level, left foot A 🔵
      - (Ex:) See PDX Collection 1365
    - **S96.129** Laceration of muscle and tendon of long extensor muscle of toe at ankle and foot level, unspecified foot A 🔵
      - (Ex:) See PDX Collection 1366

- **S96.19** Other specified injury of muscle and tendon of long extensor muscle of toe at ankle and foot level
  - **S96.191** Other specified injury of muscle and tendon of long extensor muscle of toe at ankle and foot level, right foot
  - **S96.192** Other specified injury of muscle and tendon of long extensor muscle of toe at ankle and foot level, left foot
  - **S96.199** Other specified injury of muscle and tendon of long extensor muscle of toe at ankle and foot level, unspecified foot
- **S96.2** Injury of intrinsic muscle and tendon at ankle and foot level
  - **S96.20** Unspecified injury of intrinsic muscle and tendon at ankle and foot level
    - **S96.201** Unspecified injury of intrinsic muscle and tendon at ankle and foot level, right foot
    - **S96.202** Unspecified injury of intrinsic muscle and tendon at ankle and foot level, left foot
    - **S96.209** Unspecified injury of intrinsic muscle and tendon at ankle and foot level, unspecified foot
  - **S96.21** Strain of intrinsic muscle and tendon at ankle and foot level
    - **S96.211** Strain of intrinsic muscle and tendon at ankle and foot level, right foot
    - **S96.212** Strain of intrinsic muscle and tendon at ankle and foot level, left foot
    - **S96.219** Strain of intrinsic muscle and tendon at ankle and foot level, unspecified foot
  - **S96.22** Laceration of intrinsic muscle and tendon at ankle and foot level
    - **S96.221** Laceration of intrinsic muscle and tendon at ankle and foot level, right foot A 🔵
      - (Ex:) See PDX Collection 1364
    - **S96.222** Laceration of intrinsic muscle and tendon at left ankle and foot level, left foot A 🔵
      - (Ex:) See PDX Collection 1365
    - **S96.229** Laceration of intrinsic muscle and tendon at ankle and foot level, unspecified foot A 🔵
      - (Ex:) See PDX Collection 1366
  - **S96.29** Other specified injury of intrinsic muscle and tendon at ankle and foot level
    - **S96.291** Other specified injury of intrinsic muscle and tendon at ankle and foot level, right foot
    - **S96.292** Other specified injury of intrinsic muscle and tendon at ankle and foot level, left foot
    - **S96.299** Other specified injury of intrinsic muscle and tendon at ankle and foot level, unspecified foot

● S96.8　Injury of other specified muscles and tendons at ankle and foot level

● S96.80　Unspecified injury of other specified muscles and tendons at ankle and foot level

● S96.801　Unspecified injury of other specified muscles and tendons at ankle and foot level, right foot

● S96.802　Unspecified injury of other specified muscles and tendons at ankle and foot level, left foot

● S96.809　Unspecified injury of other specified muscles and tendons at ankle and foot level, unspecified foot

● S96.81　Strain of other specified muscles and tendons at ankle and foot level

● S96.811　Strain of other specified muscles and tendons at ankle and foot level, right foot

● S96.812　Strain of other specified muscles and tendons at ankle and foot level, left foot

● S96.819　Strain of other specified muscles and tendons at ankle and foot level, unspecified foot

● S96.82　Laceration of other specified muscles and tendons at ankle and foot level

● S96.821　Laceration of other specified muscles and tendons at ankle and foot level, right foot A 🦠
Ⓔⓧ See PDX Collection 1364

● S96.822　Laceration of other specified muscles and tendons at ankle and foot level, left foot A 🦠
Ⓔⓧ See PDX Collection 1365

● S96.829　Laceration of other specified muscles and tendons at ankle and foot level, unspecified foot A 🦠
Ⓔⓧ See PDX Collection 1366

● S96.89　Other specified injury of other specified muscles and tendons at ankle and foot level

● S96.891　Other specified injury of other specified muscles and tendons at ankle and foot level, right foot

● S96.892　Other specified injury of other specified muscles and tendons at ankle and foot level, left foot

● S96.899　Other specified injury of other specified muscles and tendons at ankle and foot level, unspecified foot

● S96.9　Injury of unspecified muscle and tendon at ankle and foot level

● S96.90　Unspecified injury of unspecified muscle and tendon at ankle and foot level

● S96.901　Unspecified injury of unspecified muscle and tendon at ankle and foot level, right foot

● S96.902　Unspecified injury of unspecified muscle and tendon at ankle and foot level, left foot

● S96.909　Unspecified injury of unspecified muscle and tendon at ankle and foot level, unspecified foot

● S96.91　Strain of unspecified muscle and tendon at ankle and foot level

● S96.911　Strain of unspecified muscle and tendon at ankle and foot level, right foot

● S96.912　Strain of unspecified muscle and tendon at ankle and foot level, left foot

● S96.919　Strain of unspecified muscle and tendon at ankle and foot level, unspecified foot

● S96.92　Laceration of unspecified muscle and tendon at ankle and foot level

● S96.921　Laceration of unspecified muscle and tendon at ankle and foot level, right foot A 🦠
Ⓔⓧ See PDX Collection 1364

● S96.922　Laceration of unspecified muscle and tendon at ankle and foot level, left foot A 🦠
Ⓔⓧ See PDX Collection 1365

● S96.929　Laceration of unspecified muscle and tendon at ankle and foot level, unspecified foot A 🦠
Ⓔⓧ See PDX Collection 1366

● S96.99　Other specified injury of unspecified muscle and tendon at ankle and foot level

● S96.991　Other specified injury of unspecified muscle and tendon at ankle and foot level, right foot

● S96.992　Other specified injury of unspecified muscle and tendon at ankle and foot level, left foot

● S96.999　Other specified injury of unspecified muscle and tendon at ankle and foot level, unspecified foot

● S97　Crushing injury of ankle and foot

Use additional code(s) for all associated injuries

The appropriate 7th character is to be added to each code from category S97

> A　initial encounter
> D　subsequent encounter
> S　sequela

● S97.0　Crushing injury of ankle

X ● S97.00　Crushing injury of unspecified ankle

X ● S97.01　Crushing injury of right ankle

X ● S97.02　Crushing injury of left ankle

● S97.1　Crushing injury of toe

● S97.10　Crushing injury of unspecified toe(s)

● S97.101　Crushing injury of unspecified right toe(s)

● S97.102　Crushing injury of unspecified left toe(s)

● S97.109　Crushing injury of unspecified toe(s)
Crushing injury of toe NOS

● S97.11　Crushing injury of great toe

● S97.111　Crushing injury of right great toe

● S97.112　Crushing injury of left great toe

● S97.119　Crushing injury of unspecified great toe

● S97.12　Crushing injury of lesser toe(s)

● S97.121　Crushing injury of right lesser toe(s)

● S97.122　Crushing injury of left lesser toe(s)

● S97.129　Crushing injury of lesser toe(s), unspecified toe(s)

● S97.8　Crushing injury of foot

X ● S97.80　Crushing injury of foot, unspecified side
Crushing injury of foot NOS

X ● S97.81　Crushing injury of right foot

X ● S97.82　Crushing injury of left foot

N Newborn Age: 0　　**P** Pediatric Age: 0–17　　**M** Maternity DX: 9–64　　**A** Adult Age: 15–124　　♀ Females Only　　♂ Males Only

🦠 Complication\Comorbidity　　🦠 Major C\C　　Ⓔⓧ CC/MCC Exclusions　　🦠 Hospital-Acquired Condition　　🦠 Hierarchical Condition Category

1429

● S98　Traumatic amputation of ankle and foot

An amputation not identified as partial or complete should be coded to complete

The appropriate 7th character is to be added to each code from category S98

> A　initial encounter
> D　subsequent encounter
> S　sequela

● S98.0　Traumatic amputation of foot at ankle level
　● S98.01　Complete traumatic amputation of foot at ankle level
　　● S98.011　Complete traumatic amputation of right foot at ankle level A 🔧, A, D, S 🔧
　　　(Ex:) See PDX Collection 1333
　　● S98.012　Complete traumatic amputation of left foot at ankle level A 🔧, A, D, S 🔧
　　　(Ex:) See PDX Collection 1334
　　● S98.019　Complete traumatic amputation of unspecified foot at ankle level A 🔧, A, D, S 🔧
　　　(Ex:) See PDX Collection 1335
　● S98.02　Partial traumatic amputation of foot at ankle level
　　● S98.021　Partial traumatic amputation of right foot at ankle level A 🔧, A, D, S 🔧
　　　(Ex:) See PDX Collection 1333
　　● S98.022　Partial traumatic amputation of left foot at ankle level A 🔧, A, D, S 🔧
　　　(Ex:) See PDX Collection 1334
　　● S98.029　Partial traumatic amputation of unspecified foot at ankle level A 🔧, A, D, S 🔧
　　　(Ex:) See PDX Collection 1335

● S98.1　Traumatic amputation of one toe
　● S98.11　Complete traumatic amputation of great toe
　　● S98.111　Complete traumatic amputation of right great toe A, D, S 🔧
　　● S98.112　Complete traumatic amputation of left great toe A, D, S 🔧
　　● S98.119　Complete traumatic amputation of unspecified great toe A, D, S 🔧
　● S98.12　Partial traumatic amputation of great toe
　　● S98.121　Partial traumatic amputation of right great toe A, D, S 🔧
　　● S98.122　Partial traumatic amputation of left great toe A, D, S 🔧
　　● S98.129　Partial traumatic amputation of unspecified great toe A, D, S 🔧
　● S98.13　Complete traumatic amputation of one lesser toe
　　Traumatic amputation of toe NOS
　　● S98.131　Complete traumatic amputation of one right lesser toe A, D, S 🔧
　　● S98.132　Complete traumatic amputation of one left lesser toe A, D, S 🔧
　　● S98.139　Complete traumatic amputation of one unspecified lesser toe A, D, S 🔧
　● S98.14　Partial traumatic amputation of one lesser toe
　　● S98.141　Partial traumatic amputation of one right lesser toe A, D, S 🔧
　　● S98.142　Partial traumatic amputation of one left lesser toe A, D, S 🔧
　　● S98.149　Partial traumatic amputation of one unspecified lesser toe A, D, S 🔧

● S98.2　Traumatic amputation of two or more lesser toes
　● S98.21　Complete traumatic amputation of two or more lesser toes
　　● S98.211　Complete traumatic amputation of two or more right lesser toes A, D, S 🔧
　　● S98.212　Complete traumatic amputation of two or more left lesser toes A, D, S 🔧
　　● S98.219　Complete traumatic amputation of two or more unspecified lesser toes A, D, S 🔧
　● S98.22　Partial traumatic amputation of two or more lesser toes
　　● S98.221　Partial traumatic amputation of two or more right lesser toes A, D, S 🔧
　　● S98.222　Partial traumatic amputation of two or more left lesser toes A, D, S 🔧
　　● S98.229　Partial traumatic amputation of two or more unspecified lesser toes A, D, S 🔧

● S98.3　Traumatic amputation of midfoot
　● S98.31　Complete traumatic amputation of midfoot
　　● S98.311　Complete traumatic amputation of right midfoot A 🔧, A, D, S 🔧
　　　(Ex:) See PDX Collection 1333
　　● S98.312　Complete traumatic amputation of left midfoot A 🔧, A, D, S 🔧
　　　(Ex:) See PDX Collection 1334
　　● S98.319　Complete traumatic amputation of unspecified midfoot A 🔧, A, D, S 🔧
　　　(Ex:) See PDX Collection 1335
　● S98.32　Partial traumatic amputation of midfoot
　　● S98.321　Partial traumatic amputation of right midfoot A 🔧, A, D, S 🔧
　　　(Ex:) See PDX Collection 1333
　　● S98.322　Partial traumatic amputation of left midfoot A 🔧, A, D, S 🔧
　　　(Ex:) See PDX Collection 1334
　　● S98.329　Partial traumatic amputation of unspecified midfoot A 🔧, A, D, S 🔧
　　　(Ex:) See PDX Collection 1335

● S98.9　Traumatic amputation of foot, level unspecified
　● S98.91　Complete traumatic amputation of foot, level unspecified
　　● S98.911　Complete traumatic amputation of right foot, level unspecified A 🔧, A, D, S 🔧
　　　(Ex:) See PDX Collection 1333
　　● S98.912　Complete traumatic amputation of left foot, level unspecified A 🔧, A, D, S 🔧
　　　(Ex:) See PDX Collection 1334
　　● S98.919　Complete traumatic amputation of unspecified foot, level unspecified A 🔧, A, D, S 🔧
　　　(Ex:) See PDX Collection 1335
　● S98.92　Partial traumatic amputation of foot, level unspecified
　　● S98.921　Partial traumatic amputation of right foot, level unspecified A 🔧, A, D, S 🔧
　　　(Ex:) See PDX Collection 1333
　　● S98.922　Partial traumatic amputation of left foot, level unspecified A 🔧, A, D, S 🔧
　　　(Ex:) See PDX Collection 1334
　　● S98.929　Partial traumatic amputation of unspecified foot, level unspecified A 🔧, A, D, S 🔧
　　　(Ex:) See PDX Collection 1335

▶ New　🔸 Revised　deleted Deleted　Excludes 1　Excludes 2　Includes　Use additional　Code first　Code also　Key words

OGCR Official Guidelines　● Unacceptable Principal Diagnosis　X Assign placeholder X　● Use Additional Character(s)　▷ Manifestation Code　Coding Clinic

● **S99**   **Other and unspecified injuries of ankle and foot**
      Coding Clinic: 2016, Q4, P68

● **S99.0**   **Physeal fracture of calcaneus**

      The appropriate 7th character is to be added to each code from subcategories S99.0

A	initial encounter for closed fracture
B	initial encounter for open fracture
D	subsequent encounter for fracture with routine healing
G	subsequent encounter for fracture with delayed healing
K	subsequent encounter for fracture with nonunion
P	subsequent encounter for fracture with malunion
S	sequela

   ● **S99.00**   **Unspecified** physeal fracture of calcaneus

      ● **S99.001**   Unspecified physeal fracture of **right** calcaneus

      ● **S99.002**   Unspecified physeal fracture of **left** calcaneus

      ● **S99.009**   Unspecified physeal fracture of **unspecified** calcaneus

   ● **S99.01**   **Salter-Harris Type I** physeal fracture of calcaneus
        Coding Clinic: 2016, Q4, P69

      ● **S99.011**   Salter-Harris Type I physeal fracture of **right** calcaneus

      ● **S99.012**   Salter-Harris Type I physeal fracture of **left** calcaneus

      ● **S99.019**   Salter-Harris Type I physeal fracture of **unspecified** calcaneus

   ● **S99.02**   **Salter-Harris Type II** physeal fracture of calcaneus
        Coding Clinic: 2016, Q4, P69

      ● **S99.021**   Salter-Harris Type II physeal fracture of **right** calcaneus

      ● **S99.022**   Salter-Harris Type II physeal fracture of **left** calcaneus

      ● **S99.029**   Salter-Harris Type II physeal fracture of **unspecified** calcaneus

   ● **S99.03**   **Salter-Harris Type III** physeal fracture of calcaneus
        Coding Clinic: 2016, Q4, P69

      ● **S99.031**   Salter-Harris Type III physeal fracture of **right** calcaneus

      ● **S99.032**   Salter-Harris Type III physeal fracture of **left** calcaneus

      ● **S99.039**   Salter-Harris Type III physeal fracture of **unspecified** calcaneus

   ● **S99.04**   **Salter-Harris Type IV** physeal fracture of calcaneus
        Coding Clinic: 2016, Q4, P69

      ● **S99.041**   Salter-Harris Type IV physeal fracture of **right** calcaneus

      ● **S99.042**   Salter-Harris Type IV physeal fracture of **left** calcaneus

      ● **S99.049**   Salter-Harris Type IV physeal fracture of **unspecified** calcaneus

   ● **S99.09**   **Other** physeal fracture of calcaneus
        Coding Clinic: 2016, Q4, P69

      ● **S99.091**   Other physeal fracture of **right** calcaneus

      ● **S99.092**   Other physeal fracture of **left** calcaneus

      ● **S99.099**   Other physeal fracture of **unspecified** calcaneus

● **S99.1**   **Physeal fracture of metatarsal**

      The appropriate 7th character is to be added to each code from subcategories S99.1

A	initial encounter for closed fracture
B	initial encounter for open fracture
D	subsequent encounter for fracture with routine healing
G	subsequent encounter for fracture with delayed healing
K	subsequent encounter for fracture with nonunion
P	subsequent encounter for fracture with malunion
S	sequela

   ● **S99.10**   **Unspecified** physeal fracture of metatarsal

      ● **S99.101**   Unspecified physeal fracture of **right** metatarsal

      ● **S99.102**   Unspecified physeal fracture of **left** metatarsal

      ● **S99.109**   Unspecified physeal fracture of **unspecified** metatarsal

   ● **S99.11**   **Salter-Harris Type I** physeal fracture of metatarsal
        Coding Clinic: 2016, Q4, P69

      ● **S99.111**   Salter-Harris Type I physeal fracture of **right** metatarsal

      ● **S99.112**   Salter-Harris Type I physeal fracture of **left** metatarsal
          Coding Clinic: 2018, Q1, P3

      ● **S99.119**   Salter-Harris Type I physeal fracture of **unspecified** metatarsal

   ● **S99.12**   **Salter-Harris Type II** physeal fracture of metatarsal
        Coding Clinic: 2016, Q4, P69

      ● **S99.121**   Salter-Harris Type II physeal fracture of **right** metatarsal

      ● **S99.122**   Salter-Harris Type II physeal fracture of **left** metatarsal

      ● **S99.129**   Salter-Harris Type II physeal fracture of **unspecified** metatarsal

   ● **S99.13**   **Salter-Harris Type III** physeal fracture of metatarsal
        Coding Clinic: 2016, Q4, P69

      ● **S99.131**   Salter-Harris Type III physeal fracture of **right** metatarsal

      ● **S99.132**   Salter-Harris Type III physeal fracture of **left** metatarsal

      ● **S99.139**   Salter-Harris Type III physeal fracture of **unspecified** metatarsal

   ● **S99.14**   **Salter-Harris Type IV** physeal fracture of metatarsal
        Coding Clinic: 2016, Q4, P69

      ● **S99.141**   Salter-Harris Type IV physeal fracture of **right** metatarsal

      ● **S99.142**   Salter-Harris Type IV physeal fracture of **left** metatarsal

      ● **S99.149**   Salter-Harris Type IV physeal fracture of **unspecified** metatarsal

   ● **S99.19**   **Other** physeal fracture of metatarsal
        Coding Clinic: 2016, Q4, P69

      ● **S99.191**   Other physeal fracture of **right** metatarsal

      ● **S99.192**   Other physeal fracture of **left** metatarsal

      ● **S99.199**   Other physeal fracture of **unspecified** metatarsal

CHAPTER 19 (S00–T88)

| N | Newborn Age: 0 | P | Pediatric Age: 0–17 | M | Maternity DX: 9–64 | A | Adult Age: 15–124 | ♀ Females Only | ♂ Males Only |

Complication\Comorbidity   Major C\C   (Ex) CC/MCC Exclusions   Hospital-Acquired Condition   Hierarchical Condition Category

1431

CHAPTER 19 (S00-T88)

● S99.2   Physeal fracture of phalanx of toe

The appropriate 7th character is to be added to each code from subcategories S99.2

A	initial encounter for closed fracture
B	initial encounter for open fracture
D	subsequent encounter for fracture with routine healing
G	subsequent encounter for fracture with delayed healing
K	subsequent encounter for fracture with nonunion
P	subsequent encounter for fracture with malunion
S	sequela

  ● S99.20   Unspecified physeal fracture of phalanx of toe

    ● S99.201   Unspecified physeal fracture of phalanx of right toe

    ● S99.202   Unspecified physeal fracture of phalanx of right toe

    ● S99.209   Unspecified physeal fracture of phalanx of unspecified toe

  ● S99.21   Salter-Harris Type I physeal fracture of phalanx of toe
        Coding Clinic: 2016, Q4, P69

    ● S99.211   Salter-Harris Type I physeal fracture of phalanx of right toe

    ● S99.212   Salter-Harris Type I physeal fracture of phalanx of left toe

    ● S99.219   Salter-Harris Type I physeal fracture of phalanx of unspecified toe

  ● S99.22   Salter-Harris Type II physeal fracture of phalanx of toe
        Coding Clinic: 2016, Q4, P69

    ● S99.221   Salter-Harris Type II physeal fracture of phalanx of right toe

    ● S99.222   Salter-Harris Type II physeal fracture of phalanx of left toe

    ● S99.229   Salter-Harris Type II physeal fracture of phalanx of unspecified toe

  ● S99.23   Salter-Harris Type III physeal fracture of phalanx of toe
        Coding Clinic: 2016, Q4, P69

    ● S99.231   Salter-Harris Type III physeal fracture of phalanx of right toe

    ● S99.232   Salter-Harris Type III physeal fracture of phalanx of left toe

    ● S99.239   Salter-Harris Type III physeal fracture of phalanx of unspecified toe

  ● S99.24   Salter-Harris Type IV physeal fracture of phalanx of toe
        Coding Clinic: 2016, Q4, P69

    ● S99.241   Salter-Harris Type IV physeal fracture of phalanx of right toe

    ● S99.242   Salter-Harris Type IV physeal fracture of phalanx of left toe

    ● S99.249   Salter-Harris Type IV physeal fracture of phalanx of unspecified toe

  ● S99.29   Other physeal fracture of phalanx of toe
        Coding Clinic: 2016, Q4, P69

    ● S99.291   Other physeal fracture of phalanx of right toe

    ● S99.292   Other physeal fracture of phalanx of left toe

    ● S99.299   Other physeal fracture of phalanx of unspecified toe

● S99.8   Other specified injuries of ankle and foot

The appropriate 7th character is to be added to each code from subcategory S99.8

A	initial encounter
D	subsequent encounter
S	sequela

  ● S99.81   Other specified injuries of ankle

    ● S99.811   Other specified injuries of right ankle

    ● S99.812   Other specified injuries of left ankle

    ● S99.819   Other specified injuries of unspecified ankle

  ● S99.82   Other specified injuries of foot

    ● S99.821   Other specified injuries of right foot

    ● S99.822   Other specified injuries of left foot

    ● S99.829   Other specified injuries of unspecified foot

● S99.9   Unspecified injury of ankle and foot

The appropriate 7th character is to be added to each code from subcategory S99.9

A	initial encounter
D	subsequent encounter
S	sequela

  ● S99.91   Unspecified injury of ankle

    ● S99.911   Unspecified injury of right ankle

    ● S99.912   Unspecified injury of left ankle

    ● S99.919   Unspecified injury of unspecified ankle

  ● S99.92   Unspecified injury of foot

    ● S99.921   Unspecified injury of right foot

    ● S99.922   Unspecified injury of left foot

    ● S99.929   Unspecified injury of unspecified foot

INJURY, POISONING AND CERTAIN OTHER CONSEQUENCES OF EXTERNAL CAUSES (T07-T88)

INJURIES INVOLVING MULTIPLE BODY REGIONS (T07)

Excludes1   burns and corrosions (T20-T32)
frostbite (T33-T34)
insect bite or sting, venomous (T63.4)
sunburn (L55.-)

X ● T07   Unspecified multiple injuries

The appropriate 7th character is to be added to code T07

A	initial encounter
D	subsequent encounter
S	sequela

Excludes1   injury NOS (T14.90)

INJURY OF UNSPECIFIED BODY REGION (T14)

● T14   Injury of unspecified body region

The appropriate 7th character is to be added to each code from category T14

A	initial encounter
D	subsequent encounter
S	sequela

Excludes1   multiple unspecified injuries (T07)

  X ● T14.8   Other injury of unspecified body region

    Abrasion NOS   Skin injury NOS
    Contusion NOS   Vascular injury NOS
    Crush injury NOS   Wound NOS
    Fracture NOS

  ● T14.9   Unspecified injury

    X ● T14.90   Injury, unspecified
         Injury NOS

    X ● T14.91   Suicide attempt A, D, S 🔊
         Attempted suicide NOS

▶ New   ➠ Revised   ~~deleted~~ Deleted   Excludes 1   Excludes 2   Includes   Use additional   Code first   Code also   Key words
OGCR Official Guidelines   ● Unacceptable Principal Diagnosis   X Assign placeholder X   ● Use Additional Character(s)   ▶ Manifestation Code   Coding Clinic

EFFECTS OF FOREIGN BODY ENTERING THROUGH NATURAL ORIFICE (T15-T19)

Excludes2   foreign body accidentally left in operation wound (T81.5-)
foreign body in penetrating wound - see open wound by body region
residual foreign body in soft tissue (M79.5)
splinter, without open wound - see superficial injury by body region

● **T15   Foreign body on external eye**

Excludes2   foreign body in penetrating wound of orbit and eye ball (S05.4-, S05.5-)
open wound of eyelid and periocular area (S01.1-)
retained foreign body in eyelid (H02.8-)
retained (old) foreign body in penetrating wound of orbit and eye ball (H05.5-, H44.6-, H44.7-)
superficial foreign body of eyelid and periocular area (S00.25-)

The appropriate 7th character is to be added to each code from category T15

A	initial encounter
D	subsequent encounter
S	sequela

● **T15.0   Foreign body in cornea**
  X● **T15.00**   Foreign body in cornea, unspecified eye
  X● **T15.01**   Foreign body in cornea, right eye
  X● **T15.02**   Foreign body in cornea, left eye
● **T15.1   Foreign body in conjunctival sac**
  X● **T15.10**   Foreign body in conjunctival sac, unspecified eye
  X● **T15.11**   Foreign body in conjunctival sac, right eye
  X● **T15.12**   Foreign body in conjunctival sac, left eye
● **T15.8   Foreign body in other and multiple parts of external eye**
  Foreign body in lacrimal punctum
  X● **T15.80**   Foreign body in other and multiple parts of external eye, unspecified eye
  X● **T15.81**   Foreign body in other and multiple parts of external eye, right eye
  X● **T15.82**   Foreign body in other and multiple parts of external eye, left eye
● **T15.9   Foreign body on external eye, part unspecified**
  X● **T15.90**   Foreign body on external eye, part unspecified, unspecified eye
  X● **T15.91**   Foreign body on external eye, part unspecified, right eye
  X● **T15.92**   Foreign body on external eye, part unspecified, left eye

● **T16   Foreign body in ear**
Includes   foreign body in auditory canal
The appropriate 7th character is to be added to each code from category T16

A	initial encounter
D	subsequent encounter
S	sequela

  X● **T16.1**   Foreign body in right ear
  X● **T16.2**   Foreign body in left ear
  X● **T16.9**   Foreign body in ear, unspecified ear

● **T17   Foreign body in respiratory tract**
The appropriate 7th character is to be added to each code from category T17

A	initial encounter
D	subsequent encounter
S	sequela

  X● **T17.0**   Foreign body in nasal sinus
  X● **T17.1**   Foreign body in nostril
    Foreign body in nose NOS
  ● **T17.2**   Foreign body in pharynx
    Foreign body in nasopharynx
    Foreign body in throat NOS
    ● **T17.20**   Unspecified foreign body in pharynx
      ● **T17.200**   Unspecified foreign body in pharynx causing asphyxiation
      ● **T17.208**   Unspecified foreign body in pharynx causing other injury
    ● **T17.21**   Gastric contents in pharynx
      Aspiration of gastric contents into pharynx
      Vomitus in pharynx
      ● **T17.210**   Gastric contents in pharynx causing asphyxiation
      ● **T17.218**   Gastric contents in pharynx causing other injury
    ● **T17.22**   Food in pharynx
      Bones in pharynx
      Seeds in pharynx
      ● **T17.220**   Food in pharynx causing asphyxiation
      ● **T17.228**   Food in pharynx causing other injury
    ● **T17.29**   Other foreign object in pharynx
      ● **T17.290**   Other foreign object in pharynx causing asphyxiation
      ● **T17.298**   Other foreign object in pharynx causing other injury
  ● **T17.3**   Foreign body in larynx
    ● **T17.30**   Unspecified foreign body in larynx
      ● **T17.300**   Unspecified foreign body in larynx causing asphyxiation
      ● **T17.308**   Unspecified foreign body in larynx causing other injury
    ● **T17.31**   Gastric contents in larynx
      Aspiration of gastric contents into larynx
      Vomitus in larynx
      ● **T17.310**   Gastric contents in larynx causing asphyxiation
      ● **T17.318**   Gastric contents in larynx causing other injury
    ● **T17.32**   Food in larynx
      Bones in larynx
      Seeds in larynx
      ● **T17.320**   Food in larynx causing asphyxiation
      ● **T17.328**   Food in larynx causing other injury
    ● **T17.39**   Other foreign object in larynx
      ● **T17.390**   Other foreign object in larynx causing asphyxiation
      ● **T17.398**   Other foreign object in larynx causing other injury
  ● **T17.4**   Foreign body in trachea
    (Ex:) For category T17.4 CC codes: See PDX Collection 1373
    ● **T17.40**   Unspecified foreign body in trachea
      ● **T17.400**   Unspecified foreign body in trachea causing asphyxiation A
      ● **T17.408**   Unspecified foreign body in trachea causing other injury A

● **T17.41** Gastric contents in trachea
　　　　Aspiration of gastric contents into trachea
　　　　Vomitus in trachea

　　● **T17.410** Gastric contents in trachea causing asphyxiation A 🔧

　　● **T17.418** Gastric contents in trachea causing other injury A 🔧

● **T17.42** Food in trachea
　　　　Bones in trachea
　　　　Seeds in trachea

　　● **T17.420** Food in trachea causing asphyxiation A 🔧

　　● **T17.428** Food in trachea causing other injury A 🔧

● **T17.49** Other foreign object in trachea

　　● **T17.490** Other foreign object in trachea causing asphyxiation A 🔧

　　● **T17.498** Other foreign object in trachea causing other injury A 🔧

● **T17.5** Foreign body in bronchus
　　Ⓔ **For category T17.5 CC codes:** See PDX Collection 1374

　　● **T17.50** Unspecified foreign body in bronchus

　　　　● **T17.500** Unspecified foreign body in bronchus causing asphyxiation A 🔧

　　　　● **T17.508** Unspecified foreign body in bronchus causing other injury A 🔧

　　● **T17.51** Gastric contents in bronchus
　　　　　　Aspiration of gastric contents into bronchus
　　　　　　Vomitus in bronchus

　　　　● **T17.510** Gastric contents in bronchus causing asphyxiation A 🔧

　　　　● **T17.518** Gastric contents in bronchus causing other injury A 🔧

　　● **T17.52** Food in bronchus
　　　　　　Bones in bronchus
　　　　　　Seeds in bronchus

　　　　● **T17.520** Food in bronchus causing asphyxiation A 🔧

　　　　● **T17.528** Food in bronchus causing other injury A 🔧

　　● **T17.59** Other foreign object in bronchus

　　　　● **T17.590** Other foreign object in bronchus causing asphyxiation A 🔧

　　　　● **T17.598** Other foreign object in bronchus causing other injury A 🔧

● **T17.8** Foreign body in other parts of respiratory tract
　　　　Foreign body in bronchioles
　　　　Foreign body in lung
　　Ⓔ **For category T17.8 CC codes:** See PDX Collection 1374

　　● **T17.80** Unspecified foreign body in other parts of respiratory tract

　　　　● **T17.800** Unspecified foreign body in other parts of respiratory tract causing asphyxiation A 🔧

　　　　● **T17.808** Unspecified foreign body in other parts of respiratory tract causing other injury A 🔧

　　● **T17.81** Gastric contents in other parts of respiratory tract
　　　　　　Aspiration of gastric contents into other parts of respiratory tract
　　　　　　Vomitus in other parts of respiratory tract

　　　　● **T17.810** Gastric contents in other parts of respiratory tract causing asphyxiation A 🔧

　　　　● **T17.818** Gastric contents in other parts of respiratory tract causing other injury A 🔧

● **T17.82** Food in other parts of respiratory tract
　　　　Bones in other parts of respiratory tract
　　　　Seeds in other parts of respiratory tract

　　● **T17.820** Food in other parts of respiratory tract causing asphyxiation A 🔧

　　● **T17.828** Food in other parts of respiratory tract causing other injury A 🔧

● **T17.89** Other foreign object in other parts of respiratory tract

　　● **T17.890** Other foreign object in other parts of respiratory tract causing asphyxiation A 🔧

　　● **T17.898** Other foreign object in other parts of respiratory tract causing other injury A 🔧

● **T17.9** Foreign body in respiratory tract, part unspecified

　　● **T17.90** Unspecified foreign body in respiratory tract, part unspecified

　　　　● **T17.900** Unspecified foreign body in respiratory tract, part unspecified causing asphyxiation

　　　　● **T17.908** Unspecified foreign body in respiratory tract, part unspecified causing other injury

　　● **T17.91** Gastric contents in respiratory tract, part unspecified
　　　　　　Aspiration of gastric contents into respiratory tract, part unspecified
　　　　　　Vomitus in trachea respiratory tract, part unspecified

　　　　● **T17.910** Gastric contents in respiratory tract, part unspecified causing asphyxiation

　　　　● **T17.918** Gastric contents in respiratory tract, part unspecified causing other injury

　　● **T17.92** Food in respiratory tract, part unspecified
　　　　　　Bones in respiratory tract, part unspecified
　　　　　　Seeds in respiratory tract, part unspecified

　　　　● **T17.920** Food in respiratory tract, part unspecified causing asphyxiation

　　　　● **T17.928** Food in respiratory tract, part unspecified causing other injury

　　● **T17.99** Other foreign object in respiratory tract, part unspecified

　　　　● **T17.990** Other foreign object in respiratory tract, part unspecified in causing asphyxiation
　　　　　　Coding Clinic: 2019, Q3, P15

　　　　● **T17.998** Other foreign object in respiratory tract, part unspecified causing other injury

● **T18** Foreign body in alimentary tract
　　Excludes2 foreign body in pharynx (T17.2-)

　　The appropriate 7th character is to be added to each code from category T18

A	initial encounter
D	subsequent encounter
S	sequela

　X ● **T18.0** Foreign body in mouth

　X ● **T18.1** Foreign body in esophagus
　　Excludes2 foreign body in respiratory tract (T17.-)

　　● **T18.10** Unspecified foreign body in esophagus

　　　　● **T18.100** Unspecified foreign body in esophagus causing compression of trachea
　　　　　　Unspecified foreign body in esophagus causing obstruction of respiration

　　　　● **T18.108** Unspecified foreign body in esophagus causing other injury

● T18.11   **Gastric contents** in esophagus
           Vomitus in esophagus
    ● T18.110   **Gastric contents** in esophagus **causing compression of trachea**
                Gastric contents in esophagus causing obstruction of respiration
    ● T18.118   **Gastric contents** in esophagus **causing other injury**
● T18.12   **Food** in esophagus
           Bones in esophagus
           Seeds in esophagus
    ● T18.120   **Food** in esophagus **causing compression of trachea**
                Food in esophagus causing obstruction of respiration
    ● T18.128   **Food** in esophagus **causing other injury**
● T18.19   **Other foreign object** in esophagus
    ● T18.190   **Other foreign object** in esophagus **causing compression of trachea**
                Other foreign body in esophagus causing obstruction of respiration
                Coding Clinic: 2015, Q1, P24
    ● T18.198   **Other foreign object** in esophagus **causing other injury**
                Coding Clinic: 2015, Q1, P24
X ● T18.2   Foreign body in **stomach**
X ● T18.3   Foreign body in **small intestine**
X ● T18.4   Foreign body in **colon**
X ● T18.5   Foreign body in **anus and rectum**
            Foreign body in rectosigmoid (junction)
X ● T18.8   Foreign body in **other parts** of alimentary tract
X ● T18.9   Foreign body of alimentary tract, **part unspecified**
            Foreign body in digestive system NOS
            Swallowed foreign body NOS

● T19   Foreign body in **genitourinary tract**
    Excludes2   complications due to implanted mesh (T83.7-)
                    mechanical complications of contraceptive device (intrauterine) (vaginal) (T83.3-)
                    presence of contraceptive device (intrauterine) (vaginal) (Z97.5)

    The appropriate 7th character is to be added to each code from category T19

A	initial encounter
D	subsequent encounter
S	sequela

X ● T19.0   Foreign body in **urethra**
X ● T19.1   Foreign body in **bladder**
X ● T19.2   Foreign body in **vulva and vagina** ♀
X ● T19.3   Foreign body in **uterus** ♀
X ● T19.4   Foreign body in **penis** ♂
X ● T19.8   Foreign body in **other parts** of genitourinary tract
X ● T19.9   Foreign body in genitourinary tract, **part unspecified**

BURNS AND CORROSIONS (T20-T32)

Includes   burns (thermal) from electrical heating appliances
               burns (thermal) from electricity
               burns (thermal) from flame
               burns (thermal) from friction
               burns (thermal) from hot air and hot gases
               burns (thermal) from hot objects
               burns (thermal) from lightning
               burns (thermal) from radiation chemical
               burn [corrosion] (external) (internal) scalds

Excludes2 erythema [dermatitis] ab igne (L59.0)
               radiation-related disorders of the skin and subcutaneous tissue (L55-L59)
               sunburn (L55.-)

OGCR Section I.C.19.d.

Burns and Corrosions

The ICD-10-CM makes a distinction between burn and corrosions. The burn codes are for thermal burns, except sunburns, that come from a heat source, such as a fire or hot appliance. The burn codes are also for burns resulting from electricity and radiation. Corrosions are burns due to chemicals. The guidelines for burns and corrosions are the same.

Current burns (T20-T25) are classified by depth, extent and by agent (X code). Burns are classified by depth as first degree (erythema), second degree (blistering), and third degree (full-thickness involvement). Burns of the eye and internal organs (T26-T28) are classified by site, but not by degree.

1) Sequencing of burn and related condition codes

Sequence first the code that reflects the highest degree of burn when more than one burn is present.

a. When the reason for the admission or encounter is for treatment of external multiple burns, sequence first the code that reflects the burn of the highest degree.

b. When a patient has both internal and external burns, the circumstances of admission govern the selection of the principal diagnosis or first-listed diagnosis.

c. When a patient is admitted for burn injuries and other related conditions such as smoke inhalation and/or respiratory failure, the circumstances of admission govern the selection of the principal or first-listed diagnosis.

2) Burns of the same local site

Classify burns of the same local site (three-character category level, T20-T28) but of different degrees to the subcategory identifying the highest degree recorded in the diagnosis.

BURNS AND CORROSIONS OF EXTERNAL BODY SURFACE, SPECIFIED BY SITE (T20-T25)

Includes   burns and corrosions of first degree [erythema]
               burns and corrosions of second degree [blisters] [epidermal loss]
               burns and corrosions of third degree [deep necrosis of underlying tissue] [full-thickness skin loss]

Use additional code from category T31 or T32 to identify extent of body surface involved

● T20   Burn and corrosion of head, face, and neck
    Excludes2   burn and corrosion of ear drum (T28.41, T28.91)
                    burn and corrosion of eye and adnexa (T26.-)
                    burn and corrosion of mouth and pharynx (T28.0)

    The appropriate 7th character is to be added to each code from category T20

A	initial encounter
D	subsequent encounter
S	sequela

● T20.0   Burn of **unspecified degree** of head, face, and neck
          Use additional external cause code to identify the source, place and intent of the burn (X00-X19, X75-X77, X96-X98, Y92)
    X ● T20.00   Burn of unspecified degree of head, face, and neck, **unspecified site**
    ● T20.01   Burn of unspecified degree of **ear** [any part, except ear drum]
               Excludes2   burn of ear drum (T28.41-)
        ● T20.011   Burn of unspecified degree of **right ear** [any part, except ear drum]
        ● T20.012   Burn of unspecified degree of **left ear** [any part, except ear drum]
        ● T20.019   Burn of unspecified degree of **unspecified** ear [any part, except ear drum]

CHAPTER 19 (S00-T88)

N Newborn Age: 0   **P** Pediatric Age: 0–17   **M** Maternity DX: 9–64   **A** Adult Age: 15–124   ♀ Females Only   ♂ Males Only
🔹 Complication\Comorbidity   🔹 Major C\C   Ex) CC/MCC Exclusions   🔹 Hospital-Acquired Condition   🔹 Hierarchical Condition Category

1435

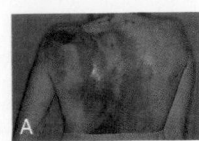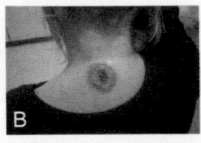

Figure 19-15 A. Second-degree burn. **B.** Third-degree burn. (A. From Black J, Hawks J: Medical-Surgical Nursing: Clinical Management for Positive Outcomes, 8e, Saunders, 2008. B. From Marx J, Hockberger R, Walls R: Rosen's Emergency Medicine - Concepts and Clinical Practice, 7e, Mosby, 2009)

X● T20.02   Burn of unspecified degree of lip(s)

X● T20.03   Burn of unspecified degree of chin

X● T20.04   Burn of unspecified degree of nose (septum)

X● T20.05   Burn of unspecified degree of scalp [any part]

X● T20.06   Burn of unspecified degree of forehead and cheek

X● T20.07   Burn of unspecified degree of neck

X● T20.09   Burn of unspecified degree of multiple sites of head, face, and neck

● T20.1   Burn of first degree of head, face, and neck

Use additional external cause code to identify the source, place and intent of the burn (X00-X19, X75-X77, X96-X98, Y92)

X● T20.10   Burn of first degree of head, face, and neck, unspecified site

● T20.11   Burn of first degree of ear [any part, except ear drum]

Excludes2   burn of ear drum (T28.41-)

● T20.111   Burn of first degree of right ear [any part, except ear drum]

● T20.112   Burn of first degree of left ear [any part, except ear drum]

● T20.119   Burn of first degree of unspecified ear [any part, except ear drum]

X● T20.12   Burn of first degree of lip(s)

X● T20.13   Burn of first degree of chin

X● T20.14   Burn of first degree of nose (septum)

X● T20.15   Burn of first degree of scalp [any part]

X● T20.16   Burn of first degree of forehead and cheek

X● T20.17   Burn of first degree of neck

X● T20.19   Burn of first degree of multiple sites of head, face, and neck

● T20.2   Burn of second degree of head, face, and neck

Use additional external cause code to identify the source, place and intent of the burn (X00-X19, X75-X77, X96-X98, Y92)

X● T20.20   Burn of second degree of head, face, and neck, unspecified site

● T20.21   Burn of second degree of ear [any part, except ear drum]

Excludes2   burn of ear drum (T28.41-)

● T20.211   Burn of second degree of right ear [any part, except ear drum]

● T20.212   Burn of second degree of left ear [any part, except ear drum]

● T20.219   Burn of second degree of unspecified ear [any part, except ear drum]

X● T20.22   Burn of second degree of lip(s)

X● T20.23   Burn of second degree of chin

X● T20.24   Burn of second degree of nose (septum)

X● T20.25   Burn of second degree of scalp [any part]
Coding Clinic: 2015, Q1, P19

X● T20.26   Burn of second degree of forehead and cheek

X● T20.27   Burn of second degree of neck

X● T20.29   Burn of second degree of multiple sites of head, face, and neck

● T20.3   Burn of third degree of head, face, and neck

Use additional external cause code to identify the source, place and intent of the burn (X00-X19, X75-X77, X96-X98, Y92)

X● T20.30   Burn of third degree of head, face, and neck, unspecified site A 🔾, A 🔾
(Ex) See PDX Collection 1375

● T20.31   Burn of third degree of ear [any part, except ear drum]

Excludes2   burn of ear drum (T28.41-)

(Ex) For category T20.31 CC codes: See PDX Collection 1376

● T20.311   Burn of third degree of right ear [any part, except ear drum] A 🔾, A 🔾

● T20.312   Burn of third degree of left ear [any part, except ear drum] A 🔾, A 🔾
Coding Clinic: 2015, Q1, P18

● T20.319   Burn of third degree of unspecified ear [any part, except ear drum] A 🔾, A 🔾

X● T20.32   Burn of third degree of lip(s) A 🔾, A 🔾
(Ex) See PDX Collection 1377

X● T20.33   Burn of third degree of chin A 🔾, A 🔾
(Ex) See PDX Collection 1378

X● T20.34   Burn of third degree of nose (septum) A 🔾, A 🔾
(Ex) See PDX Collection 1379

X● T20.35   Burn of third degree of scalp [any part] A 🔾, A 🔾
(Ex) See PDX Collection 1380

X● T20.36   Burn of third degree of forehead and cheek A 🔾, A 🔾
(Ex) See PDX Collection 1381

X● T20.37   Burn of third degree of neck A 🔾, A 🔾
(Ex) See PDX Collection 1382

X● T20.39   Burn of third degree of multiple sites of head, face, and neck A 🔾, A 🔾
(Ex) See PDX Collection 1383

● T20.4   Corrosion of unspecified degree of head, face, and neck

Code first (T51-T65) to identify chemical and intent

Use additional external cause code to identify place (Y92)

X● T20.40   Corrosion of unspecified degree of head, face, and neck, unspecified site

● T20.41   Corrosion of unspecified degree of ear [any part, except ear drum]

Excludes2   corrosion of ear drum (T28.91-)

● T20.411   Corrosion of unspecified degree of right ear [any part, except ear drum]

● T20.412   Corrosion of unspecified degree of left ear [any part, except ear drum]

● T20.419   Corrosion of unspecified degree of unspecified ear [any part, except ear drum]

X● T20.42   Corrosion of unspecified degree of lip(s)

X● T20.43   Corrosion of unspecified degree of chin

X● T20.44   Corrosion of unspecified degree of nose (septum)

X● T20.45   Corrosion of unspecified degree of scalp [any part]

X● T20.46   Corrosion of unspecified degree of forehead and cheek

X● T20.47   Corrosion of unspecified degree of neck

X● T20.49   Corrosion of unspecified degree of multiple sites of head, face, and neck

▶ New   ⇒ Revised   ~~deleted~~ Deleted   Excludes 1   Excludes 2   Includes   Use additional   Code first   Code also   Key words
OGCR Official Guidelines   ● Unacceptable Principal Diagnosis   X Assign placeholder X   ● Use Additional Character(s)   ▶ Manifestation Code   **Coding Clinic**

●T20.5   **Corrosion of** first degree **of head, face, and neck**
> *Code first (T51-T65) to identify chemical and intent*
> Use additional external cause code to identify
> place (Y92)

X● T20.50   **Corrosion of first degree of head, face, and neck,** unspecified **site**

●T20.51   **Corrosion of first degree of** ear **[any part, except ear drum]**

> **Excludes2**   corrosion of ear drum (T28.91-)

● T20.511   **Corrosion of first degree of** right **ear [any part, except ear drum]**

● T20.512   **Corrosion of first degree of** left **ear [any part, except ear drum]**

● T20.519   **Corrosion of first degree of** unspecified **ear [any part, except ear drum]**

X● T20.52   **Corrosion of first degree of** lip(s)

X● T20.53   **Corrosion of first degree of** chin

X● T20.54   **Corrosion of first degree of** nose (septum)

X● T20.55   **Corrosion of first degree of** scalp [any part]

X● T20.56   **Corrosion of first degree of** forehead and cheek

X● T20.57   **Corrosion of first degree of** neck

X● T20.59   **Corrosion of first degree of** multiple sites **of head, face, and neck**

●T20.6   **Corrosion of** second degree **of head, face, and neck**
> *Code first (T51-T65) to identify chemical and intent*
> Use additional external cause code to identify
> place (Y92)

X● T20.60   **Corrosion of second degree of head, face, and neck,** unspecified site

●T20.61   **Corrosion of second degree of** ear **[any part, except ear drum]**

> **Excludes2**   corrosion of ear drum (T28.91-)

● T20.611   **Corrosion of second degree of** right **ear [any part, except ear drum]**

● T20.612   **Corrosion of second degree of** left **ear [any part, except ear drum]**

● T20.619   **Corrosion of second degree of** unspecified **ear [any part, except ear drum]**

X● T20.62   **Corrosion of second degree of** lip(s)

X● T20.63   **Corrosion of second degree of** chin

X● T20.64   **Corrosion of second degree of** nose (septum)

X● T20.65   **Corrosion of second degree of** scalp [any part]

X● T20.66   **Corrosion of second degree of** forehead and cheek

X● T20.67   **Corrosion of second degree of** neck

X● T20.69   **Corrosion of second degree of** multiple sites **of head, face, and neck**

●T20.7   **Corrosion of** third degree **of head, face, and neck**
> *Code first (T51-T65) to identify chemical and intent*
> Use additional external cause code to identify
> place (Y92)

X● T20.70   **Corrosion of third degree of head, face, and neck,** unspecified **site** A 🔵, A 🔷
> ⒺⓍ See PDX Collection 1375

●T20.71   **Corrosion of third degree of** ear **[any part, except ear drum]**

> **Excludes2**   corrosion of ear drum (T28.91-)
> ⒺⓍ For category T20.71 CC codes: See PDX Collection 1376

● T20.711   **Corrosion of third degree of** right **ear [any part, except ear drum]** A 🔵, A 🔷

● T20.712   **Corrosion of third degree of** left **ear [any part, except ear drum]** A 🔵, A 🔷

● T20.719   **Corrosion of third degree of** unspecified **ear [any part, except ear drum]** A 🔵, A 🔷

X● T20.72   **Corrosion of third degree of** lip(s) A 🔵, A 🔷
> ⒺⓍ See PDX Collection 1377

X● T20.73   **Corrosion of third degree of** chin A 🔵, A 🔷
> ⒺⓍ See PDX Collection 1378

X● T20.74   **Corrosion of third degree of** nose (septum) A 🔵, A 🔷
> ⒺⓍ See PDX Collection 1379

X● T20.75   **Corrosion of third degree of** scalp [any part] A 🔵, A 🔷
> ⒺⓍ See PDX Collection 1380

X● T20.76   **Corrosion of third degree of** forehead and cheek A 🔵, A 🔷
> ⒺⓍ See PDX Collection 1381

X● T20.77   **Corrosion of third degree of** neck A 🔵, A 🔷
> ⒺⓍ See PDX Collection 1382

X● T20.79   **Corrosion of third degree of** multiple sites **of head, face, and neck** A 🔵, A 🔷
> ⒺⓍ See PDX Collection 1383

●T21   **Burn and corrosion of trunk**

> **Includes**   burns and corrosion of hip region
> **Excludes2**   burns and corrosion of axilla (T22.- with fifth character 4)
> burns and corrosion of scapular region (T22.- with fifth character 6)
> burns and corrosion of shoulder (T22.- with fifth character 5)

> The appropriate 7th character is to be added to each code from category T21

> | | |
> |---|---|
> | A | initial encounter |
> | D | subsequent encounter |
> | S | sequela |

●T21.0   **Burn of** unspecified degree **of trunk**
> Use additional external cause code to identify the source, place and intent of the burn (X00-X19, X75-X77, X96-X98, Y92)

X● T21.00   **Burn of unspecified degree of trunk,** unspecified **site**

X● T21.01   **Burn of unspecified degree of** chest wall
> Burn of unspecified degree of breast

X● T21.02   **Burn of unspecified degree of** abdominal wall
> Burn of unspecified degree of flank
> Burn of unspecified degree of groin

X● T21.03   **Burn of unspecified degree of** upper back
> Burn of unspecified degree of interscapular region

X● T21.04   **Burn of unspecified degree of** lower back

X● T21.05   **Burn of unspecified degree of** buttock
> Burn of unspecified degree of anus

X● T21.06   **Burn of unspecified degree of** male genital region ♂
> Burn of unspecified degree of penis
> Burn of unspecified degree of scrotum
> Burn of unspecified degree of testis

X● T21.07   **Burn of unspecified degree of** female genital region ♀
> Burn of unspecified degree of labium (majus) (minus)
> Burn of unspecified degree of perineum
> Burn of unspecified degree of vulva

> **Excludes2**   burn of vagina (T28.3)

X● T21.09   **Burn of unspecified degree of** other site **of trunk**

| N | Newborn Age: 0 | P | Pediatric Age: 0–17 | M | Maternity DX: 9–64 | A | Adult Age: 15–124 | ♀ | Females Only | ♂ | Males Only |

🔵 Complication\Comorbidity   🔷 Major C\C   ⒺⓍ CC/MCC Exclusions   🔵 Hospital-Acquired Condition   🔵 Hierarchical Condition Category

CHAPTER 19 (S00-T88)

1437

● **T21.1   Burn of first degree of trunk**

    Use additional external cause code to identify the source, place and intent of the burn (X00-X19, X75-X77, X96-X98, Y92)

X ● **T21.10   Burn of first degree of trunk, unspecified site**

X ● **T21.11   Burn of first degree of chest wall**
    Burn of first degree of breast

X ● **T21.12   Burn of first degree of abdominal wall**
    Burn of first degree of flank
    Burn of first degree of groin

X ● **T21.13   Burn of first degree of upper back**
    Burn of first degree of interscapular region

X ● **T21.14   Burn of first degree of lower back**

X ● **T21.15   Burn of first degree of buttock**
    Burn of first degree of anus

X ● **T21.16   Burn of first degree of male genital region ♂**
    Burn of first degree of penis
    Burn of first degree of scrotum
    Burn of first degree of testis

X ● **T21.17   Burn of first degree of female genital region ♀**
    Burn of first degree of labium (majus) (minus)
    Burn of first degree of perineum
    Burn of first degree of vulva

      Excludes2   burn of vagina (T28.3)

X ● **T21.19   Burn of first degree of other site of trunk**

● **T21.2   Burn of second degree of trunk**

    Use additional external cause code to identify the source, place and intent of the burn (X00-X19, X75-X77, X96-X98, Y92)

X ● **T21.20   Burn of second degree of trunk, unspecified site**

X ● **T21.21   Burn of second degree of chest wall**
    Burn of second degree of breast

X ● **T21.22   Burn of second degree of abdominal wall**
    Burn of second degree of flank
    Burn of second degree of groin

X ● **T21.23   Burn of second degree of upper back**
    Burn of second degree of interscapular region

X ● **T21.24   Burn of second degree of lower back**

X ● **T21.25   Burn of second degree of buttock**
    Burn of second degree of anus

X ● **T21.26   Burn of second degree of male genital region ♂**
    Burn of second degree of penis
    Burn of second degree of scrotum
    Burn of second degree of testis

X ● **T21.27   Burn of second degree of female genital region ♀**
    Burn of second degree of labium (majus) (minus)
    Burn of second degree of perineum
    Burn of second degree of vulva

      Excludes2   burn of vagina (T28.3)

X ● **T21.29   Burn of second degree of other site of trunk**

● **T21.3   Burn of third degree of trunk**

    Use additional external cause code to identify the source, place and intent of the burn (X00-X19, X75-X77, X96-X98, Y92)

X ● **T21.30   Burn of third degree of trunk, unspecified site** A ⬤, A ⬤
    (Ex:) See PDX Collection 1384

X ● **T21.31   Burn of third degree of chest wall** A ⬤, A ⬤
    Burn of third degree of breast
    (Ex:) See PDX Collection 1385
    Coding Clinic: 2016, Q2, P6

X ● **T21.32   Burn of third degree of abdominal wall** A ⬤, A ⬤
    Burn of third degree of flank
    Burn of third degree of groin
    (Ex:) See PDX Collection 1386

X ● **T21.33   Burn of third degree of upper back** A ⬤, A ⬤
    Burn of third degree of interscapular region
    (Ex:) See PDX Collection 1387

X ● **T21.34   Burn of third degree of lower back** A ⬤, A ⬤
    (Ex:) See PDX Collection 1387

X ● **T21.35   Burn of third degree of buttock** A ⬤, A ⬤
    Burn of third degree of anus
    (Ex:) See PDX Collection 1387

X ● **T21.36   Burn of third degree of male genital region ♂** A ⬤, A ⬤
    Burn of third degree of penis
    Burn of third degree of scrotum
    Burn of third degree of testis
    (Ex:) See PDX Collection 1388

X ● **T21.37   Burn of third degree of female genital region ♀** A ⬤, A ⬤
    Burn of third degree of labium (majus) (minus)
    Burn of third degree of perineum
    Burn of third degree of vulva

      Excludes2   burn of vagina (T28.3)
    (Ex:) See PDX Collection 1388

X ● **T21.39   Burn of third degree of other site of trunk** A ⬤, A ⬤
    (Ex:) See PDX Collection 1384

● **T21.4   Corrosion of unspecified degree of trunk**

    Code first (T51-T65) to identify chemical and intent
    Use additional external cause code to identify place (Y92)

X ● **T21.40   Corrosion of unspecified degree of trunk, unspecified site**

X ● **T21.41   Corrosion of unspecified degree of chest wall**
    Corrosion of unspecified degree of breast

X ● **T21.42   Corrosion of unspecified degree of abdominal wall**
    Corrosion of unspecified degree of flank
    Corrosion of unspecified degree of groin

X ● **T21.43   Corrosion of unspecified degree of upper back**
    Corrosion of unspecified degree of interscapular region

X ● **T21.44   Corrosion of unspecified degree of lower back**

X ● **T21.45   Corrosion of unspecified degree of buttock**
    Corrosion of unspecified degree of anus

X ● **T21.46   Corrosion of unspecified degree of male genital region ♂**
    Corrosion of unspecified degree of penis
    Corrosion of unspecified degree of scrotum
    Corrosion of unspecified degree of testis

X ● **T21.47   Corrosion of unspecified degree of female genital region ♀**
    Corrosion of unspecified degree of labium (majus) (minus)
    Corrosion of unspecified degree of perineum
    Corrosion of unspecified degree of vulva

      Excludes2   corrosion of vagina (T28.8)

X ● **T21.49   Corrosion of unspecified degree of other site of trunk**

● T21.5   **Corrosion of first degree of trunk**

     Code first (T51-T65) to identify chemical and intent

     Use additional external cause code to identify place (Y92)

X ● **T21.50**   **Corrosion of first degree of trunk, unspecified site**

X ● **T21.51**   **Corrosion of first degree of chest wall**
     Corrosion of first degree of breast

X ● **T21.52**   **Corrosion of first degree of abdominal wall**
     Corrosion of first degree of flank
     Corrosion of first degree of groin

X ● **T21.53**   **Corrosion of first degree of upper back**
     Corrosion of first degree of interscapular region

X ● **T21.54**   **Corrosion of first degree of lower back**

X ● **T21.55**   **Corrosion of first degree of buttock**
     Corrosion of first degree of anus

X ● **T21.56**   **Corrosion of first degree of male genital region ♂**
     Corrosion of first degree of penis
     Corrosion of first degree of scrotum
     Corrosion of first degree of testis

X ● **T21.57**   **Corrosion of first degree of female genital region ♀**
     Corrosion of first degree of labium (majus) (minus)
     Corrosion of first degree of perineum
     Corrosion of first degree of vulva
     Excludes2   corrosion of vagina (T28.8)

X ● **T21.59**   **Corrosion of first degree of other site of trunk**

● T21.6   **Corrosion of second degree of trunk**

     Code first (T51-T65) to identify chemical and intent

     Use additional external cause code to identify place (Y92)

X ● **T21.60**   **Corrosion of second degree of trunk, unspecified site**

X ● **T21.61**   **Corrosion of second degree of chest wall**
     Corrosion of second degree of breast

X ● **T21.62**   **Corrosion of second degree of abdominal wall**
     Corrosion of second degree of flank
     Corrosion of second degree of groin

X ● **T21.63**   **Corrosion of second degree of upper back**
     Corrosion of second degree of interscapular region

X ● **T21.64**   **Corrosion of second degree of lower back**

X ● **T21.65**   **Corrosion of second degree of buttock**
     Corrosion of second degree of anus

X ● **T21.66**   **Corrosion of second degree of male genital region ♂**
     Corrosion of second degree of penis
     Corrosion of second degree of scrotum
     Corrosion of second degree of testis

X ● **T21.67**   **Corrosion of second degree of female genital region ♀**
     Corrosion of second degree of labium (majus) (minus)
     Corrosion of second degree of perineum
     Corrosion of second degree of vulva
     Excludes2   corrosion of vagina (T28.8)

X ● **T21.69**   **Corrosion of second degree of other site of trunk**

● T21.7   **Corrosion of third degree of trunk**

     Code first (T51-T65) to identify chemical and intent

     Use additional external cause code to identify place (Y92)

X ● **T21.70**   **Corrosion of third degree of trunk, unspecified site** A 🔖, A 🔖
     (Ex:) See PDX Collection 1384

X ● **T21.71**   **Corrosion of third degree of chest wall** A 🔖, A 🔖
     Corrosion of third degree of breast
     (Ex:) See PDX Collection 1385

X ● **T21.72**   **Corrosion of third degree of abdominal wall** A 🔖, A 🔖
     Corrosion of third degree of flank
     Corrosion of third degree of groin
     (Ex:) See PDX Collection 1386

X ● **T21.73**   **Corrosion of third degree of upper back** A 🔖, A 🔖
     Corrosion of third degree of interscapular region
     (Ex:) See PDX Collection 1387

X ● **T21.74**   **Corrosion of third degree of lower back** A 🔖, A 🔖
     (Ex:) See PDX Collection 1387

X ● **T21.75**   **Corrosion of third degree of buttock** A 🔖, A 🔖
     Corrosion of third degree of anus
     (Ex:) See PDX Collection 1387

X ● **T21.76**   **Corrosion of third degree of male genital region ♂** A 🔖, A 🔖
     Corrosion of third degree of penis
     Corrosion of third degree of scrotum
     Corrosion of third degree of testis
     (Ex:) See PDX Collection 1388

X ● **T21.77**   **Corrosion of third degree of female genital region ♀** A 🔖, A 🔖
     Corrosion of third degree of labium (majus) (minus)
     Corrosion of third degree of perineum
     Corrosion of third degree of vulva
     Excludes2   corrosion of vagina (T28.8)
     (Ex:) See PDX Collection 1388

X ● **T21.79**   **Corrosion of third degree of other site of trunk** A 🔖, A 🔖
     (Ex:) See PDX Collection 1384

● T22   **Burn and corrosion of shoulder and upper limb, except wrist and hand**

     Excludes2   burn and corrosion of interscapular region (T21.-)
                     burn and corrosion of wrist and hand (T23.-)

     The appropriate 7th character is to be added to each code from category T22

A	initial encounter
D	subsequent encounter
S	sequela

● T22.0   **Burn of unspecified degree of shoulder and upper limb, except wrist and hand**

     Use additional external cause code to identify the source, place and intent of the burn (X00-X19, X75-X77, X96-X98, Y92)

X ● **T22.00**   **Burn of unspecified degree of shoulder and upper limb, except wrist and hand, unspecified site**

● **T22.01**   **Burn of unspecified degree of forearm**

     ● **T22.011**   **Burn of unspecified degree of right forearm**

     ● **T22.012**   **Burn of unspecified degree of left forearm**

     ● **T22.019**   **Burn of unspecified degree of unspecified forearm**

N Newborn Age: 0   **P** Pediatric Age: 0–17   **M** Maternity DX: 9–64   **A** Adult Age: 15–124   ♀ Females Only   ♂ Males Only

🔖 Complication\Comorbidity   🔖 Major C\C   (Ex:) CC/MCC Exclusions   🔖 Hospital-Acquired Condition   🔖 Hierarchical Condition Category

1439

- ● T22.02   Burn of unspecified degree of elbow
  - ● T22.021   Burn of unspecified degree of right elbow
  - ● T22.022   Burn of unspecified degree of left elbow
  - ● T22.029   Burn of unspecified degree of unspecified elbow
- ● T22.03   Burn of unspecified degree of upper arm
  - ● T22.031   Burn of unspecified degree of right upper arm
  - ● T22.032   Burn of unspecified degree of left upper arm
  - ● T22.039   Burn of unspecified degree of unspecified upper arm
- ● T22.04   Burn of unspecified degree of axilla
  - ● T22.041   Burn of unspecified degree of right axilla
  - ● T22.042   Burn of unspecified degree of left axilla
  - ● T22.049   Burn of unspecified degree of unspecified axilla
- ● T22.05   Burn of unspecified degree of shoulder
  - ● T22.051   Burn of unspecified degree of right shoulder
  - ● T22.052   Burn of unspecified degree of left shoulder
  - ● T22.059   Burn of unspecified degree of unspecified shoulder
- ● T22.06   Burn of unspecified degree of scapular region
  - ● T22.061   Burn of unspecified degree of right scapular region
  - ● T22.062   Burn of unspecified degree of left scapular region
  - ● T22.069   Burn of unspecified degree of unspecified scapular region
- ● T22.09   Burn of unspecified degree of multiple sites of shoulder and upper limb, except wrist and hand
  - ● T22.091   Burn of unspecified degree of multiple sites of right shoulder and upper limb, except wrist and hand
  - ● T22.092   Burn of unspecified degree of multiple sites of left shoulder and upper limb, except wrist and hand
  - ● T22.099   Burn of unspecified degree of multiple sites of unspecified shoulder and upper limb, except wrist and hand
- ● T22.1   Burn of first degree of shoulder and upper limb, except wrist and hand

  Use additional external cause code to identify the source, place and intent of the burn (X00-X19, X75-X77, X96-X98, Y92)
  - X● T22.10   Burn of first degree of shoulder and upper limb, except wrist and hand, unspecified site
  - ● T22.11   Burn of first degree of forearm
    - ● T22.111   Burn of first degree of right forearm
    - ● T22.112   Burn of first degree of left forearm
    - ● T22.119   Burn of first degree of unspecified forearm
  - ● T22.12   Burn of first degree of elbow
    - ● T22.121   Burn of first degree of right elbow
    - ● T22.122   Burn of first degree of left elbow
    - ● T22.129   Burn of first degree of unspecified elbow

- ● T22.13   Burn of first degree of upper arm
  - ● T22.131   Burn of first degree of right upper arm
  - ● T22.132   Burn of first degree of left upper arm
  - ● T22.139   Burn of first degree of unspecified upper arm
- ● T22.14   Burn of first degree of axilla
  - ● T22.141   Burn of first degree of right axilla
  - ● T22.142   Burn of first degree of left axilla
  - ● T22.149   Burn of first degree of unspecified axilla
- ● T22.15   Burn of first degree of shoulder
  - ● T22.151   Burn of first degree of right shoulder
  - ● T22.152   Burn of first degree of left shoulder
  - ● T22.159   Burn of first degree of unspecified shoulder
- ● T22.16   Burn of first degree of scapular region
  - ● T22.161   Burn of first degree of right scapular region
  - ● T22.162   Burn of first degree of left scapular region
  - ● T22.169   Burn of first degree of unspecified scapular region
- ● T22.19   Burn of first degree of multiple sites of shoulder and upper limb, except wrist and hand
  - ● T22.191   Burn of first degree of multiple sites of right shoulder and upper limb, except wrist and hand
  - ● T22.192   Burn of first degree of multiple sites of left shoulder and upper limb, except wrist and hand
  - ● T22.199   Burn of first degree of multiple sites of unspecified shoulder and upper limb, except wrist and hand
- ● T22.2   Burn of second degree of shoulder and upper limb, except wrist and hand

  Use additional external cause code to identify the source, place and intent of the burn (X00-X19, X75-X77, X96-X98, Y92)
  - X● T22.20   Burn of second degree of shoulder and upper limb, except wrist and hand, unspecified site
  - ● T22.21   Burn of second degree of forearm
    - ● T22.211   Burn of second degree of right forearm
    - ● T22.212   Burn of second degree of left forearm
    - ● T22.219   Burn of second degree of unspecified forearm
  - ● T22.22   Burn of second degree of elbow
    - ● T22.221   Burn of second degree of right elbow
    - ● T22.222   Burn of second degree of left elbow
    - ● T22.229   Burn of second degree of unspecified elbow
  - ● T22.23   Burn of second degree of upper arm
    - ● T22.231   Burn of second degree of right upper arm
    - ● T22.232   Burn of second degree of left upper arm
    - ● T22.239   Burn of second degree of unspecified upper arm
  - ● T22.24   Burn of second degree of axilla
    - ● T22.241   Burn of second degree of right axilla
    - ● T22.242   Burn of second degree of left axilla
    - ● T22.249   Burn of second degree of unspecified axilla

CHAPTER 19 (S00-T88)

● **T22.25**   Burn of second degree of shoulder
    ● **T22.251**   Burn of second degree of right shoulder
    ● **T22.252**   Burn of second degree of left shoulder
    ● **T22.259**   Burn of second degree of unspecified shoulder

● **T22.26**   Burn of second degree of scapular region
    ● **T22.261**   Burn of second degree of right scapular region
    ● **T22.262**   Burn of second degree of left scapular region
    ● **T22.269**   Burn of second degree of unspecified scapular region

● **T22.29**   Burn of second degree of multiple sites of shoulder and upper limb, except wrist and hand
    ● **T22.291**   Burn of second degree of multiple sites of right shoulder and upper limb, except wrist and hand
    ● **T22.292**   Burn of second degree of multiple sites of left shoulder and upper limb, except wrist and hand
    ● **T22.299**   Burn of second degree of multiple sites of unspecified shoulder and upper limb, except wrist and hand

● **T22.3**   Burn of third degree of shoulder and upper limb, except wrist and hand

> Use additional external cause code to identify the source, place and intent of the burn (X00-X19, X75-X77, X96-X98, Y92)

X ● **T22.30**   Burn of third degree of shoulder and upper limb, except wrist and hand, unspecified site A 🪙, A 🪙
> (Ex) See PDX Collection 1389

● **T22.31**   Burn of third degree of forearm
> (Ex) For category T22.31 CC codes: See PDX Collection 1390
    ● **T22.311**   Burn of third degree of right forearm A 🪙, A 🪙
    ● **T22.312**   Burn of third degree of left forearm A 🪙, A 🪙
    ● **T22.319**   Burn of third degree of unspecified forearm A 🪙, A 🪙

● **T22.32**   Burn of third degree of elbow
> (Ex) For category T22.32 CC codes: See PDX Collection 1391
    ● **T22.321**   Burn of third degree of right elbow A 🪙, A 🪙
    ● **T22.322**   Burn of third degree of left elbow A 🪙, A 🪙
    ● **T22.329**   Burn of third degree of unspecified elbow A 🪙, A 🪙

● **T22.33**   Burn of third degree of upper arm
> (Ex) For category T22.33 CC codes: See PDX Collection 1392
    ● **T22.331**   Burn of third degree of right upper arm A 🪙, A 🪙
    ● **T22.332**   Burn of third degree of left upper arm A 🪙, A 🪙
    ● **T22.339**   Burn of third degree of unspecified upper arm A 🪙, A 🪙

● **T22.34**   Burn of third degree of axilla
> (Ex) For category T22.34 CC codes: See PDX Collection 1393
    ● **T22.341**   Burn of third degree of right axilla A 🪙, A 🪙
    ● **T22.342**   Burn of third degree of left axilla A 🪙, A 🪙
    ● **T22.349**   Burn of third degree of unspecified axilla A 🪙, A 🪙

● **T22.35**   Burn of third degree of shoulder
> (Ex) For category T22.35 CC codes: See PDX Collection 1394
    ● **T22.351**   Burn of third degree of right shoulder A 🪙, A 🪙
    ● **T22.352**   Burn of third degree of left shoulder A 🪙, A 🪙
    ● **T22.359**   Burn of third degree of unspecified shoulder A 🪙, A 🪙

● **T22.36**   Burn of third degree of scapular region
> (Ex) For category T22.36 CC codes: See PDX Collection 1395
    ● **T22.361**   Burn of third degree of right scapular region A 🪙, A 🪙
    ● **T22.362**   Burn of third degree of left scapular region A 🪙, A 🪙
    ● **T22.369**   Burn of third degree of unspecified scapular region A 🪙, A 🪙

● **T22.39**   Burn of third degree of multiple sites of shoulder and upper limb, except wrist and hand
> (Ex) For category T22.39 CC codes: See PDX Collection 1389
    ● **T22.391**   Burn of third degree of multiple sites of right shoulder and upper limb, except wrist and hand A 🪙, A 🪙
    ● **T22.392**   Burn of third degree of multiple sites of left shoulder and upper limb, except wrist and hand A 🪙, A 🪙
    ● **T22.399**   Burn of third degree of multiple sites of unspecified shoulder and upper limb, except wrist and hand A 🪙, A 🪙

● **T22.4**   Corrosion of unspecified degree of shoulder and upper limb, except wrist and hand

> *Code first (T51-T65) to identify chemical and intent*
> Use additional external cause code to identify place (Y92)

X ● **T22.40**   Corrosion of unspecified degree of shoulder and upper limb, except wrist and hand, unspecified site

● **T22.41**   Corrosion of unspecified degree of forearm
    ● **T22.411**   Corrosion of unspecified degree of right forearm
    ● **T22.412**   Corrosion of unspecified degree of left forearm
    ● **T22.419**   Corrosion of unspecified degree of unspecified forearm

● **T22.42**   Corrosion of unspecified degree of elbow
    ● **T22.421**   Corrosion of unspecified degree of right elbow
    ● **T22.422**   Corrosion of unspecified degree of left elbow
    ● **T22.429**   Corrosion of unspecified degree of unspecified elbow

● **T22.43**   Corrosion of unspecified degree of upper arm
    ● **T22.431**   Corrosion of unspecified degree of right upper arm
    ● **T22.432**   Corrosion of unspecified degree of left upper arm
    ● **T22.439**   Corrosion of unspecified degree of unspecified upper arm

● **T22.44**   Corrosion of unspecified degree of axilla
    ● **T22.441**   Corrosion of unspecified degree of right axilla
    ● **T22.442**   Corrosion of unspecified degree of left axilla
    ● **T22.449**   Corrosion of unspecified degree of unspecified axilla

N Newborn Age: 0   **P** Pediatric Age: 0–17   **M** Maternity DX: 9–64   **A** Adult Age: 15–124   ♀ Females Only   ♂ Males Only

🪙 Complication\Comorbidity   🪙 Major C\C   (Ex) CC/MCC Exclusions   🪙 Hospital-Acquired Condition   🪙 Hierarchical Condition Category

1441

CHAPTER 19 (S00-T88)

● **T22.45**   Corrosion of unspecified degree of shoulder
- ● **T22.451**   Corrosion of unspecified degree of right shoulder
- ● **T22.452**   Corrosion of unspecified degree of left shoulder
- ● **T22.459**   Corrosion of unspecified degree of unspecified shoulder

● **T22.46**   Corrosion of unspecified degree of scapular region
- ● **T22.461**   Corrosion of unspecified degree of right scapular region
- ● **T22.462**   Corrosion of unspecified degree of left scapular region
- ● **T22.469**   Corrosion of unspecified degree of unspecified scapular region

● **T22.49**   Corrosion of unspecified degree of multiple sites of shoulder and upper limb, except wrist and hand
- ● **T22.491**   Corrosion of unspecified degree of multiple sites of right shoulder and upper limb, except wrist and hand
- ● **T22.492**   Corrosion of unspecified degree of multiple sites of left shoulder and upper limb, except wrist and hand
- ● **T22.499**   Corrosion of unspecified degree of multiple sites of unspecified shoulder and upper limb, except wrist and hand

● **T22.5**   Corrosion of first degree of shoulder and upper limb, except wrist and hand

Code first (T51-T65) to identify chemical and intent

Use additional external cause code to identify place (Y92)

- X ● **T22.50**   Corrosion of first degree of shoulder and upper limb, except wrist and hand unspecified site
- ● **T22.51**   Corrosion of first degree of forearm
  - ● **T22.511**   Corrosion of first degree of right forearm
  - ● **T22.512**   Corrosion of first degree of left forearm
  - ● **T22.519**   Corrosion of first degree of unspecified forearm
- ● **T22.52**   Corrosion of first degree of elbow
  - ● **T22.521**   Corrosion of first degree of right elbow
  - ● **T22.522**   Corrosion of first degree of left elbow
  - ● **T22.529**   Corrosion of first degree of unspecified elbow
- ● **T22.53**   Corrosion of first degree of upper arm
  - ● **T22.531**   Corrosion of first degree of right upper arm
  - ● **T22.532**   Corrosion of first degree of left upper arm
  - ● **T22.539**   Corrosion of first degree of unspecified upper arm
- ● **T22.54**   Corrosion of first degree of axilla
  - ● **T22.541**   Corrosion of first degree of right axilla
  - ● **T22.542**   Corrosion of first degree of left axilla
  - ● **T22.549**   Corrosion of first degree of unspecified axilla

● **T22.55**   Corrosion of first degree of shoulder
- ● **T22.551**   Corrosion of first degree of right shoulder
- ● **T22.552**   Corrosion of first degree of left shoulder
- ● **T22.559**   Corrosion of first degree of unspecified shoulder

● **T22.56**   Corrosion of first degree of scapular region
- ● **T22.561**   Corrosion of first degree of right scapular region
- ● **T22.562**   Corrosion of first degree of left scapular region
- ● **T22.569**   Corrosion of first degree of unspecified scapular region

● **T22.59**   Corrosion of first degree of multiple sites of shoulder and upper limb, except wrist and hand
- ● **T22.591**   Corrosion of first degree of multiple sites of right shoulder and upper limb, except wrist and hand
- ● **T22.592**   Corrosion of first degree of multiple sites of left shoulder and upper limb, except wrist and hand
- ● **T22.599**   Corrosion of first degree of multiple sites of unspecified shoulder and upper limb, except wrist and hand

● **T22.6**   Corrosion of second degree of shoulder and upper limb, except wrist and hand

Code first (T51-T65) to identify chemical and intent

Use additional external cause code to identify place (Y92)

- X ● **T22.60**   Corrosion of second degree of shoulder and upper limb, except wrist and hand, unspecified site
- ● **T22.61**   Corrosion of second degree of forearm
  - ● **T22.611**   Corrosion of second degree of right forearm
  - ● **T22.612**   Corrosion of second degree of left forearm
  - ● **T22.619**   Corrosion of second degree of unspecified forearm
- ● **T22.62**   Corrosion of second degree of elbow
  - ● **T22.621**   Corrosion of second degree of right elbow
  - ● **T22.622**   Corrosion of second degree of left elbow
  - ● **T22.629**   Corrosion of second degree of unspecified elbow
- ● **T22.63**   Corrosion of second degree of upper arm
  - ● **T22.631**   Corrosion of second degree of right upper arm
  - ● **T22.632**   Corrosion of second degree of left upper arm
  - ● **T22.639**   Corrosion of second degree of unspecified upper arm
- ● **T22.64**   Corrosion of second degree of axilla
  - ● **T22.641**   Corrosion of second degree of right axilla
  - ● **T22.642**   Corrosion of second degree of left axilla
  - ● **T22.649**   Corrosion of second degree of unspecified axilla

● **T22.65** Corrosion of second degree of shoulder
    ● **T22.651** Corrosion of second degree of right shoulder
    ● **T22.652** Corrosion of second degree of left shoulder
    ● **T22.659** Corrosion of second degree of unspecified shoulder

● **T22.66** Corrosion of second degree of scapular region
    ● **T22.661** Corrosion of second degree of right scapular region
    ● **T22.662** Corrosion of second degree of left scapular region
    ● **T22.669** Corrosion of second degree of unspecified scapular region

● **T22.69** Corrosion of second degree of multiple sites of shoulder and upper limb, except wrist and hand
    ● **T22.691** Corrosion of second degree of multiple sites of right shoulder and upper limb, except wrist and hand
    ● **T22.692** Corrosion of second degree of multiple sites of left shoulder and upper limb, except wrist and hand
    ● **T22.699** Corrosion of second degree of multiple sites of unspecified shoulder and upper limb, except wrist and hand

● **T22.7** Corrosion of third degree of shoulder and upper limb, except wrist and hand

Code first (T51-T65) to identify chemical and intent
Use additional external cause code to identify place (Y92)

X ● **T22.70** Corrosion of third degree of shoulder and upper limb, except wrist and hand, unspecified site A 🐾, A 🐾
    (Ex:) See PDX Collection 1389

● **T22.71** Corrosion of third degree of forearm
    (Ex:) For category T22.71 CC codes: See PDX Collection 1390
    ● **T22.711** Corrosion of third degree of right forearm A 🐾, A 🐾
    ● **T22.712** Corrosion of third degree of left forearm A 🐾, A 🐾
    ● **T22.719** Corrosion of third degree of unspecified forearm A 🐾, A 🐾

● **T22.72** Corrosion of third degree of elbow
    (Ex:) For category T22.72 CC codes: See PDX Collection 1391
    ● **T22.721** Corrosion of third degree of right elbow A 🐾, A 🐾
    ● **T22.722** Corrosion of third degree of left elbow A 🐾, A 🐾
    ● **T22.729** Corrosion of third degree of unspecified elbow A 🐾, A 🐾

● **T22.73** Corrosion of third degree of upper arm
    (Ex:) For category T22.73 CC codes: See PDX Collection 1392
    ● **T22.731** Corrosion of third degree of right upper arm A 🐾, A 🐾
    ● **T22.732** Corrosion of third degree of left upper arm A 🐾, A 🐾
    ● **T22.739** Corrosion of third degree of unspecified upper arm A 🐾, A 🐾

● **T22.74** Corrosion of third degree of axilla
    (Ex:) For category T22.74 CC codes: See PDX Collection 1393
    ● **T22.741** Corrosion of third degree of right axilla A 🐾, A 🐾
    ● **T22.742** Corrosion of third degree of left axilla A 🐾, A 🐾
    ● **T22.749** Corrosion of third degree of unspecified axilla A 🐾, A 🐾

● **T22.75** Corrosion of third degree of shoulder
    (Ex:) For category T22.75 CC codes: See PDX Collection 1394
    ● **T22.751** Corrosion of third degree of right shoulder A 🐾, A 🐾
    ● **T22.752** Corrosion of third degree of left shoulder A 🐾, A 🐾
    ● **T22.759** Corrosion of third degree of unspecified shoulder A 🐾, A 🐾

● **T22.76** Corrosion of third degree of scapular region
    (Ex:) For category T22.76 CC codes: See PDX Collection 1395
    ● **T22.761** Corrosion of third degree of right scapular region A 🐾, A 🐾
    ● **T22.762** Corrosion of third degree of left scapular region A 🐾, A 🐾
    ● **T22.769** Corrosion of third degree of unspecified scapular region A 🐾, A 🐾

● **T22.79** Corrosion of third degree of multiple sites of shoulder and upper limb, except wrist and hand
    (Ex:) For category T22.79 CC codes: See PDX Collection 1389
    ● **T22.791** Corrosion of third degree of multiple sites of right shoulder and upper limb, except wrist and hand A 🐾, A 🐾
    ● **T22.792** Corrosion of third degree of multiple sites of left shoulder and upper limb, except wrist and hand A 🐾, A 🐾
    ● **T22.799** Corrosion of third degree of multiple sites of unspecified shoulder and upper limb, except wrist and hand A 🐾, A 🐾

● **T23** Burn and corrosion of wrist and hand

The appropriate 7th character is to be added to each code from category T23

A	initial encounter
D	subsequent encounter
S	sequela

● **T23.0** Burn of unspecified degree of wrist and hand

Use additional external cause code to identify the source, place and intent of the burn (X00-X19, X75-X77, X96-X98, Y92)

    ● **T23.00** Burn of unspecified degree of hand, unspecified site
        ● **T23.001** Burn of unspecified degree of right hand, unspecified site
        ● **T23.002** Burn of unspecified degree of left hand, unspecified site
        ● **T23.009** Burn of unspecified degree of unspecified hand, unspecified site

    ● **T23.01** Burn of unspecified degree of thumb (nail)
        ● **T23.011** Burn of unspecified degree of right thumb (nail)
        ● **T23.012** Burn of unspecified degree of left thumb (nail)
        ● **T23.019** Burn of unspecified degree of unspecified thumb (nail)

    ● **T23.02** Burn of unspecified degree of single finger (nail) except thumb
        ● **T23.021** Burn of unspecified degree of single right finger (nail) except thumb
        ● **T23.022** Burn of unspecified degree of single left finger (nail) except thumb
        ● **T23.029** Burn of unspecified degree of unspecified single finger (nail) except thumb

N Newborn Age: 0   **P** Pediatric Age: 0–17   **M** Maternity DX: 9–64   **A** Adult Age: 15–124   ♀ Females Only   ♂ Males Only

🐾 Complication\Comorbidity   🐾 Major C\C   (Ex:) CC/MCC Exclusions   🐾 Hospital-Acquired Condition   🐾 Hierarchical Condition Category

1443

CHAPTER 19 (S00-T88)

● T23.03   Burn of unspecified degree of multiple fingers (nail), not including thumb

  ● T23.031   Burn of unspecified degree of multiple right fingers (nail), not including thumb

  ● T23.032   Burn of unspecified degree of multiple left fingers (nail), not including thumb

  ● T23.039   Burn of unspecified degree of unspecified multiple fingers (nail), not including thumb

● T23.04   Burn of unspecified degree of multiple fingers (nail), including thumb

  ● T23.041   Burn of unspecified degree of multiple right fingers (nail), including thumb

  ● T23.042   Burn of unspecified degree of multiple left fingers (nail), including thumb

  ● T23.049   Burn of unspecified degree of unspecified multiple fingers (nail), including thumb

● T23.05   Burn of unspecified degree of palm

  ● T23.051   Burn of unspecified degree of right palm

  ● T23.052   Burn of unspecified degree of left palm

  ● T23.059   Burn of unspecified degree of unspecified palm

● T23.06   Burn of unspecified degree of back of hand

  ● T23.061   Burn of unspecified degree of back of right hand

  ● T23.062   Burn of unspecified degree of back of left hand

  ● T23.069   Burn of unspecified degree of back of unspecified hand

● T23.07   Burn of unspecified degree of wrist

  ● T23.071   Burn of unspecified degree of right wrist

  ● T23.072   Burn of unspecified degree of left wrist

  ● T23.079   Burn of unspecified degree of unspecified wrist

● T23.09   Burn of unspecified degree of multiple sites of wrist and hand

  ● T23.091   Burn of unspecified degree of multiple sites of right wrist and hand

  ● T23.092   Burn of unspecified degree of multiple sites of left wrist and hand

  ● T23.099   Burn of unspecified degree of multiple sites of unspecified wrist and hand

● T23.1   Burn of first degree of wrist and hand

Use additional external cause code to identify the source, place and intent of the burn (X00-X19, X75-X77, X96-X98, Y92)

  ● T23.10   Burn of first degree of hand, unspecified site

    ● T23.101   Burn of first degree of right hand, unspecified site

    ● T23.102   Burn of first degree of left hand, unspecified site

    ● T23.109   Burn of first degree of unspecified hand, unspecified site

● T23.11   Burn of first degree of thumb (nail)

  ● T23.111   Burn of first degree of right thumb (nail)

  ● T23.112   Burn of first degree of left thumb (nail)

  ● T23.119   Burn of first degree of unspecified thumb (nail)

● T23.12   Burn of first degree of single finger (nail) except thumb

  ● T23.121   Burn of first degree of single right finger (nail) except thumb

  ● T23.122   Burn of first degree of single left finger (nail) except thumb

  ● T23.129   Burn of first degree of unspecified single finger (nail) except thumb

● T23.13   Burn of first degree of multiple fingers (nail), not including thumb

  ● T23.131   Burn of first degree of multiple right fingers (nail), not including thumb

  ● T23.132   Burn of first degree of multiple left fingers (nail), not including thumb

  ● T23.139   Burn of first degree of unspecified multiple fingers (nail), not including thumb

● T23.14   Burn of first degree of multiple fingers (nail), including thumb

  ● T23.141   Burn of first degree of multiple right fingers (nail), including thumb

  ● T23.142   Burn of first degree of multiple left fingers (nail), including thumb

  ● T23.149   Burn of first degree of unspecified multiple fingers (nail), including thumb

● T23.15   Burn of first degree of palm

  ● T23.151   Burn of first degree of right palm

  ● T23.152   Burn of first degree of left palm

  ● T23.159   Burn of first degree of unspecified palm

● T23.16   Burn of first degree of back of hand

  ● T23.161   Burn of first degree of back of right hand

  ● T23.162   Burn of first degree of back of left hand

  ● T23.169   Burn of first degree of back of unspecified hand

● T23.17   Burn of first degree of wrist

  ● T23.171   Burn of first degree of right wrist

  ● T23.172   Burn of first degree of left wrist

  ● T23.179   Burn of first degree of unspecified wrist

● T23.19   Burn of first degree of multiple sites of wrist and hand

  ● T23.191   Burn of first degree of multiple sites of right wrist and hand

  ● T23.192   Burn of first degree of multiple sites of left wrist and hand

  ● T23.199   Burn of first degree of multiple sites of unspecified wrist and hand

▶ New   ⇒ Revised   ~~deleted~~ Deleted   Excludes 1   Excludes 2   Includes   Use additional   Code first   Code also   Key words

OGCR Official Guidelines   ● Unacceptable Principal Diagnosis   X Assign placeholder X   ● Use Additional Character(s)   ▷ Manifestation Code   **Coding Clinic**

● **T23.2**   Burn of second degree of wrist and hand

Use additional external cause code to identify the source, place and intent of the burn (X00-X19, X75-X77, X96-X98, Y92)

- ● **T23.20**   Burn of second degree of hand, unspecified site
  - ● **T23.201**   Burn of second degree of right hand, unspecified site
  - ● **T23.202**   Burn of second degree of left hand, unspecified site
  - ● **T23.209**   Burn of second degree of unspecified hand, unspecified site
- ● **T23.21**   Burn of second degree of thumb (nail)
  - ● **T23.211**   Burn of second degree of right thumb (nail)
  - ● **T23.212**   Burn of second degree of left thumb (nail)
  - ● **T23.219**   Burn of second degree of unspecified thumb (nail)
- ● **T23.22**   Burn of second degree of single finger (nail) except thumb
  - ● **T23.221**   Burn of second degree of single right finger (nail) except thumb
  - ● **T23.222**   Burn of second degree of single left finger (nail) except thumb
  - ● **T23.229**   Burn of second degree of unspecified single finger (nail) except thumb
- ● **T23.23**   Burn of second degree of multiple fingers (nail), not including thumb
  - ● **T23.231**   Burn of second degree of multiple right fingers (nail), not including thumb
  - ● **T23.232**   Burn of second degree of multiple left fingers (nail), not including thumb
  - ● **T23.239**   Burn of second degree of unspecified multiple fingers (nail), not including thumb
- ● **T23.24**   Burn of second degree of multiple fingers (nail), including thumb
  - ● **T23.241**   Burn of second degree of multiple right fingers (nail), including thumb
  - ● **T23.242**   Burn of second degree of multiple left fingers (nail), including thumb
  - ● **T23.249**   Burn of second degree of unspecified multiple fingers (nail), including thumb
- ● **T23.25**   Burn of second degree of palm
  - ● **T23.251**   Burn of second degree of right palm
  - ● **T23.252**   Burn of second degree of left palm
  - ● **T23.259**   Burn of second degree of unspecified palm
- ● **T23.26**   Burn of second degree of back of hand
  - ● **T23.261**   Burn of second degree of back of right hand
  - ● **T23.262**   Burn of second degree of back of left hand
  - ● **T23.269**   Burn of second degree of back of unspecified hand
- ● **T23.27**   Burn of second degree of wrist
  - ● **T23.271**   Burn of second degree of right wrist
  - ● **T23.272**   Burn of second degree of left wrist
  - ● **T23.279**   Burn of second degree of unspecified wrist
- ● **T23.29**   Burn of second degree of multiple sites of wrist and hand
  - ● **T23.291**   Burn of second degree of multiple sites of right wrist and hand
  - ● **T23.292**   Burn of second degree of multiple sites of left wrist and hand
  - ● **T23.299**   Burn of second degree of multiple sites of unspecified wrist and hand

● **T23.3**   Burn of third degree of wrist and hand

Use additional external cause code to identify the source, place and intent of the burn (X00-X19, X75-X77, X96-X98, Y92)

- ● **T23.30**   Burn of third degree of hand, unspecified site
  - (Ex) For category T23.30 CC codes: See PDX Collection 1396
  - ● **T23.301**   Burn of third degree of right hand, unspecified site A 🔖, A 🔖
    Coding Clinic: 2015, Q1, P19
  - ● **T23.302**   Burn of third degree of left hand, unspecified site A 🔖, A 🔖
    Coding Clinic: 2016, Q2, P5
  - ● **T23.309**   Burn of third degree of unspecified hand, unspecified site A 🔖, A 🔖
- ● **T23.31**   Burn of third degree of thumb (nail)
  - (Ex) For category T23.31 CC codes: See PDX Collection 1397
  - ● **T23.311**   Burn of third degree of right thumb (nail) A 🔖, A 🔖
  - ● **T23.312**   Burn of third degree of left thumb (nail) A 🔖, A 🔖
  - ● **T23.319**   Burn of third degree of unspecified thumb (nail) A 🔖, A 🔖
- ● **T23.32**   Burn of third degree of single finger (nail) except thumb
  - (Ex) For category T23.32 CC codes: See PDX Collection 1398
  - ● **T23.321**   Burn of third degree of single right finger (nail) except thumb A 🔖, A 🔖
  - ● **T23.322**   Burn of third degree of single left finger (nail) except thumb A 🔖, A 🔖
  - ● **T23.329**   Burn of third degree of unspecified single finger (nail) except thumb A 🔖, A 🔖
- ● **T23.33**   Burn of third degree of multiple fingers (nail), not including thumb
  - (Ex) For category T23.33 CC codes: See PDX Collection 1399
  - ● **T23.331**   Burn of third degree of multiple right fingers (nail), not including thumb A 🔖, A 🔖
  - ● **T23.332**   Burn of third degree of multiple left fingers (nail), not including thumb A 🔖, A 🔖
  - ● **T23.339**   Burn of third degree of unspecified multiple fingers (nail), not including thumb A 🔖, A 🔖
- ● **T23.34**   Burn of third degree of multiple fingers (nail), including thumb
  - (Ex) For category T23.34 CC codes: See PDX Collection 1400
  - ● **T23.341**   Burn of third degree of multiple right fingers (nail), including thumb A 🔖, A 🔖
  - ● **T23.342**   Burn of third degree of multiple left fingers (nail), including thumb A 🔖, A 🔖
  - ● **T23.349**   Burn of third degree of unspecified multiple fingers (nail), including thumb A 🔖, A 🔖
- ● **T23.35**   Burn of third degree of palm
  - (Ex) For category T23.35 CC codes: See PDX Collection 1401
  - ● **T23.351**   Burn of third degree of right palm A 🔖, A 🔖
  - ● **T23.352**   Burn of third degree of left palm A 🔖, A 🔖
  - ● **T23.359**   Burn of third degree of unspecified palm A 🔖, A 🔖
- ● **T23.36**   Burn of third degree of back of hand
  - (Ex) For category T23.36 CC codes: See PDX Collection 1402
  - ● **T23.361**   Burn of third degree of back of right hand A 🔖, A 🔖
  - ● **T23.362**   Burn of third degree of back of left hand A 🔖, A 🔖
  - ● **T23.369**   Burn of third degree of back of unspecified hand A 🔖, A 🔖

CHAPTER 19 (S00-T88)

N Newborn Age: 0   **P** Pediatric Age: 0–17   **M** Maternity DX: 9–64   **A** Adult Age: 15–124   ♀ Females Only   ♂ Males Only

🔖 Complication\Comorbidity   🔖 Major C\C   (Ex) CC/MCC Exclusions   🔖 Hospital-Acquired Condition   🔖 Hierarchical Condition Category

1445

● **T23.37**   Burn of third degree of wrist
     (Ex) For category T23.37 CC codes: See PDX Collection 1403
  ● **T23.371**   Burn of third degree of right wrist A , A
  ● **T23.372**   Burn of third degree of left wrist A , A
  ● **T23.379**   Burn of third degree of unspecified wrist A , A
● **T23.39**   Burn of third degree of multiple sites of wrist and hand
     (Ex) For category T23.39 CC codes: See PDX Collection 1396
  ● **T23.391**   Burn of third degree of multiple sites of right wrist and hand A , A
  ● **T23.392**   Burn of third degree of multiple sites of left wrist and hand A , A
  ● **T23.399**   Burn of third degree of multiple sites of unspecified wrist and hand A , A

● **T23.4**   Corrosion of unspecified degree of wrist and hand
   Code first (T51-T65) to identify chemical and intent
   Use additional external cause code to identify place (Y92)
  ● **T23.40**   Corrosion of unspecified degree of hand, unspecified site
    ● **T23.401**   Corrosion of unspecified degree of right hand, unspecified site
    ● **T23.402**   Corrosion of unspecified degree of left hand, unspecified site
    ● **T23.409**   Corrosion of unspecified degree of unspecified hand, unspecified site
  ● **T23.41**   Corrosion of unspecified degree of thumb (nail)
    ● **T23.411**   Corrosion of unspecified degree of right thumb (nail)
    ● **T23.412**   Corrosion of unspecified degree of left thumb (nail)
    ● **T23.419**   Corrosion of unspecified degree of unspecified thumb (nail)
  ● **T23.42**   Corrosion of unspecified degree of single finger (nail) except thumb
    ● **T23.421**   Corrosion of unspecified degree of single right finger (nail) except thumb
    ● **T23.422**   Corrosion of unspecified degree of single left finger (nail) except thumb
    ● **T23.429**   Corrosion of unspecified degree of unspecified single finger (nail) except thumb
  ● **T23.43**   Corrosion of unspecified degree of multiple fingers (nail), not including thumb
    ● **T23.431**   Corrosion of unspecified degree of multiple right fingers (nail), not including thumb
    ● **T23.432**   Corrosion of unspecified degree of multiple left fingers (nail), not including thumb
    ● **T23.439**   Corrosion of unspecified degree of unspecified multiple fingers (nail), not including thumb
  ● **T23.44**   Corrosion of unspecified degree of multiple fingers (nail), including thumb
    ● **T23.441**   Corrosion of unspecified degree of multiple right fingers (nail), including thumb
    ● **T23.442**   Corrosion of unspecified degree of multiple left fingers (nail), including thumb
    ● **T23.449**   Corrosion of unspecified degree of unspecified multiple fingers (nail), including thumb

● **T23.45**   Corrosion of unspecified degree of palm
  ● **T23.451**   Corrosion of unspecified degree of right palm
  ● **T23.452**   Corrosion of unspecified degree of left palm
  ● **T23.459**   Corrosion of unspecified degree of unspecified palm
● **T23.46**   Corrosion of unspecified degree of back of hand
  ● **T23.461**   Corrosion of unspecified degree of back of right hand
  ● **T23.462**   Corrosion of unspecified degree of back of left hand
  ● **T23.469**   Corrosion of unspecified degree of back of unspecified hand
● **T23.47**   Corrosion of unspecified degree of wrist
  ● **T23.471**   Corrosion of unspecified degree of right wrist
  ● **T23.472**   Corrosion of unspecified degree of left wrist
  ● **T23.479**   Corrosion of unspecified degree of unspecified wrist
● **T23.49**   Corrosion of unspecified degree of multiple sites of wrist and hand
  ● **T23.491**   Corrosion of unspecified degree of multiple sites of right wrist and hand
  ● **T23.492**   Corrosion of unspecified degree of multiple sites of left wrist and hand
  ● **T23.499**   Corrosion of unspecified degree of multiple sites of unspecified wrist and hand

● **T23.5**   Corrosion of first degree of wrist and hand
   Code first (T51-T65) to identify chemical and intent
   Use additional external cause code to identify place (Y92)
  ● **T23.50**   Corrosion of first degree of hand, unspecified site
    ● **T23.501**   Corrosion of first degree of right hand, unspecified site
    ● **T23.502**   Corrosion of first degree of left hand, unspecified site
    ● **T23.509**   Corrosion of first degree of unspecified hand, unspecified site
  ● **T23.51**   Corrosion of first degree of thumb (nail)
    ● **T23.511**   Corrosion of first degree of right thumb (nail)
    ● **T23.512**   Corrosion of first degree of left thumb (nail)
    ● **T23.519**   Corrosion of first degree of unspecified thumb (nail)
  ● **T23.52**   Corrosion of first degree of single finger (nail) except thumb
    ● **T23.521**   Corrosion of first degree of single right finger (nail) except thumb
    ● **T23.522**   Corrosion of first degree of single left finger (nail) except thumb
    ● **T23.529**   Corrosion of first degree of unspecified single finger (nail) except thumb
  ● **T23.53**   Corrosion of first degree of multiple fingers (nail), not including thumb
    ● **T23.531**   Corrosion of first degree of multiple right fingers (nail), not including thumb
    ● **T23.532**   Corrosion of first degree of multiple left fingers (nail), not including thumb
    ● **T23.539**   Corrosion of first degree of unspecified multiple fingers (nail), not including thumb

▶ New   ⇒ Revised   ~~deleted~~ Deleted   Excludes 1   Excludes 2   Includes   Use additional   Code first   Code also   Key words
OGCR Official Guidelines   ● Unacceptable Principal Diagnosis   X Assign placeholder X   ● Use Additional Character(s)   ▶ Manifestation Code   Coding Clinic

● T23.54   Corrosion of first degree of multiple fingers (nail), including thumb
- ● T23.541   Corrosion of first degree of multiple right fingers (nail), including thumb
- ● T23.542   Corrosion of first degree of multiple left fingers (nail), including thumb
- ● T23.549   Corrosion of first degree of unspecified multiple fingers (nail), including thumb

● T23.55   Corrosion of first degree of palm
- ● T23.551   Corrosion of first degree of right palm
- ● T23.552   Corrosion of first degree of left palm
- ● T23.559   Corrosion of first degree of unspecified palm

● T23.56   Corrosion of first degree of back of hand
- ● T23.561   Corrosion of first degree of back of right hand
- ● T23.562   Corrosion of first degree of back of left hand
- ● T23.569   Corrosion of first degree of back of unspecified hand

● T23.57   Corrosion of first degree of wrist
- ● T23.571   Corrosion of first degree of right wrist
- ● T23.572   Corrosion of first degree of left wrist
- ● T23.579   Corrosion of first degree of unspecified wrist

● T23.59   Corrosion of first degree of multiple sites of wrist and hand
- ● T23.591   Corrosion of first degree of multiple sites of right wrist and hand
- ● T23.592   Corrosion of first degree of multiple sites of left wrist and hand
- ● T23.599   Corrosion of first degree of multiple sites of unspecified wrist and hand

● T23.6   Corrosion of second degree of wrist and hand
Code first (T51-T65) to identify chemical and intent
Use additional external cause code to identify place (Y92)

● T23.60   Corrosion of second degree of hand, unspecified site
- ● T23.601   Corrosion of second degree of right hand, unspecified site
- ● T23.602   Corrosion of second degree of left hand, unspecified site
- ● T23.609   Corrosion of second degree of unspecified hand, unspecified site

● T23.61   Corrosion of second degree of thumb (nail)
- ● T23.611   Corrosion of second degree of right thumb (nail)
- ● T23.612   Corrosion of second degree of left thumb (nail)
- ● T23.619   Corrosion of second degree of unspecified thumb (nail)

● T23.62   Corrosion of second degree of single finger (nail) except thumb
- ● T23.621   Corrosion of second degree of single right finger (nail) except thumb
- ● T23.622   Corrosion of second degree of single left finger (nail) except thumb
- ● T23.629   Corrosion of second degree of unspecified single finger (nail) except thumb

● T23.63   Corrosion of second degree of multiple fingers (nail), not including thumb
- ● T23.631   Corrosion of second degree of multiple right fingers (nail), not including thumb
- ● T23.632   Corrosion of second degree of multiple left fingers (nail), not including thumb
- ● T23.639   Corrosion of second degree of unspecified multiple fingers (nail), not including thumb

● T23.64   Corrosion of second degree of multiple fingers (nail), including thumb
- ● T23.641   Corrosion of second degree of multiple right fingers (nail), including thumb
- ● T23.642   Corrosion of second degree of multiple left fingers (nail), including thumb
- ● T23.649   Corrosion of second degree of unspecified multiple fingers (nail), including thumb

● T23.65   Corrosion of second degree of palm
- ● T23.651   Corrosion of second degree of right palm
- ● T23.652   Corrosion of second degree of left palm
- ● T23.659   Corrosion of second degree of unspecified palm

● T23.66   Corrosion of second degree of back of hand
- ● T23.661   Corrosion of second degree back of right hand
- ● T23.662   Corrosion of second degree back of left hand
- ● T23.669   Corrosion of second degree back of unspecified hand

● T23.67   Corrosion of second degree of wrist
- ● T23.671   Corrosion of second degree of right wrist
- ● T23.672   Corrosion of second degree of left wrist
- ● T23.679   Corrosion of second degree of unspecified wrist

● T23.69   Corrosion of second degree of multiple sites of wrist and hand
- ● T23.691   Corrosion of second degree of multiple sites of right wrist and hand
- ● T23.692   Corrosion of second degree of multiple sites of left wrist and hand
- ● T23.699   Corrosion of second degree of multiple sites of unspecified wrist and hand

● T23.7   Corrosion of third degree of wrist and hand
Code first (T51-T65) to identify chemical and intent
Use additional external cause code to identify place (Y92)

● T23.70   Corrosion of third degree of hand, unspecified site
    (Ex) **For category T23.70 CC codes:** See PDX Collection 1396
- ● T23.701   Corrosion of third degree of right hand, unspecified site A 🅒, A 🅜
- ● T23.702   Corrosion of third degree of left hand, unspecified site A 🅒, A 🅜
- ● T23.709   Corrosion of third degree of unspecified hand, unspecified site A 🅒, A 🅜

N Newborn Age: 0   **P** Pediatric Age: 0–17   **M** Maternity DX: 9–64   **A** Adult Age: 15–124   ♀ Females Only   ♂ Males Only

🅒 Complication\Comorbidity   🅜 Major C\C   (Ex) CC/MCC Exclusions   🅗 Hospital-Acquired Condition   🅗 Hierarchical Condition Category

1447

● **T23.71**   Corrosion of third degree of thumb (nail)
    (Ex) **For category T23.71 CC codes:** See PDX Collection 1397

    ● **T23.711**   Corrosion of third degree of right thumb (nail) A 🔖, A 🔖

    ● **T23.712**   Corrosion of third degree of left thumb (nail) A 🔖, A 🔖

    ● **T23.719**   Corrosion of third degree of unspecified thumb (nail) A 🔖, A 🔖

● **T23.72**   Corrosion of third degree of single finger (nail) except thumb
    (Ex) **For category T23.72 CC codes:** See PDX Collection 1398

    ● **T23.721**   Corrosion of third degree of single right finger (nail) except thumb A 🔖, A 🔖

    ● **T23.722**   Corrosion of third degree of single left finger (nail) except thumb A 🔖, A 🔖

    ● **T23.729**   Corrosion of third degree of unspecified single finger (nail) except thumb A 🔖, A 🔖

● **T23.73**   Corrosion of third degree of multiple fingers (nail), not including thumb
    (Ex) **For category T23.73 CC codes:** See PDX Collection 1399

    ● **T23.731**   Corrosion of third degree of multiple right fingers (nail), not including thumb A 🔖, A 🔖

    ● **T23.732**   Corrosion of third degree of multiple left fingers (nail), not including thumb A 🔖, A 🔖

    ● **T23.739**   Corrosion of third degree of unspecified multiple fingers (nail), not including thumb A 🔖, A 🔖

● **T23.74**   Corrosion of third degree of multiple fingers (nail), including thumb
    (Ex) **For category T23.74 CC codes:** See PDX Collection 1400

    ● **T23.741**   Corrosion of third degree of multiple right fingers (nail), including thumb A 🔖, A 🔖

    ● **T23.742**   Corrosion of third degree of multiple left fingers (nail), including thumb A 🔖, A 🔖

    ● **T23.749**   Corrosion of third degree of unspecified multiple fingers (nail), including thumb A 🔖, A 🔖

● **T23.75**   Corrosion of third degree of palm
    (Ex) **For category T23.75 CC codes:** See PDX Collection 1401

    ● **T23.751**   Corrosion of third degree of right palm A 🔖, A 🔖

    ● **T23.752**   Corrosion of third degree of left palm A 🔖, A 🔖

    ● **T23.759**   Corrosion of third degree of unspecified palm A 🔖, A 🔖

● **T23.76**   Corrosion of third degree of back of hand
    (Ex) **For category T23.76 CC codes:** See PDX Collection 1402

    ● **T23.761**   Corrosion of third degree of back of right hand A 🔖, A 🔖

    ● **T23.762**   Corrosion of third degree of back of left hand A 🔖, A 🔖

    ● **T23.769**   Corrosion of third degree of back of unspecified hand A 🔖, A 🔖

● **T23.77**   Corrosion of third degree of wrist
    (Ex) **For category T23.77 CC codes:** See PDX Collection 1403

    ● **T23.771**   Corrosion of third degree of right wrist A 🔖, A 🔖

    ● **T23.772**   Corrosion of third degree of left wrist A 🔖, A 🔖

    ● **T23.779**   Corrosion of third degree of unspecified wrist A 🔖, A 🔖

● **T23.79**   Corrosion of third degree of multiple sites of wrist and hand
    (Ex) **For category T23.79 CC codes:** See PDX Collection 1396

    ● **T23.791**   Corrosion of third degree of multiple sites of right wrist and hand A 🔖, A 🔖

    ● **T23.792**   Corrosion of third degree of multiple sites of left wrist and hand A 🔖, A 🔖

    ● **T23.799**   Corrosion of third degree of multiple sites of unspecified wrist and hand A 🔖, A 🔖

● **T24**   Burn and corrosion of lower limb, except ankle and foot

    Excludes2   burn and corrosion of ankle and foot (T25.-)
                 burn and corrosion of hip region (T21.-)

    The appropriate 7th character is to be added to each code from category T24

A	initial encounter
D	subsequent encounter
S	sequela

● **T24.0**   Burn of unspecified degree of lower limb, except ankle and foot

    Use additional external cause code to identify the source, place and intent of the burn (X00-X19, X75-X77, X96-X98, Y92)

    ● **T24.00**   Burn of unspecified degree of unspecified site of lower limb, except ankle and foot

       ● **T24.001**   Burn of unspecified degree of unspecified site of right lower limb, except ankle and foot

       ● **T24.002**   Burn of unspecified degree of unspecified site of left lower limb, except ankle and foot

       ● **T24.009**   Burn of unspecified degree of unspecified site of unspecified lower limb, except ankle and foot

    ● **T24.01**   Burn of unspecified degree of thigh

       ● **T24.011**   Burn of unspecified degree of right thigh

       ● **T24.012**   Burn of unspecified degree of left thigh

       ● **T24.019**   Burn of unspecified degree of unspecified thigh

    ● **T24.02**   Burn of unspecified degree of knee

       ● **T24.021**   Burn of unspecified degree of right knee

       ● **T24.022**   Burn of unspecified degree of left knee

       ● **T24.029**   Burn of unspecified degree of unspecified knee

    ● **T24.03**   Burn of unspecified degree of lower leg

       ● **T24.031**   Burn of unspecified degree of right lower leg

       ● **T24.032**   Burn of unspecified degree of left lower leg

       ● **T24.039**   Burn of unspecified degree of unspecified lower leg

    ● **T24.09**   Burn of unspecified degree of multiple sites of lower limb, except ankle and foot

       ● **T24.091**   Burn of unspecified degree of multiple sites of right lower limb, except ankle and foot

       ● **T24.092**   Burn of unspecified degree of multiple sites of left lower limb, except ankle and foot

       ● **T24.099**   Burn of unspecified degree of multiple sites of unspecified lower limb, except ankle and foot

▶ New   ⇨ Revised   ~~deleted~~ Deleted   Excludes 1   Excludes 2   Includes   Use additional   Code first   Code also   Key words

OGCR Official Guidelines   ● Unacceptable Principal Diagnosis   X Assign placeholder X   ◗ Use Additional Character(s)   ▶ Manifestation Code   **Coding Clinic**

● **T24.1**   Burn of first degree of lower limb, except ankle and foot

> Use additional external cause code to identify the source, place and intent of the burn (X00-X19, X75-X77, X96-X98, Y92)

   ● **T24.10**   Burn of first degree of unspecified site of lower limb, except ankle and foot

     ● **T24.101**   Burn of first degree of unspecified site of right lower limb, except ankle and foot

     ● **T24.102**   Burn of first degree of unspecified site of left lower limb, except ankle and foot

     ● **T24.109**   Burn of first degree of unspecified site of unspecified lower limb, except ankle and foot

   ● **T24.11**   Burn of first degree of thigh

     ● **T24.111**   Burn of first degree of right thigh

     ● **T24.112**   Burn of first degree of left thigh

     ● **T24.119**   Burn of first degree of unspecified thigh

   ● **T24.12**   Burn of first degree of knee

     ● **T24.121**   Burn of first degree of right knee

     ● **T24.122**   Burn of first degree of left knee

     ● **T24.129**   Burn of first degree of unspecified knee

   ● **T24.13**   Burn of first degree of lower leg

     ● **T24.131**   Burn of first degree of right lower leg

     ● **T24.132**   Burn of first degree of left lower leg

     ● **T24.139**   Burn of first degree of unspecified lower leg

   ● **T24.19**   Burn of first degree of multiple sites of lower limb, except ankle and foot

     ● **T24.191**   Burn of first degree of multiple sites of right lower limb, except ankle and foot

     ● **T24.192**   Burn of first degree of multiple sites of left lower limb, except ankle and foot

     ● **T24.199**   Burn of first degree of multiple sites of unspecified lower limb, except ankle and foot

● **T24.2**   Burn of second degree of lower limb, except ankle and foot

> Use additional external cause code to identify the source, place and intent of the burn (X00-X19, X75-X77, X96-X98, Y92)

   ● **T24.20**   Burn of second degree of unspecified site of lower limb, except ankle and foot

     ● **T24.201**   Burn of second degree of unspecified site of right lower limb, except ankle and foot

     ● **T24.202**   Burn of second degree of unspecified site of left lower limb, except ankle and foot

     ● **T24.209**   Burn of second degree of unspecified site of unspecified lower limb, except ankle and foot

   ● **T24.21**   Burn of second degree of thigh

     ● **T24.211**   Burn of second degree of right thigh

     ● **T24.212**   Burn of second degree of left thigh

     ● **T24.219**   Burn of second degree of unspecified thigh

   ● **T24.22**   Burn of second degree of knee

     ● **T24.221**   Burn of second degree of right knee

     ● **T24.222**   Burn of second degree of left knee

     ● **T24.229**   Burn of second degree of unspecified knee

● **T24.23**   Burn of second degree of lower leg

     ● **T24.231**   Burn of second degree of right lower leg

     ● **T24.232**   Burn of second degree of left lower leg

     ● **T24.239**   Burn of second degree of unspecified lower leg

   ● **T24.29**   Burn of second degree of multiple sites of lower limb, except ankle and foot

     ● **T24.291**   Burn of second degree of multiple sites of right lower limb, except ankle and foot

     ● **T24.292**   Burn of second degree of multiple sites of left lower limb, except ankle and foot

     ● **T24.299**   Burn of second degree of multiple sites of unspecified lower limb, except ankle and foot

● **T24.3**   Burn of third degree of lower limb, except ankle and foot

> Use additional external cause code to identify the source, place and intent of the burn (X00-X19, X75-X77, X96-X98, Y92)

   ● **T24.30**   Burn of third degree of unspecified site of lower limb, except ankle and foot
> (Ex) **For category T24.30 CC codes:** See PDX Collection 1404

     ● **T24.301**   Burn of third degree of unspecified site of right lower limb, except ankle and foot A 🦠, A 🦠

     ● **T24.302**   Burn of third degree of unspecified site of left lower limb, except ankle and foot A 🦠, A 🦠

     ● **T24.309**   Burn of third degree of unspecified site of unspecified lower limb, except ankle and foot A 🦠, A 🦠

   ● **T24.31**   Burn of third degree of thigh
> (Ex) **For category T24.31 CC codes:** See PDX Collection 1405

     ● **T24.311**   Burn of third degree of right thigh A 🦠, A 🦠

     ● **T24.312**   Burn of third degree of left thigh A 🦠, A 🦠

     ● **T24.319**   Burn of third degree of unspecified thigh A 🦠, A 🦠

   ● **T24.32**   Burn of third degree of knee
> (Ex) **For category T24.32 CC codes:** See PDX Collection 1406

     ● **T24.321**   Burn of third degree of right knee A 🦠, A 🦠

     ● **T24.322**   Burn of third degree of left knee A 🦠, A 🦠

     ● **T24.329**   Burn of third degree of unspecified knee A 🦠, A 🦠

   ● **T24.33**   Burn of third degree of lower leg
> (Ex) **For category T24.33 CC codes:** See PDX Collection 1407

     ● **T24.331**   Burn of third degree of right lower leg A 🦠, A 🦠

     ● **T24.332**   Burn of third degree of left lower leg A 🦠, A 🦠

     ● **T24.339**   Burn of third degree of unspecified lower leg A 🦠, A 🦠

   ● **T24.39**   Burn of third degree of multiple sites of lower limb, except ankle and foot
> (Ex) **For category T24.39 CC codes:** See PDX Collection 1404

     ● **T24.391**   Burn of third degree of multiple sites of right lower limb, except ankle and foot A 🦠, A 🦠
> **Coding Clinic: 2016, Q2, P5**

     ● **T24.392**   Burn of third degree of multiple sites of left lower limb, except ankle and foot A 🦠, A 🦠

     ● **T24.399**   Burn of third degree of multiple sites of unspecified lower limb, except ankle and foot A 🦠, A 🦠

N Newborn Age: 0   **P** Pediatric Age: 0–17   **M** Maternity DX: 9–64   **A** Adult Age: 15–124   ♀ Females Only   ♂ Males Only

🦠 Complication\Comorbidity   🦠 Major C\C   (Ex) CC/MCC Exclusions   🦠 Hospital-Acquired Condition   🦠 Hierarchical Condition Category

● **T24.4** Corrosion of unspecified degree of lower limb, except ankle and foot

Code first (T51-T65) to identify chemical and intent
Use additional external cause code to identify place (Y92)

● **T24.40** Corrosion of unspecified degree of unspecified site of lower limb, except ankle and foot

● **T24.401** Corrosion of unspecified degree of unspecified site of right lower limb, except ankle and foot

● **T24.402** Corrosion of unspecified degree of unspecified site of left lower limb, except ankle and foot

● **T24.409** Corrosion of unspecified degree of unspecified site of unspecified lower limb, except ankle and foot

● **T24.41** Corrosion of unspecified degree of thigh

● **T24.411** Corrosion of unspecified degree of right thigh

● **T24.412** Corrosion of unspecified degree of left thigh

● **T24.419** Corrosion of unspecified degree of unspecified thigh

● **T24.42** Corrosion of unspecified degree of knee

● **T24.421** Corrosion of unspecified degree of right knee

● **T24.422** Corrosion of unspecified degree of left knee

● **T24.429** Corrosion of unspecified degree of unspecified knee

● **T24.43** Corrosion of unspecified degree of lower leg

● **T24.431** Corrosion of unspecified degree of right lower leg

● **T24.432** Corrosion of unspecified degree of left lower leg

● **T24.439** Corrosion of unspecified degree of unspecified lower leg

● **T24.49** Corrosion of unspecified degree of multiple sites of lower limb, except ankle and foot

● **T24.491** Corrosion of unspecified degree of multiple sites of right lower limb, except ankle and foot

● **T24.492** Corrosion of unspecified degree of multiple sites of left lower limb, except ankle and foot

● **T24.499** Corrosion of unspecified degree of multiple sites of unspecified lower limb, except ankle and foot

● **T24.5** Corrosion of first degree of lower limb, except ankle and foot

Code first (T51-T65) to identify chemical and intent
Use additional external cause code to identify place (Y92)

● **T24.50** Corrosion of first degree of unspecified site of lower limb, except ankle and foot

● **T24.501** Corrosion of first degree of unspecified site of right lower limb, except ankle and foot

● **T24.502** Corrosion of first degree of unspecified site of left lower limb, except ankle and foot

● **T24.509** Corrosion of first degree of unspecified site of unspecified lower limb, except ankle and foot

● **T24.51** Corrosion of first degree of thigh

● **T24.511** Corrosion of first degree of right thigh

● **T24.512** Corrosion of first degree of left thigh

● **T24.519** Corrosion of first degree of unspecified thigh

● **T24.52** Corrosion of first degree of knee

● **T24.521** Corrosion of first degree of right knee

● **T24.522** Corrosion of first degree of left knee

● **T24.529** Corrosion of first degree of unspecified knee

● **T24.53** Corrosion of first degree of lower leg

● **T24.531** Corrosion of first degree of right lower leg

● **T24.532** Corrosion of first degree of left lower leg

● **T24.539** Corrosion of first degree of unspecified lower leg

● **T24.59** Corrosion of first degree of multiple sites of lower limb, except ankle and foot

● **T24.591** Corrosion of first degree of multiple sites of right lower limb, except ankle and foot

● **T24.592** Corrosion of first degree of multiple sites of left lower limb, except ankle and foot

● **T24.599** Corrosion of first degree of multiple sites of unspecified lower limb, except ankle and foot

● **T24.6** Corrosion of second degree of lower limb, except ankle and foot

Code first (T51-T65) to identify chemical and intent
Use additional external cause code to identify place (Y92)

● **T24.60** Corrosion of second degree of unspecified site of lower limb, except ankle and foot

● **T24.601** Corrosion of second degree of unspecified site of right lower limb, except ankle and foot

● **T24.602** Corrosion of second degree of unspecified site of left lower limb, except ankle and foot

● **T24.609** Corrosion of second degree of unspecified site of unspecified lower limb, except ankle and foot

● **T24.61** Corrosion of second degree of thigh

● **T24.611** Corrosion of second degree of right thigh

● **T24.612** Corrosion of second degree of left thigh

● **T24.619** Corrosion of second degree of unspecified thigh

● **T24.62** Corrosion of second degree of knee

● **T24.621** Corrosion of second degree of right knee

● **T24.622** Corrosion of second degree of left knee

● **T24.629** Corrosion of second degree of unspecified knee

● **T24.63** Corrosion of second degree of lower leg

● **T24.631** Corrosion of second degree of right lower leg

● **T24.632** Corrosion of second degree of left lower leg

● **T24.639** Corrosion of second degree of unspecified lower leg

● T24.69 Corrosion of second degree of multiple sites of lower limb, except ankle and foot

    ● T24.691 Corrosion of second degree of multiple sites of right lower limb, except ankle and foot

    ● T24.692 Corrosion of second degree of multiple sites of left lower limb, except ankle and foot

    ● T24.699 Corrosion of second degree of multiple sites of unspecified lower limb, except ankle and foot

● T24.7 Corrosion of third degree of lower limb, except ankle and foot

    Code first (T51-T65) to identify chemical and intent

    Use additional external cause code to identify place (Y92)

  ● T24.70 Corrosion of third degree of unspecified site of lower limb, except ankle and foot
      (Ex) For category T24.70 CC codes: See PDX Collection 1404

    ● T24.701 Corrosion of third degree of unspecified site of right lower limb, except ankle and foot A 🦠, A 🦠

    ● T24.702 Corrosion of third degree of unspecified site of left lower limb, except ankle and foot A 🦠, A 🦠

    ● T24.709 Corrosion of third degree of unspecified site of unspecified lower limb, except ankle and foot A 🦠, A 🦠

  ● T24.71 Corrosion of third degree of thigh
      (Ex) For category T24.71 CC codes: See PDX Collection 1405

    ● T24.711 Corrosion of third degree of right thigh A 🦠, A 🦠

    ● T24.712 Corrosion of third degree of left thigh A 🦠, A 🦠

    ● T24.719 Corrosion of third degree of unspecified thigh A 🦠, A 🦠

  ● T24.72 Corrosion of third degree of knee
      (Ex) For category T24.72 CC codes: See PDX Collection 1406

    ● T24.721 Corrosion of third degree of right knee A 🦠, A 🦠

    ● T24.722 Corrosion of third degree of left knee A 🦠, A 🦠

    ● T24.729 Corrosion of third degree of unspecified knee A 🦠, A 🦠

  ● T24.73 Corrosion of third degree of lower leg
      (Ex) For category T24.73 CC codes: See PDX Collection 1407

    ● T24.731 Corrosion of third degree of right lower leg A 🦠, A 🦠

    ● T24.732 Corrosion of third degree of left lower leg A 🦠, A 🦠

    ● T24.739 Corrosion of third degree of unspecified lower leg A 🦠, A 🦠

  ● T24.79 Corrosion of third degree of multiple sites of lower limb, except ankle and foot
      (Ex) For category T24.79 CC codes: See PDX Collection 1404

    ● T24.791 Corrosion of third degree of multiple sites of right lower limb, except ankle and foot A 🦠, A 🦠

    ● T24.792 Corrosion of third degree of multiple sites of left lower limb, except ankle and foot A 🦠, A 🦠

    ● T24.799 Corrosion of third degree of multiple sites of unspecified lower limb, except ankle and foot A 🦠, A 🦠

● T25 Burn and corrosion of ankle and foot

  The appropriate 7th character is to be added to each code from category T25

  | | |
  A   initial encounter
  D   subsequent encounter
  S   sequela

● T25.0 Burn of unspecified degree of ankle and foot

  Use additional external cause code to identify the source, place and intent of the burn (X00-X19, X75-X77, X96-X98, Y92)

  ● T25.01 Burn of unspecified degree of ankle

    ● T25.011 Burn of unspecified degree of right ankle

    ● T25.012 Burn of unspecified degree of left ankle

    ● T25.019 Burn of unspecified degree of unspecified ankle

  ● T25.02 Burn of unspecified degree of foot

    Excludes2 burn of unspecified degree of toe(s) (nail) (T25.03-)

    ● T25.021 Burn of unspecified degree of right foot

    ● T25.022 Burn of unspecified degree of left foot

    ● T25.029 Burn of unspecified degree of unspecified foot

  ● T25.03 Burn of unspecified degree of toe(s) (nail)

    ● T25.031 Burn of unspecified degree of right toe(s) (nail)

    ● T25.032 Burn of unspecified degree of left toe(s) (nail)

    ● T25.039 Burn of unspecified degree of unspecified toe(s) (nail)

  ● T25.09 Burn of unspecified degree of multiple sites of ankle and foot

    ● T25.091 Burn of unspecified degree of multiple sites of right ankle and foot

    ● T25.092 Burn of unspecified degree of multiple sites of left ankle and foot

    ● T25.099 Burn of unspecified degree of multiple sites of unspecified ankle and foot

● T25.1 Burn of first degree of ankle and foot

  Use additional external cause code to identify the source, place and intent of the burn (X00-X19, X75-X77, X96-X98, Y92)

  ● T25.11 Burn of first degree of ankle

    ● T25.111 Burn of first degree of right ankle

    ● T25.112 Burn of first degree of left ankle

    ● T25.119 Burn of first degree of unspecified ankle

  ● T25.12 Burn of first degree of foot

    Excludes2 burn of first degree of toe(s) (nail) (T25.13-)

    ● T25.121 Burn of first degree of right foot

    ● T25.122 Burn of first degree of left foot

    ● T25.129 Burn of first degree of unspecified foot

  ● T25.13 Burn of first degree of toe(s) (nail)

    ● T25.131 Burn of first degree of right toe(s) (nail)

    ● T25.132 Burn of first degree of left toe(s) (nail)

    ● T25.139 Burn of first degree of unspecified toe(s) (nail)

N Newborn Age: 0   P Pediatric Age: 0–17   M Maternity DX: 9–64   A Adult Age: 15–124   ♀ Females Only   ♂ Males Only

🦠 Complication\Comorbidity   🦠 Major C\C   (Ex) CC/MCC Exclusions   🦠 Hospital-Acquired Condition   🦠 Hierarchical Condition Category

1451

● **T25.19**   Burn of first degree of multiple sites of ankle and foot
     ● **T25.191**   Burn of first degree of multiple sites of right ankle and foot
     ● **T25.192**   Burn of first degree of multiple sites of left ankle and foot
     ● **T25.199**   Burn of first degree of multiple sites of unspecified ankle and foot

● **T25.2**   Burn of second degree of ankle and foot
     Use additional external cause code to identify the source, place and intent of the burn (X00-X19, X75-X77, X96-X98, Y92)
     ● **T25.21**   Burn of second degree of ankle
       ● **T25.211**   Burn of second degree of right ankle
       ● **T25.212**   Burn of second degree of left ankle
       ● **T25.219**   Burn of second degree of unspecified ankle
     ● **T25.22**   Burn of second degree of foot
       Excludes2   burn of second degree of toe(s) (nail) (T25.23-)
       ● **T25.221**   Burn of second degree of right foot
       ● **T25.222**   Burn of second degree of left foot
       ● **T25.229**   Burn of second degree of unspecified foot
     ● **T25.23**   Burn of second degree of toe(s) (nail)
       ● **T25.231**   Burn of second degree of right toe(s) (nail)
       ● **T25.232**   Burn of second degree of left toe(s) (nail)
       ● **T25.239**   Burn of second degree of unspecified toe(s) (nail)
     ● **T25.29**   Burn of second degree of multiple sites of ankle and foot
       ● **T25.291**   Burn of second degree of multiple sites of right ankle and foot
       ● **T25.292**   Burn of second degree of multiple sites of left ankle and foot
       ● **T25.299**   Burn of second degree of multiple sites of unspecified ankle and foot

● **T25.3**   Burn of third degree of ankle and foot
     Use additional external cause code to identify the source, place and intent of the burn (X00-X19, X75-X77, X96-X98, Y92)
     ● **T25.31**   Burn of third degree of ankle
       (Ex:) **For category T25.31 CC codes:** See PDX Collection 1408
       ● **T25.311**   Burn of third degree of right ankle A 🔖, A 🔖
       ● **T25.312**   Burn of third degree of left ankle A 🔖, A 🔖
       ● **T25.319**   Burn of third degree of unspecified ankle A 🔖, A 🔖
     ● **T25.32**   Burn of third degree of foot
       Excludes2   burn of third degree of toe(s) (nail) (T25.33-)
       (Ex:) **For category T25.32 CC codes:** See PDX Collection 1409
       ● **T25.321**   Burn of third degree of right foot A 🔖, A 🔖
       ● **T25.322**   Burn of third degree of left foot A 🔖, A 🔖
       ● **T25.329**   Burn of third degree of unspecified foot A 🔖, A 🔖

● **T25.33**   Burn of third degree of toe(s) (nail)
     (Ex:) **For category T25.33 CC codes:** See PDX Collection 1410
     ● **T25.331**   Burn of third degree of right toe(s) (nail) A 🔖, A 🔖
     ● **T25.332**   Burn of third degree of left toe(s) (nail) A 🔖, A 🔖
     ● **T25.339**   Burn of third degree of unspecified toe(s) (nail) A 🔖, A 🔖

● **T25.39**   Burn of third degree of multiple sites of ankle and foot
     (Ex:) **For category T25.39 CC codes:** See PDX Collection 1404
     ● **T25.391**   Burn of third degree of multiple sites of right ankle and foot A 🔖, A 🔖
     ● **T25.392**   Burn of third degree of multiple sites of left ankle and foot A 🔖, A 🔖
     ● **T25.399**   Burn of third degree of multiple sites of unspecified ankle and foot A 🔖, A 🔖

● **T25.4**   Corrosion of unspecified degree of ankle and foot
     Code first (T51-T65) to identify chemical and intent
     Use additional external cause code to identify place (Y92)
     ● **T25.41**   Corrosion of unspecified degree of ankle
       ● **T25.411**   Corrosion of unspecified degree of right ankle
       ● **T25.412**   Corrosion of unspecified degree of left ankle
       ● **T25.419**   Corrosion of unspecified degree of unspecified ankle
     ● **T25.42**   Corrosion of unspecified degree of foot
       Excludes2   corrosion of unspecified degree of toe(s) (nail) (T25.43-)
       ● **T25.421**   Corrosion of unspecified degree of right foot
       ● **T25.422**   Corrosion of unspecified degree of left foot
       ● **T25.429**   Corrosion of unspecified degree of unspecified foot
     ● **T25.43**   Corrosion of unspecified degree of toe(s) (nail)
       ● **T25.431**   Corrosion of unspecified degree of right toe(s) (nail)
       ● **T25.432**   Corrosion of unspecified degree of left toe(s) (nail)
       ● **T25.439**   Corrosion of unspecified degree of unspecified toe(s) (nail)
     ● **T25.49**   Corrosion of unspecified degree of multiple sites of ankle and foot
       ● **T25.491**   Corrosion of unspecified degree of multiple sites of right ankle and foot
       ● **T25.492**   Corrosion of unspecified degree of multiple sites of left ankle and foot
       ● **T25.499**   Corrosion of unspecified degree of multiple sites of unspecified ankle and foot

● **T25.5**   Corrosion of first degree of ankle and foot
     Code first (T51-T65) to identify chemical and intent
     Use additional external cause code to identify place (Y92)
     ● **T25.51**   Corrosion of first degree of ankle
       ● **T25.511**   Corrosion of first degree of right ankle
       ● **T25.512**   Corrosion of first degree of left ankle
       ● **T25.519**   Corrosion of first degree of unspecified ankle

● **T25.52**   Corrosion of first degree of foot

     Excludes2   corrosion of first degree of toe(s) (nail) (T25.53-)

   ● **T25.521**   Corrosion of first degree of right foot

   ● **T25.522**   Corrosion of first degree of left foot

   ● **T25.529**   Corrosion of first degree of unspecified foot

● **T25.53**   Corrosion of first degree of toe(s) (nail)

   ● **T25.531**   Corrosion of first degree of right toe(s) (nail)

   ● **T25.532**   Corrosion of first degree of left toe(s) (nail)

   ● **T25.539**   Corrosion of first degree of unspecified toe(s) (nail)

● **T25.59**   Corrosion of first degree of multiple sites of ankle and foot

   ● **T25.591**   Corrosion of first degree of multiple sites of right ankle and foot

   ● **T25.592**   Corrosion of first degree of multiple sites of left ankle and foot

   ● **T25.599**   Corrosion of first degree of multiple sites of unspecified ankle and foot

● **T25.6**   Corrosion of second degree of ankle and foot

     Code first (T51-T65) *to identify chemical and intent*

     Use additional external cause code to identify place (Y92)

  ● **T25.61**   Corrosion of second degree of ankle

   ● **T25.611**   Corrosion of second degree of right ankle

   ● **T25.612**   Corrosion of second degree of left ankle

   ● **T25.619**   Corrosion of second degree of unspecified ankle

  ● **T25.62**   Corrosion of second degree of foot

     Excludes2   corrosion of second degree of toe(s) (nail) (T25.63-)

   ● **T25.621**   Corrosion of second degree of right foot

   ● **T25.622**   Corrosion of second degree of left foot

   ● **T25.629**   Corrosion of second degree of unspecified foot

  ● **T25.63**   Corrosion of second degree of toe(s) (nail)

   ● **T25.631**   Corrosion of second degree of right toe(s) (nail)

   ● **T25.632**   Corrosion of second degree of left toe(s) (nail)

   ● **T25.639**   Corrosion of second degree of unspecified toe(s) (nail)

  ● **T25.69**   Corrosion of second degree of multiple sites of ankle and foot

   ● **T25.691**   Corrosion of second degree of right ankle and foot

   ● **T25.692**   Corrosion of second degree of left ankle and foot

   ● **T25.699**   Corrosion of second degree of unspecified ankle and foot

● **T25.7**   Corrosion of third degree of ankle and foot

     Code first (T51-T65) *to identify chemical and intent*

     Use additional external cause code to identify place (Y92)

  ● **T25.71**   Corrosion of third degree of ankle

     (Ex) **For category T25.71 CC codes:** See PDX Collection 1408

   ● **T25.711**   Corrosion of third degree of right ankle A 🅒, A 🅜

   ● **T25.712**   Corrosion of third degree of left ankle A 🅒, A 🅜

   ● **T25.719**   Corrosion of third degree of unspecified ankle A 🅒, A 🅜

● **T25.72**   Corrosion of third degree of foot

     Excludes2   corrosion of third degree of toe(s) (nail) (T25.73-)

     (Ex) **For category T25.72 CC codes:** See PDX Collection 1409

   ● **T25.721**   Corrosion of third degree of right foot A 🅒, A 🅜

   ● **T25.722**   Corrosion of third degree of left foot A 🅒, A 🅜

   ● **T25.729**   Corrosion of third degree of unspecified foot A 🅒, A 🅜

● **T25.73**   Corrosion of third degree of toe(s) (nail)

     (Ex) **For category T25.73 CC codes:** See PDX Collection 1410

   ● **T25.731**   Corrosion of third degree of right toe(s) (nail) A 🅒, A 🅜

   ● **T25.732**   Corrosion of third degree of left toe(s) (nail) A 🅒, A 🅜

   ● **T25.739**   Corrosion of third degree of unspecified toe(s) (nail) A 🅒, A 🅜

● **T25.79**   Corrosion of third degree of multiple sites of ankle and foot

     (Ex) **For category T25.79 CC codes:** See PDX Collection 1404

   ● **T25.791**   Corrosion of third degree of multiple sites of right ankle and foot A 🅒, A 🅜

   ● **T25.792**   Corrosion of third degree of multiple sites of left ankle and foot A 🅒, A 🅜

   ● **T25.799**   Corrosion of third degree of multiple sites of unspecified ankle and foot A 🅒, A 🅜

BURNS AND CORROSIONS CONFINED TO EYE AND INTERNAL ORGANS (T26-T28)

● **T26**   Burn and corrosion confined to eye and adnexa

     The appropriate 7th character is to be added to each code from category T26

A	initial encounter
D	subsequent encounter
S	sequela

  ● **T26.0**   Burn of eyelid and periocular area

     Use additional external cause code to identify the source, place and intent of the burn (X00-X19, X75-X77, X96-X98, Y92)

   X ● **T26.00**   Burn of unspecified eyelid and periocular area

   X ● **T26.01**   Burn of right eyelid and periocular area

   X ● **T26.02**   Burn of left eyelid and periocular area

  ● **T26.1**   Burn of cornea and conjunctival sac

     Use additional external cause code to identify the source, place and intent of the burn (X00-X19, X75-X77, X96-X98, Y92)

   X ● **T26.10**   Burn of cornea and conjunctival sac, unspecified eye

   X ● **T26.11**   Burn of cornea and conjunctival sac, right eye

   X ● **T26.12**   Burn of cornea and conjunctival sac, left eye

  ● **T26.2**   Burn with resulting rupture and destruction of eyeball

     Use additional external cause code to identify the source, place and intent of the burn (X00-X19, X75-X77, X96-X98, Y92)

   X ● **T26.20**   Burn with resulting rupture and destruction of unspecified eyeball A 🅒, A 🅜

     (Ex) See PDX Collection 3235

   X ● **T26.21**   Burn with resulting rupture and destruction of right eyeball A 🅒, A 🅜

     (Ex) See PDX Collection 3236

   X ● **T26.22**   Burn with resulting rupture and destruction of left eyeball A 🅒, A 🅜

     (Ex) See PDX Collection 3237

N Newborn Age: 0   **P** Pediatric Age: 0–17   **M** Maternity DX: 9–64   **A** Adult Age: 15–124   ♀ Females Only   ♂ Males Only

🅒 Complication\Comorbidity   🅜 Major C\C   (Ex) CC/MCC Exclusions   🅗 Hospital-Acquired Condition   🅗 Hierarchical Condition Category

1453

● **T26.3**   Burns of other specified parts of eye and adnexa

Use additional external cause code to identify the source, place and intent of the burn (X00-X19, X75-X77, X96-X98, Y92)

X● **T26.30**   Burns of other specified parts of unspecified eye and adnexa

X● **T26.31**   Burns of other specified parts of right eye and adnexa

X● **T26.32**   Burns of other specified parts of left eye and adnexa

● **T26.4**   Burn of eye and adnexa, part unspecified

Use additional external cause code to identify the source, place and intent of the burn (X00-X19, X75-X77, X96-X98, Y92)

X● **T26.40**   Burn of unspecified eye and adnexa, part unspecified

X● **T26.41**   Burn of right eye and adnexa, part unspecified

X● **T26.42**   Burn of left eye and adnexa, part unspecified

● **T26.5**   Corrosion of eyelid and periocular area

Code first (T51-T65) to identify chemical and intent

Use additional external cause code to identify place (Y92)

X● **T26.50**   Corrosion of unspecified eyelid and periocular area

X● **T26.51**   Corrosion of right eyelid and periocular area

X● **T26.52**   Corrosion of left eyelid and periocular area

● **T26.6**   Corrosion of cornea and conjunctival sac

Code first (T51-T65) to identify chemical and intent

Use additional external cause code to identify place (Y92)

X● **T26.60**   Corrosion of cornea and conjunctival sac, unspecified eye

X● **T26.61**   Corrosion of cornea and conjunctival sac, right eye

X● **T26.62**   Corrosion of cornea and conjunctival sac, left eye

● **T26.7**   Corrosion with resulting rupture and destruction of eyeball

Code first (T51-T65) to identify chemical and intent

Use additional external cause code to identify place (Y92)

X● **T26.70**   Corrosion with resulting rupture and destruction of unspecified eyeball A, A
(Ex:) See PDX Collection 3238

X● **T26.71**   Corrosion with resulting rupture and destruction of right eyeball A, A
(Ex:) See PDX Collection 3239

X● **T26.72**   Corrosion with resulting rupture and destruction of left eyeball A, A
(Ex:) See PDX Collection 3240

● **T26.8**   Corrosions of other specified parts of eye and adnexa

Code first (T51-T65) to identify chemical and intent

Use additional external cause code to identify place (Y92)

X● **T26.80**   Corrosions of other specified parts of unspecified eye and adnexa

X● **T26.81**   Corrosions of other specified parts of right eye and adnexa

X● **T26.82**   Corrosions of other specified parts of left eye and adnexa

● **T26.9**   Corrosion of eye and adnexa, part unspecified

Code first (T51-T65) to identify chemical and intent

Use additional external cause code to identify place (Y92)

X● **T26.90**   Corrosion of unspecified eye and adnexa, part unspecified

X● **T26.91**   Corrosion of right eye and adnexa, part unspecified

X● **T26.92**   Corrosion of left eye and adnexa, part unspecified

● **T27**   Burn and corrosion of respiratory tract

Use additional external cause code to identify the source and intent of the burn (X00-X19, X75-X77, X96-X98)

Use additional external cause code to identify place (Y92)

The appropriate 7th character is to be added to each code from category T27

A	initial encounter
D	subsequent encounter
S	sequela

(Ex:) For category T27 CC codes: See PDX Collection 1411

X● **T27.0**   Burn of larynx and trachea A, A

X● **T27.1**   Burn involving larynx and trachea with lung A, A

X● **T27.2**   Burn of other parts of respiratory tract A, A
Burn of thoracic cavity

X● **T27.3**   Burn of respiratory tract, part unspecified A, A

X● **T27.4**   Corrosion of larynx and trachea A, A
Code first (T51-T65) to identify chemical and intent

X● **T27.5**   Corrosion involving larynx and trachea with lung A, A
Code first (T51-T65) to identify chemical and intent

X● **T27.6**   Corrosion of other parts of respiratory tract A, A
Code first (T51-T65) to identify chemical and intent

X● **T27.7**   Corrosion of respiratory tract, part unspecified A, A
Code first (T51-T65) to identify chemical and intent

● **T28**   Burn and corrosion of other internal organs

Use additional external cause code to identify the source and intent of the burn (X00-X19, X75-X77, X96-X98)

Use additional external cause code to identify place (Y92)

The appropriate 7th character is to be added to each code from category T28

A	initial encounter
D	subsequent encounter
S	sequela

X● **T28.0**   Burn of mouth and pharynx

X● **T28.1**   Burn of esophagus A, A
(Ex:) See PDX Collection 1412

X● **T28.2**   Burn of other parts of alimentary tract A, A
(Ex:) See PDX Collection 1413

X● **T28.3**   Burn of internal genitourinary organs

X● **T28.4**   Burns of other and unspecified internal organs

     X● **T28.40**   Burn of unspecified internal organ

     ● **T28.41**   Burn of ear drum

         ● **T28.411**   Burn of right ear drum

         ● **T28.412**   Burn of left ear drum

         ● **T28.419**   Burn of unspecified ear drum

     X● **T28.49**   Burn of other internal organ

X● **T28.5**   Corrosion of mouth and pharynx
Code first (T51-T65) to identify chemical and intent

X● **T28.6**   Corrosion of esophagus A, A
Code first (T51-T65) to identify chemical and intent
(Ex:) See PDX Collection 1412

X● **T28.7**   Corrosion of other parts of alimentary tract A, A
Code first (T51-T65) to identify chemical and intent
(Ex:) See PDX Collection 1413

X● **T28.8**   Corrosion of internal genitourinary organs
Code first (T51-T65) to identify chemical and intent

● **T28.9**   Corrosions of other and unspecified internal organs
Code first (T51-T65) to identify chemical and intent

     X● **T28.90**   Corrosions of unspecified internal organs

     ● **T28.91**   Corrosions of ear drum

         ● **T28.911**   Corrosions of right ear drum

         ● **T28.912**   Corrosions of left ear drum

         ● **T28.919**   Corrosions of unspecified ear drum

     X● **T28.99**   Corrosions of other internal organs

▶ New   ⇒ Revised   ~~deleted~~ Deleted   Excludes 1   Excludes 2   Includes   Use additional   Code first   Code also   Key words

OGCR Official Guidelines   ● Unacceptable Principal Diagnosis   X Assign placeholder X   ● Use Additional Character(s)   ▶ Manifestation Code   **Coding Clinic**

OGCR Section I.C.19.d.5.

Assign separate code for each burn site

When coding burns, assign separate codes for each burn site. Category T30, Burn and corrosion, body region unspecified is extremely vague and should rarely be used.

BURNS AND CORROSIONS OF MULTIPLE AND UNSPECIFIED BODY REGIONS (T30-T32)

● **T30 Burn and corrosion, body region unspecified**

     T30.0 Burn of unspecified body region, unspecified degree
         This code is not for inpatient use. Code to specified site and degree of burns
         Burn NOS
         Multiple burns NOS

     T30.4 Corrosion of unspecified body region, unspecified degree
         This code is not for inpatient use. Code to specified site and degree of corrosion
         Corrosion NOS
         Multiple corrosion NOS

● **T31 Burns classified according to extent of body surface involved**

     Note: This category is to be used as the primary code only when the site of the burn is unspecified. It should be used as a supplementary code with categories T20-T25 when the site is specified.

     (Ex) **For category T31 CC codes: See PDX Collection 1414**

     T31.0 Burns involving less than 10% of body surface

●   **T31.1 Burns involving 10-19% of body surface**

         T31.10 Burns involving 10-19% of body surface with 0% to 9% third degree burns 🄲 🄼🄲
             Burns involving 10-19% of body surface NOS

         T31.11 Burns involving 10-19% of body surface with 10-19% third degree burns 🄲 🄼🄲 🄷🄲🄲

●   **T31.2 Burns involving 20-29% of body surface**

         T31.20 Burns involving 20-29% of body surface with 0% to 9% third degree burns 🄲 🄼🄲
             Burns involving 20-29% of body surface NOS

         T31.21 Burns involving 20-29% of body surface with 10-19% third degree burns 🄲 🄼🄲 🄷🄲🄲

         T31.22 Burns involving 20-29% of body surface with 20-29% third degree burns 🄲 🄼🄲 🄷🄲🄲

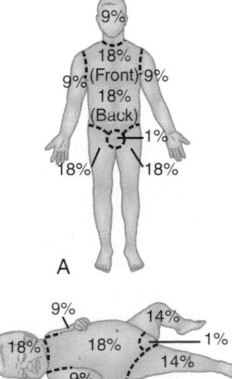

Figure 19-16 Rule of nines: percentages of total body area. (From Marx: Rosen's Emergency Medicine: Concepts and Clinical Practice, ed 6, Mosby, 2006)

● **T31.3 Burns involving 30-39% of body surface**

     T31.30 Burns involving 30-39% of body surface with 0% to 9% third degree burns 🄲 🄼🄲
         Burns involving 30-39% of body surface NOS

     T31.31 Burns involving 30-39% of body surface with 10-19% third degree burns 🄲 🄼🄲 🄷🄲🄲

     T31.32 Burns involving 30-39% of body surface with 20-29% third degree burns 🄲 🄼🄲 🄷🄲🄲

     T31.33 Burns involving 30-39% of body surface with 30-39% third degree burns 🄲 🄼🄲 🄷🄲🄲

● **T31.4 Burns involving 40-49% of body surface**

     T31.40 Burns involving 40-49% of body surface with 0% to 9% third degree burns 🄲 🄼🄲
         Burns involving 40-49% of body surface NOS

     T31.41 Burns involving 40-49% of body surface with 10-19% third degree burns 🄲 🄼🄲 🄷🄲🄲

     T31.42 Burns involving 40-49% of body surface with 20-29% third degree burns 🄲 🄼🄲 🄷🄲🄲

     T31.43 Burns involving 40-49% of body surface with 30-39% third degree burns 🄲 🄼🄲 🄷🄲🄲

     T31.44 Burns involving 40-49% of body surface with 40-49% third degree burns 🄲 🄼🄲 🄷🄲🄲

● **T31.5 Burns involving 50-59% of body surface**

     T31.50 Burns involving 50-59% of body surface with 0% to 9% third degree burns 🄲 🄼🄲
         Burns involving 50-59% of body surface NOS

     T31.51 Burns involving 50-59% of body surface with 10-19% third degree burns 🄲 🄼🄲 🄷🄲🄲

     T31.52 Burns involving 50-59% of body surface with 20-29% third degree burns 🄲 🄼🄲 🄷🄲🄲

     T31.53 Burns involving 50-59% of body surface with 30-39% third degree burns 🄲 🄼🄲 🄷🄲🄲

     T31.54 Burns involving 50-59% of body surface with 40-49% third degree burns 🄲 🄼🄲 🄷🄲🄲

     T31.55 Burns involving 50-59% of body surface with 50-59% third degree burns 🄲 🄼🄲 🄷🄲🄲

● **T31.6 Burns involving 60-69% of body surface**

     T31.60 Burns involving 60-69% of body surface with 0% to 9% third degree burns 🄲 🄼🄲
         Burns involving 60-69% of body surface NOS

     T31.61 Burns involving 60-69% of body surface with 10-19% third degree burns 🄲 🄼🄲 🄷🄲🄲

     T31.62 Burns involving 60-69% of body surface with 20-29% third degree burns 🄲 🄼🄲 🄷🄲🄲

     T31.63 Burns involving 60-69% of body surface with 30-39% third degree burns 🄲 🄼🄲 🄷🄲🄲

     T31.64 Burns involving 60-69% of body surface with 40-49% third degree burns 🄲 🄼🄲 🄷🄲🄲

     T31.65 Burns involving 60-69% of body surface with 50-59% third degree burns 🄲 🄼🄲 🄷🄲🄲

     T31.66 Burns involving 60-69% of body surface with 60-69% third degree burns 🄲 🄼🄲 🄷🄲🄲

● **T31.7 Burns involving 70-79% of body surface**

     T31.70 Burns involving 70-79% of body surface with 0% to 9% third degree burns 🄲 🄼🄲
         Burns involving 70-79% of body surface NOS

     T31.71 Burns involving 70-79% of body surface with 10-19% third degree burns 🄲 🄼🄲 🄷🄲🄲

     T31.72 Burns involving 70-79% of body surface with 20-29% third degree burns 🄲 🄼🄲 🄷🄲🄲

     T31.73 Burns involving 70-79% of body surface with 30-39% third degree burns 🄲 🄼🄲 🄷🄲🄲

     T31.74 Burns involving 70-79% of body surface with 40-49% third degree burns 🄲 🄼🄲 🄷🄲🄲

     T31.75 Burns involving 70-79% of body surface with 50-59% third degree burns 🄲 🄼🄲 🄷🄲🄲

     T31.76 Burns involving 70-79% of body surface with 60-69% third degree burns 🄲 🄼🄲 🄷🄲🄲

     T31.77 Burns involving 70-79% of body surface with 70-79% third degree burns 🄲 🄼🄲 🄷🄲🄲

N Newborn Age: 0   **P** Pediatric Age: 0–17   **M** Maternity DX: 9–64   **A** Adult Age: 15–124   ♀ Females Only   ♂ Males Only

🄲 Complication\Comorbidity   🄼🄲 Major C\C   (Ex) CC/MCC Exclusions   🄷🄰🄲 Hospital-Acquired Condition   🄷🄲🄲 Hierarchical Condition Category

1455

● **T31.8**   **Burns involving 80-89% of body surface**

    T31.80   Burns involving 80-89% of body surface with 0% to 9% third degree burns
       Burns involving 80-89% of body surface NOS

    T31.81   Burns involving 80-89% of body surface with 10-19% third degree burns

    T31.82   Burns involving 80-89% of body surface with 20-29% third degree burns

    T31.83   Burns involving 80-89% of body surface with 30-39% third degree burns

    T31.84   Burns involving 80-89% of body surface with 40-49% third degree burns

    T31.85   Burns involving 80-89% of body surface with 50-59% third degree burns

    T31.86   Burns involving 80-89% of body surface with 60-69% third degree burns

    T31.87   Burns involving 80-89% of body surface with 70-79% third degree burns

    T31.88   Burns involving 80-89% of body surface with 80-89% third degree burns

● **T31.9**   **Burns involving 90% or more of body surface**

    T31.90   Burns involving 90% or more of body surface with 0% to 9% third degree burns
       Burns involving 90% or more of body surface NOS

    T31.91   Burns involving 90% or more of body surface with 10-19% third degree burns

    T31.92   Burns involving 90% or more of body surface with 20-29% third degree burns

    T31.93   Burns involving 90% or more of body surface with 30-39% third degree burns

    T31.94   Burns involving 90% or more of body surface with 40-49% third degree burns

    T31.95   Burns involving 90% or more of body surface with 50-59% third degree burns

    T31.96   Burns involving 90% or more of body surface with 60-69% third degree burns

    T31.97   Burns involving 90% or more of body surface with 70-79% third degree burns

    T31.98   Burns involving 90% or more of body surface with 80-89% third degree burns

    T31.99   Burns involving 90% or more of body surface with 90% or more third degree burns

● **T32**   **Corrosions classified according to extent of body surface involved**

    Note: This category is to be used as the primary code only when the site of the corrosion is unspecified. It may be used as a supplementary code with categories T20-T25 when the site is specified.

    Ex: **For category T32 CC codes:** See PDX Collection 1414

    T32.0   Corrosions involving less than 10% of body surface

● **T32.1**   **Corrosions involving 10-19% of body surface**

    T32.10   Corrosions involving 10-19% of body surface with 0% to 9% third degree corrosion
       Corrosions involving 10-19% of body surface NOS

    T32.11   Corrosions involving 10-19% of body surface with 10-19% third degree corrosion

● **T32.2**   **Corrosions involving 20-29% of body surface**

    T32.20   Corrosions involving 20-29% of body surface with 0% to 9% third degree corrosion

    T32.21   Corrosions involving 20-29% of body surface with 10-19% third degree corrosion

    T32.22   Corrosions involving 20-29% of body surface with 20-29% third degree corrosion

● **T32.3**   **Corrosions involving 30-39% of body surface**

    T32.30   Corrosions involving 30-39% of body surface with 0% to 9% third degree corrosion

    T32.31   Corrosions involving 30-39% of body surface with 10-19% third degree corrosion

    T32.32   Corrosions involving 30-39% of body surface with 20-29% third degree corrosion

    T32.33   Corrosions involving 30-39% of body surface with 30-39% third degree corrosion

● **T32.4**   **Corrosions involving 40-49% of body surface**

    T32.40   Corrosions involving 40-49% of body surface with 0% to 9% third degree corrosion

    T32.41   Corrosions involving 40-49% of body surface with 10-19% third degree corrosion

    T32.42   Corrosions involving 40-49% of body surface with 20-29% third degree corrosion

    T32.43   Corrosions involving 40-49% of body surface with 30-39% third degree corrosion

    T32.44   Corrosions involving 40-49% of body surface with 40-49% third degree corrosion

● **T32.5**   **Corrosions involving 50-59% of body surface**

    T32.50   Corrosions involving 50-59% of body surface with 0% to 9% third degree corrosion

    T32.51   Corrosions involving 50-59% of body surface with 10-19% third degree corrosion

    T32.52   Corrosions involving 50-59% of body surface with 20-29% third degree corrosion

    T32.53   Corrosions involving 50-59% of body surface with 30-39% third degree corrosion

    T32.54   Corrosions involving 50-59% of body surface with 40-49% third degree corrosion

    T32.55   Corrosions involving 50-59% of body surface with 50-59% third degree corrosion

● **T32.6**   **Corrosions involving 60-69% of body surface**

    T32.60   Corrosions involving 60-69% of body surface with 0% to 9% third degree corrosion

    T32.61   Corrosions involving 60-69% of body surface with 10-19% third degree corrosion

    T32.62   Corrosions involving 60-69% of body surface with 20-29% third degree corrosion

    T32.63   Corrosions involving 60-69% of body surface with 30-39% third degree corrosion

    T32.64   Corrosions involving 60-69% of body surface with 40-49% third degree corrosion

    T32.65   Corrosions involving 60-69% of body surface with 50-59% third degree corrosion

    T32.66   Corrosions involving 60-69% of body surface with 60-69% third degree corrosion

● **T32.7**   **Corrosions involving 70-79% of body surface**

    T32.70   Corrosions involving 70-79% of body surface with 0% to 9% third degree corrosion

    T32.71   Corrosions involving 70-79% of body surface with 10-19% third degree corrosion

    T32.72   Corrosions involving 70-79% of body surface with 20-29% third degree corrosion

    T32.73   Corrosions involving 70-79% of body surface with 30-39% third degree corrosion

    T32.74   Corrosions involving 70-79% of body surface with 40-49% third degree corrosion

    T32.75   Corrosions involving 70-79% of body surface with 50-59% third degree corrosion

    T32.76   Corrosions involving 70-79% of body surface with 60-69% third degree corrosion

    T32.77   Corrosions involving 70-79% of body surface with 70-79% third degree corrosion

● **T32.8**   Corrosions involving 80-89% of body surface

    T32.80   Corrosions involving 80-89% of body surface with 0% to 9% third degree corrosion 🦠 🦠

    T32.81   Corrosions involving 80-89% of body surface with 10-19% third degree corrosion 🦠 🦠 🦠

    T32.82   Corrosions involving 80-89% of body surface with 20-29% third degree corrosion 🦠 🦠 🦠

    T32.83   Corrosions involving 80-89% of body surface with 30-39% third degree corrosion 🦠 🦠 🦠

    T32.84   Corrosions involving 80-89% of body surface with 40-49% third degree corrosion 🦠 🦠 🦠

    T32.85   Corrosions involving 80-89% of body surface with 50-59% third degree corrosion 🦠 🦠 🦠

    T32.86   Corrosions involving 80-89% of body surface with 60-69% third degree corrosion 🦠 🦠 🦠

    T32.87   Corrosions involving 80-89% of body surface with 70-79% third degree corrosion 🦠 🦠 🦠

    T32.88   Corrosions involving 80-89% of body surface with 80-89% third degree corrosion 🦠 🦠 🦠

● **T32.9**   Corrosions involving 90% or more of body surface

    T32.90   Corrosions involving 90% or more of body surface with 0% to 9% third degree corrosion 🦠 🦠

    T32.91   Corrosions involving 90% or more of body surface with 10-19% third degree corrosion 🦠 🦠 🦠

    T32.92   Corrosions involving 90% or more of body surface with 20-29% third degree corrosion 🦠 🦠 🦠

    T32.93   Corrosions involving 90% or more of body surface with 30-39% third degree corrosion 🦠 🦠 🦠

    T32.94   Corrosions involving 90% or more of body surface with 40-49% third degree corrosion 🦠 🦠 🦠

    T32.95   Corrosions involving 90% or more of body surface with 50-59% third degree corrosion 🦠 🦠 🦠

    T32.96   Corrosions involving 90% or more of body surface with 60-69% third degree corrosion 🦠 🦠 🦠

    T32.97   Corrosions involving 90% or more of body surface with 70-79% third degree corrosion 🦠 🦠 🦠

    T32.98   Corrosions involving 90% or more of body surface with 80-89% third degree corrosion 🦠 🦠 🦠

    T32.99   Corrosions involving 90% or more of body surface with 90% or more third degree corrosion 🦠 🦠 🦠

FROSTBITE (T33-T34)

> **Excludes2**   hypothermia and other effects of reduced temperature (T68, T69.-)

● **T33**   Superficial frostbite

> **Includes**   frostbite with partial thickness skin loss

The appropriate 7th character is to be added to each code from category T33

> A   initial encounter
> D   subsequent encounter
> S   sequela

● **T33.0**   Superficial frostbite of head

    (Ex) **For category T33.0 CC codes:** See PDX Collection 1415

    ● **T33.01**   Superficial frostbite of ear

       ● **T33.011**   Superficial frostbite of right ear A 🦠, A 🦠

       ● **T33.012**   Superficial frostbite of left ear A 🦠, A 🦠

       ● **T33.019**   Superficial frostbite of unspecified ear A 🦠, A 🦠

X ● **T33.02**   Superficial frostbite of nose A 🦠, A 🦠

X ● **T33.09**   Superficial frostbite of other part of head A 🦠, A 🦠

X ● **T33.1**   Superficial frostbite of neck A 🦠, A 🦠

    (Ex) See PDX Collection 1415

X ● **T33.2**   Superficial frostbite of thorax A 🦠, A 🦠

    (Ex) See PDX Collection 1416

X ● **T33.3**   Superficial frostbite of abdominal wall, lower back and pelvis A 🦠, A 🦠

    (Ex) See PDX Collection 1416

● **T33.4**   Superficial frostbite of arm

> **Excludes2**   superficial frostbite of wrist and hand (T33.5-)

    (Ex) **For category T33.4 CC codes:** See PDX Collection 1416

    X ● **T33.40**   Superficial frostbite of unspecified arm A 🦠, A 🦠

    X ● **T33.41**   Superficial frostbite of right arm A 🦠, A 🦠

    X ● **T33.42**   Superficial frostbite of left arm A 🦠, A 🦠

● **T33.5**   Superficial frostbite of wrist, hand, and fingers

    (Ex) **For category T33.5 CC codes:** See PDX Collection 1417

    ● **T33.51**   Superficial frostbite of wrist

       ● **T33.511**   Superficial frostbite of right wrist A 🦠, A 🦠

       ● **T33.512**   Superficial frostbite of left wrist A 🦠, A 🦠

       ● **T33.519**   Superficial frostbite of unspecified wrist A 🦠, A 🦠

    ● **T33.52**   Superficial frostbite of hand

> **Excludes2**   superficial frostbite of fingers (T33.53-)

       ● **T33.521**   Superficial frostbite of right hand A 🦠, A 🦠

       ● **T33.522**   Superficial frostbite of left hand A 🦠, A 🦠

       ● **T33.529**   Superficial frostbite of unspecified hand A 🦠, A 🦠

    ● **T33.53**   Superficial frostbite of finger(s)

       ● **T33.531**   Superficial frostbite of right finger(s) A 🦠, A 🦠

       ● **T33.532**   Superficial frostbite of left finger(s) A 🦠, A 🦠

       ● **T33.539**   Superficial frostbite of unspecified finger(s) A 🦠, A 🦠

● **T33.6**   Superficial frostbite of hip and thigh

    (Ex) **For category T33.6 CC codes:** See PDX Collection 1416

    X ● **T33.60**   Superficial frostbite of unspecified hip and thigh A 🦠, A 🦠

    X ● **T33.61**   Superficial frostbite of right hip and thigh A 🦠, A 🦠

    X ● **T33.62**   Superficial frostbite of left hip and thigh A 🦠, A 🦠

● **T33.7**   Superficial frostbite of knee and lower leg

> **Excludes2**   superficial frostbite of ankle and foot (T33.8-)

    (Ex) **For category T33.7 CC codes:** See PDX Collection 1416

    X ● **T33.70**   Superficial frostbite of unspecified knee and lower leg A 🦠, A 🦠

    X ● **T33.71**   Superficial frostbite of right knee and lower leg A 🦠, A 🦠

    X ● **T33.72**   Superficial frostbite of left knee and lower leg A 🦠, A 🦠

● **T33.8**   Superficial frostbite of ankle, foot, and toe(s)

    (Ex) **For category T33.8 CC codes:** See PDX Collection 1418

    ● **T33.81**   Superficial frostbite of ankle

       ● **T33.811**   Superficial frostbite of right ankle A 🦠, A 🦠

       ● **T33.812**   Superficial frostbite of left ankle A 🦠, A 🦠

       ● **T33.819**   Superficial frostbite of unspecified ankle A 🦠, A 🦠

N Newborn Age: 0   **P** Pediatric Age: 0–17   **M** Maternity DX: 9–64   **A** Adult Age: 15–124   ♀ Females Only   ♂ Males Only

🦠 Complication\Comorbidity   🦠 Major C\C   (Ex) CC/MCC Exclusions   🦠 Hospital-Acquired Condition   🦠 Hierarchical Condition Category

1457

● T33.82 Superficial frostbite of foot
  ● T33.821 Superficial frostbite of right foot A 🪙, A 🪙
  ● T33.822 Superficial frostbite of left foot A 🪙, A 🪙
  ● T33.829 Superficial frostbite of unspecified foot A 🪙, A 🪙
● T33.83 Superficial frostbite of toe(s)
  ● T33.831 Superficial frostbite of right toe(s) A 🪙, A 🪙
  ● T33.832 Superficial frostbite of left toe(s) A 🪙, A 🪙
  ● T33.839 Superficial frostbite of unspecified toe(s) A 🪙, A 🪙
● T33.9 Superficial frostbite of other and unspecified sites
  (Ex) For category T33.9 CC codes: See PDX Collection 1416
X ● T33.90 Superficial frostbite of unspecified sites A 🪙, A 🪙
  Superficial frostbite NOS
X ● T33.99 Superficial frostbite of other sites A 🪙, A 🪙
  Superficial frostbite of leg NOS
  Superficial frostbite of trunk NOS

● T34 Frostbite with tissue necrosis
The appropriate 7th character is to be added to each code from category T34

> A initial encounter
> D subsequent encounter
> S sequela

● T34.0 Frostbite with tissue necrosis of head
  (Ex) For category T34.0 CC codes: See PDX Collection 1415
● T34.01 Frostbite with tissue necrosis of ear
  ● T34.011 Frostbite with tissue necrosis of right ear A 🪙, A 🪙
  ● T34.012 Frostbite with tissue necrosis of left ear A 🪙, A 🪙
  ● T34.019 Frostbite with tissue necrosis of unspecified ear A 🪙, A 🪙
X ● T34.02 Frostbite with tissue necrosis of nose A 🪙, A 🪙
X ● T34.09 Frostbite with tissue necrosis of other part of head A 🪙, A 🪙
X ● T34.1 Frostbite with tissue necrosis of neck A 🪙, A 🪙
  (Ex) See PDX Collection 1415
X ● T34.2 Frostbite with tissue necrosis of thorax A 🪙, A 🪙
  (Ex) See PDX Collection 1416
X ● T34.3 Frostbite with tissue necrosis of abdominal wall, lower back and pelvis A 🪙, A 🪙
  (Ex) See PDX Collection 1416
● T34.4 Frostbite with tissue necrosis of arm
  Excludes2 frostbite with tissue necrosis of wrist and hand (T34.5-)
  (Ex) For category T34.4 CC codes: See PDX Collection 1416
X ● T34.40 Frostbite with tissue necrosis of unspecified arm A 🪙, A 🪙
X ● T34.41 Frostbite with tissue necrosis of right arm A 🪙, A 🪙
X ● T34.42 Frostbite with tissue necrosis of left arm A 🪙, A 🪙
● T34.5 Frostbite with tissue necrosis of wrist, hand, and finger(s)
  (Ex) For category T34.5 CC codes: See PDX Collection 1417
● T34.51 Frostbite with tissue necrosis of wrist
  ● T34.511 Frostbite with tissue necrosis of right wrist A 🪙, A 🪙
  ● T34.512 Frostbite with tissue necrosis of left wrist A 🪙, A 🪙
  ● T34.519 Frostbite with tissue necrosis of unspecified wrist A 🪙, A 🪙

● T34.52 Frostbite with tissue necrosis of hand
  Excludes2 frostbite with tissue necrosis of finger(s) (T34.53-)
  ● T34.521 Frostbite with tissue necrosis of right hand A 🪙, A 🪙
  ● T34.522 Frostbite with tissue necrosis of left hand A 🪙, A 🪙
  ● T34.529 Frostbite with tissue necrosis of unspecified hand A 🪙, A 🪙
● T34.53 Frostbite with tissue necrosis of finger(s)
  ● T34.531 Frostbite with tissue necrosis of right finger(s) A 🪙, A 🪙
  ● T34.532 Frostbite with tissue necrosis of left finger(s) A 🪙, A 🪙
  ● T34.539 Frostbite with tissue necrosis of unspecified finger(s) A 🪙, A 🪙
● T34.6 Frostbite with tissue necrosis of hip and thigh
  (Ex) For category T34.6 CC codes: See PDX Collection 1416
X ● T34.60 Frostbite with tissue necrosis of unspecified hip and thigh A 🪙, A 🪙
X ● T34.61 Frostbite with tissue necrosis of right hip and thigh A 🪙, A 🪙
X ● T34.62 Frostbite with tissue necrosis of left hip and thigh A 🪙, A 🪙
● T34.7 Frostbite with tissue necrosis of knee and lower leg
  Excludes2 frostbite with tissue necrosis of ankle and foot (T34.8-)
  (Ex) For category T34.7 CC codes: See PDX Collection 1416
X ● T34.70 Frostbite with tissue necrosis of unspecified knee and lower leg A 🪙, A 🪙
X ● T34.71 Frostbite with tissue necrosis of right knee and lower leg A 🪙, A 🪙
X ● T34.72 Frostbite with tissue necrosis of left knee and lower leg A 🪙, A 🪙
● T34.8 Frostbite with tissue necrosis of ankle, foot, and toe(s)
  (Ex) For category T34.8 CC codes: See PDX Collection 1418
● T34.81 Frostbite with tissue necrosis of ankle
  ● T34.811 Frostbite with tissue necrosis of right ankle A 🪙, A 🪙
  ● T34.812 Frostbite with tissue necrosis of left ankle A 🪙, A 🪙
  ● T34.819 Frostbite with tissue necrosis of unspecified ankle A 🪙, A 🪙
● T34.82 Frostbite with tissue necrosis of foot
  ● T34.821 Frostbite with tissue necrosis of right foot A 🪙, A 🪙
  ● T34.822 Frostbite with tissue necrosis of left foot A 🪙, A 🪙
  ● T34.829 Frostbite with tissue necrosis of unspecified foot A 🪙, A 🪙
● T34.83 Frostbite with tissue necrosis of toe(s)
  ● T34.831 Frostbite with tissue necrosis of right toe(s) A 🪙, A 🪙
  ● T34.832 Frostbite with tissue necrosis of left toe(s) A 🪙, A 🪙
  ● T34.839 Frostbite with tissue necrosis of unspecified toe(s) A 🪙, A 🪙
● T34.9 Frostbite with tissue necrosis of other and unspecified sites
  (Ex) For category T34.9 CC codes: See PDX Collection 1416
X ● T34.90 Frostbite with tissue necrosis of unspecified sites A 🪙, A 🪙
  Frostbite with tissue necrosis NOS
X ● T34.99 Frostbite with tissue necrosis of other sites A 🪙, A 🪙
  Frostbite with tissue necrosis of leg NOS
  Frostbite with tissue necrosis of trunk NOS

▶ New   ⮕ Revised   ~~deleted~~ Deleted   Excludes 1   Excludes 2   Includes   Use additional   Code first   Code also   Key words
OGCR Official Guidelines   ● Unacceptable Principal Diagnosis   X Assign placeholder X   ● Use Additional Character(s)   ▶ Manifestation Code   Coding Clinic

OGCR See Section I.C.19.e.

Adverse Effects, Poisoning, Underdosing and Toxic Effects

Codes in categories T36-T65 are combination codes that include the substance that was taken as well as the intent. No additional external cause code is required for poisonings, toxic effects, adverse effects and underdosing codes.

POISONING BY, ADVERSE EFFECTS OF AND UNDERDOSING OF DRUGS MEDICAMENTS AND BIOLOGICAL SUBSTANCES (T36-T50)

Includes　　adverse effect of correct substance properly administered
poisoning by overdose of substance
poisoning by wrong substance given or taken in error
underdosing by (inadvertently) (deliberately) taking less substance than prescribed or instructed

Code first, for adverse effects, the nature of the adverse effect, such as:
adverse effect NOS (T88.7)
aspirin gastritis (K29.-)
blood disorders (D56-D76)
contact dermatitis (L23-L25)
dermatitis due to substances taken internally (L27.-)
nephropathy (N14.0-N14.2)

Note:　The drug giving rise to the adverse effect should be identified by use of codes from categories T36-T50 with fifth or sixth character 5.

Use additional code(s) to specify:
manifestations of poisoning
underdosing or failure in dosage during medical and surgical care (Y63.6, Y63.8-Y63.9)
underdosing of medication regimen (Z91.12-, Z91.13-)

Excludes1　toxic reaction to local anesthesia in pregnancy (O29.3-)

Excludes2　abuse and dependence of psychoactive substances (F10-F19)
abuse of non-dependence-producing substances (F55.-)
drug reaction and poisoning affecting newborn (P00-P96)
immunodeficiency due to drugs (D84.821)
pathological drug intoxication (inebriation) (F10-F19)

● **T36**　Poisoning by, adverse effect of and underdosing of systemic antibiotics

Excludes1　antineoplastic antibiotics (T45.1-)
locally applied antibiotic NEC (T49.0)
topically used antibiotic for ear, nose and throat (T49.6)
topically used antibiotic for eye (T49.5)

The appropriate 7th character is to be added to each code from category T36

A	initial encounter
D	subsequent encounter
S	sequela

● **T36.0**　Poisoning by, adverse effect of and underdosing of penicillins
　● **T36.0X**　Poisoning by, adverse effect of and underdosing of penicillins
　　● **T36.0X1**　Poisoning by penicillins, accidental (unintentional)
　　　　Poisoning by penicillins NOS
　　● **T36.0X2**　Poisoning by penicillins, intentional self-harm A, S 🐾
　　● **T36.0X3**　Poisoning by penicillins, assault
　　● **T36.0X4**　Poisoning by penicillins, undetermined
　　●● **T36.0X5**　Adverse effect of penicillins
　　●● **T36.0X6**　Underdosing of penicillins

● **T36.1**　Poisoning by, adverse effect of and underdosing of cephalosporins and other betalactam antibiotics
　● **T36.1X**　Poisoning by, adverse effect of and underdosing of cephalosporins and other beta-lactam antibiotics
　　● **T36.1X1**　Poisoning by cephalosporins and other beta-lactam antibiotics, accidental (unintentional)
　　　　Poisoning by cephalosporins and other beta-lactam antibiotics NOS
　　● **T36.1X2**　Poisoning by cephalosporins and other beta-lactam antibiotics, intentional self-harm A, S 🐾
　　● **T36.1X3**　Poisoning by cephalosporins and other beta-lactam antibiotics, assault
　　● **T36.1X4**　Poisoning by cephalosporins and other beta-lactam antibiotics, undetermined
　　●● **T36.1X5**　Adverse effect of cephalosporins and other beta-lactam antibiotics
　　●● **T36.1X6**　Underdosing of cephalosporins and other beta-lactam antibiotics

● **T36.2**　Poisoning by, adverse effect of and underdosing of chloramphenicol group
　● **T36.2X**　Poisoning by, adverse effect of and underdosing of chloramphenicol group
　　● **T36.2X1**　Poisoning by chloramphenicol group, accidental (unintentional)
　　　　Poisoning by chloramphenicol group NOS
　　● **T36.2X2**　Poisoning by chloramphenicol group, intentional self-harm A, S 🐾
　　● **T36.2X3**　Poisoning by chloramphenicol group, assault
　　● **T36.2X4**　Poisoning by chloramphenicol group, undetermined
　　●● **T36.2X5**　Adverse effect of chloramphenicol group
　　●● **T36.2X6**　Underdosing of chloramphenicol group

● **T36.3**　Poisoning by, adverse effect of and underdosing of macrolides
　● **T36.3X**　Poisoning by, adverse effect of and underdosing of macrolides
　　● **T36.3X1**　Poisoning by macrolides, accidental (unintentional)
　　　　Poisoning by macrolides NOS
　　● **T36.3X2**　Poisoning by macrolides, intentional self-harm A, S 🐾
　　● **T36.3X3**　Poisoning by macrolides, assault
　　● **T36.3X4**　Poisoning by macrolides, undetermined
　　●● **T36.3X5**　Adverse effect of macrolides
　　●● **T36.3X6**　Underdosing of macrolides

● **T36.4**　Poisoning by, adverse effect of and underdosing of tetracyclines
　● **T36.4X**　Poisoning by, adverse effect of and underdosing of tetracyclines
　　● **T36.4X1**　Poisoning by tetracyclines, accidental (unintentional)
　　　　Poisoning by tetracyclines NOS
　　● **T36.4X2**　Poisoning by tetracyclines, intentional self-harm A, S 🐾
　　● **T36.4X3**　Poisoning by tetracyclines, assault
　　● **T36.4X4**　Poisoning by tetracyclines, undetermined
　　●● **T36.4X5**　Adverse effect of tetracyclines
　　●● **T36.4X6**　Underdosing of tetracyclines

CHAPTER 19 (S00-T88)

N Newborn Age: 0　　**P** Pediatric Age: 0–17　　**M** Maternity DX: 9–64　　**A** Adult Age: 15–124　　♀ Females Only　　♂ Males Only

🐾 Complication\Comorbidity　　🐾 Major C\C　　(Ex) CC/MCC Exclusions　　🐾 Hospital-Acquired Condition　　🐾 Hierarchical Condition Category

1459

● **T36.5** Poisoning by, adverse effect of and underdosing of aminoglycosides
     Poisoning by, adverse effect of and underdosing of streptomycin

   ● **T36.5X** Poisoning by, adverse effect of and underdosing of aminoglycosides

     ● **T36.5X1** Poisoning by aminoglycosides, accidental (unintentional)
        Poisoning by aminoglycosides NOS

     ● **T36.5X2** Poisoning by aminoglycosides, intentional self-harm A, S 🛇

     ● **T36.5X3** Poisoning by aminoglycosides, assault

     ● **T36.5X4** Poisoning by aminoglycosides, undetermined

     ●● **T36.5X5** Adverse effect of aminoglycosides

     ●● **T36.5X6** Underdosing of aminoglycosides

● **T36.6** Poisoning by, adverse effect of and underdosing of rifampicins

   ● **T36.6X** Poisoning by, adverse effect of and underdosing of rifampicins

     ● **T36.6X1** Poisoning by rifampicins, accidental (unintentional)
        Poisoning by rifampicins NOS

     ● **T36.6X2** Poisoning by rifampicins, intentional self-harm A, S 🛇

     ● **T36.6X3** Poisoning by rifampicins, assault

     ● **T36.6X4** Poisoning by rifampicins, undetermined

     ●● **T36.6X5** Adverse effect of rifampicins

     ●● **T36.6X6** Underdosing of rifampicins

● **T36.7** Poisoning by, adverse effect of and underdosing of antifungal antibiotics, systemically used

   ● **T36.7X** Poisoning by, adverse effect of and underdosing of antifungal antibiotics, systemically used

     ● **T36.7X1** Poisoning by antifungal antibiotics, systemically used, accidental (unintentional)
        Poisoning by antifungal antibiotics, systemically used NOS

     ● **T36.7X2** Poisoning by antifungal antibiotics, systemically used, intentional self-harm A, S 🛇

     ● **T36.7X3** Poisoning by antifungal antibiotics, systemically used, assault

     ● **T36.7X4** Poisoning by antifungal antibiotics, systemically used, undetermined

     ●● **T36.7X5** Adverse effect of antifungal antibiotics, systemically used

     ●● **T36.7X6** Underdosing of antifungal antibiotics, systemically used

● **T36.8** Poisoning by, adverse effect of and underdosing of other systemic antibiotics

   ● **T36.8X** Poisoning by, adverse effect of and underdosing of other systemic antibiotics

     ● **T36.8X1** Poisoning by other systemic antibiotics, accidental (unintentional)
        Poisoning by other systemic antibiotics NOS

     ● **T36.8X2** Poisoning by other systemic antibiotics, intentional self-harm A, S 🛇

     ● **T36.8X3** Poisoning by other systemic antibiotics, assault

     ● **T36.8X4** Poisoning by other systemic antibiotics, undetermined

     ●● **T36.8X5** Adverse effect of other systemic antibiotics
        Coding Clinic: 2017, Q1, P39

     ●● **T36.8X6** Underdosing of other systemic antibiotics

● **T36.9** Poisoning by, adverse effect of and underdosing of unspecified systemic antibiotic

   X● **T36.91** Poisoning by unspecified systemic antibiotic, accidental (unintentional)
     Poisoning by systemic antibiotic NOS

   X● **T36.92** Poisoning by unspecified systemic antibiotic, intentional self-harm A, S 🛇

   X● **T36.93** Poisoning by unspecified systemic antibiotic, assault

   X● **T36.94** Poisoning by unspecified systemic antibiotic, undetermined

   ●X● **T36.95** Adverse effect of unspecified systemic antibiotic

   ●X● **T36.96** Underdosing of unspecified systemic antibiotic

● **T37** Poisoning by, adverse effect of and underdosing of other systemic anti-infectives and antiparasitics

   Excludes1 anti-infectives topically used for ear, nose and throat (T49.6-)
     anti-infectives topically used for eye (T49.5-)
     locally applied anti-infectives NEC (T49.0-)

   The appropriate 7th character is to be added to each code from category T37

     | | |
     A   initial encounter
     D   subsequent encounter
     S   sequela

   ● **T37.0** Poisoning by, adverse effect of and underdosing of sulfonamides

     ● **T37.0X** Poisoning by, adverse effect of and underdosing of sulfonamides

       ● **T37.0X1** Poisoning by sulfonamides, accidental (unintentional)
         Poisoning by sulfonamides NOS

       ● **T37.0X2** Poisoning by sulfonamides, intentional self-harm A, S 🛇

       ● **T37.0X3** Poisoning by sulfonamides, assault

       ● **T37.0X4** Poisoning by sulfonamides, undetermined

       ●● **T37.0X5** Adverse effect of sulfonamides

       ●● **T37.0X6** Underdosing of sulfonamides

   ● **T37.1** Poisoning by, adverse effect of and underdosing of antimycobacterial drugs

     Excludes1 rifampicins (T36.6-) streptomycin (T36.5-)

     ● **T37.1X** Poisoning by, adverse effect of and underdosing of antimycobacterial drugs

       ● **T37.1X1** Poisoning by antimycobacterial drugs, accidental (unintentional)
         Poisoning by antimycobacterial drugs NOS

       ● **T37.1X2** Poisoning by antimycobacterial drugs, intentional self-harm A, S 🛇

       ● **T37.1X3** Poisoning by antimycobacterial drugs, assault

       ● **T37.1X4** Poisoning by antimycobacterial drugs, undetermined

       ●● **T37.1X5** Adverse effect of antimycobacterial drugs

       ●● **T37.1X6** Underdosing of antimycobacterial drugs

▶ New   ⇒ Revised   ~~deleted~~ Deleted   Excludes 1   Excludes 2   Includes   Use additional   Code first   Code also   Key words

OGCR Official Guidelines   ● Unacceptable Principal Diagnosis   X Assign placeholder X   ● Use Additional Character(s)   ▶ Manifestation Code   **Coding Clinic**

● **T37.2   Poisoning by, adverse effect of and underdosing of antimalarials and drugs acting on other blood protozoa**

     | Excludes1 | hydroxyquinoline derivatives (T37.8-)

  ● **T37.2X   Poisoning by, adverse effect of and underdosing of antimalarials and drugs acting on other blood protozoa**

    ● **T37.2X1   Poisoning by antimalarials and drugs acting on other blood protozoa, accidental (unintentional)**
        Poisoning by antimalarials and drugs acting on other blood protozoa NOS

    ● **T37.2X2   Poisoning by antimalarials and drugs acting on other blood protozoa, intentional self-harm A, S** 🦠

    ● **T37.2X3   Poisoning by antimalarials and drugs acting on other blood protozoa, assault**

    ● **T37.2X4   Poisoning by antimalarials and drugs acting on other blood protozoa, undetermined**

    ●● **T37.2X5   Adverse effect of antimalarials and drugs acting on other blood protozoa**

    ●● **T37.2X6   Underdosing of antimalarials and drugs acting on other blood protozoa**

● **T37.3   Poisoning by, adverse effect of and underdosing of other antiprotozoal drugs**

  ● **T37.3X   Poisoning by, adverse effect of and underdosing of other antiprotozoal drugs**

    ● **T37.3X1   Poisoning by other antiprotozoal drugs, accidental (unintentional)**
        Poisoning by other antiprotozoal drugs NOS

    ● **T37.3X2   Poisoning by other antiprotozoal drugs, intentional self-harm A, S** 🦠

    ● **T37.3X3   Poisoning by other antiprotozoal drugs, assault**

    ● **T37.3X4   Poisoning by other antiprotozoal drugs, undetermined**

    ●● **T37.3X5   Adverse effect of other antiprotozoal drugs**

    ●● **T37.3X6   Underdosing of other antiprotozoal drugs**

● **T37.4   Poisoning by, adverse effect of and underdosing of anthelminthics**

  ● **T37.4X   Poisoning by, adverse effect of and underdosing of anthelminthics**

    ● **T37.4X1   Poisoning by anthelminthics, accidental (unintentional)**
        Poisoning by anthelminthics NOS

    ● **T37.4X2   Poisoning by anthelminthics, intentional self-harm A, S** 🦠

    ● **T37.4X3   Poisoning by anthelminthics, assault**

    ● **T37.4X4   Poisoning by anthelminthics, undetermined**

    ●● **T37.4X5   Adverse effect of anthelminthics**

    ●● **T37.4X6   Underdosing of anthelminthics**

● **T37.5   Poisoning by, adverse effect of and underdosing of antiviral drugs**

     | Excludes1 | amantadine (T42.8-)
                cytarabine (T45.1-)

  ● **T37.5X   Poisoning by, adverse effect of and underdosing of antiviral drugs**

    ● **T37.5X1   Poisoning by antiviral drugs, accidental (unintentional)**
        Poisoning by antiviral drugs NOS

    ● **T37.5X2   Poisoning by antiviral drugs, intentional self-harm A, S** 🦠

    ● **T37.5X3   Poisoning by antiviral drugs, assault**

    ● **T37.5X4   Poisoning by antiviral drugs, undetermined**

    ●● **T37.5X5   Adverse effect of antiviral drugs**

    ●● **T37.5X6   Underdosing of antiviral drugs**

● **T37.8   Poisoning by, adverse effect of and underdosing of other specified systemic anti-infectives and antiparasitics**
    Poisoning by, adverse effect of and underdosing of hydroxyquinoline derivatives

     | Excludes1 | antimalarial drugs (T37.2-)

  ● **T37.8X   Poisoning by, adverse effect of and underdosing of other specified systemic anti-infectives and antiparasitics**

    ● **T37.8X1   Poisoning by other specified systemic anti-infectives and antiparasitics, accidental (unintentional)**
        Poisoning by other specified systemic anti-infectives and antiparasitics NOS

    ● **T37.8X2   Poisoning by other specified systemic anti-infectives and antiparasitics, intentional self-harm A, S** 🦠

    ● **T37.8X3   Poisoning by other specified systemic anti-infectives and antiparasitics, assault**

    ● **T37.8X4   Poisoning by other specified systemic anti-infectives and antiparasitics, undetermined**

    ●● **T37.8X5   Adverse effect of other specified systemic anti-infectives and antiparasitics**

    ●● **T37.8X6   Underdosing of other specified systemic anti-infectives and antiparasitics**

● **T37.9   Poisoning by, adverse effect of and underdosing of unspecified systemic anti-infective and antiparasitics**

  X● **T37.91   Poisoning by unspecified systemic anti-infective and antiparasitics, accidental (unintentional)**
      Poisoning by, adverse effect of and underdosing of systemic anti-infective and antiparasitics NOS

  X● **T37.92   Poisoning by unspecified systemic anti-infective and antiparasitics, intentional self-harm A, S** 🦠

  X● **T37.93   Poisoning by unspecified systemic anti-infective and antiparasitics, assault**

  X● **T37.94   Poisoning by unspecified systemic anti-infective and antiparasitics, undetermined**

  ●X● **T37.95   Adverse effect of unspecified systemic anti-infective and antiparasitic**

  ●X● **T37.96   Underdosing of unspecified systemic anti-infectives and antiparasitics**

N Newborn Age: Ø   **P** Pediatric Age: Ø–17   **M** Maternity DX: 9–64   **A** Adult Age: 15–124   ♀ Females Only   ♂ Males Only

🦠 Complication\Comorbidity   🦠 Major C\C   (Ex) CC/MCC Exclusions   🦠 Hospital-Acquired Condition   🦠 Hierarchical Condition Category

1461

● T38   Poisoning by, adverse effect of and underdosing of hormones and their synthetic substitutes and antagonists, not elsewhere classified

> **Excludes1**   mineralocorticoids and their antagonists (T50.0-)
> oxytocic hormones (T48.0-)
> parathyroid hormones and derivatives (T50.9-)

The appropriate 7th character is to be added to each code from category T38

> A   initial encounter
> D   subsequent encounter
> S   sequela

● T38.0   Poisoning by, adverse effect of and underdosing of glucocorticoids and synthetic analogues

> **Excludes1**   glucocorticoids, topically used (T49.-)

● T38.0X   Poisoning by, adverse effect of and underdosing of glucocorticoids and synthetic analogues

● T38.0X1   Poisoning by glucocorticoids and synthetic analogues, accidental (unintentional)
> Poisoning by glucocorticoids and synthetic analogues NOS

● T38.0X2   Poisoning by glucocorticoids and synthetic analogues, intentional self-harm A, S 🔖

● T38.0X3   Poisoning by glucocorticoids and synthetic analogues, assault

● T38.0X4   Poisoning by glucocorticoids and synthetic analogues, undetermined

●● T38.0X5   Adverse effect of glucocorticoids and synthetic analogues

●● T38.0X6   Underdosing of glucocorticoids and synthetic analogues

● T38.1   Poisoning by, adverse effect of and underdosing of thyroid hormones and substitutes

● T38.1X   Poisoning by, adverse effect of and underdosing of thyroid hormones and substitutes

● T38.1X1   Poisoning by thyroid hormones and substitutes, accidental (unintentional)
> Poisoning by thyroid hormones and substitutes NOS

● T38.1X2   Poisoning by thyroid hormones and substitutes, intentional self-harm A, S 🔖

● T38.1X3   Poisoning by thyroid hormones and substitutes, assault

● T38.1X4   Poisoning by thyroid hormones and substitutes, undetermined

●● T38.1X5   Adverse effect of thyroid hormones and substitutes

●● T38.1X6   Underdosing of thyroid hormones and substitutes

● T38.2   Poisoning by, adverse effect of and underdosing of antithyroid drugs

● T38.2X   Poisoning by, adverse effect of and underdosing of antithyroid drugs

● T38.2X1   Poisoning by antithyroid drugs, accidental (unintentional)
> Poisoning by antithyroid drugs NOS

● T38.2X2   Poisoning by antithyroid drugs, intentional self-harm A, S 🔖

● T38.2X3   Poisoning by antithyroid drugs, assault

● T38.2X4   Poisoning by antithyroid drugs, undetermined

●● T38.2X5   Adverse effect of antithyroid drugs

●● T38.2X6   Underdosing of antithyroid drugs

● T38.3   Poisoning by, adverse effect of and underdosing of insulin and oral hypoglycemic [antidiabetic] drugs

● T38.3X   Poisoning by, adverse effect of and underdosing of insulin and oral hypoglycemic [antidiabetic] drugs

● T38.3X1   Poisoning by insulin and oral hypoglycemic [antidiabetic] drugs, accidental (unintentional)
> Poisoning by insulin and oral hypoglycemic [antidiabetic] drugs NOS

● T38.3X2   Poisoning by insulin and oral hypoglycemic [antidiabetic] drugs, intentional self-harm

● T38.3X3   Poisoning by insulin and oral hypoglycemic [antidiabetic] drugs, assault A, S 🔖

● T38.3X4   Poisoning by insulin and oral hypoglycemic [antidiabetic] drugs, undetermined

●● T38.3X5   Adverse effect of insulin and oral hypoglycemic [antidiabetic] drugs

●● T38.3X6   Underdosing of insulin and oral hypoglycemic [antidiabetic] drugs

● T38.4   Poisoning by, adverse effect of and underdosing of oral contraceptives
> Poisoning by, adverse effect of and underdosing of multiple- and single-ingredient oral contraceptive preparations

● T38.4X   Poisoning by, adverse effect of and underdosing of oral contraceptives

● T38.4X1   Poisoning by oral contraceptives, accidental (unintentional)
> Poisoning by oral contraceptives NOS

● T38.4X2   Poisoning by oral contraceptives, intentional self-harm A, S 🔖

● T38.4X3   Poisoning by oral contraceptives, assault

● T38.4X4   Poisoning by oral contraceptives, undetermined

●● T38.4X5   Adverse effect of oral contraceptives

●● T38.4X6   Underdosing of oral contraceptives

● T38.5   Poisoning by, adverse effect of and underdosing of other estrogens and progestogens
> Poisoning by, adverse effect of and underdosing of estrogens and progestogens mixtures and substitutes

● T38.5X   Poisoning by, adverse effect of and underdosing of other estrogens and progestogens

● T38.5X1   Poisoning by other estrogens and progestogens, accidental (unintentional)
> Poisoning by other estrogens and progestogens NOS

● T38.5X2   Poisoning by other estrogens and progestogens, intentional self-harm A, S 🔖

● T38.5X3   Poisoning by other estrogens and progestogens, assault

● T38.5X4   Poisoning by other estrogens and progestogens, undetermined

●● T38.5X5   Adverse effect of other estrogens and progestogens

●● T38.5X6   Underdosing of other estrogens and progestogens

▶ New   ⮕ Revised   ~~deleted~~ Deleted   Excludes 1   Excludes 2   Includes   Use additional   Code first   Code also   Key words

OGCR Official Guidelines   ● Unacceptable Principal Diagnosis   X Assign placeholder X   ● Use Additional Character(s)   ▸ Manifestation Code   **Coding Clinic**

● T38.6   Poisoning by, adverse effect of and underdosing of antigonadotrophins, antiestrogens, antiandrogens, not elsewhere classified

    Poisoning by, adverse effect of and underdosing of tamoxifen

   ● T38.6X   Poisoning by, adverse effect of and underdosing of antigonadotrophins, antiestrogens, antiandrogens, not elsewhere classified

     ● T38.6X1   Poisoning by antigonadotrophins, antiestrogens, antiandrogens, not elsewhere classified, accidental (unintentional)

        Poisoning by antigonadotrophins, antiestrogens, antiandrogens, not elsewhere classified NOS

     ● T38.6X2   Poisoning by antigonadotrophins, antiestrogens, antiandrogens, not elsewhere classified, intentional self-harm A, S 🦠

     ● T38.6X3   Poisoning by antigonadotrophins, antiestrogens, antiandrogens, not elsewhere classified, assault

     ● T38.6X4   Poisoning by antigonadotrophins, antiestrogens, antiandrogens, not elsewhere classified, undetermined

     ●● T38.6X5   Adverse effect of antigonadotrophins, antiestrogens, antiandrogens, not elsewhere classified

     ●● T38.6X6   Underdosing of antigonadotrophins, antiestrogens, antiandrogens, not elsewhere classified

● T38.7   Poisoning by, adverse effect of and underdosing of androgens and anabolic congeners

   ● T38.7X   Poisoning by, adverse effect of and underdosing of androgens and anabolic congeners

     ● T38.7X1   Poisoning by androgens and anabolic congeners, accidental (unintentional)

        Poisoning by androgens and anabolic congeners NOS

     ● T38.7X2   Poisoning by androgens and anabolic congeners, intentional self-harm A, S 🦠

     ● T38.7X3   Poisoning by androgens and anabolic congeners, assault

     ● T38.7X4   Poisoning by androgens and anabolic congeners, undetermined

     ●● T38.7X5   Adverse effect of androgens and anabolic congeners

     ●● T38.7X6   Underdosing of androgens and anabolic congeners

● T38.8   Poisoning by, adverse effect of and underdosing of other and unspecified hormones and synthetic substitutes

   ● T38.80   Poisoning by, adverse effect of and underdosing of unspecified hormones and synthetic substitutes

     ● T38.801   Poisoning by unspecified hormones and synthetic substitutes, accidental (unintentional)

        Poisoning by unspecified hormones and synthetic substitutes NOS

     ● T38.802   Poisoning by unspecified hormones and synthetic substitutes, intentional self-harm A, S 🦠

     ● T38.803   Poisoning by unspecified hormones and synthetic substitutes, assault

     ●● T38.804   Poisoning by unspecified hormones and synthetic substitutes, undetermined

     ●● T38.805   Adverse effect of unspecified hormones and synthetic substitutes

     ●● T38.806   Underdosing of unspecified hormones and synthetic substitutes

   ● T38.81   Poisoning by, adverse effect of and underdosing of anterior pituitary [adenohypophyseal] hormones

     ● T38.811   Poisoning by anterior pituitary [adenohypophyseal] hormones, accidental (unintentional)

        Poisoning by anterior pituitary [adenohypophyseal] hormones NOS

     ● T38.812   Poisoning by anterior pituitary [adenohypophyseal] hormones, intentional self-harm A, S 🦠

     ● T38.813   Poisoning by anterior pituitary [adenohypophyseal] hormones, assault

     ● T38.814   Poisoning by anterior pituitary [adenohypophyseal] hormones, undetermined

     ●● T38.815   Adverse effect of anterior pituitary [adenohypophyseal] hormones

     ●● T38.816   Underdosing of anterior pituitary [adenohypophyseal] hormones

   ● T38.89   Poisoning by, adverse effect of and underdosing of other hormones and synthetic substitutes

     ● T38.891   Poisoning by other hormones and synthetic substitutes, accidental (unintentional)

        Poisoning by other hormones and synthetic substitutes NOS

     ● T38.892   Poisoning by other hormones and synthetic substitutes, intentional self-harm A, S 🦠

     ● T38.893   Poisoning by other hormones and synthetic substitutes, assault

     ● T38.894   Poisoning by other hormones and synthetic substitutes, undetermined

     ●● T38.895   Adverse effect of other hormones and synthetic substitutes

     ●● T38.896   Underdosing of other hormones and synthetic substitutes

● T38.9   Poisoning by, adverse effect of and underdosing of other and unspecified hormone antagonists

   ● T38.90   Poisoning by, adverse effect of and underdosing of unspecified hormone antagonists

     ● T38.901   Poisoning by unspecified hormone antagonists, accidental (unintentional)

        Poisoning by unspecified hormone antagonists NOS

     ● T38.902   Poisoning by unspecified hormone antagonists, intentional self-harm A, S 🦠

     ● T38.903   Poisoning by unspecified hormone antagonists, assault

     ● T38.904   Poisoning by unspecified hormone antagonists, undetermined

     ●● T38.905   Adverse effect of unspecified hormone antagonists

     ●● T38.906   Underdosing of unspecified hormone antagonists

CHAPTER 19 (S00-T88)

N   Newborn Age: 0   P   Pediatric Age: 0–17   M   Maternity DX: 9–64   A   Adult Age: 15–124   ♀   Females Only   ♂   Males Only

🦠 Complication\Comorbidity   🦠 Major C\C   (Ex) CC/MCC Exclusions   🦠 Hospital-Acquired Condition   🦠 Hierarchical Condition Category

1463

- ● T38.99   Poisoning by, adverse effect of and underdosing of other hormone antagonists
  - ● T38.991   Poisoning by other hormone antagonists, accidental (unintentional)
    - Poisoning by other hormone antagonists NOS
  - ● T38.992   Poisoning by other hormone antagonists, intentional self-harm A, S ⓡⓒ
  - ● T38.993   Poisoning by other hormone antagonists, assault
  - ● T38.994   Poisoning by other hormone antagonists, undetermined
  - ●● T38.995   Adverse effect of other hormone antagonists
  - ●● T38.996   Underdosing of other hormone antagonists

- ● T39   Poisoning by, adverse effect of and underdosing of nonopioid analgesics, antipyretics and antirheumatics

  The appropriate 7th character is to be added to each code from category T39

A	initial encounter
D	subsequent encounter
S	sequela

  - ● T39.0   Poisoning by, adverse effect of and underdosing of salicylates
    - ● T39.01   Poisoning by, adverse effect of and underdosing of aspirin
      - Poisoning by, adverse effect of and underdosing of acetylsalicylic acid
      - ● T39.011   Poisoning by aspirin, accidental (unintentional)
      - ● T39.012   Poisoning by aspirin, intentional self-harm A, S ⓡⓒ
      - ● T39.013   Poisoning by aspirin, assault
      - ● T39.014   Poisoning by aspirin, undetermined
      - ●● T39.015   Adverse effect of aspirin
        - Coding Clinic: 2016, Q1, P15
      - ●● T39.016   Underdosing of aspirin
    - ● T39.09   Poisoning by, adverse effect of and underdosing of other salicylates
      - ● T39.091   Poisoning by salicylates, accidental (unintentional)
        - Poisoning by salicylates NOS
      - ● T39.092   Poisoning by salicylates, intentional self-harm A, S ⓡⓒ
      - ● T39.093   Poisoning by salicylates, assault
      - ● T39.094   Poisoning by salicylates, undetermined
      - ●● T39.095   Adverse effect of salicylates
      - ●● T39.096   Underdosing of salicylates
  - ● T39.1   Poisoning by, adverse effect of and underdosing of 4-Aminophenol derivatives
    - ● T39.1X   Poisoning by, adverse effect of and underdosing of 4-Aminophenol derivatives
      - ● T39.1X1   Poisoning by 4-Aminophenol derivatives, accidental (unintentional)
        - Poisoning by 4-Aminophenol derivatives NOS
      - ● T39.1X2   Poisoning by 4-Aminophenol derivatives, intentional self-harm A, S ⓡⓒ
      - ● T39.1X3   Poisoning by 4-Aminophenol derivatives, assault
      - ● T39.1X4   Poisoning by 4-Aminophenol derivatives, undetermined
      - ●● T39.1X5   Adverse effect of 4-Aminophenol derivatives
      - ●● T39.1X6   Underdosing of 4-Aminophenol derivatives

- ● T39.2   Poisoning by, adverse effect of and underdosing of pyrazolone derivatives
  - ● T39.2X   Poisoning by, adverse effect of and underdosing of pyrazolone derivatives
    - ● T39.2X1   Poisoning by pyrazolone derivatives, accidental (unintentional)
      - Poisoning by pyrazolone derivatives NOS
    - ● T39.2X2   Poisoning by pyrazolone derivatives, intentional self-harm A, S ⓡⓒ
    - ● T39.2X3   Poisoning by pyrazolone derivatives, assault
    - ● T39.2X4   Poisoning by pyrazolone derivatives, undetermined
    - ●● T39.2X5   Adverse effect of pyrazolone derivatives
    - ●● T39.2X6   Underdosing of pyrazolone derivatives
- ● T39.3   Poisoning by, adverse effect of and underdosing of other nonsteroidal anti-inflammatory drugs [NSAID]
  - ● T39.31   Poisoning by, adverse effect of and underdosing of propionic acid derivatives
    - Poisoning by, adverse effect of and underdosing of fenoprofen
    - Poisoning by, adverse effect of and underdosing of flurbiprofen
    - Poisoning by, adverse effect of and underdosing of ibuprofen
    - Poisoning by, adverse effect of and underdosing of ketoprofen
    - Poisoning by, adverse effect of and underdosing of naproxen
    - Poisoning by, adverse effect of and underdosing of oxaprozin
    - ● T39.311   Poisoning by propionic acid derivatives, accidental (unintentional)
    - ● T39.312   Poisoning by propionic acid derivatives, intentional self-harm A, S ⓡⓒ
    - ● T39.313   Poisoning by propionic acid derivatives, assault
    - ● T39.314   Poisoning by propionic acid derivatives, undetermined
    - ●● T39.315   Adverse effect of propionic acid derivatives
    - ●● T39.316   Underdosing of propionic acid derivatives
  - ● T39.39   Poisoning by, adverse effect of and underdosing of other nonsteroidal anti-inflammatory drugs [NSAID]
    - ● T39.391   Poisoning by other nonsteroidal anti-inflammatory drugs [NSAID], accidental (unintentional)
      - Poisoning by other nonsteroidal anti-inflammatory drugs NOS
    - ● T39.392   Poisoning by other nonsteroidal anti-inflammatory drugs [NSAID], intentional self-harm A, S ⓡⓒ
    - ● T39.393   Poisoning by other nonsteroidal anti-inflammatory drugs [NSAID], assault
    - ● T39.394   Poisoning by other nonsteroidal anti-inflammatory drugs [NSAID], undetermined
    - ●● T39.395   Adverse effect of other nonsteroidal anti-inflammatory drugs [NSAID]
    - ●● T39.396   Underdosing of other nonsteroidal anti-inflammatory drugs [NSAID]

▶ New   ⇒ Revised   ~~deleted~~ Deleted   Excludes 1   Excludes 2   Includes   Use additional   Code first   Code also   Key words

OGCR Official Guidelines   ● Unacceptable Principal Diagnosis   X Assign placeholder X   ● Use Additional Character(s)   ▷ Manifestation Code   Coding Clinic

- **T39.4** Poisoning by, adverse effect of and underdosing of antirheumatics, not elsewhere classified
  - **Excludes1** poisoning by, adverse effect of and underdosing of glucocorticoids (T38.0-)
    poisoning by, adverse effect of and underdosing of salicylates (T39.0-)
  - **T39.4X** Poisoning by, adverse effect of and underdosing of antirheumatics, not elsewhere classified
    - **T39.4X1** Poisoning by antirheumatics, not elsewhere classified, accidental (unintentional)
      Poisoning by antirheumatics, not elsewhere classified NOS
    - **T39.4X2** Poisoning by antirheumatics, not elsewhere classified, intentional self-harm A, S
    - **T39.4X3** Poisoning by antirheumatics, not elsewhere classified, assault
    - **T39.4X4** Poisoning by antirheumatics, not elsewhere classified, undetermined
    - **T39.4X5** Adverse effect of antirheumatics, not elsewhere classified
    - **T39.4X6** Underdosing of antirheumatics, not elsewhere classified
- **T39.8** Poisoning by, adverse effect of and underdosing of other nonopioid analgesics and antipyretics, not elsewhere classified
  - **T39.8X** Poisoning by, adverse effect of and underdosing of other nonopioid analgesics and antipyretics, not elsewhere classified
    - **T39.8X1** Poisoning by other nonopioid analgesics and antipyretics, not elsewhere classified, accidental (unintentional)
      Poisoning by other nonopioid analgesics and antipyretics, not elsewhere classified NOS
    - **T39.8X2** Poisoning by other nonopioid analgesics and antipyretics, not elsewhere classified, intentional self-harm A, S
    - **T39.8X3** Poisoning by other nonopioid analgesics and antipyretics, not elsewhere classified, assault
    - **T39.8X4** Poisoning by other nonopioid analgesics and antipyretics, not elsewhere classified, undetermined
    - **T39.8X5** Adverse effect of other nonopioid analgesics and antipyretics, not elsewhere classified
    - **T39.8X6** Underdosing of other nonopioid analgesics and antipyretics, not elsewhere classified
- **T39.9** Poisoning by, adverse effect of and underdosing of unspecified nonopioid analgesic, antipyretic and antirheumatic
  - **T39.91** Poisoning by unspecified nonopioid analgesic, antipyretic and antirheumatic, accidental (unintentional)
    Poisoning by nonopioid analgesic, antipyretic and antirheumatic NOS
  - **T39.92** Poisoning by unspecified nonopioid analgesic, antipyretic and antirheumatic, intentional self-harm A, S
  - **T39.93** Poisoning by unspecified nonopioid analgesic, antipyretic and antirheumatic, assault
  - **T39.94** Poisoning by unspecified nonopioid analgesic, antipyretic and antirheumatic, undetermined

- **T39.95** Adverse effect of unspecified nonopioid analgesic, antipyretic and antirheumatic
- **T39.96** Underdosing of unspecified nonopioid analgesic, antipyretic and antirheumatic
- **T40** Poisoning by, adverse effect of and underdosing of narcotics and psychodysleptics [hallucinogens]
  - **Excludes2** drug dependence and related mental and behavioral disorders due to psychoactive substance use (F10.-F19.-)
  - The appropriate 7th character is to be added to each code from category T40

    | A | initial encounter |
    | D | subsequent encounter |
    | S | sequela |

  - **T40.0** Poisoning by, adverse effect of and underdosing of opium
    - **T40.0X** Poisoning by, adverse effect of and underdosing of opium
      - **T40.0X1** Poisoning by opium, accidental (unintentional)
        Poisoning by opium NOS
      - **T40.0X2** Poisoning by opium, intentional self-harm A, S
      - **T40.0X3** Poisoning by opium, assault ·
      - **T40.0X4** Poisoning by opium, undetermined
      - **T40.0X5** Adverse effect of opium
      - **T40.0X6** Underdosing of opium
  - **T40.1** Poisoning by and adverse effect of heroin
    - **T40.1X** Poisoning by and adverse effect of heroin
      - **T40.1X1** Poisoning by heroin, accidental (unintentional)
        Poisoning by heroin NOS
      - **T40.1X2** Poisoning by heroin, intentional self-harm A, S
      - **T40.1X3** Poisoning by heroin, assault
      - **T40.1X4** Poisoning by heroin, undetermined
  - **T40.2** Poisoning by, adverse effect of and underdosing of other opioids
    - **T40.2X** Poisoning by, adverse effect of and underdosing of other opioids
      - **T40.2X1** Poisoning by other opioids, accidental (unintentional)
        Poisoning by other opioids NOS
      - **T40.2X2** Poisoning by other opioids, intentional self-harm A, S
      - **T40.2X3** Poisoning by other opioids, assault
      - **T40.2X4** Poisoning by other opioids, undetermined
      - **T40.2X5** Adverse effect of other opioids
      - **T40.2X6** Underdosing of other opioids
  - **T40.3** Poisoning by, adverse effect of and underdosing of methadone
    - **T40.3X** Poisoning by, adverse effect of and underdosing of methadone
      - **T40.3X1** Poisoning by methadone, accidental (unintentional)
        Poisoning by methadone NOS
      - **T40.3X2** Poisoning by methadone, intentional self-harm A, S
      - **T40.3X3** Poisoning by methadone, assault
      - **T40.3X4** Poisoning by methadone, undetermined
      - **T40.3X5** Adverse effect of methadone
      - **T40.3X6** Underdosing of methadone

CHAPTER 19 (S00-T88)

CHAPTER 19 (S00–T88)

● T40.4   Poisoning by, adverse effect of and underdosing of other synthetic narcotics
  ● T40.41   Poisoning by, adverse effect of and underdosing of fentanyl or fentanyl analogs
     T40.411   Poisoning by fentanyl or fentanyl analogs, accidental (unintentional)
     T40.412   Poisoning by fentanyl or fentanyl analogs, intentional self-harm
     T40.413   Poisoning by fentanyl or fentanyl analogs, assault
     T40.414   Poisoning by fentanyl or fentanyl analogs, undetermined
     ● T40.415   Adverse effect of fentanyl or fentanyl analogs
     ● T40.416   Underdosing of fentanyl or fentanyl analogs
  ● T40.42   Poisoning by, adverse effect of and underdosing of tramadol
     T40.421   Poisoning by tramadol, accidental (unintentional)
     T40.422   Poisoning by tramadol, intentional self-harm
     T40.423   Poisoning by tramadol, assault
     T40.424   Poisoning by tramadol, undetermined
     ● T40.425   Adverse effect of tramadol
     ● T40.426   Underdosing of tramadol
  ● T40.49   Poisoning by, adverse effect of and underdosing of other synthetic narcotics
     T40.491   Poisoning by other synthetic narcotics, accidental (unintentional)
     T40.492   Poisoning by other synthetic narcotics, intentional self-harm
     T40.493   Poisoning by other synthetic narcotics, assault
     T40.494   Poisoning by other synthetic narcotics, undetermined
     ● T40.495   Adverse effect of other synthetic narcotics
     ● T40.496   Underdosing of other synthetic narcotics
● T40.5   Poisoning by, adverse effect of and underdosing of cocaine
  ● T40.5X   Poisoning by, adverse effect of and underdosing of cocaine
     ● T40.5X1   Poisoning by cocaine, accidental (unintentional)
       Poisoning by cocaine NOS
       Coding Clinic: 2016, Q2, P9
     ● T40.5X2   Poisoning by cocaine, intentional self-harm A, S 🔁
     ● T40.5X3   Poisoning by cocaine, assault
     ● T40.5X4   Poisoning by cocaine, undetermined
     ●● T40.5X5   Adverse effect of cocaine
     ●● T40.5X6   Underdosing of cocaine
● T40.6   Poisoning by, adverse effect of and underdosing of other and unspecified narcotics
  ● T40.60   Poisoning by, adverse effect of and underdosing of unspecified narcotics
     ● T40.601   Poisoning by unspecified narcotics, accidental (unintentional)
       Poisoning by narcotics NOS
     ● T40.602   Poisoning by unspecified narcotics, intentional self-harm A, S 🔁
     ● T40.603   Poisoning by unspecified narcotics, assault
     ● T40.604   Poisoning by unspecified narcotics, undetermined
     ●● T40.605   Adverse effect of unspecified narcotics
     ●● T40.606   Underdosing of unspecified narcotics

● T40.69   Poisoning by, adverse effect of and underdosing of other narcotics
  ● T40.691   Poisoning by other narcotics, accidental (unintentional)
     Poisoning by other narcotics NOS
  ● T40.692   Poisoning by other narcotics, intentional self-harm A, S 🔁
  ● T40.693   Poisoning by other narcotics, assault
  ● T40.694   Poisoning by other narcotics, undetermined
  ●● T40.695   Adverse effect of other narcotics
  ●● T40.696   Underdosing of other narcotics
● T40.7   Poisoning by, adverse effect of and underdosing of cannabis (derivatives)
  ▶● T40.71   Poisoning by, adverse effect of and underdosing of cannabis (derivatives)
    ▶ T40.711   Poisoning by cannabis, accidental (unintentional)
    ▶ T40.712   Poisoning by cannabis, intentional self-harm
    ▶ T40.713   Poisoning by cannabis, assault
    ▶ T40.714   Poisoning by cannabis, undetermined
    ▶ T40.715   Adverse effect of cannabis
    ▶ T40.716   Underdosing of cannabis
  ▶● T40.72   Poisoning by, adverse effect of and underdosing of synthetic cannabinoids
    ▶ T40.721   Poisoning by synthetic cannabinoids, accidental (unintentional)
    ▶ T40.722   Poisoning by synthetic cannabinoids, intentional self-harm
    ▶ T40.723   Poisoning by synthetic cannabinoids, assault
    ▶ T40.724   Poisoning by synthetic cannabinoids, undetermined
    ▶ T40.725   Adverse effect of synthetic cannabinoids
    ▶ T40.726   Underdosing of synthetic cannabinoids
  ~~T40.7X~~   ~~Poisoning by, adverse effect of and underdosing of cannabis (derivatives)~~
     ~~T40.7X1~~   ~~Poisoning by cannabis (derivatives), accidental (unintentional)~~
       ~~Poisoning by cannabis NOS~~
       ~~Coding Clinic: 2020, Q1, P8~~
     ~~T40.7X2~~   ~~Poisoning by cannabis (derivatives), intentional self-harm A, S~~
     ~~T40.7X3~~   ~~Poisoning by cannabis (derivatives), assault~~
     ~~T40.7X4~~   ~~Poisoning by cannabis (derivatives), undetermined~~
     ~~T40.7X5~~   ~~Adverse effect of cannabis (derivatives)~~
     ~~T40.7X6~~   ~~Underdosing of cannabis (derivatives)~~
● T40.8   Poisoning by and adverse effect of lysergide [LSD]
  ● T40.8X   Poisoning by and adverse effect of lysergide [LSD]
     ● T40.8X1   Poisoning by lysergide [LSD], accidental (unintentional)
       Poisoning by lysergide [LSD] NOS
     ● T40.8X2   Poisoning by lysergide [LSD], intentional self-harm A, S 🔁
     ● T40.8X3   Poisoning by lysergide [LSD], assault
     ● T40.8X4   Poisoning by lysergide [LSD], undetermined
● T40.9   Poisoning by, adverse effect of and underdosing of other and unspecified psychodysleptics [hallucinogens]
  ● T40.90   Poisoning by, adverse effect of and underdosing of unspecified psychodysleptics [hallucinogens]
     ● T40.901   Poisoning by unspecified psychodysleptics [hallucinogens], accidental (unintentional)

▶ New   ⇛ Revised   ~~deleted~~ Deleted   Excludes 1   Excludes 2   Includes   Use additional   Code first   Code also   Key words
OGCR Official Guidelines   ● Unacceptable Principal Diagnosis   X Assign placeholder X   ● Use Additional Character(s)   ▶ Manifestation Code   **Coding Clinic**

● T40.902 Poisoning by unspecified
psychodysleptics [hallucinogens],
intentional self-harm A, S 🐷

● T40.903 Poisoning by unspecified
psychodysleptics [hallucinogens],
assault

● T40.904 Poisoning by unspecified
psychodysleptics [hallucinogens],
undetermined

●● T40.905 Adverse effect of unspecified
psychodysleptics [hallucinogens]

●● T40.906 Underdosing of unspecified
psychodysleptics [hallucinogens]

● T40.99 Poisoning by, adverse effect of and underdosing
of other psychodysleptics [hallucinogens]

● T40.991 Poisoning by other psychodysleptics
[hallucinogens], accidental
(unintentional)
Poisoning by other psychodysleptics
[hallucinogens] NOS

● T40.992 Poisoning by other psychodysleptics
[hallucinogens], intentional self-harm
A, S 🐷

● T40.993 Poisoning by other psychodysleptics
[hallucinogens], assault

● T40.994 Poisoning by other psychodysleptics
[hallucinogens], undetermined

●● T40.995 Adverse effect of other
psychodysleptics [hallucinogens]

●● T40.996 Underdosing of other
psychodysleptics [hallucinogens]

● T41 Poisoning by, adverse effect of and underdosing of anesthetics
and therapeutic gases

Excludes1 benzodiazepines (T42.4-)
cocaine (T40.5-)
complications of anesthesia during pregnancy
(O29.-)
complications of anesthesia during labor and
delivery (O74.-)
complications of anesthesia during the
puerperium (O89.-) opioids (T40.0-T40.2)

The appropriate 7th character is to be added to each code from
category T41

A	initial encounter
D	subsequent encounter
S	sequela

● T41.0 Poisoning by, adverse effect of and underdosing of
inhaled anesthetics

Excludes1 oxygen (T41.5-)

● T41.0X Poisoning by, adverse effect of and
underdosing of inhaled anesthetics

● T41.0X1 Poisoning by inhaled anesthetics,
accidental (unintentional)
Poisoning by inhaled anesthetics NOS

● T41.0X2 Poisoning by inhaled anesthetics,
intentional self-harm A, S 🐷

● T41.0X3 Poisoning by inhaled anesthetics,
assault

● T41.0X4 Poisoning by inhaled anesthetics,
undetermined

●● T41.0X5 Adverse effect of inhaled anesthetics

●● T41.0X6 Underdosing of inhaled anesthetics

● T41.1 Poisoning by, adverse effect of and underdosing of
intravenous anesthetics
Poisoning by, adverse effect of and underdosing of
thiobarbiturates

● T41.1X Poisoning by, adverse effect of and
underdosing of intravenous anesthetics

● T41.1X1 Poisoning by intravenous anesthetics,
accidental (unintentional)
Poisoning by intravenous
anesthetics NOS

● T41.1X2 Poisoning by intravenous anesthetics,
intentional self-harm A, S 🐷

● T41.1X3 Poisoning by intravenous anesthetics,
assault

● T41.1X4 Poisoning by intravenous anesthetics,
undetermined

●● T41.1X5 Adverse effect of intravenous
anesthetics

●● T41.1X6 Underdosing of intravenous anesthetics

● T41.2 Poisoning by, adverse effect of and underdosing of other
and unspecified general anesthetics

● T41.20 Poisoning by, adverse effect of and
underdosing of unspecified general anesthetics

● T41.201 Poisoning by unspecified general
anesthetics, accidental (unintentional)
Poisoning by general anesthetics NOS

● T41.202 Poisoning by unspecified general
anesthetics, intentional self-harm
A, S 🐷

● T41.203 Poisoning by unspecified general
anesthetics, assault

● T41.204 Poisoning by unspecified general
anesthetics, undetermined

●● T41.205 Adverse effect of unspecified general
anesthetics
Coding Clinic: 2016, Q4, P73

●● T41.206 Underdosing of unspecified general
anesthetics

● T41.29 Poisoning by, adverse effect of and
underdosing of other general anesthetics

● T41.291 Poisoning by other general anesthetics,
accidental (unintentional)
Poisoning by other general
anesthetics NOS

● T41.292 Poisoning by other general anesthetics,
intentional self-harm A, S 🐷

● T41.293 Poisoning by other general
anesthetics, assault

● T41.294 Poisoning by other general
anesthetics, undetermined

●● T41.295 Adverse effect of other general
anesthetics

●● T41.296 Underdosing of other general
anesthetics

● T41.3 Poisoning by, adverse effect of and underdosing of local
anesthetics
Cocaine (topical)

Excludes2 poisoning by cocaine used as a central
nervous system stimulant (T40.5X1-
T40.5X4)

● T41.3X Poisoning by, adverse effect of and
underdosing of local anesthetics

● T41.3X1 Poisoning by local anesthetics,
accidental (unintentional)
Poisoning by local anesthetics NOS

● T41.3X2 Poisoning by local anesthetics,
intentional self-harm A, S 🐷

● T41.3X3 Poisoning by local anesthetics, assault

● T41.3X4 Poisoning by local anesthetics,
undetermined

●● T41.3X5 Adverse effect of local anesthetics

●● T41.3X6 Underdosing of local anesthetics

● T41.4 Poisoning by, adverse effect of and underdosing of
unspecified anesthetic

X● T41.41 Poisoning by unspecified anesthetic, accidental
(unintentional)
Poisoning by anesthetic NOS

X● T41.42 Poisoning by unspecified anesthetic,
intentional self-harm A, S 🐷

X● T41.43 Poisoning by unspecified anesthetic, assault

X● T41.44 Poisoning by unspecified anesthetic,
undetermined

CHAPTER 19 (S00-T88)

● X ● **T41.45** Adverse effect of unspecified anesthetic

● X ● **T41.46** Underdosing of unspecified anesthetics

● **T41.5** Poisoning by, adverse effect of and underdosing of therapeutic gases

  ● **T41.5X** Poisoning by, adverse effect of and underdosing of therapeutic gases

    ● **T41.5X1** Poisoning by therapeutic gases, accidental (unintentional)
         Poisoning by therapeutic gases NOS

    ● **T41.5X2** Poisoning by therapeutic gases, intentional self-harm A, S 🔖

    ● **T41.5X3** Poisoning by therapeutic gases, assault

    ● **T41.5X4** Poisoning by therapeutic gases, undetermined

    ● ● **T41.5X5** Adverse effect of therapeutic gases

    ● ● **T41.5X6** Underdosing of therapeutic gases

● **T42** Poisoning by, adverse effect of and underdosing of antiepileptic, sedative-hypnotic and antiparkinsonism drugs

  Excludes2   drug dependence and related mental and behavioral disorders due to psychoactive substance use (F10.--F19.-)

  The appropriate 7th character is to be added to each code from category T42

A	initial encounter
D	subsequent encounter
S	sequela

● **T42.0** Poisoning by, adverse effect of and underdosing of hydantoin derivatives

  ● **T42.0X** Poisoning by, adverse effect of and underdosing of hydantoin derivatives

    ● **T42.0X1** Poisoning by hydantoin derivatives, accidental (unintentional)
         Poisoning by hydantoin derivatives NOS

    ● **T42.0X2** Poisoning by hydantoin derivatives, intentional self-harm A, S 🔖

    ● **T42.0X3** Poisoning by hydantoin derivatives, assault

    ● **T42.0X4** Poisoning by hydantoin derivatives, undetermined

    ● ● **T42.0X5** Adverse effect of hydantoin derivatives

    ● ● **T42.0X6** Underdosing of hydantoin derivatives

● **T42.1** Poisoning by, adverse effect of and underdosing of iminostilbenes
     Poisoning by, adverse effect of and underdosing of carbamazepine

  ● **T42.1X** Poisoning by, adverse effect of and underdosing of iminostilbenes

    ● **T42.1X1** Poisoning by iminostilbenes, accidental (unintentional)
         Poisoning by iminostilbenes NOS

    ● **T42.1X2** Poisoning by iminostilbenes, intentional self-harm A, S 🔖

    ● **T42.1X3** Poisoning by iminostilbenes, assault

    ● **T42.1X4** Poisoning by iminostilbenes, undetermined

    ● ● **T42.1X5** Adverse effect of iminostilbenes

    ● ● **T42.1X6** Underdosing of iminostilbenes

● **T42.2** Poisoning by, adverse effect of and underdosing of succinimides and oxazolidinediones

  ● **T42.2X** Poisoning by, adverse effect of and underdosing of succinimides and oxazolidinediones

    ● **T42.2X1** Poisoning by succinimides and oxazolidinediones, accidental (unintentional)
         Poisoning by succinimides and oxazolidinediones NOS

    ● **T42.2X2** Poisoning by succinimides and oxazolidinediones, intentional self-harm A, S 🔖

    ● **T42.2X3** Poisoning by succinimides and oxazolidinediones, assault

    ● **T42.2X4** Poisoning by succinimides and oxazolidinediones, undetermined

    ● ● **T42.2X5** Adverse effect of succinimides and oxazolidinediones

    ● ● **T42.2X6** Underdosing of succinimides and oxazolidinediones

● **T42.3** Poisoning by, adverse effect of and underdosing of barbiturates

  Excludes1   poisoning by, adverse effect of and underdosing of thiobarbiturates (T41.1-)

  ● **T42.3X** Poisoning by, adverse effect of and underdosing of barbiturates

    ● **T42.3X1** Poisoning by barbiturates, accidental (unintentional)
         Poisoning by barbiturates NOS

    ● **T42.3X2** Poisoning by barbiturates, intentional self-harm A, S 🔖

    ● **T42.3X3** Poisoning by barbiturates, assault

    ● **T42.3X4** Poisoning by barbiturates, undetermined

    ● ● **T42.3X5** Adverse effect of barbiturates

    ● ● **T42.3X6** Underdosing of barbiturates

● **T42.4** Poisoning by, adverse effect of and underdosing of benzodiazepines

  ● **T42.4X** Poisoning by, adverse effect of and underdosing of benzodiazepines

    ● **T42.4X1** Poisoning by benzodiazepines, accidental (unintentional)
         Poisoning by benzodiazepines NOS

    ● **T42.4X2** Poisoning by benzodiazepines, intentional self-harm A, S 🔖

    ● **T42.4X3** Poisoning by benzodiazepines, assault

    ● **T42.4X4** Poisoning by benzodiazepines, undetermined

    ● ● **T42.4X5** Adverse effect of benzodiazepines

    ● ● **T42.4X6** Underdosing of benzodiazepines

● **T42.5** Poisoning by, adverse effect of and underdosing of mixed antiepileptics

  ● **T42.5X** Poisoning by, adverse effect of and underdosing of antiepileptics

    ● **T42.5X1** Poisoning by mixed antiepileptics, accidental (unintentional)
         Poisoning by mixed antiepileptics NOS

    ● **T42.5X2** Poisoning by mixed antiepileptics, intentional self-harm A, S 🔖

    ● **T42.5X3** Poisoning by mixed antiepileptics, assault

    ● **T42.5X4** Poisoning by mixed antiepileptics, undetermined

    ● ● **T42.5X5** Adverse effect of mixed antiepileptics

    ● ● **T42.5X6** Underdosing of mixed antiepileptics

▶ New   ⇒ Revised   ~~deleted~~ Deleted   Excludes 1   Excludes 2   Includes   Use additional   Code first   Code also   Key words

OGCR Official Guidelines   ● Unacceptable Principal Diagnosis   X Assign placeholder X   ● Use Additional Character(s)   ▶ Manifestation Code   **Coding Clinic**

● **T42.6** Poisoning by, adverse effect of and underdosing of other antiepileptic and sedative-hypnotic drugs
  Poisoning by, adverse effect of and underdosing of methaqualone
  Poisoning by, adverse effect of and underdosing of valproic acid
  Excludes1   poisoning by, adverse effect of and underdosing of carbamazepine (T42.1-)

● **T42.6X** Poisoning by, adverse effect of and underdosing of other antiepileptic and sedative-hypnotic drugs
  ● **T42.6X1** Poisoning by other antiepileptic and sedative-hypnotic drugs, accidental (unintentional)
    Poisoning by other antiepileptic and sedative-hypnotic drugs NOS
  ● **T42.6X2** Poisoning by other antiepileptic and sedative-hypnotic drugs, intentional self-harm A, S 🔶
  ● **T42.6X3** Poisoning by other antiepileptic and sedative-hypnotic drugs, assault
  ● **T42.6X4** Poisoning by other antiepileptic and sedative-hypnotic drugs, undetermined
  ●● **T42.6X5** Adverse effect of other antiepileptic and sedative-hypnotic drugs
  ●● **T42.6X6** Underdosing of other antiepileptic and sedative-hypnotic drugs

● **T42.7** Poisoning by, adverse effect of and underdosing of unspecified antiepileptic and sedative-hypnotic drugs
  X● **T42.71** Poisoning by unspecified antiepileptic and sedative-hypnotic drugs, accidental (unintentional)
    Poisoning by antiepileptic and sedative-hypnotic drugs NOS
  X● **T42.72** Poisoning by unspecified antiepileptic and sedative-hypnotic drugs, intentional self-harm A, S 🔶
  X● **T42.73** Poisoning by unspecified antiepileptic and sedative-hypnotic drugs, assault
  X● **T42.74** Poisoning by unspecified antiepileptic and sedative-hypnotic drugs, undetermined
  ●X● **T42.75** Adverse effect of unspecified antiepileptic and sedative-hypnotic drugs
  ●X● **T42.76** Underdosing of unspecified antiepileptic and sedative-hypnotic drugs

● **T42.8** Poisoning by, adverse effect of and underdosing of antiparkinsonism drugs and other central muscle-tone depressants
  Poisoning by, adverse effect of and underdosing of amantadine
  ● **T42.8X** Poisoning by, adverse effect of and underdosing of antiparkinsonism drugs and other central muscle-tone depressants
    ● **T42.8X1** Poisoning by antiparkinsonism drugs and other central muscle-tone depressants, accidental (unintentional)
      Poisoning by antiparkinsonism drugs and other central muscle-tone depressants NOS
    ● **T42.8X2** Poisoning by antiparkinsonism drugs and other central muscle-tone depressants, intentional self-harm A, S 🔶
    ● **T42.8X3** Poisoning by antiparkinsonism drugs and other central muscle-tone depressants, assault
    ● **T42.8X4** Poisoning by antiparkinsonism drugs and other central muscle-tone depressants, undetermined

  ●● **T42.8X5** Adverse effect of antiparkinsonism drugs and other central muscle-tone depressants
  ●● **T42.8X6** Underdosing of antiparkinsonism drugs and other central muscle-tone depressants

● **T43** Poisoning by, adverse effect of and underdosing of psychotropic drugs, not elsewhere classified
  Excludes1   appetite depressants (T50.5-)
    barbiturates (T42.3-)
    benzodiazepines (T42.4-)
    methaqualone (T42.6-)
    psychodysleptics [hallucinogens] (T40.7-T40.9-)
  Excludes2   drug dependence and related mental and behavioral disorders due to psychoactive substance use (F10.--F19.-)

  The appropriate 7th character is to be added to each code from category T43

A	initial encounter
D	subsequent encounter
S	sequela

  ● **T43.0** Poisoning by, adverse effect of and underdosing of tricyclic and tetracyclic antidepressants
    ● **T43.01** Poisoning by, adverse effect of and underdosing of tricyclic antidepressants
      ● **T43.011** Poisoning by tricyclic antidepressants, accidental (unintentional)
        Poisoning by tricyclic antidepressants NOS
      ● **T43.012** Poisoning by tricyclic antidepressants, intentional self-harm A, S 🔶
      ● **T43.013** Poisoning by tricyclic antidepressants, assault
      ● **T43.014** Poisoning by tricyclic antidepressants, undetermined
      ●● **T43.015** Adverse effect of tricyclic antidepressants
      ●● **T43.016** Underdosing of tricyclic antidepressants
    ● **T43.02** Poisoning by, adverse effect of and underdosing of tetracyclic antidepressants
      ● **T43.021** Poisoning by tetracyclic antidepressants, accidental (unintentional)
        Poisoning by tetracyclic antidepressants NOS
      ● **T43.022** Poisoning by tetracyclic antidepressants, intentional self-harm A, S 🔶
      ● **T43.023** Poisoning by tetracyclic antidepressants, assault
      ● **T43.024** Poisoning by tetracyclic antidepressants, undetermined
      ●● **T43.025** Adverse effect of tetracyclic antidepressants
      ●● **T43.026** Underdosing of tetracyclic antidepressants

  ● **T43.1** Poisoning by, adverse effect of and underdosing of monoamine-oxidase-inhibitor antidepressants
    ● **T43.1X** Poisoning by, adverse effect of and underdosing of monoamine-oxidase-inhibitor antidepressants
      ● **T43.1X1** Poisoning by monoamine-oxidase-inhibitor antidepressants, accidental (unintentional)
        Poisoning by monoamine-oxidase-inhibitor antidepressants NOS
      ● **T43.1X2** Poisoning by monoamine-oxidase-inhibitor antidepressants, intentional self-harm A, S 🔶

N Newborn Age: 0   P Pediatric Age: 0–17   M Maternity DX: 9–64   A Adult Age: 15–124   ♀ Females Only   ♂ Males Only
Complication\Comorbidity   Major C\C   (Ex) CC/MCC Exclusions   Hospital-Acquired Condition   Hierarchical Condition Category   1469

CHAPTER 19 (S00-T88)

● T43.1X3 Poisoning by monoamine-oxidase-inhibitor antidepressants, assault
● T43.1X4 Poisoning by monoamine-oxidase-inhibitor antidepressants, undetermined
●● T43.1X5 Adverse effect of monoamine-oxidase-inhibitor antidepressants
●● T43.1X6 Underdosing of monoamine-oxidase-inhibitor antidepressants
● T43.2 Poisoning by, adverse effect of and underdosing of other and unspecified antidepressants
　● T43.20 Poisoning by, adverse effect of and underdosing of unspecified antidepressants
　　● T43.201 Poisoning by unspecified antidepressants, accidental (unintentional)
　　　Poisoning by antidepressants NOS
　　● T43.202 Poisoning by unspecified antidepressants, intentional self-harm A, S 🞔
　　● T43.203 Poisoning by unspecified antidepressants, assault
　　● T43.204 Poisoning by unspecified antidepressants, undetermined
　　●● T43.205 Adverse effect of unspecified antidepressants
　　　Antidepressant discontinuation syndrome
　　●● T43.206 Underdosing of unspecified antidepressants
　● T43.21 Poisoning by, adverse effect of and underdosing of selective serotonin and norepinephrine reuptake inhibitors
　　Poisoning by, adverse effect of and underdosing of SSNRI antidepressants
　　● T43.211 Poisoning by selective serotonin and norepinephrine reuptake inhibitors, accidental (unintentional)
　　● T43.212 Poisoning by selective serotonin and norepinephrine reuptake inhibitors, intentional self-harm A, S 🞔
　　● T43.213 Poisoning by selective serotonin and norepinephrine reuptake inhibitors, assault
　　● T43.214 Poisoning by selective serotonin and norepinephrine reuptake inhibitors, undetermined
　　●● T43.215 Adverse effect of selective serotonin and norepinephrine reuptake inhibitors
　　●● T43.216 Underdosing of selective serotonin and norepinephrine reuptake inhibitors
　● T43.22 Poisoning by, adverse effect of and underdosing of selective serotonin reuptake inhibitors
　　Poisoning by, adverse effect of and underdosing of SSRI antidepressants
　　● T43.221 Poisoning by selective serotonin reuptake inhibitors, accidental (unintentional)
　　● T43.222 Poisoning by selective serotonin reuptake inhibitors, intentional self-harm A, S 🞔
　　● T43.223 Poisoning by selective serotonin reuptake inhibitors, assault
　　● T43.224 Poisoning by selective serotonin reuptake inhibitors, undetermined
　　●● T43.225 Adverse effect of selective serotonin reuptake inhibitors
　　●● T43.226 Underdosing of selective serotonin reuptake inhibitors

● T43.29 Poisoning by, adverse effect of and underdosing of other antidepressants
　● T43.291 Poisoning by other antidepressants, accidental (unintentional)
　　Poisoning by other antidepressants NOS
　● T43.292 Poisoning by other antidepressants, intentional self-harm A, S 🞔
　● T43.293 Poisoning by other antidepressants, assault
　● T43.294 Poisoning by other antidepressants, undetermined
　●● T43.295 Adverse effect of other antidepressants
　●● T43.296 Underdosing of other antidepressants
● T43.3 Poisoning by, adverse effect of and underdosing of phenothiazine antipsychotics and neuroleptics
　● T43.3X Poisoning by, adverse effect of and underdosing of phenothiazine antipsychotics and neuroleptics
　　● T43.3X1 Poisoning by phenothiazine antipsychotics and neuroleptics, accidental (unintentional)
　　　Poisoning by phenothiazine antipsychotics and neuroleptics NOS
　　● T43.3X2 Poisoning by phenothiazine antipsychotics and neuroleptics, intentional self-harm A, S 🞔
　　● T43.3X3 Poisoning by phenothiazine antipsychotics and neuroleptics, assault
　　● T43.3X4 Poisoning by phenothiazine antipsychotics and neuroleptics, undetermined
　　●● T43.3X5 Adverse effect of phenothiazine antipsychotics and neuroleptics
　　●● T43.3X6 Underdosing of phenothiazine antipsychotics and neuroleptics
● T43.4 Poisoning by, adverse effect of and underdosing of butyrophenone and thiothixene neuroleptics
　● T43.4X Poisoning by, adverse effect of and underdosing of butyrophenone and thiothixene neuroleptics
　　● T43.4X1 Poisoning by butyrophenone and thiothixene neuroleptics, accidental (unintentional)
　　　Poisoning by butyrophenone and thiothixene neuroleptics NOS
　　● T43.4X2 Poisoning by butyrophenone and thiothixene neuroleptics, intentional self-harm A, S 🞔
　　● T43.4X3 Poisoning by butyrophenone and thiothixene neuroleptics, assault
　　● T43.4X4 Poisoning by butyrophenone and thiothixene neuroleptics, undetermined
　　●● T43.4X5 Adverse effect of butyrophenone and thiothixene neuroleptics
　　●● T43.4X6 Underdosing of butyrophenone and thiothixene neuroleptics

● T43.5   **Poisoning by, adverse effect of and underdosing of other and unspecified antipsychotics and neuroleptics**

     Excludes1   poisoning by, adverse effect of and underdosing of rauwolfia (T46.5-)

   ● T43.50   **Poisoning by, adverse effect of and underdosing of unspecified antipsychotics and neuroleptics**

     ● T43.501   **Poisoning by unspecified antipsychotics and neuroleptics, accidental (unintentional)**
       Poisoning by antipsychotics and neuroleptics NOS

     ● T43.502   **Poisoning by unspecified antipsychotics and neuroleptics, intentional self-harm** A, S 🝆

     ● T43.503   **Poisoning by unspecified antipsychotics and neuroleptics, assault**

     ● T43.504   **Poisoning by unspecified antipsychotics and neuroleptics, undetermined**

     ●● T43.505   **Adverse effect of unspecified antipsychotics and neuroleptics**

     ●● T43.506   **Underdosing of unspecified antipsychotics and neuroleptics**

   ● T43.59   **Poisoning by, adverse effect of and underdosing of other antipsychotics and neuroleptics**

     ● T43.591   **Poisoning by other antipsychotics and neuroleptics, accidental (unintentional)**
       Poisoning by other antipsychotics and neuroleptics NOS

     ● T43.592   **Poisoning by other antipsychotics and neuroleptics, intentional self-harm** A, S 🝆
       Coding Clinic: 2017, Q1, P40

     ● T43.593   **Poisoning by other antipsychotics and neuroleptics, assault**

     ● T43.594   **Poisoning by other antipsychotics and neuroleptics, undetermined**

     ●● T43.595   **Adverse effect of other antipsychotics and neuroleptics**

     ●● T43.596   **Underdosing of other antipsychotics and neuroleptics**

● T43.6   **Poisoning by, adverse effect of and underdosing of psychostimulants**

     Excludes1   poisoning by, adverse effect of and underdosing of cocaine (T40.5-)

   ● T43.60   **Poisoning by, adverse effect of and underdosing of unspecified psychostimulant**

     ● T43.601   **Poisoning by unspecified psychostimulants, accidental (unintentional)**
       Poisoning by psychostimulants NOS

     ● T43.602   **Poisoning by unspecified psychostimulants, intentional self-harm** A, S 🝆

     ● T43.603   **Poisoning by unspecified psychostimulants, assault**

     ● T43.604   **Poisoning by unspecified psychostimulants, undetermined**

     ●● T43.605   **Adverse effect of unspecified psychostimulants**

     ●● T43.606   **Underdosing of unspecified psychostimulants**

   ● T43.61   **Poisoning by, adverse effect of and underdosing of caffeine**

     ● T43.611   **Poisoning by caffeine, accidental (unintentional)**
       Poisoning by caffeine NOS

     ● T43.612   **Poisoning by caffeine, intentional self-harm** A, S 🝆

     ● T43.613   **Poisoning by caffeine, assault**

     ● T43.614   **Poisoning by caffeine, undetermined**

     ●● T43.615   **Adverse effect of caffeine**

     ●● T43.616   **Underdosing of caffeine**

   ● T43.62   **Poisoning by, adverse effect of and underdosing of amphetamines**
     Poisoning by, adverse effect of and underdosing of methamphetamines

     ● T43.621   **Poisoning by amphetamines, accidental (unintentional)**
       Poisoning by amphetamines NOS

     ● T43.622   **Poisoning by amphetamines, intentional self-harm** A, S 🝆

     ● T43.623   **Poisoning by amphetamines, assault**

     ● T43.624   **Poisoning by amphetamines, undetermined**

     ●● T43.625   **Adverse effect of amphetamines**

     ●● T43.626   **Underdosing of amphetamines**

   ● T43.63   **Poisoning by, adverse effect of and underdosing of methylphenidate**

     ● T43.631   **Poisoning by methylphenidate, accidental (unintentional)**
       Poisoning by methylphenidate NOS

     ● T43.632   **Poisoning by methylphenidate, intentional self-harm** A, S 🝆

     ● T43.633   **Poisoning by methylphenidate, assault**

     ● T43.634   **Poisoning by methylphenidate, undetermined**

     ●● T43.635   **Adverse effect of methylphenidate**

     ●● T43.636   **Underdosing of methylphenidate**

   ● T43.64   **Poisoning by ecstasy**
     Poisoning by MDMA
     Poisoning by 3,4-methylenedioxymethamphetamine

     ● T43.641   **Poisoning by ecstasy, accidental (unintentional)**
       Poisoning by ecstasy NOS
       Coding Clinic: 2018, Q4, P31

     ● T43.642   **Poisoning by ecstasy, intentional self-harm** A, S 🝆

     ● T43.643   **Poisoning by ecstasy, assault**

     ● T43.644   **Poisoning by ecstasy, undetermined**

   ● T43.69   **Poisoning by, adverse effect of and underdosing of other psychostimulants**

     ● T43.691   **Poisoning by other psychostimulants, accidental (unintentional)**
       Poisoning by other psychostimulants NOS

     ● T43.692   **Poisoning by other psychostimulants, intentional self-harm** A, S 🝆

     ● T43.693   **Poisoning by other psychostimulants, assault**

     ● T43.694   **Poisoning by other psychostimulants, undetermined**

     ●● T43.695   **Adverse effect of other psychostimulants**

     ●● T43.696   **Underdosing of other psychostimulants**

● T43.8   **Poisoning by, adverse effect of and underdosing of other psychotropic drugs**

   ● T43.8X   **Poisoning by, adverse effect of and underdosing of other psychotropic drugs**

     ● T43.8X1   **Poisoning by other psychotropic drugs, accidental (unintentional)**
       Poisoning by other psychotropic drugs NOS

     ● T43.8X2   **Poisoning by other psychotropic drugs, intentional self-harm** A, S 🝆

N   Newborn Age: 0   **P**   Pediatric Age: 0–17   **M**   Maternity DX: 9–64   **A**   Adult Age: 15–124   ♀   Females Only   ♂   Males Only

🝆   Complication\Comorbidity   🝆   Major C\C   (Ex)   CC/MCC Exclusions   🝆   Hospital-Acquired Condition   🝆   Hierarchical Condition Category

● T43.8X3 Poisoning by other psychotropic drugs, assault

● T43.8X4 Poisoning by other psychotropic drugs, undetermined

●● T43.8X5 Adverse effect of other psychotropic drugs

●● T43.8X6 Underdosing of other psychotropic drugs

● T43.9 Poisoning by, adverse effect of and underdosing of unspecified psychotropic drug

X● T43.91 Poisoning by unspecified psychotropic drug, accidental (unintentional)
　　　　　Poisoning by psychotropic drug NOS

X● T43.92 Poisoning by unspecified psychotropic drug, intentional self-harm A, S 🪙

X● T43.93 Poisoning by unspecified psychotropic drug, assault

X● T43.94 Poisoning by unspecified psychotropic drug, undetermined

●X● T43.95 Adverse effect of unspecified psychotropic drug

●X● T43.96 Underdosing of unspecified psychotropic drug

● T44 Poisoning by, adverse effect of and underdosing of drugs primarily affecting the autonomic nervous system

The appropriate 7th character is to be added to each code from category T44

A	initial encounter
D	subsequent encounter
S	sequela

● T44.0 Poisoning by, adverse effect of and underdosing of anticholinesterase agents

● T44.0X Poisoning by, adverse effect of and underdosing of anticholinesterase agents

● T44.0X1 Poisoning by anticholinesterase agents, accidental (unintentional)
　　　　　Poisoning by anticholinesterase agents NOS

● T44.0X2 Poisoning by anticholinesterase agents, intentional self-harm A, S 🪙

● T44.0X3 Poisoning by anticholinesterase agents, assault

● T44.0X4 Poisoning by anticholinesterase agents, undetermined

●● T44.0X5 Adverse effect of anticholinesterase agents

●● T44.0X6 Underdosing of anticholinesterase agents

● T44.1 Poisoning by, adverse effect of and underdosing of other parasympathomimetics [cholinergics]

● T44.1X Poisoning by, adverse effect of and underdosing of other parasympathomimetics [cholinergics]

● T44.1X1 Poisoning by other parasympathomimetics [cholinergics], accidental (unintentional)
　　　　　Poisoning by other parasympathomimetics [cholinergics] NOS

● T44.1X2 Poisoning by other parasympathomimetics [cholinergics], intentional self-harm A, S 🪙

● T44.1X3 Poisoning by other parasympathomimetics [cholinergics], assault

● T44.1X4 Poisoning by other parasympathomimetics [cholinergics], undetermined

●● T44.1X5 Adverse effect of other parasympathomimetics [cholinergics]

●● T44.1X6 Underdosing of other parasympathomimetics [cholinergics]

● T44.2 Poisoning by, adverse effect of and underdosing of ganglionic blocking drugs

● T44.2X Poisoning by, adverse effect of and underdosing of ganglionic blocking drugs

● T44.2X1 Poisoning by ganglionic blocking drugs, accidental (unintentional)
　　　　　Poisoning by ganglionic blocking drugs NOS

● T44.2X2 Poisoning by ganglionic blocking drugs, intentional self-harm A, S 🪙

● T44.2X3 Poisoning by ganglionic blocking drugs, assault

● T44.2X4 Poisoning by ganglionic blocking drugs, undetermined

●● T44.2X5 Adverse effect of ganglionic blocking drugs

●● T44.2X6 Underdosing of ganglionic blocking drugs

● T44.3 Poisoning by, adverse effect of and underdosing of other parasympatholytics [anticholinergics and antimuscarinics] and spasmolytics
　　　　Poisoning by, adverse effect of and underdosing of papaverine

● T44.3X Poisoning by, adverse effect of and underdosing of other parasympatholytics [anticholinergics and antimuscarinics] and spasmolytics

● T44.3X1 Poisoning by other parasympatholytics [anticholinergics and antimuscarinics] and spasmolytics, accidental (unintentional)
　　　　　Poisoning by other parasympatholytics [anticholinergics and antimuscarinics] and spasmolytics NOS

● T44.3X2 Poisoning by other parasympatholytics [anticholinergics and antimuscarinics] and spasmolytics, intentional self-harm A, S 🪙

● T44.3X3 Poisoning by other parasympatholytics [anticholinergics and antimuscarinics] and spasmolytics, assault

● T44.3X4 Poisoning by other parasympatholytics [anticholinergics and antimuscarinics] and spasmolytics, undetermined

●● T44.3X5 Adverse effect of other parasympatholytics [anticholinergics and antimuscarinics] and spasmolytics

●● T44.3X6 Underdosing of other parasympatholytics [anticholinergics and antimuscarinics] and spasmolytics

▶ New　　⟹ Revised　　d̶e̶l̶e̶t̶e̶d̶ Deleted　　Excludes 1　　Excludes 2　　Includes　　Use additional　　Code first　　Code also　　Key words

OGCR Official Guidelines　● Unacceptable Principal Diagnosis　X Assign placeholder X　● Use Additional Character(s)　▷ Manifestation Code　Coding Clinic

● **T44.4 Poisoning by, adverse effect of and underdosing of predominantly alpha-adrenoreceptor agonists**
  Poisoning by, adverse effect of and underdosing of metaraminol

  ● **T44.4X Poisoning by, adverse effect of and underdosing of predominantly alpha-adrenoreceptor agonists**

    ● **T44.4X1 Poisoning by predominantly alpha-adrenoreceptor agonists, accidental (unintentional)**
      Poisoning by predominantly alpha-adrenoreceptor agonists NOS

    ● **T44.4X2 Poisoning by predominantly alpha-adrenoreceptor agonists, intentional self-harm A, S** 🔒

    ● **T44.4X3 Poisoning by predominantly alpha-adrenoreceptor agonists, assault**

    ● **T44.4X4 Poisoning by predominantly alpha-adrenoreceptor agonists, undetermined**

    ●● **T44.4X5 Adverse effect of predominantly alpha-adrenoreceptor agonists**

    ●● **T44.4X6 Underdosing of predominantly alpha-adrenoreceptor agonists**

● **T44.5 Poisoning by, adverse effect of and underdosing of predominantly beta-adrenoreceptor agonists**
  Excludes1 poisoning by, adverse effect of and underdosing of beta-adrenoreceptor agonists used in asthma therapy (T48.6-)

  ● **T44.5X Poisoning by, adverse effect of and underdosing of predominantly beta-adrenoreceptor agonists**

    ● **T44.5X1 Poisoning by predominantly beta-adrenoreceptor agonists, accidental (unintentional)**
      Poisoning by predominantly beta-adrenoreceptor agonists NOS

    ● **T44.5X2 Poisoning by predominantly beta-adrenoreceptor agonists, intentional self-harm A, S** 🔒

    ● **T44.5X3 Poisoning by predominantly beta-adrenoreceptor agonists, assault**

    ● **T44.5X4 Poisoning by predominantly beta-adrenoreceptor agonists, undetermined**

    ●● **T44.5X5 Adverse effect of predominantly beta-adrenoreceptor agonists**

    ●● **T44.5X6 Underdosing of predominantly beta-adrenoreceptor agonists**

● **T44.6 Poisoning by, adverse effect of and underdosing of alpha-adrenoreceptor antagonists**
  Excludes1 poisoning by, adverse effect of and underdosing of ergot alkaloids (T48.0)

  ● **T44.6X Poisoning by, adverse effect of and underdosing of alpha-adrenoreceptor antagonists**

    ● **T44.6X1 Poisoning by alpha-adrenoreceptor antagonists, accidental (unintentional)**
      Poisoning by alpha-adrenoreceptor antagonists NOS

    ● **T44.6X2 Poisoning by alpha-adrenoreceptor antagonists, intentional self-harm A, S** 🔒

    ● **T44.6X3 Poisoning by alpha-adrenoreceptor antagonists, assault**

    ● **T44.6X4 Poisoning by alpha-adrenoreceptor antagonists, undetermined**

    ●● **T44.6X5 Adverse effect of alpha-adrenoreceptor antagonists**

    ●● **T44.6X6 Underdosing of alpha-adrenoreceptor antagonists**

● **T44.7 Poisoning by, adverse effect of and underdosing of beta-adrenoreceptor antagonists**

  ● **T44.7X Poisoning by, adverse effect of and underdosing of beta-adrenoreceptor antagonists**

    ● **T44.7X1 Poisoning by beta-adrenoreceptor antagonists, accidental (unintentional)**
      Poisoning by beta-adrenoreceptor antagonists NOS

    ● **T44.7X2 Poisoning by beta-adrenoreceptor antagonists, intentional self-harm A, S** 🔒

    ● **T44.7X3 Poisoning by beta-adrenoreceptor antagonists, assault**

    ● **T44.7X4 Poisoning by beta-adrenoreceptor antagonists, undetermined**

    ●● **T44.7X5 Adverse effect of beta-adrenoreceptor antagonists**

    ●● **T44.7X6 Underdosing of beta-adrenoreceptor antagonists**

● **T44.8 Poisoning by, adverse effect of and underdosing of centrally-acting and adrenergic-neuron-blocking agents**
  ~~Excludes1 poisoning by, adverse effect of and underdosing of clonidine (T46.5)~~
  ~~poisoning by, adverse effect of and underdosing of guanethidine (T46.5)~~

  ▶ **Excludes2** poisoning by, adverse effect of and underdosing of clonidine (T46.5)
  ▶ poisoning by, adverse effect of and underdosing of guanethidine (T46.5)

  ● **T44.8X Poisoning by, adverse effect of and underdosing of centrally-acting and adrenergic-neuron-blocking agents**

    ● **T44.8X1 Poisoning by centrally-acting and adrenergic-neuron-blocking agents, accidental (unintentional)**
      Poisoning by centrally-acting and adrenergic-neuron-blocking agents NOS

    ● **T44.8X2 Poisoning by centrally-acting and adrenergic-neuron-blocking agents, intentional self-harm A, S** 🔒

    ● **T44.8X3 Poisoning by centrally-acting and adrenergic-neuron-blocking agents, assault**

    ● **T44.8X4 Poisoning by centrally-acting and adrenergic-neuron-blocking agents, undetermined**

    ●● **T44.8X5 Adverse effect of centrally-acting and adrenergic-neuron-blocking agents**

    ●● **T44.8X6 Underdosing of centrally-acting and adrenergic-neuron-blocking agents**

● **T44.9 Poisoning by, adverse effect of and underdosing of other and unspecified drugs primarily affecting the autonomic nervous system**
  Poisoning by, adverse effect of and underdosing of drug stimulating both alpha and beta adrenoreceptors

  ● **T44.90 Poisoning by, adverse effect of and underdosing of unspecified drugs primarily affecting the autonomic nervous system**

    ● **T44.901 Poisoning by unspecified drugs primarily affecting the autonomic nervous system, accidental (unintentional)**
      Poisoning by unspecified drugs primarily affecting the autonomic nervous system NOS

    ● **T44.902 Poisoning by unspecified drugs primarily affecting the autonomic nervous system, intentional self-harm A, S** 🔒

    ● **T44.903 Poisoning by unspecified drugs primarily affecting the autonomic nervous system, assault**

N Newborn Age: 0 **P** Pediatric Age: 0–17 **M** Maternity DX: 9–64 **A** Adult Age: 15–124 ♀ Females Only ♂ Males Only
🔒 Complication\Comorbidity 🔒 Major C\C (Ex) CC/MCC Exclusions 🔒 Hospital-Acquired Condition 🔒 Hierarchical Condition Category

CHAPTER 19 (S00-T88)

1473

CHAPTER 19 (S00-T88)

● T44.904 Poisoning by unspecified drugs primarily affecting the autonomic nervous system, undetermined

●● T44.905 Adverse effect of unspecified drugs primarily affecting the autonomic nervous system

●● T44.906 Underdosing of unspecified drugs primarily affecting the autonomic nervous system

● T44.99 Poisoning by, adverse effect of and underdosing of other drugs primarily affecting the autonomic nervous system

● T44.991 Poisoning by other drug primarily affecting the autonomic nervous system, accidental (unintentional)
Poisoning by other drugs primarily affecting the autonomic nervous system NOS

● T44.992 Poisoning by other drug primarily affecting the autonomic nervous system, intentional self-harm A, S 🔖

● T44.993 Poisoning by other drug primarily affecting the autonomic nervous system, assault

● T44.994 Poisoning by other drug primarily affecting the autonomic nervous system, undetermined

●● T44.995 Adverse effect of other drug primarily affecting the autonomic nervous system

●● T44.996 Underdosing of other drug primarily affecting the autonomic nervous system

● T45 Poisoning by, adverse effect of and underdosing of primarily systemic and hematological agents, not elsewhere classified

The appropriate 7th character is to be added to each code from category T45

A	initial encounter
D	subsequent encounter
S	sequela

● T45.0 Poisoning by, adverse effect of and underdosing of antiallergic and antiemetic drugs

Excludes1   poisoning by, adverse effect of and underdosing of phenothiazine-based neuroleptics (T43.3)

● T45.0X Poisoning by, adverse effect of and underdosing of antiallergic and antiemetic drugs

● T45.0X1 Poisoning by antiallergic and antiemetic drugs, accidental (unintentional)
Poisoning by antiallergic and antiemetic drugs NOS

● T45.0X2 Poisoning by antiallergic and antiemetic drugs, intentional self-harm A, S 🔖

● T45.0X3 Poisoning by antiallergic and antiemetic drugs, assault

● T45.0X4 Poisoning by antiallergic and antiemetic drugs, undetermined

●● T45.0X5 Adverse effect of antiallergic and antiemetic drugs

●● T45.0X6 Underdosing of antiallergic and antiemetic drugs

● T45.1 Poisoning by, adverse effect of and underdosing of antineoplastic and immunosuppressive drugs

Excludes1   poisoning by, adverse effect of and underdosing of tamoxifen (T38.6)

● T45.1X Poisoning by, adverse effect of and underdosing of antineoplastic and immunosuppressive drugs

● T45.1X1 Poisoning by antineoplastic and immunosuppressive drugs, accidental (unintentional)
Poisoning by antineoplastic and immunosuppressive drugs NOS

● T45.1X2 Poisoning by antineoplastic and immunosuppressive drugs, intentional self-harm A, S 🔖

● T45.1X3 Poisoning by antineoplastic and immunosuppressive drugs, assault

● T45.1X4 Poisoning by antineoplastic and immunosuppressive drugs, undetermined

●● T45.1X5 Adverse effect of antineoplastic and immunosuppressive drugs
Coding Clinic: 2019, Q2, P25, 28; Q1, P17, 21

●● T45.1X6 Underdosing of antineoplastic and immunosuppressive drugs

● T45.2 Poisoning by, adverse effect of and underdosing of vitamins

Excludes2   poisoning by, adverse effect of and underdosing of nicotinic acid (derivatives) (T46.7)
poisoning by, adverse effect of and underdosing of iron (T45.4)
poisoning by, adverse effect of and underdosing of vitamin K (T45.7)

● T45.2X Poisoning by, adverse effect of and underdosing of vitamins

● T45.2X1 Poisoning by vitamins, accidental (unintentional)
Poisoning by vitamins NOS

● T45.2X2 Poisoning by vitamins, intentional self-harm A, S 🔖

● T45.2X3 Poisoning by vitamins, assault

● T45.2X4 Poisoning by vitamins, undetermined

●● T45.2X5 Adverse effect of vitamins

●● T45.2X6 Underdosing of vitamins

Excludes1   vitamin deficiencies (E50-E56)

● T45.3 Poisoning by, adverse effect of and underdosing of enzymes

● T45.3X Poisoning by, adverse effect of and underdosing of enzymes

● T45.3X1 Poisoning by enzymes, accidental (unintentional)
Poisoning by enzymes NOS

● T45.3X2 Poisoning by enzymes, intentional self-harm A, S 🔖

● T45.3X3 Poisoning by enzymes, assault

● T45.3X4 Poisoning by enzymes, undetermined

●● T45.3X5 Adverse effect of enzymes

●● T45.3X6 Underdosing of enzymes

● **T45.4**   **Poisoning by, adverse effect of and underdosing of iron and its compounds**

　　● **T45.4X**   Poisoning by, adverse effect of and underdosing of iron and its compounds

　　　　● **T45.4X1**   Poisoning by iron and its compounds, accidental (unintentional)
　　　　　　　　Poisoning by iron and its compounds NOS

　　　　● **T45.4X2**   Poisoning by iron and its compounds, intentional self-harm A, S 🏷

　　　　● **T45.4X3**   Poisoning by iron and its compounds, assault

　　　　● **T45.4X4**   Poisoning by iron and its compounds, undetermined

　　　　●● **T45.4X5**   Adverse effect of iron and its compounds

　　　　●● **T45.4X6**   Underdosing of iron and its compounds
　　　　　　　　Excludes1   iron deficiency (E61.1)

● **T45.5**   **Poisoning by, adverse effect of and underdosing of anticoagulants and antithrombotic drugs**

　　● **T45.51**   Poisoning by, adverse effect of and underdosing of anticoagulants

　　　　● **T45.511**   Poisoning by anticoagulants, accidental (unintentional)
　　　　　　　　Poisoning by anticoagulants NOS

　　　　● **T45.512**   Poisoning by anticoagulants, intentional self-harm A, S 🏷

　　　　● **T45.513**   Poisoning by anticoagulants, assault

　　　　● **T45.514**   Poisoning by anticoagulants, undetermined

　　　　●● **T45.515**   Adverse effect of anticoagulants
　　　　　　　　Coding Clinic: 2021, Q1, P5; 2016, Q1, P14; 2013, Q2, P35

　　　　●● **T45.516**   Underdosing of anticoagulants

　　● **T45.52**   Poisoning by, adverse effect of and underdosing of antithrombotic drugs
　　　　　Poisoning by, adverse effect of and underdosing of antiplatelet drugs

　　　　Excludes2   poisoning by, adverse effect of and underdosing of aspirin (T39.01-)
　　　　　　　　poisoning by, adverse effect of and underdosing of acetylsalicylic acid (T39.01-)

　　　　● **T45.521**   Poisoning by antithrombotic drugs, accidental (unintentional)
　　　　　　　　Poisoning by antithrombotic drug NOS

　　　　● **T45.522**   Poisoning by antithrombotic drugs, intentional self-harm A, S 🏷

　　　　● **T45.523**   Poisoning by antithrombotic drugs, assault

　　　　● **T45.524**   Poisoning by antithrombotic drugs, undetermined

　　　　●● **T45.525**   Adverse effect of antithrombotic drugs
　　　　　　　　Coding Clinic: 2016, Q1, P15

　　　　●● **T45.526**   Underdosing of antithrombotic drugs

● **T45.6**   **Poisoning by, adverse effect of and underdosing of fibrinolysis-affecting drugs**

　　● **T45.60**   Poisoning by, adverse effect of and underdosing of unspecified fibrinolysis-affecting drugs

　　　　● **T45.601**   Poisoning by unspecified fibrinolysis-affecting drugs, accidental (unintentional)
　　　　　　　　Poisoning by fibrinolysis-affecting drug NOS

　　　　● **T45.602**   Poisoning by unspecified fibrinolysis-affecting drugs, intentional self-harm A, S 🏷

　　　　● **T45.603**   Poisoning by unspecified fibrinolysis-affecting drugs, assault

　　　　● **T45.604**   Poisoning by unspecified fibrinolysis-affecting drugs, undetermined

　　　　●● **T45.605**   Adverse effect of unspecified fibrinolysis-affecting drugs

　　　　●● **T45.606**   Underdosing of unspecified fibrinolysis-affecting drugs

　　● **T45.61**   Poisoning by, adverse effect of and underdosing of thrombolytic drugs

　　　　● **T45.611**   Poisoning by thrombolytic drug, accidental (unintentional)
　　　　　　　　Poisoning by thrombolytic drug NOS

　　　　● **T45.612**   Poisoning by thrombolytic drug, intentional self-harm A, S 🏷

　　　　● **T45.613**   Poisoning by thrombolytic drug, assault

　　　　● **T45.614**   Poisoning by thrombolytic drug, undetermined

　　　　●● **T45.615**   Adverse effect of thrombolytic drugs
　　　　　　　　Coding Clinic: 2017, Q2, P10

　　　　●● **T45.616**   Underdosing of thrombolytic drugs

　　● **T45.62**   Poisoning by, adverse effect of and underdosing of hemostatic drugs

　　　　● **T45.621**   Poisoning by hemostatic drug, accidental (unintentional)
　　　　　　　　Poisoning by hemostatic drug NOS

　　　　● **T45.622**   Poisoning by hemostatic drug, intentional self-harm A, S 🏷

　　　　● **T45.623**   Poisoning by hemostatic drug, assault

　　　　● **T45.624**   Poisoning by hemostatic drug, undetermined

　　　　●● **T45.625**   Adverse effect of hemostatic drug

　　　　●● **T45.626**   Underdosing of hemostatic drugs

　　● **T45.69**   Poisoning by, adverse effect of and underdosing of other fibrinolysis-affecting drugs

　　　　● **T45.691**   Poisoning by other fibrinolysis-affecting drugs, accidental (unintentional)
　　　　　　　　Poisoning by other fibrinolysis-affecting drug NOS

　　　　● **T45.692**   Poisoning by other fibrinolysis-affecting drugs, intentional self-harm A, S 🏷

　　　　● **T45.693**   Poisoning by other fibrinolysis-affecting drugs, assault

　　　　● **T45.694**   Poisoning by other fibrinolysis-affecting drugs, undetermined

　　　　●● **T45.695**   Adverse effect of other fibrinolysis-affecting drugs

　　　　●● **T45.696**   Underdosing of other fibrinolysis-affecting drugs

CHAPTER 19 (S00-T88)

N Newborn Age: 0   **P** Pediatric Age: 0–17   **M** Maternity DX: 9–64   **A** Adult Age: 15–124   ♀ Females Only   ♂ Males Only

🏷 Complication\Comorbidity   🏷 Major C\C   (Ex) CC/MCC Exclusions   🏷 Hospital-Acquired Condition   🏷 Hierarchical Condition Category

1475

● T45.7   Poisoning by, adverse effect of and underdosing
of anticoagulant antagonists, vitamin K and other
coagulants

● T45.7X   Poisoning by, adverse effect of and
underdosing of anticoagulant antagonists,
vitamin K and other coagulants

● T45.7X1   Poisoning by anticoagulant
antagonists, vitamin K and other
coagulants, accidental (unintentional)
Poisoning by anticoagulant
antagonists, vitamin K and
other coagulants NOS

● T45.7X2   Poisoning by anticoagulant
antagonists, vitamin K and other
coagulants, intentional self-harm
A, S ✿

● T45.7X3   Poisoning by anticoagulant
antagonists, vitamin K and other
coagulants, assault

● T45.7X4   Poisoning by anticoagulant
antagonists, vitamin K and other
coagulants, undetermined

●● T45.7X5   Adverse effect of anticoagulant
antagonists, vitamin K and other
coagulants

●● T45.7X6   Underdosing of anticoagulant
antagonist, vitamin K and other
coagulants
Excludes1   vitamin K deficiency
(E56.1)

● T45.8   Poisoning by, adverse effect of and underdosing of other
primarily systemic and hematological agents
Poisoning by, adverse effect of and underdosing of liver
preparations and other antianemic agents
Poisoning by, adverse effect of and underdosing of
natural blood and blood products
Poisoning by, adverse effect of and underdosing of
plasma substitute
Excludes2   poisoning by, adverse effect of and
underdosing of immunoglobulin
(T50.Z1)
poisoning by, adverse effect of and
underdosing of iron (T45.4)
transfusion reactions (T80.-)

● T45.8X   Poisoning by, adverse effect of and
underdosing of other primarily systemic and
hematological agents

● T45.8X1   Poisoning by other primarily systemic
and hematological agents, accidental
(unintentional)
Poisoning by other primarily
systemic and hematological
agents NOS

● T45.8X2   Poisoning by other primarily systemic
and hematological agents, intentional
self-harm A, S ✿

● T45.8X3   Poisoning by other primarily systemic
and hematological agents, assault

● T45.8X4   Poisoning by other primarily
systemic and hematological agents,
undetermined

●● T45.8X5   Adverse effect of other primarily
systemic and hematological agents
Coding Clinic: 2016, Q4, P42

●● T45.8X6   Underdosing of other primarily
systemic and hematological agents

● T45.9   Poisoning by, adverse effect of and underdosing of
unspecified primarily systemic and hematological agent

X● T45.91   Poisoning by unspecified primarily systemic
and hematological agent, accidental
(unintentional)
Poisoning by primarily systemic and
hematological agent NOS

X● T45.92   Poisoning by unspecified primarily systemic
and hematological agent, intentional self-harm
A, S ✿

X● T45.93   Poisoning by unspecified primarily systemic
and hematological agent, assault

X● T45.94   Poisoning by unspecified primarily systemic
and hematological agent, undetermined

●X● T45.95   Adverse effect of unspecified primarily
systemic and hematological agent

●X● T45.96   Underdosing of unspecified primarily systemic
and hematological agent

● T46   Poisoning by, adverse effect of and underdosing of agents
primarily affecting the cardiovascular system
Excludes1   poisoning by, adverse effect of and underdosing
of metaraminol (T44.4)
The appropriate 7th character is to be added to each code from
category T46

A	initial encounter
D	subsequent encounter
S	sequela

● T46.0   Poisoning by, adverse effect of and underdosing of
cardiac-stimulant glycosides and drugs of similar action

● T46.0X   Poisoning by, adverse effect of and
underdosing of cardiac-stimulant glycosides
and drugs of similar action

● T46.0X1   Poisoning by cardiac-stimulant
glycosides and drugs of similar
action, accidental (unintentional)
Poisoning by cardiac-stimulant
glycosides and drugs of similar
action NOS

● T46.0X2   Poisoning by cardiac-stimulant
glycosides and drugs of similar
action, intentional self-harm A, S ✿

● T46.0X3   Poisoning by cardiac-stimulant
glycosides and drugs of similar
action, assault

● T46.0X4   Poisoning by cardiac-stimulant
glycosides and drugs of similar
action, undetermined

●● T46.0X5   Adverse effect of cardiac-stimulant
glycosides and drugs of similar action

●● T46.0X6   Underdosing of cardiac-stimulant
glycosides and drugs of similar action

● T46.1   Poisoning by, adverse effect of and underdosing of
calcium-channel blockers

● T46.1X   Poisoning by, adverse effect of and
underdosing of calcium-channel blockers

● T46.1X1   Poisoning by calcium-channel
blockers, accidental (unintentional)
Poisoning by calcium-channel
blockers NOS

● T46.1X2   Poisoning by calcium-channel
blockers, intentional self-harm
A, S ✿

● T46.1X3   Poisoning by calcium-channel
blockers, assault

● T46.1X4   Poisoning by calcium-channel
blockers, undetermined

●● T46.1X5   Adverse effect of calcium-channel
blockers

●● T46.1X6   Underdosing of calcium-channel
blockers

● **T46.2**   **Poisoning by, adverse effect of and underdosing of other antidysrhythmic drugs, not elsewhere classified**

    Excludes1   poisoning by, adverse effect of and underdosing of beta-adrenoreceptor antagonists (T44.7-)

   ● **T46.2X**   **Poisoning by, adverse effect of and underdosing of other antidysrhythmic drugs**

     ● **T46.2X1**   **Poisoning by other antidysrhythmic drugs, accidental (unintentional)**
        Poisoning by other antidysrhythmic drugs NOS

     ● **T46.2X2**   **Poisoning by other antidysrhythmic drugs, intentional self-harm A, S** 🐞

     ● **T46.2X3**   **Poisoning by other antidysrhythmic drugs, assault**

     ● **T46.2X4**   **Poisoning by other antidysrhythmic drugs, undetermined**

     ●● **T46.2X5**   **Adverse effect of other antidysrhythmic drugs**

     ●● **T46.2X6**   **Underdosing of other antidysrhythmic drugs**

● **T46.3**   **Poisoning by, adverse effect of and underdosing of coronary vasodilators**

    Poisoning by, adverse effect of and underdosing of dipyridamole

    Excludes1   poisoning by, adverse effect of and underdosing of calcium-channel blockers (T46.1)

   ● **T46.3X**   **Poisoning by, adverse effect of and underdosing of coronary vasodilators**

     ● **T46.3X1**   **Poisoning by coronary vasodilators, accidental (unintentional)**
        Poisoning by coronary vasodilators NOS

     ● **T46.3X2**   **Poisoning by coronary vasodilators, intentional self-harm A, S** 🐞

     ● **T46.3X3**   **Poisoning by coronary vasodilators, assault**

     ● **T46.3X4**   **Poisoning by coronary vasodilators, undetermined**

     ●● **T46.3X5**   **Adverse effect of coronary vasodilators**

     ●● **T46.3X6**   **Underdosing of coronary vasodilators**

● **T46.4**   **Poisoning by, adverse effect of and underdosing of angiotensin-converting-enzyme inhibitors**

   ● **T46.4X**   **Poisoning by, adverse effect of and underdosing of angiotensin-converting-enzyme inhibitors**

     ● **T46.4X1**   **Poisoning by angiotensin-converting-enzyme inhibitors, accidental (unintentional)**
        Poisoning by angiotensin-converting-enzyme inhibitors NOS

     ● **T46.4X2**   **Poisoning by angiotensin-converting-enzyme inhibitors, intentional self-harm A, S** 🐞

     ● **T46.4X3**   **Poisoning by angiotensin-converting-enzyme inhibitors, assault**

     ● **T46.4X4**   **Poisoning by angiotensin-converting-enzyme inhibitors, undetermined**

     ●● **T46.4X5**   **Adverse effect of angiotensin-converting-enzyme inhibitors**

     ●● **T46.4X6**   **Underdosing of angiotensin-converting-enzyme inhibitors**

● **T46.5**   **Poisoning by, adverse effect of and underdosing of other antihypertensive drugs**

    Excludes2   poisoning by, adverse effect of and underdosing of beta-adrenoreceptor antagonists (T44.7)
          poisoning by, adverse effect of and underdosing of calcium-channel blockers (T46.1)
          poisoning by, adverse effect of and underdosing of diuretics (T50.0-T50.2)

   ● **T46.5X**   **Poisoning by, adverse effect of and underdosing of other antihypertensive drugs**

     ● **T46.5X1**   **Poisoning by other antihypertensive drugs, accidental (unintentional)**
        Poisoning by other antihypertensive drugs NOS

     ● **T46.5X2**   **Poisoning by other antihypertensive drugs, intentional self-harm A, S** 🐞

     ● **T46.5X3**   **Poisoning by other antihypertensive drugs, assault**

     ● **T46.5X4**   **Poisoning by other antihypertensive drugs, undetermined**

     ●● **T46.5X5**   **Adverse effect of other antihypertensive drugs**

     ●● **T46.5X6**   **Underdosing of other antihypertensive drugs**

● **T46.6**   **Poisoning by, adverse effect of and underdosing of antihyperlipidemic and antiarteriosclerotic drugs**

   ● **T46.6X**   **Poisoning by, adverse effect of and underdosing of antihyperlipidemic and antiarteriosclerotic drugs**

     ● **T46.6X1**   **Poisoning by antihyperlipidemic and antiarteriosclerotic drugs, accidental (unintentional)**
        Poisoning by antihyperlipidemic and antiarteriosclerotic drugs NOS

     ● **T46.6X2**   **Poisoning by antihyperlipidemic and antiarteriosclerotic drugs, intentional self-harm A, S** 🐞

     ● **T46.6X3**   **Poisoning by antihyperlipidemic and antiarteriosclerotic drugs, assault**

     ● **T46.6X4**   **Poisoning by antihyperlipidemic and antiarteriosclerotic drugs, undetermined**

     ●● **T46.6X5**   **Adverse effect of antihyperlipidemic and antiarteriosclerotic drugs**

     ●● **T46.6X6**   **Underdosing of antihyperlipidemic and antiarteriosclerotic drugs**

● **T46.7**   **Poisoning by, adverse effect of and underdosing of peripheral vasodilators**

    Poisoning by, adverse effect of and underdosing of nicotinic acid (derivatives)

    Excludes1   poisoning by, adverse effect of and underdosing of papaverine (T44.3)

   ● **T46.7X**   **Poisoning by, adverse effect of and underdosing of peripheral vasodilators**

     ● **T46.7X1**   **Poisoning by peripheral vasodilators, accidental (unintentional)**
        Poisoning by peripheral vasodilators NOS

     ● **T46.7X2**   **Poisoning by peripheral vasodilators, intentional self-harm A, S** 🐞

     ● **T46.7X3**   **Poisoning by peripheral vasodilators, assault**

     ● **T46.7X4**   **Poisoning by peripheral vasodilators, undetermined**

     ●● **T46.7X5**   **Adverse effect of peripheral vasodilators**

     ●● **T46.7X6**   **Underdosing of peripheral vasodilators**

CHAPTER 19 (S00-T88)

N Newborn Age: 0   **P** Pediatric Age: 0–17   **M** Maternity DX: 9–64   **A** Adult Age: 15–124   ♀ Females Only   ♂ Males Only

🐞 Complication\Comorbidity   🐞 Major C\C   (Ex) CC/MCC Exclusions   🐞 Hospital-Acquired Condition   🐞 Hierarchical Condition Category

1477

● T46.8   Poisoning by, adverse effect of and underdosing of antivaricose drugs, including sclerosing agents

  ● T46.8X   Poisoning by, adverse effect of and underdosing of antivaricose drugs, including sclerosing agents

    ● T46.8X1   Poisoning by antivaricose drugs, including sclerosing agents, accidental (unintentional)

      Poisoning by antivaricose drugs, including sclerosing agents NOS

    ● T46.8X2   Poisoning by antivaricose drugs, including sclerosing agents, intentional self-harm A, S 🕮

    ● T46.8X3   Poisoning by antivaricose drugs, including sclerosing agents, assault

    ● T46.8X4   Poisoning by antivaricose drugs, including sclerosing agents, undetermined

    ●● T46.8X5   Adverse effect of antivaricose drugs, including sclerosing agents

    ●● T46.8X6   Underdosing of antivaricose drugs, including sclerosing agents

● T46.9   Poisoning by, adverse effect of and underdosing of other and unspecified agents primarily affecting the cardiovascular system

  ● T46.90   Poisoning by, adverse effect of and underdosing of unspecified agents primarily affecting the cardiovascular system

    ● T46.901   Poisoning by unspecified agents primarily affecting the cardiovascular system, accidental (unintentional)

    ● T46.902   Poisoning by unspecified agents primarily affecting the cardiovascular system, intentional self-harm A, S 🕮

    ● T46.903   Poisoning by unspecified agents primarily affecting the cardiovascular system, assault

    ● T46.904   Poisoning by unspecified agents primarily affecting the cardiovascular system, undetermined

    ●● T46.905   Adverse effect of unspecified agents primarily affecting the cardiovascular system

    ●● T46.906   Underdosing of unspecified agents primarily affecting the cardiovascular system

  ● T46.99   Poisoning by, adverse effect of and underdosing of other agents primarily affecting the cardiovascular system

    ● T46.991   Poisoning by other agents primarily affecting the cardiovascular system, accidental (unintentional)

    ● T46.992   Poisoning by other agents primarily affecting the cardiovascular system, intentional self-harm A, S 🕮

    ● T46.993   Poisoning by other agents primarily affecting the cardiovascular system, assault

    ● T46.994   Poisoning by other agents primarily affecting the cardiovascular system, undetermined

    ●● T46.995   Adverse effect of other agents primarily affecting the cardiovascular system

    ●● T46.996   Underdosing of other agents primarily affecting the cardiovascular system

● T47   Poisoning by, adverse effect of and underdosing of agents primarily affecting the gastrointestinal system

  The appropriate 7th character is to be added to each code from category T47

A	initial encounter
D	subsequent encounter
S	sequela

● T47.0   Poisoning by, adverse effect of and underdosing of histamine H2-receptor blockers

  ● T47.0X   Poisoning by, adverse effect of and underdosing of histamine H2-receptor blockers

    ● T47.0X1   Poisoning by histamine H2-receptor blockers, accidental (unintentional)

      Poisoning by histamine H2-receptor blockers NOS

    ● T47.0X2   Poisoning by histamine H2-receptor blockers, intentional self-harm A, S 🕮

    ● T47.0X3   Poisoning by histamine H2-receptor blockers, assault

    ● T47.0X4   Poisoning by histamine H2-receptor blockers, undetermined

    ●● T47.0X5   Adverse effect of histamine H2-receptor blockers

    ●● T47.0X6   Underdosing of histamine H2-receptor blockers

● T47.1   Poisoning by, adverse effect of and underdosing of other antacids and anti-gastric-secretion drugs

  ● T47.1X   Poisoning by, adverse effect of and underdosing of other antacids and anti-gastric-secretion drugs

    ● T47.1X1   Poisoning by other antacids and anti-gastric-secretion drugs, accidental (unintentional)

      Poisoning by other antacids and anti-gastric-secretion drugs NOS

    ● T47.1X2   Poisoning by other antacids and anti-gastric-secretion drugs, intentional self-harm A, S 🕮

    ● T47.1X3   Poisoning by other antacids and anti-gastric-secretion drugs, assault

    ● T47.1X4   Poisoning by other antacids and anti-gastric-secretion drugs, undetermined

    ●● T47.1X5   Adverse effect of other antacids and anti-gastric-secretion drugs

    ●● T47.1X6   Underdosing of other antacids and anti-gastric-secretion drugs

● T47.2   Poisoning by, adverse effect of and underdosing of stimulant laxatives

  ● T47.2X   Poisoning by, adverse effect of and underdosing of stimulant laxatives

    ● T47.2X1   Poisoning by stimulant laxatives, accidental (unintentional)

      Poisoning by stimulant laxatives NOS

    ● T47.2X2   Poisoning by stimulant laxatives, intentional self-harm A, S 🕮

    ● T47.2X3   Poisoning by stimulant laxatives, assault

    ● T47.2X4   Poisoning by stimulant laxatives, undetermined

    ●● T47.2X5   Adverse effect of stimulant laxatives

    ●● T47.2X6   Underdosing of stimulant laxatives

▶ New   ⇒ Revised   ~~deleted~~ Deleted   Excludes 1   Excludes 2   Includes   Use additional   Code first   Code also   Key words

OGCR Official Guidelines   ● Unacceptable Principal Diagnosis   X Assign placeholder X   ● Use Additional Character(s)   ▶ Manifestation Code   Coding Clinic

● **T47.3**   Poisoning by, adverse effect of and underdosing of saline and osmotic laxatives

   ● **T47.3X**   Poisoning by and adverse effect of saline and osmotic laxatives

     ● **T47.3X1**   Poisoning by saline and osmotic laxatives, accidental (unintentional)
         Poisoning by saline and osmotic laxatives NOS

     ● **T47.3X2**   Poisoning by saline and osmotic laxatives, intentional self-harm

     ● **T47.3X3**   Poisoning by saline and osmotic laxatives, assault A, S 🐾

     ● **T47.3X4**   Poisoning by saline and osmotic laxatives, undetermined

     ●● **T47.3X5**   Adverse effect of saline and osmotic laxatives

     ●● **T47.3X6**   Underdosing of saline and osmotic laxatives

● **T47.4**   Poisoning by, adverse effect of and underdosing of other laxatives

   ● **T47.4X**   Poisoning by, adverse effect of and underdosing of other laxatives

     ● **T47.4X1**   Poisoning by other laxatives, accidental (unintentional)
         Poisoning by other laxatives NOS

     ● **T47.4X2**   Poisoning by other laxatives, intentional self-harm A, S 🐾

     ● **T47.4X3**   Poisoning by other laxatives, assault

     ● **T47.4X4**   Poisoning by other laxatives, undetermined

     ●● **T47.4X5**   Adverse effect of other laxatives

     ●● **T47.4X6**   Underdosing of other laxatives

● **T47.5**   Poisoning by, adverse effect of and underdosing of digestants

   ● **T47.5X**   Poisoning by, adverse effect of and underdosing of digestants

     ● **T47.5X1**   Poisoning by digestants, accidental (unintentional)
         Poisoning by digestants NOS

     ● **T47.5X2**   Poisoning by digestants, intentional self-harm A, S 🐾

     ● **T47.5X3**   Poisoning by digestants, assault

     ● **T47.5X4**   Poisoning by digestants, undetermined

     ●● **T47.5X5**   Adverse effect of digestants

     ●● **T47.5X6**   Underdosing of digestants

● **T47.6**   Poisoning by, adverse effect of and underdosing of antidiarrheal drugs

     Excludes2   poisoning by, adverse effect of and underdosing of systemic antibiotics and other anti-infectives (T36-T37)

   ● **T47.6X**   Poisoning by, adverse effect of and underdosing of antidiarrheal drugs

     ● **T47.6X1**   Poisoning by antidiarrheal drugs, accidental (unintentional)
         Poisoning by antidiarrheal drugs NOS

     ● **T47.6X2**   Poisoning by antidiarrheal drugs, intentional self-harm A, S 🐾

     ● **T47.6X3**   Poisoning by antidiarrheal drugs, assault

     ● **T47.6X4**   Poisoning by antidiarrheal drugs, undetermined

     ●● **T47.6X5**   Adverse effect of antidiarrheal drugs

     ●● **T47.6X6**   Underdosing of antidiarrheal drugs

● **T47.7**   Poisoning by, adverse effect of and underdosing of emetics

   ● **T47.7X**   Poisoning by, adverse effect of and underdosing of emetics

     ● **T47.7X1**   Poisoning by emetics, accidental (unintentional)
         Poisoning by emetics NOS

     ● **T47.7X2**   Poisoning by emetics, intentional self-harm A, S 🐾

     ● **T47.7X3**   Poisoning by emetics, assault

     ● **T47.7X4**   Poisoning by emetics, undetermined

     ●● **T47.7X5**   Adverse effect of emetics

     ●● **T47.7X6**   Underdosing of emetics

● **T47.8**   Poisoning by, adverse effect of and underdosing of other agents primarily affecting gastrointestinal system

   ● **T47.8X**   Poisoning by, adverse effect of and underdosing of other agents primarily affecting gastrointestinal system

     ● **T47.8X1**   Poisoning by other agents primarily affecting gastrointestinal system, accidental (unintentional)
         Poisoning by other agents primarily affecting gastrointestinal system NOS

     ● **T47.8X2**   Poisoning by other agents primarily affecting gastrointestinal system, intentional self-harm A, S 🐾

     ● **T47.8X3**   Poisoning by other agents primarily affecting gastrointestinal system, assault

     ● **T47.8X4**   Poisoning by other agents primarily affecting gastrointestinal system, undetermined

     ●● **T47.8X5**   Adverse effect of other agents primarily affecting gastrointestinal system

     ●● **T47.8X6**   Underdosing of other agents primarily affecting gastrointestinal system

● **T47.9**   Poisoning by, adverse effect of and underdosing of unspecified agents primarily affecting the gastrointestinal system

   X● **T47.91**   Poisoning by unspecified agents primarily affecting the gastrointestinal system, accidental (unintentional)
     Poisoning by agents primarily affecting the gastrointestinal system NOS

   X● **T47.92**   Poisoning by unspecified agents primarily affecting the gastrointestinal system, intentional self-harm A, S 🐾

   X● **T47.93**   Poisoning by unspecified agents primarily affecting the gastrointestinal system, assault

   X● **T47.94**   Poisoning by unspecified agents primarily affecting the gastrointestinal system, undetermined

   ●X● **T47.95**   Adverse effect of unspecified agents primarily affecting the gastrointestinal system

   ●X● **T47.96**   Underdosing of unspecified agents primarily affecting the gastrointestinal system

N Newborn Age: 0   **P** Pediatric Age: 0–17   **M** Maternity DX: 9–64   **A** Adult Age: 15–124   ♀ Females Only   ♂ Males Only

🐾 Complication\Comorbidity   🐾 Major C\C   (Ex) CC/MCC Exclusions   🐾 Hospital-Acquired Condition   🐾 Hierarchical Condition Category

1479

● **T48**   **Poisoning by, adverse effect of and underdosing of agents primarily acting on smooth and skeletal muscles and the respiratory system**

> The appropriate 7th character is to be added to each code from category T48

> | | |
> |---|---|
> | A | initial encounter |
> | D | subsequent encounter |
> | S | sequela |

● **T48.0**   **Poisoning by, adverse effect of and underdosing of oxytocic drugs**

> **Excludes1**   poisoning by, adverse effect of and underdosing of estrogens, progestogens and antagonists (T38.4-T38.6)

  ● **T48.0X**   Poisoning by, adverse effect of and underdosing of oxytocic drugs

    ● **T48.0X1**   Poisoning by oxytocic drugs, accidental (unintentional)
> Poisoning by oxytocic drugs NOS

    ● **T48.0X2**   Poisoning by oxytocic drugs, intentional self-harm A, S 🏀

    ● **T48.0X3**   Poisoning by oxytocic drugs, assault

    ● **T48.0X4**   Poisoning by oxytocic drugs, undetermined

    ●● **T48.0X5**   Adverse effect of oxytocic drugs

    ●● **T48.0X6**   Underdosing of oxytocic drugs

● **T48.1**   **Poisoning by, adverse effect of and underdosing of skeletal muscle relaxants [neuromuscular blocking agents]**

  ● **T48.1X**   Poisoning by, adverse effect of and underdosing of skeletal muscle relaxants [neuromuscular blocking agents]

    ● **T48.1X1**   Poisoning by skeletal muscle relaxants [neuromuscular blocking agents], accidental (unintentional)
> Poisoning by skeletal muscle relaxants [neuromuscular blocking agents] NOS

    ● **T48.1X2**   Poisoning by skeletal muscle relaxants [neuromuscular blocking agents], intentional self-harm A, S 🏀

    ● **T48.1X3**   Poisoning by skeletal muscle relaxants [neuromuscular blocking agents], assault

    ● **T48.1X4**   Poisoning by skeletal muscle relaxants [neuromuscular blocking agents], undetermined

    ●● **T48.1X5**   Adverse effect of skeletal muscle relaxants [neuromuscular blocking agents]

    ●● **T48.1X6**   Underdosing of skeletal muscle relaxants [neuromuscular blocking agents]

● **T48.2**   **Poisoning by, adverse effect of and underdosing of other and unspecified drugs acting on muscles**

  ● **T48.20**   Poisoning by, adverse effect of and underdosing of unspecified drugs acting on muscles

    ● **T48.201**   Poisoning by unspecified drugs acting on muscles, accidental (unintentional)
> Poisoning by unspecified drugs acting on muscles NOS

    ● **T48.202**   Poisoning by unspecified drugs acting on muscles, intentional self-harm A, S 🏀

    ● **T48.203**   Poisoning by unspecified drugs acting on muscles, assault

    ● **T48.204**   Poisoning by unspecified drugs acting on muscles, undetermined

    ●● **T48.205**   Adverse effect of unspecified drugs acting on muscles

    ●● **T48.206**   Underdosing of unspecified drugs acting on muscles

● **T48.29**   Poisoning by, adverse effect of and underdosing of other drugs acting on muscles

    ● **T48.291**   Poisoning by other drugs acting on muscles, accidental (unintentional)
> Poisoning by other drugs acting on muscles NOS

    ● **T48.292**   Poisoning by other drugs acting on muscles, intentional self-harm A, S 🏀

    ● **T48.293**   Poisoning by other drugs acting on muscles, assault

    ● **T48.294**   Poisoning by other drugs acting on muscles, undetermined

    ●● **T48.295**   Adverse effect of other drugs acting on muscles

    ●● **T48.296**   Underdosing of other drugs acting on muscles

● **T48.3**   **Poisoning by, adverse effect of and underdosing of antitussives**

  ● **T48.3X**   Poisoning by, adverse effect of and underdosing of antitussives

    ● **T48.3X1**   Poisoning by antitussives, accidental (unintentional)
> Poisoning by antitussives NOS

    ● **T48.3X2**   Poisoning by antitussives, intentional self-harm A, S 🏀

    ● **T48.3X3**   Poisoning by antitussives, assault

    ● **T48.3X4**   Poisoning by antitussives, undetermined

    ●● **T48.3X5**   Adverse effect of antitussives

    ●● **T48.3X6**   Underdosing of antitussives

● **T48.4**   **Poisoning by, adverse effect of and underdosing of expectorants**

  ● **T48.4X**   Poisoning by, adverse effect of and underdosing of expectorants

    ● **T48.4X1**   Poisoning by expectorants, accidental (unintentional)
> Poisoning by expectorants NOS

    ● **T48.4X2**   Poisoning by expectorants, intentional self-harm A, S 🏀

    ● **T48.4X3**   Poisoning by expectorants, assault

    ● **T48.4X4**   Poisoning by expectorants, undetermined

    ●● **T48.4X5**   Adverse effect of expectorants

    ●● **T48.4X6**   Underdosing of expectorants

● **T48.5**   **Poisoning by, adverse effect of and underdosing of other anti-common-cold drugs**

> Poisoning by, adverse effect of and underdosing of decongestants

> **Excludes2**   poisoning by, adverse effect of and underdosing of antipyretics, NEC (T39.9-)
> poisoning by, adverse effect of and underdosing of non-steroidal antiinflammatory drugs (T39.3-)
> poisoning by, adverse effect of and underdosing of salicylates (T39.0-)

  ● **T48.5X**   Poisoning by, adverse effect of and underdosing of other anti-common-cold drugs

    ● **T48.5X1**   Poisoning by other anti-common-cold drugs, accidental (unintentional)
> Poisoning by other anti-common-cold drugs NOS

    ● **T48.5X2**   Poisoning by other anti-common-cold drugs, intentional self-harm A, S 🏀

    ● **T48.5X3**   Poisoning by other anti-common-cold drugs, assault

    ● **T48.5X4**   Poisoning by other anti-common-cold drugs, undetermined

    ●● **T48.5X5**   Adverse effect of other anti-common-cold drugs

    ●● **T48.5X6**   Underdosing of other anti-common-cold drugs

● T48.6 **Poisoning by, adverse effect of and underdosing of antiasthmatics, not elsewhere classified**
Poisoning by, adverse effect of and underdosing of beta-adrenoreceptor agonists used in asthma therapy

Excludes 1 poisoning by, adverse effect of and underdosing of beta-adrenoreceptor agonists not used in asthma therapy (T44.5)
poisoning by, adverse effect of and underdosing of anterior pituitary [adenohypophyseal] hormones (T38.8)

● T48.6X **Poisoning by, adverse effect of and underdosing of antiasthmatics**

● T48.6X1 Poisoning by antiasthmatics, accidental (unintentional)
Poisoning by antiasthmatics NOS

● T48.6X2 Poisoning by antiasthmatics, intentional self-harm A, S 🐾

● T48.6X3 Poisoning by antiasthmatics, assault

● T48.6X4 Poisoning by antiasthmatics, undetermined

●● T48.6X5 Adverse effect of antiasthmatics

●● T48.6X6 Underdosing of antiasthmatics

● T48.9 **Poisoning by, adverse effect of and underdosing of other and unspecified agents primarily acting on the respiratory system**

● T48.90 **Poisoning by, adverse effect of and underdosing of unspecified agents primarily acting on the respiratory system**

● T48.901 Poisoning by unspecified agents primarily acting on the respiratory system, accidental (unintentional)

● T48.902 Poisoning by unspecified agents primarily acting on the respiratory system, intentional self-harm A, S 🐾

● T48.903 Poisoning by unspecified agents primarily acting on the respiratory system, assault

● T48.904 Poisoning by unspecified agents primarily acting on the respiratory system, undetermined

●● T48.905 Adverse effect of unspecified agents primarily acting on the respiratory system

●● T48.906 Underdosing of unspecified agents primarily acting on the respiratory system

● T48.99 **Poisoning by, adverse effect of and underdosing of other agents primarily acting on the respiratory system**

● T48.991 Poisoning by other agents primarily acting on the respiratory system, accidental (unintentional)

● T48.992 Poisoning by other agents primarily acting on the respiratory system, intentional self-harm A, S 🐾

● T48.993 Poisoning by other agents primarily acting on the respiratory system, assault

● T48.994 Poisoning by other agents primarily acting on the respiratory system, undetermined

●● T48.995 Adverse effect of other agents primarily acting on the respiratory system

●● T48.996 Underdosing of other agents primarily acting on the respiratory system

● T49 **Poisoning by, adverse effect of and underdosing of topical agents primarily affecting skin and mucous membrane and by ophthalmological, otorhinorlaryngological and dental drugs**

Includes poisoning by, adverse effect of and underdosing of glucocorticoids, topically used

The appropriate 7th character is to be added to each code from category T49

> A initial encounter
> D subsequent encounter
> S sequela

● T49.0 **Poisoning by, adverse effect of and underdosing of local antifungal, anti-infective and anti-inflammatory drugs**

● T49.0X **Poisoning by, adverse effect of and underdosing of local antifungal, anti-infective and anti-inflammatory drugs**

● T49.0X1 Poisoning by local antifungal, anti-infective and anti-inflammatory drugs, accidental (unintentional)
Poisoning by local antifungal, anti-infective and anti-inflammatory drugs NOS

● T49.0X2 Poisoning by local antifungal, anti-infective and anti-inflammatory drugs, intentional self-harm A, S 🐾

● T49.0X3 Poisoning by local antifungal, anti-infective and anti-inflammatory drugs, assault

● T49.0X4 Poisoning by local antifungal, anti-infective and anti-inflammatory drugs, undetermined

●● T49.0X5 Adverse effect of local antifungal, anti-infective and anti-inflammatory drugs

●● T49.0X6 Underdosing of local antifungal, anti-infective and anti-inflammatory drugs

● T49.1 **Poisoning by, adverse effect of and underdosing of antipruritics**

● T49.1X **Poisoning by, adverse effect of and underdosing of antipruritics**

● T49.1X1 Poisoning by antipruritics, accidental (unintentional)
Poisoning by antipruritics NOS

● T49.1X2 Poisoning by antipruritics, intentional self-harm A, S 🐾

● T49.1X3 Poisoning by antipruritics, assault

● T49.1X4 Poisoning by antipruritics, undetermined

●● T49.1X5 Adverse effect of antipruritics

●● T49.1X6 Underdosing of antipruritics

● T49.2 **Poisoning by, adverse effect of and underdosing of local astringents and local detergents**

● T49.2X **Poisoning by, adverse effect of and underdosing of local astringents and local detergents**

● T49.2X1 Poisoning by local astringents and local detergents, accidental (unintentional)
Poisoning by local astringents and local detergents NOS

● T49.2X2 Poisoning by local astringents and local detergents, intentional self-harm A, S 🐾

● T49.2X3 Poisoning by local astringents and local detergents, assault

● T49.2X4 Poisoning by local astringents and local detergents, undetermined

●● T49.2X5 Adverse effect of local astringents and local detergents

●● T49.2X6 Underdosing of local astringents and local detergents

N Newborn Age: 0   **P** Pediatric Age: 0–17   **M** Maternity DX: 9–64   **A** Adult Age: 15–124   ♀ Females Only   ♂ Males Only

🐾 Complication\Comorbidity   🐾 Major C\C   (Ex) CC/MCC Exclusions   🐾 Hospital-Acquired Condition   🐾 Hierarchical Condition Category

CHAPTER 19 (S00–T88)

1481

● T49.3   Poisoning by, adverse effect of and underdosing of emollients, demulcents and protectants

    ● T49.3X   Poisoning by, adverse effect of and underdosing of emollients, demulcents and protectants

        ● T49.3X1   Poisoning by emollients, demulcents and protectants, accidental (unintentional)
                 Poisoning by emollients, demulcents and protectants NOS

        ● T49.3X2   Poisoning by emollients, demulcents and protectants, intentional self-harm A, S 🔖

        ● T49.3X3   Poisoning by emollients, demulcents and protectants, assault

        ● T49.3X4   Poisoning by emollients, demulcents and protectants, undetermined

        ●● T49.3X5   Adverse effect of emollients, demulcents and protectants

        ●● T49.3X6   Underdosing of emollients, demulcents and protectants

● T49.4   Poisoning by, adverse effect of and underdosing of keratolytics, keratoplastics, and other hair treatment drugs and preparations

    ● T49.4X   Poisoning by, adverse effect of and underdosing of keratolytics, keratoplastics, and other hair treatment drugs and preparations

        ● T49.4X1   Poisoning by keratolytics, keratoplastics, and other hair treatment drugs and preparations, accidental (unintentional)
                 Poisoning by keratolytics, keratoplastics, and other hair treatment drugs and preparations NOS

        ● T49.4X2   Poisoning by keratolytics, keratoplastics, and other hair treatment drugs and preparations, intentional self-harm A, S 🔖

        ● T49.4X3   Poisoning by keratolytics, keratoplastics, and other hair treatment drugs and preparations, assault

        ● T49.4X4   Poisoning by keratolytics, keratoplastics, and other hair treatment drugs and preparations, undetermined

        ●● T49.4X5   Adverse effect of keratolytics, keratoplastics, and other hair treatment drugs and preparations

        ●● T49.4X6   Underdosing of keratolytics, keratoplastics, and other hair treatment drugs and preparations

● T49.5   Poisoning by, adverse effect of and underdosing of ophthalmological drugs and preparations

    ● T49.5X   Poisoning by, adverse effect of and underdosing of ophthalmological drugs and preparations

        ● T49.5X1   Poisoning by ophthalmological drugs and preparations, accidental (unintentional)
                 Poisoning by ophthalmological drugs and preparations NOS

        ● T49.5X2   Poisoning by ophthalmological drugs and preparations, intentional self-harm A, S 🔖

        ● T49.5X3   Poisoning by ophthalmological drugs and preparations, assault

        ● T49.5X4   Poisoning by ophthalmological drugs and preparations, undetermined

        ●● T49.5X5   Adverse effect of ophthalmological drugs and preparations

        ●● T49.5X6   Underdosing of ophthalmological drugs and preparations

● T49.6   Poisoning by, adverse effect of and underdosing of otorhinolaryngological drugs and preparations

    ● T49.6X   Poisoning by, adverse effect of and underdosing of otorhinolaryngological drugs and preparations

        ● T49.6X1   Poisoning by otorhinolaryngological drugs and preparations, accidental (unintentional)
                 Poisoning by otorhinolaryngological drugs and preparations NOS

        ● T49.6X2   Poisoning by otorhinolaryngological drugs and preparations, intentional self-harm A, S 🔖

        ● T49.6X3   Poisoning by otorhinolaryngological drugs and preparations, assault

        ● T49.6X4   Poisoning by otorhinolaryngological drugs and preparations, undetermined

        ●● T49.6X5   Adverse effect of otorhinolaryngological drugs and preparations

        ●● T49.6X6   Underdosing of otorhinolaryngological drugs and preparations

● T49.7   Poisoning by, adverse effect of and underdosing of dental drugs, topically applied

    ● T49.7X   Poisoning by, adverse effect of and underdosing of dental drugs, topically applied

        ● T49.7X1   Poisoning by dental drugs, topically applied, accidental (unintentional)
                 Poisoning by dental drugs, topically applied NOS

        ● T49.7X2   Poisoning by dental drugs, topically applied, intentional self-harm A, S 🔖

        ● T49.7X3   Poisoning by dental drugs, topically applied, assault

        ● T49.7X4   Poisoning by dental drugs, topically applied, undetermined

        ●● T49.7X5   Adverse effect of dental drugs, topically applied

        ●● T49.7X6   Underdosing of dental drugs, topically applied

● T49.8   Poisoning by, adverse effect of and underdosing of other topical agents
       Poisoning by, adverse effect of and underdosing of spermicides

    ● T49.8X   Poisoning by, adverse effect of and underdosing of other topical agents

        ● T49.8X1   Poisoning by other topical agents, accidental (unintentional)
                 Poisoning by other topical agents NOS

        ● T49.8X2   Poisoning by other topical agents, intentional self-harm A, S 🔖

        ● T49.8X3   Poisoning by other topical agents, assault

        ● T49.8X4   Poisoning by other topical agents, undetermined

        ●● T49.8X5   Adverse effect of other topical agents

        ●● T49.8X6   Underdosing of other topical agents

● T49.9   Poisoning by, adverse effect of and underdosing of unspecified topical agent

    X● T49.91   Poisoning by unspecified topical agent, accidental (unintentional)

    X● T49.92   Poisoning by unspecified topical agent, intentional self-harm A, S 🔖

    X● T49.93   Poisoning by unspecified topical agent, assault

    X● T49.94   Poisoning by unspecified topical agent, undetermined

    ●X● T49.95   Adverse effect of unspecified topical agent

    ●X● T49.96   Underdosing of unspecified topical agent

▶ New   ⇒ Revised   ~~deleted~~ Deleted   Excludes 1   Excludes 2   Includes   Use additional   Code first   Code also   Key words

OGCR Official Guidelines   ● Unacceptable Principal Diagnosis   X Assign placeholder X   ● Use Additional Character(s)   ▶ Manifestation Code   **Coding Clinic**

● **T50 Poisoning by, adverse effect of and underdosing of diuretics and other and unspecified drugs, medicaments and biological substances**

> The appropriate 7th character is to be added to each code from category T50

> A   initial encounter
> D   subsequent encounter
> S   sequela

● **T50.0 Poisoning by, adverse effect of and underdosing of mineralocorticoids and their antagonists**

  ● **T50.0X Poisoning by, adverse effect of and underdosing of mineralocorticoids and their antagonists**

    ● **T50.0X1 Poisoning by mineralocorticoids and their antagonists, accidental (unintentional)**
> Poisoning by mineralocorticoids and their antagonists NOS

    ● **T50.0X2 Poisoning by mineralocorticoids and their antagonists, intentional self-harm A, S** 🅷

    ● **T50.0X3 Poisoning by mineralocorticoids and their antagonists, assault**

    ● **T50.0X4 Poisoning by mineralocorticoids and their antagonists, undetermined**

    ●● **T50.0X5 Adverse effect of mineralocorticoids and their antagonists**

    ●● **T50.0X6 Underdosing of mineralocorticoids and their antagonists**

● **T50.1 Poisoning by, adverse effect of and underdosing of loop [high-ceiling] diuretics**

  ● **T50.1X Poisoning by, adverse effect of and underdosing of loop [high-ceiling] diuretics**

    ● **T50.1X1 Poisoning by loop [high-ceiling] diuretics, accidental (unintentional)**
> Poisoning by loop [high-ceiling] diuretics NOS

    ● **T50.1X2 Poisoning by loop [high-ceiling] diuretics, intentional self-harm A, S** 🅷

    ● **T50.1X3 Poisoning by loop [high-ceiling] diuretics, assault**

    ● **T50.1X4 Poisoning by loop [high-ceiling] diuretics, undetermined**

    ●● **T50.1X5 Adverse effect of loop [high-ceiling] diuretics**

    ●● **T50.1X6 Underdosing of loop [high-ceiling] diuretics**

● **T50.2 Poisoning by, adverse effect of and underdosing of carbonic-anhydrase inhibitors, benzothiadiazides and other diuretics**

> Poisoning by, adverse effect of and underdosing of acetazolamide

  ● **T50.2X Poisoning by, adverse effect of and underdosing of carbonic-anhydrase inhibitors, benzothiadiazides and other diuretics**

    ● **T50.2X1 Poisoning by carbonic-anhydrase inhibitors, benzothiadiazides and other diuretics, accidental (unintentional)**
> Poisoning by carbonic-anhydrase inhibitors, benzothiadiazides and other diuretics NOS

    ● **T50.2X2 Poisoning by carbonic-anhydrase inhibitors, benzothiadiazides and other diuretics, intentional self-harm A, S** 🅷

    ● **T50.2X3 Poisoning by carbonic-anhydrase inhibitors, benzothiadiazides and other diuretics, assault**

    ● **T50.2X4 Poisoning by carbonic-anhydrase inhibitors, benzothiadiazides and other diuretics, undetermined**

    ●● **T50.2X5 Adverse effect of carbonic-anhydrase inhibitors, benzothiadiazides and other diuretics**

    ●● **T50.2X6 Underdosing of carbonic-anhydrase inhibitors, benzothiadiazides and other diuretics**

● **T50.3 Poisoning by, adverse effect of and underdosing of electrolytic, caloric and water-balance agents**

> Poisoning by, adverse effect of and underdosing of oral rehydration salts

  ● **T50.3X Poisoning by, adverse effect of and underdosing of electrolytic, caloric and water-balance agents**

    ● **T50.3X1 Poisoning by electrolytic, caloric and water-balance agents, accidental (unintentional)**
> Poisoning by electrolytic, caloric and water-balance agents NOS

    ● **T50.3X2 Poisoning by electrolytic, caloric and water-balance agents, intentional self-harm A, S** 🅷

    ● **T50.3X3 Poisoning by electrolytic, caloric and water-balance agents, assault**

    ● **T50.3X4 Poisoning by electrolytic, caloric and water-balance agents, undetermined**

    ●● **T50.3X5 Adverse effect of electrolytic, caloric and water-balance agents**

    ●● **T50.3X6 Underdosing of electrolytic, caloric and water-balance agents**

● **T50.4 Poisoning by, adverse effect of and underdosing of drugs affecting uric acid metabolism**

  ● **T50.4X Poisoning by, adverse effect of and underdosing of drugs affecting uric acid metabolism**

    ● **T50.4X1 Poisoning by drugs affecting uric acid metabolism, accidental (unintentional)**
> Poisoning by drugs affecting uric acid metabolism NOS

    ● **T50.4X2 Poisoning by drugs affecting uric acid metabolism, intentional self-harm A, S** 🅷

    ● **T50.4X3 Poisoning by drugs affecting uric acid metabolism, assault**

    ● **T50.4X4 Poisoning by drugs affecting uric acid metabolism, undetermined**

    ●● **T50.4X5 Adverse effect of drugs affecting uric acid metabolism**

    ●● **T50.4X6 Underdosing of drugs affecting uric acid metabolism**

● **T50.5 Poisoning by, adverse effect of and underdosing of appetite depressants**

  ● **T50.5X Poisoning by, adverse effect of and underdosing of appetite depressants**

    ● **T50.5X1 Poisoning by appetite depressants, accidental (unintentional)**
> Poisoning by appetite depressants NOS

    ● **T50.5X2 Poisoning by appetite depressants, intentional self-harm A, S** 🅷

    ● **T50.5X3 Poisoning by appetite depressants, assault**

    ● **T50.5X4 Poisoning by appetite depressants, undetermined**

    ●● **T50.5X5 Adverse effect of appetite depressants**

    ●● **T50.5X6 Underdosing of appetite depressants**

N   Newborn Age: 0   P   Pediatric Age: 0–17   M   Maternity DX: 9–64   A   Adult Age: 15–124   ♀   Females Only   ♂   Males Only

🅒 Complication\Comorbidity   🅜 Major C\C   (Ex) CC/MCC Exclusions   🅗 Hospital-Acquired Condition   🅗 Hierarchical Condition Category

1483

● T50.6   Poisoning by, adverse effect of and underdosing of antidotes and chelating agents

     Poisoning by, adverse effect of and underdosing of alcohol deterrents

     ● T50.6X   Poisoning by, adverse effect of and underdosing of antidotes and chelating agents

        ● T50.6X1   Poisoning by antidotes and chelating agents, accidental (unintentional)

            Poisoning by antidotes and chelating agents NOS

        ● T50.6X2   Poisoning by antidotes and chelating agents, intentional self-harm A, S 🐾

        ● T50.6X3   Poisoning by antidotes and chelating agents, assault

        ● T50.6X4   Poisoning by antidotes and chelating agents, undetermined

        ●● T50.6X5   Adverse effect of antidotes and chelating agents

        ●● T50.6X6   Underdosing of antidotes and chelating agents

● T50.7   Poisoning by, adverse effect of and underdosing of analeptics and opioid receptor antagonists

     ● T50.7X   Poisoning by, adverse effect of and underdosing of analeptics and opioid receptor antagonists

        ● T50.7X1   Poisoning by analeptics and opioid receptor antagonists, accidental (unintentional)

            Poisoning by analeptics and opioid receptor antagonists NOS

        ● T50.7X2   Poisoning by analeptics and opioid receptor antagonists, intentional self-harm A, S 🐾

        ● T50.7X3   Poisoning by analeptics and opioid receptor antagonists, assault

        ● T50.7X4   Poisoning by analeptics and opioid receptor antagonists, undetermined

        ●● T50.7X5   Adverse effect of analeptics and opioid receptor antagonists

        ●● T50.7X6   Underdosing of analeptics and opioid receptor antagonists

● T50.8   Poisoning by, adverse effect of and underdosing of diagnostic agents

     ● T50.8X   Poisoning by, adverse effect of and underdosing of diagnostic agents

        ● T50.8X1   Poisoning by diagnostic agents, accidental (unintentional)

            Poisoning by diagnostic agents NOS

        ● T50.8X2   Poisoning by diagnostic agents, intentional self-harm A, S 🐾

        ● T50.8X3   Poisoning by diagnostic agents, assault

        ● T50.8X4   Poisoning by diagnostic agents, undetermined

        ●● T50.8X5   Adverse effect of diagnostic agents

        ●● T50.8X6   Underdosing of diagnostic agents

● T50.A   Poisoning by, adverse effect of and underdosing of bacterial vaccines

     ● T50.A1   Poisoning by, adverse effect of and underdosing of pertussis vaccine, including combinations with a pertussis component

        ● T50.A11   Poisoning by pertussis vaccine, including combinations with a pertussis component, accidental (unintentional)

        ● T50.A12   Poisoning by pertussis vaccine, including combinations with a pertussis component, intentional self-harm A, S 🐾

        ● T50.A13   Poisoning by pertussis vaccine, including combinations with a pertussis component, assault

        ● T50.A14   Poisoning by pertussis vaccine, including combinations with a pertussis component, undetermined

        ●● T50.A15   Adverse effect of pertussis vaccine, including combinations with a pertussis component

        ●● T50.A16   Underdosing of pertussis vaccine, including combinations with a pertussis component

     ● T50.A2   Poisoning by, adverse effect of and underdosing of mixed bacterial vaccines without a pertussis component

        ● T50.A21   Poisoning by mixed bacterial vaccines without a pertussis component, accidental (unintentional)

        ● T50.A22   Poisoning by mixed bacterial vaccines without a pertussis component, intentional self-harm A, S 🐾

        ● T50.A23   Poisoning by mixed bacterial vaccines without a pertussis component, assault

        ● T50.A24   Poisoning by mixed bacterial vaccines without a pertussis component, undetermined

        ●● T50.A25   Adverse effect of mixed bacterial vaccines without a pertussis component

        ●● T50.A26   Underdosing of mixed bacterial vaccines without a pertussis component

     ● T50.A9   Poisoning by, adverse effect of and underdosing of other bacterial vaccines

        ● T50.A91   Poisoning by other bacterial vaccines, accidental (unintentional)

        ● T50.A92   Poisoning by other bacterial vaccines, intentional self-harm A, S 🐾

        ● T50.A93   Poisoning by other bacterial vaccines, assault

        ● T50.A94   Poisoning by other bacterial vaccines, undetermined

        ●● T50.A95   Adverse effect of other bacterial vaccines

        ●● T50.A96   Underdosing of other bacterial vaccines

● T50.B   Poisoning by, adverse effect of and underdosing of viral vaccines

     ● T50.B1   Poisoning by, adverse effect of and underdosing of smallpox vaccines

        ● T50.B11   Poisoning by smallpox vaccines, accidental (unintentional)

        ● T50.B12   Poisoning by smallpox vaccines, intentional self-harm A, S 🐾

        ● T50.B13   Poisoning by smallpox vaccines, assault

        ● T50.B14   Poisoning by smallpox vaccines, undetermined

        ●● T50.B15   Adverse effect of smallpox vaccines

        ●● T50.B16   Underdosing of smallpox vaccines

▶ New   ⇒ Revised   deleted Deleted   Excludes 1   Excludes 2   Includes   Use additional   Code first   Code also   Key words

OGCR Official Guidelines   ● Unacceptable Principal Diagnosis   X Assign placeholder X   ● Use Additional Character(s)   ▶ Manifestation Code   Coding Clinic

● **T50.B9**   Poisoning by, adverse effect of and underdosing of other viral vaccines

    ● **T50.B91**   Poisoning by other viral vaccines, accidental (unintentional)

    ● **T50.B92**   Poisoning by other viral vaccines, intentional self-harm A, S 🦠

    ● **T50.B93**   Poisoning by other viral vaccines, assault

    ● **T50.B94**   Poisoning by other viral vaccines, undetermined

    ●● **T50.B95**   Adverse effect of other viral vaccines
          Coding Clinic: 2021, Q1, P43-44

    ●● **T50.B96**   Underdosing of other viral vaccines

● **T50.Z**   Poisoning by, adverse effect of and underdosing of other vaccines and biological substances

    ● **T50.Z1**   Poisoning by, adverse effect of and underdosing of immunoglobulin

       ● **T50.Z11**   Poisoning by immunoglobulin, accidental (unintentional)

       ● **T50.Z12**   Poisoning by immunoglobulin, intentional self-harm A, S 🦠

       ● **T50.Z13**   Poisoning by immunoglobulin, assault

       ● **T50.Z14**   Poisoning by immunoglobulin, undetermined

       ●● **T50.Z15**   Adverse effect of immunoglobulin

       ●● **T50.Z16**   Underdosing of immunoglobulin

    ● **T50.Z9**   Poisoning by, adverse effect of and underdosing of other vaccines and biological substances

       ● **T50.Z91**   Poisoning by other vaccines and biological substances, accidental (unintentional)

       ● **T50.Z92**   Poisoning by other vaccines and biological substances, intentional self-harm A, S 🦠

       ● **T50.Z93**   Poisoning by other vaccines and biological substances, assault

       ● **T50.Z94**   Poisoning by other vaccines and biological substances, undetermined

       ●● **T50.Z95**   Adverse effect of other vaccines and biological substances
          Coding Clinic: 2020, Q1, P19

       ●● **T50.Z96**   Underdosing of other vaccines and biological substances

● **T50.9**   Poisoning by, adverse effect of and underdosing of other and unspecified drugs, medicaments and biological substances

    ● **T50.90**   Poisoning by, adverse effect of and underdosing of unspecified drugs, medicaments and biological substances

       ● **T50.901**   Poisoning by unspecified drugs, medicaments and biological substances, accidental (unintentional)
          Coding Clinic: 2015, Q1, P21

       ● **T50.902**   Poisoning by unspecified drugs, medicaments and biological substances, intentional self-harm A, S 🦠

       ● **T50.903**   Poisoning by unspecified drugs, medicaments and biological substances, assault

       ● **T50.904**   Poisoning by unspecified drugs, medicaments and biological substances, undetermined

       ● **T50.905**   Adverse effect of unspecified drugs, medicaments and biological substances

       ● **T50.906**   Underdosing of unspecified drugs, medicaments and biological substances

● **T50.91**   Poisoning by, adverse effect of and underdosing of multiple unspecified drugs, medicaments and biological substances
     Multiple drug ingestion NOS
       Code also any specific drugs, medicaments and biological substances

    ● **T50.911**   Poisoning by multiple unspecified drugs, medicaments and biological substances, accidental (unintentional)

    ● **T50.912**   Poisoning by multiple unspecified drugs, medicaments and biological substances, intentional self-harm

    ● **T50.913**   Poisoning by multiple unspecified drugs, medicaments and biological substances, assault

    ● **T50.914**   Poisoning by multiple unspecified drugs, medicaments and biological substances, undetermined

    ● **T50.915**   Adverse effect of multiple unspecified drugs, medicaments and biological substances

    ● **T50.916**   Underdosing of multiple unspecified drugs, medicaments and biological substances

● **T50.99**   Poisoning by, adverse effect of and underdosing of other drugs, medicaments and biological substances

    ● **T50.991**   Poisoning by other drugs, medicaments and biological substances, accidental (unintentional)

    ● **T50.992**   Poisoning by other drugs, medicaments and biological substances, intentional self-harm A, S 🦠

    ● **T50.993**   Poisoning by other drugs, medicaments and biological substances, assault

    ● **T50.994**   Poisoning by other drugs, medicaments and biological substances, undetermined

    ● **T50.995**   Adverse effect of other drugs, medicaments and biological substances

    ● **T50.996**   Underdosing of other drugs, medicaments and biological substances

TOXIC EFFECTS OF SUBSTANCES CHIEFLY NONMEDICINAL AS TO SOURCE (T51-T65)

Note: When no intent is indicated code to accidental. Undetermined intent is only for use when there is specific documentation in the record that the intent of the toxic effect cannot be determined.

Use additional code(s): for all associated manifestations of toxic effect, such as:
respiratory conditions due to external agents (J60-J70)
personal history of foreign body fully removed (Z87.821)
to identify any retained foreign body, if applicable (Z18.-)

Excludes1   contact with and (suspected) exposure to toxic substances (Z77.-)

N Newborn Age: 0   **P** Pediatric Age: 0-17   **M** Maternity DX: 9-64   **A** Adult Age: 15-124   ♀ Females Only   ♂ Males Only

🦠 Complication\Comorbidity   🦠 Major C\C   (Ex) CC/MCC Exclusions   🦠 Hospital-Acquired Condition   🦠 Hierarchical Condition Category

1485

● **T51**   **Toxic effect of alcohol**

The appropriate 7th character is to be added to each code from category T51

A	initial encounter
D	subsequent encounter
S	sequela

● **T51.0**   **Toxic effect of ethanol**

Toxic effect of ethyl alcohol

Excludes2   acute alcohol intoxication or 'hangover' effects (F10.129, F10.229, F10.929)
drunkenness (F10.129, F10.229, F10.929)
pathological alcohol intoxication (F10.129, F10.229, F10.929)

● **T51.0X**   **Toxic effect of ethanol**

● **T51.0X1**   **Toxic effect of ethanol, accidental (unintentional)**

Toxic effect of ethanol NOS

● **T51.0X2**   **Toxic effect of ethanol, intentional self-harm A, S** 🅒

● **T51.0X3**   **Toxic effect of ethanol, assault**

● **T51.0X4**   **Toxic effect of ethanol, undetermined**

● **T51.1**   **Toxic effect of methanol**

Toxic effect of methyl alcohol

● **T51.1X**   **Toxic effect of methanol**

● **T51.1X1**   **Toxic effect of methanol, accidental (unintentional)**

Toxic effect of methanol NOS

● **T51.1X2**   **Toxic effect of methanol, intentional self-harm A, S** 🅒

● **T51.1X3**   **Toxic effect of methanol, assault**

● **T51.1X4**   **Toxic effect of methanol, undetermined**

● **T51.2**   **Toxic effect of 2-Propanol**

Toxic effect of isopropyl alcohol

● **T51.2X**   **Toxic effect of 2-Propanol**

● **T51.2X1**   **Toxic effect of 2-Propanol, accidental (unintentional)**

Toxic effect of 2-Propanol NOS

● **T51.2X2**   **Toxic effect of 2-Propanol, intentional self-harm A, S** 🅒

● **T51.2X3**   **Toxic effect of 2-Propanol, assault**

● **T51.2X4**   **Toxic effect of 2-Propanol, undetermined**

● **T51.3**   **Toxic effect of fusel oil**

Toxic effect of amyl alcohol
Toxic effect of butyl [1-butanol] alcohol
Toxic effect of propyl [1-propanol] alcohol

● **T51.3X**   **Toxic effect of fusel oil**

● **T51.3X1**   **Toxic effect of fusel oil, accidental (unintentional)**

Toxic effect of fusel oil NOS

● **T51.3X2**   **Toxic effect of fusel oil, intentional self-harm A, S** 🅒

● **T51.3X3**   **Toxic effect of fusel oil, assault**

● **T51.3X4**   **Toxic effect of fusel oil, undetermined**

● **T51.8**   **Toxic effect of other alcohols**

● **T51.8X**   **Toxic effect of other alcohols**

● **T51.8X1**   **Toxic effect of other alcohols, accidental (unintentional)**

Toxic effect of other alcohols NOS

● **T51.8X2**   **Toxic effect of other alcohols, intentional self-harm A, S** 🅒

● **T51.8X3**   **Toxic effect of other alcohols, assault**

● **T51.8X4**   **Toxic effect of other alcohols, undetermined**

● **T51.9**   **Toxic effect of unspecified alcohol**

X● **T51.91**   **Toxic effect of unspecified alcohol, accidental (unintentional)**

X● **T51.92**   **Toxic effect of unspecified alcohol, intentional self-harm A, S** 🅒

X● **T51.93**   **Toxic effect of unspecified alcohol, assault**

X● **T51.94**   **Toxic effect of unspecified alcohol, undetermined**

● **T52**   **Toxic effect of organic solvents**

Excludes1   halogen derivatives of aliphatic and aromatic hydrocarbons (T53.-)

The appropriate 7th character is to be added to each code from category T52

A	initial encounter
D	subsequent encounter
S	sequela

● **T52.0**   **Toxic effects of petroleum products**

Toxic effects of gasoline [petrol]
Toxic effects of kerosene [paraffin oil]
Toxic effects of paraffin wax
Toxic effects of ether petroleum
Toxic effects of naphtha petroleum
Toxic effects of spirit petroleum

● **T52.0X**   **Toxic effects of petroleum products**

● **T52.0X1**   **Toxic effect of petroleum products, accidental (unintentional)**

Toxic effects of petroleum products NOS

● **T52.0X2**   **Toxic effect of petroleum products, intentional self-harm A, S** 🅒

● **T52.0X3**   **Toxic effect of petroleum products, assault**

● **T52.0X4**   **Toxic effect of petroleum products, undetermined**

● **T52.1**   **Toxic effects of benzene**

Excludes1   homologues of benzene (T52.2)
nitroderivatives and aminoderivatives of benzene and its homologues (T65.3)

● **T52.1X**   **Toxic effects of benzene**

● **T52.1X1**   **Toxic effect of benzene, accidental (unintentional)**

Toxic effects of benzene NOS

● **T52.1X2**   **Toxic effect of benzene, intentional self-harm A, S** 🅒

● **T52.1X3**   **Toxic effect of benzene, assault**

● **T52.1X4**   **Toxic effect of benzene, undetermined**

● **T52.2**   **Toxic effects of homologues of benzene**

Toxic effects of toluene [methylbenzene]
Toxic effects of xylene [dimethylbenzene]

● **T52.2X**   **Toxic effects of homologues of benzene**

● **T52.2X1**   **Toxic effect of homologues of benzene, accidental (unintentional)**

Toxic effects of homologues of benzene NOS

● **T52.2X2**   **Toxic effect of homologues of benzene, intentional self-harm A, S** 🅒

● **T52.2X3**   **Toxic effect of homologues of benzene, assault**

● **T52.2X4**   **Toxic effect of homologues of benzene, undetermined**

● **T52.3**   **Toxic effects of glycols**

● **T52.3X**   **Toxic effects of glycols**

● **T52.3X1**   **Toxic effect of glycols, accidental (unintentional)**

Toxic effects of glycols NOS

● **T52.3X2**   **Toxic effect of glycols, intentional self-harm A, S** 🅒

● **T52.3X3**   **Toxic effect of glycols, assault**

● **T52.3X4**   **Toxic effect of glycols, undetermined**

▶ New   ⇒ Revised   ~~deleted~~ Deleted   Excludes 1   Excludes 2   Includes   Use additional   Code first   Code also   Key words

OGCR Official Guidelines   ● Unacceptable Principal Diagnosis   X Assign placeholder X   ● Use Additional Character(s)   ▶ Manifestation Code   **Coding Clinic**

● T52.4   Toxic effects of ketones
   ● T52.4X   Toxic effects of ketones
     ● T52.4X1   Toxic effect of ketones, accidental (unintentional)
         Toxic effects of ketones NOS
     ● T52.4X2   Toxic effect of ketones, intentional self-harm A, S 🦠
     ● T52.4X3   Toxic effect of ketones, assault
     ● T52.4X4   Toxic effect of ketones, undetermined

● T52.8   Toxic effects of other organic solvents
   ● T52.8X   Toxic effects of other organic solvents
     ● T52.8X1   Toxic effect of other organic solvents, accidental (unintentional)
         Toxic effects of other organic solvents NOS
     ● T52.8X2   Toxic effect of other organic solvents, intentional self-harm A, S 🦠
     ● T52.8X3   Toxic effect of other organic solvents, assault
     ● T52.8X4   Toxic effect of other organic solvents, undetermined

● T52.9   Toxic effects of unspecified organic solvent
   X ● T52.91   Toxic effect of unspecified organic solvent, accidental (unintentional)
   X ● T52.92   Toxic effect of unspecified organic solvent, intentional self-harm A, S 🦠
   X ● T52.93   Toxic effect of unspecified organic solvent, assault
   X ● T52.94   Toxic effect of unspecified organic solvent, undetermined

● T53   Toxic effect of halogen derivatives of aliphatic and aromatic hydrocarbons

   The appropriate 7th character is to be added to each code from category T53

   | | |
   A   initial encounter
   D   subsequent encounter
   S   sequela

● T53.0   Toxic effects of carbon tetrachloride
     Toxic effects of tetrachloromethane
   ● T53.0X   Toxic effects of carbon tetrachloride
     ● T53.0X1   Toxic effect of carbon tetrachloride, accidental (unintentional)
         Toxic effects of carbon tetrachloride NOS
     ● T53.0X2   Toxic effect of carbon tetrachloride, intentional self-harm A, S 🦠
     ● T53.0X3   Toxic effect of carbon tetrachloride, assault
     ● T53.0X4   Toxic effect of carbon tetrachloride, undetermined

● T53.1   Toxic effects of chloroform
     Toxic effects of trichloromethane
   ● T53.1X   Toxic effects of chloroform
     ● T53.1X1   Toxic effect of chloroform, accidental (unintentional)
         Toxic effects of chloroform NOS
     ● T53.1X2   Toxic effect of chloroform, intentional self-harm A, S 🦠
     ● T53.1X3   Toxic effect of chloroform, assault
     ● T53.1X4   Toxic effect of chloroform, undetermined

● T53.2   Toxic effects of trichloroethylene
     Toxic effects of trichloroethene
   ● T53.2X   Toxic effects of trichloroethylene
     ● T53.2X1   Toxic effect of trichloroethylene, accidental (unintentional)
         Toxic effects of trichloroethylene NOS
     ● T53.2X2   Toxic effect of trichloroethylene, intentional self-harm A, S 🦠
     ● T53.2X3   Toxic effect of trichloroethylene, assault
     ● T53.2X4   Toxic effect of trichloroethylene, undetermined

● T53.3   Toxic effects of tetrachloroethylene
     Toxic effects of perchloroethylene
     Toxic effect of tetrachloroethene
   ● T53.3X   Toxic effects of tetrachloroethylene
     ● T53.3X1   Toxic effect of tetrachloroethylene, accidental (unintentional)
         Toxic effects of tetrachloroethylene NOS
     ● T53.3X2   Toxic effect of tetrachloroethylene, intentional self-harm A, S 🦠
     ● T53.3X3   Toxic effect of tetrachloroethylene, assault
     ● T53.3X4   Toxic effect of tetrachloroethylene, undetermined

● T53.4   Toxic effects of dichloromethane
     Toxic effects of methylene chloride
   ● T53.4X   Toxic effects of dichloromethane
     ● T53.4X1   Toxic effect of dichloromethane, accidental (unintentional)
         Toxic effects of dichloromethane NOS
     ● T53.4X2   Toxic effect of dichloromethane, intentional self-harm A, S 🦠
     ● T53.4X3   Toxic effect of dichloromethane, assault
     ● T53.4X4   Toxic effect of dichloromethane, undetermined

● T53.5   Toxic effects of chlorofluorocarbons
   ● T53.5X   Toxic effects of chlorofluorocarbons
     ● T53.5X1   Toxic effect of chlorofluorocarbons, accidental (unintentional)
         Toxic effects of chlorofluorocarbons NOS
     ● T53.5X2   Toxic effect of chlorofluorocarbons, intentional self-harm A, S 🦠
     ● T53.5X3   Toxic effect of chlorofluorocarbons, assault
     ● T53.5X4   Toxic effect of chlorofluorocarbons, undetermined

● T53.6   Toxic effects of other halogen derivatives of aliphatic hydrocarbons
   ● T53.6X   Toxic effects of other halogen derivatives of aliphatic hydrocarbons
     ● T53.6X1   Toxic effect of other halogen derivatives of aliphatic hydrocarbons, accidental (unintentional)
         Toxic effects of other halogen derivatives of aliphatic hydrocarbons NOS
     ● T53.6X2   Toxic effect of other halogen derivatives of aliphatic hydrocarbons, intentional self-harm A, S 🦠
     ● T53.6X3   Toxic effect of other halogen derivatives of aliphatic hydrocarbons, assault
     ● T53.6X4   Toxic effect of other halogen derivatives of aliphatic hydrocarbons, undetermined

N Newborn Age: 0   **P** Pediatric Age: 0–17   **M** Maternity DX: 9–64   **A** Adult Age: 15–124   ♀ Females Only   ♂ Males Only

🦠 Complication\Comorbidity   🦠 Major C\C   (Ex) CC/MCC Exclusions   🦠 Hospital-Acquired Condition   🦠 Hierarchical Condition Category

1487

● **T53.7** **Toxic effects of other halogen derivatives of aromatic hydrocarbons**

● **T53.7X** **Toxic effects of other halogen derivatives of aromatic hydrocarbons**

● **T53.7X1** Toxic effect of other halogen derivatives of aromatic hydrocarbons, accidental (unintentional)
Toxic effects of other halogen derivatives of aromatic hydrocarbons NOS

● **T53.7X2** Toxic effect of other halogen derivatives of aromatic hydrocarbons, intentional self-harm A, S 🔖

● **T53.7X3** Toxic effect of other halogen derivatives of aromatic hydrocarbons, assault

● **T53.7X4** Toxic effect of other halogen derivatives of aromatic hydrocarbons, undetermined

● **T53.9** **Toxic effects of unspecified halogen derivatives of aliphatic and aromatic hydrocarbons**

X● **T53.91** Toxic effect of unspecified halogen derivatives of aliphatic and aromatic hydrocarbons, accidental (unintentional)

X● **T53.92** Toxic effect of unspecified halogen derivatives of aliphatic and aromatic hydrocarbons, intentional self-harm A, S 🔖

X● **T53.93** Toxic effect of unspecified halogen derivatives of aliphatic and aromatic hydrocarbons, assault

X● **T53.94** Toxic effect of unspecified halogen derivatives of aliphatic and aromatic hydrocarbons, undetermined

● **T54** **Toxic effect of corrosive substances**

The appropriate 7th character is to be added to each code from category T54

A	initial encounter
D	subsequent encounter
S	sequela

● **T54.0** **Toxic effects of phenol and phenol homologues**

● **T54.0X** **Toxic effects of phenol and phenol homologues**

● **T54.0X1** Toxic effect of phenol and phenol homologues, accidental (unintentional)
Toxic effects of phenol and phenol homologues NOS

● **T54.0X2** Toxic effect of phenol and phenol homologues, intentional self-harm A, S 🔖

● **T54.0X3** Toxic effect of phenol and phenol homologues, assault

● **T54.0X4** Toxic effect of phenol and phenol homologues, undetermined

● **T54.1** **Toxic effects of other corrosive organic compounds**

● **T54.1X** **Toxic effects of other corrosive organic compounds**

● **T54.1X1** Toxic effect of other corrosive organic compounds, accidental (unintentional)
Toxic effects of other corrosive organic compounds NOS

● **T54.1X2** Toxic effect of other corrosive organic compounds, intentional self-harm A, S 🔖

● **T54.1X3** Toxic effect of other corrosive organic compounds, assault

● **T54.1X4** Toxic effect of other corrosive organic compounds, undetermined

● **T54.2** **Toxic effects of corrosive acids and acid-like substances**
Toxic effects of hydrochloric acid
Toxic effects of sulfuric acid

● **T54.2X** **Toxic effects of corrosive acids and acid-like substances**

● **T54.2X1** Toxic effect of corrosive acids and acid-like substances, accidental (unintentional)
Toxic effects of corrosive acids and acid-like substances NOS

● **T54.2X2** Toxic effect of corrosive acids and acid-like substances, intentional self-harm A, S 🔖

● **T54.2X3** Toxic effect of corrosive acids and acid-like substances, assault

● **T54.2X4** Toxic effect of corrosive acids and acid-like substances, undetermined

● **T54.3** **Toxic effects of corrosive alkalis and alkali-like substances**
Toxic effects of potassium hydroxide
Toxic effects of sodium hydroxide

● **T54.3X** **Toxic effects of corrosive alkalis and alkali-like substances**

● **T54.3X1** Toxic effect of corrosive alkalis and alkali-like substances, accidental (unintentional)
Toxic effects of corrosive alkalis and alkali-like substances NOS

● **T54.3X2** Toxic effect of corrosive alkalis and alkali-like substances, intentional self-harm A, S 🔖

● **T54.3X3** Toxic effect of corrosive alkalis and alkali-like substances, assault

● **T54.3X4** Toxic effect of corrosive alkalis and alkali-like substances, undetermined

● **T54.9** **Toxic effects of unspecified corrosive substance**

X● **T54.91** Toxic effect of unspecified corrosive substance, accidental (unintentional)

X● **T54.92** Toxic effect of unspecified corrosive substance, intentional self-harm A, S 🔖

X● **T54.93** Toxic effect of unspecified corrosive substance, assault

X● **T54.94** Toxic effect of unspecified corrosive substance, undetermined

● **T55** **Toxic effect of soaps and detergents**

The appropriate 7th character is to be added to each code from category T55

A	initial encounter
D	subsequent encounter
S	sequela

● **T55.0** **Toxic effect of soaps**

● **T55.0X** **Toxic effect of soaps**

● **T55.0X1** Toxic effect of soaps, accidental (unintentional)
Toxic effect of soaps NOS

● **T55.0X2** Toxic effect of soaps, intentional self-harm A, S 🔖

● **T55.0X3** Toxic effect of soaps, assault

● **T55.0X4** Toxic effect of soaps, undetermined

● **T55.1** **Toxic effect of detergents**

● **T55.1X** **Toxic effect of detergents**

● **T55.1X1** Toxic effect of detergents, accidental (unintentional)
Toxic effect of detergents NOS

● **T55.1X2** Toxic effect of detergents, intentional self-harm A, S 🔖

● **T55.1X3** Toxic effect of detergents, assault

● **T55.1X4** Toxic effect of detergents, undetermined

● **T56   Toxic effect of metals**

     Includes   toxic effects of fumes and vapors of metals
                   toxic effects of metals from all sources, except
                   medicinal substances

     Use additional code to identify any retained metal foreign
       body, if applicable (Z18.0-, T18.1-)

     Excludes1   arsenic and its compounds (T57.0)
                   manganese and its compounds (T57.2)

     The appropriate 7th character is to be added to each code from
     category T56

         A   initial encounter
         D   subsequent encounter
         S   sequela

● **T56.0   Toxic effects of lead and its compounds**

   ● **T56.0X   Toxic effects of lead and its compounds**

     ● **T56.0X1   Toxic effect of lead and
              its compounds, accidental
              (unintentional)**
                 Toxic effects of lead and its
                     compounds NOS

     ● **T56.0X2   Toxic effect of lead and its
              compounds, intentional
              self-harm A, S** 🐾

     ● **T56.0X3   Toxic effect of lead and its
              compounds, assault**

     ● **T56.0X4   Toxic effect of lead and its
              compounds, undetermined**

● **T56.1   Toxic effects of mercury and its compounds**

   ● **T56.1X   Toxic effects of mercury and its compounds**

     ● **T56.1X1   Toxic effect of mercury and
              its compounds, accidental
              (unintentional)**
                 Toxic effects of mercury and its
                     compounds NOS

     ● **T56.1X2   Toxic effect of mercury and its
              compounds, intentional
              self-harm A, S** 🐾

     ● **T56.1X3   Toxic effect of mercury and its
              compounds, assault**

     ● **T56.1X4   Toxic effect of mercury and its
              compounds, undetermined**

● **T56.2   Toxic effects of chromium and its compounds**

   ● **T56.2X   Toxic effects of chromium and its compounds**

     ● **T56.2X1   Toxic effect of chromium and
              its compounds, accidental
              (unintentional)**
                 Toxic effects of chromium and its
                     compounds NOS

     ● **T56.2X2   Toxic effect of chromium and its
              compounds, intentional self-harm
              A, S** 🐾

     ● **T56.2X3   Toxic effect of chromium and its
              compounds, assault**

     ● **T56.2X4   Toxic effect of chromium and its
              compounds, undetermined**

● **T56.3   Toxic effects of cadmium and its compounds**

   ● **T56.3X   Toxic effects of cadmium and its compounds**

     ● **T56.3X1   Toxic effect of cadmium and
              its compounds, accidental
              (unintentional)**
                 Toxic effects of cadmium and its
                     compounds NOS

     ● **T56.3X2   Toxic effect of cadmium and its
              compounds, intentional self-harm
              A, S** 🐾

     ● **T56.3X3   Toxic effect of cadmium and its
              compounds, assault**

     ● **T56.3X4   Toxic effect of cadmium and its
              compounds, undetermined**

● **T56.4   Toxic effects of copper and its compounds**

   ● **T56.4X   Toxic effects of copper and its compounds**

     ● **T56.4X1   Toxic effect of copper and
              its compounds, accidental
              (unintentional)**
                 Toxic effects of copper and its
                     compounds NOS

     ● **T56.4X2   Toxic effect of copper and its
              compounds, intentional
              self-harm A, S** 🐾

     ● **T56.4X3   Toxic effect of copper and its
              compounds, assault**

     ● **T56.4X4   Toxic effect of copper and its
              compounds, undetermined**

● **T56.5   Toxic effects of zinc and its compounds**

   ● **T56.5X   Toxic effects of zinc and its compounds**

     ● **T56.5X1   Toxic effect of zinc and
              its compounds, accidental
              (unintentional)**
                 Toxic effects of zinc and its
                     compounds NOS

     ● **T56.5X2   Toxic effect of zinc and its
              compounds, intentional
              self-harm A, S** 🐾

     ● **T56.5X3   Toxic effect of zinc and its
              compounds, assault**

     ● **T56.5X4   Toxic effect of zinc and its
              compounds, undetermined**

● **T56.6   Toxic effects of tin and its compounds**

   ● **T56.6X   Toxic effects of tin and its compounds**

     ● **T56.6X1   Toxic effect of tin and its compounds,
              accidental (unintentional)**
                 Toxic effects of tin and its
                     compounds NOS

     ● **T56.6X2   Toxic effect of tin and its compounds,
              intentional self-harm A, S** 🐾

     ● **T56.6X3   Toxic effect of tin and its compounds,
              assault**

     ● **T56.6X4   Toxic effect of tin and its compounds,
              undetermined**

● **T56.7   Toxic effects of beryllium and its compounds**

   ● **T56.7X   Toxic effects of beryllium and its compounds**

     ● **T56.7X1   Toxic effect of beryllium and
              its compounds, accidental
              (unintentional)**
                 Toxic effects of beryllium and its
                     compounds NOS

     ● **T56.7X2   Toxic effect of beryllium and its
              compounds, intentional self-harm
              A, S** 🐾

     ● **T56.7X3   Toxic effect of beryllium and its
              compounds, assault**

     ● **T56.7X4   Toxic effect of beryllium and its
              compounds, undetermined**

● **T56.8   Toxic effects of other metals**

   ● **T56.81   Toxic effect of thallium**

     ● **T56.811   Toxic effect of thallium, accidental
              (unintentional)**
                 Toxic effect of thallium NOS

     ● **T56.812   Toxic effect of thallium, intentional
              self-harm A, S** 🐾

     ● **T56.813   Toxic effect of thallium, assault**

     ● **T56.814   Toxic effect of thallium,
              undetermined**

   ● **T56.89   Toxic effects of other metals**

     ● **T56.891   Toxic effect of other metals, accidental
              (unintentional)**
                 Toxic effects of other metals NOS

     ● **T56.892   Toxic effect of other metals,
              intentional self-harm A, S** 🐾

CHAPTER 19 (S00-T88)

N Newborn Age: 0   **P** Pediatric Age: 0–17   **M** Maternity DX: 9–64   **A** Adult Age: 15–124   ♀ Females Only   ♂ Males Only

🐾 Complication\Comorbidity   🐾 Major C\C   (Ex) CC/MCC Exclusions   🐾 Hospital-Acquired Condition   🐾 Hierarchical Condition Category

1489

CHAPTER 19 (SØØ-T88)

● T56.893 Toxic effect of other metals, assault

● T56.894 Toxic effect of other metals, undetermined

● T56.9 Toxic effects of unspecified metal

X ● T56.91 Toxic effect of unspecified metal, accidental (unintentional)

X ● T56.92 Toxic effect of unspecified metal, intentional self-harm A, S 🩹

X ● T56.93 Toxic effect of unspecified metal, assault

X ● T56.94 Toxic effect of unspecified metal, undetermined

● T57 Toxic effect of other inorganic substances

The appropriate 7th character is to be added to each code from category T57

A	initial encounter
D	subsequent encounter
S	sequela

● T57.Ø Toxic effect of arsenic and its compounds

● T57.ØX Toxic effect of arsenic and its compounds

● T57.ØX1 Toxic effect of arsenic and its compounds, accidental (unintentional)
Toxic effect of arsenic and its compounds NOS

● T57.ØX2 Toxic effect of arsenic and its compounds, intentional self-harm A, S 🩹

● T57.ØX3 Toxic effect of arsenic and its compounds, assault

● T57.ØX4 Toxic effect of arsenic and its compounds, undetermined

● T57.1 Toxic effect of phosphorus and its compounds

Excludes1 organophosphate insecticides (T6Ø.Ø)

● T57.1X Toxic effect of phosphorus and its compounds

● T57.1X1 Toxic effect of phosphorus and its compounds, accidental (unintentional)
Toxic effect of phosphorus and its compounds NOS

● T57.1X2 Toxic effect of phosphorus and its compounds, intentional self-harm A, S 🩹

● T57.1X3 Toxic effect of phosphorus and its compounds, assault

● T57.1X4 Toxic effect of phosphorus and its compounds, undetermined

● T57.2 Toxic effect of manganese and its compounds

● T57.2X Toxic effect of manganese and its compounds

● T57.2X1 Toxic effect of manganese and its compounds, accidental (unintentional)
Toxic effect of manganese and its compounds NOS

● T57.2X2 Toxic effect of manganese and its compounds, intentional self-harm A, S 🩹

● T57.2X3 Toxic effect of manganese and its compounds, assault

● T57.2X4 Toxic effect of manganese and its compounds, undetermined

● T57.3 Toxic effect of hydrogen cyanide

● T57.3X Toxic effect of hydrogen cyanide

● T57.3X1 Toxic effect of hydrogen cyanide, accidental (unintentional)
Toxic effect of hydrogen cyanide NOS

● T57.3X2 Toxic effect of hydrogen cyanide, intentional self-harm A, S 🩹

● T57.3X3 Toxic effect of hydrogen cyanide, assault

● T57.3X4 Toxic effect of hydrogen cyanide, undetermined

● T57.8 Toxic effect of other specified inorganic substances

● T57.8X Toxic effect of other specified inorganic substances

● T57.8X1 Toxic effect of other specified inorganic substances, accidental (unintentional)
Toxic effect of other specified inorganic substances NOS

● T57.8X2 Toxic effect of other specified inorganic substances, intentional self-harm A, S 🩹

● T57.8X3 Toxic effect of other specified inorganic substances, assault

● T57.8X4 Toxic effect of other specified inorganic substances, undetermined

● T57.9 Toxic effect of unspecified inorganic substance

X ● T57.91 Toxic effect of unspecified inorganic substance, accidental (unintentional)

X ● T57.92 Toxic effect of unspecified inorganic substance, intentional self-harm A, S 🩹

X ● T57.93 Toxic effect of unspecified inorganic substance, assault

X ● T57.94 Toxic effect of unspecified inorganic substance, undetermined

● T58 Toxic effect of carbon monoxide

Includes asphyxiation from carbon monoxide
toxic effect of carbon monoxide from all sources

The appropriate 7th character is to be added to each code from category T58

A	initial encounter
D	subsequent encounter
S	sequela

● T58.Ø Toxic effect of carbon monoxide from motor vehicle exhaust
Toxic effect of exhaust gas from gas engine
Toxic effect of exhaust gas from motor pump

X ● T58.Ø1 Toxic effect of carbon monoxide from motor vehicle exhaust, accidental (unintentional)

X ● T58.Ø2 Toxic effect of carbon monoxide from motor vehicle exhaust, intentional self-harm A, S 🩹

X ● T58.Ø3 Toxic effect of carbon monoxide from motor vehicle exhaust, assault

X ● T58.Ø4 Toxic effect of carbon monoxide from motor vehicle exhaust, undetermined

● T58.1 Toxic effect of carbon monoxide from utility gas
Toxic effect of acetylene
Toxic effect of gas NOS used for lighting, heating, cooking
Toxic effect of water gas

X ● T58.11 Toxic effect of carbon monoxide from utility gas, accidental (unintentional)

X ● T58.12 Toxic effect of carbon monoxide from utility gas, intentional self-harm A, S 🩹

X ● T58.13 Toxic effect of carbon monoxide from utility gas, assault

X ● T58.14 Toxic effect of carbon monoxide from utility gas, undetermined

▶ New ⟹ Revised ~~deleted~~ Deleted Excludes 1 Excludes 2 Includes Use additional Code first Code also Key words
OGCR Official Guidelines ● Unacceptable Principal Diagnosis X Assign placeholder X ● Use Additional Character(s) ▷ Manifestation Code Coding Clinic

● T58.2 Toxic effect of carbon monoxide from incomplete
           combustion of other domestic fuels
           Toxic effect of carbon monoxide from incomplete
              combustion of coal, coke, kerosene, wood
  ● T58.2X Toxic effect of carbon monoxide from
             incomplete combustion of other domestic fuels
    ● T58.2X1 Toxic effect of carbon monoxide
                from incomplete combustion of
                other domestic fuels, accidental
                (unintentional)
    ● T58.2X2 Toxic effect of carbon monoxide from
                incomplete combustion of other
                domestic fuels, intentional self-harm
                A, S 🏥
    ● T58.2X3 Toxic effect of carbon monoxide from
                incomplete combustion of other
                domestic fuels, assault
    ● T58.2X4 Toxic effect of carbon monoxide from
                incomplete combustion of other
                domestic fuels, undetermined
● T58.8 Toxic effect of carbon monoxide from other source
           Toxic effect of carbon monoxide from blast furnace gas
           Toxic effect of carbon monoxide from fuels in industrial
              use
           Toxic effect of carbon monoxide from kiln vapor
  ● T58.8X Toxic effect of carbon monoxide from other
             source
    ● T58.8X1 Toxic effect of carbon monoxide
                from other source, accidental
                (unintentional)
    ● T58.8X2 Toxic effect of carbon monoxide from
                other source, intentional self-harm
                A, S 🏥
    ● T58.8X3 Toxic effect of carbon monoxide from
                other source, assault
    ● T58.8X4 Toxic effect of carbon monoxide from
                other source, undetermined
● T58.9 Toxic effect of carbon monoxide from unspecified source
   X ● T58.91 Toxic effect of carbon monoxide from
                unspecified source, accidental (unintentional)
   X ● T58.92 Toxic effect of carbon monoxide from
                unspecified source, intentional self-harm
                A, S 🏥
   X ● T58.93 Toxic effect of carbon monoxide from
                unspecified source, assault
   X ● T58.94 Toxic effect of carbon monoxide from
                unspecified source, undetermined

● T59 Toxic effect of other gases, fumes and vapors
   Includes   aerosol propellants
   Excludes1 chlorofluorocarbons (T53.5)
   The appropriate 7th character is to be added to each code from
      category T59

A	initial encounter
D	subsequent encounter
S	sequela

● T59.0 Toxic effect of nitrogen oxides
  ● T59.0X Toxic effect of nitrogen oxides
    ● T59.0X1 Toxic effect of nitrogen oxides,
                accidental (unintentional)
                Toxic effect of nitrogen oxides NOS
    ● T59.0X2 Toxic effect of nitrogen oxides,
                intentional self-harm A, S 🏥
    ● T59.0X3 Toxic effect of nitrogen oxides, assault
    ● T59.0X4 Toxic effect of nitrogen oxides,
                undetermined

● T59.1 Toxic effect of sulfur dioxide
  ● T59.1X Toxic effect of sulfur dioxide
    ● T59.1X1 Toxic effect of sulfur dioxide,
                accidental (unintentional)
                Toxic effect of sulfur dioxide NOS
    ● T59.1X2 Toxic effect of sulfur dioxide,
                intentional self-harm A, S 🏥
    ● T59.1X3 Toxic effect of sulfur dioxide, assault
    ● T59.1X4 Toxic effect of sulfur dioxide,
                undetermined
● T59.2 Toxic effect of formaldehyde
  ● T59.2X Toxic effect of formaldehyde
    ● T59.2X1 Toxic effect of formaldehyde,
                accidental (unintentional)
                Toxic effect of formaldehyde NOS
    ● T59.2X2 Toxic effect of formaldehyde,
                intentional self-harm A, S 🏥
    ● T59.2X3 Toxic effect of formaldehyde, assault
    ● T59.2X4 Toxic effect of formaldehyde,
                undetermined
● T59.3 Toxic effect of lacrimogenic gas
           Toxic effect of tear gas
  ● T59.3X Toxic effect of lacrimogenic gas
    ● T59.3X1 Toxic effect of lacrimogenic gas,
                accidental (unintentional)
                Toxic effect of lacrimogenic gas NOS
    ● T59.3X2 Toxic effect of lacrimogenic gas,
                intentional self-harm A, S 🏥
    ● T59.3X3 Toxic effect of lacrimogenic gas,
                assault
    ● T59.3X4 Toxic effect of lacrimogenic gas,
                undetermined
● T59.4 Toxic effect of chlorine gas
  ● T59.4X Toxic effect of chlorine gas
    ● T59.4X1 Toxic effect of chlorine gas, accidental
                (unintentional)
                Toxic effect of chlorine gas NOS
    ● T59.4X2 Toxic effect of chlorine gas,
                intentional self-harm A, S 🏥
    ● T59.4X3 Toxic effect of chlorine gas, assault
    ● T59.4X4 Toxic effect of chlorine gas,
                undetermined
● T59.5 Toxic effect of fluorine gas and hydrogen fluoride
  ● T59.5X Toxic effect of fluorine gas and hydrogen fluoride
    ● T59.5X1 Toxic effect of fluorine gas and
                hydrogen fluoride, accidental
                (unintentional)
                Toxic effect of fluorine gas and
                   hydrogen fluoride NOS
    ● T59.5X2 Toxic effect of fluorine gas and
                hydrogen fluoride, intentional
                self-harm A, S 🏥
    ● T59.5X3 Toxic effect of fluorine gas and
                hydrogen fluoride, assault
    ● T59.5X4 Toxic effect of fluorine gas and
                hydrogen fluoride, undetermined
● T59.6 Toxic effect of hydrogen sulfide
  ● T59.6X Toxic effect of hydrogen sulfide
    ● T59.6X1 Toxic effect of hydrogen sulfide,
                accidental (unintentional)
                Toxic effect of hydrogen sulfide NOS
    ● T59.6X2 Toxic effect of hydrogen sulfide,
                intentional self-harm A, S 🏥
    ● T59.6X3 Toxic effect of hydrogen sulfide,
                assault
    ● T59.6X4 Toxic effect of hydrogen sulfide,
                undetermined

● T59.7   Toxic effect of carbon dioxide

  ● T59.7X   Toxic effect of carbon dioxide

    ● T59.7X1   Toxic effect of carbon dioxide, accidental (unintentional)
         Toxic effect of carbon dioxide NOS

    ● T59.7X2   Toxic effect of carbon dioxide, intentional self-harm A, S 🐾

    ● T59.7X3   Toxic effect of carbon dioxide, assault

    ● T59.7X4   Toxic effect of carbon dioxide, undetermined

● T59.8   Toxic effect of other specified gases, fumes and vapors

  ● T59.81   Toxic effect of smoke
     Smoke inhalation

     Excludes2   toxic effect of cigarette (tobacco) smoke (T65.22-)

    ● T59.811   Toxic effect of smoke, accidental (unintentional)
         Toxic effect of smoke NOS

    ● T59.812   Toxic effect of smoke, intentional self-harm A, S 🐾

    ● T59.813   Toxic effect of smoke, assault

    ● T59.814   Toxic effect of smoke, undetermined

  ● T59.89   Toxic effect of other specified gases, fumes and vapors

    ● T59.891   Toxic effect of other specified gases, fumes and vapors, accidental (unintentional)

    ● T59.892   Toxic effect of other specified gases, fumes and vapors, intentional self-harm A, S 🐾

    ● T59.893   Toxic effect of other specified gases, fumes and vapors, assault

    ● T59.894   Toxic effect of other specified gases, fumes and vapors, undetermined

● T59.9   Toxic effect of unspecified gases, fumes and vapors

   X ● T59.91   Toxic effect of unspecified gases, fumes and vapors, accidental (unintentional)

   X ● T59.92   Toxic effect of unspecified gases, fumes and vapors, intentional self-harm A, S 🐾

   X ● T59.93   Toxic effect of unspecified gases, fumes and vapors, assault

   X ● T59.94   Toxic effect of unspecified gases, fumes and vapors, undetermined

● T60   Toxic effect of pesticides

   Includes   toxic effect of wood preservatives

   The appropriate 7th character is to be added to each code from category T60

     A   initial encounter
     D   subsequent encounter
     S   sequela

● T60.0   Toxic effect of organophosphate and carbamate insecticides

  ● T60.0X   Toxic effect of organophosphate and carbamate insecticides

    ● T60.0X1   Toxic effect of organophosphate and carbamate insecticides, accidental (unintentional)
         Toxic effect of organophosphate and carbamate insecticides NOS

    ● T60.0X2   Toxic effect of organophosphate and carbamate insecticides, intentional self-harm A, S 🐾

    ● T60.0X3   Toxic effect of organophosphate and carbamate insecticides, assault

    ● T60.0X4   Toxic effect of organophosphate and carbamate insecticides, undetermined

● T60.1   Toxic effect of halogenated insecticides

   Excludes1   chlorinated hydrocarbon (T53.-)

  ● T60.1X   Toxic effect of halogenated insecticides

    ● T60.1X1   Toxic effect of halogenated insecticides, accidental (unintentional)
         Toxic effect of halogenated insecticides NOS

    ● T60.1X2   Toxic effect of halogenated insecticides, intentional self-harm A, S 🐾

    ● T60.1X3   Toxic effect of halogenated insecticides, assault

    ● T60.1X4   Toxic effect of halogenated insecticides, undetermined

● T60.2   Toxic effect of other insecticides

  ● T60.2X   Toxic effect of other insecticides

    ● T60.2X1   Toxic effect of other insecticides, accidental (unintentional)
         Toxic effect of other insecticides NOS

    ● T60.2X2   Toxic effect of other insecticides, intentional self-harm A, S 🐾

    ● T60.2X3   Toxic effect of other insecticides, assault

    ● T60.2X4   Toxic effect of other insecticides, undetermined

● T60.3   Toxic effect of herbicides and fungicides

  ● T60.3X   Toxic effect of herbicides and fungicides

    ● T60.3X1   Toxic effect of herbicides and fungicides, accidental (unintentional)
         Toxic effect of herbicides and fungicides NOS

    ● T60.3X2   Toxic effect of herbicides and fungicides, intentional self-harm A, S 🐾

    ● T60.3X3   Toxic effect of herbicides and fungicides, assault

    ● T60.3X4   Toxic effect of herbicides and fungicides, undetermined

● T60.4   Toxic effect of rodenticides

   Excludes1   strychnine and its salts (T65.1)
         thallium (T56.81-)

  ● T60.4X   Toxic effect of rodenticides

    ● T60.4X1   Toxic effect of rodenticides, accidental (unintentional)
         Toxic effect of rodenticides NOS

    ● T60.4X2   Toxic effect of rodenticides, intentional self-harm A, S 🐾

    ● T60.4X3   Toxic effect of rodenticides, assault

    ● T60.4X4   Toxic effect of rodenticides, undetermined

● T60.8   Toxic effect of other pesticides

  ● T60.8X   Toxic effect of other pesticides

    ● T60.8X1   Toxic effect of other pesticides, accidental (unintentional)
         Toxic effect of other pesticides NOS

    ● T60.8X2   Toxic effect of other pesticides, intentional self-harm A, S 🐾

    ● T60.8X3   Toxic effect of other pesticides, assault

    ● T60.8X4   Toxic effect of other pesticides, undetermined

● T60.9   Toxic effect of unspecified pesticide

   X ● T60.91   Toxic effect of unspecified pesticide, accidental (unintentional)

   X ● T60.92   Toxic effect of unspecified pesticide, intentional self-harm A, S 🐾

   X ● T60.93   Toxic effect of unspecified pesticide, assault

   X ● T60.94   Toxic effect of unspecified pesticide, undetermined

▶ New   ⇒ Revised   ~~deleted~~ Deleted   Excludes 1   Excludes 2   Includes   Use additional   Code first   Code also   Key words

1492   OGCR Official Guidelines   ● Unacceptable Principal Diagnosis   X Assign placeholder X   ● Use Additional Character(s)   ▶ Manifestation Code   Coding Clinic

● T61 Toxic effect of noxious substances eaten as seafood

> Excludes1 allergic reaction to food, such as:
>> anaphylactic reaction or shock due to adverse
>> food reaction (T78.0-)
>> bacterial foodborne intoxications (A05.-)
>> dermatitis (L23.6, L25.4, L27.2)
>> food protein-induced enterocolitis syndrome
>> (K52.21)
>> food protein-induced enteropathy (K52.22)
>> gastroenteritis (noninfective) (K52.29)
>> toxic effect of aflatoxin and other mycotoxins
>> (T64)
>> toxic effect of cyanides (T65.0-)
>> toxic effect of harmful algae bloom (T65.82-)
>> toxic effect of hydrogen cyanide (T57.3-)
>> toxic effect of mercury (T56.1-)
>> toxic effect of red tide (T65.82-)

The appropriate 7th character is to be added to each code from
category T61

> A   initial encounter
> D   subsequent encounter
> S   sequela

● T61.0 Ciguatera fish poisoning

  X● T61.01 Ciguatera fish poisoning, accidental
  (unintentional)

  X● T61.02 Ciguatera fish poisoning, intentional self-harm
  A, S 🅗

  X● T61.03 Ciguatera fish poisoning, assault

  X● T61.04 Ciguatera fish poisoning, undetermined

● T61.1 Scombroid fish poisoning
  Histamine-like syndrome

  X● T61.11 Scombroid fish poisoning, accidental
  (unintentional)

  X● T61.12 Scombroid fish poisoning, intentional
  self-harm A, S 🅗

  X● T61.13 Scombroid fish poisoning, assault

  X● T61.14 Scombroid fish poisoning, undetermined

● T61.7 Other fish and shellfish poisoning

  ● T61.77 Other fish poisoning

    ● T61.771 Other fish poisoning, accidental
    (unintentional)

    ● T61.772 Other fish poisoning, intentional
    self-harm A, S 🅗

    ● T61.773 Other fish poisoning, assault

    ● T61.774 Other fish poisoning, undetermined

  ● T61.78 Other shellfish poisoning

    ● T61.781 Other shellfish poisoning, accidental
    (unintentional)

    ● T61.782 Other shellfish poisoning, intentional
    self-harm A, S 🅗

    ● T61.783 Other shellfish poisoning, assault

    ● T61.784 Other shellfish poisoning,
    undetermined

● T61.8 Toxic effect of other seafood

  ● T61.8X Toxic effect of other seafood

    ● T61.8X1 Toxic effect of other seafood,
    accidental (unintentional)

    ● T61.8X2 Toxic effect of other seafood,
    intentional self-harm A, S 🅗

    ● T61.8X3 Toxic effect of other seafood, assault

    ● T61.8X4 Toxic effect of other seafood,
    undetermined

● T61.9 Toxic effect of unspecified seafood

  X● T61.91 Toxic effect of unspecified seafood, accidental
  (unintentional)

  X● T61.92 Toxic effect of unspecified seafood, intentional
  self-harm A, S 🅗

  X● T61.93 Toxic effect of unspecified seafood, assault

  X● T61.94 Toxic effect of unspecified seafood,
  undetermined

● T62 Toxic effect of other noxious substances eaten as food

> Excludes1 allergic reaction to food, such as:
>> anaphylactic shock (reaction) due to adverse
>> food reaction (T78.0-)
>> dermatitis (L23.6, L25.4, L27.2)
>> food protein-induced enterocolitis syndrome
>> (K52.21)
>> food protein-induced enteropathy (K52.22)
>> gastroenteritis (noninfective) (K52.29)
>> bacterial food borne intoxications (A05.-)
>> toxic effect of aflatoxin and other mycotoxins
>> (T64)
>> toxic effect of cyanides (T65.0-)
>> toxic effect of hydrogen cyanide (T57.3)
>> toxic effect of mercury (T56.1-)

The appropriate 7th character is to be added to each code from
category T62

> A   initial encounter
> D   subsequent encounter
> S   sequela

● T62.0 Toxic effect of ingested mushrooms

  ● T62.0X Toxic effect of ingested mushrooms

    ● T62.0X1 Toxic effect of ingested mushrooms,
    accidental (unintentional)
      Toxic effect of ingested mushrooms
      NOS

    ● T62.0X2 Toxic effect of ingested mushrooms,
    intentional self-harm A, S 🅗

    ● T62.0X3 Toxic effect of ingested mushrooms,
    assault

    ● T62.0X4 Toxic effect of ingested mushrooms,
    undetermined

● T62.1 Toxic effect of ingested berries

  ● T62.1X Toxic effect of ingested berries

    ● T62.1X1 Toxic effect of ingested berries,
    accidental (unintentional)
      Toxic effect of ingested berries NOS

    ● T62.1X2 Toxic effect of ingested berries,
    intentional self-harm A, S 🅗

    ● T62.1X3 Toxic effect of ingested berries,
    assault

    ● T62.1X4 Toxic effect of ingested berries,
    undetermined

● T62.2 Toxic effect of other ingested (parts of) plant(s)

  ● T62.2X Toxic effect of other ingested (parts of) plant(s)

    ● T62.2X1 Toxic effect of other ingested (parts
    of) plant(s), accidental (unintentional)
      Toxic effect of other ingested (parts
      of) plant(s) NOS

    ● T62.2X2 Toxic effect of other ingested (parts
    of) plant(s), intentional self-harm
    A, S 🅗

    ● T62.2X3 Toxic effect of other ingested (parts
    of) plant(s), assault

    ● T62.2X4 Toxic effect of other ingested (parts
    of) plant(s), undetermined

CHAPTER 19 (S00-T88)

N Newborn Age: 0   P Pediatric Age: 0–17   M Maternity DX: 9–64   A Adult Age: 15–124   ♀ Females Only   ♂ Males Only

🅒 Complication\Comorbidity   🅜 Major C\C   (Ex:) CC/MCC Exclusions   🅗 Hospital-Acquired Condition   🅗 Hierarchical Condition Category

1493

● T62.8   Toxic effect of other specified noxious substances eaten as food

   ● T62.8X   Toxic effect of other specified noxious substances eaten as food

      ● T62.8X1   Toxic effect of other specified noxious substances eaten as food, accidental (unintentional)

          Toxic effect of other specified noxious substances eaten as food NOS

      ● T62.8X2   Toxic effect of other specified noxious substances eaten as food, intentional self-harm A, S 🐾

      ● T62.8X3   Toxic effect of other specified noxious substances eaten as food, assault

      ● T62.8X4   Toxic effect of other specified noxious substances eaten as food, undetermined

● T62.9   Toxic effect of unspecified noxious substance eaten as food

   X ● T62.91   Toxic effect of unspecified noxious substance eaten as food, accidental (unintentional)

       Toxic effect of unspecified noxious substance eaten as food NOS

   X ● T62.92   Toxic effect of unspecified noxious substance eaten as food, intentional self-harm A, S 🐾

   X ● T62.93   Toxic effect of unspecified noxious substance eaten as food, assault

   X ● T62.94   Toxic effect of unspecified noxious substance eaten as food, undetermined

● T63   Toxic effect of contact with venomous animals and plants

   Includes   bite or touch of venomous animal
              pricked or stuck by thorn or leaf

   Excludes2   ingestion of toxic animal or plant (T61.-, T62.-)

   The appropriate 7th character is to be added to each code from category T63

       A   initial encounter
       D   subsequent encounter
       S   sequela

  ● T63.0   Toxic effect of snake venom

   ● T63.00   Toxic effect of unspecified snake venom

      ● T63.001   Toxic effect of unspecified snake venom, accidental (unintentional)

          Toxic effect of unspecified snake venom NOS

      ● T63.002   Toxic effect of unspecified snake venom, intentional self-harm A, S 🐾

      ● T63.003   Toxic effect of unspecified snake venom, assault

      ● T63.004   Toxic effect of unspecified snake venom, undetermined

   ● T63.01   Toxic effect of rattlesnake venom

      ● T63.011   Toxic effect of rattlesnake venom, accidental (unintentional)

          Toxic effect of rattlesnake venom NOS

      ● T63.012   Toxic effect of rattlesnake venom, intentional self-harm A, S 🐾

      ● T63.013   Toxic effect of rattlesnake venom, assault

      ● T63.014   Toxic effect of rattlesnake venom, undetermined

● T63.02   Toxic effect of coral snake venom

      ● T63.021   Toxic effect of coral snake venom, accidental (unintentional)

          Toxic effect of coral snake venom NOS

      ● T63.022   Toxic effect of coral snake venom, intentional self-harm A, S 🐾

      ● T63.023   Toxic effect of coral snake venom, assault

      ● T63.024   Toxic effect of coral snake venom, undetermined

  ● T63.03   Toxic effect of taipan venom

      ● T63.031   Toxic effect of taipan venom, accidental (unintentional)

          Toxic effect of taipan venom NOS

      ● T63.032   Toxic effect of taipan venom, intentional self-harm A, S 🐾

      ● T63.033   Toxic effect of taipan venom, assault

      ● T63.034   Toxic effect of taipan venom, undetermined

  ● T63.04   Toxic effect of cobra venom

      ● T63.041   Toxic effect of cobra venom, accidental (unintentional)

          Toxic effect of cobra venom NOS

      ● T63.042   Toxic effect of cobra venom, intentional self-harm A, S 🐾

      ● T63.043   Toxic effect of cobra venom, assault

      ● T63.044   Toxic effect of cobra venom, undetermined

  ● T63.06   Toxic effect of venom of other North and South American snake

      ● T63.061   Toxic effect of venom of other North and South American snake, accidental (unintentional)

          Toxic effect of venom of other North and South American snake NOS

      ● T63.062   Toxic effect of venom of other North and South American snake, intentional self-harm A, S 🐾

      ● T63.063   Toxic effect of venom of other North and South American snake, assault

      ● T63.064   Toxic effect of venom of other North and South American snake, undetermined

  ● T63.07   Toxic effect of venom of other Australian snake

      ● T63.071   Toxic effect of venom of other Australian snake, accidental (unintentional)

          Toxic effect of venom of other Australian snake NOS

      ● T63.072   Toxic effect of venom of other Australian snake, intentional self-harm A, S 🐾

      ● T63.073   Toxic effect of venom of other Australian snake, assault

      ● T63.074   Toxic effect of venom of other Australian snake, undetermined

  ● T63.08   Toxic effect of venom of other African and Asian snake

      ● T63.081   Toxic effect of venom of other African and Asian snake, accidental (unintentional)

          Toxic effect of venom of other African and Asian snake NOS

      ● T63.082   Toxic effect of venom of other African and Asian snake, intentional self-harm A, S 🐾

      ● T63.083   Toxic effect of venom of other African and Asian snake, assault

      ● T63.084   Toxic effect of venom of other African and Asian snake, undetermined

● T63.09   Toxic effect of venom of other snake
   ● T63.091   Toxic effect of venom of other snake, accidental (unintentional)
       Toxic effect of venom of other snake NOS
   ● T63.092   Toxic effect of venom of other snake, intentional self-harm A, S 🐾
   ● T63.093   Toxic effect of venom of other snake, assault
   ● T63.094   Toxic effect of venom of other snake, undetermined

● T63.1   Toxic effect of venom of other reptiles
  ● T63.11   Toxic effect of venom of gila monster
   ● T63.111   Toxic effect of venom of gila monster, accidental (unintentional)
       Toxic effect of venom of gila monster NOS
   ● T63.112   Toxic effect of venom of gila monster, intentional self-harm A, S 🐾
   ● T63.113   Toxic effect of venom of gila monster, assault
   ● T63.114   Toxic effect of venom of gila monster, undetermined
  ● T63.12   Toxic effect of venom of other venomous lizard
   ● T63.121   Toxic effect of venom of other venomous lizard, accidental (unintentional)
       Toxic effect of venom of other venomous lizard NOS
   ● T63.122   Toxic effect of venom of other venomous lizard, intentional self-harm A, S 🐾
   ● T63.123   Toxic effect of venom of other venomous lizard, assault
   ● T63.124   Toxic effect of venom of other venomous lizard, undetermined
  ● T63.19   Toxic effect of venom of other reptiles
   ● T63.191   Toxic effect of venom of other reptiles, accidental (unintentional)
       Toxic effect of venom of other reptiles NOS
   ● T63.192   Toxic effect of venom of other reptiles, intentional self-harm A, S 🐾
   ● T63.193   Toxic effect of venom of other reptiles, assault
   ● T63.194   Toxic effect of venom of other reptiles, undetermined

● T63.2   Toxic effect of venom of scorpion
  ● T63.2X   Toxic effect of venom of scorpion
   ● T63.2X1   Toxic effect of venom of scorpion, accidental (unintentional)
       Toxic effect of venom of scorpion NOS
   ● T63.2X2   Toxic effect of venom of scorpion, intentional self-harm A, S 🐾
   ● T63.2X3   Toxic effect of venom of scorpion, assault
   ● T63.2X4   Toxic effect of venom of scorpion, undetermined

● T63.3   Toxic effect of venom of spider
  ● T63.30   Toxic effect of unspecified spider venom
   ● T63.301   Toxic effect of unspecified spider venom, accidental (unintentional)
   ● T63.302   Toxic effect of unspecified spider venom, intentional self-harm A, S 🐾
   ● T63.303   Toxic effect of unspecified spider venom, assault
   ● T63.304   Toxic effect of unspecified spider venom, undetermined

● T63.31   Toxic effect of venom of black widow spider
   ● T63.311   Toxic effect of venom of black widow spider, accidental (unintentional)
   ● T63.312   Toxic effect of venom of black widow spider, intentional self-harm A, S 🐾
   ● T63.313   Toxic effect of venom of black widow spider, assault
   ● T63.314   Toxic effect of venom of black widow spider, undetermined
● T63.32   Toxic effect of venom of tarantula
   ● T63.321   Toxic effect of venom of tarantula, accidental (unintentional)
   ● T63.322   Toxic effect of venom of tarantula, intentional self-harm A, S 🐾
   ● T63.323   Toxic effect of venom of tarantula, assault
   ● T63.324   Toxic effect of venom of tarantula, undetermined
● T63.33   Toxic effect of venom of brown recluse spider
   ● T63.331   Toxic effect of venom of brown recluse spider, accidental (unintentional)
   ● T63.332   Toxic effect of venom of brown recluse spider, intentional self-harm A, S 🐾
   ● T63.333   Toxic effect of venom of brown recluse spider, assault
   ● T63.334   Toxic effect of venom of brown recluse spider, undetermined
● T63.39   Toxic effect of venom of other spider
   ● T63.391   Toxic effect of venom of other spider, accidental (unintentional)
   ● T63.392   Toxic effect of venom of other spider, intentional self-harm A, S 🐾
   ● T63.393   Toxic effect of venom of other spider, assault
   ● T63.394   Toxic effect of venom of other spider, undetermined

● T63.4   Toxic effect of venom of other arthropods
  ● T63.41   Toxic effect of venom of centipedes and venomous millipedes
   ● T63.411   Toxic effect of venom of centipedes and venomous millipedes, accidental (unintentional)
   ● T63.412   Toxic effect of venom of centipedes and venomous millipedes, intentional self-harm A, S 🐾
   ● T63.413   Toxic effect of venom of centipedes and venomous millipedes, assault
   ● T63.414   Toxic effect of venom of centipedes and venomous millipedes, undetermined
  ● T63.42   Toxic effect of venom of ants
   ● T63.421   Toxic effect of venom of ants, accidental (unintentional)
   ● T63.422   Toxic effect of venom of ants, intentional self-harm A, S 🐾
   ● T63.423   Toxic effect of venom of ants, assault
   ● T63.424   Toxic effect of venom of ants, undetermined
  ● T63.43   Toxic effect of venom of caterpillars
   ● T63.431   Toxic effect of venom of caterpillars, accidental (unintentional)
   ● T63.432   Toxic effect of venom of caterpillars, intentional self-harm A, S 🐾
   ● T63.433   Toxic effect of venom of caterpillars, assault
   ● T63.434   Toxic effect of venom of caterpillars, undetermined

N Newborn Age: 0   **P** Pediatric Age: 0–17   **M** Maternity DX: 9–64   **A** Adult Age: 15–124   ♀ Females Only   ♂ Males Only

🐾 Complication\Comorbidity   🐾 Major C\C   (Ex) CC/MCC Exclusions   🐾 Hospital-Acquired Condition   🐾 Hierarchical Condition Category

1495

CHAPTER 19 (S00-T88)

● T63.44   Toxic effect of venom of bees
- ● T63.441   Toxic effect of venom of bees, accidental (unintentional)
- ● T63.442   Toxic effect of venom of bees, intentional self-harm A, S 🔖
- ● T63.443   Toxic effect of venom of bees, assault
- ● T63.444   Toxic effect of venom of bees, undetermined

● T63.45   Toxic effect of venom of hornets
- ● T63.451   Toxic effect of venom of hornets, accidental (unintentional)
- ● T63.452   Toxic effect of venom of hornets, intentional self-harm A, S 🔖
- ● T63.453   Toxic effect of venom of hornets, assault
- ● T63.454   Toxic effect of venom of hornets, undetermined

● T63.46   Toxic effect of venom of wasps
Toxic effect of yellow jacket
- ● T63.461   Toxic effect of venom of wasps, accidental (unintentional)
- ● T63.462   Toxic effect of venom of wasps, intentional self-harm A, S 🔖
- ● T63.463   Toxic effect of venom of wasps, assault
- ● T63.464   Toxic effect of venom of wasps, undetermined

● T63.48   Toxic effect of venom of other arthropod
- ● T63.481   Toxic effect of venom of other arthropod, accidental (unintentional)
- ● T63.482   Toxic effect of venom of other arthropod, intentional self-harm A, S 🔖
- ● T63.483   Toxic effect of venom of other arthropod, assault
- ● T63.484   Toxic effect of venom of other arthropod, undetermined

● T63.5   Toxic effect of contact with venomous fish
> **Excludes2**   poisoning by ingestion of fish (T61.-)

● T63.51   Toxic effect of contact with stingray
- ● T63.511   Toxic effect of contact with stingray, accidental (unintentional)
- ● T63.512   Toxic effect of contact with stingray, intentional self-harm A, S 🔖
- ● T63.513   Toxic effect of contact with stingray, assault
- ● T63.514   Toxic effect of contact with stingray, undetermined

● T63.59   Toxic effect of contact with other venomous fish
- ● T63.591   Toxic effect of contact with other venomous fish, accidental (unintentional)
- ● T63.592   Toxic effect of contact with other venomous fish, intentional self-harm A, S 🔖
- ● T63.593   Toxic effect of contact with other venomous fish, assault
- ● T63.594   Toxic effect of contact with other venomous fish, undetermined

● T63.6   Toxic effect of contact with other venomous marine animals
> **Excludes1**   sea-snake venom (T63.09)
>
> **Excludes2**   poisoning by ingestion of shellfish (T61.78-)

⇒● T63.61   Toxic effect of contact with Portuguese Man-o-war
Toxic effect of contact with bluebottle
- ⇒● T63.611   Toxic effect of contact with Portuguese Man-o-war, accidental (unintentional)
- ⇒● T63.612   Toxic effect of contact with Portuguese Man-o-war, intentional self-harm A, S 🔖

- ⇒● T63.613   Toxic effect of contact with Portuguese Man-o-war, assault
- ⇒● T63.614   Toxic effect of contact with Portuguese Man-o-war, undetermined

● T63.62   Toxic effect of contact with other jellyfish
- ● T63.621   Toxic effect of contact with other jellyfish, accidental (unintentional)
- ● T63.622   Toxic effect of contact with other jellyfish, intentional self-harm A, S 🔖
- ● T63.623   Toxic effect of contact with other jellyfish, assault
- ● T63.624   Toxic effect of contact with other jellyfish, undetermined

● T63.63   Toxic effect of contact with sea anemone
- ● T63.631   Toxic effect of contact with sea anemone, accidental (unintentional)
- ● T63.632   Toxic effect of contact with sea anemone, intentional self-harm A, S 🔖
- ● T63.633   Toxic effect of contact with sea anemone, assault
- ● T63.634   Toxic effect of contact with sea anemone, undetermined

● T63.69   Toxic effect of contact with other venomous marine animals
- ● T63.691   Toxic effect of contact with other venomous marine animals, accidental (unintentional)
- ● T63.692   Toxic effect of contact with other venomous marine animals, intentional self-harm A, S 🔖
- ● T63.693   Toxic effect of contact with other venomous marine animals, assault
- ● T63.694   Toxic effect of contact with other venomous marine animals, undetermined

● T63.7   Toxic effect of contact with venomous plant

● T63.71   Toxic effect of contact with venomous marine plant
- ● T63.711   Toxic effect of contact with venomous marine plant, accidental (unintentional)
- ● T63.712   Toxic effect of contact with venomous marine plant, intentional self-harm A, S 🔖
- ● T63.713   Toxic effect of contact with venomous marine plant, assault
- ● T63.714   Toxic effect of contact with venomous marine plant, undetermined

● T63.79   Toxic effect of contact with other venomous plant
- ● T63.791   Toxic effect of contact with other venomous plant, accidental (unintentional)
- ● T63.792   Toxic effect of contact with other venomous plant, intentional self-harm A, S 🔖
- ● T63.793   Toxic effect of contact with other venomous plant, assault
- ● T63.794   Toxic effect of contact with other venomous plant, undetermined

● T63.8   Toxic effect of contact with other venomous animals

● T63.81   Toxic effect of contact with venomous frog
> **Excludes1**   contact with nonvenomous frog (W62.0)
- ● T63.811   Toxic effect of contact with venomous frog, accidental (unintentional)
- ● T63.812   Toxic effect of contact with venomous frog, intentional self-harm A, S 🔖
- ● T63.813   Toxic effect of contact with venomous frog, assault
- ● T63.814   Toxic effect of contact with venomous frog, undetermined

▶ New   ⇒ Revised   ~~deleted~~ Deleted   Excludes1   Excludes2   Includes   Use additional   Code first   Code also   Key words

1496   OGCR Official Guidelines   ● Unacceptable Principal Diagnosis   X Assign placeholder X   ● Use Additional Character(s)   ▶ Manifestation Code   Coding Clinic

● **T63.82**   Toxic effect of contact with venomous toad

    Excludes1   contact with nonvenomous toad (W62.1)

   ● **T63.821**   Toxic effect of contact with venomous toad, accidental (unintentional)

   ● **T63.822**   Toxic effect of contact with venomous toad, intentional self-harm A, S 🐾

   ● **T63.823**   Toxic effect of contact with venomous toad, assault

   ● **T63.824**   Toxic effect of contact with venomous toad, undetermined

● **T63.83**   Toxic effect of contact with other venomous amphibian

    Excludes1   contact with nonvenomous amphibian (W62.9)

   ● **T63.831**   Toxic effect of contact with other venomous amphibian, accidental (unintentional)

   ● **T63.832**   Toxic effect of contact with other venomous amphibian, intentional self-harm A, S 🐾

   ● **T63.833**   Toxic effect of contact with other venomous amphibian, assault

   ● **T63.834**   Toxic effect of contact with other venomous amphibian, undetermined

● **T63.89**   Toxic effect of contact with other venomous animals

   ● **T63.891**   Toxic effect of contact with other venomous animals, accidental (unintentional)

   ● **T63.892**   Toxic effect of contact with other venomous animals, intentional self-harm A, S 🐾

   ● **T63.893**   Toxic effect of contact with other venomous animals, assault

   ● **T63.894**   Toxic effect of contact with other venomous animals, undetermined

● **T63.9**   Toxic effect of contact with unspecified venomous animal

   X● **T63.91**   Toxic effect of contact with unspecified venomous animal, accidental (unintentional)

   X● **T63.92**   Toxic effect of contact with unspecified venomous animal, intentional self-harm A, S 🐾

   X● **T63.93**   Toxic effect of contact with unspecified venomous animal, assault

   X● **T63.94**   Toxic effect of contact with unspecified venomous animal, undetermined

● **T64**   Toxic effect of aflatoxin and other mycotoxin food contaminants

The appropriate 7th character is to be added to each code from category T64

A	initial encounter
D	subsequent encounter
S	sequela

● **T64.0**   Toxic effect of aflatoxin

   X● **T64.01**   Toxic effect of aflatoxin, accidental (unintentional)

   X● **T64.02**   Toxic effect of aflatoxin, intentional self-harm A, S 🐾

   X● **T64.03**   Toxic effect of aflatoxin, assault

   X● **T64.04**   Toxic effect of aflatoxin, undetermined

● **T64.8**   Toxic effect of other mycotoxin food contaminants

   X● **T64.81**   Toxic effect of other mycotoxin food contaminants, accidental (unintentional)

   X● **T64.82**   Toxic effect of other mycotoxin food contaminants, intentional self-harm A, S 🐾

   X● **T64.83**   Toxic effect of other mycotoxin food contaminants, assault

   X● **T64.84**   Toxic effect of other mycotoxin food contaminants, undetermined

● **T65**   Toxic effect of other and unspecified substances

The appropriate 7th character is to be added to each code from category T65

A	initial encounter
D	subsequent encounter
S	sequela

● **T65.0**   Toxic effect of cyanides

    Excludes1   hydrogen cyanide (T57.3-)

   ● **T65.0X**   Toxic effect of cyanides

     ● **T65.0X1**   Toxic effect of cyanides, accidental (unintentional)

      Toxic effect of cyanides NOS

     ● **T65.0X2**   Toxic effect of cyanides, intentional self-harm A, S 🐾

     ● **T65.0X3**   Toxic effect of cyanides, assault

     ● **T65.0X4**   Toxic effect of cyanides, undetermined

● **T65.1**   Toxic effect of strychnine and its salts

   ● **T65.1X**   Toxic effect of strychnine and its salts

     ● **T65.1X1**   Toxic effect of strychnine and its salts, accidental (unintentional)

      Toxic effect of strychnine and its salts NOS

     ● **T65.1X2**   Toxic effect of strychnine and its salts, intentional self-harm A, S 🐾

     ● **T65.1X3**   Toxic effect of strychnine and its salts, assault

     ● **T65.1X4**   Toxic effect of strychnine and its salts, undetermined

● **T65.2**   Toxic effect of tobacco and nicotine

    Excludes2   nicotine dependence (F17.-)

   ● **T65.21**   Toxic effect of chewing tobacco

     ● **T65.211**   Toxic effect of chewing tobacco, accidental (unintentional)

      Toxic effect of chewing tobacco NOS

     ● **T65.212**   Toxic effect of chewing tobacco, intentional self-harm A, S 🐾

     ● **T65.213**   Toxic effect of chewing tobacco, assault

     ● **T65.214**   Toxic effect of chewing tobacco, undetermined

   ● **T65.22**   Toxic effect of tobacco cigarettes

     Toxic effect of tobacco smoke

     Use additional code for exposure to second hand tobacco smoke (Z57.31, Z77.22)

     ● **T65.221**   Toxic effect of tobacco cigarettes, accidental (unintentional)

      Toxic effect of tobacco cigarettes NOS

     ● **T65.222**   Toxic effect of tobacco cigarettes, intentional self-harm A, S 🐾

     ● **T65.223**   Toxic effect of tobacco cigarettes, assault

     ● **T65.224**   Toxic effect of tobacco cigarettes, undetermined

   ● **T65.29**   Toxic effect of other tobacco and nicotine

     ● **T65.291**   Toxic effect of other tobacco and nicotine, accidental (unintentional)

      Toxic effect of other tobacco and nicotine NOS

     ● **T65.292**   Toxic effect of other tobacco and nicotine, intentional self-harm A, S 🐾

     ● **T65.293**   Toxic effect of other tobacco and nicotine, assault

     ● **T65.294**   Toxic effect of other tobacco and nicotine, undetermined

N Newborn Age: 0   **P** Pediatric Age: 0–17   **M** Maternity DX: 9–64   **A** Adult Age: 15–124   ♀ Females Only   ♂ Males Only

🐾 Complication\Comorbidity   🐾 Major C\C   (Ex) CC/MCC Exclusions   🐾 Hospital-Acquired Condition   🐾 Hierarchical Condition Category

1497

● T65.3 Toxic effect of nitroderivatives and aminoderivatives of benzene and its homologues
    Toxic effect of anilin [benzenamine]
    Toxic effect of nitrobenzene
    Toxic effect of trinitrotoluene

● T65.3X Toxic effect of nitroderivatives and aminoderivatives of benzene and its homologues

● T65.3X1 Toxic effect of nitroderivatives and aminoderivatives of benzene and its homologues, accidental (unintentional)
    Toxic effect of nitroderivatives and aminoderivatives of benzene and its homologues NOS

● T65.3X2 Toxic effect of nitroderivatives and aminoderivatives of benzene and its homologues, intentional self-harm A, S 🎾

● T65.3X3 Toxic effect of nitroderivatives and aminoderivatives of benzene and its homologues, assault

● T65.3X4 Toxic effect of nitroderivatives and aminoderivatives of benzene and its homologues, undetermined

● T65.4 Toxic effect of carbon disulfide

● T65.4X Toxic effect of carbon disulfide

● T65.4X1 Toxic effect of carbon disulfide, accidental (unintentional)
    Toxic effect of carbon disulfide NOS

● T65.4X2 Toxic effect of carbon disulfide, intentional self-harm A, S 🎾

● T65.4X3 Toxic effect of carbon disulfide, assault

● T65.4X4 Toxic effect of carbon disulfide, undetermined

● T65.5 Toxic effect of nitroglycerin and other nitric acids and esters
    Toxic effect of 1,2,3-Propanetriol trinitrate

● T65.5X Toxic effect of nitroglycerin and other nitric acids and esters

● T65.5X1 Toxic effect of nitroglycerin and other nitric acids and esters, accidental (unintentional)
    Toxic effect of nitroglycerin and other nitric acids and esters NOS

● T65.5X2 Toxic effect of nitroglycerin and other nitric acids and esters, intentional self-harm A, S 🎾

● T65.5X3 Toxic effect of nitroglycerin and other nitric acids and esters, assault

● T65.5X4 Toxic effect of nitroglycerin and other nitric acids and esters, undetermined

● T65.6 Toxic effect of paints and dyes, not elsewhere classified

● T65.6X Toxic effect of paints and dyes, not elsewhere classified

● T65.6X1 Toxic effect of paints and dyes, not elsewhere classified, accidental (unintentional)
    Toxic effect of paints and dyes NOS

● T65.6X2 Toxic effect of paints and dyes, not elsewhere classified, intentional self-harm A, S 🎾

● T65.6X3 Toxic effect of paints and dyes, not elsewhere classified, assault

● T65.6X4 Toxic effect of paints and dyes, not elsewhere classified, undetermined

● T65.8 Toxic effect of other specified substances

● T65.81 Toxic effect of latex

● T65.811 Toxic effect of latex, accidental (unintentional)
    Toxic effect of latex NOS

● T65.812 Toxic effect of latex, intentional self-harm A, S 🎾

● T65.813 Toxic effect of latex, assault

● T65.814 Toxic effect of latex, undetermined

● T65.82 Toxic effect of harmful algae and algae toxins
    Toxic effect of (harmful) algae bloom NOS
    Toxic effect of blue-green algae bloom
    Toxic effect of brown tide
    Toxic effect of cyanobacteria bloom
    Toxic effect of Florida red tide
    Toxic effect of pfiesteria piscicida
    Toxic effect of red tide

● T65.821 Toxic effect of harmful algae and algae toxins, accidental (unintentional)
    Toxic effect of harmful algae and algae toxins NOS

● T65.822 Toxic effect of harmful algae and algae toxins, intentional self-harm A, S 🎾

● T65.823 Toxic effect of harmful algae and algae toxins, assault

● T65.824 Toxic effect of harmful algae and algae toxins, undetermined

● T65.83 Toxic effect of fiberglass

● T65.831 Toxic effect of fiberglass, accidental (unintentional)
    Toxic effect of fiberglass NOS

● T65.832 Toxic effect of fiberglass, intentional self-harm A, S 🎾

● T65.833 Toxic effect of fiberglass, assault

● T65.834 Toxic effect of fiberglass, undetermined

● T65.89 Toxic effect of other specified substances

● T65.891 Toxic effect of other specified substances, accidental (unintentional)
    Toxic effect of other specified substances NOS
    Coding Clinic: 2018, Q1, P5

● T65.892 Toxic effect of other specified substances, intentional self-harm A, S 🎾

● T65.893 Toxic effect of other specified substances, assault

● T65.894 Toxic effect of other specified substances, undetermined

● T65.9 Toxic effect of unspecified substance

X ● T65.91 Toxic effect of unspecified substance, accidental (unintentional)
    Poisoning NOS

X ● T65.92 Toxic effect of unspecified substance, intentional self-harm A, S 🎾

X ● T65.93 Toxic effect of unspecified substance, assault

X ● T65.94 Toxic effect of unspecified substance, undetermined

OTHER AND UNSPECIFIED EFFECTS OF EXTERNAL CAUSES (T66-T78)

● T66   **Radiation sickness, unspecified**

     Excludes1   specified adverse effects of radiation, such as:
         burns (T20-T31)
         leukemia (C91-C95)
         radiation gastroenteritis and colitis (K52.0)
         radiation pneumonitis (J70.0)
         radiation related disorders of the skin and
           subcutaneous tissue (L55-L59)
         sunburn (L55.-)

     The appropriate 7th character is to be added to code T66

A	initial encounter
D	subsequent encounter
S	sequela

● T67   **Effects of heat and light**

     Excludes1   erythema [dermatitis] ab igne (L59.0)
         malignant hyperpyrexia due to anesthesia (T88.3)
         radiation-related disorders of the skin and
           subcutaneous tissue (L55-L59)

     Excludes2   burns (T20-T31)
         sunburn (L55.-)
         sweat disorder due to heat (L74-L75)

     The appropriate 7th character is to be added to each code from
     category T67

A	initial encounter
D	subsequent encounter
S	sequela

X ● T67.0   **Heatstroke and sunstroke** A 🔾

     Use additional code(s) to identify any associated
         complications of heatstroke, such as:
     coma and stupor (R40.-)
     rhabdomyolysis (M62.82)
     systemic inflammatory response syndrome (R65.1-)
     (Ex) **For category T67.0 CC codes:** See PDX Collection 1419
     Coding Clinic: 2019, Q4, P18

     X ● T67.01   **Heatstroke and sunstroke** A 🔾
         Heat apoplexy
         Heat pyrexia
         Siriasis
         Thermoplegia

     X ● T67.02   **Exertional heatstroke** A 🔾
         Coding Clinic: 2019, Q4, P18

     X ● T67.09   **Other heatstroke and sunstroke** A 🔾

X ● T67.1   **Heat syncope**
     Heat collapse

X ● T67.2   **Heat cramp**

X ● T67.3   **Heat exhaustion, anhydrotic**
     Heat prostration due to water depletion

     Excludes1   heat exhaustion due to salt depletion
             (T67.4)

X ● T67.4   **Heat exhaustion due to salt depletion**
     Heat prostration due to salt (and water) depletion

X ● T67.5   **Heat exhaustion, unspecified**
     Heat prostration NOS

X ● T67.6   **Heat fatigue, transient**

X ● T67.7   **Heat edema**

X ● T67.8   **Other effects of heat and light**

X ● T67.9   **Effect of heat and light, unspecified**

X ● T68   **Hypothermia**
     Accidental hypothermia
     Hypothermia NOS

     Use additional code to identify source of exposure:
         Exposure to excessive cold of man-made origin (W93)
         Exposure to excessive cold of natural origin (X31)

     Excludes1   hypothermia following anesthesia (T88.51)
         hypothermia not associated with low
           environmental temperature (R68.0)
         hypothermia of newborn (P80.-)

     Excludes2   frostbite (T33-T34)

     The appropriate 7th character is to be added to code T68

A	initial encounter
D	subsequent encounter
S	sequela

● T69   **Other effects of reduced temperature**
     Use additional code to identify source of exposure:
         Exposure to excessive cold of man-made origin (W93)
         Exposure to excessive cold of natural origin (X31)

     Excludes2   frostbite (T33-T34)

     The appropriate 7th character is to be added to each code from
     category T69

A	initial encounter
D	subsequent encounter
S	sequela

     ● T69.0   **Immersion hand and foot**

         ● T69.01   **Immersion hand**

             ● T69.011   **Immersion hand, right hand**
             ● T69.012   **Immersion hand, left hand**
             ● T69.019   **Immersion hand, unspecified hand**

         ● T69.02   **Immersion foot**
           Trench foot
           (Ex) **For category T69.02 CC codes:** See PDX Collection 1420

             ● T69.021   **Immersion foot, right foot** A 🔾, A 🔾
             ● T69.022   **Immersion foot, left foot** A 🔾, A 🔾
             ● T69.029   **Immersion foot, unspecified foot** A 🔾, A 🔾

     X ● T69.1   **Chilblains**
     X ● T69.8   **Other specified effects of reduced temperature**
     X ● T69.9   **Effect of reduced temperature, unspecified**

● T70   **Effects of air pressure and water pressure**
     The appropriate 7th character is to be added to each code from
     category T70

A	initial encounter
D	subsequent encounter
S	sequela

     X ● T70.0   **Otitic barotrauma**
         Aero-otitis media
         Effects of change in ambient atmospheric pressure or
           water pressure on ears

     X ● T70.1   **Sinus barotrauma**
         Aerosinusitis
         Effects of change in ambient atmospheric pressure on
           sinuses

     ● T70.2   **Other and unspecified effects of high altitude**

         Excludes2   polycythemia due to high altitude (D75.1)

         X ● T70.20   **Unspecified effects of high altitude**
         X ● T70.29   **Other effects of high altitude**
           Alpine sickness
           Anoxia due to high altitude
           Barotrauma NOS
           Hypobaropathy
           Mountain sickness

CHAPTER 19 (S00-T88)

N Newborn Age: 0   **P** Pediatric Age: 0–17   **M** Maternity DX: 9–64   **A** Adult Age: 15–124   ♀ Females Only   ♂ Males Only

🔾 Complication\Comorbidity   🔾 Major C\C   (Ex) CC/MCC Exclusions   🔾 Hospital-Acquired Condition   🔾 Hierarchical Condition Category

1499

X● **T70.3** **Caisson disease [decompression sickness]** A 🔍, A 🔍
　　　　Compressed-air disease
　　　　Diver's palsy or paralysis
　　　　Ⓔⓧ See PDX Collection 1421

X● **T70.4** **Effects of high-pressure fluids**
　　　　Hydraulic jet injection (industrial)
　　　　Pneumatic jet injection (industrial)
　　　　Traumatic jet injection (industrial)

X● **T70.8** **Other effects of air pressure and water pressure**

X● **T70.9** **Effect of air pressure and water pressure, unspecified**

● **T71** **Asphyxiation**
　　　Mechanical suffocation
　　　Traumatic suffocation

　　　Excludes1 acute respiratory distress (syndrome) (J80)
　　　　　　anoxia due to high altitude (T70.2)
　　　　　　asphyxia NOS (R09.01)
　　　　　　asphyxia from carbon monoxide (T58.-)
　　　　　　asphyxia from inhalation of food or foreign body
　　　　　　　(T17.-)
　　　　　　asphyxia from other gases, fumes and vapors
　　　　　　　(T59.-)
　　　　　　respiratory distress (syndrome) in newborn
　　　　　　　(P22.-)

　　　The appropriate 7th character is to be added to each code from
　　　　category T71

A	initial encounter
D	subsequent encounter
S	sequela

　　　Ⓔⓧ For category T71 CC codes: See PDX Collection 1422

● **T71.1** **Asphyxiation due to mechanical threat to breathing**
　　　　Suffocation due to mechanical threat to breathing

　　● **T71.11** **Asphyxiation due to smothering under pillow**

　　　　● **T71.111** **Asphyxiation due to smothering
　　　　　　under pillow, accidental** A 🔍, A 🔍
　　　　　　Asphyxiation due to smothering
　　　　　　　under pillow NOS

　　　　● **T71.112** **Asphyxiation due to smothering
　　　　　　under pillow, intentional self-harm**
　　　　　　A 🔍, A 🔍, A, S 🔍

　　　　● **T71.113** **Asphyxiation due to smothering
　　　　　　under pillow, assault** A 🔍, A 🔍

　　　　● **T71.114** **Asphyxiation due to smothering
　　　　　　under pillow, undetermined** A 🔍,
　　　　　　A 🔍

　　● **T71.12** **Asphyxiation due to plastic bag**

　　　　● **T71.121** **Asphyxiation due to plastic bag,
　　　　　　accidental** A 🔍, A 🔍
　　　　　　Asphyxiation due to plastic bag
　　　　　　　NOS

　　　　● **T71.122** **Asphyxiation due to plastic bag,
　　　　　　intentional self-harm** A 🔍, A 🔍,
　　　　　　A, S 🔍

　　　　● **T71.123** **Asphyxiation due to plastic bag,
　　　　　　assault** A 🔍, A 🔍

　　　　● **T71.124** **Asphyxiation due to plastic bag,
　　　　　　undetermined** A 🔍, A 🔍

　　● **T71.13** **Asphyxiation due to being trapped in bed
　　　　linens**

　　　　● **T71.131** **Asphyxiation due to being trapped in
　　　　　　bed linens, accidental** A 🔍, A 🔍
　　　　　　Asphyxiation due to being trapped
　　　　　　　in bed linens NOS

　　　　● **T71.132** **Asphyxiation due to being trapped in
　　　　　　bed linens, intentional self-harm**
　　　　　　A 🔍, A 🔍, A, S 🔍

　● **T71.133** **Asphyxiation due to being trapped in
　　　bed linens, assault** A 🔍, A 🔍

　● **T71.134** **Asphyxiation due to being trapped in
　　　bed linens, undetermined** A 🔍, A 🔍

● **T71.14** **Asphyxiation due to smothering under another
　　person's body (in bed)**

　● **T71.141** **Asphyxiation due to smothering
　　　under another person's body (in bed),
　　　accidental** A 🔍, A 🔍
　　　Asphyxiation due to smothering
　　　　under another person's body
　　　　(in bed) NOS

　● **T71.143** **Asphyxiation due to smothering
　　　under another person's body (in bed),
　　　assault** A 🔍, A 🔍

　● **T71.144** **Asphyxiation due to smothering
　　　under another person's body (in bed),
　　　undetermined** A 🔍, A 🔍

● **T71.15** **Asphyxiation due to smothering in furniture**

　● **T71.151** **Asphyxiation due to smothering in
　　　furniture, accidental** A 🔍, A 🔍
　　　Asphyxiation due to smothering in
　　　　furniture NOS

　● **T71.152** **Asphyxiation due to smothering in
　　　furniture, intentional self-harm** A 🔍,
　　　A 🔍, A, S 🔍

　● **T71.153** **Asphyxiation due to smothering in
　　　furniture, assault** A 🔍, A 🔍

　● **T71.154** **Asphyxiation due to smothering in
　　　furniture, undetermined** A 🔍, A 🔍

● **T71.16** **Asphyxiation due to hanging**
　　Hanging by window shade cord

　　Use additional code for any associated injuries,
　　　such as:
　　crushing injury of neck (S17.-)
　　fracture of cervical vertebrae (S12.0-S12.2-)
　　open wound of neck (S11.-)

　● **T71.161** **Asphyxiation due to hanging,
　　　accidental** A 🔍, A 🔍
　　　Asphyxiation due to hanging NOS
　　　Hanging NOS

　● **T71.162** **Asphyxiation due to hanging,
　　　intentional self-harm** A 🔍, A 🔍,
　　　A, S 🔍

　● **T71.163** **Asphyxiation due to hanging, assault**
　　　A 🔍, A 🔍

　● **T71.164** **Asphyxiation due to hanging,
　　　undetermined** A 🔍, A 🔍

● **T71.19** **Asphyxiation due to mechanical**
　　Threat to breathing due to other causes

　● **T71.191** **Asphyxiation due to mechanical
　　　threat to breathing due to other
　　　causes, accidental** A 🔍, A 🔍
　　　Asphyxiation due to other causes
　　　　NOS
　　　Coding Clinic: 2016, Q4, P76

　● **T71.192** **Asphyxiation due to mechanical
　　　threat to breathing due to other
　　　causes, intentional self-harm** A 🔍,
　　　A 🔍, A, S 🔍

　● **T71.193** **Asphyxiation due to mechanical
　　　threat to breathing due to other
　　　causes, assault** A 🔍, A 🔍

　● **T71.194** **Asphyxiation due to mechanical
　　　threat to breathing due to other
　　　causes, undetermined** A 🔍, A 🔍

● **T71.2 Asphyxiation due to systemic oxygen deficiency due to low oxygen content in ambient air**
     Suffocation due to systemic oxygen deficiency due to low oxygen content in ambient air

X ● **T71.20 Asphyxiation due to systemic oxygen deficiency due to low oxygen content in ambient air due to unspecified cause** A 🔿, A 🔿

X ● **T71.21 Asphyxiation due to cave-in or falling earth** A 🔿, A 🔿
     Use additional code for any associated cataclysm (X34-X38)

● **T71.22 Asphyxiation due to being trapped in a car trunk**

     ● **T71.221 Asphyxiation due to being trapped in a car trunk, accidental** A 🔿

     ● **T71.222 Asphyxiation due to being trapped in a car trunk, intentional self-harm** A 🔿, A, S 🔿

     ● **T71.223 Asphyxiation due to being trapped in a car trunk, assault** A 🔿

     ● **T71.224 Asphyxiation due to being trapped in a car trunk, undetermined** A 🔿

● **T71.23 Asphyxiation due to being trapped in a (discarded) refrigerator**

     ● **T71.231 Asphyxiation due to being trapped in a (discarded) refrigerator, accidental** A 🔿

     ● **T71.232 Asphyxiation due to being trapped in a (discarded) refrigerator, intentional self-harm** A 🔿, A, S 🔿

     ● **T71.233 Asphyxiation due to being trapped in a (discarded) refrigerator, assault** A 🔿

     ● **T71.234 Asphyxiation due to being trapped in a (discarded) refrigerator, undetermined** A 🔿

X ● **T71.29 Asphyxiation due to being trapped in other low oxygen environment** A 🔿, A 🔿

X ● **T71.9 Asphyxiation due to unspecified cause** A 🔿, A 🔿
     Suffocation (by strangulation) due to unspecified cause
     Suffocation NOS
     Systemic oxygen deficiency due to low oxygen content in ambient air due to unspecified cause
     Systemic oxygen deficiency due to mechanical threat to breathing due to unspecified cause
     Traumatic asphyxia NOS

● **T73 Effects of other deprivation**
     The appropriate 7th character is to be added to each code from category T73

A	initial encounter
D	subsequent encounter
S	sequela

X ● **T73.0 Starvation**
     Deprivation of food

X ● **T73.1 Deprivation of water**

X ● **T73.2 Exhaustion due to exposure**

X ● **T73.3 Exhaustion due to excessive exertion**
     Exhaustion due to overexertion

X ● **T73.8 Other effects of deprivation**

X ● **T73.9 Effect of deprivation, unspecified**

● **T74 Adult and child abuse, neglect and other maltreatment, confirmed**
     Use additional code, if applicable, to identify any associated current injury
     Use additional external cause code to identify perpetrator, if known (Y07.-)

     Excludes1 abuse and maltreatment in pregnancy (O9A.3-, O9A.4-, O9A.5-)
            adult and child maltreatment, suspected (T76.-)

     The appropriate 7th character is to be added to each code from category T74

A	initial encounter
D	subsequent encounter
S	sequela

(Ex) For category T74 CC codes unless otherwise indicated: See PDX Collection 1423

● **T74.0 Neglect or abandonment, confirmed**

X ● **T74.01 Adult neglect or abandonment, confirmed** A 🔿   A

X ● **T74.02 Child neglect or abandonment, confirmed** A 🔿   P

● **T74.1 Physical abuse, confirmed**
     Excludes2 sexual abuse (T74.2-)

X ● **T74.11 Adult physical abuse, confirmed** A 🔿   A

X ● **T74.12 Child physical abuse, confirmed** A 🔿   P
     Excludes2 shaken infant syndrome (T74.4)

● **T74.2 Sexual abuse, confirmed**
     Rape, confirmed
     Sexual assault, confirmed

X ● **T74.21 Adult sexual abuse, confirmed** A 🔿   A

X ● **T74.22 Child sexual abuse, confirmed** A 🔿   P

● **T74.3 Psychological abuse, confirmed**
     Bullying and intimidation, confirmed
     Intimidation through social media, confirmed

X ● **T74.31 Adult psychological abuse, confirmed**   A

X ● **T74.32 Child psychological abuse, confirmed** A 🔿   P

X ● **T74.4 Shaken infant syndrome** A 🔿   P

● **T74.5 Forced sexual exploitation, confirmed**

X ● **T74.51 Adult forced sexual exploitation, confirmed** 🔿   P

X ● **T74.52 Child sexual exploitation, confirmed** 🔿   P

● **T74.6 Forced labor exploitation, confirmed**

X ● **T74.61 Adult forced labor exploitation, confirmed** 🔿   P

X ● **T74.62 Child forced labor exploitation, confirmed** 🔿   P

● **T74.9 Unspecified maltreatment, confirmed**

X ● **T74.91 Unspecified adult maltreatment, confirmed** A 🔿   A
     (Ex) See PDX Collection 1424

X ● **T74.92 Unspecified child maltreatment, confirmed** A 🔿   P

● **T75 Other and unspecified effects of other external causes**
     Excludes1 adverse effects NEC (T78.-)
     Excludes2 burns (electric) (T20-T31)
     The appropriate 7th character is to be added to each code from category T75

A	initial encounter
D	subsequent encounter
S	sequela

● **T75.0 Effects of lightning**
     Struck by lightning

X ● **T75.00 Unspecified effects of lightning**
     Struck by lightning NOS

X ● **T75.01 Shock due to being struck by lightning**

X ● **T75.09 Other effects of lightning**
     Use additional code for other effects of lightning

N Newborn Age: Ø   **P** Pediatric Age: Ø–17   **M** Maternity DX: 9–64   **A** Adult Age: 15–124   ♀ Females Only   ♂ Males Only

🔿 Complication\Comorbidity   🔿 Major C\C   (Ex) CC/MCC Exclusions   🔿 Hospital-Acquired Condition   🔿 Hierarchical Condition Category

CHAPTER 19 (SØØ-T88)

1501

X● **T75.1**   Unspecified effects of drowning and nonfatal submersion A ⓒ, A ⓒ
     Immersion
     Excludes1   specified effects of drowning code to effects
     ⒺⓍ See PDX Collection 1425

● **T75.2**   Effects of vibration
   X● **T75.20**   Unspecified effects of vibration
   X● **T75.21**   Pneumatic hammer syndrome
   X● **T75.22**   Traumatic vasospastic syndrome
   X● **T75.23**   Vertigo from infrasound
       Excludes1   vertigo NOS (R42)
   X● **T75.29**   Other effects of vibration

X● **T75.3**   Motion sickness
     Airsickness   Travel sickness
     Seasickness
     Use additional external cause code to identify vehicle or type of motion (Y92.81-, Y93.5-)

X● **T75.4**   Electrocution
     Shock from electric current
     Shock from electroshock gun (taser)

● **T75.8**   Other specified effects of external causes
   X● **T75.81**   Effects of abnormal gravitation [G] forces
   X● **T75.82**   Effects of weightlessness
   X● **T75.89**   Other specified effects of external causes

● **T76**   Adult and child abuse, neglect and other maltreatment, suspected
     Use additional code, if applicable, to identify any associated current injury
     Excludes1   adult and child maltreatment, confirmed (T74.-)
                 suspected abuse and maltreatment in pregnancy (O9A.3-, O9A.4-, O9A.5-)
                 suspected adult physical abuse, ruled out (Z04.71)
                 suspected adult sexual abuse, ruled out (Z04.41)
                 suspected child physical abuse, ruled out (Z04.72)
                 suspected child sexual abuse, ruled out (Z04.42)

     The appropriate 7th character is to be added to each code from category T76

A	initial encounter
D	subsequent encounter
S	sequela

     ⒺⓍ **For category T76 CC codes unless otherwise indicated:** See PDX Collection 1423
     Coding Clinic: 2016, Q4, P129

● **T76.0**   Neglect or abandonment, suspected
   X● **T76.01**   Adult neglect or abandonment, suspected A ⓒ   A
   X● **T76.02**   Child neglect or abandonment, suspected A ⓒ   P

● **T76.1**   Physical abuse, suspected
   X● **T76.11**   Adult physical abuse, suspected A ⓒ   A
   X● **T76.12**   Child physical abuse, suspected A ⓒ   P
       Coding Clinic: 2019, Q2, P12

● **T76.2**   Sexual abuse, suspected
     Rape, suspected
     Excludes1   alleged abuse, ruled out (Z04.7)
   X● **T76.21**   Adult sexual abuse, suspected A ⓒ   A
   X● **T76.22**   Child sexual abuse, suspected A ⓒ   P

● **T76.3**   Psychological abuse, suspected
     Bullying and intimidation, suspected
     Intimidation through social media, suspected
   X● **T76.31**   Adult psychological abuse, suspected   A
   X● **T76.32**   Child psychological abuse, suspected A ⓒ   P

● **T76.5**   Forced sexual exploitation, suspected
   X● **T76.51**   Adult forced sexual exploitation, suspected ⓒ   P
   X● **T76.52**   Child sexual exploitation, suspected ⓒ   P

● **T76.6**   Forced labor exploitation, suspected
   X● **T76.61**   Adult forced labor exploitation, suspected ⓒ   P
   X● **T76.62**   Child forced labor exploitation, suspected ⓒ   P

● **T76.9**   Unspecified maltreatment, suspected
   X● **T76.91**   Unspecified adult maltreatment, suspected A ⓒ   A
       ⒺⓍ See PDX Collection 1424
   X● **T76.92**   Unspecified child maltreatment, suspected A ⓒ   P

● **T78**   Adverse effects, not elsewhere classified
     Excludes2   complications of surgical and medical care NEC (T80-T88)
     The appropriate 7th character is to be added to each code from category T78

A	initial encounter
D	subsequent encounter
S	sequela

     ⒺⓍ **For category T78 CC codes:** See PDX Collection 1426

● **T78.0**   Anaphylactic reaction due to food
     Anaphylactic reaction due to adverse food reaction
     Anaphylactic shock or reaction due to nonpoisonous foods
     Anaphylactoid reaction due to food
   X● **T78.00**   Anaphylactic reaction due to unspecified food A ⓒ
   X● **T78.01**   Anaphylactic reaction due to peanuts A ⓒ
   X● **T78.02**   Anaphylactic reaction due to shellfish (crustaceans) A ⓒ
   X● **T78.03**   Anaphylactic reaction due to other fish A ⓒ
   X● **T78.04**   Anaphylactic reaction due to fruits and vegetables A ⓒ
   X● **T78.05**   Anaphylactic reaction due to tree nuts and seeds A ⓒ
       Excludes2   anaphylactic reaction due to peanuts (T78.01)
   X● **T78.06**   Anaphylactic reaction due to food additives A ⓒ
   X● **T78.07**   Anaphylactic reaction due to milk and dairy products A ⓒ
   X● **T78.08**   Anaphylactic reaction due to eggs A ⓒ
   X● **T78.09**   Anaphylactic reaction due to other food products A ⓒ

X● **T78.1**   Other adverse food reactions, not elsewhere classified
     Use additional code to identify the type of reaction, if applicable
     Excludes1   anaphylactic reaction or shock due to adverse food reaction (T78.0-)
                 anaphylactic reaction due to food (T78.0-)
                 bacterial food borne intoxications (A05.-)
     Excludes2   allergic and dietetic gastroenteritis and colitis (K52.29)
                 allergic rhinitis due to food (J30.5)
                 dermatitis due to food in contact with skin (L23.6, L24.6, L25.4)
                 dermatitis due to ingested food (L27.2)
                 food protein-induced enterocolitis syndrome (K52.21)
                 food protein-induced enteropathy (K52.22)

X● **T78.2**   Anaphylactic shock, unspecified A ⓒ
     Occurs when allergic response triggers large quantities of histamines, prostaglandins, leukotrienes resulting in systemic vasodilation
     Allergic shock
     Anaphylactic reaction
     Anaphylaxis
     Excludes1   anaphylactic reaction or shock due to adverse effect of correct medicinal substance properly administered (T88.6)
                 anaphylactic reaction or shock due to adverse food reaction (T78.0-)
                 anaphylactic reaction or shock due to serum (T80.5-)
     ⒺⓍ See PDX Collection 3291

▶ New   ⇒ Revised   ~~deleted~~ Deleted   Excludes 1   Excludes 2   Includes   Use additional   Code first   Code also   Key words
OGCR Official Guidelines   ● Unacceptable Principal Diagnosis   X Assign placeholder X   ● Use Additional Character(s)   ▶ Manifestation Code   **Coding Clinic**

X● **T78.3** **Angioneurotic edema**
        Allergic angioedema
        Giant urticaria
        Vascular disorder resulting from abnormalities of autonomic
          nervous system fibers supplying blood vessels
        Quincke's edema
        Excludes1   serum urticaria (T80.6-)
                   urticaria (L50.-)

● **T78.4** **Other and unspecified allergy**
        Excludes1   specified types of allergic reaction
                    such as:
                  allergic diarrhea (K52.29)
                  allergic gastroenteritis and colitis
                    (K52.29)
                  dermatitis (L23-L25, L27.-)
                  food protein-induced enterocolitis
                    syndrome (K52.21)
                  food protein-induced enteropathy
                    (K52.22)
                  hay fever (J30.1)

    X● **T78.40** **Allergy, unspecified**
            Allergic reaction NOS
            Hypersensitivity NOS

    X● **T78.41** **Arthus phenomenon**
            Arthus reaction

    X● **T78.49** **Other allergy**
            Coding Clinic: 2021, Q1, P42

X● **T78.8** **Other adverse effects, not elsewhere classified**

CERTAIN EARLY COMPLICATIONS OF TRAUMA (T79)

● **T79** **Certain early complications of trauma, not elsewhere classified**
      Excludes2   acute respiratory distress syndrome (J80)
                  complications occurring during or following
                    medical procedures (T80-T88)
                  complications of surgical and medical care NEC
                    (T80-T88)
                  newborn respiratory distress syndrome (P22.0)

      The appropriate 7th character is to be added to each code from
      category T79

A	initial encounter
D	subsequent encounter
S	sequela

X● **T79.0** **Air embolism (traumatic)** A 🔹, A 🔹
        Excludes1   air embolism complicating abortion
                    or ectopic or molar pregnancy
                    (O00-O07, O08.2)
                  air embolism complicating pregnancy,
                    childbirth and the puerperium
                    (O88.0)
                  air embolism following infusion,
                    transfusion, and therapeutic injection
                    (T80.0)
                  air embolism following procedure NEC
                    (T81.7-)
      (Ex) See PDX Collection 1427

X● **T79.1** **Fat embolism (traumatic)** A 🔹, A 🔹
        Excludes1   fat embolism complicating:
                    abortion or ectopic or molar pregnancy
                    (O00-O07, O08.2)
                  pregnancy, childbirth and the
                    puerperium (O88.8)
      (Ex) See PDX Collection 1428

X● **T79.2** **Traumatic secondary and recurrent hemorrhage and seroma** A 🔹, A 🔹
      (Ex) See PDX Collection 1429

X● **T79.4** **Traumatic shock** A 🔹, A 🔹
        Shock (immediate) (delayed) following injury
        Excludes1   anaphylactic shock due to adverse food
                    reaction (T78.0-)
                  anaphylactic shock due to correct
                    medicinal substance properly
                    administered (T88.6)
                  anaphylactic shock due to serum (T80.5-)
                  anaphylactic shock NOS (T78.2)
                  ~~anesthetic shock (T88.2)~~
                  electric shock (T75.4)
                  nontraumatic shock NEC (R57.-)
                  obstetric shock (O75.1)
                  postprocedural shock (T81.1-)
                  septic shock (R65.21)
                  shock complicating abortion or ectopic or
                    molar pregnancy (O00-O07, O08.3)
              ▶ shock due to anesthesia (T88.2)
                  shock due to lightning (T75.01)
                  shock NOS (R57.9)
      (Ex) See PDX Collection 1430

X● **T79.5** **Traumatic anuria** A 🔹, A 🔹
        Crush syndrome
        Renal failure following crushing
      (Ex) See PDX Collection 1431

X● **T79.6** **Traumatic ischemia of muscle** A 🔹
        Traumatic rhabdomyolysis
        Volkmann's ischemic contracture
        Excludes2   anterior tibial syndrome (M76.8)
                  compartment syndrome (traumatic)
                    (T79.A-)
                  nontraumatic ischemia of muscle (M62.2-)

X● **T79.7** **Traumatic subcutaneous emphysema** A 🔹, A 🔹
        Excludes2   emphysema NOS (J43)
                  emphysema (subcutaneous) resulting
                    from a procedure (T81.82)
      (Ex) See PDX Collection 1432

● **T79.A** **Traumatic compartment syndrome**
        Excludes1   fibromyalgia (M79.7)
                  nontraumatic compartment syndrome
                    (M79.A-)
        Excludes2   traumatic ischemic infarction of muscle
                  (T79.6)
      (Ex) **For category T79.A CC codes unless otherwise indicated:** See PDX
        Collection 1433

    X● **T79.A0** **Compartment syndrome, unspecified** A 🔹
            Compartment syndrome NOS
            (Ex) See PDX Collection 3980

    ● **T79.A1** **Traumatic compartment syndrome of upper extremity**
            Traumatic compartment syndrome of shoulder,
              arm, forearm, wrist, hand, and fingers

       ● **T79.A11** **Traumatic compartment syndrome of right upper extremity** A 🔹, A 🔹
                 (Ex) See PDX Collection 3982

       ● **T79.A12** **Traumatic compartment syndrome of left upper extremity** A 🔹, A 🔹
                 (Ex) See PDX Collection 3984

       ● **T79.A19** **Traumatic compartment syndrome of unspecified upper extremity** A 🔹, A 🔹
                 (Ex) See PDX Collection 3985

N Newborn Age: 0   **P** Pediatric Age: 0–17   **M** Maternity DX: 9–64   **A** Adult Age: 15–124   ♀ Females Only   ♂ Males Only

🔹 Complication\Comorbidity   🔹 Major C\C   (Ex) CC/MCC Exclusions   🔹 Hospital-Acquired Condition   🔹 Hierarchical Condition Category

● **T79.A2**   **Traumatic compartment syndrome of lower extremity**
Traumatic compartment syndrome of hip, buttock, thigh, leg, foot, and toes

● **T79.A21**   Traumatic compartment syndrome of right lower extremity A 🔵, A 🔵
(Ex) See PDX Collection 3980

● **T79.A22**   Traumatic compartment syndrome of left lower extremity A 🔵, A 🔵
(Ex) See PDX Collection 3982

● **T79.A29**   Traumatic compartment syndrome of unspecified lower extremity A 🔵

X● **T79.A3**   Traumatic compartment syndrome of abdomen A 🔵, A 🔵
(Ex) See PDX Collection 1434

X● **T79.A9**   Traumatic compartment syndrome of other sites A 🔵, A 🔵
(Ex) See PDX Collection 896

X ● **T79.8**   Other early complications of trauma A 🔵

X ● **T79.9**   Unspecified early complication of trauma A 🔵

COMPLICATIONS OF SURGICAL AND MEDICAL CARE NOT ELSEWHERE CLASSIFIED (T80-T88)

Use additional code for adverse effect, if applicable, to identify drug (T36-T50 with fifth or sixth character 5)

Use additional code(s) to identify the specified condition resulting from the complication.

Use additional code to identify devices involved and details of circumstances (Y62-Y82)

Excludes2   any encounters with medical care for postprocedural conditions in which no complications are present, such as:
artificial opening status (Z93.-)
closure of external stoma (Z43.-)
fitting and adjustment of external prosthetic device (Z44.-)
burns and corrosions from local applications and irradiation (T20-T32)
complications of surgical procedures during pregnancy, childbirth and the puerperium (O00-O9A)
mechanical complication of respirator [ventilator] (J95.850)
poisoning and toxic effects of drugs and chemicals (T36-T65 with fifth or sixth character 1-4 or 6)
postprocedural fever (R50.82)
specified complications classified elsewhere, such as:
cerebrospinal fluid leak from spinal puncture (G97.0)
colostomy malfunction (K94.0-)
disorders of fluid and electrolyte imbalance (E86-E87)
functional disturbances following cardiac surgery (I97.0-I97.1)
intraoperative and postprocedural complications of specified body systems (D78.-, E36.-, E89.-, G97.3-, G97.4, H59.3-, H59.-, H95.2-, H95.3, I97.-, I97.5, J95.6-, J95.7, K91.6-, L76.-, M96.-, N99.-)
ostomy complications (J95.0-, K94.-, N99.5-)
postgastric surgery syndromes (K91.1)
postlaminectomy syndrome NEC (M96.1)
postmastectomy lymphedema syndrome (I97.2)
postsurgical blind-loop syndrome (K91.2)
ventilator associated pneumonia (J95.851)

● **T80**   **Complications following infusion, transfusion and therapeutic injection**

Includes   complications following perfusion

Excludes2   bone marrow transplant rejection (T86.01)
febrile nonhemolytic transfusion reaction (R50.84)
fluid overload due to transfusion (E87.71)
posttransfusion purpura (D69.51)
transfusion associated circulatory overload (TACO) (E87.71)
transfusion (red blood cell) associated hemochromatosis (E83.111)
transfusion related acute lung injury (TRALI) (J95.84)

The appropriate 7th character is to be added to each code from category T80

A	initial encounter
D	subsequent encounter
S	sequela

X● **T80.0**   **Air embolism** following infusion, transfusion and therapeutic injection A 🔵, A 🔵
(Ex) See PDX Collection 1435

X● **T80.1**   **Vascular complications** following infusion, transfusion and therapeutic injection A 🔵
Use additional code to identify the vascular complication

Excludes2   extravasation of vesicant agent (T80.81-)
infiltration of vesicant agent (T80.81-)
vascular complications specified as due to prosthetic devices, implants and grafts (T82.8- T83.8-, T84.8-, T85.8-)
postprocedural vascular complications (T81.7-)
(Ex) See PDX Collection 1436

● **T80.2**   **Infections** following infusion, transfusion and therapeutic injection
Use additional code to identify the specific infection, such as:
sepsis (A41.9)
Use additional code (R65.2-) to identify severe sepsis, if applicable

Excludes2   infections specified as due to prosthetic devices, implants and grafts (T82.6-T82.7, T83.5-T83.6, T84.5-T84.7, T85.7)
postprocedural infections (T81.44)
(Ex) For category T80.2 CC codes: See PDX Collection 948
Coding Clinic: 2018, Q4, P89

● **T80.21**   **Infection due to central venous catheter**
Infection due to pulmonary artery catheter (Swan-Ganz catheter)
Coding Clinic: 2019, Q1, P13-14; 2018, Q4, P89

● **T80.211**   **Bloodstream infection due to central venous catheter** A 🔵, A 🔵
Catheter-related bloodstream infection (CRBSI) NOS
Central line-associated bloodstream infection (CLABSI)
Bloodstream infection due to Hickman catheter
Bloodstream infection due to peripherally inserted central catheter (PICC)
Bloodstream infection due to portacath (port-a-cath)
Bloodstream infection due to pulmonary artery catheter
Bloodstream infection due to triple lumen catheter
Bloodstream infection due to umbilical venous catheter
Coding Clinic: 2018, Q4, P89

▶ New   ⇒ Revised   deleted Deleted   Excludes 1   Excludes 2   Includes   Use additional   Code first   Code also   Key words

OGCR Official Guidelines   ● Unacceptable Principal Diagnosis   X Assign placeholder X   ● Use Additional Character(s)   ▶ Manifestation Code   Coding Clinic

● T80.212   **Local infection due to central venous catheter** A 🅒, A 🅗
     Exit or insertion site infection
     Local infection due to Hickman catheter
     Local infection due to peripherally inserted central catheter (PICC)
     Local infection due to portacath (port-a-cath)
     Local infection due to pulmonary artery catheter
     Local infection due to triple lumen catheter
     Local infection due to umbilical venous catheter
     Port or reservoir infection
     Tunnel infection

● T80.218   **Other infection due to central venous catheter** A 🅒, A 🅗
     Other central line-associated infection
     Other infection due to Hickman catheter
     Other infection due to peripherally inserted central catheter (PICC)
     Other infection due to portacath (port-a-cath)
     Other infection due to pulmonary artery catheter
     Other infection due to triple lumen catheter
     Other infection due to umbilical venous catheter

● T80.219   **Unspecified infection due to central venous catheter** A 🅒, A 🅗
     Central line-associated infection NOS
     Unspecified infection due to Hickman catheter
     Unspecified infection due to peripherally inserted central catheter (PICC)
     Unspecified infection due to portacath (port-a-cath)
     Unspecified infection due to pulmonary artery catheter
     Unspecified infection due to triple lumen catheter
     Unspecified infection due to umbilical venous catheter

X ● T80.22   **Acute infection following transfusion, infusion, or injection of blood and blood products** A 🅒

X ● T80.29   **Infection following other infusion, transfusion and therapeutic injection** A 🅒

● T80.3   **ABO incompatibility reaction due to transfusion of blood or blood products**

     Excludes1   minor blood group antigens reactions (Duffy) (E) (K) (Kell) (Kidd) (Lewis) (M) (N) (P) (S) (T80.A-)
     (Ex) **For category T80.3 CC codes:** See PDX Collection 1437

X ● T80.30   **ABO incompatibility reaction due to transfusion of blood or blood products, unspecified** A 🅒, A 🅗
     ABO incompatibility blood transfusion NOS
     Reaction to ABO incompatibility from transfusion NOS

● T80.31   **ABO incompatibility with hemolytic transfusion reaction**

   ● T80.310   **ABO incompatibility with acute hemolytic transfusion reaction** A 🅒, A 🅗
     ABO incompatibility with hemolytic transfusion reaction less than 24 hours after transfusion
     Acute hemolytic transfusion reaction (AHTR) due to ABO incompatibility

   ● T80.311   **ABO incompatibility with delayed hemolytic transfusion reaction** A 🅒, A 🅗
     ABO incompatibility with hemolytic transfusion reaction 24 hours or more after transfusion
     Delayed hemolytic transfusion reaction (DHTR) due to ABO incompatibility

   ● T80.319   **ABO incompatibility with hemolytic transfusion reaction, unspecified** A 🅒, A 🅗
     ABO incompatibility with hemolytic transfusion reaction at unspecified time after transfusion
     Hemolytic transfusion reaction (HTR) due to ABO incompatibility NOS

X ● T80.39   **Other ABO incompatibility reaction due to transfusion of blood or blood products** A 🅒, A 🅗
     Delayed serologic transfusion reaction (DSTR) from ABO incompatibility
     Other ABO incompatible blood transfusion
     Other reaction to ABO incompatible blood transfusion

● T80.4   **Rh incompatibility reaction due to transfusion of blood or blood products**
     Reaction due to incompatibility of Rh antigens (C) (c) (D) (E) (e)
     (Ex) **For category T80.4 CC codes unless otherwise indicated:** See PDX Collection 1437

X ● T80.40   **Rh incompatibility reaction due to transfusion of blood or blood products, unspecified** A 🅒
     Reaction due to Rh factor in transfusion NOS
     Rh incompatible blood transfusion NOS

● T80.41   **Rh incompatibility with hemolytic transfusion reaction**

   ● T80.410   **Rh incompatibility with acute hemolytic transfusion reaction** A 🅒
     Acute hemolytic transfusion reaction (AHTR) due to Rh incompatibility
     Rh incompatibility with hemolytic transfusion reaction less than 24 hours after transfusion

   ● T80.411   **Rh incompatibility with delayed hemolytic transfusion reaction** A 🅒
     Delayed hemolytic transfusion reaction (DHTR) due to Rh incompatibility
     Rh incompatibility with hemolytic transfusion reaction 24 hours or more after transfusion

   ● T80.419   **Rh incompatibility with hemolytic transfusion reaction, unspecified** A 🅒
     Rh incompatibility with hemolytic transfusion reaction at unspecified time after transfusion
     Hemolytic transfusion reaction (HTR) due to Rh incompatibility NOS

X ● T80.49   **Other Rh incompatibility reaction due to transfusion of blood or blood products** A 🅒
     Delayed serologic transfusion reaction (DSTR) from Rh incompatibility
     Other reaction to Rh incompatible blood transfusion
     (Ex) See PDX Collection 3991

CHAPTER 19 (S00-T88)

● **T80.A** **Non-ABO incompatibility** reaction due to transfusion of **blood or blood products**
Reaction due to incompatibility of minor antigens (Duffy) (Kell) (Kidd) (Lewis) (M) (N) (P) (S)
Ⓔ *For category T80.A CC codes unless otherwise indicated: See PDX Collection 1438*

X● **T80.A0** **Non-ABO incompatibility reaction due to transfusion of blood or blood products, unspecified** A 🖰
Non-ABO antigen incompatibility reaction from transfusion NOS
Ⓔ *See PDX Collection 3993*

● **T80.A1** **Non-ABO incompatibility with hemolytic transfusion reaction**

● **T80.A10** **Non-ABO incompatibility with acute hemolytic transfusion reaction** A 🖰
Acute hemolytic transfusion reaction (AHTR) due to non-ABO incompatibility
Non-ABO incompatibility with hemolytic transfusion reaction less than 24 hours after transfusion

● **T80.A11** **Non-ABO incompatibility with delayed hemolytic transfusion reaction** A 🖰
Delayed hemolytic transfusion reaction (DHTR) due to non-ABO incompatibility
Non-ABO incompatibility with hemolytic transfusion reaction 24 or more hours after transfusion

● **T80.A19** **Non-ABO incompatibility with hemolytic transfusion reaction, unspecified** A 🖰
Hemolytic transfusion reaction (HTR) due to non-ABO incompatibility NOS
Non-ABO incompatibility with hemolytic transfusion reaction at unspecified time after transfusion
Ⓔ *See PDX Collection 3997*

X● **T80.A9** **Other non-ABO incompatibility reaction due to transfusion of blood or blood products** A 🖰
Delayed serologic transfusion reaction (DSTR) from non-ABO incompatibility
Other reaction to non-ABO incompatible blood transfusion
Ⓔ *See PDX Collection 1437*

● **T80.5** **Anaphylactic reaction due to serum**
Allergic reaction due to serum
Anaphylactic shock due to serum
Anaphylactoid reaction due to serum
Anaphylaxis due to serum

Excludes1   ABO incompatibility reaction due to transfusion of blood or blood products (T80.3-)
allergic reaction or shock NOS (T78.2)
anaphylactic reaction or shock NOS (T78.2)
anaphylactic reaction or shock due to adverse effect of correct medicinal substance properly administered (T88.6)
other serum reaction (T80.6-)
Ⓔ *For category T80.5 CC codes: See PDX Collection 1439*

X● **T80.51** **Anaphylactic reaction due to administration of blood and blood products** A 🖰

X● **T80.52** **Anaphylactic reaction due to vaccination** A 🖰
Coding Clinic: 2021, Q1, P43

X● **T80.59** **Anaphylactic reaction due to other serum** A 🖰

● **T80.6** **Other serum reactions**
Intoxication by serum   Serum sickness
Protein sickness   Serum urticaria
Serum rash

Excludes2   serum hepatitis (B16-B19)
Ⓔ *For category T80.6 CC codes unless otherwise indicated: See PDX Collection 1439*

X● **T80.61** **Other serum reaction due to administration of blood and blood products** A 🖰

X● **T80.62** **Other serum reaction due to vaccination** A 🖰
Coding Clinic: 2021, Q1, P42

X● **T80.69** **Other serum reaction due to other serum** A 🖰
Code also, if applicable, arthropathy in hypersensitivity reactions classified elsewhere (M36.4)
Ⓔ *See PDX Collection 1440*

● **T80.8** **Other complications following infusion, transfusion and therapeutic injection**

● **T80.81** **Extravasation of vesicant agent**
Infiltration of vesicant agent
Ⓔ *For category T80.81 CC codes: See PDX Collection 1439*

● **T80.810** **Extravasation of vesicant antineoplastic chemotherapy** A 🖰
Infiltration of vesicant antineoplastic chemotherapy

● **T80.818** **Extravasation of other vesicant agent** A 🖰
Infiltration of other vesicant agent

▶**T80.82 Complication of immune effector cellular therapy**
▶Complication of chimeric antigen receptor (CAR-T) cell therapy
▶Complication of IEC therapy

▶**Excludes2**   complication of bone marrow transplant (T86.0)
▶complication of stem cell transplant (T86.5)

▶Use additional code to identify the specific complication, such as:
▶cytokine release syndrome (D89.83-)
▶immune effector cell-associated neurotoxicity syndrome (G92.0-)

X● **T80.89** **Other complications following infusion, transfusion and therapeutic injection**
Delayed serologic transfusion reaction (DSTR), unspecified incompatibility
Use additional code to identify graft-versus-host reaction, if applicable, (D89.81-)

● **T80.9** **Unspecified complication following infusion, transfusion and therapeutic injection**

X● **T80.90** **Unspecified complication following infusion and therapeutic injection**

● **T80.91** **Hemolytic transfusion reaction, unspecified incompatibility**

Excludes1   ABO incompatibility with hemolytic transfusion reaction (T80.31-)
Non-ABO incompatibility with hemolytic transfusion reaction (T80.A1-)
Rh incompatibility with hemolytic transfusion reaction (T80.41-)
Ⓔ *For category T80.91 CC codes: See PDX Collection 1437*

● **T80.910** **Acute hemolytic transfusion reaction, unspecified incompatibility** A 🖰

● **T80.911** **Delayed hemolytic transfusion reaction, unspecified incompatibility** A 🖰

● **T80.919** **Hemolytic transfusion reaction, unspecified incompatibility, unspecified as acute or delayed** A 🖰
Hemolytic transfusion reaction NOS

X● **T80.92** **Unspecified transfusion reaction**
Transfusion reaction NOS

▶ New   ▥ Revised   deleted Deleted   Excludes 1   Excludes 2   Includes   Use additional   Code first   Code also   Key words
OGCR Official Guidelines   ● Unacceptable Principal Diagnosis   X Assign placeholder X   ● Use Additional Character(s)   ▶ Manifestation Code   Coding Clinic

● T81   **Complications of procedures, not elsewhere classified**

> Use additional code for adverse effect, if applicable, to identify drug (T36-T50 with fifth or sixth character 5)
>
> **Excludes2**   complications following immunization (T88.0-T88.1)
>> complications following infusion, transfusion and therapeutic injection (T80.-)
>> complications of transplanted organs and tissue (T86.-)
>> poisoning and toxic effects of drugs and chemicals (T36-T65 with fifth or sixth character 1-4 or 6)
>> specified complications classified elsewhere, such as:
>>> complication of prosthetic devices, implants and grafts (T82-T85)
>>> dermatitis due to drugs and medicaments (L23.3, L24.4, L25.1, L27.0-L27.1)
>>> endosseous dental implant failure (M27.6-)
>>> floppy iris syndrome (IFIS) (intraoperative) H21.81
>>> intraoperative and postprocedural complications of specific body system (D78.-, E36.-, E89.-, G97.3-, G97.4, H59.3-, H59.-, H95.2-, H95.3, I97.4-, I97.5, J95, K91.-, L76.-, M96.-, N99.-)
>>> ostomy complications (J95.0-, K94.-, N99.5-)
>>> plateau iris syndrome (post-iridectomy) (postprocedural) H21.82

> **Coding Clinic: 2019, Q2, P21-22; 2016, Q4, P29**

> The appropriate 7th character is to be added to each code from category T81

> | | |
> |---|---|
> | A | initial encounter |
> | D | subsequent encounter |
> | S | sequela |

● **T81.1   Postprocedural shock**

> Shock during or resulting from a procedure, not elsewhere classified
>
> **Excludes1**   anaphylactic shock NOS (T78.2)
>> anaphylactic shock due to correct substance properly administered (T88.6)
>> anaphylactic shock due to serum (T80.5-)
>> ~~anesthetic shock (T88.2)~~
>> electric shock (T75.4)
>> obstetric shock (O75.1)
>> septic shock (R65.21)
>> ▶shock due to anesthesia (T88.2)
>> shock following abortion or ectopic or molar pregnancy (O00-O07, O08.3)
>> traumatic shock (T79.4)

> (Ex) **For category T81.1 CC codes:** See PDX Collection 1441

X ● **T81.10   Postprocedural shock unspecified** A 🦠

> Collapse NOS during or resulting from a procedure, not elsewhere classified
> Postprocedural failure of peripheral circulation
> Postprocedural shock NOS

X ● **T81.11   Postprocedural cardiogenic shock** A 🦠, A 🦠

● X ● **T81.12   Postprocedural septic shock** A 🦠, A 🦠

> Postprocedural endotoxic shock resulting from a procedure, not elsewhere classified
> Postprocedural gram-negative shock resulting from a procedure, not elsewhere classified
>
> *Code first underlying infection*
> Use additional code, to identify any associated acute organ dysfunction, if applicable

X ● **T81.19   Other postprocedural shock** A 🦠

> Postprocedural hypovolemic shock
> **Coding Clinic: 2021, Q1, P14**

● **T81.3   Disruption of wound, not elsewhere classified**

> Disruption of any suture materials or other closure methods
>
> **Excludes1**   breakdown (mechanical) of permanent sutures (T85.612)
>> displacement of permanent sutures (T85.622)
>> disruption of cesarean delivery wound (O90.0)
>> disruption of perineal obstetric wound (O90.1)
>> mechanical complication of permanent sutures NEC (T85.692)

> (Ex) **For category T81.3 CC codes:** See PDX Collection 1442

X ● **T81.30   Disruption of wound, unspecified** A 🦠

> Disruption of wound NOS

X ● **T81.31   Disruption of external operation (surgical) wound, not elsewhere classified** A 🦠

> **Excludes1**   dehiscence of amputation stump (T87.81)
> Dehiscence of operation wound NOS
> Disruption of operation wound NOS
> Disruption or dehiscence of closure of cornea
> Disruption or dehiscence of closure of mucosa
> Disruption or dehiscence of closure of skin and subcutaneous tissue
> Full-thickness skin disruption or dehiscence
> Superficial disruption or dehiscence of operation wound
> **Coding Clinic: 2015, Q1, P20**

X ● **T81.32   Disruption of internal operation (surgical) wound, not elsewhere classified** A 🦠

> Deep disruption or dehiscence of operation wound NOS
> Disruption or dehiscence of closure of internal organ or other internal tissue
> Disruption or dehiscence of closure of muscle or muscle flap
> Disruption or dehiscence of closure of ribs or rib cage
> Disruption or dehiscence of closure of skull or craniotomy
> Disruption or dehiscence of closure of sternum or sternotomy
> Disruption or dehiscence of closure of tendon or ligament
> Disruption or dehiscence of closure of superficial or muscular fascia
> **Coding Clinic: 2017, Q3, P4**

X ● **T81.33   Disruption of traumatic injury wound repair** A 🦠

> Disruption or dehiscence of closure of traumatic laceration (external) (internal)

N Newborn Age: 0   **P** Pediatric Age: 0–17   **M** Maternity DX: 9–64   **A** Adult Age: 15–124   ♀ Females Only   ♂ Males Only

🦠 Complication\Comorbidity   🦠 Major C\C   (Ex) CC/MCC Exclusions   🦠 Hospital-Acquired Condition   🦠 Hierarchical Condition Category

1507

CHAPTER 19 (S00-T88)

CHAPTER 19 (S00-T88)

● **T81.4**   **Infection following a procedure** A ⓒ

     Use additional code to identify infection

     Use additional code (R65.2-) to identify severe sepsis, if applicable

     Excludes2   bleb associated endophthalmitis (H59.4-)

                infection due to infusion, transfusion and therapeutic injection (T80.2-)

                infection due to prosthetic devices, implants and grafts (T82.6-T82.7, T83.5-T83.6, T84.5-T84.7, T85.7)

                obstetric surgical wound infection (O86.0-)

                postprocedural fever NOS (R50.82)

                postprocedural retroperitoneal abscess (K68.11)

X ● **T81.40**   **Infection following a procedure, unspecified** A ⓒ, A ⓠ

            (Ex:) See PDX Collection 805

X ● **T81.41**   **Infection following a procedure, superficial incisional surgical site** A ⓒ, A ⓠ

            Subcutaneous abscess following a procedure

            Stitch abscess following a procedure

            (Ex:) See PDX Collection 805

            Coding Clinic: 2018, Q4, P34

X ● **T81.42**   **Infection following a procedure, deep incisional surgical site** A ⓒ, A ⓠ

            Intra-muscular abscess following a procedure

            (Ex:) See PDX Collection 805

X ● **T81.43**   **Infection following a procedure, organ and space surgical site** A ⓒ, A ⓠ

            Intra-abdominal abscess following a procedure

            Subphrenic abscess following a procedure

            (Ex:) See PDX Collection 805

X ● **T81.44**   **Sepsis following a procedure** A ⓒ, A ⓠ, A ⓠ

            Use additional code to identify the sepsis

            (Ex:) See PDX Collection 805

X ● **T81.49**   **Infection following a procedure, other surgical site** A ⓒ, A ⓠ

            (Ex:) See PDX Collection 805

            Coding Clinic: 2015, Q4, P37

● **T81.5**   **Complications of foreign body accidentally left in body following procedure**

            (Ex:) **For category T81.5 CC codes:** See PDX Collection 1443

   ● **T81.50**   **Unspecified complication of foreign body accidentally left in body following procedure**

     ● **T81.500**   Unspecified complication of foreign body accidentally left in body following **surgical operation** A ⓒ, A ⓠ

     ● **T81.501**   Unspecified complication of foreign body accidentally left in body following **infusion or transfusion** A ⓒ, A ⓠ

     ● **T81.502**   Unspecified complication of foreign body accidentally left in body following **kidney dialysis** A ⓒ, A ⓠ, A, D, S ⓠ

     ● **T81.503**   Unspecified complication of foreign body accidentally left in body following **injection or immunization** A ⓒ, A ⓠ

     ● **T81.504**   Unspecified complication of foreign body accidentally left in body following **endoscopic examination** A ⓒ, A ⓠ

     ● **T81.505**   Unspecified complication of foreign body accidentally left in body following **heart catheterization** A ⓒ, A ⓠ

     ● **T81.506**   Unspecified complication of foreign body accidentally left in body following **aspiration, puncture or other catheterization** A ⓒ, A ⓠ

     ● **T81.507**   Unspecified complication of foreign body accidentally left in body following **removal of catheter or packing** A ⓒ, A ⓠ

     ● **T81.508**   Unspecified complication of foreign body accidentally left in body following **other procedure** A ⓒ, A ⓠ

     ● **T81.509**   Unspecified complication of foreign body accidentally left in body following **unspecified procedure** A ⓒ, A ⓠ

   ● **T81.51**   **Adhesions** due to foreign body accidentally left in body following procedure

     ● **T81.510**   **Adhesions due to foreign body accidentally left in body following surgical operation** A ⓒ, A ⓠ

     ● **T81.511**   **Adhesions due to foreign body accidentally left in body following infusion or transfusion** A ⓒ, A ⓠ

     ● **T81.512**   **Adhesions due to foreign body accidentally left in body following kidney dialysis** A ⓒ, A ⓠ, A, D, S ⓠ

     ● **T81.513**   **Adhesions due to foreign body accidentally left in body following injection or immunization** A ⓒ, A ⓠ

     ● **T81.514**   **Adhesions due to foreign body accidentally left in body following endoscopic examination** A ⓒ, A ⓠ

     ● **T81.515**   **Adhesions due to foreign body accidentally left in body following heart catheterization** A ⓒ, A ⓠ

     ● **T81.516**   **Adhesions due to foreign body accidentally left in body following aspiration, puncture or other catheterization** A ⓒ, A ⓠ

     ● **T81.517**   **Adhesions due to foreign body accidentally left in body following removal of catheter or packing** A ⓒ, A ⓠ

     ● **T81.518**   **Adhesions due to foreign body accidentally left in body following other procedure** A ⓒ, A ⓠ

     ● **T81.519**   **Adhesions due to foreign body accidentally left in body following unspecified procedure** A ⓒ, A ⓠ

   ● **T81.52**   **Obstruction** due to foreign body accidentally left in body following procedure

     ● **T81.520**   **Obstruction due to foreign body accidentally left in body following surgical operation** A ⓒ, A ⓠ

     ● **T81.521**   **Obstruction due to foreign body accidentally left in body following infusion or transfusion** A ⓒ, A ⓠ

     ● **T81.522**   **Obstruction due to foreign body accidentally left in body following kidney dialysis** A ⓒ, A ⓠ, A, D, S ⓠ

     ● **T81.523**   **Obstruction due to foreign body accidentally left in body following injection or immunization** A ⓒ, A ⓠ

     ● **T81.524**   **Obstruction due to foreign body accidentally left in body following endoscopic examination** A ⓒ, A ⓠ

     ● **T81.525**   **Obstruction due to foreign body accidentally left in body following heart catheterization** A ⓒ, A ⓠ

▶ New   ⇒ Revised   ~~deleted~~ Deleted   Excludes 1   Excludes 2   Includes   Use additional   Code first   Code also   Key words

OGCR Official Guidelines   ● Unacceptable Principal Diagnosis   X Assign placeholder X   ● Use Additional Character(s)   ▶ Manifestation Code   **Coding Clinic**

● T81.526   Obstruction due to foreign body accidentally left in body following aspiration, puncture or other catheterization A ⬤, A ⬤

● T81.527   Obstruction due to foreign body accidentally left in body following removal of catheter or packing A ⬤, A ⬤

● T81.528   Obstruction due to foreign body accidentally left in body following other procedure A ⬤, A ⬤

● T81.529   Obstruction due to foreign body accidentally left in body following unspecified procedure A ⬤, A ⬤

● T81.53   Perforation due to foreign body accidentally left in body following procedure

● T81.530   Perforation due to foreign body accidentally left in body following surgical operation A ⬤, A ⬤

● T81.531   Perforation due to foreign body accidentally left in body following infusion or transfusion A ⬤, A ⬤

● T81.532   Perforation due to foreign body accidentally left in body following kidney dialysis A ⬤, A ⬤, A, D, S ⬤

● T81.533   Perforation due to foreign body accidentally left in body following injection or immunization A ⬤, A ⬤

● T81.534   Perforation due to foreign body accidentally left in body following endoscopic examination A ⬤, A ⬤

● T81.535   Perforation due to foreign body accidentally left in body following heart catheterization A ⬤, A ⬤

● T81.536   Perforation due to foreign body accidentally left in body following aspiration, puncture or other catheterization A ⬤, A ⬤

● T81.537   Perforation due to foreign body accidentally left in body following removal of catheter or packing A ⬤, A ⬤

● T81.538   Perforation due to foreign body accidentally left in body following other procedure A ⬤, A ⬤

● T81.539   Perforation due to foreign body accidentally left in body following unspecified procedure A ⬤, A ⬤

● T81.59   Other complications of foreign body accidentally left in body following procedure

Excludes2   obstruction or perforation due to prosthetic devices and implants intentionally left in body (T82.0-T82.5, T83.0-T83.4, T83.7, T84.0-T84.4, T85.0-T85.6)

● T81.590   Other complications of foreign body accidentally left in body following surgical operation A ⬤, A ⬤

● T81.591   Other complications of foreign body accidentally left in body following infusion or transfusion A ⬤, A ⬤

● T81.592   Other complications of foreign body accidentally left in body following kidney dialysis A ⬤, A ⬤, A, D, S ⬤

● T81.593   Other complications of foreign body accidentally left in body following injection or immunization A ⬤, A ⬤

● T81.594   Other complications of foreign body accidentally left in body following endoscopic examination A ⬤, A ⬤

● T81.595   Other complications of foreign body accidentally left in body following heart catheterization A ⬤, A ⬤

● T81.596   Other complications of foreign body accidentally left in body following aspiration, puncture or other catheterization A ⬤, A ⬤

● T81.597   Other complications of foreign body accidentally left in body following removal of catheter or packing A ⬤, A ⬤

● T81.598   Other complications of foreign body accidentally left in body following other procedure A ⬤, A ⬤

● T81.599   Other complications of foreign body accidentally left in body following unspecified procedure A ⬤, A ⬤

● T81.6   Acute reaction to foreign substance accidentally left during a procedure

Excludes2   complications of foreign body accidentally left in body cavity or operation wound following procedure (T81.5-)

(Ex) For category T81.6 CC codes: See PDX Collection 1444

X● T81.60   Unspecified acute reaction to foreign substance accidentally left during a procedure A ⬤, A ⬤

X● T81.61   Aseptic peritonitis due to foreign substance accidentally left during a procedure A ⬤, A ⬤
Chemical peritonitis

X● T81.69   Other acute reaction to foreign substance accidentally left during a procedure A ⬤, A ⬤

● T81.7   Vascular complications following a procedure, not elsewhere classified
Air embolism following procedure NEC
Phlebitis or thrombophlebitis resulting from a procedure

Excludes1   embolism complicating abortion or ectopic or molar pregnancy (O00-O07, O08.2)
embolism complicating pregnancy, childbirth and the puerperium (O88.-)
traumatic embolism (T79.0)

Excludes2   embolism due to prosthetic devices, implants and grafts (T82.8, T83.81, T84.8-, T85.1-)
embolism following infusion, transfusion and therapeutic injection (T80.0)

Coding Clinic: 2019, Q2, P23

● T81.71   Complication of artery following a procedure, not elsewhere classified
Coding Clinic: 2019, Q2, P22

● T81.710   Complication of mesenteric artery following a procedure, not elsewhere classified A ⬤
(Ex) See PDX Collection 1445

● T81.711   Complication of renal artery following a procedure, not elsewhere classified A ⬤
(Ex) See PDX Collection 1445

● T81.718   Complication of other artery following a procedure, not elsewhere classified A ⬤
(Ex) See PDX Collection 1446
Coding Clinic: 2019, Q2, P22-23

● T81.719   Complication of unspecified artery following a procedure, not elsewhere classified A ⬤
(Ex) See PDX Collection 1446

X● T81.72   Complication of vein following a procedure, not elsewhere classified A ⬤
(Ex) See PDX Collection 1446
Coding Clinic: 2019, Q2, P22

N Newborn Age: 0   P Pediatric Age: 0–17   M Maternity DX: 9–64   A Adult Age: 15–124   ♀ Females Only   ♂ Males Only
⬤ Complication\Comorbidity   ⬤ Major C\C   (Ex) CC/MCC Exclusions   ⬤ Hospital-Acquired Condition   ⬤ Hierarchical Condition Category

CHAPTER 19 (S00-T88)

1509

● **T81.8** Other complications of procedures, not elsewhere classified

     Excludes2 hypothermia following anesthesia (T88.51)

               malignant hyperpyrexia due to anesthesia (T88.3)

X● **T81.81** Complication of inhalation therapy

X● **T81.82** Emphysema (subcutaneous) resulting from a procedure

X● **T81.83** Persistent postprocedural fistula A 🅒
     (Ex:) See PDX Collection 1447
     Coding Clinic: 2017, Q3, P3-5

X● **T81.89** Other complications of procedures, not elsewhere classified

     Use additional code to specify complication, such as:
         postprocedural delirium (F05)

X● **T81.9** Unspecified complication of procedure

● **T82** Complications of cardiac and vascular prosthetic devices, implants and grafts

     Excludes2 failure and rejection of transplanted organs and tissue (T86.-)

     The appropriate 7th character is to be added to each code from category T82

> A   initial encounter
> D   subsequent encounter
> S   sequela

● **T82.0** Mechanical complication of heart valve prosthesis
     Mechanical complication of artificial heart valve

     Excludes1 mechanical complication of biological heart valve graft (T82.22-)
     (Ex:) **For category T82.0 CC codes:** See PDX Collection 1448

X● **T82.01** Breakdown (mechanical) of heart valve prosthesis A 🅒

X● **T82.02** Displacement of heart valve prosthesis A 🅒
     Malposition of heart valve prosthesis

X● **T82.03** Leakage of heart valve prosthesis A 🅒

X● **T82.09** Other mechanical complication of heart valve prosthesis A 🅒
     Obstruction (mechanical) of heart valve prosthesis
     Perforation of heart valve prosthesis
     Protrusion of heart valve prosthesis

● **T82.1** Mechanical complication of cardiac electronic device
     (Ex:) **For category T82.1 CC codes unless otherwise indicated:** See PDX Collection 1449

● **T82.11** Breakdown (mechanical) of cardiac electronic device

     ● **T82.110** Breakdown (mechanical) of cardiac electrode A 🅒

     ● **T82.111** Breakdown (mechanical) of cardiac pulse generator (battery) A 🅒

     ● **T82.118** Breakdown (mechanical) of other cardiac electronic device A 🅒
         (Ex:) See PDX Collection 1450

     ● **T82.119** Breakdown (mechanical) of unspecified cardiac electronic device A 🅒
         (Ex:) See PDX Collection 3241

● **T82.12** Displacement of cardiac electronic device
     Malposition of cardiac electronic device

     ● **T82.120** Displacement of cardiac electrode A 🅒

     ● **T82.121** Displacement of cardiac pulse generator (battery) A 🅒

● **T82.128** Displacement of other cardiac electronic device A 🅒
     (Ex:) See PDX Collection 1450

● **T82.129** Displacement of unspecified cardiac electronic device A 🅒
     (Ex:) See PDX Collection 3242

● **T82.19** Other mechanical complication of cardiac electronic device
     Leakage of cardiac electronic device
     Obstruction of cardiac electronic device
     Perforation of cardiac electronic device
     Protrusion of cardiac electronic device

     ● **T82.190** Other mechanical complication of cardiac electrode A 🅒

     ● **T82.191** Other mechanical complication of cardiac pulse generator (battery) A 🅒

     ● **T82.198** Other mechanical complication of other cardiac electronic device A 🅒
         (Ex:) See PDX Collection 1450

     ● **T82.199** Other mechanical complication of unspecified cardiac device A 🅒
         (Ex:) See PDX Collection 3243

● **T82.2** Mechanical complication of coronary artery bypass graft and biological heart valve graft

     Excludes1 mechanical complication of artificial heart valve prosthesis (T82.0-)

● **T82.21** Mechanical complication of coronary artery bypass graft
     (Ex:) **For category T82.21 CC codes:** See PDX Collection 1451

     ● **T82.211** Breakdown (mechanical) of coronary artery bypass graft A 🅒

     ● **T82.212** Displacement of coronary artery bypass graft A 🅒
         Malposition of coronary artery bypass graft

     ● **T82.213** Leakage of coronary artery bypass graft A 🅒

     ● **T82.218** Other mechanical complication of coronary artery bypass graft A 🅒
         Obstruction, mechanical of coronary artery bypass graft
         Perforation of coronary artery bypass graft
         Protrusion of coronary artery bypass graft

● **T82.22** Mechanical complication of biological heart valve graft
     (Ex:) **For category T82.22 CC codes:** See PDX Collection 1450

     ● **T82.221** Breakdown (mechanical) of biological heart valve graft A 🅒

     ● **T82.222** Displacement of biological heart valve graft A 🅒
         Malposition of biological heart valve graft

     ● **T82.223** Leakage of biological heart valve graft A 🅒

     ● **T82.228** Other mechanical complication of biological heart valve graft A 🅒
         Obstruction of biological heart valve graft
         Perforation of biological heart valve graft
         Protrusion of biological heart valve graft

● **T82.3**   **Mechanical complication of other vascular grafts**
   (Ex:) *For category T82.3 CC codes: See PDX Collection 1452*

   ● **T82.31**   **Breakdown** (mechanical) of other vascular grafts

     ● T82.310   Breakdown (mechanical) of **aortic (bifurcation) graft (replacement)** A 🅒, A 🅜

     ● T82.311   Breakdown (mechanical) of **carotid arterial graft (bypass)** A 🅒, A 🅜

     ● T82.312   Breakdown (mechanical) of **femoral arterial graft (bypass)** A 🅒, A 🅜

     ● T82.318   Breakdown (mechanical) of **other vascular grafts** A 🅒, A 🅜

     ● T82.319   Breakdown (mechanical) of **unspecified vascular grafts** A 🅒, A 🅜

   ● **T82.32**   **Displacement** of other vascular grafts
     Malposition of other vascular grafts

     ● T82.320   Displacement of **aortic (bifurcation) graft (replacement)** A 🅒, A 🅜

     ● T82.321   Displacement of **carotid arterial graft (bypass)** A 🅒, A 🅜

     ● T82.322   Displacement of **femoral arterial graft (bypass)** A 🅒, A 🅜

     ● T82.328   Displacement of **other vascular grafts** A 🅒, A 🅜

     ● T82.329   Displacement of **unspecified vascular grafts** A 🅒, A 🅜

   ● **T82.33**   **Leakage** of other vascular grafts

     ● T82.330   Leakage of **aortic (bifurcation) graft (replacement)** A 🅒, A 🅜

     ● T82.331   Leakage of **carotid arterial graft (bypass)** A 🅒, A 🅜

     ● T82.332   Leakage of **femoral arterial graft (bypass)** A 🅒, A 🅜

     ● T82.338   Leakage of **other vascular grafts** A 🅒, A 🅜

     ● T82.339   Leakage of **unspecified vascular graft** A 🅒, A 🅜

   ● **T82.39**   **Other** mechanical complication of other vascular grafts
     Obstruction (mechanical) of other vascular grafts
     Perforation of other vascular grafts
     Protrusion of other vascular grafts

     ● T82.390   Other mechanical complication of **aortic (bifurcation) graft (replacement)** A 🅒, A 🅜

     ● T82.391   Other mechanical complication of **carotid arterial graft (bypass)** A 🅒, A 🅜

     ● T82.392   Other mechanical complication of **femoral arterial graft (bypass)** A 🅒, A 🅜

     ● T82.398   Other mechanical complication of **other vascular grafts** A 🅒, A 🅜

     ● T82.399   Other mechanical complication of **unspecified vascular grafts** A 🅒, A 🅜

● **T82.4**   **Mechanical complication of vascular dialysis catheter**
   Mechanical complication of hemodialysis catheter
   Excludes1   mechanical complication of intraperitoneal dialysis catheter (T85.62)
   (Ex:) *For category T82.4 CC codes: See PDX Collection 1452*

   X● **T82.41**   **Breakdown** (mechanical) of vascular dialysis catheter A 🅒, A, D, S 🅜

   X● **T82.42**   **Displacement** of vascular dialysis catheter A 🅒, A, D, S 🅜
     Malposition of vascular dialysis catheter

   X● **T82.43**   **Leakage** of vascular dialysis catheter A 🅒, A, D, S 🅜

X● **T82.49**   **Other** complication of vascular dialysis catheter A 🅒, A, D, S 🅜
   Obstruction (mechanical) of vascular dialysis catheter
   Perforation of vascular dialysis catheter
   Protrusion of vascular dialysis catheter

● **T82.5**   **Mechanical complication of other cardiac and vascular devices and implants**
   Excludes2   mechanical complication of epidural and subdural infusion catheter (T85.61)
   (Ex:) *For category T82.5 CC codes unless otherwise indicated: See PDX Collection 1452*

   ● **T82.51**   **Breakdown** (mechanical) of other cardiac and vascular devices and implants

     ● T82.510   Breakdown (mechanical) of **surgically created arteriovenous fistula** A 🅒, A 🅜

     ● T82.511   Breakdown (mechanical) of **surgically created arteriovenous shunt** A 🅒, A 🅜

     ● T82.512   Breakdown (mechanical) of **artificial heart** A 🅒
      (Ex:) *See PDX Collection 1450*

     ● T82.513   Breakdown (mechanical) of **balloon (counterpulsation) device** A 🅒, A 🅜

     ● T82.514   Breakdown (mechanical) of **infusion catheter** A 🅒, A 🅜

     ● T82.515   Breakdown (mechanical) of **umbrella device** A 🅒, A 🅜

     ● T82.518   Breakdown (mechanical) of **other** cardiac and vascular devices and implants A 🅒, A 🅜

     ● T82.519   Breakdown (mechanical) of **unspecified** cardiac and vascular devices and implants A 🅒
      (Ex:) *See PDX Collection 1453*

   ● **T82.52**   **Displacement** of other cardiac and vascular devices and implants
     Malposition of other cardiac and vascular devices and implants

     ● T82.520   Displacement of **surgically created arteriovenous fistula** A 🅒, A 🅜

     ● T82.521   Displacement of **surgically created arteriovenous shunt** A 🅒, A 🅜

     ● T82.522   Displacement of **artificial heart** A 🅒
      (Ex:) *See PDX Collection 1450*

     ● T82.523   Displacement of **balloon (counterpulsation) device** A 🅒, A 🅜

     ● T82.524   Displacement of **infusion catheter** A 🅒, A 🅜
      Coding Clinic: 2019, Q3, P15

     ● T82.525   Displacement of **umbrella device** A 🅒, A 🅜

     ● T82.528   Displacement of **other** cardiac and vascular devices and implants A 🅒, A 🅜

     ● T82.529   Displacement of **unspecified** cardiac and vascular devices and implants A 🅒

   ● **T82.53**   **Leakage** of other cardiac and vascular devices and implants

     ● T82.530   Leakage of **surgically created arteriovenous fistula** A 🅒, A 🅜

     ● T82.531   Leakage of **surgically created arteriovenous shunt** A 🅒, A 🅜

     ● T82.532   Leakage of **artificial heart** A 🅒
      (Ex:) *See PDX Collection 1450*

     ● T82.533   Leakage of **balloon (counterpulsation) device** A 🅒, A 🅜

     ● T82.534   Leakage of **infusion catheter** A 🅒, A 🅜

| N | Newborn Age: 0 | P | Pediatric Age: 0–17 | M | Maternity DX: 9–64 | A | Adult Age: 15–124 | ♀ Females Only | ♂ Males Only |

🅒 Complication\Comorbidity   🅜 Major C\C   (Ex:) CC/MCC Exclusions   🅗 Hospital-Acquired Condition   🅗 Hierarchical Condition Category

1511

CHAPTER 19 (S00–T88)

● T82.535 Leakage of umbrella device A 🅒, A 🅡🅒

● T82.538 Leakage of other cardiac and vascular devices and implants A 🅒, A 🅡🅒

● T82.539 Leakage of unspecified cardiac and vascular devices and implants A 🅒
   Ⓔ⑀ See PDX Collection 1453

● T82.59 Other mechanical complication of other cardiac and vascular devices and implants
   Obstruction (mechanical) of other cardiac and vascular devices and implants
   Perforation of other cardiac and vascular devices and implants
   Protrusion of other cardiac and vascular devices and implants

  ● T82.590 Other mechanical complication of surgically created arteriovenous fistula A 🅒, A 🅡🅒

  ● T82.591 Other mechanical complication of surgically created arteriovenous shunt A 🅒, A 🅡🅒

  ● T82.592 Other mechanical complication of artificial heart A 🅒
     Ⓔ⑀ See PDX Collection 1450

  ● T82.593 Other mechanical complication of balloon (counterpulsation) device A 🅒, A 🅡🅒

  ● T82.594 Other mechanical complication of infusion catheter A 🅒, A 🅡🅒
     Ⓔ⑀ See PDX Collection 1450

  ● T82.595 Other mechanical complication of umbrella device A 🅒, A 🅡🅒

  ● T82.598 Other mechanical complication of other cardiac and vascular devices and implants A 🅒, A 🅡🅒
     Ⓔ⑀ See PDX Collection 1450

  ● T82.599 Other mechanical complication of unspecified cardiac and vascular devices and implants A 🅒
     Ⓔ⑀ See PDX Collection 1453

X● T82.6 Infection and inflammatory reaction due to cardiac valve prosthesis A 🅒, A 🅡🅒, A 🅡🅒
   Use additional code to identify infection
   Ⓔ⑀ See PDX Collection 1454

X● T82.7 Infection and inflammatory reaction due to other cardiac and vascular devices, implants and grafts A 🅒, A 🅡🅒
   Use additional code to identify infection
   Ⓔ⑀ See PDX Collection 1454
   Coding Clinic: 2019, Q1, P13-14; 2018, Q4, P89

● T82.8 Other specified complications of cardiac and vascular prosthetic devices, implants and grafts

  ● T82.81 Embolism due to cardiac and vascular prosthetic devices, implants and grafts
     Coding Clinic: 2016, Q4, P70

    ● T82.817 Embolism due to cardiac prosthetic devices, implants and grafts A 🅒
       Ⓔ⑀ See PDX Collection 1455
       Coding Clinic: 2016, Q4, P70; 2015, Q1, P20

    ● T82.818 Embolism due to vascular prosthetic devices, implants and grafts A 🅒, A 🅡🅒
       Ⓔ⑀ See PDX Collection 1454

  ● T82.82 Fibrosis due to cardiac and vascular prosthetic devices, implants and grafts
     Coding Clinic: 2016, Q4, P70

    ● T82.827 Fibrosis due to cardiac prosthetic devices, implants and grafts A 🅒
       Ⓔ⑀ See PDX Collection 1455

    ● T82.828 Fibrosis due to vascular prosthetic devices, implants and grafts A 🅒, A 🅡🅒
       Ⓔ⑀ See PDX Collection 1454

● T82.83 Hemorrhage due to cardiac and vascular prosthetic devices, implants and grafts
   Coding Clinic: 2016, Q4, P70

  ● T82.837 Hemorrhage due to cardiac prosthetic devices, implants and grafts A 🅒

  ● T82.838 Hemorrhage due to vascular prosthetic devices, implants and grafts A 🅒, A 🅡🅒
     Ⓔ⑀ See PDX Collection 1454

● T82.84 Pain due to cardiac and vascular prosthetic devices, implants and grafts
   Coding Clinic: 2016, Q4, P70

  ● T82.847 Pain due to cardiac prosthetic devices, implants and grafts A 🅒
     Ⓔ⑀ See PDX Collection 1455

  ● T82.848 Pain due to vascular prosthetic devices, implants and grafts A 🅒, A 🅡🅒
     Ⓔ⑀ See PDX Collection 1454

● T82.85 Stenosis due to cardiac and vascular prosthetic devices, implants and grafts

  ● T82.855 Stenosis of coronary artery stent A 🅒
     In-stent stenosis (restenosis) of coronary artery stent
     Restenosis of coronary artery stent
     Ⓔ⑀ See PDX Collection 1455
     Coding Clinic: 2016, Q4, P70

  ● T82.856 Stenosis of peripheral vascular stent A 🅒, A 🅡🅒
     In-stent stenosis (restenosis) of peripheral vascular stent
     Restenosis of peripheral vascular stent
     Ⓔ⑀ See PDX Collection 1454
     Coding Clinic: 2016, Q4, P70

  ● T82.857 Stenosis of other cardiac prosthetic devices, implants and grafts A 🅒
     Ⓔ⑀ See PDX Collection 1455
     Coding Clinic: 2016, Q4, P70

  ● T82.858 Stenosis of other vascular prosthetic devices, implants and grafts A 🅒, A 🅡🅒
     Ⓔ⑀ See PDX Collection 1454
     Coding Clinic: 2016, Q4, P70

● T82.86 Thrombosis of cardiac and vascular prosthetic devices, implants and grafts

  ● T82.867 Thrombosis due to cardiac prosthetic devices, implants and grafts A 🅒
     Ⓔ⑀ See PDX Collection 1455

  ● T82.868 Thrombosis due to vascular prosthetic devices, implants and grafts A 🅒, A 🅡🅒
     Ⓔ⑀ See PDX Collection 1454

● T82.89 Other specified complication of cardiac and vascular prosthetic devices, implants and grafts

  ● T82.897 Other specified complication of cardiac prosthetic devices, implants and grafts A 🅒
     Ⓔ⑀ See PDX Collection 1455
     Coding Clinic: 2019, Q2, P32-33

  ● T82.898 Other specified complication of vascular prosthetic devices, implants and grafts A 🅒, A 🅡🅒
     Ⓔ⑀ See PDX Collection 1454

X● T82.9 Unspecified complication of cardiac and vascular prosthetic device, implant and graft A 🅒
   Ⓔ⑀ See PDX Collection 1455

▶ New   ⇒ Revised   deleted Deleted   Excludes 1   Excludes 2   Includes   Use additional   Code first   Code also   Key words
OGCR Official Guidelines   ● Unacceptable Principal Diagnosis   X Assign placeholder X   ● Use Additional Character(s)   ▸ Manifestation Code   Coding Clinic

● **T83** **Complications of genitourinary prosthetic devices, implants and grafts**

> **Excludes2**　failure and rejection of transplanted organs and tissue (T86.-)
>
> The appropriate 7th character is to be added to each code from category T83
>
> | | |
> |---|---|
> | A | initial encounter |
> | D | subsequent encounter |
> | S | sequela |
>
> (Ex) **For category T83 CC codes:** See PDX Collection 1456
> **Coding Clinic: 2016, Q4, P70-71**

● **T83.0** **Mechanical complication of** urinary catheter

> **Excludes2**　complications of stoma of urinary tract (N99.5-)
>
> **Coding Clinic: 2016, Q4, P70**

　● **T83.01** **Breakdown (mechanical) of urinary catheter**

　　● **T83.010** **Breakdown (mechanical) of** cystostomy catheter A 🅒, A 🅜

　　● **T83.011** **Breakdown (mechanical) of** indwelling urethral catheter A 🅜

　　● **T83.012** **Breakdown (mechanical) of** nephrostomy catheter A 🅜

　　● **T83.018** **Breakdown (mechanical) of other** urinary catheter A 🅜
　　　　　Breakdown (mechanical) of Hopkins catheter
　　　　　Breakdown (mechanical) of ileostomy catheter
　　　　　Breakdown (mechanical) urostomy catheter

　● **T83.02** **Displacement of urinary catheter**
　　　Malposition of urinary catheter

　　● **T83.020** **Displacement of** cystostomy catheter A 🅒, A 🅜

　　● **T83.021** **Displacement of** indwelling urethral catheter A 🅜

　　● **T83.022** **Displacement of** nephrostomy catheter A 🅜

　　● **T83.028** **Displacement of other** urinary catheter A 🅜
　　　　　Displacement of Hopkins catheter
　　　　　Displacement of ileostomy catheter
　　　　　Displacement of urostomy catheter

　● **T83.03** **Leakage of urinary catheter**

　　● **T83.030** **Leakage of** cystostomy catheter A 🅒, A 🅜

　　● **T83.031** **Leakage of** indwelling urethral catheter A 🅜

　　● **T83.032** **Leakage of** nephrostomy catheter A 🅜

　　● **T83.038** **Leakage of other** urinary catheter A 🅜
　　　　　Leakage of Hopkins catheter
　　　　　Leakage of ileostomy catheter
　　　　　Leakage of urostomy catheter

　● **T83.09** **Other mechanical complication of urinary catheter**
　　　Obstruction (mechanical) of urinary catheter
　　　Perforation of urinary catheter
　　　Protrusion of urinary catheter

　　● **T83.090** **Other mechanical complication of** cystostomy catheter A 🅒, A 🅜

　　● **T83.091** **Other mechanical complication of** indwelling urethral catheter A 🅜

　　● **T83.092** **Other mechanical complication of** nephrostomy catheter A 🅜

　　● **T83.098** **Other mechanical complication of** other urinary catheter A 🅜
　　　　　Other mechanical complication of Hopkins catheter
　　　　　Other mechanical complication of ileostomy catheter
　　　　　Other mechanical complication of urostomy catheter

● **T83.1** **Mechanical complication of** other urinary devices and implants

> **Coding Clinic: 2016, Q4, P70**

　● **T83.11** **Breakdown (mechanical) of other urinary devices and implants**

　　● **T83.110** **Breakdown (mechanical) of urinary electronic stimulator device** A 🅒, A 🅜

　　　　> **Excludes2**　Breakdown (mechanical) of electrode (lead) for sacral nerve neurostimulator (T85.111)
　　　　> Breakdown (mechanical) of implanted electronic sacral neurostimulator, pulse generator or receiver (T85.113)

　　● **T83.111** **Breakdown (mechanical) of implanted urinary sphincter** A 🅒, A 🅜

　　● **T83.112** **Breakdown (mechanical) of indwelling ureteral stent** A 🅒, A 🅜

　　● **T83.113** **Breakdown (mechanical) of other urinary stents** A 🅒, A 🅜
　　　　　Breakdown (mechanical) of ileal conduit stent
　　　　　Breakdown (mechanical) of nephroureteral stent

　　● **T83.118** **Breakdown (mechanical) of other urinary devices and implants** A 🅒, A 🅜

　● **T83.12** **Displacement of other urinary devices and implants**
　　　Malposition of other urinary devices and implants

　　● **T83.120** **Displacement of urinary electronic stimulator device** A 🅒, A 🅜

　　　　> **Excludes2**　Displacement of electrode (lead) for sacral nerve neurostimulator (T85.121)
　　　　> Displacement of implanted electronic sacral neurostimulator, pulse generator or receiver (T85.123)

　　● **T83.121** **Displacement of implanted urinary sphincter** A 🅒, A 🅜

　　● **T83.122** **Displacement of indwelling ureteral stent** A 🅒, A 🅜

　　● **T83.123** **Displacement of other urinary stents** A 🅒, A 🅜
　　　　　Displacement of ileal conduit stent
　　　　　Displacement of nephroureteral stent

　　● **T83.128** **Displacement of other urinary devices and implants** A 🅒, A 🅜

N Newborn Age: 0　**P** Pediatric Age: 0–17　**M** Maternity DX: 9–64　**A** Adult Age: 15–124　♀ Females Only　♂ Males Only

🅒 Complication\Comorbidity　🅜 Major C\C　(Ex) CC/MCC Exclusions　🅗 Hospital-Acquired Condition　🅗 Hierarchical Condition Category

1513

● **T83.19** **Other mechanical complication of other urinary devices and implants**
  Leakage of other urinary devices and implants
  Obstruction (mechanical) of other urinary devices and implants
  Perforation of other urinary devices and implants
  Protrusion of other urinary devices and implants

- ● **T83.190** **Other mechanical complication of urinary electronic stimulator device** A 🪙, A 🪙
  - **Excludes2**   Other mechanical complication of electrode (lead) for sacral nerve neurostimulator (T85.191)
    Other mechanical complication of implanted electronic sacral neurostimulator, pulse generator or receiver (T85.193)

- ● **T83.191** **Other mechanical complication of implanted urinary sphincter** A 🪙, A 🪙

- ● **T83.192** **Other mechanical complication of indwelling ureteral stent** A 🪙, A 🪙

- ● **T83.193** **Other mechanical complication of other urinary stent** A 🪙, A 🪙
  Other mechanical complication of ileal conduit stent
  Other mechanical complication of nephroureteral stent

- ● **T83.198** **Other mechanical complication of other urinary devices and implants** A 🪙, A 🪙

● **T83.2** **Mechanical complication of graft of urinary organ**
  Coding Clinic: 2016, Q4, P70

- X ● **T83.21** **Breakdown (mechanical) of graft of urinary organ** A 🪙, A 🪙

- X ● **T83.22** **Displacement of graft of urinary organ** A 🪙, A 🪙
  Malposition of graft of urinary organ

- X ● **T83.23** **Leakage of graft of urinary organ** A 🪙, A 🪙

- X ● **T83.24** **Erosion of graft of urinary organ** A 🪙, A 🪙
  Coding Clinic: 2016, Q4, P70

- X ● **T83.25** **Exposure of graft of urinary organ** A 🪙, A 🪙
  Coding Clinic: 2016, Q4, P70

- X ● **T83.29** **Other mechanical complication of graft of urinary organ** A 🪙, A 🪙
  Obstruction (mechanical) of graft of urinary organ
  Perforation of graft of urinary organ
  Protrusion of graft of urinary organ

● **T83.3** **Mechanical complication of intrauterine contraceptive device**

- X ● **T83.31** **Breakdown (mechanical) of intrauterine contraceptive device** ♀

- X ● **T83.32** **Displacement of intrauterine contraceptive device** ♀
  Malposition of intrauterine contraceptive device
  Missing string of intrauterine contraceptive device

X ● **T83.39** **Other mechanical complication of intrauterine contraceptive device** ♀
  Leakage of intrauterine contraceptive device
  Obstruction (mechanical) of intrauterine contraceptive device
  Perforation of intrauterine contraceptive device
  Protrusion of intrauterine contraceptive device

● **T83.4** **Mechanical complication of other prosthetic devices, implants and grafts of genital tract**
  Coding Clinic: 2016, Q4, P71

- ● **T83.41** **Breakdown (mechanical) of other prosthetic devices, implants and grafts of genital tract**

  - ● **T83.410** **Breakdown (mechanical) of implanted penile prosthesis** ♂ A 🪙, A 🪙
    Breakdown (mechanical) of penile prosthesis cylinder
    Breakdown (mechanical) of penile prosthesis pump
    Breakdown (mechanical) of penile prosthesis reservoir

  - ● **T83.411** **Breakdown (mechanical) of implanted testicular prosthesis** A 🪙, A 🪙

  - ● **T83.418** **Breakdown (mechanical) of other prosthetic devices, implants and grafts of genital tract** A 🪙, A 🪙

- ● **T83.42** **Displacement of other prosthetic devices, implants and grafts of genital tract**
  Malposition of other prosthetic devices, implants and grafts of genital tract

  - ● **T83.420** **Displacement of implanted penile prosthesis** ♂ A 🪙, A 🪙
    Displacement of penile prosthesis cylinder
    Displacement of penile prosthesis pump
    Displacement of penile prosthesis reservoir

  - ● **T83.421** **Displacement of implanted testicular prosthesis** A 🪙, A 🪙

  - ● **T83.428** **Displacement of other prosthetic devices, implants and grafts of genital tract** A 🪙, A 🪙
    Coding Clinic: 2018, Q1, P6

- ● **T83.49** **Other mechanical complication of other prosthetic devices, implants and grafts of genital tract**
  Leakage of other prosthetic devices, implants and grafts of genital tract
  Obstruction, mechanical of other prosthetic devices, implants and grafts of genital tract
  Perforation of other prosthetic devices, implants and grafts of genital tract
  Protrusion of other prosthetic devices, implants and grafts of genital tract

  - ● **T83.490** **Other mechanical complication of implanted penile prosthesis** ♂ A 🪙, A 🪙
    Other mechanical complication of penile prosthesis cylinder
    Other mechanical complication of penile prosthesis pump
    Other mechanical complication of penile prosthesis reservoir

  - ● **T83.491** **Other mechanical complication of implanted testicular prosthesis** A 🪙, A 🪙

  - ● **T83.498** **Other mechanical complication of other prosthetic devices, implants and grafts of genital tract** A 🪙, A 🪙

▶ New   ⇒ Revised   ~~deleted~~ Deleted   Excludes 1   Excludes 2   Includes   Use additional   Code first   Code also   Key words
OGCR Official Guidelines   ● Unacceptable Principal Diagnosis   X Assign placeholder X   ● Use Additional Character(s)   ▶ Manifestation Code   **Coding Clinic**

● **T83.5** **Infection and inflammatory reaction due to prosthetic device, implant and graft in** urinary system

Use additional code to identify infection

(Ex:) **For category T83.5 CC codes unless otherwise indicated:** See PDX Collection 1458

Coding Clinic: 2016, Q4, P71

● **T83.51** **Infection and inflammatory reaction due to** urinary catheter

Excludes2 complications of stoma of urinary tract (N99.5-)

● **T83.510** **Infection and inflammatory reaction due to** cystostomy catheter A 🝛, A 🝛

● **T83.511** **Infection and inflammatory reaction due to** indwelling urethral catheter A 🝛, A 🝛

(Ex:) See PDX Collection 1457

● **T83.512** **Infection and inflammatory reaction due to** nephrostomy catheter A 🝛, A 🝛

● **T83.518** **Infection and inflammatory reaction due to** other urinary catheter A 🝛, A 🝛

Infection and inflammatory reaction due to Hopkins catheter

Infection and inflammatory reaction due to ileostomy catheter

Infection and inflammatory reaction due to urostomy catheter

● **T83.59** **Infection and inflammatory reaction due to prosthetic device, implant and graft in urinary system**

● **T83.590** **Infection and inflammatory reaction due to implanted urinary neurostimulation device** A 🝛, A 🝛

Excludes2 Infection and inflammatory reaction due to electrode lead of sacral nerve neurostimulator (T85.732)

Infection and inflammatory reaction due to pulse generator or receiver of sacral nerve neurostimulator (T85.734)

● **T83.591** **Infection and inflammatory reaction due to** implanted urinary sphincter A 🝛, A 🝛

● **T83.592** **Infection and inflammatory reaction due to** indwelling ureteral stent A 🝛, A 🝛

● **T83.593** **Infection and inflammatory reaction due to** other urinary stents A 🝛, A 🝛

Infection and inflammatory reaction due to ileal conduit stents

Infection and inflammatory reaction due to nephroureteral stent

● **T83.598** **Infection and inflammatory reaction due to** other prosthetic device, implant and graft in urinary system A 🝛, A 🝛

● **T83.6** **Infection and inflammatory reaction due to prosthetic device, implant and graft in** genital tract

Use additional code to identify infection

(Ex:) **For category T83.6:** See PDX Collection 1458

Coding Clinic: 2016, Q4, P71

● **T83.61** **Infection and inflammatory reaction due to** implanted penile prosthesis A 🝛, A 🝛

Infection and inflammatory reaction due to penile prosthesis cylinder

Infection and inflammatory reaction due to penile prosthesis pump

Infection and inflammatory reaction due to penile prosthesis reservoir

● **T83.62** **Infection and inflammatory reaction due to** implanted testicular prosthesis A 🝛, A 🝛

● **T83.69** **Infection and inflammatory reaction due to** other prosthetic device, implant and graft in genital tract A 🝛, A 🝛

● **T83.7** **Complications due to** implanted mesh and other prosthetic materials

(Ex:) **For Category T83.7 CC codes unless otherwise indicated:** See PDX Collection 1456

Coding Clinic: 2016, Q4, P71

● **T83.71** Erosion **of implanted mesh and other prosthetic materials to surrounding organ or tissue**

Coding Clinic: 2016, Q4, P71

● **T83.711** **Erosion of implanted** vaginal **mesh to surrounding organ or tissue** ♀ A 🝛

Erosion of implanted vaginal mesh into pelvic floor muscles

Coding Clinic: 2016, Q4, P71

● **T83.712** **Erosion of implanted** urethral **mesh to surrounding organ or tissue** A 🝛, A 🝛

Erosion of implanted female urethral sling

Erosion of implanted male urethral sling

Erosion of implanted urethral mesh into pelvic floor muscles

● **T83.713** **Erosion of implanted** urethral bulking agent **to surrounding organ or tissue** A 🝛, A 🝛

● **T83.714** **Erosion of implanted** ureteral bulking agent **to surrounding organ or tissue** A 🝛, A 🝛

● **T83.718** **Erosion of** other implanted mesh **to organ or tissue** A 🝛, A 🝛

Coding Clinic: 2016, Q4, P71

● **T83.719** **Erosion of** other prosthetic materials **to surrounding organ or tissue** A 🝛, A 🝛

Coding Clinic: 2016, Q4, P71

● **T83.72** Exposure **of implanted mesh and other prosthetic materials into surrounding organ or tissue**

Extrusion of implanted mesh

Coding Clinic: 2016, Q4, P71

● **T83.721** **Exposure of implanted** vaginal **mesh into vagina** ♀ A 🝛

Exposure of implanted vaginal mesh through vaginal wall

● **T83.722** **Exposure of implanted** urethral **mesh into urethra** A 🝛, A 🝛

Exposure of implanted female urethral sling

Exposure of implanted male urethral sling

Exposure of implanted urethral mesh through urethral wall

● **T83.723** **Exposure of implanted** urethral bulking agent **into urethra** A 🝛, A 🝛

● **T83.724** **Exposure of implanted** ureteral bulking agent **into ureter** A 🝛, A 🝛

N Newborn Age: 0　　**P** Pediatric Age: 0–17　　**M** Maternity DX: 9–64　　**A** Adult Age: 15–124　　♀ Females Only　　♂ Males Only

🝛 Complication\Comorbidity　　🝛 Major C\C　　(Ex:) CC/MCC Exclusions　　🝛 Hospital-Acquired Condition　　🝛 Hierarchical Condition Category

1515

T83.728   Exposure of other implanted mesh into organ or tissue A 🔵, A 🔵
Coding Clinic: 2016, Q4, P71

T83.729   Exposure of other prosthetic materials into organ or tissue A 🔵, A 🔵
Coding Clinic: 2016, Q4, P71

X● T83.79   Other specified complications due to other genitourinary prosthetic materials A 🔵, A 🔵
Ex: See PDX Collection 1458

● T83.8   Other specified complications of genitourinary prosthetic devices, implants and grafts
Ex: For category T83.8 CC codes: See PDX Collection 1458

X● T83.81   Embolism due to genitourinary prosthetic devices, implants and grafts A 🔵, A 🔵

X● T83.82   Fibrosis due to genitourinary prosthetic devices, implants and grafts A 🔵, A 🔵

X● T83.83   Hemorrhage due to genitourinary prosthetic devices, implants and grafts A 🔵, A 🔵

X● T83.84   Pain due to genitourinary prosthetic devices, implants and grafts A 🔵, A 🔵

X● T83.85   Stenosis due to genitourinary prosthetic devices, implants and grafts A 🔵, A 🔵

X● T83.86   Thrombosis due to genitourinary prosthetic devices, implants and grafts A 🔵, A 🔵

X● T83.89   Other specified complication of genitourinary prosthetic devices, implants and grafts A 🔵, A 🔵

X● T83.9   Unspecified complication of genitourinary prosthetic device, implant and graft A 🔵, A 🔵
Ex: See PDX Collection 1458

● T84   Complications of internal orthopedic prosthetic devices, implants and grafts

Excludes2   failure and rejection of transplanted organs and tissues (T86.-)
     fracture of bone following insertion of orthopedic implant, joint prosthesis or bone plate (M96.6)

The appropriate 7th character is to be added to each code from category T84

A	initial encounter
D	subsequent encounter
S	sequela

Ex: For category T84 CC codes unless otherwise indicated: See PDX Collection 911

● T84.0   Mechanical complication of internal joint prosthesis

● T84.01   Broken internal joint prosthesis
Breakage (fracture) of prosthetic joint
Broken prosthetic joint implant

Excludes1   periprosthetic joint implant fracture (M97.-)

Coding Clinic: 2016, Q4, P42

● T84.010   Broken internal right hip prosthesis A 🔵, A 🔵

● T84.011   Broken internal left hip prosthesis A 🔵, A 🔵

● T84.012   Broken internal right knee prosthesis A 🔵, A 🔵

● T84.013   Broken internal left knee prosthesis A 🔵, A 🔵

● T84.018   Broken internal joint prosthesis, other site A 🔵, A 🔵
Use additional code to identify the joint (Z96.6-)

● T84.019   Broken internal joint prosthesis, unspecified site A 🔵, A 🔵

● T84.02   Dislocation of internal joint prosthesis
Instability of internal joint prosthesis
Subluxation of internal joint prosthesis

● T84.020   Dislocation of internal right hip prosthesis A 🔵, A 🔵

● T84.021   Dislocation of internal left hip prosthesis A 🔵, A 🔵
Coding Clinic: 2019, Q2, P27

● T84.022   Instability of internal right knee prosthesis A 🔵, A 🔵

● T84.023   Instability of internal left knee prosthesis A 🔵, A 🔵

● T84.028   Dislocation of other internal joint prosthesis A 🔵, A 🔵
Use additional code to identify the joint (Z96.6-)

● T84.029   Dislocation of unspecified internal joint prosthesis A 🔵, A 🔵

● T84.03   Mechanical loosening of internal prosthetic joint
Aseptic loosening of prosthetic joint

● T84.030   Mechanical loosening of internal right hip prosthetic joint A 🔵, A 🔵

● T84.031   Mechanical loosening of internal left hip prosthetic joint A 🔵, A 🔵

● T84.032   Mechanical loosening of internal right knee prosthetic joint A 🔵, A 🔵

● T84.033   Mechanical loosening of internal left knee prosthetic joint A 🔵, A 🔵

● T84.038   Mechanical loosening of other internal prosthetic joint A 🔵, A 🔵
Use additional code to identify the joint (Z96.6-)

● T84.039   Mechanical loosening of unspecified internal prosthetic joint A 🔵, A 🔵

● T84.05   Periprosthetic osteolysis of internal prosthetic joint
Use additional code to identify major osseous defect, if applicable (M89.7-)

● T84.050   Periprosthetic osteolysis of internal prosthetic right hip joint A 🔵, A 🔵

● T84.051   Periprosthetic osteolysis of internal prosthetic left hip joint A 🔵, A 🔵

● T84.052   Periprosthetic osteolysis of internal prosthetic right knee joint A 🔵, A 🔵

● T84.053   Periprosthetic osteolysis of internal prosthetic left knee joint A 🔵, A 🔵

● T84.058   Periprosthetic osteolysis of other internal prosthetic joint A 🔵, A 🔵
Use additional code to identify the joint (Z96.6-)

● T84.059   Periprosthetic osteolysis of unspecified internal prosthetic joint A 🔵, A 🔵

● T84.06   Wear of articular bearing surface of internal prosthetic joint

● T84.060   Wear of articular bearing surface of internal prosthetic right hip joint A 🔵, A 🔵

● T84.061   Wear of articular bearing surface of internal prosthetic left hip joint A 🔵, A 🔵

● T84.062   Wear of articular bearing surface of internal prosthetic right knee joint A 🔵, A 🔵

● T84.063   Wear of articular bearing surface of internal prosthetic left knee joint A 🔵, A 🔵

● T84.068   Wear of articular bearing surface of other internal prosthetic joint A 🔵, A 🔵
Use additional code to identify the joint (Z96.6-)

● T84.069   Wear of articular bearing surface of unspecified internal prosthetic joint A 🔵, A 🔵

CHAPTER 19 (S00-T88)

▶ New   ⇒ Revised   ~~deleted~~ Deleted   Excludes 1   Excludes 2   Includes   Use additional   Code first   Code also   Key words
OGCR Official Guidelines   ● Unacceptable Principal Diagnosis   X Assign placeholder X   ● Use Additional Character(s)   ▶ Manifestation Code   Coding Clinic

● **T84.09   Other mechanical complication** of internal joint prosthesis

  Prosthetic joint implant failure NOS

  ● **T84.090   Other mechanical complication of internal right hip prosthesis**
  A 🔗, A 🔗

  Coding Clinic: 2019, Q1, P20

  ● **T84.091   Other mechanical complication of internal left hip prosthesis** A 🔗, A 🔗

  ● **T84.092   Other mechanical complication of internal right knee prosthesis**
  A 🔗, A 🔗

  ● **T84.093   Other mechanical complication of internal left knee prosthesis**
  A 🔗, A 🔗

  ● **T84.098   Other mechanical complication of other internal joint prosthesis**
  A 🔗, A 🔗

  Use additional code to identify the joint (Z96.6-)

  ● **T84.099   Other mechanical complication of unspecified internal joint prosthesis**
  A 🔗, A 🔗

● **T84.1   Mechanical complication of internal fixation device of bones of limb**

  Excludes2   mechanical complication of internal fixation device of bones of feet (T84.2-)

  mechanical complication of internal fixation device of bones of fingers (T84.2-)

  mechanical complication of internal fixation device of bones of hands (T84.2-)

  mechanical complication of internal fixation device of bones of toes (T84.2-)

  ● **T84.11   Breakdown (mechanical) of internal fixation device of bones of limb**

    ● **T84.110   Breakdown (mechanical) of internal fixation device of right humerus**
    A 🔗, A 🔗

    ● **T84.111   Breakdown (mechanical) of internal fixation device of left humerus**
    A 🔗, A 🔗

    ● **T84.112   Breakdown (mechanical) of internal fixation device of bone of right forearm** A 🔗, A 🔗

    ● **T84.113   Breakdown (mechanical) of internal fixation device of bone of left forearm**
    A 🔗, A 🔗

    ● **T84.114   Breakdown (mechanical) of internal fixation device of right femur**
    A 🔗, A 🔗

    ● **T84.115   Breakdown (mechanical) of internal fixation device of left femur** A 🔗, A 🔗

    ● **T84.116   Breakdown (mechanical) of internal fixation device of bone of right lower leg** A 🔗, A 🔗

    ● **T84.117   Breakdown (mechanical) of internal fixation device of bone of left lower leg** A 🔗, A 🔗

    ● **T84.119   Breakdown (mechanical) of internal fixation device of unspecified bone of limb** A 🔗, A 🔗

  ● **T84.12   Displacement of internal fixation device of bones of limb**

    Malposition of internal fixation device of bones of limb

    ● **T84.120   Displacement of internal fixation device of right humerus** A 🔗, A 🔗

    ● **T84.121   Displacement of internal fixation device of left humerus** A 🔗, A 🔗

  ● **T84.122   Displacement of internal fixation device of bone of right forearm**
  A 🔗, A 🔗

  ● **T84.123   Displacement of internal fixation device of bone of left forearm**
  A 🔗, A 🔗

  ● **T84.124   Displacement of internal fixation device of right femur** A 🔗, A 🔗

  ● **T84.125   Displacement of internal fixation device of left femur** A 🔗, A 🔗

  ● **T84.126   Displacement of internal fixation device of bone of right lower leg**
  A 🔗, A 🔗

  ● **T84.127   Displacement of internal fixation device of bone of left lower leg**
  A 🔗, A 🔗

  ● **T84.129   Displacement of internal fixation device of unspecified bone of limb**
  A 🔗, A 🔗

● **T84.19   Other mechanical complication** of internal fixation device of bones of limb

  Obstruction (mechanical) of internal fixation device of bones of limb

  Perforation of internal fixation device of bones of limb

  Protrusion of internal fixation device of bones of limb

  ● **T84.190   Other mechanical complication of internal fixation device of right humerus** A 🔗, A 🔗

  ● **T84.191   Other mechanical complication of internal fixation device of left humerus** A 🔗, A 🔗

  ● **T84.192   Other mechanical complication of internal fixation device of bone of right forearm** A 🔗, A 🔗

  ● **T84.193   Other mechanical complication of internal fixation device of bone of left forearm** A 🔗, A 🔗

  ● **T84.194   Other mechanical complication of internal fixation device of right femur**
  A 🔗, A 🔗

  ● **T84.195   Other mechanical complication of internal fixation device of left femur**
  A 🔗, A 🔗

  ● **T84.196   Other mechanical complication of internal fixation device of bone of right lower leg** A 🔗, A 🔗

  ● **T84.197   Other mechanical complication of internal fixation device of bone of left lower leg** A 🔗, A 🔗

  ● **T84.199   Other mechanical complication of internal fixation device of unspecified bone of limb** A 🔗, A 🔗

● **T84.2   Mechanical complication of internal fixation device of other bones**

  ● **T84.21   Breakdown (mechanical) of internal fixation device of other bones**

    ● **T84.210   Breakdown (mechanical) of internal fixation device of bones of hand and fingers** A 🔗, A 🔗

    ● **T84.213   Breakdown (mechanical) of internal fixation device of bones of foot and toes** A 🔗, A 🔗

    ● **T84.216   Breakdown (mechanical) of internal fixation device of vertebrae** A 🔗, A 🔗

    ● **T84.218   Breakdown (mechanical) of internal fixation device of other bones**
    A 🔗, A 🔗

N Newborn Age: 0   P Pediatric Age: 0–17   M Maternity DX: 9–64   A Adult Age: 15–124   ♀ Females Only   ♂ Males Only

🔗 Complication\Comorbidity   🔗 Major C\C   (Ex) CC/MCC Exclusions   🔗 Hospital-Acquired Condition   🔗 Hierarchical Condition Category

1517

● **T84.22** **Displacement** of internal fixation device of other bones
    Malposition of internal fixation device of other bones
    ● **T84.220** Displacement of internal fixation device of bones of hand and fingers A 🔄, A 🔄
    ● **T84.223** Displacement of internal fixation device of bones of foot and toes A 🔄, A 🔄
    ● **T84.226** Displacement of internal fixation device of vertebrae A 🔄, A 🔄
    ● **T84.228** Displacement of internal fixation device of other bones A 🔄, A 🔄

● **T84.29** Other mechanical complication of internal fixation device of other bones
    Obstruction (mechanical) of internal fixation device of other bones
    Perforation of internal fixation device of other bones
    Protrusion of internal fixation device of other bones
    ● **T84.290** Other mechanical complication of internal fixation device of bones of hand and fingers A 🔄, A 🔄
    ● **T84.293** Other mechanical complication of internal fixation device of bones of foot and toes A 🔄, A 🔄
    ● **T84.296** Other mechanical complication of internal fixation device of vertebrae A 🔄, A 🔄
    ● **T84.298** Other mechanical complication of internal fixation device of other bones A 🔄, A 🔄

● **T84.3** Mechanical complication of other bone devices, implants and grafts
    Excludes2   other complications of bone graft (T86.83-)

● **T84.31** **Breakdown** (mechanical) of other bone devices, implants and grafts
    ● **T84.310** Breakdown (mechanical) of electronic bone stimulator A 🔄, A 🔄
    ● **T84.318** Breakdown (mechanical) of other bone devices, implants and grafts A 🔄, A 🔄

● **T84.32** **Displacement** of other bone devices, implants and grafts
    Malposition of other bone devices, implants and grafts
    ● **T84.320** Displacement of electronic bone stimulator A 🔄, A 🔄
    ● **T84.328** Displacement of other bone devices, implants and grafts A 🔄, A 🔄

● **T84.39** Other mechanical complication of other bone devices, implants and grafts
    Obstruction (mechanical) of other bone devices, implants and grafts
    Perforation of other bone devices, implants and grafts
    Protrusion of other bone devices, implants and grafts
    ● **T84.390** Other mechanical complication of electronic bone stimulator A 🔄, A 🔄
    ● **T84.398** Other mechanical complication of other bone devices, implants and grafts A 🔄, A 🔄

● **T84.4** Mechanical complication of other internal orthopedic devices, implants and grafts
    ● **T84.41** **Breakdown** (mechanical) of other internal orthopedic devices, implants and grafts
      ● **T84.410** Breakdown (mechanical) of muscle and tendon graft A 🔄, A 🔄
      ● **T84.418** Breakdown (mechanical) of other internal orthopedic devices, implants and grafts A 🔄, A 🔄

    ● **T84.42** Displacement of other internal orthopedic devices, implants and grafts
      Malposition of other internal orthopedic devices, implants and grafts
      ● **T84.420** Displacement of muscle and tendon graft A 🔄, A 🔄
      ● **T84.428** Displacement of other internal orthopedic devices, implants and grafts A 🔄, A 🔄

    ● **T84.49** Other mechanical complication of other internal orthopedic devices, implants and grafts
      Mechanical complication of other internal orthopedic devices, implants and grafts NOS
      Obstruction (mechanical) of other internal orthopedic devices, implants and grafts
      Perforation of other internal orthopedic devices, implants and grafts
      Protrusion of other internal orthopedic devices, implants and grafts
      ● **T84.490** Other mechanical complication of muscle and tendon graft A 🔄, A 🔄
      ● **T84.498** Other mechanical complication of other internal orthopedic devices, implants and grafts A 🔄, A 🔄

● **T84.5** Infection and inflammatory reaction due to internal joint prosthesis
    Use additional code to identify infection
    (Ex:) **For category T84.5 CC codes:** See PDX Collection 1459
    Coding Clinic: 2015, Q1, P16

    X ● **T84.50** Infection and inflammatory reaction due to unspecified internal joint prosthesis A 🔄, A 🔄
      Coding Clinic: 2015, Q1, P3

    X ● **T84.51** Infection and inflammatory reaction due to internal right hip prosthesis A 🔄, A 🔄
      Coding Clinic: 2015, Q4, P36

    X ● **T84.52** Infection and inflammatory reaction due to internal left hip prosthesis A 🔄, A 🔄
      Coding Clinic: 2015, Q1, P16-17

    X ● **T84.53** Infection and inflammatory reaction due to internal right knee prosthesis A 🔄, A 🔄

    X ● **T84.54** Infection and inflammatory reaction due to internal left knee prosthesis A 🔄, A 🔄
      Coding Clinic: 2019, Q3, P16

    X ● **T84.59** Infection and inflammatory reaction due to other internal joint prosthesis A 🔄, A 🔄

● **T84.6** Infection and inflammatory reaction due to internal fixation device
    Use additional code to identify infection
    (Ex:) **For category T84.6 CC codes:** See PDX Collection 1459

    X ● **T84.60** Infection and inflammatory reaction due to internal fixation device of unspecified site A 🔄, A 🔄

    ● **T84.61** Infection and inflammatory reaction due to internal fixation device of arm
      ● **T84.610** Infection and inflammatory reaction due to internal fixation device of right humerus A 🔄, A 🔄, A 🔄
      ● **T84.611** Infection and inflammatory reaction due to internal fixation device of left humerus A 🔄, A 🔄, A 🔄
      ● **T84.612** Infection and inflammatory reaction due to internal fixation device of right radius A 🔄, A 🔄, A 🔄

CHAPTER 19 (S00-T88)

● T84.613   Infection and inflammatory reaction due to internal fixation device of left radius A ⬤, A ⬤, A ⬤

● T84.614   Infection and inflammatory reaction due to internal fixation device of right ulna A ⬤, A ⬤, A ⬤

● T84.615   Infection and inflammatory reaction due to internal fixation device of left ulna A ⬤, A ⬤, A ⬤

● T84.619   Infection and inflammatory reaction due to internal fixation device of unspecified bone of arm A ⬤, A ⬤, A ⬤

● T84.62   Infection and inflammatory reaction due to internal fixation device of leg

● T84.620   Infection and inflammatory reaction due to internal fixation device of right femur A ⬤, A ⬤

● T84.621   Infection and inflammatory reaction due to internal fixation device of left femur A ⬤, A ⬤

● T84.622   Infection and inflammatory reaction due to internal fixation device of right tibia A ⬤, A ⬤

● T84.623   Infection and inflammatory reaction due to internal fixation device of left tibia A ⬤, A ⬤

● T84.624   Infection and inflammatory reaction due to internal fixation device of right fibula A ⬤, A ⬤

● T84.625   Infection and inflammatory reaction due to internal fixation device of left fibula A ⬤, A ⬤

● T84.629   Infection and inflammatory reaction due to internal fixation device of unspecified bone of leg A ⬤, A ⬤

X● T84.63   Infection and inflammatory reaction due to internal fixation device of spine A ⬤, A ⬤, A ⬤

X● T84.69   Infection and inflammatory reaction due to internal fixation device of other site A ⬤, A ⬤, A ⬤

● T84.7   Infection and inflammatory reaction due to other internal orthopedic prosthetic devices, implants and grafts A ⬤, A ⬤, A ⬤

Use additional code to identify infection
Ex: See PDX Collection 1459

● T84.8   Other specified complications of internal orthopedic prosthetic devices, implants and grafts
Ex: For category T84.8 CC codes: See PDX Collection 1459

X● T84.81   Embolism due to internal orthopedic prosthetic devices, implants and grafts A ⬤, A ⬤

X● T84.82   Fibrosis due to internal orthopedic prosthetic devices, implants and grafts A ⬤, A ⬤

X● T84.83   Hemorrhage due to internal orthopedic prosthetic devices, implants and grafts A ⬤, A ⬤

X● T84.84   Pain due to internal orthopedic prosthetic devices, implants and grafts A ⬤, A ⬤

X● T84.85   Stenosis due to internal orthopedic prosthetic devices, implants and grafts A ⬤, A ⬤

X● T84.86   Thrombosis due to internal orthopedic prosthetic devices, implants and grafts A ⬤, A ⬤

X● T84.89   Other specified complication of internal orthopedic prosthetic devices, implants and grafts A ⬤, A ⬤

X● T84.9   Unspecified complication of internal orthopedic prosthetic device, implant and graft A ⬤, A ⬤
Ex: See PDX Collection 1459

● T85   Complications of other internal prosthetic devices, implants and grafts

Excludes2   failure and rejection of transplanted organs and tissue (T86.-)

The appropriate 7th character is to be added to each code from category T85

A	initial encounter
D	subsequent encounter
S	sequela

Coding Clinic: 2016, Q4, P71

● T85.0   Mechanical complication of ventricular intracranial (communicating) shunt
Ex: For category T85.0 CC codes: See PDX Collection 1460

X● T85.01   Breakdown (mechanical) of ventricular intracranial (communicating) shunt A ⬤, A ⬤

X● T85.02   Displacement of ventricular intracranial (communicating) shunt A ⬤, A ⬤
Malposition of ventricular intracranial (communicating) shunt

X● T85.03   Leakage of ventricular intracranial (communicating) shunt A ⬤, A ⬤

X● T85.09   Other mechanical complication of ventricular intracranial (communicating) shunt A ⬤, A ⬤
Obstruction (mechanical) of ventricular intracranial (communicating) shunt
Perforation of ventricular intracranial (communicating) shunt
Protrusion of ventricular intracranial (communicating) shunt

● T85.1   Mechanical complication of implanted electronic stimulator of nervous system
Ex: For category T85.1 CC codes: See PDX Collection 1460
Coding Clinic: 2016, Q4, P71

● T85.11   Breakdown (mechanical) of implanted electronic stimulator of nervous system

● T85.110   Breakdown (mechanical) of implanted electronic neurostimulator of brain electrode (lead) A ⬤, A ⬤

● T85.111   Breakdown (mechanical) of implanted electronic neurostimulator of peripheral nerve electrode (lead) A ⬤, A ⬤
Breakdown of electrode (lead) for cranial nerve neurostimulators
Breakdown of electrode (lead) for gastric neurostimulator
Breakdown of electrode (lead) for sacral nerve neurostimulator
Breakdown of electrode (lead) for vagal nerve neurostimulators

● T85.112   Breakdown (mechanical) of implanted electronic neurostimulator of spinal cord electrode (lead) A ⬤, A ⬤

● T85.113   Breakdown (mechanical) of implanted electronic neurostimulator, generator A ⬤, A ⬤
Breakdown (mechanical) of implanted electronic neurostimulator generator, brain, peripheral, gastric, spinal
Breakdown (mechanical) of implanted electronic sacral neurostimulator, pulse generator or receiver

● T85.118   Breakdown (mechanical) of other implanted electronic stimulator of nervous system A ⬤, A ⬤

CHAPTER 19 (S00-T88)

● **T85.12 Displacement of implanted electronic stimulator of nervous system**
Malposition of implanted electronic stimulator of nervous system

● **T85.120 Displacement of implanted electronic neurostimulator of brain electrode (lead) A 🔵, A 🔵**

● **T85.121 Displacement of implanted electronic neurostimulator of peripheral nerve electrode (lead) A 🔵, A 🔵**
Displacement of electrode (lead) for cranial nerve neurostimulators
Displacement of electrode (lead) for gastric neurostimulator
Displacement of electrode (lead) for sacral nerve neurostimulator
Displacement of electrode (lead) for vagal nerve neurostimulators

● **T85.122 Displacement of implanted electronic neurostimulator of spinal cord electrode (lead) A 🔵, A 🔵**

● **T85.123 Displacement of implanted electronic neurostimulator, generator A 🔵, A 🔵**
Displacement of implanted electronic neurostimulator generator, brain, peripheral, gastric, spinal
Displacement of implanted electronic sacral neurostimulator, pulse generator or receiver

● **T85.128 Displacement of other implanted electronic stimulator of nervous system A 🔵, A 🔵**

● **T85.19 Other mechanical complication of implanted electronic stimulator of nervous system**
Leakage of implanted electronic stimulator of nervous system
Obstruction (mechanical) of implanted electronic stimulator of nervous system
Perforation of implanted electronic stimulator of nervous system
Protrusion of implanted electronic stimulator of nervous system

● **T85.190 Other mechanical complication of implanted electronic neurostimulator of brain electrode (lead) A 🔵, A 🔵**

● **T85.191 Other mechanical complication of implanted electronic neurostimulator of peripheral nerve electrode (lead) A 🔵, A 🔵**
Other mechanical complication of electrode (lead) for cranial nerve neurostimulators
Other mechanical complication of electrode (lead) for gastric neurostimulator
Other mechanical complication of electrode (lead) for sacral nerve neurostimulator
Other mechanical complication of electrode (lead) for vagal nerve neurostimulators

● **T85.192 Other mechanical complication of implanted electronic neurostimulator of spinal cord electrode (lead) A 🔵, A 🔵**

● **T85.193 Other mechanical complication of implanted electronic neurostimulator, generator A 🔵, A 🔵**
Other mechanical complication of implanted electronic neurostimulator generator, brain, peripheral, gastric, spinal
Other mechanical complication of implanted electronic sacral neurostimulator, pulse generator or receiver

● **T85.199 Other mechanical complication of other implanted electronic stimulator of nervous system A 🔵, A 🔵**

● **T85.2 Mechanical complication of intraocular lens**
Ⓔ⃝ **For category T85.2 CC codes:** See PDX Collection 1461

X ● **T85.21 Breakdown (mechanical) of intraocular lens A 🔵**

X ● **T85.22 Displacement of intraocular lens A 🔵**
Malposition of intraocular lens

X ● **T85.29 Other mechanical complication of intraocular lens A 🔵**
Obstruction (mechanical) of intraocular lens
Perforation of intraocular lens
Protrusion of intraocular lens

● **T85.3 Mechanical complication of other ocular prosthetic devices, implants and grafts**
Excludes2 other complications of corneal graft (T86.84-)
Ⓔ⃝ **For category T85.3 CC codes:** See PDX Collection 1462

● **T85.31 Breakdown (mechanical) of other ocular prosthetic devices, implants and grafts**

● **T85.310 Breakdown (mechanical) of prosthetic orbit of right eye A 🔵**

● **T85.311 Breakdown (mechanical) of prosthetic orbit of left eye A 🔵**

● **T85.318 Breakdown (mechanical) of other ocular prosthetic devices, implants and grafts**

● **T85.32 Displacement of other ocular prosthetic devices, implants and grafts**
Malposition of other ocular prosthetic devices, implants and grafts

● **T85.320 Displacement of prosthetic orbit of right eye A 🔵**

● **T85.321 Displacement of prosthetic orbit of left eye A 🔵**

● **T85.328 Displacement of other ocular prosthetic devices, implants and grafts**

● **T85.39 Other mechanical complication of other ocular prosthetic devices, implants and grafts**
Obstruction (mechanical) of other ocular prosthetic devices, implants and grafts
Perforation of other ocular prosthetic devices, implants and grafts
Protrusion of other ocular prosthetic devices, implants and grafts

● **T85.390 Other mechanical complication of prosthetic orbit of right eye A 🔵**

● **T85.391 Other mechanical complication of prosthetic orbit of left eye A 🔵**

● **T85.398 Other mechanical complication of other ocular prosthetic devices, implants and grafts**

▶ New   ⇒ Revised   ~~deleted~~ Deleted   Excludes 1   Excludes 2   Includes   Use additional   Code first   Code also   Key words
OGCR Official Guidelines   ● Unacceptable Principal Diagnosis   X Assign placeholder X   ● Use Additional Character(s)   ▌ Manifestation Code   Coding Clinic

● **T85.4**   **Mechanical complication of breast prosthesis and implant**
     Ⓔⓧ **For category T85.4 CC codes:** See PDX Collection 1463

X● **T85.41**   **Breakdown (mechanical) of breast prosthesis and implant** A ℚ

X● **T85.42**   **Displacement of breast prosthesis and implant** A ℚ
       Malposition of breast prosthesis and implant

X● **T85.43**   **Leakage of breast prosthesis and implant** A ℚ

X● **T85.44**   **Capsular contracture of breast implant** A ℚ

X● **T85.49**   **Other mechanical complication of breast prosthesis and implant** A ℚ
       Obstruction (mechanical) of breast prosthesis and implant
       Perforation of breast prosthesis and implant
       Protrusion of breast prosthesis and implant

● **T85.5**   **Mechanical complication of gastrointestinal prosthetic devices, implants and grafts**
     Ⓔⓧ **For category T85.5 CC codes:** See PDX Collection 1464

● **T85.51**   **Breakdown (mechanical) of gastrointestinal prosthetic devices, implants and grafts**

   ● **T85.510**   **Breakdown (mechanical) of bile duct prosthesis** A ℚ

   ● **T85.511**   **Breakdown (mechanical) of esophageal anti-reflux device** A ℚ

   ● **T85.518**   **Breakdown (mechanical) of other gastrointestinal prosthetic devices, implants and grafts** A ℚ

● **T85.52**   **Displacement of gastrointestinal prosthetic devices, implants and grafts**
       Malposition of gastrointestinal prosthetic devices, implants and grafts

   ● **T85.520**   **Displacement of bile duct prosthesis** A ℚ

   ● **T85.521**   **Displacement of esophageal anti-reflux device** A ℚ

   ● **T85.528**   **Displacement of other gastrointestinal prosthetic devices, implants and grafts** A ℚ

● **T85.59**   **Other mechanical complication of gastrointestinal prosthetic devices, implants and**
       Obstruction, mechanical of gastrointestinal prosthetic devices, implants and grafts
       Perforation of gastrointestinal prosthetic devices, implants and grafts
       Protrusion of gastrointestinal prosthetic devices, implants and grafts

   ● **T85.590**   **Other mechanical complication of bile duct prosthesis** A ℚ

   ● **T85.591**   **Other mechanical complication of esophageal anti-reflux device** A ℚ

   ● **T85.598**   **Other mechanical complication of other gastrointestinal prosthetic devices, implants and grafts** A ℚ

● **T85.6**   **Mechanical complication of other specified internal and external prosthetic devices, implants and grafts**
     Coding Clinic: 2016, Q4, P71

● **T85.61**   **Breakdown (mechanical) of other specified internal prosthetic devices, implants and grafts**

   ● **T85.610**   **Breakdown (mechanical) of cranial or spinal infusion catheter** A ℚ
       Breakdown (mechanical) of epidural infusion catheter
       Breakdown (mechanical) of intrathecal infusion catheter
       Breakdown (mechanical) of subarachnoid infusion catheter
       Breakdown (mechanical) of subdural infusion catheter
       Ⓔⓧ See PDX Collection 1465

   ● **T85.611**   **Breakdown (mechanical) of intraperitoneal dialysis catheter** A ℚ, A, D, S ℚ
       Excludes1   mechanical complication of vascular dialysis catheter (T82.4-)
       Ⓔⓧ See PDX Collection 1466

   ● **T85.612**   **Breakdown (mechanical) of permanent sutures** A ℚ
       Excludes1   mechanical complication of permanent (wire) suture used in bone repair (T84.1-T84.2)
       Ⓔⓧ See PDX Collection 1467

   ● **T85.613**   **Breakdown (mechanical) of artificial skin graft and decellularized allodermis** A ℚ
       Failure of artificial skin graft and decellularized allodermis
       Non-adherence of artificial skin graft and decellularized allodermis
       Poor incorporation of artificial skin graft and decellularized allodermis
       Shearing of artificial skin graft and decellularized allodermis
       Ⓔⓧ See PDX Collection 1468

   ● **T85.614**   **Breakdown (mechanical) of insulin pump** A ℚ
       Ⓔⓧ See PDX Collection 1469

   ● **T85.615**   **Breakdown (mechanical) of other nervous system device, implant or graft** A ℚ, A ℚ
       Breakdown (mechanical) of intrathecal infusion pump
       Ⓔⓧ See PDX Collection 1467

   ● **T85.618**   **Breakdown (mechanical) of other specified internal prosthetic devices, implants and grafts** A ℚ
       Ⓔⓧ See PDX Collection 1467

CHAPTER 19 (S00-T88)

N Newborn Age: 0   **P** Pediatric Age: 0–17   **M** Maternity DX: 9–64   **A** Adult Age: 15–124   ♀ Females Only   ♂ Males Only

ℚ Complication\Comorbidity   ℚ Major C\C   Ⓔⓧ CC/MCC Exclusions   ℚ Hospital-Acquired Condition   ℚ Hierarchical Condition Category   **1521**

CHAPTER 19 (SØØ-T88)

● **T85.62 Displacement of other specified internal prosthetic devices, implants and grafts**
Malposition of other specified internal prosthetic devices, implants and grafts

    ● **T85.620 Displacement of cranial or spinal infusion catheter** A 🦠
Displacement of epidural infusion catheter
Displacement of intrathecal infusion catheter
Displacement of subarachnoid infusion catheter
Displacement of subdural infusion catheter
(Ex:) See PDX Collection 1465

    ● **T85.621 Displacement of intraperitoneal dialysis catheter** A 🦠, A, D, S 🦠
> **Excludes1** mechanical complication of vascular dialysis catheter (T82.4-)
(Ex:) See PDX Collection 1466

    ● **T85.622 Displacement of permanent sutures** A 🦠
> **Excludes1** mechanical complication of permanent (wire) suture used in bone repair (T84.1-T84.2)
(Ex:) See PDX Collection 1467

    ● **T85.623 Displacement of artificial skin graft and decellularized allodermis** A 🦠
Dislodgement of artificial skin graft and decellularized allodermis
(Ex:) See PDX Collection 1468

    ● **T85.624 Displacement of insulin pump** A 🦠
(Ex:) See PDX Collection 1469

    ● **T85.625 Displacement of other nervous system device, implant or graft** A 🦠, A 🦠
Displacement of intrathecal infusion pump
(Ex:) See PDX Collection 1467

    ● **T85.628 Displacement of other specified internal prosthetic devices, implants and grafts** A 🦠
(Ex:) See PDX Collection 1467
Coding Clinic: 2015, Q1, P15

● **T85.63 Leakage of other specified internal prosthetic devices, implants and grafts**

    ● **T85.630 Leakage of cranial or spinal infusion catheter** A 🦠
Leakage of epidural infusion catheter
Leakage of intrathecal infusion catheter
Leakage of subdural infusion catheter
Leakage of subarachnoid infusion catheter
(Ex:) See PDX Collection 1465

    ● **T85.631 Leakage of intraperitoneal dialysis catheter** A 🦠, A, D, S 🦠
> **Excludes1** mechanical complication of vascular dialysis catheter (T82.4)
(Ex:) See PDX Collection 1466

    ● **T85.633 Leakage of insulin pump** A 🦠
(Ex:) See PDX Collection 1469

    ● **T85.635 Leakage of other nervous system device, implant or graft** A 🦠, A 🦠
Leakage of intrathecal infusion pump
(Ex:) See PDX Collection 1467

    ● **T85.638 Leakage of other specified internal prosthetic devices, implants and grafts** A 🦠
(Ex:) See PDX Collection 1467

● **T85.69 Other mechanical complication of other specified internal prosthetic devices, implants and grafts**
Obstruction, mechanical of other specified internal prosthetic devices, implants and grafts
Perforation of other specified internal prosthetic devices, implants and grafts
Protrusion of other specified internal prosthetic devices, implants and grafts

    ● **T85.690 Other mechanical complication of cranial or spinal infusion catheter** A 🦠
Other mechanical complication of epidural infusion catheter
Other mechanical complication of intrathecal infusion catheter
Other mechanical complication of subarachnoid infusion catheter
Other mechanical complication of subdural infusion catheter
(Ex:) See PDX Collection 1465

    ● **T85.691 Other mechanical complication of intraperitoneal dialysis catheter** A 🦠, A, D, S 🦠
> **Excludes1** mechanical complication of vascular dialysis catheter (T82.4)
(Ex:) See PDX Collection 1466

    ● **T85.692 Other mechanical complication of permanent sutures** A 🦠
> **Excludes1** mechanical complication of permanent (wire) suture used in bone repair (T84.1-T84.2)
(Ex:) See PDX Collection 1467

    ● **T85.693 Other mechanical complication of artificial skin graft and decellularized allodermis** A 🦠
(Ex:) See PDX Collection 1468

    ● **T85.694 Other mechanical complication of insulin pump** A 🦠
(Ex:) See PDX Collection 1469

    ● **T85.695 Other mechanical complication of other nervous system device, implant or graft** A 🦠, A 🦠
Other mechanical complication of intrathecal infusion pump
(Ex:) See PDX Collection 1467

    ● **T85.698 Other mechanical complication of other specified internal prosthetic devices, implants and grafts** A 🦠
Mechanical complication of nonabsorbable surgical material NOS
(Ex:) See PDX Collection 1467

▶ New   ⇒ Revised   ~~deleted~~ Deleted   Excludes 1   Excludes 2   Includes   Use additional   Code first   Code also   Key words
OGCR Official Guidelines   ● Unacceptable Principal Diagnosis   X Assign placeholder X   ● Use Additional Character(s)   🦠 Manifestation Code   **Coding Clinic**

● **T85.7   Infection and inflammatory reaction due to other internal prosthetic devices, implants and grafts**

> Use additional code to identify infection
>
> (Ex:) **For category T85.7 CC codes unless otherwise indicated:** See PDX Collection 1470
>
> Coding Clinic: 2016, Q4, P72

X● **T85.71   Infection and inflammatory reaction due to peritoneal dialysis catheter** A 🔵, A, D, S 🔴

> (Ex:) See PDX Collection 1467

X● **T85.72   Infection and inflammatory reaction due to insulin pump** A 🔵, A 🔴

● **T85.73   Infection and inflammatory reaction due to nervous system devices, implants and graft**

   ● **T85.730   Infection and inflammatory reaction due to ventricular intracranial (communicating) shunt** A 🔵, A 🔴

   ● **T85.731   Infection and inflammatory reaction due to implanted electronic neurostimulator of brain, electrode (lead)** A 🔵, A 🔴

   ● **T85.732   Infection and inflammatory reaction due to implanted electronic neurostimulator of peripheral nerve, electrode (lead)** A 🔵, A 🔴

> Infection and inflammatory reaction due to electrode (lead) for cranial nerve neurostimulators
>
> Infection and inflammatory reaction due to electrode (lead) for gastric neurostimulator
>
> Infection and inflammatory reaction due to electrode (lead) for sacral nerve neurostimulator
>
> Infection and inflammatory reaction due to electrode (lead) for vagal nerve neurostimulators

   ● **T85.733   Infection and inflammatory reaction due to implanted electronic neurostimulator of spinal cord, electrode (lead)** A 🔵, A 🔴

   ● **T85.734   Infection and inflammatory reaction due to implanted electronic neurostimulator, generator** A 🔵, A 🔴

> Generator pocket infection

   ● **T85.735   Infection and inflammatory reaction due to cranial or spinal infusion catheter** A 🔵, A 🔴

> Infection and inflammatory reaction due to epidural catheter
>
> Infection and inflammatory reaction due to intrathecal infusion catheter
>
> Infection and inflammatory reaction due to subarachnoid catheter
>
> Infection and inflammatory reaction due to subdural catheter

   ● **T85.738   Infection and inflammatory reaction due to other nervous system device, implant or graft** A 🔵, A 🔴

> Infection and inflammatory reaction due to intrathecal infusion pump

X● **T85.79   Infection and inflammatory reaction due to other internal prosthetic devices, implants and grafts** A 🔵, A 🔴

> Coding Clinic: 2016, Q4, P72

● **T85.8   Other specified complications of internal prosthetic devices, implants and grafts, not elsewhere classified**

> (Ex:) **For category T85.8 CC codes:** See PDX Collection 1470
>
> Coding Clinic: 2016, Q4, P72

● **T85.81   Embolism due to internal prosthetic devices, implants and grafts, not elsewhere classified**

   ● **T85.810   Embolism due to nervous system prosthetic devices, implants and grafts** A, D 🔵, A 🔴

   ● **T85.818   Embolism due to other internal prosthetic devices, implants and grafts**

● **T85.82   Fibrosis due to internal prosthetic devices, implants and grafts, not elsewhere classified**

   ● **T85.820   Fibrosis due to nervous system prosthetic devices, implants and grafts** A, D 🔵, A 🔴

   ● **T85.828   Fibrosis due to other internal prosthetic devices, implants and grafts**

● **T85.83   Hemorrhage due to internal prosthetic devices, implants and grafts, not elsewhere classified**

   ● **T85.830   Hemorrhage due to nervous system prosthetic devices, implants and grafts** A, D 🔵, A 🔴

   ● **T85.838   Hemorrhage due to other internal prosthetic devices, implants and grafts**

● **T85.84   Pain due to internal prosthetic devices, implants and grafts, not elsewhere classified**

   ● **T85.840   Pain due to nervous system prosthetic devices, implants and grafts** A, D 🔵, A 🔴

   ● **T85.848   Pain due to other internal prosthetic devices, implants and grafts**

● **T85.85   Stenosis due to internal prosthetic devices, implants and grafts, not elsewhere classified**

   ● **T85.850   Stenosis due to nervous system prosthetic devices, implants and grafts** A, D 🔵, A 🔴

   ● **T85.858   Stenosis due to other internal prosthetic devices, implants and grafts**

● **T85.86   Thrombosis due to internal prosthetic devices, implants and grafts, not elsewhere classified**

   ● **T85.860   Thrombosis due to nervous system prosthetic devices, implants and grafts** A, D 🔵, A 🔴

   ● **T85.868   Thrombosis due to other internal prosthetic devices, implants and grafts**

● **T85.89   Other specified complication of internal prosthetic devices, implants and grafts, not elsewhere classified**

> Coding Clinic: 2016, Q4, P72

   ● **T85.890   Other specified complication of nervous system prosthetic devices, implants and grafts** A, D 🔵, A 🔴

   ● **T85.898   Other specified complication of other internal prosthetic devices, implants and grafts**

X● **T85.9   Unspecified complication of internal prosthetic device, implant and graft**

> Complication of internal prosthetic device, implant and graft NOS

N Newborn Age: 0   **P** Pediatric Age: 0–17   **M** Maternity DX: 9–64   **A** Adult Age: 15–124   ♀ Females Only   ♂ Males Only

🔵 Complication\Comorbidity   🔴 Major C\C   (Ex:) CC/MCC Exclusions   Hospital-Acquired Condition   Hierarchical Condition Category

1523

CHAPTER 19 (S00–T88)

CHAPTER 19 (S00-T88)

● **T86**   **Complications of transplanted organs and tissue**

     Use additional code to identify other transplant complications, such as:

         graft-versus-host disease (D89.81-)

         malignancy associated with organ transplant (C80.2)

         post-transplant lymphoproliferative disorders (PTLD) (D47.Z1)

    ● **T86.0**   **Complications of bone marrow transplant**

        (Ex) **For category T86.0 CC codes:** See PDX Collection 514

       T86.00   **Unspecified** complication of bone marrow transplant

       T86.01   Bone marrow transplant **rejection**

       T86.02   Bone marrow transplant **failure**

       T86.03   Bone marrow transplant **infection**

       T86.09   **Other** complications of bone marrow transplant

    ● **T86.1**   **Complications of kidney transplant**

        (Ex) **For category T86.1 CC codes:** See PDX Collection 1471

       T86.10   **Unspecified** complication of kidney transplant

       T86.11   Kidney transplant **rejection**

       T86.12   Kidney transplant **failure**

         Coding Clinic: 2013, Q1, P24

       T86.13   Kidney transplant **infection**

         Use additional code to specify infection

       T86.19   **Other** complication of kidney transplant

         Coding Clinic: 2019, Q2, P7

    ● **T86.2**   **Complications of heart transplant**

       Excludes1   complication of:

         ⟹ artificial heart device (T82.5-)

         ⟹ heart-lung transplant (T86.3-)

       (Ex) **For category T86.2 CC codes:** See PDX Collection 1472

       T86.20   **Unspecified** complication of heart transplant

       T86.21   Heart transplant **rejection**

       T86.22   Heart transplant **failure**

       T86.23   Heart transplant **infection**

         Use additional code to specify infection

      ● T86.29   **Other complications of heart transplant**

        T86.290   **Cardiac allograft vasculopathy**

         Excludes1   atherosclerosis of coronary arteries (I25.75-, I25.76-, I25.81-)

        T86.298   **Other** complications of heart transplant

    ● **T86.3**   **Complications of heart-lung transplant**

        (Ex) **For category T86.3 CC codes:** See PDX Collection 1472

       T86.30   **Unspecified** complication of heart-lung transplant

         CC when PDx is its own CC

       T86.31   Heart-lung transplant **rejection**

         CC when PDx is its own CC

       T86.32   Heart-lung transplant **failure**

         CC when PDx is its own CC

       T86.33   Heart-lung transplant **infection**

         Use additional code to specify infection

         CC when PDx is its own CC

       T86.39   **Other complications of heart-lung transplant**

         CC when PDx is its own CC

    ● **T86.4**   **Complications of liver transplant**

        (Ex) **For category T86.4 CC codes:** See PDX Collection 1473

       T86.40   **Unspecified complication of liver transplant**

       T86.41   Liver transplant **rejection**

       T86.42   Liver transplant **failure**

       T86.43   Liver transplant **infection**

         Use additional code to identify infection, such as:

           Cytomegalovirus (CMV) infection (B25.-)

       T86.49   **Other complications of liver transplant**

    ● **T86.5**   **Complications of stem cell transplant**

        Complications from stem cells from peripheral blood

        Complications from stem cells from umbilical cord

        (Ex) See PDX Collection 1474

    ● **T86.8**   **Complications of other transplanted organs and tissues**

      ● **T86.81**   **Complications of lung transplant**

        Excludes1   complication of heart-lung transplant (T86.3-)

        (Ex) **For category T86.81 CC codes:** See PDX Collection 1475

        T86.810   Lung transplant **rejection**

        T86.811   Lung transplant **failure**

        T86.812   Lung transplant **infection**

          Use additional code to specify infection

        T86.818   **Other** complications of lung transplant

          Coding Clinic: 2019, Q2, P7

        T86.819   **Unspecified** complication of lung transplant

      ● **T86.82**   **Complications of skin graft (allograft) (autograft)**

        Excludes2   complication of artificial skin graft (T85.693)

        (Ex) **For category T86.82 CC codes:** See PDX Collection 1476

        T86.820   Skin graft (allograft) **rejection**

        T86.821   Skin graft (allograft) (autograft) **failure**

        T86.822   Skin graft (allograft) (autograft) **infection**

          Use additional code to specify infection

        T86.828   **Other** complications of skin graft (allograft) (autograft)

        T86.829   **Unspecified** complication of skin graft (allograft) (autograft)

      ● **T86.83**   **Complications of bone graft**

        Excludes2   mechanical complications of bone graft (T84.3-)

        (Ex) **For category T86.83 CC codes:** See PDX Collection 1477

        T86.830   Bone graft **rejection**

        T86.831   Bone graft **failure**

        T86.832   Bone graft **infection**

          Use additional code to specify infection

        T86.838   **Other** complications of bone graft

        T86.839   **Unspecified** complication of bone graft

▶ New   ⟹ Revised   ~~deleted~~ Deleted   Excludes 1   Excludes 2   Includes   Use additional   Code first   Code also   Key words

OGCR Official Guidelines   ● Unacceptable Principal Diagnosis   X Assign placeholder X   ● Use Additional Character(s)   ▌ Manifestation Code   **Coding Clinic**

● T86.84   Complications of corneal transplant
            Excludes2   mechanical complications of
                             corneal graft (T85.3-)
            (Ex:) **For category T86.84 CC codes unless otherwise
            indicated:** See PDX Collection 1479

● T86.840   Corneal transplant rejection 🅒
            (Ex:) See PDX Collection 4016

            T86.8401   Corneal transplant
                        rejection, right eye 🅒
            T86.8402   Corneal transplant
                        rejection, left eye 🅒
            T86.8403   Corneal transplant
                        rejection, bilateral 🅒
            T86.8409   Corneal transplant
                        rejection, unspecified eye 🅒

● T86.841   Corneal transplant failure 🅒
            (Ex:) See PDX Collection 4016

            T86.8411   Corneal transplant failure,
                        right eye 🅒
            T86.8412   Corneal transplant failure,
                        left eye 🅒
            T86.8413   Corneal transplant failure,
                        bilateral 🅒
            T86.8419   Corneal transplant failure,
                        unspecified eye 🅒

● T86.842   Corneal transplant infection 🅒🅒
            Use additional code to specify
            infection
            (Ex:) See PDX Collection 4022

            T86.8421   Corneal transplant
                        infection, right eye 🅒
            T86.8422   Corneal transplant
                        infection, left eye 🅒
            T86.8423   Corneal transplant
                        infection, bilateral 🅒
            T86.8429   Corneal transplant
                        infection, unspecified eye 🅒

● T86.848   Other complications of corneal
            transplant 🅒
            (Ex:) See PDX Collection 4022

            T86.8481   Other complications of
                        corneal transplant, right
                        eye 🅒
            T86.8482   Other complications of
                        corneal transplant, left
                        eye 🅒
            T86.8483   Other complications of
                        corneal transplant,
                        bilateral 🅒
            T86.8489   Other complications of
                        corneal transplant,
                        unspecified eye 🅒

● T86.849   Unspecified complication of corneal
            transplant 🅒
            (Ex:) See PDX Collection 4022

            T86.8491   Unspecified complication of
                        corneal transplant, right
                        eye 🅒
            T86.8492   Unspecified complication of
                        corneal transplant, left
                        eye 🅒
            T86.8493   Unspecified complication of
                        corneal transplant,
                        bilateral 🅒
            T86.8499   Unspecified complication of
                        corneal transplant,
                        unspecified eye 🅒

● T86.85   Complication of intestine transplant
            (Ex:) **For category T86.85 CC codes:** See PDX Collection 495

            T86.850   Intestine transplant rejection 🅒🅒
            T86.851   Intestine transplant failure 🅒🅒
            T86.852   Intestine transplant infection 🅒🅒
                        Use additional code to specify
                        infection
            T86.858   Other complications of intestine
                        transplant 🅒🅒
            T86.859   Unspecified complication of intestine
                        transplant 🅒🅒

● T86.89   Complications of other transplanted tissue
            Transplant failure or rejection of pancreas
            (Ex:) **For category T86.89 CC codes:** See PDX Collection 1480

            T86.890   Other transplanted tissue rejection 🅒
            T86.891   Other transplanted tissue failure 🅒
            T86.892   Other transplanted tissue infection 🅒
                        Use additional code to specify
                        infection
            T86.898   Other complications of other
                        transplanted tissue 🅒
            T86.899   Unspecified complication of other
                        transplanted tissue 🅒

● T86.9   Complication of unspecified transplanted organ and
            tissue
            (Ex:) **For category T86.9 CC codes:** See PDX Collection 495

            T86.90   Unspecified complication of unspecified
                        transplanted organ and tissue 🅒
            T86.91   Unspecified transplanted organ and tissue
                        rejection 🅒
            T86.92   Unspecified transplanted organ and tissue
                        failure 🅒
            T86.93   Unspecified transplanted organ and tissue
                        infection 🅒
                        Use additional code to specify infection
            T86.99   Other complications of unspecified
                        transplanted organ and tissue 🅒

● T87   Complications peculiar to reattachment and amputation
    ● T87.0   Complications of reattached (part of) upper extremity
                (Ex:) **For category T87.0 CC codes:** See PDX Collection 1481

        ● T87.0X   Complications of reattached (part of) upper
                    extremity
                    T87.0X1   Complications of reattached (part of)
                                right upper extremity 🅒🅒
                    T87.0X2   Complications of reattached (part of)
                                left upper extremity 🅒🅒
                    T87.0X9   Complications of reattached (part of)
                                unspecified upper extremity 🅒🅒

    ● T87.1   Complications of reattached (part of) lower extremity
                (Ex:) **For category T87.1 CC codes:** See PDX Collection 1482

        ● T87.1X   Complications of reattached (part of) lower
                    extremity
                    T87.1X1   Complications of reattached (part of)
                                right lower extremity 🅒🅒
                    T87.1X2   Complications of reattached (part of)
                                left lower extremity 🅒🅒
                    T87.1X9   Complications of reattached (part of)
                                unspecified lower extremity 🅒🅒

      T87.2   Complications of other reattached body part 🅒🅒
                (Ex:) See PDX Collection 1483

    ● T87.3   Neuroma of amputation stump
                T87.30   Neuroma of amputation stump, unspecified
                            extremity 🅒
                T87.31   Neuroma of amputation stump, right upper
                            extremity 🅒
                T87.32   Neuroma of amputation stump, left upper
                            extremity 🅒

N Newborn Age: 0   **P** Pediatric Age: 0–17   **M** Maternity DX: 9–64   **A** Adult Age: 15–124   ♀ Females Only   ♂ Males Only

🅒 Complication\Comorbidity   🅒 Major C\C   (Ex:) CC/MCC Exclusions   🅒 Hospital-Acquired Condition   🅒 Hierarchical Condition Category

1525

T87.33   **Neuroma of amputation stump, right lower extremity** 🔖

T87.34   **Neuroma of amputation stump, left lower extremity** 🔖

● **T87.4   Infection of amputation stump**

(Ex:) **For category T87.4 CC codes: See PDX Collection 1484**

T87.40   **Infection of amputation stump, unspecified extremity** 🔖 🔖

T87.41   **Infection of amputation stump, right upper extremity** 🔖 🔖

T87.42   **Infection of amputation stump, left upper extremity** 🔖 🔖

T87.43   **Infection of amputation stump, right lower extremity** 🔖 🔖

T87.44   **Infection of amputation stump, left lower extremity** 🔖 🔖

● **T87.5   Necrosis of amputation stump**

T87.50   **Necrosis of amputation stump, unspecified extremity** 🔖

T87.51   **Necrosis of amputation stump, right upper extremity** 🔖

T87.52   **Necrosis of amputation stump, left upper extremity** 🔖

T87.53   **Necrosis of amputation stump, right lower extremity** 🔖

T87.54   **Necrosis of amputation stump, left lower extremity** 🔖

● **T87.8   Other complications of amputation stump**

T87.81   **Dehiscence of amputation stump** 🔖

T87.89   **Other complications of amputation stump** 🔖
Amputation stump contracture
Amputation stump contracture of next proximal joint
Amputation stump flexion
Amputation stump edema
Amputation stump hematoma

Excludes2   phantom limb syndrome (G54.6-G54.7)

T87.9   **Unspecified complications of amputation stump** 🔖

● **T88   Other complications of surgical and medical care, not elsewhere classified**

Excludes2   complication following infusion, transfusion and therapeutic injection (T80.-)
complication following procedure NEC (T81.-)
complications of anesthesia in labor and delivery (O74.-)
complications of anesthesia in pregnancy (O29.-)
complications of anesthesia in puerperium (O89.-)
complications of devices, implants and grafts (T82-T85)
complications of obstetric surgery and procedure (O75.4)
dermatitis due to drugs and medicaments (L23.3, L24.4, L25.1, L27.0-L27.1)
poisoning and toxic effects of drugs and chemicals (T36-T65 with fifth or sixth character 1-4 or 6)
specified complications classified elsewhere

The appropriate 7th character is to be added to each code from category T88

A	initial encounter
D	subsequent encounter
S	sequela

X ● **T88.0   Infection following immunization** A 🔖
Sepsis following immunization
(Ex:) See PDX Collection 948
Coding Clinic: 2019, Q1, P14;2018, Q4, P90

X ● **T88.1   Other complications following immunization, not elsewhere classified** A 🔖
Generalized vaccinia
Rash following immunization

Excludes1   vaccinia not from vaccine (B08.011)

Excludes2   anaphylactic shock due to serum (T80.5-)
other serum reactions (T80.6-)
postimmunization arthropathy (M02.2)
postimmunization encephalitis (G04.02)
postimmunization fever (R50.83)

(Ex:) See PDX Collection 1485

X ● **T88.2   Shock due to anesthesia** A 🔖

Use additional code for adverse effect, if applicable, to identify drug (T41.- with fifth or sixth character 5)

Excludes1   complications of anesthesia (in):
labor and delivery (O74.-)
pregnancy (O29.-)
puerperium (O89.-)
postprocedural shock NOS (T81.1-)

(Ex:) See PDX Collection 1441

X ● **T88.3   Malignant hyperthermia due to anesthesia** A 🔖

Use additional code for adverse effect, if applicable, to identify drug (T41.- with fifth or sixth character 5)

(Ex:) See PDX Collection 1486

X ● **T88.4   Failed or difficult intubation**

● **T88.5   Other complications of anesthesia**

Use additional code for adverse effect, if applicable, to identify drug (T41.- with fifth or sixth character 5)
Coding Clinic: 2016, Q4, P72

X ● **T88.51   Hypothermia following anesthesia**

X ● **T88.52   Failed moderate sedation during procedure**
Failed conscious sedation during procedure

Excludes2   personal history of failed moderate sedation (Z92.83)

X ● **T88.53   Unintended awareness under general anesthesia during procedure**

Excludes2   personal history of unintended awareness under general anesthesia (Z92.84)

Coding Clinic: 2016, Q4, P72-73

X ● **T88.59   Other complications of anesthesia**

X ● **T88.6   Anaphylactic reaction due to adverse effect of correct drug or medicament properly administered** A 🔖
Anaphylactic shock due to adverse effect of correct drug or medicament properly administered
Anaphylactoid reaction NOS

Use additional code for adverse effect, if applicable, to identify drug (T36-T50 with fifth or sixth character 5)

Excludes1   anaphylactic reaction due to serum (T80.5-)
anaphylactic shock or reaction due to adverse food reaction (T78.0-)

(Ex:) See PDX Collection 3292
Coding Clinic: 2020, Q1, P18

X ● **T88.7   Unspecified adverse effect of drug or medicament**
Drug hypersensitivity NOS
Drug reaction NOS

Use additional code for adverse effect, if applicable, to identify drug (T36-T50 with fifth or sixth character 5)

Excludes1   specified adverse effects of drugs and medicaments (A00-R94 and T80-T88.6, T88.8)

X ● **T88.8   Other specified complications of surgical and medical care, not elsewhere classified**
Use additional code to identify the complication

X ● **T88.9   Complication of surgical and medical care, unspecified**

▶ New   ⟹ Revised   ~~deleted~~ Deleted   Excludes 1   Excludes 2   Includes   Use additional   Code first   Code also   Key words

OGCR Official Guidelines   ● Unacceptable Principal Diagnosis   X Assign placeholder X   🔖 Use Additional Character(s)   ▌ Manifestation Code   **Coding Clinic**

CHAPTER 20

EXTERNAL CAUSES OF MORBIDITY (V00-Y99)

OGCR Chapter-Specific Coding Guidelines

20. **Chapter 20: External Causes of Morbidity (V00-Y99)**
The external causes of morbidity codes should never be sequenced as the first-listed or principal diagnosis.

External cause codes are intended to provide data for injury research and evaluation of injury prevention strategies. These codes capture how the injury or health condition happened (cause), the intent (unintentional or accidental; or intentional, such as suicide or assault), the place where the event occurred the activity of the patient at the time of the event, and the person's status (e.g., civilian, military).

There is no national requirement for mandatory ICD-10-CM external cause code reporting. Unless a provider is subject to a state-based external cause code reporting mandate or these codes are required by a particular payer, reporting of ICD-10-CM codes in Chapter 20, External Causes of Morbidity, is not required. In the absence of a mandatory reporting requirement, providers are encouraged to voluntarily report external cause codes, as they provide valuable data for injury research and evaluation of injury prevention strategies.

a. **General External Cause Coding Guidelines**

1) **Used with any code in the range of A00.0-T88.9, Z00-Z99**
An external cause code may be used with any code in the range of A00.0-T88.9, Z00-Z99, classification that represents a health condition due to an external cause. Though they are most applicable to injuries, they are also valid for use with such things as infections or diseases due to an external source, and other health conditions, such as a heart attack that occurs during strenuous physical activity.

2) **External cause code used for length of treatment**
Assign the external cause code, with the appropriate 7th character (initial encounter, subsequent encounter or sequela) for each encounter for which the injury or condition is being treated.

Most categories in Chapter 20 have a 7th character requirement for each applicable code. Most categories in this chapter have three 7th character values: A, initial encounter, D, subsequent encounter and S, sequela. While the patient may be seen by a new or different provider over the course of treatment for an injury or condition, assignment of the 7th character for external cause should match the 7th character of the code assigned for the associated injury or condition for the encounter.

3) **Use the full range of external cause codes**
Use the full range of external cause codes to completely describe the cause, the intent, the place of occurrence and if applicable, the activity of the patient at the time of the event, and the patient's status, for all injuries, and other health conditions due to an external cause.

4) **Assign as many external cause codes as necessary**
Assign as many external cause codes as necessary to fully explain each cause. If only one external code can be recorded, assign the code most related to the principal diagnosis.

5) **The selection of the appropriate external cause code**
The selection of the appropriate external cause code is guided by the Alphabetic Index of External Causes and by Inclusion and Exclusion notes in the Tabular List.

6) **External cause code can never be a principal diagnosis**
An external cause code can never be a principal (first-listed) diagnosis.

7) **Combination external cause codes**
Certain of the external cause codes are combination codes that identify sequential events that result in an injury, such as a fall which results in striking against an object. The injury may be due to either event or both. The combination external cause code used should correspond to the sequence of events regardless of which caused the most serious injury.

8) **No external cause code needed in certain circumstances**
No external cause code from Chapter 20 is needed if the external cause and intent are included in a code from another chapter (e.g., T36.0X1- Poisoning by penicillins, accidental (unintentional)).

b. **Place of Occurrence Guideline**
Codes from category Y92, Place of occurrence of the external cause, are secondary codes for use after other external cause codes to identify the location of the patient at the time of injury or other condition.

Generally, a place of occurrence code is assigned only once, at the initial encounter for treatment. However, in the rare instance that a new injury occurs during hospitalization, an additional place of occurrence code may be assigned. No 7th characters are used for Y92. Only one code from Y92 should be recorded on a medical record.

Do not use place of occurrence code Y92.9 if the place is not stated or is not applicable.

c. **Activity Code**
Assign a code from category Y93, Activity code, to describe the activity of the patient at the time the injury or other health condition occurred.

An activity code is used only once, at the initial encounter for treatment. Only one code from Y93 should be recorded on a medical record.

The activity codes are not applicable to poisonings, adverse effects, misadventures or sequela.

Do not assign Y93.9, Unspecified activity, if the activity is not stated.

A code from category Y93 is appropriate for use with external cause and intent codes if identifying the activity provides additional information about the event.

d. **Place of Occurrence, Activity, and Status Codes Used with Other External Cause Code**
When applicable, place of occurrence, activity, and external cause status codes are sequenced after the main external cause code(s). Regardless of the number of external cause codes assigned, there should be only one place of occurrence code, one activity code, and one external cause status code assigned to an encounter.

e. If the Reporting Format Limits the Number of External Cause Codes

If the reporting format limits the number of external cause codes that can be used in reporting clinical data, report the code for the cause/intent most related to the principal diagnosis. If the format permits capture of additional external cause codes, the cause/intent, including medical misadventures, of the additional events should be reported rather than the codes for place, activity, or external status.

f. Multiple External Cause Coding Guidelines

More than one external cause code is required to fully describe the external cause of an illness or injury. The assignment of external cause codes should be sequenced in the following priority:

If two or more events cause separate injuries, an external cause code should be assigned for each cause. The first-listed external cause code will be selected in the following order:

External codes for child and adult abuse take priority over all other external cause codes.

See Section I.C.19., Child and Adult abuse guidelines.

External codes for terrorism events take priority over all other external cause codes except child and adult abuse.

External cause codes for cataclysmic events take priority over all other external cause codes except child and adult abuse and terrorism.

External cause codes for transport accidents take priority over all other external cause codes except cataclysmic events, child and adult abuse and terrorism.

Activity and external cause status codes are assigned following all causal (intent) external cause codes.

The first-listed external cause code should correspond to the cause of the most serious diagnosis due to an assault, accident, or self-harm, following the order of hierarchy listed above.

g. Child and Adult Abuse Guideline

Adult and child abuse, neglect and maltreatment are classified as assault. Any of the assault codes may be used to indicate the external cause of any injury resulting from the confirmed abuse.

For confirmed cases of abuse, neglect and maltreatment, when the perpetrator is known, a code from Y07, Perpetrator of maltreatment and neglect, should accompany any other assault codes.

See Section I.C.19. Adult and child abuse, neglect and other maltreatment

h. Unknown or Undetermined Intent Guideline

If the intent (accident, self-harm, assault) of the cause of an injury or other condition is unknown or unspecified, code the intent as accidental intent. All transport accident categories assume accidental intent.

1) Use of undetermined intent

External cause codes for events of undetermined intent are only for use if the documentation in the record specifies that the intent cannot be determined.

i. Sequelae (Late Effects) of External Cause Guidelines

1) Sequelae external cause codes

Sequela are reported using the external cause code with the 7th character "S" for sequela. These codes should be used with any report of a late effect or sequela resulting from a previous injury.

See Section I.B.10. Sequela, (Late Effects).

2) Sequela external cause code with a related current injury

A sequela external cause code should never be used with a related current nature of injury code.

3) Use of sequela external cause codes for subsequent visits

Use a late effect external cause code for subsequent visits when a late effect of the initial injury is being treated. Do not use a late effect external cause code for subsequent visits for follow-up care (e.g., to assess healing, to receive rehabilitative therapy) of the injury when no late effect of the injury has been documented.

j. Terrorism Guidelines

1) Cause of injury identified by the Federal Government (FBI) as terrorism

When the cause of an injury is identified by the Federal Government (FBI) as terrorism, the first-listed external cause code should be a code from category Y38, Terrorism. The definition of terrorism employed by the FBI is found at the inclusion note at the beginning of category Y38. Use additional code for place of occurrence (Y92.-). More than one Y38 code may be assigned if the injury is the result of more than one mechanism of terrorism.

2) Cause of an injury is suspected to be the result of terrorism

When the cause of an injury is suspected to be the result of terrorism a code from category Y38 should not be assigned. Suspected cases should be classified as assault.

3) Code Y38.9, Terrorism, secondary effects

Assign code Y38.9, Terrorism, secondary effects, for conditions occurring subsequent to the terrorist event. This code should not be assigned for conditions that are due to the initial terrorist act.

It is acceptable to assign code Y38.9 with another code from Y38 if there is an injury due to the initial terrorist event and an injury that is a subsequent result of the terrorist event.

k. External cause status

A code from category Y99, External cause status, should be assigned whenever any other external cause code is assigned for an encounter, including an Activity code, except for the events noted below. Assign a code from category Y99, External cause status, to indicate the work status of the person at the time the event occurred. The status code indicates whether the event occurred during military activity, whether a non-military person was at work, whether an individual including a student or volunteer was involved in a non-work activity at the time of the causal event.

A code from Y99, External cause status, should be assigned, when applicable, with other external cause codes, such as transport accidents and falls. The external cause status codes are not applicable to poisonings, adverse effects, misadventures or late effects.

Do not assign a code from category Y99 if no other external cause codes (cause, activity) are applicable for the encounter.

An external cause status code is used only once, at the initial encounter for treatment. Only one code from Y99 should be recorded on a medical record.

Do not assign code Y99.9, Unspecified external cause status, if the status is not stated.

CHAPTER 20

EXTERNAL CAUSES OF MORBIDITY (V00-Y99)

Note: This chapter permits the classification of environmental events and circumstances as the cause of injury, and other adverse effects. Where a code from this section is applicable, it is intended that it shall be used secondary to a code from another chapter of the Classification indicating the nature of the condition. Most often, the condition will be classifiable to Chapter 19, Injury, poisoning and certain other consequences of external causes (S00-T88). Other conditions that may be stated to be due to external causes are classified in Chapters 1 to 18. For these conditions, codes from Chapter 20 should be used to provide additional information as to the cause of the condition.

This chapter contains the following blocks:

V00-X58	Accidents
V00-V99	Transport accidents
V00-V09	Pedestrian injured in transport accident
V10-V19	Pedal cycle rider injured in transport accident
V20-V29	Motorcycle rider injured in transport accident
V30-V39	Occupant of three-wheeled motor vehicle injured in transport accident
V40-V49	Car occupant injured in transport accident
V50-V59	Occupant of pick-up truck or van injured in transport accident
V60-V69	Occupant of heavy transport vehicle injured in transport accident
V70-V79	Bus occupant injured in transport accident
V80-V89	Other land transport accidents
V90-V94	Water transport accidents
V95-V97	Air and space transport accidents
V98-V99	Other and unspecified transport accidents
W00-X58	Other external causes of accidental injury
W00-W19	Slipping, tripping, stumbling and falls
W20-W49	Exposure to inanimate mechanical forces
W50-W64	Exposure to animate mechanical forces
W65-W74	Accidental non-transport drowning and submersion
W85-W99	Exposure to electric current, radiation and extreme ambient air temperature and pressure
X00-X08	Exposure to smoke, fire and flames
X10-X19	Contact with heat and hot substances
X30-X39	Exposure to forces of nature
X50	Overexertion and strenuous or repetitive movements
X52, X58	Accidental exposure to other specified factors
X71-X83	Intentional self-harm
X92-Y09	Assault
Y21-Y33	Event of undetermined intent
Y35-Y38	Legal intervention, operations of war, military operations, and terrorism
Y62-Y84	Complications of medical and surgical care
Y62-Y69	Misadventures to patients during surgical and medical care
Y70-Y82	Medical devices associated with adverse incidents in diagnostic and therapeutic use
Y83-Y84	Surgical and other medical procedures as the cause of abnormal reaction of the patient, or of later complication, without mention of misadventure at the time of the procedure
Y90-Y99	Supplementary factors related to causes of morbidity classified elsewhere

ACCIDENTS (V00-X58)

TRANSPORT ACCIDENTS (V00-V99)

Note: This section is structured in 12 groups. Those relating to land transport accidents (V00-V89) reflect the victim's mode of transport and are subdivided to identify the victim's 'counterpart' or the type of event. The vehicle of which the injured person is an occupant is identified in the first two characters since it is seen as the most important factor to identify for prevention purposes. A transport accident is one in which the vehicle involved must be moving or running or in use for transport purposes at the time of the accident.

Use additional code to identify:
Airbag injury (W22.1)
Type of street or road (Y92.4-)
Use of cellular telephone and other electronic equipment at the time of the transport accident (Y93.C-)

Excludes1 agricultural vehicles in stationary use or maintenance (W31.-)
assault by crashing of motor vehicle (Y03.-)
automobile or motor cycle in stationary use or maintenance - code to type of accident
crashing of motor vehicle, undetermined intent (Y32)
intentional self-harm by crashing of motor vehicle (X82)

Excludes2 transport accidents due to cataclysm (X34-X38)

Note: Definitions related to transport accidents:

(a) A transport accident (V00-V99) is any accident involving a device designed primarily for, or used at the time primarily for, conveying persons or good from one place to another.

(b) A public highway [trafficway] or street is the entire width between property lines (or other boundary lines) of land open to the public as a matter of right or custom for purposes of moving persons or property from one place to another. A roadway is that part of the public highway designed, improved and customarily used for vehicular traffic.

(c) A traffic accident is any vehicle accident occurring on the public highway [i.e., originating on, terminating on, or involving a vehicle partially on the highway]. A vehicle accident is assumed to have occurred on the public highway unless another place is specified, except in the case of accidents involving only off-road motor vehicles, which are classified as nontraffic accidents unless the contrary is stated.

(d) A nontraffic accident is any vehicle accident that occurs entirely in any place other than a public highway.

(e) A pedestrian is any person involved in an accident who was not at the time of the accident riding in or on a motor vehicle, railway train, streetcar or animal-drawn or other vehicle, or on a pedal cycle or animal. This includes, a person changing a tire, working on a parked car, or a person on foot. It also includes the user of a pedestrian conveyance such as a baby stroller, ice-skates, skis, sled, roller skates, a skateboard, nonmotorized or motorized wheelchair, motorized mobility scooter, or nonmotorized scooter.

(f) A driver is an occupant of a transport vehicle who is operating or intending to operate it.

(g) A passenger is any occupant of a transport vehicle other than the driver, except a person traveling on the outside of the vehicle.

(h) A person on the outside of a vehicle is any person being transported by a vehicle but not occupying the space normally reserved for the driver or passengers, or the space intended for the transport of property. This includes a person travelling on the bodywork, bumper, fender, roof, running board or step of a vehicle, as well as, hanging on the outside of the vehicle.

(i) A pedal cycle is any land transport vehicle operated solely by nonmotorized pedals including a bicycle or tricycle.

(j) A pedal cyclist is any person riding a pedal cycle or in a sidecar or trailer attached to a pedal cycle.

N Newborn Age: 0   **P** Pediatric Age: 0-17   **M** Maternity DX: 9-64   **A** Adult Age: 15-124   ♀ Females Only   ♂ Males Only

Complication\Comorbidity   Major C\C   (Ex) CC/MCC Exclusions   Hospital-Acquired Condition   Hierarchical Condition Category

1529

(k) A motorcycle is a two-wheeled motor vehicle with one or two riding saddles and sometimes with a third wheel for the support of a sidecar. The sidecar is considered part of the motorcycle. This includes a moped, motor scooter, or motorized bicycle.

(l) A motorcycle rider is any person riding a motorcycle or in a sidecar or trailer attached to the motorcycle.

(m) A three-wheeled motor vehicle is a motorized tricycle designed primarily for on-road use. This includes a motor-driven tricycle, a motorized rickshaw, or a three-wheeled motor car.

(n) A car [automobile] is a four-wheeled motor vehicle designed primarily for carrying up to 7 persons. A trailer being towed by the car is considered part of the car. It does not include a van or minivan—see definition (o)

(o) A pick-up truck or van is a four or six-wheeled motor vehicle designed for carrying passengers as well as property or cargo weighing less than the local limit for classification as a heavy goods vehicle, and not requiring a special driver's license. This includes a minivan and a sport-utility vehicle (SUV).

(p) A heavy transport vehicle is a motor vehicle designed primarily for carrying property, meeting local criteria for classification as a heavy goods vehicle in terms of weight and requiring a special driver's license.

(q) A bus (coach) is a motor vehicle designed or adapted primarily for carrying more than 10 passengers, and requiring a special driver's license.

(r) A railway train or railway vehicle is any device, with or without freight or passenger cars coupled to it, designed for traffic on a railway track. This includes subterranean (subways) or elevated trains.

(s) A streetcar is a device designed and used primarily for transporting passengers within a municipality, running on rails, usually subject to normal traffic control signals, and operated principally on a right-of-way that forms part of the roadway. This includes a tram or trolley that runs on rails. A trailer being towed by a streetcar is considered part of the streetcar.

(t) A special vehicle mainly used on industrial premises is a motor vehicle designed primarily for use within the buildings and premises of industrial or commercial establishments. This includes battery-powered airport passenger vehicles or baggage/mail trucks, forklifts, coal-cars in a coal mine, logging cars and trucks used in mines or quarries.

(u) A special vehicle mainly used in agriculture is a motor vehicle designed specifically for use in farming and agriculture (horticulture), to work the land, tend and harvest crops and transport materials on the farm. This includes harvesters, farm machinery and tractor and trailers.

(v) A special construction vehicle is a motor vehicle designed specifically for use on construction and demolition sites. This includes bulldozers, diggers, earth levellers, dump trucks, backhoes, front-end loaders, pavers, and mechanical shovels.

(w) A special all-terrain vehicle is a motor vehicle of special design to enable it to negotiate over rough or soft terrain, snow or sand. Examples of special design are high construction, special wheels and tires, tracks, and support on a cushion of air. This includes snow mobiles, all-terrain vehicles (ATV), and dune buggies. It does not include passenger vehicle designated as sport utility vehicles (SUV).

(x) A watercraft is any device designed for transporting passengers or goods on water. This includes motor or sail boats, ships, and hovercraft.

(y) An aircraft is any device for transporting passengers or goods in the air. This includes hot-air balloons, gliders, helicopters and airplanes.

(z) A military vehicle is any motorized vehicle operating on a public roadway owned by the military and being operated by a member of the military.

PEDESTRIAN INJURED IN TRANSPORT ACCIDENT (V00-V09)

Includes   person changing tire on transport vehicle
person examining engine of vehicle broken down in (on side of) road

Excludes1   fall due to non-transport collision with other person (W03)
pedestrian on foot falling (slipping) on ice and snow (W00.-)
struck or bumped by another person (W51)

● **V00   Pedestrian conveyance accident**

Use additional place of occurrence and activity external cause codes, if known (Y92.-, Y93.-)

Excludes1   collision with another person without fall (W51)
fall due to person on foot colliding with another person on foot (W03)
fall from non-moving wheelchair, nonmotorized scooter and motorized mobility scooter without collision (W05.-)
pedestrian (conveyance) collision with other land transport vehicle (V01-V09)
pedestrian on foot falling (slipping) on ice and snow (W00.-)

The appropriate 7th character is to be added to each code from category V00

A	initial encounter
D	subsequent encounter
S	sequela

● **V00.0   Pedestrian on foot injured in collision with pedestrian conveyance**

X● **V00.01   Pedestrian on foot injured in collision with roller-skater**

X● **V00.02   Pedestrian on foot injured in collision with skateboarder**

● **V00.03 Pedestrian on foot injured in collision with standing micro-mobility pedestrian conveyance**

     V00.031   Pedestrian on foot injured in collision with rider of standing electric scooter

     V00.038   Pedestrian on foot injured in collision with rider of other standing micro-mobility pedestrian conveyance
Pedestrian on foot injured in collision with rider of hoverboard
Pedestrian on foot injured in collision with rider of segway

X● **V00.09   Pedestrian on foot injured in collision with other pedestrian conveyance**

● **V00.1   Rolling-type pedestrian conveyance accident**

Excludes1   accident with baby stroller (V00.82-)
accident with wheelchair (powered) (V00.81-)
accident with motorized mobility scooter (V00.83-)

● **V00.11   In-line roller-skate accident**

● **V00.111   Fall from in-line roller-skates**

● **V00.112   In-line roller-skater colliding with stationary object**

● **V00.118   Other in-line roller-skate accident**

Excludes1   roller-skater collision with other land transport vehicle (V01-V09 with 5th character 1)

● **V00.12   Non-in-line roller-skate accident**

● V00.121   Fall from non-in-line roller-skates

● V00.122   Non-in-line roller-skater colliding with stationary object

● V00.128   Other non-in-line roller-skating accident

> **Excludes1**   roller-skater collision with other land transport vehicle (V01-V09 with 5th character 1)

● V00.13   Skateboard accident

● V00.131   Fall from skateboard

● V00.132   Skateboarder colliding with stationary object

● V00.138   Other skateboard accident

> **Excludes1**   skateboarder collision with other land transport vehicle (V01-V09 with 5th character 2)

● V00.14   Scooter (nonmotorized) accident

> **Excludes1**   motor scooter accident (V20-V29)

● V00.141   Fall from scooter (nonmotorized)

● V00.142   Scooter (nonmotorized) colliding with stationary object

● V00.148   Other scooter (nonmotorized) accident

> **Excludes1**   scooter (non-motorized) collision with other land transport vehicle (V01-V09 with fifth character 9)

● V00.15   Heelies accident
Rolling shoe
Wheeled shoe
Wheelies accident

● V00.151   Fall from heelies

● V00.152   Heelies colliding with stationary object

● V00.158   Other heelies accident

● V00.18   Accident on other rolling-type pedestrian conveyance

● V00.181   Fall from other rolling-type pedestrian conveyance

● V00.182   Pedestrian on other rolling-type pedestrian conveyance colliding with stationary object

● V00.188   Other accident on other rolling-type pedestrian conveyance

● V00.2   Gliding-type pedestrian conveyance accident

● V00.21   Ice-skates accident

● V00.211   Fall from ice-skates

● V00.212   Ice-skater colliding with stationary object

● V00.218   Other ice-skates accident

> **Excludes1**   ice-skater collision with other land transport vehicle (V01-V09 with 5th character 9)

● V00.22   Sled accident

● V00.221   Fall from sled

● V00.222   Sledder colliding with stationary object

● V00.228   Other sled accident

> **Excludes1**   sled collision with other land transport vehicle (V01-V09 with 5th character 9)

● V00.28   Other gliding-type pedestrian conveyance accident

● V00.281   Fall from other gliding-type pedestrian conveyance

● V00.282   Pedestrian on other gliding-type pedestrian conveyance colliding with stationary object

● V00.288   Other accident on other gliding-type pedestrian conveyance

> **Excludes1**   gliding-type pedestrian conveyance collision with other land transport vehicle (V01-V09 with 5th character 9)

● V00.3   Flat-bottomed pedestrian conveyance accident

● V00.31   Snowboard accident

● V00.311   Fall from snowboard

● V00.312   Snowboarder colliding with stationary object

● V00.318   Other snowboard accident

> **Excludes1**   snowboarder collision with other land transport vehicle (V01-V09 with 5th character 9)

● V00.32   Snow-ski accident

● V00.321   Fall from snow-skis
Coding Clinic: 2015, Q1, P12

● V00.322   Snow-skier colliding with stationary object

● V00.328   Other snow-ski accident

> **Excludes1**   snow-skier collision with other land transport vehicle (V01-V09 with 5th character 9)

● V00.38   Other flat-bottomed pedestrian conveyance accident

● V00.381   Fall from other flat-bottomed pedestrian conveyance

● V00.382   Pedestrian on other flat-bottomed pedestrian conveyance colliding with stationary object

● V00.388   Other accident on other flat-bottomed pedestrian conveyance

● V00.8   Accident on other pedestrian conveyance

● V00.81   Accident with wheelchair (powered)

● V00.811   Fall from moving wheelchair (powered)

> **Excludes1**   fall from non-moving wheelchair (W05.0)

● V00.812   Wheelchair (powered) colliding with stationary object

● V00.818   Other accident with wheelchair (powered)

● V00.82   Accident with baby stroller

● V00.821   Fall from baby stroller

● V00.822   Baby stroller colliding with stationary object

● V00.828   Other accident with baby stroller

N Newborn Age: 0   **P** Pediatric Age: 0–17   **M** Maternity DX: 9–64   **A** Adult Age: 15–124   ♀ Females Only   ♂ Males Only

Complication\Comorbidity   Major C\C   (Ex) CC/MCC Exclusions   Hospital-Acquired Condition   Hierarchical Condition Category   **1531**

CHAPTER 20 (V00-Y99)

● **V00.83   Accident with motorized mobility scooter**

   ● **V00.831   Fall from motorized mobility scooter**

       Excludes 1   fall from non-moving motorized mobility scooter (W05.2)

   ● **V00.832   Motorized mobility scooter colliding with stationary object**

   ● **V00.838   Other accident with motorized mobility scooter**

● **V00.84   Accident with standing micro-mobility pedestrian conveyance**

   V00.841   Fall from standing electric scooter

   V00.842   Pedestrian on standing electric scooter colliding with stationary object

   V00.848   Other accident with standing micro-mobility pedestrian conveyance
       Accident with hoverboard
       Accident with segway

● **V00.89   Accident on other pedestrian conveyance**

   ● **V00.891   Fall from other pedestrian conveyance**

   ● **V00.892   Pedestrian on other pedestrian conveyance colliding with stationary object**

   ● **V00.898   Other accident on other pedestrian conveyance**

       Excludes 1   other pedestrian (conveyance) collision with other land transport vehicle (V01-V09 with 5th character 9)

● **V01   Pedestrian injured in collision with pedal cycle**

The appropriate 7th character is to be added to each code from category V01

    A   initial encounter
    D   subsequent encounter
    S   sequela

● **V01.0   Pedestrian injured in collision with pedal cycle in nontraffic accident**

   X ● **V01.00   Pedestrian on foot injured in collision with pedal cycle in nontraffic accident**
       Pedestrian NOS injured in collision with pedal cycle in nontraffic accident

   X ● **V01.01   Pedestrian on roller-skates injured in collision with pedal cycle in nontraffic accident**

   X ● **V01.02   Pedestrian on skateboard injured in collision with pedal cycle in nontraffic accident**

   ● **V01.03   Pedestrian on standing micro-mobility pedestrian conveyance injured in collision with pedal cycle in nontraffic accident**

       V01.031   Pedestrian on standing electric scooter injured in collision with pedal cycle in nontraffic accident

       V01.038   Pedestrian on other standing micro-mobility pedestrian conveyance injured in collision with pedal cycle in nontraffic accident
          Pedestrian on hoverboard injured in collision with pedal cycle in nontraffic accident
          Pedestrian on segway injured in collision with pedal cycle in nontraffic accident

   X ● **V01.09   Pedestrian with other conveyance injured in collision with pedal cycle in nontraffic accident**
       Pedestrian with baby stroller injured in collision with pedal cycle in nontraffic accident
       Pedestrian in wheelchair (powered) injured in collision with pedal cycle in nontraffic accident
       Pedestrian in motorized mobility scooter injured in collision with pedal cycle in nontraffic accident
       Pedestrian on ice-skates injured in collision with pedal cycle in nontraffic accident
       Pedestrian on nonmotorized scooter injured in collision with pedal cycle in nontraffic accident
       Pedestrian on sled injured in collision with pedal cycle in nontraffic accident
       Pedestrian on snowboard injured in collision with pedal cycle in nontraffic accident
       Pedestrian on snow-skis injured in collision with pedal cycle in nontraffic accident

● **V01.1   Pedestrian injured in collision with pedal cycle in traffic accident**

   X ● **V01.10   Pedestrian on foot injured in collision with pedal cycle in traffic accident**
       Pedestrian NOS injured in collision with pedal cycle in traffic accident

   X ● **V01.11   Pedestrian on roller-skates injured in collision with pedal cycle in traffic accident**

   X ● **V01.12   Pedestrian on skateboard injured in collision with pedal cycle in traffic accident**

   ● **V01.13   Pedestrian on standing micro-mobility pedestrian conveyance injured in collision with pedal cycle in traffic accident**

       V01.131   Pedestrian on standing electric scooter injured in collision with pedal cycle in traffic accident

       V01.138   Pedestrian on other standing micro-mobility pedestrian conveyance injured in collision with pedal cycle in traffic accident
          Pedestrian on hoverboard injured in collision with pedal cycle in traffic accident
          Pedestrian on segway injured in collision with pedal cycle in traffic accident

   X ● **V01.19   Pedestrian with other conveyance injured in collision with pedal cycle in traffic accident**
       Pedestrian with baby stroller injured in collision with pedal cycle in traffic accident
       Pedestrian in wheelchair (powered) injured in collision with pedal cycle in traffic accident
       Pedestrian in motorized mobility scooter injured in collision with pedal cycle in traffic accident
       Pedestrian on ice-skates injured in collision with pedal cycle in traffic accident
       Pedestrian on nonmotorized scooter injured in collision with pedal cycle in traffic accident
       Pedestrian on sled injured in collision with pedal cycle in traffic accident
       Pedestrian on snowboard injured in collision with pedal cycle in traffic accident
       Pedestrian on snow-skis injured in collision with pedal cycle in traffic accident

▶ New   ⇒ Revised   ~~deleted~~ Deleted   Excludes 1   Excludes 2   Includes   Use additional   Code first   Code also   Key words

OGCR Official Guidelines   ● Unacceptable Principal Diagnosis   X Assign placeholder X   ● Use Additional Character(s)   ▶ Manifestation Code   **Coding Clinic**

● **V01.9**   **Pedestrian injured in collision with pedal cycle, unspecified whether traffic or nontraffic accident**

    X ● **V01.90**   **Pedestrian on foot injured in collision with pedal cycle, unspecified whether traffic or nontraffic accident**

        Pedestrian NOS injured in collision with pedal cycle, unspecified whether traffic or nontraffic accident

    X ● **V01.91**   **Pedestrian on roller-skates injured in collision with pedal cycle, unspecified whether traffic or nontraffic accident**

    X ● **V01.92**   **Pedestrian on skateboard injured in collision with pedal cycle, unspecified whether traffic or nontraffic accident**

    ● **V01.93**   **Pedestrian on standing micro-mobility pedestrian conveyance injured in collision with pedal cycle, unspecified whether traffic or nontraffic accident**

        V01.931   **Pedestrian on standing electric scooter injured in collision with pedal cycle, unspecified whether traffic or nontraffic accident**

        V01.938   **Pedestrian on other standing micro-mobility pedestrian conveyance injured in collision with pedal cycle, unspecified whether traffic or nontraffic accident**

           Pedestrian on hoverboard injured in collision with pedal cycle, unspecified whether traffic or nontraffic accident

           Pedestrian on segway injured in collision with pedal cycle, unspecified whether traffic or nontraffic accident

    X ● **V01.99**   **Pedestrian with other conveyance injured in collision with pedal cycle, unspecified whether traffic or nontraffic accident**

        Pedestrian with baby stroller injured in collision with pedal cycle, unspecified whether traffic or nontraffic accident

        Pedestrian in wheelchair (powered) injured in collision with pedal cycle, unspecified whether traffic or nontraffic accident

        Pedestrian in motorized mobility scooter injured in collision with pedal cycle, unspecified whether traffic or nontraffic accident

        Pedestrian on ice-skates injured in collision with pedal cycle unspecified, whether traffic or nontraffic accident

        Pedestrian on nonmotorized scooter injured in collision with pedal cycle, unspecified whether traffic or nontraffic accident

        Pedestrian on sled injured in collision with pedal cycle unspecified, whether traffic or nontraffic accident

        Pedestrian on snowboard injured in collision with pedal cycle, unspecified whether traffic or nontraffic accident

        Pedestrian on snow-skis injured in collision with pedal cycle, unspecified whether traffic or nontraffic accident

● **V02**   **Pedestrian injured in collision with two- or three-wheeled motor vehicle**

    The appropriate 7th character is to be added to each code from category V02

A	initial encounter
D	subsequent encounter
S	sequela

● **V02.0**   **Pedestrian injured in collision with two- or three-wheeled motor vehicle in nontraffic accident**

    X ● **V02.00**   **Pedestrian on foot injured in collision with two- or three-wheeled motor vehicle in nontraffic accident**

        Pedestrian NOS injured in collision with two- or three-wheeled motor vehicle in nontraffic accident

    X ● **V02.01**   **Pedestrian on roller-skates injured in collision with two- or three-wheeled motor vehicle in nontraffic accident**

    X ● **V02.02**   **Pedestrian on skateboard injured in collision with two- or three-wheeled motor vehicle in nontraffic accident**

    ● **V02.03**   **Pedestrian on standing micro-mobility pedestrian conveyance injured in collision with two- or three-wheeled motor vehicle in nontraffic accident**

        V02.031   **Pedestrian on standing electric scooter injured in collision with two- or three-wheeled motor vehicle in nontraffic accident**

        V02.038   **Pedestrian on other standing micro-mobility pedestrian conveyance injured in collision with two- or three-wheeled motor vehicle in nontraffic accident**

           Pedestrian on hoverboard injured in collision with two-or three wheeled motor vehicle in nontraffic accident

           Pedestrian on segway injured in collision with two- or three-wheeled motor vehicle in nontraffic accident

    X ● **V02.09**   **Pedestrian with other conveyance injured in collision with two- or three-wheeled motor vehicle in nontraffic accident**

        Pedestrian with baby stroller injured in collision with two- or three-wheeled motor vehicle in nontraffic accident

        Pedestrian on ice-skates injured in collision with two- or three-wheeled motor vehicle in nontraffic accident

        Pedestrian in wheelchair (powered) injured in collision with two- or three-wheeled motor vehicle in nontraffic accident

        Pedestrian in motorized mobility scooter injured in collision with two- or three-wheeled motor vehicle in nontraffic accident

        Pedestrian on nonmotorized scooter injured in collision with two- or three-wheeled motor vehicle in nontraffic accident

        Pedestrian on sled injured in collision with two- or three-wheeled motor vehicle in nontraffic accident

        Pedestrian on snowboard injured in collision with two- or three-wheeled motor vehicle in nontraffic accident

        Pedestrian on snow-skis injured in collision with two- or three-wheeled motor vehicle in nontraffic accident

CHAPTER 20 (V00-Y99)

N Newborn Age: 0   **P** Pediatric Age: 0–17   **M** Maternity DX: 9–64   **A** Adult Age: 15–124   ♀ Females Only   ♂ Males Only

Complication\Comorbidity   Major C\C   (Ex) CC/MCC Exclusions   Hospital-Acquired Condition   Hierarchical Condition Category   **1533**

CHAPTER 20 (V00-Y99)

● **V02.1**   Pedestrian injured in collision with two- or three-wheeled motor vehicle in traffic accident

X● **V02.10**   Pedestrian on foot injured in collision with two- or three-wheeled motor vehicle in traffic accident

Pedestrian NOS injured in collision with two- or three-wheeled motor vehicle in traffic accident

X● **V02.11**   Pedestrian on roller-skates injured in collision with two- or three-wheeled motor vehicle in traffic accident

X● **V02.12**   Pedestrian on skateboard injured in collision with two- or three-wheeled motor vehicle in traffic accident

● **V02.13**   Pedestrian on standing micro-mobility pedestrian conveyance injured in collision with two- or three-wheeled motor vehicle in traffic accident

     V02.131   Pedestrian on standing electric scooter injured in collision with two- or three-wheeled motor vehicle in traffic accident

     V02.138   Pedestrian on other standing micro-mobility pedestrian conveyance injured in collision with two- or three-wheeled motor vehicle in traffic accident

Pedestrian on hoverboard injured in collision with two-or three wheeled motor vehicle in traffic accident

Pedestrian on segway injured in collision with two- or three-wheeled motor vehicle in traffic accident

X● **V02.19**   Pedestrian with other conveyance injured in collision with two- or three-wheeled motor vehicle in traffic accident

Pedestrian with baby stroller injured in collision with two- or three-wheeled motor vehicle in traffic accident

Pedestrian in wheelchair (powered) injured in collision with two- or three-wheeled motor vehicle in traffic accident

Pedestrian in motorized mobility scooter injured in collision with two- or three-wheeled motor vehicle in traffic accident

Pedestrian on ice-skates injured in collision with two- or three-wheeled motor vehicle in traffic accident

Pedestrian on nonmotorized scooter injured in collision with two- or three-wheeled motor vehicle in traffic accident

Pedestrian on sled injured in collision with two- or three-wheeled motor vehicle in traffic accident

Pedestrian on snowboard injured in collision with two- or three-wheeled motor vehicle in traffic accident

Pedestrian on snow-skis injured in collision with two- or three-wheeled motor vehicle in traffic accident

● **V02.9**   Pedestrian injured in collision with two- or three-wheeled motor vehicle, unspecified whether traffic or nontraffic accident

X● **V02.90**   Pedestrian on foot injured in collision with two- or three-wheeled motor vehicle, unspecified whether traffic or nontraffic accident

Pedestrian NOS injured in collision with two- or three-wheeled motor vehicle, unspecified whether traffic or nontraffic accident

X● **V02.91**   Pedestrian on roller-skates injured in collision with two- or three-wheeled motor vehicle, unspecified whether traffic or nontraffic accident

X● **V02.92**   Pedestrian on skateboard injured in collision with two- or three-wheeled motor vehicle, unspecified whether traffic or nontraffic accident

● **V02.93**   Pedestrian on standing micro-mobility pedestrian conveyance injured in collision with two-or three-wheeled motor vehicle, unspecified whether traffic or nontraffic accident

     V02.931   Pedestrian on standing electric scooter injured in collision with two- or three wheeled motor vehicle, unspecified whether traffic or nontraffic accident

     V02.938   Pedestrian on other standing micro-mobility pedestrian conveyance injured in collision with two- or three wheeled motor vehicle, unspecified whether traffic or nontraffic accident

Pedestrian on hoverboard injured in collision with two-three-wheeled motor vehicle, unspecified whether traffic or nontraffic accident

Pedestrian on segway injured in collision with two- or three wheeled motor vehicle, unspecified whether traffic or nontraffic accident

X● **V02.99**   Pedestrian with other conveyance injured in collision with two- or three-wheeled motor vehicle, unspecified whether traffic or nontraffic accident

Pedestrian with baby stroller injured in collision with two- or three-wheeled motor vehicle, unspecified whether traffic or nontraffic accident

Pedestrian in wheelchair (powered) injured in collision with two- or three-wheeled motor vehicle, unspecified whether traffic or nontraffic accident

Pedestrian in motorized mobility scooter injured in collision with two- or three-wheeled motor vehicle, unspecified whether traffic or nontraffic accident

Pedestrian on ice-skates injured in collision with two- or three-wheeled motor vehicle, unspecified whether traffic or nontraffic accident

Pedestrian on nonmotorized scooter injured in collision with two- or three-wheeled motor vehicle, unspecified whether traffic or nontraffic accident

Pedestrian on sled injured in collision with two- or three-wheeled motor vehicle, unspecified whether traffic or nontraffic accident

Pedestrian on snowboard injured in collision with two- or three-wheeled motor vehicle, unspecified whether traffic or nontraffic accident

Pedestrian on snow-skis injured in collision with two- or three-wheeled motor vehicle, unspecified whether traffic or nontraffic accident

● **V03**   Pedestrian injured in collision with car, pick-up truck or van

▶ New   ⇒ Revised   ~~deleted~~ Deleted   Excludes 1   Excludes 2   Includes   Use additional   Code first   Code also   Key words

OGCR Official Guidelines   ● Unacceptable Principal Diagnosis   X Assign placeholder X   ● Use Additional Character(s)   ▶ Manifestation Code   **Coding Clinic**

The appropriate 7th character is to be added to each code from category V03

A	initial encounter
D	subsequent encounter
S	sequela

● **V03.0** Pedestrian injured in collision with car, pick-up truck or van in nontraffic accident

    X● **V03.00** Pedestrian on foot injured in collision with car, pick-up truck or van in nontraffic accident
           Pedestrian NOS injured in collision with car, pick-up truck or van in nontraffic accident

    X● **V03.01** Pedestrian on roller-skates injured in collision with car, pick-up truck or van in nontraffic accident

    X● **V03.02** Pedestrian on skateboard injured in collision with car, pick-up truck or van in nontraffic accident

    ● **V03.03** Pedestrian on standing micro-mobility pedestrian conveyance injured in collision with car, pick-up or van in nontraffic accident

         V03.031 Pedestrian on standing electric scooter injured in collision with car, pick-up or van in nontraffic accident

         V03.038 Pedestrian on other standing micro-mobility pedestrian conveyance injured in collision with car, pick-up or van in nontraffic accident
           Pedestrian on hoverboard injured in collision with car, pick-up or van in nontraffic accident
           Pedestrian on segway injured in collision with car, pick-up or van in nontraffic accident

    X● **V03.09** Pedestrian with other conveyance injured in collision with car, pick-up truck or van in nontraffic accident
        Pedestrian with baby stroller injured in collision with car, pick-up truck or van in nontraffic accident
        Pedestrian in wheelchair (powered) injured in collision with car, pick-up truck or van in nontraffic accident
        Pedestrian in motorized mobility scooter injured in collision with car, pick-up truck or van in nontraffic accident
        Pedestrian on ice-skates injured in collision with car, pick-up truck or van in nontraffic accident
        Pedestrian on nonmotorized scooter injured in collision with car, pick-up truck or van in nontraffic accident
        Pedestrian on sled injured in collision with car, pick-up truck or van in nontraffic accident
        Pedestrian on snowboard injured in collision with car, pick-up truck or van in nontraffic accident
        Pedestrian on snow-skis injured in collision with car, pick-up truck or van in nontraffic accident

● **V03.1** Pedestrian injured in collision with car, pick-up truck or van in traffic accident

    X● **V03.10** Pedestrian on foot injured in collision with car, pick-up truck or van in traffic accident
           Pedestrian NOS injured in collision with car, pick-up truck or van in traffic accident

    X● **V03.11** Pedestrian on roller-skates injured in collision with car, pick-up truck or van in traffic accident

    X● **V03.12** Pedestrian on skateboard injured in collision with car, pick-up truck or van in traffic accident

    ● **V03.13** Pedestrian on standing micro-mobility pedestrian conveyance injured in collision with car, pick-up or van in traffic accident

         V03.131 Pedestrian on standing electric scooter injured in collision with car, pick-up or van in traffic accident

         V03.138 Pedestrian on other standing micro-mobility pedestrian conveyance injured in collision with car, pick-up or van in traffic accident
           Pedestrian on hoverboard injured in collision with car, pick-up or van in traffic accident
           Pedestrian on segway injured in collision with car, pick-up or van in traffic accident

    X● **V03.19** Pedestrian with other conveyance injured in collision with car, pick-up truck or van in traffic accident
        Pedestrian with baby stroller injured in collision with car, pick-up truck or van in traffic accident
        Pedestrian in wheelchair (powered) injured in collision with car, pick-up truck or van in traffic accident
        Pedestrian in motorized mobility scooter injured in collision with car, pick-up truck or van in traffic accident
        Pedestrian on ice-skates injured in collision with car, pick-up truck or van in traffic accident
        Pedestrian on nonmotorized scooter injured in collision with car, pick-up truck or van in traffic accident
        Pedestrian on sled injured in collision with car, pick-up truck or van in traffic accident
        Pedestrian on snowboard injured in collision with car, pick-up truck or van in traffic accident
        Pedestrian on snow-skis injured in collision with car, pick-up truck or van in traffic accident

● **V03.9** Pedestrian injured in collision with car, pick-up truck or van, unspecified whether traffic or nontraffic accident

    X● **V03.90** Pedestrian on foot injured in collision with car, pick-up truck or van, unspecified whether traffic or nontraffic accident
           Pedestrian NOS injured in collision with car, pick-up truck or van, unspecified whether traffic or nontraffic accident

    X● **V03.91** Pedestrian on roller-skates injured in collision with car, pick-up truck or van, unspecified whether traffic or nontraffic accident

    X● **V03.92** Pedestrian on skateboard injured in collision with car, pick-up truck or van, unspecified whether traffic or nontraffic accident

CHAPTER 20 (V00-Y99)

N   Newborn Age: 0   P   Pediatric Age: 0–17   M   Maternity DX: 9–64   A   Adult Age: 15–124   ♀ Females Only   ♂ Males Only

🖢 Complication\Comorbidity   🖢 Major C\C   (Ex) CC/MCC Exclusions   🖢 Hospital-Acquired Condition   🖢 Hierarchical Condition Category

1535

● **V03.93** **Pedestrian on standing micro-mobility pedestrian conveyance injured in collision with car, pick-up or van, unspecified whether traffic or nontraffic accident**

    V03.931 **Pedestrian on standing electric scooter injured in collision with car, pick-up or van, unspecified whether traffic or nontraffic accident**

    V03.938 **Pedestrian on other standing micro-mobility pedestrian conveyance injured in collision with car, pick-up or van, unspecified whether traffic or nontraffic accident**

        Pedestrian on hoverboard injured in collision with car, pick-up or van, unspecified whether traffic or nontraffic accident

        Pedestrian on segway injured in collision with car, pick-up or van, unspecified whether traffic or nontraffic accident

X● **V03.99** **Pedestrian with other conveyance injured in collision with car, pick-up truck or van, unspecified whether traffic or nontraffic accident**

    Pedestrian with baby stroller injured in collision with car, pick-up truck or van, unspecified whether traffic or nontraffic accident

    Pedestrian in wheelchair (powered) injured in collision with car, pick-up truck or van, unspecified whether traffic or nontraffic accident

    Pedestrian in motorized mobility scooter injured in collision with car, pick-up truck or van, unspecified whether traffic or nontraffic accident

    Pedestrian on ice-skates injured in collision with car, pick-up truck or van, unspecified whether traffic or nontraffic accident

    Pedestrian on nonmotorized scooter injured in collision with car, pick-up truck or van, unspecified whether traffic or nontraffic accident

    Pedestrian on sled injured in collision with car, pick-up truck or van in nontraffic accident

    Pedestrian on snowboard injured in collision with car, pick-up truck or van, unspecified whether traffic or nontraffic accident

    Pedestrian on snow-skis injured in collision with car, pick-up truck or van, unspecified whether traffic or nontraffic accident

● **V04** **Pedestrian injured in collision with heavy transport vehicle or bus**

    Excludes1   pedestrian injured in collision with military vehicle (V09.01, V09.21)

    The appropriate 7th character is to be added to each code from category V04

A	initial encounter
D	subsequent encounter
S	sequela

● **V04.0** **Pedestrian injured in collision with heavy transport vehicle or bus in nontraffic accident**

    X● **V04.00** **Pedestrian on foot injured in collision with heavy transport vehicle or bus in nontraffic accident**

        Pedestrian NOS injured in collision with heavy transport vehicle or bus in nontraffic accident

X● **V04.01** **Pedestrian on roller-skates injured in collision with heavy transport vehicle or bus in nontraffic accident**

X● **V04.02** **Pedestrian on skateboard injured in collision with heavy transport vehicle or bus in nontraffic accident**

● **V04.03** **Pedestrian on standing micro-mobility pedestrian conveyance injured in collision with heavy transport vehicle or bus in nontraffic accident**

    V04.031 **Pedestrian on standing electric scooter injured in collision with heavy transport vehicle or bus in nontraffic accident**

    V04.038 **Pedestrian on other standing micro-mobility pedestrian conveyance injured in collision with heavy transport vehicle or bus in nontraffic accident**

        Pedestrian on hoverboard injured in collision with heavy transport vehicle or bus in nontraffic accident

        Pedestrian on segway injured in collision with heavy transport vehicle or bus in nontraffic accident

X● **V04.09** **Pedestrian with other conveyance injured in collision with heavy transport vehicle or bus in nontraffic accident**

    Pedestrian with baby stroller injured in collision with heavy transport vehicle or bus in nontraffic accident

    Pedestrian in wheelchair (powered) injured in collision with heavy transport vehicle or bus in nontraffic accident

    Pedestrian in motorized mobility scooter injured in collision with heavy transport vehicle or bus in nontraffic accident

    Pedestrian on ice-skates injured in collision with heavy transport vehicle or bus in nontraffic accident

    Pedestrian on nonmotorized scooter injured in collision with heavy transport vehicle or bus in nontraffic accident

    Pedestrian on sled injured in collision with heavy transport vehicle or bus in nontraffic accident

    Pedestrian on snowboard injured in collision with heavy transport vehicle or bus in nontraffic accident

    Pedestrian on snow-skis injured in collision with heavy transport vehicle or bus in nontraffic accident

● **V04.1** **Pedestrian injured in collision with heavy transport vehicle or bus in traffic accident**

    X● **V04.10** **Pedestrian on foot injured in collision with heavy transport vehicle or bus in traffic accident**

        Pedestrian NOS injured in collision with heavy transport vehicle or bus in traffic accident

    X● **V04.11** **Pedestrian on roller-skates injured in collision with heavy transport vehicle or bus in traffic accident**

    X● **V04.12** **Pedestrian on skateboard injured in collision with heavy transport vehicle or bus in traffic accident**

    ● **V04.13** **Pedestrian on standing micro-mobility pedestrian conveyance injured in collision with heavy transport vehicle or bus in traffic accident**

        V04.131 **Pedestrian on standing electric scooter injured in collision with heavy transport vehicle or bus in traffic accident**

V04.138   Pedestrian on other standing micro-mobility pedestrian conveyance injured in collision with heavy transport vehicle or bus in traffic accident
> Pedestrian on hoverboard injured in collision with heavy transport vehicle or bus in traffic accident
> Pedestrian on segway injured in collision with heavy transport vehicle or bus in traffic accident

X● V04.19   Pedestrian with other conveyance injured in collision with heavy transport vehicle or bus in traffic accident
> Pedestrian with baby stroller injured in collision with heavy transport vehicle or bus in traffic accident
> Pedestrian in wheelchair (powered) injured in collision with heavy transport vehicle or bus in traffic accident
> Pedestrian in motorized mobility scooter injured in collision with heavy transport vehicle or bus in traffic accident
> Pedestrian on ice-skates injured in collision with heavy transport vehicle or bus in traffic accident
> Pedestrian on nonmotorized scooter injured in collision with heavy transport vehicle or bus in traffic accident
> Pedestrian on sled injured in collision with heavy transport vehicle or bus in traffic accident
> Pedestrian on snowboard injured in collision with heavy transport vehicle or bus in traffic accident
> Pedestrian on snow-skis injured in collision with heavy transport vehicle or bus in traffic accident

● V04.9   Pedestrian injured in collision with heavy transport vehicle or bus, unspecified whether traffic or nontraffic accident

X● V04.90   Pedestrian on foot injured in collision with heavy transport vehicle or bus, unspecified whether traffic or nontraffic accident
> Pedestrian NOS injured in collision with heavy transport vehicle or bus, unspecified whether traffic or nontraffic accident

X● V04.91   Pedestrian on roller-skates injured in collision with heavy transport vehicle or bus, unspecified whether traffic or nontraffic accident

X● V04.92   Pedestrian on skateboard injured in collision with heavy transport vehicle or bus, unspecified whether traffic or nontraffic accident

● V04.93   Pedestrian on standing micro-mobility pedestrian conveyance injured in collision with heavy transport vehicle or bus, unspecified whether traffic or nontraffic accident

V04.931   Pedestrian on standing electric scooter injured in collision with heavy transport vehicle or bus, unspecified whether traffic or nontraffic accident

V04.938   Pedestrian on other standing micro-mobility pedestrian conveyance injured in collision with heavy transport vehicle or bus, unspecified whether traffic or nontraffic accident
> Pedestrian on hoverboard injured in collision with heavy transport vehicle or bus, unspecified whether traffic or nontraffic accident
> Pedestrian on segway injured in collision with heavy transport vehicle or bus, unspecified whether traffic or nontraffic accident

X● V04.99   Pedestrian with other conveyance injured in collision with heavy transport vehicle or bus, unspecified whether traffic or nontraffic accident
> Pedestrian with baby stroller injured in collision with heavy transport vehicle or bus, unspecified whether traffic or nontraffic accident
> Pedestrian in wheelchair (powered) injured in collision with heavy transport vehicle or bus, unspecified whether traffic or nontraffic accident
> Pedestrian in motorized mobility scooter injured in collision with heavy transport vehicle or bus, unspecified whether traffic or nontraffic accident
> Pedestrian on ice-skates injured in collision with heavy transport vehicle or bus, unspecified whether traffic or nontraffic accident
> Pedestrian on nonmotorized scooter injured in collision with heavy transport vehicle or bus, unspecified whether traffic or nontraffic accident
> Pedestrian on sled injured in collision with heavy transport vehicle or bus, unspecified whether traffic or nontraffic accident
> Pedestrian on snowboard injured in collision with heavy transport vehicle or bus, unspecified whether traffic or nontraffic accident
> Pedestrian on snow-skis injured in collision with heavy transport vehicle or bus, unspecified whether traffic or nontraffic accident

● V05   Pedestrian injured in collision with railway train or railway vehicle

The appropriate 7th character is to be added to each code from category V05

A	initial encounter
D	subsequent encounter
S	sequela

● V05.0   Pedestrian injured in collision with railway train or railway vehicle in nontraffic accident

X● V05.00   Pedestrian on foot injured in collision with railway train or railway vehicle in nontraffic accident
> Pedestrian NOS injured in collision with railway train or railway vehicle in nontraffic accident

X● V05.01   Pedestrian on roller-skates injured in collision with railway train or railway vehicle in nontraffic accident

X● V05.02   Pedestrian on skateboard injured in collision with railway train or railway vehicle in nontraffic accident

● V05.03   Pedestrian on standing micro-mobility pedestrian conveyance injured in collision with railway train or railway vehicle in nontraffic accident

V05.031   Pedestrian on standing electric scooter injured in collision with railway train or railway vehicle in nontraffic accident

V05.038   Pedestrian on other standing micro-mobility pedestrian conveyance injured in collision with railway train or railway vehicle in nontraffic accident
> Pedestrian on hoverboard injured in collision with railway train or railway vehicle in nontraffic accident
> Pedestrian on segway injured in collision with railway train or railway vehicle in nontraffic accident

N Newborn Age: 0   **P** Pediatric Age: 0–17   **M** Maternity DX: 9–64   **A** Adult Age: 15–124   ♀ Females Only   ♂ Males Only

🔖 Complication\Comorbidity   🔖 Major C\C   (Ex) CC/MCC Exclusions   🔖 Hospital-Acquired Condition   🔖 Hierarchical Condition Category

1537

CHAPTER 20 (V00-Y99)

X ● **V05.09** **Pedestrian with other conveyance injured in collision with railway train or railway vehicle in nontraffic accident**
Pedestrian with baby stroller injured in collision with railway train or railway vehicle in nontraffic accident
Pedestrian in wheelchair (powered) injured in collision with railway train or railway vehicle in nontraffic accident
Pedestrian in motorized mobility scooter injured in collision with railway train or railway vehicle in nontraffic accident
Pedestrian on ice-skates injured in collision with railway train or railway vehicle in nontraffic accident
Pedestrian on nonmotorized scooter injured in collision with railway train or railway vehicle in nontraffic accident
Pedestrian on sled injured in collision with railway train or railway vehicle in nontraffic accident
Pedestrian on snowboard injured in collision with railway train or railway vehicle in nontraffic accident
Pedestrian on snow-skis injured in collision with railway train or railway vehicle in nontraffic accident

● **V05.1** **Pedestrian injured in collision with railway train or railway vehicle in traffic accident**

X ● **V05.10** **Pedestrian on foot injured in collision with railway train or railway vehicle in traffic accident**
Pedestrian NOS injured in collision with railway train or railway vehicle in traffic accident

X ● **V05.11** **Pedestrian on roller-skates injured in collision with railway train or railway vehicle in traffic accident**

X ● **V05.12** **Pedestrian on skateboard injured in collision with railway train or railway vehicle in traffic accident**

● **V05.13** **Pedestrian on standing micro-mobility pedestrian conveyance injured in collision with railway train or railway vehicle in traffic accident**

V05.131 **Pedestrian on standing electric scooter injured in collision with railway train or railway vehicle in traffic accident**

V05.138 **Pedestrian on other standing micro-mobility pedestrian conveyance injured in collision with railway train or railway vehicle in traffic accident**
Pedestrian on hoverboard injured in collision with railway train or railway vehicle in traffic accident
Pedestrian on segway injured in collision with railway train or railway vehicle in traffic accident

X ● **V05.19** **Pedestrian with other conveyance injured in collision with railway train or railway vehicle in traffic accident**
Pedestrian with baby stroller injured in collision with railway train or railway vehicle in traffic accident
Pedestrian in wheelchair (powered) injured in collision with railway train or railway vehicle in traffic accident
Pedestrian in motorized mobility scooter injured in collision with railway train or railway vehicle in traffic accident
Pedestrian on ice-skates injured in collision with railway train or railway vehicle in traffic accident
Pedestrian on nonmotorized scooter injured in collision with railway train or railway vehicle in traffic accident
Pedestrian on sled injured in collision with railway train or railway vehicle in traffic accident
Pedestrian on snowboard injured in collision with railway train or railway vehicle in traffic accident
Pedestrian on snow-skis injured in collision with railway train or railway vehicle in traffic accident

● **V05.9** **Pedestrian injured in collision with railway train or railway vehicle, unspecified whether traffic or nontraffic accident**

X ● **V05.90** **Pedestrian on foot injured in collision with railway train or railway vehicle, unspecified whether traffic or nontraffic accident**
Pedestrian NOS injured in collision with railway train or railway vehicle, unspecified whether traffic or nontraffic accident

X ● **V05.91** **Pedestrian on roller-skates injured in collision with railway train or railway vehicle, unspecified whether traffic or nontraffic accident**

X ● **V05.92** **Pedestrian on skateboard injured in collision with railway train or railway vehicle, unspecified whether traffic or nontraffic accident**

● **V05.93** **Pedestrian on standing micro-mobility pedestrian conveyance injured in collision with railway train or railway vehicle, unspecified whether traffic or nontraffic accident**

V05.931 **Pedestrian on standing electric scooter injured in collision with railway train or railway vehicle, unspecified whether traffic or nontraffic accident**

V05.938 **Pedestrian on other standing micro-mobility pedestrian conveyance injured in collision with railway train or railway vehicle, unspecified whether traffic or nontraffic accident**
Pedestrian on hoverboard injured in collision with railway train or railway vehicle, unspecified whether traffic or nontraffic accident
Pedestrian on segway injured in collision with railway train or railway vehicle, unspecified whether traffic or nontraffic accident

X● **V05.99** **Pedestrian with** other **conveyance injured in collision with railway train or railway vehicle, unspecified whether traffic or nontraffic accident**

> Pedestrian with baby stroller injured in collision with railway train or railway vehicle, unspecified whether traffic or nontraffic
>
> Pedestrian in wheelchair (powered) injured in collision with railway train or railway vehicle, unspecified whether traffic or nontraffic
>
> Pedestrian in motorized mobility scooter injured in collision with railway train or railway vehicle, unspecified whether traffic or nontraffic
>
> Pedestrian on ice-skates injured in collision with railway train or railway vehicle, unspecified whether traffic or nontraffic
>
> Pedestrian on nonmotorized scooter injured in collision with railway train or railway vehicle, unspecified whether traffic or nontraffic
>
> Pedestrian on sled injured in collision with railway train or railway vehicle, unspecified whether traffic or nontraffic
>
> Pedestrian on snowboard injured in collision with railway train or railway vehicle, unspecified whether traffic or nontraffic
>
> Pedestrian on snow-skis injured in collision with railway train or railway vehicle, unspecified whether traffic or nontraffic

●**V06** **Pedestrian injured in collision with other nonmotor vehicle**

Includes   collision with animal-drawn vehicle, animal being ridden, nonpowered streetcar

Excludes1   pedestrian injured in collision with pedestrian conveyance (V00.0-)

The appropriate 7th character is to be added to each code from category V06

A	initial encounter
D	subsequent encounter
S	sequela

●**V06.0** **Pedestrian injured in collision with other nonmotor vehicle in** nontraffic accident

X● **V06.00** **Pedestrian on** foot **injured in collision with other nonmotor vehicle in nontraffic accident**

> Pedestrian NOS injured in collision with other nonmotor vehicle in nontraffic accident

X● **V06.01** **Pedestrian on** roller-skates **injured in collision with other nonmotor vehicle in nontraffic accident**

X● **V06.02** **Pedestrian on** skateboard **injured in collision with other nonmotor vehicle in nontraffic accident**

●**V06.03** **Pedestrian on standing micro-mobility pedestrian conveyance injured in collision with other nonmotor vehicle in nontraffic accident**

V06.031 **Pedestrian on standing electric scooter injured in collision with other nonmotor vehicle in nontraffic accident**

V06.038 **Pedestrian on other standing micro-mobility pedestrian conveyance injured in collision with other nonmotor vehicle in nontraffic accident**

> Pedestrian on hoverboard injured in collision with other nonmotor vehicle in nontraffic accident
>
> Pedestrian on segway injured in collision with other nonmotor vehicle in nontraffic accident

X● **V06.09** **Pedestrian with** other **conveyance injured in collision with other nonmotor vehicle in nontraffic accident**

> Pedestrian with baby stroller injured in collision with other nonmotor vehicle in nontraffic accident
>
> Pedestrian in wheelchair (powered) injured in collision with other nonmotor vehicle in nontraffic accident
>
> Pedestrian in motorized mobility scooter injured in collision with other nonmotor vehicle in nontraffic accident
>
> Pedestrian on ice-skates injured in collision with other nonmotor vehicle in nontraffic accident
>
> Pedestrian on nonmotorized scooter injured in collision with other nonmotor vehicle in nontraffic accident
>
> Pedestrian on sled injured in collision with other nonmotor vehicle in nontraffic accident
>
> Pedestrian on snowboard injured in collision with other nonmotor vehicle in nontraffic accident
>
> Pedestrian on snow-skis injured in collision with other nonmotor vehicle in nontraffic accident

●**V06.1** **Pedestrian injured in collision with other nonmotor vehicle in** traffic accident

X● **V06.10** **Pedestrian on** foot **injured in collision with other nonmotor vehicle in traffic accident**

> Pedestrian NOS injured in collision with other nonmotor vehicle in traffic accident

X● **V06.11** **Pedestrian on** roller-skates **injured in collision with other nonmotor vehicle in traffic accident**

X● **V06.12** **Pedestrian on** skateboard **injured in collision with other nonmotor vehicle in traffic accident**

●**V06.13** **Pedestrian on standing micro-mobility pedestrian conveyance injured in collision with other nonmotor vehicle in traffic accident**

V06.131 **Pedestrian on standing electric scooter injured in collision with other nonmotor vehicle in traffic accident**

V06.138 **Pedestrian on other standing micro-mobility pedestrian conveyance injured in collision with other nonmotor vehicle in traffic accident**

> Pedestrian on hoverboard injured in collision with other nonmotor vehicle in traffic accident
>
> Pedestrian on segway injured in collision with other nonmotor vehicle in traffic accident

X● **V06.19** **Pedestrian with** other **conveyance injured in collision with other nonmotor vehicle in traffic accident**

> Pedestrian with baby stroller injured in collision with other nonmotor vehicle in nontraffic accident
>
> Pedestrian in wheelchair (powered) injured in collision with other nonmotor vehicle in traffic accident
>
> Pedestrian in motorized mobility scooter injured in collision with other nonmotor vehicle in traffic accident
>
> Pedestrian on ice-skates injured in collision with other nonmotor vehicle in traffic accident
>
> Pedestrian on nonmotorized scooter injured in collision with other nonmotor vehicle in traffic accident
>
> Pedestrian on sled injured in collision with other nonmotor vehicle in traffic accident
>
> Pedestrian on snowboard injured in collision with other nonmotor vehicle in traffic accident
>
> Pedestrian on snow-skis injured in collision with other nonmotor vehicle in traffic accident

CHAPTER 20 (V00-Y99)

N   Newborn Age: 0   P   Pediatric Age: 0–17   M   Maternity DX: 9–64   A   Adult Age: 15–124   ♀ Females Only   ♂ Males Only

🔹 Complication\Comorbidity   🔹 Major C\C   (Ex) CC/MCC Exclusions   🔹 Hospital-Acquired Condition   🔹 Hierarchical Condition Category

1539

● V06.9   Pedestrian injured in collision with other nonmotor vehicle, unspecified whether traffic or nontraffic accident

   X ● V06.90   Pedestrian on foot injured in collision with other nonmotor vehicle, unspecified whether traffic or nontraffic accident
        Pedestrian NOS injured in collision with other nonmotor vehicle, unspecified whether traffic or nontraffic accident

   X ● V06.91   Pedestrian on roller-skates injured in collision with other nonmotor vehicle, unspecified whether traffic or nontraffic accident

   X ● V06.92   Pedestrian on skateboard injured in collision with other nonmotor vehicle, unspecified whether traffic or nontraffic accident

   ● V06.93   Pedestrian on standing micro-mobility pedestrian conveyance injured in collision with other nonmotor vehicle, unspecified whether traffic or nontraffic accident

      V06.931   Pedestrian on standing electric scooter injured in collision with other nonmotor vehicle, unspecified whether traffic or nontraffic accident

      V06.938   Pedestrian on other standing micro-mobility pedestrian conveyance injured in collision with other nonmotor vehicle, unspecified whether traffic or nontraffic accident
        Pedestrian on hoverboard injured in collision with other nonmotor, unspecified whether traffic or nontraffic accident
        Pedestrian on segway injured in collision with other nonmotor vehicle, unspecified whether traffic or nontraffic accident

   X ● V06.99   Pedestrian with other conveyance injured in collision with other nonmotor vehicle, unspecified whether traffic or nontraffic accident
        Pedestrian with baby stroller injured in collision with other nonmotor vehicle, unspecified whether traffic or nontraffic accident
        Pedestrian in wheelchair (powered) injured in collision with other nonmotor vehicle, unspecified whether traffic or nontraffic accident
        Pedestrian in motorized mobility scooter injured in collision with other nonmotor vehicle, unspecified whether traffic or nontraffic accident
        Pedestrian on ice-skates injured in collision with other nonmotor vehicle, unspecified whether traffic or nontraffic accident
        Pedestrian on nonmotorized scooter injured in collision with other nonmotor vehicle, unspecified whether traffic or nontraffic accident
        Pedestrian on sled injured in collision with other nonmotor vehicle, unspecified whether traffic or nontraffic accident
        Pedestrian on snowboard injured in collision with other nonmotor vehicle, unspecified whether traffic or nontraffic accident
        Pedestrian on snow-skis injured in collision with other nonmotor vehicle, unspecified whether traffic or nontraffic accident

● V09   Pedestrian injured in other and unspecified transport accidents
   The appropriate 7th character is to be added to each code from category V09

     A   initial encounter
     D   subsequent encounter
     S   sequela

   ● V09.0   Pedestrian injured in nontraffic accident involving other and unspecified motor vehicles

     X ● V09.00   Pedestrian injured in nontraffic accident involving unspecified motor vehicles

     X ● V09.01   Pedestrian injured in nontraffic accident involving military vehicle

     X ● V09.09   Pedestrian injured in nontraffic accident involving other motor vehicles
         Pedestrian injured in nontraffic accident by special vehicle

   X ● V09.1   Pedestrian injured in unspecified nontraffic accident

   ● V09.2   Pedestrian injured in traffic accident involving other and unspecified motor vehicles

     X ● V09.20   Pedestrian injured in traffic accident involving unspecified motor vehicles

     X ● V09.21   Pedestrian injured in traffic accident involving military vehicle

     X ● V09.29   Pedestrian injured in traffic accident involving other motor vehicles

   X ● V09.3   Pedestrian injured in unspecified traffic accident

   X ● V09.9   Pedestrian injured in unspecified transport accident

PEDAL CYCLE RIDER INJURED IN TRANSPORT ACCIDENT (V10-V19)

Includes   any non-motorized vehicle, excluding an animal-drawn vehicle, or a sidecar or trailer attached to the pedal cycle

Excludes2   rupture of pedal cycle tire (W37.0)

● V10   Pedal cycle rider injured in collision with pedestrian or animal

   Excludes1   pedal cycle rider collision with animal-drawn vehicle or animal being ridden (V16.-)

   The appropriate 7th character is to be added to each code from category V10

     A   initial encounter
     D   subsequent encounter
     S   sequela

   X ● V10.0   Pedal cycle driver injured in collision with pedestrian or animal in nontraffic accident

   X ● V10.1   Pedal cycle passenger injured in collision with pedestrian or animal in nontraffic accident

   X ● V10.2   Unspecified pedal cyclist injured in collision with pedestrian or animal in nontraffic accident

   X ● V10.3   Person boarding or alighting a pedal cycle injured in collision with pedestrian or animal

   X ● V10.4   Pedal cycle driver injured in collision with pedestrian or animal in traffic accident

   X ● V10.5   Pedal cycle passenger injured in collision with pedestrian or animal in traffic accident

   X ● V10.9   Unspecified pedal cyclist injured in collision with pedestrian or animal in traffic accident

▶ New   ➡ Revised   ~~deleted~~ Deleted   Excludes 1   Excludes 2   Includes   Use additional   Code first   Code also   Key words
OGCR Official Guidelines   ● Unacceptable Principal Diagnosis   X Assign placeholder X   ● Use Additional Character(s)   ▶ Manifestation Code   Coding Clinic

● **V11**   Pedal cycle rider injured in collision with other pedal cycle

The appropriate 7th character is to be added to each code from category V11

> A   initial encounter
> D   subsequent encounter
> S   sequela

X● **V11.0**   Pedal cycle driver injured in collision with other pedal cycle in nontraffic accident

X● **V11.1**   Pedal cycle passenger injured in collision with other pedal cycle in nontraffic accident

X● **V11.2**   Unspecified pedal cyclist injured in collision with other pedal cycle in nontraffic accident

X● **V11.3**   Person boarding or alighting a pedal cycle injured in collision with other pedal cycle

X● **V11.4**   Pedal cycle driver injured in collision with other pedal cycle in traffic accident

X● **V11.5**   Pedal cycle passenger injured in collision with other pedal cycle in traffic accident

X● **V11.9**   Unspecified pedal cyclist injured in collision with other pedal cycle in traffic accident

● **V12**   Pedal cycle rider injured in collision with two- or three-wheeled motor vehicle

The appropriate 7th character is to be added to each code from category V12

> A   initial encounter
> D   subsequent encounter
> S   sequela

X● **V12.0**   Pedal cycle driver injured in collision with two- or three-wheeled motor vehicle in nontraffic accident

X● **V12.1**   Pedal cycle passenger injured in collision with two- or three-wheeled motor vehicle in nontraffic accident

X● **V12.2**   Unspecified pedal cyclist injured in collision with two- or three-wheeled motor vehicle in nontraffic accident

X● **V12.3**   Person boarding or alighting a pedal cycle injured in collision with two- or three-wheeled motor vehicle

X● **V12.4**   Pedal cycle driver injured in collision with two- or three-wheeled motor vehicle in traffic accident

X● **V12.5**   Pedal cycle passenger injured in collision with two- or three-wheeled motor vehicle in traffic accident

X● **V12.9**   Unspecified pedal cyclist injured in collision with two- or three-wheeled motor vehicle in traffic accident

● **V13**   Pedal cycle rider injured in collision with car, pick-up truck or van

The appropriate 7th character is to be added to each code from category V13

> A   initial encounter
> D   subsequent encounter
> S   sequela

X● **V13.0**   Pedal cycle driver injured in collision with car, pick-up truck or van in nontraffic accident

X● **V13.1**   Pedal cycle passenger injured in collision with car, pick-up truck or van in nontraffic accident

X● **V13.2**   Unspecified pedal cyclist injured in collision with car, pick-up truck or van in nontraffic accident

X● **V13.3**   Person boarding or alighting a pedal cycle injured in collision with car, pick-up truck or van

X● **V13.4**   Pedal cycle driver injured in collision with car, pick-up truck or van in traffic accident

X● **V13.5**   Pedal cycle passenger injured in collision with car, pick-up truck or van in traffic accident

X● **V13.9**   Unspecified pedal cyclist injured in collision with car, pick-up truck or van in traffic accident

● **V14**   Pedal cycle rider injured in collision with heavy transport vehicle or bus

> **Excludes1**   pedal cycle rider injured in collision with military vehicle (V19.81)

The appropriate 7th character is to be added to each code from category V14

> A   initial encounter
> D   subsequent encounter
> S   sequela

X● **V14.0**   Pedal cycle driver injured in collision with heavy transport vehicle or bus in nontraffic accident

X● **V14.1**   Pedal cycle passenger injured in collision with heavy transport vehicle or bus in nontraffic accident

X● **V14.2**   Unspecified pedal cyclist injured in collision with heavy transport vehicle or bus in nontraffic accident

X● **V14.3**   Person boarding or alighting a pedal cycle injured in collision with heavy transport vehicle or bus

X● **V14.4**   Pedal cycle driver injured in collision with heavy transport vehicle or bus in traffic accident

X● **V14.5**   Pedal cycle passenger injured in collision with heavy transport vehicle or bus in traffic accident

X● **V14.9**   Unspecified pedal cyclist injured in collision with heavy transport vehicle or bus in traffic accident

● **V15**   Pedal cycle rider injured in collision with railway train or railway vehicle

The appropriate 7th character is to be added to each code from category V15

> A   initial encounter
> D   subsequent encounter
> S   sequela

X● **V15.0**   Pedal cycle driver injured in collision with railway train or railway vehicle in nontraffic accident

X● **V15.1**   Pedal cycle passenger injured in collision with railway train or railway vehicle in nontraffic accident

X● **V15.2**   Unspecified pedal cyclist injured in collision with railway train or railway vehicle in nontraffic accident

X● **V15.3**   Person boarding or alighting a pedal cycle injured in collision with railway train or railway vehicle

X● **V15.4**   Pedal cycle driver injured in collision with railway train or railway vehicle in traffic accident

X● **V15.5**   Pedal cycle passenger injured in collision with railway train or railway vehicle in traffic accident

X● **V15.9**   Unspecified pedal cyclist injured in collision with railway train or railway vehicle in traffic accident

● **V16**   Pedal cycle rider injured in collision with other nonmotor vehicle

> **Includes**   collision with animal-drawn vehicle, animal being ridden, streetcar

The appropriate 7th character is to be added to each code from category V16

> A   initial encounter
> D   subsequent encounter
> S   sequela

X● **V16.0**   Pedal cycle driver injured in collision with other nonmotor vehicle in nontraffic accident

X● **V16.1**   Pedal cycle passenger injured in collision with other nonmotor vehicle in nontraffic accident

X● **V16.2**   Unspecified pedal cyclist injured in collision with other nonmotor vehicle in nontraffic accident

X● **V16.3**   Person boarding or alighting a pedal cycle injured in collision with other nonmotor vehicle in nontraffic accident

X● **V16.4**   Pedal cycle driver injured in collision with other nonmotor vehicle in traffic accident

CHAPTER 20 (V00-Y99)

N Newborn Age: 0   **P** Pediatric Age: 0–17   **M** Maternity DX: 9–64   **A** Adult Age: 15–124   ♀ Females Only   ♂ Males Only

🅒 Complication\Comorbidity   🅒 Major C\C   (Ex) CC/MCC Exclusions   🅒 Hospital-Acquired Condition   🅒 Hierarchical Condition Category

1541

X● **V16.5** Pedal cycle passenger injured in collision with other nonmotor vehicle in traffic accident

X● **V16.9** Unspecified pedal cyclist injured in collision with other nonmotor vehicle in traffic accident

● **V17** Pedal cycle rider injured in collision with fixed or stationary object

The appropriate 7th character is to be added to each code from category V17

> A   initial encounter
> D   subsequent encounter
> S   sequela

X● **V17.0** Pedal cycle driver injured in collision with fixed or stationary object in nontraffic accident

X● **V17.1** Pedal cycle passenger injured in collision with fixed or stationary object in nontraffic accident

X● **V17.2** Unspecified pedal cyclist injured in collision with fixed or stationary object in nontraffic accident

X● **V17.3** Person boarding or alighting a pedal cycle injured in collision with fixed or stationary object

X● **V17.4** Pedal cycle driver injured in collision with fixed or stationary object in traffic accident

X● **V17.5** Pedal cycle passenger injured in collision with fixed or stationary object in traffic accident

X● **V17.9** Unspecified pedal cyclist injured in collision with fixed or stationary object in traffic accident

● **V18** Pedal cycle rider injured in noncollision transport accident

Includes fall or thrown from pedal cycle (without antecedent collision)
overturning pedal cycle NOS
overturning pedal cycle without collision

The appropriate 7th character is to be added to each code from category V18

> A   initial encounter
> D   subsequent encounter
> S   sequela

X● **V18.0** Pedal cycle driver injured in noncollision transport accident in nontraffic accident

X● **V18.1** Pedal cycle passenger injured in noncollision transport accident in nontraffic accident

X● **V18.2** Unspecified pedal cyclist injured in noncollision transport accident in nontraffic accident

X● **V18.3** Person boarding or alighting a pedal cycle injured in noncollision transport accident

X● **V18.4** Pedal cycle driver injured in noncollision transport accident in traffic accident

X● **V18.5** Pedal cycle passenger injured in noncollision transport accident in traffic accident

X● **V18.9** Unspecified pedal cyclist injured in noncollision transport accident in traffic accident

● **V19** Pedal cycle rider injured in other and unspecified transport accidents

The appropriate 7th character is to be added to each code from category V19

> A   initial encounter
> D   subsequent encounter
> S   sequela

● **V19.0** Pedal cycle driver injured in collision with other and unspecified motor vehicles in nontraffic accident

X● **V19.00** Pedal cycle driver injured in collision with unspecified motor vehicles in nontraffic accident

X● **V19.09** Pedal cycle driver injured in collision with other motor vehicles in nontraffic accident

● **V19.1** Pedal cycle passenger injured in collision with other and unspecified motor vehicles in nontraffic accident

X● **V19.10** Pedal cycle passenger injured in collision with unspecified motor vehicles in nontraffic accident

X● **V19.19** Pedal cycle passenger injured in collision with other motor vehicles in nontraffic accident

● **V19.2** Unspecified pedal cyclist injured in collision with other and unspecified motor vehicles in nontraffic accident

X● **V19.20** Unspecified pedal cyclist injured in collision with unspecified motor vehicles in nontraffic accident
Pedal cycle collision NOS, nontraffic

X● **V19.29** Unspecified pedal cyclist injured in collision with other motor vehicles in nontraffic accident

X● **V19.3** Pedal cyclist (driver) (passenger) injured in unspecified nontraffic accident
Pedal cycle accident NOS, nontraffic
Pedal cyclist injured in nontraffic accident NOS

● **V19.4** Pedal cycle driver injured in collision with other and unspecified motor vehicles in traffic accident

X● **V19.40** Pedal cycle driver injured in collision with unspecified motor vehicles in traffic accident

X● **V19.49** Pedal cycle driver injured in collision with other motor vehicles in traffic accident

● **V19.5** Pedal cycle passenger injured in collision with other and unspecified motor vehicles in traffic accident

X● **V19.50** Pedal cycle passenger injured in collision with unspecified motor vehicles in traffic accident

X● **V19.59** Pedal cycle passenger injured in collision with other motor vehicles in traffic accident

● **V19.6** Unspecified pedal cyclist injured in collision with other and unspecified motor vehicles in traffic accident

X● **V19.60** Unspecified pedal cyclist injured in collision with unspecified motor vehicles in traffic accident
Pedal cycle collision NOS (traffic)

X● **V19.69** Unspecified pedal cyclist injured in collision with other motor vehicles in traffic accident

● **V19.8** Pedal cyclist (driver) (passenger) injured in other specified transport accidents

X● **V19.81** Pedal cyclist (driver) (passenger) injured in transport accident with military vehicle

X● **V19.88** Pedal cyclist (driver) (passenger) injured in other specified transport accidents

X● **V19.9** Pedal cyclist (driver) (passenger) injured in unspecified traffic accident
Pedal cycle accident NOS

MOTORCYCLE RIDER INJURED IN TRANSPORT ACCIDENT (V20-V29)

Includes moped motorcycle with sidecar motorized bicycle motor scooter

Excludes 1 three-wheeled motor vehicle (V30-V39)

● **V20** Motorcycle rider injured in collision with pedestrian or animal

Excludes 1 motorcycle rider collision with animal-drawn vehicle or animal being ridden (V26.-)

The appropriate 7th character is to be added to each code from category V20

> A   initial encounter
> D   subsequent encounter
> S   sequela

X● **V20.0** Motorcycle driver injured in collision with pedestrian or animal in nontraffic accident

X● **V20.1** Motorcycle passenger injured in collision with pedestrian or animal in nontraffic accident

X● **V20.2** Unspecified motorcycle rider injured in collision with pedestrian or animal in nontraffic accident

X● **V20.3** Person boarding or alighting a motorcycle injured in collision with pedestrian or animal

X● **V20.4** Motorcycle driver injured in collision with pedestrian or animal in traffic accident

X● **V20.5** Motorcycle passenger injured in collision with pedestrian or animal in traffic accident

X● **V20.9** Unspecified motorcycle rider injured in collision with pedestrian or animal in traffic accident

● **V21** Motorcycle rider injured in collision with pedal cycle

The appropriate 7th character is to be added to each code from category V21

A	initial encounter
D	subsequent encounter
S	sequela

X● **V21.0** Motorcycle driver injured in collision with pedal cycle in nontraffic accident

X● **V21.1** Motorcycle passenger injured in collision with pedal cycle in nontraffic accident

X● **V21.2** Unspecified motorcycle rider injured in collision with pedal cycle in nontraffic accident

X● **V21.3** Person boarding or alighting a motorcycle injured in collision with pedal cycle

X● **V21.4** Motorcycle driver injured in collision with pedal cycle in traffic accident

X● **V21.5** Motorcycle passenger injured in collision with pedal cycle in traffic accident

X● **V21.9** Unspecified motorcycle rider injured in collision with pedal cycle in traffic accident

● **V22** Motorcycle rider injured in collision with two- or three-wheeled motor vehicle

The appropriate 7th character is to be added to each code from category V22

A	initial encounter
D	subsequent encounter
S	sequela

X● **V22.0** Motorcycle driver injured in collision with two- or three-wheeled motor vehicle in nontraffic accident

X● **V22.1** Motorcycle passenger injured in collision with two- or three-wheeled motor vehicle in nontraffic accident

X● **V22.2** Unspecified motorcycle rider injured in collision with two- or three-wheeled motor vehicle in nontraffic accident

X● **V22.3** Person boarding or alighting a motorcycle injured in collision with two- or three-wheeled motor vehicle

X● **V22.4** Motorcycle driver injured in collision with two- or three-wheeled motor vehicle in traffic accident

X● **V22.5** Motorcycle passenger injured in collision with two- or three-wheeled motor vehicle in traffic accident

X● **V22.9** Unspecified motorcycle rider injured in collision with two- or three-wheeled motor vehicle in traffic accident

● **V23** Motorcycle rider injured in collision with car, pick-up truck or van

The appropriate 7th character is to be added to each code from category V23

A	initial encounter
D	subsequent encounter
S	sequela

X● **V23.0** Motorcycle driver injured in collision with car, pick-up truck or van in nontraffic accident

X● **V23.1** Motorcycle passenger injured in collision with car, pick-up truck or van in nontraffic accident

X● **V23.2** Unspecified motorcycle rider injured in collision with car, pick-up truck or van in nontraffic accident

X● **V23.3** Person boarding or alighting a motorcycle injured in collision with car, pick-up truck or van

X● **V23.4** Motorcycle driver injured in collision with car, pick-up truck or van in traffic accident

X● **V23.5** Motorcycle passenger injured in collision with car, pick-up truck or van in traffic accident

X● **V23.9** Unspecified motorcycle rider injured in collision with car, pick-up truck or van in traffic accident

● **V24** Motorcycle rider injured in collision with heavy transport vehicle or bus

> **Excludes1**   motorcycle rider injured in collision with military vehicle (V29.81)

The appropriate 7th character is to be added to each code from category V24

A	initial encounter
D	subsequent encounter
S	sequela

X● **V24.0** Motorcycle driver injured in collision with heavy transport vehicle or bus in nontraffic accident

X● **V24.1** Motorcycle passenger injured in collision with heavy transport vehicle or bus in nontraffic accident

X● **V24.2** Unspecified motorcycle rider injured in collision with heavy transport vehicle or bus in nontraffic accident

X● **V24.3** Person boarding or alighting a motorcycle injured in collision with heavy transport vehicle or bus

X● **V24.4** Motorcycle driver injured in collision with heavy transport vehicle or bus in traffic accident

X● **V24.5** Motorcycle passenger injured in collision with heavy transport vehicle or bus in traffic accident

X● **V24.9** Unspecified motorcycle rider injured in collision with heavy transport vehicle or bus in traffic accident

● **V25** Motorcycle rider injured in collision with railway train or railway vehicle

The appropriate 7th character is to be added to each code from category V25

A	initial encounter
D	subsequent encounter
S	sequela

X● **V25.0** Motorcycle driver injured in collision with railway train or railway vehicle in nontraffic accident

X● **V25.1** Motorcycle passenger injured in collision with railway train or railway vehicle in nontraffic accident

X● **V25.2** Unspecified motorcycle rider injured in collision with railway train or railway vehicle in nontraffic accident

X● **V25.3** Person boarding or alighting a motorcycle injured in collision with railway train or railway vehicle

X● **V25.4** Motorcycle driver injured in collision with railway train or railway vehicle in traffic accident

X● **V25.5** Motorcycle passenger injured in collision with railway train or railway vehicle in traffic accident

X● **V25.9** Unspecified motorcycle rider injured in collision with railway train or railway vehicle in traffic accident

N Newborn Age: 0   **P** Pediatric Age: 0–17   **M** Maternity DX: 9–64   **A** Adult Age: 15–124   ♀ Females Only   ♂ Males Only

🅒 Complication\Comorbidity   🅒 Major C\C   (Ex) CC/MCC Exclusions   🅗 Hospital-Acquired Condition   🅗 Hierarchical Condition Category

1543

CHAPTER 20 (V00-Y99)

● **V26**   **Motorcycle rider injured in collision with other nonmotor vehicle**

> **Includes**   collision with animal-drawn vehicle, animal being ridden, streetcar

> The appropriate 7th character is to be added to each code from category V26

> | A | initial encounter |
> |---|---|
> | D | subsequent encounter |
> | S | sequela |

X● **V26.0**   Motorcycle driver injured in collision with other nonmotor vehicle in nontraffic accident

X● **V26.1**   Motorcycle passenger injured in collision with other nonmotor vehicle in nontraffic accident

X● **V26.2**   Unspecified motorcycle rider injured in collision with other nonmotor vehicle in nontraffic accident

X● **V26.3**   Person boarding or alighting a motorcycle injured in collision with other nonmotor vehicle

X● **V26.4**   Motorcycle driver injured in collision with other nonmotor vehicle in traffic accident

X● **V26.5**   Motorcycle passenger injured in collision with other nonmotor vehicle in traffic accident

X● **V26.9**   Unspecified motorcycle rider injured in collision with other nonmotor vehicle in traffic accident

● **V27**   **Motorcycle rider injured in collision with fixed or stationary object**

> The appropriate 7th character is to be added to each code from category V27

> | A | initial encounter |
> |---|---|
> | D | subsequent encounter |
> | S | sequela |

X● **V27.0**   Motorcycle driver injured in collision with fixed or stationary object in nontraffic accident

X● **V27.1**   Motorcycle passenger injured in collision with fixed or stationary object in nontraffic accident

X● **V27.2**   Unspecified motorcycle rider injured in collision with fixed or stationary object in nontraffic accident

X● **V27.3**   Person boarding or alighting a motorcycle injured in collision with fixed or stationary object

X● **V27.4**   Motorcycle driver injured in collision with fixed or stationary object in traffic accident

X● **V27.5**   Motorcycle passenger injured in collision with fixed or stationary object in traffic accident

X● **V27.9**   Unspecified motorcycle rider injured in collision with fixed or stationary object in traffic accident

● **V28**   **Motorcycle rider injured in noncollision transport accident**

> **Includes**   fall or thrown from motorcycle (without antecedent collision)
> overturning motorcycle NOS
> overturning motorcycle without collision

> The appropriate 7th character is to be added to each code from category V28

> | A | initial encounter |
> |---|---|
> | D | subsequent encounter |
> | S | sequela |

X● **V28.0**   Motorcycle driver injured in noncollision transport accident in nontraffic accident

X● **V28.1**   Motorcycle passenger injured in noncollision transport accident in nontraffic accident

X● **V28.2**   Unspecified motorcycle rider injured in noncollision transport accident in nontraffic accident

X● **V28.3**   Person boarding or alighting a motorcycle injured in noncollision transport accident

X● **V28.4**   Motorcycle driver injured in noncollision transport accident in traffic accident

X● **V28.5**   Motorcycle passenger injured in noncollision transport accident in traffic accident

X● **V28.9**   Unspecified motorcycle rider injured in noncollision transport accident in traffic accident

● **V29**   **Motorcycle rider injured in other and unspecified transport accidents**

> The appropriate 7th character is to be added to each code from category V29

> | A | initial encounter |
> |---|---|
> | D | subsequent encounter |
> | S | sequela |

Coding Clinic: 2015, Q3, P20

● **V29.0**   Motorcycle driver injured in collision with other and unspecified motor vehicles in nontraffic accident

    X● **V29.00**   Motorcycle driver injured in collision with unspecified motor vehicles in nontraffic accident

    X● **V29.09**   Motorcycle driver injured in collision with other motor vehicles in nontraffic accident

● **V29.1**   Motorcycle passenger injured in collision with other and unspecified motor vehicles in nontraffic accident

    X● **V29.10**   Motorcycle passenger injured in collision with unspecified motor vehicles in nontraffic accident

    X● **V29.19**   Motorcycle passenger injured in collision with other motor vehicles in nontraffic accident

● **V29.2**   Unspecified motorcycle rider injured in collision with other and unspecified motor vehicles in nontraffic accident

    X● **V29.20**   Unspecified motorcycle rider injured in collision with unspecified motor vehicles in nontraffic accident
> Motorcycle collision NOS, nontraffic

    X● **V29.29**   Unspecified motorcycle rider injured in collision with other motor vehicles in nontraffic accident

X● **V29.3**   Motorcycle rider (driver) (passenger) injured in unspecified nontraffic accident
> Motorcycle accident NOS, nontraffic
> Motorcycle rider injured in nontraffic accident NOS

● **V29.4**   Motorcycle driver injured in collision with other and unspecified motor vehicles in traffic accident

    X● **V29.40**   Motorcycle driver injured in collision with unspecified motor vehicles in traffic accident

    X● **V29.49**   Motorcycle driver injured in collision with other motor vehicles in traffic accident

● **V29.5**   Motorcycle passenger injured in collision with other and unspecified motor vehicles in traffic accident

    X● **V29.50**   Motorcycle passenger injured in collision with unspecified motor vehicles in traffic accident

    X● **V29.59**   Motorcycle passenger injured in collision with other motor vehicles in traffic accident

● **V29.6**   Unspecified motorcycle rider injured in collision with other and unspecified motor vehicles in traffic accident

    X● **V29.60**   Unspecified motorcycle rider injured in collision with unspecified motor vehicles in traffic accident
> Motorcycle collision NOS (traffic)

    X● **V29.69**   Unspecified motorcycle rider injured in collision with other motor vehicles in traffic accident

● **V29.8**   Motorcycle rider (driver) (passenger) injured in other specified transport accidents

    X● **V29.81**   Motorcycle rider (driver) (passenger) injured in transport accident with military vehicle

    X● **V29.88**   Motorcycle rider (driver) (passenger) injured in other specified transport accidents

X● **V29.9**   Motorcycle rider (driver) (passenger) injured in unspecified traffic accident
> Motorcycle accident NOS

▶ New   ⇒ Revised   ~~deleted~~ Deleted   Excludes 1   Excludes 2   Includes   Use additional   Code first   Code also   Key words

OGCR Official Guidelines   ● Unacceptable Principal Diagnosis   X Assign placeholder X   ● Use Additional Character(s)   ▶ Manifestation Code   **Coding Clinic**

OCCUPANT OF THREE-WHEELED MOTOR VEHICLE INJURED IN TRANSPORT ACCIDENT (V30-V39)

Includes　motorized tricycle
motorized rickshaw
three-wheeled motor car

Excludes1　all-terrain vehicles (V86.-)
motorcycle with sidecar (V20-V29)
vehicle designed primarily for off-road use (V86.-)

● **V30**　Occupant of three-wheeled motor vehicle injured in collision with pedestrian or animal

　Excludes1　three-wheeled motor vehicle collision with animal-drawn vehicle or animal being ridden (V36.-)

　The appropriate 7th character is to be added to each code from category V30

A	initial encounter
D	subsequent encounter
S	sequela

X● **V30.0**　Driver of three-wheeled motor vehicle injured in collision with pedestrian or animal in nontraffic accident

X● **V30.1**　Passenger in three-wheeled motor vehicle injured in collision with pedestrian or animal in nontraffic accident

X● **V30.2**　Person on outside of three-wheeled motor vehicle injured in collision with pedestrian or animal in nontraffic accident

X● **V30.3**　Unspecified occupant of three-wheeled motor vehicle injured in collision with pedestrian or animal in nontraffic accident

X● **V30.4**　Person boarding or alighting a three-wheeled motor vehicle injured in collision with pedestrian or animal

X● **V30.5**　Driver of three-wheeled motor vehicle injured in collision with pedestrian or animal in traffic accident

X● **V30.6**　Passenger in three-wheeled motor vehicle injured in collision with pedestrian or animal in traffic accident

X● **V30.7**　Person on outside of three-wheeled motor vehicle injured in collision with pedestrian or animal in traffic accident

X● **V30.9**　Unspecified occupant of three-wheeled motor vehicle injured in collision with pedestrian or animal in traffic accident

● **V31**　Occupant of three-wheeled motor vehicle injured in collision with pedal cycle

　The appropriate 7th character is to be added to each code from category V31

A	initial encounter
D	subsequent encounter
S	sequela

X● **V31.0**　Driver of three-wheeled motor vehicle injured in collision with pedal cycle in nontraffic accident

X● **V31.1**　Passenger in three-wheeled motor vehicle injured in collision with pedal cycle in nontraffic accident

X● **V31.2**　Person on outside of three-wheeled motor vehicle injured in collision with pedal cycle in nontraffic accident

X● **V31.3**　Unspecified occupant of three-wheeled motor vehicle injured in collision with pedal cycle in nontraffic accident

X● **V31.4**　Person boarding or alighting a three-wheeled motor vehicle injured in collision with pedal cycle

X● **V31.5**　Driver of three-wheeled motor vehicle injured in collision with pedal cycle in traffic accident

X● **V31.6**　Passenger in three-wheeled motor vehicle injured in collision with pedal cycle in traffic accident

X● **V31.7**　Person on outside of three-wheeled motor vehicle injured in collision with pedal cycle in traffic accident

X● **V31.9**　Unspecified occupant of three-wheeled motor vehicle injured in collision with pedal cycle in traffic accident

● **V32**　Occupant of three-wheeled motor vehicle injured in collision with two- or three-wheeled motor vehicle

　The appropriate 7th character is to be added to each code from category V32

A	initial encounter
D	subsequent encounter
S	sequela

X● **V32.0**　Driver of three-wheeled motor vehicle injured in collision with two- or three-wheeled motor vehicle in nontraffic accident

X● **V32.1**　Passenger in three-wheeled motor vehicle injured in collision with two- or three-wheeled motor vehicle in nontraffic accident

X● **V32.2**　Person on outside of three-wheeled motor vehicle injured in collision with two- or three-wheeled motor vehicle in nontraffic accident

X● **V32.3**　Unspecified occupant of three-wheeled motor vehicle injured in collision with two- or three-wheeled motor vehicle in nontraffic accident

X● **V32.4**　Person boarding or alighting a three-wheeled motor vehicle injured in collision with two- or three-wheeled motor vehicle

X● **V32.5**　Driver of three-wheeled motor vehicle injured in collision with two- or three-wheeled motor vehicle in traffic accident

X● **V32.6**　Passenger in three-wheeled motor vehicle injured in collision with two- or three-wheeled motor vehicle in traffic accident

X● **V32.7**　Person on outside of three-wheeled motor vehicle injured in collision with two- or three-wheeled motor vehicle in traffic accident

X● **V32.9**　Unspecified occupant of three-wheeled motor vehicle injured in collision with two- or three-wheeled motor vehicle in traffic accident

● **V33**　Occupant of three-wheeled motor vehicle injured in collision with car, pick-up truck or van

　The appropriate 7th character is to be added to each code from category V33

A	initial encounter
D	subsequent encounter
S	sequela

X● **V33.0**　Driver of three-wheeled motor vehicle injured in collision with car, pick-up truck or van in nontraffic accident

X● **V33.1**　Passenger in three-wheeled motor vehicle injured in collision with car, pick-up truck or van in nontraffic accident

X● **V33.2**　Person on outside of three-wheeled motor vehicle injured in collision with car, pick-up truck or van in nontraffic accident

X● **V33.3**　Unspecified occupant of three-wheeled motor vehicle injured in collision with car, pick-up truck or van in nontraffic accident

X● **V33.4**　Person boarding or alighting a three-wheeled motor vehicle injured in collision with car, pick-up truck or van

X● **V33.5**　Driver of three-wheeled motor vehicle injured in collision with car, pick-up truck or van in traffic accident

X● **V33.6**　Passenger in three-wheeled motor vehicle injured in collision with car, pick-up truck or van in traffic accident

X● **V33.7**　Person on outside of three-wheeled motor vehicle injured in collision with car, pick-up truck or van in traffic accident

X● **V33.9**　Unspecified occupant of three-wheeled motor vehicle injured in collision with car, pick-up truck or van in traffic accident

CHAPTER 20 (V00-Y99)

N Newborn Age: 0　　**P** Pediatric Age: 0–17　　**M** Maternity DX: 9–64　　**A** Adult Age: 15–124　　♀ Females Only　　♂ Males Only

⬡ Complication\Comorbidity　　⬡ Major C\C　　(Ex) CC/MCC Exclusions　　⬡ Hospital-Acquired Condition　　⬡ Hierarchical Condition Category

1545

● **V34** Occupant of three-wheeled motor vehicle injured in collision with heavy transport vehicle or bus

> **Excludes1**　occupant of three-wheeled motor vehicle injured in collision with military vehicle (V39.81)

> The appropriate 7th character is to be added to each code from category V34

> | | |
> |---|---|
> | A | initial encounter |
> | D | subsequent encounter |
> | S | sequela |

X● **V34.0** Driver of three-wheeled motor vehicle injured in collision with heavy transport vehicle or bus in nontraffic accident

X● **V34.1** Passenger in three-wheeled motor vehicle injured in collision with heavy transport vehicle or bus in nontraffic accident

X● **V34.2** Person on outside of three-wheeled motor vehicle injured in collision with heavy transport vehicle or bus in nontraffic accident

X● **V34.3** Unspecified occupant of three-wheeled motor vehicle injured in collision with heavy transport vehicle or bus in nontraffic accident

X● **V34.4** Person boarding or alighting a three-wheeled motor vehicle injured in collision with heavy transport vehicle or bus

X● **V34.5** Driver of three-wheeled motor vehicle injured in collision with heavy transport vehicle or bus in traffic accident

X● **V34.6** Passenger in three-wheeled motor vehicle injured in collision with heavy transport vehicle or bus in traffic accident

X● **V34.7** Person on outside of three-wheeled motor vehicle injured in collision with heavy transport vehicle or bus in traffic accident

X● **V34.9** Unspecified occupant of three-wheeled motor vehicle injured in collision with heavy transport vehicle or bus in traffic accident

● **V35** Occupant of three-wheeled motor vehicle injured in collision with railway train or railway vehicle

> The appropriate 7th character is to be added to each code from category V35

> | | |
> |---|---|
> | A | initial encounter |
> | D | subsequent encounter |
> | S | sequela |

X● **V35.0** Driver of three-wheeled motor vehicle injured in collision with railway train or railway vehicle in nontraffic accident

X● **V35.1** Passenger in three-wheeled motor vehicle injured in collision with railway train or railway vehicle in nontraffic accident

X● **V35.2** Person on outside of three-wheeled motor vehicle injured in collision with railway train or railway vehicle in nontraffic accident

X● **V35.3** Unspecified occupant of three-wheeled motor vehicle injured in collision with railway train or railway vehicle in nontraffic accident

X● **V35.4** Person boarding or alighting a three-wheeled motor vehicle injured in collision with railway train or railway vehicle

X● **V35.5** Driver of three-wheeled motor vehicle injured in collision with railway train or railway vehicle in traffic accident

X● **V35.6** Passenger in three-wheeled motor vehicle injured in collision with railway train or railway vehicle in traffic accident

X● **V35.7** Person on outside of three-wheeled motor vehicle injured in collision with railway train or railway vehicle in traffic accident

X● **V35.9** Unspecified occupant of three-wheeled motor vehicle injured in collision with railway train or railway vehicle in traffic accident

● **V36** Occupant of three-wheeled motor vehicle injured in collision with other nonmotor vehicle

> **Includes**　collision with animal-drawn vehicle, animal being ridden, streetcar

> The appropriate 7th character is to be added to each code from category V36

> | | |
> |---|---|
> | A | initial encounter |
> | D | subsequent encounter |
> | S | sequela |

X● **V36.0** Driver of three-wheeled motor vehicle injured in collision with other nonmotor vehicle in nontraffic accident

X● **V36.1** Passenger in three-wheeled motor vehicle injured in collision with other nonmotor vehicle in nontraffic accident

X● **V36.2** Person on outside of three-wheeled motor vehicle injured in collision with other nonmotor vehicle in nontraffic accident

X● **V36.3** Unspecified occupant of three-wheeled motor vehicle injured in collision with other nonmotor vehicle in nontraffic accident

X● **V36.4** Person boarding or alighting a three-wheeled motor vehicle injured in collision with other nonmotor vehicle

X● **V36.5** Driver of three-wheeled motor vehicle injured in collision with other nonmotor vehicle in traffic accident

X● **V36.6** Passenger in three-wheeled motor vehicle injured in collision with other nonmotor vehicle in traffic accident

X● **V36.7** Person on outside of three-wheeled motor vehicle injured in collision with other nonmotor vehicle in traffic accident

X● **V36.9** Unspecified occupant of three-wheeled motor vehicle injured in collision with other nonmotor vehicle in traffic accident

● **V37** Occupant of three-wheeled motor vehicle injured in collision with fixed or stationary object

> The appropriate 7th character is to be added to each code from category V37

> | | |
> |---|---|
> | A | initial encounter |
> | D | subsequent encounter |
> | S | sequela |

X● **V37.0** Driver of three-wheeled motor vehicle injured in collision with fixed or stationary object in nontraffic accident

X● **V37.1** Passenger in three-wheeled motor vehicle injured in collision with fixed or stationary object in nontraffic accident

X● **V37.2** Person on outside of three-wheeled motor vehicle injured in collision with fixed or stationary object in nontraffic accident

X● **V37.3** Unspecified occupant of three-wheeled motor vehicle injured in collision with fixed or stationary object in nontraffic accident

X● **V37.4** Person boarding or alighting a three-wheeled motor vehicle injured in collision with fixed or stationary object

X● **V37.5** Driver of three-wheeled motor vehicle injured in collision with fixed or stationary object in traffic accident

X● **V37.6** Passenger in three-wheeled motor vehicle injured in collision with fixed or stationary object in traffic accident

X● **V37.7** Person on outside of three-wheeled motor vehicle injured in collision with fixed or stationary object in traffic accident

X● **V37.9** Unspecified occupant of three-wheeled motor vehicle injured in collision with fixed or stationary object in traffic accident

▶ New　⟱ Revised　deleted Deleted　Excludes 1　Excludes 2　Includes　Use additional　Code first　Code also　Key words
OGCR Official Guidelines　● Unacceptable Principal Diagnosis　X Assign placeholder X　● Use Additional Character(s)　▶ Manifestation Code　Coding Clinic

● **V38**   **Occupant of three-wheeled motor vehicle injured in noncollision transport accident**

    Includes   fall or thrown from three-wheeled motor vehicle
               overturning of three-wheeled motor vehicle NOS
               overturning of three-wheeled motor vehicle
                 without collision

    The appropriate 7th character is to be added to each code from category V38

> A   initial encounter
> D   subsequent encounter
> S   sequela

X● **V38.0**   Driver of three-wheeled motor vehicle injured in noncollision transport accident in nontraffic accident

X● **V38.1**   Passenger in three-wheeled motor vehicle injured in noncollision transport accident in nontraffic accident

X● **V38.2**   Person on outside of three-wheeled motor vehicle injured in noncollision transport accident in nontraffic accident

X● **V38.3**   Unspecified occupant of three-wheeled motor vehicle injured in noncollision transport accident in nontraffic accident

X● **V38.4**   Person boarding or alighting a three-wheeled motor vehicle injured in noncollision transport accident

X● **V38.5**   Driver of three-wheeled motor vehicle injured in noncollision transport accident in traffic accident

X● **V38.6**   Passenger in three-wheeled motor vehicle injured in noncollision transport accident in traffic accident

X● **V38.7**   Person on outside of three-wheeled motor vehicle injured in noncollision transport accident in traffic accident

X● **V38.9**   Unspecified occupant of three-wheeled motor vehicle injured in noncollision transport accident in traffic accident

● **V39**   **Occupant of three-wheeled motor vehicle injured in other and unspecified transport accidents**

    The appropriate 7th character is to be added to each code from category V39

> A   initial encounter
> D   subsequent encounter
> S   sequela

● **V39.0**   Driver of three-wheeled motor vehicle injured in collision with other and unspecified motor vehicles in nontraffic accident

    X● **V39.00**   Driver of three-wheeled motor vehicle injured in collision with unspecified motor vehicles in nontraffic accident

    X● **V39.09**   Driver of three-wheeled motor vehicle injured in collision with other motor vehicles in nontraffic accident

● **V39.1**   Passenger in three-wheeled motor vehicle injured in collision with other and unspecified motor vehicles in nontraffic accident

    X● **V39.10**   Passenger in three-wheeled motor vehicle injured in collision with unspecified motor vehicles in nontraffic accident

    X● **V39.19**   Passenger in three-wheeled motor vehicle injured in collision with other motor vehicles in nontraffic accident

● **V39.2**   Unspecified occupant of three-wheeled motor vehicle injured in collision with other and unspecified motor vehicles in nontraffic accident

    X● **V39.20**   Unspecified occupant of three-wheeled motor vehicle injured in collision with unspecified motor vehicles in nontraffic accident
       Collision NOS involving three-wheeled motor vehicle, nontraffic

    X● **V39.29**   Unspecified occupant of three-wheeled motor vehicle injured in collision with other motor vehicles in nontraffic accident

X● **V39.3**   Occupant (driver) (passenger) of three-wheeled motor vehicle injured in unspecified nontraffic accident
       Accident NOS involving three-wheeled motor vehicle, nontraffic
       Occupant of three-wheeled motor vehicle injured in nontraffic accident NOS

● **V39.4**   Driver of three-wheeled motor vehicle injured in collision with other and unspecified motor vehicles in traffic accident

    X● **V39.40**   Driver of three-wheeled motor vehicle injured in collision with unspecified motor vehicles in traffic accident

    X● **V39.49**   Driver of three-wheeled motor vehicle injured in collision with other motor vehicles in traffic accident

● **V39.5**   Passenger in three-wheeled motor vehicle injured in collision with other and unspecified motor vehicles in traffic accident

    X● **V39.50**   Passenger in three-wheeled motor vehicle injured in collision with unspecified motor vehicles in traffic accident

    X● **V39.59**   Passenger in three-wheeled motor vehicle injured in collision with other motor vehicles in traffic accident

● **V39.6**   Unspecified occupant of three-wheeled motor vehicle injured in collision with other and unspecified motor vehicles in traffic accident

    X● **V39.60**   Unspecified occupant of three-wheeled motor vehicle injured in collision with unspecified motor vehicles in traffic accident
       Collision NOS involving three-wheeled motor vehicle (traffic)

    X● **V39.69**   Unspecified occupant of three-wheeled motor vehicle injured in collision with other motor vehicles in traffic accident

● **V39.8**   Occupant (driver) (passenger) of three-wheeled motor vehicle injured in other specified transport accidents

    X● **V39.81**   Occupant (driver) (passenger) of three-wheeled motor vehicle injured in transport accident with military vehicle

    X● **V39.89**   Occupant (driver) (passenger) of three-wheeled motor vehicle injured in other specified transport accidents

X● **V39.9**   Occupant (driver) (passenger) of three-wheeled motor vehicle injured in unspecified traffic accident
       Accident NOS involving three-wheeled motor vehicle

CAR OCCUPANT INJURED IN TRANSPORT ACCIDENT (V40-V49)

    Includes   a four-wheeled motor vehicle designed primarily for carrying passengers
              automobile (pulling a trailer or camper)

    Excludes1   bus (V50-V59)
               minibus (V50-V59)
               minivan (V50-V59)
               motorcoach (V70-V79)
               pick-up truck (V50-V59)
               sport utility vehicle (SUV) (V50-V59)

● **V40**   **Car occupant injured in collision with pedestrian or animal**

    Excludes1   car collision with animal-drawn vehicle or animal being ridden (V46.-)

    The appropriate 7th character is to be added to each code from category V40

> A   initial encounter
> D   subsequent encounter
> S   sequela

X● **V40.0**   Car driver injured in collision with pedestrian or animal in nontraffic accident

X● **V40.1**   Car passenger injured in collision with pedestrian or animal in nontraffic accident

N Newborn Age: 0   **P** Pediatric Age: 0–17   **M** Maternity DX: 9–64   **A** Adult Age: 15–124   ♀ Females Only   ♂ Males Only

  Complication\Comorbidity   Major C\C   (Ex:) CC/MCC Exclusions   Hospital-Acquired Condition   Hierarchical Condition Category

1547

X ● **V40.2** Person on outside of car injured in collision with pedestrian or animal in nontraffic accident

X ● **V40.3** Unspecified car occupant injured in collision with pedestrian or animal in nontraffic accident

X ● **V40.4** Person boarding or alighting a car injured in collision with pedestrian or animal

X ● **V40.5** Car driver injured in collision with pedestrian or animal in traffic accident

X ● **V40.6** Car passenger injured in collision with pedestrian or animal in traffic accident

X ● **V40.7** Person on outside of car injured in collision with pedestrian or animal in traffic accident

X ● **V40.9** Unspecified car occupant injured in collision with pedestrian or animal in traffic accident

● **V41** Car occupant injured in collision with pedal cycle

The appropriate 7th character is to be added to each code from category V41

A	initial encounter
D	subsequent encounter
S	sequela

X ● **V41.0** Car driver injured in collision with pedal cycle in nontraffic accident

X ● **V41.1** Car passenger injured in collision with pedal cycle in nontraffic accident

X ● **V41.2** Person on outside of car injured in collision with pedal cycle in nontraffic accident

X ● **V41.3** Unspecified car occupant injured in collision with pedal cycle in nontraffic accident

X ● **V41.4** Person boarding or alighting a car injured in collision with pedal cycle

X ● **V41.5** Car driver injured in collision with pedal cycle in traffic accident

X ● **V41.6** Car passenger injured in collision with pedal cycle in traffic accident

X ● **V41.7** Person on outside of car injured in collision with pedal cycle in traffic accident

X ● **V41.9** Unspecified car occupant injured in collision with pedal cycle in traffic accident

● **V42** Car occupant injured in collision with two- or three-wheeled motor vehicle

The appropriate 7th character is to be added to each code from category V42

A	initial encounter
D	subsequent encounter
S	sequela

X ● **V42.0** Car driver injured in collision with two- or three-wheeled motor vehicle in nontraffic accident

X ● **V42.1** Car passenger injured in collision with two- or three-wheeled motor vehicle in nontraffic accident

X ● **V42.2** Person on outside of car injured in collision with two- or three-wheeled motor vehicle in nontraffic accident

X ● **V42.3** Unspecified car occupant injured in collision with two- or three-wheeled motor vehicle in nontraffic accident

X ● **V42.4** Person boarding or alighting a car injured in collision with two- or three-wheeled motor vehicle

X ● **V42.5** Car driver injured in collision with two- or three-wheeled motor vehicle in traffic accident

X ● **V42.6** Car passenger injured in collision with two- or three-wheeled motor vehicle in traffic accident

X ● **V42.7** Person on outside of car injured in collision with two- or three-wheeled motor vehicle in traffic accident

X ● **V42.9** Unspecified car occupant injured in collision with two- or three-wheeled motor vehicle in traffic accident

● **V43** Car occupant injured in collision with car, pick-up truck or van

The appropriate 7th character is to be added to each code from category V43

A	initial encounter
D	subsequent encounter
S	sequela

● **V43.0** Car driver injured in collision with car, pick-up truck or van in nontraffic accident

X ● **V43.01** Car driver injured in collision with sport utility vehicle in nontraffic accident

X ● **V43.02** Car driver injured in collision with other type car in nontraffic accident

X ● **V43.03** Car driver injured in collision with pick-up truck in nontraffic accident

X ● **V43.04** Car driver injured in collision with van in nontraffic accident

● **V43.1** Car passenger injured in collision with car, pick-up truck or van in nontraffic accident

X ● **V43.11** Car passenger injured in collision with sport utility vehicle in nontraffic accident

X ● **V43.12** Car passenger injured in collision with other type car in nontraffic accident

X ● **V43.13** Car passenger injured in collision with pick-up truck in nontraffic accident

X ● **V43.14** Car passenger injured in collision with van in nontraffic accident

● **V43.2** Person on outside of car injured in collision with car, pick-up truck or van in nontraffic accident

X ● **V43.21** Person on outside of car injured in collision with sport utility vehicle in nontraffic accident

X ● **V43.22** Person on outside of car injured in collision with other type car in nontraffic accident

X ● **V43.23** Person on outside of car injured in collision with pick-up truck in nontraffic accident

X ● **V43.24** Person on outside of car injured in collision with van in nontraffic accident

● **V43.3** Unspecified car occupant injured in collision with car, pick-up truck or van in nontraffic accident

X ● **V43.31** Unspecified car occupant injured in collision with sport utility vehicle in nontraffic accident

X ● **V43.32** Unspecified car occupant injured in collision with other type car in nontraffic accident

X ● **V43.33** Unspecified car occupant injured in collision with pick-up truck in nontraffic accident

X ● **V43.34** Unspecified car occupant injured in collision with van in nontraffic accident

● **V43.4** Person boarding or alighting a car injured in collision with car, pick-up truck or van

X ● **V43.41** Person boarding or alighting a car injured in collision with sport utility vehicle

X ● **V43.42** Person boarding or alighting a car injured in collision with other type car

X ● **V43.43** Person boarding or alighting a car injured in collision with pick-up truck

X ● **V43.44** Person boarding or alighting a car injured in collision with van

● **V43.5** Car driver injured in collision with car, pick-up truck or van in traffic accident

X ● **V43.51** Car driver injured in collision with sport utility vehicle in traffic accident

X ● **V43.52** Car driver injured in collision with other type car in traffic accident

X ● **V43.53** Car driver injured in collision with pick-up truck in traffic accident

X ● **V43.54** Car driver injured in collision with van in traffic accident

▶ New   ⇒ Revised   ~~deleted~~ Deleted   Excludes 1   Excludes 2   Includes   Use additional   Code first   Code also   Key words

OGCR Official Guidelines   ● Unacceptable Principal Diagnosis   X Assign placeholder X   ● Use Additional Character(s)   ▷ Manifestation Code   **Coding Clinic**

● V43.6   Car passenger injured in collision with car, pick-up truck or van in traffic accident

X● V43.61   Car passenger injured in collision with sport utility vehicle in traffic accident
Coding Clinic: 2015, Q1, P5-7

X● V43.62   Car passenger injured in collision with other type car in traffic accident

X● V43.63   Car passenger injured in collision with pick-up truck in traffic accident

X● V43.64   Car passenger injured in collision with van in traffic accident

● V43.7   Person on outside of car injured in collision with car, pick-up truck or van in traffic accident

X● V43.71   Person on outside of car injured in collision with sport utility vehicle in traffic accident

X● V43.72   Person on outside of car injured in collision with other type car in traffic accident

X● V43.73   Person on outside of car injured in collision with pick-up truck in traffic accident

X● V43.74   Person on outside of car injured in collision with van in traffic accident

● V43.9   Unspecified car occupant injured in collision with car, pick-up truck or van in traffic accident

X● V43.91   Unspecified car occupant injured in collision with sport utility vehicle in traffic accident

X● V43.92   Unspecified car occupant injured in collision with other type car in traffic accident

X● V43.93   Unspecified car occupant injured in collision with pick-up truck in traffic accident

X● V43.94   Unspecified car occupant injured in collision with van in traffic accident

● V44   Car occupant injured in collision with heavy transport vehicle or bus

Excludes1   car occupant injured in collision with military vehicle (V49.81)

The appropriate 7th character is to be added to each code from category V44

A   initial encounter
D   subsequent encounter
S   sequela

X● V44.0   Car driver injured in collision with heavy transport vehicle or bus in nontraffic accident

X● V44.1   Car passenger injured in collision with heavy transport vehicle or bus in nontraffic accident

X● V44.2   Person on outside of car injured in collision with heavy transport vehicle or bus in nontraffic accident

X● V44.3   Unspecified car occupant injured in collision with heavy transport vehicle or bus in nontraffic accident

X● V44.4   Person boarding or alighting a car injured in collision with heavy transport vehicle or bus

X● V44.5   Car driver injured in collision with heavy transport vehicle or bus in traffic accident

X● V44.6   Car passenger injured in collision with heavy transport vehicle or bus in traffic accident

X● V44.7   Person on outside of car injured in collision with heavy transport vehicle or bus in traffic accident

X● V44.9   Unspecified car occupant injured in collision with heavy transport vehicle or bus in traffic accident

● V45   Car occupant injured in collision with railway train or railway vehicle

The appropriate 7th character is to be added to each code from category V45

A   initial encounter
D   subsequent encounter
S   sequela

X● V45.0   Car driver injured in collision with railway train or railway vehicle in nontraffic accident

X● V45.1   Car passenger injured in collision with railway train or railway vehicle in nontraffic accident

X● V45.2   Person on outside of car injured in collision with railway train or railway vehicle in nontraffic accident

X● V45.3   Unspecified car occupant injured in collision with railway train or railway vehicle in nontraffic accident

X● V45.4   Person boarding or alighting a car injured in collision with railway train or railway vehicle

X● V45.5   Car driver injured in collision with railway train or railway vehicle in traffic accident

X● V45.6   Car passenger injured in collision with railway train or railway vehicle in traffic accident

X● V45.7   Person on outside of car injured in collision with railway train or railway vehicle in traffic accident

X● V45.9   Unspecified car occupant injured in collision with railway train or railway vehicle in traffic accident

● V46   Car occupant injured in collision with other nonmotor vehicle

Includes   collision with animal-drawn vehicle, animal being ridden, streetcar

The appropriate 7th character is to be added to each code from category V46

A   initial encounter
D   subsequent encounter
S   sequela

X● V46.0   Car driver injured in collision with other nonmotor vehicle in nontraffic accident

X● V46.1   Car passenger injured in collision with other nonmotor vehicle in nontraffic accident

X● V46.2   Person on outside of car injured in collision with other nonmotor vehicle in nontraffic accident

X● V46.3   Unspecified car occupant injured in collision with other nonmotor vehicle in nontraffic accident

X● V46.4   Person boarding or alighting a car injured in collision with other nonmotor vehicle

X● V46.5   Car driver injured in collision with other nonmotor vehicle in traffic accident

X● V46.6   Car passenger injured in collision with other nonmotor vehicle in traffic accident

X● V46.7   Person on outside of car injured in collision with other nonmotor vehicle in traffic accident

X● V46.9   Unspecified car occupant injured in collision with other nonmotor vehicle in traffic accident

● V47   Car occupant injured in collision with fixed or stationary object

The appropriate 7th character is to be added to each code from category V47

A   initial encounter
D   subsequent encounter
S   sequela

Coding Clinic: 2016, Q4, P73

X● V47.0   Car driver injured in collision with fixed or stationary object in nontraffic accident

X● V47.1   Car passenger injured in collision with fixed or stationary object in nontraffic accident

X● V47.2   Person on outside of car injured in collision with fixed or stationary object in nontraffic accident

X● V47.3   Unspecified car occupant injured in collision with fixed or stationary object in nontraffic accident

X● V47.4   Person boarding or alighting a car injured in collision with fixed or stationary object

X● V47.5   Car driver injured in collision with fixed or stationary object in traffic accident

X● V47.6   Car passenger injured in collision with fixed or stationary object in traffic accident

X● V47.7   Person on outside of car injured in collision with fixed or stationary object in traffic accident

X● V47.9   Unspecified car occupant injured in collision with fixed or stationary object in traffic accident

CHAPTER 20 (V00-Y99)

● **V48**   **Car occupant injured in noncollision transport accident**

     Includes   overturning car NOS
                    overturning car without collision

     The appropriate 7th character is to be added to each code from category V48

A	initial encounter
D	subsequent encounter
S	sequela

X● **V48.0**   Car driver injured in noncollision transport accident in nontraffic accident

X● **V48.1**   Car passenger injured in noncollision transport accident in nontraffic accident

X● **V48.2**   Person on outside of car injured in noncollision transport accident in nontraffic accident

X● **V48.3**   Unspecified car occupant injured in noncollision transport accident in nontraffic accident

X● **V48.4**   Person boarding or alighting a car injured in noncollision transport accident

X● **V48.5**   Car driver injured in noncollision transport accident in traffic accident

X● **V48.6**   Car passenger injured in noncollision transport accident in traffic accident

X● **V48.7**   Person on outside of car injured in noncollision transport accident in traffic accident

X● **V48.9**   Unspecified car occupant injured in noncollision transport accident in traffic accident

● **V49**   **Car occupant injured in other and unspecified transport accidents**

     The appropriate 7th character is to be added to each code from category V49

A	initial encounter
D	subsequent encounter
S	sequela

● **V49.0**   Driver injured in collision with other and unspecified motor vehicles in nontraffic accident

     X● **V49.00**   Driver injured in collision with unspecified motor vehicles in nontraffic accident

     X● **V49.09**   Driver injured in collision with other motor vehicles in nontraffic accident

● **V49.1**   Passenger injured in collision with other and unspecified motor vehicles in nontraffic accident

     X● **V49.10**   Passenger injured in collision with unspecified motor vehicles in nontraffic accident

     X● **V49.19**   Passenger injured in collision with other motor vehicles in nontraffic accident

● **V49.2**   Unspecified car occupant injured in collision with other and unspecified motor vehicles in nontraffic accident

     X● **V49.20**   Unspecified car occupant injured in collision with unspecified motor vehicles in nontraffic accident
          Car collision NOS, nontraffic

     X● **V49.29**   Unspecified car occupant injured in collision with other motor vehicles in nontraffic accident

X● **V49.3**   Car occupant (driver) (passenger) injured in unspecified nontraffic accident
      Car accident NOS, nontraffic
      Car occupant injured in nontraffic accident NOS

● **V49.4**   Driver injured in collision with other and unspecified motor vehicles in traffic accident

     X● **V49.40**   Driver injured in collision with unspecified motor vehicles in traffic accident

     X● **V49.49**   Driver injured in collision with other motor vehicles in traffic accident

● **V49.5**   Passenger injured in collision with other and unspecified motor vehicles in traffic accident

     X● **V49.50**   Passenger injured in collision with unspecified motor vehicles in traffic accident

     X● **V49.59**   Passenger injured in collision with other motor vehicles in traffic accident

● **V49.6**   Unspecified car occupant injured in collision with other and unspecified motor vehicles in traffic accident

     X● **V49.60**   Unspecified car occupant injured in collision with unspecified motor vehicles in traffic accident
          Car collision NOS (traffic)

     X● **V49.69**   Unspecified car occupant injured in collision with other motor vehicles in traffic accident

● **V49.8**   Car occupant (driver) (passenger) injured in other specified transport accidents

     X● **V49.81**   Car occupant (driver) (passenger) injured in transport accident with military vehicle

     X● **V49.88**   Car occupant (driver) (passenger) injured in other specified transport accidents

X● **V49.9**   Car occupant (driver) (passenger) injured in unspecified traffic accident
      Car accident NOS
      Coding Clinic: 2015, Q1, P11

OCCUPANT OF PICK-UP TRUCK OR VAN INJURED IN TRANSPORT ACCIDENT (V50-V59)

     Includes   a four- or six-wheel motor vehicle designed primarily for carrying passengers and property but weighing less than the local limit for classification as a heavy goods vehicle
                  minibus
                  minivan
                  sport utility vehicle (SUV)
                  truck
                  van

     Excludes 1   heavy transport vehicle (V60-V69)

● **V50**   **Occupant of pick-up truck or van injured in collision with pedestrian or animal**

     Excludes 1   pick-up truck or van collision with animal-drawn vehicle or animal being ridden (V56.-)

     The appropriate 7th character is to be added to each code from category V50

A	initial encounter
D	subsequent encounter
S	sequela

X● **V50.0**   Driver of pick-up truck or van injured in collision with pedestrian or animal in nontraffic accident

X● **V50.1**   Passenger in pick-up truck or van injured in collision with pedestrian or animal in nontraffic accident

X● **V50.2**   Person on outside of pick-up truck or van injured in collision with pedestrian or animal in nontraffic accident

X● **V50.3**   Unspecified occupant of pick-up truck or van injured in collision with pedestrian or animal in nontraffic accident

X● **V50.4**   Person boarding or alighting a pick-up truck or van injured in collision with pedestrian or animal

X● **V50.5**   Driver of pick-up truck or van injured in collision with pedestrian or animal in traffic accident

X● **V50.6**   Passenger in pick-up truck or van injured in collision with pedestrian or animal in traffic accident

X● **V50.7**   Person on outside of pick-up truck or van injured in collision with pedestrian or animal in traffic accident

X● **V50.9**   Unspecified occupant of pick-up truck or van injured in collision with pedestrian or animal in traffic accident

---

► New   ⇒ Revised   ~~deleted~~ Deleted   Excludes 1   Excludes 2   Includes   Use additional   Code first   Code also   Key words

OGCR Official Guidelines   ● Unacceptable Principal Diagnosis   X Assign placeholder X   ● Use Additional Character(s)   ⟩ Manifestation Code   Coding Clinic

● **V51**   **Occupant of pick-up truck or van injured in collision with pedal cycle**

The appropriate 7th character is to be added to each code from category V51

A	initial encounter
D	subsequent encounter
S	sequela

X● **V51.0**   Driver of pick-up truck or van injured in collision with pedal cycle in nontraffic accident

X● **V51.1**   Passenger in pick-up truck or van injured in collision with pedal cycle in nontraffic accident

X● **V51.2**   Person on outside of pick-up truck or van injured in collision with pedal cycle in nontraffic accident

X● **V51.3**   Unspecified occupant of pick-up truck or van injured in collision with pedal cycle in nontraffic accident

X● **V51.4**   Person boarding or alighting a pick-up truck or van injured in collision with pedal cycle

X● **V51.5**   Driver of pick-up truck or van injured in collision with pedal cycle in traffic accident

X● **V51.6**   Passenger in pick-up truck or van injured in collision with pedal cycle in traffic accident

X● **V51.7**   Person on outside of pick-up truck or van injured in collision with pedal cycle in traffic accident

X● **V51.9**   Unspecified occupant of pick-up truck or van injured in collision with pedal cycle in traffic accident

● **V52**   **Occupant of pick-up truck or van injured in collision with two- or three-wheeled motor vehicle**

The appropriate 7th character is to be added to each code from category V52

A	initial encounter
D	subsequent encounter
S	sequela

X● **V52.0**   Driver of pick-up truck or van injured in collision with two- or three-wheeled motor vehicle in nontraffic accident

X● **V52.1**   Passenger in pick-up truck or van injured in collision with two- or three-wheeled motor vehicle in nontraffic accident

X● **V52.2**   Person on outside of pick-up truck or van injured in collision with two- or three-wheeled motor vehicle in nontraffic accident

X● **V52.3**   Unspecified occupant of pick-up truck or van injured in collision with two- or three-wheeled motor vehicle in nontraffic accident

X● **V52.4**   Person boarding or alighting a pick-up truck or van injured in collision with two- or three-wheeled motor vehicle

X● **V52.5**   Driver of pick-up truck or van injured in collision with two- or three-wheeled motor vehicle in traffic accident

X● **V52.6**   Passenger in pick-up truck or van injured in collision with two- or three-wheeled motor vehicle in traffic accident

X● **V52.7**   Person on outside of pick-up truck or van injured in collision with two- or three-wheeled motor vehicle in traffic accident

X● **V52.9**   Unspecified occupant of pick-up truck or van injured in collision with two- or three-wheeled motor vehicle in traffic accident

● **V53**   **Occupant of pick-up truck or van injured in collision with car, pick-up truck or van**

The appropriate 7th character is to be added to each code from category V53

A	initial encounter
D	subsequent encounter
S	sequela

X● **V53.0**   Driver of pick-up truck or van injured in collision with car, pick-up truck or van in nontraffic accident

X● **V53.1**   Passenger in pick-up truck or van injured in collision with car, pick-up truck or van in nontraffic accident

X● **V53.2**   Person on outside of pick-up truck or van injured in collision with car, pick-up truck or van in nontraffic accident

X● **V53.3**   Unspecified occupant of pick-up truck or van injured in collision with car, pick-up truck or van in nontraffic accident

X● **V53.4**   Person boarding or alighting a pick-up truck or van injured in collision with car, pick-up truck or van

X● **V53.5**   Driver of pick-up truck or van injured in collision with car, pick-up truck or van in traffic accident

X● **V53.6**   Passenger in pick-up truck or van injured in collision with car, pick-up truck or van in traffic accident

X● **V53.7**   Person on outside of pick-up truck or van injured in collision with car, pick-up truck or van in traffic accident

X● **V53.9**   Unspecified occupant of pick-up truck or van injured in collision with car, pick-up truck or van in traffic accident

● **V54**   **Occupant of pick-up truck or van injured in collision with heavy transport vehicle or bus**

    Excludes 1   occupant of pick-up truck or van injured in collision with military vehicle (V59.81)

The appropriate 7th character is to be added to each code from category V54

A	initial encounter
D	subsequent encounter
S	sequela

X● **V54.0**   Driver of pick-up truck or van injured in collision with heavy transport vehicle or bus in nontraffic accident

X● **V54.1**   Passenger in pick-up truck or van injured in collision with heavy transport vehicle or bus in nontraffic accident

X● **V54.2**   Person on outside of pick-up truck or van injured in collision with heavy transport vehicle or bus in nontraffic accident

X● **V54.3**   Unspecified occupant of pick-up truck or van injured in collision with heavy transport vehicle or bus in nontraffic accident

X● **V54.4**   Person boarding or alighting a pick-up truck or van injured in collision with heavy transport vehicle or bus

X● **V54.5**   Driver of pick-up truck or van injured in collision with heavy transport vehicle or bus in traffic accident

X● **V54.6**   Passenger in pick-up truck or van injured in collision with heavy transport vehicle or bus in traffic accident

X● **V54.7**   Person on outside of pick-up truck or van injured in collision with heavy transport vehicle or bus in traffic accident

X● **V54.9**   Unspecified occupant of pick-up truck or van injured in collision with heavy transport vehicle or bus in traffic accident

N Newborn Age: 0   **P** Pediatric Age: 0–17   **M** Maternity DX: 9–64   **A** Adult Age: 15–124   ♀ Females Only   ♂ Males Only

🔹 Complication\Comorbidity   🔹 Major C\C   (Ex) CC/MCC Exclusions   🔹 Hospital-Acquired Condition   🔹 Hierarchical Condition Category   **1551**

● **V55**   **Occupant of pick-up truck or van injured in collision with railway train or railway vehicle**

The appropriate 7th character is to be added to each code from category V55

A	initial encounter
D	subsequent encounter
S	sequela

X● **V55.0**   Driver of pick-up truck or van injured in collision with railway train or railway vehicle in nontraffic accident

X● **V55.1**   Passenger in pick-up truck or van injured in collision with railway train or railway vehicle in nontraffic accident

X● **V55.2**   Person on outside of pick-up truck or van injured in collision with railway train or railway vehicle in nontraffic accident

X● **V55.3**   Unspecified occupant of pick-up truck or van injured in collision with railway train or railway vehicle in nontraffic accident

X● **V55.4**   Person boarding or alighting a pick-up truck or van injured in collision with railway train or railway vehicle

X● **V55.5**   Driver of pick-up truck or van injured in collision with railway train or railway vehicle in traffic accident

X● **V55.6**   Passenger in pick-up truck or van injured in collision with railway train or railway vehicle in traffic accident

X● **V55.7**   Person on outside of pick-up truck or van injured in collision with railway train or railway vehicle in traffic accident

X● **V55.9**   Unspecified occupant of pick-up truck or van injured in collision with railway train or railway vehicle in traffic accident

● **V56**   **Occupant of pick-up truck or van injured in collision with other nonmotor vehicle**

     Includes   collision with animal-drawn vehicle, animal being ridden, streetcar

The appropriate 7th character is to be added to each code from category V56

A	initial encounter
D	subsequent encounter
S	sequela

X● **V56.0**   Driver of pick-up truck or van injured in collision with other nonmotor vehicle in nontraffic accident

X● **V56.1**   Passenger in pick-up truck or van injured in collision with other nonmotor vehicle in nontraffic accident

X● **V56.2**   Person on outside of pick-up truck or van injured in collision with other nonmotor vehicle in nontraffic accident

X● **V56.3**   Unspecified occupant of pick-up truck or van injured in collision with other nonmotor vehicle in nontraffic accident

X● **V56.4**   Person boarding or alighting a pick-up truck or van injured in collision with other nonmotor vehicle

X● **V56.5**   Driver of pick-up truck or van injured in collision with other nonmotor vehicle in traffic accident

X● **V56.6**   Passenger in pick-up truck or van injured in collision with other nonmotor vehicle in traffic accident

X● **V56.7**   Person on outside of pick-up truck or van injured in collision with other nonmotor vehicle in traffic accident

X● **V56.9**   Unspecified occupant of pick-up truck or van injured in collision with other nonmotor vehicle in traffic accident

● **V57**   **Occupant of pick-up truck or van injured in collision with fixed or stationary object**

The appropriate 7th character is to be added to each code from category V57

A	initial encounter
D	subsequent encounter
S	sequela

X● **V57.0**   Driver of pick-up truck or van injured in collision with fixed or stationary object in nontraffic accident

X● **V57.1**   Passenger in pick-up truck or van injured in collision with fixed or stationary object in nontraffic accident

X● **V57.2**   Person on outside of pick-up truck or van injured in collision with fixed or stationary object in nontraffic accident

X● **V57.3**   Unspecified occupant of pick-up truck or van injured in collision with fixed or stationary object in nontraffic accident

X● **V57.4**   Person boarding or alighting a pick-up truck or van injured in collision with fixed or stationary object

X● **V57.5**   Driver of pick-up truck or van injured in collision with fixed or stationary object in traffic accident

X● **V57.6**   Passenger in pick-up truck or van injured in collision with fixed or stationary object in traffic accident

X● **V57.7**   Person on outside of pick-up truck or van injured in collision with fixed or stationary object in traffic accident

X● **V57.9**   Unspecified occupant of pick-up truck or van injured in collision with fixed or stationary object in traffic accident

● **V58**   **Occupant of pick-up truck or van injured in noncollision transport accident**

     Includes   overturning pick-up truck or van NOS
                overturning pick-up truck or van without collision

The appropriate 7th character is to be added to each code from category V58

A	initial encounter
D	subsequent encounter
S	sequela

X● **V58.0**   Driver of pick-up truck or van injured in noncollision transport accident in nontraffic accident

X● **V58.1**   Passenger in pick-up truck or van injured in noncollision transport accident in nontraffic accident

X● **V58.2**   Person on outside of pick-up truck or van injured in noncollision transport accident in nontraffic accident

X● **V58.3**   Unspecified occupant of pick-up truck or van injured in noncollision transport accident in nontraffic accident

X● **V58.4**   Person boarding or alighting a pick-up truck or van injured in noncollision transport accident

X● **V58.5**   Driver of pick-up truck or van injured in noncollision transport accident in traffic accident

X● **V58.6**   Passenger in pick-up truck or van injured in noncollision transport accident in traffic accident

X● **V58.7**   Person on outside of pick-up truck or van injured in noncollision transport accident in traffic accident

X● **V58.9**   Unspecified occupant of pick-up truck or van injured in noncollision transport accident in traffic accident

▶ New   ⇢ Revised   ~~deleted~~ Deleted   Excludes 1   Excludes 2   Includes   Use additional   Code first   Code also   Key words

1552   OGCR Official Guidelines   ● Unacceptable Principal Diagnosis   X Assign placeholder X   ● Use Additional Character(s)   ▶ Manifestation Code   **Coding Clinic**

● **V59** **Occupant of pick-up truck or van injured in other and unspecified transport accidents**

     The appropriate 7th character is to be added to each code from category V59

> A   initial encounter
> D   subsequent encounter
> S   sequela

● **V59.0** **Driver of pick-up truck or van injured in collision with other and unspecified motor vehicles in nontraffic accident**

   X● **V59.00** Driver of pick-up truck or van injured in collision with unspecified motor vehicles in nontraffic accident

   X● **V59.09** Driver of pick-up truck or van injured in collision with other motor vehicles in nontraffic accident

● **V59.1** **Passenger in pick-up truck or van injured in collision with other and unspecified motor vehicles in nontraffic accident**

   X● **V59.10** Passenger in pick-up truck or van injured in collision with unspecified motor vehicles in nontraffic accident

   X● **V59.19** Passenger in pick-up truck or van injured in collision with other motor vehicles in nontraffic accident

● **V59.2** **Unspecified occupant of pick-up truck or van injured in collision with other and unspecified motor vehicles in nontraffic accident**

   X● **V59.20** Unspecified occupant of pick-up truck or van injured in collision with unspecified motor vehicles in nontraffic accident

         Collision NOS involving pick-up truck or van, nontraffic

   X● **V59.29** Unspecified occupant of pick-up truck or van injured in collision with other motor vehicles in nontraffic accident

   X● **V59.3** Occupant (driver) (passenger) of pick-up truck or van injured in unspecified nontraffic accident

         Accident NOS involving pick-up truck or van, nontraffic

         Occupant of pick-up truck or van injured in nontraffic accident NOS

● **V59.4** **Driver of pick-up truck or van injured in collision with other and unspecified motor vehicles in traffic accident**

   X● **V59.40** Driver of pick-up truck or van injured in collision with unspecified motor vehicles in traffic accident

   X● **V59.49** Driver of pick-up truck or van injured in collision with other motor vehicles in traffic accident

● **V59.5** **Passenger in pick-up truck or van injured in collision with other and unspecified motor vehicles in traffic accident**

   X● **V59.50** Passenger in pick-up truck or van injured in collision with unspecified motor vehicles in traffic accident

   X● **V59.59** Passenger in pick-up truck or van injured in collision with other motor vehicles in traffic accident

● **V59.6** **Unspecified occupant of pick-up truck or van injured in collision with other and unspecified motor vehicles in traffic accident**

   X● **V59.60** Unspecified occupant of pick-up truck or van injured in collision with unspecified motor vehicles in traffic accident

         Collision NOS involving pick-up truck or van (traffic)

   X● **V59.69** Unspecified occupant of pick-up truck or van injured in collision with other motor vehicles in traffic accident

   X● **V59.8** Occupant (driver) (passenger) of pick-up truck or van injured in other specified transport accidents

   X● **V59.81** Occupant (driver) (passenger) of pick-up truck or van injured in transport accident with military vehicle

   X● **V59.88** Occupant (driver) (passenger) of pick-up truck or van injured in other specified transport accidents

   X● **V59.9** Occupant (driver) (passenger) of pick-up truck or van injured in unspecified traffic accident

         Accident NOS involving pick-up truck or van

OCCUPANT OF HEAVY TRANSPORT VEHICLE INJURED IN TRANSPORT ACCIDENT (V60-V69)

Includes	18 wheeler armored car panel truck
Excludes1	bus motorcoach

● **V60** **Occupant of heavy transport vehicle injured in collision with pedestrian or animal**

     Excludes1   heavy transport vehicle collision with animal-drawn vehicle or animal being ridden (V66.-)

     The appropriate 7th character is to be added to each code from category V60

> A   initial encounter
> D   subsequent encounter
> S   sequela

   X● **V60.0** Driver of heavy transport vehicle injured in collision with pedestrian or animal in nontraffic accident

   X● **V60.1** Passenger in heavy transport vehicle injured in collision with pedestrian or animal in nontraffic accident

   X● **V60.2** Person on outside of heavy transport vehicle injured in collision with pedestrian or animal in nontraffic accident

   X● **V60.3** Unspecified occupant of heavy transport vehicle injured in collision with pedestrian or animal in nontraffic accident

   X● **V60.4** Person boarding or alighting a heavy transport vehicle injured in collision with pedestrian or animal

   X● **V60.5** Driver of heavy transport vehicle injured in collision with pedestrian or animal in traffic accident

   X● **V60.6** Passenger in heavy transport vehicle injured in collision with pedestrian or animal in traffic accident

   X● **V60.7** Person on outside of heavy transport vehicle injured in collision with pedestrian or animal in traffic accident

   X● **V60.9** Unspecified occupant of heavy transport vehicle injured in collision with pedestrian or animal in traffic accident

● **V61** **Occupant of heavy transport vehicle injured in collision with pedal cycle**

     The appropriate 7th character is to be added to each code from category V61

> A   initial encounter
> D   subsequent encounter
> S   sequela

   X● **V61.0** Driver of heavy transport vehicle injured in collision with pedal cycle in nontraffic accident

   X● **V61.1** Passenger in heavy transport vehicle injured in collision with pedal cycle in nontraffic accident

   X● **V61.2** Person on outside of heavy transport vehicle injured in collision with pedal cycle in nontraffic accident

   X● **V61.3** Unspecified occupant of heavy transport vehicle injured in collision with pedal cycle in nontraffic accident

   X● **V61.4** Person boarding or alighting a heavy transport vehicle injured in collision with pedal cycle while boarding or alighting

   X● **V61.5** Driver of heavy transport vehicle injured in collision with pedal cycle in traffic accident

N Newborn Age: 0   **P** Pediatric Age: 0–17   **M** Maternity DX: 9–64   **A** Adult Age: 15–124   ♀ Females Only   ♂ Males Only

Complication\Comorbidity   Major C\C   (Ex) CC/MCC Exclusions   Hospital-Acquired Condition   Hierarchical Condition Category

1553

X● **V61.6** Passenger in heavy transport vehicle injured in collision with pedal cycle in traffic accident

X● **V61.7** Person on outside of heavy transport vehicle injured in collision with pedal cycle in traffic accident

X● **V61.9** Unspecified occupant of heavy transport vehicle injured in collision with pedal cycle in traffic accident

● **V62** Occupant of heavy transport vehicle injured in collision with two- or three-wheeled motor vehicle

The appropriate 7th character is to be added to each code from category V62

> A initial encounter
> D subsequent encounter
> S sequela

X● **V62.0** Driver of heavy transport vehicle injured in collision with two- or three-wheeled motor vehicle in nontraffic accident

X● **V62.1** Passenger in heavy transport vehicle injured in collision with two- or three-wheeled motor vehicle in nontraffic accident

X● **V62.2** Person on outside of heavy transport vehicle injured in collision with two- or three-wheeled motor vehicle in nontraffic accident

X● **V62.3** Unspecified occupant of heavy transport vehicle injured in collision with two- or three-wheeled motor vehicle in nontraffic accident

X● **V62.4** Person boarding or alighting a heavy transport vehicle injured in collision with two- or three-wheeled motor vehicle

X● **V62.5** Driver of heavy transport vehicle injured in collision with two- or three-wheeled motor vehicle in traffic accident

X● **V62.6** Passenger in heavy transport vehicle injured in collision with two- or three-wheeled motor vehicle in traffic accident

X● **V62.7** Person on outside of heavy transport vehicle injured in collision with two- or three-wheeled motor vehicle in traffic accident

X● **V62.9** Unspecified occupant of heavy transport vehicle injured in collision with two- or three-wheeled motor vehicle in traffic accident

● **V63** Occupant of heavy transport vehicle injured in collision with car, pick-up truck or van

The appropriate 7th character is to be added to each code from category V63

> A initial encounter
> D subsequent encounter
> S sequela

X● **V63.0** Driver of heavy transport vehicle injured in collision with car, pick-up truck or van in nontraffic accident

X● **V63.1** Passenger in heavy transport vehicle injured in collision with car, pick-up truck or van in nontraffic accident

X● **V63.2** Person on outside of heavy transport vehicle injured in collision with car, pick-up truck or van in nontraffic accident

X● **V63.3** Unspecified occupant of heavy transport vehicle injured in collision with car, pick-up truck or van in nontraffic accident

X● **V63.4** Person boarding or alighting a heavy transport vehicle injured in collision with car, pick-up truck or van

X● **V63.5** Driver of heavy transport vehicle injured in collision with car, pick-up truck or van in traffic accident

X● **V63.6** Passenger in heavy transport vehicle injured in collision with car, pick-up truck or van in traffic accident

X● **V63.7** Person on outside of heavy transport vehicle injured in collision with car, pick-up truck or van in traffic accident

X● **V63.9** Unspecified occupant of heavy transport vehicle injured in collision with car, pick-up truck or van in traffic accident

● **V64** Occupant of heavy transport vehicle injured in collision with heavy transport vehicle or bus

> **Excludes1** occupant of heavy transport vehicle injured in collision with military vehicle (V69.81)

The appropriate 7th character is to be added to each code from category V64

> A initial encounter
> D subsequent encounter
> S sequela

X● **V64.0** Driver of heavy transport vehicle injured in collision with heavy transport vehicle or bus in nontraffic accident

X● **V64.1** Passenger in heavy transport vehicle injured in collision with heavy transport vehicle or bus in nontraffic accident

X● **V64.2** Person on outside of heavy transport vehicle injured in collision with heavy transport vehicle or bus in nontraffic accident

X● **V64.3** Unspecified occupant of heavy transport vehicle injured in collision with heavy transport vehicle or bus in nontraffic accident

X● **V64.4** Person boarding or alighting a heavy transport vehicle injured in collision with heavy transport vehicle or bus while boarding or alighting

X● **V64.5** Driver of heavy transport vehicle injured in collision with heavy transport vehicle or bus in traffic accident

X● **V64.6** Passenger in heavy transport vehicle injured in collision with heavy transport vehicle or bus in traffic accident

X● **V64.7** Person on outside of heavy transport vehicle injured in collision with heavy transport vehicle or bus in traffic accident

X● **V64.9** Unspecified occupant of heavy transport vehicle injured in collision with heavy transport vehicle or bus in traffic accident

● **V65** Occupant of heavy transport vehicle injured in collision with railway train or railway vehicle

The appropriate 7th character is to be added to each code from category V65

> A initial encounter
> D subsequent encounter
> S sequela

X● **V65.0** Driver of heavy transport vehicle injured in collision with railway train or railway vehicle in nontraffic accident

X● **V65.1** Passenger in heavy transport vehicle injured in collision with railway train or railway vehicle in nontraffic accident

X● **V65.2** Person on outside of heavy transport vehicle injured in collision with railway train or railway vehicle in nontraffic accident

X● **V65.3** Unspecified occupant of heavy transport vehicle injured in collision with railway train or railway vehicle in nontraffic accident

X● **V65.4** Person boarding or alighting a heavy transport vehicle injured in collision with railway train or railway vehicle

X● **V65.5** Driver of heavy transport vehicle injured in collision with railway train or railway vehicle in traffic accident

X● **V65.6** Passenger in heavy transport vehicle injured in collision with railway train or railway vehicle in traffic accident

X● **V65.7** Person on outside of heavy transport vehicle injured in collision with railway train or railway vehicle in traffic accident

X● **V65.9** Unspecified occupant of heavy transport vehicle injured in collision with railway train or railway vehicle in traffic accident

▶ New ⮕ Revised ~~deleted~~ Deleted │ Excludes 1 │ Excludes 2 │ Includes │ Use additional │ Code first │ Code also │ Key words

OGCR Official Guidelines ● Unacceptable Principal Diagnosis X Assign placeholder X ● Use Additional Character(s) ▶ Manifestation Code **Coding Clinic**

● V66 Occupant of heavy transport vehicle injured in collision with other nonmotor vehicle

> **Includes**   collision with animal-drawn vehicle, animal being ridden, streetcar

The appropriate 7th character is to be added to each code from category V66

A	initial encounter
D	subsequent encounter
S	sequela

X● V66.0 Driver of heavy transport vehicle injured in collision with other nonmotor vehicle in nontraffic accident

X● V66.1 Passenger in heavy transport vehicle injured in collision with other nonmotor vehicle in nontraffic accident

X● V66.2 Person on outside of heavy transport vehicle injured in collision with other nonmotor vehicle in nontraffic accident

X● V66.3 Unspecified occupant of heavy transport vehicle injured in collision with other nonmotor vehicle in nontraffic accident

X● V66.4 Person boarding or alighting a heavy transport vehicle injured in collision with other nonmotor vehicle

X● V66.5 Driver of heavy transport vehicle injured in collision with other nonmotor vehicle in traffic accident

X● V66.6 Passenger in heavy transport vehicle injured in collision with other nonmotor vehicle in traffic accident

X● V66.7 Person on outside of heavy transport vehicle injured in collision with other nonmotor vehicle in traffic accident

X● V66.9 Unspecified occupant of heavy transport vehicle injured in collision with other nonmotor vehicle in traffic accident

● V67 Occupant of heavy transport vehicle injured in collision with fixed or stationary object

The appropriate 7th character is to be added to each code from category V67

A	initial encounter
D	subsequent encounter
S	sequela

X● V67.0 Driver of heavy transport vehicle injured in collision with fixed or stationary object in nontraffic accident

X● V67.1 Passenger in heavy transport vehicle injured in collision with fixed or stationary object in nontraffic accident

X● V67.2 Person on outside of heavy transport vehicle injured in collision with fixed or stationary object in nontraffic accident

X● V67.3 Unspecified occupant of heavy transport vehicle injured in collision with fixed or stationary object in nontraffic accident

X● V67.4 Person boarding or alighting a heavy transport vehicle injured in collision with fixed or stationary object

X● V67.5 Driver of heavy transport vehicle injured in collision with fixed or stationary object in traffic accident

X● V67.6 Passenger in heavy transport vehicle injured in collision with fixed or stationary object in traffic accident

X● V67.7 Person on outside of heavy transport vehicle injured in collision with fixed or stationary object in traffic accident

X● V67.9 Unspecified occupant of heavy transport vehicle injured in collision with fixed or stationary object in traffic accident

● V68 Occupant of heavy transport vehicle injured in noncollision transport accident

> **Includes**   overturning heavy transport vehicle NOS
> overturning heavy transport vehicle without collision

The appropriate 7th character is to be added to each code from category V68

A	initial encounter
D	subsequent encounter
S	sequela

X● V68.0 Driver of heavy transport vehicle injured in noncollision transport accident in nontraffic accident

X● V68.1 Passenger in heavy transport vehicle injured in noncollision transport accident in nontraffic accident

X● V68.2 Person on outside of heavy transport vehicle injured in noncollision transport accident in nontraffic accident

X● V68.3 Unspecified occupant of heavy transport vehicle injured in noncollision transport accident in nontraffic accident

X● V68.4 Person boarding or alighting a heavy transport vehicle injured in noncollision transport accident

X● V68.5 Driver of heavy transport vehicle injured in noncollision transport accident in traffic accident

X● V68.6 Passenger in heavy transport vehicle injured in noncollision transport accident in traffic accident

X● V68.7 Person on outside of heavy transport vehicle injured in noncollision transport accident in traffic accident

X● V68.9 Unspecified occupant of heavy transport vehicle injured in noncollision transport accident in traffic accident

● V69 Occupant of heavy transport vehicle injured in other and unspecified transport accidents

The appropriate 7th character is to be added to each code from category V69

A	initial encounter
D	subsequent encounter
S	sequela

● V69.0 Driver of heavy transport vehicle injured in collision with other and unspecified motor vehicles in nontraffic accident

    X● V69.00 Driver of heavy transport vehicle injured in collision with unspecified motor vehicles in nontraffic accident

    X● V69.09 Driver of heavy transport vehicle injured in collision with other motor vehicles in nontraffic accident

● V69.1 Passenger in heavy transport vehicle injured in collision with other and unspecified motor vehicles in nontraffic accident

    X● V69.10 Passenger in heavy transport vehicle injured in collision with unspecified motor vehicles in nontraffic accident

    X● V69.19 Passenger in heavy transport vehicle injured in collision with other motor vehicles in nontraffic accident

● V69.2 Unspecified occupant of heavy transport vehicle injured in collision with other and unspecified motor vehicles in nontraffic accident

    X● V69.20 Unspecified occupant of heavy transport vehicle injured in collision with unspecified motor vehicles in nontraffic accident
        Collision NOS involving heavy transport vehicle, nontraffic

    X● V69.29 Unspecified occupant of heavy transport vehicle injured in collision with other motor vehicles in nontraffic accident

CHAPTER 20 (V00-Y99)

X● **V69.3** Occupant (driver) (passenger) of heavy transport vehicle injured in unspecified nontraffic accident
     Accident NOS involving heavy transport vehicle, nontraffic
     Occupant of heavy transport vehicle injured in nontraffic accident NOS

● **V69.4** Driver of heavy transport vehicle injured in collision with other and unspecified motor vehicles in traffic accident

     X● **V69.40** Driver of heavy transport vehicle injured in collision with unspecified motor vehicles in traffic accident

     X● **V69.49** Driver of heavy transport vehicle injured in collision with other motor vehicles in traffic accident

● **V69.5** Passenger in heavy transport vehicle injured in collision with other and unspecified motor vehicles in traffic accident

     X● **V69.50** Passenger in heavy transport vehicle injured in collision with unspecified motor vehicles in traffic accident

     X● **V69.59** Passenger in heavy transport vehicle injured in collision with other motor vehicles in traffic accident

● **V69.6** Unspecified occupant of heavy transport vehicle injured in collision with other and unspecified motor vehicles in traffic accident

     X● **V69.60** Unspecified occupant of heavy transport vehicle injured in collision with unspecified motor vehicles in traffic accident
         Collision NOS involving heavy transport vehicle (traffic)

     X● **V69.69** Unspecified occupant of heavy transport vehicle injured in collision with other motor vehicles in traffic accident

● **V69.8** Occupant (driver) (passenger) of heavy transport vehicle injured in other specified transport accidents

     X● **V69.81** Occupant (driver) (passenger) of heavy transport vehicle injured in transport accidents with military vehicle

     X● **V69.88** Occupant (driver) (passenger) of heavy transport vehicle injured in other specified transport accidents

X● **V69.9** Occupant (driver) (passenger) of heavy transport vehicle injured in unspecified traffic accident
     Accident NOS involving heavy transport vehicle

BUS OCCUPANT INJURED IN TRANSPORT ACCIDENT (V70-V79)

Includes	motorcoach
Excludes1	minibus (V50-V59)

● **V70** Bus occupant injured in collision with pedestrian or animal

Excludes1	bus collision with animal-drawn vehicle or animal being ridden (V76.-)

The appropriate 7th character is to be added to each code from category V70

A	initial encounter
D	subsequent encounter
S	sequela

X● **V70.0** Driver of bus injured in collision with pedestrian or animal in nontraffic accident

X● **V70.1** Passenger on bus injured in collision with pedestrian or animal in nontraffic accident

X● **V70.2** Person on outside of bus injured in collision with pedestrian or animal in nontraffic accident

X● **V70.3** Unspecified occupant of bus injured in collision with pedestrian or animal in nontraffic accident

X● **V70.4** Person boarding or alighting from bus injured in collision with pedestrian or animal

X● **V70.5** Driver of bus injured in collision with pedestrian or animal in traffic accident

X● **V70.6** Passenger on bus injured in collision with pedestrian or animal in traffic accident

X● **V70.7** Person on outside of bus injured in collision with pedestrian or animal in traffic accident

X● **V70.9** Unspecified occupant of bus injured in collision with pedestrian or animal in traffic accident

● **V71** Bus occupant injured in collision with pedal cycle

The appropriate 7th character is to be added to each code from category V71

A	initial encounter
D	subsequent encounter
S	sequela

X● **V71.0** Driver of bus injured in collision with pedal cycle in nontraffic accident

X● **V71.1** Passenger on bus injured in collision with pedal cycle in nontraffic accident

X● **V71.2** Person on outside of bus injured in collision with pedal cycle in nontraffic accident

X● **V71.3** Unspecified occupant of bus injured in collision with pedal cycle in nontraffic accident

X● **V71.4** Person boarding or alighting from bus injured in collision with pedal cycle

X● **V71.5** Driver of bus injured in collision with pedal cycle in traffic accident

X● **V71.6** Passenger on bus injured in collision with pedal cycle in traffic accident

X● **V71.7** Person on outside of bus injured in collision with pedal cycle in traffic accident

X● **V71.9** Unspecified occupant of bus injured in collision with pedal cycle in traffic accident

● **V72** Bus occupant injured in collision with two- or three-wheeled motor vehicle

The appropriate 7th character is to be added to each code from category V72

A	initial encounter
D	subsequent encounter
S	sequela

X● **V72.0** Driver of bus injured in collision with two- or three-wheeled motor vehicle in nontraffic accident

X● **V72.1** Passenger on bus injured in collision with two- or three-wheeled motor vehicle in nontraffic accident

X● **V72.2** Person on outside of bus injured in collision with two- or three-wheeled motor vehicle in nontraffic accident

X● **V72.3** Unspecified occupant of bus injured in collision with two- or three-wheeled motor vehicle in nontraffic accident

X● **V72.4** Person boarding or alighting from bus injured in collision with two- or three-wheeled motor vehicle

X● **V72.5** Driver of bus injured in collision with two- or three-wheeled motor vehicle in traffic accident

X● **V72.6** Passenger on bus injured in collision with two- or three-wheeled motor vehicle in traffic accident

X● **V72.7** Person on outside of bus injured in collision with two- or three-wheeled motor vehicle in traffic accident

X● **V72.9** Unspecified occupant of bus injured in collision with two- or three-wheeled motor vehicle in traffic accident

▶ New   ⇥ Revised   ~~deleted~~ Deleted   Excludes 1   Excludes 2   Includes   Use additional   Code first   Code also   Key words

OGCR Official Guidelines   ● Unacceptable Principal Diagnosis   X Assign placeholder X   ● Use Additional Character(s)   ▶ Manifestation Code   **Coding Clinic**

● V73 **Bus occupant injured in collision with car, pick-up truck or van**

The appropriate 7th character is to be added to each code from category V73

> A   initial encounter
> D   subsequent encounter
> S   sequela

X ● **V73.0** Driver of bus injured in collision with car, pick-up truck or van in nontraffic accident

X ● **V73.1** Passenger on bus injured in collision with car, pick-up truck or van in nontraffic accident

X ● **V73.2** Person on outside of bus injured in collision with car, pick-up truck or van in nontraffic accident

X ● **V73.3** Unspecified occupant of bus injured in collision with car, pick-up truck or van in nontraffic accident

X ● **V73.4** Person boarding or alighting from bus injured in collision with car, pick-up truck or van

X ● **V73.5** Driver of bus injured in collision with car, pick-up truck or van in traffic accident

X ● **V73.6** Passenger on bus injured in collision with car, pick-up truck or van in traffic accident

X ● **V73.7** Person on outside of bus injured in collision with car, pick-up truck or van in traffic accident

X ● **V73.9** Unspecified occupant of bus injured in collision with car, pick-up truck or van in traffic accident

● V74 **Bus occupant injured in collision with heavy transport vehicle or bus**

Excludes1 bus occupant injured in collision with military vehicle (V79.81)

The appropriate 7th character is to be added to each code from category V74

> A   initial encounter
> D   subsequent encounter
> S   sequela

X ● **V74.0** Driver of bus injured in collision with heavy transport vehicle or bus in nontraffic accident

X ● **V74.1** Passenger on bus injured in collision with heavy transport vehicle or bus in nontraffic accident

X ● **V74.2** Person on outside of bus injured in collision with heavy transport vehicle or bus in nontraffic accident

X ● **V74.3** Unspecified occupant of bus injured in collision with heavy transport vehicle or bus in nontraffic accident

X ● **V74.4** Person boarding or alighting from bus injured in collision with heavy transport vehicle or bus

X ● **V74.5** Driver of bus injured in collision with heavy transport vehicle or bus in traffic accident

X ● **V74.6** Passenger on bus injured in collision with heavy transport vehicle or bus in traffic accident

X ● **V74.7** Person on outside of bus injured in collision with heavy transport vehicle or bus in traffic accident

X ● **V74.9** Unspecified occupant of bus injured in collision with heavy transport vehicle or bus in traffic accident

● V75 **Bus occupant injured in collision with railway train or railway vehicle**

The appropriate 7th character is to be added to each code from category V75

> A   initial encounter
> D   subsequent encounter
> S   sequela

X ● **V75.0** Driver of bus injured in collision with railway train or railway vehicle in nontraffic accident

X ● **V75.1** Passenger on bus injured in collision with railway train or railway vehicle in nontraffic accident

X ● **V75.2** Person on outside of bus injured in collision with railway train or railway vehicle in nontraffic accident

X ● **V75.3** Unspecified occupant of bus injured in collision with railway train or railway vehicle in nontraffic accident

X ● **V75.4** Person boarding or alighting from bus injured in collision with railway train or railway vehicle

X ● **V75.5** Driver of bus injured in collision with railway train or railway vehicle in traffic accident

X ● **V75.6** Passenger on bus injured in collision with railway train or railway vehicle in traffic accident

X ● **V75.7** Person on outside of bus injured in collision with railway train or railway vehicle in traffic accident

X ● **V75.9** Unspecified occupant of bus injured in collision with railway train or railway vehicle in traffic accident

● V76 **Bus occupant injured in collision with other nonmotor vehicle**

Includes collision with animal-drawn vehicle, animal being ridden, streetcar

The appropriate 7th character is to be added to each code from category V76

> A   initial encounter
> D   subsequent encounter
> S   sequela

X ● **V76.0** Driver of bus injured in collision with other nonmotor vehicle in nontraffic accident

X ● **V76.1** Passenger on bus injured in collision with other nonmotor vehicle in nontraffic accident

X ● **V76.2** Person on outside of bus injured in collision with other nonmotor vehicle in nontraffic accident

X ● **V76.3** Unspecified occupant of bus injured in collision with other nonmotor vehicle in nontraffic accident

X ● **V76.4** Person boarding or alighting from bus injured in collision with other nonmotor vehicle

X ● **V76.5** Driver of bus injured in collision with other nonmotor vehicle in traffic accident

X ● **V76.6** Passenger on bus injured in collision with other nonmotor vehicle in traffic accident

X ● **V76.7** Person on outside of bus injured in collision with other nonmotor vehicle in traffic accident

X ● **V76.9** Unspecified occupant of bus injured in collision with other nonmotor vehicle in traffic accident

● V77 **Bus occupant injured in collision with fixed or stationary object**

The appropriate 7th character is to be added to each code from category V77

> A   initial encounter
> D   subsequent encounter
> S   sequela

X ● **V77.0** Driver of bus injured in collision with fixed or stationary object in nontraffic accident

X ● **V77.1** Passenger on bus injured in collision with fixed or stationary object in nontraffic accident

X ● **V77.2** Person on outside of bus injured in collision with fixed or stationary object in nontraffic accident

X ● **V77.3** Unspecified occupant of bus injured in collision with fixed or stationary object in nontraffic accident

X ● **V77.4** Person boarding or alighting from bus injured in collision with fixed or stationary object

X ● **V77.5** Driver of bus injured in collision with fixed or stationary object in traffic accident

X ● **V77.6** Passenger on bus injured in collision with fixed or stationary object in traffic accident

X ● **V77.7** Person on outside of bus injured in collision with fixed or stationary object in traffic accident

X ● **V77.9** Unspecified occupant of bus injured in collision with fixed or stationary object in traffic accident

CHAPTER 20 (V00-Y99)

● **V78**   **Bus occupant injured in noncollision transport accident**

> **Includes**   overturning bus NOS
> overturning bus without collision

The appropriate 7th character is to be added to each code from category V78

> A   initial encounter
> D   subsequent encounter
> S   sequela

X● **V78.0**   Driver of bus injured in noncollision transport accident in nontraffic accident

X● **V78.1**   Passenger on bus injured in noncollision transport accident in nontraffic accident

X● **V78.2**   Person on outside of bus injured in noncollision transport accident in nontraffic accident

X● **V78.3**   Unspecified occupant of bus injured in noncollision transport accident in nontraffic accident

X● **V78.4**   Person boarding or alighting from bus injured in noncollision transport accident

X● **V78.5**   Driver of bus injured in noncollision transport accident in traffic accident

X● **V78.6**   Passenger on bus injured in noncollision transport accident in traffic accident

X● **V78.7**   Person on outside of bus injured in noncollision transport accident in traffic accident

X● **V78.9**   Unspecified occupant of bus injured in noncollision transport accident in traffic accident

● **V79**   **Bus occupant injured in other and unspecified transport accidents**

The appropriate 7th character is to be added to each code from category V79

> A   initial encounter
> D   subsequent encounter
> S   sequela

● **V79.0**   Driver of bus injured in collision with other and unspecified motor vehicles in nontraffic accident

X● **V79.00**   Driver of bus injured in collision with unspecified motor vehicles in nontraffic accident

X● **V79.09**   Driver of bus injured in collision with other motor vehicles in nontraffic accident

● **V79.1**   Passenger on bus injured in collision with other and unspecified motor vehicles in nontraffic accident

X● **V79.10**   Passenger on bus injured in collision with unspecified motor vehicles in nontraffic accident

X● **V79.19**   Passenger on bus injured in collision with other motor vehicles in nontraffic accident

● **V79.2**   Unspecified bus occupant injured in collision with other and unspecified motor vehicles in nontraffic accident

X● **V79.20**   Unspecified bus occupant injured in collision with unspecified motor vehicles in nontraffic accident
> Bus collision NOS, nontraffic

X● **V79.29**   Unspecified bus occupant injured in collision with other motor vehicles in nontraffic accident

X● **V79.3**   Bus occupant (driver) (passenger) injured in unspecified nontraffic accident
> Bus accident NOS, nontraffic
> Bus occupant injured in nontraffic accident NOS

● **V79.4**   Driver of bus injured in collision with other and unspecified motor vehicles in traffic accident

X● **V79.40**   Driver of bus injured in collision with unspecified motor vehicles in traffic accident

X● **V79.49**   Driver of bus injured in collision with other motor vehicles in traffic accident

● **V79.5**   Passenger on bus injured in collision with other and unspecified motor vehicles in traffic accident

X● **V79.50**   Passenger on bus injured in collision with unspecified motor vehicles in traffic accident

X● **V79.59**   Passenger on bus injured in collision with other motor vehicles in traffic accident

● **V79.6**   Unspecified bus occupant injured in collision with other and unspecified motor vehicles in traffic accident

X● **V79.60**   Unspecified bus occupant injured in collision with unspecified motor vehicles in traffic accident
> Bus collision NOS (traffic)

X● **V79.69**   Unspecified bus occupant injured in collision with other motor vehicles in traffic accident

● **V79.8**   Bus occupant (driver) (passenger) injured in other specified transport accidents

X● **V79.81**   Bus occupant (driver) (passenger) injured in transport accidents with military vehicle

X● **V79.88**   Bus occupant (driver) (passenger) injured in other specified transport accidents

X● **V79.9**   Bus occupant (driver) (passenger) injured in unspecified traffic accident
> Bus accident NOS

OTHER LAND TRANSPORT ACCIDENTS (V80-V89)

● **V80**   **Animal-rider or occupant of animal-drawn vehicle injured in transport accident**

The appropriate 7th character is to be added to each code from category V80

> A   initial encounter
> D   subsequent encounter
> S   sequela

● **V80.0**   Animal-rider or occupant of animal drawn vehicle injured by fall from or being thrown from animal or animal-drawn vehicle in noncollision accident

● **V80.01**   Animal-rider injured by fall from or being thrown from animal in noncollision accident

● **V80.010**   Animal-rider injured by fall from or being thrown from horse in noncollision accident

● **V80.018**   Animal-rider injured by fall from or being thrown from other animal in noncollision accident

X● **V80.02**   Occupant of animal-drawn vehicle injured by fall from or being thrown from animal-drawn vehicle in noncollision accident
> Overturning animal-drawn vehicle NOS
> Overturning animal-drawn vehicle without collision

● **V80.1**   Animal-rider or occupant of animal-drawn vehicle injured in collision with pedestrian or animal

> **Excludes1**   animal-rider or animal-drawn vehicle collision with animal-drawn vehicle or animal being ridden (V80.7)

X● **V80.11**   Animal-rider injured in collision with pedestrian or animal

X● **V80.12**   Occupant of animal-drawn vehicle injured in collision with pedestrian or animal

● **V80.2**   Animal-rider or occupant of animal-drawn vehicle injured in collision with pedal cycle

X● **V80.21**   Animal-rider injured in collision with pedal cycle

X● **V80.22**   Occupant of animal-drawn vehicle injured in collision with pedal cycle

▶ New   ⇒ Revised   ~~deleted~~ Deleted   Excludes 1   Excludes 2   Includes   Use additional   Code first   Code also   Key words
OGCR Official Guidelines   ● Unacceptable Principal Diagnosis   X Assign placeholder X   ● Use Additional Character(s)   ▶ Manifestation Code   Coding Clinic
1558

● **V80.3** Animal-rider or occupant of animal-drawn vehicle injured in collision with two- or three-wheeled motor vehicle

   X● **V80.31** Animal-rider injured in collision with two- or three-wheeled motor vehicle

   X● **V80.32** Occupant of animal-drawn vehicle injured in collision with two- or three-wheeled motor vehicle

● **V80.4** Animal-rider or occupant of animal-drawn vehicle injured in collision with car, pick-up truck, van, heavy transport vehicle or bus

    Excludes1   animal-rider injured in collision with military vehicle (V80.910)

                occupant of animal-drawn vehicle injured in collision with military vehicle (V80.920)

   X● **V80.41** Animal-rider injured in collision with car, pick-up truck, van, heavy transport vehicle or bus

   X● **V80.42** Occupant of animal-drawn vehicle injured in collision with car, pick-up truck, van, heavy transport vehicle or bus

● **V80.5** Animal-rider or occupant of animal-drawn vehicle injured in collision with other specified motor vehicle

   X● **V80.51** Animal-rider injured in collision with other specified motor vehicle

   X● **V80.52** Occupant of animal-drawn vehicle injured in collision with other specified motor vehicle

● **V80.6** Animal-rider or occupant of animal-drawn vehicle injured in collision with railway train or railway vehicle

   X● **V80.61** Animal-rider injured in collision with railway train or railway vehicle

   X● **V80.62** Occupant of animal-drawn vehicle injured in collision with railway train or railway vehicle

● **V80.7** Animal-rider or occupant of animal-drawn vehicle injured in collision with other nonmotor vehicles

   ● **V80.71** Animal-rider or occupant of animal-drawn vehicle injured in collision with animal being ridden

      ● **V80.710** Animal-rider injured in collision with other animal being ridden

      ● **V80.711** Occupant of animal-drawn vehicle injured in collision with animal being ridden

   ● **V80.72** Animal-rider or occupant of animal-drawn vehicle injured in collision with other animal-drawn vehicle

      ● **V80.720** Animal-rider injured in collision with animal-drawn vehicle

      ● **V80.721** Occupant of animal-drawn vehicle injured in collision with other animal-drawn vehicle

   ● **V80.73** Animal-rider or occupant of animal-drawn vehicle injured in collision with streetcar

      ● **V80.730** Animal-rider injured in collision with streetcar

      ● **V80.731** Occupant of animal-drawn vehicle injured in collision with streetcar

   ● **V80.79** Animal-rider or occupant of animal-drawn vehicle injured in collision with other nonmotor vehicles

      ● **V80.790** Animal-rider injured in collision with other nonmotor vehicles

      ● **V80.791** Occupant of animal-drawn vehicle injured in collision with other nonmotor vehicles

● **V80.8** Animal-rider or occupant of animal-drawn vehicle injured in collision with fixed or stationary object

   X● **V80.81** Animal-rider injured in collision with fixed or stationary object

   X● **V80.82** Occupant of animal-drawn vehicle injured in collision with fixed or stationary object

● **V80.9** Animal-rider or occupant of animal-drawn vehicle injured in other and unspecified transport accidents

   ● **V80.91** Animal-rider injured in other and unspecified transport accidents

      ● **V80.910** Animal-rider injured in transport accident with military vehicle

      ● **V80.918** Animal-rider injured in other transport accident

      ● **V80.919** Animal-rider injured in unspecified transport accident

          Animal rider accident NOS

   ● **V80.92** Occupant of animal-drawn vehicle injured in other and unspecified transport accidents

      ● **V80.920** Occupant of animal-drawn vehicle injured in transport accident with military vehicle

      ● **V80.928** Occupant of animal-drawn vehicle injured in other transport accident

      ● **V80.929** Occupant of animal-drawn vehicle injured in unspecified transport accident

          Animal-drawn vehicle accident NOS

● **V81** Occupant of railway train or railway vehicle injured in transport accident

    Includes   derailment of railway train or railway vehicle

                person on outside of train

    Excludes1   streetcar (V82.-)

    The appropriate 7th character is to be added to each code from category V81

A	initial encounter
D	subsequent encounter
S	sequela

   X● **V81.0** Occupant of railway train or railway vehicle injured in collision with motor vehicle in nontraffic accident

      Excludes1   occupant of railway train or railway vehicle injured due to collision with military vehicle (V81.83)

   X● **V81.1** Occupant of railway train or railway vehicle injured in collision with motor vehicle in traffic accident

      Excludes1   occupant of railway train or railway vehicle injured due to collision with military vehicle (V81.83)

   X● **V81.2** Occupant of railway train or railway vehicle injured in collision with or hit by rolling stock

   X● **V81.3** Occupant of railway train or railway vehicle injured in collision with other object

        Railway collision NOS

   X● **V81.4** Person injured while boarding or alighting from railway train or railway vehicle

   X● **V81.5** Occupant of railway train or railway vehicle injured by fall in railway train or railway vehicle

   X● **V81.6** Occupant of railway train or railway vehicle injured by fall from railway train or railway vehicle

   X● **V81.7** Occupant of railway train or railway vehicle injured in derailment without antecedent collision

N Newborn Age: 0   **P** Pediatric Age: 0–17   **M** Maternity DX: 9–64   **A** Adult Age: 15–124   ♀ Females Only   ♂ Males Only

🅒 Complication\Comorbidity   🅒 Major C\C   Ⓔ CC/MCC Exclusions   🅗 Hospital-Acquired Condition   🅗 Hierarchical Condition Category

1559

● V81.8   **Occupant of railway train or railway vehicle injured in other specified railway accidents**

    X ● V81.81   **Occupant of railway train or railway vehicle injured due to explosion or fire on train**

    X ● V81.82   **Occupant of railway train or railway vehicle injured due to object falling onto train**

         Occupant of railway train or railway vehicle injured due to falling earth onto train

         Occupant of railway train or railway vehicle injured due to falling rocks onto train

         Occupant of railway train or railway vehicle injured due to falling snow onto train

         Occupant of railway train or railway vehicle injured due to falling trees onto train

    X ● V81.83   **Occupant of railway train or railway vehicle injured due to collision with military vehicle**

    X ● V81.89   **Occupant of railway train or railway vehicle injured due to other specified railway accident**

   X ● V81.9   **Occupant of railway train or railway vehicle injured in unspecified railway accident**

        Railway accident NOS

● V82   **Occupant of powered streetcar injured in transport accident**

   Includes   interurban electric car
            person on outside of streetcar
            tram (car)
            trolley (car)

   Excludes1   bus (V70-V79)
            motorcoach (V70-V79)
            nonpowered streetcar (V76.-)
            train (V81.-)

The appropriate 7th character is to be added to each code from category V82

    A   initial encounter
    D   subsequent encounter
    S   sequela

   X ● V82.0   **Occupant of streetcar injured in collision with motor vehicle in nontraffic accident**

   X ● V82.1   **Occupant of streetcar injured in collision with motor vehicle in traffic accident**

   X ● V82.2   **Occupant of streetcar injured in collision with or hit by rolling stock**

   X ● V82.3   **Occupant of streetcar injured in collision with other object**

      Excludes1   collision with animal-drawn vehicle or animal being ridden (V82.8)

   X ● V82.4   **Person injured while boarding or alighting from streetcar**

   X ● V82.5   **Occupant of streetcar injured by fall in streetcar**

      Excludes1   fall in streetcar:
               while boarding or alighting (V82.4)
               with antecedent collision (V82.0-V82.3)

   X ● V82.6   **Occupant of streetcar injured by fall from streetcar**

      Excludes1   fall from streetcar:
               while boarding or alighting (V82.4)
               with antecedent collision (V82.0-V82.3)

   X ● V82.7   **Occupant of streetcar injured in derailment without antecedent collision**

      Excludes1   occupant of streetcar injured in derailment with antecedent collision (V82.0-V82.3)

   X ● V82.8   **Occupant of streetcar injured in other specified transport accidents**

        Streetcar collision with military vehicle
        Streetcar collision with train or nonmotor vehicles

   X ● V82.9   **Occupant of streetcar injured in unspecified traffic accident**

        Streetcar accident NOS

● V83   **Occupant of special vehicle mainly used on industrial premises injured in transport accident**

   Includes   battery-powered airport passenger vehicle
            battery-powered truck (baggage) (mail)
            coal-car in mine
            forklift (truck)
            logging car
            self-propelled industrial truck
            station baggage truck (powered)
            tram, truck, or tub (powered) in mine or quarry

   Excludes1   special construction vehicles (V85.-)
            special industrial vehicle in stationary use or maintenance (W31.-)

The appropriate 7th character is to be added to each code from category V83

    A   initial encounter
    D   subsequent encounter
    S   sequela

   X ● V83.0   **Driver of special industrial vehicle injured in traffic accident**

   X ● V83.1   **Passenger of special industrial vehicle injured in traffic accident**

   X ● V83.2   **Person on outside of special industrial vehicle injured in traffic accident**

   X ● V83.3   **Unspecified occupant of special industrial vehicle injured in traffic accident**

   X ● V83.4   **Person injured while boarding or alighting from special industrial vehicle**

   X ● V83.5   **Driver of special industrial vehicle injured in nontraffic accident**

   X ● V83.6   **Passenger of special industrial vehicle injured in nontraffic accident**

   X ● V83.7   **Person on outside of special industrial vehicle injured in nontraffic accident**

   X ● V83.9   **Unspecified occupant of special industrial vehicle injured in nontraffic accident**

        Special-industrial-vehicle accident NOS

● V84   **Occupant of special vehicle mainly used in agriculture injured in transport accident**

   Includes   self-propelled farm machinery
            tractor (and trailer)

   Excludes1   animal-powered farm machinery accident (W30.8-)
            contact with combine harvester (W30.0)
            special agricultural vehicle in stationary use or maintenance (W30.-)

The appropriate 7th character is to be added to each code from category V84

    A   initial encounter
    D   subsequent encounter
    S   sequela

   X ● V84.0   **Driver of special agricultural vehicle injured in traffic accident**

   X ● V84.1   **Passenger of special agricultural vehicle injured in traffic accident**

   X ● V84.2   **Person on outside of special agricultural vehicle injured in traffic accident**

   X ● V84.3   **Unspecified occupant of special agricultural vehicle injured in traffic accident**

   X ● V84.4   **Person injured while boarding or alighting from special agricultural vehicle**

   X ● V84.5   **Driver of special agricultural vehicle injured in nontraffic accident**

   X ● V84.6   **Passenger of special agricultural vehicle injured in nontraffic accident**

   X ● V84.7   **Person on outside of special agricultural vehicle injured in nontraffic accident**

   X ● V84.9   **Unspecified occupant of special agricultural vehicle injured in nontraffic accident**

        Special-agricultural vehicle accident NOS

▶ New   ⇒ Revised   ~~deleted~~ Deleted   Excludes 1   Excludes 2   Includes   Use additional   Code first   Code also   Key words

OGCR Official Guidelines   ● Unacceptable Principal Diagnosis   X Assign placeholder X   ● Use Additional Character(s)   ▷ Manifestation Code   Coding Clinic

● **V85   Occupant of special construction vehicle injured in transport accident**

> **Includes**   bulldozer
> digger
> dump truck
> earth-leveller
> mechanical shovel
> road-roller

> **Excludes1**   special industrial vehicle (V83.-)
> special construction vehicle in stationary use or maintenance (W31.-)

The appropriate 7th character is to be added to each code from category V85

> A   initial encounter
> D   subsequent encounter
> S   sequela

X● **V85.0   Driver of special construction vehicle injured in traffic accident**

X● **V85.1   Passenger of special construction vehicle injured in traffic accident**

X● **V85.2   Person on outside of special construction vehicle injured in traffic accident**

X● **V85.3   Unspecified occupant of special construction vehicle injured in traffic accident**

X● **V85.4   Person injured while boarding or alighting from special construction vehicle**

X● **V85.5   Driver of special construction vehicle injured in nontraffic accident**

X● **V85.6   Passenger of special construction vehicle injured in nontraffic accident**

X● **V85.7   Person on outside of special construction vehicle injured in nontraffic accident**

X● **V85.9   Unspecified occupant of special construction vehicle injured in nontraffic accident**
> Special-construction-vehicle accident NOS

● **V86   Occupant of special all-terrain or other off-road motor vehicle, injured in transport accident**

> **Excludes1**   special all-terrain vehicle in stationary use or maintenance (W31.-)
> sport-utility vehicle (V50-V59)
> three-wheeled motor vehicle designed for on-road use (V30-V39)

The appropriate 7th character is to be added to each code from category V86

> A   initial encounter
> D   subsequent encounter
> S   sequela

● **V86.0   Driver of special all-terrain or other off-road motor vehicle injured in traffic accident**

X● **V86.01   Driver of ambulance or fire engine injured in traffic accident**

X● **V86.02   Driver of snowmobile injured in traffic accident**

X● **V86.03   Driver of dune buggy injured in traffic accident**

X● **V86.04   Driver of military vehicle injured in traffic accident**

X● **V86.05   Driver of 3- or 4-wheeled all-terrain vehicle (ATV) injured in traffic accident**

X● **V86.06   Driver of dirt bike or motor/cross bike injured in traffic accident**

X● **V86.09   Driver of other off-road special all-terrain or other off-road vehicle injured in traffic accident**
> Driver of go cart injured in traffic accident
> Driver of golf cart injured in traffic accident

● **V86.1   Passenger of special all-terrain or other off-road motor vehicle injured in traffic accident**

X● **V86.11   Passenger of ambulance or fire engine injured in traffic accident**

X● **V86.12   Passenger of snowmobile injured in traffic accident**

X● **V86.13   Passenger of dune buggy injured in traffic accident**

X● **V86.14   Passenger of military vehicle injured in traffic accident**

X● **V86.15   Passenger of 3- or 4-wheeled all-terrain vehicle (ATV) injured in traffic accident**

X● **V86.16   Passenger of dirt bike or motor/cross bike injured in traffic accident**

X● **V86.19   Passenger of other off-road special all-terrain or other off-road off-road motor vehicle injured in traffic accident**
> Passenger of go cart injured in traffic accident
> Passenger of golf cart injured in traffic accident

● **V86.2   Person on outside of special all-terrain or other off-road motor vehicle injured in traffic accident**

X● **V86.21   Person on outside of ambulance or fire engine injured in traffic accident**

X● **V86.22   Person on outside of snowmobile injured in traffic accident**

X● **V86.23   Person on outside of dune buggy injured in traffic accident**

X● **V86.24   Person on outside of military vehicle injured in traffic accident**

X● **V86.25   Person on outside of 3- or 4-wheeled all-terrain vehicle (ATV) injured in traffic accident**

X● **V86.26   Person on outside of dirt bike or motor/cross bike injured in traffic accident**

X● **V86.29   Person on outside of other special all-terrain or other off-road motor vehicle injured in traffic accident**
> Person on outside of go cart in traffic accident
> Person on outside of golf cart injured in traffic accident

● **V86.3   Unspecified occupant of special all-terrain or other off-road motor vehicle injured in traffic accident**

X● **V86.31   Unspecified occupant of ambulance or fire engine injured in traffic accident**

X● **V86.32   Unspecified occupant of snowmobile injured in traffic accident**

X● **V86.33   Unspecified occupant of dune buggy injured in traffic accident**

X● **V86.34   Unspecified occupant of military vehicle injured in traffic accident**

X● **V86.35   Unspecified occupant of 3- or 4-wheeled all-terrain vehicle (ATV) injured in traffic accident**

X● **V86.36   Unspecified occupant of dirt bike or motor/cross bike injured in traffic accident**

X● **V86.39   Unspecified occupant of other special all-terrain or other off-road motor vehicle injured in traffic accident**
> Unspecified occupant of go cart injured in traffic accident
> Unspecified occupant of golf cart injured in traffic accident

● **V86.4   Person injured while boarding or alighting from special all-terrain or other off-road motor vehicle**

X● **V86.41** Person injured while boarding or alighting from ambulance or fire engine

X● **V86.42** Person injured while boarding or alighting from snowmobile

X● **V86.43** Person injured while boarding or alighting from dune buggy

X● **V86.44** Person injured while boarding or alighting from military vehicle

X● **V86.45** Person injured while boarding or alighting from a 3- or 4-wheeled all-terrain vehicle (ATV)

X● **V86.46** Person injured while boarding or alighting from a dirt bike or motor/cross bike

X● **V86.49** Person injured while boarding or alighting from other special all-terrain or other off-road motor vehicle

     Person injured while boarding or alighting from go cart

     Person injured while boarding or alighting from golf cart

● **V86.5** Driver of special all-terrain or other off-road motor vehicle injured in nontraffic accident

X● **V86.51** Driver of ambulance or fire engine injured in nontraffic accident

X● **V86.52** Driver of snowmobile injured in nontraffic accident

X● **V86.53** Driver of dune buggy injured in nontraffic accident

X● **V86.54** Driver of military vehicle injured in nontraffic accident

X● **V86.55** Driver of 3- or 4-wheeled all-terrain vehicle (ATV) injured in nontraffic accident

X● **V86.56** Driver of dirt bike or motor/cross bike injured in nontraffic accident

X● **V86.59** Driver of other off-road special all-terrain or other off-road motor vehicle injured in nontraffic accident

     Driver of go cart injured in nontraffic accident

     Driver of golf cart injured in nontraffic accident

● **V86.6** Passenger of special all-terrain or other off-road motor vehicle injured in nontraffic accident

X● **V86.61** Passenger of ambulance or fire engine injured in nontraffic accident

X● **V86.62** Passenger of snowmobile injured in nontraffic accident

X● **V86.63** Passenger of dune buggy injured in nontraffic accident

X● **V86.64** Passenger of military vehicle injured in nontraffic accident

X● **V86.65** Passenger of 3- or 4-wheeled all-terrain vehicle (ATV) injured in nontraffic accident

X● **V86.66** Passenger of dirt bike or motor/cross bike injured in nontraffic accident

X● **V86.69** Passenger of other special all-terrain or other off-road vehicle injured in nontraffic accident

     Passenger of go cart injured in nontraffic accident

     Passenger of golf cart injured in nontraffic accident

● **V86.7** Person on outside of special all-terrain or other off-road motor vehicle injured in nontraffic accident

X● **V86.71** Person on outside of ambulance or fire engine injured in nontraffic accident

X● **V86.72** Person on outside of snowmobile injured in nontraffic accident

X● **V86.73** Person on outside of dune buggy injured in nontraffic accident

X● **V86.74** Person on outside of military vehicle injured in nontraffic accident

X● **V86.75** Person on outside of 3- or 4-wheeled all-terrain vehicle (ATV) injured in nontraffic accident

X● **V86.76** Person on outside of dirt bike or motor/cross bike injured in nontraffic accident

X● **V86.79** Person on outside of other special all-terrain or other off-road motor vehicles injured in nontraffic accident

     Person on outside of go cart injured in nontraffic accident

     Person on outside of golf cart injured in nontraffic accident

● **V86.9** Unspecified occupant of special all-terrain or other off-road motor vehicle injured in nontraffic accident

X● **V86.91** Unspecified occupant of ambulance or fire engine injured in nontraffic accident

X● **V86.92** Unspecified occupant of snowmobile injured in nontraffic accident

X● **V86.93** Unspecified occupant of dune buggy injured in nontraffic accident

X● **V86.94** Unspecified occupant of military vehicle injured in nontraffic accident

X● **V86.95** Unspecified occupant of 3- or 4-wheeled all-terrain vehicle (ATV) injured in nontraffic accident

X● **V86.96** Unspecified occupant of dirt bike or motor/cross bike injured in nontraffic accident

X● **V86.99** Unspecified occupant of other special all-terrain or other off-road motor vehicle injured in nontraffic accident

     Off-road motor-vehicle accident NOS

     Other motor-vehicle accident NOS

     Unspecified occupant of go cart injured in nontraffic accident

     Unspecified occupant of golf cart injured in nontraffic accident

     Unspecified occupant of race car injured in nontraffic accident

● **V87** Traffic accident of specified type but victim's mode of transport unknown

> **Excludes1**   collision involving:
>   pedal cycle (V10-V19)
>   pedestrian (V01-V09)

The appropriate 7th character is to be added to each code from category V87

A	initial encounter
D	subsequent encounter
S	sequela

X● **V87.0** Person injured in collision between car and two- or three-wheeled powered vehicle (traffic)

X● **V87.1** Person injured in collision between other motor vehicle and two- or three-wheeled motor vehicle (traffic)

X● **V87.2** Person injured in collision between car and pick-up truck or van (traffic)

X● **V87.3** Person injured in collision between car and bus (traffic)

X● **V87.4** Person injured in collision between car and heavy transport vehicle (traffic)

X● **V87.5** Person injured in collision between heavy transport vehicle and bus (traffic)

X● **V87.6** Person injured in collision between railway train or railway vehicle and car (traffic)

X● **V87.7** Person injured in collision between other specified motor vehicles (traffic)

X● **V87.8** Person injured in other specified noncollision transport accidents involving motor vehicle (traffic)

X● **V87.9** Person injured in other specified (collision) (noncollision) transport accidents involving nonmotor vehicle (traffic)

● **V88** Nontraffic accident of specified type but victim's mode of transport unknown

> **Excludes1**   collision involving:

▶ New   ⇒ Revised   ~~deleted~~ Deleted   Excludes 1   Excludes 2   Includes   Use additional   Code first   Code also   Key words

OGCR Official Guidelines   ● Unacceptable Principal Diagnosis   X Assign placeholder X   ● Use Additional Character(s)   ▶ Manifestation Code   **Coding Clinic**

pedal cycle (V10-V19)
pedestrian (V01-V09)

The appropriate 7th character is to be added to each code from category V88

A	initial encounter
D	subsequent encounter
S	sequela

X● **V88.0** **Person injured in collision between car and two- or three-wheeled motor vehicle, nontraffic**

X● **V88.1** **Person injured in collision between other motor vehicle and two- or three-wheeled motor vehicle, nontraffic**

X● **V88.2** **Person injured in collision between car and pick-up truck or van, nontraffic**

X● **V88.3** **Person injured in collision between car and bus, nontraffic**

X● **V88.4** **Person injured in collision between car and heavy transport vehicle, nontraffic**

X● **V88.5** **Person injured in collision between heavy transport vehicle and bus, nontraffic**

X● **V88.6** **Person injured in collision between railway train or railway vehicle and car, nontraffic**

X● **V88.7** **Person injured in collision between other specified motor vehicle, nontraffic**

X● **V88.8** **Person injured in other specified noncollision transport accidents involving motor vehicle, nontraffic**

X● **V88.9** **Person injured in other specified (collision) (noncollision) transport accidents involving nonmotor vehicle, nontraffic**

● **V89** **Motor- or nonmotor-vehicle accident, type of vehicle unspecified**

The appropriate 7th character is to be added to each code from category V89

A	initial encounter
D	subsequent encounter
S	sequela

X● **V89.0** **Person injured in unspecified motor-vehicle accident, nontraffic**
Motor-vehicle accident NOS, nontraffic

X● **V89.1** **Person injured in unspecified nonmotor-vehicle accident, nontraffic**
Nonmotor-vehicle accident NOS (nontraffic)

X● **V89.2** **Person injured in unspecified motor-vehicle accident, traffic**
Motor-vehicle accident [MVA] NOS
Road (traffic) accident [RTA] NOS

X● **V89.3** **Person injured in unspecified nonmotor-vehicle accident, traffic**
Nonmotor-vehicle traffic accident NOS

X● **V89.9** **Person injured in unspecified vehicle accident**
Collision NOS

WATER TRANSPORT ACCIDENTS (V90-V94)

● **V90** **Drowning and submersion due to accident to watercraft**

Excludes1   civilian water transport accident involving military watercraft (V94.81-)
fall into water not from watercraft (W16.-)
military watercraft accident in military or war operations (Y36.0-, Y37.0-)
water-transport–related drowning or submersion without accident to watercraft (V92.-)

The appropriate 7th character is to be added to each code from category V90

A	initial encounter
D	subsequent encounter
S	sequela

● **V90.0** **Drowning and submersion due to watercraft overturning**

X● **V90.00** **Drowning and submersion due to merchant ship overturning**

X● **V90.01** **Drowning and submersion due to passenger ship overturning**
Drowning and submersion due to ferry-boat overturning
Drowning and submersion due to liner overturning

X● **V90.02** **Drowning and submersion due to fishing boat overturning**

X● **V90.03** **Drowning and submersion due to other powered watercraft overturning**
Drowning and submersion due to hovercraft (on open water) overturning
Drowning and submersion due to jet ski overturning

X● **V90.04** **Drowning and submersion due to sailboat overturning**

X● **V90.05** **Drowning and submersion due to canoe or kayak overturning**

X● **V90.06** **Drowning and submersion due to (nonpowered) inflatable craft overturning**

X● **V90.08** **Drowning and submersion due to other unpowered watercraft overturning**
Drowning and submersion due to windsurfer overturning

X● **V90.09** **Drowning and submersion due to unspecified watercraft overturning**
Drowning and submersion due to boat NOS overturning
Drowning and submersion due to ship NOS overturning
Drowning and submersion due to watercraft NOS overturning

● **V90.1** **Drowning and submersion due to watercraft sinking**

X● **V90.10** **Drowning and submersion due to merchant ship sinking**

X● **V90.11** **Drowning and submersion due to passenger ship sinking**
Drowning and submersion due to ferry-boat sinking
Drowning and submersion due to liner sinking

X● **V90.12** **Drowning and submersion due to fishing boat sinking**

X● **V90.13** **Drowning and submersion due to other powered watercraft sinking**
Drowning and submersion due to hovercraft (on open water) sinking
Drowning and submersion due to jet ski sinking

X● **V90.14** **Drowning and submersion due to sailboat sinking**

X● **V90.15** **Drowning and submersion due to canoe or kayak sinking**

CHAPTER 20 (V00-Y99)

N Newborn Age: 0   **P** Pediatric Age: 0–17   **M** Maternity DX: 9–64   **A** Adult Age: 15–124   ♀ Females Only   ♂ Males Only

🝖 Complication\Comorbidity   🝖 Major C\C   (Ex) CC/MCC Exclusions   🝖 Hospital-Acquired Condition   🝖 Hierarchical Condition Category   1563

X● **V90.16** Drowning and submersion due to (nonpowered) inflatable craft sinking

X● **V90.18** Drowning and submersion due to other unpowered watercraft sinking

X● **V90.19** Drowning and submersion due to unspecified watercraft sinking
Drowning and submersion due to boat NOS sinking
Drowning and submersion due to ship NOS sinking
Drowning and submersion due to watercraft NOS sinking

● **V90.2** Drowning and submersion due to falling or jumping from burning watercraft

X● **V90.20** Drowning and submersion due to falling or jumping from burning merchant ship

X● **V90.21** Drowning and submersion due to falling or jumping from burning passenger ship
Drowning and submersion due to falling or jumping from burning ferry-boat
Drowning and submersion due to falling or jumping from burning liner

X● **V90.22** Drowning and submersion due to falling or jumping from burning fishing boat

X● **V90.23** Drowning and submersion due to falling or jumping from other burning powered watercraft
Drowning and submersion due to falling and jumping from burning hovercraft (on open water)
Drowning and submersion due to falling and jumping from burning jet ski

X● **V90.24** Drowning and submersion due to falling or jumping from burning sailboat

X● **V90.25** Drowning and submersion due to falling or jumping from burning canoe or kayak

X● **V90.26** Drowning and submersion due to falling or jumping from burning (nonpowered) inflatable craft

X● **V90.27** Drowning and submersion due to falling or jumping from burning water-skis

X● **V90.28** Drowning and submersion due to falling or jumping from other burning unpowered watercraft
Drowning and submersion due to falling and jumping from burning surf-board
Drowning and submersion due to falling and jumping from burning windsurfer

X● **V90.29** Drowning and submersion due to falling or jumping from unspecified burning watercraft
Drowning and submersion due to falling or jumping from burning boat NOS
Drowning and submersion due to falling or jumping from burning ship NOS
Drowning and submersion due to falling or jumping from burning watercraft NOS

● **V90.3** Drowning and submersion due to falling or jumping from crushed watercraft

X● **V90.30** Drowning and submersion due to falling or jumping from crushed merchant ship

X● **V90.31** Drowning and submersion due to falling or jumping from crushed passenger ship
Drowning and submersion due to falling and jumping from crushed ferry-boat
Drowning and submersion due to falling and jumping from crushed liner

X● **V90.32** Drowning and submersion due to falling or jumping from crushed fishing boat

X● **V90.33** Drowning and submersion due to falling or jumping from other crushed powered watercraft
Drowning and submersion due to falling and jumping from crushed hovercraft

Drowning and submersion due to falling and jumping from crushed jet ski

X● **V90.34** Drowning and submersion due to falling or jumping from crushed sailboat

X● **V90.35** Drowning and submersion due to falling or jumping from crushed canoe or kayak

X● **V90.36** Drowning and submersion due to falling or jumping from crushed (nonpowered) inflatable craft

X● **V90.37** Drowning and submersion due to falling or jumping from crushed water-skis

X● **V90.38** Drowning and submersion due to falling or jumping from other crushed unpowered watercraft
Drowning and submersion due to falling and jumping from crushed surf-board
Drowning and submersion due to falling and jumping from crushed windsurfer

X● **V90.39** Drowning and submersion due to falling or jumping from crushed unspecified watercraft
Drowning and submersion due to falling and jumping from crushed boat NOS
Drowning and submersion due to falling and jumping from crushed ship NOS
Drowning and submersion due to falling and jumping from crushed watercraft NOS

● **V90.8** Drowning and submersion due to other accident to watercraft

X● **V90.80** Drowning and submersion due to other accident to merchant ship

X● **V90.81** Drowning and submersion due to other accident to passenger ship
Drowning and submersion due to other accident to ferry-boat
Drowning and submersion due to other accident to liner

X● **V90.82** Drowning and submersion due to other accident to fishing boat

X● **V90.83** Drowning and submersion due to other accident to other powered watercraft
Drowning and submersion due to other accident to hovercraft (on open water)
Drowning and submersion due to other accident to jet ski

X● **V90.84** Drowning and submersion due to other accident to sailboat

X● **V90.85** Drowning and submersion due to other accident to canoe or kayak

X● **V90.86** Drowning and submersion due to other accident to (nonpowered) inflatable craft

X● **V90.87** Drowning and submersion due to other accident to water-skis

X● **V90.88** Drowning and submersion due to other accident to other unpowered watercraft
Drowning and submersion due to other accident to surf-board
Drowning and submersion due to other accident to windsurfer

X● **V90.89** Drowning and submersion due to other accident to unspecified watercraft
Drowning and submersion due to other accident to boat NOS
Drowning and submersion due to other accident to ship NOS
Drowning and submersion due to other accident to watercraft NOS

● **V91** Other injury due to accident to watercraft
Includes   any injury except drowning and submersion as a result of an accident to watercraft

CHAPTER 20 (V00-Y99)

Excludes1   civilian water transport accident involving military watercraft (V94.81-)
military watercraft accident in military or war operations (Y36, Y37.-)

Excludes2   drowning and submersion due to accident to watercraft (V90.-)

The appropriate 7th character is to be added to each code from category V91

A	initial encounter
D	subsequent encounter
S	sequela

● **V91.0   Burn due to watercraft on fire**

     Excludes1   burn from localized fire or explosion on board ship without accident to watercraft (V93.-)

X ● **V91.00   Burn due to merchant ship on fire**

X ● **V91.01   Burn due to passenger ship on fire**
     Burn due to ferry-boat on fire
     Burn due to liner on fire

X ● **V91.02   Burn due to fishing boat on fire**

X ● **V91.03   Burn due to other powered watercraft on fire**
     Burn due to hovercraft (on open water) on fire
     Burn due to jet ski on fire

X ● **V91.04   Burn due to sailboat on fire**

X ● **V91.05   Burn due to canoe or kayak on fire**

X ● **V91.06   Burn due to (nonpowered) inflatable craft on fire**

X ● **V91.07   Burn due to water-skis on fire**

X ● **V91.08   Burn due to other unpowered watercraft on fire**

X ● **V91.09   Burn due to unspecified watercraft on fire**
     Burn due to boat NOS on fire
     Burn due to ship NOS on fire
     Burn due to watercraft NOS on fire

● **V91.1   Crushed between watercraft and other watercraft or other object due to collision**
     Crushed by lifeboat after abandoning ship in a collision
     Note: Select the specified type of watercraft that the victim was on at the time of the collision.

X ● **V91.10   Crushed between merchant ship and other watercraft or other object due to collision**

X ● **V91.11   Crushed between passenger ship and other watercraft or other object due to collision**
     Crushed between ferry-boat and other watercraft or other object due to collision
     Crushed between liner and other watercraft or other object due to collision

X ● **V91.12   Crushed between fishing boat and other watercraft or other object due to collision**

X ● **V91.13   Crushed between other powered watercraft and other watercraft or other object due to collision**
     Crushed between hovercraft (on open water) and other watercraft or other object due to collision
     Crushed between jet ski and other watercraft or other object due to collision

X ● **V91.14   Crushed between sailboat and other watercraft or other object due to collision**

X ● **V91.15   Crushed between canoe or kayak and other watercraft or other object due to collision**

X ● **V91.16   Crushed between (nonpowered) inflatable craft and other watercraft or other object due to collision**

X ● **V91.18   Crushed between other unpowered watercraft and other watercraft or other object due to collision**

Crushed between surfboard and other watercraft or other object due to collision
Crushed between windsurfer and other watercraft or other object due to collision

X ● **V91.19   Crushed between unspecified watercraft and other watercraft or other object due to collision**
     Crushed between boat NOS and other watercraft or other object due to collision
     Crushed between ship NOS and other watercraft or other object due to collision
     Crushed between watercraft NOS and other watercraft or other object due to collision

● **V91.2   Fall due to collision between watercraft and other watercraft or other object**
     Fall while remaining on watercraft after collision
     Note: Select the specified type of watercraft that the victim was on at the time of the collision.

     Excludes1   crushed between watercraft and other watercraft and other object due to collision (V91.1-)
drowning and submersion due to falling from crushed watercraft (V90.3-)

X ● **V91.20   Fall due to collision between merchant ship and other watercraft or other object**

X ● **V91.21   Fall due to collision between passenger ship and other watercraft or other object**
     Fall due to collision between ferry-boat and other watercraft or other object
     Fall due to collision between liner and other watercraft or other object

X ● **V91.22   Fall due to collision between fishing boat and other watercraft or other object**

X ● **V91.23   Fall due to collision between other powered watercraft and other watercraft or other object**
     Fall due to collision between hovercraft (on open water) and other watercraft or other object
     Fall due to collision between jet ski and other watercraft or other object

X ● **V91.24   Fall due to collision between sailboat and other watercraft or other object**

X ● **V91.25   Fall due to collision between canoe or kayak and other watercraft or other object**

X ● **V91.26   Fall due to collision between (nonpowered) inflatable craft and other watercraft or other object**

X ● **V91.29   Fall due to collision between unspecified watercraft and other watercraft or other object**
     Fall due to collision between boat NOS and other watercraft or other object
     Fall due to collision between ship NOS and other watercraft or other object
     Fall due to collision between watercraft NOS and other watercraft or other object

● **V91.3   Hit or struck by falling object due to accident to watercraft**
     Hit or struck by falling object (part of damaged watercraft or other object) after falling or jumping from damaged watercraft

     Excludes2   drowning or submersion due to fall or jumping from damaged watercraft (V90.2-, V90.3-)

X ● **V91.30   Hit or struck by falling object due to accident to merchant ship**

X ● **V91.31   Hit or struck by falling object due to accident to passenger ship**
     Hit or struck by falling object due to accident to ferry-boat
     Hit or struck by falling object due to accident to liner

X ● **V91.32   Hit or struck by falling object due to accident to fishing boat**

N Newborn Age: 0   **P** Pediatric Age: 0–17   **M** Maternity DX: 9–64   **A** Adult Age: 15–124   ♀ Females Only   ♂ Males Only

Complication\Comorbidity   Major C\C   (Ex:) CC/MCC Exclusions   Hospital-Acquired Condition   Hierarchical Condition Category

1565

X● **V91.33** **Hit or struck by falling object due to accident to other powered watercraft**
    Hit or struck by falling object due to accident to hovercraft (on open water)
    Hit or struck by falling object due to accident to jet ski

X● **V91.34** **Hit or struck by falling object due to accident to sailboat**

X● **V91.35** **Hit or struck by falling object due to accident to canoe or kayak**

X● **V91.36** **Hit or struck by falling object due to accident to (nonpowered) inflatable craft**

X● **V91.37** **Hit or struck by falling object due to accident to water-skis**
    Hit by water-skis after jumping off of waterskis

X● **V91.38** **Hit or struck by falling object due to accident to other unpowered watercraft**
    Hit or struck by surf-board after falling off damaged surf-board
    Hit or struck by object after falling off damaged windsurfer

X● **V91.39** **Hit or struck by falling object due to accident to unspecified watercraft**
    Hit or struck by falling object due to accident to boat NOS
    Hit or struck by falling object due to accident to ship NOS
    Hit or struck by falling object due to accident to watercraft NOS

● **V91.8** **Other injury due to other accident to watercraft**

X● **V91.80** **Other injury due to other accident to merchant ship**

X● **V91.81** **Other injury due to other accident to passenger ship**
    Other injury due to other accident to ferry-boat
    Other injury due to other accident to liner

X● **V91.82** **Other injury due to other accident to fishing boat**

X● **V91.83** **Other injury due to other accident to other powered watercraft**
    Other injury due to other accident to hovercraft (on open water)
    Other injury due to other accident to jet ski

X● **V91.84** **Other injury due to other accident to sailboat**

X● **V91.85** **Other injury due to other accident to canoe or kayak**

X● **V91.86** **Other injury due to other accident to (nonpowered) inflatable craft**

X● **V91.87** **Other injury due to other accident to water-skis**

X● **V91.88** **Other injury due to other accident to other unpowered watercraft**
    Other injury due to other accident to surf-board
    Other injury due to other accident to windsurfer

X● **V91.89** **Other injury due to other accident to unspecified watercraft**
    Other injury due to other accident to boat NOS
    Other injury due to other accident to ship NOS
    Other injury due to other accident to watercraft NOS

● **V92** **Drowning and submersion due to accident on board watercraft, without accident to watercraft**

Excludes1 civilian water transport accident involving military watercraft (V94.81-)
    drowning or submersion due to accident to watercraft (V90-V91)
    drowning or submersion of diver who voluntarily jumps from boat not involved in an accident (W16.711, W16.721)
    fall into water without watercraft (W16.-)
    military watercraft accident in military or war operations (Y36, Y37)

The appropriate 7th character is to be added to each code from category V92

A	initial encounter
D	subsequent encounter
S	sequela

● **V92.0** **Drowning and submersion due to fall off watercraft**
    Drowning and submersion due to fall from gangplank of watercraft
    Drowning and submersion due to fall overboard watercraft

    Excludes2 hitting head on object or bottom of body of water due to fall from watercraft (V94.0-)

X● **V92.00** **Drowning and submersion due to fall off merchant ship**

X● **V92.01** **Drowning and submersion due to fall off passenger ship**
    Drowning and submersion due to fall off ferry-boat
    Drowning and submersion due to fall off liner

X● **V92.02** **Drowning and submersion due to fall off fishing boat**

X● **V92.03** **Drowning and submersion due to fall off other powered watercraft**
    Drowning and submersion due to fall off hovercraft (on open water)
    Drowning and submersion due to fall off jet ski

X● **V92.04** **Drowning and submersion due to fall off sailboat**

X● **V92.05** **Drowning and submersion due to fall off canoe or kayak**

X● **V92.06** **Drowning and submersion due to fall off (nonpowered) inflatable craft**

X● **V92.07** **Drowning and submersion due to fall off water-skis**

    Excludes1 drowning and submersion due to falling off burning water-skis (V90.27)
        drowning and submersion due to falling off crushed water-skis (V90.37)
        hit by boat while water-skiing NOS (V94.X)

X● **V92.08** **Drowning and submersion due to fall off other unpowered watercraft**

Drowning and submersion due to fall off surf-board

Drowning and submersion due to fall off windsurfer

> **Excludes1**   drowning and submersion due to fall off burning unpowered watercraft (V90.28)
>
> drowning and submersion due to fall off crushed unpowered watercraft (V90.38)
>
> drowning and submersion due to fall off damaged unpowered watercraft (V90.88)
>
> drowning and submersion due to rider of nonpowered watercraft being hit by other watercraft (V94.-)
>
> other injury due to rider of nonpowered watercraft being hit by other watercraft (V94.-)

X● **V92.09**   **Drowning and submersion due to fall off unspecified watercraft**

Drowning and submersion due to fall off boat NOS

Drowning and submersion due to fall off ship

Drowning and submersion due to fall off watercraft NOS

●**V92.1**   **Drowning and submersion due to being thrown overboard by motion of watercraft**

> **Excludes1**   drowning and submersion due to fall off surf-board (V92.08)
>
> drowning and submersion due to fall off water-skis (V92.07)
>
> drowning and submersion due to fall off windsurfer (V92.08)

X● **V92.10**   **Drowning and submersion due to being thrown overboard by motion of merchant ship**

X● **V92.11**   **Drowning and submersion due to being thrown overboard by motion of passenger ship**

Drowning and submersion due to being thrown overboard by motion of ferry-boat

Drowning and submersion due to being thrown overboard by motion of liner

X● **V92.12**   **Drowning and submersion due to being thrown overboard by motion of fishing boat**

X● **V92.13**   **Drowning and submersion due to being thrown overboard by motion of other powered watercraft**

Drowning and submersion due to being thrown overboard by motion of hovercraft

X● **V92.14**   **Drowning and submersion due to being thrown overboard by motion of sailboat**

X● **V92.15**   **Drowning and submersion due to being thrown overboard by motion of canoe or kayak**

X● **V92.16**   **Drowning and submersion due to being thrown overboard by motion of (nonpowered) inflatable craft**

X● **V92.19**   **Drowning and submersion due to being thrown overboard by motion of unspecified watercraft**

Drowning and submersion due to being thrown overboard by motion of boat NOS

Drowning and submersion due to being thrown overboard by motion of ship NOS

Drowning and submersion due to being thrown overboard by motion of watercraft NOS

●**V92.2**   **Drowning and submersion due to being washed overboard from watercraft**

Code first any associated cataclysm (X37.0-)

X● **V92.20**   **Drowning and submersion due to being washed overboard from merchant ship**

X● **V92.21**   **Drowning and submersion due to being washed overboard from passenger ship**

Drowning and submersion due to being washed overboard from ferry-boat

Drowning and submersion due to being washed overboard from liner

X● **V92.22**   **Drowning and submersion due to being washed overboard from fishing boat**

X● **V92.23**   **Drowning and submersion due to being washed overboard from other powered watercraft**

Drowning and submersion due to being washed overboard from hovercraft (on open water)

Drowning and submersion due to being washed overboard from jet ski

X● **V92.24**   **Drowning and submersion due to being washed overboard from sailboat**

X● **V92.25**   **Drowning and submersion due to being washed overboard from canoe or kayak**

X● **V92.26**   **Drowning and submersion due to being washed overboard from (nonpowered) inflatable craft**

X● **V92.27**   **Drowning and submersion due to being washed overboard from water-skis**

> **Excludes1**   drowning and submersion due to fall off water-skis (V92.07)

X● **V92.28**   **Drowning and submersion due to being washed overboard from other unpowered watercraft**

Drowning and submersion due to being washed overboard from surf-board

Drowning and submersion due to being washed overboard from windsurfer

X● **V92.29**   **Drowning and submersion due to being washed overboard from unspecified watercraft**

Drowning and submersion due to being washed overboard from boat NOS

Drowning and submersion due to being washed overboard from ship NOS

Drowning and submersion due to being washed overboard from watercraft NOS

●**V93**   **Other injury due to accident on board watercraft, without accident to watercraft**

> **Excludes1**   civilian water transport accident involving military watercraft (V94.81-)
>
> other injury due to accident to watercraft (V91.-)
>
> military watercraft accident in military or war operations (Y36, Y37.-)

> **Excludes2**   drowning and submersion due to accident on board watercraft, without accident to watercraft (V92.-)

The appropriate 7th character is to be added to each code from category V93

> A   initial encounter
> D   subsequent encounter
> S   sequela

●**V93.0**   **Burn due to localized fire on board watercraft**

> **Excludes1**   burn due to watercraft on fire (V91.0-)

X● **V93.00**   **Burn due to localized fire on board merchant vessel**

X● **V93.01**   **Burn due to localized fire on board passenger vessel**

Burn due to localized fire on board ferry-boat

Burn due to localized fire on board liner

X● **V93.02**   **Burn due to localized fire on board fishing boat**

X● **V93.03**   **Burn due to localized fire on board other powered watercraft**

N Newborn Age: 0   **P** Pediatric Age: 0–17   **M** Maternity DX: 9–64   **A** Adult Age: 15–124   ♀ Females Only   ♂ Males Only

✿ Complication\Comorbidity   ✿ Major C\C   (Ex:) CC/MCC Exclusions   ✿ Hospital-Acquired Condition   ✿ Hierarchical Condition Category   1567

Burn due to localized fire on board hovercraft
Burn due to localized fire on board jet ski

X● **V93.04** **Burn due to localized fire on board** sailboat

X● **V93.09** **Burn due to localized fire on board** unspecified watercraft
Burn due to localized fire on board boat NOS
Burn due to localized fire on board ship NOS
Burn due to localized fire on board watercraft NOS

● **V93.1** **Other burn on board watercraft**
Burn due to source other than fire on board watercraft

Excludes1 burn due to watercraft on fire (V91.0-)

X● **V93.10** **Other burn on board** merchant vessel

X● **V93.11** **Other burn on board** passenger vessel
Other burn on board ferry-boat
Other burn on board liner

X● **V93.12** **Other burn on board** fishing boat

X● **V93.13** **Other burn on board** other powered watercraft
Other burn on board hovercraft
Other burn on board jet ski

X● **V93.14** **Other burn on board** sailboat

X● **V93.19** **Other burn on board** unspecified watercraft
Other burn on board boat NOS
Other burn on board ship NOS
Other burn on board watercraft NOS

● **V93.2** **Heat exposure on board watercraft**

Excludes1 exposure to man-made heat not aboard watercraft (W92)
exposure to natural heat while on board watercraft (X30)
exposure to sunlight while on board watercraft (X32)

Excludes2 burn due to fire on board watercraft (V93.0-)

X● **V93.20** **Heat exposure on board** merchant ship

X● **V93.21** **Heat exposure on board** passenger ship
Heat exposure on board ferry-boat
Heat exposure on board liner

X● **V93.22** **Heat exposure on board** fishing boat

X● **V93.23** **Heat exposure on board** other powered watercraft
Heat exposure on board hovercraft

X● **V93.24** **Heat exposure on board** sailboat

X● **V93.29** **Heat exposure on board** unspecified watercraft
Heat exposure on board boat NOS
Heat exposure on board ship NOS
Heat exposure on board watercraft NOS

● **V93.3** **Fall on board watercraft**

Excludes1 fall due to collision of watercraft (V91.2-)

X● **V93.30** **Fall on board** merchant ship

X● **V93.31** **Fall on board** passenger ship
Fall on board ferry-boat
Fall on board liner

X● **V93.32** **Fall on board** fishing boat

X● **V93.33** **Fall on board** other powered watercraft
Fall on board hovercraft (on open water)
Fall on board jet ski

X● **V93.34** **Fall on board** sailboat

X● **V93.35** **Fall on board** canoe or kayak

X● **V93.36** **Fall on board (nonpowered)** inflatable craft

X● **V93.38** **Fall on board** other unpowered watercraft

X● **V93.39** **Fall on board** unspecified watercraft
Fall on board boat NOS
Fall on board ship NOS
Fall on board watercraft NOS

● **V93.4** **Struck by falling object on board watercraft**
Hit by falling object on board watercraft

Excludes1 struck by falling object due to accident to watercraft (V91.3)

X● **V93.40** **Struck by falling object on** merchant ship

X● **V93.41** **Struck by falling object on** passenger ship
Struck by falling object on ferry-boat
Struck by falling object on liner

X● **V93.42** **Struck by falling object on** fishing boat

X● **V93.43** **Struck by falling object on** other powered watercraft
Struck by falling object on hovercraft

X● **V93.44** **Struck by falling object on** sailboat

X● **V93.48** **Struck by falling object on** other unpowered watercraft

X● **V93.49** **Struck by falling object on** unspecified watercraft

● **V93.5** **Explosion on board watercraft**
Boiler explosion on steamship

Excludes2 fire on board watercraft (V93.0-)

X● **V93.50** **Explosion on board** merchant ship

X● **V93.51** **Explosion on board** passenger ship
Explosion on board ferry-boat
Explosion on board liner

X● **V93.52** **Explosion on board** fishing boat

X● **V93.53** **Explosion on board** other powered watercraft
Explosion on board hovercraft
Explosion on board jet ski

X● **V93.54** **Explosion on board** sailboat

X● **V93.59** **Explosion on board** unspecified watercraft
Explosion on board boat NOS
Explosion on board ship NOS
Explosion on board watercraft NOS

● **V93.6** **Machinery accident on board watercraft**

Excludes1 machinery explosion on board watercraft (V93.4-)
machinery fire on board watercraft (V93.0-)

X● **V93.60** **Machinery accident on board** merchant ship

X● **V93.61** **Machinery accident on board** passenger ship
Machinery accident on board ferry-boat
Machinery accident on board liner

X● **V93.62** **Machinery accident on board** fishing boat

X● **V93.63** **Machinery accident on board** other powered watercraft
Machinery accident on board hovercraft

X● **V93.64** **Machinery accident on board** sailboat

X● **V93.69** **Machinery accident on board** unspecified watercraft
Machinery accident on board boat NOS
Machinery accident on board ship NOS
Machinery accident on board watercraft NOS

● **V93.8** **Other injury due to other accident on board watercraft**
Accidental poisoning by gases or fumes on watercraft

X● **V93.80** **Other injury due to other accident on board** merchant ship

X● **V93.81** **Other injury due to other accident on board** passenger ship
Other injury due to other accident on board ferry-boat
Other injury due to other accident on board liner

X● **V93.82** **Other injury due to other accident on board** fishing boat

X● **V93.83** **Other injury due to other accident on board** other powered watercraft

▶ New　⟹ Revised　~~deleted~~ Deleted　Excludes 1　Excludes 2　Includes　Use additional　Code first　Code also　Key words
OGCR Official Guidelines　● Unacceptable Principal Diagnosis　X Assign placeholder X　● Use Additional Character(s)　▷ Manifestation Code　Coding Clinic

Other injury due to other accident on board hovercraft

Other injury due to other accident on board jet ski

X● **V93.84**   **Other injury due to other accident on board sailboat**

X● **V93.85**   **Other injury due to other accident on board canoe or kayak**

X● **V93.86**   **Other injury due to other accident on board (nonpowered) inflatable craft**

X● **V93.87**   **Other injury due to other accident on board water-skis**

Hit or struck by object while waterskiing

X● **V93.88**   **Other injury due to other accident on board other unpowered watercraft**

Hit or struck by object while surfing

Hit or struck by object while on board windsurfer

X● **V93.89**   **Other injury due to other accident on board unspecified watercraft**

Other injury due to other accident on board boat NOS

Other injury due to other accident on board ship NOS

Other injury due to other accident on board watercraft NOS

● **V94**   **Other and unspecified water transport accidents**

    Excludes1   military watercraft accidents in military or war operations (Y36, Y37)

The appropriate 7th character is to be added to each code from category V94

A	initial encounter
D	subsequent encounter
S	sequela

X● **V94.0**   **Hitting object or bottom of body of water due to fall from watercraft**

    Excludes2   drowning and submersion due to fall from watercraft (V92.0-)

● **V94.1**   **Bather struck by watercraft**

Swimmer hit by watercraft

X● **V94.11**   **Bather struck by powered watercraft**

X● **V94.12**   **Bather struck by nonpowered watercraft**

● **V94.2**   **Rider of nonpowered watercraft struck by other watercraft**

X● **V94.21**   **Rider of nonpowered watercraft struck by other nonpowered watercraft**

Canoer hit by other nonpowered watercraft

Surfer hit by other nonpowered watercraft

Windsurfer hit by other nonpowered watercraft

X● **V94.22**   **Rider of nonpowered watercraft struck by powered watercraft**

Canoer hit by motorboat

Surfer hit by motorboat

Windsurfer hit by motorboat

● **V94.3**   **Injury to rider of (inflatable) watercraft being pulled behind other watercraft**

X● **V94.31**   **Injury to rider of (inflatable) recreational watercraft being pulled behind other watercraft**

Injury to rider of inner-tube pulled behind motor boat

X● **V94.32**   **Injury to rider of non-recreational watercraft being pulled behind other watercraft**

Injury to occupant of dingy being pulled behind boat or ship

Injury to occupant of life-raft being pulled behind boat or ship

X● **V94.4**   **Injury to barefoot water-skier**

Injury to person being pulled behind boat or ship

● **V94.8**   **Other water transport accident**

● **V94.81**   **Water transport accident involving military watercraft**

● **V94.810**   **Civilian watercraft involved in water transport accident with military watercraft**

Passenger on civilian watercraft injured due to accident with military watercraft

● **V94.811**   **Civilian in water injured by military watercraft**

● **V94.818**   **Other water transport accident involving military watercraft**

X● **V94.89**   **Other water transport accident**

X● **V94.9**   **Unspecified water transport accident**

Water transport accident NOS

AIR AND SPACE TRANSPORT ACCIDENTS (V95-V97)

    Excludes1   military aircraft accidents in military or war operations (Y36, Y37)

● **V95**   **Accident to powered aircraft causing injury to occupant**

The appropriate 7th character is to be added to each code from category V95

A	initial encounter
D	subsequent encounter
S	sequela

● **V95.0**   **Helicopter accident injuring occupant**

X● **V95.00**   **Unspecified helicopter accident injuring occupant**

X● **V95.01**   **Helicopter crash injuring occupant**

X● **V95.02**   **Forced landing of helicopter injuring occupant**

X● **V95.03**   **Helicopter collision injuring occupant**

Helicopter collision with any object, fixed, movable or moving

X● **V95.04**   **Helicopter fire injuring occupant**

X● **V95.05**   **Helicopter explosion injuring occupant**

X● **V95.09**   **Other helicopter accident injuring occupant**

● **V95.1**   **Ultralight, microlight or powered-glider accident injuring occupant**

X● **V95.10**   **Unspecified ultralight, microlight or powered-glider accident injuring occupant**

X● **V95.11**   **Ultralight, microlight or powered-glider crash injuring occupant**

X● **V95.12**   **Forced landing of ultralight, microlight or powered-glider injuring occupant**

X● **V95.13**   **Ultralight, microlight or powered-glider collision injuring occupant**

Ultralight, microlight or powered-glider collision with any object, fixed, movable or moving

X● **V95.14**   **Ultralight, microlight or powered-glider fire injuring occupant**

X● **V95.15**   **Ultralight, microlight or powered-glider explosion injuring occupant**

X● **V95.19**   **Other ultralight, microlight or powered-glider accident injuring occupant**

● **V95.2**   **Other private fixed-wing aircraft accident injuring occupant**

N   Newborn Age: 0   P   Pediatric Age: 0–17   M   Maternity DX: 9–64   A   Adult Age: 15–124   ♀   Females Only   ♂   Males Only

🅒 Complication\Comorbidity   🅜 Major C\C   ⒺⓍ CC/MCC Exclusions   🅗 Hospital-Acquired Condition   🅗 Hierarchical Condition Category

1569

X ● **V95.20**   **Unspecified** accident to other private fixed-wing aircraft, injuring occupant

X ● **V95.21**   Other private fixed-wing aircraft **crash** injuring occupant

X ● **V95.22**   **Forced landing** of other private fixed-wing aircraft injuring occupant

X ● **V95.23**   Other private fixed-wing aircraft **collision** injuring occupant
     Other private fixed-wing aircraft collision with any object, fixed, movable or moving

X ● **V95.24**   Other private fixed-wing aircraft **fire** injuring occupant

X ● **V95.25**   Other private fixed-wing aircraft **explosion** injuring occupant

X ● **V95.29**   **Other** accident to other private fixed-wing aircraft injuring occupant

● **V95.3**   **Commercial fixed-wing aircraft** accident injuring occupant

X ● **V95.30**   **Unspecified** accident to commercial fixed-wing aircraft injuring occupant

X ● **V95.31**   Commercial fixed-wing aircraft **crash** injuring occupant

X ● **V95.32**   **Forced landing** of commercial fixed-wing aircraft injuring occupant

X ● **V95.33**   Commercial fixed-wing aircraft **collision** injuring occupant
     Commercial fixed-wing aircraft collision with any object, fixed, movable or moving

X ● **V95.34**   Commercial fixed-wing aircraft **fire** injuring occupant

X ● **V95.35**   Commercial fixed-wing aircraft **explosion** injuring occupant

X ● **V95.39**   **Other** accident to commercial fixed-wing aircraft injuring occupant

● **V95.4**   **Spacecraft** accident injuring occupant

X ● **V95.40**   **Unspecified** spacecraft accident injuring occupant

X ● **V95.41**   Spacecraft **crash** injuring occupant

X ● **V95.42**   **Forced landing** of spacecraft injuring occupant

X ● **V95.43**   Spacecraft **collision** injuring occupant
     Spacecraft collision with any object, fixed, moveable or moving

X ● **V95.44**   Spacecraft **fire** injuring occupant

X ● **V95.45**   Spacecraft **explosion** injuring occupant

X ● **V95.49**   **Other** spacecraft accident injuring occupant

X ● **V95.8**   **Other** powered aircraft accidents injuring occupant

X ● **V95.9**   **Unspecified** aircraft accident injuring occupant
     Aircraft accident NOS
     Air transport accident NOS

● **V96**   **Accident to nonpowered aircraft causing injury to occupant**
     The appropriate 7th character is to be added to each code from category V96

> A   initial encounter
> D   subsequent encounter
> S   sequela

● **V96.0**   **Balloon** accident injuring occupant

X ● **V96.00**   **Unspecified** balloon accident injuring occupant

X ● **V96.01**   **Balloon crash** injuring occupant

X ● **V96.02**   **Forced landing** of balloon injuring occupant

X ● **V96.03**   Balloon **collision** injuring occupant
     Balloon collision with any object, fixed, moveable or moving

X ● **V96.04**   Balloon **fire** injuring occupant

X ● **V96.05**   Balloon **explosion** injuring occupant

X ● **V96.09**   **Other** balloon accident injuring occupant

● **V96.1**   **Hang-glider** accident injuring occupant

X ● **V96.10**   **Unspecified** hang-glider accident injuring occupant

X ● **V96.11**   Hang-glider **crash** injuring occupant

X ● **V96.12**   **Forced landing** of hang-glider injuring occupant

X ● **V96.13**   Hang-glider **collision** injuring occupant
     Hang-glider collision with any object, fixed, moveable or moving

X ● **V96.14**   Hang-glider **fire** injuring occupant

X ● **V96.15**   Hang-glider **explosion** injuring occupant

X ● **V96.19**   **Other** hang-glider accident injuring occupant

● **V96.2**   **Glider** (nonpowered) accident injuring occupant

X ● **V96.20**   **Unspecified** glider (nonpowered) accident injuring occupant

X ● **V96.21**   Glider (nonpowered) **crash** injuring occupant

X ● **V96.22**   **Forced landing** of glider (nonpowered) injuring occupant

X ● **V96.23**   Glider (nonpowered) **collision** injuring occupant
     Glider (nonpowered) collision with any object, fixed, moveable or moving

X ● **V96.24**   Glider (nonpowered) **fire** injuring occupant

X ● **V96.25**   Glider (nonpowered) **explosion** injuring occupant

X ● **V96.29**   **Other** glider (nonpowered) accident injuring occupant

X ● **V96.8**   **Other** nonpowered-aircraft accidents injuring occupant
     Kite carrying a person accident injuring occupant

X ● **V96.9**   **Unspecified** nonpowered-aircraft accident injuring occupant
     Nonpowered-aircraft accident NOS

● **V97**   **Other specified air transport accidents**
     The appropriate 7th character is to be added to each code from category V97

> A   initial encounter
> D   subsequent encounter
> S   sequela

X ● **V97.0**   **Occupant of aircraft injured in other specified air transport accidents**
     Fall in, on or from aircraft in air transport accident
     Excludes1   accident while boarding or alighting aircraft (V97.1)

X ● **V97.1**   **Person injured while boarding or alighting from aircraft**

● **V97.2**   **Parachutist accident**

X ● **V97.21**   Parachutist **entangled in object**
     Parachutist landing in tree

X ● **V97.22**   Parachutist **injured on landing**

X ● **V97.29**   **Other** parachutist accident

● **V97.3**   **Person on ground injured in air transport accident**

X ● **V97.31**   **Hit by object falling from aircraft**
     Hit by crashing aircraft
     Injured by aircraft hitting house
     Injured by aircraft hitting car

X ● **V97.32**   **Injured by rotating propeller**

X ● **V97.33**   **Sucked into jet engine**

X ● **V97.39**   **Other injury to person on ground due to air transport accident**

● **V97.8**   **Other air transport accidents, not elsewhere classified**

▶ New   ⇛ Revised   ~~deleted~~ Deleted   Excludes 1   Excludes 2   Includes   Use additional   Code first   Code also   Key words

OGCR Official Guidelines   ● Unacceptable Principal Diagnosis   X Assign placeholder X   ● Use Additional Character(s)   ▷ Manifestation Code   **Coding Clinic**

Excludes1   aircraft accident NOS (V95.9)
exposure to changes in air pressure during ascent or descent (W94.-)

● **V97.81**   **Air transport accident involving military aircraft**

  ● **V97.810**   **Civilian aircraft involved in air transport accident with military aircraft**

     Passenger in civilian aircraft injured due to accident with military aircraft

  ● **V97.811**   **Civilian injured by military aircraft**

  ● **V97.818**   **Other air transport accident involving military aircraft**

X● **V97.89**   **Other air transport accidents, not elsewhere classified**

     Injury from machinery on aircraft

OTHER AND UNSPECIFIED TRANSPORT ACCIDENTS (V98-V99)

Excludes1   vehicle accident, type of vehicle unspecified (V89.-)

● **V98**   **Other specified transport accidents**

The appropriate 7th character is to be added to each code from category V98

A	initial encounter
D	subsequent encounter
S	sequela

X● **V98.0**   **Accident to, on or involving cable-car, not on rails**
Caught or dragged by cable-car, not on rails
Fall or jump from cable-car, not on rails
Object thrown from or in cable-car, not on rails

X● **V98.1**   **Accident to, on or involving land-yacht**

X● **V98.2**   **Accident to, on or involving ice yacht**

X● **V98.3**   **Accident to, on or involving ski lift**
Accident to, on or involving ski chair-lift
Accident to, on or involving ski lift with gondola

X● **V98.8**   **Other specified transport accidents**

X● **V99**   **Unspecified transport accident**

The appropriate 7th character is to be added to code V99

A	initial encounter
D	subsequent encounter
S	sequela

OTHER EXTERNAL CAUSES OF ACCIDENTAL INJURY (W00-X58)

SLIPPING, TRIPPING, STUMBLING AND FALLS (W00-W19)

Excludes1   assault involving a fall (Y01-Y02)
fall from animal (V80.-)
fall (in) (from) machinery (in operation) (W28-W31)
fall (in) (from) transport vehicle (V01-V99)
intentional self-harm involving a fall (X80-X81)

Excludes2   at risk for fall (history of fall) Z91.81
fall (in) (from) burning building (X00.-)
fall into fire (X00-X04, X08)

● **W00**   **Fall due to ice and snow**

Includes   pedestrian on foot falling (slipping) on ice and snow

Excludes1   fall on (from) ice and snow involving pedestrian conveyance (V00.-)
fall from stairs and steps not due to ice and snow (W10.-)

The appropriate 7th character is to be added to each code from category W00

A	initial encounter
D	subsequent encounter
S	sequela

X● **W00.0**   **Fall on same level due to ice and snow**
Coding Clinic: 2016, Q2, P5

X● **W00.1**   **Fall from stairs and steps due to ice and snow**

X● **W00.2**   **Other fall from one level to another due to ice and snow**

X● **W00.9**   **Unspecified fall due to ice and snow**

● **W01**   **Fall on same level from slipping, tripping and stumbling**

Includes   fall on moving sidewalk

Excludes1   fall due to bumping (striking) against object (W18.0-)
fall in shower or bathtub (W18.2-)
fall on same level NOS (W18.30)
fall on same level from slipping, tripping and stumbling due to ice or snow (W00.0)
fall off or from toilet (W18.1-)
slipping, tripping and stumbling NOS (W18.40)
slipping, tripping and stumbling without falling (W18.4-)

The appropriate 7th character is to be added to each code from category W01

A	initial encounter
D	subsequent encounter
S	sequela

X● **W01.0**   **Fall on same level from slipping, tripping and stumbling without subsequent striking against object**
Falling over animal

● **W01.1**   **Fall on same level from slipping, tripping and stumbling with subsequent striking against object**

  X● **W01.10**   **Fall on same level from slipping, tripping and stumbling with subsequent striking against unspecified object**

  ● **W01.11**   **Fall on same level from slipping, tripping and stumbling with subsequent striking against sharp object**

    ● **W01.110**   **Fall on same level from slipping, tripping and stumbling with subsequent striking against sharp glass**

    ● **W01.111**   **Fall on same level from slipping, tripping and stumbling with subsequent striking against power tool or machine**

    ● **W01.118**   **Fall on same level from slipping, tripping and stumbling with subsequent striking against other sharp object**

    ● **W01.119**   **Fall on same level from slipping, tripping and stumbling with subsequent striking against unspecified sharp object**

N Newborn Age: 0   **P** Pediatric Age: 0–17   **M** Maternity DX: 9–64   **A** Adult Age: 15–124   ♀ Females Only   ♂ Males Only

Complication\Comorbidity   Major C\C   (Ex) CC/MCC Exclusions   Hospital-Acquired Condition   Hierarchical Condition Category

1571

CHAPTER 20 (V00-Y99)

● **W01.19 Fall on same level from slipping, tripping and stumbling with subsequent striking against other object**

  ● **W01.190 Fall on same level from slipping, tripping and stumbling with subsequent striking against furniture**

Coding Clinic: 2021, Q1, P5

  ● **W01.198 Fall on same level from slipping, tripping and stumbling with subsequent striking against other object**

X● **W03 Other fall on same level due to collision with another person**

Fall due to non-transport collision with other person

Excludes1   collision with another person without fall (W51)
crushed or pushed by a crowd or human stampede (W52)
fall involving pedestrian conveyance (V00-V09)
fall due to ice or snow (W00)
fall on same level NOS (W18.30)

The appropriate 7th character is to be added to code W03

A	initial encounter
D	subsequent encounter
S	sequela

Coding Clinic: 2015, Q1, P9-10; 2012, Q4, P108

X● **W04 Fall while being carried or supported by other persons**

Accidentally dropped while being carried

The appropriate 7th character is to be added to code W04

A	initial encounter
D	subsequent encounter
S	sequel

● **W05 Fall from non-moving wheelchair, nonmotorized scooter and motorized mobility scooter**

Excludes1   fall from moving wheelchair (powered) (V00.811)
fall from moving motorized mobility scooter (V00.831)
fall from nonmotorized scooter (V00.141)

The appropriate 7th character is to be added to each code from category W05

A	initial encounter
D	subsequent encounter
S	sequela

  X● **W05.0 Fall from non-moving wheelchair**

Coding Clinic: 2019, Q2, P27

  X● **W05.1 Fall from non-moving nonmotorized scooter**

  X● **W05.2 Fall from non-moving motorized mobility scooter**

X● **W06 Fall from bed**

The appropriate 7th character is to be added to code W06

A	initial encounter
D	subsequent encounter
S	sequela

X● **W07 Fall from chair**

The appropriate 7th character is to be added to code W07

A	initial encounter
D	subsequent encounter
S	sequela

X● **W08 Fall from other furniture**

The appropriate 7th character is to be added to code W08

A	initial encounter
D	subsequent encounter
S	sequela

● **W09 Fall on and from playground equipment**

Excludes1   fall involving recreational machinery (W31)

The appropriate 7th character is to be added to each code from category W09

A	initial encounter
D	subsequent encounter
S	sequela

X● **W09.0 Fall on or from playground slide**

X● **W09.1 Fall from playground swing**

X● **W09.2 Fall on or from jungle gym**

X● **W09.8 Fall on or from other playground equipment**

● **W10 Fall on and from stairs and steps**

Excludes1   fall from stairs and steps due to ice and snow (W00.1)

The appropriate 7th character is to be added to each code from category W10

A	initial encounter
D	subsequent encounter
S	sequela

X● **W10.0 Fall (on) (from) escalator**

X● **W10.1 Fall (on) (from) sidewalk curb**

X● **W10.2 Fall (on) (from) incline**

Fall (on) (from) ramp

X● **W10.8 Fall (on) (from) other stairs and steps**

X● **W10.9 Fall (on) (from) unspecified stairs and steps**

X● **W11 Fall on and from ladder**

The appropriate 7th character is to be added to code W11

A	initial encounter
D	subsequent encounter
S	sequela

X● **W12 Fall on and from scaffolding**

The appropriate 7th character is to be added to code W12

A	initial encounter
D	subsequent encounter
S	sequela

● **W13 Fall from, out of or through building or structure**

The appropriate 7th character is to be added to each code from category W13

A	initial encounter
D	subsequent encounter
S	sequela

X● **W13.0 Fall from, out of or through balcony**

Fall from, out of or through railing

X● **W13.1 Fall from, out of or through bridge**

X● **W13.2 Fall from, out of or through roof**

X● **W13.3 Fall through floor**

X● **W13.4 Fall from, out of or through window**

   Excludes2   fall with subsequent striking against sharp glass (W01.110-)

X● **W13.8 Fall from, out of or through other building or structure**

Fall from, out of or through viaduct
Fall from, out of or through wall
Fall from, out of or through flag-pole

X● **W13.9 Fall from, out of or through building, not otherwise specified**

Excludes1   collapse of a building or structure (W20.-)
fall or jump from burning building or structure (X00.-)

▶ New   ⇒ Revised   ~~deleted~~ Deleted   Excludes 1   Excludes 2   Includes   Use additional   Code first   Code also   Key words

OGCR Official Guidelines   ● Unacceptable Principal Diagnosis   X Assign placeholder X   ● Use Additional Character(s)   ▶ Manifestation Code   Coding Clinic

X● **W14   Fall from tree**

The appropriate 7th character is to be added to code W14

A	initial encounter
D	subsequent encounter
S	sequela

X● **W15   Fall from cliff**

The appropriate 7th character is to be added to code W15

A	initial encounter
D	subsequent encounter
S	sequela

● **W16   Fall, jump or diving into water**

> **Excludes1**   accidental non-watercraft drowning and
> submersion not involving fall (W65-W74)
> effects of air pressure from diving (W94.-)
> fall into water from watercraft (V90-V94)
> hitting an object or against bottom when falling
> from watercraft (V94.0)
>
> **Excludes2**   striking or hitting diving board (W21.4)

The appropriate 7th character is to be added to each code from
category W16

A	initial encounter
D	subsequent encounter
S	sequela

● **W16.0   Fall into swimming pool**

Fall into swimming pool NOS

> **Excludes1**   fall into empty swimming pool (W17.3)

   ● **W16.01   Fall into swimming pool striking water surface**

     ● **W16.011   Fall into swimming pool striking water surface causing drowning and submersion**

> **Excludes1**   drowning and submersion while in swimming pool without fall (W67)

     ● **W16.012   Fall into swimming pool striking water surface causing other injury**

   ● **W16.02   Fall into swimming pool striking bottom**

     ● **W16.021   Fall into swimming pool striking bottom causing drowning and submersion**

> **Excludes1**   drowning and submersion while in swimming pool without fall (W67)

     ● **W16.022   Fall into swimming pool striking bottom causing other injury**

   ● **W16.03   Fall into swimming pool striking wall**

     ● **W16.031   Fall into swimming pool striking wall causing drowning and submersion**

> **Excludes1**   drowning and submersion while in swimming pool without fall (W67)

     ● **W16.032   Fall into swimming pool striking wall causing other injury**

● **W16.1   Fall into natural body of water**

Fall into lake
Fall into open sea
Fall into river
Fall into stream

   ● **W16.11   Fall into natural body of water striking water surface**

     ● **W16.111   Fall into natural body of water striking water surface causing drowning and submersion**

> **Excludes1**   drowning and submersion while in natural body of water without fall (W69)

     ● **W16.112   Fall into natural body of water striking water surface causing other injury**

   ● **W16.12   Fall into natural body of water striking bottom**

     ● **W16.121   Fall into natural body of water striking bottom causing drowning and submersion**

> **Excludes1**   drowning and submersion while in natural body of water without fall (W69)

     ● **W16.122   Fall into natural body of water striking bottom causing other injury**

   ● **W16.13   Fall into natural body of water striking side**

     ● **W16.131   Fall into natural body of water striking side causing drowning and submersion**

> **Excludes1**   drowning and submersion while in natural body of water without fall (W69)

     ● **W16.132   Fall into natural body of water striking side causing other injury**

● **W16.2   Fall in (into) filled bathtub or bucket of water**

   ● **W16.21   Fall in (into) filled bathtub**

> **Excludes1**   fall into empty bathtub (W18.2)

     ● **W16.211   Fall in (into) filled bathtub causing drowning and submersion**

> **Excludes1**   drowning and submersion while in filled bathtub without fall (W65)

     ● **W16.212   Fall in (into) filled bathtub causing other injury**

   ● **W16.22   Fall in (into) bucket of water**

     ● **W16.221   Fall in (into) bucket of water causing drowning and submersion**

     ● **W16.222   Fall in (into) bucket of water causing other injury**

CHAPTER 20 (V00-Y99)

N Newborn Age: 0   **P** Pediatric Age: 0–17   **M** Maternity DX: 9–64   **A** Adult Age: 15–124   ♀ Females Only   ♂ Males Only

Complication\Comorbidity   Major C\C   (Ex) CC/MCC Exclusions   Hospital-Acquired Condition   Hierarchical Condition Category

1573

● W16.3   **Fall into other water**
     Fall into fountain
     Fall into reservoir

● W16.31   **Fall into other water striking water surface**

● W16.311   **Fall into other water striking water surface causing drowning and submersion**
     Excludes1   drowning and submersion while in other water without fall (W73)

● W16.312   **Fall into other water striking water surface causing other injury**

● W16.32   **Fall into other water striking bottom**

● W16.321   **Fall into other water striking bottom causing drowning and submersion**
     Excludes1   drowning and submersion while in other water without fall (W73)

● W16.322   **Fall into other water striking bottom causing other injury**

● W16.33   **Fall into other water striking wall**

● W16.331   **Fall into other water striking wall causing drowning and submersion**
     Excludes1   drowning and submersion while in other water without fall (W73)

● W16.332   **Fall into other water striking wall causing other injury**

● W16.4   **Fall into unspecified water**

X ● W16.41   **Fall into unspecified water causing drowning and submersion**

X ● W16.42   **Fall into unspecified water causing other injury**

● W16.5   **Jumping or diving into swimming pool**

● W16.51   **Jumping or diving into swimming pool striking water surface**

● W16.511   **Jumping or diving into swimming pool striking water surface causing drowning and submersion**
     Excludes1   drowning and submersion while in swimming pool without jumping or diving (W67)

● W16.512   **Jumping or diving into swimming pool striking water surface causing other injury**

● W16.52   **Jumping or diving into swimming pool striking bottom**

● W16.521   **Jumping or diving into swimming pool striking bottom causing drowning and submersion**
     Excludes1   drowning and submersion while in swimming pool without jumping or diving (W67)

● W16.522   **Jumping or diving into swimming pool striking bottom causing other injury**

● W16.53   **Jumping or diving into swimming pool striking wall**

● W16.531   **Jumping or diving into swimming pool striking wall causing drowning and submersion**
     Excludes1   drowning and submersion while in swimming pool without jumping or diving (W67)

● W16.532   **Jumping or diving into swimming pool striking wall causing other injury**

● W16.6   **Jumping or diving into natural body of water**
     Jumping or diving into lake
     Jumping or diving into open sea
     Jumping or diving into river
     Jumping or diving into stream

● W16.61   **Jumping or diving into natural body of water striking water surface**

● W16.611   **Jumping or diving into natural body of water striking water surface causing drowning and submersion**
     Excludes1   drowning and submersion while in natural body of water without jumping or diving (W69)

● W16.612   **Jumping or diving into natural body of water striking water surface causing other injury**

● W16.62   **Jumping or diving into natural body of water striking bottom**

● W16.621   **Jumping or diving into natural body of water striking bottom causing drowning and submersion**
     Excludes1   drowning and submersion while in natural body of water without jumping or diving (W69)

● W16.622   **Jumping or diving into natural body of water striking bottom causing other injury**

● W16.7   **Jumping or diving from boat**
     Excludes1   fall from boat into water - see watercraft accident (V90-V94)

● W16.71   **Jumping or diving from boat striking water surface**

● W16.711   **Jumping or diving from boat striking water surface causing drowning and submersion**

● W16.712   **Jumping or diving from boat striking water surface causing other injury**

● W16.72   **Jumping or diving from boat striking bottom**

● W16.721   **Jumping or diving from boat striking bottom causing drowning and submersion**

● W16.722   **Jumping or diving from boat striking bottom causing other injury**

▶ New   ⇒ Revised   ~~deleted~~ Deleted   Excludes 1   Excludes 2   Includes   Use additional   Code first   Code also   Key words

OGCR Official Guidelines   ● Unacceptable Principal Diagnosis   X Assign placeholder X   ● Use Additional Character(s)   ▷ Manifestation Code   **Coding Clinic**

● **W16.8 Jumping or diving into other water**
        Jumping or diving into fountain
        Jumping or diving into reservoir
    ● **W16.81 Jumping or diving into other water striking water surface**
        ● **W16.811 Jumping or diving into other water striking water surface causing drowning and submersion**
           Excludes1   drowning and submersion while in other water without jumping or diving (W73)
        ● **W16.812 Jumping or diving into other water striking water surface causing other injury**
    ● **W16.82 Jumping or diving into other water striking bottom**
        ● **W16.821 Jumping or diving into other water striking bottom causing drowning and submersion**
           Excludes1   drowning and submersion while in other water without jumping or diving (W73)
        ● **W16.822 Jumping or diving into other water striking bottom causing other injury**
    ● **W16.83 Jumping or diving into other water striking wall**
        ● **W16.831 Jumping or diving into other water striking wall causing drowning and submersion**
           Excludes1   drowning and submersion while in other water without jumping or diving (W73)
        ● **W16.832 Jumping or diving into other water striking wall causing other injury**
    ● **W16.9 Jumping or diving into unspecified water**
     X ● **W16.91 Jumping or diving into unspecified water causing drowning and submersion**
     X ● **W16.92 Jumping or diving into unspecified water causing other injury**

◐ **W17 Other fall from one level to another**
      The appropriate 7th character is to be added to each code from category W17

A	initial encounter
D	subsequent encounter
S	sequela

  X ● **W17.0 Fall into well**
  X ● **W17.1 Fall into storm drain or manhole**
  X ● **W17.2 Fall into hole**
        Fall into pit
  X ● **W17.3 Fall into empty swimming pool**
        Excludes1   fall into filled swimming pool (W16.0-)
  X ● **W17.4 Fall from dock**
    ● **W17.8 Other fall from one level to another**
     X ● **W17.81 Fall down embankment (hill)**
     X ● **W17.82 Fall from (out of) grocery cart**
         Fall due to grocery cart tipping over
     X ● **W17.89 Other fall from one level to another**
         Fall from cherry picker
         Fall from lifting device
         Fall from mobile elevated work platform [MEWP]
         Fall from sky lift
         Coding Clinic: 2015, Q2, P6

● **W18 Other slipping, tripping and stumbling and falls**
      The appropriate 7th character is to be added to each code from category W18

A	initial encounter
D	subsequent encounter
S	sequela

    ● **W18.0 Fall due to bumping against object**
        Striking against object with subsequent fall
        Excludes1   fall on same level due to slipping, tripping, or stumbling with subsequent striking against object (W01.1-)
     X ● **W18.00 Striking against unspecified object with subsequent fall**
     X ● **W18.01 Striking against sports equipment with subsequent fall**
     X ● **W18.02 Striking against glass with subsequent fall**
     X ● **W18.09 Striking against other object with subsequent fall**
    ● **W18.1 Fall from or off toilet**
     X ● **W18.11 Fall from or off toilet without subsequent striking against object**
         Fall from (off) toilet NOS
     X ● **W18.12 Fall from or off toilet with subsequent striking against object**
   X ● **W18.2 Fall in (into) shower or empty bathtub**
        Excludes1   fall in full bathtub causing drowning or submersion (W16.21-)
    ● **W18.3 Other and unspecified fall on same level**
     X ● **W18.30 Fall on same level, unspecified**
     X ● **W18.31 Fall on same level due to stepping on an object**
         Fall on same level due to stepping on an animal
         Excludes1   slipping, tripping and stumbling without fall due to stepping on animal (W18.41)
     X ● **W18.39 Other fall on same level**
    ● **W18.4 Slipping, tripping and stumbling without falling**
        Excludes1   collision with another person without fall (W51)
     X ● **W18.40 Slipping, tripping and stumbling without falling, unspecified**
     X ● **W18.41 Slipping, tripping and stumbling without falling due to stepping on object**
         Slipping, tripping and stumbling without falling due to stepping on animal
         Excludes1   slipping, tripping and stumbling with fall due to stepping on animal (W18.31)
     X ● **W18.42 Slipping, tripping and stumbling without falling due to stepping into hole or opening**
     X ● **W18.43 Slipping, tripping and stumbling without falling due to stepping from one level to another**
     X ● **W18.49 Other slipping, tripping and stumbling without falling**

X ● **W19 Unspecified fall**
      Accidental fall NOS
      The appropriate 7th character is to be added to code W19

A	initial encounter
D	subsequent encounter
S	sequela

      Coding Clinic: 2021, Q2, P5; 2012, Q4, P95

N Newborn Age: 0   **P** Pediatric Age: 0–17   **M** Maternity DX: 9–64   **A** Adult Age: 15–124   ♀ Females Only   ♂ Males Only

🔲 Complication\Comorbidity   🔲 Major C\C   (Ex) CC/MCC Exclusions   🔲 Hospital-Acquired Condition   🔲 Hierarchical Condition Category

EXPOSURE TO INANIMATE MECHANICAL FORCES (W20-W49)

> **Excludes1**   assault (X92-Y09)
> contact or collision with animals or persons
>   (W50-W64)
> exposure to inanimate mechanical forces
>   involving military or war operations (Y36.-,
>   Y37.-)
> intentional self-harm (X71-X83)

Coding Clinic: 2016, Q4, P129

● **W20   Struck by thrown, projected or falling object**
> *Code first any associated:*
> cataclysm (X34-X39)
> lightning strike (T75.00)

> **Excludes1**   falling object in machinery accident (W24,
>   W28-W31)
> falling object in transport accident (V01-V99)
> object set in motion by explosion (W35-W40)
> object set in motion by firearm (W32-W34)
> struck by thrown sports equipment (W21.-)

The appropriate 7th character is to be added to each code from
category W20

> A   initial encounter
> D   subsequent encounter
> S   sequela

X● **W20.0   Struck by falling object in cave-in**
> **Excludes2**   asphyxiation due to cave-in (T71.21)

X● **W20.1   Struck by object due to collapse of building**
> **Excludes1**   struck by object due to collapse of
>   burning building (X00.2, X02.2)

X● **W20.8   Other cause of strike by thrown, projected or falling
object**
> **Excludes1**   struck by thrown sports equipment
>   (W21.-)

● **W21   Striking against or struck by sports equipment**
> **Excludes1**   assault with sports equipment (Y08.0-)
> striking against or struck by sports equipment
>   with subsequent fall (W18.01)

The appropriate 7th character is to be added to each code from
category W21

> A   initial encounter
> D   subsequent encounter
> S   sequela

● **W21.0   Struck by hit or thrown ball**
X● **W21.00   Struck by hit or thrown ball, unspecified type**
X● **W21.01   Struck by football**
X● **W21.02   Struck by soccer ball**
X● **W21.03   Struck by baseball**
X● **W21.04   Struck by golf ball**
X● **W21.05   Struck by basketball**
X● **W21.06   Struck by volleyball**
X● **W21.07   Struck by softball**
X● **W21.09   Struck by other hit or thrown ball**
● **W21.1   Struck by bat, racquet or club**
X● **W21.11   Struck by baseball bat**
X● **W21.12   Struck by tennis racquet**
X● **W21.13   Struck by golf club**
X● **W21.19   Struck by other bat, racquet or club**
● **W21.2   Struck by hockey stick or puck**
● **W21.21   Struck by hockey stick**
● **W21.210   Struck by ice hockey stick**
● **W21.211   Struck by field hockey stick**

● **W21.22   Struck by hockey puck**
● **W21.220   Struck by ice hockey puck**
● **W21.221   Struck by field hockey puck**
● **W21.3   Struck by sports foot wear**
X● **W21.31   Struck by shoe cleats**
> Stepped on by shoe cleats
X● **W21.32   Struck by skate blades**
> Skated over by skate blades
X● **W21.39   Struck by other sports foot wear**
X● **W21.4   Striking against diving board**
> Use additional code for subsequent falling into water, if
> applicable (W16.-)
● **W21.8   Striking against or struck by other sports equipment**
X● **W21.81   Striking against or struck by football helmet**
X● **W21.89   Striking against or struck by other sports
equipment**
X● **W21.9   Striking against or struck by unspecified sports
equipment**

● **W22   Striking against or struck by other objects**
> **Excludes1**   striking against or struck by object with
>   subsequent fall (W18.09)

The appropriate 7th character is to be added to each code from
category W22

> A   initial encounter
> D   subsequent encounter
> S   sequela

● **W22.0   Striking against stationary object**
> **Excludes1**   striking against stationary sports
>   equipment (W21.8)
X● **W22.01   Walked into wall**
X● **W22.02   Walked into lamppost**
X● **W22.03   Walked into furniture**
● **W22.04   Striking against wall of swimming pool**
● **W22.041   Striking against wall of swimming
pool causing drowning and
submersion**
> **Excludes1**   drowning and
>   submersion
>   while swimming
>   without striking
>   against wall
>   (W67)

● **W22.042   Striking against wall of swimming
pool causing other injury**
X● **W22.09   Striking against other stationary object**
● **W22.1   Striking against or struck by automobile airbag**
X● **W22.10   Striking against or struck by unspecified
automobile airbag**
X● **W22.11   Striking against or struck by driver side
automobile airbag**
X● **W22.12   Striking against or struck by front passenger
side automobile airbag**
X● **W22.19   Striking against or struck by other automobile
airbag**
X● **W22.8   Striking against or struck by other objects**
> Striking against or struck by object NOS
> **Excludes1**   struck by thrown, projected or falling
>   object (W20.-)

▶ New   ⇒ Revised   ~~deleted~~ Deleted   Excludes 1   Excludes 2   Includes   Use additional   Code first   Code also   Key words
OGCR Official Guidelines   ● Unacceptable Principal Diagnosis   X Assign placeholder X   ● Use Additional Character(s)   ▌ Manifestation Code   Coding Clinic

● **W23 Caught, crushed, jammed or pinched in or between objects**

     Excludes1   injury caused by cutting or piercing instruments (W25-W27)

                  injury caused by firearms malfunction (W32.1, W33.1-, W34.1-)

                  injury caused by lifting and transmission devices (W24.-)

                  injury caused by machinery (W28-W31)

                  injury caused by nonpowered hand tools (W27.-)

                  injury caused by transport vehicle being used as a means of transportation (V01-V99)

                  injury caused by struck by thrown, projected or falling object (W20.-)

     The appropriate 7th character is to be added to each code from category W23

A	initial encounter
D	subsequent encounter
S	sequela

   X● **W23.0 Caught, crushed, jammed, or pinched between moving objects**

   X● **W23.1 Caught, crushed, jammed, or pinched between stationary objects**

● **W24 Contact with lifting and transmission devices, not elsewhere classified**

     Excludes1   transport accidents (V01-V99)

     The appropriate 7th character is to be added to each code from category W24

A	initial encounter
D	subsequent encounter
S	sequela

   X● **W24.0 Contact with lifting devices, not elsewhere classified**

       Contact with chain hoist

       Contact with drive belt

       Contact with pulley (block)

   X● **W24.1 Contact with transmission devices, not elsewhere classified**

       Contact with transmission belt or cable

X● **W25 Contact with sharp glass**

     Code first any associated:

       injury due to flying glass from explosion or firearm discharge (W32-W40)

       transport accident (V00-V99)

     ➡**Excludes1**   fall on same level due to slipping, tripping and stumbling with subsequent striking against sharp glass (W01.110-)

               ➡striking against sharp glass with subsequent fall (W18.02-)

     ➡**Excludes2**   glass embedded in skin (W45.-)

     The appropriate 7th character is to be added to code W25

A	initial encounter
D	subsequent encounter
S	sequela

● **W26 Contact with other sharp objects**

     ➡**Excludes2**   sharp object(s) embedded in skin (W45.-)

     The appropriate 7th character is to be added to each code from category W26

A	initial encounter
D	subsequent encounter
S	sequela

     Coding Clinic: 2016, Q4, P73

   X● **W26.0 Contact with knife**

       Excludes1   contact with electric knife (W29.1)

   X● **W26.1 Contact with sword or dagger**

   X● **W26.2 Contact with edge of stiff paper**

       Paper cut

       Coding Clinic: 2016, Q4, P73

   X● **W26.8 Contact with other sharp object(s), not elsewhere classified**

       Contact with tin can lid

       Coding Clinic: 2016, Q4, P73

   X● **W26.9 Contact with unspecified sharp object(s)**

       Coding Clinic: 2016, Q4, P73

● **W27 Contact with nonpowered hand tool**

     The appropriate 7th character is to be added to each code from category W27

A	initial encounter
D	subsequent encounter
S	sequela

   X● **W27.0 Contact with workbench tool**

       Contact with auger

       Contact with axe

       Contact with chisel

       Contact with handsaw

       Contact with screwdriver

   X● **W27.1 Contact with garden tool**

       Contact with hoe

       Contact with nonpowered lawn mower

       Contact with pitchfork

       Contact with rake

   X● **W27.2 Contact with scissors**

   X● **W27.3 Contact with needle (sewing)**

       Excludes1   contact with hypodermic needle (W46.-)

   X● **W27.4 Contact with kitchen utensil**

       Contact with fork

       Contact with ice-pick

       Contact with can-opener NOS

   X● **W27.5 Contact with paper-cutter**

   X● **W27.8 Contact with other nonpowered hand tool**

       Contact with nonpowered sewing machine

       Contact with shovel

X● **W28 Contact with powered lawn mower**

     Powered lawn mower (commercial) (residential)

     Excludes1   contact with nonpowered lawn mower (W27.1)

     Excludes2   exposure to electric current (W86.-)

     The appropriate 7th character is to be added to code W28

A	initial encounter
D	subsequent encounter
S	sequela

● **W29 Contact with other powered hand tools and household machinery**

     Excludes1   contact with commercial machinery (W31.82)

               contact with hot household appliance (X15)

               contact with nonpowered hand tool (W27.-)

               exposure to electric current (W86)

     The appropriate 7th character is to be added to each code from category W29

A	initial encounter
D	subsequent encounter
S	sequela

   X● **W29.0 Contact with powered kitchen appliance**

       Contact with blender

       Contact with can-opener

       Contact with garbage disposal

       Contact with mixer

   X● **W29.1 Contact with electric knife**

   X● **W29.2 Contact with other powered household machinery**

       Contact with electric fan

       Contact with powered dryer (clothes) (powered) (spin)

       Contact with washing-machine

       Contact with sewing machine

N Newborn Age: 0   **P** Pediatric Age: 0–17   **M** Maternity DX: 9–64   **A** Adult Age: 15–124   ♀ Females Only   ♂ Males Only

🅒 Complication\Comorbidity   🅒 Major C\C   (Ex) CC/MCC Exclusions   🅒 Hospital-Acquired Condition   🅒 Hierarchical Condition Category

1577

X● **W29.3 Contact with powered garden and outdoor hand tools and machinery**
     Contact with chainsaw
     Contact with edger
     Contact with garden cultivator (tiller)
     Contact with hedge trimmer
     Contact with other powered garden tool
     Excludes1   contact with powered lawn mower (W28)

X● **W29.4 Contact with nail gun**

X● **W29.8 Contact with other powered hand tools and household machinery**
     Contact with do-it-yourself tool NOS

● **W30 Contact with agricultural machinery**
     Includes   animal-powered farm machine
     Excludes1   agricultural transport vehicle accident (V01-V99)
          explosion of grain store (W40.8)
          exposure to electric current (W86.-)

     The appropriate 7th character is to be added to each code from category W30

          A   initial encounter
          D   subsequent encounter
          S   sequela

X● **W30.0 Contact with combine harvester**
     Contact with reaper
     Contact with thresher

X● **W30.1 Contact with power take-off devices (PTO)**

X● **W30.2 Contact with hay derrick**

X● **W30.3 Contact with grain storage elevator**
     Excludes1   explosion of grain store (W40.8)

● **W30.8 Contact with other specified agricultural machinery**

X● **W30.81 Contact with agricultural transport vehicle in stationary use**
     Contact with agricultural transport vehicle under repair, not on public roadway
     Excludes1   agricultural transport vehicle accident (V01-V99)

X● **W30.89 Contact with other specified agricultural machinery**

X● **W30.9 Contact with unspecified agricultural machinery**
     Contact with farm machinery NOS

● **W31 Contact with other and unspecified machinery**
     Excludes1   contact with agricultural machinery (W30.-)
          contact with machinery in transport under own power or being towed by a vehicle (V01-V99)
          exposure to electric current (W86)

     The appropriate 7th character is to be added to each code from category W31

          A   initial encounter
          D   subsequent encounter
          S   sequela

X● **W31.0 Contact with mining and earth-drilling machinery**
     Contact with bore or drill (land) (seabed)
     Contact with shaft hoist
     Contact with shaft lift
     Contact with undercutter

X● **W31.1 Contact with metalworking machines**
     Contact with abrasive wheel
     Contact with forging machine
     Contact with lathe
     Contact with mechanical shears
     Contact with metal drilling machine
     Contact with milling machine
     Contact with power press
     Contact with rolling-mill
     Contact with metal sawing machine

X● **W31.2 Contact with powered woodworking and forming machines**
     Contact with band saw
     Contact with bench saw
     Contact with circular saw
     Contact with molding machine
     Contact with overhead plane
     Contact with powered saw
     Contact with radial saw
     Contact with sander
     Excludes1   nonpowered woodworking tools (W27.0)

X● **W31.3 Contact with prime movers**
     Contact with gas turbine
     Contact with internal combustion engine
     Contact with steam engine
     Contact with water driven turbine

● **W31.8 Contact with other specified machinery**

X● **W31.81 Contact with recreational machinery**
     Contact with roller-coaster

X● **W31.82 Contact with other commercial machinery**
     Contact with commercial electric fan
     Contact with commercial kitchen appliances
     Contact with commercial powered dryer (clothes) (powered) (spin)
     Contact with commercial washing-machine
     Contact with commercial sewing machine
     Excludes1   contact with household machinery (W29.-)
          contact with powered lawn mower (W28)

X● **W31.83 Contact with special construction vehicle in stationary use**
     Contact with special construction vehicle under repair, not on public roadway
     Excludes1   special construction vehicle accident (V01-V99)

X● **W31.89 Contact with other specified machinery**

X● **W31.9 Contact with unspecified machinery**
     Contact with machinery NOS

● **W32 Accidental handgun discharge and malfunction**
     Includes   accidental discharge and malfunction of gun for single hand use
          accidental discharge and malfunction of pistol
          accidental discharge and malfunction of revolver
          handgun discharge and malfunction NOS
     Excludes1   accidental airgun discharge and malfunction (W34.010, W34.110)
          accidental BB gun discharge and malfunction (W34.010, W34.110)
          accidental pellet gun discharge and malfunction (W34.010, W34.110)
          accidental shotgun discharge and malfunction (W33.01, W33.11)
          assault by handgun discharge (X93)
          handgun discharge involving legal intervention (Y35.0-)
          handgun discharge involving military or war operations (Y36.4-)
          intentional self-harm by handgun discharge (X72)
          Very pistol discharge and malfunction (W34.09, W34.19)

     The appropriate 7th character is to be added to each code from category W32

          A   initial encounter
          D   subsequent encounter
          S   sequela

X● **W32.0 Accidental handgun discharge**

X● **W32.1 Accidental handgun malfunction**
     Injury due to explosion of handgun (parts)
     Injury due to malfunction of mechanism or component of handgun
     Injury due to recoil of handgun
     Powder burn from handgun

▶ New   ⇒ Revised   ~~deleted~~ Deleted   Excludes 1   Excludes 2   Includes   Use additional   Code first   Code also   Key words
OGCR Official Guidelines   ● Unacceptable Principal Diagnosis   X Assign placeholder X   ● Use Additional Character(s)   ▶ Manifestation Code   **Coding Clinic**

● **W33 Accidental rifle, shotgun and larger firearm discharge and malfunction**

> **Includes**   rifle, shotgun and larger firearm discharge and malfunction NOS
>
> **Excludes1**   accidental airgun discharge and malfunction (W34.010, W34.110)
> accidental BB gun discharge and malfunction (W34.010, W34.110)
> accidental handgun discharge and malfunction (W32.-)
> accidental pellet gun discharge and malfunction (W34.010, W34.110)
> assault by rifle, shotgun and larger firearm discharge (X94)
> firearm discharge involving legal intervention (Y35.0-)
> firearm discharge involving military or war operations (Y36.4-)
> intentional self-harm by rifle, shotgun and larger firearm discharge (X73)
>
> The appropriate 7th character is to be added to each code from category W33
>
> | A | initial encounter |
> | D | subsequent encounter |
> | S | sequela |

● **W33.0 Accidental rifle, shotgun and larger firearm discharge**

X● **W33.00 Accidental discharge of unspecified larger firearm**
Discharge of unspecified larger firearm NOS

X● **W33.01 Accidental discharge of shotgun**
Discharge of shotgun NOS

X● **W33.02 Accidental discharge of hunting rifle**
Discharge of hunting rifle NOS

X● **W33.03 Accidental discharge of machine gun**
Discharge of machine gun NOS

X● **W33.09 Accidental discharge of other larger firearm**
Discharge of other larger firearm NOS

● **W33.1 Accidental rifle, shotgun and larger firearm malfunction**
Injury due to explosion of rifle, shotgun and larger firearm (parts)
Injury due to malfunction of mechanism or component of rifle, shotgun and larger firearm
Injury due to piercing, cutting, crushing or pinching due to (by) slide trigger mechanism, scope or other gun part
Injury due to recoil of rifle, shotgun and larger firearm
Powder burn from rifle, shotgun and larger firearm

X● **W33.10 Accidental malfunction of unspecified larger firearm**
Malfunction of unspecified larger firearm NOS

X● **W33.11 Accidental malfunction of shotgun**
Malfunction of shotgun NOS

X● **W33.12 Accidental malfunction of hunting rifle**
Malfunction of hunting rifle NOS

X● **W33.13 Accidental malfunction of machine gun**
Malfunction of machine gun NOS

X● **W33.19 Accidental malfunction of other larger firearm**
Malfunction of other larger firearm NOS

● **W34 Accidental discharge and malfunction from other and unspecified firearms and guns**

> The appropriate 7th character is to be added to each code from category W34
>
> | A | initial encounter |
> | D | subsequent encounter |
> | S | sequela |

● **W34.0 Accidental discharge from other and unspecified firearms and guns**

X● **W34.00 Accidental discharge from unspecified firearms or gun**
Discharge from firearm NOS
Gunshot wound NOS
Shot NOS
Coding Clinic: 2015, Q1, P17

● **W34.01 Accidental discharge of gas, air or spring-operated guns**

● **W34.010 Accidental discharge of airgun**
Accidental discharge of BB gun
Accidental discharge of pellet gun

● **W34.011 Accidental discharge of paintball gun**
Accidental injury due to paintball discharge

● **W34.018 Accidental discharge of other gas, air or spring-operated gun**

X● **W34.09 Accidental discharge from other specified firearms**
Accidental discharge from Very pistol [flare]

● **W34.1 Accidental malfunction from other and unspecified firearms and guns**

X● **W34.10 Accidental malfunction from unspecified firearms or gun**
Firearm malfunction NOS

● **W34.11 Accidental malfunction of gas, air or spring-operated guns**

● **W34.110 Accidental malfunction of airgun**
Accidental malfunction of BB gun
Accidental malfunction of pellet gun

● **W34.111 Accidental malfunction of paintball gun**
Accidental injury due to paintball gun malfunction

● **W34.118 Accidental malfunction of other gas, air or spring-operated gun**

X● **W34.19 Accidental malfunction from other specified firearms**
Accidental malfunction from Very pistol [flare]

X● **W35 Explosion and rupture of boiler**

> **Excludes1**   explosion and rupture of boiler on watercraft (V93.4)
>
> The appropriate 7th character is to be added to code W35
>
> | A | initial encounter |
> | D | subsequent encounter |
> | S | sequela |

● **W36 Explosion and rupture of gas cylinder**

> The appropriate 7th character is to be added to each code from category W36
>
> | A | initial encounter |
> | D | subsequent encounter |
> | S | sequela |

X● **W36.1 Explosion and rupture of aerosol can**

X● **W36.2 Explosion and rupture of air tank**

X● **W36.3 Explosion and rupture of pressurized-gas tank**

X● **W36.8 Explosion and rupture of other gas cylinder**

X● **W36.9 Explosion and rupture of unspecified gas cylinder**

CHAPTER 20 (V00-Y99)

N Newborn Age: 0   P Pediatric Age: 0–17   M Maternity DX: 9–64   A Adult Age: 15–124   ♀ Females Only   ♂ Males Only
● Complication\Comorbidity   ◐ Major C\C   (Ex) CC/MCC Exclusions   Hospital-Acquired Condition   Hierarchical Condition Category

1579

● **W37**   **Explosion and rupture of pressurized tire, pipe or hose**
     The appropriate 7th character is to be added to each code from category W37

A	initial encounter
D	subsequent encounter
S	sequela

X● **W37.0**   **Explosion of bicycle tire**

X● **W37.8**   **Explosion and rupture of other pressurized tire, pipe or hose**

X● **W38**   **Explosion and rupture of other specified pressurized devices**
     The appropriate 7th character is to be added to code W38

A	initial encounter
D	subsequent encounter
S	sequela

X● **W39**   **Discharge of firework**
     The appropriate 7th character is to be added to code W39

A	initial encounter
D	subsequent encounter
S	sequela

● **W40**   **Explosion of other materials**
     Excludes1   assault by explosive material (X96)
                     explosion involving legal intervention (Y35.1-)
                     explosion involving military or war operations (Y36.0-, Y36.2-)
                     intentional self-harm by explosive material (X75)
     The appropriate 7th character is to be added to each code from category W40

A	initial encounter
D	subsequent encounter
S	sequela

X● **W40.0**   **Explosion of blasting material**
     Explosion of blasting cap
     Explosion of detonator
     Explosion of dynamite
     Explosion of explosive (any) used in blasting operations

X● **W40.1**   **Explosion of explosive gases**
     Explosion of acetylene
     Explosion of butane
     Explosion of coal gas
     Explosion in mine NOS
     Explosion of explosive gas
     Explosion of fire damp
     Explosion of gasoline fumes
     Explosion of methane
     Explosion of propane

X● **W40.8**   **Explosion of other specified explosive materials**
     Explosion in dump NOS
     Explosion in factory NOS
     Explosion in grain store
     Explosion in munitions
       Excludes1   explosion involving legal intervention (Y35.1-)
                       explosion involving military or war operations (Y36.0-, Y36.2-)

X● **W40.9**   **Explosion of unspecified explosive materials**
     Explosion NOS

● **W42**   **Exposure to noise**
     The appropriate 7th character is to be added to each code from category W42

A	initial encounter
D	subsequent encounter
S	sequela

X● **W42.0**   **Exposure to supersonic waves**

X● **W42.9**   **Exposure to other noise**
     Exposure to sound waves NOS

● **W45**   **Foreign body or object entering through skin**
     Includes   foreign body or object embedded in skin
                 nail embedded in skin
     Excludes2   contact with hand tools (nonpowered) (powered) (W27-W29)
                 contact with other sharp object(s) (W26.-)
                 contact with sharp glass (W25.-)
                 struck by objects (W20-W22)
     The appropriate 7th character is to be added to each code from category W45

A	initial encounter
D	subsequent encounter
S	sequela

X● **W45.0**   **Nail entering through skin**

X● **W45.8**   **Other foreign body or object entering through skin**
     Splinter in skin NOS

● **W46**   **Contact with hypodermic needle**
     The appropriate 7th character is to be added to each code from category W46

A	initial encounter
D	subsequent encounter
S	sequela

X● **W46.0**   **Contact with hypodermic needle**
     Hypodermic needle stick NOS

X● **W46.1**   **Contact with contaminated hypodermic needle**

● **W49**   **Exposure to other inanimate mechanical forces**
     Includes   exposure to abnormal gravitational [G] forces
                 exposure to inanimate mechanical forces NEC
     Excludes1   exposure to inanimate mechanical forces involving military or war operations (Y36.-, Y37.-)
     The appropriate 7th character is to be added to each code from category W49

A	initial encounter
D	subsequent encounter
S	sequela

● **W49.0**   **Item causing external constriction**
   X● **W49.01**   **Hair causing external constriction**
   X● **W49.02**   **String or thread causing external constriction**
   X● **W49.03**   **Rubber band causing external constriction**
   X● **W49.04**   **Ring or other jewelry causing external constriction**
   X● **W49.09**   **Other item causing external constriction**
X● **W49.9**   **Exposure to other inanimate mechanical forces**

EXPOSURE TO ANIMATE MECHANICAL FORCES (W50-W64)

     Excludes1   toxic effect of contact with venomous animals and plants (T63.-)

● **W50**   **Accidental hit, strike, kick, twist, bite or scratch by another person**
     Includes   hit, strike, kick, twist, bite, or scratch by another person NOS
     Excludes1   assault by bodily force (Y04)
                 struck by objects (W20-W22)
     The appropriate 7th character is to be added to each code from category W50

A	initial encounter
D	subsequent encounter
S	sequela

X● **W50.0**   **Accidental hit or strike by another person**
     Hit or strike by another person NOS

X● **W50.1**   **Accidental kick by another person**
     Kick by another person NOS

▶ New   ⇒ Revised   ~~deleted~~ Deleted   Excludes 1   Excludes 2   Includes   Use additional   Code first   Code also   Key words

OGCR Official Guidelines   ● Unacceptable Principal Diagnosis   X Assign placeholder X   ● Use Additional Character(s)   ▶ Manifestation Code   Coding Clinic

X● **W50.2** **Accidental** twist **by another person**
    Twist by another person NOS
    Coding Clinic: 2015, Q1, P8

X● **W50.3** **Accidental** bite **by another person**
    Human bite
    Bite by another person NOS

X● **W50.4** **Accidental** scratch **by another person**
    Scratch by another person NOS

X● **W51** **Accidental striking against or bumped into by another person**

    Excludes1   assault by striking against or bumping into by
        another person (Y04.2)
        fall due to collision with another person (W03)

    The appropriate 7th character is to be added to code W51

A	initial encounter
D	subsequent encounter
S	sequela

X● **W52** **Crushed, pushed or stepped on by crowd or human stampede**
    Crushed, pushed or stepped on by crowd or human stampede
        with or without fall

    The appropriate 7th character is to be added to code W52

A	initial encounter
D	subsequent encounter
S	sequela

● **W53** **Contact with rodent**

    Includes   contact with saliva, feces or urine of rodent

    The appropriate 7th character is to be added to each code from
    category W53

A	initial encounter
D	subsequent encounter
S	sequela

  ● **W53.0** **Contact with** mouse
    X● **W53.01** **Bitten by mouse**
    X● **W53.09** **Other contact with mouse**

  ● **W53.1** **Contact with** rat
    X● **W53.11** **Bitten by rat**
    X● **W53.19** **Other contact with rat**

  ● **W53.2** **Contact with** squirrel
    X● **W53.21** **Bitten by squirrel**
    X● **W53.29** **Other contact with squirrel**

  ● **W53.8** **Contact with** other rodent
    X● **W53.81** **Bitten by other rodent**
    X● **W53.89** **Other contact with other rodent**

● **W54** **Contact with** dog

    Includes   contact with saliva, feces or urine of dog

    The appropriate 7th character is to be added to each code from
    category W54

A	initial encounter
D	subsequent encounter
S	sequela

  X● **W54.0** **Bitten by dog**
  X● **W54.1** **Struck by dog**
    Knocked over by dog
  X● **W54.8** **Other contact with dog**

● **W55** **Contact with other mammals**

    Includes   contact with saliva, feces or urine of mammal
    Excludes1   animal being ridden - see transport accidents
        bitten or struck by dog (W54)
        bitten or struck by rodent (W53.-)
        contact with marine mammals (W56.X-)

    The appropriate 7th character is to be added to each code from
    category W55

A	initial encounter
D	subsequent encounter
S	sequela

  ● **W55.0** **Contact with** cat
    X● **W55.01** **Bitten by cat**
    X● **W55.03** **Scratched by cat**
    X● **W55.09** **Other contact with cat**

  ● **W55.1** **Contact with** horse
    X● **W55.11** **Bitten by horse**
    X● **W55.12** **Struck by horse**
    X● **W55.19** **Other contact with horse**

  ● **W55.2** **Contact with** cow
    Contact with bull
    X● **W55.21** **Bitten by cow**
    X● **W55.22** **Struck by cow**
        Gored by bull
    X● **W55.29** **Other contact with cow**

  ● **W55.3** **Contact with** other hoof stock
    Contact with goats
    Contact with sheep
    X● **W55.31** **Bitten by other hoof stock**
    X● **W55.32** **Struck by other hoof stock**
        Gored by goat
        Gored by ram
    X● **W55.39** **Other contact with other hoof stock**

  ● **W55.4** **Contact with** pig
    X● **W55.41** **Bitten by pig**
    X● **W55.42** **Struck by pig**
    X● **W55.49** **Other contact with pig**

  ● **W55.5** **Contact with** raccoon
    X● **W55.51** **Bitten by raccoon**
    X● **W55.52** **Struck by raccoon**
    X● **W55.59** **Other contact with raccoon**

  ● **W55.8** **Contact with** other mammals
    X● **W55.81** **Bitten by other mammals**
    X● **W55.82** **Struck by other mammals**
    X● **W55.89** **Other contact with other mammals**

● **W56** **Contact with nonvenomous marine animal**

    Excludes1   contact with venomous marine animal (T63.-)

    The appropriate 7th character is to be added to each code from
    category W56

A	initial encounter
D	subsequent encounter
S	sequela

  ● **W56.0** **Contact with** dolphin
    X● **W56.01** **Bitten by dolphin**
    X● **W56.02** **Struck by dolphin**
    X● **W56.09** **Other contact with dolphin**

  ● **W56.1** **Contact with** sea lion
    X● **W56.11** **Bitten by sea lion**
    X● **W56.12** **Struck by sea lion**
    X● **W56.19** **Other contact with sea lion**

CHAPTER 20 (V00-Y99)

N Newborn Age: 0   P Pediatric Age: 0–17   M Maternity DX: 9–64   A Adult Age: 15–124   ♀ Females Only   ♂ Males Only

Complication\Comorbidity   Major C\C   (Ex:) CC/MCC Exclusions   Hospital-Acquired Condition   Hierarchical Condition Category

● W56.2   Contact with orca
     Contact with killer whale
   X● W56.21   **Bitten by orca**
   X● W56.22   **Struck by orca**
   X● W56.29   **Other contact with orca**
● W56.3   Contact with other marine mammals
   X● W56.31   **Bitten by other marine mammals**
   X● W56.32   **Struck by other marine mammals**
   X● W56.39   **Other contact with other marine mammals**
● W56.4   Contact with shark
   X● W56.41   **Bitten by shark**
   X● W56.42   **Struck by shark**
   X● W56.49   **Other contact with shark**
● W56.5   Contact with other fish
   X● W56.51   **Bitten by other fish**
   X● W56.52   **Struck by other fish**
   X● W56.59   **Other contact with other fish**
● W56.8   Contact with other nonvenomous marine animals
   X● W56.81   **Bitten by other nonvenomous marine animals**
   X● W56.82   **Struck by other nonvenomous marine animals**
   X● W56.89   **Other contact with other nonvenomous marine animals**

X● W57   **Bitten or stung by nonvenomous insect and other nonvenomous arthropods**
   Excludes1   contact with venomous insects and arthropods (T63.2-, T63.3-, T63.4-)
   The appropriate 7th character is to be added to code W57

A	initial encounter
D	subsequent encounter
S	sequela

● W58   Contact with crocodile or alligator
   The appropriate 7th character is to be added to each code from category W58

A	initial encounter
D	subsequent encounter
S	sequela

   ● W58.0   Contact with alligator
     X● W58.01   **Bitten by alligator**
     X● W58.02   **Struck by alligator**
     X● W58.03   **Crushed by alligator**
     X● W58.09   **Other contact with alligator**
   ● W58.1   Contact with crocodile
     X● W58.11   **Bitten by crocodile**
     X● W58.12   **Struck by crocodile**
     X● W58.13   **Crushed by crocodile**
     X● W58.19   **Other contact with crocodile**

● W59   Contact with other nonvenomous reptiles
   Excludes1   contact with venomous reptile (T63.0-, T63.1-)
   The appropriate 7th character is to be added to each code from category W59

A	initial encounter
D	subsequent encounter
S	sequela

   ● W59.0   Contact with nonvenomous lizards
     X● W59.01   **Bitten by nonvenomous lizards**
     X● W59.02   **Struck by nonvenomous lizards**
     X● W59.09   **Other contact with nonvenomous lizards**
       Exposure to nonvenomous lizards

● W59.1   Contact with nonvenomous snakes
   X● W59.11   **Bitten by nonvenomous snake**
   X● W59.12   **Struck by nonvenomous snake**
   X● W59.13   **Crushed by nonvenomous snake**
   X● W59.19   **Other contact with nonvenomous snake**
● W59.2   Contact with turtles
   Excludes1   contact with tortoises (W59.8-)
   X● W59.21   **Bitten by turtle**
   X● W59.22   **Struck by turtle**
   X● W59.29   **Other contact with turtle**
     Exposure to turtles
● W59.8   Contact with other nonvenomous reptiles
   X● W59.81   **Bitten by other nonvenomous reptiles**
   X● W59.82   **Struck by other nonvenomous reptiles**
   X● W59.83   **Crushed by other nonvenomous reptiles**
   X● W59.89   **Other contact with other nonvenomous reptiles**

X● W60   **Contact with nonvenomous plant thorns and spines and sharp leaves**
   Excludes1   contact with venomous plants (T63.X7-)
   The appropriate 7th character is to be added to code W60

A	initial encounter
D	subsequent encounter
S	sequela

● W61   Contact with birds (domestic) (wild)
   Includes   contact with excreta of birds
   The appropriate 7th character is to be added to each code from category W61

A	initial encounter
D	subsequent encounter
S	sequela

   ● W61.0   Contact with parrot
     X● W61.01   **Bitten by parrot**
     X● W61.02   **Struck by parrot**
     X● W61.09   **Other contact with parrot**
       Exposure to parrots
   ● W61.1   Contact with macaw
     X● W61.11   **Bitten by macaw**
     X● W61.12   **Struck by macaw**
     X● W61.19   **Other contact with macaw**
       Exposure to macaws
   ● W61.2   Contact with other psittacines
     X● W61.21   **Bitten by other psittacines**
     X● W61.22   **Struck by other psittacines**
     X● W61.29   **Other contact with other psittacines**
       Exposure to other psittacines
   ● W61.3   Contact with chicken
     X● W61.32   **Struck by chicken**
     X● W61.33   **Pecked by chicken**
     X● W61.39   **Other contact with chicken**
       Exposure to chickens
   ● W61.4   Contact with turkey
     X● W61.42   **Struck by turkey**
     X● W61.43   **Pecked by turkey**
     X● W61.49   **Other contact with turkey**
   ● W61.5   Contact with goose
     X● W61.51   **Bitten by goose**
     X● W61.52   **Struck by goose**
     X● W61.59   **Other contact with goose**

● W61.6   Contact with duck
     X ● W61.61   **Bitten by duck**
     X ● W61.62   **Struck by duck**
     X ● W61.69   **Other contact with duck**
● W61.9   Contact with other birds
     X ● W61.91   **Bitten by other birds**
     X ● W61.92   **Struck by other birds**
     X ● W61.99   **Other contact with other birds**
                 Contact with bird NOS

● W62   Contact with nonvenomous amphibians
     Excludes1   contact with venomous amphibians
                     (T63.81-R63.83)

     The appropriate 7th character is to be added to each code from
         category W62

A	initial encounter
D	subsequent encounter
S	sequela

     X ● W62.0   **Contact with nonvenomous frogs**
     X ● W62.1   **Contact with nonvenomous toads**
     X ● W62.9   **Contact with other nonvenomous amphibians**

X ● W64   Exposure to other animate mechanical forces
     Includes   exposure to nonvenomous animal NOS
     Excludes1   contact with venomous animal (T63.-)
     The appropriate 7th character is to be added to code W64

A	initial encounter
D	subsequent encounter
S	sequela

ACCIDENTAL NON-TRANSPORT DROWNING AND SUBMERSION (W65-W74)

     Excludes1   accidental drowning and submersion due to fall
                   into water (W16.-)
                   accidental drowning and submersion due to
                   water transport accident (V90.-, V92.-)
     Excludes2   accidental drowning and submersion due to
                   cataclysm (X34-X39)

X ● W65   Accidental drowning and submersion while in bathtub
     Excludes1   accidental drowning and submersion due to fall
                   in (into) bathtub (W16.211)
     The appropriate 7th character is to be added to code W65

A	initial encounter
D	subsequent encounter
S	sequela

X ● W67   Accidental drowning and submersion while in swimming pool
     Excludes1   accidental drowning and submersion due to fall
                   into swimming pool (W16.011, W16.021,
                   W16.031)
                   accidental drowning and submersion due
                   to striking into wall of swimming pool
                   (W22.041)
     The appropriate 7th character is to be added to code W67

A	initial encounter
D	subsequent encounter
S	sequela

X ● W69   Accidental drowning and submersion while in natural water
         Accidental drowning and submersion while in lake
         Accidental drowning and submersion while in open sea
         Accidental drowning and submersion while in river
         Accidental drowning and submersion while in stream
     Excludes1   accidental drowning and submersion due to
                   fall into natural body of water (W16.111,
                   W16.121, W16.131)
     The appropriate 7th character is to be added to code W69

A	initial encounter
D	subsequent encounter
S	sequela

X ● W73   Other specified cause of accidental non-transport drowning and submersion
         Accidental drowning and submersion while in quenching tank
         Accidental drowning and submersion while in reservoir
     Excludes1   accidental drowning and submersion due to
                   fall into other water (W16.311, W16.321,
                   W16.331)
     The appropriate 7th character is to be added to code W73

A	initial encounter
D	subsequent encounter
S	sequela

X ● W74   Unspecified cause of accidental drowning and submersion
         Drowning NOS
     The appropriate 7th character is to be added to code W74

A	initial encounter
D	subsequent encounter
S	sequela

EXPOSURE TO ELECTRIC CURRENT, RADIATION AND EXTREME AMBIENT AIR TEMPERATURE AND PRESSURE (W85-W99)

     Excludes1   exposure to:
                   failure in dosage of radiation or temperature
                   during surgical and medical care
                   (Y63.2-Y63.5)
                   lightning (T75.0-)
                   natural cold (X31)
                   natural heat (X30)
                   natural radiation NOS (X39)
                   radiological procedure and radiotherapy
                   (Y84.2)
                   sunlight (X32)

X ● W85   Exposure to electric transmission lines
         Broken power line
     The appropriate 7th character is to be added to code W85

A	initial encounter
D	subsequent encounter
S	sequela

● W86   Exposure to other specified electric current
     The appropriate 7th character is to be added to each code from
         category W86

A	initial encounter
D	subsequent encounter
S	sequela

     X ● W86.0   **Exposure to domestic wiring and appliances**
     X ● W86.1   **Exposure to industrial wiring, appliances and electrical machinery**
           Exposure to conductors
           Exposure to control apparatus
           Exposure to electrical equipment and machinery
           Exposure to transformers

CHAPTER 20 (V00-Y99)

X● **W86.8**   **Exposure to other electric current**
    Exposure to wiring and appliances in or on farm (not farmhouse)
    Exposure to wiring and appliances outdoors
    Exposure to wiring and appliances in or on public building
    Exposure to wiring and appliances in or on residential institutions
    Exposure to wiring and appliances in or on schools

● **W88**   **Exposure to ionizing radiation**
    Excludes1   exposure to sunlight (X32)

The appropriate 7th character is to be added to each code from category W88

A	initial encounter
D	subsequent encounter
S	sequela

X● **W88.0**   **Exposure to X-rays**
X● **W88.1**   **Exposure to radioactive isotopes**
X● **W88.8**   **Exposure to other ionizing radiation**

● **W89**   **Exposure to man-made visible and ultraviolet light**
    Includes   exposure to welding light (arc)
    Excludes2   exposure to sunlight (X32)

The appropriate 7th character is to be added to each code from category W89

A	initial encounter
D	subsequent encounter
S	sequela

X● **W89.0**   **Exposure to welding light (arc)**
X● **W89.1**   **Exposure to tanning bed**
X● **W89.8**   **Exposure to other man-made visible and ultraviolet light**
X● **W89.9**   **Exposure to unspecified man-made visible and ultraviolet light**

● **W90**   **Exposure to other nonionizing radiation**
    Excludes2   exposure to sunlight (X32)

The appropriate 7th character is to be added to each code from category W90

A	initial encounter
D	subsequent encounter
S	sequela

X● **W90.0**   **Exposure to radiofrequency**
X● **W90.1**   **Exposure to infrared radiation**
X● **W90.2**   **Exposure to laser radiation**
X● **W90.8**   **Exposure to other nonionizing radiation**

X● **W92**   **Exposure to excessive heat of man-made origin**

The appropriate 7th character is to be added to code W92

A	initial encounter
D	subsequent encounter
S	sequela

● **W93**   **Exposure to excessive cold of man-made origin**

The appropriate 7th character is to be added to each code from category W93

A	initial encounter
D	subsequent encounter
S	sequela

   ● **W93.0**   **Contact with or inhalation of dry ice**
     X● **W93.01**   **Contact with dry ice**
     X● **W93.02**   **Inhalation of dry ice**

● **W93.1**   **Contact with or inhalation of liquid air**
   X● **W93.11**   **Contact with liquid air**
     Contact with liquid hydrogen
     Contact with liquid nitrogen
   X● **W93.12**   **Inhalation of liquid air**
     Inhalation of liquid hydrogen
     Inhalation of liquid nitrogen

X● **W93.2**   **Prolonged exposure in deep freeze unit or refrigerator**
X● **W93.8**   **Exposure to other excessive cold of man-made origin**

● **W94**   **Exposure to high and low air pressure and changes in air pressure**

The appropriate 7th character is to be added to each code from category W94

A	initial encounter
D	subsequent encounter
S	sequela

X● **W94.0**   **Exposure to prolonged high air pressure**
● **W94.1**   **Exposure to prolonged low air pressure**
   X● **W94.11**   **Exposure to residence or prolonged visit at high altitude**
   X● **W94.12**   **Exposure to other prolonged low air pressure**
● **W94.2**   **Exposure to rapid changes in air pressure during ascent**
   X● **W94.21**   **Exposure to reduction in atmospheric pressure while surfacing from deep-water diving**
   X● **W94.22**   **Exposure to reduction in atmospheric pressure while surfacing from underground**
   X● **W94.23**   **Exposure to sudden change in air pressure in aircraft during ascent**
   X● **W94.29**   **Exposure to other rapid changes in air pressure during ascent**
● **W94.3**   **Exposure to rapid changes in air pressure during descent**
   X● **W94.31**   **Exposure to sudden change in air pressure in aircraft during descent**
   X● **W94.32**   **Exposure to high air pressure from rapid descent in water**
   X● **W94.39**   **Exposure to other rapid changes in air pressure during descent**

X● **W99**   **Exposure to other man-made environmental factors**

The appropriate 7th character is to be added to code W99

A	initial encounter
D	subsequent encounter
S	sequela

EXPOSURE TO SMOKE, FIRE AND FLAMES (X00-X08)

   Excludes1   arson (X97)
   Excludes2   explosions (W35-W40)
     lightning (T75.0-)
     transport accident (V01-V99)

● **X00**   **Exposure to uncontrolled fire in building or structure**
    Includes   conflagration in building or structure
    Code first any associated cataclysm
    Excludes2   exposure to ignition or melting of nightwear (X05)
     exposure to ignition or melting of other clothing and apparel (X06.-)
     exposure to other specified smoke, fire and flames (X08.-)

The appropriate 7th character is to be added to each code from category X00

A	initial encounter
D	subsequent encounter
S	sequela

X● **X00.0**   **Exposure to flames in uncontrolled fire in building or structure**
    Coding Clinic: 2016, Q2, P5-6; 2015, Q1, P19

X● **X00.1**   **Exposure to smoke in uncontrolled fire in building or structure**

▶ New   ⇒ Revised   ~~deleted~~ Deleted   Excludes 1   Excludes 2   Includes   Use additional   Code first   Code also   Key words

OGCR Official Guidelines   ● Unacceptable Principal Diagnosis   X Assign placeholder X   ● Use Additional Character(s)   ▶ Manifestation Code   Coding Clinic

X ● **X00.2** **Injury due to collapse** of burning building or structure in uncontrolled fire

       Excludes1   injury due to collapse of building not on fire (W20.1)

X ● **X00.3** **Fall from** burning building or structure in uncontrolled fire

X ● **X00.4** **Hit by object** from burning building or structure in uncontrolled fire

X ● **X00.5** **Jump from** burning building or structure in uncontrolled fire

X ● **X00.8** **Other** exposure to uncontrolled fire in building or structure

● **X01** **Exposure to uncontrolled fire, not in building or structure**

       Includes   exposure to forest fire

The appropriate 7th character is to be added to each code from category X01

A	initial encounter
D	subsequent encounter
S	sequela

X ● **X01.0** **Exposure to flames** in uncontrolled fire, not in building or structure

X ● **X01.1** **Exposure to smoke** in uncontrolled fire, not in building or structure

X ● **X01.3** **Fall** due to uncontrolled fire, not in building or structure

X ● **X01.4** **Hit by object** due to uncontrolled fire, not in building or structure

X ● **X01.8** **Other** exposure to uncontrolled fire, not in building or structure

● **X02** **Exposure to controlled fire in building or structure**

       Includes   exposure to fire in fireplace exposure to fire in stove

The appropriate 7th character is to be added to each code from category X02

A	initial encounter
D	subsequent encounter
S	sequela

X ● **X02.0** **Exposure to flames** in controlled fire in building or structure

X ● **X02.1** **Exposure to smoke** in controlled fire in building or structure

X ● **X02.2** **Injury due to collapse** of burning building or structure in controlled fire

       Excludes1   injury due to collapse of building not on fire (W20.1)

X ● **X02.3** **Fall from** burning building or structure in controlled fire

X ● **X02.4** **Hit by object** from burning building or structure in controlled fire

X ● **X02.5** **Jump from** burning building or structure in controlled fire

X ● **X02.8** **Other** exposure to controlled fire in building or structure

● **X03** **Exposure to controlled fire, not in building or structure**

       Includes   exposure to bon fire exposure to camp fire exposure to trash fire

The appropriate 7th character is to be added to each code from category X03

A	initial encounter
D	subsequent encounter
S	sequela

X ● **X03.0** **Exposure to flames** in controlled fire, not in building or structure
       Coding Clinic: 2015, Q1, P19

X ● **X03.1** **Exposure to smoke** in controlled fire, not in building or structure

X ● **X03.3** **Fall** due to controlled fire, not in building or structure

X ● **X03.4** **Hit by object** due to controlled fire, not in building or structure

X ● **X03.8** **Other** exposure to controlled fire, not in building or structure

X ● **X04** **Exposure to ignition of highly flammable material**

       Exposure to ignition of gasoline
       Exposure to ignition of kerosene
       Exposure to ignition of petrol

       Excludes2   exposure to ignition or melting of nightwear (X05)

                     exposure to ignition or melting of other clothing and apparel (X06)

The appropriate 7th character is to be added to code X04

A	initial encounter
D	subsequent encounter
S	sequela

Coding Clinic: 2016, Q2, P4

X ● **X05** **Exposure to ignition or melting of nightwear**

       Excludes2   exposure to uncontrolled fire in building or structure (X00.-)

                     exposure to uncontrolled fire, not in building or structure (X01.-)

                     exposure to controlled fire in building or structure (X02.-)

                     exposure to controlled fire, not in building or structure (X03.-)

                     exposure to ignition of highly flammable materials (X04.-)

The appropriate 7th character is to be added to code X05

A	initial encounter
D	subsequent encounter
S	sequela

● **X06** **Exposure to ignition or melting of other clothing and apparel**

       Excludes2   exposure to uncontrolled fire in building or structure (X00.-)

                     exposure to uncontrolled fire, not in building or structure (X01.-)

                     exposure to controlled fire in building or structure (X02.-)

                     exposure to controlled fire, not in building or structure (X03.-)

                     exposure to ignition of highly flammable materials (X04.-)

The appropriate 7th character is to be added to each code from category X06

A	initial encounter
D	subsequent encounter
S	sequela

X ● **X06.0** **Exposure to ignition** of plastic jewelry

X ● **X06.1** **Exposure to melting** of plastic jewelry

X ● **X06.2** **Exposure to ignition** of other clothing and apparel

X ● **X06.3** **Exposure to melting** of other clothing and apparel

● **X08** **Exposure to other specified smoke, fire and flames**

The appropriate 7th character is to be added to each code from category X08

A	initial encounter
D	subsequent encounter
S	sequela

● **X08.0** **Exposure to bed fire**
       Exposure to mattress fire

X ● **X08.00** **Exposure to bed fire** due to **unspecified** burning material

X ● **X08.01** **Exposure to bed fire** due to burning **cigarette**
       Coding Clinic: 2015, Q1, P19

X ● **X08.09** **Exposure to bed fire** due to **other** burning material

---

N Newborn Age: 0   **P** Pediatric Age: 0–17   **M** Maternity DX: 9–64   **A** Adult Age: 15–124   ♀ Females Only   ♂ Males Only

🔾 Complication\Comorbidity   🔾 Major C\C   (Ex) CC/MCC Exclusions   🔾 Hospital-Acquired Condition   ● Hierarchical Condition Category

● X08.1   **Exposure to sofa fire**
X● X08.10   Exposure to sofa fire due to unspecified burning material
X● X08.11   Exposure to sofa fire due to burning cigarette
X● X08.19   Exposure to sofa fire due to other burning material
● X08.2   **Exposure to other furniture fire**
X● X08.20   Exposure to other furniture fire due to unspecified burning material
X● X08.21   Exposure to other furniture fire due to burning cigarette
X● X08.29   Exposure to other furniture fire due to other burning material
X● X08.8   **Exposure to other specified smoke, fire and flames**

CONTACT WITH HEAT AND HOT SUBSTANCES (X10-X19)

Excludes1   exposure to excessive natural heat (X30)
               exposure to fire and flames (X00-X08)

● X10   **Contact with hot drinks, food, fats and cooking oils**
The appropriate 7th character is to be added to each code from category X10

A	initial encounter
D	subsequent encounter
S	sequela

X● X10.0   **Contact with hot drinks**
X● X10.1   **Contact with hot food**
X● X10.2   **Contact with fats and cooking oils**

● X11   **Contact with hot tap-water**
Includes   contact with boiling tap-water
          contact with boiling water NOS
Excludes1   contact with water heated on stove (X12)
The appropriate 7th character is to be added to each code from category X11

A	initial encounter
D	subsequent encounter
S	sequela

X● X11.0   **Contact with hot water in bath or tub**
Excludes1   contact with running hot water in bath or tub (X11.1)
X● X11.1   **Contact with running hot water**
Contact with hot water running out of hose
Contact with hot water running out of tap
X● X11.8   **Contact with other hot tap-water**
Contact with hot water in bucket
Contact with hot tap-water NOS

X● X12   **Contact with other hot fluids**
Contact with water heated on stove
Excludes1   hot (liquid) metals (X18)
The appropriate 7th character is to be added to code X12

A	initial encounter
D	subsequent encounter
S	sequela

● X13   **Contact with steam and other hot vapors**
The appropriate 7th character is to be added to each code from category X13

A	initial encounter
D	subsequent encounter
S	sequela

X● X13.0   **Inhalation of steam and other hot vapors**
X● X13.1   **Other contact with steam and other hot vapors**

● X14   **Contact with hot air and other hot gases**
The appropriate 7th character is to be added to each code from category X14

A	initial encounter
D	subsequent encounter
S	sequela

X● X14.0   **Inhalation of hot air and gases**
X● X14.1   **Other contact with hot air and other hot gases**

● X15   **Contact with hot household appliances**
Excludes1   contact with heating appliances (X16)
         contact with powered household appliances (W29.-)
         exposure to controlled fire in building or structure due to household appliance (X02.8)
         exposure to household appliances electrical current (W86.0)
The appropriate 7th character is to be added to each code from category X15

A	initial encounter
D	subsequent encounter
S	sequela

X● X15.0   **Contact with hot stove (kitchen)**
X● X15.1   **Contact with hot toaster**
X● X15.2   **Contact with hotplate**
X● X15.3   **Contact with hot saucepan or skillet**
X● X15.8   **Contact with other hot household appliances**
Contact with cooker
Contact with kettle
Contact with light bulbs

X● X16   **Contact with hot heating appliances, radiators and pipes**
Excludes1   contact with powered appliances (W29.-)
         exposure to controlled fire in building or structure due to appliance (X02.8)
         exposure to industrial appliances electrical current (W86.1)
The appropriate 7th character is to be added to code X16

A	initial encounter
D	subsequent encounter
S	sequela

X● X17   **Contact with hot engines, machinery and tools**
Excludes1   contact with hot heating appliances, radiators and pipes (X16)
         contact with hot household appliances (X15)
The appropriate 7th character is to be added to code X17

A	initial encounter
D	subsequent encounter
S	sequela

X● X18   **Contact with other hot metals**
Contact with liquid metal
The appropriate 7th character is to be added to code X18

A	initial encounter
D	subsequent encounter
S	sequela

X● X19   **Contact with other heat and hot substances**
Excludes1   objects that are not normally hot, e.g., an object made hot by a house fire (X00-X08)
The appropriate 7th character is to be added to code X19

A	initial encounter
D	subsequent encounter
S	sequela

▶ New   ⇒ Revised   ~~deleted~~ Deleted   Excludes 1   Excludes 2   Includes   Use additional   Code first   Code also   Key words
OGCR Official Guidelines   ● Unacceptable Principal Diagnosis   X Assign placeholder X   ● Use Additional Character(s)   ▶ Manifestation Code   Coding Clinic

CHAPTER 20 (V00-Y99)

EXPOSURE TO FORCES OF NATURE (X30-X39)

X● **X30 Exposure to excessive natural heat**
Exposure to excessive heat as the cause of sunstroke
Exposure to heat NOS

Excludes1 excessive heat of man-made origin (W92)
exposure to man-made radiation (W89)
exposure to sunlight (X32)
exposure to tanning bed (W89)

The appropriate 7th character is to be added to code X30

A	initial encounter
D	subsequent encounter
S	sequela

X● **X31 Exposure to excessive natural cold**
Excessive cold as the cause of chilblains NOS
Excessive cold as the cause of immersion foot or hand
Exposure to cold NOS
Exposure to weather conditions

Excludes1 cold of man-made origin (W93.-)
contact with or inhalation of dry ice (W93.-)
contact with or inhalation of liquefied gas (W93.-)

The appropriate 7th character is to be added to code X31

A	initial encounter
D	subsequent encounter
S	sequela

X● **X32 Exposure to sunlight**

Excludes1 man-made radiation (tanning bed) (W89)

Excludes2 radiation-related disorders of the skin and subcutaneous tissue (L55-L59)

The appropriate 7th character is to be added to code X32

A	initial encounter
D	subsequent encounter
S	sequela

X● **X34 Earthquake**

Excludes2 tidal wave (tsunami) due to earthquake (X37.41)

The appropriate 7th character is to be added to code X34

A	initial encounter
D	subsequent encounter
S	sequela

X● **X35 Volcanic eruption**

Excludes2 tidal wave (tsunami) due to volcanic eruption (X37.41)

The appropriate 7th character is to be added to code X35

A	initial encounter
D	subsequent encounter
S	sequela

●**X36 Avalanche, landslide and other earth movements**

Includes victim of mudslide of cataclysmic nature

Excludes1 earthquake (X34)

Excludes2 transport accident involving collision with avalanche or landslide not in motion (V01-V99)

The appropriate 7th character is to be added to each code from category X36

A	initial encounter
D	subsequent encounter
S	sequela

X● **X36.0 Collapse of dam or man-made structure causing earth movement**

X● **X36.1 Avalanche, landslide, or mudslide**

●**X37 Cataclysmic storm**
The appropriate 7th character is to be added to each code from category X37

A	initial encounter
D	subsequent encounter
S	sequela

X● **X37.0 Hurricane**
Storm surge   Typhoon

X● **X37.1 Tornado**
Cyclone   Twister

X● **X37.2 Blizzard (snow) (ice)**

X● **X37.3 Dust storm**

● **X37.4 Tidalwave**

X● **X37.41 Tidal wave due to earthquake or volcanic eruption**
Tidal wave NOS
Tsunami

X● **X37.42 Tidal wave due to storm**

X● **X37.43 Tidal wave due to landslide**

X● **X37.8 Other cataclysmic storms**
Cloudburst
Torrential rain

Excludes2 flood (X38)

X● **X37.9 Unspecified cataclysmic storm**
Storm NOS

Excludes1 collapse of dam or man-made structure causing earth movement (X36.0)

X● **X38 Flood**
Flood arising from remote storm
Flood of cataclysmic nature arising from melting snow
Flood resulting directly from storm

Excludes1 collapse of dam or man-made structure causing earth movement (X36.0)
tidal wave NOS (X37.41)
tidal wave caused by storm (X37.42)

The appropriate 7th character is to be added to code X38

A	initial encounter
D	subsequent encounter
S	sequela

●**X39 Exposure to other forces of nature**
The appropriate 7th character is to be added to each code from category X39

A	initial encounter
D	subsequent encounter
S	sequela

● **X39.0 Exposure to natural radiation**

Excludes1 contact with and (suspected) exposure to radon and other naturally occurring radiation (Z77.123)
exposure to man-made radiation (W88-W90)
exposure to sunlight (X32)

X● **X39.01 Exposure to radon**

X● **X39.08 Exposure to other natural radiation**

X● **X39.8 Other exposure to forces of nature**

N Newborn Age: 0   **P** Pediatric Age: 0–17   **M** Maternity DX: 9–64   **A** Adult Age: 15–124   ♀ Females Only   ♂ Males Only

Complication\Comorbidity   Major C\C   (Ex:) CC/MCC Exclusions   Hospital-Acquired Condition   Hierarchical Condition Category

1587

OVEREXERTION AND STRENUOUS OR REPETITIVE MOVEMENTS (X50)

●X50   Overexertion and strenuous or repetitive movements

The appropriate 7th character is to be added to each code from category X50

A	initial encounter
D	subsequent encounter
S	sequela

Coding Clinic: 2016, Q4, P73-74

X●X50.0   Overexertion from strenuous movement or load
Lifting heavy objects
Lifting weights
Coding Clinic: 2016, Q4, P74

X●X50.1   Overexertion from prolonged static or awkward postures
Prolonged bending
Prolonged kneeling
Prolonged reaching
Prolonged sitting
Prolonged standing
Prolonged twisting
Static bending
Static kneeling
Static reaching
Static sitting
Static standing
Static twisting

X●X50.3   Overexertion from repetitive movements
Use of hand as hammer
Excludes2   Overuse from prolonged static or awkward postures (X50.1)
Coding Clinic: 2016, Q4, P74

X●X50.9   Other and unspecified overexertion or strenuous movements or postures
Contact pressure
Contact stress

ACCIDENTAL EXPOSURE TO OTHER SPECIFIED FACTORS (X52, X58)

X●X52   Prolonged stay in weightless environment
Weightlessness in spacecraft (simulator)
The appropriate 7th character is to be added to code X52

A	initial encounter
D	subsequent encounter
S	sequela

X●X58   Exposure to other specified factors
Accident NOS
Exposure NOS
The appropriate 7th character is to be added to code X58

A	initial encounter
D	subsequent encounter
S	sequela

INTENTIONAL SELF-HARM (X71-X83)

Purposely self-inflicted injury
Suicide (attempted)

●X71   Intentional self-harm by drowning and submersion
The appropriate 7th character is to be added to each code from category X71

A	initial encounter
D	subsequent encounter
S	sequela

X●X71.0   Intentional self-harm by drowning and submersion while in bathtub A, D, S 🖐

X●X71.1   Intentional self-harm by drowning and submersion while in swimming pool A, D, S 🖐

X●X71.2   Intentional self-harm by drowning and submersion after jump into swimming pool A, D, S 🖐

X●X71.3   Intentional self-harm by drowning and submersion in natural water A, D, S 🖐

X●X71.8   Other intentional self-harm by drowning and submersion A, D, S 🖐

X●X71.9   Intentional self-harm by drowning and submersion, unspecified A, D, S 🖐

X●X72   Intentional self-harm by handgun discharge A, D, S 🖐
Intentional self-harm by gun for single hand use
Intentional self-harm by pistol
Intentional self-harm by revolver
Excludes1   Very pistol (X74.8)
The appropriate 7th character is to be added to code X72

A	initial encounter
D	subsequent encounter
S	sequela

●X73   Intentional self-harm by rifle, shotgun and larger firearm discharge
Excludes1   airgun (X74.01)
The appropriate 7th character is to be added to each code from category X73

A	initial encounter
D	subsequent encounter
S	sequela

X●X73.0   Intentional self-harm by shotgun discharge A, D, S 🖐

X●X73.1   Intentional self-harm by hunting rifle discharge A, D, S 🖐

X●X73.2   Intentional self-harm by machine gun discharge A, D, S 🖐

X●X73.8   Intentional self-harm by other larger firearm discharge A, D, S 🖐

X●X73.9   Intentional self-harm by unspecified larger firearm discharge A, D, S 🖐

●X74   Intentional self-harm by other and unspecified firearm and gun discharge
The appropriate 7th character is to be added to each code from category X74

A	initial encounter
D	subsequent encounter
S	sequela

●X74.0   Intentional self-harm by gas, air or spring-operated guns

X●X74.01   Intentional self-harm by airgun A, D, S 🖐
Intentional self-harm by BB gun discharge
Intentional self-harm by pellet gun discharge

X●X74.02   Intentional self-harm by paintball gun A, D, S 🖐

X●X74.09   Intentional self-harm by other gas, air or spring-operated gun A, D, S 🖐

X●X74.8   Intentional self-harm by other firearm discharge A, D, S 🖐
Intentional self-harm by Very pistol [flare] discharge

X●X74.9   Intentional self-harm by unspecified firearm discharge A, D, S 🖐

X●X75   Intentional self-harm by explosive material A, D, S 🖐
The appropriate 7th character is to be added to code X75

A	initial encounter
D	subsequent encounter
S	sequela

X●X76   Intentional self-harm by smoke, fire and flames A, D, S 🖐
The appropriate 7th character is to be added to code X76

A	initial encounter
D	subsequent encounter
S	sequela

▶ New   ⇒ Revised   ~~deleted~~ Deleted   Excludes 1   Excludes 2   Includes   Use additional   Code first   Code also   Key words

OGCR Official Guidelines   ● Unacceptable Principal Diagnosis   X Assign placeholder X   ● Use Additional Character(s)   ▶ Manifestation Code   Coding Clinic

● X77   **Intentional self-harm by steam, hot vapors and hot objects**

    The appropriate 7th character is to be added to each code from category X77

A	initial encounter
D	subsequent encounter
S	sequela

X ● X77.0   **Intentional self-harm by** steam or hot vapors **A, D, S** 🐾
X ● X77.1   **Intentional self-harm by** hot tap water **A, D, S** 🐾
X ● X77.2   **Intentional self-harm by** other hot fluids **A, D, S** 🐾
X ● X77.3   **Intentional self-harm by** hot household appliances **A, D, S** 🐾
X ● X77.8   **Intentional self-harm by** other hot objects **A, D, S** 🐾
X ● X77.9   **Intentional self-harm by** unspecified hot objects **A, D, S** 🐾

● X78   **Intentional self-harm by sharp object**

    The appropriate 7th character is to be added to each code from category X78

A	initial encounter
D	subsequent encounter
S	sequela

X ● X78.0   **Intentional self-harm by** sharp glass **A, D, S** 🐾
X ● X78.1   **Intentional self-harm by** knife **A, D, S** 🐾
X ● X78.2   **Intentional self-harm by** sword or dagger **A, D, S** 🐾
X ● X78.8   **Intentional self-harm by** other sharp object **A, D, S** 🐾
X ● X78.9   **Intentional self-harm by** unspecified sharp object **A, D, S** 🐾

X ● X79   **Intentional self-harm by blunt object A, D, S** 🐾

    The appropriate 7th character is to be added to code X79

A	initial encounter
D	subsequent encounter
S	sequela

X ● X80   **Intentional self-harm by jumping from a high place A, D, S** 🐾
    Intentional fall from one level to another
    The appropriate 7th character is to be added to code X80

A	initial encounter
D	subsequent encounter
S	sequela

● X81   **Intentional self-harm by jumping or lying in front of moving object**

    The appropriate 7th character is to be added to each code from category X81

A	initial encounter
D	subsequent encounter
S	sequela

X ● X81.0   **Intentional self-harm by jumping or lying in front of** motor vehicle **A, D, S** 🐾
X ● X81.1   **Intentional self-harm by jumping or lying in front of** (subway) train **A, D, S** 🐾
X ● X81.8   **Intentional self-harm by jumping or lying in front of** other moving object **A, D, S** 🐾

● X82   **Intentional self-harm by crashing of motor vehicle**

    The appropriate 7th character is to be added to each code from category X82

A	initial encounter
D	subsequent encounter
S	sequela

X ● X82.0   **Intentional collision of motor vehicle with** other motor vehicle **A, D, S** 🐾
X ● X82.1   **Intentional collision of motor vehicle with** train **A, D, S** 🐾

X ● X82.2   **Intentional collision of motor vehicle with** tree **A, D, S** 🐾
X ● X82.8   **Other intentional self-harm by crashing of motor vehicle A, D, S** 🐾

● X83   **Intentional self-harm by other specified means**

    Excludes1   intentional self-harm by poisoning or contact with toxic substance - see Table of Drugs and Chemicals

    The appropriate 7th character is to be added to each code from category X83

A	initial encounter
D	subsequent encounter
S	sequela

X ● X83.0   **Intentional self-harm by** crashing of aircraft **A, D, S** 🐾
X ● X83.1   **Intentional self-harm by** electrocution **A, D, S** 🐾
X ● X83.2   **Intentional self-harm by** exposure to extremes of cold **A, D, S** 🐾
X ● X83.8   **Intentional self-harm by** other specified means **A, D, S** 🐾

ASSAULT (X92-Y09)

    Includes   homicide injuries inflicted by another person with intent to injure or kill, by any means

    Excludes1   injuries due to legal intervention (Y35.-)
                injuries due to operations of war (Y36.-)
                injuries due to terrorism (Y38.-)

● X92   **Assault by drowning and submersion**

    The appropriate 7th character is to be added to each code from category X92

A	initial encounter
D	subsequent encounter
S	sequela

X ● X92.0   **Assault by drowning and submersion while in** bathtub
X ● X92.1   **Assault by drowning and submersion while in** swimming pool
X ● X92.2   **Assault by drowning and submersion after** push into swimming pool
X ● X92.3   **Assault by drowning and submersion in** natural water
X ● X92.8   **Other assault by drowning and submersion**
X ● X92.9   **Assault by drowning and submersion,** unspecified

X ● X93   **Assault by** handgun discharge
    Assault by discharge of gun for single hand use
    Assault by discharge of pistol
    Assault by discharge of revolver

    Excludes1   Very pistol (X95.8)

    The appropriate 7th character is to be added to code X93

A	initial encounter
D	subsequent encounter
S	sequela

● X94   **Assault by rifle, shotgun and larger firearm discharge**

    Excludes1   airgun (X95.01)

    The appropriate 7th character is to be added to each code from category X94

A	initial encounter
D	subsequent encounter
S	sequela

X ● X94.0   **Assault by** shotgun
X ● X94.1   **Assault by** hunting rifle
X ● X94.2   **Assault by** machine gun
X ● X94.8   **Assault by** other larger firearm discharge
X ● X94.9   **Assault by** unspecified larger firearm discharge

CHAPTER 20 (V00-Y99)

N Newborn Age: 0   **P** Pediatric Age: 0–17   **M** Maternity DX: 9–64   **A** Adult Age: 15–124   ♀ Females Only   ♂ Males Only
🐾 Complication\Comorbidity   🐾 Major C\C   (Ex) CC/MCC Exclusions   🐾 Hospital-Acquired Condition   🐾 Hierarchical Condition Category

1589

CHAPTER 20 (V00-Y99)

● X95   **Assault by other and unspecified firearm and gun discharge**

The appropriate 7th character is to be added to each code from category X95

A	initial encounter
D	subsequent encounter
S	sequela

● X95.0   **Assault by gas, air or spring-operated guns**

X● X95.01   **Assault by** airgun **discharge**
Assault by BB gun discharge
Assault by pellet gun discharge

X● X95.02   **Assault by** paintball gun **discharge**

X● X95.09   **Assault by** other gas, air or spring-operated gun

X● X95.8   **Assault by** other firearm discharge
Assault by very pistol [flare] discharge

X● X95.9   **Assault by** unspecified firearm discharge
Coding Clinic: 2016, Q3, P24

● X96   **Assault by explosive material**

Excludes1   incendiary device (X97)
terrorism involving explosive material (Y38.2-)

The appropriate 7th character is to be added to each code from category X96

A	initial encounter
D	subsequent encounter
S	sequela

X● X96.0   **Assault by** antipersonnel **bomb**

Excludes1   antipersonnel bomb use in military or war (Y36.2-)

X● X96.1   **Assault by** gasoline **bomb**
X● X96.2   **Assault by** letter **bomb**
X● X96.3   **Assault by** fertilizer **bomb**
X● X96.4   **Assault by** pipe **bomb**
X● X96.8   **Assault by** other specified explosive
X● X96.9   **Assault by** unspecified **explosive**

X● X97   **Assault by smoke, fire and flames**
Assault by arson
Assault by cigarettes
Assault by incendiary device

The appropriate 7th character is to be added to code X97

A	initial encounter
D	subsequent encounter
S	sequela

● X98   **Assault by steam, hot vapors and hot objects**

The appropriate 7th character is to be added to each code from category X98

A	initial encounter
D	subsequent encounter
S	sequela

X● X98.0   **Assault by** steam or hot vapors
X● X98.1   **Assault by** hot tap water
X● X98.2   **Assault by** hot fluids
X● X98.3   **Assault by** hot household appliances
X● X98.8   **Assault by** other hot objects
X● X98.9   **Assault by** unspecified hot objects

● X99   **Assault by sharp object**

Excludes1   assault by strike by sports equipment (Y08.0-)

The appropriate 7th character is to be added to each code from category X99

A	initial encounter
D	subsequent encounter
S	sequela

X● X99.0   **Assault by** sharp glass
X● X99.1   **Assault by** knife
X● X99.2   **Assault by** sword or dagger
X● X99.8   **Assault by** other sharp object
X● X99.9   **Assault by** unspecified sharp object
Assault by stabbing NOS

X● Y00   **Assault by blunt object**

Excludes1   assault by strike by sports equipment (Y08.0)

The appropriate 7th character is to be added to code Y00

A	initial encounter
D	subsequent encounter
S	sequela

X● Y01   **Assault by pushing from high place**

The appropriate 7th character is to be added to code Y01

A	initial encounter
D	subsequent encounter
S	sequela

● Y02   **Assault by pushing or placing victim in front of moving object**

The appropriate 7th character is to be added to each code from category Y02

A	initial encounter
D	subsequent encounter
S	sequela

X● Y02.0   **Assault by pushing or placing victim in front of** motor vehicle

X● Y02.1   **Assault by pushing or placing victim in front of** (subway) train

X● Y02.8   **Assault by pushing or placing victim in front of** other moving object

● Y03   **Assault by crashing of motor vehicle**

The appropriate 7th character is to be added to each code from category Y03

A	initial encounter
D	subsequent encounter
S	sequela

X● Y03.0   **Assault by being** hit or run over **by motor vehicle**
X● Y03.8   Other **assault by crashing of motor vehicle**

● Y04   **Assault by bodily force**

Excludes1   assault by:
submersion (X92.-)
use of weapon (X93-X95, X99, Y00)

The appropriate 7th character is to be added to each code from category Y04

A	initial encounter
D	subsequent encounter
S	sequela

X● Y04.0   **Assault by unarmed** brawl or fight
X● Y04.1   **Assault by human** bite
X● Y04.2   **Assault by** strike **against or bumped into by another person**
X● Y04.8   **Assault by** other bodily force
Assault by bodily force NOS

▶ New   ➡ Revised   ~~deleted~~ Deleted   Excludes 1   Excludes 2   Includes   Use additional   Code first   Code also   Key words

OGCR Official Guidelines   ● Unacceptable Principal Diagnosis   X Assign placeholder X   ● Use Additional Character(s)   ▶ Manifestation Code   **Coding Clinic**

OGCR Section I.C.19.f.

Adult and child abuse, neglect and other maltreatment

Sequence first the appropriate code from categories T74 or T76 for abuse, neglect and other maltreatment, followed by any accompanying mental health or injury code(s).

If the documentation in the medical record states abuse or neglect it is coded as confirmed (T74.-). It is coded as suspected if it is documented as suspected (T76.-).

For cases of confirmed abuse or neglect an external cause code from the assault section (X92-Y09) should be added to identify the cause of any physical injuries. A perpetrator code (Y07) should be added when the perpetrator of the abuse is known. For suspected cases of abuse or neglect, do not report external cause or perpetrator code.

If a suspected case of abuse, neglect or mistreatment is ruled out during an encounter code Z04.71, Encounter for examination and observation following alleged physical adult abuse, ruled out, or code Z04.72, Encounter for examination and observation following alleged adult rape, should be used, not a code from T76.

If a suspected case of alleged rape or sexual abuse is ruled out during an encounter code Z04.41, Encounter for examination and observation following alleged adult rape or code Z04.42, Encounter for examination and observation following alleged child rape should be used, not a code from T76.

● **Y07**   **Perpetrator of assault, maltreatment and neglect**

> **Note:** Codes from this category are for use only in cases of confirmed abuse (T74.-)
>
> Selection of the correct perpetrator code is based on the relationship between the perpetrator and the victim

> **Includes**   perpetrator of abandonment
> perpetrator of emotional neglect
> perpetrator of mental cruelty
> perpetrator of physical abuse
> perpetrator of physical neglect
> perpetrator of sexual abuse
> perpetrator of torture

Coding Clinic: 2016, Q4, P129

● **Y07.0**   **Spouse or partner, perpetrator of maltreatment and neglect**

> Spouse or partner, perpetrator of maltreatment and neglect against spouse or partner

     Y07.01   **Husband, perpetrator of maltreatment and neglect**

     Y07.02   **Wife, perpetrator of maltreatment and neglect**

     Y07.03   **Male partner, perpetrator of maltreatment and neglect**

     Y07.04   **Female partner, perpetrator of maltreatment and neglect**

● **Y07.1**   **Parent (adoptive) (biological), perpetrator of maltreatment and neglect**

     Y07.11   **Biological father, perpetrator of maltreatment and neglect**

     Y07.12   **Biological mother, perpetrator of maltreatment and neglect**

     Y07.13   **Adoptive father, perpetrator of maltreatment and neglect**

     Y07.14   **Adoptive mother, perpetrator of maltreatment and neglect**

● **Y07.4**   **Other family member, perpetrator of maltreatment and neglect**

   ● Y07.41   **Sibling, perpetrator of maltreatment and neglect**

> **Excludes1**   stepsibling, perpetrator of maltreatment and neglect (Y07.435, Y07.436)

     Y07.410   **Brother, perpetrator of maltreatment and neglect**

     Y07.411   **Sister, perpetrator of maltreatment and neglect**

● Y07.42   **Foster parent, perpetrator of maltreatment and neglect**

     Y07.420   **Foster father, perpetrator of maltreatment and neglect**

     Y07.421   **Foster mother, perpetrator of maltreatment and neglect**

● Y07.43   **Stepparent or stepsibling, perpetrator of maltreatment and neglect**

     Y07.430   **Stepfather, perpetrator of maltreatment and neglect**

     Y07.432   **Male friend of parent (co-residing in household), perpetrator of maltreatment and neglect**

     Y07.433   **Stepmother, perpetrator of maltreatment and neglect**

     Y07.434   **Female friend of parent (co-residing in household), perpetrator of maltreatment and neglect**

     Y07.435   **Stepbrother, perpetrator or maltreatment and neglect**

     Y07.436   **Stepsister, perpetrator of maltreatment and neglect**

● Y07.49   **Other family member, perpetrator of maltreatment and neglect**

     Y07.490   **Male cousin, perpetrator of maltreatment and neglect**

     Y07.491   **Female cousin, perpetrator of maltreatment and neglect**

     Y07.499   **Other family member, perpetrator of maltreatment and neglect**

● **Y07.5**   **Non-family member, perpetrator of maltreatment and neglect**

     Y07.50   **Unspecified non-family member, perpetrator of maltreatment and neglect**

● Y07.51   **Daycare provider, perpetrator of maltreatment and neglect**

     Y07.510   **At-home childcare provider, perpetrator of maltreatment and neglect**

     Y07.511   **Daycare center childcare provider, perpetrator of maltreatment and neglect**

     Y07.512   **At-home adultcare provider, perpetrator of maltreatment and neglect**

     Y07.513   **Adultcare center provider, perpetrator of maltreatment and neglect**

     Y07.519   **Unspecified daycare provider, perpetrator of maltreatment and neglect**

● Y07.52   **Healthcare provider, perpetrator of maltreatment and neglect**

     Y07.521   **Mental health provider, perpetrator of maltreatment and neglect**

     Y07.528   **Other therapist or healthcare provider, perpetrator of maltreatment and neglect**

> Nurse perpetrator of maltreatment and neglect
> Occupational therapist perpetrator of maltreatment and neglect
> Physical therapist perpetrator of maltreatment and neglect
> Speech therapist perpetrator of maltreatment and neglect

     Y07.529   **Unspecified healthcare provider, perpetrator of maltreatment and neglect**

N Newborn Age: 0   **P** Pediatric Age: 0–17   **M** Maternity DX: 9–64   **A** Adult Age: 15–124   ♀ Females Only   ♂ Males Only

Complication\Comorbidity   Major C\C   (Ex) CC/MCC Exclusions   Hospital-Acquired Condition   Hierarchical Condition Category

1591

CHAPTER 20 (V00-Y99)

Y07.53 Teacher or instructor, perpetrator of maltreatment and neglect

　Coach, perpetrator of maltreatment and neglect

Y07.59 Other non-family member, perpetrator of maltreatment and neglect

Y07.6 Multiple perpetrators of maltreatment and neglect

Y07.9 Unspecified perpetrator of maltreatment and neglect

● **Y08** Assault by other specified means

The appropriate 7th character is to be added to each code from category Y08

A	initial encounter
D	subsequent encounter
S	sequela

● **Y08.0** Assault by strike by sport equipment

X● **Y08.01** Assault by strike by hockey stick

X● **Y08.02** Assault by strike by baseball bat

X● **Y08.09** Assault by strike by other specified type of sport equipment

● **Y08.8** Assault by other specified means

X● **Y08.81** Assault by crashing of aircraft

X● **Y08.89** Assault by other specified means

● **Y09** Assault by unspecified means

Assassination (attempted) NOS
Homicide (attempted) NOS
Manslaughter (attempted) NOS
Murder (attempted) NOS

EVENT OF UNDETERMINED INTENT (Y21-Y33)

Undetermined intent is only for use when there is specific documentation in the record that the intent of the injury cannot be determined. If no such documentation is present, code to accidental (unintentional)

● **Y21** Drowning and submersion, undetermined intent

The appropriate 7th character is to be added to each code from category Y21

A	initial encounter
D	subsequent encounter
S	sequela

X● **Y21.0** Drowning and submersion while in bathtub, undetermined intent

X● **Y21.1** Drowning and submersion after fall into bathtub, undetermined intent

X● **Y21.2** Drowning and submersion while in swimming pool, undetermined intent

X● **Y21.3** Drowning and submersion after fall into swimming pool, undetermined intent

X● **Y21.4** Drowning and submersion in natural water, undetermined intent

X● **Y21.8** Other drowning and submersion, undetermined intent

X● **Y21.9** Unspecified drowning and submersion, undetermined intent

X● **Y22** Handgun discharge, undetermined intent

Discharge of gun for single hand use, undetermined intent
Discharge of pistol, undetermined intent
Discharge of revolver, undetermined intent

Excludes2 very pistol (Y24.8)

The appropriate 7th character is to be added to code Y22

A	initial encounter
D	subsequent encounter
S	sequela

● **Y23** Rifle, shotgun and larger firearm discharge, undetermined intent

Excludes2 airgun (Y24.0)

The appropriate 7th character is to be added to each code from category Y23

A	initial encounter
D	subsequent encounter
S	sequela

X● **Y23.0** Shotgun discharge, undetermined intent

X● **Y23.1** Hunting rifle discharge, undetermined intent

X● **Y23.2** Military firearm discharge, undetermined intent

X● **Y23.3** Machine gun discharge, undetermined intent

X● **Y23.8** Other larger firearm discharge, undetermined intent

X● **Y23.9** Unspecified larger firearm discharge, undetermined intent

● **Y24** Other and unspecified firearm discharge, undetermined intent

The appropriate 7th character is to be added to each code from category Y24

A	initial encounter
D	subsequent encounter
S	sequela

X● **Y24.0** Airgun discharge, undetermined intent

BB gun discharge, undetermined intent
Pellet gun discharge, undetermined intent

X● **Y24.8** Other firearm discharge, undetermined intent

Paintball gun discharge, undetermined intent
Very pistol [flare] discharge, undetermined intent

X● **Y24.9** Unspecified firearm discharge, undetermined intent

X● **Y25** Contact with explosive material, undetermined intent

The appropriate 7th character is to be added to code Y25

A	initial encounter
D	subsequent encounter
S	sequela

X● **Y26** Exposure to smoke, fire and flames, undetermined intent

The appropriate 7th character is to be added to code Y26

A	initial encounter
D	subsequent encounter
S	sequela

● **Y27** Contact with steam, hot vapors and hot objects, undetermined intent

The appropriate 7th character is to be added to each code from category Y27

A	initial encounter
D	subsequent encounter
S	sequela

X● **Y27.0** Contact with steam and hot vapors, undetermined intent

X● **Y27.1** Contact with hot tap water, undetermined intent

X● **Y27.2** Contact with hot fluids, undetermined intent

X● **Y27.3** Contact with hot household appliance, undetermined intent

X● **Y27.8** Contact with other hot objects, undetermined intent

X● **Y27.9** Contact with unspecified hot objects, undetermined intent

● **Y28** Contact with sharp object, undetermined intent

The appropriate 7th character is to be added to each code from category Y28

A	initial encounter
D	subsequent encounter
S	sequela

X● **Y28.0** Contact with sharp glass, undetermined intent

X● **Y28.1** Contact with knife, undetermined intent

X ● Y28.2   Contact with sword or dagger, undetermined intent
X ● Y28.8   Contact with other sharp object, undetermined intent
X ● Y28.9   Contact with unspecified sharp object, undetermined intent

X ● Y29   Contact with blunt object, undetermined intent
> The appropriate 7th character is to be added to code Y29
>
> | | |
> |---|---|
> | A | initial encounter |
> | D | subsequent encounter |
> | S | sequela |

X ● Y30   Falling, jumping or pushed from a high place, undetermined intent
> Victim falling from one level to another, undetermined intent
> The appropriate 7th character is to be added to code Y30
>
> | | |
> |---|---|
> | A | initial encounter |
> | D | subsequent encounter |
> | S | sequela |

X ● Y31   Falling, lying or running before or into moving object, undetermined intent
> The appropriate 7th character is to be added to code Y31
>
> | | |
> |---|---|
> | A | initial encounter |
> | D | subsequent encounter |
> | S | sequela |

X ● Y32   Crashing of motor vehicle, undetermined intent
> The appropriate 7th character is to be added to code Y32
>
> | | |
> |---|---|
> | A | initial encounter |
> | D | subsequent encounter |
> | S | sequela |

X ● Y33   Other specified events, undetermined intent
> The appropriate 7th character is to be added to code Y33
>
> | | |
> |---|---|
> | A | initial encounter |
> | D | subsequent encounter |
> | S | sequela |

LEGAL INTERVENTION, OPERATIONS OF WAR, MILITARY OPERATIONS, AND TERRORISM (Y35-Y38)

● Y35   Legal intervention
> **Includes**   any injury sustained as a result of an encounter with any law enforcement official, serving in any capacity at the time of the encounter, whether on-duty or off-duty. Includes: injury to law enforcement official, suspect and bystander
>
> The appropriate 7th character is to be added to each code from category Y35
>
> | | |
> |---|---|
> | A | initial encounter |
> | D | subsequent encounter |
> | S | sequela |

● Y35.0   Legal intervention involving firearm discharge
  ● Y35.00   Legal intervention involving unspecified firearm discharge
> Legal intervention involving gunshot wound
> Legal intervention involving shot NOS

    ● Y35.001   Legal intervention involving unspecified firearm discharge, law enforcement official injured
    ● Y35.002   Legal intervention involving unspecified firearm discharge, bystander injured

● Y35.003   Legal intervention involving unspecified firearm discharge, suspect injured
● Y35.009   Legal intervention involving unspecified firearm discharge, unspecified person injured

● Y35.01   Legal intervention involving injury by machine gun
  ● Y35.011   Legal intervention involving injury by machine gun, law enforcement official injured
  ● Y35.012   Legal intervention involving injury by machine gun, bystander injured
  ● Y35.013   Legal intervention involving injury by machine gun, suspect injured
  ● Y35.019   Legal intervention involving injury by machine gun, unspecified person injured

● Y35.02   Legal intervention involving injury by handgun
  ● Y35.021   Legal intervention involving injury by handgun, law enforcement official injured
  ● Y35.022   Legal intervention involving injury by handgun, bystander injured
  ● Y35.023   Legal intervention involving injury by handgun, suspect injured
  ● Y35.029   Legal intervention involving injury by handgun, unspecified person injured

● Y35.03   Legal intervention involving injury by rifle pellet
  ● Y35.031   Legal intervention involving injury by rifle pellet, law enforcement official injured
  ● Y35.032   Legal intervention involving injury by rifle pellet, bystander injured
  ● Y35.033   Legal intervention involving injury by rifle pellet, suspect injured
  ● Y35.039   Legal intervention involving injury by rifle pellet, unspecified person injured

● Y35.04   Legal intervention involving injury by rubber bullet
  ● Y35.041   Legal intervention involving injury by rubber bullet, law enforcement official injured
  ● Y35.042   Legal intervention involving injury by rubber bullet, bystander injured
  ● Y35.043   Legal intervention involving injury by rubber bullet, suspect injured
  ● Y35.049   Legal intervention involving injury by rubber bullet, unspecified person injured

● Y35.09   Legal intervention involving other firearm discharge
  ● Y35.091   Legal intervention involving other firearm discharge, law enforcement official injured
  ● Y35.092   Legal intervention involving other firearm discharge, bystander injured
  ● Y35.093   Legal intervention involving other firearm discharge, suspect injured
  ● Y35.099   Legal intervention involving other firearm discharge, unspecified person injured

---

N Newborn Age: 0   **P** Pediatric Age: 0–17   **M** Maternity DX: 9–64   **A** Adult Age: 15–124   ♀ Females Only   ♂ Males Only

🔷 Complication\Comorbidity   🔷 Major C\C   (Ex) CC/MCC Exclusions   🔷 Hospital-Acquired Condition   🔷 Hierarchical Condition Category

1593

● Y35.1   Legal intervention involving explosives
   ● Y35.10   Legal intervention involving unspecified explosives
     ● Y35.101   Legal intervention involving unspecified explosives, law enforcement official injured
     ● Y35.102   Legal intervention involving unspecified explosives, bystander injured
     ● Y35.103   Legal intervention involving unspecified explosives, suspect injured
     ● Y35.109   Legal intervention involving unspecified explosives, unspecified person injured
   ● Y35.11   Legal intervention involving injury by dynamite
     ● Y35.111   Legal intervention involving injury by dynamite, law enforcement official injured
     ● Y35.112   Legal intervention involving injury by dynamite, bystander injured
     ● Y35.113   Legal intervention involving injury by dynamite, suspect injured
     ● Y35.119   Legal intervention involving injury by dynamite, unspecified person injured
   ● Y35.12   Legal intervention involving injury by explosive shell
     ● Y35.121   Legal intervention involving injury by explosive shell, law enforcement official injured
     ● Y35.122   Legal intervention involving injury by explosive shell, bystander injured
     ● Y35.123   Legal intervention involving injury by explosive shell, suspect injured
     ● Y35.129   Legal intervention involving other explosives, unspecified person injured
   ● Y35.19   Legal intervention involving other explosives
         Legal intervention involving injury by grenade
         Legal intervention involving injury by mortar bomb
     ● Y35.191   Legal intervention involving other explosives, law enforcement official injured
     ● Y35.192   Legal intervention involving other explosives, bystander injured
     ● Y35.193   Legal intervention involving other explosives, suspect injured
     ● Y35.199   Legal intervention involving other explosives, unspecified person injured
● Y35.2   Legal intervention involving gas
         Legal intervention involving asphyxiation by gas
         Legal intervention involving poisoning by gas
   ● Y35.20   Legal intervention involving unspecified gas
     ● Y35.201   Legal intervention involving unspecified gas, law enforcement official injured
     ● Y35.202   Legal intervention involving unspecified gas, bystander injured
     ● Y35.203   Legal intervention involving unspecified gas, suspect injured
     ● Y35.209   Legal intervention involving unspecified gas, unspecified person injured

● Y35.21   Legal intervention involving injury by tear gas
     ● Y35.211   Legal intervention involving injury by tear gas, law enforcement official injured
     ● Y35.212   Legal intervention involving injury by tear gas, bystander injured
     ● Y35.213   Legal intervention involving injury by tear gas, suspect injured
     ● Y35.219   Legal intervention involving injury by tear gas, unspecified person injured
   ● Y35.29   Legal intervention involving other gas
     ● Y35.291   Legal intervention involving other gas, law enforcement official injured
     ● Y35.292   Legal intervention involving other gas, bystander injured
     ● Y35.293   Legal intervention involving other gas, suspect injured
     ● Y35.299   Legal intervention involving other gas, unspecified person injured
● Y35.3   Legal intervention involving blunt objects
         Legal intervention involving being hit or struck by blunt object
   ● Y35.30   Legal intervention involving unspecified blunt objects
     ● Y35.301   Legal intervention involving unspecified blunt objects, law enforcement official injured
     ● Y35.302   Legal intervention involving unspecified blunt objects, bystander injured
     ● Y35.303   Legal intervention involving unspecified blunt objects, suspect injured
     ● Y35.309   Legal intervention involving unspecified blunt objects, unspecified person injured
   ● Y35.31   Legal intervention involving baton
     ● Y35.311   Legal intervention involving baton, law enforcement official injured
     ● Y35.312   Legal intervention involving baton, bystander injured
     ● Y35.313   Legal intervention involving baton, suspect injured
     ● Y35.319   Legal intervention involving baton, unspecified person injured
   ● Y35.39   Legal intervention involving other blunt objects
     ● Y35.391   Legal intervention involving other blunt objects, law enforcement official injured
     ● Y35.392   Legal intervention involving other blunt objects, bystander injured
     ● Y35.393   Legal intervention involving other blunt objects, suspect injured
     ● Y35.399   Legal intervention involving other blunt objects, unspecified person injured
● Y35.4   Legal intervention involving sharp objects
         Legal intervention involving being cut by sharp objects
         Legal intervention involving being stabbed by sharp objects
   ● Y35.40   Legal intervention involving unspecified sharp objects
     ● Y35.401   Legal intervention involving unspecified sharp objects, law enforcement official injured
     ● Y35.402   Legal intervention involving unspecified sharp objects, bystander injured

▶ New   ⇒ Revised   ~~deleted~~ Deleted   Excludes 1   Excludes 2   Includes   Use additional   Code first   Code also   Key words
OGCR Official Guidelines   ● Unacceptable Principal Diagnosis   X Assign placeholder X   ● Use Additional Character(s)   ▶ Manifestation Code   Coding Clinic

● Y35.403   Legal intervention involving unspecified sharp objects, suspect injured

● Y35.409   Legal intervention involving unspecified sharp objects, unspecified person injured

● Y35.41   Legal intervention involving bayonet

　　● Y35.411   Legal intervention involving bayonet, law enforcement official injured

　　● Y35.412   Legal intervention involving bayonet, bystander injured

　　● Y35.413   Legal intervention involving bayonet, suspect injured

　　● Y35.419   Legal intervention involving bayonet, unspecified person injured

● Y35.49   Legal intervention involving other sharp objects

　　● Y35.491   Legal intervention involving other sharp objects, law enforcement official injured

　　● Y35.492   Legal intervention involving other sharp objects, bystander injured

　　● Y35.493   Legal intervention involving other sharp objects, suspect injured

　　● Y35.499   Legal intervention involving other sharp objects, unspecified person injured

● Y35.8   Legal intervention involving other specified means

　● Y35.81   Legal intervention involving manhandling

　　● Y35.811   Legal intervention involving manhandling, law enforcement official injured

　　● Y35.812   Legal intervention involving manhandling, bystander injured

　　● Y35.813   Legal intervention involving manhandling, suspect injured

　　● Y35.819   Legal intervention involving manhandling, unspecified person injured

　● Y35.83   Legal intervention involving a conducted energy device
　　　Electroshock device (taser)
　　　Stun gun

　　● Y35.831   Legal intervention involving a conducted energy device, law enforcement official injured

　　● Y35.832   Legal intervention involving a conducted energy device, bystander injured

　　● Y35.833   Legal intervention involving a conducted energy device, suspect injured

　　● Y35.839   Legal intervention involving a conducted energy device, unspecified person injured

　● Y35.89   Legal intervention involving other specified means

　　● Y35.891   Legal intervention involving other specified means, law enforcement official injured

　　● Y35.892   Legal intervention involving other specified means, bystander injured

　　● Y35.893   Legal intervention involving other specified means, suspect injured
　　　　Coding Clinic: 2018, Q1, P5

▶● Y35.899   Legal intervention involving other specified means, unspecified person injured

● Y35.9   Legal intervention, means unspecified

X ● Y35.91   Legal intervention, means unspecified, law enforcement official injured

X ● Y35.92   Legal intervention, means unspecified, bystander injured

X ● Y35.93   Legal intervention, means unspecified, suspect injured

X ● Y35.99   Legal intervention, means unspecified, unspecified person injured

● Y36   Operations of war

Includes	injuries to military personnel and civilians caused by war, civil insurrection, and peacekeeping missions
Excludes1	injury to military personnel occurring during peacetime military operations (Y37.-)
	military vehicles involved in transport accidents with non-military vehicle during peacetime (V09.01, V09.21, V19.81, V29.81, V39.81, V49.81, V59.81, V69.81, V79.81)

The appropriate 7th character is to be added to each code from category Y36

A	initial encounter
D	subsequent encounter
S	sequela

● Y36.0   War operations involving explosion of marine weapons
　　Weapons and military watercraft

　● Y36.00   War operations involving explosion of unspecified marine weapon
　　　War operations involving underwater blast NOS

　　● Y36.000   War operations involving explosion of unspecified marine weapon, military personnel

　　● Y36.001   War operations involving explosion of unspecified marine weapon, civilian

　● Y36.01   War operations involving explosion of depth-charge

　　● Y36.010   War operations involving explosion of depth-charge, military personnel

　　● Y36.011   War operations involving explosion of depth-charge, civilian

　● Y36.02   War operations involving explosion of marine mine
　　　War operations involving explosion of marine mine, at sea or in harbor

　　● Y36.020   War operations involving explosion of marine mine, military personnel

　　● Y36.021   War operations involving explosion of marine mine, civilian

　● Y36.03   War operations involving explosion of sea-based artillery shell

　　● Y36.030   War operations involving explosion of sea-based artillery shell, military personnel

　　● Y36.031   War operations involving explosion of sea-based artillery shell, civilian

　● Y36.04   War operations involving explosion of torpedo

　　● Y36.040   War operations involving explosion of torpedo, military personnel

　　● Y36.041   War operations involving explosion of torpedo, civilian

CHAPTER 20 (V00-Y99)

N Newborn Age: 0   **P** Pediatric Age: 0–17   **M** Maternity DX: 9–64   **A** Adult Age: 15–124   ♀ Females Only   ♂ Males Only

🝆 Complication\Comorbidity   🝆 Major C\C   (Ex) CC/MCC Exclusions   🝆 Hospital-Acquired Condition   🝆 Hierarchical Condition Category

1595

● **Y36.05** War operations involving accidental detonation of onboard marine weapons
   ● **Y36.050** War operations involving accidental detonation of onboard marine weapons, military personnel
   ● **Y36.051** War operations involving accidental detonation of onboard marine weapons, civilian
● **Y36.09** War operations involving explosion of other marine weapons
   ● **Y36.090** War operations involving explosion of other marine weapons, military personnel
   ● **Y36.091** War operations involving explosion of other marine weapons, civilian
● **Y36.1** War operations involving destruction of aircraft
   ● **Y36.10** War operations involving unspecified destruction of aircraft
      ● **Y36.100** War operations involving unspecified destruction of aircraft, military personnel
      ● **Y36.101** War operations involving unspecified destruction of aircraft, civilian
   ● **Y36.11** War operations involving destruction of aircraft due to enemy fire or explosives
      War operations involving destruction of aircraft due to air to air missile
      War operations involving destruction of aircraft due to explosive placed on aircraft
      War operations involving destruction of aircraft due to rocket propelled grenade [RPG]
      War operations involving destruction of aircraft due to small arms fire
      War operations involving destruction of aircraft due to surface to air missile
      ● **Y36.110** War operations involving destruction of aircraft due to enemy fire or explosives, military personnel
      ● **Y36.111** War operations involving destruction of aircraft due to enemy fire or explosives, civilian
   ● **Y36.12** War operations involving destruction of aircraft due to collision with other aircraft
      ● **Y36.120** War operations involving destruction of aircraft due to collision with other aircraft, military personnel
      ● **Y36.121** War operations involving destruction of aircraft due to collision with other aircraft, civilian
   ● **Y36.13** War operations involving destruction of aircraft due to onboard fire
      ● **Y36.130** War operations involving destruction of aircraft due to onboard fire, military personnel
      ● **Y36.131** War operations involving destruction of aircraft due to onboard fire, civilian
   ● **Y36.14** War operations involving destruction of aircraft due to accidental detonation of onboard munitions and explosives
      ● **Y36.140** War operations involving destruction of aircraft due to accidental detonation of onboard munitions and explosives, military personnel
      ● **Y36.141** War operations involving destruction of aircraft due to accidental detonation of onboard munitions and explosives, civilian

● **Y36.19** War operations involving other destruction of aircraft
   ● **Y36.190** War operations involving other destruction of aircraft, military personnel
   ● **Y36.191** War operations involving other destruction of aircraft, civilian
● **Y36.2** War operations involving other explosions and fragments
   Excludes1 war operations involving explosion of aircraft (Y36.1-)
                 war operations involving explosion of marine weapons (Y36.0-)
                 war operations involving explosion of nuclear weapons (Y36.5-)
                 war operations involving explosion occurring after cessation of hostilities (Y36.8-)
   ● **Y36.20** War operations involving unspecified explosion and fragments
      War operations involving air blast NOS
      War operations involving blast NOS
      War operations involving blast fragments NOS
      War operations involving blast wave NOS
      War operations involving blast wind NOS
      War operations involving explosion NOS
      War operations involving explosion of bomb NOS
      ● **Y36.200** War operations involving unspecified explosion and fragments, military personnel
      ● **Y36.201** War operations involving unspecified explosion and fragments, civilian
   ● **Y36.21** War operations involving explosion of aerial bomb
      ● **Y36.210** War operations involving explosion of aerial bomb, military personnel
      ● **Y36.211** War operations involving explosion of aerial bomb, civilian
   ● **Y36.22** War operations involving explosion of guided missile
      ● **Y36.220** War operations involving explosion of guided missile, military personnel
      ● **Y36.221** War operations involving explosion of guided missile, civilian
   ● **Y36.23** War operations involving explosion of improvised explosive device [IED]
      War operations involving explosion of person-borne improvised explosive device [IED]
      War operations involving explosion of vehicle-borne improvised explosive device [IED]
      War operations involving explosion of roadside improvised explosive device [IED]
      ● **Y36.230** War operations involving explosion of improvised explosive device [IED], military personnel
      ● **Y36.231** War operations involving explosion of improvised explosive device [IED], civilian
   ● **Y36.24** War operations involving explosion due to accidental detonation and discharge of own munitions or munitions launch device
      ● **Y36.240** War operations involving explosion due to accidental detonation and discharge of own munitions or munitions launch device, military personnel
      ● **Y36.241** War operations involving explosion due to accidental detonation and discharge of own munitions or munitions launch device, civilian

▶ New   ⇒ Revised   ~~deleted~~ Deleted   Excludes 1   Excludes 2   Includes   Use additional   Code first   Code also   Key words
OGCR Official Guidelines   ● Unacceptable Principal Diagnosis   X Assign placeholder X   ● Use Additional Character(s)   ▷ Manifestation Code   **Coding Clinic**

● Y36.25   War operations involving fragments from munitions
     ● Y36.250   War operations involving fragments from munitions, military personnel
     ● Y36.251   War operations involving fragments from munitions, civilian
● Y36.26   War operations involving fragments of improvised explosive device [IED]
     War operations involving fragments of person-borne improvised explosive device [IED]
     War operations involving fragments of vehicle-borne improvised explosive device [IED]
     War operations involving fragments of roadside improvised explosive device [IED]
     ● Y36.260   War operations involving fragments of improvised explosive device [IED], military personnel
     ● Y36.261   War operations involving fragments of improvised explosive device [IED], civilian
● Y36.27   War operations involving fragments from weapons
     ● Y36.270   War operations involving fragments from weapons, military personnel
     ● Y36.271   War operations involving fragments from weapons, civilian
● Y36.29   War operations involving other explosions and fragments
     War operations involving explosion of grenade
     War operations involving explosions of land mine
     War operations involving shrapnel NOS
     ● Y36.290   War operations involving other explosions and fragments, military personnel
     ● Y36.291   War operations involving other explosions and fragments, civilian
● Y36.3   War operations involving fires, conflagrations and hot substances
     War operations involving smoke, fumes, and heat from fires, conflagrations and hot substances
     Excludes1   war operations involving fires and conflagrations aboard military aircraft (Y36.1-)
         war operations involving fires and conflagrations aboard military watercraft (Y36.0-)
         war operations involving fires and conflagrations caused indirectly by conventional weapons (Y36.2-)
         war operations involving fires and thermal effects of nuclear weapons (Y36.53-)
     ● Y36.30   War operations involving unspecified fire, conflagration and hot substance
         ● Y36.300   War operations involving unspecified fire, conflagration and hot substance, military personnel
         ● Y36.301   War operations involving unspecified fire, conflagration and hot substance, civilian
     ● Y36.31   War operations involving gasoline bomb
         War operations involving incendiary bomb
         War operations involving petrol bomb
         ● Y36.310   War operations involving gasoline bomb, military personnel
         ● Y36.311   War operations involving gasoline bomb, civilian

● Y36.32   War operations involving incendiary bullet
     ● Y36.320   War operations involving incendiary bullet, military personnel
     ● Y36.321   War operations involving incendiary bullet, civilian
● Y36.33   War operations involving flamethrower
     ● Y36.330   War operations involving flamethrower, military personnel
     ● Y36.331   War operations involving flamethrower, civilian
● Y36.39   War operations involving other fires, conflagrations and hot substances
     ● Y36.390   War operations involving other fires, conflagrations and hot substances, military personnel
     ● Y36.391   War operations involving other fires, conflagrations and hot substances, civilian
● Y36.4   War operations involving firearm discharge and other forms of conventional warfare
     ● Y36.41   War operations involving rubber bullets
         ● Y36.410   War operations involving rubber bullets, military personnel
         ● Y36.411   War operations involving rubber bullets, civilian
     ● Y36.42   War operations involving firearms pellets
         ● Y36.420   War operations involving firearms pellets, military personnel
         ● Y36.421   War operations involving firearms pellets, civilian
     ● Y36.43   War operations involving other firearms discharge
         War operations involving bullets NOS
         Excludes1   war operations involving munitions fragments (Y36.25-)
             war operations involving incendiary bullets (Y36.32-)
         ● Y36.430   War operations involving other firearms discharge, military personnel
         ● Y36.431   War operations involving other firearms discharge, civilian
     ● Y36.44   War operations involving unarmed hand to hand combat
         Excludes1   war operations involving combat using blunt or piercing object (Y36.45-)
             war operations involving intentional restriction of air and airway (Y36.46-)
             war operations involving unintentional restriction of air and airway (Y36.47-)
         ● Y36.440   War operations involving unarmed hand to hand combat, military personnel
         ● Y36.441   War operations involving unarmed hand to hand combat, civilian
     ● Y36.45   War operations involving combat using blunt or piercing object
         ● Y36.450   War operations involving combat using blunt or piercing object, military personnel
         ● Y36.451   War operations involving combat using blunt or piercing object, civilian

CHAPTER 20 (V00-Y99)

● **Y36.46**   War operations involving intentional restriction of air and airway
- ● **Y36.460**   War operations involving intentional restriction of air and airway, military personnel
- ● **Y36.461**   War operations involving intentional restriction of air and airway, civilian

● **Y36.47**   War operations involving unintentional restriction of air and airway
- ● **Y36.470**   War operations involving unintentional restriction of air and airway, military personnel
- ● **Y36.471**   War operations involving unintentional restriction of air and airway, civilian

● **Y36.49**   War operations involving other forms of conventional warfare
- ● **Y36.490**   War operations involving other forms of conventional warfare, military personnel
- ● **Y36.491**   War operations involving other forms of conventional warfare, civilian

● **Y36.5**   War operations involving nuclear weapons
War operations involving dirty bomb NOS

● **Y36.50**   War operations involving unspecified effect of nuclear weapon
- ● **Y36.500**   War operations involving unspecified effect of nuclear weapon, military personnel
- ● **Y36.501**   War operations involving unspecified effect of nuclear weapon, civilian

● **Y36.51**   War operations involving direct blast effect of nuclear weapon
War operations involving blast pressure of nuclear weapon
- ● **Y36.510**   War operations involving direct blast effect of nuclear weapon, military personnel
- ● **Y36.511**   War operations involving direct blast effect of nuclear weapon, civilian

● **Y36.52**   War operations involving indirect blast effect of nuclear weapon
War operations involving being thrown by blast of nuclear weapon
War operations involving being struck or crushed by blast debris of nuclear weapon
- ● **Y36.520**   War operations involving indirect blast effect of nuclear weapon, military personnel
- ● **Y36.521**   War operations involving indirect blast effect of nuclear weapon, civilian

● **Y36.53**   War operations involving thermal radiation effect of nuclear weapon
War operations involving direct heat from nuclear weapon
War operation involving fireball effects from nuclear weapon
- ● **Y36.530**   War operations involving thermal radiation effect of nuclear weapon, military personnel
- ● **Y36.531**   War operations involving thermal radiation effect of nuclear weapon, civilian

● **Y36.54**   War operation involving nuclear radiation effects of nuclear weapon
War operation involving acute radiation exposure from nuclear weapon
War operation involving exposure to immediate ionizing radiation from nuclear weapon
War operation involving fallout exposure from nuclear weapon
War operation involving secondary effects of nuclear weapons
- ● **Y36.540**   War operation involving nuclear radiation effects of nuclear weapon, military personnel
- ● **Y36.541**   War operation involving nuclear radiation effects of nuclear weapon, civilian

● **Y36.59**   War operation involving other effects of nuclear weapons
- ● **Y36.590**   War operation involving other effects of nuclear weapons, military personnel
- ● **Y36.591**   War operation involving other effects of nuclear weapons, civilian

● **Y36.6**   War operations involving biological weapons
- ● **Y36.6X**   War operations involving biological weapons
  - ● **Y36.6X0**   War operations involving biological weapons, military personnel
  - ● **Y36.6X1**   War operations involving biological weapons, civilian

● **Y36.7**   War operations involving chemical weapons and other forms of unconventional warfare
    Excludes 1   war operations involving incendiary devices (Y36.3-, Y36.5-)
- ● **Y36.7X**   War operations involving chemical weapons and other forms of unconventional warfare
  - ● **Y36.7X0**   War operations involving chemical weapons and other forms of unconventional warfare, military personnel
  - ● **Y36.7X1**   War operations involving chemical weapons and other forms of unconventional warfare, civilian

● **Y36.8**   War operations occurring after cessation of hostilities
War operations classifiable to categories Y36.0-Y36.8 but occurring after cessation of hostilities
- ● **Y36.81**   Explosion of mine placed during war operations but exploding after cessation of hostilities
  - ● **Y36.810**   Explosion of mine placed during war operations but exploding after cessation of hostilities, military personnel
  - ● **Y36.811**   Explosion of mine placed during war operations but exploding after cessation of hostilities, civilian

- ● **Y36.82**   Explosion of bomb placed during war operations but exploding after cessation of hostilities
  - ● **Y36.820**   Explosion of bomb placed during war operations but exploding after cessation of hostilities, military personnel
  - ● **Y36.821**   Explosion of bomb placed during war operations but exploding after cessation of hostilities, civilian

▶ New   ⇒ Revised   ~~deleted~~ Deleted   Excludes 1   Excludes 2   Includes   Use additional   Code first   Code also   Key words

OGCR Official Guidelines   ● Unacceptable Principal Diagnosis   X Assign placeholder X   ● Use Additional Character(s)   ▶ Manifestation Code   **Coding Clinic**

● Y36.88   Other war operations occurring after cessation of hostilities
- ● Y36.880   Other war operations occurring after cessation of hostilities, military personnel
- ● Y36.881   Other war operations occurring after cessation of hostilities, civilian

● Y36.89   Unspecified war operations occurring after cessation of hostilities
- ● Y36.890   Unspecified war operations occurring after cessation of hostilities, military personnel
- ● Y36.891   Unspecified war operations occurring after cessation of hostilities, civilian

● Y36.9   Other and unspecified war operations
- X ● Y36.90   War operations, unspecified
- X ● Y36.91   War operations involving unspecified weapon of mass destruction [WMD]
- X ● Y36.92   War operations involving friendly fire

● Y37   Military operations

Includes	Injuries to military personnel and civilians occurring during peacetime on military property and during routine military exercises and operations
Excludes1	military aircraft involved in aircraft accident with civilian aircraft (V97.81-)
	military vehicles involved in transport accident with civilian vehicle (V09.01, V09.21, V19.81, V29.81, V39.81, V49.81, V59.81, V69.81, V79.81)
	military watercraft involved in water transport accident with civilian watercraft (V94.81-)
	war operations (Y36.-)

The appropriate 7th character is to be added to each code from category Y37

A	initial encounter
D	subsequent encounter
S	sequela

● Y37.0   Military operations involving explosion of marine weapons

- ● Y37.00   Military operations involving explosion of unspecified marine weapon
  Military operations involving underwater blast NOS
  - ● Y37.000   Military operations involving explosion of unspecified marine weapon, military personnel
  - ● Y37.001   Military operations involving explosion of unspecified marine weapon, civilian

- ● Y37.01   Military operations involving explosion of depth-charge
  - ● Y37.010   Military operations involving explosion of depth-charge, military personnel
  - ● Y37.011   Military operations involving explosion of depth-charge, civilian

- ● Y37.02   Military operations involving explosion of marine mine
  Military operations involving explosion of marine mine, at sea or in harbor
  - ● Y37.020   Military operations involving explosion of marine mine, military personnel
  - ● Y37.021   Military operations involving explosion of marine mine, civilian

● Y37.03   Military operations involving explosion of sea-based artillery shell
- ● Y37.030   Military operations involving explosion of sea-based artillery shell, military personnel
- ● Y37.031   Military operations involving explosion of sea-based artillery shell, civilian

● Y37.04   Military operations involving explosion of torpedo
- ● Y37.040   Military operations involving explosion of torpedo, military personnel
- ● Y37.041   Military operations involving explosion of torpedo, civilian

● Y37.05   Military operations involving accidental detonation of onboard marine weapons
- ● Y37.050   Military operations involving accidental detonation of onboard marine weapons, military personnel
- ● Y37.051   Military operations involving accidental detonation of onboard marine weapons, civilian

● Y37.09   Military operations involving explosion of other marine weapons
- ● Y37.090   Military operations involving explosion of other marine weapons, military personnel
- ● Y37.091   Military operations involving explosion of other marine weapons, civilian

● Y37.1   Military operations involving destruction of aircraft

- ● Y37.10   Military operations involving unspecified destruction of aircraft
  - ● Y37.100   Military operations involving unspecified destruction of aircraft, military personnel
  - ● Y37.101   Military operations involving unspecified destruction of aircraft, civilian

- ● Y37.11   Military operations involving destruction of aircraft due to enemy fire or explosives
  Military operations involving destruction of aircraft due to air to air missile
  Military operations involving destruction of aircraft due to explosive placed on aircraft
  Military operations involving destruction of aircraft due to rocket propelled grenade [RPG]
  Military operations involving destruction of aircraft due to small arms fire
  Military operations involving destruction of aircraft due to surface to air missile
  - ● Y37.110   Military operations involving destruction of aircraft due to enemy fire or explosives, military personnel
  - ● Y37.111   Military operations involving destruction of aircraft due to enemy fire or explosives, civilian

- ● Y37.12   Military operations involving destruction of aircraft due to collision with other aircraft
  - ● Y37.120   Military operations involving destruction of aircraft due to collision with other aircraft, military personnel
  - ● Y37.121   Military operations involving destruction of aircraft due to collision with other aircraft, civilian

CHAPTER 20 (V00-Y99)

● Y37.13   Military operations involving destruction of aircraft due to onboard fire

     ● Y37.130   Military operations involving destruction of aircraft due to onboard fire, military personnel

     ● Y37.131   Military operations involving destruction of aircraft due to onboard fire, civilian

● Y37.14   Military operations involving destruction of aircraft due to accidental detonation of onboard munitions and explosives

     ● Y37.140   Military operations involving destruction of aircraft due to accidental detonation of onboard munitions and explosives, military personnel

     ● Y37.141   Military operations involving destruction of aircraft due to accidental detonation of onboard munitions and explosives, civilian

● Y37.19   Military operations involving other destruction of aircraft

     ● Y37.190   Military operations involving other destruction of aircraft, military personnel

     ● Y37.191   Military operations involving other destruction of aircraft, civilian

● Y37.2   Military operations involving other explosions and fragments

     Excludes1   military operations involving explosion of aircraft (Y37.1-)

                   military operations involving explosion of marine weapons (Y37.0-)

                   military operations involving explosion of nuclear weapons (Y37.5-)

● Y37.20   Military operations involving unspecified explosion and fragments

     Military operations involving air blast NOS

     Military operations involving blast NOS

     Military operations involving blast fragments NOS

     Military operations involving blast wave NOS

     Military operations involving blast wind NOS

     Military operations involving explosion NOS

     Military operations involving explosion of bomb NOS

     ● Y37.200   Military operations involving unspecified explosion and fragments, military personnel

     ● Y37.201   Military operations involving unspecified explosion and fragments, civilian

● Y37.21   Military operations involving explosion of aerial bomb

     ● Y37.210   Military operations involving explosion of aerial bomb, military personnel

     ● Y37.211   Military operations involving explosion of aerial bomb, civilian

● Y37.22   Military operations involving explosion of guided missile

     ● Y37.220   Military operations involving explosion of guided missile, military personnel

     ● Y37.221   Military operations involving explosion of guided missile, civilian

● Y37.23   Military operations involving explosion of improvised explosive device [IED]

     Military operations involving explosion of person-borne improvised explosive device [IED]

     Military operations involving explosion of vehicle-borne improvised explosive device [IED]

     Military operations involving explosion of roadside improvised explosive device [IED]

     ● Y37.230   Military operations involving explosion of improvised explosive device [IED], military personnel

     ● Y37.231   Military operations involving explosion of improvised explosive device [IED], civilian

● Y37.24   Military operations involving explosion due to accidental detonation and discharge of own munitions or munitions launch device

     ● Y37.240   Military operations involving explosion due to accidental detonation and discharge of own munitions or munitions launch device, military personnel

     ● Y37.241   Military operations involving explosion due to accidental detonation and discharge of own munitions or munitions launch device, civilian

● Y37.25   Military operations involving fragments from munitions

     ● Y37.250   Military operations involving fragments from munitions, military personnel

     ● Y37.251   Military operations involving fragments from munitions, civilian

● Y37.26   Military operations involving fragments of improvised explosive device [IED]

     Military operations involving fragments of person-borne improvised explosive device [IED]

     Military operations involving fragments of vehicle-borne improvised explosive device [IED]

     Military operations involving fragments of roadside improvised explosive device [IED]

     ● Y37.260   Military operations involving fragments of improvised explosive device [IED], military personnel

     ● Y37.261   Military operations involving fragments of improvised explosive device [IED], civilian

● Y37.27   Military operations involving fragments from weapons

     ● Y37.270   Military operations involving fragments from weapons, military personnel

     ● Y37.271   Military operations involving fragments from weapons, civilian

● Y37.29   Military operations involving other explosions and fragments

     Military operations involving explosion of grenade

     Military operations involving explosions of land mine

     Military operations involving shrapnel NOS

     ● Y37.290   Military operations involving other explosions and fragments, military personnel

     ● Y37.291   Military operations involving other explosions and fragments, civilian

▶ New   ⇒ Revised   deleted Deleted   Excludes 1   Excludes 2   Includes   Use additional   Code first   Code also   Key words

OGCR Official Guidelines   ● Unacceptable Principal Diagnosis   X Assign placeholder X   ● Use Additional Character(s)   ▸ Manifestation Code   **Coding Clinic**

● **Y37.3   Military operations involving fires, conflagrations and hot substances**
> Military operations involving smoke, fumes, and heat from fires, conflagrations and hot substances

> Excludes1   military operations involving fires and conflagrations aboard military aircraft (Y37.1-)
> military operations involving fires and conflagrations aboard military watercraft (Y37.0-)
> military operations involving fires and conflagrations caused indirectly by conventional weapons (Y37.2-)
> military operations involving fires and thermal effects of nuclear weapons (Y36.53-)

● **Y37.30   Military operations involving unspecified fire, conflagration and hot substance**
  ● **Y37.300   Military operations involving unspecified fire, conflagration and hot substance, military personnel**
  ● **Y37.301   Military operations involving unspecified fire, conflagration and hot substance, civilian**

● **Y37.31   Military operations involving gasoline bomb**
> Military operations involving incendiary bomb
> Military operations involving petrol bomb
  ● **Y37.310   Military operations involving gasoline bomb, military personnel**
  ● **Y37.311   Military operations involving gasoline bomb, civilian**

● **Y37.32   Military operations involving incendiary bullet**
  ● **Y37.320   Military operations involving incendiary bullet, military personnel**
  ● **Y37.321   Military operations involving incendiary bullet, civilian**

● **Y37.33   Military operations involving flamethrower**
  ● **Y37.330   Military operations involving flamethrower, military personnel**
  ● **Y37.331   Military operations involving flamethrower, civilian**

● **Y37.39   Military operations involving other fires, conflagrations and hot substances**
  ● **Y37.390   Military operations involving other fires, conflagrations and hot substances, military personnel**
  ● **Y37.391   Military operations involving other fires, conflagrations and hot substances, civilian**

● **Y37.4   Military operations involving firearm discharge and other forms of conventional warfare**
● **Y37.41   Military operations involving rubber bullets**
  ● **Y37.410   Military operations involving rubber bullets, military personnel**
  ● **Y37.411   Military operations involving rubber bullets, civilian**

● **Y37.42   Military operations involving firearms pellets**
  ● **Y37.420   Military operations involving firearms pellets, military personnel**
  ● **Y37.421   Military operations involving firearms pellets, civilian**

● **Y37.43   Military operations involving other firearms discharge**
> Military operations involving bullets NOS
> Excludes1   military operations involving munitions fragments (Y37.25-)
> military operations involving incendiary bullets (Y37.32-)
  ● **Y37.430   Military operations involving other firearms discharge, military personnel**
  ● **Y37.431   Military operations involving other firearms discharge, civilian**

● **Y37.44   Military operations involving unarmed hand to hand combat**
> Excludes1   military operations involving combat using blunt or piercing object (Y37.45-)
> military operations involving intentional restriction of air and airway (Y37.46-)
> military operations involving unintentional restriction of air and airway (Y37.47-)
  ● **Y37.440   Military operations involving unarmed hand to hand combat, military personnel**
  ● **Y37.441   Military operations involving unarmed hand to hand combat, civilian**

● **Y37.45   Military operations involving combat using blunt or piercing object**
  ● **Y37.450   Military operations involving combat using blunt or piercing object, military personnel**
  ● **Y37.451   Military operations involving combat using blunt or piercing object, civilian**

● **Y37.46   Military operations involving intentional restriction of air and airway**
  ● **Y37.460   Military operations involving intentional restriction of air and airway, military personnel**
  ● **Y37.461   Military operations involving intentional restriction of air and airway, civilian**

● **Y37.47   Military operations involving unintentional restriction of air and airway**
  ● **Y37.470   Military operations involving unintentional restriction of air and airway, military personnel**
  ● **Y37.471   Military operations involving unintentional restriction of air and airway, civilian**

● **Y37.49   Military operations involving other forms of conventional warfare**
  ● **Y37.490   Military operations involving other forms of conventional warfare, military personnel**
  ● **Y37.491   Military operations involving other forms of conventional warfare, civilian**

● **Y37.5   Military operations involving nuclear weapons**
> Military operation involving dirty bomb NOS
● **Y37.50   Military operations involving unspecified effect of nuclear weapon**
  ● **Y37.500   Military operations involving unspecified effect of nuclear weapon, military personnel**
  ● **Y37.501   Military operations involving unspecified effect of nuclear weapon, civilian**

● **Y37.51   Military operations involving direct blast effect of nuclear weapon**
> Military operations involving blast pressure of nuclear weapon
  ● **Y37.510   Military operations involving direct blast effect of nuclear weapon, military personnel**
  ● **Y37.511   Military operations involving direct blast effect of nuclear weapon, civilian**

N Newborn Age: 0   **P** Pediatric Age: 0–17   **M** Maternity DX: 9–64   **A** Adult Age: 15–124   ♀ Females Only   ♂ Males Only

Complication\Comorbidity   Major C\C   (Ex) CC/MCC Exclusions   Hospital-Acquired Condition   Hierarchical Condition Category

CHAPTER 20 (V00-Y99)

● Y37.52   Military operations involving indirect blast effect of nuclear weapon
Military operations involving being thrown by blast of nuclear weapon
Military operations involving being struck or crushed by blast debris of nuclear weapon

● Y37.520   Military operations involving indirect blast effect of nuclear weapon, military personnel

● Y37.521   Military operations involving indirect blast effect of nuclear weapon, civilian

● Y37.53   Military operations involving thermal radiation effect of nuclear weapon
Military operations involving direct heat from nuclear weapon
Military operation involving fireball effects from nuclear weapon

● Y37.530   Military operations involving thermal radiation effect of nuclear weapon, military personnel

● Y37.531   Military operations involving thermal radiation effect of nuclear weapon, civilian

● Y37.54   Military operation involving nuclear radiation effects of nuclear weapon
Military operation involving acute radiation exposure from nuclear weapon
Military operation involving exposure to immediate ionizing radiation from nuclear weapon
Military operation involving fallout exposure from nuclear weapon
Military operation involving secondary effects of nuclear weapons

● Y37.540   Military operation involving nuclear radiation effects of nuclear weapon, military personnel

● Y37.541   Military operation involving nuclear radiation effects of nuclear weapon, civilian

● Y37.59   Military operation involving other effects of nuclear weapons

● Y37.590   Military operation involving other effects of nuclear weapons, military personnel

● Y37.591   Military operation involving other effects of nuclear weapons, civilian

● Y37.6   Military operations involving biological weapons

● Y37.6X   Military operations involving biological weapons

● Y37.6X0   Military operations involving biological weapons, military personnel

● Y37.6X1   Military operations involving biological weapons, civilian

● Y37.7   Military operations involving chemical weapons and other forms of unconventional warfare

Excludes1   military operations involving incendiary devices (Y36.3-, Y36.5-)

● Y37.7X   Military operations involving chemical weapons and other forms of unconventional warfare

● Y37.7X0   Military operations involving chemical weapons and other forms of unconventional warfare, military personnel

● Y37.7X1   Military operations involving chemical weapons and other forms of unconventional warfare, civilian

● Y37.9   Other and unspecified military operations

X● Y37.90   Military operations, unspecified

X● Y37.91   Military operations involving unspecified weapon of mass destruction [WMD]

X● Y37.92   Military operations involving friendly fire

● Y38   Terrorism
These codes are for use to identify injuries resulting from the unlawful use of force or violence against persons or property to intimidate or coerce a government, the civilian population, or any segment thereof, in furtherance of political or social objective

Use additional code for place of occurrence (Y92.-)

The appropriate 7th character is to be added to each code from category Y38

A	initial encounter
D	subsequent encounter
S	sequela

● Y38.0   Terrorism involving explosion of marine weapons
Terrorism involving depth-charge
Terrorism involving marine mine
Terrorism involving mine NOS, at sea or in harbor
Terrorism involving sea-based artillery shell
Terrorism involving torpedo
Terrorism involving underwater blast

● Y38.0X   Terrorism involving explosion of marine weapons

● Y38.0X1   Terrorism involving explosion of marine weapons, public safety official injured

● Y38.0X2   Terrorism involving explosion of marine weapons, civilian injured

● Y38.0X3   Terrorism involving explosion of marine weapons, terrorist injured

● Y38.1   Terrorism involving destruction of aircraft
Terrorism involving aircraft burned
Terrorism involving aircraft exploded
Terrorism involving aircraft being shot down
Terrorism involving aircraft used as a weapon

● Y38.1X   Terrorism involving destruction of aircraft

● Y38.1X1   Terrorism involving destruction of aircraft, public safety official injured

● Y38.1X2   Terrorism involving destruction of aircraft, civilian injured

● Y38.1X3   Terrorism involving destruction of aircraft, terrorist injured

● Y38.2   Terrorism involving other explosions and fragments
Terrorism involving antipersonnel (fragments) bomb
Terrorism involving blast NOS
Terrorism involving explosion NOS
Terrorism involving explosion of breech block
Terrorism involving explosion of cannon block
Terrorism involving explosion (fragments) of artillery shell
Terrorism involving explosion (fragments) of bomb
Terrorism involving explosion (fragments) of grenade
Terrorism involving explosion (fragments) of guided missile
Terrorism involving explosion (fragments) of land mine
Terrorism involving explosion of mortar bomb
Terrorism involving explosion of munitions
Terrorism involving explosion (fragments) of rocket
Terrorism involving explosion (fragments) of shell
Terrorism involving shrapnel
Terrorism involving mine NOS, on land

Excludes1   terrorism involving explosion of nuclear weapon (Y38.5)
terrorism involving suicide bomber (Y38.81)

● Y38.2X   Terrorism involving other explosions and fragments

● Y38.2X1   Terrorism involving other explosions and fragments, public safety official injured

● Y38.2X2   Terrorism involving other explosions and fragments, civilian injured

● Y38.2X3   Terrorism involving other explosions and fragments, terrorist injured

▶ New   ⇒ Revised   ~~deleted~~ Deleted   Excludes 1   Excludes 2   Includes   Use additional   Code first   Code also   Key words
OGCR Official Guidelines   ● Unacceptable Principal Diagnosis   X Assign placeholder X   ● Use Additional Character(s)   ▷ Manifestation Code   **Coding Clinic**

● Y38.3   Terrorism involving fires, conflagration and hot
          substances
              Terrorism involving conflagration NOS
              Terrorism involving fire NOS
              Terrorism involving petrol bomb
              Excludes1   terrorism involving fire or heat of nuclear
                             weapon (Y38.5)
  ● Y38.3X Terrorism involving fires, conflagration and hot
            substances
      ● Y38.3X1   Terrorism involving fires,
                  conflagration and hot substances,
                  public safety official injured
      ● Y38.3X2   Terrorism involving fires,
                  conflagration and hot substances,
                  civilian injured
      ● Y38.3X3   Terrorism involving fires,
                  conflagration and hot substances,
                  terrorist injured

● Y38.4   Terrorism involving firearms
              Terrorism involving carbine bullet
              Terrorism involving machine gun bullet
              Terrorism involving pellets (shotgun)
              Terrorism involving pistol bullet
              Terrorism involving rifle bullet
              Terrorism involving rubber (rifle) bullet
  ● Y38.4X Terrorism involving firearms
      ● Y38.4X1   Terrorism involving firearms, public
                  safety official injured
      ● Y38.4X2   Terrorism involving firearms, civilian
                  injured
      ● Y38.4X3   Terrorism involving firearms, terrorist
                  injured

● Y38.5   Terrorism involving nuclear weapons
              Terrorism involving blast effects of nuclear weapon
              Terrorism involving exposure to ionizing radiation from
                  nuclear weapon
              Terrorism involving fireball effect of nuclear weapon
              Terrorism involving heat from nuclear weapon
  ● Y38.5X Terrorism involving nuclear weapons
      ● Y38.5X1   Terrorism involving nuclear weapons,
                  public safety official injured
      ● Y38.5X2   Terrorism involving nuclear weapons,
                  civilian injured
      ● Y38.5X3   Terrorism involving nuclear weapons,
                  terrorist injured

● Y38.6   Terrorism involving biological weapons
              Terrorism involving anthrax
              Terrorism involving cholera
                  A serious, often deadly, infectious disease of the small
                  intestine
              Terrorism involving smallpox
  ● Y38.6X Terrorism involving biological weapons
      ● Y38.6X1   Terrorism involving biological
                  weapons, public safety official
                  injured
      ● Y38.6X2   Terrorism involving biological
                  weapons, civilian injured
      ● Y38.6X3   Terrorism involving biological
                  weapons, terrorist injured

● Y38.7   Terrorism involving chemical weapons
              Terrorism involving gases, fumes, chemicals
              Terrorism involving hydrogen cyanide
              Terrorism involving phosgene
              Terrorism involving sarin
  ● Y38.7X Terrorism involving chemical weapons
      ● Y38.7X1   Terrorism involving chemical
                  weapons, public safety official
                  injured
      ● Y38.7X2   Terrorism involving chemical
                  weapons, civilian injured
      ● Y38.7X3   Terrorism involving chemical
                  weapons, terrorist injured

● Y38.8   Terrorism involving other and unspecified means
  ● Y38.80 Terrorism involving unspecified means
              Terrorism NOS
  ● Y38.81 Terrorism involving suicide bomber
      ● Y38.811   Terrorism involving suicide bomber,
                  public safety official injured
      ● Y38.812   Terrorism involving suicide bomber,
                  civilian injured
  ● Y38.89 Terrorism involving other means
              Terrorism involving drowning and submersion
              Terrorism involving lasers
              Terrorism involving piercing or stabbing
                  instruments
      ● Y38.891   Terrorism involving other means,
                  public safety official injured
      ● Y38.892   Terrorism involving other means,
                  civilian injured
      ● Y38.893   Terrorism involving other means,
                  terrorist injured

● Y38.9   Terrorism, secondary effects
              Note: This code is for use to identify conditions
                  occurring subsequent to a terrorist attack not those
                  that are due to the initial terrorist attack.
  ● Y38.9X Terrorism, secondary effects
      ● Y38.9X1   Terrorism, secondary effects, public
                  safety official injured
      ● Y38.9X2   Terrorism, secondary effects, civilian
                  injured categories

COMPLICATIONS OF MEDICAL AND SURGICAL CARE (Y62-Y84)

Includes   complications of medical devices surgical
               and medical procedures as the cause of
               abnormal reaction of the patient, or of
               later complication, without mention of
               misadventure at the time of the procedure

MISADVENTURES TO PATIENTS DURING SURGICAL AND MEDICAL CARE (Y62-Y69)

Excludes1   surgical and medical procedures as the cause of
               abnormal reaction of the patient, without
               mention of misadventure at the time of the
               procedure (Y83-Y84)

● Y62   Failure of sterile precautions during surgical and medical care
    Y62.0   Failure of sterile precautions during surgical operation
    Y62.1   Failure of sterile precautions during infusion or
            transfusion
    Y62.2   Failure of sterile precautions during kidney dialysis and
            other perfusion 🔖
    Y62.3   Failure of sterile precautions during injection or
            immunization
    Y62.4   Failure of sterile precautions during endoscopic
            examination
    Y62.5   Failure of sterile precautions during heart
            catheterization
    Y62.6   Failure of sterile precautions during aspiration, puncture
            and other catheterization
    Y62.8   Failure of sterile precautions during other surgical and
            medical care
    Y62.9   Failure of sterile precautions during unspecified surgical
            and medical care

● Y63   Failure in dosage during surgical and medical care
    Excludes2   accidental overdose of drug or wrong drug given
                   in error (T36-T50)
    Y63.0   Excessive amount of blood or other fluid given during
            transfusion or infusion
    Y63.1   Incorrect dilution of fluid used during infusion
    Y63.2   Overdose of radiation given during therapy

N Newborn Age: Ø   **P** Pediatric Age: Ø–17   **M** Maternity DX: 9–64   **A** Adult Age: 15–124   ♀ Females Only   ♂ Males Only

🔖 Complication\Comorbidity   🔖 Major C\C   (Ex) CC/MCC Exclusions   🔖 Hospital-Acquired Condition   🔖 Hierarchical Condition Category

1603

CHAPTER 20 (V00-Y99)

Y63.3   Inadvertent exposure of patient to radiation during medical care

Y63.4   Failure in dosage in electroshock or insulin-shock therapy

Y63.5   Inappropriate temperature in local application and packing

Y63.6   Underdosing and nonadministration of necessary drug, medicament or biological substance

Y63.8   Failure in dosage during other surgical and medical care

Y63.9   Failure in dosage during unspecified surgical and medical care

● Y64   Contaminated medical or biological substances

Y64.0   Contaminated medical or biological substance, transfused or infused

Y64.1   Contaminated medical or biological substance, injected or used for immunization

Y64.8   Contaminated medical or biological substance administered by other means

Y64.9   Contaminated medical or biological substance administered by unspecified means
     Administered contaminated medical or biological substance NOS

● Y65   Other misadventures during surgical and medical care

Y65.0   Mismatched blood in transfusion

Y65.1   Wrong fluid used in infusion

Y65.2   Failure in suture or ligature during surgical operation

Y65.3   Endotracheal tube wrongly placed during anesthetic procedure

Y65.4   Failure to introduce or to remove other tube or instrument

● Y65.5   Performance of wrong procedure (operation)

   ● Y65.51   Performance of wrong procedure (operation) on correct patient
       Wrong device implanted into correct surgical site

       Excludes1   performance of correct procedure (operation) on wrong side or body part (Y65.53)
       MCE: Wrong procedure performed

   ● Y65.52   Performance of procedure (operation) on patient not scheduled for surgery
       Performance of procedure (operation) intended for another patient
       Performance of procedure (operation) on wrong patient
       MCE: Wrong procedure performed

   ● Y65.53   Performance of correct procedure (operation) on wrong side or body part
       Performance of correct procedure (operation) on wrong side
       Performance of correct procedure (operation) on wrong site
       MCE: Wrong procedure performed

Y65.8   Other specified misadventures during surgical and medical care
     Coding Clinic: 2019, Q2, P24

Y66   Nonadministration of surgical and medical care
     Premature cessation of surgical and medical care

     Excludes1   DNR status (Z66)
       palliative care (Z51.5)

Y69   Unspecified misadventure during surgical and medical care

MEDICAL DEVICES ASSOCIATED WITH ADVERSE INCIDENTS IN DIAGNOSTIC AND THERAPEUTIC USE (Y70-Y82)

Includes   breakdown or malfunction of medical devices (during use) (after implantation) (ongoing use)

Excludes2   later complications following use of medical devices without breakdown or malfunctioning of device (Y83-Y84)
     misadventure to patients during surgical and medical care, classifiable to (Y62-Y69)
     surgical and other medical procedures as the cause of abnormal reaction of the patient, or of later complication, without mention of misadventure at the time of the procedure (Y83-Y84)

● Y70   Anesthesiology devices associated with adverse incidents

Y70.0   Diagnostic and monitoring anesthesiology devices associated with adverse incidents

Y70.1   Therapeutic (nonsurgical) and rehabilitative anesthesiology devices associated with adverse incidents

Y70.2   Prosthetic and other implants, materials and accessory anesthesiology devices associated with adverse incidents

Y70.3   Surgical instruments, materials and anesthesiology devices (including sutures) associated with adverse incidents

Y70.8   Miscellaneous anesthesiology devices associated with adverse incidents, not elsewhere classified

● Y71   Cardiovascular devices associated with adverse incidents

Y71.0   Diagnostic and monitoring cardiovascular devices associated with adverse incidents

Y71.1   Therapeutic (nonsurgical) and rehabilitative cardiovascular devices associated with adverse incidents

Y71.2   Prosthetic and other implants, materials and accessory cardiovascular devices associated with adverse incidents

Y71.3   Surgical instruments, materials and cardiovascular devices (including sutures) associated with adverse incidents

Y71.8   Miscellaneous cardiovascular devices associated with adverse incidents, not elsewhere classified

● Y72   Otorhinolaryngological devices associated with adverse incidents

Y72.0   Diagnostic and monitoring otorhinolaryngological devices associated with adverse incidents

Y72.1   Therapeutic (nonsurgical) and rehabilitative otorhinolaryngological devices associated with adverse incidents

Y72.2   Prosthetic and other implants, materials and accessory otorhinolaryngological devices associated with adverse incidents

Y72.3   Surgical instruments, materials and otorhinolaryngological devices (including sutures) associated with adverse incidents

Y72.8   Miscellaneous otorhinolaryngological devices associated with adverse incidents, not elsewhere classified

● Y73   Gastroenterology and urology devices associated with adverse incidents

Y73.0   Diagnostic and monitoring gastroenterology and urology devices associated with adverse incidents

Y73.1   Therapeutic (nonsurgical) and rehabilitative gastroenterology and urology devices associated with adverse incidents

Y73.2   Prosthetic and other implants, materials and accessory gastroenterology and urology devices associated with adverse incidents

Y73.3 Surgical instruments, materials and gastroenterology and urology devices (including sutures) associated with adverse incidents

Y73.8 Miscellaneous gastroenterology and urology devices associated with adverse incidents, not elsewhere classified

● Y74 General hospital and personal-use devices associated with adverse incidents

Y74.0 Diagnostic and monitoring general hospital and personal-use devices associated with adverse incidents

Y74.1 Therapeutic (nonsurgical) and rehabilitative general hospital and personal-use devices associated with adverse incidents

Y74.2 Prosthetic and other implants, materials and accessory general hospital and personal-use devices associated with adverse incidents

Y74.3 Surgical instruments, materials and general hospital and personal-use devices (including sutures) associated with adverse incidents

Y74.8 Miscellaneous general hospital and personal-use devices associated with adverse incidents, not elsewhere classified

● Y75 Neurological devices associated with adverse incidents

Y75.0 Diagnostic and monitoring neurological devices associated with adverse incidents

Y75.1 Therapeutic (nonsurgical) and rehabilitative neurological devices associated with adverse incidents

Y75.2 Prosthetic and other implants, materials and neurological devices associated with adverse incidents

Y75.3 Surgical instruments, materials and neurological devices (including sutures) associated with adverse incidents

Y75.8 Miscellaneous neurological devices associated with adverse incidents, not elsewhere classified

● Y76 Obstetric and gynecological devices associated with adverse incidents

Y76.0 Diagnostic and monitoring obstetric and gynecological devices associated with adverse incidents ♀

Y76.1 Therapeutic (nonsurgical) and rehabilitative obstetric and gynecological devices associated with adverse incidents ♀

Y76.2 Prosthetic and other implants, materials and accessory obstetric and gynecological devices associated with adverse incidents ♀

Y76.3 Surgical instruments, materials and obstetric and gynecological devices (including sutures) associated with adverse incidents ♀

Y76.8 Miscellaneous obstetric and gynecological devices associated with adverse incidents, not elsewhere classified ♀

● Y77 Ophthalmic devices associated with adverse incidents

Y77.0 Diagnostic and monitoring ophthalmic devices associated with adverse incidents

● Y77.1 Therapeutic (nonsurgical) and rehabilitative ophthalmic devices associated with adverse incidents

Y77.11 Contact lens associated with adverse incidents
Rigid gas permeable contact lens associated with adverse incidents
Soft (hydrophilic) contact lens associated with adverse incidents

Y77.19 Other therapeutic (nonsurgical) and rehabilitative ophthalmic devices associated with adverse incidents

Y77.2 Prosthetic and other implants, materials and accessory ophthalmic devices associated with adverse incidents

Y77.3 Surgical instruments, materials and ophthalmic devices (including sutures) associated with adverse incidents

Y77.8 Miscellaneous ophthalmic devices associated with adverse incidents, not elsewhere classified

● Y78 Radiological devices associated with adverse incidents

Y78.0 Diagnostic and monitoring radiological devices associated with adverse incidents

Y78.1 Therapeutic (nonsurgical) and rehabilitative radiological devices associated with adverse incidents

Y78.2 Prosthetic and other implants, materials and accessory radiological devices associated with adverse incidents

Y78.3 Surgical instruments, materials and radiological devices (including sutures) associated with adverse incidents

Y78.8 Miscellaneous radiological devices associated with adverse incidents, not elsewhere classified

● Y79 Orthopedic devices associated with adverse incidents

Y79.0 Diagnostic and monitoring orthopedic devices associated with adverse incidents

Y79.1 Therapeutic (nonsurgical) and rehabilitative orthopedic devices associated with adverse incidents

Y79.2 Prosthetic and other implants, materials and accessory orthopedic devices associated with adverse incidents

Y79.3 Surgical instruments, materials and orthopedic devices (including sutures) associated with adverse incidents

Y79.8 Miscellaneous orthopedic devices associated with adverse incidents, not elsewhere classified

● Y80 Physical medicine devices associated with adverse incidents

Y80.0 Diagnostic and monitoring physical medicine devices associated with adverse incidents

Y80.1 Therapeutic (nonsurgical) and rehabilitative physical medicine devices associated with adverse incidents

Y80.2 Prosthetic and other implants, materials and accessory physical medicine devices associated with adverse incidents

Y80.3 Surgical instruments, materials and physical medicine devices (including sutures) associated with adverse incidents

Y80.8 Miscellaneous physical medicine devices associated with adverse incidents, not elsewhere classified

● Y81 General- and plastic-surgery devices associated with adverse incidents

Y81.0 Diagnostic and monitoring general- and plastic-surgery devices associated with adverse incidents

Y81.1 Therapeutic (nonsurgical) and rehabilitative general- and plastic-surgery devices associated with adverse incidents

Y81.2 Prosthetic and other implants, materials and accessory general- and plastic-surgery devices associated with adverse incidents

Y81.3 Surgical instruments, materials and general- and plastic-surgery devices (including sutures) associated with adverse incidents

Y81.8 Miscellaneous general- and plastic-surgery devices associated with adverse incidents, not elsewhere classified

● Y82 Other and unspecified medical devices associated with adverse incidents

Y82.8 Other medical devices associated with adverse incidents

Y82.9 Unspecified medical devices associated with adverse incidents

CHAPTER 20 (V00-Y99)

SURGICAL AND OTHER MEDICAL PROCEDURES AS THE CAUSE OF ABNORMAL REACTION OF THE PATIENT, OR OF LATER COMPLICATION, WITHOUT MENTION OF MISADVENTURE AT THE TIME OF THE PROCEDURE (Y83-Y84)

> **Excludes1**   misadventures to patients during surgical and medical care, classifiable to (Y62-Y69)
>
> **Excludes2**   breakdown or malfunctioning of medical device (after implantation) (during procedure) (ongoing use) (Y70-Y82)

● **Y83**   Surgical operation and other surgical procedures as the cause of abnormal reaction of the patient, or of later complication, without mention of misadventure at the time of the procedure

     Y83.0   Surgical operation with transplant of whole organ as the cause of abnormal reaction of the patient, or of later complication, without mention of misadventure at the time of the procedure

     Y83.1   Surgical operation with implant of artificial internal device as the cause of abnormal reaction of the patient, or of later complication, without mention of misadventure at the time of the procedure

     Y83.2   Surgical operation with anastomosis, bypass or graft as the cause of abnormal reaction of the patient, or of later complication, without mention of misadventure at the time of the procedure

     Y83.3   Surgical operation with formation of external stoma as the cause of abnormal reaction of the patient, or of later complication, without mention of misadventure at the time of the procedure

     Y83.4   Other reconstructive surgery as the cause of abnormal reaction of the patient, or of later complication, without mention of misadventure at the time of the procedure

     Y83.5   Amputation of limb(s) as the cause of abnormal reaction of the patient, or of later complication, without mention of misadventure at the time of the procedure

     Y83.6   Removal of other organ (partial) (total) as the cause of abnormal reaction of the patient, or of later complication, without mention of misadventure at the time of the procedure

     Y83.8   Other surgical procedures as the cause of abnormal reaction of the patient, or of later complication, without mention of misadventure at the time of the procedure

     Y83.9   Surgical procedure, unspecified as the cause of abnormal reaction of the patient, or of later complication, without mention of misadventure at the time of the procedure

● **Y84**   Other medical procedures as the cause of abnormal reaction of the patient, or of later complication, without mention of misadventure at the time of the procedure

     Y84.0   Cardiac catheterization as the cause of abnormal reaction of the patient, or of later complication, without mention of misadventure at the time of the procedure

     Y84.1   Kidney dialysis as the cause of abnormal reaction of the patient, or of later complication, without mention of misadventure at the time of the procedure

     Y84.2   Radiological procedure and radiotherapy as the cause of abnormal reaction of the patient, or of later complication, without mention of misadventure at the time of the procedure
         Coding Clinic: 2019, Q1, P21; 2017, Q1, P34

     Y84.3   Shock therapy as the cause of abnormal reaction of the patient, or of later complication, without mention of misadventure at the time of the procedure

     Y84.4   Aspiration of fluid as the cause of abnormal reaction of the patient, or of later complication, without mention of misadventure at the time of the procedure

     Y84.5   Insertion of gastric or duodenal sound as the cause of abnormal reaction of the patient, or of later complication, without mention of misadventure at the time of the procedure

     Y84.6   Urinary catheterization as the cause of abnormal reaction of the patient, or of later complication, without mention of misadventure at the time of the procedure

     Y84.7   Blood-sampling as the cause of abnormal reaction of the patient, or of later complication, without mention of misadventure at the time of the procedure

     Y84.8   Other medical procedures as the cause of abnormal reaction of the patient, or of later complication, without mention of misadventure at the time of the procedure
         Coding Clinic: 2021, Q1, P5

     Y84.9   Medical procedure, unspecified as the cause of abnormal reaction of the patient, or of later complication, without mention of misadventure at the time of the procedure

SUPPLEMENTARY FACTORS RELATED TO CAUSES OF MORBIDITY CLASSIFIED ELSEWHERE (Y90-Y99)

Note: These categories may be used to provide supplementary information concerning causes of morbidity. They are not to be used for single-condition coding.

● **Y90**   Evidence of alcohol involvement determined by blood alcohol level
     Code first any associated alcohol related disorders (F10)

     Y90.0   Blood alcohol level of less than 20 mg/100 ml

     Y90.1   Blood alcohol level of 20-39 mg/100 ml

     Y90.2   Blood alcohol level of 40-59 mg/100 ml

     Y90.3   Blood alcohol level of 60-79 mg/100 ml

     Y90.4   Blood alcohol level of 80-99 mg/100 ml

     Y90.5   Blood alcohol level of 100-119 mg/100 ml

     Y90.6   Blood alcohol level of 120-199 mg/100 ml

     Y90.7   Blood alcohol level of 200-239 mg/100 ml

     Y90.8   Blood alcohol level of 240 mg/100 ml or more

     Y90.9   Presence of alcohol in blood, level not specified

OGCR Section I.C.20.b.

Place of Occurrence Guideline

Codes from category Y92, Place of occurrence of the external cause, are secondary codes for use after other external cause codes to identify the location of the patient at the time of injury or other condition.

Generally, a place of occurrence code is assigned only once, at the initial encounter for treatment. However, in the rare instance that a new injury occurs during hospitalization, an additional place of occurrence code may be assigned. No 7th characters are used for Y92. Only one code from Y92 should be recorded on a medical record.

Do not use place of occurrence code Y92.9 if the place is not stated or is not applicable.

● **Y92**   Place of occurrence of the external cause
     The following category is for use, when relevant, to identify the place of occurrence of the external cause. Use in conjunction with an activity code.
     Place of occurrence should be recorded only at the initial encounter for treatment

     ● **Y92.0**   Non-institutional (private) residence as the place of occurrence of the external cause

> **Excludes1**   abandoned or derelict house (Y92.89)
> home under construction but not yet occupied (Y92.6-)
> institutional place of residence (Y92.1-)

         ● **Y92.00**   Unspecified non-institutional (private) residence as the place of occurrence of the external cause

             Y92.000   Kitchen of unspecified non-institutional (private) residence as the place of occurrence of the external cause

             Y92.001   Dining room of unspecified non-institutional (private) residence as the place of occurrence of the external cause

Y92.002   **Bathroom** of unspecified non-institutional (private) residence as the place of occurrence of the external cause

Y92.003   **Bedroom** of unspecified non-institutional (private) residence as the place of occurrence of the external cause

Y92.007   **Garden or yard** of unspecified non-institutional (private) residence as the place of occurrence of the external cause

Y92.008   **Other place** in unspecified non-institutional (private) residence as the place of occurrence of the external cause

Y92.009   **Unspecified place** in unspecified non-institutional (private) residence as the place of occurrence of the external cause

     Home (NOS) as the place of occurrence of the external cause
     Coding Clinic: 2021, Q2, P5

● Y92.01   **Single-family non-institutional (private) house** as the place of occurrence of the external cause
     Farmhouse as the place of occurrence of the external cause

     Excludes1   barn (Y92.71)
               chicken coop or hen house (Y92.72)
               farm field (Y92.73)
               orchard (Y92.74)
               single family mobile home or trailer (Y92.02-)
               slaughter house (Y92.86)

Y92.010   **Kitchen** of single-family (private) house as the place of occurrence of the external cause

Y92.011   **Dining room** of single-family (private) house as the place of occurrence of the external cause

Y92.012   **Bathroom** of single-family (private) house as the place of occurrence of the external cause

Y92.013   **Bedroom** of single-family (private) house as the place of occurrence of the external cause

Y92.014   **Private driveway** to single-family (private) house as the place of occurrence of the external cause

Y92.015   **Private garage** of single-family (private) house as the place of occurrence of the external cause

Y92.016   **Swimming pool** in single-family (private) house or garden as the place of occurrence of the external cause

Y92.017   **Garden or yard** in single-family (private) house as the place of occurrence of the external cause

Y92.018   **Other place** in single-family (private) house as the place of occurrence of the external cause

Y92.019   **Unspecified** place in single-family (private) house as the place of occurrence of the external cause

● Y92.02   **Mobile home** as the place of occurrence of the external cause

Y92.020   **Kitchen** in mobile home as the place of occurrence of the external cause

Y92.021   **Dining room** in mobile home as the place of occurrence of the external cause

Y92.022   **Bathroom** in mobile home as the place of occurrence of the external cause

Y92.023   **Bedroom** in mobile home as the place of occurrence of the external cause

Y92.024   **Driveway** of mobile home as the place of occurrence of the external cause

Y92.025   **Garage** of mobile home as the place of occurrence of the external cause

Y92.026   **Swimming pool** of mobile home as the place of occurrence of the external cause

Y92.027   **Garden or yard** of mobile home as the place of occurrence of the external cause

Y92.028   **Other place** in mobile home as the place of occurrence of the external cause

Y92.029   **Unspecified** place in mobile home as the place of occurrence of the external cause

● Y92.03   **Apartment** as the place of occurrence of the external cause
     Condominium as the place of occurrence of the external cause
     Co-op apartment as the place of occurrence of the external cause

Y92.030   **Kitchen** in apartment as the place of occurrence of the external cause

Y92.031   **Bathroom** in apartment as the place of occurrence of the external cause

Y92.032   **Bedroom** in apartment as the place of occurrence of the external cause

Y92.038   **Other place** in apartment as the place of occurrence of the external cause

Y92.039   **Unspecified** place in apartment as the place of occurrence of the external cause

● Y92.04   **Boarding-house** as the place of occurrence of the external cause

Y92.040   **Kitchen** in boarding-house as the place of occurrence of the external cause

Y92.041   **Bathroom** in boarding-house as the place of occurrence of the external cause

Y92.042   **Bedroom** in boarding-house as the place of occurrence of the external cause

Y92.043   **Driveway** of boarding-house as the place of occurrence of the external cause

Y92.044   **Garage** of boarding-house as the place of occurrence of the external cause

Y92.045   **Swimming pool** of boarding-house as the place of occurrence of the external cause

Y92.046   **Garden or yard** of boarding-house as the place of occurrence of the external cause

CHAPTER 20 (V00-Y99)

N   Newborn Age: 0   P   Pediatric Age: 0–17   M   Maternity DX: 9–64   A   Adult Age: 15–124   ♀   Females Only   ♂   Males Only

Complication\Comorbidity   Major C\C   (Ex)   CC/MCC Exclusions   Hospital-Acquired Condition   Hierarchical Condition Category   1607

CHAPTER 20 (V00-Y99)

Y92.048   Other place in boarding-house as the place of occurrence of the external cause

Y92.049   Unspecified place in boarding-house as the place of occurrence of the external cause

● Y92.09   Other non-institutional residence as the place of occurrence of the external cause

Y92.090   Kitchen in other non-institutional residence as the place of occurrence of the external cause

Y92.091   Bathroom in other non-institutional residence as the place of occurrence of the external cause

Y92.092   Bedroom in other non-institutional residence as the place of occurrence of the external cause

Y92.093   Driveway of other non-institutional residence as the place of occurrence of the external cause

Y92.094   Garage of other non-institutional residence as the place of occurrence of the external cause

Y92.095   Swimming pool of other non-institutional residence as the place of occurrence of the external cause

Y92.096   Garden or yard of other non-institutional residence as the place of occurrence of the external cause

Y92.098   Other place in other non-institutional residence as the place of occurrence of the external cause

Y92.099   Unspecified place in other non-institutional residence as the place of occurrence of the external cause
     Coding Clinic: 2017, Q2, P10

● Y92.1   Institutional (nonprivate) residence as the place of occurrence of the external cause

Y92.10   Unspecified residential institution as the place of occurrence of the external cause

● Y92.11   Children's home and orphanage as the place of occurrence of the external cause

Y92.110   Kitchen in children's home and orphanage as the place of occurrence of the external cause

Y92.111   Bathroom in children's home and orphanage as the place of occurrence of the external cause

Y92.112   Bedroom in children's home and orphanage as the place of occurrence of the external cause

Y92.113   Driveway of children's home and orphanage as the place of occurrence of the external cause

Y92.114   Garage of children's home and orphanage as the place of occurrence of the external cause

Y92.115   Swimming pool of children's home and orphanage as the place of occurrence of the external cause

Y92.116   Garden or yard of children's home and orphanage as the place of occurrence of the external cause

Y92.118   Other place in children's home and orphanage as the place of occurrence of the external cause

Y92.119   Unspecified place in children's home and orphanage as the place of occurrence of the external cause

● Y92.12   Nursing home as the place of occurrence of the external cause
     Home for the sick as the place of occurrence of the external cause
     Hospice as the place of occurrence of the external cause

Y92.120   Kitchen in nursing home as the place of occurrence of the external cause

Y92.121   Bathroom in nursing home as the place of occurrence of the external cause

Y92.122   Bedroom in nursing home as the place of occurrence of the external cause

Y92.123   Driveway of nursing home as the place of occurrence of the external cause

Y92.124   Garage of nursing home as the place of occurrence of the external cause

Y92.125   Swimming pool of nursing home as the place of occurrence of the external cause

Y92.126   Garden or yard of nursing home as the place of occurrence of the external cause

Y92.128   Other place in nursing home as the place of occurrence of the external cause

Y92.129   Unspecified place in nursing home as the place of occurrence of the external cause
     Coding Clinic: 2017, Q2, P10

● Y92.13   Military base as the place of occurrence of the external cause

     Excludes1   military training grounds (Y92.83)

Y92.130   Kitchen on military base as the place of occurrence of the external cause

Y92.131   Mess hall on military base as the place of occurrence of the external cause

Y92.133   Barracks on military base as the place of occurrence of the external cause

Y92.135   Garage on military base as the place of occurrence of the external cause

Y92.136   Swimming pool on military base as the place of occurrence of the external cause

Y92.137   Garden or yard on military base as the place of occurrence of the external cause

Y92.138   Other place on military base as the place of occurrence of the external cause

Y92.139   Unspecified place military base as the place of occurrence of the external cause

● Y92.14   Prison as the place of occurrence of the external cause

Y92.140   Kitchen in prison as the place of occurrence of the external cause

Y92.141   Dining room in prison as the place of occurrence of the external cause

Y92.142   Bathroom in prison as the place of occurrence of the external cause

Y92.143   Cell of prison as the place of occurrence of the external cause

Y92.146 Swimming pool of prison as the place of occurrence of the external cause

Y92.147 Courtyard of prison as the place of occurrence of the external cause

Y92.148 Other place in prison as the place of occurrence of the external cause

Y92.149 Unspecified place in prison as the place of occurrence of the external cause

● **Y92.15** Reform school as the place of occurrence of the external cause

Y92.150 Kitchen in reform school as the place of occurrence of the external cause

Y92.151 Dining room in reform school as the place of occurrence of the external cause

Y92.152 Bathroom in reform school as the place of occurrence of the external cause

Y92.153 Bedroom in reform school as the place of occurrence of the external cause

Y92.154 Driveway of reform school as the place of occurrence of the external cause

Y92.155 Garage of reform school as the place of occurrence of the external cause

Y92.156 Swimming pool of reform school as the place of occurrence of the external cause

Y92.157 Garden or yard of reform school as the place of occurrence of the external cause

Y92.158 Other place in reform school as the place of occurrence of the external cause

Y92.159 Unspecified place in reform school as the place of occurrence of the external cause

● **Y92.16** School dormitory as the place of occurrence of the external cause

Excludes1 reform school as the place of occurrence of the external cause (Y92.15-)
school buildings and grounds as the place of occurrence of the external cause (Y92.2-)
school sports and athletic areas as the place of occurrence of the external cause (Y92.3-)

Y92.160 Kitchen in school dormitory as the place of occurrence of the external cause

Y92.161 Dining room in school dormitory as the place of occurrence of the external cause

Y92.162 Bathroom in school dormitory as the place of occurrence of the external cause

Y92.163 Bedroom in school dormitory as the place of occurrence of the external cause

Y92.168 Other place in school dormitory as the place of occurrence of the external cause

Y92.169 Unspecified place in school dormitory as the place of occurrence of the external cause

● **Y92.19** Other specified residential institution as the place of occurrence of the external cause

Y92.190 Kitchen in other specified residential institution as the place of occurrence of the external cause

Y92.191 Dining room in other specified residential institution as the place of occurrence of the external cause

Y92.192 Bathroom in other specified residential institution as the place of occurrence of the external cause

Y92.193 Bedroom in other specified residential institution as the place of occurrence of the external cause

Y92.194 Driveway of other specified residential institution as the place of occurrence of the external cause

Y92.195 Garage of other specified residential institution as the place of occurrence of the external cause

Y92.196 Pool of other specified residential institution as the place of occurrence of the external cause

Y92.197 Garden or yard of other specified residential institution as the place of occurrence of the external cause

Y92.198 Other place in other specified residential institution as the place of occurrence of the external cause
Coding Clinic: 2017, Q2, P11

Y92.199 Unspecified place in other specified residential institution as the place of occurrence of the external cause
Coding Clinic: 2017, Q2, P10

● **Y92.2** School, other institution and public administrative area as the place of occurrence of the external cause
Building and adjacent grounds used by the general public or by a particular group of the public

Excludes1 building under construction as the place of occurrence of the external cause (Y92.6)
residential institution as the place of occurrence of the external cause (Y92.1)
school dormitory as the place of occurrence of the external cause (Y92.16-)
sports and athletics area of schools as the place of occurrence of the external cause (Y92.3-)

● **Y92.21** School (private) (public) (state) as the place of occurrence of the external cause

Y92.210 Daycare center as the place of occurrence of the external cause

Y92.211 Elementary school as the place of occurrence of the external cause
Kindergarten as the place of occurrence of the external cause

Y92.212 Middle school as the place of occurrence of the external cause

Y92.213 High school as the place of occurrence of the external cause
Coding Clinic: 2012, Q4, P108

Y92.214 College as the place of occurrence of the external cause
University as the place of occurrence of the external cause

Y92.215 Trade school as the place of occurrence of the external cause

Y92.218 Other school as the place of occurrence of the external cause

Y92.219 Unspecified school as the place of occurrence of the external cause

CHAPTER 20 (V00-Y99)

Y92.22 Religious institution as the place of occurrence of the external cause

Church as the place of occurrence of the external cause

Mosque as the place of occurrence of the external cause

Synagogue as the place of occurrence of the external cause

● **Y92.23** Hospital as the place of occurrence of the external cause

Excludes1 ambulatory (outpatient) health services establishments (Y92.53-)

home for the sick as the place of occurrence of the external cause (Y92.12-)

hospice as the place of occurrence of the external cause (Y92.12-)

nursing home as the place of occurrence of the external cause (Y92.12-)

Y92.230 Patient room in hospital as the place of occurrence of the external cause

Y92.231 Patient bathroom in hospital as the place of occurrence of the external cause

Y92.232 Corridor of hospital as the place of occurrence of the external cause

Y92.233 Cafeteria of hospital as the place of occurrence of the external cause

Y92.234 Operating room of hospital as the place of occurrence of the external cause

Y92.238 Other place in hospital as the place of occurrence of the external cause

Y92.239 Unspecified place in hospital as the place of occurrence of the external cause

● **Y92.24** Public administrative building as the place of occurrence of the external cause

Y92.240 Courthouse as the place of occurrence of the external cause

Y92.241 Library as the place of occurrence of the external cause

Y92.242 Post office as the place of occurrence of the external cause

Y92.243 City hall as the place of occurrence of the external cause

Y92.248 Other public administrative building as the place of occurrence of the external cause

● **Y92.25** Cultural building as the place of occurrence of the external cause

Y92.250 Art gallery as the place of occurrence of the external cause

Y92.251 Museum as the place of occurrence of the external cause

Y92.252 Music hall as the place of occurrence of the external cause

Y92.253 Opera house as the place of occurrence of the external cause

Y92.254 Theater (live) as the place of occurrence of the external cause

Y92.258 Other cultural public building as the place of occurrence of the external cause

Y92.26 Movie house or cinema as the place of occurrence of the external cause

Y92.29 Other specified public building as the place of occurrence of the external cause

Assembly hall as the place of occurrence of the external cause

Clubhouse as the place of occurrence of the external cause

● **Y92.3** Sports and athletics area as the place of occurrence of the external cause

● **Y92.31** Athletic court as the place of occurrence of the external cause

Excludes1 tennis court in private home or garden (Y92.09)

Y92.310 Basketball court as the place of occurrence of the external cause

Y92.311 Squash court as the place of occurrence of the external cause

Y92.312 Tennis court as the place of occurrence of the external cause

Y92.318 Other athletic court as the place of occurrence of the external cause

● **Y92.32** Athletic field as the place of occurrence of the external cause

Y92.320 Baseball field as the place of occurrence of the external cause

Y92.321 Football field as the place of occurrence of the external cause

Y92.322 Soccer field as the place of occurrence of the external cause

Y92.328 Other athletic field as the place of occurrence of the external cause

Cricket field as the place of occurrence of the external cause

Hockey field as the place of occurrence of the external cause

● **Y92.33** Skating rink as the place of occurrence of the external cause

Y92.330 Ice skating rink (indoor) (outdoor) as the place of occurrence of the external cause

Y92.331 Roller skating rink as the place of occurrence of the external cause

Y92.34 Swimming pool (public) as the place of occurrence of the external cause

Excludes1 swimming pool in private home or garden (Y92.016)

Y92.39 Other specified sports and athletic area as the place of occurrence of the external cause

Golf-course as the place of occurrence of the external cause

Gymnasium as the place of occurrence of the external cause

Riding-school as the place of occurrence of the external cause

Stadium as the place of occurrence of the external cause

● **Y92.4** Street, highway and other paved roadways as the place of occurrence of the external cause

Excludes1 private driveway of residence (Y92.014, Y92.024, Y92.043, Y92.093, Y92.113, Y92.123, Y92.154, Y92.194)

● **Y92.41** Street and highway as the place of occurrence of the external cause

Y92.410 Unspecified street and highway as the place of occurrence of the external cause

Road NOS as the place of occurrence of the external cause

Y92.411 Interstate highway as the place of occurrence of the external cause

Freeway as the place of occurrence of the external cause

Motorway as the place of occurrence of the external cause

Y92.412 Parkway as the place of occurrence of the external cause

Y92.413 State road as the place of occurrence of the external cause

▶ New   ⇒ Revised   ~~deleted~~ Deleted   Excludes 1   Excludes 2   Includes   Use additional   Code first   Code also   Key words

OGCR Official Guidelines   ● Unacceptable Principal Diagnosis   X Assign placeholder X   ● Use Additional Character(s)   ▌ Manifestation Code   **Coding Clinic**

Y92.414   **Local residential or business street** as the place of occurrence of the external cause

Y92.415   **Exit ramp or entrance ramp** of street or highway as the place of occurrence of the external cause

● Y92.48   **Other paved roadways** as the place of occurrence of the external cause

Y92.480   **Sidewalk** as the place of occurrence of the external cause

Y92.481   **Parking lot** as the place of occurrence of the external cause

Y92.482   **Bike path** as the place of occurrence of the external cause

Y92.488   **Other** paved roadways as the place of occurrence of the external cause

● Y92.5   **Trade and service area** as the place of occurrence of the external cause

     Excludes1   garage in private home (Y92.015)
                       schools and other public administration buildings (Y92.2-)

● Y92.51   **Private commercial establishments** as the place of occurrence of the external cause

Y92.510   **Bank** as the place of occurrence of the external cause

Y92.511   **Restaurant or café** as the place of occurrence of the external cause

Y92.512   **Supermarket, store or market** as the place of occurrence of the external cause

Y92.513   **Shop (commercial)** as the place of occurrence of the external cause

● Y92.52   **Service areas** as the place of occurrence of the external cause

Y92.520   **Airport** as the place of occurrence of the external cause

Y92.521   **Bus station** as the place of occurrence of the external cause

Y92.522   **Railway station** as the place of occurrence of the external cause

Y92.523   **Highway rest stop** as the place of occurrence of the external cause

Y92.524   **Gas station** as the place of occurrence of the external cause

              Petroleum station as the place of occurrence of the external cause
              Service station as the place of occurrence of the external cause

● Y92.53   **Ambulatory health services establishments** as the place of occurrence of the external cause

Y92.530   **Ambulatory surgery center** as the place of occurrence of the external cause

              Outpatient surgery center, including that connected with a hospital as the place of occurrence of the external cause
              Same day surgery center, including that connected with a hospital as the place of occurrence of the external cause

Y92.531   **Health care provider office** as the place of occurrence of the external cause

              Physician office as the place of occurrence of the external cause

Y92.532   **Urgent care center** as the place of occurrence of the external cause

Y92.538   **Other** ambulatory health services establishments as the place of occurrence of the external cause
              Coding Clinic: 2019, Q1, P21

Y92.59   **Other trade areas** as the place of occurrence of the external cause

         Office building as the place of occurrence of the external cause
         Casino as the place of occurrence of the external cause
         Garage (commercial) as the place of occurrence of the external cause
         Hotel as the place of occurrence of the external cause
         Radio or television station as the place of occurrence of the external cause
         Shopping mall as the place of occurrence of the external cause
         Warehouse as the place of occurrence of the external cause

● Y92.6   **Industrial and construction area** as the place of occurrence of the external cause

Y92.61   **Building [any] under construction** as the place of occurrence of the external cause

Y92.62   **Dock or shipyard** as the place of occurrence of the external cause

         Dockyard as the place of occurrence of the external cause
         Dry dock as the place of occurrence of the external cause
         Shipyard as the place of occurrence of the external cause

Y92.63   **Factory** as the place of occurrence of the external cause

         Factory building as the place of occurrence of the external cause
         Factory premises as the place of occurrence of the external cause
         Industrial yard as the place of occurrence of the external cause

Y92.64   **Mine or pit** as the place of occurrence of the external cause

         Mine as the place of occurrence of the external cause

Y92.65   **Oil rig** as the place of occurrence of the external cause

         Pit (coal) (gravel) (sand) as the place of occurrence of the external cause

Y92.69   **Other** specified industrial and construction area as the place of occurrence of the external cause

         Gasworks as the place of occurrence of the external cause
         Power-station (coal) (nuclear) (oil) as the place of occurrence of the external cause
         Tunnel under construction as the place of occurrence of the external cause
         Workshop as the place of occurrence of the external cause

● Y92.7   **Farm** as the place of occurrence of the external cause
         Ranch as the place of occurrence of the external cause

     Excludes1   farmhouse and home premises of farm (Y92.01-)

Y92.71   **Barn** as the place of occurrence of the external cause

Y92.72   **Chicken coop** as the place of occurrence of the external cause

         Hen house as the place of occurrence of the external cause

Y92.73   **Farm field** as the place of occurrence of the external cause

Y92.74   **Orchard** as the place of occurrence of the external cause

Y92.79   **Other farm location** as the place of occurrence of the external cause

N Newborn Age: 0   **P** Pediatric Age: 0–17   **M** Maternity DX: 9–64   **A** Adult Age: 15–124   ♀ Females Only   ♂ Males Only

Complication\Comorbidity   Major C\C   (Ex.) CC/MCC Exclusions   Hospital-Acquired Condition   Hierarchical Condition Category

1611

● Y92.8   **Other places** as the place of occurrence of the external cause

   ● Y92.81   **Transport vehicle** as the place of occurrence of the external cause

     Excludes1   transport accidents (V00-V99)

     Y92.810   **Car** as the place of occurrence of the external cause

     Y92.811   **Bus** as the place of occurrence of the external cause

     Y92.812   **Truck** as the place of occurrence of the external cause

     Y92.813   **Airplane** as the place of occurrence of the external cause

     Y92.814   **Boat** as the place of occurrence of the external cause

     Y92.815   **Train** as the place of occurrence of the external cause

     Y92.816   **Subway car** as the place of occurrence of the external cause

     Y92.818   **Other transport vehicle** as the place of occurrence of the external cause

   ● Y92.82   **Wilderness area**

     Y92.820   **Desert** as the place of occurrence of the external cause

     Y92.821   **Forest** as the place of occurrence of the external cause

     Y92.828   **Other wilderness area** as the place of occurrence of the external cause

       Swamp as the place of occurrence of the external cause

       Mountain as the place of occurrence of the external cause

       Marsh as the place of occurrence of the external cause

       Prairie as the place of occurrence of the external cause

   ● Y92.83   **Recreation area** as the place of occurrence of the external cause

     Y92.830   **Public park** as the place of occurrence of the external cause

     Y92.831   **Amusement park** as the place of occurrence of the external cause

     Y92.832   **Beach** as the place of occurrence of the external cause

       Seashore as the place of occurrence of the external cause

     Y92.833   **Campsite** as the place of occurrence of the external cause

     Y92.834   **Zoological garden (zoo)** as the place of occurrence of the external cause

     Y92.838   **Other recreation area** as the place of occurrence of the external cause

   Y92.84   **Military training ground** as the place of occurrence of the external cause

   Y92.85   **Railroad track** as the place of occurrence of the external cause

   Y92.86   **Slaughter house** as the place of occurrence of the external cause

   Y92.89   **Other** specified places as the place of occurrence of the external cause

       Derelict house as the place of occurrence of the external cause

OGCR Section I.C.20.b.

Do not use place of occurrence code Y92.9 if the place is not stated or is not applicable.

Y92.9   **Unspecified** place or not applicable

OGCR See Section I.C.20.c.

Activity Code

Assign a code from category Y93, Activity code, to describe the activity of the patient at the time the injury or other health condition occurred.

An activity code is used only once, at the initial encounter for treatment. Only one code from Y93 should be recorded on a medical record.

The activity codes are not applicable to poisonings, adverse effects, misadventures or sequela.

Do not assign Y93.9, Unspecified activity, if the activity is not stated.

A code from category Y93 is appropriate for use with external cause and intent codes if identifying the activity provides additional information about the event.

● Y93   **Activity codes**

   Note: Category Y93 is provided for use to indicate the activity of the person seeking healthcare for an injury or health condition, such as a heart attack while shoveling snow, which resulted from, or was contributed to, by the activity. These codes are appropriate for use for both acute injuries, such as those from Chapter 19, and conditions that are due to the long-term, cumulative effects of an activity, such as those from Chapter 13. They are also appropriate for use with external cause codes for cause and intent if identifying the activity provides additional information on the event. These codes should be used in conjunction with codes for external cause status (Y99) and place of occurrence (Y92).

   This section contains the following broad activity categories:

     Y93.0   Activities involving walking and running

     Y93.1   Activities involving water and water craft

     Y93.2   Activities involving ice and snow

     Y93.3   Activities involving climbing, rappelling, and jumping off

     Y93.4   Activities involving dancing and other rhythmic movement

     Y93.5   Activities involving other sports and athletics played individually

     Y93.6   Activities involving other sports and athletics played as a team or group

     Y93.7   Activities involving other specified sports and athletics

     Y93.A   Activities involving other cardiorespiratory exercise

     Y93.B   Activities involving other muscle strengthening exercises

     Y93.C   Activities involving computer technology and electronic devices

     Y93.D   Activities involving arts and handcrafts

     Y93.E   Activities involving personal hygiene and interior property and clothing maintenance

     Y93.F   Activities involving caregiving

     Y93.G   Activities involving food preparation, cooking and grilling

     Y93.H   Activities involving exterior property and land maintenance, building and construction

     Y93.I   Activities involving roller coasters and other types of external motion

     Y93.J   Activities involving playing musical instrument

     Y93.K   Activities involving animal care

     Y93.8   Activities, other specified

     Y93.9   Activity, unspecified

● Y93.0   **Activities involving walking and running**

     Excludes1   Activity, walking an animal (Y93.K1)

       Activity, walking or running on a treadmill (Y93.A1)

   Y93.01   **Activity, walking, marching and hiking**

     Activity, walking, marching and hiking on level or elevated terrain

     Excludes1   activity, mountain climbing (Y93.31)

   Y93.02   **Activity, running**

▶ New   ⇒ Revised   ~~deleted~~ Deleted   Excludes 1   Excludes 2   Includes   Use additional   Code first   Code also   Key words

OGCR Official Guidelines   ● Unacceptable Principal Diagnosis   X Assign placeholder X   ● Use Additional Character(s)   ▶ Manifestation Code   **Coding Clinic**

● **Y93.1** **Activities involving water and water craft**
     Excludes1   activities involving ice (Y93.2-)
   Y93.11 **Activity,** swimming
   Y93.12 **Activity,** springboard and platform diving
   Y93.13 **Activity,** water polo
   Y93.14 **Activity,** water aerobics and water exercise
   Y93.15 **Activity,** underwater diving and snorkeling
       Activity, SCUBA diving
   Y93.16 **Activity,** rowing, canoeing, kayaking, rafting and tubing
       Activity, canoeing, kayaking, rafting and tubing in calm and turbulent water
   Y93.17 **Activity,** water skiing and wake boarding
   Y93.18 **Activity,** surfing, windsurfing and boogie boarding
       Activity, water sliding
   Y93.19 **Activity,** other involving water and watercraft
       Activity involving water NOS
       Activity, parasailing
       Activity, water survival training and testing

● **Y93.2** **Activities involving ice and snow**
     Excludes1   activity, shoveling ice and snow (Y93.H1)
   Y93.21 **Activity,** ice skating
       Activity, figure skating (singles) (pairs)
       Activity, ice dancing
     Excludes1   activity, ice hockey (Y93.22)
   Y93.22 **Activity,** ice hockey
   Y93.23 **Activity,** snow (alpine) (downhill) skiing, snowboarding, sledding, tobogganing and snow tubing
     Excludes1   activity, cross country skiing (Y93.24)
   Y93.24 **Activity,** cross country skiing
       Activity, nordic skiing
   Y93.29 **Activity,** other activity involving ice and snow
       Activity, activity involving ice and snow NOS

● **Y93.3** **Activities involving climbing, rappelling and jumping off**
     Excludes1   activity, hiking on level or elevated terrain (Y93.01)
           activity, jumping rope (Y93.56)
           activity, trampoline jumping (Y93.44)
   Y93.31 **Activity,** mountain climbing, rock climbing and wall climbing
   Y93.32 **Activity,** rappelling
   Y93.33 **Activity,** BASE jumping
       Activity, building, Antenna, Span, Earth jumping
   Y93.34 **Activity,** bungee jumping
   Y93.35 **Activity,** hang gliding
   Y93.39 **Activity,** other activity involving climbing, rappelling and jumping off

● **Y93.4** **Activities involving dancing and other rhythmic movement**
     Excludes1   activity, martial arts (Y93.75)
   Y93.41 **Activity,** dancing
       Coding Clinic: 2012, Q4, P108
   Y93.42 **Activity,** yoga
   Y93.43 **Activity,** gymnastics
       Activity, rhythmic gymnastics
     Excludes1   activity, trampolining (Y93.44)
   Y93.44 **Activity,** trampolining
   Y93.45 **Activity,** cheerleading
   Y93.49 **Activity,** other involving dancing and other rhythmic movements

● **Y93.5** **Activities involving other sports and athletics played individually**
     Excludes1   activity, dancing (Y93.41)
           activity, gymnastic (Y93.43)
           activity, trampolining (Y93.44)
           activity, yoga (Y93.42)
   Y93.51 **Activity,** roller skating (inline) and skateboarding
   Y93.52 **Activity,** horseback riding
   Y93.53 **Activity,** golf
   Y93.54 **Activity,** bowling
   Y93.55 **Activity,** bike riding
   Y93.56 **Activity,** jumping rope
   Y93.57 **Activity,** non-running track and field events
     Excludes1   activity, running (any form) (Y93.02)
   Y93.59 **Activity,** other involving other sports and athletics played individually
     Excludes1   activities involving climbing, rappelling, and jumping (Y93.3-)
           activities involving ice and snow (Y93.2-)
           activities involving walking and running (Y93.0-)
           activities involving water and watercraft (Y93.1-)

● **Y93.6** **Activities involving other sports and athletics played as a team or group**
     Excludes1   activity, ice hockey (Y93.22)
           activity, water polo (Y93.13)
   Y93.61 **Activity,** American tackle football
       Activity, football NOS
   Y93.62 **Activity,** American flag or touch football
   Y93.63 **Activity,** rugby
   Y93.64 **Activity,** baseball
       Activity, softball
   Y93.65 **Activity,** lacrosse and field hockey
       Coding Clinic: 2015, Q1, P9
   Y93.66 **Activity,** soccer
   Y93.67 **Activity,** basketball
       Coding Clinic: 2019, Q4, P18
   Y93.68 **Activity,** volleyball (beach) (court)
   Y93.6A **Activity,** physical games generally associated with school recess, summer camp and children
       Activity, capture the flag
       Activity, dodge ball
       Activity, four square
       Activity, kickball
   Y93.69 **Activity,** other involving other sports and athletics played as a team or group
       Cricket

● **Y93.7** **Activities involving other specified sports and athletics**
   Y93.71 **Activity,** boxing
   Y93.72 **Activity,** wrestling
   Y93.73 **Activity,** racquet and hand sports
       Activity, handball
       Activity, racquetball
       Activity, squash
       Activity, tennis
   Y93.74 **Activity,** frisbee
       Activity, ultimate frisbee
   Y93.75 **Activity,** martial arts
       Activity, combatives
   Y93.79 **Activity,** other specified sports and athletics
     Excludes1   sports and athletics activities specified in categories Y93.0-Y93.6

CHAPTER 20 (V00-Y99)

N   Newborn Age: 0   P   Pediatric Age: 0–17   M   Maternity DX: 9–64   A   Adult Age: 15–124   ♀ Females Only   ♂ Males Only

🅒 Complication\Comorbidity   🅜 Major C\C   (Ex) CC/MCC Exclusions   🅗 Hospital-Acquired Condition   🅗🅒 Hierarchical Condition Category

1613

● **Y93.A   Activities involving other cardiorespiratory exercise**
Activities involving physical training

    Y93.A1   Activity, exercise machines primarily for cardiorespiratory conditioning
        Activity, elliptical and stepper machines
        Activity, stationary bike
        Activity, treadmill

    Y93.A2   Activity, calisthenics
        Activity, jumping jacks
        Activity, warm up and cool down

    Y93.A3   Activity, aerobic and step exercise

    Y93.A4   Activity, circuit training

    Y93.A5   Activity, obstacle course
        Activity, challenge course
        Activity, confidence course

    Y93.A6   Activity, grass drills
        Activity, guerilla drills

    Y93.A9   Activity, other involving other cardiorespiratory exercise

        Excludes1   activities involving cardiorespiratory exercise specified in categories Y93.0-Y93.7

● **Y93.B   Activity involving other muscle strengthening exercises**

    Y93.B1   Activity, exercise machines primarily for muscle strengthening

    Y93.B2   Activity, push-ups, pull-ups, sit-ups

    Y93.B3   Activity, free weights
        Activity, barbells
        Activity, dumbbells

    Y93.B4   Activity, pilates

    Y93.B9   Activity, other involving other muscle strengthening exercises

        Excludes1   activities involving muscle strengthening specified in categories Y93.0-Y93.A

● **Y93.C   Activities involving computer technology and electronic devices**

    Excludes1   activity, electronic musical keyboard or instruments (Y93.J-)

    Y93.C1   Activity, computer keyboarding
        Activity, electronic game playing using keyboard or other stationary device

    Y93.C2   Activity, hand held interactive electronic device
        Activity, cellular telephone and communication device
        Activity, electronic game playing using interactive device

        Excludes1   activity, electronic game playing using keyboard or other stationary device (Y93.C1)

    Y93.C9   Activity, other involving computer technology and electronic devices

● **Y93.D   Activities involving arts and handcrafts**

    Excludes1   activities involving playing musical instrument (Y93.J-)

    Y93.D1   Knitting and crocheting

    Y93.D2   Sewing

    Y93.D3   Furniture building and finishing
        Furniture repair

    Y93.D9   Activity, other involving arts and handcrafts

● **Y93.E   Activities involving personal hygiene and interior property and clothing maintenance**

    Excludes1   activities involving cooking and grilling (Y93.G-)
        activities involving exterior property and land maintenance, building and construction (Y93.H-)
        activity involving caregiving (Y93.F-)
        activity, dishwashing (Y93.G1)
        activity, food preparation (Y93.G1)
        activity, gardening (Y93.H2)

    Y93.E1   Activity, personal bathing and showering

    Y93.E2   Activity, laundry

    Y93.E3   Activity, vacuuming

    Y93.E4   Activity, ironing

    Y93.E5   Activity, floor mopping and cleaning

    Y93.E6   Activity, residential relocation
        Activity, packing up and unpacking involved in moving to a new residence

    Y93.E8   Activity, other personal hygiene activity

    Y93.E9   Activity, other household maintenance

● **Y93.F   Activities involving person providing caregiving**
Activity involving the provider of caregiving

    Y93.F1   Activity, caregiving involving bathing

    Y93.F2   Activity, caregiving involving lifting
        Coding Clinic: 2016, Q4, P74

    Y93.F9   Activity, other caregiving

● **Y93.G   Activities involving food preparation, cooking and grilling**

    Y93.G1   Activity, food preparation and clean up
        Activity, dishwashing

    Y93.G2   Activity, grilling and smoking food

    Y93.G3   Activity, cooking and baking
        Activity, use of stove, oven and microwave oven

    Y93.G9   Activity, other activity involving cooking and grilling

● **Y93.H   Activities involving property and land maintenance, building and construction**

    Y93.H1   Activity, digging, shoveling and raking
        Activity, dirt digging
        Activity, raking leaves
        Activity, snow shoveling

    Y93.H2   Activity, gardening and landscaping
        Activity, pruning, trimming shrubs, weeding

    Y93.H3   Activity, building and construction

    Y93.H9   Activity, other activity involving property and land maintenance, building and construction

● **Y93.I   Activities involving roller coasters and other types of external motion**

    Y93.I1   Activity, rollercoaster riding

    Y93.I9   Activity, other involving external motion

● **Y93.J   Activities involving playing musical instrument**
Activity involving playing electric musical instrument

    Y93.J1   Activity, piano playing
        Activity, musical keyboard (electronic) playing

    Y93.J2   Activity, drum and other percussion instrument playing

    Y93.J3   Activity, string instrument playing

    Y93.J4   Activity, winds and brass instrument playing

● **Y93.K**   **Activities involving animal care**

> **Excludes1**   activity, horseback riding (Y93.52)

     Y93.K1   **Activity, walking an animal**

     Y93.K2   **Activity, milking an animal**

     Y93.K3   **Activity, grooming and shearing an animal**

     Y93.K9   **Activity, other activity involving animal care**

● **Y93.8**   **Other activity**

> Coding Clinic: 2016, Q4, P74

     Y93.81   **Activity, refereeing a sports activity**

     Y93.82   **Activity, spectator at an event**

     Y93.83   **Activity, rough housing and horseplay**

> Coding Clinic: 2015, Q1, P8

     Y93.84   **Activity, sleeping**

     Y93.85   **Activity, choking game**

> Activity, blackout game
> Activity, fainting game
> Activity, pass out game
> Coding Clinic: 2016, Q4, P74-76

     Y93.89   **Activity, other specified**

OGCR   See Section I.C.20.c.

> Do not assign Y93.9, Unspecified activity, if the activity is not stated.

● **Y93.9**   **Activity, unspecified**

Y95   **Nosocomial condition**

● **Y99**   **External cause status**

> **Note:** A single code from category Y99 should be used in conjunction with the external cause code(s) assigned to a record to indicate the status of the person at the time the event occurred.
> Coding Clinic: 2016, Q4, P74

   Y99.0   **Civilian activity done for income or pay**

> Civilian activity done for financial or other compensation
>
> **Excludes1**   military activity (Y99.1)
>   volunteer activity (Y99.2)

   Y99.1   **Military activity**

> **Excludes1**   activity of off duty military personnel (Y99.8)

   Y99.2   **Volunteer activity**

> **Excludes1**   activity of child or other family member assisting in compensated work of other family member (Y99.8)

   Y99.8   **Other external cause status**

> Activity NEC
> Activity of child or other family member assisting in compensated work of other family member
> Hobby not done for income
> Leisure activity
> Off-duty activity of military personnel
> Recreation or sport not for income or while a student
> Student activity
>
> **Excludes1**   civilian activity done for income or compensation (Y99.0)
>   military activity (Y99.1)
> Coding Clinic: 2012, Q4, P108

   Y99.9   **Unspecified external cause status**

N   Newborn Age: 0   **P**   Pediatric Age: 0–17   **M**   Maternity DX: 9–64   **A**   Adult Age: 15–124   ♀   Females Only   ♂   Males Only

Complication\Comorbidity   Major C\C   (Ex)   CC/MCC Exclusions   Hospital-Acquired Condition   Hierarchical Condition Category

1615

CHAPTER 20 (V00-Y99)

CHAPTER 21

FACTORS INFLUENCING HEALTH STATUS AND CONTACT WITH HEALTH SERVICES (Z00-Z99)

OGCR Chapter-Specific Coding Guidelines

21. **Chapter 21: Factors influencing health status and contact with health services (Z00-Z99)**
Note: The chapter specific guidelines provide additional information about the use of Z codes for specified encounters.

a. Use of Z codes in any healthcare setting
Z codes are for use in any healthcare setting. Z codes may be used as either a first-listed (principal diagnosis code in the inpatient setting) or secondary code, depending on the circumstances of the encounter. Certain Z codes may only be used as first-listed or principal diagnosis.

b. Z Codes indicate a reason for an encounter
Z codes are not procedure codes. A corresponding procedure code must accompany a Z code to describe any procedure performed.

c. Categories of Z Codes

1) Contact/Exposure
Category Z20 indicates contact with, and suspected exposure to, communicable diseases. These codes are for patients who do not show any sign or symptom of a disease but are suspected to have been exposed to it by close personal contact with an infected individual or are in an area where a disease is epidemic.

Category Z77, Other contact with and (suspected) exposures hazardous to health, indicates contact with and suspected exposures hazardous to health.

Contact/exposure codes may be used as a first-listed code to explain an encounter for testing, or, more commonly, as a secondary code to identify a potential risk.

2) Inoculations and vaccinations
Code Z23 is for encounters for inoculations and vaccinations. It indicates that a patient is being seen to receive a prophylactic inoculation against a disease. Procedure codes are required to identify the actual administration of the injection and the type(s) of immunizations given. Code Z23 may be used as a secondary code if the inoculation is given as a routine part of preventive health care, such as a well-baby visit.

3) Status
Status codes indicate that a patient is either a carrier of a disease or has the sequelae or residual of a past disease or condition. This includes such things as the presence of prosthetic or mechanical devices resulting from past treatment. A status code is informative, because the status may affect the course of treatment and its outcome. A status code is distinct from a history code. The history code indicates that the patient no longer has the condition.

A status code should not be used with a diagnosis code from one of the body system chapters, if the diagnosis code includes the information provided by the status code. For example, code Z94.1, Heart transplant status, should not be used with a code from subcategory T86.2, Complications of heart transplant. The status code does not provide additional information. The complication code indicates that the patient is a heart transplant patient.

For encounters for weaning from a mechanical ventilator, assign a code from subcategory J96.1, Chronic respiratory failure, followed by code Z99.11, Dependence on respirator [ventilator] status.

The status Z codes/categories are:

Z14	Genetic carrier

Genetic carrier status indicates that a person carries a gene, associated with a particular disease, which may be passed to offspring who may develop that disease. The person does not have the disease and is not at risk of developing the disease.

Z15	Genetic susceptibility to disease Genetic susceptibility indicates that a person has a gene that increases the risk of that person developing the disease.

Codes from category Z15 should not be used as principal or first-listed codes. If the patient has the condition to which he/she is susceptible, and that condition is the reason for the encounter, the code for the current condition should be sequenced first. If the patient is being seen for follow-up after completed treatment for this condition, and the condition no longer exists, a follow-up

code should be sequenced first, followed by the appropriate personal history and genetic susceptibility codes. If the purpose of the encounter is genetic counseling associated with procreative management, code Z31.5, Encounter for genetic counseling, should be assigned as the first-listed code, followed by a code from category Z15. Additional codes should be assigned for any applicable family or personal history.

Z16	Resistance to antimicrobial drugs

This code indicates that a patient has a condition that is resistant to antimicrobial drug treatment. Sequence the infection code first.

Z17	Estrogen receptor status
Z18	Retained foreign body fragments
Z19	Hormone sensitivity malignancy status
Z21	Asymptomatic HIV infection status This code indicates that a patient has tested positive for HIV but has manifested no signs or symptoms of the disease.
Z22	Carrier of infectious disease Carrier status indicates that a person harbors the specific organisms of a disease without manifest symptoms and is capable of transmitting the infection.
Z28.3	Underimmunization status
Z33.1	Pregnant state, incidental This code is a secondary code only for use when the pregnancy is in no way complicating the reason for visit. Otherwise, a code from the obstetric chapter is required.
Z66	Do not resuscitate

This code may be used when it is documented by the provider that a patient is on do not resuscitate status at any time during the stay.

Z67	Blood type
Z68	Body mass index (BMI)

BMI codes should only be assigned when the associated diagnosis (such as overweight or obesity) meets the definition of a reportable diagnosis (see Section III, Reporting Additional Diagnoses). Do not assign BMI codes during pregnancy. See Section I.B.14 for BMI documentation by clinicians other than the patient's provider.

Z74.01	Bed confinement status
Z76.82	Awaiting organ transplant status
Z78	Other specified health status

Code Z78.1, Physical restraint status, may be used when it is documented by the provider that a patient has been put in restraints during the current encounter. Please note that this code should not be reported when it is documented by the provider that a patient is temporarily restrained during a procedure.

Z79	Long-term (current) drug therapy

Codes from this category indicate a patient's continuous use of a prescribed drug (including such things as aspirin therapy) for the long-term treatment of a condition or for prophylactic use. It is not for use for patients who have addictions to drugs. This subcategory is not for use of medications for detoxification or maintenance programs to prevent withdrawal symptoms in patients with drug dependence (e.g., methadone maintenance for opiate dependence). Assign the appropriate code for the drug dependence instead.

Assign a code from Z79 if the patient is receiving a medication for an extended period as a prophylactic measure (such as for the prevention of deep vein thrombosis) or as treatment of a chronic condition (such as arthritis) or a disease requiring a lengthy course of treatment (such as cancer). Do not assign a code from category Z79 for medication being administered for a brief period of time to treat an acute illness or injury (such as a course of antibiotics to treat acute bronchitis).

Z88	Allergy status to drugs, medicaments and biological substances Except: Z88.9, Allergy status to unspecified drugs, medicaments and biological substances status
Z89	Acquired absence of limb
Z90	Acquired absence of organs, not elsewhere classified
Z91.0-	Allergy status, other than to drugs and biological substances
Z92.82	Status post administration of tPA (rtPA) in a different facility within the last 24 hours prior to admission to a current facility Assign code Z92.82, Status post administration of tPA (rtPA) in a different facility within the last 24 hours prior to admission to current

facility, as a secondary diagnosis when a patient is received by transfer into a facility and documentation indicates they were administered tissue plasminogen activator (tPA) within the last 24 hours prior to admission to the current facility. This guideline applies even if the patient is still receiving the tPA at the time they are received into the current facility. The appropriate code for the condition for which the tPA was administered (such as cerebrovascular disease or myocardial infarction) should be assigned first. Code Z92.82 is only applicable to the receiving facility record and not to the transferring facility record.

Z93   Artificial opening status
Z94   Transplanted organ and tissue status
Z95   Presence of cardiac and vascular implants and grafts
Z96   Presence of other functional implants
Z97   Presence of other devices
Z98   Other postprocedural states

Assign code Z98.85, Transplanted organ removal status, to indicate that a transplanted organ has been previously removed. This code should not be assigned for the encounter in which the transplanted organ is removed. The complication necessitating removal of the transplant organ should be assigned for that encounter.

See Section I.C.19. for information on the coding of organ transplant complications.

Z99   Dependence on enabling machines and devices, not elsewhere classified

Note: Categories Z89-Z90 and Z93-Z99 are for use only if there are no complications or malfunctions of the organ or tissue replaced, the amputation site or the equipment on which the patient is dependent.

4) History (of)

There are two types of history Z codes, personal and family. Personal history codes explain a patient's past medical condition that no longer exists and is not receiving any treatment, but that has the potential for recurrence, and therefore may require continued monitoring.

Family history codes are for use when a patient has a family member(s) who has had a particular disease that causes the patient to be at higher risk of also contracting the disease.

Personal history codes may be used in conjunction with follow-up codes and family history codes may be used in conjunction with screening codes to explain the need for a test or procedure. History codes are also acceptable on any medical record regardless of the reason for visit. A history of an illness, even if no longer present, is important information that may alter the type of treatment ordered.

The history Z code categories are:

Z80   Family history of primary malignant neoplasm
Z81   Family history of mental and behavioral disorders
Z82   Family history of certain disabilities and chronic diseases (leading to disablement)
Z83   Family history of other specific disorders
Z84   Family history of other conditions
Z85   Personal history of malignant neoplasm
Z86   Personal history of certain other diseases
Z87   Personal history of other diseases and conditions
Z91.4-   Personal history of psychological trauma, not elsewhere classified
Z91.5   Personal history of self-harm
Z91.81   History of falling
Z91.82   Personal history of military deployment
Z92   Personal history of medical treatment Except: Z92.0, Personal history of contraception Except: Z92.82, Status post administration of tPA (rtPA) in a different facility within the last 24 hours prior to admission to a current facility

5) Screening

Screening is the testing for disease or disease precursors in seemingly well individuals so that early detection and treatment can be provided for those who test positive for the disease (e.g., screening mammogram).

The testing of a person to rule out or confirm a suspected diagnosis because the patient has some sign or symptom is a diagnostic examination, not a screening. In these cases, the sign or symptom is used to explain the reason for the test.

A screening code may be a first-listed code if the reason for the visit is specifically the screening exam. It may also be used as an additional code if the screening is done during an office visit for other health problems. A screening code is not necessary if the screening is inherent to a routine examination, such as a pap smear done during a routine pelvic examination.

Should a condition be discovered during the screening then the code for the condition may be assigned as an additional diagnosis.

The Z code indicates that a screening exam is planned. A procedure code is required to confirm that the screening was performed.

The screening Z codes/categories:

Z11   Encounter for screening for infectious and parasitic diseases
Z12   Encounter for screening for malignant neoplasms
Z13   Encounter for screening for other diseases and disorders Except: Z13.9, Encounter for screening, unspecified
Z36   Encounter for antenatal screening for mother

6) Observation

There are three observation Z code categories. They are for use in very limited circumstances when a person is being observed for a suspected condition that is ruled out. The observation codes are not for use if an injury or illness or any signs or symptoms related to the suspected condition are present. In such cases the diagnosis/symptom code is used with the corresponding external cause code.

The observation codes are to be used as principal diagnosis only. The only exception to this is when the principal diagnosis is required to be a code from category Z38, Liveborn infants according to place of birth and type of delivery. Then a code from category Z05, Encounter for observation and evaluation of newborn for suspected diseases and conditions ruled out, is sequenced after the Z38 code. Additional codes may be used in addition to the observation code but only if they are unrelated to the suspected condition being observed.

Codes from subcategory Z03.7 Encounter for suspected maternal and fetal conditions ruled out, may either be used as a first-listed or as an additional code assignment depending on the case. They are for use in very limited circumstances on a maternal record when an encounter is for a suspected maternal or fetal condition that is ruled out during that encounter (for example, a maternal or fetal condition may be suspected due to an abnormal test result). These codes should not be used when the condition is confirmed. In those cases, the confirmed condition should be coded. In addition, these codes are not for use if an illness or any signs or symptoms related to the suspected condition or problem are present. In such cases the diagnosis/symptom code is used.

Additional codes may be used in addition to the code from subcategory Z03.7, but only if they are unrelated to the suspected condition being evaluated.

Codes from subcategory Z03.7 may not be used for encounters for antenatal screening of mother. *See Section I.C.21. Screening.*

For encounters for suspected fetal condition that are inconclusive following testing and evaluation, assign the appropriate code from category O35, O36, O40 or O41.

The observation Z code categories:

Z03   Encounter for medical observation for suspected diseases and conditions ruled out
Z04   Encounter for examination and observation for other reasons Except: Z04.9, Encounter for examination and observation for unspecified reason
Z05   Encounter for observation and evaluation of newborn for suspected diseases and conditions ruled out

7) Aftercare

Aftercare visit codes cover situations when the initial treatment of a disease has been performed and the patient requires continued care during the healing or recovery phase, or for the long-term consequences of the disease. The aftercare Z code should not be used if treatment is directed at a current, acute disease. The diagnosis code is to be used in these cases.

Exceptions to this rule are codes Z51.0, Encounter for antineoplastic radiation therapy, and codes from subcategory Z51.1, Encounter for antineoplastic chemotherapy and immunotherapy. These codes are to be first-listed, followed by the diagnosis code when a patient's encounter is solely

to receive radiation therapy, chemotherapy, or immunotherapy for the treatment of a neoplasm. If the reason for the encounter is more than one type of antineoplastic therapy, code Z51.0 and a code from subcategory Z51.1 may be assigned together, in which case one of these codes would be reported as a secondary diagnosis.

The aftercare Z codes should also not be used for aftercare for injuries. For aftercare of an injury, assign the acute injury code with the appropriate 7th character (for subsequent encounter).

The aftercare codes are generally first-listed to explain the specific reason for the encounter. An aftercare code may be used as an additional code when some type of aftercare is provided in addition to the reason for admission and no diagnosis code is applicable. An example of this would be the closure of a colostomy during an encounter for treatment of another condition.

Aftercare codes should be used in conjunction with other aftercare codes or diagnosis codes to provide better detail on the specifics of an aftercare encounter visit, unless otherwise directed by the classification. Should a patient receive multiple types of antineoplastic therapy during the same encounter, code Z51.0, Encounter for antineoplastic radiation therapy, and codes from subcategory Z51.1, Encounter for antineoplastic chemotherapy and immunotherapy, may be used together on a record. The sequencing of multiple aftercare codes depends on the circumstances of the encounter.

Certain aftercare Z code categories need a secondary diagnosis code to describe the resolving condition or sequelae. For others, the condition is included in the code title.

Additional Z code aftercare category terms include fitting and adjustment, and attention to artificial openings.

Status Z codes may be used with aftercare Z codes to indicate the nature of the aftercare. For example code Z95.1, Presence of aortocoronary bypass graft, may be used with code Z48.812, Encounter for surgical aftercare following surgery on the circulatory system, to indicate the surgery for which the aftercare is being performed. A status code should not be used when the aftercare code indicates the type of status, such as using Z43.0, Encounter for attention to tracheostomy, with Z93.0, Tracheostomy status.

The aftercare Z category/codes:

Z42	Encounter for plastic and reconstructive surgery following medical procedure or healed injury
Z43	Encounter for attention to artificial openings
Z44	Encounter for fitting and adjustment of external prosthetic device
Z45	Encounter for adjustment and management of implanted device
Z46	Encounter for fitting and adjustment of other devices
Z47	Orthopedic aftercare
Z48	Encounter for other postprocedural aftercare
Z49	Encounter for care involving renal dialysis
Z51	Encounter for other aftercare and medical care

8) Follow-up

The follow-up codes are used to explain continuing surveillance following completed treatment of a disease, condition, or injury. They imply that the condition has been fully treated and no longer exists. They should not be confused with aftercare codes, or injury codes with a 7th character for subsequent encounter, that explain ongoing care of a healing condition or its sequelae. Follow-up codes may be used in conjunction with history codes to provide the full picture of the healed condition and its treatment. The follow-up code is sequenced first, followed by the history code.

A follow-up code may be used to explain multiple visits. Should a condition be found to have recurred on the follow-up visit, then the diagnosis code for the condition should be assigned in place of the follow-up code.

The follow-up Z code categories:

Z08	Encounter for follow-up examination after completed treatment for malignant neoplasm
Z09	Encounter for follow-up examination after completed treatment for conditions other than malignant neoplasm
Z39	Encounter for maternal postpartum care and examination

9) Donor

Codes in category Z52, Donors of organs and tissues, are used for living individuals who are donating blood or other body tissue.

These codes are only for individuals donating for others, not for self-donations. They are not used to identify cadaveric donations.

10) Counseling

Counseling Z codes are used when a patient or family member receives assistance in the aftermath of an illness or injury, or when support is required in coping with family or social problems.

The counseling Z codes/categories:

Z30.0-	Encounter for general counseling and advice on contraception
Z31.5	Encounter for procreative genetic counseling
Z31.6-	Encounter for general counseling and advice on procreation
Z32.2	Encounter for childbirth instruction
Z32.3	Encounter for childcare instruction
Z69	Encounter for mental health services for victim and perpetrator of abuse
Z70	Counseling related to sexual attitude, behavior and orientation
Z71	Persons encountering health services for other counseling and medical advice, not elsewhere classified
Z76.81	Expectant mother prebirth pediatrician visit

11) Encounters for Obstetrical and Reproductive Services

See Section I.C.15. Pregnancy, Childbirth, and the Puerperium, for further instruction on the use of these codes.

Z codes for pregnancy are for use in those circumstances when none of the problems or complications included in the codes from the Obstetrics chapter exist (a routine prenatal visit or postpartum care). Codes in category Z34, Encounter for supervision of normal pregnancy, are always first listed and are not to be used with any other code from the OB chapter.

Codes in category Z3A, Weeks of gestation, may be assigned to provide additional information about the pregnancy. Category Z3A codes should not be assigned for pregnancies with abortive outcomes (categories O00-O08), elective termination of pregnancy (code Z33.2), nor for postpartum conditions, as category Z3A is not applicable to these conditions. The date of the admission should be used to determine weeks of gestation for inpatient admissions that encompass more than one gestational week.

The outcome of delivery, category Z37, should be included on all maternal delivery records. It is always a secondary code. Codes in category Z37 should not be used on the newborn record.

Z codes for family planning (contraceptive) or procreative management and counseling should be included on an obstetric record either during the pregnancy or the postpartum stage, if applicable.

Z codes/categories for obstetrical and reproductive services:

Z30	Encounter for contraceptive management
Z31	Encounter for procreative management
Z32.2	Encounter for childbirth instruction
Z32.3	Encounter for childcare instruction
Z33	Pregnant state
Z34	Encounter for supervision of normal pregnancy
Z36	Encounter for antenatal screening of mother
Z3A	Weeks of gestation
Z37	Outcome of delivery
Z39	Encounter for maternal postpartum care and examination
Z76.81	Expectant mother prebirth pediatrician visit

12) Newborns and Infants

See Section I.C.16. Newborn (Perinatal) Guidelines, for further instruction on the use of these codes.

Newborn Z codes/categories:

Z76.1	Encounter for health supervision and care of foundling
Z00.1-	Encounter for routine child health examination
Z38	Liveborn infants according to place of birth and type of delivery

13) Routine and administrative examinations

The Z codes allow for the description of encounters for routine examinations, such as, a general check-up, or, examinations for administrative purposes, such as, a pre-employment physical. The codes are not to be used if the examination is for diagnosis of a suspected condition or for treatment purposes. In such cases the diagnosis code is used. During a routine exam, should a diagnosis

or condition be discovered, it should be coded as an additional code. Pre-existing and chronic conditions and history codes may also be included as additional codes as long as the examination is for administrative purposes and not focused on any particular condition.

Some of the codes for routine health examinations distinguish between "with" and "without" abnormal findings. Code assignment depends on the information that is known at the time the encounter is being coded. For example, if no abnormal findings were found during the examination, but the encounter is being coded before test results are back, it is acceptable to assign the code for "without abnormal findings." When assigning a code for "with abnormal findings," additional code(s) should be assigned to identify the specific abnormal finding(s).

Pre-operative examination and pre-procedural laboratory examination Z codes are for use only in those situations when a patient is being cleared for a procedure or surgery and no treatment is given.

The Z codes/categories for routine and administrative examinations:

Z00	Encounter for general examination without complaint, suspected or reported diagnosis
Z01	Encounter for other special examination without complaint, suspected or reported diagnosis
Z02	Encounter for administrative examination Except: Z02.9, Encounter for administrative examinations, unspecified
Z32.0-	Encounter for pregnancy test

14) Miscellaneous Z codes

The miscellaneous Z codes capture a number of other health care encounters that do not fall into one of the other categories. Certain of these codes identify the reason for the encounter; others are for use as additional codes that provide useful information on circumstances that may affect a patient's care and treatment.

Prophylactic Organ Removal

For encounters specifically for prophylactic removal of an organ (such as prophylactic removal of breasts due to a genetic susceptibility to cancer or a family history of cancer), the principal or first-listed code should be a code from category Z40, Encounter for prophylactic surgery, followed by the appropriate codes to identify the associated risk factor (such as genetic susceptibility or family history).

If the patient has a malignancy of one site and is having prophylactic removal at another site to prevent either a new primary malignancy or metastatic disease, a code for the malignancy should also be assigned in addition to a code from subcategory Z40.0, Encounter for prophylactic surgery for risk factors related to malignant neoplasms. A Z40.0 code should not be assigned if the patient is having organ removal for treatment of a malignancy, such as the removal of the testes for the treatment of prostate cancer.

Miscellaneous Z codes/categories:

Z28	Immunization not carried out Except: Z28.3, Underimmunization status
Z29	Encounter for other prophylactic measures
Z40	Encounter for prophylactic surgery
Z41	Encounter for procedures for purposes other than remedying health state Except: Z41.9, Encounter for procedure for purposes other than remedying health state, unspecified
Z53	Persons encountering health services for specific procedures and treatment, not carried out
Z55	Problems related to education and literacy
Z56	Problems related to employment and unemployment
Z57	Occupational exposure to risk factors
Z58	Problems related to physical environment
Z59	Problems related to housing and economic circumstances
Z60	Problems related to social environment
Z62	Problems related to upbringing
Z63	Other problems related to primary support group, including family circumstances
Z64	Problems related to certain psychosocial circumstances
Z65	Problems related to other psychosocial circumstances
Z72	Problems related to lifestyle Note: These codes should be assigned only when the documentation specifies that the patient has an associated problem
Z73	Problems related to life management difficulty

Z74	Problems related to care provider dependency Except: Z74.01, Bed confinement status
Z75	Problems related to medical facilities and other health care
Z76.0	Encounter for issue of repeat prescription
Z76.3	Healthy person accompanying sick person
Z76.4	Other boarder to healthcare facility
Z76.5	Malingerer [conscious simulation]
Z91.1-	Patient's noncompliance with medical treatment and regimen
Z91.83	Wandering in diseases classified elsewhere
Z91.84-	Oral health risk factors
Z91.89	Other specified personal risk factors, not elsewhere classified

See Section I.B.14 for Z55-Z65 Persons with potential health hazards related to socioeconomic and psychosocial circumstances, documentation by clinicians other than the patient's provider.

15) Nonspecific Z codes

Certain Z codes are so non-specific, or potentially redundant with other codes in the classification, that there can be little justification for their use in the inpatient setting. Their use in the outpatient setting should be limited to those instances when there is no further documentation to permit more precise coding. Otherwise, any sign or symptom or any other reason for visit that is captured in another code should be used.

Nonspecific Z codes/categories:

Z02.9	Encounter for administrative examinations, unspecified
Z04.9	Encounter for examination and observation for unspecified reason
Z13.9	Encounter for screening, unspecified
Z41.9	Encounter for procedure for purposes other than remedying health state, unspecified
Z52.9	Donor of unspecified organ or tissue
Z86.59	Personal history of other mental and behavioral disorders
Z88.9	Allergy status to unspecified drugs, medicaments and biological substances status
Z92.0	Personal history of contraception

16) Z Codes That May Only Be Principal/First-Listed Diagnosis

The following Z codes/categories may only be reported as the principal/first listed diagnosis, except when there are multiple encounters on the same day and the medical records for the encounters are combined:

Z00	Encounter for general examination without complaint, suspected or reported diagnosis Except: Z00.6
Z01	Encounter for other special examination without complaint, suspected or reported diagnosis
Z02	Encounter for administrative examination
Z03	Encounter for medical observation for suspected diseases and conditions ruled out
Z04	Encounter for examination and observation for other reasons
Z33.2	Encounter for elective termination of pregnancy
Z31.81	Encounter for male factor infertility in female patient
Z31.83	Encounter for assisted reproductive fertility procedure cycle
Z31.84	Encounter for fertility preservation procedure
Z34	Encounter for supervision of normal pregnancy
Z39	Encounter for maternal postpartum care and examination
Z38	Liveborn infants according to place of birth and type of delivery
Z40	Encounter for prophylactic surgery
Z42	Encounter for plastic and reconstructive surgery following medical procedure or healed injury
Z51.0	Encounter for antineoplastic radiation therapy
Z51.1-	Encounter for antineoplastic chemotherapy and immunotherapy
Z52	Donors of organs and tissues Except: Z52.9, Donor of unspecified organ or tissue
Z76.1	Encounter for health supervision and care of foundling
Z76.2	Encounter for health supervision and care of other healthy infant and child
Z99.12	Encounter for respirator [ventilator] dependence during power failure

CHAPTER 21

FACTORS INFLUENCING HEALTH STATUS AND CONTACT WITH HEALTH SERVICES (Z00-Z99)

Note: Z codes represent reasons for encounters. A corresponding procedure code must accompany a Z code if a procedure is performed. Categories Z00-Z99 are provided for occasions when circumstances other than a disease, injury or external cause classifiable to categories A00-Y89 are recorded as "diagnoses" or "problems." This can arise in two main ways:

(a) When a person who may or may not be sick encounters the health services for some specific purpose, such as to receive limited care or service for a current condition, to donate an organ or tissue, to receive prophylactic vaccination (immunization), or to discuss a problem which is in itself not a disease or injury.

(b) When some circumstance or problem is present which influences the person's health status but is not in itself a current illness or injury.

This chapter contains the following blocks:

Z00-Z13	Persons encountering health services for examination
Z14-Z15	Genetic carrier and genetic susceptibility to disease
Z16	Resistance to antimicrobial drugs
Z17	Estrogen receptor status
Z18	Retained foreign body fragments
Z19	Hormone sensitivity malignancy status
Z20-Z29	Persons with potential health hazards related to communicable diseases
Z30-Z39	Persons encountering health services in circumstances related to reproduction
Z40-Z53	Encounters for other specific health care
Z55-Z65	Persons with potential health hazards related to socioeconomic and psychosocial circumstances
Z66	Do not resuscitate status
Z67	Blood type
Z68	Body mass index (BMI)
Z69-Z76	Persons encountering health services in other circumstances
Z77-Z99	Persons with potential health hazards related to family and personal history and certain conditions influencing health status

PERSONS ENCOUNTERING HEALTH SERVICES FOR EXAMINATIONS (Z00-Z13)

Note: Nonspecific abnormal findings disclosed at the time of these examinations are classified to categories R70-R94.

> **Excludes1** examinations related to pregnancy and reproduction (Z30-Z36, Z39.-)

● **Z00**   **Encounter for general examination without complaint, suspected or reported diagnosis**

> **Excludes1** encounter for examination for administrative purposes (Z02.-)

> **Excludes2** encounter for pre-procedural examinations (Z01.81-)
> special screening examinations (Z11-Z13)

● **Z00.0**   **Encounter for general adult medical examination**
Encounter for adult periodic examination (annual) (physical) and any associated laboratory and radiologic examinations

> **Excludes1** encounter for examination of sign or symptom - code to sign or symptom
> general health check-up of infant or child (Z00.12.-)

Coding Clinic: 2016, Q4, P131

  ● **Z00.00**   **Encounter for general adult medical examination without abnormal findings**   A
Encounter for adult health check-up NOS
Coding Clinic: 2017, Q4, P95; 2016, Q1, P37

  ● **Z00.01**   **Encounter for general adult medical examination with abnormal findings**   A
Use additional code to identify abnormal findings
Coding Clinic: 2016, Q1, P36

● **Z00.1**   **Encounter for newborn, infant and child health examinations**

  ● **Z00.11**   **Newborn health examination**
Health check for child under 29 days old
Use additional code to identify any abnormal findings

> **Excludes1** health check for child over 28 days old (Z00.12-)

    ● **Z00.110**   **Health examination for newborn under 8 days old**   N
Health check for newborn under 8 days old

    ● **Z00.111**   **Health examination for newborn 8 to 28 days old**   N
Health check for newborn 8 to 28 days old
Newborn weight check

  ● **Z00.12**   **Encounter for routine child health examination**
Immunizations appropriate for age
Health check (routine) for child over 28 days old
Routine developmental screening of infant or child
Routine vision and hearing testing

> **Excludes1** health check for child under 29 days old (Z00.11-)
> health supervision of foundling or other healthy infant or child (Z76.1-Z76.2)
> newborn health examination (Z00.11-)

    ● **Z00.121**   **Encounter for routine child health examination with abnormal findings** P
Use additional code to identify abnormal findings
Coding Clinic: 2017, Q4, P95; 2016, Q1, P34-35

    ● **Z00.129**   **Encounter for routine child health examination without abnormal findings**   P
Encounter for routine child health examination NOS
Coding Clinic: 2016, Q1, P34

● **Z00.2**   **Encounter for examination for period of rapid growth in childhood**   P

● **Z00.3**   **Encounter for examination for adolescent development state**   P
Encounter for puberty development state

● **Z00.5**   **Encounter for examination of potential donor of organ and tissue**

  Z00.6   **Encounter for examination for normal comparison and control in clinical research program**
Examination of participant or control in clinical research program

● **Z00.7**   **Encounter for examination for period of delayed growth in childhood**

  ● **Z00.70**   **Encounter for examination for period of delayed growth in childhood without abnormal findings**   P

  ● **Z00.71**   **Encounter for examination for period of delayed growth in childhood with abnormal findings**   P
Use additional code to identify abnormal findings

● **Z00.8**   **Encounter for other general examination**
Encounter for health examination in population surveys

▶ New   ⟹ Revised   ~~deleted~~ Deleted   Excludes 1   Excludes 2   Includes   Use additional   Code first   Code also   Key words

OGCR Official Guidelines   ● Unacceptable Principal Diagnosis   X Assign placeholder X   ● Use Additional Character(s)   ▶ Manifestation Code   Coding Clinic

● **Z01** Encounter for other special examination without complaint, suspected or reported diagnosis

  Includes   routine examination of specific system

  Note: Codes from category Z01 represent the reason for the encounter. A separate procedure code is required to identify any examinations or procedures performed.

  Excludes1   encounter for examination for administrative purposes (Z02.-)
  encounter for examination for suspected conditions, proven not to exist (Z03.-)
  encounter for laboratory and radiologic examinations as a component of general medical examinations (Z00.0-)
  encounter for laboratory, radiologic and imaging examinations for sign(s) and symptom(s) - code to the sign(s) or symptom(s)

  Excludes2   screening examinations (Z11-Z13)

● **Z01.0** Encounter for examination of eyes and vision

  Excludes1   examination for driving license (Z02.4)

  Z01.00 Encounter for examination of eyes and vision without abnormal findings
  Encounter for examination of eyes and vision NOS

  Z01.01 Encounter for examination of eyes and vision with abnormal findings
  Use additional code to identify abnormal findings
  Coding Clinic: 2016, Q4, P21

  ● **Z01.02** Encounter for examination of eyes and vision following failed vision screening

    ➡**Excludes1**   encounter for examination of eyes and vision with abnormal findings (Z01.01)
    ➡encounter for examination of eyes and vision without abnormal findings (Z01.00)

    ● **Z01.020** Encounter for examination of eyes and vision following failed vision screening without abnormal findings

    ● **Z01.021** Encounter for examination of eyes and vision following failed vision screening with abnormal findings
    Use additional code to identify abnormal findings

● **Z01.1** Encounter for examination of ears and hearing

  ● **Z01.10** Encounter for examination of ears and hearing without abnormal findings
  Encounter for examination of ears and hearing NOS
  Coding Clinic: 2016, Q4, P25

  ● **Z01.11** Encounter for examination of ears and hearing with abnormal findings
  Coding Clinic: 2016, Q3, P18

    ● **Z01.110** Encounter for hearing examination following failed hearing screening
    Coding Clinic: 2016, Q3, P18-19

    ● **Z01.118** Encounter for examination of ears and hearing with other abnormal findings
    Use additional code to identify abnormal findings
    Coding Clinic: 2016, Q3, P17

  ● **Z01.12** Encounter for hearing conservation and treatment

● **Z01.2** Encounter for dental examination and cleaning

  ● **Z01.20** Encounter for dental examination and cleaning without abnormal findings
  Encounter for dental examination and cleaning NOS

  ● **Z01.21** Encounter for dental examination and cleaning with abnormal findings
  Use additional code to identify abnormal findings

● **Z01.3** Encounter for examination of blood pressure

  ● **Z01.30** Encounter for examination of blood pressure without abnormal findings
  Encounter for examination of blood pressure NOS

  ● **Z01.31** Encounter for examination of blood pressure with abnormal findings
  Use additional code to identify abnormal findings

● **Z01.4** Encounter for gynecological examination

  Excludes2   pregnancy examination or test (Z32.0-)
  routine examination for contraceptive maintenance (Z30.4-)

  ● **Z01.41** Encounter for routine gynecological examination
  Encounter for general gynecological examination with or without cervical smear
  Encounter for gynecological examination (general) (routine) NOS
  Encounter for pelvic examination (annual) (periodic)
  Use additional code:
    for screening for human papillomavirus, if applicable (Z11.51)
    for screening vaginal pap smear, if applicable (Z12.72)
    to identify acquired absence of uterus, if applicable (Z90.71-)

    Excludes1   gynecologic examination status-post hysterectomy for malignant condition (Z08)
    screening cervical pap smear not a part of a routine gynecological examination (Z12.4)

    Z01.411 Encounter for gynecological examination (general) (routine) with abnormal findings ♀
    Use additional code to identify any abnormal findings

    Z01.419 Encounter for gynecological examination (general) (routine) without abnormal findings ♀

  Z01.42 Encounter for cervical smear to confirm findings of recent normal smear following initial abnormal smear ♀

● **Z01.8** Encounter for other specified special examinations

  ● **Z01.81** Encounter for preprocedural examinations
  Encounter for preoperative examinations
  Encounter for radiological and imaging examinations as part of preprocedural examination

    Z01.810 Encounter for preprocedural cardiovascular examination

    Z01.811 Encounter for preprocedural respiratory examination

    ● **Z01.812** Encounter for preprocedural laboratory examination
    Blood and urine tests prior to treatment or procedure
    Coding Clinic: 2021, Q1, P38

    ● **Z01.818** Encounter for other preprocedural examination
    Encounter for preprocedural examination NOS
    Encounter for examinations prior to antineoplastic chemotherapy

  ● **Z01.82** Encounter for allergy testing
  Excludes1   encounter for antibody response examination (Z01.84)

  ● **Z01.83** Encounter for blood typing
  Encounter for Rh typing

N Newborn Age: 0   **P** Pediatric Age: 0–17   **M** Maternity DX: 9–64   **A** Adult Age: 15–124   ♀ Females Only   ♂ Males Only

🔖 Complication\Comorbidity   🔖 Major C\C   (Ex) CC/MCC Exclusions   🔖 Hospital-Acquired Condition   🔖 Hierarchical Condition Category

1621

CHAPTER 21 (Z00-Z99)

● **Z01.84** **Encounter for antibody response examination**
Encounter for immunity status testing
> **Excludes1** encounter for allergy testing (Z01.82)

● **Z01.89** **Encounter for other specified special examinations**

● **Z02** **Encounter for administrative examination**

● **Z02.0** **Encounter for examination for admission to educational institution**
Encounter for examination for admission to preschool (education)
Encounter for examination for re-admission to school following illness or medical treatment

Z02.1 **Encounter for pre-employment examination**

● **Z02.2** **Encounter for examination for admission to residential institution**
> **Excludes1** examination for admission to prison (Z02.89)

Z02.3 **Encounter for examination for recruitment to armed forces**

● **Z02.4** **Encounter for examination for driving license**

● **Z02.5** **Encounter for examination for participation in sport**
> **Excludes1** blood-alcohol and blood-drug test (Z02.83)

● **Z02.6** **Encounter for examination for insurance purposes**

● **Z02.7** **Encounter for issue of medical certificate**
> **Excludes1** encounter for general medical examination (Z00-Z01, Z02.0-Z02.6, Z02.8-Z02.9)

● **Z02.71** **Encounter for disability determination**
Encounter for issue of medical certificate of incapacity
Encounter for issue of medical certificate of invalidity

● **Z02.79** **Encounter for issue of other medical certificate**

● **Z02.8** **Encounter for other administrative examinations**

Z02.81 **Encounter for paternity testing**

● **Z02.82** **Encounter for adoption services**

Z02.83 **Encounter for blood-alcohol and blood-drug test**
Use additional code for findings of alcohol or drugs in blood (R78.-)

● **Z02.89** **Encounter for other administrative examinations**
Encounter for examination for admission to prison
Encounter for examination for admission to summer camp
Encounter for immigration examination
Encounter for naturalization examination
Encounter for premarital examination
> **Excludes1** health supervision of foundling or other healthy infant or child (Z76.1-Z76.2)

● **Z02.9** **Encounter for administrative examinations, unspecified**

Observation

There are three observation Z code categories. They are for use in very limited circumstances when a person is being observed for a suspected condition that is ruled out. The observation codes are not for use if an injury or illnesss or any signs or symptoms related to the suspected condition are present. In such cases the diagnosis/symptom code is used with the corresponding external cause code.

The observation codes are to be used as principal diagnosis only. The only exception to this is when the principal diagnosis is required to be a code from category Z38, Liveborn infants according to place of birth and type of delivery. Then a code from category Z05, Encounter for observation and evaluation of newborn for suspected diseases and conditions ruled out, is sequenced after the Z38 code. Additional codes may be used in addition to the observation code but only if they are unrelated to the suspected condition being observed.

Codes from subcategory Z03.7 Encounter for suspected maternal and fetal conditions ruled out, may either be used as a first listed or as an additional code assignment depending on the case. They are for use in very limited circumstances on a maternal record when an encounter is for a suspected maternal or fetal condition that is ruled out during that encounter (for example, a maternal or fetal condition may be suspected due to an abnormal test result). These codes should not be used when the condition is confirmed. In those cases, the confirmed condition should be coded. In addition, these codes are not for use if an illness or any signs or symptoms related to the suspected condition or problem are present. In such cases the diagnosis/symptom code is used.

Additional codes may be used in addition to the code from subcategory Z03.7, but only if they are unrelated to the suspected condition being evaluated.

Codes from subcategory Z03.7 may not be used for encounters for antenatal screening of mother. *See Section I.C.21. Screening.*

For encounters for suspected fetal condition that are inconclusive following testing and evaluation, assign the appropriate code from category O35, O36, O40 or O41.

The observation Z code categories:

Z03 Encounter for medical observation for suspected diseases and conditions ruled out

Z04 Encounter for examination and observation for other reasons Except: Z04.9, Encounter for examination and observation for unspecified reason

Z05 Encounter for observation and evaluation of newborn for suspected diseases and conditions ruled out

● **Z03** **Encounter for medical observation for suspected diseases and conditions ruled out**
This category is to be used when a person without a diagnosis is suspected of having an abnormal condition, without signs or symptoms, which requires study, but after examination and observation, is ruled out. This category is also for use for administrative and legal observation status.
> **Excludes1** contact with and (suspected) exposures hazardous to health (Z77.-)
> encounter for observation and evaluation of newborn for suspected diseases and conditions ruled out (Z05.-)
> person with feared complaint in whom no diagnosis is made (Z71.1)
> signs or symptoms under study - code to signs or symptoms

Z03.6 **Encounter for observation for suspected toxic effect from ingested substance ruled out**
Encounter for observation for suspected adverse effect from drug
Encounter for observation for suspected poisoning

CHAPTER 21 (Z00-Z99)

● Z03.7   Encounter for suspected maternal and fetal conditions ruled out
　　Encounter for suspected maternal and fetal conditions not found
　　Excludes1   known or suspected fetal anomalies affecting management of mother, not ruled out (O26.-, O35.-, O36.-, O40.-, O41.-)

　● Z03.71   Encounter for suspected problem with amniotic cavity and membrane ruled out ♀   **M**
　　　Encounter for suspected oligohydramnios ruled out
　　　Encounter for suspected polyhydramnios ruled out

　● Z03.72   Encounter for suspected placental problem ruled out ♀   **M**

　● Z03.73   Encounter for suspected fetal anomaly ruled out ♀   **M**
　　　Coding Clinic: 2016, Q4, P6

　● Z03.74   Encounter for suspected problem with fetal growth ruled out ♀   **M**

　● Z03.75   Encounter for suspected cervical shortening ruled out ♀   **M**

　● Z03.79   Encounter for other suspected maternal and fetal conditions ruled out ♀   **M**
　　　Coding Clinic: 2016, Q4, P7

● Z03.8   Encounter for observation for other suspected diseases and conditions ruled out

　● Z03.81   Encounter for observation for suspected exposure to biological agents ruled out

　　Z03.810   Encounter for observation for suspected exposure to anthrax ruled out

　　Z03.818   Encounter for observation for suspected exposure to other biological agents ruled out

　● Z03.82   Encounter for observation for suspected foreign body ruled out
　　Excludes1   retained foreign body (Z18.-)
　　　retained foreign body in eyelid (H02.81)
　　　residual foreign body in soft tissue (M79.5)
　　Excludes2   confirmed foreign body ingestion or aspiration including:
　　　foreign body in alimentary tract (T18)
　　　foreign body in ear (T16)
　　　foreign body on external eye (T15)
　　　foreign body in respiratory tract (T17)

　　● Z03.821   Encounter for observation for suspected ingested foreign body ruled out

　　● Z03.822   Encounter for observation for suspected aspirated (inhaled) foreign body ruled out

　　● Z03.823   Encounter for observation for suspected inserted (injected) foreign body ruled out
　　　Encounter for observation for suspected inserted (injected) foreign body in eye ruled out
　　　Encounter for observation for suspected inserted (injected) foreign body in orifice ruled out
　　　Encounter for observation for suspected inserted (injected) foreign body in skin ruled out

　　Z03.89   Encounter for observation for other suspected diseases and conditions ruled out

● Z04   Encounter for examination and observation for other reasons
　　Includes   encounter for examination for medicolegal reasons
　　This category is to be used when a person without a diagnosis is suspected of having an abnormal condition, without signs or symptoms, which requires study, but after examination and observation, is ruled-out. This category is also for use for administrative and legal observation status.

　Z04.1   Encounter for examination and observation following transport accident
　　Excludes1   encounter for examination and observation following work accident (Z04.2)
　　　Coding Clinic: 2019, Q2, P11

　Z04.2   Encounter for examination and observation following work accident

　Z04.3   Encounter for examination and observation following other accident

● Z04.4   Encounter for examination and observation following alleged rape
　　Encounter for examination and observation of victim following alleged rape
　　Encounter for examination and observation of victim following alleged sexual abuse
　　Coding Clinic: 2016, Q4, P129

　　Z04.41   Encounter for examination and observation following alleged adult rape   **A**
　　　Suspected adult rape, ruled out
　　　Suspected adult sexual abuse, ruled out

　　Z04.42   Encounter for examination and observation following alleged child rape   **P**
　　　Suspected child rape, ruled out
　　　Suspected child sexual abuse, ruled out

　Z04.6   Encounter for general psychiatric examination, requested by authority

● Z04.7   Encounter for examination and observation following alleged physical abuse

　　Z04.71   Encounter for examination and observation following alleged adult physical abuse   **A**
　　　Suspected adult physical abuse, ruled out
　　　Excludes1   confirmed case of adult physical abuse (T74.-)
　　　encounter for examination and observation following alleged adult sexual abuse (Z04.41)
　　　suspected case of adult physical abuse, not ruled out (T76.-)

　　Z04.72   Encounter for examination and observation following alleged child physical abuse   **P**
　　　Suspected child physical abuse, ruled out
　　　Excludes1   confirmed case of child physical abuse (T74.-)
　　　encounter for examination and observation following alleged child sexual abuse (Z04.42)
　　　suspected case of child physical abuse, not ruled out (T76.-)

● Z04.8   Encounter for examination and observation for other specified reasons
　　Encounter for examination and observation for request for expert evidence

　　Z04.81   Encounter for examination and observation of victim following forced sexual exploitation

　　Z04.82   Encounter for examination and observation of victim following forced labor exploitation

　　Z04.89   Encounter for examination and observation for other specified reasons

● Z04.9   Encounter for examination and observation for unspecified reason
　　Encounter for observation NOS

CHAPTER 21 (Z00-Z99)

N Newborn Age: 0   **P** Pediatric Age: 0–17   **M** Maternity DX: 9–64   **A** Adult Age: 15–124   ♀ Females Only   ♂ Males Only

🔷 Complication\Comorbidity   🔷 Major C\C   (Ex) CC/MCC Exclusions   🔷 Hospital-Acquired Condition   🔷 Hierarchical Condition Category

1623

● Z05   Encounter for observation and evaluation of newborn for suspected diseases and conditions ruled out

> This category is to be used for newborns, within the neonatal period (the first 28 days of life), who are suspected of having an abnormal condition, but without signs or symptoms, and which, after examination and observation, is ruled out.
>
> Coding Clinic: 2019, Q2, P11; 2016, Q4, P54, 77, 126-127, 130

Z05.0   Observation and evaluation of newborn for suspected cardiac condition ruled out   N

Z05.1   Observation and evaluation of newborn for suspected infectious condition ruled out   N
> Coding Clinic: 2019, Q2, P11

Z05.2   Observation and evaluation of newborn for suspected neurological condition ruled out   N

Z05.3   Observation and evaluation of newborn for suspected respiratory condition ruled out   N

● Z05.4   Observation and evaluation of newborn for suspected genetic, metabolic or immunologic condition ruled out

> **Z05.41**   Observation and evaluation of newborn for suspected genetic condition ruled out   N
> Coding Clinic: 2016, Q4, P55
>
> **Z05.42**   Observation and evaluation of newborn for suspected metabolic condition ruled out   N
>
> **Z05.43**   Observation and evaluation of newborn for suspected immunologic condition ruled out   N

Z05.5   Observation and evaluation of newborn for suspected gastrointestinal condition ruled out   N

Z05.6   Observation and evaluation of newborn for suspected genitourinary condition ruled out   N

● Z05.7   Observation and evaluation of newborn for suspected skin, subcutaneous, musculoskeletal and connective tissue condition ruled out

> **Z05.71**   Observation and evaluation of newborn for suspected skin and subcutaneous tissue condition ruled out   N
>
> **Z05.72**   Observation and evaluation of newborn for suspected musculoskeletal condition ruled out   N
>
> **Z05.73**   Observation and evaluation of newborn for suspected connective tissue condition ruled out   N

Z05.8   Observation and evaluation of newborn for other specified suspected condition ruled out   N

Z05.9   Observation and evaluation of newborn for unspecified suspected condition ruled out   N

OGCR   See Section II.C.21.c.8.

> The follow-up codes are used to explain continuing surveillance following completed treatment of a disease, condition, or injury. They imply that the condition has been fully treated and no longer exists. They should not be confused with aftercare codes, or injury codes with 7th character "D," that explain ongoing care of a healing condition or its sequelae. Follow-up codes may be used in conjunction with history codes to provide the full picture of the healed condition and its treatment. The follow-up code is sequenced first, followed by the history code.
>
> A follow-up code may be used to explain multiple visits. Should a condition be found to have recurred on the follow-up visit, then the diagnosis code for the condition should be assigned in place of the follow-up code.
>
> The follow-up Z code categories:
>
> Z08   Encounter for follow-up examination after completed treatment for malignant neoplasm
>
> Z09   Encounter for follow-up examination after completed treatment for conditions other than malignant neoplasm
>
> Z39   Encounter for maternal postpartum care and examination

● Z08   Encounter for follow-up examination after completed treatment for malignant neoplasm
> Medical surveillance following completed treatment
>
> Use additional code to identify any acquired absence of organs (Z90.-)
>
> Use additional code to identify the personal history of malignant neoplasm (Z85.-)
>
> **Excludes1**   aftercare following medical care (Z43-Z49, Z51)

● Z09   Encounter for follow-up examination after completed treatment for conditions other than malignant neoplasm
> Medical surveillance following completed treatment
>
> ⇒ Use additional code to identify any applicable history of disease code (Z86.-, Z87.-)
>
> **Excludes1**   aftercare following medical care (Z43-Z49, Z51)
> surveillance of contraception (Z30.4-)
> surveillance of prosthetic and other medical devices (Z44-Z46)
>
> Coding Clinic: 2021, Q1, P33; 2017, Q1, P9; 2015, Q1, P8

OGCR   Section II.C.21.c.5.

> Screening
>
> Screening is the testing for disease or disease precursors in seemingly well individuals so that early detection and treatment can be provided for those who test positive for the disease (e.g., screening mammogram).
>
> The testing of a person to rule out or confirm a suspected diagnosis because the patient has some sign or symptom is a diagnostic examination, not a screening. In these cases, the sign or symptom is used to explain the reason for the test.
>
> A screening code may be a first listed code if the reason for the visit is specifically the screening exam. It may also be used as an additional code if the screening is done during an office visit for other health problems. A screening code is not necessary if the screening is inherent to a routine examination, such as a pap smear done during a routine pelvic examination.
>
> Should a condition be discovered during the screening then the code for the condition may be assigned as an additional diagnosis.
>
> The Z code indicates that a screening exam is planned. A procedure code is required to confirm that the screening was performed.
>
> The screening Z codes/categories:
>
> Z11   Encounter for screening for infectious and parasitic diseases
>
> Z12   Encounter for screening for malignant neoplasms
>
> Z13   Encounter for screening for other diseases and disorders
> Except: Z13.9, Encounter for screening, unspecified
>
> Z36   Encounter for antenatal screening for mother

● Z11   Encounter for screening for infectious and parasitic diseases
> Screening is the testing for disease or disease precursors in asymptomatic individuals so that early detection and treatment can be provided for those who test positive for the disease.
>
> **Excludes1**   encounter for diagnostic examination - code to sign or symptom

● Z11.0   Encounter for screening for intestinal infectious diseases
> Encounter for screening for active tuberculosis disease

● Z11.1   Encounter for screening for respiratory tuberculosis

● Z11.2   Encounter for screening for other bacterial diseases

● Z11.3   Encounter for screening for infections with a predominantly sexual mode of transmission
> **Excludes2**   encounter for screening for human immunodeficiency virus [HIV] (Z11.4)
> encounter for screening for human papillomavirus (Z11.51)

● Z11.4   Encounter for screening for human immunodeficiency virus [HIV]

▶ New   ⇒ Revised   ~~deleted~~ Deleted   Excludes 1   Excludes 2   Includes   Use additional   Code first   Code also   Key words

OGCR Official Guidelines   ● Unacceptable Principal Diagnosis   X Assign placeholder X   ● Use Additional Character(s)   ▶ Manifestation Code   Coding Clinic

● **Z11.5 Encounter for screening for other viral diseases**
     Excludes2 encounter for screening for viral intestinal disease (Z11.0)
  ● **Z11.51 Encounter for screening for human papillomavirus (HPV)**
  ● **Z11.52 Encounter for screening for COVID-19**
       Coding Clinic: 2021, Q1, P37, 42
  ● **Z11.59 Encounter for screening for other viral diseases**
       Coding Clinic: 2021, Q1, P37

● **Z11.6 Encounter for screening for other protozoal diseases and helminthiases**
     Diseases or infestations caused by parasitic worms
     Excludes2 encounter for screening for protozoal intestinal disease (Z11.0)

   Z11.7 Encounter for testing for latent tuberculosis infection

● **Z11.8 Encounter for screening for other infectious and parasitic diseases**
     Encounter for screening for chlamydia
     Encounter for screening for rickettsial
     Encounter for screening for spirochetal
     Encounter for screening for mycoses

● **Z11.9 Encounter for screening for infectious and parasitic diseases, unspecified**

● **Z12 Encounter for screening for malignant neoplasms**
     Screening is the testing for disease or disease precursors in asymptomatic individuals so that early detection and treatment can be provided for those who test positive for the disease.
     Use additional code to identify any family history of malignant neoplasm (Z80.-)
     Excludes1 encounter for diagnostic examination - code to sign or symptom

● **Z12.0 Encounter for screening for malignant neoplasm of stomach**

● **Z12.1 Encounter for screening for malignant neoplasm of intestinal tract**
  ● **Z12.10 Encounter for screening for malignant neoplasm of intestinal tract, unspecified**
  ● **Z12.11 Encounter for screening for malignant neoplasm of colon**
     Encounter for screening colonoscopy NOS
     Coding Clinic: 2018, Q1, P7; 2017, Q1, P8-9
  ● **Z12.12 Encounter for screening for malignant neoplasm of rectum**
  ● **Z12.13 Encounter for screening for malignant neoplasm of small intestine**

● **Z12.2 Encounter for screening for malignant neoplasm of respiratory organs**

● **Z12.3 Encounter for screening for malignant neoplasm of breast**
  ● **Z12.31 Encounter for screening mammogram for malignant neoplasm of breast**
     Excludes1 inconclusive mammogram (R92.2)
     Coding Clinic: 2015, Q1, P24
  ● **Z12.39 Encounter for other screening for malignant neoplasm of breast**

● **Z12.4 Encounter for screening for malignant neoplasm of cervix ♀**
     Encounter for screening pap smear for malignant neoplasm of cervix
     Excludes1 when screening is part of general gynecological examination (Z01.4-)
     Excludes2 encounter for screening for human papillomavirus (Z11.51)

   Z12.5 Encounter for screening for malignant neoplasm of prostate ♂

● **Z12.6 Encounter for screening for malignant neoplasm of bladder**

● **Z12.7 Encounter for screening for malignant neoplasm of other genitourinary organs**
  ● **Z12.71 Encounter for screening for malignant neoplasm of testis ♂**
  ● **Z12.72 Encounter for screening for malignant neoplasm of vagina ♀**
     Vaginal pap smear status - post hysterectomy for non-malignant condition
     Use additional code to identify acquired absence of uterus (Z90.71-)
     Excludes1 vaginal pap smear status - post hysterectomy for malignant conditions (Z08)
  ● **Z12.73 Encounter for screening for malignant neoplasm of ovary ♀**
  ● **Z12.79 Encounter for screening for malignant neoplasm of other genitourinary organs**

● **Z12.8 Encounter for screening for malignant neoplasm of other sites**
  ● **Z12.81 Encounter for screening for malignant neoplasm of oral cavity**
  ● **Z12.82 Encounter for screening for malignant neoplasm of nervous system**
  ● **Z12.83 Encounter for screening for malignant neoplasm of skin**
  ● **Z12.89 Encounter for screening for malignant neoplasm of other sites**
     Coding Clinic: 2021, Q1, P15

● **Z12.9 Encounter for screening for malignant neoplasm, site unspecified**

● **Z13 Encounter for screening for other diseases and disorders**
     Screening is the testing for disease or disease precursors in asymptomatic individuals so that early detection and treatment can be provided for those who test positive for the disease.
     Excludes1 encounter for diagnostic examination - code to sign or symptom

● **Z13.0 Encounter for screening for diseases of the blood and blood-forming organs and certain disorders involving the immune mechanism**

● **Z13.1 Encounter for screening for diabetes mellitus**

● **Z13.2 Encounter for screening for nutritional, metabolic and other endocrine disorders**
  ● **Z13.21 Encounter for screening for nutritional disorder**
  ● **Z13.22 Encounter for screening for metabolic disorder**
    ● **Z13.220 Encounter for screening for lipoid disorders**
       Encounter for screening for cholesterol level
       Encounter for screening for hypercholesterolemia
       Encounter for screening for hyperlipidemia
    ● **Z13.228 Encounter for screening for other metabolic disorders**
  ● **Z13.29 Encounter for screening for other suspected endocrine disorder**
     ~~**Excludes1** encounter for screening for diabetes mellitus (Z13.1)~~
     ▶**Excludes2** encounter for screening for diabetes mellitus (Z13.1)

● **Z13.3 Encounter for screening examination for mental health and behavioral disorders**
  ● **Z13.30 Encounter for screening examination for mental health and behavioral disorders, unspecified**
  ● **Z13.31 Encounter for screening for depression**
     Encounter for screening for depression, adult
     Encounter for screening for depression for child or adolescent

N Newborn Age: 0   **P** Pediatric Age: 0–17   **M** Maternity DX: 9–64   **A** Adult Age: 15–124   ♀ Females Only   ♂ Males Only

Complication\Comorbidity   Major C\C   (Ex) CC/MCC Exclusions   Hospital-Acquired Condition   Hierarchical Condition Category   **1625**

CHAPTER 21 (Z00-Z99)

● Z13.32　Encounter for screening for maternal depression ♀
　　　　Encounter for screening for perinatal depression

● Z13.39　Encounter for screening examination for other mental health and behavioral disorders
　　　　Encounter for screening for alcoholism
　　　　Encounter for screening for intellectual disabilities

● Z13.4　Encounter for screening for certain developmental disorders in childhood　　　　　　P
　　　　Encounter for development testing of infant or child
　　　　Encounter for screening for developmental handicaps in early childhood
　　　Excludes2　encounter for routine child health examination (Z00.12-)

● Z13.40　Encounter for screening for unspecified developmental delays

● Z13.41　Encounter for autism screening

● Z13.42　Encounter for screening for global developmental delays (milestones)
　　　　Encounter for screening for developmental handicaps in early childhood

● Z13.49　Encounter for screening for other developmental delays

● Z13.5　Encounter for screening for eye and ear disorders
　　　Excludes2　encounter for general hearing examination (Z01.1-)
　　　　　　encounter for general vision examination (Z01.0-)
　　　Coding Clinic: 2016, Q3, P17

● Z13.6　Encounter for screening for cardiovascular disorders

● Z13.7　Encounter for screening for genetic and chromosomal anomalies
　　　Excludes1　genetic testing for procreative management (Z31.4-)

● Z13.71　Encounter for nonprocreative screening for genetic disease carrier status

● Z13.79　Encounter for other screening for genetic and chromosomal anomalies

● Z13.8　Encounter for screening for other specified diseases and disorders
　　　Excludes2　screening for malignant neoplasms (Z12.-)

● Z13.81　Encounter for screening for digestive system disorders

　● Z13.810　Encounter for screening for upper gastrointestinal disorder

　● Z13.811　Encounter for screening for lower gastrointestinal disorder
　　　　Excludes1　encounter for screening for intestinal infectious disease (Z11.0)

　● Z13.818　Encounter for screening for other digestive system disorders

● Z13.82　Encounter for screening for musculoskeletal disorder

　● Z13.820　Encounter for screening for osteoporosis

　● Z13.828　Encounter for screening for other musculoskeletal disorder

● Z13.83　Encounter for screening for respiratory disorder NEC
　　　Excludes1　encounter for screening for respiratory tuberculosis (Z11.1)

● Z13.84　Encounter for screening for dental disorders

● Z13.85　Encounter for screening for nervous system disorders

　● Z13.850　Encounter for screening for traumatic brain injury

　● Z13.858　Encounter for screening for other nervous system disorders

● Z13.88　Encounter for screening for disorder due to exposure to contaminants
　　　Excludes1　those exposed to contaminants without suspected disorders (Z57-Z77.-)

● Z13.89　Encounter for screening for other disorder
　　　　Encounter for screening for genitourinary disorders

● Z13.9　Encounter for screening, unspecified

GENETIC CARRIER AND GENETIC SUSCEPTIBILITY TO DISEASE (Z14-Z15)

● Z14　Genetic carrier

● Z14.0　Hemophilia A carrier

　● Z14.01　Asymptomatic hemophilia A carrier

　● Z14.02　Symptomatic hemophilia A carrier

● Z14.1　Cystic fibrosis carrier

● Z14.8　Genetic carrier of other disease

● Z15　Genetic susceptibility to disease
　　　Excludes1　chromosomal anomalies (Q90-Q99)
　　　Includes　confirmed abnormal gene
　　　Use additional code, if applicable, for any associated family history of the disease (Z80-Z84)

● Z15.0　Genetic susceptibility to malignant neoplasm
　　　Code first if applicable, any current malignant neoplasm (C00-C75, C81-C96)
　　　Use additional code, if applicable, for any personal history of malignant neoplasm (Z85.-)

　● Z15.01　Genetic susceptibility to malignant neoplasm of breast

　● Z15.02　Genetic susceptibility to malignant neoplasm of ovary ♀

　● Z15.03　Genetic susceptibility to malignant neoplasm of prostate ♂

　● Z15.04　Genetic susceptibility to malignant neoplasm of endometrium ♀

　● Z15.09　Genetic susceptibility to other malignant neoplasm
　　　　Coding Clinic: 2021, Q1, P15

● Z15.8　Genetic susceptibility to other disease

　● Z15.81　Genetic susceptibility to multiple endocrine neoplasia [MEN]
　　　　Excludes1　multiple endocrine neoplasia [MEN] syndromes (E31.2-)

　● Z15.89　Genetic susceptibility to other disease

RESISTANCE TO ANTIMICROBIAL DRUGS (Z16)

● Z16　Resistance to antimicrobial drugs
　　　Note: The codes in this category are provided for use as additional codes to identify the resistance and non-responsiveness of a condition to antimicrobial drugs.
　　　Code first the infection
　　　Excludes1　Methicillin resistant Staphylococcus aureus infection (A49.02)
　　　　　　Methicillin resistant Staphylococcus aureus pneumonia (J15.212)
　　　　　　Sepsis due to Methicillin resistant Staphylococcus aureus (A41.02)

▶ New　⇒ Revised　~~deleted~~ Deleted　Excludes 1　Excludes 2　Includes　Use additional　Code first　Code also　Key words
OGCR Official Guidelines　● Unacceptable Principal Diagnosis　X Assign placeholder X　● Use Additional Character(s)　▷ Manifestation Code　Coding Clinic

● **Z16.1**   **Resistance to** beta lactam antibiotics
- ● **Z16.10**   **Resistance to** unspecified beta lactam antibiotics 🅒
  - (Ex) See PDX Collection 3496
- ● **Z16.11**   **Resistance to** penicillins 🅒
  - Resistance to amoxicillin
  - Resistance to ampicillin
  - (Ex) See PDX Collection 3497
- ● **Z16.12**   Extended spectrum beta lactamase (ESBL) resistance 🅒
  - **Excludes2**   Methicillin resistant Staphylococcus aureus infection in diseases classified elsewhere (B95.62)
  - (Ex) See PDX Collection 3454
- ● **Z16.19**   **Resistance to** other specified beta lactam antibiotics 🅒
  - Resistance to cephalosporins
  - (Ex) See PDX Collection 3498

● **Z16.2**   **Resistance to** other antibiotics
- ● **Z16.20**   **Resistance to** unspecified antibiotic 🅒
  - Resistance to antibiotics NOS
  - (Ex) See PDX Collection 3485
- ● **Z16.21**   **Resistance to** vancomycin 🅒
  - (Ex) See PDX Collection 3455
- ● **Z16.22**   **Resistance to** vancomycin related antibiotics 🅒
  - (Ex) See PDX Collection 3486
- ● **Z16.23**   **Resistance to** quinolones and fluoroquinolones 🅒
  - (Ex) See PDX Collection 3487
- ● **Z16.24**   **Resistance to** multiple antibiotics 🅒
  - (Ex) See PDX Collection 3456
- ● **Z16.29**   **Resistance to** other single specified antibiotic 🅒
  - Resistance to aminoglycosides
  - Resistance to macrolides
  - Resistance to sulfonamides
  - Resistance to tetracyclines
  - (Ex) See PDX Collection 3488

● **Z16.3**   **Resistance to** other antimicrobial drugs
- **Excludes1**   resistance to antibiotics (Z16.1-, Z16.2-)
- ● **Z16.30**   **Resistance to** unspecified antimicrobial drugs 🅒
  - Drug resistance NOS
  - (Ex) See PDX Collection 3489
- ● **Z16.31**   **Resistance to** antiparasitic drug(s) 🅒
  - Resistance to quinine and related compounds
  - (Ex) See PDX Collection 3490
- ● **Z16.32**   **Resistance to** antifungal drug(s) 🅒
  - (Ex) See PDX Collection 3491
- ● **Z16.33**   **Resistance to** antiviral drug(s) 🅒
  - (Ex) See PDX Collection 3492
- ● **Z16.34**   **Resistance to** antimycobacterial drug(s)
  - Resistance to tuberculostatics
  - ● **Z16.341**   **Resistance to** single antimycobacterial drug 🅒
    - Resistance to antimycobacterial drug NOS
    - (Ex) See PDX Collection 3493
  - ● **Z16.342**   **Resistance to** multiple antimycobacterial drugs 🅒
    - (Ex) See PDX Collection 3494
- ● **Z16.35**   **Resistance to** multiple antimicrobial drugs 🅒
  - **Excludes1**   Resistance to multiple antibiotics only (Z16.24)
  - (Ex) See PDX Collection 3495
- ● **Z16.39**   **Resistance to** other specified antimicrobial drug 🅒
  - (Ex) See PDX Collection 3457

ESTROGEN RECEPTOR STATUS (Z17)

● **Z17**   Estrogen receptor status
- *Code first malignant neoplasm of breast (C50.-)*
- ● **Z17.0**   Estrogen receptor positive status [ER+]
- ● **Z17.1**   Estrogen receptor negative status [ER-]

RETAINED FOREIGN BODY FRAGMENTS (Z18)

● **Z18**   Retained foreign body fragments
- **Includes**   embedded fragment (status)
  - embedded splinter (status)
  - retained foreign body status
- **Excludes1**   artificial joint prosthesis status (Z96.6-)
  - foreign body accidentally left during a procedure (T81.5-)
  - foreign body entering through orifice (T15-T19)
  - in situ cardiac device (Z95.-)
  - organ or tissue replaced by means other than transplant (Z96.-, Z97.-)
  - organ or tissue replaced by transplant (Z94.-)
  - personal history of retained foreign body fully removed Z87.821
  - superficial foreign body (non-embedded splinter) - code to superficial foreign body, by site
- ● **Z18.0**   Retained radioactive fragments
  - ● **Z18.01**   Retained depleted uranium fragments
  - ● **Z18.09**   Other retained radioactive fragments
    - Other retained depleted isotope fragments
    - Retained nontherapeutic radioactive fragments
- ● **Z18.1**   Retained metal fragments
  - **Excludes1**   retained radioactive metal fragments (Z18.01-Z18.09)
  - ● **Z18.10**   Retained metal fragments, unspecified
    - Retained metal fragment NOS
  - ● **Z18.11**   Retained magnetic metal fragments
  - ● **Z18.12**   Retained nonmagnetic metal fragments
- ● **Z18.2**   Retained plastic fragments
  - Acrylics fragments
  - Diethylhexylphthalates fragments
  - Isocyanate fragments
- ● **Z18.3**   Retained organic fragments
  - ● **Z18.31**   Retained animal quills or spines
  - ● **Z18.32**   Retained tooth
  - ● **Z18.33**   Retained wood fragments
  - ● **Z18.39**   Other retained organic fragments
- ● **Z18.8**   Other specified retained foreign body
  - ● **Z18.81**   Retained glass fragments
  - ● **Z18.83**   Retained stone or crystalline fragments
    - Retained concrete or cement fragments
  - ● **Z18.89**   Other specified retained foreign body fragments
    - Coding Clinic: 2016, Q3, P24
- ● **Z18.9**   Retained foreign body fragments, unspecified material

HORMONE SENSITIVITY MALIGNANCY STATUS (Z19)

● **Z19**   Hormone sensitivity malignancy status
- *Code first* malignant neoplasm —*see* Table of Neoplasms, by site, malignant
- Coding Clinic: 2016, Q4, P129
- **Z19.1**   Hormone sensitive malignancy status
  - Coding Clinic: 2016, Q4, P76
- **Z19.2**   Hormone resistant malignancy status
  - Castrate resistant prostate malignancy status
  - Coding Clinic: 2016, Q4, P76

CHAPTER 21 (Z00-Z99)

N   Newborn Age: 0   P   Pediatric Age: 0–17   M   Maternity DX: 9–64   A   Adult Age: 15–124   ♀   Females Only   ♂   Males Only

🅒   Complication\Comorbidity   🅒   Major C\C   (Ex)   CC/MCC Exclusions   🅒   Hospital-Acquired Condition   🅒   Hierarchical Condition Category

PERSONS WITH POTENTIAL HEALTH HAZARDS RELATED TO COMMUNICABLE DISEASES (Z20-Z29)

● **Z20** **Contact with and (suspected) exposure to communicable diseases**

> **Excludes1** carrier of infectious disease (Z22.-)
> diagnosed current infectious or parasitic disease - see Alphabetic Index

> **Excludes2** personal history of infectious and parasitic diseases (Z86.1-)

> Coding Clinic: 2021, Q1, P37

● **Z20.0** **Contact with and (suspected) exposure to intestinal infectious diseases**

> **Z20.01** Contact with and (suspected) exposure to intestinal infectious diseases due to Escherichia coli (E. coli)

> ● **Z20.09** Contact with and (suspected) exposure to other intestinal infectious diseases

● **Z20.1** Contact with and (suspected) exposure to tuberculosis

● **Z20.2** Contact with and (suspected) exposure to infections with a predominantly sexual mode of transmission

● **Z20.3** Contact with and (suspected) exposure to rabies

● **Z20.4** Contact with and (suspected) exposure to rubella

Z20.5 Contact with and (suspected) exposure to viral hepatitis

Z20.6 Contact with and (suspected) exposure to human immunodeficiency virus [HIV]

> **Excludes1** asymptomatic human immunodeficiency virus [HIV]
> HIV infection status (Z21)

● **Z20.7** Contact with and (suspected) exposure to pediculosis, acariasis and other infestations

● **Z20.8** Contact with and (suspected) exposure to other communicable diseases

> ● **Z20.81** Contact with and (suspected) exposure to other bacterial communicable diseases

>> ● **Z20.810** Contact with and (suspected) exposure to anthrax

>> **Z20.811** Contact with and (suspected) exposure to meningococcus

>> ● **Z20.818** Contact with and (suspected) exposure to other bacterial communicable diseases

> ● **Z20.82** Contact with and (suspected) exposure to other viral communicable diseases

>> **Z20.820** Contact with and (suspected) exposure to varicella

>> ● **Z20.821** Contact with and (suspected) exposure to Zika virus

>> ● **Z20.822** Contact with and (suspected) exposure to COVID-19
>> Contact with and (suspected) exposure to SARS-CoV-2
>> Coding Clinic: 2021, Q1, P37-39, 42

>> **Z20.828** Contact with and (suspected) exposure to other viral communicable diseases
>> Coding Clinic: 2021, Q1, P37-39; 2016, Q4, P6-7, 121

> ● **Z20.89** Contact with and (suspected) exposure to other communicable diseases

● **Z20.9** Contact with and (suspected) exposure to unspecified communicable disease

● **Z21** **Asymptomatic human immunodeficiency virus [HIV] infection status** ⊛

> HIV positive NOS

> *Code first* Human immunodeficiency virus [HIV] disease complicating pregnancy, childbirth and the puerperium, if applicable (O98.7-)

> **Excludes1** acquired immunodeficiency syndrome (B20)
> contact with human immunodeficiency virus [HIV] (Z20.6)
> exposure to human immunodeficiency virus [HIV] (Z20.6)
> human immunodeficiency virus [HIV] disease (B20)
> inconclusive laboratory evidence of human immunodeficiency virus [HIV] (R75)

> MCE: Questionable admission when principal dx
> Coding Clinic: 2019, Q1, P10-11

● **Z22** **Carrier of infectious disease**

> **Includes** colonization status
> suspected carrier

> **Excludes2** carrier of viral hepatitis (B18.-)

● **Z22.0** Carrier of typhoid

● **Z22.1** Carrier of other intestinal infectious diseases

● **Z22.2** Carrier of diphtheria

● **Z22.3** Carrier of other specified bacterial diseases

> ● **Z22.31** Carrier of bacterial disease due to meningococci

> ● **Z22.32** Carrier of bacterial disease due to staphylococci

>> ● **Z22.321** Carrier or suspected carrier of Methicillin susceptible Staphylococcus aureus
>> MSSA colonization

>> ● **Z22.322** Carrier or suspected carrier of Methicillin resistant Staphylococcus aureus
>> MRSA colonization

> ● **Z22.33** Carrier of bacterial disease due to streptococci

>> ● **Z22.330** Carrier of Group B streptococcus

>>> **Excludes1** Carrier of streptococcus group B (GBS) complicating pregnancy, childbirth and the puerperium (O99.82-)

>> ● **Z22.338** Carrier of other streptococcus

> ● **Z22.39** Carrier of other specified bacterial diseases

● **Z22.4** Carrier of infections with a predominantly sexual mode of transmission

● **Z22.6** Carrier of human T-lymphotropic virus type-1 [HTLV-1] infection

● **Z22.7** Latent tuberculosis
> Latent tuberculosis infection (LTBI)

> **Excludes1** nonspecific reaction to cell mediated immunity measurement of gamma interferon antigen response without active tuberculosis (R76.12)
> nonspecific reaction to tuberculin skin test without active tuberculosis (R76.11)

● **Z22.8** Carrier of other infectious diseases

● **Z22.9** Carrier of infectious disease, unspecified

● **Z23** **Encounter for immunization**

> *Code first* any routine childhood examination

> **Note:** Procedure codes are required to identify the types of immunizations given.

> ▶ Code also, if applicable, encounter for immunization safety counseling (Z71.85)

● **Z28   Immunization not carried out and underimmunization status**

> **Includes**   vaccination not carried out

▶ Code also, if applicable, encounter for immunization safety counseling (Z71.85)

● **Z28.0   Immunization not carried out because of contraindication**

● **Z28.01   Immunization not carried out because of acute illness of patient**

● **Z28.02   Immunization not carried out because of chronic illness or condition of patient**

● **Z28.03   Immunization not carried out because of immune compromised state of patient**

● **Z28.04   Immunization not carried out because of patient allergy to vaccine or component**

● **Z28.09   Immunization not carried out because of other contraindication**

● **Z28.1   Immunization not carried out because of patient decision for reasons of belief or group pressure**

Immunization not carried out because of religious belief

● **Z28.2   Immunization not carried out because of patient decision for other and unspecified reason**

● **Z28.20   Immunization not carried out because of patient decision for unspecified reason**

● **Z28.21   Immunization not carried out because of patient refusal**

● **Z28.29   Immunization not carried out because of patient decision for other reason**

● **Z28.3   Underimmunization status**

Delinquent immunization status
Lapsed immunization schedule status

● **Z28.8   Immunization not carried out for other reason**

● **Z28.81   Immunization not carried out due to patient having had the disease**

● **Z28.82   Immunization not carried out because of caregiver refusal**

Immunization not carried out because of guardian refusal
Immunization not carried out because of parent refusal

> **Excludes1**   immunization not carried out because of caregiver refusal because of religious belief (Z28.1)

● **Z28.83   Immunization not carried out due to unavailability of vaccine**

Delay in delivery of vaccine
Lack of availability of vaccine
Manufacturer delay of vaccine

● **Z28.89   Immunization not carried out for other reason**

● **Z28.9   Immunization not carried out for unspecified reason**

● **Z29   Encounter for other prophylactic measures**

> **Excludes1**   desensitization to allergens (Z51.6)
> prophylactic surgery (Z40.-)

Coding Clinic: 2016, Q4, P130

● **Z29.1   Encounter for prophylactic immunotherapy**

Encounter for administration of immunoglobulin

Coding Clinic: 2016, Q4, P78-79

● **Z29.11   Encounter for prophylactic immunotherapy for respiratory syncytial virus (RSV)**

● **Z29.12   Encounter for prophylactic antivenin**

● **Z29.13   Encounter for prophylactic Rho(D) immune globulin**

Coding Clinic: 2019, Q3, P5

● **Z29.14   Encounter for prophylactic rabies immune globin**

● **Z29.3   Encounter for prophylactic fluoride administration**

Coding Clinic: 2016, Q4, P79

● **Z29.8   Encounter for other specified prophylactic measures**

Coding Clinic: 2016, Q4, P79

● **Z29.9   Encounter for prophylactic measures, unspecified**

Coding Clinic: 2016, Q4, P79

PERSONS ENCOUNTERING HEALTH SERVICES IN CIRCUMSTANCES RELATED TO REPRODUCTION (Z30-Z39)

● **Z30   Encounter for contraceptive management**

● **Z30.0   Encounter for general counseling and advice on contraception**

● **Z30.01   Encounter for initial prescription of contraceptives**

> **Excludes1**   encounter for surveillance of contraceptives (Z30.4-)

● **Z30.011   Encounter for initial prescription of contraceptive pills ♀**

● **Z30.012   Encounter for prescription of emergency contraception ♀**

Encounter for postcoital contraception

● **Z30.013   Encounter for initial prescription of injectable contraceptive ♀**

● **Z30.014   Encounter for initial prescription of intrauterine contraceptive device ♀**

> **Excludes1**   encounter for insertion of intrauterine contraceptive device (Z30.430, Z30.432)

● **Z30.015   Encounter for initial prescription of vaginal ring hormonal contraceptive ♀**

Coding Clinic: 2016, Q4, P78

● **Z30.016   Encounter for initial prescription of transdermal patch hormonal contraceptive device**

Coding Clinic: 2016, Q4, P78

● **Z30.017   Encounter for initial prescription of implantable subdermal contraceptive**

Coding Clinic: 2016, Q4, P78

● **Z30.018   Encounter for initial prescription of other contraceptives ♀**

Encounter for initial prescription of barrier contraception
Encounter for initial prescription of diaphragm

● **Z30.019   Encounter for initial prescription of contraceptives, unspecified ♀**

● **Z30.02   Counseling and instruction in natural family planning to avoid pregnancy**

● **Z30.09   Encounter for other general counseling and advice on contraception**

Encounter for family planning advice NOS

● **Z30.2   Encounter for sterilization**

● **Z30.4   Encounter for surveillance of contraceptives**

● **Z30.40   Encounter for surveillance of contraceptives, unspecified**

● **Z30.41   Encounter for surveillance of contraceptive pills ♀**

Encounter for repeat prescription for contraceptive pill

● **Z30.42   Encounter for surveillance of injectable contraceptive ♀**

● **Z30.43   Encounter for surveillance of intrauterine contraceptive device**

● **Z30.430   Encounter for insertion of intrauterine contraceptive device ♀**

● **Z30.431   Encounter for routine checking of intrauterine contraceptive device ♀**

● **Z30.432   Encounter for removal of intrauterine contraceptive device ♀**

● **Z30.433   Encounter for removal and reinsertion of intrauterine contraceptive device ♀**

Encounter for replacement of intrauterine contraceptive device

● **Z30.44   Encounter for surveillance of vaginal ring hormonal contraceptive device ♀**

Coding Clinic: 2016, Q4, P78

N Newborn Age: 0   **P** Pediatric Age: 0–17   **M** Maternity DX: 9–64   **A** Adult Age: 15–124   ♀ Females Only   ♂ Males Only

🔖 Complication\Comorbidity   🔖 Major C\C   (Ex) CC/MCC Exclusions   🔖 Hospital-Acquired Condition   🔖 Hierarchical Condition Category

Z30.45 **Encounter for surveillance of** transdermal patch **hormonal contraceptive device** ♀
Coding Clinic: 2016, Q4, P78

Z30.46 **Encounter for surveillance of** implantable subdermal contraceptive ♀
Encounter for checking, reinsertion or removal of implantable subdermal contraceptive
Coding Clinic: 2016, Q4, P78

Z30.49 **Encounter for surveillance of** other contraceptives ♀
Encounter for surveillance of barrier contraception
Encounter for surveillance of diaphragm

Z30.8 **Encounter for** other contraceptive management
Encounter for postvasectomy sperm count
Encounter for routine examination for contraceptive maintenance
Excludes1 sperm count following sterilization reversal (Z31.42)
sperm count for fertility testing (Z31.41)

Z30.9 **Encounter for contraceptive management,** unspecified

Z31 **Encounter for procreative management**
~~Excludes1 complications associated with artificial fertilization (N98.-)~~
~~female infertility (N97.-)~~
~~male infertility (N46.-)~~

▶**Excludes2** complications associated with artificial fertilization (N98.-)
female infertility (N97.-)
male infertility (N46.-)

Z31.0 **Encounter for** reversal of previous sterilization

Z31.4 **Encounter for procreative** investigation and testing
Excludes1 postvasectomy sperm count (Z30.8)

Z31.41 **Encounter for** fertility testing
Encounter for fallopian tube patency testing
Encounter for sperm count for fertility testing

Z31.42 Aftercare following sterilization reversal
Sperm count following sterilization reversal

Z31.43 **Encounter for** genetic testing of female **for procreative management**
Use additional code for recurrent pregnancy loss, if applicable (N96, O26.2-)
Excludes1 nonprocreative genetic testing (Z13.7-)

Z31.430 **Encounter of female for testing for genetic disease carrier status for procreative management** ♀

Z31.438 **Encounter for** other genetic testing of female for procreative management ♀

Z31.44 **Encounter for** genetic testing of male **for procreative management**
Excludes1 nonprocreative genetic testing (Z13.7-)

Z31.440 **Encounter of male for testing for genetic disease carrier status for procreative management** ♂

Z31.441 **Encounter for testing of male partner of patient with** recurrent pregnancy loss ♂   A

Z31.448 **Encounter for** other genetic testing of male for procreative management ♂   A

Z31.49 **Encounter for** other procreative investigation and testing

Z31.5 **Encounter for procreative genetic counseling**

Z31.6 **Encounter for general counseling and advice on procreation**

Z31.61 **Procreative counseling and advice using** natural family planning

Z31.62 **Encounter for** fertility preservation counseling
Encounter for fertility preservation counseling prior to cancer therapy
Encounter for fertility preservation counseling prior to surgical removal of gonads

Z31.69 **Encounter for** other general counseling and advice on procreation

Z31.7 **Encounter for procreative management and counseling for gestational carrier** ♀
Excludes1 pregnant state, gestational carrier (Z33.3)
Coding Clinic: 2016, Q4, P78

Z31.8 **Encounter for other procreative management**

Z31.81 **Encounter for** male factor **infertility in female patient** ♀

Z31.82 **Encounter for Rh incompatibility status** ♀
Coding Clinic: 2015, Q3, P40

Z31.83 **Encounter for** assisted reproductive fertility procedure cycle ♀
Patient undergoing in vitro fertilization cycle
Use additional code to identify the type of infertility
Excludes1 pre-cycle diagnosis and testing - code to reason for encounter

Z31.84 **Encounter for** fertility preservation procedure
Encounter for fertility preservation procedure prior to cancer therapy
Encounter for fertility preservation procedure prior to surgical removal of gonads

Z31.89 **Encounter for** other procreative management

Z31.9 **Encounter for procreative management,** unspecified

Z32 **Encounter for pregnancy test and childbirth and childcare instruction**

Z32.0 **Encounter for** pregnancy test

Z32.00 **Encounter for pregnancy test,** result unknown ♀
Encounter for pregnancy test NOS

Z32.01 **Encounter for pregnancy test, result** positive ♀ M

Z32.02 **Encounter for pregnancy test, result** negative ♀

Z32.2 **Encounter for** childbirth instruction

Z32.3 **Encounter for** childcare instruction
Encounter for prenatal or postpartum childcare instruction

Z33 **Pregnant state**

Z33.1 **Pregnant state,** incidental ♀   M
Pregnancy NOS
Pregnant state NOS
Excludes1 complications of pregnancy (O00-O9A)
pregnant state, gestational carrier (Z33.3)

Z33.2 **Encounter for** elective termination of pregnancy ♀   M
Excludes1 early fetal death with retention of dead fetus (O02.1)
late fetal death (O36.4)
spontaneous abortion (O03)
Coding Clinic: 2016, Q4, P130

Z33.3 **Pregnant state, gestational carrier** ♀
Excludes1 encounter for procreative management and counseling for gestational carrier (Z31.7)
Coding Clinic: 2016, Q4, P78

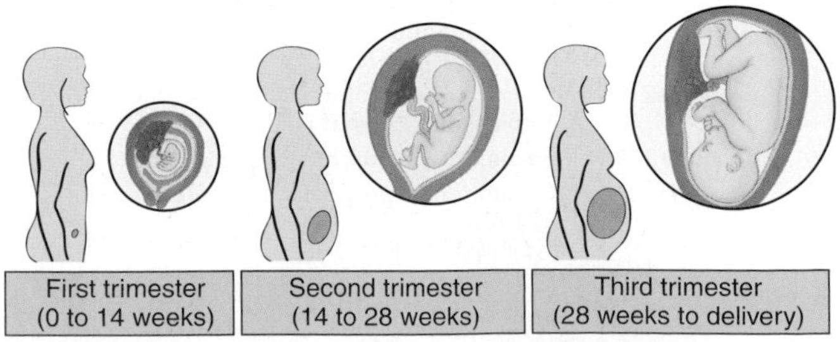

Figure 21-1 Trimesters. (From Shiland, Betsy J. Medical Terminology & Anatomy for ICD-10 Coding, ed 2, Mosby, 2015)

| First trimester (0 to 14 weeks) | Second trimester (14 to 28 weeks) | Third trimester (28 weeks to delivery) |

▶ New   ⮞ Revised   ~~deleted~~ Deleted   Excludes 1   Excludes 2   Includes   Use additional   Code first   Code also   Key words

OGCR Official Guidelines   ● Unacceptable Principal Diagnosis   X Assign placeholder X   ● Use Additional Character(s)   ▶ Manifestation Code   Coding Clinic

● Z34   Encounter for supervision of normal pregnancy

       Excludes1   any complication of pregnancy (O00-O9A)
                      encounter for pregnancy test (Z32.0-)
                      encounter for supervision of high risk pregnancy (O09.-)

       Coding Clinic: 2016, Q4, P6

  ● Z34.0 Encounter for supervision of normal first pregnancy

    ● Z34.00 Encounter for supervision of normal first pregnancy, unspecified trimester ♀   M

    ● Z34.01 Encounter for supervision of normal first pregnancy, first trimester ♀   M

    ● Z34.02 Encounter for supervision of normal first pregnancy, second trimester ♀   M

    ● Z34.03 Encounter for supervision of normal first pregnancy, third trimester ♀   M

  ● Z34.8 Encounter for supervision of other normal pregnancy

    ● Z34.80 Encounter for supervision of other normal pregnancy, unspecified trimester ♀   M

    ● Z34.81 Encounter for supervision of other normal pregnancy, first trimester ♀   M

    ● Z34.82 Encounter for supervision of other normal pregnancy, second trimester ♀   M

    ● Z34.83 Encounter for supervision of other normal pregnancy, third trimester ♀   M

  ● Z34.9 Encounter for supervision of normal pregnancy, unspecified

    ● Z34.90 Encounter for supervision of normal pregnancy, unspecified, unspecified trimester ♀   M

    ● Z34.91 Encounter for supervision of normal pregnancy, unspecified, first trimester ♀   M

    ● Z34.92 Encounter for supervision of normal pregnancy, unspecified, second trimester ♀   M

    ● Z34.93 Encounter for supervision of normal pregnancy, unspecified, third trimester ♀   M

● Z36   Encounter for antenatal screening of mother ♀

       Includes   Encounter for placental sample (taken vaginally)
                      Screening is the testing for disease or disease precursors in asymptomatic individuals so that early detection and treatment can be provided for those who test positive for the disease.

       Excludes1   diagnostic examination - code to sign or symptom
                      encounter for suspected maternal and fetal conditions ruled out (Z03.7-)
                      suspected fetal condition affecting management of pregnancy - code to condition in Chapter 15

       Excludes2   abnormal findings on antenatal screening of mother (O28.-)
                      genetic counseling and testing (Z31.43-, Z31.5)
                      routine prenatal care (Z34)

  Z36.0 Encounter for antenatal screening for chromosomal anomalies ♀   M

  Z36.1 Encounter for antenatal screening for raised alphafetoprotein level ♀   M
       Encounter for antenatal screening for elevated maternal serum alphafetoprotein level

  Z36.2 Encounter for other antenatal screening follow-up ♀   M
       Non-visualized anatomy on a previous scan

  Z36.3 Encounter for antenatal screening for malformations ♀ M
       Screening for a suspected anomaly

  Z36.4 Encounter for antenatal screening for fetal growth retardation ♀   M
       Intrauterine growth restriction (IUGR)/small-for-dates

  Z36.5 Encounter for antenatal screening for isoimmunization ♀   M

  ● Z36.8 Encounter for other antenatal screening

    Z36.81 Encounter for antenatal screening for hydrops fetalis ♀   M

    Z36.82 Encounter for antenatal screening for nuchal translucency ♀   M

    Z36.83 Encounter for fetal screening for congenital cardiac abnormalities ♀   M

    Z36.84 Encounter for antenatal screening for fetal lung maturity ♀   M

    Z36.85 Encounter for antenatal screening for Streptococcus B ♀   M

    Z36.86 Encounter for antenatal screening for cervical length ♀   M
          Screening for risk of pre-term labor

    Z36.87 Encounter for antenatal screening for uncertain dates ♀

    Z36.88 Encounter for antenatal screening for fetal macrosomia ♀   M
          Screening for large-for-dates

    Z36.89 Encounter for other specified antenatal screening ♀   M

    Z36.8A Encounter for antenatal screening for other genetic defects ♀   M

  Z36.9 Encounter for antenatal screening, unspecified ♀   M

● Z3A Weeks of gestation

    Note: Codes from category Z3A are for use, only on the maternal record, to indicate the weeks of gestation of the pregnancy, if known.

    ▶Code first ~~complications of pregnancy, childbirth and the puerperium (O09-O9A)~~ obstetric condition or encounter for delivery (O09-O60, O80-O82)

    Coding Clinic: 2016, Q4, P130; 2013, Q2, P33

  ● Z3A.0 Weeks of gestation of pregnancy, unspecified or less than 10 weeks

    ● Z3A.00 Weeks of gestation of pregnancy not specified ♀   M

    ● Z3A.01 Less than 8 weeks gestation of pregnancy ♀   M

    ● Z3A.08 8 weeks gestation of pregnancy ♀   M

    ● Z3A.09 9 weeks gestation of pregnancy ♀   M

  ● Z3A.1 Weeks of gestation of pregnancy, weeks 10-19

    ● Z3A.10 10 weeks gestation of pregnancy ♀   M

    ● Z3A.11 11 weeks gestation of pregnancy ♀   M

    ● Z3A.12 12 weeks gestation of pregnancy ♀   M

    ● Z3A.13 13 weeks gestation of pregnancy ♀   M

    ● Z3A.14 14 weeks gestation of pregnancy ♀   M

    ● Z3A.15 15 weeks gestation of pregnancy ♀   M

    ● Z3A.16 16 weeks gestation of pregnancy ♀   M
          Coding Clinic: 2016, Q4, P5

    ● Z3A.17 17 weeks gestation of pregnancy ♀   M

    ● Z3A.18 18 weeks gestation of pregnancy ♀   M
          Coding Clinic: 2019, Q2, P11

    ● Z3A.19 19 weeks gestation of pregnancy ♀   M

  ● Z3A.2 Weeks of gestation of pregnancy, weeks 20-29

    ● Z3A.20 20 weeks gestation of pregnancy ♀   M
          Coding Clinic: 2016, Q4, P6

    ● Z3A.21 21 weeks gestation of pregnancy ♀   M

    ● Z3A.22 22 weeks gestation of pregnancy ♀   M
          Coding Clinic: 2016, Q4, P6

    ● Z3A.23 23 weeks gestation of pregnancy ♀   M

    ● Z3A.24 24 weeks gestation of pregnancy ♀   M

    ● Z3A.25 25 weeks gestation of pregnancy ♀   M

    ● Z3A.26 26 weeks gestation of pregnancy ♀   M

    ● Z3A.27 27 weeks gestation of pregnancy ♀   M

    ● Z3A.28 28 weeks gestation of pregnancy ♀   M

CHAPTER 21 (Z00-Z99)

N Newborn Age: 0   **P** Pediatric Age: 0–17   **M** Maternity DX: 9–64   **A** Adult Age: 15–124   ♀ Females Only   ♂ Males Only

Complication\Comorbidity   Major C\C   (Ex) CC/MCC Exclusions   Hospital-Acquired Condition   Hierarchical Condition Category

1631

● Z3A.29 29 weeks gestation of pregnancy ♀   M
● Z3A.3 Weeks of gestation of pregnancy, weeks 30-39
  ● Z3A.30 30 weeks gestation of pregnancy ♀   M
  ● Z3A.31 31 weeks gestation of pregnancy ♀   M
  ● Z3A.32 32 weeks gestation of pregnancy ♀   M
            Coding Clinic: 2016, Q4, P6
  ● Z3A.33 33 weeks gestation of pregnancy ♀   M
  ● Z3A.34 34 weeks gestation of pregnancy ♀   M
  ● Z3A.35 35 weeks gestation of pregnancy ♀   M
  ● Z3A.36 36 weeks gestation of pregnancy ♀   M
  ● Z3A.37 37 weeks gestation of pregnancy ♀   M
  ● Z3A.38 38 weeks gestation of pregnancy ♀   M
            Coding Clinic: 2016, Q2, P34
  ● Z3A.39 39 weeks gestation of pregnancy ♀   M
● Z3A.4 Weeks of gestation of pregnancy, weeks 40 or greater
  ● Z3A.40 40 weeks gestation of pregnancy ♀   M
  ● Z3A.41 41 weeks gestation of pregnancy ♀   M
  ● Z3A.42 42 weeks gestation of pregnancy ♀   M
  ● Z3A.49 Greater than 42 weeks gestation of
            pregnancy ♀   M

● Z37 Outcome of delivery
       This category is intended for use as an additional code to
          identify the outcome of delivery on the mother's record. It
          is not for use on the newborn record.
       Excludes1 stillbirth (P95)
● Z37.0 Single live birth ♀   M
         Coding Clinic: 2016, Q2, P34
● Z37.1 Single stillbirth ♀   M
● Z37.2 Twins, both liveborn ♀   M
● Z37.3 Twins, one liveborn and one stillborn ♀   M
● Z37.4 Twins, both stillborn ♀   M
● Z37.5 Other multiple births, all liveborn
  ● Z37.50 Multiple births, unspecified, all liveborn ♀   M
  ● Z37.51 Triplets, all liveborn ♀   M
  ● Z37.52 Quadruplets, all liveborn ♀   M
  ● Z37.53 Quintuplets, all liveborn ♀   M
  ● Z37.54 Sextuplets, all liveborn ♀   M
  ● Z37.59 Other multiple births, all liveborn ♀   M
● Z37.6 Other multiple births, some liveborn
  ● Z37.60 Multiple births, unspecified, some liveborn ♀ M
  ● Z37.61 Triplets, some liveborn ♀   M
  ● Z37.62 Quadruplets, some liveborn ♀   M
  ● Z37.63 Quintuplets, some liveborn ♀   M
  ● Z37.64 Sextuplets, some liveborn ♀   M
  ● Z37.69 Other multiple births, some liveborn ♀   M
● Z37.7 Other multiple births, all stillborn ♀   M
● Z37.9 Outcome of delivery, unspecified ♀   M
         Multiple birth NOS
         Single birth NOS

● Z38 Liveborn infants according to place of birth and type of delivery
       This category is for use as the principal code on the initial record
          of a newborn baby. It is to be used for the initial birth
          record only. It is not to be used on the mother's record.
       Coding Clinic: 2017, Q2, P6-7; 2016, Q4, P126-127, 130; 2015, Q2, P15
● Z38.0 Single liveborn infant, born in hospital
         Single liveborn infant, born in birthing center or other
            health care facility
         Coding Clinic: 2017, Q2, P5-7
  ● Z38.00 Single liveborn infant, delivered vaginally   N
            Coding Clinic: 2018, Q4, P26; 2016, Q4, P7, 55
  ● Z38.01 Single liveborn infant, delivered by cesarean   N
            Coding Clinic: 2017, Q2, P7; 2016, Q3, P18
  Z38.1 Single liveborn infant, born outside hospital   N
  Z38.2 Single liveborn infant, unspecified as to place of birth   N
         Single liveborn infant NOS

● Z38.3 Twin liveborn infant, born in hospital
  Z38.30 Twin liveborn infant, delivered vaginally   N
  Z38.31 Twin liveborn infant, delivered by cesarean   N
  Z38.4 Twin liveborn infant, born outside hospital   N
  Z38.5 Twin liveborn infant, unspecified as to place of birth   N
● Z38.6 Other multiple liveborn infant, born in hospital
  Z38.61 Triplet liveborn infant, delivered vaginally   N
  Z38.62 Triplet liveborn infant, delivered by cesarean   N
  Z38.63 Quadruplet liveborn infant, delivered
          vaginally   N
  Z38.64 Quadruplet liveborn infant, delivered by
          cesarean   N
  Z38.65 Quintuplet liveborn infant, delivered
          vaginally   N
  Z38.66 Quintuplet liveborn infant, delivered by
          cesarean   N
  Z38.68 Other multiple liveborn infant, delivered
          vaginally   N
  Z38.69 Other multiple liveborn infant, delivered by
          cesarean   N
  Z38.7 Other multiple liveborn infant, born outside hospital   N
  Z38.8 Other multiple liveborn infant, unspecified as to place
         of birth   N

● Z39 Encounter for maternal postpartum care and examination
  Z39.0 Encounter for care and examination of mother
         immediately after delivery ♀   M
         Care and observation in uncomplicated cases when the
            delivery occurs outside a healthcare facility
         Excludes1 care for postpartum complication - see
                    Alphabetic index
● Z39.1 Encounter for care and examination of lactating
         mother ♀   M
         Encounter for supervision of lactation
         Excludes1 disorders of lactation (O92.-)
● Z39.2 Encounter for routine postpartum follow-up ♀   M

ENCOUNTERS FOR OTHER SPECIFIC HEALTH CARE (Z40-Z53)

Categories Z40-Z53 are intended for use to indicate a reason
for care. They may be used for patients who have already been
treated for a disease or injury, but who are receiving aftercare or
prophylactic care, or care to consolidate the treatment, or to deal
with a residual state

Excludes2 follow-up examination for medical surveillance
           after treatment (Z08-Z09)

● Z40 Encounter for prophylactic surgery
       Excludes1 organ donations (Z52.-)
                  therapeutic organ removal - code to condition
       Coding Clinic: 2016, Q4, P79
● Z40.0 Encounter for prophylactic surgery for risk factors
         related to malignant neoplasms
         Admission for prophylactic organ removal
         Use additional code to identify risk factor
  Z40.00 Encounter for prophylactic removal of
          unspecified organ
  Z40.01 Encounter for prophylactic removal of breast
  Z40.02 Encounter for prophylactic removal of
          ovary(s) ♀
          Encounter for prophylactic removal of ovary(s)
             and fallopian tube(s)
  Z40.03 Encounter for prophylactic removal of fallopian
          tube(s) ♀
  Z40.09 Encounter for prophylactic removal of other
          organ
● Z40.8 Encounter for other prophylactic surgery
● Z40.9 Encounter for prophylactic surgery, unspecified

▶ New   ⇒ Revised   ~~deleted~~ Deleted   Excludes 1   Excludes 2   Includes   Use additional   Code first   Code also   Key words
OGCR Official Guidelines   ● Unacceptable Principal Diagnosis   X Assign placeholder X   ● Use Additional Character(s)   ▶ Manifestation Code   Coding Clinic

● **Z41**   **Encounter for procedures for purposes other than remedying health state**

    Z41.1   Encounter for cosmetic surgery

        Encounter for cosmetic breast implant

        Encounter for cosmetic procedure

        Excludes 1   encounter for plastic and reconstructive surgery following medical procedure or healed injury (Z42.-)

                 encounter for post-mastectomy breast implantation (Z42.1)

    Z41.2   Encounter for routine and ritual male circumcision ♂

●   **Z41.3**   Encounter for ear piercing

    Z41.8   Encounter for other procedures for purposes other than remedying health state

●   **Z41.9**   Encounter for procedure for purposes other than remedying health state, unspecified

● **Z42**   **Encounter for plastic and reconstructive surgery following medical procedure or healed injury**

    Excludes 1   encounter for cosmetic plastic surgery (Z41.1)

            encounter for plastic surgery for treatment of current injury - code to relevent injury

    Z42.1   Encounter for breast reconstruction following mastectomy   **A**

        Excludes 1   deformity and disproportion of reconstructed breast (N65.1-)

    Z42.8   Encounter for other plastic and reconstructive surgery following medical procedure or healed injury

        Coding Clinic: 2017, Q1, P42

● **Z43**   **Encounter for attention to artificial openings**

    Includes   closure of artificial openings

          passage of sounds or bougies through artificial openings

          reforming artificial openings

          removal of catheter from artificial openings

          toilet or cleansing of artificial openings

    Excludes 1   complications of external stoma (J95.0-, K94.-, N99.5-)

    Excludes 2   fitting and adjustment of prosthetic and other devices (Z44-Z46)

    Z43.0   Encounter for attention to tracheostomy 🅒

    Z43.1   Encounter for attention to gastrostomy 🅒 🅜

        Excludes 2   artificial opening status only, without need for care (Z93.-)

        (Ex:) See PDX Collection 1487

    Z43.2   Encounter for attention to ileostomy 🅒

        Coding Clinic: 2016, Q3, P5

    Z43.3   Encounter for attention to colostomy 🅒

    Z43.4   Encounter for attention to other artificial openings of digestive tract 🅒

    Z43.5   Encounter for attention to cystostomy 🅒

    Z43.6   Encounter for attention to other artificial openings of urinary tract 🅒

        Encounter for attention to nephrostomy

        Encounter for attention to ureterostomy

        Encounter for attention to urethrostomy

    Z43.7   Encounter for attention to artificial vagina

    Z43.8   Encounter for attention to other artificial openings 🅒

●   **Z43.9**   Encounter for attention to unspecified artificial opening 🅒

● **Z44**   **Encounter for fitting and adjustment of external prosthetic device**

    Includes   removal or replacement of external prosthetic device

    Excludes 1   malfunction or other complications of device - see Alphabetical Index presence of prosthetic device (Z97.-)

●   **Z44.0**   Encounter for fitting and adjustment of artificial arm

●   **Z44.00**   Encounter for fitting and adjustment of unspecified artificial arm

        Z44.001   Encounter for fitting and adjustment of unspecified right artificial arm

        Z44.002   Encounter for fitting and adjustment of unspecified left artificial arm

        Z44.009   Encounter for fitting and adjustment of unspecified artificial arm, unspecified arm

●   **Z44.01**   Encounter for fitting and adjustment of complete artificial arm

        Z44.011   Encounter for fitting and adjustment of complete right artificial arm

        Z44.012   Encounter for fitting and adjustment of complete left artificial arm

        Z44.019   Encounter for fitting and adjustment of complete artificial arm, unspecified arm

●   **Z44.02**   Encounter for fitting and adjustment of partial artificial arm

        Z44.021   Encounter for fitting and adjustment of partial artificial right arm

        Z44.022   Encounter for fitting and adjustment of partial artificial left arm

        Z44.029   Encounter for fitting and adjustment of partial artificial arm, unspecified arm

●   **Z44.1**   Encounter for fitting and adjustment of artificial leg

●   **Z44.10**   Encounter for fitting and adjustment of unspecified artificial leg

        Z44.101   Encounter for fitting and adjustment of unspecified right artificial leg 🅒

        Z44.102   Encounter for fitting and adjustment of unspecified left artificial leg 🅒

        Z44.109   Encounter for fitting and adjustment of unspecified artificial leg, unspecified leg 🅒

●   **Z44.11**   Encounter for fitting and adjustment of complete artificial leg

        Z44.111   Encounter for fitting and adjustment of complete right artificial leg 🅒

        Z44.112   Encounter for fitting and adjustment of complete left artificial leg 🅒

        Z44.119   Encounter for fitting and adjustment of complete artificial leg, unspecified leg 🅒

●   **Z44.12**   Encounter for fitting and adjustment of partial artificial leg

        Z44.121   Encounter for fitting and adjustment of partial artificial right leg 🅒

        Z44.122   Encounter for fitting and adjustment of partial artificial left leg 🅒

        Z44.129   Encounter for fitting and adjustment of partial artificial leg, unspecified leg 🅒

●   **Z44.2**   Encounter for fitting and adjustment of artificial eye

        Excludes 1   mechanical complication of ocular prosthesis (T85.3)

    Z44.20   Encounter for fitting and adjustment of artificial eye, unspecified

    Z44.21   Encounter for fitting and adjustment of artificial right eye

    Z44.22   Encounter for fitting and adjustment of artificial left eye

●   **Z44.3**   Encounter for fitting and adjustment of external breast prosthesis

        Excludes 1   complications of breast implant (T85.4-)

                 encounter for adjustment or removal of breast implant (Z45.81-)

                 encounter for initial breast implant insertion for cosmetic breast augmentation (Z41.1)

                 encounter for breast reconstruction following mastectomy (Z42.1)

    Z44.30   Encounter for fitting and adjustment of external breast prosthesis, unspecified breast

    Z44.31   Encounter for fitting and adjustment of external right breast prosthesis

    Z44.32   Encounter for fitting and adjustment of external left breast prosthesis

N Newborn Age: 0   **P** Pediatric Age: 0–17   **M** Maternity DX: 9–64   **A** Adult Age: 15–124   ♀ Females Only   ♂ Males Only

🅒 Complication\Comorbidity   🅜 Major C\C   (Ex:) CC/MCC Exclusions   🅗 Hospital-Acquired Condition   🅒 Hierarchical Condition Category

1633

CHAPTER 21 (Z00-Z99)

Z44.8   Encounter for fitting and adjustment of other external prosthetic devices

● Z44.9   Encounter for fitting and adjustment of unspecified external prosthetic device

● **Z45**   **Encounter for adjustment and management of implanted device**

     Includes   removal or replacement of implanted device

     Excludes1   malfunction or other complications of device - see Alphabetical Index

     Excludes2   encounter for fitting and adjustment of non-implanted device (Z46.-)

● Z45.0   Encounter for adjustment and management of cardiac device

     ● Z45.01   Encounter for adjustment and management of cardiac pacemaker

         Encounter for adjustment and management of cardiac resynchronization therapy pacemaker (CRT-P)

         Excludes1   encounter for adjustment and management of automatic implantable cardiac defibrillator with synchronous cardiac pacemaker (Z45.02)

         Z45.010   **Encounter for checking and testing of cardiac pacemaker pulse generator [battery]**

             Encounter for replacing cardiac pacemaker pulse generator [battery]

             MCE: Questionable admission when principal dx

         Z45.018   **Encounter for adjustment and management of other part of cardiac pacemaker**

             Excludes1   presence of other part of cardiac pacemaker (Z95.0)

             Excludes2   presence of prosthetic and other devices (Z95.1-Z95.5, Z95.811-Z97)

             MCE: Questionable admission when principal dx

     Z45.02   **Encounter for adjustment and management of automatic implantable cardiac defibrillator**

         Encounter for adjustment and management of automatic implantable cardiac defibrillator with synchronous cardiac pacemaker

         Encounter for adjustment and management of cardiac resynchronization therapy defibrillator (CRT-D)

         MCE: Questionable admission when principal dx

     Z45.09   **Encounter for adjustment and management of other cardiac device**

         MCE: Questionable admission when principal dx

Z45.1   Encounter for adjustment and management of infusion pump

Z45.2   Encounter for adjustment and management of vascular access device

     Encounter for adjustment and management of vascular catheters

     Excludes1   encounter for adjustment and management of renal dialysis catheter (Z49.01)

● Z45.3   Encounter for adjustment and management of implanted devices of the special senses

     Z45.31   **Encounter for adjustment and management of implanted visual substitution device**

     ● Z45.32   **Encounter for adjustment and management of implanted hearing device**

         Excludes1   encounter for fitting and adjustment of hearing aide (Z46.1)

Z45.320   **Encounter for adjustment and management of bone conduction device**

Z45.321   **Encounter for adjustment and management of cochlear device**

Z45.328   **Encounter for adjustment and management of other implanted hearing device**

● Z45.4   Encounter for adjustment and management of implanted nervous system device

     Z45.41   **Encounter for adjustment and management of cerebrospinal fluid drainage device**

         Encounter for adjustment and management of cerebral ventricular (communicating) shunt

     Z45.42   **Encounter for adjustment and management of neuropacemaker**

         Encounter for adjustment and management of brain neurostimulator

         Encounter for adjustment and management of gastric neurostimulator

         Encounter for adjustment and management of peripheral nerve neurostimulator

         Encounter for adjustment and management of sacral nerve neurostimulator

         Encounter for adjustment and management of spinal cord neurostimulator

         Encounter for adjustment and management of vagus nerve neurostimulator

     Z45.49   **Encounter for adjustment and management of other implanted nervous system device**

● Z45.8   Encounter for adjustment and management of other implanted devices

     ● Z45.81   **Encounter for adjustment or removal of breast implant**

         Encounter for elective implant exchange (different material) (different size)

         ⇒ Encounter for removal of tissue expander with or without synchronous insertion of permanent implant

         Excludes1   complications of breast implant (T85.4-)

             encounter for initial breast implant insertion for cosmetic breast augmentation (Z41.1)

             encounter for breast reconstruction following mastectomy (Z42.1)

         Z45.811   **Encounter for adjustment or removal of right breast implant**

         Z45.812   **Encounter for adjustment or removal of left breast implant**

         Z45.819   **Encounter for adjustment or removal of unspecified breast implant**

     ● Z45.82   **Encounter for adjustment or removal of myringotomy device (stent) (tube)**

     ● Z45.89   **Encounter for adjustment and management of other implanted devices**

● Z45.9   Encounter for adjustment and management of unspecified implanted device

● **Z46**   **Encounter for fitting and adjustment of other devices**

     Includes   removal or replacement of other device

     Excludes1   malfunction or other complications of device - see Alphabetical Index

     Excludes2   encounter for fitting and management of implanted devices (Z45.-)

     issue of repeat prescription only (Z76.0)

     presence of prosthetic and other devices (Z95-Z97)

▶ New   ⇒ Revised   ~~deleted~~ Deleted   Excludes 1   Excludes 2   Includes   Use additional   Code first   Code also   Key words

OGCR Official Guidelines   ● Unacceptable Principal Diagnosis   X Assign placeholder X   ● Use Additional Character(s)   ▶ Manifestation Code   **Coding Clinic**

● **Z46.0** **Encounter for fitting and adjustment of spectacles and contact lenses**

● **Z46.1** **Encounter for fitting and adjustment of hearing aid**
> **Excludes1** encounter for adjustment and management of implanted hearing device (Z45.32-)

Z46.2 **Encounter for fitting and adjustment of other devices related to nervous system and special senses**
> **Excludes2** encounter for adjustment and management of implanted nervous system device (Z45.4-)
> encounter for adjustment and management of implanted visual substitution device (Z45.31)

Z46.3 **Encounter for fitting and adjustment of dental prosthetic device**
> Encounter for fitting and adjustment of dentures

● **Z46.4** **Encounter for fitting and adjustment of orthodontic device**

● **Z46.5** **Encounter for fitting and adjustment of other gastrointestinal appliance and device**
> **Excludes1** encounter for attention to artificial openings of digestive tract (Z43.1-Z43.4)

　● **Z46.51** **Encounter for fitting and adjustment of gastric lap band**

　● **Z46.59** **Encounter for fitting and adjustment of other gastrointestinal appliance and device**

● **Z46.6** **Encounter for fitting and adjustment of urinary device**
> **Excludes2** attention to artificial openings of urinary tract (Z43.5, Z43.6)

● **Z46.8** **Encounter for fitting and adjustment of other specified devices**

　● **Z46.81** **Encounter for fitting and adjustment of insulin pump**
> Encounter for insulin pump instruction and training
> Encounter for insulin pump titration

　Z46.82 **Encounter for fitting and adjustment of non-vascular catheter**

　● **Z46.89** **Encounter for fitting and adjustment of other specified devices**
> Encounter for fitting and adjustment of wheelchair

● **Z46.9** **Encounter for fitting and adjustment of unspecified device**

● **Z47** **Orthopedic aftercare**
> **Excludes1** aftercare for healing fracture - code to fracture with 7th character D

Z47.1 **Aftercare following joint replacement surgery**
> Use additional code to identify the joint (Z96.6-)
> Coding Clinic: 2020, Q1, P23-24

Z47.2 **Encounter for removal of internal fixation device**
> **Excludes1** encounter for adjustment of internal fixation device for fracture treatment - code to fracture with appropriate 7th character
> encounter for removal of external fixation device - code to fracture with 7th character D
> infection or inflammatory reaction to internal fixation device (T84.6-)
> mechanical complication of internal fixation device (T84.1-)

● **Z47.3** **Aftercare following explantation of joint prosthesis**
> Aftercare following explantation of joint prosthesis, staged procedure
> Encounter for joint prosthesis insertion following prior explantation of joint prosthesis
> Coding Clinic: 2020, Q1, P23; 2015, Q1, P17

Z47.31 **Aftercare following explantation of shoulder joint prosthesis**
> **Excludes1** acquired absence of shoulder joint following prior explantation of shoulder joint prosthesis (Z89.23-)
> shoulder joint prosthesis explantation status (Z89.23-)

Z47.32 **Aftercare following explantation of hip joint prosthesis**
> **Excludes1** acquired absence of hip joint following prior explantation of hip joint prosthesis (Z89.62-)
> hip joint prosthesis explantation status (Z89.62-)
> Coding Clinic: 2015, Q1, P17

Z47.33 **Aftercare following explantation of knee joint prosthesis**
> **Excludes1** acquired absence of knee joint following prior explantation of knee prosthesis (Z89.52-)
> knee joint prosthesis explantation status (Z89.52-)

● **Z47.8** **Encounter for other orthopedic aftercare**

Z47.81 **Encounter for orthopedic aftercare following surgical amputation**
> Use additional code to identify the limb amputated (Z89.-)

Z47.82 **Encounter for orthopedic aftercare following scoliosis surgery**

Z47.89 **Encounter for other orthopedic aftercare**
> Coding Clinic: 2015, Q1, P8

● **Z48** **Encounter for other postprocedural aftercare**
> **Excludes1** encounter for aftercare following injury - code to Injury, by site, with appropriate 7th character for subsequent encounter
> encounter for follow-up examination after completed treatment (Z08-Z09)
> **Excludes2** encounter for attention to artificial openings (Z43.-)
> encounter for fitting and adjustment of prosthetic and other devices (Z44-Z46)

● **Z48.0** **Encounter for attention to dressings, sutures and drains**
> **Excludes1** encounter for planned postprocedural wound closure (Z48.1)

　● **Z48.00** **Encounter for change or removal of nonsurgical wound dressing**
> Encounter for change or removal of wound dressing NOS

　● **Z48.01** **Encounter for change or removal of surgical wound dressing**
> Coding Clinic: 2019, Q2, P33; 2015, Q4, P38

　● **Z48.02** **Encounter for removal of sutures**
> Encounter for removal of staples
> Coding Clinic: 2015, Q1, P6

　Z48.03 **Encounter for change or removal of drains**

Z48.1 **Encounter for planned postprocedural wound closure**
> **Excludes1** encounter for attention to dressings and sutures (Z48.0-)

● **Z48.2** **Encounter for aftercare following organ transplant**

Z48.21 **Encounter for aftercare following heart transplant** 🅒 🅒
> CC when PDx is its own CC
> (Ex) See PDX Collection 3287

Z48.22 **Encounter for aftercare following kidney transplant** 🅒
> CC when PDx is its own CC
> (Ex) See PDX Collection 3288

Z48.23 **Encounter for aftercare following liver transplant** 🅒 🅒
> CC when PDx is its own CC
> (Ex) See PDX Collection 3289

N Newborn Age: 0 　 **P** Pediatric Age: 0–17 　 **M** Maternity DX: 9–64 　 **A** Adult Age: 15–124 　 ♀ Females Only 　 ♂ Males Only

🅒 Complication\Comorbidity 　 🅒 Major C\C 　 (Ex) CC/MCC Exclusions 　 🅒 Hospital-Acquired Condition 　 🅒 Hierarchical Condition Category

1635

Z48.24 Encounter for aftercare following lung transplant 🏷️ 🏷️
  CC when PDx is its own CC
  (Ex) See PDX Collection 3290

● **Z48.28** Encounter for aftercare following multiple organ transplant

  Z48.280 Encounter for aftercare following heart-lung transplant 🏷️ 🏷️
    CC when PDx is its own CC
    (Ex) See PDX Collection 3285

  Z48.288 Encounter for aftercare following multiple organ transplant

● **Z48.29** Encounter for aftercare following other organ transplant

  Z48.290 Encounter for aftercare following bone marrow transplant 🏷️ 🏷️
    CC when PDx is its own CC
    (Ex) See PDX Collection 3286

  Z48.298 Encounter for aftercare following other organ transplant

Z48.3 Aftercare following surgery for neoplasm
  Use additional code to identify the neoplasm

● **Z48.8** Encounter for other specified postprocedural aftercare

● **Z48.81** Encounter for surgical aftercare following surgery on specified body systems
  These codes identify the body system requiring aftercare. They are for use in conjunction with other aftercare codes to fully explain the aftercare encounter. The condition treated should also be coded if still present.

  Excludes1 aftercare for injury - code the injury with 7th character D
  aftercare following surgery for neoplasm (Z48.3)

  Excludes2 aftercare following organ transplant (Z48.2-)
  orthopedic aftercare (Z47.-)

  Z48.810 Encounter for surgical aftercare following surgery on the sense organs

  Z48.811 Encounter for surgical aftercare following surgery on the nervous system

    Excludes2 encounter for surgical aftercare following surgery on the sense organs (Z48.810)

  Z48.812 Encounter for surgical aftercare following surgery on the circulatory system
    Coding Clinic: 2012, Q4, P96

  Z48.813 Encounter for surgical aftercare following surgery on the respiratory system
    Coding Clinic: 2019, Q2, P33

  Z48.814 Encounter for surgical aftercare following surgery on the teeth or oral cavity

  Z48.815 Encounter for surgical aftercare following surgery on the digestive system
    Coding Clinic: 2015, Q4, P38

  Z48.816 Encounter for surgical aftercare following surgery on the genitourinary system

    Excludes1 encounter for aftercare following sterilization reversal (Z31.42)

  Z48.817 Encounter for surgical aftercare following surgery on the skin and subcutaneous tissue
    Coding Clinic: 2015, Q1, P6

  Z48.89 Encounter for other specified surgical aftercare

● **Z49** Encounter for care involving renal dialysis
  Code also associated end stage renal disease (N18.6)

  ● **Z49.0** Preparatory care for renal dialysis
    Encounter for dialysis instruction and training

    ● **Z49.01** Encounter for fitting and adjustment of extracorporeal dialysis catheter 🏷️
      Removal or replacement of renal dialysis catheter
      Toilet or cleansing of renal dialysis catheter

    ● **Z49.02** Encounter for fitting and adjustment of peritoneal dialysis catheter 🏷️

  ● **Z49.3** Encounter for adequacy testing for dialysis

    ● **Z49.31** Encounter for adequacy testing for hemodialysis 🏷️

    ● **Z49.32** Encounter for adequacy testing for peritoneal dialysis 🏷️
      Encounter for peritoneal equilibration test

● **Z51** Encounter for other aftercare and medical care
  Code also condition requiring care

  Excludes1 follow-up examination after treatment (Z08-Z09)
  Coding Clinic: 2017, Q1, P49; 2016, Q4, P130

  Z51.0 Encounter for antineoplastic radiation therapy
    Coding Clinic: 2017, Q4, P103

  ● **Z51.1** Encounter for antineoplastic chemotherapy and immunotherapy

    Excludes2 encounter for chemotherapy and immunotherapy for nonneoplastic condition-code to condition

    Z51.11 Encounter for antineoplastic chemotherapy
      Coding Clinic: 2015, Q3, P19

    Z51.12 Encounter for antineoplastic immunotherapy

  Z51.5 Encounter for palliative care
    Coding Clinic: 2017, Q1, P48-49

  ● **Z51.6** Encounter for desensitization to allergens
    Coding Clinic: 2016, Q4, P77-79

  ● **Z51.8** Encounter for other specified aftercare

    Excludes1 holiday relief care (Z75.5)

    Z51.81 Encounter for therapeutic drug level monitoring
      Code also any long-term (current) drug therapy (Z79.-)

      Excludes1 encounter for blood-drug test for administrative or medicolegal reasons (Z02.83)

    ● **Z51.89** Encounter for other specified aftercare
      MCE: This code may be considered "acceptable" when a secondary diagnosis is also coded on the record.
      Coding Clinic: 2012, Q4, P96-97

● **Z52** Donors of organs and tissues

  Includes autologous and other living donors
  Excludes1 cadaveric donor - omit code
  examination of potential donor (Z00.5)
  Coding Clinic: 2012, Q4, P100

  ● **Z52.0** Blood donor

    ● **Z52.00** Unspecified blood donor
      ● **Z52.000** Unspecified donor, whole blood
      ● **Z52.001** Unspecified donor, stem cells
      ● **Z52.008** Unspecified donor, other blood

    ● **Z52.01** Autologous blood donor
      ● **Z52.010** Autologous donor, whole blood
      ● **Z52.011** Autologous donor, stem cells
      ● **Z52.018** Autologous donor, other blood

● Z52.09   **Other blood donor**
     Volunteer donor
     ● Z52.090   Other blood donor, whole blood
     ● Z52.091   Other blood donor, stem cells
     ● Z52.098   Other blood donor, other blood
● Z52.1   **Skin donor**
     Z52.10   Skin donor, unspecified
     Z52.11   Skin donor, autologous
     Z52.19   Skin donor, other
● Z52.2   **Bone donor**
     Z52.20   Bone donor, unspecified
     Z52.21   Bone donor, autologous
     Z52.29   Bone donor, other
Z52.3   **Bone marrow donor**
Z52.4   **Kidney donor**
Z52.5   **Cornea donor**
Z52.6   **Liver donor**
     Coding Clinic: 2012, Q4, P100
● Z52.8   **Donor of other specified organs or tissues**
     ● Z52.81   Egg (Oocyte) donor
         ● Z52.810   Egg (Oocyte) donor under age 35, anonymous recipient ♀
             Egg donor under age 35 NOS
         ● Z52.811   Egg (Oocyte) donor under age 35, designated recipient ♀
         ● Z52.812   Egg (Oocyte) donor age 35 and over, anonymous recipient ♀
             Egg donor age 35 and over NOS
         ● Z52.813   Egg (Oocyte) donor age 35 and over, designated recipient ♀
         ● Z52.819   Egg (Oocyte) donor, unspecified ♀
     Z52.89   Donor of other specified organs or tissues
Z52.9   **Donor of unspecified organ or tissue**
     Donor NOS

● Z53   **Persons encountering health services for specific procedures and treatment, not carried out**
● Z53.0   **Procedure and treatment not carried out because of contraindication**
     ● Z53.01   Procedure and treatment not carried out due to patient smoking
     ● Z53.09   Procedure and treatment not carried out because of other contraindication
● Z53.1   **Procedure and treatment not carried out because of patient's decision for reasons of belief and group pressure**
● Z53.2   **Procedure and treatment not carried out because of patient's decision for other and unspecified reasons**
     ● Z53.20   Procedure and treatment not carried out because of patient's decision for unspecified reasons
     ● Z53.21   Procedure and treatment not carried out due to patient leaving prior to being seen by health care provider
     ● Z53.29   Procedure and treatment not carried out because of patient's decision for other reasons
● Z53.3   **Procedure converted to open procedure**
     Coding Clinic: 2016, Q4, P79
     ● Z53.31   Laparoscopic surgical procedure converted to open procedure
         Coding Clinic: 2016, Q4, P100
     ● Z53.32   Thoracoscopic surgical procedure converted to open procedure
     ● Z53.33   Arthroscopic surgical procedure converted to open procedure
     ● Z53.39   Other specified procedure converted to open procedure
● Z53.8   **Procedure and treatment not carried out for other reasons**
● Z53.9   **Procedure and treatment not carried out, unspecified reason**

PERSONS WITH POTENTIAL HEALTH HAZARDS RELATED TO SOCIOECONOMIC AND PSYCHOSOCIAL CIRCUMSTANCES (Z55-Z65)

● Z55   **Problems related to education and literacy**
     Excludes1   disorders of psychological development (F80-F89)
● Z55.0   **Illiteracy and low-level literacy**
● Z55.1   **Schooling unavailable and unattainable**
● Z55.2   **Failed school examinations**
● Z55.3   **Underachievement in school**
● Z55.4   **Educational maladjustment and discord with teachers and classmates**
▶● Z55.5   **Less than a high school diploma**
     ▶No general equivalence degree (GED)
● Z55.8   **Other problems related to education and literacy**
     Problems related to inadequate teaching
● Z55.9   **Problems related to education and literacy, unspecified**
     Academic problems NOS

● Z56   **Problems related to employment and unemployment**
     Excludes2   occupational exposure to risk factors (Z57.-)
                    problems related to housing and economic circumstances (Z59.-)
● Z56.0   **Unemployment, unspecified**
● Z56.1   **Change of job**   **A**
● Z56.2   **Threat of job loss**
● Z56.3   **Stressful work schedule**
● Z56.4   **Discord with boss and workmates**
● Z56.5   **Uncongenial work environment**
     Difficult conditions at work
● Z56.6   **Other physical and mental strain related to work**
● Z56.8   **Other problems related to employment**
     ● Z56.81   Sexual harassment on the job
     ● Z56.82   Military deployment status
         Individual (civilian or military) currently deployed in theater or in support of military war, peacekeeping and humanitarian operations
     ● Z56.89   Other problems related to employment
● Z56.9   **Unspecified problems related to employment**
     Occupational problems NOS

● Z57   **Occupational exposure to risk factors**
● Z57.0   **Occupational exposure to noise**
● Z57.1   **Occupational exposure to radiation**
● Z57.2   **Occupational exposure to dust**
● Z57.3   **Occupational exposure to other air contaminants**
     ● Z57.31   Occupational exposure to environmental tobacco smoke
         Excludes2   exposure to environmental tobacco smoke (Z77.22)
     ● Z57.39   Occupational exposure to other air contaminants
● Z57.4   **Occupational exposure to toxic agents in agriculture**
     Occupational exposure to solids, liquids, gases or vapors in agriculture
● Z57.5   **Occupational exposure to toxic agents in other industries**
     Occupational exposure to solids, liquids, gases or vapors in other industries
● Z57.6   **Occupational exposure to extreme temperature**
● Z57.7   **Occupational exposure to vibration**
● Z57.8   **Occupational exposure to other risk factors**
● Z57.9   **Occupational exposure to unspecified risk factor**

▶● Z58   **Problems related to physical environment**
     ▶**Excludes2**   occupational exposure (Z57.-)
▶● Z58.6   **Inadequate drinking-water supply**
     ▶Lack of safe drinking water
         ▶**Excludes2**   deprivation of water (T73.1)

▶● Z59   **Problems related to housing and economic circumstances**
     Excludes2   problems related to upbringing (Z62.-)

N Newborn Age: 0	P Pediatric Age: 0–17	M Maternity DX: 9–64	A Adult Age: 15–124	♀ Females Only	♂ Males Only

🅒 Complication\Comorbidity   🅜 Major C\C   (Ex) CC/MCC Exclusions   🅗 Hospital-Acquired Condition   🅗 Hierarchical Condition Category

CHAPTER 21 (Z00-Z99)

➡️● **Z59.0**   **Homelessness**
> ● **Z59.00 Homelessness unspecified**
> ● **Z59.01 Sheltered homelessness**
>> ▶ Doubled up
>> ▶ Living in a shelter such as: motel, scattered site housing, temporary or transitional living situation
> ● **Z59.02 Unsheltered homelessness**
>> ▶ Residing in place not meant for human habitation such as: abandoned buildings, cars, parks, sidewalk
>> ▶ Residing on the street

● **Z59.1**   **Inadequate housing**
Lack of heating
Restriction of space
Technical defects in home preventing adequate care
Unsatisfactory surroundings
> **Excludes1**   problems related to the natural and physical environment (Z77.1-)

● **Z59.2**   **Discord with neighbors, lodgers and landlord**

● **Z59.3**   **Problems related to living in residential institution**
Boarding-school resident
> **Excludes1**   institutional upbringing (Z62.2)

➡️● **Z59.4**   **Lack of adequate food** ~~and safe drinking water~~
~~Inadequate drinking water supply~~
~~Excludes1   effects of hunger (T73.0)~~
~~inappropriate diet or eating habits (Z72.4)~~
~~malnutrition (E40-E46)~~
> ▶ **Excludes2**   deprivation of food (T73.0)
>> ▶ effects of hunger (T73.0)
>> ▶ inappropriate diet or eating habits (Z72.4)
>> ▶ malnutrition (E40-E46)
> ● **Z59.41 Food insecurity**
> ● **Z59.48 Other specified lack of adequate food**
>> ▶ Inadequate food
>> ▶ Lack of food

● **Z59.5**   **Extreme poverty**

● **Z59.6**   **Low income**

● **Z59.7**   **Insufficient social insurance and welfare support**

➡️● **Z59.8**   **Other problems related to housing and economic circumstances**
~~Foreclosure on loan~~
~~Isolated dwelling~~
~~Problems with creditors~~
> ● **Z59.81 Housing instability, housed**
>> ▶ Foreclosure on home loan
>> ▶ Past due on rent or mortgage
>> ▶ Unwanted multiple moves in the last 12 months
>> ● **Z59.811 Housing instability, housed, with risk of homelessness**
>>> ▶ Imminent risk of homelessness
>> ● **Z59.812 Housing instability, housed, homelessness in past 12 months**
>> ● **Z59.819 Housing instability, housed unspecified**
> ● **Z59.89 Other problems related to housing and economic circumstances**
>> ▶ Foreclosure on loan
>> ▶ Isolated dwelling
>> ▶ Problems with creditors

● **Z59.9**   **Problem related to housing and economic circumstances, unspecified**

● **Z60**   **Problems related to social environment**

● **Z60.0**   **Problems of adjustment to life-cycle transitions**
Empty nest syndrome
Phase of life problem
Problem with adjustment to retirement [pension]

● **Z60.2**   **Problems related to living alone**

● **Z60.3**   **Acculturation difficulty**
Problem with migration
Problem with social transplantation

● **Z60.4**   **Social exclusion and rejection**

Exclusion and rejection on the basis of personal characteristics, such as unusual physical appearance, illness or behavior.
> **Excludes1**   target of adverse discrimination such as for racial or religious reasons (Z60.5)

● **Z60.5**   **Target of (perceived) adverse discrimination and persecution**
> **Excludes1**   social exclusion and rejection (Z60.4)

● **Z60.8**   **Other problems related to social environment**

● **Z60.9**   **Problem related to social environment, unspecified**

● **Z62**   **Problems related to upbringing**
> **Includes**   current and past negative life events in childhood
current and past problems of a child related to upbringing
> **Excludes2**   maltreatment syndrome (T74.-)
problems related to housing and economic circumstances (Z59.-)

● **Z62.0**   **Inadequate parental supervision and control**

● **Z62.1**   **Parental overprotection**

● **Z62.2**   **Upbringing away from parents**
> **Excludes1**   problems with boarding school (Z59.3)
> ● **Z62.21**   **Child in welfare custody**   **P**
>> Child in care of non-parental family member
>> Child in foster care
>> **Excludes2**   problem for parent due to child in welfare custody (Z63.5)
> ● **Z62.22**   **Institutional upbringing**
>> Child living in orphanage or group home
> ● **Z62.29**   **Other upbringing away from parents**

● **Z62.3**   **Hostility towards and scapegoating of child**   **P**

● **Z62.6**   **Inappropriate (excessive) parental pressure**

● **Z62.8**   **Other specified problems related to upbringing**
> ● **Z62.81**   **Personal history of abuse in childhood**
>> ● **Z62.810**   **Personal history of physical and sexual abuse in childhood**
>>> **Excludes1**   current child physical abuse (T74.12, T76.12)
>>> current child sexual abuse (T74.22, T76.22)
>> ● **Z62.811**   **Personal history of psychological abuse in childhood**
>>> **Excludes1**   current child psychological abuse (T74.32, T76.32)
>> ● **Z62.812**   **Personal history of neglect in childhood**
>>> **Excludes1**   current child neglect (T74.02, T76.02)
>> ● **Z62.813**   **Personal history of forced labor or sexual exploitation in childhood**
>> ● **Z62.819**   **Personal history of unspecified abuse in childhood**
>>> **Excludes1**   current child abuse NOS (T74.92, T76.92)
> ● **Z62.82**   **Parent-child conflict**
>> ● **Z62.820**   **Parent-biological child conflict**
>>> Parent-child problem NOS
>> ● **Z62.821**   **Parent-adopted child conflict**
>> ● **Z62.822**   **Parent-foster child conflict**
> ● **Z62.89**   **Other specified problems related to upbringing**
>> ● **Z62.890**   **Parent-child estrangement NEC**
>> ● **Z62.891**   **Sibling rivalry**
>> ● **Z62.898**   **Other specified problems related to upbringing**

● **Z62.9**   **Problem related to upbringing, unspecified**

▶ New   ➡️ Revised   ~~deleted~~ Deleted   Excludes 1   Excludes 2   Includes   Use additional   Code first   Code also   Key words

1638   OGCR Official Guidelines   ● Unacceptable Principal Diagnosis   X Assign placeholder X   ● Use Additional Character(s)   ▶ Manifestation Code   **Coding Clinic**

● **Z63**   **Other problems related to primary support group, including family circumstances**
   > **Excludes2**   maltreatment syndrome (T74.-, T76)
   > parent-child problems (Z62.-)
   > problems related to negative life events in childhood (Z62.-)
   > problems related to upbringing (Z62.-)

● **Z63.0**   **Problems in relationship with spouse or partner**
   Relationship distress with spouse or intimate partner
   > **Excludes1**   counseling for spousal or partner abuse problems (Z69.1)
   > counseling related to sexual attitude, behavior, and orientation (Z70.-)

● **Z63.1**   **Problems in relationship with in-laws**

● **Z63.3**   **Absence of family member**
   > **Excludes1**   absence of family member due to disappearance and death (Z63.4)
   > absence of family member due to separation and divorce (Z63.5)

   ● **Z63.31**   **Absence of family member due to military deployment**
      Individual or family affected by other family member being on military deployment
      > **Excludes1**   family disruption due to return of family member from military deployment (Z63.71)

   ● **Z63.32**   **Other absence of family member**

● **Z63.4**   **Disappearance and death of family member**
   Assumed death of family member
   Bereavement

● **Z63.5**   **Disruption of family by separation and divorce**
   Marital estrangement

● **Z63.6**   **Dependent relative needing care at home**

● **Z63.7**   **Other stressful life events affecting family and household**

   ● **Z63.71**   **Stress on family due to return of family member from military deployment**
      Individual or family affected by family member having returned from military deployment (current or past conflict)

   ● **Z63.72**   **Alcoholism and drug addiction in family**

   ● **Z63.79**   **Other stressful life events affecting family and household**
      Anxiety (normal) about sick person in family
      Health problems within family
      Ill or disturbed family member
      Isolated family

● **Z63.8**   **Other specified problems related to primary support group**
   Family discord NOS
   Family estrangement NOS
   High expressed emotional level within family
   Inadequate family support NOS
   Inadequate or distorted communication within family

● **Z63.9**   **Problem related to primary support group, unspecified**
   Relationship disorder NOS

● **Z64**   **Problems related to certain psychosocial circumstances**

● **Z64.0**   **Problems related to unwanted pregnancy** ♀

● **Z64.1**   **Problems related to multiparity** ♀

● **Z64.4**   **Discord with counselors**
   Discord with probation officer
   Discord with social worker

● **Z65**   **Problems related to other psychosocial circumstances**

● **Z65.0**   **Conviction in civil and criminal proceedings without imprisonment**

● **Z65.1**   **Imprisonment and other incarceration**

● **Z65.2**   **Problems related to release from prison**

● **Z65.3**   **Problems related to other legal circumstances**
   Arrest
   Child custody or support proceedings
   Litigation
   Prosecution

● **Z65.4**   **Victim of crime and terrorism**
   Victim of torture

● **Z65.5**   **Exposure to disaster, war and other hostilities**
   > **Excludes1**   target of perceived discrimination or persecution (Z60.5)

● **Z65.8**   **Other specified problems related to psychosocial circumstances**
   Religious or spiritual problem

● **Z65.9**   **Problem related to unspecified psychosocial circumstances**

DO NOT RESUSCITATE STATUS (Z66)

● **Z66**   **Do not resuscitate**
   DNR status

BLOOD TYPE (Z67)

● **Z67**   **Blood type**
   Coding Clinic: 2015, Q3, P40

   ● **Z67.1**   **Type A blood**
      ● **Z67.10**   **Type A blood, Rh positive**
      ● **Z67.11**   **Type A blood, Rh negative**

   ● **Z67.2**   **Type B blood**
      ● **Z67.20**   **Type B blood, Rh positive**
      ● **Z67.21**   **Type B blood, Rh negative**

   ● **Z67.3**   **Type AB blood**
      ● **Z67.30**   **Type AB blood, Rh positive**
      ● **Z67.31**   **Type AB blood, Rh negative**

   ● **Z67.4**   **Type O blood**
      ● **Z67.40**   **Type O blood, Rh positive**
      ● **Z67.41**   **Type O blood, Rh negative**

   ● **Z67.9**   **Unspecified blood type**
      ● **Z67.90**   **Unspecified blood type, Rh positive**
      ● **Z67.91**   **Unspecified blood type, Rh negative**
         Coding Clinic: 2015, Q3, P40

BODY MASS INDEX [BMI] (Z68)

OGCR Section I.B.14.

> **General Coding Guidelines**
>
> 14. Documentation for BMI, Depth of Non-pressure ulcers, Pressure Ulcer Stages, Coma Scale, and NIH Stroke Scale
>
> For the Body Mass Index (BMI), depth of non-pressure chronic ulcers, pressure ulcer stage, coma scale, and NIH stroke scale (NIHSS) codes, code assignment may be based on medical record documentation from clinicians who are not the patient's provider (i.e., physician or other qualified healthcare practitioner legally accountable for establishing the patient's diagnosis), since this information is typically documented by other clinicians involved in the care of the patient (e.g., a dietitian often documents the BMI, a nurse often documents the pressure ulcer stages, and an emergency medical technician often documents the coma scale). However, the associated diagnosis (such as overweight, obesity, acute stroke, or pressure ulcer) must be documented by the patient's provider. If there is conflicting medical record documentation, either from the same clinician or different clinicians, the patient's attending provider should be queried for clarification.
>
> The BMI, coma scale, and NIHSS codes should only be reported as secondary diagnoses.

● **Z68**   **Body mass index [BMI]**
   Kilograms per meters squared
   Note: BMI adult codes are for use for persons 20 years of age or older.
   BMI pediatric codes are for use for persons 2-19 years of age.
   These percentiles are based on the growth charts published by the Centers for Disease Control and Prevention (CDC)
   Coding Clinic: 2018, Q4, P81; 2016, Q4, P129

● **Z68.1**   **Body mass index [BMI] 19.9 or less, adult** 🖤   **A**
   (Ex:) See PDX Collection 1493
   Coding Clinic: 2017, Q1, P39

N Newborn Age: 0	P Pediatric Age: 0–17	M Maternity DX: 9–64	A Adult Age: 15–124	♀ Females Only	♂ Males Only
🖤 Complication\Comorbidity	🖤 Major C\C	(Ex:) CC/MCC Exclusions	🖤 Hospital-Acquired Condition	🖤 Hierarchical Condition Category	

CHAPTER 21 (Z00-Z99)

CHAPTER 21 (Z00-Z99)

● **Z68.2**   Body mass index [BMI] 20-29, adult
  - ● **Z68.20**   Body mass index [BMI] 20.0-20.9, adult   A
  - ● **Z68.21**   Body mass index [BMI] 21.0-21.9, adult   A
  - ● **Z68.22**   Body mass index [BMI] 22.0-22.9, adult   A
  - ● **Z68.23**   Body mass index [BMI] 23.0-23.9, adult   A
  - ● **Z68.24**   Body mass index [BMI] 24.0-24.9, adult   A
  - ● **Z68.25**   Body mass index [BMI] 25.0-25.9, adult   A
  - ● **Z68.26**   Body mass index [BMI] 26.0-26.9, adult   A
  - ● **Z68.27**   Body mass index [BMI] 27.0-27.9, adult   A
  - ● **Z68.28**   Body mass index [BMI] 28.0-28.9, adult   A
  - ● **Z68.29**   Body mass index [BMI] 29.0-29.9, adult   A

● **Z68.3**   Body mass index [BMI] 30-39, adult
  - ● **Z68.30**   Body mass index [BMI] 30.0-30.9, adult   A
  - ● **Z68.31**   Body mass index [BMI] 31.0-31.9, adult   A
  - ● **Z68.32**   Body mass index [BMI] 32.0-32.9, adult   A
  - ● **Z68.33**   Body mass index [BMI] 33.0-33.9, adult   A
  - ● **Z68.34**   Body mass index [BMI] 34.0-34.9, adult   A
  - ● **Z68.35**   Body mass index [BMI] 35.0-35.9, adult   A
  - ● **Z68.36**   Body mass index [BMI] 36.0-36.9, adult   A
  - ● **Z68.37**   Body mass index [BMI] 37.0-37.9, adult   A
  - ● **Z68.38**   Body mass index [BMI] 38.0-38.9, adult   A
  - ● **Z68.39**   Body mass index [BMI] 39.0-39.9, adult   A

● **Z68.4**   Body mass index [BMI] 40 or greater, adult
  Ex: For category Z68.4 CC codes: See PDX Collection 1494
  - ● **Z68.41**   Body mass index [BMI] 40.0-44.9, adult ⊘ 🔴   A
  - ● **Z68.42**   Body mass index [BMI] 45.0-49.9, adult ⊘ 🔴   A
  - ● **Z68.43**   Body mass index [BMI] 50.0-59.9, adult ⊘ 🔴   A
  - ● **Z68.44**   Body mass index [BMI] 60.0-69.9, adult ⊘ 🔴   A
  - ● **Z68.45**   Body mass index [BMI] 70 or greater, adult ⊘ 🔴   A

● **Z68.5**   Body mass index [BMI] pediatric
  Coding Clinic: 2018, Q4, P81
  - ● **Z68.51**   Body mass index [BMI] pediatric, less than 5th percentile for age
    Coding Clinic: 2018, Q4, P82
  - ● **Z68.52**   Body mass index [BMI] pediatric, 5th percentile to less than 85th percentile for age
  - ● **Z68.53**   Body mass index [BMI] pediatric, 85th percentile to less than 95th percentile for age
  - ● **Z68.54**   Body mass index [BMI] pediatric, greater than or equal to 95th percentile for age

PERSONS ENCOUNTERING HEALTH SERVICES IN OTHER CIRCUMSTANCES (Z69-Z76)

● **Z69**   Encounter for mental health services for victim and perpetrator of abuse
  Includes   counseling for victims and perpetrators of abuse

● **Z69.0**   Encounter for mental health services for child abuse problems
  - ● **Z69.01**   Encounter for mental health services for parental child abuse
    - **Z69.010**   Encounter for mental health services for victim of parental child abuse   P
      Encounter for mental health services for victim of child abuse by parent
      Encounter for mental health services for victim of child neglect by parent
      Encounter for mental health services for victim of child psychological abuse by parent
      Encounter for mental health services for victim of child sexual abuse by parent

- ● **Z69.011**   Encounter for mental health services for perpetrator of parental child abuse
    Encounter for mental health services for perpetrator of parental child neglect
    Encounter for mental health services for perpetrator of parental child psychological abuse
    Encounter for mental health services for perpetrator of parental child sexual abuse
    Excludes1   encounter for mental health services for non-parental child abuse (Z69.02-)

  - ● **Z69.02**   Encounter for mental health services for non-parental child abuse
    - **Z69.020**   Encounter for mental health services for victim of non-parental child abuse   P
      Encounter for mental health services for victim of non-parental child neglect
      Encounter for mental health services for victim of non-parental child psychological abuse
      Encounter for mental health services for victim of non-parental child sexual abuse
    - ● **Z69.021**   Encounter for mental health services for perpetrator of non- parental child abuse
      Encounter for mental health services for perpetrator of non-parental child neglect
      Encounter for mental health services for perpetrator of non-parental child psychological abuse
      Encounter for mental health services for perpetrator of non-parental child sexual abuse

● **Z69.1**   Encounter for mental health services for spousal or partner abuse problems
  - ● **Z69.11**   Encounter for mental health services for victim of spousal or partner abuse
    Encounter for mental health services for victim of spouse or partner neglect
    Encounter for mental health services for victim of spouse or partner psychological abuse
    Encounter for mental health services for victim of spouse or partner violence, physical
  - ● **Z69.12**   Encounter for mental health services for perpetrator of spousal or partner abuse
    Encounter for mental health services for perpetrator of spouse or partner neglect
    Encounter for mental health services for perpetrator of spouse or partner psychological abuse
    Encounter for mental health services for perpetrator of spouse or partner violence, physical
    Encounter for mental health services for perpetrator of spouse or partner violence, sexual

● **Z69.8**   Encounter for mental health services for victim or perpetrator of other abuse
  - ● **Z69.81**   Encounter for mental health services for victim of other abuse
    Encounter for mental health services for victim of non-spousal adult abuse
    Encounter for mental health services for victim of spouse or partner violence, sexual
    Encounter for rape victim counseling
  - ● **Z69.82**   Encounter for mental health services for perpetrator of other abuse
    Encounter for mental health services for perpetrator of non-spousal adult abuse

▶ New   ⇒ Revised   ~~deleted~~ Deleted   Excludes 1   Excludes 2   Includes   Use additional   Code first   Code also   Key words
OGCR Official Guidelines   ● Unacceptable Principal Diagnosis   X Assign placeholder X   ● Use Additional Character(s)   ▷ Manifestation Code   Coding Clinic

● **Z70 Counseling related to sexual attitude, behavior and orientation**
> **Includes** encounter for mental health services for sexual attitude, behavior and orientation
> **Excludes2** contraceptive or procreative counseling (Z30-Z31)

● **Z70.0 Counseling related to sexual attitude**
● **Z70.1 Counseling related to patient's sexual behavior and orientation**
> Patient concerned regarding impotence
> Patient concerned regarding non-responsiveness
> Patient concerned regarding promiscuity
> Patient concerned regarding sexual orientation

● **Z70.2 Counseling related to sexual behavior and orientation of third party**
> Advice sought regarding sexual behavior and orientation of child
> Advice sought regarding sexual behavior and orientation of partner
> Advice sought regarding sexual behavior and orientation of spouse

● **Z70.3 Counseling related to combined concerns regarding sexual attitude, behavior and orientation**
● **Z70.8 Other sex counseling**
> Encounter for sex education
● **Z70.9 Sex counseling, unspecified**

● **Z71 Persons encountering health services for other counseling and medical advice, not elsewhere classified**
> **Excludes2** contraceptive or procreation counseling (Z30-Z31)
> sex counseling (Z70.-)

● **Z71.0 Person encountering health services to consult on behalf of another person**
> Person encountering health services to seek advice or treatment for non-attending third party
> **Excludes2** anxiety (normal) about sick person in family (Z63.7)
> expectant (adoptive) parent(s) pre-birth pediatrician visit (Z76.81)

● **Z71.1 Person with feared health complaint in whom no diagnosis is made**
> Person encountering health services with feared condition which was not demonstrated
> Person encountering health services in which problem was normal state
> "Worried well"
> **Excludes1** medical observation for suspected diseases and conditions proven not to exist (Z03.-)
> Coding Clinic: 2016, Q4, P7

● **Z71.2 Person consulting for explanation of examination or test findings**
● **Z71.3 Dietary counseling and surveillance**
> Use additional code for any associated underlying medical condition
> Use additional code to identify body mass index (BMI), if known (Z68.-)
● **Z71.4 Alcohol abuse counseling and surveillance**
> Use additional code for alcohol abuse or dependence (F10.-)
> ● **Z71.41 Alcohol abuse counseling and surveillance of alcoholic**
> ● **Z71.42 Counseling for family member of alcoholic**
> Counseling for significant other, partner, or friend of alcoholic
● **Z71.5 Drug abuse counseling and surveillance**
> Use additional code for drug abuse or dependence (F11-F16, F18-F19)
> ● **Z71.51 Drug abuse counseling and surveillance of drug abuser**
> ● **Z71.52 Counseling for family member of drug abuser**
> Counseling for significant other, partner, or friend of drug abuser

● **Z71.6 Tobacco abuse counseling**
> Use additional code for nicotine dependence (F17.-)
● **Z71.7 Human immunodeficiency virus [HIV] counseling**
● **Z71.8 Other specified counseling**
> **Excludes2** counseling for contraception (Z30.0-)
> ● **Z71.81 Spiritual or religious counseling**
> ● **Z71.82 Exercise counseling**
> **Z71.83 Encounter for nonprocreative genetic counseling**
> > **Excludes1** counseling for procreative genetics (Z31.5)
> > counseling for procreative management (Z31.6)
> **Z71.84 Encounter for health counseling related to travel**
> > Encounter for health risk and safety counseling for (international) travel
> > Code also, if applicable, encounter for immunization (Z23)
> > **Excludes2** encounter for administrative examination (Z02.-)
> > encounter for other special examination without complaint, suspected or reported diagnosis (Z01.-)
> ▶**Z71.85 Encounter for immunization safety counseling**
> > ▶Encounter for vaccine product safety counseling
> > ▶Code also, if applicable, encounter for immunization (Z23)
> > ▶Code also, if applicable, immunization not carried out (Z28.-)
> > ▶**Excludes1** encounter for health counseling related to travel (Z71.84)
> ● **Z71.89 Other specified counseling**
● **Z71.9 Counseling, unspecified**
> Encounter for medical advice NOS

● **Z72 Problems related to lifestyle**
> **Excludes2** problems related to life-management difficulty (Z73.-)
> problems related to socioeconomic and psychosocial circumstances (Z55-Z65)
> Coding Clinic: 2016, Q4, P130
● **Z72.0 Tobacco use**
> Tobacco use NOS
> **Excludes1** history of tobacco dependence (Z87.891)
> nicotine dependence (F17.2-)
> tobacco dependence (F17.2-)
> tobacco use during pregnancy (O99.33-)
● **Z72.3 Lack of physical exercise**
● **Z72.4 Inappropriate diet and eating habits**
> **Excludes1** behavioral eating disorders of infancy or childhood (F98.2.-F98.3)
> eating disorders (F50.-)
> lack of adequate food (Z59.48)
> malnutrition and other nutritional deficiencies (E40-E64)
● **Z72.5 High risk sexual behavior**
> Promiscuity
> **Excludes1** paraphilias (F65)
> ● **Z72.51 High risk heterosexual behavior**
> ● **Z72.52 High risk homosexual behavior**
> ● **Z72.53 High risk bisexual behavior**
● **Z72.6 Gambling and betting**
> **Excludes1** compulsive or pathological gambling (F63.0)
● **Z72.8 Other problems related to lifestyle**
> ● **Z72.81 Antisocial behavior**
> > **Excludes1** conduct disorders (F91.-)

N Newborn Age: 0   P Pediatric Age: 0–17   M Maternity DX: 9–64   A Adult Age: 15–124   ♀ Females Only   ♂ Males Only
Complication\Comorbidity   Major C\C   (Ex) CC/MCC Exclusions   Hospital-Acquired Condition   Hierarchical Condition Category
CHAPTER 21 (Z00-Z99)   1641

Z72.810   **Child and adolescent** antisocial behavior   P
   Antisocial behavior (child) (adolescent) without manifest psychiatric disorder
   Delinquency NOS
   Group delinquency
   Offenses in the context of gang membership
   Stealing in company with others
   Truancy from school

Z72.811   **Adult antisocial behavior**   A
   Adult antisocial behavior without manifest psychiatric disorder

Z72.82   **Problems related to sleep**

Z72.820   **Sleep deprivation**
   Lack of adequate sleep
   Excludes1   insomnia (G47.0-)

Z72.821   **Inadequate sleep hygiene**
   Bad sleep habits
   Irregular sleep habits
   Unhealthy sleep wake schedule
   Excludes1   insomnia (F51.0-, G47.0-)

Z72.89   **Other problems related to lifestyle**
   Self-damaging behavior

Z72.9   **Problem related to lifestyle, unspecified**

Z73   Problems related to life management difficulty
   Excludes2   problems related to socioeconomic and psychosocial circumstances (Z55-Z65)

Z73.0   **Burn-out**

Z73.1   **Type A behavior pattern**

Z73.2   **Lack of relaxation and leisure**

Z73.3   **Stress, not elsewhere classified**
   Physical and mental strain NOS
   Excludes1   stress related to employment or unemployment (Z56.-)

Z73.4   **Inadequate social skills, not elsewhere classified**

Z73.5   **Social role conflict, not elsewhere classified**

Z73.6   **Limitation of activities due to disability**
   Excludes1   care-provider dependency (Z74.-)

Z73.8   **Other problems related to life management difficulty**

Z73.81   **Behavioral insomnia of childhood**

Z73.810   **Behavioral insomnia of childhood, sleep-onset association type**   P

Z73.811   **Behavioral insomnia of childhood, limit setting type**   P

Z73.812   **Behavioral insomnia of childhood, combined type**   P

Z73.819   **Behavioral insomnia of childhood, unspecified type**   P

Z73.82   **Dual sensory impairment**

Z73.89   **Other problems related to life management difficulty**

Z73.9   **Problem related to life management difficulty, unspecified**

Z74   Problems related to care provider dependency
   Excludes2   dependence on enabling machines or devices NEC (Z99.-)

Z74.0   **Reduced mobility**

Z74.01   **Bed confinement status**
   Bedridden

Z74.09   **Other reduced mobility**
   Chairridden
   Reduced mobility NOS
   Excludes2   wheelchair dependence (Z99.3)

Z74.1   **Need for assistance with personal care**

Z74.2   **Need for assistance at home and no other household member able to render care**

Z74.3   **Need for continuous supervision**

Z74.8   **Other problems related to care provider dependency**

Z74.9   **Problem related to care provider dependency, unspecified**

Z75   Problems related to medical facilities and other health care

Z75.0   **Medical services not available in home**
   Excludes1   no other household member able to render care (Z74.2)

Z75.1   **Person awaiting admission to adequate facility elsewhere**

Z75.2   **Other waiting period for investigation and treatment**

Z75.3   **Unavailability and inaccessibility of health care facilities**
   Excludes1   bed unavailable (Z75.1)

Z75.4   **Unavailability and inaccessibility of other helping agencies**

Z75.5   **Holiday relief care**

Z75.8   **Other problems related to medical facilities and other health care**

Z75.9   **Unspecified problem related to medical facilities and other health care**

Z76   Persons encountering health services in other circumstances

Z76.0   **Encounter for issue of repeat prescription**
   Encounter for issue of repeat prescription for appliance
   Encounter for issue of repeat prescription for medicaments
   Encounter for issue of repeat prescription for spectacles
   Excludes2   issue of medical certificate (Z02.7) repeat prescription for contraceptive (Z30.4-)

Z76.1   **Encounter for health supervision and care of foundling**

Z76.2   **Encounter for health supervision and care of other healthy infant and child**   P
   Encounter for medical or nursing care or supervision of healthy infant under circumstances such as adverse socioeconomic conditions at home
   Encounter for medical or nursing care or supervision of healthy infant under circumstances such as awaiting foster or adoptive placement
   Encounter for medical or nursing care or supervision of healthy infant under circumstances such as maternal illness
   Encounter for medical or nursing care or supervision of healthy infant under circumstances such as number of children at home preventing or interfering with normal care

Z76.3   **Healthy person accompanying sick person**

Z76.4   **Other boarder to healthcare facility**
   Excludes1   homelessness (Z59.0-)

Z76.5   **Malingerer [conscious simulation]**
   Person feigning illness (with obvious motivation)
   Excludes1   factitious disorder (F68.1-, F68.A) peregrinating patient (F68.1-)

● **Z76.8**   **Persons encountering health services in other specified circumstances**

    ● **Z76.81**   **Expectant parent(s) prebirth pediatrician visit**
         Pre-adoption pediatrician visit for adoptive parent(s)

    ● **Z76.82**   **Awaiting organ transplant status**
         Patient waiting for organ availability

    ● **Z76.89**   **Persons encountering health services in other specified circumstances**
         Persons encountering health services NOS

PERSONS WITH POTENTIAL HEALTH HAZARDS RELATED TO FAMILY AND PERSONAL HISTORY AND CERTAIN CONDITIONS INFLUENCING HEALTH STATUS (Z77-Z99)

Code also any follow-up examination (Z08-Z09)

● **Z77**   **Other contact with and (suspected) exposures hazardous to health**

     Includes   contact with and (suspected) exposures to potential hazards to health

     Excludes2   contact with and (suspected) exposure to communicable diseases (Z20.-)
         exposure to (parental) (environmental) tobacco smoke in the perinatal period (P96.81)
         newborn affected by noxious substances transmitted via placenta or breast milk (P04.-)
         occupational exposure to risk factors (Z57.-)
         retained foreign body (Z18.-)
         retained foreign body fully removed (Z87.821)
         toxic effects of substances chiefly nonmedicinal as to source (T51-T65)

● **Z77.0**   **Contact with and (suspected) exposure to hazardous, chiefly nonmedicinal, chemicals**

    ● **Z77.01**   **Contact with and (suspected) exposure to hazardous metals**

        ● **Z77.010**   **Contact with and (suspected) exposure to arsenic**

        ● **Z77.011**   **Contact with and (suspected) exposure to lead**

        ● **Z77.012**   **Contact with and (suspected) exposure to uranium**
             Excludes1   retained depleted uranium fragments (Z18.01)

        ● **Z77.018**   **Contact with and (suspected) exposure to other hazardous metals**
             Contact with and (suspected) exposure to chromium compounds
             Contact with and (suspected) exposure to nickel dust

    ● **Z77.02**   **Contact with and (suspected) exposure to hazardous aromatic compounds**

        ● **Z77.020**   **Contact with and (suspected) exposure to aromatic amines**

        ● **Z77.021**   **Contact with and (suspected) exposure to benzene**

        ● **Z77.028**   **Contact with and (suspected) exposure to other hazardous aromatic compounds**
             Aromatic dyes NOS
             Polycyclic aromatic hydrocarbons

    ● **Z77.09**   **Contact with and (suspected) exposure to other hazardous, chiefly nonmedicinal, chemicals**

        ● **Z77.090**   **Contact with and (suspected) exposure to asbestos**

        ● **Z77.098**   **Contact with and (suspected) exposure to other hazardous, chiefly nonmedicinal, chemicals**
             Dyes NOS

● **Z77.1**   **Contact with and (suspected) exposure to environmental pollution and hazards in the physical environment**

    ● **Z77.11**   **Contact with and (suspected) exposure to environmental pollution**

        ● **Z77.110**   **Contact with and (suspected) exposure to air pollution**

        ● **Z77.111**   **Contact with and (suspected) exposure to water pollution**

        ● **Z77.112**   **Contact with and (suspected) exposure to soil pollution**

        ● **Z77.118**   **Contact with and (suspected) exposure to other environmental pollution**

    ● **Z77.12**   **Contact with and (suspected) exposure to hazards in the physical environment**

        ● **Z77.120**   **Contact with and (suspected) exposure to mold (toxic)**

        ● **Z77.121**   **Contact with and (suspected) exposure to harmful algae and algae toxins**
             Contact with and (suspected) exposure to (harmful) algae bloom NOS
             Contact with and (suspected) exposure to blue-green algae bloom
             Contact with and (suspected) exposure to brown tide
             Contact with and (suspected) exposure to cyanobacteria bloom
             Contact with and (suspected) exposure to Florida red tide
             Contact with and (suspected) exposure to pfiesteria piscicida
             Contact with and (suspected) exposure to red tide

        ● **Z77.122**   **Contact with and (suspected) exposure to noise**

        ● **Z77.123**   **Contact with and (suspected) exposure to radon and other naturally occurring radiation**
             Excludes2   radiation exposure as the cause of a confirmed condition (W88-W90, X39.0-)
                     radiation sickness NOS (T66)

        ● **Z77.128**   **Contact with and (suspected) exposure to other hazards in the physical environment**

● **Z77.2**   **Contact with and (suspected) exposure to other hazardous substances**

    ● **Z77.21**   **Contact with and (suspected) exposure to potentially hazardous body fluids**

    ● **Z77.22**   **Contact with and (suspected) exposure to environmental tobacco smoke (acute) (chronic)**
         Exposure to second hand tobacco smoke (acute) (chronic)
         Passive smoking (acute) (chronic)
         Excludes1   nicotine dependence (F17.-)
                     tobacco use (Z72.0)
         Excludes2   occupational exposure to environmental tobacco smoke (Z57.31)

    ● **Z77.29**   **Contact with and (suspected) exposure to other hazardous substances**
         Coding Clinic: 2016, Q2, P34

N Newborn Age: 0   **P** Pediatric Age: 0–17   **M** Maternity DX: 9–64   **A** Adult Age: 15–124   ♀ Females Only   ♂ Males Only

Complication\Comorbidity   Major C\C   (Ex) CC/MCC Exclusions   Hospital-Acquired Condition   Hierarchical Condition Category   **1643**

CHAPTER 21 (Z00-Z99)

CHAPTER 21 (Z00-Z99)

- **Z77.9 Other contact with and (suspected) exposures hazardous to health**

- **Z78 Other specified health status**
  - **Excludes2**   asymptomatic human immunodeficiency virus [HIV] infection status (Z21)
    postprocedural status (Z93-Z99)
    sex reassignment status (Z87.890)
  - **Z78.0 Asymptomatic menopausal state ♀**   A
    Menopausal state NOS
    Postmenopausal status NOS
    - **Excludes2**   symptomatic menopausal state (N95.1)
  - **Z78.1 Physical restraint status**
    - **Excludes1**   physical restraint due to a procedure - omit code
  - **Z78.9 Other specified health status**

- **Z79 Long term (current) drug therapy**
  - **Includes**   long term (current) drug use for prophylactic purposes
  - Code also any therapeutic drug level monitoring (Z51.81)
  - **Excludes2**   drug abuse and dependence (F11-F19)
    drug use complicating pregnancy, childbirth, and the puerperium (O99.32-)
  - **Z79.0 Long term (current) use of anticoagulants and antithrombotics/antiplatelets**
    - **Excludes2**   long term (current) use of aspirin (Z79.82)
    - Coding Clinic: 2021, Q1, P12-13
    - **Z79.01 Long term (current) use of anticoagulants**
      - Coding Clinic: 2021, Q1, P5
    - **Z79.02 Long term (current) use of antithrombotics/antiplatelets**
  - **Z79.1 Long term (current) use of non-steroidal anti-inflammatories (NSAID)**
    - **Excludes2**   long term (current) use of aspirin (Z79.82)
  - **Z79.2 Long term (current) use of antibiotics**
  - **Z79.3 Long term (current) use of hormonal contraceptives**
    Long term (current) use of birth control pill or patch
  - **Z79.4 Long term (current) use of insulin** 🔖
    - ~~**Excludes1**   long term (current) use of oral antidiabetic drugs (Z79.84)~~
      ~~long term (current) use of oral hypoglycemic drugs (Z79.84)~~
    - ▶ **Excludes2**   long term (current) use of oral hypoglycemic drugs (Z79.84)
      ▶ long term (current) use of oral antidiabetic drugs (Z79.84)
  - **Z79.5 Long term (current) use of steroids**
    - **Z79.51 Long term (current) use of inhaled steroids**
    - **Z79.52 Long term (current) use of systemic steroids**
  - **Z79.8 Other long term (current) drug therapy**
    - **Z79.81 Long term (current) use of agents affecting estrogen receptors and estrogen levels**
      - *Code first, if applicable:*
        malignant neoplasm of breast (C50.-)
        malignant neoplasm of prostate (C61)
      - Use additional code, if applicable, to identify:
        estrogen receptor positive status (Z17.0)
        family history of breast cancer (Z80.3)
        genetic susceptibility to malignant neoplasm (cancer) (Z15.0-)
        personal history of breast cancer (Z85.3)
        personal history of prostate cancer (Z85.46)
        postmenopausal status (Z78.0)
      - **Excludes1**   hormone replacement therapy (Z79.890)

- **Z79.810 Long term (current) use of selective estrogen receptor modulators (SERMs)**
  Long term (current) use of raloxifene (Evista)
  Long term (current) use of tamoxifen (Nolvadex)
  Long term (current) use of toremifene (Fareston)
- **Z79.811 Long term (current) use of aromatase inhibitors**
  Long term (current) use of anastrozole (Arimidex)
  Long term (current) use of exemestane (Aromasin)
  Long term (current) use of letrozole (Femara)
- **Z79.818 Long term (current) use of other agents affecting estrogen receptors and estrogen levels**
  Long term (current) use of estrogen receptor downregulators
  Long term (current) use of fulvestrant (Faslodex)
  Long term (current) use of gonadotropin-releasing hormone (GnRH) agonist
  Long term (current) use of goserelin acetate (Zoladex)
  Long term (current) use of leuprolide acetate (leuprorelin) (Lupron)
  Long term (current) use of megestrol acetate (Megace)
- **Z79.82 Long term (current) use of aspirin**
- **Z79.83 Long term (current) use of bisphosphonates**
  - Coding Clinic: 2016, Q4, P42
- **Z79.84 Long term (current) use of oral hypoglycemic drugs**
  Long term (current) use of oral antidiabetic drugs
  - **Excludes2**   long term (current) use of insulin (Z79.4)
  - Coding Clinic: 2016, Q4, P76, 121-122, 126
- **Z79.89 Other long term (current) drug therapy**
  - **Z79.890 Hormone replacement therapy**
  - **Z79.891 Long term (current) use of opiate analgesic**
    Long term (current) use of methadone for pain management
    - **Excludes1**   methadone use NOS (F11.9-)
      use of methadone for treatment of heroin addiction (F11.2-)
  - **Z79.899 Other long term (current) drug therapy**
    - Coding Clinic: 2015, Q4, P34, Q3, P21

- **Z80 Family history of primary malignant neoplasm**
  - **Z80.0 Family history of malignant neoplasm of digestive organs**
    Conditions classifiable to C15-C26
    - Coding Clinic: 2018, Q1, P7
  - **Z80.1 Family history of malignant neoplasm of trachea, bronchus and lung**
    Conditions classifiable to C33-C34

▶ New   ⟹ Revised   ~~deleted~~ Deleted   Excludes 1   Excludes 2   Includes   Use additional   Code first   Code also   Key words

OGCR Official Guidelines   ● Unacceptable Principal Diagnosis   X Assign placeholder X   ● Use Additional Character(s)   � Manifestation Code   Coding Clinic

● Z80.2   Family history of malignant neoplasm of other respiratory and intrathoracic organs
           Conditions classifiable to C30-C32, C37-C39

● Z80.3   Family history of malignant neoplasm of breast
           Conditions classifiable to C50.-

● Z80.4   Family history of malignant neoplasm of genital organs
           Conditions classifiable to C51-C63

    ● Z80.41   Family history of malignant neoplasm of ovary

    ● Z80.42   Family history of malignant neoplasm of prostate

    ● Z80.43   Family history of malignant neoplasm of testis

    ● Z80.49   Family history of malignant neoplasm of other genital organs

● Z80.5   Family history of malignant neoplasm of urinary tract
           Conditions classifiable to C64-C68

    ● Z80.51   Family history of malignant neoplasm of kidney

    ● Z80.52   Family history of malignant neoplasm of bladder

    ● Z80.59   Family history of malignant neoplasm of other urinary tract organ

● Z80.6   Family history of leukemia
           Conditions classifiable to C91-C95

● Z80.7   Family history of other malignant neoplasms of lymphoid, hematopoietic and related tissues
           Conditions classifiable to C81-C90, C96.-

● Z80.8   Family history of malignant neoplasm of other organs or systems
           Conditions classifiable to C00-C14, C40-C49, C69-C79

● Z80.9   Family history of malignant neoplasm, unspecified
           Conditions classifiable to C80.1

● Z81   Family history of mental and behavioral disorders

● Z81.0   Family history of intellectual disabilities
           Conditions classifiable to F70-F79

● Z81.1   Family history of alcohol abuse and dependence
           Conditions classifiable to F10.-

● Z81.2   Family history of tobacco abuse and dependence
           Conditions classifiable to F17.-

● Z81.3   Family history of other psychoactive substance abuse and dependence
           Conditions classifiable to F11-F16, F18-F19

● Z81.4   Family history of other substance abuse and dependence
           Conditions classifiable to F55

● Z81.8   Family history of other mental and behavioral disorders
           Conditions classifiable elsewhere in F01-F99

● Z82   Family history of certain disabilities and chronic diseases (leading to disablement)

● Z82.0   Family history of epilepsy and other diseases of the nervous system
           Conditions classifiable to G00-G99

● Z82.1   Family history of blindness and visual loss
           Conditions classifiable to H54.-

● Z82.2   Family history of deafness and hearing loss
           Conditions classifiable to H90-H91

● Z82.3   Family history of stroke
           Conditions classifiable to I60-I64

● Z82.4   Family history of ischemic heart disease and other diseases of the circulatory system
           ⟹Conditions classifiable to I00-I5A, I65-I99

    ● Z82.41   Family history of sudden cardiac death

    ● Z82.49   Family history of ischemic heart disease and other diseases of the circulatory system

● Z82.5   Family history of asthma and other chronic lower respiratory diseases
           Conditions classifiable to J40-J47

           Excludes2   family history of other diseases of the respiratory system (Z83.6)

● Z82.6   Family history of arthritis and other diseases of the musculoskeletal system and connective tissue
           Conditions classifiable to M00-M99

    ● Z82.61   Family history of arthritis

    ● Z82.62   Family history of osteoporosis

    ● Z82.69   Family history of other diseases of the musculoskeletal system and connective tissue

● Z82.7   Family history of congenital malformations, deformations and chromosomal abnormalities
           Conditions classifiable to Q00-Q99

    ● Z82.71   Family history of polycystic kidney

    ● Z82.79   Family history of other congenital malformations, deformations and chromosomal abnormalities

● Z82.8   Family history of other disabilities and chronic diseases leading to disablement, not elsewhere classified

● Z83   Family history of other specific disorders

           Excludes2   contact with and (suspected) exposure to communicable disease in the family (Z20.-)

● Z83.0   Family history of human immunodeficiency virus [HIV] disease
           Conditions classifiable to B20

● Z83.1   Family history of other infectious and parasitic diseases
           Conditions classifiable to A00-B19, B25-B94, B99

● Z83.2   Family history of diseases of the blood and blood-forming organs and certain disorders involving the immune mechanism
           Conditions classifiable to D50-D89

● Z83.3   Family history of diabetes mellitus
           Conditions classifiable to E08-E13

● Z83.4   Family history of other endocrine, nutritional and metabolic diseases
           Conditions classifiable to E00-E07, E15-E88

    ● Z83.41   Family history of multiple endocrine neoplasia [MEN] syndrome

    ● Z83.42   Family history of familial hypercholesterolemia
                Coding Clinic: 2016, Q4, P77

    ● Z83.43   Family history of other disorder of lipoprotein metabolism and other lipidemias

        ● Z83.430   Family history of elevated lipoprotein(a)
                     Family history of elevated Lp(a)

        ● Z83.438   Family history of other disorder of lipoprotein metabolism and other lipidemia
                     Family history of familial combined hyperlipidemia

    ● Z83.49   Family history of other endocrine, nutritional and metabolic diseases

● Z83.5   Family history of eye and ear disorders

    ● Z83.51   Family history of eye disorders
                Conditions classifiable to H00-H53, H55-H59

                Excludes2   family history of blindness and visual loss (Z82.1)

        ● Z83.511   Family history of glaucoma

        ● Z83.518   Family history of other specified eye disorder

    ● Z83.52   Family history of ear disorders
                Conditions classifiable to H60-H83, H92-H95

                Excludes2   family history of deafness and hearing loss (Z82.2)

● Z83.6   Family history of other diseases of the respiratory system
           Conditions classifiable to J00-J39, J60-J99

           Excludes2   family history of asthma and other chronic lower respiratory diseases (Z82.5)

N Newborn Age: 0   P Pediatric Age: 0–17   M Maternity DX: 9–64   A Adult Age: 15–124   ♀ Females Only   ♂ Males Only

🅒 Complication\Comorbidity   🅜 Major C\C   (Ex) CC/MCC Exclusions   🅗 Hospital-Acquired Condition   🅗 Hierarchical Condition Category

1645

CHAPTER 21 (Z00-Z99)

● **Z83.7   Family history of diseases of the digestive system**
Conditions classifiable to K00-K93

  ● **Z83.71   Family history of colonic polyps**

  Excludes2   family history of malignant neoplasm of digestive organs (Z80.0)
  Coding Clinic: 2021, Q1, P15

  ● **Z83.79   Family history of other diseases of the digestive system**

● **Z84   Family history of other conditions**

  ● **Z84.0   Family history of diseases of the skin and subcutaneous tissue**
  Conditions classifiable to L00-L99

  ● **Z84.1   Family history of disorders of kidney and ureter**
  Conditions classifiable to N00-N29

  ● **Z84.2   Family history of other diseases of the genitourinary system**
  Conditions classifiable to N30-N99
  Coding Clinic: 2016, Q4, P77

  ● **Z84.3   Family history of consanguinity**

  ● **Z84.8   Family history of other specified conditions**

    ● **Z84.81   Family history of carrier of genetic disease**
    Coding Clinic: 2021, Q1, P15

    ● **Z84.82   Family history of sudden infant death syndrome**
    Family history of SIDS

    ● **Z84.89   Family history of other specified conditions**

● **Z85   Personal history of malignant neoplasm**

  Code first any follow-up examination after treatment of malignant neoplasm (Z08)

  Use additional code to identify:
  alcohol use and dependence (F10.-)
  exposure to environmental tobacco smoke (Z77.22)
  history of tobacco dependence (Z87.891)
  occupational exposure to environmental tobacco smoke (Z57.31)
  tobacco dependence (F17.-)
  tobacco use (Z72.0)

  Excludes2   personal history of benign neoplasm (Z86.01-)
  personal history of carcinoma-in-situ (Z86.00-)

  ● **Z85.0   Personal history of malignant neoplasm of digestive organs**

    ● **Z85.00   Personal history of malignant neoplasm of unspecified digestive organ**

    ● **Z85.01   Personal history of malignant neoplasm of esophagus**
    Conditions classifiable to C15

    ● **Z85.02   Personal history of malignant neoplasm of stomach**

      ● **Z85.020   Personal history of malignant carcinoid tumor of stomach**
      Conditions classifiable to C7A.092

      ● **Z85.028   Personal history of other malignant neoplasm of stomach**
      Conditions classifiable to C16

    ● **Z85.03   Personal history of malignant neoplasm of large intestine**

      ● **Z85.030   Personal history of malignant carcinoid tumor of large intestine**
      Conditions classifiable to C7A.022-C7A.025, C7A.029

      ● **Z85.038   Personal history of other malignant neoplasm of large intestine**
      Conditions classifiable to C18

    ● **Z85.04   Personal history of malignant neoplasm of rectum, rectosigmoid junction, and anus**

      ● **Z85.040   Personal history of malignant carcinoid tumor of rectum**
      Conditions classifiable to C7A.026

      ● **Z85.048   Personal history of other malignant neoplasm of rectum, rectosigmoid junction, and anus**
      Conditions classifiable to C19-C21

    ● **Z85.05   Personal history of malignant neoplasm of liver**
    Conditions classifiable to C22

    ● **Z85.06   Personal history of malignant neoplasm of small intestine**

      ● **Z85.060   Personal history of malignant carcinoid tumor of small intestine**
      Conditions classifiable to C7A.01-

      ● **Z85.068   Personal history of other malignant neoplasm of small intestine**
      Conditions classifiable to C17

    ● **Z85.07   Personal history of malignant neoplasm of pancreas**
    Conditions classifiable to C25

    ● **Z85.09   Personal history of malignant neoplasm of other digestive organs**

  ● **Z85.1   Personal history of malignant neoplasm of trachea, bronchus and lung**

    ● **Z85.11   Personal history of malignant neoplasm of bronchus and lung**

      ● **Z85.110   Personal history of malignant carcinoid tumor of bronchus and lung**
      Conditions classifiable to C7A.090

      ● **Z85.118   Personal history of other malignant neoplasm of bronchus and lung**
      Conditions classifiable to C34

    ● **Z85.12   Personal history of malignant neoplasm of trachea**
    Conditions classifiable to C33

  ● **Z85.2   Personal history of malignant neoplasm of other respiratory and intrathoracic organs**

    ● **Z85.20   Personal history of malignant neoplasm of unspecified respiratory organ**

    ● **Z85.21   Personal history of malignant neoplasm of larynx**
    Conditions classifiable to C32

    ● **Z85.22   Personal history of malignant neoplasm of nasal cavities, middle ear, and accessory sinuses**
    Conditions classifiable to C30-C31

    ● **Z85.23   Personal history of malignant neoplasm of thymus**

      ● **Z85.230   Personal history of malignant carcinoid tumor of thymus**
      Conditions classifiable to C7A.091

      ● **Z85.238   Personal history of other malignant neoplasm of thymus**
      Conditions classifiable to C37

    ● **Z85.29   Personal history of malignant neoplasm of other respiratory and intrathoracic organs**

  ● **Z85.3   Personal history of malignant neoplasm of breast**
  Conditions classifiable to C50.-

  ● **Z85.4   Personal history of malignant neoplasm of genital organs**
  Conditions classifiable to C51-C63

    ● **Z85.40   Personal history of malignant neoplasm of unspecified female genital organ ♀**

● **Z85.41**   Personal history of malignant neoplasm of cervix uteri ♀

● **Z85.42**   Personal history of malignant neoplasm of other parts of uterus ♀

● **Z85.43**   Personal history of malignant neoplasm of ovary ♀

● **Z85.44**   Personal history of malignant neoplasm of other female genital organs ♀

● **Z85.45**   Personal history of malignant neoplasm of unspecified male genital organ ♂

● **Z85.46**   Personal history of malignant neoplasm of prostate ♂

● **Z85.47**   Personal history of malignant neoplasm of testis ♂

● **Z85.48**   Personal history of malignant neoplasm of epididymis ♂

● **Z85.49**   Personal history of malignant neoplasm of other male genital organs ♂

● **Z85.5**   Personal history of malignant neoplasm of urinary tract
Conditions classifiable to C64-C68

● **Z85.50**   Personal history of malignant neoplasm of unspecified urinary tract organ

● **Z85.51**   Personal history of malignant neoplasm of bladder

● **Z85.52**   Personal history of malignant neoplasm of kidney

     Excludes1   personal history of malignant neoplasm of renal pelvis (Z85.53)

● **Z85.520**   Personal history of malignant carcinoid tumor of kidney
Conditions classifiable to C7A.093

● **Z85.528**   Personal history of other malignant neoplasm of kidney
Conditions classifiable to C64

● **Z85.53**   Personal history of malignant neoplasm of renal pelvis

● **Z85.54**   Personal history of malignant neoplasm of ureter

● **Z85.59**   Personal history of malignant neoplasm of other urinary tract organ

● **Z85.6**   Personal history of leukemia
Conditions classifiable to C91-C95

     Excludes1   leukemia in remission C91.0-C95.9 with 5th character 1

● **Z85.7**   Personal history of other malignant neoplasms of lymphoid, hematopoietic and related tissues

● **Z85.71**   Personal history of Hodgkin lymphoma
Conditions classifiable to C81

● **Z85.72**   Personal history of non-Hodgkin lymphomas
Conditions classifiable to C82-C85

● **Z85.79**   Personal history of other malignant neoplasms of lymphoid, hematopoietic and related tissues
Conditions classifiable to C88-C90, C96

     Excludes1   multiple myeloma in remission (C90.01)
plasma cell leukemia in remission (C90.11)
plasmacytoma in remission (C90.21)

● **Z85.8**   Personal history of malignant neoplasms of other organs and systems
Conditions classifiable to C00-C14, C40-C49, C69-C75, C7A.098, C76-C79

● **Z85.81**   Personal history of malignant neoplasm of lip, oral cavity, and pharynx
Conditions classifiable to C00-C14

● **Z85.810**   Personal history of malignant neoplasm of tongue

● **Z85.818**   Personal history of malignant neoplasm of other sites of lip, oral cavity, and pharynx

● **Z85.819**   Personal history of malignant neoplasm of unspecified site of lip, oral cavity, and pharynx

● **Z85.82**   Personal history of malignant neoplasm of skin

● **Z85.820**   Personal history of malignant melanoma of skin
Conditions classifiable to C43

● **Z85.821**   Personal history of Merkel cell carcinoma
Conditions classifiable to C4A

● **Z85.828**   Personal history of other malignant neoplasm of skin
Conditions classifiable to C44

● **Z85.83**   Personal history of malignant neoplasm of bone and soft tissue
Conditions classifiable to C40-C41; C45-C49

● **Z85.830**   Personal history of malignant neoplasm of bone

● **Z85.831**   Personal history of malignant neoplasm of soft tissue

     Excludes2   personal history of malignant neoplasm of skin (Z85.82-)

● **Z85.84**   Personal history of malignant neoplasm of eye and nervous tissue
Conditions classifiable to C69-C72

● **Z85.840**   Personal history of malignant neoplasm of eye

● **Z85.841**   Personal history of malignant neoplasm of brain

● **Z85.848**   Personal history of malignant neoplasm of other parts of nervous tissue

● **Z85.85**   Personal history of malignant neoplasm of endocrine glands
Conditions classifiable to C73-C75

● **Z85.850**   Personal history of malignant neoplasm of thyroid

● **Z85.858**   Personal history of malignant neoplasm of other endocrine glands

● **Z85.89**   Personal history of malignant neoplasm of other organs and systems
Conditions classifiable to C7A.098, C76, C77-C79

● **Z85.9**   Personal history of malignant neoplasm, unspecified
Conditions classifiable to C7A.00, C80.1

● **Z86**   Personal history of certain other diseases
Code first any follow-up examination after treatment (Z09)

● **Z86.0**   Personal history of in-situ and benign neoplasms and neoplasms of uncertain behavior

     Excludes2   personal history of malignant neoplasms (Z85.-)

● **Z86.00**   Personal history of in-situ neoplasm
Conditions classifiable to D00-D09

● **Z86.000**   Personal history of in-situ neoplasm of breast
Conditions classifiable to D05

● **Z86.001**   Personal history of in-situ neoplasm of cervix uteri ♀
Conditions classifiable to D06
Personal history of cervical intraepithelial neoplasia III [CIN III]

N Newborn Age: 0   **P** Pediatric Age: 0–17   **M** Maternity DX: 9–64   **A** Adult Age: 15–124   ♀ Females Only   ♂ Males Only

🖇 Complication\Comorbidity   🖇 Major C\C   (Ex) CC/MCC Exclusions   🖇 Hospital-Acquired Condition   🖇 Hierarchical Condition Category

1647

CHAPTER 21 (Z00-Z99)

CHAPTER 21 (Z00-Z99)

- ● Z86.002　**Personal history of in-situ neoplasm of other and unspecified genital organs**
  Conditions classifiable to D07
  Personal history of high-grade prostatic intraepithelial neoplasia III [HGPIN III]
  Personal history of vaginal intraepithelial neoplasia III [VAIN III]
  Personal history of vulvar intraepithelial neoplasia III [VIN III]
- ● Z86.003　**Personal history of in-situ neoplasm of oral cavity, esophagus and stomach**
  Conditions classifiable to D00
- ● Z86.004　**Personal history of in-situ neoplasm of other and unspecified digestive organs**
  Conditions classifiable to D01
  Personal history of anal intraepithelial neoplasia (AIN III)
- ● Z86.005　**Personal history of in-situ neoplasm of middle ear and respiratory system**
  Conditions classifiable to D02
- ● Z86.006　**Personal history of melanoma in-situ**
  Conditions classifiable to D03
  Excludes2　sites other than skin - code to personal history of in-situ neoplasm of the site
- ● Z86.007　**Personal history of in-situ neoplasm of skin**
  Conditions classifiable to D04
  Personal history of carcinoma in situ of skin
- ● Z86.008　**Personal history of in-situ neoplasm of other site**
  Conditions classifiable to D09
- ● Z86.01　**Personal history of benign neoplasm**
  Coding Clinic: 2017, Q1, P14
  - ● Z86.010　**Personal history of colonic polyps**
    Coding Clinic: 2021, Q1, P15; 2017, Q1, P9, P14
  - ● Z86.011　**Personal history of benign neoplasm of the brain**
  - ● Z86.012　**Personal history of benign carcinoid tumor**
  - ● Z86.018　**Personal history of other benign neoplasm**
    Coding Clinic: 2017, Q1, P14
- ● Z86.03　**Personal history of neoplasm of uncertain behavior**
- ● Z86.1　**Personal history of infectious and parasitic diseases**
  Conditions classifiable to A00-B89, B99
  Excludes1　personal history of infectious diseases specific to a body system sequelae of infectious and parasitic diseases (B90-B94)
  Coding Clinic: 2016, Q4, P5
  - ● Z86.11　**Personal history of tuberculosis**
  - ● Z86.12　**Personal history of poliomyelitis**
  - ● Z86.13　**Personal history of malaria**
  - ● Z86.14　**Personal history of Methicillin resistant Staphylococcus aureus infection**
    Personal history of MRSA infection
  - ● Z86.15　**Personal history of latent tuberculosis infection**
  - ● Z86.16　**Personal history of COVID-19**
    Coding Clinic: 2021, Q1, P34-35, 40-42, 44, 46
    ▶ **Excludes1**　post COVID-19 condition (U09.9)

- ● Z86.19　**Personal history of other infectious and parasitic diseases**
  Coding Clinic: 2021, Q1, P34-35, 40-41
- ● Z86.2　**Personal history of diseases of the blood and blood-forming organs and certain disorders involving the immune mechanism**
  Conditions classifiable to D50-D89
- ● Z86.3　**Personal history of endocrine, nutritional and metabolic diseases**
  Conditions classifiable to E00-E88
  - ● Z86.31　**Personal history of diabetic foot ulcer**
    Excludes2　current diabetic foot ulcer (E08.621, E09.621, E10.621, E11.621, E13.621)
  - ● Z86.32　**Personal history of gestational diabetes** ♀
    Personal history of conditions classifiable to O24.4-
    Excludes1　gestational diabetes mellitus in current pregnancy (O24.4-)
  - ● Z86.39　**Personal history of other endocrine, nutritional and metabolic disease**
    Coding Clinic: 2020, Q1, P13
- ● Z86.5　**Personal history of mental and behavioral disorders**
  Conditions classifiable to F40-F59
  - ● Z86.51　**Personal history of combat and operational stress reaction**　A
  - ● Z86.59　**Personal history of other mental and behavioral disorders**
- ● Z86.6　**Personal history of diseases of the nervous system and sense organs**
  Conditions classifiable to G00-G99, H00-H95
  - ● Z86.61　**Personal history of infections of the central nervous system**
    Personal history of encephalitis
    Personal history of meningitis
  - ● Z86.69　**Personal history of other diseases of the nervous system and sense organs**
    Coding Clinic: 2016, Q4, P25
- ● Z86.7　**Personal history of diseases of the circulatory system**
  Conditions classifiable to I00-I99
  Excludes2　old myocardial infarction (I25.2)
  personal history of anaphylactic shock (Z87.892)
  postmyocardial infarction syndrome (I24.1)
  - ● Z86.71　**Personal history of venous thrombosis and embolism**
    - ● Z86.711　**Personal history of pulmonary embolism**
    - ● Z86.718　**Personal history of other venous thrombosis and embolism**
  - ● Z86.72　**Personal history of thrombophlebitis**
  - ● Z86.73　**Personal history of transient ischemic attack (TIA), and cerebral infarction without residual deficits**
    Personal history of prolonged reversible ischemic neurological deficit (PRIND)
    Personal history of stroke NOS without residual deficits
    Excludes1　personal history of traumatic brain injury (Z87.820)
    sequelae of cerebrovascular disease (I69.-)
    Coding Clinic: 2012, Q4, P3
  - ● Z86.74　**Personal history of sudden cardiac arrest**
    Personal history of sudden cardiac death successfully resuscitated
  - ● Z86.79　**Personal history of other diseases of the circulatory system**
    Coding Clinic: 2020, Q1, P13

▶ New　⇒ Revised　d̶e̶l̶e̶t̶e̶d̶ Deleted　Excludes 1　Excludes 2　Includes　Use additional　Code first　Code also　Key words

1648　OGCR Official Guidelines　● Unacceptable Principal Diagnosis　X Assign placeholder X　● Use Additional Character(s)　▶ Manifestation Code　Coding Clinic

- **Z87   Personal history of other diseases and conditions**
  Code first any follow-up examination after treatment (Z09)
  - **Z87.0   Personal history of diseases of the respiratory system**
    Conditions classifiable to J00-J99
    - **Z87.01   Personal history of pneumonia (recurrent)**
    - **Z87.09   Personal history of other diseases of the respiratory system**
  - **Z87.1   Personal history of diseases of the digestive system**
    Conditions classifiable to K00-K93
    - **Z87.11   Personal history of peptic ulcer disease**
    - **Z87.19   Personal history of other diseases of the digestive system**
      Coding Clinic: 2017, Q1, P14
  - **Z87.2   Personal history of diseases of the skin and subcutaneous tissue**
    Conditions classifiable to L00-L99
    - **Excludes2**   personal history of diabetic foot ulcer (Z86.31)
  - **Z87.3   Personal history of diseases of the musculoskeletal system and connective tissue**
    Conditions classifiable to M00-M99
    - **Excludes2**   personal history of (healed) traumatic fracture (Z87.81)
    - **Z87.31   Personal history of (healed) nontraumatic fracture**
      - **Z87.310   Personal history of (healed) osteoporosis fracture**
        Personal history of (healed) fragility fracture
        Personal history of (healed) collapsed vertebra due to osteoporosis
      - **Z87.311   Personal history of (healed) other pathological fracture**
        Personal history of (healed) collapsed vertebra NOS
        - **Excludes2**   personal history of osteoporosis fracture (Z87.310)
      - **Z87.312   Personal history of (healed) stress fracture**
        Personal history of (healed) fatigue fracture
    - **Z87.39   Personal history of other diseases of the musculoskeletal system and connective tissue**
  - **Z87.4   Personal history of diseases of genitourinary system**
    Conditions classifiable to N00-N99
    - **Z87.41   Personal history of dysplasia of the female genital tract**
      - **Excludes1**   personal history of intraepithelial neoplasia III of female genital tract (Z86.001, Z86.008)
        personal history of malignant neoplasm of female genital tract (Z85.40-Z85.44)
      - **Z87.410   Personal history of cervical dysplasia ♀**
      - **Z87.411   Personal history of vaginal dysplasia ♀**
      - **Z87.412   Personal history of vulvar dysplasia ♀**
    - **Z87.42   Personal history of other diseases of the female genital tract ♀**

- **Z87.43   Personal history of diseases of male genital organs**
  - **Z87.430   Personal history of prostatic dysplasia ♂**
    - **Excludes1**   personal history of malignant neoplasm of prostate (Z85.46)
  - **Z87.438   Personal history of other diseases of male genital organs ♂**
- **Z87.44   Personal history of diseases of urinary system**
  - **Excludes1**   personal history of malignant neoplasm of cervix uteri (Z85.41)
  - **Z87.440   Personal history of urinary (tract) infections**
  - **Z87.441   Personal history of nephrotic syndrome**
  - **Z87.442   Personal history of urinary calculi**
    Personal history of kidney stones
  - **Z87.448   Personal history of other diseases of urinary system**
- **Z87.5   Personal history of complications of pregnancy, childbirth and the puerperium**
  Conditions classifiable to O00-O9A
  - **Excludes2**   recurrent pregnancy loss (N96)
  - **Z87.51   Personal history of pre-term labor ♀**
    - **Excludes1**   current pregnancy with history of pre-term labor (O09.21-)
  - **Z87.59   Personal history of other complications of pregnancy, childbirth and the puerperium ♀**
    Personal history of trophoblastic disease
- **Z87.7   Personal history of (corrected) congenital malformations**
  Conditions classifiable to Q00-Q89 that have been repaired or corrected
  - **Excludes1**   congenital malformations that have been partially corrected or repair but which still require medical treatment - code to condition
  - **Excludes2**   other postprocedural states (Z98.-)
    personal history of medical treatment (Z92.-)
    presence of cardiac and vascular implants and grafts (Z95.-)
    presence of other devices (Z97.-)
    presence of other functional implants (Z96.-)
    transplanted organ and tissue status (Z94.-)
  - **Z87.71   Personal history of (corrected) congenital malformations of genitourinary system**
    - **Z87.710   Personal history of (corrected) hypospadias ♂**
    - **Z87.718   Personal history of other specified (corrected) congenital malformations of genitourinary system**
  - **Z87.72   Personal history of (corrected) congenital malformations of nervous system and sense organs**
    - **Z87.720   Personal history of (corrected) congenital malformations of eye**
    - **Z87.721   Personal history of (corrected) congenital malformations of ear**
    - **Z87.728   Personal history of other specified (corrected) congenital malformations of nervous system and sense organs**

CHAPTER 21 (Z00-Z99)

- ● Z87.73 Personal history of (corrected) congenital malformations of digestive system
  - ● Z87.730 Personal history of (corrected) cleft lip and palate
  - ● Z87.738 Personal history of other specified (corrected) congenital malformations of digestive system
- ● Z87.74 Personal history of (corrected) congenital malformations of heart and circulatory system
- ● Z87.75 Personal history of (corrected) congenital malformations of respiratory system
- ● Z87.76 Personal history of (corrected) congenital malformations of integument, limbs and musculoskeletal system
- ● Z87.79 Personal history of other (corrected) congenital malformations
  - ● Z87.790 Personal history of (corrected) congenital malformations of face and neck
  - ● Z87.798 Personal history of other (corrected) congenital malformations
- ● Z87.8 Personal history of other specified conditions
  - ➡ **Excludes2** personal history of self harm (Z91.5-)
  - ● Z87.81 Personal history of (healed) traumatic fracture
    - **Excludes2** personal history of (healed) nontraumatic fracture (Z87.31-)
  - ● Z87.82 Personal history of other (healed) physical injury and trauma
    - Conditions classifiable to S00-T88, except traumatic fractures
    - ● Z87.820 Personal history of traumatic brain injury
      - **Excludes1** personal history of transient ischemic attack (TIA), and cerebral infarction without residual deficits (Z86.73)
    - ● Z87.821 Personal history of retained foreign body fully removed
    - ● Z87.828 Personal history of other (healed) physical injury and trauma
  - ● Z87.89 Personal history of other specified conditions
    - Z87.890 Personal history of sex reassignment
    - ● Z87.891 Personal history of nicotine dependence
      - **Excludes1** current nicotine dependence (F17.2-)
      - Coding Clinic: 2017, Q2, P27
    - ● Z87.892 Personal history of anaphylaxis
      - Code also allergy status such as: allergy status to drugs, medicaments and biological substances (Z88.-) allergy status, other than to drugs and biological substances (Z91.0-)
    - ● Z87.898 Personal history of other specified conditions
      - Coding Clinic: 2013, Q1, P21
- ● Z88 Allergy status to drugs, medicaments and biological substances
  - **Excludes2** allergy status, other than to drugs and biological substances (Z91.0-)
  - ● Z88.0 Allergy status to penicillin
  - ● Z88.1 Allergy status to other antibiotic agents
  - ● Z88.2 Allergy status to sulfonamides
    - Coding Clinic: 2015, Q3, P23
- ● Z88.3 Allergy status to other anti-infective agents
- ● Z88.4 Allergy status to anesthetic agent
- ● Z88.5 Allergy status to narcotic agent
- ● Z88.6 Allergy status to analgesic agent
- ● Z88.7 Allergy status to serum and vaccine
- ● Z88.8 Allergy status to other drugs, medicaments and biological substances
- ● Z88.9 Allergy status to unspecified drugs, medicaments and biological substances
- ● Z89 Acquired absence of limb
  - **Includes** amputation status / postprocedural loss of limb / post-traumatic loss of limb
  - **Excludes1** acquired deformities of limbs (M20-M21) / congenital absence of limbs (Q71-Q73)
  - ● Z89.0 Acquired absence of thumb and other finger(s)
    - ● Z89.01 Acquired absence of thumb
      - ● Z89.011 Acquired absence of right thumb
      - ● Z89.012 Acquired absence of left thumb
      - ● Z89.019 Acquired absence of unspecified thumb
    - ● Z89.02 Acquired absence of other finger(s)
      - **Excludes2** acquired absence of thumb (Z89.01-)
      - ● Z89.021 Acquired absence of right finger(s)
      - ● Z89.022 Acquired absence of left finger(s)
      - ● Z89.029 Acquired absence of unspecified finger(s)
  - ● Z89.1 Acquired absence of hand and wrist
    - ● Z89.11 Acquired absence of hand
      - ● Z89.111 Acquired absence of right hand
      - ● Z89.112 Acquired absence of left hand
      - ● Z89.119 Acquired absence of unspecified hand
    - ● Z89.12 Acquired absence of wrist
      - Disarticulation at wrist
      - ● Z89.121 Acquired absence of right wrist
      - ● Z89.122 Acquired absence of left wrist
      - ● Z89.129 Acquired absence of unspecified wrist
  - ● Z89.2 Acquired absence of upper limb above wrist
    - ● Z89.20 Acquired absence of upper limb, unspecified level
      - ● Z89.201 Acquired absence of right upper limb, unspecified level
      - ● Z89.202 Acquired absence of left upper limb, unspecified level
      - ● Z89.209 Acquired absence of unspecified upper limb, unspecified level
        - Acquired absence of arm NOS
    - ● Z89.21 Acquired absence of upper limb below elbow
      - ● Z89.211 Acquired absence of right upper limb below elbow
      - ● Z89.212 Acquired absence of left upper limb below elbow
      - ● Z89.219 Acquired absence of unspecified upper limb below elbow
    - ● Z89.22 Acquired absence of upper limb above elbow
      - Disarticulation at elbow
      - ● Z89.221 Acquired absence of right upper limb above elbow
      - ● Z89.222 Acquired absence of left upper limb above elbow
      - ● Z89.229 Acquired absence of unspecified upper limb above elbow

- Z89.23   Acquired absence of shoulder
  Acquired absence of shoulder joint following explantation of shoulder joint prosthesis, with or without presence of antibiotic-impregnated cement spacer
  - Z89.231   Acquired absence of right shoulder
  - Z89.232   Acquired absence of left shoulder
  - Z89.239   Acquired absence of unspecified shoulder
- Z89.4   Acquired absence of toe(s), foot, and ankle
  - Z89.41   Acquired absence of great toe
    - Z89.411   Acquired absence of right great toe 🦠
    - Z89.412   Acquired absence of left great toe 🦠
    - Z89.419   Acquired absence of unspecified great toe 🦠
  - Z89.42   Acquired absence of other toe(s)
    Excludes2   acquired absence of great toe (Z89.41-)
    - Z89.421   Acquired absence of other right toe(s) 🦠
    - Z89.422   Acquired absence of other left toe(s) 🦠
    - Z89.429   Acquired absence of other toe(s), unspecified side 🦠
  - Z89.43   Acquired absence of foot
    - Z89.431   Acquired absence of right foot 🦠
    - Z89.432   Acquired absence of left foot 🦠
    - Z89.439   Acquired absence of unspecified foot 🦠
  - Z89.44   Acquired absence of ankle
    Disarticulation of ankle
    - Z89.441   Acquired absence of right ankle 🦠
    - Z89.442   Acquired absence of left ankle 🦠
    - Z89.449   Acquired absence of unspecified ankle 🦠
- Z89.5   Acquired absence of leg below knee
  - Z89.51   Acquired absence of leg below knee
    - Z89.511   Acquired absence of right leg below knee 🦠
    - Z89.512   Acquired absence of left leg below knee 🦠
    - Z89.519   Acquired absence of unspecified leg below knee 🦠
  - Z89.52   Acquired absence of knee
    Acquired absence of knee joint following explantation of knee joint prosthesis, with or without presence of antibiotic-impregnated cement spacer
    - Z89.521   Acquired absence of right knee
    - Z89.522   Acquired absence of left knee
    - Z89.529   Acquired absence of unspecified knee
- Z89.6   Acquired absence of leg above knee
  - Z89.61   Acquired absence of leg above knee
    Acquired absence of leg NOS
    Disarticulation at knee
    - Z89.611   Acquired absence of right leg above knee 🦠
    - Z89.612   Acquired absence of left leg above knee 🦠
    - Z89.619   Acquired absence of unspecified leg above knee 🦠
  - Z89.62   Acquired absence of hip
    Acquired absence of hip joint following explantation of hip joint prosthesis, with or without presence of antibiotic-impregnated cement spacer
    Disarticulation at hip

- Z89.621   Acquired absence of right hip joint
- Z89.622   Acquired absence of left hip joint
- Z89.629   Acquired absence of unspecified hip joint
- Z89.9   Acquired absence of limb, unspecified
- Z90   Acquired absence of organs, not elsewhere classified
  Includes   postprocedural or post-traumatic loss of body part NEC
  Excludes1   congenital absence - see Alphabetical Index
  Excludes2   postprocedural absence of endocrine glands (E89.-)
  - Z90.0   Acquired absence of part of head and neck
    - Z90.01   Acquired absence of eye
    - Z90.02   Acquired absence of larynx
    - Z90.09   Acquired absence of other part of head and neck
      Acquired absence of nose
      Excludes2   teeth (K08.1)
  - Z90.1   Acquired absence of breast and nipple
    - Z90.10   Acquired absence of unspecified breast and nipple
    - Z90.11   Acquired absence of right breast and nipple
    - Z90.12   Acquired absence of left breast and nipple
    - Z90.13   Acquired absence of bilateral breasts and nipples
  - Z90.2   Acquired absence of lung [part of]
  - Z90.3   Acquired absence of stomach [part of]
  - Z90.4   Acquired absence of other specified parts of digestive tract
    - Z90.41   Acquired absence of pancreas
      Code also exocrine pancreatic insufficiency (K86.81)
      Use additional code to identify any associated: diabetes mellitus, postpancreatectomy (E13.-)
      insulin use (Z79.4)
      - Z90.410   Acquired total absence of pancreas
        Acquired absence of pancreas NOS
      - Z90.411   Acquired partial absence of pancreas
    - Z90.49   Acquired absence of other specified parts of digestive tract
  - Z90.5   Acquired absence of kidney
  - Z90.6   Acquired absence of other parts of urinary tract
    Acquired absence of bladder
  - Z90.7   Acquired absence of genital organ(s)
    Excludes1   personal history of sex reassignment (Z87.890)
    Excludes2   female genital mutilation status (N90.81-)
    - Z90.71   Acquired absence of cervix and uterus
      - Z90.710   Acquired absence of both cervix and uterus ♀
        Acquired absence of uterus NOS
        Status post total hysterectomy
      - Z90.711   Acquired absence of uterus with remaining cervical stump ♀
        Status post partial hysterectomy with remaining cervical stump
      - Z90.712   Acquired absence of cervix with remaining uterus ♀
    - Z90.72   Acquired absence of ovaries
      - Z90.721   Acquired absence of ovaries, unilateral ♀
      - Z90.722   Acquired absence of ovaries, bilateral ♀
    - Z90.79   Acquired absence of other genital organ(s)

N Newborn Age: 0   **P** Pediatric Age: 0–17   **M** Maternity DX: 9–64   **A** Adult Age: 15–124   ♀ Females Only   ♂ Males Only

🦠 Complication\Comorbidity   🦠 Major C\C   (Ex) CC/MCC Exclusions   🦠 Hospital-Acquired Condition   🦠 Hierarchical Condition Category   **1651**

CHAPTER 21 (Z00-Z99)

CHAPTER 21 (Z00-Z99)

● **Z90.8   Acquired absence of other organs**
    ● **Z90.81   Acquired absence of spleen**
    ● **Z90.89   Acquired absence of other organs**

● **Z91   Personal risk factors, not elsewhere classified**
    Excludes2   contact with and (suspected) exposures hazardous to health (Z77.-)
        exposure to pollution and other problems related to physical environment (Z77.1-)
        female genital mutilation status (N90.81-)
        occupational exposure to risk factors (Z57.-)
        personal history of physical injury and trauma (Z87.81, Z87.82-)

  ● **Z91.0   Allergy status, other than to drugs and biological substances**
    Excludes2   allergy status to drugs, medicaments, and biological substances (Z88.-)

    ● **Z91.01   Food allergy status**
      Excludes2   food additives allergy status (Z91.02)
      ● **Z91.010   Allergy to peanuts**
      ● **Z91.011   Allergy to milk products**
        Excludes1   lactose intolerance (E73.-)
      ● **Z91.012   Allergy to eggs**
      ● **Z91.013   Allergy to seafood**
        Allergy to shellfish
        Allergy to octopus or squid ink
      ▶● **Z91.014   Allergy to mammalian meats**
        ▶Allergy to beef
        ▶Allergy to lamb
        ▶Allergy to pork
        ▶Allergy to red meats
      ● **Z91.018   Allergy to other foods**
        Allergy to nuts other than peanuts
    ● **Z91.02   Food additives allergy status**
    ● **Z91.03   Insect allergy status**
      ● **Z91.030   Bee allergy status**
      ● **Z91.038   Other insect allergy status**
    ● **Z91.04   Nonmedicinal substance allergy status**
      ● **Z91.040   Latex allergy status**
        Latex sensitivity status
      ● **Z91.041   Radiographic dye allergy status**
        Allergy status to contrast media used for diagnostic X-ray procedure
      ● **Z91.048   Other nonmedicinal substance allergy status**
    ● **Z91.09   Other allergy status, other than to drugs and biological substances**

  ● **Z91.1   Patient's noncompliance with medical treatment and regimen**
    ● **Z91.11   Patient's noncompliance with dietary regimen**
    ● **Z91.12   Patient's intentional underdosing of medication regimen**
      Code first underdosing of medication (T36-T50) with fifth or sixth character 6
      Excludes1   adverse effect of prescribed drug taken as directed - code to adverse effect
        poisoning (overdose) - code to poisoning
      ● **Z91.120   Patient's intentional underdosing of medication regimen due to financial hardship**
      ● **Z91.128   Patient's intentional underdosing of medication regimen for other reason**

    ● **Z91.13   Patient's unintentional underdosing of medication regimen**
      Code first underdosing of medication (T36-T50) with fifth or sixth character 6
      Excludes1   adverse effect of prescribed drug taken as directed - code to adverse effect
        poisoning (overdose) - code to poisoning
      ● **Z91.130   Patient's unintentional underdosing of medication regimen due to age-related debility**
      ● **Z91.138   Patient's unintentional underdosing of medication regimen for other reason**
    ● **Z91.14   Patient's other noncompliance with medication regimen**
      Patient's underdosing of medication NOS
    ● **Z91.15   Patient's noncompliance with renal dialysis** 🖦
    ● **Z91.19   Patient's noncompliance with other medical treatment and regimen**
      Nonadherence to medical treatment

  ● **Z91.4   Personal history of psychological trauma, not elsewhere classified**
    ● **Z91.41   Personal history of adult abuse**
      Excludes2   personal history of abuse in childhood (Z62.81-)
      ● **Z91.410   Personal history of adult physical and sexual abuse**   A
        Excludes1   current adult physical abuse (T74.11, T76.11)
          current adult sexual abuse (T74.21, T76.11)
      ● **Z91.411   Personal history of adult psychological abuse**   A
      ● **Z91.412   Personal history of adult neglect**   A
        Excludes1   current adult neglect (T74.01, T76.01)
      ● **Z91.419   Personal history of unspecified adult abuse**   A
    ● **Z91.42   Personal history of forced labor or sexual exploitation**
    ● **Z91.49   Other personal history of psychological trauma, not elsewhere classified**

  ⇒● **Z91.5   Personal history of self-harm**
    ~~Personal history of parasuicide~~
    ~~Personal history of self-poisoning~~
    ~~Personal history of suicide attempt~~
    ▶Code also mental health disorder, if known
    ▶● **Z91.51   Personal history of suicidal behavior**
      ▶Personal history of parasuicide
      ▶Personal history of self-poisoning
      ▶Personal history of suicide attempt
    ▶● **Z91.52   Personal history of nonsuicidal self-harm**
      ▶Personal history of nonsuicidal self-injury
      ▶Personal history of self-inflicted injury without suicidal intent
      ▶Personal history of self-mutilation

  ● **Z91.8   Other specified personal risk factors, not elsewhere classified**
    ● **Z91.81   History of falling**
      At risk for falling

▶ New   ⇒ Revised   ~~deleted~~ Deleted   Excludes 1   Excludes 2   Includes   Use additional   Code first   Code also   Key words

OGCR Official Guidelines   ● Unacceptable Principal Diagnosis   X Assign placeholder X   ● Use Additional Character(s)   ▷ Manifestation Code   **Coding Clinic**

● **Z91.82**   **Personal history of military deployment**   A
              Individual (civilian or military) with past
                  history of military war, peacekeeping and
                  humanitarian deployment (current or past
                  conflict)
              Returned from military deployment

▷ **Z91.83**   *Wandering in diseases classified elsewhere*
              Code first underlying disorder such as:
                  Alzheimer's disease (G30.-)
                  autism or pervasive developmental disorder
                      (F84.-)
                  intellectual disabilities (F70-F79)
                  unspecified dementia with behavioral
                      disturbance (F03.9-)

● **Z91.84**   **Oral health risk factors**
   ● **Z91.841**   **Risk for dental caries, low**
   ● **Z91.842**   **Risk for dental caries, moderate**
   ● **Z91.843**   **Risk for dental caries, high**
   ● **Z91.849**   **Unspecified risk for dental caries**

● **Z91.89**   **Other specified personal risk factors, not
              elsewhere classified**
              Coding Clinic: 2017, Q1, P46

● **Z92**   **Personal history of medical treatment**
         Excludes2   postprocedural states (Z98.-)

● **Z92.0**   **Personal history of contraception**
         Excludes1   counseling or management of current
                      contraceptive practices (Z30.-)
                  long term (current) use of contraception
                      (Z79.3)
                  presence of (intrauterine) contraceptive
                      device (Z97.5)

● **Z92.2**   **Personal history of drug therapy**
         Excludes2   long term (current) drug therapy (Z79.-)
   ● **Z92.21**   **Personal history of antineoplastic
              chemotherapy**
   ● **Z92.22**   **Personal history of monoclonal drug therapy**
   ● **Z92.23**   **Personal history of estrogen therapy**
   ● **Z92.24**   **Personal history of steroid therapy**
      ● **Z92.240**   **Personal history of inhaled steroid
                  therapy**
      ● **Z92.241**   **Personal history of systemic steroid
                  therapy**
                  Personal history of steroid therapy
                      NOS
   ➠● **Z92.25**   **Personal history of immunosuppression
              therapy**
              Excludes2   personal history of steroid
                          therapy (Z92.24)
   ● **Z92.29**   **Personal history of other drug therapy**

● **Z92.3**   **Personal history of irradiation**
              Personal history of exposure to therapeutic radiation
         Excludes1   exposure to radiation in the physical
                      environment (Z77.12)
                  occupational exposure to radiation
                      (Z57.1)

● **Z92.8**   **Personal history of other medical treatment**
              Coding Clinic: 2016, Q4, P72
   ● **Z92.81**   **Personal history of extracorporeal membrane
              oxygenation (ECMO)**
   ● **Z92.82**   **Status post administration of tPA (rtPA) in a
              different facility within the last 24 hours prior
              to admission to current facility**
              *Code first condition requiring tPA administration,
                  such as:*
                  acute cerebral infarction (I63.-)
                  acute myocardial infarction (I21.-, I22.-)

● **Z92.83**   **Personal history of failed moderate sedation**
              Personal history of failed conscious sedation
              Excludes2   failed moderate sedation during
                          procedure (T88.52)
● **Z92.84**   **Personal history of unintended awareness
              under general anesthesia**
              Excludes2   unintended awareness under
                          general anesthesia during
                          procedure (T88.53)
              Coding Clinic: 2016, Q4, P72, 77

▷● **Z92.85** **Personal history of cellular therapy**
   ▷● **Z92.850** **Personal history of Chimeric Antigen
                  Receptor T-cell therapy**
                  ▷Personal history of CAR T-cell
                      therapy
   ▷● **Z92.858** **Personal history of other cellular
                  therapy**
   ▷● **Z92.859** **Personal history of cellular therapy,
                  unspecified**

▷● **Z92.86** **Personal history of gene therapy**

● **Z92.89**   **Personal history of other medical treatment**
              Coding Clinic: 2020, Q1, P18

● **Z93**   **Artificial opening status**
         Excludes1   artificial openings requiring attention or
                      management (Z43.-)
                  complications of external stoma (J95.0-, K94.-,
                      N99.5-)

● **Z93.0**   **Tracheostomy status** 🅗🅒
● **Z93.1**   **Gastrostomy status** 🅗🅒
● **Z93.2**   **Ileostomy status** 🅗🅒
● **Z93.3**   **Colostomy status** 🅗🅒
● **Z93.4**   **Other artificial openings of gastrointestinal tract
              status** 🅗🅒
● **Z93.5**   **Cystostomy status** 🅗🅒
   ● **Z93.50**   **Unspecified cystostomy status** 🅗🅒
   ● **Z93.51**   **Cutaneous-vesicostomy status** 🅗🅒
   ● **Z93.52**   **Appendico-vesicostomy status** 🅗🅒
   ● **Z93.59**   **Other cystostomy status** 🅗🅒
● **Z93.6**   **Other artificial openings of urinary tract status** 🅗🅒
              Nephrostomy status
              Ureterostomy status
              Urethrostomy status
● **Z93.8**   **Other artificial opening status** 🅗🅒
● **Z93.9**   **Artificial opening status, unspecified** 🅗🅒

● **Z94**   **Transplanted organ and tissue status**
         Includes   organ or tissue replaced by heterogenous or
                      homogenous transplant
         Excludes1   complications of transplanted organ or tissue -
                      see Alphabetical Index
         Excludes2   presence of vascular grafts (Z95.-)
● **Z94.0**   **Kidney transplant status** 🅒
              (Ex) See PDX Collection 1489
● **Z94.1**   **Heart transplant status** 🅒 🅗🅒
              Excludes1   artificial heart status (Z95.812)
                          heart-valve replacement status
                              (Z95.2-Z95.4)
              (Ex) See PDX Collection 1488
● **Z94.2**   **Lung transplant status** 🅒 🅗🅒
              (Ex) See PDX Collection 1491
● **Z94.3**   **Heart and lungs transplant status** 🅒 🅗🅒
              CC when PDx is its own CC
              (Ex) See PDX Collection 1488

CHAPTER 21 (Z00-Z99)

N Newborn Age: Ø   **P** Pediatric Age: Ø–17   **M** Maternity DX: 9–64   **A** Adult Age: 15–124   ♀ Females Only   ♂ Males Only

🅒 Complication\Comorbidity   🅜🅒 Major C\C   (Ex) CC/MCC Exclusions   🅗 Hospital-Acquired Condition   🅗🅒 Hierarchical Condition Category   **1653**

● **Z94.4**   Liver transplant status 🔲 🔲
     (Ex:) See PDX Collection 1490

● **Z94.5**   Skin transplant status
     Autogenous skin transplant status

● **Z94.6**   Bone transplant status

● **Z94.7**   Corneal transplant status

● **Z94.8**   Other transplanted organ and tissue status

     ● **Z94.81**   Bone marrow transplant status 🔲 🔲
         (Ex:) See PDX Collection 3282

     ● **Z94.82**   Intestine transplant status 🔲 🔲
         (Ex:) See PDX Collection 1495

     ● **Z94.83**   Pancreas transplant status 🔲 🔲
         (Ex:) See PDX Collection 1496

     ● **Z94.84**   Stem cells transplant status 🔲 🔲
         (Ex:) See PDX Collection 3284

     ● **Z94.89**   Other transplanted organ and tissue status

● **Z94.9**   Transplanted organ and tissue status, unspecified

● **Z95**   **Presence of cardiac and vascular implants and grafts**
     Excludes2   complications of cardiac and vascular devices, implants and grafts (T82.-)

● **Z95.0**   Presence of cardiac pacemaker
     Presence of cardiac resynchronization therapy (CRT-P) pacemaker
     Excludes1   adjustment or management of cardiac device (Z45.0-)
         adjustment or management of cardiac pacemaker (Z45.0)
         presence of automatic (implantable) cardiac defibrillator with synchronous cardiac pacemaker (Z95.810)
     Coding Clinic: 2019, Q1, P33

● **Z95.1**   Presence of aortocoronary bypass graft
     Presence of coronary artery bypass graft

● **Z95.2**   Presence of prosthetic heart valve
     Presence of heart valve NOS

● **Z95.3**   Presence of xenogenic heart valve

● **Z95.4**   Presence of other heart-valve replacement

● **Z95.5**   Presence of coronary angioplasty implant and graft
     Excludes1   coronary angioplasty status without implant and graft (Z98.61)

● **Z95.8**   Presence of other cardiac and vascular implants and grafts

     ● **Z95.81**   Presence of other cardiac implants and grafts
         (Ex:) For category Z95.81 CC codes: See PDX Collection 1498

         ● **Z95.810**   Presence of automatic (implantable) cardiac defibrillator
             Presence of automatic (implantable) cardiac defibrillator with synchronous cardiac pacemaker
             Presence of cardiac resynchronization therapy defibrillator (CRT-D)
             Presence of cardioverter-defribrillator (ICD)

         ● **Z95.811**   Presence of heart assist device 🔲 🔲
         ● **Z95.812**   Presence of fully implantable artificial heart 🔲 🔲

         ● **Z95.818**   Presence of other cardiac implants and grafts

     ● **Z95.82**   Presence of other vascular implants and grafts

         ● **Z95.820**   Peripheral vascular angioplasty status with implants and grafts
             Excludes1   peripheral vascular angioplasty without implant and graft (Z98.62)

         ● **Z95.828**   Presence of other vascular implants and grafts
             Presence of intravascular prosthesis NEC

● **Z95.9**   Presence of cardiac and vascular implant and graft, unspecified

● **Z96**   **Presence of other functional implants**
     Excludes2   complications of internal prosthetic devices, implants and grafts (T82-T85)
         fitting and adjustment of prosthetic and other devices (Z44-Z46)

● **Z96.0**   Presence of urogenital implants

● **Z96.1**   Presence of intraocular lens
     Presence of pseudophakia

● **Z96.2**   Presence of otological and audiological implants

     ● **Z96.20**   Presence of otological and audiological implant, unspecified

     ● **Z96.21**   Cochlear implant status

     ● **Z96.22**   Myringotomy tube(s) status

     ● **Z96.29**   Presence of other otological and audiological implants
         Presence of bone-conduction hearing device
         Presence of eustachian tube stent
         Stapes replacement

● **Z96.3**   Presence of artificial larynx

● **Z96.4**   Presence of endocrine implants

     ● **Z96.41**   Presence of insulin pump (external) (internal)

     ● **Z96.49**   Presence of other endocrine implants

● **Z96.5**   Presence of tooth-root and mandibular implants

● **Z96.6**   Presence of orthopedic joint implants

     ● **Z96.60**   Presence of unspecified orthopedic joint implant

     ● **Z96.61**   Presence of artificial shoulder joint

         ● **Z96.611**   Presence of right artificial shoulder joint

         ● **Z96.612**   Presence of left artificial shoulder joint

         ● **Z96.619**   Presence of unspecified artificial shoulder joint

     ● **Z96.62**   Presence of artificial elbow joint

         ● **Z96.621**   Presence of right artificial elbow joint

         ● **Z96.622**   Presence of left artificial elbow joint

         ● **Z96.629**   Presence of unspecified artificial elbow joint

     ● **Z96.63**   Presence of artificial wrist joint

         ● **Z96.631**   Presence of right artificial wrist joint

         ● **Z96.632**   Presence of left artificial wrist joint

         ● **Z96.639**   Presence of unspecified artificial wrist joint

     ● **Z96.64**   Presence of artificial hip joint
         Hip-joint replacement (partial) (total)

         ● **Z96.641**   Presence of right artificial hip joint
             Coding Clinic: 2016, Q3, P17

         ● **Z96.642**   Presence of left artificial hip joint
             Coding Clinic: 2015, Q1, P16

         ● **Z96.643**   Presence of artificial hip joint, bilateral

         ● **Z96.649**   Presence of unspecified artificial hip joint

▶ New   ⟹ Revised   ~~deleted~~ Deleted   Excludes 1   Excludes 2   Includes   Use additional   Code first   Code also   Key words
OGCR Official Guidelines   ● Unacceptable Principal Diagnosis   X Assign placeholder X   ● Use Additional Character(s)   ▶ Manifestation Code   Coding Clinic

● **Z96.65** Presence of artificial knee joint
   ● **Z96.651** Presence of right artificial knee joint
   ● **Z96.652** Presence of left artificial knee joint
      Coding Clinic: 2019, Q3, P16
   ● **Z96.653** Presence of artificial knee joint, bilateral
   ● **Z96.659** Presence of unspecified artificial knee joint
● **Z96.66** Presence of artificial ankle joint
   ● **Z96.661** Presence of right artificial ankle joint
   ● **Z96.662** Presence of left artificial ankle joint
   ● **Z96.669** Presence of unspecified artificial ankle joint
● **Z96.69** Presence of other orthopedic joint implants
   ● **Z96.691** Finger-joint replacement of right hand
   ● **Z96.692** Finger-joint replacement of left hand
   ● **Z96.693** Finger-joint replacement, bilateral
   ● **Z96.698** Presence of other orthopedic joint implants
● **Z96.7** Presence of other bone and tendon implants
      Presence of skull plate
● **Z96.8** Presence of other specified functional implants
   ● **Z96.81** Presence of artificial skin
   ● **Z96.82** Presence of neurostimulator
      Presence of brain neurostimulator
      Presence of gastric neurostimulator
      Presence of peripheral nerve neurostimulator
      Presence of sacral nerve neurostimulator
      Presence of spinal cord neurostimulator
      Presence of vagus nerve neurostimulator
   ● **Z96.89** Presence of other specified functional implants
● **Z96.9** Presence of functional implant, unspecified

● **Z97** Presence of other devices
   Excludes2 fitting and adjustment of prosthetic and other devices (Z44-Z46)
               presence of cerebrospinal fluid drainage device (Z98.2)

● **Z97.0** Presence of artificial eye
● **Z97.1** Presence of artificial limb (complete) (partial)
   ● **Z97.10** Presence of artificial limb (complete) (partial), unspecified
   ● **Z97.11** Presence of artificial right arm (complete) (partial)
   ● **Z97.12** Presence of artificial left arm (complete) (partial)
   ● **Z97.13** Presence of artificial right leg (complete) (partial)
   ● **Z97.14** Presence of artificial left leg (complete) (partial)
   ● **Z97.15** Presence of artificial arms, bilateral (complete) (partial)
   ● **Z97.16** Presence of artificial legs, bilateral (complete) (partial)
● **Z97.2** Presence of dental prosthetic device (complete) (partial)
      Presence of dentures (complete) (partial)
● **Z97.3** Presence of spectacles and contact lenses
● **Z97.4** Presence of external hearing-aid
● **Z97.5** Presence of (intrauterine) contraceptive device ♀
   Excludes1 checking, reinsertion or removal of implantable subdermal contraceptive (Z30.46)
               checking, reinsertion or removal of intrauterine contraceptive device (Z30.43-)
● **Z97.8** Presence of other specified devices

● **Z98** Other postprocedural states
   Excludes2 aftercare (Z43-Z49, Z51)
               follow-up medical care (Z08-Z09)
               postprocedural complication - see Alphabetical Index
● **Z98.0** Intestinal bypass and anastomosis status
   Excludes2 bariatric surgery status (Z98.84)
               gastric bypass status (Z98.84)
               obesity surgery status (Z98.84)
● **Z98.1** Arthrodesis status
● **Z98.2** Presence of cerebrospinal fluid drainage device
      Presence of CSF shunt
● **Z98.3** Post therapeutic collapse of lung status
      Code first underlying disease
● **Z98.4** Cataract extraction status
      Use additional code to identify intraocular lens implant status (Z96.1)
   Excludes1 aphakia (H27.0)
   ● **Z98.41** Cataract extraction status, right eye
   ● **Z98.42** Cataract extraction status, left eye
   ● **Z98.49** Cataract extraction status, unspecified eye
● **Z98.5** Sterilization status
   Excludes1 female infertility (N97.-)
               male infertility (N46.-)
   ● **Z98.51** Tubal ligation status ♀
   ● **Z98.52** Vasectomy status ♂   A
● **Z98.6** Angioplasty status
   ● **Z98.61** Coronary angioplasty status
      Excludes1 coronary angioplasty status with implant and graft (Z95.5)
   ● **Z98.62** Peripheral vascular angioplasty status
      Excludes1 peripheral vascular angioplasty status with implant and graft (Z95.820)
● **Z98.8** Other specified postprocedural states
      Coding Clinic: 2016, Q4, P76
   ● **Z98.81** Dental procedure status
      ● **Z98.810** Dental sealant status
      ● **Z98.811** Dental restoration status
         Dental crown status
         Dental fillings status
      ● **Z98.818** Other dental procedure status
   ● **Z98.82** Breast implant status
      Excludes1 breast implant removal status (Z98.86)
   ● **Z98.83** Filtering (vitreous) bleb after glaucoma surgery status
      Excludes1 inflammation (infection) of postprocedural bleb (H59.4-)
   ● **Z98.84** Bariatric surgery status
         Gastric banding status
         Gastric bypass status for obesity
         Obesity surgery status
      Excludes1 bariatric surgery status complicating pregnancy, childbirth, or the puerperium (O99.84)
      Excludes2 intestinal bypass and anastomosis status (Z98.0)
      Coding Clinic: 2020, Q1, P12
   ● **Z98.85** Transplanted organ removal status
         Transplanted organ previously removed due to complication, failure, rejection or infection
      Excludes1 encounter for removal of transplanted organ - code to complication of transplanted organ (T86.-)

CHAPTER 21 (Z00-Z99)

N Newborn Age: 0   P Pediatric Age: 0–17   M Maternity DX: 9–64   A Adult Age: 15–124   ♀ Females Only   ♂ Males Only

🔹 Complication\Comorbidity   🔹 Major C\C   (Ex) CC/MCC Exclusions   🔹 Hospital-Acquired Condition   🔹 Hierarchical Condition Category

1655

- **Z98.86** Personal history of breast implant removal
- **Z98.87** Personal history of in utero procedure
  - **Z98.870** Personal history of in utero procedure during pregnancy ♀
    - **Excludes2** complications from in utero procedure for current pregnancy (O35.7)
      supervision of current pregnancy with history of in utero procedure during previous pregnancy (O09.82-)
  - **Z98.871** Personal history of in utero procedure while a fetus
- **Z98.89** Other specified postprocedural states
  Coding Clinic: 2016, Q4, P76
  - **Z98.890** Other specified postprocedural states
    Personal history of surgery, not elsewhere classified
  - **Z98.891** History of uterine scar from previous surgery ♀
    - **Excludes1** Maternal care due to uterine scar from previous surgery (O34.2-)
    Coding Clinic: 2016, Q4, P52, P76

- **Z99** Dependence on enabling machines and devices, not elsewhere classified
  - ~~Excludes1~~ ~~cardiac pacemaker status (Z95.0)~~
  Coding Clinic: 2020, Q1, P11
- **Z99.0** Dependence on aspirator
- **Z99.1** Dependence on respirator
  Dependence on ventilator
  (Ex:) For category Z99.1 CC codes: See PDX Collection 759
  - **Z99.11** Dependence on respirator [ventilator] status
    Coding Clinic: 2018, Q1, P14; 2015, Q1, P21
  - **Z99.12** Encounter for respirator [ventilator] dependence during power failure
    - **Excludes1** mechanical complication of respirator [ventilator] (J95.850)
- **Z99.2** Dependence on renal dialysis
  Hemodialysis status
  Peritoneal dialysis status
  Presence of arteriovenous shunt for dialysis
  Renal dialysis status NOS
  - **Excludes1** encounter for fitting and adjustment of dialysis catheter (Z49.0-)
  - **Excludes2** noncompliance with renal dialysis (Z91.15)
  Coding Clinic: 2016, Q1, P13
- **Z99.3** Dependence on wheelchair
  Wheelchair confinement status
  Code first cause of dependence, such as:
    muscular dystrophy (G71.0-)
    obesity (E66.-)
- **Z99.8** Dependence on other enabling machines and devices
  - **Z99.81** Dependence on supplemental oxygen
    Dependence on long-term oxygen
  - **Z99.89** Dependence on other enabling machines and devices
    Dependence on machine or device NOS
    Coding Clinic: 2020, Q1, P11

▶ New ⇶ Revised ~~deleted~~ Deleted Excludes 1 Excludes 2 Includes Use additional Code first Code also Key words
OGCR Official Guidelines ● Unacceptable Principal Diagnosis X Assign placeholder X ● Use Additional Character(s) ▹ Manifestation Code Coding Clinic

CHAPTER 22

CODES FOR SPECIAL PURPOSES (U00–U85)

Note: Codes from this chapter are for use on newborn records only, never on maternal records.

This chapter contains the following blocks:

U00–U49	Provisional assignment of new diseases of uncertain etiology or emergency use

---

PROVISIONAL ASSIGNMENT OF NEW DISEASES OF UNCERTAIN ETIOLOGY OR EMERGENCY USE (U00–U49)

U07   **Emergency use of U07**

    U07.0   **Vaping-related disorder**

        Dabbing related lung damage
        Dabbing related lung injury
        E-cigarette, or vaping, product use associated lung injury [EVALI]
        Electronic cigarette related lung damage
        Electronic cigarette related lung injury

        Use additional code to identify manifestations, such as:
            abdominal pain (R10.84)
            acute respiratory distress syndrome (J80)
            diarrhea (R19.7)
            drug-induced interstitial lung disorder (J70.4)
            lipoid pneumonia (J69.1)
            weight loss (R63.4)

U07.1   **COVID-19** 🦠

    Use additional code to identify pneumonia or other manifestations

    Excludes1 coronavirus infection, unspecified (B34.2)
                coronavirus as the cause of diseases classified elsewhere (B97.2-)
                pneumonia due to SARS-associated coronavirus (J12.81)

    (Ex:) See PDX Collection 4122

    Coding Clinic: 2021, Q1, P31-33, 36, 39-40, 47, 49

● U09   **Post COVID-19 condition**

    ▶ U09.9   **Post COVID-19 condition, unspecified**

        ▶**Note: This code enables establishment of a link with COVID-19.**

            ▶This code is not to be used in cases that are still presenting with active COVID-19. However, an exception is made in cases of re-infection with COVID-19, occurring with a condition related to prior COVID-19.

        ▶Post-acute sequela of COVID-19

        ▶*Code first the specific condition related to COVID-19 if known, such as:*
            ▶chronic respiratory failure (J96.1-)
            ▶loss of smell (R43.8)
            ▶loss of taste (R43.8)
            ▶multisystem inflammatory syndrome (M35.81)
            ▶pulmonary embolism (I26.-)
            ▶pulmonary fibrosis (J84.10)

N Newborn Age: 0   **P** Pediatric Age: 0–17   **M** Maternity DX: 9–64   **A** Adult Age: 15–124   ♀ Females Only   ♂ Males Only
🦠 Complication\Comorbidity   🦠 Major C\C   (Ex:) CC/MCC Exclusions   🦠 Hospital-Acquired Condition   🦠 Hierarchical Condition Category

1657

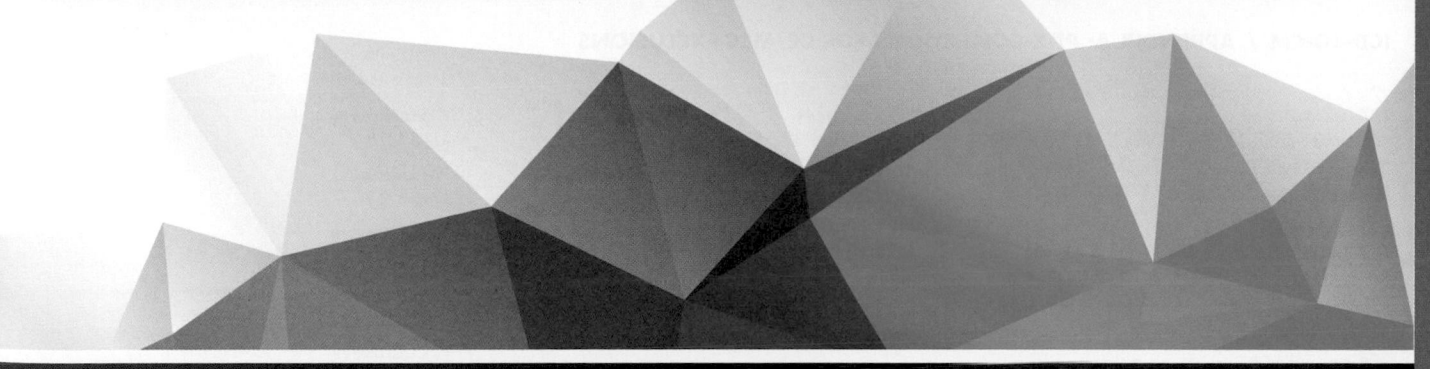

APPENDIX A

PDX Collections for CC/MCC Exclusions

FY 2022 MS-DRG Version 36

PDX Collection 2
A00.0-A00.9

PDX Collection 3
A01.00-A01.4

PDX Collection 4
A01.00-A01.09, A01.4-A02.0, A03.9-A05.2, A07.4,
A08.0-A09, A48.51-A48.52, K30, K52.1-K52.3, K52.82-K52.9,
K58.0-K58.9, K65.0, K65.2, K65.8, K68.12-K68.9,
P76.8-P77.9, P78.1, P78.3-P78.89

PDX Collection 5
A02.1, A20.7, A22.7, A26.7, A32.7, A39.2-A39.4, A40.0-A40.1,
A40.8-A41.9, A42.7, A48.2-A48.4, A48.8-A49.9, A54.86,
B00.7, B37.7, B92, B94.2-B96.89, P36.0-P36.9, P39.2,
P39.4-P39.9, R65.10-R65.20, Z16.10-Z16.39

PDX Collection 6
A02.21, A17.0-A17.1, A27.81, A39.0, A50.41, A51.41, A52.13,
A54.82, A54.84, A54.89-A54.9, A74.81-A74.9, A87.0-A87.9,
A96.2, A98.3-A98.4, B26.1, B33.24, B33.4-B33.8,
B34.1-B34.2, B34.4-B34.8, B37.5, B38.4, B45.1, B58.2,
B92, B94.2-94.9, B97.10, B97.19, B97.29, B97.5-B97.6,
B97.81-B97.89, G00.0-G03.9, G04.2, G32.89, G96.9,
G98.0-G98.8, G99.8

PDX Collection 7
A02.22, A15.0-A15.6, A15.8-A15.9, A17.9, A18.82, A18.84,
A18.89, A20.2, A21.1, A22.1, A31.0, A37.01, A37.11, A37.81,
A37.91, A42.0, A43.0, A48.1, B25.0, B39.0-B39.2, B44.0,
B58.3, B59, B67.1, J09.X1-J09.X2, J10.00-J10.1, J11.00-J11.1,
J12.0-J12.3, J12.89-J18.1, J18.8-J18.9, J22, J60, J62.0-J67.7,
J68.0-J70.4, J70.8-J70.9, J98.4, J98.8-J99, R91.1

PDX Collection 8
A02.23, A18.02, A18.09, A39.83-A39.84, A54.40,
A54.42-A54.43, A54.82, A54.84, A54.89-A54.9, B06.82,
M00.00-M02.30, M02.319, M02.329, M02.339, M02.349,
M02.359, M02.369, M02.379-M02.9, M05.40-M05.59,

M05.70-M06.09, M06.20-M06.39, M06.80-M07.69,
M11.00-M11.9, M12.10-M15.0, M15.3-M15.9, M16.2-M16.9,
M17.2-M17.9, M18.2-M18.9, M19.111-M19.93,
M24.10-M24.176, M25.00, M25.08-M25.18, M25.40-M25.676,
M25.80-M25.9, M35.2, M36.1-M36.4, R29.4

PDX Collection 9
A02.24, A18.03-A18.09, M46.20-M46.39, M86.00-M86.9

PDX Collection 10
A02.25-A02.29

PDX Collection 11
A02.8

PDX Collection 12
A02.9

PDX Collection 13
A00.1, A01.00-A01.09, A01.4-A02.0, A03.0, A03.9,
A04.7-A05.2, A06.0-A06.2, A06.9, A07.1-A07.9, A08.4-A09,
A18.32-A18.39, A18.83, A48.51-A48.52, B37.82, B82.9,
J09.X3-J09.X9, J10.2-J10.89, J11.2-J11.89, K30, K31.84,
K50.00-K51.919, K52.1-K52.3, K52.82-K55.1, K55.30-K55.33,
K55.8-K55.9, K58.0-K58.9, P70.0-P70.4, P70.9-P71.9, P72.1,
P72.9-P74.4, P74.9, P76.8-P77.9, P78.1, P78.3-P78.89, P94.0

PDX Collection 14
A02.0, A03.9-A05.0, A05.2, A07.4, A08.0-A09, J09.X3-J09.X9,
J10.2-J10.89, J11.2-J11.89, K30, K31.84, K52.1-K52.3,
K52.82-K52.9, K58.0-K58.9, K65.0, K65.2, K65.8,
K68.12-K68.9, P76.8-P77.9, P78.1, P78.3-P78.89

PDX Collection 15
A00.1, A01.00-A01.09, A01.4-A02.0, A03.9, A04.0-A04.8,
A04.9-A05.2, A06.0-A06.2, A06.9, A07.1-A09, A18.32-A18.39,
A18.83, A48.51-A48.52, B37.82, B82.9, J09.X3-J09.X9,
J10.2-J10.89, J11.2-J11.89, K30, K31.84, K50.00-K51.919,
K52.1-K52.3, K52.82-K55.1, K55.30-K55.33, K55.8-K55.9,
K58.0-K58.9, P70.0-P70.4, P70.9-P71.9, P72.1, P72.9-P74.4,
P74.9, P76.8-P77.9, P78.1, P78.3-P78.89, P94.0

PDX Collection 16
A00.1, A01.00-A01.09, A01.4-A02.0, A03.9-A05.0, A05.2,
A06.0-A06.2, A06.9, A07.1-A09, A18.32-A18.39, A18.83,
B37.82, B82.9, J09.X3-J09.X9, J10.2-J10.89, J11.2-J11.89,
K30, K31.84, K52.1-K52.3, K52.82-K52.9, K58.0-K58.9,
K65.0, K65.2, K65.8, K68.12-K68.9, P76.8-P77.9, P78.1,
P78.3-P78.89

PDX Collection 17
A00.0-A09, A48.51-A48.52

PDX Collection 18
A04.71-A04.72, A05.0-A05.2, A48.51-A48.52

PDX Collection 19
A02.0, A03.9-A05.2, A07.4, A08.0-A09, A48.51-A48.52,
J09.X3-J09.X9, J10.2-J10.89, J11.2-J11.89, K30, K31.84,
K52.1-K52.3, K52.82-K52.9, K58.0-K58.9, K65.0, K65.2,
K65.8, K68.12-K68.9, P76.8-P77.9, P78.1, P78.3-P78.89

PDX Collection 20
A06.0-A06.1, A07.4

PDX Collection 21
A02.0, A03.9-A05.0, A05.2, A06.0-A06.2, A06.9, A07.1-A09,
B82.9, J09.X3-J09.X9, J10.2-J10.89, J11.2-J11.89, K30,
K31.84, K50.00-K51.919, K52.1-K52.3, K52.82-K55.1,
K55.30-K55.33, K55.8-K55.9, K58.0-K58.9, P76.8-P77.9,
P78.1, P78.3, P78.81-P78.89

PDX Collection 22
A06.0-A06.6, A06.81-A06.89

PDX Collection 23
A06.4, K75.0

PDX Collection 24
A06.5, J85.0-J85.2

PDX Collection 25
A06.6, G06.0

PDX Collection 26
A02.0, A03.9-A05.0, A05.2, A06.0-A06.2, A06.9, A07.1-A09,
B82.9, J09.X3-J09.X9, J10.2-J10.89, J11.2-J11.89, K30,
K31.84, K52.1-K52.3, K52.82-K52.9, K58.0-K58.9

PDX Collection 27
A02.0, A03.9-A05.0, A05.2, A06.0-A06.2, A06.9, A07.1-A09,
B82.9, J09.X3-J09.X9, J10.2-J10.89, J11.2-J11.89, K30,
K31.84, K52.1-K52.3, K52.82-K52.9, K58.0-K58.9, K65.0,
K65.2, K65.8, K68.12-K68.9

PDX Collection 28
A02.0, A03.9-A05.0, A05.2, A06.0-A06.2, A06.9, A07.1-A09,
A18.32-A18.39, A18.83, B37.82, B82.9, J09.X3-J09.X9,
J10.2-J10.89, J11.2-J11.89, K30, K31.84, K52.1-K52.3,
K52.82-K52.9, K58.0-K58.9, K65.0, K65.2, K65.8,
K68.12-K68.9, P76.8-P77.9, P78.1, P78.3-P78.89

PDX Collection 29
A15.0-A15.9, A17.9, A18.82, A18.84, A18.89-A19.9, A22.1,
A31.0, A31.2-A31.9, A37.01, A37.11, A37.81, A37.91, A48.1,
A49.3-A49.9, B25.0, B44.0, B90.9, B92, B94.2-B94.9, B96.0,
B96.6-B96.89, J09.X1-J09.X2, J10.00-J10.1, J11.00-J11.1,
J12.0-J12.3, J12.89-J18.1, J18.8-J18.9, J44.9, J47.0-J70.4,
J70.8-J70.9, J98.4, R91.1

PDX Collection 30
A15.0-A17.82, A17.89-A19.9

PDX Collection 31
A15.0-A17.82, A17.89, A18.31-A18.39, A18.83, A19.0-A19.9

PDX Collection 32
A02.21, A17.0-A17.1, A17.89-A17.9, A18.82, A18.84, A18.89,
A27.81, A31.2-A31.9, A39.0, A49.3-A49.9, A50.41, A51.41,
A52.13, A54.82, A54.84, A54.89-A54.9, A87.0-A87.9, B00.3,
B02.1, B26.1, B37.5, B38.4, B45.1, B58.2, B90.0, B92,
B94.2-B94.9, B96.0, B96.6-B96.89, G00.0-G03.9, G04.2,
G32.89, G61.0, G96.9, G98.0-G98.8, G99.8

PDX Collection 33
A17.81-A17.82, A17.89-A17.9, A18.82, A18.84, A18.89,
A31.2-A31.9, A49.3-A49.9, B90.0, B92, B94.2-B94.9, B96.0,
B96.6-B96.89

PDX Collection 34
A17.89-A17.9, A18.82, A18.84, A18.89, A31.2-A31.9,
A49.3-A49.9, B90.0, B92, B94.2-B94.9, B96.0, B96.6-B96.89

PDX Collection 35
A17.9, A18.82, A18.84, A18.89, A31.2-A31.9, A49.3-A49.9,
B92, B94.2-B94.9, B96.0, B96.6-B96.89

PDX Collection 36
A18.01

PDX Collection 37
A18.02

PDX Collection 38
A18.01, A18.03

PDX Collection 39
A18.01-A18.02, A18.09

PDX Collection 40
A17.9, A18.10, A18.82, A18.84, A18.89, A31.2-A31.9,
A49.3-A49.9, B90.0, B92, B94.2-B94.9, B96.0, B96.6-B96.89

PDX Collection 41
A17.9, A18.10-A18.13, A18.82, A18.84, A18.89, A31.2-A31.9,
A49.3-A49.9, B90.0, B92, B94.2-B94.9, B96.0, B96.6-B96.89

PDX Collection 42
A17.9, A18.10, A18.82, A18.84, A18.89, A31.2-A31.9,
A49.3-A49.9, B90.1, B92, B94.2-B94.9, B96.0, B96.6-B96.89

PDX Collection 43
A17.9, A18.0, A18.16-A18.18, A18.82, A18.84, A18.89,
A31.2-A31.9, A49.3-A49.9, B90.1, B92, B94.2-B94.9, B96.0,
B96.6-B96.89

PDX Collection 44
A17.9, A18.2, A18.82, A18.84, A18.89, A31.2-A31.9,
A49.3-A49.9, B92, B94.2-B94.9, B96.0, B96.6-B96.89

PDX Collection 45
A17.9, A18.31-A18.39, A18.82-A18.84, A18.89, A31.2-A31.9,
A49.3-A49.9, B92, B94.2-B94.9, B96.0, B96.6-B96.89

PDX Collection 46
A17.9, A18.50-A18.59, A18.82, A18.84, A18.89, A31.2-A31.9,
A49.3-A49.9, B92, B94.2-B94.9, B96.0, B96.6-B96.89

PDX Collection 47
A17.9, A18.6, A18.82, A18.84, A18.89, A31.2-A31.9,
A49.3-A49.9, B92, B94.2-B94.9, B96.0, B96.6-B96.89

PDX Collection 48
A17.9, A18.7, A18.82, A18.84, A18.89, A31.2-A31.9,
A49.3-A49.9, B92, B94.2-B94.9, B96.0, B96.6-B96.89

PDX Collection 49
A17.9, A18.81-A18.82, A18.84, A18.89, A31.2-A31.9,
A49.3-A49.9, B92, B94.2-B94.9, B96.0, B96.6-B96.89

PDX Collection 50
A17.9, A18.82, A18.84-A18.85 A18.89, A31.2-A31.9,
A49.3-A49.9, B92, B94.2-B94.9, B96.0, B96.6-B96.89

PDX Collection 51
A17.9, A18.82, A18.84, A18.89, A19.0-A19.9, A31.2-A31.9,
A49.3-A49.9, B92, B94.2-B94.9, B96.0, B96.6-B96.89

PDX Collection 52
A20.0-A20.9

PDX Collection 53
A20.2, J12.81

PDX Collection 54
A20.3, A20.8

PDX Collection 55
A02.1, A20.0-A20.9, A22.7, A26.7, A32.7, A40.0-A40.1,
A40.8-A41.9, A42.7, A54.86, B37.7, P36.0-P36.9, P39.2,
P39.4-P39.9, R65.10-R65.20

PDX Collection 56
A20.9

PDX Collection 57
A21.0

PDX Collection 58
A21.1, J12.81

PDX Collection 59
A21.2, A22.1, A37.01, A37.11, A37.81, A37.91, A48.1, B25.0,
B44.0, J09.X1-J09.X2, J10.00-J10.1, J11.00-J11.1, J15.29,
J15.5-J18.0, J18.8-J18.9, J22, J60-J70.4, J70.8-J70.9, J98.4,
J98.8-J99, R91.1

PDX Collection 60
A21.3

PDX Collection 61
A21.0-A21.9

PDX Collection 62
A22.0

PDX Collection 63
A15.0-A15.9, A17.9, A18.82, A18.84, A18.89, A20.2,
A21.1-A21.2, A22.1, A31.0, A37.01, A37.11, A37.81, A37.91,
A42.0, A43.0, A48.1, B25.0, B39.0-B39.2, B44.0, B58.3,
B59, B67.1, J09.X1-J09.X2, J10.00-J10.1, J11.00-J11.1,
J12.0-J12.3, J12.81-J18.1, J18.8-J18.9, J22, J44.9,
J47.0-J70.4, J70.8-J70.9, J98.4, J98.8-J99, R91.1

PDX Collection 64
A22.2

PDX Collection 65
A22.8

PDX Collection 66
A22.0-A22.9

PDX Collection 67
A23.0-A23.9

PDX Collection 68
A24.0

PDX Collection 69
A24.1-A24.9

PDX Collection 70
A25.0-A25.9

PDX Collection 71
A02.1, A20.7, A22.7, A26.7, A32.7, A39.2-A39.4, A40.0-A40.1,
A40.8-A41.9, A42.7, A48.2-A48.4, A48.8-A49.9, A54.86,
B00.7, B3.77, B92, B94.2-B96.89, R65.10-R65.20,
Z16.10-Z16.39

PDX Collection 72
A27.0-A27.9

PDX Collection 73
A02.21, A17.0-A17.1, A27.0-A27.9, A39.0, A50.41, A51.41,
A52.13, A54.82, A54.84, A54.89-A54.9, A74.81-A74.9,
A87.0-A87.9, A96.2, A98.3-A98.4, B26.1, B33.24,
B33.4-B33.8, B34.1-B34.2, B34.4-B34.8, B37.5, B38.4,
B45.1, B58.2, B92, B94.2-B94.9, B97.10, B97.19, B97.29,
B97.5-B97.6, B97.81-B97.89, G00.0-G03.9, G04.2, G32.89,
G61.0, G96.9, G98.0-G98.8, G99.8

PDX Collection 74
A26.0, A26.8-A26.9, A28.0, A28.2-A28.9, A32.0-A32.12,
A32.81-A32.9

PDX Collection 75
A28.1, B97.21

PDX Collection 76
A30.0

PDX Collection 77
A30.1

PDX Collection 78
A30.2-A30.4

PDX Collection 79
A30.5

PDX Collection 80
A30.8

PDX Collection 81
A30.9

PDX Collection 82
A15.0-A15.9, A17.9, A18.82, A18.84, A18.89, A22.1, A31.0,
A31.2-A31.9, A37.01, A37.11, A37.81, A37.91, A48.1,
A49.3-A49.9, B25.0, B44.0, B90.0, B92, B94.2-B94.9, B96.0,
B96.6-B96.89, J09.X1-J09.X2, J10.00-J10.1, J11.00-J11.1,
J12.0-J12.3, J12.89-J18.1, J18.8-J18.9, J44.9, J47.0-J70.4,
J70.8-J70.9, J98.4, R91.1

PDX Collection 83
A31.0-A31.9

PDX Collection 84
A33, P29.0-P29.2, P29.4, P29.89-P29.9, P94.1-P94.9, P96.0,
P96.3-P96.5, P96.82-P96.89

PDX Collection 85
A34, 008.0, 008.2-008.9, 011.4, 011.5, 012.04, 012.05,
012.14, 012.15, 012.24, 012.25, 013.4, 013.5, 014.04,
014.05, 014.14, 014.15, 014.24, 014.25, 014.94, 014.95,
016.4, 016.5, 020.0-020.9, 025.10-025.3, 026.10-026.13,
026.30-026.43, 026.63-026.819, 026.841-026.86,
026.891-026.93, 029.011-029.93, 035.7XX0-035.7XX9,
044.00-044.13, 044.20-044.53, 045.8X1-045.93, 075.4,

075.81, 075.89-075.9, 080, 090.89, 099.111-099.285,
099.330-099.335, 099.350-099.355, 099.511-099.73,
099.820-099.825, 099.840-09A.53

PDX Collection 86
A35, B92, B94.2-B94.9

PDX Collection 87
A36.0-A36.9

PDX Collection 88
A36.81, A52.06, B33.20-B33.22, I00, I01.2-I01.9, I09.0, I09.9,
I23.0-I23.3, I23.6-I23.8, I40.0-I41, I51.0, I51.4, I87.8-I87.9,
I99.8-I99.9

PDX Collection 89
A37.00-A37.91

PDX Collection 90
A15.0-A15.9, A17.9, A18.82, A18.84, A18.89, A21.2,
A22.1, A31.0, A37.00-A37.91, A42.0, A43.0, A48.1, B25.0,
B39.0-B39.2, B44.0, B58.3, B59, B67.1, J09.X1-J09.X2,
J10.00-J10.1, J11.00-J11.1, J12.0-J12.3, J12.89-J18.1,
J18.8-J18.9, J22, J44.9, J47.0-J70.4, J70.8-J70.9, J98.4,
J98.8-J98.9, Q33.4, R91.1

PDX Collection 91
A38.0-A38.9, A46, J02.0, J03.00-J03.01

PDX Collection 92
A02.21, A17.0-A17.1, A27.81, A39.0, A39.89-A39.9,
A49.3-A49.9, A50.41, A51.41, A52.13, A54.82, A54.84,
A54.89-A54.9, A87.0-A87.9, B00.3, B02.1, B26.1, B37.5,
B38.4, B45.1, B58.2, B92, B94.2-B94.9, B96.0, B96.6-B96.89,
G00.0-G03.9, G04.2, G32.89, G61.0, G96.9, G98.0-G98.8,
G99.8

PDX Collection 93
A39.1, A39.89-A39.9, A49.3-A49.9, B92, B94.2-B94.9, B96.0,
B96.6-B96.89

PDX Collection 94
A02.1, A20.7, A22.7, A26.7, A32.7, A39.2-A39.4,
A39.89-A41.9, A42.7, A49.3-A49.9, A54.86, B00.7, B37.7,
B92, B94.2-B94.9, B96.0, B96.6-B96.89, R65.10 R65.20

PDX Collection 95
A39.50, A39.89-A39.9, A49.3-A49.9, B92, B94.2-B94.9, B96.0,
B96.6-B96.89

PDX Collection 96
A39.51, A39.89-A39.9, A49.3-A49.9, B92, B94.2-B94.9, B96.0,
B96.6-B96.89

PDX Collection 97
A39.52, A49.3-A49.9, B92, B94.2-B94.9, B96.0, B96.6-B96.89

PDX Collection 98
A39.53, A39.89-A39.9, A49.3-A49.9, B92, B94.2-B94.9, B96.0,
B96.6-B96.89

PDX Collection 99
A39.81, A39.89-A39.9, A49.3-A49.9, B92, B94.2-B94.9, B96.0,
B96.6-B96.89

PDX Collection 100
A39.82, A39.89-A39.9, A49.3-A49.9, B92, B94.2-B94.9, B96.0,
B96.6-B96.89

PDX Collection 101
A39.83-A39.9, A49.3-A49.9, B92, B94.2-B94.9, B96.0,
B96.6-B96.89

PDX Collection 102
A39.89-A39.9, A49.3-A49.9, B92, B94.2-B94.9, B96.0,
B96.6-B96.89

PDX Collection 103
A42.0, A42.81-A43.0, A43.8-A43.9, B47.1, J12.81

PDX Collection 104
A42.1, A42.81-A42.9, A43.8-A43.9, B47.1

PDX Collection 105
A42.2, A42.81-A42.9, A43.8-A43.9, B47.1

PDX Collection 106
A42.0-A42.2, A42.81-A43.9, B47.1-B47.9, L08.1

PDX Collection 107
A42.81-A42.9, A43.1-A43.9, B47.1, L08.1

PDX Collection 108
A44.0-A44.9, A68.0-A68.9, A69.20-A69.29, A75.0-A79.9,
B55.0-B57.5, B60.00-B609

PDX Collection 109
A48.0, B92, B94.2-B94.9

PDX Collection 110
A15.0-A15.9, A17.9, A18.82, A18.84, A18.89, A21.2, A22.1,
A31.0, A37.01, A37.11, A37.81, A37.91, A42.0, A43.0, A48.1,
B25.0, B39.0-B39.2, B44.0, B58.3, B59, B67.1, J09.X1-J09.X2,
J10.00-J10.1, J11.00-J11.1, J12.0-J12.3, J12.89-J18.1,
J18.8-J18.9, J22, J44.9, J47.0-J70.4, J70.8-J70.9, J98.4,
J98.8-J98.9, Q33.4, R91.1

PDX Collection 111
A48.3, G89.0-G89.4, R09.89, R29.700-R29.742, R41.0-R41.3,
R41.82, R41.9, R44.8-R44.9, R45.83-R45.84, R46.0-R46.89,
R52, R57.0-R57.9, R65.21, R68.0-R68.19, R68.81-R68.89, R69

PDX Collection 112
A50.01-A51.46, A51.5-A53.9

PDX Collection 113
A50.01-A51.46, A51.5-A54.85, A54.89-A58, A63.8, A64, B92,
B94.2-B94.9, M02.30-M02.39, N34.1

PDX Collection 114
A50.01-A51.46, A51.5-A53.9, A56.00-A56.8, A63.8-A64, B92,
B94.2-B94.9, N34.1

PDX Collection 115
A02.21, A17.0-A17.1, A27.81, A39.0, A50.01-A51.46,
A51.5-A53.9, A54.82, A54.84, A54.89-A54.9, A56.00-A56.8,
A63.8-A64, A87.0-A87.9, B00.3, B02.1, B26.1, B37.5, B38.4,
B45.1, B58.2, B92, B94.2-B94.9, G00.0-G03.9, G04.2, G32.89,
G61.0, G96.9, G98.0-G98.8, G99.8, N34.1

PDX Collection 116
A50.01-A51.46, A51.5-A54.85, A54.89-A58, A63.8, A64,
M02.30-M02.39, N34.1

PDX Collection 117
A02.21, A17.0-A17.1, A27.81, A39.0, A50.01-A51.46,
A51.5-A54.49, A54.5-A54.85, A54.89-A58, A63.8-A64,
A74.81-A74.9, A87.0-A87.9, A96.2, A98.3-A98.4, B26.1, B33.24,
B33.4-B33.8, B34.1-B34.2, B34.4-B34.8, B37.5, B38.4, B45.1,
B58.2, B92, B94.2-B94.9, B97.10, B97.19, B97.29, B97.5-B97.6,
B97.81-B97.89, G00.0-G03.9, G04.2, G32.89, G61.0, G96.9,
G98.0-G98.8, G99.8, M02.30-M02.39, N34.1

PDX Collection 118
A50.01-A51.46, A51.5-A54.85, A54.89-A58, A63.8, A64,
K71.0-K71.9, K73.1-K73.8, K74.0-K74.69, K75.2-K76.0,
K76.4-K76.5, K76.89-K76.9, M02.30-M02.39, N34.1

PDX Collection 119
A18.09, A50.01-A51.46, A51.5-A54.85, A54.89-A58,
A63.8, A64, A66.6, M02.30-M02.39, M84.80-M84.9,
M85.10-M85.19, M85.80-M85.89, M86.30-M86.8X9,
M89.20-M89.39, M89.50-M89.59, M89.8X0-M89.8X9, M94.1,
M94.351-M94.8X9, N34.1

PDX Collection 120
A18.50-A18.59, A50.01-A51.46, A51.5-A54.85, A54.89-A58,
A63.8-A64, H15.001-H15.009, II15.091-H15.129,
M02.30-M02.39, N34.1

PDX Collection 121
A54.00-A54.29, A54.82, A54.84, A54.89, A54.9, A56.00-A56.8,
A63.8-A64, B92, B94.-B94.9, N34.1

PDX Collection 122
A02.23, A17.9, A18.02, A18.09, A18.82, A18.84, A18.89,
A39.83-A39.84, A50.01-A51.9, A52.00-A54.89, A54.9-A58,
A63.8, A64, B06.82, M00.00-M02.9, M05.40-M05.59,
M05.70-M06.09, M06.20-M06.39, M06.80-M07.69,
M11.00-M11.9, M12.10-M15.0, M15.3-M15.9, M16.2-M16.9,
M17.2-M17.9, M18.2-M18.9, M19.111-M19.93,
M24.10-M24.176, M25.00, M25.08, M25.10-M25.18,
M25.40-M25.676, M25.80-M25.9, M35.2, M36.1-M36.4,
N34.1, R29.4

PDX Collection 123
A50.01-A51.46, A51.5-A54.85, A54.89-A58, A63.8, A64,
M02.30-M02.39, N25.81-N25.89, N34.1

PDX Collection 124
A01.00-A01.09, A39.51, A50.01-A58, A63.8-A64, A78,
B33.20-B33.22, B37.6, B40.0-B40.9, I00, I01.1-I02.0,
I05.0-I05.1, I05.2, I05.8-I08.3, I08.9-I09.1, I09.89-I09.9,
I23.0-I23.3, I23.6-I23.8, I33.0-I41, I42.4, I51.0, I51.4,
I87.8-I87.9, I99.8-I99.9, M00.00, M00.08-M00.10,
M00.18-M00.20, M00.28-M00.80, M00.88-M00.9,
M02.30-M02.39, N34.1, Q22.2, Q23.8, Q23.9, Q24.8,
T82.6XX[A]

PDX Collection 125
A18.31, A34, A50.01-A58, A63.8, A64, K35.2-K35.3, K63.4,
K63.89-K63.9, K65.1, K65.3, K65.9, K67, K86.81-K86.89,
K92.89-K92.9, M02.30-M02.39, N34.1, N73.3-N73.4, N73.6,
O08.0, O08.82, O85, O86.12, O86.81, O86.89, P78.0, R11.13,
T81.60X[A]-T81.69X[A]

PDX Collection 126
A69.1

PDX Collection 127
A70

PDX Collection 128
A17.82, A44.0-A44.9, A50.42, A52.14, A68.0-A68.9,
A69.20-A69.29, A75.0-A79.9, A81.1, A81.82-A81.89,
A83.0-A85.8, A87.2, A88.0, A88.8, A92.1-A92.8, A93.0, B00.4,
B00.82, B01.11-B01.12, B04, B06.01, B08.09, B08.20-B08.22,
B08.60-B08.79, B09, B10.01-B10.09, B26.2, B33.1, B45.0,
B45.2-B45.9, B50.9, B55.0-B57.5, B58.2, B60.00-B60.09,
B75, B97.10, B97.21, G04.00-G04.01, G04.31, G04.81-G05.4,
G37.0, G37.4-G37.5, J09.X3-J09.X9, J10.2-J10.89,
J11.2-J11.89, L44.4, M1A.10X0-M1A.19X1, P35.2-P35.9,
P37.0-P37.4, P37.8-P37.9, T56.0X1-T56.0X4[A]

PDX Collection 129
A77.0-A79.9

PDX Collection 130
A80.0-A80.39

PDX Collection 131
A17.82, A50.42, A52.14, A75.9, A79.9, A81.00-A81.9,
A83.0-A85.8, A87.2, A88.0, A88.8, A92.1-A92.2, A92.4-A92.8,
A93.0, B00.4, B00.82, B01.11-B01.12, B04, B06.01, B08.09,
B08.20-B08.22, B08.60-B08.79, B09, B10.01-B10.09,
B26.2, B33.1, B45.0, B45.2-B45.9, B58.2, B75, B97.10,
G04.00-G04.01, G04.31, G04.81-G05.4, G37.0, G37.4-G37.5,
I67.3, J09.X3-J09.X9, J10.2-J10.89, J11.2-J11.89, L44.4,
M1A.10X0-M1A.19X1, P35.2-P35.9, P37.0-P37.4, P37.8-P37.9,
T56.0X1-T56.0X4[A]

PDX Collection 132
A81.1, B92, B94.2-B94.9

PDX Collection 133
A17.82, A50.42, A52.14, A75.9, A79.9, A81.00-A81.9,
A83.0-A85.8, A87.2, A88.0, A88.8, A92.1-A92.2, A92.4-A92.8,
A93.0, B00.4, B00.82, B01.11-B01.12, B04, B06.01, B08.09,
B08.20-B08.22, B08.60-B08.79, B09, B10.01-B10.09, B26.2,
B27.00-B27.99, B33.1, B45.0, B45.2-B45.9, B58.2, B75,
G04.00-G04.01, G04.31, G04.81-G05.4, G37.0, G37.4-G37.5,
I67.3, J09.X3-J09.X9, J10.2-J10.89, J11.2-J11.89, L44.4,
M1A.10X0-M1A.19X1, P35.2-P35.9, P37.0-P37.4, P37.8-P37.9,
T56.0X1-T56.0X4[A]

PDX Collection 134
A81.00-A81.9, I67.3

PDX Collection 135
A81.00-A81.9, A92.30-A92.39, B97.21, I67.3

PDX Collection 136
A82.0-A82.9

PDX Collection 137
A17.82, A50.42, A52.14, A75.9, A79.9, A81.1, A81.82-A81.89,
A83.0-A85.8, A87.2, A88.0, A88.8, A92.1-A92.8, A93.0, B00.4,
B00.82, B01.11-B01.12, B04, B06.01, B08.09, B08.20-B08.22,
B08.60-B08.79, B09, B10.01-B10.09, B26.2, B27.00-B27.99,
B33.1, B45.0, B45.2-B45.9, B58.2, B75, B97.10-B97.21,
G04.00-G04.01, G04.31, G04.81-G04.91, G05.3-G05.4, G37.0,
G37.4-G37.5, J09.X3-J09.X9, J10.2-J10.89, J11.2-J11.89,
L44.4, M1A.10X0-M1A.19X1, P35.2-P35.9, P37.0-P37.9,
T56.0X1-T56.0X4[A]

PDX Collection 138
A17.82, A50.42, A52.14, A75.9, A79.9, A81.1, A81.82-A81.89,
A83.0-A85.8, A87.2, A88.0, A88.8, A92.1-A92.8, A93.0, B00.4,
B00.82, B01.11-B01.12, B04, B06.01, B08.09, B08.20-B08.22,
B08.60-B08.79, B09, B10.01-B10.09, B26.2, B27.00-B27.99,
B33.1, B45.0, B45.2-B45.9, B58.2, B75, B97.10-B97.21,
G04.00-G04.01, G04.31, G04.81-G04.91, G05.3-G05.4, G37.0,
G37.4-G37.5, H66.40-H66.43, J09.X3-J09.X9, J10.2-J10.89,
J11.2-J11.89, L44.4, M1A.10X0-M1A.19X1, M32.0-M32.9,
P35.2-P35.9, P37.0-P37.9, T56.0X1-T56.0X4[A]

PDX Collection 139
A17.82, A50.42, A52.14, A75.9, A79.9, A81.1, A81.82-A81.89,
A83.0-A86, A87.2, A88.0, A88.8-A89, A92.1-A92.2,
A92.4-A92.8, A93.0, B00.4, B00.82, B01.11-B01.12, B04,
B06.01, B08.09, B08.20-B08.22, B08.60-B08.79, B09,
B10.01-B10.09, B26.2, B27.00-B27.99, B33.1, B45.0,
B45.2-B45.9, B58.2, B75, B97.10, G04.00-G04.01, G04.31,
G04.81-G04.91, G05.3-G05.4, G37.0, G37.4-G37.5,
H66.40-H66.43, J09. X3-J09.X9, J10.2-J10.89, J11.2-J11.89,
L44.4, M1A.10X0-M1A.19X1, M32.0-M32.9, P35.2-P35.9,
P37.0-P37.9, T56.0X1-T56.0X4[A]

PDX Collection 140
A02.21, A17.0-A17.1, A27.81, A39.0, A50.41, A51.41, A52.13,
A54.82-A54.84, A54.89-A54.9, A74.81-A74.9, A87.0-A87.9,
A96.2, A98.3-A98.4, B26.1, B33.24, B33.4-B33.8,
B34.1-B34.8, B37.5, B38.4, B45.1, B58.2, B92, B94.2-B94.9,
B97.10, B97.19, B97.29, B97.5-B97.6, B97.81-B97.89,
G00.0-G03.9, G04.2, G32.89, G61.0, G96.9, G98.0-G98.8,
G99.8

PDX Collection 141
A02.21, A17.0-A17.1, A27.81, A39.0, A50.41, A51.41, A52.13,
A54.82-A54.84, A54.89-A54.9, A74.81-A74.9, A87.0-A87.9,
A92.30-A92.39, A96.2, A98.3-A98.4, B26.1, B33.24,
B33.4-B33.8, B34.1-B34.8, B37.5, B38.4, B45.1, B58.2, B92,
B94.2-B94.9, B97.10, B97.19, B97.21-B97.29, B97.5-B97.6,
B97.81-B97.89, G00.0-G03.9, G04.2, G32.89, G61.0, G96.9,
G98.0-G98.8, G99.8

PDX Collection 142
A90

PDX Collection 143
A91, A92.0-A94, A98.0-A98.2, A98.8-A99, B33.1

PDX Collection 144
A17.82, A50.42, A52.14, A75.9, A79.9, A81.1, A81.82-A81.89,
A83.0-A85.8, A87.2, A88.0, A88.8, A91-A94, A98.0-A98.2,
A98.8-A99, B00.4, B00.82, B01.11-B01.12, B04, B06.01,
B08.09, B08.20-B08.22, B08.60-B08.79, B09, B10.01-B10.09,
B26.2, B27.00-B27.99, B33.1, B45.0, B45.2-B45.9,
B58.2, B75, B97.10, B97.21, G04.00-G04.01, G04.31,
G04.81-G04.91, G05.3-G05.4, G37.0, G37.4-G37.5,
J09.X3-J09.X9, J10.2-J10.89, J11.2-J11.89, L44.4,
M1A.10X0-M1A.19X1, P35.2-P35.9, P37.0-P37.9,
T56.0X1-T56.0X4[A]

PDX Collection 145
A17.82, A50.42, A52.14, A75.9, A79.9, A81.1, A81.82-A81.89,
A83.0-A85.8, A87.2, A88.0, A88.8, A91, A92.0-A92.2,
A92.39, A92.4-A94, A98.0-A98.2, A98.8-A99, B00.4, B00.82,
B01.11-B01.12, B04, B06.01, B08.09, B08.20-B08.22,
B08.60-B08.79, B09, B10.01-B10.09, B26.2, B27.00-B27.99,
B33.1, B45.0, B45.2-B45.9, B58.2, B75, B97.10,
G04.00-G04.01, G04.31, G04.81-G04.91, G05.3-G05.4, G37.0,
G37.4-G37.5, J09.X3-J09.X9, J10.2-J10.89, J11.2-J11.89,
L44.4, P35.2-P35.9, P37.0-P37.9

PDX Collection 146
A95.0-A95.9

PDX Collection 147
A74.81-A74.9, A88.1, A96.0-A96.9, A98.3-A98.5, B25.8-B25.9,
B33.24-B34.2, B34.4-B34.8, B97.0-B97.89

PDX Collection 148
A17.9, A18.10-A18.11, A18.13, A18.82, A18.84, A18.89,
A54.21, A54.29, A54.82, A54.84, A54.89-A54.9, A59.00,
A59.8-A59.9, A98.5, B37.41-B37.49, B97.21, E08.21-E08.29,
E08.618-E08.638, E08.649-E08.8, E09.21-E09.29,
E09.618-E09.638, E09.649-E09.8, E10.21-E10.29,
E10.618-E10.638, E10.649, E10.69-E10.8, E11.21-E11.29,
E11.618-E11.638, E11.649, E11.69-E11.8, E13.21-E13.29,
E13.618-E13.638, E13.649-E13.8, M10.30-M10.39,
N00.0-N11.0, N11.8-N13.39, N13.6, N14.0-N17.9, N19,
N25.0-N26.1, N26.9-N27.9, N28.1-N29, N36.41-N36.43,
N36.8-N36.9, N39.8-N39.9, R31.0-R31.9

PDX Collection 149
B00.2

PDX Collection 150
A02.21, A17.0-A17.1, A27.81, A39.0, A50.41, A51.41,
A52.13, A54.82, A54.84, A54.89-A54.9, A87.0-A87.9, B00.3,
B00.82-B00.9, B02.1, B10.81-B10.89, B26.1, B37.5, B38.4,
B45.1, B58.2, B92, B94.2-B94.9, G00.0-G03.9, G04.2, G32.89,
G61.0, G96.9, G98.0-G98.8, G99.8

PDX Collection 151
B00.4, B00.82-B00.9, B10.01-B10.89, B92, B94.2-B94.9

PDX Collection 152
B00.50-B00.59, B00.89-B00.9, B10.81-B10.89

PDX Collection 153
A02.1, A20.7, A22.7, A26.7, A32.7, A39.2-A39.4, A40.0-A41.9,
A42.7, A54.86, B00.7, B00.82-B00.9, B10.81-B10.89, B37.7,
B92, B94.2-B94.9, R65.10-R65.20

PDX Collection 154
B00.3, B00.81-B00.9, B10.81-B10.89, B92, B94.2-B94.9

PDX Collection 155
A74.81-A74.9, A96.2, A98.3-A98.4, B00.82-B00.9, B01.12,
B02.24, B10.81-B10.89, B33.24, B33.4-B33.8, B34.1-B34.2,
B34.4-B34.8, B92, B94.2-B94.9, B97.10, B97.19, B97.29,
B97.5-B97.6, B97.81-B97.89, G04.00-G04.01, G04.31,
G04.81-G04.89, G05.3-G05.4, G37.3

PDX Collection 156
A74.81-A74.9, A96.2, A98.3-A98.4, B00.82-B00.9,
B10.81-B10.89, B33.24, B33.4-B33.8, B34.1-B34.2,
B34.4-B34.8, B92, B94.2-B94.9, B97.10, B97.19, B97.29,
B97.5-B97.6, B97.81-B97.89

PDX Collection 157
A74.81-A74.9, A96.2, A98.3-A98.4, B01.0, B01.12,
B01.81-B01.9, B08.04, B33.24, B33.4-B33.8, B34.1-B34.2,
B34.4-B34.8, B92, B94.2-B94.9, B97.10, B97.19, B97.29,
B97.5-B97.6, B97.81

PDX Collection 158
A74.81-A74.9, A96.2, A98.3-A98.4, B01.0-B01.12,
B01.81-B01.9, B08.04, B33.24, B33.4-B33.8, B34.1-B34.2,
B34.4-B34.8, B92, B94.2-B94.9, B97.10, B97.19, B97.29,
B97.5-B97.6, B97.81-B97.89

PDX Collection 159
A74.81-A74.9, A96.2, A98.3-A98.4, B00.82, B01.0, B01.12,
B01.81-B01.9, B02.24, B08.04, B33.24, B33.4-B33.8,
B34.1-B34.2, B34.4-B34.8, B92, B94.2-B94.9, B97.10, B97.19,
B97.29, B97.5-B97.6, B97.81-B97.89, G04.00-G04.01,
G04.31, G04.81-G04.89, G05.3-G05.4, G37.3

PDX Collection 160
A74.81-A74.9, A96.2, A98.3-A98.4, B01.0, B01.12-B01.9,
B08.04, B33.24, B33.4-B33.8, B34.1-B34.2, B34.4-B34.8, B92,
B94.2-B94.9, B97.10, B97.19, B97.29, B97.5-B97.6, B97.81

PDX Collection 161
A74.81-A74.9, A96.2, A98.3-A98.4, B00.3, B00.82-B00.9,
B02.0-B02.29, B02.7-B02.9, B10.81-B10.89, B33.24,
B33.4-B33.8, B34.1-B34.2, B34.4-B34.8, B92, B94.2-B94.9,
B97.10, B97.19, B97.29, B97.5-B97.6, B97.81-B97.89

PDX Collection 162
A02.21, A17.0-A17.1, A27.81, A39.0, A50.41, A51.41, A52.13,
A54.82, A54.84, A54.89-A54.9, A74.81-A74.9, A87.0-A87.9,
A96.2, A98.3-A98.4, B00.3, B00.82-B00.9, B02.0-B02.29,
B02.7-B02.9, B10.81-B10.89, B26.1, B33.24, B33.4, B33.8,
B34.1-B34.2, B34.4-B34.8, B37.5, B38.4, B45.1, B58.2, B92,
B94.2-B94.9, B97.10, B97.19, B97.29, B97.5-B97.6, B97.81,
G00.0-G03.9, G04.2, G32.89, G61.0, G96.9, G98.0-G98.8,
G99.8

PDX Collection 163
A74.81-A74.9, A96.2, A98.3-A98.4, B00.3, B00.82-B00.9,
B01.12, B02.0-B02.29, B02.7-B02.9, B10.81-B10.89, B33.24,
B33.4-B33.8, B34.1-B34.2, B34.4-B34.8, B92, B94.2-B94.9,
B97.10, B97.19, B97.29, B97.5-B97.6, B97.81-B97.89,
G04.00-G04.01, G04.31, G04.81-G04.89, G05.3-G05.4, G37.3

PDX Collection 164
B02.30-B02.39

PDX Collection 165
A60.00-A60.9, A74.81-A74.9, A96.2, A98.3-A98.4,
B00.0-B00.2, B00.4-B00.9, B02.0-B02.9, B10.01-B10.89,
B33.24, B33.4-B33.8, B34.1-B34.2, B34.4, B34.8, B92,
B94.2-B94.9, B97.10, B97.19, B97.29, B97.5-B97.6,
B97.81-B97.89

PDX Collection 166
B01.0-B01.9, B03, B08.010-B08.04

PDX Collection 167
B04, B08.010-B08.011, B08.09, B08.3, B08.60-B08.79, B09,
L44.4

PDX Collection 168
A74.81-A74.9, A96.2, A98.3-A98.4, B05.0-B05.1, B05.4,
B05.89-B05.9, B33.24, B33.4-B33.8, B34.1-B34.2,
B34.4-B34.8, B92, B94.2-B94.9, B97.10, B97.19, B97.29,
B97.5-B97.6, B97.81-B97.89

PDX Collection 169
A74.81-A74.9, A96.2, A98.3-A98.4, B05.1, B05.4,
B05.89-B05.9, B33.24, B33.4-B33.8, B34.1-B34.2,
B34.4-B34.8, B92, B94.2-B94.9, B97.10, B97.19, B97.29,
B97.5-B97.6, B97.81-B97.89

PDX Collection 170
A74.81-A74.9, A96.2, A98.3-A98.4, B05.1-B05.2, B05.4,
B05.89-B05.9, B33.24, B33.4-B33.8, B34.1-B34.2,
B34.4-B34.8, B92, B94.2-B94.9, B97.10, B97.19, B97.29,
B97.5-B97.6, B97.81-B97.89

PDX Collection 171
A74.81-A74.9, A96.2, A98.3-A98.4, B05.1, B05.4,
B05.81-B05.9, B33.24, B33.4-B33.8, B34.1-B34.2,
B34.4-B34.8, B92, B94.2-B94.9, B97.10, B97.19, B97.29,
B97.5-B97.6, B97.81-B97.89

PDX Collection 172
A74.81-A74.9, A96.2, A98.3-A98.4, B05.1, B05.4,
B05.81-B05.9, B06.00-B06.81, B06.89-B06.9, B33.24,
B33.4-B33.8, B34.1-B34.2, B34.4-B34.8, B92, B94.2-B94.9,
B97.10, B97.19, B97.29, B97.5-B97.6, B97.81-B97.89

PDX Collection 173
A74.81-A74.9, A96.2, A98.3-A98.4, B05.1, B05.4,
B05.81-B05.9, B06.81-B06.82, B06.89-B06.9, B33.24,
B33.4-B33.8, B34.1-B34.2, B34.4-B34.8, B92, B94.2-B94.9,
B97.10, B97.19, B97.29, B97.5-B97.6, B97.81-B97.89

PDX Collection 174
B08.3, B34.3

PDX Collection 175
A74.81-A74 9, A96.2, A98.3-A98.4, B15.0 B19.9, B33.24,
B33.4-B33.8, B34.1-B34.2, B34.4-B34.8, B92, B94.2-B94.9,
B97.10, B97.19, B97.29, B97.5-B97.6, B97.81-B97.89

PDX Collection 176
B20, B92, B94.2-B94.9

PDX Collection 177
B25.2, K85.00-K86.1, K86.81-K86.9

PDX Collection 178
A96.0 A96.9, A98.3-A98.5, B25.0-B25.9, B33.24-B34.2,
B34.4-B34.8, B97.0-B97.32, B97.39, B97.5-B97.89

PDX Collection 179
A74.81-A74.9, A96.2, A98.3-A98.4, B26.0, B26.82-B26.83,
B26.85-B26.9, B33.24, B33.4-B33.8, B34.1-B34.8, B92,
B94.2-B94.9, B97.10, B97.19, B97.29, B97.5-B97.6,
B97.81-B97.89

PDX Collection 180
A02.21, A17.0-A17.1, A27.81, A39.0, A50.41, A51.41,
A52.13, A54.82, A54.84, A54.89-A54.9, A74.81-A74.9,
A87.0-A87.9, A96.2, A98.3-A98.4, B00.3, B02.1, B26.1,
B26.82-B26.83, B26.85-B26.9, B33.24, B33.4-B33.8,
B34.1-B34.2, B34.4-B34.8, B37.5, B38.4, B45.1, B58.2, B92,
B94.2, B94.8-B94.9, B97.10, B97.19, B97.29, B97.5-B97.6,
B97.81-B97.89, G00.0-G03.9, G04.2, G32.89, G61.0, G96.9,
G98.0-G98.8, G99.8

PDX Collection 181
A74.81-A74.9, A96.2, A98.3-A98.4, B26.2, B26.82-B26.83,
B26.85-B26.9, B33.24, B33.4, B33.8, B34.1-B34.2,
B34.4-B34.8, B92, B94.2, B94.8-B94.9, B97.10, B97.19,
B97.29, B97.5-B97.6, B97.81-B97.89

PDX Collection 182
A74.81-A74.9, A96.2, A98.3-A98.4, B26.3, B26.82-B26.83,
B26.85-B26.9, B33.24, B33.4, B33.8, B34.1-B34.2,
B34.4-B34.8, B92, B94.2, B94.8-B94.9, B97.10, B97.19,
B97.29, B97.5-B97.6, B97.81-B97.89

PDX Collection 183
A74.81-A74.9, A96.2, A98.3-A98.4, B26.81-B26.83,
B26.85-B26.9, B33.24, B33.4, B33.8, B34.1-B34.2,

B34.4-B34.8, B92, B94.2, B94.8-B94.9, B97.10, B97.19,
B97.29, B97.5-B97.6, B97.81-B97.89

PDX Collection 184
A74.81-A74.9, A96.2, A98.3-A98.4, B26.82-B26.83,
B26.85-B26.9, B33.24, B33.4, B33.8, B34.1-B34.2,
B34.4-B34.8, B92, B94.2, B94.8-B94.9, B97.10, B97.19,
B97.29, B97.5-B97.6, B97.81-B97.89

PDX Collection 185
A74.81-A74.9, A96.2, A98.3-A98.4, B26.82-B26.9, B33.24,
B33.4, B33.8, B34.1 B34.2, B34.4-B34.8, B92, B94.2,
B94.8-B94.9, B97.10, B97.19, B97.29, B97.5-B97.6,
B97.81-B97.89

PDX Collection 186
A52.06, B33.20-B33.22, I00, I01.2-I01.9, I09.0, I09.9,
I23.0-I23.3, I23.6-I23.8, I40.0-I41, I51.0, I51.4, I87.8-I87.9,
I99.8-I99.9

PDX Collection 187
A01.00-A01.09, A39.51, A52.03, A78, B33.21, B37.6,
B40.0-B40.9, I00, I01.1, I01.8-I02.0, I05.0-I07.9, I08.1-I08.3,
I08.9, I09.1, I09.89-I09.9, I33.0-I39, I42.4, I87.8-I87.9,
I99.8-I99.9, Q22.2, Q23.8-Q23.9, Q24.8, T82.6XXA

PDX Collection 188
B33.23, I01.0, I09.2, I30.0-I30.9, I31.3-I32, I87.8-I87.9,
I99.8-I99.9

PDX Collection 189
A74.81-A74.9, A88.1, A96.0-A96.9, A98.3-A98.5,
B19.20-B19.21, B25.8-B25.9, B33.24, B33.3-B34.2,
B34.4-B34.8, B97.0-B97.89

PDX Collection 190
B37.0-B37.9, B48.3, B49, B92, B94.2-B94.9

PDX Collection 191
B37.1, B37.41-B37.82, B37.84-B37.9, N25.81-N25.89

PDX Collection 192
A02.21, A17.0-A17.1, A27.81, A39.0, A50.41, A51.41,
A52.13, A54.82, A54.84, A54.89-A54.9, A87.0-A87.9, B00.3,
B02.1, B26.1, B37.0-B38 4, B45.1, B48.3, B49, B58.2, B92,
B94.2-B94.9, G00.0-G03.9, G04.2, G32.89, G61.0, G96.9,
G98.0, G98.8-G99.8

PDX Collection 193
A02.1, A20.7, A22.7, A26.7, A32.7, A39.2-A39.4, A40.0-A40.1,
A40.8-A41.9, A42.7, A48.2-A48.4, A48.8-A49.9, A54.86,
B00.7, B37.0-B37.9, B48.3, B49, B92, B94.2-B96.89,
R65.10-R65.20, Z16.10-Z16.39

PDX Collection 194
B37.1, B37.5-B37.82, B37.84-B37.9

PDX Collection 195
B38.0-B38.2, B38.7, B38.89-B38.9, B48.3, B49, B92,
B94.2-B94.9

PDX Collection 196
B38.0-B39.9

PDX Collection 197
B38.0-B38.9

PDX Collection 198
A02.21, A17.0-A17.1, A27.81, A39.0, A50.41, A51.41, A52.13,
A54.82, A54.84, A54.89-A54.9, A87.0-A87.9, B00.3, B02.1,
B26.1, B37.5, B38.4-B38.87, B38.89-B38.9, B45.1, B48.3,
B49, B58.2, B92, B94.2-B94.9, G00.0-G03.9, G04.2, G32.89,
G61.0, G96.9, G98.0, G98.8-G99.8

PDX Collection 199
B38.7, B38.89-B38.9, B48.3, B49, B92, B94.2-B94.9

PDX Collection 200
A22.1, A37.01-A37.11, A37.81, A37.9, A48.1, B25.0,
B39.0-B39.4, B39.9-B44.0, B48.3, B49, B92, B94.2-B94.9,
J09.X1-J09.X2, J10.00-J10.1, J11.00-J11.1, J12.0-J12.3,

J12.89-J18.1, J18.8-J18.9, J44.9, J47.0-J47.9, J60-J70.4,
J70.8-J70.9, J98.4, R91.1

PDX Collection 201
B38.0-B39.4

PDX Collection 202
B40.0-B40.9, B48.3, B49, B92, B94.2-B94.9

PDX Collection 203
B41.0-B41.9, B48.3, B49, B92, B94.2-B94.9

PDX Collection 204
B44.1-B44.7, B44.89-B44.9, B48.3-B48.4, B49, B92,
B94.2-B94.9

PDX Collection 205
B44.81, J22, J98.8-J98.9

PDX Collection 206
B45.0, B45.2-B45.9, B48.3, B49, B92, B94.2-B94.9

PDX Collection 207
A02.21, A17.0-A17.1, A27.81, A39.0, A50.41, A51.41,
A52.13, A54.82, A54.84, A54.89-A54.9, A87.0-A87.9, B00.3,
B02.1, B26.1, B37.5, B38.4, B45.1, B58.2, E08.40-E08.49,
E08.618-E08.638, E08.649-E08.8, E09.40-E09.49,
E09.618-E09.638, E09.649-E09.8, E10.40-E10.49,
E10.618-E10.638, E10.649, E10.69, E10.8, E11.40-E11.49,
E11.618-E11.638, E11.649, E11.69-E11.8, E13.40-E13.49,
E13.618-E13.638, E13.649-E13.69, E13.8, G00.0-G03.9,
G04.2, G32.89, G61.0, G96.9, G98.0-G98.8, G99.8

PDX Collection 208
B46.0-B46.9, B48.3, B49, B92, B94.2-B94.9

PDX Collection 209
B47.0, B48.3, B49, B92, B94.2-B94.9

PDX Collection 210
A42.81-A42.9, A43.8-A43.9, B47.1-B47.9

PDX Collection 211
B48.2-B48.3, B49, B92, B94.2-B94.9

PDX Collection 212
B48.3, B49

PDX Collection 213
B48.3, B48.8-B49, B92, B94.2-B94.9

PDX Collection 214
B50.0-B57.5

PDX Collection 215
A44.0 A44.9, A68.0-A68.9, A69.20-A69.29, B50.0-B57.5,
B60.00-B60.09

PDX Collection 216
A17.9, A18.10-A18.13, A18.84, A18.89, A54.21,
A54.29, A54.82, A54.84, A54.89-A54.9, A59.00, A59.8-A59.9,
B37.41-B37.49, B50.0-B57.5, E08.21-E08.29, E08.618,
E08.620-E08.638, E08.649-E08.8, E09.21-E09.29,
E09.618-E09.638, E09.649-E09.8, E10.21-E10.29,
E10.618-E10.638, E10.649, E10.69-E10.8, E11.21-E11.29,
E11.618 E11.638, E11.649, E11.69-E11.8, E13.21-E13.29,
E13.618-E13.638, E13.649-E13.8, E88.3, M10.30-M10.39,
N00.0-N11.0, N11.8-N13.39, N13.6, N14.0-N19, N25.0-N26.1,
N26.9-N27.9, N28.1 N29, N36.41-N36.43, N36.8-N36.9,
N39.8-N39.9, R31.0-R31.9

PDX Collection 217
B50.0-B57.5, B97.21

PDX Collection 218
A44.0-A44.9, A68.0-A68.9, A69.20-A69.29, A75.0-A79.9,
B50.0-B57.5, B60.00-B60.09

PDX Collection 219
B57.0, B57.2, B92, B94.2-B94.9

PDX Collection 220
B58.00, B58.82-B58.9, B92, B94.2-B94.9

PDX Collection 221
B58.00-B58.01, B58.82-B58.9, B92, B94.2-B94.4

PDX Collection 222
B58.00, B58.09, B58.82-B58.9, B92, B94.2-B94.9

PDX Collection 223
B58.00, B58.1, B58.82-B58.9, B92, B94.2-B94.9

PDX Collection 224
B58.00, B58.2, B58.82-B58.9, B92, B94.2-B94.9

PDX Collection 225
A22.1, A37.01, A37.11, A37.81, A37.91, A48.1, B25.0, B44.0, B58.00, B58.3, B58.82-B58.9, B92, B94.2-B94.9, J09.X1-J09.X2, J10.00-J10.1, J11.00-J11.1, J12.0-J12.3, J12.89-J18.1, J18.8-J18.9, J44.9, J47.0-J70.4, J70.8-J70.9, J98.4, R91.1

PDX Collection 226
B58.00, B58.81-B58.9, B92, B94.2-B94.9

PDX Collection 227
B58.9

PDX Collection 228
A22.1, A37.01, A37.11, A37.81, A37.91, A48.1, B25.0, B44.0, B59, B92, B94.2-B94.9, J09.X1-J09.X2, J10.00-J10.1, J11.00-J11.1, J12.0-J12.3, J12.89-J15.20, J15.211-J18.1, J18.8-J18.9, J44.9, J47.0-J70.4, J70.8-J70.9, J98.4, R91.1

PDX Collection 229
B59, B60.10-B60.11, B60.19-B64, B89, B99.8-B99.9, L94.6, M35.2

PDX Collection 230
B65.0-B65.9

PDX Collection 231
B66.0-B66.9

PDX Collection 232
B67.0, B67.8-B67.99

PDX Collection 233
B67.1, B67.8-B67.99, J12.81

PDX Collection 234
B67.2, B67.32-B67.39, B67.8-B67.99

PDX Collection 235
B67.31, B67.8-B67.99

PDX Collection 236
B67.4, B67.8-B67.99

PDX Collection 237
B67.5, B67.8-B67.99

PDX Collection 238
B67.61-B67.69, B67.8-B67.99

PDX Collection 239
B67.7-B67.99

PDX Collection 240
B67.8-B67.99

PDX Collection 241
A00.1, A01.00-A01.09, A01.4-A02.0, A03.9-A05.2, A06.0-A06.2, A06.9, A07.1-A09, A18.32-A18.39, A18.83, A48.51-A48.52, B37.82, B68.0-B71.9, B82.9, J09.X3-J09.X9, J10.2-J10.89, J11.2-J11.89, K30, K31.84, K52.1-K52.3, K52.82-K52.9, K58.0-K58.9, P76.8-P77.9, P78.1, P78.3-P78.89

PDX Collection 242
B68.0-B71.9

PDX Collection 243
B72-B74.9

PDX Collection 244
A17.82, A50.42, A52.14, A75.9, A79.9, A81.1, A81.82-A81.89, A83.0-A85.8, A87.2, A88.0, A88.8, A92.1-A92.8, A93.0, B00.4, B00.82, B01.11-B01.12, B04, B06.01, B08.09, B08.20-B08.22, B08.60-B08.79, B09, B10.01-B10.09, B26.2, B33.1, B45.0,

B45.2-B45.9, B58.2, B75, B97.10, B97.21, G04.00-G04.01, G04.31, G04.81-G05.4, G37.0, G37.4-G37.5, J09.X3-J09.X9, J10.2-J10.89, J11.2-J11.89, L44.4, M1A.10X0-M1A.10X1, M1A.1110-M1A.19X1, P35.2-P35.9, P37.0-P37.4, P37.8-P37.9, T56.0X1-T56.0X4[A]

PDX Collection 245
B76.0-B76.9

PDX Collection 246
B77.0-B78.0, B78.7-B82.0

PDX Collection 247
A15.0-A15.6, A15.8-A15.9, A17.9, A18.82, A18.84, A18.89, A21.2, A22.1, A31.0, A37.01, A37.11, A37.81, A37.91, A42.0, A43.0, A48.1, B25.0, B39.0-B39.2, B44.0, B58.3, B59, B67.1, B77.0-B78.0, B78.7-B82.0, J09.X1-J09.X2, J10.00-J10.1, J11.00-J11.1, J12.0-J12.3, J12.89-J18.1, J18.8-J18.9, J22, J44.9, J47.0-J70.4, J70.8-J70.9, J98.4, J98.8-J99, Q33.4, R91.1

PDX Collection 248
B77.0-B78.0, B78.7-B83.3, B83.8-B83.9

PDX Collection 249
A15.0-A15.6, A15.8-A15.9, A17.9, A18.82, A18.84, A18.89, A21.2, A22.1, A31.0, A37.01, A37.11, A37.81, A37.91, A42.0, A43.0, A48.1, B25.0, B34.1-B34.2, B34.4-B34.8, B39.0-B39.2, B44.0, B58.3, B59, B67.1, B97.19-B97.29, B97.5-B97.6, B97.81-B97.89, J09.X1-J09.X2, J10.00-J10.1, J11.00-J11.1, J12.0-J12.3, J12.89-J15.20, J15.211-J18.1, J18.8-J18.9, J22, J44.9, J47.0-J70.4, J70.8-J70.9, J98.4, J98.8-J99, Q33.4, R91.1

PDX Collection 250
A74.81, A74.9, B33.3-B33.4, B34.1-B34.2, B34.4-B34.8, B97.10, B97.19-B97.29, B97.31-B97.39, B97.5-B97.6, B97.81-B97.89

PDX Collection 251
A74.81, A74.9, B33.3-B33.4, B34.1-B34.2, B34.4-B34.8, B97.10, B97.19-B97.39, B97.5-B97.6, B97.81, B97.89

PDX Collection 252
A74.81, A74.9, B20, B33.3-B33.4, B34.1-B34.2, B34.4, B34.8, B97.10, B97.19-B97.39, B97.5-B97.6, B97.81, B97.89

PDX Collection 253
C15.3-C15.9, C26.0, C26.9, C45.7-C45.9, C46.4, C76.8, C7A.00, C7A.098-C7B.00, C7B.1, C80.0-C80.2, D49.0, D49.81-D49.9

PDX Collection 254
C16.0-C16.9, C26.0, C26.9, C45.7-C45.9, C46.4, C49.A2, C76.8, C7A.00, C7A.092, C7A.094-C7B.00, C7B.1, C80.0-C80.2, D49.0, D49.81-D49.9

PDX Collection 255
C17.0, C17.8-C17.9, C26.0, C26.9, C45.7-C45.9, C46.4, C76.8, C7A.00-C7A.010, C7A.019, C7A.098-C7B.00, C7B.1, C80.0-C80.2, D49.0, D49.81-D49.9

PDX Collection 256
C17.1, C17.8-C17.9, C26.0, C26.9, C45.7-C45.9, C46.4, C76.8, C7A.00, C7A.011, C7A.019, C7A.098, C7A.1-C7B.00, C7B.1, C80.0-C80.2, D49.0, D49.81-D49.9

PDX Collection 257
C17.2, C17.8-C17.9, C26.0, C26.9, C45.7-C45.9, C46.4, C76.8, C7A.00, C7A.012-C7A.019, C7A.098, C7A.1-C7B.00, C7B.1, C80.0-C80.2, D49.0, D49.81-D49.9

PDX Collection 258
C17.3-C17.9, C26.0, C26.9, C45.7-C45.9, C46.4, C76.8, C7A.00, C7A.019, C7A.098-C7B.00, C7B.1, C80.0-C80.2, D49.0, D49.81-D49.9

PDX Collection 259
C17.8-C17.9, C26.0, C26.9, C45.7-C45.9, C46.4, C76.8, C7A.00, C7A.019, C7A.098, C7A.1-C7B.00, C7B.1, C80.0-C80.2, D49.0, D49.81-D49.9

PDX Collection 260
C18.0, C18.8-C18.9, C26.0-C26.9, C45.7-C45.9, C46.4, C76.8, C7A.00, C7A.021, C7A.029, C7A.098-C7B.00, C7B.1, C80.0-C80.2, D49.0, D49.81-D49.9

PDX Collection 261
C18.1, C18.8-C18.9, C26.0, C26.9, C45.7-C45.9, C46.4, C76.8, C7A.00, C7A.020, C7A.029, C7A.098, C7A.1-C7B.00, C7B.1, C80.0-C80.2, D49.0, D49.81-D49.9

PDX Collection 262
C18.2, C18.8-C18.9, C26.0, C26.9, C45.7-C45.9, C46.4, C76.8, C7A.00, C7A.022, C7A.029, C7A.098, C7A.1-C7B.00, C7B.1, C80.0-C80.2, D49.0, D49.81-D49.9

PDX Collection 263
C18.3, C18.8-C18.9, C26.0, C26.9, C45.7-C45.9, C46.4, C76.8, C7A.00, C7A.029, C7A.098-C7B.00, C7B.1, C80.0-C80.2, D49.0, D49.81-D49.9

PDX Collection 264
C18.4, C18.8-C18.9, C26.0, C26.9, C45.7-C45.9, C46.4, C76.8, C7A.00, C7A.023, C7A.029, C7A.098, C7A.1-C7B.00, C7B.1, C80.0-C80.2, D49.0, D49.81-D49.9

PDX Collection 265
C18.5, C18.8-C18.9, C26.0, C26.9, C45.7-C45.9, C46.4, C76.8, C7A.00, C7A.029, C7A.098-C7B.00, C7B.1, C80.0-C80.2, D49.0, D49.81-D49.9

PDX Collection 266
C18.6, C18.8-C18.9, C26.0, C26.9, C45.7-C45.9, C46.4, C76.8, C7A.00, C7A.024, C7A.029, C7A.098-C7B.00, C7B.1, C80.0-C80.2, D49.0, D49.81-D49.9

PDX Collection 267
C18.7-C18.9, C26.0, C26.9, C45.7-C45.9, C46.4, C76.8, C7A.00, C7A.025, C7A.029, C7A.098, C7A.1-C7B.00, C7B.1, C80.0-C80.2, D49.0, D49.81-D49.9

PDX Collection 268
C18.8-C18.9, C26.0, C26.9, C45.7-C45.9, C46.4, C76.8, C7A.00, C7A.029, C7A.098, C7A.1-C7B.00, C7B.1, C80.0-C80.2, D49.0, D49.81-D49.9

PDX Collection 269
C19, C21.2-C21.8, C26.0, C26.9, C45.7-C45.9, C46.4, C76.8, C7A.00, C7A.098, C7A.1-C7B.00, C7B.1, C80.0-C80.2, D49.0, D49.81-D49.9

PDX Collection 270
C20, C21.2-C21.8, C26.0, C26.9, C45.7-C45.9, C46.4, C76.8, C7A.00, C7A.026, C7A.098, C7A.1-C7B.00, C7B.1, C80.0-C80.2, D49.0, D49.81-D49.9

PDX Collection 271
C21.0-C21.8, C26.0, C26.9, C45.7-C45.9, C46.4, C76.8, C7A.00, C7A.098, C7A.1-C7B.00, C7B.1, C80.0-C80.2, D49.0, D49.81-D49.9

PDX Collection 272
C21.2-C21.8, C26.0, C26.9, C45.7-C45.9, C46.4, C76.8, C7A.00, C7A.098, C7A.1-C7B.00, C7B.1, C80.0-C80.2, D49.0, D49.81-D49.9

PDX Collection 273
C22.0-C22.9, C26.0, C26.9, C45.7-C45.9, C46.4, C76.8, C7A.00, C7A.098, C7A.1-C7B.00, C7B.1, C80.0-C80.2, D49.0, D49.81-D49.9

PDX Collection 274
C23, C24.8-C24.9, C26.0, C26.9, C45.7-C45.9, C46.4, C76.8, C7A.00, C7A.098, C7A.1-C7B.00, C7B.1, C8.00-C8.02, D49.0, D49.81-D49.9

PDX Collection 275
C24.0, C24.8-C24.9, C26.0, C26.9, C45.7-C45.9, C46.4, C76.8, C7A.00, C7A.098-C7B.00, C7B.1, C80.0-C80.2, D49.0, D49.81-D49.9

PDX Collection 276
C24.1, C24.8-C24.9, C26.0, C26.9, C45.7-C45.9, C46.4, C76.8, C7A.00, C7A.098, C7A.1, C7A.8, C7B.00, C7B.1, C80.0-C80.2, D49.0, D49.81-D49.9

PDX Collection 277
C24.8-C24.9, C26.0, C26.9, C45.7-C45.9, C46.4, C76.8, C7A.00, C7A.098-C7A.8, C7B.00, C7B.1, C80.0-C80.2, D49.0, D49.81-D49.9

PDX Collection 278
C25.0-C26.0, C26.9, C45.7-C45.9, C46.4, C76.8, C7A.00, C7A.098, C7A.1-C7B.00, C7B.1, C8.00-C80.2, D49.0, D49.81-D49.9

PDX Collection 279
C33, C34.00-C34.92, C39.9, C45.7-C45.9, C46.50-C46.52, C76.1, C76.8, C78.00-C78.1, C78.30-C78.39, C7A.00, C7A.090, C7A.098-C7B.00, C7B.1, C80.0-C80.2, D49.1, D49.81-D49.9

PDX Collection 280
C34.00-C34.02, C34.80-C34.92, C39.9, C45.7-C45.9, C46.50-C46.52, C76.8, C7A.00, C7A.090, C7A.098, C7A.1-C7B.00, C7B.1, C80.0-C80.2, D49.1, D49.81-D49.9

PDX Collection 281
C34.10-C34.12, C34.80-C34.92, C39.9, C45.7-C45.9, C46.50-C46.52, C76.8, C7A.00, C7A.090, C7A.098-C7B.00, C7B.1, C80.0-C80.2, D49.1, D49.81-D49.9

PDX Collection 282
C34.2, C34.80-C34.92, C39.9, C45.7-C45.9, C46.50-C46.52, C76.8, C7A.00, C7A.090, C7A.098-C7B.00, C7B.1, C80.0-C80.2, D49.1, D49.81-D49.9

PDX Collection 283
C34.30-C34.92, C39.9, C45.7-C45.9, C46.50-C46.52, C76.8, C7A.00, C7A.090, C7A.098-C7B.00, C7B.1, C80.0-C80.2, D49.1, D49.81-D49.9

PDX Collection 284
C34.80-C34.92, C39.9, C45.7-C45.9, C46.50-C46.52, C76.8, C7A.00, C7A.090, C7A.098-C7B.00, C7B.1, C80.0-C80.2, D49.1, D49.81-D49.9

PDX Collection 285
C37, C7A.091

PDX Collection 286
C38.0, C45.2

PDX Collection 287
C38.1-C38.3, C38.8, C39.9, C45.7-C45.9, C76.0, C7A.00, C7A.098-C7B.00, C7B.1, C80.0-C80.2, D49.1, D49.81-D49.9

PDX Collection 288
C38.4, C39.9, C45.0, C45.7-C45.9, C76.8, C7A.00, C7A.098, C7A.1-C7B.00, C7B.1, C80.0-C80.2, D49.1, D49.81-D49.9

PDX Collection 289
C40.00-C40.02, C40.80-C40.92, C41.9, Z51.0

PDX Collection 290
C40.10-C40.12, C40.80-C40.92, C41.9, Z51.0

PDX Collection 291
C40.20-C40.22, C40.80-C40.92, C41.9, Z51.0

PDX Collection 292
C40.30-C40.92, C41.9, Z51.0

PDX Collection 293
C40.00-C41.9, Z51.0

PDX Collection 294
C40.80-C41.0, C41.9, Z51.0

PDX Collection 295
C40.80-C40.92, C41.1, C41.9, Z51.0

PDX Collection 296
C40.80-C40.9, C41.2, C41.9, Z51.0

PDX Collection 297
C40.80-C40.92, C41.3, C41.9, Z51.0

PDX Collection 298
C40.80-C40.92, C41.4-C41.9, Z51.0

PDX Collection 299
C45.1, C48.0-C48.8, Z51.0

PDX Collection 300
C46.0, C46.7-C46.9, Z51.0

PDX Collection 301
C46.1, C46.7-C46.9, Z51.0

PDX Collection 302
C46.2, C46.7-C46.9, Z51.0

PDX Collection 303
C45.7-C45.9, C46.3, C76.8-C77.9, C7A.00, C7A.098-C7B.01, C7B.1, C80.0-C80.2, D49.81-D49.9

PDX Collection 304
C46.4, C46.7-C46.9, Z51.0

PDX Collection 305
C46.0-C46.9, Z51.0

PDX Collection 306
C45.7-C46.9, C51.0-C72.9, C76.0-C79.9, C7A.00, C7A.093, C7A.098-C7B.8, C80.0-C80.2, D00.00-D02.4, D04.0-D09.9, D37.01-D44.9, D48.0-D49.9, Z51.0

PDX Collection 308
C48.0, Z51.0

PDX Collection 309
C45.9, C56.1-C57.4, C76.3, C79.60-C79.62, C7A.00, C7A.098-C7B.00, C7B.1, C80.0-C80.2

PDX Collection 310
C45.7-C45.9, C64.1-C65.9, C68.8-C68.9, C76.8, C7A.00, C7A.093, C7A.098-C7B.00, C7B.1, C80.0-C80.2, D49.511-D49.59, D49.81-D49.9

PDX Collection 311
C45.7-C45.9, C66.1-C66.9, C68.8-C68.9, C76.8, C7A.00, C7A.098, C7A.1-C7B.00, C7B.1, C80.0-C80.2, D49.511-D49.59, D49.81-D49.9

PDX Collection 312
C68.0-C68.9, C79.82

PDX Collection 313
C6.41-C66.9, C68.0-C68.9, C76.3, C79.00-C79.19, C7A.093

PDX Collection 314
C45.7-C45.9, C70.0, C70.9, C72.9, C76.8, C7A.00, C7A.098-C7B.00, C7B.1, C80.0-C80.2, D49.6-D49.9

PDX Collection 315
C45.7-C45.9, C70.1, C72.9, C76.8, C7A.00, C7A.098-C7B.00, C7B.1, C80.0-C80.2, D49.6-D49.9

PDX Collection 316
C45.7-C45.9, C70.0, C70.9-C71.9, C72.20-C72.9, C76.8, C7A.00, C7A.098-C7B.00, C7B.1, C80.0-C80.2, D49.6-D49.9

PDX Collection 317
C45.7-C45.9, C72.0-C72.1, C72.9, C76.8, C7A.00, C7A.098, C7A.1-C7B.00, C7B.1, C80.0-C80.2, D49.6-D49.9

PDX Collection 318
C45.7-C45.9, C72.20-C72.9, C76.8, C7A.00, C7A.098-C7B.00, C7B.1, C80.0-C80.2, D49.6-D49.9

PDX Collection 319
C45.7-C45.9, C70.0-C72.9, C76.8, C79.31-C79.49, C7A.00, C7A.098-C7B.00, C7B.1, C80.0-C80.2, D49.6-D49.9

PDX Collection 320
C45.7-C45.9, C74.00-C74.92, C75.9, C76.2, C76.8, C79.70-C79.72, C7A.00, C7A.098-C7B.00, C7B.1, C80.0-C80.2

PDX Collection 321
C75.0, C75.8-C75.9

PDX Collection 322
C75.1-C75.2, Z51.0

PDX Collection 323
C75.3, Z51.0

PDX Collection 324
C75.4, C75.8-C75.9

PDX Collection 325
C75.4-C75.9

PDX Collection 326
C74.00-C75.9

PDX Collection 327
C45.7-C45.9, C76.8, C78.00-C78.39, C79.89-C79.9, C7A.00, C7A.098-C7B.00, C7B.09-C7B.8, C80.0-C80.2, D49.81-D49.9

PDX Collection 328
C45.7-C45.9, C76.8, C78.1, C78.30-C78.39, C79.89-C79.9, C7A.00, C7A.098-C7B.00, C7B.09-C7B.8, C80.0-C80.2, D49.81-D49.9

PDX Collection 329
C45.7-C45.9, C76.8, C78.2-C78.39, C79.89-C79.9, C7A.00, C7A.098-C7B.00, C7B.09-C7B.8, C80.0-C80.2, D49.81-D49.9, J91.0

PDX Collection 330
C45.7-C45.9, C76.8, C78.00-C78.39, C79.89-C79.9, C7A.00, C7A.098-C7B.00, C7B.09-C7B.8, C80.0-C80.2, D49.81-D49.9

PDX Collection 331
C45.7-C45.9, C76.8, C78.4, C78.80-C78.89, C79.89-C79.9, C7A.00, C7A.098-C7B.00, C7B.09-C7B.8, C80.0-C80.2, D49.81-D49.9

PDX Collection 332
C45.7-C45.9, C76.8, C78.5, C78.80-C78.89, C79.89-C79.9, C7A.00, C7A.098-C7B.00, C7B.09-C7B.8, C80.0-C80.2, D49.81-D49.9

PDX Collection 333
C45.7-C45.9, C76.8, C78.6, C78.80-C78.89, C79.89-C79.9, C7A.00, C7A.098-C7B.00, C7B.04-C7B.8, C80.0-C80.2, D49.81-D49.9

PDX Collection 334
C45.7-C45.9, C76.8, C78.7-C78.89, C79.89-C79.9, C7A.00, C7A.098-C7A.8, C7B.00, C7B.02, C7B.09-C7B.8, C80.0-C80.2, D49.81-D4.99

PDX Collection 335
C45.7-C45.9, C76.8, C78.4-C78.89, C79.89-C79.9, C7A.00, C7A.098-C7B.00, C7B.02, C7B.04-C7B.8, C80.0-C80.2, D49.81-D49.9

PDX Collection 336
C45.7-C45.9, C76.8, C79.00-C79.19, C79.89-C79.9, C7A.00, C7A.098-C7B.00, C7B.09-C7B.8, C80.0-C80.2, D49.81-D49.9

PDX Collection 337
C45.7-C45.9, C76.8, C79.2, C79.89-C79.9, C7A.00, C7A.098-C7B.00, C7B.09-C7B.8, C80.0-C80.2, D49.81-D49.9

PDX Collection 338
C45.7-C45.9, C76.8, C79.31, C79.89-C79.9, C7A.00, C7A.098-C7B.00, C7B.09-C7B.8, C80.0-C80.2, D49.81-D49.9

PDX Collection 339
C45.7-C45.9, C76.8, C79.32-C79.49, C79.89-C79.9, C7A.00, C7A.098-C7B.00, C7B.09-C7B.8, C80.0-C80.2, D49.81-D49.9

PDX Collection 340
C45.7-C45.9, C76.8, C79.51-C79.52, C79.89-C79.9, C7A.00, C7A.098-C7B.00, C7B.03, C7B.09-C7B.8, C80.0-C80.2, D49.81-D49.9

PDX Collection 341
C45.7-C45.9, C76.8, C79.60-C79.62, C79.89-C79.9, C7A.00, C7A.098-C7B.00, C7B.09-C7B.8, C80.0-C80.2, D49.81-D49.9

PDX Collection 342
C45.7-C45.9, C76.8, C79.70-C79.72, C79.89-C79.9, C7A.00, C7A.098-C7B.00, C7B.09-C7B.8, C80.0-C80.2, D49.81-D49.9

PDX Collection 343
C45.7-C45.9, C76.8, C79.81, C79.89-C79.9, C7A.00, C7A.098-C7B.00, C7B.09-C7B.8, C80.0-C80.2, D49.81-D49.9

PDX Collection 344
C45.7-C45.9, C76.8, C79.82-C79.9, C7A.00, C7A.098-C7B.00, C7B.09-C7B.8, C80.0-C80.2, D49.81-D49.9

PDX Collection 345
C45.7-C45.9, C76.8, C79.89-C79.9, C7A.00, C7A.098-C7B.00, C7B.09, C7B.1-C7B.8, C80.0-C80.2, D49.81-D49.9

PDX Collection 346
C45.7-C45.9, C76.8, C79.89-C79.9, C7A.00-C7B.00, C7B.09-C7B.8, C80.0-C80.2, D49.81-D49.9

PDX Collection 347
C17.0, C17.8-C17.9, C26.0, C26.9, C45.7-C45.9, C46.4, C76.8, C7A.00-C7B.00, C7B.1, C80.0-C80.2, D49.0, D49.81-D49.9

PDX Collection 348
C17.1, C17.8-C17.9, C26.0, C26.9, C45.7-C45.9, C46.4, C76.8, C7A.00-C7B.00, C7B.1, C80.0-C80.2, D49.0, D49.81-D49.9

PDX Collection 349
C17.2, C17.8-C17.9, C26.0, C26.9, C45.7-C45.9, C46.4, C76.8, C7A.00-C7B.00, C7B.1, C80.0-C80.2, D49.0, D49.81-D49.9

PDX Collection 350
C17.8-C17.9, C26.0, C26.9, C45.7-C45.9, C46.4, C76.8, C7A.00-C7B.00, C7B.1, C80.0-C80.2, D49.0, D49.81-D49.9

PDX Collection 351
C18.1, C18.8-C18.9, C26.0, C26.9, C45.7-C45.9, C46.4, C76.8, C7A.00-C7B.00, C7B.1, C80.0-C80.2, D49.0, D49.81-D49.9

PDX Collection 352
C18.0, C18.8-C18.9, C26.0, C26.9, C45.7-C45.9, C46.4, C76.8, C7A.00-C7B.00, C7B.1, C80.0-C80.2, D49.0, D49.81-D49.9

PDX Collection 353
C18.2, C18.8-C18.9, C26.0, C26.9, C45.7-C45.9, C46.4, C76.8, C7A.00-C7B.00, C7B.1, C80.0-C80.2, D49.0, D49.81-D49.9

PDX Collection 354
C18.4, C18.8-C18.9, C26.0, C26.9, C45.7-C45.9, C46.4, C76.8, C7A.00-C7B.00, C7B.1, C80.0-C80.2, D49.0, D49.81-D49.9

PDX Collection 355
C18.6, C18.8-C18.9, C26.0, C26.9, C45.7-C45.9, C46.4, C76.8, C7A.00-C7B.00, C7B.1, C80.0-C80.2, D49.0, D49.81-D49.9

PDX Collection 356
C18.7-C18.9, C26.0, C26.9, C45.7-C45.9, C46.4, C76.8, C7A.00-C7B.00, C7B.1, C80.0-C80.2, D49.0, D49.81-D49.9

PDX Collection 357
C20, C21.2-C21.8, C26.0, C26.9, C45.7-C45.9, C46.4, C76.8, C7A.00-C7B.00, C7B.1, C80.0-C80.2, D49.0, D49.81-D49.9

PDX Collection 358
C18.8-C18.9, C26.0, C26.9, C45.7-C45.9, C46.4, C76.8, C7A.00-C7B.00, C7B.1, C80.0-C80.2, D49.0, D49.81-D49.9

PDX Collection 359
C34.80-C34.92, C39.9, C45.7-C45.9, C46.50-C46.52, C76.8, C7A.00-C7B.00, C7B.1, C80.0-C80.2, D49.1, D49.81-D49.9

PDX Collection 360
C37, C7A.00-C7A.8

PDX Collection 361
C16.0-C16.9, C26.0, C26.9, C45.7-C45.9, C46.4, C49.A2, C76.8, C7A.00-C7B.00, C7B.1, C80.0-C80.2, D49.0, D49.81-D49.9

PDX Collection 362
C45.7-C45.9, C64.1-C65.9, C68.8-C68.9, C76.8, C7A.00-C7B.00, C7B.1, C80.0-C80.2, D49.511-D49.59, D49.81-D49.9

PDX Collection 363
C45.7-C45.9, C46.3, C76.8-C77.9, C7A.00, C7A.098-C7B.8, C80.0-C80.2, D49.81-D49.9

PDX Collection 364
C45.7-C45.9, C76.8, C78.7-C78.89, C79.89-C79.9, C7A.00, C7A.098-C7B.8, C80.0-C80.2, D49.81-D49.9

PDX Collection 365
C45.7-C45.9, C76.8, C79.51-C79.52, C79.89-C79.9, C7A.00, C7A.098-C7B.8, C80.0-C80.2, D49.81-D49.9

PDX Collection 366
C45.7-C45.9, C76.8, C78.6, C78.80-C78.89, C79.89-C79.9, C7A.00, C7A.098-C7B.8, C80.0-C80.2, D49.81-D49.9

PDX Collection 367
C45.7-C45.9, C76.8, C79.89-C79.9, C7A.00, C7A.098-C7B.8, C80.0-C80.2, D49.81-D49.9

PDX Collection 368
C81.00-C81.09, C81.40-C81.49, C81.90, C81.98, D49.81-D49.9

PDX Collection 369
C81.00-C81.01, C81.08-C81.09, C81.40-C81.41, C81.48-C81.49, C81.90-C81.91, C81.98, D49.81-D49.9

PDX Collection 370
C81.00-C81.02, C81.08-C81.09, C81.40-C81.42, C81.48-C81.49, C81.90-C81.92, C81.98, D49.81-D49.9

PDX Collection 371
C81.00, C81.03, C81.08-C81.09, C81.40, C81.43, C81.48-C81.49, C81.90, C81.93, C81.98, D49.81-D49.9

PDX Collection 372
C81.00, C81.04, C81.08-C81.09, C81.40, C81.44, C81.48-C81.49, C81.90, C81.94, C81.98, D49.81-D49.9

PDX Collection 373
C81.00, C81.05, C81.08-C81.09, C81.40, C81.45, C81.48-C81.49, C81.90, C81.95, C81.98, D49.81-D49.9

PDX Collection 374
C81.00, C81.06, C81.08-C81.09, C81.40, C81.46, C81.48-C81.49, C81.90, C81.96, C81.98, D49.81-D49.9

PDX Collection 375
C81.00, C81.07-C81.09, C81.40, C81.47-C81.49, C81.90, C81.97-C81.98, D49.81-D49.9

PDX Collection 376
C81.10-C81.19, C81.90, C81.98, D49.81-D49.9

PDX Collection 377
C81.10-C81.11, C81.18-C81.19, C81.90-C81.91, C81.98, D49.81-D49.9

PDX Collection 378
C81.10, C81.12, C81.18-C81.19, C81.90, C81.92, C81.98, D49.81-D49.9

PDX Collection 379
C81.10, C81.13, C81.18-C81.19, C81.90, C81.93, C81.98, D49.81-D49.9

PDX Collection 380
C81.10, C81.14, C81.18-C81.19, C81.90, C81.94, C81.98, D49.81-D49.9

PDX Collection 381
C81.10, C81.15, C81.18-C81.19, C81.90, C81.95, C81.98, D49.81-D49.9

PDX Collection 382
C81.10, C81.16, C81.18-C81.19, C81.90, C81.96, C81.98, D49.81-D49.9

PDX Collection 383
C81.10, C81.17-C81.19, C81.90, C81.97-C81.98, D49.81-D49.9

PDX Collection 384
C81.20-C81.29, C81.90, C81.98, D49.81-D49.9

PDX Collection 385
C81.20-C81.21, C81.28-C81.29, C81.90-C81.91, C81.98, D49.81-D49.9

PDX Collection 386
C81.20, C81.22, C81.28-C81.29, C81.90, C81.92, C81.98, D49.81-D49.9

PDX Collection 387
C81.20, C81.23, C81.28-C81.29, C81.90, C81.93, C81.98, D49.81-D49.9

PDX Collection 388
C81.20, C81.24, C81.28-C81.29, C81.90, C81.94, C81.98, D49.81-D49.9

PDX Collection 389
C81.20, C81.25, C81.28-C81.29, C81.90, C81.95, C81.98, D49.81-D49.9

PDX Collection 390
C81.20, C81.26, C81.28-C81.29, C81.90, C81.96, C81.98, D49.81-D49.9

PDX Collection 391
C81.20, C81.27, C81.28-C81.29, C81.90, C81.97, C81.98, D49.81-D49.9

PDX Collection 392
C81.30-C81.39, C81.90, C81.98, D49.81-D49.9

PDX Collection 393
C81.30-C81.31, C81.38-C81.39, C81.90-C81.91, C81.98, D49.81-D49.

PDX Collection 394
C81.30, C81.32, C81.38-C81.39, C81.90, C81.92, C81.98, D49.81-D49.9

PDX Collection 395
C81.30, C81.33, C81.38-C81.39, C81.90, C81.93, C81.98, D49.81-D49.9

PDX Collection 396
C81.30, C81.34, C81.38-C81.39, C81.90, C81.94, C81.98, D49.81-D49.9

PDX Collection 397
C81.30, C81.35, C81.38-C81.39, C81.90, C81.95, C81.98, D49.81-D49.9

PDX Collection 398
C81.30, C81.36, C81.38-C81.39, C81.90, C81.96, C81.98, D49.81-D49.9

PDX Collection 399
C81.30, C81.37, C81.38-C81.39, C81.90, C81.97, C81.98, D49.81-D49.9

PDX Collection 400
C81.30-C81.39, C81.98, D49.81-D49.9

PDX Collection 401
C81.70-C81.79, C81.90, C81.98, D49.81-D49.9

PDX Collection 402
C81.70-C81.71, C81.78-C81.79, C81.90-C81.91, C81.98, D49.81-D49.9

PDX Collection 403
C81.70, C81.72, C81.78-C81.79, C81.90, C81.92, C81.98, D49.81-D49.9

PDX Collection 404
C81.70, C81.73, C81.78-C81.79, C81.90, C81.93, C81.98, D49.81-D49.9

PDX Collection 405
C81.70, C81.74, C81.78-C81.79, C81.90, C81.94, C81.98, D49.81-D49.9

PDX Collection 406
C81.70, C81.75, C81.78-C81.79, C81.90, C81.95, C81.98,
D49.81-D49.9

PDX Collection 407
C81.70, C81.76, C81.78-C81.79, C81.90, C81.96, C81.98,
D49.81-D49.9

PDX Collection 408
C81.70, C81.77, C81.78-C81.79, C81.90, C81.97, C81.98,
D49.81-D49.9

PDX Collection 409
C81.90-C81.98, D49.81-D49.9

PDX Collection 410
C81.90-C81.91, C81.98, D49.81-D49.9

PDX Collection 411
C81.90, C81.92, C81.98, D49.81-D49.9

PDX Collection 412
C81.90, C81.93, C81.98, D49.81-D49.9

PDX Collection 413
C81.90, C81.94, C81.98, D49.81-D49.9

PDX Collection 414
C81.90, C81.95, C81.98, D49.81-D49.9

PDX Collection 415
C81.90, C81.96, C81.98, D49.81-D49.9

PDX Collection 416
C81.90, C81.97-C81.98, D49.81-D49.9

PDX Collection 417
C82.00-C82.50, C82.59-C82.99, C83.10, C83.19, C84.40,
C84.49, C84.60, C84.69-C84.70, C84.79, C84.A0, C84.A9,
C84.Z0, C84.Z9, C84.90, C84.99-C85.10, C85.19-C85.20,
C85.29-C85.80, C85.89-C85.90, C85.99, C86.4, C88.4, C96.4,
C96.9, C96.Z, D49.81-D49.9

PDX Collection 418
C82.00-C82.01, C82.08-C82.11, C82.18-C82.21,
C82.28-C82.31, C82.38-C82.41, C82.48-C82.49, C82.51,
C82.60-C82.61, C82.68-C82.81, C82.88-C82.91,
C82.98-C82.99, C83.11, C84.41, C84.61, C84.71, C84.A1,
C84.Z1, C84.91, C85.11, C85.21, C85.81, C85.91, C86.0,
D49.81-D49.9

PDX Collection 419
C82.00, C82.02, C82.08-C82.10, C82.12, C82.18-C82.20,
C82.22, C82.28-C82.30, C82.32, C82.38-C82.40, C82.42,
C82.48-C82.49, C82.52, C82.60, C82.62, C82.68-C82.80,
C82.82, C82.88-C82.90, C82.92, C82.98-C82.99, C83.12,
C84.42, C84.62, C84.72, C84.92, C84.A2, C84.Z2, C85.12,
C85.22, C85.82, C85.92, D49.81-D49.9

PDX Collection 420
C82.00, C82.03, C82.08-C82.10, C82.13, C82.18-C82.20,
C12.23, C82.28-C82.30, C82.33, C82.38-C82.40, C82.43,
C82.48-C82.49, C82.53, C82.60, C82.63, C82.68-C82.80,
C82.83, C82.88-C82.90, C82.93, C82.98-C82.99, C83.13,
C84.43, C84.63, C84.73, C84.93, C04.A3, C84.Z3, C85.13,
C85.23, C85.83, C85.93, C86.2, C86.3, D49.81-D49.9

PDX Collection 421
C82.00, C82.04, C82.08-C82.10, C82.14, C82.18-C82.20,
C82.24, C82.28-C82.30, C82.34, C82.38-C82.40, C82.44,
C82.48-C82.49, C82.54, C82.60, C82.64, C82.68-C82.80,
C82.84, C82.88-C82.90, C82.94, C82.98-C82.99, C83.14,
C84.44, C84.64, C84.74, C84.94, C84.A4, C84.Z4, C85.14,
C85.24, C85.84, C85.94, D49.81-D49.9

PDX Collection 422
C82.00, C82.05, C82.08-C82.10, C82.15, C82.18-C82.20,
C82.25, C82.28-C82.30, C82.35, C82.38-C82.40, C82.45,
C82.48-C82.49, C82.55, C82.60, C82.65, C82.68-C82.80,
C82.85, C82.88-C82.90, C82.95, C82.98-C82.99, C83.15,

C84.45, C84.65, C84.75, C84.95, C84.A5, C84.Z5, C85.15,
C85.25, C85.85, C85.95, D49.81-D49.9

PDX Collection 423
C82.00, C82.06, C82.08-C82.10, C82.16, C82.18-C82.20,
C82.26, C82.28-C82.30, C82.36, C82.38-C82.40, C82.46,
C82.48-C82.49, C82.56, C82.60, C82.66, C82.68-C82.80,
C82.86, C82.88-C82.90, C82.96, C82.98-C82.99, C83.16,
C84.46, C84.66, C84.76, C84.96, C84.A6, C84.Z6, C85.16,
C85.26, C85.86, C85.96, D49.81-D49.9

PDX Collection 424
C82.00, C82.07, C82.08-C82.10, C82.17-C82.20,
C82.27-C82.30, C82.37-C82.40, C82.47-C82.49, C82.57,
C82.60, C82.67-C82.80, C82.87-C82.90, C82.97-C82.99,
C83.17, C84.47, C84.67, C84.77, C84.97, C84.A7, C84.Z7,
C85.17, C85.27, C85.87, C85.97, C86.1, D49.81-D49.9

PDX Collection 425
C82.00-C82.49, C82.58, C82.60-C82.99, C83.18, C84.48,
C84.68, C84.78, C84.98, C84.A8, C84.Z8, C85.18, C85.28,
C85.88, C85.98, D49.81-D49.9

PDX Collection 426
C82.50-C82.59, C83.10-C83.19, C84.40-C84.49,
C84.60-C84.79, C84.90-C84.99, C84.A0-C84.Z9, C85.10-C86.4,
C88.4, C96.4, C96.9, C96.Z, D49.81-D49.9

PDX Collection 427
C82.50-C82.51, C82.58-C82.59, C83.10-C83.11,
C83.18-C83.19, C84.40-C84.41, C84.48-C84.61,
C84.68-C84.71, C84.78-C84.79, C84.90-C84.91,
C84.98-C84.99, C84.A0-C84.A1, C84.A8-C84.A9,
C84.Z0-C84.Z1, C84.Z8-C84.Z9, C85.10-C85.11, C85.18-C85.21,
C85.28-C85.81, C85.88-C85.91, C85.98-C85.99, C86.0, C86.4,
C88.4, D49.81-D49.9

PDX Collection 428
C82.50, C82.52, C82.58-C82.59, C83.10, C83.12,
C83.18-C83.19, C84.40, C84.42, C84.48-C84.60, C84.62,
C84.68-C84.70, C84.72, C84.78-C84.79, C84.90, C84.92,
C84.98-C84.99, C84.A0, C84.A2, C84.A8-C84.A9, C04.Z0,
C84.Z2, C84.Z8-C84.Z9, C05.10, C85.12, C85.18-C85.20,
C85.22, C85.28-C85.80, C85.82, C85.88-C85.90, C85.92,
C85.98-C85.99, C86.4, C88.4, D49.81-D49.9

PDX Collection 429
C82.50, C82.53, C82.58-C82.59, C83.10, C83.13,
C83.18-C83.19, C84.40, C84.43, C84.48-C84.60, C84.63,
C84.68-C84.70, C84.73, C84.78-C84.79, C84.90, C84.93,
C84.98-C84.99, C84.A0, C84.A3, C84.A8-C84.A9, C84.Z0,
C84.Z3, C84.Z8-C84.Z9, C85.10, C85.13, C85.18-C85.20,
C85.22, C85.28-C85.80, C85.83, C85.88-C85.90, C85.93,
C85.98-C85.99, C86.2-C86.4, C88.4, D49.81-D49.9

PDX Collection 430
C82.50, C82.54, C82.58-C82.59, C83.10, C83.14,
C83.18-C83.19, C84.40, C84.44, C84.48-C84.60, C84.64,
C84.68-C84.70, C84.74, C84.78-C84.79, C84.90, C84.94,
C84.98-C84.99, C84.A0, C84.A4, C84.A8-C84.A9, C84.Z0,
C84.Z4, C84.Z8-C84.Z9, C85.10, C85.14, C85.18-C85.20,
C85.24, C85.28-C85.80, C85.84, C85.88-C85.90, C85.94,
C85.98-C85.99, C86.4, C88.4, D49.81-D49.9

PDX Collection 431
C82.50, C82.55, C82.58-C82.59, C83.10, C83.15,
C83.18-C83.19, C84.40, C84.45, C84.48-C84.60, C84.65,
C84.68-C84.70, C84.75, C84.78-C84.79, C84.90, C84.95,
C84.98-C84.99, C84.A0, C84.A5, C84.A8-C84.A9, C84.Z0,
C84.Z5, C84.Z8-C84.Z9, C85.10, C85.15, C85.18-C85.20,
C85.25, C85.28-C85.80, C85.85, C85.88-C85.90, C85.95,
C85.98-C85.99, C86.4, C88.4, D49.81-D49.9

PDX Collection 432
C82.50, C82.56, C82.58-C82.59, C83.10, C83.16,
C83.18-C83.19, C84.40, C84.46, C84.48-C84.60, C84.66,

C84.68-C84.70, C84.76, C84.78-C84.79, C84.90, C84.96,
C84.98-C84.99, C84.A0, C84.A6, C84.A8-C84.A9, C84.Z0,
C84.Z6, C84.Z8-C84.Z9, C85.10, C85.16, C85.18-C85.20,
C85.26, C85.28-C85.80, C85.86, C85.88-C85.90, C85.96,
C85.98-C85.99, C86.4, C88.4, D49.81-D49.9

PDX Collection 433
C82.50, C82.57, C82.58-C82.59, C83.10, C83.17,
C83.18-C83.19, C84.40, C84.47-C84.49, C84.60, C84.67,
C84.68-C84.69, C84.70, C84.77, C84.78-C84.79, C84.90,
C84.97-C84.99, C84.A0, C84.A7-C84.A9, C84.Z0, C84.Z7,
C84.Z8-C84.Z9, C85.10, C85.17-C85.20, C85.27-C85.29,
C85.80, C85.87-C85.90, C85.97-C85.99, C86.1, C86.4, C88.4,
D49.81-D49.9

PDX Collection 434
C82.50-C82.59, C83.10-C83.19, C84.40-C84.49,
C84.60-C84.79, C84.90-C84.99, C84.A0-C84.Z9, C85.10-C86.4,
C88.4, D49.81-D49.9

PDX Collection 435
C83.00-C83.09, C83.80-C83.99, C86.5-C86.6, D49.81-D49.9

PDX Collection 436
C83.00-C83.01, C83.08-C83.09, C83.80-C83.81,
C83.88-C83.91, C83.98-C83.99, C86.5-C86.6, D49.81-D49.9

PDX Collection 437
C83.00, C83.02, C83.08-C83.09, C83.80, C83.82,
C83.88-C83.89, C83.90, C83.92, C83.98-C83.99, C86.5-C86.6,
D49.81-D49.9

PDX Collection 438
C83.00, C83.03, C83.00-C83.09, C83.80, C83.83,
C83.88-C83.89, C83.90, C83.93, C83.98-C83.99, C86.5-C86.6,
D49.81-D49.9

PDX Collection 439
C83.00, C83.04, C83.08-C83.09, C83.80, C83.84,
C83.88-C83.89, C83.90, C83.94, C83.98-C83.99, C86.5-C86.6,
D49.81-D49.9

PDX Collection 440
C83.00, C83.05, C83.08-C83.09, C83.00, C83.85,
C83.88-C83.89, C83.90, C83.95, C83.98-C83.99, C86.5-C86.6,
D49.81-D49.9

PDX Collection 441
C83.00, C83.06, C83.08-C83.09, C83.80, C83.86,
C83.88-C83.89, C83.90, C83.96, C83.98-C83.99, C86.5-C86.6,
D49.81-D49.9

PDX Collection 442
C83.00, C83.07-C83.09, C83.80, C83.87-C83.89, C83.90,
C83.97-C83.99, C86.5-C86.6, D49.81-D49.9

PDX Collection 443
C83.30-C83.39, D49.81-D49.9

PDX Collection 444
C83.30-C83.31, C83.38-C83.39, D49.81-D49.9

PDX Collection 445
C83.30, C83.32, C83.38-C83.39, D49.81-D49.9

PDX Collection 446
C83.30, C83.33, C83.38-C83.39, D49.81-D49.9

PDX Collection 447
C83.30, C83.34, C83.38-C83.39, D49.81-D49.9

PDX Collection 448
C83.30, C83.35, C83.38-C83.39, D49.81-D49.9

PDX Collection 449
C83.30, C83.36, C83.38-C83.39, D49.81-D49.9

PDX Collection 450
C83.30, C83.37-C83.39, D49.81-D49.9

PDX Collection 451
C83.50-C83.59, D49.81-D49.9

PDX Collection 452
C83.50-C83.51, C83.58-C83.59, D49.81-D49.9

PDX Collection 453
C83.50, C83.52, C83.58-C83.59, D49.81-D49.9

PDX Collection 454
C83.50, C83.53, C83.58-C83.59, D49.81-D49.9

PDX Collection 455
C83.50, C83.54, C83.58-C83.59, D49.81-D49.9

PDX Collection 456
C83.50, C83.55, C83.58-C83.59, D49.81-D49.9

PDX Collection 457
C83.50, C83.56, C83.58-C83.59, D49.81-D49.9

PDX Collection 458
C83.50, C83.57-C83.59, D49.81-D49.9

PDX Collection 459
C83.70-C83.79, D49.81-D49.9

PDX Collection 460
C83.70-C83.71, C83.78-C83.79, D49.81-D49.9

PDX Collection 461
C83.70, C83.72, C83.78-C83.79, D49.81-D49.9

PDX Collection 462
C83.70, C83.73, C83.78-C83.79, D49.81-D49.9

PDX Collection 463
C83.70, C83.74, C83.78-C83.79, D49.81-D49.9

PDX Collection 464
C83.70, C83.75, C83.78-C83.79, D49.81-D49.9

PDX Collection 465
C83.70, C83.76, C83.78-C83.79, D49.81-D49.9

PDX Collection 466
C83.70, C83.77-C83.79, D49.81-D49.9

PDX Collection 467
C82.50, C82.59, C83.10, C83.19, C84.00-C84.09, C84.40, C84.49, C84.60, C84.69-C84.70, C84.79, C84.90, C84.99, C84.A0, C84.A9-C84.Z0, C84.Z9, C85.10, C85.19-C85.20, C85.29-C85.80, C85.89-C85.90, C85.99, C86.4, C88.4, C96.4, C96.9, C96.Z, D49.81-D49.9

PDX Collection 468
C82.51, C83.11, C84.00-C84.01, C84.08-C84.09, C84.41, C84.61, C84.71, C84.91, C84.A1, C84.Z1, C85.11, C85.21, C85.81, C85.91, C86.0, D49.81-D49.9

PDX Collection 469
C82.52, C83.12, C84.00, C84.02, C84.08-C84.09, C84.42, C84.62, C84.72, C84.92, C84.A2, C84.Z2, C85.12, C85.22, C85.82, C85.92, D49.81-D49.9

PDX Collection 470
C82.53, C83.13, C84.00, C84.03, C84.08-C84.09, C84.43, C84.63, C84.73, C84.93, C84.A3, C84.Z3, C85.13, C85.23, C85.83, C85.93, C86.2-C86.3, D49.81-D49.9

PDX Collection 471
C82.54, C83.14, C84.00, C84.04, C84.08-C84.09, C84.44, C84.64, C84.74, C84.94, C84.A4, C84.Z4, C85.14, C85.24, C85.84, C85.94, D49.81-D49.9

PDX Collection 472
C82.55, C83.15, C84.00, C84.05, C84.08-C84.09, C84.45, C84.65, C84.75, C84.95, C84.A5, C84.Z5, C85.15, C85.25, C85.85, C85.95, D49.81-D49.9

PDX Collection 473
C82.56, C83.16, C84.00, C84.06, C84.08-C84.09, C84.46, C84.66, C84.76, C84.96, C84.A6, C84.Z6, C85.16, C85.26, C85.86, C85.96, D49.81-D49.9

PDX Collection 474
C82.57, C83.17, C84.00, C84.07, C84.08-C84.09, C84.47, C84.67, C84.77, C84.97, C84.A7, C84.Z7, C85.17, C85.27, C85.87, C85.97, D49.81-D49.9

PDX Collection 475
C82.58, C83.18, C84.00-C84.09, C84.48, C84.68, C84.78, C84.98, C84.A8, C84.Z8, C85.18, C85.28, C85.88, C85.98, D49.81-D49.9

PDX Collection 476
C82.50, C82.59, C83.10, C83.19, C84.10-C84.19, C84.40, C84.49-C84.60, C84.69-C84.70, C84.79, C84.90, C84.99, C84.A0, C84.A9-C84.Z0, C84.Z9, C85.10, C85.19-C85.20, C85.29-C85.80, C85.89-C85.90, C85.99, C86.4, C88.4, C96.4, C96.9, C96.Z, D49.81-D49.9

PDX Collection 477
C82.51, C83.11, C84.10-C84.11, C84.18-C84.19, C84.41, C84.61, C84.71, C84.91, C84.A1, C84.Z1, C85.11, C85.21, C85.81, C85.91, C86.0, D49.81-D49.9

PDX Collection 478
C82.52, C83.12, C84.10, C84.12, C84.18-C84.19, C84.42, C84.62, C84.72, C84.92, C84.A2, C84.Z2, C85.12, C85.22, C85.82, C85.92, D49.81-D49.9

PDX Collection 479
C82.53, C83.13, C84.10, C84.13, C84.18-C84.19, C84.43, C84.63, C84.73, C84.93, C84.A3, C84.Z3, C85.13, C85.23, C85.83, C85.93, C86.2-C86.3, D49.81-D49.9

PDX Collection 480
C82.54, C83.14, C84.10, C84.14, C84.18-C84.19, C84.44, C84.64, C84.74, C84.94, C84.A4, C84.Z4, C85.14, C85.24, C85.84, C85.94, D49.81-D49.9

PDX Collection 481
C82.55, C83.15, C84.10, C84.15, C84.18-C84.19, C84.45, C84.65, C84.75, C84.95, C84.A5, C84.Z5, C85.15, C85.25, C85.85, C85.95, D49.81-D49.9

PDX Collection 482
C82.56, C83.16, C84.10, C84.16, C84.18-C84.19, C84.46, C84.66, C84.76, C84.96, C84.A6, C84.Z6, C85.16, C85.26, C85.86, C85.96, D49.81-D49.9

PDX Collection 483
C82.57, C83.17, C84.10, C84.17-C84.19, C84.47, C84.67, C84.77, C84.97, C84.A7, C84.Z7, C85.17, C85.27, C85.87, C85.97, C86.1, D49.81-D49.9

PDX Collection 484
C82.58, C83.18, C84.10-C84.19, C84.48, C84.68, C84.78, C84.98, C84.A8, C84.Z8, C85.18, C85.28, C85.88, C85.98, D49.81-D49.9

PDX Collection 485
C88.2-C88.3, C88.8-C90.02, C90.10-C90.12, C90.20-C90.22, C90.30-C90.32, C91.00-C91.02, C91.10-C91.12, C91.30-C91.32, C91.50-C91.52, C91.60-C91.62, C91.90-C91.92, C91.A0-C91.A2, C91.Z0-C91.Z2, C92.00-C92.02, C92.10-C92.12, C92.20-C92.22, C92.30-C92.32, C92.40-C92.42, C92.50-C92.52, C92.60-C92.62, C92.90-C92.92, C92.A0-C92.A2, C92.Z0-C92.Z2, C93.00-C93.02, C93.10-C93.12, C93.30-C93.32, C93.90-C93.92, C93.Z0-C93.Z2, C94.00-C94.02, C94.20-C94.22, C94.30-C94.32, C94.80-C94.82, C95.00-C95.02, C95.10-C95.12, C95.90-C95.92, D49.81-D49.9

PDX Collection 486
C88.2-C88.3, C88.8-C90.02, C90.10-C90.12, C90.20-C90.22, C90.30-C90.32, C91.00-C91.02, C91.10-C91.12, C91.30-C91.32, C91.40-C91.42, C91.50-C91.52, C91.60-C91.62, C91.90-C91.92,
C91.A0-C91.A2, C91.Z0-C91.Z2, C92.00-C92.02, C92.10-C92.12, C92.20-C92.22, C92.30-C92.32, C92.40-C92.42, C92.50-C92.52, C92.60-C92.62, C92.90-C92.92, C92.A0-C92.A2, C92.Z0-C92.Z2, C93.00-C93.02, C93.10-C93.12, C93.30-C93.32, C93.90-C93.92, C93.Z0-C93.Z2, C94.00-C94.02, C94.20-C94.22, C94.30-C94.32, C94.40-C94.42, C94.6, C94.80-C94.82, C95.00-C95.02, C95.10-C95.12, C95.90-C95.92, D45-D46.22, D46.4, D46.9, D46.A-D46.Z, D47.01-D47.09, D47.3, D47.9, D47.Z2, D47.Z9, D48.7-D48.9, D49.81-D49.9

PDX Collection 487
C82.50, C82.59, C83.10, C83.19, C84.40, C84.49-C84.60, C84.69-C84.70, C84.79, C84.90, C84.99, C84.A0, C84.A9-C84.Z0, C84.Z9, C85.10, C85.19-C85.20, C85.29-C85.80, C85.89-C85.90, C85.99, C86.4, C88.4, C91.40-C91.42, C96.4, C96.9, C96.Z, D49.81-D49.9

PDX Collection 488
C88.2-C88.3, C88.8-C88.9, C90.10-C90.11, C90.20-C90.21, C90.30-C90.31, C91.00-C91.02, C91.10-C91.12, C91.30-C91.32, C91.40-C91.42, C91.50-C91.52, C91.60-C91.62, C91.90-C91.92, C91.A0-C91.A2, C91.Z0-C91.Z2, C92.00-C92.02, C92.10-C92.12, C92.20-C92.22, C92.30-C92.32, C92.40-C92.42, C92.50-C92.52, C92.60-C92.62, C92.90-C92.92, C92.A0-C92.A2, C92.Z0-C92.Z2, C93.00-C93.02, C93.10-C93.12, C93.30-C93.32, C93.90-C93.92, C93.Z0-C93.Z2, C94.00-C94.02, C94.20-C94.22, C94.30-C94.32, C94.40-C94.42, C94.6, C94.80-C94.82, C95.00-C95.02, C95.10-C95.12, C95.90-C95.92, D45-D46.22, D46.4, D46.9, D46.A-D46.Z, D47.01-D47.1, D47.3, D47.9, D47.Z2, D47.Z9, D48.7-D48.9

PDX Collection 489
C82.50, C82.59, C83.10, C83.19, C84.40, C84.49-C84.60, C84.69-C84.70, C84.79, C84.90, C84.99, C84.A0, C84.A9-C84.Z0, C84.Z9, C85.10, C85.19-C85.20, C85.29-C85.80, C85.89-C85.90, C85.99, C86.4, C88.4, C96.0, C96.4, C96.9, C96.Z, D49.81-D49.9

PDX Collection 490
C82.50, C82.59, C83.10, C83.19, C84.40, C84.49-C84.60, C84.69-C84.70, C84.79, C84.90, C84.99, C84.A0, C84.A9-C84.Z0, C84.Z9, C85.10, C85.19-C85.20, C85.29-C85.80, C85.89-C85.90, C85.99, C86.4, C88.4, C96.20-C96.29, C96.4, C96.9, C96.Z, D49.81-D49.9

PDX Collection 491
C96.4, C96.9, C96.Z, D49.81-D49.9

PDX Collection 492
E71.310-E71.32, E71.40-E71.548, E80.3-E80.7, E88.40-E88.49, H49.811-H49.819

PDX Collection 493
C82.50, C82.59, C83.10, C83.19, C84.40, C84.49-C84.60, C84.69-C84.70, C84.79, C84.90, C84.99, C84.A0, C84.A9-C84.Z0, C84.Z9, C85.10, C85.19-C85.20, C85.29-C85.80, C85.89-C85.90, C85.99, C86.4, C88.4, C96.4, C96.9, C96.A, C96.Z, D49.81-D49.9

PDX Collection 494
C88.8, C94.40-C94.42, C94.6, D45-D46.22, D46.4, D46.9, D46.A-D46.C, D46.Z, D47.01-D47.1, D47.3, D47.9, D47.Z2, D47.Z9, D75.81, Z51.0

PDX Collection 495
D47.Z1, D78.81-D78.89, E89.810-E89.89, H59.011-H59.019, H59.031-H59.099, H59.811-H59.89, H95.811-H95.89, I97.3, M96.89, N98.1-N98.9, T86.850-T86.99

PDX Collection 496

PDX Collection 497
D50.0-D64.9, D75.9, P61.2-P61.4

PDX Collection 498
D50.0-D64.9, D75.9, P61.2-P61.4

PDX Collection 499
D50.0-D64.9, D69.3-D69.49, D75.9, P61.2-P61.4

PDX Collection 500
D60.0-D60.9, D61.1-D64.9, D70.0-D70.9, D72.810-D72.820, D72.823, D72.825-D77 829, D75.9-D76.3, P61.2

PDX Collection 501
D47.4, D50.0-D64.9, D68.312, D68.51-D68.69, D75.81, D75.89-D75.9, D75.A, D77, D89.2, T79.2XX[A]

PDX Collection 502
D47.4, D65-D69.9, D75.81-D75.9, D75.A, D77, D89.2

PDX Collection 503
D47.4, D65-D69.9, D75.82-D75.9, D75.A, D77, D89.2

PDX Collection 504
D47.4, D68.311-D68.318, D68.51-D68.69, D70.0-D72.9, D73.81, D75.81, D77, D89.2

PDX Collection 505
D47.4, D68.312, D68.51-D68.69, D70.0-D72.9, D73.81, D75.81, D75.89-D77, D89.2

PDX Collection 506
D56.4, D58.2-D59.2, D59.4-D59.9, D64.4-D64.9, D74.0-D74.9, D75.9

PDX Collection 507
D60.0-D60 9, D61.1-D61.9, D65, D69.3-D70.9, D72.818-D72.819, D75.82, D75.9, D76.3

PDX Collection 508
D78.01-D78.02, D78.21-D78.89, H95.811-H95.89, I85.01, I85.11, I97.3, K21.9, K22.8, K23-K25.0, K25.2, K25.4, K25.6, K26.0, K26.2, K26.4, K26.6, K27.0, K27.2, K27.4, K27.6, K28.0, K28.2, K28.4, K28.6, K29.01, K29.21, K29.31, K29.41, K29.51, K29.61, K29.71, K29.81, K29.91, K31.811, K55.21, K57.01, K57.11, K57.13, K57.21, K57.31, K57.33, K57.41, K57.51, K57.53, K57.81, K57.91, K57.93, K62.5, K92.0-K92.2, M96.89, N98.1-N98.9, P54.1-P54.3, T81.10X-T81.19X[A], T81.82X[A], T81.89X-T81.9XX[A]

PDX Collection 509
D78.11-D78.12, D78.81-D78.89, E36.11-E36.8, E89.810-E89.89, G96 11, G97 41-G97.49, H59.011 H59.019, H59.031-H59.099, H59.211-H59.229, H59.811-H59.89, H95.31-H95.32, H95.811-H95.89, I97.3, I97.51-I97.52, J95.71-J95.72, K91.71-K91.72, L76.11-L76.12, L76.81-L76.82, M96.820-M96.821, M96.89, N98.1-N98.9, N99.71-N99.72, T81.82X[A], T81.89X-T81.9XX[A]

PDX Collection 510
D78.81-D78.89, H95.811-H95.89, I97.3, M96.89, N98.1-N98.9, T81.82X[A], T81.89X-T81.9XX[A]

PDX Collection 511
D80.0, D80.3-D81.4, D81.6-D81.7, D81.89-D84.0, D84.8-D84.9, D89.3-D89.9

PDX Collection 512
D80.0-D81.2, D81.4, D81.6-D81.7, D81.89-D84.0, D84.8-D84.9, D89.3-D89.9

PDX Collection 513
D81.30-D81.39, D81.5, D81.810, D84.1, E76.01-E76.9, E79.1-E80.29, E80.4-E80.7, E88.81

PDX Collection 514
D78.81-D78.89, D89.810-D89.813, E89.810-E89.89, H59.011-H59.019, H59.031-H59.099, H59.811-H59.89, H95.811-H95.89, I97.3, M96.89, N98.1-N98.9, T86.00-T86.09

PDX Collection 515
B15.0-B19.9, E03.5, E08.00-E08.59, E08.618-E09.59, E09.618-E10.59, E10.618-E10.649, E10.69-E11.59, E11.618-E11.649, E11.69-E13.59, E13.618-E16.2, E89.1, G32.89, G89.0-G89.4, G93.81-G93.9, G96.9, G98.0-G98.8, G99.8, I60.00-I62.9, K72.91, R29.700-R29.742, R40.0-R40.2124, R40.2210-R40.2224, R40.2310-R40.2324, R40.2340-R40.2344, R40.3-R41.3, R41.82, R41.9-R42, R44.8-R44.9, R45.83-R45.84, R46.0-R46.89, R52, R55, R68.0-R68.83, R68.89-R69, S02.0XX-S02.19X[A,B], S02.91X, S06.0X1[A], S06.0X9-S06.9X9[A]

PDX Collection 516
A17.9, A18.81-A18.82, A18.84, A18.89, E00.0-E03.4, E03.8-E07.1, E07.89-E07.9, E30.9, E34.1, E34.50-E35, E89.0

PDX Collection 517
E06.0-E06.9

PDX Collection 518
E08.00-E08.59, E08.618-E09.59, E09.618-E10.52, E10.59, E10.618-E10.649, E10.69-E11.59, E11.618-E11.649, E11.69-E13.59, E13.618-E16.2, E30.9, E34.1, E34.8-E35, E89.1

PDX Collection 519
G89.0-G89.4, I70.261-I70.269, I96, R41.0-R41.3, R41.82, R41.9, R44.8-R44.9, R45.83-R45.84, R46.0-R46.89, R52, R68.0-R68.19, R68.81-R68.83, R68.89-R69

PDX Collection 520
E08.00-E08.59, E08.618-E09.59, E09.618-E10.59, E10.618-E10.649, E10.69-E11.59, E11.618-E11.649, E11.69-E13.59, E13.618-E16.2, E30.9, E34.1, E34.50-E35, E89.1

PDX Collection 521
E22.1-E22.9

PDX Collection 522
E22.0-E23.7, E24.1, E30.9, E34.1, E34.4, E34.8-E35, E89.3

PDX Collection 523
E22.0-E23.7, E24.1, E30.9, E34.1, E34.4-E35, E89.3

PDX Collection 524
E22.1-E23.7, E24.1, E30.9, E34.1, E34.50-E35, E89.3

PDX Collection 525
E24.0, E24.2-E26.9, E30.9, E34.1, E34.50-E35

PDX Collection 526
A17.9, A18.7, A18.82, A18.84, A18.89, E27.0-E27.9, E30.9, E34.1, E34.50-E35, E89.6

PDX Collection 527
E30.9, E32.0-E32.9, E34.1, E34.50-E35

PDX Collection 528
E30.9, E34.0-E34.2, E34.50-E35

PDX Collection 529
E36.01-E36.02, E36.8, E89.810-E89.89, H95.811-H95.89, I85.01, I85.11, I97.3, K21.9, K22.8, K23-K25.0, K25.2, K25.4, K25.6, K26.0, K26.2, K26.4, K26.6, K27.0, K27.2, K27.4, K27.6, K28.0, K28.2, K28.4, K28.6, K29.01, K29.21, K29.31, K29.41, K29.51, K29.61, K29.71, K29.81, K29.91, K31.811, K55.21, K57.01, K57.11, K57.13, K57.21, K57.31, K57.33, K57.41, K57.51, K57.53, K57.81, K57.91, K57.93, K62.5, K92.0-K92.2, M96.89, N98.1-N98.9, P54.1-P54.3, T81.10X-T81.19X[A], T81.82XA, T81.89X-T81.9XX[A]

PDX Collection 530
E40-E46, E64.0

PDX Collection 531
D81.818-D81.819, E51.11-E53.9, E56.0, E56.8-E63.9, E64.8-E64.9

PDX Collection 532
E55.0-E63.9, E64.3-E64.9, M83.0-M83.9

PDX Collection 533
E66.2, I27.0-I27.81, I27.83, I27.89-I27.9

PDX Collection 534
C88.0, D47.2, D89.0-D89.1, E70.0-E71.30, E72.00-E72.02, E72.04-E74.9, E75.21-E75.249, E75.3, E75.5-E75.6, E77.0-E78.70, E78.79-E78.9, E88.02-E88.2, E88.89

PDX Collection 535
C96.5-C96.6, E71.32-E71.548, E80.3, E88.40-E88.49, E88.89, H49.811-H49.819

PDX Collection 536
C96.5-C96.6, E71.310-E71.448, E71.548, E80.3-E80.7, E88.40-E88.49, E88.89, H49.811-H49.819

PDX Collection 537
E75.00-E75.19, E75.4, E84.2, G13.2-G13.8, G30.0-G31.82, G31.84-G31.9, G91.4, G94

PDX Collection 538
E75.00-E75.19, E75.23, E75.25-E75.29, E75.4, F84.2, G13.2-G13.8, G31.2-G31.82, G32.89, G91.4, G93.81, G93.89-G94, G96.9, G98.0-G98.8, G99.8

PDX Collection 539
D81.30-D81.39, D81.5, D81.810, D84.1, E76.01-E76.9, E79.1-E80.29, E80.4-E80.7, E85.0, E85.9, E88.81

PDX Collection 540
E78.71-E78.72, Q87.2-Q87.89, Q89.8, Q99.2

PDX Collection 541
E84.0-E84.9

PDX Collection 542
E85.0-E85.9, E88.81

PDX Collection 543
E86.0-E87.8

PDX Collection 544
E08.21-E08.29, E09.21-E09.29, E88.3, N00.0-N01.9, N02.8-N02.9, N04.7-N05.1, N05.6-N06.1, N06.6-N07.1, N07.6-N08, N14.0-N15.0, N15.8-N17.9

PDX Collection 545
C96.5-C96.6, E71.310-E71.548, E80.3-E80.7, E88.89, H49.819

PDX Collection 546
E36.8, E89.810-E89.89, H95.811-H95.89, I97.3, M96.89, N98.1-N98.9, T81.82XA, T81.89X-T81.9XX[A]

PDX Collection 547
F01 51

PDX Collection 548
F02.81, F03.91

PDX Collection 549
F05, R45.851

PDX Collection 550
F02.80-F02.81, F04-F06.8, F10.10-F11.19, F11.21-F13.19, F13.21-F14.19, F14.21-F15.19, F15.21-F16.19, F16.21-F17.209, F17.213-F17.219, F17.223-F17.229, F17.293-F18.19, F18.21-F19.19, F19.21-F19.99, F53-F55.8, R78.0

PDX Collection 551
F07.0-F07.81, F07.9-F09, F20.0-F51.03, F51.12, F51.19, F51.3-F51.9, F52.5, F54, F59-F63.2, F63.81-F63.9, F68.10-F80.4, F80.82-F84.0, F84.3-F99, G44.201-G44.229, H93.25, R45.1-R45.2, R45.5-R45.82, R45.86-R45.87

PDX Collection 552
F30.13, F30.2, F31.13-F31.2, F31.4-F31.5, F31.63-F31.64

PDX Collection 553
F31.13-F31.2, F31.63-F31.64

PDX Collection 554
F31.13-F31.2, F31.4-F31.5, F31.63-F31.64

PDX Collection 555
F32.0-F32.3, F33.0-F33.40, F33.9

PDX Collection 556
F45.9, F50.00-F50.9, F59, F98.21-F98.3

PDX Collection 557
F50.00-F50.9, F98.21-F98.29

PDX Collection 558
F72-F73

PDX Collection 559
A02.21, A17.0-A17.1, A27.81, A39.0, A50.41, A51.41, A52.13, A54.82, A54.84, A54.89-A54.9, A87.0-A87.9, B00.3, B02.1, B26.1, B37.5, B38.4, B45.1, B58.2, G00.0-G03.9, G04.2, G32.89, G61.0, G96.9, G98.0-G98.8, G99.8

PDX Collection 560
A02.21, A17.0-A17.1, A17.82, A27.81, A39.0, A50.41-A50.42, A51.41, A52.13-A52.14, A54.82, A54.84, A54.89-A54.9, A81.1, A81.82-A81.89, A83.0-A85.8, A87.0-A88.0, A88.8, A92.1-A92.8, A93.0, A96.2, A98.3-A98.4, B00.3-B00.4, B00.89-B01.11, B01.81-B02.23, B02.29, B02.7-B02.9, B04, B06.01, B08.04-B08.09, B08.20-B08.22, B08.60-B08.79, B09-B10.89, B26.1-B26.2, B27.00-B27.99, B33.1, B33.24, B33.4-B33.8, B34.1-B34.2, B34.4, B34.8, B37.5, B38.4, B45.1-B58.2, B92, B94.2, B94.8-B94.9, B97.10, B97.19-B97.29, B97.5-B97.6, B97.81-B97.89, G00.0-G04.01, G04.2, G04.31, G04.81-G05.4, G32.89, G37.0, G37.4-G37.5, G61.0, G96.9, G98.0-G98.8, G99.8, J09.X3-J09.X9, J10.2-J10.89, J11.2-J11.89, L44.4, P35.2-P35.9, P37.0-P37.4, P37.8-P37.9

PDX Collection 561
G04.1, G11.0-G12.9, G32.0-G37.3, G37.5-G37.9, G80.0-G80.2, G80.4-G80.9, G81.00-G83.9, G90.01-G90.09, G90.2, G90.4, G90.50-G90.9, G92, G93.40-G93.49, G93.81, G93.89-G95.9, G96.9, G98.0-G99.8, I67.83, R53.2

PDX Collection 562
A17.82, A28.1, A50.42, A52.14, A75.9, A79.9, A81.1, A81.82-A81.89, A83.0-A85.8, A87.2, A88.0, A88.8, A92.1-A92.8, A93.0, B00.4, B00.82, B01.11-B01.12, B04, B06.01, B08.09, B08.20-B08.22, B08.60-B08.79, B09, B10.01-B10.09, B26.2, B27.00-B27.99, B33.1, B45.0, B45.2-B45.9, B54, B58.2, B75, B97.10, B97.21, G04.00-G04.01, G04.31, G04.81-G05.4, G37.0, G37.4-G37.5, H66.40-H66.43, J09.X3-J09.X9, J10.2-J10.89, J11.2-J11.89, L44.4, M1A.10X0-M1A.19X1, M32.0-M32.9, P35.2-P35.9, P37.0-P37.9, T56.0X1-T56.0X4[A]

PDX Collection 563
A06.6, A17.81, E08.40-E08.49, E08.618-E08.638, E08.649-E08.8, E09.40-E09.49, E09.618-E09.638, E09.649-E09.8, E10.40-E10.49, E10.618-E10.638, E10.649, E10.69-E10.8, E11.40-E11.49, E11.618-E11.638, E11.649, E11.69-E11.8, E13.40-E13.49, E13.618-E13.638, E13.649-E13.8, G06.0-G08, G93.81, G93.89-G93.9

PDX Collection 564
A06.6, A17.81, E08.40-A08.49, E08.618-E08.638, E08.649-E08.8, E09.40-E09.49, E09.618-E09.638, E09.649-E09.8, E10.40-E10.49, E10.618-E10.638, E10.649, E10.69-E10.8, E11.40-E11.49, E11.618-E11.638, E11.649, E11.69-E11.8, E13.40-E13.49, E13.618-E13.638, E13.649-E13.8, G06.1

PDX Collection 565
A06.6, A17.81, E08.40-E08.49, E08.618-E08.638, E08.649-E08.8, E09.40-E09.49, E09.618-E09.638, E09.649-E09.8, E10.40-E10.49, E10.618-E10.638, E10.649, E10.69-E10.8, E11.40-E11.49, E11.618-E11.638, E11.649, E11.69-E11.8, E13.40-E13.49, E13.618-E13.638, E13.649-E13.8, G06.0-G06.2, G07-G08

PDX Collection 566
G04.1, G10, G20, G21.11-G21.9, G32.89-G37.9, G80.0-G80.2, G80.4-G80.9, G82.20-G83.0, G92, G93.1, G93.40-G93.6, G93.81, G93.89-G93.9, G96.9, G98.0-G98.8, G99.8, I67.83, R53.2

PDX Collection 567
G04.1, G10-G12.9, G21.0, G23.0-G25.79, G25.82-G26, G32.0-G37.9, G80.0-G83.9, G90.01-G90.09, G90.2-G90.9, G92-G93.1, G93.40-G93.49, G93.81, G93.89-G95.9, G96.9, G98.0-G99.8, I67.83, R53.2

PDX Collection 568
G04.1, G10-G12.9, G21.0, G23.0-G25.79, G25.82-G26, G32.0-G37.3, G37.5-G37.9, G80.0-G83.9, G90.01-G90.09, G90.2-G90.9, G92, G93.1, G93.40-G93.49, G93.81, G93.89-G93.9, G95.0-G95.9, G96.12-G96.9, G97.1, G98.0-G99.8, I67.83, R53.2

PDX Collection 569
G11.0-G11.9, G32.81

PDX Collection 570
E08.40-E08.49, E08.618-E08.638, E08.649-E08.8, E09.40-E09.49, E09.618-E09.638, E09.649-E09.8, E10.40-E10.49, E10.618-E10.638, E10.649, E10.69-E10.8, E11.40-E11.49, E11.618-E11.638, E11.649, E11.69-E11.8, E13.40-E13.49, E13.618-E13.638, E13.649-E13.8, G11.3, G11.8-G12.9, G32.0, G32.89, G90.01-G90.09, G90.2, G90.4, G90.50-G90.9, G95.0-G95.9, G96.9, G98.0-G99.8

PDX Collection 571
G10, G21.0, G23.0-G25.79, G25.82-G26, G80.3, G81.00-G81.94, G90.3, G93.2, G93.40-G93.49, I67.83

PDX Collection 572
G20, G21.11-G21.9

PDX Collection 573
G20, G21.11-G21.9, G90.01-G90.09, G90.3, G93.40-G93.49, I67.83

PDX Collection 574
G20, G21.11-G21.9, G24.8, G25.70-G25.79, G25.89-G26, G80.3, G93.40, G93.41-G93.49, I67.83

PDX Collection 575
G04.1, G10, G12.22, G20-G21.9, G24.01-G25.79, G25.82-G26, G32.89-G37.2, G37.5-G37.9, G80.0-G80.9, G82.20-G83.0, G92, G93.1, G93.40-G93.6, G93.81, G93.89-G93.9, G96.9, G98.0-G98.8, G99.8, I67.83, R53.2

PDX Collection 576
G04.1, G11.3, G11.8-G12.9, G32.0, G32.89-G37.3, G37.5-G37.9, G80.0-G83.9, G90.01-G90.09, G90.2, G90.4-G90.9, G93.1, G93.40-G93.49, G95.0-G96.9, G97.1, G98.0-G99.8, I67.83, R53.2

PDX Collection 577
G36.0, G93.40-G93.49, I67.83

PDX Collection 578
G04.1, G10-G12.9, G21.0, G24.01-G25.79, G25.82-G26, G32.0-G37.3, G37.5, G37.8-G37.9, G80.0-G83.9, G90.01-G90.09, G90.2, G90.4-G90.9, G92, G93.40-G93.49, G93.81, G93.89-G95.9, G96.9, G98.0-G99.8, I67.83, R53.2

PDX Collection 579
A92.30-A92.39, B97.21, G37.5, G93.40-G93.49, I67.83

PDX Collection 580
A02.21, A17.0-A27.81, A39.0, A50.41, A51.41, A52.13, A54.82, A54.84, A54.89-A54.9, A87.0-A87.9, A96.2, A98.3-A98.4, B00.3, B00.89-B00.9, B02.0-B02.29, B02.7-B02.9, B10.81-B10.89, B26.1, B33.24-B33.8, B34.1-B34.2, B34.4-B34.8, B37.5, B38.4, B45.1, B58.2, B92, B94.2-B94.9, B97.10, B97.19, B97.29, B97.5-B97.6, B97.81-B97.89, E08.40-E08.49, E09.40-E0955555.49, E10.40-E10.49, E11.40-E11.49, E13.40-E13.49, G00.0-G03.9,

PDX Collection 581
G04.1-G04.2, G11.3, G11.8-G12.9, G32.0, G32.89-G37.3, G37.5-G37.9, G61.0, G80.0-G80.2, G80.4-G83.9, G90.01-G90.09, G90.2, G90.4-G90.9, G93.1, G93.40-G93.49, G95.0-G95.9, G96.12-G96.9, G97.1, G98.0-G99.8, I67.83, R53.2

PDX Collection 581
G32.89, G40.001-G40.319, G40.401-G40.919, G40.A01-G40.B19, G93.40-G93.49, G93.9, G96.9, G98.0-G98.8, G99.8, I67.83, R56.1

PDX Collection 582
E08.40-E08.49, E09.40-E09.49, E10.40-E10.49, E11.40-E11.49, E13.40-E13.49, G32.89, G40.001-G40.319, G40.401-G40.919, G40.A01-G40.A19, G40.B01-G40.B19, G93.81, G93.89-G93.9, G96.9, G98.8, G99.8, R56.1

PDX Collection 583
E08.40-E08.49, E08.618-E08.638, E08.649-E08.8, E09.40-E09.49, E09.618-E09.638, E09.649-E09.8, E10.40-E10.49, E10.618-E10.638, E10.649, E10.69-E10.8, E11.40-E11.49, E11.618-E11.638, E11.649, E11.69-E11.8, E13.40-E13.49, E13.618-E13.638, E13.649-E13.8, G32.89, G40.001-G40.319, G40.401-G40.419, G40.42, G40.501-G40.919, G40.A01-G40.B19, G93.3.89-G93.9, G96.9, G98.0-G98.8, G99.8, R56.1

PDX Collection 584
G43.601-G43.619, I63.00-I66.9

PDX Collection 585
G43.601-G43.619, I63.00-I66.9

PDX Collection 586
E08.51-E08.59, E08.618-E08.638, E08.649-E08.8, E09.51-E09.59, E09.618-E09.638, E09.649-E09.8, E10.51-E10.59, E10.618-E10.638, E10.649, E10.69-E10.8, E11.51-E11.59, E11.618-E11.638, E11.649, E11.69, E11.8, E13.51-E13.59, E13.618-E13.638, E13.649-E13.8, G45.0-G45.2, G45.8-G46.2, I63.00-I63.039, I63.09, I63.139, I63.19-I63.239, I63.29, I65.01-I65.9, I67.841-I67.848, I87.8-I87.9, I99.8-I99.9

PDX Collection 587
G45.3, H34.00-H34.9

PDX Collection 588
E11.42, G13.0, G13.1, G50.0-G65.2, M34.83

PDX Collection 589
G51.0-G54.5, G54.8-G60.9, G61.81-G61.89, G62.81-G62.89, G64

PDX Collection 590
G51.0-G54.5, G54.8-G60.9, G61.81-G61.9, G62.81, G62.89-G62.9, G64

PDX Collection 591
E08.40-E08.49, E08.618-E08.638, E08.649-E08.8, E09.40-E09.49, E09.618-E09.638, E09.649-E09.8, E10.40-E10.49, E10.618-E10.638, E10.649, E10.69-E10.8, E11.40-E11.49, E11.618-E11.638, E11.649, E11.69-E11.8, E13.40-E13.49, E13.618-E13.638, E13.649-E13.8, G32.89, G70.00-G70.01, G70.80-G70.81, G73.1-G73.3

PDX Collection 593
G32.89, G70.00-G71.02, G71.11-G72.3, G72.81-G73.7, G96.8-G96.9, G98.0-G98.8, G99.8

PDX Collection 594
G70.1-G72.3, G72.81-G73.7

PDX Collection 595
E08.40-E08.49, E08.618-E08.638, E08.649-E08.8, E09.40-E09.49, E09.618-E09.638, E09.649-E09.8, E10.40-E10.49, E10.618-E10.638, E10.649, E10.69-E10.8, E11.40-E11.49, E11.618-E11.638, E11.649, E11.69-E11.8, E13.40-E13.49, E13.618-E13.638, E13.649-E13.8, G04.1, G80.0-G80.2, G80.4-G83.9, G90.1, G93.81, G93.89-G93.9,

G96.9, G98.0-G98.8, G99.8, Q06.0-Q06.1, Q06.3,
Q06.8-Q06.9, Q07.8-Q07.9, R53.2

PDX Collection 596
G80.1, G93.40-G93.49, I67.83

PDX Collection 597
G80.2, G93.40-G93.49, I67.83

PDX Collection 598
G20, G21.11-G21.9, G25.70-G25.79, G25.89-G26,
G80.0-G80.9, G93.40-G93.49, I67.83

PDX Collection 599
G32.89, G82.50-G83.0, G83.5-G83.9, G96.9, G98.0-G98.8,
G99.8, R53.2

PDX Collection 600
G04.1, G32.89, G82.20-G82.54, G83.10-G83.14, G83.4-G83.9,
G96.8-G96.9, G98.8-G99.8, R53.2

PDX Collection 601
G04.1, G32.89, G80.0-G83.9, G92, G93.40-G93.49, G93.81,
G93.89-G93.9, G96.9, G98.0-G98.8, G99.8, I67.83, R53.2

PDX Collection 602
G90.50-G90.59

PDX Collection 603
E08.40-E08.49, E09.40-E09.49, E10.40-E10.49, E11.40-E11.49,
E13.40-E13.49, G04.1, G11.3, G11.8-G12.9, G32.0,
G32.89-G37.3, G37.5-G37.9, G80.0-G80.2, G80.4-G83.9,
G90.01-G90.09, G90.2, G90.4-G90.9, G93.1, G93.40-G93.49,
G95.0-G95.9, G96.12-G96.9, G97.1, G98.0-G99.8, I67.83,
R53.2

PDX Collection 604
G91.0-G91.3, G91.8-G91.9

PDX Collection 605
E08.40-E08.49, E08.618-E08.638, E08.649-E08.8,
E09.40-E09.49, E09.618-E09.638, E09.649-E09.8,
E10.40-E10.49, E10.618-E10.638, E10.649, E10.69-E10.8,
E11.40-E11.49, E11.618-E11.638, E11.649, E11.69-E11.8,
E13.40-E13.49, E13.618-E13.638, E13.649-E13.8,
C13.2-G13.8, G31.2, G31.83-G31.9, G90.1, G91.0-G91.9,
G93.81, G93.89-G94, Q03.0-Q03.9, Q04.4-Q04.8,
Q05.0-Q05.4, Q05.9-Q06.1, Q06.3, Q06.8-Q06.9,
Q07.02-Q07.9

PDX Collection 606
A17.82, A17.9, A18.82, A18.84, A18.89, A39.81, A50.42,
A52.14, A83.0-A85.1, A85.8-A86, A88.8-A89, B00.4,
B01.11, B10.01-B10.09, B26.2, B58.2, E08.40-E08.49,
E08.618-E08.638, E08.649-E08.8, E09.40-E09.49,
F09.618-E09.638, E09.649-E09.8, E10.40-E10.49,
E10.618-E10.638, E10.649, E10.69-E10.8, E11.40-E11.49,
E11.618-E11.638, E11.649, E11.69-E11.8, E13.40-E13.49,
E13.618-E13.638, E13.649-E13.8, G04.00-G04.01, G04.31,
G04.81-G05.4, G32.89, G37.3-G37.4, G92, G93.40-G93.49,
G93.81, G93.89-G93.9, G96.9, G98.0-G98.8, G99.8, I67.83

PDX Collection 607
E08.40-E08.49, E08.618-E08.638, E08.649-E08.8,
E09.40-E09.49, E09.618-E09.638, E09.649-E09.8,
E10.40-E10.49, E10.618-E10.638, E10.649, E10.69-E10.8,
[11.40-E11.49, E11.618-E11.638, E11.649, E11.69-E11.8,
E13.40-E13.49, E13.618-E13.638, E13.649-E13.8, G32.89,
G93.1-G93.2, G96.9, G98.0-G98.8, G99.8

PDX Collection 608
G21.0, G83.5, G93.40-G93.49, I67.83

PDX Collection 609
G21.0, G83.5, G93.40-G93.49, I67.83

PDX Collection 610
G21.0, G83.5, G93.40, G93.41, I67.83

PDX Collection 611
G81.90, G93.5, G93.82

PDX Collection 612
G93.6, G93.82

PDX Collection 613
G93.7

PDX Collection 614
G04.1, G11.3, G11.8-G12.9, G32.0, G32.89-G37.3,
G37.5-G37.9, G80.0-G80.2, G80.4-G83.9, G90.01-G90.09,
G90.2, G90.4-G90.9, G93.40-G93.49, G93.81, G93.89-G93.9,
G95.0-G95.9, G96.12-G96.9, G97.1, G98.0-G99.8, I67.83,
R53.2

PDX Collection 615
E08.40-E08.49, E09.40-E09.49, E10.40-E10.49, E13.40-E13.49,
G04.1, G11.3-G12.9, G32.0, G32.89, G35-G37.9, G80.0-G83.9,
G90.01, G90.09, G90.2, G90.4-G90.9, G93.1, G93.40-G93.49,
G95.11-G95.9, G96.12-G96.9, G97.1, G98.0-G99.8, I67.83,
R53.2

PDX Collection 617
D78.81-D78.89, E36.8, E89.810-E89.89, G97.0, G97.2-G97.32,
G97.81-G97.84, H59.011-H59.019, H59.031-H59.099,
H59.811-H59.89, H95.811-H95.89, I97.3, I97.810-I97.821,
L76.81-L76.82, M96.89, N98.1-N98.9, T81.82XA,
T81.89X-T81.9XX[A]

PDX Collection 618
G97.0, G97.2-G97.32, G97.81-G97.84, H95.811-H95.89,
I97.3, I97.810-I97.821, M96.89, N98.1-N98.9, T81.82XA,
T81.89X-T81.9XX[A]

PDX Collection 619
97.51-G97.52, G97.61-G97.64, H95.811-H95.89, I85.01,
I85.11, I97.3, K21.9, K22.8, K23-K25.0, K25.2, K25.4, K25.6,
K26.0, K26.2, K26.4, K26.6, K27.0, K27.2, K27.4, K27.6,
K28.0, K28.2, K28.4, K28.6, K29.01, K29.21, K29.31, K29.41,
K29.51, K29.61, K29.71, K29.81, K29.91, K31.811, K55.21,
K57.01, K57.11, K57.13, K57.21, K57.31, K57.33, K57.41,
K57.51, K57.53, K57.81, K57.91, K57.93, K62.5, K92.0 K92.2,
M96.89, N98.1-N98.9, P54.1 P54.3, I81.10X-T01.19X[A],
T81.82X-T81.9XX[A]

PDX Collection 620
G90.01, G90.09, G90.2, G90.50-G90.9, G93.40-G93.49,
G99.0, I67.83

PDX Collection 621
H05.00-H05.049

PDX Collection 622
A02.24, A17.9, A18.03-A18.09, A18.82, A18.84, A18.89,
H05.021-H05.029, M46.20-M46.39, M86.00-M86.9

PDX Collection 623
A02.24, A17.9, A18.03-A18.09, A18.82, A18.84, A18.89,
H05.031-H05.039, M46.20-M46.39, M86.00-M86.9

PDX Collection 624
A18.54, H20.00-H20.9

PDX Collection 625
H20.051-H20.059, H21.331-H21.339, H33.121-H33.129,
H44.001-H44.029, H44.121-H44.129, H44.19

PDX Collection 626
H30.001-H30.93

PDX Collection 627
H31.301-H32

PDX Collection 628
H33.001-H33.119, H33.191-H33.8, H35.70-H35.739

PDX Collection 629
H35.60-H35.63, H35.81-H35.89

PDX Collection 630
H40.211-H40.219

PDX Collection 631
H16.241-H16.249, H21.331-H21.339, H33.121-H33.129,
H44.001-H44.19

PDX Collection 632
H44.111-H44.119, H44.131-H44.139

PDX Collection 633
H46.00-H46.9

PDX Collection 634
A17.9, A18.50-A18.59, A18.82, A18.84, A18.89, A39.82,
E08.311-E08.39, E08.618-E08.638, E08.649-E08.8,
E09.311-E09.39, E09.618-E09.638, E09.649-E09.8,
E10.311-E10.39, E10.618-E10.638, E10.649, E10.69-E10.8,
E11.311-E11.39, E11.618-E11.638, E11.649, E11.69-E11.8,
E13.311-E13.39, E13.618-E13.638, E13.649-E13.8,
H47.10-H47.13, H47.231-H47.239, H47.331-H47.339,
H57.8-H57.9, H59.40-H59.43, Q11.3, Q15.8-Q15.9

PDX Collection 635
H47.41-H47.539

PDX Collection 636
H47.611-H47.9

PDX Collection 637
H53.10-H53.139, H53.16, R44.1, R48.3

PDX Collection 638
H59.011-H59.019, H59.031-H59.099, H59.811-H59.89,
H95.811-H95.89, I97.3, M96.89, N98.1-N98.9, T81.82XA,
T81.89X-T81.9XX[A]

PDX Collection 639
II59.011-H59.019, H59.031-H59.129, H59.311-H59.329,
H59.331-H59.369, H59.811-H59.89, H95.811 H95.89, I85.01,
I85.11, I97.3, K21.9, K22.8, K23-K25.0, K25.2, K25.4, K25.6,
K26.0, K26.2, K26.4, K26.6, K27.0, K27.2, K27.4, K27.6,
K28.0, K28.2, K28.4, K28.6, K29.01, K29.21, K29.31, K29.41,
K29.51, K29.61, K29.71, K29.81, K29.91, K31.811, K55.21,
K57.01, K57.11, K57.13, K57.21, K57.31, K57.33, K57.41,
K57.51, K57.53, K57.81, K57.91, K57.93, K62.5, K92.0-K92.2,
M96.89, N98.1-N98.9, P54.1 P54.3, T81.10X-T81 19X[A],
T81.82X[A], T81.89X-T81.9XX[A]

PDX Collection 640
H60.20-H60.23, H70.001-H70.13

PDX Collection 641
A17.9, A18.6, A18.82, A18.84, A18.89, H70.001-H70.213,
H70.219-H70.93, H75.00-H75.83, H93.8X1-H93.93,
H94.80-H95.199, Q16.1, Q16.9, Q17.3-Q17.9

PDX Collection 642
H95.21-H95.22, H95.41-H95.89, I85.01, I85.11, I97.3,
K21.9, K22.8, K23-K25.2, K25.4, K25.6, K26.0, K26.2, K26.4,
K26.6, K27.0, K27.2, K27.4, K27.6, K28.0, K28.2, K28.4,
K28.6, K29.01, K29.21, K29.31, K29.41, K29.51, K29.61,
K29.71, K29.81, K29.91, K31.811, K55.21, K57.01, K57.11,
K57.13, K57.21, K57.31, K57.33, K57.41, K57.51, K57.53,
K57.81, K57.91, K57.93, K62.5, K92.0-K92.2, M96.89,
N98.1-N98.9, P54.1-P54.3, T81.10X-T81.19X[A], T81.82XA,
T81.89X-T81.9XX[A]

PDX Collection 643
D78.81-D78.89, E36.8, E89.810-E89.89, H59.011-H59.019,
H59.031-H59.099, H59.811-H59.89, H95.811-H95.89,
I97.3, L76.81-L76.82, M96.89, N98.1-N98.9, T81.82XA,
T81.89X-T81.9XX[A]

PDX Collection 644
A01.00-A01.09, A39.51, A52.03, A78, B33.21, B37.6, I00,
I01.1, I01.8-I02.0, I05.0-I07.9, I08.1-I08.3, I08.9, I09.1,
I09.89-I09.9, I33.0-I39, I42.4, I87.8-I87.9, I99.8-I99.9, Q22.2,
Q23.8-Q23.9, Q24.8, T82.6XXA

PDX Collection 645
I01.0-I09.9, I50.20-I50.43

PDX Collection 646
I01.0-I09.9

PDX Collection 647
I00, I01.2-I01.9, I09.0, I09.9, I23.0-I23.3, I23.6-I23.8,
I40.0-I41, I51.0, I51.4, I87.8-I87.9, I99.8-I99.9

PDX Collection 648
I09.81, I09.9, I11.0, I50.1-I50.9, I87.8-I87.9, I99.8-I99.9

PDX Collection 649
I10-I16.9, I87.8-I87.9, I99.8-I99.9, N18.6, N26.2

PDX Collection 650
I10-I16.9, I87.8-I87.9, I99.8-I99.9, N26.2

PDX Collection 651
I09.81, I11.0, I13.0, I13.2, I20.0-I22.9, I24.0, I24.8-I24.9,
I25.5-I25.6, I25.82-I25.83, I25.89-I25.9, I50.1, I50.810-I50.9,
I87.8-I87.9, I99.8-I99.9, R57.0, R57.9

PDX Collection 652
I20.0-I22.9, I24.0, I24.8-I24.9, I25.5-I25.6, I25.89-I25.9,
I87.8-I87.9, I99.8-I99.9

PDX Collection 653
I21.01-I22.9, I87.8-I87.9, I99.8-I99.9

PDX Collection 655
I23.0-I23.4, I23.6-I23.8, I51.0-I51.1, I87.8-I87.9, I99.8-I99.9

PDX Collection 656
I23.0-I23.3, I23.5-I23.8, I51.0, I51.2, I87.8-I87.9, I99.8-I99.9

PDX Collection 657
I20.0-I22.9, I24.0-I24.9, I25.5-I25.6, I25.89-I25.9,
I87.8-I87.9, I99.8-I99.9

PDX Collection 658
I24.0-I24.9, I87.8-I87.9, I99.8-I99.9

PDX Collection 659
I25.3-I25.41

PDX Collection 660
I25.42, I67.0, I77.2-I77.3, I77.5-I77.6, I77.70, I77.75-I77.79,
I77.89-I77.9, M31.8-M31.9

PDX Collection 661
I09.381, I11.0, I13.0, I13.2, I20.0-I22.9, I24.0, I24.8-I25.119,
I25.5-I25.739, I25.760-I25.799, I25.812-I25.9, I50.1,
I50.810-I50.9, I87.8-I87.9, I99.8-I99.9, R57.0, R57.9

PDX Collection 662
I25.10-I25.119, I25.700-I25.739, I25.760-I25.799,
I25.812-I25.84

PDX Collection 663
I09.81, I11.0, I13.0, I13.2, I20.0-I22.9, I24.0, I24.8-I25.119,
I25.5-I25.799, I25.811-I25.9, I50.1, I50.810-I50.9,
I87.8-I87.9, I99.8-I99.9, R57.0, R57.9

PDX Collection 664
I25.10-I25.119, I25.700-I25.799, I25.811-I25.84

PDX Collection 665
I09.81, I11.0, I13.0, I13.2, I20.0-I22.9, I24.0, I24.8-I25.119,
I25.5-I25.760, I25.790-I25.799, I25.811, I25.82-I25.9, I50.1,
I50.810-I50.9, I87.8-I87.9, I99.8-I99.9, R57.0, R57.9

PDX Collection 666
I25.10-I25.119, I25.700-I25.759, I25.790-I25.799,
I25.811-I25.812, I25.82-I25.84

PDX Collection 667
I26.01-I26.99, I27.20-I27.9, I74.01-I74.10, I74.19,
I87.8-I87.9, I99.8-I99.9

PDX Collection 668
I26.01-I26.99, I27.82, I74.01-I74.10, I74.19, I87.8-I87.9,
I99.8-I99.9, T80.0XX[A], T81.718A, T81.72XA,
T82.817-T82.818[A]

PDX Collection 669
I26.01-I26.99, I27.82, I74.01-I74.10, I74.19, I87.8-I87.9,
I99.8-I99.9

PDX Collection 670
I26.01-I26.99, I27.82, I74.01-I74.10, I74.19,
I87.8-I87.9, I99.8-I99.9, T80.0XXA, T81.718A, T81.72XA,
T82.817-T82.818[A]

PDX Collection 671
E66.2, I27.0, I27.20-I27.9, I28.8-I28.9, I87.8-I87.9,
I99.8-I99.9

PDX Collection 672
I28.0-I28.9

PDX Collection 673
I01.0, I09.2, I30.0-I30.9, I31.3-I32, I87.8-I87.9, I99.8-I99.9

PDX Collection 674
I31.0-I31.9, I87.8, I99.8-I99.9

PDX Collection 675
I01.1, I08.1-I08.3, I09.1, I33.0-I33.9, I38-I39, I87.8-I87.9,
I99.8-I99.9

PDX Collection 676
I38-I39, I87.8-I87.9, I99.8-I99.9

PDX Collection 677
I01.2, I09.0, I23.0-I23.3, I23.6-I23.8, I40.0-I41, I51.0, I51.4,
I87.8-I87.9, I99.8-I99.9

PDX Collection 678
I09.81, I11.0, I13.0, I13.2, I25.10-I25.119, I25.5-I25.799,
I25.811-I25.9, I42.0-I44.1, I44.30-I44.39, I45.2-I45.4,
I45.81-I45.89, I48.0-I49.1, I49.3-I49.8, I50.1, I50.810-I50.9,
I87.8-I87.9, I99.8-I99.9, Q24.6, R00.0-R00.2, R57.0, R57.9

PDX Collection 679
I44.0-I49.02, I49.2, I49.8, I87.8-I87.9, I99.8-I99.9, R00.1

PDX Collection 680
I46.2-I49.02, I49.2, I87.8-I87.9, I99.8-I99.9

PDX Collection 681
I09.81, I11.0, I50.1-I50.9, I87.8-I87.9, I99.8-I99.9

PDX Collection 682
I09.81, I11.0, I50.1-I50.9, I87.8-I87.9, I99.8-I99.9, J81.0

PDX Collection 683
I09.81, I11.0, I50.1-I50.9, I51.81, I51.9-I52, I87.8-I87.9,
I99.8-I99.9

PDX Collection 684
E03.5, G93.82, I60.00-I62.9, I87.8-I87.9, I99.8-I99.9,
R40.0-R40.2224, R40.2310-R40.2324, R40.2340-R40.2344,
R40.3-R40.4, S02.0XX[A,B], S02.101-S02.102[A,B],
S02.109[A,B], S02.110-S02.19X[A,B], S02.91X[A,B],
S06.0X0-S06.0X1[A], S06.0X9-S06.9X9[A]

PDX Collection 689
I77.2-I77.3, I77.5-I77.6, I77.79, I77.89-I77.9, M31.8-M31.9

PDX Collection 690
E08.51-E08.59, E08.618-E08.638, E08.649-E08.8,
E09.51-E09.59, E09.618-E09.638, E09.649-E09.8,
E10.51-E10.59, E10.618-E10.638, E10.649, E10.69-E10.8,
E11.51-E11.59, E11.618-E11.638, E11.649, E11.69-E11.8,
E13.51-E13.59, E13.618-E13.638, E13.649-E13.8, I67.4,
I87.8-I87.9, I99.8-I99.9

PDX Collection 691
E08.51-E08.59, E08.618-E08.638, E08.649-E08.8,
E09.51-E09.59, E09.618-E09.638, E09.649-E09.8,
E10.51-E10.59, E10.618-E10.638, E10.649, E10.69-E10.8,
E11.51-E11.59, E11.618-E11.638, E11.649, E11.69-E11.8,
E13.51-E13.59, E13.618-E13.638, E13.649-E13.8, I67.5,
I87.8-I87.9, I99.8-I99.9

PDX Collection 692
E08.51-E08.59, E08.618-E08.638, E08.649-E08.8,
E09.51-E09.59, E09.618-E09.638, E09.649-E09.8,
E10.51-E10.59, E10.618-E10.638, E10.649, E10.69-E10.8,
E11.51-E11.59, E11.618-E11.638, E11.649, E11.69-E11.8,
E13.51-E13.59, E13.618-E13.638, E13.649-E13.8, I67.6,
I87.8-I87.9, I99.8-I99.9

PDX Collection 693
E08.51-E08.59, E08.618-E08.638, E08.649-E08.8,
E09.51-E09.59, E09.618-E09.638, E09.649-E09.8,
E10.51-E10.59, E10.618-E10.638, E10.649, E10.69-E10.8,
E11.51-E11.59, E11.618-E11.638, E11.649, E11.69-E11.8,
E13.51-E13.59, E13.618-E13.638, E13.649-E13.8, I67.7, I68.2,
I87.8-I87.9, I99.8-I99.9

PDX Collection 694
E08.51-E08.59, E08.618-E08.638, E08.649-E08.8,
E09.51-E09.59, E09.618-E09.638, E09.649-E09.8,
E10.51-E10.59, E10.618-E10.638, E10.649, E10.69-E10.8,
E11.51-E11.59, E11.618-E11.638, E11.649, E11.69-E11.8,
E13.51-E13.59, E13.618-E13.638, E13.649-E13.8,
G45.0-G45.2, G45.8-G46.2, I60.00-I62.9, I63.30-I63.9,
I66.01-I66.9, I67.81-I67.85, I67.841-I67.89, I87.8-I87.9,
I99.8-I99.9

PDX Collection 695
I69.051-I69.052, I69.151-I69.152, I69.251-I69.252,
I69.351-I69.352, I69.851-I69.852, I69.951-I69.952

PDX Collection 696
I69.053-I69.054, I69.153-I69.154, I69.253-I69.254,
I69.353-I69.354, I69.853-I69.854, I69.953-I69.954

PDX Collection 697
I69.059, I69.159, I69.259, I69.359, I69.859, I69.959

PDX Collection 698
I70.231-I70.25, L44.8-L45, L94.2, L94.4, L97.101-L97.929,
L98.411-L98.499, L98.7, L98.7-L99

PDX Collection 699
I70.92, I73.81-I74.19, .I74.2-I77.2, I77.5-I77.6,
I77.810-I77.819, I79.1-I79.8, M31.8-M31.9

PDX Collection 700
E08.51-E08.59, E08.618-E08.638, E08.649-E08.8,
E09.51-E09.59, E09.618-E09.638, E09.649, E09.65-E09.8,
E10.51-E10.59, E10.618-E10.638, E10.649, E10.69-E10.8,
E11.51-E11.59, E11.618-E11.638, E11.649, E11.69-E11.8,
E13.51-E13.59, E13.618-E13.638, E13.649-E13.8,
I71.00-I71.9, I77.810-I77.819, I79.0, I87.8-I87.9, I99.8-I99.9

PDX Collection 701
E08.51-E08.59, E08.618-E08.638, E08.649-E08.8,
E09.51-E09.59, E09.618-E09.638, E09.649, E09.65-E09.8,
E10.51-E10.59, E10.618-E10.638, E10.649, E10.69-E10.8,
E11.51-E11.59, E11.618-E11.638, E11.649, E11.69-E11.8,
E13.51-E13.59, E13.618-E13.638, E13.649-E13.8, I74.11,
I74.8-I74.9, I76, I87.8-I87.9, I99.8-I99.9

PDX Collection 702
E08.51-E08.59, E08.618-E08.638, E08.649-E08.8,
E09.51-E09.59, E09.618-E09.638, E09.649, E09.65-E09.8,
E10.51-E10.59, E10.618-E10.638, E10.649, E10.69-E10.8,
E11.51-E11.59, E11.618-E11.638, E11.649, E11.69-E11.8,
E13.51-E13.59, E13.618-E13.638, E13.649-E13.8, I74.2,
I74.8-I74.9, I76, I87.8-I87.9, I99.8-I99.9

PDX Collection 703
E08.51-E08.59, E08.618-E08.638, E08.649-E08.8,
E09.51-E09.59, E09.618-E09.638, E09.649, E09.65-E09.8,
E10.51-E10.59, E10.618-E10.638, E10.649, E10.69-E10.8,
E11.51-E11.59, E11.618-E11.638, E11.649, E11.69-E11.8,
E13.51-E13.59, E13.618-E13.638, E13.649-E13.8, I74.3-I74.4,
I74.8-I74.9, I76, I87.8-I87.9, I99.8-I99.9

PDX Collection 704
E08.51-E08.59, E08.618-E08.638, E08.649-E08.8,
E09.51-E09.59, E09.618-E09.638, E09.649, E09.65-E09.8,
E10.51-E10.59, E10.618-E10.638, E10.649, E10.69-E10.8,
E11.51-E11.59, E11.618-E11.638, E11.649, E11.69-E11.8,
E13.51-E13.59, E13.618-E13.638, E13.649-E13.8, I74.5-I74.9,
I76, I87.8-I87.9, I99.8-I99.9

PDX Collection 705
E08.51-E08.59, E08.618-E08.638, E08.649-E08.8,
E09.51-E09.59, E09.618-E09.638, E09.649, E09.65-E09.8,
E10.51-E10.59, E10.618-E10.638, E10.649, E10.69-E10.8,
E11.51-E11.59, E11.618-E11.638, E11.649, E11.69-E11.8,
E13.51-E13.59, E13.618-E13.638, E13.649-E13.8, I74.8-I74.9,
I76, I87.8-I87.9, I99.8-I99.9

PDX Collection 706
E08.51-E08.59, E08.618-E08.638, E08.649-E08.8,
E09.51-E09.59, E09.618-E09.638, E09.649, E09.65-E09.8,
E10.51-E10.59, E10.618-E10.638, E10.649, E10.69-E10.8,
E11.51-E11.59, E11.618-E11.638, E11.649, E11.69-E11.8,
E13.51-E13.59, E13.618-E13.638, E13.649-E13.8,
I74.8-I75.019, I76, I87.8-I87.9, I99.8-I99.9

PDX Collection 707
E08.51-E08.59, E08.618-E08.638, E08.649-E08.8,
E09.51-E09.59, E09.618-E09.638, E09.649, E09.65-E09.8,
E10.51-E10.59, E10.618-E10.638, E10.649, E10.69-E10.8,
E11.51-E11.59, E11.618-E11.638, E11.649, E11.69-E11.8,
E13.51-E13.59, E13.618-E13.638, E13.649-E13.8, I74.8-I74.9,
I75.021-I75.029, I76, I87.8-I87.9, I99.8-I99.9

PDX Collection 708
E08.51-E08.59, E08.618-E08.638, E08.649-E08.8,
E09.51-E09.59, E09.618-E09.638, E09.649, E09.65-E09.8,
E10.51-E10.59, E10.618-E10.638, E10.649, E10.69-E10.8,
E11.51-E11.59, E11.618-E11.638, E11.649, E11.69-E11.8,
E13.51-E13.59, E13.618-E13.638, E13.649-E13.8, I74.8-I74.9,
I75.81, I76, I87.8-I87.9, I99.8-I99.9

PDX Collection 709
E08.51-E08.59, E08.618-E08.638, E08.649-E08.8,
E09.51-E09.59, E09.618-E09.638, E09.649, E09.65-E09.8,
E10.51-E10.59, E10.618-E10.638, E10.649, E10.69-E10.8,
E11.51-E11.59, E11.618-E11.638, E11.649, E11.69-E11.8,
E13.51-E13.59, E13.618-E13.638, E13.649-E13.8, I74.8-I74.9,
I75.89, I76, I87.8-I87.9, I99.8-I99.9

PDX Collection 710
I25.42, I67.0, I77.2, I77.70, I77.72-I77.79

PDX Collection 711
I77.4

PDX Collection 712
I77.5, M31.8-M31.9

PDX Collection 713
E08.51-E08.59, E08.618-E08.638, E08.649-E08.8,
E09.51-E09.59, E09.618-E09.638, E09.649, E09.65-E09.8,
E10.51-E10.59, E10.618-E10.638, E10.649, E10.69-E10.8,
E11.51-E11.59, E11.618-E11.638, E11.649, E11.69-E11.8,
E13.51-E13.59, E13.618-E13.638, E13.649-E13.8,
I80.00-I80.9, I87.8-I87.9, I99.8-I99.9

PDX Collection 714
E08.51-E08.59, E08.618-E08.638, E08.649-E08.8,
E09.51-E09.59, E09.618-E09.638, E09.649, E09.65-E09.8,
E10.51-E10.59, E10.618-E10.638, E10.649, E10.69-E10.8,
E11.51-E11.59, E11.618-E11.638, E11.649, E11.69-E11.8,
E13.51-E13.59, E13.618-E13.638, E13.649-E13.8, I81,
I82.210-I82.291, I82.401-I82.729, I82.811-I82.91,
I82.A11-I82.C29, I87.8-I87.9, I99.8-I99.9

PDX Collection 715
E08.51-E08.59, E08.618-E08.638, E08.649-E08.8,
E09.51-E09.59, E09.618-E09.638, E09.649, E09.65-E09.8,

E10.51-E10.59, E10.618-E10.638, E10.649, E10.69-E10.8,
E11.51-E11.59, E11.618-E11.638, E11.649, E11.69-E11.8,
E13.51-E13.59, E13.618-E13.638, E13.649-E13.8, I82.0,
I82.210-I82.291, I82.401-I82.729, I82.811-I82.91,
I82.A11-I82.C29, I87.8-I87.9, I99.8-I99.9

PDX Collection 716
E08.51-E08.59, E08.618-E08.638, E08.649-E08.8,
E09.51-E09.59, E09.618-E09.638, E09.649, E09.65-E09.8,
E10.51-E10.59, E10.618-E10.638, E10.649, E10.69-E10.8,
E11.51-E11.59, E11.618-E11.638, E11.649, E11.69-E11.8,
E13.51-E13.59, E13.618-E13.638, E13.649-E13.8, I82.1,
I82.210-I82.291, I82.401-I82.729, I82.811-I82.91,
I82.A11-I82.C29, I87.8-I87.9, I99.8-I99.9

PDX Collection 717
E08.51-E08.59, E08.618-E08.638, E08.649-E08.8,
E09.51-E09.59, E09.618-E09.638, E09.649, E09.65-E09.8,
E10.51-E10.59, E10.618-E10.638, E10.649, E10.69-E10.8,
E11.51-E11.59, E11.618-E11.638, E11.649, E11.69-E11.8,
E13.51-E13.59, E13.618-E13.638, E13.649-E13.8,
I82.210-I82.291, I82.401-I82.729, I82.811-I82.91,
I82.A11-I82.C29, I87.8-I87.9, I99.8-I99.9

PDX Collection 718
E08.51-E08.59, E08.618-E08.638, E08.649-E08.8,
E09.51-E09.59, E09.618-E09.638, E09.649, E09.65-E09.8,
E10.51-E10.59, E10.618-E10.638, E10.649, E10.69-E10.8,
E11.51-E11.59, E11.618-E11.638, E11.649, E11.69-E11.8,
E13.51-E13.59, E13.618-E13.638, E13.649-E13.8,
I82.210-I82.291, I82.401-I82.729, I82.811-I82.91,
I82.A11-I82.C29, I87.8-I87.9, I99.8-I99.9

PDX Collection 719
E08.51-E08.59, E08.618-E08.638, E08.649-E08.8,
E09.51-E09.59, E09.618-E09.638, E09.649, E09.65-E09.8,
E10.51-E10.59, E10.618-E10.638, E10.649, E10.69-E10.8,
E11.51-E11.59, E11.618-E11.638, E11.649, E11.69-E11.8,
E13.51-E13.59, E13.618-E13.638, E13.649-E13.8,
I82.210-I82.291, I82.3, I82.401-I82.729, I82.811-I82.91,
I82.A11-I82.C29, I87.8-I87.9, I99.8-I99.9

PDX Collection 720
I83.001-I83.229, I83.90-I83.93

PDX Collection 721
E16.4, I85.00-I85.01, I85.11, I87.8-I87.9, I99.8-I99.9, K22.6,
K25.0-K28.9, K29.01, K29.21, K29.31, K29.41, K29.51,
K29.61, K29.71, K29.81, K29.91, K31.811, K92.0-K92.2

PDX Collection 722
E16.4, I85.01, I85.11, I87.8-I87.9, I99.8-I99.9,
K22.10-K22.11, K22.6-K22.70, K22.710-K22.719,
K25.0-K28.9, K29.01, K29.21, K29.31, K29.41, K29.51,
K29.61, K29.71, K29.81, K29.91, K31.811, K55.21, K57.01,
K57.11, K57.13, K57.21, K57.31, K57.33, K57.41, K57.51,
K57.53, K57.81, K57.91, K57.93, K62.5, K92.0-K92.2

PDX Collection 723
E16.4, I85.01, I85.10-I85.11, I87.8-I87.9, I99.8-I99.9, K22.6,
K25.0-K28.9, K29.01, K29.21, K29.31, K29.41, K29.51,
K29.61, K29.71, K29.81, K29.91, K31.811, K92.0-K92.2

PDX Collection 724
I85.01, I85.11, I87.8-I87.9, I99.8-I99.9

PDX Collection 726
I87.1

PDX Collection 728
D78.81-D78.89, E36.8, E89.810-E89.89, H59.011-H59.019,
H59.031-H59.099, H59.811-H59.89, H95.811-H95.89,
I97.110-I97.191, I97.3, I97.710-I97.791, I97.88-I97.89,
L76.81-L76.82, M96.89, N98.1-N98.9, T81.82XA,
T81.89X-T81.9XX[A]

PDX Collection 729
H95.811-H95.89, I85.01, I85.11, I97.3-I97.42,
I97.610-I97.648, K21.9, K22.8, K23-K25.0, K25.2, K25.4,
K25.6, K26.0, K26.2, K26.4, K26.6, K27.0, K27.2, K27.4,
K27.6, K28.0, K28.2, K28.4, K28.6, K29.01, K29.21,
K29.31, K29.41, K29.51, K29.61, K29.71, K29.81, K29.91,
K31.811, K55.21, K57.01, K57.11, K57.13, K57.21, K57.31,
K57.33, K57.41, K57.51, K57.53, K57.81, K57.91, K57.93,
K62.5, K92.0-K92.2, M96.89, N98.1-N98.9, P54.1-P54.3,
T81.10X-T81.19X[A], T81.82XA, T81.89X-T81.9XX[A]

PDX Collection 730
A15.8-A15.9, A17.9, A18.82, A18.84, A18.89, J04.10-J04.2,
J05.10-J05.11, J22, J98.8-J98.9

PDX Collection 731
A15.8-A15.9, A17.9, A18.82, A18.84, A18.89, J04.0-J04.2,
J04.31, J05.10-J05.11, J22, J98.8-J98.9

PDX Collection 732
J04.31, J05.10-J05.11

PDX Collection 733
A15.0-A15.6, A15.8-A15.9, A17.9, A18.82, A18.84, A18.89,
A21.2, A22.1, A31.0, A37.01, A37.11, A37.81, A37.91, A42.0,
A43.0, A48.1, B25.0, B39.0-B39.2, B44.0, B58.3, B59, B67.1,
J09.X1-J09.X2, J10.00-J10.1, J11.00-J11.1, J12.0-J12.3,
J12.89-J18.1, J18.8-J18.9, J22, J44.0-J44.9, J45.21-J45.22,
J45.31-J45.32, J45.41-J45.42, J45.51-J45.902, J47.0-J70.4,
J70.8-J70.9, J98.4, J98.8-J99, Q33.4, R91.1

PDX Collection 734
A15.0-A15.6, A15.8-A15.9, A17.9, A18.82, A18.84, A18.89,
A20.2, A21.1, A22.1, A31.0, A37.01, A37.11, A37.81, A37.91,
A42.0, A43.0, A48.1, B25.0, B39.0-B39.2, B44.0, B58.3,
B59, B67.1, J09.X1-J09.X2, J10.00-J10.1, J11.00-J11.1,
J12.0-J12.3, J12.81-J18.1, J18.8-J18.9, J22, J60-J70.4,
J70.8-J70.9, J98.4, J98.8-J99, R91.1

PDX Collection 735
A15.0-A15.6, A15.8-A15.9, A17.9, A18.82, A18.84, A18.89,
A21.2, A22.1, A31.0, A37.01, A37.11, A37.81, A37.91, A42.0,
A43.0, A48.1, B25.0, B39.0-B39.2, B44.0, B58.3, B59, B67.1,
J09.X1-J09.X2, J10.00-J10.1, J11.00-J11.1, J12.0-J12.3,
J12.81-J18.1, J18.8-J18.9, J22, J44.9, J47.0-J70.4,
J70.8-J70.9, J98.4, J98.8-J99, Q33.4, R91.1

PDX Collection 736
J18.2, J22, J81.1, J98.4, J98.8-J99, R91.1

PDX Collection 737
J21.0

PDX Collection 738
J20.0-J21.9

PDX Collection 739
J22, J36, J98.8-J98.9

PDX Collection 740
J22, J39.0-J39.1, J98.8-J98.9

PDX Collection 741
J10.08, J41.1-J42, J44.0-J44.1

PDX Collection 742
J10.08, J22, J45.20-J45.998, J98.4, J98.8-J99, R91.1

PDX Collection 743
A17.9, A18.82, A18.84, A18.89, J09.X2, J10.08, J11.1, J44.9,
J47.0-J47.1, J68.1, J68.4-J68.9, Q33.4

PDX Collection 744
J22, J80, J96.00-J96.92, J98.8-J98.9, R09.2

PDX Collection 745
I09.81, I50.1-I50.9, J22, J81.0, J98.8-J98.9

PDX Collection 747
A15.0-A15.6, A15.8-A15.9, A17.9, A18.82, A18.84, A18.89,
J22, J44.9, J47.0-J70.4, J70.8-J70.9, J84.01-J84.82,
J84.89-J84.9, J98.4, J98.8-J99, Q33.4, R91.1

PDX Collection 748
J84.83-J84.848, P22.0-P28.5, P28.89-P29.2, P29.4,
P29.89-P29.9, P84, P94.1-P96.0, P96.3-P96.5, P96.82-P96.89

PDX Collection 749
A06.5, A15.0-A15.6, A15.8-A15.9, A17.9, A18.82, A18.84,
A18.89, J22, J85.0-J85.2, J98.8-J98.9

PDX Collection 750
J22, J85.3, J98.8-J98.9

PDX Collection 751
J22, J86.0-J86.9, J98.4, J98.8-J99, R91.1

PDX Collection 752
A15.0-A15.6, A15.8-A15.9, A17.9, A18.82, A18.84, A18.89,
J22, J90-J92.9, J94.0-J94.9, J98.4, J98.8-J99, R09.1, R91.1

PDX Collection 753
C45.7-C45.9, C76.8, C78.2-C78.39, C79.89-C79.9, C7A.00,
C7A.098, C7A.1-C7B.00, C7B.09-C7B.8, C80.0-C80.2,
D49.81-D49.9, J90-J91.0, J94.0, J94.2

PDX Collection 754
J22, J93.0-J93.9, J95.811-J95.812, J98.4, J98.8-J99, R91.1

PDX Collection 755
J22, J39.8, J95.00-J95.09, J98.01-J98.09, J98.8-J98.9

PDX Collection 756
J22, J95.1-J95.3, J95.821-J95.822, J98.8-J98.9

PDX Collection 757
D78.81-D78.89, E36.8, E89.810-E89.89, H59.011-H59.019,
H59.031-H59.099, H59.811-H59.89, H95.811-H95.89, I97.3,
J95.4-J95.5, J95.84, J95.851-J95.89, L76.81-L76.82, M96.89,
N98.1-N98.9, T81.82XA, T81.89X-T81.9XX[A]

PDX Collection 758
H95.811-H95.89, I85.01, I85.11, I97.3, J95.61-J95.62,
J95.830-J95.831, J95.860-J95.863, K21.9, K22.8,
K23-K25.0, K25.2, K25.4, K25.6, K26.0, K26.2, K26.4,
K26.6, K27.0, K27.2, K27.4, K27.6, K28.0, K28.2, K28.4,
K28.6, K29.01, K29.21, K29.31, K29.41, K29.51, K29.61,
K29.71, K29.81, K29.91, K31.811, K55.21, K57.01, K57.11,
K57.13, K57.21, K57.31, K57.33, K57.41, K57.51, K57.53,
K57.81, K57.91, K57.93, K62.5, K92.0-K92.2, M96.89,
N98.1-N98.9, P54.1-P54.3, T81.10X-T81.19X[A], T81.82XA,
T81.89X-T81.9XX[A]

PDX Collection 759
J95.850, Z99.0-Z99.12, Z99.81-Z99.89

PDX Collection 760
J22, J98.11-J98.19, J98.8-J98.9

PDX Collection 761
K00.0-K08.9, M26.00-M26.9, M27.61-M27.69

PDX Collection 762
K11.0-K11.9, K31.89-K31.9, K92.81, R68.2

PDX Collection 763
K12.1-K12.39, K14.0, K14.2

PDX Collection 764
K22.10-K22.11, K22.8-K23, K31.82

PDX Collection 765
E16.4, I85.01, K22.10-K22.11, K22.6-K22.719, K25.0-K28.9,
K29.01, K29.21, K29.31, K29.41, K29.51, K29.61, K29.71,
K29.81, K29.91, K31.811, K31.89-K31.9, K55.21, K57.01,
K57.11, K57.13, K57.21, K57.31, K57.33, K57.41, K57.51,
K57.53, K57.81, K57.91, K57.93, K62.5, K92.0-K92.81

PDX Collection 766
K21.9, K22.3, K22.6, K22.8-K23

PDX Collection 767
E16.4, I85.01, K21.9, K22.10-K22.11, K22.3, K22.6-K28.9,
K29.01, K29.21, K29.31, K29.41, K29.51, K29.61, K29.71,
K29.81, K29.91, K31.811, K55.21, K57.01, K57.11, K57.13,
K57.21, K57.31, K57.33, K57.41, K57.51, K57.53, K57.81,
K57.91, K57.93, K62.5, K92.0-K92.2

PDX Collection 768
E16.4, I85.01, K22.10-K22.11, K22.6-K22.719, K25.0-K28.9,
K29.01, K29.21, K29.31, K29.41, K29.51, K29.61, K29.71,
K29.81, K29.91, K31.5, K31.811, K31.89-K31.9, K55.21,
K57.01, K57.11, K57.13, K57.21, K57.31, K57.33,
K57.41, K57.51, K57.53, K57.81, K57.91, K57.93, K62.5,
K92.0-K92.81

PDX Collection 769
E16.4, I85.01, K22.6, K25.0-K28.9, K29.01, K29.21, K29.31,
K29.41, K29.51, K29.61, K29.71, K29.81, K29.91, K31.5,
K31.811, K31.82, K31.89-K31.9, K55.21, K57.01, K57.11,
K57.13, K57.21, K57.31, K57.33, K57.41, K57.51, K57.53,
K57.81, K57.91, K57.93, K62.5, K92.0-K92.81

PDX Collection 770
E16.4, I85.01, K22.10-K22.11, K22.6-K22.719, K25.0-K28.9,
K29.01, K29.21, K29.31, K29.41, K29.51, K29.61, K29.71,
K29.81, K29.91, K31.811, K55.21, K57.01, K57.11, K57.13,
K57.21, K57.31, K57.33, K57.41, K57.51, K57.53, K57.81,
K57.91, K57.93, K62.5, K92.0-K92.2

PDX Collection 771
K31.0

PDX Collection 772
K30-K31.1, K31.5, K31.84, Q38.5, Q40.0, Q40.8-Q41.9,
Q43.4-Q43.9

PDX Collection 773
K31.5, Q38.5, Q40.8-Q41.9, Q43.4-Q43.9

PDX Collection 774
K31.6, Q38.5, Q40.8-Q40.9, Q43.4-Q43.9

PDX Collection 775
E16.4, I85.01, K22.10-K22.11, K22.6-K22.719, K25.0-K28.9,
K29.01, K29.21, K29.31, K29.41, K29.51, K29.61, K29.71,
K29.81, K29.91, K31.811, K31.82, K55.21, K57.01, K57.11,
K57.13, K57.21, K57.31, K57.33, K57.41, K57.51, K57.53,
K57.81, K57.91, K57.93, K62.5, K92.0-K92.2

PDX Collection 776
K31.89-K38.9, K92.81

PDX Collection 777
K31.89-K31.9, K40.00-K40.91, K45.0, K45.8-K46.0, K92.81

PDX Collection 778
K31.89-K31.9, K41.00-K41.91, K45.0, K45.8-K46.0, K92.81

PDX Collection 779
K31.89-K31.9, K41.10-K41.21, K41.40-K41.91, K45.0,
K45.8-K46.0, K92.81

PDX Collection 780
K42.0-K42.1, K43.0-K43.1, K43.3-K43.4, K43.6-K43.7, K45.0,
K45.8-K46.0

PDX Collection 781
K31.89-K31.9, K42.0-K43.9, K45.0, K45.8-K46.0, K46.9,
K92.81

PDX Collection 782
K44.0-K46.0

PDX Collection 783
K40.00-K46.9

PDX Collection 784
K31.89-K31.9, K40.00-K46.9, K92.81

PDX Collection 785
K50.00-K51.919

PDX Collection 786
K50.00-K50.919

PDX Collection 787
K51.00-K51.919

PDX Collection 788
K52.0

PDX Collection 789
K52.1

PDX Collection 790
K55.011-K55.1, K55.30-K55.33

PDX Collection 791
K55.011-K55.069, K55.1, K55.30-K55.33, K55.8-K55.9

PDX Collection 792
K56.0-K56.3, K56.49-K56.7, K63.4, K63.89-K63.9,
K91.30-K91.32, K92.89-K92.9, R11.13

PDX Collection 793
K57.00-K57.13

PDX Collection 794
K57.20-K57.93

PDX Collection 795
K58.0-K58.9, K59.1-K59.9, K91.0-K91.1

PDX Collection 796
K61.0-K61.4

PDX Collection 797
K62.6

PDX Collection 798
K63.0

PDX Collection 799
K63.1

PDX Collection 800
K63.2

PDX Collection 801
K63.3

PDX Collection 802
E16.4, I85.01, K22.10-K22.11, K22.6-K22.719, K25.0-K28.9,
K29.01, K29.21, K29.31, K29.41, K29.51, K29.61, K29.71,
K29.81, K29.91, K31.811, K55.21, K57.01, K57.11, K57.13,
K57.21, K57.31, K57.33, K57.41, K57.51, K57.53, K57.81,
K57.91, K57.93, K62.5, K63.81, K92.0-K92.2

PDX Collection 803
K63.4, K63.89-K63.9, K65.0-K65.9, K67, K68.19-K68.9,
K92.89-K92.9, R11.13

PDX Collection 804
K66.1

PDX Collection 805
D78.81-D78.89, E36.8, E89.810-E89.89, H59.011-H59.019,
H59.031-H59.099, H59.811-H59.89, H95.811-H95.89, I97.3,
K68.11, L76.81-L76.82, M96.89, N98.1-N98.9, T81.40-T81.49,
T81.82XA, T81.89X-T81.9XX[A]

PDX Collection 806
K68.12, M60.00-M60.19, M61.00-M61.19, M61.30-M61.59,
M62.3, M62.50-M62.59, M62.84, M62.89, M72.6

PDX Collection 807
K72.91, K76.5, K76.89-K76.9 K72.00-K72.01, K76.2-K76.3,
K76.5, K76.89-K76.9

PDX Collection 808
K72.00-K72.01, K76.2-K76.3, K76.5, K76.89-K76.9

PDX Collection 809
A06.4, K75.0-K75.1, K76.5, K76.89-K76.9

PDX Collection 810
K72.91, K76.5-K76.6, K76.89-K76.9

PDX Collection 811
K76.5, K76.7, K76.89-K76.9

PDX Collection 812
K80.00-K80.21, K80.40, K80.44, K80.62-K80.63,
K80.66-K80.67, K80.80, K81.0-K81.9, K82.9, K83.5-K83.9,
K87

PDX Collection 813
K80.00-K80.21, K80.62-K80.63, K80.66-K80.67, K80.80,
K81.0-K81.9, K82.9, K83.5-K83.9, K87

PDX Collection 814
K83.09, K83.5-K83.9, K87

PDX Collection 815
K80.30-K80.71, K80.81-K81.9, K83.5-K83.9, K87

PDX Collection 816
K80.62-K80.63, K81.0-K81.9, K82.9, K83.5-K83.9, K87

PDX Collection 817
K80.66-K80.67, K81.0-K81.9, K82.9, K83.5-K83.9, K87

PDX Collection 818
K80.00, K80.12, K80.62-K80.63, K80.66-K80.67, K81.0-K81.9,
K82.9, K83.5-K83.9, K87

PDX Collection 819
K81.0-K81.9, K82.9, K83.5-K83.9, K87

PDX Collection 820
K82.0-K82.9, K83.5-K83.9, K87

PDX Collection 821
K80.31, K80.33, K80.35, K80.37, K80.41, K80.43, K80.45,
K80.47, K80.51, K80.81, K83.1, K83.5-K83.9, K87,
Q44.2-Q44.3

PDX Collection 822
K83.2-K83.3, K83.5-K83.9, K87

PDX Collection 823
B25.2, E16.8, K85.00-K86.9

PDX Collection 824
K86.2-K86.9

PDX Collection 825
E84.19, K90.0-K90.49, K90.89-K90.9, K91.2

PDX Collection 826
K90.81

PDX Collection 827
K90.3-K90.49, K90.89-K90.9, K91.2

PDX Collection 828
D78.81-D78.89, E36.8, E89.810-E89.89, H59.011-H59.019,
H59.031-H59.099, H59.811-H59.89, H95.811-H95.89,
I97.3, K91.81-K91.83, K91.850-K91.89, K94.20-K95.89,
L76.81-L76.82, M96.89, N98.1-N98.9, T81.710A, T81.82XA,
T81.89X-T81.9XX[A]

PDX Collection 829
H95.811-H95.89, I85.01, I85.11, I97.3, K21.9, K22.8,
K23-K25.0, K25.2, K25.4, K25.6, K26.0, K26.2, K26.4,
K26.6, K27.0, K27.2, K27.4, K27.6, K28.0, K28.2, K28.4,
K28.6, K29.01, K29.21, K29.31, K29.41, K29.51, K29.61,
K29.71, K29.81, K29.91, K31.811, K55.21, K57.01,
K57.11, K57.13, K57.21, K57.31, K57.33, K57.41, K57.51,
K57.53, K57.81, K57.91, K57.93, K62.5, K91.61-K91.62,
K91.840-K91.841, K91.870-K91.873, K92.0-K92.2, M96.89,
N98.1-N98.9, P54.1-P54.3, T81.10X-T81.19X[A], T81.82XA,
T81.89X-T81.9XX[A]

PDX Collection 830
K94.00-K94.19

PDX Collection 831
D78.81-D78.89, E36.8, E89.810-E89.89, H59.011-H59.019,
H59.031-H59.099, H59.811-H59.89, H95.811-H95.89,
I97.3, K91.81-K91.83, K91.850-K91.89, K94.00-K95.89,
L76.81-L76.82, M96.89, N98.1-N98.9, T81.710A, T81.82XA,
T81.89X-T81.9XX[A]

PDX Collection 832
A17.9, A18.4, A18.82, A18.84, A18.89, A48.2-A48.4,
A48.8-A49.9, B78.1, B95.0-B96.89, E83.2, L02.11,
L02.811-L02.818, L02.91, L03.221-L03.222, L03.811-L03.91,
L08.0-L08.9, L44.8-L45, L73.2, L88, L92.8, L94.2, L94.4,
L98.0, L98.3, L98.7, L98.8, L99, Z16.10-Z16.39

PDX Collection 833
A17.9, A18.4, A18.82, A18.84, A18.89, A48.2-A48.4,
A48.8-A49.9, B78.1, B95.0-B96.89, E83.2, L02.211-L02.219,
L02.811-L02.818, L02.91, L03.311-L03.316, L03.319-L03.326,
L03.329-L03.91, L08.0, L08.81-L08.9, L44.8-L45, L73.2,
L88, L92.8, L94.2, L94.4, L98.0, L98.3, L98.7, L98.8, L99,
Z16.10-Z16.39

PDX Collection 834
A17.9, A18.4, A18.82, A18.84, A18.89, A48.2-A48.4,
A48.8-A49.9, B78.1, B95.0-B96.89, E83.2, L02.31,
L02.811-L02.818, L02.91, L03.317, L03.327, L03.811-L03.91,
L08.0, L08.81-L08.9, L44.8-L45, L73.2, L88, L92.8, L94.2,
L94.4, L98.0, L98.3, L98.7, L98.8, L99, Z16.10-Z16.39

PDX Collection 835
A17.9, A18.4, A18.82, A18.84, A18.89, A48.2-A48.4,
A48.8-A49.9, B78.1, B95.0-B96.89, E83.2, L02.411-L02.414,
L02.811-L02.818, L02.91, L03.111-L03.114, L03.121-L03.124,
L03.811-L03.91, L08.0, L08.81-L08.9, L44.8-L45, L73.2,
L88, L92.8, L94.2, L94.4, L98.0, L98.3, L98.7, L98.8, L99,
Z16.10-Z16.39

PDX Collection 836
A17.9, A18.4, A18.82, A18.84, A18.89, A48.2-A48.4,
A48.8-A49.9, B78.1, B95.0-B96.89, E83.2, L02.415-L02.419,
L02.811-L02.818, L02.91, L03.115-L03.119, L03.125-L03.129,
L03.811-L03.91, L08.0, L08.81-L08.9, L44.8-L45, L73.2,
L88, L92.8, L94.2, L94.4, L98.0, L98.3, L98.7, L98.8, L99,
Z16.10-Z16.39

PDX Collection 837
A17.9, A18.4, A18.82, A18.84, A18.89, A48.2-A48.4,
A48.8-A49.9, B78.1, B95.0-B96.89, E83.2, L02.511-L02.519,
L02.811-L02.818, L02.91, L03.811-L03.91, L08.0,
L08.81-L08.9, L44.8-L45, L73.2, L88, L92.8, L94.2, L94.4,
L98.0, L98.3, L98.7, L98.8, L99, Z16.10-Z16.39

PDX Collection 838
A17.9, A18.4, A18.82, A18.84, A18.89, A48.2-A48.4,
A48.8-A49.9, B78.1, B95.0-B96.89, E83.2, L02.611-L02.619,
L02.811-L02.818, L02.91, L03.811-L03.91, L08.0,
L08.81-L08.9, L44.8-L45, L73.2, L88, L92.8, L94.2, L94.4,
L98.0, L98.3, L98.7, L98.8, L99, Z16.10-Z16.39

PDX Collection 839
A17.9, A18.4, A18.82, A18.84, A18.89, A48.2-A48.4,
A48.8-A49.9, B78.1, B95.0-B96.89, E83.2, L02.811-L02.818,
L02.91, L03.811-L03.91, L08.0, L08.81-L08.9, L44.8-L45,
L73.2, L88, L92.8, L94.2, L94.4, L98.0, L98.3, L98.7, L98.8,
L99, Z16.10-Z16.39

PDX Collection 840
A17.9, A18.4, A18.82, A18.84, A18.89, A48.2-A48.4,
A48.8-A49.9, B78.1, B95.0-B96.89, E83.2, L02.811-L02.818,
L02.91, L03.211, L03.213, L03.811-L03.91, L08.0,
L08.81-L08.9, L44.8-L45, L73.2, L88, L92.8, L94.2, L94.4,
L98.0, L98.3, L98.7, L98.8, L99, Z16.10-Z16.39

PDX Collection 841
L05.01-L05.92, L44.8-L45, L94.2, L94.4, L98.7, L98.8, L99

PDX Collection 842
L10.0-L10.9, L12.0-L12.1, L12.8-L12.9, L13.8-L14, L44.8-L45,
L94.2, L94.4, L98.7, L98.8, L99

PDX Collection 843
L00, L12.30-L12.35, L26, L30.4, L44.8-L45, L51.0-L54,
L71.0-L71.9, L92.0, L93.0-L93.2, L94.2, L94.4, L95.1, L98.2,
L98.7, L98.8, L99

PDX Collection 844
L49.3

PDX Collection 845
L49.4

PDX Collection 846
L49.5

PDX Collection 847
L49.6

PDX Collection 848
L49.7

PDX Collection 849
L49.8

PDX Collection 850
L49.9

PDX Collection 851
L12.30-L12.35, L44.8-L45, L51.0-L53.3, L71.0-L71.9,
L93.0-L93.2, L94.2, L94.4, L98.7, L98.8, L99

PDX Collection 852
H95.811-H95.89, I85.01, I85.11, I97.3, K21.9, K22.8, K23,
K25.0, K25.2, K25.4, K25.6, K26.0, K26.2, K26.4, K26.6,
K27.0, K27.2, K27.4, K27.6, K28.0, K28.2, K28.4, K28.6,
K29.01, K29.21, K29.31, K29.41, K29.51, K29.61, K29.71,
K29.81, K29.91, K31.811, K55.21, K57.01, K57.11, K57.13,
K57.21, K57.31, K57.33, K57.41, K57.51, K57.53, K57.81,
K57.91, K57.93, K62.5, K92.0-K92.2, L76.01-L76.02,
L76.21-L76.82, M96.89, N98.1-N98.9, P54.1-P54.3,
T81.10X-T81.19X[A], I81.82XA, T81.89X-T81.9XX[A]

PDX Collection 853
L08.0, L08.81, L88

PDX Collection 854
L89.000-L89.96, L97.101-L97.929, L98.411-L98.499

PDX Collection 855
A17.9, A18.02, A18.09, A18.82, A18.84, A18.89,
A39.83-A39.84, A54.40, A54.42-A54.43, A54.82, A54.84,
A54.89-A54.9, B06.82, M00.00-M02.30, M02.319, M02.329,
M02.339, M02.349, M02.359, M02.369, M02.379-M02.9,
M05.40-M05.59, M05.70-M06.09, M06.20-M07.69,
M11.00-M11.9, M12.10-M15.0, M15.3-M15.9, M16.2-M16.9,
M17.2-M17.9, M18.2-M19.93, M24.10-M24.176, M25.00,
M25.08-M25.18, M25.40-M25.676, M25.80-M25.9, M35.2,
M36.1-M36.4, R26.2, R29.4

PDX Collection 856
A17.9, A18.02, A18.09, A18.82, A18.84, A18.89,
A39.83-A39.84, A54.40, A54.42-A54.43, A54.82, A54.84,
A54.89-A54.9, B06.82, M00.00-M02.30, M02.319,
M02.38-M02.819, M02.88-M02.9, M05.40-M05.59,
M05.70-M06.09, M06.20-M07.69, M11.00-M11.9,
M11.20-M11.219, M11.28-M11.819, M11.88-M11.9,
M12.10-M15.0, M15.3-M15.9, M19.011-M19.019,
M19.111-M19.119, M19.211-M19.219, M19.90-M19.93,
M24.10-M24.119, M25.00, M25.011-M25.019,
M25.08-M25.119, M25.18, M25.40-M25.419,
M25.48-M25.519, M25.541-M25.549, M25.60-M25.619,
M25.80-M25.819, M25.9, M35.2, M36.1-M36.4, R26.2

PDX Collection 857
A17.9, A18.02, A18.09, A18.82, A18.84, A18.89,
A39.83-A39.84, A54.40, A54.42-A54.43, A54.82, A54.84,
A54.89-A54.9, B06.82, M00.00-M02.30, M02.329,
M02.38-M02.80, M02.821-M02.829, M02.88-M02.9,
M05.40-M05.59, M05.70-M07.60, M07.621-M07.629,
M07.68-M07.69, M11.00, M11.021-M11.029,

M11.08-M11.10, M11.121-M11.129, M11.18-M11.20,
M11.221-M11.229, M11.28-M11.80, M11.821-M11.829,
M11.88-M11.9, M12.10, M12.121-M12.129, M12.18-M12.20,
M12.221-M12.229, M12.28-M12.30, M12.321-M12.329,
M12.38-M12.40, M12.421-M12.429, M12.48-M12.50,
M12.521-M12.529, M12.58-M12.80, M12.821-M12.829,
M12.88-M12.9, M13.0-M13.10, M13.121-M13.129, M13.80,
M13.821-M13.829, M13.88-M13.89, M14.60-M15.9,
M19.021-M19.029, M19.121-M19.129, M19.221-M19.229,
M19.90-M19.93, M24.10, M24.121-M24.129, M25.00,
M25.021-M25.029, M25.08-M25.10, M25.121-M25.129,
M25.18, M25.40, M25.421-M25.429, M25.48-M25.50,
M25.521-M25.529, M25.541-M25.549, M25.60,
M25.621-M25.629, M25.80, M25.821-M25.829, M25.9,
M35.2, M36.1-M36.4, R26.2

PDX Collection 858
A17.9, A18.02, A18.09, A18.82, A18.84, A18.89,
A39.83-A39.84, A54.40, A54.42-A54.43, A54.82, A54.84,
A54.89-A54.9, B06.82, M00.00-M02.30, M02.339,
M02.38-M02.80, M02.831-M02.839, M02.88-M02.9,
M05.40-M05.59, M05.70-M07.60, M07.631-M07.639,
M07.68-M07.69, M11.00, M11.031-M11.039,
M11.08-M11.10, M11.131-M11.139, M11.18-M11.20,
M11.231-M11.239, M11.28-M11.80, M11.831-M11.839,
M11.88-M11.9, M12.10, M12.131-M12.139, M12.18-M12.20,
M12.231-M12.239, M12.28-M12.30, M12.331-M12.339,
M12.38-M12.40, M12.431-M12.439, M12.48-M12.50,
M12.531-M12.539, M12.58-M12.80, M12.831-M12.839,
M12.88-M12.9, M13.0-M13.10, M13.131-M13.139, M13.80,
M13.831-M13.839, M13.88-M15.9, M19.031-M19.039,
M19.131-M19.139, M19.231-M19.239, M19.90-M19.93,
M24.10, M24.131-M24.139, M25.00, M25.031-M25.039,
M25.08-M25.10, M25.131-M25.139, M25.18, M25.40,
M25.431-M25.439, M25.48-M25.50, M25.531-M25.539,
M25.541-M25.549, M25.60, M25.631-M25.639, M25.80,
M25.831-M25.839, M25.9, M35.2, M36.1-M36.4, R26.2

PDX Collection 859
A17.9, A18.02, A18.09, A18.82, A18.84, A18.89,
A39.83-A39.84, A54.40, A54.42-A54.43, A54.82, A54.84,
A54.89-A54.9, B06.82, M00.00, M00.041-M00.049,
M00.08-M00.10, M00.141-M00.149, M00.18-M00.20,
M00.241-M00.249, M00.28-M00.80, M00.841-M00.849,
M00.88-M01.X0, M01, X41-M01.X49, M01.X8-M02.10,
M02.141-M02.149, M02.18-M02.30, M02.349,
M02.38-M02.80, M02.841-M02.849, M02.88-M02.9,
M05.40-M05.59, M05.70-M06.09, M06.20-M07.60,
M07.641-M07.649, M07.68-M07.69, M11.00,
M11.041-M11.049, M11.08-M11.10, M11.141-M11.149,
M11.18-M11.20, M11.241-M11.249, M11.28-M11.80,
M11.841-M11.849, M11.88-M11.9, M12.10,
M12.141-M12.149, M12.18-M12.20, M12.241-M12.249,
M12.28-M12.30, M12.341-M12.349, M12.38-M12.40,
M12.441-M12.449, M12.48-M12.50, M12.541-M12.549,
M12.58-M12.80, M12.841-M12.849, M12.88-M13.10,
M13.141-M13.149, M13.80, M13.841-M13.849,
M13.88-M15.9, M18.0-M18.9, M19.041-M19.049,
M19.141-M19.149, M19.241-M19.249, M19.90-M19.93,
M24.10, M24.141-M24.149, M25.00, M25.041-M25.049,
M25.08-M25.10, M25.141-M25.149, M25.18, M25.40,
M25.441-M25.449, M25.48-M25.50, M25.541-M25.549,
M25.60, M25.641-M25.649, M25.80, M25.841-M25.849,
M25.9, M35.2, M36.1-M36.4, R26.2

PDX Collection 860
A17.9, A18.02, A18.09, A18.82, A18.84, A18.89,
A39.83-A39.84, A54.40, A54.42-A54.43, A54.82, A54.84,
A54.89-A54.9, B06.82, M00.00, M00.051-M00.059,
M00.08-M00.10, M00.151-M00.159, M00.18-M00.20,
M00.251-M00.259, M00.28-M00.29, M00.80,

M00.851-M00.859, M00.88-M00.9, M01.X0,
M01.X51-M01.X59 , M01.X8-M02.10, M02.151-M02.159,
M02.18-M02.30, M02.359, M02.38-M02.80, M02.851-M02.9,
M05.40-M05.59, M05.70-M06.09, M06.20-M06.39,
M06.80-M07.60, M07.651-M07.659, M07.68-M07.69, M11.00,
M11.051-M11.059, M11.08-M11.10, M11.151-M11.159,
M11.18-M11.20, M11.251-M11.259, M11.28-M11.80,
M11.851-M11.859, M11.88-M12.10, M12.151-M12.159,
M12.18-M12.20, M12.251-M12.259, M12.28-M12.30,
M12.351-M12.359, M12.38-M12.40, M12.451-M12.459,
M12.48-M12.50, M12.551-M12.559, M12.58-M12.80,
M12.851-M12.859, M12.88-M13.10, M13.151-M13.159,
M13.80, M13.851-M13.859, M13.88-M15.0, M15.3-M16.9,
M19.90-M19.93, M24.10, M24.151-M24.159, M25.00,
M25.051-M25.059, M25.08-M25.10, M25.151-M25.159,
M25.18, M25.40, M25.451-M25.459, M25.48-M25.559,
M25.60, M25.651-M25.659, M25.80, M25.851-M25.859,
M25.9, M35.2, M36.1-M36.4, R26.2, R29.4

PDX Collection 861
A17.9, A18.02, A18.09, A18.82, A18.84, A18.89,
A39.83-A39.84, A54.40, A54.42-A54.43, A54.82, A54.84,
A54.89-A54.9, B06.82, M00.00, M00.061-M00.069,
M00.08-M00.10, M00.161-M00.169, M00.18-M00.20,
M00.261-M00.269, M00.28-M00.29, M00.80,
M00.861-M00.869, M00.88-M00.9, M01.X0,
M01.X61-M01.X69, M01.X8-M02.10, M02.161-M02.169,
M02.18-M02.30, M02.369, M02.38-M02.80,
M02.861-M02.869, M02.88-M02.9, M05.40-M05.59,
M05.70-M06.09, M06.20-M06.39, M06.80-M07.60,
M07.661-M07.669, M07.68-M07.69, M11.00,
M11.061-M11.069, M11.08-M11.10, M11.161-M11.169,
M11.18-M11.20, M11.261-M11.269, M11.28-M11.80,
M11.861-M11.869, M11.88-M12.10, M12.161-M12.169,
M12.18-M12.20, M12.261-M12.269, M12.28-M12.30,
M12.361-M12.369, M12.38-M12.40, M12.461-M12.469,
M12.48-M12.50, M12.561-M12.569, M12.58-M12.80,
M12.861-M12.869, M12.88-M13.10, M13.161-M13.169,
M13.80, M13.861-M13.869, M13.88-M15.0, M15.3-M15.9,
M17.0-M17.9, M19.90-M19.93, M24.10, M25.00,
M25.061-M25.069, M25.08-M25.10, M25.161-M25.169,
M25.18, M25.40, M25.461-M25.469, M25.48-M25.50,
M25.541-M25.549, M25.561-M25.569, M25.60,
M25.661-M25.669, M25.80, M25.861-M25.869, M25.9,
M35.2, M36.1-M36.4, R26.2

PDX Collection 862
A17.9, A18.02, A18.09, A18.82, A18.84, A18.89,
A39.83-A39.84, A54.40, A54.42-A54.43, A54.82, A54.84,
A54.89-A54.9, B06.82, M00.00, M00.071-M00.079,
M00.08-M00.10, M00.171-M00.179, M00.18-M00.20,
M00.271-M00.279, M00.28-M00.29, M00.80,
M00.871-M00.879, M00.88-M00.9, M01.X0,
M01.X71-M01.X79, M01.X8-M02.10, M02.171-M02.179,
M02.18-M02.9, M05.40-M05.59, M05.70-M06.09,
M06.20-M06.39, M06.80-M07.60, M07.671-M07.679,
M07.68-M07.69, M11.00, M11.071-M11.079, M11.08-M11.10,
M11.171-M11.179, M11.18-M11.20, M11.271-M11.279,
M11.28-M11.80, M11.871-M11.879, M11.88-M11.9, M12.10,
M12.171-M12.179, M12.18-M12.20, M12.271-M12.279,
M12.28-M12.30, M12.371-M12.379, M12.38-M12.40,
M12.471-M12.479, M12.48-M12.50, M12.571-M12.579,
M12.58-M12.80, M12.871-M12.879, M12.88-M13.10,
M13.171-M13.179, M13.80, M13.871-M13.879,
M13.88-M15.0, M15.3-M15.9, M19.071-M19.079,
M19.171-M19.179, M19.271-M19.279, M19.90-M19.93,
M24.10, M24.171-M24.176, M25.00, M25.071-M25.10,
M25.171-M25.18, M25.40, M25.471-M25.50,
M25.541-M25.549, M25.571-M25.60, M25.671-M25.676,
M25.80, M25.871-M25.9, M35.2, M36.1-M36.4, R26.2

PDX Collection 863
A02.23, A17.9, A18.02, A18.09, A18.82, A18.84, A18.89,
A39.83-A39.84, A54.40, A54.42-A54.43, A54.82, A54.84,
A54.89-A54.9, B06.82, M00.00, M00.011-M02.30,
M02.319, M02.329, M02.339, M02.349, M02.359, M02.369,
M02.379, M02.38-M02.9, M05.40-M05.59, M05.70-M07.69,
M11.00-M15.0, M15.3-M15.9, M16.2-M16.9, M17.2-M17.9,
M18.2-M18.9, M19.111-M19.93, M24.10-M24.176, M25.00,
M25.08-M25.18, M25.40-M25.676, M25.80-M25.9, M35.2,
M36.1-M36.4, R29.4

PDX Collection 864
A02.23, A17.9, A18.02, A18.09, A18.82, A18.84, A18.89,
A39.83-A39.84, A54.40, A54.42-A54.43, A54.82, A54.84,
A54.89-A54.9, B06.82, M00.00, M00.011-M02.30,
M02.319, M02.329, M02.339, M02.349, M02.359, M02.369,
M02.379, M02.38-M02.9, M05.40-M05.59, M05.70-M07.69,
M11.00-M15.0, M15.3-M15.9, M16.2-M16.9, M17.2-M17.9,
M18.2-M18.9, M19.111-M19.93, M24.10-M24.176, M25.00,
M25.08-M25.18, M25.40-M25.676, M25.80-M25.9, M35.2,
M36.1-M36.4, R29.4

PDX Collection 865
A02.23, A17.9, A18.02, A18.09, A18.82, A18.84, A18.89,
A39.83-A39.84, A54.40, A54.42-A54.43, A54.82, A54.84,
A54.89-A54.9, B06.82, M00.00, M00.011-M02.30,
M02.319, M02.329, M02.339, M02.349, M02.359, M02.369,
M02.379, M02.38-M02.9, M05.40-M05.59, M05.70-M07.69,
M11.00-M15.0, M15.3-M15.9, M16.2-M16.9, M17.2-M17.9,
M18.2-M18.9, M19.111-M19.93, M24.10-M24.176, M25.00,
M25.08-M25.18, M25.40-M25.676, M25.80-M25.9, M35.2,
M36.1-M36.4, R29.4

PDX Collection 867
E08.40-E08.49, E08.618-E08.638, E08.649-E08.8,
E09.40-E09.49, E09.618-E09.638, E09.649-E09.8,
E10.40-E10.49, E10.618-E10.638, E10.649, E10.69-E10.8,
E11.40-E11.49, E11.618-E11.638, E11.649, E11.69-E11.8,
E13.40-E13.49, E13.618-E13.638, E13.649-E13.8, G32.89,
G70.00-G72.3, G72.81-G73.7, G96.8-G96.9, G98.0-G98.8,
G99.8

PDX Collection 868
M25.00-M25.08, T79.A11A-T79.A29A

PDX Collection 869
M25.00-M25.039, M25.08, T79.A11-T79.A19[A]

PDX Collection 870
M25.00-M25.029, M25.08, T79.A11-T79.A19[A]

PDX Collection 871
M25.00-M25.049, M25.08, T79.A11-T79.A19[A]

PDX Collection 872
M25.00, M25.031-M25.049, M25.08, T79.A11-T79.A19[A]

PDX Collection 873
M25.00, M25.061-M25.08, T79.A21-T79.A29[A]

PDX Collection 874
E08.51-E08.59, E08.618-E08.638, E08.649-E08.8,
E09.51-E09.59, E09.618-E09.638, E09.649-E09.8,
E10.51-E10.59, E10.618-E10.638, E10.649, E10.69-E10.8,
E11.51-E11.59, E11.618-E11.638, E11.649, E11.69-E11.8,
E13.51-E13.59, E13.618-E13.638, E13.649-E13.8, I87.8-I87.9,
I99.8-I99.9, M30.0-M31.7

PDX Collection 875
I87.8-I87.9, I99.8-I99.9, M30.0-M31.7

PDX Collection 876
M33.00-M33.19, M33.90-M33.99, M36.0

PDX Collection 877
E08.40-E08.49, E08.618-E08.638, E08.649-E08.8,
E09.40-E09.49, E09.618-E09.638, E09.649-E09.8,
E10.40-E10.49, E10.618-E10.638, E10.649, E10.69-E10.8,

E11.40-E11.49, E11.618-E11.638, E11.649, E11.69-E11.8,
E13.40-E13.49, E13.618-E13.638, E13.649-E13.8, G32.89,
G70.00-G72.3, G72.81-G73.7, G96.8-G96.9, G98.0-G98.8,
G99.8, M33.00-M33.19, M33.90-M33.99, M36.0

PDX Collection 878
M33.20-M33.29

PDX Collection 879
E08.40-E08.49, E08.618-E08.638, E08.649-E08.8,
E09.40-E09.49, E09.618-E09.638, E09.649-E09.8,
E10.40-E10.49, E10.618-E10.638, E10.649, E10.69-E10.8,
E11.40-E11.49, E11.618-E11.638, E11.649, E11.69-E11.8,
E13.40-E13.49, E13.618-E13.638, E13.649-E13.8, G32.89,
G70.00-G72.3, G72.81-G73.7, G96.9, G98.0-G98.8, G99.8,
M33.20-M33.29

PDX Collection 880
G72.41-G72.49, M35.1, M35.5, M35.81-M35.89

PDX Collection 881
A02.24, A17.9, A18.03, A18.09, A18.82, A18.84, A18.89,
M46.20-M46.39, M86.00-M86.9

PDX Collection 882
A17.9, A18.01, A18.03, A18.09, A18.82, A18.84, A18.89,
M46.20-M46.39, M86.00-M86.9

PDX Collection 883
M47.011-M47.029, M47.11-M47.13, M47.21-M47.23,
M47.811-M47.813, M47.891-M47.893

PDX Collection 884
M25.78, M47.011-M47.16, M47.20-M47.9, M48.10-M48.38,
M48.9

PDX Collection 885
M47.14-M47.15

PDX Collection 886
M46.40, M46.46-M46.49, M47.16, M47.26-M47.28,
M47.816-M47.818, M47.896-M47.898, M51.06, M51.26-M51.27,
M51.36-M51.37, M51.46-M51.47, M51.86-M51.9

PDX Collection 887
M48.30-M48.38

PDX Collection 888
M48.40X-M48.58X[A], M80.00X-M80.88X[A],
M84.30X-M84.68X[A], M84.750-M84.759[A]

PDX Collection 889
M50.00-M50.03, M50.20-M50.23

PDX Collection 890
M51.04-M51.05, M51.24-M51.25

PDX Collection 891
M51.06, M51.24-M51.25

PDX Collection 892
K68.12, M60.000-M60.19, M61.00-M61.19, M61.30-M61.59,
M62.3, M62.50-M62.59, M62.82, M62.84, M62.89, M72.6

PDX Collection 894
M70.80-M70.99, M79.81-M79.A29, R29.898,
S75.801-S75.899[A], S85.201-S85.899[A],
S95.001-S95.099[A], S95.201-S95.899[A]

PDX Collection 895
M79.A3, S31.001A, S31.011A, S31.021A, S31.031A,
S31.041A, S31.051-S31.159[A], S31.600-S31.659[A],
S31.831-S31.839[A], S36.00X-S37.599[A],
S37.812-S37.99X[A], S38.3XX[A], S39.021-S39.023[A],
T07.XXX-T14.91X[A], T79.8XX-T79.9XX[A]

PDX Collection 896
S31.001A, S31.011A, S31.021A, S31.031A, S31.041A,
S31.051A, S31.600-S31.659[A], S36.81X-S36.899[A],
T79.A9X[A]

PDX Collection 897
M80.00X-M80.88X[K,P], M84.30X-M84.68X[K,P],
M84.750-M84.759[K,P], S02.0XX-S02.92X[K],
S12.000-S12.691[K], S22.000-S22.9XX[K],
S32.000-S32.9XX[K], S42.001-S42.92X[K,P],
S49.001-S49.199[K,P], S52.001-S52.92X[K,M,N,P,Q,R],
S59.001-S59.299[K,P], S62.001-S62.92X[K,P],
S72.001-S72.92X[K,M,N,P,Q,R], S79.001-S79.199[K,P],
S82.001-S82.92X[K,M,N,P,Q,R], S89.001-S89.399[K,P],
S92.001-S92.919[K,P]

PDX Collection 898
A17.9, A18.03-A18.09, A18.82, A18.84, A18.89,
M46.20-M46.39, M86.00-M86.9

PDX Collection 899
A17.9, A18.03-A18.09, A18.82, A18.84, A18.89,
M46.20-M46.39, M86.00, M86.08-M86.10, M86.18-M86.20,
M86.219, M86.28-M86.319, M86.38-M86.419,
M86.48-M86.519, M86.58-M86.619, M86.68-M86.8X1,
M86.8X8-M86.9

PDX Collection 900
A17.9, A18.03-A18.09, A18.82, A18.84, A18.89,
M46.20-M46.39, M86.00, M86.08-M86.10, M86.18-M86.20,
M86.229, M86.28-M86.30, M86.321-M86.329,
M86.38-M86.40, M86.421-M86.429, M86.48-M86.50,
M86.521-M86.529, M86.58-M86.60, M86.621-M86.629,
M86.68-M86.69, M86.8X0, M86.8X2, M86.8X8-M86.9

PDX Collection 901
A17.9, A18.03-A18.09, A18.82, A18.84, A18.89,
M46.20-M46.39, M86.00, M86.08-M86.10, M86.18-M86.20,
M86.239, M86.28-M86.30, M86.331-M86.339,
M86.38-M86.40, M86.431-M86.439, M86.48-M86.50,
M86.531-M86.539, M86.58-M86.60, M86.631-M86.639,
M86.68-M86.8X0, M86.8X3, M86.8X8-M86.9

PDX Collection 902
A17.9, A18.03-A18.09, A18.82, A18.84, A18.89,
M46.20-M46.39, M86.00, M86.08-M86.10, M86.18-M86.20,
M86.249, M86.28-M86.30, M86.341-M86.349,
M86.38-M86.40, M86.441-M86.449, M86.48-M86.50,
M86.541-M86.549, M86.58-M86.60, M86.41-M86.649,
M86.68-M86.69, M86.8X0, M86.8X4, M86.8X8-M86.9

PDX Collection 903
A17.9, A18.03-A18.09, A18.82, A18.84, A18.89,
M46.20-M46.39, M86.00, M86.08-M86.10, M86.18-M86.20,
M86.259, M86.28-M86.30, M86.351-M86.359,
M86.38-M86.40, M86.451-M86.459, M86.48-M86.50,
M86.551-M86.559, M86.58-M86.60, M86.651-M86.659,
M86.68-M86.8X0, M86.8X5, M86.8X8-M86.9

PDX Collection 904
A17.9, A18.03-A18.09, A18.82, A18.84, A18.89,
M46.20-M46.39, M86.00, M86.08-M86.10, M86.18-M86.20,
M86.269, M86.28-M86.30, M86.361-M86.369,
M86.38-M86.40, M86.461-M86.469, M86.48-M86.50,
M86.561-M86.569, M86.58-M86.60, M86.661-M86.669,
M86.68-M86.8X0, M86.8X6, M86.8X8-M86.9

PDX Collection 905
A17.9, A18.03-A18.09, A18.82, A18.84, A18.89,
M46.20-M46.39, M86.00, M86.08-M86.10, M86.18-M86.20,
M86.279, M86.28-M86.30, M86.371-M86.379,
M86.38-M86.40, M86.471-M86.479, M86.48-M86.50,
M86.571-M86.579, M86.58-M86.60, M86.671-M86.679,
M86.68-M86.8X0, M86.8X7-M86.9

PDX Collection 906
M46.20-M46.39, M86.30-M86.9, M88.0-M88.9,
M90.60-M90.69

PDX Collection 907
M87.00-M87.9, M90.50-M90.59

PDX Collection 908
M87.00-M87.9, M90.50-M90.59

PDX Collection 909
M87.00-M87.9, M90.50-M90.59

PDX Collection 910
M87.00, M87.031-M87.819, M87.831-M87.849,
M87.861-M87.9, M90.50, M90.521-M90.549,
M90.561-M90.59

PDX Collection 911
D78.81, D78.89, E36.8, E89.810-E89.89, H59.011-H59.019,
H59.031-H59.819, H59.88-H59.89, H95.811-H95.89,
I97.3, L76.81-L76.82, M96.621-M96.69, M96.89,
M97.01X-M97.9XX[A], N98.1-N98.9, T81.82XA,
T81.89X-T81.9XX[A], T84.010-T84.039[A],
T84.050-T84.9XX[A]

PDX Collection 912
H95.811-H95.89, I85.01, I85.11, I97.3, K21.9, K22.8,
K23-K25.2, K25.4, K25.6, K26.0, K26.2, K26.4, K26.6,
K27.0, K27.2, K27.4, K27.6, K28.0, K28.2, K28.4, K28.6,
K29.01, K29.21, K29.31, K29.41, K29.51, K29.61, K29.71,
K29.81, K29.91, K31.811, K55.21, K57.01, K57.11, K57.13,
K57.21, K57.31, K57.33, K57.41, K57.51, K57.53, K57.81,
K57.91, K57.93, K62.5, K92.0-K92.2, M96.810-M96.811,
M96.830-M96.89, N98.1-N98.9, P54.1-P54.3,
T81.10X-T81.19X[A], T81.82XA, T81.89X-T81.9XX[A]

PDX Collection 913
M99.10-M99.11, S03.8XX-S03.9XX[A], S12.000-S12.691[A,B],
S12.9XX-S13.4XX[A], S13.8XX[A], S14.0XX-S14.108[A],
S14.111-S14.118[A], S14.121-S14.128[A],
S14.131-S14.138[A], S14.141-S14.148[A],
S14.151-S14.158[A], S16.1XX[A], S29.011-S29.019[A],
S38.3XX[A], S39.011-S39.013[A], T07.XXX-T14.91X[A],
T79.A0X-T79.9XX[A]

PDX Collection 914
M99.18, S43.201-S43.226[A]

PDX Collection 915
A17.9, A18.10-A18.11, A18.13, A18.82, A18.84,
A18.89, A54.21, A54.29, A54.82, A54.84, A54.89-A54.9,
A59.00, A59.8-A59.9, B37.41-B37.49, E08.21-E08.29,
E08.618-E08.638, E08.649, E08.65-E08.8, E09.21-E09.29,
E09.618-E09.638, E09.649-E09.8, E10.21-E10.29,
E10.618-E10.638, E10.649, E10.69-E10.8, E11.21-E11.29,
E11.618-E11.638, E11.649, E11.69-E11.8, E13.21-E13.29,
E13.618-E13.638, E13.649-wE13.69, E13.8, E88.3,
M10.30-M10.39, N00.0-N07.A, N10, N11.10, N11.8, N11.9,
N13.0-N13.39, N13.6, N14.0-N19, N25.0-N27.9, N28.1-N29,
N36.41-N36.43, N36.8-N36.9, N39.8-N39.9, R31.0-R31.9

PDX Collection 916
A17.9, A18.10-A18.11, A18.13, A18.82, A18.84, A18.89,
A54.21, A54.29, A54.82, A54.84, A54.89-A54.9, A59.00,
A59.8-A59.9, B37.41-B37.49, E08.21-E08.29, E09.21-E09.29,
E88.3, M10.30-M10.39, N00.0-N13.39, N13.6, N14.0-N19,
N25.0-N27.9, N28.1-N29, N36.41-N36.43, N36.8-N36.9,
N39.8-N39.9, R31.0-R31.9

PDX Collection 917
A17.9, A18.10-A18.11, A18.13, A18.82, A18.84,
A18.89, A54.21, A54.29, A54.82, A54.84, A54.89-A54.9,
A59.00, A59.8-A59.9, B37.41-B37.49, E08.21-E08.29,
E08.618-E08.638, E08.649, E08.65-E08.8, E09.21-E09.29,
E09.618-E09.638, E09.649-E09.8, E10.21-E10.29,
E10.618-E10.638, E10.649, E10.69-E10.8, E11.21-E11.29,
E11.618-E11.638, E11.649, E11.69-E11.8, E13.21-E13.29,
E13.618-E13.638, E13.649-E13.69, E13.8, M10.30-M10.39,
N00.0-N13.39, N13.6, N14.0-N19, N25.0-N27.9, N28.1-N29,
N36.41-N36.43, N36.8-N36.9, N39.8-N39.9, R31.0-R31.9

PDX Collection 918
A17.9, A18.10-A18.11, A18.13, A18.82, A18.84, A18.89,
A54.21, A54.29, A54.82, A54.84, A54.89-A54.9, A59.00,
A59.8-A59.9, A98.5, B37.41-B37.49, E08.21-E08.29,
E08.618-E08.638, E08.649, E08.65-E08.8, E09.21-E09.29,
E09.618-E09.638, E09.649-E09.8, E10.21-E10.29,
E10.618-E10.638, E10.649, E10.69-E10.8, E11.21-E11.29,
E11.618-E11.638, E11.649, E11.69-E11.8, E13.21-E13.29,
E13.618-E13.638, E13.649-E13.69, E13.8, M10.30-M10.39,
N00.0-N13.39, N13.6, N14.0-N19, N25.0-N27.9, N28.1-N29,
N36.41-N36.43, N36.8-N36.9, N39.8-N39.9, R31.0-R31.9

PDX Collection 919
A17.9, A18.10-A18.11, A18.13, A18.82, A18.84,
A18.89, A54.21, A54.29, A54.82, A54.84, A54.89-A54.9,
A59.00, A59.8-A59.9, B37.41-B37.49, E08.21-E08.29,
E08.618-E08.638, E08.649, E08.65-E08.8, E09.21-E09.29,
E09.618-E09.638, E09.649-E09.8, E10.21-E10.29,
E10.618-E10.638, E10.649, E10.69-E10.8, E11.21-E11.29,
E11.618-E11.638, E11.649, E11.69-E11.8, E13.21-E13.29,
E13.618-E13.638, E13.649-E13.69, E13.8, M10.30-M10.39,
N00.0-N13.39, N13.6, N14.0-N19, N25.0-N27.9, N28.1-N29,
N36.41-N36.43, N36.8-N36.9, N39.0, N39.8-N39.9,
R31.0-R31.9, R82.71

PDX Collection 920
N11.1, N13.4-N13.5, N13.8-N13.9, N28.82, N28.89-N30.91,
N32.89-N33, N36.41-N36.43, N36.8-N36.9, N39.0,
N39.8-N39.9, Q62.4-Q62.8, Q64.10-Q64.19, Q64.8-Q64.9,
R31.0-R31.9, R82.71, Z90.6

PDX Collection 921
A17.9, A18.10-A18.11, A18.13, A18.82, A18.84, A18.89,
A54.21, A54.29, A54.82, A54.84, A54.89-A54.9, A59.00,
A59.8-A59.9, A98.5, B37.41-B37.49, E08.21-E08.29,
E08.618-E08.638, E08.649, E08.65-E08.8, E09.21-E09.29,
E09.618-E09.638, E09.649-E09.8, E10.21-E10.29,
E10.618-E10.638, E10.649, E10.69-E10.8, E11.21-E11.29,
E11.618-E11.638, E11.649, E11.69-E11.8, E13.21-E13.29,
E13.618-E13.638, E13.649-E13.69, E13.8, M10.30-M10.39,
N00.0-N13.39, N13.6, N14.0-N19, N25.0-N27.9, N28.1-N29,
N36.41-N36.43, N36.8-N36.9, N39.8-N39.9, O23.01-O23.03,
O23.11-O23.13, O23.21-O23.23, O23.31-O23.33,
O23.41-O23.43, O23.511-O23.513, O23.521-O23.523,
O23.591-O23.593, O23.91-O23.93, O86.11, O86.13-O86.29,
R31.0-R31.9

PDX Collection 923
N11.1, N13.4-N13.5, N13.8-N13.9, N28.82, N28.89-N30.91,
N32.89-N33, N36.41-N36.43, N36.8-N36.9, N39.0,
N39.8-N39.9, Q62.4-Q62.8, Q64.10-Q64.19, Q64.8-Q64.9,
R31.0-R31.9, R82.71

PDX Collection 924
E08.21-E08.29, E08.618-E08.638, E08.649-E08.8,
E09.21-E09.29, E09.618-E09.638, E09.649-E09.8,
E10.21-E10.29, E10.618-E10.638, E10.649, E10.69-E10.8,
E11.21-E11.29, E11.618-E11.638, E11.649, E11.69-E11.8,
E13.21-E13.29, E13.618-E13.638, E13.649-E13.8, E88.3,
M10.30-M10.39, N00.0-N13.39, N13.6, N14.0-N19,
N25.0-N27.9, N28.1-N29, N36.41-N36.43, N36.8-N36.9,
N39.8-N39.9, Q60.0-Q62.39, Q63.0-Q63.9, Q64.8-Q64.9,
R31.0-R31.9

PDX Collection 925
E08.21-E08.29, E08.618-E08.638, E08.649-E08.8,
E09.21-E09.29, E09.618-E09.638, E09.649-E09.8,
E10.21-E10.29, E10.618-E10.638, E10.649, E10.69-E10.8,
E11.21-E11.29, E11.618-E11.638, E11.649, E11.69-E11.8,
E13.21-E13.29, E13.618-E13.638, E13.649-E13.8, E88.3,
M10.30-M10.39, N00.0-N13.39, N13.6, N14.0-N19,
N25.0-N27.9, N28.1-N29, N36.41-N36.43, N36.8-N36.9,
N39.8-N39.9, R31.0-R31.9

PDX Collection 926
E08.21-E08.29, E08.618-E08.638, E08.649-E08.8,
E09.21-E09.29, E09.618-E09.638, E09.649-E09.8,
E10.21-E10.29, E10.618-E10.638, E10.649, E10.69-E10.8,
E11.21-E11.29, E11.618-E11.638, E11.649, E11.69-E11.8,
E13.21-E13.29, E13.618-E13.638, E13.649-E13.8,
M10.30-M10.39, N00.0-N13.39, N13.6, N14.0-N19,
N25.0-N27.9, N28.1-N29, N36.41-N36.43, N36.8-N36.9,
N39.8-N39.9, Q60.0-Q62.39, Q63.0-Q63.9, Q64.8-Q64.9,
R31.0-R31.9

PDX Collection 927
E08.21-E08.29, E08.618-E08.638, E08.649-E08.8,
E09.21-E09.29, E09.618-E09.638, E09.649-E09.8,
E10.21-E10.29, E10.618-E10.638, E10.649, E10.69-E10.8,
E11.21-E11.29, E11.618-E11.638, E11.649, E11.69-E11.8,
E13.21-E13.29, E13.618-E13.638, E13.649-E13.8, I12.9,
M10.30-M10.39, N00.0-N13.39, N13.6, N14.0-N19,
N25.0-N27.9, N28.1-N29, N36.41-N36.43, N36.8-N36.9,
N39.8-N39.9, Q60.0-Q62.39, Q63.0-Q63.9, Q64.8-Q64.9,
R31.0-R31.9

PDX Collection 928
N11.1, N13.4-N13.5, N13.8-N13.9, N20.0-N22, N28.82,
N28.89-N29, N36.41-N36.43, N36.8-N36.9, N39.8-N39.9,
R31.0-R31.9

PDX Collection 929
A17.9, A18.10-A18.11, A18.13, A18.82, A18.84, A18.89,
A54.21, A54.29, A54.82, A54.84, A54.89-A54.9, A59.00,
A59.8-A59.9, A98.5, B37.41-B37.49, E08.21-E08.29,
E08.618-E08.638, E08.649, E08.65-E08.8, E09.21-E09.29,
E09.618-E09.638, E09.649-E09.8, E10.21-E10.29,
E10.618-E10.638, E10.649, E10.69-E10.8, E11.21-E11.29,
E11.618-E11.638, E11.649, E11.69-E11.8, E13.21-E13.29,
E13.618-E13.638, E13.649-E13.69, E13.8, M10.30-M10.39,
N00.0-N13.39, N13.6, N14.0-N19, N25.0-N27.9, N28.1-N29,
N36.41-N36.43, N36.8-N36.9, N39.8-N39.9, R31.0-R31.9

PDX Collection 930
A17.9, A18.10-A18.11, A18.13, A18.82, A18.84, A18.89,
A54.21, A54.29, A54.82, A54.84, A54.89-A54.9, A59.00,
A59.8-A59.9, A98.5, B37.41-B37.49, E08.21-E08.29,
E08.618-E08.638, E08.649, E08.65-E08.8, E09.21-E09.29,
E09.618-E09.638, E09.649-E09.8, E10.21-E10.29,
E10.618-E10.638, E10.649, E10.69-E10.8, E11.21-E11.29,
E11.618-E11.638, E11.649, E11.69-E11.8, E13.21-E13.29,
E13.618-E13.638, E13.649-E13.69, E13.8, M10.30-M10.39,
N00.0-N13.39, N13.6, N14.0-N19, N25.0-N27.9, N28.1-N29,
N36.41-N36.43, N36.8-N36.9, N39.8-N39.9, R31.0-R31.9

PDX Collection 931
N13.70-N13.739, N28.0, N28.9-N29

PDX Collection 932
A17.9, A18.10, A18.12-A18.13, A18.82, A18.84, A18.89,
A54.00-A54.02, A54.09-A54.1, A54.82, A54.84, A54.89-A54.9,
A59.00, A59.8-A59.9, B37.41-B37.49, N11.1, N13.4-N13.5,
N13.8-N13.9, N28.82, N28.89-N30.91, N32.89-N33,
N36.41-N36.43, N36.8-N36.9, N39.0, N39.8-N39.9,
R31.0-R31.9, R82.71

PDX Collection 933
A54.00-A54.02, A54.09-A54.1, A54.82, A54.84, A54.89-A54.9,
N32.1-N32.2, N32.89-N33, N36.41-N36.43, N36.8-N36.9,
N39.8-N39.9, R30.0, R30.9, R31.0-R31.9

PDX Collection 934
A54.00-A54.02, A54.09-A54.1, A54.82, A54.84, A54.89-A54.9,
A59.00, A59.03, A59.8-A59.9, B37.41-B37.49, N13.9,
N34.0-N34.3, N35.111-N35.9, N36.41-N36.43, N36.8-N39.0,
N39.8-N39.9, N44.1-N44.8, N47.6, N48.1-N48.9, N49.1-N49.9,
N50.3-N50.89, N51, N53.11-N53.9, Q54.0-Q55.9, Q64.0,
Q64.2-Q64.9, R30.0, R30.9-R31.9, R82.71

PDX Collection 935
N13.9, N34.0, N34.2-N36.43, N36.5-N37, N39.8-N39.9,
N44.1-N44.8, N47.6, N48.1-N48.9, N49.1-N49.9, N50.3-N50.89,
N51, N53.11-N53.9, N99.110-N99.115, Q54.0-Q55.21,
Q55.23-Q55.9, Q64.0, Q64.8-Q64.9, R30.0, R30.9-R31.9

PDX Collection 936
A54.82, A54.84, A54.89-A54.9, A59.00, A59.8-A59.9,
B37.41-B37.49, N10, N11.9-N13.39, N13.6, N13.9, N15.1,
N28.82, N28.84-N30.91, N34.1, N36.41-N36.43, N36.8-N36.9,
N39.0, N39.8-N39.9, N99.511, R30.0, R30.9-R31.9, T83.511A

PDX Collection 937
A18.14, A54.22, A54.82, A54.84, A54.89-A54.9, A59.00,
A59.02, A59.8-A59.9, B37.41-B37.49, N40.0-N42.9

PDX Collection 938
A59.00, A59.8-A59.9, B37.41-B37.49, N43.0-N43.3

PDX Collection 939
N44.00-N44.04

PDX Collection 940
A54.23, A54.82, A54.84, A54.89-A54.9, A59.00, A59.8-A59.9,
B26.0, B37.41-B37.49, N45.1-N45.4

PDX Collection 941
N47.6, N48.0-N48.9, N52.01-N52.9

PDX Collection 942
A17.9, A18.10, A18.16-A18.18, A18.82, A18.84, A18.89,
A54.03, A54.24, A54.82, A54.84, A54.89-A54.9, A59.00,
A59.8-A59.9, B37.41-B37.49, N70.01-N71.9, N73.0-N74,
N75.9, N76.5, N76.81-N76.89, N90.810-N90.818,
N94.818-N94.9, N96, Q55.0-Q55.4, Q55.7-Q55.9

PDX Collection 943
A17.9, A18.10, A18.16-A18.18, A18.82, A18.84, A18.89,
A54.03, A54.24, A54.82, A54.84, A54.89-A54.9, A59.00,
A59.8-A59.9, B37.41-B37.49, N70.01-N71.9, N72, N73.0-N74,
N75.9, N76.5, N76.81-N76.89, N85.8-N85.9, N90.810-N90.818,
N94.818-N94.9, N96, Q55.0-Q55.4, Q55.7-Q55.9

PDX Collection 944
A17.9, A18.10, A18.16-A18.18, A18.82, A18.84, A18.89,
A59.00-A59.01, A59.8-A59.9, B37.3-B37.49, N75.0-N77.1,
N84.3, N90.3, N90.60-N90.9, N94.810-N94.9, N96,
Q55.0-Q55.4, Q55.7-Q55.9

PDX Collection 945
N72, N75.9, N76.5, N76.81-N76.89

PDX Collection 946
N82.0-N82.9

PDX Collection 947
N83.00-N83.53, N83.6-N83.9, N99.83

PDX Collection 948
N98.0, T80.211-T80.29X[A], T82.7XXA, T88.0XXA

PDX Collection 949
D78.81-D78.89, E36.8, E89.810-E89.89, H59.011-H59.019,
H59.031-H59.099, H59.811-H59.89, H95.811-H95.89,
I97.3, L76.81-L76.82, M96.89, N32.89, N33, N98.1-N98.9,
N99.510-N99.518, T81.82XA, T81.89X-T81.9XX[A], T83.010A,
T83.020A, T83.030A, T83.090A, T83.110-T83.29X[A],
T83.410-T83.69X[A], T83.712-T83.714[A], T83.718A,
T83.719A, T83.722-T83.724[A], T83.728-T83.9XX[A],
T85.310-T85.311[A], T85.320-T85.321[A],
T85.390-T85.391[A], T85.510-T85.9XX[A], T85.810D,
T85.820D, T85.830D, T85.840D, T85.850D, T85.860D,
T85.890D, T86.820-T86.829

PDX Collection 950
D78.81-D78.89, E36.8, E89.810-E89.89,
H59.011-H59.019, H59.031-H59.099, H59.811-H59.89,
H95.811-H95.89, I97.3, L76.81-L76.82, M96.89,
N32.89, N33, N39.0, N98.1-N98.9, N99.510-N99.518,
R82.71, T81.82XA, T81.89X-T81.9XX[A], T83.010A,

T83.020A, T83.030A, T83.090A, T83.110-T83.29X[A], T83.410-T83.69X[A], T83.712-T83.714[A], T83.718A, T83.719A, T83.722-T83.724[A], T83.728-T83.9XX[A], T85.310-T85.311[A], T85.320-T85.321[A], T85.390-T85.391[A], T85.510-T85.9XX[A], T85.810D, T85.820D, T85.830D, T85.840D, T85.850D, T85.860D, T85.890D

PDX Collection 951
D78.81-D78.89, E36.8, E89.810-E89.89, H59.011-H59.019, H59.031-H59.099, H59.811-H59.89, H95.811-H95.89, I97.3, L76.81-L76.82, M96.89, N32.89, N33, N98.1-N98.9, N99.510-N99.518, T81.82XA, T81.89X-T81.9XX[A], T83.010A, T83.020A, T83.030A, T83.090A, T83.110-T83.29X[A], T83.410-T83.69X[A], T83.712-T83.714[A], T83.718A, T83.719A, T83.722A-T83.724A, T83.728-T83.9XX[A]

PDX Collection 952
H95.811-H95.89, I85.01, I85.11, I97.3, K21.9, K22.8, K23-K25.0, K25.2, K25.4, K25.6, K26.0, K26.2, K26.4, K26.6, K27.0, K27.2, K27.4, K27.6, K28.0, K28.2, K28.4, K28.6, K29.01, K29.21, K29.31, K29.41, K29.51, K29.61, K29.71, K29.81, K29.91, K31.811, K55.21, K57.01, K57.11, K57.13, K57.21, K57.31, K57.33, K57.41, K57.51, K57.53, K57.81, K57.91, K57.93, K62.5, K92.0-K92.2, M96.89, N98.1-N98.9, N99.61-N99.62, N99.820-N99.821, N99.840-N99.843, P54.1-P54.3, T81.10X-T81.19X[A], T81.82XA, T81.89X-T81.9XX[A]

PDX Collection 953
O00.00-O00.91

PDX Collection 954
O03.0-O07.4, O11.4-O11.5, O12.04-O12.05, O12.14-O12.15, O12.24-O12.25, O13.4-O13.5, O14.04-O14.05, O14.14-O14.15, O14.24-O14.25, O14.94-O14.95, O16.4-O16.5, O20.0-O20.9, O25.10-O25.3, O26.10-O26.13, O26.30-O26.43, O26.63, O26.711-O26.819, O26.841-O26.86, O26.891-O26.93, O29.011-O29.5X3, O44.63

PDX Collection 956
O03.0-O07.4, O11.4, O11.5, O12.04, O12.05, O12.14, O12.15, O12.24, O12.25, O13.4, O13.5, O14.04, O14.05, O14.14, O14.15, O14.24, O14.25, O14.94, O14.95, O16.4, O16.5, O20.0-O20.9, O25.10-O25.3, O26.10-O26.13, O26.30-O26.43, O26.63-O26.819, O26.841-O26.86, O26.891-O26.93, O29.011-O29.93, O35.7XX0-O35.7XX9, O44.00-O44.13, O44.20-O44.53, O45.8X1-O45.93, O75.4, O75.81, O75.89-O75.9, O80, O90.89, O99.111-O99.285, O99.330-O99.335, O99.350-O99.355, O99.511-O99.73, O99.820-O99.825, O99.840-O9A.53, Z33.2

PDX Collection 957
O03.0-O07.4, O11.4, O11.5, O12.04, O12.05, O12.14, O12.15, O12.24, O12.25, O13.4, O13.5, O14.04, O14.05, O14.14, O14.15, O14.24, O14.25, O14.94, O14.95, O16.4, O16.5, O20.0-O20.9, O25.10-O25.3, O26.10-O26.13, O26.30-O26.43, O26.63-O26.819, O26.841-O26.86, O26.891-O26.93, O29.011-O29.93, O35.7XX0-O35.7XX9, O44.00-O44.13, O44.20-O44.53, O45.8X1-O45.93, O75.4, O75.81, O75.89-O75.9, O80, O90.89, O99.111-O99.285, O99.330-O99.335, O99.350-O99.355, O99.511-O99.73, O99.820-O99.825, O99.840-O9A.53, Z33.2

PDX Collection 958
O03.0-O07.4, O11.4, O11.5, O12.04, O12.05, O12.14, O12.15, O12.24, O12.25, O13.4, O13.5, O14.04, O14.05, O14.14, O14.15, O14.24, O14.25, O14.94, O14.95, O16.4, O16.5, O20.0-O20.9, O25.10-O25.3, O26.10-O26.13, O26.30-O026.43, O26.63-O26.819, O26.841-O26.86, O26.891-O26.93, O29.011-O29.93, O35.7XX0-O35.7XX9, O44.00-O44.13, O44.20-O44.53, O45.8X1-O45.93, O75.4, O75.81, O75.89-O75.9, O80, O90.89, O99.111-O99.285,

O99.330-O99.335, O99.350-O99.355, O99.511-O99.73, O99.820-O99.825, O99.840-O9A.53, Z33.2

PDX Collection 959
O03.0-O07.4, O11.4, O11.5, O12.04, O12.05, O12.14, O12.15, O12.24, O12.25, O13.4, O13.5, O14.04, O14.05, O14.14, O14.15, O14.24, O14.25, O14.94, O14.95, O16.4, O16.5, O20.0-O20.9, O25.10-O25.3, O26.10-O26.13, O26.30-O26.43, O26.63-O26.819, O26.841-O26.86, O26.891-O26.93, O29.011-O29.93, O35.7XX0-O35.7XX9, O44.00-O44.13, O44.20-O44.53, O45.8X1-O45.93, O75.4, O75.81, O75.89-O75.9, O80, O90.89, O99.111-O99.285, O99.330-O99.335, O99.350-O99.355, O99.511-O99.73, O99.820-O99.825, O99.840-O9A.53, Z33.2

PDX Collection 960
O03.0-O07.4, O11.4, O11.5, O12.04, O12.05, O12.14, O12.15, O12.24, O12.25, O13.4, O13.5, O14.04, O14.05, O14.14, O14.15, O14.24, O14.25, O14.94, O14.95, O16.4, O16.5, O20.0-O20.9, O25.10-O25.3, O26.10-O26.13, O26.30-O26.43, O26.63-O26.819, O26.841-O26.86, O26.891-O26.93, O29.011-O29.93, O35.7XX0-O35.7XX9, O44.00-O44.13, O44.20-O44.53, O45.8X1-O45.93, O75.4, O75.81, O75.89-O75.9, O80, O90.89, O99.111-O99.285, O99.330-O99.335, O99.350-O99.355, O99.511-O99.73, O99.820-O99.825, O99.840-O9A.53, Z33.2

PDX Collection 961
O03.0-O07.4, O11.4, O11.5, O12.04, O12.05, O12.14, O12.15, O12.24, O12.25, O13.4, O13.5, O14.04, O14.05, O14.14, O14.15, O14.24, O14.25, O14.94, O14.95, O16.4, O16.5, O20.0-O20.9, O25.10-O25.3, O26.10-O26.13, O26.30-O26.43, O26.63-O26.819, O26.841-O26.86, O26.891-O26.93, O29.011-O29.93, O35.7XX0-O35.7XX9, O44.00-O44.13, O44.20-O44.53, O45.8X1-O45.93, O75.4, O75.81, O75.89-O75.9, O80, O90.89, O99.111-O99.285, O99.330-O99.335, O99.350-O99.355, O99.511-O99.73, O99.820-O99.825, O99.840-O9A.53, Z33.2

PDX Collection 962
O08.1-O08.81, O08.83-O08.9, O11.4, O11.5, O12.04, O12.05, O12.14, O12.15, O12.24, O12.25, O13.4, O13.5, O14.04, O14.05, O14.14, O14.15, O14.24, O14.25, O14.94, O14.95, O16.4, O16.5, O20.0-O20.9, O25.10-O25.3, O26.10-O26.13, O26.30-O26.43, O26.63-O26.819, O26.841-O26.86, O26.891-O26.93, O29.011-O29.93, O35.7XX0-O35.7XX9, O44.00-O44.13, O44.20-O44.53, O45.8X1-O45.93, O75.4, O75.81, O75.89-O75.9, O80, O90.89, O99.111-O99.285, O99.330-O99.335, O99.350-O99.355, O99.511-O99.73, O99.820-O99.825, O99.840-O9A.53

PDX Collection 963
O08.2-O08.81, O08.83-O08.9, O11.4, O11.5, O12.04, O12.05, O12.14, O12.15, O12.24, O12.25, O13.4, O13.5, O14.04, O14.05, O14.14, O14.15, O14.24, O14.25, O14.94, O14.95, O16.4, O16.5, O20.0-O20.9, O25.10-O25.3, O26.10-O26.13, O26.30-O26.43, O26.63-O26.819, O26.841-O26.86, O26.891-O26.93, O29.011-O29.93, O35.7XX0-O35.7XX9, O44.00-O44.13, O44.20-O44.53, O45.8X1-O45.93, O75.4, O75.81, O75.89-O75.9, O80, O90.89, O99.111-O99.285, O99.330-O99.335, O99.350-O99.355, O99.511-O99.73, O99.820-O99.825, O99.840-O9A.53

PDX Collection 964
O10.011-O12.03, O12.04, O12.05, O12.14, O12.15, O12.20-O16.9, O25.10-O26.13, O26.30-O26.43, O26.63-O26.819, O26.841-O26.86, O26.891-O26.93, O29.011-O29.93, O35.7XX0-O35.7XX9, O75.4, O75.81, O75.89-O75.9, O80, O90.89, O99.111-O99.285, O99.330-O99.335, O99.350-O99.355, O99.511-O99.73, O99.820-O99.825, O99.840-O9A.53

PDX Collection 965
O11.5, O12.05, O12.11-O12.13, O12.15, O12.21-O12.23, O12.25, O13.5, O14.05, O14.15, O14.25, O14.95, O16.5, O26.831-O26.833, O90.89

PDX Collection 966
O11.4, O11.5, O12.04, O12.05, O12.14, O12.15, O12.24, O12.25, O13.4, O13.5, O14.04, O14.05, O14.14, O14.15, O14.24, O14.25, O14.94, O14.95, O16.4, O16.5, O20.0-O20.9, O25.10-O25.3, O26.10-O26.13, O26.30-O26.43, O26.63-O26.819, O26.841-O26.86, O26.891-O26.93, O29.011-O29.93, O35.7XX0-O35.7XX9, O44.00-O44.13, O44.20-O44.53, O75.4, O75.81, O75.89-O75.9, O80, O90.89, O99.111-O99.119, O99.12-O99.285, O99.330-O99.335, O99.350-O99.355, O99.511-O99.73, O99.820-O99.825, O99.840-O9A.53

PDX Collection 967
O11.4, O11.5, O12.04, O12.05, O12.14, O12.15, O12.24, O12.25, O13.4, O13.5, O14.04, O14.05, O14.14, O14.15, O14.24, O14.25, O14.94, O14.95, O16.4, O16.5, O22.20-O22.93, O25.10-O25.3, O26.10-O26.13, O26.30-O26.43, O26.63-O26.819, O26.841-O26.86, O26.891-O26.93, O29.011-O29.93, O35.7XX0-O35.7XX9, O75.4, O75.81, O75.89-O75.9, O80, O87.0-O87.9, O90.89, O99.111-O99.119, O99.12-O99.285, O99.330-O99.335, O99.350-O99.355, O99.511-O99.73, O99.820-O99.825, O99.840-O9A.53

PDX Collection 968
O11.4, O11.5, O12.04, O12.05, O12.14, O12.15, O12.24, O12.25, O13.4, O13.5, O14.04, O14.05, O14.14, O14.15, O14.24, O14.25, O14.94, O14.95, O16.4, O16.5, O23.00-O23.93, O25.10-O25.3, O26.10-O26.13, O26.30-O26.43, O26.63-O26.819, O26.841-O26.86, O26.891-O26.93, O29.011-O29.93, O35.7XX0-O35.7XX9, O75.4, O75.81, O75.89-O75.9, O80, O86.11, O86.13-O86.29, O90.89, O99.111-O99.285, O99.330-O99.335, O99.350-O99.355, O99.511-O99.73, O99.820-O99.825, O99.840-O9A.53

PDX Collection 969
O11.4, O11.5, O12.04, O12.05, O12.14, O12.15, O12.24, O12.25, O13.4, O13.5, O14.04, O14.05, O14.14, O14.15, O14.24, O14.25, O14.94, O14.95, O16.4, O16.5, O24.011-O24.33, O24.811-O25.3, O26.10-O26.13, O26.30-O26.43, O26.63-O26.819, O26.841-O26.86, O26.891-O26.93, O29.011-O29.93, O35.7XX0-O35.7XX9, O75.4, O75.81, O75.89-O75.9, O80, O90.89, O99.111-O99.285, O99.330-O99.335, O99.350-O99.355, O99.511-O99.73, O99.820-O99.825, O99.840-O9A.53

PDX Collection 972
O11.4, O11.5, O12.04, O12.05, O12.14, O12.15, O12.24, O12.25, O13.4, O13.5, O14.04, O14.05, O14.14, O14.15, O14.24, O14.25, O14.94, O14.95, O16.4, O16.5, O25.10-O25.3, O26.10-O26.13, O26.30-O26.43, O26.611-O26.819, O26.841-O26.86, O26.891-O26.93, O29.011-O29.93, O35.7XX0-O35.7XX9, O75.4, O75.81, O75.89-O75.9, O80, O90.89, O99.111-O99.285, O99.330-O99.335, O99.350-O99.355, O99.511-O99.73, O99.820-O99.825, O99.840-O9A.53

PDX Collection 973
O26.872-O26.879, O34.31-O34.33

PDX Collection 976
O30.001-O30.019, O30.031-O31.23X9, O31.31X0-O32.9XX9, O80

PDX Collection 977
O33.0

PDX Collection 978
O36.0110-O36.0139, O36.0910-O36.0939

PDX Collection 979
O36.4XXØ-O36.4XX9

PDX Collection 982
O41.Ø1XØ-O41.Ø3X9

PDX Collection 983
O41.1Ø1Ø-O41.1Ø39, O41.121Ø-O41.1239,
O41.141Ø-O41.1439

PDX Collection 988
O11.4, O11.5, O12.Ø4, O12.Ø5, O12.14, O12.15, O12.24, O12.25,
O13.4, O13.5, O14.Ø4, O14.Ø5, O14.14, O14.15, O14.24, O14.25,
O14.94, O14.95, O16.4, O16.5, O25.1Ø-O25.3, O26.1Ø-O26.13,
O26.3Ø-O26.43, O26.63-O26.819, O26.841-O26.86,
O26.891-O26.93, O29.Ø11-O29.93, O35.7XXØ-O35.7XX9,
O36.812Ø-O36.8199, O63.9, O71.ØØ-O71.1, O71.5, O71.81,
O71.89-O71.9, O75.4, O75.81, O75.89-O75.9, O8Ø, O9Ø.89,
O99.111-O99.285, O99.33Ø-O99.335, O99.35Ø-O99.355,
O99.511-O99.73, O99.82Ø-O99.825, O99.84Ø-O9A.53

PDX Collection 989
O68, O76, PØ3.811

PDX Collection 991
O11.4, O11.5, O12.Ø4, O12.Ø5, O12.14, O12.15, O12.24, O12.25,
O13.4, O13.5, O14.Ø4, O14.Ø5, O14.14, O14.15, O14.24, O14.25,
O14.94, O14.95, O16.4, O16.5, O25.1Ø-O25.3, O26.1Ø-O26.13,
O26.3Ø-O26.43, O26.63-O26.819, O26.841-O26.86,
O26.891-O26.93, O29.Ø11-O29.93, O35.7XXØ-O35.7XX9,
O36.812Ø-O36.8199, O7Ø.3, O71.ØØ-O71.1, O71.5, O71.81,
O71.89-O71.9, O75.4, O75.81, O75.89-O75.9, O8Ø, O9Ø.89,
O99.111-O99.285, O99.33Ø-O99.335, O99.35Ø-O99.355,
O99.511-O99.73, O99.82Ø-O99.825, O99.84Ø-O9A.53

PDX Collection 992
O11.4, O11.5, O12.Ø4, O12.Ø5, O12.14, O12.15, O12.24, O12.25,
O13.4, O13.5, O14.Ø4, O14.Ø5, O14.14, O14.15, O14.24, O14.25,
O14.94, O14.95, O16.4, O16.5, O25.1Ø-O25.3, O26.1Ø-O26.13,
O26.3Ø-O26.43, O26.63-O26.819, O26.841-O26.86,
O26.891-O26.93, O29.Ø11-O29.93, O35.7XXØ-O35.7XX9,
O36.812Ø-O36.8199, O7Ø.2Ø-O7Ø.23, O7Ø.4, O71.ØØ-O71.1,
O71.5, O71.81, O71.89-O71.9, O75.4, O75.81, O75.89-O75.9,
O8Ø, O9Ø.89, O99.111-O99.285, O99.33Ø-O99.335,
O99.35Ø-O99.355, O99.511-O99.73, O99.82Ø-O99.825,
O99.84Ø-O9A.53

PDX Collection 993
O11.4, O11.5, O12.Ø4, O12.Ø5, O12.14, O12.15, O12.24, O12.25,
O13.4, O13.5, O14.Ø4, O14.Ø5, O14.14, O14.15, O14.24, O14.25,
O14.94, O14.95, O16.4, O16.5, O25.1Ø-O25.3, O26.1Ø-O26.13,
O26.3Ø-O26.43, O26.63-O26.819, O26.841-O26.86,
O26.891-O26.93, O29.Ø11-O29.93, O35.7XXØ-O35.7XX9,
O36.812Ø-O36.8199, O71.ØØ-O71.1, O71.5, O71.81,
O71.89-O71.9, O75.4, O75.81, O75.89-O75.9, O8Ø, O9Ø.89,
O99.111-O99.285, O99.33Ø-O99.335, O99.35Ø-O99.355,
O99.511-O99.73, O99.82Ø-O99.825, O99.84Ø-O9A.53

PDX Collection 994
O11.4, O11.5, O12.Ø4, O12.Ø5, O12.14, O12.15, O12.24,
O12.25, O13.4, O13.5, O14.Ø4, O14.Ø5, O14.14,
O14.15, O14.24, O14.25, O14.94, O14.95, O16.4,
O16.5, O25.1Ø-O25.3, O26.1Ø-O26.13, O26.3Ø-O26.43,
O26.63-O26.819, O26.841-O26.86, O26.891-O26.93,
O29.Ø11-O29.93, O35.7XXØ-O35.7XX9, O36.812Ø-O36.8199,
O71.ØØ-O71.2, O71.5, O71.81, O71.89-O71.9, O75.4,
O75.81, O75.89-O75.9, O8Ø, O9Ø.89, O99.111-O99.285,
O99.33Ø-O99.335, O99.35Ø-O99.355, O99.511-O99.73,
O99.82Ø-O99.825, O99.84Ø-O9A.53

PDX Collection 995
O11.4, O11.5, O12.Ø4, O12.Ø5, O12.14, O12.15, O12.24,
O12.25, O13.4, O13.5, O14.Ø4, O14.Ø5, O14.14,
O14.15, O14.24, O14.25, O14.94, O14.95, O16.4,
O16.5, O25.1Ø-O25.3, O26.1Ø-O26.13, O26.3Ø-O26.43,

O26.63-O26.819, O26.841-O26.86, O26.891-O26.93,
O29.Ø11-O29.93, O35.7XXØ-O35.7XX9, O36.812Ø-O36.8199,
O71.ØØ-O71.1, O71.3, O71.5, O71.81, O71.89-O71.9, O75.4,
O75.81, O75.89-O75.9, O8Ø, O9Ø.89, O99.111-O99.285,
O99.33Ø-O99.335, O99.35Ø-O99.355, O99.511-O99.73,
O99.82Ø-O99.825, O99.84Ø-O9A.53

PDX Collection 996
O11.4, O11.5, O12.Ø4, O12.Ø5, O12.14, O12.15, O12.24,
O12.25, O13.4, O13.5, O14.Ø4, O14.Ø5, O14.14,
O14.15, O14.24, O14.25, O14.94, O14.95, O16.4,
O16.5, O25.1Ø-O25.3, O26.1Ø-O26.13, O26.3Ø-O26.43,
O26.63-O26.819, O26.841-O26.86, O26.891-O26.93,
O29.Ø11-O29.93, O35.7XXØ-O35.7XX9, O36.812Ø-O36.8199,
O71.ØØ-O71.1, O71.4, O71.5, O71.81, O71.89-O71.9, O75.4,
O75.81, O75.89-O75.9, O8Ø, O9Ø.89, O99.111-O99.285,
O99.33Ø-O99.335, O99.35Ø-O99.355, O99.511-O99.73,
O99.82Ø-O99.825, O99.84Ø-O9A.53

PDX Collection 997
O11.4, O11.5, O12.Ø4, O12.Ø5, O12.14, O12.15, O12.24,
O12.25, O13.4, O13.5, O14.Ø4, O14.Ø5, O14.14,
O14.15, O14.24, O14.25, O14.94, O14.95, O16.4,
O16.5, O25.1Ø-O25.3, O26.1Ø-O26.13, O26.3Ø-O26.43,
O26.63-O26.819, O26.841-O26.86, O26.891-O26.93,
O29.Ø11-O29.93, O35.7XXØ-O35.7XX9, O36.812Ø-O36.8199,
O71.ØØ-O71.1, O71.5-O71.6, O71.81, O71.89-O71.9, O75.4,
O75.81, O75.89-O75.9, O8Ø, O9Ø.89, O99.111-O99.285,
O99.33Ø-O99.335, O99.35Ø-O99.355, O99.511-O99.73,
O99.82Ø-O99.825, O99.84Ø-O9A.53

PDX Collection 998
O11.4, O11.5, O12.Ø4, O12.Ø5, O12.14, O12.15, O12.24,
O12.25, O13.4, O13.5, O14.Ø4, O14.Ø5, O14.14,
O14.15, O14.24, O14.25, O14.94, O14.95, O16.4,
O16.5, O25.1Ø-O25.3, O26.1Ø-O26.13, O26.3Ø-O26.43,
O26.63-O26.819, O26.841-O26.86, O26.891-O26.93,
O29.Ø11-O29.93, O35.7XXØ-O35.7XX9, O36.812Ø-O36.8199,
O71.ØØ-O71.1, O71.5, O71.7, O71.81, O71.89-O71.9, O75.4,
O75.81, O75.89-O75.9, O8Ø, O9Ø.89, O99.111-O99.285,
O99.33Ø-O99.335, O99.35Ø-O99.355, O99.511-O99.73,
O99.82Ø-O99.825, O99.84Ø-O9A.53

PDX Collection 999
O11.4, O11.5, O12.Ø4, O12.Ø5, O12.14, O12.15, O12.24,
O12.25, O13.4, O13.5, O14.Ø4, O14.Ø5, O14.14,
O14.15, O14.24, O14.25, O14.94, O14.95, O16.4,
O16.5, O25.1Ø-O25.3, O26.1Ø-O26.13, O26.3Ø-O26.43,
O26.63-O26.819, O26.841-O26.86, O26.891-O26.93,
O29.Ø11-O29.93, O35.7XXØ-O35.7XX9, O36.812Ø-O36.8199,
O71.ØØ-O71.1, O71.5, O71.81, O71.89-O71.9, O72.Ø, O75.4,
O75.81, O75.89-O75.9, O8Ø, O9Ø.89, O99.111-O99.285,
O99.33Ø-O99.335, O99.35Ø-O99.355, O99.511-O99.73,
O99.82Ø-O99.825, O99.84Ø-O9A.53

PDX Collection 1000
O11.4, O11.5, O12.Ø4, O12.Ø5, O12.14, O12.15, O12.24,
O12.25, O13.4, O13.5, O14.Ø4, O14.Ø5, O14.14,
O14.15, O14.24, O14.25, O14.94, O14.95, O16.4,
O16.5, O25.1Ø-O25.3, O26.1Ø-O26.13, O26.3Ø-O26.43,
O26.63-O26.819, O26.841-O26.86, O26.891-O26.93,
O29.Ø11-O29.93, O35.7XXØ-O35.7XX9, O36.812Ø-O36.8199,
O71.ØØ-O71.1, O71.5, O71.81, O71.89-O71.9, O72.1, O75.4,
O75.81, O75.89-O75.9, O8Ø, O9Ø.89, O99.111-O99.285,
O99.33Ø-O99.335, O99.35Ø-O99.355, O99.511-O99.73,
O99.82Ø-O99.825, O99.84Ø-O9A.53

PDX Collection 1001
O11.4, O11.5, O12.Ø4, O12.Ø5, O12.14, O12.15, O12.24,
O12.25, O13.4, O13.5, O14.Ø4, O14.Ø5, O14.14,
O14.15, O14.24, O14.25, O14.94, O14.95, O16.4,
O16.5, O25.1Ø-O25.3, O26.1Ø-O26.13, O26.3Ø-O26.43,
O26.63-O26.819, O26.841-O26.86, O26.891-O26.93,

O29.Ø11-O29.93, O35.7XXØ-O35.7XX9, O36.812Ø-O36.8199,
O71.ØØ-O71.1, O71.5, O71.81, O71.89-O71.9, O72.2, O75.4,
O75.81, O75.89-O75.9, O8Ø, O9Ø.89, O99.111-O99.285,
O99.33Ø-O99.335, O99.35Ø-O99.355, O99.511-O99.73,
O99.82Ø-O99.825, O99.84Ø-O9A.53

PDX Collection 1002
O11.4, O11.5, O12.Ø4, O12.Ø5, O12.14, O12.15, O12.24,
O12.25, O13.4, O13.5, O14.Ø4, O14.Ø5, O14.14,
O14.15, O14.24, O14.25, O14.94, O14.95, O16.4,
O16.5, O25.1Ø-O25.3, O26.1Ø-O26.13, O26.3Ø-O26.43,
O26.63-O26.819, O26.841-O26.86, O26.891-O26.93,
O29.Ø11-O29.93, O35.7XXØ-O35.7XX9, O75.1, O75.4,
O75.81, O75.89-O75.9, O8Ø, O9Ø.89, O99.111-O99.285,
O99.33Ø-O99.335, O99.35Ø-O99.355, O99.511-O99.73,
O99.82Ø-O99.825, O99.84Ø-O9A.53

PDX Collection 1003
O75.2

PDX Collection 1004
O11.4, O11.5, O12.Ø4, O12.Ø5, O12.14, O12.15, O12.24,
O12.25, O13.4, O13.5, O14.Ø4, O14.Ø5, O14.14,
O14.15, O14.24, O14.25, O14.94, O14.95, O16.4,
O16.5, O25.1Ø-O25.3, O26.1Ø-O26.13, O26.3Ø-O26.43,
O26.63-O26.819, O26.841-O26.86, O26.891-O26.93,
O29.Ø11-O29.93, O35.7XXØ-O35.7XX9, O75.3-O75.4,
O75.81, O75.89-O75.9, O8Ø, O9Ø.89, O99.111-O99.285,
O99.33Ø-O99.335, O99.35Ø-O99.355, O99.511-O99.73,
O99.82Ø-O99.825, O99.84Ø-O9A.53

PDX Collection 1005
O11.4, O11.5, O12.Ø4, O12.Ø5, O12.14, O12.15, O12.24,
O12.25, O13.4, O13.5, O14.Ø4, O14.Ø5, O14.14,
O14.15, O14.24, O14.25, O14.94, O14.95, O16.4,
O16.5, O25.1Ø-O25.3, O26.1Ø-O26.13, O26.3Ø-O26.43,
O26.63-O26.819, O26.841-O26.86, O26.891-O26.93,
O26.899-O26.93, O29.Ø11-O29.93, O35.7XXØ-O35.7XX9,
O75.4, O75.81, O75.89, O75.9, O8Ø, O85, O86.Ø4,
O86.12, O86.81-O86.89, O9Ø.89, O99.111-O99.285,
O99.33Ø-O99.335, O99.35Ø-O99.355, O99.511-O99.73,
O99.82Ø-O99.825, O99.84Ø-O9A.53

PDX Collection 1006
O11.4, O11.5, O12.Ø4, O12.Ø5, O12.14, O12.15, O12.24,
O12.25, O13.4, O13.5, O14.Ø4, O14.Ø5, O14.14,
O14.15, O14.24, O14.25, O14.94, O14.95, O16.4,
O16.5, O22.2Ø-O22.93, O25.1Ø-O25.3, O26.1Ø-O26.13,
O26.3Ø-O26.43, O26.63-O26.819, O26.841-O26.86,
O26.891-O26.93, O29.Ø11-O29.93, O35.7XXØ-O35.7XX9,
O75.4, O75.81, O75.89-O75.9, O8Ø, O86.4-O87.9, O9Ø.89,
O99.111-O99.285, O99.33Ø-O99.335, O99.35Ø-O99.355,
O99.511-O99.73, O99.82Ø-O99.825, O99.84Ø-O9A.53

PDX Collection 1008
O11.4, O11.5, O12.Ø4, O12.Ø5, O12.14, O12.15, O12.24,
O12.25, O13.4, O13.5, O14.Ø4, O14.Ø5, O14.14,
O14.15, O14.24, O14.25, O14.94, O14.95, O16.4,
O16.5, O25.1Ø-O25.3, O26.1Ø-O26.13, O26.3Ø-O26.43,
O26.63-O26.819, O26.841-O26.86, O26.891-O26.93,
O29.Ø11-O29.93, O35.7XXØ-O35.7XX9, O75.4, O75.81,
O75.89-O75.9, O8Ø, O9Ø.3, O99.111-O99.285,
O99.33Ø-O99.335, O99.35Ø-O99.73, O99.82Ø-O99.825,
O99.84Ø-O9A.53

PDX Collection 1009
O11.4, O11.5, O12.Ø4, O12.Ø5, O12.14, O12.15, O12.24,
O12.25, O13.4, O13.5, O14.Ø4, O14.Ø5, O14.14,
O14.15, O14.24, O14.25, O14.94, O14.95, O16.4,
O16.5, O25.1Ø-O25.3, O26.1Ø-O26.13, O26.3Ø-O26.43,
O26.63-O26.819, O26.841-O26.86, O26.891-O26.93,
O29.Ø11-O29.93, O35.7XXØ-O35.7XX9, O75.4, O75.81,
O75.89-O75.9, O8Ø, O9Ø.4, O9Ø.89, O99.111-O99.285,

O99.330-O99.335, O99.350-O99.355, O99.511-O99.73, O99.820-O99.825, O99.840-O9A.53

PDX Collection 1011
O11.4, O11.5, O12.04, O12.05, O12.14, O12.15, O12.24, O12.25, O13.4, O13.5, O14.04, O14.05, O14.14, O14.15, O14.24, O14.25, O14.94, O14.95, O16.4, O16.5, O25.10-O25.3, O26.10-O26.13, O26.30-O26.43, O26.63-O26.819, O26.841-O26.86, O26.891-O26.93, O29.011-O29.93, O35.7XX0-O35.7XX9, O75.4, O75.81, O75.89-O75.9, O80, O90.89, O98.011-O98.03, O99.111-O99.285, O99.330-O99.335, O99.350-O99.355, O99.511-O99.73, O99.820-O99.825, O99.840-O9A.53

PDX Collection 1012
O26.11-O26.13, O26.31-O26.33, O26.41-O26.43, O26.63-O26.713, O26.72-O26.813, O26.86, O26.891-O26.893, O26.90-O26.93, O29.011-O29.013, O29.021-O29.023, O29.091-O29.093, O29.111-O29.113, O29.121-O29.123, O29.191-O29.193, O29.211-O29.213, O29.291-O29.293, O29.3X1-O29.3X3, O29.41-O29.5X3, O29.61-O29.8X3, O29.91-O29.93, O35.7XX0-O35.7XX9, O98.111-O98.33, O99.351-O99.353, O99.355

PDX Collection 1013
O98.411-O98.613, O98.711-O98.93, O99.830-O99.835

PDX Collection 1014
O11.4, O11.5, O12.04, O12.05, O12.14, O12.15, O12.24, O12.25, O13.4, O13.5, O14.04, O14.05, O14.14, O14.15, O14.24, O14.25, O14.94, O14.95, O16.4, O16.5, O25.10-O25.3, O26.10-O26.13, O26.30-O26.43, O26.63-O26.819, O26.841-O26.86, O26.891-O26.93, O29.011-O29.93, O35.7XX0-O35.7XX9, O75.4, O75.81, O75.89-O75.9, O80, O90.89, O98.411-O98.93, O99.111-O99.285, O99.330-O99.335, O99.350-O99.355, O99.511-O99.73, O99.820-O9A.53

PDX Collection 1015
O11.4, O11.5, O12.04, O12.05, O12.14, O12.15, O12.24, O12.25, O13.4, O13.5, O14.04, O14.05, O14.14, O14.15, O14.24, O14.25, O14.94, O14.95, O16.4, O16.5, O25.10-O25.3, O26.10-O26.13, O26.30-O26.43, O26.63-O26.819, O26.841-O26.86, O26.891-O26.93, O29.011-O29.93, O35.7XX0-O35.7XX9, O75.4, O75.81, O75.89-O75.9, O80, O90.89, O98.611-O98.63, O99.111-O99.285, O99.330-O99.335, O99.350-O99.355, O99.511-O99.73, O99.820-O9A.53

PDX Collection 1016
O25.11-O25.3, O99.281-O99.285, O99.355, O99.511-O99.513, O99.52-O99.613, O99.62-O99.713, O99.72-O99.73, O99.820-O99.825, O9A.111-O9A.113, O9A.12-O9A.213, O9A.22-O9A.313, O9A.32-O9A.413, O9A.42-O9A.513, O9A.52-O9A.53

PDX Collection 1017
O25.10, O99.199, O99.280, O99.519, O99.619, O99.719, O9A.119, O9A.219, O9A.319, O9A.419, O9A.519

PDX Collection 1019
O11.4, O11.5, O12.04, O12.05, O12.14, O12.15, O12.24, O12.25, O13.4, O13.5, O14.04, O14.05, O14.14, O14.15, O14.24, O14.25, O14.94, O14.95, O16.4, O16.5, O25.10-O25.3, O26.10-O26.13, O26.30-O26.43, O26.63-O26.819, O26.841-O26.86, O26.891-O26.93, O29.011-O29.93, O35.7XX0-O35.7XX9, O75.4, O75.81, O75.89-O75.9, O80, O90.3, O90.89, O99.111-O99.285, O99.330-O99.335, O99.350-O99.73, O99.820-O99.825, O99.840-O9A.53

PDX Collection 1020
P10.0-P10.1, P10.4-P11.2, P11.9, P15.0-P15.9, P29.0-P29.2, P29.4, P29.89-P29.9, P52.4, P52.6-P52.9, P94.1-P94.9, P96.0, P96.3-P96.5, P96.82-P96.89

PDX Collection 1021
P10.2-P10.3, P29.0-P29.2, P29.4, P29.89-P29.9, P50.0-P50.9, P52.0-P52.3, P52.5, P53-P54.0, P54.6-P54.9, P60-P61.9, P94.1-P94.9, P96.0, P96.3-P96.5, P96.82-P96.89

PDX Collection 1022
P10.2-P10.3, P29.0-P29.2, P29.4, P29.89-P29.9, P50.0-P50.9, P52.0-P52.3, P52.5, P53-P54.0, P54.6-P54.9, P60-P61.9, P91.2, P94.1-P94.9, P96.0, P96.3-P96.5, P96.82-P96.89

PDX Collection 1023
P10.0-P10.1, P10.4-P11.2, P11.9-P12.2, P15.0-P15.9, P29.0-P29.2, P29.4, P29.89-P29.9, P52.4, P52.6-P52.9, P94.1-P94.9, P96.0, P96.3-P96.5, P96.82-P96.89

PDX Collection 1024
P22.8-P22.9, P28.2-P28.4, P28.81-P28.9, R06.81, R23.0

PDX Collection 1025
P22.8-P22.9, P28.2-P28.4, P28.81-P28.9, R06.81

PDX Collection 1026
P22.8-P22.9, P28.2-P28.4, P28.81-P28.9, R06.81

PDX Collection 1027
P22.1-P22.9, P24.00, P24.10, P24.20, P24.30, P24.80, P28.2-P28.5, P28.81-P28.9, P29.81, R06.81, R09.2

PDX Collection 1028
I27.0, I27.20-I27.81, I27.83-I27.9, P29.38

PDX Collection 1029
P29.81

PDX Collection 1030
P29.0-P29.2, P29.4, P29.89-P35.9, P37.0-P37.4, P37.8-P37.9, P94.1-P94.9, P96.0, P96.3-P96.5, P96.82-P96.89

PDX Collection 1031
P29.0-P29.2, P29.4, P29.89-P29.9, P36.0-P36.9, P37.5, P38.1-P39.9, P53, P60-P61.9, P94.1-P94.9, P96.0, P96.3-P96.5, P96.82-P96.89

PDX Collection 1032
P39.0, P39.2, P39.4-P39.9

PDX Collection 1033
A02.1, A20.7, A22.7, A39.2-A39.4, A40.9-A41.59, A41.81-A41.9, A42.7, A48.2, A48.4, A48.8-A49.9, B00.7, B92, B94.2-B96.89, P39.2-P39.9, P95, P96.9, R78.81

PDX Collection 1034
A49.9, N10-N11.0, N11.8-N12, N13.6, N15.1, N28.82, N28.84-N30.31, N30.80-N30.91, N36.9-N39.0, N39.9, N99.511, P39.2, P39.4-P39.9, R30.0, R30.9, T83.511A

PDX Collection 1035
P29.0-P29.2, P29.4, P29.89-P29.9, P53, P60-P61.9, P94.1-P96.0, P96.3-P96.5, P96.82-P96.89

PDX Collection 1036
P29.0-P29.2, P29.4, P29.89-P29.9, P50.0-P50.9, P53-P54.9, P60-P61.9, P94.1-P96.0, P96.3-P96.5, P96.82-P96.89

PDX Collection 1037
P29.0-P29.2, P29.4, P29.89-P29.9, P55.0-P57.0, P94.1-P96.0, P96.3-P96.5, P96.82-P96.89

PDX Collection 1038
P29.0-P29.2, P29.4, P29.89-P29.9, P57.8-P59.9, P94.1-P96.0, P96.3-P96.5, P96.82-P96.89

PDX Collection 1039
D50.0-D55.9, D56.4, D57.00-D57.3, D57.80-D64.9, D75.9, P61.2-P61.4

PDX Collection 1040
D50.1-D53.9, D56.4, D57.00-D57.20, D57.3, D57.811-D57.819, D58.2, D59.0-D59.19, D59.3, D60.0-D61.9, D63.0-D64.9, D75.9, P61.5, P61.8-P61.9

PDX Collection 1041
P29.0-P29.2, P29.4, P29.89-P29.9, P70.0-P71.9, P72.1, P72.9-P74.4, P74.9, P94.0-P94.9, P96.0, P96.3-P96.5, P96.82-P96.89

PDX Collection 1042
P70.0-P70.4, P70.9-P71.9, P72.1, P72.9-P74.41, P74.5-P74.8, P94.0

PDX Collection 1043
P76.0-P78.9

PDX Collection 1044
P29.0-P29.2, P29.4-P29.9, P76.0-P78.9, P94.1-P96.0, P96.3-P96.5, P96.82-P96.89

PDX Collection 1045
P83.0, P83.30-P83.39

PDX Collection 1046
P29.0-P29.2, P29.4, P29.89-P29.9, P83.2, P94.1-P96.0, P96.3-P96.5, P96.82-P96.89

PDX Collection 1047
P80.0-P83.0, P83.30-P83.39

PDX Collection 1048
P29.0-P29.2, P29.4, P29.89-P29.9, P90, P91.811-P91.9, P94.1-P96.0, P96.3-P96.5, P96.82-P96.89

PDX Collection 1049
P90-P91.1, P91.3-P91.5, P91.811-P91.9

PDX Collection 1050
P84, P91.60-P91.63

PDX Collection 1051
P92.01-P92.09

PDX Collection 1052
P93.0-P93.8, P96.1-P96.2

PDX Collection 1053
Q00.0-Q00.2

PDX Collection 1054
Q01.0-Q02, Q04.0-Q04.8

PDX Collection 1055
Q04.4-Q04.8

PDX Collection 1057
E78.71-E78.72, I23.0-I23.3, I23.6-I23.8, I51.0, P29.30-P29.38, Q20.0-Q21.9, Q23.8-Q23.9, Q24.8-Q24.9, Q27.30, Q27.4, Q28.0-Q28.1, Q28.8-Q28.9, Q87.1-Q87.89, Q89.7-Q89.8, Q99.2

PDX Collection 1058
E78.71-E78.72, I23.0-I23.3, I23.6-I23.8, I51.0, Q20.0-Q20.9, Q21.1-Q21.9, Q23.8-Q23.9, Q24.8-Q24.9, Q27.30, Q27.4, Q28.0-Q28.1, Q28.8-Q28.9, Q87.2-Q87.3, Q87.5-Q87.89, Q89.7-Q89.8

PDX Collection 1060
E78.71-E78.72, Q20.9, Q22.0-Q22.3, Q23.8-Q23.9, Q24.8-Q24.9, Q27.30, Q27.4, Q28.0-Q28.1, Q28.8-Q28.9, Q87.2-Q87.3, Q87.5-Q87.89, Q89.7-Q89.8

PDX Collection 1061
E78.71-E78.72, P29.30-P29.38, Q20.9, Q22.4-Q23.9, Q24.8-Q24.9, Q27.30, Q27.4, Q28.0-Q28.1, Q28.8-Q28.9, Q87.2-Q87.89, Q89.7-Q89.8, Q99.2

PDX Collection 1062
E78.71-E78.72, Q20.9, Q23.8-Q24.4, Q24.8-Q24.9, Q27.30, Q27.4, Q28.0-Q28.1, Q28.8-Q28.9, Q87.2-Q87.3, Q87.5-Q87.89, Q89.7-Q89.8

PDX Collection 1064
Q20.9, Q23.8-Q23.9, Q24.5, Q24.8-Q24.9

PDX Collection 1066
Q25.0, Q27.30, Q27.4, Q28.0-Q28.1, Q28.8

PDX Collection 1067
E78.71-E78.72, Q25.1-Q25.3, Q27.30, Q27.4, Q28.0-Q28.1, Q28.8-Q28.9, Q87.2-Q87.3, Q87.5-Q87.89, Q89.7-Q89.8

PDX Collection 1069
E78.71-E78.72, Q25.1-Q25.49, Q25.8-Q25.9, Q27.30, Q27.4, Q28.0-Q28.1, Q28.8-Q28.9, Q87.2-Q87.3, Q87.5-Q87.89, Q89.7-Q89.8

PDX Collection 1070
Q25.5-Q25.79, Q27.30, Q27.4, Q28.0-Q28.1, Q28.8-Q28.9

PDX Collection 1071
Q26.0-Q26.1, Q26.8, Q27.30, Q27.4, Q28.0-Q28.1, Q28.8-Q28.9

PDX Collection 1072
Q26.2, Q27.30, Q27.4, Q28.0-Q28.1, Q28.8-Q28.9

PDX Collection 1073
Q26.3-Q26.4, Q27.30, Q27.4, Q28.0-Q28.1, Q28.8-Q28.9

PDX Collection 1074
Q26.9, Q27.30, Q27.4, Q28.0-Q28.1, Q28.8-Q28.9

PDX Collection 1075
Q20.0-Q20.8, Q21.0-Q21.9, Q27.30, Q27.4, Q28.0-Q28.1, Q28.8

PDX Collection 1076
Q27.30, Q27.4, Q28.0-Q28.9

PDX Collection 1077
Q20.0-Q28.9

PDX Collection 1078
J39.8, J45.990, J98.09, Q31.1-Q32.4, Q34.0-Q34.9

PDX Collection 1079
Q33.0-Q34.9

PDX Collection 1080
J44.9, J47.0-J47.9, J68.1, J68.4-J68.9, Q33.4

PDX Collection 1081
Q39.0-Q39.9, Q45.8-Q45.9

PDX Collection 1082
Q39.5-Q39.9, Q45.8-Q45.9

PDX Collection 1083
Q41.0-Q41.9, Q45.8-Q45.9

PDX Collection 1084
Q42.0-Q42.9, Q45.8-Q45.9

PDX Collection 1085
Q43.1-Q43.2, Q45.8-Q45.9

PDX Collection 1086
Q43.3-Q43.9

PDX Collection 1087
Q41.0-Q43.9

PDX Collection 1088
Q44.0-Q44.7

PDX Collection 1089
Q44.2-Q44.3, Q45.8-Q45.9

PDX Collection 1090
Q44.0-Q44.1, Q44.4-Q44.7

PDX Collection 1091
Q45.0-Q45.9

PDX Collection 1092
N13.9, Q60.0-Q60.6

PDX Collection 1093
N13.9, Q61.00, Q61.9

PDX Collection 1094
N13.9, Q61.01

PDX Collection 1095
N13.9, Q61.02, Q61.5-Q61.8

PDX Collection 1096
N13.9, Q61.11-Q61.3

PDX Collection 1097
N13.9, Q61.4

PDX Collection 1098
N13.9, Q62.0-Q62.2, Q62.39

PDX Collection 1099
N13.9, Q64.10-Q64.19, Q64.8-Q64.9

PDX Collection 1100
N13.9, Q64.2-Q64.39, Q64.8-Q64.9

PDX Collection 1101
Q67.5, Q76.3, Q76.425-Q76.429

PDX Collection 1102
Q67.6-Q67.8, Q68.1, Q74.3

PDX Collection 1103
Q76.5-Q76.9, Q77.2

PDX Collection 1104
Q77.3, Q77.6, Q78.0-Q78.3, Q78.5-Q78.9

PDX Collection 1105
Q40.1, Q79.0-Q79.1

PDX Collection 1106
Q79.2-Q79.59

PDX Collection 1108
Q85.1-Q85.9, Q89.7, Q89.9

PDX Collection 1109
Q85.8-Q85.9, Q89.9

PDX Collection 1111
Q89.01-Q89.09, Q89.9

PDX Collection 1112
Q89.3, Q89.7, Q89.9

PDX Collection 1113
Q89.4-Q89.7, Q89.9

PDX Collection 1114
Q90.0-Q99.1, Q99.8-Q99.9

PDX Collection 1115
Q90.0-Q99.1, Q99.8-Q99.9

PDX Collection 1116
Q90.0-Q99.1, Q99.8-Q99.9

PDX Collection 1117
Q90.0-Q99.1, Q99.8-Q99.9

PDX Collection 1118
Q90.0-Q99.1, Q99.8-Q99.9

PDX Collection 1119
R04.2-R04.9, R09.3, R68.13

PDX Collection 1120
J22, J80, J96.00-J96.92, J98.8-J98.9, R06.3, R06.81, R09.2

PDX Collection 1121
G89.0-G89.4, J80, J96.00-J96.92, R09.01-R09.02, R09.2, R29.700-R29.742, R41.0-R41.3, R41.82, R41.9, R44.8-R44.9, R45.83-R45.84, R46.0-R46.89, R52, R68.0-R68.19, R68.81-R68.83, R68.89-R69

PDX Collection 1122
P57.8-P59.9, R17, R23.8-R23.9

PDX Collection 1123
G89.0-G89.4, R18.0-R19.09, R19.30-R19.37, R29.700-R29.742, R41.0-R41.3, R41.82, R41.9, R44.8-R44.9, R45.83-R45.84, R46.0-R46.89, R52, R68.0-R68.19, R68.81-R68.83, R68.89-R69

PDX Collection 1124
A33, A35, G10-G11.2, G11.4, G20-G25.79, G25.82-G26, G32.81, G80.3, G81.10-G81.14, G89.0-G89.4, G90.3, R29.0, R29.700-R29.742, R41.0-R41.3, R41.82, R41.9, R44.8-R44.9, R45.83-R45.84, R46.0-R46.89, R52, R68.0-R68.19, R68.81-R68.83, R68.89-R69

PDX Collection 1125
R29.1, R29.810

PDX Collection 1126
R29.5, R29.810

PDX Collection 1127
R30.1, R39.0, R39.2-R39.9

PDX Collection 1128
R29.3, R29.6-R29.890, R29.90-R29.91, R41.4

PDX Collection 1129
G89.0-G89.4, R29.700-R29.742, R41.0-R41.3, R41.82, R41.9-R42, R44.0, R44.2-R44.9, R45.83-R45.84, R46.0-R46.89, R52, R68.0-R68.19, R68.81-R68.83, R68.89-R69

PDX Collection 1130
F05, R45.851

PDX Collection 1131
F80.1, F80.81, I62.00-I66.9, R47.01-R47.9, R49.0-R49.9

PDX Collection 1132
G32.89, G40.001-G40.319, G40.401-G40.919, G40.A01-G40.B19, G89.0-G89.4, G93.81, G93.89-G93.9, G96.9, G98.0-G98.8, P90, P91.811-P91.9, R29.700-R29.742, R41.0-R41.3, R41.82, R41.9, R44.8-R44.9, R45.83-R45.84, R46.0-R46.89, R52, R56.00-R56.9, R68.0-R68.19, R68.81-R68.83, R68.89-R69

PDX Collection 1133
G89.0-G89.4, R09.89, R29.700-R29.742, R41.0-R41.3, R41.82, R41.9, R44.8-R44.9, R45.83-R45.84, R46.0-R46.89, R52, R57.0-R57.9, R65.21, R68.0-R68.19, R68.81-R68.83, R68.89-R69

PDX Collection 1134
G89.0-G89.4, R29.700-R29.742, R41.0-R41.3, R41.82, R41.9, R44.8-R44.9, R45.83-R45.84, R46.0-R46.89, R52, R64, R68.0-R68.19, R68.81-R68.83, R68.89-R69

PDX Collection 1136
B34.9, E07.81, G89.0-G89.4, R29.700-R29.742, R41.0-R41.3, R41.82, R41.9, R44.8-R44.9, R45.83-R45.84, R46.0-R46.89, R52, R68.0-R68.19, R68.81-R68.83, R68.89-R69, R70.1, R77.0-R77.9, R78.1-R78.6, R78.81, R78.9, R79.1-R79.89, R97.20, R97.21

PDX Collection 1137
G89.0-G89.4, R29.700-R29.742, R41.0-R41.3, R41.82, R41.9, R44.8-R44.9, R45.83-R45.84, R46.0-R46.89, R52, R68.0-R68.19, R68.81-R68.83, R68.89-R69, R82.0, R82.5-R82.998

PDX Collection 1138
G89.0-G89.4, R29.700-R29.742, R41.0-R41.3, R41.82, R41.9, R44.8-R44.9, R45.83-R45.84, R46.0-R46.89, R52, R68.0-R68.19, R68.81-R68.83, R68.89-R69, R82.1, R82.3, R82.5-R82.998

PDX Collection 1139
S01.101-S01.159[A], S05.20X-S05.8X9[A], S05.91X-S05.92X[A], S38.3XXA, T07.XXX-T14.91X[A], T79.A0X-T79.9XX[A]

PDX Collection 1140
S01.90X-S01.95X[A], S02.0XX-S02.19X[A,B,S], S02.2XX-S02.82X[S], S02.91X[A,B,S], S02.92XS, S06.0X0-S07.9XX[A], S08.89XA, S09.10X-S09.19X[A], S09.8XX-S09.90X[A], S09.92X-S09.93X[A], S16.8XX-S19.9XX[A], S38.3XX[A], T07.XXX-T14.91X[A], T79.A0XA-T79.9XX[A]

PDX Collection 1141
S01.90X-S01.95X[A], S02.0XX-S02.2XX[A,B,S], S02.30X-S02.413[S], S02.42X-S02.82X[S], S02.91X[A,B,S], S02.92XS, S06.0X0-S07.9XX[A], S08.89XA, S09.10X-S09.19X[A], S09.8XX-S09.90X[A], S09.92X-S09.93X[A], S16.8XX-S19.9XX[A], S38.3XXA, S92.811-S92.819[A,B], T07.XXX-T14.91X[A], T79.A0X-T79.8XX[A]

PDX Collection 1142
S01.90X-S01.95X[A], S02.0XX[A,B,S], S02.101-S02.2XX[A,B,S], S02.30X-S02.32X[A,B,S], S02.400-S02.413[S], S02.42X[A,B,S], S02.5XX-S02.69X[S], S02.80X-S02.92X[A,B,S], S06.0X0-S07.9XX[A], S08.89XA, S09.10X-S09.19X[A], S09.8XX-S09.919X[A], S09.8XX-S09.90X-S09.3X[A], S16.8XX-S19.9XX[A], S38.3XX[A], T07.XXX-T14.91X[A], T79.8XX-T79.9XX[A], T79.A0X-T79.A9X[A]

PDX Collection 1143
S01.90X- S01.95X[A], S02.0XX[A,B,S], S02.101-S02.413[A,B,S], S02.42XS, S02.5XXS, S02.600[A,B,S]-S02.69X[A,B,S], S02.80[S]-S02.85X[S], S02.91[A,B,S], S02.92XS, S06.0X0-S07.9XX[A], S08.89X[A], S09.10X-S09.19X[A], S09.8XX-S09.90X[A], S09.92X-S09.93X[A], S16.8XX-S19.9XX[A], S38.3XXA, T07.XXX-T14.91X[A], T79.8XX-T79.9XX[A], T79.A0X-T79.A9X[A]

PDX Collection 1144
S04.011-S04.049[A], S04.811-S04.9XX[A]

PDX Collection 1145
S04.10X-S04.12X[A], S04.811-S04.9XX[A]

PDX Collection 1146
S04.20X-S04.22X[A], S04.811-S04.9XX[A]

PDX Collection 1147
S04.30X-S04.32X[A], S04.811-S04.9XX[A]

PDX Collection 1148
S04.40X-S04.42X[A], S04.811-S04.9XX[A]

PDX Collection 1149
S04.50X-S04.52X[A], S04.811-S04.9XX[A]

PDX Collection 1150
S04.60X-S04.62X[A], S04.811-S04.9XX[A]

PDX Collection 1151
S04.70X-S04.9XX[A]

PDX Collection 1152
S04.811-S04.9XX[A]

PDX Collection 1153
S01.101-S01.159[A], S05.20X-S05.8X9[A], S05.91X-S05.92X[A], S38.3XXA, T07.XXX-T14.91X[A], T79.8XX-T79.9XX[A]

PDX Collection 1154
S01.90X-S01.95X[A], S02.0XX-S02.19X[A,B,S], S02.2XX-S02.85X[S], S02.91X[A,B,S], S02.92XS, S06.0X0-S07.9XX[A], S08.89X-S09.19X[A], S09.8X-S09.90X[A]. S09.92X-S09.93X[A], S16.8XX-S19.9XX[A], S38.3XXA. T07.XXX-T14.91X[A], T79.A0X-T79.9XX[A]

PDX Collection 1155
G93.6, G93.82, S01.90X-S01.95X[A], S02.0XX-S02.19X[A,B,S], S02.2XXS-S02.85X[S], S02.91X[A,B,S], S02.92X[S], S06.0X0-S07.9XX[A], S08.89X-S09.19X[A], S09.8XX-S09.90X[A], S09.92X-S09.93X[A], S16.8XX-S19.9XX[A], S38.3XX[A], T07.XXX-T14.91X[A], T79.8XX-T79.9XX[A], T79.A0X-T79.A9X[A]

PDX Collection 1156
S01.90X-S01.95X[A], S02.0XX-S02.92X[S], S07.0XX-S07.9XX[A], S08.89X-S09.19X[A], S09.8XX-S09.90X[A], S09.92X-S09.93X[A], S16.8XX-S19.9XX[A], T07.XXX-T14.91X[A], T79.8XX-T79.9XX[A], T79.A0X-T79.A9X[A]

PDX Collection 1157
S09.0XXA, S15.101-S15.199[A], S15.8XX-S15.9XX[A], T07.XXX-T14.91X[A], T79.8XX-T79.9XX[A], T79.A0X-T79.A9X[A]

PDX Collection 1158
S01.301-S01.359[A], S08.111-S08.129[A], S09.20X-S09.399[A], S09.91X[A], S38.3XX[A], T07.XXX-T14.91X[A], T79.8XX-T79.9XX[A]

PDX Collection 1159
S11.011-S11.039[A], S11.80X-S11.95X[A], S13.4XXA, S13.8XX[A], S16.1XX-S16.2XX[A], S38.3XX[A], T07.XXX-T14.91X[A], T79.8XX-T79.9XX[A], T79.A0X-T79.A9X[A]

PDX Collection 1160
S11.10X-S11.15X[A], S11.80X-S11.95X[A], S13.4XX[A], S13.8XXA, S16.1XX-S16.2XX[A], S38.3XXA, T07.XXX-T14.91X[A], T79.8XX-T79.9XX[A]

PDX Collection 1161
S11.10X-S11.15X[A], S11.80X-S11.95X[A], S13.4XX[A], S13.8XXA, S16.1XX-S16.2XX[A], S38.3XXA, T07.XXX-T14.91X[A], T79.8XX-T79.9XX[A], T79.A0X-T79.A9X[A]

PDX Collection 1162
S11.20X-S11.95X[A], S13.4XXA, S13.8XXA, S16.1XX-S16.2XX[A], S38.3XX[A], T07.XXX-T14.91X[A], T79.8XX-T79.9XX[A]

PDX Collection 1163
S11.20X-S11.95X[A], S13.4XX[A], S13.8XXA, S16.1XX-S16.2XX[A], S38.3XXA, T07.XXX-T14.91X[A], T79.8XX-T79.9XX[A], T79.A0X-T79.A9X[A]

PDX Collection 1164
M48.40X-M48.58X[S], M80.08X[S], M80.88X[S], M84.350[S], M84.454[S], M84.550[S], M84.58X[S], M84.650[S], M99.10-M99.11, M99.15-M99.17, M99.19, S03.1XX[A], S03.8XX-S03.9XX[A], S12.000-S12.691[A,B,S], S12.8XXS, S12.9XX[A,S], S13.0XX-S13.4XX[A], S13.8XX-S14.159[A], S16.1XXA, S22.000-S22.9XX[S], S23.20X-S23.29X[A], S23.9XX[A], S24.109A, S24.119A, S24.139A, S24.149A, S24.159A, S29.001-S29.019[A], S29.091-S29.9XX[A], S32.000-S32.9XX[S], S33.30X-S33.39X[A], S33.9XXA, S38.1XXA, S38.3XX-S39.013[A], S39.091-S39.94X[A], T07.XXX-T14.91X[A], T79.8XX-T79.9XX[A], T79.A0X-T79.A9X[A]

PDX Collection 1165
S03.8XX-S03.9XX[A], S12.8XXA, S29.011-S29.019[A], S38.3XXA, S39.011-S39.013[A], T07.XXX-T14.91X[A], T79.8XX-T79.9XX[A], T79.A0X-T79.A9X[A]

PDX Collection 1166
M48.40X-M48.58X[S], M80.08XS, M80.88XS, M84.350S, M84.454S, M84.550S, M84.58XS, M84.650S, M99.10-M99.11, M99.15-M99.17, M99.19, S03.1XXA, S12.000-S12.691[A,B,S], S12.8X[S, S12.9XX[A, S], S13.0XX-S13.29X[A], S13.9XX-S14.159[A], S22.000-S22.9XX[S], S23.20X-S23.29X[A], S23.9XXA, S24.109A, S24.119A, S24.139A, S24.149A, S24.159A, S29.001-S29.009[A], S29.091-S29.9XX[A], S32.000-S32.9XX[S], S33.30X-S33.39X[A], S33.9XXA, S38.1XXA, S39.001-S39.003[A], S39.091-S39.94X[A], T07.XXX-T14.91X[A], T79.8XX-T79.9XX[A], T79.A0X-T79.A9X[A]

PDX Collection 1167
S09.0XXA, S15.009A, S15.02[A, S15.099-S15.199[A], S15.8XX-S15.9XX[A], T07.XXX-T14.91X[A], T79.8XX-T79.9XX[A], T79.A0X-T79.A9X[A]

PDX Collection 1168
S21.101-S21.159[A], S21.301-S21.95X[A], S23.3XX[A], S23.8XX[A], S27.50X-S27.69X[A], S27.892A-S28.1XX[A], S29.021A, S29.029A, S38.3XXA, T07.XXX-T14.91X[A], T79.7XXA, T79.8XX-T79.9XX[A], T79.A0X-T79.A9X[A]

PDX Collection 1169
S21.101-S21.159[A], S21.301A-S21.95X[A], S27.50X-S27.69X[A], S27.892-S27.9XX[A], S28.1XXA, S29.021A, S29.029A, S38.3XXA, T07.XXX-T14.91X[A], T79.7XXA, T79.8XX-T79.9XX[A], T79.A0X-T79.A9X[A]

PDX Collection 1170
S21.101A-S21.159[A], S21.301-S21.95X[A], S27.0XX-S27.2XX[A], S27.309A, S27.329A, S27.339A, S27.409A, S27.50X-S27.69X[A], S27.803A, S27.892-S28.1XX[A], S29.021A, S29.029A, S38.3XXA, T07.XXX-T14.91X[A], T79.7XXA, T79.8XX-T79.9XX[A], T79.A0X-T79.A9X[A]

PDX Collection 1171
M48.40X-M48.58X[S], M80.08XS, M80.88XS, M83.50S, M84.454S, M84.550S, M84.58XS, M84.650S, M99.12, M99.15-M99.17, M99.19, S03.1XXA, S03.8XX-S03.9XX[A], S12.000-S12.9XX[S], S13.9XXA, S14.109A, S14.119A, S14.129A, S14.139A, S14.149A, S14.159A, S22.000-S22.089[A,B,S], S22.20XS-S23.3XX[A], S23.8XX-S24.159[A], S29.001-S29.019[A], S29.091-S29.9XX[A], S32.000-S32.9XX[S], S32.9XXS, S33.30X-S33.39X[A], S33.9XXA, S38.1XXA, S38.3XXA, S39.001-S39.013[A], S39.091-S39.94X[A], T07.XXX-T14.91X[A], T79.8XX-T79.9XX[A], T79.A0X-T79.A9X[A]

PDX Collection 1172
S03.8XX-S03.9XX[A], S22.20X-S22.24X[A,B], S22.5XX[A,B], S29.011-S29.019[A], S38.3XXA, S39.011-S39.013[A], T07.XXX-T14.91X[A], T79.8XX-T79.9XX[A], T79.A0X-T79.A9X[A]

PDX Collection 1173
S03.8XX-S03.9XX[A], S22.20X-S22.5XX[A,B], S29.011-S29.019[A], S38.3XXA, S39.011-S39.013[A], T07.XXX-T14.91X[A], T79.8XX-T79.9XX[A], T79.A0X-T79.A9X[A]

PDX Collection 1174
S03.8XX-S03.9XX[A], S22.31X-S22.5XX[A,B], S29.011-S29.019[A], S38.3XX[A], S39.011-S39.013[A], T07.XXX-T14.91X[A], T79.8XX-T79.9XX[A], T79.A0X-T79.A9X[A]

PDX Collection 1175
S03.8XX-S03.9XX[A], S22.20X-S22.5XX[A,B], S29.011-S29.019[A], S38.3XXA, S39.011-S39.013[A], T07.XXX-T14.91X[A], T79.8XX-T79.9XX[A], T79.A0X-T79.A9X[A]

PDX Collection 1176
M80.00X-M80.019[A], M80.041A-M80.049[A], M80.80X-M80.819[A], M80.841-M80.849[A], M84.40X-M84.419[A], M84.441-M84.446[A], M84.454A, M84.474-M84.519[A], M84.541-M84.550[A], M84.574-M84.576[A], M84.60X-M84.619[A], M84.641-M84.650[A], M84.674-M84.68X[A], S03.8XX-S03.9XX[A], S22.9XX-S22.9XX[A,B], S29.011-S29.019[A], S32.301-S32.9XX[A,B], S33.4XX[A], S33.6XX-S33.8XX[A], S38.3XXA, S39.011-S39.013[A], S73.001-S73.199[A], S76.001-S76.019[A], S76.091-S76.119[A], S76.191-S76.219[A],

S76.291-S76.319[A], S76.391-S76.819[A],
S76.891-S76.919[A], S76.991-S76.999[A],
S79.811-S79.929[A], T07.XXX-T14.91X[A],
T79.8XX-T79.9XX[A], T79.A9X[A]

PDX Collection 1177
M48.40X-M48.58X[S], M80.08X[S], M80.88XS,
M84.350S, M84.454S, M84.550S, M84.58S, M84.650S,
M99.15-M99.17, M99.19, S03.1XXA, S12.000-S12.9XX[S],
S13.9XXA, S14.109A, S14.119A, S14.129A,
S14.139A, S14.149A, S14.159A, S22.000-S22.9XX[S],
S23.20X-S23.29X[A], S23.9XX-S24.159[A],
S29.001-S29.009[A], S29.091-S29.9XX[A],
S32.000-S32.9XX[S], S33.30X-S33.39X[A], S33.9XXA,
S38.1XXA, S39.001-S39.003[A], S39.091-S39.94X[A],
T07.XXX-T14.91X[A], T79.8XX-T79.9XX[A],
T79.A0X-T79.A9X[A]

PDX Collection 1178
S25.00XA-S25.09X[A], T07.XXX-T14.91X[A],
T79.8XX-T79.9XX[A], T79.A0X-T79.A9X[A]

PDX Collection 1179
S25.101-S25.199[A], T07.XXX-T14.91X[A],
T79.8XX-T79.9XX[A], T79.A0X-T79.A9X[A]

PDX Collection 1180
S25.20X-S25.29X[A], T07.XXX-T14.91X[A],
T79.8XX-T79.9XX[A], T79.A0X-T79.A9X[A]

PDX Collection 1181
S25.301-S25.399[A], T07.XXX-T14.91X[A],
T79.8XX-T79.9XX[A], T79.A0X-T79.A9X[A]

PDX Collection 1182
S25.401-S25.499[A], T07.XXX-T14.91X[A],
T79.8XX-T79.9XX[A], T79.A0X-T79.A9X[A]

PDX Collection 1183
S25.401[A]-S25.499[A], T07.XXX-T14.91X[A],
T79.A0X[A]-T79.9XX[A]

PDX Collection 1184
S25.501-S25.899[A]

PDX Collection 1185
S25.00X-S25.99X[A]

PDX Collection 1186
S21.301-S21.459[A], S26.00X-S26.99X[A],
S27.50X-S27.69X[A], S27.892-S27.9XX[A],
T07.XXX-T14.91X[A]

PDX Collection 1187
S21.101-S21.159[A], S21.301-S21.95X[A],
S26.00X-S26.99X[A], S27.50X-S27.69X[A],
S27.892-S27.9XX[A], S28.1XX[A], S29.021A, S29.029A,
S38.3XXA, T07.XXX-T14.91X[A], T79.7XX-T79.9XX[A],
T79.A0X-T79.A9X[A]

PDX Collection 1188
S21.101-S21.159[A], S21.301-S21.95X[A],
S27.0XX-S27.399[A], S27.50X-S27.69X[A],
S27.892-S27.9XX[A], S28.1XXA, S29.021A, S29.029A,
S38.3XX[A], T07.XXX-T14.91X[A], T79.7XX-T79.9XX[A],
T79.A0X-T79.A9X[A]

PDX Collection 1189
S21.101-S21.159[A], S21.301-S21.95X[A],
S27.301-S27.399[A], S27.50X-S27.69X[A],
S27.892-S27.9XX[A], S28.1XXA, S29.021A, S29.029A,
S38.3XXA, T07.XXX-T14.91X[A], T79.7XX-T79.9XX[A],
T79.A9XA

PDX Collection 1190
S21.101-S21.159[A], S21.301-S21.95X[A],
S27.301-S27.399[A], S27.50X-S27.69X[A],
S27.892-S27.9XX[A], S28.1XXA, S29.021A, S29.029A,

S38.3XXA, T07.XXX-T14.91X[A], T79.7XX-T79.9XX[A],
T79.A0X-T79.A9X[A]

PDX Collection 1191
S21.101-S21.159[A], S21.301-S21.95X[A],
S27.401-S27.69X[A], S27.892-S27.9XX[A], S28.1XXA,
S29.021A, S29.029A, S38.3XXA, T07.XXX-T14.91X[A],
T79.7XX-T79.9XX[A], T79.A0X-T79.A9X[A]

PDX Collection 1192
S21.101-S21.159[A], S21.301-S21.95X[A],
S27.50X-S27.809[A], S27.892-S27.9XX[A], S28.1XXA,
S29.021A, S29.029A, S38.3XXA, T07.XXX-T14.91X[A],
T79.7XX-T79.9XX[A], T79.A9XA

PDX Collection 1193
S21.101-S21.159[A], S21.301-S21.95X[A],
S27.50X-S27.69X[A], S27.812-S27.9XX[A], S28.1XXA,
S29.021A, S29.029A, S38.3XXA, T07.XXX-T14.91X[A],
T79.7XX-T79.9XX[A], T79.A0X-T79.A9X[A]

PDX Collection 1194
S21.101-S21.159[A], S21.301-S21.95X[A],
S27.50X-S27.69X[A], S27.892-S27.9XX[A], S28.1XXA,
S29.021A, S29.029A, S38.3XXA, T07.XXX-T14.91X[A],
T79.7XX-T79.9XX[A], T79.A3X-T79.A9X[A]

PDX Collection 1195
S31.001[A], S31.011[A], S31.021[A], S31.031[A], S31.041[A],
S31.051[A], S31.100-S31.159[A], S31.600-S31.659[A],
S31.831-S31.839[A], S36.81X-S36.99X[A],
S38.3XXA, S39.021-S39.023[A], T07.XXX-T14.91X[A],
T79.8XX-T79.9XX[A], T79.A0X-T79.A9X[A]

PDX Collection 1196
M48.40X-M48.58X[S], M80.08XS, M80.88XS,
M84.350S, M84.454S, M84.550S, M84.58XS, M84.650S,
M99.13, M99.15-M99.17, M99.19, S03.1XXA,
S03.8XX-S03.9XX[A], S12.000-S12.9XX[S], S13.9XXA,
S14.109A, S14.119A, S14.129A, S14.139A, S14.149A,
S14.159A, S22.000-S22.9XX[S], S23.20X-S23.29X[A],
S23.9XXA, S24.109A, S24.119A, S24.139A, S24.149A,
S24.159A, S29.001-S29.019[A], S29.091-S29.9XX[A],
S32.000-S32.059[A,B,S], S32.10X-S32.9XX[S],
S33.0XX-S33.141[A], S33.30X-S33.39X[A],
S33.5XXA, S33.9X[A, S34.01XA, S34.101-S34.129[A],
S38.1XXA, S38.3XX-S39.013[A], S39.091-S39.94X[A],
T07.XXX-T14.91X[A], T79.8XX-T79.9XX[A],
T79.A0X-T79.A9X[A]

PDX Collection 1197
M48.40X-M48.58X[S], M80.08XS, M80.88XS, M84.350S,
M84.454S, M84.550S, M84.58XS, M84.650S, M99.14-M99.17,
M99.19, S03.1XXA, S03.8XX-S03.9XX[A], S12.000-S12.9XX[S],
S13.9XXA, S14.109A, S14.119A, S14.129A, S14.139A,
S14.149A, S14.159A, S22.000-S22.9XX[S], S23.20XA,
S23.29XA, S23.9XXA, S24.109A, S24.119A,
S24.139A, S24.149A, S24.159A, S29.001-S29.019[A],
S29.091-S29.9XX[A], S32.000-S32.059[S],
S32.10X-S32.2XX[A,B,S], S32.301-S32.9XX[S],
S33.2XX-S33.4XX[A], S33.6XX-S33.9XX[A],
S34.02X[A], S34.131-S34.3XX[A], S38.1XXA,
S38.3XXA, S39.001-S39.013[A], S39.091-39.94X[A],
T07.XXX-T14.91X[A], T79.8XX-T79.9XX[A],
T79.A0X-T79.A9X[A]

PDX Collection 1198
M48.40X-M48.58X[A], M80.00X-M80.88X[A],
M84.30X-M84.68X[A], M84.750-M84.759[A],
S03.8XX-S03.9XX[A], S22.9XX[A,B], S29.011-S29.019[A],
S32.301-S32.399[A,B], S32.810-S32.9XX[A,B], S33.4XXA,
S33.6XX-S33.8XX[A], S38.3XXA, S39.011-S39.013[A],
S73.001-S73.199[A], S76.001-S76.019[A],
S76.091-S76.119[A], S76.191-S76.219[A],

S76.291-S76.319[A], S76.391-S76.819[A],
S76.891-S76.919[A], S76.991-S76.999[A],
S79.811-S79.929[A], T07.XXX-T14.91X[A],
T79.8XX-T79.9XX[A], T79.A0X-T79.A9X[A]

PDX Collection 1199
M48.40X-M48.58X[A], M80.00X-M80.88X[A],
M84.30X-M84.68X[A], M84.750-M84.759[A],
S03.8XX-S03.9XX[A], S22.9XX[A,B], S29.011-S29.019[A],
S32.401-S32.499[A,B], S32.810-S32.811[A,B],
S32.89X-S32.9XX[A,B], S33.4XXA, S33.6XX-S33.8XX[A],
S38.3XXA, S39.011-S39.013[A], S73.001-S73.199[A],
S76.001-S76.019[A], S76.091-S76.119[A],
S76.191-S76.219[A], S76.291-S76.319[A],
S76.391-S76.819[A], S76.891-S76.919[A],
S76.991-S76.999[A], S79.811-S79.829[A],
S79.911-S79.929[A], T07.XXX-T14.91X[A],
T79.8XX-T79.9XX[A], T79.A0X-T79.A9X[A]

PDX Collection 1200
S03.8XX-S03.9XX[A], S22.9XX[A,B], S29.011-S29.019[A],
S32.401-S32.499[A,B], S32.810-S32.811[A,B],
S32.89X-S32.9XX[A,B], S33.4XXA, S33.6XX-S33.8XX[A],
S38.3XXA, S39.011-S39.013[A], S73.001-S73.199[A],
S76.001-S76.019[A], S76.091-S76.119[A], S76.191-S76.219[A],
S76.291-S76.319[A], S76.391-S76.819[A], S76.891-S76.919[A],
S76.991-S76.999[A], S79.811-S79.929[A], T07.XXX-T14.91X[A],
T79.A0X-T79.A9X[A], T79.8XX-T79.9XX[A]

PDX Collection 1201
M48.40X-M48.58X[A], M80.00X-M80.88X[A],
M84.30X-M84.68X[A], M84.750-M84.759[A],
S03.8XX-S03.9XX[A], S22.9XX[A,B], S29.011-S29.019[A],
S32.501-S32.599[A,B], S32.810-S32.811[A,B],
S32.89X-S32.9XX[A,B], S33.4XXA, S33.6XX-S33.8XX[A],
S38.3XX-S39.013[A], S73.001-S73.199[A], S76.001-S76.019[A],
S76.091-S76.119[A], S76.191-S76.219[A], S76.291-S76.319[A],
S76.391-S76.819[A], S76.891-S76.919[A], S76.991-S76.999[A],
S79.811-S79.929[A], T07.XXX-T14.91X[A],T79.A0X-T79.A9X[A],
T79.8XX-T79.9XX[A]

PDX Collection 1202
S32.601-S32.699[A]

PDX Collection 1203
M48.40X-M48.58X[A], M80.00X-M80.88X[A],
M84.30X-M84.68X[A], M84.750-M84.759[A],
S03.8XX-S03.9XX[A], S22.9XX[A,B], S29.011-S29.019[A],
S32.601-S32.811[A,B], S32.89X-S32.9XX[A,B], S33.4XX[A],
S33.6XX-S33.8XX[A], S38.3XXA, S39.011-S39.013[A],
S73.001-S73.199[A], S76.001-S76.019[A], S76.091-S76.119[A],
S76.191-S76.219[A], S76.291-S76.319[A], S76.391-S76.819[A],
S76.891-S76.919[A], S76.991-S76.999[A], S79.811-S79.929[A],
T07.XXX-T14.91X[A], T79.A0X-T79.A9X[A], T79.8XX-T79.9XX[A]

PDX Collection 1204
M48.40X-M48.58X[A], M80.00X-M80.88X[A],
M84.30X-M84.68X[A], M84.750-M84.759[A],
S03.8XX-S03.9XX[A], S22.9XX[A,B], S29.011-S29.019[A],
S32.301-S32.811[A,B], S32.89X-S32.9XX[A,B], S33.4XXA,
S33.6XX-S33.8XX[A], S38.3XXA, S39.011-S39.013[A],
S73.001-S73.199[A], S76.001-S76.019[A], S76.091-S76.119[A],
S76.191-S76.219[A], S76.291-S76.319[A], S76.391-S76.819[A],
S76.891-S76.919[A], S76.991-S76.999[A], S79.811-S79.929[A],
T07.XXX-T14.91X[A], T79.A0X-T79.A9X[A], T79.8XX-T79.9XX[A]

PDX Collection 1205
S32.82XB, S32.89XA

PDX Collection 1206
M48.40X-M48.58X[A], M80.00X-M80.88X[A],
M84.30X-M84.68X[A], M84.750-M84.759[A],
S03.8XX-S03.9XX[A], S22.9XX[A,B], S29.011-S29.019[A],
S32.301-S32.9XX[A,B], S33.4XXA, S33.6XX-S33.8XX[A],
S38.3XXA, S39.011-S39.013[A], S73.001-S73.199[A],

S76.001-S76.019[A], S76.091-S76.119[A], S76.191-S76.219[A], 76.291-S76.319[A], S76.391-S76.819[A], S76.891-S76.919[A], S76.991-S76.999[A], S79.811-S79.929[A], T07.XXX-T14.91X[A], T79.A0X-T79.A9X[A], T79.8XX-T79.A9X[A]

PDX Collection 1207
M48.40X-M48.58X[S], M80.08XS, M80.88XS, M84.350S, M84.454S, M84.550S, M84.58XS, M84.650S, M99.15-M99.17, M99.19, S03.1XXA, S12.000-S12.9XX[S], S13.9XXA, S14.109A, S14.119A, S14.129A, S14.139A, S14.149A, S14.159A, S22.000-S22.9XX[S], S23.20XA, S23.29XA, S23.9XXA, S24.109A, S24.119A, S24.139A, S24.149A, S24.159A, S29.001-S29.009[A], S29.091-S29.9XX[A], S32.000-S32.9XX[S], S33.30X-S33.39X[A], S33.9XX-S34.01X[A], S34.101-S34.129[A], S38.1XX[A], S39.001-S39.003[A], S39.091-S39.94X[A], T07.XXX-T14.91X[A], T79.A0X-T79.A9X[A], T79.8XX-T79.A9X[A]

PDX Collection 1208
M48.40X-M48.58X[S], M80.08XS, M80.88XS, M84.350S, M84.454S, M84.550S, M84.58XS, M84.650S, M99.15-M99.17, M99.19, S03.1XXA, S12.000-S12.9XX[S], S13.9XXA, S14.109A, S14.119A, S14.129A, S14.139A, S14.149A, S14.159A, S22.000-S22.9XX[S], S23.20X-S23.29X[A], S23.9XXA, S24.109A, S24.119A, S24.139A, S24.149A, S24.159A, S29.001-S29.009[A], S29.091-S29.9XX[A], S32.000-S32.9XX[S], S33.30X-S33.39X[A], S33.9XXA, S34.02XA, S34.131-S34.139[A], S34.3XXA, S38.1XXA, S39.001-S39.003[A], S39.091-S39.94X[A], T07.XXX-T14.91X[A], T79.A0X-T79.A9X[A], T79.8XX-T79.A9X[A]

PDX Collection 1209
S35.00X-S35.09X[A], S35.8X1-S35.99X[A], T07.XXX-T14.91X[A], T79.A0X-T79.A9X[A], T79.8XX-T79.A9X[A]

PDX Collection 1210
S35.10X-S35.19X[A], S35.8X1-S35.99X[A], T07.XXX-T14 91X[A], T79.A0X-T79.A9X[A], T79.8XX-T79.A9X[A]

PDX Collection 1211
S35.211-S35.219[A], S35.8X1-S35.99X[A], T07.XXX-T14.91X[A], T79.A0X-T79.A9X[A], T79.8XX-T79.A9X[A]

PDX Collection 1212
S35.221-S35.229[A], S35.8X1-S35.99X[A], T07.XXX-T14.91X[A], T79.A0X-T79.A9X[A], T79.8XX-T79.A9X[A]

PDX Collection 1213
S35.231-S35.239[A], S35.8X1-S35.99X[A], T07.XXX-T14.91X[A], T79.A0X-T79.A9X[A], T79.8XX-T79.A9X[A]

PDX Collection 1214
S35.291[A], S35.8X1-S35.99X[A], T07.XXX-T14.91X[A], 1/9.8XX-T79.9XX[A], T79.A0XA, T79.A3X-T79.A9X[A]

PDX Collection 1215
S35.292-S35.298[A], S35.8X1-S35.99X[A], T07.XXX-T14.91X[A], T79.A0X-T79.A9X[A], T79.8XX-T79.9XX[A]

PDX Collection 1216
S35.299A, S35.8X1-S35.99X[A], T07.XXX-T14.91X[A], T79.A0X-T79.A9X[A], T79.8XX-T79.9XX[A]

PDX Collection 1217
S35.311-S35.319[A], S35.8X1-S35.99X[A], T07.XXX-T14.91X[A], T79.A0X-T79.A9X[A], T79.8XX-T79.9XX[A]

PDX Collection 1218
S35.321-S35.329[A], S35.8X1-S35.99X[A], T07.XXX-T14.91X[A], T79.A0X-T79.A9X[A], T79.8XX-T79.9XX[A]

PDX Collection 1219
S35.331-S35.339[A], S35.8X1-S35.99X[A], T07.XXX-T14.91X[A], T79.A0X-T79.A9X[A], T79.8XX-T79.9XX[A]

PDX Collection 1220
S35.341-S35.349[A], S35.8X1-S35.99X[A], T07.XXX-T14.91X[A], T79.A0X-T79.A9X[A], T79.8XX-T79.9XX[A]

PDX Collection 1221
S35.401-S35.403[A], S35.411-S35.413[A], S35.491-S35.493[A], S35.8X1-S35.99X[A], T07.XXX-T14.91X[A], T79.A0X-T79.A9X[A], T79.8XX-T79.9XX[A]

PDX Collection 1222
S35.404-S35.406[A], S35.414-S35.416[A], S35.494-S35.496[A], S35.8X1-S35.99X[A], T07.XXX-T14.91X[A], T79.A0X-T79.A9X[A], T79.8XX-T79.9XX[A]

PDX Collection 1223
S35.50X-S35.516[A], S35.59X-S35.99X[A], T07.XXX-T14.91X[A], T79.A0X-T79.A9X[A], T79.8XX-T79.9XX[A]

PDX Collection 1224
S35.50X-S35.513[A], S35.59X-S35.99X[A], T07.XXX-T14.91X[A], T79.A0X-T79.A9X[A], T79.8XX-T79.9XX[A]

PDX Collection 1225
S35.50XA, S35.514-S35.516[A], S35.59X-S35.99X[A], T07.XXX-T14.91X[A], T79.A0X-T79.A9X[A], T79.8XX-T79.9XX[A]

PDX Collection 1226
S35.50XA, S35.531-S35.533[A], S35.59X-S35.99X[A], T07.XXX-T14.91X[A], T79.8XX-T79.9XX[A], T79.A0X[A], T79.A3X-T79.A9X[A]

PDX Collection 1227
S35.50X[A], S35.534-S35.536[A], S35.59X-S35.99X[A], T07.XXX-T14.91X[A], T79.8XX-T79.9XX[A], T79.A0XA, T79.A3X-T79.A9X[A]

PDX Collection 1228
S35.8X1-S35.99X[A], T07.XXX-T14 91X[A], T79.8XX-T79.9XX[A], T79.A0XA, T79.A3X-T79.A9X[A]

PDX Collection 1229
S35.00X-S35.99X[A], T07.XXX-T14.91X[A], T79.8XX-T79.9XX[A], T79.A0XA, T79.A3X-T79.A9X[A]

PDX Collection 1230
S31.001A, S31.011A, S31.021A, S31.031A, S31.041A, S31.051A, S31.100-S31.159[A], S31.600-S31.659[A], S31.831-S31.839[A], S36.00X-S36.09[A], S36.81X-S36.99X[A], S38.3XXA, S39.021-S39 023[A], T07.XXX-T14.91X[A], T79.8XX-T79.9XX[A], T79.A0X-T79.A9X[A]

PDX Collection 1231
S31.001A, S31.011A, S31.021A, S31.031A, S31.041A, S31.051A, S31.100-S31.159[A], S31.600-S31.659[A], S31.831-S31.839[A], S36.112-S36.119[A], S36.81X-S36.99X[A], S38.3XXA, S39.021-S39.023[A], T07.XXX-T14.91X[A], T79.8XX-T79.9XX[A], T79.A0X-T79.A9X[A]

PDX Collection 1232
S31.001A, S31.011A, S31.021A, S31.031A, S31.041A, S31.051A, S31.100-S31.159[A], S31.600-S31.659[A], S31.831-S31.839[A], S36.122-S36.13X[A], S36.81X-S36.99X[A], S38.3XXA, S39.021-S39.023[A],

T07.XXX-T14.91X[A], T79.8XX-T79.9XX[A], T79.A0X-T79.A9X[A]

PDX Collection 1233
M79.A3, S31.001A, S31.011A, S31.021A, S31.031A, S31.041A, S31.051A, S31.100-S31.159[A], S31.600-S31.659[A], S31.831-S31.839[A], S36.200-S36.299[A], S36.81X-S36.99X[A], S38.3XX[A], S39.021-S39.023[A], T07.XXX-T14.91X[A], T79.8XX-T79.9XX[A], T79.A3X-T79.A9X[A]

PDX Collection 1234
M79.A3, S31.001A, S31.011A, S31.021A, S31.031A, S31.041A, S31.051A, S31.100-S31.159[A], S31.600-S31.659[A], S31.831-S31.839[A], S36.30X-S36.39X[A], S36.81X-S36.99X[A], S38.3XXA, S39.021-S39.023[A], T07.XXX-T14.91X[A], T79.8XX-T799.XX[A], T79.A3X-T79.A9X[A]

PDX Collection 1235
M79.A3, S31.001A, S31.011A, S31.021A, S31.031A, S31.041A, S31.051A, S31.100-S31.159[A], S31.600-S31.659[A], S31.831-S31.839[A], S36.400-S36.499[A], S36.81X-S36.99X[A], S38.3XXA, S39.021-S39.023[A], T07.XXX-T14.91X[A], T79.8XX-T79.9XX[A], T79.A3X-T79.A9X[A]

PDX Collection 1236
M79.A3, S31.001A, S31.011A, S31.021A, S31.031A, S31.041A, S31.051A, S31.100-S31.159[A], S31.600-S31.659[A], S31.831-S31.839[A], S36.500-S36.99X[A], S38.3XXA, S39.021-S39.023[A], T07.XXX-T14.91X[A], T79.8XX-T79.9XX[A], T79.A3X-179.A9X[A]

PDX Collection 1237
S31.001A, S31.011A, S31.021A, S31 031A, S31.041A, S31.051A, S31.100-S31.159[A], S31.600-S31.659[A], S31.831-S31.839[A], S36.81X-S37.099[A], S38.3XXA, S39.021-S39.023[A], T07.XXX-T14.91X[A], T79.8XX-T79.9XX[A], T79.A0X-T79.A9X[A]

PDX Collection 1238
S31.001A, S31.011A, S31.021A, S31.031A, S31.041A, S31.051A, S31.100-S31.159[A], S31.600-S31.659[A], S31.831-S31.839[A], S36.81X-S36.99X[A], S37.10X-S37.19X[A], S37.401-S37.599[A], S37.822-S37.99X[A], S38.3XXA, S39.021-S39.023[A], T07.XXX-T14.91X[A], T79.8XX-T79.9XX[A], T79.A0X-T79.A9X[A]

PDX Collection 1239
S31.001A, S31.011A, S31.021A, S31.031A, S31.041A, S31.051A, S31.100-S31.159[A], S31.600-S31.659[A], S31.831-S31.839[A], S36.81X-S36.99X[A], S37.20X-S37.599[A], S37.822-S37.99X[A], S38.3XXA, S39.021-S39.023[A], T07.XXX-T14.91X[A], T79.8XX-T79.9XX[A], T79.A0X-T79.A9X[A]

PDX Collection 1240
S31.001A, S31.011A, S31.021A, S31.031A, S31.041A, S31.051A, S31.100-S31.159[A], S31.600-S31.659[A], S31.831-S31.839[A], S36.81X-S36.99X[A], S37.401-S37.69X[A], S37.822-S37.99X[A], S38.3XXA, S39.021-S39.023[A], T07.XXX-T14.91X[A], T79.8XX-T79.9XX[A], T79.A0X-T79.A9X[A]

PDX Collection 1241
S31.001A, S31.011A, S31.021A, S31.031A, S31.041A, S31.051A, S31.100-S31.159[A], S31.600-S31.659[A], S31.831-S31.839[A], S36.81X-S36.99X[A], S37.812-S37.819[A], S38.3XXA, S39.021-S39.023[A], T07.XXX-T14.91X[A], T79.8XX-T79.9XX[A], T79.A0X-T79.A9X[A]

PDX Collection 1242
S31.001A, S31.011A, S31.021A, S31.031A, S31.041A, S31.051A, S31.100-S31.159[A], S31.600-S31.659[A], S31.831-S31.839[A], S36.81X-S36.99X[A], S37.401-S37.599[A], S37.822-S37.99X[A], S38.3XXA, S39.021-S39.023[A], T07.XXX-T14.91X[A], T79.8XX-T79.9XX[A], T79.A0X-T79.A9X[A]

PDX Collection 1243
S42.001-S42.036[A,B], S62.90XB

PDX Collection 1244
S42.101-S42.199[A,B], S62.90XB

PDX Collection 1245
S42.201[A,B], S42.202B, S42.209-S42.211[A,B], S42.212[B], S42.213-S42.214[A,B], S42.215[B], S42.216-S42.221[A,B], S42.222[B], S42.223-S42.224[A,B], S42.225[B], S42.226-S42.231[A,B], S42.232[B], S42.239-S42.241[A,B], S42.242[B], S42.249-S42.251[A,B], S42.252[B], S42.253-S42.254[A,B], S42.255[B], S42.256-S42.261[A,B], S42.262[B], S42.263-S42.264[A,B], S42.265[B], S42.266[A,B], S42.271A, S42.279A, S42.291[A,B], S42.292B, S42.293-S42.294[A,B], S42.295B, S42.296-S42.301[A,B], S42.302B, S42.309[A,B], S42.311A, S42.319A, S42.321[A,B], S42.322B, S42.323-S42.324[A,B], S42.325B, S42.326-S42.331[A,B], S42.332B, S42.333-S42.334[A,B], S42.335B, S42.336-S42.341[A,B], S42.342B, S42.343-S42.344[A,B], S42.345B, S42.346-S42.351[A,B], S42.352B, S42.353-S42.354[A,B], S42.355B, S42.356-S42.361[A,B], S42.362B, S42.363-S42.364[A,B], S42.365B, S42.366-S42.391[A,B], S42.392B, S42.399-S42.401[A,B], S42.402B, S42.409-S42.411[A,B], S42.412B, S42.413-S42.414[A,B], S42.415B, S42.416-S42.421[A,B], S42.422B, S42.423-S42.424[A,B], S42.425B, S42.426-S42.431[A,B], S42.432B, S42.433-S42.434[A,B], S42.435B, S42.436-S42.441[A,B], S42.442B, S42.443-S42.444[A,B], S42.445B, S42.446-S42.447[A,B], S42.448B, S42.449-S42.451[A,B], S42.452B, S42.453-S42.454[A,B], S42.455B, S42.456-S42.461[A,B], S42.462B, S42.463-S42.464[A,B], S42.465B, S42.466-S42.471[A,B], S42.472B, S42.473-S42.474[A,B], S42.475B, S42.476[A,B], S42.481A, S42.489A, S42.491[A,B], S42.492B, S42.493-S42.494[A,B], S42.495B, S42.496-S42.92X[A,B], S49.001A, S49.009-S49.011[A], S49.019-S49.021[A], S49.029-S49.031[A], S49.039-S49.041[A], S49.049-S49.091[A], S49.099-S49.101[A], S49.109-S49.111[A], S49.119-S49.121[A], S49.129-S49.131[A], S49.139-S49.141[A], S49.149-S49.191[A], S49.199A

PDX Collection 1246
S42.201-S42.266[B], S42.291-S42.296[B], S42.301-S42.309[A,B], S42.311-S42.319[A], S42.321-S42.476[A,B], S42.481-S42.489[A], S42.491-S42.92X[A,B], S49.101-S49.199[A], S62.90X[B]

PDX Collection 1247
S42.201B, S42.202-S42.209[A,B], S42.211B, S42.212-S42.213[A,B], S42.214B, S42.215-S42.216[A,B], S42.221B, S42.222-S42.223[A,B], S42.224B, S42.225-S42.226[A,B], S42.231B, S42.232-S42.239[A,B], S42.241B, S42.242-S42.249[A,B], S42.251B, S42.252-S42.253[A,B], S42.254B, S42.255-S42.256[A,B], S42.261B, S42.262-S42.263[A,B], S42.264B, S42.265-S42.266[A,B], S42.272-S42.279[A], S42.291B, S42.292-S42.293[A,B], S42.294B, S42.295-S42.296[A,B], S42.301B, S42.302-S42.309[A,B], S42.312-S42.319[A], S42.321B, S42.322-S42.323[A,B], S42.324B, S42.325-S42.326[A,B], S42.331B, S42.332-S42.333[A,B], S42.334B, S42.335-S42.336[A,B], S42.341B, S42.342-S42.343[A,B], S42.344B, S42.345-S42.346[A,B], S42.351B, S42.352-S42.353[A,B], S42.354B,

S42.355-S42.356[A,B], S42.361B, S42.362-S42.363[A,B], S42.364B, S42.365-S42.366[A,B], S42.391B, S42.392-S42.399[A,B], S42.401B, S42.402-S42.409[A,B], S42.411B, S42.412-S42.413[A,B], S42.414B, S42.415-S42.416[A,B], S42.421B, S42.422-S42.423[A,B], S42.424B, S42.425-S42.426[A,B], S42.431B, S42.432-S42.433[A,B], S42.434B, S42.435-S42.436[A,B], S42.441B, S42.442-S42.443[A,B], S42.444B, S42.445-S42.446[A,B], S42.447B, S42.448-S42.449[A,B], S42.451B, S42.452-S42.453[A,B], S42.454B, S42.455-S42.456[A,B], S42.461B, S42.462-S42.463[A,B], S42.464B, S42.465-S42.466[A,B], S42.471B, S42.472-S42.473[A,B], S42.474B, S42.475-S42.476[A,B], S42.482-S42.489[A], S42.491B, S42.492-S42.493[A,B], S42.494B, S42.495-S42.92X[A,B], S49.002-S49.009[A], S49.012-S49.019[A], S49.022-S49.029[A], S49.032-S49.039[A], S49.042-S49.049[A], S49.092-S49.099[A], S49.102-S49.109[A], S49.112-S49.119[A], S49.122-S49.129[A], S49.132-S49.139[A], S49.142-S49.149[A], S49.192-S49.199[A]

PDX Collection 1248
S42.201-S42.266[A,B], S42.271-S42.279[A], S42.291-S42.309[A,B], S42.311-S42.319[A], S42.321-S42.476[A,B], S42.481-S42.489[A], S42.491-S42.92X[A,B], S49.001-S49.199[A]

PDX Collection 1249
S42.311A, S42.319-S42.321[A], S42.323-S42.324[A], S42.326-S42.331[A], S42.333-S42.334[A], S42.336-S42.341[A], S42.343-S42.344[A], S42.346-S42.351[A], S42.353-S42.354[A], S42.356-S42.361[A], S42.363-S42.364[A], S42.366-S42.391[A], S42.399A

PDX Collection 1250
S42.312-S42.319[A], S42.322-S42.323[A], S42.325-S42.326[A], S42.332-S42.333[A], S42.335-S42.336[A], S42.342-S42.343[A], S42.345-S42.346[A], S42.352-S42.353[A], S42.355-S42.356[A], S42.362-S42.363[A], S42.365-S42.366[A], S42.392-S42.399[A]

PDX Collection 1251
S42.311-S42.399[A]

PDX Collection 1252
M99.18, S43.201A, S43.203-S43.204[A], S43.206A, S43.211A, S43.213-S43.214[A], S43.216A, S43.221A, S43.223-S43.224[A], S43.226A

PDX Collection 1253
M99.18, S43.202-S43.203[A], S43.205-S43.206[A], S43.212-S43.213[A], S43.215-S43.216[A], S43.222-S43.223[A], S43.225-S43.226[A]

PDX Collection 1254
S45.001A, S45.009-S45.011[A], S45.019-S45.091[A], S45.099A, S45.301A, S45.309-S45.311[A], S45.319-S45.391[A], S45.399-S45.801[A], S45.809-S45.811[A], S45.819-S45.891[A], S45.899-S45.901[A], S45.909-S45.911[A], S45.919-S45.991[A], S45.999[A], S55.201A, S55.209-S55.211[A], S55.219-S55.291[A], S55.299-S55.801[A], S55.809-S55.811[A], S55.819-S55.891[A], S55.899-S55.901[A], S55.909-S55.911[A], S55.919-S55.991[A], S55.999A, S65.801A, S65.809-S65.811[A], S65.819-S65.891[A], S65.899-S65.901[A], S65.909-S65.911[A], S65.919-S65.991[A], S65.999A

PDX Collection 1255
S45.002-S45.009[A], S45.012-S45.019[A], S45.092-S45.099[A], S45.302-S45.309[A], S45.312-S45.319[A], S45.392-S45.399[A],

S45.802-S45.809[A], S45.812-S45.819[A], S45.892-S45.899[A], S45.902-S45.909[A], S45.912-S45.919[A], S45.992-S45.999[A], S55.202-S55.209[A], S55.212-S55.219[A], S55.292-S55.299[A], S55.802-S55.809[A], S55.812-S55.819[A], S55.892-S55.899[A], S55.902-S55.909[A], S55.912-S55.919[A], S55.992-S55.999[A], S65.802-S65.809[A], S65.812-S65.819[A], S65.892-S65.899[A], S65.902-S65.909[A], S65.912-S65.919[A], S65.992-S65.999[A]

PDX Collection 1256
S45.001-S45.099[A], S45.301-S45.399[A], S45.801-S45.999[A], S55.201-S55.999[A], S65.801-S65.999[A]

PDX Collection 1257
S45.101A, S45.109-S45.111[A], S45.119-S45.191[A], S45.199-S45.201[A], S45.209A-S45.211[A], S45.219-S45.291[A], S45.299-S45.301[A], S45.309-S45.311[A], S45.319-S45.391[A], S45.399-S45.801[A], S45.809-S45.811[A], S45.819-S45.891[A], S45.899-S45.901[A], S45.909-S45.911[A], S45.919-S45.991[A], S45.999A, S55.201[A], S55.209-S55.211[A], S55.219-S55.291[A], S55.299-S55.801[A], S55.809-S55.811[A], S55.819-S55.891[A], S55.899-S55.901[A], S55.909-S55.911[A], S55.919-S55.991[A], S55.999A, S65.801A, S65.809-S65.811[A], S65.819-S65.891[A], S65.899-S65.901[A], S65.909-S65.911[A], S65.919-S65.991[A], S65.999A

PDX Collection 1258
S45.102-S45.109[A], S45.112-S45.119[A], S45.192-S45.199[A], S45.202-S45.209[A], S45.212-S45.219[A], S45.292-S45.299[A], S45.302-S45.309[A], S45.312-S45.319[A], S45.392-S45.399[A], S45.802-S45.809[A], S45.812-S45.819[A], S45.892-S45.899[A], S45.902-S45.909[A], S45.912-S45.919[A], S45.992-S45.999[A], S55.202-S55.209[A], S55.212-S55.219[A], S55.292-S55.299[A], S55.802-S55.809[A], S55.812-S55.819[A], S55.892-S55.899[A], S55.902-S55.909[A], S55.912-S55.919[A], S55.992-S55.999[A], S65.802-S65.809[A], S65.812-S65.819[A], S65.892-S65.899[A], S65.902-S65.909[A], S65.912-S65.919[A], S65.992-S65.999[A]

PDX Collection 1259
S45.101-S45.999[A], S55.201-S55.999[A], S65.801-S65.999[A]

PDX Collection 1260
S45.301A, S45.309-S45.311[A], S45.319-S45.391[A], S45.399-S45.801[A], S45.809-S45.811[A], S45.819-S45.891[A], S45.899-S45.901[A], S45.909-S45.911[A], S45.919-S45.991[A], S45.999A, S55.001A, S55.009-S55.011[A], S55.019-S55.091[A], S55.099A, S55.201A, S55.209-S55.211[A], S55.219-S55.291[A], S55.299-S55.801[A], S55.809-S55.811[A], S55.819-S55.891[A], S55.899-S55.901[A], S55.909-S55.911[A], S55.919-S55.991[A], S55.999A, S65.001A, S65.009-S65.011[A], S65.019-S65.091[A], S65.099A, S65.201A, S65.209-S65.211[A], S65.219-S65.291[A], S65.299-S65.301[A], S65.309-S65.311[A], S65.319-S65.391[A], S65.399-S65.401[A], S65.409-S65.411[A], S65.419-S65.491[A], S65.499-S65.500[A], S65.502A, S65.504A, S65.506A, S65.508-S65.510[A], S65.512A, S65.514A, S65.516A,

S65.518-S65.590[A], S65.592A, S65.594A, S65.596A,
S65.598-S65.801[A], S65.809-S65.811[A],
S65.819-S65.891[A], S65.899-S65.901[A],
S65.909-S65.911[A], S65.919-S65.991[A], S65.999A

PDX Collection 1261
S45.302-S45.309[A], S45.312-S45.319[A],
S45.392-S45.399[A], S45.802-S45.809[A],
S45.812-S45.819[A], S45.892-S45.899[A],
S45.902-S45.909[A], S45.912-S45.919[A],
S45.992-S45.999[A], S55.002 S55.009[A],
S55.012-S55.019[A], S55.092-S55.099[A],
S55.202-S55.209[A], S55.212-S55.219[A],
S55.292-S55.299[A], S55.802-S55.809[A],
S55.812-S55.819[A], S55.892-S55.899[A],
S55.902-S55.909[A], S55.912-S55.919[A],
S55.992-S55.999[A], S65.002-S65.009[A],
S65.012-S65.019[A], S65.092-S65.099[A],
S65.202-S65.209[A], S65.212-S65.219[A],
S65.292-S65.299[A], S65.302-S65.309[A],
S65.312-S65.319[A]. S65.392-S65.399[A],
S65.402-S65.409[A], S65.412-S65.419[A],
S65.492-S65.499[A], S65.501A, S65.503A, S65.505A,
S65.507-S65.509[A], S65.511A, S65.513A, S65.515A,
S65.517-S65.519[A], S65.591A, S65.593A, S65.595A,
S65.597-S65.599[A], S65.802-S65.809[A],
S65.812-S65.819[A], S65.892-S65.899[A],
S65.902-S65.909[A], S65.912-S65.919[A],
S65.992-S65.999[A]

PDX Collection 1262
S45.301-S45.999[A], S55.001-S55.099[A],
S55.201-S55.999[A], S65.001-S65.099[A],
S65.201-S65.999[A]

PDX Collection 1263
S41.001A, S41.009-S41.011[A], S41.019-S41.021[A],
S41.029-S41.031[A], S41.039-S41.041[A],
S41.049-S41.051[A], S41.059-S41.101[A],
S41.109 S41.111[A], S41.119-S41.121[A],
S41.129-S41.131[A], S41.139-S41.141[A],
S41.149-S41.151[A], S41.159A, S46.021A, S46.029A,
S46.121A, S46.129A, S46.221A, S46.229A, S46.321A,
S46.329A, S46.821A, S46.829A, S46.921A, S46.929A

PDX Collection 1264
S41.002-S41.009[A], S41.012-S41.019[A],
S41.022-S41.029[A], S41.032-S41.039[A],
S41.042-S41.049[A], S41.052-S41.059[A],
S41.102-S41.109[A], S41.112-S41.119[A],
S41.122-S41.129[A], S41.132-S41.139[A],
S41.142-S41.149[A], S41.152-S41.159[A],
S46.022-S46.029[A], S46.122-S46.129[A],
S46.222-S46.229[A], S46.322-S46.329[A],
S46.822-S46.829[A], S46.922-S46.929[A]

PDX Collection 1265
S41.001-S41.159[A], S46.021-S46.029[A],
S46.121-S46.129[A], S46.221-S46.229[A],
S46.321-S46.329[A], S46.821-S46.829[A],
S46.921 S46.929[A]

PDX Collection 1266
S41.001A, S41.009-S41.011[A], S41.019-S41.021[A],
S41.029-S41.031[A], S41.039-S41.041[A], S41.049-S41.051[A],
S41.059-S41.101[A], S41.109-S41.111[A], S41.119-S41.121[A],
S41.129-S41.131[A], S41.139-S41.141[A], S41.149-S41.151[A],
S41.159A, S46.021A, S46.029A, S46.121A, S46.129A, S46.221A,
S46.229A, S46.321A, S46.329A, S46.821A, S46.829A, S46.921A,
S46.929A, S48.011A, S48.019-S48.021[A], S48.029-S48.111[A],
S48.119-S48.121[A], S48.129-S48.911[A], S48.919-S48.921[A],
S48.929A, S51.001A, S51.009-S51.011[A], S51.019-S51.021[A],
S51.029-S51.031[A], S51.039-S51.041[A], S51.049-S51.051[A],

S51.059-S51.801[A], S51.809-S51.811[A], S51.819-S51.821[A],
S51.829-S51.831[A], S51.839-S51.841[A], S51.849-S51.851[A],
S51.859A, S56.021A, S56.029A, S56.121A, S56.123A, S56.125A,
S56.127A, S56.129A, S56.221A, S56.229A, S56.321A, S56.329A,
S56.421A, S56.423A, S56.425A, S56.427A, S56.429A, S56.521A,
S56.529A, S56.821A, S56.829A, S56.921A, S56.929A, S58.011A,
S58.019-S58.021[A], S58.029-S58.111[A], S58.119-S58.121[A],
S58.129-S58.911[A], S58.919-S58.921[A], S58.929A, S61.001A,
S61.009-S61.011[A], S61.019-S61.021[A], S61.029-S61.031[A],
S61.039-S61.041[A], S61.049-S61.051[A], S61.059-S61.101[A],
S61.109-S61.111[A], S61.119-S61.121[A], S61.129-S61.131[A],
S61.139-S61.141[A], S61.149-S61.151[A], S61.159-S61.200[A],
S61.202A, S61.204A, S61.206A, S61.208-S61.210[A],
S61.212A, S61.214A, S61.216A, S61.218-S61.220[A], S61.222A,
S61.224A, S61.226A, S61.228-S61.230[A], S61.232A,
S61.234A, S61.236A, S61.238-S61.240[A], S61.242A,
S61.244A, S61.246A, S61.248-S61.250[A], S61.252A, S61.254A,
S61.256A, S61.258-S61.300[A], S61.302A, S61.304A,
S61.306A, S61.308-S61.310[A], S61.312A, S61.314A,
S61.316A, S61.318-S61.320[A], S61.322A, S61.324A,
S61.326A, S61.328-S61.330[A], S61.332A, S61.334A,
S61.336A, S61.338-S61.340[A], S61.342A, S61.344A,
S61.346A, S61.348-S61.350[A], S61.352A, S61.354A, S61.356A,
S61.358-S61.401[A], S61.409-S61.411[A], S61.419-S61.421[A],
S61.429-S61.431[A], S61.439-S61.441[A], S61.449-S61.451[A],
S61.459-S61.501[A], S61.509-S61.511[A], S61.519-S61.521[A],
S61.529-S61.531[A], S61.539-S61.541[A], S61.549-S61.551[A],
S61.559A, S66.021A, S66.029A, S66.120A, S66.122A, S66.124A,
S66.126A, S66.128-S66.129[A], S66.221A, S66.229A, S66.320A,
S66.322A, S66.324A, S66.326A, S66.328-S66.329[A],
S66.421A, S66.429A, S66.520A, S66.522A, S66.524A, S66.526A,
S66.528-S66.529[A], S66.821A, S66.829A, S66.921A, S66.929A,
S68.011A, S68.019-S68.021[A], S68.029-S68.110[A],
S68.112A, S68.114A, S68.116A, S68.118-S68.120[A], S68.122A,
S68.124A, S68.126A, S68.128-S68.411[A], S68.419-S68.421[A],
S68.429-S68.511[A], S68.519-S68.521[A], S68.529-S68.610[A],
S68.612A, S68.614A, S68.616A, S68.618-S68.620[A], S68.622A,
S68.624A, S68.626A, S68.628 S68.711[A], S68.719-S68.721[A],
S68.729[A], T07.XXX-T14.91X[A], T79.A0X-T79.9XX[A]

PDX Collection 1267
S41.002-S41.009[A], S41.012 S41.019[A], S41.022-S41.029[A],
S41.032-S41.039[A], S41.042-S41.049[A], S41.052-S41.059[A],
S41.102-S41.109[A], S41.112-S41.119[A], S41.122-S41.129[A],
S41.132-S41.139[A], S41.142-S41.149[A], S41.152 S41.159[A],
S46.022-S46.029[A], S46.122-S46.129[A], S46.222-S46.229[A],
S46.322-S46.329[A], S46.822-S46.829[A], S46.922-S46.929[A],
S48.012-S48.019[A], S48.022-S48.029[A], S48.112-S48.119[A],
S48.122-S48.129[A], S48.912-S48.919[A], S48.922-S48.929[A],
S51.002-S51.009[A], S51.012-S51.019[A], S51.022-S51.029[A],
S51.032-S51.039[A], S51.042-S51.049[A], S51.052-S51.059[A],
S51.802-S51.809[A], S51.812-S51.819[A], S51.822-S51.829[A],
S51.832-S51.839[A], S51.842-S51.849[A], S51.852-S51.859[A],
S56.022-S56.029[A], S56.122A, S56.124A, S56.126A,
S56.128-S56.129[A], S56.222-S56.229[A], S56.322-S56.329[A],
S56.422A, S56.424A, S56.426A, S56.428-S56.429[A],
S56.522-S56.529[A], S56.822-S56.829[A], S56.922-S56.929[A],
S58.012-S58.019[A], S58.022-S58.029[A], S58.112-S58.119[A],
S58.122-S58.129[A], S58.912-S58.919[A], S58.922-S58.929[A],
S61.002-S61.009[A], S61.012-S61.019[A], S61.022-S61.029[A],
S61.032-S61.039[A], S61.042-S61.049[A], S61.052-S61.059[A],
S61.102-S61.109[A], S61.112-S61.119[A], S61.122-S61.129[A].
S61.132-S61.139[A], S61.142-S61.149[A], S61.152-S61.159[A],
S61.201A, S61.203A, S61.205A, S61.207-S61.209[A],
S61.211A, S61.213A, S61.215A, S61.217-S61.219[A], S61.221A,
S61.223A, S61.225A, S61.227-S61.229[A], S61.231A,
S61.233A, S61.235A, S61.237-S61.239[A], S61.241A, S61.243A,
S61.245A, S61.247-S61.249[A], S61.251A, S61.253A,
S61.255A, S61.257-S61.259[A], S61.301A, S61.303A,

S61.305A, S61.307-S61.309[A], S61.311A, S61.313A,
S61.315A, S61.317-S61.319[A], S61.321A, S61.323A,
S61.325A, S61.327-S61.329[A], S61.331A, S61.333A,
S61.335A, S61.337-S61.339[A], S61.341A, S61.343A, S61.345A,
S61.347-S61.349[A], S61.351A, S61.353A, S61.355A,
S61.357-S61.359[A], S61.402-S61.409[A], S61.412-S61.419[A],
S61.422-S61.429[A], S61.432-S61.439[A], S61.442-S61.449[A],
S61.452-S61.459[A], S61.502-S61.509[A], S61.512-S61.519[A],
S61.522-S61.529[A], S61.532-S61.539[A], S61.542-S61.549[A],
S61.552-S61.559[A], S66.022-S66.029[A], S66.121[A],
S66.123A, S66.125A, S66.127-S66.129[A], S66.222-S66.229[A],
S66.321A, S66.323A, S66.325A, S66.327-S66.329[A],
S66.422-S66.429[A], S66.521A, S66.523A, S66.525A,
S66.527-S66.529[A], S66.822-S66.829[A], S66.922-S66.929[A],
S68.012-S68.019[A], S68.022-S68.029[A], S68.111A, S68.113A,
S68.115A, S68.117-S68.119[A], S68.121A, S68.123A, S68.125A,
S68.127-S68.129[A], S68.412-S68.419[A], S68.422-S68.429[A],
S68.512-S68.519[A], S68.522-S68.529[A], S68.611A, S68.613A,
S68.615A, S68.617-S68.619[A], S68.621A, S68.623A, S68.625A,
S68.627-S68.629[A], S68.712-S68.719[A], S68.722-S68.729[A],
T07.XXX-T14.91X[A], T79.A0X-T79.9XX[A]

PDX Collection 1268
S41.001-S41.159[A], S46.021-S46.029[A],
S46.121-S46.129[A], S46.221-S46.229[A],
S46.321-S46.329[A], S46.821-S46.829[A],
S46.921-S46.929[A], S48.011-S48.929[A],
S51.001-S51.859[A], S56.021-S56.029[A],
S56.121-S56.129[A], S56.221-S56.229[A],
S56.321-S56.329[A], S56.421-S56.479[A],
S56.521-S56.529[A], S56.821-S56.829[A],
S56.921-S56.929[A], S58.011-S58.929[A],
S61.001-S61.559[A], S66.021 S66.029[A],
S66.120-S66.129[A], S66.221-S66.229[A],
S66.320-S66.329[A], S66.421-S66.429[A],
S66.520-S66.529[A], S66.821-S66.829[A],
S66.921-S66.929[A], S68.011-S68.729[A],
T07.XXX-T14.91X[A], T79.A0X-T79.9XX[A]

PDX Collection 1269
S52.001-S52.009[B,C], S52.021-S52.109[B,C],
S52.121-S52.189[B,C], S52.201-S52.209[A,B,C],
S52.211-S52.219[A], S52.221-S52.266[A,B,C],
S52.271-S52.279[B,C], S52.281-S52.309[A,B,C],
S52.311-S52.319[A], S52.321-S52.516[A,B,C],
S52.531-S52.616[A,B,C], S52.691-S52.92X[A,B,C],
S59.001-S59.099[A], S59.201-S59.299[A], S62.90XB

PDX Collection 1270
S52.001 [A,B,C], S52.002[B,C], S52.009 [A,B,C],
S52.011[A], S52.019[A], S52.021[A,B,C], S52.022[B,C],
S52.023 S52.024[A,B,C], S52.025[B,C], S52.026-S52.031[A,B,C],
S52.032[B,C], S52.033-S52.034[A,B,C], S52.035[B,C],
S52.036-S52.041[A,B,C], S52.042[B,C], S52.043-S52.044[A,B,C],
S52.045[B,C], S52.046-S52.091[A,B,C], S52.092[B,C],
S52.099-S52.101[A,B,C], S52.102[B,C], S52.109[A,B,C],
S52.111A, S52.119A, S52.121[A,B,C], S52.122[B,C],
S52.123-S52.124[A,B,C], S52.125[B,C], S52.126-S52.131[A,B,C],
S52.132[B,C], S52.133 S52.134[A,B,C], S52.135[B, C],
S52.136-S52.181[A,B,C], S52.182[B,C], S52.189-S52.201[A,B,C],
S52.202[B,C], S52.209[A,B,C], S52.211A, S52.219A,
S52.221[A,C], S52.222[B,C], S52.223-S52.224[A,B,C],
S52.225[B,C], S52.226-S52.231[C], S52.232[B,C],
S52.233-S52.234[A,B,C], S52.235[B,C], S52.236-S52.241[C],
S52.242[B,C], S52.243-S52.244[A,B,C], S52.245[B,C],
S52.246-S52.251[A,B,C], S52.252[B,C], S52.253-S52.254[A,B,C],
S52.255[B,C], S52.256-S52.261[A,B,C], S52.262[BC],
S52.263-S52.264[A,B,C], S52.265[B,C], S52.266-S52.271[A,B,C],
S52.272[B,C], S52.279-S52.281[A,B,C], S52.282[B,C],
S52.283-S52.291[A,B,C], S52.292[B,C], S52.299-S52.301[A,B,C],
S52.302[B,C], S52.309[A,B,C], S52.311A, S52.319A,

S52.321[A,B,C], S52.322[B,C], S52.323-S52.324[A,B,C], S52.325[B,C], S52.326-S52.331[A,B,C], S52.332[B,C], S52.333-S52.334[A,B,C], S52.335[B,C], S52.336-S52.341[A,B,C], S52.342[B,C], S52.343-S52.344[A,B,C], S52.345[B,C], S52.346-S52.351[A,B,C], S52.352[B,C], S52.353-S52.354[A,B,C], S52.355[B,C], S52.356-S52.361[A,B,C], S52.362[B,C], S52.363-S52.364[A,B,C], S52.365[B,C], S52.366-S52.371[A,B,C], S52.372[B,C], S52.379-S52.381[A,B,C], S52.382[B,C], S52.389-S52.391[A,B,C], S52.392[B,C], S52.399-S52.501[A,B,C], S52.502[B,C], S52.509-S52.511[A,B,C], S52.512[B,C], S52.513-S52.514[A,B,C], S52.515[B,C], S52.16[A,B,C], S52.521[A], S52.529[A], S52.531[A,B,C], S52.532[B,C], S52.539-S52.541[A,B,C], S52.542[B,C], S52.549-S52.551[A,B,C], S52.552[B,C], S52.559-S52.561[A,B,C], S52.562[B,C], S52.569-S52.571[A,B,C], S52.572[B,C], S52.579-S52.591[A,B,C], S52.592[B,C], S52.599-S52.601[A,B,C], S52.602[B,C], S52.609-S52.611[A,B,C], S52.612[B,C], S52.613-S52.614[A,B,C], S52.615[B,C], S52.616[A,B,C], S52.621[A], S52.629A, S52.691[A,B,C], S52.692[B,C], S52.699-S52.92X[A,B,C], S59.001A, S59.009-S59.011[A], S59.019-S59.021[A], S59.029-S59.031[A], S59.039-S59.041[A], S59.049-S59.091[A], S59.099-S59.101[A], S59.109-S59.111[A], S59.119-S59.121[A], S59.129-S59.131[A], S59.139-S59.141[A], S59.149-S59.191[A], S59.199-S59.201[A], S59.209-S59.211[A], S59.219-S59.221[A], S59.229-S59.231[A], S59.239-S59.241[A], S59.249-S59.291[A], S59.299A

PDX Collection 1271

S52.001[B,C], S52.002-S52.009[A,B,C], S52.012-S52.019[A], S52.021[B,C], S52.022-S52.023[A,B,C], S52.024[B,C], S52.025-S52.026[A,B,C], S52.031[B,C], S52.032-S52.033[A,B,C], S52.034[B,C], S52.035-S52.036[A,B,C], S52.041[B,C], S52.042-S52.043[A,B,C], S52.044[B,C], S52.045-S52.046[A,B,C], S52.091[B,C], S52.092-S52.099[A,B,C], S52.101[B,C], S52.102-S52.109[A,B,C], S52.112-S52.119[A], S52.121[B,C], S52.122-S52.123[A,B,C], S52.124[B,C], S52.125-S52.126[A,B,C], S52.131[B,C], S52.132-S52.133[A,B,C], S52.134[B,C], S52.135-S52.136[A,B,C], S52.181[B,C], S52.182-S52.189[A,B,C], S52.201[B,C], S52.202-S52.209[A,B,C], S52.212-S52.219[A], S52.221[B,C], S52.222-S52.223[A,B,C], S52.224[B,C], S52.225-S52.226[A,B,C], S52.231[B,C], S52.232-S52.233[A,B,C], S52.234[B,C], S52.235-S52.236[A,B,C], S52.241[B,C], S52.242-S52.243[A,B,C], S52.244[B,C], S52.245-S52.246[A,B,C], S52.251[B,C], S52.252-S52.253[A,B,C], S52.254[B,C], S52.255-S52.256[A,B,C], S52.261[B,C], S52.262-S52.263[A,B,C], S52.264[B,C], S52.265-S52.266[A,B,C], S52.271[B,C], S52.272-S52.279[A,B,C], S52.281[B,C], S52.282-S52.283[A,B,C], S52.291[B,C], S52.292-S52.299[A,B,C], S52.301[B,C], S52.302-S52.309[A,B,C], S52.312-S52.319[A], S52.321[B,C], S52.322-S52.323[A,B,C], S52.324[B,C], S52.325-S52.326[A,B,C], S52.331[B,C], S52.332-S52.333[A,B,C], S52.334[B,C], S52.335-S52.336[A,B,C], S52.341[B,C], S52.342-S52.343[A,B,C], S52.344[B,C], S52.345-S52.346[A,B,C], S52.351[B,C], S52.352-S52.353[A,B,C], S52.354[B,C], S52.355-S52.356[A,B,C], S52.361[B,C], S52.362-S52.363[A,B,C], S52.364[B,C], S52.365-S52.366[A,B,C], S52.371[B,C], S52.372-S52.379[A,B,C], S52.381[B,C], S52.382-S52.389[A,B,C], S52.391[B,C], S52.392-S52.399[A,B,C], S52.501[B,C], S52.502-S52.509[A,B,C], S52.511[B,C], S52.512-S52.513[A,B,C], S52.514[B,C], S52.515-S52.516[A,B,C], S52.522-S52.529[A], S52.531[B,C], S52.532-S52.539[A,B,C], S52.541[B,C], S52.542-S52.549[A,B,C], S52.551[B,C], S52.552-S52.559[A,B,C], S52.561[B,C], S52.562-S52.569[A,B,C], S52.571[B,C], S52.572-S52.579[A,B,C], S52.591[B,C], S52.592-S52.599[A,B,C], S52.601[B,C], S52.602-S52.609[A,B,C], S52.611[B,C], S52.612-S52.613[A,B,C], S52.614[B,C], S52.615-S52.616[A,B,C], S52.622-S52.629[A], S52.691[B,C], S52.692-S52.92X[A,B,C], S59.002-S59.009[A], S59.012-S59.019[A], S59.022-S59.029[A], S59.032-S59.039[A], S59.042-S59.049[A], S59.092-S59.099[A], S59.102-S59.109[A],

S59.112-S59.119[A], S59.122-S59.129[A], S59.132-S59.139[A], S59.142-S59.149[A], S59.192-S59.199[A], S59.202-S59.209[A], S59.212-S59.219[A], S59.222-S59.229[A], S59.232-S59.239[A], S59.242-S59.249[A], S59.292-S59.299[A]

PDX Collection 1272

S52.001-S52.009[A,B,C], S52.011-S52.019[A], S52.021-S52.109[A,B,C], S52.111-S52.119[A], S52.121-S52.209[A,B,C], S52.211-S52.219[A], S52.221-S52.309[A,B,C], S52.311-S52.319[A], S52.321-S52.516[A,B,C], S52.521-S52.529[A], S52.531-S52.616[A,B,C], S52.621-S52.629[A], S52.691-S52.92X[A,B,C], S59.001-S59.299[A]

PDX Collection 1273

S52.001-S52.009[BC], S52.021-S52.109[BC], S52.121-S52.189[BC], S52.201-S52.209[ABC], S52.211-S52.219[A], S52.221-S52.266[ABC], S52.271-S52.279[BC], S52.281-S52.309[ABC], S52.311-S52.319[A], S52.321-S52.516[ABC], S52.531-S52.549[BC], S52.551-S52.616[ABC], S52.691-S52.92X[ABC], S59.001-S59.099[A], S59.201-S59.299[A], S62.90XB

PDX Collection 1274

S45.301A, S45.309-S45.311[A], S45.319-S45.391[A], S45.399-S45.801[A], S45.809-S45.811[A], S45.819-S45.891[A], S45.899-S45.901[A], S45.909-S45.911[A], S45.919-S45.991[A], S45.999A, S55.001A, S55.009-S55.011[A], S55.019-S55.091[A], S55.099A, S55.201A, S55.209-S55.211[A], S55.219-S55.291[A], S55.299-S55.801[A], S55.809-S55.811[A], S55.819-S55.891[A], S55.899-S55.901[A], S55.909-S55.911[A], S55.919-S55.991[A], S55.999A, S65.001A, S65.009-S65.011[A], S65.019-S65.091[A], S65.099A, S65.801A, S65.809-S65.811[A], S65.819-S65.891[A], S65.899-S65.901[A], S65.909-S65.911[A], S65.919-S65.991[A], S65.999A

PDX Collection 1275

S45.302-S45.309[A], S45.312-S45.319[A], S45.392-S45.399[A], S45.802-S45.809[A], S45.812-S45.819[A], S45.892-S45.899[A], S45.902-S45.909[A], S45.912-S45.919[A], S45.992-S45.999[A], S55.002-S55.009[A], S55.012-S55.019[A], S55.092-S55.099[A], S55.202-S55.209[A], S55.212-S55.219[A], S55.292-S55.299[A], S55.802-S55.809[A], S55.812-S55.819[A], S55.892-S55.899[A], S55.902-S55.909[A], S55.912-S55.919[A], S55.992-S55.999[A], S65.002-S65.009[A], S65.012-S65.019[A], S65.092-S65.099[A], S65.802-S65.809[A] S65.812-S65.819[A], S65.892-S65.899[A], S65.902-S65.909[A], S65.912-S65.919[A], S65.992-S65.999[A]

PDX Collection 1276

S45.301-S45.999[A], S55.001-S55.099[A], S55.201-S55.999[A], S65.001-S65.099[A], S65.801-S65.999[A]

PDX Collection 1277

S45.301A, S45.309-S45.311[A], S45.319-S45.391[A], S45.399-S45.801[A], S45.809-S45.811[A], S45.819-S45.891[A], S45.899-S45.901[A], S45.909-S45.911[A], S45.919-S45.991[A], S45.999A, S55.101A, S55.109-S55.111[A], S55.119-S55.191[A], S55.199-S55.201[A], S55.209-S55.211[A], S55.219-S55.291[A], S55.299-S55.801[A], S55.809-S55.811[A], S55.819-S55.891[A], S55.899-S55.901[A], S55.909-S55.911[A], S55.919-S55.991[A], S55.999A, S65.101A,

S65.109-S65.111[A], S65.119-S65.191[A], S65.199A, S65.801A, S65.809-S65.811[A], S65.819-S65.891[A], S65.899-S65.901[A], S65.909-S65.911[A], S65.919-S65.991[A], S65.999A

PDX Collection 1278

S45.302-S45.309[A], S45.312-S45.319[A], S45.392-S45.399[A], S45.802-S45.809[A], S45.812-S45.819[A], S45.892-S45.899[A], S45.902-S45.909[A], S45.912-S45.919[A], S45.992-S45.999[A], S55.102-S55.109[A], S55.112-S55.119[A], S55.192-S55.199[A], S55.202-S55.209[A], S55.212-S55.219[A], S55.292-S55.299[A], S55.802A-S55.809[A], S55.812-S55.819[A], S55.892-S55.899[A], S55.902-S55.909[A], S55.912-S55.919[A], S55.992-S55.999[A], S65.102-S65.109[A], S55.112-S65.119[A], S65.192-S65.199[A], S65.802-S65.809[A], S65.812-S65.819[A], S65.892-S65.899[A], S65.902-S65.909[A], S65.912-S65.919[A], S65.992-S65.999[A]

PDX Collection 1279

S45.301-S45.999[A], S55.101-S55.999[A], S65.101-S65.199[A], S65.801-S65.999[A]

PDX Collection 1280

S51.001[A], S51.009-S51.011[A], S51.019-S51.021[A], S51.029-S51.031[A], S51.039-S51.041[A], S51.049-S51.051[A], S51.059-S51.801[A], S51.809-S51.811[A], S51.819-S51.821[A], S51.829-S51.831[A], S51.839-S51.841[A], S51.849-S51.851[A], S51.859A, S56.021A, S56.029A, S56.121A, S56.123A, S56.125A, S56.127A, S56.129A, S56.221A, S56.229A, S56.321A, S56.329A, S56.421A, S56.423A, S56.425A, S56.427A, S56.429A, S56.521A, S56.529A, S56.821A, S56.829A, S56.921A, S56.929A, S61.501A, S61.509-S61.511[A], S61.519-S61.521[A], S61.529-S61.531[A], S61.539-S61.541[A], S61.549-S61.551[A], S61.559A

PDX Collection 1281

S51.002-S51.009[A], S51.012-S51.019[A], S51.022-S51.029[A], S51.032-S51.039[A], S51.042-S51.049[A], S51.052-S51.059[A], S51.802-S51.809[A], S51.812-S51.819[A], S51.822-S51.829[A], S51.832-S51.839[A], S51.842-S51.849[A], S51.852-S51.859[A], S56.022-S56.029[A], S56.122A, S56.124A, S56.126A, S56.128-S56.129[A], S56.222-S56.229[A], S56.322-S56.329[A], S56.422A, S56.424A, S56.426A, S56.428-S56.429[A], S56.522-S56.529[A], S56.822-S56.829[A], S56.922-S56.929[A], S61.502-S61.509[A], S61.512-S61.519[A], S61.522-S61.529[A], S61.532-S61.539[A], S61.542-S61.549[A], S61.552-S61.559[A]

PDX Collection 1282

S51.001-S51.859[A], S56.021-S56.029[A], S56.121-S56.129[A], S56.221-S56.229[A], S56.321-S56.329[A], S56.421-S56.429[A], S56.521-S56.529[A], S56.821-S56.829[A], S56.921-S56.929[A], S61.501-S61.559[A]

PDX Collection 1283

S62.001-S62.186[A,B]

PDX Collection 1284

S62.201-S62.399[B], S62.90X[A]

PDX Collection 1285

S62.501-S62.669[A,B], S62.90XA, S62.91X-S62.92X[A,B]

PDX Collection 1286
S42.201-S42.266[A,B], S42.271-S42.279[A],
S42.291-S42.309[A,B], S42.311-S42.319[A],
S42.321-S42.476[A,B], S42.481-S42.489[A],
S42.491-S42.92X[A,B], S49.001-S49.199[A],
S52.001-S52.009[A,B,C], S52.021-S52.109[A,B,C],
S52.121-S52.209[A,B,C], S52.211-S52.219[A],
S52.221-S52.309[A,B,C], S52.311-S52.319[A],
S52.321-S52.616[A,B,C], S52.691-S52.92X[A,B,C],
S59.001-S59.299[A], S62.001-S62.92X[A,B]

PDX Collection 1287
S62.501-S62.669[A,B], S62.90X[B], S62.91X-S62.92X[A,B]

PDX Collection 1288
S45.301[A], S45.309-S45.311[A], S45.319-S45.391[A],
S45.399-S45.801[A], S45.809-S45.811[A],
S45.819-S45.891[A], S45.899-S45.901[A],
S45.909-S45.911[A], S45.919-S45.991[A], S45.999A,
S55.201A, S55.209-S55.211[A], S55.219-S55.291[A],
S55.299-S55.801[A], S55.809-S55.811[A],
S55.819-S55.891[A], S55.899-S55.901[A],
S55.909-S55.911[A], S55.919-S55.991[A], S55.999[A],
S65.201A, S65.209-S65.211[A], S65.219-S65.291[A],
S65.299-S65.301[A], S65.309-S65.311[A], S65.319-
S65.391[A], S65.399A, S65.801A, S65.809-S65.811[A],
S65.819-S65.891[A], S65.899-S65.901[A],
S65.909-S65.911[A], S65.919-S65.991[A], S65.999A

PDX Collection 1289
S45.302-S45.309[A], S45.312-S45.319[A],
S45.392-S45.399[A], S45.802-S45.809[A],
S45.812-S45.819[A], S45.892-S45.899[A],
S45.902-S45.909[A], S45.912-S45.919[A],
S45.992-S45.999[A], S55.202-S55.209[A],
S55.212-S55.219[A], S55.292-S55.299[A],
S55.802-S55.809[A], S55.812-S55.819[A],
S55.892-S55.899[A], S55.902-S55.909[A],
S55.912-S55.919[A], S55.992-S55.999[A],
S65.202-S65.209[A], S65.212-S65.219[A],
S65.292-S65.299[A], S65.302-S65.309[A],
S65.312-S65.319[A], S65.392-S65.399[A],
S65.802-S65.809[A], S65.812-S65.819[A],
S65.892-S65.899[A], S65.902-S65.909[A],
S65.912-S65.919[A], S65.992-S65.999[A]

PDX Collection 1290
S45.301-S45.999[A], S55.201-S55.999[A],
S65.201-S65.399[A], S65.801-S65.999

PDX Collection 1291
S45.301A, S45.309-S45.311[A], S45.319-S45.391[A],
S45.399-S45.801[A], S45.809-S45.811[A],
S45.819-S45.891[A], S45.899-S45.901[A],
S45.909-S45.911[A], S45.919-S45.991[A], S45.999A,
S55.201A, S55.209-S55.211[A], S55.219-S55.291[A],
S55.299-S55.801[A], S55.809-S55.811[A],
S55.819-S55.891[A], S55.899-S55.901[A],
S55.909-S55.911[A], S55.919-S55.991[A], S55.999A,
S65.401A, S65.409-S65.411[A], S65.419-S65.491[A],
S65.499-S65.500[A], S65.502A, S65.504A, S65.506A,
S65.508-S65.510[A], S65.512A, S65.514A, S65.516A,
S65.518-S65.590[A], S65.592A, S65.594A, S65.596A,
S65.598-S65.801[A], S65.809-S65.811[A],
S65.819-S65.891[A], S65.899-S65.901[A],
S65.909-S65.911[A], S65.919-S65.991[A], S65.999A

PDX Collection 1292
S45.302-S45.309[A], S45.312-S45.319[A],
S45.392-S45.399[A], S45.802-S45.809[A],
S45.812-S45.819[A], S45.892-S45.899[A],
S45.902-S45.909[A], S45.912-S45.919[A],
S45.992-S45.999[A], S55.202-S55.209[A],

S55.212-S55.219[A], S55.292-S55.299[A],
S55.802-S55.809[A], S55.812-S55.819[A],
S55.892-S55.899[A], S55.902-S55.909[A],
S55.912-S55.919[A], S55.992-S55.999[A],
S65.402-S65.409[A], S65.412-S65.419[A],
S65.492-S65.499[A], S65.501A, S65.503A, S65.505A,
S65.507-S65.509[A], S65.511A, S65.513A, S65.515A,
S65.517-S65.519[A], S65.591A, S65.593A, S65.595A,
S65.597-S65.599[A], S65.802-S65.809[A],
S65.812-S65.819[A], S65.892-S65.899[A],
S65.902-S65.909[A], S65.912A, S65.919A, S65.992A,
S65.999A

PDX Collection 1293
S45.301-S45.999[A], S55.201-S55.999[A],
S65.401-S65.999[A]

PDX Collection 1294
S61.401A, S61.409-S61.411[A], S61.419-S61.421[A],
S61.429-S61.431[A], S61.439-S61.441[A],
S61.449-S61.451[A], S61.459A, S66.021A,
S66.029A, S66.120A, S66.122A, S66.124A, S66.126A,
S66.128-S66.129[A], S66.221A, S66.229A, S66.320A,
S66.322A, S66.324A, S66.326A, S66.328-S66.329[A],
S66.421A, S66.429A, S66.520A, S66.522A, S66.524A,
S66.526A, S66.528-S66.529[A], S66.821A, S66.829A,
S66.921A, S66.929A

PDX Collection 1295
S61.402-S61.409[A], S61.412-S61.419[A],
S61.422-S61.429[A], S61.432-S61.439[A],
S61.442-S61.449[A], S61.452-S61.459[A],
S66.022-S66.029[A], S66.121A, S66.123A, S66.125A,
S66.127-S66.129[A], S66.222-S66.229[A],
S66.321A, S66.323A, S66.325[A], S66.327-S66.329A,
S66.422-S66.429[A], S66.521A, S66.523A, S66.525A,
S66.527-S66.529[A], S66.822-S66.829[A],
S66.922-S66.929[A]

PDX Collection 1296
S61.401-S61.459[A], S66.021-S66.029[A],
S66.120-S66.129[A], S66.221-S66.229[A],
S66.320-S66.329[A], S66.421-S66.429[A],
S66.520-S66.529[A], S66.821-S66.829[A],
S66.921-S66.929[A]

PDX Collection 1297
M48.40X-M48.58X[A], M80.00X-M80.88X[A],
M84.30X-M84.68X[A], M84.750-M84.759[A],
S03.8XX-S03.9XX[A], S29.011-S29.019[A],
S38.3XXA, S39.011-S39.013[A], S72.001[A,B,C],
S72.002[B,C], S72.009-S72.011[A,B,C],
S72.012[B,C], S72.019-S72.021[A,B,C],
S72.022[B,C], S72.023-S72.024[A,B,C],
S72.025[B,C], S72.026-S72.031[A,B,C],
S72.032[B,C], S72.033-S72.034[A,B,C],
S72.035[B,C], S72.036-S72.041[A,B,C],
S72.042[B,C], S72.043-S72.044[A,B,C],
S72.045[B,C], S72.046-S72.051[A,B,C],
S72.052[B,C], S72.059-S72.061[A,B,C],
S72.062[B,C], S72.063-S72.064[A,B,C],
S72.065[B,C], S72.066-S72.091[A,B,C],
S72.092[B,C], S72.099-S72.101[A,B,C],
S72.102[B,C], S72.109-S72.111[A,B,C],
S72.112[B,C], S72.113-S72.114[A,B,C],
S72.115[B,C], S72.116-S72.121[A,B,C],
S72.122[B,C], S72.123-S72.124[A,B,C],
S72.125[B,C], S72.126-S72.131[A,B,C],
S72.132[B,C], S72.133-S72.134[A,B,C],
S72.135[B,C], S72.136-S72.141[A,B,C],
S72.142[B,C], S72.143-S72.144[A,B,C],
S72.145[B,C], S72.146-S72.301[A,B,C],

S72.302[B,C], S72.309-S72.321[A,B,C],
S72.322[B,C], S72.323-S72.324[A,B,C], S72.325[B,C],
S72.326-S72.331[A,B,C], S72.332[B,C],
S72.333-S72.334[A,B,C], S72.335[B,C],
S72.336-S72.341[A,B,C], S72.342[B,C],
S72.343-S72.344[A,B,C], S72.345[B,C],
S72.346-S72.351[A,B,C], S72.352[B,C],
S72.353-S72.354[A,B,C], S72.355[B,C],
S72.356-S72.361[A,B,C], S72.362[B,C],
S72.363-S72.364[A,B,C], S72.365[B,C],
S72.366-S72.391[A,B,C], S72.392[B,C],
S72.399-S72.401[A,B,C], S72.402[B,C],
S72.409-S72.411[A,B,C], S72.412[B,C],
S72.413-S72.414[A,B,C], S72.415[B,C],
S72.416-S72.421[A,B,C], S72.422[B,C],
S72.423-S72.424[A,B,C], S72.425[B,C],
S72.426-S72.431[A,B,C], S72.432[B,C],
S72.433-S72.434[A,B,C], S72.435[B,C],
S72.436-S72.441[A,B,C], S72.442[B,C],
S72.443-S72.444[A,B,C], S72.445[B,C],
S72.446-S72.451[A,B,C], S72.452[B,C],
S72.453-S72.454[A,B,C], S72.455[B,C],
S72.456-S72.461[A,B,C], S72.462[B,C],
S72.463-S72.464[A,B,C], S72.465[B,C], S72.466[A,B,C],
S72.471A, S72.479A, S72.491[A,B,C], S72.492[B,C],
S72.499-S72.92X[A,B,C], S73.101A, S73.109-S73.111[A],
S73.119-S73.121[A], S73.129-S73.191[A], S73.199A,
S76.001A, S76.009-S76.011[A], S76.019A, S76.091A,
S76.099-S76.101[A], S76.109-S76.111[A],
S76.119A, S76.191A, S76.199-S76.201[A],
S76.209-S76.211[A], S76.219A, S76.291A,
S76.299-S76.301[A], S76.309-S76.311[A], S76.319A,
S76.391A, S76.399-S76.801[A], S76.809-S76.811[A],
S76.819A, S76.891A, S76.899-S76.901[A],
S76.909-S76.911[A], S76.919A, S76.991A, S76.999A,
S79.001A, S79.009-S79.011[A], S79.019-S79.091[A],
S79.099-S79.101[A], S79.109-S79.111[A],
S79.119-S79.121[A], S79.129-S79.131[A],
S79.139-S79.141[A], S79.149-S79.191[A],
S79.199-S79.811[A], S79.819-S79.821[A],
S79.829-S79.911[A], S79.919-S79.921[A], S79.929A,
S82.90X-S82.92X[A,B,C], T07.XXX-T14.91X[A],
T79.A0X-T79.9XX[A]

PDX Collection 1298
M48.40X-M48.58X[A], M80.00X-M80.88X[A],
M84.30X-M84.68X[A], M84.750-M84.759[A],
S03.8XX-S03.9XX[A], S29.011-S29.019[A], S38.3XX[A],
S39.011-S39.013[A], S72.001-S72.466[A,B,C],
S72.471-S72.479[A], S72.491-S72.92X[A,B,C],
S73.101-S73.199[A], S76.001-S76.019[A],
S76.091-S76.119[A], S76.191-S76.219[A],
S76.291-S76.319[A], S76.391-S76.819[A],
S76.891-S76.919[A], S76.991-S76.999[A],
S79.001-S79.929[A], S82.90X-S82.92X[A,B,C],
T07.XXX-T14.91X[A], T79.A0X-T79.9XX[A]

PDX Collection 1299
M48.40X-M48.58X[A], M80.00X-M80.88X[A],
M84.30X-M84.68X[A], M84.750-M84.759[A],
S03.8XX-S03.9XX[A], S29.011-S29.019[A], S38.3XXA,
S39.011-S39.013[A], S72.001[B,C], S72.002-S72.009[A,B,C],
S72.011[B,C], S72.012-S72.019[A,B,C],
S72.021[B,C], S72.022-S72.023[A,B,C],
S72.024[B,C], S72.025-S72.026[A,B,C],
S72.031[B,C], S72.032-S72.033[A,B,C],
S72.034[B,C], S72.035-S72.036[A,B,C],
S72.041[B,C], S72.042-S72.043[A,B,C],
S72.044[B,C], S72.045-S72.046[A,B,C],
S72.051[B,C], S72.052-S72.059[A,B,C],

S72.061[B,C], S72.062-S72.063[A,B,C],
S72.064[B,C], S72.065-S72.066[A,B,C],
S72.091[B,C], S72.092-S72.099[A,B,C],
S72.101[B,C], S72.102-S72.109[A,B,C],
S72.111[B,C], S72.112-S72.113[A,B,C],
S72.114[B,C], S72.115-S72.116[A,B,C],
S72.121[B,C], S72.122-S72.123[A,B,C],
S72.124[B,C], S72.125-S72.126[A,B,C],
S72.131[B,C], S72.132-S72.133[A,B,C],
S72.134[B,C], S72.135-S72.136[A,B,C],
S72.141[B,C], S72.142-S72.143[C], S72.144[B,C],
S72.145-S72.146[A,B,C], S72.21X-S72.26X[A,B,C],
S72.301[B,C], S72.302-S72.309[A,B,C],
S72.321[B,C], S72.322-S72.323[A,B,C], S72.324[B,C],
S72.325-S72.326[A,B,C], S72.331[B,C],
S72.332-S72.333[A,B,C], S72.334[B,C],
S72.335-S72.336[A,B,C], S72.341[B,C],
S72.342-S72.343[A,B,C], S72.344[B,C],
S72.345-S72.346[A,B,C], S72.351[B,C],
S72.352-S72.353[A,B,C], S72.354[B,C],
S72.355-S72.356[A,B,C], S72.361[B,C],
S72.362-S72.363[A,B,C], S72.364[B,C],
S72.365-S72.366[A,B,C], S72.391[B,C],
S72.392-S72.399[A,B,C], S72.401[B,C],
S72.402-S72.409[A,B,C], S72.411[B,C],
S72.412-S72.413[A,B,C], S72.414[B,C],
S72.415-S72.416[A,B,C], S72.421[B,C],
S72.422-S72.423[A,B,C], S72.424[B,C],
S72.425-S72.426[A,B,C], S72.431[B,C],
S72.432-S72.433[A,B,C], S72.434[B,C],
S72.435-S72.436[A,B,C], S72.441[B,C],
S72.442-S72.443[A,B,C], S72.444[B,C],
S72.445-S72.446[A,B,C], S72.451[B,C],
S72.452-S72.453[A,B,C], S72.454[B,C],
S72.455-S72.456[A,B,C], S72.461[B,C],
S72.462-S72.463[A,B,C], S72.464[B,C],
S72.465-S72.466[A,B,C], S72.472-S72.479[A], S72.491[B,C],
S72.492-S72.92X[A,B,C], S73.102-S73.109[A],
S73.112-S73.119[A], S73.122-S73.129[A],
S73.192-S73.199[A], S76.002-S76.009[A],
S76.012-S76.019[A], S76.092-S76.099[A],
S76.102-S76.109[A], S76.112-S76.119[A],
S76.192-S76.199[A], S76.202-S76.209[A],
S76.212-S76.219[A], S76.292-S76.299[A],
S76.302-S76.309[A], S76.312-S76.319[A],
S76.392-S76.399[A], S76.802-S76.809[A],
S76.812-S76.819[A], S76.892-S76.899[A],
S76.902-S76.909[A], S76.912-S76.919[A],
S76.992-S76.999[A], S79.002-S79.009[A],
S79.012-S79.019[A], S79.092-S79.099[A],
S79.102-S79.109[A], S79.112-S79.119[A],
S79.122-S79.129[A], S79.132-S79.139[A],
S79.142-S79.149[A], S79.192-S79.199[A],
S79.812-S79.819[A], S79.822-S79.829[A],
S79.912-S79.919[A], S79.922-S79.929[A],
S82.90X-S82.92X[A,B,C], T07.XXX-T14.91X[A], T79.8XXA
T79.A0X-T79.9XX[A]

PDX Collection 1300

M80.00X-M80.019[A], M80.041-M80.059[A],
M80.80X-M80.819[A], M80.841-M80.859[A],
M84.40X-M84.419[A], M84.441-M84.459[A],
M84.474-M84.519[A], M84.541-M84.559[A],
M84.574-M84.576[A], M84.60X-M84.619[A],
M84.641-M84.659[A], M84.674-M84.68X[A],
M84.750-M84.759[A], S03.8XX-S03.9XX[A],
S29.011-S29.019[A], S38.3XX[A], S39.011-S39.013[A],
S72.001[A,B,C], S72.002[B,C], S72.009-S72.011[A,B,C],
S72.012[B,C], S72.019-S72.021[A,B,C],

S72.022[B,C], S72.023-S72.024[A,B,C],
S72.025[B,C], S72.026-S72.031[A,B,C],
S72.032[B,C], S72.033-S72.034[A,B,C],
S72.035[B,C], S72.036-S72.041[A,B,C],
S72.042[B,C], S72.043-S72.044[A,B,C],
S72.045[B,C], S72.046-S72.051[A,B,C],
S72.052[B,C], S72.059-S72.061[A,B,C], S72.062[B,C],
S72.063-S72.064[A,B,C], S72.065[B,C],
S72.066-S72.091[A,B,C], S72.092[B,C],
S72.099-S72.101[C], S72.102[B,C], S72.109-S72.111[A,B,C],
S72.112[B,C], S72.113-S72.114[A,B,C],
S72.115[B,C], S72.116-S72.121[A,B,C],
S72.122[B,C], S72.123-S72.124[A,B,C],
S72.125[B,C], S72.126-S72.131[A,B,C],
S72.132[B,C], S72.133-S72.134[A,B,C],
S72.135[B,C], S72.136-S72.141[A,B,C],
S72.142[B,C], S72.143-S72.144[A,B,C],
S72.145[B,C], S72.146-S72.301[A,B,C],
S72.302[B,C], S72.309-S72.321[A,B,C],
S72.322[B,C], S72.323-S72.324[A,B,C],
S72.325[B,C], S72.326-S72.331[A,B,C],
S72.332[B,C], S72.333-S72.334[A,B,C],
S72.335[B,C], S72.336-S72.341[A,B,C],
S72.342[B,C], S72.343-S72.344[A,B,C],
S72.345[B,C], S72.346-S72.351[A,B,C],
S72.352[B,C], S72.353-S72.354[A,B,C],
S72.355[B,C], S72.356-S72.361[A,B,C],
S72.362[B,C], S72.363-S72.364[A,B,C],
S72.365[B,C], S72.366-S72.391[A,B,C],
S72.392[B,C], S72.399-S72.401[A,B,C],
S72.402[B,C], S72.409-S72.411[A,B,C],
S72.412[B,C], S72.413-S72.414[A,B,C], S72.415[B,C],
S72.416-S72.421[A,B,C], S72.422[B,C],
S72.423-S72.424[A,B,C], S72.425[B,C],
S72.426-S72.431[A,B,C], S72.432[B,C],
S72.433-S72.434[A,B,C], S72.435[B,C],
S72.436-S72.441[A,B,C], S72.442[B,C],
S72.443-S72.444[A,B,C], S72.445[B,C],
S72.446-S72.451[A,B,C], S72.452[B,C],
S72.453-S72.454[A,B,C], S72.455[B,C],
S72.456-S72.461[A,B,C], S72.462[B,C],
S72.463-S72.464[A,B,C], S72.465[B,C], S72.466[A,B,C],
S72.471A, S72.479A, S72.491[A,B,C], S72.492[B,C],
S72.499-S72.92X[A,B,C], S73.101A, S73.109-S73.111[A],
S73.119-S73.121[A], S73.129-S73.191[A], S73.199A,
S76.001A, S76.009-S76.011[A], S76.019A, S76.091A,
S76.099-S76.101[A], S76.109-S76.111[A],
S76.119A, S76.191A, S76.199-S76.201[A],
S76.209-S76.211[A], S76.219A, S76.291A,
S76.299-S76.301[A], S76.309-S76.311[A], S76.319A,
S76.391A, S76.399-S76.801[A], S76.809-S76.811[A],
S76.819A, S76.891A, S76.899-S76.901[A],
S76.909-S76.911[A], S76.919A, S76.991A, S76.999A,
S79.001A, S79.009-S79.011[A], S79.019-S79.091[A],
S79.099-S79.101[A], S79.109-S79.111[A],
S79.119-S79.121[A], S79.129-S79.131[A],
S79.139-S79.141[A], S79.149-S79.191[A],
S79.199-S79.811[A], S79.819-S79.821[A],
S79.829-S79.911[A], S79.919-S79.921[A], S79.929A,
S82.90X-S82.92X[A,B,C], T07.XXX-T14.91X[A],
T79.A9X-T79.9XX[A]

PDX Collection 1301

M80.00X-M80.019[A], M80.041-M80.059[A],
M80.80X-M80.819[A], M80.841-M80.859[A],
M84.40X-M84.419[A], M84.441-M84.459[A],
M84.474-M84.519[A], M84.541-M84.559[A],
M84.574-M84.576[A], M84.60X-M84.619[A],
M84.641-M84.659[A], M84.674-M84.68X[A],

M84.750-M84.759[A], S03.8XX-S03.9XX[A],
S29.011-S29.019[A], S38.3XXA, S39.011-S39.013[A],
S72.001-S72.466[A,B,C], S72.471-S72.479[A],
S72.491-S72.92X[A,B,C], S73.101-S73.199[A],
S76.001-S76.019[A], S76.091-S76.119[A],
S76.191-S76.219[A], S76.291-S76.319[A],
S76.391-S76.819[A], S76.891-S76.919[A],
S76.991-S76.999[A], S79.001-S79.929[A],
S82.90X-S82.92X[A,B,C], T07.XXX-T14.91X[A],
T79.A9X-T79.9XX[A]

PDX Collection 1302

M80.00X-M80.019[A], M80.041-M80.059[A],
M80.80X-M80.819[A], M80.841-M80.859[A],
M84.40X-M84.419[A], M84.441-M84.459[A],
M84.474-M84.519[A], M84.541-M84.559[A],
M84.574-M84.576[A], M84.60X-M84.619[A],
M84.641-M84.659[A], M84.674-M84.68X[A],
M84.750-M84.759[A], S03.8XX-S03.9XX[A],
S29.011-S29.019[A], S38.3XX[A], S39.011-S39.013[A],
S72.001[B,C], S72.002-S72.009[A,B,C],
S72.011[B,C], S72.012-S72.019[A,B,C],
S72.021[B,C], S72.022-S72.023[A,B,C],
S72.024[B,C], S72.025-S72.026[A,B,C],
S72.031[B,C], S72.032-S72.033[A,B,C],
S72.034[B,C], S72.035-S72.036[A,B,C],
S72.041[B,C], S72.042-S72.043[A,B,C],
S72.044[B,C], S72.045-S72.046[A,B,C],
S72.051[B,C], S72.052-S72.059[A,B,C],
S72.061[B,C], S72.062-S72.063[A,B,C],
S72.064[B,C], S72.065-S72.066[A,B,C],
S72.091[B,C], S72.092-S72.099[A,B,C],
S72.101[B,C], S72.102-S72.109[A,B,C],
S72.111[B,C], S72.112-S72.113[A,B,C], S72.114[B,C],
S72.115-S72.116[A,B,C], S72.121[B,C],
S72.122-S72.123[A,B,C], S72.124[B,C],
S72.125-S72.126[A,B,C], S72.131[B,C],
S72.132-S72.133[A,B,C], S72.134[B,C],
S72.135-S72.136[A,B,C], S72.141[B,C],
S72.142-S72.143[A,B,C], S72.144[B,C],
S72.145-S72.146[A,B,C], S72.21X-S72.26X[A,B,C],
S72.301[B,C], S72.302-S72.309[A,B,C],
S72.321[B,C], S72.322-S72.323[A,B,C],
S72.324[B,C], S72.325-S72.326[A,B,C], S72.331[B,C],
S72.332-S72.333[A,B,C], S72.334[B,C],
S72.335-S72.336[A,B,C], S72.341[B,C],
S72.342-S72.343[A,B,C], S72.344[B,C],
S72.345-S72.346[A,B,C], S72.351[B,C],
S72.352-S72.353[A,B,C], S72.354[B,C],
S72.355-S72.356[A,B,C], S72.361[B,C],
S72.362-S72.363[A,B,C], S72.364[B,C],
S72.365-S72.366[A,B,C], S72.391[B,C],
S72.392-S72.399[A,B,C], S72.401[B,C],
S72.402-S72.409[A,B,C], S72.411[B,C],
S72.412-S72.413[A,B,C], S72.414[B,C],
S72.415-S72.416[A,B,C], S72.421[B,C],
S72.422-S72.423[A,B,C], S72.424[B,C],
S72.425-S72.426[A,B,C], S72.431[B,C],
S72.432-S72.433[A,B,C], S72.434[B,C],
S72.435-S72.436[A,B,C], S72.441[B,C],
S72.442-S72.443[A,B,C], S72.444[B,C],
S72.445-S72.446[A,B,C], S72.451[B,C],
S72.452-S72.453[A,B,C], S72.454[B,C],
S72.455-S72.456[A,B,C], S72.461[B,C],
S72.462-S72.463[A,B,C], S72.464[B,C],
S72.465-S72.466[A,B,C], S72.472-S72.479[A], S72.491[B,C],
S72.492-S72.92X[A,B,C], S73.102-S73.109[A],
S73.112-S73.119[A], S73.122-S73.129[A],
S73.192-S73.199[A], S76.002-S76.009[A],

S76.012-S76.019[A], S76.092-S76.099[A],
S76.102-S76.109[A], S76.112-S76.119[A],
S76.192-S76.199[A], S76.202-S76.209[A],
S76.212-S76.219[A], S76.292-S76.299[A],
S76.302-S76.309[A], S76.312-S76.319[A],
S76.392-S76.399[A], S76.802-S76.809[A],
S76.812-S76.819[A], S76.892-S76.899[A],
S76.902-S76.909[A], S76.912-S76.919[A],
S76.992-S76.999[A], S79.002-S79.009[A],
S79.012-S79.019[A], S79.092-S79.099[A],
S79.102-S79.109[A], S79.112-S79.119[A],
S79.122-S79.129[A], S79.132-S79.139[A],
S79.142-S79.149[A], S79.192-S79.199[A],
S79.812-S79.819[A], S79.822-S79.829[A],
S79.912-S79.919[A], S79.922-S79.929[A],
S82.90X-S82.92X[A,B,C], T07.XXX-T14.91X[A],
T79.A9X-T79.9XX[A],

PDX Collection 1303
M80.00X-M80.019[A], M80.041-M80.059[A],
M80.80X-M80.819[A], M80.841-M80.859[A],
M84.40X-M84.419[A], M84.441-M84.459[A],
M84.474-M84.519[A], M84.541-M84.559[A],
M84.574-M84.619[A], M84.641-M84.659[A],
M84.674-M84.68X[A], M84.750-M84.759[A],
S03.8XX-S03.9XX[A], S29.011-S29.019[A], S38.3XXA,
S39.011-S39.013[A], S72.491-S72.499[B,C],
S73.101-S73.199[A], S76.001-S76.019[A],
S76.091-S76.119[A], S76.191-S76.219[A],
S76.291-S76.319[A], S76.391-S76.819[A],
S76.891-S76.919[A], S76.991-S76.999[A],
S79.811-S79.929[A], S82.001-S82.099[A,B,C],
S82.90X-S82.92X[A,B,C], T07.XXX-T14.91X[A],
T79.A9X-T79.9XX[A]

PDX Collection 1304
M99.16-M99.17, M99.19, S03.1XXA, S33.30X-S33.39X[A],
S73.001A, S73.003-S73.004[A], S73.006A, S73.041A,
S73.043-S73.044[A], S73.046A

PDX Collection 1305
M99.16-M99.17, M99.19, S03.1XXA, S33.30X-S33.39X[A],
S73.002-S73.003[A], S73.005-S73.006[A],
S73.042-S73.043[A], S73.045-S73.046[A]

PDX Collection 1306
M99.16-M99.17, M99.19, S03.1XXA, S33.30X-S33.39X[A],
S73.001-S73.006[A], S73.041-S73.046[A]

PDX Collection 1307
M99.16-M99.17, M99.19, S03.1XXA, S33.30X-S33.39X[A],
S73.011A, S73.013-S73.014[A], S73.016A

PDX Collection 1308
M99.16-M99.17, M99.19, S03.1XXA, S33.30X-S33.39X[A],
S73.012-S73.013[A], S73.015-S73.016[A]

PDX Collection 1309
M99.16-M99.17, M99.19, S03.1XXA, S33.30X-S33.39X[A],
S73.011-S73.016[A]

PDX Collection 1310
M99.16-M99.17, M99.19, S03.1XXA, S33.30X-S33.39X[A],
S73.021A, S73.023-S73.024[A], S73.026A

PDX Collection 1311
M99.16-M99.17, M99.19, S03.1XXA, S33.30X-S33.39X[A],
S73.022-S73.023[A], S73.025-S73.026[A]

PDX Collection 1312
M99.16-M99.17, M99.19, S03.1XXA, S33.30X-S33.39X[A],
S73.021-S73.026[A]

PDX Collection 1313
M99.16-M99.17, M99.19, S03.1XXA, S33.30X-S33.39X[A],
S73.031A, S73.033-S73.034[A], S73.036A

PDX Collection 1314
M99.16-M99.17, M99.19, S03.1XXA, S33.30X-S33.39X[A],
S73.032-S73.033[A], S73.035-S73.036[A]

PDX Collection 1315
M99.16-M99.17, M99.19, S03.1XXA, S33.30X-S33.39X[A],
S73.031-S73.036[A]

PDX Collection 1316
S75.001A, S75.009-S75.021[A], S75.029-S75.091[A],
S75.099A, S75.801A, S75.809-S75.811[A],
S75.819-S75.891[A], S75.899-S75.901[A],
S75.909-S75.911[A], S75.919-S75.991[A], S75.999A,
S85.201A, S85.209-S85.211[A], S85.219-S85.291[A],
S85.299A, S85.801A, S85.809-S85.811[A],
S85.819-S85.891[A], S85.899-S85.901[A],
S85.909-S85.911[A], S85.919-S85.991[A], S85.999A,
S95.001A, S95.009-S95.011[A], S95.019-S95.091[A],
S95.099A, S95.201A, S95.209-S95.211[A],
S95.219-S95.291[A], S95.299-S95.801[A],
S95.809-S95.811[A], S95.819-S95.891[A],
S95.899-S95.901[A], S95.909-S95.911[A],
S95.919-S95.991[A], S95.99[A]

PDX Collection 1317
S75.002-S75.009[A], S75.012-S75.019[A],
S75.022-S75.029[A], S75.092A, S75.099A,
S75.802-S75.809[A], S75.812-S75.819[A],
S75.892-S75.899[A], S75.902-S75.909[A],
S75.912-S75.919[A], S75.992-S75.999[A],
S85.202-S85.209[A], S85.212-S85.219[A],
S85.292-S85.299[A], S85.802-S85.809[A],
S85.812-S85.819[A], S85.892-S85.899[A],
S85.902-S85.909[A], S85.912-S85.919[A],
S85.992-S85.999[A], S95.002-S95.009[A],
S95.012-S95.019[A], S95.092-S95.099[A],
S95.202-S95.209[A], S95.212-S95.219[A],
S95.292-S95.299[A], S95.802-S95.809[A],
S95.812-S95.819[A], S95.892-S95.899[A],
S95.902-S95.909[A], S95.912-S95.919[A],
S95.992-S95.999[A]

PDX Collection 1318
S75.001-S75.099[A], S75.801-S75.999[A],
S85.201-S85.299[A], S85.801-S85.999[A],
S95.001-S95.099[A], S95.201-S95.999[A]

PDX Collection 1319
S75.101A, S75.109-S75.111[A], S75.119-S75.121[A],
S75.129-S75.191[A], S75.199[A], S75.801A,
S75.809-S75.811[A], S75.819-S75.891[A],
S75.899-S75.901[A], S75.909-S75.911[A],
S75.919-S75.991[A], S75.999[A], S85.201A,
S85.209-S85.211[A], S85.219-S85.291[A], S85.299A,
S85.801A, S85.809-S85.811[A], S85.819-S85.891[A],
S85.899-S85.901[A], S85.909-S85.911[A],
S85.919-S85.991[A], S85.999A, S95.001A,
S95.009-S95.011[A], S95.019-S95.091[A], S95.099A,
S95.201A, S95.209-S95.211[A], S95.219-S95.291[A],
S95.299-S95.801[A], S95.809-S95.811[A],
S95.819-S95.891[A], S95.899-S95.901[A],
S95.909-S95.911[A], S95.919-S95.991[A], S95.999A

PDX Collection 1320
S75.102-S75.109[A], S75.112-S75.119[A],
S75.122-S75.129[A], S75.192-S75.199[A],
S75.802-S75.809[A], S75.812-S75.819[A],
S75.892-S75.899[A], S75.902-S75.909[A],
S75.912-S75.919[A], S75.992-S75.999[A],
S85.202-S85.209[A], S85.212-S85.219[A],
S85.292-S85.299[A], S85.802-S85.809[A],
S85.812-S85.819[A], S85.892-S85.899[A],
S85.902-S85.909[A], S85.912-S85.919[A],

S85.992-S85.999[A], S95.002-S95.009[A],
S95.012-S95.019[A], S95.092-S95.099[A],
S95.202-S95.209[A], S95.212-S95.219[A],
S95.292-S95.299[A], S95.802-S95.809[A],
S95.812-S95.819[A], S95.892-S95.899[A],
S95.902-S95.909[A], S95.912-S95.919[A],
S95.992-S95.999[A]

PDX Collection 1321
S75.101-S75.199[A], S75.801-S75.999[A],
S85.201-S85.299[A], S85.801-S85.999[A],
S95.001-S95.099[A], S95.201-S95.999[A]

PDX Collection 1322
S75.201A, S75.209-S75.211[A], S75.219-S75.221[A],
S75.229-S75.291[A], S75.299-S75.801[A],
S75.809-S75.811[A], S75.819-S75.891[A],
S75.899-S75.901[A], S75.909-S75.911[A],
S75.919-S75.991[A], S75.999A, S85.201A, S85.209A,
S85.211A, S85.219-S85.291[A], S85.299-S85.301[A],
S85.309-S85.311[A], S85.319-S85.391[A],
S85.399-S85.401[A], S85.409-S85.411[A],
S85.419-S85.491[A], S85.499A, S85.801A, S85.809A,
S85.811A, S85.819-S85.891[A], S85.899-S85.901[A],
S85.909-S85.911[A], S85.919-S85.991[A], S85.999A,
S95.001A, S95.009-S95.011[A], S95.019-S95.091[A],
S95.099A, S95.201A, S95.209-S95.211[A],
S95.219-S95.291[A], S95.299-S95.801[A],
S95.809-S95.811[A], S95.819-S95.891[A],
S95.899-S95.901[A], S95.909-S95.911[A],
S95.919-S95.991[A], S95.999A

PDX Collection 1323
S75.202-S75.209[A], S75.212-S75.219[A],
S75.222-S75.229[A], S75.292-S75.299[A],
S75.802-S75.809[A], S75.812-S75.819[A],
S75.892-S75.899[A], S75.902-S75.909[A],
S75.912-S75.919[A], S75.992-S75.999[A],
S85.202-S85.209[A], S85.212-S85.219[A],
S85.292-S85.299[A], S85.302-S85.309[A],
S85.312-S85.319[A], S85.392-S85.399[A],
S85.402-S85.409[A], S85.412-S85.419[A],
S85.492-S85.499[A], S85.802-S85.809[A],
S85.812-S85.819[A], S85.892-S85.899[A],
S85.902-S85.909[A], S85.912-S85.919[A],
S85.992-S85.999[A], S95.002-S95.009[A],
S95.012-S95.019[A], S95.092-S95.099[A],
S95.202-S95.209[A], S95.212-S95.219[A],
S95.292-S95.299[A], S95.802-S95.809[A],
S95.812-S95.819[A], S95.892-S95.899[A],
S95.902-S95.909[A], S95.912-S95.919[A],
S95.992-S95.999[A]

PDX Collection 1324
S75.201-S75.999[A], S85.201-S85.499[A],
S85.801-S85.999[A], S95.001-S95.099[A],
S95.201-S95.999[A]

PDX Collection 1325
M79.A21-M79.A29, S75.001A, S75.009-S75.011[A],
S75.019-S75.021[A], S75.029-S75.091[A],
S75.099-S75.101[A], S75.109-S75.111[A],
S75.119-S75.121[A], S75.129-S75.191[A],
S75.199-S75.201[A], S75.209-S75.211[A],
S75.219-S75.221[A], S75.229-S75.291[A],
S75.299-S75.801[A], S75.809-S75.891[A],
S75.899-S75.901[A], S75.909-S75.911[A],
S75.919-S75.991[A], S75.999A, S85.001A,
S85.009-S85.011[A], S85.019-S85.091[A],
S85.099-S85.101[A], S85.109-S85.111[A],
S85.119-S85.121[A], S85.129-S85.131[A],
S85.139-S85.141[A], S85.149-S85.151[A],

S85.159-S85.161[A], S85.169-S85.171[A],
S85.179-S85.181[A], S85.189-S85.201[A],
S85.209-S85.211[A], S85.219-S85.291[A],
S85.299-S85.301[A], S85.309-S85.311[A],
S85.319-S85.391[A], S85.399-S85.401[A],
S85.409-S85.411[A], S85.419-S85.491[A],
S85.499-S85.501[A], S85.509-S85.511[A],
S85.519-S85.591[A], S85.599-S85.801[A],
S85.809-S85.811[A], S85.819-S85.891[A],
S85.899-S85.901[A], S85.909-S85.911[A],
S85.919-S85.991[A], S85.999A, S95.001A,
S95.009-S95.011[A], S95.019A, S95.091A,
S95.099-S95.101[A], S95.109-S95.111[A], S95
119-S95.191[A], S95.199-S95.201[A], S95.209-S95.211[A],
S95.219-S95.291[A], S95.299-S95.801[A],
S95.809-S95.811[A], S95.819-S95.891[A],
S95.899-S95.901[A], S95.909-S95.911[A],
S95.919-S95.991[A], S95.999A

PDX Collection 1326
M79.A21-M79.A29, S75.002-S75.009[A], S75.012-S75.019[A],
S75.022-S75.029[A], S75.092-S75.099[A],
S75.102-S75.109[A], S75.112-S75.119[A],
S75.122-S75.129[A], S75.192-S75.199[A],
S75.202-S75.209[A], S75.212-S75.219[A],
S75.222-S75.229[A], S75.292-S75.299[A],
S75.802-S75.809[A], S75.812-S75.819[A],
S75.892-S75.899[A], S75.902-S75.909[A],
S75.912-S75.919[A], S75.992-S75.999[A],
S85.002-S85.009[A], S85.012-S85.019[A],
S85.092-S85.099[A], S85.102-S85.109[A],
S85.112-S85.119[A], S85.122-S85.129[A],
S85.132-S85.139[A], S85.142-S85.149[A],
S85.152-S85.159[A], S85.162-S85.169[A],
S85.172-S85.179[A], S85.182-S85.189[A],
S85.202-S85.209[A], S85.212-S85.219[A],
S85.292-S85.299[A], S85.302-S85.309[A],
S85.312-S85.319[A], S85.392-S85.399[A],
S85.402-S85.409[A], S85.412-S85.419[A],
S85.492-S85.499[A], S85.502-S85.509[A],
S85.512-S85.519[A], S85.592-S85.599[A],
S85.802-S85.809[A], S85.812-S85.819[A],
S85.892-S85.899[A], S85.902-S85.909[A],
S85.912-S85.919[A], S85.992-S85.999[A],
S95.002-S95.009[A], S95.012-S95.019[A],
S95.092-S95.099[A], S95.102-S95.109[A],
S95.112-S95.119[A], S95.192-S95.199[A],
S95.202-S95.209[A], S95.212-S95.219[A],
S95.292-S95.299[A], S95.802-S95.809[A],
S95.812-S95.819[A], S95.892-S95.899[A],
S95.902-S95.909[A], S95.912-S95.919[A],
S95.992-S95.999[A]

PDX Collection 1327
M79.A21-M79.A29, S75.001-S75.999[A], S85.001-S85.999[A],
S95.001-S95.999[A]

PDX Collection 1328
S71.001A, S71.009-S71.011[A], S71.019-S71.021[A],
S71.029-S71.031[A], S71.039-S71.041[A],
S71.049-S71.051[A], S71.059-S71.101[A],
S71.109-S71.111[A], S71.119-S71.121[A],
S71.129-S71.131[A], S71.139-S71.141[A],
S71.149-S71.151[A], S71.159A, S76.021A, S76.029A,
S76.121A, S76.129A, S76.221A, S76.229A, S76.321A,
S76.329A, S76.821A, S76.829A, S76.921A, S76.929A

PDX Collection 1329
S71.002-S71.009[A], S71.012-S71.019[A],
S71.022-S71.029[A], S71.032-S71.039[A],
S71.042-S71.049[A], S71.052-S71.059[A],

S71.102-S71.109[A], S71.112-S71.119[A],
S71.122-S71.129[A], S71.132-S71.139[A],
S71.142-S71.149[A], S71.152-S71.159[A],
S76.022-S76.029[A], S76.122-S76.129[A],
S76.222-S76.229[A], S76.322-S76.329[A],
S76.822-S76.829[A], S76.922-S76.929[A]

PDX Collection 1330
S71.001-S71.159[A], S76.021-S76.029[A],
S76.121-S76.129[A], S76.221-S76.229[A],
S76.321-S76.329[A], S76.821-S76.829[A],
S76.921-S76.929[A]

PDX Collection 1331
S77.00X-S77.02X[A], S77.20X-S77.22X[A]

PDX Collection 1332
S77.10X-S77.22X[A]

PDX Collection 1333
S71.001A, S71.009-S71.011[A], S71.019-S71.021[A],
S71.029-S71.031[A], S71.039-S71.041[A],
S71.049-S71.051[A], S71.059-S71.101[A],
S71.109-S71.111[A], S71.119-S71.121[A],
S71.129-S71.131[A], S71.139-S71.141[A],
S71.149-S71.151[A], S71.159A, S76.021A, S76.029A,
S76.121A, S76.129A, S76.221A, S76.229A, S76.321A,
S76.329A, S76.821A, S76.829A, S76.921A, S76.929A,
S78.011A, S78.019-S78.021[A], S78.029-S78.111[A],
S78.119-S78.121[A], S78.129-S78.911[A],
S78.919-S78.921[A], S78.929A, S81.001A,
S81.009-S81.011[A], S81.019-S81.021[A],
S81.029-S81.031[A], S81.039-S81.041[A],
S81.049-S81.051[A], S81.059-S81.801[A],
S81.809-S81.811[A], S81.819-S81.821[A],
S81.829-S81.831[A], S81.839-S81.841[A],
S81.849-S81.851[A], S81.859A, S86.021A, S86.029A,
S86.121A, S86.129A, S86.221A, S86.229A, S86.321A,
S86.329A, S86.821A, S86.829A, S86.921A, S86.929A,
S88.011A, S88.019-S88.021[A], S88.029-S88.111[A],
S88.119-S88.121[A], S88.129-S88.911[A],
S88.919-S88.921[A], S88.929A, S91.001A,
S91.009-S91.011[A], S91.019-S91.021[A],
S91.029-S91.031[A], S91.039-S91.041[A],
S91.049-S91.051[A], S91.059-S91.101[A],
S91.103-S91.104[A], S91.106-S91.111[A],
S91.113-S91.114[A], S91.116-S91.121[A],
S91.123-S91.124[A], S91.126-S91.131[A],
S91.133-S91.134[A], S91.136-S91.141[A],
S91.143-S91.144[A], S91.146-S91.151[A],
S91.153-S91.154[A], S91.156-S91.201[A],
S91.203-S91.204[A], S91.206-S91.211[A],
S91.213-S91.214[A], S91.216-S91.221[A],
S91.223-S91.224[A], S91.226-S91.231[A],
S91.233-S91.234[A], S91.236-S91.241[A],
S91.243-S91.244[A], S91.246-S91.251[A],
S91.253-S91.254[A], S91.256-S91.301[A],
S91.309-S91.311[A], S91.319-S91.321[A],
S91.329-S91.331[A], S91.339-S91.341[A],
S91.349-S91.351[A], S91.359A, S96.021A,
S96.029A, S96.121A, S96.129A, S96.221A, S96.229A,
S96.821A, S96.829A, S96.921A, S96.929A, S98.011A,
S98.019-S98.021[A], S98.029-S98.111[A],
S98.119-S98.121[A], S98.129-S98.131[A],
S98.139-S98.141[A], S98.149-S98.211[A],
S98.219-S98.221[A], S98.229-S98.311[A],
S98.319-S98.321[A], S98.329-S98.911[A],
S98.919-S98.921[A], S98.929[A], T07.XXX-T14.91X[A],
T79.8XX-T79.9XX[A], T79.A0X-T79.A9X[A]

PDX Collection 1334
S71.002-S71.009[A],
S71.012-S71.019[A], S71.022-S71.029[A],
S71.032-S71.039[A], S71.042-S71.049[A],
S71.052-S71.059[A], S71.102-S71.109[A],
S71.112-S71.119[A], S71.122-S71.129[A],
S71.132-S71.139[A], S71.142-S71.149[A],
S71.152-S71.159[A], S76.022-S76.029[A],
S76.122-S76.129[A], S76.222-S76.229[A],
S76.322-S76.329[A], S76.822-S76.829[A],
S76.922-S76.929[A], S78.012-S78.019[A],
S78.022-S78.029[A], S78.112-S78.119[A],
S78.122-S78.129[A], S78.912-S78.919[A],
S78.922-S78.929[A], S81.002-S81.009[A],
S81.012-S81.019[A], S81.022-S81.029[A],
S81.032-S81.039[A], S81.042-S81.049[A],
S81.052-S81.059[A], S81.802-S81.809[A],
S81.812-S81.819[A], S81.822-S81.829[A],
S81.832-S81.839[A], S81.842-S81.849[A],
S81.852-S81.859[A], S86.022-S86.029[A],
S86.122-S86.129[A], S86.222-S86.229[A],
S86.322-S86.329[A], S86.822-S86.829[A],
S86.922-S86.929[A], S88.012-S88.019[A],
S88.022-S88.029[A], S88.112-S88.119[A],
S88.122-S88.129[A], S88.912-S88.919[A],
S88.922-S88.929[A], S91.002-S91.009[A],
S91.012-S91.019[A], S91.022-S91.029[A],
S91.032-S91.039[A], S91.042-S91.049[A],
S91.052-S91.059[A], S91.102-S91.103[A],
S91.105-S91.109[A], S91.112-S91.113[A],
S91.115-S91.119[A], S91.122-S91.123[A],
S91.125-S91.129[A], S91.132-S91.133[A],
S91.135-S91.139[A], S91.142-S91.143[A],
S91.145-S91.149[A], S91.152-S91.153[A],
S91.155-S91.159[A], S91.202-S91.203[A],
S91.205-S91.209[A], S91.212-S91.213[A],
S91.215-S91.219[A], S91.222-S91.223[A],
S91.225-S91.229[A], S91.232-S91.233[A],
S91.235-S91.239[A], S91.242-S91.243[A],
S91.245-S91.249[A], S91.252-S91.253[A],
S91.255-S91.259[A], S91.302-S91.309[A],
S91.312-S91.319[A], S91.322-S91.329[A],
S91.332-S91.339[A], S91.342-S91.349[A],
S91.352-S91.359[A], S96.022-S96.029[A],
S96.122-S96.129[A], S96.222-S96.229[A],
S96.822-S96.829[A], S96.922-S96.929[A],
S98.012-S98.019[A], S98.022-S98.029[A],
S98.112-S98.119[A], S98.122-S98.129[A],
S98.132-S98.139[A], S98.142-S98.149[A],
S98.212-S98.219[A], S98.222-S98.229[A],
S98.312-S98.319[A], S98.322-S98.329[A],
S98.912-S98.919[A], S98.922-S98.929[A],
T07.XXX-T14.91X[A], T79.8XX-T79.9XX[A],
T79.A0X-T79.A9X[A]

PDX Collection 1335
S71.001-S71.159[A], S76.021-S76.029[A],
S76.121-S76.129[A], S76.221-S76.229[A],
S76.321-S76.329[A], S76.821-S76.829[A],
S76.921-S76.929[A], S78.011-S78.929[A],
S81.001-S81.859[A], S86.021-S86.029[A],
S86.121-S86.129[A], S86.221-S86.229[A],
S86.321-S86.329[A], S86.821-S86.829[A],
S86.921-S86.929[A], S88.011-S88.929[A],
S91.001-S91.359[A], S96.021-S96.029[A],
S96.121-S96.129[A], S96.221-S96.229[A],
S96.821-S96.829[A], S96.921-S96.929[A],
S98.011-S98.929[A], T07.XXX-T14.91X[A],
T79.8XX-T79.9XX[A], T79.A0X-T79.A9X[A]

PDX Collection 1336
S82.001-S82.099[A,B,C]

PDX Collection 1337
M80.00X-M80.019[A], M80.041-M80.049[A],
M80.80X-M80.819[A], M80.841-M80.849[A],
M84.40X-M84.419[A], M84.441-M84.446[A],
M84.454A, M84.474-M84.519[A], M84.541-M84.550[A],
M84.574-M84.576[A], M84.60X-M84.619[A],
M84.641-M84.650[A], M84.674-M84.68X[A],
S03.8XX-S03.9XX[A], S29.011-S29.019[A],
S38.3XXA, S39.011-S39.013[A], S73.101-S73.199[A],
S76.001-S76.019[A], S76.091-S76.119[A],
S76.191-S76.219[A], S76.291-S76.319[A],
S76.391-S76.819[A], S76.891-S76.919[A],
S76.991-S76.999[A], S79.811-S79.929[A],
S82.001-S82.099[B,C], S82.101-S82.156[A,B,C],
S82.191-S82.299[A,B,C], S82.401-S82.499[A,B,C],
S82.831-S82.839[A,B,C], S82.861-S82.866[A,B,C],
S82.90X-S82.92X[A,B,C], S89.001-S89.099[A],
S89.201-S89.299[A], T07.XXX-T14.91X[A],
T79.8XX-T79.9XX[A], T79.A9XA

PDX Collection 1338
S82.001[B,C], S82.002-S82.009[A,B,C], S82.011[B,C],
S82.012-S82.013[A,B,C], S82.014-S82.021[B,C],
S82.022-S82.023[A,B,C], S82.024[B,C],
S82.025-S82.026[A,B,C], S82.031-S82.033[A,B,C],
S82.034[B,C], S82.035-S82.036[A,B,C],
S82.041[B,C], S82.042-S82.043[A,B,C], S82.044[B,C],
S82.045-S82.046[A,B,C], S82.091[B,C],
S82.092-S82.099[A,B,C]

PDX Collection 1339
S82.001-S82.099[A,B,C]

PDX Collection 1340
M80.00X-M80.019[A], M80.041-M80.049[A],
M80.061-M80.819[A], M80.841-M80.849[A],
M80.861-M80.879[A], M84.40X-M84.419[A],
M84.441-M84.446[A], M84.454A, M84.461-M84.519[A],
M84.541-M84.550[A], M84.561-M84.619[A],
M84.641-M84.650[A], M84.661-M84.68X[A],
S03.8XX-S03.9XX[A], S29.011-S29.019[A], S38.3XXA,
S39.011-S39.013[A], S73.101A, S73.109-S73.111[A],
S73.119-S73.121[A], S73.129-S73.191[A],
S73.199[A], S76.001[A], S76.009-S76.011[A],
S76.019A, S76.091A, S76.099-S76.101[A],
S76.109-S76.111[A], S76.119A, S76.191A,
S76.199-S76.201[A], S76.209-S76.211[A], S76.219A,
S76.291A, S76.299-S76.301[A], S76.309-S76.311[A],
S76.319A, S76.391A, S76.399-S76.801[A],
S76.809-S76.811[A], S76.819A, S76.891A,
S76.899-S76.901[A], S76.909-S76.911[A], S76.919A,
S76.991A, S76.999A, S79.811A, S79.819-S79.821[A],
S79.829A, S79.911A, S79.919-S79.921[A], S79.929A,
S82.101[A,B,C], S82.102[B,C], S82.109-S82.111[A,B,C],
S82.112[B,C], S82.113-S82.114[A,B,C], S82.115[B,C],
S82.116-S82.121[A,B,C], S82.122[B,C],
S82.123-S82.124[A,B,C], S82.125[B,C],
S82.126-S82.131[A,B,C], S82.132[B,C],
S82.133-S82.134[A,B,C], S82.135[B,C],
S82.136-S82.141[A,B,C], S82.142[B,C],
S82.143-S82.144[A,B,C], S82.145[B,C],
S82.146-S82.151[A,B,C], S82.152[B,C],
S82.153-S82.154[A,B,C], S82.155[B,C], S82.156[A,B,C],
S82.191[A,B,C], S82.192[B,C], S82.199-S82.201[A,B,C],
S82.202[B,C], S82.209-S82.221[A,B,C],
S82.222[B,C], S82.223-S82.224[A,B,C], S82.225[B,C],
S82.226-S82.231[A,B,C], S82.232[B,C],
S82.233-S82.234[A,B,C], S82.235[B,C],
S82.236-S82.241[A,B,C], S82.242[B,C],

S82.243-S82.244[A,B,C], S82.245[B,C],
S82.246-S82.251[A,B,C], S82.252[B,C],
S82.253-S82.254[A,B,C], S82.255[B,C],
S82.256-S82.261[A,B,C], S82.262[B,C],
S82.263-S82.264[A,B,C], S82.265[B,C],
S82.266-S82.291[A,B,C], S82.292[B,C], S82.299[A,B,C],
S82.401[A,B,C], S82.402[B,C], S82.409-S82.421[A,B,C],
S82.422[B,C], S82.423-S82.424[A,B,C], S82.425[B,C],
S82.426-S82.431[A,B,C], S82.432[B,C],
S82.433 S82.434[A,B,C], S82.435[B,C],
S82.436-S82.441[A,B,C], S82.442[B,C],
S82.443-S82.444[A,B,C], S82.445[B,C],
S82.446-S82.451[A,B,C], S82.452[B,C],
S82.453-S82.454[A,B,C], S82.455[B,C],
S82.456-S82.461[A,B,C], S82.462[B,C],
S82.463-S82.464[A,B,C], S82.465[B,C],
S82.466-S82.491[A,B,C], S82.492[B,C], S82.499[A,B,C],
S82.831[A,B,C], S82.831-S82.832[B,C], S82.839[A,B,C],
S82.861[A,B,C], S82.862[B,C], S82.863-S82.864[A,B,C],
S82.865[B,C], S82.866[A,B,C], S82.90X-S82.92X[A,B,C],
S89.001A, S89.009-S89.011[A], S89.019-S89.021[A],
S89.029-S89.031[A], S89.039-S89.041[A],
S89.049-S89.091[A], S89.099A, S89.201A,
S89.209-S89.211[A], S89.219-S89.221[A],
S89.229-S89.291[A], S89.299A, T07.XXX-T14.91X[A],
T79.8XX-T79.9XX[A], T79.A9XA

PDX Collection 1341
M80.00X-M80.019[A], M80.041-M80.049[A],
M80.061-M80.819[A], M80.841-M80.849[A],
M80.861-M80.879[A], M84.40X-M84.419[A],
M84.441-M84.446[A], M84.454A, M84.461-M84.519[A],
M84.541-M84.550[A], M84.561-M84.619[A],
M84.641 M84.650[A], M84.661-M84.68X[A],
S03.8XX-S03.9XX[A], S29.011-S29.019[A],
S38.3XXA, S39.011-S39.013[A], S73.101-S73.199[A],
S76.001-S76.019[A], S76.091-S76.119[A],
S76.191-S76.219[A], S76.291-S76.319[A],
S76.391 S76.819[A], S76.891-S76.919[A],
S76.991-S76.999[A], S79.811-S79.929[A],
S82.101-S82.156[A,B,C], S82.191-S82.299[A,B,C],
S82.401-S82.499[A,B,C], S82.831-S82.839[A,B,C],
S82.861 S82.866[A,B,C], S82.90X-S82.92X[A,B,C],
S89.001-S89.099[A], S89.201-S89.299[A],
T07.XXX T14.91X[A], T79.8XX-T79.9XX[A], T79.A9XA

PDX Collection 1342
M80.00X-M80.019[A], M80.041-M80.049[A],
M80.061-M80.819[A], M80.841-M80.849[A],
M80.861-M80.879[A], M84.40X-M84.419[A],
M84.441-M84.446[A], M84.454A, M84.461-M84.519[A],
M84.541-M84.550[A], M84.561-M84.619[A],
M84.641-M84.650[A], M84.661-M84.68X[A],
S03.8XX-S03.9XX[A], S29.011-S29.019[A],
S38.3XXA, S39.011-S39.013[A], S73.102-S73.109[A],
S73.112-S73.119[A], S73.122-S73.129[A],
S73.192-S73.199[A], S76.002-S76.009[A],
S76.012-S76.019[A], S76.092-S76.099[A],
S76.102-S76.109[A], S76.112-S76.119[A],
S76.192-S76.199[A], S76.202-S76.209[A],
S76.212-S76.219[A], S76.292-S76.299[A],
S76.302-S76.309[A], S76.312-S76.319[A],
S76.392-S76.399[A], S76.802-S76.809[A],
S76.812-S76.819[A], S76.892-S76.899[A],
S76.902-S76.909[A], S76.912-S76.919[A],
S76.992-S76.999[A], S79.812-S79.819[A],
S79.822-S79.829[A], S79.912-S79.919[A],
S79.922-S79.929[A], S82.101[B,C], S82.102-S82.109[A,B,C],
S82.111[B,C], S82.112-S82.113[A,B,C], S82.114[B,C],
S82.115-S82.116[A,B,C], S82.121[B,C],

S82.122-S82.123[A,B,C], S82.124[B,C],
S82.125-S82.126[A,B,C], S82.131[B,C],
S82.132-S82.133[A,B,C], S82.134[B,C],
S82.135-S82.136[A,B,C], S82.141[B,C],
S82.142-S82.143[A,B,C], S82.144[B,C],
S82.145-S82.146[A,B,C], S82.151[B,C],
S82.152-S82.153[A,B,C], S82.154[B,C],
S82.155-S82.156[A,B,C], S82.191[B,C],
S82.192-S82.199[A,B,C], S82.201[B,C],
S82.202-S82.209[A,B,C], S82.221[B,C],
S82.222-S82.223[A,B,C], S82.224[B,C],
S82.225-S82.226[A,B,C], S82.231[B,C],
S82.232-S82.233[A,B,C], S82.234[B,C],
S82.235-S82.236[A,B,C], S82.241[B,C],
S82.242-S82.243[A,B,C], S82.244[B,C],
S82.245-S82.246[A,B,C], S82.251[B,C],
S82.252-S82.253[A,B,C], S82.254[B,C],
S82.255-S82.256[A,B,C], S82.261[B,C],
S82.262-S82.263[A,B,C], S82.264[B,C],
S82.265-S82.266[A,B,C], S82.291[B,C],
S82.292-S82.299[A,B,C], S82.401[B,C],
S82.402-S82.409[A,B,C], S82.421[B,C],
S82.422-S82.423[A,B,C], S82.424[B,C],
S82.425-S82.426[A,B,C], S82.431[B,C],
S82.432-S82.433[A,B,C], S82.434[B,C],
S82.435-S82.436[A,B,C], S82.441[B,C],
S82.442-S82.443[A,B,C], S82.444[B,C],
S82.445-S82.446[A,B,C], S82.451[B,C],
S82.452-S82.453[A,B,C], S82.454[B,C],
S82.455-S82.456[A,B,C], S82.461[B,C],
S82.462-S82.463[A,B,C], S82.464[B,C],
S82.465-S82.466[A,B,C], S82.491[B,C],
S82.492-S82.499[A,B,C], S82.831[B,C],
S82.832-S82.839[A,B,C], S82.861[B,C],
S82.862-S82.863[A,B,C], S82.864[B,C],
S82.865-S82.866[A,B,C], S82.90X-S82.92X[A,B,C],
S89.002-S89.009[A], S89.012 S89.019[A],
S89.022-S89.029[A], S09.032-S89.039[A],
S89.042-S89.049[A], S89.092-S89.099[A],
S89.202-S89.209[A], S89.212-S89.219[A],
S89.222-S89.229[A], S89.292-S89.299[A],
T07.XXX-T14.91X[A], T79.8XX-T79.9XX[A], T79.A9XA

PDX Collection 1343
S82.101[A,B,C], S82.102[B,C], S82.109-S82.111[A,B,C],
S82.112[A,B], S82.113-S82.114[A,B,C],
S82.115[B,C], S82.116-S82.121[A,B,C], S82.122[B,C],
S82.123-S82.124[A,B,C], S82.125[B,C],
S82.126-S82.131[A,B,C], S82.132[B,C],
S82.133-S82.134[A,B,C], S82.135[B,C],
S82.136-S82.141[A,B,C], S82.142[B,C],
S82.143-S82.144[A,B,C], S82.145[B,C],
S82.146-S82.151[A,B,C], S82.152[B,C],
S82.153-S82.154[A,B,C], S82.155[B,C],
S82.156[A,B,C], S82.161A, S82.169A, S82.191[A,B,C],
S82.192[B,C], S82.199-S82.201[A,B,C],
S82.202[B,C], S82.209-S82.221[A,B,C],
S82.222[B,C], S82.223-S82.224[A,B,C], S82.225[B,C],
S82.226-S82.231[A,B,C], S82.232[B,C],
S82.233-S82.234[A,B,C], S82.235[B,C],
S82.236-S82.241[A,B,C], S82.242[B,C],
S82.243-S82.244[A,B,C], S82.245[B,C],
S82.246-S82.251[A,B,C], S82.252[B,C],
S82.253-S82.254[A,B,C], S82.255[B,C],
S82.256-S82.261[A,B,C], S82.262[B,C],
S82.263-S82.264[A,B,C], S82.265[B,C],
S82.266-S82.291[A,B,C], S82.292[B,C],
S82.299[A,B,C], S82.311A, S82.319A, S82.401[A,B,C],
S82.402[B,C], S82.409-S82.421[A,B,C],

S82.422[B,C], S82.423-S82.424[A,B,C], S82.425[B,C],
S82.426-S82.431[A,B,C], S82.432[B,C],
S82.433-S82.434[A,B,C], S82.435[B,C],
S82.436-S82.441[A,B,C], S82.442[B,C],
S82.443-S82.444[A,B,C], S82.445[B,C],
S82.446-S82.451[A,B,C], S82.452[B,C],
S82.453-S82.454[A,B,C], S82.455[B,C],
S82.456-S82.461[A,B,C], S82.462[B,C],
S82.463-S82.464[A,B,C], S82.465[B,C],
S82.466-S82.491[A,B,C], S82.492[B,C], S82.499[A,B,C],
S82.811A, S82.819-S82.821[A], S82.829[A], S82.831[A,B,C],
S82.832[B,C], S82.839[A,B,C], S82.861[A,B,C],
S82.862[B,C], S82.863-S82.864[A,B,C], S82.865[B,C],
S82.866[A,B,C], S89.001A, S89.009-S89.011[A],
S89.019-S89.021[A], S89.029-S89.031[A],
S89.039-S89.041[A], S89.049-S89.091[A], S89.099A,
S89.201A, S89.209-S89.211[A], S89.219-S89.221[A],
S89.229-S89.291[A], S89.299A

PDX Collection 1344
S82.101[B,C], S82.102-S82.109[A,B,C],
S82.111[B,C], S82.112-S82.113[A,B,C],
S82.114[B,C], S82.115-S82.116[A,B,C], S82.121[B,C],
S82.122-S82.123[A,B,C], S82.124[B,C],
S82.125-S82.126[A,B,C], S82.131[B,C],
S82.132-S82.133[A,B,C], S82.134[B,C],
S82.135-S82.136[A,B,C], S82.141[B,C],
S82.142-S82.143[A,B,C], S82.144[B,C],
S82.145-S82.146[A,B,C], S82.151[B,C],
S82.152-S82.153[A,B,C], S82.154[B,C],
S82.155-S82.156[A,B,C], S82.162-S82.169[A],
S82.191[B,C], S82.192-S82.199[A],
S82.201[B,C], S82.202-S82.209[A,B,C],
S82.221[B,C], S82.222-S82.223[A,B,C], S82.224[B,C],
S82.225-S82.226[A,B,C], S82.231[B,C],
S82.232-S82.233[A,B,C], S82.234[B,C],
S82.235-S82.236[A,B,C], S82.241[B,C],
S82.242-S82.243[A,B,C], S82.244[B,C],
S82.245-S82.246[A,B,C], S82.251[B,C],
S82.252-S82.253[A,B,C], S82.254[B,C],
S82.255-S82.256[A,B,C], S82.261[B,C],
S82.262-S82.263[A,B,C], S82.264[B,C],
S82.265-S82.266[A,B,C], S82.291[B,C],
S82.292-S82.299[A,B,C], S82.312-S82.319[A],
S82.401[B,C], S82.402-S82.409[A,B,C],
S82.421[B,C], S82.422-S82.423[A,B,C], S82.424[B,C],
S82.425-S82.426[A,B,C], S82.431[B,C],
S82.432-S82.433[A,B,C], S82.434[B,C],
S82.435-S82.436[A,B,C], S82.441[B,C],
S82.442-S82.443[A,B,C], S82.444[B,C],
S82.445-S82.446[A,B,C], S82.451[B,C],
S82.452-S82.453[A,B,C], S82.454[B,C],
S82.455-S82.456[A,B,C], S82.461[B,C],
S82.462-S82.463[A,B,C], S82.464[B,C],
S82.465-S82.466[A,B,C], S82.491[B,C],
S82.492-S82.499[A,B,C], S82.812-S82.819[A],
S82.822-S82.829[A], S82.831[B,C], S82.832-S82.839[A,B,C],
S82.861[B,C], S82.862-S82.863[A,B,C], S82.864[B,C],
S82.865-S82.866[A,B,C], S89.002-S89.009[A],
S89.012-S89.019[A], S89.022-S89.029[A],
S89.032-S89.039[A], S89.042-S89.049[A],
S89.092-S89.099[A], S89.202-S89.209[A],
S89.212-S89.219[A], S89.222-S89.229[A],
S89.292-S89.299[A]

PDX Collection 1345
S82.101-S82.156[A,B,C], S82.161-S82.169[A],
S82.191-S82.299[A,B,C], S82.311-S82.319[A],
S82.401-S82.499[A,B,C], S82.811-S82.829[A],

S82.831-S82.839[A,B,C], S82.861-S82.866[A,B,C],
S89.001-S89.099[A], S89.201-S89.299[A]

PDX Collection 1346
M80.00X-M80.019[A], M80.041-M80.049[A],
M80.061-M80.819[A], M80.841-M80.849[A],
M80.861-M80.879[A], M84.40X-M84.419[A],
M84.441-M84.446[A], M84.454[A], M84.461-M84.519[A],
M84.541-M84.550[A], M84.561-M84.576[A],
M84.60X-M84.619[A], M84.641-M84.650[A],
M84.661-M84.68X[A], S03.8XX-S03.9XX[A],
S29.011-S29.019[A], S38.3XXA, S39.011-S39.013[A],
S73.101A, S73.109-S73.111[A], S73.119-S73.121[A],
S73.129-S73.191[A], S73.199A, S76.001A,
S76.009-S76.011[A], S76.019A, S76.091A,
S76.099-S76.101[A], S76.109-S76.111[A],
S76.119A, S76.191A, S76.199-S76.201[A],
S76.209-S76.211[A], S76.219A, S76.291A,
S76.299-S76.301[A], S76.309-S76.311[A], S76.319A,
S76.391A, S76.399-S76.801[A], S76.809-S76.811[A],
S76.819A, S76.891A, S76.899-S76.901[A],
S76.909-S76.911[A], S76.919A, S76.991A, S76.999A,
S79.811A, S79.819-S79.821[A], S79.829-S79.911[A],
S79.919-S79.921[A], S79.929A, S82.101[A,B,C],
S82.102[B,C], S82.109-S82.111[A,B,C],
S82.112[B,C], S82.113-S82.114[A,B,C], S82.115[B,C],
S82.116-S82.121[A,B,C], S82.122[B,C],
S82.123-S82.124[A,B,C], S82.125[B,C],
S82.126-S82.131[A,B,C], S82.132[B,C],
S82.133-S82.134[A,B,C], S82.135[B,C],
S82.136-S82.141[A,B,C], S82.142[B,C],
S82.143-S82.144[A,B,C], S82.145[B,C],
S82.146-S82.151[A,B,C], S82.152[B,C],
S82.153-S82.154[A,B,C], S82.155[B,C],
S82.156[A,B,C], S82.161A, S82.169A, S82.191[A,B,C],
S82.192[B,C], S82.199-S82.201[A,B,C],
S82.202[B,C], S82.209-S82.221[A,B,C],
S82.222[B,C], S82.223-S82.224[A,B,C], S82.225[B,C],
S82.226-S82.231[A,B,C], S82.232[B,C],
S82.233-S82.234[A,B,C], S82.235[B,C],
S82.236-S82.241[A,B,C], S82.242[B,C],
S82.243-S82.244[A,B,C], S82.245[B,C],
S82.246-S82.251[A,B,C], S82.252[B,C],
S82.253-S82.254[A,B,C], S82.255[B,C],
S82.256-S82.261[A,B,C], S82.262[B,C,],
S82.263-S82.264[A,B,C], S82.265[B,C],
S82.266-S82.291[A,B,C], S82.292[B,C],
S82.299[A,B,C], S82.311A, S82.319A, S82.401[A,B,C],
S82.402[B,C], S82.409-S82.421[A,B,C],
S82.422[B,C], S82.423-S82.424[A,B,C], S82.425[B,C],
S82.426-S82.431[A,B,C], S82.432[B,C],
S82.433-S82.434[A,B,C], S82.435[B,C],
S82.436-S82.441[A,B,C], S82.442[B,C],
S82.443-S82.444[A,B,C], S82.445[B,C],
S82.446-S82.451[A,B,C], S82.452[B,C,],
S82.453-S82.454[A,B,C], S82.455[B,C],
S82.456-S82.461[A,B,C], S82.462[B,C],
S82.463-S82.464[A,B,C], S82.465[B,C],
S82.466-S82.491[A,B,C], S82.492[B,C], S82.499[A,B,C],
S82.811A, S82.819-S82.821[A], S82.829A, S82.831[A,B,C],
S82.832[B,C], S82.839[A,B,C], S82.861[A,B,C], S82.862[B,C],
S82.863-S82.864[A,B,C], S82.865[B,C], S82.866[A,B,C],
S82.90X-S82.92X[A,B,C], S89.001A, S89.009-S89.011[A],
S89.019-S89.021[A], S89.029-S89.031[A],
S89.039-S89.041[A], S89.049-S89.091[A],
S89.099A, S89.201A, S89.209A, S89.211-S89.219[A],
S89.221-S89.229[A], S89.291-S89.299[A],
T07.XXX-T14.91X[A], T79.A9X-T79.9XX[A]

PDX Collection 1347
M80.00X-M80.019[A], M80.041-M80.049[A],
M80.061-M80.819[A], M80.841-M80.849[A],
M80.861-M80.879[A], M84.40X-M84.419[A],
M84.441-M84.446[A], M84.454A, M84.461-M84.519[A],
M84.541-M84.550[A], M84.561-M84.576[A],
M84.60X-M84.619[A], M84.641-M84.650[A],
M84.661-M84.68X[A], S03.8XX-S03.9XX[A],
S29.011-S29.019[A], S38.3XXA, S39.011-S39.013[A],
S73.101-S73.199[A], S76.001-S76.019[A],
S76.091-S76.119[A], S76.191-S76.219[A],
S76.291-S76.319[A], S76.391-S76.819[A],
S76.891-S76.919[A], S76.991-S76.999[A],
S79.811-S79.929[A], S82.301-S82.309[A,B,C],
S82.391-S82.399[A,B,C], S82.51X-S82.56X[B,C],
S82.61X-S82.66X[A,B,C], S82.841-S82.856[A,B,C],
S82.871-S82.876[B,C], S82.891-S82.92X[A,B,C],
S89.101-S89.199[A], S89.301-S89.399[A],
T07.XXX-T14.91X[A], T79.A9X-T79.9XX[A]

PDX Collection 1348
S72.001-S72.92X[A,B,C], S79.001-S79.199[A],
S82.001-S82.156[A,B,C], S82.191-S82.309[A,B,C],
S82.391-S82.66X[A,B,C], S82.831-S82.92X[A,B,C],
S89.001-S89.399[A], S92.001-S92.599[A,B],
S92.811-S92.919[A,B]

PDX Collection 1349
S75.801A, S75.809-S75.811[A], S75.819-S75.891[A],
S75.899-S75.901[A], S75.909-S75.911[A],
S75.919-S75.991[A], S75.999A, S85.001A,
S85.009-S85.011[A], S85.019-S85.091[A], S85.099A,
S85.201A, S85.209-S85.211[A], S85.219-S85.291[A],
S85.299A, S85.801A, S85.809-S85.811[A],
S85.819-S85.891[A], S85.899-S85.901[A],
S85.909-S85.911[A], S85.919-S85.991[A], S85.999A,
S95.001A, S95.009-S95.011[A], S95.019-S95.091[A],
S95.099-S95.201[A], S95.209-S95.211[A],
S95.219-S95.291[A], S95.299-S95.801[A],
S95.809-S95.811[A], S95.819-S95.891[A],
S95.899-S95.901[A], S95.909-S95.911[A],
S95.919-S95.991[A], S95.999A

PDX Collection 1350
S75.802-S75.809[A], S75.812-S75.819[A],
S75.892-S75.899[A], S75.902-S75.909[A],
S75.912-S75.919[A], S75.992-S75.999[A],
S85.002-S85.009[A], S85.012-S85.019[A],
S85.092-S85.099[A], S85.202-S85.209[A],
S85.212-S85.219[A], S85.292-S85.299[A],
S85.802-S85.809[A], S85.812-S85.819[A],
S85.892-S85.899[A], S85.902-S85.909[A],
S85.912-S85.919[A], S85.992-S85.999[A],
S95.002-S95.009[A], S95.012-S95.019[A],
S95.092-S95.099[A], S95.202-S95.209[A],
S95.212-S95.219[A], S95.292-S95.299[A],
S95.802-S95.809[A], S95.812-S95.819[A],
S95.892-S95.899[A], S95.902-S95.909[A],
S95.912-S95.919[A], S95.992-S95.999[A]

PDX Collection 1351
S75.801A-S75.999[A], S85.001-S85.099[A],
S85.201-S85.299[A], S85.801-S85.999[A],
S95.001-S95.009[A], S95.201-S95.999[A]

PDX Collection 1352
S75.801A, S75.809-S75.811[A], S75.819-S75.891[A],
S75.899-S75.901[A], S75.909-S75.911[A],
S75.919-S75.991[A], S75.999A, S85.101A,
S85.109-S85.111[A], S85.119-S85.121[A], S85.129A,
S85.201A, S85.209-S85.211[A], S85.219-S85.291[A],

S85.299A, S85.801A, S85.809-S85.811[A],
S85.819-S85.891[A], S85.899-S85.901[A],
S85.909-S85.911[A], S85.919-S85.991[A], S85.999A,
S95.001A, S95.009-S95.011[A], S95.019-S95.091[A],
S95.099-S95.201[A], S95.209-S95.211[A],
S95.219-S95.291[A], S95.299-S95.801[A],
S95.809-S95.811[A], S95.819-S95.891[A],
S95.899-S95.901[A], S95.909-S95.911[A],
S95.919-S95.991[A], S95.999A

PDX Collection 1353
S75.802-S75.809[A], S75.812-S75.819[A],
S75.892-S75.899[A], S75.902-S75.909[A],
S75.912-S75.919[A], S75.992-S75.999[A],
S85.102-S85.109[A], S85.112-S85.119[A],
S85.122-S85.129[A], S85.202-S85.209[A],
S85.212-S85.219[A], S85.292-S85.299[A],
S85.802-S85.809[A], S85.812-S85.819[A],
S85.892-S85.899[A], S85.902-S85.909[A],
S85.912-S85.919[A], S85.992-S85.999[A],
S95.002-S95.009[A], S95.012-S95.019[A],
S95.092-S95.099[A], S95.202-S95.209[A],
S95.212-S95.219[A], S95.292-S95.299[A],
S95.802-S95.809[A], S95.812-S95.819[A],
S95.892-S95.899[A], S95.902-S95.909[A],
S95.912-S95.919[A], S95.992-S95.999[A]

PDX Collection 1354
S75.801-S75.999[A], S85.101-S85.129[A],
S85.201-S85.299[A], S85.801-S85.999[A],
S95.001-S95.099[A], S95.201-S95.999[A]

PDX Collection 1355
S75.801A, S75.809-S75.811[A], S75.819-S75.891[A],
S75.899-S75.901[A], S75.909-S75.911[A],
S75.919-S75.991[A], S75.999A, S85.131A,
S85.139-S85.141[A], S85.149-S85.151[A], S85.159A,
S85.201A, S85.209-S85.211[A], S85.219-S85.291[A],
S85.299A, S85.801A, S85.809-S85.811[A],
S85.819-S85.891[A], S85.899-S85.901[A],
S85.909-S85.911[A], S85.919-S85.991[A], S85.999A,
S95.001A, S95.009-S95.011[A], S95.019-S95.091[A],
S95.099-S95.201[A], S95.209-S95.211[A],
S95.219-S95.291[A], S95.299-S95.801[A],
S95.809-S95.811[A], S95.819-S95.891[A],
S95.899-S95.901[A], S95.909-S95.911[A],
S95.919-S95.991[A], S95.999A

PDX Collection 1356
S75.802-S75.809[A], S75.812-S75.819[A],
S75.892-S75.899[A], S75.902-S75.909[A],
S75.912-S75.919[A], S75.992-S75.999[A],
S85.132-S85.139[A], S85.142-S85.149[A],
S85.152-S85.159[A], S85.202-S85.209[A],
S85.212-S85.219[A], S85.292-S85.299[A],
S85.802-S85.809[A], S85.812-S85.819[A],
S85.892-S85.899[A], S85.902-S85.909[A],
S85.912-S85.919[A], S85.992-S85.999[A],
S95.002-S95.009[A], S95.012-S95.019[A],
S95.092-S95.099[A], S95.202-S95.209[A],
S95.212-S95.219[A], S95.292-S95.299[A],
S95.802-S95.809[A], S95.812-S95.819[A],
S95.892-S95.899[A], S95.902-S95.909[A],
S95.912-S95.919[A], S95.992-S95.999[A]

PDX Collection 1357
S75.801-S75.999[A], S85.131-S85.159[A],
S85.201-S85.299[A], S85.801-S85.999[A],
S95.001-S95.099[A], S95.201-S95.999[A]

PDX Collection 1358
S75.801A, S75.809-S75.811[A], S75.819-S75.891[A],
S75.899-S75.901[A], S75.909-S75.911[A],

S75.919-S75.991[A], S75.999A, S85.161A,
S85.169-S85.171[A], S85.179-S85.181[A], S85.189A,
S85.201A, S85.209-S85.211[A], S85.219-S85.291[A],
S85.299A, S85.801A, S85.809-S85.811[A],
S85.819-S85.891[A], S85.899-S85.901[A],
S85.909-S85.911[A], S85.919-S85.991[A], S85.999A,
S95.001A, S95.009-S95.011[A], S95.019-S95.091[A],
S95.099-S95.201[A], S95.209-S95.211[A],
S95.219-S95.291[A], S95.299-S95.801[A],
S95.809-S95.811[A], S95.819-S95.891[A],
S95.899-S95.901[A], S95.909-S95.911[A],
S95.919-S95.991[A], S95.999A

PDX Collection 1359
S75.802-S75.809[A], S75.812-S75.819[A],
S75.892-S75.899[A], S75.902-S75.909[A],
S75.912-S75.919[A], S75.992-S75.999[A],
S85.162-S85.169[A], S85.172-S85.179[A],
S85.182-S85.189[A], S85.202-S85.209[A],
S85.212-S85.219[A], S85.292-S85.299[A],
S85.802-S85.809[A], S85.812-S85.819[A],
S85.892-S85.899[A], S85.902-S85.909[A],
S85.912-S85.919[A], S85.992-S85.999[A],
S95.002-S95.009[A], S95.012-S95.019[A],
S95.092-S95.099[A], S95.202-S95.209[A],
S95.212-S95.219[A], S95.292-S95.299[A],
S95.802-S95.809[A], S95.812-S95.819[A],
S95.892-S95.899[A], S95.902-S95.909[A],
S95.912-S95.919[A], S95.992-S95.999[A]

PDX Collection 1360
S75.801-S75.999[A], S85.161-S85.189[A],
S85.201-S85.299[A], S85.801-S85.999[A],
S95.001-S95.099[A], S95.201-S95.999[A]

PDX Collection 1361
S75.801[A], S75.809-S75.811[A], S75.819-S75.891[A],
S75.899-S75.901[A], S75.909-S75.911[A],
S75.919-S75.991[A], S75.999A, S85.201A,
S85.209-S85.211[A], S85.219-S85.291[A], S85.299A,
S85.501A, S85.509-S85.511[A], S85.519-S85.591[A],
S85.599A, S85.801A, S85.809-S85.811[A],
S85.819-S85.891[A], S85.899-S85.901[A],
S85.909-S85.911[A], S85.919-S85.991[A], S85.999A,
S95.001A, S95.009-S95.011[A], S95.019-S95.091[A],
S95.099-S95.201[A], S95.209-S95.211[A],
S95.219-S95.291[A], S95.299-S95.801[A],
S95.809-S95.811[A], S95.819-S95.891[A],
S95.899-S95.901[A], S95.909-S95.911[A],
S95.919-S95.991[A], S95.999A

PDX Collection 1362
S75.802-S75.809[A], S75.812-S75.819[A],
S75.892-S75.899[A], S75.902-S75.909[A],
S75.912-S75.919[A], S75.992-S75.999[A],
S85.202-S85.209[A], S85.212-S85.219[A],
S85.292-S85.299[A], S85.502-S85.509[A],
S85.512-S85.519[A], S85.592-S85.599[A],
S85.802-S85.809[A], S85.812-S85.819[A],
S85.892-S85.899[A], S85.902-S85.909[A],
S85.912-S85.919[A], S85.992-S85.999[A],
S95.002-S95.009[A], S95.012-S95.019[A],
S95.092-S95.099[A], S95.202-S95.209[A],
S95.212-S95.219[A], S95.292-S95.299[A],
S95.802-S95.809[A], S95.812-S95.819[A],
S95.892-S95.899[A], S95.902-S95.909[A],
S95.912-S95.919[A], S95.992-S95.999[A]

PDX Collection 1363
S75.801-S75.999[A], S85.201-S85.299[A],
S85.501-S85.599[A], S85.801-S85.999[A],
S95.001-S95.099[A], S95.201-S95.999[A]

PDX Collection 1364
S81.001A, S81.009-S81.011[A], S81.019-S81.021[A],
S81.029-S81.031[A], S81.039-S81.041[A],
S81.049-S81.051[A], S81.059-S81.801[A],
S81.809-S81.811[A], S81.819-S81.821[A],
S81.829-S81.831[A], S81.839-S81.841[A],
S81.849-S81.851[A], S81.859A, S86.021A, S86.029A,
S86.121A, S86.129A, S86.221A, S86.229A, S86.321A,
S86.329A, S86.821A, S86.829-S86.921[A], S86.929A,
S91.001A, S91.009A, S91.011A, S91.019-S91.021[A],
S91.029-S91.031[A], S91.039-S91.041[A],
S91.049-S91.051[A], S91.059A, S96.021A, S96.029A,
S96.121A, S96.129A, S96.221A, S96.229A, S96.821A,
S96.829A, S96.921A, S96.929A

PDX Collection 1365
S81.002-S81.009[A], S81.012-S81.019[A],
S81.022-S81.029[A], S81.032-S81.039[A],
S81.042-S81.049[A], S81.052-S81.059[A],
S81.802-S81.809[A], S81.812-S81.819[A],
S81.822-S81.829[A], S81.832-S81.839[A],
S81.842-S81.849[A], S81.852-S81.859[A],
S86.022-S86.029[A], S86.122-S86.129[A],
S86.222-S86.229[A], S86.322-S86.329[A],
S86.822-S86.829[A], S86.922-S86.929[A],
S91.002-S91.009[A], S91.012-S91.019[A],
S91.022-S91.029[A], S91.032-S91.039[A],
S91.042-S91.049[A], S91.052-S91.059[A],
S96.022-S96.029[A], S96.122-S96.129[A],
S96.222-S96.229[A], S96.822-S96.829[A],
S96.922-S96.929[A]

PDX Collection 1366
S81.001-S81.859[A], S86.021-S86.029[A],
S86.121-S86.129[A], S86.221-S86.229[A],
S86.321-S86.329[A], S86.821-S86.829[A],
S86.921-S86.929[A], S91.001-S91.059[A],
S96.021-S96.029[A], S96.121-S96.129[A],
S96.221-S96.229[A], S96.821-S96.829[A],
S96.921-S96.929[A]

PDX Collection 1367
M80.00X-M80.019[A], M80.041-M80.049[A],
M80.061-M80.819[A], M80.841-M80.849[A],
M80.861-M80.879[A], M84.40X-M84.419[A],
M84.441-M84.446[A], M84.454A, M84.461-M84.519[A],
M84.541-M84.550[A], M84.561-M84.576[A],
M84.60X-M84.619[A], M84.641-M84.650[A],
M84.661-M84.68X[A], S03.8XX-S03.9XX[A],
S29.011-S29.019[A], S38.3XXA, S39.011-S39.013[A],
S73.101-S73.199[A], S76.001-S76.019[A],
S76.091-S76.219[A], S76.291-S76.319[A],
S76.391-S76.819[A], S76.891-S76.919[A],
S76.991-S76.999[A], S79.811-S79.929[A],
S82.90X-S82.92X[A,B,C], S92.001-S92.066[B],
S92.101-S92.356[A,B], S92.811-S92.819[A,B],
S92.901-S92.909[A,B], T07.XXX-T14.91X[A],
T79.A9X-T79.9XX[A]

PDX Collection 1368
M80.00X-M80.019[A], M80.041-M80.049[A],
M80.80X-M80.819[A], M80.841-M80.849[A],
M84.40X-M84.419[A], M84.441-M84.446[A],
M84.454A, M84.474-M84.519[A], M84.541-M84.550[A],
M84.574-M84.576[A], M84.60X-M84.619[A],
M84.641-M84.650[A], M84.674-M84.68X[A],
S03.8XX-S03.9XX[A], S29.011-S29.019[A],
S38.3XXA, S39.011-S39.013[A], S73.101-S73.199[A],
S76.001-S76.019[A], S76.091-S76.219[A],
S76.291-S76.319[A], S76.391-S76.819[A],
S76.891-S76.919[A], S76.991-S76.999[A],
S79.821-S79.929[A], S82.90X-S82.92X[A,B,C],

S92.001-S92.066[B], S92.101-S92.356[A,B],
S92.811-S92.819[A,B], S92.901-S92.909[A,B],
T07.XXX-T14.91X[A], T79.A9X-T79.9XX[A]

PDX Collection 1369
S92.001-S92.919[A,B]

PDX Collection 1370
S75.801A, S75.809-S75.811[A], S75.819-S75.891[A],
S75.899-S75.901[A], S75.909-S75.911[A],
S75.919-S75.991[A], S75.999A, S85.201A,
S85.209-S85.211[A], S85.219-S85.291[A], S85.299A,
S85.801A, S85.809-S85.811[A], S85.819-S85.891[A],
S85.899-S85.901[A], S85.909-S85.911[A],
S85.919-S85.991[A], S85.999A, S95.001A,
S95.009-S95.011[A], S95.019-S95.091[A],
S95.099-S95.201[A], S95.209-S95.211[A],
S95.219-S95.291[A], S95.299-S95.801[A],
S95.809-S95.811[A], S95.819-S95.891[A],
S95.899-S95.901[A], S95.909-S95.911[A],
S95.919-S95.991[A], S95.999A

PDX Collection 1371
S75.802-S75.809[A], S75.812-S75.819[A],
S75.892-S75.899[A], S75.902-S75.909[A],
S75.912-S75.919[A], S75.992-S75.999[A],
S85.202-S85.209[A], S85.212-S85.219[A],
S85.292-S85.299[A], S85.802-S85.809[A],
S85.812-S85.819[A], S85.892-S85.899[A],
S85.902-S85.909[A], S85.912-S85.919[A],
S85.992-S85.999[A], S95.002-S95.009[A],
S95.012-S95.019[A], S95.092-S95.099[A],
S95.102-S95.109[A], S95.112-S95.119[A],
S95.192-S95.199[A], S95.202-S95.209[A],
S95.212-S95.219[A], S95.292-S95.299[A],
S95.802-S95.809[A], S95.812-S95.819[A],
S95.892-S95.899[A], S95.902-S95.909[A],
S95.912-S95.919[A], S95.992-S95.999[A]

PDX Collection 1372
S75.801-S75.999[A], S85.201-S85.299[A],
S85.801-S85.999[A], S95.001-S95.099[A],
S95.101-S95.999[A]

PDX Collection 1373
T17.400-T17.498[A]

PDX Collection 1374
T17.400-T17.998[A]

PDX Collection 1375
T20.30XA, T20.39XA, T20.70XA, T20.79XA

PDX Collection 1376
T20.311-T20.319[A], T20.39XA, T20.711-T20.719[A],
T20.79XA

PDX Collection 1377
T20.32XA, T20.39XA, T20.72XA, T20.79XA

PDX Collection 1378
T20.33XA, T20.39XA, T20.73XA, T20.79XA

PDX Collection 1379
T20.34XA, T20.39XA, T20.74XA, T20.79XA

PDX Collection 1380
T20.35XA, T20.39XA, T20.75XA, T20.79XA

PDX Collection 1381
T20.36XA, T20.39XA, T20.76XA, T20.79XA

PDX Collection 1382
T20.37X-T20.39X[A], T20.77X-T20.79X[A]

PDX Collection 1383
T20.30X-T20.39X[A], T20.70X-T20.79X[A]

PDX Collection 1384
T21.30XA, T21.39XA, T21.70XA, T21.79XA

PDX Collection 1385
T21.30X-T21.31X[A], T21.39XA, T21.70X-T21.71X[A],
T21.79XA

PDX Collection 1386
T21.30XA, T21.32XA, T21.39XA, T21.70XA, T21.72XA,
T21.79XA

PDX Collection 1387
T21.30XA, T21.33X-T21.35X[A], T21.39XA, T21.70XA,
T21.73X-T21.75X[A], T21.79XA

PDX Collection 1388
T21.30XA, T21.36X-T21.39X[A], T21.70XA,
T21.76X-T21.79X[A]

PDX Collection 1389
T22.30XA, T22.391-T22.399[A], T22.70XA,
T22.791-T22.799[A]

PDX Collection 1390
T22.30X-T22.319[A], T22.391-T22.399[A],
T22.70X-T22.719[A], T22.791-T22.799[A]

PDX Collection 1391
T22.30XA, T22.321-T22.329[A], T22.391-T22.399[A],
T22.70XA, T22.721-T22.729[A], T22.791-T22.799[A]

PDX Collection 1392
T22.30XA, T22.331-T22.339[A], T22.391-T22.399[A],
T22.70XA, T22.731-T22.739[A], T22.791-T22.799[A]

PDX Collection 1393
T22.30XA, T22.341-T22.349[A], .T22.391-T22.399[A],
T22.70XA, T22.741-T22.749[A], T22.791-T22.799[A]

PDX Collection 1394
T22.30XA, T22.351-T22.359[A], T22.391-T22.399[A],
T22.70XA, T22.751-T22.759[A], T22.791-T22.799[A]

PDX Collection 1395
T22.30XA, T22.361-T22.369[A], T22.391-T22.399[A],
T22.70XA, T22.761-T22.769[A], T22.791-T22.799[A]

PDX Collection 1396
T23.301-T23.309[A], T23.391-T23.399[A],
T23.701-T23.709[A], T23.791-T23.799[A]

PDX Collection 1397
T23.301-T23.319[A], T23.391-T23.399[A],
T23.701-T23.719[A], T23.791-T23.799[A]

PDX Collection 1398
T23.301-T23.309[A], T23.321-T23.329[A],
T23.391-T23.399[A], T23.701-T23.709[A],
T23.721-T23.729[A], T23.791-T23.799[A]

PDX Collection 1399
T23.301-T23.309[A], T23.331-T23.339[A],
T23.391-T23.399[A], T23.701-709[A], T23.731-T23.739[A],
T23.791-T23.799[A]

PDX Collection 1400
T23.301-T23.309[A], T23.341-T23.349[A],
T23.391-T23.399[A], T23.701-T23.709[A],
T23.741-T23.749[A], T23.791-T23.799[A]

PDX Collection 1401
T23.301-T23.309[A], T23.351-T23.359[A],
T23.391-T23.399[A], T23.701-T23.709[A],
T23.751-T23.759[A], T23.791-T23.799[A]

PDX Collection 1402
T23.301-T23.309[A], T23.361-T23.369[A],
T23.391-T23.399[A], T23.701-T23.709[A],
T23.761-T23.769[A], T23.791-T23.799[A]

PDX Collection 1403
T23.301-123.309[A], T23.371-T23.379[A],
T23.391-T23.399[A], T23.701-T23.709[A],
T23.771-T23.779[A], T23.791-T23.799[A]

PDX Collection 1404
T24.301-T24.309[A], T24.391-T24.399[A],
T24.701-T24.709[A], T24.791-T24.799[A],
T25.391-T25.399[A], T25.791-T25.799[A]

PDX Collection 1405
T24.301-T24.309[A], T24.311-T24.319[A],
T24.391-T24.399[A], T24.701-T24.709-T24.719[A],
T24.791-T24.799[A], T25.391-T25.399[A],
T25.791-T25.799[A]

PDX Collection 1406
T24.301-T24.309[A], T24.321-T24.329[A],
T24.391-T24.399[A], T24.701-T24.709[A],
T24.721-T24.729[A], T24.791-T24.799[A],
T25.391-T25.399[A], T25.791-T25.799[A]

PDX Collection 1407
T24.301-T24.309[A], T24.331-T24.339[A],
T24.391-T24.399[A], T24.701-T24.709[A],
T24.731-T24.739[A], T24.791-T24.799[A],
T25.391-T25.399[A], T25.791-T25.799[A]

PDX Collection 1408
T24.301-T24.309[A], T24.391-T24.399[A],
T24.701-T24.709[A], T24.791-T24.799[A],
T25.311-T25.319[A], T25.391-T25.399[A],
T25.711-T25.719[A], T25.791-T25.799[A]

PDX Collection 1409
T24.301-T24.309[A], T24.391-T24.399[A],
T24.701-T24.709[A], T24.791-T24.799[A],
T25.321-T25.329[A], T25.391-T25.399[A],
T25.721-T25.729[A], T25.791-T25.799[A]

PDX Collection 1410
T24.301-T24.309[A], T24.391-T24.399[A],
T24.701-T24.709[A], T24.791-T24.799[A],
T25.331-T25.339[A], T25.391-T25.399[A],
T25.731-T25.739[A], T25.791-T25.799[A]

PDX Collection 1411
T27.0XX-T27.7XX[A], T28.3XX-T28.49X[A],
T28.8XX-T28.99X[A]

PDX Collection 1412
T28.1XXA, T28.3XX-T28.49X[A], T28.6XXA,
T28.8XX-T28.99X[A]

PDX Collection 1413
T28.2XX-T28.49X[A], T28.7XX-T28.99X[A]

PDX Collection 1414
T31.0-T32.99

PDX Collection 1415
T33.011-T33.42X[A], T33.60X-T33.72X[A],
T33.90X-T34.42X[A], T34.60X-T34.72X[A],
T34.90X-T34.99X[A]

PDX Collection 1416
T33.011-T34.99X[A], T69.021-T69.029[A]

PDX Collection 1417
T33.2XX-T33.72X[A], T33.90X-T33.99X[A],
T34.2XX-T34.72X[A], T34.90X-T34.99X[A]

PDX Collection 1418
T33.2XX-T33.42X[A], T33.60X-T33.99X[A],
T34.2XX-T34.42X[A], T34.60X-T34.99X[A]

PDX Collection 1419
T67.01X-T67.9XX[A]

PDX Collection 1420
T33.2XX-T33.42X[A], T33.60X-T33.72X[A],
T33.90X-T33.99X[A], T34.2XX-T34.42X[A],
T34.60X-T34.72X[A], T34.90X-T34.99X[A],
T69.021-T69.029[A]

PDX Collection 1421
T70.3XX-T70.9XX[A]

PDX Collection 1422
T71.111-T71.9XX[A]

PDX Collection 1423
T74.01X-T74.92X[A], T76.01X-T76.92X[A]

PDX Collection 1424
T74.91XA, T76.91XA

PDX Collection 1425
T75.1XXA

PDX Collection 1426
T78.00X-T78.09X[A]

PDX Collection 1427
D78.81-D78.89, E36.8, E89.810-E89.89, H59.011-H59.019,
H59.031-H59.039, H59.091-H59.099, H59.811-H59.89,
H95.811-H95.89, I97.3, L76.81-L76.82, M96.89, N98.1-N98.9,
T07.XXX-T14.91X[A], T79.0XXA, T79.A0X-T79.9XX[A],
T80.0XXA, T81.82XA, T81.89X-T81.9XX[A]

PDX Collection 1428
D78.81-D78.89, E36.8, E89.810-E89.89, H59.011-H59.019,
H59.031-H59.039, H59.091-H59.099, H59.811-H59.89,
H95.811-H95.89, I97.3, L76.81-L76.82, M96.89, N98.1-N98.9,
T07.XXX-T14.91X[A], T79.0XX[A], T79.A0X-T79.9XX[A],
T81.82XA, T81.89X-T81.9XX[A]

PDX Collection 1429
D78.81-D78.89, E36.8, E89.810-E89.89, H59.011-H59.019,
H59.031-H59.039, H59.091-H59.099, H59.811-H59.89,
H95.811-H95.89, I97.3, L76.81-L76.82, M96.89, N98.1-N98.9,
T07.XXX-T14.91X[A], T79.2XXA, T79.A0X-T79.9XX[A],
T81.82X-T81.9XX[A]

PDX Collection 1430
D78.81-D78.89, E36.8, E89.810-E89.89, H59.011-H59.019,
H59.031-H59.039, H59.091-H59.099, H59.811-H59.89,
H95.811-H95.89, I97.3, L76.81-L76.82, M96.89, N98.1-N98.9,
T07.XXX-T14.91X[A], T79.4XXA, T79.A0X-T79.9XX[A],
T81.82X-T81.9XX[A]

PDX Collection 1431
D78.01-D78.02, D78.21-D78.22, D78.31-D78.34,
D78.81-D78.89, E36.01-E36.02, E36.8, E89.810-E89.89,
G97.51-G97.52, G97.61-G97.64, H59.011-H59.019,
H59.031-H59.039, H59.091-H59.099, H59.111-H59.129,
H59.311-H59.329, H59.331-H59.369, H59.811-H59.819,
H59.88-H59.89, H95.21-H95.22, H95.41-H95.42,
H95.51-H92.52, H95.551-H95.554, H95.811-H95.819,
H95.88-H95.89, I97.3-I97.42, I97.610-I97.648,
J95.61-J95.62, J95.830-J95.831, J95.860-J95.863,
K91.61-K91.62, K91.840-K91.841, K91.870-K91.873,
L76.01-L76.02, L76.21-L76.22, L76.31-L76.34, L76.81-L76.82,
M96.810-M96.811, M96.830-M96.89, N98.1-N98.9,
N99.61-N99.62, N99.820-N99.821, N99.840-N99.843,
T07.XXX-T14.91X[A], T79.5XXA, T79.A0X-T79.9XX[A],
T81.10X-T81.19X[A], T81.82X-T81.9XX[A], T88.2XXA

PDX Collection 1432
D78.01-D78.09, E36.0, E09.810-E09.89, H59.011-H59.019,
H59.031-H59.039, H59.091-H59.099, H59.811-H59.89,
H95.811-H95.89, I97.3, L76.81-L76.82, M96.89,
N98.1-N98.9, S21.101-S21.159[A], S21.301-S21.459[A],
S21.90X-S21.95X[A], S27.0XX-S27.399[A],
S27.50X-S27.809[A], S27.892-S27.9XX[A],
S28.1XX[A], S29.021-S29.029[A], T07.XXX-T14.91X[A],
T79.7XX-T79.9XX[A], T81.82X-T81.9XX[A]

PDX Collection 1433
M70.80-M70.99, M79.81-M79.9, R29.898, T79.A29A

PDX Collection 1434
S31.001A, S31.011A, S31.021A, S31.031A, S31.041A,
S31.051A, S31.100-S31.159[A], S31.600-S31.659[A],
S31.831-S31.839[A], S36.00X-S37.599[A],
S37.812-S37.99X[A], S38.3XXA, S39.021-S39.023[A],
T07.XXX-T14.91X[A], T79.8XX-T79.9XX[A], T79.A3XA

PDX Collection 1435
T79.0XXA, T80.0XXA

PDX Collection 1436
T80.1XXA, T80.810-T80.818[A], T80.90XA

PDX Collection 1437
T80.30X-T80.A9X[A], T80.910-T80.92X[A]

PDX Collection 1438
T80.30X-T80.419[A], T80.910-T80.92X[A], T80.A19A,
T80.A9XA

PDX Collection 1439
T80.51X-T80.69X[A]

PDX Collection 1440
T80.61X-T80.69X[A]

PDX Collection 1441
D78.01-D78.02, D78.21-D78.22, D78.31-D78.34,
D78.81-D78.89, E36.01-E36.02, E36.8, E89.810-E89.89,
G97.51-G97.52, G97.61-G97.64, H59.011-H59.019,
H59.031-H59.039, H59.091-H59.099, H59.111-H59.129,
H59.311-H59.369, H59.331-H59.349, H59.811-H59.819,
H59.88-H59.89, H95.21-H95.22, H95.41-H95.42,
H59.51-H59.54, H95.811-H95.819, H95.88-H95.89,
I97.3-I97.42, I97.610-I97.648, J95.61-J95.62,
J95.830-J95.831, J95.860-J95.863, K91.61-K91.62,
K91.840-K91.841, K91.870-K91.873, L76.01-L76.02,
L76.21-L76.22, L76.31-L76.34, L76.81-L76.82,
M96.810-M96.811, M96.830-M96.89, N98.1-N98.9,
N99.61-N99.62, N99.820-N99.821, N99.840-N99.843,
T79.4XXA, T81.10X-T81.19X[A], T81.82X-T81.9XX[A],
T88.2XXA

PDX Collection 1442
D78.81-D78.89, E36.8, E89.810-E89.89, H59.011-H59.019,
H59.031-H59.039, H59.091-H59.099, H59.811-H59.89,
H95.811-H95.89, I97.3, L76.81-L76.82, M96.89, N98.1-N98.9,
T81.30X-T81.33X[A], T81.82X-T81.9XX[A]

PDX Collection 1443
D78.81-D78.89, E36.8, E89.810-E89.89, H59.011-H59.019,
H59.031-H59.039, H59.091-H59.099, H59.811-H59.89,
H95.811-H95.89, I97.3, L76.81-L76.82, M96.89, N98.1-N98.9,
T81.500-T81.599[A], T81.82X-T81.9XX[A]

PDX Collection 1444
D78.81-D78.89, E36.8, E89.810-E89.89, H59.011-H59.019,
H59.031-H59.039, H59.091-H59.099, H59.811-H59.89,
H95.811-H95.89, I97.3, L76.81-L76.82, M96.89, N98.1-N98.9,
T81.60X-T81.69X[A], T81.82X-T81.9XX[A]

PDX Collection 1445
D78.81-D78.89, E36.8, E89.810-E89.89, H59.011-H59.019,
H59.031-H59.039, H59.091-H59.099, H59.811-H59.89,
H95.811-H95.89, I97.3, L76.81-L76.82, M96.89, N98.1-N98.9,
T81.710-T81.72X[A], T81.82X-T81.9XX[A]

PDX Collection 1446
D78.81-D78.89, E36.8, E89.810-E89.89, H59.011-H59.019,
H59.031-H59.039, H59.091-H59.099, H59.811-H59.89,
H95.811-H95.89, I97.3, L76.81-L76.82, M96.89, N98.1-N98.9,
T81.718-T81.72X[A], T81.82X-T81.9XX[A]

PDX Collection 1447
D78.81-D78.89, E36.8, E89.810-E89.89, H59.011-H59.019,
H59.031-H59.039, H59.091-H59.099, H59.811-H59.89,
H95.811-H95.89, I97.3, L76.81-L76.82, M96.89, N98.1-N98.9,
T81.82X-T81.9XX[A]

PDX Collection 1448
D78.81-D78.89, E36.8, E89.810-E89.89, H59.011-H59.019,
H59.031-H59.039, H59.091-H59.099, H59.811-H59.89,
H95.811-H95.89, I97.3, L76.81-L76.82, M96.89, N98.1-N98.9,
T81.82X-T81.9XX[A], T82.01X-T82.09X[A]

PDX Collection 1449
D78.81-D78.89, E36.8, E89.810-E89.89, H59.011-H59.019,
H59.031-H59.039, H59.091-H59.099, H59.811-H59.89,
H95.811-H95.89, I97.3, L76.81-L76.82, M96.89,
N98.1-N98.9, T81.82X-T81.9XX[A], T82.110-T82.111[A],
T82.120-T82.121[A], T82.190-T82.191[A]

PDX Collection 1450
D78.81-D78.89, E36.8, E89.810-E89.89, H59.011-H59.019,
H59.031-H59.039, H59.091-H59.099, H59.811-H59.89,
H95.811-H95.89, I97.3, L76.81-L76.82, M96.89, N98.1-N98.9,
T81.82X-T81.9XX[A], T82.118A, T82.128A, T82.198A,
T82.221-T82.228[A], T82.512A, T82.522A, T82.532A,
T82.592A, T82.594A, T82.598A

PDX Collection 1451
D78.81-D78.89, E36.8, E89.810-E89.89, H59.011-H59.019,
H59.031-H59.039, H59.091-H59.099, H59.811-H59.89,
H95.811-H95.89, I97.3, L76.81-L76.82, M96.89, N98.1-N98.9,
T81.82X-T81.9XX[A], T82.211-T82.218[A]

PDX Collection 1452
D78.81-D78.89, E36.8, E89.810-E89.89, H59.011-H59.019,
H59.031-H59.039, H59.091-H59.099, H59.811-H59.89,
H95.811-H95.89, I97.3, L76.81-L76.82, M96.89,
N98.1-N98.9, T81.82X-T81.9XX[A], T82.310-T82.538[A],
T82.590-T82.595[A]

PDX Collection 1453
D78.81-D78.89, E36.8, E89.810-E89.89, H59.011-H59.019,
H59.031-H59.039, H59.091-H59.099, H59.811-H59.89,
H95.811-H95.89, I97.3, L76.81-L76.82, M96.89,
N98.1-N98.9, T81.82X-T81.9XX[A], T82.519A, T82.539A,
T82.599-T82.9XX[A], T85.9XXA

PDX Collection 1454
D78.81-D78.89, E36.8, E89.810-E89.89, H59.011-H59.019,
H59.031-H59.039, H59.091-H59.099, H59.811-H59.89,
H95.811-H95.89, I97.3, L76.81-L76.82, M96.89,
N98.1-N98.9, T81.82X-T81.9XX[A], T82.01X-T82.118[A],
T82.120-T82.128[A], T82.190-T82.198[A],
T82.211-T82.9XX[A], T85.310-T85.311[A],
T85.320-T85.321[A], T85.390-T85.391[A],
T85.510-T85.738[A], T85.7XXA, T85.810[A,D], T85.820[A,D],
T85.830[A,D], T85.840[A,D], T85.850[A,D], T85.860[A,D],
T85.890[A,D], T86.820-T86.829

PDX Collection 1455
D78.81-D78.89, E36.8, E89.810-E89.89, H59.011-H59.019,
H59.031-H59.039, H59.091-H59.099, H59.811-H59.89,
H95.811-H95.89, I97.3, L76.81-L76.82, M96.89,
N98.1-N98.9, T81.82X-T81.9XX[A], T82.01X-T82.118[A],
T82.120-T82.128[A], T82.190-T82.198[A],
T82.221-T82.9XX[A], T85.310-T85.311[A],
T85.320-T85.321[A], T85.390-T85.391[A],
T85.510-T85.738[A], T85.79XA, 85.810[A,D], T85.820[A,D],
T85.830[A,D], T85.840[A,D], T85.850[A,D], T85.860[A,D],
T85.890[A,D], T85.9XXA, T86.820-T86.829

PDX Collection 1456
D78.81-D78.89, E36.8, E89.810-E89.89, H59.011-H59.019,
H59.031-H59.039, H59.091-H59.099, H59.811-H59.89,
H95.811-H95.89, I97.3, L76.81-L76.82, M96.89, N98.1-N98.9,
N99.510-N99.518, T81.82A, T81.89-T81.9[A], T83.010A,
T83.020A, T83.030A, T83.090A, T83.110-T83.29X[A],
T83.410-T83.69[A], T83.712-T83.714[A], T83.718A, T83.719A,
T83.722-T83.724[A], T83.728-T83.9XX[A]

PDX Collection 1457
D78.81-D78.89, E36.8, E89.810-E89.89, H59.011-H59.019, H59.031-H59.039, H59.091-H59.099, H59.811-H59.89, H95.811-H95.89, I97.3, L76.81-L76.82, M96.89, N98.1-N98.9, N99.510-N99.518, R82.71, T81.82X-T81.9XX[A], T83.010A, T83.020A, T83.030A, T83.090A, T83.110-T83.29X[A], T83.410-T83.498[A], T83.510-T83.518[A], T83.590-T83.598[A], T83.61X-T83.69X[A], T83.712-T83.719[A], T83.722-T83.729[A], T83.79XA, T83.81X-T83.9XX[A], T85.310-T85.311[A], T85.320-T85.321[A], T85.390-T85.391[A], T85.510-T85.79X[A], T85.810[A,D], T85.820[A,D], T85.830[A,D], T85.840[A,D], T85.850[A,D], T85.860[A,D], T850.890[A,D], T85.9XXA

PDX Collection 1458
D78.81-D78.89, E36.8, E89.810-E89.89, H59.011-H59.019, H59.031-H59.039, H59.091-H59.099, H59.811-H59.89, H95.811-H95.89, I97.3, L76.81-L76.82, M96.89, N39.0, N98.1-N98.9, N99.510-N99.518, T81.82X-T81.9XX[A], T83.010A, T83.020A, T83.030A, T83.090A, T83.110-T83.29X[A], T83.410-T83.498[A], T83.510-T83.518[A], T83.590-T83.598[A], T83.61X-T83.69X[A], T83.712-T83.719[A], T83.722-T83.729[A], T83.79XA, T83.81X-T83.9XX[A], T85.310-T85.738[A], T85.79XA, T85.810[A,D], T85.820[A,D], T85.830[A,D], T85.840[A,D], T85.850[A,D], T85.860[A,D], T850.890[A,D], T85.9XXA, T86.820-T86.829

PDX Collection 1459
D78.81-D78.89, E36.8, E89.810-E89.89, H59.011-H59.019, H59.031-H59.039, H59.091-H59.099, H59.811-H59.89, H95.811-H95.89, I97.3, L76.81-L76.82, M96.621-M96.69, M96.89, M97.01X-M97.02X[A], M97.11X-M97.12X[A], M97.21X-M97.22X[A], M97.31X-M97.32X[A], M97.41X-M97.42X[A], M97.8XXA, M97.9XXA, N98.1-N98.9, T81.82X-T81.9XX[A], T84.010-T84.039[A], T84.050-T84.9XX[A], T85.310-T85.311[A], T85.320-T85.321[A], T85.390-T85.391[A], T85.510-T85.738[A], T85.79XA, T85.810[A,D], T85.820[A,D], T85.830[A,D], T85.840[A,D], T85.850[A,D], T85.860[A,D], T85.890[A,D],T85.9XXA, T86.820-T86.829

PDX Collection 1460
D78.81-D78.89, E36.8, E89.810-E89.89, H59.011-H59.019, H59.031-H59.039, H59.091-H59.099, H59.811-H59.89, H95.811-H95.89, I97.3, L76.81-L76.82, M96.89, N98.1-N98.9, T81.82X-T81.9XX[A], T85.01X-T85.199[A]

PDX Collection 1461
D78.81-D78.89, E89.810-E89.89, H59.011-H59.019, H59.031-H59.039, H59.091-H59.099, H59.811-H59.89, H95.811-H95.89, I97.3, M96.89, N98.1-N98.9, T85.21X-T85.29X[A]

PDX Collection 1462
H59.011-H59.019, H59.031-H59.819, H59.88-H59.89, H95.811-H95.89, I97.3, M96.89, N98.1-N98.9, T85.310-T85.311[A], T85.320-T85.321[A], T85.390-T85.391[A], T85.612A, T85.615A, T85.618A, T85.622A, T85.625A, T85.628A, T85.635A, T85.638A, T85.692A, T85.695A, T85.698-T85.738[A], T85.79XA, T85.810[A,D], T85.820[A,D], T85.830[A,D], T85.840[A,D], T85.850[A,D], T85.860[A,D], T85.890[A,D], T85.9XX[A]

PDX Collection 1463
D78.81-D78.89, E89.810-E89.89, H59.011-H59.019, H59.031-H59.039, H59.091-H59.099, H59.811-H59.89, H95.811-H95.89, I97.3, M96.89, N98.1-N98.9, T85.41X-T85.49X[A]

PDX Collection 1464
H95.811-H95.89, I97.3, M96.89, N98.1-N98.9, T85.510-T85.598[A], T85.612A, T85.615A, T85.618A,

T85.622A, T85.625A,T85.628A, T85.635A, T85.638A, T85.692A, T85.695A, T85.698-T85.738[A], T85.79XA, T85.810[A,D], T85.820[A,D], T85.830[A,D], T85.840[A,D], T85.850[A,D], T85.860[A,D], T85.890[A,D], T85.9XXA

PDX Collection 1465
H95.811-H95.89, I97.3, M96.89, N98.1-N98.9, T85.610A, T85.612A, T85.615A, T85.618-T85.620A, T85.622A, T85.625A, T85.628-T85.630A, T85.635A, T85.638-T85.690[A], T85.692A, T85.695A, T85.698-T85.738[A], T85.79XA, T85.810[A,D], T85.820[A,D], T85.830[A,D], T85.840[A,D], T85.850[A,D], T85.860[A,D], T85.890[A,D], T85.9XXA

PDX Collection 1466
H95.811-H95.89, I97.3, M96.89, N98.1-N98.9, T85.611-T85.612[A], T85.614-T85.618[A], T85.621-T85.622[A], T85.624-T85.628[A], T85.631-T85.638[A], T85.691-T85.692[A], T85.694-T85.738[A], T85.79XA, T85.810[A,D], T85.820[A,D], T85.830[A,D], T85.840[A,D], T85.850[A,D], T85.860[A,D], T85.890[A,D], T85.9XXA

PDX Collection 1467
D78.81-D78.89, E89.810-E89.89, H59.011-H59.019, H59.031-H59.039, H59.091-H59.099, H59.811-H59.89, H95.811-H95.89, I97.3, M96.89, N98.1-N98.9, T85.310-T85.311[A], T85.320-T85.321[A], T85.390-T85.391[A], T85.510-T85.738A, T85.79XA, T85.810[A,D], T85.820[A,D], T85.830[A,D], T85.840[A,D], T85.850[A,D], T85.860[A,D], T85.890[A,D], T85.9XXA

PDX Collection 1468
H95.811-H95.89, I97.3, M96.89, N98.1-N98.9, T85.612-T85.613[A], T85.615A, T85.618[A], T85.622-T85.623[A], T85.625A, T85.628[A], T85.635A, T85.638[A], T85.692-T85.693[A], T85.695A, T85.698-T85.738[A], T85.79XA, T85.810[A,D], T85.820[A,D], T85.830[A,D], T85.840[A,D], T85.850[A,D], T85.860[A,D], T85.890[A,D], T85.9XXA, T86.820-T86.829

PDX Collection 1469
H95.811-H95.89, I97.3, M96.621-M96.89, M97.01X-M97.9XX[A], N98.1-N98.9, N99.510-N99.518, T81.82X-T81.9XX[A], T82.01X-T82.118[A], T82.120-T82.128[A], T82.192-T82.198[A], T82.211-T83.010[A], T83.020[A], T83.030[A], T83.090A, T83.110-T83.29X[A], T83.410-T83.69X[A], T83.712-T83.714[A], T83.718A, T83.719A, T83.722-T83.724[A], T83.728-T83.9XX[A], T84.010-T84.039[A], T84.050-T85.29X[A], T85.41X-T85.49X[A], T85.611-T85.618[A], T85.621-T85.622[A], T85.624-T85.628[A], T85.631-T85.638[A], T85.691-T85.692[A], T85.694-T85.738[A], T85.79XA, T85.810[A,D], T85.820[A,D], T85.830[A,D], T85.840[A,D], T85.850[A,D], T85.860[A,D], T85.890[A,D], T85.9XXA, T86.820-T86.829

PDX Collection 1470
D78.81-D78.89, E36.8, E89.810-E89.89, H59.011-H59.019, H59.031-H59.039, H59.091-H59.099, H59.811-H59.89, H95.811-H95.89, I97.3, L76.81-L76.82, M96.621-M96.89, M97.01X-M97.9XX[A], N98.1-N98.9, N99.510-N99.518, T81.82X-T81.9XX[A], T82.01X-T82.118[A], T82.120-T82.128[A], T82.192-T82.198[A], T82.211-T83.29X[A], T83.410-T83.69X[A], T83.712-T83.714[A], T83.718A, T83.719A, T83.722-T83.724[A], T83.728-T83.9XX[A], T84.010-T84.039[A], T84.050-T85.738[A], T85.79XA, T85.810[A,D], T85.820[A,D], T85.830[A,D], T85.840[A,D], T85.850[A,D], T85.860[A,D], T85.890[A,D], T85.9XXA, T86.820-T86.829

PDX Collection 1471
D78.81-D78.89, E89.810-E89.89, H59.011-H59.019, H59.031-H59.039, H59.091-H59.099, H59.811-H59.89, H95.811-H95.89, I97.3, M96.89, N98.1-N98.9, T86.10-T86.19

PDX Collection 1472
D78.81-D78.89, E89.810-E89.89, H59.011-H59.019, H59.031-H59.039, H59.091-H59.099, H59.811-H59.89, H95.811-H95.89, I97.3, M96.89, N98.1-N98.9, T86.20-T86.39

PDX Collection 1473
D78.81-D78.89, E89.810-E89.89, H59.011-H59.019, H59.031-H59.039, H59.091-H59.099, H59.811-H59.89, H95.811-H95.89, I97.3, M96.89, N98.1-N98.9, T86.40-T86.49

PDX Collection 1474
D78.81-D78.89, E89.810-E89.89, H59.011-H59.019, H59.031-H59.039, H59.091-H59.099, H59.811-H59.89, H95.811-H95.89, I97.3, M96.89, N98.1-N98.9, T86.5, T86.830-T86.839

PDX Collection 1475
D78.81-D78.89, E89.810-E89.89, H59.011-H59.019, H59.031-H59.039, H59.091-H59.099, H59.811-H59.89, H95.811-H95.89, I97.3, M96.89, N98.1-N98.9, T86.810-T86.819

PDX Collection 1476
D78.81-D78.89, E89.810-E89.89, H59.011-H59.019, H59.031-H59.039, H59.091-H59.099, H59.811-H59.89, H95.811-H95.89, I97.3, M96.89, N98.1-N98.9, T85.613A, T85.623A, T85.693A, T86.820-T86.829

PDX Collection 1477
H95.811-H95.89, I97.3, M96.89, N98.1-N98.9, T86.5, T86.830-T86.839

PDX Collection 1480
D78.81-D78.89, E89.810-E89.89, H59.011-H59.019, H59.031-H59.039, H59.091-H59.099, H59.811-H59.89, H95.811-H95.89, I97.3, M96.89, N98.1-N98.9, T86.890-T86.899

PDX Collection 1481
D78.81-D78.89, E36.8, E89.810-E89.89, H59.011-H59.019, H59.031-H59.039, H59.091-H59.099, H59.811-H59.89, H95.811-H95.89, I97.3, L76.81-L76.82, M96.89, N98.1-N98.9, T81.82X-T81.9XX[A], T87.0X1-T87.0X9

PDX Collection 1482
D78.81-D78.89, E36.8, E89.810-E89.89, H59.011-H59.019, H59.031-H59.039, H59.091-H59.099, H59.811-H59.89, H95.811-H95.89, I97.3, L76.81-L76.82, M96.89, N98.1-N98.9, T81.82X-T81.9XX[A], T87.1X1-T87.1X9

PDX Collection 1483
D78.81-D78.89, E36.8, E89.810-E89.89, H59.011-H59.019, H59.031-H59.039, H59.091-H59.099, H59.811-H59.89, H95.811-H95.89, I97.3, L76.81-L76.82, M96.89, N98.1-N98.9, T81.82X-T81.9XX[A], T87.2

PDX Collection 1484
D78.81-D78.89, E36.8, E89.810-E89.89, H59.011-H59.019, H59.031-H59.039, H59.091-H59.099, H59.811-H59.89, H95.811-H95.89, I97.3, L76.81-L76.82, M96.89, N98.1-N98.9, T81.82X-T81.9XX[A], T87.40-T87.9

PDX Collection 1485
T88.1XXA

PDX Collection 1486
D78.01-D78.02, D78.21-D78.89, E36.01-E36.02, E36.8, E89.810-E89.89, G97.51-G97.52, G97.61-G97.64, H59.011-H59.019, H59.031-H59.039, H59.091 H59.099, H59.111-H59.129, H59.311-H59.329, H59.331-H59.369, H59.811-H59.89, H95.21-H95.22, H95.41-H95.42, H95.51-H95.54, H95.811-H95.89, I97.3-I97.42, I97.610-I97.648, J95.61-J95.62, J95.830-J95.831,

J95.860-J95.863, K91.61-K91.62, K91.840-K91.841,
K91.870-K91.873, L76.01-L76.02, L76.21-L76.22,
L76.31-L76.34, L76.81-L76.82, M96.810-M96.811,
M96.830-M96.89, N98.1-N98.9, N99.61-N99.62,
N99.820-N99.821, T79.4XXA, T81.10X-T81.19X[A], T81.82XA,
T81.89X-T81.9XX[A], T88.2XX-T88.3XX[A]

PDX Collection 1487
Z43.1

PDX Collection 1488
D47.Z1, T86.20-T86.39, T86.850-I86.859, I86.90-I86.99,
Z94.1, Z94.3, Z94.89-Z94.9

PDX Collection 1489
D47.Z1, T86.10-T86.19, T86.850-T86.859, T86.90-T86.99,
Z94.0, Z94.89-Z94.9

PDX Collection 1490
D47.Z1, T86.40-T86.49, T86.850-T86.859, T86.90-T86.99,
Z94.4, Z94.89, Z94.9

PDX Collection 1491
D47.Z1, T86.810-T86.819, T86.850-T86.859, T86.90-T86.99,
Z94.2, Z94.89-Z94.9

PDX Collection 1493
E66.01-E66.1, E66.8-E66.9, Z68.1-Z68.54

PDX Collection 1494
E65-E66.1, E66.8-E66.9, Z68.1-Z68.54

PDX Collection 1495
D47.Z1, T86.830-T86.839, T86.90-T86.99, Z94.82,
Z94.89-Z94.9

PDX Collection 1496
D47.Z1, T86.850 T86.859, T86.890-T86.99, Z94.83, Z94.9

PDX Collection 1498
D47.Z1, T86.20-T86.39, T86.850-T86.99, Z94.1, Z94.3,
Z95.811-Z95.812

PDX Collection 2025
I09.81, I50.1-I50.43, I50.810-I50.814, I50.82-I50.9,
I87.8-I87.9, I99.8-I99.9, J81.0

PDX Collection 2029
T74.01X-T74.12X[A], T74.21X-T74.22X[A,D,S],
T74.31X-T74.4XX[A], T74.51X-T74.92X[A,D,S],
T76.01X-T76.12X[A], T76.21X-T76.22X[A,D,S],
T76.31X-T76.32X[A], T76.51X-T76.92X[A,D,S]

PDX Collection 2030
T74.01X-T74.12X[A], T74.21X-T74.22X[A,D,S],
T74.31X-T74.4XX[A], T74.51X-T74.92X[A,D,S],
T76.01X-T76.12X[A], T76.21X-T76.22X[A,D,S],
T76.31X-T76.32X[A], T76.51X-T76.92X[A,D,S]

PDX Collection 2031
T74.01X-T74.12X[A], T74.21X-T74.22X[A,D,S],
T74.31X-T74.4XX[A], T74.51X-T74.92X[A,D,S],
T76.01X-T76.12X[A], T76.21X-T76.22X[A,D,S],
T76.31X-T76.32X[A], T76.51X-T76.92X[A,D,S]

PDX Collection 2032
T74.01X-T74.12X[A], T74.21X-T74.22X[A,D,S],
T74.31X-T74.4XX[A], T74.51X-T74.92X[A,D,S],
T76.01X-T76.12X[A], T76.21X-T76.22X[A,D,S],
T76.31X-T76.32X[A], T76.51X-T76.92X[A,D,S]

PDX Collection 2033
T74.01X-T74.12X[A], T74.21X-T74.22X[A],
T74.31X-T74.4XX[A], T74.51X-T74.92X[A,D,S],
T76.01X-T76.12X[A], T76.21X-T76.22X[A,D,S],
T76.31X-T76.32X[A], T76.51X-T76.92X[A,D,S]

PDX Collection 2034
C88.0, D47.2, D89.0-D89.1, E70.0-E71.30, E72.00-E72.02,
E72.04-E74.9, E75.21-E75.22, E75.240-E75.3, E75.5-E75.6,
E77.0-E78.70, E78.79-E78.9, E88.02-E88.2

PDX Collection 2919
A17.9, A18.10-A18.11, A18.13, A18.82, A18.84, A18.89,
A18.21, A18.29, A54.21, A54.29, A54.82, A54.84,
A54.89-A54.9, A59.00, A59.8-A59.9, B37.41-B37.49,
E08.21-E08.29, E08.618-E08.638, E08.649-E08.8,
E09.21-E09.29, E09.618-E09.638, E0.9649-E09.8,
E10.21-E10.29, E10.618-E10.638, E10.649, E10.69-E10.8,
E11.21-E11.29, E11.618-E11.638, E11.649, E11.69-E11..8,
E13.21-E13.29, E13.618-E13.638, E13.649-E13.8,
M10.30-M10.39, N00.0-N11.0, N11.8-N13.39, N13.6,
N14.0-N19, N25.0-N26.1, N26.9-N27.9, N28.1, N28.81-N29,
N36.41-N36.43, N36.8-N36.9, N39.0, N39.8-N39.9,
R31.0-R31.9, R82.71

PDX Collection 2932
A17.9, A18.10, A18.12-A18.13, A18.82, A18.84, A18.89,
A54.00-A54.02, A54.09-A54.1, A54.82, A54.84, A54.89-A54.9,
A59.00, A59.8- A59.9, B37.41-B37.49, N11.1, N13.4-N13.5,
N13.8-N13.9, N28.82, N28.89-N30.91, N32.89-N33,
N36.41-N36.43, N36.8-N36.9, N39.0, N39.8-N39.9,
R31.0-R31.9, R82.71

PDX Collection 2979
Q87.11-Q87.19

PDX Collection 3209
A17.83

PDX Collection 3210
A40.3

PDX Collection 3211
A51.49

PDX Collection 3212
B25.1

PDX Collection 3213
C81.99

PDX Collection 3214
E72.03

PDX Collection 3215
F11.20

PDX Collection 3216
F13.20

PDX Collection 3217
F14.20

PDX Collection 3218
F15.20

PDX Collection 3219
F16.20

PDX Collection 3220
F18.20

PDX Collection 3221
F19.20

PDX Collection 3222
G04.02

PDX Collection 3223
G04.30

PDX Collection 3224
G04.32

PDX Collection 3225
G04.39

PDX Collection 3226
I25.810

PDX Collection 3227
J98.51

PDX Collection 3228
J98.59

PDX Collection 3229
K77

PDX Collection 3230
L02.01

PDX Collection 3231
L03.212

PDX Collection 3232
M35.81

PDX Collection 3233
M96.0

PDX Collection 3234
S22.49X[B]

PDX Collection 3235
T26.20X[A]

PDX Collection 3236
T26.21X[A]

PDX Collection 3237
T26.22X[A]

PDX Collection 3238
T26.70X[A]

PDX Collection 3239
T26.81X[A]

PDX Collection 3240
T26.72X[A]

PDX Collection 3241
T82.119[A]

PDX Collection 3242
T82.129[A]

PDX Collection 3243
T82.199[A]

PDX Collection 3244
C47.0, Z51.0

PDX Collection 3245
C47.10, Z51.0

PDX Collection 3246
C47.11, Z51.0

PDX Collection 3247
C47.12, Z51.0

PDX Collection 3248
C47.20, Z51.0

PDX Collection 3249
C47.21, Z51.0

PDX Collection 3250
C47.22, Z51.0

PDX Collection 3251
C47.3, Z51.0

PDX Collection 3252
C47.4, Z51.0

PDX Collection 3253
C47.5, Z51.0

PDX Collection 3254
C47.6, Z51.0

PDX Collection 3255
C47.8, Z51.0

PDX Collection 3256
C47.9, Z51.0

PDX Collection 3257
C49.0, Z51.0

PDX Collection 3258
C49.10, Z51.0

PDX Collection 3259
C49.11, Z51.0

PDX Collection 3260
C49.12, Z51.0

PDX Collection 3261
C49.20, Z51.0

PDX Collection 3262
C49.21, Z51.0

PDX Collection 3263
C49.22, Z51.0

PDX Collection 3264
C49.3, Z51.0

PDX Collection 3265
C49.4, Z51.0

PDX Collection 3266
C49.5, Z51.0

PDX Collection 3267
C49.6, Z51.0

PDX Collection 3268
C49.8, Z51.0

PDX Collection 3269
C49.9, Z51.0

PDX Collection 3270
C49.A0, Z51.0

PDX Collection 3271
C49.A1, Z51.0

PDX Collection 3272
C49.A3, Z51.0

PDX Collection 3273
C49.A4, Z51.0

PDX Collection 3274
C49.A5 Z51.0

PDX Collection 3275
C49.A9, Z51.0

PDX Collection 3276
K70.41, K72.91, K76.5, K76.89-K76.9

PDX Collection 3277
K72.11, K72.91, K76.5, K76.89-K76.9

PDX Collection 3278
M70.80-M70.99, M79.81-M79.9, M79.A11, R29.898, S45.301-S45.899[A], S55.201-S55.899[A], S65.801-S65.899[A]

PDX Collection 3279
M70.80-M70.99, M79.81- M79.9, M79.A12, R29.898, S45.301-S45.899[A], S55.201-S55.899[A], S65.801-S65.899[A]

PDX Collection 3280
M70.80-M70.99, M79.81-M79.9, M79.A19, R29.898, S45.301-S45.899[A], S55.201-S55.899[A], S65.801-S65.899[A]

PDX Collection 3281
M79.A9, S31.001[A], S31.031[A]. S31.041[A], S31.051[A], S31.600-S31.659[A], S36.81X[A], S36892-S36.899[A]

PDX Collection 3282
D47.Z1, D89.810-D89.813, T86.00-T86.09, T86.850-T86.859, T86.90-T86.99, Z94.81, Z94.9

PDX Collection 3284
D47.Z1, T86.850-T86.859, T86.90-T86.99, Z94.84, Z94.9

PDX Collection 3285
D47.Z1, T86.20-T86.39, T86.850-T86.859, T86.90-T86.99, Z48.280, Z94.1, Z94.3, Z94.89-Z94.9

PDX Collection 3286
D47Z1, D89.810-D89.813, T86.00-T86.09, T86.850-T86.859, T86.90-T86.99, Z48.290, Z94.9

PDX Collection 3287
D47.Z1, T86.20-T86.39, T86.850-T86.859, T86.90-T86.99, Z48.21, Z94.1, Z94.3, Z94.89-Z94.9

PDX Collection 3288
D47.Z1, T86.10-T86.19, T86.850-T86.859, T86.90-T86.99, Z94.0, Z94.89-Z94.9

PDX Collection 3289
D47.Z1, T86.40-T86.49, T86.850-T86.859, T86.90-T86.99, Z48.23, Z94.4, Z94.89-Z94.9

PDX Collection 3290
D47.Z1, T86.810-T86.819, T86.850-T86.859, T86.90-T86.99, Z48.24, Z94.2, Z94.89-Z94.9

PDX Collection 3291
T78.00X-T78.09X[A], T78.2XX[A]

PDX Collection 3292
T78.00X-T78.09X[A], T88.6XX[A]

PDX Collection 3300
I70.231-I70.25, I70.331, L44.8-L45, L94.2, L94.4, L97.101-L97.929, L98.411-L98.499, L98.7-L99

PDX Collection 3301
I70.231-I70.25, I70.332, L44.8-L45, L94.2, L94.4, L97.101-L97.929, L98.411-L98.499, L98.7-L99

PDX Collection 3302
I70.231-I70.25, I70.333, L44.8-L45, L94.2, L94.4, L97.101-L97.929, L98.411-L98.499, L98.7-L99

PDX Collection 3303
I70.231-I70.25, I70.334, L44.8-L45, L94.2, L94.4, L97.101-L97.929, L98.411-L98.499, L98.7-L99

PDX Collection 3304
I70.231-I70.25, I70.338, L44.8-L45, L94.2, L94.4, L97.101-L97.929, L98.411-L98.499, L98.7-L99

PDX Collection 3305
I70.231-I70.25, I70.331, L44.8-L45, L94.2, L94.4, L97.101-L97.929, L98.411-L98.499, L98.7-L99

PDX Collection 3306
I70.231-I70.25, I70.341, L44.8-L45, L94.2, L94.4, L97.101-L97.929, L98.411-L98.499, L98.7-L99

PDX Collection 3307
I70.231-I70.25, I70.342, L44.8-L45, L94.2, L94.4, L97.101-L97.929, L98.411-L98.499, L98.7-L99

PDX Collection 3308
I70.231-I70.25, I70.343, L44.8-L45, L94.2, L94.4, L97.101-L97.929, L98.411-L98.499, L98.7-L99

PDX Collection 3309
I70.231-I70.25, I70.344, L44.8-L45, L94.2, L94.4, L97.101-L97.929, L98.411-L98.499, L98.7-L99

PDX Collection 3310
I70.231-I70.25, I70.348, L44.8-L45, L94.2, L94.4, L97.101-L97.929, L98.411-L98.499, L98.7-L99

PDX Collection 3311
I70.231-I70.25, I70.349, L44.8-L45, L94.2, L94.4, L97.101-L97.929, L98.411-L98.499, L98.7-L99

PDX Collection 3312
G89.0-G89.4, I70.261-I70.269, I70.361, I96, R29.700-R29.742, R41.0-R41.3, R41.82, R41.9, R44.8-R44.9, R45.83-R45.84, R46.0-R46.89, R52, R68.0-R68.19, R68.81-R69

PDX Collection 3313
G89.0-G89.4, I70.261-I70.269, I70.362, I96, R29.700-R29.742, R41.0-R41.3, R41.82, R41.9, R44.8-R44.9, R45.83-R45.84, R46.0-R46.89, R52, R68.0-R68.19, R68.81-R69

PDX Collection 3314
G89.0-G89.4, I70.261-I70.269, I70.368, I96, R29.700-R29.742, R41.0-R41.3, R41.82, R41.9, R44.8-R44.9, R45.83-R45.84, R46.0-R46.89, R52, R68.0-R68.19, R68.81-R69

PDX Collection 3315
G89.0-G89.4, I70.261-I70.269, I70.361, I96, R29.700-R29.742, R41.0-R41.3, R41.82, R41.9, R44.8-R44.9, R45.83-R45.84, R46.0-R46.89, R52, R68.0-R68.19, R68.81-R69

PDX Collection 3316
G89.0-G89.4, I70.261-I70.269, I70.369, I96, R29.700-R29.742, R41.0-R41.3, R41.82, R41.9, R44.8-R44.9, R45.83-R45.84, R46.0-R46.89, R52, R68.0-R68.19, R68.81-R69

PDX Collection 3317
I70.231-I70.25, I70.431, L44.8-L45, L94.2, L94.4, L97.101-L97.929, L98.411-L98.499, L98.7-L99

PDX Collection 3318
I70.231-I70.25, I70.432, L44.8-L45, L94.2, L94.4, L97.101-L97.929, L98.411-L98.499, L98.7-L99

PDX Collection 3319
I70.231-I70.25, I70.433, L44.8-L45, L94.2, L94.4, L97.101-L97.929, L98.411-L98.499, L98.7-L99

PDX Collection 3320
I70.231-I70.25, I70.434, L44.8-L45, L94.2, L94.4, L97.101-L97.929, L98.411-L98.499, L98.7-L99

PDX Collection 3321
I70.231-I70.25, I70.438, L44.8-L45, L94.2, L94.4, L97.101-L97.929, L98.411-L98.499, L98.7-L99

PDX Collection 3322
I70.231-I70.25, I70.439, L44.8-L45, L94.2, L94.4, L97.101-L97.929, L98.411-L98.499, L98.7-L99

PDX Collection 3323
I70.231-I70.25, I70.441, L44.8-L45, L94.2, L94.4, L97.101-L97.929, L98.411-L98.499, L98.7-L99

PDX Collection 3324
I70.231-I70.25, I70.442, L44.8-L45, L94.2, L94.4, L97.101-L97.929, L98.411-L98.499, L98.7-L99

PDX Collection 3325
I70.231-I70.25, I70.443, L44.8-L45, L94.2, L94.4, L97.101-L97.929, L98.411-L98.499, L98.7-L99

PDX Collection 3326
I70.231-I70.25, I70.444, L44.8-L45, L94.2, L94.4, L97.101-L97.929, L98.411-L98.499, L98.7-L99

PDX Collection 3327
I70.231-I70.25, I70.448, L44.8-L45, L94.2, L94.4, L97.101-L97.929, L98.411-L98.499, L98.7-L99

PDX Collection 3328
I70.231-I70.25, I70.449, L44.8-L45, L94.2, L94.4, L97.101-L97.929, L98.411-L98.499, L98.7-L99

PDX Collection 3329
G89.0-G89.4, I70.261-I70.269, I70.461, I96, R29.700-R29.742, R41.0-R41.3, R41.82, R41.9, R44.8-R44.9, R45.83-R45.84, R46.0-R46.89, R52, R68.0-R68.19, R68.81-R69

PDX Collection 3330
G89.0-G89.4, I70.261-I70.269, I70.462, I96, R29.700-R29.742, R41.0-R41.3, R41.82, R41.9, R44.8-R44.9, R45.83-R45.84, R46.0-R46.89, R52, R68.0-R68.19, R68.81-R69

PDX Collection 3331
G89.0-G89.4, I70.261-I70.269, I70.463, I96,
R29.700-R29.742, R41.0-R41.3, R41.82, R41.9, R44.8-R44.9,
R45.83-R45.84, R46.0-R46.89, R52, R68.0-R68.19,
R68.81-R69

PDX Collection 3332
G89.0-G89.4, I70.261-I70.269, I70.468, I96,
R29.700-R29.742, R41.0-R41.3, R41.82, R41.9, R44.8-R44.9,
R45.83-R45.84, R46.0-R46.89, R52, R68.0-R68.19,
R68.81-R69

PDX Collection 3333
G89.0-G89.4, I70.261-I70.269, I70.469, I96,
R29.700-R29.742, R41.0-R41.3, R41.82, R41.9, R44.8-R44.9,
R45.83-R45.84, R46.0-R46.89, R52, R68.0-R68.19,
R68.81-R69

PDX Collection 3334
I70.231-I70.25, I70.531, L44.8-L45, L94.2, L94.4,
L97.101-L97.929, L98.411-L98.499, L98.7-L99

PDX Collection 3335
I70.231-I70.25, I70.532, L44.8-L45, L94.2, L94.4,
L97.101-L97.929, L98.411-L98.499, L98.7-L99

PDX Collection 3336
I70.231-I70.25, I70.533, L44.8-L45, L94.2, L94.4,
L97.101-L97.929, L98.411-L98.499, L98.7-L99

PDX Collection 3337
I70.231-I70.25, I70.534, L44.8-L45, L94.2, L94.4,
L97.101-L97.929, L98.411-L98.499, L98.7-L99

PDX Collection 3338
I70.231-I70.25, I70.538, L44.8-L45, L94.2, L94.4,
L97.101-L97.929, L98.411-L98.499, L98.7-L99

PDX Collection 3339
I70.231-I70.25, I70.539, L44.8-L45, L94.2, L94.4,
L97.101-L97.929, L98.411-L98.499, L98.7-L99

PDX Collection 3340
I70.231-I70.25, I70.541, L44.8-L45, L94.2, L94.4,
L97.101-L97.929, L98.411-L98.499, L98.7-L99

PDX Collection 3341
I70.231-I70.25, I70.542, L44.8-L45, L94.2, L94.4,
L97.101-L97.929, L98.411-L98.499, L98.7-L99

PDX Collection 3342
I70.231-I70.25, I70.543, L44.8-L45, L94.2, L94.4,
L97.101-L97.929, L98.411-L98.499, L98.7-L99

PDX Collection 3343
I70.231-I70.25, I70.544, L44.8-L45, L94.2, L94.4,
L97.101-L97.929, L98.411-L98.499, L98.7-L99

PDX Collection 3344
I70.231-I70.25, I70.548, L44.8-L45, L94.2, L94.4,
L97.101-L97.929, L98.411-L98.499, L98.7-L99

PDX Collection 3345
I70.231-I70.25, I70.549, L44.8-L45, L94.2, L94.4,
L97.101-L97.929, L98.411-L98.499, L98.7-L99

PDX Collection 3346
G89.0-G89.4, I70.261-I70.269, I70.561, I96,
R29.700-R29.742, R41.0-R41.3, R41.82, R41.9, R44.8-R44.9,
R45.83-R45.84, R46.0-R46.89, R52, R68.0-R68.19,
R68.81-R69

PDX Collection 3347
G89.0-G89.4, I70.261-I70.269, I70.562, I96,
R29.700-R29.742, R41.0-R41.3, R41.82, R41.9, R44.8-R44.9,
R45.83-R45.84, R46.0-R46.89, R52, R68.0-R68.19,
R68.81-R69

PDX Collection 3348
G89.0-G89.4, I70.261-I70.269, I70.563, I96,
R29.700-R29.742, R41.0-R41.3, R41.82, R41.9, R44.8-R44.9,

R45.83-R45.84, R46.0-R46.89, R52, R68.0-R68.19,
R68.81-R69

PDX Collection 3349
G89.0-G89.4, I70.261-I70.269, I70.568, I96,
R29.700-R29.742, R41.0-R41.3, R41.82, R41.9, R44.8-R44.9,
R45.83-R45.84, R46.0-R46.89, R52, R68.0-R68.19,
R68.81-R69

PDX Collection 3350
G89.0-G89.4, I70.261-I70.269, I70.469, I96,
R29.700-R29.742, R41.0-R41.3, R41.82, R41.9, R44.8-R44.9,
R45.83-R45.84, R46.0-R46.89, R52, R68.0-R68.19,
R68.81-R69

PDX Collection 3351
I70.231-I70.25, I70.631, L44.8-L45, L94.2, L94.4,
L97.101-L97.929, L98.411-L98.499, L98.7-L99

PDX Collection 3352
I70.231-I70.25, I70.632, L44.8-L45, L94.2, L94.4,
L97.101-L97.929, L98.411-L98.499, L98.7-L99

PDX Collection 3353
I70.231-I70.25, I70.633, L44.8-L45, L94.2, L94.4,
L97.101-L97.929, L98.411-L98.499, L98.7-L99

PDX Collection 3354
I70.231-I70.25, I70.634, L44.8-L45, L94.2, L94.4,
L97.101-L97.929, L98.411-L98.499, L98.7-L99

PDX Collection 3355
I70.231-I70.25, I70.638, L44.8-L45, L94.2, L94.4,
L97.101-L97.929, L98.411-L98.499, L98.7-L99

PDX Collection 3356
I70.231-I70.25, I70.639, L44.8-L45, L94.2, L94.4,
L97.101-L97.929, L98.411-L98.499, L98.7-L99

PDX Collection 3357
I70.231-I70.25, I70.641, L44.8-L45, L94.2, L94.4,
L97.101-L97.929, L98.411-L98.499, L98.7-L99

PDX Collection 3358
I70.231-I70.25, I70.642, L44.8-L45, L94.2, L94.4,
L97.101-L97.929, L98.411-L98.499, L98.7-L99

PDX Collection 3359
I70.231-I70.25, I70.643, L44.8-L45, L94.2, L94.4,
L97.101-L97.929, L98.411-L98.499, L98.7-L99

PDX Collection 3360
I70.231-I70.25, I70.644, L44.8-L45, L94.2, L94.4,
L97.101-L97.929, L98.411-L98.499, L98.7-L99

PDX Collection 3361
I70.231-I70.25, I70.648, L44.8-L45, L94.2, L94.4,
L97.101-L97.929, L98.411-L98.499, L98.7-L99

PDX Collection 3362
I70.231-I70.25, I70.649, L44.8-L45, L94.2, L94.4,
L97.101-L97.929, L98.411-L98.499, L98.7-L99

PDX Collection 3363
G89.0-G89.4, I70.261-I70.269, I70.661, I96,
R29.700-R29.742, R41.0-R41.3, R41.82, R41.9, R44.8-R44.9,
R45.83-R45.84, R46.0-R46.89, R52, R68.0-R68.19,
R68.81-R69

PDX Collection 3364
G89.0-G89.4, I70.261-I70.269, I70.662, I96,
R29.700-R29.742, R41.0-R41.3, R41.82, R41.9, R44.8-R44.9,
R45.83-R45.84, R46.0-R46.89, R52, R68.0-R68.19,
R68.81-R69

PDX Collection 3365
G89.0-G89.4, I70.261-I70.269, I70.663, I96,
R29.700-R29.742, R41.0-R41.3, R41.82, R41.9, R44.8-R44.9,
R45.83-R45.84, R46.0-R46.89, R52, R68.0-R68.19,
R68.81-R69

PDX Collection 3366
G89.0-G89.4, I70.261-I70.269, I70.668, I96,
R29.700-R29.742, R41.0-R41.3, R41.82, R41.9, R44.8-R44.9,
R45.83-R45.84, R46.0-R46.89, R52, R68.0-R68.19,
R68.81-R69

PDX Collection 3367
G89.0-G89.4, I70.261-I70.269, I70.669, I96,
R29.700-R29.742, R41.0-R41.3, R41.82, R41.9, R44.8-R44.9,
R45.83-R45.84, R46.0-R46.89, R52, R68.0-R68.19,
R68.81-R69

PDX Collection 3368
I70.231-I70.25, I70.731, L44.8-L45, L94.2, L94.4,
L97.101-L97.929, L98.411-L98.499, L98.7-L99

PDX Collection 3369
I70.231-I70.25, I70.732, L44.8-L45, L94.2, L94.4,
L97.101-L97.929, L98.411-L98.499, L98.7-L99

PDX Collection 3370
I70.231-I70.25, I70.733, L44.8-L45, L94.2, L94.4,
L97.101-L97.929, L98.411-L98.499, L98.7-L99

PDX Collection 3371
I70.231-I70.25, I70.734, L44.8-L45, L94.2, L94.4,
L97.101-L97.929, L98.411-L98.499, L98.7-L99

PDX Collection 3372
I70.231-I70.25, I70.738, L44.8-L45, L94.2, L94.4,
L97.101-L97.929, L98.411-L98.499, L98.7-L99

PDX Collection 3373
I70.231-I70.25, I70.739, L44.8-L45, L94.2, L94.4,
L97.101-L97.929, L98.411-L98.499, L98.7-L99

PDX Collection 3374
I70.231-I70.25, I70.741, L44.8-L45, L94.2, L94.4,
L97.101-L97.929, L98.411-L98.499, L98.7-L99

PDX Collection 3375
I70.231-I70.25, I70.742, L44.8-L45, L94.2, L94.4,
L97.101-L97.929, L98.411-L98.499, L98.7-L99

PDX Collection 3376
I70.231-I70.25, I70.743, L44.8-L45, L94.2, L94.4,
L97.101-L97.929, L98.411-L98.499, L98.7-L99

PDX Collection 3377
I70.231-I70.25, I70.744, L44.8-L45, L94.2, L94.4,
L97.101-L97.929, L98.411-L98.499, L98.7-L99

PDX Collection 3378
I70.231-I70.25, I70.748, L44.8-L45, L94.2, L94.4,
L97.101-L97.929, L98.411-L98.499, L98.7-L99

PDX Collection 3379
I70.231-I70.25, I70.749, L44.8-L45, L94.2, L94.4,
L97.101-L97.929, L98.411-L98.499, L98.7-L99

PDX Collection 3380
G89.0-G89.4, I70.261-I70.269, I70.761, I96,
R29.700-R29.742, R41.0-R41.3, R41.82, R41.9, R44.8-R44.9,
R45.83-R45.84, R46.0-R46.89, R52, R68.0-R68.19,
R68.81-R69

PDX Collection 3381
G89.0-G89.4, I70.261-I70.269, I70.762, I96,
R29.700-R29.742, R41.0-R41.3, R41.82, R41.9, R44.8-R44.9,
R45.83-R45.84, R46.0-R46.89, R52, R68.0-R68.19,
R68.81-R69

PDX Collection 3382
G89.0-G89.4, I70.261-I70.269, I70.763, I96,
R29.700-R29.742, R41.0-R41.3, R41.82, R41.9, R44.8-R44.9,
R45.83-R45.84, R46.0-R46.89, R52, R68.0-R68.19,
R68.81-R69

PDX Collection 3383
G89.0-G89.4, I70.261-I70.269, I70.768, I96,
R29.700-R29.742, R41.0-R41.3, R41.82, R41.9, R44.8-R44.9,

R45.83-R45.84, R46.0-R46.89, R52, R68.0-R68.19,
R68.81-R69

PDX Collection 3384
G89.0-G89.4, I70.261-I70.269, I70.769, I96, R29.700-R29.742,
R41.0-R41.3, R41.82, R41.9, R44.8-R44.9, R45.83-R45.84,
R46.0-R46.89, R52, R68.0-R68.19, R68.81-R69

PDX Collection 3385
G89.0-G89.4, I70.261-I70.269, I73.01, I96, R29.700-R29.742,
R41.0-R41.3, R41.82, R41.9, R44.8-R44.9, R45.83-R45.84,
R46.0-R46.89, R52, R68.0-R68.19, R68.81-R69

PDX Collection 3386
I77.2-I77.3, I77.5-I77.6, I77.71, I77.89-I77.9, M31.9-M31.9

PDX Collection 3387
I80.00-I80.9, I87.011

PDX Collection 3388
I80.00-I80.9, I87.012

PDX Collection 3389
I80.00-I80.9, I87.013

PDX Collection 3390
I80.00-I80.9, I87.019

PDX Collection 3391
I80.00-I80.9, I87.031

PDX Collection 3392
I80.00-I80.9, I87.032

PDX Collection 3393
I80.00-I80.9, I87.033

PDX Collection 3394
I80.00-I80.9, I87.039

PDX Collection 3395
I83.001-I83.229, I83.90-I83.93, I87.2, I87.311, I87.8-I87.9,
I99.8-I99.9

PDX Collection 3396
I83.001-I83.229, I83.90-I83.93, I87.2, I87.312, I87.8-I87.9,
I99.8-I99.9

PDX Collection 3397
I83.001-I83.229, I83.90-I83.93, I87.2, I87.313, I87.8-I87.9,
I99.8-I99.9

PDX Collection 3398
I83.001-I83.229, I83.90-I83.93, I87.2, I87.319, I87.8-I87.9,
I99.8-I99.9

PDX Collection 3399
I83.001-I83.229, I83.90-I83.93, I87.2, I87.331, I87.8-I87.9,
I99.8-I99.9

PDX Collection 3400
I83.001-I83.229, I83.90-I83.93, I87.2, I87.332, I87.8-I87.9,
I99.8-I99.9

PDX Collection 3401
I83.001-I83.229, I83.90-I83.93, I87.2, I87.333, I87.8-I87.9,
I99.8-I99.9

PDX Collection 3402
I83.001-I83.229, I83.90-I83.93, I87.2, I87.339, I87.8-I87.9,
I99.8-I99.9

PDX Collection 3403
E08.40-E08.49, E08.618-E08.638, E08.649-E08.8,
E09.40-E09.49, E09.618-E09.638, E09.649-E09.8,
E10.40-E10.49, E10.618-E10.638, E10.649, E10.69-E10.8,
E11.40-E11.49, E11.618-E11.638, E11.649, E11.69-E11.8,
E13.40-E13.49, E13.618-E13.638, E13.649, E13.65-E13.8,
G32.89, G70.00-G72.3, G72.81-G73.7, G96.8-G96.9,
G98.0-G98.8, G99.8, M34.82

PDX Collection 3404
E08.40-E08.49, E08.618-E08.638, E08.649-E08.8,
E09.40-E09.49, E09.618-E09.638, E09.649-E09.8,

E10.40-E10.49, E10.618-E10.638, E10.649, E10.69-E10.8,
E11.40-E11.49, E11.618-E11.638, E11.649, E11.69-E11.8,
E13.40-E13.49, E13.618-E13.638, E13.649, E13.65-E13.8,
G32.89, G70.00-G72.3, G72.81-G73.7, G96.8-G96.9,
G98.0-G98.8, G99.8, M35.03

PDX Collection 3405
S09.0XX[A], S15.001[A], S15.009[A], T07.
XXX[A], T14.8XX-T14.91X[A], T79.8XX-T79.9XX[A],
T79.A0X-T79.A9X[A]

PDX Collection 3406
S09.0XX[A], S15.002[A], S15.009[A], S15.029[A],
S15.099[A], S15.101-S15.199[A], S15.8XX-S15.9XX[A], T07.
XXX[A], T14.8XX

PDX Collection 3407
S09.0XX[A], S15.009-S15.011[A], S15.029[A], S15.099[A],
S15.101-S15.199[A], S15.8XX-S15.9XX[A], T07.XXX[A],
T14.8XX[A] -T14.91X[A], T79.8XX-T79.9XX[A]

PDX Collection 3408
S09.0XX[A], S15.009[A], S15.012[A], S15.9XX[A], T07.
XXX[A], T14.8XX-T14.91X[A], T79.8XX-T79.9XX[A], T79.
A0X[A], T79.A11- T79.A9X[A]

PDX Collection 3409
S09.0XX[A], S15.009[A], S15.019[A], S15.029[A],
S15.099[A], S15.101-S15.199[A], S15.8XX-S15.9XX[A], T07.
XXX[A], T14.8XX[A]

PDX Collection 3410
S09.0XX[A], S15.009[A], S15.021[A], S15.029[A],
S15.099[A], S15.101-S15.199[A], S15.8XX-S15.9XX[A],
T07.XXX[A], T14.8XX-T14.91X[A], T79.8XX-T79.9XX[A],
T79.A0X-T79.A9X[A]

PDX Collection 3411
S09.0XX[A], S15.009[A], S15.022[A], S15.9XX[A], T07.
XXX[A], T14.8XX-T14.91X[A], T79.8XX-T79.9XX[A],
T79.A0X-T79.A9X[A]

PDX Collection 3412
S09.0XX[A], S15.009[A], S15.029[A], S15.091[A],
S15.099[A], S15.101-S15.199[A], S15.8XX-S15.9XX[A], T07.
XXX[A], T14.8XX[A], T79.A12-T79.A9X[A]

PDX Collection 3413
S09.0XX[A], S15.009[A], S15.029[A], S15.92[A],
S15.099[A], S15.101-S15.199[A], S15.8XX-S15.9XX[A],
T07.XXX[A], T14.8XX-T14.91X[A], T79.8XX-T79.9XX[A],
T79.A0X-T79.A9X[A]

PDX Collection 3414
S15.101-S15.199[A], S15.201[A], S15.8XX-S15.9XX[A],
T07.XXX[A], T14.8XX-T14.91X[A], T79.8XX-T79.9XX[A],
T79.A0X-T79.A9X[A]

PDX Collection 3415
S09.0XX[A], S15.101-S15.199[A], S15.202[A],
S15.8XX-S15.9XX[A], T07.XXX[A], T14.8XX-T14.91X[A],
T79.8XX-T79.9XX[A], T79.A0X-T79.A9X[A]

PDX Collection 3416
S09.0XX[A], S15.101-S15.199[A], S15.209[A],
S15.8XX-S15.9XX[A], T07.XXX[A], T14.8XX-T14.91X[A],
T79.8XX-T79.9XX[A], T79.A0X-T79.A9X[A]

PDX Collection 3417
S09.0XX[A], S15.101-S15.199[A], S15.211[A],
S15.8XX-S15.9XX[A], T07.XXX[A], T14.8XX-T14.91X[A],
T79.8XX-T79.9XX[A], T79.A0X-T79.A9X[A]

PDX Collection 3418
S09.0XX[A], S15.101-S15.199[A], S15.212[A],
S15.8XX-S15.9XX[A], T07.XXX[A], T14.8XX-T14.91X[A],
T79.8XX-T79.9XX[A], T79.A0X-T79.A9X[A]

PDX Collection 3419
S09.0XX[A], S15.101-S15.199[A], S15.219[A],
S15.8XX-S15.9XX[A], T07.XXX[A], T14.8XX-T14.91X[A],
T79.8XX-T79.9XX[A], T79.A0X-T79.A9X[A]

PDX Collection 3420
S09.0XX[A], S15.101-S15.199[A], S15.221[A],
S15.8XX-S15.9XX[A], T07.XXX[A], T14.8XX-T14.91X[A],
T79.8XX-T79.9XX[A], T79.A0X-T79.A9X[A]

PDX Collection 3421
S09.0XX[A], S15.101-S15.199[A], S15.222[A],
S15.8XX-S15.9XX[A], T07.XXX[A], T14.8XX-T14.91X[A],
T79.8XX-T79.9XX[A], T79.A0X-T79.A9X[A]

PDX Collection 3422
S09.0XX[A], S15.101-S15.199[A], S15.229[A],
S15.8XX-S15.9XX[A], T07.XXX[A], T14.8XX-T14.91X[A],
T79.8XX-T79.9XX[A], T79.A0X-T79.A9X[A]

PDX Collection 3423
S09.0XX[A], S15.101-S15.199[A], S15.291[A],
S15.8XX-S15.9XX[A], T07.XXX[A], T14.8XX-T14.91X[A],
T79.8XX-T79.9XX[A], T79.A0X-T79.A9X[A]

PDX Collection 3424
S09.0XX[A], S15.101-S15.199[A], S15.292[A],
S15.8XX-S15.9XX[A], T07.XXX[A], T14.8XX-T14.91X[A],
T79.8XX-T79.9XX[A], T79.A0X-T79.A9X[A]

PDX Collection 3425
S09.0XX[A], S15.101-S15.199[A], S15.299[A],
S15.8XX-S15.9XX[A], T07.XXX[A], T14.8XX-T14.91X[A],
T79.8XX-T79.9XX[A], T79.A0X-T79.A9X[A]

PDX Collection 3426
S09.0XX[A], S15.101-S15.199[A], S15.301[A],
S15.8XX-S15.9XX[A], T07.XXX[A], T14.8XX-T14.91X[A],
T79.8XX-T79.9XX[A], T79.A0X-T79.A9X[A]

PDX Collection 3427
S09.0XX[A], S15.101-S15.199[A], S15.302[A],
S15.8XX-S15.9XX[A], T07.XXX[A], T14.8XX-T14.91X[A],
T79.8XX-T79.9XX[A], T79.A0X-T79.A9X[A]

PDX Collection 3428
S09.0XX[A], S15.101-S15.199[A], S15.309[A],
S15.8XX-S15.9XX[A], T07.XXX[A], T14.8XX-T14.91X[A],
T79.8XX-T79.9XX[A], T79.A0X-T79.A9X[A]

PDX Collection 3429
S09.0XX[A], S15.101-S15.199[A], S15.311[A],
S15.8XX-S15.9XX[A], T07.XXX[A], T14.8XX-T14.91X[A],
T79.8XX-T79.9XX[A], T79.A0X-T79.A9X[A]

PDX Collection 3430
S09.0XX[A], S15.101-S15.199[A], S15.312[A],
S15.8XX-S15.9XX[A], T07.XXX[A], T14.8XX-T14.91X[A],
T79.8XX-T79.9XX[A], T79.A0X-T79.A9X[A]

PDX Collection 3431
S09.0XX[A], S15.101-S15.199[A], S15.319A],
S15.8XX-S15.9XX[A], T07.XXX[A], T14.8XX-T14.91X[A],
T79.8XX-T79.9XX[A], T79.A0X-T79.A9X[A]

PDX Collection 3432
S09.0XX[A], S15.101-S15.199[A], S15.321[A],
S15.8XX-S15.9XX[A], T07.XXX[A], T14.8XX-T14.91X[A],
T79.8XX-T79.9XX[A], T79.A0X-T79.A9X[A]

PDX Collection 3433
S09.0XX[A], S15.101-S15.199[A], S15.322[A],
S15.8XX-S15.9XX[A], T07.XXX[A], T14.8XX-T14.91X[A],
T79.8XX-T79.9XX[A], T79.A0X-T79.A9X[A]

PDX Collection 3434
S09.0XX[A], S15.101-S15.199[A], S15.329[A],
S15.8XX-S15.9XX[A], T07.XXX[A], T14.8XX-T14.91X[A],
T79.8XX-T79.9XX[A], T79.A0X-T79.A9X[A]

PDX Collection 3435
S09.0XX[A], S15.101-S15.199[A], S15.391[A],
S15.8XX-S15.9XX[A], T07.XXX[A], T14.8XX-T14.91X[A],
T79.8XX-T79.9XX[A], T79.A0X-T79.A9X[A]

PDX Collection 3436
S09.0XX[A], S15.101-S15.199[A], S15.392[A],
S15.8XX-S15.9XX[A], T07.XXX[A], T14.8XX-T14.91X[A],
T79.8XX-T79.9XX[A], T79.A0X-T79.A9X[A]

PDX Collection 3437
S09.0XX[A], S15.101-S15.199[A], S15.399[A],
S15.8XX-S15.9XX[A], T07.XXX[A], T14.8XX-T14.91X[A],
T79.8XX-T79.9XX[A], T79.A0X-T79.A9X[A]

PDX Collection 3453
D62, D64.4-D64.9, R71.0

PDX Collection 3454
Z16.12

PDX Collection 3455
Z16.21

PDX Collection 3456
Z16.24

PDX Collection 3457
Z16.39

PDX Collection 3458
P70.0-P71.9, P72.1, P72.9, P74.0-P74.49, P94.0

PDX Collection 3459
P70.0-P72.1, P72.9, P74.0-P74.49, P74.9, P94.0

PDX Collection 3460
P70.0-P71.9, P72.1-P72.2, P72.9, P74.0-P74.49, P74.9, P94.0

PDX Collection 3461
P70.0-P71.9, P72.1, P72.8-P72.9, P74.0-P74.49, P74.9, P94.0

PDX Collection 3462
P70.0-P71.9, P72.1, P72.9, P74.0-P74.5, P74.9, P94.0

PDX Collection 3463
P70.0-P71.9, P72.1, P72.9, P74.0-P74.49, P74.6, P74.9, P94.0

PDX Collection 3464
P70.0-P71.9, P72.1, P74.0-P74.49, P74.8-P74.9, P94.0

PDX Collection 3467
Q79.60-Q79.69

PDX Collection 3485
Z16.20

PDX Collection 3486
Z16.22

PDX Collection 3487
Z16.23

PDX Collection 3488
Z16.29

PDX Collection 3489
Z16.30

PDX Collection 3490
Z16.31

PDX Collection 3491
Z16.32

PDX Collection 3492
Z16.33

PDX Collection 3493
Z16.341

PDX Collection 3494
Z16.342

PDX Collection 3495
Z16.35

PDX Collection 3496
Z16.10

PDX Collection 3497
Z16.11

PDX Collection 3498
Z16.19

PDX Collection 3499
E78.71-E78.72, Q87.11-Q87.89, Q89.8, Q99.2

PDX Collection 3500
E78.71-E78.72, I23.0-I23.8, I40.0-I41, I51.0-I51.2, I51.4,
I87.8-I87.9, I97.0-I97.191, I99.8-I99.9, P29.30-P29.38,
Q20.0-Q21.9, Q23.8-Q23.9, Q24.8-Q24.9, Q27.30, Q27.4,
Q28.0-Q28.1, Q28.8-Q28.9, Q87.11-Q87.89, Q89.7-Q89.8,
Q99.2

PDX Collection 3501
E78.01-E78.72, G90.1, Q05.0-Q06.3, Q06.8-Q07.9,
Q87.11-Q87.89, Q89.7-Q89.8, Q22.9

PDX Collection 3502
E78.71-E78.72, I23.0-I23.3, I23.6-I23.8, I51.0, P29.30-P29.38,
Q20.0-Q21.9, Q23.8-Q23.9, Q24.8-Q24.9, Q27.30, Q27.4,
Q28.0-Q28.1, Q28.8-Q28.9, Q87.11-Q87.89, Q89.7-Q89.8,
Q99.2

PDX Collection 3503
E78.71-E78.72, P29.30-P29.38, Q20.9, Q22.0-Q22.3,
Q23.8-Q23.9, Q24.8-Q24.9, Q27.30, Q27.4, Q28.0-Q28.1,
Q28.8-Q28.9, Q87.11-Q87.89, Q89.7-Q89.8, Q99.2

PDX Collection 3504
E78.71-E78.72, P29.30-P29.38, Q20.9, Q22.4-Q23.9,
Q24.8-Q24.9, Q27.30, Q27.4, Q28.0-Q28.1, Q28.8-Q28.9,
Q87.11-Q87.89, Q89.7-Q89.8, Q99.2

PDX Collection 3505
E78.71-E78.72, P29.30-P29.38, Q20.9, Q23.8-Q23.9,
Q24.2-Q24.9, Q27.30, Q27.4, Q28.0-Q28.1, Q28.8-Q28.9,
Q87.11-Q87.89, Q89.7-Q89.8, Q99.2

PDX Collection 3506
E78.71-E78.72, P29.30-P29.38, Q20.9, Q23.8-Q23.9, Q24.6,
Q24.8-Q24.9, Q27.30, Q27.4, Q28.0-Q28.1, Q28.8-Q28.9,
Q87.11-Q87.89, Q89.7-Q89.8, Q99.2

PDX Collection 3507
E78.71-E78.72, P29.30-P29.38, Q25.1, Q25.21-Q25.3,
Q27.30, Q27.4, Q28.0-Q28.1, Q28.8-Q28.9, Q87.11-Q87.89,
Q89.7-Q89.8, Q99.2

PDX Collection 3508
E78.71-E78.72, Q85.8-Q85.9, Q87.11-Q87.89, Q89.7-Q89.2,
Q99.2

PDX Collection 3556
F11.222

PDX Collection 3557
F11.259

PDX Collection 3558
F11.281

PDX Collection 3559
F11.282

PDX Collection 3560
F11.288

PDX Collection 3561
F13.259

PDX Collection 3562
F13.26

PDX Collection 3563
F13.280

PDX Collection 3564
F13.281

PDX Collection 3565
F13.282

PDX Collection 3566
F13.288

PDX Collection 3567
F14.222

PDX Collection 3568
F14.229

PDX Collection 3569
F14.259

PDX Collection 3570
F14.280

PDX Collection 3571
F14.281

PDX Collection 3572
F14.282

PDX Collection 3573
F14.288

PDX Collection 3574
F15.222

PDX Collection 3575
F15.259

PDX Collection 3576
F15.280

PDX Collection 3577
F15.281

PDX Collection 3578
F15.282

PDX Collection 3579
F15.288

PDX Collection 3580
F16.259

PDX Collection 3581
F16.280

PDX Collection 3582
F16.283

PDX Collection 3583
F16.288

PDX Collection 3584
F18.259

PDX Collection 3585
F18.280

PDX Collection 3586
F18.288

PDX Collection 3587
F19.222

PDX Collection 3588
F19.259

PDX Collection 3589
F19.26

PDX Collection 3590
F19.280

PDX Collection 3591
F19.281

PDX Collection 3592
F19.282

PDX Collection 3593
F19.288

PDX Collection 3594
F23

PDX Collection 3595
I16.1

PDX Collection 3596
I16.9

PDX Collection 3597
I25.791

PDX Collection 3598
I25.798

PDX Collection 3599
I25.799

PDX Collection 3600
J94.8

PDX Collection 3601
S06.370[A]

PDX Collection 3602
S06.380[A]

PDX Collection 3604
A15.0-A15.6, A15.8-A15.9, A17.9, A18.82, A18.84, A18.89, A21.2, A22.1, A31.0, A37.01, A37.11, A37.81, A37.91, A42.0, A43.0, A48.1, B25.0, B39.-B39.2, B44.0, B58.3, B59, B67.1, J09.X1-J09.X2, J10.00-J10.1, J11.00-J11.1, J12.0-J12.3, J12.89-J12.9, J13-J18.1, J18.8-J18.9, J22, J44.9, J47.0-J70.4, J70.8-J70.9, J98.4, J98.8-J99, Q33.4, R91.1, U07.0

PDX Collection 3605
G43.601-G43.619, I63.00-I63.119, I63.12-I63.212, I65.23, I65.29, I65.8-I65.9, I87.8-I87.9, I99.8-I99.9

PDX Collection 3606
G43.601-G43.619, I63.00-I63.2, I63.031-I63.039, I63.09-I63.12, I63.131-I63.212, I65.23, I65.29, I65.8-I65.9, I87.8-I87.9, I99.8-I99.9

PDX Collection 3607
G43.601-G43.619, I63.00-I63.2, I63.031-I63.039, I63.09-I63.12, I63.131-I63.212, I65.23, I65.29, I65.8-I65.9, I87.8-I87.9, I99.8-I99.9

PDX Collection 3608
G43.601-G43.619, I63.30, I63.311-I63.6, I63.81-I63.9, I66.01-I66.3, I66.8-I66.9, I87.8-I87.9, I99.8-I99.9

PDX Collection 3610
A17.82, A50.42, A52.14, A75.9, A79.9, A81.1, A81.82-A81.89, A83.0-A84.1, A84.81-A85.8, A87.2, A88.0, A88.8, A91, A92.0-A92.2, A92.30, A92.4-A94, A98.0-A99, B00.4, B00.82, B01.11-B01.12, B04, B06.01, B08.09, B08.20-B08.22, B08.61-B09, B10.01-B10.09, B26.2, B27.00-B27.19, B27.80-B27.99, B33.1, B45.0-B45.9, B58.2, B75, B97.10, G04.00-G04.01, G04.31, G04.81-G04.91, G05.3-G05.4, G37.0, G37.4-G37.5, J09.X3-J09.X9, J10.2, J10.81-J10.89, J11.2, J11.81-J11.89, L44.4, P35.2-P35.9, P37.0-P37.9

PDX Collection 3612
A17.82, A50.42, A52.14, A75.9, A79.9, A81.1, A81.82-A81.89, A83.0-A84.1, A84.81-A85.8, A87.2, A88.0, A88.8, A91, A92.0-A92.2, A92.31, A92.4-A94, A98.0-A99, B00.4, B00.82, B01.11-B01.12, B04, B06.01, B08.09, B08.20-B08.22, B08.60-B09, B10.01-B10.09, B26.2, B27.00-B27.19, B27.80-B27.99, B33.1, B45.0-B45.9, B58.2, B75, B97.10, G04.00-G04.01, G04.31, G04.81-G04.91, G05.3-G05.4, G37.0, G37.4-G37.5, J09.X3-J09.X9, J10.2, J10.81-J10.89, J11.2, J11.81-J11.89, L44.4, P35.2-P35.9, P37.0-P37.9

PDX Collection 3614
A17.82, A50.42, A52.14, A75.9, A79.9, A81.1, A81.82-A81.89, A83.0-A84.1, A84.81-A85.8, A87.2, A88.0, A88.8, A91, A92.0-A92.2, A92.32, A92.4-A94, A98.0-A99, B00.4, B00.82, B01.11-B01.12, B04, B06.01, B08.09, B08.20-B08.22, B08.60-B09, B10.01-B10.09, B26.2, B27.00-B27.19, B27.80-B27.99, B33.1, B45.0-B45.9, B58.2, B75, B97.10, G04.00-G04.01, G04.31, G04.81-G04.91, G05.3-G05.4, G37.0, G37.4-G37.5, J09.X3-J09.X9, J10.2, J10.81-J10.89, J11.2, J11.81-J11.89, L44.4, P35.2-P35.9, P37.0-P37.9

PDX Collection 3616
C96.5, E71.310-E71.318, E71.32, E71.40-E71.548, E80.4-E80.7, E88.40-E88.49, H49.811-H49.819

PDX Collection 3618
C96.6, E71.310-E71.318, E71.32, E71.40-E71.548, E80.4-E80.7, E88.40-E88.49, H49.811-H49.819

PDX Collection 3619
C88.2-C88.9, C90.10-C90.31, C91.00-C91.92, C91.A0-C91.A2, C91.Z0-C91.Z2, C92.00-C92.92, C92.A0-C92.A2, C92.Z0-C92.Z2, C93.00-C93.92, C93.Z0-C93.Z2, C94.00-C94.42, C94.6, C94.80-C95.92, D45, D46.0-D46.Z, D47.01-D47.09, D47.1-D47.Z9, D48.7-D48.9, D75.81

PDX Collection 3621
D60.0-D60.9, D61.1-D61.3, D61.810-D61.818, D61.82-D61.9, D65, D69.3, D69.41-D69.49, D69.51-D69.59, D69.6-D69.9, D70.0-D70.9, D72.818-D72.819, D75.82, D75.9, D76.1

PDX Collection 3623
D60.0-D60.9, D61.1-D61.3, D61.810-D61.818, D61.82-D61.9, D65, D69.3, D69.41-D69.49, D69.51-D69.59, D69.6-D69.9, D70.0-D70.9, D72.818-D72.819, D75.82, D75.9, D76.2

PDX Collection 3626
E08.52, G89.0, G89.11-G89.4, I70.261-I70.269, I96, R29.700-R29.742, R41.0-R41.3, R41.82, R41.9, R44.8-R44.9, R45.43-R45.84, R46.0-R46.89, R52, R68.0-R68.19, R68.81-R69

PDX Collection 3628
E09.52, G89.0, G89.11-G89.4, I70.261-I70.269, I96, R29.700-R29.742, R41.0-R41.3, R41.82, R41.9, R44.8-R44.9, R45.43-R45.84, R46.0-R46.89, R52, R68.0-R68.19, R68.81-R69

PDX Collection 3630
E10.52, G89.0, G89.11-G89.4, I70.261-I70.269, I96, R29.700-R29.742, R41.0-R41.3, R41.82, R41.9, R44.8-R44.9, R45.43-R45.84, R46.0-R46.89, R52, R68.0-R68.19, R68.81-R69

PDX Collection 3632
E11.52, G89.0, G89.11-G89.4, I70.261-I70.269, I96, R29.700-R29.742, R41.0-R41.3, R41.82, R41.9, R44.8-R44.9, R45.43-R45.84, R46.0-R46.89, R52, R68.0-R68.19, R68.81-R69

PDX Collection 3634
E13.52, G89.0, G89.11-G89.4, I70.261-I70.269, I96, R29.700-R29.742, R41.0-R41.3, R41.82, R41.9, R44.8-R44.9, R45.43-R45.84, R46.0-R46.89, R52, R68.0-R68.19, R68.81-R69

PDX Collection 3636
C96.5-C96.6, E71.310-E71.529, E71.53, E71.540-E71.548, E80.3, E88.40-E88.49, E88.89, H49.811-H49.819

PDX Collection 3638
C96.5-C96.6, E71.311-E71.529, E71.53, E71.540-E71.548, E80.3, E88.40-E88.49, E88.89, H49.811-H49.819

PDX Collection 3640
C96.5-C96.6, E71.312-E71.529, E71.53, E71.540-E71.548, E80.3, E88.40-E88.49, E88.89, H49.811-H49.819

PDX Collection 3642
C96.5-C96.6, E71.313-E71.529, E71.53, E71.540-E71.548, E80.3, E88.40-E88.49, E88.89, H49.811-H49.819

PDX Collection 3644
C96.5-C96.6, E71.314-E71.529, E71.53, E71.540-E71.548, E80.3, E88.40-E88.49, E88.89, H49.811-H49.819

PDX Collection 3646
C96.5-C96.6, E71.318-E71.529, E71.53, E71.540-E71.548, E80.3, E88.40-E88.49, E88.89, H49.811-H49.819

PDX Collection 3648
E71.310-E71.529, E71.53, E71.540-E71.548, E80.4-E80.7, E88.40-E88.49, E88.89, H49.811-H49.819

PDX Collection 3650
C96.5-C96.6, E71.310-E71.318, E71.32-E71.39, E71.40-E71.448, E71.50, E80.4-E80.7, E88.40-E88.49, E88.89, H49.811-H49.819

PDX Collection 3652
C96.5-C96.6, E71.310-E71.318, E71.32-E71.448, E71.510, E80.3-E80.7, E88.40-E88.49, E88.89, H49.811-H49.819

PDX Collection 3654
C96.5-C96.6, E71.310-E71.318, E71.32-E71.448, E71.511, E80.3-E80.7, E88.40-E88.49, E88.89, H49.811-H49.819

PDX Collection 3656
C96.5-C96.6, E71.310-E71.318, E71.32-E71.448, E71.518, E80.3-E80.7, E88.40-E88.49, E88.89, H49.811-H49.819

PDX Collection 3658
C96.5-C96.6, E71.310-E71.318, E71.32-E71.448, E71.520, E80.3-E80.7, E88.40-E88.49, E88.89, H49.811-H49.819

PDX Collection 3660
C96.5-C96.6, E71.310-E71.318, E71.32-E71.448, E71.521, E80.3-E80.7, E88.40-E88.49, E88.89, H49.811-H49.819

PDX Collection 3662
C96.5-C96.6, E71.310-E71.318, E71.32-E71.448, E71.522, E80.3-E80.7, E88.40-E88.49, E88.89, H49.811-H49.819

PDX Collection 3664
C96.5-C96.6, E71.310-E71.318, E71.32-E71.448, E71.528, E80.3-E80.7, E88.40-E88.49, E88.89, H49.811-H49.819

PDX Collection 3666
C96.5-C96.6, E71.310-E71.318, E71.32-E71.448, E71.529, E80.3-E80.7, E88.40-E88.49, E88.89, H49.811-H49.819

PDX Collection 3668
C96.5-C96.6, E71.310-E71.318, E71.32-E71.448, E71.53, E80.3-E80.7, E88.40-E88.49, E88.89, H49.811-H49.819

PDX Collection 3670
C96.5-C96.6, E71.310-E71.318, E71.32-E71.448, E71.540, E80.3-E80.7, E88.40-E88.49, E88.89, H49.811-H49.819

PDX Collection 3672
C96.5-C96.6, E71.310-E71.318, E71.32-E71.448, E71.541, E80.3-E80.7, E88.40-E88.49, E88.89, H49.811-H49.819

PDX Collection 3674
C96.5-C96.6, E71.310-E71.318, E71.32-E71.448, E71.542, E80.3-E80.7, E88.40-E88.49, E88.89, H49.811-H49.819

PDX Collection 3676
C96.5-C96.6, E71.310-E71.318, E71.32-E71.448, E71.50-E71.529, E71.53, E71.540-E71.548, E80.3-E80.7, E88.40, E88.89

PDX Collection 3678
C96.5-C96.6, E71.310-E71.318, E71.32-E71.448, E71.50-E71.529, E71.53, E71.540-E71.548, E80.3-E80.7, E88.41, E88.89

PDX Collection 3680
C96.5-C96.6, E71.310-E71.318, E71.32-E71.448, E71.50-E71.529, E71.53, E71.540-E71.548, E80.3-E80.7, E88.42, E88.89

PDX Collection 3682
C96.5-C96.6, E71.310-E71.318, E71.32-E71.448, E71.50-E71.529, E71.53, E71.540-E71.548, E80.3-E80.7, E88.49, E88.89

PDX Collection 3685
G20, G21.11-G21.19, G21.2-G21.9, G23.0, G90.01, G90.09, G93.40-G93.49, I67.83

PDX Collection 3687
G20, G21.11-G21.19, G21.2-G21.9, G23.1, G90.01, G90.09, G93.40-G93.49, I67.83

PDX Collection 3689
G20, G21.11-G21.19, G21.2-G21.9, G23.2, G90.01, G90.09, G93.40-G93.49, I67.83

PDX Collection 3691
G20, G21.11-G21.19, G21.2-G21.9, G23.8, G90.01, G90.09, G93.40-G93.49, I67.83

PDX Collection 3693
G20, G21.11-G21.19, G21.2-G21.9, G23.9, G90.01, G90.09, G93.40-G93.49, I67.83

PDX Collection 3695
G20, G21.11-G21.19, G21.2-G21.9, G24.02, G25.70-G25.79, G25.89-G26, G80.3, G93.40-G93.49, I67.83

PDX Collection 3697
G20, G21.11-G21.19, G21.2-G21.9, G24.09, G25.70-G25.79, G25.89-G26, G80.3, G93.40-G93.49, I67.83

PDX Collection 3699
G20, G21.11-G21.19, G21.2-G21.9, G24.2, G25.70-G25.79, G25.89-G26, G80.3, G93.40-G93.49, I67.83

PDX Collection 3702
A92.30-A92.39, B97.21, G37.0, G93.40-G93.49, I67.83

PDX Collection 3704
G21.0, G83.5, G93.40-G93.49

PDX Collection 3706
C96.5-C96.6, E71.310-E71.318, E71.32-E71.448, E71.50-E71.529, E71.53, E71.540-E71.548, E80.3-E80.7, E88.89, H49.811

PDX Collection 3708
C96.5-C96.6, E71.310-E71.318, E71.32-E71.448, E71.50-E71.529, E71.53, E71.540-E71.548, E80.3-E80.7, E88.89, H49.812

PDX Collection 3710
C96.5-C96.6, E71.310-E71.318, E71.32-E71.448, E71.50-E71.529, E71.53, E71.540-E71.548, E80.3-E80.7, E88.89, H49.813

PDX Collection 3712
I09.81, I11.0, I13.0-I13.2, I20.1-I22.9, I24.0-I24.9, I25.110, I25.5-I25.6, I25.82-I25.9, I50.1, I50.811-I50.814, I50.82-I50.9, I87.8-I87.9, I99.8 I99.9, R57.0, R57.9

PDX Collection 3714
I09.81, I11.0, I13.0-I13.2, I20.1-I22.9, I24.0-I24.9, I25.110, I25.5-I25.6, I25.700, I25.82-I25.9, I50.1, I50.810-I50.814, I50.82-I50.9, I87.8-I87.9, I99.8-I99.9, R57.0, R57.9

PDX Collection 3717
I25.10, I25.110-I25.119, I25.700-I25.739, I25.750-I25.759, I25.761, I25.790-I25.799, I25.811, I25.82-I25.84

PDX Collection 3719
I25.10, I25.110-I25.119, I25.700-I25.739, I25.750-I25.759, I25.768, I25.790-I25.799, I25.811, I25.82-I25.84

PDX Collection 3721
I25.10, I25.110-I25.119, I25.700-I25.739, I25.750-I25.759, I25.769, I25.790-I25.799, I25.811, I25.82-I25.84

PDX Collection 3723
I09.81, I11.0, I13.0-I13.2, I20.1-I22.9, I24.0-I24.9, I25.5-I25.6, I25.790, I25.82-I25.9, I50.1, I50.810-I50.814, I50.82-I50.9, I87.8-I87.9, I99.8-I99.9, R57.0, R57.9

PDX Collection 3725
I67.0, I77.2-I77.6, I77.89-I77.9, M31.8-M31.9

PDX Collection 3727
I77.2-I77.6, I77.70, I77.89-I77.9, M31.8-M31.9

PDX Collection 3729
I77.2-I77.6, I77.72, I77.89-I77.9, M31.8-M31.9

PDX Collection 3731
I77.2-I77.6, I77.73, I77.89-I77.9, M31.8-M31.9

PDX Collection 3732
I77.2-I77.6, I77.74, I77.89-I77.9, M31.8-M31.9

PDX Collection 3734
I77.2-I77.6, I77.75, I77.89-I77.9, M31.8-M31.9

PDX Collection 3736
I77.2-I77.6, I77.76, I77.89-I77.9, M31.8-M31.9

PDX Collection 3738
I77.2-I77.6, I77.77, I77.89-I77.9, M31.8-M31.9

PDX Collection 3742
K71.11, K72.91, K76.5, K76.89-K76.9

PDX Collection 3744
K80.30, K83.01-K83.09, K83.5, K83.8-K83.9, K87

PDX Collection 3746
K80.32, K83.01-K83.09, K83.5, K83.8-K83.9, K87

PDX Collection 3748
K80.34, K83.01-K83.09, K83.5, K83.8-K83.9, K87

PDX Collection 3750
K80.36, K83.01-K83.09, K83.5, K83.8-K83.9, K87

PDX Collection 3752
A02.23, A17.9, A18.02-A18.09, A18.82-A18.89, A39.83-A39.84, A54.40-A54.43, A54.82-A54.9, B06.82, M00.00-M00.9, M01.X0-M01.X9, M02.00-M02.9, M05.40-M06.9, M07.60-M07.69, M11.011-M15.9, M16.2-M16.9, M17.2-M17.9, M18.2-M18.9, M19.111-M19.149, M19.171-M19.179, M19.211-M19.249, M19.271-M19.279, M19.90-M19.93, M24.10-M24.159, M24.171-M24.176, M25.00-M25.176, M25.18, M24.40-M25.676, M25.80-M25.879, M25.9, M35.2, M36.1-M36.4, R92.4

PDX Collection 3754
A02.23, A17.9, A18.02-A18.09, A18.82-A18.89, A39.83-A39.84, A54.40-A54.43, A54.82-A54.9, B06.82, M00.00-M00.9, M01.X0-M01.X9, M02.00-M02.9, M05.40 M06.9, M07.60-M07.69, M11.00-M15.9, M16.2-M16.9, M17.2-M17.9, M18.2-M18.9, M19.111-M19.149, M19.171-M19.179, M19.211-M19.249, M19.271-M19.279, M19.90-M19.93, M24.10-M24.159, M24.171-M24.176, M25.00-M25.176, M25.18, M24.40-M25.676, M25.80-M25.879, M25.9, M35.2, M36.1-M36.4, R92.4

PDX Collection 3756
A02.23, A17.9, A18.02-A18.09, A18.82-A18.89, A39.83-A39.84, A54.40-A54.43, A54.82-A54.9, B06.82, M00.00-M00.29, M00.8-M00.9, M01.X0-M01.X9, M02.00-M02.9, M05.40-M06.9, M07.60-M07.69, M11.00-M15.9, M16.2-M16.9, M17.2-M17.9, M18.2-M18.9, M19.111-M19.149, M19.171-M19.179, M19.211-M19.249, M19.271-M19.279, M19.90-M19.93, M24.10-M24.159, M24.171-M24.176, M25.00-M25.176, M25.18, M24.40-M25.676, M25.80-M25.879, M25.9, M35.2, M36.1-M36.4, R92.4

PDX Collection 3758
A02.23, A17.9, A18.02-A18.09, A18.82-A18.89, A39.83-A39.84, A54.40-A54.43, A54.82-A54.9, B06.82, M00.00-M00.29, M00.80-M00.9, M01.X0-M01.X9, M02.00-M02.9, M05.40-M06.9, M07.60-M07.69, M11.00-M15.9, M16.2-M16.9, M17.2-M17.9, M18.2-M18.9, M19.111-M19.149, M19.171-M19.179, M19.211-M19.249, M19.271-M19.279, M19.90-M19.93, M24.10-M24.159, M24.171-M24.176, M25.00-M25.176, M25.18, M24.40-M25.676, M25.80-M25.879, M25.9, M35.2, M36.1-M36.4, R92.4

PDX Collection 3760
A02.23, A17.9, A18.02-A18.09, A18.82-A18.89, A39.83-A39.84, A54.40-A54.43, A54.82-A54.9, B06.82, M00.00-M00.29, M00.80-M00.9, M01.X0-M01.X9, M02.00-M02.9, M05.40-M06.9, M07.60-M07.69, M11.00-M15.9, M16.2-M16.9, M17.2-M17.9, M18.2-M18.9, M19.111-M19.149, M19.171-M19.179, M19.211-M19.249, M19.271-M19.279, M19.90-M19.93, M24.10-M24.159, M24.171-M24.176, M25.00-M25.176, M25.18, M24.40-M25.676, M25.80-M25.879, M25.9, M35.2, M36.1-M36.4, R92.4

PDX Collection 3762
A02.23, A17.9, A18.02-A18.09, A18.82-A18.89, A39.83-A39.84, A54.40-A54.43, A54.82-A54.9, B06.82, M00.00-M00.29, M00.80-M00.9, M01.X0-M01.X9, M02.00-M02.9, M05.40-M06.9, M07.60-M07.69, M11.00-M15.9, M16.2-M16.9, M17.2-M17.9, M18.2-M18.9, M19.111-M19.149, M19.171-M19.179, M19.211-M19.249, M19.271-M19.279, M19.90-M19.93, M24.10-M24.159, M24.171-M24.176, M25.00-M25.176, M25.18, M24.40-M25.676, M25.80-M25.879, M25.9, M35.2, M36.1-M36.4, R92.4

PDX Collection 3764
A02.23, A17.9, A18.02-A18.09, A18.82-A18.89, A39.83-A39.84, A54.40-A54.43, A54.82-A54.9, B06.82, M00.00-M00.29, M00.80-M00.9, M01.X0-M01.X9, M02.00-M02.9, M05.40-M06.9, M07.60-M07.69, M11.00-M15.9, M16.2-M16.9, M17.2-M17.9, M18.2-M18.9, M19.111-M19.149, M19.171-M19.179, M19.211-M19.249, M19.271-M19.279, M19.90-M19.93, M24.10-M24.159, M24.171-M24.176, M25.00-M25.176, M25.18, M24.40-M25.676, M25.80-M25.879, M25.9, M35.2, M36.1-M36.4, R92.4

PDX Collection 3766
A02.23, A17.9, A18.02-A18.09, A18.82-A18.89, A39.83-A39.84, A54.40-A54.43, A54.82-A54.9, B06.82, M00.00-M00.29, M00.80-M00.9, M01.X0-M01.X9, M02.00-M02.9, M05.40-M06.9, M07.60-M07.69, M11.00-M15.9, M16.2-M16.9, M17.2-M17.9, M18.2-M18.9, M19.111-M19.149, M19.171-M19.179, M19.211-M19.249, M19.271-M19.279, M19.90-M19.93, M24.10-M24.159, M24.171-M24.176, M25.00-M25.176, M25.18, M24.40-M25.676, M25.80-M25.879, M25.9, M35.2, M36.1-M36.4, R92.4

PDX Collection 3768
A02.23, A17.9, A18.02-A18.09, A18.82-A18.89, A39.83-A39.84, A54.40-A54.43, A54.82-A54.9, B06.82, M00.00-M00.29, M00.80-M00.9, M01.X0-M01.X9, M02.00-M02.9, M05.40-M06.9, M07.60-M07.69, M11.00-M15.9, M16.2-M16.9, M17.2-M17.9, M18.2-M18.9, M19.111-M19.149, M19.171-M19.179, M19.211-M19.249, M19.271-M19.279, M19.90-M19.93, M24.10-M24.159, M24.171-M24.176, M25.00-M25.176, M25.18, M24.40-M25.676, M25.80-M25.879, M25.9, M35.2, M36.1-M36.4, R92.4

PDX Collection 3770
A02.23, A17.9, A18.02-A18.09, A18.82-A18.89, A39.83-A39.84, A54.40-A54.43, A54.82-A54.9, B06.82, M00.00-M00.29, M00.80-M00.9, M01.X0-M01.X9, M02.00-M02.9, M05.40-M06.9, M07.60-M07.69, M11.00-M15.9, M16.2-M16.9, M17.2-M17.9, M18.2-M18.9, M19.111-M19.149, M19.171-M19.179, M19.211-M19.249, M19.271-M19.279, M19.90-M19.93, M24.10-M24.159, M24.171-M24.176, M25.00-M25.176, M25.18, M24.40-M25.676, M25.80-M25.879, M25.9, M35.2, M36.1-M36.4, R92.4

PDX Collection 3772
A02.23, A17.9, A18.02-A18.09, A18.82-A18.89, A39.83-A39.84, A54.40-A54.43, A54.82-A54.9, B06.82, M00.00-M00.29, M00.80-M00.9,

M01.X0-M01.X9, M02.00-M02.9, M05.40-M06.9,
M07.60-M07.69, M11.00-M15.9, M16.2-M16.9, M17.2-M17.9,
M18.2-M18.9, M19.111-M19.149, M19.171-M19.179,
M19.211-M19.249, M19.271-M19.279, M19.90-M19.93,
M24.10-M24.159, M24.171-M24.176, M25.00-M25.176,
M25.18, M24.40-M25.676, M25.80-M25.879, M25.9, M35.2,
M36.1-M36.4, R92.4

PDX Collection 3774

A02.23, A17.9, A18.02-A18.09, A18.82-A18.89,
A39.83-A39.84, A54.40-A54.43, A54.82-A54.9,
B06.82, M00.00-M00.29, M00.80-M00.9,
M01.X0-M01.X9, M02.00-M02.9, M05.40-M06.9,
M07.60-M07.69, M11.00-M15.9, M16.2-M16.9, M17.2-M17.9,
M18.2-M18.9, M19.111-M19.149, M19.171-M19.179,
M19.211-M19.249, M19.271-M19.279, M19.90-M19.93,
M24.10-M24.159, M24.171-M24.176, M25.00-M25.176,
M25.18, M24.40-M25.676, M25.80-M25.879, M25.9, M35.2,
M36.1-M36.4, R92.4

PDX Collection 3776

A02.23, A17.9, A18.02-A18.09, A18.82-A18.89,
A39.83-A39.84, A54.40-A54.43, A54.82-A54.9,
B06.82, M00.00-M00.29, M00.80-M00.9,
M01.X0-M01.X9, M02.00-M02.9, M05.40-M06.9,
M07.60-M07.69, M11.00-M15.9, M16.2-M16.9, M17.2-M17.9,
M18.2-M18.9, M19.111-M19.149, M19.171-M19.179,
M19.211-M19.249, M19.271-M19.279, M19.90-M19.93,
M24.10-M24.159, M24.171-M24.176, M25.00-M25.176,
M25.18, M24.40-M25.676, M25.80-M25.879, M25.9, M35.2,
M36.1-M36.4, R92.4

PDX Collection 3778

A02.23, A17.9, A18.02-A18.09, A18.82-A18.89,
A39.83-A39.84, A54.40-A54.43, A54.82-A54.9,
B06.82, M00.00-M00.29, M00.80-M00.9,
M01.X0-M01.X9, M02.00-M02.9, M05.40-M06.9,
M07.60-M07.69, M11.00-M15.9, M16.2-M16.9, M17.2-M17.9,
M18.2-M18.9, M19.111-M19.149, M19.171-M19.179,
M19.211-M19.249, M19.271-M19.279, M19.90-M19.93,
M24.10-M24.159, M24.171-M24.176, M25.00-M25.176,
M25.18, M24.40-M25.676, M25.80-M25.879, M25.9, M35.2,
M36.1-M36.4, R92.4

PDX Collection 3780

E08.40-E08.49, E08.618, E08.620-E08.628, E08.630, E08.638,
E08.649, E08.65, E08.69, E08.8, E09.40-E09.49, E09.618,
E09.620-E09.628, E09.630, E09.638, E09.649, E09.65, E09.69,
E09.8, E10.40-E10.49, E10.618, E10.620-E10.628, E10.630,
E10.638, E10.649, E10.69, E10.8, E11.40-E11.49, E11.618,
E11.620-E11.628, E11.630, E11.638, E11.649, E11.69, E11.8,
E13.40-E13.49, E13.618, E13.620-E13.628, E13.630, E13.638,
E13.649,E13.65, E13.69, E13.8, G32.89, G70.00-G70.2,
G70.80-G71.29, G71.3, G71.8-G72.3, G72.81-G72.9, G73.1,
G73.3, G73.7, G96.9, G98.0, G98.8, M05.40

PDX Collection 3782

E08.40-E08.49, E08.618, E08.620-E08.628, E08.630, E08.638,
E08.649, E08.65, E08.69, E08.8, E09.40-E09.49, E09.618,
E09.620-E09.628, E09.630, E09.638, E09.649, E09.65, E09.69,
E09.8, E10.40-E10.49, E10.618, E10.620-E10.628, E10.630,
E10.638, E10.649, E10.69, E10.8, E11.40-E11.49, E11.618,
E11.620-E11.628, E11.630, E11.638, E11.649, E11.69, E11.8,
E13.40-E13.49, E13.618, E13.620-E13.628, E13.630, E13.638,
E13.649, E13.65, E13.69, E13.8, G32.89, G70.00-G70.2,
G70.80-G71.29, G71.3, G71.8-G72.3, G72.81-G72.9, G73.1,
G73.3, G73.7, G96.9, G98.0, G98.8, M05.411

PDX Collection 3784

E08.40-E08.49, E08.618, E08.620-E08.628, E08.630, E08.638,
E08.649, E08.65, E08.69, E08.8, E09.40-E09.49, E09.618,
E09.620-E09.628, E09.630, E09.638, E09.649, E09.65, E09.69,
E09.8, E10.40-E10.49, E10.618, E10.620-E10.628, E10.630,

E10.638, E10.649, E10.69, E10.8, E11.40-E11.49, E11.618,
E11.620-E11.628, E11.630, E11.638, E11.649, E11.69, E11.8,
E13.40-E13.49, E13.618, E13.620-E13.628, E13.630, E13.638,
E13.649, E13.65, E13.69, E13.8, G32.89, G70.00-G70.2,
G70.80-G71.29, G71.3, G71.8-G72.3, G72.81-G72.9, G73.1,
G73.3, G73.7, G96.9, G98.0, G98.8, M05.412

PDX Collection 3786

E08.40-E08.49, E08.618, E08.620-E08.628, E08.630, E08.638,
E08.649, E08.65, E08.69, E08.8, E09.40-E09.49, E09.618,
E09.620-E09.628, E09.630, E09.638, E09.649, E09.65, E09.69,
E09.8, E10.40-E10.49, E10.618, E10.620-E10.628, E10.630,
E10.638, E10.649, E10.69, E10.8, E11.40-E11.49, E11.618,
E11.620-E11.628, E11.630, E11.638, E11.649, E11.69, E11.8,
E13.40-E13.49, E13.618, E13.620-E13.628, E13.630, E13.638,
E13.649, E13.65, E13.69, E13.8, G32.89, G70.00-G70.2,
G70.80-G71.29, G71.3, G71.8-G72.3, G72.81-G72.9, G73.1,
G73.3, G73.7, G96.9, G98.0, G98.8, M05.419

PDX Collection 3788

E08.40-E08.49, E08.618, E08.620-E08.628, E08.630, E08.638,
E08.649, E08.65, E08.69, E08.8, E09.40-E09.49, E09.618,
E09.620-E09.628, E09.630, E09.638, E09.649, E09.65, E09.69,
E09.8, E10.40-E10.49, E10.618, E10.620-E10.628, E10.630,
E10.638, E10.649, E10.69, E10.8, E11.40-E11.49, E11.618,
E11.620-E11.628, E11.630, E11.638, E11.649, E11.69, E11.8,
E13.40-E13.49, E13.618, E13.620-E13.628, E13.630, E13.638,
E13.649, E13.65, E13.69, E13.8, G32.89, G70.00-G70.2,
G70.80-G71.29, G71.3, G71.8-G72.3, G72.81-G72.9, G73.1,
G73.3, G73.7, G96.9, G98.0, G98.8, M05.421

PDX Collection 3790

E08.40-E08.49, E08.618, E08.620-E08.628, E08.630, E08.638,
E08.649, E08.65, E08.69, E08.8, E09.40-E09.49, E09.618,
E09.620-E09.628, E09.630, E09.638, E09.649, E09.65, E09.69,
E09.8, E10.40-E10.49, E10.618, E10.620-E10.628, E10.630,
E10.638, E10.649, E10.69, E10.8, E11.40-E11.49, E11.618,
E11.620-E11.628, E11.630, E11.638, E11.649, E11.69, E11.8,
E13.40-E13.49, E13.618, E13.620-E13.628, E13.630, E13.638,
E13.649, E13.65, E13.69, E13.8, G32.89, G70.00-G70.2,
G70.80-G71.29, G71.3, G71.8-G72.3, G72.81-G72.9, G73.1,
G73.3, G73.7, G96.9, G98.0, G98.8, M05.422

PDX Collection 3792

E08.40-E08.49, E08.618, E08.620-E08.628, E08.630, E08.638,
E08.649, E08.65, E08.69, E08.8, E09.40-E09.49, E09.618,
E09.620-E09.628, E09.630, E09.638, E09.649, E09.65, E09.69,
E09.8, E10.40-E10.49, E10.618, E10.620-E10.628, E10.630,
E10.638, E10.649, E10.69, E10.8, E11.40-E11.49, E11.618,
E11.620-E11.628, E11.630, E11.638, E11.649, E11.69, E11.8,
E13.40-E13.49, E13.618, E13.620-E13.628, E13.630, E13.638,
E13.649, E13.65, E13.69, E13.8, G32.89, G70.00-G70.2,
G70.80-G71.29, G71.3, G71.8-G72.3, G72.81-G72.9, G73.1,
G73.3, G73.7, G96.9, G98.0, G98.8, M05.429

PDX Collection 3794

E08.40-E08.49, E08.618, E08.620-E08.628, E08.630, E08.638,
E08.649, E08.65, E08.69, E08.8, E09.40-E09.49, E09.618,
E09.620-E09.628, E09.630, E09.638, E09.649, E09.65, E09.69,
E09.8, E10.40-E10.49, E10.618, E10.620-E10.628, E10.630,
E10.638, E10.649, E10.69, E10.8, E11.40-E11.49, E11.618,
E11.620-E11.628, E11.630, E11.638, E11.649, E11.69, E11.8,
E13.40-E13.49, E13.618, E13.620-E13.628, E13.630, E13.638,
E13.649, E13.65, E13.69, E13.8, G32.89, G70.00-G70.2,
G70.80-G71.29, G71.3, G71.8-G72.3, G72.81-G72.9, G73.1,
G73.3, G73.7, G96.9, G98.0, G98.8, M05.431

PDX Collection 3796

E08.40-E08.49, E08.618, E08.620-E08.628, E08.630, E08.638,
E08.649, E08.65, E08.69, E08.8, E09.40-E09.49, E09.618,
E09.620-E09.628, E09.630, E09.638, E09.649, E09.65, E09.69,
E09.8, E10.40-E10.49, E10.618, E10.620-E10.628, E10.630,
E10.638, E10.649, E10.69, E10.8, E11.40-E11.49, E11.618,

E11.620-E11.628, E11.630, E11.638, E11.649, E11.69, E11.8,
E13.40-E13.49, E13.618, E13.620-E13.628, E13.630, E13.638,
E13.649, E13.65, E13.69, E13.8, G32.89, G70.00-G70.2,
G70.80-G71.29, G71.3, G71.8-G72.3, G72.81-G72.9, G73.1,
G73.3, G73.7, G96.9, G98.0, G98.8, M05.432

PDX Collection 3798

E08.40-E08.49, E08.618, E08.620-E08.628, E08.630, E08.638,
E08.649, E08.65, E08.69, E08.8, E09.40-E09.49, E09.618,
E09.620-E09.628, E09.630, E09.638, E09.649, E09.65, E09.69,
E09.8, E10.40-E10.49, E10.618, E10.620-E10.628, E10.630,
E10.638, E10.649, E10.69, E10.8, E11.40-E11.49, E11.618,
E11.620-E11.628, E11.630, E11.638, E11.649, E11.69, E11.8,
E13.40-E13.49, E13.618, E13.620-E13.628, E13.630, E13.638,
E13.649, E13.65, E13.69, E13.8, G32.89, G70.00-G70.2,
G70.80-G71.29, G71.3, G71.8-G72.3, G72.81-G72.9, G73.1,
G73.3, G73.7, G96.9, G98.0, G98.8, M05.439

PDX Collection 3800

E08.40-E08.49, E08.618, E08.620-E08.628, E08.630, E08.638,
E08.649, E08.65, E08.69, E08.8, E09.40-E09.49, E09.618,
E09.620-E09.628, E09.630, E09.638, E09.649, E09.65, E09.69,
E09.8, E10.40-E10.49, E10.618, E10.620-E10.628, E10.630,
E10.638, E10.649, E10.69, E10.8, E11.40-E11.49, E11.618,
E11.620-E11.628, E11.630, E11.638, E11.649, E11.69, E11.8,
E13.40-E13.49, E13.618, E13.620-E13.628, E13.630, E13.638,
E13.649, E13.65, E13.69, E13.8, G32.89, G70.00-G70.2,
G70.80-G71.29, G71.3, G71.8-G72.3, G72.81-G72.9, G73.1,
G73.3, G73.7, G96.9, G98.0, G98.8, M05.441

PDX Collection 3802

E08.40-E08.49, E08.618, E08.620-E08.628, E08.630, E08.638,
E08.649, E08.65, E08.69, E08.8, E09.40-E09.49, E09.618,
E09.620-E09.628, E09.630, E09.638, E09.649, E09.65, E09.69,
E09.8, E10.40-E10.49, E10.618, E10.620-E10.628, E10.630,
E10.638, E10.649, E10.69, E10.8, E11.40-E11.49, E11.618,
E11.620-E11.628, E11.630, E11.638, E11.649, E11.69, E11.8,
E13.40-E13.49, E13.618, E13.620-E13.628, E13.630, E13.638,
E13.649, E13.65, E13.69, E13.8, G32.89, G70.00-G70.2,
G70.80-G71.29, G71.3, G71.8-G72.3, G72.81-G72.9, G73.1,
G73.3, G73.7, G96.9, G98.0, G98.8, M05.442

PDX Collection 3804

E08.40-E08.49, E08.618, E08.620-E08.628, E08.630, E08.638,
E08.649, E08.65, E08.69, E08.8, E09.40-E09.49, E09.618,
E09.620-E09.628, E09.630, E09.638, E09.649, E09.65, E09.69,
E09.8, E10.40-E10.49, E10.618, E10.620-E10.628, E10.630,
E10.638, E10.649, E10.69, E10.8, E11.40-E11.49, E11.618,
E11.620-E11.628, E11.630, E11.638, E11.649, E11.69, E11.8,
E13.40-E13.49, E13.618, E13.620-E13.628, E13.630, E13.638,
E13.649, E13.65, E13.69, E13.8, G32.89, G70.00-G70.2,
G70.80-G71.29, G71.3, G71.8-G72.3, G72.81-G72.9, G73.1,
G73.3, G73.7, G96.9, G98.0, G98.8, M05.449

PDX Collection 3806

E08.40-E08.49, E08.618, E08.620-E08.628, E08.630, E08.638,
E08.649, E08.65, E08.69, E08.8, E09.40-E09.49, E09.618,
E09.620-E09.628, E09.630, E09.638, E09.649, E09.65, E09.69,
E09.8, E10.40-E10.49, E10.618, E10.620-E10.628, E10.630,
E10.638, E10.649, E10.69, E10.8, E11.40-E11.49, E11.618,
E11.620-E11.628, E11.630, E11.638, E11.649, E11.69, E11.8,
E13.40-E13.49, E13.618, E13.620-E13.628, E13.630, E13.638,
E13.649, E13.65, E13.69, E13.8, G32.89, G70.00-G70.2,
G70.80-G71.29, G71.3, G71.8-G72.3, G72.81-G72.9, G73.1,
G73.3, G73.7, G96.9, G98.0, G98.8, M05.451

PDX Collection 3808

E08.40-E08.49, E08.618, E08.620-E08.628, E08.630, E08.638,
E08.649, E08.65, E08.69, E08.8, E09.40-E09.49, E09.618,
E09.620-E09.628, E09.630, E09.638, E09.649, E09.65, E09.69,
E09.8, E10.40-E10.49, E10.618, E10.620-E10.628, E10.630,
E10.638, E10.649, E10.69, E10.8, E11.40-E11.49, E11.618,
E11.620-E11.628, E11.630, E11.638, E11.649, E11.69, E11.8,

E13.40-E13.49, E13.618, E13.620-E13.628, E13.630, E13.638, E13.649, E13.65, E13.69, E13.8, G32.89, G70.00-G70.2, G70.80-G71.29, G71.3, G71.8-G72.3, G72.81-G72.9, G73.1, G73.3, G73.7, G96.9, G98.0, G98.8, M05.452

PDX Collection 3810
E08.40-E08.49, E08.618, E08.620-E08.628, E08.630, E08.638, E08.649, E08.65, E08.69, E08.8, E09.40-E09.49, E09.618, E09.620-E09.628, E09.630, E09.638, E09.649, E09.65, E09.69, E09.8, E10.40-E10.49, E10.618, E10.620-E10.628, E10.630, E10.638, E10.649, E10.69, E10.8, E11.40-E11.49, E11.618, E11.620-E11.628, E11.630, E11.638, E11.649, E11.69, E11.8, E13.40-E13.49, E13.618, E13.620-E13.628, E13.630, E13.638, E13.649, E13.65, E13.69, E13.8, G32.89, G70.00-G70.2, G70.80-G71.29, G71.3, G71.8-G72.3, G72.81-G72.9, G73.1, G73.3, G73.7, G96.9, G98.0, G98.8, M05.459

PDX Collection 3812
E08.40-E08.49, E08.618, E08.620-E08.628, E08.630, E08.638, E08.649, E08.65, E08.69, E08.8, E09.40-E09.49, E09.618, E09.620-E09.628, E09.630, E09.638, E09.649, E09.65, E09.69, E09.8, E10.40-E10.49, E10.618, E10.620-E10.628, E10.630, E10.638, E10.649, E10.69, E10.8, E11.40-E11.49, E11.618, E11.620-E11.628, E11.630, E11.638, E11.649, E11.69, E11.8, E13.40-E13.49, E13.618, E13.620-E13.628, E13.630, E13.638, E13.649, E13.65, E13.69, E13.8, G32.89, G70.00-G70.2, G70.80-G71.29, G71.3, G71.8-G72.3, G72.81-G72.9, G73.1, G73.3, G73.7, G96.9, G98.0, G98.8, M05.461

PDX Collection 3814
E08.40-E08.49, E08.618, E08.620-E08.628, E08.630, E08.638, E08.649, E08.65, E08.69, E08.8, E09.40-E09.49, E09.618, E09.620-E09.628, E09.630, E09.638, E09.649, E09.65, E09.69, E09.8, E10.40-E10.49, E10.618, E10.620-E10.628, E10.630, E10.638, E10.649, E10.69, E10.8, E11.40-E11.49, E11.618, E11.620-E11.628, E11.630, E11.638, E11.649, E11.69, E11.8, E13.40-E13.49, E13.618, E13.620-E13.628, E13.630, E13.638, E13.649, E13.65, E13.69, E13.8, G32.89, G70.00-G70.2, G70.80-G71.29, G71.3, G71.8-G72.3, G72.81-G72.9, G73.1, G73.3, G73.7, G96.9, G98.0, G98.8, M05.462

PDX Collection 3816
E08.40-E08.49, E08.618, E08.620-E08.628, E08.630, E08.638, E08.649, E08.65, E08.69, E08.8, E09.40-E09.49, E09.618, E09.620-E09.628, E09.630, E09.638, E09.649, E09.65, E09.69, E09.8, E10.40-E10.49, E10.618, E10.620-E10.628, E10.630, E10.638, E10.649, E10.69, E10.8, E11.40-E11.49, E11.618, E11.620-E11.628, E11.630, E11.638, E11.649, E11.69, E11.8, E13.40-E13.49, E13.618, E13.620-E13.628, E13.630, E13.638, E13.649, E13.65, E13.69, E13.8, G32.89, G70.00-G70.2, G70.80-G71.29, G71.3, G71.8-G72.3, G72.81-G72.9, G73.1, G73.3, G73.7, G96.9, G98.0, G98.8, M05.469

PDX Collection 3818
E08.40-E08.49, E08.618, E08.620-E08.628, E08.630, E08.638, E08.649, E08.65, E08.69, E08.8, E09.40-E09.49, E09.618, E09.620-E09.628, E09.630, E09.638, E09.649, E09.65, E09.69, E09.8, E10.40-E10.49, E10.618, E10.620-E10.628, E10.630, E10.638, E10.649, E10.69, E10.8, E11.40-E11.49, E11.618, E11.620-E11.628, E11.630, E11.638, E11.649, E11.69, E11.8, E13.40-E13.49, E13.618, E13.620-E13.628, E13.630, E13.638, E13.649, E13.65, E13.69, E13.8, G32.89, G70.00-G70.2, G70.80-G71.29, G71.3, G71.8-G72.3, G72.81-G72.9, G73.1, G73.3, G73.7, G96.9, G98.0, G98.8, M05.471

PDX Collection 3820
E08.40-E08.49, E08.618, E08.620-E08.628, E08.630, E08.638, E08.649, E08.65, E08.69, E08.8, E09.40-E09.49, E09.618, E09.620-E09.628, E09.630, E09.638, E09.649, E09.65, E09.69, E09.8, E10.40-E10.49, E10.618, E10.620-E10.628, E10.630, E10.638, E10.649, E10.69, E10.8, E11.40-E11.49, E11.618, E11.620-E11.628, E11.630, E11.638, E11.649, E11.69, E11.8, E13.40-E13.49, E13.618, E13.620-E13.628, E13.630, E13.638,

E13.649, E13.65, E13.69, E13.8, G32.89, G70.00-G70.2, G70.80-G71.29, G71.3, G71.8-G72.3, G72.81-G72.9, G73.1, G73.3, G73.7, G96.9, G98.0, G98.8, M05.472

PDX Collection 3822
E08.40-E08.49, E08.618, E08.620-E08.628, E08.630, E08.638, E08.649, E08.65, E08.69, E08.8, E09.40-E09.49, E09.618, E09.620-E09.628, E09.630, E09.638, E09.649, E09.65, E09.69, E09.8, E10.40-E10.49, E10.618, E10.620-E10.628, E10.630, E10.638, E10.649, E10.69, E10.8, E11.40-E11.49, E11.618, E11.620-E11.628, E11.630, E11.638, E11.649, E11.69, E11.8, E13.40-E13.49, E13.618, E13.620-E13.628, E13.630, E13.638, E13.649, E13.65, E13.69, E13.8, G32.89, G70.00-G70.2, G70.80-G71.29, G71.3, G71.8-G72.3, G72.81-G72.9, G73.1, G73.3, G73.7, G96.9, G98.0, G98.8, M05.479

PDX Collection 3825
I38-I39, I87.8-I87.9, I99.8-I99.9, M32.11

PDX Collection 3827
I01.0, I09.2, I30.0-I03.0, I30.8-I30.9, I31.3-I31.4, I31.8-I31.9, I32, I87.8-I87.9I99.8-I99.9, M32.12

PDX Collection 3829
M70.80-M70.979, M70.99, M79.81, M79.89-M79.9, M79.A21, S75.801A-S75.819A, S75.892A, S75.899A, S85.201A-S85.219A, S85.291A-S85.819A, S85.891A-S85.892A, S85.899A, S95.001A-S95.019A, S95.091A-S95.219A, S95.291A-S95819A, S95.891A-S95.899A

PDX Collection 3831
M70.80-M70.979, M70.98-M70.99, M79.81, M79.89-M79.9, M79.A22, S75.801A-S75.819A, S75.891A-S75.892A, S75.899A, S85.201A-S85.219A, S85.291A-S85.819A, S85.891A-S85.892A, S85.899A, S95.001A-S95.019A, S95.091A-S95.219A, S95.291A-S95.819A, S95.891A-S95.899A

PDX Collection 3833
A17.9, A18.03, A18.09, A18.82, A18.84, A18.89, M46.20-M46.39, M86.00, M86.011, M86.08-M86.10, M86.18-M86.419, M86.48-M86.519, M86.58-M86.619, M86.68-M86.69, M86.8X0-M86.9

PDX Collection 3835
A17.9, A18.03, A18.09, A18.82, A18.84, A18.89, M46.20-M46.39, M86.00, M86.012, M86.08-M86.10, M86.18-M86.319, M86.38-M86.519, M86.58-M86.619, M86.68-M86.69, M86.8X0-M86.9

PDX Collection 3837
A17.9, A18.03, A18.09, A18.82, A18.84, A18.89, M46.20-M46.39, M86.00, M86.019, M86.08-M86.10, M86.18-M86.319, M86.38-M86.519, M86.58-M86.619, M86.68-M86.69, M86.8X0-M86.9

PDX Collection 3839
A17.9, A18.03, A18.09, A18.82, A18.84, A18.89, M46.20-M46.39, M86.00, M86.021, M86.08-M86.10, M86.18-M86.429, M86.38-M86.529, M86.58-M86.629, M86.68-M86.69, M86.8X0-M86.9

PDX Collection 3841
A17.9, A18.03, A18.09, A18.82, A18.84, A18.89, M46.20-M46.39, M86.00, M86.022, M86.08-M86.10, M86.18-M86.329, M86.38-M86.529, M86.58-M86.619, M86.68-M86.69, M86.8X0-M86.9

PDX Collection 3843
A17.9, A18.03, A18.09, A18.82, A18.84, A18.89, M46.20-M46.39, M86.00, M86.029, M86.08-M86.10, M86.18-M86.429, M86.48-M86.529, M86.58-M86.629, M86.68-M86.69, M86.8X0-M86.9

PDX Collection 3845
A17.9, A18.03, A18.09, A18.82, A18.84, A18.89, M46.20-M46.39, M86.00, M86.031, M86.08-M86.10, M86.18-M86.339, M86.38-M86.439, M86.48-M86.539,

M86.58-M86.59, M86.60, M86.631-M86.639, M86.68-M86.69, M86.8X0-M86.9

PDX Collection 3847
A17.9, A18.03, A18.09, A18.82, A18.84, A18.89, M46.20-M46.39, M86.00, M86.032, M86.08-M86.10, M86.18-M86.339, M86.38-M86.439, M86.48-M86.539, M86.58-M86.59, M86.60, M86.631-M86.639, M86.68-M86.69, M86.8X0-M86.9

PDX Collection 3849
A17.9, A18.03, A18.09, A18.82, A18.84, A18.89, M46.20-M46.39, M86.00, M86.039, M86.08-M86.10, M86.18-M86.339, M86.38-M86.439, M86.48-M86.539, M86.58-M86.59, M86.60, M86.631-M86.639, M86.68-M86.69, M86.8X0-M86.9

PDX Collection 3851
A17.9, A18.03, A18.09, A18.82, A18.84, A18.89, M46.20-M46.39, M86.00, M86.041, M86.08-M86.10, M86.18-M86.30, M86.341-M86.349, M86.38-M86.449, M86.48-M86.50, M86.541-M86.549, M86.58-M86.60, M86.641-M86.649, M86.68-M86.69, M86.8X0-M86.9

PDX Collection 3853
A17.9, A18.03, A18.09, A18.82, A18.84, A18.89, M46.20-M46.39, M86.00, M86.042, M86.08-M86.10, M86.18-M86.30, M86.341-M86.349, M86.38-M86.449, M86.48-M86.50, M86.541-M86.549, M86.58-M86.60, M86.641-M86.649, M86.68-M86.69, M86.8X0-M86.9

PDX Collection 3855
A17.9, A18.03, A18.09, A18.82, A18.84, A18.89, M46.20-M46.39, M86.00, M86.049, M86.08-M86.10, M86.18-M86.30, M86.341-M86.349, M86.38-M86.449, M86.48-M86.50, M86.541-M86.549, M86.58-M86.60, M86.641-M86.649, M86.68-M86.69, M86.8X0-M86.9

PDX Collection 3857
A17.9, A18.03, A18.09, A18.82, A18.84, A18.89, M46.20-M46.39, M86.00, M86.051, M86.08-M86.10, M86.18-M86.30, M86.351-M86.359, M86.38-M86.40, M86.451-M86.459, M86.48-M86.50, M86.551-M86.559, M86.58-M86.60, M86.651-M86.659, M86.68-M86.69, M86.8X0-M86.9

PDX Collection 3859
A17.9, A18.03, A18.09, A18.82, A18.84, A18.89, M46.20-M46.39, M86.00, M86.052, M86.08-M86.10, M86.18-M86.30, M86.351-M86.359, M86.38-M86.40, M86.451-M86.459, M86.48-M86.50, M86.551-M86.559, M86.58-M86.60, M86.651-M86.659, M86.68-M86.69, M86.8X0-M86.9

PDX Collection 3861
A17.9, A18.03, A18.09, A18.82, A18.84, A18.89, M46.20-M46.39, M86.00, M86.059, M86.08-M86.10, M86.18-M86.30, M86.351-M86.359, M86.38-M86.40, M86.451-M86.459, M86.48-M86.50, M86.551-M86.559, M86.58-M86.60, M86.651-M86.659, M86.68-M86.69, M86.8X0-M86.9

PDX Collection 3863
A17.9, A18.03, A18.09, A18.82, A18.84, A18.89, M46.20-M46.39, M86.00, M86.061, M86.08-M86.10, M86.18-M86.30, M86.361-M86.369, M86.38-M86.40, M86.461-M86.469, M86.48-M86.50, M86.561-M86.569, M86.58-M86.60, M86.661-M86.669, M86.68-M86.69, M86.8X0-M86.9

PDX Collection 3865
A17.9, A18.03, A18.09, A18.82, A18.84, A18.89, M46.20-M46.39, M86.00, M86.062, M86.08-M86.10, M86.18-M86.30, M86.361-M86.369, M86.38-M86.40, M86.461-M86.469, M86.48-M86.50, M86.561-M86.569,

M86.58-M86.60, M86.661-M86.669, M86.68-M86.69,
M86.8X0-M86.9

PDX Collection 3867
A17.9, A18.03, A18.09, A18.82, A18.84, A18.89,
M46.20-M46.39, M86.00, M86.069, M86.08-M86.10,
M86.18-M86.30, M86.361-M86.369, M86.38-M86.40,
M86.461-M86.469, M86.48-M86.50, M86.561-M86.569,
M86.58-M86.60, M86.661-M86.669, M86.68-M86.69,
M86.8X0-M86.9

PDX Collection 3869
A17.9, A18.03, A18.09, A18.82, A18.84, A18.89,
M46.20-M46.39, M86.00, M86.071, M86.08-M86.10,
M86.18-M86.30, M86.371-M86.379, M86.38-M86.40,
M86.471-M86.479, M86.48-M86.50, M86.571-M86.579,
M86.58-M86.60, M86.671-M86.679, M86.68-M86.69,
M86.8X0-M86.9

PDX Collection 3871
A17.9, A18.03, A18.09, A18.82, A18.84, A18.89,
M46.20-M46.39, M86.00, M86.072, M86.08-M86.10,
M86.18-M86.30, M86.371-M86.379, M86.38-M86.40,
M86.471-M86.479, M86.48-M86.50, M86.571-M86.579,
M86.58-M86.60, M86.671-M86.679, M86.68-M86.69,
M86.8X0-M86.9

PDX Collection 3873
A17.9, A18.03, A18.09, A18.82, A18.84, A18.89,
M46.20-M46.39, M86.00, M86.079, M86.08-M86.10,
M86.18-M86.30, M86.371-M86.379, M86.38-M86.40,
M86.471-M86.479, M86.48-M86.50, M86.571-M86.579,
M86.58-M86.60, M86.671-M86.679, M86.68-M86.69,
M86.8X0-M86.9

PDX Collection 3875
A17.9, A18.03, A18.09, A18.82, A18.84, A18.89,
M46.20-M46.39, M86.00, M86.08-M86.10, M86.111,
M86.18-M86.319, M86.38-M86.419, M86.48-M86.519,
M86.58-M86.619, M86.68-M86.69, M86.8X0-M86.9

PDX Collection 3877
A17.9, A18.03, A18.09, A18.82, A18.84, A18.89,
M46.20-M46.39, M86.00, M86.08-M86.10, M86.112,
M86.18-M86.319, M86.38-M86.419, M86.48-M86.519,
M86.58-M86.619, M86.68-M86.69, M86.8X0-M86.9

PDX Collection 3879
A17.9, A18.03, A18.09, A18.82, A18.84, A18.89,
M46.20-M46.39, M86.00, M86.08-M86.10, M86.119,
M86.18-M86.319, M86.38-M86.419, M86.48-M86.519,
M86.58-M86.619, M86.68-M86.69, M86.8X0-M86.9

PDX Collection 3881
A17.9, A18.03, A18.09, A18.82, A18.84, A18.89,
M46.20-M46.39, M86.00, M86.08-M86.10, M86.121,
M86.18-M86.30, M86.321, M86.329, M86.38-M86.40,
M86.421-M86.429, M86.48-M86.50, M86.521-M86.529,
M86.58-M86.60, M86.621-M86.629, M86.68-M86.69,
M86.8X0-M86.9

PDX Collection 3883
A17.9, A18.03, A18.09, A18.82, A18.84, A18.89,
M46.20-M46.39, M86.00, M86.08-M86.10, M86.122,
M86.18-M86.30, M86.321, M86.329, M86.38-M86.40,
M86.421-M86.429, M86.48-M86.50, M86.521-M86.529,
M86.58-M86.60, M86.621-M86.629, M86.68-M86.69,
M86.8X0-M86.9

PDX Collection 3885
A17.9, A18.03, A18.09, A18.82, A18.84, A18.89,
M46.20-M46.39, M86.00, M86.08-M86.10, M86.129,
M86.18-M86.30, M86.321, M86.329, M86.38-M86.40,
M86.421-M86.429, M86.48-M86.50, M86.521-M86.529,
M86.58-M86.60, M86.621-M86.629, M86.68-M86.69,
M86.8X0-M86.9

PDX Collection 3887
A17.9, A18.03, A18.09, A18.82, A18.84, A18.89,
M46.20-M46.39, M86.00, M86.08-M86.10, M86.131,
M86.18-M86.30, M86.331, M86.339, M86.38-M86.40,
M86.431-M86.439, M86.48-M86.50, M86.531-M86.539,
M86.58-M86.60, M86.631-M86.639, M86.68-M86.69,
M86.8X0-M86.9

PDX Collection 3889
A17.9, A18.03, A18.09, A18.82, A18.84, A18.89,
M46.20-M46.39, M86.00, M86.08-M86.10, M86.132,
M86.18-M86.30, M86.331, M86.339, M86.38-M86.40,
M86.431-M86.439, M86.48-M86.50, M86.531-M86.539,
M86.58-M86.60, M86.631-M86.639, M86.68-M86.69,
M86.8X0-M86.9

PDX Collection 3891
A17.9, A18.03, A18.09, A18.82, A18.84, A18.89,
M46.20-M46.39, M86.00, M86.08-M86.10, M86.139,
M86.18-M86.30, M86.331, M86.339, M86.38-M86.40,
M86.431-M86.439, M86.48-M86.50, M86.531-M86.539,
M86.58-M86.60, M86.631-M86.639, M86.68-M86.69,
M86.8X0-M86.9

PDX Collection 3893
A17.9, A18.03, A18.09, A18.82, A18.84, A18.89,
M46.20-M46.39, M86.00, M86.08-M86.10, M86.141,
M86.18-M86.30, M86.341, M86.349, M86.38-M86.40,
M86.441-M86.449, M86.48-M86.50, M86.541-M86.549,
M86.58-M86.60, M86.641-M86.649, M86.68-M86.69,
M86.8X0-M86.9

PDX Collection 3895
A17.9, A18.03, A18.09, A18.82, A18.84, A18.89,
M46.20-M46.39, M86.00, M86.08-M86.10, M86.142,
M86.18-M86.30, M86.341, M86.349, M86.38-M86.40,
M86.441-M86.449, M86.48-M86.50, M86.541-M86.549,
M86.58-M86.60, M86.641-M86.649, M86.68-M86.69,
M86.8X0-M86.9

PDX Collection 3897
A17.9, A18.03, A18.09, A18.82, A18.84, A18.89,
M46.20-M46.39, M86.00, M86.08-M86.10, M86.149,
M86.18-M86.30, M86.341, M86.349, M86.38-M86.40,
M86.441-M86.449, M86.48-M86.50, M86.541-M86.549,
M86.58-M86.60, M86.641-M86.649, M86.68-M86.69,
M86.8X0-M86.9

PDX Collection 3899
A17.9, A18.03, A18.09, A18.82, A18.84, A18.89,
M46.20-M46.39, M86.00, M86.08-M86.10, M86.151,
M86.18-M86.30, M86.351, M86.359, M86.38-M86.40,
M86.451-M86.459, M86.48-M86.50, M86.551-M86.559,
M86.58-M86.60, M86.651-M86.659, M86.68-M86.69,
M86.8X0-M86.9

PDX Collection 3901
A17.9, A18.03, A18.09, A18.82, A18.84, A18.89,
M46.20-M46.39, M86.00, M86.08-M86.10, M86.152,
M86.18-M86.30, M86.351, M86.359, M86.38-M86.40,
M86.451-M86.459, M86.48-M86.50, M86.551-M86.559,
M86.58-M86.60, M86.651-M86.659, M86.68-M86.69,
M86.8X0-M86.9

PDX Collection 3903
A17.9, A18.03, A18.09, A18.82, A18.84, A18.89,
M46.20-M46.39, M86.00, M86.08-M86.10, M86.159,
M86.18-M86.30, M86.351, M86.359, M86.38-M86.40,
M86.451-M86.459, M86.48-M86.50, M86.551-M86.559,
M86.58-M86.60, M86.651-M86.659, M86.68-M86.69,
M86.8X0-M86.9

PDX Collection 3905
A17.9, A18.03, A18.09, A18.82, A18.84, A18.89,
M46.20-M46.39, M86.00, M86.08-M86.10, M86.161,

M86.18-M86.30, M86.361, M86.369, M86.38-M86.40,
M86.461-M86.469, M86.48-M86.50, M86.561-M86.569,
M86.58-M86.60, M86.661-M86.669, M86.68-M86.69,
M86.8X0-M86.9

PDX Collection 3907
A17.9, A18.03, A18.09, A18.82, A18.84, A18.89,
M46.20-M46.39, M86.00, M86.08-M86.10, M86.162,
M86.18-M86.30, M86.361, M86.369, M86.38-M86.40,
M86.461-M86.469, M86.48-M86.50, M86.561-M86.569,
M86.58-M86.60, M86.661-M86.669, M86.68-M86.69,
M86.8X0-M86.9

PDX Collection 3909
A17.9, A18.03, A18.09, A18.82, A18.84, A18.89,
M46.20-M46.39, M86.00, M86.08-M86.10, M86.169,
M86.18-M86.30, M86.361, M86.369, M86.38-M86.40,
M86.461-M86.469, M86.48-M86.50, M86.561-M86.569,
M86.58-M86.60, M86.661-M86.669, M86.68-M86.69,
M86.8X0-M86.9

PDX Collection 3911
A17.9, A18.03, A18.09, A18.82, A18.84, A18.89,
M46.20-M46.39, M86.00, M86.08-M86.10, M86.171,
M86.18-M86.30, M86.371, M86.379, M86.38-M86.40,
M86.471-M86.479, M86.48-M86.50, M86.571-M86.579,
M86.58-M86.60, M86.671-M86.679, M86.68-M86.69,
M86.8X0-M86.9

PDX Collection 3913
A17.9, A18.03, A18.09, A18.82, A18.84, A18.89,
M46.20-M46.39, M86.00, M86.08-M86.10, M86.172,
M86.18-M86.30, M86.371, M86.379, M86.38-M86.40,
M86.471-M86.479, M86.48-M86.50, M86.571-M86.579,
M86.58-M86.60, M86.671-M86.679, M86.68-M86.69,
M86.8X0-M86.9

PDX Collection 3915
A17.9, A18.03, A18.09, A18.82, A18.84, A18.89,
M46.20-M46.39, M86.00, M86.08-M86.10, M86.179,
M86.18-M86.30, M86.371, M86.379, M86.38-M86.40,
M86.471-M86.479, M86.48-M86.50, M86.571-M86.579,
M86.58-M86.60, M86.671-M86.679, M86.68-M86.69,
M86.8X0-M86.9

PDX Collection 3917
A17.9, A18.03, A18.09, A18.82, A18.84, A18.89,
M46.20-M46.39, M86.00, M86.08-M86.10, M86.18-M86.319,
M86.38-M86.40, M86.411-M86.419, M86.48-M86.519,
M86.58-M86.619, M86.68-M86.69, M86.8X0-M86.9

PDX Collection 3919
A17.9, A18.03, A18.09, A18.82, A18.84, A18.89,
M46.20-M46.39, M86.00, M86.08-M86.10, M86.18-M86.221,
M86.28-M86.30, M86.321-M86.329, M86.38-M86.40,
M86.421-M86.429, M86.48-M86.50, M86.521-M86.529,
M86.58-M86.619, M86.68-M86.69, M86.8X0-M86.9

PDX Collection 3921
A17.9, A18.03, A18.09, A18.82, A18.84, A18.89,
M46.20-M46.39, M86.00, M86.08-M86.10, M86.18-M86.221,
M86.28-M86.329, M86.38-M86.40, M86.421-M86.429,
M86.48-M86.50, M86.521-M86.529, M86.58-M86.60,
M86.621-M86.629, M86.68-M86.69, M86.8X0-M86.9

PDX Collection 3923
A17.9, A18.03, A18.09, A18.82, A18.84, A18.89,
M46.20-M46.39, M86.00, M86.08-M86.10, M86.18-M86.20,
M86.222, M86.28-M86.30, M86.321-M86.329,
M86.38-M86.40, M86.429, M86.48-M86.50,
M86.521-M86.529, M86.58-M86.60, M86.621-M86.629,
M86.68-M86.69, M86.8X0-M86.9

PDX Collection 3925
A17.9, A18.03, A18.09, A18.82, A18.84, A18.89,
M46.20-M46.39, M86.00, M86.08-M86.10, M86.18-M86.20,

M86.231, M86.28-M86.30, M86.331-M86.339,
M86.38-M86.40, M86.431-M86.439, M86.48-M86.50,
M86.531-M86.539, M86.58-M86.60, M86.631-M86.639,
M86.68-M86.69, M86.8X0-M86.9

PDX Collection 3927
A17.9, A18.03, A18.09, A18.82, A18.84, A18.89,
M46.20-M46.39, M86.00, M86.08-M86.10, M86.18-M86.20,
M86.232, M86.28-M86.30, M86.331-M86.339,
M86.38-M86.40, M86.431-M86.439, M86.48-M86.50,
M86.531-M86.539, M86.58-M86.60, M86.631-M86.639,
M86.68-M86.69, M86.8X0-M86.9

PDX Collection 3929
A17.9, A18.03, A18.09, A18.82, A18.84, A18.89,
M46.20-M46.39, M86.00, M86.08-M86.10, M86.18-M86.20,
M86.241, M86.28-M86.30, M86.341-M86.349,
M86.38-M86.40, M86.441-M86.449, M86.48-M86.50,
M86.541-M86.549, M86.58-M86.60, M86.641-M86.649,
M86.68-M86.69, M86.8X0-M86.9

PDX Collection 3931
A17.9, A18.03, A18.09, A18.82, A18.84, A18.89,
M46.20-M46.39, M86.00, M86.08-M86.10, M86.18-M86.20,
M86.242, M86.28-M86.30, M86.341-M86.349,
M86.38-M86.40, M86.441-M86.449, M86.48-M86.50,
M86.541-M86.549, M86.58-M86.60, M86.641-M86.649,
M86.68-M86.69, M86.8X0-M86.9

PDX Collection 3933
A17.9, A18.03, A18.09, A18.82, A18.84, A18.89,
M46.20-M46.39, M86.00, M86.08-M86.10, M86.18-M86.20,
M86.251, M86.28-M86.30, M86.351-M86.359,
M86.38-M86.40, M86.451-M86.459, M86.48-M86.50,
M86.551-M86.559, M86.58-M86.60, M86.651-M86.659,
M86.68-M86.69, M86.8X0-M86.9

PDX Collection 3935
A17.9, A18.03, A18.09, A18.82, A18.84, A18.89,
M46.20-M46.39, M86.00, M86.08-M86.10, M86.18-M86.20,
M86.252, M86.28-M86.30, M86.351-M86.359,
M86.38-M86.40, M86.451-M86.459, M86.48-M86.50,
M86.551-M86.559, M86.58-M86.60, M86.651-M86.659,
M86.68-M86.69, M86.8X0-M86.9

PDX Collection 3937
A17.9, A18.03, A18.09, A18.82, A18.84, A18.89,
M46.20-M46.39, M86.00, M86.08-M86.10, M86.18-M86.20,
M86.261, M86.28-M86.30, M86.361-M86.369,
M86.38-M86.40, M86.461-M86.469, M86.48-M86.50,
M86.561-M86.569, M86.58-M86.60, M86.661-M86.669,
M86.68-M86.69, M86.8X0-M86.9

PDX Collection 3939
A17.9, A18.03, A18.09, A18.82, A18.84, A18.89,
M46.20-M46.39, M86.00, M86.08-M86.10, M86.18-M86.20,
M86.262, M86.28-M86.30, M86.361-M86.369,
M86.38-M86.40, M86.461-M86.469, M86.48-M86.50,
M86.561-M86.569, M86.58-M86.60, M86.661-M86.669,
M86.68-M86.69, M86.8X0-M86.9

PDX Collection 3941
A17.9, A18.03, A18.09, A18.82, A18.84, A18.89,
M46.20-M46.39, M86.00, M86.08-M86.10, M86.18-M86.20,
M86.271, M86.28-M86.30, M86.371-M86.379,
M86.38-M86.40, M86.471-M86.479, M86.48-M86.50,
M86.571-M86.579, M86.58-M86.60, M86.671-M86.679,
M86.68-M86.69, M86.8X0-M86.9

PDX Collection 3943
A17.9, A18.03, A18.09, A18.82, A18.84, A18.89,
M46.20-M46.39, M86.00, M86.08-M86.10, M86.18-M86.20,
M86.272, M86.28-M86.30, M86.371-M86.379,
M86.38-M86.40, M86.471-M86.479, M86.48-M86.50,

M86.571-M86.579, M86.58-M86.60, M86.671-M86.679,
M86.68-M86.69, M86.8X0-M86.9

PDX Collection 3945
O25.11-O25.13, O25.2-O25.3, O99.111, O99.281-O99.285,
O99.511-O99.513, O99.52-O99.53, O99.611-O99.613,
O99.62-O99.63, O99.711-O99.713, O99.72-O99.73, O99.820,
O99.824-O99.825, O9A.111-O9A.113, O9A.12-O9A.13,
O9A.211-O9A.213, O9A.22-O9A.23, O9A.311-O9A.313,
O9A.32-O9A.33, O9A.411-O9A.413, O9A.42-O9A.43,
O9A.511-O9A.513, O9A.52-O9A.53

PDX Collection 3947
O25.11-O25.13, O25.2-O25.3, O99.112, O99.281-O99.285,
O99.511-O99.513, O99.52-O99.53, O99.611-O99.613,
O99.62-O99.63, O99.711-O99.713, O99.72-O99.73, O99.820,
O99.824-O99.825, O9A.111-O9A.113, O9A.12-O9A.13,
O9A.211-O9A.213, O9A.22-O9A.23, O9A.311-O9A.313,
O9A.32-O9A.33, O9A.411-O9A.413, O9A.42-O9A.43,
O9A.511-O9A.513, O9A.52-O9A.53

PDX Collection 3949
O25.11-O25.13, O25.2-O25.3, O99.113, O99.281-O99.285,
O99.511-O99.513, O99.52-O99.53, O99.611-O99.613,
O99.62-O99.63, O99.711-O99.713, O99.72-O99.73, O99.820,
O99.824-O99.825, O9A.111-O9A.113, O9A.12-O9A.13,
O9A.211-O9A.213, O9A.22-O9A.23, O9A.311-O9A.313,
O9A.32-O9A.33, O9A.411-O9A.413, O9A.42-O9A.43,
O9A.511-O9A.513, O9A.52-O9A.53

PDX Collection 3952
O25.11-O25.13, O25.2-O25.3, O99.13, O99.281-O99.285,
O99.511-O99.513, O99.52-O99.53, O99.611-O99.613,
O99.62-O99.63, O99.711-O99.713, O99.72-O99.73, O99.820,
O99.824-O99.825, O9A.111-O9A.113, O9A.12-O9A.13,
O9A.211-O9A.213, O9A.22-O9A.23, O9A.311-O9A.313,
O9A.32-O9A.33, O9A.411-O9A.413, O9A.42-O9A.43,
O9A.511-O9A.513, O9A.52-O9A.53

PDX Collection 3954
O25.11-O25.13, O25.2-O25.3, O99.112, O99.281-O99.285,
O99.511-O99.513, O99.52-O99.53, O99.611-O99.613,
O99.62-O99.63, O99.711-O99.713, O99.72-O99.73, O99.820,
O99.824-O99.825, O9A.111-O9A.113, O9A.12-O9A.13,
O9A.211-O9A.213, O9A.22-O9A.23, O9A.311-O9A.313,
O9A.32-O9A.33, O9A.411-O9A.413, O9A.42-O9A.43,
O9A.511-O9A.513, O9A.52-O9A.53

PDX Collection 3956
O25.11-O25.13, O25.2-O25.3, O99.281-O99.285, O99.354,
O99.511-O99.513, O99.52-O99.53, O99.611-O99.613,
O99.62-O99.63, O99.711-O99.713, O99.72-O99.73, O99.820,
O99.824-O99.825, O9A.111-O9A.113, O9A.12-O9A.13,
O9A.211-O9A.213, O9A.22-O9A.23, O9A.311-O9A.313,
O9A.32-O9A.33, O9A.411-O9A.413, O9A.42-O9A.43,
O9A.511-O9A.513, O9A.52-O9A.53

PDX Collection 3959
I27.0, I27.20-I27.29, I27.81-I27.9, P29.30

PDX Collection 3961
P38.1, P39.2-P39.9

PDX Collection 3963
P38.9, P39.2-P39.9

PDX Collection 3966
N13.9, Q62.0, Q62.10-Q62.12, Q62.2, Q62.31, Q62.39

PDX Collection 3968
N13.9, Q62.0, Q62.10-Q62.12, Q62.2, Q62.32, Q62.39

PDX Collection 3970
Q90.0-Q93.4, Q93.81, Q93.88, Q95.0-Q99.9

PDX Collection 3972
Q90.0-Q93.4, Q93.7, Q93.81, Q93.88, Q95.0-Q99.9

PDX Collection 3974
Q90.0-Q93.4, Q93.81, Q93.88-Q93.89, Q95.0-Q99.9

PDX Collection 3977
G93.6, G93.82, S06.1X0A

PDX Collection 3979
S32.8XXA, S32.89XA

PDX Collection 3980
S31.001A- S31.051A, S31.601A-S31.659A,
S36.892A-S36.899A, T79.A0XA

PDX Collection 3982
M70.80-M70.99, M79.81-M79.9, R29.898, T79.A11A

PDX Collection 3984
M70.80-M70.99, M79.81-M79.9, R29.898, T79.A12A

PDX Collection 3985
M70.80-M70.99, M79.81-M79.9, R29.898, T79.A19A

PDX Collection 3987
M70.80-M70.99, M79.81-M79.9, R29.898, T79.A21A

PDX Collection 3989
M70.80-M70.99, M79.81-M79.9, R29.898, T79.A22A

PDX Collection 3991
T80.30XA, T80.310A-T80.319A, T80.39XA, T80.410A-T80.419A,
T80.49XA, T80.910A-T80.919A, T80.92XA, T80.A9XA

PDX Collection 3993
T80.30XA, T80.310A-T80.319A, T80.39XA, T80.410A-T80.419A,
T80.49XA, T80.910A-T80.919A, T80.92XA, T80.A0XA, T80.A9XA

PDX Collection 3995
T80.30XA, T80.310A-T80.319A, T80.39XA-T80.40XA,
T80.410A-T80.419A, T80.910A-T80.919A, T80.92XA, T80.A1XA,
T80.A9XA

PDX Collection 3997
T80.30XA, T80.310A-T80.319A, T80.39XA-T80.40XA,
T80.410A-T80.419A, T80.910A-T80.919A, T80.92XA, T80.A11A,
T80.A9XA

PDX Collection 3998
F02.80-F02.81, F04-F10.29, F10.920-F11.90, F11.920-F12.13,
F12.150-F12.159, F12.180, F12.188-F12.23, F12.250-F12.259,
F12.280-F12.29, F12.90, F12.920-F12.93, F12.950-F12.959,
F12.80, F12.988, F12.99, F13.10-F13.159, F13.180-F13.29,
F13.90-, F13.920-F14.159, F14.180-F14.259, F14.280-F14.29,
F14.90-F14.959, F14.980-F15.159, F15.180-F15.259,
F15.280-F15.959, F15.980-F15.99, F16.11-F16.159,
F16.180-F16.259, F16.280-F16.90, F16.920-F16.929,
F16.94-F16.959, F16.980-F16.988, F16.99, F17.203-F17.229,
F17.293-F17.299, F18.10-F18.129, F18.14-F18.229,
F18.24-F18.259, F18.27-F18.29, F18.90-F18.929,
F18.94-F18.959, F18.97-F19.159, F19.16-F19.29, F19.90,
F19.920-F19.99, F53.0-F53.1, F55.0-F55.8, R78.0

PDX Collection 3999
O11.4-O11.5, O12.04-O12.05, O12.14-O12.15,
O12.24-O12.25, O13.4-O13.5, O14.04-O14.05,
O14.14-O14.15, O14.24-O14.25, O14.94-O14.95,
O16.4-O16.5, O24.011-O24.019, O24.02-O24.03,
O24.111-O24.33, O24.811-O24.83, O24.911-O24.93,
O25.41-O25.3, O26.10-O26.13, O26.30-O26.43, O26.63,
O26.711-O26.73, O26.811-O26.819, O26.841-O26.86,
O26.891-O26.93, O29.011-O29.029, O29.091-O29.099,
O29.111-O29.129, O29.191-O29.219, O29.291-O29.299,
O29.3X1-O29.3X9, O29.41-O29.43, O29.5X1-O29.5X9,
O29.60-O29.63, O29.8X1-O29.8X9, O29.90-O29.93,
O35.7XX0-O35.7XX9, O75.4, O75.81-O75.9, O80, O90.89,
O99.111-O99.13, O99.210-O99.215, O99.281-O99.285,
O99.330-O99.335, O99.350-O99.355, O99.511-O99.53,
O99.611-O99.63, O99.711-O99.73, O99.820-O99.825,
O99.840-O99.845, O99.891-O99.892, O9A.111-O9A.13,
O9A.211-O9A.23, O9A.311-O9A.319, O9A.32-O9A.33,

O9A.411-O9A.419, O9A.42-O9A.43, O9A.511-O9A.519,
O9A.52-O9A.53

PDX Collection 4000

O11.4-O11.5, O12.04-O12.05, O12.14-O12.15,
O12.24-O12.25, O13.4-O13.5, O14.04-O14.05,
O14.14-O14.15, O14.24-O14.25, O14.94-O14.95,
O16.4-O16.5, O24.011-O24.019, O24.02-O24.03,
O24.111-O24.33, O24.311-O24.33, O24.811-O24.83,
O24.911-O24.93, O25.41-O25.3, O26.10-O26.13,
O26.30-O26.43, O26.63, O26.711-O26.73, O26.811-O26.819,
O26.841-O26.86, O26.891-O26.93, O29.011-O29.029,
O29.091-O29.099, O29.111-O29.129, O29.191-O29.219,
O29.291-O29.299, O29.3X1-O29.3X9, O29.41-O29.43,
O29.5X1-O29.5X9, O29.60-O29.63, O29.8X1-O29.8X9,
O29.90-O29.93, O35.7XX0-O35.7XX9, O75.4, O75.81-O75.9,
O80, O90.89, O99.111-O99.13, O99.210-O99.215,
O99.281-O99.285, O99.330-O99.335, O99.350-O99.355,
O99.511-O99.53, O99.611-O99.63, O99.711-O99.73,
O99.820-O99.825, O99.840-O99.845, O99.891-O99.892,
O9A.111-O9A.13, O9A.211-O9A.23, O9A.311-O9A.319,
O9A.32-O9A.33, O9A.411-O9A.419, O9A.42-O9A.43,
O9A.511-O9A.519, O9A.52-O9A.53

PDX Collection 4001

N00.0-N08, N11.8-N12, N17.0-N17.9

PDX Collection 4002

O11.4-O11.5, O12.04-O12.05, O12.14-O12.15,
O12.24-O12.25, O13.4-O13.5, O14.04-O14.05,
O14.14-O14.15, O14.24-O14.25, O14.94-O14.95,
O16.4-O16.5, O25.10-O25.13, O25.2-O25.3, O26.10-O26.13,
O26.30-O26.43, O26.63, O26.711-O26.73, O26.811-O26.819,
O26.841-O26.86, O26.891-O26.93, O29.011-O29.029,
O29.091-O29.099, O29.111-O29.129, O29.191-O29.219,
O29.291-O29.299, O29.3X1-O29.3X9, O29.41-O29.43,
O29.5X1-O29.5X9, O29.60-O29.63, O29.8X1-O29.8X9,
O29.90-O29.93, O35.7XX0-O35.7XX9, O75.4, O75.81-O75.9,
O80, O90.89, O99.111-O99.13, O99.210-O99.215,
O99.281-O99.285, O99.330-O99.335, O99.350-O99.355,
O99.511-O99.53, O99.611-O99.63, O99.711-O99.73,
O99.820-O99.825, O99.840-O99.845, O99.891-O99.892,
O9A.111-O9A.13, O9A.211-O9A.23, O9A.311-O9A.319,
O9A.32-O9A.33, O9A.411-O9A.419, O9A.42-O9A.43,
O9A.511-O9A.519, O9A.52-O9A.53

PDX Collection 4003

O11.4-O11.5, O12.04-O12.05, O12.14-O12.15,
O12.24-O12.25, O13.4-O13.5, O14.04-O14.05,
O14.14-O14.15, O14.24-O14.25, O14.94-O14.95,
O16.4-O16.5, O24.011-O24.019, O24.02-O24.03,
O24.111-O24.33, O24.311-O24.33, O24.811-O24.83,
O24.911-O24.93, O25.10-O25.13, O25.2-O25.3,
O26.10-O26.13, O26.30-O26.43, O26.63, O26.711-O26.73,
O26.811-O26.819, O26.841-O26.86, O26.891-O26.93,
O29.011-O29.029, O29.091-O29.099, O29.111-O29.129,
O29.191-O29.219, O29.291-O29.299, O29.3X1-O29.3X9,
O29.41-O29.43, O29.5X1-O29.5X9, O29.60-O29.63,
O29.8X1-O29.8X9, O29.90-O29.93, O35.7XX0-O35.7XX9,
O75.4, O75.81-O75.9, O80, O90.89, O99.111-O99.13,
O99.210-O99.215, O99.281-O99.285, O99.330-O99.335,
O99.350-O99.355, O99.511-O99.53, O99.611-O99.63,
O99.711-O99.73, O99.820-O99.825, O99.840-O99.845,
O99.891-O99.892, O9A.111-O9A.13, O9A.211-O9A.23,
O9A.311-O9A.319, O9A.32-O9A.33, O9A.411-O9A.419,
O9A.42-O9A.43, O9A.511-O9A.519, O9A.52-O9A.53

PDX Collection 4004

O11.4-O11.5, O12.04-O12.05, O12.14-O12.15,
O12.24-O12.25, O13.4-O13.5, O14.04-O14.05,
O16.4-O16.5, O24.011-O24.019, O24.02-O24.03,

O24.111-O24.33, O24.311-O24.33, O24.811-O24.83,
O24.911-O24.93, O25.10-O25.13, O25.2-O25.3,
O26.10-O26.13, O26.30-O26.43, O26.63, O26.711-O26.73,
O26.811-O26.819, O26.841-O26.86, O26.891-O26.93,
O29.011-O29.029, O29.091-O29.099, O29.111-O29.129,
O29.191-O29.219, O29.291-O29.299, O29.3X1-O29.3X9,
O29.41-O29.43, O29.5X1-O29.5X9, O29.60-O29.63,
O29.8X1-O29.8X9, O29.90-O29.93, O35.7XX0-O35.7XX9,
O75.4, O75.81-O75.9, O80, O90.89, O99.111-O99.13,
O99.210-O99.215, O99.281-O99.285, O99.330-O99.335,
O99.350-O99.355, O99.511-O99.53, O99.611-O99.63,
O99.711-O99.73, O99.820-O99.825, O99.840-O99.845,
O99.891-O99.892, O9A.111-O9A.13, O9A.211-O9A.23,
O9A.311-O9A.319, O9A.32-O9A.33, O9A.411-O9A.419,
O9A.42-O9A.43, O9A.511-O9A.519, O9A.52-O9A.53

PDX Collection 4005

O11.4-O11.5, O12.04-O12.05, O12.14-O12.15,
O12.24-O12.25, O13.4-O13.5, O14.04-O14.05,
O14.14-O14.15, O14.24-O14.25, O14.94-O14.95,
O16.4-O16.5, O25.10-O25.13, O25.2-O25.3, O26.10-O26.13,
O26.30-O26.43, O26.63, O26.711-O26.73, O26.811-O26.819,
O26.841-O26.86, O26.891-O26.93, O29.011-O29.029,
O29.091-O29.099, O29.111-O29.129, O29.191-O29.219,
O29.291-O29.299, O29.3X1-O29.3X9, O29.41-O29.43,
O29.5X1-O29.5X9, O29.60-O29.63, O29.8X1-O29.8X9,
O29.90-O29.93, O35.7XX0-O35.7XX9, O75.4, O75.81-O75.9,
O80, O90.89, O99.111-O99.13, O99.210-O99.215,
O99.281-O99.285, O99.330-O99.335, O99.350-O99.355,
O99.511-O99.53, O99.611-O99.63, O99.711-O99.73,
O99.820-O99.825, O99.840-O99.845, O99.891-O99.892,
O9A.111-O9A.13, O9A.211-O9A.23, O9A.311-O9A.319,
O9A.32-O9A.33, O9A.411-O9A.419, O9A.42-O9A.43,
O9A.511-O9A.519, O9A.52-O9A.53

PDX Collection 4006

O11.4-O11.5, O12.04-O12.05, O12.14-O12.15,
O12.24-O12.25, O13.4-O13.5, O14.04-O14.05,
O14.14-O14.15, O14.24-O14.25, O14.94-O14.95,
O16.4-O16.5, O25.10-O25.13, O25.2-O25.3, O26.10-O26.13,
O26.30-O26.43, O26.63, O26.711-O26.73, O26.811-O26.819,
O26.841-O26.86, O26.891-O26.93, O29.011-O29.029,
O29.091-O29.099, O29.111-O29.129, O29.191-O29.219,
O29.291-O29.299, O29.3X1-O29.3X9, O29.41-O29.43,
O29.5X1-O29.5X9, O29.60-O29.63, O29.8X1-O29.8X9,
O29.90-O29.93, O35.7XX0-O35.7XX9, O75.4, O75.81-O75.9,
O80, O90.89, O99.111-O99.13, O99.210-O99.215,
O99.281-O99.285, O99.330-O99.335, O99.350-O99.355,
O99.511-O99.53, O99.611-O99.63, O99.711-O99.73,
O99.820-O99.825, O99.840-O99.845, O99.891-O99.892,
O9A.111-O9A.13, O9A.211-O9A.23, O9A.311-O9A.319,
O9A.32-O9A.33, O9A.411-O9A.419, O9A.42-O9A.43,
O9A.511-O9A.519, O9A.52-O9A.53

PDX Collection 4007

G32.89, G40.001-G40.019, G40.101-G40.119,
G40.201-G40.219, G40.301-G40.319, G40.401-G40.419,
G40.42, G40.501, G40.509, G40.801-G40.804,
G40.811-G40.814, G40.821-G40.824, G40.833-G40.834,
G40.89, G40.901, G40.909, G40.911, G40.919,
G40.B01-G40.B19

PDX Collection 4008

O11.4-O11.5, O12.04-O12.05, O12.14-O12.15,
O12.24-O12.25, O13.4-O13.5, O14.04-O14.05,
O14.14-O14.15, O14.24-O14.25, O14.94-O14.95,
O16.4-O16.5, O25.10-O25.13, O25.2-O25.3, O26.10-O26.13,
O26.30-O26.43, O26.63, O26.611-O26.619, O26.62-O26.63,
O26.711-O26.73, O26.811-O26.819, O26.841-O26.86,
O26.891-O26.93, O29.011-O29.029, O29.091-O29.099,
O29.111-O29.129, O29.191-O29.219, O29.291-O29.299,

O29.3X1-O29.3X9, O29.41-O29.43, O29.5X1-O29.5X9,
O29.60-O29.63, O29.8X1-O29.8X9, O29.90-O29.93,
O35.7XX0-O35.7XX9, O75.4, O75.81-O75.9, O80, O90.89,
O99.111-O99.13, O99.210-O99.215, O99.281-O99.285,
O99.330-O99.335, O99.350-O99.355, O99.511-O99.53,
O99.611-O99.63, O99.711-O99.73, O99.820-O99.825,
O99.840-O99.845, O99.891-O99.892, O9A.111-O9A.13,
O9A.211-O9A.23, O9A.311-O9A.319, O9A.32-O9A.33,
O9A.411-O9A.419, O9A.42-O9A.43, O9A.511-O9A.519,
O9A.52-O9A.53

PDX Collection 4009

F02.80-F02.81, F04-F10.29, F10.920-F11.90,
F11.920-F12.129, F12.150-F12.159, F12.180, F12.188-F12.23,
F12.250-F12.259, F12.280-F12.29, F12.90, F12.920-F12.93,
F12.950-F12.959, F12.80, F12.988, F12.99, F13.10-F13.159,
F13.180-F13.29, F13.90, F13.920-F14.159, F14.180-F14.259,
F14.280-F14.29, F14.90-F14.959, F14.980-F15.159,
F15.180-F15.259, F15.280-F15.959, F15.980-F15.99,
F16.11-F16.159, F16.180-F16.259, F16.280-F16.90,
F16.920-F16.929, F16.94-F16.959, F16.980-F16.988, F16.99,
F17.203-F17.229, F17.293-F17.299, F18.10-F18.129,
F18.14-F18.229, F18.24-F18.259, F18.27-F18.29,
F18.90-F18.929, F18.94-F18.959, F18.97-F19.159,
F19.16-F19.29, F19.90, F19.920-F19.99, F53.0-F53.1,
F55.0-F55.8, R78.0

PDX Collection 4010

O11.4-O11.5, O12.04-O12.05, O12.14-O12.15,
O12.24-O12.25, O13.4-O13.5, O14.04-O14.05,
O14.14-O14.15, O14.24-O14.25, O14.94-O14.95,
O16.4-O16.5, O25.10-O25.13, O25.2-O25.3, O26.10-O26.13,
O26.30-O26.43, O26.63, O26.711-O26.73, O26.811-O26.819,
O26.841-O26.86, O26.891-O26.93, O29.011-O29.029,
O29.091-O29.099, O29.111-O29.129, O29.191-O29.219,
O29.291-O29.299, O29.3X1-O29.3X9, O29.41-O29.43,
O29.5X1-O29.5X9, O29.60-O29.63, O29.8X1-O29.8X9,
O29.90-O29.93, O35.7XX0-O35.7XX9, O75.4, O75.81-O75.9,
O80, O90.89, O99.111-O99.13, O99.210-O99.215,
O99.281-O99.285, O99.330-O99.335, O99.350-O99.355,
O99.511-O99.53, O99.611-O99.63, O99.711-O99.73,
O99.820-O99.825, O99.840-O99.845, O99.891-O99.892,
O9A.111-O9A.13, O9A.211-O9A.23, O9A.311-O9A.319,
O9A.32-O9A.33, O9A.411-O9A.419, O9A.42-O9A.43,
O9A.511-O9A.519, O9A.52-O9A.53

PDX Collection 4011

O11.4-O11.5, O12.04-O12.05, O12.14-O12.15,
O12.24-O12.25, O13.4-O13.5, O14.04-O14.05,
O14.14-O14.15, O14.24-O14.25, O14.94-O14.95,
O16.4-O16.5, O25.10-O25.13, O25.2-O25.3, O26.10-O26.13,
O26.30-O26.43, O26.63, O26.611-O26.619, O26.62-O26.63,
O26.711-O26.73, O26.811-O26.819, O26.841-O26.86,
O26.891-O26.93, O29.011-O29.029, O29.091-O29.099,
O29.111-O29.129, O29.191-O29.219, O29.291-O29.299,
O29.3X1-O29.3X9, O29.41-O29.43, O29.5X1-O29.5X9,
O29.60-O29.63, O29.8X1-O29.8X9, O29.90-O29.93,
O35.7XX0-O35.7XX9, O75.4, O75.81-O75.9, O80, O90.89,
O99.111-O99.13, O99.210-O99.215, O99.281-O99.285,
O99.330-O99.335, O99.350-O99.355, O99.511-O99.53,
O99.611-O99.63, O99.711-O99.73, O99.820-O99.825,
O99.840-O99.845, O99.891-O99.892, O9A.111-O9A.13,
O9A.211-O9A.23, O9A.311-O9A.319, O9A.32-O9A.33,
O9A.411-O9A.419, O9A.42-O9A.43, O9A.511-O9A.519,
O9A.52-O9A.53

PDX Collection 4012

O11.4-O11.5, O12.04-O12.05, O12.14-O12.15,
O12.24-O12.25, O13.4-O13.5, O14.04-O14.05,
O14.14-O14.15, O14.24-O14.25, O14.94-O14.95,
O16.4-O16.5, O25.10-O25.13, O25.2-O25.3, O26.10-O26.13,

O26.30-O26.43, O26.63, O26.611-O26.619, O26.62-O26.63,
O26.711-O26.73, O26.811-O26.819, O26.841-O26.86,
O26.891-O26.93, O29.011-O29.029, O29.091-O29.099,
O29.111-O29.129, O29.191-O29.219, O29.291-O29.299,
O29.3X1-O29.3X9, O29.41-O29.43, O29.5X1-O29.5X9,
O29.60-O29.63, O29.8X1-O29.8X9, O29.90-O29.93,
O35.7XX0-O35.7XX9, O75.4, O75.81-O75.9, O80, O90.89,
O99.111-O99.13, O99.210-O99.215, O99.281-O99.285,
O99.330-O99.335, O99.350-O99.355, O99.511-O99.53,
O99.611-O99.63, O99.711-O99.73, O99.820-O99.825,
O99.840-O99.845, O99.891-O99.892, O9A.111-O9A.13,
O9A.211-O9A.23, O9A.311-O9A.319, O9A.32-O9A.33,
O9A.411-O9A.419, O9A.42-O9A.43, O9A.511-O9A.519,
O9A.52-O9A.53

PDX Collection 4013
O11.4-O11.5, O12.04-O12.05, O12.14-O12.15,
O12.24-O12.25, O13.4-O13.5, O14.04-O14.05,
O14.14-O14.15, O14.24-O14.25, O14.94-O14.95,
O16.4-O16.5, O25.10-O25.13, O25.2-O25.3, O26.10-O26.13,
O26.30-O26.43, O26.63, O26.611-O26.619, O26.62-O26.63,
O26.711-O26.73, O26.811-O26.819, O26.841-O26.86,
O26.891-O26.93, O29.011-O29.029, O29.091-O29.099,
O29.111-O29.129, O29.191-O29.219, O29.291-O29.299,
O29.3X1-O29.3X9, O29.41-O29.43, O29.5X1-O29.5X9,
O29.60-O29.63, O29.8X1-O29.8X9, O29.90-O29.93,
O35.7XX0-O35.7XX9, O75.4, O75.81-O75.9, O80, O90.89,
O99.111-O99.13, O99.210-O99.215, O99.281-O99.285,
O99.330-O99.335, O99.350-O99.355, O99.511-O99.53,
O99.611-O99.63, O99.711-O99.73, O99.820-O99.825,
O99.840-O99.845, O99.891-O99.892, O9A.111-O9A.13,
O9A.211-O9A.23, O9A.311-O9A.319, O9A.32-O9A.33,
O9A.411-O9A.419, O9A.42-O9A.43, O9A.511-O9A.519,
O9A.52-O9A.53

PDX Collection 4014
A02.23, A17.9, A18.02, A18.09, A18.82-A18.89,
A39.83-A39.84, A54.40-A54.43, A54.81 A54.9,
M00.00-M00.29, M00.80-M00.9,
M01.X0-M01.X9, M02.00-M02.39, M02.80-M02.9,
M05.40-M05.479, M05.50-M05.59, M05.70-M06.0A,
M06.20-M06.39, M06.80-M06.9, M07.60-M07.69,
M11.00-M13.89, M14.60-M14.69, M14.80-M14.89,
M15.0-M16.9, M17.2-M17.9, M18.2-M18.9, M19.111-M19.149,
M19.171-M19.179, M19.211-M19.249, M19.271-M19.279,
M19.90 M19.93, M24.10-M24.176, M25.00-M25.18,
M25.40-M25.48, M25.50-M25.579, M25.611-M25.676,
M25.80-M25.9, M35.2, M36.1-M36.4, R29.4

PDX Collection 4015
A17.9, A18.10-A18.13, A18.82, A18.84, A18.89, A54.21,
A54.29, A54.82-A54.9, A59.00, A59.8-A59.9, B37.41-B37.49,
E08.21-F08.29, E09.21-E09.29, M10.30-M10.39, N00.0-N08,
N10, N11.0-N13.39, N13.6, N14.0-N14.4, N15.0-N19,
N25.0-N25.1, N25.81-N25.9, N26 1-N79, N36.41-N36.43,
N36.8-N36.9, N39.0, N39.8-N39.9, R31.0-R31.19, R31.9,
R82.71

PDX Collection 4016
T86.8401-T86.8419

PDX Collection 4017
O26.11-O26.43, O26.63, O26.711-O26.73,
O26.811-O26.813, O26.86, O26.891-O26.893,
O26.90-O26.93, O29.011-O29.013, O29.021-O29.023,
O29.091-O29.093, O29.211-O29.213, O29.3X1-O29.3X3,
O29.41-O29.43, O29.5X1-O29.5X3, O29.62-O29.63,
O29.8X1-O29.8X3, O29.91-O29.93, O35.7XX0-O35.7XX9,
O98.111-O98.119, O98.12-O98.13, O98.211-O98.219,
O98.23, O98.311-O98.319, O98.32-O98.33, O99.351-O99..55,
O98.891

PDX Collection 4019
F02.80-F02.81, F04-F10.29, F10.920-F11.90,
F11.920-F12.129, F12.150-F12.159, F12.180, F12.188-F12.23,
F12.250-F12.259, F12.280-F12.29, F12.90, F12.920-F12.93,
F12.950-F12.959, F12.980, F12.988, F12.99, F13.10-F13.159,
F13.180-F13.29, F13.90, F13.920-F14.159, F14.180-F14.259,
F14.280-F14.29, F14.90-F14.959, F14.980-F15.159,
F15.180-F15.259, F15.280-F15.959, F15.980-F15.99,
F16.10-F16.159, F16.180-F16.259, F16.280-F16.90,
F16.920-F16.929, F16.94-F16.959, F16.980-F16.988, F16.99,
F17.203-F17.229, F17.293-F17.299, F18.10-F18.129,
F18.14-F18.229, F18.24-F18.259, F18.27-F18.29,
F18.90-F18.929, F18.94-F18.959, F18.97-F19.159,
F19.16-F19.29, F19.90, F19.920-F19.99, F53.0-F53.1,
F55.0-F55.8, R78.0

PDX Collection 4020
O11.4-O11.5, O12.04-O12.05, O12.14-O12.15,
O12.24-O12.25, O13.4-O13.5, O14.04-O14.05,
O14.14-O14.15, O14.24-O14.25, O14.94-O14.95,
O16.4-O16.5, O25.10-O25.13, O25.2-O25.3, O26.10-O26.13,
O26.30-O26.43, O26.63, O26.711-O26.73, O26.811-O26.819,
O26.841-O26.86, O26.891-O26.93, O29.011-O29.029,
O29.091-O29.099, O29.111-O29.129, O29.191-O29.219,
O29.291-O29.299, O29.3X1-O29.3X9, O29.41-O29.43,
O29.5X1-O29.5X9, O29.60-O29.63, O29.8X1-O29.8X9,
O29.90-O29.93, O29.011-O29.029, O29.92-O29.129,
O29.191-O29.219, O29.292-O29.299, O29.3X1-O29.3X9,
O29.40-O29.43, O29.5X1-O29.5X9, O29.60-O29.63,
O29.8X1-O29.8X9, O29.90-O29.93, O35.7XX0-O35.7XX9,
O75.4, O75.81-O75.9, O80, O88.011-O88.03,
O88.111-O88.13, O88.212-O88.219, O88.22-O88.23,
O88.311-O88.33, O88.811-O88.83, O90.89, O99.111-O99.13,
O99.210-O99.215, O99.280-O99.285, O99.330-O99.335,
O99.350-O99.355, O99.511-O99.53, O99.611-O99.63,
O99.711-O99.73, O99.820-O99.825, O99.840-O99.845,
O99.893, O9A.111-O9A.13, O9A.211-O9A.23,
O9A.311 O9A.319, O9A.32-O9A.33, O9A.411-O9A 419,
O9A.42-O9A.43, O9A.511-O9A.519, O9A.52-O9A.53

PDX Collection 4021
O11.4 O11.5, O12.04-O12.05, O12.14-O12.15,
O12.24-O12.25, O13.4-O13.5, O14.04-O14.05,
O14.14-O14.15, O14.24-O14.25, O14.94-O14.95,
O16.4-O16.5, O25.10-O25.13, O25.2-O25.3, O26.10-O26.13,
O26.30-O26.43, O26.63, O26.711-O26.73, O26.811-O26.819,
O26.841-O26.86, O26.891-O26.93, O29.011-O29.029,
O29.091-O29.099, O29.111-O29.129, O29.191-O29.219,
O29.291-O29.299, O29.3X1-O29.3X9, O29.40-O29.43,
O29.5X1-O29.5X9, O29.60-O29.63, O29.8X1-O29.8X9,
O29.90-O29.93, O35.7XX0-O35.7XX9, O75.4, O75.81-O75.9,
O80, O88.011-O88.03, O88.111-O88.13, O88.212-O88.219,
O88.22-O88.23, O88.311-O88.33, O88.811-O88.83, O90.89,
O99.111-O99.13, O99.210-O99.215, O99.280-O99.285,
O99.330-O99.335, O99.350-O99.355, O99.511-O99.53,
O99.611-O99.63, O99.711-O99.73, O99.820-O99.825,
O99.840-O99.845, O99.892, O9A.111-O9A.13,
O9A.211-O9A.23, O9A.311-O9A.319, O9A.32-O9A.33,
O9A.411-O9A.419, O9A.42-O9A.43, O9A.511-O9A.519,
O9A.52-O9A.53

PDX Collection 4022
T86.8421-T86.8429, T86.8481- T86.8489, T86.8491- T86.8499

PDX Collection 4023
O11.4-O11.5, O12.04-O12.05, O12.14-O12.15,
O12.24-O12.25, O13.4-O13.5, O14.04-O14.05,
O14.14-O14.15, O14.24-O14.25, O14.94-O14.95,
O16.4-O16.5, O25.10-O25.13, O25.2-O25.3, O26.10-O26.13,
O26.30-O26.43, O26.63, O26.711-O26.73, O26.811-O26.819,
O26.841-O26.86, O26.891-O26.93, O29.011-O29.029,
O29.092-O29.099, O29.111-O29.129, O29.191-O29.219,

O29.291-O29.299, O29.3X1-O29.3X9, O29.40-O29.43,
O29.5X1-O29.5X9, O29.60-O29.63, O29.8X1-O29.8X9,
O29.90-O29.93, O35.7XX0-O35.7XX9, O75.4, O75.81-O75.9,
O80, O90.89, O99.111-O99.13, O99.210-O99.215,
O99.280-O99.285, O99.320-O99.325, O99.330-O99.335,
O99.350-O99.355, O99.511-O99.53, O99.611-O99.63,
O99.711-O99.73, O99.820-O99.825, O99.840-O99.845,
O99.891, O9A.111-O9A.13, O9A.211-O9A.23,
O9A.311-O9A.319, O9A.32-O9A.33, O9A.411-O9A.419,
O9A.42-O9A.43, O9A.511-O9A.519, O9A.52-O9A.53

PDX Collection 4024
O11.4-O11.5, O12.04-O12.05, O12.14-O12.15,
O12.24-O12.25, O13.4-O13.5, O14.04-O14.05,
O14.14-O14.15, O14.24-O14.25, O14.94-O14.95,
O16.4-O16.5, O25.10-O25.13, O25.2-O25.3, O26.10-O26.13,
O26.30-O26.43, O26.63, O26.711-O26.73, O26.811-O26.819,
O26.841-O26.86, O26.891-O26.93, O29.011-O29.029,
O29.091-O29.099, O29.111-O29.129, O29.191-O29.219,
O29.291-O29.299, O29.3X1-O29.3X9, O29.40-O29.43,
O29.5X1-O29.5X9, O29.60-O29.63, O29.8X1-O29.8X9,
O29.90-O29.93, O35.7XX0-O35.7XX9, O75.4, O75.81-O75.9,
O80, O90.89, O99.111-O99.13, O99.210-O99.215,
O99.280-O99.285, O99.320-O99.325, O99.330-O99.335,
O99.350-O99.355, O99.511-O99.53, O99.611-O99.63,
O99.711-O99.73, O99.820-O99.825, O99.840-O99.845,
O99.891-O99.892, O9A.111-O9A.13, O9A.211-O9A.23,
O9A.311-O9A.319, O9A.32-O9A.33, O9A.411-O9A.419,
O9A.42-O9A.43, O9A.511-O9A.519, O9A.52-O9A.53

PDX Collection 4025
O11.4-O11.5, O12.04-O12.05, O12.14-O12.15,
O12.24-O12.25, O13.4-O13.5, O14.04-O14.05,
O14.14-O14.15, O14.24-O14.25, O14.94-O14.95,
O16.4-O16.5, O25.10-O25.13, O25.2-O25.3, O26.10-O26.13,
O26.30-O26.43, O26.63, O26.711-O26.73, O26.811-O26.819,
O26.841-O26.86, O26.891-O26.93, O29.011-O29.029,
O29.091-O29.099, O29.111-O29.129, O29.191-O29.219,
O29.291-O29.299, O29.3X1 O29.3X9, O29.40-O29.43,
O29.5X1-O29.5X9, O29.60-O29.63, O29.8X1-O29.8X9,
O29.90-O29.93, O35.7XX0-O35.7XX9, O75.4, O75.81-O75.9,
O80, O90.89, O99.111-O99.13, O99.210-O99.215,
O99.280-O99.285, O99.320-O99.325, O99.330-O99.335,
O99.350-O99.355, O99.511-O99.53, O99.611-O99.63,
O99.711-O99.73, O99.820-O99.825, O99.840-O99.845,
O99.892, O9A.111-O9A.13, O9A.211-O9A.23,
O9A.311-O9A.319, O9A.32-O9A.33, O9A.411-O9A.419,
O9A.42-O9A.43, O9A.511-O9A.519, O9A.52-O9A.53

PDX Collection 4026
O11.4-O11.5, O12.04-O12.05, O12.14-O12.15,
O12.24-O12.25, O13.4-O13.5, O14.04-O14.05,
O14.14-O14.15, O14.24-O14.25, O14.94-O14.95,
O16.4-O16.5, O25.10-O25.13, O25.2-O25.3, O26.10-O26.13,
O26.30-O26.43, O26.63, O26.711-O26.73, O26.811-O26.819,
O26.841-O26.86, O26.891-O26.93, O29.011-O29.029,
O29.091-O29.099, O29.111-O29.129, O29.191-O29.219,
O29.291-O29.299, O29.3X1-O29.3X9, O29.40-O29.43,
O29.5X1-O29.5X9, O29.60-O29.63, O29.8X1-O29.8X9,
O29.90-O29.93, O35.7XX0-O35.7XX9, O75.4, O75.81-O75.9,
O80, O90.89, O99.111-O99.13, O99.210-O99.215,
O99.280-O99.285, O99.320-O99.325, O99.330-O99.335,
O99.350-O99.355, O99.511-O99.53, O99.611-O99.63,
O99.711-O99.73, O99.820-O99.825, O99.840-O99.845,
O99.893, O9A.111-O9A.13, O9A.211-O9A.23,
O9A.311-O9A.319, O9A.32-O9A.33, O9A.411-O9A.419,
O9A.42-O9A.43, O9A.511-O9A.519, O9A.52-O9A.53

PDX Collection 4027

D47.4, D50.0-D53.9, D55.0-D57.459, D57.80-D57.819, D58.0-D61.3, D61.810-D64.4, D64.81-D64.9, D68.312, D68.51-D68.69, D75.81-D75.A, D77, D89.2

PDX Collection 4028

D56.4-D57.459, D57.80-D57.819

PDX Collection 4029

D59.0-D59.9

PDX Collection 4030

O11.4-O11.5, O12.04-O12.05, O12.14-O12.15, O12.24-O12.25, O13.4-O13.5, O14.04-O14.05, O14.14-O14.15, O14.24-O14.25, O14.94-O14.95, O16.4-O16.5, O25.10-O25.13, O25.2-O25.3, O26.10-O26.13, O26.30-O26.43, O26.63, O26.711-O26.73, O26.811-O26.819, O26.841-O26.86, O26.891-O26.93, O29.011-O29.029, O29.091-O29.099, O29.111-O29.129, O29.191-O29.219, O29.291-O29.299, O29.3X1-O29.3X9, O29.40-O29.43, O29.5X1-O29.5X9, O29.60-O29.63, O29.8X1-O29.8X9, O29.90-O29.93, O35.7XX0-O35.7XX9, O75.4, O75.81-O75.9, O80, O88.011-O88.33, O88.811-O88.83, O90.89, O99.111-O99.13, O99.210-O99.215, O99.280-O99.285, O99.330-O99.335, O99.350-O99.355, O99.511-O99.53, O99.611-O99.63, O99.711-O99.73, O99.820-O99.825, O99.840-O99.845, O99.891-O99.892, O9A.111-O9A.13, O9A.211-O9A.23, O9A.311-O9A.319, O9A.32-O9A.33, O9A.411-O9A.419, O9A.42-O9A.43, O9A.511-O9A.519, O9A.52-O9A.53

PDX Collection 4031

O11.4-O11.5, O12.04-O12.05, O12.14-O12.15, O12.24-O12.25, O13.4-O13.5, O14.04-O14.05, O14.14-O14.15, O14.24-O14.25, O14.94-O14.95, O16.4-O16.5, O25.10-O25.13, O25.2-O25.3, O26.10-O26.13, O26.30-O26.43, O26.63, O26.711-O26.73, O26.811-O26.819, O26.841-O26.86, O26.891-O26.93, O29.011-O29.029, O29.091-O29.099, O29.111-O29.129, O29.191-O29.219, O29.291-O29.299, O29.3X1-O29.3X9, O29.40-O29.43, O29.5X1-O29.5X9, O29.60-O29.63, O29.8X1-O29.8X9, O29.90-O29.93, O35.7XX0-O35.7XX9, O75.4, O75.81-O75.9, O80, O88.011-O88.33, O88.811-O88.83, O90.89, O99.111-O99.13, O99.210-O99.215, O99.280-O99.285, O99.330-O99.335, O99.350-O99.355, O99.511-O99.53, O99.611-O99.63, O99.711-O99.73, O99.820-O99.825, O99.840-O99.845, O99.891, O9A.111-O9A.13, O9A.211-O9A.23, O9A.311-O9A.319, O9A.32-O9A.33, O9A.411-O9A.419, O9A.42-O9A.43, O9A.511-O9A.519, O9A.52-O9A.53

PDX Collection 4032

D47.4, D50.0-D53.9, D55.0-D57.419, D57.80-D57.819, D58.0-D61.3, D61.810-D64.4, D64.81-D64.9, D68.312, D68.51-D68.69, D75.81-D75.A, D77, D89.2

PDX Collection 4033

O11.4-O11.5, O12.04-O12.05, O12.14-O12.15, O12.24-O12.25, O13.4-O13.5, O14.04-O14.05, O14.14-O14.15, O14.24-O14.25, O14.94-O14.95, O16.4-O16.5, O25.10-O25.13, O25.2-O25.3, O26.10-O26.13, O26.30-O26.43, O26.63, O26.711-O26.73, O26.811-O26.819, O26.841-O26.86, O26.891-O26.93, O29.011-O29.029, O29.091-O29.099, O29.111-O29.129, O29.191-O29.219, O29.291-O29.299, O29.3X1-O29.3X9, O29.40-O29.43, O29.5X1-O29.5X9, O29.60-O29.63, O29.8X1-O29.8X9, O29.90-O29.93, O35.7XX0-O35.7XX9, O47.00-O47.9, O60.00-O60.03, O60.10X0-O60.14X9, O60.20X0-O60.20X9, O60.22X0-O60.23X9, O75.4, O75.81-O75.9, O80, O90.89, O99.111-O99.13, O99.210-O99.215, O99.280-O99.285, O99.330-O99.335, O99.350-O99.355, O99.511-O99.53, O99.611-O99.63, O99.711-O99.73, O99.820-O99.825, O99.840-O99.845, O99.892, O9A.111-O9A.13,

O9A.211-O9A.23, O9A.311-O9A.319, O9A.32-O9A.33, O9A.411-O9A.419, O9A.42-O9A.43, O9A.511-O9A.519, O9A.52-O9A.53

PDX Collection 4034

O11.4-O11.5, O12.04-O12.05, O12.14-O12.15, O12.24-O12.25, O13.4-O13.5, O14.04-O14.05, O14.14-O14.15, O14.24-O14.25, O14.94-O14.95, O16.4-O16.5, O25.10-O25.13, O25.2-O25.3, O26.10-O26.13, O26.30-O26.43, O26.63, O26.711-O26.73, O26.811-O26.819, O26.841-O26.86, O26.891-O26.93, O29.011-O29.029, O29.091-O29.099, O29.111-O29.129, O29.191-O29.219, O29.291-O29.299, O29.3X1-O29.3X9, O29.40-O29.43, O29.5X1-O29.5X9, O29.60-O29.63, O29.8X1-O29.8X9, O29.90-O29.93, O35.7XX0-O35.7XX9, O75.4, O75.81-O75.9, O80, O90.89, O98.011-O98.03, O99.111-O99.13, O99.210-O99.215, O99.280-O99.285, O99.330-O99.335, O99.350-O99.355, O99.511-O99.53, O99.611-O99.63, O99.711-O99.73, O99.820-O99.825, O99.840-O99.845, O99.891-O99.892, O9A.111-O9A.13, O9A.211-O9A.23, O9A.311-O9A.319, O9A.32-O9A.33, O9A.411-O9A.419, O9A.42-O9A.43, O9A.511-O9A.519, O9A.52-O9A.53

PDX Collection 4035

O11.4-O11.5, O12.04-O12.05, O12.14-O12.15, O12.24-O12.25, O13.4-O13.5, O14.04-O14.05, O14.14-O14.15, O14.24-O14.25, O14.94-O14.95, O16.4-O16.5, O25.10-O25.13, O25.2-O25.3, O26.10-O26.13, O26.30-O26.43, O26.63, O26.711-O26.73, O26.811-O26.819, O26.841-O26.86, O26.891-O26.93, O29.011-O29.029, O29.091-O29.099, O29.111-O29.129, O29.191-O29.219, O29.291-O29.299, O29.3X1-O29.3X9, O29.40-O29.43, O29.5X1-O29.5X9, O29.60-O29.63, O29.8X1-O29.8X9, O29.90-O29.93, O35.7XX0-O35.7XX9, O75.4, O75.81-O75.9, O80, O90.89, O98.011-O98.03, O99.111-O99.13, O99.210-O99.215, O99.280-O99.285, O99.330-O99.335, O99.350-O99.355, O99.511-O99.53, O99.611-O99.63, O99.711-O99.73, O99.820-O99.825, O99.840-O99.845, O99.891, O9A.111-O9A.13, O9A.211-O9A.23, O9A.311-O9A.319, O9A.32-O9A.33, O9A.411-O9A.419, O9A.42-O9A.43, O9A.511-O9A.519, O9A.52-O9A.53

PDX Collection 4036

O11.4-O11.5, O12.04-O12.05, O12.14-O12.15, O12.24-O12.25, O13.4-O13.5, O14.04-O14.05, O14.14-O14.15, O14.24-O14.25, O14.94-O14.95, O16.4-O16.5, O25.10-O25.13, O25.2-O25.3, O26.10-O26.13, O26.30-O26.43, O26.63, O26.711-O26.73, O26.811-O26.819, O26.841-O26.86, O26.891-O26.93, O29.011-O29.029, O29.091-O29.099, O29.111-O29.129, O29.191-O29.219, O29.291-O29.299, O29.3X1-O29.3X9, O29.40-O29.43, O29.5X1-O29.5X9, O29.60-O29.63, O29.8X1-O29.8X9, O29.90-O29.93, O35.7XX0-O35.7XX9, O75.4, O75.81-O75.9, O80, O86.11-O86.29, O90.89, O99.111-O99.13, O99.210-O99.215, O99.280-O99.285, O99.330-O99.335, O99.350-O99.355, O99.511-O99.53, O99.611-O99.63, O99.711-O99.73, O99.820-O99.825, O99.840-O99.845, O99.893, O9A.111-O9A.13, O9A.211-O9A.23, O9A.311-O9A.319, O9A.32-O9A.33, O9A.411-O9A.419, O9A.42-O9A.43, O9A.511-O9A.519, O9A.52-O9A.53

PDX Collection 4037

O11.4-O11.5, O12.04-O12.05, O12.14-O12.15, O12.24-O12.25, O13.4-O13.5, O14.04-O14.05, O14.14-O14.15, O14.24-O14.25, O14.94-O14.95, O16.4-O16.5, O25.10-O25.13, O25.2-O25.3, O26.10-O26.13, O26.30-O26.43, O26.63, O26.711-O26.73, O26.811-O26.819, O26.841-O26.86, O26.891-O26.93, O29.011-O29.029, O29.091-O29.099, O29.111-O29.129, O29.191-O29.219, O29.291-O29.299, O29.3X1-O29.3X9, O29.40-O29.43, O29.5X1-O29.5X9, O29.60-O29.63, O29.8X1-O29.8X9,

O29.90-O29.93, O35.7XX0-O35.7XX9, O75.4, O75.81-O75.9, O80, O90.3, O90.89, O98.011-O98.03, O99.111-O99.13, O99.210-O99.215, O99.280-O99.285, O99.330-O99.335, O99.350-O99.355, O99.511-O99.53, O99.611-O99.63, O99.711-O99.73, O99.820-O99.825, O99.840-O99.845, O99.892, O9A.111-O9A.13, O9A.211-O9A.23, O9A.311-O9A.319, O9A.32-O9A.33, O9A.411-O9A.419, O9A.42-O9A.43, O9A.511-O9A.519, O9A.52-O9A.53

PDX Collection 4038

O11.4-O11.5, O12.04-O12.05, O12.14-O12.15, O12.24-O12.25, O13.4-O13.5, O14.04-O14.05, O14.14-O14.15, O14.24-O14.25, O14.94-O14.95, O16.4-O16.5, O25.10-O25.13, O25.2-O25.3, O26.10-O26.13, O26.30-O26.43, O26.63, O26.711-O26.73, O26.811-O26.819, O26.841-O26.86, O26.891-O26.93, O29.011-O29.029, O29.091-O29.099, O29.111-O29.129, O29.191-O29.219, O29.291-O29.299, O29.3X1-O29.3X9, O29.40-O29.43, O29.5X1-O29.5X9, O29.60-O29.63, O29.8X1-O29.8X9, O29.90-O29.93, O35.7XX0-O35.7XX9, O75.4, O75.81-O75.9, O80, O90.3, O90.89, O98.011-O98.03, O99.111-O99.13, O99.210-O99.215, O99.280-O99.285, O99.330-O99.335, O99.350-O99.355, O99.511-O99.53, O99.611-O99.63, O99.711-O99.73, O99.820-O99.825, O99.840-O99.845, O99.893, O9A.111-O9A.13, O9A.211-O9A.23, O9A.311-O9A.319, O9A.32-O9A.33, O9A.411-O9A.419, O9A.42-O9A.43, O9A.511-O9A.519, O9A.52-O9A.53

PDX Collection 4039

O11.4-O11.5, O12.04-O12.05, O12.14-O12.15, O12.24-O12.25, O13.4-O13.5, O14.04-O14.05, O14.14-O14.15, O14.24-O14.25, O14.94-O14.95, O16.4-O16.5, O25.10-O25.13, O25.2-O25.3, O26.10-O26.13, O26.30-O26.43, O26.63, O26.711-O26.73, O26.811-O26.819, O26.841-O26.86, O26.891-O26.93, O29.011-O29.029, O29.091-O29.099, O29.111-O29.129, O29.191-O29.219, O29.291-O29.299, O29.3X1-O29.3X9, O29.40-O29.43, O29.5X1-O29.5X9, O29.60-O29.63, O29.8X1-O29.8X9, O29.90-O29.93, O35.7XX0-O35.7XX9, O75.4, O75.81-O75.9, O80, O85, O86.04, O86.12, O86.81-O86.89, O90.89, O98.011-O98.03, O99.111-O99.13, O99.210-O99.215, O99.280-O99.285, O99.330-O99.335, O99.350-O99.355, O99.511-O99.53, O99.611-O99.63, O99.711-O99.73, O99.820-O99.825, O99.840-O99.845, O99.893, O9A.111-O9A.13, O9A.211-O9A.23, O9A.311-O9A.319, O9A.32-O9A.33, O9A.411-O9A.419, O9A.42-O9A.43, O9A.511-O9A.519, O9A.52-O9A.53

PDX Collection 4040

O11.4-O11.5, O12.04-O12.05, O12.14-O12.15, O12.24-O12.25, O13.4-O13.5, O14.04-O14.05, O14.14-O14.15, O14.24-O14.25, O14.94-O14.95, O16.4-O16.5, O25.10-O25.13, O25.2-O25.3, O26.10-O26.13, O26.30-O26.43, O26.63, O26.711-O26.73, O26.811-O26.819, O26.841-O26.86, O26.891-O26.93, O29.011-O29.029, O29.091-O29.099, O29.111-O29.129, O29.191-O29.219, O29.291-O29.299, O29.3X1-O29.3X9, O29.40-O29.43, O29.5X1-O29.5X9, O29.60-O29.63, O29.8X1-O29.8X9, O29.90-O29.93, O35.7XX0-O35.7XX9, O75.4, O75.81-O75.9, O80, O85, O86.04, O86.12, O86.81-O86.89, O90.89, O98.011-O98.03, O99.111-O99.13, O99.210-O99.215, O99.280-O99.285, O99.330-O99.335, O99.350-O99.355, O99.511-O99.53, O99.611-O99.63, O99.711-O99.73, O99.820-O99.825, O99.840-O99.845, O99.892, O9A.111-O9A.13, O9A.211-O9A.23, O9A.311-O9A.319, O9A.32-O9A.33, O9A.411 O9A.419, O9A.42-O9A.43, O9A.511-O9A.519, O9A.52-O9A.53

PDX Collection 4041

O11.4-O11.5, O12.04-O12.05, O12.14-O12.15, O12.24-O12.25, O13.4-O13.5, O14.04-O14.05,

014.14-014.15, 014.24-014.25, 014.94-014.95,
016.4-016.5, 025.10-025.13, 025.2-025.3, 026.10-026.13,
026.30-026.43, 026.63, 026.711-026.73, 026.811-026.819,
026.841-026.86, 026.891-026.93, 029.011-029.029,
029.091-029.099, 029.111-029.129, 029.191-029.219,
029.291-029.299, 029.3X1-029.3X9, 029.40-029.43,
029.5X1-029.5X9, 029.60-029.63, 029.8X1-029.8X9,
029.90-029.93, 035.7XX0-035.7XX9, 075.4, 075.81-075.9,
080, 087.0-087.9, 090.89, 098.011-098.03,099.111-099.13,
099.210-099.215, 099.280-099.285, 099.330-099.335,
099.350-099.355, 099.511-099.53, 099.611-099.63,
099.711-099.73, 099.820-099.825, 099.840-099.845,
099.893, 09A.111-09A.13, 09A.211-09A.23,
09A.311-09A.319, 09A.32-09A.33, 09A.411-09A.419,
09A.42-09A.43, 09A.511-09A.519, 09A.52-09A.53

PDX Collection 4042
010.011-010.03, 010.111-010.13, 010.211-010.23,
010.311-010.33, 010.411-010.43, 010.911-010.93,
011.1-012.05, 012.14-012.15, 012.20-012.25,
013.1-014.05, 014.10-014.15, 014.20-014.25,
014.90-014.95, 015.00-015.03, 015.1-015.9, 016.1-016.9,
025.10-025.13, 025.2-025.3, 026.00-026.3, 026.10-026.13,
026.30-026.43, 026.63, 026.711-026.73, 026.811-026.819,
026.841-026.86, 026.891-026.93, 029.011-029.029,
029.091-029.099, 029.111-029.129, 029.191-029.219,
029.291-029.299, 029.3X1-029.3X9, 029.40-029.43,
029.5X1-029.5X9, 029.60-029.63, 029.8X1-029.8X9,
029.90-029.93, 035.7XX0-035.7XX9, 075.4, 075.81-075.9,
080, 090.89, 099.111-099.13, 099.210-099.215,
099.280-099.285, 099.330-099.335, 099.350-099.355,
099.511-099.53, 099.611-099.63, 099.711-099.73,
099.820-099.825, 099.840-099.845, 099.891,
09A.111-09A.13, 09A.211-09A.23, 09A.311-09A.319,
09A.32-09A.33, 09A.411-09A.419, 09A.42-09A.43,
09A.511-09A.519, 09A.52-09A.53

PDX Collection 4043
010.011-010.03, 010.111-010.13, 010.211 010.23,
010.311-010.33, 010.411-010.43, 010.911-010.93,
011.1-012.05, 012.14-012.15, 012.20-012.25,
013.1-014.05, 014.10-014.15, 014.20-014.25,
014.90-014.95, 015.00-015.03, 015.1-015.9, 016.1-016.9,
025.10-025.13, 025.2-025.3, 026.00-026.3, 026.10-026.13,
026.30-026.43, 026.63, 026.711-026.73, 026.811-026.819,
026.841-026.86, 026.891-026.93, 029.011-029.029,
029.091-029.099, 029.111-029.129, 029.191-029.219,
029.291-029.299, 029.3X1-029.3X9, 029.40-029.43,
029.5X1-029.5X9, 029.60-029.63, 029.8X1-029.8X9,
029.90-029.93, 035.7XX0-035.7XX9, 075.4, 075.81-075.9,
080, 090.89, 099.111-099.13, 099.210-099.215,
099.280-099.285, 099.330-099.335, 099.350-099.355,
099.511-099.53, 099.611-099.63, 099.711-099.73,
099.820-099.825, 099.840-099.845, 099.892,
09A.111-09A.13, 09A.211-09A.23, 09A.311-09A.319,
09A.32-09A.33, 09A.411-09A.419, 09A.42-09A.43,
09A.511-09A.519, 09A.52-09A.53

PDX Collection 4044
G96.00-G96.09

PDX Collection 4045
E70.81-E70.89, E74.810-E74.89

PDX Collection 4046
M80.0AXA, M80.0AXK, M80.0AXP, M80.8AXA, M80.8AXK,
M80.8AXP

PDX Collection 4047
A17.9, A18.10-A18.13, A18.82, A18.84, A18.89, A54.21,
A54.29, A54.82-A54.9, A59.00, A59.8-A59.9, B37.41-B37.49,
E08.21-E08.29, E09.21-E09.29, M10.30-M10.39, N00.0-N08,
N10, N11.0-N13.39, N13.6, N14.0-N14.4, N15.0-N19,

N25.0-N25.1, N25.81-N25.9, N26.1-N29, N36.41-N36.43,
N36.8-N36.9, N39.0, N39.8-N39.9, R31.0-R31.19, R31.9,
R82.71

PDX Collection 4048
G04.1, G10, G11.0-G12.9, G21.0, G23.0-G23.9

PDX Collection 4049
A17.81, A28.1, A50.42, A52.14, A75.9, A79.9, A81.1,
A81.82-A81.89, A83.0-A84.1, A84.81-A85.8, A87.2, A88.8,
A92 1-A92.2, A92.30-A93.0, B00.4, B00.82, B01.11-B01.12,
B04, B06.01, B08.09, B08.20-B08.22, B08.60-B09,
B10.01-B10.09, B26.2, B27.00-B27.19, B27.80-B27.99, B33.1,
B45.0-B45.9, B58.2, B75, B97.10, B97.21, G04.00-G04.01,
G04.31, G04.81-G04.91, G05.3-G05.4, G37.0, G37.4-G37.5,
H66.40-H66.43, J09.X3-J09.X9, J10.2, J10.81-J10.89,
J11.2, J11.81-J11.89, L44.4, M1A.10X0-M1A.10X1,
M1A.1110-M1A.19X1, M32.0-M32.9, P35.2-P35.9,
P37.0-P37.9, T56.0X1A- T56.0X4A

PDX Collection 4050
011.4-011.5, 012.04-012.05, 012.14-012.15,
012.24-012.25, 013.4-013.5, 014.04-014.05,
014.14-014.15, 014.24-014.25, 014.94-014.95,
016.4-016.5, 025.10-025.13, 025.2-025.3, 026.10-026.13,
026.30-026.43, 026.63, 026.711-026.73, 026.811-026.819,
026.841-026.86, 026.891-026.93, 029.011-029.029,
029.091-029.099, 029.111-029.129, 029.191-029.219,
029.291-029.299, 029.3X1-029.3X9, 029.40-029.43,
029.5X1-029.5X9, 029.60-029.63, 029.8X1-029.8X9,
029.90-029.93, 035.7XX0-035.7XX9, 047.00-047.03,
047.0-047.9, 060.00-060.03, 060.10X1-060.14X9,
060.20X1 060.23X9, 075.4, 075.81-075.9, 080,
099.111-099.13, 099.210-099.215, 099.280-099.285,
099.330-099.335, 099.350-099.355, 099.511-099.53,
099.611-099.63, 099.711-099.73, 099.820-099.825,
099.840-099.845, 099.891, 09A.111-09A.13,
09A.211-09A.23, 09A.311-09A.319, 09A.32-09A.33,
09A.411-09A.419, 09A.42-09A.43, 09A.511-09A.519,
09A.52-09A.53

PDX Collection 4051
011.4-011.5, 012.04-012.05, 012.14-012.15,
012.24-012.25, 013.4-013.5, 014.04-014.05,
014.14-014.15, 014.24-014.25, 014.94-014.95,
016.4-016.5, 025.10-025.13, 025.2-025.3, 026.10-026.13,
026.30-026.43, 026.63, 026.711 026.73, 026.811-026.819,
026.841-026.86, 026.891-026.93, 029.011-029.029,
029.091-029.099, 029.111-029.129, 029.191-029.219,
029.291-029.299, 029.3X1-029.3X9, 029.40-029.43,
029.5X1-029.5X9, 029.60-029.63, 029.8X1-029.8X9,
029.90-029.93, 035.7XX0-035.7XX9, 047.00-047.03,
047.0-047.9, 060.00-060.03, 060.10X1-060.14X9,
060.20X1-060.23X9, 075.4, 075.81-075.9, 080,
099.111-099.13, 099.210-099.215, 099.280-099.285,
099.330-099.335, 099.350-099.355, 099.511-099.53,
099.611-099.63, 099.711-099.73, 099.820-099.825,
099.840-099.845, 099.891-099.892, 09A.111-09A.13,
09A.211-09A.23, 09A.311-09A.319, 09A.32-09A.33,
09A.411-09A.419, 09A.42-09A.43, 09A.511-09A.519,
09A.52-09A.53

PDX Collection 4052
011.4-011.5, 012.04-012.05, 012.14-012.15,
012.24-012.25, 013.4-013.5, 014.04-014.05,
014.14-014.15, 014.24-014.25, 014.94-014.95,
016.4-016.5, 025.10-025.13, 025.2-025.3, 026.10-026.13,
026.30-026.43, 026.63, 026.711-026.73, 026.811-026.819,
026.841-026.86, 026.891-026.93, 029.011-029.029,
029.091-029.099, 029.111-029.129, 029.191-029.219,
029.291-029.299, 029.3X1-029.3X9, 029.40-029.43,
029.5X1-029.5X9, 029.60-029.63, 029.8X1-029.8X9,

029.90-029.93, 035.7XX0-035.7XX9, 075.4, 075.81-075.9,
080, 086.11-086.29, 099.111-099.13, 099.210-099.215,
099.280-099.285, 099.330-099.335, 099.350-099.355,
099.511-099.53, 099.611-099.63, 099.711-099.73,
099.820-099.825, 099.840-099.845, 099.891,
09A.111-09A.13, 09A.211-09A.23, 09A.311-09A.319,
09A.32-09A.33, 09A.411-09A.419, 09A.42-09A.43,
09A.511-09A.519, 09A.52-09A.53

PDX Collection 4053
011.4-011.5, 012.04-012.05, 012.14-012.15,
012.24-012.25, 013.4-013.5, 014.04-014.05,
014.14-014.15, 014.24-014.25, 014.94-014.95,
016.4-016.5, 025.10-025.13, 025.2-025.3, 026.10-026.13,
026.30-026.43, 026.63, 026.711-026.73, 026.811-026.819,
026.841-026.86, 026.891-026.93, 029.011-029.029,
029.091-029.099, 029.111-029.129, 029.191-029.219,
029.291-029.299, 029.3X1-029.3X9, 029.40-029.43,
029.5X1-029.5X9, 029.60-029.63, 029.8X1-029.8X9,
029.90-029.93, 035.7XX0-035.7XX9, 075.4, 075.81-075.9,
080, 086.11-086.29, 090.89, 099.111-099.13,
099.210-099.215, 099.280-099.285, 099.330-099.335,
099.350-099.355, 099.511-099.53, 099.611-099.63,
099.711-099.73, 099.820-099.825, 099.840-099.845,
099.891-099.892, 09A.111-09A.13, 09A.211-09A.23,
09A.311-09A.319, 09A.32-09A.33, 09A.411-09A.419,
09A.42-09A.43, 09A.511-09A.519, 09A.52-09A.53

PDX Collection 4054
011.4-011.5, 012.04-012.05, 012.14-012.15,
012.24-012.25, 013.4-013.5, 014.04-014.05,
014.14-014.15, 014.24-014.25, 014.94-014.95,
016.4-016.5, 025.10-025.13, 025.2-025.3, 026.10-026.13,
026.30-026.43, 026.63, 026.711-026.73, 026.811 026.819,
026.841-026.86, 026.891-026.93, 029.011-029.029,
029.091-029.099, 029.111-029.129, 029.191-029.219,
029.291-029.299, 029.3X1-029.3X9, 029.40-029.43,
029.5X1-029.5X9, 029.60-029.63, 029.8X1-029.8X9,
029.90-029.93, 035.7XX0-035.7XX9, 075.4, 075.81-075.9,
080, 090.89, 099.111-099.13, 099.210-099.215,
099.280-099.285, 099.330-099.335, 099.350-099.355,
099.511-099.53, 099.611-099.63, 099.711-099.73,
099.820-099.825, 099.840-099.845, 099.891,
09A.111-09A.13, 09A.211-09A.23, 09A.311-09A.319,
09A.32-09A.33, 09A.411-09A.419, 09A.42-09A.43,
09A.511 09A.519, 09A.52-09A.53

PDX Collection 4055
G71.00-G71.29, G96.9, G98.8, G99.8

PDX Collection 4056
D80.0, D80.3-D84.0, D84.81-D84.9, D89.3-D89.49,
D89.82-D89.9

PDX Collection 4057
A81.89, A83.0-A84.1, A84.81-A85.8, A87.2, A88.0, A88.8

PDX Collection 4058
D56.4-D57.459, D57.80-D57.819

PDX Collection 4059
010.011-010.03, 010.111-010.13, 010.211-010.23,
010.311-010.33, 010.411-010.43, 010.911-010.93,
011.1-012.05, 012.14-012.15, 012.20-012.25,
013.1-014.05, 014.10-014.15, 014.20-014.25,
014.90-014.95, 015.00-015.03, 015.1-015.9, 016.1-016.9,
025.10-025.13, 025.2-025.3, 026.00-026.3, 026.10-026.13,
026.30-026.43, 026.63, 026.711-026.73, 026.811-026.819,
026.841-026.86, 026.891-026.93, 029.011-029.029,
029.091-029.099, 029.111-029.129, 029.191-029.219,
029.291-029.299, 029.3X1-029.3X9, 029.40-029.43,
029.5X1-029.5X9, 029.60-029.63, 029.8X1-029.8X9,
029.90-029.93, 035.7XX0-035.7XX9, 075.4, 075.81-075.9,
080, 090.89, 099.111-099.13, 099.210-099.215,

O99.280-O99.285, O99.330-O99.335, O99.350-O99.355,
O99.511-O99.53, O99.611-O99.63, O99.711-O99.73,
O99.820-O99.825, O99.840-O99.845, O99.892,
O9A.111-O9A.13, O9A.211-O9A.23, O9A.311-O9A.319,
O9A.32-O9A.33, O9A.411-O9A.419, O9A.42-O9A.43,
O9A.511-O9A.519, O9A.52-O9A.53

PDX Collection 4060
O10.011-O10.03, O10.111-O10.13, O10.211-O10.23,
O10.311-O10.33, O10.411-O10.43, O10.911-O10.93,
O11.1-O12.05, O12.14-O12.15, O12.20-O12.25,
O13.1-O14.05, O14.10-O14.15, O14.20-O14.25,
O14.90-O14.95, O15.00-O15.03, O15.1-O15.9, O16.1-O16.9,
O25.10-O25.13, O25.2-O25.3, O26.00-O26.3, O26.10-O26.13,
O26.30-O26.43, O26.63, O26.711-O26.73, O26.811-O26.819,
O26.841-O26.86, O26.891-O26.93, O29.011-O29.029,
O29.091-O29.099, O29.111-O29.129, O29.191-O29.219,
O29.291-O29.299, O29.3X1-O29.3X9, O29.40-O29.43,
O29.5X1-O29.5X9, O29.60-O29.63, O29.8X1-O29.8X9,
O29.90-O29.93, O35.7XX0-O35.7XX9, O75.4, O75.81-O75.9,
O80, O90.89, O99.111-O99.13, O99.210-O99.215,
O99.280-O99.285, O99.330-O99.335, O99.350-O99.355,
O99.511-O99.53, O99.611-O99.63, O99.711-O99.73,
O99.820-O99.825, O99.840-O99.845, O99.891,
O9A.111-O9A.13, O9A.211-O9A.23, O9A.311-O9A.319,
O9A.32-O9A.33, O9A.411-O9A.419, O9A.42-O9A.43,
O9A.511-O9A.519, O9A.52-O9A.53

PDX Collection 4061
O10.011-O10.03, O10.111-O10.13, O10.211-O10.23,
O10.311-O10.33, O10.411-O10.43, O10.911-O10.93,
O11.1-O12.05, O12.14-O12.15, O12.20-O12.25,
O13.1-O14.05, O14.10-O14.15, O14.20-O14.25,
O14.90-O14.95, O15.00-O15.03, O15.1-O15.9, O16.1-O16.9,
O25.10-O25.13, O25.2-O25.3, O26.00-O26.3, O26.10-O26.13,
O26.30-O26.43, O26.63, O26.711-O26.73, O26.811-O26.819,
O26.841-O26.86, O26.891-O26.93, O29.011-O29.029,
O29.091-O29.099, O29.111-O29.129, O29.191-O29.219,
O29.291-O29.299, O29.3X1-O29.3X9, O29.40-O29.43,
O29.5X1-O29.5X9, O29.60-O29.63, O29.8X1-O29.8X9,
O29.90-O29.93, O35.7XX0-O35.7XX9, O44.00-O44.53,
O45.8X1-O45.8X3, O45.91-O45.93, O75.4, O75.81-O75.9,
O80, O90.89, O99.111-O99.13, O99.210-O99.215,
O99.280-O99.285, O99.330-O99.335, O99.350-O99.355,
O99.511-O99.53, O99.611-O99.63, O99.711-O99.73,
O99.820-O99.825, O99.840-O99.845, O99.891,
O9A.111-O9A.13, O9A.211-O9A.23, O9A.311-O9A.319,
O9A.32-O9A.33, O9A.411-O9A.419, O9A.42-O9A.43,
O9A.511-O9A.519, O9A.52-O9A.53

PDX Collection 4062
O10.011-O10.03, O10.111-O10.13, O10.211-O10.23,
O10.311-O10.33, O10.411-O10.43, O10.911-O10.93,
O11.1-O12.05, O12.14-O12.15, O12.20-O12.25,
O13.1-O14.05, O14.10-O14.15, O14.20-O14.25,
O14.90-O14.95, O15.00-O15.03, O15.1-O15.9, O16.1-O16.9,
O25.10-O25.13, O25.2-O25.3, O26.00-O26.3, O26.10-O26.13,
O26.30-O26.43, O26.63, O26.711-O26.73, O26.811-O26.819,
O26.841-O26.86, O26.891-O26.93, O29.011-O29.029,
O29.091-O29.099, O29.111-O29.129, O29.191-O29.219,
O29.291-O29.299, O29.3X1-O29.3X9, O29.40-O29.43,
O29.5X1-O29.5X9, O29.60-O29.63, O29.8X1-O29.8X9,
O29.90-O29.93, O35.7XX0-O35.7XX9, O44.00-O44.53,
O45.8X1-O45.8X3, O45.91-O45.93, O75.4, O75.81-O75.9,
O80, O90.89, O99.111-O99.13, O99.210-O99.215,
O99.280-O99.285, O99.330-O99.335, O99.350-O99.355,
O99.511-O99.53, O99.611-O99.63, O99.711-O99.73,
O99.820-O99.825, O99.840-O99.845, O99.891-O99.892,
O9A.111-O9A.13, O9A.211-O9A.23, O9A.311-O9A.319,
O9A.32-O9A.33, O9A.411-O9A.419, O9A.42-O9A.43,
O9A.511-O9A.519, O9A.52-O9A.53

PDX Collection 4063
O10.011-O10.03, O10.111-O10.13, O10.211-O10.23,
O10.311-O10.33, O10.411-O10.43, O10.911-O10.93,
O11.1-O12.05, O12.14-O12.15, O12.20-O12.25,
O13.1-O14.05, O14.10-O14.15, O14.20-O14.25,
O14.90-O14.95, O15.00-O15.03, O15.1-O15.9, O16.1-O16.9,
O25.10-O25.13, O25.2-O25.3, O26.00-O26.3, O26.10-O26.13,
O26.30-O26.43, O26.63, O26.711-O26.73, O26.811-O26.819,
O26.841-O26.86, O26.891-O26.93, O29.011-O29.029,
O29.091-O29.099, O29.111-O29.129, O29.191-O29.219,
O29.291-O29.299, O29.3X1-O29.3X9, O29.40-O29.43,
O29.5X1-O29.5X9, O29.60-O29.63, O29.8X1-O29.8X9,
O29.90-O29.93, O35.7XX0-O35.7XX9, O75.4, O75.81-O75.9,
O80, O90.89, O99.111-O99.13, O99.210-O99.215,
O99.280-O99.285, O99.330-O99.335, O99.350-O99.355,
O99.511-O99.53, O99.611-O99.63, O99.711-O99.73,
O99.820-O99.825, O99.840-O99.845, O99.893,
O9A.111-O9A.13, O9A.211-O9A.23, O9A.311-O9A.319,
O9A.32-O9A.33, O9A.411-O9A.419, O9A.42-O9A.43,
O9A.511-O9A.519, O9A.52-O9A.53

PDX Collection 4064
A44.0-A44.9, A68.0-A68.9, A69.20, A75.0-A75.9,
A77.0-A77.49, A77.8-A78, A79.0-A79.1, A79.81-A79.9,
B50.0-B54, B60.00-B60.09

PDX Collection 4065
O11.4-O11.5, O12.04-O12.05, O12.14-O12.15,
O12.24-O12.25, O13.4-O13.5, O14.04-O14.05,
O14.14-O14.15, O14.24-O14.25, O14.94-O14.95,
O16.4-O16.5, O25.10-O25.13, O25.2-O25.3, O26.10-O26.13,
O26.30-O26.43, O26.63, O26.711-O26.73, O26.811-O26.819,
O26.841-O26.86, O26.891-O26.93, O29.011-O29.029,
O29.091-O29.099, O29.111-O29.129, O29.191-O29.219,
O29.291-O29.299, O29.3X1-O29.3X9, O29.40-O29.43,
O29.5X1-O29.5X9, O29.60-O29.63, O29.8X1-O29.8X9,
O29.90-O29.93, O35.7XX0-O35.7XX9, O75.4, O75.81-O75.9,
O80, O90.89, O99.111-O99.13, O99.210-O99.215,
O99.280-O99.285, O99.330-O99.335, O99.350-O99.355,
O99.511-O99.53, O99.611-O99.63, O99.711-O99.73,
O99.820-O99.825, O99.840-O99.845, O99.892,
O9A.111-O9A.13, O9A.211-O9A.23, O9A.311-O9A.319,
O9A.32-O9A.33, O9A.411-O9A.419, O9A.42-O9A.43,
O9A.511-O9A.519, O9A.52-O9A.53

PDX Collection 4066
J82.81-J82.89

PDX Collection 4067
O11.4-O11.5, O12.04-O12.05, O12.14-O12.15,
O12.24-O12.25, O13.4-O13.5, O14.04-O14.05,
O14.14-O14.15, O14.24-O14.25, O14.94-O14.95,
O16.4-O16.5, O25.10-O25.13, O25.2-O25.3, O26.10-O26.13,
O26.30-O26.43, O26.63, O26.711-O26.73, O26.811-O26.819,
O26.841-O26.86, O26.891-O26.93, O29.011-O29.029,
O29.091-O29.099, O29.111-O29.129, O29.191-O29.219,
O29.291-O29.299, O29.3X1-O29.3X9, O29.40-O29.43,
O29.5X1-O29.5X9, O29.60-O29.63, O29.8X1-O29.8X9,
O29.90-O29.93, O35.7XX0-O35.7XX9, O75.4, O75.81-O75.9,
O80, O90.89, O98.62-O98.63,
O99.111-O99.13, O99.210-O99.215, O99.280-O99.285,
O99.330-O99.335, O99.350-O99.355, O99.511-O99.53,
O99.611-O99.63, O99.711-O99.73, O99.820-O99.825,
O99.840-O99.845, O99.892, O9A.111-O9A.13,
O9A.211-O9A.23, O9A.311-O9A.319, O9A.32-O9A.33,
O9A.411-O9A.419, O9A.42-O9A.43, O9A.511-O9A.519,
O9A.52-O9A.53

PDX Collection 4068
E08.40-E08.49, E09.40-E09.49, E10.40-E10.49, E11.40-E11.49,
E13.40-E13.49, G04.1, G11.3-G12.9, G32.0, G32.89,
G35, G36.0-G80.9, G81.00-G81.14, G81.90-G81.94,
G82.20-G82.22, G82.50-G82.54, G83.0-G83.5, G83.81-G83.9,

G90.01, G90.09, G90.2-G90.59, G90.8-G90.9, G93.1,
G93.40-G93.49, G95.0-G95.29, G95.81-G95.9, G96.12,
G96.191-G96.9, G97.1, G98.0, G98.8, G90.0, G99.2, G99.8,
I67.83, R53.2

PDX Collection 4069
N00.0-N08, N11.8-N12, N17.0-N17.9

PDX Collection 4070
N00.0-N08, N11.8-N12, N17.0-N17.9

PDX Collection 4072
G97.0-G97.84, I97.810-I97.821

PDX Collection 4073
A81.89, A83.0-A84.1, A84.81-A85.8, A87.2, A88.0, A88.8,
A92.1-A92.2, A92.30-A93.0, B00.4, B00.82, B01.11-B01.12

PDX Collection 4074
D56.4-D57.459, D57.80-D57.819

PDX Collection 4075
F02.80-F02.81, F04-F10.29, F10.920-F11.90, F11.920-F12.13,
F12.150-F12.159, F12.180, F12.188-F12.23, F12.250-F12.259,
F12.280-F12.29, F12.90, F12.920-F12.93, F12.950-F12.959,
F12.80, F12.988, F12.99, F13.10-F13.159, F13.180-F13.29,
F13.90-, F13.920-F14.159, F14.180-F14.259, F14.280-F14.29,
F14.90-F14.959, F14.980-F15.159, F15.180-F15.259,
F15.280-F15.959, F15.980-F15.99, F16.10-F16.159,
F16.180-F16.259, F16.280-F16.90, F16.920-F16.929,
F16.94-F16.959, F16.980-F16.988, F16.99, F17.203-F17.229,
F17.293-F17.299, F18.10-F18.129, F18.14-F18.229,
F18.24-F18.259, F18.27-F18.29, F18.90-F18.929,
F18.94-F18.959, F18.97-F19.159, F19.16-F19.29, F19.90,
F19.920-F19.99, F53.0-F53.1, F55.0-F55.8, R78.0

PDX Collection 4076
F02.80-F02.81, F04-F10.29, F10.920-F11.90, F11.920-F12.13,
F12.150-F12.159, F12.180, F12.188-F12.23, F12.250-F12.259,
F12.280-F12.29, F12.90, F12.920-F12.93, F12.950-F12.959,
F12.80, F12.988, F12.99, F13.10-F13.159, F13.180-F13.29,
F13.90-, F13.920-F14.159, F14.180-F14.259, F14.280-F14.29,
F14.90-F14.959, F14.980-F15.159, F15.180-F15.259,
F15.280-F15.959, F15.980-F15.99, F16.10-F16.159,
F16.180-F16.259, F16.280-F16.90, F16.920-F16.929,
F16.94-F16.959, F16.980-F16.988, F16.99, F17.203-F17.229,
F17.293-F17.299, F18.10-F18.129, F18.14-F18.229,
F18.24-F18.259, F18.27-F18.29, F18.90-F18.929,
F18.94-F18.959, F18.97-F19.159, F19.16-F19.29, F19.90,
F19.920-F19.99, F53.0-F53.1, F55.0-F55.8, R78.0

PDX Collection 4077
F02.80-F02.81, F04-F10.29, F10.920-F11.90, F11.920-F12.13,
F12.150-F12.159, F12.180, F12.188-F12.23, F12.250-F12.259,
F12.280-F12.29, F12.90, F12.920-F12.93, F12.950-F12.959,
F12.80, F12.988, F12.99, F13.10-F13.159, F13.180-F13.29,
F13.90-, F13.920-F14.159, F14.180-F14.259, F14.280-F14.29,
F14.90-F14.959, F14.980-F15.159, F15.180-F15.259,
F15.280-F15.959, F15.980-F15.99, F16.10-F16.159,
F16.180-F16.259, F16.280-F16.90, F16.920-F16.929,
F16.94-F16.959, F16.980-F16.988, F16.99, F17.203-F17.229,
F17.293-F17.299, F18.10-F18.129, F18.14-F18.229,
F18.24-F18.259, F18.27-F18.29, F18.90-F18.929,
F18.94-F18.959, F18.97-F19.159, F19.16-F19.29, F19.90,
F19.920-F19.99, F53.0-F53.1, F55.0-F55.8, R78.0

PDX Collection 4078
F02.80-F02.81, F04-F10.29, F10.920-F11.90, F11.920-F12.13,
F12.150-F12.159, F12.180, F12.188-F12.23, F12.250-F12.259,
F12.280-F12.29, F12.90, F12.920-F12.93, F12.950-F12.959,
F12.80, F12.988, F12.99, F13.10-F13.159, F13.180-F13.29,
F13.90-, F13.920-F14.159, F14.180-F14.259, F14.280-F14.29,
F14.90-F14.959, F14.980-F15.159, F15.180-F15.259,
F15.280-F15.959, F15.980-F15.99, F16.10-F16.159,
F16.180-F16.259, F16.280-F16.90, F16.920-F16.929,

F16.94-F16.959, F16.980-F16.988, F16.99, F17.203-F17.229,
F17.293-F17.299, F18.10-F18.129, F18.14-F18.229,
F18.24-F18.259, F18.27-F18.29, F18.90-F18.929,
F18.94-F18.959, F18.97-F19.159, F19.16-F19.29, F19.90,
F19.920-F19.99, F53.0-F53.1, F55.0-F55.8, R78.0

PDX Collection 4079
E16.4, I85.01, K20.81, K20.91, K21.9, K22.10-K22.11,
K22.3, K22.6, K27.0-K28.9, K29.01, K29.21, K29.31, K29.41,
K29.51, K29.61, K29.71, K29.81, K29.91, K31.811

PDX Collection 4080
F02.80-F02.81, F04-F10.29, F10.920-F11.90, F11.920-F12.13,
F12.150-F12.159, F12.180, F12.188-F12.23, F12.250-F12.259,
F12.280-F12.29, F12.90, F12.920-F12.93, F12.950-F12.959,
F12.80, F12.988, F12.99, F13.10-F13.159, F13.180-F13.29,
F13.90-, F13.920-F14.159, F14.180-F14.259, F14.280-F14.29,
F14.90-F14.959, F14.980-F15.159, F15.180-F15.259,
F15.280-F15.959, F15.980-F15.99, F16.10-F16.159,
F16.180-F16.259, F16.280-F16.90, F16.920-F16.929,
F16.94-F16.959, F16.980-F16.988, F16.99, F17.203-F17.229,
F17.293-F17.299, F18.10-F18.129, F18.14-F18.229,
F18.24-F18.259, F18.27-F18.29, F18.90-F18.929,
F18.94-F18.959, F18.97-F19.159, F19.16-F19.29, F19.90,
F19.920-F19.99, F53.0-F53.1, F55.0-F55.8, R78.0

PDX Collection 4081
F02.80-F02.81, F04-F10.29, F10.920-F11.90, F11.920-F12.13,
F12.150-F12.159, F12.180, F12.188-F12.23, F12.250-F12.259,
F12.280-F12.29, F12.90, F12.920-F12.93, F12.950-F12.959,
F12.80, F12.988, F12.99, F13.10-F13.159, F13.180-F13.29,
F13.90-, F13.920-F14.159, F14.180-F14.259, F14.280-F14.29,
F14.90-F14.959, F14.980-F15.159, F15.180-F15.259,
F15.280-F15.959, F15.980-F15.99, F16.10-F16.159,
F16.180-F16.259, F16.280-F16.90, F16.920-F16.929,
F16.94-F16.959, F16.980-F16.988, F16.99, F17.203-F17.229,
F17.293-F17.299, F18.10-F18.129, F18.14-F18.229,
F18.24-F18.259, F18.27-F18.29, F18.90-F18.929,
F18.94-F18.959, F18.97-F19.159, F19.16-F19.29, F19.90,
F19.920-F19.99, F53.0-F53.1, F55.0-F55.8, R78.0

PDX Collection 4082
E70.81-E70.89, E72.50-E72.59, E72.81-E72.9, E73.0-E73.9,
E74.00-E74.29, E74.31-E74.4, E74.810-E74.9, E75.21-E75.22,
E75.240-E75.249, E75.3, E75.5-E75.6, E77.0-E77.9

PDX Collection 4083
P91.021-P91.029

PDX Collection 4084
M48.40XA-M48.58XA, M80.00XA, M80.011A-M80.019A,
M80.021A-M80.029A, M80.031A-M80.039A,
M80.041A-M80.049A, M80.051A-M80.059A,
M80.061A-M80.069A, M80.071A-M80.079A, M80.0AXA,
M80.08XA, M80.0AXK, M80.0AXP, M80.80XA, M80.811A-
M80.819A, M80.821A- M80.829A, M80.831A- M80.839A,
M80.841A- M80.849A, M80.851A- M80.859A,
M80.861A- M80.869A, M80.871A- M80.879A, M80.8AXA,
M80.8AXK, M80.8AXP, M84.30XA, M84.311A-M84.319A,
M84.321A-M84.329A, M84.331A-M84.339A,
M84.341A-M84.346A, M84.350A-M84.359A,
M84.361A-M84.369A, M84.371A-M84.379A, M84.38XA,
M84.40XA, M84.411A-M84.419A, M84.421A-M84.429A,
M84.431A-M84.439A, M84.441A-M84.446A,
M84.450A-M84.459A, M84.461A-M84.469A,
M84.471A-M84.479A, M84.48XA

PDX Collection 4085
M48.40XA-M48.58XA, M80.00XA, M80.011A- M80.019A,
M80.021A-M80.029A, M80.031A-M80.039A,
M80.041A-M80.049A, M80.051A-M80.059A,
M80.061A-M80.069A, M80.071A-M80.079A, M80.08XA,
M80.0AXA, M80.0AXK, M80.0AXP, M80.80XA, M80.811A-
M80.819A, M80.821A- M80.829A, M80.831A- M80.839A,

M80.841A- M80.849A, M80.851A- M80.859A,
M80.861A- M80.869A, M80.871A- M80.879A, M80.8AXA,
M80.8AXK, M80.8AXP, M84.30XA, M84.311A-M84.319A,
M84.321A-M84.329A, M84.331A-M84.339A,
M84.341A-M84.346A, M84.350A-M84.359A,
M84.361A-M84.369A, M84.371A-M84.379A, M84.38XA,
M84.40XA, M84.411A-M84.419A, M84.421A-M84.429A,
M84.431A-M84.439A, M84.441A-M84.446A,
M84.450A-M84.459A, M84.461A-M84.469A,
M84.471A-M84.479A, M84.48XA

PDX Collection 4086
M80.00XP, M80.011K, M80.011P, M80.012K, M80.012P,
M80.019K, M80.019P, M80.021K, M80.021P,
M80.022K, M80.022P, M80.029K, M80.029P, M80.031K,
M80.031P, M80.032K, M80.032P, M80.039K, M80.039P,
M80.041K, M80.041P, M80.042K, M80.042P, M80.049K,
M80.049P, M80.051K, M80.051P, M80.052K, M80.052P,
M80.059K, M80.059P, M80.061K, M80.061P, M80.062K,
M80.062P, M80.069K, M80.069P, M80.071K, M80.071P,
M80.072K, M80.072P, M80.079K, M80.079P, M80.08XK,
M80.08XP, M80.0AXA, M80.0AXK, M80.0AXP, M80.80XK,
M80.80XP, M80.811K, M80.811P, M80.812K, M80.812P,
M80.819K, M80.819P, M80.821K, M80.821P, M80.822K,
M80.822P, M80.829K, M80.829P, M80.831K, M80.831P,
M80.832K, M80.832P, M80.839K, M80.839P, M80.841K,
M80.841P, M80.842K, M80.842P, M80.849K, M80.849P,
M80.851K, M80.851P, M80.852K, M80.852P, M80.859K,
M80.859P, M80.861K, M80.861P, M80.862K, M80.862P,
M80.869K, M80.869P, M80.871K, M80.871P, M80.872K,
M80.872P, M80.879K, M80.879P, M80.88XK, M80.88XP,
M80.8AXA, M80.8AXK, M80.8AXP, M84.30XK, M84.30XP,
M84.311K, M84.311P, M84.312K, M84.312P, M84.319K,
M84.319P, M84.321K, M84.321P, M84.322K, M84.322P,
M84.329K, M84.329P, M84.331K, M84.331P, M84.332K,
M84.332P, M84.333K, M84.333P, M84.334K, M84.334P,
M84.339K, M84.339P, M84.341K, M84.341P, M84.342K,
M84.342P, M84.343K, M84.343P, M84.344K, M84.344P,
M84.346K, M84.346P, M84.350K, M84.350P, M84.351K,
M84.351P, M84.352K, M84.352P, M84.353K, M84.353P,
M84.359K, M84.359P, M84.361K, M84.361P, M84.362K,
M84.362P, M84.363K, M84.363P, M84.364K, M84.364P,
M84.369K, M84.369P, M84.371K, M84.371P, M84.372K,
M84.372P, M84.373K, M84.373P, M84.374K, M84.374P,
M84.375K, M84.375P, M84.376K, M84.376P, M84.377K,
M84.377P, M84.378K, M84.378P, M84.379K, M84.379P,
M84.38XK, M84.38XP, M84.40XK, M84.40XP, M84.411K,
M84.411P, M84.412K, M84.412P, M84.419K, M84.419P,
M84.421K, M84.421P, M84.422K, M84.422P, M84.429K,
M84.429P, M84.431K, M84.431P, M84.432K, M84.432P,
M84.433K, M84.433P, M84.434K, M84.434P, M84.439K,
M84.439P, M84.441K, M84.441P, M84.442K, M84.442P,
M84.443K, M84.443P, M84.444K, M84.444P, M84.445K,
M84.445P, M84.446K, M84.446P, M84.451K, M84.451P,
M84.452K, M84.452P, M84.453K, M84.453P, M84.454K,
M84.454P, M84.459K, M84.459P, M84.461K, M84.461P,
M84.462K, M84.462P, M84.463K, M84.463P, M84.464K,
M84.464P, M84.469K, M84.469P, M84.471K, M84.471P,
M84.472K, M84.472P, M84.473K, M84.473P, M84.474K,
M84.474P, M84.475K, M84.475P, M84.476K, M84.476P,
M84.477K, M84.477P, M84.478K, M84.478P, M84.479K,
M84.479P, M84.48XK, M84.48XP, X84.50XK, M84.50XP,
M84.511K, M84.511P, M84.512K, M84.512P, M84.519K,
M84.519P, M84.521K, M84.521P, M84.522K, M84.522P,
M84.529K, M84.529P, M84.531K, M84.531P, M84.532K,
M84.532P, M84.533K, M84.533P, M84.534K, M84.534P,
M84.539K, M84.539P, M84.541K, M84.541P, M84.542K,
M84.542P, M84.543K, M84.543P, M84.544K, M84.544P,
M84.545K, M84.545P, M84.546K, M84.546P, M84.551K,

M84.551P, M84.552K, M84.552P, M84.553K, M84.553P,
M84.554K, M84.554P, M84.559K, M84.559P, M84.561K,
M84.561P, M84.562K, M84.562P, M84.563K, M84.563P,
M84.564K, M84.564P, M84.569K, M84.569P, M84.571K,
M84.571P, M84.572K, M84.572P, M84.573K, M84.573P,
M84.574K, M84.574P, M84.575K, M84.575P, M84.576K,
M84.576P, M84.58XK, M84.58XP, M84.60XK, M84.60XP,
M84.611K, M84.611P, M84.612K, M84.612P, M84.619K,
M84.619P, M84.621K, M84.621P, M846522K, M84.622P,
M84.629K, M84.629P, M84.631K, M84.631P, M84.632K,
M84.632P, M84.633K, M84.633P, M84.634K, M84.634P,
M84.639K, M84.639P, M84.641K, M84.641P, M84.642K,
M84.642P, M84.649K, M84.649P, M84.651K, M84.651P,
M84.652K, M84.652P, M84.653K, M84.653P, M84.659K,
M84.659P, M84.661K, M84.661P, M84.662K, M84.662P,
M84.663K, M84.663P, M84.664K, M84.664P, M84.669K,
M84.669P, M84.671K, M84.671P, M84.672K, M84.672P,
M84.673K, M84.673P, M84.674K, M84.674P, M84.675K,
M84.675P, M84.676K, M84.676P, M84.68XK, M84.68XP

PDX Collection 4087
E70.81-E70.89, E72.50-E72.59, E72.81-E74.4, E74.810-E74.9,
E75.21-E75.22, E75.240-E75.249, E75.3, E75.5-E75.6,
E77.0-E77.9

PDX Collection 4088
E70.81-E70.89, E72.50-E72.59, E72.81-E74.4, E74.810-E74.9,
E75.21-E75.22, E75.240-E75.249, E75.3, E75.5-E75.6,
E77.0-E77.9

PDX Collection 4089
E70.81-E70.89, E72.50-E72.59, E72.81-E74.4, E74.810-E74.9,
E75.21-E75.22, E75.240-E75.249, E75.3, E75.5-E75.6,
E77.0-E77.9

PDX Collection 4122
U07.1

PDX Collection 4123
D89.831-D89.839

PDX Collection 4125
M35.81-M35.89

PDX Collection 4128
J12.82

PDX Collection 4090
U07.1

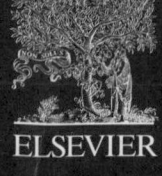
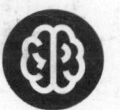
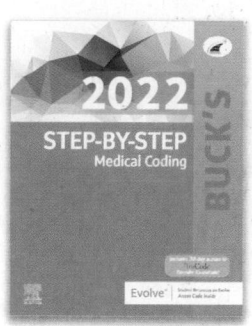

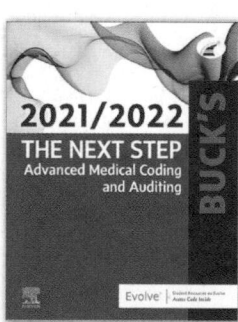
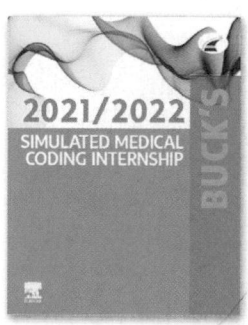
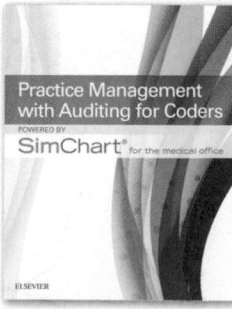
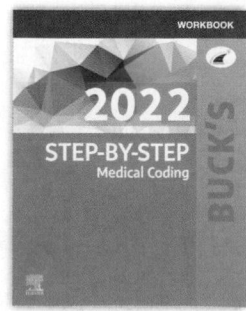